INFECTIOUS DISEASES

INTERNAL MEDICINE

MISCELLANEOUS

NEPHROLOGY

NEUROLOGY

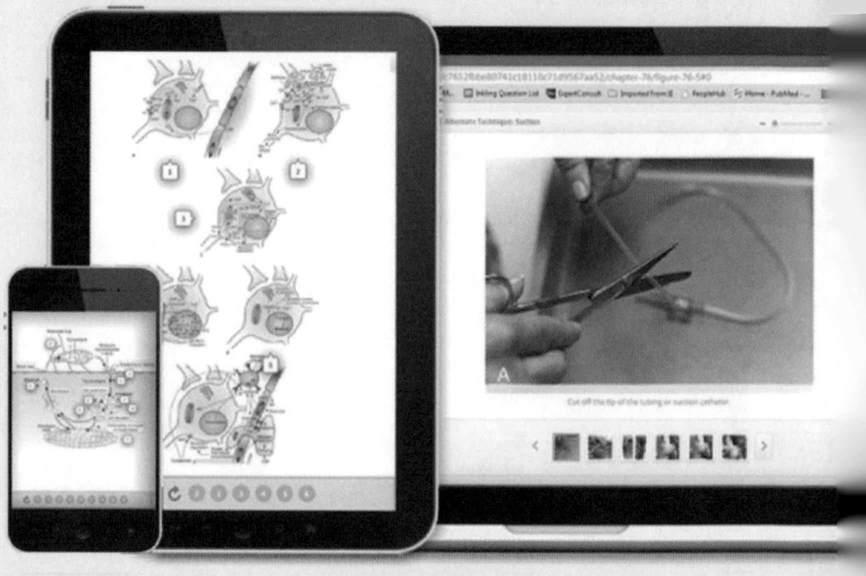

2022 Ferri's CLINICAL ADVISOR

FRED F. FERRI, MD, FACP
Clinical Professor
Department of Medicine
Warren Alpert Medical School
Brown University
Providence, Rhode Island

ELSEVIER

Elsevier
1600 John F. Kennedy Blvd.
Ste 1600
Philadelphia, PA 19103-2899

FERRI'S CLINICAL ADVISOR 2022 ISBN: 978-0-323-75570-2

Notice

Practitioners and researchers must always rely on their own experience and knowledge in evaluating and using any information, methods, compounds or experiments described herein. Because of rapid advances in the medical sciences, in particular, independent verification of diagnoses and drug dosages should be made. To the fullest extent of the law, no responsibility is assumed by Elsevier, authors, editors or contributors for any injury and/or damage to persons or property as a matter of products liability, negligence or otherwise, or from any use or operation of any methods, products, instructions, or ideas contained in the material herein.

International Standard Book Number: 978-0-323-75570-2

Publisher: Sarah Barth
Senior Content Development Specialist: Mary Hegeler
Publishing Services Manager: Catherine Jackson
Senior Project Manager: Kate Mannix
Design Direction: Bridget Hoette

Printed in the United States

Last digit is the print number: 9 8 7 6 5 4 3 2 1

Section Editors

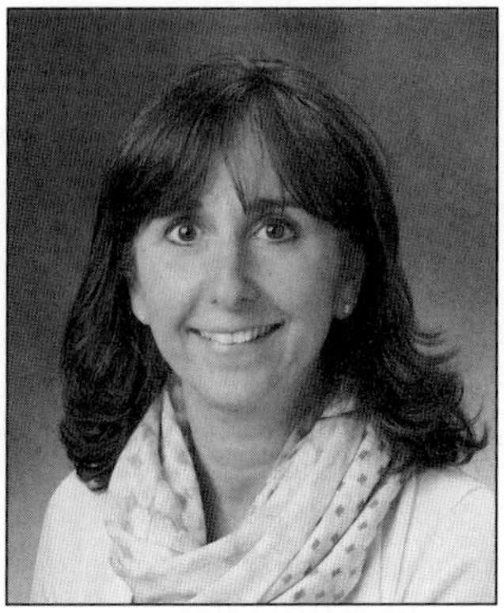

Cindy W. Christian, MD
Anthony A. Latini Chair in Child Abuse and Neglect Prevention
Children's Hospital of Philadelphia;
Professor of Pediatrics
University of Pennsylvania, Perelman School of Medicine
Philadelphia, Pennsylvania

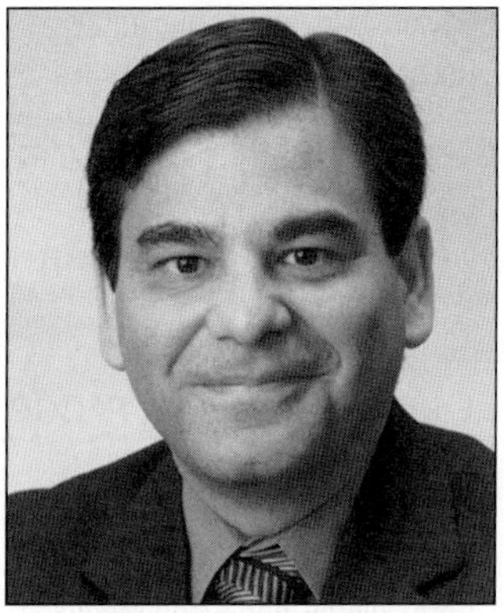

Glenn G. Fort, MD, MPH, FACP, FIDSA
Clinical Associate Professor of Medicine
Warren Alpert Medical School of Brown University;
Chief, Infectious Diseases
Our Lady of Fatima Hospital and Landmark Medical Center
Providence, Rhode Island

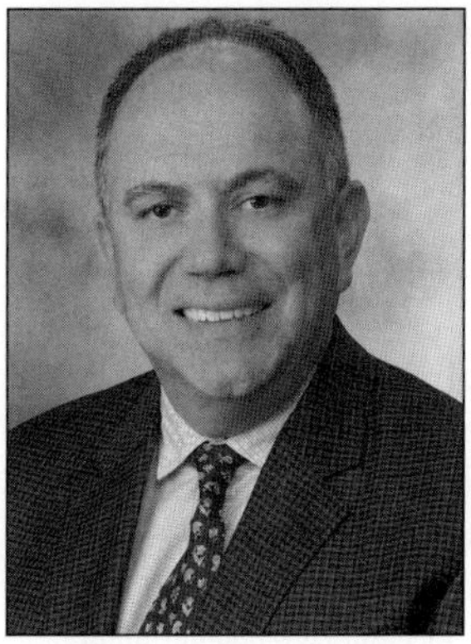

Manuel F. DaSilva, MD
Associate Professor
Director, Medical Student Education
Department of Orthopedic Surgery
Warren Alpert Medical School of Brown University
Providence, Rhode Island

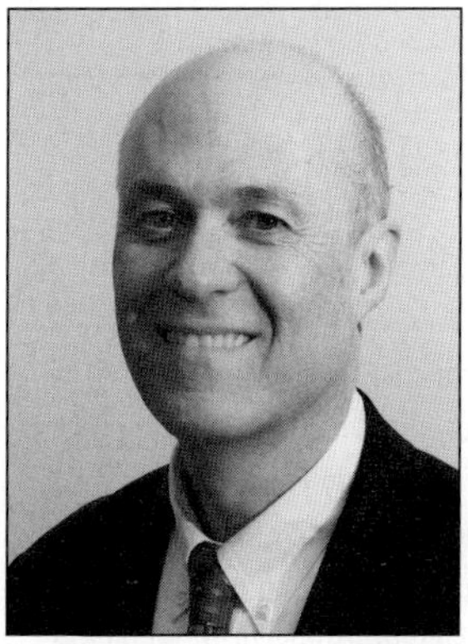

Gregory L. Fricchione, MD
Associate Chief of Psychiatry
Director, Benson Henry Institute for Mind Body Medicine
Director, Pierce Division of Global Psychiatry
Massachusetts General Hospital
Mind Body Medical Institute Professor of Psychiatry
Harvard Medical School
Boston, Massachusetts

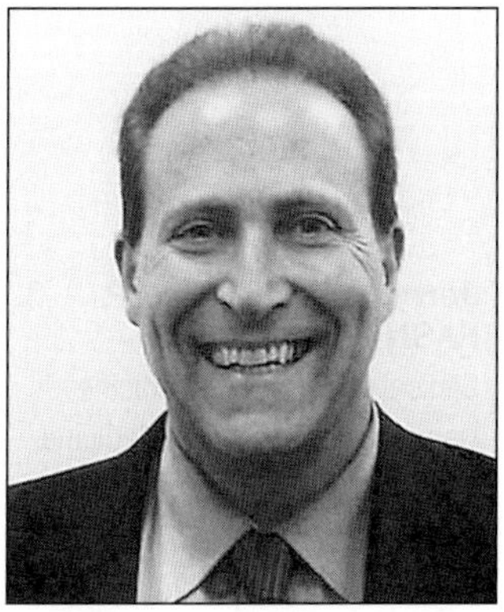

Fred F. Ferri, MD, FACP
Clinical Professor
Department of Medicine
Warren Alpert Medical School of Brown University
Providence, Rhode Island

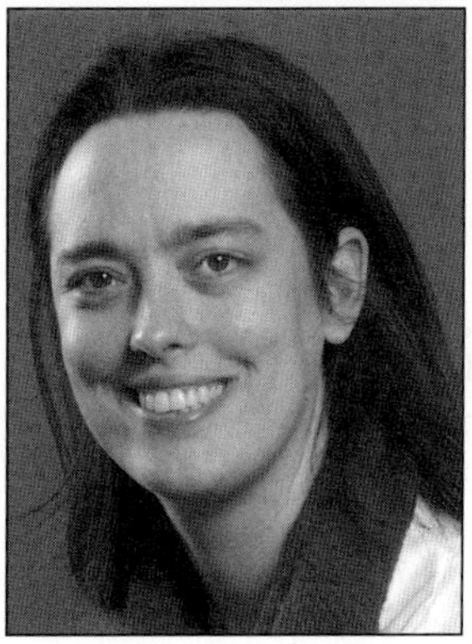

Corey Elam Goldsmith, MD
Assistant Professor of Neurology
Neurology Residency Program Director
Baylor College of Medicine
Chief of Neurology Outpatient Clinics
Ben Taub Hospital—Harris Health System
Houston, Texas

Section Editors

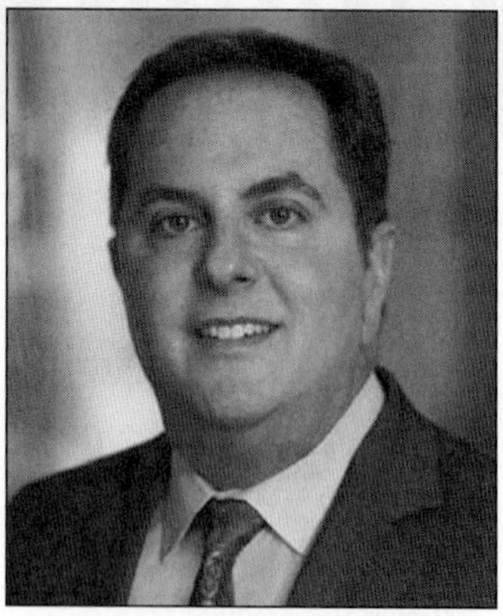

Joseph S. Kass, MD, JD, FAAN
Associate Dean of Student Affairs
Professor of Neurology, Psychiatry, and Medical Ethics
Director, Alzheimer's Disease and Memory Disorders Center
Baylor College of Medicine
Houston, Texas

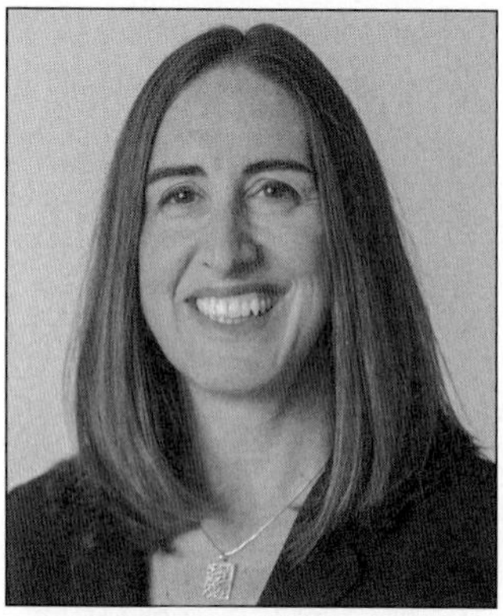

Lorriana Leard, MD, FACCP
Professor of Clinical Medicine
Vice Chief, Clinical Operations
Division of Pulmonary, Critical Care, Allergy, and Sleep Medicine
University of California San Francisco
San Francisco, California

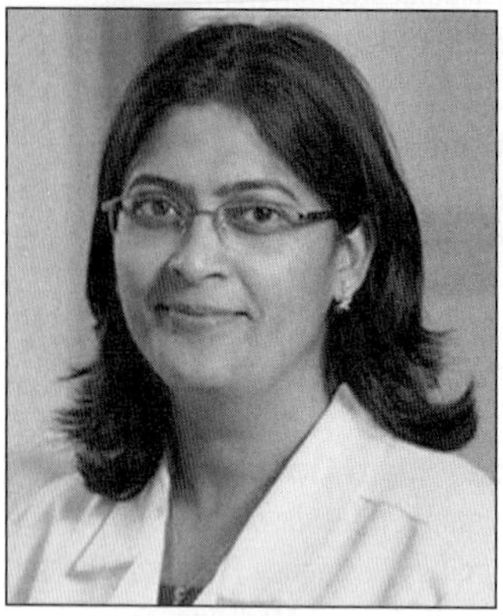

Bharti Rathore, MD
Program Director, Hematology/Oncology Fellowship
Roger Williams Medical Center
Providence, Rhode Island;
Assistant Professor of Medicine
Boston University School of Medicine
Boston, Massachusetts

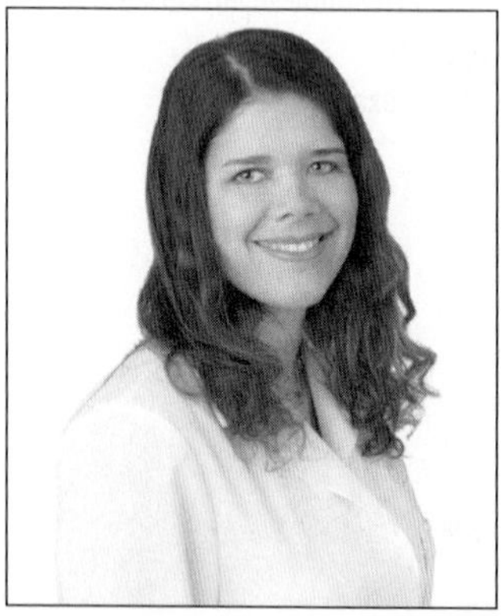

Daphne Scaramangas-Plumley, MD
Rheumatologist
Attune Health
Cedars-Sinai Medical Center
Beverly Hills, California

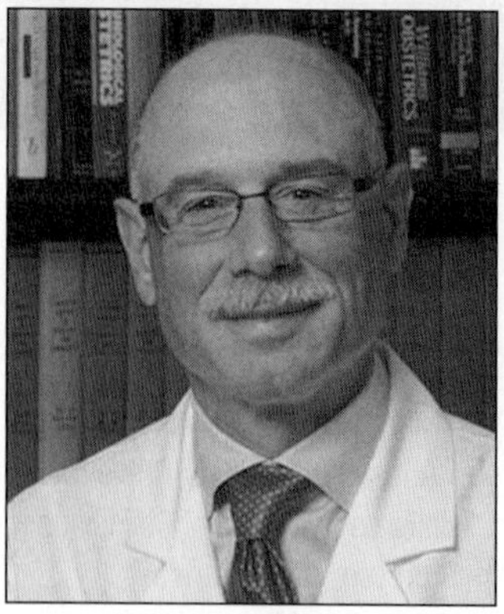

Anthony Sciscione, DO
Professor of Obstetrics and Gynecology
Jefferson Medical College
Philadelphia, Pennsylvania;
Residency Program Director
Director of Maternal-Fetal Medicine
Department of Obstetrics and Gynecology
Christiana Care Health System
Newark, Delaware

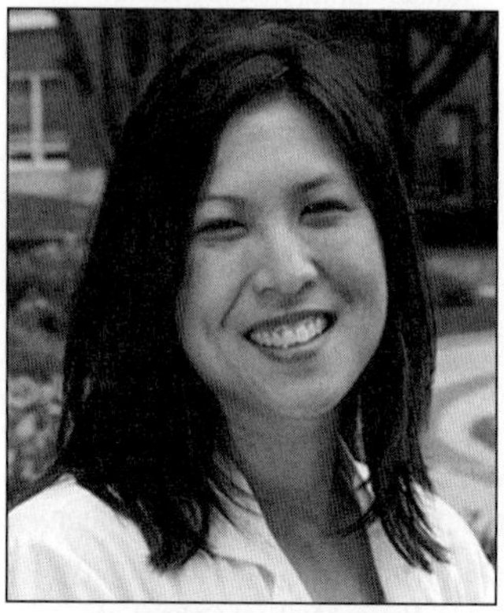

Iris L. Tong, MD
Associate Professor
Department of Medicine
Warren Alpert Medical School of Brown University;
Attending Physician
Women's Primary Care
Women's Medicine Collaborative
Providence, Rhode Island

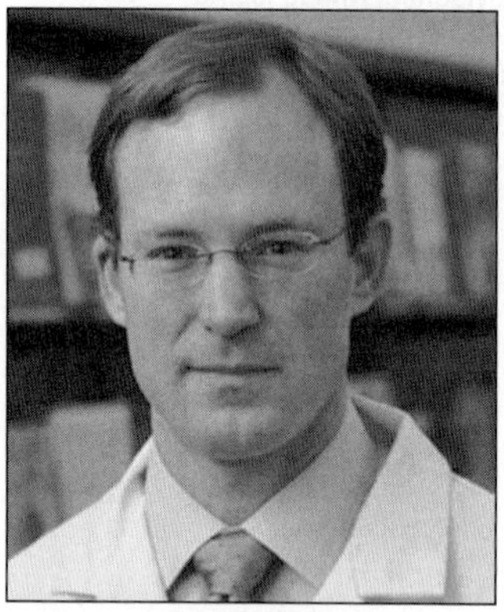

John Wylie, MD, FACC
Director, Cardiac Electrophysiology
Steward Health Care System;
Associate Professor of Medicine
Tufts University School of Medicine
St. Elizabeth's Medical Center
Boston, Massachusetts

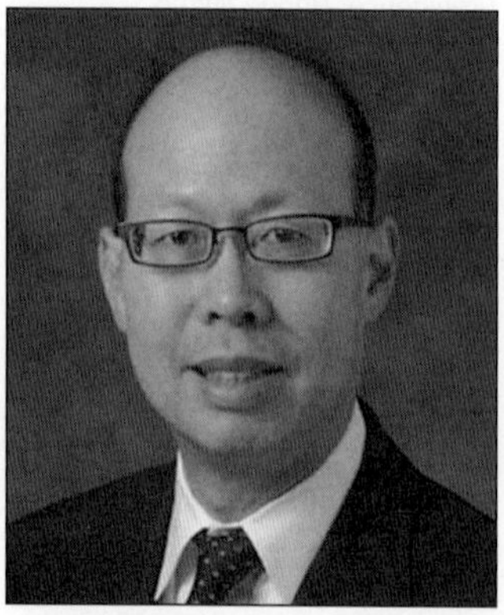

Jerry Yee, MD, MACP, FASN, FNKF
Clinical Professor of Medicine
Department of Internal Medicine
Wayne State University School of Medicine;
Division Head, Nephrology and Hypertension
Henry Ford Hospital
Detroit, Michigan

Contributors

Rebecca A. Abelman, MD
Clinical Fellow, Division of Infectious Diseases
University of California San Francisco
San Francisco, CA

Alexandra Abrams-Downey, MD
Professor, Medicine
Icahn School of Medicine at Mount Sinai
New York, NY

Emily Adams, PMP
Open Door Health Clinic
Providence, RI

Maxwell Eyram Afari, MD
Attending Physician
Advanced Heart Failure and Transplant Cardiologist
Cardiovascular Medicine
Maine Medical Center
Portland, ME

Shanice Akoto, MD, MPH
Obstetrics and Gynecology Resident
Christiana Care Health System
Newark, DE

MHD Hussam Al Jandali, MD
Nephrology Fellow
Division of Nephrology and Hypertension
Henry Ford Hospital
Detroit, MI

Maad M. Alhudairy, MD, MAS
Internal Medicine Resident
St. Elizabeth's Medical Center
Tufts University School of Medicine
Boston, MA

Tanya Ali, MD
Clinical Assistant Professor of Medicine
Warren Alpert Medical School of Brown University
Providence, RI

Narges Alipanah-Lechner, MD
Fellow
Pulmonary and Critical Care Medicine
University of California San Francisco
San Francisco, CA

Stephanie M. Allen, MS
Baylor College of Medicine
Houston, TX

Ihab Alomari, MD, FACC
Interventional Cardiologist
Associate Professor of Medicine
University of California Irvine
Orange, CA

Erin Alpert-Rathhauser, MD
Pediatric Resident
Pediatrics
NYU School of Medicine
New York, NY

Ilana Ander, BA
Clinical Research Coordinator
Psychiatry
Massachusetts General Hospital
Boston, MA

Maria Andrievskaya, MD
Nephrology Fellow
Henry Ford Hospital
Detroit, MI

Kathryn Taylor Anilowski, MS, PT, CLT-LANA
Physical Therapist
Kinder Touch Lymphedema Center
Saratoga Springs, NY

AnnGene Anthony, MD, MPH, FAAFP
Teaching Faculty
HMH Mountainside Family Medicine Residency Program
Assistant Professor of Family Medicine
Associate Clerkship Director/Site Director - Family Medicine Clerkship
Hackensack Meridian School of Medicine
Nutley, NJ

Joe Aoun, MD
Cardiovascular Medicine Fellow
Houston Methodist DeBakey Heart and Vascular Center
Houston, TX

Zuhal Arzomand, MD
Rheumatologist
Northern Virginia Arthritis and Rheumatology
Alexandria, VA

Ali Ashtiani, MD
Interventional Cardiology Fellow
University of California Irvine
Irvine, CA

Daniel K. Asiedu, MD, PhD, FACP
Staff Physician
Coastal Medical, Inc.
Lincoln, RI

Artem Astsaturov, MD
Cardiology Fellow
Steward St. Elizabeth's Medical Center
Brighton, MA

Sudeep K. Aulakh, MD
Director Ambulatory Education, Internal Medicine Residency
UMASS Medical School-Baystate
Springfield, MA

Contributors

Rupali Avasare, MD
Assistant Professor of Medicine
Division of Nephrology and Hypertension
Oregon Health & Science University
Portland, OR

Sarah Aziz, DO
Rowan University School of Osteopathic Medicine
Stratford, NJ

Tania B. Babar, MD
Electrophysiologist
Department of Electrophysiology
Charleston Area Medical Center
Charleston, WV

Emelia Argyropoulos Bachman, MD
Assistant Professor of Clinical Obstetrics and Gynecology
Division of Reproductive Endocrinology and Infertility
Hospital of the University of Pennsylvania
Philadelphia, PA

Ashika Bains, MD, MS
Clinical Fellow, Consultation-Liaison Psychiatry
Massachusetts General Hospital
Boston, MA

T. Caroline Bank, MD
Obstetrics and Gynecology Resident
Christiana Care Health System
Newark, DE

Brenda Banwell, MD
Chief, Division of Neurology
Neurology and Pediatrics
Children's Hospital of Philadelphia
Philadelphia, PA

Trace Barrett, MD
Assistant Professor
Division of Cardiovascular Medicine
University of Vermont Medical Center
Burlington, VT

Ailin Barseghian, MD
Associate Clinical Professor
University of California Irvine
Internal Medicine, Division of Cardiology
Orange, CA

Craig L. Basman, MD
Structural Heart Disease Attending and Interventionalist
Cardiothoracic Surgery
Lenox Hill Hospital, Northwell Health
New York, NY

Hasnain Bawaadam, MD, MPH
Interventional Pulmonary Fellow
Division of Pulmonary, Critical Care, Allergy, and Sleep Medicine
University of California San Francisco
San Francisco, CA

Noor Beckwith, MD
Senior Resident
Psychiatry
Massachusetts General Hospital
Boston, MA

Ren Belcher, MD
Psychiatry Resident
Massachusetts General Hospital and McLean Hospital
Clinical Fellow in Psychiatry
Harvard Medical School
Boston, MA

Jennifer Bell, MD
Advanced Heart Failure Fellow
New York Presbyterian/Columbia Medical Center
New York, NY

Amy L. Bellinghausen, MD
Post-Doctoral Fellow
Division of Pulmonary, Critical Care, Sleep Medicine and Physiology
University of California San Diego
San Diego, CA

Deanna Benner, MSN, APRN
Nurse Practitioner
Christiana Care Health System
Obstetrics and Gynecology
Newark, DE

Nicole M. Benson, MD
Attending Psychiatrist, Child and Adolescent Psychiatry
Massachusetts General Hospital and McLean Hospital
Instructor in Psychiatry
Harvard Medical School
Boston, MA

Michael Bergen, MD
Orthopedic Surgery Resident
Warren Alpert Medical School of Brown University
Providence, RI

Agatha Berger, MD
Faculty
Obstetrics and Gynecology
Christiana Care Health System
Newark, DE

Arnaldo A. Berges, MD
Director, Division of Inpatient Psychiatry
Rhode Island Hospital
Providence, RI

Carol Berkowitz, MD
Chief, Division of General Pediatrics
Harbor-UCLA Medical Center
Torrance, CA
Distinguished Professor of Pediatrics
David Geffen School of Medicine at UCLA

Kristin Bevington, MD, MEd
Psychiatry Resident
Massachusetts General Hospital
Boston, MA,
McLean Hospital
Belmont, MA

Vicky H. Bhagat, MD, MPH
Gastroenterology Fellow
Robert Wood Johnson University Hospital
New Brunswick, NJ

Harikrashna B. Bhatt, MD
Assistant Professor
Endocrinology
Warren Alpert Medical School of Brown University
Providence, RI

Prachi H. Bhuptani, MA
Clinical Psychology Resident
Warren Alpert Medical School of Brown University
Providence, RI

Courtney Clark Bilodeau, MD, FACP
Assistant Professor, Obstetric Medicine
Warren Alpert Medical School of Brown University
Attending Physician, Internal Medicine
Women's Medicine Collaborative, Miriam Hospital
Providence, RI

Stefani Bissonette, MD
Obstetrics and Gynecology Resident
Christiana Care Health System
Newark, DE

Ghamar Bitar, MD
Obstetrics and Gynecology Resident
Christiana Care Hospital
Newark, DE

Craig Blakeney, MD
Emergency Medicine Physician
University of Tennessee Health Science Center
Memphis, TN

Brad Blankenhorn, MD
Attending Physician
Orthopaedic Surgery
Warren Alpert Medical School of Brown University
Rhode Island Hospital
Providence, RI

Brian Block, MD
Assistant Professor
Division of Pulmonary, Critical Care, Allergy, and Sleep Medicine
University of California San Francisco
San Francisco, CA

Christopher P. Blomberg, DO
Cardiovascular Medicine
Southern Maine Health Care/Maine Health
Biddeford, ME

Abigail N. Boduch, MD
Orthopaedic Surgery
Warren Alpert Medical School of Brown University
Providence, RI

Steven L. Bokshan, MD
Orthopedics
Warren Alpert Medical School of Brown University
Providence, RI

Christina M. Bortz, MD
Assistant Professor of Medicine, Clinical Educator
Warren Alpert Medical School of Brown University
Providence, RI

Alexandre Boulos, MD, MPH
Orthopaedic Surgery Resident
Warren Alpert Medical School of Brown University
Providence, RI

Tara C. Bouton, MD, MPH, TM
Assistant Professor of Medicine
Section of Infectious Disease
Boston Medical Center
Boston University School of Medicine
Boston, MA

Mary E. Bove, MD
Attending Physician
Children's Hospital of Philadelphia - Care Network
Philadelphia, PA

Lynn A. Bowlby, MD
Medical Director, Duke Outpatient Clinic
Duke University Medical Center
Durham, NC

Amanda Box, MD, MS
Assistant Professor of Emergency Medicine
University of Tennessee Health Science Center
Memphis, TN

Mark F. Brady, MD, MPH, MMSc
Assistant Professor
Emergency Medicine
University of Tennessee Health Science Center
Memphis, TN

Russell E. Bratman, MD
Fellow, Division of Endocrinology
Warren Alpert Medical School of Brown University
Providence, RI

Keith Brennan, MD
Geriatric Medicine
Stony Brook University
Stony Brook, NY

Amy Bridges, MD
Assistant Professor, Faculty
Emergency Medicine
University of Tennessee Health Science Center
Memphis, TN

Emily Brown, MD
Attending in Child Abuse Pediatrics
Professor of Pediatrics
Seattle Children's Hospital
University of Washington School of Medicine
Seattle, WA

Jeffrey Budzyn, MD
Urology Resident
Vattikuti Urology Institute
Henry Ford Health System
Detroit, MI

Eric Bui, MD, PhD
Professor of Psychiatry
Caen University Hospital
Caen, France
Psychiatrist
Massachusetts General Hospital
Boston, MA

Contributors

Christine Burke, MD
Obstetrics and Gynecology Resident
Christiana Care Health System
Newark, DE

Katerina L. Byanova, MD, MS
Clinical Fellow
Division of Pulmonary, Critical Care, Allergy and Sleep Medicine
University of California San Francisco
San Francisco, CA

Kate Cahill, MD
Assistant Professor of Medicine, Clinician Educator
Division of General Internal Medicine
Warren Alpert Medical School of Brown University
Providence, RI

Katherine Canty, MD
Fellow, Child Abuse Pediatrics
Harbor-UCLA Medical Center
Torrance, CA

Damon Cao, MD
Nephrology Fellow
Division of Nephrology and Hypertension
Henry Ford Hospital
Detroit, MI

Andrew Caraganis, MD
Internal Medicine
Boston University School of Medicine
Roger Williams Medical Center
Providence, RI

Randy S. Carpenter, BA
MD Candidate (MS2)
University of Tennessee Health Science Center
Memphis, TN

Eugene Carragee, MD
Resident Physician
Anesthesia and Perioperative Care
University of California San Francisco
San Francisco, CA

Ashlie Sewdass Carter, MD
Obstetrics and Gynecology Resident
Christiana Care Health System
Newark, DE

Ana Castaneda-Guarderas, MD
Assistant Professor
Emergency Medicine
University of Tennessee Regional One Physicians
Memphis, TN

Jorge J. Castillo, MD
Clinical Director, Bing Center for Waldenström Macroglobulinemia, Dana-Farber Cancer Institute
Associate Professor, Harvard Medical School
Boston, MA

Andreea M. Catana, MD
Co-director of Liver Tumor Program
Gastroenterology and Hepatology
Beth Israel Deaconess Medical Center
Harvard Medical School
Boston, MA

Carolina S. Cerezo, MD, FAAP
Associate Professor of Pediatrics
Warren Alpert Medical School of Brown University
Division Chief, Pediatric Gastroenterology, Nutrition & Liver Diseases
Hasbro Children's/Rhode Island Hospital
Providence, RI

Philip A. Chan, MD, MS
Associate Professor
Warren Alpert Medical School of Brown University
Providence, RI

Lucy Y. Chang, MD, MSci
Assistant Clinical Professor
Pediatrics
NYU Langone Hospital/Bellevue Hospital Center
New York, NY

Arlene Chapman, MD
Professor of Medicine
Chief, Section of Nephrology
University of Chicago
Chicago, IL

Anjulika Chawla, MD
Associate Medical Director
Bluebird Bio, Inc.
Cambridge, MA

Hrak Chemchirian, MD
Steward St. Elizabeth's Medical Center
Tufts University School of Medicine
Boston, MA

Vicky Cheng, MD
Assistant Professor
Endocrinology
Warren Alpert Medical School of Brown University
Providence, RI

Tracy Cherian, BA
University of Tennessee Regional One Physicians
Memphis, TN

Robin Chin, MD
Pediatric Resident
Children's Hospital of Philadelphia
Philadelphia, PA

Roxana Chis, MD
Gastroenterology Fellow
University of Toronto
Toronto, Ontario, Canada

Chandrika Chitturi, MD
Senior Staff
Nephrology and Hypertension
Henry Ford Hospital
Detroit, MI

Dana Ricci Chofay, MD
Assistant Professor of Medicine and Medical Science
Warren Alpert Medical School of Brown University
Providence, RI

George Cholankeril, MD
Transplant Hepatology
University of Tennessee Health Science Center
Memphis, TN

Rosann Cholankeril, MD
Boston University School of Medicine
Roger Williams Medical Center
Providence, RI

Stella T. Chou, MD
Associate Professor of Pediatrics
Division of Hematology
Children's Hospital of Philadelphia
Philadelphia, PA

Aruj Choudhry, MD
Clinical Hepatology Fellow
Division of Gastroenterology and Hepatology
Beth Israel Deaconess Medical Center
Harvard Medical School
Boston, MA

Shivali Choxi, MD
General Pediatrician
NYU Grossman School of Medicine
New York, NY

Cindy W. Christian, MD
Anthony A. Latini Chair in Child Abuse and Neglect Prevention
Children's Hospital of Philadelphia
Professor, Pediatrics
Perelman School of Medicine
University of Pennsylvania
Philadelphia, PA

Winona Chua, MD
Clinical Associate Professor of Pediatrics
Perelman School of Medicine
University of Pennsylvania
Philadelphia, PA

Seth Clark, MD, MPH
Addiction Medicine Physician, Assistant Professor
Department of Medicine and Psychiatry and Human Behavior
Warren Alpert Medical School of Brown University
Providence, RI

Karl T. Clebak, MD, FAAFP
Assistant Professor, Program Director
Family and Community Medicine Residency Program
Penn State Health M. S. Hershey Medical Center
Hershey, PA

Debbie L. Cohen, MD
Professor of Medicine
Renal Electrolyte and Hypertension Division
Perelman School of Medicine, University of Pennsylvania
Philadelphia, PA

Lisa Cohen, PharmD
Associate Professor of Pharmacy
University of Rhode Island
Kingston, RI

Phillip D. Cohen, MD
General Pediatrics Resident
Children's Hospital of Philadelphia
Philadelphia, PA

Zachary Cohn, MD
Fellow Physician
Hematology/Oncology
University of Massachusetts
Worcester, MA

Morgan Congdon, MD, MPH
Clinical Instructor of Pediatrics
Children's Hospital of Philadelphia
Philadelphia, PA

Maria Constantinou, MD
Clinical Assistant Professor of Medicine
Warren Alpert Medical School of Brown University
Medical Oncologist
Lifespan Cancer
Providence, RI

Eddie L. Copelin II, MD, MHA
Internal Medicine
Boston University School of Medicine
Roger Williams Medical Center
Providence, RI

James Earl Corley III, MD
Chief Resident, Emergency Medicine
University of Tennessee Health Science Center
Memphis, TN

Rebecca Craine, MSEd, CCC-SLP
Speech Language Pathologist, Rehabilitation
Bradley Hospital
East Providence, RI

Patricia Cristofaro, MD
Assistant Professor
Internal Medicine and Infectious Diseases
Warren Alpert Medical School of Brown University
Providence, RI

Tess Crouss, MD
Fellow
Cooper University Health Care
Female Pelvic Medicine and Reconstructive Surgery
Camden, NJ

Aristides I. Cruz, MD
Orthopaedic Surgery
Warren Alpert Medical School of Brown University
Providence, RI

Joanne Szczygiel Cunha, MD
Director, Rheumatology Fellowship Program
Assistant Professor of Medicine
Division of Rheumatology
Warren Alpert Medical School of Brown University
Providence Veterans Affairs Medical Center
Providence, RI

Karlene Cunningham, PhD
Clinical Assistant Professor
Psychiatry and Behavioral Medicine
Brody School of Medicine, East Carolina University
Greenville, NC

Chase Currier, BS
Medical Scribe
Massachusetts General Hospital
Boston, MA

Contributors

Alicia J. Curtin, PhD
Assistant Professor
Division of Geriatrics
Warren Alpert Medical School of Brown University
Providence, RI

Joseph Cusano, MD
Orthopedic Surgery Resident
Warren Alpert Medical School of Brown University/Rhode Island Hospital
Providence, RI

Ganary Dabiri, MD, PhD
Staff Dermatologist
Roger Williams Medical Center
Providence, RI

Lynn Dado, MD
Attending Physician, Primary Care
Henry Ford Internal Medicine Group
Bloomfield Hills, MI

Deepan S. Dalal, MD, MPH
Assistant Professor
Warren Alpert Medical School of Brown University
School of Medicine and School of Public Health
Department of Medicine (Rheumatology) and Department of Health Services, Policy and Practices
Providence, RI

Gerhard H. Daly, MD, MSc
Interventional Cardiology Fellow
St. Elizabeth's Medical Center
Boston, MA

Shivang U. Danak, MD
St. George's University
Detroit, MI

Rituparna Das, MD
Assistant Professor, Neurology
Baylor College of Medicine
Houston, TX

Manuel F. DaSilva, MD
Associate Professor
Director Medical Student Education
Orthopedics
Warren Alpert Medical School of Brown University
Providence, RI

Natasha Dave, MD
Division of Nephrology
Bruce W. Carter VA Medical Center
Miami, FL

Mackenzie Davis, MD
Clinical Fellow in Psychiatry
Harvard Medical School
Adult Psychiatry Residency
Massachusetts General Hospital/McLean Hospital
Boston, MA

Alison Dedent, MD
Clinical Instructor
Pulmonary and Critical Care Medicine
University of California San Francisco
San Francisco, CA

John Denninger, MD, PhD
Director in Clinical Research
Department of Psychiatry, Benson-Henry Institute for Mind Body Medicine
Massachusetts General Hospital
Boston, MA

Colette Desrochers, MD
Primary Care Attending Physician
Children's Hospital of Philadelphia
Associate Professor of Pediatrics in the Associated Faculty of the Perelman School of Medicine
Philadelphia, PA

Jacquelyn Detweiler, DO, FAAP
Attending Physician
Children's Hospital of Philadelphia
Philadelphia, PA

Erin Pete Devon, MD
Assistant Professor of Clinical Pediatrics
Children's Hospital of Philadelphia
Perelman School of Medicine, University of Pennsylvania
Philadelphia, PA

Ashwini U. Dhokte, MD
Resident Physician
Christiana Care Hospital
Newark, DE

Joseph A. Diaz, MD, MPH
Associate Professor of Medicine
Warren Alpert Medical School of Brown University
Providence, RI

Kevin J. DiSilvestro, MD
Department of Orthopaedic Surgery
Warren Alpert Medical School of Brown University
Providence, RI

Thomas H. Dohlman, MD
Cornea Service
Massachusetts Eye and Ear Infirmary
Harvard Medical School
Boston, MA

Stephen Dolter, MD
Pediatric Hospitalist
Children's Hospital and Medical Center
Pediatric Hospital Medicine
Omaha, NE

David J. Domenichini, MD
Clinical Instructor, Endocrinology and Metabolism
Hartford Hospital
University of Connecticut Health Center
West Hartford, CT

Kathleen Doo, MD, MHPE
Clinical Faculty
Pulmonary, Sleep and Critical Care Medicine
Kaiser Permanente East Bay
Oakland, CA

James H. Dove, MD
Orthopedic Surgery Resident
Warren Alpert Medical School of Brown University
Providence, RI

Carol Duh-Leong, MD
Clinical Assistant Professor
NYU Grossman School of Medicine
New York, NY

Andrew P. Duker, MD
Associate Professor, Movement Disorders Division
Director, Department of Neurology and Rehabilitation Medicine
University of Cincinnati College of Medicine
Cincinnati, OH

Shashank Dwivedi, MD
Orthopedic Surgery Resident
Warren Alpert Medical School of Brown University/Rhode Island Hospital
Providence, RI

Myles Dworkin, MD
Orthopedic Surgery Resident
Warren Alpert Medical School of Brown University
Providence, RI

Christine Eisenhower, PharmD
Clinical Assistant Professor
Pharmacy Practice
University of Rhode Island College of Pharmacy
Kingston, RI

Amani A. Elghafri, MD, MSc, MEd
Internal Medicine Resident
UCSF Fresno
Fresno, CA

Pamela Ellsworth, MD
Chief, Division of Pediatric Urology
Professor of Urology
Nemours Children's Hospital
University of Central Florida College of Medicine
Orlando, FL

Alan Epstein, MD
Roger Williams Medical Center
Providence, RI

Patricio Sebastian Espinosa, MD, MPH, FAAN
Associate Professor of Neurology
Neurology Residency Program Director
Neurology Department - Marcus Neuroscience Institute
Boca Raton Regional Hospital
Charles E. Schmidt College of Medicine
Florida Atlantic University
Boca Raton, FL

Andrew R. Evans, MD
Assistant Professor of Orthopedic Surgery
Co-director, Division of Orthopedic Traumatology
Warren Alpert Medical School of Brown University/Rhode Island Hospital
Providence, RI

Eileen Everly, MD
Attending Physician
General Pediatrics
Children's Hospital of Philadelphia
Philadelphia, PA

Mark D. Faber, MD
Division Head, Nephrology and Hypertension
Senior Staff Physician
Henry Ford Hospital
Detroit, MI

Mary Fabio, MD
Attending Physician
Children's Hospital of Philadelphia
Clinical Assistant Professor of Pediatrics
Perelman School of Medicine, University of Pennsylvania
Philadelphia, PA

Evan Facer, DO
Pediatric Infectious Diseases Fellow
UPMC Children's Hospital of Pittsburgh
Pittsburgh, PA

Paul Fadale, MD
Orthopaedic Surgery
Warren Alpert Medical School of Brown University
Providence, RI

Matthew J. Fagan, MD, FACOG
Attending Physician, Director of Undergraduate Medical Education
Obstetrics and Gynecology
Christiana Care Health System
Newark, DE

Jon Farkas, MD
Pediatric Hospital Medicine Attending
NYU School of Medicine
New York, NY

Erica Farrand, MD
Assistant Professor
Pulmonary and Critical Care Medicine
University of California San Francisco
San Francisco, CA

Kevin Fay, MD
Fellow, Critical Care Medicine
Jefferson Northeast Hospital
Philadelphia, PA

Carlos Fernandez-Robles, MD, MBA
Clinical Director, Center for Psychiatric Oncology and Behavioral Sciences
Associate Director, Somatic Therapies Service
Assistant Professor of Psychiatry
Massachusetts General Hospital/Harvard Medical School
Boston, MA

Jason D. Ferreira, MD
Clinical Assistant Professor of Medicine
Gastroenterology
Warren Alpert Medical School of Brown University
University Gastroenterology, LLC/Miriam Hospital
Providence, RI

Fred F. Ferri, MD
Clinical Professor
Department of Medicine
Warren Alpert Medical School of Brown University
Providence, RI

Heather Ferri, DO
Department of Medicine
Warren Alpert Medical School of Brown University
Rhode Island Hospital
Providence, RI

Staci A. Fischer, MD
Clinical Learning Environment Review Field Representative Team Leader
Accreditation Council for Graduate Medical Education
Chicago, IL

Contributors

Yaneve Fonge, MD
Obstetrics and Gynecology Resident
Christiana Care Health System
Newark, DE

Kellie C. Forbes, MD
Obstetrics and Gynecology Resident
Christiana Care
Newark, DE

Michelle Forcier, MD, MPH
Professor of Pediatrics
Warren Alpert Medical School of Brown University
Providence, RI

Sydney Ford, MD, MPH
Obstetrics and Gynecology Resident
Christiana Care Health System
Newark, DE

Frank G. Fort, MD, FACS, RPHS
Medical Director
Capital Region Vein Centre
Schenectady, NY

Glenn G. Fort, MD, MPH
Clinical Associate Professor of Medicine
Warren Alpert Medical School of Brown University
Providence, RI

Justin F. Fraser, MD
Assistant Professor of Cerebrovascular, Endovascular, and Skull Base Surgery
Neurosurgery
University of Kentucky
Lexington, KY

Gregory L. Fricchione, MD
Associate Chief of Psychiatry
Director, Benson Henry Institute for Mind Body Medicine
Director, Pierce Division of Global Psychiatry
Massachusetts General Hospital
Mind Body Medical Institute Professor of Psychiatry
Harvard Medical School
Boston, MA

Michael Friedman, MD
Clinical Associate Professor
Psychiatry and Human Behavior; Neurology
Warren Alpert Medical School of Brown University
Providence, RI

Daniel R. Frisch, MD
Associate Professor of Medicine
Division of Cardiology, Electrophysiology Section
Thomas Jefferson University Hospital
Philadelphia, PA

Mark Fusunyan, MD
Department of Psychiatry
Massachusetts General Hospital
Boston, MA

Anthony Gallo, MD
Director of ECT Service
Rhode Island Hospital
Clinical Assistant Professor
Warren Alpert Medical School of Brown University
Providence, RI

Rimmy Garg, MD
Resident, Internal Medicine
Warren Alpert Medical School of Brown University
Providence, RI

Arturo Gasga, MD
Internal Medicine Resident
University of California San Francisco
San Francisco, CA

Tatiana Londoño Gentile, MD
Attending Physician
General Pediatrics
Children's Hospital of Philadelphia
Philadelphia, PA

Yaron B. Gesthalter, MD
Assistant Professor of Medicine
Co-director of Interventional Pulmonary Medicine
Division of Pulmonary and Critical Care Medicine
University of California San Francisco
San Francisco, CA

Mostafa Ghanim, MD
Cardiology Fellow
MercyOne North Iowa Medical Center
Mason City, IA

Armen S. Ghazarian, MD
Resident Physician, Internal Medicine
University of California Irvine Medical Center
Orange, CA

Nisha H. Gidwani, MD
Associate Clinical Professor
Division of Pulmonary, Critical Care, Allergy, and Sleep Medicine
University of California San Francisco
San Francisco, CA

Joseph Gil, MD
Orthopaedic Surgery
Warren Alpert Medical School of Brown University
Providence, RI

Dimitri Gitelmaker, MD
Internal Medicine Resident
Roger Williams Medical Center
Boston University School of Medicine
Providence, RI

Mark Godding, MD
Internal Medicine Resident
Warren Alpert Medical School of Brown University
Providence, RI

Alla Goldburt, MD
Assistant Clinical Professor, Family Medicine
Warren Alpert Medical School of Brown University
Providence, RI

Danielle Goldfarb, MD
Assistant Professor of Neurology and Psychiatry
University of Arizona College of Medicine
Phoenix, AZ

Corey Goldsmith, MD
Assistant Professor of Neurology
Baylor College of Medicine
Houston, TX

Maheswara Satya Gangadhara Rao Golla, MD
Interventional Cardiologist
Parkersburg Cardiology Associate
Camden Clark Medical Center
Parkersburg, WV

Helen B. Gomez, MD
Obstetrics and Gynecology Resident
Christiana Care Health System
Newark, DE

Avi D. Goodman, MD
Orthopedic Trauma Fellow
Department of Orthopedics
Warren Alpert Medical School of Brown University
Providence, RI

Paul Gordon, MD
Clinical Assistant Professor of Medicine
Division of Cardiology
Warren Alpert Medical School of Brown University
Providence, RI

John A. Gray, MD, PhD
Assistant Professor
Department of Neurology, Center for Neuroscience
University of California Davis
Davis, CA

Morgan Greenfield, MD
Attending Physician
Pediatrics
Children's Hospital of Philadelphia
Philadelphia, PA

Lindsey Anne Grisham, MD
Emergency Medicine Resident
University of Tennessee Health Science Center
Memphis, TN

Patan Gultawatvichai, MD
Assistant Professor
Division of Hematology-Oncology
University of Massachusetts Medical School
Worcester, MA

David Guo, MD
Urologist
Kaiser Permanente Hospital
Santa Clara, CA

Priya Sarin Gupta, MD, MPH
Adolescent Medicine Fellow
Division of General Pediatrics and Adolescent Medicine
Johns Hopkins Hospital
Baltimore, MD

Brittany Guttadauria, MD
Pediatrics Resident
Children's Hospital of Philadelphia
Philadelphia, PA

Herodes Guzman, MD, MPH
General Pediatrics Resident
Children's Hospital of Philadelphia
Philadelphia, PA

Nawaz K. A. Hack, MD
Assistant Professor of Neurology
F. Edward Hébert School of Medicine, Uniformed Services University of the Health Sciences
Bethesda, MD

Sajeev Handa, MD, SFHM
Chief of Hospital Medicine and Director of Clinical Integration
Lifespan Physician Group
Clinical Assistant Professor of Medicine and Neurology
Warren Alpert Medical School of Brown University
Providence, RI

Nikolas Harbord, MD
Associate Professor of Medicine
Division of Nephrology
Mount Sinai School of Medicine
New York, NY

Erica Hardy, MD, MMS
Director, Division of Infectious Disease
Women and Infants Hospital
Clinical Assistant Professor of Medicine and Obstetrics and Gynecology
Divisions of Infectious Disease and Obstetric Medicine
Warren Alpert Medical School of Brown University
Providence, RI

Colin J. Harrington, MD
Professor of Psychiatry and Human Behavior
Professor of Medical Science
Professor of Medicine
Warren Alpert Medical School of Brown University
Providence, RI

Nathan Hartvigsen, MD
Co-director, Intensive Clinical Program
Home Base, A Red Sox Foundation and Massachusetts General Hospital Program
Charlestown, MA;
Clinical Instructor in Psychiatry
Harvard Medical School
Massachusetts General Hospital Law and Psychiatry Service
Boston, MA

Sonia A. Havele, MD
Resident Physician
Children's Hospital of Philadelphia
Philadelphia, PA

Don Hayes Jr., MD, MS, MEd
Professor
Departments of Pediatrics, Internal Medicine, Surgery, Epidemiology
Ohio State University
Columbus, OH

Jaspreet K. Hehar, DO
Endocrinology Fellow
Diabetes and Bone and Mineral Disorders
Henry Ford Health System
Detroit, MI

Rachel Wright Heinle, MD, FACOG
Attending Physician
Obstetrics and Gynecology
Christiana Care Health System
Newark, DE

Leesha A. Helm, MD, MPH
Assistant Professor
Family and Community Medicine
Penn State Medical Center
Hershey, PA

Matthew F. Helm, MD
Assistant Professor
Dermatology
Penn State Medical Center
Hershey, PA

Ruth B. Hennebery, MD
Obstetrics and Gynecology Resident
Christiana Care Health System
Wilmington, DE

Jyothsna I. Herek, MD
Senior Staff Physician
Nephrology and Hypertension
Henry Ford Hospital
Detroit, MI

Melissa A. Hewson, MD
Attending Physician
General Pediatrics
Children's Hospital of Philadelphia
Philadelphia, PA

Margaret R. Hines, MD
Clinical Fellow
Female Pelvic Medicine and Reconstructive Surgery
Urogynecology
Baylor Scott and White
Temple, TX

Katherine Hladky, MD
Obstetrics and Gynecology
Christiana Care Health System
Newark, DE

Ashley Hodges, MD
Obstetrics and Gynecology Resident
Christiana Care Health System
Newark, DE

R. Scott Hoffman, MD
Ophthalmologist
Assistant Clinical Professor
University of Louisville School of Medicine
Doctors Eye Institute and University of Louisville Ophthalmology
Louisville, KY

Dawn Hogan, MD
Clinical Assistant Professor of Family Medicine
Warren Alpert Medical School of Brown University
Providence, RI

Jennifer J. Holiman, MSN, APRN, PMHNP-BC
Nurse Practitioner
Geriatric Psychiatry
McLean Hospital
Belmont, MA

N. Wilson Holland, MD
Associate Professor of Medicine
Division of Geriatrics and Gerontology
Emory University School of Medicine;
Acting Designated Learning Officer
Atlanta Veterans Administration Medical Center
Atlanta, GA

Karima A. Holmes, MD
Psychiatry Resident
Massachusetts General Hospital and McLean Hospital
Boston, MA

Siri M. Holton, MD
Physician
Obstetrics and Gynecology
Christiana Care Health System
Newark, DE

Austin Hoy, MD
Fellow, Hand and Upper Extremity
Department of Orthopedics
Warren Alpert Medical School of Brown University
Providence, RI

Raymond Hsu, MD
Assistant Professor of Orthopedic Surgery
Warren Alpert Medical School of Brown University
Providence, RI

Elena Huang, MD, FAAP
Attending Physician
Children's Hospital of Philadelphia, Primary Care Network
Associate Professor of Pediatrics
Perelman School of Medicine at the University of Pennsylvania
Philadelphia, PA

Lawrence Huang, MD, FCCP, ATSF
Professor of Medicine
Division of Pulmonary and Critical Care Medicine and HIV, Infectious Diseases
Global Medicine Division
University of California San Francisco
San Francisco, CA

Anne L. Hume, PharmD
Professor of Pharmacy
Department of Pharmacy Practice
University of Rhode Island
Kingston, RI

Zilla Hussain, MD
Gastroenterologist
Lifespan Physicians Group at Rhode Island Hospital
Providence, RI

Donny V. Huynh, MD
Staff Physician
McLeod Oncology and Hematology at Seacoast
McLeod Regional Medical Center
Little River, SC

Sarah Hyder, MD
Assistant Professor of Medicine
Director of Endoscopic Ultrasound
Warren Alpert Medical School of Brown University
Lifespan Physician Group
Providence, RI

Dina A. Ibrahim, MD
Hospitalist
Yale New Haven Hospital
Yale University
New Haven, CT

Zainab Ibrahim, MD
Orthopaedic Surgery
Warren Alpert Medical School of Brown University
Providence, RI

Caitlin Ingraham, MD
Obstetrics and Gynecology Resident
Christiana Care Health System
Newark, DE

Nicholas J. Inman, MD
Emergency Medicine Resident
University of Tennessee Health Science Center
Memphis, TN

Louis F. Insalaco, MD
Department of Otolaryngology
Mass Eye and Ear, Stoneham
Harvard Medical School
Stoneham, MA

Ana Ivkovic, MD
Staff Psychiatrist
Massachusetts General Hospital
Boston, MA

Ashley A. Jacobson, MD
Emergency Medicine Resident
Mayo Clinic
Rochester, MN

S. Hammad Jafri, MD, MMSCI
Department of Cardiology
Warren Alpert Medical School of Brown University
Providence, RI

Koyal Jain, MD, MPH
Assistant Professor of Medicine
Division of Nephrology and Hypertension
University of North Carolina at Chapel Hill
Chapel Hill, NC

Vanita B. D. Jain, MD
Delaware Center for Maternal and Fetal Medicine
Medical Director, High Risk Unit (PSCU) and Clinic
Christiana Care Health Systems
Newark, DE;
Clinical Assistant Professor
Sidney Kimmel School of Medicine
Thomas Jefferson University
Philadelphia, PA

Fariha Jamal, MD
Assistant Professor of Neurology
Baylor College of Medicine
Michael E. DeBakey VA Medical Center
Houston, TX

Marcus L. Jamil, MD
Urology Resident
Vattikuti Urology Institute
Henry Ford Health System
Detroit, MI

Robert H. Janigian, Jr., MD
Clinical Associate Professor of Surgery
Warren Alpert Medical School of Brown University
Providence, RI

Sonia Jasuja, MD
Fellow Physician
Division of Pulmonary and Critical Care Medicine
University of California Los Angeles
Los Angeles, CA

Noelle Marie Javier, MD
Associate Professor of Medicine
Brookdale Department of Geriatrics and Palliative Care
Icahn School of Medicine at Mount Sinai
New York, NY

Derek R. Jenkins, MD
Assistant Professor
Orthopaedic Surgery
Division of Adult Reconstruction
Warren Alpert Medical School of Brown University
Providence, RI

Vybhav Jetty, MD, MHA
Cardiology Fellow
St. Elizabeth's Medical Center
Boston, MA

Lillian Jin, MD, MPH
Resident Physician
Children's Hospital of Philadelphia
Philadelphia, PA

Katie Johnson, MD
Fellow in Child Abuse Pediatrics
Seattle Children's Hospital
Washington School of Medicine
Seattle, WA

Michael P. Johnson, MD
MDVIP Affiliate Physician
Internal Medicine
Providence, RI

Angad Jolly, PhD
Baylor College of Medicine
Houston, TX

Rebecca Jonas, MD
Neurohospitalist
Departments of Medicine and Neurological Surgery
Thomas Jefferson University Hospital
Philadelphia, PA

Matthew C. Jones, MD, MS
Orthopaedic Surgery Fellow
Warren Alpert Medical School of Brown University
Providence, RI

Priyanka Joshi, MD
Pediatric Resident
Children's Hospital of Philadelphia
Philadelphia, PA

Shyam Joshi, MD
Assistant Professor of Medicine
Section of Allergy and Immunology
Oregon Health and Science University
Portland, OR

Joshua Justice, MD
Assistant Professor
Emergency Medicine
University of Tennessee Health Science Center
Memphis, TN

Vanji Karthikeyan, MD
Senior Staff
Division of Nephrology
Henry Ford Hospital
Detroit, MI

Joseph S. Kass, MD, JD, FAAN
Associate Dean of Student Affairs
Professor of Neurology, Psychiatry, and Medical Ethics
Director, Alzheimer's Disease and Memory Disorders Center
Baylor College of Medicine;
Chief of Neurology
Director of Comprehensive Stroke Program
Ben Taub General Hospital
Houston, TX

Naomi R. Kass, BA
Rice University
Houston, TX

Zain Kassam, MD
Cardiology Fellow
Lenox Hill Hospital, Northwell Health
New York, NY

Julia Katarincic, MD
Associate Professor
Orthopedic Surgery
Warren Alpert School of Medicine of Brown University
Providence, RI

Bhavika Kaul, MD
Clinical Instructor
Pulmonary and Critical Care Medicine
University of California San Francisco
San Francisco, CA

Gurmehr Kaur, MD
Psychiatry Resident
University of Arizona College of Medicine
Phoenix, AZ

Ali Kazim, MD
Chief of Psychiatry
VA Health Care System
Phoenix, AZ

Sudad Kazzaz, MD
Baylor College of Medicine
Houston, TX

Sachin Kedar, MBBS, MD
Associate Professor
Neurological Sciences, Ophthalmology and Visual Sciences
University of Nebraska Medical School and Truhlsen Eye Institute
Omaha, NE

Vasken Keleshian, MD
General Cardiology Fellow
University of California Irvine
Orange, CA

Dennis Keselman, MD
Child Neurology Resident
Children's Hospital of Philadelphia
Philadelphia, PA

Rizwan Khan, MD
Fellow in Cardiology
St. Elizabeth's Medical Center
Tufts University School of Medicine
Boston, MA

Sarthak Khare, MD
Cardiology Fellow
St. Elizabeth's Medical Center
Boston, MA

Hussain R. Khawaja, MD, FACP
Assistant Professor of Medicine, Clinician Educator
General Internal Medicine
Warren Alpert Medical School of Brown University/Rhode Island Hospital
Providence, RI

Robert M. Kirchner, MD
Cardiology Fellow
Warren Alpert Medical School of Brown University
Providence, RI

Samuel I. Kohrman, MD
Clinical Fellow, Consultation-Liaison Psychiatry
Massachusetts General Hospital
Boston, MA

Erna Milunka Kojic, MD
Professor, Department of Medicine
Mount Sinai School of Medicine
New York, NY

Aravind Rao Kokkirala, MD, FACC
Division of Cardiology
Warren Alpert Medical School of Brown University
Providence Veterans Affairs Medical Center
Providence, RI

Yuval Konstantino, MD
Soroka University Medical Center
Cardiology
Faculty of Health Sciences
Ben Gurion University of the Negev
Beer-Sheva, Israel

Nelson Kopyt, DO
Chief of Nephrology
Lehigh Valley Hospital
Allentown, PA

Lindsay R. Kosinski, MD
Orthopaedic Surgery Resident
Warren Alpert Medical School of Brown University/Rhode Island Hospital
Providence, RI

Savan Kothadia, MD
House Staff, Internal Medicine
Rhode Island Hospital
Providence, RI

Ioannis Koulouridis, MD, MS
Cardiology Fellow
St Elizabeth's Medical Center
Boston, MA

Natalija Kovacevic, MD
Urology Resident
Vattikuti Urology Institute
Henry Ford Health System
Detroit, MI

Timothy R. Kreider, MD, PhD
Assistant Professor, Psychiatry
Donald and Barbara Zucker School of Medicine at Hofstra/Northwell
Hemstead, NY

Prashanth Krishnamohan, MBBS, MD
Neurocritical Care
Stanford University
Stanford, CA

Van S. Krueger, MD
Department of Orthopedic Surgery
Warren Alpert Medical School of Brown University
Providence, RI

Lalathaksha Kumbar, MD
Senior Staff Physician
Nephrology and Hypertension
Henry Ford Hospital
Detroit, MI

Eren O. Kuris, MD
Assistant Professor, Orthopaedic Surgery
Warren Alpert Medical School of Brown University/Rhode Island Hospital
Providence, RI

David I. Kurss, MD, FACOG, NCMP
Attending Physician
Women's Wellness Center of Western New York
Invision Health
Amherst, NY;
Clinical Assistant Professor
School of Medicine, Obstetrics and Gynecology
State University of New York at Buffalo
Buffalo, NY

Michael Kutschke, MD
Orthopedic Surgery Resident
Warren Alpert Medical School of Brown University
Providence, RI

Ann S. LaCasce, MD, MMSc
Associate Professor of Medicine, Medical Oncology
Harvard Medical School;
Institute Physician, Medical Oncology
Dana-Farber Cancer Institute
Boston, MA

Uyen T. Lam, MD
St. Elizabeth's Medical Center
Tufts University School of Medicine
Boston, MA

Ajibike Lapite, MD, MPTM
Resident Physician
Children's Hospital of Philadelphia
Philadelphia, PA

Julianna Lau, MD
Pediatric Resident
Children's Hospital of Philadelphia
Philadelphia, PA

Lorriana E. Leard, MD
Professor of Clinical Medicine
Vice Chief of Clinical Operations
Pulmonary, Critical Care, Allergy, and Sleep Medicine
University of California San Francisco
San Francisco, CA

David A. Leavitt, MD
Associate Director of Endourology
Director of Laser Surgery
Vattikuti Urology Institute
Henry Ford Hospital Health System
Detroit, MI

Hyun Lee, MD
Resident, Internal Medicine
Warren Alpert Medical School of Brown University
Providence, RI

Kachiu C. Lee, MD, MPH
Department of Dermatology
Warren Alpert Medical School of Brown University
Providence, RI

Yvonne Lee, MD
Rheumatology Fellow
Cedars-Sinai Medical Center
Beverly Hills, CA

Nicholas J. Lemme, MD
Orthopedics Resident
Warren Alpert Medical School of Brown University/Rhode Island Hospital
Providence, RI

René Lento, PhD
Clinical Psychologist and Director of Addiction Services
MGH Home Base Program, Psychiatry
Massachusetts General Hospital
Boston, MA

James G. Levins, MD
Orthopedic Surgery Resident
Warren Alpert Medical School of Brown University
Providence, RI

Jian Li, MD, PhD
Clinical Assistant Professor
Internal Medicine, Hypertension and Nephrology
Wayne State University School of Medicine
Henry Ford Hospital
Detroit, MI

Suqing Li, MD
Gastroenterology Fellow
Gastroenterology and Hepatology
University of Toronto
Toronto, Ontario, Canada

Leora Lieberman, MD
General Pediatrics Resident
Children's Hospital of Philadelphia
Philadelphia, PA

Donita D. Lightner, MD
Assistant Professor of Pediatric Neurology
Department of Neurology
University of Kentucky
Lexington, KY

Erica Lin, MD
Fellow
Division of Pulmonary, Critical Care and Sleep Medicine
University of California San Diego
La Jolla, CA

Cynthia Longjohn, MD
House Staff, Pediatric Resident
Pediatrics
NYU Langone Hospital/Bellevue Hospital Center
New York, NY

Gabriela López, PhD
Center for Alcohol and Addiction Studies (CAAS)
Warren Alpert Medical School of Brown University
Providence, RI

Kito Akin Lord, MD, MBA
Assistant Professor
Emergency Medicine
University of Tennessee Health Science Center
Memphis, TN

Elizabeth A. Lowenhaupt, MD
Associate Professor of Psychiatry
Medical Sciences and Pediatrics
Rhode Island Hospital
Providence, RI

Curtis (Trey) Lee Lowery III, PhD, MD
Emergency Medicine Resident
University of Tennessee Health Science Center
Memphis, TN

David J. Lucier Jr., MD, MBA, MPH
Director of Quality and Patient Safety
Hospital Medicine, Division of General Internal Medicine
Massachusetts General Hospital
Boston, MA

Michelle C. Maciag, MD
Physician and Instructor
Allergy and Immunology
Boston Children's Hospital
Harvard Medical School
Boston, MA

Rachel L. MacLean, MD
Psychiatry Resident
Massachusetts General Hospital/McLean Hospital
Boston, MA

Elizabeth N. Madva, MD
Consultation-Liaison Psychiatry Fellow
Massachusetts General Hospital
Harvard Medical School
Boston, MA

Abiramy Maheswaran, MD
Fellow Physician
Hematology/Oncology
University of Massachusetts
Worcester, MA

Shefali Majmudar, DO
Rheumatologist
Division of Rheumatology
Jackson Medical Center
Miami, FL

Gretchen Makai, MD
Director, Division of Minimally Invasive Gynecologic Surgery
Obstetrics and Gynecology
Christiana Care Health System
Newark, DE

Katherine Malcolm, MD, MPH
Fellow, Division of Pulmonary, Critical Care, Allergy, and Sleep Medicine
University of California San Francisco
San Francisco, CA

Pieusha Malhotra, MD, MPH
Assistant Professor
Division of Allergy, Immunology, and Rheumatology
Rutgers New Jersey School of Medicine
Newark, NJ

Eishita Manjrekar, PhD
Clinical Director, Psychology and Psychiatry
Lifestance Health
Los Angeles, CA

Stephen E. Maracaccio, MD
Orthopaedic Surgery
Warren Alpert Medical School of Brown University
Providence, RI

Charles Masaki, MD, PhD
Chief Resident and Clinical Fellow in Psychiatry
Massachusetts General Hospital/McLean Hospital
Boston, MA

Maitreyi Mazumdar, MD, MPH, MSc
Associate Professor of Neurology
Boston Children's Hospital
Harvard Medical School
Boston, MA

Peter J. Mazzaglia, MD
Endocrine Surgeon
Department of Surgery
Rhode Island Hospital
Providence, RI

Nadine Mbuyi, MD
Assistant Professor of Medicine
Division of Rheumatology
The George Washington University School of Medicine and Health Sciences
Washington, DC

Russell J. McCulloh, MD
Division Chief, Pediatric Hospital Medicine
Children's Hospital and Medical Center
Omaha, NE;
Physician, Infectious Diseases and Hospital Medicine
Department of Pediatrics
Children's Mercy Kansas City
Kansas City, MO

Christopher McDonald, MD
Orthopedic Surgery
Warren Alpert Medical School of Brown University/Rhode Island Hospital
Providence, RI

Alexandra McGowen, MD
Emergency Medicine Resident
University of Tennessee Health Science Center
Memphis, TN

Barbara McGuirk, MD
Director of Surgery
Reproductive Associates of Delaware
Newark, DE

Kelly McNamara, MD
Attending Generalist Physician
Obstetrics and Gynecology
Christiana Care
Newark, DE

Jorge Mercado, MD
Assistant Professor of Medicine
Pulmonary and Critical Care Medicine Division
NYU School of Medicine;
Co-chief of Pulmonary & Critical Care Section; Director of Bronchoscopy
NYU Langone Brooklyn
New York, NY

Scott J. Merrill, MD
Obstetrics and Gynecology Resident
Christiana Care Hospital, Inc.
Newark, DE

Jennifer B. Merriman, MD
Division of Maternal-Fetal Medicine
Intermountain Healthcare
Murray, UT

Rory Merritt, MD, MEHP
Assistant Dean of Medicine - PLME Advising
Assistant Professor of Emergency Medicine
Warren Alpert Medical School of Brown University
Providence, RI

Robin Metcalfe-Klaw, MD
Obstetrics and Gynecology Resident
Christiana Care
Newark, DE

Marian G. Michaels, MD, MPH
Professor of Pediatrics and Surgery
Pediatric Infectious Diseases
UPMC Children's Hospital of Pittsburgh
Pittsburgh, PA

Gaetane Michaud, MD
Professor of Medicine and Cardiothoracic Surgery
NYU Langone Health;
Section Chief, Interventional Pulmonology
Division of Pulmonary, Critical Care & Sleep Medicine
NYU Langone Medical Center
New York, NY

Jeremy Michel, MD, MHS
Assistant Professor of Pediatrics
Perelman School of Medicine, University of Pennsylvania
Philadelphia, PA

Brian D. Mikolasko, MD
Assistant Professor of Medicine
Warren Alpert Medical School of Brown University
Providence, RI

May Min, MD
Fellow, Division of Gastroenterology
Warren Alpert Medical School of Brown University
Providence, RI

Taro Minami, MD
Associate Professor of Medicine, Clinician Educator
Warren Alpert Medical School of Brown University
Providence, RI;
Director, Simulation and Ultrasound Training
Division of Pulmonary, Critical Care and Sleep Medicine
Memorial Hospital of Rhode Island
Pawtucket, RI

Jared D. Minkel, PhD
Clinical Assistant Professor of Psychiatry and Human Behavior
Warren Alpert Medical School of Brown University
Providence, RI

Farhan A. Mirza, MD
Neurosurgery Resident
University of Kentucky
Lexington, KY

Hetal D. Mistry, MD
Internal Medicine Resident
Warren Alpert Medical School of Brown University
Providence, RI

Rei Mitsuyama, MD
Internal Medicine Resident
Warren Alpert Medical School of Brown University/Rhode Island Hospital
Providence, RI

Jacob Modest, MD
Department of Orthopaedic Surgery
Warren Alpert Medical School of Brown University/Rhode Island Hospital
Providence, RI

Marc Monachese, MD
Gastroenterology Fellow
University of Toronto
Toronto, Ontario, Canada

Ethan Monhollon, MD
Emergency Medicine Resident
University of Tennessee Health Science Center
Memphis, TN

Philippe Montgrain, MD
Professor of Medicine
Division of Pulmonary, Critical Care and Sleep Medicine
University of California San Diego
La Jolla, CA

Eveline Mordehai, MD
Resident Physician
Anesthesiology
Rhode Island Hospital
Providence, RI

Leah Morelli, MD
Psychiatry Resident
Massachusetts General Hospital
Boston, MA

Aleem I. Mughal, MD, FHRS
Cardiac Electrophysiologist
Department of Electrophysiology
Heart Center of North Texas
Fort Worth, TX

Contributors

Marjan Mujib, MD
Cardiologist
Penn Medicine Lancaster General Health
Lancaster, PA

Shiva Kumar R. Mukkamalla, MD, MPH
Attending Physician
Hematology and Medical Oncology
Presbyterian Rust Cancer Care
Rio Rancho, NM

Katherine M. Mullersman, MD
Psychiatry Resident
Massachusetts General Hospital/McLean Hospital
Boston, MA

Omar Nadeem, MD
Instructor in Medicine
Hematologic Malignancies, Medical Oncology
Harvard Medical School
Dana-Farber Cancer Institute
Boston, MA

Hussain Mohammad H. Naseri, MD
Physician
Hematology/Oncology
MercyOne Waterloo Cancer Center
Waterloo, IA

Uzma Nasir, MD
Assistant Professor
Clinical Anesthesia and Pain Management
SUNY at Stony Brook University Hospital
VA Hospital
Northport, NY

Adrienne B. Neithardt, MD
Associate Physician
Reproductive Endocrinology and Infertility
Reproductive Associates of Delaware
Newark, DE

Samantha Ni, MD
Emergency Medicine Resident
University of Tennessee Health Science Center
Memphis, TN

Mladen Nisavic, MD
Attending Physician
Consultation-Liaison Service, Acute Psychiatry Service
Massachusetts General Hospital
Boston, MA

Natalie Nokoff, MD, MSCS
Assistant Professor
Department of Pediatrics, Division of Endocrinology
University of Colorado
Anschutz Medical Campus
Aurora, CO

James E. Novak, MD, PhD
Senior Staff
Program Director, Nephrology Fellowship
Nephrology and Hypertension
Henry Ford Hospital
Detroit, MI

Chloe Mander Nunneley, MD
Baylor College of Medicine
Houston, TX

Emily E. Nuss, MD
Obstetrics and Gynecology Resident
Christiana Care Health System
Newark, DE

Ryan M. O'Donnell, MD
Orthopaedic Resident
Warren Alpert Medical School of Brown University/Rhode Island Hospital
Providence, RI

Adam J. Olszewski, MD
Associate Professor of Medicine
Hematology-Oncology
Warren Alpert Medical School of Brown University/Rhode Island Hospital
Providence, RI

Henry K. Onyeaka, MD, MPH
Resident Physician
Psychiatry
Massachusetts General Hospital/McLean Hospital
Boston, MA

Lindsay M. Orchowski, PhD
Associate Professor (Research)
Psychiatry and Human Behavior
Warren Alpert Medical School of Brown University/Rhode Island Hospital
Providence, RI

Sebastian Orman, MD
Orthopaedic Surgery Resident
Warren Alpert Medical School of Brown University
Lifespan
Providence, RI

Ashley D. Osborne, MD
Fellow Physician
Neonatal and Perinatal Medicine
Children's Hospital of Philadelphia
Philadelphia, PA

Brett D. Owens, MD
Surgeon, Orthopedic Sports Medicine
Complex Shoulder and Knee Specialist
Warren Alpert Medical School of Brown University
Providence, RI

Ayotomide Oyelakin, MD, MPH
Child and Adolescent Psychiatry Fellow
Massachusetts General Hospital/McLean Hospital;
Clinical Fellow
Harvard Medical School
Boston, MA

Paolo G. Pace, MASc, MD
Internal Medicine Resident
Roger Williams Medical Center
Providence, RI

Alexa Papaila, MD, MPH
Internal Medicine Resident
Warren Alpert Medical School of Brown University
Providence, RI

Lisa Pappas-Taffer, MD
Assistant Professor of Clinical Dermatology
Perelman School of Medicine, University of Pennsylvania
Philadelphia, PA

Marco Pares, MD
Baylor College of Medicine
Houston, TX

Mihir Parikh, MD
Instructor in Medicine
Thoracic Surgery and Interventional Pulmonology
Beth Israel Deaconess Medical Center
Harvard Medical School
Boston, MA

Shivani Parikh, MD
Resident Physician
Obstetrics and Gynecology
Trihealth
Cincinnati, OH

Michael T. Partin, MD
Assistant Professor
Family and Community Medicine
Penn State Health M. S. Hershey Medical Center
Hershey, PA

Birju B. Patel, MD
Assistant Professor of Medicine
Division of Geriatrics and Gerontology
Emory University School of Medicine
Atlanta Veterans Affairs Medical Center
Atlanta, GA

Devan D. Patel, MD
Orthopedic Surgery Resident
Warren Alpert Medical School of Brown University
Providence, RI

Melissa D. Patel, MD, MPH
Associate Professor of Clinical Pediatrics
University of Pennsylvania School of Medicine;
Section Chief, Pediatric Hospital Medicine
Children's Hospital of Philadelphia
Philadelphia, PA

Nima R. Patel, MD, MS
Residency Program Director and Division Director Obstetrics and Gynecology
Obstetrics and Gynecology, Minimally Invasive Surgery
TriHealth
Cincinnati, OH

Pranav M. Patel, MD, FACC, FAHA, FSCAI
Professor of Medicine and Biomedical Engineering
Chief, Division of Cardiology
University of California Irvine
Irvine, CA;
Director of Cardiac Cath Lab and Cardiac Care Unit
University of California Irvine Medical Center
Orange, CA

Shivani K. Patel, MD
Rheumatologist
Internal Medicine/Rheumatology
St. Jude Heritage Medical Center
Fullerton, CA

Shyam A. Patel, MD
Orthopaedic Trauma Fellow
Orthopaedic Surgery
Warren Alpert Medical School of Brown University/Rhode Island Hospital
Providence, RI

Brett Patrick, MD
University of Tennessee Health Science Center
Memphis, TN

Shreedhar Paudel, MD, MPH
Psychiatrist
Massachusetts General Hospital;
Instructor in Psychiatry
Harvard Medical School
Boston, MA

Grace Rebecca Paul, MBBS, MD
Assistant Professor of Pediatrics
Division of Pulmonary and Sleep Medicine
Nationwide Children's Hospital
Columbus, OH

E. Scott Paxton, MD
Assistant Professor
Orthopedic Surgery
Warren Alpert Medical School of Brown University
Providence, RI

Ethan Pearlstein, MD
Internal Medicine Resident
Warren Alpert Medical School of Brown University
Rhode Island Hospital
Providence, RI

Alexander Peck, DO
Fellow in Rheumatology
Cedars-Sinai Medical Center
Los Angeles, CA

Mark Perazella, MD
Professor of Medicine
Division of Nephrology
Yale University School of Medicine
New Haven, CT

David L. Perez, MD, MMSc
Assistant Professor of Neurology
Departments of Neurology and Psychiatry
Massachusetts General Hospital
Harvard Medical School
Boston, MA

Courtney Pfeuti, MD
Obstetrics and Gynecology Resident
Christiana Care
Newark, DE

Lily C. Pham, MD
Neuro-Oncology Fellow
MD Anderson Cancer Center
Houston, TX

Long Pham, MD
Rheumatologist
Cedars-Sinai Medical Group
Los Angeles, CA

Katharine A. Phillips, MD
Professor of Psychiatry
DeWitt Wallace Senior Scholar
Residency Research Director
Department of Psychiatry
Weill Cornell Medical College;
Attending Psychiatrist
New York-Presbyterian Hospital/Weill Cornell Medical Center
New York, NY

Contributors

Oliver W. Phillips, MD
Neurology Chief Resident
Warren Alpert Medical School of Brown University
Providence, RI

Quan Phung, MD
Resident Physician
Internal Medicine
Warren Alpert Medical School of Brown University
Providence, RI

Wendy A. Plante, PhD
Clinical Associate Professor of Psychiatry and Human Behavior
Warren Alpert Medical School of Brown University;
Assistant Director of Child Psychology
Hasbro Children's/Rhode Island Hospital
Providence, RI

Kevin V. Plumley, MD, MPH
Urgentologist
Kaiser West LA
Los Angeles, CA

Nathan Praschan, MD, MPH
Administrative Chief Resident
Adult Psychiatry Residency
Massachusetts General Hospital/McLean Hospital
Boston, MA

Rohini Prashar, MD
Senior Staff
Division of Nephrology
Henry Ford Hospital
Detroit, MI

Amanda Pressman, MD
Assistant Professor of Medicine
Division of Gastroenterology
Warren Alpert Medical School of Brown University;
Gastroenterologist
Women's Medicine Collaborative
Director of Motility
Gastroenterology
Lifespan
Providence, RI

Margaret Priestly, MD
Senior Medical Director, Pediatric Intensive Care Unit
Anesthesiology and Critical Care Medicine
Children's Hospital of Philadelphia
Philadelphia, PA

Diana Punko, MD, MS
Fellow in Consultation-Liaison Psychiatry
Division of Psychiatry and Medicine
Massachusetts General Hospital
Boston, MA

Imran Puthawala, MD
Hematology/Oncology Fellow
University of Massachusetts Memorial Medical Center
Worcester, MA

Imrana Qawi, MD
Assistant Professor, Medicine
Pulmonary and Critical Care Medicine Division
Tufts Medical Center
Boston, MA

Michele Quan, MD, MPH
Fellow Physician
Division of Pulmonary, Critical Care, Hyperbaric, Allergy and Sleep Medicine
Loma Linda University Health
Loma Linda, CA

Nadia Quijije, MD
Attending Consultation Psychiatrist
Massachusetts General Hospital;
Instructor in Psychiatry
Harvard Medical School
Boston, MA

Matthew Quinn, MD
Orthopaedic Resident
Warren Alpert Medical School of Brown University/Rhode Island Hospital
Providence, RI

Gregory S. Rachu, MD, MPH
Assistant Professor of Medicine
Division of Geriatrics and Palliative Medicine
Warren Alpert Medical School of Brown University
Providence, RI

Jeremy E. Raducha, MD
Orthopedic Surgery Resident
Warren Alpert Medical School of Brown University
Providence, RI

Samaan Rafeq, MD
Clinical Associate Professor of Medicine and Cardiothoracic Surgery
New York University School of Medicine;
Chief, Interventional Pulmonology
Associate Section Chief, Pulmonary, Critical Care and Sleep Medicine
NYU Langone Health
New York, NY

Gina Ranieri, DO
Obstetrics and Gynecology Resident
Christiana Care Health System
Newark, DE

Bharti Rathore, MD
Program Director, Hematology/Oncology Fellowship
Roger Williams Medical Center
Providence, RI;
Assistant Professor of Medicine
Boston University School of Medicine
Boston, MA

Ritesh Rathore, MD
Associate Professor
Boston University School of Medicine;
Director, Hematology/Oncology
Roger Williams Medical Center
Providence, RI

Neha P. Raukar, MD, MS
Consultant, Emergency Medicine
Mayo Clinic
Rochester, MN

John L. Reagan, MD
Assistant Professor of Medicine
Warren Alpert Medical School of Brown University
Providence, RI

Bharathi V. Reddy, MD
Associate Professor of Medicine
Section of Nephrology
University of Chicago
Chicago, IL

Snigdha T. Reddy, MD
Senior Staff, Nephrology
Division of Nephrology and Hypertension
Henry Ford Hospital
Detroit, MI

Griffin Reed, MD
Internal Medicine Resident
Warren Alpert Medical School of Brown University
Providence, RI

Anthony M. Reginato, PhD, MD
Director, Division of Rheumatology
Associate Professor of Medicine
Warren Alpert School of Medicine at Brown University
Rhode Island Hospital
Providence, RI

James P. Reichart, MD
Department of Medicine
Lehigh Valley Health Network
Allentown, PA

Michaela B. Reinhart, MD
Pediatrics-Medical Genetics Resident
Children's Hospital of Philadelphia
Philadelphia, PA

Judith A. Restrepo, MD
Attending in Consultation-Liaison Psychiatry
Massachusetts General Hospital;
Instructor in Psychiatry
Harvard Medical School
Boston, MA

Victor I. Reus, MD
Distinguished Professor of Psychiatry
Psychiatry and Behavioral Sciences
University of California San Francisco School of Medicine
UCSF Weill Institute for Neurosciences
San Francisco, CA

Alexis Revet, MD
Assistant Professor of Child and Adolescent Psychiatry
Toulouse University Hospital & UMR1027 INSERM – University Toulouse-III-Paul-Sabatier
Toulouse, France

Candice Reyes, MD, RhMSUS
Associate Clinical Professor of Medicine
Rheumatology
University of California San Francisco
Fresno, CA

Harlan G. Rich, MD, FACP, AGAF
Associate Professor of Medicine and Medical Science
Warren Alpert Medical School of Brown University;
Clinical Director, Division of Gastroenterology
Brown Medicine/Brown Physicians, Inc.;
Medical Director
Brown Medicine Endoscopy Center
Providence, RI

Rocco J. Richards, MD
University of Pittsburgh Medical Center
Pittsburgh, PA

Sheyla Richards, MD
Resident Physician
Children's Hospital of Philadelphia
Philadelphia, PA

Nathan Riddell, MD
Interventional Cardiologist
Merrimack Valley Cardiology
Lowell General Hospital
Lowell, MA

Giulia Righi, PhD
Assistant Professor of Psychiatry and Human Behavior (Research)
Warren Alpert Medical School of Brown University
Providence, RI

Alvaro M. Rivera, MD
Internal Medicine
Roger Williams Medical Center
Providence, RI

Lauren Davis Rivera, MD, MSEd
Obstetrics and Gynecology Resident
Christiana Care Health Services
Newark, DE

Amy E. Riviere, DO, MA
Cardiovascular Disease Fellow
Maine Medical Center
Portland, ME

Todd F. Roberts, MD, FRCP(C)
Medical Director, Leukemia, Hematopoietic Cell Transplantation and Immunotherapy Program
Roger Williams Medical Center
Providence, RI

Melena Robertson, DO
Pediatric Infectious Disease Fellow
Pediatric Infectious Diseases
University of Pittsburgh Medical Center
Pittsburgh, PA

Alejandra E. Morfin Rodriguez, MD
Resident and Clinical Fellow
Psychiatry
Massachusetts General Hospital/ McLean Hospital
Harvard Medical School
Boston, MA

Perla M. Romero Gómez, MD
Research Fellow, Psychiatry
Massachusetts General Hospital
Boston, MA

Julie L. Roth, MD
Associate Professor of Neurology
Warren Alpert Medical School of Brown University
Providence, RI

Breton Roussel, MD
Gastroenterology Fellow
Rhode Island Hospital
Providence, RI

Amity Rubeor, DO, CAQSM
Assistant Professor, Family Medicine
Warren Alpert Medical School of Brown University
Providence, RI

David Rubin, MD
Director, Child and Adolescent Psychiatry Residency Training
Executive Director, MGH Psychiatry Academy
Director, Postgraduate Medical Education
Department of Psychiatry
Massachusetts General Hospital/McLean Hospital;
Lecturer in Psychiatry
Harvard Medical School
Boston, MA

Kelly Ruhstaller, MD
Christiana Care Health Systems
Newark, DE

Firrah Saeed, MD
Internal Medicine Resident
Warren Alpert Medical School of Brown University/Rhode Island Hospital
Providence, RI

Javeryah Safi, MD
Clinical Associate
Pulmonary and Critical Care Medicine
Tufts University;
Pulmonary and Critical Care Medicine
St. Elizabeth's Medical Center
Boston, MA

Emily Saks, MD, MSCE
Physician
Female Pelvic Medicine and Reconstructive Surgery
Christiana Care Health System
Newark, DE

Jeffrey W. Sall, PhD, MD
Professor and James P. Livingston Endowed Chair
Anesthesia and Perioperative Care
University of California San Francisco
San Francisco, CA

Milagros Samaniego-Picota, MD
Director, Kidney and Pancreas Transplantation
Transplantation Institute
Henry Ford Hospital
Detroit, MI

Wesley M. Sanders, PhD
Staff Psychologist, Home Base
Massachusetts General Hospital
Boston, MA

Lekshmi Santhosh, MD, MAEd
Assistant Professor of Clinical Medicine
Pulmonary and Critical Care Medicine Fellowship Associate Program Director
Division of Pulmonary, Critical Care, Allergy, and Sleep Medicine
University of California San Francisco
San Francisco, CA

Linda Herrera Santos, MD, PhD
Adult Psychiatry Resident
Massachusetts General Hospital
Boston, MA

Jinendra Satiya, MD
Clinical Hepatology Fellow
Gastroenterology and Hepatology
Beth Israel Deaconess Medical Center
Harvard Medical School
Boston, MA

Hemant K. Satpathy, MD
Fellow, Maternal Fetal Medicine
Obstetrics and Gynecology
Emory University
Atlanta, GA

Ruby K. Satpathy, MD
Cardiology Fellow
Department of Internal Medicine
Creighton University
Omaha, NE

Emily Sauck, DO, MBA
Resident Physician
Obstetrics and Gynecology
Christiana Care
Newark, DE

Syeda M. Sayeed, MD
Attending Physician
Rheumatology
South Coast Health
Fall River, MA

Leah Saylor, DO
Obstetrics and Gynecology Resident
TriHealth
Cincinnati, OH

Daphne Scaramangas-Plumley, MD
Rheumatologist
Attune Health
Cedars-Sinai Medical Center
Department of Rheumatology
Los Angeles, CA

Paul J. Scheel, Jr., MD, MBA, MPH
Associate Vice Chancellor for Clinical Affairs
CEO Faculty Practice Plan
Washington University
St. Louis, MO

Bradley Schlussel, MD
Rheumatologist
Trumbull Rheumatology - Bridgeport Hospital
Trumbull, CT

Kristina Schnitzer, MD
Psychiatrist, Schizophrenia Clinical and Research Program
Massachusetts General Hospital;
Instructor
Harvard Medical School
Boston, MA

Anthony Sciscione, DO
Professor, Obstetrics and Gynecology
Jefferson Medical College
Philadelphia, PA;
Residency Program Director
Director of Maternal-Fetal Medicine
Obstetrics and Gynecology
Christiana Care Health System
Newark, DE

Christina D. Scully, MD
Clinical Assistant Professor of Psychiatry and Human Behavior
Clinical Assistant Professor of Medical Science
Warren Alpert Medical School of Brown University
Providence, RI

Richard E. Seeber II, MD
Psychiatry Resident
Massachusetts General Hospital/McLean Hospital
Boston, MA

Katarzyna Gilek-Seibert, MD, RhMUS
Program Director, Rheumatology Division and Fellowship Training Program
Boston University Affiliated Roger Williams Medical Center
Providence, RI

Peter J. Sell, DO
Associate Professor
University of Massachusetts Medical School
UMass Memorial Medical Center
Worcester, MA

Rachel Sewell, MD
Pediatrics Resident
University of Colorado Anschutz Medical Campus
Aurora, CO

Hesham Shaban, MD
Senior Staff Physician
Nephrology and Hypertension
Henry Ford Hospital System
Detroit, MI

Ankur Shah, MD
Assistant Professor of Medicine
Kidney Disease and Hypertension
Warren Alpert Medical School of Brown University
Providence, RI

Animesh Sharma, MD
Assistant Professor of Pediatrics
Pediatric Endocrinology
Children's Hospital of Colorado
Aurora, CO

Esseim Sharma, MD
Cardiology Fellow
Warren Alpert Medical School of Brown University
Providence, RI

Gargi Priamvada Sharma, MD
Adult Nephrology Fellow
Division of Nephrology and Hypertension
University of North Carolina, UNC Kidney Center
Chapel Hill, NC

Yuvraj Sharma, MD
Senior Staff
Nephrology and Hypertension
Henry Ford Hospital
Detroit, MI

Lydia Sharp, MD
Assistant Professor
Neurology
Baylor College of Medicine
Houston, TX

Alexander Sherman, MD
Fellow Physician
Pulmonary and Critical Care Medicine
University of California Los Angeles
Los Angeles, CA

Jessica E. Shill, MD
Senior Staff Physician
Endocrinology, Diabetes and Bone and Mineral Disorders
Henry Ford Health System
Detroit, MI;
Clinical Associate Professor of Medicine
Wayne State University School of Medicine
Detroit, MI

Philip A. Shlossman, MD
Associate Director, Maternal and Fetal Medicine
Obstetrics and Gynecology
Christiana Hospital
Newark, DE

Asha Shrestha, MD
Rheumatologist
CareMount Medical
Mount Kisco, NY

Khawja A. Siddiqui, MD
Neuro-ICU Fellow
Neurology
Baylor College of Medicine
Houston, TX

Alyssa Siegel, MD
Attending Physician, General Pediatrics
Children's Hospital of Philadelphia;
Clinical Assistant Professor
Perelman School of Medicine at the University of Pennsylvania
Philadelphia, PA

Mark Sigman, MD
Professor and Chair
Department of Urology
Warren Alpert Medical School of Brown University
Providence, RI

Harinder P. Singh, MD
Assistant Professor
Pulmonary and Critical Care Medicine
Carney Hospital
Tufts University
Boston, MA

Vikas Singh, MD
Adult Nephrology Fellow
Nephrology and Hypertension
University of North Carolina, UNC Kidney Center
Chapel Hill, NC

Jerome L. Slate, MD, FCCP
Pulmonologist
Mount Auburn Hospital
Lexington, MA

Brett Slingsby, MD
Child Abuse Pediatrician
Assistant Professor of Pediatrics, Clinician Educator
Warren Alpert Medical School of Brown University
Providence, RI

Alexandra H. Smick, MD
Obstetrics and Gynecology Resident
TriHealth
Cincinnati, OH

Jeanette G. Smith, MD
Assistant Professor
Department of Medicine
Warren Alpert Medical School of Brown University
Providence, RI

Jonathan H. Smith, MD
Assistant Professor
Neurology
University of Kentucky
Lexington, KY

Matthew J. Smith, MD
Physical Medicine and Rehabilitation
Warren Alpert Medical School of Brown University
Rhode Island Hospital
Providence, RI

Vivek Soi, MD
Associate Clinical Professor
Nephrology
Wayne State University School of Medicine
Detroit, MI

Rebecca Soinski, MD
Rheumatologist
Women's Medicine Collaborative
Providence, RI

Maria E. Soler, MD, MPH, MBA
Director, Education Division and OB Triage
Obstetrics and Gynecology
Christiana Care Health System
Newark, DE

Sandeep Soman, MD
Associate Division Head
Nephrology and Hypertension
Henry Ford Hospital
Detroit, MI

Emily Sorg, MD
Attending Psychiatrist
Avery D. Weisman Psychiatric Consultation Service
MA General Hospital;
Instructor of Psychiatry
Harvard Medical School
Boston, MA

Timothy T. Spear, MD, PhD
General Pediatrics Resident
Children's Hospital of Philadelphia
Philadelphia, PA

C. John Sperati, MD, MHS
Associate Professor of Medicine
Division of Nephrology
Johns Hopkins University School of Medicine
Baltimore, MD

Diana Stern, MD
Psychiatry Resident
Massachusetts General Hospital/McLean Hospital
Boston, MA

Ella Stern, MD
Obstetrics and Gynecology Resident
Christiana Care Health Services
Newark, DE

Philip Stockwell, MD
Assistant Professor of Medicine
Division of Cardiology
Warren Alpert Medical School of Brown University
Providence, RI

Padmaja Sudhakar, MBBS
Assistant Professor
Neurology
University of Kentucky
Lexington, KY

Edward Suh, MD, MPH
Assistant Professor
Anesthesiology
Warren Alpert Medical School of Brown University/Rhode Island Hospital
Providence, RI

Jennifer K. Sun, MD, PhD
Internal Medicine-Pediatrics Resident
Children's Hospital of Philadelphia
Hospital of the University of Pennsylvania
Philadelphia, PA

Stephanie Sutter, MD
Resident Physician
Anesthesia and Perioperative Care
University of California San Francisco
San Francisco, CA

Joseph Sweeney, MD, FACP, FRCPath
Professor, Laboratory Medicine and Pathology
Warren Alpert Medical School of Brown University
Providence, RI

Simone Sweeney, MD
Physician, Women's Health
Obstetrics and Gynecology
Christiana Care Health System
Newark, DE

Maher Tabba, MD, FACP, FCCP
Associate Professor of Medicine and Surgery
Chief, Section of Interventional Pulmonology
Division of Pulmonary and Critical Care and Sleep Medicine
Tufts University School of Medicine
Boston, MA

Kaoru Takasaki, MD
Fellow, Pediatrics
Divisions of Hematology and Oncology
Children's Hospital of Philadelphia
Philadelphia, PA

Ryosuke Takei, MD
Attending Physician
General Pediatrics, Hospital Medicine
Children's Hospital of Philadelphia
Philadelphia, PA

Dominick Tammaro, MD
Associate Professor, Internal Medicine
Program Director, Internal Medicine Residency
Warren Alpert Medical School of Brown University/Rhode Island Hospital
Providence, RI

Laren Tan, MD
Associate Professor of Medicine
Pulmonary, Critical Care, Hyperbaric, Allergy and Sleep Medicine
Loma Linda University Health
Loma Linda, CA

Alan Taylor, MD
Assistant Program Director, Emergency Medicine
University of Tennessee Health Science Center
Memphis, TN

Tahir Tellioglu, MD
Clinical Instructor in Psychiatry
Harvard Medical School;
Addiction Psychiatrist
Massachusetts General Hospital
Boston, MA

Edward J. Testa, MD
Orthopedic Surgery Resident
Warren Alpert Medical School of Brown University
Providence, RI

Anthony G. Thomas, DO, FACP
Assistant Professor of Medicine
Medical Oncology/Hematology
Warren Alpert Medical School of Brown University
The Miriam Hospital
Lifespan Cancer Institute
Providence, RI

Andrew P. Thome Jr., MD
Orthopedic Surgery Resident
Warren Alpert Medical School of Brown University/Rhode Island Hospital
Providence, RI

Alexandra Meyer Tien, MD
Assistant Clinical Professor of Family Medicine
Warren Alpert Medical School of Brown University
Providence, RI

David Robbins Tien, MD
Associate Clinical Professor of Surgery (Ophthalmology)
Warren Alpert Medical School of Brown University
Providence, RI

Anna-Marie Tierney, MD
Attending Physician
Children's Hospital of Philadelphia
Philadelphia, PA

Patrick Tiffany, MD
Pediatrics Resident
Colorado University School of Medicine
Aurora, CO

Helen Toma, MD, MSPH
Obstetrics and Gynecology Resident
Christiana Care Health System
Newark, DE

Thomas M. Triplett, MD
Assistant Professor
Emergency Medicine
University of Tennessee Health Science Center;
Simulation Director, Site Director for Regional One Health
Memphis, TN

Hirsh D. Trivedi, MD
Gastroenterology and Hepatology Fellow
Beth Israel Deaconess Medical Center
Harvard Medical School
Boston, MA

Vrinda Trivedi, MBBS
Division of Cardiology
Warren Alpert Medical School of Brown University
Providence, RI

Margaret Tryforos, MD
Family Medicine
Care New England Primary Care Medical Group/Kent Hospital
Pawtucket, RI

Gal Tsaban, MD, MPH
Department of Internal Medicine
Soroka University Medical Center;
School of Public Health
Faculty of Health Sciences
Ben Gurion University of the Negev
Beer-Sheva, Israel

Joseph R. Tucci, MD, FACP, FACE
Professor of Medicine
Boston University School of Medicine;
Director, Division of Endocrinology
Roger Williams Medical Center/Boston University School of Medicine;
Adjunct Professor of Medicine
Warren Alpert Medical School at Brown University
Providence, RI

Junior Uduman, MD
Senior Staff Physician
Nephrology and Hypertension
Henry Ford Hospital
Detroit, MI

Sean H. Uiterwyk, MD
Clinical Assistant Professor
Community and Family Medicine
Geisel School of Medicine at Dartmouth
Hanover, NH;
White River Family Practice
White River Junction, VT

Rebecca Ukaegbu, MD
Psychiatry Resident
Massachusetts General Hospital/McLean Hospital
Boston, MA

Kausik Umanth, MD, MS, FASN
Associate Professor of Medicine
Wayne State University;
Section Head, Clinical Research
Nephrology and Hypertension
Henry Ford Hospital
Detroit, MI

Bryant Uy, MPH, PA-C
Physician Assistant
Attune Health, Rheumatology
Beverly Hills, CA

Babak Vakili, MD
Clinical Associate Professor
Obstetrics and Gynecology
Drexel University College of Medicine
Philadelphia, PA;
Vice-Chair, Gynecologic Surgery
Obstetrics and Gynecology
Christiana Care Health System
Newark, DE

Emily Van Kirk, MD
Internal Medicine
Roger Williams Medical Center
Providence, RI

Jennifer E. Vaughan, MD
Fellow
Neurology and Rehabilitation Medicine
University of Cincinnati College of Medicine
Cincinnati, OH

Aida Venado, MD, MAS
Assistant Professor of Medicine
Pulmonary, Critical Care, Allergy, and Sleep Medicine
University of California San Francisco
San Francisco, CA

Shilpa Vijayakumar, MD
Division of Cardiology
Warren Alpert Medical School of Brown University
Providence, RI

Kathryn G. Vollum, MD
Obstetrics and Gynecology Resident
Christiana Care
Newark, DE

Ethan Vorel, MD
Pediatrics Resident
Children's Hospital of Philadelphia
Philadelphia, PA

Kimberly Vu, MD
Internal Medicine Resident
University of California Irvine Medical Center
Orange, CA

Emil Stefan Vutescu, MD
Orthopaedic Surgery Resident
Warren Alpert Medical School of Brown University/Rhode Island Hospital
Providence, RI

J. Richard Walker III, MD, MS, FACEP
Associate Professor of Emergency Medicine
Program Director and Chair of Emergency Medicine Department
University of Tennessee Health Science Center
Memphis, TN

Ryan Walsh, MD
Emergency Medicine Resident
University of Tennessee Health Science Center
Memphis, TN

Ifeanyi Walson, DO
Psychiatry and Behavioral Medicine Resident
Brody School of Medicine
East Carolina University
Greenville, NC

Angela Wang, MD
Clinical Professor of Medicine
Medical Director, Pulmonary Outpatient Services
Pulmonary, Critical Care, Sleep Medicine and Physiology
University of California San Diego
San Diego, CA

Danielle Wang, MD
Rheumatology Fellow
Cedars-Sinai Medical Center
Los Angeles, CA

Evelyn R. Wang, MD
General Pediatrics Resident
Children's Hospital of Philadelphia
Philadelphia, PA

Jarey H. Wang, MD, PhD
Baylor College of Medicine
Houston, TX

Ming-Jin Wang, DO
Oncology Fellow
Division of Hematology Oncology
University of Massachusetts
Worcester, MA

Stephani C. Wang, MD
General Cardiology Fellow
University of California Irvine
Orange, CA

Tisha Wang, MD
Associate Professor of Clinical Medicine
Pulmonary and Critical Care Medicine
University of California Los Angeles
Los Angeles, CA

Ryan Watson, MD
Interventional and Structural Cardiology Fellow
Division of Cardiology
Brigham and Women's Hospital
Boston, MA

Manuel Shayne Weekley, MD
Associate Professor of Emergency Medicine
University of Tennessee Health Science Center
Regional One Health
Memphis, TN

Marc S. Weinberg, MD, PhD
Resident Psychiatrist
Massachusetts General Hospital/McLean Hospital
Boston, MA

Max Weiss, MD
Clinical Cardiac Electrophysiology Fellow
Cardiovascular Diseases
University of Michigan
Ann Arbor, MI

Mary-Beth Walesko, MS, APRN-BC, WCC
Nurse Practitioner
Geriatrics and Palliative Medicine
Care New England Medical Group
Warwick, RI

Adrienne Werth, MD
Obstetrics and Gynecology Resident
Christiana Care Health System
Newark, DE

Matthew J. White, DO
Rheumatologist
Dartmouth-Hitchcock Medical Center
Lebanon, NH

Patrick Williamson, BS
University of Tennessee Health Science Center College of Medicine
Memphis, TN

John P. Wincze, PhD
Clinical Professor Emeritus
Psychiatry and Human Behavior
Warren Alpert Medical School of Brown University
Providence, RI

Jared M. Winikor, MD
Attending Physician
Pediatrics
Children's Hospital of Philadelphia
Philadelphia, PA

Bryce Wininger, MD
Attending Psychiatrist
Massachusetts General Hospital
Harvard Medical School
Boston, MA

Marlene Fishman Wolpert, MPH, CIC, FAPIC
Long-Term Care Infection Preventionist
The Miriam Hospital;
Independent Consultant
Providence, RI

Sariya Wongsaengsak, MD
Internal Medicine Resident
Texas Tech University Health Sciences Center School of Medicine
Lubbock, TX

John Wylie, MD, FACC
Director, Cardiac Electrophysiology
Steward Health Care System;
Associate Professor of Medicine
Tufts University School of Medicine
St. Elizabeth's Medical Center
Boston, MA

Tzu-Ching (Teddy) Wu, MD, MPH
Assistant Professor of Neurology
University of Texas Medical School at Houston;
Director of Telemedicine
Mischer Neuroscience Institute
Houston, TX

Anna Yang, MD
Assistant Professor of Emergency Medicine
University of Tennessee Health Sciences Center
Memphis, TN

Nicole B. Yang, MD
Instructor in Medicine
Harvard Medical School;
Rheumatology, Inflammation, and Immunity
Brigham and Women's Hospital
Boston, MA

Jerry Yee, MD
Division Head
Department of Nephrology and Hypertension
Henry Ford Hospital
Detroit, MI

Gemini Yesodharan, MD
Cardiology Fellow
St. Elizabeth's Medical Center
Brighton, MA

Jia Yi, MD
Adult Nephrology Fellow
Nephrology and Hypertension
Chapel Hill, NC

Agustin G. Yip, MD, PhD
McLean Hospital
Harvard Medical School
Belmont, MA

Robert J. York, MD
University of Tennessee Regional One Physicians
Emergency Medicine Department
Memphis, TN

John Q. Young, MD, MPP, PhD
Professor and Vice Chair for Education, Department of Psychiatry
Donald and Barbara Zucker School of Medicine at Hofstra/Northwell
Hemstead, NY

Shane Young, MD
Emergency Medicine Resident
University of Tennessee Health Science Center
Memphis, TN

Reem Yusufani, MD
Nephrology Fellow
Nephrology and Hypertension
Henry Ford Hospital
Detroit, MI

Caroline Zahm, MD
Cardiology Fellow
St. Elizabeth's Medical Center
Boston, MA

Anna V. Zdroik, DO
Physician
Obstetrics and Gynecology
TriHealth
Cincinnati, OH

Talia Zenlea, MD
Assistant Professor of Medicine
Associate Program Director
Gastroenterology
University of Toronto
Toronto, Canada

Diana Zhou, MD
University of Tennessee Health Science Center, School of Medicine
Memphis, TN

B. Shoshana Zia, MD, PhD
Clinical Instructor
Pulmonary, Critical Care and Sleep Medicine
University of California San Francisco
San Francisco, CA

Navid Ziaie, MD
Internal Medicine Resident
Oregon Health and Science University
Portland, OR

Mark Zimmerman, MD
Director, Outpatient Psychiatry and Partial Hospital Program
Rhode Island Hospital;
Professor, Psychiatry and Human Behavior
Warren Alpert Medical School of Brown University
Providence, RI

Rachel Zipursky, MD
Resident Physician
Children's Hospital of Philadelphia
Philadelphia, PA

Joshua W. Zollman, MD
Psychiatry Resident
Massachusetts General Hospital/McLean Hospital
Boston, MA

Danylo Zorin, MD
Cardiology Fellow
St. Elizabeth's Medical Center
Boston, MA

Aline N. Zouk, MD
Fellow
New York University School of Medicine
New York, NY

Olivia Zurek, MD
Attending Psychiatrist
Massachusetts General Hospital
Boston, MA

To my sons, Dr. Vito F. Ferri and Dr. Christopher A. Ferri, and my daughter-in-law, Dr. Heather A. Ferri, for their help and constant support, and to my wife, Christina, for her patience during manuscript preparation. A special thanks to all the readers who have personally commented on the merits of this book and through their suggestions have helped make this product a bestseller in the medical field.

Fred F. Ferri, MD, FACP
Clinical Professor
Department of Medicine
Warren Alpert Medical School of Brown University
Providence, Rhode Island

Preface

This book is intended to be a clear and concise reference for physicians and allied health professionals. Its user-friendly format is designed to provide a fast and efficient way to identify important clinical information and to offer practical guidance in patient management. The book is divided into five sections and an appendix, each with emphasis on clinical information.

The tremendous success of the previous editions and the enthusiastic comments from numerous colleagues have brought about several positive changes over time. Each section has been significantly expanded from prior editions, bringing the total number of medical topics covered in this book to more than 1200. New illustrations, tables, and boxes have been added to this edition to enhance recollection of clinically important facts. The expedited claims submission and reimbursement ICD-10CM codes are included in all topics.

Section I describes in detail 1,000 medical disorders and diseases—including 30 new topics this edition—arranged alphabetically and presented in outline format for ease of retrieval. Topics with an accompanying algorithm are identified with an ALG icon; similarly, those topics with an accompanying online Patient Teaching Guide (PTG) are identified with a PTG symbol. Throughout the text, key quick-access information is consistently highlighted, with clinical photographs to further illustrate selected medical conditions, and relevant ICD-10CM codes listed. Most references focus on current peer-reviewed journal articles rather than outdated textbooks and old review articles.

Topics in **Section I** use the following structured approach:

1. Basic Information (Definition, Synonyms, ICD-10CM Codes, Epidemiology & Demographics, Physical Findings & Clinical Presentation, Etiology)
2. Diagnosis (Differential Diagnosis, Workup, Laboratory Tests, Imaging Studies)
3. Treatment (Nonpharmacologic Therapy, Acute General Rx, Chronic Rx, Disposition, Referral)
4. Pearls & Considerations (Comments, Suggested Readings)

Section II includes the differential diagnosis, etiology, and classification of signs and symptoms. This practical section allows the user investigating a physical complaint or abnormal laboratory value to follow a "workup" leading to a diagnosis. The physician can then easily look up the presumptive diagnosis in Section I for information specific to that illness. Several new signs and symptoms have been added to this section for the 2022 edition.

Section III includes more than 150 clinical algorithms to guide and expedite the patient's workup and therapy. For the 2022 edition, we have continued to update algorithms and colorize online versions for improved readability. Physicians describe this section as particularly valuable in today's managed-care environment.

Section IV includes normal laboratory values and interpretation of results of commonly ordered laboratory tests. By providing interpretation of abnormal results, this section facilitates the diagnosis of medical disorders and further adds to the comprehensive "one-stop" nature of our text. New illustrations and tables have been added for this edition.

Section V focuses on preventive medicine. Information here includes screening recommendations for major diseases and disorders, patient counseling, and immunization and chemoprophylaxis recommendations.

The **Appendix** is divided into nine major sections. Appendix I contains extensive information on complementary and alternative medicine (CAM), including Common Herbs in Integrated Medicine as well as Herbal Activities Against Pain and Chronic Diseases. With this material, we aim to lessen the current scarcity of exposure of allopathic and osteopathic physicians to the diversity of CAM therapies. Appendix II focuses on nutrition, with an emphasis on dietary supplements, vitamins, and minerals. Appendix III deals with diagnosis and treatment of acute poisoning. Appendix IV is a guide on impairment and disability evaluation. Appendix V focuses on the protection of travelers. Appendix VI is new for this edition and addresses care of the transgender patient. Appendix VII—available in the online version of *Ferri's Clinical Advisor*—is a repository of practical patient instruction sheets, organized alphabetically, and covers the majority of topics in this book. These guides can be easily customized and printed and serve as valuable tools for improving physician-patient communication, patient satisfaction, and ultimately quality of care. Appendix VIII and IX offer guidance related to palliative care and preoperative evaluation, respectively.

I believe that we have produced a state-of-the-art information system with significant differences from existing texts. The information offered in all five sections and patient education guides could be sold separately based on their content, yet are available under a single cover, offering the reader tremendous value. I hope that the *Clinical Advisor*'s user-friendly approach, numerous unique features, and yearly updates will make this book a valuable medical reference, not only to primary care physicians but also to physicians in other specialties, medical students, and allied health professionals.

Fred F. Ferri, MD, FACP
Clinical Professor
Department of Medicine
Warren Alpert Medical School of Brown University
Providence, Rhode Island

Note: Comments from readers are always appreciated and can be forwarded directly to Dr. Ferri at fred_ferri@brown.edu.

Ferri's Clinical Advisor 2022—How to Use This Book

Mouse icon: Indicates content with additional references, figures, or tables available at ExpertConsult.com.

PTG PTG icon: Indicates an accompanying Patient Teaching Guide available at ExpertConsult.com. Many additional PTGs are available online that are not connected to topics in Section I.

ALG ALG icon: Indicates a topic with an accompanying algorithm.

Contents

Detailed Contents

SECTION I Diseases and Disorders

Additional Topics Available at ExpertConsult.com

SECTION II **Differential Diagnosis**

Detailed Contents

SECTION III **Clinical Algorithms**

Additional Algorithms Content Available at ExpertConsult.com

SECTION IV Laboratory Tests and Interpretation of Results

Detailed Contents

SECTION V Clinical Practice Guidelines

APPENDIX I Complementary and Alternative Medicine

APPENDIX II Nutrition

APPENDIX III Acute Poisoning

SECTION I

Diseases and Disorders

BASIC INFORMATION

DEFINITION

An abdominal aortic aneurysm (AAA) is a focal full-thickness dilation of the abdominal aortic artery to at least 1.5 times the diameter measured at the level of the renal arteries, or exceeding the normal diameter of the abdominal aorta by 50%. The normal diameter at the renal arteries is 2 cm (range 1.4 to 3.0 cm), and a diameter 3 cm or larger is generally considered aneurysmal.

ICD-10CM CODES

I71.4 Abdominal aortic aneurysm, without rupture

I71.3 Abdominal aortic aneurysm, ruptured

EPIDEMIOLOGY & DEMOGRAPHICS

- Approximately 15,000 deaths/yr in the U.S. are attributed to AAA.
- AAA is predominantly a disease of older adults, affecting men more than women (4:1).
- The prevalence rate ranges from 4% to 8% in men aged 65 to 80 in developed countries.
- Clinically important AAAs ≥4 cm are present in 1% of men between age 55 and 64; and the prevalence rate increases by 2% to 4% per decade thereafter.
- The peak incidence is among men approximately 70 yr old.
- The frequency is much higher in smokers than in nonsmokers (8:1); and the risk decreases with smoking cessation.
- Risk factors for AAA are similar to those for other atherosclerotic cardiovascular diseases. They include age, Caucasian race, smoking, male gender, family history, hypertension, hyperlipidemia, peripheral vascular disease, and aneurysm of other large vessels.
- AAA is two to four times more common in first-degree male relatives of known AAA patients.
- A decreased risk of AAA is associated with female gender, non-Caucasian race, and diabetes.
- Rupture of the AAA occurs in 1% to 3% of men age 65 or older.
  1. Rupture is the 10th leading cause of death in men older than age 55.
  2. Mortality from rupture is 70% to 95%.
  3. Risk factors for rupture include cardiac or renal transplants, severe obstructive lung disease, uncontrolled blood pressure, female sex, and ongoing tobacco use.
- A recent decline in incidence and prevalence of AAA and related mortality has been attributed to reductions in tobacco use. Reported prevalence rates in males 60 yr and older in the U.S. is estimated to be roughly now 1% to 4%. However, AAA are at least 9× more common than thoracic aortic aneurysms.

ETIOLOGY

Exact etiology is unknown and is likely multifactorial.

- Degenerative:
  1. Alterations in vascular wall biology leading to a loss of vascular structural proteins and wall strength.
  2. The most common association is atherosclerosis. It is uncertain whether atherosclerosis causes or results from AAAs.
  3. Tobacco use: >90% of people who develop an AAA have smoked at some point in their lives.
- Inherited: Familial clusters are common. High familial prevalence rate is notable in male individuals. The nature of the genetic disorder is unclear but may be linked to alpha-1-antitrypsin deficiency or X-linked mutation. Connective tissue disorders, such as Marfan syndrome and Ehlers-Danlos syndrome, have also been strongly associated with AAA.
- Inflammatory: AAA is a progressive inflammatory disease of the artery walls. Activated B lymphocytes promote AAA by producing immunoglobulins, cytokines, and matrix metalloproteinases (MMPs), resulting in the activation of macrophages, mast cells (MCs), and complement pathways that lead to the degradation of collagen and matrix proteins and to aortic wall remodeling.
- Infection, mycotic: Syphilis, *Salmonella.*

NATURAL HISTORY

- AAAs tend to develop in the infrarenal aorta and to expand, on average, at a rate of 0.2 to 0.5 cm per yr.
- The risk of aneurysmal rupture is largely influenced by aneurysm size, rate of expansion, and sex. Other factors associated with increased risk for rupture include continued smoking, uncontrolled hypertension, and increased wall stress.
- Higher tension in the abdominal aorta (together with histopathologic changes such as accumulation of foam cells, cholesterol crystals, and matrix metalloproteinases) renders the abdominal aortic wall more susceptible to dilation and subsequent rupture.
- The 5-yr rupture rate of asymptomatic AAAs is 25% to 40% for aneurysms >5.0 cm in diameter, 1% to 7% for AAAs 4.0 to 5.0 cm, and nearly 0% for AAAs <4.0 cm. The likelihood that an aneurysm will rupture is increased in aneurysms with a diameter >5.5 cm; this size also demonstrates a faster rate of expansion (>0.5 cm over 6 mo) and is more likely to be found in those who continue to smoke and in females.
- Mortality rate after rupture can be as high as 90% because most patients do not reach the hospital in time for surgical repair. Of those who reach the hospital, the mortality rate is still 50%, compared with the 1% to 4% mortality rate for elective repair of a nonruptured AAA.

SCREENING AND MONITORING

- The U.S. Preventive Services Task Force (USPSTF) recommends one-time screening for AAA by ultrasonography in men ages 65 to 75 who have a history of smoking, and selectively offer men 65 yr of age or older who have never smoked but haver certain risk factors, including family history of AAA in a parent or sibling. These populations have been shown to have a higher prevalence of AAA, and selectively screening this group has been shown to decrease AAA-specific mortality.
- The USPSTF has found little benefit in repeat screening in men with a negative ultrasound and has determined that men over the age of 75 are unlikely to benefit from screening. It was also concluded that the current evidence is insufficient to assess the balance of the harms and benefits of screening for AAA in women ages 65 to 75 who have ever smoked or with family history of AAA.
- The Society for Vascular Surgery recommends one-time ultrasonography screening for AAAs in men aged 55 yr or older with a family history of AAA, all men aged 65 yr or older, and women aged 65 yr or older who have smoked or have a family history of AAA.
- The Society for Vascular Surgery Guidelines recommend monitoring by ultrasound or CT scan should be performed every 6 mo for patients with AAAs measuring 5.0 to 5.4 cm in diameter, every 12 mo for AAAs measuring 4.0 to 4.9 cm in diameter, and every 3 yr for AAAs 3.0 to 3.9 cm in diameter.

PHYSICAL FINDINGS & CLINICAL PRESENTATION

- Most aneurysms are asymptomatic and incidentally discovered on imaging studies; however, symptomatic aneurysms are at an increased risk for rupture.
- Physical examination has a sensitivity of 76% for detecting AAAs >5 cm and only 29% for AAAs 3.0 to 3.9 cm. The accuracy of the physical examination is markedly diminished by obese body habitus.
- Symptomatic patients may present with abdominal, back, flank, or groin pain.
- A pulsatile epigastric mass that may or may not be tender may be present.
- Abdominal bruits can be present in case of renal or visceral arterial stenosis.
- Common iliac arteries can be aneurysmal and palpable in the lower abdominal quadrants. In addition, prominent femoral and popliteal pulses warrant an abdominal ultrasound and lower extremity ultrasound.
- Early satiety, nausea, and vomiting may be caused by compression of adjacent bowel.
- Venous thrombosis or insufficiency may occur from iliocaval venous compression.
- Thromboembolization can cause lower extremity pain and discoloration.
- Ureteral obstruction and hydronephrosis can cause flank and groin pain and lead to obstructive renal failure.

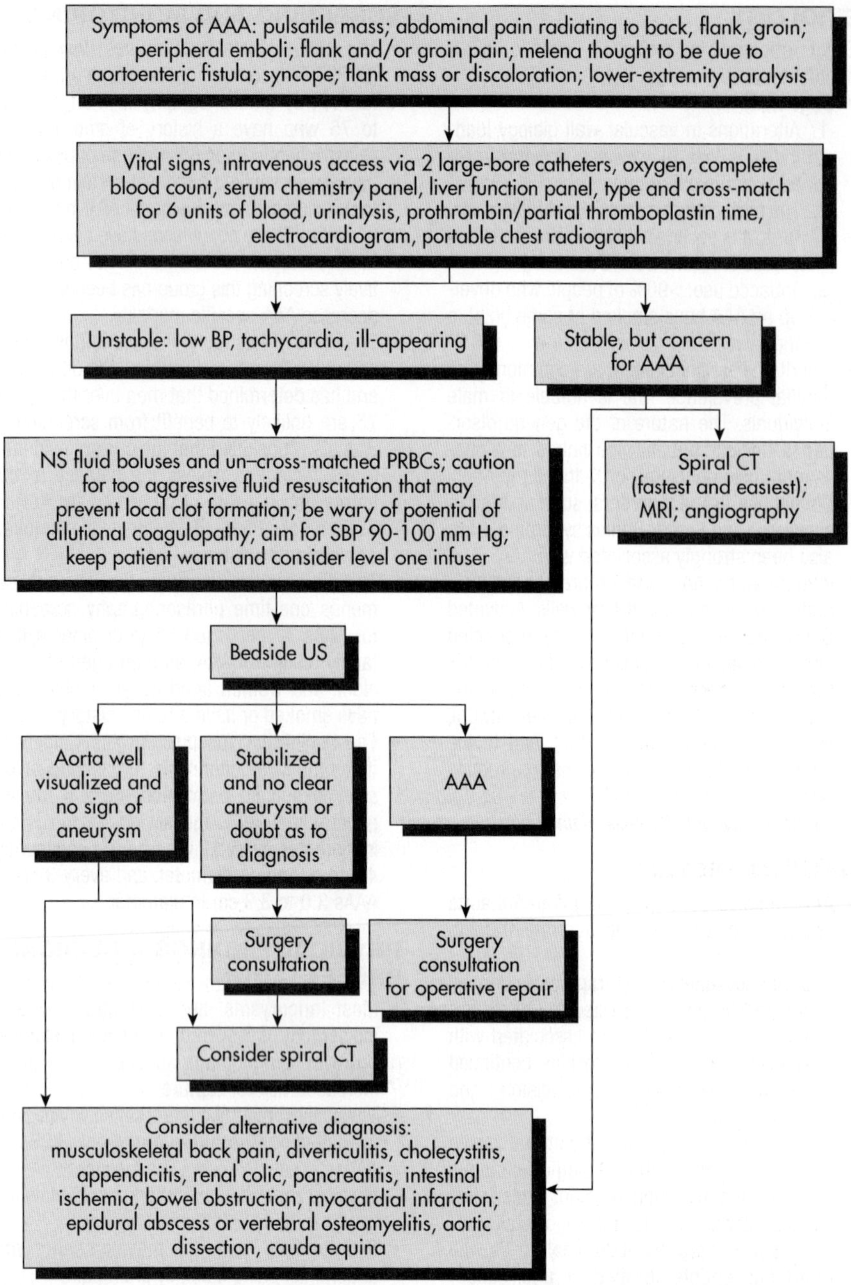

FIG. 1 Algorithm for the diagnosis and treatment of abdominal aortic aneurysms *(AAAs).* *BP,* Blood pressure; *CT,* computed tomography; *MRI,* magnetic resonance imaging; *NS,* normal saline; *PRBCs,* packed red blood cells; *SBP,* systolic blood pressure; *US,* ultrasonography. (From Adams JG et al: *Emergency medicine, clinical essentials,* ed 2, Philadelphia, 2013, Elsevier.)

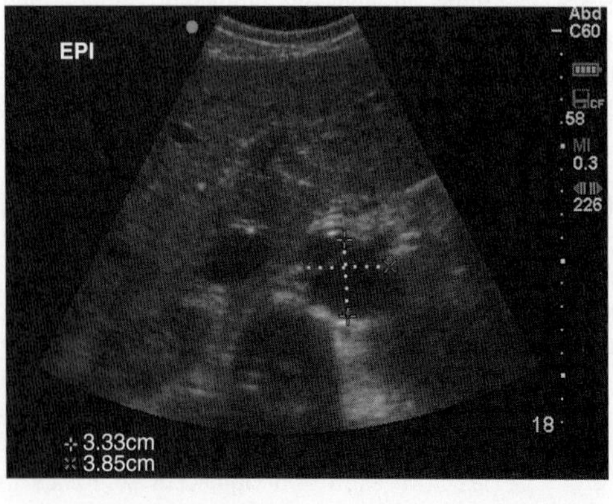

FIG. 2 Transverse image of an abdominal aortic aneurysm. Note the measurements of 3.33 × 3.85 cm. The inferior vena cava is seen to the patient's right of the aorta, and the vertebral body is seen below the two vessels. Note also that there appears to be an echogenic flap within the aorta, possibly representing an aortic dissection. (From Adams JG et al: *Emergency medicine, clinical essentials,* ed 2, Philadelphia, 2013, Elsevier.)

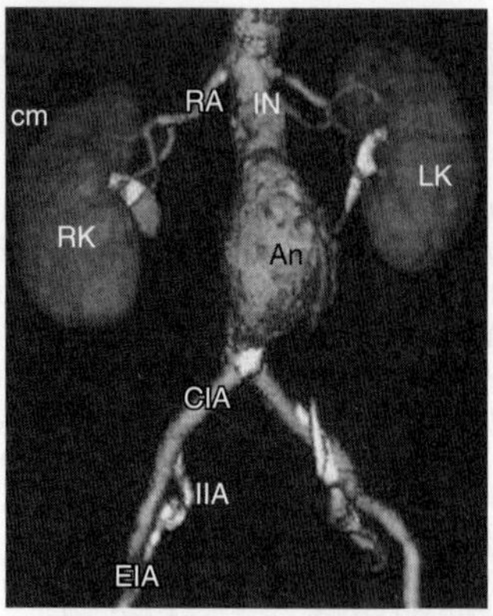

FIG. 3 Three-dimensional computed tomography image illustrates the presence of an infrarenal abdominal aortic aneurysm. *An,* Aneurysm; *CIA,* common iliac artery; *EIA,* external iliac artery; *IIA,* internal iliac artery; *IN,* infrarenal neck; *LK,* left kidney; *RA,* renal artery; *RK,* right kidney. (From Townsend CM et al [eds]: *Sabiston textbook of surgery,* ed 17, Philadelphia, 2004, Saunders.)

- Rupture classically presents as a triad of abdominal or back pain, hypotension, and a pulsatile abdominal mass in 50% of patients.
- Acute blood loss may lead to myocardial infarction; arteriovenous fistulas may present as heart failure; aortoenteric fistulas may present as hematemesis or melena associated with abdominal and back pain.

Dx DIAGNOSIS

DIFFERENTIAL DIAGNOSIS

Almost 75% of patients with AAA are asymptomatic, and the condition is discovered on routine examination or serendipitously when ordering studies for other symptoms. Diagnosis of AAA should be considered in the differential of the following symptoms: Abdominal pain, back pain, and/or pulsatile abdominal mass. The differential diagnosis includes peptic ulcer disease, mesenteric ischemia, renal calculi, pyelonephritis, and diverticulitis.

LABORATORY TESTS

Not routinely indicated. For suspected infected or inflammatory aneurysms, WBC, ESR/CRP, and blood cultures can be considered. An elevated D-dimer may indicate a thrombus within the aneurysm. Fig. 1 describes an algorithm for the diagnosis and treatment of abdominal aortic aneurysms.

IMAGING STUDIES

- Abdominal ultrasound (Fig. 2) has nearly 100% sensitivity and specificity in identifying an aneurysm and estimating the size to within 0.3 to 0.4 cm. It is not accurate in estimating the extension to the renal arteries or the iliac arteries.
- Computed tomography (CT) (Fig. 3) scan is recommended for preoperative aneurysm imaging and estimates the size of the AAA to within 0.3 mm. There are no false-negative

results, and the scan can identify extension to renal vessels with more precision than ultrasound. It is the imaging modality of choice for symptomatic AAA. Intravenous contrast is not required to establish a diagnosis of ruptured AAA. CT can also detect the integrity of the wall (Fig. 4) and exclude rupture.

- Magnetic resonance angiography (MRA) may also be used and is at least as accurate as CT.
- Plain radiographs may show the outline of an aneurysm in calcified aortas. This is an insensitive test for diagnosing AAA.
- Diagnostic aortography has essentially been replaced by other noninvasive imaging modalities such as CT or MR angiography. Intraoperative angiography is still used for determining treatment options and postprocedure efficacy (Fig. 5).
- Endovascular aneurysm repair (EVAR) needs close and lifelong imaging surveillance of the aneurysm site for the timely detection of possible complications, including endoleaks, graft migration, fractures, graft infection, and enlargement of aneurysm sac size with eventual rupture. The rate of complications after EVAR is approximately 30% with 2% to 3% of these requiring reintervention. Contrast-enhanced computed tomography (CTA) is considered the gold standard in EVAR follow-up (Fig. 6), but it is accompanied with radiation burden and renal injury because of the use of contrast media. In the past 2 decades, several studies have shown the role of contrast-enhanced ultrasonography (CEUS) in post-EVAR surveillance, with very good diagnostic performance, absence of renal impairment, and no radiation, accompanied by low costs, in comparison with CTA. In numerous prospective studies and meta-analyses, the detection and characterization of endoleaks with CEUS is comparable to that of CTA imaging.

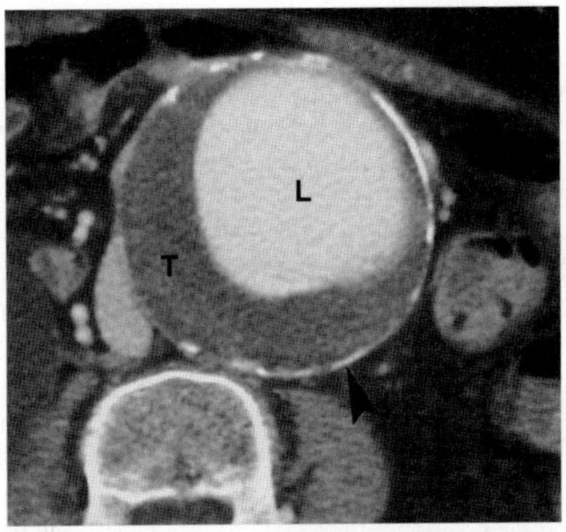

FIG. 4 Aneurysm of the abdominal aorta. A large aortic aneurysm is evident. The aorta exceeds 5 cm in diameter. A large amount of thrombus *(T)* partially surrounds the contrast-enhanced patent lumen *(L)*. Note the atherosclerotic calcification (*arrowhead*) in the wall of the aneurysm.

Rx TREATMENT

NONPHARMACOLOGIC THERAPY

- Despite lack of data substantiating reduction in expansion rate through treatment of cardiac risk factors, nonpharmacologic treatment continues to focus on risk factor modification (most importantly smoking cessation, diet, and exercise). Of note, moderate exercise does not increase the rate of aneurysm expansion or the risk of rupture.
- Serial studies have shown that expansion rates are faster in current smokers than in former smokers. Patients with known AAA or a family history of aneurysms should be advised to stop smoking and be offered smoking cessation interventions.
- Definitive treatment depends on the size of the aneurysm (see "Chronic Rx").

ACUTE GENERAL Rx

- Acute symptomatic or ruptured AAA can be treated with open surgical repair (OSR) or EVAR. The choice is determined by anatomic considerations, operative risks, and availability of regular patient follow-up for EVAR.
- Emergent open repair has been the traditional method of treatment. However, multiple trials have shown lower mortality and shorter hospital stay with EVAR. More centers are increasingly using endovascular repair for patients who fit certain anatomic and physiologic criteria.
- A recent Cochrane meta-analysis involving pooled data for four trials comparing EVAR versus open repair for ruptured abdominal aortic aneurysm failed to show a difference in 30-day mortality between EVAR versus open repair. There was a higher incidence of reintervention for patients undergoing EVAR, although interventions to deal with procedural complications were generally less invasive and involved catheter-based approaches.
- The major limitations for EVAR include anatomical issues such as tortuosity or small caliber iliac arteries and inability to follow up patients to exclude late failure of stent-grafts and development of endoleaks.

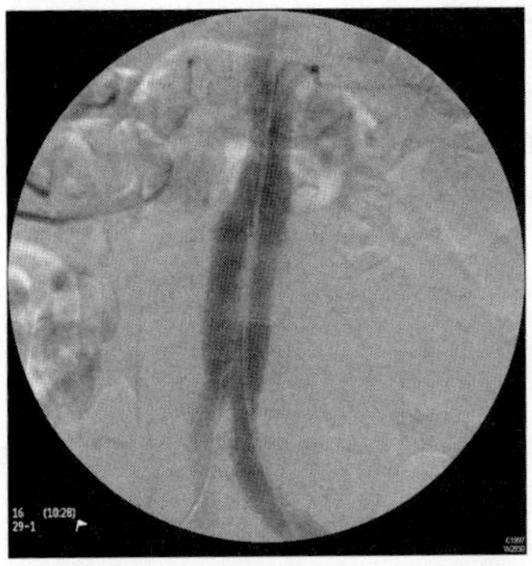

FIG. 6 Completion digital subtraction angiogram following endovascular aneurysm repair. (From Fillit HM: *Brocklehurst's textbook of geriatric medicine and gerontology,* ed 8, Philadelphia, 2017, Elsevier.)

CHRONIC Rx

- Blood pressure and fasting lipids should be monitored and controlled as recommended for patients with atherosclerotic disease. Statins are associated with decreased mortality after successful AAA repair, and are recommended for those with known AAA to reduce the progression of atherosclerosis and overall cardiovascular risk.
- The most commonly used predictor of rupture is the maximum diameter of the AAA.
- Long-term beta-blocker therapy has slowed the rate of aortic dilation and decreased the incidence of aortic complications in patients with Marfan syndrome. Several studies have also suggested that beta-blocker therapy may reduce the rate of expansion and risk of rupture; however, conclusive evidence is lacking.
- A recent multicenter study of 5362 patients with AAA found no significant association between AAA progression and the use of statins, beta-blockers, angiotensin-converting enzyme inhibitors, or angiotensin II receptor blockers.
- Antibiotics such as doxycycline and roxithromycin have been shown to limit the expansion of small AAAs.
- AAA repair to eliminate the risk for rupture should be performed for patients with infrarenal or juxtarenal AAA of approximately 5.5 cm or larger in diameter. Repair in females can be considered at diameters larger than 5 cm. Additionally, AAAs with a rate of enlargement greater than 0.5 cm over 6 mo should be considered for repair. All patients who are symptomatic should undergo repair, regardless of size. Timing of repair in symptomatic unruptured AAA is still under debate.
- There is no clear advantage to early repair (open or endovascular) for small asymptomatic AAAs (less than 5.5 cm). Several studies have shown no significant difference in

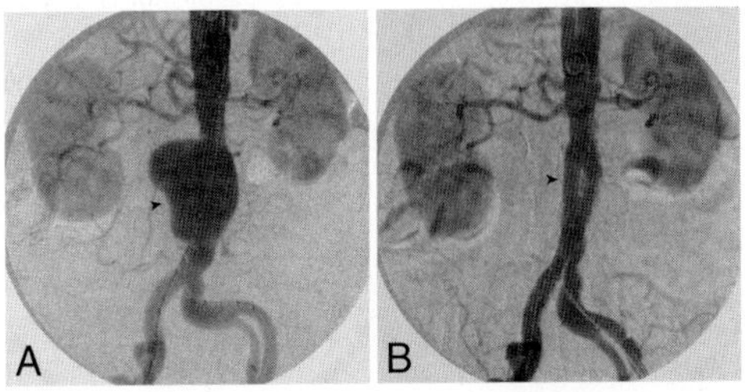

FIG. 5 A, Conventional catheter angiography with bilateral marked catheters in place demonstrates a large, lobulated, infrarenal aortic aneurysm (*arrowhead*) with a 4-cm proximal neck suitable for endovascular repair. **B,** An image after endovascular repair demonstrates complete exclusion of the aneurysm (*arrowhead*) with no endoleak and preservation of the renal and hypogastric arteries. (From Soto JA, Lucey BC: *Emergency radiology: the requisites*, ed 2, Philadelphia, 2017, Elsevier.)

all-cause mortality or AAA-related mortality with early treatment (EVAR vs. OSR) compared with surveillance for small AAAs.

- Percutaneous, endovascular, stent-anchored grafts placed with the patient under local anesthesia have provided an alternative approach for patients with favorable anatomy. In patients who have undergone EVAR, long-term surveillance is required to assess for an endoleak, stent migration, change in aneurysm size, and need for re-intervention.
- EVAR with proximally fenestrated grafts is an alternative to open repair in the management of juxtarenal aortic aneurysms and short-neck abdominal aortic aneurysms (the "neck" is the distance from the lowest main renal artery to the beginning of the aneurysm). Contemporary literature shows it is a safe and efficacious treatment, particularly for those deemed surgically high risk.
- Randomized trials and meta-analyses comparing EVAR with OSR have shown that EVAR is associated with lower 30-day mortality and MI rates, shorter hospital stays, and better health-related quality of life up to 12 mo postoperatively. However, EVAR also has increased rates of graft-related complications and is more costly. Additionally, a recent meta-analysis showed that 5 to 9 yr postoperatively, EVAR is associated with higher all-cause mortality, reintervention, and secondary rupture rates compared with OSR. Over >10 yr, EVAR is associated with higher reintervention and secondary rupture rates.
- Based on current data, less than 2% of endovascular repairs require open conversion, and approximately half of all early endoleaks resolve spontaneously within a period of 30 days.
- Open surgical repair of AAAs is the preferred approach for patients with a long life expectancy.
- Endovascular AAA repair is the preferred approach for most patients with a reasonable life expectancy and suitable anatomy.
- For patients with limited life expectancy, elective AAA repair is not recommended.
- Surveillance for endovascular AAA repair has typically involved use of periodic CT scans, but abdominal ultrasound is gaining widespread adoption for postprocedure monitoring. Surveillance is recommended to occur 1 and 12 mo postoperatively and then annually thereafter.
- In high-risk patients undergoing AAA repair, specifically those with coronary artery disease or those with more than one clinical risk factor based on the American Heart Association (AHA) guidelines, preoperative administration of beta-blockers titrated to a goal heart rate of 60 have been shown to decrease incidence of death from cardiac causes or nonfatal myocardial infarctions. Beta-blockers initiated within 24 hr of the procedure have not shown an advantage; however beta-blockers the patient is already taking should be continued.
- Patients with chronic obstructive pulmonary disease (COPD) are at higher risk for major clinical complications, particularly if the COPD is suboptimally managed or if it is present in conjunction with cardiac or renal disease. Smoking cessation for 2 mo before surgery has also been shown to decrease pulmonary morbidity.
- Renal dysfunction is a strong predictor of mortality, showing up to as high as 41% mortality in those with impaired renal function compared with 6% in those without renal dysfunction.

REFERRAL

- Vascular surgical referral should be made in asymptomatic patients with AAAs that are approximately 4.5 cm.
- In patients with an expansion rate of 0.5 cm over 6 mo, it is reasonable to offer repair, although small studies have shown that using expansion as a criterion for surgical referral is of unclear benefit.
- It is important to optimize any comorbid conditions before surgical referral.

PEARLS & CONSIDERATIONS

- FDA recommendation to avoid prescribing fluoroquinolones to patients with AAA. Observational studies have shown that fluoroquinolones may increase the risk of occurrence of aortic aneurysm or dissection.
- Repairing asymptomatic AAAs smaller than 5.5 cm has not been shown to improve survival because the risk of rupture is lower than the risk of surgery.
- The results from multiple trials to date demonstrate no advantage to immediate repair for small AAA (4.0 to 5.5 cm), regardless of whether open or endovascular repair is used and, at least for open repair, regardless of patient age and AAA diameter. Thus, neither immediate open nor immediate endovascular repair of small AAAs is supported by the currently available evidence.
- Five-yr survival remains poor after elective AAA repair despite advances in short-term outcomes and is associated with AAA diameter and patient age at the time of surgery. Research in this field should attempt to improve the life expectancy of patients with repaired AAA and to optimize patient selection.

COMMENTS

- Most AAAs are infrarenal. This is thought to be due in part to decreased lamellar structural proteins in the vascular wall below the renal arteries leading to decreased vascular wall strength.
- Surgical risk is increased in patients with coexisting coronary artery disease, pulmonary disease, or chronic renal failure. Evaluation for ischemia and aggressive perioperative hemodynamic monitoring help identify high-risk patients and decrease postoperative complications.
- It is estimated that AAAs at <5 cm expand at a rate of 0.2 to 0.3 cm/yr, and AAAs at >5 cm expand at a rate of 0.3 to 0.5 cm/yr.

SUGGESTED READINGS

Available at ExpertConsult.com

RELATED CONTENT

Abdominal Aortic Aneurysm (Patient Information)

AUTHORS: **Armen S. Ghazarian, MD,** and **Pranav M. Patel, MD, FACC, FAHA, FSCAI**

BASIC INFORMATION

DEFINITION

Abnormal uterine bleeding (AUB) describes uterine bleeding that is abnormal in regularity, quantity, frequency, or duration, in the nonpregnant person. Historically, AUB was described as in Table 1. The term "dysfunctional uterine bleeding" was applied when no clear etiology could be identified. These terms have fallen out of favor. In 2011, the FIGO Working Group on Menstrual Disorders released a classification system intended to simplify these definitions. It is known by the acronym PALM-COEIN, which is further described later. This classification system divides the causes of AUB into two groups: structural (PALM) and nonstructural (COEIN). Today, AUB is described according to these criteria.

A normal menstrual cycle is typically described as lasting 21 to 35 days with 5 days of bleeding per cycle. Total blood loss for normal menses is thought to be less than 80 ml.

SYNONYMS

AUB
Dysfunctional uterine bleeding

ICD-10CM CODES

N91.5 Oligomenorrhea, unspecified
N92.0 Excessive and frequent menstruation with regular cycle
N92.1 Excessive and frequent menstruation with irregular cycle
N92.5 Other specified irregular menstruation
N93.8 Other specified abnormal uterine and vaginal bleeding
N93.9 Abnormal uterine and vaginal bleeding, unspecified

EPIDEMIOLOGY & DEMOGRAPHICS

- One third of outpatient visits to the gynecologist are for AUB.
- Most cases of AUB result from structural (uterine) pathology (the PALM portion of the acronym).
- Up to 20% of women presenting with heavy menstrual bleeding will be found to have a coagulopathy or underlying bleeding disorder.

PHYSICAL FINDINGS & CLINICAL PRESENTATION

- The clinical presentation of AUB is variable. Although many patients complain of the abnormality of their cycles, some will present with symptoms of anemia, with AUB being elicited only with a careful history. Patients may note recent weight gain or on examination, may have other findings (as noted later) suggestive of the etiology for their bleeding.
- Physical findings depend on the etiology. For example, an enlarged or irregular uterine contour may suggest fibroids, or a polyp may be seen on the cervix during a speculum examination.
- A thorough physical and pelvic examination should be done to exclude the other causes of abnormal bleeding, such as thyroid or endocrine diseases.

TABLE 1 Definitions of Abnormal Uterine Bleeding

Term	Description
Oligomenorrhea	Bleeding at intervals greater than 35 days
Polymenorrhea	Bleeding at intervals less than 21 days
Hypermenorrhea (menorrhagia)	Excessive flow or bleeding with normal intervals
Metrorrhagia	Bleeding between menses
Menometrorrhagia	Excessive flow or duration with periods and between periods
Withdrawal bleeding	Bleeding after the withdrawal of hormones

From Crum CP et al: *Diagnostic gynecologic and obstetric pathology,* ed 3, Philadelphia, 2018, Elsevier.

TABLE 2 Causes of Abnormal Uterine Bleeding

Age (yr)	Differential Diagnosis
Prepubertal	Precocious puberty (hypothalamic, pituitary, ovarian)
Adolescence	• Immature hypothalamic-pituitary axis (transient) • Pregnancy • Disorders in folliculogenesis (transient) • Sexually transmitted infections • Hematologic disorders (von Willebrand disease, hemophilias, factors VII, XI)
Third and fourth decades	• Oral contraceptive pill-related • Pregnancy or postpartum • Benign organic lesions (polyps, leiomyomata, endometritis) • Anovulatory cycle
Fifth decade	• Anovulatory or altered cycle • Benign organic lesions (polyps, adenomyosis, leiomyomata, or endometritis) • Neoplasia
Sixth decade	• Hormone replacement therapy • Benign organic lesions (polyps, adenomyosis, leiomyomata, endometritis) • Atrophy • Neoplasia

From Crum CP et al: *Diagnostic gynecologic and obstetric pathology,* ed 3, Philadelphia, 2018, Elsevier.

ETIOLOGY

- Table 2 describes many of the various causes of AUB. The causes of AUB in the fourth and fifth decade are summarized in Table 3.
- Endocrinopathies, including hyperprolactinemia, hyperthyroidism, and hypothyroidism, may also contribute to heavy or irregular menstrual bleeding.

DIAGNOSIS

DIFFERENTIAL DIAGNOSIS

- PALM–COEIN:
  1. Polyps (AUB-P)
  2. Adenomyosis (AUB-A)
  3. Leiomyoma (AUB-L)
  4. Malignancy/hyperplasia (AUB-M)
  5. Coagulopathy (AUB-C; most commonly von Willebrand disease)
  6. Ovulatory dysfunction (AUB-O; most commonly polycystic ovarian syndrome)
  7. Endometrial (AUB-E)
  8. Iatrogenic (AUB-I; e.g., anticoagulants, hormonal contraception, and some herbal remedies)
  9. Not yet classified (AUB-N)
- Anatomic nonuterine causes:
  1. Cervix: Cervical neoplasia, cervicitis
  2. Vagina: Vaginal neoplasia, adhesions, trauma, foreign body, atrophic vaginitis, infections, condyloma
  3. Vulva: Vulvar trauma, infections, neoplasia, condyloma, dystrophy, varices
  4. Urinary tract: Urethral caruncle, diverticulum, hematuria, neoplasia
  5. Gastrointestinal tract: Hemorrhoids, anal fissure, colorectal lesions or neoplasia

TABLE 3 Causes of Abnormal Uterine Bleeding in the Fourth and Fifth Decades

Cause	Differential Diagnosis
Anovulation	• Endometrial polyp • Basalis
Endometrial polyp	• Basalis/lower uterine segment • Tangentially sectioned functionalis • Atypical polypoid adenomyoma • Adenomyomatous polyp • Intraendometrial leiomyoma • Adenosarcoma
Chronic endometritis	• Late menstrual endometrium • Postpartum/postabortal endometrium • Cervical tissue (plasma cells) • Menstrual endometrium • Lymphoproliferative disorder
Submucosal leiomyoma	• Progestin/tamoxifen therapy • Endometrial polyp • Stromal neoplasm

From Crum CP et al: *Diagnostic gynecologic and obstetric pathology,* ed 3, Philadelphia, 2018, Elsevier.

- Systemic diseases/effects:
  1. Exogenous hormone intake: Hormone replacement therapy
  2. Medications
  3. Coagulopathies: Von Willebrand disease, thrombocytopenia, hepatic failure
  4. Endocrinopathies: Thyroid disorder, hyperprolactinemia, diabetes mellitus
  5. Renal diseases: Generally causing acquired coagulopathy
  6. Impaired nutritional status: Anorexia/bulimia, excessive exercise

WORKUP

- Detailed history:
  1. Age of menarche
  2. Prior menstrual characteristics
  3. Severity of bleeding is important to discern, but can be difficult for patients to describe objectively. Asking specifics regarding size of tampon/pads used, frequency of changing menstrual products, use of concomitant tampons and pads, and saturating clothes can be useful to estimate severity
  4. Review of systems, including symptoms of anemia, hyper- or hypothyroidism, hyperprolactinemia
  5. Surgical and medical history suggestive of other causes/contributors
  6. Family history of bleeding disorders, gynecologic conditions such as uterine fibroids, endometriosis, or neoplasia
- Thorough physical examination, including a pelvic examination (bimanual and speculum) to exclude causes mentioned above:
  1. Includes thyroid, breast, liver, skin (e.g., presence or absence of ecchymotic lesions)
  2. Patient habitus: Obese and hirsute (e.g., polycystic ovarian disease) or underweight (e.g., anorexia nervosa or excessive exercise)
  3. Presence or absence of vulvar, vaginal, or cervical lesions; uterine (fibroid) or ovarian tumors; urethral caruncles or diverticula; hemorrhoids; anal fissures; colorectal lesions
  4. Complete pelvic exam to identify lesions and the size and shape of the uterus

LABORATORY TESTS (AS INDICATED BY HISTORY AND PHYSICAL)

- Pregnancy test (blood or urine)
- Complete blood count
- Targeted screening for bleeding disorders when indicated per history or physical exam:
  1. Prothrombin/INR and partial thromboplastin (or PFA-100 assay) if coagulopathy is suspected
  2. von Willebrand panel, particularly in women with heavy bleeding since menarche if initial testing suggests coagulopathy
- Iron studies
- TSH level
- *Chlamydia trachomatis* testing, and other STI testing if desired/indicated
- Endometrial biopsy or dilation and curettage: First line in patients over 45. It should also be performed in younger patients with history of unopposed estrogen exposure (such as in obesity or PCOS), or in patients who have failed medical management and have persistent AUB
- Pap smear if indicated
- Stool testing for occult blood
- Urinalysis for hematuria

IMAGING STUDIES

- Pelvic ultrasound, including measurement of endometrial thickness in the postmenopausal woman and assessment of myometrial or endometrial defects. This is considered first line.
- Fluid contrast ultrasound (also called saline sonogram, sonohysterogram, or saline infusion sonogram) may be indicated if the endometrium appears thickened or irregular. It distends the uterine cavity so that "filling defects" of the endometrium can be assessed for possible endometrial polyp, uterine fibroid, or neoplasm.
- Hysteroscopy may be performed to assess intracavitary fibroids or polyps.
- Magnetic resonance imaging may help better characterize large fibroids or uterine pathology, and can be particularly helpful in diagnosing adenomyosis.

Rx TREATMENT

NONPHARMACOLOGIC THERAPY

- Increase dietary iron intake or consider PO iron supplementation for anemia.
- Initiate lifestyle changes, including weight loss, exercise, and low-carb diet, if indicated.

ACUTE THERAPY

- Progestins:
  1. Medroxyprogesterone acetate (oral), 20 mg PO tid daily for 7 days
  2. Combined oral contraceptives (containing 35 mcg ethinyl estradiol): One tablet tid for 7 days; patient should then continue on oral contraceptives daily
  3. Tranexamic acid, 1.3 g PO or 10 mg/kg IV (max 600 mg per dose), tid for 5 days
- Estrogens:
  1. Conjugated equine estrogen 25 mg IV every 4 to 6 hr for a maximum of 24 hr
- Nonpharmacologic:
  1. Intrauterine tamponade with 26F Foley catheter inflated with 30 cc saline

CHRONIC THERAPY

- Progestins:
  1. Medroxyprogesterone acetate 10 mg daily for 12 days, then cyclically to induce monthly withdrawal bleeding, or can be continued daily
  2. Norethindrone 2.5 to 10 mg daily for 12 days each mo, or can be continued daily, or 0.35 mg daily (marketed as the "mini-pill")
  3. Depo-Provera 150 mg IM every 3 mo
  4. Combined hormonal contraceptives, one tablet daily either cyclically or continuously using only active pills (or patch or ring)
  5. Levonorgestrel-releasing intrauterine device - Mirena IUD has an FDA indication for heavy menstrual bleeding
- Others:
  1. Antiprostaglandins: Ibuprofen or naproxen sodium can reduce bleeding by 40%
  2. Danazol: Suppresses estrogen and progesterone receptors in the endometrium, leading to endometrial atrophy and reduced menstrual loss, but is rarely used due to side-effect profile (androgenism, menopause-like symptoms, weight gain, acne)
  3. Gonadotropin-releasing hormone (GnRH) analogues; often used to reduce bleeding, and ameliorate anemia and preparation for a surgical procedure
  4. Tranexamic acid is an antifibrinolytic agent FDA approved for cyclic heavy menstrual bleeding. Dosage in normal renal function is 3900 mg daily (650 mg tablets, 2 tablets tid) for up to 5 days during menses
- Surgical treatment:
  1. Dilation and curettage
  2. Operative hysteroscopy
  3. Endometrial ablation
  4. Uterine artery embolization
  5. Hysterectomy for definitive management

DISPOSITION

Can consider cyclical treatment on birth control pills or Provera for several cycles, then discontinue pill and watch patient for onset of regular menses. However, if the patient does not desire pregnancy, cycle management with a hormonal contraceptive or placement of LNG-IUD are commonly used.

REFERRAL

To gynecologist in case of failure of treatment.

PEARLS & CONSIDERATIONS

- Don't forget a pregnancy test!
- Up to 20% of patients with AUB will have an underlying bleeding disorder.
- Endometrial sampling is a first-line test in patients over age 45 with new AUB.

COMMENTS

Patient education material may be obtained from the American College of Obstetricians and Gynecologists, 409 12th Street SW, Washington, DC 20024-2188; phone 202-638-5577.

SUGGESTED READING

Available at ExpertConsult.com

RELATED CONTENT

Abnormal Uterine Bleeding (Patient Information)
Endometrial Cancer (Related Key Topic)
Heavy Menstrual Bleeding (Menorrhagia) (Related Key Topic)
Uterine Fibroids (Related Key Topic)

AUTHORS: **Sydney Ford, MD, MPH,** and **Siri M. Holton, MD**

BASIC INFORMATION

DEFINITION

Abruptio placentae is the separation of placenta from the uterine wall before delivery of the fetus. The condition occurs in approximately 1% of pregnancies. There are three classes of abruption (Fig. 1) based on maternal and fetal status, including an assessment of uterine contractions, quantity of bleeding, fetal heart rate monitoring, and abnormal coagulation studies (fibrinogen, prothrombin time, partial thromboplastin time).

- Grade I: Mild vaginal bleeding, uterine irritability, stable vital signs, reassuring fetal heart rate, normal coagulation profile (fibrinogen 450 mg/dl). Approximately half of abruptions are grade I.
- Grade II: Moderate vaginal bleeding, hypertonic uterine contractions, orthostatic blood pressure measurements, unfavorable fetal status, fibrinogen 150 to 250 mg. Approximately a quarter of abruptions are grade II.
- Grade III: Severe bleeding (may be concealed), hypertonic uterine contractions, overt signs of hypovolemic shock, fetal death, thrombocytopenia, fibrinogen <150 mg/dl. Approximately a quarter of abruptions are grade III.

SYNONYM

Premature separation of placenta

ICD-10CM CODES	
045.8X1	Other premature separation of placenta, first trimester
045.8X2	Other premature separation of placenta, second trimester
045.8X3	Other premature separation of placenta, third trimester
045.8X9	Other premature separation of placenta, unspecified trimester
045.91	Premature separation of placenta, unspecified, first trimester
045.92	Premature separation of placenta, unspecified, second trimester
045.93	Premature separation of placenta, unspecified, third trimester

EPIDEMIOLOGY & DEMOGRAPHICS

INCIDENCE (IN U.S.): 9.6 per 1000 births; 80% occur before the onset of labor.

PREVALENCE: 5% to 17%, some studies showing a 5- to 10-fold increase in risk; with two prior episodes, 25%.

RISK FACTORS: Hypertension (greatest association), trauma, polyhydramnios, multifetal gestation, smoking, use of cocaine, chorioamnionitis, preterm premature rupture of membranes. Table 1 summarizes placental abruption risk factors.

PHYSICAL FINDINGS & CLINICAL PRESENTATION

- Triad of uterine bleeding (concealed or per vagina), hypertonic uterine contractions or signs of preterm labor, and evidence of fetal compromise exists.
- More than 80% of cases have external bleeding; 20% of cases have no bleeding but have indirect evidence of abruption, such as failed tocolysis for preterm labor.
- Tetanic uterine contractions are found in only 17%.

ETIOLOGY

- Primary etiology: Unknown
- Hypertension: Found in 40% to 50% of grade III abruptions
- Rapid decompression of uterine cavity, as can occur in polyhydramnios or multifetal gestation
- Blunt external trauma (motor vehicle accident, spousal abuse)

Dx DIAGNOSIS

DIFFERENTIAL DIAGNOSIS

- Placenta previa
- Cervical or vaginal trauma
- Labor
- Cervical cancer
- Rupture of membranes
- The differential diagnosis of vaginal bleeding in pregnancy is described in Section III

WORKUP

- Placental abruption is primarily a clinical diagnosis that is supported by laboratory, radiographic (Fig. 2), and pathologic studies.
- Initial assessment should evaluate for the source of bleeding, ruling out placenta previa that may contraindicate any type of vaginal examination (e.g., pelvic speculum examination).
- Continuous fetal heart monitoring is indicated for all viable gestations (60% incidence of fetal distress in labor); may show early signs of maternal hypovolemia (late decelerations or fetal tachycardia) before overt maternal vital sign changes.
- Actual amount of blood loss is often greater than initially perceived because of the possibility of concealed retroplacental bleeding and apparent "normal" vital signs. The relative hypervolemia of pregnancy initially protects the patient until late in the course of bleeding, when abrupt and sudden cardiovascular collapse can occur.

LABORATORY TESTS

- Baseline serum hemoglobin helps quantify blood loss and establish baseline values for serial comparisons during expectant management.
- Coagulation profile: Platelets, fibrinogen, prothrombin, and partial thromboplastin time. Diffuse intravascular coagulation can develop with severe abruption. If fibrinogen is <150 mg/dl, estimated blood loss is approximately 2000 ml; if fibrinogen is <100 mg/dl, consider fresh frozen plasma to prevent further bleeding.
- Type and antibody screen is important to identify Rh-negative patients who need Rh immune globulin.

IMAGING STUDIES

Ultrasound should include fetal presentation and status, amniotic fluid volume, placental location, as well as any evidence of hematoma (retroplacental, subchorionic, or preplacental) (Fig. 3).

Rx TREATMENT

ACUTE GENERAL Rx

- Stabilization of the mother is the first priority.
- Treatment depends on gestational age of the fetus, severity of the abruption, and maternal status.
- Initial assessment for signs of maternal hemodynamic compromise or hemorrhagic shock; large-bore intravenous access, with crystalloid fluid resuscitation using a replacement of 3 ml lactated Ringer solution for every 1 ml estimated blood loss.

TABLE 1 Placental Abruption Risk Factors

Increasing parity or maternal age
Cigarette smoking
Cocaine abuse
Trauma
Maternal hypertension
Preterm premature rupture of membranes
Rapid uterine decompression associated with multiple gestation and polyhydramnios
Inherited or acquired thrombophilia
Uterine malformations or fibroids
Placental abnormalities or ischemia
Prior abruption

From Gabbe SG: *Obstetrics*, ed 6, Philadelphia, 2012, Saunders.

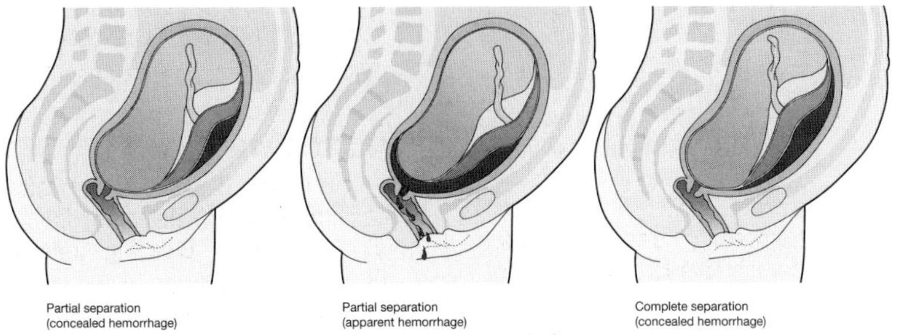

FIG. 1 Classification of placental abruption. (From Magowan BA: *Clinical obstetrics & gynecology*, ed 4, 2019, Elsevier.)

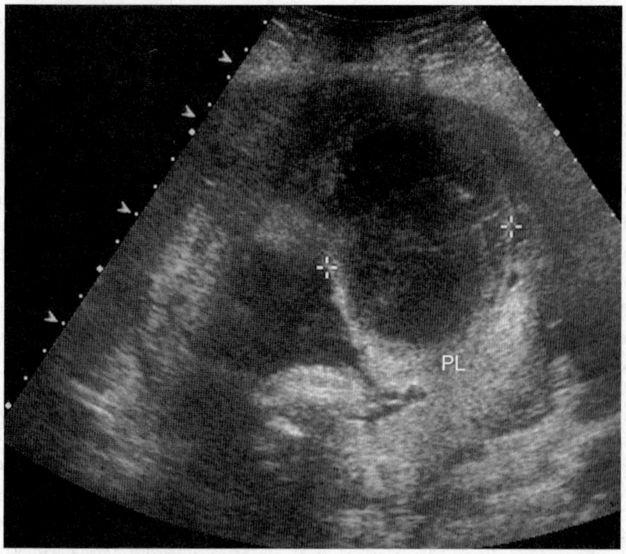

FIG. 2 Placental abruption. Transabdominal sonogram of the placenta *(PL)* with a hematoma *(calipers)* lifting the placenta away from the uterine wall. (From Rumack CM et al [eds]: *Diagnostic ultrasound*, ed 4, Philadelphia, 2011, Mosby.)

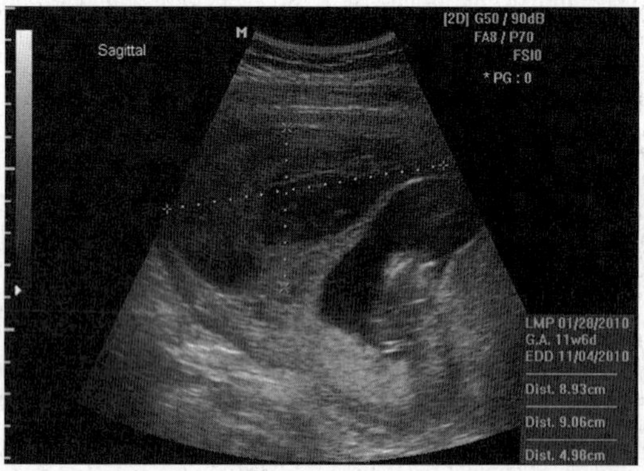

FIG. 3 Ultrasonic image of a subchorionic abruption. (Courtesy K. Francois; from Gabbe SG: *Obstetrics*, ed 6, Philadelphia, 2012, Saunders.)

- Indwelling Foley catheter to monitor urine output and maternal volume status, with a goal of 30 ml/hr urine output.
- Assess fetal status and gestational age by sonogram and continuous fetal heart rate monitoring.
- Because of the unpredictable nature of abruptions, cross-matched blood should be made available during the initial resuscitation period.

CHRONIC Rx

- In the term fetus, delivery is indicated.
- In the preterm fetus, consider betamethasone 12.5 mg IM q24h for two doses and then delivery, depending on the severity of the abruption and the likelihood of fetal complications from preterm birth.
- Cesarean section should be reserved for cases of fetal distress or for standard obstetric indications. While cesarean delivery may be needed to stabilize the fetal and/or maternal status, the mother's coagulation status may complicate the procedure and availability of blood products may be critical.
- In cases of maternal stability and fetal prematurity, expectant management can occur in the setting of close follow-up, including regular evaluation of fetal growth and reassuring antenatal testing.

DISPOSITION

Because of the unpredictable nature of abruptions, expectant management should occur only under controlled circumstances.

REFERRAL

Abruptio placentae places mother and fetus in a high-risk situation and should be managed by a qualified obstetrician in a facility with capability for neonatal and maternal resuscitation, for supporting a preterm infant if delivery is indicated at an early gestational age, and for performing emergency cesarean sections.

RELATED CONTENT

Abruptio Placentae (Patient Information)
Premature Labor (Related Key Topic)
Vaginal Bleeding during Pregnancy (Related Key Topic)

AUTHOR: **Kelly Ruhstaller, MD**

BASIC INFORMATION

DEFINITION

Absence seizures are a type of generalized seizure characterized by brief episodes of staring with impairment of consciousness (absence). They usually last no more than 20 to 30 sec. The onset and the end of the seizures are sudden. Usually the patients are not aware of them and resume the activity they were performing before the seizure. The electroencephalogram signature of absence seizures consists of a generalized 3-Hz spike and slow wave discharges.

SYNONYMS

Childhood absence epilepsy
Seizures, absence

ICD-10CM CODE

G40.309 Generalized idiopathic epilepsy and epileptic syndromes, not intractable, without status epilepticus

EPIDEMIOLOGY & DEMOGRAPHICS

INCIDENCE: 1 to 10 cases per 100,000 population
PREVALENCE: Represents up to 18% of all pediatric epilepsy syndromes
PREDOMINANT SEX & AGE: More common in girls than in boys, absences typically begin between 4 and 8 yr
PEAK INCIDENCE: 6 to 7 yr

PHYSICAL FINDINGS & CLINICAL PRESENTATION

- Patients with absence seizures usually have normal physical and neurologic examinations.
- During the seizures, the patients are unresponsive and can have motor phenomena (automatisms, eye blinks, mouth and hand movements).
- Absence seizures are not associated with postictal confusion.
- They may be triggered by hyperventilation associated with activity.
- Tonic clonic seizures are not usually a feature of this syndrome. If the patient also experiences tonic clonic seizures, other etiologies should be investigated, such as juvenile absence epilepsy, juvenile myoclonic epilepsy, complex partial seizures, etc.

ETIOLOGY

Genetic

DIAGNOSIS

DIFFERENTIAL DIAGNOSIS

- Juvenile absence epilepsy
- Juvenile myoclonic epilepsy
- Complex partial seizures
- Focal seizures with altered consciousness (Table E1)
- Nonepileptic spells comprised of staring

WORKUP

- EEG with hyperventilation and photic stimulation is crucial in the diagnosis.
- Ambulatory EEG and video EEG are recommended for patients with diagnostic uncertainty.

LABORATORY TESTS

No specific studies needed

IMAGING STUDIES

- MRI of the brain should be performed in all epilepsy patients, especially if the EEG does not show the typical characteristic of absence seizures (3-Hz spike and slow wave discharges).
- CT scans of the head should be avoided in children due to unnecessary exposure to radiation and low yield of the test except when MRI cannot be obtained.

TREATMENT

The medication of choice based on the best current evidence available is ethosuximide, followed by valproic acid and lamotrigine.

NONPHARMACOLOGIC THERAPY

Not applicable

GENERAL Rx

- Ethosuximide: Initial dose: 10 mg/kg/day; then after 7 days, 20 mg/kg
- Divalproex sodium (Depakote): Initial dose: 5 to 10 mg/kg/day (divided bid), maximum dose: 60 mg/kg/day
- Lamotrigine (Lamictal): Dose for patients on no other antiepileptic drugs. Wk 1 and 2: 0.3 mg/kg/day. Wk 3 and 4: 0.6 mg/kg/day. Wk 5 onward: Increase every 1 to 2 wk by 0.6 mg/kg/day. Maintenance: 4.5 to 7.5 mg/kg/day. Warning: Should be used with caution due to the potential for toxicity and Stevens-Johnson syndrome. Patients on other antiepileptic drugs can also have severe adverse reactions (e.g., valproate can cause increased levels of lamotrigine, and lamotrigine must be titrated much more slowly in patients on valproate therapy)

CHRONIC Rx

- Children with recurrent seizures require chronic treatment.
- If children are seizure-free for a period of 1 to 2 yr, a trial on no medications should be considered; children typically outgrow childhood absence seizures.

COMPLEMENTARY & ALTERNATIVE MEDICINE

Not applicable

DISPOSITION

- Response to treatment is excellent.
- Absence seizures tend to remit in teenage yr.
- Epilepsy can be considered as resolved once 10 yr have elapsed since the last event, including 5 yr free from medications.

REFERRAL

Patients with epilepsy and seizures should be referred for a consultation by a neurologist, preferably one specializing in epilepsy.

PEARLS & CONSIDERATIONS

COMMENTS

- Absence seizures can be present in other epilepsy syndromes.
- Valproate should be avoided in girls and women with childbearing potential due to the risk of teratogenicity.
- Carbamazepine and phenytoin should be avoided in the treatment of absence seizures, since these medications may worsen seizures and could provoke absence status epilepticus.
- All women of childbearing age taking antiepileptic drugs should take folic acid supplementation (1 to 4 mg/day) for the prevention of neural tube defects.

PREVENTION

Sleep deprivation and alcohol consumption should be avoided.

PATIENT & FAMILY EDUCATION

Patients with ongoing seizures are forbidden to drive; check state regulations and laws regarding driving and epilepsy.

SUGGESTED READING

Available at ExpertConsult.com

RELATED CONTENT

Absence Seizures (Patient Information)

AUTHOR: **Joseph S. Kass, MD, JD, FAAN**

Acetaminophen Poisoning

BASIC INFORMATION

DEFINITION

Acetaminophen (APAP) poisoning is a disorder caused by excessive intake of APAP and is manifested by jaundice, nausea, vomiting, abdominal discomfort, and potential death from hepatic necrosis if not treated appropriately.

SYNONYM

Paracetamol poisoning

ICD-10CM CODES

T39.1	Poisoning by 4-aminophenol derivatives, accidental
X60	Intentional self-poisoning by 4-aminophenol derivatives

EPIDEMIOLOGY & DEMOGRAPHICS

- APAP is one of the most widely prescribed antipyretics and analgesics in the U.S. Potentially toxic ingestions, both intentional and unintentional, exceed 100,000 cases annually in the U.S.
- APAP toxicity is the number one cause of liver transplant in the U.S.
- Death rate is approximately one in 1000 persons. Nearly 50% of exposures occur in children ≤6 yr.
- Hepatic necrosis is most likely to occur in people who (1) are chronically malnourished, (2) regularly abuse alcohol, (3) have chronic liver disease, and (4) use other potentially hepatotoxic medications.
- Combination opioid and acetaminophen medications are an important source of APAP toxicity.

PHYSICAL FINDINGS & CLINICAL PRESENTATION

- The physical examination may vary depending on the amount of time since ingestion.
- Phase I (0 to 24 hr): Initial symptoms may be mild or absent and may consist of anorexia, diaphoresis, malaise, nausea, vomiting, lethargy, and a subclinical rise in transaminase levels.
- Phase II (24 to 72 hr): Right upper quadrant pain, vomiting, somnolence, tachycardia, jaundice, hypotension, and continued increase in transaminases.
- Phase III (72 to 96 hr): Hepatic necrosis with abdominal pain, jaundice, hepatic encephalopathy, coagulopathy, hypoglycemia, renal failure, fatality from multiorgan failure.
- Phase IV (4 days to 2 wk): Complete resolution of symptoms and resolution of organ failure.
- Table E1 summarizes the four phases/stages of acetaminophen poisoning.

ETIOLOGY

- The amount of APAP necessary for hepatic toxicity varies with the patient's body size and hepatic function. It is recommended that APAP intake should not exceed 3 to 4 g for adults and 90 mg/kg in children within a 24-hr period.
- A standardized nomogram is used to determine potential hepatic toxicity by knowing the APAP plasma level and the number of hr after ingestion. See the APAP ingestion algorithm (Fig. E1).

DIAGNOSIS

DIFFERENTIAL DIAGNOSIS

- Liver disease from alcohol abuse or viral hepatitis
- Ingestion of other hepatotoxic substances
- Bacterial/viral gastroenteritis

WORKUP

Initial workup is aimed at confirming APAP overdose with plasma APAP level and assessment of hepatic damage. A careful history should elicit the time of APAP ingestion, amount, preparation (e.g., extended release), and possible coingestants (see "Laboratory Tests").

LABORATORY TESTS

- Initial laboratory evaluation should include an initial plasma APAP level with a second level drawn approximately 4 hr after the initial ingestion. Subsequent levels can be obtained every 2 to 4 hr until the levels stabilize or decline. Levels starting from 4 hr post-ingestion should be plotted on the Rumack-Matthew nomogram (see acetaminophen ingestion algorithm [Fig. E1] to calculate potential hepatic toxicity). The nomogram cannot be used with patients who present >24 hr after ingestion, took extended-release preparations, had chronic ingestions, or when the time of ingestion is unknown.
- Transaminases (aminotransferase [AST], alanine aminotransferase [ALT]), serum glucose, bilirubin level, lipase level, prothrombin time (INR), blood urea nitrogen, creatinine, EKG, and urinalysis should be initially obtained on all patients.
- Serum and urine toxicology screens for other potential toxic substances (e.g., salicylate level, ethanol level, urine drugs of abuse screening) are also recommended on admission. Screening for infectious hepatitis should also be considered.
- Urine for β-hCG should be obtained from all women of childbearing age.

TREATMENT

NONPHARMACOLOGIC THERAPY

Consultation with a Poison Control Center is recommended for patients who have ingested a large amount of APAP and/or other toxic substances. A single toxic dose of APAP usually exceeds 7 g or 150 mg/kg in adults.

ACUTE GENERAL Rx

- Hepatotoxicity is defined as any increase in ALT or aspartate AST >1000 IU/L, and hepatic failure manifests as hepatotoxicity with hepatic encephalopathy. For those who cannot be risk stratified using the nomogram, the American College of Emergency Physicians recommends that *N*-acetylcysteine be administered without delay to those >12 yr and >8 hr after ingestion at presentation. This would include anyone with an ingestion of APAP over many days with an APAP level <20 μg/ml (with or without ALT elevation) or anyone with undetectable APAP levels with an elevated ALT and a history of excessive APAP intake.
- Administer activated charcoal 1g/kg PO if the patient is seen within 1 hr of ingestion or the clinician suspects polysubstance ingestion that delays gastric emptying.
- Determine serum acetaminophen levels 4 hr after ingestion; if in the toxic range based on the Rumack-Matthew nomogram, start *N*-acetylcysteine (NAC) either IV (Acetadote) or PO (Mucomyst). Acetylcysteine IV loading dose is 150 mg/kg ×1 diluted in 200 ml D5W over 15 to 60 min. Maintenance dose is 50 mg/kg diluted in 500 ml D5W over 4 hr, followed by 100 mg/kg diluted in 1000 ml D5W over 16 hr. The dose does not require adjustment for renal or hepatic impairment or for dialysis. Total administration time is 21 hr.
- Oral administration is 140 mg/kg PO as a loading dose, followed after 4 hr by 70 mg/kg PO q4h for a total of 18 doses. *N*-acetylcysteine therapy should be started within 24 hr of APAP overdose. Total administration time is 72 hr.
- Advantages of IV administration include more reliable absorption, fewer doses, and shorter duration of treatment. Disadvantages include cost and lower hepatic concentrations from first-pass flow as compared to oral acetylcysteine.
- Monitor APAP level; use Rumack-Matthew nomogram to trend hepatic toxicity. Repeat AST/ALT and APAP levels after 12 to 14 hr of IV acetylcysteine infusion and continue infusion longer than 16 hr if transaminases are elevated, if APAP concentration is still measurable, or if coagulopathy exists (INR >1.5 to 2.0). Patients with severe, irreversible liver failure may need to continue NAC until liver transplantation is available.
- Provide adequate IV hydration (e.g., D_5½NS at 150 ml/hr).
- Patients on IV *N*-acetylcysteine with liver failure require frequent monitoring of vital signs, oxygen saturation by pulse oximetry, and frequent blood draws. Frequent reassessment for hypoglycemia and infection is also essential.
- If APAP level is nontoxic, *N*-acetylcysteine therapy may be discontinued.

DISPOSITION

All patients with confirmed APAP poisoning will require admission, usually to an intensive care unit. Most patients (90%) will recover fully without persistent hepatic abnormalities. Hepatic failure is particularly unusual in children <6 yr.

REFERRAL

Psychiatric referral is recommended after intentional ingestions.

RELATED CONTENT

Acetaminophen Overdose (Patient Information)

AUTHOR: **Rory Merritt, MD, MEHP**

BASIC INFORMATION

DEFINITION

Achalasia is a motility disorder of the esophagus classically characterized by incomplete relaxation of the lower esophageal sphincter (LES) and aperistalsis of the esophageal smooth muscle resulting in functional obstruction of the esophagus.

SYNONYMS

Achalasia and cardiospasm
Achalasia (of cardia)
Aperistalsis of esophagus
Megaesophagus
Esophageal achalasia
Esophageal cardiospasm

ICD-10CM CODE

K22.0 Achalasia of cardia

EPIDEMIOLOGY & DEMOGRAPHICS

- Incidence has increased to approximately to 0.03 to 1.63 in 100,000 persons/yr due to studies using high-resolution esophageal manometry (HRM).
- Prevalence is around 10 per 100,000 persons.
- Although the onset of symptoms may occur at any age, incidence is typically bimodal (between 20 and 40 yr, then after 60 yr) with greater incidence in the elderly.
- Men and women are affected equally.

PHYSICAL FINDINGS & CLINICAL PRESENTATION

Symptoms:

- Dysphagia (most commonly with both solids and liquids) without oropharyngeal transfer difficulties
- Difficulty belching
- Regurgitation or vomiting of undigested food
- Chest pain and/or heartburn
- Globus
- Frequent hiccups
- Symptoms of aspiration such as nocturnal cough; possible dyspnea and pneumonia
- Weight loss
- The Eckardt symptom score (assessing dysphagia, regurgitation, retrosternal pain, and weight loss) is a fairly reliable measure of achalasia severity and may be used to assess response to therapy

Physical Exam:

- Focal lung examination abnormalities and wheezing are possible

ETIOLOGY

- Etiology is poorly understood.
- Loss of intrinsic inhibitory neurons in the myenteric plexus and smooth muscle portion of the esophagus as well as depletion of networks of interstitial cells of Cajal of the LES result in the loss of inhibitory neurotransmitters nitric oxide and vasoactive intestinal polypeptide and unopposed excitatory cholinergic activity, leading to incomplete relaxation of the LES and loss of esophageal peristalsis.
- Loss of myenteric nerve fibers is associated with lymphocytic and eosinophilic infiltrates, capillaritis, plexitis, venulitis, nerve hypertrophy, and fibrosis.
- This disorder may be caused by autoimmune degeneration of the esophageal myenteric plexus in association with several HLA class II DQ antigens. An eight amino-acid insertion in the cytoplasmic tail of HLA-DQβ1 has been identified as a strong achalasia risk factor. Antimyenteric plexus and other antineural autoantibodies have also been described. Patients with achalasia are more likely to have other autoimmune diseases.
- Abnormal immune reactions to neurotropic viruses, such as varicella zoster, measles, herpes simplex type 1, and human papilloma virus have been implicated. A host T-cell–mediated response may lead to neuronal injury; this has been suggested as the cause of types I and II achalasia (see "Imaging Studies" section).
- Achalasia is also seen in Allgrove syndrome, a rare autosomal recessive disorder caused by gene mutation on chromosome 12q13 and defined by achalasia, alacrima, autonomic disturbance, and acetylcholine insensitivity. Neurons in this syndrome may be susceptible to oxidative injury.
- Recent studies suggest that type III achalasia (see "Imaging Studies" section) is associated with myenteric inflammation but not neuronal loss; downregulation of nitric oxide synthase expression and increased cholinergic sensitivity are cytokine-mediated.
- A type III achalasia pattern has been described in chronic daily opiate users.

DIAGNOSIS

DIFFERENTIAL DIAGNOSIS

- Primary achalasia:
  1. Idiopathic
- Secondary achalasia:
  1. Chagas disease
  2. Vagal injury or surgery, including fundoplication
  3. Achalasia-like esophageal dilation has been described after laparoscopic gastric banding
- Pseudoachalasia (diseases that may mimic achalasia):
  1. Esophageal cancer
  2. Infiltrating gastric cancer
  3. Oat cell and bronchogenic lung cancer
  4. Lymphoma
  5. Amyloidosis
  6. Paraneoplastic syndrome
- Angina
- Bulimia
- Anorexia nervosa
- Gastric bezoar
- Gastritis
- Peptic ulcer disease
- Postvagotomy dysmotility
- Esophageal disease (Table 1):
  1. Gastroesophageal reflux disease
  2. Sarcoidosis
  3. Amyloidosis
  4. Esophageal stricture
  5. Esophageal webs and rings
  6. Scleroderma
  7. Barrett esophagus
  8. Esophagitis
  9. Diffuse esophageal spasm

TABLE 1 Esophageal Motor Disorders

	Achalasia	Scleroderma	Diffuse Esophageal Spasm
Symptoms	Dysphagia Regurgitation of nonacidic material	Gastroesophageal reflux disease Dysphagia	Substernal chest pain (angina-like) Dysphagia with pain
Radiographic appearance	Dilated, fluid-filled esophagus Distal *bird-beak* stricture	Aperistaltic esophagus Free reflux Peptic stricture	Simultaneous noncoordinated contractions
Manometric findings	High resting pressure	Low resting pressure	Normal pressure
Lower esophageal sphincter	Incomplete or abnormal relaxation with swallow		
Body	Low-amplitude, simultaneous contractions after swallowing	Low-amplitude peristaltic contractions or no peristalsis	Some peristalsis Diffuse and simultaneous nonperistaltic contractions, occasionally high amplitude

From Andreoli TE et al: *Andreoli and Carpenter's Cecil essentials of medicine*, ed 8, Philadelphia, 2010, Saunders.

WORKUP

- Physical examination and laboratory analyses to rule out other causes (Fig. E1, Table 2) and assess complications
- Imaging studies, manometry, and endoscopy (may be supportive or complementary)

LABORATORY TESTS

- Assessment of nutritional status
- Complete blood count; ECG and/or stress test if diagnosis is in doubt
- Serologic assays for *Trypanosoma cruzi* (Chagas disease) in appropriate individuals

IMAGING STUDIES

Barium swallow with fluoroscopy (particularly a timed barium esophagogram) may demonstrate:

- Uncoordinated or absent esophageal contractions (loss of peristalsis)
- An acutely tapered contrast column ("bird's beak"; Fig. E2)
- Dilation of the distal esophagus (smooth muscle portion)
- Esophageal air-fluid level with evidence of poor esophageal emptying
- Late-stage changes include tortuosity, angulation, dilated megaesophagus, retained food, and secretions

Manometry is considered the "gold standard" test to confirm the diagnosis. High-resolution manometry (HRM) or high-resolution esophageal pressure topography (HREPT) has defined subsets of patients with achalasia who may have different responses to medical or surgical therapies and prognoses.

- In classic achalasia (type I achalasia), conventional manometric abnormalities include low-amplitude disorganized contractions/aperistalsis, incomplete or absent LES relaxation (with residual pressure >10 mm Hg) after swallow, and high resting LES pressure.
- A subset of patients with "vigorous achalasia" may have high-amplitude, long-duration, simultaneous esophageal contractions. This term is now thought to be imprecise because of a newer classification of the disease.
- Unlike type I achalasia, type II achalasia shows panesophageal pressurization to greater than 30 mm Hg with ≥20% of test swallows, and type III achalasia shows spastic, lumen-obliterating contractions of the distal esophagus with ≥20% of swallows. This technique uses the integrated relaxation pressure (IRP) >15 mm Hg to define better the failure of esophagogastric junction relaxation. HRM also utilizes the distal contraction integral (DCI) to define hypercontractile vs. weak swallows vs. failed peristalsis. The distal latency (DL) defines premature contractions, seen with diffuse esophageal spasm and type III achalasia.
- HREPT has also defined an achalasia variant described as esophagogastric junction outflow obstruction, where the IRP is >15 mm Hg, but peristalsis is present. Some are associated with secondary causes; a small percentage may progress to achalasia; and, in many, the natural history is unclear and response to therapy is variable.
- Direct visualization by endoscopy, including careful visualization of the esophagogastric junction and cardia, should be performed to exclude other causes of dysphagia, including "functional esophagogastric junction obstruction," strictures, secondary causes of achalasia (including infiltrating cancers), and pseudoachalasia.
- Functional luminal imaging probe (FLIP) technology is a new technique that can measure compliance and distensibility across the esophagogastric junction and may demonstrate both impaired LES relaxation and response to achalasia therapy.

Rx TREATMENT

NONPHARMACOLOGIC THERAPY

- Achalasia is treatable but incurable. The goals of therapy are to decrease LES pressure to relieve the functional obstruction, relieve symptoms, and prevent progression to a dilated esophagus, also referred to as a megaesophagus. Treatment does not improve esophageal peristalsis.
- Pneumatic dilation (PD) uses a fixed-diameter and high-pressure dilating balloon across the LES under fluoroscopic visualization to disrupt the muscle fibers and may benefit 50% to 93% of patients. Most protocols use a graded dilation approach, starting with a 30-mm balloon and repeating if required with a 35-mm or 40-mm balloon. Studies show this may be more effective in females, older patients, and HRM type II patients. Esophageal rupture or perforation is a rare complication (2% to 4%) that may be managed conservatively in stable patients with a small perforation. There is currently no standardized protocol for PD.
- Surgical: Laparoscopic, or less commonly, open Heller esophagomyotomy (HM) is effective (90%). Approximately 35% of patients undergoing surgery will develop reflux disease. As a result, some surgeons will perform an anterior Dor or posterior Toupet antireflux repair (fundoplication) as part of the surgical procedure. Studies suggest this may be more effective in men and younger patients. An observational study has suggested that those with prior endoscopic treatment before myotomy may not do as well as those who have a primary myotomy.
- A large European study suggested that patients may expect similar medium-term outcomes from myotomy and balloon dilation. A meta-analysis suggests better long-term durability of myotomy, while balloon dilation may be more cost-effective. About 20% to 30% of patients undergoing either therapy may require retreatment within 5 to 7 yr.
- Endoscopic submucosal myotomy (per-oral endoscopic myotomy [POEM]) has a high success rate comparable to laparoscopic HM (particularly in HRM type III patients in whom a longer myotomy, tailored to the length of the diseased segment, improves outcome), few adverse events (which can include pneumomediastinum, pneumothorax, pneumoperitoneum, pleural effusion, pneumonia, and bleeding), and exceedingly rare mortality. Since no antireflux procedure is performed, there is a modest risk (up to 53%) of developing pathologic reflux. This should only be performed at high-volume centers. A randomized multicenter study showed a higher treatment success rate for POEM at 2 yr when compared with pneumatic dilation.
- FLIP and timed barium esophagogram may help determine response to therapy.
- Esophagectomy has been performed in patients with end-stage achalasia with a dilated, often sigmoid-shaped or megaesophagus, who have failed myotomy or pneumatic dilation.
- Self-expanding metal stents (SEMS) have been studied as a temporary treatment in a few studies with low-quality evidence and are not currently recommended. Patients with SEMS often reported chest pain and regurgitation.

ACUTE GENERAL Rx

- Medications may be useful for short-term symptom relief and in patients with refractory chest pain. They should only be considered in patients unable to receive, or who are scheduled for, more definitive procedures. LES pressure may be lowered by up to 50% through sublingual use of long-acting nitrates (e.g., isosorbide dinitrate 5 to 20 mg) or calcium channel blockers (e.g., nifedipine 10 to 30 mg). Side effects are common and duration of relief tends to be short. Sildenafil was shown to be effective in a few small, short-term studies but it is generally not recommended. Anticholinergics such as atropine and theophylline are less commonly used.
- Botulinum toxin (BT) injection will benefit up to 85% of patients by inhibiting acetylcholine release from cholinergic nerve endings and blocking the unopposed cholinergic stimulation of the LES, without impacting the myogenic tone. Up to half will require repeat injections by 6 mo. A few studies have suggested that repeated injections may have diminished efficacy and can lead to fibrosis, complicating subsequent attempts at surgical therapy. Studies have identified age >40 and type II or III achalasia to have more favorable response to BT injections. BT is recommended as first-line therapy for patients who may not be candidates for surgical options.
- Many patients will require proton pump inhibitor therapy for gastroesophageal reflux after effective disruption of the LES.
- For patients with weight loss secondary to achalasia, studies regarding dietary modification as adjunctive treatment are underway to help improve weight after intervention.

TABLE 2 Chicago Classification of Esophageal Motility Disorders

Diagnosis	Diagnostic Criteria
Achalasia	
Type I	100% failed peristalsis, mean IRP >10 mm Hg
Type II	No esophageal contraction and panesophageal pressurization with ≥20% of swallows; mean IRP >10 mm Hg
Type III	Premature contractions with ≥20% of swallows, mean IRP ≥17 mm Hg
EGJ outflow obstruction	Mean IRP ≥15 mm Hg; mix of normal, weak, rapid, hypertensive, failed peristalsis or panesophageal pressurization
Motility Disorders	(Patterns not observed in normal individuals)
Distal esophageal spasm	Mean IRP <17 mm Hg, ≥20% premature contractions
Hypercontractile esophagus (jackhammer esophagus)	At least one swallow DCI >8000 mm Hg·s·cm
Absent peristalsis	Mean IRP ≤10 mm Hg, 100% failed peristalsis
Peristaltic Abnormality	(Defined by exceeding statistical limits of normal)
Weak peristalsis	Mean IRP <15 mm Hg and ≥20% swallows with large breaks (≥5 cm) or ≥30% with small breaks (2-5 cm) in the 20-mm Hg isobaric contour Or DCI of 150-450 mm Hg·s·cm in ≥30% test swallows
Frequent failed peristalsis	>30%, but <100% of swallows with failed peristalsis
Rapid peristalsis	Rapid contraction with ≥20% of swallows, DL >4.5 s
Hypertensive peristalsis (nutcracker esophagus)	Mean DCI >5000 mm Hg·s·cm, but not meeting criteria for hypercontractile esophagus
Normal	Not achieving any of the above diagnostic criteria

DCI, Distal contractile interval; *DL,* distal latency; *EGJ,* esophagogastric junction; *IRP,* integrated relaxation pressure.
From Feldman M et al: *Sleisenger and Fortran's gastrointestinal and liver disease*, ed 10, Philadelphia, 2016, Saunders.

- Future therapies, including neural cell transplantation and electrical stimulation, are currently under investigation but likely yr away from implementation.

PEARLS & CONSIDERATIONS

COMMENTS

- Medication has a limited role in treatment.
- Botulinum toxin is transiently effective in improving symptoms.
- Pneumatic dilation, surgical myotomy, and POEM provide more durable long-term responses and are the treatment of choice for most patients. Botulinum toxin should be considered primarily in patients too elderly or ill to be considered for these other therapies.
- Patients with achalasia may be at long-term risk of squamous cell carcinoma of the esophagus and non–reflux-associated esophagitis. Treated patients may be at long-term risk for reflux esophagitis, Barrett esophagus, and adenocarcinoma. Endoscopic surveillance is not routinely recommended in these patients.

RELATED CONTENT

Achalasia (Patient Information)
Dysphagia (Related Key Topic)

SUGGESTED READINGS

Available at ExpertConsult.com

AUTHORS: **Firrah Saeed, MD** and **Harlan G. Rich, MD, FACP, AGAF**

BASIC INFORMATION

DEFINITION

Acne vulgaris is a chronic disorder of the pilosebaceous apparatus caused by abnormal desquamation of follicular epithelium leading to obstruction of the pilosebaceous canal, resulting in inflammation and subsequent formation of papules, pustules, nodules, comedones, and scarring. Based on their appearance, the acne lesions can be divided into inflammatory (presence of papules, pustules, and nodules) or noninflammatory (open and closed comedones) For inflammatory acne, lesions can be classified as papulopustular, nodular, or both. The American Academy of Dermatology classification scheme for acne denotes the following three levels:

1. Mild acne: Characterized by the presence of comedones (Figs. E1 and E2) (noninflammatory lesions), few papules and pustules (generally <10), but no nodules.
2. Moderate acne: Presence of several to many papules and pustules (10 to 40) along with comedones (10 to 40). The presence of >40 papules and pustules along with larger, deeper nodular inflamed lesions (Figs. E3 and E4) (up to five) denotes moderately severe acne.
3. Severe acne: Presence of numerous or extensive papules and pustules as well as many nodular lesions (Fig. E5).

SYNONYM

Acne

ICD-10CM CODES	
L70.0	Acne vulgaris
L70.1	Acne conglobata
L70.2	Acne varioliformis
L70.3	Acne tropica
L70.4	Infantile acne
L70.5	Acne excoriee des jeunes filles
L70.8	Other acne
L70.9	Acne, unspecified
L73.0	Acne keloid

EPIDEMIOLOGY & DEMOGRAPHICS

- Acne is the most common skin disease in the U.S. Increased incidence due to prolonged wearing of masks during COVID-19 pandemic.
- It is most common in teenagers, with 85% of all teenagers being affected to some degree.
- Highest incidence between ages of 15 and 18 yr in both genders.
- Involution of the disease usually occurs before age 25 yr, but 26% of women and 12% of men will continue to have clinical acne until the mid-40s.

PHYSICAL FINDINGS & CLINICAL PRESENTATION

- Open comedones (blackheads), closed comedones (whiteheads)
- Greasiness (oily skin)
- Presence of scars from prior acne cysts
- Various stages of development and severity may be present concomitantly
- Common distribution of acne: Face, back, and upper chest
- Inflammatory papules, pustules, and ectatic pores

ETIOLOGY

- Acne vulgaris is a follicular disease, with the principal abnormality being comedone formation.
- Overactivity of the sebaceous glands and blockage in the ducts. The obstruction leads to the formation of comedones, which can become inflamed because of overgrowth of *Propionibacterium acnes.*
- Exacerbated by environmental factors (hot, humid, tropical climate), medications (e.g., iodine in cough mixtures, hair greases), industrial exposure to halogenated hydrocarbons.
- Mechanical or frictional forces can aggravate existing acne (e.g., excessive washing by some patients to help rid them of their blackheads or oiliness).

DIAGNOSIS

DIFFERENTIAL DIAGNOSIS (TABLE 1)

- Gram-negative folliculitis
- Staphylococcal pyoderma
- Acne rosacea
- Drug eruption
- Sebaceous hyperplasia
- Angiofibromas, basal cell carcinomas, osteoma cutis
- Occupational exposures to oils or grease
- Steroid acne
- Hidradenitis suppurativa
- Perioral dermatitis
- Pseudofolliculitis barbae
- Miliaria
- Seborrheic dermatitis

WORKUP

History and physical examination:

- Inquire about previous treatment
- Careful drug history (including all OTC products)
- Family history, history of cyclic menstrual flares
- History of use of cosmetics and cleansers
- Oral contraceptive use
- Use of medications that may worsen acne such as corticosteroids, anabolic steroids, lithium, neuroleptics, cyclosporine
- Consider the possibility of hyperandrogenic state in all women (hirsutism, irregular menses, androgenic alopecia) or children (seborrhea, acanthosis nigricans, onset of acne between ages 1 and 7 yr and no obvious external factors)

LABORATORY TESTS

- Laboratory evaluation is generally not helpful. Patients who are candidates for therapy with isotretinoin should have baseline liver enzymes, cholesterol, and triglycerides checked because this medication may result in elevation of lipids and liver enzymes.
- A negative serum pregnancy test or two negative urine pregnancy tests should also be obtained in females 1 wk before initiation of isotretinoin; it is also imperative to maintain effective contraception during and 1 mo after therapy with isotretinoin ends because of its teratogenic effects. Pregnancy status should be rechecked at monthly visits.
- If hyperandrogenism is suspected in female patients, levels of dehydroepiandrosterone sulfate (DHEAS), testosterone (total and free), and androstenedione should be measured. For women with regular menstrual cycles, serum androgen measurements generally are not necessary.

TREATMENT

NONPHARMACOLOGIC THERAPY

- Blue light (ClearLight therapy system) can be used for treatment of moderate inflammatory acne vulgaris. Light in the violet/blue range can cause bacterial death by a photoreaction in which porphyrins react with oxygen to generate reactive oxygen species, which damage the cell membranes of *P. acnes.* Treatment usually consists of 15-min exposures twice weekly for 4 wk. Phototherapy may be effective for short-term treatment of acne, but long-term efficacy and how it compares with conventional acne therapy is unclear.
- Diet: In obese patients, dietary counseling is recommended. A high-glycemic or high-dairy diet may worsen acne, although the strength of its influence is controversial.

ACUTE GENERAL Rx

Treatment generally varies with the type of lesions (comedones, papules, pustules, cystic lesions) and the severity of acne. Table 2 summarizes an acne treatment algorithm. First-line treatment for mild acne vulgaris includes benzoyl peroxide, a topical retinoid, or a combination of topical medications, including topical antibiotics. Use of topical treatments for 6 to 8 wk is required to judge their efficacy. Table E3 describes prescription topical therapies for acne.

- Comedones (noninflammatory acne) can be treated with retinoids or retinoid analogs. Topical retinoids are comedolytic and work by normalizing follicular keratinization. Commonly available agents are Adapalene (Differin, 0.1% gel or cream, applied once or twice daily), tazarotene (Tazorac 0.1% cream or gel applied daily), tretinoin (Retin-A 0.1% cream or 0.025 gel applied once daily), tretinoin microsphere (Retin-A Micro, 0.1% gel, applied at bedtime). Tretinoin is inactivated by ultraviolet light and oxidized by benzoyl peroxide; therefore, it should only be applied at night and not used concomitantly with benzoyl peroxide.
- Tretinoin is pregnancy category C and tazarotene is pregnancy category X. Salicylic acid preparations (e.g., Neutrogena 2% wash) have keratolytic and antiinflammatory properties and are also useful in the treatment of comedones. Large, open comedones (blackheads) should be expressed.
- Patients should be reevaluated after 4 to 6 wk.
- Benzoyl peroxide gel (2.5% or 5%) may be added if the comedones become inflamed or form pustules. The most common adverse effects are dryness, erythema, and peeling.

TABLE 1 Differential Diagnosis of Acne

Closed	Open
ACNE VULGARIS – COMEDONAL	
• Milia • Osteoma cutis • Sebaceous hyperplasia • Pseudoacne of the nasal crease • Syringomas • Trichoepitheliomas* • Trichodiscomas, fibrofolliculomas • Eruptive vellus hair cysts[†], steatocystoma multiplex[†] • Colloid milia • Acne exacerbated by systemic corticosteroids[‡] or anabolic steroids • Contact acne (occupational, pomade, cosmetica, mechanica; chloracne) • Follicular mucinosis • Follicular mycosis fungoides	• Contact acne (see Closed) • Acne exacerbated by systemic corticosteroids[‡] or anabolic steroids • Trichostasis spinulosa (see inset) • Favre–Racouchot syndrome • Pseudoacne of the nasal crease • Nevus comedonicus • Basaloid follicular hamartoma syndrome • Familial dyskeratotic comedones • Dowling–Degos disease • Radiation-induced comedones • Molluscum-induced comedones • Childhood flexural comedones (often a single double-orifice lesion) • Dilated pore of Winer (single lesion) • Trichofolliculoma (usually a single lesion) • Follicular spines – in settings such as trichodysplasia spinulosa[§], type VI pityriasis rubra pilaris[§], multiple myeloma, demodicosis[§], follicular mucinosis, and drug-induced (e.g., BRAF inhibitors, cyclosporine[§], acitretin)
Acne vulgaris – inflammatory	
• Rosacea • Perioral/periorificial dermatitis • Demodicosis (adults > children[§]) • Folliculitis – culture-negative (normal flora), staphylococcal, gram-negative, eosinophilic[§], *Pityrosporum* • Acne/acneiform eruptions due to topical or systemic corticosteroids[‡], anabolic steroids, or other medications (e.g. lithium, EGFR inhibitors) • Pseudofolliculitis barbae, acne keloidalis nuchae • Pseudoacne of the nasal crease • Furuncle/carbuncle • Idiopathic facial aseptic granuloma (in children) • Neutrophilic dermatoses and neutrophilic eccrine hidradenitis	• Keratosis pilaris • Trichodysplasia spinulosa (viral-associated trichodysplasia)[§] • Lupus miliaris disseminatus faciei • Psychogenic (neurotic) excoriations, factitial lesions • Follicular mucinosis • Follicular mycosis fungoides • Tinea faciei • Molluscum contagiosum (especially inflamed lesions) • Angiofibromas • Dowling–Degos disease (especially the Haber syndrome variant) • Cutaneous Rosai-Dorfman disease • Granulomatosis with polyangiitis (Wegener granulomatosis) • Syndromes associated with acne, e.g., PAPA, (PA)PASH, SAPHO, Apert syndrome
Neonatal acne (neonatal cephalic pustulosis)	
• Sebaceous hyperplasia • Milia • Miliaria rubra (especially pustular variant)	• Candidal infection • Papulopustular eruption of hyper-IgE syndrome • Vesiculopustular eruption of transient myeloproliferative disorder
Solid facial edema secondary to acne vulgaris	
• Solid facial edema secondary to rosacea • Melkersson-Rosenthal syndrome, sarcoidosis (e.g., Heerfordt syndrome), lepromatous leprosy • Lymphoma (B- or T-cell), leukemia cutis, angiosarcoma • Scleromyxedema, myxedema, self-healing (juvenile) cutaneous mucinosis • Autoimmune connective tissue disease (e.g., dermatomyositis, lupus erythematosus, Still disease)	• Angioedema (lasts <24-72 hr), C1 esterase inhibitor deficiency (lasts 2-3 days), blepharochalasis/Ascher syndrome • Sweet syndrome or cellulitis – more abrupt onset • Superior vena caval obstruction • Lymphatic malformation • Pachydermoperiostosis and other genetic disorders with coarse facies • Other – trichinosis, primary systemic amyloidosis

EGFR, Epidermal growth factor receptor; *PAPA*, pyogenic arthritis, pyoderma gangrenosum, and acne conglobata; *(PA)PASH*, (pyogenic arthritis), pyoderma gangrenosum, acne, and suppurative hidradenitis; *SAPHO*, synovitis, acne, pustulosis, hyperostosis, and osteitis.

*Early or small-sized.

[†]In the differential diagnosis of cystic lesions of the trunk.

[‡]Can also lead to rosacea-like picture.

[§]Often in the setting of HIV infection and/or other immunocompromised states, including trichodysplasia spinulosa in patients receiving cyclosporine.

From Bolognia J: Dermatology, ed 4, 2018, Elsevier.

- Topical antibiotics (erythromycin, clindamycin lotions or pads) can also be used in patients with significant inflammation. They reduce *P. acnes* in the pilosebaceous follicle and have some anti-inflammatory effects. The combination of 5% benzoyl peroxide and 3% erythromycin (Benzamycin) or 1% clindamycin with 5% benzoyl peroxide (BenzaClin) is highly effective in patients who have a mixture of comedonal and inflammatory acne lesions.
- Fixed-dose combinations of clindamycin phosphate 1.2% and tretinoin 0.025% are available (Veltin gel, Ziana) and are more effective than either product used alone; however, they are much more expensive than the individual generic components.
- Pustular acne can be treated with tretinoin and benzoyl peroxide gel applied on alternate evenings; drying agents (sulfacetamide-sulfa lotions [Novacet, Sulfacet]) are also effective when used in combination with benzoyl peroxide; oral antibiotics (doxycycline 100 mg qd or erythromycin 1 g qd given in 2 to 3 divided doses) are effective in patients with moderate to severe pustular acne. Patients not responding well to these antibiotics can be switched to minocycline 50 to 100 mg bid. Table E4 summarizes oral antibiotics for acne vulgaris.
- Patients with nodular cystic acne and those with moderate to severe inflammatory acne unresponsive to topical drugs can be treated with systemic agents: Antibiotics (erythromycin, tetracycline, doxycycline, minocycline), isotretinoin (available on a restricted basis), or oral contraceptives. Periodic intralesional triamcinolone (Kenalog) injections by a dermatologist are also effective. The possibility of endocrinopathy should be considered in patients responding poorly to therapy.
- Isotretinoin is the most effective drug available for treatment of severe nodulocystic acne. It is indicated for acne resistant to antibiotic therapy and severe acne. It inhibits *P. acne's* colonization by reducing sebum production and has anti-inflammatory and keratolytic effects. It is available only on a restricted basis. Dosage is 0.5 to 1 mg/kg/day in 2 divided doses (maximum of 2 mg/kg/day); duration of therapy is generally 20 wk to reach a cumulative dose ≥120 mg/kg for severe cystic acne. Before using this medication patients should undergo baseline laboratory evaluation (see "Laboratory Tests"). This drug is absolutely contraindicated during pregnancy because of its teratogenicity. It should be used with caution in patients with history of depression. Physicians, distributors, pharmacies, and patients must register in the iPLEDGE program (www.ipledgeprogram.com) before using isotretinoin.
- Azelaic acid is a bacteriostatic dicarboxylic acid used to normalize keratinization and reduce inflammation. It can be used in pregnant women.
- Oral contraceptives reduce androgen levels and therefore sebum production. They

TABLE 2 Acne Treatment Algorithm

Therapy	SEVERITY (LESION TYPE) Mild (Comedonal)	Mild (Inflammatory/ Mixed)	Moderate (Inflammatory/Mixed)	Severe (Inflammatory/ Mixed)	Severe (Nodular/ Scarring)
*Initial therapy options**,†	Topical retinoid BP Salicylic acid cleanser	BP/retinoid combo BP/antibiotic combo Antibiotic/retinoid combo + BP	BP/retinoid combo BP/antibiotic combo ± topical retinoid Antibiotic/retinoid combo + BP ± oral antibiotic	BP/retinoid combo + oral antibioticBP/antibiotic combo + topical retinoid + oral antibiotic Antibiotic/retinoid combo + BP + oral antibiotic	Isotretinoin
*Alternative therapy options**,†,‡	Add BP or retinoid if not already prescribed BP/antibiotic combo BP/retinoid combo Antibiotic/retinoid combo	Substitute another combo product Add missing component (i.e., topical retinoid, BP, topical antibiotic) Change type, strength, or formulation of topical retinoid	Substitute another combo product Add missing component (i.e., topical retinoid, BP, topical antibiotic, oral antibiotic) Change type, strength, or formulation of topical retinoid Consider hormonal therapy for females Consider oral isotretinoin	Consider changing oral antibiotic Consider isotretinoin Consider hormonal therapy for females	Consider hormonal therapy for females
Maintenance therapy	Topical retinoid or BP/retinoid combo	Topical retinoid or BP/ retinoid combo	Topical retinoid or BP/retinoid combo	Topical retinoid or BP/retinoid combo	Topical retinoid or BP/ retinoid combo

BP, Benzoyl peroxide.
*If combination products not available to patient, consider substitution of individual components as separate prescriptions.
†Topical dapsone may be considered in place of topical antibiotic.
‡If needed as determined by physician assessment and patient satisfaction.
Modified from Zaenglein AL, Thiboutot DM: Expert committee recommendations for acne management, *Pediatrics* 118(3):1188-99, 2006; Thiboutot D et al: New insights into the management of acne: an update from the Global Alliance to Improve Outcomes in Acne Group, *J Am Acad Dermatol* 60:S1-50, 2009; Eichenfield LF et al: Evidence-based recommendations for the diagnosis and treatment of pediatric acne, *Pediatrics* 131(3):S163-86, 2013; Thiboutot DM, Gollnick HP: Treatment considerations for inflammatory acne: clinical evidence for adapalene 0.1% in combination therapies, *J Drugs Dermatol* 5(8):785-94, 2006; Gollnick H et al: Management of acne: a report from a Global Alliance to Improve Outcomes in Acne, *J Am Acad Dermatol* 49(Suppl. 1):S1-37, 2003.

represent a useful adjunctive therapy for all types of acne in women and adolescent girls. Commonly used agents are norgestimate/ethinyl estradiol (Ortho Tri-Cyclen) and drospirenone/ethinyl estradiol (Yasmin).

REFERRAL

Referral for intralesional injection and dermabrasion should be considered in patients with severe acne unresponsive to conventional therapy. Table E5 summarizes alternative treatments for acne vulgaris.

PEARLS & CONSIDERATIONS

- Gram-negative folliculitis should be suspected if inflammatory acne worsens after several mo of oral antibiotic therapy.
- Acne may worsen during the first 3 to 4 wk of retinoid therapy before improving.
- Tips for topical acne therapy are summarized in Table 6.

COMMENTS

Indications for systemic therapy of acne are:
- Painful deep papules or nodules.
- Extensive lesions.
- Active acne with severe scarring or hyperpigmentation.
- Patient's morale.

Patients should be educated that in most cases acne can be controlled but not cured and that at least 4 to 6 wk of initial therapy should be required before significant improvement is noted.

TABLE 6 Tips for Topical Acne Therapy

Improve adherence—often compromised due to patients having busy schedules or quitting when the response is not rapid	• Simplify the regimen: Once daily when possible; consider combination products (e.g., benzoyl peroxide + adapalene or clindamycin; tretinoin + clindamycin), especially in less motivated adolescents • Inform patients that it will take 6-8 wk of treatment for substantial improvement • Ask specifically about adherence: "Out of 7 nights, how many times do you apply the medication?"
Educate on proper use	• In general, topical medications (especially retinoids) should be used to the entire acne-prone region rather than as "spot treatment" of individual lesions • Provide instructions on where to apply the medication and how much to use
Minimize irritation—most common in adolescents with atopic dermatitis and adults	• Note that using too much medication or applying it too frequently can increase irritation • Devise a gradual initial approach to improve tolerance in patients with sensitive skin; for example, a single agent may be used for the first 2-3 wk (starting every other day for retinoids), followed by slow introduction of a second medication (e.g., transitioning from alternate days to daily) • Advise to avoid harsh scrubs and other irritating agents (e.g., toners, acne products that are not part of the regimen) • Suggest use of a noncomedogenic sensitive skin moisturizer if dryness occurs
Avoid exacerbation	• Review all skin care products and cosmetics; having patients bring everything that they apply to their face to a visit may help to determine the source of problems • Advise noncomedogenic products (e.g., moisturizers, sunscreens, make-up) and to avoid having oily hair or using pomades that may contribute to acne • Instruct patients not to pick or manipulate lesions
Reinforce the plan—patients often forget what is recommended and are bombarded by advertising and false information about acne	• Provide a written handout with your specific instructions • Recommend additional reliable educational resources about acne and its treatment (e.g., www.aad.org/public/diseases/acne# www.webmd.com/skin-problems-and-treatments/acne/default.htm)

- The negative psychological effect of acne may be severe and long-lasting.

SUGGESTED READINGS

Available at ExpertConsult.com

RELATED CONTENT

Acne (Patient Information)

AUTHORS: **Lillian Jin, MD, MPH,** and **Jacquelyn Detweiler, DO, FAAP**

BASIC INFORMATION

DEFINITION

Acoustic neuroma is a benign proliferation of the Schwann cells that cover the vestibular branch of the eighth cranial nerve (CN VIII). Symptoms are commonly a result of compression of the acoustic branch of CN VIII, the facial nerve (CN VII), and the trigeminal nerve (CN V). The glossopharyngeal nerve (CN IX) and vagus nerve (CN X) are less commonly involved. In extreme cases, compression of the brain stem may lead to obstruction of cerebrospinal fluid (CSF) outflow and elevated intracranial pressure (ICP).

SYNONYMS

Vestibular schwannoma
Acoustic schwannoma

ICD-10CM CODE
D33.3 Benign neoplasm of cranial nerves

EPIDEMIOLOGY & DEMOGRAPHICS

Overall incidence is approximately 1 in 100,000 person-yr with a higher incidence in patients with neurofibromatosis type 2 (NF2). In the U.S., there are about 3000 new cases of acoustic neuroma diagnosed each yr. The tumor most commonly presents in the fifth and sixth decades.

PHYSICAL FINDINGS & CLINICAL PRESENTATION

- Most frequently unilateral hearing loss and/or tinnitus. Also balance problems, vertigo, facial pain (trigeminal neuralgia) and weakness, difficulty swallowing, fullness or pain of the involved ear. Headache may occur.
- With elevated ICP, patients may also have vomiting, fever, and visual changes.
- Hearing loss is the most common presenting complaint and is usually high frequency.

ETIOLOGY

The etiology is incompletely understood, but long-term exposure to acoustic trauma has been implicated. Bilateral acoustic neuromas may be inherited in an autosomal-dominant manner as part of NF2. This disease is associated with a defect on chromosome 22q1. Childhood exposure to low-dose radiation for benign head and neck conditions may increase risk for acoustic neuromas. There is inconclusive evidence to link chronic exposure to radiofrequency radiation from cellular telephone use and the risk for developing brain tumors.

DIAGNOSIS

DIFFERENTIAL DIAGNOSIS

- Benign positional vertigo
- Menière disease
- Trigeminal neuralgia
- Cerebellar disease
- Normal-pressure hydrocephalus
- Presbycusis
- Glomus tumors
- Vertebrobasilar insufficiency
- Ototoxicity from medications
- Other tumors:
  1. Meningioma, glioma
  2. Facial nerve schwannoma
  3. Cavernous hemangioma
  4. Metastatic tumors

WORKUP

- A detailed neurologic examination with special attention to the cranial nerves is crucial.
- Rinne and Weber tests help determine conductive or sensorineural hearing loss.
- Common office balance tests (i.e., Romberg, Dix-Hallpike) are typically normal.
- Otoscopic evaluation may help rule out other causes of hearing loss.

LABORATORY TESTS

- Audiometry is useful, often showing asymmetric, sensorineural, high-frequency hearing loss.
- CSF protein may be elevated.

IMAGING STUDIES

- MRI with gadolinium (Fig. 1) is the preferred test. It can detect tumors as small as 2 mm in diameter.
- High-resolution CT scan with and without contrast can detect tumors 1 cm in diameter or larger.
- Treatment decisions should be based on the size of the tumor, rate of growth (older patients tend to have slower-growing tumors), degree of neurologic deficit, desire to preserve hearing, life expectancy, age of the patient, and surgical risk. A combination of treatments can also be used.

TREATMENT

NONPHARMACOLOGIC THERAPY

- Surgery is the definitive treatment. Choice of approach (middle cranial fossa, translabyrinthine, or retromastoid suboccipital) may vary depending on the size of the tumor, amount of residual hearing desired, and degree of surgical risk that can be tolerated. Partial resection is sometimes undertaken to minimize the risk of injury to nearby structures. Intraoperative facial nerve monitoring is recommended.
- Radiation therapy (stereotactic radiotherapy, stereotactic radiosurgery, or proton beam radiotherapy) is useful for tumors <3 cm in diameter or for those in whom surgery is not an option. Radiotherapy after partial resection has also been used to minimize complications.
- Age alone is not a contraindication to surgery.

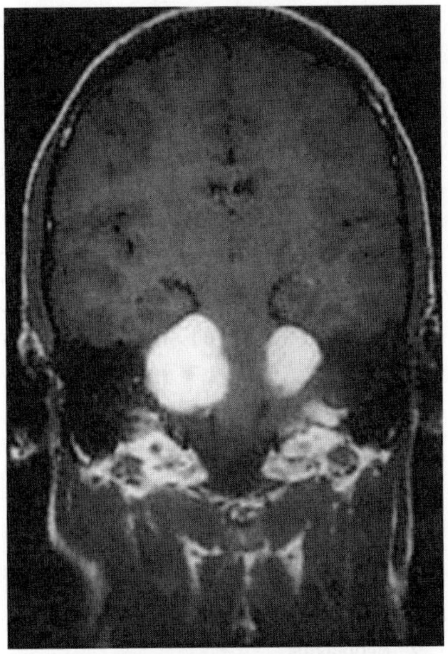

FIG. 1 Magnetic resonance imaging with enhancement shows bilateral acoustic neuromas. Coronal view. (From Kanski JJ, Bowling B: *Clinical ophthalmology, a systematic approach*, ed 7, Philadelphia, 2011, Saunders.)

GENERAL Rx

- Bevacizumab, an antivascular endothelial growth factor (VEGF) monoclonal antibody, has been shown to improve hearing and reduce the volume of growing acoustic neuromas in some neurofibromatosis type 2 patients.
- Observation with MRI every 6 to 12 mo may be appropriate for frail patients with small tumors, but risk of unrecoverable hearing loss may increase if surgery is delayed. Also, progressive hearing loss may occur despite absence of growth on subsequent imaging.

DISPOSITION

Hearing can be preserved at near-preoperative levels in more than two thirds of patients with small- to medium-sized tumors. Occurrence of secondary radiation-related tumors following radiosurgery is rare. There are no standard posttreatment follow-up recommendations. Therefore, an individualized approach to follow-up imaging and audiometry is recommended.

REFERRAL

Prompt referral to an otolaryngologist or neurosurgeon who is facile with all three surgical approaches is recommended.

PEARLS & CONSIDERATIONS

COMMENTS

- Presents most commonly as unilateral, sensorineural hearing loss.
- Treatment outcomes are excellent, with surgical cure rates greater than 95%.
- Of those who are managed with observation only, approximately half have continued enlargement, and approximately one-fifth eventually have a surgical intervention.

PATIENT & FAMILY EDUCATION

Acoustic Neuroma Association: https://www.anausa.org/

SUGGESTED READINGS
Available at ExpertConsult.com

RELATED CONTENT

Acoustic Neuroma (Patient Information)
Tinnitus (Related Key Topic)

AUTHOR: **Courtney Clark Bilodeau, MD, FACP**

BASIC INFORMATION

DEFINITION

Acquired immunodeficiency syndrome (AIDS) is a disorder caused by infection with the human immunodeficiency virus (HIV) and marked by progressive deterioration of the cellular immune system, leading to secondary (opportunistic) infections and/or malignancies.

SYNONYM

AIDS

ICD-10CM CODE
B20 Human immunodeficiency virus [HIV] disease

EPIDEMIOLOGY & DEMOGRAPHICS

INCIDENCE (IN U.S.):
- The estimated number of persons diagnosed with AIDS in the U.S. is approximately 18,000/yr.
- There is a disproportionate number of new AIDS cases among Black/African Americans and Latino/Hispanic Americans compared with white Americans.
- The majority of all new AIDS diagnoses are among gay, bisexual, or other men who have sex with men (MSM).

PREVALENCE (IN U.S.): The cumulative number of AIDS diagnoses in the U.S. exceeds 1.2 million.

PREDOMINANT SEX: Men constitute approximately 75% of incident AIDS diagnoses in the U.S.; more than half of AIDS diagnoses occur in MSM.

PREDOMINANT AGE: The predominant age group diagnosed with AIDS is 25 to 59 yr of age.

PEAK INCIDENCE: Ages 25 to 59 yr

GENETICS:
- Familial disposition: Although there is no proven genetic predisposition, individuals with deletions in the *CCR5* gene are less susceptible to HIV infection with macrophage tropic virus (the predominant virus in sexual transmission) and may progress to AIDS more slowly.
- Congenital infection:
  1. HIV is transmittable from an infected mother to the fetus in utero in as many as 30% of pregnancies if untreated.
  2. No specific congenital malformations associated with infection; low birth weight and spontaneous abortion are possible.

PHYSICAL FINDINGS & CLINICAL PRESENTATION

- Nonspecific findings: Fever, weight loss, anorexia
- Specific syndromes:
  1. Seen in association with specific opportunistic infections and malignancies. These include:
     a. Opportunistic infections:
        (1) Disseminated strongyloidiasis
        (2) Disseminated toxoplasmosis, cryptococcosis, histoplasmosis, cytomegalovirus (CMV), herpes simplex virus (HSV), or mycobacterial disease (most common is mycobacterium avium complex)
        (3) *Candida* esophagitis or bronchopulmonary disease
        (4) Chronic cryptosporidiosis diarrhea
        (5) *Pneumocystis jiroveci* pneumonia (PJP)
        (6) Extensive pulmonary and extrapulmonary tuberculosis (TB)
        (7) Recurrent pneumonia or other bacterial infections
        (8) Progressive multifocal leukoencephalopathy (PML)
     b. AIDS-related neoplasms:
        (1) Kaposi sarcoma
        (2) Primary brain lymphoma
        (3) Invasive cervical carcinoma
        (4) High-grade B-cell non-Hodgkin lymphoma, Burkitt lymphoma, undifferentiated non-Hodgkin lymphoma, or immunoblastic lymphoma
  2. Most common:
     a. Respiratory infections (*Pneumocystis jiroveci* [formerly known as *Pneumocystis carinii*] pneumonia, TB, bacterial pneumonia, fungal infection)
     b. CNS infections (toxoplasmosis, TB)
     c. GI (cryptosporidiosis, isosporiasis, CMV); Sections II and III describe organisms associated with diarrhea in patients with AIDS
     d. Eye infections (CMV, toxoplasmosis)
     e. Kaposi sarcoma (cutaneous or visceral) or lymphoma (nodal or extranodal)
- Possibly asymptomatic
- Diagnosis of AIDS if the CD4 cell count is <200 or <14% of total lymphocyte in the presence of proven HIV infection, even in the absence of other infections
- The various manifestations of HIV infection are described in Section II

ETIOLOGY

- Caused by infection with HIV-1 or HIV-2 (less common).
- HIV is transmitted by sexual contact, needle-sharing (during injection drug use), transfusion of contaminated blood or blood products, and from infected mother to fetus or neonate.

DIAGNOSIS

DIFFERENTIAL DIAGNOSIS

- Other wasting illnesses mimicking the nonspecific features of AIDS:
  1. TB
  2. Neoplasms
  3. Disseminated fungal infection
  4. Malabsorption syndromes
  5. Depression
- Other disorders associated with dementia or demyelination producing encephalopathy, myelopathy, or neuropathy

WORKUP

Prompt evaluation of respiratory, CNS, and GI complaints. Fig. 1 illustrates a syndromic approach to suspected opportunistic infection in HIV.

LABORATORY TESTS

- HIV antibody testing. See "Human Immunodeficiency Virus" topic for the updated surveillance case definition for HIV infection
- CD4 cell count: Performed to determine the degree of immunodeficiency
- Viral load assay: To plan long-term antiviral therapy and to follow progression and success of treatment (i.e., HIV RNA PCR)
- CSF examination: For meningitis or neurologic disease (if indicated)
- Serologic tests for syphilis, hepatitis A, hepatitis B, hepatitis C, and toxoplasmosis
- Testing for other sexually transmitted infections (STIs) such as syphilis, gonorrhea, and chlamydia
- Genotypic resistance testing: Used to assess for primary resistance in naïve patients and secondary resistance in patients failing a regimen
- Eye exam: To evaluate for CMV retinitis in patients with CD4 counts <50 cells/mm^3
- Cryptococcal antigen: Part of the evaluation in AIDS patients with CD4 counts <100 cells/mm^3 who have fever, diffuse pneumonia, or evidence of meningitis
- Evaluation for infection with mycobacterium (TB or MAI) including a tuberculin skin test (TST) or interferon-gamma release assay (IGRA), sputum cultures, chest radiograph, and blood cultures for acid-fast bacteria, depending on clinical presentation

IMAGING STUDIES

- MRI or CT of head for encephalopathy or focal CNS complications (e.g., toxoplasmosis [Fig. E2], lymphoma)
- Chest radiography or CT to aid in the diagnosis of *Pneumocystis jiroveci* pneumonia (PJP), TB, or bacterial pneumonia

TREATMENT

The most important aspect in management of AIDS due to HIV infection is the timely initiation of antiretroviral therapy.

NONPHARMACOLOGIC THERAPY

- Maintain adequate caloric intake.
- Encourage good oral hygiene and regular dental care.
- Avoid high-risk behaviors that increase the risk of other potential pathogens—use condoms, avoid sharing needles, etc.
- Update vaccines—particularly Tdap (tetanus, diphtheria, and pertussis), pneumococcal, meningococcal, and hepatitis A/B vaccines along with annual influenza vaccines.

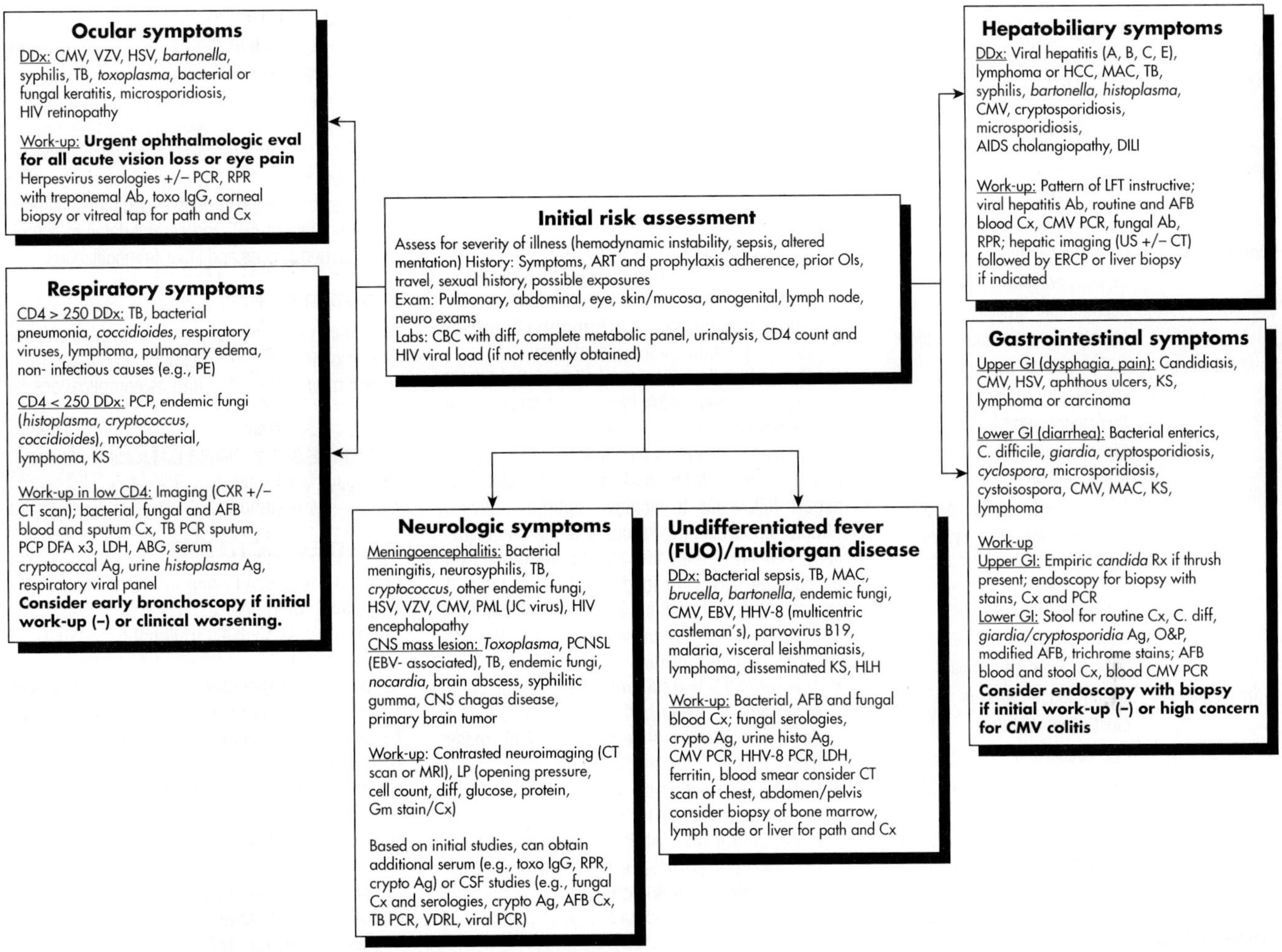

FIG. 1 Syndromic approach to suspected opportunistic infection in HIV. *AFB*, acid-fast bacilli; *ABG*, arterial blood gas; *ART*, antiretroviral therapy; *CBC*, complete blood count; *CMV*, cytomegalovirus; *DFA*, direct fluorescent antibody; *DILI*, drug-induced liver injury; *EBV*, Epstein–Barr virus; *ERCP*, endoscopic retrograde cholangiopancreatography; *FUO*, fever of unknown origin; *HCC*, hepatocellular carcinoma; *HHV-8*, human herpes virus 8; *HLH*, hemophagocytic lymphohistiocytosis; *HSV*, herpes simplex virus; *KS*, Kaposi sarcoma; *LDH*, lactate dehydrogenase; *LP*, lumbar puncture; *MAC*, *Mycobacterium avium* complex; *O&P*, ova and parasite; *PCNSL*, primary CNS lymphoma; *PCP*, *Pneumocystis* pneumonia; *PCR*, polymerase chain reaction; *PE*, pulmonary embolism; *PML*, progressive multifocal leukoencephalopathy; *RPR*, rapid plasma reagin; *TB*, tuberculosis; *US*, ultrasound; *VDRL*, Venereal Disease Research Laboratory test; *VZV*, varicella-zoster virus. (From Spec A, et al: *Comprehensive review of infectious diseases*, 2020, Elsevier.)

- Avoid administration of any live attenuated vaccines that may be a risk to these immunocompromised patients (e.g., MMR, varicella). (See "Section V" for immunization schedules for HIV-infected children.)
- When feasible, avoid activities that might increase risk of exposure to opportunistic infections (e.g., cleaning out a cat litter box [toxoplasmosis], getting scratched by a cat [*Bartonella* infections], exposure to pet reptiles [salmonellosis], traveling to developing countries [cryptosporidiosis, tuberculosis], eating undercooked foods and drinking from unsafe water supplies, etc.). A description of enteropathogens causing infections in HIV-infected patients is provided in Table 1.

ACUTE GENERAL Rx

Acute management of opportunistic infections is summarized in Table 2 and reviewed elsewhere in this text under specific AIDS-related disorders. For management of AIDS-related malignancies, please refer to the specific malignancy elsewhere in this text.

CHRONIC Rx

For all HIV-infected patients, particularly those meeting the case definition of AIDS:
- Preventive therapy for *Pneumocystis jiroveci* pneumonia and *Mycobacterium avium* (see specific chapters elsewhere in this text). With appropriate antiretroviral therapy, many patients experience substantial restoration of cellular immune function. Preventive therapy for *Pneumocystis jiroveci* can be safely stopped if the CD4 cell count rises above 200 for at least 3 mo.
- Based on the Department of Health and Human Services (DHHS) Guidelines, active antiretroviral therapy (ART) should be started regardless of CD4 cell count. Individuals with CD4 cell counts <350 and especially CD4 cell counts <200 should be strongly encouraged to start ART in a timely fashion.
- ART usually includes three-drug combinations of:
  1. Nucleoside reverse transcriptase inhibitors (NRTI): Tenofovir disoproxil fumarate (TDF), tenofovir alafenamide fumarate (TAF), lamivudine (3TC), emtricitabine (FTC), and abacavir (ABC). Older drugs such as zidovudine (AZT), didanosine (ddI), and stavudine (d4T) are generally not recommended.
  2. Protease inhibitors (PI): Darunavir (preferred) or atazanavir.
  3. Nonnucleoside reverse transcriptase inhibitors (NNRTI): Nevirapine, efavirenz (EFV), etravirine, doravirine, and rilpivirine
  4. Integrase inhibitors: Raltegravir, elvitegravir, bictegravir, and dolutegravir
  5. Others: Maraviroc, enfuvirtide, and ibalizumab

The medications ritonavir or cobicistat are usually used in combination with other protease inhibitors or integrase inhibitors to obtain more sustained drug levels. Usual

TABLE 1 Organisms That Cause Gastrointestinal Tract Infections in Patients With HIV/AIDS

	ORGANISMS
Esophagus	*Candida albicans*[a]
	Cytomegalovirus[a]
	Herpes simplex virus[a]
Hepatobiliary	Cytomegalovirus
	Cryptosporidium[a]
	Hepatotropic viruses
	Mycobacterium avium complex[a]
Small intestine	*Campylobacter* species
	Cytomegalovirus[a]
	Cryptosporidium[a]
	Giardia lamblia[a]
	Isospora belli[a]
	Mycobacterium avium complex[a]
	Microsporidia[a] (*Enterocytozoon bieneusi* and *Encephalitozoon intestinalis*)
	Salmonella species[a]
	Enteroaggregative *E. coli*
	Strongyloides stercoralis
Large intestine	*Campylobacter* species
	Clostridium difficile
	Cytomegalovirus[a]
	Entamoeba histolytica
	Herpes simplex virus[a]
	Salmonella species[a]
	Enteroaggregative *E. coli*
	Shigella species

[a] Diseases of the gastrointestinal tract that fulfill the Centers for Disease Control and Prevention surveillance case definition of AIDS.

From Cherry JD et al: *Feigin and Cherry's pediatric infectious diseases,* ed 8, Philadelphia, 2019, Elsevier.

initial dosing regimens include two NRTIs and an NNRTI or PI or integrase inhibitor. Currently, integrase inhibitors are recommended as first-line drugs because of tolerability. Examples of initial regimens recommended by the guidelines:

1. Bictegravir/tenofovir alafenamide/emtricitabine
2. Dolutegravir/abacavir/lamivudine (in patients who are HLA-B*5701 NEGATIVE)
3. Dolutegravir plus tenofovir/emtricitabine*
4. Raltegravir plus tenofovir/emtricitabine*
5. Elvitegravir/cobicistat/tenofovir/emtricitabine (certain clinical situations)
6. Darunavir/ritonavir or darunavir/cobicistat plus tenofovir/emtricitabine (certain clinical situations)

All these drugs have unique and class-specific side effects and require careful and expert follow-up to achieve optimal antiviral effects, ensure compliance, and maintain efficacy. Antiviral response should be monitored by baseline HIV viral load and CD4 count and repeat measurement at 2 wk and 4 wk into treatment and then periodically (3-6 mo) to ensure viral suppression.

- The approach to a patient with CNS signs and symptoms is described in Fig. 3, and Fig. 4 describes the management of CNS mass lesions.
- Genotypic resistance testing is strongly encouraged for all patients initiating treatment and for any patient failing antiretroviral therapy. Poor adherence to therapy, however, often underlies virologic failure.

*Tenofovir-based formulations can include tenofovir disoproxil fumarate (TDF) or tenofovir alafenamide (TAF).

DISPOSITION

The outlook for HIV has changed radically since the advent of ART from an essentially fatal disease to a chronic medical illness compatible with long-term survival and remarkably good quality of life. Patients should be aggressively treated for severe illnesses as outcomes following ICU admissions remain good. This is accomplished through expert and continuous follow-up, use of ART, and careful detail to compliance to medications and lifestyle modification.

REFERRAL

All patients with HIV should be referred to a physician knowledgeable and experienced in the management of the disease and its complications.

SUGGESTED READINGS

Available at ExpertConsult.com

RELATED CONTENT

Acquired Immunodeficiency Syndrome (AIDS) (Patient Information)
Candidiasis, Cutaneous (Related Key Topic)
Candidiasis, Invasive (Related Key Topic)
Cryptosporidium Infection (Related Key Topic)
Cytomegalovirus Infection (Related Key Topic)
Herpes Simplex (Related Key Topic)
Histoplasmosis (Related Key Topic)
HIV-Associated Cognitive Dysfunction (Related Key Topic)
Human Immunodeficiency Virus (Related Key Topic)
Kaposi Sarcoma (Related Key Topic)
Pneumonia, *pneumocystis jiroveci (carinii)* (Related Key Topic)
Progressive Multifocal Leukoencephalopathy (Related Key Topic)
Toxoplasmosis (Related Key Topic)
Tuberculosis, Pulmonary (Related Key Topic)

AUTHOR: **Philip A. Chan, MD, MS**

TABLE 2 Treatment of AIDS-Associated Opportunistic Infections

Opportunistic Infection	Preferred Therapy	Alternative Therapy	Other Comments
PJP	• Patients who develop PJP despite TMP-SMX prophylaxis can usually be treated with standard doses of TMP-SMX. • Duration of PJP treatment: 21 days. • *For Moderate to Severe PJP:* • TMP-SMX: (TMP 15-20 mg and SMX 75-100 mg/kg/day) IV given q6h or q8h, may switch to PO after clinical improvement. • *For Mild to Moderate PJP:* • TMP-SMX: (TMP 15-20 mg and SMX 75-100 mg/kg/day), given PO in 3 divided doses, *or* • TMP-SMX: (160 mg/800 mg or DS) 2 tablets PO tid. • *Secondary Prophylaxis, after completion of PJP treatment:* • TMP-SMX DS: 1 tablet PO daily *or* • TMP-SMX (80 mg/400 mg or SS): 1 tablet PO daily.	*For Moderate to Severe PJP:* • Pentamidine 4 mg/kg IV daily infused over ≥60 minutes; can reduce dose to 3 mg/kg IV daily because of toxicities, *or* • Primaquine 30 mg (base) PO daily + (clindamycin 600 mg q6h IV or 900 mg IV q8h) or (clindamycin 300 mg PO q6h or 450 mg PO q8h). • *For Mild to Moderate PJP:* • Dapsone 100 mg PO daily + TMP 5 mg/kg PO tid, *or* • Primaquine 30 mg (base) PO daily + (clindamycin 300 mg PO q6h or 450 mg PO q8h), *or* • Atovaquone 750 mg PO bid with food. • *Secondary Prophylaxis, after completion of PJP treatment:* • TMP-SMX DS: 1 tablet PO tiw, *or* • Dapsone 100 mg PO daily, *or* • Dapsone 50 mg PO daily + (pyrimethamine 50 mg + leucovorin 25 mg) PO weekly, *or* • (Dapsone 200 mg + pyrimethamine 75 mg + leucovorin 25 mg) PO weekly, *or* • Aerosolized pentamidine 300 mg monthly via Respirgard II nebulizer, *or* • Atovaquone 1500 mg PO daily, *or* • (Atovaquone 1500 mg + pyrimethamine 25 mg + leucovorin 10 mg) PO daily.	*Indications for Adjunctive Corticosteroids:* • Pa_{O_2} <70 mm Hg at room air, *or* • Alveolar-arterial O_2 gradient >35 mm Hg. • *Prednisone Doses (beginning as early as possible and within 72 hours of PJP therapy):* • Days 1-5: 40 mg PO bid. • Days 6-10: 40 mg PO daily. • Days 11-21: 20 mg PO daily. • IV methylprednisolone can be administered as 75% of prednisone dose. • Benefit of corticosteroid if started after 72 hours of treatment is unknown, but some clinicians will use it for moderate-to-severe PJP. • Whenever possible, patients should be tested for G6PD before use of dapsone or primaquine. Alternative therapy should be used in patients found to have G6PD deficiency. • Patients who are receiving pyrimethamine/sulfadiazine for treatment or suppression of toxoplasmosis do not require additional PJP prophylaxis. • If TMP-SMX is discontinued because of a mild adverse reaction, reinstitution should be considered after the reaction resolves. The dose can be increased gradually (desensitization) or be reduced, or the frequency can be modified. • TMP-SMX should be permanently discontinued in patients with possible or definite Stevens–Johnson syndrome or toxic epidermal necrosis.
Toxoplasma gondii encephalitis	*Treatment of Acute Infection:* • Pyrimethamine 200 mg PO 1 time, followed by weight-based therapy: • If <60 kg, pyrimethamine 50 mg PO once daily + sulfadiazine 1000 mg PO q6h + leucovorin 10-25 mg PO once daily. • If ≥60 kg, pyrimethamine 75 mg PO once daily + sulfadiazine 1500 mg PO q6h + leucovorin 10-25 mg PO once daily. • Leucovorin dose can be increased to 50 mg daily or bid. • *Duration for Acute Therapy:* • At least 6 wk; longer duration if clinical or radiologic disease is extensive or response is incomplete at 6 wk. • *Chronic Maintenance Therapy:* • Pyrimethamine 25-50 mg PO daily + sulfadiazine 2000-4000 mg PO daily (in 2-4 divided doses) + leucovorin 10-25 mg PO daily (AI). • *After collecting specimen for culture and molecular diagnostic tests, empiric TB treatment should be started in individuals with clinical and radiographic presentation suggestive of TB.* • *Initial Phase (2 mo, given daily):* • *INH + [RIF or RFB] + PZA + EMB.*	*Treatment of Acute Infection:* • Pyrimethamine (leucovorin)* + clindamycin 600 mg IV or PO q6h *or* • TMP-SMX (TMP 5 mg/kg and SMX 25 mg/kg) IV or PO bid, *or* • Atovaquone 1500 mg PO bid with food + pyrimethamine (leucovorin), *or* • Atovaquone 1500 mg PO bid with food + sulfadiazine 1000-1500 mg PO q6h (weight-based dosing, as in preferred therapy) *or* • Atovaquone 1500 mg PO bid with food, *or* • Pyrimethamine (leucovorin)* + azithromycin 900-1200 mg PO daily. • *Chronic Maintenance Therapy:* • Clindamycin 600 mg PO q8h + (pyrimethamine 25-50 mg + leucovorin 10-25 mg) PO daily *or* • TMP-SMX DS 1 tablet bid, *or* • Atovaquone 750-1500 mg PO bid + (pyrimethamine 25 mg + leucovorin 10 mg) PO daily, *or* • Atovaquone 750-1500 mg PO bid + sulfadiazine 2000-4000 mg PO daily (in 2-4 divided doses), *or* • Atovaquone 750-1500 mg PO bid with food.	• Adjunctive corticosteroids (e.g., dexamethasone) should only be administered when clinically indicated to treat mass effect associated with focal lesions or associated edema; discontinue as soon as clinically feasible. • Anticonvulsants should be administered to patients with a history of seizures and continued through acute treatment but should not be used as seizure prophylaxis. • If clindamycin is used in place of sulfadiazine, additional therapy must be added to prevent PCP.

Continued

TABLE 2 Treatment of AIDS-Associated Opportunistic Infections—cont'd

Opportunistic Infection	Preferred Therapy	Alternative Therapy	Other Comments
Mycobacterium tuberculosis disease (TB)	• *Continuation Phase:* • INH + (RIF or RFB) daily. • *Total Duration of Therapy (for drug-susceptible TB):* • Pulmonary TB: 6 mo. • Pulmonary TB and culture-positive after 2 mo of TB treatment: 9 mo. • Extrapulmonary TB with CNS infection: 9-12 mo. • Extrapulmonary TB with bone or joint involvement: 6-9 mo. • Extrapulmonary TB in other sites: 6 mo. • Total duration of therapy should be based on number of doses received, not on calendar time.	*Treatment for Drug-Resistant TB* • *Resistant to INH:* • (RIF or RFB) + EMB + PZA + (moxifloxacin or levofloxacin) for 2 mo; followed by (RIF or RFB) + EMB + (moxifloxacin or levofloxacin) for 7 mo. *Treatment for Drug-Resistant TB* • *Resistant to INH:* • (RIF or RFB) + EMB + PZA + (moxifloxacin or levofloxacin) for 2 mo; followed by (RIF or RFB) + EMB + (moxifloxacin or levofloxacin) for 7 mo. • *Resistant to Rifamycins ± Other Drugs:* • Regimen and duration of treatment should be individualized based on resistance pattern, clinical and microbiologic responses, and in close consultation with experienced specialists.	• Adjunctive corticosteroid improves survival for TB meningitis and pericarditis. See text for drug, dose, and duration recommendations. • RIF *is not recommended* for patients receiving HIV PI because of its induction of PI metabolism. • RFB is a less potent CYP3A4 inducer than RIF and is preferred in patients receiving PIs. • Once-weekly rifapentine can result in development of rifamycin resistance in HIV-infected patients and *is not recommended.* • Therapeutic drug monitoring should be considered in patients receiving rifamycin and interacting ART. • Paradoxical IRIS that is not severe can be treated with NSAIDs without a change in TB or HIV therapy. • For severe IRIS reaction, consider prednisone and taper over 4 wk based on clinical symptoms. For example: • *If receiving RIF:* Prednisone 1.5 mg/kg/day for 2 wk, then 0.75 mg/kg/day for 2 wk. • *If receiving RFB:* Prednisone 1.0 mg/kg/day for 2 wk, then 0.5 mg/kg/day for 2 wk. • A more gradual tapering schedule over a few mo may be necessary for some patients.
Disseminated MAC disease	*At Least 2 Drugs as Initial Therapy with:* • Clarithromycin 500 mg PO bid + ethambutol 15 mg/kg PO daily, *or* • Azithromycin 500-600 mg + ethambutol 15 mg/kg PO daily if drug interaction or intolerance precludes the use of clarithromycin. • *Duration:* • At least 12 mo of therapy, can discontinue if no signs and symptoms of MAC disease and sustained (>6 mo) CD4 count >100 cells/μl in response to ART.	• Addition of a third or fourth drug should be considered for patients with advanced immunosuppression (CD4 counts <50 cells/μl), high mycobacterial loads (>2 log CFU/ml of blood), or in the absence of effective ART. *Third or Fourth Drug Options May Include:* • RFB 300 mg PO daily (dosage adjustment may be necessary based on drug interactions), *or* • Amikacin 10-15 mg/kg IV daily, *or* • Streptomycin 1 g IV or IM daily, *or* • Moxifloxacin 400 mg PO daily or levofloxacin 500 mg PO daily.	• Testing of susceptibility to clarithromycin and azithromycin is recommended. • NSAIDs can be used for patients who experience moderate to severe symptoms attributed to IRIS. • If IRIS symptoms persist, short-term (4-8 wk) systemic corticosteroids (equivalent to 20-40 mg prednisone) can be used.
Bacterial respiratory diseases *(with focus on pneumonia)*	Empiric antibiotic therapy should be initiated promptly for patients presenting with clinical and radiographic evidence consistent with bacterial pneumonia. The recommendations listed are suggested empiric therapy. The regimen should be modified as needed once microbiologic results are available. *Empiric Outpatient Therapy:* • A PO β-lactam + a PO macrolide (azithromycin or clarithromycin). • *Preferred β-lactams*: High-dose amoxicillin or amoxicillin/clavulanate. • *Alternative β-lactams*: Cefpodoxime or cefuroxime, *or* • *For penicillin-allergic patients:* Levofloxacin 750 mg PO once daily, or moxifloxacin 400 mg PO once daily. • *Duration:* 7-10 days (a minimum of 5 days). Patients should be afebrile for 48-72 hours and clinically stable before stopping antibiotics. • *Empiric Therapy for Non-ICU Hospitalized Patients:*	*Empiric Outpatient Therapy:* • A PO β-lactam + PO doxycycline. • Preferred β-lactams: High-dose amoxicillin or amoxicillin/clavulanate. • Alternative β-lactams: Cefpodoxime or cefuroxime. • *Empiric Therapy for Non-ICU Hospitalized Patients:* • An IV β-lactam + doxycycline. • *Empiric Therapy for ICU Patients:* • *For penicillin-allergic patients:* Aztreonam IV + (levofloxacin 750 mg IV once daily or moxifloxacin 400 mg IV once daily). *Empiric Therapy for Patients at Risk of Pseudomonas Pneumonia:*	• Fluoroquinolones should be used with caution in patients in whom TB is suspected but is not being treated. • Empiric therapy with a macrolide alone is not routinely recommended because of increasing pneumococcal resistance. • Patients receiving a macrolide for MAC prophylaxis should not receive macrolide monotherapy for empiric treatment of bacterial pneumonia. • For patients begun on IV antibiotic therapy, switching to PO should be considered when they are clinically improved and able to tolerate oral medications. • Chemoprophylaxis can be considered for patients with frequent recurrences of serious bacterial pneumonia.

TABLE 2 Treatment of AIDS-Associated Opportunistic Infections—cont'd

Opportunistic Infection	Preferred Therapy	Alternative Therapy	Other Comments
	• An IV β-lactam + a macrolide (azithromycin or clarithromycin). • *Preferred β-lactams:* Ceftriaxone, cefotaxime, *or* ampicillin-sulbactam. • *For penicillin-allergic patients:* • Levofloxacin, 750 mg IV once daily, *or* moxifloxacin, 400 mg IV once daily. • *Empiric Therapy for ICU Patients:* • An IV β-lactam + IV azithromycin, *or* • An IV β-lactam + (levofloxacin 750 mg IV once daily or moxifloxacin 400 mg IV once daily). • *Preferred β-lactams*: Ceftriaxone, cefotaxime, or ampicillin-sulbactam. • *Empiric Therapy for Patients at Risk of* Pseudomonas *Pneumonia:* • An IV antipneumococcal, antipseudomonal β-lactam + ciprofloxacin 400 mg IV q8-12h or levofloxacin 750 mg IV once daily. • *Preferred β-lactams*: Piperacillin-tazobactam, cefepime, imipenem, or meropenem. • *Empiric Therapy for Patients at Risk for Methicillin-Resistant* Staphylococcus aureus *Pneumonia:* • Add vancomycin IV or linezolid (IV or PO) to the baseline regimen. • Addition of clindamycin to vancomycin (but not to linezolid) can be considered for severe necrotizing pneumonia to minimize bacterial toxin production.	• Above β-lactam + an aminoglycoside + (levofloxacin 750 mg IV once daily or moxifloxacin 400 mg IV once daily), *or* • *For penicillin-allergic patients*: Replace the β-lactam with aztreonam. • An IV antipneumococcal, antipseudomonal β-lactam + an aminoglycoside + azithromycin, *or*	• Clinicians should be cautious about using antibiotics to prevent recurrences because of the potential for developing drug resistance and drug toxicities.
Bacterial enteric infections *Empiric therapy pending definitive diagnosis*	• Diagnostic fecal specimens should be obtained before initiation of empiric antibiotic therapy. • Empiric antibiotic therapy is indicated for patients with advanced HIV (CD4 count <200 cells/µl or concomitant AIDS-defining illnesses), with clinically severe diarrhea (>6 stools/day), and/or accompanying fever or chills. • *Empiric Therapy:* • Ciprofloxacin 500-750 mg PO (or 400 mg IV) q12h. • Therapy should be adjusted based on the results of diagnostic workup. • For patients with chronic diarrhea (>14 days) without severe clinical signs, empiric antibiotics therapy is not necessary; can withhold treatment until a diagnosis is made.	*Empiric Therapy:* • Ceftriaxone 1 g IV q24h, *or* • Cefotaxime 1 g IV q8h.	• Hospitalization with IV antibiotics should be considered in patients with marked nausea, vomiting, diarrhea, electrolyte abnormalities, acidosis, and blood pressure instability. • Oral or IV rehydration if indicated. • Antimotility agents should be avoided if there is concern about inflammatory diarrhea, including *Clostridium difficile*–associated diarrhea. • If no clinical response after 5-7 days, consider follow-up stool culture with antibiotic susceptibility testing or alternative diagnostic tests (e.g., toxin assays, molecular testing), alternative diagnosis, or antibiotic resistance.
Salmonellosis	All HIV-infected patients with salmonellosis should be treated because of high risk of bacteremia.		
	• Ciprofloxacin 500-750 mg PO (or 400 mg IV) q12h, if susceptible. • *Duration of Therapy:* • *For gastroenteritis without bacteremia:* • If CD4 count ≥200 cells/µl: 7-14 days. • If CD4 count <200 cells/µl: 2-6 wk. *For gastroenteritis with bacteremia:* • If CD4 count ≥200/µl: 14 days; longer duration if bacteremia persists or if the infection is complicated (e.g., if metastatic foci of infection are present). • If CD4 count <200 cells/µl: 2-6 wk. *Secondary Prophylaxis Should Be Considered for:* • Patients with recurrent *Salmonella* gastroenteritis ± bacteremia, *or* • Patients with CD4 <200 cells/µl with severe diarrhea.	• Levofloxacin 750 mg (PO or IV) q24h, *or* • Moxifloxacin 400 mg (PO or IV) q24h, *or* • TMP, 160 mg-SMX 800 mg (PO or IV) q12h, or • Ceftriaxone 1 g IV q24h, *or* • Cefotaxime 1 g IV q8h.	• Oral or IV rehydration if indicated. • Antimotility agents should be avoided. • The role of long-term secondary prophylaxis in patients with recurrent *Salmonella* bacteremia is not well established. Must weigh benefit against risks of long-term antibiotic exposure. • Effective ART may reduce the frequency, severity, and recurrence of *Salmonella* infections.

Continued

TABLE 2 Treatment of AIDS-Associated Opportunistic Infections—cont'd

Opportunistic Infection	Preferred Therapy	Alternative Therapy	Other Comments
Mucocutaneous candidiasis	*For Oropharyngeal Candidiasis; Initial Episodes (for 7-14 days):* • *Oral Therapy* • Fluconazole 100 mg PO daily, *or* • *Topical Therapy* • Clotrimazole troches, 10 mg PO 5 times daily, *or* • Miconazole mucoadhesive buccal 50-mg tablet—apply to mucosal surface over the canine fossa once daily (do not swallow, chew, or crush). *For Esophageal Candidiasis (for 14-21 days):* • Fluconazole 100 mg (up to 400 mg) PO or IV daily, *or* • Itraconazole oral solution 200 mg PO daily. *For Uncomplicated Vulvovaginal Candidiasis:* • Oral fluconazole 150 mg for 1 dose, *or* • Topical azoles (clotrimazole, butoconazole, miconazole, tioconazole, or terconazole) for 3-7 days. *For Severe or Recurrent Vulvovaginal Candidiasis:* • Fluconazole 100-200 mg PO daily for ≥7 days, *or* • Topical antifungal ≥7 days.	*For Oropharyngeal Candidiasis; Initial Episodes (for 7-14 days):* • *Oral Therapy* • Itraconazole oral solution 200 mg PO daily, *or* • Posaconazole oral solution 400 mg PO bid for 1 day, then 400 mg daily. • *Topical Therapy* • Nystatin suspension 4-6 ml qid or 1-2 flavored pastilles 4-5 times daily. *For Esophageal Candidiasis (for 14-21 days):* • Voriconazole 200 mg PO or IV bid, *or* • Posaconazole 400 mg PO bid, *or* • Anidulafungin 100 mg IV 1 time, then 50 mg IV daily, *or* • Caspofungin 50 mg IV daily, *or* • Micafungin 150 mg IV daily, *or* • Amphotericin B deoxycholate 0.6 mg/kg IV daily, *or* • Lipid formulation of amphotericin B 3-4 mg/kg IV daily. *For Uncomplicated Vulvovaginal Candidiasis:* • Itraconazole oral solution 200 mg PO daily for 3-7 days.	• Chronic or prolonged use of azoles may promote development of resistance. • Higher relapse rate for esophageal candidiasis is seen with echinocandins than with fluconazole use. • Suppressive therapy is usually not recommended unless patients have frequent or severe recurrences. *If Decision Is to Use Suppressive Therapy:* *Oropharyngeal Candidiasis:* • Fluconazole 100 mg PO daily or tiw. • Itraconazole oral solution 200 mg PO daily. *Esophageal Candidiasis:* • Fluconazole 100-200 mg PO daily. • Posaconazole 400 mg PO bid. *Vulvovaginal Candidiasis:* • Fluconazole 150 mg PO once weekly.
Cryptococcosis	*Cryptococcal Meningitis* • *Induction Therapy (for at least 2 wk, followed by consolidation therapy):* • Liposomal amphotericin B 3-4 mg/kg IV daily + flucytosine 25 mg/kg PO qid. (NOTE: Flucytosine dose should be adjusted in patients with renal dysfunction.) • *Consolidation Therapy (for at least 8 wk followed by maintenance therapy):* • Fluconazole 400 mg PO (or IV) daily. • *Maintenance Therapy:* • Fluconazole 200 mg PO daily for at least 12 mo. *For Non-CNS, Extrapulmonary Cryptococcosis and Diffuse Pulmonary Disease:* • Treatment same as for cryptococcal meningitis. *Non-CNS Cryptococcosis With Mild to Moderate Symptoms and Focal Pulmonary Infiltrates:* • Fluconazole, 400 mg PO daily for 12 mo.	*Cryptococcal Meningitis* • *Induction Therapy (for at least 2 wk, followed by consolidation therapy):* • Amphotericin B deoxycholate 0.7 mg/kg IV daily + flucytosine 25 mg/kg PO qid, *or* • Amphotericin B lipid complex 5 mg/kg IV daily + flucytosine 25 mg/kg PO qid, *or* • Liposomal amphotericin B 3-4 mg/kg IV daily + fluconazole 800 mg PO or IV daily, *or* • Amphotericin B deoxycholate 0.7 mg/kg IV daily + fluconazole 800 mg PO or IV daily, *or* • Fluconazole 400-800 mg PO or IV daily + flucytosine 25 mg/kg PO qid, *or* • Fluconazole 1200 mg PO or IV daily. • *Consolidation Therapy (for at least 8 wk followed by maintenance therapy):* • Itraconazole 200 mg PO bid for 8 wk—less effective than fluconazole. • *Maintenance Therapy:* • No alternative therapy recommendation.	• Addition of flucytosine to amphotericin B has been associated with more rapid sterilization of CSF and decreased risk for subsequent relapse. • Patients receiving flucytosine should have either blood levels monitored (peak level 2 hours after dose should be 30-80 μg/ml) or close monitoring of blood counts for development of cytopenia. Dosage should be adjusted in patients with renal insufficiency. • Opening pressure should always be measured when an LP is performed. Repeated LPs or CSF shunting are essential to effectively manage increased intracranial pressure. • Corticosteroids and mannitol are ineffective in reducing intracranial pressure and are *not* recommended. • Some specialists recommend a brief course of corticosteroid for management of severe IRIS symptoms.

TABLE 2 Treatment of AIDS-Associated Opportunistic Infections—cont'd

Opportunistic Infection	Preferred Therapy	Alternative Therapy	Other Comments
Histoplasmosis	*Moderately Severe to Severe Disseminated Disease Induction Therapy (for at least 2 wk or until clinically improved):* • Liposomal amphotericin B 3 mg/kg IV daily. • *Maintenance Therapy:* • Itraconazole 200 mg PO tid for 3 days, then 200 mg PO bid. *Less Severe Disseminated Disease* • Induction and Maintenance Therapy: • Itraconazole 200 mg PO tid for 3 days, then 200 mg PO bid. • *Duration of Therapy:* • At least 12 mo. *Meningitis* • *Induction Therapy (4-6 wk):* • Liposomal amphotericin B 5 mg/kg/day. • *Maintenance Therapy:* • Itraconazole 200 mg PO bid to tid for ≥1 yr and until resolution of abnormal CSF findings. • *Long-Term Suppression Therapy:* • *For patients with severe disseminated or CNS infection after completion of at least 12 mo of therapy; and those who relapse despite appropriate therapy* • Itraconazole 200 mg PO daily.	*Moderately Severe to Severe Disseminated Disease Induction Therapy (for at least 2 wk or until clinically improved):* • Amphotericin B lipid complex 3 mg/kg IV daily, *or* • Amphotericin B cholesteryl sulfate complete 3 mg/kg IV daily. • *Alternatives to Itraconazole for Maintenance Therapy or Treatment of Less Severe Disease:* • Voriconazole 400 mg PO bid for 1 day, then 200 mg bid, *or* • Posaconazole 400 mg PO bid. • Fluconazole 800 mg PO daily. *Meningitis* • No alternative therapy recommendation. • *Long-Term Suppression Therapy:* • Fluconazole 400 mg PO daily.	• Itraconazole, posaconazole, and voriconazole may have significant interactions with certain ARV agents. These interactions are complex and can be bidirectional. • Therapeutic drug monitoring and dosage adjustment may be necessary to ensure triazole antifungal and ARV efficacy and to reduce concentration-related toxicities. • Random serum concentration of itraconazole + hydroxyitraconazole should be >1 μg/ml. • Clinical experience with voriconazole or posaconazole in the treatment of histoplasmosis is limited. • Acute pulmonary histoplasmosis in HIV-infected patients with CD4 counts >300 cells/μl should be managed as nonimmunocompromised host.
Coccidioidomycosis	*Clinically Mild Infections (e.g., focal pneumonia):* • Fluconazole 400 mg PO daily *or* • Itraconazole 200 mg PO bid. *Severe, Nonmeningeal Infection (diffuse pulmonary infection or severely ill patients with extrathoracic, disseminated disease):* • Amphotericin B deoxycholate 0.7-1.0 mg/kg IV daily. • Lipid formulation amphotericin B 4-6 mg/kg IV daily. • Duration of therapy: Continue until clinical improvement, then switch to an azole. *Meningeal Infections:* • Fluconazole 400-800 mg IV or PO daily. • *Chronic Suppressive Therapy:* • Fluconazole 400 mg PO daily, *or* • Itraconazole 200 mg PO bid.	*Mild Infections (focal pneumonia) for patients who failed to respond to fluconazole or itraconazole:* • Posaconazole 200 mg PO bid, *or* • Voriconazole 200 mg PO bid. *Severe, Nonmeningeal Infection (diffuse pulmonary infection or severely ill patients with extrathoracic, disseminated disease):* • Some specialists will add a triazole (fluconazole or itraconazole, with itraconazole preferred for bone disease) 400 mg per day to amphotericin B therapy and continue triazole once amphotericin B is stopped. *Meningeal Infections:* • Itraconazole 200 mg PO tid for 3 days, then 200 mg PO bid, *or* • Posaconazole 200 mg PO bid, *or* • Voriconazole 200-400 mg PO bid, *or* • Intrathecal amphotericin B deoxycholate, when triazole antifungals are ineffective. • *Chronic Suppressive Therapy:* • Posaconazole 200 mg PO bid, *or* • Voriconazole 200 mg PO bid.	• Some patients with meningitis may develop hydrocephalus and require CSF shunting. • Therapy should be continued indefinitely in patients with diffuse pulmonary or disseminated diseases because relapse can occur in 25%-33% of HIV-negative patients. It can also occur in HIV-infected patients with CD4 counts >250 cells/μL. • Therapy should be lifelong in patients with meningeal infections because relapse occurs in 80% of HIV-infected patients after discontinuation of triazole therapy. • Itraconazole, posaconazole, and voriconazole may have significant interactions with certain ARV agents. These interactions are complex and can be bidirectional. Therapeutic drug monitoring and dosage adjustment may be necessary to ensure triazole antifungal and antiretroviral efficacy and to reduce concentration-related toxicities. • Intrathecal amphotericin B should be given only in consultation with a specialist and should be administered by an individual with experience with the technique.
Aspergillosis, invasive	*Preferred Therapy:* • Voriconazole 6 mg/kg IV q12h for 1 day, then 4 mg/kg IV q12h, followed by voriconazole 200 mg PO q12h after clinical improvement. • *Duration of Therapy:* • Until CD4 cell count >200 cells/μl and the infection appears to be resolved.	*Alternative Therapy:* • Lipid formulation of amphotericin B 5 mg/kg IV daily, *or* • Amphotericin B deoxycholate 1 mg/kg IV daily, *or* • Caspofungin 70 mg IV 1 time, then 50 mg IV daily, *or* • Micafungin 100-150 mg IV daily, *or* • Anidulafungin 200 mg IV 1 time, then 100 mg IV daily, *or* • Posaconazole 200 mg PO qid, then, after condition improved, 400 mg PO bid.	• Potential for significant pharmacokinetic interactions between certain ARV agents and voriconazole; they should be used cautiously in these situations. Consider therapeutic drug monitoring and dosage adjustment if necessary.

Continued

TABLE 2 Treatment of AIDS-Associated Opportunistic Infections—cont'd

Opportunistic Infection	Preferred Therapy	Alternative Therapy	Other Comments
CMV disease	*CMV Retinitis Induction Therapy for Immediate Sight-Threatening Lesions (adjacent to the optic nerve or fovea)* • Consult ophthalmologist; ganciclovir implant no longer available: • Ganciclovir 5 mg/kg IV q12h for 14-21 days followed by Valganciclovir 900 mg PO bid. *For Small Peripheral Lesions:* • Valganciclovir 900 mg PO bid for 14-21 days. • One dose of intravitreal ganciclovir can be administered immediately after diagnosis until steady-state plasma ganciclovir concentration is achieved with oral valganciclovir. • *Chronic Maintenance (secondary prophylaxis):* • Valganciclovir 900 mg PO daily (for small peripheral lesion). *CMV Esophagitis or Colitis:* • Ganciclovir 5 mg/kg IV q12h; may switch to valganciclovir 900 mg PO q12h once patient can tolerate oral therapy.	*CMV Retinitis Induction Therapy:* • Ganciclovir 5 mg/kg IV q12h for 14-21 days, *or* • Foscarnet 90 mg/kg IV q12h or 60 mg q8h for 14-21 days, *or* • Cidofovir 5 mg/kg/wk IV for 2 wk; saline hydration before and after therapy and probenecid, 2 g PO 3 hours before dose, followed by 1 g PO 2 hours and 8 hours after the dose (total of 4 g). (Note: This regimen should be avoided in patients with sulfa allergy because of cross-hypersensitivity with probenecid.) • *Chronic Maintenance (secondary prophylaxis):* • Ganciclovir 5 mg/kg IV 5-7 times weekly, *or*	• The choice of therapy for CMV retinitis should be individualized, based on location and severity of the lesions, level of immunosuppression, and other factors (e.g., concomitant medications and ability to adhere to treatment). • The choice of chronic maintenance therapy (route of administration and drug choices) should be made in consultation with an ophthalmologist. Considerations should include the anatomic location of the retinal lesion, vision in the contralateral eye, the patients' immunologic and virologic status, and response to ART.
	• Duration: 21-42 days or until symptoms have resolved. • Maintenance therapy is usually not necessary but should be considered after relapses. *Well-Documented, Histologically Confirmed CMV Pneumonia:* • Experience for treating CMV pneumonitis in HIV patients is limited. Use of IV ganciclovir or IV foscarnet is reasonable (doses same as for CMV retinitis). • The optimal duration of therapy and the role of oral valganciclovir have not been established. • *CMV Neurologic Disease* • Note: Treatment should be initiated promptly. • Ganciclovir 5 mg/kg IV q12h + (foscarnet 90 mg/kg IV q12h or 60 mg/kg IV q8h) to stabilize disease and maximize response; continue until symptomatic improvement and resolution of neurologic symptoms. • The optimal duration of therapy and the role of oral valganciclovir have not been established.	• Foscarnet 90-120 mg/kg IV once daily, *or* • Cidofovir 5 mg/kg IV every other wk with saline hydration and probenecid as above. *CMV Esophagitis or Colitis:* • Foscarnet 90 mg/kg IV q12h or 60 mg/kg q8h for patients with treatment-limiting toxicities to ganciclovir or with ganciclovir resistance, *or* • Valganciclovir 900 mg PO q12h in milder disease and if able to tolerate PO therapy, *or* • For mild cases, if ART can be initiated without delay, consider withholding CMV therapy. • Duration: 21-42 days or until symptoms have resolved.	• Patients with CMV retinitis who discontinue maintenance therapy should undergo regular eye examinations for early detection of relapse IRU—optimally every 3 mo and then annually after immune reconstitution. • IRU may develop in the setting of immune reconstitution. • *Treatment of IRU:* • Periocular corticosteroid or short courses of systemic steroid. • Initial therapy in patients with CMV retinitis, esophagitis, colitis, and pneumonitis should include initiation or optimization of ART.
HSV disease	*Orolabial Lesions (for 5-10 days):* • Valacyclovir 1 g PO bid *or* • Famciclovir 500 mg PO bid *or* • Acyclovir 400 mg PO tid. *Initial or Recurrent Genital HSV (for 5-14 days):* • Valacyclovir 1 g PO bid, *or* • Famciclovir 500 mg PO bid, *or* • Acyclovir 400 mg PO tid. *Severe Mucocutaneous HSV:* • Initial therapy acyclovir 5 mg/kg IV q8h • After lesions begin to regress, change to PO therapy as previously. Continue until lesions are completely healed. • *Chronic Suppressive Therapy for Patients With Severe Recurrences of Genital Herpes or for Patients Who Want to Minimize Frequency of Recurrences:* • Valacyclovir 500 mg PO bid. • Famciclovir 500 mg PO bid. • Acyclovir 400 mg PO bid. • Continue indefinitely regardless of CD4 cell count.	*For Acyclovir-Resistant HSV* • *Preferred Therapy:* • Foscarnet 80-120 mg/kg/day IV in 2-3 divided doses until clinical response. • *Alternative Therapy* • IV cidofovir (dosage as in CMV retinitis), *or* • Topical trifluridine, *or* • Topical cidofovir, *or* • Topical imiquimod. • *Duration of Therapy:* • 21-28 days or longer.	• Patients with HSV infections can be treated with episodic therapy when symptomatic lesions occur, or with daily suppressive therapy to prevent recurrences. • Topical formulations of trifluridine and cidofovir are not commercially available. • Extemporaneous compounding of topical products can be prepared using trifluridine ophthalmic solution and the IV formulation of cidofovir.

TABLE 2 Treatment of AIDS-Associated Opportunistic Infections—cont'd

Opportunistic Infection	Preferred Therapy	Alternative Therapy	Other Comments
VZV disease	*Primary Varicella Infection (Chickenpox):* • *Uncomplicated Cases (for 5-7 days):* • Valacyclovir 1 g PO tid *or* • Famciclovir 500 mg PO tid. • *Severe or Complicated Cases:* • Acyclovir 10-15 mg/kg IV q8h for 7-10 days. • May switch to oral valacyclovir, famciclovir, or acyclovir after defervescence if no evidence of visceral involvement. *Herpes Zoster (Shingles) Acute Localized Dermatomal:* • For 7-10 days; consider longer duration if lesions are slow to resolve. • Valacyclovir 1 g PO tid *or* • Famciclovir 500 mg tid. *Extensive Cutaneous Lesion or Visceral Involvement:* • Acyclovir 10-15 mg/kg IV q8h until clinical improvement is evident. • May switch to PO therapy (valacyclovir, famciclovir, or acyclovir) after clinical improvement (i.e., when no new vesicle formation or improvement of signs and symptoms of visceral VZV), to complete a 10- to 14-day course. *Progressive Outer Retinal Necrosis:* • Ganciclovir 5 mg/kg + foscarnet 90 mg/kg IV q12h + ganciclovir 2 mg/0.05 ml ± foscarnet 1.2 mg/0.05 ml intravitreal injection twice weekly *or* • Initiate or optimize ART. *Acute Retinal Necrosis:* • Acyclovir 10 mg/kg IV q8h for 10-14 days, followed by valacyclovir 1 g PO tid for 6 wk.	*Primary Varicella Infection (Chickenpox):* • *Uncomplicated Cases (for 5-7 days):* • Acyclovir 800 mg PO 5 times/day. *Herpes Zoster (Shingles)* • Acute Localized Dermatomal: • For 7-10 days; consider longer duration if lesions are slow to resolve. • Acyclovir 800 mg PO 5 times/day.	• In managing VZV retinitis: Consultation with an ophthalmologist experienced in management of VZV retinitis is strongly recommended. • Duration of therapy for VZV retinitis is not well defined and should be determined based on clinical, virologic, immunologic, and ophthalmologic responses. • Optimization of ART is recommended for serious and difficult-to-treat VZV infections (e.g., retinitis, encephalitis).
Progressive multifocal leukoencephalopathy (JC virus infections)	• There is no specific antiviral therapy for JC virus infection. The main treatment approach is to reverse the immunosuppression caused by HIV. • Initiate ART immediately in ART-naïve patients. • Optimize ART in patients who develop PML in phase of HIV viremia on ART.	None.	• Corticosteroids may be used for PML-IRIS characterized by contrast enhancement, edema, or mass effect and with clinical deterioration.

AIDS, Acquired immunodeficiency syndrome; *ART,* antiretroviral therapy; *ARV,* antiretroviral; bid, twice a day; *CD4,* CD4 T lymphocyte cell; *CFU,* colony-forming unit; *CMV,* cytomegalovirus; *CNS,* central nervous system; *CSF,* cerebrospinal fluid; *CYP3A4,* cytochrome P-450 3A4; *DS,* double strength; *EMB,* ethambutol; *G6PD,* glucose-6-phosphate dehydrogenase; *HIV,* human immunodeficiency virus; *HSV,* herpes simplex virus; *ICU,* intensive care unit; *IM,* intramuscular; *INH,* isoniazid; *IRIS,* immune reconstitution inflammatory syndrome; *IRU,* immune recovery uveitis; *IV,* intravenous; *JC,* John Cunningham (virus); *LP,* lumbar puncture; *MAC, Mycobacterium avium* complex; *NSAID,* nonsteroidal antiinflammatory drugs; *PCP, Pneumocystis* pneumonia; *PI,* protease inhibitor; *PJP, Pneumocystis jiroveci* pneumonia; *PML,* progressive multifocal leukoencephalopathy; *PO,* oral; *PZA,* pyrazinamide; *qid,* four times a day; *RFB,* rifabutin; *RIF,* rifampin; *SS,* single strength; *TB,* tuberculosis; *tid,* three times daily; *tiw,* three times weekly; *TMP-SMX,* trimethoprim-sulfamethoxazole; *VZV,* varicella zoster virus.

Quality of Evidence for the Recommendation:

I: One or more randomized trials with clinical outcomes and/or validated laboratory endpoints

II: One or more well-designed, nonrandomized trials or observational cohort studies with long-term clinical outcomes

III: Expert opinion

* Pyrimethamine and leucovorin doses are the same as for preferred therapy.

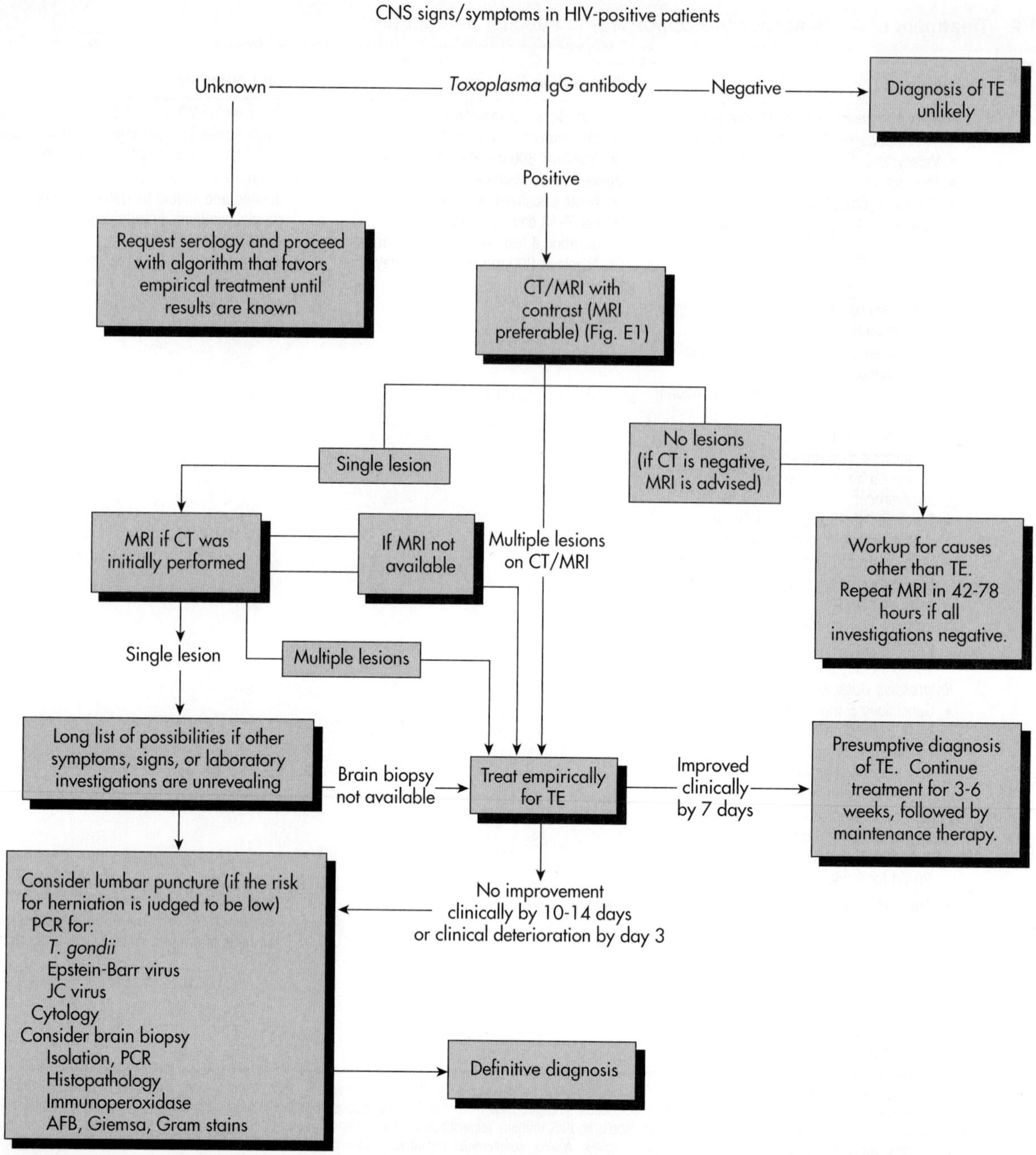

FIG. 3 Diagnostic approach and management algorithm for human immunodeficiency virus *(HIV)*–infected patients with central nervous system *(CNS)* symptoms or signs that might potentially be toxoplasmic encephalitis *(TE).* *AFB*, Acid-fast bacilli; *CT*, computed tomography; *IgG*, immunoglobulin G; *MRI*, magnetic resonance imaging; *PCR*, polymerase chain reaction. (From Bennett JE et al: *Mandell, Douglas, and Bennett's principles and practice of infectious diseases*, ed 8, Philadelphia, 2015, Saunders.)

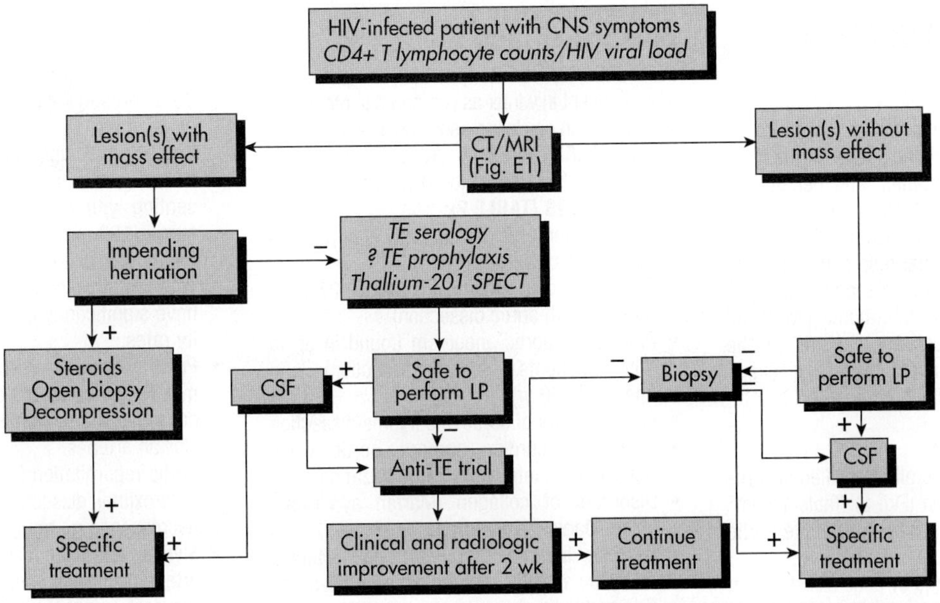

FIG. 4 Management of the human immunodeficiency virus *(HIV)* type 1–infected patient with central nervous system *(CNS)* mass lesions. The elements in italics represent data that contribute to the decision-making process (see text for details). *CSF,* Cerebrospinal fluid; *CT,* computed tomography; *LP,* lumbar puncture; *MRI,* magnetic resonance imaging; *SPECT,* single-photon emission computed tomography; *TE, Toxoplasma* encephalitis. (From Bennett JE et al: *Mandell, Douglas, and Bennett's principles and practice of infectious diseases,* ed 8, Philadelphia, 2015, Saunders.)

Acute Aortic Syndromes

BASIC INFORMATION

DEFINITION

Acute aortic syndromes are a spectrum of aortic pathologies that include aortic dissection, intramural hematomas, and penetrating atherosclerotic ulcers. Aortic dissections are the most common and occur when blood passes through an intimal tear, separating the intima from the medial layers and creating a false lumen. Intramural hematoma (IMH) and penetrating aortic ulcer are variants of the classically described aortic dissection. Fig. 1 illustrates acute aortic syndromes.

CLASSIFICATION

Aortic dissection is generally classified according to anatomic location (Fig. 2). Table 1 summarizes classification schemes of acute aortic dissection.

- Stanford (more commonly used classification system): Type A ascending aorta (proximal), type B descending aorta (distal)
- DeBakey: Type I ascending and descending aorta, type II ascending aorta, type III descending aorta
- Aortic dissection can also be classified by acuity of presentation: Hyperacute (<24 hr), acute (2 to 7 days), subacute (8 to 30 days), and chronic (>30 days). The overall survival rate is inversely related to time of presentation, with the highest survival rate in the hyperacute group and the lowest survival rate in the chronic group.

SYNONYMS

Aortic dissection
Dissecting aortic aneurysm
AAS

ICD-10CM CODES

I71.00	Dissection of unspecified site of aorta
I71.01	Dissection of thoracic aorta
I71.02	Dissection of abdominal aorta
I71.03	Dissection of thoracoabdominal aorta

EPIDEMIOLOGY & DEMOGRAPHICS

INCIDENCE: 2.6 to 3.5 per 100,000 person-yr; more frequent in winter as compared to other seasons, although no clear reason has been identified.

PREDOMINANT SEX & AGE: Males (65%) females (35%), ages 60 to 80 yr; mean = 63 yr

RISK FACTORS (TABLE 2):

- Hypertension (found in up to 77% of patients with aortic dissection)
- Atherosclerosis (found in up to 27% of patients with aortic dissection)
- Preexisting aortic aneurysm (found in up to 16% of patients with aortic dissection)
- Age (60 to 80 yr)
- Family history of aortic aneurysms/dissection
- History of cardiac surgery, aortic valve replacement, intraaortic catheterization
- Disorders of collagen (Marfan syndrome, Ehlers-Danlos syndrome)
- Vascular inflammation (giant cell arteritis, Takayasu arteritis, rheumatoid arthritis, syphilitic aortitis)
- Aortic coarctation, bicuspid aortic valve
- Turner syndrome
- Cocaine abuse (usually within 12 hours of last use of cocaine)
- Trauma
- Pregnancy and delivery
- Fluoroquinolone use[1]
- Table 3 summarizes genetically triggered conditions associated with aortic dissection

PHYSICAL FINDINGS & CLINICAL PRESENTATION

- Sudden onset of severe sharp, tearing, or ripping chest, back, or abdominal pain. However, painless dissection occurs in approximately 6.4% of cases.
- Anterior chest pain (79% type A, 63% type B)
- Back pain, abdominal pain (43% type A, 64% type B)
- Syncope (19% type A, 3% type B), generally secondary to cardiac tamponade or stroke
- Congestive heart failure (CHF)
- May present with hypertension (28% for type A, 66% in type B dissection), although 25% present with hypotension (systolic blood pressure <100 mm Hg), which can indicate bleeding, cardiac tamponade, or severe aortic regurgitation. Patients presenting with very high systolic blood pressure (>180 mm Hg for type A, >200 mm Hg for type B dissection), as well as in those with systolic blood pressure <=100 mm Hg, have significantly higher in-hospital mortality rates.
- Pulse and blood pressure differentials (>20 mm Hg between arms) in 19% to 31% of cases caused by partial compression of subclavian arteries
- Aortic regurgitation in 18% to 50% of cases of proximal dissection, often with diastolic decrescendo murmur
- Myocardial ischemia caused by coronary artery occlusion, most commonly involving the right coronary artery
- Stroke in 5% to 10% of patients (secondary to dissection into or decreased blood flow to the carotids)
- Mesenteric ischemia occurs in 3% to 5% of cases, with external compression, flap prolapse, or involvement of arterial ostia
- Horner syndrome (ptosis, miosis, anhidrosis)
- Vocal cord paralysis or hoarse voice (caused by compression of the left recurrent laryngeal nerve)

ETIOLOGY

Genetics, in addition to other risk factors (see Tables 4, 5, 6, and 7), contribute to the development of aortic aneurysms and dissection.

DIAGNOSIS

DIFFERENTIAL DIAGNOSIS

- Known as the great imitator: Pulmonary embolism, acute coronary syndrome, aortic stenosis/insufficiency, nondissecting aneurysm, pericarditis, cholecystitis, peptic ulcer disease, pancreatitis, musculoskeletal pain
- Consider aortic dissection in patients with unexplained stroke, chest pain, syncope, acute-onset CHF, abdominal pain, back pain, and malperfusion of extremities or internal organs. Acute aortic syndromes may be associated with nonspecific signs and symptoms; a high clinical index of suspicion is necessary to detect the disease early in its course as nearly two thirds of patients under medical care are not diagnosed prior to death.
- In an emergency situation, a rapid yet comprehensive workup is crucial to reduce diagnostic time delay. This should include clinical assessment, laboratory data (D-dimer and troponin), chest x-ray, electrocardiogram (ECG), and aortic imaging in the appropriate patient.
- The Aortic Dissection Detection Risk Score (ADD-RS) can be a useful tool in diagnosing aortic dissection in the emergency room setting. ADD-RS is based on the presence of one

[1]Gopalakrishnan C et al: Association of fluoroquinolones with the risk of aortic aneurysm or aortic dissection. *JAMA Intern Med* 180(12):1596-1605, 2020.

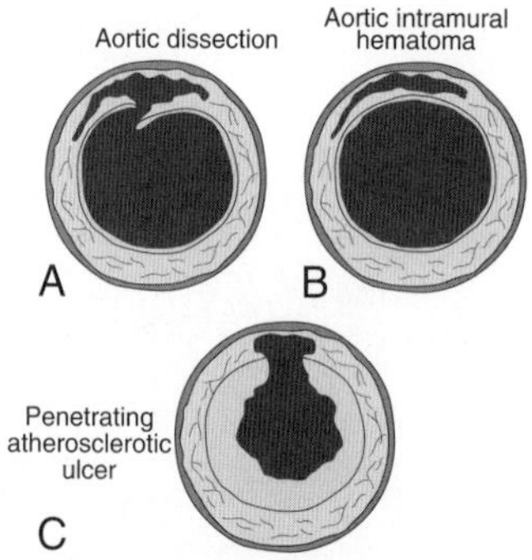

FIG. 1 Acute aortic syndromes. A, Classic aortic dissection. There is a tear in the intima with blood entering the media and a dissecting cleavage plane propagating for variable distances anterograde (and occasionally retrograde) throughout the aortic wall. **B,** Aortic intramural hematoma (IMH). A spontaneous hemorrhage of the vasa vasorum leads to bleeding within the media in the absence of an intimal tear or intimal flap. **C,** Penetrating atherosclerotic aortic ulcer (PAU). An ulcerated aortic plaque ruptures into the media, leading to an outpouching or ulceration in the aortic wall. This may be associated with IMH formation, pseudoaneurysm, or a focal, thick-walled aortic dissection. (From Zipes DP: *Braunwald's heart disease, a textbook of cardiovascular medicine,* ed 11, Philadelphia, 2019, Elsevier.)

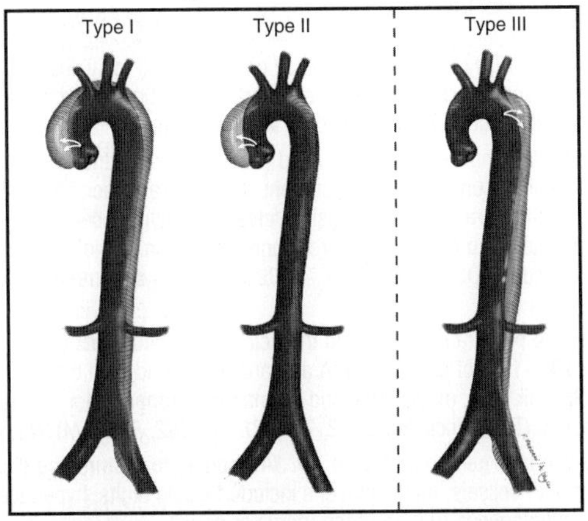

FIG. 2 Classification schemes of acute aortic dissection. (From Mann DL et al: *Braunwald's heart disease,* ed 10, Philadelphia, 2015, Elsevier.)

TABLE 1 Classification Schemes of Acute Aortic Dissection

DeBakey Classification	
Type I	Originates in the ascending aorta and extends at least to the aortic arch and often to the descending aorta (and beyond)
Type II	Originates in the ascending aorta and confined to this segment
Type III	Originates in the descending aorta, usually just distal to the left subclavian artery, and extends distally
Stanford Classification	
Type A	Dissections involving the ascending aorta (with or without extension into the descending aorta)
Type B	Dissections not involving the ascending aorta

From Mann DL et al: *Braunwald's heart disease,* ed 10, Philadelphia, 2015, Elsevier.

TABLE 2 Risk Factors for Aortic Dissection

Hypertension
Heritable or genetic thoracic aortic disease and syndromes
- Marfan syndrome
- Loeys-Dietz syndrome
- Familial thoracic aortic aneurysm syndromes
- Vascular Ehlers-Danlos syndrome
- Turner syndrome

Congenital diseases/syndromes
- Bicuspid aortic valve
- Coarctation of the aorta
- Tetralogy of Fallot

Atherosclerosis
- Penetrating atherosclerotic ulcer

Trauma, blunt or iatrogenic
- Catheter/guidewire
- Intra-aortic balloon pump
- Aortic/vascular surgery
- Motor vehicle accident
- Coronary artery bypass grafting/aortic valve replacement/TAVR
- Thoracic endovascular aneurysm repair (TEVAR)

Cocaine/methamphetamine use
Inflammatory/infectious diseases
- Giant cell arteritis
- Takayasu arteritis
- Behçet syndrome
- Aortitis
- Syphilis

Pregnancy (with underlying aortopathy)
Weightlifting (with underlying aortopathy)

TAVR, Transcatheter aortic valve replacement.
From Zipes DP: *Braunwald's heart disease, a textbook of cardiovascular medicine,* ed 11, Philadelphia, 2019, Elsevier.

or more of the clinical risk markers outlined in Table 8. A high ADD-RS effectively stratifies the risk for acute aortic dissection (score 0 is low risk, score 1 is intermediate risk, and score ≥2 is high risk). Score 0 has 95.6% certainty in ruling out aortic dissection.
- The addition of D-dimer to ADD-RS may further improve diagnostic performance of each of these when used alone for ruling out acute aortic dissection or other acute aortic syndromes. Among low- to intermediate-risk patients (ADD-RS <2), a negative D-dimer (<500 mg/dl) can rule out aortic dissection with 99.7% certainty. Among high-risk patients (ADD-RS ≥2), D-dimer is not discriminatory and requires conclusive imaging.

WORKUP

ECG: Helpful to rule out MI, although dissection can lead to coronary ischemia.

LABORATORY TESTS

- D-dimer has a high negative predictive value in dissection, but lacks specificity in the setting of acute aortic dissection. However, a negative D-dimer does not rule out intramural hematoma or penetrating aortic ulcer.
- Soluble ST2, a novel biomarker, may have superior diagnostic performance over D-dimer in discriminating acute aortic dissection from other acute chest pain syndromes. At a cutoff level of 34.6 ng/ml, the sensitivity and specificity for acute aortic dissection were 99.1% and 84.9%, respectively.
- Several other biomarkers with different diagnostic windows can be used in the diagnosis of aortic dissection:
  1. Smooth muscle myosin heavy chain protein (released from damaged medial smooth muscle) can be used to detect proximal aortic dissections (91% sensitivity and 93% specificity). Myosin heavy chains will peak within 3 hr of dissection and clear within 24 hr of aortic injury.
  2. CK-BB isoenzyme also peaks within 6 hr of dissection.
  3. Calponin, a smooth muscle troponin counterpart, increases in aortic dissection with a wider diagnostic window when compared to smooth muscle myosin heavy chain and CK-BB.
  4. C-reactive protein, fibrinogen and soluble elastin fragments are under investigation.

IMAGING STUDIES

- Multidetector CT (Fig. E3) is considered the gold standard, but its use may be limited in patients with renal failure as it involves the use of intravenous contrast.
- Transesophageal echocardiography (TEE), multidetector CT, and MRI are all highly sensitive (98%-100%) and specific (95%-98%). Test of choice depends on clinical circumstances and hospital availability.
- TEE is study of choice in unstable patients with type A dissection but is operator dependent.
- MRI has high sensitivity and specificity but limited availability; not suitable for unstable patients; contraindicated with noncompatible pacemakers, metal devices.
- With medium or high pretest probability, a second diagnostic test should be done if the first is negative.
- Coronary computed tomographic angiography (CTA) may be an alternative and useful diagnostic study when evaluating for pulmonary embolism, acute coronary syndrome, and aortic dissection.
- Aortography rarely done, as less sensitive than TEE, CT, or MRI.
- Chest radiograph may show widened mediastinum (52% in type A dissections and 39% in type B dissections) and displacement of aortic intimal calcium. It is normal in 29%-36% of patients with aortic dissection.
- Although the diagnostic sensitivity of transthoracic echocardiography is suboptimal (31%-55%), it is useful in assessing potential high-risk features or complications, such as pericardial effusion, and making other potential diagnoses. A negative transthoracic

TABLE 3 Genetically Triggered Conditions Associated with Aortic Dissection

Marfan syndrome (MFS)	Autosomal dominant disorder of connective tissue caused by *FBN1* mutation; incidence of 1 in ≈5000 individuals; multisystem manifestations, including ectopia lentis; mitral valve prolapse, aortic root aneurysm, aortic dissection; skeletal features (pectus deformities, scoliosis, arachnodactyly, hyperflexibility, tall stature, elongated fingers and toes); dural ectasia; spontaneous pneumothorax
Loeys-Dietz syndrome (LDS)	Autosomal dominant disorder caused by mutations in *TGFBR1* and *TGFBR2*, associated with aneurysms and dissections involving the aorta and branch vessels, often at relatively small diameters and young age; manifestations include craniofacial features (hypertelorism, craniosynostosis, cleft palate, bifid or broad uvula), bluish sclera, arterial tortuosity, velvety and hyperlucent skin, easily visible veins, clubfeet, skeletal abnormalities; phenotypes may vary, including those with more pronounced craniofacial features and those with more cutaneous features; ectopia lentis has not been described in LDS; mutations in *TGFB2* lead to a syndrome with an overlap in clinical features of LDS and MFS
Familial thoracic aortic aneurysm (FTAA) syndromes	Autosomal dominant disorders with variable expression and penetrance leading to thoracic aortic aneurysms (TAAs) and dissections at variable ages in families; *ACTA2* mutations occur in 10%-15% of cases of FTAA and are associated with bicuspid aortic valve (BAV) disease, cerebral aneurysms, livedo reticularis, iris flocculi, PDA, moyamoya, and premature coronary artery disease; gene mutations causing familial thoracic aortic aneurysm and dissection (TAAD) include *ACTA2, TGFBR1, TGFBR2, FBN1, MYH11, MYLK, TGFB2, SMAD3*
Vascular Ehlers-Danlos syndrome (vEDS)	Autosomal dominant disorder of collagen synthesis caused by a gene mutation in *COL3A1* leading to rupture and dissection of the aorta (usually the descending and abdominal aorta) and branch vessels; manifestations include flexible digits, hyperlucent skin with visible veins, varicose veins, typical facial appearance, and spontaneous rupture of the uterus or bowel
Bicuspid aortic valve (BAV)	Congenital condition affecting ≈1% of the population, familial in ≈9% of cases; often associated with dilation of the ascending aorta and carries increased risk for aortic dissection; gene mutations include *NOTCH1* and loci at 15q, 18q, 5q, and 13q; may be associated with FTAA
Turner syndrome (TS)	Genetic disorder affecting 1 in 2000 live-born girls and caused by complete or partial loss of the second sex chromosome (XO, Xp); women with TS often have BAV and aortic coarctation; associated with ascending aortic dilation for body size and increased risk for aortic dissection, especially when associated with BAV, hypertension, and coarctation
Aneurysms-osteoarthritis syndrome	Autosomal dominant genetic disorder resulting from mutations in the *SMAD3* gene and associated with premature osteoarthritis, osteochondritis dissecans, skeletal features, aortic aneurysms, branch vessel aneurysms, and arterial tortuosity; overlap with LDS phenotype

From Mann DL et al: *Braunwald's heart disease,* ed 10, Philadelphia, 2015, Elsevier.

TABLE 4 Ascending Thoracic Aortic Aneurysms

Degenerative	Associated with atherosclerosis
Inheritable/connective tissue	Marfan syndrome
	Ehlers-Danlos syndrome
	Loeys-Dietz syndrome
	Turner syndrome
	Osteogenesis imperfecta
	Rheumatoid arthritis
	Bicuspid aortic valve
	Aneurysm of sinus of Valsalva
Arteritis	Giant cell
	Takayasu
	Behçet disease
	Relapsing polychondritis
Infectious	Syphilis
	Mycotic aneurysms

From Soto JA, Lucey BC: *Emergency radiology, the requisites,* ed 2, Philadelphia, 2017, Elsevier.

TABLE 5 Aortic Arch Aneurysms

Degenerative	Resulting from atherosclerosis
Arteritis	Giant cell
	Takayasu
	Behçet disease
Infectious	Syphilis

From Soto JA, Lucey BC: *Emergency radiology, the requisites,* ed 2, Philadelphia, 2017, Elsevier.

echocardiography, however, does not exclude aortic dissection.

Rx TREATMENT

- Urgent surgical consultation should be obtained for all thoracic aortic dissection regardless of anatomic location. Table 9 summarizes size threshold for prophylactic aortic root or ascending aortic aneurysm resection for various conditions.
- Proximal dissections (acute type A) require emergent surgery to prevent rupture or pericardial effusion.
- Distal dissections (Stanford type B) are usually treated medically unless distal organ involvement or impending rupture occurs.

1. Surgical intervention for distal dissections is reserved for patients who have a complicated course, including occlusion of a major aortic branch, propagation of the dissection, enlarging aneurysm, and evidence of aortic rupture.
2. Thoracic endovascular aortic repair (TEVAR) is a less invasive option for complicated type B aortic dissections and is associated with lower short- and midterm mortality than medical therapy. Indications for thoracic endovascular aortic repair for type B aortic dissection are summarized in Table 10.
3. For acute type B dissections, in-hospital mortality in patients managed surgically has been reported to be 33.9% versus those managed with endovascular treatment at 10.6%.
4. Independent predictors of complication and mortality in distal dissections include periaortic hematoma and descending aortic diameter >5.5 cm, partial false lumen thrombosis, primary tear >10 mm, one entry tear, and false lumen >22 mm.
5. There is ongoing debate about a possible beneficial role of TEVAR for uncomplicated type B dissections. Data suggest that 30% of uncomplicated type B dissections will progress to an aneurysm.

ACUTE GENERAL Rx

- Admit to ICU for monitoring.
- Target systolic blood pressure 100-120 mm Hg; heart rate <60 beats/min to reduce aortic wall stress. Treatment with beta-blockers has been associated with improved survival in all patients with acute aortic dissections.
- IV beta-blockers are cornerstones of treatment, but multiple medications may be needed.

TABLE 6 Descending Thoracic Aortic Aneurysm

Degenerative	Resulting from atherosclerosis
	Focal pseudoaneurysm resulting from a penetrating aortic ulcer
Arteritis	Giant cell
	Takayasu
	Behçet disease
Inherited/connective tissue	Marfan syndrome
	Ductus aneurysm
	Loeys-Dietz syndrome
Infectious	Mycotic aneurysms
Traumatic	Posttraumatic pseudoaneurysms
	Chronic aortic transection

From Soto JA, Lucey BC: *Emergency radiology, the requisites*, ed 2, Philadelphia, 2017, Elsevier.

TABLE 7 Crawford Classification of Thoracoabdominal Aneurysms

I	Descending thoracic aorta to suprarenal aorta
II	Proximal descending thoracic aorta to infrarenal aorta (below the diaphragm)
III	Mid descending thoracic aorta to infrarenal aorta
IV	Supravisceral aorta to infrarenal aorta

From Soto JA, Lucey BC: *Emergency radiology, the requisites*, ed 2, Philadelphia, 2017, Elsevier.

TABLE 8 Aortic Dissection Detection Risk Score (ADD-RS)

Clinical risk markers*	Score
High-risk condition such as Marfan syndrome, family history of aortic disease, known aortic valve disease, known thoracic aortic aneurysm, or previous aortic manipulation, including cardiac surgery.	1
Pain in the chest, back, or abdomen described as abrupt, of severe intensity, or a ripping/tearing sensation.	1
Physical examination findings of perfusion deficit, including pulse deficit, systolic blood pressure difference, or focal neurologic deficit, or with aortic diastolic murmur and hypotension/shock.	1

*Presence of ≥1 marker within each of these groups is given a score of 1 with a maximum cumulative score of 3 if all three are present.

Modified from Erbel R et al: 2014 ESC guidelines on the diagnosis and treatment of aortic diseases: document covering acute and chronic aortic diseases of the thoracic and abdominal aorta of the adult. The Task Force for the Diagnosis and Treatment of Aortic Diseases of the European Society of Cardiology (ESC), *Eur Heart J* 35:2873-926, 2014; Hiratzka LF et al: 2010 ACCF/AHA/AATS/ACR/ASA/SCA/SCAI/SIR/STS/SVM guidelines for the diagnosis and management of patients with thoracic aortic disease, *Circulation* 121:e266-369, 2010; and Hiratzka et al: Surgery for aortic dilatation in patients with bicuspid aortic valves: a statement of clarification from the American College of Cardiology/American Heart Association Task Force on Clinical Practice Guidelines, *J Am Coll Cardiol* 67:724-31, 2016.

1. Propranolol 1 mg every 3-5 min, metoprolol 5 mg IV every 5 min, or labetalol 20 mg IV, then 20-80 mg every 10 min, followed by nitroprusside 0.3-10 mcg/kg/min.
2. Vasodilators should not be used without beta-blockade as they can induce reflex sympathetic stimulation and increase aortic shear stress.
3. IV calcium channel blockers with negative inotropy (i.e., verapamil, diltiazem) may be used if beta-blockers are contraindicated.

- Pain control, often with morphine.

CHRONIC Rx

- Chronic aortic dissection (>2 wk) managed with aggressive blood pressure control; target <120/80 mm Hg in most patients
- Statin therapy to reduce low-density lipoprotein <70 mg/dl
- Tobacco cessation
- Minimize strenuous physical activity such as heavy lifting
- Serial imaging of the aorta, with multidetector CT or MRI should be performed at presentation, at 1, 3, 6, and 12 months given the higher risk of instability early on, followed by yearly clinical and imaging follow-up
- As stated above, endovascular repair should be considered in complicated chronic type B dissections, i.e., when the aortic diameter exceeds 5.5 cm, when there is uncontrolled pain or blood pressure, or when there is rapid growth of the dissecting aneurysm (>4 mm per yr).

DISPOSITION

- 90% mortality rate is within 2 wk for an untreated type A dissection.
- Proximal dissection is a surgical emergency. Time is critical; mortality rate is 1%-3% per hour, approaching 70% after 48 hr.
- Overall, in-hospital mortality rate is 22% with proximal dissections (27% treated surgically and 56% treated medically) and 10%-17% with distal dissections.
- Table 11 summarizes suggested imaging surveillance of asymptomatic thoracic aortic aneurysms.

REFERRAL

For ICU management and surgical intervention

PEARLS & CONSIDERATIONS

- Blood pressure control is essential; beta-blocker is first-line medication.
- Proximal dissection is a surgical emergency.
- Cardiac tamponade is not uncommon in patients with acute type A aortic dissection. Syncope, altered mental status, and a widened mediastinum on chest radiograph on presentation suggest tamponade, which warrants urgent operative therapy.
- Surgery for acute type A aortic dissection in patients ≥70 yr old can be performed with acceptable outcomes.

OTHER ACUTE AORTIC SYNDROMES

ACUTE INTRAMURAL HEMATOMA:

- Acute intramural hematoma occurs when the vasa vasorum ruptures within the medial wall. It does not involve an intimal tearing unless a dissection develops.
- About 10% to 20% of patients with suspected aortic dissection will be found to have acute intramural hematoma.
- The key imaging findings are the absence of intimal tear and absence of blood flow into a false lumen.
- Echocardiography shows crescentic or circumferential thickening of aortic wall without an intimal flap.
- About 8% to 16% of patients with intramural hematoma will evolve into aortic dissection.
- Similar to aortic dissections, in-hospital mortality is significantly worse among patients with Type A intramural hematomas compared to Type B.

PENETRATING ATHEROSCLEROTIC ULCER:

- Penetrating atherosclerotic ulcers occur in the setting of extensive aortic atherosclerosis and hypertension.
- These are seen mostly in older adults and occurs in descending aorta in over 90% of cases.
- There is an ulceration of atheroma that disrupts the internal elastic lamina and extends into the media and allows hematoma formation.
- There is potential for extensive intramural hematoma, pseudoaneurysm or complete rupture of aorta.

The general principles of the treatment of acute intramural hematomas and penetrating atherosclerotic ulcers are similar to acute aortic dissection.

TABLE 9 Size Threshold for Prophylactic Aortic Root or Ascending Aortic Aneurysm Resection for Various Conditions

Condition	Size Threshold*
Degenerative aneurysm	≥5.5 cm
Bicuspid aortic valve	≥5.5 cm
Bicuspid aortic valve with risk factors or low surgical risk†	≥5.0 cm
Bicuspid aortic valve requiring aortic valve replacement	>4.5 cm
Marfan syndrome	≥5.0 cm
Marfan syndrome with risk factors‡	>4.5 cm
Loeys-Dietz syndrome§	4.0-4.5 cm
Familial thoracic aortic aneurysm syndromes¶	4.5-5.0 cm
Turner syndrome	>2.5 cm/m²

*Lower thresholds for intervention may be considered according to body surface area in patients of small stature or in the case of rapid growth of the aorta. Age, body size, rapid growth, family history, risk of surgery, and patient and physician wishes may influence aortic size threshold.

†Family history of aortic dissection or aortic growth rate of 0.5 cm or more per yr or if the patient is at low surgical risk (<4%) and the surgery is performed by an experienced aortic surgical team in a center with established expertise in these procedures. Other risk factors for aortic dissection include coarctation of the aorta, hypertension, and the root phenotype of bicuspid aortic valve.

‡Family history of aortic dissection or rapid aortic growth (>3 mm/yr), or severe aortic or mitral regurgitation. If pregnancy desired, consider prophylactic aortic surgery for aortic diameter of 4.0-4.5 cm.

§It is reasonable to consider surgical repair of the aorta in adults with Loeys-Dietz syndrome or a confirmed *TGFBR1* or *TGFBR2* mutation with aortic diameter of 4.2 cm or more by transesophageal echocardiogram or 4.4-4.6 or more by CT or MRI. Aortic surgery at smaller diameters may be recommended when there are severe craniofacial features, rapid growth, or a family history of aortic dissection.

¶Surgical thresholds vary depending on the specific gene mutation involved. TAA caused by *ACTA2*, *SMAD3*, and *MYLK* may lead to aortic dissection at relatively small aortic diameters.

From Zipes DP: *Braunwald's heart disease, a textbook of cardiovascular medicine,* ed 11, Philadelphia, 2019, Elsevier.

TABLE 10 Indications for Thoracic Endovascular Aortic Repair for Type B Aortic Dissection*

Rupture
Impending rupture
Malperfusion
Hemorrhagic pleural effusion
Refractory pain
Refractory hypertension
Aneurysmal dilation (>55 mm)
Rapid increase in diameter
Recurrent symptoms

*Or open surgical repair if anatomy is unsuitable for TEVAR.

From Zipes DP: *Braunwald's heart disease, a textbook of cardiovascular medicine,* ed 11, Philadelphia, 2019, Elsevier.

SUGGESTED READINGS

Available at ExpertConsult.com

RELATED CONTENT

Aortic Dissection (Patient Information)

AUTHORS: **Marjan Mujib, MD,** and **Philip Stockwell, MD**

TABLE 11 Suggested Imaging Surveillance of Asymptomatic Thoracic Aortic Aneurysms*

Initial Discovery of Aneurysm	Repeated Imaging at 6 Months to Document Stability
Degenerative aneurysm†	
3.5-4.4 cm	Annual imaging
4.5-5.4 cm	Annual to biannual imaging
MFS, BAV with TAA, and familial TAA	
3.5-4.4 cm	Annual imaging
4.5-5.0 cm	Biannual imaging
LDS‡	
<4 cm	At least annual imaging
>4 cm	Biannual imaging

BAV, Bicuspid aortic valve; *LDS,* Loeys-Dietz syndrome; *MFS,* Marfan syndrome; *TAA,* thoracic aortic aneurysm.

*For aneurysms growing rapidly, more frequent imaging is recommended. Management of TAA must take into account the family history, age, body size, sex, rate of aneurysm growth, and underlying disease.

†For relatively small degenerative aneurysms found by imaging to be stable from year to year, imaging may be performed every 2-3 yr (Hiratzka et al).

‡Some recommend surgery for aortic root dimensions larger than 4 cm in adults with LDS, whereas the American College of Cardiology/American Heart Association guidelines for thoracic aortic disease recommend prophylactic surgery at 4.2 cm by TEE and 4.4-4.6 cm by CT or MRI (Hiratzka et al).

From Hiratzka LF et al: 2010 ACCF/AHA/AATS/ACR/ASA/SCA/SCAI/SIR/STS/SVM guidelines for the diagnosis and management of patients with thoracic aortic disease: a report of the American College of Cardiology Foundation/American Heart Association Task Force on Practice Guidelines, American Association for Thoracic Surgery, American College of Radiology, American Stroke Association, Society of Cardiovascular Anesthesiologists, Society for Cardiovascular Angiography and Interventions, Society of Interventional Radiology, Society of Thoracic Surgeons, and Society for Vascular Medicine, *Circulation* 121:e266, 2010; Mann DL et al: *Braunwald's heart disease,* ed 10, Philadelphia, 2015, Elsevier.

BASIC INFORMATION

DEFINITION

Acute bronchitis is a self-limited inflammation of trachea and bronchi.

SYNONYM

Chest cold

ICD-10CM CODE

J20.9 Acute bronchitis, unspecified

EPIDEMIOLOGY & DEMOGRAPHICS

- Highest incidence in smokers, older adults, and young children and during winter months.
- In the U.S. there are nearly 30 million ambulatory visits annually for cough, leading to more than 12 million diagnoses of "bronchitis."
- Acute lower respiratory tract infection is the most common condition treated in primary care.

PHYSICAL FINDINGS & CLINICAL PRESENTATION

- In most cases, acute bronchitis begins with signs and symptoms typical of the common cold syndrome (nasal congestion, sore throat), followed shortly by the onset of cough
- Cough, usually worse in the morning, often productive; mainly caused by transient bronchial hyperresponsiveness
- Low-grade fever
- Substernal discomfort worsened by coughing
- Postnasal drip, pharyngeal injection
- Rhonchi that may clear after cough, occasional wheezing
- Various host factors (age, immune status, smoking, underlying medical conditions) can influence illness severity and clinical presentation
- In mild cases, the illness lasts only 7 to 10 days, whereas in others, cough may persist for up to 3 wk or longer

ETIOLOGY

- Viral infections are the leading cause of bronchitis (rhinovirus, influenza virus, adenovirus, respiratory syncytial virus)
- Atypical organisms *(Mycoplasma, Chlamydia pneumoniae)*
- Bacterial infections *(Bordetella pertussis, Haemophilus influenzae, Moraxella, Streptococcus pneumoniae)*
- Table 1 summarizes viral and bacterial causes of acute bronchitis

DIAGNOSIS

DIFFERENTIAL DIAGNOSIS

- Pneumonia
- Asthma
- Sinusitis
- Bronchiolitis
- Aspiration
- Cystic fibrosis
- Pharyngitis
- Cough secondary to medications
- Neoplasm (elderly patients)
- Influenza
- Allergic aspergillosis
- Gastroesophageal reflux disease
- Congestive heart failure (in elderly patients)
- Bronchogenic neoplasm

WORKUP

Seldom necessary (e.g., to rule out pneumonia, neoplasm)

LABORATORY TESTS

Laboratory tests are generally not necessary.

IMAGING STUDIES

Chest x-ray is usually reserved for patients with suspected pneumonia, influenza, or underlying chronic obstructive pulmonary disease (COPD) and no improvement with therapy.

TREATMENT

NONPHARMACOLOGIC THERAPY

- Avoidance of tobacco and other pulmonary irritants
- Increased fluid intake
- Use of vaporizer to increase room humidity

ACUTE GENERAL Rx

- Therapy is generally symptomatic and directed at relief of cough and wheezing.
- Inhaled bronchodilators (e.g., albuterol, metaproterenol) PRN for 1 to 2 wk in patients with wheezing or troublesome cough. Inhaled albuterol has been proven effective in reducing the duration of cough in adults with uncomplicated acute bronchitis.

TABLE 1 Viral and Bacterial Causes of Acute Bronchitis

Pathogen	Seasonality	Comments
Influenza viruses	Winter	Local epidemics last 6-8 wk during which clinical illness of cough and fever has high predictive value; laboratory diagnosis readily available; early neuraminidase inhibitor therapy effective
Rhinoviruses	Fall and spring	Most frequent cause of common cold syndrome; immunity is serotype specific
Coronaviruses	Winter to spring	Cause common cold syndrome; newer strains are difficult to culture and require RT-PCR for diagnosis
Adenoviruses	Yr round, winter epidemics	High attack rates in closed populations such as persons living in military barracks or college dormitories; serotype-specific immunity
Respiratory syncytial virus (RSV)	Late fall to early spring	Attack rates approach 75% in neonates, 3%-5% in adults; associated with wheezing in all age groups; rapid antigen test accurate in children but requires culture or RT-PCR to diagnose in adults
Human metapneumovirus (hMPV)	Winter to early spring	Associated with wheezing in adults and in infants; difficult to isolate in tissue culture and often requires RT-PCR
Parainfluenza viruses	Fall to winter	Similar to RSV and hMPV, parainfluenza viruses primarily pediatric pathogens but can cause severe acute disease in some adults
Measles virus	Yr round	Can cause respiratory disease in malnourished children; illness causes transient immune suppression
Mycoplasma pneumoniae	Yr round, fall outbreaks	Long incubation period (10-21 days) results in staggered epidemic pattern in families; nonproductive persistent cough typical; diagnosed by IgM serology; treated with macrolide, quinolone, or tetracycline antibiotics
Chlamydia pneumoniae	Yr round	Associated with sinusitis; diagnosis by RT-PCR not readily available
Bordetella pertussis	Yr round	Severe illness in nonimmunized children; illness milder in partially immune adults; can be associated with prolonged cough; adults often reservoir for epidemics; early therapy with antibiotics can reduce spread

RT-PCR, Reverse-transcriptase polymerase chain reaction.
From Bennett JE et al: *Mandell, Douglas, and Bennett's principles and practice of infectious diseases,* ed 8, Philadelphia, 2015, Saunders.

- Cough suppression with dextromethorphan and guaifenesin is commonly recommended; addition of codeine for cough suppression if cough is severe and is significantly interrupting patient's sleep pattern.
- Use of antibiotics (TMP-SMX, amoxicillin, doxycycline, cefuroxime) for acute bronchitis is generally not indicated; should be considered only in patients with concomitant COPD and purulent sputum or in patients with suspected pertussis. In the few cases of acute bronchitis caused by *B. pertussis* or atypical bacteria such as *C. pneumoniae* or *Mycoplasma pneumoniae,* early use of macrolide antibiotics is reasonable.
- Antibiotics are overused in patients with acute bronchitis (70% to 90% of office visits for acute bronchitis result in treatment with antibiotics); this practice pattern is contributing to increases in resistant organisms.
- Trials have shown that there are no significant differences in patients receiving antibiotics compared with those receiving placebo in overall clinical improvements or limitations in work or other activities. There was a significant increase in adverse effects in the antibiotic group, particularly gastrointestinal symptoms.[1]

CHRONIC Rx

Avoidance of tobacco and other pulmonary irritants.

DISPOSITION

- Complete recovery within 7 to 10 days in most patients.
- Patients should be informed to expect to have a cough for 10 to 14 days after the visit.

REFERRAL

For pulmonary function testing only in patients with recurrent bronchitis and suspected underlying pulmonary disease.

PEARLS & CONSIDERATIONS

COMMENTS

- Patients are more likely to receive prescriptions for antibiotics from mid- or late-career physicians with high patient volumes and from physicians who were trained outside of Canada or the U.S.[2] Intervention studies reveal that patient and physician education are effective in reducing the use of antibiotic therapy. No offer or delayed offer of antibiotics for acute uncomplicated lower respiratory tract infection is acceptable, is associated with little difference in symptom resolution, and is likely to reduce antibiotic use and beliefs in the effectiveness of antibiotics.
- It is helpful to refer to acute bronchitis as a "chest cold." Patients should be informed that antibiotics are probably not going to be beneficial and may result in significant side effects.

RELATED CONTENT

Acute Bronchitis (Patient Information)

AUTHOR: **Fred F. Ferri, MD**

[1] Smith SM, Smucny J, Fahey T: Antibiotics for acute bronchitis, *JAMA* 312:2678, 2014.

[2] Silverman M et al: Antibiotic prescribing for nonbacterial acute upper respiratory infections in elderly persons. *Ann Intern Med* 166:765-774, 2017.

BASIC INFORMATION

Acute coronary syndrome (ACS) represents a spectrum of clinical disorders that results from a sudden and unpredictable decrease of blood flow to the myocardium. ACS is a formidable disease that incurs high, and in some cases immediate, mortality. This syndrome is usually due to interaction of vulnerable atherosclerotic plaque in the coronary arteries with that of activated clotting factors and platelets in the systemic circulation. In the modern era, management of ACS involves highly protocolized and systematic care of both procedural and medical therapies guided toward restoring blood flow to the heart. The spectrum of ACS is predominated by two important subtypes: ST-elevation myocardial infarction (STEMI) and non–ST-elevation myocardial infarction (NSTEMI). The third category of ACS is called unstable angina (UA) and falls within the NSTEMI subtype. The type of ACS dictates the timing of reperfusion, with STEMI being the most severe and always emergent. In this spectrum, UA and NSTEMI are represented by an abnormal electrocardiogram (ECG) without the presence of ST-segment elevation in the appropriate clinical setting (i.e., chest discomfort). NSTEMI is additionally characterized by positive cardiac biomarkers. STEMI is characterized by ST-segment elevation or presumed new left bundle branch block on ECG, similarly in the appropriate clinical setting. ACS should be thought of as a continuous spectrum as UA will often progress to a myocardial infarction if left untreated (Table 1). Because of this continuum, the 2014 American College of Cardiology/American Heart Association (ACC/AHA) guidelines have grouped UA and NSTEMI into a single category called non–ST-elevation ACS (NSTE-ACS).

SYNONYMS

ACS
Unstable angina
NSTEMI
STEMI
Acute myocardial infarction

ICD-10CM CODES

I20.0	Unstable angina
I21.0-I21.3	ST elevation (STEMI)
I21.4	Non-ST elevation (NSTEMI) myocardial infarction
I24.9	Acute ischemic heart disease, unspecified

EPIDEMIOLOGY & DEMOGRAPHICS

INCIDENCE: In the U.S., cardiovascular disease accounts for approximately 640,000 deaths each yr. The estimated annual incidence of heart attack in the U.S. is 600,000 new attacks and 200,000 recurrent attacks. Approximately 70% of myocardial infarctions are listed as NSTEMI, with the remainder being listed as STEMI. Patients with NSTE-ACS have more cardiac and noncardiac comorbidities than patients with STEMI. The underlying etiology, atherosclerotic coronary artery disease (CAD), remains the number one cause of mortality.

PREDOMINANT SEX AND AGE: In evaluating chest pain, male gender and older age are important clinical factors that can identify ACS as a potential cause. In the U.S., the median age at ACS presentation is 68 yr (interquartile range 56 to 79), and the male-to-female ratio is approximately 3:2. In a 2005-2011 study sponsored by National Heart, Lung, and Blood Institute, the average age-adjusted first MI or fatal coronary heart disease rates per 1000 population in patients age 35 to 84 yr of age were 3.7 for white men, 5.9 for black men, 2.1 for white women, and 4.0 for black women. As noted in this study, heart disease affects African Americans disproportionately. Heart disease is also the leading cause of death in women, surpassing all forms of cancer.

RISK FACTORS: Hypertension, diabetes mellitus, dyslipidemia, tobacco use, and family history of premature CAD (CAD in a male first-degree relative younger than 55 yr or a female younger than 65 yr) are all associated risk factors for CAD. There are also female-specific risk factors for CAD, including disorders of pregnancy and early onset of menopause. Refer to the topic "Angina Pectoris" for an extensive list of risk factors. Presence of these risk factors causes damage to the vascular endothelium and progression of atherosclerotic coronary artery plaques.

PHYSICAL FINDINGS & CLINICAL PRESENTATION

- Symptoms often, but not always, include chest discomfort described as a pressure that may radiate to the shoulders, neck, jaw, or back. Typical angina is substernal in location, brought on by emotional or physical stress, and relieved with rest and/or nitroglycerin. The pain and discomfort associated with an ACS event is often diffuse rather than localized. It is often associated with diaphoresis.
- Women, diabetics, the elderly (>75 yr old), and postoperative patients often have an atypical presentation for ACS.
- Unstable angina has three typical presentations:
  1. Rest angina: Angina occurring at rest and prolonged usually for longer than 20 minutes.
  2. New-onset angina: New-onset angina of at least Canadian Cardiovascular Society (CCS) class III symptoms (Table 2).
  3. Increasing angina: Previously diagnosed angina that has become distinctly more frequent, longer in duration, or lower in threshold (i.e., increased by ≥1 CCS class to at least CCS class III severity).
- "Anginal equivalents" may include dyspnea, nausea, vomiting, and fatigue.
- ECG for NSTE-ACS may reveal transient ST-segment elevation, ST-segment depression, and/or new T-wave inversion. ECG for definition of STEMI will reveal at least 1-mm ST-segment elevation in two contiguous leads or new left bundle branch block in the appropriate clinical presentation.
- Physical examination findings alone are insufficient for the diagnosis of ACS. The physical examination may provide clues as to alternative diagnoses, such as aortic dissection (differences in pulse and blood pressure between the arms, murmur of aortic regurgitation), aortic stenosis, pericarditis (friction rub), cardiac tamponade (pulsus paradoxus), and pneumothorax (differential breath sounds.) In ACS it is important to assess the patient's hemodynamic stability, as signs of heart failure may be present. These signs include elevated jugular venous pressure (JVP), presence of an S3 gallop, rales, and to a lesser extent, peripheral edema. The degree of heart failure with MI can be represented by the Killip classification, with the greater the Killip classification, the greater the mortality noted:
  1. Killip Class 1 is no heart failure.
  2. Killip Class 2 includes individuals with rales, elevated JVP, and S3 on examination.
  3. Killip Class 3 includes individuals with frank pulmonary edema.
  4. Killip Class 4 describes individuals in cardiogenic shock or hypotension with evidence of vasoconstriction noted.

ETIOLOGY

Atherosclerotic CAD is the underlying etiology. The hallmark of ACS is the vulnerable atherosclerotic plaque, which typically has a thin fibrous cap and a large lipid core. This vulnerable plaque can spontaneously rupture, which leads to platelet activation and aggregation and a systemic inflammatory cascade,

TABLE 1 Acute Coronary Syndromes

	Spectrum of Acute Coronary Syndrome		
	Unstable Angina	**NSTEMI**	**STEMI**
Chest discomfort	1	1	1
Cardiac biomarkers	2	1	1
ECG changes	TWI and/or ST depression	TWI and/or ST depression	ST elevation or presumed new left bundle branch block
Pathophysiology	Partial/transient thrombotic occlusion	Partial/transient thrombotic occlusion	Complete thrombotic occlusion

ECG, Electrocardiogram; *NSTEMI,* non–ST-segment elevation myocardial infarction; *STEMI,* ST-segment myocardial infarction; *TWI,* T-wave inversion.

TABLE 2 Grading of Angina Pectoris According to CCS Classification

Class	Description of Stage
I	"Ordinary physical activity does not cause ... angina," such as walking or climbing stairs. Angina occurs with strenuous, rapid, or prolonged exertion at work or recreation.
II	"Slight limitation of ordinary activity." Angina occurs on walking or climbing stairs rapidly; walking uphill; walking or stair climbing after meals; in cold, in wind, or under emotional stress; or only during the few hours after awakening. Angina occurs on walking 0.2 blocks on the level and climbing 0.1 flight of ordinary stairs at a normal pace and under normal conditions.
III	"Marked limitations of ordinary physical activity." Angina occurs on walking 1-2 blocks on the level and climbing 1 flight of stairs under normal conditions and at a normal pace.
IV	"Inability to carry on any physical activity without discomfort—anginal symptoms may be present at rest."

Adapted with permission from Campeau L. Grading of angina pectoris (letter), *Circulation* 54:522-523, 1976. © 1976, American Heart Association, Inc.

From Braunwald E et al: ACC/AHA guidelines for the management of patients with unstable angina and non–ST-segment elevation myocardial infarction. A report of the American College of Cardiology/American Heart Association Task Force on Practice Guidelines (Committee on the Management of Patients With Unstable Angina), *J Am Coll Cardiol* 36:970-1062, 2000.

leading to thrombus formation. STEMI typically results from complete thrombotic occlusion of a coronary artery, whereas NSTE-ACS often has partial occlusion. Angiographically, it is often the intermediate coronary artery lesions (30% to 50% diameter vessel stenosis) that lead to subtotal or total vessel occlusion in two thirds of STEMI cases.

Dx DIAGNOSIS

DIFFERENTIAL DIAGNOSIS

Chest pain mimicking ACS may be the result of various underlying disorders, some of which are also accompanied by ECG changes and/or cardiac biomarker release. Examples include acute pulmonary embolism, acute aortic dissection, pericarditis, myocarditis, costochondritis, pneumonia, tension pneumothorax, perforating ulcer, or Boerhaave syndrome. Refer to topics "Angina Pectoris," "Coronary Artery Syndrome," and "Myocardial Infarction" for extensive differential diagnoses of chest pain.

WORKUP

Focused history and physical exam, 12-lead ECG, cardiac biomarkers, and chest radiograph (CXR). Initial biomarkers may not be positive early in the disease process. Often serial biomarkers are drawn every 6 to 8 hr for a total of three sets for the purposes of ruling out myocardial infarction (MI), or until peak to determine the severity of an established MI. Echocardiogram may reveal new regional wall motion abnormalities or newly depressed LV function or aneurysm formation. Fig. 1 summarizes the evaluation of patients for acute coronary syndrome.

LABORATORY TESTS:

- Biomarkers and, in particular, the rising and/or falling pattern play an important role in the early detection and diagnosis of acute coronary syndrome (ACS). While troponin is essential to the diagnosis of acute myocardial infarction, other markers have demonstrated utility in the setting of acute chest pain and ACS. CK-MB and myoglobin are two traditional markers that are frequently used in combination with troponin and will be elevated in the setting of NSTEMI or STEMI. See Fig. E2, *A* for timing of release of each biomarker. Troponin is the most sensitive biomarker for cardiac myocyte damage and also predicts 42-day mortality in ACS. Troponin is considered the gold standard biomarker for diagnosis of myocardial infarction (Fig. E2, *B*). Newer troponin assays have the ability to detect troponin levels at thresholds approximately 100 times lower than older assays. These assays allow for improved sensitivity in diagnosis or exclusion of acute myocardial infarction.
- Creatinine kinase-myocardial band (CK-MB) is the cardiac specific isoform of creatinine kinase (CK) and is found in high concentrations in the myocardium. After an acute myocardial injury, CK-MB levels peak within 4 to 6 hr. Its shorter half-life leads to normal values within 24 to 48 hr after an event. As such, CK-MB is especially useful when assessing a patient for possible reinfarction given troponin levels can remain elevated up to 14 days or more after an acute myocardial infarction.
- Myocardial infarction is not always the cause of elevated troponin levels. Any form of myocardial injury can cause elevation in troponin. Cardiac conditions that cause supply-demand mismatch without acute coronary obstruction, including arrhythmias, hypotension/hypertension, heart failure, and myocarditis, are a few examples that can lead to elevated levels. Noncardiac conditions including renal failure, sepsis, respiratory failure, and neurological diseases, may similarly lead to elevations in troponin.
- Meanwhile, other biomarkers also have significant prognostic value. Testing for B-type natriuretic peptide (BNP) can help risk-stratify mortality in patients presenting with ACS. Notably, a BNP >80 portends a high risk of death at initial presentation of a STEMI.

RISK MODELS & RISK SCORES

Risk models and scores such as TIMI (see "Risk Assessment" in "Myocardial Infarction" topic), PURSUIT, and GRACE based on clinical, ECG, and laboratory data at presentation help to discriminate patients at high risk versus low risk for short- and intermediate-term adverse outcomes (Fig. E2, *C*). These risk stratification models are helpful in determining the timing and strategy of treatment.

IMAGING STUDIES

- A CXR to assist in evaluating for volume overload and possible widened mediastinum, which could be indicative of an aortic dissection. CXR can be useful in assessing for pneumonia, pneumothorax, intraperitoneal free air, and other noncardiac causes of chest pain.
- In patients for whom ECG and cardiac biomarkers are nondiagnostic but they have high clinical suspicion for ACS, an echocardiogram may be helpful to assess left ventricular (LV) function and regional wall motion abnormalities.
- Coronary CT angiography can be performed in patients with suspected ACS but with a normal 12-lead EKG, negative troponin, and no history of coronary artery disease (Class IIa).
- Cardiac stress testing (treadmill ECG, imaging stress studies using echocardiography or nuclear modalities) is helpful in further risk stratification of these patients. (See "Coronary Artery Syndrome" in Section I.)
- Coronary angiogram/cardiac catheterization will reveal coronary artery luminal irregularities/stenotic lesions. In patients with ACS who undergo coronary angiography, approximately 25% will have one vessel disease, 25% will have two vessel disease, 25% will have three vessel disease, 10% will have left main disease, and 15% will have coronary stenosis of <50% or normal coronaries.

Rx TREATMENT

The overall goal for patients with ACS is to relieve myocardial ischemia and to prevent recurrent cardiovascular events. This is achieved by targeting both vulnerable coronary plaque and activated clotting factors and platelets in the blood. Revascularization, whether it is chemical (i.e., thrombolysis) or mechanical (i.e., percutaneous coronary intervention [PCI]), is needed to prevent further events and improve flow within the coronary artery lumen. In the modern era, PCI has improved outcomes for patients presenting with ACS. For patients with STEMI, time from onset of ischemia to revascularization guides the reperfusion strategy. STEMI patients presenting to a hospital with PCI capability should be treated with primary PCI within 90 min of first medical contact (Figs. 3 and 4). At non–PCI-capable hospitals where the first medical contact to PCI is more than 120 min, thrombolytic therapy should be given to eligible patients within the first 12 hr after symptom

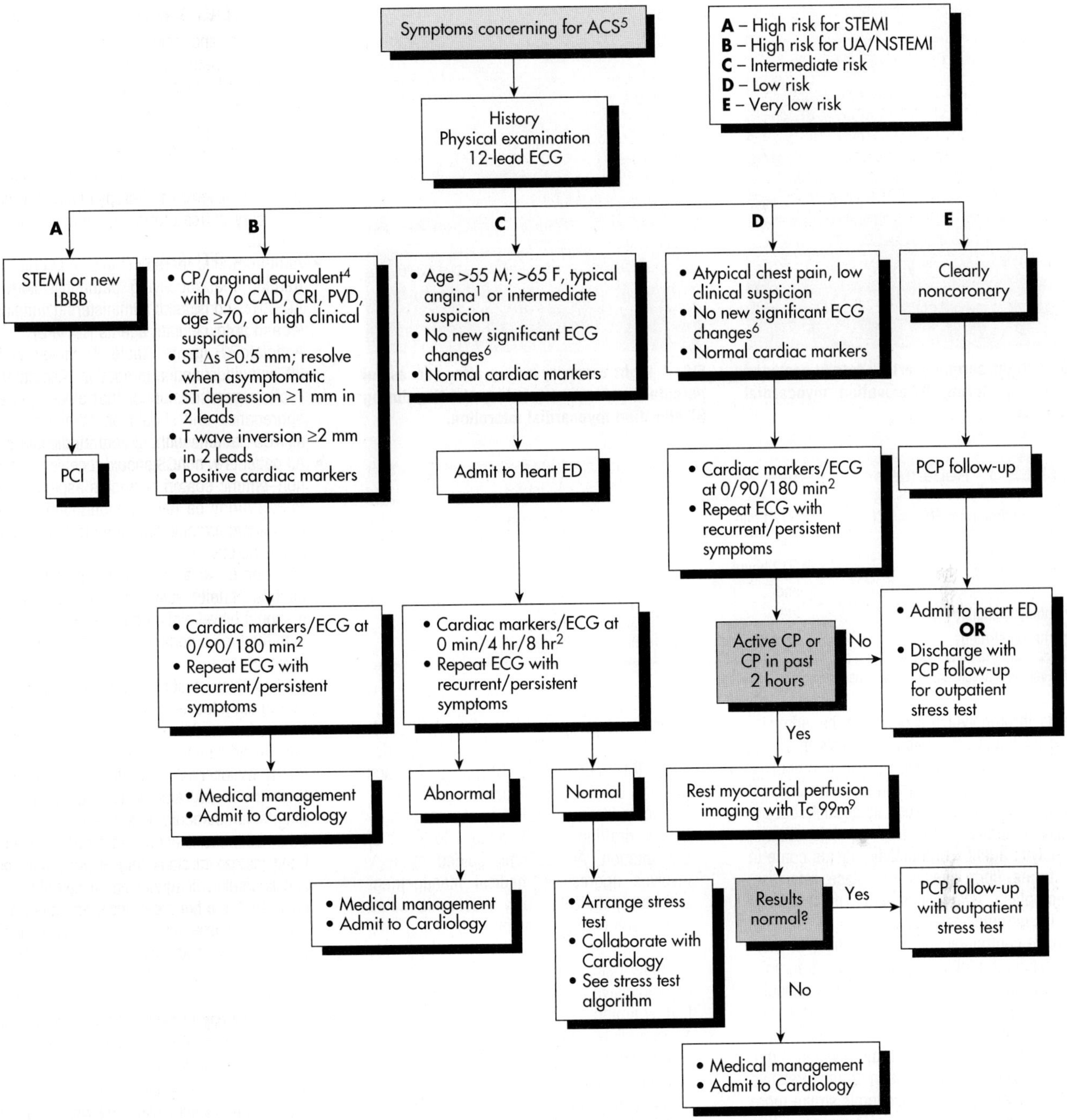

DEFINITIONS:

[1]**Typical angina:**
(1) Substernal chest pain or discomfort that is (2) provoked by exertion or emotional stress and (3) relieved by rest and/or nitroglycerin

[2]**Cardiac marker timing:** Based on symptom onset; in cases of uncertainty assume symptom onset at ED arrival

[3]**ECG normal:** No significant ST depression/T wave inversions, BBB, LVH with repolarization, conduction defect, digoxin effect

[4]**Anginal equivalent:**
- Any symptoms that the physician feels may represent ACS
- Exertional dyspnea—most common anginal equivalent symptom

[5]**ACS:**
- STE-ACS—1 mm ST elevation in 2 leads
- NSTE-ACS
  - NSTEMI—positive cardiac biomarkers
  - Unstable angina—ischemia with negative biomarkers

[6]**New significant ECG changes:**
- ST Δs ≥0.5 mm; resolve when asymptomatic
- ST depression ≥1 mm in 2 leads
- T wave inversion ≥2 mm in 2 leads

[7]**Regadenoson** is preferred agent for chemical nuclear stress test. Technetium Tc-99m tetrofosmin is the preferred tracer.

FIG. 1 Evaluation of patients for acute coronary syndrome *(ACS)*. *CAD*, Coronary artery disease; *CP*, chest pain; *CRI*, chronic renal insufficiency; *ECG*, electrocardiogram; *ED*, emergency department; *h/o*, history of; *LBBB*, left bundle branch block; *NSTE*, non–ST-segment elevation; *NSTEMI*, non–ST-segment elevation myocardial infarction; *PCP*, primary care physician; *PVD*, peripheral vascular disease; *STE*, ST-segment elevation; *STEMI*, ST-segment elevation myocardial infarction; *UA*, unstable angina. (From Adams JG et al: *Emergency medicine, clinical essentials*, ed 2, Philadelphia, 2013, Elsevier.)

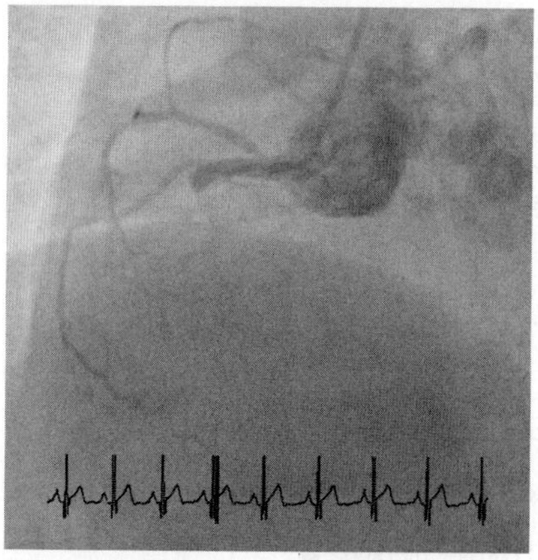

FIG. 3 Right coronary artery totally occluded proximally during ST-elevation myocardial infarction.

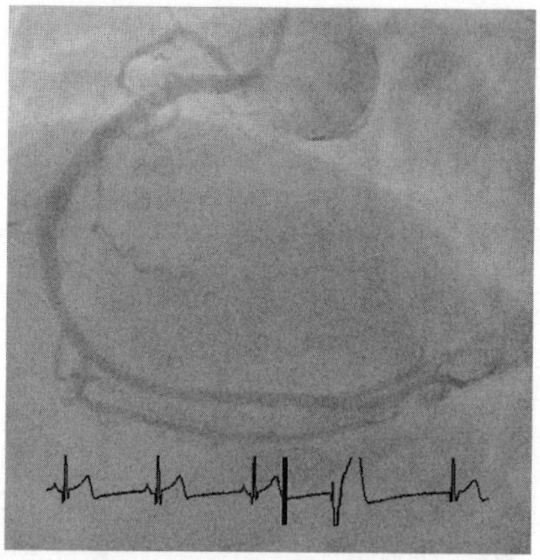

FIG. 4 Right coronary artery after successful percutaneous coronary artery stenting during ST-elevation myocardial infarction.

TABLE 3 Reperfusion Strategies

Anticipated time from FMC to PCI	>120 min	<120 min
	and	or
Symptom duration?	<12 hours	<24 hours
	and	or
Thrombolytic eligible?	YES	NO
Reperfusion strategy	Thrombolytics and transfer	Primary PCI

FMC, First medical contact; *PCI,* percutaneous coronary intervention.

onset; thrombolytics should not be administered 24 hours after initial diagnosis of STEMI (Table 3). In patients who receive thrombolytic agents, coronary angiography can be done at a receiving hospital as soon as possible but not within the first 2 to 3 hr after administration of fibrinolytic agent. Thrombolytic agents come in two forms, fibrin specific (alteplase, reteplase, tenecteplase, staphylokinase) and nonfibrin specific (streptokinase, anistreplase, urokinase). Absolute contraindications to thrombolytic therapy include the following: History of intracranial hemorrhage, known structural cerebral vascular lesion, known intracranial neoplasm, ischemic stroke within 3 mo, suspected aortic dissection, active bleeding, head trauma within 3 mo, or intracranial surgery within 2 mo. Relative contraindications include ischemic stroke more than 3 mo prior, dementia, major surgery within 3 wk, current oral anticoagulant therapy, and traumatic or prolonged CPR. Antithrombotic therapy is needed to reduce thrombus burden, prevent further thrombosis, and improve coronary artery flow.

NONPHARMACOLOGIC THERAPY

- STEMI is a medical emergency and requires immediate reperfusion therapy; the best outcomes are seen with cardiac catheterization with primary PCI. Guidelines call for a goal door-to-balloon time of ≤90 min.
- Patients with NSTE-ACS should be risk stratified in conjunction with the cardiology consult service. Risk scores such as the TIMI and GRACE scores can be used to decide between an early invasive strategy and an ischemia-guided strategy. Overall, an early invasive strategy is associated with better outcomes in patients with higher risk (i.e., TIMI score >3 or GRACE >140) and involves cardiac catheterization followed by revascularization with PCI or coronary artery bypass grafting (CABG) within 4 to 24 hr of presentation. An ischemia-guided strategy involves aggressive medical management and revascularization only if ischemia recurs or is documented on noninvasive testing. This should only be reserved for selected patients with low-risk scores (TIMI score 0 to 2). The early invasive strategy can be further stratified by timing:
  1. Immediate (within 2 hr): Patients with refractory or recurrent angina despite optimal initial treatment, signs or symptoms of heart failure, new or worsening mitral regurgitation, hemodynamic instability, sustained ventricular tachycardia or ventricular fibrillation
  2. Early (within 24 hr): No characteristics from the immediate category but new ST-segment depression, a GRACE risk score >140 or temporal change in troponin
  3. Delayed invasive (25 to 72 hr): None of the immediate or early characteristics but renal insufficiency, left ventricular ejection fraction of <40%, early post-infarct angina, history of PCI within the past 6 mo, prior coronary artery bypass graft, GRACE risk score of 109 to 140, or TIMI score of 2 or more
- Continuous ECG monitoring is recommended for all ACS patients. Supplemental oxygen should be administered to patients with arterial oxygen saturation of less than 90%, respiratory distress, or other high-risk features of hypoxemia. Finger pulse oximetry should be utilized to assess arterial oxygen saturation.

ACUTE GENERAL Rx

- Table 4 is a summary of recommendations for standard medical therapy in the early hospital care phase of management of patients with NSTE-ACS.
- Antithrombotic therapy (Table 5) is critical in treating the underlying pathophysiology of ACS. This consists of administering antiplatelet and anticoagulant agents (Table 6).
- Antiplatelet agents (Table 7) inhibit platelet activation and aggregation. Aspirin is a cyclooxygenase inhibitor that blocks platelet aggregation and should be administered to all ACS patients without contraindications.
- All patients with ACS should receive full-dose non–enteric-coated chewable aspirin of 162 to 325 mg to establish a high blood level for its antiplatelet effects. Thereafter, daily dose of 81 mg should be continued indefinitely.
- Clopidogrel is a thienopyridine agent that inhibits platelet activation and aggregation. It should be administered in all ACS patients, with the timing dependent on the clinical scenario and management strategy. It requires a loading dose of 300 to 600 mg followed by 75 mg daily. It should be discontinued at least 5 days before CABG. If a patient is unable to take aspirin in the setting of hypersensitivity or major gastrointestinal intolerance, a loading dose of clopidogrel followed by daily maintenance should be started.
- Other antiplatelet agents that can be substituted instead of clopidogrel include prasugrel and ticagrelor. Ticagrelor has a half-life of 12 hours with a more rapid onset and more consistent onset of action. There was a reduction in death from vascular causes, MI, and stroke in patients with NSTE-ACS over clopidogrel. This benefit is limited to patients taking aspirin 75 to 100 mg per day. Prasugrel is not recommended as the initial antiplatelet agent in patients with NSTE-ACS. Multiple studies have demonstrated an increase in bleeding in patients taking prasugrel, in particular those who are >75 yr old, low body weight (<60 kg), or with a history of cerebrovascular events. Cangrelor is an IV ADP-P2Y12 receptor antagonist that may be used initially as a load in the emergency department before an invasive strategy, given its initial action and quick platelet recovery time. As a rule, all ACS patients should have two antiplatelet agents initiated and should be continued up to 12 mo regardless of treatment strategy.
- GP IIb/IIIa inhibitors (Table 8) may be considered as an intravenous antiplatelet therapy in addition to aspirin for medium- or high-risk patients with NSTE-ACS in whom an invasive strategy is planned (Class IIb). Eptifibatide and tirofiban are preferred agents over abciximab for NSTE-ACS patients; however, for STEMI patients undergoing primary PCI, IV abciximab has the same Class IIa indication as tirofiban and eptifibatide.

TABLE 4 Summary of Recommendations for Standard Medical Therapy in the Early Hospital Care Phase of Management of Patients With Non–ST-Elevation Acute Coronary Syndromes (NSTE-ACS)

Recommendations	COR	LOE
Oxygen		
Administer supplemental oxygen only with oxygen saturation <90%, respiratory distress, or other high-risk features for hypoxemia.	I	C
Nitrates		
Administer sublingual NTG every 5 min ×3 for continuing ischemic pain and then assess need for IV NTG.	I	C
Administer IV NTG for persistent ischemia, HF, or hypertension.	I	B
Nitrates are contraindicated with recent use of a phosphodiesterase inhibitor.	III: Harm	B
Analgesic Therapy		
IV morphine sulfate may be reasonable for continued ischemic chest pain despite maximally tolerated antiischemic medications.	IIb	B
NSAIDs (except aspirin) should not be initiated and should be discontinued during hospitalization for NSTE-ACS because of the increased risk of MACE associated with their use.	III: Harm	B
Beta-Adrenergic Blockers		
Initiate oral beta blockers within the first 24 hr in the absence of HF, low-output state, risk for cardiogenic shock, or other contraindications to beta blockade.	I	A
Use of sustained-release metoprolol succinate, carvedilol, or bisoprolol is recommended for beta-blocker therapy with concomitant NSTE-ACS, *stabilized* HF, and reduced systolic function.	I	C
Reevaluate to determine subsequent eligibility in patients with initial contraindications to beta blockers.	I	C
It is reasonable to continue beta-blocker therapy in patients with normal LV function with NSTE-ACS.	IIa	C
IV beta blockers are potentially harmful when risk factors for shock are present.	III: Harm	B
Calcium Channel Blockers (CCBs)		
Administer initial therapy with nondihydropyridine CCBs with recurrent ischemia and contraindications to beta blockers in the absence of LV dysfunction, increased risk for cardiogenic shock, PR interval >0.24 sec, or second- or third-degree atrioventricular block without a cardiac pacemaker.	I	B
Administer oral nondihydropyridine calcium antagonists with recurrent ischemia after use of beta blocker and nitrates in the absence of contraindications.	I	C
CCBs are recommended for ischemic symptoms when beta blockers are not successful, are contraindicated, or cause unacceptable side effects.*	I	C
Long-acting CCBs and nitrates are recommended for patients with coronary artery spasm.	I	C
Immediate-release nifedipine is contraindicated in the absence of a beta-blocker.	III: Harm	B
Cholesterol Management		
Initiate or continue high-intensity statin therapy in patients with no contraindications.	I	A
Obtain a fasting lipid profile, preferably within 24 hr.	IIa	C

*Short-acting dihydropyridine calcium channel antagonists should be avoided.

COR, Class of recommendation; *HF*, heart failure; *IV*, intravenous; *LOE*, level of evidence; *LV*, left ventricular; *MACE*, major adverse cardiovascular events; *N/A*, not available; *NSAIDs*, nonsteroidal anti-inflammatory drugs; *NTG*, nitroglycerin.

From Amsterdam EA et al: 2014 AHA/ACC guideline for the management of patients with non–ST-elevation acute coronary syndromes: a report of the American College of Cardiology/American Heart Association task force on practice guidelines, *J Am Coll Cardiol* 64:e139-228, 2014 in Zipes DP: *Braunwald's heart disease, a textbook of cardiovascular medicine*, ed 11, Philadelphia, 2019, Elsevier.

- Anticoagulant agents should be administered to all ACS patients, irrespective of initial treatment strategy. Options include either unfractionated heparin (UFH), or low-molecular-weight heparin (enoxaparin), or factor Xa inhibitors such as fondaparinux, or direct thrombin inhibitors such as bivalirudin (Table 9).
- For STEMI, fondaparinux can be used for anticoagulation. It has been shown to decrease bleeding complications as compared with either UFH or LMWH. However, it should not be used as the sole anticoagulant in PCI because of the risk of catheter thrombosis.
- Bivalirudin is a reversible direct thrombin inhibitor and may be considered as an alternative to UFH and GP IIb/IIIa inhibitors in patients with STEMI who are undergoing primary PCI. When bivalirudin was compared to UFH plus a glycoprotein IIb/IIIa inhibitor in patients with STEMI and PCI, less bleeding and a short- and long-term reduction in cardiac events and overall mortality was observed. With bivalirudin, there is no risk of heparin-induced thrombocytopenia, less bleeding is observed, and the anticoagulant effect can be monitored during intervention by the activated clotting time. Similar results were reported in the use of bivalirudin alone in patients with UA/NSTEMI in the ACUITY trial when compared to enoxaparin/UFH with GP IIb/IIIa arms.
- Beta-blocker therapy reduces ischemia by decreasing myocardial oxygen demand and has a proven long-term mortality benefit. Oral therapy should be initiated within 24 hours of onset of ACS unless signs or symptoms of heart failure and shock are present or bradycardia precludes its use. Oral administration, titrated to a heart rate of 50 to 60 beats/min, is preferred. Intravenous beta-blockers can be administered to STEMI patients who are hypertensive or have ongoing ischemia; they should be avoided if the patients have any of the following:
  1. Signs of heart failure
  2. Evidence of a low output state
  3. Increased risk for cardiogenic shock
  4. Other relative contraindications to beta-blockade (PR interval >0.24 second, second- or third-degree heart block, active asthma, or reactive airway disease)
- Nitroglycerin is a vasodilator that should be administered to relieve chest discomfort in all ACS patients. It can be administered sublingually at first, up to 3 doses, followed by intravenous administration if symptoms persist. In the setting of an inferior STEMI, it is necessary to rule out a right ventricular (RV) infarct with a right-sided ECG before the administration of nitroglycerin. This is because RV infarcts are preload dependent and nitroglycerin decreases preload through venodilation, which leads to hypotension in this setting. This can be corrected by discontinuing nitroglycerin and starting bolus intravenous fluids. Nitrates should not be administered in patients who recently received a phosphodiesterase inhibitor. Nitroglycerin provides no mortality benefit in ACS patients.
- Oxygen should be administered to patients with signs of acute heart failure, cardiogenic shock, or an arterial oxyhemoglobin saturation of less than 90%. The 2014 ACC/AHA guidelines report no demonstrated benefit for routine use of supplemental oxygen in normoxic patients with NSTE-ACS; rather, emerging data suggest that routine use of

TABLE 5 Summary of Recommendations for Antithrombotic Therapy

Recommendations	Dosing, Special Considerations	COR	LOE
Aspirin			
Non–enteric-coated aspirin to all patients promptly after presentation	162-325 mg	I	A
Aspirin maintenance dose continued indefinitely	81-325 mg/day*	I	A
P2Y12 Inhibitors			
Clopidogrel loading dose followed by daily maintenance dose in patients unable to take aspirin	75 mg	I	B
P2Y12 inhibitor, in addition to aspirin, for up to 12 mo for patients treated initially with either an early invasive or initial ischemia-guided strategy:		I	B
• Clopidogrel	300- or 600-mg loading dose, then 75 mg/day		
• Ticagrelor	180-mg loading dose, then 90 mg twice daily		
P2Y12 inhibitor therapy (clopidogrel, prasugrel, or ticagrelor) continued for at least 12 mo in post-PCI patients treated with coronary stents	N/A	I	B
Ticagrelor in preference to clopidogrel for patients treated with an early invasive or ischemia-guided strategy	N/A	IIa	B
Glycoprotein (GP) IIb/IIIa Inhibitors			
GP IIb/IIIa inhibitor in patients treated with an early invasive strategy and DAPT with intermediate/high-risk features (e.g., positive troponin)	Preferred options are eptifibatide or tirofiban	IIb	B
Parenteral Anticoagulant and Fibrinolytic Therapy			
SC enoxaparin for duration of hospitalization or until PCI is performed	1 mg/kg SC every 12 hr (reduce dose to 1 mg/kg/day SC in patients with CrCl <30 ml/min) Initial 30-mg IV loading dose in select patients	I	A
Bivalirudin until diagnostic angiography or PCI is performed in patients with early invasive strategy only	Loading dose 0.10 mg/kg, followed by 0.25 mg/kg/hr Only provisional use of GP IIb/IIIa inhibitor in patients also treated with DAPT	I	B
SC fondaparinux for the duration of hospitalization or until PCI is performed	2.5 mg SC daily	I	B
Administer additional anticoagulant with anti-IIa activity if PCI is performed while patient is on fondaparinux	N/A	I	B
IV UFH for 48 hr or until PCI is performed	Initial loading dose 60 IU/kg (max 4000 IU) with initial infusion 12 IU/kg/hr (max 1000 IU/hr) Adjusted to therapeutic APTT range	I	B
IV fibrinolytic treatment not recommended in patients with NSTE-ACS	N/A	III: Harm	A

*The recommended maintenance dose of aspirin to be used with ticagrelor is 81 mg daily.[10]

APTT, Activated partial thromboplastin time; *COR,* class of recommendation; *CrCl,* creatinine clearance; *DAPT,* dual antiplatelet therapy; *IV,* intravenous; *LOE,* level of evidence; *max,* maximum; *N/A,* not available; *NSTE-ACS,* non–ST-elevation acute coronary syndromes; *PCI,* percutaneous coronary intervention; *SC,* subcutaneous; *UFH,* unfractionated heparin.

Modified from Amsterdam EA et al: 2014 AHA/ACC guideline for the management of patients with non–ST-elevation acute coronary syndromes: a report of the American College of Cardiology/American Heart Association task force on practice guidelines, *J Am Coll Cardiol* 64:e139-228, 2014, in Zipes DP: *Braunwald's heart disease, a textbook of cardiovascular medicine,* ed 11, Philadelphia, 2019, Elsevier.

oxygen can lead to adverse effects such as increased coronary vascular resistance, reduced coronary blood flow, and increased mortality rate.

- Morphine can be used intravenously in patients with NSTE-ACS if there is continued ischemic chest pain despite treatment with maximally tolerated antiischemic medications (Class IIb).
- Calcium channel blockers (nondihydropyridine) may be used in patients with persisting or recurrent symptoms, despite treatment with beta-blockers and nitroglycerin. They work by having negative inotropic and chronotropic effects and causing coronary vasodilation. They are especially useful when beta-blockers are contraindicated and in patients with coronary artery spasm. Calcium channel blockers should not be used in cases of severe LV dysfunction, pulmonary edema, increased risk for cardiogenic shock or advanced heart blocks.
- Patients routinely taking nonsteroidal anti-inflammatory drugs (NSAIDs) (except for aspirin), both nonselective as well as COX-2 selective agents, before ACS should discontinue those agents at the time of presentation because of the increased risks of mortality, reinfarction, hypertension, heart failure, and myocardial rupture associated with their use.
- Angiotensin-converting enzyme (ACE) inhibitors may be added and should be used within 24 hr of onset of ACS in all patients with depressed LV function (ejection fraction [EF] <40%) and those with a history of hypertension, diabetes mellitus, or stable chronic kidney disease. Angiotensin receptor blockers (ARBs) should be used in patients who are ACE inhibitor intolerant.
- Table 10 summarizes indications and cautions for adjunctive medical therapies for patients with ST-elevation myocardial infarction.
- Refer to topic "Cocaine Overdose" for treatment of cocaine-related ACS.

CHRONIC Rx

- Post-ACS medical therapy involves aspirin, statin, beta-blocker, and a second antiplatelet agent such as clopidogrel, ticagrelor, or prasugrel.
- In patients already on an oral anticoagulant for another diagnosis such as atrial fibrillation, the duration of triple therapy should be minimized. Strategies aimed at minimizing the risk of bleeding in patients treated with triple therapy (dual antiplatelet therapy and an oral anticoagulant) are summarized in Table 11. The WOEST trial showed that using clopidogrel along with an oral anticoagulant but without aspirin resulted in a significant reduction in bleeding complications with those patients on a triple therapy of oral anticoagulant, aspirin, and clopidogrel. It is a class IIB recommendation in those patients with atrial fibrillation and a CHADS-VASC score of 2 or greater after coronary revascularization to consider using clopidogrel concurrently with oral anticoagulant (Table 12) but without aspirin. Similarly, the AUGUSTUS trial in 2019 demonstrated that triple therapy (ASA, P2Y12 inhibitor, DOAC, or warfarin) was associated with substantial increases in bleeding without improved thrombotic

TABLE 6 2014 Guideline Recommendations for Antithrombotic Agents in Patients With Non–ST-Elevation Acute Coronary Syndromes

Antiplatelet Therapy

Non–enteric-coated, chewable aspirin (162-325 mg) should be given to all patients without contraindications on presentation, and a maintenance dose of aspirin (81-325 mg/day) continued indefinitely.

In patients who are unable to take aspirin because of hypersensitivity or major gastrointestinal intolerance, a loading dose of clopidogrel (300 or 600 mg) followed by a daily maintenance dose of 75 mg should be substituted.

Either clopidogrel or ticagrelor can be used initially with either an early invasive or ischemic guided strategy (COR I, LOE: B).

Ticagrelor may be preferred over clopidogrel as the initial treatment (COR IIa, LOE: B).

In patients treated with ticagrelor, the preferred aspirin maintenance dose is 81 mg/day.

Use prasugrel only in patients receiving coronary stents (COR I, LOE: B).

The use of glycoprotein IIb/IIIa receptor inhibitors is reserved mainly to the time of PCI in high-risk patients who were not adequately pretreated with P2Y12 inhibitors (COR I, LOE: A) or in those patients who were adequately pretreated with P2Y12 inhibitors but have a high-risk profile (COR IIa, LOE: B).

Clopidogrel and ticagrelor should be discontinued at least 5 days (COR I, LOE: B) and prasugrel at least 7 days (COR I, LOE: C) before major surgery.

Anticoagulant Therapy

Enoxaparin is recommended at presentation (COR I, LOE: A); other options include unfractionated heparin (UFH) (COR I, B) and fondaparinux (COR I, LOE: B). If an early invasive strategy is planned, bivalirudin (COR I, LOE: B) is also an option.

If fondaparinux is used initially, add UFH or bivalirudin just before or during PCI to prevent catheter-related thrombosis (COR I, LOE: B).

Bivalirudin is preferred over UFH plus GP IIb/IIIa inhibitor in patients undergoing PCI who are at high risk of bleeding (COR IIa, LOE: B).

It is reasonable to use enoxaparin during PCI if it was used as the initial anticoagulant (COR IIb, LOE: B).

COR, Class of recommendation; *LOE,* level of evidence; *PCI,* percutaneous coronary intervention.

Modified from Eisen A, Giugliano RP: Antiplatelet and anticoagulation treatment in patients with non–ST-segment elevation acute coronary syndrome: comparison of the updated North American and European guidelines, *Cardiol Rev* 24:170-6, 2016; and Amsterdam EA et al: 2014 AHA/ACC guideline for the management of patients with non–ST-elevation acute coronary syndromes: a report of the American College of Cardiology/American Heart Association Task Force on Practice Guidelines, *J Am Coll Cardiol* 64: e139-228, 2014, in Zipes DP: *Braunwald's heart disease, a textbook of cardiovascular medicine,* ed 11, Philadelphia, 2019, Elsevier.

TABLE 7 Pharmacologic Characteristics of Oral Antiplatelet Drugs Commonly Used in the Management of Acute Coronary Syndromes

		ADP Receptor Antagonists		
Characteristic	**Aspirin**	**Clopidogrel**	**Prasugrel**	**Ticagrelor**
Class	COX inhibitor	Thienopyridine (second generation)	Thienopyridine (third generation)	Cyclopentyl triazolopyrimidine
Target	COX-1	P2Y12	P2Y12	P2Y12
Dose	162- to 325-mg loading dose; 75-325mg/day maintenance dose	300- to 600-mg loading dose; 75mg/day maintenance dose	60-mg loading dose; 10mg/day maintenance dose	180-mg loading dose; 90 mg bid maintenance dose
Prodrug	No	Yes	Yes	No
Time to effect[a]	<1 hr	4-6 hr[b]	<1 hr	<1 hr
Drug half-life	20 min	Minutes	Minutes	12 hr
Reversible	No	No	No	Yes

ADP, Adenosine diphosphate; bid, twice daily; *COX,* cyclooxygenase.

[a]After loading dose

[b]Increased antithrombotic benefit was seen after the first hour in patients enrolled in the COMMIT trial who did not receive a loading dose, but maximum effect is not seen until after 4-6 hr.

From Hoffman R et al: *Hematology, basic principles and practice,* ed 7, Philadelphia, 2018, Elsevier.

protection compared with P2Y12 inhibitor and oral anticoagulation alone.

- Lipid lowering with statins has been evaluated in trials such as the MIRACL study, in which high-dose atorvastatin 80 mg reduced death, MI, and cardiac events at 16 wk when administered early, within 24 to 96 hr after an ACS. The A-Z trial and PROVE IT-TIMI 22 trials demonstrated benefit of early high-intensity statin therapy with LDL targets <70 mg/dl in ACS.
- ACE inhibitors may be added to treat hypertension and should be used in all patients with depressed LV function (EF <40%) or pulmonary vascular congestion. ARBs should be used in patients who are ACE inhibitor intolerant.
- An aldosterone blocker should be used in post-MI patients without significant renal dysfunction (creatinine >2.5 mg/dl in men or creatinine >2.0 mg/dl in women) or hyperkalemia (K >5.0 mEq/L) who have an ejection fraction of less than 40% and are already on therapeutic doses of an ACE inhibitor and a beta-blocker.
- Cardiac rehabilitation and a monitored exercise program should be recommended at the time of discharge.
- Aggressive risk factor management, including smoking cessation, weight loss, diet and exercise, diabetes control, and so on, for secondary prevention of future events is crucial.

REFERRAL

- All ACS patients should be cared for in conjunction with the cardiology consult service.
- When appropriate, referral to a cardiac surgeon may be necessary for CABG and heart team approach.
- At the time of discharge, patients should be referred for cardiac rehabilitation.

PEARLS & CONSIDERATIONS

COMMENTS

- ACS is common and a leading cause of mortality in the U.S.
- The diagnosis hinges on the basics—history and physical, ECG, biomarkers, and CXR.
- Remember the potentially fatal non-ACS causes of chest discomfort, which include acute pulmonary embolism and acute ascending aortic dissection.
- STEMI patients presenting to a hospital with PCI capability should be treated with primary PCI within 90 min of first medical contact.
- STEMI patients presenting to a hospital without PCI capability and who cannot be transferred to a PCI center and undergo PCI within 120 min of first medical contact should be

TABLE 8 Pharmacologic Characteristics of Intravenous Antiplatelet Drugs Used in the Management of Acute Coronary Syndrome

	GP IIb/IIIa Inhibitors			ADP Receptor Antagonists
Characteristic	**Abciximab**	**Eptifibatide**	**Tirofiban**	**Cangrelor**
Class	Fab fragment	Nonpeptide	Cyclic heptapeptide	Nonthienopyridine
Onset	Rapid	Rapid	Rapid	Rapid
Drug half-life	10-30 min	2 hours	2.5 hours	3-6 min
Reversibility of platelet inhibition	Slow	Rapid	Rapid	Rapid
Excretion	Unknown	40%-70% renal	50% renal	Dephosphorylation

ADP, Adenosine diphosphate; *GP,* glycoprotein.
From Hoffman R et al: *Hematology, basic principles and practice,* ed 7, Philadelphia, 2018, Elsevier.

TABLE 9 Pharmacologic Characteristics of Parenteral Anticoagulants Commonly Used in the Management of Patients With Acute Coronary Syndromes

	Unfractionated Heparin	**Enoxaparin**	**Bivalirudin**	**Fondaparinux**
Route of administration	IV	SC (first dose IV[a])	IV	SC (first dose IV[a])
Frequency of dosing	Continuous IV infusion	Twice daily; once daily if CrCl <30 ml/min	Continuous IV infusion	Once-daily injection
Clearance	Primarily nonrenal	Renal	Renal, proteolytic cleavage	Renal
Use in ACS patients with moderate renal impairment	Yes	Yes (dose reduction)	Yes (dose reduction)	Yes[b]
Use in ACS patients undergoing dialysis	Yes	No experience	Yes (dose reduction)	No experience[c]
Routine laboratory monitoring	Yes	No	No[d]	No
Dose	Adjust dose according to the results of the aPTT	Fixed weight adjusted	Fixed weight adjusted	Fixed
Accumulation in renal failure	No	Yes	Yes	Yes
Nonanticoagulant side effects	Allergy, HIT	HIT (rare)	—	—
Nonbleeding contraindications	Allergy, immune HIT	Allergy, immune HIT	Allergy	Allergy
Antidote	Protamine sulfate	Protamine sulfate partially reverses	No	No

ACS, Acute coronary syndromes; *aPTT,* activated partial thromboplastin time; *CrCl,* creatinine clearance; *HIT,* heparin-induced thrombocytopenia; *IV,* intravenous; *SC,* subcutaneous.
[a]The first dose of enoxaparin was given by the intravenous route in the TIMI-11B (Thrombolysis In Myocardial Infarction 11B) and EXTRACT-TIMI 25 (Enoxaparin and Thrombolysis Reperfusion for Acute Myocardial Infarction Treatment, Thrombolysis in Myocardial Infarction 25) studies. The first dose of fondaparinux was given by the intravenous route in the OASIS-6 (Optimal Antiplatelet Strategy for Interventions 6) trial.
[b]Acute coronary syndrome patients with creatinine up to 265 μmol/L were eligible for inclusion in the OASIS-5 and -6 trials (equivalent to an estimated creatinine clearance of 15-20 ml/min in a 70-kg patient who is 70 yr of age).
[c]Fondaparinux is contraindicated in patients with venous thromboembolism who have severe renal impairment.
[d]Monitoring and dose adjustment required in patients with creatinine clearance below 30 ml/min.
From Hoffman R et al: *Hematology, basic principles and practice,* ed 7, Philadelphia, 2018, Elsevier.

TABLE 10 Indications and Cautions for Adjunctive Medical Therapies for Patients With ST-Elevation Myocardial Infarction

Therapy	Indications	Cautions
Beta-adrenergic receptor–blocking agents	Oral: All patients without contraindication IV: Patients with refractory hypertension or ongoing ischemia without contraindication	Signs of congestive heart failure Low-output state Increased risk for cardiogenic shock Prolonged first-degree or high-grade atrioventricular block Reactive airways disease
Angiotensin-converting enzyme (ACE) inhibitors	Anterior myocardial infarction and LVEF ≤0.40 or congestive heart failure All patients without contraindication	Hypotension Renal failure Hyperkalemia
Angiotensin receptor–blocking agents (ARBs)	Intolerant of ACE inhibitors	Hypotension Renal failure Hyperkalemia
Statins	All patients without contraindications	With drugs metabolized via CYP3A4, fibrates Monitor for myopathy, hepatotoxicity Adjust dose for lipid targets
Nitroglycerin	Ongoing chest pain Hypertension and congestive heart failure	Suspected right ventricular infarction SBP <90 (or 30 mm Hg below baseline) Recent use of a type 5 PDE inhibitor
Oxygen	Clinically significant hypoxemia (Spo_2 <90) Congestive heart failure Dyspnea	Chronic obstructive pulmonary disease and CO_2 retention
Morphine	Pain Anxiety Pulmonary edema	Lethargic or moribund patient Hypotension Bradycardia Known hypersensitivity

IV, Intravenous; *LVEF,* left ventricular ejection fraction; *PDE,* phosphodiesterase; *SBP,* systolic blood pressure.
From Zipes DP: *Braunwald's heart disease, a textbook of cardiovascular medicine,* ed 11, Philadelphia, 2019, Elsevier.

TABLE 11 Strategies Aimed at Minimizing the Risk of Bleeding in Patients Treated With Triple Therapy (Dual Antiplatelet Therapy and an Oral Anticoagulant)

Proposed Approach	Rationale
Aspirin maintenance dose ≤100 mg/day	Higher aspirin maintenance doses increase bleeding, and there is no evidence that they improve efficacy.
PPI with a preference for agents that interfere less with CYP 2C19 (e.g., pantoprazole)	Much of the excess bleeding is from the GI tract. The use of acid-suppressive agents that interfere less with CYP 2C19 minimizes the potential for a negative interaction with clopidogrel.
Preference for a non–vitamin K antagonist oral anticoagulant	Dabigatran 110 mg twice daily and apixaban 2.5 or 5.0 mg twice daily are associated with lower rates of bleeding than warfarin.
For warfarin, use a target INR of 2-2.5	Some evidence that a restricted target INR range reduces the risk of bleeding.
Manage warfarin in a specialized anticoagulation clinic	Compared with usual care, specialist clinics achieve a higher TTR of the INR.
Minimize duration of triple therapy	The risk of bleeding is highest during the first 30 days but remains elevated with long-term treatment.
Avoid NSAIDs	NSAIDs are a common cause of upper GI bleeding.
Avoid prasugrel and ticagrelor	Prasugrel and ticagrelor cannot be recommended because they are more potent than clopidogrel and cause more bleeding.

CYP, Cytochrome P-450; *GI,* gastrointestinal; *INR,* international normalized ratio; *NSAID,* nonsteroidal antiinflammatory drug; *PPI,* proton pump inhibitor; *TTR,* time in therapeutic range.
From Hoffman R et al: *Hematology, basic principles and practice,* ed 7, Philadelphia, 2018, Elsevier.

TABLE 12 Pharmacological Characteristics of Warfarin and New Oral Anticoagulants Evaluated in Phase III Trials for the Long-Term Management of Acute Coronary Syndromes

Characteristic	Warfarin	Rivaroxaban	Apixaban
Target	VKORC1	Factor Xa	Factor Xa
Prodrug	No	No	No
Bioavailability (%)	100	80	60
Dosing	Variable, once daily	Fixed, 2.5 or 5 mg twice daily[a]	Fixed, 5 mg twice daily (2.5 mg twice daily in selected patients)
Half-life	Mean: 40 hr (range: 20-60 hr)	7-11 hr	12 hr
Renal clearance (%)	Nil	66[b]	25
Routine coagulation monitoring	Yes (INR)	No	No
Drug interactions	Multiple	Potent inhibitors of CYP3A4 and P-gp[c]	Potent inhibitors of CYP3A4 and P-gp[c]
Antidote	Yes (vitamin K, PCC, FFP)	Yes (Andexanet alfa)	Yes (Andexanet alfa)
Approved for ACS management	Yes	Yes, in Europe	No

ACS, Acute coronary syndromes; *CYP3A4,* cytochrome P-450 3A4; *FFP,* fresh frozen plasma; *fXa,* activated factor X; *INR,* international normalized ratio; *PCC,* prothrombin complex concentrates; *P-gp,* P-glycoprotein; *VKORC1,* C1 subunit of vitamin K epoxide reductase. Strategies Aimed at Minimizing the Risk of Bleeding in Patients Treated with Triple Therapy (Dual Antiplatelet Therapy and an Oral Anticoagulant).

[a]A once-daily regimen was tested in atrial fibrillation.

[b]Half of renally cleared rivaroxaban is cleared as unchanged drug and half as inactive metabolites.

[c]Potent inhibitors of both CYP3A4 and P-glycoprotein include azole antifungals (e.g., ketoconazole, itraconazole, voriconazole, posaconazole) and protease inhibitors, such as ritonavir. Potent inhibitors of CYP3A4 include azole antifungals, macrolide antibiotics (e.g., clarithromycin) and protease inhibitors (e.g., atazanavir).

From Hoffman R et al: *Hematology, basic principles and practice,* ed 7, Philadelphia, 2018, Elsevier.

treated with fibrinolytic therapy within 30 min of hospital presentation unless fibrinolytic therapy is contraindicated.

- Refer to topics "Angina Pectoris" and "Myocardial Infarction" for additional discussion of this subject matter.

SUGGESTED READINGS

Available at ExpertConsult.com

RELATED CONTENT

Acute Coronary Syndrome (Patient Information)

Angina Pectoris (Related Key Topic)
Coronary Artery Disease (Related Key Topic)
Myocardial Infarction (Related Key Topic)
Hypertension (Related Key Topic)

AUTHORS: **Vasken Keleshian, MD,** and **Pranav M. Patel, MD, FACC, FAHA, FSCAI**

BASIC INFORMATION

DEFINITION

Acute disseminated encephalomyelitis (ADEM) is an acquired demyelinating syndrome that is often believed to be post-infectious in origin and most predominant in the pediatric population. ADEM is a clinical syndrome associated with acute-onset widespread CNS inflammation. Current diagnostic criteria for ADEM include acute polyfocal neurologic deficits with the presence of encephalopathy and is supported by multifocal areas of increased T2 signal in the brain. ADEM is typically a monophasic illness. Some children experience evolution of new deficits within 90 days of onset, which is considered to represent a single ADEM event. New attacks, more than 90 days apart, can include a second ADEM event (multiphasic ADEM, MDEM), or more localized demyelination such as optic neuritis, transverse myelitis, or demyelination of other CNS regions. Chronic relapsing disease can also occur, including neuromyelitis optica spectrum disorder (NMOSD), relapsing myelin oligodendrocyte glycoprotein (MOG)-associated disease (MOGAD), or multiple sclerosis (MS). Acute hemorrhagic leukoencephalitis (AHLE) is considered a more acute variant of ADEM that typically presents with similar symptoms and neurologic signs as ADEM but with a more rapidly progressive course and has multifocal hemorrhages found on imaging.

SYNONYMS

ADEM
Postinfectious encephalomyelitis

ICD-10CM CODE
G04.0 Acute disseminated encephalitis and encephalomyelitis

EPIDEMIOLOGY & DEMOGRAPHICS

ADEM is most prevalent in school-aged children, with a mean age range at onset of 5 to 8 yr. ADEM may manifest in adulthood with a poorer prognosis relative to pediatric ADEM. ADEM is associated with preceding infection in most patients, and thus the higher frequency of infectious illness in childhood is thought to contribute to the greater likelihood of ADEM occurring in this age group. Recent comprehensive studies have not demonstrated associations between ADEM and current common vaccines.

INCIDENCE: 0.1 to 0.6 per 100,000 per yr

PREVALENCE: Prevalence studies are not available given the transient nature of this illness in the vast majority of patients.

PREDOMINANT SEX & AGE: Between 5 and 8 yr old with a slight male predominance

PEAK INCIDENCE: Winter and spring

RISK FACTORS: Preceding infection

GENETICS: Genetic studies have failed to demonstrate genetic mutations, single nucleotide polymorphisms, or human leukocyte antigen associations for sporadic ADEM.

PHYSICAL FINDINGS & CLINICAL PRESENTATION

- Many patients have fever due to a primary infectious source in the weeks preceding signs and symptoms of a demyelinating episode.
- Pediatric ADEM:
  1. A child with ADEM may first present with headache, vomiting, vision changes, gait disturbances, meningismus, and potentially seizures (seen in 1/3 of patients).
  2. The hallmark and required core symptom, as its name suggests, is encephalopathy, ranging from irritability and confusion to lethargy and coma.
  3. The spinal cord may also be affected (transverse myelitis) (Fig. 1) with resultant motor and sensory deficits as well as potential bowel and bladder dysfunction.
  4. Cranial neuropathies may be present, including optic neuritis.
  5. The progression of disease is typically very rapid and aggressive, often requiring ICU monitoring.
- Adult ADEM:
  1. No consensus on diagnostic criteria have been made to this date, but the criteria listed for pediatric patients are generally applied.
  2. Typically worse prognosis in adults compared to children.

ETIOLOGY

There is a strong suggestion that ADEM is expressed in close proximity to recent infections, most commonly ones with URI symptoms. Like other post-infectious inflammatory conditions, it has been postulated that ADEM is the result of molecular mimicry, but definitive proof is lacking.

In animal models for acquired autoimmune demyelinating diseases, Experimental Autoimmune Encephalitis (EAE), exposure of animals to myelin protein antigens, as well as an external stimulant of cell-mediated immunity (Freund's adjuvant), leads to a T cell and macrophage-mediated inflammatory infiltration and resultant demyelination. While there are many parallels between EAE and human ADEM, myelin-reactive immune cells are not easily measured nor conclusively found in the human disease, and it is not clear whether ADEM has a definitive triggering antigen exposure.

DIAGNOSIS

DIFFERENTIAL DIAGNOSIS

- Neuromyelitis optica spectrum disorder (NMOSD)
- Myelin Oligodendrocyte Glycoprotein Associated disorder (MOGAD)
- Multiple sclerosis (MS)
- Meningitis
- Brain mass
- Acute hemorrhagic leukoencephalitis (AHLE)
- CNS vasculitis
- Hemophagocytic lymphohistiocytosis (HLH)
- Inborn errors of metabolism or Mitochondrial Encephalopathy

WORKUP

- ADEM is a clinical diagnosis.
- As ADEM can either be a monophasic illness or the first manifestation of more chronic demyelinating conditions such as MS, the workup is largely centered on obtaining biomarkers for such conditions. These biomarkers are most sensitive early in the course of illness.

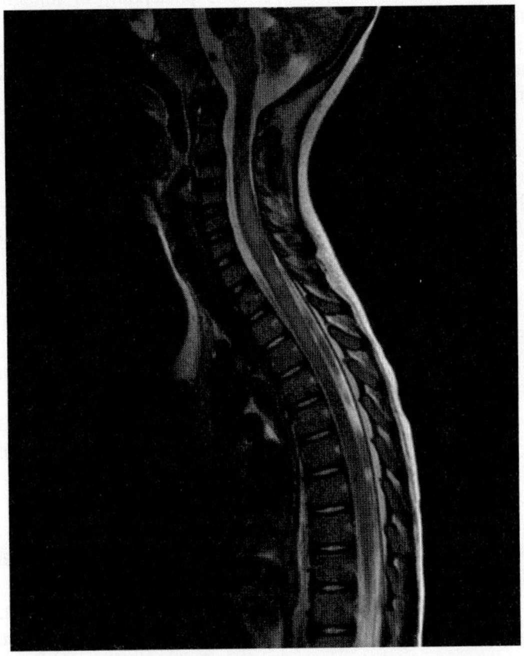

FIG 1 A 5-yr-old boy. Spinal cord sagittal T2 demonstrating extensive hyperintensities extending several spinal segments in length in the cervical and thoracic cord, consistent with longitudinally extensive transverse myelitis (LETM) in the setting of ADEM. The spinal cord is affected in one-third of ADEM patients.

Acute Disseminated Encephalomyelitis (ADEM)

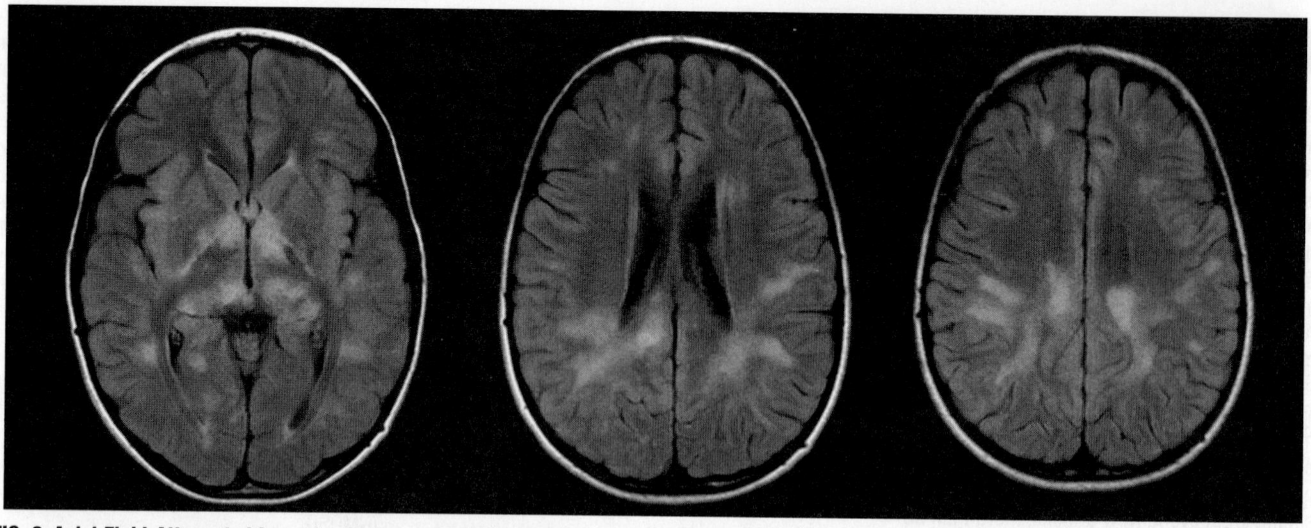

FIG. 2 Axial Fluid-Attenuated Inversion Recovery (FLAIR) images demonstrating multifocal areas of increased signal in the deep gray nuclei and in the white matter bilaterally. Lesions are "flame-like" and ill-defined.

LABORATORY TESTS

- No known marker exists for ADEM, but laboratory studies are focused on ruling out other conditions, such as a first presentation of a more chronic demyelinating condition such as MS or NMOSD or acute infection such as meningoencephalitis.
- CSF analysis:
  1. Pleocytosis due to inflammation is expected.
  2. Oligoclonal bands are rarely seen in ADEM. They are a nonspecific finding and can be found in the context of neuroimmune conditions such as multiple sclerosis, as well as in patients with antibody-associated neuroinflammatory conditions. Oligoclonal bands are also present in some intracerebral infections, as well as in some rheumatologic conditions.
- Serum studies:
  1. Oligoclonal bands: You must have paired CSF and serum in order to evaluate oligoclonal bands. The positive test is defined by the presence of >2 bands (IgG) in CSF not present in serum.
  2. Anti-MOG IgG: About half of all cases of ADEM are MOG-Ab positive, whereas almost all cases of MDEM are MOG-Ab positive.
  3. Anti-AQP4 IgG: A biomarker for NMOSD. The presence of these autoantibodies with either optic neuritis or transverse myelitis meets criteria for diagnosis of NMOSD.

IMAGING STUDIES

- Head CT is often obtained upon initial presentation to exclude other causes of neurologic disease such as space-occupying lesions. CT brain is relatively insensitive to white matter changes and can miss the features of ADEM. Brain and spine MRI with and without contrast is indicated:
  1. Brain MRI typically demonstrates disseminated T2 and FLAIR hyperintense lesions throughout the supratentorial or infratentorial white matter, the cerebral cortex, the deep gray matter, the brain stem, optic nerves. and the spinal cord.
  2. Lesions are bilateral, large, poorly demarcated and diffuse (Fig. 2).
  3. Follow-up MRI shows improvement and resolution of lesions several months following an episode of monophasic ADEM.

Rx TREATMENT

ICU admission and monitoring is required in a large percentage of patients in the setting of a rapidly progressive course, seizures, marked encephalopathy, or ventilatory dysfunction due to spinal cord or brainstem lesions.

NONPHARMACOLOGIC THERAPY

Appropriate ICU interventions in the case of increased intracranial pressure, severe encephalopathy or in ADEM patients with severe seizures.

ACUTE GENERAL Rx

- Acute anti-inflammatory therapy with intravenous corticosteroids (methylprednisolone 30 mg/kg/day, maximum of 1000 mg/day) for 3 to 5 days
- Intravenous immunoglobulin (IVIG, 2 grams/kg total divided over 2 to 5 days) or 5 to 7 plasma exchanges (PLEX) are offered to children failing to improve with corticosteroids

CHRONIC Rx

- Most patients respond to 3 to 5 days of acute corticosteroid therapy and do not require corticosteroid taper.
- Long-term steroids are not indicated, even if MOG antibodies are present.
- Chronic immunomodulatory therapy is required for children diagnosed with NMOSD, relapsing MOGAD or MS. Selection of immunomodulatory therapies should be in conjunction with pediatric neuroimmune experts.

COMPLEMENTARY & ALTERNATIVE MEDICINE

Vitamin D insufficiency is commonly noted in children with ADEM (and other CNS inflammatory disorders), and it is clinical practice to ensure adherence with nutritional recommendations for vitamin D supplementation in children (typically 400 to 1000 IU per day vitamin D3).

DISPOSITION

ICU admission and monitoring is required in a large percentage of patients in the setting of a rapidly progressive course, seizures, marked encephalopathy, or ventilatory dysfunction due to spinal cord or brainstem lesions.

REFERRAL

Neurology consultation and referral is indicated.

PEARLS & CONSIDERATIONS

COMMENTS

Relapses of ADEM or new lesions on MRI is not consistent with monophasic ADEM and instead suggests either multiphasic ADEM, MOG-associated disease, NMOSD, or MS.

SUGGESTED READINGS

Available at ExpertConsult.com

AUTHORS: **Dennis Keselman, MD,** and **Brenda Banwell, MD**

BASIC INFORMATION

DEFINITION

Acute glomerulonephritis (GN) is inflammation of the glomeruli, usually caused by deposition of immunoreactants. Clinically, patients present with blood and protein in the urine and high blood pressure. If untreated, chronic glomerular inflammation leads to progressive chronic kidney disease.

SYNONYMS

Acute nephritic syndrome
Glomerulonephritis, acute GN

ICD-10CM CODES	
N00.0	Acute nephritic syndrome with minor glomerular abnormality
N00.1	Acute nephritic syndrome with focal and segmental glomerular lesions
N00.2	Acute nephritic syndrome with diffuse membranous glomerulonephritis
N00.3	Acute nephritic syndrome with diffuse mesangial proliferative glomerulonephritis
N00.4	Acute nephritic syndrome with diffuse endocapillary proliferative glomerulonephritis
N00.5	Acute nephritic syndrome with diffuse mesangiocapillary glomerulonephritis
N00.6	Acute nephritic syndrome with dense deposit disease
N00.7	Acute nephritic syndrome with diffuse crescentic glomerulonephritis
N00.8	Acute nephritic syndrome with other morphologic changes
N00.9	Acute nephritic syndrome with unspecified morphologic changes

EPIDEMIOLOGY & DEMOGRAPHICS

- Incidence of primary glomerulonephritis (GN) varies between 0.2/100,000 cases per patient-year and 2.5/100,000 per patient-year.
- Immunoglobulin A (IgA) nephropathy is the most common form of glomerulonephritis worldwide.
- GN accounts for 23% of end-stage kidney disease cases worldwide.
- GN affects adults and children.

PHYSICAL FINDINGS & CLINICAL PRESENTATION

- Acute onset of hypertension.
- Dark, "tea-colored" urine.
- Edema (peripheral, periorbital, or pulmonary).
- Fatigue.
- Concurrent pulmonary hemorrhage and rapidly progressive decline in kidney function may indicate antineutrophil cytoplasmic antibody (ANCA) vasculitis or anti-glomerular basement membrane (anti-GBM) disease.
- Joint pains, oral ulcers, and malar rash are frequently seen with systemic lupus erythematosus (SLE).
- Palpable purpura may be seen in patients with systemic vasculitides such as IgA vasculitis (formerly, Henoch-Schönlein purpura), ANCA-associated vasculitis, SLE, or cryoglobulinemia.
- A recent history of endocarditis, cellulitis, or pharyngitis preceding urinary abnormalities may indicate infection-related glomerulonephritis.
- Hepatitis C virus infection may cause membranoproliferative glomerulonephritis (MPGN) with or without cryoglobulinemia.
- Concurrent upper respiratory tract infection (synpharyngitic infection) and gross hematuria may indicate IgA nephropathy.
- Table 1 summarizes the clinical and laboratory features of the different causes of rapidly progressive glomerulonephritis.

ETIOLOGY

- Acute GN may occur as a renal-limited disease or part of a systemic disorder. A description of target antigens is included in Table E2.
- In the past decade, the knowledge of the pathogeneses of several acute GNs has greatly expanded.
- IgA nephropathy is considered a multi-hit process that involves under-galactosylated IgA1, development of antiglycan antibodies, and deposition of immune complexes in the kidney.
- Post-streptococcal GN is now part of the broader category termed infection-related glomerulonephritis that includes IgA-dominant *Staphylococcus*-associated GN. ANCA-associated vasculitis is associated with antibodies to myeloperoxidase and proteinase 3, although not all studies have supported direct disease causation.
- Hepatitis C causes chronic immune stimulation and production of cryoglobulins that deposit in the kidney.
- Paraproteins, which are components of or whole immunoglobulins, may deposit in the kidney and cause a variety of glomerular lesions. When these paraproteins are not associated with a hematologic malignant condition, the kidney condition is termed monoclonal gammopathy of renal significance (MGRS).
- C3 glomerulopathy, composed of C3 glomerulonephritis and dense deposit disease, is caused by dysregulation of the alternative complement pathway. The alternative complement pathway is now implicated in several different GNs, including IgA nephropathy and ANCA-associated vasculitis. Identification of complement activation in these disorders portends future treatment implications.
- Thrombotic microangiopathy in the native kidney is caused by endothelial damage that can be triggered by drugs, autoimmune diseases (e.g., atypical HUS, antiphospholipid antibody disease, lupus), infection, and primary genetic disorders.
- Pathologic features of immune glomerular diseases are summarized in Table E3.

Dx DIAGNOSIS

DIFFERENTIAL DIAGNOSIS FOR HEMATURIA AND/OR PROTEINURIA, IN ADDITION TO ACUTE GLOMERULONEPHRITIS

- Urinary tract infection
- Nephrolithiasis
- Urothelial malignancy
- Polycystic kidney disease
- Acute interstitial nephritis
- Acute tubular necrosis
- Nephrotic syndrome
- Hereditary nephritis (Alport syndrome and thin basement membrane nephropathy)
- Diabetic nephropathy

WORKUP

Initial evaluation of suspected glomerulonephritis consists of laboratory testing.

LABORATORY TESTS

- Urinalysis, with albuminuria (majority of proteinuria in glomerulonephritis is albuminuria) and hematuria (dysmorphic erythrocytes and red cell casts).
- Blood urea nitrogen and serum creatinine to estimate glomerular filtration rate (GFR).
- 24-hour urine collection for total protein excretion (includes albumin plus tubular proteins) and creatinine clearance to document degree of renal dysfunction and accuracy of urine collection. Random urine (spot) specimen for evaluation of the protein-to-creatinine ratio instead of a 24-hour collection is also acceptable. Proteinuria in acute glomerulonephritis typically ranges from 500 mg/day to 3 gram/day, but nephrotic-range proteinuria (>3.5 g/day) may be present.
- Streptococcal tests (Streptozyme) and antistreptolysin O (ASO) quantitative titer (highest in 3 to 5 wk). The ASO titer is not related to severity of kidney disease, duration, or prognosis.
- Additional serologic testing, including antinuclear antibody (ANA), antibody directed against double-stranded DNA (anti-dsDNA), C3, C4, hepatitis B and C viral serologies, HIV, ANCA (myeloperoxidase and proteinase-3 antigens), anti-glomerular basement membrane (GBM) antibodies, cryoglobulins, rheumatoid factor, serum and urine protein electrophoresis with immunofixation, and serum free light chain analysis.
- Hematocrit and platelet count are decreased in thrombotic microangiopathies, although these parameters may be normal in renal-limited thrombotic microangiopathy.
- Blood cultures are obtained from any febrile patient.

IMAGING STUDIES

- Chest radiograph: If opacities are present, consider diffuse alveolar hemorrhage as occurs with ANCA-associated vasculitis and anti-GBM disease (Goodpasture disease).
- Renal ultrasound to exclude structural causes of hematuria and proteinuria. A kidney size of <9 cm in sagittal length may indicate extensive scarring and a low likelihood of reversibility.
- Echocardiogram in patients with new cardiac murmurs or positive blood cultures to rule out endocarditis and pericardial effusion.
- Kidney biopsy with light, electron, and immunofluorescence microscopy.
- Biopsy of other affected organs if systemic vasculitis is suspected.

TABLE 1 Clinical and Laboratory Features in the Different Causes of Rapidly Progressive Glomerulonephritis

Disease	Typical Clinical Features	Serologic Findings	Complement Levels	Immune Deposits in Glomerulus on Renal Biopsy
Vasculitis				Few/pauci-immune
Granulomatosis with polyangiitis (formerly, Wegener granulomatosis)	Prodrome of nasal stuffiness, blocked ears, arthralgia; then onset of hemoptysis, purpura, peripheral neuropathy	C-ANCA	Normal or increased	
Microscopic polyangiitis	Similar to granulomatosis with polyangiitis (Wegener granulomatosis) or affecting the kidneys only (renal-limited) or overlap with polyarteritis nodosa	P-ANCA	Normal or increased	
Anti-GBM disease	Macroscopic hematuria and hemoptysis	Anti-GBM antibodies	Normal or increased	Linear staining for IgG and C3
SLE (diffuse proliferative, WHO Class IV)	Previous history of SLE, marked hematuria and proteinuria, hypertension "telescoping" urinary sediment	ANA, anti-dsDNA antibodies	Low C3, low C4	Granular immune deposits
IgA disease	Persistent microscopic hematuria with episodes of synpharyngitic macroscopic hematuria, with proteinuria, hypertension	IgA (increased in about half of cases)	Normal or increased	
Poststreptococcal glomerulonephritis	At 1-3 wk after streptococcal pharyngitis or impetigo, macroscopic hematuria, edema, hypertension, oliguria	ASO, anti-DNase B antibodies	Low C3, normal C4	

ANA, Antinuclear antibody; *anti-DNase B,* anti-deoxyribonuclease B antibody; *anti-dsDNA,* anti–double-stranded DNA antibody; anti-GBM, glomerular basement membrane antibody; *ASO,* antistreptolysin O antibody; *C-ANCA,* cytoplasmic antineutrophil cytoplasmic antibody; *IgA,* immunoglobulin A; *IgG,* immunoglobin G; *P-ANCA,* perinuclear antineutrophil cytoplasmic antibody; *SLE,* systemic lupus erythematosus; *WHO,* World Health Organization.
From Ronco C et al: *Critical care nephrology,* ed 3, Philadelphia, 2019, Elsevier.

Rx TREATMENT

NONPHARMACOLOGIC THERAPY

- Low-sodium (i.e., 2 gram sodium) diet if edema or hypertension is present
- Avoidance of high-potassium foods if patient is hyperkalemic

ACUTE GENERAL Rx

- Diuretics if edema or hypertension is present.
- Correction of electrolyte abnormalities (hypocalcemia, hyperkalemia) and metabolic acidosis.
- High-dose steroids (1 mg/kg per day) for rapidly progressive glomerulonephritis.
- Additional immunosuppressive treatment with alkylating agents, calcineurin inhibitors, antimetabolites, or biologic agents may be required depending on the underlying disease.
- Treatment of streptococcal infection with penicillin (or erythromycin in penicillin-allergic patients). Hemodialysis in patients with diuretic-resistant volume overload, refractory hyperkalemia, uremic symptoms, and severe metabolic acidosis. Plasma exchange therapy for antibody removal in cases of diffuse alveolar hemorrhage or rapidly progressive glomerulonephritis is not considered a standard evidence-based treatment but is frequently considered a therapeutic option.

CHRONIC Rx

- Periodic monitoring of blood pressure, urinalysis, serum creatinine and blood urea nitrogen, serum albumin, and random urine protein-to-creatinine ratio.
- Angiotensin–converting-enzyme (ACE) inhibitors or angiotensin II type 1 receptor blockers (ARBs) to reduce proteinuri
- Lipid management with statins and fibrates as indicated
- Monitor for side effects related to immunosuppression such as infection, leukopenia and anemia, osteoporosis or osteopenia, gastrointestinal ulcers, high blood pressure, and tumors
- Routine health maintenance with vaccinations for influenza and *Pneumococcus*, age-appropriate vaccinations, and age-appropriate malignancy screening. Live vaccines are contraindicated in patients treated with immunosuppressants

DISPOSITION

- Prognosis is generally correlated to initial serum creatinine and degree of fibrosis on kidney biopsy.
- In general, prognosis is worse in patients with heavy albuminuria/proteinuria, low GFR at presentation, severe hypertension, and kidney biopsy-proven crescentic glomerulonephritis with high degree of crescents.

REFERRAL

Nephrology consultation for all patients with suspected glomerulonephritis. Urgent consultation is recommended if hyperkalemia, acidosis, or azotemia is present.

PEARLS & CONSIDERATIONS

COMMENTS

- Diagnosis of acute GN is established by kidney biopsy if the biopsy results influence the treatment plan, especially with systemic illnesses; significant proteinuria (>500 mg to 1000 mg per day); or increasing serum creatinine. Exploration for systemic illness, including infections, autoimmune disease, and malignancy is required along with careful history, physical examination, and serologic tests. Some patients with suspected GN may not require a kidney biopsy because of the success of supportive therapies (e.g., infection-related GN).
- Nephrology consultation should be obtained before initiating immunosuppressive therapy. ACE inhibitor or ARB therapy is essential for proteinuria reduction, unless contraindicated. Spironolactone has been added to ACE inhibitor treatment for greater proteinuria reduction.
- Periodic monitoring for side effects of immunosuppressive drugs and complications of corticosteroids is necessary.
- Monitor lipids and treat persistent hyperlipidemia.

SUGGESTED READINGS

Available at ExpertConsult.com

RELATED CONTENT

Glomerulonephritis (Patient Information)
Acute Kidney Injury (Related Key Topic)

AUTHOR: **Rupali Avasare, MD**

BASIC INFORMATION

DEFINITION

Acute kidney injury (AKI) is defined as a rapid impairment in kidney function that results in oliguria and retention of products in the blood normally excreted by the kidneys. The decline in kidney function can result in volume overload and dysregulation of acid-base status and electrolytes. Current consensus criteria for diagnosis of AKI requires an increase in serum creatinine of 0.3 mg/dl within 48 hr or 1.5 times baseline serum creatinine over 7 days, and/or a decline in urine in output to <0.5 ml/kg/hr for 6 to 12 hr. AKI is further graded by severity as described in Table 1.

SYNONYMS

AKI
Acute renal failure (ARF)
Acute kidney failure

ICD-10CM CODES

N17.0 Acute kidney failure with tubular necrosis
N17.1 Acute kidney failure with acute cortical necrosis
N17.2 Acute kidney failure with medullary necrosis
N17.8 Other acute kidney failure
N17.9 Acute kidney failure, unspecified
N99.0 Postprocedural (acute) (chronic) kidney failure
O90.4 Postpartum acute kidney failure

EPIDEMIOLOGY & DEMOGRAPHICS

- An estimated 20% of hospitalized patients and 60% of intensive care unit patients develop AKI.
- AKI occurs in 20% of patients with moderate sepsis and in >50% of patients with septic shock and positive blood cultures.
- Greater than 40% of hospital-associated AKI is iatrogenic.
- AKI in hospitalized patients is associated with increased hospital length-of-stay and cost.
- Most common cause of AKI in hospitalized patients is from intrinsic kidney failure due to acute tubular necrosis (ATN).
- Key risk factors for AKI include older age, preexisting chronic kidney disease, diabetes mellitus, and/or preexisting proteinuria.

PHYSICAL FINDINGS & CLINICAL PRESENTATION

- Early or mild AKI is frequently asymptomatic.
- Frequent presenting symptoms include weakness, anorexia, generalized malaise, and nausea.
- Patients may develop oliguric or nonoliguric kidney injury.
- Oliguria is defined as <400 to 500 ml of urine per 24 hr. Anuria is frequently seen in ATN or bilateral obstructive uropathy.
- Physical examination should focus on evaluation of volume status and systemic signs of kidney injury.
- Findings vary with duration and rapidity of onset of renal failure and underlying cause of AKI.
- Peripheral edema from volume overload, heart failure, liver failure, or nephrotic syndrome.
- Pulmonary edema.
- Cardiac dysrhythmias.
- Neurologic findings include altered mental status, delirium, lethargy, myoclonus, seizures, and asterixis.
- Pruritus, uremic odor.
- Flank pain.
- Painless hematuria may be seen with glomerulonephritis, whereas painful hematuria is more consistent with obstructive uropathy.
- Pericardial effusion and/or pericardial rub.
- Fever, skin rash, and arthralgia can be seen with systemic vasculitis.
- Classic triad of fever, rash, and eosinophilia in the setting of AKI strongly implicates allergic interstitial nephritis (AIN). However, the simultaneous appearance of all three manifestations occur in only 30% of cases. When AIN is considered the cause of AKI, a careful review of medications is required.

ETIOLOGY

- **Prerenal:** Inadequate renal perfusion caused by hypovolemia, congestive heart failure (impaired cardiac output), cirrhosis (fluid third-spacing), sepsis (vasodilation), abdominal compartment syndrome, or other. Sixty percent of community-acquired cases of AKI are due to prerenal conditions.
- **Postrenal:** Bladder outlet obstruction (prostatic enlargement, urethral fibrosis), ureteral obstruction (stones, bladder masses, retroperitoneal fibrosis, ureteral fibrosis), or renal vein occlusion. With two functioning kidneys, bilateral obstruction is usually required to produce significant AKI. Postrenal causes of AKI account for 5% to 15% of community-acquired AKI.
- **Intrinsic renal:** ATN, glomerulonephritis, AIN. Common causes of ATN include ischemia (e.g., hypotension or shock, postcardiac bypass, or aorta surgery), rhabdomyolysis, sepsis, drug toxicity (e.g., aminoglycosides, amphotericin, cisplatin), and iodinated radiocontrast-induced nephropathy. Contrast-induced nephropathy is the third-most common cause of new-onset AKI in hospitalized patients. However, most of these cases have multiple confounding factors and are better characterized as contrast-associated nephropathy. AIN can develop following exposure to medications, most commonly nonsteroidal anti-inflammatory drugs, antibiotics, and proton pump inhibitors. Microvascular diseases that cause AKI include thrombotic microangiopathies (e.g., thrombotic thrombocytopenic purpura, classical and atypical hemolytic uremic syndrome, or preeclampsia) and cholesterol emboli.
- Causes of AKI are listed in Table 2
- Nearly one third of AKI cases may be prevented or mitigated

TABLE 1 Kidney Disease: Improving Global Outcomes (KDIGO) Criteria for Diagnosis of Acute Kidney Injury

AKI Definition and Staging

Stage	Serum Creatinine Criteria	Urine Output Criteria
1	ΔS_{Cr} ≥0.3 mg/dl (30 μmol/L) or S_{Cr} ≥1.5, <2.0 × baseline*	UO <0.5 ml/kg per hr × 6-12 hr
2	S_{Cr} >2.0, <3.0 × baseline	UO <0.5 ml/kg per hr >12 hr
3	S_{Cr} >3.0 × baseline or	
	S_{Cr} ≥4.0 mg/dl with an acute rise ≥0.5 mg/dl (50 μmol/L) or on renal replacement therapy	UO <0.3 ml/kg per hr × 24 hr or anuria × 12 hr

AKI, Acute kidney injury; *S_{Cr},* serum creatinine; *UO,* urinary output.
*To fulfill AKI criteria, an S_{Cr} rise of ≥0.3 mg/dl must occur within 48 hr; or increase to ≥1.5 times baseline SCr is known or presumed to have occurred within previous 7 days.
Adapted from KDIGO Clinical Practice Guideline for Acute Kidney Injury, 2012.

Dx DIAGNOSIS

Table 3 summarizes useful clinical features, urinary findings, and confirmatory tests in the differential diagnosis of AKI.

DIFFERENTIAL DIAGNOSIS

Refer to "Etiology." Diagnostic tests to distinguish prerenal and renal AKI are described in Table 4. A diagnostic approach to patients with suspected AKI is shown in Fig. 1.

LABORATORY TESTS

- Elevated serum creatinine.
- Standard estimating equations for glomerular filtration rate (GFR) require steady-state creatinine levels and are not recommended to estimate GFR during AKI.
- Elevated blood urea nitrogen (BUN): BUN-to-creatinine ratio is commonly >20:1 in prerenal azotemia, postrenal azotemia, and acute glomerulonephritis.
- BUN-to-creatinine ratio is <20:1 in acute interstitial nephritis and ATN.
- Hyperkalemia, hyperphosphatemia, and metabolic acidosis are common.
- Hypocalcemia and hyponatremia or hypernatremia may occur, depending on etiology.
- Urinalysis is the initial diagnostic evaluation. Prerenal and postrenal AKI are typically characterized by a normal urinalysis. Conversely, abnormal findings should prompt further work-up for specific intrinsic causes of AKI that may require intervention. Hematuria and proteinuria imply glomerulonephritis, heavy (>3+) proteinuria is associated with nephrotic syndrome, and

TABLE 2 Etiologies of Acute Kidney Injury

Prerenal Causes (Decreased Renal Blood Flow)	Intrinsic Renal Causes	Postrenal Causes
Hypovolemia Renal losses (diuretics, osmotic agents, polyuria) Gastrointestinal losses (vomiting, diarrhea) Cutaneous losses (burns, exfoliative syndromes) Hemorrhage Pancreatitis **Decreased Cardiac Output** Congestive heart failure Pulmonary embolism Acute myocardial infarction Severe valvular heart disease Abdominal compartment syndrome Renal artery obstruction (stenosis, embolism, thrombosis, dissection) **Systemic Vasodilation** Sepsis Anaphylaxis Anesthetics Drug overdose **Afferent Arteriolar Vasoconstriction** Hypercalcemia Drugs (NSAIDs, amphotericin B, calcineurin inhibitors, norepinephrine, radiocontrast agents, aminoglycosides) Hepatorenal syndrome Efferent arteriolar vasodilation (angiotensin converting enzyme inhibitors, aldosterone receptor blockers)	**Vascular: Large and Small Vessels** Trauma Renal vein obstruction (thrombosis, ventilation with high-level PEEP, abdominal compartment syndrome) Microangiopathy (thrombotic thrombocytopenic purpura, hemolytic-uremic syndrome, disseminated intravascular coagulation, preeclampsia) Malignant hypertension Scleroderma renal crisis Transplant rejection Atheroembolic disease **Glomerular** Antiglomerular basement membrane disease (Goodpasture syndrome) Antineutrophil cytoplasmic antibody-associated glomerulonephritis (Wegener granulomatosis) Immune complex glomerulonephritis, systemic lupus erythematosus, postinfectious cryoglobulinemia, primary membranoproliferative glomerulonephritis **Tubular** Ischemic Cytotoxic Heme pigment (rhabdomyolysis, intravascular hemolysis) Crystals (tumor lysis syndrome, seizures, ethylene glycol poisoning, vitamin C megadose, acyclovir, indinavir, methotrexate) Drugs (aminoglycosides, lithium, amphotericin B, pentamidine, cisplatin, ifosfamide, radiocontrast agents), synthetic cannabinoid use **Interstitial** Drugs (penicillins, cephalosporins, NSAIDs, proton pump inhibitors, allopurinol, rifampin, indinavir, mesalamine, sulfonamides, trimethoprim) Infection (pyelonephritis, viral infection) **Systemic Disease** Sjögren syndrome, sarcoidosis, systemic lupus erythematosus, lymphoma, leukemia, tubulonephritis, uveitis	**Ureteral Obstruction** Calculus Tumor (intrinsic or extrinsic) Fibrosis Ligation during pelvic surgery **Bladder Neck Obstruction** Benign prostatic hypertrophy Prostate cancer Neurogenic bladder Tricyclic antidepressants Ganglionic blockers Bladder tumor Calculus Hemorrhage/clot **Urethral Obstruction** Strictures Tumor Phimosis Renal calcinosis Obstructed urinary catheter, ureteral stent, or ileal conduit Pelvic trauma, retroperitoneal hematoma

NSAIDs, Nonsteroidal antiinflammatory drugs; *PEEP,* positive end-expiratory pressure.
Modified from Cameron JL, Cameron AM: *Current surgical therapy,* ed 10, Philadelphia, 2011, Saunders.

leukocyturia may signify AIN. Microscopic examination of urine sediment may facilitate diagnosis: Granular casts in ATN, dysmorphic red blood cells or red blood cell casts in acute glomerulonephritis, and white blood cell casts in AIN.

- In oliguric patients, obtain urine sodium and creatinine concentrations for determination of fractional excretion of sodium: $FE_{Na} = 100\% \times (U_{Na} \times P_{Cr})/(P_{Na} \times U_{Cr})$. FE_{Na} <1% is occurs in prerenal AKI and is >1% in intrinsic AKI. FE_{Na} may be falsely elevated in patients taking diuretics or falsely low in several intrinsic renal conditions, including acute glomerulonephritis, contrast-induced nephropathy, and rhabdomyolysis.
- Fractional excretion of urea (FE_{Urea}) can be used to assess renal dysfunction in AKI. FE_{Urea} is more useful than FE_{Na} during diuretic therapy. FE_{Urea} is calculated as follows: $FE_{Urea} = 100\% \times (U_{Urea} \times P_{Cr}) / (P_{Urea} \times U_{Cr})$. If FE_{Urea} <35% prerenal acute kidney injury is likely, and if FE_{Urea} >50% intrinsic AKI is likely.
- Urinary osmolarity range of 250 mOsm/kg H_2O to 300 mOsm/kg H_2O in ATN (isosthenuria), <400 mOsm/kg H_2O in postrenal azotemia, and >500 mOsm/kg H_2O in prerenal azotemia and acute glomerulonephritis.
- In suspected glomerulonephritis (GN) (e.g., hematuria plus proteinuria), additional serologic testing may be warranted. Abnormal liver function tests and elevated inflammatory markers are nonspecific. Immune complex deposition disorders (e.g., infectious GN, lupus nephritis, cryoglobulinemic vasculitis) are characterized by decreased complement (C3, C4) levels. Specific testing includes antinuclear antibodies (lupus), antineutrophil cytoplasmic antibodies (ANCA-associated vasculitis), antiglomerular basement membrane antibodies (Goodpasture disease), and cryoglobulins. Kidney biopsy is frequently required for diagnostic confirmation.
- Creatinine phosphokinase level is indicated if rhabdomyolysis is suspected; positive blood reaction on a urine dipstick with typically few or no red blood cells by microscopy may indicate myoglobinuria from rhabdomyolysis.
- Serum free light chain analysis, serum and urine protein electrophoresis, and serum and urine immunofixation electrophoresis for suspected multiple myeloma or other plasma cell dyscrasias. Myeloma can cause AKI via a variety of mechanisms, including tubular precipitation of filtered light chains (cast nephropathy), hypercalcemia, and amyloidosis, among others.
- Kidney biopsy may be indicated in patients with intrinsic kidney failure when considering specific therapy. The major indications for kidney biopsy include the following: Differential diagnosis of nephrotic syndrome, distinguishing lupus vasculitis from other vasculitides, distinguishing lupus membranous nephropathy from idiopathic membranous nephropathy, confirmation of hereditary nephropathies based on ultrastructure, diagnosis of rapidly progressive glomerulonephritis, distinguishing AIN from ATN, and separation of primary glomerulonephritides. In addition to establishing a diagnosis, biopsy may determine renal prognosis and guide direction of management. Severe interstitial fibrosis is associated with poor renal outcomes.
- Biomarkers of kidney injury have been explored for earlier diagnosis of AKI or to separate intrinsic from prerenal causes. Candidate markers include cystatin C, neutrophil gelatinase-associated lipocalin (NGAL), kidney-injury molecule 1 (KIM-1), liver fatty acid binding protein (LFABP), and the product of tissue inhibitor of metalloproteinase-2 and insulin-like growth-factor binding protein-7 (TIMP2*IGFBP7), the first biomarker of AKI risk prediction approved in the U.S. However,

TABLE 3 Useful Clinical Features, Urinary Findings, and Confirmatory Tests in the Differential Diagnosis of Acute Kidney Injury

Cause of Acute Kidney Injury	Some Suggestive Clinical Features	Typical Urinalysis Results	Some Confirmatory Tests
Prerenal azotemia	Evidence of true volume depletion (thirst, postural or absolute hypotension and tachycardia, low jugular venous pressure, dry mucous membranes and axillae, weight loss, fluid output greater than input) or decreased effective circulatory volume (e.g., heart failure, liver failure), treatment with NSAID, diuretic, or ACE inhibitor/ARB	Hyaline casts FE_{Na} <1% U_{Na} <10 mmol/L SG >1.018	Occasionally requires invasive hemodynamic monitoring; rapid resolution of AKI with restoration of renal perfusion
Diseases Involving Large Renal Vessels			
Renal artery thrombosis	History of atrial fibrillation or recent myocardial infarction, nausea, vomiting, flank or abdominal pain	Mild proteinuria Occasionally RBCs	Elevated LDH level with normal transaminase levels, renal arteriogram, MAG3 renal scan, MRA*
Atheroembolism	Usually age >50 yr, recent manipulation of aorta, retinal plaques, subcutaneous nodules, palpable purpura, livedo reticularis	Often normal Eosinophiluria Rarely casts	Eosinophilia, hypocomplementemia, skin biopsy, renal biopsy
Renal vein thrombosis	Evidence of nephrotic syndrome or pulmonary embolism, flank pain	Proteinuria, hematuria	Inferior venacavogram, Doppler flow studies, MRV*
Diseases of Small Renal Vessels and Glomeruli			
Glomerulonephritis or vasculitis	Compatible clinical history (e.g., recent infection), sinusitis, lung hemorrhage, rash or skin ulcers, arthralgias, hypertension, edema	RBC or granular casts, RBCs, white blood cells, proteinuria	Low complement levels; positive antineutrophil cytoplasmic antibodies, anti-glomerular basement membrane antibodies, anti-streptolysin O antibodies, anti-DNase, cryoglobulins; renal biopsy
HUS/TTP	Compatible clinical history (e.g., recent gastrointestinal infection, cyclosporine, anovulants), pallor, ecchymoses, neurologic findings	May be normal, RBCs, mild proteinuria, rarely RBC or granular casts	Anemia, thrombocytopenia, schistocytes on peripheral blood smear, low haptoglobin level, increased LDH, renal biopsy
Malignant hypertension	Severe hypertension with headaches, cardiac failure, retinopathy, neurologic dysfunction, papilledema	May be normal, RBCs, mild proteinuria, rarely RBC casts	LVH by echocardiography or ECG, resolution of AKI with BP control
Ischemic or Nephrotoxic Acute Tubular Necrosis			
Ischemia	Recent hemorrhage, hypotension, surgery often in combination with vasoactive medication (e.g., ACE inhibitor, NSAID)	Muddy-brown granular or tubular epithelial cell casts FE_{Na} >1%, U_{Na} >20 mmol/L SG ≈1.010	Clinical assessment and urinalysis usually inform diagnosis
Exogenous toxin	Recent contrast medium-enhanced procedure; nephrotoxic medications; certain chemotherapeutic agents often with coexistent volume depletion, sepsis, or chronic kidney disease	Muddy-brown granular or tubular epithelial cell casts FE_{Na} >1%, U_{Na} >20 mmol/L SG ≈1.010	Clinical assessment and urinalysis usually inform diagnosis
Endogenous toxin	History suggestive of rhabdomyolysis (coma, seizures, drug abuse, trauma)	Urine supernatant tests positive for heme in absence of RBCs	Hyperkalemia, hyperphosphatemia, hypocalcemia, increased CK, myoglobin
	History suggestive of hemolysis (recent blood transfusion)	Urine supernatant pink and tests positive for heme in absence of RBCs	Hyperkalemia, hyperphosphatemia, hypocalcemia, hyperuricemia, and free circulating hemoglobin
	History suggestive of tumor lysis (recent chemotherapy), myeloma (bone pain), or ethylene glycol ingestion	Urate crystals, dipstick-negative proteinuria, oxalate crystals, respectively	Hyperuricemia, hyperkalemia, hyperphosphatemia (for tumor lysis); circulating or urinary monoclonal protein (for myeloma); toxicology screen, acidosis, osmolal gap (for ethylene glycol)
Diseases of the Tubulointerstitium			
Allergic interstitial nephritis	Recent ingestion of drug and fever, rash, loin pain, or arthralgias	White blood cell casts, white blood cells (frequently eosinophiluria), RBCs, rarely RBC casts, proteinuria (occasionally nephritic)	Systemic eosinophilia, renal biopsy
Acute bilateral pyelonephritis	Fever, flank pain and tenderness, toxic state	Leukocytes, occasionally white blood cell casts, RBCs, bacteria	Urine and blood cultures
Postrenal AKI	Abdominal and flank pain, palpable bladder	Frequently normal, hematuria if stones, prostatic hypertrophy	Plain abdominal radiography, renal ultrasonography, postvoid residual bladder volume, computed tomography, retrograde or antegrade pyelography

ACE, Angiotensin-converting enzyme; *AKI,* acute kidney injury; *ARB,* angiotensin receptor blocker; *BP,* blood pressure; *CK,* creatine kinase; *DNase,* deoxyribonuclease; *ECG,* electrocardiography; FE_{Na}, fractional excretion of sodium; *HUS,* hemolytic uremic syndrome; *LDH,* lactate dehydrogenase; *LVH,* left ventricular hypertrophy; *MAG3,* mercaptoacetyltriglycine; *MRA,* magnetic resonance angiography; *MRV,* magnetic resonance venography; *NSAID,* nonsteroidal antiinflammatory drug; *RBC,* red blood cell; *SG,* specific gravity; *TTP,* thrombotic thrombocytopenic purpura; U_{Na}, urinary sodium concentration.

*Contrast-enhanced MRA and MRV should be used with extreme caution in patients with AKI.

From Skorecki K et al: *Brenner & Rector's the kidney,* ed 10, Philadelphia, 2016, Elsevier.

TABLE 4 Diagnostic Tests to Distinguish Between Prerenal and Renal Acute Kidney Injury

Index	Prerenal Causes	Renal Causes
FE_{Na}	<1%	>2%
Urine sodium	<10 mmol/L	>40 mmol/L
Urine/plasma osmolality	>1.5	1 to 1.5
Renal failure index	<1	>2
BUN/creatinine ratio	>20	<10

BUN, Blood urea nitrogen; *FE_{Na},* fractional excretion of sodium. Calculation of FE_{Na}: (Urine sodium × Plasma creatinine)/(Plasma sodium × Serum creatinine) ×100. Renal failure index: (Urine sodium × Urine creatinine)/Plasma creatinine.
From Cameron JL, Cameron AM: *Current surgical therapy,* ed 10, Philadelphia, 2011, Saunders.

there remains little published experience with this test, and the clinical role remains undefined.

IMAGING STUDIES

- ECG for arrhythmia detection, especially in hyperkalemia: Peaked T waves in precordial leads, widening QRS interval, and/or bradycardia with AV node blockade
- Chest radiograph to detect signs of congestive heart failure and pulmonary renal syndromes, which frequently present with alveolar hemorrhage (Goodpasture disease, ANCA-associated vasculitis)
- Bladder scan to assess postvoid residual urine when urinary obstruction is suspected
- Kidney ultrasonography to determine kidney sizes (distinguishes acute from chronic kidney disease), presence of obstruction, and renal vascular status (Doppler study)

Rx TREATMENT

Management of AKI depends on the underlying etiology. Some conditions (e.g., glomerulonephritis) require specific therapy. The general focus of treatment for established AKI is supportive care and limiting additional injury. Fig. 2 illustrates an algorithm for management of AKI.

NONPHARMACOLOGIC THERAPY

- Withdraw nephrotoxic medications.
- Evaluate volume status and correct hypovolemia. Goal of therapy is to increase cardiac output and improve tissue perfusion.
- Avoid excessive fluid administration in patients who are non-volume responsive.
- Dietary modification: (1) Energy prescription of 29 to 36 Kcal/kg per day, (2) potassium restriction (60 mmol per day), (3) sodium restriction (90 mmol per day), (4) phosphorus restriction (<800 mg per day), and (5) high biological value protein 1.2 g/kg per day depending on requirement for dialysis.
- Daily weight to monitor for fluid retention (in addition to intake and output measurement).
- Modification of drug dosages or schedules of renally excreted medications. Dosing should consider the trajectory of renal function (during evolving and recovering AKI) and may require additional adjustments in patients who require dialysis.

ACUTE GENERAL Rx

- Correct electrolyte abnormalities and metabolic acidosis
- Administer loop diuretics for volume overload
- Administer vasopressors for circulatory shock or vasodilators, when appropriate, to optimize cardiac output in congestive heart failure.

Specific treatment is variable and depends on cause of AKI:

- Prerenal: IV volume expansion with isotonic solutions in hypovolemic patients or those with shock. Balanced crystalloid solutions are preferable.
- Intrinsic kidney failure: Discontinue all potential nephrotoxins and treat condition(s) causing kidney failure. In severe AIN cases, consider a trial of corticosteroids. For acute noninfectious glomerulonephritis, high-dose pulse corticosteroids are first-line therapy, typically in conjunction with other immunomodulatory therapy and plasma exchange, depending on the clinical scenario.
- Postrenal: Eliminate cause of obstruction. Immediate bladder catheter insertion for suspected bladder outlet obstruction. Percutaneous nephrostomy tubes or ureteral stents may be required for upper tract obstruction.
- Hyperkalemia-related ECG changes: IV (intravenous) calcium if electrocardiographic changes present; IV insulin and/or glucose to shift potassium into cells; and IV bicarbonate therapy when metabolic acidosis is present to shift potassium into cells. These three treatments are temporary, and definitive therapy requires potassium removal via the gastrointestinal tract (cation exchangers) or urinary tract by diuretics or dialytic therapy.

Dialysis in AKI:

- General indications for initiation of dialysis during AKI:
  1. Uremic symptoms (encephalopathy, pericarditis)
  2. Extracellular fluid volume overload refractory to medical management
  3. Severe acid-base derangement(s) refractory to medical management
  4. Significant electrolyte derangement(s) (e.g., hyperkalemia, hyponatremia) refractory to medical management
- Among critically ill patients, kidney replacement therapy may be required despite an absence of other indications. Optimal timing of initiation of dialysis remains controversial and is not solely dependent on previous metabolic parameters. Multiple recent clinical trials have not shown that early dialysis in AKI is beneficial.
- Intermittent hemodialysis (IHD) and continuous renal replacement therapy (CRRT) have similar outcomes for patients with AKI. However, CRRT is associated with greater hemodynamic stability and fluid removal compared to conventional IHD. CRRT is employed in critically ill patients with hemodynamic instability.

ADJUNCTIVE Rx

- Monitoring of renal function parameters and electrolytes.
- Renally excreted drugs are adjusted according to creatinine clearance or glomerular filtration rate to prevent further kidney damage or other medication-related toxicities.
- Prevent further renal insult with appropriate volume expansion, particularly before contrast administration, and avoid nephrotoxic agents. Volume expansion with isotonic solutions is more effective than hydration with hypotonic solutions. Isotonic saline or bicarbonate-containing solutions are effective. N-acetylcysteine does not increase the benefit of prophylactic crystalloid infusion.
- Renal function recovery (ability to discontinue dialysis) varies from 50% to 75% in AKI survivors. Preexisting CKD, longer duration of dialysis dependence, congestive heart failure, and older age are negative prognostic factors for renal function recovery.
- Overall mortality rate in AKI is nearly 25% and approaches 50% to 60% in patients who require acute dialysis.
- The combination of AKI and sepsis is associated with a mortality rate as high as 70%.

PEARLS & CONSIDERATIONS

- Patients with AKI are susceptible to infections and sepsis.
- In patients with community-acquired AKI, it is important to obtain a thorough medication history, including nonprescription medications or supplements.
- AKI survivors are at risk for development of CKD, and follow-up with monitoring of kidney function for at least 3 yr is recommended even with apparent renal recovery.

SUGGESTED READING

Available at ExpertConsult.com

RELATED CONTENT

Acute Renal Failure (Patient Information)
Chronic Kidney Disease (Related Key Topic)

AUTHOR: **Junior Uduman, MD**

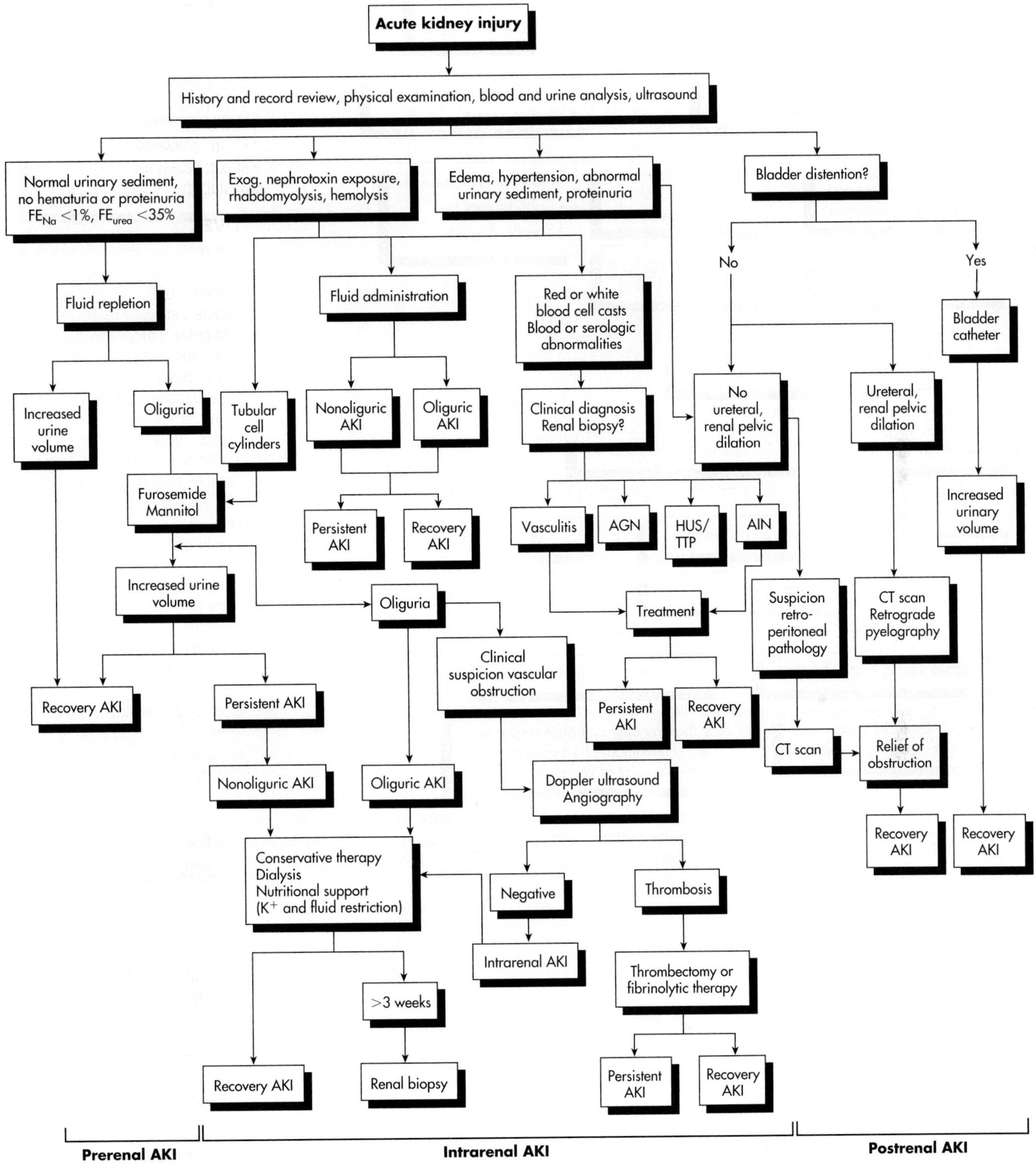

FIG. 1 Diagnostic approach to patients with suspected acute kidney injury (AKI). *AGN,* Acute glomerulonephritis; *AIN,* acute interstitial nephritis; *CT,* computed tomography; *Exog.,* exogenous; *HUS/TTP,* hemolytic-uremic syndrome/thrombotic thrombocytopenic purpura. (From Floege J et al: *Comprehensive clinical nephrology,* ed 4, Philadelphia, 2010, Saunders.)

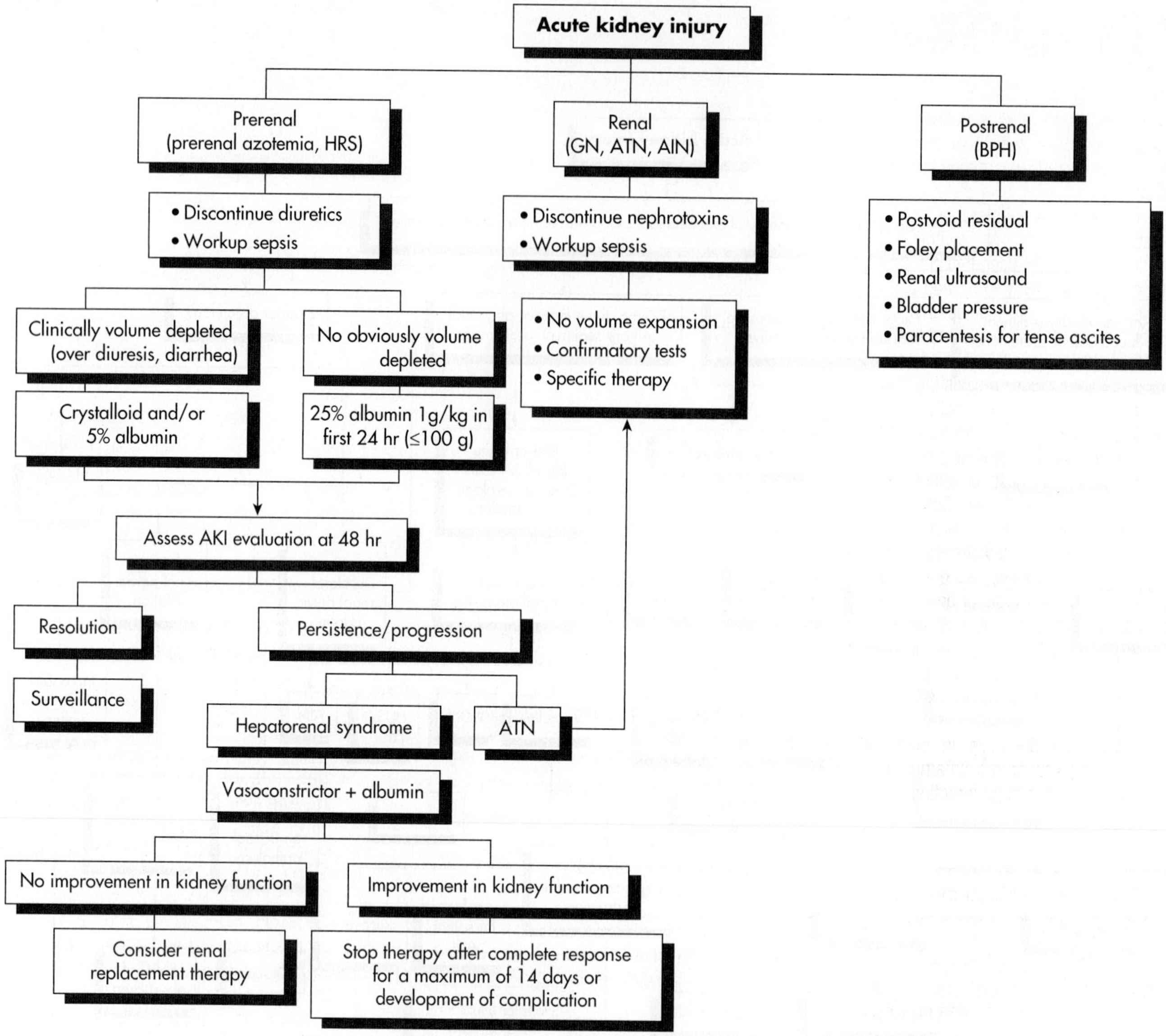

FIG. 2 Algorithm for management of acute kidney injury (AKI). *AIN,* Acute interstitial nephritis; *ATN,* acute tubular necrosis; *BPH,* benign prostatic hypertrophy; *GN,* glomerulonephritis; *HRS,* hepatorenal syndrome. (From Ronco C et al: *Critical care nephrology,* ed 3, Philadelphia, 2019, Elsevier.)

BASIC INFORMATION

DEFINITION

Acute liver failure (ALF) is defined as the rapid progression of liver dysfunction resulting in coagulopathy and altered mentation in patients without previously known liver disease. Practically, it is described as the constellation of acute severe hepatic injury (<26 wk); synthetic liver dysfunction, specifically coagulopathy (international normalized ratio [INR] >1.5); and any degree of mental alteration (encephalopathy) in a patient without preexisting cirrhosis and in the absence of acute alcoholic hepatitis. ALF can also be diagnosed in patients with preexisting liver disease, such as Wilson disease, vertically acquired hepatitis B, and autoimmune hepatitis (despite the possibility of cirrhosis in these patients), provided that diagnosis of these conditions was made within the preceding 26 wk. Box 1 summarizes classifications of acute liver failure.

"Acutely decompensated cirrhosis" refers to the development of ascites, encephalopathy, gastrointestinal hemorrhage, or any combination of these disorders in patients with cirrhosis.[1]

"Acute-on-chronic liver failure" is a syndrome characterized by the following 3 major features:

1. It occurs in the context of intense systemic inflammation
2. Frequently develops in close temporal relationship with pro-inflammatory precipitating events (e.g., infections or alcoholic hepatitis)
3. Is associated with single- or multiple-organ failure[2]

SYNONYMS

Fulminant hepatic failure
Fulminant hepatitis
Fulminant hepatic necrosis
Acute hepatic necrosis
Acute and subacute necrosis of liver
ALF

ICD-10CM CODES

K72	Hepatic failure, not elsewhere classified
K72.0	Acute and subacute hepatic failure
K72.00	Acute and subacute hepatic failure without coma
K72.01	Acute and subacute hepatic failure with coma

EPIDEMIOLOGY & DEMOGRAPHICS

INCIDENCE: Affects approximately 2000 people/yr in U.S. and 1 to 8 people per million population in the U.K.

PREDOMINANT SEX & AGE: Seen more often in women (90% of cases), often affects younger people.

RISK FACTORS:

- Intentional or inadvertent drug overdose
- Risk factors for viral hepatitis:
  1. Intravenous drug use
  2. Occupational exposure to blood or body fluids
  3. Blood transfusions
  4. Hemodialysis
  5. Intranasal cocaine use
  6. Imprisonment
  7. Travel to endemic hepatitis areas
- Previous alcohol use
- Hepatotoxic medications
- Critical illness

ETIOLOGY

- Common causes in the Western world:
  1. Acetaminophen toxicity (46%)
  2. Indeterminate (14%)
  3. Idiosyncratic drug reaction (12%)
  4. Viral hepatitis (A, B) (10%)

Other, more rare causes include alcoholic hepatitis, autoimmune hepatitis, Wilson disease, ischemic hepatopathy, Budd-Chiari syndrome, acute fatty liver of pregnancy, venoocclusive disease, toxin ingestion (e.g., mushroom poisoning [*Amanita phalloides*]), sepsis, infiltrative malignancy (breast cancer, lymphoma, myeloma, melanoma, small cell lung cancer), and other viruses (adenovirus, hepatitis E, HSV). Box 2 summarizes possible etiologies of liver failure.

CLINICIAN PRESENTATION & PHYSICAL FINDINGS

- **Clinical Presentation** Initial symptoms of ALF are mostly nonspecific and depend on the etiology of liver injury. They include fatigue, lethargy, anorexia, and nausea/vomiting. Pruritus, jaundice, and right upper quadrant abdominal pain and distention may be present. Symptoms may also be more serious and consist of severe hypotension, sepsis, and hepatic encephalopathy.
- **Physical examination** Findings include, by definition, abnormal neurologic findings of encephalopathy (see Table 1). Other findings may include jaundice, asterixis, hepatomegaly, decreased hepatic mass on percussion, and ascites. Multisystem organ failure can ensue. In rare cases, as the hepatic encephalopathy progresses, cerebral edema and increased intracranial pressure can occur, with abnormal pupillary exam findings, hypertension, bradycardia, respiratory depression (Cushing triad), and loss of brain stem reflexes. Seizures secondary to increased intracranial pressure and hypoxia can occur. Vesicular skin lesions are suggestive of herpes simplex virus (HSV).
- Family history of unexplained liver disease/cirrhosis should prompt slit lamp ocular examination for the identification of Kayser-Fleischer rings (copper rings around the iris seen in Wilson disease).

LABORATORY FINDINGS

- Coagulopathy is characteristic of patients with ALF, given decreased synthesis of clotting factors II, V, VII, IX and X by the liver. Patients with ALF typically have a prolonged prothrombin time (INR >1.5), elevated transaminases, and elevated bilirubin, and may have a low platelet count (<150,000).
- Other possible laboratory findings can include an elevated BUN/creatinine (studies show 30%

BOX 1 Classifications of Acute Liver Failure

Trey and Davidson
Fulminant hepatic failure: Development of HE within 8 wk of onset of symptoms

British Classification
Acute liver failure (includes only patients with encephalopathy)

Subclassification Depending on the Interval between the Onset of Jaundice and HE
- Hyperacute liver failure: 0-7 days
- Acute liver failure: 8-28 days
- Subacute liver failure: 29-72 days
- Late-onset acute liver failure: 56-182 days

French Classification
Acute hepatic failure: A rapidly developing impairment of liver function
Severe acute hepatic failure: Prothrombin time or factor V concentration below 50% of normal with or without HE

Subclassification
- Fulminant hepatic failure: HE within 2 wk of onset of jaundice
- Subfulminant hepatic failure: HE between 3 and 12 wk of onset of jaundice

International Association for the Study of Acute Liver Failure
Acute liver failure (occurrence of HE within 4 wk after onset of symptoms)

Subclassification
- Acute liver failure—hyperacute: Within 10 days
- Acute liver failure—fulminant: 10-30 days
- Acute liver failure—not otherwise specified
- Subacute liver failure (development of ascites and/or HE from 5 to 24 wk after onset of symptoms)

HE, Hepatic encephalopathy.
From Vincent JL et al: *Textbook of critical care*, ed 7, Philadelphia, 2017, Elsevier.

[1] Sarin SK, Choudhury A, Sharma MK et al: Acute-on-chronic liver failure: consensus recommendations of the Asian Pacific association for the study of the liver (APASL): an update, *Hepatol Int* 13:353-90, 2019.

[2] Arroyo V, Moreau R, Jalan R: Acute-on-chronic liver failure, *N Engl Med* 382:2137-45, 2020.

TABLE 1 Grades of Encephalopathy

Grade	Description
I	Changes in behavior with minimal change in level of consciousness (mild confusion, slurred speech, disordered sleep)
II	Gross disorientation, drowsiness, possibly asterixis, inappropriate behavior
III	Marked confusion (stupor), incoherent speech, sleeping most of the time but rousable to vocal stimuli
IV	Comatose, unresponsiveness to pain, decorticate or decerebrate posturing

to 50% also have acute kidney injury) and hypoglycemia (impairment of gluconeogenesis). Electrolyte disturbances, hyponatremia, hypophosphatemia, hypomagnesemia, hypokalemia, metabolic acidosis or respiratory alkalosis, elevated LDH, and elevated ammonia.

Dx DIAGNOSIS

DIFFERENTIAL DIAGNOSIS

- Severe acute hepatitis, also known as acute liver injury (including alcoholic hepatitis): Jaundice and coagulopathy without encephalopathy
- Acute on chronic liver failure (in patients with liver disease duration >26 wk)
- Cirrhosis (includes decompensated cirrhosis)
- Hepatocellular carcinoma

WORKUP (BOX 3)

- Fig. 1 describes an algorithm for evaluation of acute liver failure.
- Clinical history is critical, but in the case of patients with severe encephalopathy, the history may be limited, and efforts should be made to obtain information from the patient's family. Important history components include medication use (6-mo history of prescriptions, over-the-counter medications, herbal supplements), alcohol use, recreational drug use, prior symptoms of jaundice, onset of symptoms, history of depression and prior suicide attempts, recent travel to endemic areas of viral hepatitis, sexual exposures, previous blood transfusions, family history of liver failure/disease, history of malignancy, or hypercoagulable state.
- Physical examination should include assessing for stigmata of chronic liver disease, as their presence has different diagnostic and management implications, and mental status. Grading of hepatic encephalopathy should be performed (Table 1). Perform an asterixis maneuver, consider psychometric tests (i.e., number connection test) to detect subtle degree of encephalopathy.
- Laboratory evaluation should be targeted to assess the severity of ALF, as well as its etiology. Early testing includes complete blood count, liver function tests (LFTs) including prothrombin time and INR, bilirubin, chemistry panel (sodium, potassium, chloride, bicarbonate, BUN, creatinine, glucose, magnesium, phosphate, calcium), arterial blood gas, arterial lactate, blood type and screen, acetaminophen level, ethanol level, toxicology screen, viral hepatitis serologies (hepatitis A IgM, hepatitis B surface antigen, anti-hepatitis B core IgM, anti-hepatitis C antibody [IgM and IgG]), hepatitis C viral load (HCV RNA), anti-hepatitis E IgM and IgG, HSV-1 IgM and HSV PCR, EBV DNA PCR, CMV DNA

BOX 2 Etiologic Classification of Acute Liver Failure

Acetaminophen Toxicity
Idiosyncratic Drug Injury

Infrequent Agents
Isoniazid
Valproate
Halothane
Phenytoin
Sulfonamide
Propylthiouracil
Amiodarone
Disulfiram
Dapsone
Bromfenac
Troglitazone
Zidovudine
Lamivudine
Lamotrigine
Gatifloxacin
Methotrexate

Miscellaneous Agents
Ecstasy
Cocaine
Phencyclidine

Rare Agents
Carbamazepine
Ofloxacin
Ketoconazole
Lisinopril
Nicotinic acid
Labetalol
Etoposide
Imipramine
Interferon alfa
Flutamide
Tolcapone
Nefazodone
Oral contraceptives

Combination Agents with Enhanced Hepatotoxicity
Alcohol-acetaminophen
Trimethoprim-sulfamethoxazole
Rifampicin-isoniazid
Amoxicillin-clavulanic acid

Viral Hepatitides
Hepatitis A, B, C, D, E, G
Human herpesvirus
Cytomegalovirus
Epstein-Barr virus
Herpes simplex virus
Varicella zoster virus
Paramyxovirus
Parvovirus B19
Adenovirus
Togavirus
Parvovirus
SEN virus
TT virus
Yellow fever virus

Toxins
CCl_4
Amanita phalloides
Yellow phosphorus
Herbal products

Vascular
Ischemic
Venoocclusive disease
Budd-Chiari syndrome
Malignant infiltration
Non-Hodgkin lymphoma

Miscellaneous
Wilson disease
Autoimmune hepatitis
Acute fatty liver of pregnancy
Reye syndrome

CCl4, Carbon tetrachloride.

From Vincent JL et al: *Textbook of critical care,* ed 7, Philadelphia, 2017, Elsevier.

BOX 3 Investigations in Fulminant Hepatic Failure

Baseline essential investigations
Biochemistry
- Bilirubin, transaminases
- Alkaline phosphatase
- Albumin
- Urea and electrolytes
- Creatinine
- Calcium, phosphate
- Ammonia
- Acid-base, lactate
- Glucose

Hematology
- Full blood count, platelets
- PT, PTT
- Factors V or VII
- Blood group cross-match
  Septic screen

Omitting lumbar puncture
- Radiology
- Chest radiograph
- Abdominal ultrasound
- Head CT scan or MRI

Neurophysiology
- Electroencephalogram

Diagnostic investigations
  Serum
- Acetaminophen levels
- Cu, ceruloplasmin (>3 yr)
- Autoantibodies
- Immunoglobulins
- Amino acids
- Lactate
- Pyruvate
- Hepatitis A, B, C, E
- EBV, CMV, HSV viral loads
- Other viruses

Urine
- Toxic metabolites
- Amino acids, succinylacetone
- Organic acids
- Reducing sugars

CMV, Cytomegalovirus; *CT,* computed tomography; *EBV,* Epstein-Barr virus; *HSV,* herpes simplex virus; *PT,* prothrombin time; *PTT,* partial thromboplastin time.

From Fuhrman BP, Zimmerman JJ: *Fuhrman and Zimmerman's pediatric critical care,* ed 4, Philadelphia, 2011, Mosby.

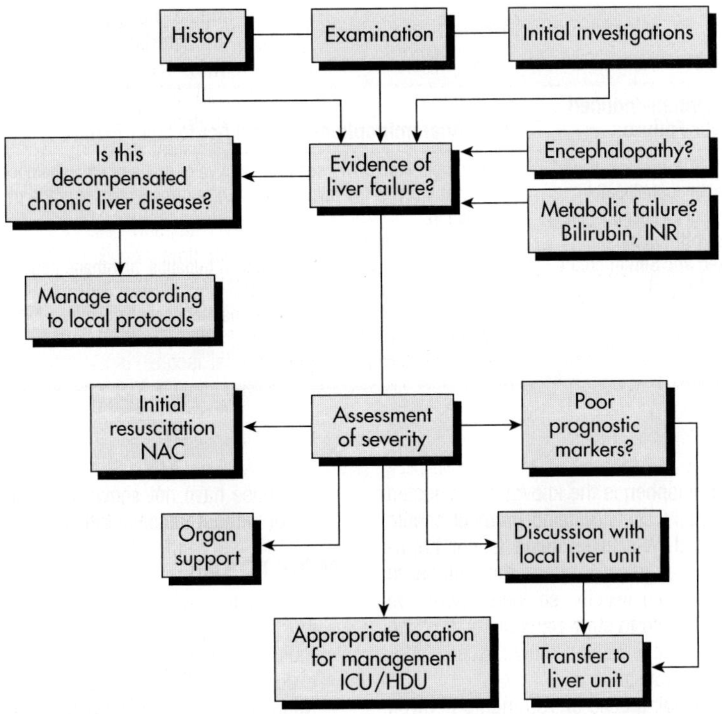

FIG. 1 Initial management of a patient presenting with liver failure. *HDU,* High-dependency unit; *ICU,* intensive care unit; *INR,* international normalized ratio; *NAC,* N-acetylcysteine. (From Parrillo JE, Dellinger RP: *Critical care medicine, principles of diagnosis and management in the adult,* ed 5, Philadelphia, 2019, Elsevier.)

PCR, anti-hepatitis D IgM and IgG, hepatitis D viral load (HDV RNA), ceruloplasmin level (as well as serum copper and 24-hr urine copper if high suspicion), pregnancy test, arterial ammonia level, autoimmune markers (ANA, ASMA, anti-LKM-1, total IgG levels), HIV-1, HIV-2, amylase, lipase. Imaging studies include abdominal ultrasound with Doppler to evaluate for Budd-Chiari syndrome, portal hypertension, hepatic congestion, and hepatic steatosis. Cirrhosis cannot be diagnosed in the setting of ALF, as the liver may appear nodular in ALF due to massive necrosis; consider cross-sectional imaging of the liver (triphasic CT, MRCP, or MRI with gadolinium). CT or MRI of the head should be considered to ensure no other causes for altered mental status.

- Prompt liver biopsy (via transjugular approach to decrease risk of bleeding) should be performed in cases in which:
  1. The etiology is unknown after the initial workup; *or*
  2. Etiology is thought to be secondary to autoimmune hepatitis, malignancy, or HSV.

COMPLICATIONS

Complications or progression of liver failure may result in cerebral edema due to increased intracranial pressure (in up to 40% of patients). Hypoglycemia and lactic acidosis are common complications of ALF, as well as acute kidney injury and pancreatitis (particularly in acetaminophen-induced ALF). Upper gastrointestinal hemorrhage is uncommon (in 1.5% of patients). Infections do occur from impaired leukocyte function (in nearly 80% patients), High-output cardiac failure can occur, as well acute respiratory distress syndrome. Hypotension occurs due to decreased oral intake as well as extravasation of fluid into extravascular space.

Rx TREATMENT (BOXES 4 AND 5)

Broadly, the treatment of acute liver failure should include:

- Identification of the etiology of liver injury, if possible, and specific treatment
- Symptomatic and supportive management and transfer to an ICU if necessary
- Early involvement of a liver specialist and transfer to a transplant center when required

NONPHARMACOLOGIC THERAPY

- Initial treatment should focus on the patient's mental status and managing encephalopathy.
  1. Grade I encephalopathy may be managed on a medical ward (neuro vital signs q4h).
  2. Grade II, III, and IV encephalopathy should be managed in ICU (with elevated head of the bed to 30 degrees). Grade III and IV encephalopathy require intubation and mechanical ventilation.
  3. Decreased stimulation is important (avoiding sedatives; dimly lit, quiet room; no audible monitor alarms).
- A liver specialist should be notified urgently, and arrangements should be made for imminent transfer to a transplant center. Early transport is important, as the patient transport risks increase or even preclude transfer in later stages of encephalopathy.

BOX 4 Management of Fulminant Hepatic Failure

No sedation except for procedures
Minimal handling
Enteric precautions until infection ruled out
Monitor:
- Heart and respiratory rate
- Arterial BP, CVP
- Core/toe temperature
- Neurologic observations
- Gastric pH (>5.0)
- Blood glucose (>4 mmol/L)
- Acid-base
- Electrolytes
- PT, PTT

Fluid balance
- 75% maintenance
- Dextrose 10%-50% (provide 6-10 mg/kg/min)
- Sodium (0.5-1 mmol/L)
- Potassium (2-4 mmol/L)

Maintain circulating volume with colloid/FFP
Coagulation support only if required
Drugs:
- Vitamin K
- H_2 antagonist
- Antacids
- Lactulose
- *N*-acetylcysteine for acetaminophen toxicity
- Broad-spectrum antibiotics
- Antifungals

Nutrition
- Enteral feeding (1-2 g protein/kg/day)
- PN if ventilated

BP, Blood pressure; *CVP,* central venous pressure; *FFP,* fresh frozen plasma; *PN,* parenteral nutrition; *PT,* prothrombin time; *PTT,* partial thromboplastin time.

From Fuhrman BP, Zimmerman JJ: *Fuhrman and Zimmerman's pediatric critical care,* ed 4, Philadelphia, 2011, Mosby.

- Nutritional support should be initiated early. A daily intake goal of 60 g of protein (or amino acids 0.8 to 1.2 g/kg/day) is recommended to prevent catabolism of protein stores. Enteral feeding should be initiated in patients with grade III or IV encephalopathy.
- Fluid support should be initiated if patient is not tolerating oral intake, or signs of hypoperfusion are present. Crystalloid solutions (normal saline in hypotensive patients, ½ normal saline + 75 mEq/L $NaCO_3$ in acidotic patients, normal saline + dextrose in hypoglycemic patients) can be used.

PHARMACOLOGIC TREATMENT

- If encephalopathy progresses and cerebral edema develops leading to increased ICP, intravenous mannitol is recommended to reduce cerebral edema transiently. Prophylactic hyperventilation is not recommended in patients with ALF.
- Phenytoin can be used to manage seizures. In patients not responding to phenytoin, short-acting benzodiazepines may be used.

BOX 5 Hepatic Replacement Therapeutic Options Available to Patients with Fulminant Hepatic Failure

Liver Transplantation
- Cadaveric transplantation
- Whole liver
- Reduced-size liver
- Split liver
- Auxiliary partial liver
- Orthotopic position
- Heterotopic position
- Auxiliary whole liver
- Living-related transplantation
- Left lateral segment
- Left lobe
- Extended left lobe
- Right lobe

Artificial Liver Assist Devices
- Non–cell-based systems
- Charcoal hemoperfusion
- High-volume plasmapheresis
- Continuous high-frequency hemodiafiltration
- Molecular adsorbent recirculating system (MARS)
- Cell-based systems (bioartificial liver assist devices)
- Primary porcine hepatocytes
- Human hepatoblastoma cells
- Extracorporeal liver assist device (ELAD)

Hepatocyte Transplantation

From Vincent JL, et al: *Textbook of critical care,* ed 6, Philadelphia, 2011, Saunders.

TABLE 2 King's College Hospital Criteria for Liver Transplantation in Acute Liver Failure

Acetaminophen-Induced Acute Liver Failure	Non–Acetaminophen-Induced Acute Liver Failure
Arterial pH <7.3 (irrespective of grade of encephalopathy) *OR* Grade III or IV encephalopathy *and* Prothrombin time >100 sec *and* Serum creatinine >3.4 mg/dl	Prothrombin time >100 sec (irrespective of grade of encephalopathy *OR* Any of three of the following variables (irrespective of grade of encephalopathy): 1. Age <10 yr or >40 yr 2. Etiology: Non-A hepatitis, non-B hepatitis, halothane hepatitis, idiosyncratic drug reactions 3. Duration of jaundice before onset of encephalopathy >7 days 4. Prothrombin time >50 sec 5. Serum bilirubin >18 mg/dl

Sec, Seconds.

- Sedative medications should also be avoided, as they are not cleared well and may mask signs of worsening encephalopathy or cerebral edema.
- Lactulose is not routinely recommended for encephalopathy treatment; neomycin should be avoided due to concerns of nephrotoxicity.
- Broad-spectrum antibiotics should be started immediately if infection is suspected. Sources usually include respiratory, urinary, and blood; there is no evidence for empiric antibiotic treatment. Antifungals should be initiated if no initial improvement with antibiotics occurs.
- In the case of persistent hypotension, norepinephrine is the initial vasopressor of choice; vasopressin can be added as a second pressor to maintain MAP >75 mm Hg. Persistent hypotension despite fluid resuscitation and pressor support should prompt concern for adrenal insufficiency.
- Patients should receive stress ulcer prophylaxis, given the risk of gastrointestinal bleeding.
- Routine correction of thrombocytopenia or INR correction are not recommended in the absence of bleeding. However, in the setting of clinical bleeding or the need for a procedure with a high bleeding risk, plasma or clotting factors are recommended. Vitamin K should be given routinely since in patients with ALF vitamin K deficiency is common.
- Part of the pharmacologic treatment will be specific to the suspected etiology of ALF.
- If acetaminophen is the known or suspected cause, an IV acetylcysteine protocol should be initiated. *N*-acetylcysteine is not harmful and dramatically alters the course in acetaminophen toxicity, so there should be a low threshold to start, particularly in young patients or those with no known cause of ALF.
- The 20-hr protocol is:
  1. Initial loading dose of 150 mg/kg IV given over 60 min followed by;
  2. 12.5 mg/kg IV/hr over 4 hr followed by;
  3. 6.25 mg/kg IV/hr for 16 hr.
- A repeat acetaminophen level and ALT should be checked at hr 18 of NAC treatment. If either the acetaminophen level or the ALT is elevated, the 16-hr portion of treatment (6.25 mg/kg) should be extended and another ALT, INR, or acetaminophen level should be checked every 12 hr. The acetylcysteine can be stopped once the acetaminophen level is undetectable, INR <2, or ALT is shown to be either normal or decreasing. Additional information on acetaminophen overdose is available in the topic "Acetaminophen Poisoning."
- *N*-acetylcysteine therapy outside of acetaminophen poisoning has been investigated and may be beneficial; however, its routine use is not currently recommended by practice guidelines and is center specific.
- Liver support systems:
  1. Liver support systems have been trialed either to support the patient until the liver recovers or as a bridge to liver transplantation.
  2. High-volume plasma exchange can improve hepatic encephalopathy and transplant-free survival in a patient ineligible for liver transplantation, but no survival benefit has been shown for a patient undergoing liver transplantation with plasma exchange compared with supportive therapy alone.
  3. The molecular absorbents recirculating system (MARS) is an artificial extracorporeal hepatic support system that allows albumin-bound toxins to be removed. But this, too, has failed to show a survival benefit in patients with ALF.
  4. Bioartificial support systems in the form of hepatocytes (human or other mammalian origin) have also been used in cartridges as part of extracorporeal systems. These have not shown any benefit, with or without transplantation.

MONITORING

- In patients with high-grade HE awaiting transplant, intracranial pressure (ICP) monitoring is recommended in centers with expertise in ICP monitoring.
- Neurologic examination every 1 to 4 hr is recommended in the absence of ICP monitoring.
- Patients with suspected acetaminophen toxicity should have LFTs monitored every 12 hr. Otherwise, LFTs can be monitored daily.
- Chemistry panels and PT/INR should be monitored every 8 to 12 hr. Correction of coagulopathy should be avoided because it can interfere with assessment of liver function. In the setting of life-threatening bleeding, fresh frozen plasma (FFP) and recombinant factor VIIa can be considered.
- Point-of-care glucose should be checked every 4 hr initially to evaluate for hypoglycemia. If hypoglycemia is detected, dextrose should be added to crystalloid solution.
- Because of the increased risk of infection, daily urine, sputum, and blood cultures, as well as chest radiographs, should be checked even in the absence of signs or symptoms of infection.

PROGNOSIS

- Overall mortality from ALF is 30% to 40% and has improved significantly over the last 20 yr.
- Transplant-free survival in ALF in the setting of acetaminophen, hepatitis A, shock liver, and pregnancy-related disease is >50%; for all other causes of ALF, transplant-free survival is <25%.
- Higher-grade hepatic encephalopathy and renal dysfunction in nonacetaminophen ALF predict worse survival.
- Multiple models have been developed to predict spontaneous recovery in ALF patients (King's College criteria, Clichy criteria, MELD score, APACHE II score).
- The King's College criteria form the basis of the model most commonly used for prognostication (Table 2).
- Transplantation:
  1. Patients with ALF are given the highest priority for liver transplantation. ALF

accounts for only 10% of the U.S. liver transplants.

2. Contraindications to listing include medical history of irreversible brain injury, psychiatric illness severe enough to affect patients' survival or likelihood of compliance with medications, active sepsis, severe medical comorbidities including malignancy, increasing dependence on ventilator/inotropic support, acute substance abuse, previous episodes of self-harm (>5 episodes), refractory mental illness, and inadequate family support.
3. For patients with alcoholic liver disease, many centers require a 6-mo abstinence period, but several transplant centers in North America and Europe have transplanted selected patients with alcoholic hepatitis who were unlikely to survive 6 mo.
4. Mortality on the waiting list is 25%; 1-yr and 5-yr survival after transplantation is 73% and 67%, respectively.
5. Various prognostic criteria used for liver transplantation in patients with fulminant hepatic failure are summarized in Box E6.

PEARLS & CONSIDERATIONS

- ALF is defined as severe hepatic injury (as evidenced by elevated liver enzymes) with INR >1.5 and hepatic encephalopathy occurring <26 wk before presentation in a patient with no prior history of liver disease.
- Close to half of ALF is caused by drug ingestion, usually acetaminophen.
- Given the potential rapidity of deterioration, referral must be made as soon as possible to a liver transplant center.
- There should be a low threshold to start *N*-acetylcysteine.
- Coagulopathy should not be corrected unless life-threatening bleeding occurs or it is recommended by the liver transplant hepatologist.

SUGGESTED READINGS

Available at ExpertConsult.com

RELATED CONTENT

Acetaminophen Poisoning (Related Key Topic)
Ascites (Related Key Topic)
Encephalopathy (Related Key Topic)
Hepatopulmonary Syndrome (Related Key Topic)
Hepatorenal Syndrome (Related Key Topic)

AUTHORS: **Marc Monachese, MD, Roxana Chis, MD,** and **Talia Zenlea, MD**

Acute Lower Gastrointestinal Bleeding

BASIC INFORMATION

DEFINITION
Acute lower gastrointestinal bleeding is defined as sudden colonic blood loss.

SYNONYMS
Acute colonic bleeding
Gastrointestinal hemorrhage
Melena
Hematochezia

ICD-10CM CODES
K62.5 Hemorrhage of rectum and anus
K92.1 Melena
K92.2 Gastrointestinal hemorrhage, unspecified

EPIDEMIOLOGY & DEMOGRAPHICS
INCIDENCE:
- Annual incidence in U.S. of lower gastrointestinal (GI) bleeding is 72/100,000.
- Annual incidence in U.S. of hospitalization is 33 to 38/100,000 (about half of that for upper GI bleeding).
- Mortality rates of 2.5% to 3.9% during hospitalization.
- Rebleeding rates of 13% to 19% at 1 yr.

PREDOMINANT SEX & AGE: 24.2/100,000 in males versus 17.2/100,000 in females.
PEAK INCIDENCE: The rate of lower GI bleeding, including that necessitating hospitalization, is higher in the elderly. The risk of lower GI bleed increases 200-fold by the 9th decade of life.
RISK FACTORS: Risk factors include use of antithrombotic agents, NSAID use, aspirin use, alcohol abuse, GI malignancy, atrial fibrillation, coagulopathies, prior GI bleed, cirrhosis, constipation, congenital malformations, radiation exposure, recent infectious illness, recent travel, abdominal aortic aneurysm (AAA) repair, and inflammatory bowel disease.

PHYSICAL FINDINGS & CLINICAL PRESENTATION
- Attention should be paid in the history to details suggesting the location and etiology of the bleed. For instance, weight loss and abdominal pain suggest inflammatory bowel disease; recent AAA repair, especially with history of a sentinel bleed, raises suspicion for aortoenteric fistula; a history of cirrhosis suggests bleeding from portal hypertension, e.g., varices. Bright red blood per rectum is typically from a brisk upper GI bleed, distal colon, or anorectal disease. Melena arises from the upper GI tract, small bowel, or proximal colon. Take a detailed medication history, noting NSAIDs or other drugs that may cause or mimic GI bleeding as well as beta blockers that may mask tachycardia in the setting of significant blood loss.
- The clinician should first and foremost check vital signs, including orthostatics, if stable. Perform ABCs as indicated. Check for pallor and signs of volume depletion, such as delayed capillary refill and skin tenting. Observe for stigmata of liver disease, such as telangiectasias and jaundice. Auscultate for bowel sounds. Absence of bowel sounds may indicate perforation. Palpate the abdomen for pain, masses, and hepatosplenomegaly. Rectal exam should be performed, noting the presence of blood, rate of bleeding, masses, fissures, hemorrhoids, tenderness, and skin changes. If no gross bleed is seen, perform hemoccult testing. Ensure that the bleeding is, in fact, gastrointestinal, excluding hematuria, vaginal bleeding, and wounds.

ETIOLOGY
Diverticulosis is the most common cause of lower GI bleeding at 30%. Internal hemorrhoids are the second most common cause, colitis (ischemia, infection, inflammatory bowel disease), diverticular bleeding, angioectasia, and rectal ulcers are less common causes. 15% of lower GI bleeds are due to upper GI bleeding.

DIAGNOSIS

DIFFERENTIAL DIAGNOSIS
- Upper GI bleed
- Diverticulosis
- Diverticulitis
- Ischemic colitis
- Postpolypectomy bleeding
- Vascular ectasias (angiodysplasia, arteriovenous malformation)
- Anal fissure
- Rectal ulcer
- Colonic polyps
- Advanced neoplasms
- Hemorrhoids
- Intussusception
- Coagulopathies
- Infectious colitis (*E. coli, Shigella, Salmonella, Giardia*)
- Autoimmune (hemolytic uremic syndrome)
- Radiation colitis or proctitis
- Aortoenteric fistula
- Vasculitis
- Inflammatory (ulcerative colitis, Crohn disease)
- Colonic varices
- Drugs (iron, NSAIDs)
- Foreign body

WORKUP
Assess vital signs and ABCs. Establish large-bore intravenous access. If the patient has significant hematochezia without hematemesis, consider performing nasogastric lavage to evaluate for upper GI bleeding. An algorithm for the management of severe hematochezia is illustrated in Fig. 1.

LABORATORY TESTS
- Complete blood count may reveal anemia and/or thrombocytopenia. The hematocrit and hemoglobin should generally be trended every 4 to 6 hr to document the status of the bleed
- Order a comprehensive metabolic panel to evaluate the following: Elevated blood urea nitrogen, which indicates reabsorption of red blood cells; elevated creatinine, which indicates poor renal perfusion; liver function tests, which could reveal liver disease that is exacerbating bleeding
- International normalized ratio, especially if patient is taking warfarin
- Partial thromboplastin time, especially if the patient is on heparin
- Type and screen/cross in anticipation of the need for blood products
- Stool studies, including white blood cell count, Gram stain, culture, and pathogen-specific testing to identify infectious etiologies
- Inflammatory markers including procalcitonin, ESR, and CRP

IMAGING STUDIES
- Computed tomography (CT) angiography (sensitivity 85.2%, specificity 92.1%) can potentially identify the location of the bleed as well as abnormal vasculature.
- Perform a tagged red blood cell scan if source is not identified on CT angiography.
- CT scan of the abdomen and pelvis may identify malignancy as the source of bleeding.
- If free air is suspected from perforation, an abdominal or chest plain film should be ordered immediately. An abdominal plain film can also identify radiopaque foreign bodies.
- Abdominal ultrasound if intussusception is suspected.
- Meckel (technetium-99) scan if Meckel diverticulum is suspected.

TREATMENT
Begin crystalloid bolus to maintain a systolic blood pressure of at least 100 mm Hg. Transfuse for hemoglobin and hematocrit of 7 and 21, respectively, or less. If the patient has coronary artery disease or multiple medical comorbidities and is older than 65 yr, the goal hemoglobin and hematocrit are 8 and 24, respectively. Platelets should be maintained above 50,000 and international normalized ratio 1.5 or less. If possible discontinue any antithrombotic agents and NSAIDs after consultation with the appropriate physician who initiated therapy.

NONPHARMACOLOGIC THERAPY
- Colonoscopy defines the colonic anatomy, can identify the source of bleeding, and allows for potential therapy.
- Endoscopy can be performed if the source of the bleed is suspected to be proximal to the ligament of Treitz.
- Anoscopy can be performed for bleeding internal hemorrhoids or other anorectal disorders.
- Balloon tamponade of esophageal or anorectal bleeds.
- Perform surgery if the source of the bleed cannot be otherwise identified, for aortoenteric fistula, or if air enema for intussusception is unsuccessful.
- Interventional radiology for embolization.
- Ablation.

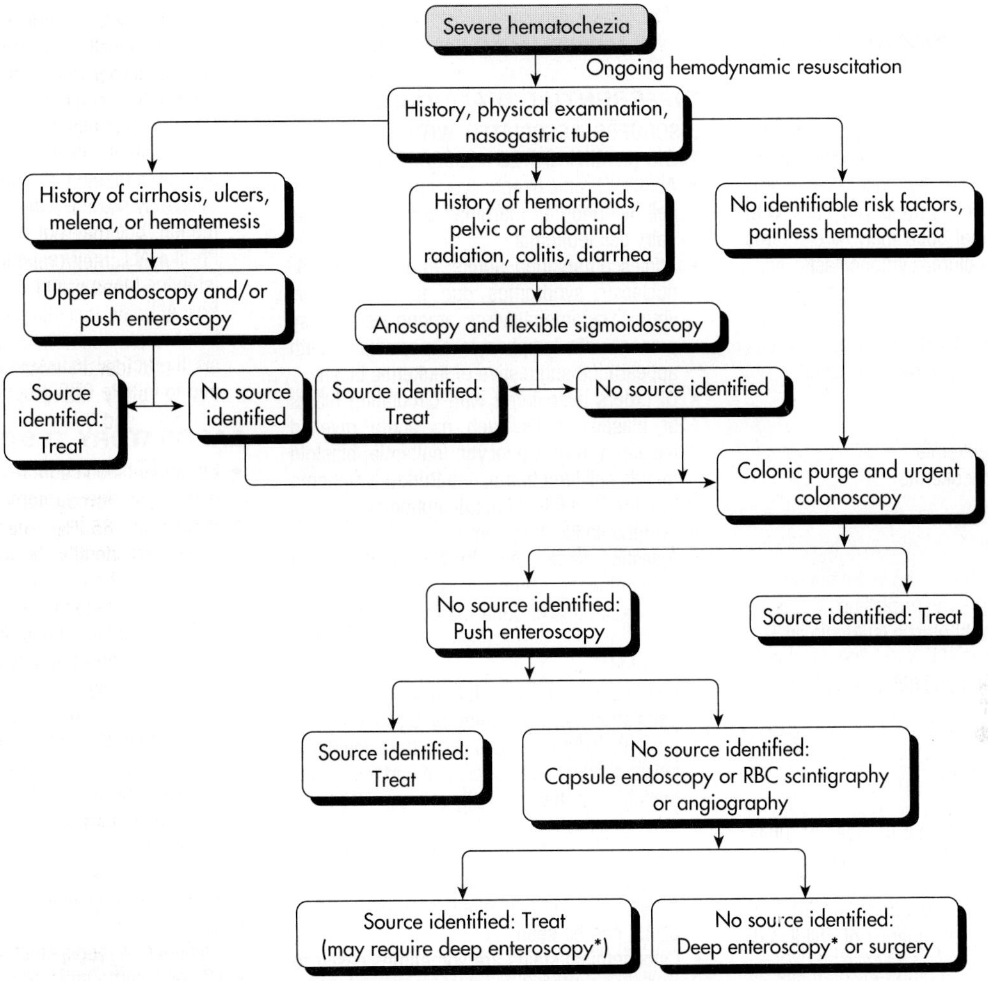

FIG. 1 Algorithm for the management of severe hematochezia modified according to patient's history. *Deep enteroscopy includes double-balloon enteroscopy, single-balloon enteroscopy, and spiral enteroscopy. *RBC,* Red blood cell. (From Feldman M et al: *Sleisenger and Fortran's gastrointestinal liver disease,* ed 10, Philadelphia, 2016, Elsevier.)

ACUTE GENERAL Rx

Proton pump inhibitor, histamine 2 blocker if suspecting UGI blood with rapid transit

CHRONIC Rx

Avoid NSAIDs and alcohol. Treat the underlying cause of the bleed, e.g., coagulopathy, portal hypertension, etc. Most patients are prescribed daily proton pump inhibitors. Fiber, stool softeners, and analgesic creams may alleviate development and/or symptoms of hemorrhoids.

DISPOSITION

Lower GI bleeding will resolve spontaneously in 80% to 85% of patients. Therefore, if the patient is hemodynamically stable without symptomatic anemia or brisk bleeding, he or she may follow up with his or her primary care physician or a gastroenterologist. However, patients with shock or other hemodynamic compromise, severe bleeding, or significant comorbidities should be admitted to the intensive care unit. These patients are at high risk for acute decompensation and as such require close monitoring and aggressive resuscitation; furthermore, they will require urgent diagnosis and intervention to stop the bleeding. Clinical factors predictive of severe colonic bleeding include aspirin use, at least two comorbid illnesses, pulse greater than 100 beats/minute, and systolic blood pressure <115 mm Hg. The overall mortality rate from colonic bleeding is 2.4% to 3.9%. Independent predictors of in-hospital mortality are age over 70 yr, intestinal ischemia, and two or more comorbidities. Inform patients that the risk of rebleeding is fairly high (13% to 19% within 1 yr) and they should continue to closely monitor their symptoms and stool for any signs of recurrence.

REFERRAL

Patients should be referred to gastroenterology for follow-up.

SUGGESTED READINGS

Available at ExpertConsult.com

RELATED CONTENT

Bleeding, Gastrointestinal (Algorithm)
Colorectal Cancer (Related Key Topic)
Diverticular Disease (Related Key Topic)
Meckel Diverticulum (Related Key Topic)

AUTHORS: **Curtis (Trey) Lee Lowery III, PhD, MD,** and **J. Richard Walker III, MD, MS, FACEP**

Acute Lymphoblastic Leukemia (PTG)

BASIC INFORMATION

DEFINITION

Acute lymphoblastic leukemia (ALL) is a malignancy of precursor B or T lymphocytes (lymphoblasts) characterized by uncontrolled proliferation of malignant lymphocytic cells with replacement of normal bone marrow elements and bone marrow failure. Lymphoblastic lymphoma is diagnosed when the disease presents in extramedullary sites (most commonly as mediastinal mass in T-cell disease) *and* less than 25% of the bone marrow is involved.

SYNONYMS

Acute lymphocytic leukemia
Acute lymphoblastic leukemia
ALL

ICD-10CM CODES

C91.00	Acute lymphoblastic leukemia not having achieved remission
C91.01	Acute lymphoblastic leukemia, in remission
C91.02	Acute lymphoblastic leukemia, in relapse

EPIDEMIOLOGY & DEMOGRAPHICS

- ALL is primarily a disease of children (peak incidence occurring at 3 to 5 yr of age).
- Overall incidence is 4.5 cases per 100,000 persons per yr; 60% are under age 20. It is the most common malignancy of childhood. (SEER database accessed 11/26/15.)
- Incidence varies according to race and ethnic group: 14.8 cases per million for blacks, 35.6 cases per million for whites, and 40.9 cases per million for Hispanics.
- Male:female ratio is 55%:45%.

PHYSICAL FINDINGS & CLINICAL PRESENTATION

- Findings consistent with bone marrow failure and peripheral cytopenias—pallor, bruising, petechiae
- Lymphadenopathy or hepatosplenomegaly
- Fever (disease related or infectious), bone pain, weakness, weight loss, mental status changes, and neurologic findings associated with central nervous system (CNS) involvement (if present)
- T-cell lymphoblastic lymphoma is usually associated with a mediastinal mass
- Table 1 summarizes the clinical presentation of acute lymphoblastic leukemia

ETIOLOGY

- Most cases are sporadic without established risk factors.
- Ionizing radiation exposure appears to be a risk factor.
- Down syndrome (trisomy 21) is associated with an approximately 3% risk of developing leukemia by age 30, predominantly ALL. ALL may be seen with other hereditary premalignancy syndromes (e.g., ataxia-telangiectasia).

DIAGNOSIS

DIFFERENTIAL DIAGNOSIS

DISORDERS ASSOCIATED WITH LYMPHOCYTOSIS (LYMPHOCYTES >5000/MCL):

- Adults: Chronic lymphocytic leukemia, mantle cell lymphoma, marginal zone lymphoma, hairy cell leukemia
- Adolescents/young adults: Infectious mononucleosis syndromes due to Epstein-Barr virus or cytomegalovirus, among others, may present with lymphocyte abnormalities with appearance suggestive of leukemic blasts
- Disorders associated with circulating blasts or blastlike cells such as acute myeloid leukemia, prolymphocytic leukemia, blastoid mantle cell lymphoma, and Burkitt lymphoma (mature B-cell leukemia/lymphoma)
- Lymphoblastic lymphoma
- Aplastic anemia; ALL may present without circulating leukemia cells and with only manifestations of bone marrow failure

WORKUP

- Identification of circulating abnormal cell population by flow cytometry. CD19 identifies most precursor B cells. Immature leukemic blasts should have *absence* of surface immunoglobulin and will usually express CD34 and stain positive for terminal deoxynucleotidyltransferase (TdT). Cytoplasmic CD3 and CD7 establish immature T-cell lineage in most cases. Aberrant myeloid markers (CD13, CD33) can be seen.
- Cytochemical stains are sometimes easier to perform and may be available sooner but are less specific. ALL blasts should be negative for myeloperoxidase and esterase stains.
- Bone marrow examination (Fig. E1).
- Genetic studies define important treatment categories, of which the most important is Philadelphia chromosome positive (Ph+) vs. Philadelphia chromosome negative (Ph–) disease, as these are treated differently. Ph status can be determined rapidly by polymerase chain reaction (PCR) or fluorescence *in situ* hybridization (FISH) and should be available within 24 to 48 hr of diagnosis. The WHO classification recognizes genetic variants of ALL as distinct syndromes (Table 2), and the clinical significance of common abnormalities is outlined in Table 3.
- Genetic profiling for "Ph-like" ALL (genetic profile similar to Ph+ disease, but no BCR/ABL abnormality) or IKZF1 (IKAROS) mutations may provide additional prognostic information, but may not be uniformly available. Ph-like ALL may respond to tyrosine kinase inhibitor therapy and may behave more like Ph+ ALL.
- Lumbar puncture is usually done at diagnosis, if practical, to assess for CNS involvement and to initiate CNS prophylactic therapy.

LABORATORY TESTS

- Complete blood count reveals normochromic, normocytic anemia, thrombocytopenia.
- Peripheral smear will usually reveal lymphoblasts, but in some cases only the marrow is involved.
- Initial blood work should also include assessment for basic organ function (creatinine, bilirubin), blood glucose (glucocorticoids are part of therapy), and spontaneous tumor lysis syndrome (K^+, Ca^{++}, $PO4^{++}$, uric acid).
- Coagulation studies (full disseminated intravascular coagulation [DIC] screen) prior to lumbar puncture.
- Studies appropriate to identifying and risk-stratifying leukemia as outlined previously.

IMAGING STUDIES

- Chest x-ray to evaluate fever and for the presence of mediastinal mass.
- CT for symptomatic complaints. Be cautious about contrast dye exposure in patients with evidence of spontaneous tumor lysis syndrome to avoid further renal injury.

TREATMENT

ACUTE GENERAL Rx

- Survival of children with ALL has improved from 10% to 90% in the last 40 yr and is a major success story of modern medical science and research. Adults have fared less well,

TABLE 1 Clinical Presentation of Acute Lymphoblastic Leukemia

Symptoms/ Signs	Etiology	Management
Fever	Disease or infection	Always conduct fever workup and provide broad antimicrobial coverage until infectious etiology is ruled out
Fatigue, pallor	Anemia (ALL infiltrating bone marrow)	Packed red blood cell transfusion (slow if anemia is severe, avoid in hyperleukocytosis)
Petechiae, bruising, bleeding	Thrombocytopenia (ALL infiltrating bone marrow)	Transfuse with platelets
Pain	Leukemia infiltrating bones/ joints, or expanding marrow cavity	Establish diagnosis and start chemotherapy
Respiratory distress/ superior vena cava syndrome	Mediastinal mass	Avoid sedation in presence of tracheal compression. Establish diagnosis as soon as possible and start chemotherapy

ALL, Acute lymphoblastic leukemia.
From Hoffman R et al: *Hematology, basic principles and practice,* ed 7, Philadelphia, 2018, Elsevier.

TABLE 2 WHO Classification of Precursor Lymphoid Neoplasms

B-lymphoblastic leukemia/lymphoma, not otherwise specified
B-lymphoblastic leukemia/lymphoma with recurrent cytogenetic abnormalities:
B-lymphoblastic leukemia/lymphoma with t(9;22)(q34;q11.2); *BCR-ABL1*
B-lymphoblastic leukemia/lymphoma with t(v*;11q23) *MLL* rearranged
B-lymphoblastic leukemia/lymphoma with t(12;21)(p13;q22); *TEL-AML1 (ETV6-RUNX1)*
B-lymphoblastic leukemia/lymphoma with hyperdiploidy
B-lymphoblastic leukemia/lymphoma with hypodiploidy
B-lymphoblastic leukemia/lymphoma with t(5;14)(q32;q32); IL3-IGH
B-lymphoblastic leukemia/lymphoma with t(1;19)(q23;p13.3); *EZA-PBX1 (TCF3-PBX-1)*
T-lymphoblastic leukemia/lymphoma
Provisional entities:
B-lymphoblastic leukemia/lymphoma *BCR/ABL1*-like
B lymphoblastic leukemia/lymphoma with iAMP21
Early T-cell precursor lymphoblastic leukemia/lymphoma

*v**, Variable gene partners; *WHO*, World Health Organization.

TABLE 3 More Common Recurrent Cytogenetic Abnormalities in B-Lymphoblastic Leukemia/Lymphoma

Abnormality	Clinical Relevance
t(9;22)(q34;q11.2); *BCR-ABL1*	Incidence approximately 3% in children, 25% in adults, rising with age; requires therapy with tyrosine kinase inhibitors
t(v*;11q23) *MLL* rearranged	Most common variant is t(4;11); often presents with very high WBC; confers worse prognosis; rare in adults; common in infant leukemia
t(12;21)(p13;q22); *TEL-AML1*	Common in children (20%-30%); rare in adults; confers improved prognosis
Hyperdiploidy	Seen in about 25% of children, less in adults; confers favorable prognosis
Hypodiploidy	Uncommon; confers worse prognosis
t(5;14)(q32;q32); *IL3-IGH*	Rare; commonly associated with eosinophilia; T-cell disease, ? neutral prognostically
t(1;19)(q23;p13.3); *TCF3-PBX1*	Incidence approximately 5%; intermediate/favorable in children, intermediate/poor in adults

*v**, Variable gene partners.
Many of these disorders also have distinct immunophenotypes by flow cytometry. Additional molecular abnormalities of recently defined relevance include mutations of *IKZF1*, which encodes a lymphoid transcription factor IKAROS, is associated with high relapse rates and gene expression profile similar to *BCR-ABL1* translocated disease. Gene expression profiling has identified a subgroup of "Philadelphia chromosome-like" acute lymphoblastic leukemia (ALL) with a gene expression similar to *BCR-ABL1* translocation associated disease, which confers worse prognosis, but which may identify new opportunities for targeted therapies.

but cure rates have also improved to about 60%-70% in standard-risk patients in recent trials. Adults in particular have benefited from tyrosine kinase inhibitor therapy for Ph+ ALL, since this disease is more common in adults and may represent 50% or more of disease in patients over 50.

- **Hyperleukocytic leukemia** (WBC >100,000/mcl) is uncommon in ALL and lymphocyte counts of 100,000 may be well tolerated. Prednisone and vincristine usually offer rapid cytoreduction and leukapheresis is rarely (but sometimes) required.
- **Tumor lysis syndrome** is common in ALL and was seen in 23% of patients in one large series. It is sometimes spontaneous—i.e., present before therapy is given—and is a potential cause of early death. Tumor lysis syndrome is caused by release of intracellular potassium, phosphate, and nucleic acids. The nucleic acids adenosine and guanosine are eventually metabolized to uric acid. Elevated potassium may cause cardiac dysrhythmia and death. Elevated uric acid may cause renal failure through renal urate crystal deposition and possibly other mechanisms. Elevated phosphates cause renal calcium phosphate deposition and kidney injury while also lowering serum calcium, which can cause cardiac dysrhythmia and spasms. Therapy is directed mainly at maintaining renal function through vigorous hydration (3 liters normal saline per day if practical, alkalinization not recommended); "forced diuresis" if necessary to maintain urine output at 2 ml/kg/h; and dialysis if necessary to control K^+, phosphates, or fluid balance. Allopurinol, up to 800 mg/day for adults, 300-450 mg/m^2/day for children, is given routinely. Rasburicase is a recombinant urate oxidase that rapidly lowers uric acid levels. The dose is 0.2 mg/kg, and one dose is usually enough. Rasburicase should be avoided in patients with G6PD deficiency. Phosphate binders are of uncertain value but are usually given. Asymptomatic hypocalcemia is not treated to avoid increasing calcium phosphate deposition. Definitions of laboratory and clinical tumor lysis and defined risk categories are outlined in Table 4.
- Numerous protocols have been used for Ph-ALL, and the specific protocol is likely to be determined by institution/physician familiarity and access to clinical trials, among other factors.
- In the 1990s and early 2000s, it was noted that adolescents and young adult (AYA) patients had better outcomes on pediatric trials than on adult trials. Consequently, this group (currently defined as ages 15-39) is now often (especially younger AYAs) treated on pediatric protocols by pediatric services or on adult "pediatric inspired" protocols.
- Therapy for Ph− ALL generally has four components:
  1. Induction therapy, typically with corticosteroids, cyclophosphamide (some regimens), vincristine, an anthracycline (doxorubicin or daunorubicin usually), and asparaginase. The CD20 directed antibody rituximab has shown benefit in patients with greater than 20% CD20 expression on their blast cells.
  2. Consolidation therapy is high-dose chemotherapy aimed at preventing relapse after remission and commonly consists of cytarabine and methotrexate in combination with other agents.
  3. Maintenance therapy is low-intensity outpatient therapy that is continued for 2 to 3 yr after completion of consolidation. Prednisone, monthly vincristine, methotrexate, and oral 6-mercaptopurine (POMP regimen) are commonly used.
  4. CNS prophylaxis is universal and is usually done with intrathecal therapy (methotrexate alone or in combination with cytarabine and hydrocortisone) administered by lumbar puncture or an Ommaya reservoir. Due to increased toxicity, cranial radiotherapy is reserved for patients with high-risk features, such as active CNS disease at diagnosis.
- Allogeneic bone marrow transplant in first remission of ALL is controversial because of improving results with current nontransplant therapies. It is usually recommended for patients in whom the likelihood of cure is considered less than 50% to 60% with chemotherapy alone, depending on age and donor availability. Autologous bone marrow transplant is rarely used in Ph-ALL. In 2008, the final results of the MRC/UKALL XII/ECOG E2993 study were published. This study evaluated the relative safety and efficacy of chemotherapy, and autologous and allogeneic transplant after first CR in Ph− patients. This was a randomized trial of 1826 patients with newly diagnosed ALL. Patients who had a matched related donor were offered an allogeneic transplant. Patients without a donor were further randomized to an autologous transplant or chemotherapy and maintenance. The key conclusions of this study were:
  1. Allogeneic transplant in first complete remission is associated with lower relapse rates versus autologous transplant or chemotherapy/maintenance therapy alone in Ph− patients.
  2. Allogeneic transplant in first complete remission improved overall survival in standard risk patients. There was a lower risk of relapse in both standard and high-risk patients. There was high

TABLE 4 Tumor Lysis Syndrome

Laboratory Tumor Lysis Syndrome[a]	
Uric acid: ≥8 mg/dl or 476 μmol/L	
Potassium: ≥6.0 mmol/L	
Phosphorus: ≥4.5 mg/dl or 1.5 mmol/L (adults), ≥6.5 mg/dl or 2.1 mmol (children)	
• Calcium: Corrected[b] Ca^{++} <7.0 mg/dl or 1.75 mmol/L or ionized Ca^{++} <1.12 mg/dl or 0.3 mmol/L, or 25% increase from baseline uric acid, potassium, phosphorus; 25% decrease for calcium	
Clinical Tumor Lysis Syndrome	
Acute kidney injury	
• Rise in serum creatinine ≥0.3 mg/dl (26.5 μmol/L)	
• Any creatinine >1.5 age-appropriate upper limit normal if no baseline available	
• Oliguria defined as urine output <0.5 ml/kg/hr for 6 hr	
Cardiac arrhythmia	
Seizure	
Symptomatic hypocalcemia (e.g., neuromuscular irritability such as tetany)	

[a]Laboratory tumor lysis syndrome present if two or more abnormalities are present within 3 days before or 7 days after therapy.
[b]Corrected calcium is measured calcium (mg/dl) + 0.8 × (4 – measured albumin g/dl).
From Arber DA et al: The 2016 revision to the World Health Organization classification of myeloid neoplasms and acute leukemia, *Blood* 127:2391-2405, 2016.

TABLE 5 Risk Factors for Treatment Failure in Recent ALL Trials

t(v*;11q23) *MLL* rearranged
Hypodiploidy
Minimal residual disease after remission or consolidation*
Philadelphia chromosome-like genomic signature (in Ph-ALL)†
Early precursor T (ETP) ALL (absent CD1a, CD8, weak CD5, myeloid or stem cell antigen expression)

ALL, Acute lymphoblastic leukemia; v*, variable gene partners.
*Measured variously after induction or consolidation therapy.
†Standardized testing for this is still in development, but it may have important treatment implications. Note also that many historic risk factors (e.g., T-cell vs B-cell disease) have not been independent risk factors in current trials.
From Roberts KG et al: Targetable kinase-activating lesions in Ph-like acute lymphoblastic leukemia, *N Engl J Med* 371(11):1005-1015, 2014.

treatment-related mortality in high-risk older patients. The increased mortality offsets the benefit of lower relapse risk for the patient group.

- The findings did not support autologous transplant as replacement therapy in any ALL group.
- Risk factors for treatment failure in recent protocols are outlined in Table 5. Prognostic factors in ALL are summarized in Tables 6 and 7.
- Therapy of Ph+ ALL consists of a tyrosine kinase inhibitor—imatinib, dasatinib, nilotinib, ponatinib have been used—with chemotherapy.
  1. 2-yr survival rates are reported at 50%-65%, with various regimens.
  2. Low-intensity induction chemotherapy with dasatinib and prednisone or imatinib, vincristine, and prednisone have resulted in remission rates of 100% and 98% and may allow for less toxicity and hospitalization at diagnosis.
  3. Allogeneic bone marrow transplant is commonly used as consolidative therapy if available but has become more controversial. Maintenance therapy with tyrosine kinase inhibitor is usually given after BMT or non-BMT therapy.
- Therapy of relapsed disease:
  1. Allogeneic bone marrow transplant is offered for relapsed disease, but relapse after BMT is common, and long-term cure rates have been low at about 20%.
  2. In 2017, the FDA approved three new therapies for relapsed ALL: Chimeric antigen receptor T cell (CAR-T) therapy, a form of targeted immunotherapy, yielded a remission rate of 90% in pediatric and young adult (under age 26 yr) patients with relapsed B-cell ALL. Chimeric antigen T cells are created by harvesting the patient's T cells, then transfecting them with lentivirus vector that inserts DNA expressing an anti-CD19 domain (the target antigen on B cells) coupled to a T cell receptor. The T cells expressing the chimeric anti-CD19/T-cell receptor specifically target CD19-expressing B cells. The CAR-T cell population is then expanded ex vivo and reinfused to the patient. About 70% of remissions were durable at 6 mo. The main side effect is cytokine release syndrome (CRS) associated with "vascular leak," hypotension, respiratory and renal insufficiency, and coagulopathy. CRS is treated with tocilizumab and anti-IL6 receptor blocking antibody. CAR-T cells for ALL have been given the generic designation tisagenlecleucel (trade name Kymriah). It currently costs $475,000 and is available at centers certified for its use.
  3. Blinatumomab is a bispecific antibody that binds CD19 and CD3, redirecting T cells to leukemia cells. It was FDA-approved for relapsed ALL, including Ph+ ALL, in adults and children. Blinatumomab is administered as a continuous infusion for 4 wk (9 μg/day wk 1, 28 μg/day thereafter), with maintenance therapy for 4 wk every 12 wk. In a large phase III trial, the remission rate was 44% (vs. 25% with chemotherapy), a small number durable. In a smaller phase II trial for Ph+ ALL, the remission rate was 36%. A small number of blinatumomab responses have been durable. Blinatumomab can also be associated with cytokine release syndrome.
- Inotuzumab ozogamicin (IO) is an antibody drug conjugate, in which chemotherapeutic agent calicheamicin is bound to an anti-CD22 antibody. In a large phase III trial, the remission rate was 81% vs. 33% for standard chemotherapy, with a median duration of 4.6 mo. Approximately 40% of IO patients were successfully bridged to transplant vs. 10% with chemotherapy. A small number of responses were durable.
- Survivorship:
  1. Survivors of childhood and adult ALL are increasingly being seen in primary care practices; as of 2006 there were estimated >50,000 survivors, likely increasing by about 2000+ per yr.
  2. Long-term complications of ALL therapy include secondary malignancy from chemotherapy (usually in first 5 to 10 yr) or from radiation: If given, no plateau in risk, congestive heart failure from anthracycline therapy (often manifesting 20 to 30 yr after treatment), osteopenia and avascular necrosis from glucocorticoid therapy, obesity, and neurocognitive defects. Key recommendations include the following:
     a. Echocardiography every 3 to 5 yr for asymptomatic congestive heart failure, more often if anthracycline exposure was >250 to 300 mg/m^2, since asymptomatic congestive heart failure may warrant therapy. This may show up decades after therapy.
     b. Screening for malignancy and endocrinopathies in pertinent radiation fields.
     c. Attention to the increased risk of obesity and metabolic derangement in survivors.
     d. Recent reviews (see references) summarizing current recommendations and guidelines are accessible online (www.survivorshipguidelines.org/pdf/LTFUGuidelines_40.pdf, www.sign.ac.uk/pdf/sign132.pdf).

SUGGESTED READINGS

Available at ExpertConsult.com

RELATED CONTENT

Acute Lymphocytic Leukemia (ALL) (Patient Information)
Tumor Lysis Syndrome (Related Key Topic)

AUTHOR: **Todd F. Roberts, MD, FRCP(C)**

TABLE 6 Prognostic Factors in Acute Lymphoblastic Leukemia

Factor	Prognosis	Clinical Application
Age		
<1 yr	MLL+ (70%-80% infants) poor outcome; MLL− same outcome as older children	MLL− do well on standard ALL therapy Potential role for FLT3 inhibitors, proteasome inhibitors, histone deacetylase inhibitors, and hypomethylating agents for MLL+
1-9 yr	Lower (standard) risk	ALL biology may change risk
>9 yr	Higher risk	ALL biology may change risk
WBC		
$<50 \times 10^9$/L	Lower (standard) risk	ALL biology may change risk
$\geq 50 \times 10^9$/L	Higher risk	ALL biology may change risk
CNS		
CNS3	Higher risk of CNS and bone marrow relapse	Therapy intensification
CNS2 Traumatic lumbar puncture with blasts	Higher risk of CNS relapse	CNS directed therapy intensification
Testicular	Higher risk	Therapy intensification
Immunophenotype		
T cell	Higher risk	Poor outcome abolished with current therapy
pre-B (cIgM+)	Standard risk	Poor outcome abolished with current therapy
Early pre-B	Standard risk	Genetics may change risk
Early T-cell precursor	Adverse prognosis	Ongoing studies exploring targeted therapies
Ploidy		
>50 (DI >1.16)	Low risk	Good response to antimetabolites
<44	Higher risk	Therapy intensification
Genetic Alterations		
t(9;22)/*BCR-ABL1*	Higher risk	ABL TKI
t(4;11)/*MLL-AF4*	Higher risk	Potential role for FLT3 inhibitors, proteasome inhibitors, histone deacetylase inhibitors, and hypomethylating agents
t(1;19)/*E2A-PBX1*	Higher risk of CNS relapse	Improved outcome with current therapy
t(12;21)/*ETV6-RUNX1*	Low risk	
IKZF1	Poor prognosis. Present in 80% Ph+ and also in Ph-like ALL	Potential role for tyrosine kinase, JAK inhibitors
NUP214-ABL1	High risk	Potential benefits from TKI
CRLF2	In half of Ph-like cases, associated with Hispanic/Latino, poor outcome	Potential role for JAK inhibitors
CREBBP	Associated with drug resistance and relapse	Potential benefit from histone deacetylase inhibitors
MRD		
Day 15 <0.01%	Excellent outcome	No benefit from 2nd delayed intensification
Slow early responders	Higher MRD = higher risk of relapse	Benefit from augmented delayed intensification
End of induction >1%	Dismal prognosis	Transplantation in first CR
4 mo after diagnosis >0.01%	Dismal outcome	Transplantation in first CR

ALL, Acute lymphoblastic leukemia; *CNS,* central nervous system; *CR,* complete remission; *DI,* deoxyribonucleic acid index; *JAK,* Janus kinase; *MLL,* mixed-lineage leukemia; *MRD,* minimal residual disease; *TKI,* tyrosine kinase inhibitor; *WBC,* white blood cell.
From Hoffman R et al: *Hematology, basic principles and practice,* ed 7, Philadelphia, 2018, Elsevier.

TABLE 7 Markers for Poor Prognosis in Adult Acute Lymphoblastic Leukemia

Established Risk Factors	
Age	>60 yr
Presenting WBC count	>30,000/μL (B-cell ALL); >100,000/μL (T-cell ALL)
Immunophenotype	Pro-B cell; early T cell[a]
Cytogenetics	t(4;11)(q21;q23) and other *MLL* rearrangements
	t(9;22)(q34;q11.2) – Philadelphia chromosome
	Hypodiploidy (<44 chromosomes)
	Complex (>5 abnormalities)
Therapy response	Time to complete remission >4 wk
MRD	≥0.01% at 3-6 mo after initiation of therapy[b]
Emerging Risk Factors	
Immunophenotype	CD20
Molecular	BAALC
	FUS
	ERG
	IKZF1[c]
	Ph-like ALL

ALL, Acute lymphoblastic leukemia; *ETP,* early T-cell precursor; *MRD,* minimal residual disease; *Ph,* Philadelphia chromosome; *WBC,* white blood cell.
[a]Initial report characterizing ETP ALL showed a poor outcome. However, subsequent studies have shown variable association with response to therapy.
[b]Different studies have used different time points for MRD assessment.
[c]Focal deletions in IKZF1 are present in up to 70% of Ph-like ALL. However, IKZF1 deletions are associated with adverse outcome irrespective of association with Ph-like phenotype.
From Hoffman R et al: *Hematology, basic principles and practice,* ed 7, Philadelphia, 2018, Elsevier.

Acute Mesenteric Ischemia

BASIC INFORMATION

DEFINITION

Acute mesenteric ischemia (AMI) is the sudden onset of intestinal hypoperfusion to all or part of the small bowel caused by emboli, arterial or venous thrombosis, vasoconstriction from low-flow states, or arterial vasospasm which ultimately leads to ischemia and secondary inflammatory changes.

SYNONYMS

AMI
Mesenteric ischemia, acute

ICD-10CM CODE

K55.0 Acute vascular disorders of intestine

EPIDEMIOLOGY & DEMOGRAPHICS

INCIDENCE:

- Accounts for 0.09% to 0.2% of all acute admissions to emergency departments.
- Mortality ranges between 50% and 80%.
- The incidence appears to be increasing. Factors for this include increased awareness among clinicians, improved diagnostic modalities, the aging of the population, and improved intensive care leading to longer survival of sicker patients.

PREDOMINANT SEX & AGE:

- AMI caused by arterial embolism or thrombosis occurs more frequently in the elderly.
- AMI due to mesenteric venous thrombosis often presents in younger age groups.

RISK FACTORS:

- Advanced age, atherosclerosis, low cardiac output (especially atrial fibrillation), severe cardiac valvular disease, intraabdominal malignancy.
- In the subgroup of cases caused by venous thrombosis, risk factors include hypercoagulable states, portal hypertension, abdominal infection, blunt trauma, pancreatitis, and portal malignancy.
- Additional risk factors for AMI caused by nonocclusive mesenteric ischemia include recent cardiac or aortic surgery, dialysis, hypovolemia, and vasoconstrictive medications (including illicit drugs such as cocaine).
- Table 1 summarizes risk factors for ischemic bowel disease.
- AMI may also occur rarely in patients with no identifiable risk factors.

GENETICS: No specific genetic predisposition but may be related to underlying factors such as cardiac disease, atherosclerosis, and hypercoagulable states.

PHYSICAL FINDINGS & CLINICAL PRESENTATION

- The classic presentation is rapid onset of severe periumbilical pain "out of proportion to physical examination findings," often followed by nausea/vomiting, diarrhea, and/or blood per rectum.
- Approximately one third of patients present with the triad of abdominal pain, fever, and hemoccult-positive stools. Nausea and vomiting are commonly associated.
- Generally patients with mesenteric venous thrombosis tend to present with less abrupt onset of abdominal pain than those with acute arterial occlusion.
- Initial abdominal examination may be normal, with no rebound or guarding, or may include minimal distention or stool positive for occult blood. An epigastric bruit may be present in some patients.
- Later in the disease course the patient may present with septic shock, gross abdominal distention, absence of bowel sounds, and peritoneal signs. In the elderly, mental status changes may occur.
- If the physical examination demonstrates signs of peritonitis, there is likely irreversible intestinal ischemia with bowel necrosis.

ETIOLOGY

Conventionally, AMI is stratified into four groups by etiology: Arterial embolism, arterial thrombosis, venous thrombosis, and nonocclusive mesenteric ischemia (NOMI). The pathophysiology behind these different etiologies is summarized in Table 2. Causes and approximate frequencies of acute mesenteric ischemia are summarized in Table 3. The pathophysiologic mechanisms that cause AMI include:

TABLE 1 Risk Factors for Ischemic Bowel Diseases*

Risk Factor	Arterial Thrombosis	Embolus	Mesenteric Vein Thrombosis	Nonobstructive Mesenteric Ischemia
Advanced age	+	+	+	+
Atherosclerosis	+			
Aortic dissection	+			
Low cardiac output	+	+		+
Congestive heart failure				+
Shock				+
Severe dehydration	+		+	
Cardiac arrhythmias, especially atrial fibrillation		+		+
Severe cardiac valvular disease		+		
Recent myocardial infarction	+			+
Intraabdominal malignancy			+	
Abdominal trauma			+	
Intraabdominal infection			+	
Intraabdominal inflammatory conditions			+	
Parasitic infection (ascariasis)			+	
Hypercoagulable states (venous thrombosis)			+	
Sickle cell anemia			+	
Recent cardiac surgery	+	+		+
Recent abdominal surgery			+	
Vascular aortic prosthetic grafts proximal to the superior mesenteric artery		+		
Hemodialysis				+
Vasculitis	+		+	
Pregnancy			+	
Decompression sickness			+	
Blast lung caused by systemic air embolism		+		
Drugs that cause constriction:				
• Digitalis				+
• Cocaine				+
• Amphetamines				+
• Pseudoephedrine				+
• Vasopressin			+†	+
Estrogen therapy			+	

*A plus sign (+) indicates that the factor is a risk for the disease subtype.
†Especially after sclerotherapy.
From Adams JG et al: *Emergency medicine, clinical essentials,* ed 2, Philadelphia, 2013, Elsevier.

TABLE 2 Pathophysiology of the Four Different Causes of Acute Mesenteric Ischemia (AMI)

Cause	Pathophysiology
Embolism	• Often in patients with atrial fibrillation • Emboli lodge 3-10 cm distal to origin of SMA, often past branching of middle colic artery • Proximal mid-jejunum is spared
Thrombosis	• Typically these patients have a history of symptomatic stenosis of mesenteric arteries • Any clinical scenario that leads to low flow or hypotension can result in acute-on-chronic arterial thrombosis • Affects the orifice of the SMA • Flush occlusion of the SMA and the entire middle gut is involved during the initial presentation
Nonocclusive	• Low flow state resulting from any type of shock or the use of vasoconstrictors • The entire bowel may be involved
Mesenteric venous thrombosis	• Thrombosis of the veins draining the intestines; SMV, IMV, splenic and portal veins among hypercoagulable patients with cancer or hypercoagulable state • Decreased venous outflow, bowel edema, distension, and decreased mesenteric perfusion

IMV, Inferior mesenteric vein; *SMA,* superior mesenteric artery; *SMV,* superior mesenteric vein.
Modified from Cameron JL, Cameron AM: *Current surgical therapy,* ed 12, Philadelphia, 2017, Elsevier.

TABLE 3 Causes and Approximate Frequencies of Acute Mesenteric Ischemia

Cause	Frequency (%)
SMA thrombosis	54-68
SMA embolus	26-32
Nonocclusive mesenteric ischemia	10
Mesenteric venous thrombosis	5
Focal segmental ischemia of the small intestine	5

SMA, Superior mesenteric artery.
From Feldman M et al: *Sleisenger and Fordtran's gastrointestinal and liver disease,* ed 10, Philadelphia, 2016, Elsevier.

- Mesenteric arterial embolism (40% to 50% of cases of AMI) typically arises from a cardiac source: Left atrium associated with cardiac dysrhythmias such as atrial fibrillation, left ventricle with global myocardial dysfunction associated with poor ejection fraction, or cardiac valves due to endocarditis. The superior mesenteric artery (SMA) is most commonly affected because of its relatively large diameter and low takeoff angle from the aorta.
- Mesenteric arterial thrombosis (20% to 35% of cases of AMI) is often seen in patients with prior progressive atherosclerotic stenosis, with superimposed abdominal trauma or infection. Many of these patients have a history consistent with chronic mesenteric ischemia (CMI), including postprandial pain, weight loss, or "food fear."
- Nonocclusive mesenteric ischemia (20% of cases of AMI) is usually a consequence of SMA vasoconstriction associated with low splanchnic blood flow as seen with hypotension, hypovolemia, vasoconstricting drugs, and hemodialysis.
- Mesenteric venous thrombosis (less than 10% of cases of AMI) may occur in the setting of hypercoagulable states (acquired or inherited), blunt trauma, abdominal infection, portal hypertension, pancreatitis, and portal malignancy. Other risk factors include intraabdominal sepsis, smoking, oral contraceptives, and liver cirrhosis. In these situations, the consequences of bowel edema and increased vascular resistance secondary to venous thrombosis result in reduced arterial blood flow, leading to bowel ischemia.
- Dissection or inflammation of the mesenteric artery accounts for less than 5% of cases of AMI.

Dx DIAGNOSIS

DIFFERENTIAL DIAGNOSIS

Initially include other causes of acute-onset abdominal pain, including perforated peptic ulcer, acute pancreatitis, and early appendicitis, as well as the varied causes of peritonitis.

WORKUP

- Early diagnosis is key, and the key to early diagnosis is a high level of clinical suspicion.
- Treatment success is related to the duration of symptoms before diagnosis. Consider early laparotomy for diagnosis in cases with a high index of suspicion when imaging is not readily available.

LABORATORY TESTS

- Classically, patients with AMI have leukocytosis, metabolic acidosis, elevated D-dimer, and elevated serum lactate; however, these laboratory test results are nonspecific, especially early in the course. Elevated lactic acid, leukocytosis, and elevated hematocrit from hemoconcentration can occur later in the course, often after progression to bowel necrosis has occurred, hence are not useful for early diagnosis.
- D-dimer has been reported to be an independent risk factor of intestinal ischemia, reflecting ongoing clot formation and endogenous degradation via fibrinolysis. Normal D-dimer testing may help rule out AMI while elevated levels are nonspecific.
- When a hypercoagulable state is suspected, workup may include proteins C and S, antithrombin III, and factor V Leiden. This will likely not affect the diagnosis of AMI but may help guide long-term therapy.
- Amylase levels may be elevated in up to 50% of individuals with intestinal ischemia; phosphate levels may be elevated in up to 80% of affected individuals.

IMAGING STUDIES

- Contrast-enhanced computed tomography (CT) has replaced conventional angiography as the gold standard imaging modality in AMI. It is more readily available and has similar sensitivity to angiography, the prior gold standard test. Computed tomographic angiography (CTA) has 95% to 100% accuracy for the diagnosis of visceral ischemic syndromes and is also useful in detecting potential sources of emboli and other pathologic processes.
- Plain CT findings are nonspecific and more often found late in the course. Portal venous gas or intramural gas may be seen after the development of gangrene (Fig. E1). In many cases, CT findings remain nonspecific even at advanced stages.
- Gadolinium-enhanced magnetic resonance imaging (MRI) can be used to detect proximal obstruction of the SMA and celiac axis, but it has less value in the evaluation of distal arterial occlusions and other intestinal findings in AMI. Magnetic resonance angiography (MRA) may be more useful in cases of mesenteric vein thrombosis causing AMI. It has also been found useful in monitoring the progress of patients with superior mesenteric venous thrombosis who are treated nonsurgically. MRA, however, takes longer than CTA to perform and can overestimate the degree of stenosis.
- Plain radiographs are not useful in AMI; plain films are normal 25% of the time in early stages. Suggestive findings may include ileus (Fig. E2), bowel wall thickening, or intramural gas. Gas in the portal veins is a sign of extensive intestinal pneumatosis and implies that bowel necrosis has developed. Free air under the diaphragm may support early surgical intervention before further radiologic evaluation.
- Ultrasound is not recommended in AMI if CT is available. Doppler ultrasound evaluation of intestinal blood flow is time consuming and is often limited by the presence of air-filled loops of bowel, body habitus, or recent intraabdominal surgery.
- Angiography may be considered if the diagnosis remains unclear after CT or MRI.

Rx TREATMENT

- The goal of treatment is to restore blood flow to ischemic bowel as rapidly as possible (Fig. E3) before the occurrence of infarction.
- Treatment varies depending on specific etiology.

NONPHARMACOLOGIC THERAPY

- Specific management will depend on patient status and most likely etiology of the ischemia. Signs of peritonitis mandate early laparotomy and resection of infarcted bowel.
- When workup is positive for major SMA embolus, embolectomy is considered standard treatment in the absence of peritoneal signs. Depending on the location and degree of occlusion of the embolus, surgical revascularization, intraarterial infusion of thrombolytics or vasodilators, or systemic anticoagulation may be considered.
- In cases of SMA thrombosis, emergency surgical revascularization is the treatment of choice. Stent placement may be a viable alternative.
- Management of NOMI is based on treatment of the underlying precipitating cause. Fluid resuscitation, optimization of cardiac output, and elimination of vasopressors remain important primary measures. Additional treatment may include systemic anticoagulation and the use of catheter-directed infusion of vasodilatory and antispasmodic agents, most commonly papaverine hydrochloride.
- In patients with mesenteric vein thrombosis, treatment depends on the presence or absence of peritoneal signs. Laparotomy and resection of infarcted bowel is indicated in more advanced cases. If there are no peritoneal signs, immediate anticoagulant therapy with heparin, and ultimately warfarin, may be adequate treatment.
- In general, percutaneous treatment with lytic therapy, balloon angioplasty, or stenting may be limited by the frequent presence of nonviable bowel, which would require laparotomy despite success with percutaneous treatment.
- A "second look" procedure is indicated in most patients, 24 to 48 hr after initial revascularization.

ACUTE GENERAL Rx

- Initial management should include hemodynamic monitoring and support, including fluid resuscitation with crystalloid and blood products, correction of acidosis, pain control (using parenteral opioids), administration of broad-spectrum antibiotics to cover gram-negative and anaerobic organisms, and gastric decompression by nasogastric tube.
- Vasopressors should be used with caution and only to avoid fluid overload and abdominal compartment syndrome. Dobutamine, low-dose dopamine, and milrinone to improve cardiac function have been shown to have less impact on mesenteric blood flow.
- In the absence of active bleeding, the use of systemic anticoagulation is usually indicated. The optimal timing of initiation is unclear.

CHRONIC Rx

Patients should be followed up in an outpatient clinical setting at regular intervals.

- Patients who receive endovascular treatment should be managed with 3 to 6 mo of clopidogrel; additionally, periodic surveillance for restenosis with duplex ultrasound or CTA is indicated.
- In the subgroup of patients with mesenteric venous thrombosis, prevention of further thrombosis is indicated. The optimal duration of anticoagulation is unclear.

DISPOSITION

- Prognosis is best in AMI due to mesenteric venous thrombosis and after surgical treatment for acute arterial embolism. It remains poor in cases of arterial thrombosis and nonocclusive ischemia.
- With delayed diagnosis, intestinal infarction—resulting in perforation or gangrenous bowel, sepsis, shock, and death—is typical.

REFERRAL

- Early surgical consultation should be considered. There should be no delay in patients with peritoneal signs.
- Surgery may also be warranted for diagnostic purposes.

PEARLS & CONSIDERATIONS

COMMENTS

- The diagnosis of AMI should be considered in any patient with acute onset of abdominal pain out of proportion to physical findings, particularly in at-risk patients.
- Early diagnosis, before intestinal infarction occurs, is critical and correlates with improved survival rates.
- The use of endovascular procedures for AMI is becoming more common and may be most appropriate for patients with ischemia that is not severe, and for those who have severe coexisting conditions that place them at high risk for complications and death associated with open surgery.

PREVENTION

Prevention of underlying factors, most notably atherosclerotic disease (smoking cessation, management of hypertension, and use of statins) is indicated for primary prevention as well as prevention of recurrence.

SUGGESTED READINGS

Available at ExpertConsult.com

RELATED CONTENT

Mesenteric Venous Thrombosis (Related Key Topic)

AUTHORS: **Firrah Saeed, MD,** and **Sarah Hyder, MD**

BASIC INFORMATION

DEFINITION

Acute myeloid leukemia (AML) is a malignancy of hematopoietic progenitor cells that would normally give rise to mature granulocytes. Strictly speaking, AML is a subset of acute nonlymphocytic leukemia (ANLL), a designation that broadly distinguishes these diseases from the biologically distinct leukemias of lymphocytic origin. ANLL includes leukemias involving the spectrum of myeloid stem cells, including precursors of granulocytes, monocytes, erythrocytes, and megakaryocytes. Acute promyelocytic leukemia is a distinct leukemia syndrome that is part of the ANLL spectrum, but that has very different treatment implications. ANLL is characterized by maturation failure of myeloid progenitors, excessive numbers of immature progenitors ("blasts"), and various degrees of bone marrow failure (neutropenia, thrombocytopenia, anemia).

SYNONYMS

Acute nonlymphocytic leukemia (ANLL)
Acute myelogenous leukemia (AML)

ICD-10CM CODES

C92.60	Acute myeloid leukemia with 11q23-abnormality not having achieved remission
C92.61	Acute myeloid leukemia with 11q23-abnormality in remission
C92.62	Acute myeloid leukemia with 11q23-abnormality in relapse
C92.90	Myeloid leukemia, unspecified, not having achieved remission
C92.91	Myeloid leukemia, unspecified in remission
C92.92	Myeloid leukemia, unspecified in relapse
C92.A0	Acute myeloid leukemia with multilineage dysplasia, not having achieved remission
C92.A1	Acute myeloid leukemia with multilineage dysplasia, in remission
C92.A2	Acute myeloid leukemia with multilineage dysplasia, in relapse
C92.Z0	Other myeloid leukemia not having achieved remission
C92.Z1	Other myeloid leukemia, in remission
C92.Z2	Other myeloid leukemia, in relapse
C92.00	Acute myeloblastic leukemia, not having achieved remission
C92.01	Acute myeloblastic leukemia, in remission
C92.02	Acute myeloblastic leukemia, in relapse

EPIDEMIOLOGY & DEMOGRAPHICS

- AML incidence rises with age:
  1. Incidence 20 to 55 yr old: 1 to 3/100,000 persons/yr
  2. Incidence 65 to 80 yr old: 11 to 20/100,000 persons/yr
- Annual incidence is 4 cases/100,000 persons/yr
- Males slightly > females; European ancestry slightly > African ancestry

PHYSICAL FINDINGS & CLINICAL PRESENTATION

Symptoms/exam findings:
- Complications of bone marrow failure:
  1. Thrombocytopenia-associated bleeding
  2. Fatigue and shortness of breath associated with anemia
  3. Infection associated with neutropenia
- Complications of leukocytosis (hyperleukocytic leukemia, WBC >100,000/mcl):
  1. Retinal hemorrhage with visual symptoms
  2. Headache and intracranial bleeding
  3. Respiratory symptoms from pulmonary involvement
- Systemic symptoms:
  1. Fatigue, fever (usually infectious, rarely tumor), bone pain (more common in ALL)
- Hemorrhagic complications of disseminated intravascular coagulation (DIC), especially with acute promyelocytic leukemia (APML).
- Physical exam will reflect consequences of cytopenias (bruising from thrombocytopenia, pallor from anemia). Enlarged lymph nodes and enlarged liver and spleen are rare. Exam is often normal.
- Rarely disease will present as skin lesions (leukemia cutis) or mass lesions (granulocytic sarcoma).
- Gum hypertrophy and organ/skin involvement is more common in monocytic leukemia.

ETIOLOGY

- Environmental/exposure related: Benzene (best documented), organic solvents (including gasoline), cigarette smoking (≥20 pack-yr 1.34 relative risk), obesity, best documented in women
- Hereditary disorders: Numerous, including Fanconi anemia, Bloom syndrome, Shwachman Diamond syndrome, Diamond Blackfan anemia, among others
- Therapy related:
  1. Alkylator (e.g., melphalan, busulfan, cisplatin) related: Typical latency 5 to 7 yr, associated with chromosome 5 and 7 abnormalities
  2. Topoisomerase II inhibitor (e.g. etoposide, doxorubicin): Typical latency 1-3 yr, associated with 11q23 (mixed lineage leukemia [MLL] gene) rearrangements
- Radiation exposures (therapeutic—generally low risk), occupational
- Antecedent hematologic disorders: Myelodysplasia, myeloproliferative disorders, aplastic anemia

DIAGNOSIS

DIFFERENTIAL DIAGNOSIS

- Disorders that can present with circulating blasts or cells with blastlike appearance:
  1. Acute myeloid leukemia/acute lymphocytic leukemia
  2. Myelodysplasia (up to 20% circulating blasts, if ≥20% = AML)
  3. Primary myelofibrosis
  4. Chronic myeloid leukemia
  5. Blastoid variant of mantle cell lymphoma
  6. Prolymphocytic leukemia
  7. Blastic plasmacytoid dendritic cell neoplasm
  8. Atypical lymphocytes of Epstein-Barr and cytomegalovirus infection may have blastlike appearance

WORKUP

The diagnostic workup consists of a morphologic assessment, immunophenotyping by flow cytometry, assessment of karyotype, and a panel of gene mutations (Fig. 1).

LABORATORY TESTS

- Complete blood counts and blood smear evaluation. Note that morphologic evaluation of blasts may suggest myeloid or lymphoid origin, but flow cytometry or cytochemistries (often faster) are needed to confirm. Auer rods are seen in blasts of myeloid origin.
- LDH is commonly elevated. Other biochemistries to assess organ function (creatinine, liver enzymes) and spontaneous tumor lysis syndrome (uric acid, potassium, phosphate, calcium).
- Coagulation studies to assess DIC. DIC is always present in APML, but can be present in ***all*** forms of acute leukemia, especially acute monocytic leukemia.
- HLA typing for possible bone marrow transplant and platelet support.
- Cytochemical stains:
  1. Myeloperoxidase can be performed in minutes, + in myeloid origin leukemia.
  2. Alpha naphthyl acetate esterase ("nonspecific esterase") stains mainly monocytic cells.
- Flow cytometry on blood and/or bone marrow (see Table E1).
- Cytogenetic studies, ideally on bone marrow, but can be done on peripheral blood. Fluorescence in situ hybridization (FISH) is often used as an adjunct to conventional chromosome analysis.
- Next Generation Sequencing (NGS) by PCR to detect specific prognostic gene mutations.
- Molecular studies to further stratify risk and prognosis, which may affect treatment choices (see Tables E2, 3, and 4). Directing this workup should be done with combined hematology and laboratory expertise and typically will consist of studies for fms-related tyrosine kinase gene (FLT3) mutations, nucleophosmin gene (NPM) mutations, and CCAAT/enhancer binding protein α gene (CEBPA) mutations. Wider molecular panels are increasingly common because of the increasing numbers of potential markers and the potential availability of targeted therapies for FLT3 mutated disease and those with isocitrate dehydrogenase mutations, among others. TP53 mutation, mutated RUNX1, and mutated ASXL1 have recently been added to the NCCN poor-risk category for AML in 2018. Table E5 summarizes common recurrent mutations in adult acute myeloid leukemia.

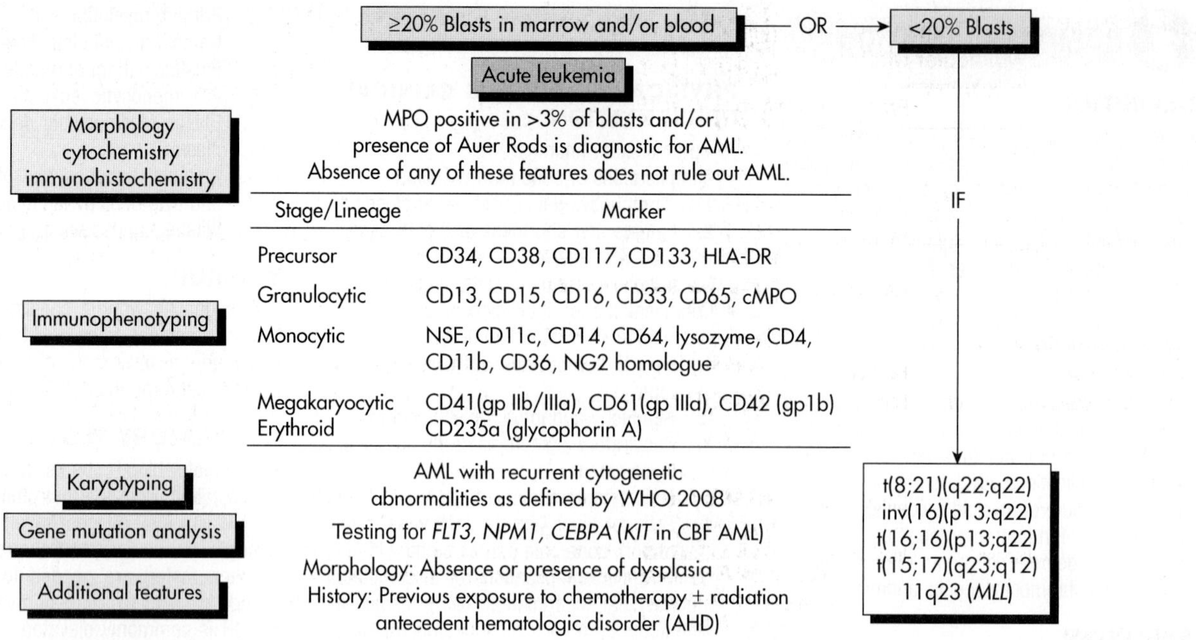

FIG. 1 Workup of acute myeloid leukemia. The diagnostic workup consists of a morphologic assessment, immunophenotyping by flow cytometry, assessment of the karyotype, and a panel of gene mutations. Whereas morphologic assessment by itself is often not sufficient to render a diagnosis, flow cytometry will confirm the lineage assignment (myeloid vs. lymphoid) and stage of differentiation in more than 95% of cases. In the remainder, either no lineage-specific antigens are expressed (acute undifferentiated leukemia) or antigens of more than one lineage are present (mixed-phenotype acute leukemia). In the latter scenario, antigens of several lineages can be found on one (biphenotypic) or separate populations of blasts (bilineal). Karyotyping and gene mutation analysis may add diagnostic information in morphologically ambiguous situations but is otherwise of more interest in determining prognosis. Additional information (exposure to previous chemotherapy and/or radiation therapy, history of an antecedent hematologic disorder, dysplasia) forms the basis for the 2008 revision of the WHO classification of AML. *AHD,* Antecedent hematologic disorder; *AML,* acute myeloid leukemia; *ANLL,* acute nonlymphocytic leukemia; *CBF,* core-binding factor; *MPO,* myeloperoxidase; *WHO,* World Health Organization. (From Hoffman R et al: *Hematology, basic principles and practice,* ed 7, Philadelphia, 2018, Elsevier.)

TABLE 3 European LeukemiaNet AML Risk Classification

Genetic Group	Subsets
Favorable	t(8;21)(q22;q22); *RUNX1-RUNX1T1*
	inv(16)(p13.1q22) or t(16;16)(p13.1;q22); *CBFB-MYH11*
	Mutated *NPM1* without *FLT3*-ITD (normal karyotype)
	Mutated *CEBPA* (normal karyotype)
Intermediate-I[a]	Mutated *NPM1* and *FLT3*-ITD (normal karyotype)
	Wild-type *NPM1* and *FLT3*-ITD (normal karyotype)
	Wild-type *NPM1* without *FLT3*-ITD (normal karyotype)
Intermediate-II	t(9;11)(p22;q23); *MLLT3-MLL*
	Cytogenetic abnormalities not classified as favorable or adverse[b]
Adverse	inv(3)(q21q26.2) or t(3;3)(q21;q26.2); *RPN1-EVI1*
	t(6;9)(p23;q34); *DEK-NUP214*
	t(v;11)(v;q23); *MLL* rearranged
	−5 or del(5q); −7; abnl(17p); complex karyotype[c]

[a]Includes all AMLs with normal karyotype except for those included in the favorable subgroup; most of these cases are associated with poor prognosis.
[b]For most abnormalities, adequate numbers have not been studied to draw firm conclusions regarding their prognostic significance.
[c]Three or more chromosome abnormalities in the absence of one of the WHO designated recurring translocations or inversions, that is, t(15;17), t(8;21), inv(16) or t(16;16), t(9;11), t(v;11)(v;q23), t(6;9), inv(3), or t(3;3).
From Hoffman R et al: *Hematology, basic principles and practice,* ed 7, Philadelphia, 2018, Elsevier.

- Formal diagnosis of acute nonlymphocytic leukemia is established if the marrow or peripheral blood blast percentage is ≥20%, unless t(8;21), inv(16), t(16;16) or t(15;17) are present, in which case the percentage of blasts may be lower.
  1. Myeloperoxidase (MPO) staining of 3% of blasts establishes myeloid lineage, but MPO may be negative in some AML cases diagnosed by flow cytometry.
  2. Specific criteria exist for diagnosing other forms of ANLL, mainly to distinguish it from myelodysplasia. The WHO AML classification is outlined in Table 6.
  3. Bone marrow findings are described in Fig. E2.

IMAGING STUDIES

- Imaging studies are typically directed to evaluating specific complaints.
- Echocardiogram or multigated acquisition scan is usually performed to verify that cardiac function is adequate to tolerate anthracycline (usually daunorubicin) therapy, with left ventricular ejection fraction (LVEF) of >50% typically considered acceptable.

Rx TREATMENT

ACUTE GENERAL Rx

- The general approach to AML is summarized in Fig. 3. Therapy of AML typically has three components:
  1. Immediate therapy to correct metabolic, infectious, or hyperleukocytic emergencies (if needed). Therapy for AML is always urgent but not always an emergency. However, treatment for APML should be considered a medical emergency to prevent catastrophic bleeding.
  2. Induction therapy, which is therapy of active disease intended to obtain remission and restore normal bone marrow function. Remission is defined as blasts <5% in the bone marrow, absolute neutrophils (ANC) of >1000/mcl, platelets >100,000/mcl, and transfusion independence. Complete remission with incomplete marrow recovery (CRi) indicates absence of leukemic blasts in the marrow but persistent cytopenias.
  3. Consolidation therapy, typically some form of intensive chemotherapy or stem

TABLE 4 Allogeneic Transplantation Guidelines for Adult Acute Myeloid Leukemia Based on Commonly Assessed Cytogenetic and Molecular Markers

AML Category	Prognostic Impact	Allogeneic Transplantation	Notes
AML-CR1: Younger Adults			
Good-risk disease			
APL	Favorable	No	APL is treatable by chemotherapy.
CBF-AML *without mKIT*	Favorable	No	t(8;21) AML with high WBC count at diagnosis may have worse prognosis.
CBF-AML *with mKIT*	Intermediate	Possible: MRD, MUD Uncertain: MMUD, UCB, haplo	
Intermediate-Risk Disease			
CN-AML *with CEBPA*	Favorable	No	Benefit likely restricted to *DM-CEBPA.*
CN-AML *with mutant NPM1 but not FLT-3-ITD*	Favorable	Possible: MRD	Emerging data suggests allogeneic HSCT benefit for this category, with reduced relapse and improved DFS in patients >40 yr.
CN-AML *with FLT-3-ITD*	Unfavorable[a]	Yes: MRD, MUD Possible[b]: MMUD, UCB, haplo	Unfavorable risk may be restricted to AML *with FLT-3-ITD allelic ratio >0.51.*
Other intermediate-risk disease	Intermediate or Unfavorable	Yes: MRD Likely acceptable[a]: MUD Possible[b]: MMUD, UCB, haplo	Likely considerable underlying clinical heterogeneity. Molecular risk profiling may further delineate risk in this category.
Poor-Risk Disease			
Monosomal karyotype *absent*	Unfavorable	Yes: MRD, MUD Likely acceptable[b]: MMUD, UCB, haplo	
Monosomal karyotype *present*	Very unfavorable	Yes: MRD, MUD Acceptable[b]: MMUD, UCB, haplo	
Abnormal 17(p)	Very unfavorable	Yes: MRD, MUD Acceptable[b]: MMUD, UCB, haplo	
AML-CR1: Older adults	Unfavorable	Yes: MRD, MUD Likely acceptable[b]: MMUD, UCB, haplo	
AML-CR1: t-AML, AML/MDS	Unfavorable	Yes: MRD, MUD Acceptable[b]: MMUD, UCB, haplo	Molecular risk profiling may supersede clinical classification of secondary AML, especially in older patients.
AML-CR2	Very unfavorable	Yes: MRD, MUD Acceptable[b]: MMUD, UCB, haplo	
AML not in remission	Very unfavorable	Yes: MRD, MUD Uncertain: MMUD, UCB, haplo	For selected patients: Good performance status, little comorbidity, lower leukemic burden; CIBMTR risk score may be useful.

AML, Acute myeloid leukemia; *APL,* acute promyelocytic leukemia; *CBF,* core binding factor; *CIBMTR,* Center for International Blood and Marrow Transplant Research; *CN,* cytogenetically normal; *CR1,* first complete remission; *CR2,* second complete remission; *haplo,* haploidentical; *MDS,* myelodysplastic syndrome; *MMUD,* mismatched unrelated donor; *MRD,* matched related donor; *MUD,* matched unrelated donor; *t-AML,* therapy-related AML; *UCB,* umbilical cord blood; *WBC,* white blood cell.
[a]If no sibling donor available.
[b]If no timely matched donor available.
From Hoffman R et al: *Hematology, basic principles and practice,* ed 7, Philadelphia, 2018, Elsevier.

cell transplant therapy intended to prevent relapse.

4. Hyperleukocytic symptoms are typically seen with WBC >100,000/ml. Leukapheresis requires catheter placement and pheresis but spares tumor lysis. Rapid cytoreduction with chemotherapy (hydroxyurea 3 to 6 g orally or cytarabine) is often adequate and easier but risks tumor lysis. Optimal management is therefore individualized.
5. Tumor lysis syndrome (TLS) is associated with a rise in uric acid, potassium, and serum phosphate, the last causing a reciprocal fall in calcium. The metabolic changes may result in renal failure, cardiac dysrhythmias, muscle spasms (due to low calcium), seizures, and death (a more detailed discussion is in the section on acute lymphocytic leukemia).
6. The mainstays of therapy for AML are medications dating from the 1970s—daunorubicin and cytarabine—with few medications having meaningful impact on therapy in the last four decades. In 2017, the U.S. FDA approved four new agents, including three targeted agents, for treatment of AML. The role of these agents and their relation to standard therapy is outlined below.
7. Induction chemotherapy typically consists of daunorubicin 60 or 90 mg/m^2 IV for 3 days and cytarabine (Ara-C) 100 or 200 mg/m^2/day as continuous infusion for 7 days ("7+3"). Success rates are 60% to 80% and have been better in recent trials. Other agents that are used include etoposide, idarubicin, fludarabine, and cladribine. Bone marrow examination is usually performed at day 14 of therapy to assess the response.
8. Gemtuzumab ozogamicin (GO, Mylotarg) is an antibody-drug conjugate binding an anti-CD33 antibody to the chemotherapeutic agent calicheamicin that was approved in 2017 for therapy of newly diagnosed CD33+ AML. In newly diagnosed AML, the use of low-dose GO when added to standard 7+3 induction had a success rate of 81%, with 2-yr relapse-free survival improving from 22.7% to 50.3% compared with standard therapy alone. The benefit was seen in favorable and intermediate-risk patients.
9. Midostaurin was also approved in 2017 for treatment of newly diagnosed AML with mutations in the fms-related tyrosine kinase 3 *(FLT3)* gene in combination with standard induction therapy. Four-yr overall survival was 51.4% in FLT3-positive patients receiving midostaurin vs. 44.3% in the placebo arm, with improved durability of remissions in patients achieving remission. The optimal use of these therapies requires rapid

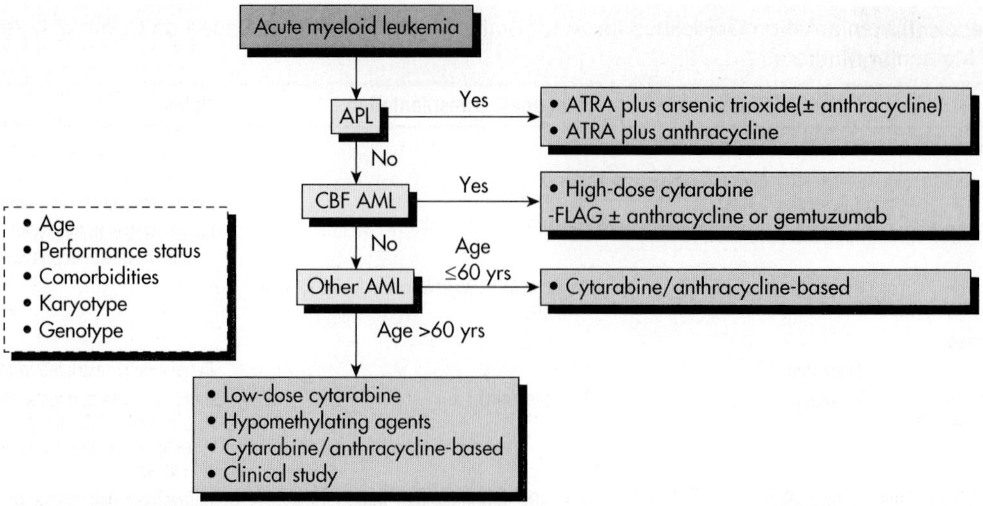

FIG. 3 General approach to acute myeloid leukemia therapy. *AML,* Acute myeloid leukemia; *APL,* acute promyelocytic leukemia; *ATRA,* all-trans retinoic acid; *CBF,* core binding factor; *FLAG,* fludarabine, cytarabine (Ara-C), and granulocyte colony-stimulating factor. (From Hoffman R et al: *Hematology, basic principles and practice,* ed 7, Philadelphia, 2018, Elsevier.)

access to genetic data at the time of diagnosis. Also approved in 2017 was CPX-351, a liposomal formulation of cytarabine and daunorubicin encapsulated in a 5:1 ratio, for patients with AML related to previous therapy (t-AML) or with AML with myelodysplasia-related change (AML-MRC). In a trial of t-AML and AML evolving from myelodysplasia or with WHO-defined myelodysplasia-related cytogenetic changes in patients ages 60 to 75 yr, CPX-351 improved survival to 9.56 mo vs. 5.95 mo with standard 7+3 induction. This overall survival was maintained out to 5 yr (18% vs. 8%).

10. Gilteritinib was FDA approved in 2018 for treatment of adult patients who have relapsed or refractory acute myeloid leukemia with a FLT3 mutation. Approval was based on an interim analysis of a trial, which included 138 adult patients with relapsed or refractory AML having an FLT3 ITD, D835, or I836 mutation. Gilteritinib was given orally at a dose of 120 mg daily until unacceptable toxicity or lack of clinical benefit. After a median follow-up of 4.6 mo, 21% of patients achieved complete remission (CR) or CR with partial hematologic recovery (CRh).
11. In 2018, the FDA granted accelerated approval to venetoclax, a BCL-2 inhibitor, in combination with azacitidine or decitabine or low-dose cytarabine for the treatment of newly diagnosed acute myeloid leukemia in adults who are age 75 yr or older, or who have comorbidities that preclude the use of intensive induction chemotherapy. The recommended venetoclax dose depends upon the combination regimen.

- Consolidation therapy is controversial. For patients managed with chemotherapy, cytarabine 3 g/m^2 for six doses is commonly used (day 1, 3, 5), but intermediate doses (1000-1500 mg/m^2) for six doses appear equally effective and less toxic. Doses above 1000 mg/m^2 are poorly tolerated in patients over 60 yr because of cerebellar toxicity. Renal insufficiency also increases the risk of cerebellar toxicity from Ara-C, which can be severe.

1. For favorable risk disease, consolidation with chemotherapy alone with two to four cycles of intermediate/high-dose cytarabine is typically given, with long-term survival of 60% to 70%.
2. For intermediate-risk and unfavorable-risk disease, first-remission allogeneic stem cell marrow transplant is often recommended if a donor is available. If not, chemotherapy consolidation chemotherapy is offered, although the optimal therapy and schedule, especially for unfavorable disease, is uncertain.
3. In the trial of GO as initial therapy, GO was also used in consolidation with high-dose cytarabine and daunorubicin.
4. The role of autologous bone marrow transplant is controversial, with some evidence of decreased relapse rates after chemotherapy but no clear benefit in overall survival.
5. Allogeneic bone marrow transplant is offered to patients with relapsed disease if a second remission can be obtained in good-risk patients. It is offered to high-risk and intermediate-risk patients in first remission if a donor is available. In 2018, most patients will be able to find a donor from either a matched related donor, matched unrelated donor, mismatched unrelated donor, haploidentical donor, or cord blood donor. The Center for International Blood and Marrow Transplant Research (CIBMTR) has published data for 12,309 patients receiving an HLA-matched sibling transplant and 15,632 patients receiving a matched unrelated donor for AML between 2002 and 2012. Their disease status at the time of transplant and the donor type were found to be the best predictors of posttransplant survival. The 3-yr probabilities of survival after HLA-matched sibling transplant in this cohort was 58% ± 1%, 50% ± 1%, and 24% ± 1% for patients with early, intermediate, and advanced disease, respectively. The probabilities of survival after an unrelated donor transplant were 49% ± 1%, 47% ± 1%, and 22% ± 1% for patient with early, intermediate, and advanced disease, respectively.
6. Enasidenib, a selective inhibitor of mutated isocitrate dehydrogenase 2 (IDH-2), was approved by the FDA in 2017 for relapsed or refractory AML with IDH-2 mutations. IDH-2 mutations are found in about 12% of AML patients. At a dose of 100 mg orally, the response rate was 40.3%, with 19.3% achieving remission, some durable. Differentiation syndrome can be seen with enasidenib, similar to therapy for APML. In November 2020, results of the phase 3 IDHENTIFY study for relapsed or refractory AML failed to meet the primary endpoint of overall survival. This study compared enasidenib and best supportive care to conventional care regimens, including best supportive care only, azacitidine and best supportive, low-dose cytarabine and best supportive care, or intermediate-dose cytarabine and best supportive care.
7. Ivosidenib, a selective inhibitor of isocitrate dehydrogenase-1 (IDH-1) mutation, was approved by the FDA in 2018 as the first treatment of adult patients with relapsed/refractory acute myeloid leukemia with an IDH-1 mutation. Approval was based on results from a phase 1, open-label, single-arm, multicenter, dose-escalation, expansion trial of adult patients in this population. The primary end point was combined complete remission and complete remission with partial hematologic improvement; the combined rate was 32.8%,

TABLE 6 Classification of Acute Myeloid Leukemia According to the Revised World Health Organization Classification (2016)

Category	Subtype/Definition*
AML with recurrent cytogenetic abnormalities	t(8;21)(q22;q22); RUNX1-RUNX1T1† inv(16)(p13.1q22); CBFB-MYH11† t(16;16)(p13.1q22); CBFB-MYH11† t(15;17)(q22;q12); PML-RARA† (= acute promyelocytic leukemia) t(9;11)(p22;q23); MLLT3-KMT2A t(6;9)(p23;q34); DEK-NUP214 inv(3)(q21q26.2); GATA2, MECOM t(3;3)(q21;q26.2); RPN1-EVI1 t(1;22)(p13q13); RBM15-MKL1 (megakaryoblastic) with mutated NPM1 with biallelic mutations of CEBPA
AML with MDS-related changes	Morphologic features of MDS, or prior history of MDS or MDS/MPN, or MDS-related karyotype, and none of the recurrent genetic abnormalities above
Therapy-related myeloid neoplasms	Late complications of cytotoxic chemotherapy (alkylating agents, topoisomerase II inhibitors) and/or ionizing radiation therapy†
AML, not otherwise specified	AML with minimal differentiation AML without maturation AML with maturation Acute myelomonocytic leukemia Acute monoblastic/monocytic leukemia Pure erythroid leukemia Acute megakaryoblastic leukemia Acute basophilic leukemia Acute panmyelosis with myelofibrosis
Myeloid Sarcoma	
Myeloid proliferations related to Down syndrome	Transient abnormal myelopoiesis Myeloid leukemia associated with Down syndrome
Blastic Plasmacytoid Dendritic Cell Neoplasm	
Acute leukemia of ambiguous lineage	Acute undifferentiated leukemia Mixed-phenotype acute leukemia with: t(9;22)(q34;q11.2); BCR-ABL1 t(v;11q23); KMT2A rearranged Mixed-phenotype acute leukemia, B/myeloid, NOS Mixed-phenotype acute leukemia, T/myeloid, NOS
Provisional entities	AML with mutated NPM1 AML with mutated CEBPA NK-cell lymphoblastic leukemia/lymphoma

AML, Acute myeloid leukemia; *MDS,* myelodysplastic syndrome; *MPN,* myeloproliferative neoplasm; *NK,* natural killer; *NOS,* not otherwise specified. For AML with recurrent genetic abnormalities, specific genes rearranged follow the chromosome rearrangement. In 2016, the *MLL* gene has been renamed *KMT2A.*
*Diagnosis of AML regardless of percentage of blasts.
†Excluded are patients with AML who have transformed from MPN.

and the median duration of remission was 8.2 mo.

8. Relapses after bone marrow transplant can sometimes be managed with donor lymphocyte infusions, adjustment of immune suppression, and chemotherapy (often low intensity). In general, outcomes are poor with posttransplant relapses.

- Treatment of older patients (>60 yr) is problematic, with cure rates of 10% to 15%. Older patients do worse because they are more likely to have high-risk features and less likely to tolerate therapy. Several models have been devised to identify variables that predict which patients may do well with conventional therapy versus those who will not (Table 7). Options for these patients include:
  1. Standard induction therapy is reasonable for patients likely to tolerate it. Even in the absence of cure, quality of life is often excellent in remission. More recent studies suggest that the early death rate (within 30 days of diagnosis) was lower for patients in their 70s and 80s receiving standard induction. There is no standardized approach to evaluating fitness for therapy; one algorithm is at www.aml-score.org/.
  2. Hypomethylating agents—decitabine and azacytidine—may be considered in patients unlikely to tolerate induction therapy. Azacytidine (75 mg/m^2 daily for 7 days every 28 days) and decitabine (20 mg/m^2 for 5 days every 28 days) are considered in older patients who are not considered appropriate for induction chemotherapy. Both are outpatient regimens, and decitabine especially is very well tolerated. Recent data with azacytidine suggest benefit in about 20% to 30% lasting 14 to 16 mo in responders, with equivalent results in low blast count (20%-30% in the bone marrow) vs. higher blast count disease.
  3. Single-agent gemtuzumab ozogamicin is an option for treatment of CD33+ AML in patients considered unfit for induction. The benefit compared to best supportive care (BSC) was mainly seen in patients with CD33 expression of greater than 80% and favorable/intermediate cytogenetics (1 yr survival 22% and 37% respectively, BSC <10%), with no benefit in patients with high-risk cytogenetics.
  4. Low-dose cytarabine 20 mg/m^2 twice daily or 40 mg/m^2 daily for 10 days subcutaneously) has shown survival benefit over hydroxyurea in low-/intermediate-risk patients.
  5. In November 2018, the FDA granted the accelerated approval to venetoclax (a bcl-2 protein inhibitor) in combination with azacitidine or decitabine or low-dose cytarabine for the treatment of newly diagnosed acute myeloid leukemia in adults who are age 75 yr or older, or who have comorbidities that preclude use of intensive induction chemotherapy. The recommended venetoclax dose depends upon the combination regimen and is described in prescribing information of venetoclax.
  6. In November 2018, the FDA approved glasdegib (a small molecule inhibitor of Sonic hedgehog pathway) in combination with low-dose cytarabine (LDAC), for newly diagnosed acute myeloid leukemia in patients who are 75 yr old or older or who have comorbidities that preclude intensive induction chemotherapy. Approval was based upon a multicenter, open-label, randomized study that randomized eligible patients 2:1 to receive glasdegib, 100 mg daily, with LDAC 20 mg subcutaneously twice daily on days 1 to 10 of a 28-day cycle or LDAC alone in 28-day cycles until disease progression or unacceptable toxicity. Efficacy was established based on an improvement in overall survival, 8.3 mo for LDAC + glasdegib versus 4.3 mo for LDAC alone. HR of 0.46 (95% CI: 0.30, 0.71; p=0.0002).
  7. Oral hydroxyurea dosed to counts and cytopenias.
  8. Best supportive care.
  9. Reduced-intensity allogeneic stem cell transplant is an option for patients in remission after standard therapy. A recent meta-analysis of studies including 749 patients over 60 receiving RIT identified a 3-yr relapse-free survival of 35%.

- **Acute Promyelocytic Leukemia (APML):** APML is a distinct leukemia syndrome with very different treatment implications. Cure rates greater than 95% have been seen in current protocols in the absence of high-risk features. It is associated with t(15;17), which translocates the PML gene to retinoic acid receptor α (PML-RARa). Uncommon variants are t(11;17) and t(5;17). Risk groups for relapse were defined in studies using retinoic acid and chemotherapy. Patients with presenting WBC >10,000/mcl were considered high

TABLE 7 Prognostic Models in Older Patients With Acute Myeloid Leukemia

Study	Outcome	Unfavorable Characteristics
Study Alliance Leukemia	Survival Disease-free survival	CD34 expression >10% WBC >20 × 10^9/L Age >65 yr LDH >700 U/L NPM1 status wild-type[a]
UK Medical Research Council	Survival	Adverse cytogenetic group Elevated WBC[b] Poor performance status[b] Older age[b] Secondary AML
Acute Leukemia French Association	Survival	High-risk cytogenetics ± Age ≥75 yr Performance status ≥2 WBC ≥50 × 10^9/L
MD Anderson Cancer Center	Remission rate Induction mortality Survival	Age ≥75 yr Secondary AML[c] AHD duration ≥6[c] (12) mo Treatment outside LAFR Unfavorable cytogenetics WBC ≥25 × 10^9/Lc Hemoglobin ≤8 g/dlc Creatinine >1.3 mg/dl Performance status >2 LDH >600 U/L[d]
Hematopoietic Cell Transplantation Comorbidity Index	Early mortality Survival	Dyspnea Coronary artery disease, CHF, MI, or EF <50% Chronic hepatitis, elevation of bilirubin and/or transaminases Cirrhosis Elevations of creatinine, dialysis, renal transplant Secondary AML Depression/anxiety requiring therapy Continued use of antimicrobial therapy after day 0 BMI >35 kg/m²

AHD, Antecedent hematologic disorder; *AML,* acute myeloid leukemia; *BMI,* body mass index; *CHF,* congestive heart failure; *EF,* ejection fraction; *LAFR,* laminar air flow room (isolation floor); *LDH,* lactate dehydrogenase; *MI,* myocardial infarction; *WBC,* white blood cell count.
[a]Favorable and high-risk groups were defined solely by cytogenetic aberrations. Above factors served to further divide the intermediate-risk group into good intermediate versus adverse intermediate.
[b]As continuous variables.
[c]Only significant for prediction of remission.
[d]Only significant for prediction of survival.
From Hoffman R et al: *Hematology, basic principles and practice,* ed 7, Philadelphia, 2018, Elsevier.

risk, patients with WBC <10,000 and platelets >40,000 were considered low risk, and all others were considered intermediate risk. In current protocols, high-risk patients receive some form of intensified therapy.

- APML is a medical emergency because of the high risk of bleeding complications.
  1. All patients with APML have DIC, caused by overexpression of annexin II (which increases generation of plasmin, degrading fibrin), elastases (which degrade fibrinogen and fibrinolytic inhibitors), and increased endothelial tissue plasminogen activator release.
  2. Early death due to hemorrhage is seen in 5% to 17% of newly diagnosed APML patients, usually intracranial or pulmonary. Risk factors include elevated WBC, increased age, and elevated creatinine.
  3. Retinoic acid rapidly stabilizes the coagulopathy of APML; consideration should be given to starting this immediately for suspected cases.
  4. Cryoprecipitate (usual dose 10 bags) to raise the fibrinogen level to 150 mg/dl and platelet transfusion to raise the count to >50,000mcl should be given as needed.
  5. Unfractionated heparin may paradoxically stop bleeding in APML by inhibiting DIC, but is rarely used in the retinoic acid treatment era.
- Diagnosis of APML.
  1. Rapid diagnosis is essential due to treatment implications.
  2. Diagnosis by classic APML blast morphology and clinical syndrome (especially DIC with low fibrinogen) is sufficient to justify starting treatment with retinoic acid pending confirmation with molecular studies. Immediate therapy with retinoic acid will rapidly stabilize the coagulopathy and help prevent catastrophic bleeding.
  3. Polymerase chain reaction for PML/RARa.
  4. FISH for t(15;17) or variants.
  5. Flow cytometry is typically distinct with lack of HLA-DR and CD34; CD13, CD33 and CD64 are usually positive.
- Therapy of APML.
  1. Emergency measures to stabilize coagulopathy as outlined previously.
  2. Patients with WBC ≤10,000 (low/intermediate risk) are treated with retinoic acid and arsenic trioxide ("differentiation therapy").
  3. Therapy of high-risk patients is less well standardized but has included intensification with cytarabine, anthracyclines, and gemtuzumab ozogamicin. A recent trial using arsenic and retinoic acid with GO demonstrated 100% 4-yr survival in high-risk patients after 30 days, emphasizing the importance of preventing early deaths in APML.
  4. Maintenance therapy for 2 yr is given in some APML protocols.
  5. Patients with high-risk disease receive central nervous system prophylaxis with intrathecal chemotherapy.
  6. Treatment of relapsed disease typically consists of autologous bone marrow transplant after obtaining second remission.
- Differentiation syndrome (DS) is a potentially fatal complication of therapy with retinoic acid and arsenic trioxide. It is associated with fever, interstitial pulmonary infiltrates, peripheral edema, pleural and pericardial effusions and renal failure; it is commonly associated with rising WBC seen in patients on differentiation therapy.
  1. Therapy for suspected differentiation syndrome is dexamethasone 10 mg/m² every 12 hr. Cytoreductive therapy (hydroxyurea, idarubicin) and stopping retinoic acid and arsenic are appropriate for inadequate response to dexamethasone.
  2. Prophylaxis for differentiation syndrome with dexamethasone 2.5 mg/m² every 12 hr has been suggested for WBC >5000 or creatinine >1.4 mg/dl. Hydroxyurea is used to keep the WBC below 10,000/mcl in some protocols.

PEARLS & CONSIDERATIONS

- The diagnosis of acute myeloid leukemia or variants is often, but not always, a medical emergency requiring rapid clinical and laboratory assessment by appropriate expertise.
- APML is a distinct clinical entity that has a high cure rate with current protocols, but which requires intensive supportive care at the time of diagnosis.

RELATED CONTENT

Acute Myelogenous Leukemia (Patient Information)

SUGGESTED READINGS

Available at ExpertConsult.com

AUTHOR: **Todd F. Roberts, MD, FRCP(C)**

BASIC INFORMATION

DEFINITION

Acute pelvic pain in women is defined as pain present in the pelvis or the bilateral lower quadrants of the abdomen that is typically noncyclic, sudden in onset, and present for less than 3 mo.

SYNONYMS

Acute lower abdominal pain
Acute suprapubic pain

ICD-10CM CODE
R10.2 Pelvic and perineal pain/acute female pelvic pain/pelvic pain, acute

EPIDEMIOLOGY & DEMOGRAPHICS

Acute pelvic pain occurs in women of all ages.

PREVALENCE: Acute pelvic pain is a very broad term with multiple etiologies, thus not lending itself to a single calculable prevalence. However, the prevalence of some of the most documented common causes in the U.S. include PID (2,500,000 women with a personal history in the U.S. as of 2015), ovarian torsion (2.7% of emergent gynecologic surgeries each year), ectopic pregnancy (0.6% to 2.1% of all pregnancies), and appendicitis (6.7% lifetime risk in women).

PREDOMINANT SEX & AGE: Women of reproductive age report the greatest amount of acute pelvic pain.

RISK FACTORS: Risk factors for acute pelvic pain depend on the etiology with the most common cause being PID. Risk factors for PID include women under the age of 25, increasing number of sexual partners, lack of condom use, recent STI treatment, or HIV-positive status.

PHYSICAL FINDINGS & CLINICAL PRESENTATION

- The history and physical examination are key to narrowing the diagnosis when a patient presents with acute pelvic pain.
- Standard thorough history-taking techniques should be employed, and the patient should be asked about location, onset, severity, radiation, exacerbating and alleviating factors, as well as the quality of the pain.
- Associated symptoms depend on the etiology; symptoms that should be inquired about include nausea, vomiting, anorexia, vaginal discharge, vaginal bleeding, dyspareunia, dysuria, hematuria, urinary frequency, fever, recent upper respiratory infection (URI) symptoms, cyclic midcycle pelvic pain, or any missed or irregular menses.
- A thorough sexual history should also be taken, including form of birth control used. Patients should also be asked about any history of ovarian cysts, uterine fibroids, recent pregnancies (including ectopic pregnancies), or other pelvic infections.
- Physical examination is focused on the abdominal and pelvic examination, as described under Workup later in this chapter.

ETIOLOGY

Etiologies of acute pelvic pain are varied and depend on the age and pregnancy status of the patient. Please see Differential Diagnosis for further information.

Dx DIAGNOSIS

DIFFERENTIAL DIAGNOSIS

The differential diagnosis of acute pelvic pain is described in Table 1

WORKUP

The workup of acute pelvic pain begins with a thorough history and physical examination including determination of pregnancy status, then targeted imaging and laboratory studies are ordered to further delineate the diagnosis.

The pelvic examination includes vaginal speculum examination with evaluation for any active vaginal bleeding, any vaginal or cervical discharge, and any vulvar or vaginal lesions and masses. Additional key components of the pelvic examinations include bimanual, rectovaginal, and rectal examinations. The bimanual and rectovaginal examinations help elucidate the size and contour of the uterus, the presence of any adnexal masses or tenderness, and whether the patient has cervical motion tenderness. Testing for gonorrhea and chlamydia should be collected via nucleic acid probe.

LABORATORY TESTS

First and foremost, one must determine the pregnancy status of the patient. The most common pregnancy-related causes of acute pelvic pain are ectopic pregnancy (approximately 1 in 7000 spontaneously conceived pregnancies and 1 in 100 pregnancies conceived via artificial reproduction) and spontaneous or threatened miscarriage. In both of these cases, the Rh status of the patient must be determined and RhoGAM administered if she is Rh negative.

Key laboratory test considerations:

- Pregnancy testing via urine or serum.
- Urinalysis will assist with the diagnosis of both acute cystitis and nephrolithiasis, and urine culture should be ordered as well when appropriate.
- Nucleic acid probes for gonorrhea and chlamydia are very sensitive and specific tests and should be collected on any patient with pelvic pain via vaginal and cervical swab.
- A cervical culture should be considered in individuals who have been recently treated with an antibiotic and have persistent pain.
- Vaginal or cervical wet mount can detect bacterial vaginosis, trichomoniasis, or a yeast infection when symptoms suggest one of these etiologies.
- CBC should be considered for suspected gastrointestinal disease, appendicitis, and pelvic infection of any kind to help determine the severity of disease.

IMAGING STUDIES

- Pelvic ultrasound is the primary imaging modality for acute pelvic pain in women that is suspected to be of gynecologic origin. Ultrasound can be used to diagnose intrauterine and ectopic pregnancy (Fig. 1), uterine fibroids, adnexal masses, nephrolithiasis, and even appendicitis, thus assisting with the diagnosis of the vast majority of the differential diagnosis of acute pelvic pain in women. However, there are limitations to the test, such as the level of

TABLE 1 Differential Diagnosis of Acute Pelvic Pain

Gynecologic Causes	Obstetric-Related Causes	Nongynecologic or Obstetric-Related Causes
PID	Intrauterine pregnancy	Appendicitis
Ruptured ovarian cyst	Ectopic pregnancy (especially with ruptured ectopic)	Urinary tract infection
Adnexal mass (typically cysts >4-5 cm in size and hemorrhagic in nature)	Heterotopic pregnancy	Nephrolithiasis
Ovarian torsion	Placental abruption	Diverticulitis
Degenerating or torsed uterine fibroid	Uterine rupture	Colitis
Mittelschmerz pain	Miscarriage	Bowel obstruction
Tubo-ovarian abscess	Gestational trophoblastic disease	Mesenteric lymphadenitis
Endometriosis	Postpartum endometritis	Inflammatory bowel disease
Dysmenorrhea	Retained products of conception	Meckel diverticulum
Malpositioned intrauterine device or uterine perforation		Constipation
Cervicitis		Hernia
Hematometra/Hematocolpos		Gastroenteritis
		Musculoskeletal dysfunction
		Trauma

PID, Pelvic inflammatory disease.

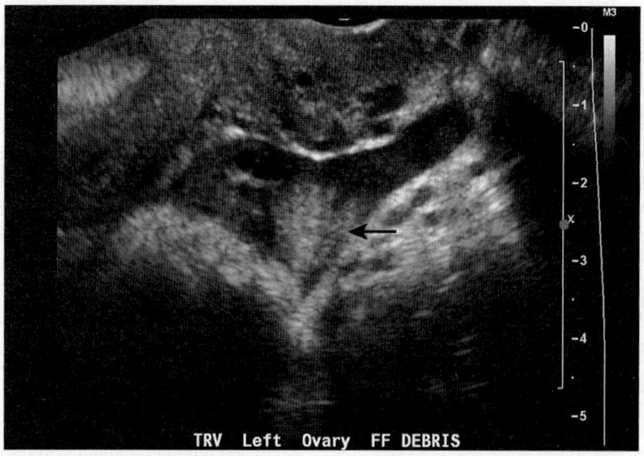

FIG. 1 A sonographic image of a 23-year-old patient with a ruptured ectopic pregnancy. The free fluid containing echogenic debris representing blood is seen in the cul-de-sac *(arrow)*. (From Soto JA, Lucey BC: *Emergency radiology, the requisites,* ed 2, Philadelphia, 2017, Elsevier.)

expertise of the individual sonographer and patient body habitus interfering with the quality of the images. Useful modes of ultrasound include transvaginal and transabdominal with the former providing greater detail and the latter and larger field of view.

- In the case of the patient with nonfocal symptoms or an inconclusive ultrasound, computed tomography (CT) of the abdomen and pelvis can be performed and should be performed with oral and IV contrast. CT is highly useful in the patient with early pelvic inflammatory disease (PID) or tubo-ovarian abscess, as well as in the nonpregnant patient with appendicitis or other gastrointestinal pathology not seen on ultrasound.
- Magnetic resonance imaging (MRI) also plays a role when CT is nondiagnostic or when CT is unable to discern whether a mass in the pelvis is of uterine or adnexal origin such as with a degenerating fibroid or when one must further characterize an ovarian mass. MRI is also extremely helpful in the pregnant patient who presents with many signs and symptoms of appendicitis but has an inconclusive ultrasound result. Pediatric patients are also excellent candidates for MRI when ultrasound is inconclusive. Lower levels of ionizing radiation and its excellent diagnostic capabilities make it a very useful test in this population.
- Review of the imaging studies should include assessment of the genitourinary system as well as the gastrointestinal system including the ureters, uterus, ovaries, and bowel with evaluation of the presence or absence of ascites, inflammation, and fluid collections.

Rx TREATMENT

NONPHARMACOLOGIC THERAPY

- The underlying cause of acute pelvic pain cannot always be diagnosed with history, exam, laboratory, and imaging studies alone. In many cases, diagnostic laparoscopy is necessary to complete the diagnosis. For example, clinically significant adnexal torsion can be present even with normal vasculature visualized on ultrasound with Doppler. Moreover, laparoscopy can reveal entirely different findings than what was clinically diagnosed as was illustrated in one study where just over half of women diagnosed with appendicitis actually had the disease.
- The practitioner should not hesitate to take the patient with unstable vital signs and suspected intraabdominal bleeding or findings suggestive of ruptured appendix to the operating room. When one's clinical suspicion is quite high for such diagnoses, laboratory data and imaging studies should be forgone to expedite getting the patient the surgical interventions she needs.

ACUTE GENERAL Rx

The initial treatment of the woman with acute pelvic pain must be tailored to the underlying cause. However, it is imperative to manage the patient's pain while workup is in progress. NSAIDs are the traditional first-line pharmacotherapy for the patient with pelvic pain of an inflammatory nature. They are highly useful in cases of endometriosis, dysmenorrhea, nonsurgical cases of ovarian masses and ruptured ovarian cysts, spontaneous miscarriage, nephrolithiasis, musculoskeletal dysfunction, and PID/tubo-ovarian abscess. Heat and ice can also be employed as needed for additional symptomatic relief in the appropriate patient. Narcotic pain medications should be reserved for select cases of refractory pain.

CHRONIC Rx

Once a diagnosis is made, treatment is based on the underlying cause of the pain. Most patients are managed on a combination of NSAID and narcotic pain medications for a short course until the pathology has resolved or after any surgical interventions. Antibiotic therapy is routinely included in the case of an infectious cause. Drainage is indicated if a tubo-ovarian abscess is present and can be performed via transabdominal, transvaginal, transgluteal, and transrectal routes depending on the location.

REFERRAL

Patients with pain lasting greater than 3 to 6 mo should be seen by a specialist in the appropriate field—gynecology, gastroenterology, general surgery, or musculoskeletal medicine—for further workup and management of their now chronic pelvic pain. Referral should also be considered when the underlying cause of pain cannot be found.

PEARLS & CONSIDERATIONS

COMMENTS

A solid knowledge of the differential diagnosis of acute pelvic pain in women and a thorough history and physical examination will lead the practitioner to the underlying cause in the vast majority of cases. But all women who present with acute pelvic pain MUST have a pregnancy test as a part of their initial workup. If imaging is needed, pelvic ultrasound is an excellent tool and should be utilized first before CT and MRI in most cases.

PREVENTION

Prevention of acute pelvic pain depends on the etiology with the most common cause being PID; the important preventative actions include minimizing risk of STIs with condom use and avoidance of multiple sexual partners.

SUGGESTED READINGS

Available at ExpertConsult.com

RELATED CONTENT

Appendicitis (Related Key Topic)
Crohn Disease (Related Key Topic)
Diverticular Disease (Diverticulosis, Diverticulitis, Diverticular Hemorrhage) (Related Key Topic)
Ectopic Pregnancy (Related Key Topic)
Endometriosis (Related Key Topic)
Endometritis (Related Key Topic)
Pelvic Inflammatory Disease (Related Key Topic)
Spontaneous Abortion (Related Key Topic)
Ulcerative Colitis (Related Key Topic)
Urinary Tract Infection (Related Key Topic)
Urolithiasis (Nephrolithiasis) (Related Key Topic)
Uterine Fibroids (Related Key Topic)

AUTHORS: **Courtney Pfeuti, MD,** and **Simone Sweeney, MD**

BASIC INFORMATION

DEFINITION

Acute respiratory distress syndrome (ARDS) is a form of noncardiogenic pulmonary edema that results from acute damage to the alveoli. It is characterized by diffuse infiltrative lung lesions with resulting interstitial and alveolar edema, severe hypoxemia, and respiratory failure. The cardinal feature of ARDS, refractory hypoxemia, is caused by formation of protein-rich alveolar edema after damage to the integrity of the lung's alveolar-capillary barrier.

The initial definition of ARDS was based on the American–European Consensus Conference (AECC) from 1994 included the following components:

1. The syndrome must present acutely
2. A ratio of Pa_{O_2} to Fi_{O_2} ≤200 regardless of the level of positive end expiratory pressure (PEEP)
3. The detection of bilateral pulmonary infiltrates on frontal chest radiograph
4. Absence of congestive heart failure (pulmonary artery wedge pressure [PAWP] ≤18 mm Hg or no clinical evidence of elevated left atrial pressure on the basis of chest radiograph or other clinical data)

The 2012 Berlin definition of ARDS (Table 1) addresses some of the limitations of the AECC definition and establishes the criteria for ARDS:

- Timing: Within 1 wk of a known clinical insult or new or worsening respiratory symptoms
- Chest imaging (chest x-ray or computed tomography [CT] scan): Bilateral opacities, not fully explained by effusions, lobar/lung collapse, or nodules
- Origin of edema: Respiratory failure not fully explained by cardiac failure or fluid overload. Need objective assessment (e.g., echocardiography) to exclude hydrostatic edema if no risk factor present
- Oxygenation (if altitude is higher than 1000 m, the correction factor should be calculated as follows: [Pa_{O_2}/Fi_{O_2} × {barometric pressure/760}]
- Mild: 200 mm Hg <Pa_{O_2}/Fi_{O_2} ≤300 mm Hg with PEEP or CPAP ≥5 cm H_2O (this may be delivered noninvasively in the mild ARDS group)
- Moderate: 100 mm Hg <Pa_{O_2}/Fi_{O_2} ≤200 mm Hg with PEEP or CPAP ≥5 cm H_2O
- Severe: Pa_{O_2}/Fi_{O_2} ≤100 mm Hg with PEEP or CPAP ≥5 cm H_2O

SYNONYMS

ARDS
Adult respiratory distress syndrome

ICD-10CM CODE

J80 Acute respiratory distress syndrome

EPIDEMIOLOGY & DEMOGRAPHICS

- More than 150,000 ARDS cases/yr in the U.S. 7.1% of all patients admitted to an intensive care unit (ICU) and 16.1% of all patients on mechanical ventilation develop ARDS.
- An international study of 50 countries revealed that 10% of those admitted to an ICU fulfilled criteria for ARDS, and of these, 93% developed it within 48 hours of admission. The study reinforced the notion that ARDS is underrecognized.
- Black, Hispanic, and other patients belonging to racial minorities in the United States were observed to exhibit significantly higher in-hospital sepsis-related respiratory failure and associated mortality.

PHYSICAL FINDINGS & CLINICAL PRESENTATION

- Signs and symptoms:
  1. Dyspnea
  2. Chest discomfort
  3. Cough
  4. Anxiety
- Physical examination:
  1. Tachypnea
  2. Tachycardia
  3. Hypertension
  4. Paradoxical breathing and use of accessory muscles
  5. Coarse crepitations or crackles of both lungs
  6. Fever may be present if infection is the underlying etiology

ETIOLOGY

- Sepsis (>40% of cases)
- Aspiration: Near-drowning, aspiration of gastric contents (>30% of cases)
- Trauma (>20% of cases)
- Pneumonia (aspiration of gastric contents and sepsis together account for more than 85% of cases of ARDS in recent clinical trials)
- Multiple transfusions, blood products
- Drugs (e.g., overdose of morphine, methadone, heroin; reaction to nitrofurantoin)
- Noxious inhalation (e.g., chlorine gas, high O_2 concentration)
- Post-resuscitation
- Cardiopulmonary bypass
- Burns
- Pancreatitis
- A history of chronic alcohol abuse significantly increases the risk of developing ARDS in critically ill patients
- Table 2 describes risk factors associated with development of ARDS

TABLE 1 2012 Berlin Definition of Acute Respiratory Distress Syndrome (All Components Must Be Present)

Timing	Within 1 wk of a known clinical insult or new/worsening respiratory symptoms		
Chest imaging	Bilateral opacities—not fully explained by effusions, lobar/lung collapse, or nodules		
Origin of edema	Respiratory failure not fully explained by cardiac failure or fluid overload; need objective assessment (e.g., echocardiography) to exclude hydrostatic edema if no risk factor for ARDS is present		
Oxygenation	*Mild ARDS*	*Moderate ARDS*	*Severe ARDS*
	200 < Pa_{O_2}/Fi_{O_2} ≤300 with PEEP or CPAP ≥5 cm H_2O	100 < Pa_{O_2}/Fi_{O_2} ≤200 PEEP ≥5 cm H_2O	Pa_{O_2}/Fi_{O_2} ≤100 with PEEP ≥5 cm H_2O

ARDS, Acute respiratory distress syndrome.
From Weinberger SE: *Principles of pulmonary medicine,* ed 7, Philadelphia, 2019, Elsevier.

TABLE 2 Risk Factors Associated With Development of Acute Lung Injury and Acute Respiratory Distress Syndrome

Direct Lung Injury	Indirect Lung Injury
Pneumonia	Sepsis
Aspiration of gastric contents	Multiple trauma
Pulmonary contusion	Cardiopulmonary bypass
Fat, amniotic fluid, or air emboli	Drug overdose
Near-drowning	Acute pancreatitis
Inhalational injury	Transfusion of blood products
Reperfusion pulmonary edema	

From Vincent JL et al: *Textbook of critical care,* ed 6, Philadelphia, 2011, Saunders.

DIAGNOSIS

DIFFERENTIAL DIAGNOSIS

- Cardiogenic pulmonary edema
- Interstitial lung disease (acute interstitial pneumonia, nonspecific interstitial pneumonia [NSIP], cryptogenic organizing pneumonia [COP], acute eosinophilic pneumonia, hypersensitivity pneumonia, pulmonary alveolar proteinosis)
- Connective tissue diseases, such as polymyositis
- Diffuse alveolar hemorrhage
- Lymphangitic carcinomatosis from T-cell or B-cell lymphomas
- Drug-induced lung diseases (amiodarone, bleomycin)

WORKUP

The search for an underlying cause should focus on treatable causes (e.g., infections such as sepsis or pneumonia).

- Arterial blood gases (ABGs)
- Hemodynamic monitoring
- Bronchoalveolar lavage (selected patients)
- Transthoracic echocardiogram

LABORATORY TESTS

- ABGs:
  1. Initially: Varying degrees of hypoxemia, generally resistant to supplemental oxygen
  2. Respiratory alkalosis, decreased P_{CO_2}
  3. Widened alveolar-arterial gradient
  4. Hypercapnia as the disease progresses
- Bronchoalveolar lavage:
  1. The most prominent finding is an increased number of polymorphonucleocytes.
  2. The presence of eosinophilia has therapeutic implications because these patients respond to corticosteroids.
- Blood and urine cultures
- Blood work:
  1. Increased or reduced white blood cell count with left shift if concomitant infectious process
  2. Normal or mildly elevated B-type natriuretic peptide level
  3. Increased lactate level if concomitant sepsis or septic shock

IMAGING STUDIES

Chest radiograph (Fig. E1).

- The initial chest radiograph might be normal in the initial hours after the precipitating event.
- Bilateral interstitial infiltrates are usually seen within 24-72 hours; they often are more prominent in the bases and periphery.
- CT scan of chest: Bilateral diffuse, dense consolidations with air bronchograms.

Rx TREATMENT

NONPHARMACOLOGIC THERAPY

Treatment of ARDS is supportive.

Hemodynamic monitoring:

- Can be used for the initial evaluation of ARDS (in ruling out cardiogenic pulmonary edema) and its subsequent management. However, a pulmonary catheter is not indicated in the routine management of ARDS. Trials have shown that clinical management involving the early use of pulmonary artery catheters in patients with ARDS did not significantly affect mortality and morbidity rates and may result in more complications as compared with a central venous catheter.
- Although no dynamic profile is diagnostic of ARDS, the presence of pulmonary edema, a high cardiac output, and a low pulmonary capillary wedge pressure (PCWP) is characteristic of ARDS.
- It is important to remember that partially treated intravascular volume overload and flash pulmonary edema can have the hemodynamic features of ARDS; filling pressures can also be elevated by increased intrathoracic pressures or with fluid administration; cardiac function can be depressed by acidosis, hypoxemia, or other factors associated with sepsis.

Ventilatory support:

- Noninvasive positive-pressure ventilation (NIPPV) (i.e., BiPAP) should only be used in selected cases in patients with hypoxic respiratory failure.
- A randomized control study showed that high-flow oxygen by nasal cannula reduced ventilator-free days and mortality compared with NIPPV in patients with hypoxemic respiratory failure without hypercapnia. Either modality should not delay intubation and mechanical ventilation initiation in patients with rapidly progressing clinical deterioration.
- Mechanical ventilation is generally necessary to maintain adequate gas exchange. Ventilatory strategy for patients with ARDS as proposed by the ARDS Network is summarized in Fig. 2. A low tidal volume and low plateau pressure ventilator strategy are recommended to avoid ventilator-induced injury. Assist-control is generally preferred initially with the following ventilator settings:
  1. F_{IO_2} 1.0 (until a lower value can be used to achieve adequate oxygenation). When possible, minimize oxygen toxicity by maintaining F_{IO_2} at <60%.
  2. Tidal volume: Set initial tidal volume at 6 ml/kg of predicted body weight (PBW). Tidal volumes are reduced from 6 ml/kg of PBW to a minimum of 4 ml/kg if plateau airway pressures exceed 30 cm of water. The concept of using PBW is based on the fact that lung size depends most strongly on height and sex; PBW normalizes the tidal volume to lung size. Aim to maintain plateau pressure (Pplat) at <30 mm HgPEEP 5 cm H_2O or greater (to increase lung volume and keep alveoli open).
  3. PEEP should be increased in small increments of 3-5 cm H_2O to achieve acceptable arterial saturation (>0.9) with nontoxic F_{IO_2} values (<0.6) and acceptable airway plateau pressures (<30-35 cm H_2O). It is important to remember that an increase in PEEP may lower cardiac output and, despite improvement in Pa_{O_2}, may actually have a negative effect on tissue oxygenation (the major determinants of tissue oxygenation are hemoglobin, percent saturation, and cardiac output). The optimal level of PEEP remains unestablished. Although higher levels of PEEP may help prevent life-threatening hypoxemia and be associated with lower hospital mortality in patients meeting criteria for ARDS, such benefit is unlikely in patients with less severe lung injury (Pa_{O_2}/F_{IO_2} >200) and a strategy of treating such patients with high PEEP levels may be harmful. A study published in 2017 demonstrated that the open lung approach increases mortality in patients with moderate to severe ARDS.
  4. Inspiratory flow: 60 L/min.
  5. Ventilatory rate: High ventilatory rates of up to 35 breaths/min are often necessary in patients with ARDS to achieve the desired minute ventilation because of their increased physiologic dead space and smaller lung volumes. Patients must be monitored for excessive intrathoracic gas trapping (auto-PEEP or intrinsic PEEP) that can depress cardiac output.
- Permissive hypercapnia: To maintain a low plateau pressure, a low tidal volume is frequently required, leading to a reduced minute ventilation and hypoventilation with consequently a respiratory acidosis (elevated PCO_2 and reduced pH). Most patients (excluding patients with cerebral edema, acute coronary syndrome, seizures, cardiac arrhythmias, and so on) can tolerate a low pH without major consequences. Bicarbonate replacement is suggested when the pH falls to below 7.20.
- Sedation: Gamma-aminobutyric acid (GABA) receptor agonists (including propofol and benzodiazepines) have traditionally been the most commonly administered sedative drugs for ICU patients. Recent trials indicate that the alpha-2 agonist dexmedetomidine (Precedex) may have distinct advantages. At comparable sedation levels, dexmedetomidine-treated patients spent less time on ventilator, experienced less delirium, and developed less tachycardia and hypertension. The most notable adverse effect of dexmedetomidine was bradycardia. The benefits of early continuous neuromuscular blockade in patients with ARDS who are receiving mechanical ventilation remains unclear. In a trial among patients with moderate-to-severe ARDS who were treated with a strategy involving a high PEEP, there was no significant difference in mortality at 90 days between patients who received an early and continuous infusion of the neuromuscular blocking agent cisatracurium and those who were treated with a usual-care approach with lighter sedation targets.
- Discontinuing ventilation/extubation: Fig. 3 is an algorithm for assessing whether a patient is ready to be liberated from mechanical ventilation and extubated.

ACUTE GENERAL Rx

Identify and treat precipitating conditions:

- Blood and urine cultures and trial of antibiotics in presumed sepsis (routine administration of antibiotics in all cases of ARDS is not recommended).
- Prompt repair of bone fractures in patients with major trauma.
- Crystalloid resuscitation in pancreatitis.
- Fluid management: In most patients with ARDS, fluid restriction is associated with better outcomes than a liberal fluid policy. Optimal fluid and hemodynamic management of patients with ARDS should be patient specific; in general, administration of crystalloids is recommended if a downward trend in PCWP is associated with diminished cardiac index, resulting in prerenal azotemia, oliguria, and relative tachycardia.
- Positioning the patient: Changes in position can improve oxygenation by improving the distribution of perfusion to ventilated lung

Ventilatory Strategy for Patients With ARDS*

Goal 1: Low Vt / P_{plat}

Initiation:

Calculate PBW
- Male:
  50 + 2.3 (height [inches] − 60)
- Female:
  45.5 + 2.3 (height [inches] − 60)

Initiate volume assist control
- start with 8 mL/kg, and ↓ to 6 mL/kg over a few hours

↓

Keep P_{plat} (based on 0.5-sec pause) < 35 cm H_2O

If P_{plat} > 30 cm H_2O, ↓ Vt by 1 mL/kg to 5 or 4 mL/kg

If P_{plat} < 25 AND Vt < 6 mL/kg, ↑ Vt by 1 mL/kg until P_{plat} > 25 cm H_2O OR Vt = 6 mL/kg

If patient severely distressed and/or breath stacking, consider ↑ Vt to 7 or 8 mL/kg, as long as P_{plat} ≤ 30 cm H_2O†

Goal 2: Adequate Oxygenation

Specific goal:

PaO_2 55-80 mm Hg

or

SpO_2 88-95%

Use only FIO_2 /PEEP combinations shown below to achieve this target
- if oxygenation is low, choose FIO_2 /PEEP combination (from FIO_2 /PEEP table) to the right
- if oxygenation is high, choose FIO_2 /PEEP combination to the left

Goal 3: Arterial pH

Goal:

pH: 7.30–7.45

Acidosis algorithm

If pH 7.15–7.30
- ↑ set rate until pH > 7.30 or $PaCO_2$ < 25 mm Hg (max RR = 35)
- if RR = 35 & pH < 7.30 $NaHCO_3$ may be given

If pH < 7.15
- ↑ set RR to 35
- if set RR = 35 & pH < 7.15, Vt may be ↑ in 1 mL/kg steps until pH > 7.15

(P_{plat} target may be exceeded)

Alkalosis algorithm

If pH > 7.45
- ↓ set RR until patient RR > set RR

(minimum set RR = 6/min)

FIO_2/PEEP Table

FIO_2	0.3	0.4	0.4	0.5	0.5	0.6	0.7	0.7	0.7	0.8	0.9	0.9	0.9	1.0
PEEP	5	5	8	8	10	10	10	12	14	14	14	16	18	18–24

*Based on ARDS Network Algorithm

†If compliance of the chest wall is markedly decreased (e.g., massive ascites), it may be reasonable or necessary (if the patient is very hypoxemic) to allow a P_{plat} >30 cm H_2O.

FIG. 2 Ventilatory strategy for patients with the acute respiratory distress syndrome (ARDS) as proposed by the ARDS Network. Several caveats should be considered in using the low tidal volume strategy. (1) Tidal volume (Vt) is based on predicted body weight (PBW), not actual body weight; PBW tends to be about 20% lower than actual body weight. (2) The protocol mandates decreases in the Vt lower than 6 ml/kg of PBW if the plateau pressure (P_{plat}) is greater than 30 cm H_2O and allows small increases in Vt if the patient is severely distressed or if there is breath stacking, as long as P_{plat} remains at 30 cm H_2O or lower. (3) Because arterial carbon dioxide (CO_2) levels will rise, pH will fall; acidosis is treated with increasingly aggressive strategies dependent on the arterial pH. (4) The protocol has no specific provisions for the patient with a stiff chest wall, which in this context refers to the rib cage and abdomen; in such patients, it seems reasonable to allow P_{plat} to increase to more than 30 cm H_2O, even though it is not mandated by the protocol; in such cases, the limit on P_{plat} may be modified on the basis of analysis of abdominal pressure, which can be estimated by measuring bladder pressure. RR = respiratory rate; SpO_2 = oxygen saturation based on pulse oximeter. FIO_2 = fraction of inspired oxygen; $PaCO_2$ = arterial partial pressure of carbon dioxide; PaO_2 = arterial partial pressure of oxygen; PBW = predicted body weight; P_{plat} = plateau pressure; PEEP = positive end-expiratory pressure; Vt = tidal volume. (From Goldman L, Shafer AI. *Goldman-Cecil Medicine*, ed 26, Elsevier, 2020.)

regions; repositioning (lateral decubitus positioning) should be attempted in patients with hypoxemia that is not responsive to other medical interventions. Placing patients with moderate and severe hypoxemia in a prone position may improve their oxygenation. A meta-analysis that included the recent trials by Guerin et al have shown that in patients with severe ARDS, early application of prolonged (over 16 hr/day) prone-positioning sessions significantly decreases 28-day and 90-day mortality.

- Corticosteroids: Routine use of corticosteroids in ARDS is not recommended; corticosteroids may be beneficial in patients with many eosinophils in the bronchoalveolar lavage fluid or in patients with severe pneumonia. Systemic infections should be ruled out or adequately treated before administration of corticosteroids. Use of methylprednisolone has not been shown to increase the rate of infectious complications but is associated with a higher rate of neuromuscular weakness. In addition, starting methylprednisolone therapy more than 2 wk after the onset of ARDS may increase the risk of death.
- Nutritional support: Nutritional support, preferably administered by the enteral route, is necessary to maintain adequate colloid oncotic pressure and intravascular volume. The use of antioxidants and dietary oil supplements is still equivocal and cannot be recommended at this time.
- Tracheostomy: Tracheostomy is warranted in patients requiring >2 wk of mechanical ventilation; discussion regarding tracheostomy should begin with patient (if alert and oriented) and/or family members/legal guardian after 5 to 7 days of ventilatory support. Early tracheostomy (within 4 days of admission to critical care) does not limit mortality and results in many unneeded procedures (Young et al, 2013).
- Some form of deep vein thrombosis prophylaxis is indicated in all patients with ARDS.
- Stress ulcer prophylaxis with sucralfate suspension (by nasogastric tube), or proton pump inhibitors (PO or IV) or H_2 blockers (PO or IV). Should be reserved for seriously ill patients who are at high risk for this complication.
- The use of surfactant remains controversial. Patients who receive surfactant have a greater improvement in gas exchange in the initial 24-hour period than patients who receive standard therapy alone; however, the use of exogenous surfactant does not improve survival.

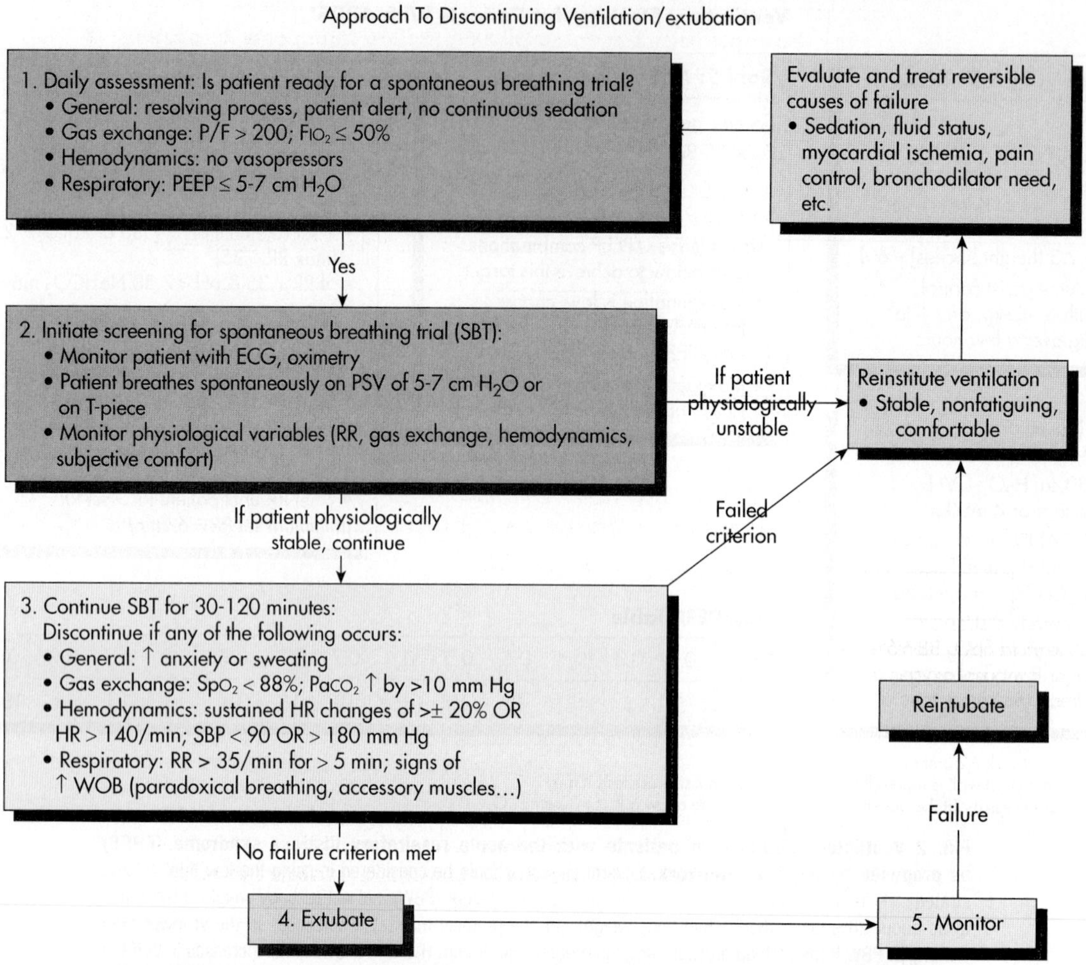

FIG. 3 Algorithm for assessing whether a patient is ready to be liberated from mechanical ventilation and extubated. ECG = electrocardiogram; HR = heart rate; $Paco_2$ = arterial partial pressure of carbon dioxide; PEEP = positive end-expiratory pressure; P/F = Pao_2/Fio_2 PSV = pressure support ventilation; RR = respiratory rate; SBP = systolic blood pressure; Spo_2 = oxygen saturation based on pulse oximeter; WOB = work of breathing. (From Goldman L, Shafer AI: *Goldman-Cecil medicine*, ed 26, Elsevier, 2020.)

- Fig. 4 illustrates the management of acute respiratory failure from acute lung injury and ARDS.

DISPOSITION

- Patients who survive ARDS are at risk of diminished functional capacity, mental illness, and decreased quality of life. Prognosis for ARDS varies with the underlying cause. Prognosis is worse in patients with chronic liver disease, nonpulmonary organ dysfunction, sepsis, and advanced age. ARDS survivors are at high risk for incident joblessness and substantial loss of wages, and 58% of those returning to work received disability.
- Elevated values of dead space fraction ([$Paco_2$ >2 $Peco_2$]/$Paco_2$; normal is <0.3) is associated with an increased risk of death.
- In ARDS, the percentage of potentially recruitable lung is variable and associated with the response to PEEP.
- Overall mortality rate varies between 32% and 45%. Most deaths are attributable to sepsis or multiorgan dysfunction rather than primary respiratory causes.
- Trials have shown that as compared with the current standard of care, a ventilator strategy using esophageal measures to estimate the transpulmonary pressure significantly improves oxygenation and compliance. Further trials will determine if this approach should be widely adopted.
- Other strategies for treatment of life-threatening refractory hypoxemia (inhaled nitric acid, extracorporeal membrane oxygenation [ECMO], high-frequency oscillatory ventilation, recruitment maneuvers) may improve oxygenation, but their impact on mortality remains unproven. Use of ECMO in combination with lung-protective ventilation was found to be beneficial as a treatment strategy early in the course of ARDS related to H1N1 infection. Extracorporeal gas exchange may allow the use of low tidal volumes and lower levels of inspired oxygen and use of higher PEEP if desired. ECMO is costly and labor-intensive. The role and proper use of ECMO for patients with ARDS have not been clearly defined.
- General indications for venovenous ECMO in severe cases of ARDS are:
  1. Severe hypoxemia (e.g., ratio of Pao_2 to Fio_2 <80 despite the application of high levels of PEEP [typically 15 to 20 cm H_2O]) for at least 6 hours in patients with potentially reversible respiratory failure
  2. Uncompensated hypercapnia with acidemia (pH <7.15) despite the best accepted standard of care for management with a ventilator
  3. Excessively high end inspiratory plateau pressure (>35 to 45 cm H_2O, according to the patient's body size) despite the best accepted standard of care for management with a ventilator

REFERRAL

Surgical referral for tracheostomy (see "Acute General Rx").

SUGGESTED READINGS

Available at ExpertConsult.com

RELATED CONTENT

Acute Respiratory Distress Syndrome (ARDS) (Patient Information)

AUTHOR: **Jorge Mercado, MD**

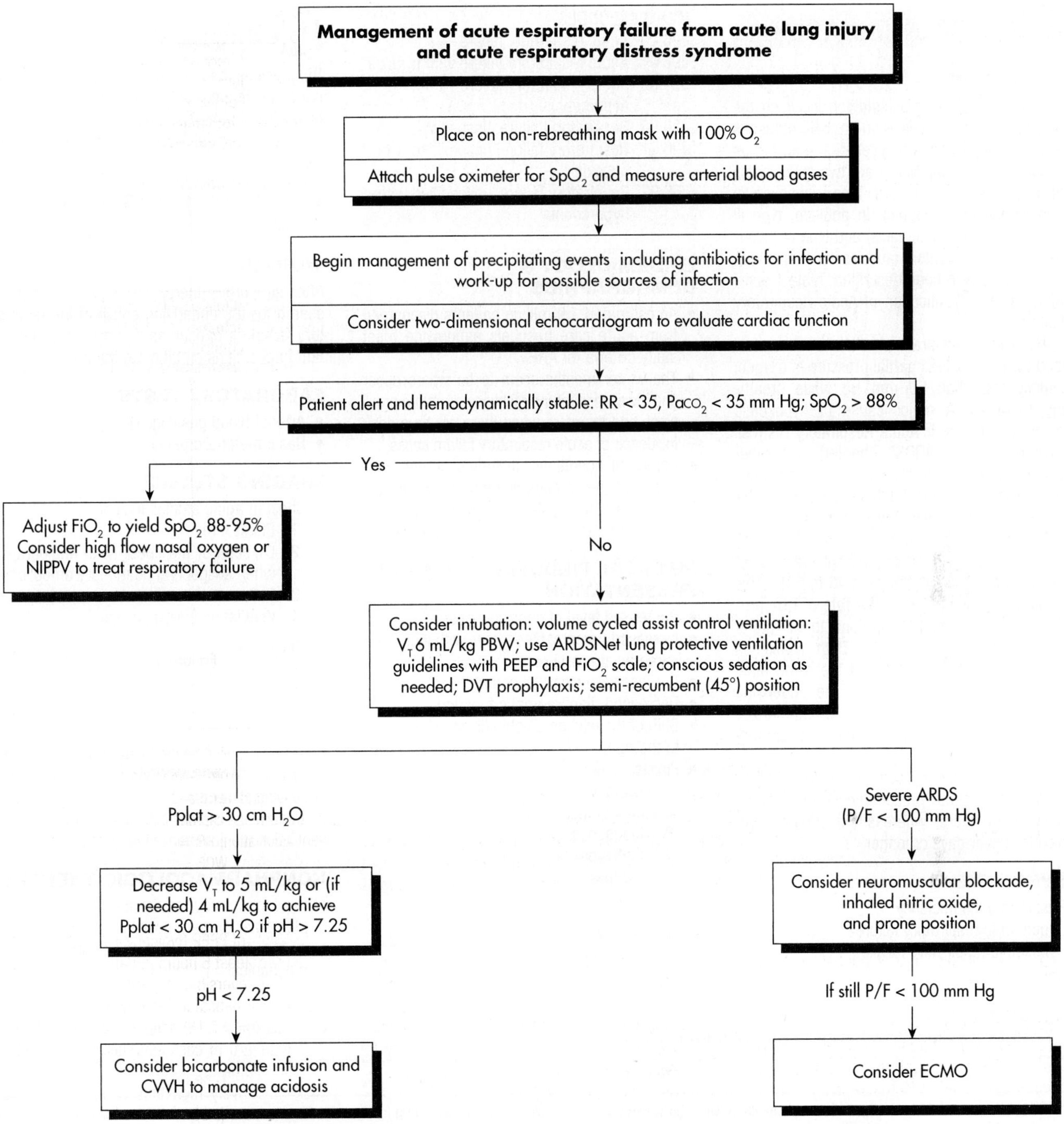

FIG. 4 Management of acute respiratory failure from acute lung injury and acute respiratory distress syndrome. CVVH = continuous venovenous hemofiltration; DVT = deep venous thrombosis; ECMO = extracorporeal membrane oxygenation; NIPPV = noninvasive positive pressure ventilation; PBW = predicted body weight; PEEP = positive end-expiration pressure; P/F = Pao_2/Fio_2 ; Pplat = plateau airway pressure; RR = respiratory rate; Spo_2 = arterial oxygen saturation; V T = tidal volume. (From Goldman L, Shafer AI: *Goldman-Cecil medicine*, ed 26, Elsevier, 2020.)

Acute Respiratory Failure (ARF)

BASIC INFORMATION

DEFINITION

Respiratory failure is a condition in which the respiratory system fails in one or both of its gas exchanging functions (oxygenation and carbon dioxide elimination). There are two major types of acute respiratory failure: Type I (hypoxemic) and type II (hypercapnic). In addition, type III (associated with atelectasis) and type IV (hypoperfusion of respiratory muscles in patients with shock) have also been described. Table 1 summarizes the classification of Acute Respiratory Failure.

Hypoxemic respiratory failure is characterized by a low arterial partial pressure of oxygen, usually less than 60 mm Hg while breathing room air. A major cause of hypoxemic respiratory failure is Acute Respiratory Distress Syndrome (see "ARDS" chapter), but other etiologies include heart failure and pneumonia. See Table 2 for list of potential etiologies for acute hypoxemic respiratory failure.

Hypercapnic respiratory failure is defined as an elevation in arterial partial pressure of carbon dioxide to greater than 45 mm Hg. This is directly proportional to the rate of CO_2 production and inversely proportional to the rate of CO_2 elimination by the lungs. Both hypoxemia and hypercapnia can occur at the same time, depending on the location of the underlying disorder and mechanism. Table 3 summarizes etiologies for acute hypercapnic respiratory failure.

Respiratory failure can be acute (ARF) or chronic. The acute presentation occurs within minutes to hours, whereas the chronic form develops over days or longer.

SYNONYMS

Respiratory insufficiency
Hypercarbic respiratory failure
Hypoxemic respiratory failure
ARF

ICD-10CM CODES

J96.00 Acute respiratory failure
J96.01 Acute respiratory failure with hypoxia
J96.02 Acute respiratory failure with hypercapnia
J96.90 Respiratory failure, unspecified
J96.91 Respiratory failure, unspecified with hypoxia
J96.92 Respiratory failure, unspecified with hypercapnia

EPIDEMIOLOGY & DEMOGRAPHICS

- An estimated 1.9 million patients discharged from acute care hospitals nationwide meet study criteria for ARF.
- The winter months seem to be where upper and lower respiratory infections are more prevalent, and therefore when there will be a peak incidence of acute respiratory failure cases.
- Comorbid conditions, including chronic disorders of the cardiac, pulmonary, neurologic, renal, hepatic systems, and the patient's advanced age elevate the risk of mortality.

PHYSICAL FINDINGS & CLINICAL PRESENTATION

- Decreased level of consciousness
- Increased cerebral blood flow, with increased intracranial pressure
- Decreased myocardial contractility
- Decreased diaphragmatic function
- Shift of the oxyhemoglobin dissociation curve to the right
- Physical signs:
  1. Dyspnea
  2. Somnolence
  3. Headaches
  4. Confusion
  5. Asterixis
  6. Coma

ETIOLOGY

See Tables 2 and 3.

DIAGNOSIS

Diagnosis is made clinically according to physical exam findings and is confirmed by arterial blood gas. Table 4 summarizes common clues obtained from the history and physical examination.

DIFFERENTIAL DIAGNOSIS

See Tables 2 and 3.

WORKUP

After supportive therapy is initiated, a careful search for the underlying cause of the respiratory failure is critical, as this may have important implications on ultimate therapy.

LABORATORY TESTS

- Arterial blood gas (Fig. 1)
- Basal metabolic panel

IMAGING STUDIES

- Chest imaging studies include:
  1. Chest x-ray
  2. CT scan of the chest (with angiography when suspecting pulmonary embolism)
  3. Chest ultrasound
  4. Ventilation perfusion scan

TREATMENT

The treatment of respiratory failure is initially supportive, aiming to determine first the acuity and/or severity of the presentation. Correction of the hypoxemia, hypercapnia, and management of the underlying etiology of the condition are essential to its treatment. Potential indications for mechanical ventilation are summarized in Table 5.

NONPHARMACOLOGIC THERAPY

- Hypoxemia may require treatment with supplemental oxygen, positive pressure support in the form of noninvasive ventilation, or mechanical ventilation.

TABLE 1 Classification of Acute Respiratory Failure

	Type I	Type II	Type III	Type IV
MECHANISM OF HYPOXEMIA	Low Fio2 ventilation/perfusion (V/Q) mismatch Shunting Reduced diffusing capacity	Hypoventilation	Shunting Hypoventilation V/Q mismatch	Hypoperfusion or inadequate oxygenation of peripheral tissues
LOCATION OF PATHOLOGICAL PROCESS	Inhaled air composition Alveolar-capillary unit Oxygen-carrying capacity of blood	Airway Central Nervous System (CNS) Neuromuscular system Chest wall	Alveolar-capillary unit collapse with regional hypoventilation	Cardiovascular system Peripheral tissues
CLINICAL SYNDROMES	Cardiogenic pulmonary edema Acute respiratory distress syndrome Pneumonia Interstitial lung disease Pulmonary embolism Pulmonary hypertension Atelectasis Alveolar hemorrhage Carbon monoxide poisoning Anatomic shunts	Chronic obstructive pulmonary disease Asthma CNS depression (intoxication) CNS trauma or injury Neuromuscular disorders Skeletal disorders Obesity-hypoventilation syndrome	Thoracic or upper abdominal surgery or trauma Inadequate postoperative analgesia Pleural tumor or inflammation Trapped lung Subdiaphragmatic tumor or inflammation Obesity	Septic (distributive) shock Hypovolemic shock Cardiogenic shock Compromised cellular oxidation Hypermetabolic states

FiO_2, Fraction of inspired oxygen.
Modified from Jean-Louis V: *Intensive care medicine: annual update 2008,* Berlin Heidelberg, 2008, Springer-Verlag.

TABLE 2 Pathophysiological Mechanisms of Acute Hypoxemic Respiratory Failure

Extrapulmonary processes including chest wall and skeletal abnormalities (hypoxic hypoxia)	Deficiency of oxygen in inspired air (high altitude, suffocation) Hypoactive hypoventilation (central nervous system trauma, drug toxicities, and neuromuscular and skeletal disorders) Upper airway obstruction leading to hypoventilation (trauma and angioedema)
Pulmonary etiologies (hypoxic hypoxia)	Hypoventilation caused by increased airway resistance (chronic obstructive pulmonary disease and asthma) Abnormal alveolar ventilation-perfusion ratio (pulmonary embolism, pneumonia, aspiration, and emphysema) Diminished diffusing capacity via the alveolar-capillary membrane (interstitial lung disease and pulmonary vascular disease) Pulmonary shunting (atelectasis, pneumonia, hepatopulmonary syndrome, and arteriovenous malformations)
Cardiac right-to-left shunts; e.g., atrial septal defect (hypoxic hypoxia)	—
Inadequate capacity of blood to transport oxygen (anemic hypoxia)	Anemia Hemoglobinopathies (methemoglobinemia and carbon monoxide poisoning)
Inadequate oxygen transport due to a circulatory defect (static hypoxia)	General circulatory deficiency or collapse (shock or cardiac failure) Localized circulatory deficiency (peripheral, cerebral, and coronary vessels)
Abnormal tissue capability for using oxygen (histotoxic hypoxia)	Late-stage irreversible shock Poisoning of cellular oxidation enzymes (cyanide or arsenic toxicity and heavy ethanol intoxication) Diminished cellular metabolic capacity for using oxygen (severe vitamin deficiencies; e.g., beri-beri)

Vincent JL et al: *Textbook of critical care*, ed 7, Philadelphia, 2017, Elsevier.

TABLE 3 Potential Causes of Acute Hypercapnic Respiratory Failure

Central Nervous System	Spinal Cord, Nerves, Muscle	Chest Wall, Thoracic Cage	Increased Dead Space
Medications (anesthetics and/or opioids) Alveolar hypoventilation Trauma Meningoencephalitis Localized tumors or vascular abnormalities of the medulla Strokes affecting medullary control centers Severe alkalosis	Medications Trauma Myasthenia gravis Guillain-Barre syndrome Electrolyte abnormalities	Trauma Kyphoscoliosis Flail chest Pleural disease Scleroderma Morbid obesity Ascites Severe ileus	Obstructive airways disorders Upper: Acute epiglottitis, foreign body aspiration, tracheal tumor Lower: COPD, asthma, cystic fibrosis

COPD, Chronic obstructive pulmonary disease.

TABLE 4 Common Clues Obtained from the History, Symptoms, and Clinical Examination Findings That Can Help in the Initial Diagnostic Workup and Management of Acute Respiratory Failure

History and Symptoms	Signs on Physical Examination	Diagnosis
Cough, sputum, secretions	Rales or wheezing	Pneumonia, chronic obstructive pulmonary disease (COPD) exacerbation, bronchiectasis
Sudden onset of shortness of breath	Normal auscultation and percussion, possible signs of leg swelling to suggest deep vein thrombosis	Pulmonary embolism
History of heavy smoking	Wheezing, rhonchi	Emphysema, chronic bronchitis
Orthopnea, chest pain, paroxysmal nocturnal dyspnea	Arrhythmia, peripheral edema, jugular venous distention, peripheral hypoperfusion	Congestive heart failure or acute coronary syndrome
Trauma, aspiration, blood transfusions	Diffuse crackles	Acute respiratory distress syndrome
History of allergies, wheezing, or airway disease	Wheezing	Asthma, COPD
Exposure to heavy metals, handling of animals, dust or other significant environmental exposures	"Velcro" rales, clubbing	Chronic interstitial lung disease
Choking, aspiration, vomiting, dental procedures	Inspiratory stridor, poor air entry	Foreign body
Drug abuse	Constricted or dilated pupils, altered mental status, skin marks, perforated nasal septum, hypersalivation, decreased respiratory frequency	Central nervous system depression, intoxication
Exposure to a new drug/chemical or foods known to be allergenic	Swollen oral mucosa and tongue; stridor or wheezing	Angioedema, anaphylaxis
Progressive muscle weakness or immobility	Sensory abnormalities	Neuromuscular disorders
Trauma, procedures, inhalational injury	Absent breath sounds unilaterally, hypertympanic, tracheal deviation	Pneumothorax
Trauma, procedures	Absent breath sounds, dull on percussion, tracheal deviation	Hemothorax

Vincent JL et al: *Textbook of critical care*, ed 7, Philadelphia, 2017, Elsevier.

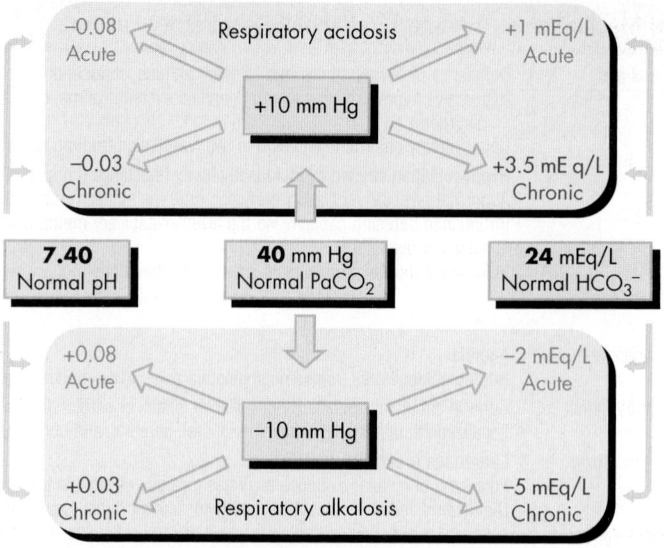

FIG. 1 Interpretation of an arterial blood gas in the setting of respiratory failure. (From Vincent JL et al: *Textbook of critical care,* ed 7, Philadelphia, 2017, Elsevier.)

- Hypercapnia may require treatment with ventilatory support, noninvasive ventilation, or mechanical ventilation. The decision for either can be difficult and is primarily based on clinical presentation, severity of symptoms, comorbidities, and level of acid base derangement, as well as mental status.
- Contraindications to noninvasive ventilation include respiratory arrest, hemodynamic or cardiac instability, or inability to protect the airway.
- Monitoring carbon dioxide levels has not been standardized, but a change in symptoms and or worsening in mental status can prompt a repeat in blood gas analysis.
- Worsening blood gas levels can be remediated with changes in the pressures on the noninvasive ventilator or by switching to a mechanical ventilator.

ACUTE GENERAL Rx

Ventilatory support, either invasive (mechanical ventilation) or noninvasive. Table 6 provides an overview of features of selected modes of mechanical ventilation. Potential advantages and disadvantages of each mode are summarized in Table 7.

REFERRAL

Pulmonologist

SUGGESTED READINGS

Available at ExpertConsult.com

RELATED CONTENT

Acute Respiratory Distress Syndrome (Related key topic)
Asthma (Related key topic)
Carbon Monoxide Poisoning (Related key topic)
Chronic Obstructive Pulmonary Disease (Related key topic)
Interstitial Lung Disease (Related key topic)
Pneumonia, Bacterial (Related key topic)
Pneumonia, Mycoplasma (Related key topic)
Pneumonia, Pneumocystis Jiroveci (Related key topic)
Pneumonia, Viral (Related key topic)
Pulmonary Embolism (Related key topic)
Pulmonary Edema (Related key topic)

AUTHOR: **Jorge Mercado, MD**

TABLE 5 Potential Indications for Mechanical Ventilation

Physiologic Mechanism	Clinical Assessment	Normal Range	Value(s)/Finding(s) Supporting Need for Mechanical Ventilation
Hypoxemia	$P(A\text{-}a)O_2$ gradient (mm Hg)	25-65	>350
	PaO_2/FIO_2 ratio	425-475	<300
	SaO_2	98%	<90% despite supplemental oxygen
Hypercarbia/inadequate alveolar ventilation	$PaCO_2$	35-45 mm Hg	Acute increase from patient's baseline pH <7.20 Mental status decline
Oxygen delivery/oxygen consumption imbalance	Elevated lactate	≤2.2 mg/dl	≥4 mg/dl despite adequate resuscitation
	Decreased mixed venous oxygen saturation	70%	<70% despite adequate acute resuscitation
Increased work of breathing	Minute ventilation	5-10 L/min	>15-20 L/min
	Dead space	0.15-0.30	≥0.5 (acute)
Inspiratory muscle weakness	NIP	80-100 cm H_2O	<20-30
	VC	60-75 ml/kg	<15-20
Acute decompensated heart failure	Jugular venous distention Pulmonary edema Decreased EF		Clinical judgment combined with the listed factors
Inadequate lung expansion	V_T (ml/kg)	5-8	<4-5
	VC (ml/kg)	60-75	<10-15
	Respiratory rate (breaths/min)	12-20	≥35

EF, Ejection fraction; *FIO_2,* fraction of inspired oxygen; *NIP,* negative inspiratory pressure; *$P(A\text{-}a)O_2$,* alveolar-arterial oxygen pressure difference; *PaO_2,* partial pressure of oxygen; *$PaCO_2$,* partial pressure of carbon dioxide; *SaO_2,* arterial oxygen saturation; *VC,* vital capacity; *V_T,* tidal volume.
From Parrillo JE, Dellinger RP: *Critical care medicine, principles of diagnosis and management in the adult,* ed 5, Philadelphia, 2019, Elsevier.

TABLE 6 Overview of Features of Selected Modes of Mechanical Ventilation

Ventilator Mode	Trigger	Control	Cycling	Inspiratory Flow
Continuous mandatory ventilation	Time	Flow or pressure	Volume or time	Selected or decelerating
Volume control/assist control (VC/AC)	Patient or time	Flow	Volume	Square, decelerating, or sinusoidal
Pressure control/assist control (PC/AC)	Patient or time	Pressure	Time	Decelerating
Synchronized intermittent mandatory ventilation	Patient or time	Pressure for patient breaths Flow (VC) or pressure (PC) for ventilator breaths	Flow for spontaneous breaths Volume or time for ventilator breaths	Decelerating for spontaneous breath Square (VC), decelerating (VC or PC), sinusoidal for spontaneous breaths
Stand-alone pressure-support ventilation	Patient	None	Flow	Decelerating

From Parrillo JE, Dellinger RP: *Critical care medicine, principles of diagnosis and management in the adult,* ed 5, Philadelphia, 2019, Elsevier.

TABLE 7 Potential Advantages and Disadvantages of Selected Modes of Mechanical Ventilation

Mode	Advantage(s)	Disadvantage(s)
Controlled mechanical ventilation	Rests muscles of respiration	Requires use of heavy sedation/neuromuscular blockade
Assist volume control	Reduced work of breathing Guarantees delivery of set tidal volume (unless peak pressure limit alarm is exceeded)	Potential adverse hemodynamic effects May lead to inappropriate hyperventilation and excessive inspiration pressures
Assist pressure control	Allows limitation of peak inspiratory pressures	Same as for assist volume control Potential hyperventilation or hypoventilation with lung resistance/compliance changes
Synchronized intermittent mandatory ventilation	Less interference with normal cardiovascular function	Increased work of breathing compared with assist control Patient may find it difficult to adjust to two different types of ventilator breaths
Stand-alone pressure-support ventilation	Patient comfort Improved patient-ventilator interaction Decreased work of breathing	Apnea alarm is only backup Variable patient tolerance

From Parrillo JE, Dellinger RP: *Critical care medicine, principles of diagnosis and management in the adult,* ed 5, Philadelphia, 2019, Elsevier.

Acute Urinary Retention (AUR)

BASIC INFORMATION

DEFINITION

An acute inability to urinate when the bladder is full. Acute urinary retention (AUR) is often, but not always, painful. The distended bladder may be palpable and percussible. Acute urinary retention is distinct from chronic urinary retention, a condition in which patients can still void but chronically retain a significant volume of urine in the bladder after voiding. Chronic urinary retention is not painful.

SYNONYMS

AUR
Urinary retention
Retaining urine

ICD-10CM CODES	
R33	Retention of urine
R33.8	Other retention of urine
R33.9	Retention of urine, unspecified

EPIDEMIOLOGY & DEMOGRAPHICS

INCIDENCE:

- One of the most common urologic emergencies.
- Typically occurs in aging men, especially those older than 60 yr. However, it may occur in any age group and in either sex.
- Over a 5-yr period, AUR will occur in 10% of men older than 70 yr and in one third of men older than 80 yr. There is a near-linear increase in age-specific incidence for men ages 40 to 80 yr.

PREVALENCE: Estimates are 40/100,000 in males and 3/100,000 in females. Prevalence increases as average lifespan increases.

GENETICS: None known.

PHYSICAL FINDINGS & CLINICAL PRESENTATION

- Acute inability to pass urine or only small amounts of urine.
- Pain and/or pressure in the lower abdomen and suprapubic region is typical. Low back pain may also occur. Pain may be absent, especially in the elderly, patients with underlying neurologic disorders and during chronic urinary retention.
- Palpable and/or percussible bladder may be detected.
- Suprapubic or bladder tenderness with deep palpation may be elicited.
- Increased urge to urinate with bladder palpation.
- Rarely, flank pain and costovertebral angle tenderness are present when high bladder pressures are transmitted to the ureters and kidney.
- Increased severity of lower urinary tract symptoms (LUTS) is associated with increased AUR risk. Patients may complain of worsening LUTS prior to episode, including increased urinary urgency, incontinence, nocturia, stranguria, hesitancy, and intermittency. These symptoms usually develop between 1 day and a few wk prior to AUR.
- Patients with cognitive deficits or inability to communicate may present with restlessness, discomfort, confusion, or delirium.
- Acute kidney injury, electrolyte abnormalities, nausea, lower extremity edema, and acute kidney injury may be present with delayed presentation.

ETIOLOGY

- Acute urinary retention may be spontaneous or precipitated by a triggering event. Spontaneous AUR may arise from the natural progression of bladder outlet obstruction, more commonly from benign prostatic hyperplasia (BPH), and less commonly from pelvic masses and urethral stricture disease. Conversely, precipitated AUR episodes have an identifiable triggering event, such as acute trauma, surgical procedures (e.g., spinal, orthopedic, and urologic), medications (e.g., over-the-counter [OTC] antihistamines and sympathomimetic agents commonly found in cough medications, anticholinergic drugs, opioids), excessive fluid intake (e.g., alcohol), urinary tract infection, central nervous system insults (e.g., strokes, hemorrhage, spinal cord injuries), and severe constipation. There is overlap between spontaneous and precipitated AUR, particularly when triggering events are superimposed on underlying obstructive risk factors.
- Urinary retention generally result from one of three categories: (1) Increased bladder outflow obstruction, as seen in BPH, urethral stricture disease, extrinsic compression from malignancy, constipation, and in gross hematuria where large clots can obstruct the urethra or bladder neck; (2) disruption of detrusor muscle innervation in association with diabetic neuropathy, spinal cord injury, progressive neurologic pathologies, and bladder contractile dysfunction and decompensation, secondary to prolonged outlet obstruction; and (3) bladder overdistension that leads to impaired contractility and may result from general anesthesia, epidural anesthesia, or anticholinergic use.
- Acute retention is often multifactorial in older patients, with an underlying obstructive risk factor and acute precipitant.
- In women, obstructive factors can include benign tumors (especially, fibroid tumors); malignant tumors of pelvic, urethral, or vaginal origin; urethral strictures and urethral meatal stenosis; postpartum vulvar edema; and labial fusion. Pelvic organ prolapse, including cystocele, rectocele, and uterine prolapse, can also lead to urinary retention.
- Infection including prostatitis, urethritis, cystitis, genital herpes, and herpes zoster may also produce AUR.
- AUR is common in the postoperative period when patients are less mobile, are constipated, or have received opioid medications.

Dx DIAGNOSIS

DIFFERENTIAL DIAGNOSIS

- AUR is typically self-evident to the cognitively intact patient and the treating physician.
- Chronic urinary retention.
- Pelvic masses, fluid collections, uterine fibroids, pregnancies, or ascites may be confused for a full bladder, particularly when using bedside ultrasonic bladder capacity-measuring instruments.

WORKUP

- History is focused on urologic symptoms: Dysuria, hematuria, baseline voiding symptoms (caliber of stream, nocturia, sensation of incomplete emptying, double-voiding, incontinence, hesitancy), past episodes of retention, surgical history (urologic and other surgical procedures, particularly recent ones), pelvic/perineal trauma, and urologic cancer.
- History should include a complete list of prescribed and over-the-counter medications, and recent medication changes.
- Review of symptoms should include presence of fever, back pain, neurologic symptoms, and rash.
- Rectal examination for masses, fecal impaction, perineal and perianal sensation, prostate size, and sphincter tone.
- Genitourinary examination in men, with special attention for meatal stenosis and phimosis or paraphimosis.
- Pelvic examination in women to assess for evidence of pelvic organ prolapse(s).
- Neurologic examination, with particular evaluation for "saddle" anesthesia (i.e., cauda equina syndrome) and pelvic sensory or motor deficits, to rule out an underlying neurologic cause.

LABORATORY TESTS

- Electrolytes, BUN, and serum creatinine.
- Urinalysis and culture, obtained via bladder or suprapubic catheterization.
- Prostate-specific antigen (PSA) testing is not helpful in AUR and may be falsely elevated after catheter placement. This test should not be routinely checked in the acute setting.

IMAGING STUDIES

- Bladder ultrasound or a bedside postvoid residual urine scan ("bladder scan") can be diagnostic. Ascites, pelvic fluid collections, body habitus, and presence of surgical implants (e.g., reservoirs for inflatable penile prostheses or artificial urinary sphincters) may confound accurate volume measurement with these devices.
- Abdominal ultrasound or computed tomography (CT) may be helpful if there is suspicion of a pelvic mass.
- CT (Fig. 1) can be helpful when high volumes are measured by a bedside bladder scan, but low volumes are returned upon bladder catheterization.

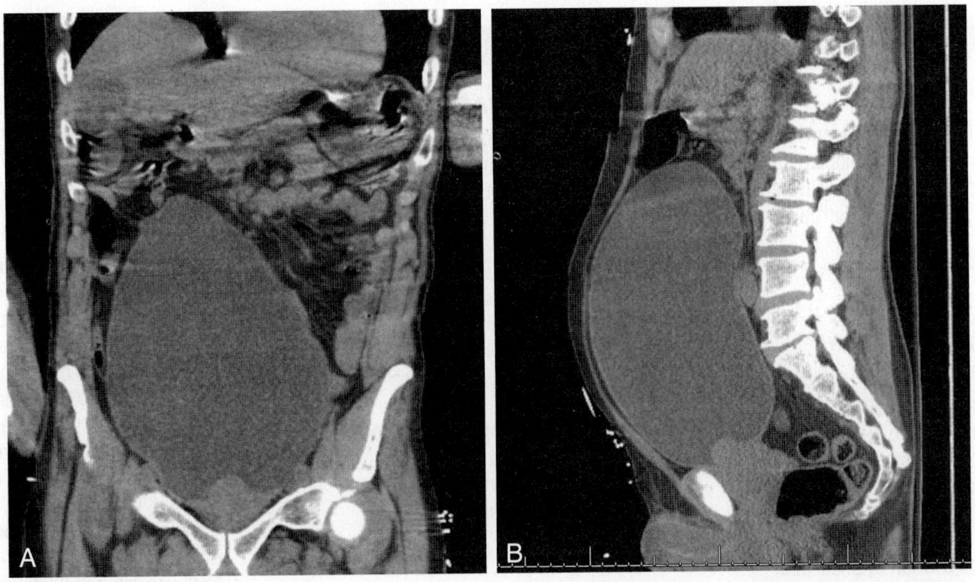

FIG. 1 Large volume urinary retention. Computed tomography images of coronal view **(A)** and sagittal view **(B)** of greatly distended bladder. The bladder extends into the mid-abdomen and above the pubic symphysis. More than 2 liters of urine were drained on bladder catheterization.

- MRI should be obtained when a spinal cord problem is suspected.
- Renal ultrasound or abdominopelvic CT may be obtained when there is kidney functional impairment and/or hydronephrosis is suspected.
- Evaluation of bladder function by urodynamic testing may be conducted after initial management, particularly in females with no evidence of anatomic obstruction, or patients with longstanding obstruction and/or other neurologic conditions that affect bladder contractility.
- X-rays are of limited utility in evaluating AUR, but may show underlying constipation.

Rx TREATMENT

ACUTE GENERAL Rx

- Prompt bladder decompression and drainage is the initial management of AUR, generally by indwelling urethral catheterization. Coude-tip (angled-tip) catheters can facilitate catheter placement in men with large prostates. Clean intermittent catheterization is an option for patients with sufficient dexterity, vision, and motivation.
- Urological consultation is advised after recent genitourinary surgery or a history of urethral stricture disease or difficult urethral catheterizations.
- When urethral catheterization is not possible or contraindicated, suprapubic catheter placement is required.
- Postdecompression hematuria may develop shortly after bladder drainage due to small vessel injury of the overstretched bladder wall. This complication is usually self-limiting.
- Monitor for postobstructive diuresis that results from a mixed osmotic and saline diuresis from salt and urea accumulation during the period of obstruction.
- Avoid and/or discontinue medications that precipitate AUR (e.g., narcotics, anticholinergics, antihistamines).

CHRONIC Rx

- A voiding trial is reasonable 5 to 7 days after relief of obstruction in most patients.
- α-blockers are effective for treatment of BPH symptoms in males. These agents increase the success rate of early catheter removal and should be initiated, unless contraindicated. There is limited evidence to suggest benefit in females.
- If feasible, discontinue medications that increase the risk of AUR.
- Correct constipation and increase patient mobility.
- Inability to void after 5 to 7 days of catheterization mandates urologic consultation, with more intensive evaluation of AUR, including possible cystoscopic evaluation and/or urodynamic studies.
- Patients who unable to void after a voiding trial can either initiate clean intermittent catheterization, often 2 to 3 times a day, or have the urinary bladder catheter replaced.

DISPOSITION

- Patients can be discharged home when close follow-up is feasible and progressive kidney injury and postobstructive diuresis are absent
- Hospital admission if sepsis; complicated urinary tract infection; acute kidney injury; severe postobstructive diuresis; hyperkalemia; acidemia or azotemia; or if AUR is from malignancy, hematuria, or spinal cord compression

REFERRAL

- Urologist, if initial bladder catheterization is unsuccessful, or in surgical scenarios of radical prostatectomy, transurethral resection of prostate, urethral stricture surgery, and other bladder/prostate surgeries
- Urologic referral for recurrent AUR in men
- Gynecologic referral is mandatory if a pelvic mass is identified as etiology of AUR in females

! PEARLS & CONSIDERATIONS

- AUR is often painful.
- Rapid bladder drainage is of paramount importance.
- Monitor for postobstructive diuresis and correct electrolyte abnormalities.
- Request urologic advice or referral for AUR after urologic surgery.

PREVENTION

- Avoid and/or treat constipation.
- Avoid and/or discontinue medications that precipitate AUR (e.g., narcotics, anticholinergics, antihistamines).
- Patients with BPH should be cautious regarding medications that may precipitate AUR, including antihistamines, sympathomimetics, sedatives, and anticholinergics. On a chronic basis, 5-α reductase inhibitors (e.g., finasteride, dutasteride) may reduce the risk of AUR in men with BPH and large prostates.

SUGGESTED READINGS

Available at ExpertConsult.com

RELATED CONTENT

Benign Prostatic Hyperplasia (Related Key Topic)

AUTHORS: **Marcus L. Jamil, MD,** and **David A. Leavitt, MD**

Adnexal Masses (ALG)

BASIC INFORMATION

DEFINITION

The adnexa refer to the region adjacent to the uterus that includes the ovary, fallopian tube, and associated structures. Masses that arise in these regions are collectively referred to as *adnexal masses.*

SYNONYM

Pelvic mass

ICD-10CM CODES	
R19.09	Other intra-abdominal and pelvic swelling, mass, and lump
C57.4	Malignant neoplasm of uterine adnexa, unspecified
N83.2	Other and unspecified ovarian cysts
N83.209	Unspecified ovarian cyst, unspecified side

EPIDEMIOLOGY & DEMOGRAPHICS

PREVALENCE: Because the etiology of adnexal masses is so broad and ranges from benign to malignant and can be gynecologic or nongynecologic in origin, a single prevalence is difficult to establish and not particularly useful in this case.

PREDOMINANT AGE: Adnexal masses can be found in females of all ages ranging from childhood to the reproductive yr to postmenopause.

RISK FACTORS: There are many risk factors for benign adnexal masses, but it is important to consider risk factors for malignancy. While age is the most important independent risk factor for ovarian cancer, family history of breast or ovarian cancer is the most important personal risk factor.

PHYSICAL FINDINGS & CLINICAL PRESENTATION

- The majority of adnexal masses are found incidentally when pelvic imaging is performed or on physical examination.
- Though less common, they are sometimes detected when a woman presents with acute or intermittent pelvic or abdominal pain.
- Urgent conditions such as adnexal torsion or ectopic pregnancy typically present with fairly specific symptoms such as severe pain or first trimester bleeding and should be evaluated immediately.

ETIOLOGY

The etiology of an adnexal mass depends on the organ from which the mass arises. Masses can be benign or malignant. They can be ovarian, tubal, or uterine in origin. Additionally, nongynecologic etiologies include masses arising from other organs in the pelvis such as the bladder, kidney, bowel, or peritoneum. Masses could also be due to cancer metastases.

DIAGNOSIS

DIFFERENTIAL DIAGNOSIS

- The differential diagnosis of adnexal masses is best divided into gynecologic and nongynecologic and then further into benign and malignant
- Gynecologic:
  1. Benign:
     a. Physiologic cyst
     b. Corpus luteal cyst
     c. Theca lutein cyst
     d. Endometrioma
     e. Cystadenoma
     f. Benign ovarian germ cell tumor (mature teratoma)
     g. Benign sex cord-stromal tumor
     h. Ectopic pregnancy
     i. Hydrosalpinx
     j. Paratubal cyst
     k. Uterine leiomyoma (pedunculated or cervical)
     l. Tuboovarian abscess
     m. Adnexal torsion
     n. Müllerian anomalies
  2. Malignant:
     a. Epithelial carcinoma
     b. Epithelial borderline carcinoma
     c. Germ cell tumor
     d. Sex-cord or stromal tumor
     e. Metastatic cancer
- Nongynecologic:
  1. Benign:
     a. Abscess: Pelvic, appendiceal, diverticular
     b. Bladder diverticulum
     c. Ureteral diverticulum
     d. Pelvic kidney
     e. Nerve sheath tumors
  2. Malignant:
     a. Bowel neoplasm
     b. Appendiceal neoplasm
     c. Retroperitoneal sarcoma
     d. Metastasis (breast, colon, lymphoma, etc.)

WORKUP

- Evaluation of an adnexal mass (Fig. 1) begins with a thorough history that considers individual patient characteristics and the physical examination.
- A detailed gynecologic history should be obtained as well as a thorough family history and review of other risk factors.
- A full set of vital signs, the general physical appearance of the patient, and the patient's symptoms should be evaluated.
- A comprehensive physical examination including palpation of lymph nodes (cervical, supraclavicular, axillary, and groin), abdominal examination, and thorough pelvic examination should be performed.
- Laboratory studies and imaging should be considered as outlined below.

LABORATORY TESTS

- A pregnancy test should be obtained on all women of reproductive age.
- If infection is suspected, CBC and cultures for gonorrhea and chlamydia should be obtained.
- Other laboratory tests that may be helpful include urinalysis and/or urine culture, fecal occult testing, and serum marker testing such as CA-125, CEA, B-hCG, AFP, and LDH if malignancy is suspected.

IMAGING STUDIES

- Transvaginal ultrasonography is the initial imaging modality of choice for evaluation of adnexal masses, including size, composition (cystic, solid, mixed), laterality, presence or absence of septations, and papillary excrescences. Abdominal ultrasonography should also be performed and can be useful if pelvic structures are distorted by prior surgery or if the mass extends above the pelvis.
- CT and MRI are not recommended for initial evaluation.
- MRI can be helpful to differentiate masses that are not ovarian in origin, especially leiomyomas.
- CT scans are most useful for evaluating metastasis if cancer is suspected, as well as ascites, pelvic or periaortic lymph node enlargement, obstructive uropathy, or an alternate primary cancer site.

TREATMENT

Treatment of adnexal masses (Fig. E2) depends on the etiology of the mass, stability of the patient, and level of suspicion for malignancy.

ACUTE GENERAL Rx

- A ruptured ectopic pregnancy or ovarian torsion is a surgical emergency and warrants immediate surgical intervention. Surgical intervention may also be necessary for nongynecologic causes of adnexal masses such as appendicitis. Table 1 summarizes indications for surgery in a patient with adnexal mass.
- Ultrasound imaging with features concerning for malignancy (mass >10 cm, papillary or solid components, irregularity, ascites, and presence of high color Doppler flow) warrants surgical intervention. Fig. E3 illustrates the management of a premenopausal woman with adnexal mass.
- Masses that appear benign but are greater than 5 cm in size are at increased risk of ovarian torsion, therefore surgical intervention needs to be considered.

CHRONIC Rx

Adnexal masses can be observed if imaging suggests benign disease or if there is a compelling reason to avoid surgical intervention. There is no established interval for ultrasound follow-up. Timing of a follow-up ultrasound should be determined on an individual basis considering patient risk factors, symptoms, menopausal status, and suspicion for malignancy. Six mo follow-up is reasonable for masses larger than

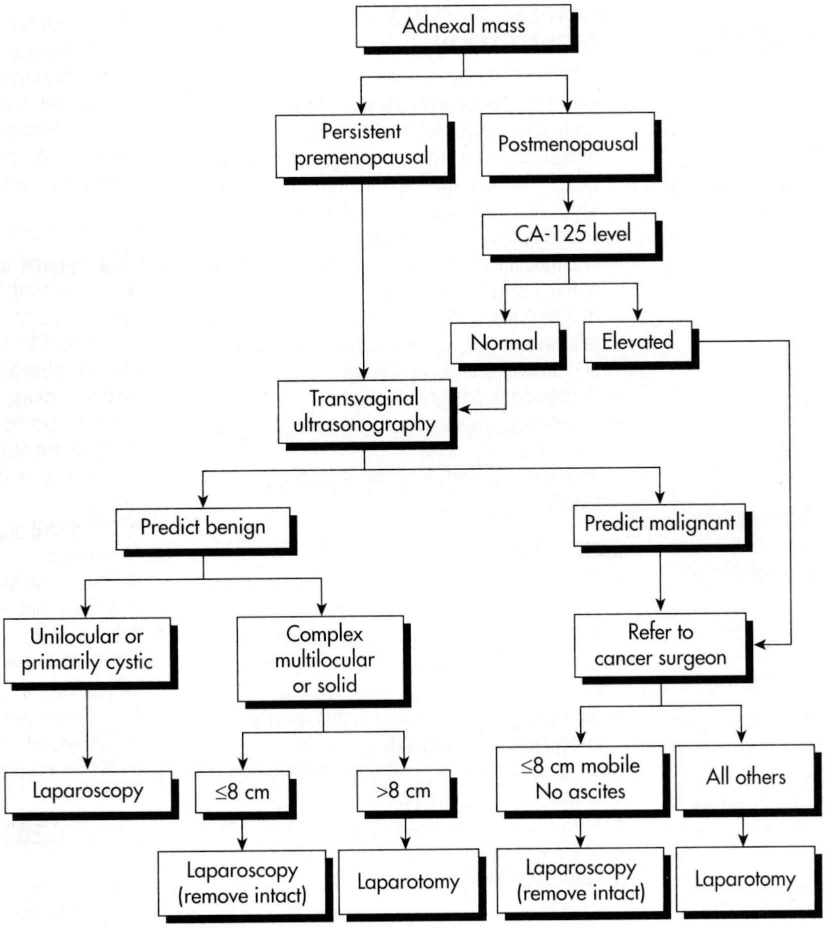

FIG. 1 Suggested management of an adnexal mass. (From Disaia PJ et al: *Clinical gynecologic oncology*, ed 9, Philadelphia, 2018, Elsevier.)

TABLE 1 Adnexal Mass: Indications for Surgery

- Ovarian cystic structure >5 cm that has been observed 6-8 wk without regression
- Any solid ovarian lesion
- Any ovarian lesion with papillary vegetation on the cyst wall
- Any adnexal mass >10 cm in diameter
- Ascites
- Palpable adnexal mass in a premenarchal or postmenopausal patient
- Torsion or rupture suspected

From Disaia PJ et al: *Clinical gynecologic oncology*, ed 9, Philadelphia, 2018, Elsevier.

5 cm, for patients who are symptomatic, or when concern for malignancy is higher. For patients who are otherwise asymptomatic, have a small mass, are premenopausal, and in whom suspicion for malignancy is low, repeat ultrasound in 1 yr is reasonable.

REFERRAL

- A referral to a gynecologic oncologist is recommended when ultrasound findings are suggestive of malignancy. Referral guidelines for women with a newly diagnosed pelvic mass are summarized in Table E2.
- A referral to general surgery or surgical oncologist should be considered if the mass is nongynecologic in origin.

SUGGESTED READINGS

Available at ExpertConsult.com

AUTHORS: **Helen Toma, MD, MSPH,** and **Kelly McNamara, MD**

Adrenal Insufficiency (PTG)

BASIC INFORMATION

DEFINITION

Adrenal insufficiency is characterized by inadequate secretion of corticosteroids resulting from partial or complete destruction of the adrenal glands (primary adrenal failure). Inadequate secretion of cortisol from the adrenals due to critical illness and pituitary insufficiency is known as secondary cortisol deficiency.

SYNONYMS

Primary adrenocortical insufficiency
Addison disease

ICD-10CM CODES

E23.3	Hypopituitarism
E27.1	Primary adrenocortical insufficiency
E27.2	Addisonian crisis
E27.3	Drug-induced adrenocortical insufficiency
E27.40	Unspecified adrenocortical insufficiency
E27.49	Other adrenocortical insufficiency

EPIDEMIOLOGY & DEMOGRAPHICS

PREVALENCE: 10 to 15 per 100,000 persons
PREDOMINANT SEX: Female:male ratio of 2:1

PHYSICAL FINDINGS & CLINICAL PRESENTATION

- Adrenal insufficiency may present insidiously with nonspecific symptoms. A high index of suspicion is required for diagnosis. About half of patients may present acutely with adrenal crises. Table 1 summarizes the clinical features of primary adrenal insufficiency
- Hyperpigmentation of skin (Figs. E1 and E2) and mucous membranes is a cardinal sign of adrenal insufficiency: More prominent in palmar creases, buccal mucosa, pressure points (elbows, knees, knuckles), perianal mucosa, and around areolas of nipples
- Hypotension, postural dizziness
- Generalized weakness, chronic fatigue, malaise, anorexia
- Amenorrhea and loss of axillary hair in females

ETIOLOGY

- Autoimmune destruction of the adrenal glands (80% of cases)
- Tuberculosis (TB) (7% to 20% of cases)
- Carcinomatous destruction of the adrenal glands, lymphoma
- Adrenal hemorrhage (anticoagulants, trauma, coagulopathies, pregnancy, sepsis)
- Adrenal infarction (antiphospholipid syndrome, arteritis, thrombosis)
- AIDS (adrenal insufficiency develops in 30% of patients with AIDS, often cytomegalovirus [CMV] adrenalitis)
- Genetic causes: Autoimmune polyglandular syndromes (APS) types 1 and 2, X-linked adrenoleukodystrophy, congenital adrenal hyperplasia
- Other: Sarcoidosis, amyloidosis, hemochromatosis, Wegener granulomatosis, postoperative, fungal infections (candidiasis, histoplasmosis)

TABLE 1 Clinical Features of Primary Adrenal Insufficiency

Feature	Frequency (%)
Symptoms	
Weakness, tiredness, fatigue	100
Anorexia	100
Gastrointestinal symptoms	92
Nausea	86
Vomiting	75
Constipation	33
Abdominal pain	31
Diarrhea	16
Salt craving	16
Postural dizziness	12
Muscle or joint pains	13
Signs	
Weight loss	100
Hyperpigmentation	94
Hypotension (<110 mm Hg systolic)	88-94
Vitiligo	10-20
Auricular calcification	5
Laboratory Findings	
Electrolyte disturbances	92
Hyponatremia	88
Hyperkalemia	64
Hypercalcemia	6
Azotemia	55
Anemia	40
Eosinophilia	17

From Melmed SZ et al: *Williams Textbook of Endocrinology*, ed 14, Philadelphia, 2019, Saunders.

Dx DIAGNOSIS

DIFFERENTIAL DIAGNOSIS

Sepsis, hypovolemic shock, acute abdomen, apathetic hyperthyroidism in the elderly, myopathies, gastrointestinal malignancy, major depression, anorexia nervosa, hemochromatosis, salt-losing nephritis, chronic infection

WORKUP

- An early morning (8 A.M.) serum cortisol <3 mcg/dl (82.8 mmol/L) is consistent with cortisol deficiency.
- If the cortisol level is 3 to 15 mcg/dl, the diagnosis can be confirmed with the rapid adrenocorticotropic hormone (ACTH) test:
  1. Give 250 mcg ACTH (Synacthen, tetracosactrin) by IV push and measure cortisol levels at 0, 30, and 60 min.
  2. An increase in serum cortisol level to peak concentration >500 nmol/L (18 mcg/dl) indicates a normal response. Cortisol level ≤18 mcg/dl at 30 or 60 min is suggestive of adrenal insufficiency.
  3. Measure plasma ACTH. A high ACTH level (>200 pg/ml [44 pmol/L]) confirms primary adrenal insufficiency.
- Critical illness-related corticosteroid insufficiency (e.g., in sepsis) is best established with the 1-mcg ACTH stimulation test in which cortisol levels are measured at baseline and 30 min after administration of ACTH. A level <25 mcg/dl (690 nmol/L) or an increment over baseline of <9 mcg (250 nmol/L) represents an inadequate adrenal response.
- Secondary adrenocortical insufficiency (caused by pituitary dysfunction) can be distinguished from primary adrenal insufficiency by the following:
  1. Normal or low plasma ACTH level after rapid ACTH.
  2. Absence of hyperpigmentation.
  3. No significant impairment of aldosterone secretion (because aldosterone secretion is under control of the renin-angiotensin system).
  4. Additional evidence of hypopituitarism (e.g., hypogonadism, hypothyroidism).

LABORATORY TESTS

- Hyponatremia, hyperkalemia
- Decreased glucose
- Increased BUN/creatinine ratio (prerenal azotemia)
- Mild normocytic, normochromic anemia, neutropenia, lymphocytosis, eosinophilia (significant dehydration may mask hyponatremia and anemia), hypercalcemia, metabolic acidosis

- A morning cortisol level >500 mmol/L (18 mcg/dl) generally excludes the diagnosis whereas a level <165 mmol/L (6 mcg/dl) is suggestive of Addison disease and a level <3 mcg/dl requires further evaluation (see "Workup")
- Additional evaluation may include 21-hydroxylase antibodies present in 90% of autoimmune adrenalitis cases. If negative, obtain CT scan of adrenal glands
- PPD or QuantiFERON Gold test to rule out TB

IMAGING STUDIES

- Imaging is not necessary for diagnosis but may help identify potential causes.
- Abdominal CT scan (Fig. 3): Small adrenal glands generally indicate either idiopathic atrophy or longstanding TB, whereas enlarged glands are suggestive of early TB or potentially treatable diseases.
- Chest radiograph may reveal a small heart (Fig. E4).
- Abdominal radiograph: Adrenal calcifications may be noted if the adrenocortical insufficiency is secondary to TB or fungal infection.

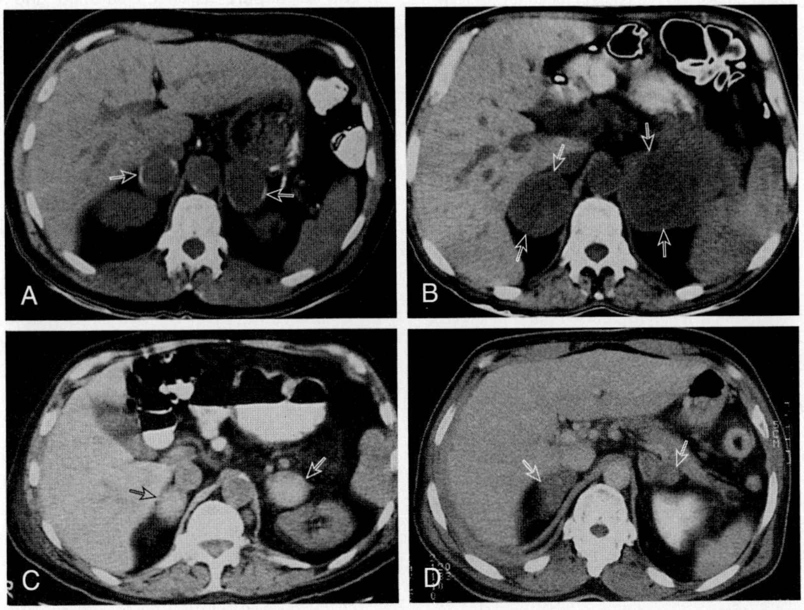

FIG. 3 Computed tomographic (CT) scans of patients with primary adrenal insufficiency. The affected adrenal glands are indicated by arrows. **A,** CT scan of a 59-yr-old man with histoplasmosis. Notice the subcapsular calcium in both glands. **B,** CT scan of a 59-yr-old man with metastatic melanoma. **C,** CT scan of an 80-yr-old man with bilateral adrenal hemorrhage resulting from anticoagulation for pulmonary emboli. **D,** Bilateral adrenal tuberculomas in a 79-yr-old man with tuberculosis affecting the urogenital tract. (**A** and **B** courtesy Dr. William D. Salmon, Jr.; **C,** courtesy Dr. Craig R. Sussman.) (From Melmed S, Polonsky KS, Larsen PR, Kronenberg HM: *Williams Textbook of Endocrinology,* ed 14, Philadelphia, 2019, Saunders.)

TABLE 2 Treatment of Acute Adrenal Insufficiency (Adrenal Crisis) in Adults

Emergency Measures

1. Establish intravenous access with a large-gauge needle.
2. Draw blood for immediate serum electrolytes and glucose and routine measurement of plasma cortisol and ACTH. Do not wait for laboratory results.
3. Infuse 2-3 L of 154 mmol/L NaCl (0.9% saline) solution, or 50 g/L (5%) dextrose in 154 mmol/L NaCl (0.9% saline) solution, as quickly as possible. Monitor for signs of fluid overload by measuring central or peripheral venous pressure and listening for pulmonary rales. Reduce infusion rate if indicated.
4. Inject intravenous hydrocortisone (100 mg immediately and every 6 hr).
5. Use supportive measures as needed.

Subacute Measures After Stabilization of the Patient

1. Continue intravenous 154 mmol/L NaCl (0.9% saline) solution at a slower rate for next 24-48 hr.
2. Search for and treat possible infectious precipitating causes of the adrenal crisis.
3. Perform a short ACTH stimulation test to confirm the diagnosis of adrenal insufficiency (if patient does not have known adrenal insufficiency).
4. Determine the type of adrenal insufficiency and its cause, if not already known.
5. Taper glucocorticoids to maintenance dosage over 1-3 days, if precipitating or complicating illness permits.
6. Begin mineralocorticoid replacement with fludrocortisone (0.1 mg by mouth daily) when saline infusion is stopped.

ACTH, Adrenocorticotropic hormone.

From Melmed S et al: *Williams Textbook of Endocrinology,* ed 14, 2019, Elsevier.

Rx TREATMENT

NONPHARMACOLOGIC THERAPY

- Perform periodic monitoring of serum electrolytes, vital signs, and body weight; liberal sodium intake is suggested.
- Periodic measurement of bone density may be helpful in identifying patients at risk for the development of osteoporosis.
- Patients should carry a MedicAlert bracelet and an emergency pack containing hydrocortisone 100-mg ampule, syringe, and needle.
- Patients and partners should be educated on how to give IM injection in case of vomiting or coma.

ACUTE GENERAL Rx

- Adrenal crisis is an acute complication of adrenal insufficiency characterized by circulatory collapse, dehydration, nausea, vomiting, hypoglycemia, and hyperkalemia. Table 2 summarizes the treatment of acute adrenal insufficiency (adrenal crisis) in adults.
  1. Draw plasma cortisol level; do not delay therapy while waiting for confirming laboratory results.
  2. Administer hydrocortisone 100 mg IV immediately and every 6 hr; if patient shows good clinical response, gradually taper dosage over 1 to 3 days and change to oral maintenance dose (usually prednisone 7.5 mg/day).
  3. Provide adequate volume replacement with D_5NS solution until hypotension, dehydration, and hypoglycemia are completely corrected. Large volumes (2-3 L) under continuous cardiac monitoring may be necessary in the first 2 to 3 hr to correct the volume deficit and hypoglycemia and to avoid further hyponatremia.
- Identify and correct any precipitating factor (e.g., sepsis, hemorrhage).

CHRONIC Rx

- Table 3 summarizes the treatment of chronic primary adrenal insufficiency in adults.
- Give hydrocortisone 15 to 20 mg PO every morning and 5 to 10 mg in late afternoon or prednisone 5 mg in morning and 2.5 mg hs.
- Give oral fludrocortisone 0.05 mg/day to 0.4 mg/day. This mineralocorticoid is necessary if the patient has primary adrenocortical insufficiency. The dose is adjusted based on the serum sodium level and the presence of postural hypotension or marked orthostasis.
- Instruct patients to increase glucocorticoid replacement in times of stress and to receive parenteral glucocorticoids if diarrhea or vomiting occurs. Typical supplementation varies from 25 mg PO qd of hydrocortisone for minor medical and

TABLE 3 Treatment of Chronic Primary Adrenal Insufficiency in Adults

Maintenance Therapy

Glucocorticoid Replacement

- Hydrocortisone 15-20 mg on awakening and 5-10 mg in early afternoon.
- Monitor clinical symptoms and morning plasma ACTH.

Mineralocorticoid Replacement

- Fludrocortisone 0.1 (0.05-0.4) mg orally.
- Liberal salt intake.
- Monitor lying and standing blood pressure and pulse, edema, serum potassium, and plasma renin activity.
- Educate patient about the disease, how to manage minor illnesses and major stresses, and how to inject steroid intramuscularly.
- Obtain MedicAlert bracelet/necklace, Emergency Medical Information card.

Treatment of Minor Febrile Illness or Stress

- Increase glucocorticoid dose twofold to threefold for the few days of illness; do not change mineralocorticoid dose.
- Contact physician if illness worsens or persists for more than 3 days or if vomiting develops.
- No extra supplementation is needed for most uncomplicated, outpatient dental procedures with local anesthesia. General anesthesia or intravenous sedation should not be used in the office.

Emergency Treatment of Severe Stress or Trauma

- Inject contents of prefilled dexamethasone (4-mg) syringe or contents of hydrocortisone hemisuccinate rapid reconstitution vial (100-mg) intramuscularly.
- Get to physician as quickly as possible.

Steroid Coverage for Illness or Surgery in Hospital

- For moderate illness, give hydrocortisone 50 mg bid PO or IV. Taper rapidly to maintenance dose as patient recovers.
- For severe illness, give hydrocortisone 100 mg IV q8h. Taper to maintenance level by decreasing by half every day. Adjust dose according to course of illness.
- For minor procedures under local anesthesia and most radiologic studies, no extra supplementation is needed.
- For moderately stressful procedures such as barium enema, endoscopy, or arteriography, give a single 100-mg IV dose of hydrocortisone just before the procedure.
- For major surgery, give hydrocortisone 100 mg IV just before induction of anesthesia and continue q8h for first 24 hr. Taper dose rapidly, decreasing by half per day, to maintenance level.

ACTH, Adrenocorticotropic hormone; *bid,* twice a day; *IV,* intravenous; *PO,* orally; *q,* every.

From Melmed S et al: *Williams Textbook of Endocrinology,* ed 14, 2019, Elsevier.

surgical stress to 50 to 100 mg IV hydrocortisone q8h for sepsis-induced hypotension or shock.

- The administration of dehydroepiandrosterone (DHEA) is controversial due to lack of robust data. It is not indicated in men but may be considered in women with primary adrenal failure. A dose of 50 mg PO qd may improve well-being and sexuality in women with adrenal insufficiency.
- Patients with concomitant hypothyroidism should be treated with glucocorticoids first before correcting hypothyroidism because correction of thyroid hormone deficiency will accelerate cortisol clearance and can precipitate adrenal crisis.
- A plan for steroid replacement in patients withdrawing from chronic corticosteroid therapy is outlined in Table 4.

SUGGESTED READINGS

Available at ExpertConsult.com

RELATED CONTENT

Addison Disease (Patient Information)

AUTHOR: **Fred F. Ferri, MD**

TABLE 4 Suggested Plan for Steroid Replacement in Patients Withdrawing From Chronic Corticosteroid Therapy

Pred Dose (mg/day)	DURATION OF GLUCOCORTICOID TREATMENT			
	≤3 WK[a]			>3 WK
≥7.5	Can stop	↓ rapidly (e.g., 2.5 mg q3-4d) THEN		
5-7.5	Can stop	↓ 1 mg q2-4 wk THEN	OR	Convert 5 mg pred to 20 mg HC, then ↓ 2.5 mg/wk to 10 mg/day THEN
<5	Can stop	↓ 1 mg q2-4 wk		After 2-3 mo HC 10 mg/day, administer SST/ITT: Pass → Withdraw Fail → Continue

HC, hydrocortisone; *ITT,* insulin tolerance test; *pred,* prednisolone; *SST,* short Synacthen test. Basal 0900h ACTH can be used to monitor for recovery of HPA axis and levels may be above the normal range ahead of a "pass" on an SST.

[a]Beware of frequent steroid courses (e.g., in asthma).

From Melmed S et al: *Williams Textbook of Endocrinology,* ed 14, 2019, Elsevier.

BASIC INFORMATION

DEFINITION

- "Moderate drinking": Moderate drinking has been defined as two standard drinks (e.g., 12 oz of beer) per day and one drink per day for women and persons older than 65 yr.
- "Hazardous" or "At-risk drinking": For men, *at-risk drinking* is defined as more than 14 drinks/wk or more than 4 drinks/occasion. For women, at-risk drinking is defined as approximately half that given for men.
- "Alcohol withdrawal": The American Psychiatric Association defines diagnostic criteria for *alcohol withdrawal* as follows:
  1. Cessation of (or reduction in) alcohol use that has been heavy and prolonged
  2. Two (or more) of the following, developing within several hours to a few days after criterion A:
     a. Autonomic hyperactivity (e.g., sweating or pulse rate >100 beats/min)
     b. Increased hand tremor
     c. Insomnia
     d. Nausea and vomiting
     e. Transient visual, tactile, or auditory hallucinations or illusions
     f. Psychomotor agitation
     g. Anxiety
     h. Grand mal seizures
  3. The symptoms in criterion B cause clinically significant distress or impairment in social, occupational, or other important areas of functioning
- The symptoms are not attributable to a general medical condition and are not better accounted for by another mental disorder.

SYNONYMS

Alcohol dependence syndrome
Substance abuse
Alcohol withdrawal syndrome
Alcoholism

ICD-10CM CODES

F10	Mental and behavioral disorders due to use of alcohol
F10.1	Mental and behavioral disorders due to use of alcohol: Harmful use
F10.2	Mental and behavioral disorders due to use of alcohol: Dependence syndrome
F10.3	Mental and behavioral disorders due to use of alcohol: Withdrawal state
F10.4	Mental and behavioral disorders due to use of alcohol: Withdrawal state with delirium
F10.5	Mental and behavioral disorders due to use of alcohol: Psychotic disorder
F10.6	Mental and behavioral disorders due to use of alcohol: Amnesic syndrome

EPIDEMIOLOGY & DEMOGRAPHICS

INCIDENCE (IN U.S.):

- The clinical history suggests alcohol problems in 15% to 20% of patients in primary care and hospitalized patients. In the U.S., alcohol use disorder generates nearly $223 billion in annual economic costs. An estimated 14% of adults in the U.S. have alcohol dependence. Alcohol accounts for 6.8% of age-standardized deaths in men and 2.2% in women.
- 20% achieve abstinence without help; 70% achieve sobriety for 1 yr.

PREVALENCE (IN U.S.): 7% of population ≥18 yr

PREDOMINANT SEX:

- Lifetime risk for males 8% to 10%
- Lifetime risk for females 3% to 5%

PEAK INCIDENCE: 20 to 40 yr. The most common age range for initial treatment of alcohol dependence is 35 to 45 yr. However, the peak period for meeting alcohol dependence criteria is ≥10 yr earlier.

GENETICS: More common with a family history of alcoholism and in patients of Irish, Scandinavian, and Native American descent

PHYSICAL FINDINGS & CLINICAL PRESENTATION

- Recurring minor trauma
- Gastrointestinal bleeding from gastritis and/or varices
- Pancreatitis (acute and chronic)
- Liver disease
- Odor of alcohol on breath
- Tremulousness
- Tachycardia
- Peripheral neuropathy
- Recent memory loss

ETIOLOGY

- Social and genetic factors important
- Risk factors:
  1. Broken homes
  2. Unemployment
  3. Divorce
  4. Recurrent depression
  5. Addiction to another substance, including tobacco
  6. Working long hours (≥55 hours/wk)

Dx DIAGNOSIS

WORKUP

- The USPSTF recommends that clinicians screen adults 18 yr and older for alcohol misuse and provide persons engaged in risky or hazardous drinking with brief behavioral counseling interventions to reduce alcohol misuse. Several screening tests (CAGE [Table 1], TWEAK, CRAFFT, AUDIT-C [Table 2]) are available. The four-item CAGE (feeling need to **C**ut down, **A**nnoyed by criticism, **G**uilty about drinking, and need for an **E**ye-opener in the morning) is the most popular screening test in primary care. A positive response should lead to further questioning. The sensitivity of the CAGE ranges from 43% to 94% and its specificity ranges from 70% to 97%. The five-item TWEAK scale (**T**olerance, **W**orry, **E**ye-openers, **A**mnesia, [**K**] cut down) and the TACE questionnaire (**T**olerance, **A**nnoyance, **C**ut down, **E**ye-opener) are designed to screen pregnant women for alcohol misuse. They detect lower levels of alcohol consumption that may pose risks during pregnancy. The CRAFFT questionnaire (riding in **C**ar with someone who was drinking, using alcohol to **R**elax, using alcohol while **A**lone, **F**orgetfulness, criticism from **F**riends and **F**amily, **T**rouble) is useful as a screening tool for adolescents. Its sensitivity is 92% and specificity 64% for alcohol use disorder. Single-question screening about alcohol consumption in a day ("When was the last time you had more than X drinks in a day?" [where X is 5 for men and 4 for women]) with the threshold set at "in the past 3 months" is 85% sensitive and 70% specific in men and 82% and 70% in women for unhealthy alcohol use. The 3-question AUDIT-C is a shorter form of the 10-item AUDIT, and the questions center on the quantity and frequency of alcohol use. It asks how often someone has had a drink containing alcohol, how many standard drinks containing alcohol one consumes on a typical day when one is drinking, and how often one has six or more drinks on one occasion. Scoring ranges from 0 to 4 on each question with a total score range of 0 to 12. A total score of 3 or higher for women and 4 or higher for men indicates alcohol use disorder and need for further assessment. Its sensitivity ranges from 85% in Hispanic women to 95% in white men.
- Laboratory evaluation (see below).

TABLE 1 CAGE Questionnaire for Alcohol Problems Screening[a]

C	Have you felt the need to **C**ut down on your drinking?
A	Have people **A**nnoyed you by criticizing your drinking?
G	Have you ever felt bad or **G**uilty about your drinking?
E	Have you had a drink first thing in the morning to steady your nerves or to get rid of a hangover (i.e., an "**E**ye opener")?

From Stern TA et al: *Massachusetts General Hospital handbook of general hospital psychiatry,* ed 7, Philadelphia, 2018, Elsevier.

TABLE 2 AUDIT-C Questionnaire for Alcohol Problems Screening[a]

Question	Score
How often did you have a drink containing alcohol in the past year?	Never (0 points) Monthly or less (1 point) 2-4 times per month (2 points) 2-3 times per week (3 points) >4 times per week (4 points)

[a]AUDIT-C is scored 0-12, with score >4 (men) and >3 (women) considered positive for problematic drinking.
From Stern TA et al: *Massachusetts General Hospital handbook of general hospital psychiatry,* ed 7, Philadelphia, 2018, Elsevier.

LABORATORY TESTS

Lab tests alone do not accurately detect alcohol problems but can help identify medical complications related to alcohol use, such as pancreatitis or cirrhosis.

- Gamma-glutamyltransferase (GGTP), generally elevated.
- Liver transaminases (alanine aminotransferase [ALT], aspartate aminotransferase [AST]), often elevated, may be normal or low in advanced liver disease.
- Low albumin level, hypophosphatemia, hypomagnesemia from malnutrition.
- Complete blood count (CBC) reveals elevated mean corpuscular volume from toxic effect of alcohol on erythrocyte development in nutritional deficiencies.
- Stool for occult blood may be positive as a result of gastritis or variceal bleeding.
- RBC folate, vitamin B_{12} level, vitamin B_6, vitamin B_1 level.

IMAGING STUDIES

Indicated only with a history of trauma. CT or ultrasound of abdomen may reveal fatty liver or cirrhosis in advanced stages.

Rx TREATMENT

NONPHARMACOLOGIC THERAPY

- Twelve-step facilitation, cognitive behavioral therapy, and motivational enhancement therapy improve the chances of recovery in patients with alcohol use disorder and dependence.
- Depression, if present, should be treated at same time alcohol is withdrawn.

ACUTE GENERAL Rx

Alcohol withdrawal syndrome (AWS) occurs when a person stops ingesting alcohol after prolonged consumption. It can result in four possible clinical patterns depending on the severity of the patient's alcohol use and the time from the patient's previous alcohol ingestion. Blood ethanol level decreases by ~20 mg/dl/hr in a normal person. Although discussed separately, these withdrawal states blend together in real life. Table 3 summarizes medications for the treatment of alcohol dependence. The cornerstone of treatment for alcohol withdrawal syndrome is the use of benzodiazepines.

- **Tremulous state** (early alcohol withdrawal, "impending DTs," "shakes," "jitters")
  1. Time interval: Usually occurs 6 to 8 hr after the last drink or 12 to 48 hr after reduction of alcohol intake; becomes most pronounced at 24 to 36 hr
  2. Manifestation: Tremors, mild agitation, insomnia, tachycardia; symptoms are relieved by alcohol
  3. Detoxification can be in the outpatient (ambulatory) or inpatient setting. Candidates for outpatient detoxification should have a reasonable support system (e.g., reliable contact person) who can monitor progress and lack of any significant comorbid conditions (e.g., suicide risk, seizure disorder, coexisting benzodiazepine dependence, prior unsuccessful outpatient detoxification, pregnancy, cirrhosis) or risk factors for severe withdrawal (age >40 yr, drinking >100 g of ethanol daily [e.g., 1 pint of liquor or eight 12-oz cans of beer, random blood alcohol concentration >200 mg/dl])
  4. Inpatient treatment:
     a. The management of alcohol withdrawal is facilitated by the use of ethanol withdrawal charts. An example of such a chart is shown in Fig. E1
     b. Admit to medical floor (private room); monitor vital signs q4h; institute seizure precautions; maintain adequate sedation
     c. Administer lorazepam as follows:
        (1) Day 1: 2 mg PO q4h while awake and not lethargic
        (2) Day 2: 1 mg PO q4h while awake and not lethargic
        (3) Day 3: 0.5 mg PO q4h while awake and not lethargic
        (4) NOTE: Hold sedation for lethargy or abnormal vital or neurologic signs. The preceding doses are only guidelines; it is best to titrate the dose case by case
     d. In patients with mild to moderate withdrawal and without history of seizures, individualized benzodiazepine administration (rather than a fixed-dose regimen) results in lower benzodiazepine administration and avoids unnecessary sedation. The Clinical Institute Withdrawal Assessment Scale for Alcohol, Revised (CIWA-Ar) scale (Box 1) can be used to measure the severity of alcohol withdrawal. It consists of 10 items: Nausea; tremor; autonomic hyperactivity; anxiety; agitation; tactile, visual, and auditory

TABLE 3 Medications for the Treatment of Alcohol Dependence*

Medication	Dose and Route	Frequency	Effects	Major Common Adverse Effects
Alcohol Withdrawal				
		Benzodiazepines†		
Chlordiazepoxide*	25-100 mg, PO/IV/IM†	Every 4-6 hr	Decreased severity of withdrawal; stabilization of vital signs; prevention of seizures and delirium tremens	Confusion, oversedation, respiratory depression
Diazepam‡	5-10 mg, PO/IV/IM†	Every 6-8 hr		
Oxazepam‡	15-30 mg, PO†	Every 6-8 hr		
Lorazepam‡	1-4 mg, PO/IV/IM†	Every 4-8 hr		
		β-Blockers		
Atenolol	25-50 mg, PO	Once a day	Improvement in vital signs	Bradycardia, hypotension
Propranolol	10-40 mg, PO	Every 6-8 hr	Reduction in craving	
		α-Agonists		
Clonidine	0.1-0.2 mg, PO	Every 6 hr	Decreased withdrawal symptoms	Hypotension, fatigue
		Antiepileptics		
Carbamazepine	200 mg, PO	Every 6-8 hr	Decreased severity of withdrawal; prevention of seizures	Dizziness, fatigue, red blood cell abnormalities
		Prevention of Relapse		
Disulfiram‡	125-500 mg, PO	Daily	Decreased alcohol use among those who relapse	Disulfiram-alcohol reaction, rash, drowsiness, peripheral neuropathy
Naltrexone‡	50 mg, PO	Daily	Increased abstinence, decreased drinking days	Nausea, abdominal pain, myalgias-arthralgias
	380 mg, IM	Every 4 wk		
Acamprosate‡	666 mg, PO	Three times a day	Increased abstinence	Diarrhea

*Most commonly used medications listed.
†Currently approved by U.S. Food and Drug Administration for the indication noted.
‡Dose and routes given for standard fixed-dose regimens, which include dose tapers over time.
From Goldman L, Schafer AI: *Goldman's Cecil medicine,* ed 24, Philadelphia, 2012, Saunders.

disturbances; headache; and disorientation. Each item is assigned a score from 0 to 7. For example, in the "agitation" category 0 indicates normal activity, and 7 indicates that the patient constantly thrashes about. For the category of "tremor," 0 indicates that tremor is not present and 7 that tremor is severe, even with arms not extended. The maximum total score is 67. Patients with mild AWS symptoms (CIWA-Ar score <8) can be monitored on an outpatient basis. Benzodiazepines are beneficial for most patients with a CIWA-AR score ≥8 and are strongly recommended in patients with substantial withdrawal symptoms (CIWA-Ar score >12). Patients with CIWA-Ar score of ≥15 should be admitted to detox unit. In-patient treatment is also recommended for patients with history of withdrawal seizures and for those with suicidal ideation and significant comorbidities

e. Beta-adrenergic blockers: Beta-blockers are useful for controlling blood pressure and tachyarrhythmias. However, they do not prevent progression to more serious symptoms of withdrawal and, if used, should not be administered alone but in conjunction with benzodiazepines. Beta-blockers should be avoided in patients with contraindications to their use (e.g., bronchospasm, bradycardia, or severe congestive heart failure). Centrally acting alpha-adrenergic agonists such as clonidine ameliorate symptoms in patients with mild to moderate withdrawal but do not reduce delirium or seizures

f. Vitamin replacement: Thiamine 100 mg IV or IM for at least 5 days plus oral multivitamins. The IV administration of glucose can precipitate Wernicke encephalopathy in alcoholics with thiamine deficiency; therefore thiamine administration should precede IV dextrose

g. Hydration PO or IV (high-caloric solution): If IV, glucose with Na+, K+, Mg2+, and phosphate replacement prn

h. Laboratory studies:
   (1) CBC, platelet count, INR
   (2) Electrolytes, glucose, blood urea nitrogen, creatinine
   (3) GGTP, ALT, AST
   (4) Phosphorus and magnesium
   (5) Serum vitamin B_{12} and folic acid (if megaloblastic features in blood smear)

i. Diagnostic imaging: Generally not necessary; if subdural hematoma is suspected (evidence of trauma, persistent lethargy), a CT scan should be ordered

j. Social rehabilitation: Group therapy such as Alcoholics Anonymous; identification and treatment of social and family problems should be initiated during the patient's hospital stay

- **Alcoholic hallucinosis:**
  1. Manifestations: Hallucinations usually are auditory, but hallucinations occasionally are visual, tactile, or olfactory; usually there is no clouding of sensorium as in delirium (clinical presentation may be mistaken for an acute schizophrenic episode). Disordered perceptions become most pronounced after 24 to 36 hr of abstinence
  2. Treatment: Same as for DTs (see "Withdrawal seizures")
- **Withdrawal seizures ("rum fits"):**
  1. Time interval: Usually occurs 7 to 30 hr after cessation of drinking, with a peak incidence between 13 and 24 hr
  2. Manifestations: Generalized convulsions with loss of consciousness; focal signs are usually absent; consider further investigation with CT scan of head and electroencephalography if clearly indicated (e.g., presence of focal neurologic deficits, prolonged postictal confusion state). In addition, in a febrile patient who is having a seizure or altered mental state, a lumbar puncture is necessary
  3. Treatment:
     a. Diazepam 2.5 mg/min IV until seizure is controlled (check for respiratory depression or hypotension) may be beneficial for prolonged seizure

BOX 1 Alcohol Withdrawal Assessment Scoring Guidelines (Revised Clinical Institute Withdrawal Assessment for Alcohol Scale)

Nausea and Vomiting (0-7)
0, none; 1, mild nausea with no vomiting; 4, intermittent nausea; 7, constant nausea, frequent dry heaves and vomiting

Tremor (0-7)
0, no tremor; 1, not visible, but can be felt fingertip to fingertip; 4, moderate, with patient's arms extended; 7, severe, even with arms not extended

Paroxysmal Sweats (0-7)
0, no sweats; 1, barely perceptible sweating, palms moist; 4, beads of sweat obvious on forehead; 7, drenching sweats

Anxiety (0-7)
0, no anxiety, patient at ease; 1, mildly anxious; 4, moderately anxious or guarded, so anxiety is inferred; 7, equivalent to acute panic states seen in severe delirium or acute schizophrenic reactions

Agitation (0-7)
0, normal activity; 1, somewhat more than normal activity; 4, moderately fidgety and restless; 7, pacing back and forth during, or constantly thrashing about

Tactile Disturbances (0-7)
Ask, "Have you experienced any itching, pins and needles sensation, burning or numbness, or a feeling of bugs crawling on or under your skin?"
0, none; 1, very mild itching, pins and needles, burning, or numbness; 2, mild itching, pins and needles, burning, or numbness; 3, moderate itching, pins and needles, burning, or numbness; 4, moderately severe tactile hallucinations; 5, severe hallucinations; 6, extremely severe hallucinations; 7, continuous hallucinations

Auditory Disturbances (0-7)
Ask, "Are you more aware of sounds around you? Are they harsh? Do they startle you? Do you hear anything that disturbs you or that you know isn't there?"
0, not present; 1, very mild harshness or ability to startle; 2, mild harshness or ability to startle; 3, moderate harshness or ability to startle; 4, moderate hallucinations; 5, severe hallucinations; 6, extremely severe hallucinations; 7, continuous hallucinations

Visual Disturbances (0-7)
Ask, "Does the light appear to be too bright? Is its color different than normal? Does it hurt your eyes? Are you seeing anything that disturbs you?"
0, not present; 1, very mild sensitivity to light; 2, mild sensitivity; 3, moderate sensitivity; 4, moderate hallucinations; 5, severe hallucinations; 6, extremely severe hallucinations; 7, continuous hallucinations

Headache (0-7)
0, not present; 1, very mild; 2, mild; 3, moderate; 4, moderately severe; 5, severe; 6, very severe; 7, extremely severe

Orientation and Clouding of Sensorium (0-4)
Ask, "What day is this? Where are you? Who am I?"
0, oriented; 1, cannot do serial additions or is uncertain about date; 2, disoriented to date by no more than 2 calendar days; 3, disoriented to date by more than 2 calendar days; 4, disoriented to place and/or person

Total Score
0-9: Absent or minimal withdrawal
10-19: Mild to moderate withdrawal
More than 20: Severe withdrawal

From Sullivan JT et al: Assessment of alcohol withdrawal: the revised clinical institute withdrawal assessment for alcohol scale (CIWA-Ar), *Br J Addict* 84:1353-1357, 1989.

activity; IV lorazepam 1 to 2 mg q2h can be used in place of diazepam. Withdrawal seizures generally are self-limited and treatment is not required; the use of phenytoin or other anticonvulsants for short-term treatment of alcohol withdrawal seizures is not recommended

b. Thiamine 100 mg IV, followed by IV dextrose, should also be administered

c. Electrolyte imbalances (increased Mg^{2+}, decreased K^+, increased or decreased Na^+, decreased PO_4^{3-}) that may exacerbate seizures should be corrected

- **DTs:**
  1. Time interval: Variable; usually occurs within 1 wk after reduction or cessation of heavy alcohol intake and persists for 1 to 3 days. Peak incidence is 72 hr and 96 hr after the cessation of alcohol consumption
  2. Manifestations: Profound confusion, tremors, vivid visual and tactile hallucinations, autonomic hyperactivity; this is the most serious clinical presentation of alcohol withdrawal (mortality rate is approximately 15% in untreated patients)
  3. Treatment:
     a. Admission to a detoxification unit where patient can be observed closely
     b. Vital signs q30min (neurologic signs, if necessary)
     c. Use of lateral decubitus or prone position if restraints are necessary
     d. NPO: Nasogastric tube for abdominal distention may be necessary but should not be routinely used
     e. Laboratory studies: Same as for early alcohol withdrawal
     f. Vigorous hydration (4 to 6 L/day): IV with glucose (Na^+, K^+, PO_4^{3-} and Mg^{2+} replacement [if patient has hypophosphatemia or hypomagnesemia])
     g. Vitamins: Thiamine 100 mg IV qd. The initial dose of thiamine should precede the administration of IV dextrose; multivitamins (may be added to the hydrating solution)
     h. Sedation: Control of agitation should be achieved with rapid-acting sedative-hypnotic agents in adequate doses to maintain light somnolence for the duration of delirium
        (1) Initially: Lorazepam 2 to 5 mg IM/IV repeated prn
        (2) Maintenance (individualized dosage): Chlordiazepoxide, 50 to 100 mg PO q4 to 6h, lorazepam 2 mg PO q4h, or diazepam 5 to 10 mg PO tid; withhold doses or decrease subsequent doses if signs of oversedation are apparent
        (3) Midazolam is also effective for managing DTs. Its rapid onset (sedation within 2 to 4 min of IV injection) and short duration of action (approximately 30 min) make it an ideal agent for titration in continuous infusion
     i. Treatment of seizures (as previously described)
     j. Diagnosis and treatment of concomitant medical, surgical, or psychiatric conditions

CHRONIC Rx

- See "Referral."
- Pharmacotherapies for alcoholism include:
  1. Acamprosate is a synthetic compound with a chemical structure similar to the neurotransmitter gamma-aminobutyric acid and the amino acid neuromodulator taurine. Its mechanism of action is not completely understood. It is indicated for the maintenance of abstinence from alcohol in patients with alcohol dependence who are abstinent at treatment initiation. It should be used only as part of a comprehensive psychosocial treatment program. It does not cause a disulfiram-like reaction as a result of ethanol ingestion. Dose is two 333-mg tablets tid. Treatment should be initiated as soon as possible after the period of alcohol withdrawal, when the patient has achieved abstinence, and should be maintained if the patient relapses. Avoid acamprosate if severe renal impairment is present.
  2. The long-acting opiate antagonist naltrexone inhibits the rewarding effects of alcohol. The starting dose is 25 mg/day, increased to 50 mg PO qd after 1 wk. An extended-release, once-monthly injection of naltrexone is also available and can be used along with psychosocial support to maintain alcohol abstinence. In patients with opioid dependence, naltrexone can precipitate acute withdrawal syndrome and should not be used at least 7 days from last opioid use. There are no established guidelines on the appropriate length of naltrexone treatment for alcohol dependence. One study recommends at least 3 mo of treatment. Avoid naltrexone if acute hepatitis, hepatic failure, or ongoing opioid use is present.
  3. Topiramate or gabapentin can be offered as second line drugs; to patients with moderate to severe alcohol use disorder topiramate might be preferable.
  4. Disulfiram (Antabuse): Dosage is 500 mg max qd for 1 to 2 wk, then 125 to 500 mg qd. It interferes with the metabolism of alcohol by inhibiting aldehyde dehydrogenase, causing an accumulation of acetaldehyde. It produces unpleasant symptoms (nausea, flushing, elevated blood pressure, headache, weakness) when alcohol is ingested. It is an older drug that is now rarely used.
  5. Avoid pharmacological treatments in pregnant or breastfeeding women.

DISPOSITION

See "Referral."

REFERRAL

- To Alcoholics Anonymous or Adult Children of Alcoholics
- Family members to Al-Anon or Al-A-Teen
- Many cities have Salvation Army Adult Rehabilitation centers; all patients accepted, regardless of ability to pay

PEARLS & CONSIDERATIONS

COMMENTS

- Relative indications for inpatient alcohol detoxification are as follows: History of DTs or withdrawal seizures, severe withdrawal symptoms, concomitant psychiatric or medical illness, pregnancy, multiple previous detoxifications, recent high levels of alcohol consumption, and lack of reliable support network.
- Detoxification is not a stand-alone treatment but should serve as a bridge to a formal treatment program for alcohol dependence.
- The cure rate for alcoholism is highly disappointing, regardless of the modality. Only those who want to be helped will be helped. An effective strategy for the primary care physician is a prominently displayed sign in the office that states, "If you think you consume too many alcoholic beverages, please discuss it with me." Those who do open up the discussion can be given the facts in a nonjudgmental way and often can be helped. All too often problem drinkers lie on the questionnaire until they face a life-threatening health issue—and even then denial often reigns supreme.
- In a recent clinical trial, patients receiving medical management with naltrexone (100 mg/day), combined behavioral intervention (CBI), or both fared better on drinking outcomes, whereas acamprosate showed no evidence of efficacy, with or without CBI. No combination produced better efficacy than naltrexone or CBI alone in the presence of medical management.

SUGGESTED READINGS

Available at ExpertConsult.com

RELATED CONTENT

Alcohol Use Disorder (Patient Information)
Drug Use Disorder (Related Key Topic)
Alcoholic Hepatitis (Related Key Topic)
Substance Use Disorder (Related Key Topic)
Wernicke Syndrome (Related Key Topic)

AUTHOR: **Fred F. Ferri, MD**

BASIC INFORMATION

DEFINITION

Alcoholic hepatitis (AH) is a severe, progressive, inflammatory, and cholestatic liver disease occurring in patients with long-term heavy alcohol use (60 to 80 g/day in men and 20 to 40 g/day in women)

SYNONYM

AH

ICD-10CM CODES
K70.10 Alcoholic hepatitis without ascites
K70.9 Alcoholic liver disease, unspecified

EPIDEMIOLOGY & DEMOGRAPHICS

- Approximately 2 million people in the U.S. (about 1% of the population) are affected by alcoholic liver disease.
- Alcoholic hepatitis accounts for 0.8% of all admissions in the U.S.
- Typical presentation age: 40 to 50 yr. Majority occurs before age 60.
- Patients with alcoholic hepatitis typically drink more than 100 g of alcohol daily for two or more decades.

PREVALENCE: Approximately 25% to 30%

PREDOMINANT SEX AND AGE: The majority of patients are males. Males are two times as likely as women to abuse alcohol. However, women develop alcoholic hepatitis after a shorter time and smaller amount of alcoholic exposure than men.

RISK FACTORS: Drinking multiple alcohol types, drinking alcohol between meal times, poor nutrition, female gender, obesity, Hispanic ethnicity, long-term ingestion of >10 to 20 g/day of alcohol in women and >20 to 40 g/day in men

GENETICS: No genetic predilection for any one race. In the U.S., however, there is increased incidence in minority groups.

PHYSICAL FINDINGS & CLINICAL PRESENTATION

Common presenting symptoms include:

- Rapid onset of jaundice
- Jaundice with duration <3 mo
- Right upper quadrant abdominal/epigastric pain
- Nausea/vomiting
- Malaise
- Low-grade fever
- Anorexia
- Abdominal distention/pain (due to ascites)
- Weight loss or malnourishment
- Proximal muscle wasting and weakness
- Complications of liver impairment (GI bleed; confusion, lethargy, ascites)

Findings on physical examination include:

- Jaundice and ascites
- Hepatomegaly, with tender liver on palpation
- Fever (first exclude other causes of fever, such as spontaneous bacterial peritonitis, urinary tract infection [UTI], pneumonia)
- Asterixis (a flapping tremor)
- Splenomegaly
- Tachycardia
- Hypotension
- Peripheral edema
- Abdominal distention with shifting dullness (ascites)
- Hepatic bruit (may occur in >50% of patients)
- With coexistent cirrhosis, look for:
  1. Gynecomastia
  2. Proximal muscles wasting
  3. Spider angiomata
  4. Altered hair distribution

DIAGNOSIS

DIFFERENTIAL DIAGNOSIS

- Hepatitis B
- Hepatitis C
- Nonalcoholic steatohepatitis (NASH)
- Chronic pancreatitis
- Drug-induced liver injury
- Hemochromatosis
- Cholangitis

WORKUP

- The standard screening test for alcohol abuse is the Alcohol Use Disorders Identification Test (AUDIT).
- A thorough and detailed history is needed.
- Relevant questions may include:
  1. When patient started drinking
  2. Number of times patient drinks per day
  3. How many yr of regular/daily drinking
  4. Types of alcohol
  5. Home or bar drinking
  6. Rehabilitation for drinking
  7. Social problems (e.g., arrest for public intoxication or driving under the influence, marital discord due to alcoholism)
  8. A typical patient may have a long history of excessive alcohol intake (>100 g of alcohol per day for at least 20 yr)

LABORATORY TESTS

The best biomarkers of harmful ethanol use are gamma glutamyltransferase (GGT), aspartate aminotransferase (AST), ethyl glucuronide (ETG), and phosphatidyl ethanol.

- Elevated transaminase (aspartate aminotransferase [AST] >45 U/L but <500 U/L; however, some patients may not have elevations in ALT, AST in early phases)
- AST: Alanine aminotransferase [ALT] ratio ≥2:1
- S-bilirubin >5 mg/dl
- Increased prothrombin time [PT]/international normalized ratio [INR]
- Elevated gamma glutamyltransferase (GGT)
- Carbohydrate-deficient transferrin (CDT) is a reliable marker for chronic alcoholism
- Elevated C-reactive protein
- Electrolyte disorder (hypokalemia, hypomagnesemia, low zinc, hypophosphatemia)
- Hypoalbuminemia
- Hyperferritinemia
- CBC (may reveal leukocytosis with bandemia or anemia or thrombocytopenia); mean corpuscular volume (MCV) may be elevated
- Screening tests to rule out other conditions include checking:
  1. Hepatitis B surface antigen (HBsAg), hepatitis B core antibody (HB_CAb) (IgM), hepatitis A antibody (IgM)
  2. Anti-hepatitis C antibody, hepatitis C ribonucleic acid (RNA)
  3. Ferritin-transferrin saturation
  4. Alpha-fetoprotein
  5. Alkaline phosphatase
- Laboratory criteria of severe alcoholic hepatitis are defined as
  1. Maddrey Discriminant Function (MDF) score >32, which is calculated as follows: MDF = 4.6× prothrombin time − control prothrombin time + total bilirubin (mg/dl)
  2. OR Model for End-Stage Liver Disease (MELD) >21
  3. AND/OR Hepatic encephalopathy

There are other models for determining severity such as the Alcohol Hepatitis Histologic Score (AHHS) or for prognostication such as the MELD + Lille combination models.

IMAGING STUDIES

Ultrasonography is the preferred imaging study. The earliest histologic change in alcoholic liver disease is macrovesicular steatosis.

LIVER BIOPSY

- Liver biopsy is rarely needed
- Useful to:
  1. Confirm the diagnosis
  2. Evaluate the effect of coexisting disease
  3. Rule out cirrhosis
  4. Exclude other diagnoses (especially other causes of liver diseases, biliary obstruction, Budd-Chiari syndrome)
- Typical histologic findings include:
  1. Micro- or macrovesicular steatosis
  2. Hepatocyte injury (ballooning degeneration and focal hepatocyte necrosis)
  3. Mallory-Denk bodies (characteristic of alcoholic hepatitis)
  4. Perivenular fibrosis
  5. Portal and lobular inflammation with neutrophils or lymphocyte infiltration

TREATMENT

An algorithm for the management of patients with alcoholic hepatitis is described in Fig. 1. Treatment can be divided into three main components:

1. Lifestyle modifications
2. Nutritional support
3. Pharmacologic therapy

LIFESTYLE MODIFICATIONS

- Abstinence from alcohol (this improves both short- and long-term survival). Fig. E2 describes the effect of subsequent alcohol intake on 5-yr survival in patients with alcoholic hepatitis.
- Nonpharmacologic methods to promote abstinence include cognitive-behavioral therapy (CBT), Alcoholic Anonymous (AA) attendance, and motivational interviewing.
- Pharmacologic aids include using naltrexone, acamprosate, or baclofen.
- Monitor abstinence with breath test or urine drug screen (for use in past 3 days) or hair

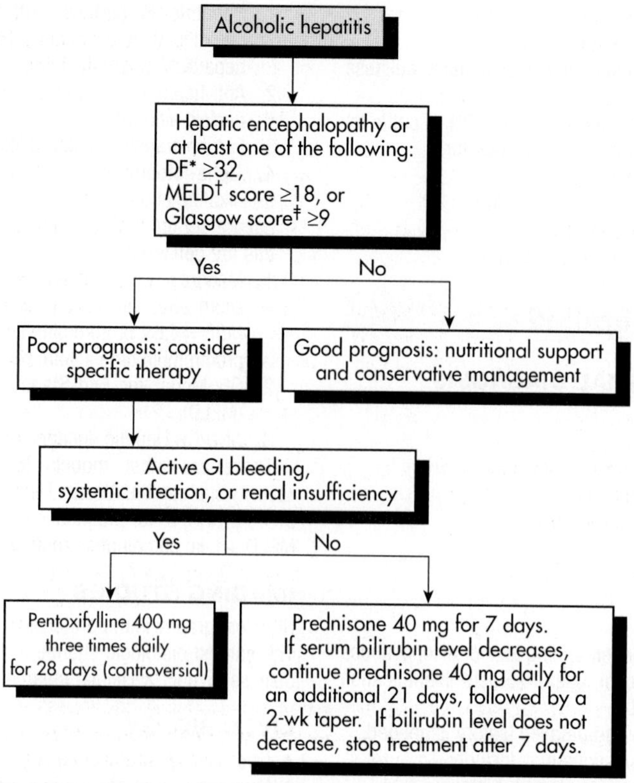

FIG. 1 Algorithm for the management of patients with alcoholic hepatitis. *The DF is calculated as follows: 4.6 (prothrombin time of patient − prothrombin time of control) + serum bilirubin level (in mg/dl). †The Model for End-Stage Liver Disease *(MELD)* score is based on the serum bilirubin level, INR, and serum creatinine level. ‡The Glasgow alcoholic hepatitis score is based on the patient's age, white blood cell count, blood urea nitrogen level, ratio of prothrombin time to a control value, and serum bilirubin level. *DF,* Discriminant function; *GI,* gastrointestinal. Online calculators for these various models are available at www.lillemodel.com. (Modified from Feldman M et al: *Sleisenger and Fordtran's gastrointestinal and liver disease,* ed 10, Philadelphia, 2016, Elsevier.)

sample analysis for ethyl glucuronide (test alcohol intake within the last few mo).
- Smoking cessation (to decrease oxidative stress).
- Treatment of substance abuse.

NUTRITIONAL SUPPORT

- Good nutrition is an essential part of treatment because many patients with alcoholic hepatitis have severe protein-calorie malnutrition as well as deficiencies of trace minerals and several vitamins.
- Nutritional support includes:
  1. Liberal vitamin supplementation (especially thiamine, folic acid, vitamin K)
  2. Mineral supplementation **(but not iron)**
  3. Calorie counting is essential. A high calorie intake (1.2 to 1.4 times the normal resting intake) may be required.
  4. Protein intake of 1.2 to 1.5 g/kg of ideal body weight per day will provide adequate support. **Exception: In patients with severe encephalopathy, protein restriction may be required.**
  5. Fluid management

PHARMACOLOGIC THERAPY

Severe alcoholic hepatitis may require treatment. Severity can be assessed by calculating the MELD score or MDF score or the Glasgow score.

- An MDF score ≥32 indicates significant or severe alcoholic hepatitis (30-day mortality of 50%).
- MELD score can easily be calculated (visit https://optn.transplant.hrsa.gov/resources/allocation-calculators/meld-calculator/). This score predicts short-term survival in patients with cirrhosis. A score >20 predicts increased short-term mortality.
- Glasgow score: Contains four variables (BUN, PT, WBC count, and bilirubin). A score ≥9 indicates increased mortality.

Indications for hospitalization include:
1. MDF ≥32
2. MELD >20
3. Glasgow score >8
4. Hepatic encephalopathy

Patients with severe alcoholic hepatitis may be treated with glucocorticosteroids (prednisolone 40 mg/day for 28 days with a 2-wk taper). Glucocorticosteroids reduce hepatic injury, suppress inflammation, and promote liver regeneration. However, not all studies have demonstrated consistent therapeutic benefits for steroids, even in high-risk patients. Prednisolone should be discontinued if bilirubin does not decrease by day 17. An alternative agent for patients with contraindications to corticosteroids is pentoxifylline. Pentoxifylline is not effective in patients who do not respond to prednisone, and data supporting its use is weak.

LIVER TRANSPLANTATION

- Usually reserved for patients with end-stage liver disease. Patients whose hepatitis is not responding to medical therapy have a 6-mo survival rate of approximately 30%. Since most hepatitis deaths occur within 2 mo, early liver transplantation is attractive and associated with higher than 80% survival at 3 yr.
- Patients with alcoholic hepatitis must be sober for at least 6 mo before they can be eligible for consideration for liver transplantation. However, transplantation candidates should not be based solely on 6 mo abstinence, and other factors, such as social support and need for rehabilitation, should be considered.

REFERRAL

Severe acute alcoholic hepatitis may require intensive care unit (ICU) care and referral to different subspecialists:
- GI/hepatology (for patients with evidence of GI hemorrhage)
- Nutritional services
- Nephrology (for acute renal failure, hepatorenal syndrome)
- Neurology (for change in mental status, seizures)
- Infectious disease (for fever/leukocytosis)

PEARLS & CONSIDERATIONS

COMMENTS

- Referral to substance abuse treatment programs may be helpful.
  1. Stress to patients that there are limited long-term drug treatments for alcoholic hepatitis.
  2. Maintaining good general nutrition is important.
  3. Advise patient about the risk of taking certain medications, especially acetaminophen.
- Periodic follow-up to monitor patient's response to check basic metabolic panel (BMP) and liver function tests (LFTs).
- Encourage alcohol abstinence. Abstinence improves long-term survival.
- If patient develops liver cirrhosis, check serum alpha-fetoprotein every 6 mo and liver ultrasound annually to rule out hepatocellular carcinoma.
- Vaccinate patient against hepatitis A and B viruses, pneumococci, influenza A virus, and routine adult vaccinations, if appropriate.

SUGGESTED READINGS

Available at ExpertConsult.com

RELATED CONTENT

Alcoholic Hepatitis (Patient Information)

AUTHOR: **Daniel K. Asiedu, MD, PHD, FACP**

BASIC INFORMATION

DEFINITION

Primary aldosteronism is a group of disorders distinguished by inappropriate, autonomous and excessive aldosterone production that results in renal sodium retention, plasma renin suppression, and secondary hypertension, classically characterized by hypokalemia and metabolic alkalosis.

SYNONYMS

Hyperaldosteronism
Conn syndrome

ICD-10CM CODES	
E26.0	Primary hyperaldosteronism
E26.01	Conn syndrome
E26.02	Glucocorticoid-remediable aldosteronism
E26.1	Secondary hyperaldosteronism
E26.9	Hyperaldosteronism, unspecified

EPIDEMIOLOGY & DEMOGRAPHICS

PREVALENCE: The prevalence of primary aldosteronism in patients with stage I, stage II, and resistant hypertension is 8.6% to 22.9%, 16.1% to 27.0%, and 17.2% to 26.8%, respectively. Recent studies suggest that the true prevalence of primary aldosteronism in hypertensive patients is three- to fivefold higher than previously recognized.[1]

GENETICS: Familial hyperaldosteronism is a subset of hyperaldosteronism with 5 known heritable forms. It should be suspected in patients with any of the following:

- Onset of hypertension before age 21 yr and a family history of hypertension
- Family history of primary aldosteronism
- Family history of stroke before age 40 yr

ETIOLOGY

- Bilateral idiopathic adrenal hyperplasia (60%-70%)
- Unilateral adenoma or Conn syndrome (30%-40%)
- Unilateral adrenal hyperplasia (2%)
- Familial hyperaldosteronism (<1%)
- Carcinoma (<0.1%)
- Ectopic production (<0.1%)

PHYSICAL FINDINGS & CLINICAL PRESENTATION

- Generally asymptomatic
- Hypertension that is often resistant
- Spontaneous hypokalemia
- Family history of early-onset hypertension or cerebrovascular accident at age <40 yr

DIAGNOSIS

DIFFERENTIAL DIAGNOSIS

- Hypokalemia from diuretic use
- Hypokalemia from vomiting and/or diarrhea
- Renovascular hypertension
- Other endocrine neoplasm (pheochromocytoma, deoxycorticosterone-producing tumor, renin-secreting tumor)

WORKUP

Primary aldosteronism is characterized by suppressed plasma renin activity (PRA) and an elevated serum aldosterone level, usually exceeding 15 ng/dl. Box 1 provides guidance on when to consider testing for primary aldosteronism. Fig. 1 describes a diagnostic approach to patients with suspected primary aldosteronism. CT, MRI, and adrenal vein sampling (AVS) are used to distinguish unilateral from bilateral increased aldosterone secretion. This distinction affects treatment options. Unilateral secretion ideally is treated surgically, and bilateral secretion is treated medically.

LABORATORY TESTS

- A 24-hour urinary excretion is the gold standard for diagnosing primary aldosteronism. The sensitivity of serum ARR to exclude primary aldosteronism is only 32%.
- Routine laboratory tests may suggest primary aldosteronism but are not diagnostic. Common abnormalities include the following:
- Spontaneous hypokalemia (9% to 37% of cases) or severe hypokalemia while receiving conventional doses of diuretics
- Possible alkalosis and hypernatremia

IMAGING STUDIES

- Adrenal CT scan (Fig. E2) is the preferred imaging technique because adrenal adenomas have a high lipid content and are better visualized on CT scan.
- MRI may be used as an alternative.

TREATMENT

NONPHARMACOLOGIC THERAPY

Regular blood pressure monitoring, low-sodium diet, tobacco avoidance, maintenance of ideal body weight, and regular exercise

ACUTE GENERAL Rx

- Control of blood pressure and hypokalemia with spironolactone, eplerenone, or amiloride
- Surgery (unilateral adrenalectomy) for aldosterone-producing adenoma (APA) or unilateral adrenal hyperplasia (UAH)

CHRONIC Rx

A mineralocorticoid receptor antagonist, spironolactone (starting dose 25 mg daily) or eplerenone (starting dose, 25 mg twice daily), is titrated upward until a mid- to high-normal serum potassium concentration is achieved without potassium supplementation. The dose is increased at 2-wk intervals. Eplerenone causes less gynecomastia in men and less menstrual irregularities in women because of greater mineralocorticoid receptor selectivity. Amiloride (starting dose, 5 mg twice daily) may be used for patients intolerant of spironolactone and eplerenone.

DISPOSITION

Treatment of primary aldosteronism with mineralocorticoid receptor antagonism or unilateral adrenalectomy resolves hypokalemia, reduces blood pressure, and improves impaired cardiac and renal function.

Hypertension persists in 40% to 65% of patients after unilateral adrenalectomy. Patients who are more likely to experience complete resolution of hypertension are younger, take 2 or fewer antihypertensive agents preoperatively, have short duration of hypertension, have no family history of hypertension, and/or have a higher plasma aldosterone concentration (PAC) to plasma renin activity (PRA) ratio.

REFERRAL

Referral to an experienced interventional radiologist for arteriovenous sampling. If lateralization occurs, surgical referral for unilateral adrenalectomy should proceed after confirmation of a unilateral APA, UAH, or carcinoma.

PEARLS & CONSIDERATIONS

- Primary aldosteronism is more common than previously thought and should be considered in all patients with apparent treatment resistant hypertension.
- There is more rapid decline in eGFR, increased LV mass, and increased relative risk of stroke, myocardial infarction, and atrial fibrillation in patients with primary aldosteronism than in patients with essential hypertension matched for age, gender, and blood pressure. Increased risk is attenuated but persists when treated with a mineralocorticoid antagonist. Adrenalectomy decreases these risks to below that of a matched essential hypertension cohort.
- Frequent monitoring of blood pressure and electrolytes after adrenalectomy is required because normalization of blood pressure after unilateral adrenalectomy may take up to 4 mo.
- Caution must be taken during interpretation of direct renin concentration (DRC) and PRA testing results because of different units used

BOX 1 Testing Considerations for Primary Aldosteronism

- Resistant hypertension
- Onset of hypertension at a young age (<20 yr)
- Hypertension with one of the following:
  Spontaneous or diuretic-induced hypokalemia
  Adrenal incidentaloma
  Sleep apnea
- Hypertension with a family history of:
  Primary aldosteronism
  Stroke before age 40 yr

[1]Brown JM et al: The unrecognized prevalence of primary aldosteronism: a cross-sectional study, Ann Intern Med 173(1):10-20, 2020.

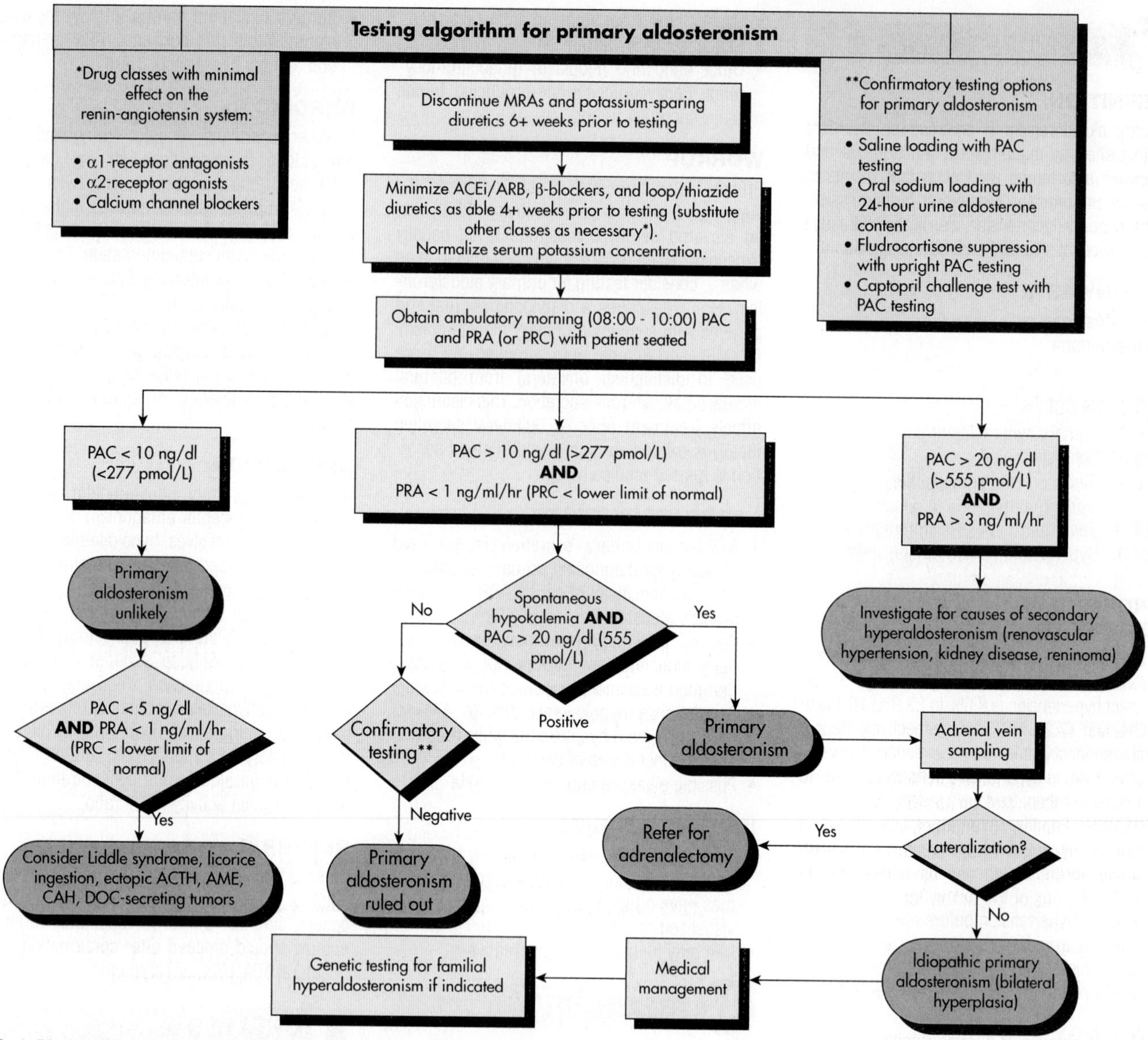

FIG. 1 Diagnostic approach to patients with suspected primary aldosteronism. The authors' preferred confirmatory test for primary aldosteronism is oral sodium loading with 300 mmol/day of sodium and 75 mmol/day of potassium for 3 days prior to a 24-hr urine collection with measurement of urine sodium, potassium, creatinine, and aldosterone secretion. Excessive urine aldosterone excretion (>12 μg/day [33 nmol/day]) in this setting is consistent with primary aldosteronism. Adrenal vein sampling shows lateralization if the lateralization index (aldosterone-to-cortisol ratio measured in an adrenal vein divided by the aldosterone-to-cortisol ratio of the contralateral adrenal vein) is >4. A lateralization index <3 indicates bilateral adrenal hyperplasia. *ACEi*, angiotensin-converting-enzyme inhibitor; *ACTH*, adrenocorticotropic hormone; *ARB*, angiotensin II receptor blocker; *AME*, Apparent mineralocorticoid excess; *CAH*, congenital adrenal hyperplasia; *DOC*, deoxycorticosterone; *MRA*, mineralocorticoid receptor antagonist; *PAC*, plasma aldosterone concentration; *PRA*, plasma renin activity; *PRC*, plasma renin concentration.

for each assay. The aldosterone-to-DRC ratio is yet to be as widely validated as the PAC-to-PRA ratio.

SUGGESTED READINGS

Available at ExpertConsult.com

RELATED CONTENT

Aldosteronism (Hyperaldosteronism, Primary) (Patient Information)
Hypertension (Related Key Topic)

AUTHORS: **Kevin S. Fay, MD,** and **Debbie L. Cohen, MD**

BASIC INFORMATION

DEFINITION

Allergic rhinitis (AR) is an immunoglobulin E (IgE)-mediated hypersensitivity response to nasally inhaled allergens that involves mucosal inflammation driven by type 2 helper T (Th2) cells that leads to sneezing, rhinorrhea, nasal pruritus, and congestion. It may be seasonal or perennial.

SYNONYMS

Hay fever
IgE-mediated rhinitis
Seasonal allergic rhinitis
SAR

ICD-10CM CODES

J30.9	Allergic rhinitis, unspecified
J30.1	Allergic rhinitis due to pollen
J30.2	Other seasonal allergic rhinitis
J30.5	Allergic rhinitis due to food
J30.8	Other allergic rhinitis
J30.81	Allergic rhinitis due to animal (dog) (cat) hair and dander
J30.89	Other allergic rhinitis

EPIDEMIOLOGY & DEMOGRAPHICS

- AR affects approximately 10% to 30% of the U.S. population and up to 40% of children. The estimated direct, indirect, intangible, and opportunity costs to the health care system are alarmingly high and have been shown to have a major impact in learning and job performance.
- Mean age of onset is 8 to 12 yr with 80% of cases developing before the age of 20. Aeroallergen sensitization typically does not occur before the age of 1.
- The prevalence of allergic rhinitis in patients presenting to their primary care provider with nasal symptoms is estimated to be between 30% and 60%.

PHYSICAL FINDINGS & CLINICAL PRESENTATION

- Compared to nonallergic rhinitis (NAR), allergic sensitization typically involves sneezing, nasal pruritus, and ocular pruritus. Both AR and NAR can involve nasal congestion, postnasal drip, and cough. Loss of or alteration of smell, sensation of plugged ears, irritability, and fatigue are other common symptoms.
- Physical findings in AR:
  1. Pale or violaceous mucosa of the turbinates caused by venous engorgement (this can help distinguish AR from viral rhinitis, where erythema is typically present)
  2. Nasal polyps
  3. Erythema of the throat, conjunctival and scleral injection
  4. Clear nasal discharge, or if the nasal passages are obstructed, rhinorrhea may be visible dripping down the posterior pharynx

ETIOLOGY

- Pollen allergens
- Dust mites, mold spores, and animal allergens:
  1. Irritants (nonallergic triggers) can often exacerbate symptoms and can be associated with both AR and NAR

DIAGNOSIS

DIFFERENTIAL DIAGNOSIS

- Infectious rhinitis/rhinosinusitis: Due to viral infections in 98% of cases, less commonly bacterial or fungal infections
- Nonallergic rhinitis (vasomotor rhinitis, rhinitis medicamentosa, gustatory rhinitis, atrophic rhinitis, drug-induced rhinitis, hormone-induced rhinitis, and nonallergic rhinitis with eosinophilia syndrome [NARES])
- Septal obstruction (e.g., deviated septum), nasal polyps, and nasal neoplasms
- Systemic diseases (e.g., Wegener granulomatosis, sarcoidosis, systemic lupus erythematous, and hypothyroidism [rare])

WORKUP

- The initial strategy is to determine whether patients should undergo diagnostic testing or receive empiric treatment.
- Testing is often unnecessary if the diagnosis is apparent. A detailed medical history is useful in identifying the culprit allergen:
  1. Spring symptoms are typically due to tree pollen sensitization.
  2. Summer symptoms are typically due to grass pollen sensitization.
  3. Fall symptoms are typically due to weed pollen sensitization.
  4. Perennial symptoms are often due to pet dander, house dust mite, or mold sensitization.
- Selected patients with AR that is not controlled with standard therapy may benefit from allergy testing to target specific allergen avoidance measures or guide immunotherapy. While both are acceptable forms of testing, the decision between skin testing and in vitro specific IgE testing is outlined in Table 1.

TABLE 1 Comparison of In Vivo Skin Testing versus In Vitro Specific IgE testing

Skin Testing	Serum Specific IgE Testing
Higher sensitivity	No patient risk (other than blood draw)
Immediate results	May be more convenient for patient
Less expensive	Preferred to skin testing in select patients: - Skin conditions (dermatographism) - Can perform while on antihistamines

TREATMENT

NONPHARMACOLOGIC THERAPY

- Reducing dust mite exposure in patients with known sensitivity by covering mattresses and pillows with dust mite-proof casings, eliminating carpeting, and removing dust mite–collecting products from the bedroom (stuffed animals, curtains, and decorative pillows).
- Use of air purifiers (HEPA standard) and HVAC filters is helpful to reduce concentrations of certain airborne allergens such as most pollens.
- Remove pets from the home, or at a minimum, keep animals out of the bedroom of patients with confirmed sensitivity to animal allergens.
- Nasal saline sprays are effective in relieving nasal dryness and congestion. Nasal irrigations are likely more effective and can be administered via various applicators available over-the-counter.

ACUTE GENERAL Rx

- For patients with AR, monotherapy with an intranasal corticosteroid is the preferred initial agent. Patients should be instructed on proper use and informed that improvement might not occur for at least 1 wk after initiation of therapy. Commonly available intranasal corticosteroids include fluticasone, mometasone, triamcinolone, beclomethasone, flunisolide, and budesonide.
- In patients with moderate to severe disease, combination therapy with an intranasal corticosteroid and an intranasal antihistamine (azelastine, olopatadine) provides greater clinical benefit than either as monotherapy.
- Montelukast should be used only when an intranasal corticosteroid (INCS) or an oral second-generation antihistamine have been ineffective or intolerable.
- Addition of oral antihistamines to intranasal corticosteroids has not been shown to provide clinical benefit, but may be useful in the treatment of ocular symptoms not controlled with intranasal therapies:
  1. Most oral first-generation antihistamines can cause considerable sedation and anticholinergic symptoms and are not recommended. The second-generation antihistamines (loratadine, fexofenadine, cetirizine, levocetirizine, desloratadine) are preferred agents, as they have similar efficacy and fewer anticholinergic or sedative effects.
  2. When rhinorrhea is the main symptom, consider intranasal ipratropium.

CHRONIC Rx

- Allergen immunotherapy is of limited benefit and is generally reserved for patients that do not have adequate response to standard medical therapy. Traditionally, subcutaneous immunotherapy (SCIT), consisting of subcutaneous injections of gradually increasing doses of allergens, has been utilized. More recently, sublingual immunotherapy (SLIT) has emerged as an alternative option, which may be safer, more convenient, and have similar efficacy in select patients. Allergists and otolaryngologists are specifically trained in the administration of both of these therapeutic options.

- Allergen immunotherapy (both SCIT and SLIT) is contraindicated in patients with severe or uncontrolled asthma or in those with a history of severe allergic reactions to these therapies. In addition, SLIT is contraindicated in patients with eosinophilic esophagitis.

DISPOSITION

The vast majority of patients experience significant symptom relief with avoidance of allergens and proper use of medications. In addition, approximately 80% of patients report improvement in allergic rhinitis symptoms in response to immunotherapy.

REFERRAL

Consider referral to an allergist or otolaryngologist for allergy testing and management in patients with moderate to severe symptoms, those who are unresponsive to therapy, and/or those who are interested in immunotherapy.

PEARLS & CONSIDERATIONS[1]

- Congestion, rhinorrhea, sneezing, and pruritus are typical of AR; congestion and anosmia are common in chronic sinusitis with nasal polyps; congestion and postnasal drainage with lack of pruritus are typical of NAR.
- Montelukast should be used rarely for AR and should be avoided in NAR due to potential neuropsychiatric side effects.

Intranasal decongestants such as oxymetazoline (Afrin) can cause rebound congestion and should be limited to short-term use. Combination with INCS in patients with severe refractory congestion should not exceed 4 wk.

[1] Dykewicz MS et al: Rhinitis 2020: a practice parameter update, *J Allergy Clin Immunol* 146(4):721-767, 2020.

RELATED CONTENT

Allergic Rhinitis (Patient Information)

SUGGESTED READINGS

Available at ExpertConsult.com

AUTHORS: **Navid Ziaie, MD,** and **Shyam Joshi, MD**

BASIC INFORMATION

DEFINITION

Alopecia is the term used to describe involuntary hair loss, typically on the scalp but can occur anywhere over the body. *Nonscarring alopecia* is hair loss without clinically apparent scarring, inflammation, or skin atrophy. *Scarring alopecia* is characterized by permanent hair loss accompanied by tissue destruction in the form of scarring, inflammation, and/or skin atrophy.

SYNONYMS

Hair loss
Balding

ICD-10CM CODES	
L63	Alopecia aerata
L63.0	Alopecia (capitis) totalis
L64	Androgenic alopecia
L64.0	Drug-induced androgenic alopecia
L64.8	Other androgenic alopecia
L64.9	Androgenic alopecia, unspecified
L65	Other nonscarring hair loss
L66	Cicatricial alopecia
L65.9	Nonscarring hair loss, unspecified
L63.8	Other alopecia areata
L65.0	Telogen effluvium

EPIDEMIOLOGY & DEMOGRAPHICS

INCIDENCE: Depends on etiology, for example:
- Alopecia areata affects 1% of the U.S. population by age 50 yr. There is a higher incidence at a younger age and both sexes are affected equally.
- Androgenetic alopecia affects males > females with 50% of Caucasian men affected by age 50 yr. Less common in Asians and African-American men, and often has later onset. By age 70, 40% of females are affected, with incidence increasing after menopause.

GENETICS: Depends on etiology, for example:
- Androgenetic alopecia is polygenic with variable penetrance and can be inherited from one or both parents.
- Certain scarring alopecias are more predominant in people with coarser hair.

ETIOLOGY

NONSCARRING:
- Failure of follicle production
- Hair shaft abnormality
- Pattern hair loss, i.e., androgenetic alopecia
- Hair breakage, i.e., trichotillomania, traction alopecia, cosmetic overprocessing
- Problem with cycling (excess shedding), i.e., telogen effluvium, anagen effluvium, loose chemotherapy anagen syndrome, alopecia areata, syphilis

SCARRING:
- Infectious: Tinea capitis with inflammation (kerion), bacterial folliculitis as in dissecting folliculitis and folliculitis decalvans
- Neoplasm: Alopecia mucinosa in cutaneous T-cell lymphoma or alopecia neoplastica due to metastatic carcinoma (breast cancer)
- Autoimmune: Chronic cutaneous lupus erythematosus
- Congenital

CLINICAL FEATURES

HISTORY: A careful history must be taken and should include time course for hair loss, the pattern of hair loss, any recent change in life situation/stresses, any associated medical conditions, new medications, any family history of hair loss, diet, hair care practices, and other skin/nail symptoms.

PHYSICAL EXAMINATION:
- General: Patient's emotional response to hair loss
- Hair/skin:
  1. Hair thinning/loss
  2. May have fine downy hairs also referred to as vellus hairs
  3. Skin may show changes consistent with inflammation, infection, and/or atrophy
  4. Women may show virilization (e.g., hirsutism)
  5. Exclamation-point hairs can be seen in alopecia areata
  6. Broken hairs of different length may be seen in traumatic alopecia
  7. Hairs that crack or crumble with palpation most often signify shaft damage due to overprocessing

Dx DIAGNOSIS

WORKUP

- Pull test: No shower for 24 hr, 60 hairs are gently pulled from the scalp, removal of 6 or more hairs is considered positive result and indicates telogen effluvium (active shedding). Look for telogen bulbs on recovered hairs to differentiate from breaking (blunt ends).
- Punch biopsy: Mandatory when suspecting scarring alopecia. Send two punches: One for vertical and one for horizontal sectioning for histopathologic analysis, preferably by a dermatopathologist.
- Trichogram: Quantifies hair loss. Pull 25 to 50 hairs and measure proportion of anagen to catagen and telogen hairs under light microscopy: 10% to 20% telogen hairs is normal, whereas >35% is highly suspicious for telogen effluvium.
- Fig. 1 illustrates a clinical approach to scalp alopecia.

LABORATORY TESTS

Initiate laboratory studies if not clear based on clinical presentation:
- CBC: Rule out Fe deficiency.
- Total Fe/ferritin: Rule out subclinical Fe deficiency.
- TSH: Rule out underlying thyroid disease.
- ANA: Screen for autoimmune disease.
- RPR: Rule out cutaneous syphilis if history suggestive of increased risk.

DIFFERENTIAL DIAGNOSIS

NONSCARRING:
- *Telogen effluvium:* This type of alopecia is usually diffuse thinning that follows significant life stress (death of loved one, high fever, severe infection, crash dieting) or change in hormones (postpartum, change in or cessation of oral contraceptives). Patient often presents with a bag of hair that has fallen out. This is caused by a large number of anagen (growing) hairs entering telogen (dying phase) simultaneously. Telogen effluvium is more common in women.
- *Androgenetic alopecia:* Gradual thinning of hair and a trend toward finer hair, which in men has a typical pattern of receding anterior bitemporal hairline resulting in an M-shaped pattern and hair loss at the vertex (Fig. E2) and in women has a typical pattern of thinning along vertex with or without frontotemporal thinning. This type of thinning is due to a combination of genetic predisposition and androgenic conversion of hair follicles into vellus-like follicles. Widening of the central hair part is often seen, leading to scalp visibility (Fig. E3). This female pattern of more diffuse hair loss is seen in 20% to 30% of adolescent males.
- *Alopecia areata:* Patches of acute hair loss (Fig. E4), typically 2 to 5 cm in diameter, with normal-appearing skin, black dots (cadaver hairs, point noir) from hair that breaks before reaching the skin's surface, and occasional "exclamation point hairs," which are evidence of hairs breaking off as they are pushed from the follicle. Fingernails may show fine pitting. On biopsy, lymphocytes surround the hair bulb and resemble a "swarm of bees," evidence of the autoimmune etiology. Patients often have positive family history. AA Universalis (AAU)—generalized loss of body hair. AA Totalis (AAT)—complete loss of scalp hair.
- *Tinea:* This type of hair loss is evident in round patches, possibly with scarring, erythema, and lymphadenopathy. This is the most common type of hair loss in children. Diagnosis can be made by scraping the erythematous edge and placing the scraping with KOH under a microscope to check for hyphae. Wood's lamp only fluoresces if tinea is caused by *Microsporum* spp.; however, the most common (in the U.S.) *Trichophyton* spp. does not fluoresce. If a kerion (severe alopecia associated with bogginess) is present, it may cause scarring.
- *Traumatic alopecia (traction alopecia):* This type of hair loss is in a pattern consistent with breaking off of hairs due to traction (hair pulling) (Fig. E5) or chemical or heating agents (hair straightening or permanent). Etiology usually becomes apparent with careful history taking and visualizing the pattern of hair loss. In trichotillomania (Fig. E6), the alopecia area has an irregular shape, scalp excoriations may present, and hairs are broken at different lengths.

SCARRING:
- *Lichen planus:* The hair loss associated with LP is typically associated with scaling and atrophy of pruritic, painful skin underlying the hair loss. This hair loss is more common in middle-aged women. While there are numerous variations in clinical presentation,

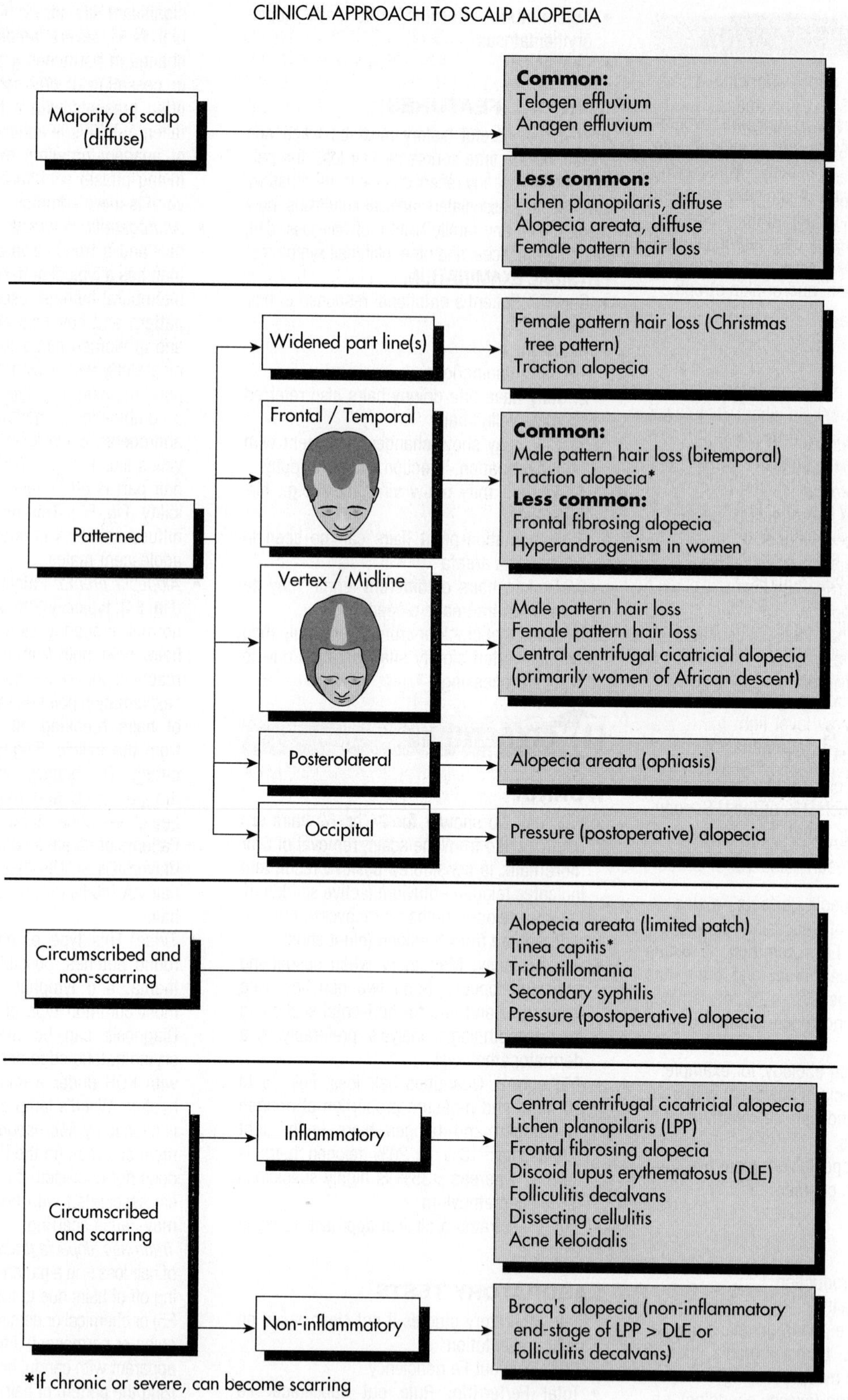

FIG. 1 Clinical approach to scalp alopecia. (From Bolognia J et al: *Dermatology*, ed 4, 2018, Elsevier.)

the general clinical picture is one of a chronic inflammatory condition of the skin, nails, mucous membranes, and/or hair. The typical skin lesions are flat topped, violaceous lesions with white lines (Wickham striae), while the typical oral lesions are milky white.

- *Chronic cutaneous (discoid) lupus erythematosus:* This type of hair loss frequently is evident in well-demarcated, erythematous plaques in chronically sun-exposed areas of skin. Lesions exhibit hypopigmentations or hyperpigmentations, atrophy, erythema, and scaling. It may be present concurrently with SLE or be the first presenting symptom of SLE, but in most cases it is a purely cutaneous condition.
- *Tinea with kerion:* A kerion represents an exuberant delayed-type hypersensitivity reaction to the tinea capitis, resulting in one (or many) inflamed boggy plaque(s) on the scalp depending on the severity of the infection.

Rx TREATMENT

- *Telogen effluvium:* Stop offending stress/medication and in 3 to 4 mo anagen recurs. Hair density should be normalized by 12 mo. Multiple medications have been shown to be an inciting factor and one should consider stopping them (these include, but are not limited to, enalapril, colchicine, levodopa, metoprolol, propranolol, oral contraceptives, and lithium). Full regrowth is expected in most cases.
- *Androgenetic alopecia:* For men, the most likely first-line treatment is oral finasteride (type II 5α-reductase inhibitor) which leads to lower levels of dihydrotestosterone. This leads to hair regrowth in about 6 mo, but with cessation, hair returns to pattern of loss within 6 to 9 mo. Topical minoxidil has shown similar results to finasteride and can be useful in partially restoring lost hair in both men and women. Dutasteride (off-label) has been shown to be superior to finasteride in a randomized trial but requires higher doses than that used for BPH. Discontinuation of minoxidil will result in loss of regrown hair often over several mo. Other options include surgical intervention with hair transplantation or hair flaps, camouflaging agents, the use of a hairpiece, or low-level light therapy. In women with elevated androgens, antiandrogens such as spironolactone, flutamide, and cimetidine may be considered.
- *Alopecia areata (AA):* Spontaneous remission occurs in patchy AA, but less commonly in AAT or AAU. Glucocorticoids (GCs) are the mainstay of treatment but have little effect on the long-term outcome of hair loss—topical GC for small patches, intralesional injection of high-potency GC, and even systemic steroids can all be temporarily effective but at the cost of glucocorticoid exposure. Induction of allergic contact dermatitis using short-contact anthralin therapy or squaric acid sensitization can be effective but tends to have significant local discomfort, thereby limiting its use. Photochemotherapy has shown some beneficial outcomes, although there is a high relapse rate after discontinuation.
- *Tinea capitis:* To effectively treat tinea capitis, oral antifungal agents must be used. Griseofulvin is considered the drug of choice in the U.S., and the recommended time course is 6 wk to several mo. Other oral agents to consider include terbinafine, itraconazole, fluconazole, and ketoconazole. If there is a kerion (area of boggy, purulent inflammation underlying the area of hair loss), the patient is at increased risk for scarring alopecia due to bacterial superinfection, and a short course of oral steroids and oral antibiotic must be considered.
- *Traumatic alopecia (traction alopecia):* First priority is stopping inciting activity/agent, ideally leading to gradual resolution of hair loss and hair regrowth.
- *Lichen planus:* Associated hair loss is often permanent; however, for symptomatic control of itching and pain, topical or oral glucocorticoids may be considered.
- *Chronic cutaneous discoid erythematosus:* The best prevention is sun protection, with SPF lotion. Treatment options center around the cautious use of topical or intralesional glucocorticoids. Hydroxychloroquine and retinoids are also used with caution.
- *Chemotherapy-induced alopecia:* Scalp cooling devices may be effective in reducing chemotherapy-induced alopecia. In a recent trial among women with stage I to II breast cancer receiving chemotherapy with taxane, anthracycline, or both, those who underwent scalp cooling were significantly more likely to have less than 50% hair loss after the fourth chemotherapy cycle compared with those who received no scalp cooling.[1]

REFERRAL

Dermatology

PATIENT & FAMILY EDUCATION

Alopecia areata: www.naaf.org

RELATED CONTENT

Alopecia (Patient Information)

SUGGESTED READINGS

Available at ExpertConsult.com

AUTHOR: **Fred F. Ferri, MD**

[1] Nangia J et al: Effect of a scalp cooling device on alopecia in women undergoing chemotherapy for breast cancer. The SCALP randomized clinical trial, *JAMA* 317(6):596-605, 2017.

BASIC INFORMATION

DEFINITION

Dementia is a syndrome characterized by progressive loss of previously acquired cognitive skills including memory, language, insight, and judgment. Alzheimer disease (AD) is thought to account for the majority (50% to 75%) of all cases of dementia.

ICD-10CM CODES

G30.0	Alzheimer disease with early onset
G30.1	Alzheimer disease with late onset
G30.8	Other Alzheimer disease
G30.9	Alzheimer disease, unspecified

EPIDEMIOLOGY & DEMOGRAPHICS

INCIDENCE: Risk doubles every 5 yr after the age of 65; above the age of 85, the annual incidence is about 10%.

PREVALENCE: Currently an estimated 5.4 million Americans have AD; 3% of the population between the ages of 65 and 74, 17% between 75 and 84, and 32% at 85 yr and older.

PREDOMINANT SEX: Female greater than male.

PHYSICAL FINDINGS & CLINICAL PRESENTATION

- Spouse or other family member, usually not the patient, notes insidious memory impairment.
- Patients have difficulties learning and retaining new information and handling complex tasks (e.g., balancing the checkbook) and have impairments in reasoning, judgment, spatial ability, and orientation (e.g., difficulty driving, getting lost away from home).
- Behavioral changes, such as mood changes and apathy, may accompany memory impairment. In later stages, patients may develop agitation and psychosis.
- Rare variants: Atypical presentations include early and severe behavioral changes, focal findings on examination, parkinsonism, hallucinations, falls, or onset of symptoms younger than the age of 65.

DIAGNOSIS

Diagnosis of AD has evolved with the development of biomarkers that indicate AD pathology *in vivo* such as brain amyloidosis and pathological tau accumulation. The National Institute on Aging (NIA) and the Alzheimer Association (AA) recommended new diagnostic criteria and guidelines for AD in 2011, and these criteria were further revised in 2018 (Tables 1 and 2). The NIA-AA criteria differed from prior DSM or NINDCS-ADRDA criteria in the following ways: (1) they recommend AD be considered a disease well before the onset of symptoms by incorporating the biomarkers in diagnosis, and (2) they define three distinct stages of AD: (1) *preclinical* AD, in which there is measurable biologic evidence of AD pathology but no symptoms; (2) *mild cognitive impairment* (MCI) due to AD, in which the patient experiences mild memory loss but no functional impairment at home or work plus biomarker evidence of AD; and (3) *dementia* due to AD, in which the patient experiences cognitive decline causing functional impairment plus biomarker evidence of AD. The 2018 NIA-AA criteria define Alzheimer disease not as three clinical syndromes but as a biologic process defined by biomarkers indicating the presence of beta amyloid (A+), pathologic tau (T+), and neurodegeneration or neuronal injury (N+). Using the ATN system and clinical status together allows an entire study population to be characterized (Fig. 1).

Although not yet commonly used in the clinic but invariably used in AD clinical trials, biomarkers transform the diagnosis of AD into one that can be established definitively while the patient is still alive. In clinical practice, the diagnosis is commonly made based on clinical history, a thorough physical and neurologic examination, and use of reliable and valid diagnostic criteria (i.e., DSM or NINDCS-ADRDA) such as the following:

- Loss of memory and one or more additional cognitive abilities (aphasia, apraxia, agnosia, or other disturbance in executive functioning)
- Impairment in social or occupational functioning that represents a decline from a previous level of functioning and results in significant disability
- Deficits that do not occur exclusively during the course of delirium
- Insidious onset and gradual progression of symptoms
- Cognitive loss documented by neuropsychologic tests
- No physical signs, neuroimaging, or laboratory evidence of other diseases that can cause dementia (i.e., metabolic abnormalities, medication or toxin effects, infection, stroke, Parkinson disease, subdural hematoma, or tumors)

Red flags for an AD diagnosis are summarized in Box 1.

TABLE 1 New Diagnostic Criteria

	Research Criteria		
Criteria for Probable Alzheimer Disease	**DSM-5 2013**	**NINCDS–ADRDA 2007**	**NIA-AA 2011**
Insidious onset	X	X	X
Onset over months to years		X	X
Progressive decline	X	X	X
Deficits are not explained by delirium or other medical or psychiatric conditions	X	X	X
Social/occupational impairment	X		X
Presence of episodic memory deficit	X	X	
Cognitive deficits in at least two domains	X		X
Neuropsychological testing required for diagnosis?	Preferably	X	Only if routine history and mental status testing are inconclusive
Abnormal PET or MRI scan		Supportive feature*	For research purposes
Genetic markers?	X Required only if there is evidence of multiple causes and no clear evidence of progression and decline in memory and another cognitive domain	Supportive feature*	For research purposes
Abnormal cerebrospinal fluid marker required?		Supportive feature*	For research purposes

DSM-5, Diagnostic and Statistical Manual of Mental Disorders, fifth edition; *MRI,* magnetic resonance imaging; *NIA-AA,* National Institute on Aging–Alzheimer's Association; *NINCDS-ADRDA,* National Institute of Neurological and Communicative Disorders and Stroke–Alzheimer's Disease and Related Disorders Association; *PET,* positron emission tomography.
*At least one supportive feature is required for diagnosis of probable AD.
From Fillit HM: *Brocklehurst's textbook of geriatric medicine and gerontology,* ed 8, Philadelphia, 2017, Elsevier.

TABLE 2 National Institute on Aging–Alzheimer's Association Criteria for Alzheimer Disease (AD)

I. Core Clinical Criteria

- Interferes with work or usual activities *and*
- Represents a decline from previous level of functioning *and*
- Not explained by delirium of psychiatric disorder
- Documented cognitive impairment by history taking and objective cognitive assessment (bedside mental status examination or neuropsychological testing)
- A minimum of two of the following domains should be impaired:
    1. Impairment in acquisition and recall of new information (symptoms—repetitive questions and/or conversations, misplaced belongings, forgetting appointments, getting lost)
    2. Impairment in reasoning of complex tasks, poor judgment (symptoms—poor safety assessment, poor financial management, poor decision making, inability to plan complex activities)
    3. Impairment in visuospatial abilities (symptoms—inability to recognizes faces or objects or finding objects in plain view, despite good visual acuity; inability to operate simple tools; inability to orient clothing to the body)
    4. Impaired language functions (speaking, reading, writing; symptoms—difficulty thinking of common words while speaking, hesitation; speech, spelling, writing errors)
    5. Changes in personality, behavior, or comportment (symptoms—uncharacteristic mood fluctuations, e.g., agitation, poor motivation, apathy, social withdrawal, decreased interest in previous activities, loss of empathy, compulsions and/or obsessions, social impairment)

II. Probable AD Dementia (meets core criteria plus the following)

- Insidious onset (gradual over months to years)
- Clear history of worsening cognition *and*
- Initial and most prominent cognitive deficits fall into two categories (all must include cognitive dysfunction in at least one other domain)
    1. Amnestic—most common presentation; impairment in learning and recall of recent information
    2. Nonamnestic
        a. Language presentation—most prominent in word finding
        b. Visuospatial presentation—most prominent in spatial cognition (object agnosia, face recognition, simultanagnosia, alexia)
        c. Executive dysfunction—impaired reasoning, judgment, problem solving
- Should not be applied if substantial cerebrovascular disease or core features of dementia with Lewy bodies (other than dementia) are present; features consistent with behavioral variant of frontotemporal dementia, primary progressive aphasia (semantic, nonfluent, or agrammatic variants), or evidence of other neurologic disease or medical comorbidity that could affect cognition
- Increased certainty if there is documented decline based on subsequent evaluations and in persons who have evidence of causative genetic mutations

III. Probable AD With Evidence of AD Pathophysiologic Process

- High probability of AD pathology if both of the following are present:
    1. β-Amyloid level is low in the cerebrospinal fluid (CSF) or there is a positive positron emission tomography (PET) scan
    2. Neuronal injury is proven with high CSF tau levels, decreased fluorodeoxyglucose-PET uptake in the temporoparietal cortex, or disproportionate atrophy in the mediobasolateral temporal lobe and medial parietal cortex on a structural MRI scan
- Intermediate probability of AD pathology if only one of the two criteria above are met (and the other is absent or negative)

IV. Possible AD Dementia (meets core clinical criteria but has the following features)

- Atypical course—sudden onset of cognitive impairment, insufficient historical details of objective cognitive decline or progressive decline
- Causally mixed presentation—evidence of cerebrovascular disease; features of dementia with Lewy bodies (other than dementia); evidence of other neurologic disease, medical comorbidity, or pharmaceutical use that could have a substantial effect on cognition

V. Possible AD with Evidence of AD Pathophysiologic Process

- High probability of AD pathology if both of the following are present:
    1. β-Amyloid level is low in the CSF or there is a positive PET scan
    2. Neuronal injury is proven with high CSF tau levels, decreased fluorodeoxyglucose-PET uptake in the temporoparietal cortex, or disproportionate atrophy in the mediobasolateral temporal lobe and medial parietal cortex on a structural MRI scan
- Uninformative unless the above criteria are met
- May also be a second pathophysiologic condition present to explain why the patient does not meet AD criteria (e.g., concomitant dementia with Lewy bodies)

VI. Pathophysiologically Proven AD Dementia

- Clinical and cognitive criteria for AD are satisfied *and* neuropathologic criteria demonstrate presence of AD pathology

VII. Dementia Unlikely to Be Due to AD

- Does not meet clinical criteria for AD dementia *or*
- Regardless of meeting clinical criteria for probable or possible AD dementia, there is sufficient evidence for an alternative diagnosis (e.g., HIV dementia, Huntington disease)
- Regardless of meeting clinical criteria for possible AD dementia, both β-amyloid and neuronal injury biomarkers are negative

Adapted from McKhann GM et al: The diagnosis of dementia due to Alzheimer's disease: recommendations from the National Institute on Aging-Alzheimer's Association workgroups on diagnostic guidelines for Alzheimer's disease, *Alzheimers Dement* 7:263-269, 2011; Albert MS et al: The diagnosis of mild cognitive impairment due to Alzheimer's disease: recommendations from the National Institute on Aging-Alzheimer's Association workgroups on diagnostic guidelines for Alzheimer's disease, *Alzheimers Dement* 7:270-279, 2011; and Sperling RA et al: Toward defining the preclinical stages of Alzheimer's disease: recommendations from the National Institute on Aging-Alzheimer's Association workgroups on diagnostic guidelines for Alzheimer's disease, *Alzheimers Dement* 7:280-292, 2011.

DIFFERENTIAL DIAGNOSIS

- Other neurodegenerative dementia (see Table 3):
    1. Primary age-related tauopathy
    2. Limbic predominant age-related TDP-43 encephalopathy (LATE)
    3. Argryphilic grain disease
    4. Frontotemporal lobar degeneration
    5. Dementia with Lewy bodies
    6. Corticobasal syndrome
    7. Progressive supranuclear palsy
- Vascular cognitive impairment disorder (vascular dementia due to multiple strokes, severe small vessel changes, chronic vasculitis, or chronic subdural hematoma)
- Subjective memory loss
- Depression (pseudodementia)
- Neoplasm (benign or malignant brain tumor, leptomeningeal disease)
- Infection (HIV-associated dementia, neurosyphilis, progressive multifocal leukoencephalopathy [PML])
- Toxic/metabolic (EtOH, hypothyroidism, vitamin B12 deficiency, mercury exposure, drug effects)
- Organ failure (hepatic encephalopathy)

WORKUP

HISTORY & GENERAL PHYSICAL EXAMINATION:

- Medication lists should always be reviewed for drugs or home remedies that may cause mental status changes, especially anticholinergic medications, benzodiazepines, opiates, barbiturates, and neuroleptics.
- Patients should be screened for depression, because it can sometimes mimic dementia but often occurs as a coexisting condition and should be treated.

		Cognitive Stage		
		Cognitively Unimpaired	**Mild Cognitive Impairment**	**Dementia**
Biomarker Profile	$A^-T^-(N)^-$	normal AD biomarkers, cognitively unimpaired	normal AD biomarkers with MCI	normal AD biomarkers with dementia
	$A^+T^-(N)^-$	Preclinical Alzheimer pathologic change	Alzheimer pathologic change with MCI	Alzheimer pathologic change with dementia
	$A^+T^+(N)^-$, $A^+T^+(N)^+$	Preclinical Alzheimer disease	Alzheimer disease with MCI (Prodromal AD)	Alzheimer disease with dementia
	$A^+T^-(N)^+$	Alzheimer and concomitant suspected non Alzheimer pathologic change, cognitively unimpaired	Alzheimer and concomitant suspected non Alzheimer pathologic change with MCI	Alzheimer and concomitant suspected non Alzheimer pathologic change with dementia
	$A^-T^+(N)^-$, $A^-T^-(N)^+$, $A^-T^+(N)^+$	non-Alzheimer pathologic change, cognitively unimpaired	non-Alzheimer pathologic change with MCI	non-Alzheimer pathologic change with dementia

FIG. 1 Descriptive nomenclature: Syndromal cognitive staging combined with biomarkers. *AD*, Alzheimer disease; *MCI*, mild cognitive impairment. NOTE: Formatting denotes three general biomarker "categories" based on biomarker profiles: Those with normal AD biomarkers (no color), those with non-AD pathologic change (dark gray), and those who are in the Alzheimer continuum (light gray). (From Clifford RJ Jr et al: NIA-AA research framework: toward a biological definition of Alzheimer's disease, *Alzheimer's & Dementia* 14:535-562, 2018.)

BOX 1 Red Flags for an Alzheimer Disease Diagnosis

- Age younger than 65 yr
- Fluctuating level of consciousness (consider toxic-metabolic encephalopathy, Lewy body dementia)
- Behavioral, emotional, or personality disturbances overshadowing cognitive impairment (consider frontotemporal dementia, HIV dementia)
- Rapidly (6-12 mo) progressive development (consider Creutzfeldt–Jakob disease, paraneoplastic limbic encephalitis, HIV dementia, frontotemporal dementia)
- Presence of physical abnormalities:
  1. Gait impairment (consider vascular dementia, HIV dementia, NPH)
  2. Lateralized signs, e.g., hemiparesis, spasticity, other corticospinal tract signs (consider vascular dementia)
  3. Movement disorders
  4. Myoclonus (consider Creutzfeldt–Jakob disease, paraneoplastic encephalitis)
  5. Rigidity, bradykinesia (parkinsonism) (consider dementia with Lewy bodies and Parkinson disease)

Modified from Kaufman DM, et al: *Kaufman's clinical neurology for psychiatrists*, ed 8, Philadelphia, 2017, Elsevier.

TABLE 3 Features Distinguishing Alzheimer Disease and Frontotemporal Dementia

Feature	Alzheimer Disease	Frontotemporal Dementia
Age at onset (yr)	>65	53 (mean)
Memory impairments	Early, pronounced	Subtle, at least initially, with preserved visual-spatial ability
Behavior abnormalities	None until middle or late stage	Early and prominent perseverative and compulsive behavior; hyperorality; impaired executive ability
Language impairment	Except for anomia, none until late stage	Paraphasias, anomia, decreased fluency
CT/MRI appearance	General atrophy, but especially parietal and temporal lobes	Frontal and temporal lobe atrophy
Histologic marker	Aβ accumulation	Tau accumulation

CT, Computed tomography; *MRI*, magnetic resonance imaging.
From Kaufman DM et al: *Kaufman's clinical neurology for psychiatrists*, ed 8, Philadelphia, 2017, Elsevier.

- On examination, look for signs of metabolic disturbance, presence of psychiatric features, or focal neurologic deficits.

MENTAL STATUS TESTING: Brief mental status testing can be done easily and quickly in the office. Commonly used cognitive tests to detect dementia include the Folstein Mini-Mental State Examination (MMSE), the Mini-Cog test, and the Montreal Cognitive Assessment. The Montreal Cognitive Assessment (MoCA, www.mocatest.org/) is a highly sensitive 30-point test that takes approximately 10 minutes to administer. Cognitive domains tested include visual-spatial, attention, verbal recall, language, abstraction, and orientation. A score of 25 points or less (26 points if the patient has less than 12 yr of education) indicates cognitive impairment. The test is available in over 35 languages, and multiple forms in English allow for repeated assessments over time. A summary of commonly used tests may be found in Table E4.

Mental status testing should include tests that assess the following cognitive functions:

- Orientation: Ask the patient to give the day, date, month, year, and place and to name the current president.
- Attention: Ask the patient to recite the months of the year forward and in reverse.
- Verbal recall: Ask the patient to remember three items; test for recall after a 1- and 5-min delay.
- Language: Ask the patient to write and then read a sentence; have the patient name both common and less common objects.
- Visual-spatial: Ask the patient to draw a clock and to set the hands of the clock at 11:10.

Patients with AD typically have trouble with verbal recall in addition to experiencing visuospatial or language deficits. Attention is usually preserved until the later stages of AD, so consider alternate diagnoses in patients who perform poorly on tests of attention. A summary of the pattern of cognitive deficits associated with different dementias and depression may be found in Table 5.

In addition to the common amnestic presentation, AD rarely presents as one of three rare nonamnestic syndromes that affect memory later in the course of the disease. These three rare presentations should also raise suspicion of another dementia type. A primary language variant presents as either logopenic expressive aphasia of progressive nonfluent aphasia and may be either a form of AD or of frontotemporal lobar degeneration. A primary visuospatial variant called posterior cortical atrophy presents with disturbances in complex visual processing and may be a form of either AD or dementia with Lewy bodies. An executive/behavioral variant presents with impaired executive function and/or behavior derangement and may represent either a frontal variant of AD or behavioral variant frontotemporal dementia.

LABORATORY TESTS (TABLE 6)

- CBC
- Serum electrolytes
- Glucose
- BUN/creatinine
- Liver and thyroid function tests
- Serum vitamin B_{12}

TABLE 5 Patterns of Cognitive Impairment by Domain and Dementia

Episodic Memory	Attention	Language	Executive	Visuospatial	BEHAVIORAL SYMPTOMS	
Alzheimer disease	(I)	Simple (P) Divided (I)	Phonemic (P) Semantic (I) Naming (I)	(I)	Simple (P) Complex (I)	Early apathy, late psychotic symptoms
Mild cognitive impairment—amnestic	Immediate and Delayed recall (I); Recognition (I)	Simple (P) Divided (P)	(P)	(P)	(P)	(P)
Vascular dementia	Immediate and Delayed recall (V) Recognition (P)	Simple (P) Divided (I)	(I)	(I)	(P)	Depression
Behavioral variant FTLD	(V)	Simple (P) Divided (I)	(I)	(I)	(P)	Disinhibition, apathy, hyperorality, inappropriate social interaction
Semantic variant PPA	(P)	(P)	(I) Comprehension (I) Fluency	(P)	(P) (I) Visual agnosia	(P)
Nonfluent variant PPA	(P)	(P)	(I) Fluency (P) Comprehension, (I) Expressive speech	(P)	(P)	(P)
Parkinson disease dementia	(V) Immediate and Delayed recall (P) recognition	(I)	(P)	(I)	(I)	Depression, possible hallucinations, psychomotor slowing
Dementia with Lewy bodies	(V) Immediate and Delayed recall (P) Recognition	(V)	(V)	(I)	(I)	Hallucinations, delusions
Depression	(V) Immediate and Delayed recall (P) Recognition +	(V)	(V) Fluency (P) Naming	I/V	(P)	Psychomotor slowing, apathy

FTLD, Frontotemporal lobar degeneration; *I*, impaired; *P*, preserved; *PPA*, primary progressive aphasia; *V*, variable.
From Fillit HM: *Brocklehurst's textbook of geriatric medicine and gerontology*, ed 8, Philadelphia, 2017, Elsevier.

TABLE 6 Laboratory Evaluation of Patients with Dementia

Type of Study	Examples
Basic studies, excluding reversible with specific indication from history for causes of dementia or examination	• Complete blood count (CBC) • Chemistry or metabolic panel (SM-17) • Thyroid function tests (thyroid-stimulating hormone [TSH]) • Vitamin B_{12}, folate levels • Computed tomography (CT) or magnetic resonance imaging (MRI) • HIV testing • Sedimentation rate • Hemoglobin A1C (Hb A1C) • Urinalysis • Chest x-ray • Urine or plasma for drugs or heavy metals
Adjuvant studies to aid diagnosis	
Other tests as indicated by history or physical or neurologic examination	• Single-photon emission computed tomography (SPECT) • Positron emission tomography (PET) • Lumbar puncture with cerebrospinal fluid for β-amyloid

From Fillit HM: *Brocklehurst's textbook of geriatric medicine and gerontology*, ed 8, Philadelphia, 2017, Elsevier.

- Syphilis serology (RPR), if supported by clinical history
- HIV screening as appropriate
- Lumbar puncture if history or signs of cancer, infectious process, or unusual clinical presentation (e.g., rapid progression of symptoms)
- EEG if there is history of seizures, episodic confusion, rapid clinical decline, or suspicion of Creutzfeldt-Jakob disease
- Apolipoprotein E genotyping, measurement of CSF tau, and amyloid, and functional imaging including positron emission tomography (PET), single-photon emission computed tomography (SPECT), or amyloid PET imaging using florbetapir (Amyvid) are not yet routinely indicated but are used in clinical trials
- Brain biopsy is usually reserved for diagnoses such as prion disease and cerebral vasculitis. Generally performed postmortem

IMAGING STUDIES

- MRI to rule out hydrocephalus, cerebrovascular disease, and mass lesions, including subdural hematoma and to look for typical patterns of neurodegeneration (i.e, regional brain atrophy) such as hippocampal atrophy. CT can be used if MRI is unobtainable.
- Amyloid PET: The FDA has approved three agents for beta-amyloid PET imaging: Florbetapir, flutemetamol, and florbetaben. As with these other imaging agents, a positive amyloid scan does not establish a diagnosis of AD or any other cognitive disorder, but a negative scan indicating sparse to no amyloid plaques is inconsistent with a neuropathological diagnosis of AD. A positive amyloid scan indicates the presence of moderate to frequent amyloid neuritic plaques; neuropathological examination has shown this amount of amyloid plaque is present in AD patients but may also be present in individuals with other types of neurologic conditions as well as in cognitively normal older adults.
- Tau PET: The FDA has approved one agent for tau imaging: Flortaucipir. Flortaucipir is used to estimate the density and distribution of aggregated tau neurofibrillary tangles in adult patients with cognitive impairment under evaluation for AD. It is not indicated for use in patients undergoing evaluation for chronic traumatic encephalopathy, which is also a tauopathy.

Rx TREATMENT

NONPHARMACOLOGIC THERAPY

- Patient safety, including risks associated with impaired driving, wandering behavior, leaving stoves unattended, and accidents, must be addressed with the patient and family early and appropriate measures implemented.
- Wandering, hoarding or hiding objects, repetitive questioning, withdrawal, and social inappropriateness often respond to behavioral therapies.
- Cognitive stimulation programs are beneficial for maintenance of cognitive function and improved self-reported quality of life in patients with mild to moderate Alzheimer disease.

ACUTE GENERAL Rx

None

CHRONIC Rx

- Symptomatic treatment of memory disturbance (Table 7):
  1. Cholinesterase inhibitors (ChEIs): Donepezil (Aricept), galantamine (Razadyne), and rivastigmine (Exelon)
     a. FDA approved for the treatment of mild to moderate AD with the exception of donepezil, which is approved for mild, moderate, and severe dementia. Common side effects include vivid dreams, bradycardia, and gastrointestinal side effects (nausea, diarrhea, and anorexia). Gastrointestinal side effects may be bothersome enough to require either a slower escalation of dosage or switching to another agent. The rivastigmine patch has lower rates of gastrointestinal side effects than the oral agents. Table 8 summarizes some instruments used to monitor clinical response of AD to pharmacologic therapy
  2. NMDA receptor antagonist: Memantine (Namenda)
     a. FDA approved for the treatment of moderate to severe AD. Common side effects include constipation, dizziness, or headache. Memantine is contraindicated in patients with renal insufficiency or history of seizures
- Symptomatic treatment of neuropsychiatric and behavioral disturbances (Table 9)
- Depression, agitation, delusions, or hallucinations may respond to medications

DISPOSITION & REFERRAL

- Patients with complex or atypical presentations or challenging management issues should be referred to a neurologist, geriatric psychiatrist, or geriatrician with expertise in dementia.
- Approximately 1 in 8 hospitalized patients with AD who develop delirium will have at least one adverse outcome (e.g., institutionalization, cognitive decline, death) associated with delirium.
- Family education and support may help reduce need for skilled nursing facility and reduce caregiver stress, depression, and burnout.

TABLE 7 Symptomatic Treatment of Memory Disturbance

	Initial Dose	Target Dose
Donepezil	5 mg qd for 4-6 wk	10 mg qd
Rivastigmine	1.5 mg bid with food, increase by 1.5 mg bid weekly	3-6 mg bid
Galantamine	4 mg bid with food, increase by 4 mg bid every 4 wk	8-12 mg bid
Memantine	5 mg qd, increase by 5 mg weekly	10 mg bid

TABLE 8 Instruments Used to Monitor Clinical Response of Alzheimer Disease (AD) to Pharmacologic Therapy

Mini-Mental State Examination
- Global measure of cognition widely used by physicians and third-party caregivers
- Assesses orientation, registration, recall, language, and attention
- Uses a 30-point scale
- Requires ≈5-10 min to complete
- Sensitivity, 80%-90%; specificity, 80%
- Administered by psychometricians, nurses, and physicians
- AD typically advances by 3 points/yr

Clock Drawing
- Global measure of cognition widely used by physicians
- Multiple scoring systems with proven validity; sensitivity, 59%; specificity, 90%
- Assesses multiple cognitive domains in a single test
- 1-2 min to complete
- Minimal training to administer

Geriatric Depression Scale
- Evaluates depressive symptoms in patients
- Requires 5 min to complete
- Very useful in assessing depression in new patients and in follow-up
- Minimal training to administer
- Ease of administration has led to rapid spread in its use

From Fillit HM: *Brocklehurst's textbook of geriatric medicine and gerontology*, ed 8, Philadelphia, 2017, Elsevier.

TABLE 9 Treatment of Behavioral and Neuropsychiatric Symptoms

	Initial Dose	Maximum Dose
Atypical Antipsychotics		
Olanzapine	2.5 mg qd to bid, may increase by 2.5 mg as needed	7.5 mg bid
Quetiapine	25 mg bid, may increase by 25 mg every 2 days	250 mg tid
Antidepressants		
Sertraline	25-50 mg qd, may increase by 25 mg every wk	200 mg qd
Escitalopram	10 mg qd, may increase after 1 wk to 20 mg qd	10 mg qd

PEARLS & CONSIDERATIONS

The physician should make a thorough search for the treatable causes of dementia. Current American Academy of Neurology practice parameters recommend:

- Treat cognitive symptoms of AD with ChEIs.
- Treat depression.
- Treat agitation and psychosis using nonpharmacological interventions first and use pharmacological interventions at the lowest possible dose if other interventions have failed.
- Encourage caregivers to participate in educational programs and support groups.

COMMENTS

- Ginkgo biloba is marketed widely as effective in delaying cognitive impairment; however, trials have shown that it is not effective in reducing the incidence of Alzheimer dementia or dementia overall.
- Higher midlife fitness levels seem to be associated with lower hazards of developing all-cause dementia later in life independent of cerebrovascular disease. Exercise also may slow the rate of functional deterioration in mild AD.
- Even moderate adherence to the MIND (the Mediterranean-DASH Intervention for Neurodegenerative Delay) diet, a hybrid of the Mediterranean and DASH diets specifically designed to optimize brain health, has been shown to reduce the incidence of AD.
- Antipsychotics should be used with extreme caution in treating dementia-related psychosis. All antipsychotics carry a warning from the FDA stating that the medication is not approved for dementia-related psychosis because elderly patients on either conventional or atypical antipsychotics experience an increased risk of death due to cardiovascular or infectious causes.
- Apolipoprotein E (APOE) is the main cholesterol-carrying molecule in the brain, and it exists in three allelic variants: E2, E3, and E4. The E3 allele is most common and has a neutral influence on developing AD, whereas the E2 allele, the rarest allele, may be protective against AD. The E4 allele increases the risk of developing AD and advances the age of first symptoms in those who experience the disease. However, neither E4 heterozygosity or homozygosity is required or sufficient to cause AD. Among Caucasians, E4 heterozygosity increases the risk of developing AD approximately threefold, whereas E4 homozygosity increases AD risk by approximately 15 times compared to the E3/E3 baseline. The APOE E4 allele is also associated with an earlier age of onset of AD. Because the benefits of genetic testing are often modest, and the tests themselves are often imprecise in identifying risk, the test is generally discouraged. Recent trials, however, reveal that the disclosure of *APOE* genotyping results to adult children of patients with AD did not result in significant short-term psychological risks. Test-related distress was reduced among those who learned that they were *APOE4* negative. Persons with high levels of emotional distress before undergoing genetic testing are more likely to have emotional difficulties after disclosure.

For additional information for patients, families, and clinicians, contact the following organizations:

- Alzheimer's Association (www.alz.org; 800-272-3900)
- Alzheimer's Disease Education and Referral Center (www.nia.nih.gov/Alzheimers; 800-438-4380)

SUGGESTED READINGS

Available at ExpertConsult.com

AUTHORS: **Naomi R. Kass, BA,** and **Joseph S. Kass, MD, JD, FAAN**

A

Diseases and Disorders

I

BASIC INFORMATION

DEFINITION

Amaurosis fugax is a temporary loss of monocular vision caused by transient retinal ischemia.

ICD-10CM CODE
G45.3 Amaurosis fugax

EPIDEMIOLOGY & DEMOGRAPHICS

INCIDENCE (IN U.S.): An uncommon but important presentation of carotid artery disease
PEAK INCIDENCE: Approximately 55 yr

PHYSICAL FINDINGS & CLINICAL PRESENTATION

- Onset is sudden, typically lasting seconds to minutes, and often accompanied by scotomas such as a shade or curtain being pulled over the front of the eye (usually downward).
- Vision loss can be complete, hemianopic, or quadrantic.
- Acute stage: Cholesterol emboli may be seen in retinal artery (*Hollenhorst plaque*).

ETIOLOGY

- Usually embolic from either the internal carotid artery or the heart
- Cardiac embolus most commonly due to atrial fibrillation
- Internal carotid artery embolus will be apparent as carotid stenosis on carotid imaging such as CT angiography, MR angiography, or carotid ultrasound
- Giant cell arteritis causing inflammation of retinal arteries
- Hyperviscosity syndromes, such as sickle cell disease, which causes ischemia in the vascular territory of the ophthalmic artery
- Hypercoagulable states
- Reversible cerebral vasoconstriction syndrome

Dx DIAGNOSIS

DIFFERENTIAL DIAGNOSIS

- Retinal migraine: In contrast to amaurosis, the onset of visual loss develops more slowly, usually over 15 to 20 min.
- Transient visual obscurations occur in the setting of papilledema due to elevated intracranial pressure; intermittent rises in intracranial pressure briefly compromise optic disc perfusion and cause transient visual loss lasting 1 to 2 seconds. The episodes may be binocular. If the visual loss persists at the time of evaluation (i.e., vision has not yet recovered), then the differential diagnosis should be broadened to include:
  1. Anterior ischemic optic neuropathy: Arteritic (classically giant cell arteritis [GCA]) or nonarteritic
  2. Central retinal vein occlusion

WORKUP

- Workup should focus on embolic sources, but GCA should always be considered.
- Careful examination of retina; embolus may be visible and confirm the diagnosis (Fig. 1).
- Auscultation of arteries for carotid bruits.
- Examination of all pulses and for temporal artery tenderness.
- Inquire about symptoms of GCA (scalp tenderness, headache, fever, jaw claudication).
- Examine for signs of hemispheric stroke resulting from intracranial atherosclerosis (contralateral limb and facial weakness or sensory loss, aphasia, etc.).

LABORATORY TESTS

- Complete blood count with erythrocyte sedimentation rate and C-reactive protein
- Serum chemistries, including lipid profile
- Cardiac enzymes and ECG
- Hypercoagulable workup is discretionary based on younger age and history

IMAGING STUDIES

- CT or MR angiography of head and neck preferred to examine carotid and intracranial vasculature. Carotid ultrasound if contraindication to MR or CT angiography
- MRI of the brain with diffusion-weighted imaging to look for infarcts, especially those presenting with focal neurologic disturbances
- Transthoracic echocardiography is indicated to screen for sources of emboli in patients with evidence of heart disease and in patients without an evident source for transient neurologic deficit. Transesophageal echocardiography is more sensitive for detecting cardiac sources of emboli (ventricular mural thrombus, atrial appendage, patent foramen ovale, aortic arch)
- Extended monitoring for atrial fibrillation if neither carotid stenosis nor giant cell arteritis is found to be the etiology

Rx TREATMENT

NONPHARMACOLOGIC THERAPY

- Diet (decrease saturated fatty acids and high-cholesterol foods)
- Exercise
- Cessation of tobacco use

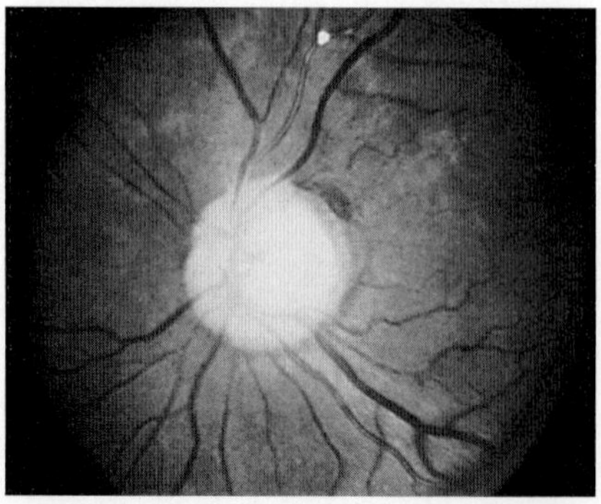

FIG. 1 A cholesterol crystal embolus lodged at an arterial bifurcation. (From Stein JH [ed]: *Internal medicine,* ed 5, St Louis, 1998, Mosby.)

ACUTE GENERAL Rx

- Investigate as an emergency
- Aspirin
- If GCA is suspected, start prednisone and refer for temporal artery biopsy within 48 hr (see "Giant Cell Arteritis" in Section I)

CHRONIC Rx

- Reduce risks by carotid endarterectomy if stenosis >50%. Carotid stenting may be performed in high-risk surgical candidates.
- Manage vascular risk factors such as hypertension, hyperlipidemia (statin therapy), diabetes, smoking cessation, etc.
- Antiplatelet therapy due to arterial atherosclerosis and postcarotid intervention; anticoagulation if etiology is atrial fibrillation.

DISPOSITION

Among patients with >50% carotid stenosis who do not undergo carotid endarterectomy, those who present with transient monocular blindness have an approximate 10% risk of stroke within 3 yr compared with an approximate 20% risk in patients who present with a hemispheric transient ischemic attack (TIA).

REFERRAL

- As with any TIA, emergent inpatient workup in a hospital that is a certified stroke center, if possible.
- If significant carotid stenosis, consider either carotid endarterectomy or carotid stenting for the following:
  1. Ipsilateral high-grade (≥70%) stenosis, but consider for ipsilateral stenosis of 50% to 69%
  2. Multiple TIAs despite medical therapy in the setting of high-grade or ulcerative disease

PEARLS & CONSIDERATIONS

- Cholesterol emboli in retinal arteries on fundoscopy confirm the diagnosis.
- Recognize that transient visual loss has multiple other causes.
- Refer to emergent evaluation like any other transient ischemic attack.

RELATED CONTENT

Amaurosis Fugax (Patient Information)
Carotid Artery Stenosis (Related Key Topic)
Giant Cell Arteritis (Related Key Topic)
Transient Ischemic Attack (Related Key Topic)

AUTHOR: **Joseph S. Kass, MD, JD, FAAN**

BASIC INFORMATION

DEFINITION

Anal cancer refers to malignant transformation of the mucosa within the anal canal and can be of squamous, neuroendocrine cancer, or adenocarcinoma subtypes.

SYNONYMS

Anal Carcinoma
Cancer of the Anal Canal
Malignant Neoplasm of Anus

ICD 10-CM CODE
C 21.1 Malignant neoplasm of anal canal

EPIDEMIOLOGY & DEMOGRAPHICS

INCIDENCE:

- Anal cancer is an uncommon cancer occurring at the rate of 1 to 2 new cases per 100,000 population. There has been a 2% to 3% annual increase in incidence over the last 3 decades in the United States.
- In 2020, an estimated 8590 new cases and 1350 deaths were expected to occur in the United States.
- Globally, an estimated 48,541 new cases and 19,129 deaths were expected due to anal cancer worldwide in 2018 as per the GLOBOCAN database.
- The median age of anal cancer is 60 yr.
- During the last 2 decades, there has been an increase in cases in young black men and older women.
- There has been an increase in locally advanced (node-positive) as well as distant-disease cases along with increased mortality in elderly patients.

RISK FACTORS: The increase in incidence of anal cancer has been noted in tandem with the HIV epidemic and the rise in the incidence of sexually transmitted diseases in the United States.

Risk factors include:

- HIV infection: Unlike other HIV-associated malignancies, the incidence of anal cancer has not decreased in the era of HAART
- Human papilloma virus (HPV) infection
- Cigarette smoking
- Sexual activity practices: MSM (men having sex with men), women with >10 partners, history of anal intercourse
- History of prior sexually transmitted diseases
- History of genital warts
- History of prior cervical cancer
- Chronic immunosuppression

PHYSICAL FINDINGS & CLINICAL PRESENTATION

- Clinical presentation of anal cancer is often related to the size and infiltration of tumor.
- Anorectal bleeding (Fig. E1) is the most common symptom.
- Anorectal pain and fullness.
- Bowel movement alteration with thin-caliber stools and sense of incomplete evacuation.
- Many patients (20% to 25%) may be asymptomatic.
- Local examination can reveal skin lesions, plaques, tumors, and background of warts.
- Digital rectal examination can reveal sphincter function, tumor location, and size. It also can help assess tumor extent and likely involvement of adjacent organs (vagina, prostate, rectum).
- Inguinal adenopathy can be noted in advanced cases.

ETIOLOGY

- Anal cancer development is strongly linked to anogenital infections with HPV, a double-stranded DNA virus. The HPV-16 and -18 genotypes are strongly linked with cancer development accounting for the large majority of cases. Most infected patients remain asymptomatic and only a few patients develop dysplasia over time. The HPV viral proteins, E6 and E7, prevent apoptosis, cause cell-cycle arrest, and contribute to genomic instability, all of which contributes to oncogenesis.
- Chronic immunosuppression in the setting of therapy for autoimmune disorders or organ transplantation is associated with increased incidence of genital warts, persistence of HPV infections, development of anal intraepithelial neoplasia (AIN), and finally anal cancer. Low CD4 counts in HIV-infected patients are a risk factor for development and progression of AIN.

DIAGNOSIS

DIFFERENTIAL DIAGNOSIS

- Anal fissures and fistulas
- Anal ulcers
- Anorectal abscess
- Chancroid
- Genital warts
- Hemorrhoids
- Extramammary Page disease

WORKUP & IMAGING STUDIES

- Local examination followed by anoscopy/proctoscopy and colonoscopy to assess extent of tumor.
- CT scans of the chest, abdomen, and pelvis to detect nodal and distant disease.
- MRI pelvis provides tumor detail, sphincter involvement analysis, and evaluation of mesorectal nodes.
- PET scans (Fig. E2, Fig. E3) are useful in detecting nodal involvement and also monitoring response to therapy.
- Biopsy of anal lesion to confirm diagnosis and type of cancer is required.
- Inguinal nodal biopsy may be required to assess for involvement with metastatic disease.
- Box E1 summarizes recommended diagnostic evaluation in patients with anal cancer.

LABORATORY TESTS

- Complete blood count
- Complete metabolic panel
- HIV testing

STAGING

Table 1 provides the TNM descriptors and stage descriptions for anal cancer.

TREATMENT

The mainstay of therapy for most cases of anal cancer is nonsurgical and includes radiotherapy delivered concurrently with systemic chemotherapy.

NONPHARMACOLOGIC THERAPY

- Early small tumors (T_1N_0 lesions) may be amenable to local surgical resection with wide margins especially when located on the anal margin.
- In some cases, a temporary colostomy is required to facilitate chemoradiotherapy for patients.
- Abdominoperineal resection (APR) is reserved for the salvage of cases of persistent cancer after definitive chemoradiotherapy or in cases of locoregional cancer recurrence.

ACUTE GENERAL Rx

- Previously, APR resulted in surgical cures in 25% to 75% of cases but was notable for up to a 35% rate of locoregional relapse, especially in cases with involved nodal disease.
- Currently, the standard of care is mitomycin and infusional 5-Fluorouracil chemotherapy administered along with pelvic radiotherapy over a 5-wk period. In cases of incomplete responses, as documented by positive biopsies, options include radiotherapy boost or salvage APR.
- This combined modality approach is superior to radiotherapy alone and results in better locoregional control, progression-free survival, overall survival, and colostomy-free survival.
- Major side effects with this approach include myelosuppression, infections, dermatologic, and gastrointestinal toxicities.
- Locoregional recurrence rates are in the range of 10% to 30% and the 5-yr survival of patients who undergo salvage APR is 40% to 60%.
- In patients with distant metastatic or nonsurgical disease (Fig. 4), the use of combination chemotherapy with regimens such as cisplatin and 5-Fluorouracil or carboplatin and weekly paclitaxel is associated with response rates in the range of 60% and overall survival in the range of 2 yr.
- Current novel approaches in metastatic disease include antiepidermal growth factor antibody therapy (cetuximab) and the immune checkpoint inhibitors (nivolumab, pembrolizumab).

CHRONIC Rx

- Colostomy care and attention to nutritional requirements is required on a long-term basis.
- Regular follow-up and examination to detect locoregional or distant recurrences is recommended.

REFERRAL

Referral to Surgical oncology, Radiation oncology, Medical oncology

PEARLS & CONSIDERATIONS

SCREENING

No formal guideline exists but high-risk individuals (chronic immunosuppression, HIV patients, cases of MSM, etc.) should be considered for routine local examination with anoscopy on a 4- to 6-mo basis along with annual anal cytology.

PREVENTION

The availability of HPV vaccination is expected to alter the landscape of anal cancer management. The currently available vaccine, Gardasil 9, is effective against nine subtypes of the HPV. Current guidelines recommend vaccination for all children ages 11 to 12 yr, girls and women ages 13 to 26 yr, boys and men ages 13 to 21 yr, and high-risk men ages 22 to 26 yr. An expanded indication now allows men and women ages 27 to 45 yr to undergo HPV vaccination.

SUGGESTED READINGS

Available at ExpertConsult.com

AUTHOR: **Ritesh Rathore, MD**

TABLE 1 TNM Descriptors and Stage Descriptions for Anal Cancer

TNM Definitions	
Tumor (T)	
T_x	Primary tumor cannot be assessed
T_0	No evidence of primary tumor
T_{is}	Carcinoma in situ (Bowen disease, high grade squamous intraepithelial lesion HSIL, anal intraepithelial neoplasia AIN II-III
T_1	Tumor 2 cm or less in greatest dimension
T_2	Tumor more than 2 cm but not more than 5 cm in greatest dimension
T_3	Tumor more than 5 cm in greatest dimension
T_4	Tumor of any size invades adjacent organ(s)*
Regional Lymph Nodes (N)	
N_x	Regional lymph nodes cannot be assessed
N_0	No regional lymph nodes metastasis
N_1	Metastasis in perirectal lymph node(s)
N_2	Metastasis in unilateral internal iliac and/or inguinal lymph node(s)
N_3	Metastasis in perirectal and inguinal lymph nodes and/or bilateral internal iliac and/or inguinal lymph nodes
Distant Metastasis (M)	
M_0	No distant metastasis
M_1	Distant metastasis

ANATOMIC STAGE/PROGNOSTIC GROUPS STAGE

Stage	T	N	M
0	T_{is}	N_0	M_0
I	T_1	N_0	M_0
II	T_2	N_0	M_0
	T_3	N_0	M_0
III_A	T_1	N_1	M_0
	T_2	N_1	M_0
	T_3	N_1	M_0
	T_4	N_0	M_0
III_B	T_4	N_1	M_0
	Any T	N_2	M_0
	Any T	N_3	M_0
IV	Any T	Any N	M_1

*Note: Direct invasion of the rectal wall, perirectal skin, subcutaneous tissue or the sphincter muscle(s) is not classified as T_4.
From Pessia B et al: *Ann Med Surg (Lond)* 55:36-46, 2020 May 12.

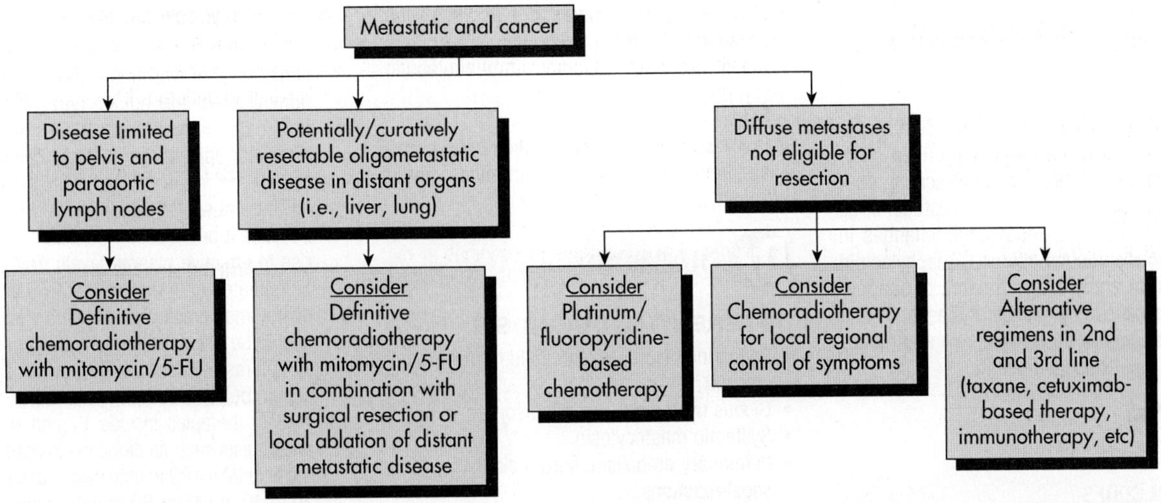

FIG. 4 Treatment algorithm: Metastatic anal cancer. *5-FU,* 5-Fluorouracil. (From Niederhuber JE: *Abeloff's Clinical Oncology*, ed 6, Philadelphia, 2020, Elsevier.)

BASIC INFORMATION

DEFINITION

Anaphylaxis is a severe allergic reaction that is rapid in onset and life-threatening. It is characterized by respiratory, cardiovascular, gastrointestinal, and cutaneous manifestations, as well as vasodilatory hemodynamic changes in response to a particular allergen. Anaphylactoid reaction is an entity closely related to anaphylaxis and is caused by release of mast cells and basophil mediators triggered by non–immunoglobulin E (IgE)-mediated events.

SYNONYM

Anaphylactoid reaction

ICD-10CM CODES	
T78.2	Anaphylactic shock, unspecified, initial encounter
T78.00XA	Anaphylactic reaction due to unspecified food, initial encounter
T80.52XA	Anaphylactic reaction due to vaccination, initial encounter
T63.94XA	Toxic effect of contact with unspecified venomous animal, undetermined, initial encounter

EPIDEMIOLOGY & DEMOGRAPHICS

INCIDENCE: The incidence of anaphylaxis in the U.S. is 50 to 2000 episodes per 100,000 persons. Lifetime prevalence is 0.05% to 2%, with a mortality rate of 1%. Anaphylaxis rates are 0.0004% for food, 0.7% to 10% for penicillin, 0.22% to 1% for contrast media, and 0.5% to 5% after insect stings. Annual mortality is nearly 2000 persons/yr in the U.S.

PHYSICAL FINDINGS & CLINICAL PRESENTATION

- Urticaria, pruritus, skin flushing, angioedema (Table E1)
- Dyspnea, cough, wheezing, shortness of breath
- Nausea, vomiting, diarrhea, difficulty swallowing
- Hypotension, tachycardia, weakness, dizziness, malaise, vascular collapse (Table E2)

ETIOLOGY

Anaphylaxis results from a sudden systematic release of histamine and other inflammatory mediators from basophils and mast cells. This causes swelling of the mucous membranes and the urticarial rash on the skin. Virtually any substance may induce anaphylaxis. In an acute setting, the cause of anaphylaxis is often unidentifiable.

- Foods and food additives: Peanuts, tree nuts, eggs, shellfish, fish, cow's milk, fruits, soy
- Medications: Antibiotics (especially penicillins and sulfa-based agents), insulin, allergen extracts, opiates, vaccines, NSAIDs, contrast media, streptokinase
- Environmental exposures: Bee or wasp sting, snake venom, fire ant venom
- Blood products: Plasma, immunoglobulin, cryoprecipitate, whole blood
- Latex
- Box 1 summarizes agents frequently associated with immune and nonimmune types of anaphylaxis

DIAGNOSIS

DIFFERENTIAL DIAGNOSIS

- Endocrine disorders (carcinoid, pheochromocytoma)
- Globus hystericus, anxiety disorder
- Systemic mastocytosis
- Pulmonary embolism, serum sickness, vasovagal reactions
- Severe asthma (the key clinical difference is the abrupt onset of symptoms in anaphylaxis versus a history of progressive worsening of symptoms)
- Scombroid poisoning
- Localized angioedema
- Septic shock or other form of vasodilatory shock
- Airway foreign body

WORKUP

Workup is aimed at ruling out other conditions that may mimic anaphylaxis. Given the potentially life-threatening nature of anaphylaxis, treatment should not be delayed. Clinical criteria for diagnosing anaphylaxis are summarized in Box 2.

LABORATORY TESTS

- Laboratory evaluation is generally not helpful because anaphylaxis is typically a clinical diagnosis.
- Elevated serum and urine histamine levels and serum tryptase levels can be useful for diagnosis of anaphylaxis, but these tests are not commonly available in the emergency setting.

IMAGING STUDIES

- Generally not helpful.
- Chest radiography for evaluation of foreign body aspiration or pulmonary pathology is indicated in patients with acute respiratory compromise.
- Consider ECG in all patients with sudden loss of consciousness or reports of chest pain or dyspnea and in any elderly patient. ECG in anaphylaxis usually reveals sinus tachycardia.

TREATMENT

NONPHARMACOLOGIC THERAPY

- Establish and protect airway. Provide supplemental O_2 if indicated.
- Intravenous (IV) access should be rapidly established, and IV fluids (i.e., normal saline) should be administered.
- Cardiac monitoring is recommended.

ACUTE GENERAL Rx

- 0.3 to 0.5 mg intramuscular epinephrine (1:1000 concentration) should be rapidly administered for adults and children >30 kg in the lateral thigh. 0.01 mg/kg intramuscular epinephrine (1:1000 concentration) should be administered for children <30 kg. Intramuscular administration is preferred because it provides more reliable and quicker rise to effective plasma levels. The dose may be repeated after approximately 5 to 15 min if symptoms persist. Patients with mild episodes should be observed for 1 hr after resolution of symptoms. Patients with severe symptoms should be observed for at least 6 hr.
- Adjunct therapies include H_1 and H_2 receptor antagonists such as diphenhydramine 25 to 50 mg IV or IM (or PO in mild cases) and famotidine 20 to 40 mg IV (or PO in mild cases). Although useful to improve cutaneous erythema and pruritus, H_1 antagonists are not as effective as epinephrine, since onset of action is 1 to 2 hr and they are not effective in reversing upper airway obstruction or improving hypotension.
- Corticosteroids are not useful in the acute episode because of their slow onset of action; however, they should be administered in most cases to prevent prolonged or recurrent anaphylaxis. Commonly used agents are prednisone, methylprednisolone 40 to 250 mg IV in adults (1 to 2 mg/kg in children), or dexamethasone.
- Aerosolized β-agonists (e.g., albuterol, 2.5 to 5.0 mg, repeat prn 20 min) are useful to control bronchospasm.
- Vasopressor therapy with IV epinephrine (1:10,000 concentration) indicated in patients with refractory hypotension/cardiovascular collapse after crystalloid resuscitation.
- Patients taking beta-blocking medications may be refractory to initial treatment; consider administration of IV glucagon.
- Table 3 summarizes drugs and other agents used in anaphylaxis therapy.
- Fig. E1 illustrates an algorithm for the management of a patient with severe anaphylaxis.

PEARLS & CONSIDERATIONS

COMMENTS

- Patient education regarding the nature of the illness and preventive measures is recommended. A documented history of previous anaphylactic episodes or known triggers is the most reliable method of identifying individuals at risk.
- Prescription for a prefilled epinephrine syringe (EpiPen or EpiPen Jr.) should be given, and the patient should be instructed on the use of this emergency kit, and to carry it with them at all times. School-aged children should keep an additional EpiPen at school with the appropriate staff.
- Patients should also be advised to carry or wear a MedicAlert ID describing substances that have caused anaphylaxis.
- Avoidance of radiologic contrast is also recommended in those who have had a prior

BOX 1 Agents Frequently Associated with Immune and Nonimmune Types of Anaphylaxis

Immunologic Mechanisms

IgE-mediated:

- Food (nuts, shellfish, fruits, etc.)
- Venoms (stinging insects)
- Medications (β-lactam antibiotics, NSAIDs, neuromuscular blocking agents, etc.)
- Natural rubber latex
- Seminal fluid
- Radiocontrast media (in some cases)

IgE-Independent

- Radiocontrast media (in most cases)
- Dextrans
- Monoclonal antibodies (Rituximab)
- Medications (β-lactam antibiotics, NSAIDs, etc.)
- Natural rubber latex
- Seminal fluid

Nonimmunologic Mechanisms

- Medications (opioids, protamine, etc.)

NSAIDs, Nonsteroidal antiinflammatory drugs.
From Parrillo JE, Dellinger RP: *Critical care medicine, principles of diagnosis and management in the adult,* ed 5, Philadelphia, 2019, Elsevier.

BOX 2 Clinical Criteria for Diagnosing Anaphylaxis

Anaphylaxis is highly likely when any one of the following three criteria is fulfilled:

1. Acute onset of an illness (minutes to several hours) with involvement of the skin, mucosal tissue, or both (e.g., generalized urticaria, itching or flushing, swollen lips/tongue/uvula) and at least one of the following:
   a. Respiratory compromise (e.g., dyspnea, wheeze/bronchospasm, stridor, reduced PEF, hypoxemia)
   b. Reduced blood pressure or associated symptoms of end-organ dysfunction (e.g., hypotonia collapse, syncope, incontinence)
   OR
2. Two or more of the following that occur rapidly after exposure to a likely allergen for that patient (minutes to several hours):
   a. Involvement of the skin-mucosal tissue (e.g., generalized urticaria, itch/flush, swollen lips/tongue/uvula)
   b. Respiratory compromise (e.g., dyspnea, wheeze/bronchospasm, stridor, reduced PEF, hypoxemia)
   c. Reduced blood pressure or associated symptoms (e.g., hypotonia collapse, syncope, incontinence)
   d. Persistent gastrointestinal symptoms (e.g., crampy abdominal pain, vomiting)
   OR
3. Reduced blood pressure after exposure to known allergen for that patient (minutes to several hours)
   a. Infants and children: Low systolic blood pressure (age-specific) or >30% decrease in systolic blood pressure
   b. Adults: Systolic blood pressure of <90 mm Hg or >30% decrease from that person's baseline

PEF, Peak expiratory flow.
From Parrillo JE, Dellinger RP: *Critical care medicine, principles of diagnosis and management in the adult,* ed 5, Philadelphia, 2019, Elsevier.

TABLE 3 Management of a Patient with Anaphylaxis

Treatment	Mechanism(s) of Effect	Dosage(s)	Comments; Adverse Reactions
PATIENT EMERGENCY MANAGEMENT (DEPENDENT ON SEVERITY OF SYMPTOMS)			
Epinephrine (adrenaline)	α_1-, β_1-, β_2-Adrenergic effects	0.01 mg/kg, up to 0.5 mg IM in lateral thigh Adrenaclick, Auvi-Q, EpiPen Jr./EpiPen: 0.15 mg IM for 8-25 kg 0.3 mg IM for 25 kg or more Epinephrine autoinjector: 0.1 mg for 7.5-15 kg 0.15 mg for 15 to 25 kg 0.3 mg for 25 kg or more	Tachycardia, hypertension, nervousness, headache, nausea, irritability, tremor
Cetirizine (liquid)	Antihistamine (competitive of H_1 receptor)	Cetirizine liquid: 5 mg/5 ml 0.25 mg/kg, up to 10 mg PO	Hypotension, tachycardia, somnolence
Alternative: Diphenhydramine	Antihistamine (competitive of H_1 receptor)	1.25 mg/kg up to 50 mg PO or IM	Hypotension, tachycardia, somnolence, paradoxic excitement
Transport to an emergency facility			
EMERGENCY PERSONNEL MANAGEMENT (DEPENDENT ON SEVERITY OF SYMPTOMS)			
Epinephrine (adrenaline)	α_1-, β_1-, β_2-Adrenergic effects	0.01 mg/kg, up to 0.5 mg IM in lateral thigh Epinephrine autoinjector: 0.1 mg for 7.5-15 kg 0.15 mg for 15 to 25 kg 0.3 mg for 25 kg or more 0.01 ml/kg/dose of 1:1,000 (vial) solution, up to 0.5 ml IM May repeat every 10-15 min For severe hypotension: 0.01 ml/kg/dose of 1:10,000 slow IV push	Tachycardia, hypertension, nervousness, headache, nausea, irritability, tremor

TABLE 3 Management of a Patient with Anaphylaxis—cont'd

Treatment	Mechanism(s) of Effect	Dosage(s)	Comments; Adverse Reactions
SUPPLEMENTAL OXYGEN AND AIRWAY MANAGEMENT			
Volume Expanders			
Crystalloids (normal saline or Ringer lactate)		30 ml/kg in 1st hr	Rate titrated against BP response If tolerated, place patient supine with legs raised
Colloids (hydroxyethyl starch)		10 ml/kg rapidly followed by slow infusion	Rate titrated against BP response If tolerated, place patient supine with legs raised
Antihistamines			
Cetirizine (liquid)	Antihistamine (competitive of H_1 receptor)	Cetirizine liquid: 5 mg/5 ml 0.25 mg/kg, up to 10 mg PO	Hypotension, tachycardia, somnolence
Alternative: Diphenhydramine	Antihistamine (competitive of H_1 receptor)	1.25 mg/kg, up to 50 mg PO, IM, or IV	Hypotension, tachycardia, somnolence, paradoxic excitement
Ranitidine	Antihistamine (competitive of H_2 receptor)	1 mg/kg, up to 50 mg IV Should be administered slowly	Headache, mental confusion
Alternative: Cimetidine	Antihistamine (competitive of H_2 receptor)	4 mg/kg, up to 200 mg IV Should be administered slowly	Headache, mental confusion
Corticosteroids			
Methylprednisolone	Antiinflammatory	Solu-Medrol (IV): 1-2 mg/kg, up to 125 mg IV Depo-Medrol (IM): 1 mg/kg, up to 80 mg IM	Hypertension, edema, nervousness, agitation
Prednisone	Antiinflammatory	1 mg/kg up, to 75 mg PO	Hypertension, edema, nervousness, agitation
Nebulized albuterol	β-Agonist	0.83 mg/ml (3 ml) via mask with O_2	Palpitations, nervousness, CNS stimulation, tachycardia; use to supplement epinephrine when bronchospasm appears unresponsive; may repeat
POSTEMERGENCY MANAGEMENT			
Antihistamine	Cetirizine (5-10 mg qd) or loratadine (5-10 mg qd) for 3 days		
Corticosteroids	*Optional:* Oral prednisone (1 mg/kg up to 75 mg) daily for 3 days		
Preventive Treatment			
Prescription for epinephrine autoinjector and antihistamine			
Provide written plan outlining patient emergency management (may download form from http://www.aap.org or http://www.foodallergy.org)			
Follow-up evaluation to determine/confirm etiology			
Immunotherapy for insect sting allergy			
Patient Education			
Instruction on avoidance of causative agent			
Information on recognizing early signs of anaphylaxis			
Stress early treatment of allergic symptoms to avoid systemic anaphylaxis			
Encourage wearing medical identification jewelry			

BP, Blood pressure; *CNS,* central nervous system; *IM,* intramuscularly; *IV,* intravenously; *PO,* orally; *qd,* every day.
From Kliegman RM: *Nelson textbook of pediatrics*, ed 21, Philadelphia, 2020, Elsevier.

reaction. However, pretreatment regimens with methylprednisolone or diphenhydramine, exist for those who have had contrast reactions in the past.

- Venom immunotherapy immediately after a sting is effective and recommended for up to 5 yr after the anaphylactic incident.

SUGGESTED READINGS

Available at ExpertConsult.com

AUTHOR: **Rory Merritt, MD, Mehp**

BASIC INFORMATION

DEFINITION

Antineutrophil cytoplasm antibody (ANCA)-associated vasculitis (AAV) describes a family of small to medium vessel systemic vasculitis that shares many overlapping features including clinical manifestations and therapies but also has distinct differences among each condition (granulomatosis with polyangiitis [GPA], microscopic polyangiitis [MPA], and eosinophilic granulomatosis with polyangiitis [EGPA]). These vasculitides are characterized by necrotizing, pauci-immune small vessel vasculitis with GPA and without MPA granulomatous inflammation. Most patients present with both renal and pulmonary involvement, but the skin, nervous system, and gastrointestinal tract can also be affected. In a limited form of GPA, disease is generally confined to the upper respiratory tract and can be managed less aggressively.

SYNONYMS

Antineutrophil cetoplasmic antibody-associated vasculitis
Antineutrophil cytoplasmic antibody positive vasculitis
Granulomatosis with polyangiitis
GPA
Wegener granulomatosis (WG)
MPA
Microscopic polyangiitis
Eosinophilic granulomatosis with polyangiitis
EGPA

ICD-10CM CODES	
I77.6	Arteritis, unspecified
M31.3	Granulomatosis with polyangiitis
M31.7	Microscopic polyangiitis
M30.1	EGPA

EPIDEMIOLOGY & DEMOGRAPHICS

INCIDENCE: 10 to 20 cases per million per year in most parts of the world
PREVALENCE: Varies between 94 to 160 per million
PREDOMINANT SEX AND AGE: Slightly higher incidence in males, peak 60 to 70 yr
PEAK INCIDENCE: Increases with age, peak 60 to 70 yr of age
RISK FACTORS: Infections (e.g., *S. aureus*), silica exposure, hydrocarbon exposure, cigarette smoking, pesticides, medications (e.g., hydralazine, minocycline, propylthiouracil, levamisole-cocaine, allopurinol)
GENETICS: Familial forms have been described but are rare; GPA associated with SNP in HLA-DP, PRTN3, SERPINA1; MPA associated with HLA-DQ polymorphisms

PHYSICAL FINDINGS & CLINICAL PRESENTATION

- Constitutional symptoms: Fever, fatigue, weight loss, myalgia, arthralgia
- Upper respiratory tract (URT): Chronic sinusitis, chronic otitis media, mastoiditis, nasal crusting, obstruction and epistaxis, nasal septal perforation, nasal lacrimal duct stenosis, saddle nose deformities (Fig. 1), tracheal and subglottic stenosis. Up to 90% of patients with GPA have one or more URT manifestations
- Eyes: Conjunctivitis, ulcerative keratosis, episcleritis or scleritis, optic neuropathy, nasolacrimal duct obstruction, retinal vasculitis, uveitis, proptosis
- Ears: Sensorineural and conductive hearing loss, otorrhea, and polychondritis
- Mouth: Chronic ulcerative lesions of the oral mucosa, "mulberry" gingivitis, can be seen in GPA
- Pulmonary: Dyspnea, hemoptysis, pleuritic chest pain. Imaging may show nodules, infiltrates, cavitary lesions, effusion, or alveolar hemorrhage
- Gastrointestinal: Ischemic abdominal pain, peritonitis, bloody diarrhea, bowel ulceration or perforation, most commonly in MPA
- Renal: Most commonly affected organ in GPA and MPA. Elevated blood pressure, edema, decreased urine output. Rapidly progressive glomerulonephritis (38% to 70%), microscopic hematuria with or without red cell casts, and proteinuria
- Nervous system: Mononeuritis multiplex and peripheral neuropathies (15% to 50% in both), meningeal inflammation (pachymeningitis), headaches, and rarely CNS involvement with seizures or strokes
- Skin: Cutaneous nodules over extensor surfaces of joints, necrotizing skin lesions (Fig. E2), palpable purpura (30% to 46%), urticaria, livedo reticularis, and digital gangrene

ETIOLOGY

Unclear etiology of this complex immune-mediated disorder. ANCAs play a major role in the pathogenesis. When PR3 and MPO are expressed on cell surfaces of neutrophils, they can cause endothelial damage as well as local tissue necrosis if activated in extravascular tissue. Other risk factors including genetic, environmental exposure to silica or certain strains of *Staphylococcus aureus* have been proposed.

DIAGNOSIS

DIFFERENTIAL DIAGNOSIS

- Other granulomatous lung diseases for GPA (e.g., sarcoidosis, lymphomatoid granulomatosis, EGPA, necrotizing bronchocentric granulomatosis). The differential diagnosis of granulomatous lung disease is described in Section II. Table 1 describes differential diagnostic features of ANCA-associated vasculitis.
- Other ANCA-associated vasculitides and systemic vasculitis.
- Goodpasture disease, other causes of glomerulonephritis (e.g., poststreptococcal nephritis)
- Neoplasms (especially lymphoproliferative disease).
- Bacterial or fungal sinusitis for GPA
- Viral infections.
- Cocaine-induced midline destructive lesions and levamisole-induced vasculitis.

WORKUP

- Thorough medical history and physical examination. Suspect GPA/MPA if patient has pulmonary and renal symptoms and is refractory to conventional treatment. Suspect GPA if sinus disease.
- Chest x-ray, laboratory evaluation, PFTs, and tissue (lung or kidney) biopsy for granulomatous lesions in GPA (Fig. E3) or nongranulomatous vasculitis in MPA.

LABORATORY TESTS

- ANCA serology: Most patients with GPA have a cytoplasmic pattern of ANCA (c-ANCA) which are predominantly directed against proteinase 3 (PR3). Whereas in MPA, the majority of patients have a perinuclear pattern (p-ANCA) directed against myeloperoxidase (MPO). Up to 15% of GPA patients have p-ANCA/MPO and about 25% of MPA patients have c-ANCA/PR3. Approximately 10% to 15% of AAV patients are ANCA negative
- CBC: Anemia, leukocytosis, thrombocytosis (>400,000/μL)
- Chemistry: Elevated serum creatinine, decreased creatinine clearance
- Urinalysis: May reveal hematuria, RBC casts, and proteinuria
- Inflammatory markers: Increased ESR, positive rheumatoid factor, and elevated C-reactive protein may be found
- Liver function, hepatitis serologies, cryoglobulins, HIV screens, ANA, C3, C4, anti-GBM, and cultures to exclude other processes with similar constitutional symptoms

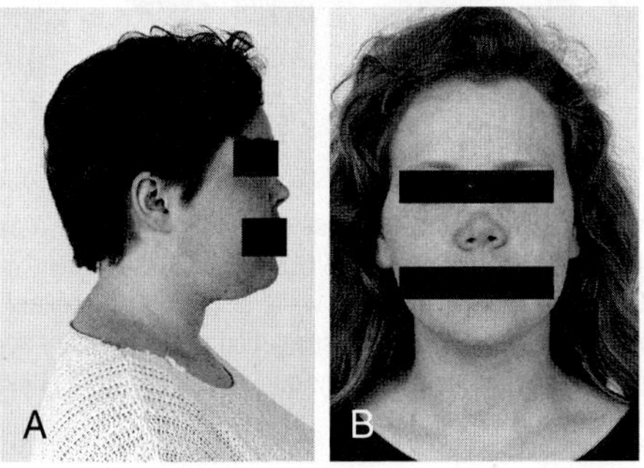

FIG. 1 Saddle-nose deformity in a patient with Wegener granulomatosis. (From *Kelley's textbook of rheumatology*, ed 8, Philadelphia, 2009, Elsevier.)

TABLE 1 Differential Diagnostic Features of the Antineutrophil Cytoplasm Antibody–Associated Vasculitides

Feature	Microscopic Polyangiitis (MPA)	GPA (Wegener Granulomatosis)	EGPA (Churg-Strauss Syndrome)	Comments
Glomerulonephritis	+++	+++	+	Progressive renal failure uncommon in EGPA
Pulmonary infiltrates or nodules	++	+++	+++	Asthma and eosinophilia in EGPA
Alveolar hemorrhage	++	++	+	
Upper airway disease	+	+++	++	Ear, nose, and throat disease usually favors GPA
Skin, purpura	+++	+	++	
Peripheral nerve involvement	+	++	+++	Often a prominent feature of EGPA
Central nervous system involvement	+	+	+	

+++, Very commonly seen; ++, seen often; +, uncommon finding; *EGPA*, eosinophilic granulomatosis with polyangiitis; *GPA*, granulomatosis with polyangiitis.
From Firestein GS et al: *Kelly's textbook of rheumatology*, ed 9, Philadelphia, 2013, Saunders.

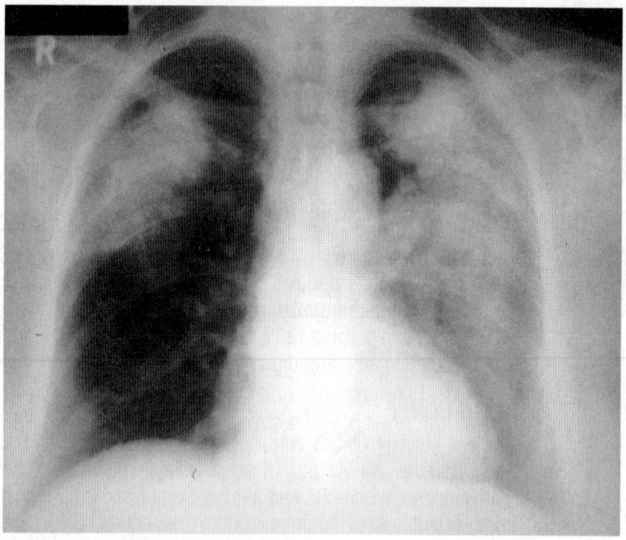

FIG. 4 Pulmonary hemorrhage in microscopic polyangiitis. (From Hochberg MC et al: *Rheumatology*, ed 5, St Louis, 2011, Mosby.)

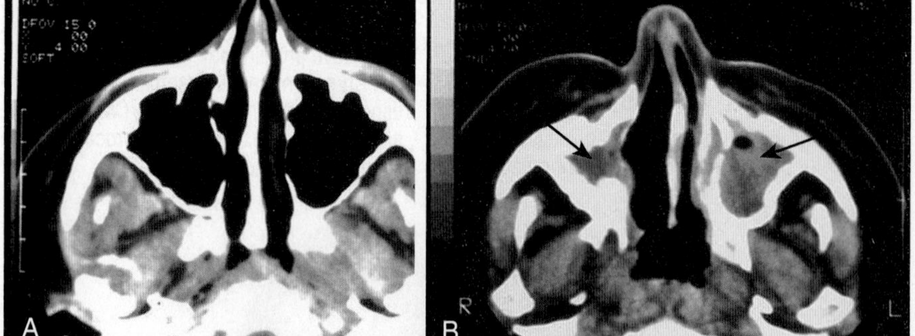

FIG. 5 Computed tomography (CT) scans of the sinuses. A, Normal maxillary sinuses in a recently diagnosed Wegener granulomatosis (WG) patient. **B,** Sinus CT scan of a patient with long-standing WG: Nasal septal deviation to the left, destruction of the medial walls of the right maxillary sinus, opacification of both sinuses with soft tissue densities *(arrows)*, and neo-ossification of all maxillary bony structures due to chronic inflammation. (From Hochberg MC et al: *Rheumatology*, ed 5, St Louis, 2011, Mosby.)

IMAGING STUDIES

- Chest radiograph: Pulmonary infiltrates, nodules, pleural effusions, and cavitary lesions (Fig. 4)
- Computed tomography of sinuses (Fig. 5), computed tomography of chest, mesenteric angiography (if renal function permits), MRI of brain depending on symptoms
- Fiber optic bronchoscopy with BAL and endoscopic ENT examination: Nasal crusting ("golden crusts") are typical on evaluation (Fig. E6)
- Electromyography/nerve conduction study: Sensorimotor peripheral neuropathy
- Biopsy of one or more affected organs should be attempted, including the lung, skin, nasopharynx, or kidneys

Rx TREATMENT

NONPHARMACOLOGIC THERAPY

- Ensure proper airway drainage
- Give nutritional counseling

ACUTE GENERAL Rx

- Immunosuppressive therapy should be considered in all patients with GPA.
- Induction therapy consists of glucocorticoid with either cyclophosphamide or rituximab. Selected patients with severe disease including alveolar hemorrhage or rapidly progressive glomerulonephritis may benefit from the addition of plasma exchange to this regimen.
- The gold standard for treatment is pulse methylprednisolone followed by prednisone 60 to 80 mg/day. Based on PEXIVAS trial, a reduced dose glucocorticoid regimen demonstrated equal efficacy as compared to the standard dose glucocorticoid regimen.
- Based on the RAVE trial, rituximab (375 mg/m^2/wk ×4 wk) appears to be more effective than traditional therapy in treating GPA/MPA that presents with disease flares and is at least as effective as traditional therapy for the induction of remission. The RITUXVAS trial concluded that a combined cyclophosphamide-rituximab regimen was not inferior to pulse cyclophosphamide alone. Both of these studies used concurrent methylprednisolone followed by prednisone. If cyclophosphamide is used, MESNA can be given to prevent cyclophosphamide-induced hemorrhagic cystitis.
- Methotrexate and glucocorticoids alone may be used with mild extrarenal disease or little to no renal involvement, or with limited sinus and upper airway involvement.
- The initial MEPEX trial demonstrated that plasma exchange in addition to cyclophosphamide and glucocorticoids may enhance renal function recovery. However, the more recent PEXIVAS trials showed no additional benefit in reducing mortality or progression to end stage renal disease with plasma exchange.
- Ongoing ADVOCATE trial of investigating the oral C5a receptor blocker, avacopan as a steroid sparing agent, in addition to rituximab or cyclophosphamide shows promising preliminary results of comparable remission rate and serious adverse events.

CHRONIC Rx

- Potentially useful agents for maintenance therapy include rituximab, methotrexate, azathioprine, and mycophenolate mofetil. The MAINRITSAN trial showed that rituximab may be preferable for maintenance therapy. A recent trial[1] demonstrated that extended therapy with biannual rituximab infusions over 18 mo is associated with a lower incidence of antineutrophil cytoplasmic antibody-associated vasculities (AAV).
- The CYCAZAREM (for azathioprine) and LEM (for leflunomide) trials showed that these agents can also be used. The WEGENT study showed oral methotrexate and azathioprine were noninferior for maintenance than intravenous cyclophosphamide.
- Maintenance therapy should generally be continued for at least 18 to 24 mo, and ultimate duration of immunosuppression is decided on a case-by-case basis.
- Mepolizumab, an anti-IL5 monoclonal antibody, is approved for the treatment of EGPA and is used in patients who are not controlled with oral steroids alone.
- Treatment with TMP-SMX (160 mg/800 mg bid) may reduce the incidence of relapses in patients with granulomatosis with polyangiitis in remission. It is also useful in preventing *Pneumocystis jiroveci* pneumonia (PJP), which occurs in 10% of patients receiving induction therapy. Dose of TMP-SMX (160 mg/800 mg) for prophylaxis is 1 tablet three times/wk. If the patient is unable to tolerate TMP-SMX, PJP prophylaxis can also be achieved with dapsone, atovaquone, or inhaled pentamidine.

[1] Charles P et al: Long-term rituximab use to maintain remission of antineutrophil cytoplasmic antibody-associated vasculitis, *Ann Intern Med* 173:179-187, 2020.

DISPOSITION

- 5-yr survival with prompt initiation and aggressive treatment is approximately 80%; without treatment 2-yr survival is 20%.
- Renal failure and pulmonary involvement are major causes of morbidity and mortality. Age over 50 yr and lack of ENT changes at diagnosis are also associated with worse outcomes and increased mortality in GPA.
- Remission rate can be achieved in the majority of patients, but relapse is frequent.

REFERRAL

- Rheumatology referral for continued treatment.
- Multidisciplinary consultation including nephrology, ENT, pulmonary, dermatology may be required depending on other organ involvement.

PEARLS & CONSIDERATIONS

COMMENTS

The goal with treatment of AAV is to achieve rapid, long-standing remission, based on induction therapy and then maintenance regimens. Without treatment there is very high mortality, and treatment is complicated by serious infections and renal disease.

PATIENT & FAMILY EDUCATION

Support can be found with the Vasculitis Foundation.

SUGGESTED READINGS

Available at ExpertConsult.com

RELATED CONTENT

Systemic Vasculitis (Related Key Topic)

AUTHORS: **Nicole B. Yang, MD, Anthony M. Reginato, PhD, MD,** and **Daphne Scaramangas-Plumley, MD**

BASIC INFORMATION

DEFINITION

Autoimmune hemolytic anemia (AIHA) is secondary to premature clearance of red blood cells (RBCs) caused by binding of autoantibodies and/or complement to RBCs. Primary AIHA comprises approximately 50% of cases, whereas secondary AIHA is usually associated with diseases or drugs. The classification of the hemolytic anemias is described in Table 1.

SYNONYMS

AIHA Autoimmune hemolytic anemia
Cold agglutinin disease
CAHA
Cold hemagglutinin disease
CHAD
CAIHA
Drug-induced hemolytic anemia
Warm autoimmune hemolytic anemia
WAHA
WAIHA

ICD-10CM CODES

D59.0	Drug-induced autoimmune hemolytic anemia
D59.1	Other autoimmune hemolytic anemias

EPIDEMIOLOGY & DEMOGRAPHICS

The annual incidence is 1 to 3 cases per 100,000 persons, with 10% mortality; most common in women <50 yr.

PHYSICAL FINDINGS & CLINICAL PRESENTATION

- Most common presentation is dyspnea and fatigue.
- Pallor, jaundice may be present.
- Tachycardia with a flow murmur may be present if anemia is pronounced.
- Patients with intravascular hemolysis may present with dark urine and back pain.
- Hepatomegaly and/or lymphadenopathy suggests an underlying lymphoproliferative disorder or malignancy; splenomegaly may indicate hypersplenism as a cause of hemolysis.
- Chronic process with multiple relapses typically seen during the course of the disease.

ETIOLOGY

- Warm antibody mediated: Almost always IgG antibodies only (often idiopathic or associated with leukemia, lymphoma [Table 2], thymoma, myeloma, viral infections [Table 3], babesiosis, and collagen-vascular disease)
- Cold antibody mediated: IgM and complement in majority of cases (often idiopathic; at times associated with infections, lymphoma, or cold agglutinin disease)
- Il-33 may have a role in promoting increasing RBC autoantibodies in AIHA
- Drug induced (Table 4): Three major mechanisms:
  1. Antibody directed against Rh complex (e.g., methyldopa)
  2. Antibody directed against RBC-drug complex (hapten induced; e.g., penicillin)
  3. Antibody directed against complex formed by drug and plasma proteins; the drug-plasma protein-antibody complex causes destruction of RBCs (innocent bystander; e.g., quinidine)

DIAGNOSIS

DIFFERENTIAL DIAGNOSIS

- Hemolytic anemia caused by membrane defects (acquired: Paroxysmal nocturnal hemoglobinuria, spur cell anemia, Wilson disease; inherited: Spherocytosis, elliptosis), hemoglobinopathies, and enzyme deficiencies (G6PD, pyruvate kinase)
- Non–immune-mediated (microangiopathic hemolytic anemias, hypersplenism, cardiac valve prosthesis, giant cavernous hemangiomas, march hemoglobinuria, physical agents, infections, heavy metals, certain drugs [nitrofurantoin, sulfonamides, ribavirin])
- Chronic lymphocytic leukemia (CLL) can cause direct antiglobulin test (DAT) positivity (15% of CLL cases) without AIHA. In a series

TABLE 1 Classification of the Hemolytic Anemias

Acquired

Environmental factors
- Antibody: Immunohemolytic anemias
- Mechanical trauma: TTP, HUS, heart valve
- Toxins, infectious agents: Malaria, etc.

Membrane defects
- Paroxysmal nocturnal hemoglobinuria
- Spur cell anemia
- Hereditary spherocytosis, etc.

Congenital

Defects of cell interior
- Hemoglobinopathies: Sickle cell, thalassemia
- Enzymopathies: G6PD deficiency, etc.

G6PD, Glucose-6-phosphate dehydrogenase; *HUS,* hemolytic-uremic syndrome; *TTP,* thrombotic thrombocytopenic purpura.
From Goldman L, Schafer AI: *Goldman's Cecil medicine,* ed 24, Philadelphia, 2012, Saunders.

TABLE 2 Secondary Autoimmune Hemolytic Anemia in Malignancies

Malignancy	Prevalence	WAIHAs	CAIHAs
MGUS	Very low	None	All
All NHL	0.23%-2.6%		
CLL	4.3%-9%	90%	10%
SMZL	10%	2/3	1/3
LPL	3%-5%	None	Most
Angioimmunoblastic T-cell lymphoma	13%	One third	Two thirds
Hodgkin lymphoma	0.19%-1.7%	All	None
Ovarian teratoma	Very low	All	None
Solid tumors	Very low	Two thirds	One third

CAIHAs, Cold antibody autoimmune hemolytic anemias; *CLL,* chronic lymphocytic leukemia; *LPL,* lymphoplasmacytic lymphoma; *MGUS,* monoclonal gammopathy with unknown significance; *NHL,* non-Hodgkin lymphoma; *SMZL,* splenic marginal zone lymphoma; *WAIHAs,* warm antibody autoimmune hemolytic anemias.
From Hoffman R et al: *Hematology, basic principles and practice,* ed 7, Philadelphia, 2018, Elsevier.

TABLE 3 Autoimmune Hemolytic Anemia after Infections

	Infection	WAIHA	CAIHA (Specificities)
Respiratory tract infections (unspecified)	—	—	+ (DL)/PCH
Viral infections (specific)	EBV	+/–	+ (anti-i)
	CMV	+	+/– (anti-i)
	Parvovirus (B19)	+ (often with PRCA)	+/– (DL)
	Varicella	+/–	+ (anti-Pr, anti-I, anti-DL)
	Rubella	—	+ (anti-Pr1) Monotypic IgM
	HIV	+	+ (anti-I, anti-i, anti-Pr)
Bacterial infections (specific)	Mycoplasma	+/–	+ (anti-I, anti-Pr)
	Brucellosis	+/–	+ (anti-I)
	Haemophilus influenzae		+ (DL)
Parasitic infections (specific)	Visceral leishmaniosis	+	—

—, Not reported; +, predominant type of autoimmune hemolytic anemia; +/–, single or few cases reported; *CAIHA,* cold antibody autoimmune hemolytic anemia; *CMV,* cytomegalovirus; *EBV,* Epstein-Barr virus; *HIV,* human immunodeficiency virus; *IgM,* immunoglobulin M; *PCH,* paroxysmal cold hemoglobinuria; *PRCA,* pure red blood cell aplasia; *WAIHA,* warm antibody autoimmune hemolytic anemia.
From Hoffman R et al: *Hematology, basic principles and practice,* ed 7, Philadelphia, 2018, Elsevier.

TABLE 4 Drug-Induced Autoimmune Hemolytic Anemia

Drug	Risk Factors	AIHA Onset	Type of AIHA	Response to Treatment	Diseases Treated
Methyldopa	Not known	Delayed	WAIHA	Resolution after withdrawal	Hypertension
IFN-α	Pretherapeutic positive DAT	Delayed (8-11 mo)	WAIHA	Resolution spontaneous or after steroids	Hepatitis C; hematologic malignancies
Efazulimab	Not known	Many mo	WAIHA	Resolution after withdrawal	Arthritis (rare)
Etanercept	Not known	Delayed	CAIHA	Resolution after rituximab	Rheumatoid arthritis (rare)
Fludarabine Cladribine Pentostatin	CLL Pretherapeutic positive DAT result	Early (median, 3-4 cycle) or delayed	WAIHA Mixed AIHA	Half of AIHA resolve after steroids	CLL Lymphomas[a] AML[a]
Bendamustin	CLL	No or only very low risk of AIHA			CLL Lymphomas
Chlorambucil	CLL	Delayed onset	WAIHA		CLL
Eculizumab	Patients with incomplete response	After treatment	CAIHA		PNH
Lenalidomide		During treatment	WAIHA	Resolution after withdrawal	One case treated for lymphoma
Checkpoint inhibitors (anti-CTLA4, anti-PD1/PD1L)		During treatment	WAIHA		Solid tumors, Hodgkin lymphoma

AIHA, Autoimmune hemolytic anemia; *AML,* acute myeloid leukemia; *CAIHA,* cold autoimmune hemolytic anemia; *CLL,* chronic lymphocytic leukemia; *DAT,* direct antiglobulin test; *IFN,* interferon; *PNH,* paroxysmal nocturnal hemoglobinuria; *WAIHA,* warm autoimmune hemolytic anemia.
[a]No or very low risk.
From Hoffman R et al: *Hematology, basic principles and practice,* ed 7, Philadelphia, 2018, Elsevier.

TABLE 5 Positive Direct Antiglobulin Test Findings, Characteristic Features of Autoantibody in Autoimmune Hemolytic Anemia

	Warm AIHA	CHAD	Mixed-AIHA	PCH	IgA AIHA
DAT	IgG or IgG + C3 or IgG + C3 + IgM	C3 or C3 + IgM	IgG + C3 + IgM	C3	Neg with polyspecific reagent Pos with anti-IgA
Antibody characteristic					
1) Antibody subclass	IgG	IgM	IgG + IgM	IgG	IgA
1) Specificity	Apparent Rh specificity (common)	I, i, Pr		P	
1) Thermal reactivity (in vitro)	Optimal at 37°C (98.6° F) by IAT	0-30° C (32-86° F) by saline agglutination	Combined	0-24° C (32-75.2° F), biphasic in nature	
1) Antibody titer at 4° C (39.2° F)	Not applicable	≥256	Usually <64 but can be >256	Usually <32	
Autoagglutination	No	Common	Common	Less common	No

AIHA, Autoimmune hemolytic anemia; *C,* complement; *CHAD,* cold hemagglutinin disease; *DAT,* direct antiglobulin test; *IAT,* indirect antiglobulin test; *Ig,* immunoglobulin; *Neg,* negative; *PCH,* Paroxysmal cold hemoglobinuria; *Pos,* positive.The determination of autospecificity is not required for diagnosis of CHAD, but confirmation of high thermal amplitude (i.e., cold autoagglutinin reacting at or above 30° C [86° F]) is essential.
From Bain BJ et al: *Dacie and Lewis practical haematology,* ed 12, Philadelphia, 2017, Elsevier.

of patients treated with fludarabine and cyclophosphamide, only 30% of patients with DAT+ disease developed AIHA after therapy; conversely, 85% of patients with AIHA were previously positive for DAT

WORKUP

Evaluation consists primarily of laboratory evaluation to confirm hemolysis and exclude other causes of the anemia. Although most cases of AIHA are idiopathic, potential causes should always be sought.

LABORATORY TESTS

- The basic features of hemolytic anemia are reticulocytosis (if no concurrent bone marrow suppression), low haptoglobin levels, elevated indirect bilirubin, and elevated LDH.
- Initial laboratory tests: Complete blood count (anemia), reticulocyte count (elevated), liver function studies (elevated indirect bilirubin, LDH), evaluation of peripheral smear (Fig. E1).
- A direct antiglobulin test (DAT, Coombs test) is initially performed with a polyspecific antibody to detect IgG or complement C3d bound to RBCs. If the DAT is positive, the diagnosis of autoimmune hemolytic anemia (AIHA) is confirmed. A positive direct Coombs test indicates presence of antibodies or complement on the surface of RBCs; positive indirect Coombs test implies presence of anti-RBC antibodies freely circulating in the patient's serum. Positive DAT findings and characteristic features of autoantibody in AIHA are summarized in Table 5. Typical serologic features of the different types of drug-induced hemolytic anemia of immunologic origin are summarized in Table 6.
- If the DAT is positive with IgG alone or with IgG + C3d, the AIHA is most likely due to warm antibody (WAIHA), whereas if the DAT is positive with C3d only, it is most likely caused by a cold antibody (CAIHA).
- Hepatitis serology, antinuclear antibody.
- Urinary tests may reveal hemosiderinuria or hemoglobinuria (documenting intravascular hemolysis).

IMAGING STUDIES

- Chest x-ray.
- CT scans of chest, abdomen, and pelvis should be considered if underlying lymphoproliferative disorder is suspected.

TABLE 6 Serologic Features of the Different Types of Drug-Induced Hemolytic Anemia of Immunologic Origin

Mechanism	Prototype drug	DAT	IAT		
			No drug	Serum + drug	Eluate + drug
Drug-dependent antibody					
C′ activation	Quin(id)ine	C′*	Neg	C′*	Neg
No C′ activation	Penicillin	IgG	Neg	IgG	IgG
Autoantibody	α-Methyldopa	IgG	IgG	NA	NA

C′, Complement; *DAT,* direct antiglobulin test; *IAT,* indirect antiglobulin test; *IgG,* immunoglobulin G; *NA,* not applicable; *Neg,* negative.
*Occasionally also IgG.
From Bain BJ et al: *Dacie and Lewis practical haematology,* ed 12, Philadelphia, 2017, Elsevier.

TABLE 7 Treatment Options for Primary and Secondary Warm Autoimmune Hemolytic Anemia and Cold Autoimmune Hemolytic Anemia

Disease or Condition	First Line	Second Line	Beyond Second Line	Last Resort
Primary AIHA	Steroids (trituximab)	Splenectomy Rituximab	Azathioprine, MMF, cyclosporine, cyclophosphamide	High-dose cyclophosphamide, alemtuzumab
B- and T-cell NHL	Steroids	Chemotherapy +/− rituximab (splenectomy in SMZL)	Other anti-CD23 antibodies/ ibrutinib	
Hodgkin lymphoma	Steroids	Chemotherapy		
Solid tumors	Steroids Surgery			
Ovarian dermoid cyst	Ovariectomy			
SLE	Steroids	Azathioprine	MMF	Rituximab Autologous SCT
Ulcerative colitis	Steroids	Azathioprine		Total colectomy
CVID	Steroids + IgG replacement			
ALPD	Steroids	MMF	Sirolimus	
Wiskott-Aldrich syndrome	Steroids	Allogeneic SCT		
Allogeneic SCT	Steroids	Rituximab*	Splenectomy T-cell infusion	
Organ transplantation	Reduction of immune suppression, steroids			
Drug induced	Withdrawal	Steroids		
Primary CAD	Protection from cold exposure	Rituximab Chlorambucil	Fludarabine + rituximab	Eculizumab,† bortezomib†
PCH	Supportive treatment (postinfectious)	Rituximab* (chronic)		

AIHA, Autoimmune hemolytic anemia; *ALPD,* autoimmune lymphoproliferative disorders; *CAD,* cold agglutinin disease; *CVID,* common variable immune deficiency; *IgG,* immunoglobulin G; *MMF,* mycophenolate mofetil; *NHL,* non-Hodgkin lymphoma; *PCH,* paroxysmal cold hemoglobinuria; *SCT,* stem cell transplantation; *SLE,* systemic lupus erythematosus; *SMZL,* splenic marginal zone lymphoma.
*Early second-line treatment because of known poor response to steroids.
†Off-label use in single cases.
From Hoffman R et al: *Hematology, basic principles and practice,* ed 7, Philadelphia, 2018, Saunders.

Rx TREATMENT

NONPHARMACOLOGIC THERAPY

- Discontinuation of any potentially offending drugs
- Plasmapheresis and exchange transfusion for severe life-threatening cases only
- Avoid cold exposure in patients with cold antibody AIHA

ACUTE GENERAL Rx

- Warm AIHA:
  1. Prednisone 1 to 2 mg/kg/day in divided doses is initially used in warm antibody AIHA. After achieving a sustained response, tapering should be initiated after 2 to 3 wk and completed over a period of 3 to 6 mo.
  2. Two randomized controlled trials have demonstrated improved outcomes and duration of response with the combined upfront use of steroids and rituximab, and this is also another standard option in clinical use.
  3. For patients relapsing or refractory to initial steroid therapy, the use of rituximab has in most cases replaced the use of splenectomy.
  4. Splenectomy now is more often used in patients refractory to both corticosteroids and rituximab.
  5. Immunosuppressive drugs and/or immunoglobulins are recommended after failure of the above approaches to produce an adequate remission.
  6. Danazol, used in conjunction with corticosteroids, may be useful in some cases of warm AIHA.
  7. Immunosuppressive drugs (azathioprine, cyclophosphamide) may be useful in warm antibody AIHA but are indicated only in multiply relapsed or refractory cases.
- Cold AIHA:
  1. Corticosteroids are generally ineffective in cold antibody AIHA, and response rates are much lower than those seen with warm AIHA.
  2. Therapy of underlying lymphoproliferative disorder or infection is recommended.
  3. In primary cold agglutin disease, the use of rituximab plus bendamustine chemotherapy regimen is considered a standard approach in fit patients; rituximab alone is used in elderly patients.
  4. In severe cases, IVIG therapy or plasmapheresis can be used as a temporary bridge until more effective therapies achieve durable responses.
  5. Complement-directed therapy with eculizumab can also be considered in severe cases.
  6. Splenectomy is not effective as the sensitized RBCs are mainly removed in the liver.
- Table 7 summarizes treatment options for primary and secondary warm autoimmune

TABLE 8 Second-Line Treatment Options after Steroids

Treatment	Dosing and Application	Side Effects	Precautions
Splenectomy (acute)	Preferentially laparoscopic	Infections, thrombosis	Postoperative thromboprophylaxis
Splenectomy (long term)	—	Infections Venous thrombosis	Vaccination, patient information
Rituximab	375 mg/m^2 on days 1, 8, 15, and 22 IV	Infusional reactions Infections	Premedication with antihistamines (and steroids)
Danazol	200-400/day PO	Hepatotoxicity	None
Cyclophosphamide	PO or IV Dose adjusted to neutrophil count	Neutropenia Mutagenesis	Neutrophil count monitoring, bladder protection after high doses
Azathioprine	2.0-3.mg/kg/day PO Dose adjusted to neutrophil count	Neutropenia	Neutrophil count monitoring; avoid interaction with other drugs (e.g., allopurinol)
MFF	1-2 × 1 g/day PO	Gastrointestinal	
Cyclosporine	PO Dose adjusted to blood levels (Target 200-400 ng/ml)	Nephrotoxicity Gum hyperplasia	Monitoring of CyA levels and creatinine
Alemtuzumab	SC (variable doses)	Neutropenia	Anti-infectious prophylaxis
Complement inhibition with eculizumab, TNT009		Infections	Vaccination

CyA, Cyclosporine A; *IV,* intravenous; *MMF,* mycophenolate mofetil; *PO,* oral; *SC,* subcutaneous.
From Hoffman R et al: *Hematology, basic principles and practice,* ed 7, Philadelphia, 2018, Elsevier.

hemolytic anemia and cold autoimmune hemolytic anemia. Second-line treatment options after steroids are described in Table 8.

DISPOSITION

Prognosis is generally good unless anemia is associated with underlying disorder with a poor prognosis (e.g., leukemia, myeloma).

REFERRAL

- Hematology referral in all cases of AIHA
- Surgical referral for splenectomy in refractory cases of warm AIHA

PEARLS & CONSIDERATIONS

COMMENTS

- The direct antiglobulin test demonstrates the presence of antibodies or complement on the surface of RBCs and is the hallmark of autoimmune hemolysis.
- Warm AIHA is often associated with autoimmune diseases, whereas cold AIHA often follows viral infections (e.g., mononucleosis) and *Mycoplasma pneumoniae* infections.
- HIV can induce both warm and cold AIHA.
- Hemolytic anemia is a common autoimmune complication of hematopoietic stem cell transplantation occurring in up to 6% of patients as a late complication (median 202 days); it presents as either warm or cold AIHA.

SUGGESTED READINGS

Available at ExpertConsult.com

AUTHOR: **Bharti Rathore, MD**

BASIC INFORMATION

DEFINITION

Inflammatory anemia, also known as *anemia of chronic disease (ACD),* is a disorder of iron homeostasis (Table 1) promoted by hepcidin-25 in response to an inflammatory condition.

SYNONYMS

Inflammatory anemia
Anemia of chronic disease
ACD

ICD-10CM CODES

D63.8	Anemia in chronic diseases classified elsewhere
D63.0	Anemia in neoplastic disease
D64.8	Anemia, unspecified

EPIDEMIOLOGY & DEMOGRAPHICS

PREVALENCE:

- Second-most prevalent anemia after iron deficiency anemia:
  1. Around 11% of men and 10% of women ages 65 to 85 yr
  2. >20% of adults older than 85 yr

PATHOPHYSIOLOGY (FIG. 1)

Iron is carried in the bloodstream shelled by a hollow protein called transferrin (<0.2% of total iron body content) or at the core of hemoglobin in RBCs (60% of total iron body content). It is mainly stored (15% to 30% of total iron body content) inside the liver, spleen, and skeletal muscle as ferritin and in lysosomes as hemosiderin. The rest of the iron body content is trapped in myoglobin in skeletal muscle and cytochromes in mitochondria. In clinical practice, ferritin is a surrogate for iron stores, and total iron binding capacity (TIBC) is a surrogate for transferrin and the carrying capacity of iron.

Cells involved in the response to inflammatory insults cause the release of cytokines, such as IL-6, which stimulates hepatic release of hepcidin. Hepcidin is a circulating protein that blocks ferroportin, an iron channel responsible for the exit of iron from enterocytes (and thus gastrointestinal absorption) and macrophages (which accumulate iron from engulfed senescent blood cells). IL-1 and TNF-alpha stimulate IFN-gamma release by marrow stromal cells, which in turn suppress the erythroid response to erythropoietin (EPO). In chronic kidney disease, ACD is a consequence of decreased production of EPO and decreased renal clearance of hepcidin. The low availability of serum iron causes iron deficiency in the bone marrow compartment and decreased reticulocyte levels.

TABLE 1 Suspected Causes of Anemia of Chronic Disease

Shortened erythrocyte survival
Block in reuse of iron by erythrocyte
Direct inhibition of erythropoiesis
Relative deficiency of erythropoietin

From Hoffman R et al: *Hematology, basic principles and practice,* ed 7, Philadelphia, 2018, Elsevier.

CLINICAL PRESENTATION

- Besides fatigue, shortness of breath, and generalized weakness from the anemia itself, it is important to consider other complaints if the underlying diagnosis is unknown, such as weight loss (malignancy, chronic infections, connective tissue diseases), anorexia, nausea, paresthesias, pleuritic chest pain, weight gain (CKD), diarrhea, bloody stools, abdominal pain, oral ulcers (IBD), and fevers (HIV, chronic infections).
- Physical findings may include pallor, lymphadenopathy, stigmatas of connective tissue diseases (malar rash, sclerodactyly), palpable or visible masses, and localized findings for infection or malignancy.

DIAGNOSIS

Isolated ACD:

- CBC with differential: Normocytic, normochromic, moderate (Hb rarely <8 g/dl) anemia
- Hypoproliferative anemia (low reticulocyte index; corrected reticulocyte count <2%)

Iron studies:

- Low iron concentration as in IDA (iron deficiency anemia)
- Normal/high ferritin (>35 mg/dl) in ACD as it is an acute phase reactant (Fig. 2)
- Low/normal TIBC (as opposed to IDA) and low transferrin saturation (as in IDA)
- Normal soluble transferrin receptor (sTfR, high in IDA)

Combined ACD/IDA:

- If normal to high ferritin, sTfR/log ferritin ratio <1 defines isolated ACD, and ratio >2 defines combined IDA/ACD

ETIOLOGY

- Malignancy
- CKD (patients with CKD stage IV [GFR<30 ml/min] should be screened for ACD)
- CHF (ACD is the main cause of anemia in CHF patients)
- Chronic infections
- Anemia of critical illness (develops within days)
- Connective tissue diseases

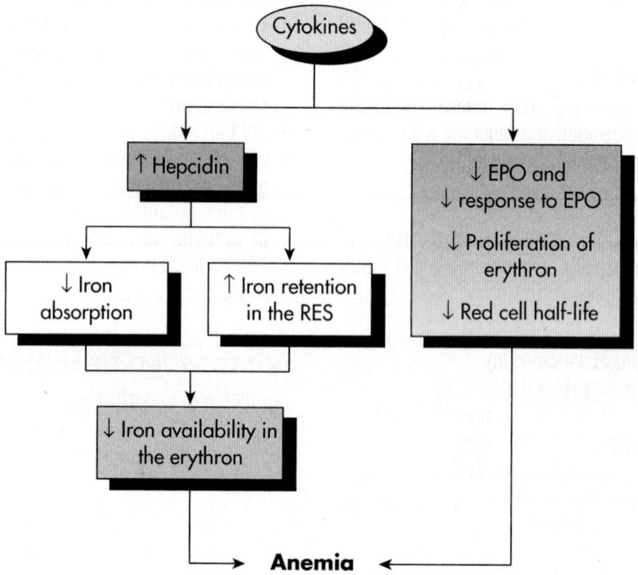

FIG. 1 Pathophysiologic factors associated with the development of anemia of chronic disease. *EPO,* Erythropoietin; *RES,* reticuloendothelial system. (From Hoffman R et al: *Hematology, basic principles and practice,* ed 7, Philadelphia, 2018, Elsevier.)

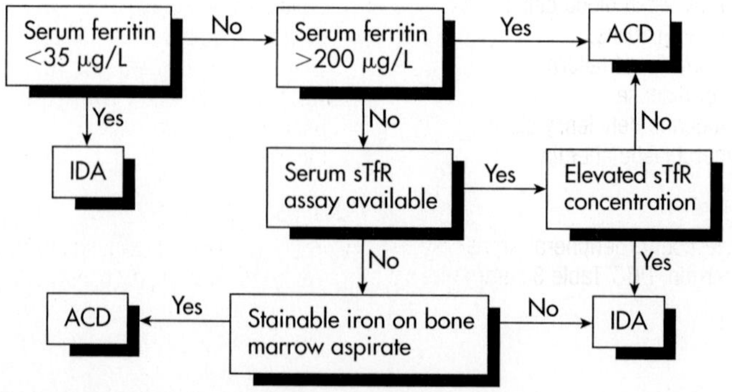

FIG. 2 Differential diagnosis of anemia with low serum iron. *ACD,* Anemia of chronic disease; *IDA,* iron deficiency anemia; *sTfR,* soluble transferrin receptor.

TABLE 2 Laboratory Features in Microcytic Hypochromic Anemias

	Serum Iron	Serum TIBC	% Saturation	MARROW % Sideroblasts	MARROW Iron Stores	Serum Ferritin	ZPP	Hb A_2	Hb F
Iron deficiency	↓	↑	↓	↓	↓	↓	↑	N-↓	N
β-Thalassemia trait	N (↑)	N	N	N	N-↑	N-↑	N	↑	N-↑
ACD	↓	N-↓	↓	↓	N-↑	N-↑	↑	N	N
Sideroblastic anemia	↑	↓	↑	↑	↑	↑	↑ (↓)	N	N-↑

ACD, Anemia of chronic disease; *Hb,* hemoglobin; *N,* normal; *TIBC,* total iron-binding capacity; *ZPP,* zinc protoporphyrins; ↓, decreased; ↑, increased.
McPherson RA, Pincus MR: *Henry's clinical diagnosis and management by laboratory methods,* ed 23, Philadelphia, 2017, Elsevier.

TABLE 3 Laboratory Characteristics of ACD, IDA, and IDA with Inflammation

	Anemia of Chronic Disease (ACD)	Iron Deficiency Anemia (IDA)	IDA with Inflammation
Mean corpuscular volume (MCV)	72-100 fL	<85 fL	<100 fL
Mean corpuscular hemoglobin concentration (MCHC)	<36 g/dl	<32 g/dl	<32 g/dl
Serum iron	Decreased	Decreased	Decreased
Serum total iron-binding capacity (TIBC)	Typical below mid-normal range	Elevated	Less than upper limit of normal range
Transferrin saturation*	2%-20%	<15% (usually <10%)	<15%
Serum ferritin	>35 μg/L	<35 μg/L	>35 μg/L, <200μg/L
Serum soluble transferrin receptor concentration (sTfR)	Normal (may be increased if serum ferritin >200 μg/L)	Increased	Increased
TfR index (sTfR/log ferritin)	<1	>2	>2
Hepcidin	High	Low	Normal
Stainable iron in bone marrow	Present	Absent	Absent

*Serum iron/TIBC * 100.

DIFFERENTIAL DIAGNOSIS

- Liver injury (increases ferritin):
  1. Iron deficiency anemia:
     a. Other causes of normocytic anemia or microcytic anemia (Table 2)
     b. Red blood cell loss or destruction:
        (1) Acute blood loss
        (2) Hypersplenism
        (3) Hemolysis
     c. Decreased red blood cell production:
        (1) Primary causes:
           (a) Bone marrow hypoplasia or aplasia
           (b) Myeloproliferative disease
           (c) Pure red blood cell aplasia
     d. Secondary causes:
        (1) Chronic renal failure
        (2) Liver disease
        (3) Endocrine deficiency states
        (4) Sideroblastic anemia

WORKUP

CBC, reticulocyte count, peripheral smear (Fig. E3), iron level, ferritin, TIBC. Table 3 summarizes characteristic findings in inflammatory anemia. Characteristic bone marrow findings of increased iron stores in stromal histiocytes and impaired erythroid iron incorporation are shown in Fig. E4.

Rx TREATMENT

Treat the underlying disorder/disease.

ACUTE GENERAL Rx

- The treatment of inflammatory anemia is directed primarily at treatment of underlying conditions, which can improve symptoms and facilitate hemoglobin recovery.
- Blood transfusion is usually reserved for severe anemia (with Hb level <7 g/dl or <8 g/dl in patients with cardiac disease), especially if complicated with ongoing bleeding.

CHRONIC Rx

- Erythropoiesis-stimulating agents (ESA) (epoetin alfa and darbepoetin alfa) are FDA approved for use in patients with anemia resulting from:
  1. Chronic kidney disease
  2. Chemotherapy
  3. Zidovudine therapy
- A 1998 study, the Normal Hematocrit Cardiac Trial (NHCT), showed a nonsignificant increase in the combined endpoint death and nonfatal MI in patients with goal hematocrit of 33% versus 27%. Subsequent studies (CHOIR, CREATE, and TREAT) showed that higher doses and higher hematocrit targets were associated with increased cardiovascular events
- ESA dose should be individualized for each patient, and the lowest sufficient dose to reduce blood transfusions should be used. A hemoglobin target of approximately 10 g% is widely acceptable. Iron deficiency should be ruled out before ESA is started. After starting ESA therapy, ASH/ASCO guidelines recommend periodic monitoring of iron status. When there is no or suboptimal response to oral therapy, parenteral iron therapy should be considered before concluding that a patient is nonresponsive to iron therapy
- The hepcidin–ferroportin axis is the target of development of novel agents of which the most promising are hypoxia-induced factor modulators. HIF is a transcription factor that promotes expression of erythropoietin. HIF is upregulated by inhibition of PHD. Small molecule inhibitors of prolyl hydroxylase domain dioxygenases (HIF-PHI [prolyl hydroxylase inhibitor]) stimulate the production of endogenous erythropoietin and improve iron metabolism. The clinical development of three oral agents targeting this axis–daprodustat, roxadustat, and vadadustat–has now completed randomized clinical development and led to approvals in Asia

SUGGESTED READINGS
Available at ExpertConsult.com

AUTHOR: **Bharti Rathore, MD**

BASIC INFORMATION

DEFINITION

Anemia is defined as a hemoglobin level 2 standard deviations below normal for age and sex. Iron deficiency anemia is anemia resulting from inadequate iron supplementation or excessive blood loss.

ICD-10CM CODES

D50.0	Iron deficiency anemia secondary to blood loss (chronic)
D50.8	Other iron deficiency anemias
D50.9	Iron deficiency anemia, unspecified
O99.019	Anemia complicating pregnancy, unspecified trimester

EPIDEMIOLOGY & DEMOGRAPHICS

- Dietary iron deficiency occurs often in infants as a result of unsupplemented milk diets. It is also commonly seen in women during their reproductive years, as a result of heavy menstrual periods, and during pregnancy (increased demand).
- Iron deficiency is the most common nutritional deficiency worldwide.
- The prevalence of iron deficiency is greatest among toddlers ages 1 to 2 yr (7%) from inadequate intake and female individuals ages 12 to 49 yr (9%-16%) from menstrual losses.
- The prevalence of iron deficiency is 2% in adult men, 9% to 12% in non-Hispanic white women, and 20% in black and Mexican American women.
- GI cancer is diagnosed in 10% of elderly patients with iron deficiency anemia.

PHYSICAL FINDINGS & CLINICAL PRESENTATION

- Most patients have normal examination results.
- Skin pallor and conjunctival pallor may be present.
- Signs and symptoms specific for iron deficiency are koilonychias, pica, pagophagia, blue sclera, glossitis, and angular stomatitis (Fig. E1).
- Patients with severe anemia can have palpitations, headache, weakness, dizziness, and easy fatigability.

ETIOLOGY

- Blood loss from GI or menstrual bleeding (genitourinary blood loss less often the cause)
- Dietary iron deficiency (rare in adults)
- Poor iron absorption in patients with gastric or small-bowel surgery
- Repeated phlebotomy
- Increased requirements (e.g., during pregnancy)
- Other: Traumatic hemolysis (abnormally functioning cardiac valves), idiopathic pulmonary hemosiderosis (iron sequestration in pulmonary macrophages), paroxysmal nocturnal hemoglobinuria (intravascular hemolysis)
- The most common cause worldwide is hookworm infection

DIAGNOSIS

DIFFERENTIAL DIAGNOSIS

- Anemia of chronic disease
- Sideroblastic anemia
- Thalassemia trait
- Lead poisoning

WORKUP

Diagnostic workup consists primarily of laboratory evaluation. Table 1 describes laboratory studies differentiating the most common microcytic anemias. Most patients with iron deficiency anemia are asymptomatic in the early stages. With progressive anemia, the major symptoms are fatigue, dizziness, exertional dyspnea, pagophagia (ice eating), and pica. Patient history may also suggest GI blood loss (melena, hematochezia, hemoptysis).

LABORATORY TESTS

- Laboratory results vary with the stage of deficiency.
- Absent iron marrow stores and decreased serum ferritin are the initial abnormalities.
- Decreased serum iron and increased total iron-binding capacity (TIBC) are the next abnormalities.
- Hypochromic microcytic anemia is present with significant iron deficiency.
- Peripheral smear in patients with iron deficiency generally reveals microcytic hypochromic red blood cells (Fig. E2) with a wide area of central pallor, anisocytosis, and poikilocytosis when severe.
- Laboratory abnormalities consistent with iron deficiency are low serum ferritin level, increased RBC distribution width with values generally >15, low mean corpuscular volume, low mean corpuscular hemoglobin, increased TIBC, and low serum iron.
- In patients diagnosed with iron deficiency anemia, a GI workup including an upper endoscopy and colonoscopy is recommended to look for source of iron loss.

TREATMENT

The goal of therapy is to supply sufficient iron to correct the low hemoglobin and replenish iron stores.

NONPHARMACOLOGIC THERAPY

Patients should be instructed to consume foods that contain large amounts of iron, such as liver, red meat, and legumes.

ACUTE GENERAL Rx

- Iron supplementation will result in reticulocytosis and will generally increase hemoglobin levels by 0.5 to 1 g per wk.
- Treatment consists of ferrous sulfate 325 mg PO daily for 3 to 6 mo. Doses higher than 325 mg/day are poorly tolerated. Calcium supplements can decrease iron absorption; therefore, these medications should be staggered. Supplemental vitamin C can increase oral absorption.
- Parenteral iron therapy is reserved for patients with poor tolerance, noncompliance with oral preparations, or malabsorption. Indications for intravenous iron therapy are summarized in Table 2.
- Transfusion of packed RBCs is indicated in patients with severe symptomatic anemia.

CHRONIC Rx

Patients should be instructed to continue their iron supplements for at least 6 mo or longer to correct depleted body iron stores.

DISPOSITION

- Most patients respond rapidly to iron supplementation with improvement in CBC and general well-being (Table 3). GI side effects from oral iron therapy are common and may require decreased dosage to once every other day or to change to parenteral iron.

TABLE 1 Laboratory Studies Differentiating the Most Common Microcytic Anemias

Study	Iron Deficiency Anemia	α or β Thalassemia	Anemia of Chronic Disease
Hemoglobin	Decreased	Decreased	Decreased
MCV	Decreased	Decreased	Normal-decreased
RDW	Increased	Normal	Normal-increased
RBC	Decreased	Normal-increased	Normal-decreased
Serum ferritin	Decreased	Normal	Increased
Total Fe binding capacity	Increased	Normal	Decreased
Transferrin saturation	Decreased	Normal	Decreased
FEP	Increased	Normal	Increased
Transferrin receptor	Increased	Normal	Increased
Reticulocyte hemoglobin concentration	Decreased	Normal	Normal-decreased

Fe, Ferritin; *FEP,* free erythrocyte protoporphyrin; *MCV,* mean corpuscular volume; *RBC,* red blood cell; *RDW,* red cell distribution width.

From Kliegman RM et al: *Nelson Textbook of Pediatrics,* ed 19, Philadelphia, 2011, Saunders.

TABLE 2 Indications for Intravenous Iron Therapy

Accepted Indications
- Oral iron intolerance
- Oral iron refractoriness, including iron refractory iron deficiency anemia (IRIDA)
- Need for a quick recovery: e.g., severe anemia of pregnancy
- Chronic bleeding not manageable with oral iron
- Concurrently with erythropoiesis-stimulating agents in chronic kidney disease
- Gastrointestinal disorders (inflammatory bowel disease, acute flares)
- Substitution for blood transfusions when not accepted by patient

Novel Proposed Indications
- Iron deficiency in chronic heart failure
- Perioperative anemia (transfusion sparing strategy)
- Anemia of chronic kidney disease before treatment with erythropoiesis-stimulating agents
- Persistent anemia after erythropoiesis-stimulating agents in cancer patients on chemotherapy

From Goldman L, Shafer AI: *Goldman-Cecil Medicine,* ed 26. 2019, Elsevier.

TABLE 3 Responses to Iron Therapy in Iron Deficiency Anemia

Time after Iron Administration	Response
12-24 hr	Replacement of intracellular iron enzymes; subjective improvement; decreased irritability; increased appetite
36-48 hr	Initial bone marrow response; erythroid hyperplasia
48-72 hr	Reticulocytosis, peaking at 5-7 days
4-30 days	Increase in hemoglobin level
1-3 mo	Repletion of stores

From Kliegman RM et al: *Nelson Textbook of Pediatrics,* ed 19, Philadelphia, 2011, Saunders.

TABLE 4 Differential Diagnosis of Microcytic Anemia That Fails to Respond to Oral Iron

Poor compliance (true intolerance of iron is uncommon)
Incorrect dose or medication
Malabsorption of administered iron
Ongoing blood loss including gastrointestinal, menstrual, and pulmonary
Concurrent infection or inflammatory disorder inhibiting the response to iron
Concurrent vitamin B_{12} or folate deficiency
Diagnosis other than iron deficiency:
- Thalassemias
- Hemoglobin C and E disorders
- Anemia of chronic disease
- Lead poisoning
- Sickle thalassemias, hemoglobin SC disease
- Rare microcytic anemias

From Kliegman RM et al: *Nelson Textbook of Pediatrics,* ed 19, Philadelphia, 2011, Saunders.

- A differential diagnosis of microcytic anemia that fails to respond to oral iron is described in Table 4.

REFERRAL

GI referral for evaluation of GI malignancy is recommended in all patients with iron deficiency and suspected GI blood loss.

PEARLS & CONSIDERATIONS

COMMENTS

- Iron deficiency may impair aerobic performance and worsen symptoms in patients with heart failure. Treatment with IV iron in patients with chronic heart failure and iron deficiency has been shown to improve symptoms, quality of life, and functional capacity.
- If the diagnosis of iron deficiency anemia is made, locating the suspected site of iron loss is mandatory.

RELATED CONTENT

Algorithm for Diagnosis of Anemias (Algorithm in Section III)
Anemia (Patient Information)

AUTHOR: **Fred F. Ferri, MD**

BASIC INFORMATION

DEFINITION

Pernicious anemia (PA) is an autoimmune disease resulting from antibodies against gastric intrinsic factor and gastric parietal cells.

SYNONYMS

Megaloblastic anemia resulting from vitamin B_{12} deficiency
Addison-Biermer anemia

ICD-10CM CODES

D51.0	Vitamin B_{12} deficiency anemia due to intrinsic factor deficiency
D51.8	Other vitamin B_{12} deficiency anemias
D51.9	Vitamin B_{12} deficiency anemia, unspecified
D51.1	Vitamin B_{12} deficiency anemia due to selective vitamin B_{12} malabsorption with proteinuria

EPIDEMIOLOGY & DEMOGRAPHICS

- Increased incidence in females and older adults (40 to 70 yr)
- More frequent in patients of northern European ancestry
- Overall prevalence of undiagnosed PA after age 60 yr is 1.9%
- Prevalence is higher in women (2.7%), particularly in black women (4.3%)
- Associated with other autoimmune diseases (e.g., type 1 diabetes mellitus, Graves disease, Addison disease), along with possible *Helicobacter pylori* association

PHYSICAL FINDINGS & CLINICAL PRESENTATION

- Mucosal pallor and/or glossitis
- Angular cheilosis
- Mild jaundice (representative of intramedullary hemolysis of megaloblastic cells); "lemon yellow" skin due to pallor and jaundice
- Peripheral sensory neuropathy with paresthesias initially and absent reflexes in advanced disease
- Delirium or dementia
- Worsening weakness and possible subacute combined degeneration of spinal cord (Fig. E1)
- Loss of proprioception and an unsteady gait
- Gastrointestinal symptoms including anorexia, pyrosis, nausea, and vomiting
- Possible splenomegaly and mild hepatomegaly

ETIOLOGY

- Parietal cell antibodies are present in >70% of patients, while intrinsic factor antibodies are noted in >50% of patients.
- Atrophic gastric mucosa (Fig. E2) with achlorhydria.
- Inborn errors of cobalamin-cofactor synthesis are rare. Fig. E3 illustrates the components and mechanism of cobalamin absorption. An etiopathophysiologic classification of cobalamin deficiency is described in Section II.

DIAGNOSIS

DIFFERENTIAL DIAGNOSIS

- Nutritional vitamin B_{12} deficiency
- Malabsorption (e.g., celiac disease)
- Chronic alcoholism (multifactorial)
- Chronic gastritis related to *H. pylori* infection
- Folic acid deficiency
- Myelodysplasia
- Thyroid abnormalities
- Atrophic gastritis
- Paraproteinemias
- Gastrectomy or use of H2 blockers
- Insufficient pancreatic enzymes (Zollinger-Ellison syndrome, chronic pancreatitis, post-Whipple procedure)

TABLE 1 Stepwise Approach to the Diagnosis of Cobalamin and Folate Deficiency

Megaloblastic Anemia or Neurologic-Psychiatric Manifestations Consistent With Cobalamin Deficiency *Plus* Test Results on Serum Cobalamin and Serum Folate

Cobalamin[a] (pg/ml)	Folate[b] (ng/ml)	Provisional Diagnosis	Proceed with Metabolites?[c]
>300	>4	Cobalamin or folate deficiency is unlikely	No
<200	>4	Consistent with cobalamin deficiency	No
200-300	>4	Rule out cobalamin deficiency	Yes
>300	<2	Consistent with folate deficiency	No
<200	<2	Consistent with (1) combined cobalamin plus folate deficiency or (2) isolated folate deficiency	Yes
>300	2-4	Consistent with (1) folate deficiency or (2) an anemia unrelated to vitamin deficiency	Yes

Test Results on Metabolites: Serum Methylmalonic Acid and Total Homocysteine

Methylmalonic Acid (Normal, 70-270 nM)	Total Homocysteine (Normal, 5-14 μM)	Diagnosis
Increased	Increased	Cobalamin deficiency confirmed; folate deficiency still possible (i.e., combined cobalamin plus folate deficiency possible)
Normal	Increased	Folate deficiency is likely
Normal	Normal	Cobalamin and folate deficiency is excluded

[a]Serum cobalamin levels: Abnormally low, <200 pg/ml; clinically relevant low-normal range, 200-300 pg/ml.
[b]Serum folate levels: Abnormally low, <2 ng/ml; clinically relevant low-normal range, 2-4 ng/ml.
[c]Any frozen-over sample from serum folate/cobalamin determination can be subjected to metabolite tests.
From Hoffman R et al: *Hematology, basic principles and practice*, ed 7, Philadelphia, 2018, Saunders.

WORKUP

- The clinical presentation of PA varies with the stage. Initially, patients may be asymptomatic. In advanced stages patients may have impaired memory, depression, gait disturbances, paresthesias, and generalized weakness.
- Investigation consists primarily of laboratory evaluation. Table 1 describes a step-wise approach to the diagnosis of cobalamin and folate deficiency.
- Endoscopy and biopsy for atrophic gastritis may be performed in selected cases.
- Diagnosis is crucial because failure to treat may result in irreversible neurologic deficits.

LABORATORY TESTS

- Complete blood count generally reveals macrocytic anemia, thrombocytopenia, and mild leukopenia with hypersegmented neutrophils (Fig. E4).
- Mean corpuscular volume (MCV) is significantly elevated in advanced stages.
- Reticulocyte count is low to normal.
- False low serum cobalamin levels can occur in patients who are pregnant or taking oral contraceptives, have multiple myeloma, have transcobalamin I (TCI) deficiency, have severe folic acid deficiency, or are taking large doses of ascorbic acid. False high normal levels in patients with cobalamin deficiency can occur in several conditions including hepatomas, severe liver disease, or monoblastic leukemias (Table 2).
- The absence of anemia or macrocytosis does not exclude the diagnosis of cobalamin deficiency. Anemia is absent in 20% of patients with cobalamin deficiency, and macrocytosis is absent in >30% of patients at the time of diagnosis. Macrocytosis can be masked by concurrent iron deficiency, anemia of chronic disease, or thalassemia trait.
- Laboratory tests used for detecting cobalamin deficiency in patients with normal vitamin B_{12} levels include serum and urinary methylmalonic acid (MMA) level (elevated), total homocysteine level (elevated), and intrinsic factor antibody (positive). Cobalamin is a cofactor for the enzymes L-methylmalonyl coenzyme A mutase and methionine synthase. Inadequate levels of cobalamin will thus result in increased MMA and homocysteine levels. Plasma MMA levels can also be used to differentiate cobalamin deficiency from folate deficiency because patients with folate deficiency have normal or mild elevations of MMA levels.
- An increased concentration of plasma MMA does not predict clinical manifestations of vitamin B_{12} deficiency and should not be used as the only marker for diagnosis of B_{12} deficiency.

TABLE 2 Serum Cobalamin: False-Positive and False-Negative Test Results

Falsely Low Serum Cobalamin in the Absence of True Cobalamin Deficiency

- Folate deficiency (one third of patients)
- Multiple myeloma
- TCI deficiency
- Megadose vitamin C therapy
- Pregnancy
- Oral contraceptives

Falsely Raised Cobalamin Levels in the Presence of a True Deficiency[a]

- Cobalamin binders (TCI and II) increased (e.g., myeloproliferative states, hepatomas, and fibrolamellar hepatic tumors)
- TCII-producing macrophages are activated (e.g., autoimmune diseases, monoblastic leukemias and lymphomas)
- Release of cobalamin from hepatocytes (e.g., active liver disease)
- High serum anti-IF antibody titer

IF, Intrinsic factor; *TC,* transcobalamin.

[a]Although a low serum cobalamin level is not synonymous with cobalamin deficiency, 5% of patients with true cobalamin deficiency have low-normal cobalamin levels, a potentially serious problem because the patient's underlying cobalamin deficiency will progress if uncorrected.

From Hoffman R et al: *Hematology, basic principles and practice,* ed 6, Philadelphia, 2013, Saunders.

- Additional laboratory abnormalities can include elevated lactate dehydrogenase, direct hyperbilirubinemia, and decreased haptoglobin, due to rapid destruction of red blood cells
- Bone marrow aspirate is not necessary to diagnose cobalamin deficiency. It may show giant C-shaped neutrophil bands and megaloblastic normoblasts (Fig. E5).
- Schilling test: No longer used. It was historically used to identify the locus of cobalamin malabsorption and the cause of cobalamin deficiency.

Rx TREATMENT

NONPHARMACOLOGIC THERAPY

Avoid folic acid supplementation without proper vitamin B_{12} supplementation. Folic acid supplementation alone may result in hematologic remission in patients with vitamin B_{12} deficiency but will not treat or prevent neurologic manifestations.

ACUTE GENERAL Rx

Traditional therapy of cobalamin deficiency consists of intramuscular (IM) or deep subcutaneous (SC) injections of vitamin B_{12} 1000 mcg/day for 1 wk, followed by 1000 mcg/mo, indefinitely. Monitor response and increase dosing if serum B_{12} levels decline.

CHRONIC Rx

- Parenteral vitamin B_{12} 1000 mcg/mo or intranasal cyanocobalamin 500 mcg/wk for the remainder of life.
- In patients who have no nervous system involvement, intranasal cyanocobalamin may be used in place of parenteral cyanocobalamin after hematologic parameters have returned to normal range. Macrocytosis correction can be noted during the first mo of treatment. The initial dose of intranasal cyanocobalamin is 1 spray (500 mcg) in one nostril once per wk. Nasal cyanocobalamin is expensive.
- Oral cobalamin (1000 to 2000 mcg/day) is also being effective in mild cases of pernicious anemia because approximately 1% of an oral dose is absorbed by passive diffusion, a pathway that does not require intrinsic factor. Cost for 1 mo of therapy is approximately $5. Consider returning to IM vitamin B_{12} supplementation if decline recurs.

DISPOSITION

Anemia generally resolves with appropriate cobalamin replacement therapy. Neurologic deficits, on the other hand, may be corrected only if treated early on.

REFERRAL

Gastroenterology referral for endoscopy on diagnosis of PA followed by periodic surveillance endoscopies to rule out gastric adenocarcinoma or carcinoid tumors.

PEARLS & CONSIDERATIONS

COMMENTS

- Early manifestations of negative cobalamin balance are increased serum methylmalonic acid and total homocysteine levels. This occurs when the total cobalamin in serum is still in the low-normal range.
- Vitamin B_{12} deficiency that is allowed to progress for longer than 3 mo may produce permanent degenerative lesions of the spinal cord (e.g., subacute combined degeneration of spinal cord).
- Vitamin B_{12} deficiency may suppress signs of polycythemia vera; treatment of B_{12} deficiency may unmask this disorder.
- Blunted or impeded therapeutic response to vitamin B_{12} may be due to concurrent iron or folic acid deficiency, uremia, infections, or use of drugs with bone marrow suppressant properties. Causes of megaloblastosis not responding to therapy with cobalamin or folate are summarized in Table 3.
- Drugs that interfere with B_{12} absorption include metformin, colchicine, neomycin, and aminosalicylic acid.
- Patients must understand that cobalamin replacement therapy is lifelong.
- Self-injection of vitamin B_{12} may be taught in selected patients. Cost of monthly injections is less than $10.
- Patients who have had bariatric surgery should receive 1 mg of oral vitamin B_{12} per day indefinitely.

TABLE 3 Causes of Megaloblastosis Not Responding to Therapy with Cobalamin or Folate

Wrong Diagnosis

Combined folate and cobalamin deficiencies being treated with only one vitamin

Associated iron deficiency

Associated hemoglobinopathy (e.g., sickle cell disease, thalassemia)

Associated anemia of chronic disease

Associated hypothyroidism

From Hoffman R et al: *Hematology, basic principles and practice,* ed 7, Philadelphia, 2018, Elsevier.

SUGGESTED READINGS

Available at ExpertConsult.com

RELATED CONTENT

Pernicious Anemia (Patient Information)

AUTHOR: **Shiva Kumar R. Mukkamalla, MD, MPH**

BASIC INFORMATION

DEFINITION

Angina pectoris is a term used to describe a clinical syndrome, typically characterized by chest, jaw, shoulder, back or arm discomfort that is caused by myocardial ischemia. This is most commonly related to atheromatous plaque in one or more than one large epicardial coronary artery; however, myocardial ischemia may occur in the absence of obstructive coronary artery disease (CAD), such as uncontrolled hypertension, microvascular disease, valvular heart disease, hypertrophic cardiomyopathy, coronary spasm, or endothelial dysfunction. Any situation that causes an imbalance in myocardial oxygen supply and demand can cause an angina syndrome. Angina can be classified as follows:

- Chronic stable angina, stable ischemic heart disease (SIHD), or chronic coronary artery disease:
  1. Predictable. Usually follows a precipitating event (e.g., climbing stairs, sexual intercourse, a heavy meal, emotional stress, cold weather)
  2. Generally has the same severity as previous attacks; relieved by rest or by the customary dose of sublingual nitroglycerin
  3. Caused by a fixed coronary artery obstruction secondary to atherosclerosis. The presence of one or more obstructions in major coronary arteries is likely; the severity of stenosis is usually >70%
- Unstable (rest, recent onset, crescendo angina; will be reviewed under Acute Coronary Syndrome):
  1. Rest angina: Angina occurring at rest and usually prolonged >20 min, occurring within 1 wk of presentation
  2. Recent onset: Angina of at least CCS Class III severity occurring less than 2 mo after the onset of the symptoms
  3. Crescendo angina: Previously diagnosed angina that is distinctly more frequent, longer in duration, or lower in threshold (i.e., increased by >1 CCS class within 2 mo of initial presentation to at least CCS Class III severity)
- Prinzmetal variant:
  1. Occurs at rest, common after cold exposure
  2. Cyclical in nature
  3. EKG finding of episodic ST-segment elevations
  4. Caused by coronary artery spasm with or without superimposed CAD
  5. Patients are more likely to develop ventricular arrhythmias
- Microvascular angina (syndrome X):
  1. Refers to patients with angina symptoms, positive exercise test, normal coronary angiograms and no coronary spasm. Defective endothelium-dependent dilation in the coronary microcirculation contributes to the altered regulation of myocardial perfusion and the ischemic manifestations in these patients
  2. Patients with chest pain and normal or nonobstructive coronary angiograms are predominantly women, and many have a prognosis that is not as benign as commonly thought (2% risk of death or myocardial infarction [MI] at 30 days of follow-up)
- Refractory angina:
  1. Refers to patients whom, despite optimal medical therapy with at least maximal doses, or as tolerated of two antianginal medications, in addition to aspirin, aggressive risk factor modification, such as smoking cessation, adequate control of hypertension, diabetes, and hyperlipidemia, still have both angina and objective evidence of ischemia
- Other:
  1. Angina due to aortic stenosis and idiopathic hypertrophic subaortic stenosis, cocaine-induced coronary vasoconstriction

FUNCTIONAL CLASSIFICATION

Stable angina should be classified using a grading system. The most commonly adopted is that of the Canadian Cardiovascular Society (CCS):

- Class I: Ordinary physical activity, such as walking or climbing stairs, does not cause angina. Angina occurs with strenuous, rapid, or prolonged exertion at work or recreation.
- Class II: Slight limitation of ordinary activity. Angina occurs on walking or climbing stairs rapidly; walking uphill; walking or stair climbing after meals, in cold, in wind, or under emotional stress; or only during the few hr after awakening. Angina occurs on walking more than two level blocks and climbing more than one flight of ordinary stairs at a normal pace and in normal conditions.
- Class III: Marked limitations of ordinary physical activity. Angina occurs on walking one to two level blocks and climbing one flight of stairs in normal conditions and at a normal pace.
- Class IV: Inability to carry on any physical activity without discomfort; anginal symptoms may be present at rest.

ICD-10CM CODES

I20.1	Angina pectoris with documented spasm
I20.8	Other forms of angina pectoris
I20.9	Angina pectoris, unspecified
I25.110	Atherosclerotic heart disease of native coronary artery with unstable angina pectoris
I25.111	Atherosclerotic heart disease of native coronary artery with angina pectoris with documented spasm
I25.118	Atherosclerotic heart disease of native coronary artery with other forms of angina pectoris
I25.119	Atherosclerotic heart disease of native coronary artery with unspecified angina pectoris
I25.700	Atherosclerosis of coronary artery bypass graft(s), unspecified, with unstable angina pectoris
I25.790	Atherosclerosis of other coronary artery bypass graft(s) with unstable angina pectoris
I25.791	Atherosclerosis of other coronary artery bypass graft(s) with angina pectoris with documented spasm
I25.798	Atherosclerosis of other coronary artery bypass graft(s) with other forms of angina pectoris
I25.799	Atherosclerosis of other coronary artery bypass graft(s) with unspecified angina pectoris

EPIDEMIOLOGY & DEMOGRAPHICS

- It is estimated that one in three adults in the U.S. (about 81 million) has some form of cardiovascular disease. Based on the NHANES survey 2007 to 2010, an estimated 15.4 million have coronary heart disease of which 7.8 million have angina.
- Angina is most common in middle-aged and elderly men. Among persons 60 to 79 yr of age, approximately 25% of men and 16% of women have coronary heart disease, and these figures rise to 37% and 23% among men and women >80 yr of age, respectively.
- The incidence of coronary heart disease and angina in women after menopause is similar to that of men.
- Although the survival rate has steadily improved over time, SIHD remains the number one cause of death in men and women (27% of deaths).
- The initial manifestation of ischemic heart disease is angina pectoris in 50%, and about 50% of patients presenting to the hospital with acute coronary syndrome have preceding angina.
- Two older population-based studies from Olmstead County, MN, and Framingham, MA, showed annual rate of myocardial infarction in patients with symptomatic angina of 3% to 3.5%/yr.
- Within 12 mo of initial diagnosis, 10% to 20% of patients with diagnosis of stable angina progress to MI or unstable angina.

PHYSICAL FINDINGS & CLINICAL PRESENTATION

- The assessment of chest pain should include quality, location, severity, and duration of pain; radiation; associated symptoms; provocative factors; and alleviating factors. Anginal pain can be described as "squeezing," "griplike," "suffocating," and "heavy," but it is rarely sharp or stabbing and typically does not vary with position or respiration. The classic Levine sign is placing a clenched fist over the precordium to describe the pain. Many patients do not, however, describe angina as frank pain but as tightness, pressure, or discomfort. Other patients, in particular women and older adults, can present with atypical symptoms such as nausea, vomiting, midepigastric discomfort, sharp (atypical) chest pain, dizziness, or syncope.

- Ischemic pain of more than 20 minutes' duration should raise concern for possible acute coronary syndrome.
- Women are more likely than men to report atypical chest pain or discomfort (65% reported on Women's Ischemic Syndrome Evaluation [WISE] study).
- Elderly and diabetics may report symptoms other than chest pain, such as dyspnea, fatigue, or diaphoresis.

ETIOLOGY

RISK FACTORS:

- Advanced age
- Male sex
- Genetic predisposition, family history of premature coronary artery disease (CAD) in first-degree relatives (men younger than 55 yr of age, and women younger than 65 yr of age)
- Smoking (risk of first MI is increased by near threefold)
- Hypertension
- Hyperlipidemia
- Impaired glucose tolerance or diabetes mellitus
- History of stroke or peripheral arterial disease
- Chronic kidney disease (CKD)
- Metabolic syndrome
- Physical inactivity
- Obesity (body mass index >30% over ideal). A higher body mass index during childhood is also associated with an increased risk of coronary heart disease (CHD) in adulthood
- Entities that cause increased oxygen demand include hyperthermia (particularly if accompanied by volume contraction), hyperthyroidism, and cocaine or methamphetamine abuse
- Cocaine is used by >5 million Americans regularly and is responsible for >64,000 emergency department (ED) evaluations yearly to rule out myocardial ischemia. Cocaine causes sympathomimetic toxicity and not only increases myocardial oxygen demand but also induces coronary vasospasm and can cause infarction in young patients. Long-term cocaine use can cause premature development of SIHD
- Severe uncontrolled hypertension causes increased myocardial oxygen demand and decreased subendocardial perfusion that increases LV wall tension. Hypertrophic cardiomyopathy and aortic stenosis can induce even more severe LV hypertrophy and resultant wall tension
- Other causes of increased myocardial oxygen demand are ventricular or supraventricular tachycardias. Ambulatory monitoring may be required to diagnose these
- Entities that limit myocardial oxygen supply such as anemia may cause angina when the hemoglobin drops to <9 g/dl, and ST-T-wave changes (depression or inversion) can occur at levels <7 g/dl
- Hypoxemia resulting from pulmonary disease (e.g., pneumonia, asthma, chronic obstructive pulmonary disease, pulmonary hypertension, interstitial fibrosis, or obstructive sleep apnea) can also precipitate angina
- Polycythemia, leukemia, thrombocytosis, and hypergammaglobulinemia
- Oral contraceptive and HRT use
- Coronary artery calcium is associated with an increased risk of MI
- Long-term use of nonsteroidal antiinflammatory drugs (NSAIDs)
- Exposure to air pollution from traffic (dilute diesel exhaust) promotes myocardial ischemia and is associated with adverse cardiovascular events
- Low serum folate levels required for conversion of homocysteine to methionine are associated with an increased risk of fatal CHD. Hyperhomocysteinemia has a toxic effect on vascular endothelium and interferes with proliferation of arterial wall smooth muscle cells. Elevated plasma homocysteine level is a strong and independent risk factor for CHD events, especially in patients with type 2 diabetes mellitus
- Elevated levels of highly sensitive C-reactive protein (hs-CRP, cardio CRP). Diseases associated with systemic inflammation can lead to accelerated atherosclerosis
- Depression
- Vasculitis
- Elevated levels of lipoprotein-associated phospholipase A_2
- Elevated fibrinogen levels
- Low level of red blood cell glutathione peroxidase-1 activity
- Radiation therapy

Dx DIAGNOSIS

DIFFERENTIAL DIAGNOSIS

- **Nonischemic cardiovascular:** Aortic dissection, pericarditis
- **Pulmonary:** Pulmonary embolism, pneumothorax, pneumonia, pleuritis
- **Gastrointestinal:** Esophageal, esophagitis, spasm, reflux, biliary colic, cholecystitis, choledocholithiasis, cholangitis, peptic ulcer, pancreatitis
- **Chest wall:** Costochondritis, fibrositis, rib fracture, sternoclavicular arthritis, herpes zoster (before the rash)
- **Psychiatric:** Anxiety disorders, hyperventilation, panic disorder, primary anxiety, affective disorders (i.e., depression), somatoform disorders, thought disorders (i.e., fixed delusions)

WORKUP

- In patients with chest pain, the probability of CAD should be estimated on the basis of patient age, sex, cardiovascular risk factors, and pain characteristics.
- The most important diagnostic element is the history. Chest pain or left arm pain or discomfort occurring with exertion and relieved by rest in a patient with cardiovascular risk factors is consistent with a high likelihood of CAD.
- In assessing the likelihood of underlying SIHD it is helpful to classify the chest pain as typical angina, atypical angina, and/or noncardiac chest pain.
- Typical angina, (definite) will have the following three features: (1) Substernal chest discomfort with a characteristic quality and duration, (2) provoked by exertion or emotional stress, and (3) relieved by rest and/or sublingual nitroglycerin (NTG).
- Atypical angina, (probable) will have two of the above listed three features.
- Noncardiac chest pain will have one or none of the previously listed features.
- Physical examination may be completely normal in many patients; however, certain findings may be helpful in the assessment of the patient with suspected SIHD. Some findings may identify consequences of ischemia or possible causes of the anginal syndrome other than CAD. The presence of hypertension, arcus senilis, xanthelasma, carotid or peripheral bruits, and a prominent S4 are all physical signs that could raise concern for the presence of CAD. A murmur of mitral regurgitation may be a marker of an ischemic cardiomyopathy or transient ischemia. A murmur suggestive of hypertrophic cardiomyopathy or aortic stenosis may suggest a cause of angina other than CAD.
- The ultimate goal for an SIHD patient's evaluation is to identify high-risk coronary artery disease patients with minimal use of resources. In general, four common steps would help a clinician to assess high feature of SIHD. Those are (1) CAD risk assessment based on various classical risk factors, (2) functional capacity and stress test result, (3) LV and RV function, and (4) coronary anatomy. Every patient does not need each of the modalities. One should classify stable angina without history of CAD patients to low, intermediate, and high pretest probability or likelihood for CAD after assessment of comorbidities. Consider functional capacity and stress test (ETT, ETT-MIBI, or Stress echo) for low and intermediate pretest probability patients. Exercise testing (Fig. 1) is preferred to pharmacologic stress tests when possible. Functional capacity and stress test results categorize SIHD patients based on their risk of annual mortality. Patients with an estimated annual mortality of <1% classify as low risk, 1% to 3% are considered as intermediate risk, and >3% annual mortality belongs to high-risk patient population (please see "Coronary Artery Disease" chapter).

LABORATORY TESTS

- Screen for hypertension, diabetes, and hyperlipidemia per routine guidelines.
- Electrocardiogram should be obtained during pain and when the patient is free of any discomfort. A normal resting electrocardiogram is not unusual in patients with SIHD; in patients who present with chest pain, 1% to 6% who have an acute MI will have a normal or nondiagnostic electrocardiogram.
- Chest x-ray PA and lateral, if symptoms suggestive of heart failure, pericardial disease, aortic aneurysm/dissection.
- Cardio-CRP (hs-CRP): Its elevation is a relatively moderate predictor of CHD, and it adds prognostic information to that conveyed by the Framingham risk score.

EXERCISE TESTING AND IMAGING STUDIES (PLEASE SEE "CORONARY ARTERY DISEASE" CHAPTER, FIG. 1)

- Exercise testing is used for diagnosis as well as prognosis of SIHD. If the patient is physically capable to perform at least moderate physical exercise, exercise stress testing (Fig. 1) is useful because of the important prognostic information obtained from exercise performance and the hemodynamic response. Risk stratification based on noninvasive testing is summarized in Table 1. Patients who have an intermediate likelihood of CAD, as patients in a low-risk or high-likelihood category are more likely to have a false-positive or false-negative result, respectively. Risk assessment is also indicated in patients with SIHD who are being considered for revascularization of known coronary stenosis of unclear physiological significance. The exercise treadmill test is contraindicated in patients with presence of ST depression >0.5 mm or WPW syndrome or LBBB or pacemaker rhythm in baseline ECG.
- Stress echocardiography or stress testing with myocardial perfusion imaging may be employed when baseline electrocardiographic abnormalities are present that render the electrocardiographic response to exercise uninterpretable. Stress echocardiography has the advantage of higher specificity and a lower cost. Stress radionuclide perfusion imaging has a higher sensitivity, particularly for single-vessel coronary disease, and has a higher technical success rate. When the patient is unable to exercise adequately, pharmacologic stress testing

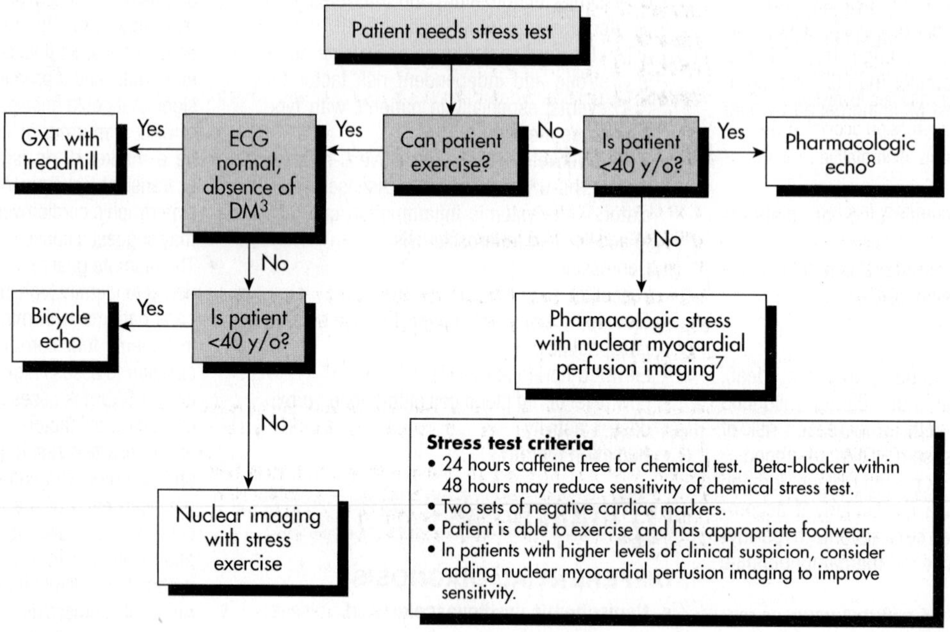

DEFINITIONS:

[1]**Typical angina:**
(1) Substernal chest pain or discomfort that is (2) provoked by exertion or emotional stress and (3) relieved by rest and/or nitroglycerin

[2]**Cardiac marker timing:** based on symptom onset; in cases of uncertainty assume symptom onset at ED arrival

[3]**ECG normal:** no significant ST depression/T wave inversions, BBB, LVH with repolarization, conduction defect, digoxin effect

[4]**Anginal equivalent:**
- Any symptoms that the physician feels may represent ACS
- Exertional dyspnea—most common anginal equivalent symptom

[5]**ACS:**
- STE-ACS—1 mm ST elevation in 2 leads
- NSTE-ACS
  - NSTEMI—positive cardiac biomarkers
  - Unstable angina—ischemia with negative biomarkers

[6]**New significant ECG changes:**
- ST Δs ≥ 0.5 mm; resolve when asymptomatic
- ST depression ≥1 mm in 2 leads
- T wave inversion ≥2 mm in 2 leads

[7]**Regadenoson** is preferred agent for chemical nuclear stress test. Technetium Tc 99m tetrofosmin is the preferred tracer.

FIG. 1 Stress test algorithm. *ACS,* Acute coronary syndrome; *BBB,* bundle branch block; *DM,* diabetes mellitus; *ECG,* electrocardiogram; *echo,* echocardiography; *ED,* emergency department; *GTX,* graded exercise test; *LVH,* left ventricular hypertrophy; *NSTE,* non–ST-segment elevation; *NSTEMI,* NSTE myocardial infarction; *STE,* ST-segment elevation; *y/o,* years old. (From Adams JG et al: *Emergency medicine: clinical essentials,* ed 2, Philadelphia, 2013, Saunders.)

TABLE 1 Risk Stratification Based on Noninvasive Testing

High Risk (>3% Annual Risk for Death or Myocardial Infarction)
1. Severe resting left ventricular dysfunction (LVEF <35%) not readily explained by noncoronary causes
2. Resting perfusion abnormalities involving ≥10% of the myocardium without previous known MI
3. High-risk stress findings on the ECG, including:
   - ≥2-mm ST-segment depression at low workload or persisting into recovery
   - Exercise-induced ST-segment elevation
   - Exercise-induced VT/VF
4. Severe stress-induced LV dysfunction (peak exercise LVEF <45% or drop in LVEF with stress ≥10%)
5. Stress-induced perfusion abnormalities encumbering ≥10% of the myocardium or stress segmental scores indicating multiple vascular territories with abnormalities
6. Stress-induced LV dilation
7. Inducible wall motion abnormality (involving >2 segments or 2 coronary beds)
8. Wall motion abnormality developing at a low dose of dobutamine (≤10 mg/kg/min) or at a low heart rate (<120 beats/min)
9. Multivessel obstructive CAD (≥70% stenosis) or left main stenosis (≥50% stenosis) on CCTA

Intermediate Risk (1%-3% Annual Risk for Death or Myocardial Infarction)
1. Mild to moderate resting LV dysfunction (LVEF of 35%-49%) not readily explained by noncoronary causes
2. Resting perfusion abnormalities involving 5%-9.9% of the myocardium in patients without a history or previous evidence of MI
3. ≥1-mm ST-segment depression occurring with exertional symptoms
4. Stress-induced perfusion abnormalities encumbering 5%-9.9% of the myocardium or stress segmental scores indicating 1 vascular territory with abnormalities but without LV dilation
5. Small wall motion abnormality involving 1-2 segments and only 1 coronary bed
6. 1-vessel CAD with ≥70% stenosis or moderate CAD stenosis (50%-69% stenosis) in ≥2 arteries on CCTA

Low Risk (<1% Annual Risk for Death or Myocardial Infarction)
1. Low-risk treadmill score (score ≥5) or no new ST-segment changes or exercise-induced chest pain symptoms when achieving maximal levels of exercise
2. Normal or small myocardial perfusion defect at rest or with stress encumbering <5% of the myocardium*
3. Normal stress or no change in limited resting wall motion abnormalities during stress
4. No coronary stenosis >50% on CCTA

CCTA, Cardiac computed tomography angiography; *LVEF,* left ventricular ejection fraction; *VF,* ventricular fibrillation; *VT,* ventricular tachycardia.
Assessment of coronary artery calcium (CAC) can also be used to contribute to risk assessment.
*Although the published data are limited, patients with these findings will probably not be at low risk in the presence of either a high-risk treadmill score or severe resting LV dysfunction (LVEF <35%).
Modified from Fihn SD et al: ACCF/AHA/ACP/AATS/PCNA/SCAI/STS guideline for the diagnosis and management of patients with stable ischemic heart disease: a report of the American College of Cardiology Foundation/American Heart Association Task Force on Practice Guidelines, and the American College of Physicians, American Association for Thoracic Surgery, Preventive Cardiovascular Nurses Association, Society for Cardiovascular Angiography and Interventions, and Society of Thoracic Surgeons, *Circulation* 126:e354, 2012; in Zipes DP: *Braunwald's heart disease, a textbook of cardiovascular medicine,* ed 11, Philadelphia, 2019, Elsevier.

(i.e., dobutamine, adenosine, regadenoson) may be used with these imaging modalities.
- A good predictor of risk for a patient with stable angina is the Duke treadmill score, which incorporates the patient's functional status (METS or time in minutes during the Bruce protocol), ST-segment depression in millimeters, and an angina index (yes or no). Patients with favorable Duke scores (>5) have a 5-yr survival rate of >97%; this is independent of other factors such as coronary anatomy and LV function.
- Echocardiography is indicated in patients with murmurs suggestive of aortic stenosis, hypertrophic cardiomyopathy, mitral regurgitation, mitral valve prolapse, previous MI, pathological Q waves, complex ventricular arrhythmias, heart failure, hypertension, diabetes, and abnormal EKG.
- Cardiac computed tomography (CCTA; Fig. 2) is useful for the detection of subclinical CAD in asymptomatic patients with an intermediate Framingham 10-yr risk estimate of 10% to 20%. Detects and quantifies coronary calcium and evaluates the lumen and wall of the coronary artery. CCTA can be useful as a first-line test for risk assessment in patients with SIHD who are unable to exercise to an adequate workload regardless of interpretability of ECG. Also can be used when a functional test has an indeterminate result and to assess bypass graft patency or patency of previous stents >3 mm diameter. CCTA CT cost and radiation exposure are limiting factors to recommending widespread routine use of this marker. CCTA has an excellent negative predictive value to rule out severe CAD in the setting of active chest pain evaluation in the emergency room (ROMICAT-II trial). In 2018 the SCOT-HEART trial showed coronary CTA resulted in a lower risk of nonfatal myocardial infarction than standard care alone (ETT) in stable angina patients.
- Coronary artery calcium (CAC) score is a strong predictor of incidence of CAD and provides predictive information in patients with low to intermediate pretest probability of CAD beyond that provided by standard risk factors. A score below 100 indicates low risk, and a score above 400 high risk.
- Cardiac magnetic resonance imaging (CMRA), in addition to its use for diagnosis of arrhythmogenic right ventricular dysplasia, can also be used to assess myocardial perfusion and viability as well as function in patients unable to exercise. Additional studies are needed to determine the cost effectiveness of these studies in patients with ischemic cardiomyopathy.
- Invasive coronary angiography remains the gold standard for the identification of clinically significant CAD. Angiography is performed to define the location and extent of coronary disease; indicated in selected patients who are candidates for coronary revascularization (either coronary artery bypass graft [CABG] surgery or angioplasty).

Rx TREATMENT

FIVE FUNDAMENTAL OVERLAPPING STRATEGIES ARE RECOMMENDED

- Patient education: Support active participation of patients in the decision-making process of their treatment.
- Management of comorbid conditions that contribute or worsen SIHD.
- Aggressive modification of preventable risk factors such as smoking cessation, weight reduction in obese patients, regular aerobic exercise program (at least 30 to 60 min/day for 5 days a wk), correction of folate deficiency, reduced intake of saturated fats (to <7% of total calories) and trans fatty acids (to <1% of total calories), low-sodium diet (<2 g/day), and teaching importance of medication adherence. Whole grains as the main form of carbohydrates, an abundance of fruits and vegetables, and adequate omega-3 fatty acids are optimal for prevention of SIHD.

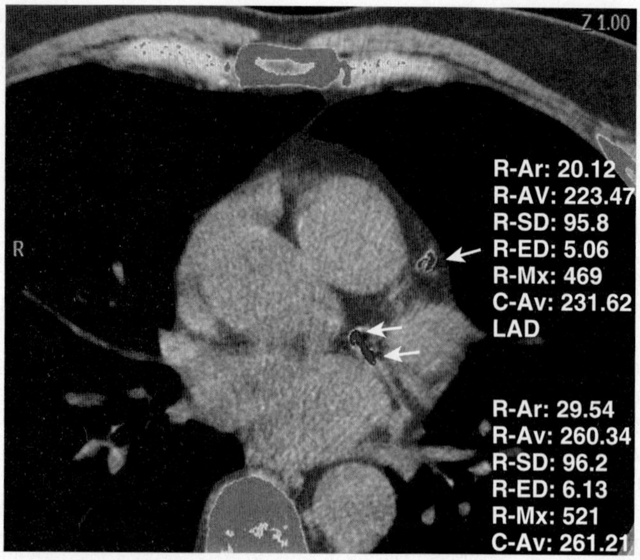

FIG. 2 Example of coronary artery calcium scoring in which calcified foci are identified within the left anterior descending *(orange; single arrow)* and left circumflex *(pink outlined in blue; double arrow)* coronary arteries. The region's area *(R-Ar)* and its average density in Hounsfield units *(R-Av)* are displayed and used in the area-density calcium scoring calculation. (From Bonow RO et al: *Heart disease,* ed 9, Philadelphia, 2012, Saunders.)

- Evidence-based pharmacologic management to improve quality of life and survival.
- Use appropriate revascularization procedures to improve survival and long-term outcomes in selected patients.

PHARMACOLOGIC THERAPY (PLEASE SEE "CORONARY ARTERY DISEASE" CHAPTER)

Treatment can be classified based on medications that prevent MI and death.

- Aspirin reduces cardiovascular mortality and morbidity rates by 20% to 25% among patients with CAD. Appropriate dose is 75 to 162 mg/day in the absence of contraindications. It inhibits the enzyme cyclooxygenase and synthesis of thromboxane A2 and reduces the risk of adverse cardiovascular events by 33% in patients with unstable angina. Patients intolerant to aspirin can be treated with clopidogrel or can undergo aspirin desensitization. Clopidogrel irreversibly blocks the P2Y12 adenosine diphosphate receptor on the platelet surface, thereby interrupting platelet activation and aggregation. Clopidogrel can be combined with ASA in high-risk patients with SIHD with low risk for bleeding complications or can be given alone in patients that are aspirin intolerant. Dose is 75 mg/day.
- Ticagrelor, the newest CTPT inhibitor (P2Y12 antagonist), in the PEGASUS-TIMI-54 reduced the risk of death, cardiovascular MI, or stroke in patients after 1 yr of MI. However, it is associated with an increased risk of bleeding when compared to placebo.
- Dipyridamole is not recommended as an antiplatelet therapy for the treatment of patients with SIHD.
- Beta-adrenergic blockers, which prevent MI and death, are first-line therapy in the management of angina pectoris. They achieve their major antianginal effect by decreasing myocardial oxygen demand in reducing heart rate and systolic blood pressure product, AV nodal conduction, and myocardial contractility, in this manner contributing to a reduction in angina onset, with improvement in the ischemic threshold during exercise and during the usual daily activities. Absent contraindications, they should be regarded as initial therapy for stable angina for all patients. Their dose should generally be adjusted to reduce the resting heart rate to 55 to 60 beats/min. Despite the difference among the available beta-blockers, they all seem to be equally efficacious in SIHD. Beta-blockers recommended for at least 2 to 3 yr after MI, and lifelong for patients with LV ejection fraction of <40% with heart failure or prior MI.
- Nitrates cause venodilation and relaxation of vascular smooth muscle; the decreased venous return from venodilation decreases diastolic ventricular wall tension (preload) and thereby reduces mechanical activity (and myocardial oxygen consumption) during systole. Relaxation of vascular smooth muscle increases coronary blood flow and reduces systemic pressure. Dilatation of the arterial wall will not be affected by plaque, but independent of an intact endothelium, leads to reduced resistance across the obstructed lumen. Nitroglycerin contributes to coronary blood flow redistribution by augmenting collateral flow and lowering ventricular diastolic pressure from areas of normal perfusion to ischemic zones. Nitroglycerin also has demonstrated antithrombotic and antiplatelet effects. Sublingual nitroglycerin or nitroglycerin spray should be prescribed to all patients with SIHD for immediate angina relief. Tolerance to nitrates can be minimized by avoiding sustained blood levels with a daily nitrate-free period (e.g., omission of bedtime dose of oral isosorbide dinitrate or 12 hr on/12 hr off transdermal nitroglycerin therapy). Nitrates are relatively contraindicated in patients with hypertrophic obstructive cardiomyopathy, and should also be avoided in patients with severe aortic stenosis. Nitrates should not be used within 24 hr of sildenafil (Viagra) or vardenafil (Levitra) or within 48 hr of tadalafil (Cialis) because of the potential for hypotension.
- Calcium channel blockers are antiischemic medications that have no proven mortality benefit in SIHD. They improve myocardial oxygen supply by decreasing coronary vascular resistance and augmenting epicardial conduit vessel and systemic arterial blood flow. Myocardial demand is decreased by a reduction in myocardial contractility, systemic vascular resistance, and arterial pressure. They are first-line treatment when beta-blockers are contraindicated. They play a major role in preventing and terminating myocardial ischemia induced by coronary artery spasm. They are particularly effective in treating microvascular angina. All classes of calcium channel blockers reduce anginal episodes, increase exercise duration, and reduce use of sublingual nitroglycerin in patients with effort-induced angina. Short-acting calcium channel blockers should be avoided. Calcium channel blockers (particularly nondihydropyridine) should generally also be avoided in patients with CHF secondary to systolic dysfunction due to its negative inotropic effect.
- Ranolazine, which has been tested in four different studies with a total of 1737 patients (MARISA, CARISA, RAN080, and ERICA), inhibits the late inward sodium current, indirectly reducing the sodium-dependent calcium current during ischemic conditions and leading to improvement in ventricular diastolic

tension and oxygen consumption. It seems to increase the efficiency of energy production in the heart, maintaining cardiac function. Its antianginal and antiischemic effects do not depend on reductions in heart rate or blood pressure. It is indicated for treatment of chronic angina that is inadequately controlled with other antianginals. It represents a new class of drugs known as metabolic modulators and can be useful when prescribed as substitute for beta-blockers or in combination with them for relief of symptoms when initial treatment with beta-blockers is not successful or is contraindicated. Side effects include prolongation of QT interval. Low doses of diltiazem and verapamil should be used with ranolazine. The extended-release preparation reduces the frequency of angina, improves exercise performance, and delays the development of exercise-induced angina and ST-segment depression.

- Angiotensin-converting enzyme (ACE) inhibition through changes in the physiologic balance between angiotensin II and bradykinin could contribute to the reductions in LV and vascular hypertrophy, atherosclerosis progression, plaque rupture, and thrombosis; the favorable changes in cardiac hemodynamics; and the improved myocardial oxygen supply/demand. It has been shown to be effective in reducing cardiovascular death, MI, and stroke in patients who are at risk for or who had vascular disease. They are indicated in patients with hypertension, diabetes, LVEF <40%, and CKD. Angiotensin receptor blockers (ARBs) can be given to patients with SIHD who are intolerant to ACEI and qualify for them.
- Use of high-intensity statin drugs is recommended in all patients with CAD. In late 2018 the American College of Cardiology (ACC) recommended an LDL goal of <70 mg/dl for secondary prevention of atherosclerotic cardiovascular disease. There is no LDL goal for primary prevention. The FDA approved PCSK9 (proprotein convertase subtilisin/kexin type 9) inhibitors (Alirocumab and Evolocumab) for heterozygous familial hypercholesterolemia in those who maximally tolerated statins. Newer 2018 lipid guidelines suggested starting PCSK9 inhibitor in very-high-risk atherosclerotic cardiovascular disease patients who did not meet the LDL goal on high-intensity statin and ezetimibe. One should always consider adding ezetimibe to high-intensity statin prior to initiation of PCSK9 inhibitor due to cost issues.
- Influenza vaccine is recommended for patients with SIHD on annual basis to prevent all-cause mortality, morbidity, and hospitalization caused by the exacerbation of underlying medical conditions produced by influenza.

NEW MODALITIES FOR THE TREATMENT OF CHRONIC STABLE ANGINA PECTORIS

- Although a significant amount of progress has been made in the management of CAD with percutaneous coronary intervention (PCI) and CABG, many patients with the condition require additional therapeutic modalities for relief of symptoms and improvement in quality of life. This group of patients includes those with diffuse CAD who are not suitable for revascularization, patients with previous multiple PCIs or CABG limiting the chances for further revascularization, the lack of vascular conduits for CABG, severe left ventricular systolic dysfunction in patients with previous CABG or PCI, and comorbidities that would render the patients at high risk for revascularization.
- The following pharmacologic agents have been used for the management of stable angina in combination with the standard protocol of nitrates, beta-blockers, calcium channel blockers, and ranolazine: High-dose statin therapy, trimetazidine, perhexiline, nicorandil, allopurinol, ivabradine, fasudil, and testosterone.
- Other, nonpharmacologic modalities that are highly experimental include stem cell therapy, therapeutic angiogenesis, and mechanical therapies like external counterpulsation, spinal cord stimulation, transmyocardial laser revascularization, and coronary sinus reducing device.
- In TACT (Trial to Assess Chelation Therapy), Ethylenediaminetetraacetic acid (EDTA) intravenous infusion resulted significant decrease in total mortality, recurrent MI, stroke, coronary revascularization, or hospitalization for angina. Thus, chelation therapy was upgraded from Class III (not recommended) to Class IIb in the 2014 SIHD guidelines. Allopurinol, a xanthine oxidase inhibitor, was shown to reduce myocardial oxygen demand per unit of cardiac output in patients with heart failure in a small crossover study of 65 patients given 600 mg of allopurinol daily for 6 wk. Allopurinol increased the median time to ST depression from 232 sec at baseline to 393 sec. Further and larger studies are necessary to recommend allopurinol as an adjunctive therapy for stable angina.
- Testosterone improves endothelial dysfunction and may be an effective antianginal agent. However, given the potential side effects, additional trials are necessary to recommend testosterone as an adjunctive drug for chronic angina.

The value of enhanced external counterpulsation(EECP) was assessed with the MUST-EECP trial, which randomly assigned 139 outpatients with angina, documented CAD, and a positive stress test to 35 hr of active EECP. The results indicated the following regarding EECP: (1) Was well tolerated; (2) exercise duration increased in both groups; (3) active EECP patients had a significant increase in time to 1-mm ST-segment depression, while there was no change in the inactive group; (4) more patients undergoing active EECP had a decrease in angina episodes, and fewer had an increase in angina symptoms compared with the active group. These data corroborate similar data from multicenter registries. The American Heart Association, American College of Cardiology, Society for Cardiovascular Angiography and Interventions, American Thoracic Society, and Society of Thoracic Surgeons focused update states that EECP may be considered for relief of refractory angina.

The following treatments have NOT been shown to be beneficial in reducing cardiovascular risk or improving clinical outcomes: Estrogen therapy, vitamin C, vitamin E, and beta-carotene supplementation; treatment of elevated homocysteine with folate or vitamins B_6 and B_{12}; chelation therapy; garlic; coenzyme Q10; selenium; and chromium.

REFERRAL

Revascularization:

- Revascularization methods should be formulated taking into consideration improved survival or improved symptoms. Revascularization includes either percutaneous coronary intervention (balloon angioplasty and stenting) or CABG. However, note that although the role of PCI is unquestionable in the presence of an acute myocardial infarction, its role is not so clear in stable CAD. The utilization of PCI for stable CAD was reduced by 51.7% from 2007 to 2011, and hospitals with higher volumes of PCI had the largest reduction of these procedures.
- **To improve survival:**
  1. Perform CABG for patients with significant (>50% diameter stenosis) left main coronary artery stenosis, more than 70% diameter stenosis in proximal left anterior descending artery (LAD), or more than 70% diameter stenosis in three major epicardial vessels, >70% diameter stenosis in two major coronary arteries with severe or extensive myocardial ischemia, and in patients with mild to moderate LV systolic dysfunction (EF 35% to 50%) and significant multivessel CAD. Left internal mammary artery (LIMA) graft improves survival when used to bypass a proximal LAD artery stenosis. CABG is recommended in preference to PCI to improve survival in patients with multivessel CAD with Syntax score of >22 and multivessel CAD with diabetes, particularly if a LIMA graft to LAD is used.
  2. PCI is reasonable as an alternative to CABG in selected stable patients (low or intermediate SYNTAX score and[or] high STS score) with unprotected left main CAD, low risk of PCI procedural complications, and a high likelihood of good long-term outcome *and* clinical characteristics that predict a significantly increased risk of adverse surgical outcomes (e.g., STS-predicted risk of operative mortality >5).
- **To improve symptoms:** CABG or PCI to improve symptoms is beneficial in patients with one or more significant (>70% diameter) coronary artery stenosis amenable to revascularization and unacceptable angina despite maximal medical treatment, or in whom increasing medical therapy cannot be implemented because of medication contraindications, adverse effects, or patient preferences.

In 2017, ORBITA trial showed no significant improvement in angina score after PCI for optimally treated stable angina patients. However, 85% of study patients in placebo group underwent PCI within 6 wk after ORBITA trial completed. In 2020, the Ischemia trial showed no benefit with routine invasive therapy compared to conservative treatment in moderate to severe ischemia patients. However, this study excludes patients with ACS, severe and frequent symptoms, EF <35%, and left main stenosis. Hybrid coronary revascularization: LIMA-to-LAD artery grafting and of >1 non-LAD coronary artery can be used in patients who have an unfavorable aorta, have poor target vessels for CABG, have unsuitable graft conduits, or have unfavorable LAD for PCI.

- Compared with percutaneous coronary intervention (PCI), CABG is more effective in relieving angina and leads to fewer repeated revascularizations but has a higher risk for procedural stroke. Survival to 10 yr is similar for both procedures.
- Angioplasty and coronary stents (Fig. E3).
- PCI has an established place in treating angina but is not superior to intensive medical therapy to prevent MI and death in symptomatic or asymptomatic patients. Patients selected for PCI should also be candidates for CABG. Approximately 80% of patients show immediate benefit after PCI. The development of coronary stents has increased the number of patients who can be treated in the cardiac laboratory. Cardiac stents (Fig. E4) are currently used in nearly 95% of all patients with PCI lesions. The rate of restenosis is reduced by placing a stent electively in primary atheromatous lesions. The major limitations of stenting are subacute thrombosis, restenosis within the stent, bleeding complications when antiplatelets are used after stenting, and higher cost. The combination of aspirin and P2Y12 antagonists is effective in preventing coronary stent thrombosis and the duration of therapy depends on whether bare metal stents (BMS) or drug-eluting stents (DES) are used. Duration of dual antiplatelet therapy can be as short as 4 wk for BMS, but 6 to 12 mo of therapy is generally required for DES. This difference in duration is due to the lack of endothelium proliferation in DES initially. New drug-eluting stents with thin struts releasing Limus-family analogs from durable polymers have lowered the risk of stent thrombosis compared with early-generation stents releasing sirolimus or paclitaxel. Current evidence supports the use of drug-eluting stents in most clinical settings without safety concerns (unless there are contraindications to use of dual antiplatelet therapy).

PEARLS & CONSIDERATIONS

COMMENTS

- Although nitrate responsiveness is usually an integral part of a diagnostic strategy for SIHD, recent reports question its value and conclude that in a general population admitted for chest pain, relief of pain after nitroglycerin treatment does not predict active CAD and should not be used to guide diagnosis in the acute care setting.
- CABG is associated with higher long-term survival rates and lower rates of repeat revascularization than PCI and stenting; however, patients often prefer stenting because it is less invasive, involves a shorter hospital stay, and has a lower in-hospital mortality rate.

SUGGESTED READINGS

Available at: ExpertConsult.com

RELATED CONTENT

Angina (Patient Information)
Unstable Angina (Patient Information)
Acute Coronary Syndrome (Related Key Topic)
Coronary Artery Disease (Related Key Topic)
Myocardial Infarction (Related Key Topic)

AUTHOR: **Maheswara Satya Gangadhara Rao Golla, MD**

BASIC INFORMATION

DEFINITION

- The mucocutaneous swelling caused by the release of vasoactive mediators is called urticaria and angioedema.
- Urticaria causes edema of the superficial dermis.
- Angioedema is the physical manifestation of transient increases in vascular permeability and involves the deep layers of the dermis and the subcutaneous tissue.

SYNONYMS

Angioneurotic edema
HAE (hereditary angioedema)

ICD-10CM CODES

T78.3	Angioedema
D84.1	Angioedema, hereditary

EPIDEMIOLOGY & DEMOGRAPHICS

INCIDENCE: 100 to 3000/100,000 persons (for urticaria and angioedema)

LIFETIME PREVALENCE: Approximately 20% of the population experiences urticaria and/or angioedema at some time during life. The prevalence of hereditary angioedema is 1 case per 50,000 persons.

DEMOGRAPHICS:

- Race: Slightly more common among African Americans.
- Sex: More occurrences in women than men.
- Angioedema commonly occurs after adolescence in the third decade of life.
- Angioedema can occur together with urticaria (40%) or alone (20%); the remaining 40% have urticaria alone.
- The mean age of onset of hereditary angioedema with C1 inhibitor is 8 to 12 yr and rarely occurs before 1 yr of age.

PHYSICAL FINDINGS & CLINICAL PRESENTATION

- Angioedema may be acute or chronic:
  1. Acute angioedema is defined as symptoms lasting 6 wk
  2. Chronic angioedema is defined as symptoms lasting >6 wk
- Urticaria is commonly known as "hives" and is:
  1. Pruritic
  2. Palpable and well demarcated
  3. Erythematous
  4. Millimeters to centimeters in size
  5. Multiple in number
  6. Fades within 12 to 24 hr
  7. Reappears at other sites
- Angioedema is characterized by the following:
  1. Nonpruritic
  2. Burning
  3. Not well demarcated
  4. Involves eyelids, lips (Fig. 1), tongue, and extremities
  5. Can involve the upper airway, causing respiratory distress
  6. Can involve the gastrointestinal tract, leading to cyclic abdominal pain, nausea, vomiting, and diarrhea
  7. Resolves slowly

ETIOLOGY

- Angioedema, with or without urticaria, is classified as acquired (allergic or idiopathic) or hereditary.
- Angioedema is primarily caused by mast cell activation and degranulation with release of vasoactive mediators (e.g., histamine, serotonin, bradykinins), resulting in postcapillary venule inflammation, vascular leakage, and edema in the deep layers of the dermis and subcutaneous tissue.
- Pathologically, angioedema has both immunologic- and nonimmunologic-mediated mechanisms (Fig. 2).
  1. Immunoglobulin E–mediated angioedema may result from antigen exposure (e.g., foods [milk, eggs, peanuts, shellfish, tomatoes, chocolate, sulfites] or drugs [penicillin, aspirin, nonsteroidal anti-inflammatory drugs, phenytoin, sulfonamides, recombinant tissue plasminogen activator]).
  2. Complement-mediated angioedema involving immune complex mechanisms can also lead to mast cell activation that manifests as serum sickness.
  3. Hereditary angioedema is an autosomal-dominant disease caused by a deficiency of or mutation in C1 esterase inhibitor (C1-INH). C1-INH is a protease inhibitor normally present in high concentrations in the plasma. C1-INH serves many functions, one of which is to inhibit plasma kallikrein, a protease that cleaves kininogen and releases bradykinin. Deficient C1-INH activity results in excess concentration of kininogen and the subsequent release of kinin mediators. Hereditary angioedema types I and II are phenotypically indistinguishable. Type I hereditary angioedema with C1 inhibitor deficiency accounts for 85% of cases of hereditary angioedema, type II accounts for 15% of cases. Both types are characterized by low serum C_4 levels from activation of the complement cascade, for which C1 inhibitor is a key regulatory protein. Patients with type II have normal antigen levels but low C1 inhibitor function as a result of mutations affecting the reactive loop of the molecule.[1]
  4. Acquired angioedema is usually associated with other diseases, most commonly B-cell lymphoproliferative disorders, but may also result from the formation of autoantibodies directed against C1 inhibitor protein.
  5. Other causes of angioedema include infection (e.g., herpes simplex, hepatitis B, Coxsackie A and B, *Streptococcus, Candida, Ascaris,* and *Strongyloides*), insect bites and stings, stress, physical factors (e.g., cold, exercise, pressure, and vibration), connective tissue diseases (e.g., systemic lupus erythematosus, Henoch-Schönlein purpura), and idiopathic causes. Angiotensin-converting enzyme (ACE) inhibitors can increase kinin activity and lead to angioedema.

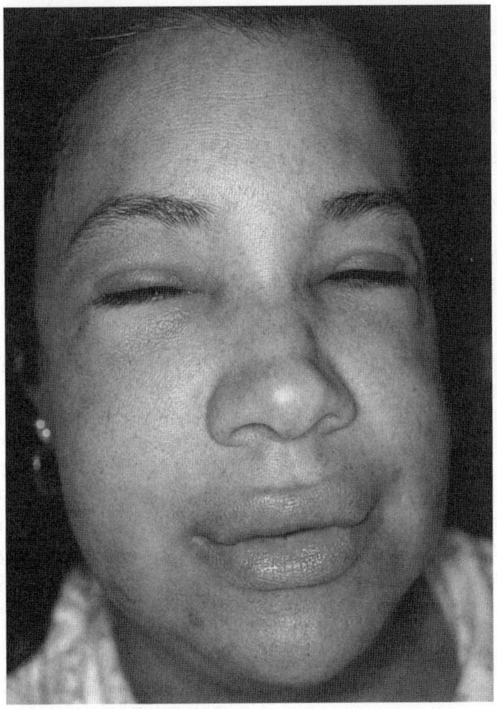

FIG. 1 Angioedema. The swelling is deeper than wheals and may affect mucosal surfaces. Note the swelling of the lips and periorbital region and the lack of erythema. (From Bolognia J et al: *Dermatology,* ed 4, London, 2018, Elsevier Limited.)

[1] Busse PJ, Christiansen SC: Hereditary angioedema, N *Engl J Med* 382:1136-48, 2020.

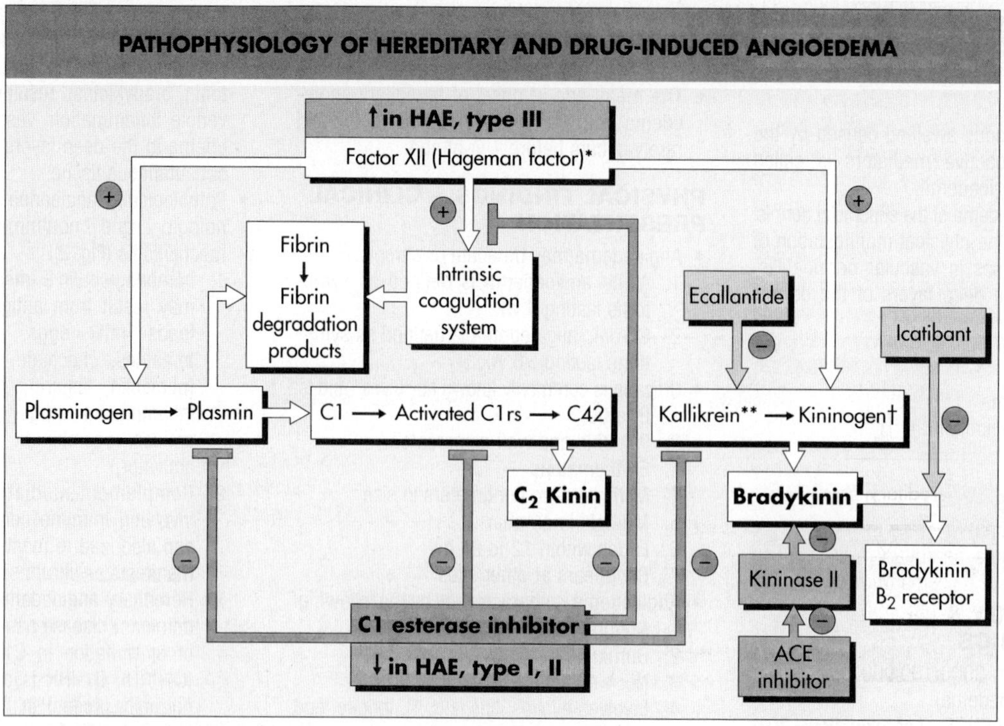

FIG. 2 Pathophysiology of hereditary and drug-induced angioedema. Angiotensin-converting enzyme *(ACE)* inhibitor-induced urticaria is believed to result from the inhibition of endogenous kininase and a subsequent increase in bradykinin. Icatibant and ecallantide have been approved for the emergency treatment of hereditary angioedema *(HAE)* as alternatives to C1 esterase inhibitor (C1-INH) concentrate (derived from human plasma) or recombinant C1-INH (derived from milk of transgenic rabbits). Icatibant, a decapeptide, is a specific bradykinin B2 receptor antagonist. Ecallantide, a 60-amino acid recombinant protein, selectively inhibits kallikrein. Off label, icatibant has been used to treat ACE inhibitor-induced angioedema. Two forms of C1-INH, one of which is administered intravenously and the other subcutaneously, are approved for prevention of attacks. At the time of writing, twice-monthly administration of lanadelumab, a human monoclonal antibody that inhibits plasma kallikrein, is under investigation for prevention of attacks. *The active form of factor XII (Hageman factor) is XIIa. **Kallikrein is formed from prekallikrein. †High-molecular-weight. (From Bolognia J et al: *Dermatology,* ed 4, London, 2018, Elsevier Limited.)

Dx DIAGNOSIS

A detailed history and physical examination usually establish the diagnosis of angioedema. Extensive laboratory testing is of limited value.

DIFFERENTIAL DIAGNOSIS

- Cellulitis
- Arthropod bite
- Hypothyroidism
- Contact dermatitis
- Atopic dermatitis
- Mastocytosis
- Granulomatous cheilitis
- Bullous pemphigoid
- Urticaria pigmentosa
- Anaphylaxis
- Erythema multiforme
- Epiglottitis
- Peritonsillar abscess

WORKUP

- An extensive workup searching for the cause of angioedema is often unrevealing (90%).
- Workup, including diagnostic blood tests and allergy testing, is performed according to results of the history and physical examination. Fig. 3 illustrates an algorithm for the diagnosis of angioedema.

LABORATORY TESTS

- Complete blood count, erythrocyte sedimentation rate, and urinalysis are sometimes helpful as part of the initial evaluation.
- Stools for ova and parasites.
- Serology testing.
- C4 levels are usually reduced in acquired and hereditary angioedema (occurring without urticaria). If C4 levels are low, C1-INH levels and activity should be obtained. There are isolated reports of hereditary angioedema with normal C4 levels but reduced C1-INH levels.
- Skin and radioallergosorbent testing may be done if food allergies are suspected.
- Skin biopsy is usually done in patients with chronic angioedema refractory to corticosteroid treatment.

Rx TREATMENT

NONPHARMACOLOGIC THERAPY

- Eliminate the offending agent
- Avoid triggering factors (e.g., cold, stress)
- Cold compresses to affected areas

ACUTE GENERAL Rx

- Acute life-threatening angioedema involving the larynx is treated with:
  1. Epinephrine 0.3 mg in a solution of 1:1000 given SC
  2. Diphenhydramine 25 to 50 mg IV or IM
  3. Cimetidine 300 mg IV or ranitidine 50 mg IV
  4. Methylprednisolone 125 mg IV
- Mainstay therapy in nonhereditary angioedema is H_1 antihistamines:
  1. Diphenhydramine 25 to 50 mg q6h
  2. Chlorpheniramine 4 mg q6h
  3. Hydroxyzine 10 to 25 mg q6h
  4. Cetirizine 5 to 10 mg qd
  5. Loratadine 10 mg qd
  6. Fexofenadine 60 mg qd
- H_2 antihistamines can be added to H_1 antihistamines:
  1. Cimetidine 400 mg bid
  2. Famotidine 20 mg bid
- Tricyclic antidepressants:
  1 Doxepin 25 to 50 mg qd

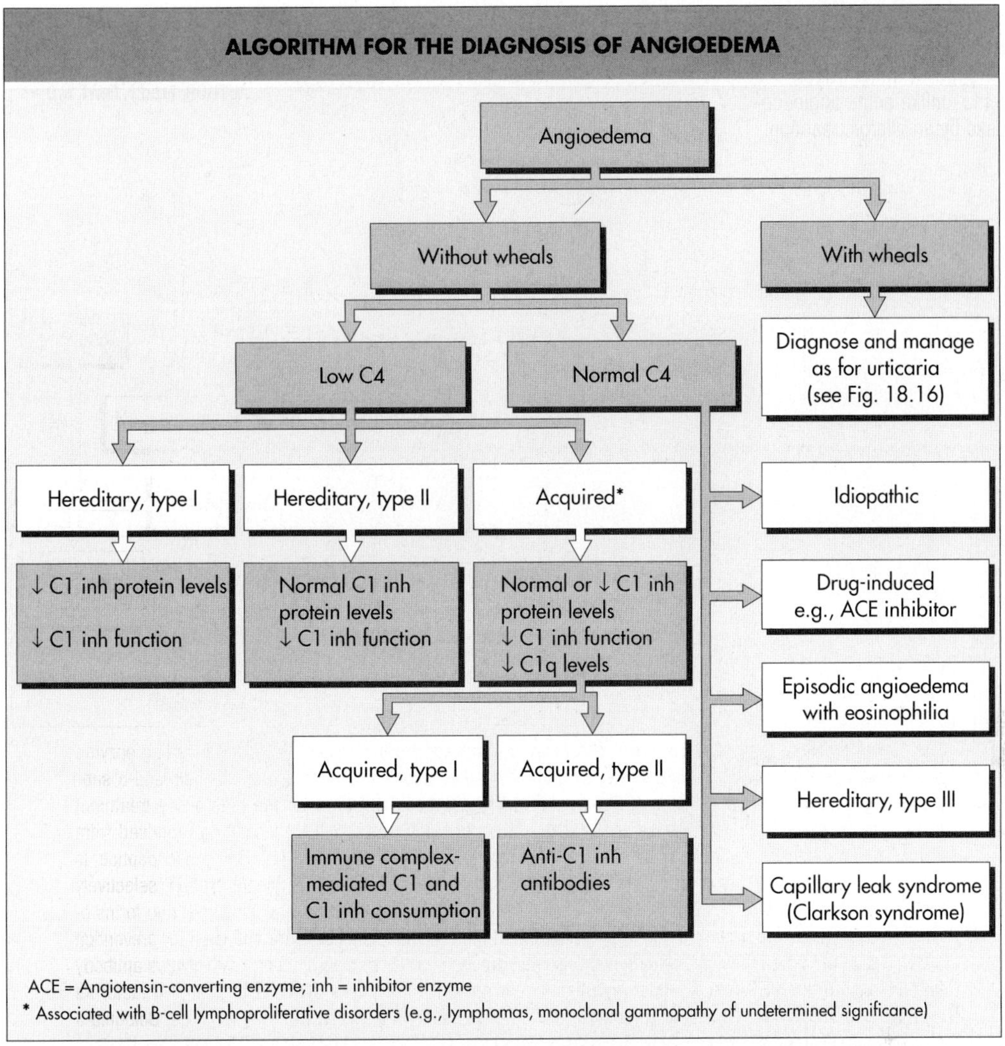

FIG. 3 Algorithm for the diagnosis of angioedema. Episodic angioedema with hypereosinophilia, along with weight gain and fever, is known as Gleich syndrome. (From Bolognia J et al: *Dermatology,* ed 4, London, 2018, Elsevier Limited.)

- Corticosteroids are rarely required for symptomatic relief of acute angioedema.
- Antihistamines are probably ineffective in acute hereditary angioedema.
- Purified plasma-derived C1-INH replacement therapy is effective and safe in treating acute attacks of hereditary angioedema caused by C1 inhibitor deficiency. Cost is a limiting factor. Acute attacks can be managed with plasma-derived or recombinant preparations of C1 inhibitor, with ecallantide, a specific plasma kallikrein inhibitor, or with the use of the B2 bradykinin-receptor antagonist icatibant.

CHRONIC Rx

- Chronic angioedema is treated as described under "Acute General Rx." Corticosteroids are used more often in chronic nonhereditary angioedema.
- Prednisone 1 mg/kg/day for 5 days and then tapered over a period of weeks.
- Androgens (danazol, stanozolol, oxandrolone, methyltestosterone) and antifibrinolytic agents can be used for the treatment of chronic hereditary angioedema, which does not respond to antihistamines or corticosteroids but these agents are associated with many adverse effects.
- Long-term prophylaxis with intravenous plasma-derived C1 inhibitors (Cinryze, Berinert) are safe and effective and may be used in patients who have frequent or severe attacks. Cost can be a limiting factor. A twice-weekly subcutaneous formulation (Haegarda/CSL830, CSL Behring) is approved by the FDA to treat type I and type II hereditary angioedema. Icatibant is a bradykinin-receptor antagonist effective in hereditary angioedema. Lanadelumab is a kallikrein inhibitor shown in preliminary studies to reduce attack frequency, although it is not yet FDA approved.

DISPOSITION

- Antihistamines achieve symptomatic relief in more than 80% of patients with nonhereditary acute angioedema.
- In chronic nonhereditary angioedema, corticosteroids are given in addition to antihistamines.
- A small percentage of people will have recurrence of symptoms after steroid treatment.
- Chronic angioedema can last for mo and even yr.

REFERRAL

Consultation with dermatologist and allergist is recommended in patients with chronic angioedema, hereditary angioedema, and recurring angioedema.

PEARLS & CONSIDERATIONS

ACE inhibitors can cause angioedema up to many months after initiation. There are multiple case reports and case series of angiotensin receptor blocker (ARB)–induced angioedema, although the risk is substantially less than that of ACE inhibitors. (Incidence rates per 1000 person-yr are 4.38 cases for ACE inhibitors, 1.66 cases for ARBs.) The incidence rate is also very high for the direct renin inhibitor aliskiren (4.67).

COMMENTS

- Identifying a cause for angioedema in patients is often difficult and met with frustration.
- Chronic angioedema, unlike acute angioedema, is rarely caused by an allergic reaction.

SUGGESTED READINGS

Available at ExpertConsult.com

RELATED CONTENT

Angioedema (Patient Information)

AUTHOR: **Fred F. Ferri, MD**

BASIC INFORMATION

DEFINITION

Ankylosing spondylitis (AS) is a type of inflammatory arthritis involving the sacroiliac joints and axial skeleton characterized by ankylosis and enthesitis (inflammation at tendon insertions). It is one of a family of overlapping syndromes called seronegative spondyloarthropathies (SpA) that includes reactive arthritis (formerly Reiter syndrome), psoriatic spondylitis, and enteropathic arthritis.

SYNONYM

Marie-Strümpell disease

ICD-10CM CODES

M45.9 Ankylosing spondylitis of unspecified sites in spine
M08.1 Juvenile ankylosing spondylitis
M45.0 Ankylosing spondylitis of multiple sites in spine
M45.1 Ankylosing spondylitis of occipito-atlanto-axial region
M45.2 Ankylosing spondylitis of cervical region
M45.3 Ankylosing spondylitis of cervicothoracic region
M45.4 Ankylosing spondylitis of thoracic region
M45.5 Ankylosing spondylitis of thoracolumbar region
M45.6 Ankylosing spondylitis lumbar region
M45.7 Ankylosing spondylitis of lumbosacral region
M45.8 Ankylosing spondylitis sacral and sacrococcygeal region

EPIDEMIOLOGY & DEMOGRAPHICS

PREVALENCE: Between 0.1% and 1% of the population. Varies with prevalence of HLA-B27 and ethnicity. Much higher in those with positive family history of spondyloarthropathy.
PREDOMINANT SEX: Male:female ratio 2 to 3:1
PREDOMINANT AGE: 15 to 35 yr, usually symptoms present before age 45

PHYSICAL FINDINGS & CLINICAL PRESENTATION

- Prolonged morning back stiffness of insidious onset lasting more than 3 mo
- Bilateral sacroiliac joint tenderness (sacroiliitis)
- Inflammatory back pain; often improves with exercise and is worse with rest
- Limited lumbar spine motion
- Tenderness at tendon insertion sites, especially the Achilles tendons and plantar fascia
- Loss of chest expansion reflecting rib cage involvement
- Possible to have peripheral joint arthritis, usually involving lower extremities
- In advanced cases the typical posture consists of compensatory hyperextension of neck, fixed flexion of hips, and compensatory flexion of knees (Fig. 1)
- There is an increased incidence of iritis and uveitis (30% to 40% lifetime prevalence)
- Other extra-skeletal manifestations include effects on the cardiovascular system (aortic insufficiency, cardiovascular disease) and lungs (pulmonary fibrosis). There is also an increased risk for osteoporosis

ETIOLOGY

Genetic factors, particularly HLA-B27, play an important role in susceptibility to the spondyloarthropathies. Infectious triggers have been implicated in some cases. Tumor necrosis factor is important in the inflammatory response.

DIAGNOSIS

DIFFERENTIAL DIAGNOSIS

- Diffuse idiopathic skeletal hyperostosis (Forestier disease)

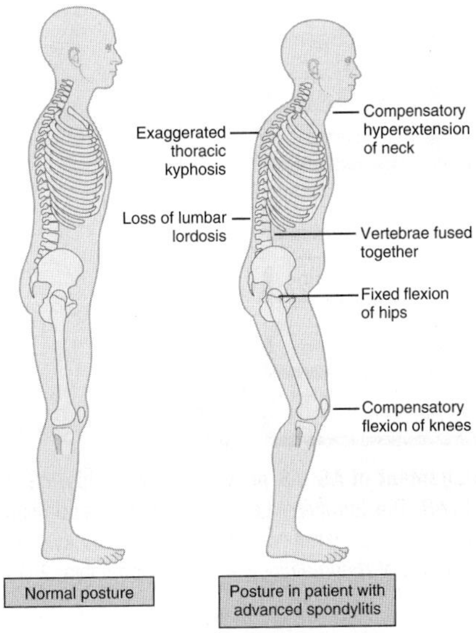

FIG. 1 Ankylosing spondylitis. Typical posture in advanced cases compared with normal posture. (From Ballinger A: *Kumar & Clark's essentials of clinical medicine,* ed 6, Edinburgh, 2012, Saunders.)

- Noninflammatory back pain (a clinical algorithm for the evaluation of back pain is described in Section III)
- Table 1 compares ankylosing spondylitis and related disorders

LABORATORY TESTS

- Elevated sedimentation rate, C-reactive protein
- Mild hyperchromic anemia
- Demonstration of inflammatory sacroiliitis by radiography or MRI is diagnostic for most patients, although some patients may meet criteria for "nonradiographic spondyloarthropathy" based on compelling clinical evaluation
- HLA-B27 antigen is not useful in the evaluation of noninflammatory back pain because it is present in up to 10% of the normal population (varies based on ethnicity)

IMAGING STUDIES

- Classic feature is bilateral sacroiliitis on pelvic radiographs (modified NY criteria).
- Vertebral bodies lose anterior concave shape and become square.
- With progression, calcification of the annulus fibrosus and paravertebral ligaments develops, giving rise to the so-called *bamboo spine* (Figs. E2 through Fig. E6).
- Severe diskovertebral erosions and destruction may occur (Andersson lesion, Fig. 7).
- MRI (Fig. E8) may be useful in detecting early inflammatory lesions and is especially helpful when the history is suggestive but radiographs are equivocal; can see bone marrow edema, fatty metaplasia, sacroiliitis, erosions, shiny corners.

TREATMENT

NONPHARMACOLOGIC THERAPY

- Exercises primarily to maintain flexibility and aerobic activity are important (Fig. E9).
- Postural training:
  1. Patients must be instructed on spinal extension exercises to avoid fusion in a flexed position.

TABLE 1 Comparison of Ankylosing Spondylitis and Related Disorders

Feature	Ankylosing Spondylitis	Psoriatic Arthritis	Reactive Arthritis	Enteropathic Arthropathy
Gender (male:female)	2-3:1	1:1	1:1	1:1
Age of onset	<40 yr	35-55 yr	20-40 yr	Any age
Sacroiliitis or spondylitis (%)	100	~20	~40	<20
Symmetry of sacroiliitis	Symmetrical	Asymmetrical	Asymmetrical	Symmetrical
Peripheral arthritis (%)	~25	95	90	5-20
Distribution	Axial and lower limbs	Variable	Lower limbs	Variable
HLA-B27 positivity (%)	85-95	25-60*	30-70	7-70†
Uveitis	0-40	~20	~50	<15

*60% when spondylitis is present.
†60% when spondylitis is present.
From Hochberg MC: *Rheumatology,* ed 7, Philadelphia, 2019, Elsevier.

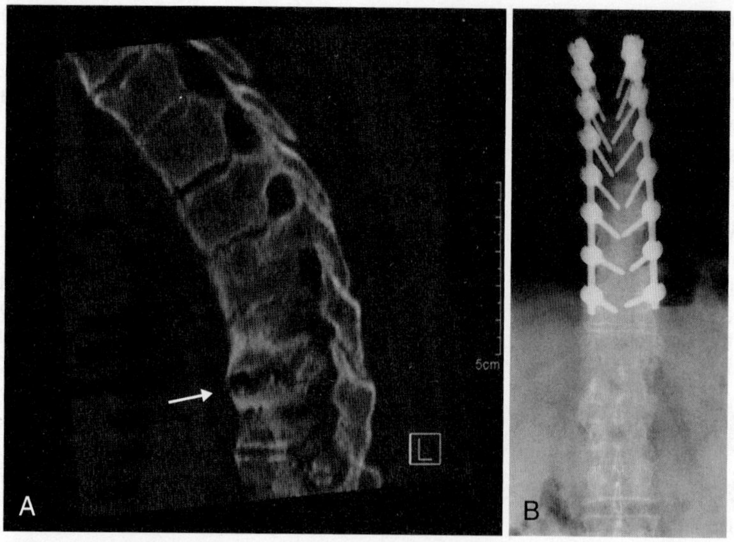

FIG. 7 Severe Andersson lesion (diskovertebral erosions and destruction) (**A,** *arrow*) of the thoracic spine in a patient with ankylosing spondylitis resulting in instability and severe pain, which was treated with a fusion operation **(B)**. (From Hochberg MC: *Rheumatology,* ed 7, Philadelphia, 2019, Elsevier.)

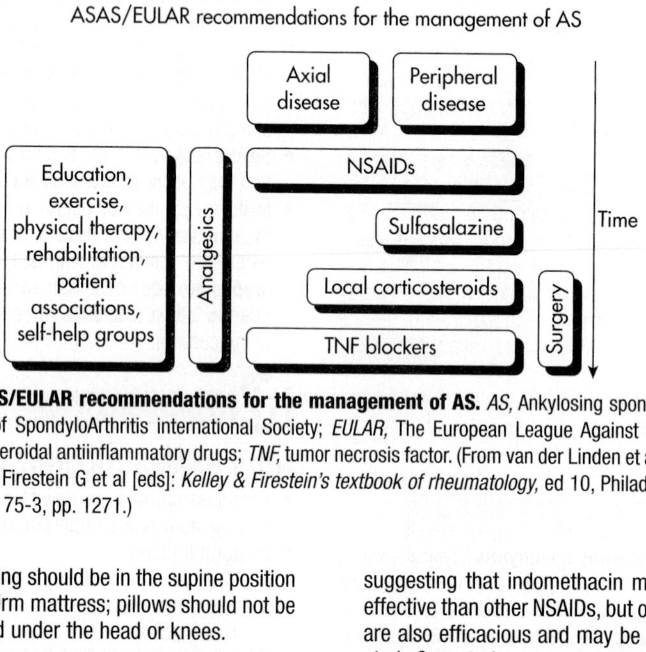

FIG. 10 ASAS/EULAR recommendations for the management of AS. *AS,* Ankylosing spondylitis; *ASAS,* Assessment of SpondyloArthritis international Society; *EULAR,* The European League Against Rheumatism; *NSAIDs,* nonsteroidal antiinflammatory drugs; *TNF,* tumor necrosis factor. (From van der Linden et al: Ankylosing spondylitis. In Firestein G et al [eds]: *Kelley & Firestein's textbook of rheumatology,* ed 10, Philadelphia, 2017, Elsevier, Table 75-3, pp. 1271.)

2. Sleeping should be in the supine position on a firm mattress; pillows should not be placed under the head or knees.

PHARMACOLOGIC THERAPY

- NSAIDs: Patients with ankylosing spondylitis should be trialed on full-dose continuous NSAID therapy. There is anecdotal evidence suggesting that indomethacin may be more effective than other NSAIDs, but other NSAIDs are also efficacious and may be better tolerated. One study suggested that continuous NSAID therapy may retard the radiographic progression of ankylosing spondylitis, but data are conflicting.
- Sulfasalazine may be efficacious in patients with peripheral arthritis.
- Numerous controlled trials have shown that tumor necrosis factor (TNF) antagonists such as etanercept, infliximab, and adalimumab are very effective for relieving symptoms of spinal inflammatory arthritis. Anti-TNF therapy should be recommended for patients whose symptoms are not completely controlled with NSAIDs, and it can result in dramatic improvement in symptoms, range of motion of the spine, and quality of life for these patients. There is evidence suggesting that anti-TNF therapy slows the radiographic progression of the disease. Etanercept should generally be avoided if history of uveitis.
- Secukinumab, an anti-interleukin-17A monoclonal antibody, has been approved for treating AS. Ixekizumab, another IL-17A antibody, was also approved in 2019.
- Fig. 10 shows American College of Rheumatology (ACR)/The European League Against Rheumatism (EULAR) recommendations for management.

DISPOSITION

Most patients have a normal life span but many can suffer significant disability from loss of spinal mobility.

REFERRAL

All patients with seronegative spondyloarthropathy should be referred to a rheumatologist for further evaluation and treatment.

PEARLS & CONSIDERATIONS

A family history of seronegative spondyloarthropathy increases the specificity of testing for HLA-B27. Surgical osteotomy may benefit selected patients with severe spinal deformity. Recent data suggest that men with AS have increased risk of vascular mortality.

SUGGESTED READINGS

Available at ExpertConsult.com

RELATED CONTENT

Ankylosing Spondylitis (Patient Information)

AUTHOR: **Daphne Scaramangas-Plumley, MD**

BASIC INFORMATION

DEFINITION

Antiphospholipid antibody syndrome (APS), the most common acquired thrombophilia, is characterized by clinical features of arterial or venous thrombosis and/or pregnancy morbidity *as well as* the persistence of at least one type of antiphospholipid autoantibody (aPL). aPLs are antibodies directed against anionic phospholipids and phospholipid-binding protein cofactors. These autoantibodies lead to stimulation of procoagulant factors and inhibition of the fibrinolytic system. This further triggers downstream pathways, including MTOR upregulation, Toll-like receptor signaling, and activation of vascular endothelium, monocytes, neutrophils, platelets, complement, and proinflammatory cytokines.

Three types of aPLs have been characterized:
- Anticardiolipin antibodies (detected in approximately 23% to 44% of patients)
- Lupus anticoagulants (detected in approximately 34% of patients)
- Anti-β2-glycoprotein-I (anti-β2-GPI) antibodies (detected in approximately 20% of patients)

APS can be a primary condition or secondary to a rheumatic disease, with the most common being systemic lupus erythematosus (SLE). APS can affect all organ systems and includes venous and arterial thrombosis, recurrent fetal losses, and cytopenias, including thrombocytopenia and microangiopathic hemolytic anemia.

SYNONYM

Antiphospholipid syndrome

ICD-10CM CODE
D68.61 Antiphospholipid syndrome

EPIDEMIOLOGY & DEMOGRAPHICS

PREVALENCE:
- Up to 5% of healthy individuals without a history of thrombosis have positive aPLs.
- aPL are positive in approximately 13% of patients with stroke, 11% with myocardial infarction, 10% of patients with DVT, and 6% of patients with pregnancy complications.
- Nearly 20% of women under 50 who have a cerebrovascular accident (CVA) test positive for aPLs.
- 10% to 15% of women with recurrent miscarriages have aPLs.
- aPLs without APS can be seen in patients with certain medications, infections, malignancies, and autoimmune conditions.

PREDOMINANT AGE: Young to middle-aged adults

RISK FACTORS:
- Underlying SLE and collagen-vascular diseases; other autoimmune disorders, including rheumatoid arthritis, Sjögren syndrome, Behçet syndrome, primary immune thrombocytopenia (also known as idiopathic thrombocytopenic purpura), AIDS.
- However, most individuals are otherwise healthy and have no underlying medical condition.

Thrombotic risk is increased by the presence of other etiologies of systemic hypercoagulability, including genetic thrombophilia as well as acquired risk factors such as oral contraceptive use, pregnancy, smoking, prolonged immobilization, malignancy, and hyperlipidemia

PROGNOSIS:
- 91% survival at 10-yr follow-up
- 71% success rate in pregnancy with recommended therapies; prematurity and intrauterine growth restriction are common complications

GENETICS: Some APS-positive families exist, and human leukocyte antigen (HLA) studies have suggested associations with HLA DR7, DR4, and Dqw7+Drw53.

PHYSICAL FINDINGS & CLINICAL PRESENTATION

No pathognomonic findings on examination; Table 1 summarizes other features suggesting the presence of antiphospholipid antibodies, including abnormal findings consistent with ischemia or infarction.
- Thrombosis (Fig. E1): Patients with APS are at risk for both venous and arterial thromboses. Venous thromboses are more common, occurring as the initial manifestation of APS in approximately 30% of APS patients. The most common site for deep vein thrombosis is the calf, but thromboses may also occur in the renal, hepatic, axillary, subclavian, vena cava, and retinal veins. The most common site of arterial thrombosis are the cerebral vessels, followed by the coronary, renal, mesenteric, and bypass arteries. Recurrent thrombosis is common with APS.
- Commonly involved organ systems include:
  1. Central nervous system: Stroke, transient ischemic attack, migraine, multi-infarct dementia, epilepsy, movement disorders, transverse myelopathy, retinal venous or arterial occlusion.
  2. Pulmonary: Pulmonary embolism and infarction, pulmonary hypertension, acute respiratory distress syndrome, diffuse alveolar hemorrhage.
  3. Cardiology: Libman-Sacks endocarditis, intracardiac thrombosis, coronary artery disease, myocardial infarction, valvulopathy, left ventricular diastolic dysfunction.
  4. Gastrointestinal: Abdominal pain, gastrointestinal bleed secondary to esophageal/mesenteric ischemia, splenic or pancreatic infarction, hepatic vein thrombosis, Budd-Chiari syndrome.
  5. Renal: Hypertension, renal infarct, renal artery or vein thrombosis, acute renal failure, glomerular damage including membranous nephropathy, minimal change disease, and pauci-immune glomerulonephritis.
  6. Hematology: Thrombocytopenia, hemolytic anemia.
  7. Endocrine: Addison disease secondary to adrenal hemorrhage and, less frequently, thrombosis.
  8. Cutaneous: Livedo reticularis, cutaneous necrosis, skin ulcerations, phlegmasia cerulea dolens, gangrene of digits (Fig. E2).
  9. Obstetric: Recurrent spontaneous abortion, premature delivery, fetal growth restriction, preeclampsia/eclampsia, abruptio placentae
  10. Vascular: Deep venous thrombosis, arterial thrombosis in extremities, superficial thrombophlebitis, amaurosis fugax
- **Catastrophic APS** (CAPS) (Table 2): CAPS is a rapidly progressive multiorgan thrombotic disease. Approximately 1% of APS is CAPS; approximately 45% of patients with CAPS do not present as APS initially. To make the diagnosis of catastrophic APS, four criteria must be satisfied:
  1. Evidence of involvement of three or more organs, systems, and/or tissues. The most common symptoms are abdominal pain, dyspnea, neurologic symptoms, chest pain, and skin rash.
  2. Development of manifestations simultaneously or in ≤1 wk.
  3. Confirmation by histopathology of small-vessel occlusion in at least one organ or tissue.
  4. Laboratory confirmation of the presence of aPL.

TABLE 1 Other Features Suggesting the Presence of Antiphospholipid Antibodies

Clinical
Livedo reticularis
Thrombocytopenia (usually 50,000-100,000 platelets/mm^3)
Autoimmune hemolytic anemia
Cardiac valve disease (vegetations or thickening)
Multiple sclerosis–like syndrome, chorea, or other myelopathy

From Firestein GS et al: *Kelley's textbook of rheumatology*, ed 9, Philadelphia, 2013, Saunders.

ETIOLOGY/PATHOPHYSIOLOGY

- Endothelial cells are activated by aPLs causing upregulation of adhesion and procoagulant molecules such as tissue factor and von Willebrand factor.
- Table 3 and Box 1 summarize proposed pathogenic mechanisms of antiphospholipid syndrome. Mechanisms of pregnancy loss in antiphospholipid syndrome are summarized in Box 2.
- Monocyte activation by aPLs yields expression of inflammatory cytokines and additional tissue factor, contributing to the procoagulant state.
- Neutrophil activation by aPLs via complement is proposed to cause the release of neutrophil extracellular traps leading to increased thrombin.
- aPL binding to glycoprotein 1b and ApoE receptor 2 causes platelet activation and increased platelet adhesion.

TABLE 2 Differential Diagnosis of Catastrophic Antiphospholipid Syndrome (CAPS)

Laboratory Abnormalities	CAPS	TTP	DIC
Microangiopathic hemolytic anemia	–	+	+
Thrombocytopenia	+	+	+
Fibrinogen/FDP	Normal/Normal	Normal/Increased	Decreased/Increased
Anticardiolipin antibody	+	–	–
Lupus anticoagulant	+	–	–

DIC, Disseminated intravascular coagulation; *FDP,* fibrin degradation products; *TTP,* time to progression.

TABLE 3 Proposed Pathogenic Mechanisms of Antiphospholipid Syndrome

I. aPL-mediated promotion of tissue factor expression
   A. Direct injury and subsequent anti-β2-GPI binding on endothelial cells
   B. Signaling via annexin A2/TLR4/apoER2 inducing proadhesive prothrombotic phenotype
   C. Induction of adhesion molecules and tissue factor on endothelial cells and cytokine release
I. Activation of platelets and monocytes by aPL antibodies
   A. Activation of platelets via apoER2′, GPIbα, and/or β2 GPI-platelet factor 4 interaction
   B. Interference of β2 GPI in regulating vWF-mediated platelet adhesion
   C. Activation of monocytes results in increased tissue factor, VEGF, cytokine expression
   D. Activation of monocytes causes mitochondrial dysfunction and oxidative stress
I. Inhibition of endogenous anticoagulant and fibrinolytic mechanisms
   A. Disruption of the annexin A5 anticoagulant shield
   B. Interference with fibrinolysis via annexin A2, β2 GPI cofactor activity, autoactivation of XIIa, direct inhibition of plasmin and increase of PAI-1
   C. Inhibition of the protein C pathway: Decreased activation of protein C, barrier of APC proteolysis of factor Va and VIIIa, prevention of protein C and EPCR binding
   D. Interference with tissue factor pathway inhibitor
I. aPL-mediated activation of complement
   A. Antibodies against β2 GP–HLA-DR7 complexes on cell surfaces trigger complement-mediated cytotoxicity
I. Direct activation of trophoblasts and endometrial cells by aPL antibodies
   A. Abnormal trophoblast proliferation, migration and invasiveness, increased trophoblast apoptosis, and reduced secretion of HCG and adhesion molecules
   B. Disruption in the differentiation of decidual endometrial cells
   C. Disruption of maternal spiral artery transformation and maturation
I. Other mechanisms
   A. mTORC pathway–mediated vasculopathy
   B. Release in procoagulant microparticles by endothelial cells and platelets

APC, Activated protein C; *aPL,* antiphospholipid; *apoER2,* apolipoprotein E receptor 2; *EPCR,* endothelial cell protein C receptor; *β2 GPI,* β2-glycoprotein I; *HCG,* human chorionic gonadotropin; *HLA,* human leukocyte antigen; *mTORC,* mammalian target of rapamycin complex; *PAI-1,* plasminogen activator inhibitor 1; *TLR,* Toll-like receptor; *VEGF,* vascular endothelial growth factor; *vWF,* von Willebrand factor.
From Hoffman R et al: *Hematology, basic principles and practice,* ed 7, Philadelphia, 2018, Elsevier.

BOX 1 Mechanisms of Thrombosis in Antiphospholipid Syndrome

- Interaction between antiphospholipid antibodies and cells (endothelial cells, monocytes, platelets)
- Activation of cell signaling pathways
- Transcription of procoagulant factors (tissue factor) and adhesion molecules
- Complement activation
- Impaired nitric oxide production
- Antiphospholipid antibody inactivation of fibrinolysis
- Heightened release and decreased degradation of NETs

NET, Neutrophil extracellular trap.

- aPL binding decreases activation of antithrombin and protein C, while also reducing the ability of activated protein C to inactivate coagulation factors V and VIII.
- aPL binding to annexin A2 (tissue plasminogen activator receptor) contributes to the prothrombotic state seen in APS.
- The mammalian target of rapamycin complex (mTORC) has been shown to be involved in endothelial activation and in regulating expression of tissue factor and IL-8 in monocytes.
- Toll-like receptors 4 and 7 and triggering of the innate immune system are involved in endothelial activation and the development of the prothrombotic state.
- Autoantibodies against other antigens, such as phosphatidylserine, phosphatidyl ethanolamine, and other complexes have been identified in APS patients, but their clinical significance has yet to be elucidated.

Dx DIAGNOSIS

DIFFERENTIAL DIAGNOSIS

Other hypercoagulable states (inherited or acquired):

- Inherited: Antithrombin III, protein C and protein S deficiencies, factor V Leiden, prothrombin gene mutation
- Acquired: Malignancy, heparin-induced thrombocytopenia, myeloproliferative syndromes
- Alternate causes of recurrent pregnancy loss should also be considered (e.g., anatomic or chromosomal abnormalities)

WORKUP

Diagnostic criteria of APS include at least one clinical criterion and at least one laboratory criterion.

- Clinical (Box 3):
  1. Venous, arterial, or small vessel thrombosis *or*
  2. Morbidity with pregnancy, defined as:
     a. Unexplained fetal death at ≥10 wk gestation *or*
     b. ≥1 premature births before 34 wk gestation secondary to eclampsia, preeclampsia, or severe placental insufficiency *or*
     c. ≥3 unexplained spontaneous abortions before 10 wk gestation.
- Laboratory:
  1. Lupus anticoagulant present in plasma on two or more occasions at least 12 wk apart, *or*
  2. Anticardiolipin antibody, IgG or IgM present in serum or plasma at >40 MP or GPL units (titer), or >99th percentile on two or more occasions at least 12 wk apart, *or*
  3. Anti-β2-GPI antibodies present in serum or plasma at >99th percentile on two or more occasions at least 12 wk apart
- Screening tests:
  1. Partial thromboplastin time (PTT): Elevated. Activated PTT prolongation indicating either the presence of a clotting factor deficiency, or the presence of an inhibitor such as a lupus anticoagulant.
  2. Mixing study: Normal plasma is incubated with the patient's plasma. In cases of clotting factor deficiencies, the PTT will correct. If an inhibitor is present as in the case with APS, the PTT will not correct.
  3. Dilute Russell viper venom time: Elevated. Laboratory clotting requires the addition of phospholipids and calcium to plasma samples. Antiphospholipid antibodies bind the phospholipids in the

BOX 2 Mechanisms of Pregnancy Loss in Antiphospholipid Syndrome

- Intraplacental thrombosis
- Impaired trophoblastic invasion and hormone production
- Activation of the complement system
- Defective placentation due to interference of anti–β2-GPI with trophoblast growth and differentiation
- Displacement of annexin A5 by IgG antiphospholipid antibody–β_2-GPI complexes

β_2-GPI, β_2-Glycoprotein I; *IgG,* immunoglobulin.

BOX 3 Preliminary Criteria for Classification of Antiphospholipid Syndrome

Clinical criteria

Vascular thrombosis

One or more clinical events of arterial, venous, or small-vessel thrombosis in any tissue or organ. Thrombosis must be confirmed by Doppler ultrasonography, other imaging, or histopathologic analysis, with the exception of superficial venous thrombosis. The histopathologic study does not have to demonstrate significant evidence of inflammation of the blood vessel.

Pregnancy morbidity

- One or more unexplained deaths of morphologically normal fetuses at 10 or more wk of gestation, with a normal fetal morphology confirmed by ultrasound or direct examination of the fetus.
- One or more premature births of a morphologically normal newborn at 34 wk of gestation or before caused by
  - Severe preeclampsia or eclampsia defined according to current standards, or
  - Recognized placental insufficiency
- Three or more consecutive spontaneous abortions without explanation before 10 wk of gestation, excluding those associated with hormonal or anatomic alterations in the mother or chromosomal alterations inherited from either parent.

Laboratory criteria

The presence of at least one of the following test results:

- Lupus anticoagulant in the plasma on two or more separate occasions within a period of 12 wk, detected according to the guidelines of the International Society of Thrombosis and Haemostasis (Scientific Subcommittee on lupus anticoagulant/phospholipid-dependent antibodies).
- IgG or IgM anticardiolipin antibodies in plasma or serum in medium-high titers (more than 40 GPL or MPL units, respectively) on two or more separate occasions within a period of 12 wk, as measured by standardized ELISA.
- IgG or IgM anti–β2-GPI antibodies in the serum or plasma (in titer above the 99th percentile) on two or more separate occasions within a period of 12 wk, as measured by standardized ELISA according to recommended procedures.

ELISA, Enzyme-linked immunosorbent assay; *Ig,* immunoglobulin.
From Hochberg MC: *Rheumatology*, ed 7, Philadelphia, 2019, Elsevier.

test tube, thereby preventing clot formation. The addition of Russell viper venom to plasma results in immediate activation of Factor X (common pathway). Therefore, it will not be prolonged in intrinsic or extrinsic factor deficiencies but will be prolonged in the presence of an antiphospholipid antibody.

4. The Lupus Anticoagulant screen is the addition of Russell viper venom to plasma. In the Lupus Anticoagulant confirmatory testing, massive doses of phospholipids are added to saturate the antiphospholipid antibody, thereby correcting the prolonged PTT.

- Initial testing for presence of aPL:
  1. Anticardiolipin (aCL) ELISA antibodies (IgG or IgM), *or*
  2. Lupus anticoagulant (LA) activity identified, *or*
  3. Anti-β2-GPI ELISA antibodies (IgG or IgM).
- Confirmatory aPL testing: Repeat testing after 12 wk is required to confirm the persistence of a positive aCL, anti-β2-GPI, or LA test because transient aPL elevations can occur.
- Note that patients on anticoagulants may have falsely prolonged aPTT and interfere with the LA screening test. These patients should be tested for aCL and anti-β2-GPI antibodies, as these assays are unaffected by the presence of an anticoagulant.

LABORATORY TESTS

Diagnostic evaluation of aPLs is indicated in:

- Patient with underlying SLE or collagen-vascular disease with thrombosis. (European League Against Rheumatism [EULAR] recommendation)
- Patient with recurrent, familial, or juvenile deep vein thrombosis (DVT) or thrombosis in an unusual location (mesenteric or cerebral).
- One or more unexplained thrombotic events. Do not test those at low risk, e.g., elderly patients with other thrombotic risk factors.
- One or more specific pregnancy events such as early fetal death, premature birth due to severe preeclampsia, embryonic losses within 10 wk of gestation.
- Thrombotic complications associated with autoimmune diseases.
- Patients with an unexplained elevation in PTT, or less commonly, in PT/INR.

Rx TREATMENT

ACUTE Rx

- Initial anticoagulation with heparin or low-molecular-weight heparin (LMWH), before transitioning to a vitamin K antagonist (VKA) such as warfarin, is recommended. DOACs are not recommended due to recent studies which have shown increased risk of recurrent thromboembolism, particularly in patients with high-risk APS (positivity for all three antiphospholipid antibodies) for patients on rivaroxaban compared to warfarin.
- Standard intensity (INR 2.0 to 3.0) anticoagulation with warfarin is preferred in venous thrombosis, as prior randomized trials failed to show a decrease in recurrent thromboses with high-intensity anticoagulation (INR 3.0 to 4.0). Task-force reports have not reached a consensus regarding intensity of anticoagulation in secondary thromboprophylaxis of arterial events.
- Unfractionated heparin (UFH) is preferred if quick reversibility is needed.

PRIMARY PREVENTION

- Modifiable risk factors for thrombosis, such as smoking and immobility, should be controlled.
- Cardiovascular risk factors, such as hypertension, obesity, and hyperlipidemia, should also be addressed.
- Aspirin use for primary prevention remains controversial.
- Adding low-dose warfarin to aspirin for primary prevention seems to confer no benefit.
- Hydroxychloroquine may be useful in those patients with SLE and aPL; it has been shown to reduce the incidence of thrombotic complications in this population.
- For pregnant women with a positive test for aPL antibodies without a history of DVT or pregnancy morbidity, decision to treat with low-dose subcutaneous UFH or LMWH and/or low-dose aspirin, or to manage with surveillance should be made on an individual basis as there is no clear consensus data.

SECONDARY PREVENTION

- For men and nonpregnant women, long-term anticoagulation with warfarin, or with UFH or LMWH if warfarin is contraindicated, should be used (Table 4).
- Modifiable risk factors for thrombosis should be reduced when possible.
- For pregnant women with previously diagnosed APS:
  1. Warfarin should be discontinued before pregnancy due to its teratogenic effects.
  2. For women with APS without prior thrombosis but with pregnancy morbidities of either unexplained fetal death at ≥10 wk gestation or ≥3 unexplained spontaneous

TABLE 4 Risk Stratification and Treatment of Various Phenotypes of Antiphospholipid Syndrome

Risk	Laboratory Result	Clinical Manifestation	Treatment
High	Triple positive for LA, aCL (IgG or IgM >40 GPL) and anti-β2-GPI (IgG or IgM >99th percentile)	Venous thrombosis	Long-term vitamin K antagonist, INR 2.0-3.0
		Arterial thrombosis	Stroke: Long-term vitamin K antagonist, INR 2.0-3.0 plus low dose aspirin Myocardial infarction: Long-term vitamin K antagonist, INR 2.0-3.0 plus low-dose aspirin or Long-term vitamin K antagonist, INR 3.0-4.0 Myocardial infarction with percutaneous coronary interventions and stent placement: Long-term vitamin K antagonist, INR 2.0-3.0, low dose aspirin, and clopidogrel 75 mg per day
		Pregnant women with history of pregnancy complications or thrombotic events	Unfractionated heparin plus low-dose aspirin
		Asymptomatic	Consider anticoagulant prophylaxis for high risk situations, e.g., immobilization, surgery, air travel Consider long-term vitamin K antagonist recommended to prevent thromboembolic events Consider low-dose aspirin and possible unfractionated heparin for pregnant patients
Medium	Double positive for LA, aCL (IgG or IgM >40 GPL) or anti-β2-GPI (IgG or IgM >99th percentile) or Single positive for LA	Venous thrombosis	Long-term vitamin K antagonist, INR 2.0-3.0
		Arterial thrombosis	Long-term vitamin K antagonist, INR 2.0-3.0 plus low dose aspirin
		Pregnant women with history of pregnancy complications or thrombotic events	Unfractionated heparin plus low-dose aspirin
		Asymptomatic	No treatment, consider prophylaxis treatment in situations with increased risk: Surgery or prolonged immobilization
Low	Single positive for aCL (IgG or IgM >40 GPL) or anti-β2-GPI (IgG or IgM >99th percentile)	Venous thrombosis	Long-term vitamin K antagonist, INR 2.0-3.0
		Arterial thrombosis	Long-term vitamin K antagonist, INR 2.0-3.0
		Pregnant women with history of pregnancy complications or thrombotic events	Early miscarriage (does not meet clinical criteria for obstetric APS): Consider low-dose aspirin Late miscarriage: Unfractionated heparin plus low-dose aspirin
		Asymptomatic	No treatment; however, consider prophylaxis treatment in situations with increased risk: Surgery or prolonged immobilization

aCL, Anticardiolipin; β_2 *GPI*, β_2 -glycoprotein I; *Ig*, immunoglobulin; *INR*, international normalized ratio; *LA*, lupus anticoagulant.
Adapted from Rand, J; Wolgast L: The antiphospholipid syndrome. In *Hematology: Basic Principles and Practice*, ed 7, Philadelphia, 2018, Elsevier.

abortions before 10 wk gestation, aspirin 81 mg in combination with subcutaneous UFH or LMWH is recommended to improve pregnancy outcomes.

3. For women with APS without prior thrombosis but with pregnancy morbidity of ≥1 premature births before 34 wk gestation secondary to eclampsia, preeclampsia, or severe placental insufficiency, aspirin 81 mg is recommended to improve pregnancy outcomes.
4. For pregnant women with APS and prior thrombosis, aspirin in combination with subcutaneous UFH or LMWH should be used.
5. Pregnant patients taking LMWH should be transitioned to unfractionated heparin before delivery for ease of reversibility.
6. Hypertension, obesity, and hyperlipidemia, if present, should be controlled.

FOR CATASTROPHIC ANTIPHOSPHOLIPID ANTIBODY SYNDROME (CAPSS)

- The combination of anticoagulation with heparin products, high-dose corticosteroids, and supportive care, including debriding necrotic tissue and treating underlying infections is the mainstay of therapy.
- Patients may be transitioned to oral anticoagulation with warfarin once clinically stable.
- Plasma exchange with or without IVIG has been shown to improve mortality; however, the decision to use IVIG should be made on an individual basis (e.g., avoid in patients in whom anticoagulation has been discontinued).
- Eculizumab (monoclonal antibody against complement protein C5) and rituximab (monoclonal antibody against CD20) have been used successfully in refractory cases.
- Immunosuppressant therapy with cyclophosphamide should be considered in patients with CAPS and SLE as it has been demonstrated to decrease mortality in this group.

CHRONIC Rx

- Anticoagulation with VKAs, such as warfarin, remains the standard of care. The potential role of new oral anticoagulants in APS remains uncertain. Meta-analyses of patients with APS treated with direct oral anticoagulants demonstrate higher rates of recurrent thrombosis, which are increased up to fourfold in patients with triple positivity (positive for all three APS antibodies) (Dufrost et al. 2018). Trials involving rivaroxaban did not show noninferiority to dose adjusted VKAs for thrombotic APS, and in fact showed a nonstatistically significant near doubling of the risk for recurrent thrombosis (Ordi Ros et al. 2019).
- Duration of treatment is unknown and should be determined on an individual basis. However, in the absence of any contraindication to anticoagulation, indefinite therapy is recommended, as the lifelong recurrence rate reached nearly 30% in some studies.
- Evidence on length of therapy is unclear in provoked DVTs (prolonged hospitalization, estrogen supplementation) in patients who later test negative for aPL.
- Immunosuppressive agents such as corticosteroids and cyclophosphamide have not been shown to be effective for chronic treatment of APS.
- Limited data suggest that hydroxychloroquine may be effective in patients with APS and SLE, although efficacy in primary APS remains unproven.
- Recurrent thrombosis can occur even in the setting of "therapeutic" anticoagulation, and multiple assays have been studied to monitor the adequacy of anticoagulation in APS.
- In cases of recurrent thrombosis, hydroxychloroquine and statins (antiinflammatory and antithrombotic activity) may be considered as adjuvant therapies.

TABLE 5 Alternative Therapies for Antiphospholipid Syndrome

Treatment	Target Effect (in vitro and/or animal studies)	Results of Human Studies
Hydroxychloroquine	aPL-induced platelet activation Inhibition of aPL-mediated thrombosis in mice Protection of aPL-induced displacement of annexin A5 from phospholipid bilayers	Decreases thrombotic risk in SLE Increases survival in SLE Protective against thrombosis in aPL+ individuals Decreases aPL and/or LAC in SLE patients
Statins	Reversal of aPL-induced endothelial cell activation and TF upregulation Abrogation of enhanced thrombus formation in mice	Decrease proinflammatory and prothrombotic markers in APS Contraindicated in pregnancy
Rituximab	Blocking of B-cell activating factor, which can prevent disease onset in APS mouse model	Effective for aPL-related cytopenias Effective for catastrophic APS Increases response in APS (off-label use) RITAPS trial: Effective for some noncriteria manifestations of APS
Potential immunomodulatory approaches	Anticomplement peptidesInhibition of TF Inhibition of nuclear factor κB Inhibition of p38 MAPK Inhibition of TLR-4 Inhibition of TNF-α, or IL-6 Inhibition of apo ER2 Inhibition of mTORC Peptides mimicking domains of β_2-GPI or β_2-GPI receptor blockers Other biologics (Eculizumab Belimumab, Abatacept)	Experimental studies (MBB2: A single-chain fragment variable recognizing β_2-GP1) Eculizumab (complement-5 inhibitor): Based on case reports/series has been effective in treating CAPS, limited data in pregnancy; currently ongoing clinical trials[1]
Experimental Tx	Autologous hematopoietic stem cell transplantation	Limited data; appears to be effective and safe in APS patients

[1]Dobrowolski C, Erkan D. Treatment of antiphospholipid syndrome beyond anticoagulation. *Clin Immunol* 206:53-62, 2019.

aPL, Antiphospholipid antibody; *APS,* antiphospholipid syndrome; *β_2-GPI,* β_2-glycoprotein I; *IL-6,* interleukin-6; *LAC,* lupus anticoagulant; *MAPK,* mitogen-activated protein kinase; *mTORC,* mammalian target of rapamycin complex; *RITAPS,* rituximab in antiphospholipid syndrome; *SLE,* systemic lupus erythematosus; *TF,* tissue factor; *TLR,* Toll-like receptor; *TNF,* tumor necrosis factor.

Modified from Hochberg MC: *Rheumatology*, ed 7, Philadelphia, 2019, Elsevier

- Table 5 summarizes alternative therapies for antiphospholipid syndrome.

DISPOSITION

- APS patients have a 20% to 70% risk for recurrent thrombosis. Positivity in more than one aPL assay is associated with increased thrombotic risk.
- Initial arterial thrombosis tends to be followed by arterial events, and initial venous thrombosis tends to be followed by venous events.
- Incidence of developing catastrophic APS is approximately 1.0% among APS patients. CAPS is associated with a high mortality rate (35% to 45%, primarily due to cerebral and cardiac involvement).

REFERRAL

Referrals to hematology, rheumatology, and/or obstetric medicine should be placed when diagnosis is made.

PEARLS & CONSIDERATIONS

COMMENTS

- Observational studies show APS is associated with a 10% mortality over a 10-yr period. Causes of death included arterial and venous thrombotic events (stroke, MI), as well as infection and CAPS (Cervera et al. 2015). Cerebral features of SLE may be more related to thrombosis than inflammation and may respond better to anticoagulants than immunosuppression.

PREVENTION

Prophylaxis for asymptomatic patients with positive aPL tests without previous thrombosis:

- No routine prophylaxis is recommended.
- Questionable whether low-dose aspirin is effective.
- Antithrombotic prophylaxis for major surgery, prolonged immobilization, and pregnancy is appropriate.
- Avoid combination oral contraceptive pills in women with positive aPL tests.

RELATED CONTENT

Antiphospholipid Antibody Syndrome (Patient Information)
Deep Vein Thrombosis (Related Key Topic)
Hypercoagulable State (Related Key Topic)
Pulmonary Embolism (Related Key Topic)

SUGGESTED READINGS

Available at ExpertConsult.com

AUTHORS: **Hetal Mistry, MD,** and **John L. Reagan, MD**

Anxiety (Generalized Anxiety Disorder) (PTG)

BASIC INFORMATION

DEFINITION

Generalized anxiety disorder (GAD) is most likely to present in combination with other psychiatric and medical conditions. Based on DSM-5 criteria, individuals with GAD commonly present with excessive and disproportionately high levels of anxiety, fear, or worry for most days over at least a 6-mo period in a number of areas. The worrying must be greater than would be expected given the situation, and it must cause significant interference in functioning. The subjective anxiety must be accompanied by at least three somatic symptoms in adults and one in children (e.g., restlessness, irritability, sleep disturbance, muscle tension, difficulty concentrating, or fatigue). GAD cannot be diagnosed if it occurs only in the context of an active mood disorder, such as depression, or if the anxiety is better explained by another active anxiety disorder, such as PTSD or panic disorder.

SYNONYMS

Anxiety neurosis (former name for a subset of anxiety disorders)
Chronic anxiety
GAD

ICD-10CM CODE
F41.1 Generalized anxiety disorder
DSM-5 CODE
300.02 Generalized anxiety disorder

EPIDEMIOLOGY & DEMOGRAPHICS

INCIDENCE (IN U.S.): 6% to 9% per yr in adult primary care clinics; 1-yr incident rate per 100 persons/yr of 1.12

PREVALENCE (IN U.S.): In general population: Lifetime morbid risk of 9%; 12-mo prevalence of 2.9%; lifetime prevalence in the National Comorbidity Survey-Replication was 5.7%.

- In primary care setting: 3% (the most common anxiety disorder in this setting)

PREDOMINANT SEX: Women are more frequently affected (2:1 ratio) but may present for treatment less often (3:2 female:male).

PREDOMINANT AGE:

- 30% report onset before age 11
- 50% have onset before age 18
- Median age of onset: 30 yr

PEAK INCIDENCE: Peak incidence tends to occur later relative to other anxiety disorders, such as phobias; cumulative incidence of 4.3% by age 34 in a German community sample.

GENETICS: Concordance rates in dizygotic twins and monozygotic twins are not different (0% to 5%)

PHYSICAL FINDINGS & CLINICAL PRESENTATION

- Report of being "anxious" all of their lives
- Excessive worry, usually regarding family, finances, work, or health
- Sleep disturbance, particularly early insomnia
- Muscle tension (typically in the muscles of neck and shoulders) or headache
- Difficulty concentrating
- Daytime fatigue
- Gastrointestinal symptoms compatible with irritable bowel syndrome (one third of patients)
- Physical symptoms are the usual reason for seeking medical attention
- Comorbid psychiatric illness (e.g., dysthymia or major depression, substance use disorders (e.g., alcohol use disorder), and chronic pain conditions are frequent

ETIOLOGY

- Hypotheses include models based on neurotransmitters (catecholamines, indolamines) and developmental psychology (e.g., behavioral inhibition, neuroticism, and harm avoidance)
- Prevalence increased with a family history, increase in stress, history of physical or emotional trauma, and medical illness

Dx DIAGNOSIS

DIFFERENTIAL DIAGNOSIS

- Wide range of psychiatric and medical conditions:
  1. Cardiovascular and pulmonary disease, such as cardiac arrhythmias or COPD
  2. Hyperthyroidism, hypoglycemia
  3. Substance abuse (e.g., cocaine, amphetamines, and PCP) or withdrawal (e.g., alcohol or benzodiazepines)
  4. Other anxiety disorders (e.g., social anxiety disorder), mood disorder
  5. Intrusive thoughts in obsessive-compulsive disorder or illness anxiety disorder

WORKUP

- Screening tests may enhance detection. A screening tool often used in primary care is the GAD-2. It asks, "During the past month, have you been bothered a lot by: (1) Nerves or feeling anxious or on edge? (2) Worrying about a lot of different things?" The response to each question is given a score of 0 (not at all), 1 (several days), 2 (more than half of the days), 3 (nearly every day). A score of ≥3 has a sensitivity of 86% and a specificity of 83% for detecting GAD. A simple 7-item in-office case finding instrument, the GAD-7, includes additional questions to assess symptom severity and can be used to monitor symptoms.
- Physical examination: Additional laboratory and radiologic workup depending on presenting symptoms.
- Iatrogenic cause should be suspected if anxiety follows recent changes in medication.

Rx TREATMENT

NONPHARMACOLOGIC THERAPY

- Cognitive-behavioral therapy
- Acceptance and commitment therapy
- Relaxation training and meditative approaches
- Biofeedback
- Psychodynamic psychotherapy

PHARMACOLOGIC THERAPY

- Selective serotonin reuptake inhibitors (SSRIs) or serotonin-norepinephrine reuptake inhibitors (SNRIs)
- Azapirones (e.g., buspirone)
- Pregabalin (a GABA-analogue)
- Benzodiazepines (less favored)

ACUTE GENERAL Rx

- Acute treatment is rarely indicated because GAD is a chronic condition.
- If patients are in acute distress, the possibility of another cause, including another anxiety disorder such as panic disorder, should be considered.
- Caution in prescribing benzodiazepines because of the propensity for misuse and dependence. If used, the patient should be educated about the options and the risks.

CHRONIC Rx

- SSRIs (e.g., escitalopram) and SNRIs (e.g., venlafaxine and duloxetine) are effective typical first-line treatments with the strongest support from meta-analyses. Particularly useful if comorbid depression present. Pregabalin is also an effective first-line treatment and has been shown to have the best tolerability among first-line agents.
- Buspirone can be effective with minimal potential for tolerance or abuse. May be less effective in patients with previous benzodiazepine exposure and may require a high-dose titration.
- Benzodiazepines can be effective under close supervision; however, they have fallen out of favor as a first-line treatment given their potential for functional impairment, abuse, and dependence.
- Quetiapine may be more effective than first-line treatments at reducing anxiety symptoms, but its use is limited by comparatively poor tolerability.
- Sedating antidepressants, such as mirtazapine, may also be useful for initial insomnia secondary to anxious ruminations.

DISPOSITION

- GAD is chronic with periodic exacerbations.
- Treatment is given to reduce level of symptoms and improve functioning. Suicide risk is higher than in the general population.

REFERRAL

- For refractory symptoms
- For comorbid psychiatric conditions

PEARLS & CONSIDERATIONS

Since GAD is a risk factor for major depression, screening and early intervention for GAD (especially in women) may sometimes be helpful in reducing vulnerability to a mood disorder later in life.

SUGGESTED READINGS

Available at ExpertConsult.com

RELATED CONTENT

Anxiety (Patient Information)
Panic Disorder, with or without Agoraphobia (Related Key Topic)
Social Anxiety Disorder (Related Key Topic)

AUTHORS: **Katherine M. Mullersman, MD,** and **Joshua W. Zollman, MD**

Aortic Regurgitation

BASIC INFORMATION

DEFINITION

Aortic regurgitation (AR) is abnormal retrograde blood flow into the left ventricle from the aorta due to an inadequately closing aortic valve (AV). The inadequate closure of the valve can result from either disease of the ascending aorta (ex. Dilation) and aortic root or disease of aortic valve leaflets. In addition, it can be acute or chronic in nature.

Stages of chronic aortic regurgitation:

- Stage A = at risk of aortic insufficiency (AI) without even trace AR (e.g., bicuspid AV, AV sclerosis, diseases of the ascending aorta, history of rheumatic heart disease, or infective endocarditis)
- Stage B = progressive AI with mild to moderate AR and preserved left ventricular ejection fraction (LVEF)
- Stage C = asymptomatic severe AR with preserved (stage C1) or reduced (stage C2) LVEF
- Stage D = symptomatic severe AR

SYNONYMS

Aortic insufficiency
AI
AR

ICD-10CM CODES

I35.1	Nonrheumatic aortic (valve) insufficiency
I35.2	Nonrheumatic aortic (valve) stenosis with insufficiency
I06.1	Rheumatic aortic insufficiency
I06.2	Rheumatic aortic stenosis with insufficiency
Q23.1	Congenital insufficiency of aortic valve

EPIDEMIOLOGY & DEMOGRAPHICS

Prevalence varies with severity of AR, age, and gender, as summarized in Table 1.

- Most common cause in the developing world is rheumatic heart disease.
- Most common causes in developed countries are aortic root dilation, congenital bicuspid aortic valve, and calcific valve disease.
- Infectious endocarditis (IE) is the most frequent cause of acute AR.

TABLE 1 Prevalence of Aortic Regurgitation (AR)

Mild AR Prevalence	Male	Females
Age 50-59	3.7 %	1.9%
Age 60-69	12.1%	6%
Age 70-83	12.2%	14.6%
Moderate-Severe AR Prevalence	Male	Females
Age 50-59	0.5%	0.2%
Age 60-69	0.6%	0.8%
Age 70-83	2.2%	2.3%

From Singh JP et al: Prevalence and clinical determinants of mitral, tricuspid, and aortic regurgitation (the Framingham Heart Study), *Am J Cardiol 83:897, 1999.*

PHYSICAL FINDINGS & CLINICAL PRESENTATION

Clinical presentation varies depending on whether AR is acute or chronic. Chronic AR is well tolerated (except when secondary to IE), and patients remain asymptomatic for years. Common manifestations after significant deterioration of LVEF are dyspnea on exertion, syncope, chest pain, and congestive heart failure (CHF). The stages of chronic AR are summarized in Table 2. Acute severe AR manifests primarily with hypotension caused by a sudden fall in cardiac output and resultant cardiogenic shock. A rapid rise in left ventricular diastolic pressure results in a further decrease in coronary blood flow.

Physical findings in chronic AR:

- Widened pulse pressure (markedly increased systolic blood pressure with decreased diastolic blood pressure). Fig. 1 illustrates characteristics of the AR murmur
- Findings associated with widened pulse pressure:
  1. Bounding, "water hammer," or collapsing pulse **(*Corrigan* pulse)** can be palpated at the wrist or femoral artery and is caused by the rapid rise and sudden collapse of arterial pressure during late systole
  2. Head "bobbing" with each heart beat **(*de Musset* sign)**
  3. "Pistol shot femorals" **(*Traube* sign)** describes a loud sound over the femoral artery with systole and diastole
  4. Capillary pulsations **(*Quincke* sign)** may occur on the lips or at the base of the nail beds
- A to-and-fro intermittent femoral murmur **(*Duroziez* sign)** may be heard with slight compression of the femoral arteries. Popliteal systolic pressure increased >20 mm Hg over the brachial systolic pressure **(*Hill* sign);** a 40 to 60 mm difference represents moderate AR and >60 mm difference, severe AR
- Findings more of historical than practical interest, which are neither sensitive nor specific, include:
  1. ***Mueller* sign**—Systolic pulsations of the uvula
  2. ***Becker* sign**—Visible pulsations of the retinal arteries and pupils
  3. ***Mayne* sign**—More than a 15 mm Hg decrease in diastolic blood pressure with arm elevation from the value obtained with the arm in the standard position
  4. ***Rosenbach* sign**—Systolic pulsations of the liver
  5. ***Gerhard* sign**—Systolic pulsations of the spleen
  6. ***Landofi* sign**—Pupil dilation and constriction with each heart beat on the ocular exam

Cardiac auscultation reveals:

- Displacement of cardiac impulse downward and to the patient's left
- S_3 heard over the apex
- Decrescendo, blowing diastolic murmur heard along left sternal border
- Low-pitched apical diastolic rumble **(*Austin Flint* murmur)**—the precise etiology is uncertain, but it is generally believed to be related to increased velocity of mitral inflow consequent to the AR
- Early systolic ejection sound and systolic ejection murmur

In patients with acute aortic insufficiency both the wide pulse pressure and the large stroke volume are absent. A short, blowing diastolic murmur may be the only finding on physical examination.

ETIOLOGY

- Leaflet abnormalities:
  1. Infective endocarditis
  2. Rheumatic fibrosis (most common cause in developing countries)
  3. Trauma with valvular rupture
  4. Congenital heart disease (bicuspid aortic valve—most common cause in the U.S., sinus of Valsalva aneurysm)
  5. Myxomatous degeneration
  6. Calcific AV disease
  7. Drug-induced (fenfluramine, dexfenfluramine, pergolide, cabergoline)
  8. Systemic rheumatic disorders (ankylosing spondylitis, rheumatoid arthritis, systemic lupus erythematosus)
  9. Iatrogenic (ex. Aortic balloon valvotomy)
- Aortic root or ascending aorta abnormalities:
  1. Annuloaortic ectasia
  2. Genetic syndromes (Ehlers-Danlos, Marfan)
  3. Trauma
  4. Ankylosing spondylitis
  5. Syphilitic aortitis
  6. Systemic hypertension
  7. Aortic dissection
- Postprocedural AR, usually due to a paravalvular leak, occurs in 10% to 20% of patients undergoing transcatheter aortic valve replacement (TAVR). Patients with more than mild AR after TAVR have worse outcomes than those without AR

DIAGNOSIS

DIFFERENTIAL DIAGNOSIS

- Patent ductus arteriosus, pulmonary regurgitation, and other valvular abnormalities.
- The differential diagnosis of cardiac murmurs is described in Sections II and III.

WORKUP

- Echocardiogram, chest radiograph, electrocardiogram (ECG), cardiac magnetic resonance (CMR) imaging, and cardiac catheterization (selected patients)
- Medical history and physical examination focused on dyspnea on exertion, syncope, chest pain, and CHF

IMAGING STUDIES

- Chest radiography:
  1. Left ventricular hypertrophy (LVH) (chronic AR).
  2. Aortic dilation.
  3. Normal cardiac silhouette with pulmonary edema: Possible in patients with acute AR.

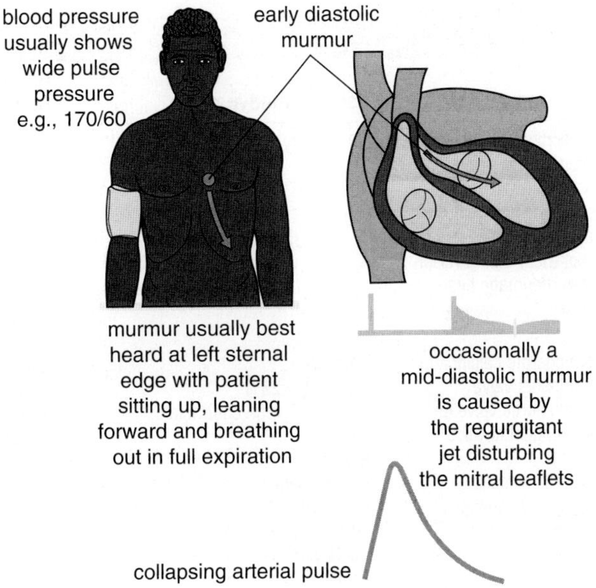

FIG. 1 Aortic regurgitation as an example of an early diastolic murmur. (From Epstein O et al: *Pocket guide to clinical examination,* ed 4, St Louis, 2009, Mosby.)

- ECG is not useful for diagnostic purposes but is commonly used in evaluation of patients with chronic AR to exclude associated arrythmia. Typical findings on an ECG are LVH as a result of volume overload.
- Echocardiography (Fig. E2) is the main imaging modality to diagnose AR and assess left ventricular size and function. Quantification of the severity of regurgitation can be made either qualitatively by Doppler vena contracta width (severe if >0.6 cm) or quantitatively by effective regurgitant orifice area (severe if >0.30 cm^2) and/or regurgitant volume (severe if >60 ml per/beat).
- Echocardiography can also be used for periodic monitoring of asymptomatic patients with normal LV systolic function and chronic AR. Based on 2014 AHA/ACC valve guideline, Mild AR is followed every 3 to 5 yr, Moderate AR is followed every 1 to 2 yr, and Severe AR should be followed every 6 to 12 mo or more frequently if there is worsening of LV dilatation.
- CMR is indicated (class 1) in patients with moderate or severe AR and suboptimal echocardiographic images for the assessment of AR severity as well as LV systolic function and volumes.
- Cardiac catheterization is indicated in selected patients to assess the degree of left ventricular dysfunction and AR when echocardiographic parameters are inconclusive, and to determine if there is coexistent coronary artery disease.
- Serial evaluation of the size and morphology of the aortic sinuses and ascending aorta by echocardiography, CMR, or CT angiography is recommended in patients with a bicuspid AV and an aortic diameter >4.0 cm, with the examination interval determined by the degree and rate of progression of aortic dilation and by family history. Patients with an aortic diameter >4.5 cm should be evaluated annually (Class 1).

Rx TREATMENT

NONPHARMACOLOGIC THERAPY

- Avoidance of competitive sports and heavy weight lifting if: Severe AR, patient is symptomatic, ejection fraction <50%, AR is associated with aortic root dilation
- Salt restriction
- Endocarditis prophylaxis is not recommended for chronic AR patients with native valves undergoing invasive procedures. However, antibiotic prophylaxis is recommended for patients with a prior history of infective endocarditis or a presence of prosthetic heart valve

ACUTE GENERAL Rx

- Emergent AV replacement (preferred) or repair for acute, severe AR
- Intraaortic balloon pump is contraindicated
- Afterload reduction: Angiotensin-converting enzyme (ACE) inhibitors and vasodilators (i.e., nitroprusside) in acute AR; diuretics for pulmonary edema
- Avoid beta-blockers that can prolong diastole
- Emergent surgical referral for cardiogenic shock

CHRONIC Rx

Management depends on whether patients are symptomatic and candidates for valve surgery. ACC/AHA guidelines for aortic valve replacement for chronic aortic regurgitation are summarized in Table 3.

- Symptomatic patients with severe AR who are candidates for valve surgery should proceed with valve replacement after medical optimization of heart failure. When surgery is contraindicated, TAVR is currently under assessment for treatment of native AR.
- Asymptomatic patients with severe AR and systolic dysfunction who are not surgical candidates should receive ACE/ARBs.
- Other medical treatments for AR are based on limited studies. Beta-blocker use is controversial but has been associated with a higher survival rate in severe AR. Vasodilatory therapies (nifedipine and enalapril) have failed to show benefit in reducing the need for or delaying AV replacement in asymptomatic, severe AR with normal systolic function, but ACE/ARB therapy may indeed benefit moderate to severe AR. Long-term vasodilator therapy with ACE inhibitors or nifedipine may be used in patients who have concomitant hypertension. There is no current definitive indication of medical therapy with afterload reduction for aortic regurgitation other than hypertension control.
- Beta-blockers in combination with ACE inhibitors are reasonable in patients with symptomatic severe AR or LV dysfunction when surgery cannot be performed because of concomitant comorbidities. In a retrospective cohort study of 756 patients with chronic AR, beta-blocker therapy was associated with decreased mortality. Patients treated with beta-blockers were more likely to be taking ACE inhibitors and dihydropyridine calcium channel blockers as well (53% vs. 40%). In the same study, patients treated with beta-blockers and undergoing AVR were also noted to have a mortality benefit.
- Diuretics and sodium restriction for CHF.

TABLE 2 Stages of Chronic Aortic Regurgitation

Stage	Definition	Valve Anatomy	Valve Hemodynamics	Hemodynamic Consequences	Symptoms
A	At risk of AR	Bicuspid aortic valve (or other congenital valve anomaly) Aortic valve sclerosis Diseases of the aortic sinuses or ascending aorta History of rheumatic fever or known rheumatic heart disease IE	AR severity none or trace	None	None
B	Progressive AR	Mild to moderate calcification of a trileaflet valve bicuspid aortic valve (or other congenital valve anomaly) Dilated aortic sinuses Rheumatic valve changes Previous IE	***Mild AR:*** Jet width <25% of LVOT vena contracta <0.3 cm RVol <30 ml/beat RF <30% ERO <0.10 cm^2 Angiography grade 1+ ***Moderate AR:*** Jet width 25-64% of LVOT Vena contracta 0.3-0.6 cm RVol 30-59 ml/beat RF 30-49% ERO 0.10-0.29 cm^2 Angiography grade 2+	Normal LV systolic function Normal LV volume or mild LV dilation	None
C	Asymptomatic severe AR	Calcific aortic valve disease Bicuspid valve (or other congenital abnormality) Dilated aortic sinuses or ascending aorta Rheumatic valve changes IE with abnormal leaflet closure or perforation	***Severe AR:*** Jet width ≥65% of LVOT Vena contracta >0.6 cm Holodiastolic flow reversal in the proximal abdominal aorta RVol ≥60 ml/beat RF ≥50% ERO ≥0.3 cm^2 Angiography grade 3+ to 4+ In addition, diagnosis of chronic severe AR requires evidence of LV dilation	*C1:* Normal LVEF (≥50%) and mild-to-moderate LV dilation (LVESD ≤50 mm) *C2:* Abnormal LV systolic function with depressed LVEF (<50%) or severe LV dilation (LVESD >50 mm or indexed LVESD >25 mm/m^2)	None; exercise testing is reasonable to confirm symptom status
D	Symptomatic severe AR	Calcific valve disease Bicuspid valve (or other congenital abnormality) Dilated aortic sinuses or ascending aorta Rheumatic valve changes Previous IE with abnormal leaflet closure or perforation	***Severe AR:*** Doppler jet width ≥65% of LVOT Vena contracta >0.6 cm Holodiastolic flow reversal in the proximal abdominal aorta RVol ≥60 ml/beat RF ≥50% ERO ≥0.3 cm^2 Angiography grade 3+ to 4+ In addition, diagnosis of chronic severe AR requires evidence of LV dilation	Symptomatic severe AR may occur with normal systolic function (LVEF ≥50%), mild-to-moderate LV dysfunction (LVEF 40%-50%), or severe LV dysfunction (LVEF <40%)Moderate-to-severe LV dilation is present	Exertional dyspnea or angina, or more severe HF symptoms

AR, Aortic regurgitation; *ERO,* effective regurgitant orifice; *HF,* heart failure; *IE,* infective endocarditis; *LV,* left ventricle; *LVEF,* left ventricular ejection fraction; *LVESD,* left ventricular end-systolic dimension; *LVOT,* left ventricular outflow tract; *RF,* regurgitant fraction; *RVol,* regurgitant volume.
From Nishimura RA et al: 2014 AHA/ACCF guideline for the management of patients with valvular heart disease: a report of the American College of Cardiology Foundation/American Heart Association Task Force on Practice Guidelines, *J Am Coll Cardiol* 63:e57, 2014. In Mann DL et al: *Braunwald's heart disease,* ed 10, Philadelphia, 2015, Elsevier.

- Comparable efficacy of losartan and atenolol was shown in curbing aortic root dilatation growth in children and young adults (6 mo to 25 yr) with Marfan syndrome with similar outcomes of aortic regurgitation severity, surgery, aortic dissection, and death at 3 yr. Fig. 3 describes a management strategy for patients with chronic severe AR.

REFERRAL

Surgical referral is reserved for the following patients:

- Patients with acute severe AR (i.e., infective endocarditis) and cardiogenic shock
- Symptomatic patients with severe AR regardless of LV systolic function (class I)
- Patients with hemodynamically stable severe AR undergoing CABG or surgery on the aorta or other heart valves
- Evidence of systolic dysfunction with left ventricular ejection fraction of less than 50% and asymptomatic patients with chronic severe AR
- Asymptomatic patients with severe AR and left ventricular ejection fraction >50%, but with left ventricular dilation:

1. Echocardiographic end-systolic dimension >50 mm (Class IIa level of evidence) *or;*
2. Echocardiographic end-diastolic dimension >65 mm with low surgical risk (Class IIb)

SUGGESTED READINGS

Available at ExpertConsult.com

RELATED CONTENT

Aortic Insufficiency (Patient Information)

AUTHOR: **Sarthak Khare, MD**

TABLE 3 American College of Cardiology/American Heart Association Guidelines for Aortic Valve Replacement (AVR) for Chronic Aortic Regurgitation (AR)

Class	Indication	LOE
I	AVR for symptomatic patients with severe AR regardless of LV systolic function (stage D).	B
	AVR for asymptomatic patients with chronic severe AR and LV systolic dysfunction (LVEF <50%) (stage C2).	B
	AVR for patients with severe AR (stage C or D) while undergoing cardiac surgery for other indications.	C
IIa	AVR is reasonable for asymptomatic patients with severe AR with normal LV systolic function (LVEF ≥50%), but severe LV dilation (stage C2, LVESD >50 mm).	B
	AVR is reasonable in patients with moderate AR (stage B) who are undergoing other cardiac surgery.	C
IIb	AVR may be considered for asymptomatic patients with severe AR and normal LV systolic function (stage C1, LVEF ≥50%) but severe LV dilation (LVEDD >65 mm) if surgical risk is low.*	C

LOE, Level of evidence; *LV,* left ventricular; *LVEDD,* LV end-diastolic dimension; *LVEF,* LV ejection fraction; *LVESD,* LV end-systolic dimension.
*Particularly in the setting of progressive LV enlargement.
From Zipes DP et al: *Braunwald's heart disease, a textbook of cardiovascular disease,* ed 11, Philadelphia, 2019, Elsevier.

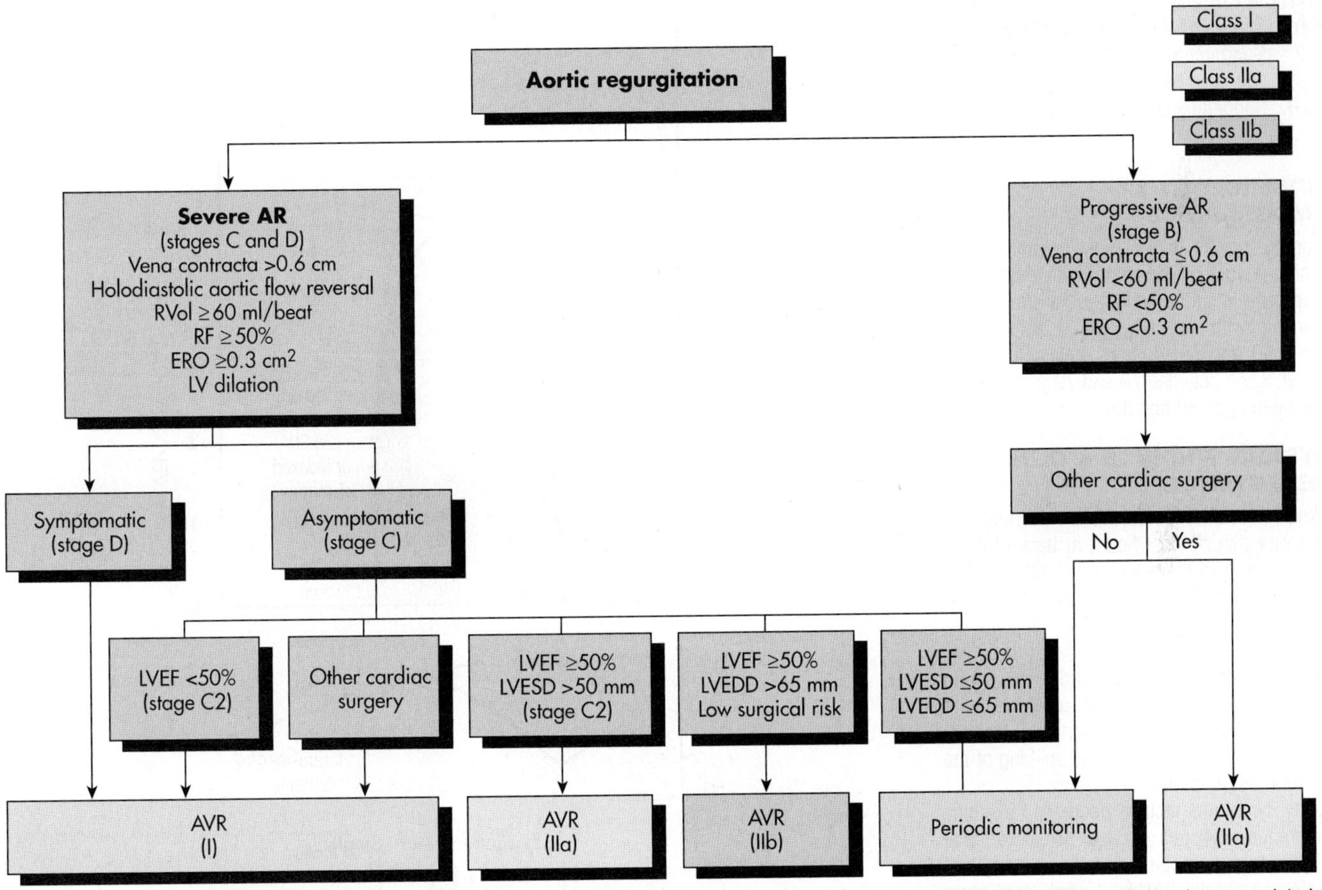

FIG. 3 Management strategy for patients with chronic severe aortic regurgitation (AR). *AVR,* Aortic valve replacement (valve repair may be appropriate in selected patients); *ERO,* effective regurgitant orifice; *LV,* left ventricle; *LVEDD,* left ventricular end-diastolic dimension; *LVEF,* left ventricular ejection fraction; *LVESD,* left ventricular end-systolic dimension; *RF,* regurgitant fraction; *RVol,* regurgitant volume. (From Zipes DP et al: *Braunwald's heart disease, a textbook of cardiovascular disease,* ed 11, Philadelphia, 2019, Elsevier.)

BASIC INFORMATION

DEFINITION

Aortic stenosis (AS) is obstruction of left ventricular systolic outflow due to aortic valve thickening/calcification generating a significant pressure gradient (aortic jet velocity of at least 2 m/sec). Symptoms typically appear when the valve orifice decreases to <1 cm^2 (normal orifice is 3 to 4 cm^2). Criteria for severe AS include a valve area <1.0 cm^2, a mean gradient >40 mm Hg, or a peak gradient >4 m/s. Doppler aortic jet velocities >5 m/sec is defined as very severe.

SYNONYMS

Aortic valve stenosis
AS

ICD-10CM CODES

I35.0	Nonrheumatic aortic (valve) stenosis
I35.2	Nonrheumatic aortic (valve) stenosis with insufficiency
Q23.0	Congenital stenosis of aortic valve

EPIDEMIOLOGY & DEMOGRAPHICS

- Aortic stenosis is the most common valve lesion in adults in North America and Europe.
- The prevalence demonstrates a strong relationship with age, affecting 0.2% between ages 50 and 59 yr, 1.3% between 60 and 69 yr, 3.9% between 70 and 79 yr, and 9.8% between ages 80 and 89.

PHYSICAL FINDINGS & CLINICAL PRESENTATION

- Harsh midsystolic, crescendo-decrescendo murmur (Fig. 1) best heard at base of heart and radiating into neck vessels; often associated with a thrill or ejection click; may also be heard well at the apex.
- Signs of severe AS include absent or diminished intensity of the second heart sound and/or slow-rising carotid upstroke with delayed amplitude (pulsus parvus et tardus), presence of S4, and a reverse splitting of the second heart sound.
- Early symptoms include decreased exercise tolerance, dyspnea on exertion, exertional dizziness or syncope, and exertional angina.
- Late symptoms include angina (secondary primarily to reduced coronary blood flow and increased total left ventricle [LV] oxygen demand), syncope, and heart failure.
- Table 1 summarizes the stages of valvular aortic stenosis.
- Pathophysiology: Antegrade velocities remain normal until the cross-sectional area of the left ventricular outflow tract (typically 3 to 4 cm^2) is reduced by roughly half. At this point, secondary to the increased resistance, the left ventricle systolic pressure starts to increase and the LV adapts with concentric hypertrophy. The hypertrophy allows for normalization of the wall stress and preservation of the ejection fraction, cardiac output, and left ventricular end diastolic pressures despite the LV/peripheral arterial system pressure gradient.
- LV hypertrophy eventually leads to LV diastolic dysfunction, which may herald early symptoms. That said, symptoms generally do not begin until stenosis becomes severe (valve area <1.0 cm^2, a mean gradient >40 mm Hg, or a peak gradient >4 m/s).
- For most patients, after becoming symptomatic, LV systolic function will begin to drop (decreased cardiac output and stroke volume) with development of signs and symptoms of overt heart failure. At this point, if a symptomatic severe AS patient does not undergo valve replacement, their mortality drastically increases.
- Acquired von Willebrand disease is seen in approximately 20% of severe AS, which can lead to GI bleeding from angiodysplasia (Heyde syndrome) that resolves after aortic valve replacement.

ETIOLOGY

- Idiopathic calcification of the aortic valve (most common cause in North America and Europe, presents at ages 60 to 80)
- Rheumatic heart disease: Characterized by commissural fusion leaving a small central orifice (most common cause worldwide)
- Progressive stenosis of congenital unicuspid or bicuspid valve (found in 1% to 2% of the population, presents at ages <30 yr for unicuspid and at ages 40 to 60 for bicuspid valves)
- Less common causes include rare metabolic disease (Fabry disease), systemic lupus erythematosus, radiation, end-stage

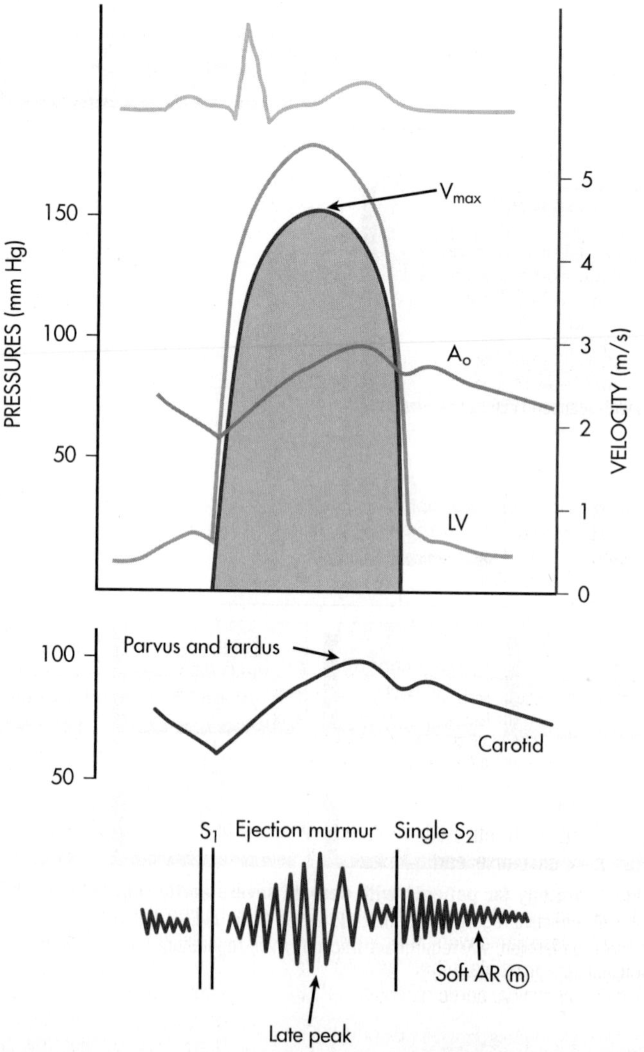

FIG. 1 Relationship between left ventricle (LV) and aortic (Ao) pressures and the Doppler aortic stenosis velocity curve (*in red*). The pressure difference between the LV and aorta in systole is four times the velocity squared (the Bernoulli equation). Thus, a maximum velocity (V_{max}) of 4.3 m/sec corresponds to a maximum LV to Ao pressure difference of 74 mm Hg and a mean systolic gradient of 44 mm Hg. On physical examination, the slow rate of rise and delayed peak in the carotid pulse (or parvus and tardus) matches the contour of the aortic pressure waveform. The murmur corresponds to the Doppler velocity curve with a harsh crescendo-decrescendo late-peaking systolic murmur, best heard at the aortic region (upper right sternal border). Often, a soft, high-pitched diastolic decrescendo murmur of aortic regurgitation also is appreciated. *AR,* Aortic regurgitation. (From Bonow et al [eds]: *Braunwald's heart disease,* ed 9, Philadelphia, 2012, Saunders.)

TABLE 1 Stages of Valvular Aortic Stenosis

Stage	Definition	Valve Anatomy	Valve Hemodynamics	Hemodynamic Consequences	Symptoms
A	**At risk of AS**	Bicuspid aortic valve (or other congenital valve anomaly) Aortic valve sclerosis	Aortic V_{max} <2 m/sec	None	None
B	**Progressive AS**	Mild to moderate leaflet calcification of a bicuspid or trileaflet valve with some reduction in systolic motion or rheumatic valve changes with commissural fusion	***Mild AS:*** Aortic V_{max} 2.0-2.9 m/sec or mean ΔP <20 mm Hg ***Moderate AS:*** Aortic V_{max} 3.0-3.9 m/sec or mean ΔP 20-39 mm Hg	Early LV diastolic dysfunction may be presentNormal LVEF	None
C	**Asymptomatic severe AS**				
C1	Asymptomatic severe AS with preserved LVEF	Severe leaflet calcification or congenital stenosis with severely reduced leaflet opening	***Severe AS:*** Aortic V_{max} ≥4 m/sec or mean ΔP ≥40 mm Hg AVA typically is ≤1 cm^2 (or AVAi ≤0.6 cm^2/m^2) Very severe AS is an aortic V_{max} ≥5 m/sec, or mean ΔP ≥60 mm Hg	LV diastolic dysfunction Mild LV hypertrophy Normal LVEF	None; exercise testing is reasonable to confirm symptom status
C2	Asymptomatic severe AS with LV dysfunction	Severe leaflet calcification or congenital stenosis with severely reduced leaflet opening	Aortic V_{max} ≥4 m/sec or mean ΔP ≥40 mm Hg AVA typically is ≤1 cm^2 (or AVAi ≤0.6 cm^2/m^2)	LVEF <50%	None
D	**Symptomatic severe AS**				
D1	Symptomatic severe high-gradient AS	Severe leaflet calcification or congenital stenosis with severely reduced leaflet opening	***Severe AS:*** Aortic V_{max} ≥4 m/sec, or mean ΔP ≥40 mm Hg AVA typically is ≤1 cm^2 (or AVAi ≤0.6 cm^2/m^2), but may be larger with mixed AS/AR	LV diastolic dysfunction LV hypertrophy Pulmonary hypertension may be present	Exertional dyspnea or decreased exercise tolerance Exertional angina Exertional syncope or presyncope
D2	Symptomatic severe low-flow/low-gradient AS with reduced LVEF	Severe leaflet calcification with severely reduced leaflet motion	AVA ≤1 cm^2 with resting aortic V_{max} <4 m/sec, or mean ΔP <40 mm Hg Dobutamine stress echo shows AVA ≤1 cm^2 with V_{max} ≥4 m/sec at any flow rate	LV diastolic dysfunction LV hypertrophy LVEF <50%	HF, angina, syncope or presyncope
D3	Symptomatic severe low-gradient AS with normal LVEF or paradoxical low-flow severe AS	Severe leaflet calcification with severely reduced leaflet motion	AVA ≤1 cm^2 with aortic V_{max} <4 m/sec, or mean ΔP <40 mm HgAVAi ≤0.6 cm^2/m^2 Stroke volume index <35 ml/m^2 Measured when the patient is normotensive (systolic BP <140 mm Hg)	Increased LV relative wall thickness Small LV chamber with low-stroke volume. Restrictive diastolic filling LVEF ≥50%	HF, angina, syncope or presyncope

AR, Aortic regurgitation; *AS,* aortic stenosis; *AVA,* aortic valve area; *AVAi,* aortic valve area indexed to body surface area; *BP,* blood pressure; *HF,* heart failure; *LV,* left ventricle; *LVEF,* left ventricular ejection fraction; *ΔP,* pressure gradient; V_{max}, maximum aortic velocity.

From Nishimura RA et al: 2014 AHA/ACCF guideline for the management of patients with valvular heart disease: a report of the American College of Cardiology Foundation/American Heart Association Task Force on Practice Guidelines. In Mann DL et al (eds): *Braunwald's heart disease*, ed 10, Philadelphia, 2015, Elsevier.

renal disease, and obstructive vegetations/endocarditis may all cause early development of AS

- Genetic variation in the LPA locus, mediated by Lp(2) levels, is associated with aortic valve calcification across multiple ethnic groups and with incidental clinical aortic stenosis

Dx DIAGNOSIS

DIFFERENTIAL DIAGNOSIS

- Hypertrophic cardiomyopathy
- Mitral regurgitation
- Ventricular septal defect
- Aortic sclerosis. Aortic stenosis is distinguished from aortic sclerosis by the degree of valve impairment. In aortic sclerosis, the valve leaflets are abnormally thickened but obstruction to outflow is absent or minimal
- Subvalvular membrane or supravalvular AS
- Stages of valvular AS
  1. Stage A = at risk of AS
  2. Stage B = progressive AS (formerly known as mild and moderate AS)
  3. Stage C = asymptomatic severe AS
  4. Stage D = symptomatic severe AS

WORKUP

- Echocardiography: The primary test for diagnosis (see "Imaging Studies")
- ECG: May demonstrate left ventricular hypertrophy and/or left atrial abnormality
- Chest radiograph: May demonstrate cardiomegaly. Poststenotic dilation of the ascending aorta may also be evident
- Cardiac catheterization in selected patients (see "Imaging Studies")
- Dobutamine challenge (for low-gradient, low-flow AS)

IMAGING STUDIES

- Doppler echocardiography: Used to evaluate structure and anatomy of the valve. Hemodynamics can easily be assessed; allows calculation of both aortic valve area and estimation of pressure gradients to determine severity of AS (Fig. 2). Furthermore, allows evaluation of the LV size and function and pulmonary pressures.
- Chest x-ray:
  1. Poststenotic dilation of the ascending aorta
  2. Calcification of aortic cusps
  3. Rounding of left ventricle (LV) apex

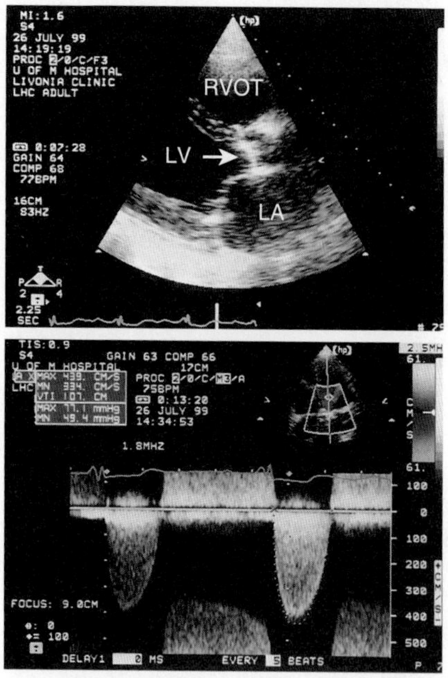

FIG. 2 Echocardiogram recorded in a patient with severe aortic stenosis. The *top panel* is a parasternal long-axis view recorded in systole. Left ventricular function is diminished. The aortic valve is markedly thickened and partially calcified. Its motion is markedly reduced, and in systole it appears that the valve occludes the orifice *(arrow)*. The *lower panel* is a continuous-wave Doppler recorded from the apex of the left ventricle along a line aimed through the stenotic aortic valve. Note the aortic stenosis signal below the zero crossing line. The peak velocity is 430 cm/sec, which corresponds to a maximum gradient of 77 mm Hg and a mean gradient of 49.4 mm Hg. *LA*, Left atrium; *LV*, left ventricle; *RVOT*, right ventricular outflow tract. (From Zipes DP et al [eds]: *Braunwald's heart disease*, ed 7, Philadelphia, 2005, Saunders.)

- ECG:
  1. Left ventricular hypertrophy (found in 80% of patients)
  2. Left atrial enlargement
  3. Atrial fibrillation (in late disease)
- Cardiac catheterization: Indicated in symptomatic patients awaiting aortic valve replacement (AVR) in order to detect coexisting coronary artery stenosis that may need bypass at the same time as aortic valve replacement. Previously, cardiac catheterization was used in symptomatic patients when noninvasive tests are inconclusive or when there is a discrepancy between noninvasive tests and clinical findings regarding severity of AS. Due to the increased risk of stroke when crossing the valve and with the advent of newer or improved imaging modalities (cardiac MR, PET-CT, TEE), there is rarely a role to directly measure the gradient across the valve.
- A CT with contrast for imaging the aorta may be needed for annular sizing, aortic measurements and if a transcatheter aortic valve replacement (TAVR) is planned, the CT scan is crucial to planning TAVR approach.
- Exercise testing: Strongly encouraged for any patient with stage C "asymptomatic" severe AS to evaluate exercise tolerance and to look for a fall in systemic blood pressure while exercising.

Rx TREATMENT

GENERAL Rx

MEDICAL:

- Once symptomatic, the mainstay of treatment is replacement of the valve. AS is a surgical disease. Fig. 3 summarizes a treatment strategy for patients with severe AS.
- Optimize loading conditions by keeping a normal volume status (gentle diuresis for volume overload as preload dependent) and controlling hypertension (HTN) but avoid vasodilators (nitrates); maintain sinus rhythm.
- In 2007, the AHA guidelines for prevention of infectious endocarditis were revised and routine antibiotic prophylaxis to undergo dental or other invasive procedures is no longer recommended, unless the patient has prior endocarditis.

INDICATIONS FOR AORTIC VALVE REPLACEMENT: Valve replacement is the treatment of choice in symptomatic patients because there is a 50% mortality rate at 2 yr with medical therapy alone. If a patient does not have a >1 yr life expectancy postprocedure or quality of life will not be improved by the aortic valve, then replacement should not be considered, but rather palliative therapies should be discussed. ACC/AHA guidelines for aortic valve replacement for aortic stenosis are summarized in Table 2.

Percutaneous aortic balloon valvuloplasty serves best as palliative therapy in severely symptomatic patients who are not surgical candidates and as a bridge to surgery in hemodynamically unstable adult patients. It is not an option in patients who are good candidates for valve replacement because restenosis occurs in most adult patients at 6 mo. Updated ACC /AHA guidelines for choice of surgical versus transcatheter treatment of aortic stenosis are summarized in Table 3.

If the patient does fulfill the intervention criteria (>1 yr life expectancy postprocedure and quality of life will be improved by the aortic valve), then replacement can be further considered.

Valve replacement is a **Class I Indication** for any patients with:

- Stage D1: Symptomatic severe AS
- Stage C2: Asymptomatic severe AS with LV ejection fraction (EF) <50%
- Stage C1 or C2: Asymptomatic severe AS undergoing CABG or surgery on the aorta or other heart valves

Valve replacement is a **Class IIa indication** for patients with:

- Stage D2: Low-flow/low gradient (with low ejection fraction <50%) with a positive low-dose dobutamine stress echo
- Stage D3: Symptomatic patients with low-flow/low gradient severe AS with a **normal LVEF** ≥50%, a valve area ≤1.0 cm^2, and a stroke volume index <35 ml/m^2
- Stage C: Asymptomatic severe AS and abnormal blood pressure response (decrease in systolic blood pressure) or decreased exercise tolerance during exercise
- Stage C: Asymptomatic patients with critical AS (peak velocity >5 m/s or mean pressure gradient >60 mm Hg) with low surgical risk
- Stage B: Patients with moderate AS who are undergoing cardiac surgery for other indications

Valve replacement is a **Class IIb indication** for patients with:

- Stage C: Asymptomatic severe AS in a low-risk patient showing rapid progression of disease (V_{max} >0.3m/s/yr).
- When deciding replacement strategy, surgical aortic valve replacement (SAVR) vs. transcatheter aortic valve replacement (TAVR), in all cases a heart team approach is a Class I indication. TAVR is a catheter-based technology that allows for implantation of a prosthetic valve without open heart surgery, decreasing recovery time and hospital stay. Historically, the replacement strategy has been driven by patient surgical risk. Primarily due to TAVR trial design, patients were classified by their STS-PROM score into four categories: Extreme surgical risk (absolute surgical contraindication), high surgical risk (STS-PROM score >8), intermediate surgical risk (STS-PROM score 4 to 8), and low surgical risk (STS-PROM score <4).
- For the **extreme surgical risk** patients and **high surgical risk** patients (STS-PROM score >8), if a TAVR approach is feasible, then the recommendation is for a TAVR strategy. In a large meta-analysis of these high-risk patients with severe AS who were candidates for surgery, transfemoral TAVR (but not transthoracic TAVR) was associated with lower mortality at 2 yr. The surgical group had double the incidence of new-onset atrial fibrillation and major bleeding, but the TAVR group had a higher rate of paravalvular regurgitation and vascular complications.
- For **intermediate surgical risk** (STS-PROM 4 to 8), if TAVR approach is feasible and there is an absence of high-risk anatomical features that would increase the risk of a transcatheter approach, then the recommendation is for a TAVR strategy. In these intermediate-risk patients, transfemoral TAVR was associated with lower mortality rates, and nontransfemoral TAVR was similar to surgical aortic valve replacement with respect to death or disabling stroke rates, as demonstrated by the same large meta-analysis of four randomized trials. The notable differences were that TAVR resulted in larger aortic valve areas and had a lower rate of acute kidney injury, severe bleeding, and new-onset atrial fibrillation, whereas surgery resulted in fewer major vascular complications and less paravalvular aortic regurgitation.
- For **low surgical risk** patients (STS-PROM <4), if the patient meets the following four criteria: >65 yr old, transcatheter approach is feasible, aortic valve is trileaflet, and there is an absence of high-risk anatomic features

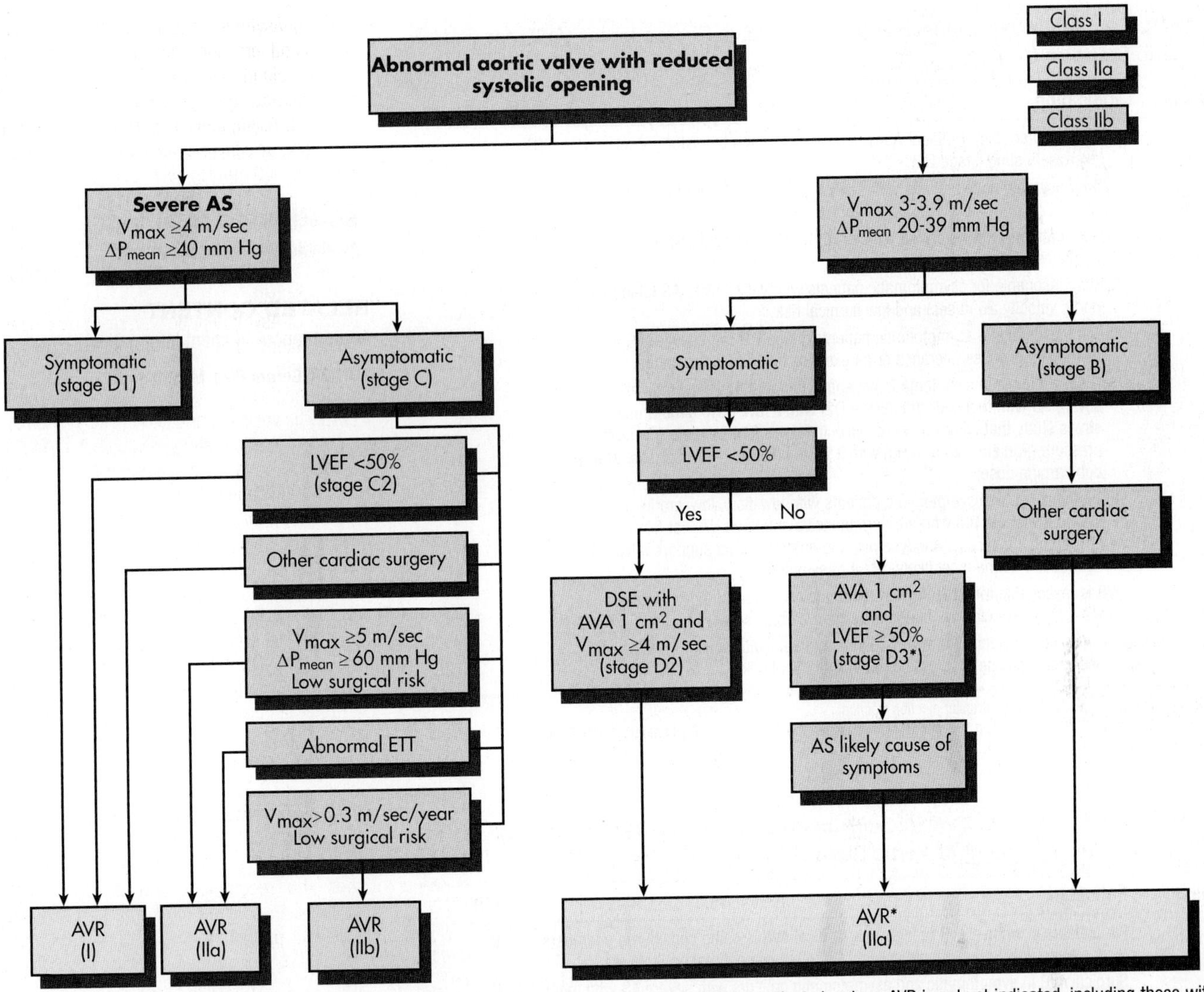

FIG. 3 Management strategy for patients with severe AS. Periodic monitoring is indicated for all patients in whom AVR is not yet indicated, including those with asymptomatic AS (stage B or C) and those with low-gradient AS (stage D2 or D3) who do not meet criteria for intervention. AVR should be considered with stage D3 AS only if valve obstruction is the most likely cause of symptoms, stroke volume index is <35 ml/m^2, indexed AVA is ≤0.6 cm^2/m^2, and data are recorded when the patient is normotensive (systolic BP <140 mm Hg). *AS,* Aortic stenosis; *AVA,* aortic valve area; *AVR,* aortic valve replacement; *BP,* blood pressure; *DSE,* dobutamine stress echocardiography; *ETT,* exercise treadmill test; *LVEF,* left ventricular ejection fraction; ΔP_{mean}, mean pressure gradient; V_{max}, maximum velocity. (From Nishimura RA et al: 2014 AHA/ACC Guideline for the management of patients with valvular heart disease: a report of the American College of Cardiology /American Heart Association Task Force on Practice Guidelines. In Mann DL et al [eds]: *Braunwald's heart disease,* ed 10, Philadelphia, 2015, Elsevier.)

that would increase the risk of transcatheter approach, then the recommendation is for a TAVR strategy. For these low-risk patients, from the PARTNER 3 trial, there was a significant lower primary endpoint (composite death, stroke, or rehospitalization at 1 yr). For patients under the age of 65 or with a bicuspid valve, a heart team approach, as with all aortic valve replacements, is strongly advised.

DISPOSITION

- The presence of even mild symptoms is an indicator of poor survival for patients with AS. The average duration of symptoms before death is angina, 5 yr; syncope, 3 yr; CHF, 2 yr.
- Approximately 75% of patients with symptomatic AS will die within 3 yr of symptom onset unless the aortic valve is replaced.

REFERRAL

- A heart team referral for valve replacement in all symptomatic AS patients (Class I indication). There are studies that are examining the presence of moderate or severe valvular calcification, together with a rapid increase in aortic jet velocity and elevated BNP, to identify patients with a very poor prognosis who should be considered for early valve replacement rather than delayed until symptoms develop. Additionally, patients with severe AS who are asymptomatic should be considered for exercise stress test to see if they are truly without symptoms (low exercise tolerance) or if the BP drops with exercise, both which would be indications for a heart team referral.
- In asymptomatic patients, Doppler echocardiography is recommended every 6 to 12 mon for severe aortic stenosis, every 1 to 2 yr for moderate disease, and every 2 to 3 yr for mild disease. Should have a low threshold to repeated echocardiogram for any change in symptoms or exam.
- Referral to cardiology should be considered in any patients with severe AS and in particular those with low-flow, low-gradient (low ejection fraction) symptomatic aortic stenosis for further workup (dobutamine stress echo).
- Balloon valvuloplasty is useful in infants and children or poor surgical candidates who do not have calcified valve apparatus; it can be done as an intermediate procedure to stabilize high-risk patients before surgery.
- Role of palliative care:
  1. If life expectancy with aortic valve replacement (SAVR or TAVR) is <1 yr **or** the patient's quality of life is unlikely to improve after aortic valve replacement

TABLE 2 ACC/AHA Guidelines for Aortic Valve Replacement (AVR) for Aortic Stenosis (AS)

Class	Indication	LOE
I	AVR with severe high-gradient AS who have symptoms by history or on exercise testing (stage D1).	B
	AVR for asymptomatic patients with severe AS (stage C2) and LVEF less than 50%.	B
	AVR for patients with severe AS (stage C or D) when undergoing other cardiac surgery.	B
IIa	AVR is reasonable for asymptomatic patients with very severe AS (stage C1, aortic velocity ≥5 m/sec) and low surgical risk.	B
	AVR is reasonable in asymptomatic patients (stage C1) with severe AS and decreased exercise tolerance or an exercise fall in blood pressure.	B
	AVR is reasonable in symptomatic patients with low-flow/low-gradient severe AS with reduced LVEF (stage D2) with a low-dose dobutamine stress study that shows an aortic velocity of 4 m/sec or more (or mean pressure gradient ≥40 mm Hg) with a valve area of 1.0 cm^2 or less at any dobutamine dose.	B
	AVR is reasonable in symptomatic patients with low-flow, low-gradient severe AS (stage D3) who are normotensive and have LVEF of 50% or greater, if clinical, hemodynamic, and anatomic data support valve obstruction as the most likely cause of symptoms.	C
	AVR is reasonable for patients with moderate AS (stage B) (aortic velocity, 3.0-3.9 m/sec) who are undergoing other cardiac surgery.	C
IIb	AVR may be considered for asymptomatic patients with severe AS (stage C1) and rapid disease progression and low surgical risk.	C

LOE, Level of evidence; *LVEF,* left ventricular ejection fraction.
Zipes DP: *Braunwald's heart disease, a textbook of cardiovascular medicine,* ed 11, Philadelphia, 2019, Elsevier.

TABLE 3 Updated ACC/AHA Guidelines for Choice of Surgical Versus Transcatheter Treatment of Aortic Stenosis (AS)

Class	Indication	LOE
I	For patients in whom TAVR or high-risk surgical AVR is being considered, members of a heart valve team should collaborate to provide optimal patient care.	C
	Surgical AVR in symptomatic and asymptomatic patients with severe AS who meet an indication for AVR (listed in Table 2) when surgical risk is low or intermediate. (*Modified 2017*)	B
	TAVR in patients who meet an indication for AVR for AS who have a prohibitive surgical risk and a predicted post-TAVR survival >12 mo. (*Modified 2017*)	A
	TAVR or surgical AVR in patients with severe AS who meet an indication for AVR and who have high surgical risk. (*Modified 2017*)	A
IIa	TAVR is a reasonable alternative to surgical AVR for symptomatic patients with severe AS and an intermediate surgical risk. (*New 2017*)	B
IIb	Percutaneous aortic balloon dilation may be considered as a bridge to surgical or transcatheter AVR in severely symptomatic patients with severe AS.	C
III	TAVR is not recommended in patients in whom the existing comorbidities would preclude the expected benefit from correction of AS.	B

ACC, American College of Cardiology; *AHA,* American Heart Association; *AVR,* aortic valve replacement; *LOE,* level of evidence; *TAVR,* transcatheter AVR.
Zipes DP: *Braunwald's heart disease, a textbook of cardiovascular medicine,* ed 11, Philadelphia, 2019, Elsevier.

(due to coexisting significant comorbidities), palliative care consultation is extremely valuable as it focuses on shared decision making as well as improving quality of life without interruption of conservative medical therapy.

SUGGESTED READINGS

Available at ExpertConsult.com

RELATED CONTENT

Aortic Stenosis (Patient Information)

AUTHOR: **Gerard Daly, MD, MSc**

BASIC INFORMATION

DEFINITION

Appendicitis is the acute inflammation of the vermiform appendix.

ICD-10CM CODES

K35.2	Acute appendicitis with generalized peritonitis
K35.3	Acute appendicitis with localized peritonitis
K35.80	Unspecified acute appendicitis
K35.89	Other acute appendicitis
K36	Other appendicitis
K37	Unspecified appendicitis

EPIDEMIOLOGY & DEMOGRAPHICS

- Appendicitis occurs in 10% of the population, most commonly between the ages of 10 and 30 yr. Median age is 22 yr. Lifetime risk is 7% to 14%.
- Approximately 300,000 appendectomies are performed in the U.S. each yr.
- It is the most common abdominal surgical emergency.
- Incidence of appendicitis has declined over the past 30 yr.
- Male:female ratio is 3:2 until mid-20s; it equalizes after age 30 yr.

PHYSICAL FINDINGS & CLINICAL PRESENTATION

- In children with abdominal pain, fever is the single most useful sign associated with appendicitis. Vomiting, rectal tenderness, and rebound tenderness along with fever are more indicative of appendicitis in children than in adults.
- Abdominal pain: Initially the pain may be epigastric or periumbilical in nearly 50% of patients; it subsequently localizes to the right lower quadrant within 12 to 18 hr. Pain can be found in back or right flank if appendix is retrocecal or in other abdominal locations if there is malrotation of the appendix.
- Pain with right thigh extension *(psoas sign)*, low-grade fever: Temperature may be >38° C if there is appendiceal perforation.
- Pain with internal rotation of the flexed right thigh *(obturator sign)* is present.
- Right lower quadrant (RLQ) pain on palpation of the left lower quadrant (LLQ) *(Rovsing sign):* Physical examination may reveal right-sided tenderness in patients with pelvic appendix.
- Point of maximum tenderness is in the RLQ *(McBurney point).*
- Nausea, vomiting, tachycardia, cutaneous hyperesthesias at the level of T12 can be present.

ETIOLOGY

Obstruction of the appendiceal lumen with subsequent vascular congestion, inflammation, and edema; common causes of obstruction are:
- Fecaliths: 30% to 35% of cases (most common in adults)
- Foreign body: 4% (fruit seeds, pinworms, tapeworms, roundworms, calculi)
- Inflammation: 50% to 60% of cases (submucosal lymphoid hyperplasia [most common etiology in children, teens])
- Neoplasms: 1% (carcinoids, metastatic disease, carcinoma)

DIAGNOSIS

DIFFERENTIAL DIAGNOSIS

- Intestinal: Regional cecal enteritis, incarcerated hernia, cecal diverticulitis, intestinal obstruction, perforated ulcer, perforated cecum, Meckel diverticulitis
- Reproductive: Ectopic pregnancy, ovarian cyst, torsion of ovarian cyst, salpingitis, tubo-ovarian abscess, mittelschmerz, endometriosis, seminal vesiculitis
- Renal: Renal and ureteral calculi, neoplasms, pyelonephritis
- Vascular: Leaking aortic aneurysm
- Psoas abscess
- Trauma
- Cholecystitis
- Mesenteric adenitis
- Table 1 summarizes the differential diagnosis of appendicitis

WORKUP

Patients with RLQ pain, nausea, vomiting, anorexia, and RLQ rebound tenderness should undergo prompt clinical and laboratory evaluation. Imaging studies are generally not necessary in typical appendicitis and generally reserved for patients with an equivocal likelihood of appendicitis. They are useful when the diagnosis is uncertain. Laparoscopy may be useful as both a diagnostic and a therapeutic modality.

LABORATORY TESTS

- Complete blood count with differential reveals leukocytosis with a left shift in 90% of patients with appendicitis. Total white blood cell (WBC) count is generally lower

TABLE 1 Differential Diagnosis of Appendicitis

Diagnosis	Findings That Help Differentiate Entity from Appendicitis
Bacterial or viral enteritis	Nausea, vomiting, and diarrhea are severe; pain usually develops after vomiting.
Epiploic appendagitis	Focal abdominal pain and tenderness without migration or progression of the pain; patients have a paucity of other GI symptoms such as anorexia or nausea. Laboratory findings are usually normal.
Mesenteric adenitis	Duration of symptoms is longer; fever is uncommon; RLQ physical findings are less marked; WBC count is usually normal.
Pyelonephritis	Pain is more likely to be felt in the right flank; high fever and rigors are common; marked pyuria or bacteriuria and urinary symptoms are present; abdominal rigidity is less marked.
Renal colic	Pain radiates to the right groin; significant hematuria; character of the pain is clearly colicky.
Acute pancreatitis	Pain and vomiting are more severe; tenderness is less well localized; serum amylase and lipase levels are elevated.
Crohn disease	History of recurrent similar attacks; diarrhea is more common; palpable mass is more common; extraintestinal manifestations may have occurred or be present.
Cholecystitis	History of prior attacks is common; pain and tenderness are greater; radiation of pain is to the right shoulder; nausea is more marked; liver biochemical tests are more likely to be abnormal.
Meckel diverticulitis	Nearly impossible to distinguish preoperatively from appendicitis.
Cecal diverticulitis	Difficult to distinguish preoperatively from appendicitis; symptoms are milder and of longer duration; CT is helpful; patients are usually older.
Sigmoid diverticulitis	Usually occurs in older patients; changes in bowel habits are more common; radiation of the pain is to the suprapubic area, not RLQ; fever and WBC count are higher.
Small bowel obstruction	History of abdominal surgery; pain is colicky; vomiting and distention are more marked; RLQ localization is uncommon.
Ectopic pregnancy	History of menstrual irregularities; characteristic progression of symptoms is absent; syncope; positive pregnancy test.
Ruptured ovarian cyst	Occurs in the middle of the menstrual cycle; pain is of sudden onset; nausea and vomiting are less common; WBC count is normal.
Ovarian torsion	Vomiting is more marked and occurs at the same time as the pain; progression of symptoms is absent; abdominal or pelvic mass often is palpable.
Acute salpingitis or tubo-ovarian abscess	Longer duration of symptoms; pain begins in the lower abdomen; often there is a history of STDs; vaginal discharge and marked cervical tenderness often are present.

CT, Computed tomography; *GI,* gastrointestinal; *IV,* intravenous; *RLQ,* right lower quadrant; *STD,* sexually transmitted disease; *WBC,* white blood cell.
From Feldman M et al: *Sleisenger and Fordtran's gastrointestinal and liver disease*, ed 10, Philadelphia, 2016, Elsevier.

than 20,000/mm³. Higher counts may be indicative of perforation. Less than 4% have a normal WBC and differential. A WBC count <10,000/mm³ decreases the likelihood of appendicitis. Low hemoglobin and hematocrit levels in an older patient should raise suspicion for gastrointestinal tract carcinoma.

- Microscopic hematuria and pyuria may occur in <20% of patients.
- Human chorionic gonadotropin to rule out pregnancy in females of reproductive age.

IMAGING STUDIES

- Multidetector computed tomography (Fig. E1) is a useful test for routine evaluation of suspected appendicitis in adults. CT of the abdomen/pelvis without contrast has a sensitivity of >90% and an accuracy >94% for acute appendicitis. A distended appendix, periappendiceal inflammation, and a thickened appendiceal wall are indicative of appendicitis. Table 2 describes CT findings of appendicitis. In children and young adults, exposure to CT radiation is of particular concern. Trials with low-dose CT (116 mGy cm) have shown that low-dose CT is not inferior to standard-dose CT (521 mGy cm) with respect to negative (unnecessary) appendectomy rates in young adults with suspected appendicitis.
- Ultrasonography (Fig. E2) has a sensitivity of 75% to 90% for the diagnosis of acute appendicitis, although it is highly operator dependent and difficult in patients with large body habitus. Ultrasound is useful, especially in pregnancy and in younger women when diagnosis is unclear. Normal ultrasonographic findings should not deter surgery if the history and physical examination are indicative of appendicitis.
- MRI of the abdomen and pelvis can also be used to accurately diagnose acute appendicitis in pregnant patients (100% sensitivity, 93.6% specificity) without exposure to ionizing radiation.

TABLE 2 Computed Tomography Findings of Appendicitis: SCALPEL Mnemonic

Term	Description
Stranding	Fat stranding suggests regional inflammation, possibly because of appendicitis.
Cecum	The appendix originates from the cecum, which should be identified first to help localize the appendix. The cecum may show wall thickening, suggesting appendicitis.
Air	Air outside of the lumen of the appendix is pathologic and suggests perforation. Air within the appendiceal wall is also abnormal.
Large	The normal appendix is <6 mm; an enlarged appendix >6 mm suggests appendicitis. Wall thickening >1 mm also suggests appendicitis.
Phlegmon	Inflammatory changes surrounding the appendix suggest a perforated appendix. A heterogeneous collection called a phlegmon may be seen. If the appendix has ruptured, a pericecal phlegmon may be the only remaining evidence, because the appendix itself may not be seen.
Enhancement	The wall of an abnormal appendix enhances with IV contrast and appears brighter than the normal bowel or the normal psoas muscle.
Lith	An appendicolith is a calcified stone sometimes found in the lumen of an inflamed appendix.

IV, Intravenous.
From Broder JS: *Diagnostic imaging for the emergency physician*, Philadelphia, 2011, Saunders.

Rx TREATMENT

NONPHARMACOLOGIC THERAPY

- Nothing by mouth
- Do not administer analgesics until the diagnosis is made

ACUTE GENERAL Rx

- Urgent appendectomy (laparoscopic or open), correction of fluid and electrolyte imbalance with vigorous IV hydration, and electrolyte replacement
- IV antibiotic prophylaxis to cover gram-negative bacilli and anaerobes (ampicillin/sulbactam 3 g IV q6h or piperacillin/tazobactam 4.5 g IV q8h in adults)

PEARLS & CONSIDERATIONS

COMMENTS

- Perforation is common (20% in adult patients). Indicators of perforation are pain lasting >24 hr, leukocytosis >20,000/mm³, temperature >102° F (38.9° C), palpable abdominal mass, and peritoneal findings.
- In general, prognosis is excellent. Mortality rate is <1% in young adults without complications; however, it exceeds 10% in elderly patients with ruptured appendix.
- In approximately 20% of patients who undergo exploratory laparotomy because of suspected appendicitis, the appendix is normal.
- An increasing amount of evidence supports the use of antibiotics instead of surgery for treating patients with uncomplicated appendicitis. A trial assessing the feasibility of nonoperative management for uncomplicated acute appendicitis in children using either IV piperacillin-tazobactam or ciprofloxacin metronidazole therapy for at least 24 hr followed by oral antibiotics for 10 days revealed that 90% of children managed nonoperatively had no progression within 30 days.[1] Another trial among patients with CT-proven, uncomplicated appendicitis revealed that antibiotic treatment did not meet the prescribed criterion for noninferiority compared with appendectomy. Most patients randomized to antibiotic treatment for uncomplicated appendicitis did not require appendectomy during the 1-yr follow-up period, and those who required appendectomy did not experience significant complications.[2] A 5-yr follow-up of antibiotic therapy for uncomplicated acute appendicitis in the APPAC randomized clinical trial revealed that among patients who were initially treated with antibiotics for uncomplicated acute appendicitis, the likelihood of late recurrence within 5 yr was 39.1%.[3] A more recent trial[5] also confirmed that antibiotics are not inferior to appendectomy on the basis of a health status questionnaire; however, in the antibiotics group nearly 3 in 10 participants had unresolved appendectomy by 90 days and those with an appendicolith had a higher risk for appendectomy and for complications. It remains to be determined whether the benefits of potentially avoiding an operation with antibiotics-first approach are outweighed by the burden to the patient related to future appendicitis episodes, more days of antibiotic therapy, lingering symptoms, and uncertainty that may affect quality of life.[4]

SUGGESTED READINGS

Available at ExpertConsult.com

RELATED CONTENT

Appendicitis (Patient Information)

AUTHOR: **Fred F. Ferri, MD**

[1]Minneci PC et al: Feasibility of a nonoperative management strategy for uncomplicated acute appendicitis in children, *J Am Coll Surg* 219:272-279, 2014.
[2]Salminen P et al: Antibiotic therapy vs appendectomy for treatment of uncomplicated acute appendicitis, the APPAC Randomized trial, *JAMA* 313(23):2340-2348, 2015.
[3]Salminen P et al: Five-year follow-up of antibiotic therapy for uncomplicated acute appendicitis in the APPAC randomized clinical trial, *JAMA* 320(12):1259-1265, 2018.
[4]Flum DR: Acute appendicitis—appendectomy or the "antibiotics first" strategy, *N Engl J Med* 372:1937-43, 2015.
[5]The CODA Collaborative: a randomized trial comparing antibiotics with appendectomy for appendicitis, *N Engl J Med* 383:1907-19, 2020.

BASIC INFORMATION

DEFINITION

Arrhythmogenic right ventricular dysplasia (ARVD) is a cardiomyopathy characterized by replacement of the normal myocardium with fibrofatty tissue, mainly of the right ventricle but also occasionally with involvement of the left ventricle. It is defined clinically by palpitations and syncope and potentially life-threatening ventricular arrhythmias.

SYNONYMS

Arrhythmogenic right ventricular cardiomyopathy
ARVC

ICD-10CM CODE

I42.8 Arrhythmogenic ventricular dysplasia

EPIDEMIOLOGY & DEMOGRAPHICS

PREVALENCE: 1:2000 to 5000 persons. It is one of the leading causes of arrhythmic cardiac arrest in young people and athletes.
PREDOMINANT SEX AND AGE: Mean age, 31 yr (range, 12 to 50 yr), predominantly male
RISK FACTORS: Family history of ARVD (present in nearly 50% of affected patients)
GENETICS:
- Autosomal dominant (most common) with variable penetrance and polymorphic phenotypic expression
- Autosomal recessive (rarely, e.g., Naxos disease)
- Several different gene mutations in desmosomal proteins
- Gene mutations can be identified in 50% of affected individuals

PHYSICAL FINDINGS & CLINICAL PRESENTATION

- ARVD can present with palpitations, syncope, and chest discomfort and less commonly sudden cardiac arrest and signs of right ventricular failure such as dyspnea, edema, and fatigue. Patients may be clinically asymptomatic for many yr.
- Cardiac arrest after physical exertion may be the initial presentation.
- Physical examination will be normal in most patients. Widely split S2 is an important diagnostic clue.

ETIOLOGY

ARVD is characterized by progressive replacement of mainly the right ventricular myocardium with fibrofatty tissue after apoptotic myocardial cell death caused by mutations of desmosomal protein.

DIAGNOSIS

A major criterion equals 2 points; a minor criterion equals 1 point. The diagnosis of ARVD is considered definite if the patient has 4 points and probable with 3 points. See Table 1 for diagnostic criteria.

DIFFERENTIAL DIAGNOSIS

- Cardiomyopathy with involvement of the right ventricle
- Uhl anomaly: Rare anomaly that presents mainly in childhood with signs and symptoms of right heart failure and characterized by a paper-thin right ventricle resulting from death of the myocytes throughout the right ventricle
- Idiopathic RV tachycardia
- Sarcoidosis
- Right ventricular infarction

WORKUP

- Initial workup includes history with focus on sudden death in the family, resting ECG, 24-Holter ECG, signal-averaged ECG, and imaging studies with echocardiography and cardiac MRI.
- ECG will have diagnostic findings in 50%-90% of patients with ARVD, including T-wave inversions in anterior precordial leads V_1 to V_6, epsilon waves, and a QRS duration longer than 110 ms in V1 or >40 ms longer in V1 than V6 (Fig. 1).
- Ventricular tachycardia (VT) with left bundle branch block pattern and frequent PVCs (>500 in 24 hr) might be detected by 24-hr Holter monitoring.
- An abnormal signal-averaged ECG is a minor diagnostic criteria.
- Echocardiography will show right ventricular dilation with regional wall motion abnormalities, aneurysms, and depressed RV function that varies with the severity of the disease.
- MRI (Fig. 2) is a noninvasive method to detect structural abnormalities (fibrofatty changes) and regional dysfunction. Cardiac MRI (CMR) is the most sensitive method to detect ARVD, but it has high false-positive rates. Cardiac CT angiogram (Fig. E3) will reveal thinning and aneurysmal dilation of the RV anterior wall and outflow tract.
- If the routine tests are not conclusive, endomyocardial biopsy and electrophysiologic testing can be considered. However, biopsies and radionuclide ventriculography are rarely performed in the U.S.

TREATMENT

No curative treatment is available. The treatment goal is focused on preventing sudden cardiac death, symptomatic treatment of right heart failure, and pharmacologic and invasive treatment of arrhythmias. Therapy with cardio-selective beta-blockers is recommended. Family members with a negative phenotype (either healthy gene carriers or those with an unknown genotype) do not need any specific treatment other than sports restriction; however, lifelong clinical assessment with the use of noninvasive tests at least every 2 yr is warranted.[1]

NONPHARMACOLOGIC THERAPY

- Avoidance of activity that may trigger ventricular tachycardia and may lead to disease progression.
- ICD implantation needs to be considered in patients who have the definite diagnosis of ARVD. Patients with unexplained syncope, advanced disease, documented ventricular arrhythmias, or a family history of sudden cardiac death or who have been resuscitated from cardiac arrest are at high risk. A subcutaneous ICD might be an alternative option instead of transvenous implantation.
- Radiofrequency catheter ablation is used in cases of refractory VT or frequent tachycardia after defibrillator placement.
- Cardiac transplantation.
- Fig. 4 describes a management algorithm for ARVD.

PHARMACOLOGIC TREATMENT

Antiarrhythmic therapy with sotalol (first-line treatment) or amiodarone, often in combination with beta-blockers, is used for tachycardia suppression.

REFERRAL

- Early cardiology and electrophysiology referral
- Consider referring for genetic counseling

PEARLS & CONSIDERATIONS

PREVENTION

All first-degree relatives should be tested if ARVD is confirmed. Sports activity increases the risk of sudden cardiac death among adolescents and young adults with ARVC. The estimated overall mortality ranges from 0.08% to 3.6% per yr.

SUGGESTED READINGS

Available at ExpertConsult.com

AUTHOR: **John Wylie, MD**

[1] Corrado D et al: Arrhythmogenic right ventricular cardiomyopathy, *N Engl J Med* 376:61-72, 2017.

TABLE 1 Global or Regional Dysfunction and Structural Alterations

Major

2D echo criteria

Regional RV akinesia, dyskinesia, or aneurysm and one of the following measured at end diastole:

- PLAX RVOT ≥32 mm or
- PSAX RVOT ≥36
- Fractional area change ≤33%
- MRI criteria

Regional RV akinesia or dyskinesia or dyssynchronous RV contraction and one of the following:

- Ratio of RV end-diastolic volume to BSA >100, <110 ml/m^2 (male) or >100 ml/m^2
- RV ejection fraction >40% ≤45%
- RV angiography criteria
- Regional RV akinesia, dyskinesia, or aneurysm

Minor

2D echo criteria

Regional RV akinesia or dyskinesia or dyssynchronous RV contraction and one of the following measured at end diastole:

- PLAX RVOT ≥29 <32 mm or
- PSAX RVOT ≥32 <36
- Fractional area change >33% ≤40%
- MRI criteria
- Regional RV akinesia or dyskinesia or dyssynchronous RV contraction and one of the following:
- Ratio of RV end-diastolic volume to BSA ≥110 ml/m^2 (male) or ≥100 ml/m^2
- RV ejection fraction ≤40%

Tissue characterization of wall

Major

Residual myocytes <60% by morphometric analysis (or <50% if estimated) with fibrous replacement of the RV free wall myocardium in >1 sample, with or without fatty replacement of tissue on endomyocardial biopsy

Minor

Residual myocytes 60%-75% by morphometric analysis (or 50%-65% if estimated), with fibrous replacement of the RV free wall myocardium in >1 sample with or without fatty replacement of tissue on endomyocardial biopsy

Repolarization abnormalities

Major

Inverted T waves in right precordial leads (V1, V2, and V3) or beyond in individuals >14 yr of age (in the absence of complete RBBB QRS ≥120 ms)

Minor

Inverted T waves in V1 and V2 in individuals >14 yr of age (in the absence of complete RBBB) or in V4, V5, and V6

Inverted T waves in leads V1, V2, V3, and V4 in individuals >14 yr of age in the presence of a complete RBBB

Depolarization or conduction abnormalities

Major

Epsilon wave (reproducible low-amplitude signals between end of QRS complex to onset of T wave) in the right precordial leads (V1-V3)

Minor

Late potentials by SAECG in ≥1 of 3 parameters in the absence of a QRSd of ≥110 ms on standard ECG

Filtered QRS ≥114 ms

Duration of terminal QRS <40 mV ≥38 ms

Root-mean-square voltage of terminal 40 ms ≤20 μV

Terminal activation duration ≥55 ms measured from the nadir of the end of the QRS, including R', in V1, V2, or V3 in absence of complete RBBB

Arrhythmias

Major

Nonsustained or sustained VT of LBBB morph with superior axis

Minor

Nonsustained or sustained VT of RVOT configuration, LBBB morph with inferior axis or of unknown axis

>500 PVCs per 24 hr (Holter)

Family history

Major

ARVD/C in first-degree relative who meets Task Force criteria

ARVD/C confirmed pathologically at autopsy or surgery in first-degree relative

Identification of pathogenic mutation categorized as associated or probably associated with ARVD/C in the patient under evaluation

Minor

History of ARVD/C in first-degree relative in whom it is not possible to determine whether the family member meets Task Force criteria

Premature sudden death (<35 yr of age) caused by suspected ARVD/C in a first-degree relative

ARVD/C confirmed pathologically or by current Task Force criteria in second-degree relative

A major criterion equals 2 points, a minor criterion 1 point. The diagnosis of arrhythmogenic right ventricular dysplasia (ARVD) is considered definite if the patient has 4 points and probable with 3 points. *BSA,* Body surface area; *ECG,* electrocardiogram; *MRI,* magnetic resonance imaging; *PLAX,* parasternal long axis; *PSAX,* parasternal short axis; *PVCs,* premature ventricular contractions; *RBBB,* right bundle branch block; *RV,* right ventricle; *RVOT,* right ventricular outflow tract; *SAECG,* signal-averaged electrocardiogram; *2D,* two dimensional; *VT,* ventricular tachycardia.

From Marcus IM: Diagnosis of arrhythmogenic right ventricular cardiomyopathy/dysplasia proposed modification of the Task Force criteria, *Circulation* 121:1533-1541, 2010.

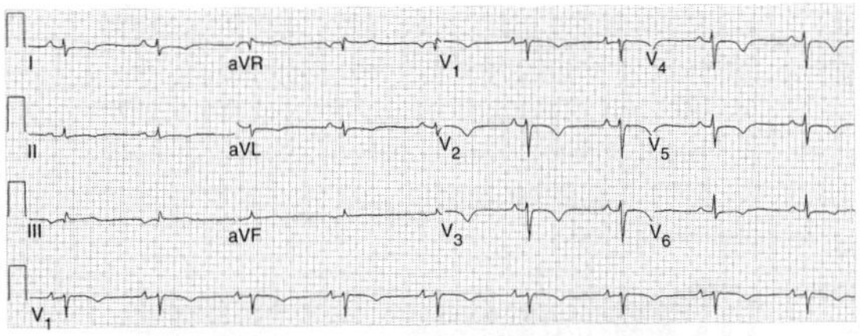

FIG. 1 Arrhythmogenic right ventricular cardiomyopathy—Epsilon wave. This 12-lead electrocardiogram tracing with lead Vfn$_{11}$ rhythm strip shows sinus rhythm with T-wave inversion over the right precordial leads. In addition, there is an epsilon wave (small deflection at the end of the QRS complex), evident in lead V_1, which is characteristic of arrhythmogenic right ventricular cardiomyopathy. *aVF,* Augmented vector foot. (From Olshansky B et al: *Arrhythmia essentials*, ed 2, Philadelphia, 2017, Elsevier.)

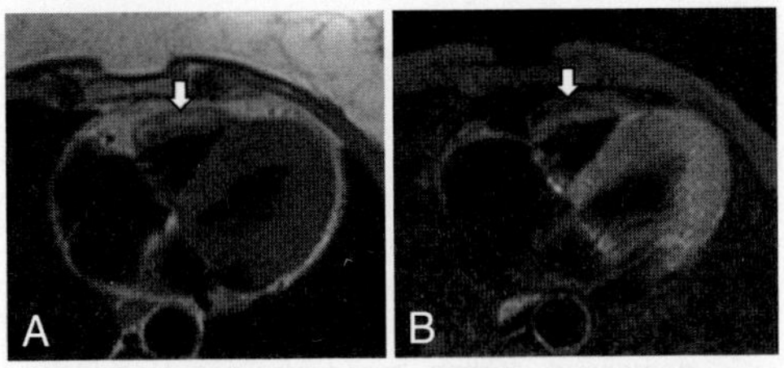

FIG. 2 Arrhythmogenic right ventricular cardiomyopathy. Spin-echo cardiovascular magnetic resonance without **(A)** and with **(B),** a fat-suppression prepulse. There is bright signal in the free wall of the right ventricle that suppresses with fat suppression *(arrows).* (From Sellke FW et al: *Sabiston & Spencer surgery of the chest*, ed 9, Philadelphia, 2016, Elsevier.)

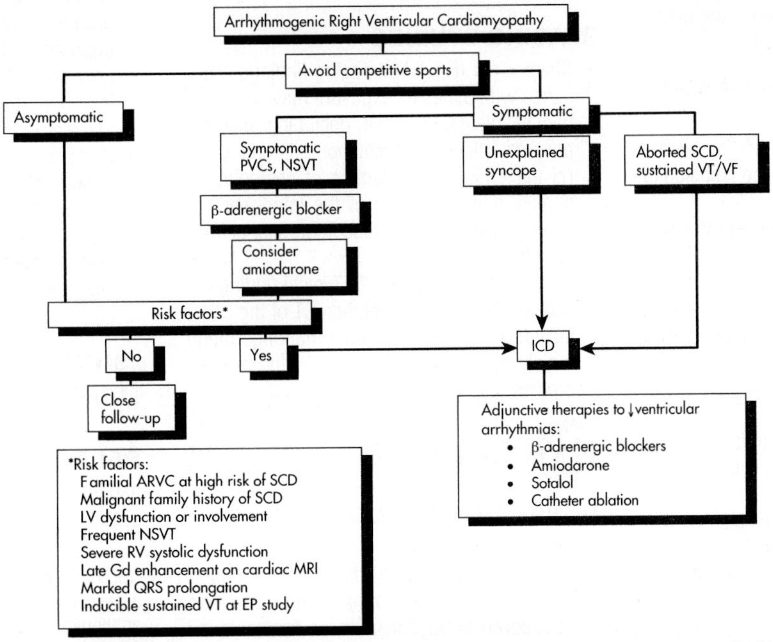

FIG. 4 Arrhythmogenic right ventricular cardiomyopathy. *ARVC,* Arrhythmogenic right ventricular cardiomyopathy; *EP,* electrophysiology; *Gd,* gadolinium; *ICD,* implantable cardiodefibrillator; *NSVT,* nonsustained ventricular tachycardia; *PVCs,* premature ventricular contractions; *SCD,* sequential compression device; *VF,* ventricular fibrillation; *VT,* ventricular tachycardia. (From Olshansky B et al: *Arrhythmia essentials*, ed 2, Philadelphia, 2017, Elsevier.)

BASIC INFORMATION

DEFINITION

Asbestosis is a slow, progressive diffuse interstitial fibrosis as a consequence of dose-related inhalation exposure to fibers of asbestos in miners, millers, workers of asbestos textiles, and insulators. Clinically, the lung involvement is characterized by bilateral diffuse interstitial fibrosis, more pronounced in the lower lobes, and pleural thickening, leading to shortness of breath and dry cough.

Asbestos exposure can lead to the spectrum of pulmonary pathology, including pulmonary fibrosis; asbestos-related pleural plaque disease (ARPD), both focal and diffuse; and malignancies (lung cancer or mesothelioma).

ICD-10CM CODE

J61 Pneumoconiosis due to asbestos and other mineral fibers

EPIDEMIOLOGY & DEMOGRAPHICS

- 5 to 10 new cases per 100,000 persons per yr in the U.S.
- Prolonged interval (20-30 yr) between exposures to inhaled fibers and clinical manifestations of disease.
- Most common in workers over age 40 yr involved in the primary extraction of asbestos from rock deposits and in those involved in the fabrication and installation of products containing asbestos (e.g., naval shipyards in World War II; installation of floor tiles, ceiling tiles, acoustic ceiling coverings, wall insulation, and pipe coverings in public buildings).
- Smokers and heavy drinkers have the greatest risk of developing this disease.

PHYSICAL FINDINGS & CLINICAL PRESENTATION

- Insidious onset of shortness of breath and dry cough with exertion is usually the first sign of asbestosis.
- Dyspnea becomes more severe as the disease advances; with time, progressively less exertion is tolerated.
- Cough is frequent and usually paroxysmal, dry, and nonproductive. Hemoptysis is rare but reported. Scant mucoid sputum may accompany the cough in the later stages of the disease.
- Fine end-respiratory crackles (rales, crepitations) are heard more predominantly in the lung bases.
- Digital clubbing, edema, and jugular venous distention may be present.
- Advanced cases may have signs of right heart failure.

ETIOLOGY/PATHOGENESIS

Inhalation of asbestos fibers. The pathogenesis of pulmonary interstitial inflammation and fibrosis is related to immune mechanisms. Asbestosis is known to be associated with positive serum antinuclear antibody (ANA) and rheumatoid factor (RF). An important role of interleukin-1beta (IL-1beta) in the pathogenesis of asbestosis and its systemic autoimmune manifestations has been reported.

Dx DIAGNOSIS

DIFFERENTIAL DIAGNOSIS

- Silicosis
- Siderosis, other pneumonoconioses
- Interstitial lung disease
- Lung cancer

WORKUP

Documentation of exposure history
Pulmonary function testing
Diagnostic imaging studies

LABORATORY TESTS

- Generally not helpful
- Arterial blood gases: May show hypoxemia and/or hypercarbia in advanced stages

Pulmonary function testing:

- Most often shows decreased vital capacity (VC), decreased total lung capacity (TLC), and decreased carbon monoxide gas transfer (DLco)
- FEV1 might be reduced in concomitant smokers

Bronchoscopy with bronchoalveolar lavage:

- Clinical utility of bronchoscopy is limited. It can be helpful in ruling out infection, or hypersensitivity pneumonitis. Asbestos bodies are found in sputum and BAL fluid of asbestos workers but utility in diagnosis of asbestos-related lung disease and progression is limited.

IMAGING STUDIES

- Chest x-ray (Fig. E1): Imaging findings associated with asbestos exposure may vary from benign pleural disease (including discrete plaques, pleural calcification, diffuse pleural thickening with blunting of costophrenic angles, and thickening of the interlobar fissure) to asbestosis (diffuse interstitial pulmonary fibrosis).
- CT scan of chest (Fig. E2): Typical findings of asbestosis on high-resolution CT of the chest include increased interstitial markings found mainly at the bases (Fig. E3). As the disease progresses, honeycombing is noted.

Rx TREATMENT

NONPHARMACOLOGIC THERAPY

- Smoking cessation
- Exercise program to maximize available lung function. Pulmonary rehabilitation can be considered in advanced cases for improved cardiopulmonary capacity
- Supplemental oxygen on a PRN basis
- Removal of patient from further asbestos fiber exposure
- Prompt identification and treatment of respiratory infections
- Pneumococcal vaccination and annual influenza vaccination

PHARMACOLOGIC THERAPY

- There is no specific pharmacologic treatment for asbestosis
- Some new data are coming out targeting IL-1beta therapy on the progression of lung fibrosis that suggest a new perspective for the treatment of systemic autoimmune features of asbestosis and, possibly, of lung involvement.[1]

DISPOSITION

- Death is usually from respiratory failure from cor pulmonale.
- Survival in patients after development of mesothelioma is 4 to 6 yr.
- Benign asbestos pleural effusions (BAPEs) are usually small and unilateral and occur yr before the onset of interstitial disease.
- Diffuse pleural thickening and asbestosis are associated with increased risks of malignant peritoneal mesothelioma beyond the risk calculated to be associated with the degree of asbestos exposure.[2]
- None of the benign pleural diseases or ARPD was associated with an increased risk of malignant pleural mesothelioma.
- Asbestos increases the risk for development of lung cancer regardless of smoking status. The joint effect of asbestos and smoking is additive and depends in part on the presence of asbestosis. Patients with a history of tobacco smoking who have diffuse parenchymal disease secondary to asbestos, have a 40-fold increased risk of lung cancer compared to never-smokers. Asbestos workers who stop smoking experience a dramatic decline in lung cancer risk, which approaches that of nonsmokers after 30 yr.
- Low-dose chest CT scanning offers an excellent opportunity to detect early-stage lung cancers in asbestos-exposed workers.
- Computed tomography is more sensitive than radiography, computed tomography without contrast generally suffices for evaluation, and PET scan (fluorodeoxyglucose-positron emission tomography) may have utility in patients with mesothelioma.

SUGGESTED READINGS

Available at ExpertConsult.com

RELATED CONTENT

Asbestosis (Patient Information)

AUTHOR: **Imrana Qawi, MD**

[1]Niccoli L et al: Systemic autoimmune disease in asbestosis rapidly responding to anti-interleukin-1beta antibody canakinumab: a case report, *BMC Musculoskelet Disord* 14(16):146, 2015.

[2]Reid A et al: The additional risk of malignant mesothelioma in former workers and residents of Wittenoom with benign pleural disease or asbestosis, *Occup Environ Med* 62:665-669, 2005.

BASIC INFORMATION

DEFINITION

Ascariasis is a parasitic infection caused by the nematode *Ascaris lumbricoides.* The majority of those infected are asymptomatic; however, clinical disease may arise from pulmonary hypersensitivity, intestinal obstruction, or nutrient depletion and other secondary complications.

SYNONYMS

Round worms
Worms

ICD-10CM CODES

B77.0	Ascariasis with intestinal complications
B77.81	Ascariasis pneumonia
B77.89	Ascariasis with other complications
B77.9	Ascariasis, unspecified

EPIDEMIOLOGY & DEMOGRAPHICS

INCIDENCE (IN U.S.):

- Unknown. Worldwide, *A. lumbricoides* is the most common helminthic infection of humans, infecting as many as 1 billion or more persons. 71% of persons at risk for infection live in Asia and the Western Pacific.
- Three times the infection rates found in blacks as in whites.

PREVALENCE (IN U.S.): Estimated at 4 million, the majority of which live in the rural southeastern part of the country; ascariasis is associated with poor sanitation.

PREDOMINANT SEX: Both sexes probably equally affected, with a possible slight female preponderance.

PREDOMINANT AGE: Most common in children from ages 2 to 10 yr old and decreases after age 15; infections tend to cluster in families.

PEAK INCIDENCE: Unknown

NEONATAL INFECTION: Probable transmission, though not specifically studied

PHYSICAL FINDINGS & CLINICAL PRESENTATION

- Most people infected with *Ascaris* are asymptomatic
- Occurs approximately 9 to 12 days after ingestion of eggs (corresponding to the larval migration through the lungs)
- Nonproductive cough
- Substernal chest discomfort
- Fever
- In patients with large worm burdens, especially children, intestinal obstruction associated with perforation, volvulus, and intussusception
- Migration of worms into the biliary tree giving clinical appearance of biliary colic and pancreatitis as well as acute appendicitis with movement into that appendage
- Rarely, infection with *A. lumbricoides* producing interstitial nephritis and acute renal failure
- In endemic areas in Asia and Africa, malabsorption of dietary proteins and vitamins as a consequence of chronic worm intestinal carriage; 1 billion people worldwide are infected with this nematode

ETIOLOGY

- Transmission is usually hand to mouth, but eggs may be ingested via transported vegetables grown in contaminated soil.
- Eggs are hatched in the small intestine, with larvae penetrating intestinal mucosa and migrating via the circulation to the lungs.
- Larval forms proceed through the alveoli, ascend the bronchial tree, and return to the intestines after swallowing, where they mature into adult worms.
- Estimated time until the female adult worm begins producing eggs is 2 to 3 mo.
- Eggs are passed out of the intestines with feces and can survive for years in warm, moist, shaded soil.
- Within human host, adult worm life span is 1 to 2 yr.

Dx DIAGNOSIS

DIFFERENTIAL DIAGNOSIS

- Radiologic manifestations and eosinophilia to be distinguished from drug hypersensitivity and Löffler syndrome.
- Table 1 compares features of major intestinal nematodes.

TABLE 1 Features of Major Intestinal Nematodes

Nematode	Transmission	Direct Person-to-Person Transmission	Geographic Distribution	Duration of Infection	Location of Adult Worm(s)	Treatment*
Ascaris lumbricoides	Ingestion of infective eggs	No	Warm, humid areas; temperate zones in warmer months	1-2 yr	Free in lumen of small bowel, primarily jejunum	Albendazole Mebendazole Pyrantel Ivermectin Levamisole Piperazine
Trichuris trichiura (whipworm)	Ingestion of infective eggs	No	Warm, humid areas; temperate zones in warmer months	1-3 yr	Anchored in superficial mucosa of cecum and colon	Albendazole Mebendazole
Necator americanus, Ancylostoma duodenale (hookworm)	Penetration of skin by filariform larvae	No	Warm, humid areas; temperate zones in warmer months	3-5 yr *(Necator)*; 1 yr *(Ancylostoma)*	Attached to mucosa of mid to upper portion of small bowel	Albendazole Mebendazole Levamisole Pyrantel
Strongyloides stercoralis	Penetration of skin or bowel mucosa by filariform larvae	Yes	Primarily warm, humid areas but can be worldwide	Lifetime of host	Embedded in mucosa of duodenum, jejunum	Ivermectin† Albendazole Thiabendazole
Enterobius vermicularis (pinworm)	Ingestion of infective eggs	Yes	Worldwide	1 mo	Free in lumen of cecum, appendix, adjacent colon	Albendazole Mebendazole Pyrantel Ivermectin Levamisole Piperazine

*Nitazoxanide has been shown to be effective in the treatment of ascariasis, trichuriasis, and enterobiasis in several trials in Mexico. Tribendimidine, which is licensed in China, was shown to be efficacious against *Ascaris* spp. and had moderate efficacy against *Strongyloides* spp. in a randomized trial.

†Drug of choice.

From Bennett et al: *Mandell, Douglas, and Bennett's principles and practice of infectious diseases*, ed 8, Philadelphia, 2015, Saunders.

LABORATORY TESTS

- Examination of the stool for *Ascaris* ova (Fig. E1).
- The World Health Organization (WHO) recommends the Kato-Katz thick smear kit for soil-transmitted helminths.
- Expectoration or fecal passage of adult worm.
- Adult male worms: 10 to 30 cm long; adult female worms: Larger than male, up to 40 cm.
- Eosinophilia: Most prominent early in the infection and subsides as the adult worm infestation established in the intestines; usually in 5% to 12% range but can be up to 50%.
- Serology: Patients develop immunoglobulin G (IgG) antibodies, but they cross react with antigens from other helminths and are not protective; thus, serology is used more for epidemiologic purposes than for individual diagnosis.
- Polymerase chain reaction (PCR) on stool samples; multiplex PCR can differentiate multiple different parasite species (*A. lumbricoides, T. trichiura,* and *N. americanus*).

IMAGING STUDIES

- Chest x-ray to reveal bilateral oval or round infiltrates of varying size (Löffler syndrome); NOTE: Infiltrates are transient and eventually resolve.
- Plain films of the abdomen and contrast studies to reveal worm masses in loops of bowel.
- Ultrasonography and endoscopic retrograde cholangiopancreatography (ERCP) to identify worms in the pancreaticobiliary tract.
- CT scan with oral contrast can also assist in the detection of GI foreign bodies such as parasites.

Rx TREATMENT

NONPHARMACOLOGIC THERAPY

Aggressive IV hydration, especially in children with fever, severe vomiting, and resultant dehydration

ACUTE GENERAL Rx

- All infected patients, including asymptomatic ones, should be treated.
  1. Albendazole: 400 mg PO × 1 dose is the first-line agent
  2. Mebendazole 100 mg PO bid × 3 days for persons >1 yr of age or mebendazole 500 mg PO × 1 dose for persons >1 yr of age (not available as 500 mg in the U.S.)
- Cure rate with these agents is 95% to 100%, but they are contraindicated in pregnancy.
- Side effects: GI discomfort, headache, and rarely leukopenia
- Alternative agent or for use in pregnancy: Pyrantel pamoate (Antiminth):
  1. Given at a dose of 11 mg/kg PO (maximum dose of 1 g/day)
  2. Considered safe for use in pregnant women
- Other alternative agents:
  1. Ivermectin: 150 to 200 mcg/kg orally once
  2. Nitazoxanide: Ages 2 to 3 yr: 100 mg/5 ml bid × 3 days, and ages 4 to 11 yr: 200 mg/10 ml bid × 3 days. Cure rates in heavy worm burden are only 50% to 80%
  3. Piperazine citrate: No longer first-line agent due to toxicity but still used in cases of intestinal or biliary obstruction, as drug paralyzes the worm, helping its expulsion. Dose: 50 to 75 mg/kg once daily up to maximum of 3.5 g for 2 days
  4. Levamisole: 2.5 mg/kg once orally is recommended by the WHO as alternative therapy, but not available in the U.S.
- Complete obstruction should be managed surgically.

DISPOSITION

Overall prognosis is good. Patients should be reevaluated in 2 to 3 mo. Reinfection is common.

REFERRAL

- To gastroenterologist in cases of visualized pancreaticobiliary tract or appendiceal obstruction
- To surgeon in cases of complete obstruction or suspected secondary complication (e.g., perforation or volvulus)

PEARLS & CONSIDERATIONS

COMMENTS

- Hepatic abscess, containing both viable and dead worms, complicating *Ascaris*-induced biliary duct disease has been documented.
- Given the known transmission of the parasite, routine hand washing with soap and proper disposal of human waste would significantly decrease the prevalence of this disease.
- Other protective measures to avoid ingestion of worm eggs:
  1. Peel or cook food.
  2. Boil drinking water.
  3. Do not place small children directly on soil.

SUGGESTED READINGS

Available at ExpertConsult.com

RELATED CONTENT

Ascariasis (Patient Information)

AUTHOR: **Glenn G. Fort, MD, MPH**

BASIC INFORMATION

DEFINITIONS

Ascites refers to a pathologic accumulation of fluid in the peritoneal cavity, most commonly caused by liver cirrhosis.

- **Diuretic-resistant ascites:** Ascites that cannot be mobilized or the early occurrence of ascites that cannot be prevented because of a lack of response to dietary sodium restriction and intensive diuretic treatment
- **Diuretic-intractable ascites:** Ascites that cannot be mobilized or the early recurrence of ascites that cannot be prevented because of the development of diuretic-induced complications that precludes the use of effective doses of diuretics
- Grade 1 (mild ascites): Ascites only detectable by ultrasound
- Grade 2 (moderate ascites): Ascites with moderate symmetrical distension of abdomen
- Grade 3 (large ascites): Ascites with marked abdominal distension

SYNONYMS

Peritoneal cavity fluid
Hydroperitoneum
Hydroperitonia
Hydrops abdominis

ICD-10CM CODES

R18	Ascites
K70.11	Alcoholic hepatitis with ascites
K70.31	Alcoholic cirrhosis of liver with ascites
K71.51	Toxic liver disease with chronic active hepatitis with ascites
R18.8	Other ascites

EPIDEMIOLOGY & DEMOGRAPHICS

Ascites is the most common complication of cirrhosis and signifies decompensation of chronic liver disease. Ascites occurs at a rate of 7% to 10% annually in cirrhotic patients. Ascites occurs in ~60% of individuals with cirrhosis within 10 yr of diagnosis. Cirrhosis is the cause of 85% of cases of ascites.

CLINICAL PRESENTATION & PHYSICAL FINDINGS

- Important information to elicit within history:
  1. History of viral hepatitis
  2. Alcoholism
  3. Intravenous drug use, intranasal cocaine use
  4. Sexual history (i.e., men who have sex with men)
  5. History of transfusions, tattoos, piercings, imprisonment
  6. Travel history and time spent in endemic regions for hepatitis
  7. Symptoms suggestive of peritoneal malignancy (e.g., weight loss, pain, palpable masses, rectal/vaginal bleeding)
  8. Other liver disease symptoms (e.g., increasing abdominal girth, jaundice, pruritus, confusion, pedal edema)
  9. Cardiac symptoms (e.g., pedal edema, shortness of breath, orthopnea, chest pain)
  10. Hypothyroid disease (fatigue, weight gain, constipation)
  11. History of ascites, prior treatment, LVP requirements and frequency
- Important physical exam findings:
  1. Protuberant abdomen (Fig. E1)
  2. Bulging flanks (can be present in obesity)
  3. Flank dullness to percussion (requires ~1500 ml of fluid)
  4. Fluid wave on abdominal exam
  5. Lower extremity edema
  6. Shifting dullness on abdominal exam
  7. Physical signs associated with liver cirrhosis: Spider angiomas, jaundice, loss of body hair, skeletal muscle wasting (sarcopenia), Dupuytren contracture, bruising, palmar erythema, gynecomastia, testicular atrophy, rectal varices, and caput medusa

ETIOLOGY

Pathophysiology of ascites (Fig. E2): Increased hepatic resistance to portal flow leads to portal hypertension. A portal pressure >12 mm Hg appears to be required for fluid retention. The splanchnic vessels respond by increased secretion of nitric oxide, causing splanchnic artery vasodilation. Vasodilation appears also to be mediated by the translocation of enteric bacteria and bacterial products. Early in the disease increased plasma volume and increased cardiac output compensate for this vasodilation. However, as the disease progresses the effective arterial blood volume decreases, causing sodium and fluid retention through activation of the renin-angiotensin system. Over time, activation of the sympathetic system causes renal vascular perfusion to decrease and may lead to hepatorenal syndrome. The change in capillary pressure causes increased permeability and retention of fluid in the abdomen.

DIAGNOSIS

DIFFERENTIAL DIAGNOSIS

- Chronic parenchymal liver disease, leading to portal hypertension
- Acute liver failure
- Noncirrhotic portal hypertension (e.g., portal vein clot)
- Peritoneal carcinomatosis
- Cardiac disease (e.g., heart failure, constrictive pericarditis)
- Hepatic venous outflow obstruction (e.g., Budd-Chiari syndrome, IVC webs)
- Protein losing enteropathy
- Peritoneal tuberculosis
- Nephrotic syndrome
- Pancreatitis

LABORATORY TESTS

- Initial evaluation should always include:
  1. Diagnostic paracentesis. Laboratory tests on fluid should include a cell count and differential, cytology, albumin, total protein, culture, and Gram stain. A serum-ascites albumin gradient (SAAG) should be calculated in all patients. The SAAG is measured by subtracting the level of albumin in the ascitic fluid from a concurrent serum albumin measurement: SAAG = serum albumin – ascites albumin
     a. If the SAAG is greater than 1.1, the cause of ascites can be attributed to portal hypertension (from cirrhosis, Budd-Chiari syndrome) or heart failure.
     b. If SAAG is less than 1.1, a nonportal hypertension etiology of ascites must be sought. Optional tests on paracentesis fluid include amylase, LDH, acid-fast bacilli, and glucose levels.
     c. Total ascitic fluid protein: assess the risk of spontaneous bacterial peritonitis (SBP). Patients with protein concentration <1.5 g/dl have an increased risk of SBP.
  2. AST, ALT, total and direct bilirubin, albumin, alkaline phosphatase, GGTP.
  3. CBC, coagulation studies.
  4. Electrolytes, BUN, creatinine.
- Causes of ascites in the normal or diseased peritoneum by SAAG are summarized in Table 1.
- Fig. 3 illustrates an algorithm for the approach to the differential diagnosis of ascites.

IMAGING STUDIES

- Abdominal ultrasound (Fig. 4) is the most sensitive measure for detecting ascitic fluid; a CT or MRI scan is a viable alternative. Doppler studies of portal and hepatic veins should be added to rule out vascular etiology.
- Endoscopy of the upper GI tract to evaluate for esophageal varices if ascites is secondary to portal hypertension.

TREATMENT

NONPHARMACOLOGIC THERAPY

- Sodium-restricted diet (88 mmol, <2 g/day)
- Fluid restriction to 1 L/day in patients with severe hyponatremia (sodium <120 mEq/L)
- Counsel on avoiding NSAIDs and discontinuation of ACE inhibitors and ARBs

ACUTE GENERAL Rx

Patients with moderate-volume ascites causing only moderate discomfort may be treated on an outpatient basis with the following diuretic regimen:

1. Spironolactone: Start at 50 to 100 mg/day and titrate up to 400 mg day every 3 to 4 days (monotherapy or combination therapy with furosemide).
2. Furosemide: Start at 40 mg/day and titrate up to 160 mg/day maximum (no role for monotherapy).

TABLE 1 Causes of Ascites in the Normal or Diseased Peritoneum by Serum-to-Ascites Albumin Gradient (SAAG)

Normal Peritoneum	
Portal Hypertension (SAAG >1.1 G/dl)	**Hypoalbuminemia (SAAG <1.1 g/dl)**
Hepatic congestion	Nephrotic syndrome
Congestive heart failure	Protein-losing enteropathy
Constrictive pericarditis	Severe malnutrition with anasarca
Tricuspid insufficiency	
Budd-Chiari syndrome	
Liver Disease	**Miscellaneous Conditions (SAAG <1.1 g/dl)**
Cirrhosis	Chylous ascites
Alcoholic hepatitis	Pancreatic ascites
Fulminant hepatic failure	Bile ascites
Massive hepatic metastases	Nephrogenic ascites
	Urine ascites
	Ovarian disease
Diseased Peritoneum (SAAG <1.1 g/dl)	
Infections	**Other Rare Conditions**
Bacterial peritonitis	Familial Mediterranean fever
Tuberculous peritonitis	Vasculitis
Fungal peritonitis	Granulomatous peritonitis
HIV-associated peritonitis	Eosinophilic peritonitis
Malignant Conditions	
Peritoneal carcinomatosis	
Primary mesothelioma	
Pseudomyxoma peritonei	
Hepatocellular carcinoma	

HIV, Human immunodeficiency virus.
From Vincent JL et al: *Textbook of critical care*, ed 7, Philadelphia, 2017, Elsevier.

3. Monitor renal function and sodium levels carefully for signs of prerenal azotemia (in patients without edema. Goal weight loss is 300 to 500 g/day; in patients with edema, goal weight loss is 800 to 1000 g/day). Furosemide alone is not recommended.
4. Measurement of the urinary sodium level can be helpful to identify noncompliance with dietary sodium restriction and diuretic therapy. Patients excreting more than 78 mmol of sodium/day (24-hour urine) and not losing weight likely have nonadherence with low Na diet. Patients with low Na excretion, less than 78 mmol daily, require up titration of diuretics and evaluation of compliance.

Patients with large-volume ascites causing marked discomfort or decrease in activities of daily living may also be treated as outpatients if there are no complications. There are two options for treatment in these patients:

1. Large-volume paracentesis
2. Diuretic therapy until loss of fluid is noted (maximum spironolactone 400 mg daily and furosemide 160 mg daily)
   a. No difference in long-term mortality rate was found; however, paracentesis is faster, more effective, and associated with fewer adverse effects
   b. Patients receiving large-volume paracentesis should receive albumin replacement therapy at the dose of 7 to 9 g/L of fluid removed if more than 5 L are taken out to prevent paracentesis-induced circulatory dysfunction (PICD). Patients with renal dysfunction or hyponatremia should receive albumin for lower volumes as well.

Table 2 summarizes primary medical therapy and adjunctive medications used to increase the efficacy of primary therapy in the treatment of ascites.

CHRONIC Rx

- 5% to 10% of patients with large-volume ascites will be refractory to high-dose diuretic treatment. Treatment strategies include repeated large-volume paracentesis with infusion of albumin every 2 to 4 wk or placement of a transjugular intrahepatic portosystemic shunt (TIPS). TIPS evaluation should include echocardiogram, assessment for hepatic encephalopathy, and characterization of liver impairment.
- Long-term albumin administration (40 g weekly) has been shown to improve mortality, reduce episodes of HE, and delay accumulation of ascites compared to standard medical therapy.
- There is limited data on use of nonselective betablockers (NSBBs) in patients with diuretic-resistant ascites. Changes in mean arterial pressure (MAP) should be carefully monitored in patients on NSBBs, and these should be dose-reduced or stopped if substantial decrease in MAP is observed or systolic blood pressure is less than 90 mm Hg.
- Discuss referral to transplant-capable center.
- Patients known to have ascites should receive a diagnostic tap if they develop any signs of SBP or on any admission to the hospital even in the absence of these signs.
- Primary prophylaxis for SBP is recommended in patients with ascitic fluid protein <1.5 g/dl along with impaired renal function (creatinine ≥1.2 mg/dl or 106 micromol/L), BUN ≥25 mg/dl or 8.9 mmol/L or Na ≤130 mEq/L or 130 mmol/L, or liver failure (Child-Pugh score ≥9 and bilirubin ≥3 mg/dl or 51 micromol/L).
- Secondary prophylaxis should be instituted in all patients who were diagnosed with SBP in the form of a daily fluoroquinolone, ciprofloxacin or norfloxacin, or double-strength trimethoprim-sulfamethoxazole.
- Patients with known ascites who develop gastrointestinal bleeding should receive intravenous ceftriaxone for 7 days to prevent bacterial infections.
- Clinical use of Vaptan agents is not currently recommended in cirrhotic patients.
- Oral midodrine 7.5 mg three times daily has been shown to increase urine volume, urine sodium, mean arterial pressure, and survival.
- Peritoneovenous shunts or surgical portosystemic shunts have poor evidence and are not recommended.
- The Automated Low-Flow Ascites pump (not approved in North America) works by transporting small amounts of fluid from the peritoneal cavity to the bladder. Studies have shown improved symptoms and reduced LVP requirements.
- Liver transplantation remains definitive management for cirrhosis with refractory ascites.
- Table 3 summarizes the management of refractory ascites.
- A treatment approach to patients with malignant ascites is described in Fig. E5.

DISPOSITION

- Development of ascites signals a shift to decompensated cirrhosis and close follow-up is required. Two-year mortality reaches 75% in refractory ascites cases.
- Monitor closely for worsening liver function and development of spontaneous bacterial peritonitis (SBP).

REFERRAL

Referral to hepatology at a transplant-capable center.

PEARLS & CONSIDERATIONS

COMMENTS

- Prevalence of SBP in patients with ascites ranges between 10% and 30%.
  1. Presence of at least 250 neutrophils per cubic millimeter of ascitic fluid is diagnostic.
  2. Gram-negative bacteria such as *E. coli* are the most common isolates.
  3. Third-generation cephalosporins are the treatment of choice.

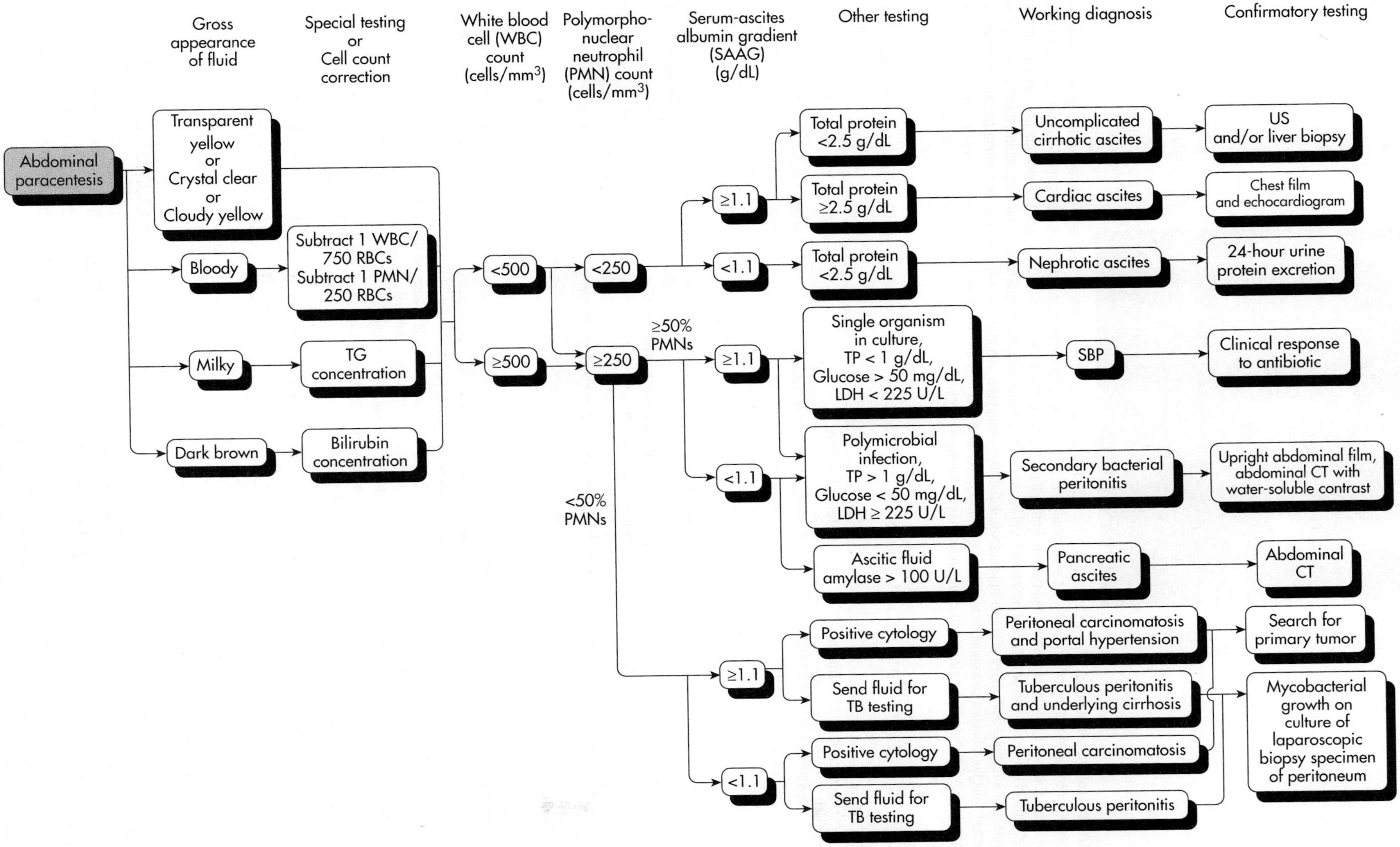

FIG. 3 Algorithm for the approach to the differential diagnosis of ascites. *CT,* Computed tomography; *LDH,* lactic dehydrogenase; *PMN,* polymorphonuclear neutrophil; *RBC,* red blood cell; *TB,* tuberculosis; *TG,* triglyceride; *TP,* total protein; *U/L,* upper and lower; *US,* ultrasound. (From Feldman M et al: *Sleisenger and Fordtran's gastrointestinal and liver disease*, ed 10, Philadelphia, 2016, Elsevier.)

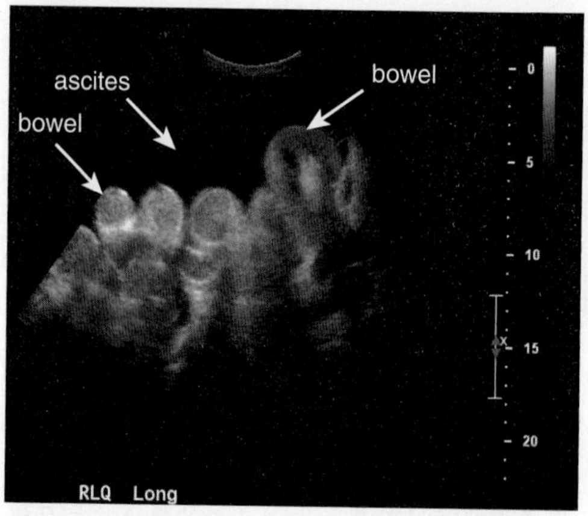

FIG. 4 Ascites, ultrasound. Ultrasound is useful for detection of ascites. Simple fluids such as ascites are excellent sound transmission media, reflecting almost no sound waves. As a consequence, they appear quite hypoechoic *(black)* on ultrasound. This view of the right lower quadrant shows loops of bowel surrounded by fluid. During the ultrasound, the bowel loops would be seen to undergo peristalsis and drift back and forth in the ascitic fluid with patient movement. Ultrasound cannot distinguish the composition of the fluid; ascites, liquid blood, liquid bile, urine, and infectious fluids have a similar appearance, with a few exceptions. Blood may coagulate and form septations within the fluid collection. Infectious fluids also frequently form loculated fluid collections that may be recognized on ultrasound, although the exact composition cannot be determined. (From Broder JS: *Diagnostic imaging for the emergency physician,* Philadelphia, 2011, Saunders.)

TABLE 2 Primary Medical Therapy and Adjunctive Medications Used to Increase the Efficacy of Primary Therapy in the Treatment of Ascites

Class	Medication	Dosing	Relevant Action	Notes
Diuretics	Spironolactone	400 mg + daily*	Aldosterone receptor antagonist	Primary therapy
	Furosemide	160 mg + daily*	Inhibits Na-K-2Cl symporter	Primary therapy
Vasoconstrictors	Octreotide	300 mcg bid*	Splanchnic vasoconstriction, inhibits RAAS	Also used in combination with midodrine to treat hepatorenal syndrome; given for first 5 days following variceal bleeding to decrease recurrence
	Midodrine	7.5 mg tid*	Inhibits RAAS	Also used in combination with octreotide and albumin to treat hepatorenal syndrome
α2-Agonist	Clonidine	0.075 mg bid*	Inhibits sympathetic outflow, inhibits RAAS	Increases sensitivity to spironolactone
Colloid	Albumin	25 g*	Increased oncotic pressure	Also utilized with large-volume paracentesis and in the treatment of hepatorenal syndrome

RAAS, Renin-angiotensin-aldosterone system

*The above doses have been derived from various studies and may not be suitable for all patients. Titration is always recommended.

From Cameron JL, Cameron AM: *Current surgical therapy,* ed 10, Philadelphia, 2011, Saunders.

TABLE 3 Management of Refractory Ascites

Definitions	Ascites that is not eliminated even with maximum diuretic therapy Ascites that is not eliminated because maximum dosages of diuretics cannot be attained, given the development of diuretic-induced complications
Recommended therapy	Total paracentesis + IV albumin (7-9 g/L of ascites removed) if >5 L removed Continue with salt restriction and diuretic therapy as tolerated
Alternative therapy	TIPS for patients who require frequent paracenteses (every 1-2 wk) and whose CTP score is ≤11 or MELD <17
Peritoneovenous shunt for patients who are not candidates for TIPS or transplant	

CTP, Child-Turcotte-Pugh; *IV,* intravenous; *MELD,* model for end-stage liver disease; *TIPS,* transjugular intrahepatic portosystemic shunt.

Data from Garcia-Tsao G, Lim JK; Members of the Veterans Affairs Hepatitis C Resource Center Program: management and treatment of patients with cirrhosis and portal hypertension: recommendations from the Department of Veterans Affairs Hepatitis C Resource Center Program and the National Hepatitis C Program, *Am J Gastroenterol,* 104:1802-1829, 2009.

From Vincent JL et al: *Textbook of critical care,* ed 7, Philadelphia, 2017, Elsevier.

4. By 1 yr, 70% of patients have recurrence of SBP and may be prophylaxed with ciprofloxacin 750 mg PO once/wk.

PREVENTION

- Prevention of liver cirrhosis through avoidance of long-term use of alcohol, immunization against hepatitis A and B, and treatment of hepatitis C
- In cirrhotic patients, following a low-sodium diet (<2 g daily)

SUGGESTED READINGS

Available at ExpertConsult.com

RELATED CONTENT

Ascites (Patient Information)
Cirrhosis (Related Key Topic)

AUTHORS: **Marc Monachese, MD, MSc, Roxana Chis, MD, MSc,** and **Talia Zenlea, MD**

BASIC INFORMATION

DEFINITION

Aspergillus spp is a ubiquitous mold most commonly found in soil, building materials, and water. *Aspergillosis* refers to several forms of a broad range of illnesses caused by infection with *Aspergillus* species. Fig. 1 illustrates the spectrum of *Aspergillus* infection.

ICD-10CM CODES

B44.0	Invasive pulmonary aspergillosis
B44.1	Other pulmonary aspergillosis
B44.2	Tonsillar aspergillosis
B44.7	Disseminated aspergillosis
B44.81	Allergic bronchopulmonary aspergillosis
B44.89	Other forms of aspergillosis
B44.9	Aspergillosis, unspecified

EPIDEMIOLOGY & DEMOGRAPHICS

INCIDENCE & PREVALENCE:

- *Aspergillus* species are ubiquitous in the environment internationally and occur as a mold found in soil. *Aspergillus fumigatus* is the most common human pathogen
- Cause a variety of illness from hypersensitivity pneumonitis to disseminated overwhelming infection in immunosuppressed patients
- Frequently cultured from hospital wards from unfiltered outside air circulating through open windows as well as water sources
- Reach the patient by airborne conidia (spores) that are small enough (2.5-3 μm) to reach the alveoli on inhalation
- Can invade the nose, paranasal sinuses, external ear, or traumatized skin

RISK FACTORS:

- The clinical syndrome depends on the underlying lung architecture, the host's immune response, and the degree of inoculum.
- Incidence of invasive aspergillosis is increasing with advances in the treatment of life-threatening diseases, such as aggressive chemotherapy or bone marrow and solid organ transplantation. Liver and lung transplant recipients are at highest risk for invasive pulmonary aspergillosis. Genetic deficiency of the soluble-pattern-recognition receptor known as long pentraxin 3 (PTX3) affects the antifungal capacity of neutrophils and may contribute to the risk of invasive aspergillosis in patients treated with hematopoietic stem-cell transplantation (HSCT).
- Patients with AIDS and a CD4 count <50/mm^3 have an increased susceptibility to invasive aspergillosis, but it is otherwise uncommon in patients with HIV.
- Pandemic influenza A (H1N1) infection may predispose immunocompromised patients to invasive aspergillosis and, rarely, in normal hosts.
- Patients with chronic granulomatous disease are at higher risk for infections with *Aspergillus* species, for example, *Aspergillus nidulans.*
- *Aspergillus nidulans* causes mostly invasive infections in patients with chronic granulomatous disease.

ETIOLOGY

- *Aspergillus fumigatus* is the usual cause.
- *Aspergillus flavus* is the second most important species, particularly in invasive disease of immunosuppressed patients and in lesions beginning in the nose and paranasal sinuses. *Aspergillus niger* can also cause invasive human infection.

ALLERGIC ASPERGILLOSIS:

- Is a hypersensitivity pneumonitis
- Presents as cough, dyspnea, fever, chills, and malaise typically 4 to 8 hours after exposure
- Repeated attacks can lead to granulomatous disease and pulmonary fibrosis

ALLERGIC BRONCHOPULMONARY ASPERGILLOSIS (ABPA):

- Symptoms occur most commonly in atopic individuals during the third and fourth decades of life
- Hypersensitivity reaction to *Aspergillus* fungal antigens present in the bronchial tree
- Results from an initial type I (immediate hypersensitivity) and type III reactions (immune complexes)
- Underdiagnosed pulmonary disorder in patients with asthma and cystic fibrosis (reported prevalence in asthmatic patients varies from 6% to 28% and in cystic fibrosis 6% to 25%)

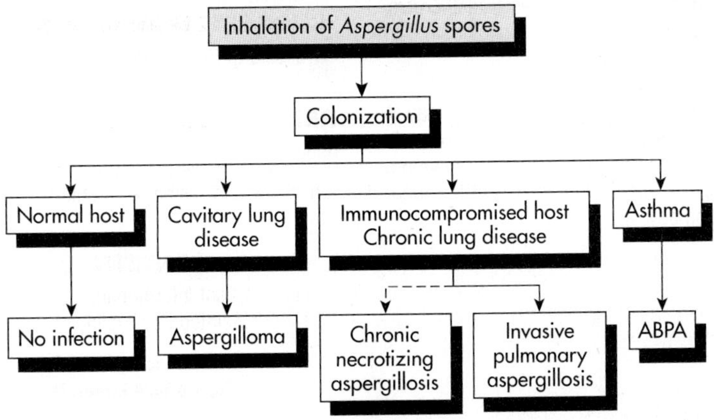

FIG. 1 The spectrum of *Aspergillus* infection. *ABPA,* Allergic bronchopulmonary aspergillosis. (From Sellke FW, del Nido PJ, Swanson SJ: *Sabiston & Spencer surgery of the chest,* ed 9, Philadelphia, 2016, Elsevier.)

ASPERGILLOMAS ("FUNGUS BALLS"):

- In the absence of invasion or significant immune response, *Aspergillus* can colonize a preexisting cavity, causing pulmonary aspergilloma.
- Forms masses of tangled hyphal elements, fibrin, and mucus.
- Patients typically have a history of chronic lung disease, tuberculosis, sarcoidosis, or emphysema.
- Manifests commonly as hemoptysis.
- Many are asymptomatic.

INVASIVE ASPERGILLOSIS:

- Patients with prolonged and profound granulocytopenia or impaired phagocytic function are predisposed to rapidly progressive *Aspergillus* pneumonia.
- Typically a necrotizing bronchopneumonia, ranging from small areas of infiltrate to intensive bilateral hemorrhagic infarction.
- Most common presentation: Unremitting fever and a new pulmonary infiltrate despite broad-spectrum antibiotic therapy in an immunosuppressed patient.
- Dyspnea and nonproductive cough are common; sudden pleuritic pain and tachycardia, sometimes with a pleural rub, may mimic pulmonary embolism; hemoptysis is uncommon.
- Chest radiograph (CXR) may reveal patchy bronchopneumonic, nodular densities, consolidation, or cavitation. High-resolution CT scan is more sensitive and specific than CXR in neutropenic patients.
- Immunocompromised patients: Invasive pulmonary *Aspergillus* (IPA) generally is acute and evolves over days to weeks; less commonly, patients with normal or only mild abnormalities of the immune system may develop a more chronic, slowly progressive form of IPA.

EXTRAPULMONARY DISSEMINATION:

- Cerebral infarction from hematogenous dissemination may occur in immunosuppressed individuals.
- Abscess formation from direct extension or invasive disease in the sinuses.
- Esophageal or gastrointestinal ulcerations may occur in the immunosuppressed host.
- Fatal perforation of the viscus or bowel infarction may occur.
- Necrotizing skin ulcers (Fig. E2).
- Osteomyelitis.
- Culture negative endocarditis in patients with abnormal or prosthetic valves who are immunosuppressed.
- Infection of an implantable cardioverter-defibrillator has been reported.

Dx DIAGNOSIS

DIFFERENTIAL DIAGNOSIS

- Tuberculosis
- Cystic fibrosis
- Carcinoma of the lung
- Eosinophilic pneumonia
- Bronchiectasis
- Sarcoidosis
- Lung abscess

WORKUP

Physical examination and laboratory data

LABORATORY TESTS

ABPA:

- Peripheral blood eosinophilia and an elevated total serum immunoglobulin E (IgE) level.
- Skin test with *Aspergillus* antigenic extract is usually positive but nonspecific.
- *Aspergillus* serum precipitating antibody is present in 70% to 100% of cases.
- Sputum cultures may be positive for *Aspergillus* spp. but are nonspecific.

ASPERGILLOMAS:

- Sputum culture
- Serum precipitating antibody

INVASIVE ASPERGILLOSIS:

- Definitive diagnosis requires the demonstration of tissue invasion (i.e., septate, acute angle branching hyphae) or a positive culture from the tissue obtained by an invasive procedure such as transbronchial biopsy.
- Sputum and nasal cultures: In high-risk patients a positive culture is strongly suggestive of invasive aspergillosis.
- Serology: The *Platelia Aspergillus* ELISA assay detects a circulating fungal antigen, galactomannan. The **Galactomannan antigen immunoassay** is often used for diagnosis. Galactomannan is a polysaccharide contained in the cell wall of *Aspergillus.* Its presence in serum or other body fluids is indicative of invasive infection, and it is recommended as an accurate marker for diagnosis in certain patient subpopulations (hematologic malignancy and hematopoietic stem cell transplantation). The sensitivity of the Galactomannan antigen immunoassay can be impaired by antifungal therapy. The β-D glucan assay can also be used to detect early infection, but is not specific for *Aspergillus* species.[1]
- Blood cultures: Usually negative (*Aspergillus* is rarely found in the blood).
- Lung biopsy is necessary for definitive diagnosis.
- Biopsy and culture of extrapulmonary lesions.
- Polymerase chain reaction assays may be employed, but their results should be interpreted in conjunction with other diagnostic tests and the clinical context.

[1] False-negative results occur in patients who are receiving antifungal agents other than fluconazole. The sensitivity of the galactomannan assay for invasive pulmonary aspergillosis is higher in brochoalveolar lavage fluid than in serum. In patients with risk factors and radiologic findings suggestive of invasive aspergillosis, a positive galactomannan confirms the diagnosis of probable invasive pulmonary aspergillosis.

IMAGING STUDIES

ABPA:

- CXRs show a variety of abnormalities, from small, patchy, fleeting infiltrates (commonly in the upper lobes) to lobar consolidation or cavitation.
- A majority of patients eventually develop central bronchiectasis.

ASPERGILLOMAS: CXR or CT scans usually show the characteristic intracavity mass (Figs. E3 and E4) partially surrounded by a crescent of air ("halo sign").

INVASIVE ASPERGILLOSIS: CXR and CT scanning may also reveal cavity formation and the halo sign. Air bronchograms typically disappear as they are filled with hemorrhagic fluid.

Rx TREATMENT

ACUTE GENERAL Rx

ABPA:

- Prednisone (0.5-1 mg/kg PO) until the CXR has cleared, followed by alternate-day therapy at 0.5 mg/kg PO (3-6 mo) plus itraconazole oral solution 2.5 mg/kg PO bid or 200 mg capsules bid for 16 wk. An alternative to itraconazole would be voriconazole 200 mg bid.
- If a patient is corticosteroid dependent, prophylaxis for the prevention of *Pneumocystis jiroveci* infection and maintenance of bone mineralization should be considered.
- Bronchodilators and physiotherapy.
- Serial CXR and serum IgE is useful in guiding treatment.

ASPERGILLOMAS:

- Controversial and problematic; the optimal treatment strategy is unknown.
- Up to 10% of aspergillomas may resolve clinically without overt pharmacologic or surgical intervention.
- Observation for asymptomatic patients.
- Surgical resection/arterial embolization for those patients with severe hemoptysis or life-threatening hemorrhage.
- For those patients at risk for marked hemoptysis with inadequate pulmonary reserve, consider itraconazole 200 to 400 mg/day PO. Voriconazole and isavuconazonium sulfate may also be used as well as transthoracic, intracavitary installation of amphotericin B in poor surgical candidates.

INVASIVE ASPERGILLOSIS:

- Voriconazole 6 mg/kg IV/PO bid on day 1 followed by 4 mg/kg IV/PO bid. Voriconazole serum concentrations need to be monitored to achieve a target range of 1.0 to 5.5 mg/L (trough on day 4).
- Isavuconazonium sulfate (prodrug of Isavuconazole) 372 mg IV/PO tid for six doses and then 372 mg IV/PO daily.

Alternative treatment:

- Amphotericin B lipid complex (ABLC) 5 mg/kg IV daily
- Liposomal amphotericin B (L-AMB) 3 to 5 mg/kg IV daily
- Posaconazole delayed-release tabs 300 mg PO for two doses, then 300 mg PO daily or posaconazole suspension 200 mgs qid, then 400 mg po bid after stabilization of disease or posaconazole 300 mg IV over 90 minutes bid for one day, then 300 mg IV daily
- Because azoles and echinocandins target different cellular sites, combination therapy may have additive activity against *Aspergillus* species

REFERRAL

To an infectious diseases specialist

PEARLS & CONSIDERATIONS

- Unlike fluconazole, the potential for drug-drug interactions with voriconazole, isavuconazole, and posaconazole is very high. Azoles may interact with drugs used for chemotherapy or immunosuppression by increasing toxicity and/or by reducing efficacy.
- Azole resistance has appeared in *Aspergillus fumigatus*; the main resistance mechanism is a point mutation of CYP51A, the gene coding for 14 alpha-sterol demethylase, the target enzyme of antifungal drugs. Global prevalence of azole resistance in *Aspergillus* is estimated to be approximately 3% to 6%.
- Agitation of hospital buildings by renovations or repairs may increase the incidence of *Aspergillus* infections in immunosuppressed individuals.
- Echinocandins should never be used as primary treatment of aspergillosis.
- *Aspergillus and Nocardia* species may co-infect.
- Use of antifungal agents in combination is discussed in Box 1.

SUGGESTED READINGS

Available at ExpertConsult.com

RELATED CONTENT

Aspergillosis (Patient Information)

AUTHOR: **Sajeev Handa, MD, SFHM**

BOX 1 Use of Antifungal Agents in Combination

The development of new antifungal drugs gives the clinician more options for prophylaxis and therapy than in previous years. There is an overall level of simplicity to the drug choices once their mechanisms of action are understood. The polyenes, including amphotericin products and the topical agent nystatin, attach onto ergosterol in the fungal cell membrane and are considered fungicidal, because cytoplasm leaks out, and individual cells die. The azoles, including fluconazole, itraconazole, voriconazole, and posaconazole, prevent the formation of new ergosterol. Azoles are considered fungistatic, because removal of the drug permits cell regrowth. Theoretically, use of an azole together with a polyene may have an overall static effect for an established infection as the ergosterol target for the fungicidal polyene is depleted. However, this combination may have advantages in terms of enhanced spectrum of activity. The echinocandins, including caspofungin, micafungin, and anidulafungin, prevent interaction of the catalytic and regulatory subunits of the β-glucan synthesis enzyme, so less β-glucan is formed for the cell wall. The scaffolding for the fungal cell wall is not maintained, and a dividing cell may burst open when trying to extend the new cell wall over daughter cells. The echinocandins are considered fungicidal for yeasts but fungistatic for molds, because drug activity is concentrated at only the tips of the extending hyphae with little effect on less metabolically active subapical compartments of the fungus. Combination therapy may have the most effect when a cell wall agent (an echinocandin) is used together with a cell membrane agent (a polyene or an azole). There is no role for three-drug therapy (an echinocandin, a polyene, and an azole). Aside from cases of cryptococcal meningitis, in which the importance of combination therapy is well established, the benefits of frontline use of combination antifungal for molds remain controversial, although active investigation continues in clinical trials. The value of combination regimens as salvage therapy for refractory mold infections remains uncertain.

From Hoffman R et al: *Hematology, basic principles and practice*, ed 7, Philadelphia, 2018, Elsevier.

BASIC INFORMATION

DEFINITION

Aspiration pneumonia refers to pulmonary infection of the lower airways and lung parenchyma resulting from entry of colonized oropharyngeal or upper gastrointestinal contents. *Aspiration pneumonia* is considered part of the continuum that also includes community- and hospital-acquired pneumonias. *Chemical pneumonitis* (or *aspiration pneumonitis*) refers to lung injury and inflammation resulting from entry of sterile substances toxic to the lower airways.

SYNONYM

Pneumonia, aspiration

ICD-10CM CODE

J69.0 Pneumonitis due to inhalation of food and vomit

EPIDEMIOLOGY & DEMOGRAPHICS

INCIDENCE (IN U.S.):
- 20% to 35% of all pneumonias
- 5% to 15% of all community-acquired pneumonias

PREVALENCE (IN U.S.): Unknown (unreliable data)

PREDOMINANT SEX: Males and females affected equally

PREDOMINANT AGE: Elderly

PEAK INCIDENCE: Elderly patients in hospitals or nursing homes

PHYSICAL FINDINGS & CLINICAL PRESENTATION

- Symptoms develop within hours to a few days after aspiration event, though anaerobic infections can have a more subacute presentation.
- Clinical presentation ranges from minimal symptoms to fulminant respiratory failure. Symptoms can include dyspnea, diffuse wheeze, cough, hypoxia, tachypnea, tachycardia, sputum production, and fever.
- Lung exam may demonstrate wheezes, crackles, or rhonchi.

ETIOLOGY

Complex interaction of etiologies, ranging from chemical (often acid) pneumonitis after aspiration of sterile gastric contents (generally not requiring antibiotic treatment) to bacterial aspiration. Risk factors for aspiration pneumonia include vomiting, decreased consciousness, poor dentition, ineffective cough reflex or glottic closure, and gastroesophageal reflux disease. Table 1 summarizes risk factors for aspiration pneumonia.

COMMUNITY-ACQUIRED ASPIRATION PNEUMONIA:
- Most patients have a mixed infection with aerobic and anaerobic bacteria. The most common bacteria are *Streptococcus pneumoniae, Staphylococcus aureus, Haemophilus influenza,* and Enterobacteriaceae. Anaerobes (*Peptostreptococcus, Fusobacterium nucleatum, Fusobacterium necrophorum, Prevotella,* and *Bacteroides* species) are less frequently isolated.
- High-risk groups: The elderly; alcoholics; IV drug users; patients who are obtunded; stroke victims; and those with esophageal disorders, seizures, periodontal disease, or recent dental manipulations

HOSPITAL-ACQUIRED ASPIRATION PNEUMONIA:
- Causative organisms:
  1. Anaerobes listed above, although in many studies gram-negative aerobes (60%) and gram-positive aerobes (20%) predominate
  2. *E. coli, P. aeruginosa, S. aureus* including MRSA, *Klebsiella, Enterobacter, Serratia, Proteus* spp., *H. influenzae, S. pneumoniae, Legionella,* and *Acinetobacter* spp. (sporadic pneumonias) in two thirds of cases
  3. Fungi, including *Candida albicans,* in <1%
- High-risk groups: Seriously ill hospitalized patients (especially patients with coma, acidosis, alcoholism, uremia, diabetes mellitus, nasogastric intubation, or recent antimicrobial therapy, who are frequently colonized with aerobic gram-negative rods); patients undergoing anesthesia; those with strokes, dementia, or swallowing disorders; the elderly; and those receiving antacids or H_2 blockers, or proton pump inhibitors (but not sucralfate).
- Hypoxic patients receiving concentrated O_2 have diminished ciliary activity, encouraging aspiration.

DIAGNOSIS

DIFFERENTIAL DIAGNOSIS

- Other necrotizing or cavitary pneumonias (especially tuberculosis, gram-negative pneumonias)
- See "Tuberculosis, Pulmonary"

WORKUP

- Chest x-ray
- Complete blood count (CBC), blood cultures
- Sputum Gram stain and culture
- Consideration of tracheal aspirate

LABORATORY TESTS

- CBC: Leukocytosis often present.
- Sputum Gram stain:
  1. Often useful when carefully prepared immediately after obtaining suctioned or expectorated specimen, examined by experienced observer.
  2. Only specimens with multiple white blood cells and rare or absent epithelial cells should be examined.
  3. Unlike nonaspiration pneumonias (e.g., pneumococcal), multiple organisms may be present.
  4. Long, slender rods suggest anaerobes, though these organisms are difficult to isolate due to frequent contamination of sputum samples with oral flora.
  5. Sputum from pneumonia caused by acid aspiration may be devoid of organisms.
  6. Cultures should be interpreted in light of morphology of visualized organisms.

IMAGING STUDIES

- Chest x-ray may be negative early in the disease course. It often reveals infiltrates in gravity-dependent lung regions. In an upright patient, infiltrates commonly affect the basal segments of the lower lobes. In a supine patient, infiltrates can involve the superior segment of the lower lobes, posterior right upper lobe, or the apicoposterior segment of the left upper lobe (Fig. 1). Chest x-ray can also demonstrate a pattern of diffuse lung involvement characteristic of the acute respiratory distress syndrome.
- Aspiration pneumonia of several days' or longer duration may reveal necrosis (especially community-acquired anaerobic pneumonias) and even cavitation with air-fluid levels, indicating lung abscess.

TREATMENT

NONPHARMACOLOGIC THERAPY

- Airway management to prevent repeated aspiration
- Ventilatory support if necessary
- Rehabilitative management: Physical, pulmonary, and dysphagia therapy combined with appropriate nutrition can reduce length of stay and mortality

ACUTE GENERAL Rx

- **Chemical pneumonitis:** Acute aspiration of acidic gastric contents without bacteria may not require antibiotic therapy; initial treatment involves airway maintenance and management of bronchospasm and airway edema. Routine adjunctive treatment with glucocorticoids is not recommended. Empiric

TABLE 1 Risk Factors for Dysphagia and Aspiration Pneumonia

Cerebrovascular disease
Ischemic stroke
Hemorrhagic stroke
Subarachnoid hemorrhage
Degenerative neurologic disease
Alzheimer disease
Multi-infarct dementia
Parkinson disease
Amyotrophic lateral sclerosis (motor neuron disease)
Multiple sclerosis
Head and neck cancer
Oropharyngeal malignancy
Oral cavity malignancy
Esophageal malignancy
Other
Scleroderma
Diabetic gastroparesis
Reflux esophagitis
Presbyesophagus
Achalasia

From Vincent JL et al: *Textbook of critical care*, ed 7, Philadelphia, 2017, Elsevier.

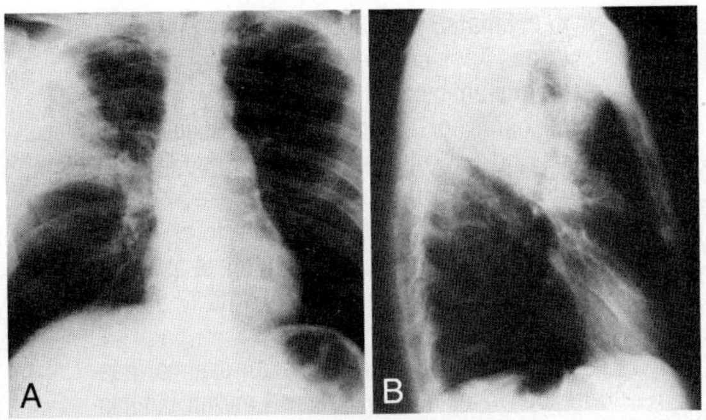

FIG. 1 Anaerobic necrotizing pneumonia following aspiration of oropharyngeal secretions. Multiple, small (<2 cm) radiolucencies are seen throughout the posterior segment of the right upper lobe on the postero-anterior **(A)** and lateral **(B)** projections. (Courtesy Michael Gotway, MD. From Mason RJ et al: *Murray & Nadel's textbook of respiratory medicine*, ed 5, Philadelphia, 2010, Saunders.)

antibiotics may be considered in severe cases, but their ongoing use should be reassessed at 48 to 72 hr.

- **Aspiration pneumonia:** Antibiotic selection depends on the site of acquisition (long-term care facility, hospital, community), which modifies risk factors for infection with multidrug-resistant pathogens. Additionally, a history of treatment with broad-spectrum antibiotics in the past 90 days warrants empiric treatment for multidrug-resistant organisms.
  1. Community-acquired aspiration pneumonia or hospital-acquired cases with low risk of multidrug-resistant pathogens: Ampicillin-sulbactam 1.5 to 3 g every 6 hr IV, or amoxicillin-clavulanate PO 875 mg twice daily, or a fluoroquinolone (levofloxacin 750 mg IV or PO) is effective. Clindamycin (450 mg oral qid or 600 mg IV every 8 hr) can be added to the other agent when the risk of predominantly anaerobic infection is high.
  2. Nursing home aspirations or hospital-acquired aspiration pneumonias with concerns for resistance: Broad-spectrum treatment with piperacillin-tazobactam 4.5 g q8h or 3.375 g q6h, cefepime 2 g q8h, levofloxacin 750 mg IV or PO once daily, imipenem 500 mg q6h or 1 g q8h, or meropenem 1 g q8h. The addition of vancomycin (15 mg/kg q12h IV) or linezolid (600 mg q12h PO or IV) is warranted if MRSA is suspected or known (e.g., documented nasal or respiratory colonization with MRSA).
     a. Knowledge of resident flora in the microenvironment of the aspiration within the hospital is crucial to intelligent antibiotic selection; consult infection control nurses or hospital epidemiologist.
     b. Confirmed *Pseudomonas* pneumonia in patients not in septic shock or at high risk of death can be treated with an antipseudomonal beta-lactam agent (piperacillin/tazobactam, cefepime, meropenem) or an antipseudomonal fluoroquinolone pending results of susceptibility testing. In severe cases, empiric two-drug combination therapy with an antipseudomonal beta-lactam agent and an antipseudomonal fluoroquinolone or an aminoglycoside is recommended. The choice of agents should be guided by the results of drug susceptibility testing when available.

DISPOSITION

Repeat chest x-ray in 6 to 8 wk in most patients.

REFERRAL

For consultation with infectious disease and/or pulmonary experts for patients with respiratory distress, hypoxia, ventilatory support, pneumonia in more than one lobe, or necrosis or cavitation on x-ray examination or for those not responding to antibiotic therapy within 2 to 3 days.

SUGGESTED READINGS

Available at ExpertConsult.com

RELATED CONTENT

Aspiration Pneumonia (Patient Information)

AUTHOR: **Narges Alipanah-Lechner, MD**

BASIC INFORMATION

DEFINITION

The National Asthma Education and Prevention Program (NAEPP) guidelines define asthma as "a chronic inflammatory disease of the airways in which many cells and cellular elements play a role: In particular mast cells, neutrophils, eosinophils, T lymphocytes, macrophages, and epithelial cells. In susceptible individuals, this inflammation causes recurrent episodes of coughing (particularly at night or early in the morning), wheezing, breathlessness, and chest tightness. The episodes are usually associated with widespread but variable airflow obstruction that is reversible either spontaneously or as a result of treatment." **Status asthmaticus,** or acute severe asthma, is a refractory state that does not respond to standard therapy such as inhaled beta-agonists or subcutaneous epinephrine. It may persist for several hours.

SYNONYMS

Bronchospasm
Reactive airway disease
Asthmatic bronchitis

ICD-10CM CODES

J45.20	Mild intermittent asthma, uncomplicated
J45.21	Mild intermittent asthma with (acute) exacerbation
J45.22	Mild intermittent asthma with status asthmaticus
J45.30	Mild persistent asthma, uncomplicated
J45.31	Mild persistent asthma with (acute) exacerbation
J45.32	Mild persistent asthma with status asthmaticus
J45.40	Moderate persistent asthma, uncomplicated
J45.41	Moderate persistent asthma with (acute) exacerbation
J45.42	Moderate persistent asthma with status asthmaticus
J45.50	Severe persistent asthma, uncomplicated
J45.51	Severe persistent asthma with (acute) exacerbation
J45.52	Severe persistent asthma with status asthmaticus
J45.901	Unspecified asthma with (acute) exacerbation
J45.902	Unspecified asthma with status asthmaticus
J45.909	Unspecified asthma, uncomplicated
J45.991	Cough variant asthma
J45.998	Other asthma

EPIDEMIOLOGY & DEMOGRAPHICS

- Asthma has been diagnosed in 7.7% of the population in the U.S., and its prevalence is steadily rising among patients older than 65 yr, African Americans, women, and persons living below the poverty level.
- It is estimated that 300 million people have asthma. An increase in prevalence to 400 million is anticipated by 2025.
- It accounts for around 440,000 hospitalizations and 1.8 million emergency department visits yearly in the U.S.
- It was previously more common in children, but given the increase of adult onset asthma, it is now more common in adults (7.5% of children vs. 7.7% of adults).
- Overall, mortality secondary to asthma has declined in the U.S. to 10.5 per 1 million, but has not changed for children aged 1 to 14 yr.
- 50% to 80% of children with asthma develop symptoms before 5 yr of age. Early childhood risk factors for asthma are described in Table 1.
- Box 1 summarizes risk factors for severe and fatal asthma in adults.

PHYSICAL FINDINGS & CLINICAL PRESENTATION

Physical examination findings vary with the stage and severity of asthma and may reveal normal lung examination results in many patients. However, some degree of wheezing and prolonged expiratory phases of respiration are seen with persistent or acute disease. Box 2 summarizes signs and symptoms of severe asthma. Physical examination during status asthmaticus may reveal:

- Tachycardia and tachypnea
- Use of accessory respiratory muscles
- Pulsus paradoxus (inspiratory decline in systolic blood pressure >10 mm Hg)
- Absence of wheezing (silent chest) or decreased wheezing can indicate worsening obstruction
- Mental status changes: Generally secondary to hypoxia and hypercapnia and constitute an indication for urgent intubation
- Paradoxical abdominal and diaphragmatic movement on inspiration (detected by palpation over the upper part of the abdomen in a semirecumbent position) indicates diaphragmatic fatigue, another sign of impending respiratory crisis

TABLE 1 Early Childhood Risk Factors for Persistent Asthma

Parental asthma
Allergy:
Atopic dermatitis (eczema)
Allergic rhinitis
Food allergy
Inhalant allergen sensitization
Food allergen sensitization
Severe lower respiratory tract infection:
Pneumonia
Bronchiolitis requiring hospitalization
Wheezing apart from colds
Male gender
Low birthweight
Environmental tobacco smoke exposure
Possible use of acetaminophen (paracetamol)
Exposure to chlorinated swimming pools
Reduced lung function at birth

From Kliegman RM et al: *Nelson textbook of pediatrics,* ed 19, Philadelphia, 2011, Saunders.

BOX 1 Risk Factors for Severe and Fatal Asthma in Adults

- History of prior nonfatal asthma attack
- Prior intubation
- Female gender
- Age >65 yr
- African American ethnicity
- Obesity
- Tobacco use
- Inhalational drug abuse
- Poorly controlled disease
- Poor recognition of dyspnea and other symptoms
- Steroid dependence
- H1N1 viral infection
- Misuse or lack of proper use of maintenance medications
- Psychiatric illness
- Lack of access to medical care
- Lack of ability to limit triggers (i.e., persistent exposure to pollutants, dust)
- Comorbid heart disease, obesity, and/or diabetes
- Bronchoalveolar lavage predominance of neutrophils, interleukin 8, and matrix metalloproteinase

From Parrillo JE, Dellinger RP: *Critical care medicine, principles of diagnosis and management in the adult,* ed 5, Philadelphia, 2019, Elsevier.

BOX 2 Signs and Symptoms of Severe Asthma

- "Tripoding"—sitting upright and leaning forward
- Diaphoresis
- Use of accessory muscles
- Asynchronous accessory muscle use
- Air trapping and hyperinflation manifesting as decreased inspiratory stroke volume and pulsus paradoxus
- Peak flow <200 L/min and/or <30% predicted*
- FEV1 <1 L/min and/or <20% predicted*
- Evidence of barotrauma:
  - Unilateral diminution in breath sounds
  - Tracheal deviation
  - Thoracic crepitus
- Signs of impending respiratory arrest:
  - Altered mentation
  - Cyanosis
  - Hypoxia
  - Hypercarbia
  - Hemodynamic instability
  - Silent chest

*These values are estimations because both peak expiratory flow rate and forced expiratory volume in 1 second (FEV_1) vary with age, gender, and height.
From Parrillo JE, Dellinger RP: *Critical care medicine, principles of diagnosis and management in the adult,* ed 5, Philadelphia, 2019, Elsevier.

- The following abnormalities in vital signs are indicative of severe asthma:
  1. Pulsus paradoxus >12 mm Hg
  2. Respiratory rate >30 breaths/min
  3. Tachycardia with heart rate >120 beats/min

ETIOLOGY

- The pathophysiology of asthma involves a complex interaction among various environmental and genetic factors. Genetic and phenotypic associations in asthma are described in Box 3.
- Allergic (atopic, extrinsic) asthma is triggered by various aeroallergens or nonallergic (nonatopic) nonspecific (e.g., dust, cigarette smoke, fumes, cold air, exercise) exposures in patients who are prone to develop IgE antibodies in response to various exposures. The pathogenesis of antigen-induced asthma is illustrated in Fig. 1.
- A longitudinal epidemiologic cohort study of a prebirth cohort observed that maternal intake of foods commonly considered allergenic (peanut and milk) was associated with a decrease in allergy and asthma in the offspring. No dietary changes during pregnancy are therefore recommended for prevention of allergies or asthma.
- A single center, randomized control trial revealed that supplementation with n-3 long-chain polyunsaturated fatty acids (LCPUFAs, fish oil-derived fatty acids) in the third trimester of pregnancy reduced the absolute risk of persistent wheeze or asthma and infections of the lower respiratory tract in offspring by approximately 7 percentage points, or one third.
- Nonallergic (intrinsic) asthma commonly manifests as adult-onset asthma in response to respiratory tract infection or psychologic stress.
- Occupational exposure to certain organic or nonorganic agents can trigger asthma.
- Evidence suggests that dampness and mold contribute to the risk of developing asthma and that remediation of these in homes reduces asthma symptoms and medication use in adults.
- Exercise-induced asthma is seen most frequently in adolescents and manifests with bronchospasm after beginning of exercise and improves with discontinuation of exercise.
- Drug-induced asthma is associated with use of NSAIDs, β-blockers, sulfites, and certain foods and beverages.
- There is a strong association of the *ADAM 33* gene with asthma and bronchial hyperresponsiveness. Experimental, genetic, and clinical studies support an important role for Type-2 inflammatory pathways in the pathogenesis of severe asthma. Atopic triggers stimulate Th2 cells to produce IL-5, IL-13, and IL-4, driving IgE synthesis, eosinophilia and airway changes. IL-5 is felt to be the most specific cytokine in eosinophil regulatory pathways. Nonatopic triggers (e.g., smoke, viruses) also have a vital role in the Type-2 inflammatory pathway. Type-2 Innate Lymphoid Cells (ILC2) produce IL-5, IL-13 through release of Damaged Associated Molecular Patterns (DAMPs) from the respiratory epithelium.

BOX 3 Genetic and Phenotypic Associations in Asthma

- ***ADAM33:*** Gene bronchoconstriction
- ***ORMDL3/GSDMB*** locus, chromosome 17q21: Childhood onset
- CpG portion of ***ACSL3:*** Associated with maternal exposure to automobile pollution
- ***IL33*** on chromosome 9
- ***IL2RB*** on chromosome 22

From Parrillo JE, Dellinger RP: *Critical care medicine, principles of diagnosis and management in the adult,* ed 5, Philadelphia, 2019, Elsevier.

Dx DIAGNOSIS

DIFFERENTIAL DIAGNOSIS

- Postinfectious bronchitis
- Rhinitis with postnasal drip
- Paradoxical vocal fold motion (vocal cord dysfunction)
- Chronic obstructive pulmonary disease (COPD)
- Gastroesophageal reflux disease (GERD)
- Pneumonia and other upper respiratory infections
- Foreign body aspiration (most frequent in younger patients)
- Anxiety disorder
- Diffuse interstitial lung disease
- Hypersensitivity pneumonitis
- Heart failure
- Pulmonary embolism

WORKUP

- Diagnosis of asthma requires documentation of airway obstruction and some degree of reversibility of the obstruction.
- For symptomatic adults and children age >5 yr who can perform spirometry, pre- and postbronchodilator spirometry is the recommended test of choice.
- Airflow reversibility is defined as increase in forced expiratory volume in 1 sec (FEV_1 by at least 12% and 200 ml) after inhaling a short-acting bronchodilator.
- The degree of reversibility measured by spirometry correlates with airway inflammation, and patients with a high degree of reversibility have a greater risk of irreversible airflow obstruction in subsequent years.

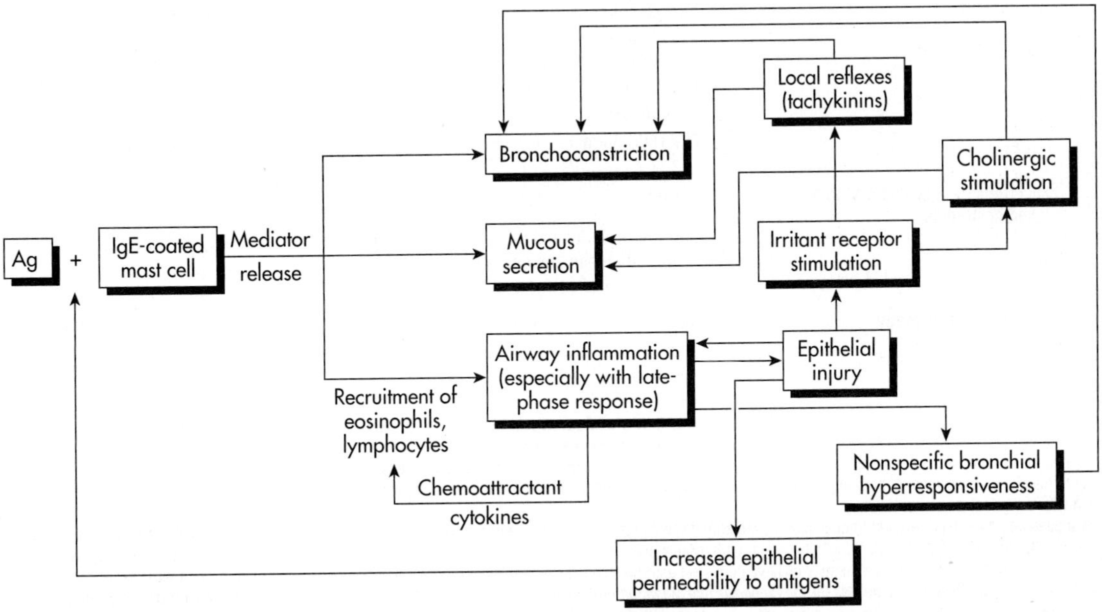

FIG. 1 Schematic diagram of events in pathogenesis of antigen-induced asthma. A hypothetical series of complex interactions is shown, focusing on bronchoconstriction, mucus secretion, and airway inflammation. *Ag,* Antigen; *IgE,* immunoglobulin E. (From Weinberger SE: *Principles of pulmonary medicine,* ed 7, Philadelphia, 2019, Elsevier.)

- For children age <5 yr, spirometry is generally not feasible. Young children with asthma symptoms should be treated as having suspected asthma after alternative diagnoses are ruled out.
- Negative spirometry results do not rule out asthma. Patients with high clinical suspicion should undergo bronchial challenge test using methacholine or other specific agents.
- The clinician should evaluate for environmental causes (e.g., house dust mites, indoor pets) and exposure to other allergens such as tobacco smoke.
- In the absence of spirometry testing, variability of peak flow measurements by a handheld device can be used to diagnose asthma.
- Fig. E2 describes an algorithm for diagnosing asthma.

After diagnosis, the severity of asthma should be classified during the initial assessment before initiating therapy. Patients are divided into four groups based on the severity of their asthma symptoms and number of exacerbations (Table 2).

- Once therapy is initiated, the emphasis for clinical management should gear toward achievement of asthma control. The level of asthma control should be used to guide decisions either to maintain or adjust therapy.
- Schedule visits at 2- to 6-wk intervals for patients who are just starting therapy or who require a step up in therapy to achieve or regain asthma control. Schedule visits at 6- to 12-mo intervals, after asthma control is achieved, to monitor whether asthma control is maintained. The interval will depend on factors such as the duration of asthma control or the level of treatment required. Consider scheduling visits at 3-mo intervals if step-down therapy is anticipated.

LABORATORY TESTS

Laboratory tests are usually not necessary, and the results can be normal if obtained during a stable period.

- Arterial blood gases (ABGs) can be used during acute bronchospasm in staging the severity of an asthmatic attack:
  1. Mild: Decreased Pao_2 and $Paco_2$, increased pH
  2. Moderate: Decreased Pao_2, normal $Paco_2$, normal pH
  3. Severe: Marked decreased Pao_2, increased $Paco_2$, and decreased pH
- Complete blood count: Leukocytosis with left shift may indicate the existence of bacterial infection. Elevated eosinophils point toward allergic component of asthma.
- Spirometry is recommended at the initial assessment and at least every 1 to 2 yr after treatment is initiated and when the symptoms and peak expiratory flow have stabilized. Spirometry as a monitoring measure may be performed more frequently, if indicated, based on severity of symptoms and the disease's lack of response to treatment.
- Peak expiratory flow rate (PEFR) can be used to assess severity of an acute exacerbation episode. Values should be compared with individual's personal best number (see "asthma action plan").
- Serum IgE and eosinophil levels help guide treatment for patients with severe persistent asthma, and they also help monitor response to treatment in the same group.
- Specific allergy testing may be helpful in a subgroup of patients.
- Fractional exhaled Nitric Oxide (FeNO) can be used to assess airway inflammation and help guide treatment as well as monitor response to treatment.

TABLE 2 Classifying Asthma Severity and Initiating Treatment in Youths ≥12 Yr and Adults (Assessing severity and initiating treatment for patients who are not currently taking long-term control medications)

		CLASSIFICATION OF ASTHMA SEVERITY (≥12 YR)			
			PERSISTENT		
Components of Severity		**Intermittent**	**Mild**	**Moderate**	**Severe**
Impairment Normal FEV_1/FVC: yr85% yr80% yr75% yr70%	Symptoms	≤2 days/wk	>2 days/wk but not daily	Daily	Throughout the day
	Nighttime awakenings	≤2×/mo	3-4×/mo	>1×/wk but not nightly	Often 7×/wk
	Short-acting $beta_2$-agonist use for symptom control (not prevention of EIB)	≤2 days/wk	>2 days/wk but not daily, and not more than 1× on any day	Daily	Several times per day
	Interference with normal activity	None	Minor limitation	Some limitation	Extremely limited
	Lung function	Normal FEV_1 between exacerbations			
		FEV_1 >80% predicted	FEV_1 >80% predicted	FEV_1 >60% but <80% predicted	FEV_1 <60% predicted
		FEV_1/FVC normal	FEV_1/FVC normal	FEV_1/FVC reduced 5%	FEV_1/FVC reduced >5%
Risk	Exacerbations requiring oral systemic corticosteroids	0-1 per yr	≥2 per yr		
		Consider severity and interval since last exacerbation. Frequency and severity may fluctuate over time for patients in any severity category. Relative annual risk of exacerbations may be related to FEV_1.			
Recommended Step for Initiating Therapy		Step 1	Step 2	Step 3	Step 4 or 5
				And consider short course of oral systemic corticosteroids	
		In 2-6 wk, evaluate level of asthma control that is achieved and adjust therapy accordingly.			

The stepwise approach is meant to assist, not replace, the clinical decision-making required to meet individual patient needs.
Level of severity is determined by assessment of both impairment and risk. Assess impairment domain by patient's/caregiver's recall of previous 2-4 wk and spirometry. Assign severity to the most severe category in which any feature occurs.
At present, there are inadequate data to correspond frequencies of exacerbations with different levels of asthma severity. In general, more frequent and intense exacerbations (e.g., requiring urgent, unscheduled care, hospitalization, or ICU admission) indicate greater underlying disease severity. For treatment purposes, patients who had ≥2 exacerbations requiring oral systemic corticosteroids in the past year may be considered the same as patients who have persistent asthma, even in the absence of impairment levels consistent with persistent asthma.
To access the complete *Expert Panel Report 3: Guidelines for the Diagnosis and Management of Asthma,* go to www.nhlbi.nih.gov/sites/default/files/media/docs/asthsumm.pdf.
EIB, Exercise-induced bronchospasm; *FEV_1,* forced expiratory volume in 1 second; *FVC,* forced vital capacity; *ICU,* intensive care unit.
From National Asthma Education and Prevention Program: *Expert panel report 3: guidelines for diagnosis and management of asthma,* National Institutes of Health, National Heart, Lung, and Blood Institute, August 2007, NIH publication 08-4051.

IMAGING STUDIES

- Chest x-ray: Usually normal, may show evidence of thoracic hyperinflation (e.g., flattening of the diaphragm, increased volume over the retrosternal air space).
- ECG: Tachycardia, nonspecific ST-T wave changes are common during an asthma attack; may also show cor pulmonale, right bundle branch block, right axial deviation, counterclockwise rotation.

Rx TREATMENT

NONPHARMACOLOGIC THERAPY

- Avoidance of triggering factors (e.g., salicylates, sulfites), environmental, or occupational triggers
- Encouragement of regular exercise (e.g., swimming)
- Patient education regarding warning signs of an attack and proper use of medications (e.g., correct use of inhalers)
- Assess asthma control with use of validated questionnaires

GENERAL Rx

The 2007 NAEPP guidelines (see Tables 2-10) provide treatment options by age groups: 0 to 4 yr, 5 to 11 yr, and >12 yr. A step-up approach is described based on the severity of symptoms.

An approach to home management of acute asthma is described in Fig. E3. Selected inhaled medications used by patients with asthma are summarized in Table 11. Short-acting beta-selective adrenergic agonists (SABAs) administered by inhalation is the most effective therapy for quick relief of asthmatic symptoms. They are recommended for use only as needed for relief of symptoms or before anticipated exposure to known triggers such as exercise. They should not be used as a single agent except for intermittent asthma symptoms. When symptoms become more frequent or more severe, step-up treatment with maintenance inhalers is recommended (see Table 4). Inhaled corticosteroids are the mainstay of treatment for maintenance therapy. Other treatment options include long-acting beta-agonist (LABA), combination of inhaled corticosteroids and LABA, leukotriene receptor antagonist (LTRA), cromolyn, zileuton, and theophylline. Oral corticosteroids are reserved as a last resort for maintenance therapy for recalcitrant cases. There are several corticosteroid/LABA combination inhalers available (fluticasone/salmeterol [Advair], budesonide/formoterol [Symbicort], mometasone/formoterol [Dulera], and ICS/LABA fluticasone furoate 200 mcg and vilanterol 25 mcg inhalation powder [Breo Ellipta]) on the market. None of these combinations is indicated for the initial treatment of asthma or for acute therapy of asthma symptoms. There is no evidence that one product is more effective than the others. A large study investigating the safety of LABA and ICS combination inhalers confirmed their long-term safety and demonstrated a reduced risk of exacerbations and improved lung function, when compared with an equivalent dose of ICS alone.

TABLE 3 Assessing Asthma Control and Adjusting Therapy in Youths ≥12 Yr and Adults

Components of Control		CLASSIFICATION OF ASTHMA CONTROL (≥12 YR)		
		Well Controlled	**Not Well Controlled**	**Very Poorly Controlled**
Impairment	Symptoms	≤2 days/wk	>2 days/wk	Throughout the day
	Nighttime awakenings	≤2×/mo	1-3×/wk	≥4/wk
	Interference with normal activity	None	Some limitation	Extremely limited
	Short-acting beta$_2$-agonist use for symptom control (not prevention of EIB)	≤2 days/wk	>2 days/wk	Several times per day
	FEV$_1$ or peak flow	>80% predicted/personal best	60%-80% predicted/personal best	<60% predicted/personal best
	Validated questionnaires			
	ATAQ	0	1-2	3-4
	ACQ	≤0.75*	≥1.5	N/A
	ACT™	≥20	16-19	≤15
Risk	Exacerbations requiring oral systemic corticosteroids	0-1 per yr	≥2 per yr	
		Consider severity and interval since last exacerbation		
	Progressive loss of lung function	Evaluation requires long-term follow-up care		
	Treatment-related adverse effects	Medication side effects can vary in intensity from none to very troublesome and worrisome. The level of intensity does not correlate to specific levels of control but should be considered in the overall assessment of risk.		
Recommended Action for Treatment		Maintain current step. Regular follow-up every 1-6 mo to maintain control. Consider step down if well controlled for at least 3 mo.	Step up 1 step and reevaluate in 2-6 wk. For side effects, consider alternative treatment options.	Consider short course of oral systemic corticosteroids. Step up 1-2 steps. Reevaluate in 2 wk. For side effects, consider alternative treatment options.

The stepwise approach is meant to assist, not replace, the clinical decision-making required to meet individual patient needs.
The level of control is based on the most severe impairment or risk category. Assess impairment domain by patient's recall of previous 2-4 wk and by spirometry or peak flow measures.
Symptom assessment for longer periods should reflect a global assessment, such as inquiring whether the patient's asthma is better or worse since the last visit.
At present, there are inadequate data to correspond frequencies of exacerbations with different levels of asthma control. In general, more frequent and intense exacerbations (e.g., requiring urgent, unscheduled care, hospitalization, or ICU admission) indicate poorer disease control. For treatment purposes, patients who had ≥2 exacerbations requiring oral systemic corticosteroids in the past year may be considered the same as patients who have not-well-controlled asthma, even in the absence of impairment levels consistent with not-well-controlled asthma.
Validated questionnaires for the impairment domain (the questionnaires do not assess lung function or the risk domain):

- ATAQ = Asthma Therapy Assessment Questionnaire
- ACQ = Asthma Control Questionnaire (user package may be obtained at www.qoltech.co.uk or juniper@qoltech.co.uk)
- ACT = Asthma Control Test™
- Minimal Important Difference: 1.0 for the ATAQ; 0.5 for the ACQ; not determined for the ACT

Before step up in therapy:

- Review adherence to medication, inhaler technique, environmental control, and comorbid conditions
- If an alternative treatment option was used in a step, discontinue and use the preferred treatment for that step

EIB, Exercise-induced bronchospasm; *FEV$_1$,* forced expiratory volume in 1 second; *ICU,* intensive care unit.
The Asthma Control Test is a trademark of QualityMetric Incorporated.
*ACQ values of 0.76-1.4 are indeterminate regarding well-controlled asthma.
From National Asthma Education and Prevention Program: *Expert panel report 3: guidelines for diagnosis and management of asthma,* National Institutes of Health, National Heart, Lung, and Blood Institute, August 2007, NIH publication 08-4051.

Various studies have showed some degree of benefit when adding a long-acting muscarinic antagonist (LAMA) to ICS + LABA in moderate to severe asthma. The LAMA tiotropium (Spiriva), which has been used for decades as a first-line treatment for COPD, is now approved for the treatment of asthma and is included in the most recent (2020) Global Initiative for Asthma (GINA) guidelines as a possible add-on at step 4. A systematic review including more than 7000 patients demonstrated the use of LAMA compared with placebo as an add-on to inhaled corticosteroids was associated with lower risk of exacerbation. Adding LAMA to a dual LABA-ICS regimen was not shown to reduce exacerbation rates but can improve lung function.

IMMUNOLOGIC TARGETS

- Dupilumab, a human monoclonal antibody to IL-4 and IL-13, is FDA approved for use in patients >12 yr with moderate to severe asthma with an eosinophilic phenotype or with oral corticosteroid–dependent asthma.
- Mepolizumab (Nucala), a monoclonal antibody to IL-5, is approved by the FDA as an add-on for patients ≥12 yr with severe eosinophilic asthma that is uncontrolled on Step 4 treatment. Mepolizumab has been shown to reduce exacerbations in patients with severe asthma who have blood eosinophil counts of 150/μL or greater. It is administered subcutaneously into the upper arm, thigh, or abdomen, 100 mg every 4 wk. Hypersensitivity reactions have been reported with mepolizumab. In addition, herpes zoster infections have led to the recommendation of the administration of the varicella zoster vaccine to adults ages 50 or older 4 wk prior to initiation of mepolizumab (unless they are at risk for disseminated zoster).
- Reslizumab, another anti-IL-5 monoclonal antibody, has a similar indication for eosinophilic asthma and uses a higher eosinophil cutoff (400 μL or greater) based on a greater predictive value for sputum eosinophilia.
- Benralizumab, a monoclonal anti-IL5 receptor alpha antibody, is an additional FDA-approved add-on treatment to consider for patients >12 yr with persistent severe eosinophilic asthma. It is administered as a subcutaneous injection every 4 wk for the first 3 doses then every 8 wk after that. Hypersensitivity reactions are more common than other anti-IL-5 antibodies and occur in about 3% of patients. Other adverse events include headache and pharyngitis.
- Omalizumab, an anti-IgE monoclonal antibody, is indicated for the treatment of moderate and severe persistent asthma with elevated IgE level, which is refractory to other treatment noted earlier. It is administered subcutaneously every 2 or 4 wk.

BRONCHIAL THERMOPLASTY

Selected patients with severe persistent asthma who have failed medical treatment may benefit from bronchial thermoplasty. This requires the insertion of a catheter via bronchoscopy and use of radiofrequency heat to reduce bronchial smooth muscle. Long-term follow-up data

TABLE 4 Stepwise Approach for Managing Asthma in Youths ≥12 Yr and Adults

Intermittent Asthma	**Persistent Asthma: Daily Medication** Consult with asthma specialist if step 4 care or higher is required. Consider consultation at step 3.					
Step 1 *Preferred:* SABA prn	**Step 2** *Preferred:* Low-dose ICS *Alternative:* Cromolyn, LTRA, nedocromil, or theophylline	**Step 3** *Preferred:* Low-dose ICS + LABA OR Medium-dose ICS *Alternative:* Low-dose ICS + either LTRA, theophylline, or zileuton	**Step 4** *Preferred:* Medium-dose ICS + LABA *Alternative:* Medium-dose ICS + either LTRA, theophylline, or zileuton	**Step 5** *Preferred:* High-dose ICS + LABA AND Consider omalizumab for patients who have allergies	**Step 6** *Preferred:* High-dose ICS + LABA + oral corticosteroid AND Consider omalizumab for patients who have allergies	↑ Step up if needed (first, check adherence, environmental control, and comorbid conditions) **Assess control** Step down if possible (and asthma is well controlled at least 3 mo) ↓

Each step: Patient education, environmental control, and management of comorbidities
Steps 2-4: Consider subcutaneous allergen immunotherapy for patients who have allergic asthma

Quick-Relief Medication for All Patients
- SABA as needed for symptoms. Intensity of treatment depends on severity of symptoms: Up to 3 treatments at 20-min intervals as needed. Short course of oral systemic corticosteroids may be needed.
- Use of SABA >2 days a wk for symptom relief (not prevention of EIB) generally indicates inadequate control and the need to step up treatment.

The stepwise approach is meant to assist, not replace, the clinical decision-making required to meet individual patient needs.
If alternative treatment is used and response is inadequate, discontinue it and use the preferred treatment before stepping up.
Zileuton is a less desirable alternative due to limited studies as adjunctive therapy and the need to monitor liver function. Theophylline requires monitoring of serum concentration levels. In step 6, before oral systemic corticosteroids are introduced, a trial of high-dose ICS + LABA + either LTRA, theophylline, or zileuton may be considered, although this approach has not been studied in clinical trials.
Steps 1, 2, and 3 preferred therapies are based on Evidence A; step 3 alternative therapy is based on Evidence A for LTRA, Evidence B for theophylline, and Evidence D for zileuton. Step 5 preferred therapy is based on Evidence B. Step 6 preferred therapy is based on (EPR-2 1997) and Evidence B for omalizumab.
Immunotherapy for steps 2-4 is based on Evidence B for house-dust mites, animal danders, and pollens; evidence is weak or lacking for molds and cockroaches. Evidence is strongest for immunotherapy with single allergens. The role of allergy in asthma is greater in children than in adults.
Clinicians who administer immunotherapy or omalizumab should be prepared and equipped to identify and treat anaphylaxis that may occur.
This information is directly abstracted from the 2007 NAEPP *Expert Panel Report 3: Guidelines for the Diagnosis and Management of Asthma* and is not intended to promote or endorse any of the listed products.
To access the complete *Expert Panel Report 3: Guidelines for the Diagnosis and Management of Asthma,* go to www.nhlbi.nih.gov/sites/default/files/media/docs/asthsumm.pdf.
EIB, Exercise-induced bronchospasm; *ICS,* inhaled corticosteroid; *LABA,* inhaled long-acting beta$_2$-agonist; *LTRA,* leukotriene receptor antagonist; *prn,* as necessary; *SABA,* inhaled short-acting beta$_2$-agonist.
From National Asthma Education and Prevention Program: *Expert panel report 3: guidelines for diagnosis and management of asthma,* National Institutes of Health, National Heart, Lung, and Blood Institute, August 2007, NIH publication 08-4051.

TABLE 5 Classifying Asthma Severity and Initiating Treatment in Children 5-11 Yr (Assessing severity and initiating treatment in children who are not currently taking long-term control medications)

Components of Severity		CLASSIFICATION OF ASTHMA SEVERITY (5-11 YR OF AGE)			
			PERSISTENT		
		Intermittent	**Mild**	**Moderate**	**Severe**
Impairment	Symptoms	≤2 days/wk	>2 days/wk but not daily	Daily	Throughout the day
	Nighttime awakenings	≤23/mo	3-4×/mo	>1×/wk but not nightly	Often 7×/wk
	Short-acting $beta_2$-agonist use for symptom control (not prevention of EIB)	≤2 days/wk	>2 days/wk but not daily	Daily	Several times per day
	Interference with normal activity	None	Minor limitation	Some limitation	Extremely limited
	Lung function	Normal FEV_1 between exacerbations			
		FEV_1 >80% predicted	FEV_1 = >80% predicted	FEV_1 60%-80% predicted	FEV_1 <60% predicted
		FEV_1/FVC >85%	FEV_1/FVC >80%	FEV_1/FVC 75%-80%	FEV_1/FVC <75%
Risk	Exacerbations requiring oral systemic corticosteroids	0-1 per yr	≥2 per yr		
		Consider severity and interval since last exacerbation. Frequency and severity may fluctuate over time for patients in any severity category.			
		Relative annual risk of exacerbations may be related to FEV_1.			
Recommended Step for Initiating Therapy		Step 1	Step 2	Step 3, medium-dose ICS option	Step 3, medium-dose ICS option, or Step 4
				And consider short course of oral systemic corticosteroids	
		In 2-6 wk, evaluate level of asthma control that is achieved and adjust therapy accordingly.			

The stepwise approach is meant to assist, not replace, the clinical decision-making required to meet individual patient needs.
Level of severity is determined by both impairment and risk. Assess impairment domain by patient's/caregiver's recall of previous 2-4 wk and spirometry. Assign severity to the most severe category in which any feature occurs.
At present, there are inadequate data to correspond frequencies of exacerbations with different levels of asthma severity. In general, more frequent and intense exacerbations (e.g., requiring urgent, unscheduled care, hospitalization, or ICU admission) indicate greater underlying disease severity. For treatment purposes, patients who had ≥2 exacerbations requiring oral systemic corticosteroids in the past year may be considered the same as patients who have persistent asthma, even in the absence of impairment levels consistent with persistent asthma.
EIB, Exercise-induced bronchospasm; *FEV_1*, forced expiratory volume in 1 second; *FVC,* forced vital capacity; *ICS,* inhaled corticosteroid; *ICU,* intensive care unit.
From National Asthma Education and Prevention Program: *Expert panel report 3: guidelines for diagnosis and management of asthma,* National Institutes of Health, National Heart, Lung, and Blood Institute, August 2007, NIH publication 08-4051.

TABLE 6 Assessing Asthma Control and Adjusting Therapy in Children 5-11 Yr

Components of Control		CLASSIFICATION OF ASTHMA CONTROL (5-11 YR OF AGE)		
		Well Controlled	**Not Well Controlled**	**Very Poorly Controlled**
Impairment	Symptoms	≤2 days/wk but not more than once on each day	>2 days/wk or multiple times on ≤2 days/wk	Throughout the day
	Nighttime awakenings	≤1×/mo	≥2×/mo	≥2×/wk
	Interference with normal activity	None	Some limitation	Extremely limited
	Short-acting $beta_2$-agonist use for symptom control (not prevention of EIB)	≤2 days/wk	>2 days/wk	Several times per day
	Lung function			
	FEV_1 or peak flow	>80% predicted/personal best	60%-80% predicted/personal best	<60% predicted/personal best
	FEV_1/FVC	>80% predicted	75%-80%	<75% predicted
Risk	Exacerbations requiring oral systemic corticosteroids	0-1 per yr	≥2 per yr	
		Consider severity and interval since last exacerbation		
	Reduction in lung growth	Evaluation requires long-term follow-up care		
	Treatment-related adverse effects	Medication side effects can vary in intensity from none to very troublesome and worrisome. The level of intensity does not correlate to specific levels of control but should be considered in the overall assessment of risk.		
Recommended Action for Treatment		Maintain current step. Regular follow-up every 1-6 mo. Consider step down if well controlled for at least 3 mo.	Step up 1 step and reevaluate in 2-6 wk. For side effects, consider alternative treatment options.	Consider short course of oral systemic corticosteroids. Step up 1-2 steps. Reevaluate in 2 wk. For side effects, consider alternative treatment options.

The stepwise approach is meant to assist, not replace, the clinical decision-making required to meet individual patient needs.
The level of control is based on the most severe impairment or risk category. Assess impairment domain by patient's/caregiver's recall of previous 2-4 wk and by spirometry or peak flow measures. Symptom assessment for longer periods should reflect a global assessment such as inquiring whether the patient's asthma is better or worse since the last visit.
At present, there are inadequate data to correspond frequencies of exacerbations with different levels of asthma control. In general, more frequent and intense exacerbations (e.g., requiring urgent, unscheduled care, hospitalization, or ICU admission) indicate poorer disease control. For treatment purposes, patients who had ≥2 exacerbations requiring oral systemic corticosteroids in the past year may be considered the same as patients who have persistent asthma, even in the absence of impairment levels consistent with persistent asthma.
Before step up in therapy:

- Review adherence to medications, inhaler technique, environmental control, and comorbid conditions.
- If an alternative treatment option was used in a step, discontinue it and use preferred treatment for that step.

EIB, Exercise-induced bronchospasm; *FEV_1*, forced expiratory volume in 1 second; *FVC,* forced vital capacity; *ICU,* intensive care unit.
From National Asthma Education and Prevention Program: *Expert panel report 3: guidelines for diagnosis and management of asthma,* National Institutes of Health, National Heart, Lung, and Blood Institute, August 2007, NIH publication 08-4051.

TABLE 7 Stepwise Approach for Managing Asthma in Children 5-11 Yr

Intermittent Asthma	Persistent Asthma: Daily Medication Consult with asthma specialist if step 4 care or higher is required. Consider consultation at step 3.					
Step 1 *Preferred:* SABA prn	**Step 2** *Preferred:* Low-dose ICS *Alternative:* Cromolyn, LTRA, nedocromil, or theophylline	**Step 3** *Preferred:* Low-dose ICS + either LABA, LTRA, or theophylline OR Medium-dose ICS	**Step 4** *Preferred:* Medium-dose ICS + LABA *Alternative:* Medium-dose ICS + either LTRA or theophylline	**Step 5** *Preferred:* High-dose ICS + LABA *Alternative:* High-dose ICS + either LTRA or theophylline	**Step 6** *Preferred:* High-dose ICS + LABA + oral corticosteroid *Alternative:* High-dose ICS + either LTRA or theophylline + oral systemic corticosteroid	↑ Step up if needed (first, check adherence, inhaler technique, environmental control, and comorbid conditions) **Assess control** Step down if possible (and asthma is well controlled at least 3 mo) ↓

Each step: Patient education, environmental control, and management of comorbidities
Steps 2-4: Consider subcutaneous allergen immunotherapy for patients who have allergic asthma

Quick-Relief Medication for All Patients
- SABA as needed for symptoms. Intensity of treatment depends on severity of symptoms: Up to 3 treatments at 20-min intervals as needed. Short course of oral systemic corticosteroids may be needed.
- Caution: Increasing use of SABA or use >2 days a wk for symptom relief (not prevention of EIB) generally indicates inadequate control and the need to step up treatment.

The stepwise approach is meant to assist, not replace, the clinical decision-making required to meet individual patient needs.
If alternative treatment is used and response is inadequate, discontinue it and use the preferred treatment before stepping up.
Theophylline is a less desirable alternative due to the need to monitor serum concentration levels.
Step 1 and step 2 medications are based on Evidence A. Step 3 ICS 1 adjunctive therapy and ICS are based on Evidence B for efficacy of each treatment and extrapolation from comparator trials in older children and adults—comparator trials are not available for this age group; steps 4-6 are based on expert opinion and extrapolation from studies in older children and adults. Immunotherapy for steps 2-4 is based on Evidence B for house-dust mites, animal danders, and pollens; evidence is weak or lacking for molds and cockroaches. Evidence is strongest for immunotherapy with single allergens. The role of allergy in asthma is greater in children than in adults. Clinicians who administer immunotherapy should be prepared and equipped to identify and treat anaphylaxis that may occur. This information is directly abstracted from the 2007 NAEPP *Expert Panel Report 3: Guidelines for the Diagnosis and Management of Asthma* and is not intended to promote or endorse any of the listed products.
EIB, Exercise-induced bronchoconstriction; *ICS,* inhaled corticosteroid; *LABA,* inhaled long-acting beta$_2$-agonist; *LTRA,* leukotriene receptor antagonist; *prn,* as necessary; *SABA,* inhaled short-acting beta$_2$-agonist.
From National Asthma Education and Prevention Program: *Expert panel report 3: guidelines for diagnosis and management of asthma,* National Institutes of Health, National Heart, Lung, and Blood Institute, August 2007, NIH publication 08-4051.

showed persistent reduction in asthma exacerbation and fewer ED visits over a period of 5 yr in carefully selected patients. FDA labeling is for "severe persistent asthma inadequately controlled on ICS + LABA."

OTHER MEDICATIONS

- Azithromycin: The AZISAST Trial randomized 109 patients on high-dose ICS/LABA (step 4 or 5 per GINA guidelines) to maintenance therapy with azithromycin or placebo. Overall, there was no benefit seen with azithromycin therapy with regard to any of the outcomes tested. However, subgroup analysis showed that patients with noneosinophilic asthma had fewer exacerbations. More data are needed, but this result suggests azithromycin may be an effective option for the neutrophilic/Th-1 phenotype (COPD is also neutrophilic).
- Immunosuppressants such as methotrexate can decrease long-term steroid requirements; however, they have significant side effects, and there is no evidence of persistent therapeutic effect after discontinuing them.

TREATMENT OF SEVERE ASTHMA (ATS/ERS GUIDELINES)

- The American Thoracic Society (ATS) classification of "severe asthma" refers to patients who require high-dose inhaled or near-continuous oral glucocorticoid treatment to maintain asthma control.
- In patients who do not achieve adequate control with the combination of a high-dose inhaled glucocorticoid and LABA, an additional controller medication such as an LTRA or LAMA is recommended.
- For patients with atopic severe asthma who have a serum IgE level of 30 to 700 IU/ml and documented sensitivity to a perennial allergen, adding omalizumab is recommended.
- For patients with severe asthma, frequent exacerbations, and an eosinophilic phenotype despite guideline-based therapy, consider add-on therapy with one of the anti-interleukin (IL)-5 antibodies, mepolizumab, reslizumab, benralizumab, or anti-IL4α receptor antibody dupilumab.
- Bronchial thermoplasty is approved for use in selected adults with severe asthma that is not well controlled with inhaled glucocorticoids and LABAs.
- Potential alternative and experimental therapies include immunomodulatory therapy and macrolide antibiotics.[a]
- In the future, treatments tailored to asthma phenotypes may improve asthma outcomes.

Treatment of status asthmaticus is as follows:

1. Oxygen generally started at 2 to 4 L/min by nasal cannula or Venti-Mask at 40% Fio$_2$; further adjustments are made according to oxygen saturations.
2. Bronchodilators: Initiate treatment with albuterol nebulizer solution (0.63 mg/3 ml, 1.25 mg/3 ml, 2.5 mg/3 ml, or 5.0 mg/ml): 2.5 to 5 mg every 20 min over the first hr, then 2.5 to 10 mg every 1 to 4 hr as needed or 10 to 15 mg/hr continuously. Other useful medications are levalbuterol nebulizer solution (0.31 mg/3 ml, 0.63 mg/3 ml, 1.25 mg/3 ml) and ipratropium nebulizer solution (0.25/ml [0.025%]).

[a] Recent trials (AMAZES) in patients who have symptomatic asthma despite inhaled maintenance therapy have shown that azithromycin 500 mg 3 times/wk reduced exacerbations and improved quality of life.

TABLE 8 Classifying Asthma Severity and Initiating Treatment in Children 0-4 Yr (Assessing severity and initiating treatment in children who are not currently taking long-term control medications)

Components of Severity		Classification of Asthma Severity (0-4 Yr of Age): Intermittent	Persistent: Mild	Persistent: Moderate	Persistent: Severe
Impairment	Symptoms	≤2 days/wk	>2 days/wk but not daily	Daily	Throughout the day
	Nighttime awakenings	0	1-2×/mo	3-4×/mo	>1×/wk
	Short-acting beta₂-agonist use for symptom control (not prevention of EIB)	≤2 days/wk	>2 days/wk but not daily	Daily	Several times per day
	Interference with normal activity	None	Minor limitation	Some limitation	Extremely limited
Risk	Exacerbations requiring oral systemic corticosteroids	0-1 per yr	≥2 exacerbations in 6 mo requiring oral systemic corticosteroids, or ≥4 wheezing episodes/1 yr lasting >1 day AND risk factors for persistent asthma.		
		Consider severity and interval since last exacerbation. Frequency and severity may fluctuate over time. Exacerbations of any severity may occur in patients in any severity category.			
Recommended Step for Initiating Therapy		Step 1	Step 2	Step 3 and consider short course of oral systemic corticosteroids	
		In 2-6 wk, depending on severity, evaluate level of asthma control that is achieved. If no clear benefit is observed in 4-6 wk, consider adjusting therapy or alternative diagnoses.			

The stepwise approach is meant to assist, not replace, the clinical decision-making required to meet individual patient needs.

Level of severity is determined by assessment of both impairment and risk. Assess impairment domain by patient's/caregiver's recall of previous 2-4 wk. Symptom assessment for longer periods should reflect a global assessment such as inquiring whether the patient's asthma is better or worse since the last visit. Assign severity to the most severe category in which any feature occurs.

At present, there are inadequate data to correspond frequencies of exacerbations with different levels of asthma severity. For treatment purposes, patients who had ≥2 exacerbations requiring oral systemic corticosteroids in the past 6 mo, or ≥4 wheezing episodes in the past year, and who have risk factors for persistent asthma may be considered the same as patients who have persistent asthma, even in the absence of impairment levels consistent with persistent asthma. To access the complete *Expert Panel Report 3: Guidelines for the Diagnosis and Management of Asthma,* go to www.nhlbi.nih.gov/sites/default/files/media/docs/asthsumm.pdf.

EIB, Exercise-induced bronchospasm.

From National Asthma Education and Prevention Program: *Expert panel report 3: guidelines for diagnosis and management of asthma,* National Institutes of Health, National Heart, Lung, and Blood Institute, August 2007, NIH publication 08-4051.

TABLE 9 Assessing Asthma Control and Adjusting Therapy in Children 0-4 Yr of Age

Components of Control		Classification of Asthma Control (0-4 Yr of Age): Well Controlled	Not Well Controlled	Very Poorly Controlled
Impairment	Symptoms	≤2 days/wk	>2 days/wk	Throughout the day
	Nighttime awakenings	≤13/mo	>1×/mo	>1×/wk
	Interference with normal activity	None	Some limitation	Extremely limited
	Short-acting beta₂-agonist use for symptom control (not prevention of EIB)	≤2 days/wk	>2 days/wk	Several times per day
Risk	Exacerbations requiring oral systemic corticosteroids	0-1 per yr	2-3 per yr	>3 per yr
	Treatment-related adverse effects	Medication side effects can vary in intensity from none to very troublesome and worrisome. The level of intensity does not correlate to specific levels of control but should be considered in the overall assessment of risk.		
Recommended Action for Treatment		Maintain current step. Regular follow-up every 1-6 mo. Consider step down if well controlled for at least 3 mo.	Step up 1 step. Reevaluate in 2-6 wk. If no clear benefit in 4-6 wk, consider alternative diagnoses or adjusting therapy. For side effects, consider alternative treatment options.	Consider short course of oral systemic corticosteroids. Step up 1-2 steps. Reevaluate in 2 wk. If no clear benefit in 4-6 wk, consider alternative diagnoses or adjusting therapy. For side effects, consider alternative treatment options.

The stepwise approach is meant to assist, not replace, the clinical decision-making required to meet individual patient needs.

The level of control is based on the most severe impairment or risk category. Assess impairment domain by caregiver's recall of previous 2-4 wk. Symptom assessment for longer periods should reflect a global assessment such as inquiring whether the patient's asthma is better or worse since the last visit.

At present, there are inadequate data to correspond frequencies of exacerbations with different levels of asthma control. In general, more frequent and intense exacerbations (e.g., requiring urgent, unscheduled care, hospitalization, or ICU admission) indicate poorer disease control. For treatment purposes, patients who had ≥2 exacerbations requiring oral systemic corticosteroids in the past year may be considered the same as patients who have not-well-controlled asthma, even in the absence of impairment levels consistent with not-well-controlled asthma.

Before step up in therapy:

- Review adherence to medications, inhaler technique, and environmental control.
- If an alternative treatment option was used in a step, discontinue it and use preferred treatment for that step.

EIB, Exercise-induced bronchospasm; *ICU,* Intensive care unit.

From National Asthma Education and Prevention Program: *Expert panel report 3: guidelines for diagnosis and management of asthma,* National Institutes of Health, National Heart, Lung, and Blood Institute, August 2007, NIH publication 08-4051.

TABLE 10 Stepwise Approach for Managing Asthma in Children 0-4 Yr

Intermittent Asthma	Persistent Asthma: Daily Medication Consult with asthma specialist if step 3 care or higher is required. Consider consultation at step 2.					↑
Step 1 *Preferred:* SABA prn	**Step 2** *Preferred:* Low-dose ICS *Alternative:* Cromolyn or montelukast	**Step 3** *Preferred:* Medium-dose ICS	**Step 4** *Preferred:* Medium-dose ICS + either LABA or montelukast	**Step 5** *Preferred:* High-dose ICS + either LABA or montelukast	**Step 6** *Preferred:* High-dose ICS + either LABA or montelukast Oral systemic corticosteroid	Step up if needed (first, check adherence, inhaler technique, and environmental control) **Assess control** Step down if possible (and asthma is well controlled at least 3 mo)
Patient Education and Environmental Control at Each Step						
Quick-Relief Medication for All Patients • SABA as needed for symptoms. Intensity of treatment depends on severity of symptoms. • With viral respiratory infection: SABA q4-6h up to 24 hr (longer with physician consult). Consider short course of oral systemic corticosteroids if exacerbation is severe or patient has history of previous severe exacerbations. • Caution: Frequent use of SABA may indicate the need to step up treatment. See text for recommendations on initiating daily long-term-control therapy.						↓

The stepwise approach is meant to assist, not replace, the clinical decision-making required to meet individual patient needs. If alternative treatment is used and response is inadequate, discontinue it and use the preferred treatment before stepping up.

If clear benefit is not observed within 4-6 wk and patient/family medication technique and adherence are satisfactory, consider adjusting therapy or alternative diagnosis.

Studies on children 0-4 yr are limited. Step 2 preferred therapy is based on Evidence A. All other recommendations are based on expert opinion and extrapolation from studies in other children.

This information is directly abstracted from the 2007 NAEPP *Expert Panel Report 3: Guidelines for the Diagnosis and Management of Asthma* and is not intended to promote or endorse any of the listed products.

ICS, Inhaled corticosteroid; *LABA,* inhaled long-acting beta$_2$-agonist; *prn,* as necessary; *SABA,* inhaled short-acting beta$_2$-agonist.

From National Asthma Education and Prevention Program: *Expert panel report 3: guidelines for diagnosis and management of asthma,* National Institutes of Health, National Heart, Lung, and Blood Institute, August 2007, NIH publication 08-4051.

- Corticosteroids:
  1. Early administration is advised, particularly in patients using steroids at home.
  2. Patients may be started on systemic corticosteroids; methylprednisolone, prednisone, or prednisolone may be used. Dose range is from 40 to 80 mg/day in one or two divided doses, generally given until peak expiratory flow reaches 70% of predicted value.
  3. Generally for corticosteroid courses <1 wk there is no need to taper the dose.
- IV hydration: Judicious use is necessary to avoid heart failure in elderly patients. Aggressive IV hydration is not recommended.
- IV antibiotics are indicated when there is suspicion of bacterial infection (e.g., infiltrate on chest radiograph, fever, or leukocytosis).
- Intubation and mechanical ventilation are indicated when previous measures fail to produce significant improvement. Table 12 summarizes treatment of life-threatening asthma.
- Discharge home from the emergency department is appropriate if the FEV_1 or PEF after treatment is 70% or greater of the personal best or predicted value and if there is sustained improvement in lung function and symptoms for at least 1 hr.

REFERRAL

Box 4 describes indications for referral to an asthma specialist.

PEARLS & CONSIDERATIONS

COMMENTS

- The differentiation of asthma from COPD can be challenging. A history of atopy and intermittent, reactive symptoms points toward a diagnosis of asthma, whereas smoking and advanced age are more indicative of COPD. Spirometry is useful in distinguishing asthma from COPD.
- In all asthma patients it is important to treat or prevent comorbid conditions (e.g., rhinosinusitis, vocal cord dysfunction, gastroesophageal reflux disease). However, despite the presumed association between asthma and GERD, trials of PPIs in patients with poorly controlled asthma did not reveal any beneficial effects.
- Inhaled low-dose corticosteroids are the single most effective therapy for adult patients with asthma who require more than an occasional use of SABAs to control their asthma.
- Stepping down inhaled corticosteroids after asthma is well controlled now has level A evidence.
- Leukotriene modifiers/receptor agonists represent a reasonable alternative in adults unable or unwilling to use corticosteroids; however, these agents are less effective than monotherapy with inhaled corticosteroids.
- Use of LABAs alone without use of a long-term asthma medication, such as an inhaled corticosteroid, is contraindicated. LABAs should also not be used in patients whose asthma is adequately controlled on low- or medium-dose inhaled corticosteroids. Continued use of LABAs may cause down-regulation of the beta-2 receptor with loss of the bronchoprotective effect from rescue therapy with a SABA.
- Patients who remain symptomatic despite inhaled corticosteroids benefit from the addition of LABAs. Trials in patients with poorly controlled asthma despite the use of inhaled glucocorticoids and LABAs have shown that the addition of tiotropium, a long-acting anticholinergic bronchodilator approved for treatment of COPD, increased the time to the

TABLE 11 Selected Inhaled Medications Used by Patients with Asthma

Generic Name	Trade Name*	Dose/Puff	Dose as Puffs	Comments
Beta-Agonist Bronchodilators†				
Albuterol-MDI‡	AccuNeb, Proair HFA, Proventil HFA, Ventolin HFA, Airomir HFA, Salamol HFA	Varies from 90-200 μg	2 puffs as needed for asthma symptoms. Can be repeated every 4 hr. 10-12 puffs in 24 hr is the maximum dose. Use of more than 6 puffs/day should prompt medical consultation for asthma control.	All are metered-dose inhalers that deliver a fixed amount of medication per puff
Albuterol-DPI	Ventolin, Asmasal, Salbulin	100 or 200 μg	1 puff as needed, otherwise same as albuterol MDI	All are dry powder inhalers that deliver a fixed amount of medication per inhalation
Albuterol solution	—	Varies from 0.63-5 mg/ml	Inhale while breathing till solution consumed. Need for more than 6 home treatments/day should prompt medical consultation.	This solution is for use with a liquid nebulizer driven by compressed gas. Mix the dose with a volume of sterile normal saline to achieve a nebulizer concentration of 0.63 mg/ml
Levalbuterol-MDI	Xopenex HFA		Same as albuterol-MDI	The isolated R-isomer of albuterol. Some studies show superiority to the racemic albuterol found in the MDIs listed above
Levalbuterol-solution	Xopenex inhalation solution	0.63 mg/ml	Same as albuterol solution.	Nebulizer solution as noted for albuterol above
Terbutaline-DPI	Bricanyl	250 or 500 μg	Same as albuterol-MDI	Dry powder inhaler, uses patient generated effort to achieve airflow to disperse and deposit medication
Terbutaline solution	Bricanyl inhalation solution	2.5 mg/ml	Same as albuterol	The per dose amount is 2 ml with sterile saline added to achieve the requisite volume for the nebulizer used
Long-Acting Anticholinergic Bronchodilator for Use in Severe Asthma				
Tiotropium bromide	Spiriva Respimat (MDI)	1.25 μg	2 puffs once/day	For patients with asthma not controlled by β-agonist and inhaled glucocorticoid treatment
Inhaled Glucocorticoids				
Beclomethasone	Beclovent, Clenil, Qvar, Asmabec	Comes in both MDI and DPI inhalers with amounts per puff varying from 50-400 μg	Adjust dose to achieve asthma control with a dose of 2 puffs twice/day. The maximum dose is two puffs twice daily of the highest strength.	Inhaled glucocorticoid with the longest use record. Although medication is generic, the inhaler type and propellant may be proprietary. Dose adjustments for patients in renal or hepatic failure are not needed.
Budesonide	Budelin, Pulmicort	Inhalers are all DPIs with amounts per dose 100-400 μg. Solution for nebulization is also available with amount of drug per treatment varies between 0.5-1.0 mg.	Adjust dose to achieve asthma control with a dose of 2 puffs twice/day. The maximum dose is two puffs twice daily of the highest strength.	Dose adjustments for patients in renal or hepatic failure are not needed.
Fluticasone propionate	Flovent, Flixotide	MDIs with 50, 125, 250 μg dose strengths as well as packets for nebulization at 0.25 and 1.0 mg/ml	With MDI, start at low concentration and adjust dose to achieve asthma control with a dose of 2 puffs twice/day. The maximum dose is two puffs twice daily of the highest strength. With nebulizer, choose a concentration that gives asthma control when used twice daily.	Dose labels on U.S. marketed inhalers are 44, 110, and 220 μg/puff. The difference is the amount loaded in the metering chamber (outside of U.S.) vs the dose leaving the inhaler (U.S.). Dose adjustments for patients in renal failure not needed. In patients with hepatic failure, patients should be carefully monitored for steroid side effects and dose adjusted appropriately.
Ciclesonide	Alvesco	MDIs delivering 40, 80, or 160 μg	With MDI, start at low concentration and adjust dose to achieve asthma control with a dose of 2 puffs twice/day. The maximum dose is two puffs twice daily of the highest strength.	Dose adjustments for patients in renal or hepatic failure are not needed.
Flunisolide	Aerospan	80 μg	Start at 2 puffs twice/day and escalate as needed. 4 puffs twice/day is maximal dose.	Dose adjustments for patients in renal or hepatic failure are not needed.
Mometasone	Asmanex HFA	100 or 200 μg in HFA form; 110 or 220 μg in DPI form	Start with 200 (220) μg once/day (P.M. dosing suggested). Max dose is 800 (880) μg once daily. Titrate dose down as control is achieved.	Dose adjustments for patients in renal failure not needed. In patients with hepatic failure, patients should be carefully monitored for steroid side effects and dose adjusted appropriately.

Continued

TABLE 11 Selected Inhaled Medications Used by Patients with Asthma—cont'd

Generic Name	Trade Name*	Dose/Puff	Dose as Puffs	Comments
Combination Inhalers Containing Both Igc and Laba§				
IGC = fluticasone propionate LABA = salmeterol	Advair, Seretide, AirFluSal, Sirdupla	Available as MDIs or DPIs. Each type contains a fixed dose of LABA with varying amounts of IGC. Exact amounts vary by inhaler type.	Start with one puff twice daily at the lowest dose of IGC that is effective for asthma control. Titrate up and down as symptom control requires. Max dose is 4 puffs of highest strength per day.	Dose adjustments for patients in renal failure not needed. In patients with hepatic failure, patients should be carefully monitored for steroid side effects and dose adjusted appropriately.
IGC = fluticasone propionate LABA = formoterol	Flutiform	Available only as MDIs. Each strength contains a fixed dose of LABA with varying amounts of IGC.	Start with two puffs twice daily at the lowest dose of IGC that is effective for asthma control. Titrate up and down as symptom control requires. Max dose is 4 puffs of highest strength per day.	Dose adjustments for patients in renal failure not needed. In patients with hepatic failure, patients should be carefully monitored for steroid side effects and dose adjusted appropriately. Not recommended for children under 12 yr.
IGC = budesonide LABA = formoterol	DuoResp, Symbicort, Bufoler	Available only as DPIs. Each strength contains a fixed dose of LABA with varying amounts of IGC. Exact amounts vary by inhaler type.	Start with one puff twice daily at the lowest dose of IGC that is effective for asthma control. Titrate up and down as symptom control requires. Max dose is 4 puffs of highest strength per day.	Dose adjustments for patients in renal or hepatic failure are not needed.
IGC = budesonide LABA = salmeterol	Busalair	Available only as DPIs. Each strength contains a fixed dose of LABA with varying amounts of IGC. Exact amounts vary by inhaler type	Start with one puff twice daily at the lowest dose of IGC that is effective for asthma control. Titrate up and down as symptom control requires. Max dose is 4 puffs of highest strength per day.	Dose adjustments for patients in renal or hepatic failure are not needed.
IGC = mometasone LABA = formoterol	Dulera	Available only as MDIs. Each strength contains a 5-μg dose of formoterol with varying amounts of IGC. Exact amounts vary by inhaler type.	Start with one puff twice daily at the lowest dose of IGC that is effective for asthma control. Titrate up and down as symptom control requires. Max dose is 4 puffs of highest strength per day.	Dose adjustments for patients in renal or hepatic failure are not needed.
IGC = beclomethasone LABA = formoterol	Fostair MDI or DPI or Fostair Inhalation Solution	All contain 6 μg of formoterol with amounts of glucocorticoid varying from 100-200 μg.	Adjust IGC dose to achieve asthma control with a dose of 2 puffs twice/day.	Not available in the U.S.
IGC = fluticasone furoate LABA = vilanterol	Relvar Ellipta or Breo Ellipta	All forms contain 25 μg of vilanterol with amount of glucocorticoid varying from 92-184 μg.	Adjust IGC dose to achieve asthma control with a dose of 2 puffs once/day.	Bronchodilator effect of vilanterol onsets in about 15 min. Dose adjustments for patients in renal failure not needed. In patients with hepatic failure, patients should be carefully monitored for steroid side effects and dose adjusted appropriately.

DPI, Dry powder inhale; *HFA*, hydrofluoroalkane; *IGC*, inhaled glucocorticoid; *LABA*, long-acting β-agonist; *MDI*, metered dose inhaler.
*Not all products marketing each medication are listed.
†All are short acting with onset of effect 5-10 min and duration of effect 4-8 hr. All patients with asthma should have a short-acting bronchodilator as a rescue inhaler to use for rescue from signs of airway obstruction.
‡The generic names albuterol and salbutamol are synonyms. Albuterol is used in the United States and salbutamol in many other countries.
§LABAs alone should not be used in patients with asthma.
From Goldman L, Shafer AI: *Goldman-Cecil medicine,* ed 26, Philadelphia, 2020, Elsevier.

first severe exacerbation and provided modest sustained bronchodilation.

- Therapy with systemic corticosteroids accelerates the resolution of acute asthma and reduces the risk of relapse. There is no evidence that doses >50 to 100 mg prednisone equivalent are beneficial.
- In patients with allergies and elevated serum immunoglobulin (Ig) E levels, use of anti-IgE therapy is beneficial.
- Bronchial thermoplasty may be considered in select patients with severe persistent asthma with recurrent exacerbations or ED visits.
- Biologic modifiers of the Th2 immune pathways (neutralizing monoclonal antibodies, receptor antagonists, soluble receptors) are potential options for the development of new treatments of severe asthma. Adjunct therapies for bronchospasm are summarized in Table 13.
- The response to treatment for asthma is characterized by wide individual variability. A functional glucocorticoid-induced transcript 1 gene *(GLCCI1)* variant is associated with substantial decrements in the response to inhaled glucocorticoids in patients with asthma. Another potential cause of the variability in response to treatment is heterogeneity in the role of interleukin-13 expression in the clinical asthma phenotype. Patients with asthma who have a certain biochemical signature are more likely to respond to an anti–interleukin-13 monoclonal antibody than those without such a signature. Identification of genetic variants can eventually lead to personalized asthma treatment. Failure of pharmacologic treatment is often due to uncontrolled comorbid conditions (tobacco, allergic rhinitis, pollutants), poor inhaler technique, or lack of adherence to prescribed medication.

SUGGESTED READINGS

Available at ExpertConsult.com

RELATED CONTENT

Asthma (Patient Information)
Asthma-COPD Overlap Syndrome (Related Key Topic)

AUTHORS: **Laren Tan, MD,** and **Michele Quan, MD, MPH**

TABLE 12 Summary of Treatment for Life-Threatening Asthma

Treatment	Dose and Frequency	Comments
Oxygen	1-3 L/min by nasal cannula Goal is to maintain oxygen saturation (Spo_2) >92% Use heated cascade humidifier to avoid dry air–induced bronchoconstriction	Transient drop in O_2 tension with beta-adrenergic therapy Avoid hyperoxia (may be associated with hypercarbia)
Bronchodilators		
$Beta_2$-selective agonists: Albuterol or salbutamol, levalbuterol	*Albuterol:* 2.5-5 mg (0.5-1 ml of 0.5% solution in 5 ml of normal saline) by nebulizer every 20 min for 3 doses total (for optimal delivery, dilute aerosols to a minimum of 3 ml at gas flow of 6-8 L/min), followed by 2.5-10 mg q1-4h as needed, or 10-15 mg/h continuously; titration based on response and severity of symptoms *Albuterol MDI,* delivered with a spacer (each spacer dose takes 1-2 min; 90 μg/puff), 4-8 puffs every 20 min for 4 hr, then q4h as needed *Albuterol:* 5-7.5 mg by jet nebulizer (each treatment takes 15-20 min) *Levalbuterol* (0.63 mg/3 ml and 1.25 mg/3 ml nebulizer): 1.25-2.5 mg every 20 min for 3 doses total, then 1.25-5 mg q1-4h as needed, or 5-7.5 mg/h continuous nebulization *Levalbuterol MDI* (45 μg/puff): 4-8 puffs every 20 min for 4 hr, followed by q1-4h as needed	$Beta_2$-selective agonists are the cornerstone of therapy Continuous nebulization used for a majority of severely ill patients In study of continuous vs. intermittent therapy in severe exacerbations (excluding life-threatening asthma), no difference noted in pulmonary function improvement or need for hospitalization Lower frequency of side effects with continuous treatment Watch for hypokalemia, tremors, tachycardia, and lactic acidosis Oral or parenteral route: Loss of $beta_2$-selectivity MDI: 4 puffs of albuterol (0.36 mg) = 2.5 mg of albuterol nebulization Levalbuterol 0.63 mg = racemic albuterol 1.25 mg for efficacy and side effects *Intubated patients:* Nebulizers are less efficient in delivering doses to lower airways (6%-10%) than MDIs (11%)
Epinephrine	*Subcutaneous epinephrine* dose for adults: 0.3-0.5 ml of a 1:1000 dilution (1 mg/ml), depending on age and weight; repeat every 20 min for 3 doses total	
Terbutaline	*Subcutaneous terbutaline,* 0.25 mg; repeat every 20 min for 3 doses total	Terbutaline is the parenteral agent of choice in pregnancy For refractory life-threatening asthma: Intravenous epinephrine (high risk for cardiac events, infarction, and arrhythmias) or racemic epinephrine may be considered
Anticholinergics		
Ipratropium (for acute severe asthma warranting visit to emergency department)	*Ipratropium bromide*: 0.5 mg by nebulizer (0.25 mg/ml) every 20 min for 3 doses, then q2-4h as needed *Ipratropium MDI* (0.018 mg/puff): 4-8 puffs per treatment every 20 min for up to 3 hr *Combinations*: Albuterol (2.5 mg/3 ml) + ipratropium (0.5 mg/3 ml): 3 ml every 20 min for 3 doses total, then as needed MDI delivering albuterol 90 μg + ipratropium 18 μg: 8 puffs every 20 min for up to 3 hr	Ipratropium: Onset of action is slow (20 min), peak effectiveness at 60-90 min, no systemic side effects, improved lung function and reduced recovery time Use a handheld mouthpiece nebulizer (contamination of the ocular area with precipitation of narrow-angle glaucoma may occur if facemask is used for delivery of anticholinergic agent) Ipratropium may be combined with nebulized albuterol dose in the emergency room; no proven benefit shown in hospitalized patients
Corticosteroids: Prednisone, prednisolone, methylprednisolone	40-80 mg/day in 1 or 2 divided doses until peak expiratory flow reaches 70% of predicted or personal best FEV_1 or PEFR <50% Methylprednisolone 40 mg IV q6h OR Hydrocortisone 200 mg IV	No advantage of higher doses No advantage of IV therapy over oral if absorption and gut transit are not impaired Total steroid course: 3-10 days, <1 wk; no need to taper steroids Inhaled steroids can be started at any time
Heliox	Helium-oxygen mixture (80-20 or 70-30) Routine use cannot be recommended at this time	Improves O_2 and aerosolized medication delivery to distal lung Decreases flow turbulence and resistance Lower gas density facilitates exhalation, reduces air trapping and intrinsic PEEP Improves pulmonary function in subgroup of patients with most severe airflow obstruction
Magnesium sulfate	2 g IV given over 20 min; may repeat Monitor magnesium levels Avoid in renal insufficiency	Bronchodilatation from inhibition of the calcium channel and decreased acetylcholine release IV and inhaled or nebulized magnesium sulfate improves pulmonary function in acute severe asthma IV magnesium widely used as adjunct therapy

FEV_1, Forced expiratory flow in 1 second; *IV,* intravenous; *MDI,* metered-dose inhaler; *PEEP,* positive end-expiratory pressure; *PEFR,* peak expiratory flow rate.
From Parrillo JE, Dellinger RP: *Critical care medicine, principles of diagnosis and management in the adult,* ed 4, Philadelphia, 2014, Elsevier.

BOX 4 Possible Indications for Referral to an Asthma Specialist

- Severe, acute asthma that has caused loss of consciousness, hypoxia, respiratory failure, convulsions, or near death
- Poorly controlled asthma as indicated by admission to a hospital, frequent need for emergency care, need for oral corticosteroids, absence from school or work, disruption of sleep, interference with quality of life
- Severe, persistent asthma requiring step 4 care (consider for patients who require step 3 care)
- Patient <3 yr who requires step 3 or 4 care (consider for patient <3 yr who requires step 2 care)
- Requirement for continuous oral corticosteroids or high-dose inhaled corticosteroids or more than two short courses of oral corticosteroids within 1 yr
- Need for additional diagnostic testing such as allergy skin testing, rhinoscopy, provocative challenge, complete pulmonary function testing, bronchoscopy
- Consideration for immunotherapy
- Need for additional education regarding asthma, complications of asthma and treatment of asthma, problems with adherence to management recommendations, or allergen avoidance
- Uncertainty of diagnosis
- Complications of asthma, including sinusitis, nasal polyposis, aspergillosis, severe rhinitis, vocal cord dysfunction, gastroesophageal reflux

Modified from National Asthma Education and Prevention Program, National Heart, Lung, and Blood Institute: *Expert Panel Report 2: guidelines for the diagnosis and management of asthma,* Bethesda, MD, 1997, National Institutes of Health, NIH publication No 97-4051.

TABLE 13 Adjunct Therapies for Bronchospasm

Nontraditional Therapy for Severe Bronchospasm	Comments
Intravenous beta$_2$-agonists	No data show any benefit in adding IV agent to nebulization Avoid IV isoproterenol owing to danger of myocardial toxicity
Oral or IV leukotriene receptor antagonists (LTRAs): Montelukast 10 mg oral daily, zafirlukast	Rapid bronchodilation in impending respiratory failure Improves pulmonary function within 10 min Oral LTRAs can be added as an adjunct in severe asthma
Noninvasive positive-pressure ventilation (NPPV)	NPPV reduces the need for endotracheal intubation in severe asthma exacerbation
Inhaled nitric oxide (NO) (adding 15 ppm to the inspiratory circuit)	Rapid improvement in ventilated patients with asthma refractory to medical treatment
Omalizumab (anti-IgE antibody)	Role in acute asthma is unstudied Improves asthma control in allergic asthmatics
General anesthetic agents: Isoflurane or halothane anesthesia IV thiopental, IV propofol, IV ketamine	Propofol relaxes the smooth muscles in arteries and veins and has bronchodilator effect
Plasma exchange (during pregnancy) Pumpless extracorporeal carbon dioxide removal Extracorporeal life support (ECLS)	Case reports of adjunct therapies; used as salvage therapy for life-threatening asthma
Glucagon	Rapid smooth muscle relaxant, short half-life; small study report
Nebulized DNase (dornase 2.5 mg via tracheal tube)	Case report of use in pregnant patient with rapid improvement
Bronchial lavage	Anecdotal reports: Exacerbates auto-PEEP, decreases oxygenation

IgE, Immunoglobulin E; *IV,* intravenous; *PEEP,* positive end-expiratory pressure.
From Parrillo JE, Dellinger RP: *Critical care medicine, principles of diagnosis and management in the adult,* ed 4, Philadelphia, 2014, Elsevier.

BASIC INFORMATION

DEFINITION

Astrocytoma is a type of neuroepithelial tumor arising from astrocytes, which are glial precursor cells. The distinction of different grades of astrocytoma provides important clinical prognostic information (Table 1). According to the World Health Organization (WHO) classification astrocytoma is classified as below based on the histopathology:

- Grade I: Pilocytic astrocytoma
- Grade II: Diffuse astrocytoma
- Grade III: Anaplastic astrocytoma
- Grade IV: Glioblastoma
- Grades III and IV are considered high-grade astrocytomas (HGAs) or malignant

SYNONYM

Astroglial neoplasms

ICD-10CM CODE
C71.9 Malignant neoplasm of brain, unspecified

EPIDEMIOLOGY & DEMOGRAPHICS

There are an estimated 24,000 new cases of primary CNS tumors in the U.S., of which astrocytomas constitute approximately 10% of cases according to the Central Brain Tumor Registry of the United States (CBTRUS). The incidence of primary CNS tumor is 6.4 cases per 100,000 persons per yr with age-adjusted death rate of 4.4 per 100,000 population, of which about 50% cases are that of glioblastoma.

PHYSICAL FINDINGS & CLINICAL PRESENTATION

The presenting symptoms of astrocytoma depend, in part, on the location of the lesion and its rate of growth. Astrocytomas classically present with any one or more of the following features:

- Headache (not frequent) are associated with mass effect
- New-onset partial or generalized seizures (<50%)
- Nausea and vomiting, fatigue, weakness
- Focal neurologic deficit (cranial nerve palsy, hemiplegia, ataxia, visual loss, language alteration, etc.)
- Change in mood, memory, or mental status
- Papilledema (rare)

ETIOLOGY

- No agent has been definitely implicated in the causation of CNS tumors, and risk factors can be identified in some patients. Farmers and petrochemical workers have been shown to have a higher incidence of primary brain tumors. Exposure to ionizing radiation to the CNS is a known risk factor for astrocytomas.
- Different hereditary syndromes are associated with increased risk and high frequency of astrocytoma.
  1. Neurofibromatosis type 1 is associated with increased frequency of astrocytoma.
  2. Inherited syndromes such as Lynch syndrome and Li-Fraumeni syndrome are associated with an increased frequency of malignant gliomas.

GENE AND CHROMOSOMAL ALTERATIONS IN ASTROCYTOMA:

- Alteration in p53, a tumor suppressor encoded by the *TP53* gene on chromosome 17p, plays a key role in the development of at least one third of all grades of astrocytoma. In addition, in high-grade astrocytomas, p53 function may be deregulated by alteration of other genes, including amplification of MDM2 or MDM4 and 9p deletions that result in loss of the p14 product of the *CDKN2A* gene.
- Mutations of isocitrate dehydrogenase 1 gene (*IDH1*) occur in a large fraction of grade II and grade III astrocytomas as well as in other gliomas. IDH-mutated tumors have a better prognosis compared with those with IDH-wild type status.
- Recently, gliomas have been defined into five molecular groups with the use of three alterations: Mutations in the *TERT* promoter, mutations in *IDH*, and codeletion of chromosome arms 1p and 19q (1p/19q codeletion).

DIAGNOSIS

A provisional diagnosis of astrocytoma is made on clinical grounds and radiographic imaging studies. Tissue pathology is needed to establish the diagnosis and to grade the astrocytoma.

DIFFERENTIAL DIAGNOSIS

The differential diagnosis is vast and includes any cause of headache, seizures, change in mental status, and focal neurologic deficits.

WORKUP

- The imaging modality of choice is contrast-enhanced MRI, which can demonstrate anatomy and pathological process in detail. CT scanning is reserved for patients who are unable or unwilling to get MRI. Biopsy with histological confirmation is required to establish a diagnosis of astrocytoma.
- Stereotactic biopsy under CT or MRI guidance has been reserved for tumors that are deeply seated, multicentric tumors or diffuse nonfocal tumors where surgical resection is not practical. Major objectives of surgical resection are to maximally remove the tumor bulk, reduce tumor-associated mass effect and elevated intracranial pressure and provide tissue for pathological analysis. The surgical resection is carried out in a manner that minimizes the risk to neurological functioning. Surgery can also rapidly reduce the tumor bulk with potential benefits in terms of mass effect, edema, and hydrocephalus.

LABORATORY TESTS

- Complete blood count
- Complete chemistry panel
- Coagulation testing (PT, PTT)

IMAGING STUDIES

MRI (Fig. 1) is the diagnostic imaging study of choice. MRI with contrast and magnetic resonance angiography are used to locate the margins of the tumor, distinguish vascular masses from tumors, detect low-grade astrocytomas (LGAs) not seen by CT scan, and provide clear views of the posterior fossa.

TREATMENT

ACUTE GENERAL Rx

- Corticosteroids (usually dexamethasone) need to be started immediately preoperatively in all primary CNS tumors unless CNS lymphoma is being suspected. Corticosteroids reduce cerebral edema and thus minimize secondary brain injury from cerebral retraction. Corticosteroids needs to be continued in the immediate postoperative period and tapered as quickly as possible. If there is increased intracranial pressure and impending herniation, patient should be started on IV mannitol, and mechanical ventilation

TABLE 1 Comparison of Astrocytoma Histopathology

	Pilocytic Astrocytoma	Diffuse Astrocytoma	Anaplastic Astrocytoma	Glioblastoma Multiforme
Malignant potential	Benign	Low grade	High grade	Very malignant
Age (approximate)	Children	Third or fourth decade	Fifth decade	Sixth decade
Location	Optic chiasm or hypothalamus > cerebellum > brainstem*	Hemispheres (cortex + white matter)	Hemispheres (cortex + white matter)	Hemispheres (cortex + white matter)
Enhancement	Mild	Mild	Moderate (ring)	Intense
Vasogenic edema	Minimal	Minimal	Moderate	Significant
Calcification	Common	Up to 20%	Occasional	Rare

*It is typically cystic with a mural nodule and located within the posterior fossa—it tends to be solid or lobulated when seen elsewhere.
From Grant LA: *Grainger & Allison's diagnostic radiology essentials,* ed 2, Philadelphia, 2019, Elsevier.

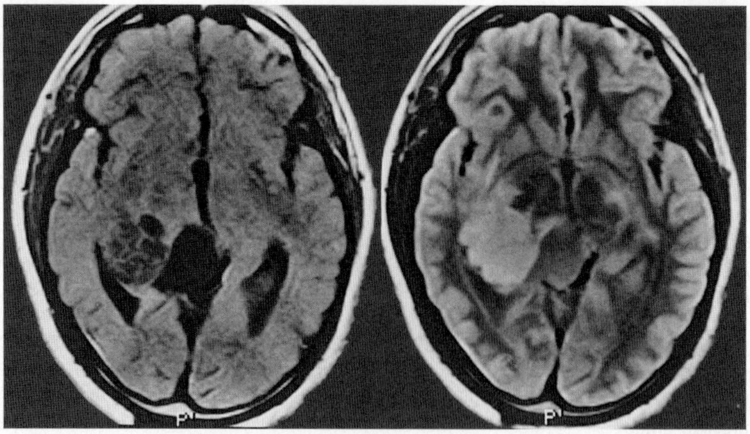

FIG. 1 Magnetic resonance image of a low-grade astrocytoma, demonstrating a hypointense right temporal lesion without contrast enhancement on T1 and hyperintense signal on T2. (From Goetz CG, Pappert EJ: *Textbook of clinical neurology,* Philadelphia, 1999, Saunders.)

with hyperventilation should be considered if there is depressed consciousness.

- The use of preoperative prophylactic anticonvulsants is less commonly indicated though the current practice pattern in the U.S. indicates widespread use.

STAGE-SPECIFIC Rx

- Grade I astrocytomas are usually indolent and circumscribed tumors. Complete surgical resection is the mainstay of therapy whenever feasible and is curative for these tumors. If complete surgical resection is not feasible due to location of tumor such as when the tumor is in optic pathway, hypothalamus, and in deep midline structures, asymptomatic patients can be observed in these cases until maximally safe resection is feasible upon progression. Unfortunately, despite aggressive near-total resection, delayed recurrence and eventual malignant transformation are common.
- In grade II astrocytoma, the extent of postoperative residual disease is an important variable for time to first relapse. Postoperative use of chemotherapy (PCV regimen or temozolomide) concurrent with radiotherapy improves progression-free survival and overall survival.
- In grade III anaplastic astrocytoma, surgical resection has shown to prolong survival and postoperative chemotherapy and radiotherapy is routinely used. Recent randomized clinical trials have established a survival benefit with the use of concurrent chemotherapy (temozolomide or nitrosoureas) for 6 to 12 mo.
- In grade IV glioblastoma, maximal surgical resection improves median survival. Randomized trials have demonstrated survival benefit with use of concurrent chemotherapy with radiotherapy followed by further 6 mo of temozolomide chemotherapy alone. The survival benefit with this approach is mostly seen in patients whose tumors have MGMT-methylated status. Unfortunately, even with chemotherapy and radiation therapy, the 2-yr survival in these patients is only 16% and long-term survival is approximately 1%.

TREATMENT OF RECURRENT DISEASE

- For grade 1 astrocytoma, re-resection should be considered. For patients who have tumors that are not amenable to resection, chemotherapy or radiotherapy can improve recurrence-free survival, although the role of chemotherapy in adults remain controversial.
- For grade 2 astrocytoma, radiation therapy can be considered in the relapsed setting if not given in the adjuvant setting. Data on use of chemotherapy in low-grade gliomas in adults is sparse. Although the results are encouraging, the number of patients treated in these studies is small and there were many methodological flaws in the studies. For recurrent grade III anaplastic astrocytoma treated with radiation therapy in the past, there is a role for chemotherapy. Nitrosoureas-based regimen and temozolomide (alkylating agent) have shown efficacy in this setting.
- Various targeted therapies are currently being studied in patients with recurrent glioblastoma. Irinotecan with bevacizumab or bevacizumab alone have been studied in a phase 2 trial, and a response rate of 38% and 28% respectively was reported in that study. Median survival was 8.7 mo and 9.2 mo, respectively.
- The PD-1 checkpoint inhibitors have been evaluated in this setting, and randomized studies have not shown any survival benefits in newly diagnosed patients. However, certain subsets of patients with recurrent GBM have demonstrated survival benefits when used in neoadjuvant approach or in hypermutated tumors.
- In the case of both recurrent and newly diagnosed glioblastoma, the use of tumor-treatment fields (TTF) devices in conjunction with the use of temozolomide chemotherapy has demonstrated a survival benefit and is approved by the FDA.

PROGNOSIS

- Grade 1 astrocytoma has a good prognosis and is usually cured with surgical resection.
- Grade 2 astrocytoma has a median survival of about 7.5 yr with treatment.
- Grade 3 anaplastic astrocytoma has a median survival of approximately 5 yr. Patients with tumors that have IDH-mutation and 1p/19q co-deletion have superior survival compared with patients without deletion.
- Median survival of glioblastoma is approximately 14 mo. Primary glioblastomas are IDH-wild type and account for 90% of cases. Secondary glioblastomas in contrast are IDH-mutated, have typically evolved from low-grade gliomas, and have a much more protracted natural course than the primary cases.

REFERRAL

A multidisciplinary consultation with a neurosurgeon, radiation oncologist, and neurooncologist is required to assist in the diagnostic workup and to provide immediate and follow-up treatment.

SUGGESTED READINGS

Available at ExpertConsult.com

RELATED CONTENT

Astrocytoma (Patient Information)
Brain Cancer (Patient Information)
Brain Neoplasm, Benign (Related Key Topic)
Brain Neoplasm, Glioblastoma (Related Key Topic)

AUTHOR: **Bharti Rathore, MD**

BASIC INFORMATION

DEFINITION

Atelectasis describes collapse of part or all of the lung with resultant volume loss. There are two major types of atelectasis.

1. Obstructive atelectasis: Most common and results from a blocked airway (e.g., mucous plug or tumor-obstructing airway) with resorption of the gas in the alveoli distal to the area of obstruction.
2. Nonobstructive atelectasis: May result from several nonobstructive etiologies, including external compression from outside the lung (e.g., pleural effusion), abnormalities in surfactant leading to increased tendency for part of the lung to collapse, reduction in size of part of the lung due to scarring, and decreased ventilation of portion of the lung.

ICD-10CM CODE
J98.11 Atelectasis

EPIDEMIOLOGY & DEMOGRAPHICS

- Postoperative patients and patients with lung or chest wall injury are at increased risk of atelectasis.
- Asbestos exposure increases risk for an entity called "rounded atelectasis."
- Occurs frequently in patients receiving mechanical ventilation.
- There is no known racial or sexual predilection for atelectasis.
- Dependent regions of the lung are more prone to atelectasis.

PHYSICAL FINDINGS & CLINICAL PRESENTATION

- Patient may be asymptomatic or may have cough, dyspnea, and decrease in oxygen saturations.
- Physical examination may disclose decreased or absent breath sounds over affected area, with dullness to percussion, decreased fremitus, and decreased vocal resonance.

ETIOLOGY

- Airway obstruction (e.g., endobronchial tumor, a lymph node, foreign bodies, mucous plug)
- Extrinsic bronchial compression (e.g., neoplasms, aneurysms of ascending aorta, enlarged left atrium)
- Pleural disease (e.g., pleural effusion, mesothelioma, rounded atelectasis, pneumothorax)
- Alveolar injury (e.g., toxic fumes, aspiration of gastric contents, infections, acute respiratory distress syndrome)
- Chest wall abnormalities (e.g., trauma, scoliosis, rib fracture, obesity)
- Impaired respiratory mechanics or decreased cough response (e.g., pain, postanesthetic effect, abdominal distention, neuromuscular disease)
- Trauma caused by shear force generated by repetitive expansion and collapse during positive-pressure ventilation (e.g., mechanical ventilation)
- Characteristic rounded atelectasis may be associated with prior asbestos exposure
- Table 1 summarizes anatomic causes of atelectasis

DIAGNOSIS

DIFFERENTIAL DIAGNOSIS

- Neoplasm (bronchogenic carcinoma must be excluded)
- Pneumonia
- Pleural effusion
- Abnormalities of brachiocephalic vein and the left pulmonary ligament

WORKUP

- Chest x-ray (Fig. 1)
- Thoracic ultrasonography
- Chest CT scan (Prone positioning CT scan with improvement or reduction in atelectasis) may be used to differentiate from other etiology
- Fiber-optic bronchoscopy (in select patients) to assess for endobronchial obstruction

IMAGING STUDIES

- Chest x-ray often suggests the diagnosis.
- Ultrasonography helps differentiate atelectasis from effusion or consolidation.
- Chest CT scan is useful in patients with suspected endobronchial neoplasm or extrinsic bronchial compression. Prone images help differentiate true consolidation from dependent atelectasis.

TABLE 1 Anatomic Causes of Atelectasis

Cause	Clinical Examples
External compression on the pulmonary parenchyma	Pleural effusion, pneumothorax, intrathoracic tumors, diaphragmatic hernia
Endobronchial obstruction completely obstructing the ingress of air	Enlarged lymph node, tumor, cardiac enlargement, foreign body, mucoid plug, broncholithiasis
Intraluminal obstruction of a bronchus	Foreign body, asthma, granulomatous tissue, tumor, secretions including mucous plugs, bronchiectasis, pulmonary abscess, chronic bronchitis, acute laryngotracheobronchitis, plastic bronchitis
Intrabronchiolar obstruction	Bronchiolitis, interstitial pneumonitis, asthma
Respiratory compromise or paralysis	Neuromuscular abnormalities, osseous deformities, overly restrictive casts and surgical dressings, defective movement of the diaphragm, or restriction of respiratory effort

From Kliegman RM: *Nelson textbook of pediatrics,* ed 21, Philadelphia, 2020, Elsevier.

TREATMENT

NONPHARMACOLOGIC THERAPY

- Deep breathing
- Mobilization of the patient: Encouraging out of bed in upright position, ambulation
- Incentive spirometry
- Tracheal suctioning in select patients (e.g., mechanical ventilation and tracheostomy)
- Mechanical airway clearance therapies for improving cough and clearance of secretions from airways:
  1. Positive expiratory pressure (PEP) devices (e.g., Acapella, Aerobika, TheraPEP)
  2. Cough assist devices
  3. Chest physiotherapy with vest therapy, frequencer, or chest wall percussion
- Fiber-optic bronchoscopy might be helpful with mucous plug aspiration, removal of foreign body, or evaluation for endobronchial and peribronchial lesions

ACUTE GENERAL Rx

- Oxygen if indicated
- Positive-pressure breathing (continuous positive airway pressure by face mask, positive end-expiratory pressure for patients on mechanical ventilation)
- Use of mucolytic agents (e.g., acetylcysteine [Mucomyst]) or hypertonic saline if due to mucous plugging
- Bronchodilator therapy in selected patients
- Pain control in postoperative and trauma cases to facilitate deeper breathing
- Pleural drainages in cases of large effusions, hemothorax, or empyema
- Treatment of atelectasis is summarized in Table 2

CHRONIC Rx

- Mechanical airway clearance therapies.
- If significant endobronchial obstruction, may need to consider debulking of obstruction or possible placement of bronchial stent.
- If external compression (e.g., pleural effusion or mass) is leading to the atelectasis, then need to drain or remove the contributing source of the compression.

DISPOSITION

Prognosis varies with the underlying etiology.

REFERRAL

- Pulmonary for bronchoscopy to evaluate for obstructing lesion as etiology for atelectasis and for possible removal of foreign body.
- Interventional pulmonology to debulk or remove endobronchial tumor or to place endobronchial stent if indicated.

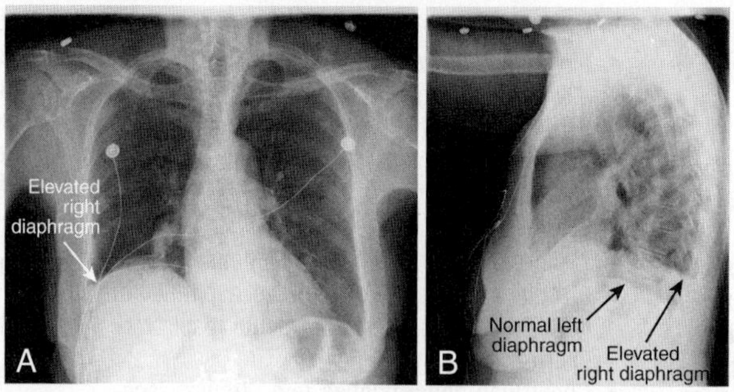

FIG. 1 Atelectasis with elevated diaphragm: An example of volume loss. The right hemidiaphragm in this patient appears elevated on both the posterior-anterior **(A)** and the lateral **(B)** views. Is this the correct interpretation of the x-ray, and if so, what is the cause? Consider the alternative interpretations. A subpulmonic pleural effusion would appear similar, as it would have the same density as liver, heart, and diaphragm and would layer over the diaphragm with the patient upright. This appears less likely in that a meniscus might be seen along the lateral chest wall with a pleural effusion but is not present here. In addition, a pleural effusion occupies space and might be expected to push the heart to the left, whereas in this case the heart may be slightly deviated to the right. Atelectasis of the lower right lung would result in volume loss, pulling the heart and hemidiaphragm into the space normally occupied by lung. This is consistent with the observed features. An infiltrate in this location could explain the x-ray findings but appears less likely for similar reasons to those cited for effusion. Some simple maneuvers could narrow the differential diagnosis. Chest ultrasound, decubitus x-ray views, or CT could identify an effusion. (From Broder JS: *Diagnostic imaging for the emergency physician,* Philadelphia, 2011, Saunders.)

TABLE 2 Treatment for Atelectasis

Cause of Atelectasis	Treatment
Pleural effusion or pneumothorax	Relieve compression
Mucous plug	Tracheal or bronchoscopic aspiration Continuous positive airway pressure
Foreign body	Bronchoscopic examination
Asthma	Bronchodilator and corticosteroid treatment Recombinant human deoxyribonuclease (off label use) Hypertonic saline with or without bronchodilator
Neuromuscular diseases	Intermittent positive pressure breathing Mechanical insufflator–exsufflator Noninvasive bilevel positive pressure ventilation
Cystic fibrosis	Airway clearance therapies Hypertonic saline with or without bronchodilator

From Kliegman RM: *Nelson textbook of pediatrics,* ed 21, Philadelphia, 2020, Elsevier.

PEARLS & CONSIDERATIONS

COMMENTS

Patients should be educated that frequent changes of position are helpful in clearing secretions. Sitting the patient upright in a chair is recommended to increase both volume and vital capacity relative to the supine position. Adequate pain control and early mobilization are paramount after surgical intervention or rib fractures.

RELATED CONTENT

Atelectasis (Patient Information)

AUTHOR: **Lorriana E. Leard, MD**

BASIC INFORMATION

DEFINITION

Atopic dermatitis is a chronic inflammatory skin disease characterized by pruritic eruptions that wax and wane, and is associated with a personal and family of allergic manifestations including food allergies, asthma, and allergic rhinoconjunctivitis (atopy). Box 1 summarizes criteria for atopic dermatitis. Modified criteria for children with atopic dermatitis are described in Box 2.

SYNONYMS

Eczema
Atopic neurodermatitis
Atopic eczema

ICD-10CM CODES

L20.9 Atopic dermatitis, unspecified
L20.89 Other atopic dermatitis

EPIDEMIOLOGY & DEMOGRAPHICS

- Prevalence is about 30% in most developed nations and exceeds 10% in many countries.
- About 50% of cases occur in the first year of life, 85% of patients experience onset of disease before age 5, and the remaining cases usually present before age 30.
- More than 50% of children with generalized atopic dermatitis eventually develop asthma and allergic rhinitis, often referred to as the "atopic march."
- Concordance in monozygotic twins is 80%.
- General risk factors include female gender, family history of atopy (especially a maternal history of eczema), high latitude (and therefore low sun exposure), and birth order (oldest are at greatest risk).
- Risk factors for developing atopic dermatitis in the first 6 mo of life include African and Asian race/ethnicity, male gender, and greater gestational age at birth.
- Consumption of a Western diet, delivery by cesarean section, exposure to antibiotics prenatally, and colonization with *Clostridium* cluster I are also associated with increased risk and suggest that alternations in the intestinal microbiome may play a role in the development of atopic dermatitis.
- Protective factors include breast feeding, dog ownership before age 1, and being raised on a farm (i.e., hygiene hypothesis).

PHYSICAL FINDINGS & CLINICAL PRESENTATION

- Atopic dermatitis presentation can be subdivided into three phases:
  1. Acute: Vesicular, crusting, weeping eruption
  2. Subacute: Dry, scaly, erythematous papules and plaques
  3. Chronic: Lichenification from repeated scratching
- The lesions are typically on the neck, face, upper trunk, and bends of elbows and knees (symmetric on flexural surfaces of extremities; Fig. E1). Atopic dermatitis lesions are usually discrete but vaguely delineated, scaly, and erythematous.
- There is dryness, thickening of the involved areas, discoloration, blistering, and oozing.
- Papular lesions are frequently found in the antecubital and popliteal fossae.
- In children, red scaling plaques are often confined to the cheeks and spare the perioral and perinasal areas (Fig. E2A,B).
- ***Hertoghe sign:*** Loss of the outer eyebrow from chronic rubbing.
- Pruritus is the most common and burdensome symptom of atopic dermatitis. Constant scratching may result in areas of hypopigmentation or hyperpigmentation (more common in black patients).
- In adults, redness and scaling on the dorsal aspect of the hands or about the fingers are the most common expression of atopic dermatitis; oozing and crusting may be present.

BOX 1 Criteria for Atopic Dermatitis

Major criteria
Must have three of the following:
1. Pruritus
2. Typical morphology and distribution
   - Flexural lichenification in adults
   - Facial and extensor involvement in infancy
3. Chronic or chronically relapsing dermatitis
4. Personal or family history of atopic disease (e.g., asthma, allergic rhinitis, atopic dermatitis)

Minor criteria
Must also have three of the following:
- Xerosis
- Ichthyosis, hyperlinear palms, or keratosis pilaris
- IgE reactivity (immediate skin test reactivity, RAST test positive)
- Elevated serum IgE
- Early age of onset
- Tendency for cutaneous infections (especially *Staphylococcus aureus* and HSV)
- Tendency to nonspecific hand/foot dermatitis
- Nipple eczema
- Cheilitis
- Recurrent conjunctivitis
- Dennie-Morgan infraorbital fold
- Keratoconus
- Anterior subcapsular cataracts
- Orbital darkening
- Facial pallor or facial erythema
- Pityriasis alba
- Itch when sweating
- Intolerance to wool and lipid solvents
- Perifollicular accentuation
- Food hypersensitivity
- Course influenced by environmental or emotional factors
- White dermatographism or delayed blanch to cholinergic agents

HSV, Herpes simplex virus; *IgE*, immunoglobulin E; *RAST*, radioallergosorbent assay.
From James WD et al: *Andrews' diseases of the skin,* ed 13, Philadelphia, 2020, Elsevier.

BOX 2 Modified Criteria for Children with Atopic Dermatitis

Essential features
1. Pruritus
2. Eczema
   - Typical morphology and age-specific pattern
   - Chronic or relapsing history

Important features
1. Early age at onset
2. Atopy
3. Personal or family history
4. IgE reactivity
5. Xerosis

Associated features
1. Atypical vascular responses (e.g., facial pallor, white dermatographism)
2. Keratosis pilaris, ichthyosis, or hyperlinear palms
3. Orbital or periorbital changes
4. Other regional findings (e.g., perioral changes, periauricular lesions)
5. Perifollicular accentuation, lichenification, or prurigo lesions

IgE, Immunoglobulin E.
From James WD et al: *Andrews' diseases of the skin,* ed 13, Philadelphia, 2020, Elsevier.

TABLE 1 Associated Features of Atopic Dermatitis ("Atopic Stigmata")

Xerosis	• Important feature that is present in most patients with AD • Often most prominent on the lower legs; may be generalized • Dry skin with fine scale in areas without clinically apparent inflammation • Typically worse during the winter • Impaired epidermal barrier function from decreased water content in the stratum corneum leads to easier entry of irritants, which can promote pruritus and initiate an inflammatory response
Ichthyosis vulgaris	• Autosomal semidominant disorder with incomplete penetrance caused by mutations in the filaggrin gene *(FLG)* • ~15% of patients with AD have moderate-to-severe ichthyosis vulgaris; conversely, >50% of patients with ichthyosis vulgaris have AD • Excessive fine, whitish to brown scaling that favors the lower legs (especially the shins) and spares the flexures
Keratosis pilaris	• Common condition that affects >40% of patients with AD and ~75% of those with ichthyosis vulgaris • Onset typically in childhood; may improve after puberty (especially facial involvement) • Affects the lateral aspect of the upper arms, thighs, and lateral cheeks (especially in children) > trunk and extensor aspects of the distal extremities • Keratotic follicular papules, often with a rim of erythema or a background of patchy erythema (especially on the cheeks) • The *keratosis pilaris rubra (KPR)* variant features numerous tiny, "grain-like" follicular papules superimposed on prominent confluent erythema; often widespread on face & ears > trunk & proximal extremities, and tends to persist after puberty; presence of erythema rather than hyperpigmentation differentiates KPR from erythromelanosis follicularis faciei et colli, and a lack of atrophy in KPR differentiates it from keratosis pilaris atrophicans • Keratolytic agents and topical retinoids are sometimes used to decrease the hyperkeratotic component, but the benefit is limited and these agents can be irritating, especially in AD patients; treatment with vascular lasers (e.g., pulsed dye laser) can sometimes improve associated erythema
Palmar and plantar hyperlinearity	• Increased prominence of the palmar and, less often, plantar creases • Associated with ichthyosis vulgaris and *FLG* mutations
Dennie–Morgan lines	• Symmetric, prominent horizontal fold(s) (single or double) just beneath the margin of the lower lid, originating at or near the inner canthus and extending one-half to two-thirds the width of the lid
Periorbital darkening ("allergic shiners")	• Skin around the eyes appears gray to violet–brown, while the rest of the facial skin is rather pale • Periorbital edema and lichenification may also be seen
Anterior neck folds	• Horizontal folds across the middle of the anterior neck
Hertoghe sign	• Absence or thinning of the lateral eyebrows
White dermographism	• Stroking the skin leads to a white streak that reflects excessive vasoconstriction • Most apparent on the forehead • Midfacial pallor and a delayed blanch response represent additional manifestations of aberrant vascular reactivity in patients with atopic dermatitis
Follicular prominence	• "Goose bump-like" appearance of the skin, most often on the trunk • More commonly observed in children with darkly pigmented skin

AD, Atopic dermatitis.
From Bolognia J: *Dermatology*, ed 4, 2018, Elsevier.

- Secondary skin infections may be present (*Staphylococcus aureus,* dermatophytosis, herpes simplex).
- Associated features of atopic dermatitis (atopic stigmata) are summarized in Table 1.

ETIOLOGY

- The pathogenesis of atopic dermatitis is multifactorial, involving immunologic, genetic, and environmental factors that disrupt the epidermis.
- Barrier defect activates T-lymphocytes, leading to a cycle of inflammation mediated by multiple signals; filaggrin mutations, elevated T-lymphocyte activation, defective cell immunity, and B-cell IgE overproduction may all play a significant role.

Dx DIAGNOSIS

DIFFERENTIAL DIAGNOSIS

- Scabies
- Psoriasis
- Dermatitis herpetiform
- Contact dermatitis
- Photosensitivity
- Seborrheic dermatitis
- Candidiasis, tinea
- Lichen simplex chronicus
- Other: Xerosis, impetigo, Wiskott-Aldrich syndrome, phenylketonuria, ichthyosis, HIV dermatitis, nonnummular eczema, histiocytosis X, malignancies (T-cell lymphoma/mycosis fungoides, Letterer-Siwe disease), graft-versus-host disease, metabolic and nutritional deficiencies (zinc, niacin, pyridoxine deficiencies)
- Table 2 summarizes characteristics and clinical features of disorders in the differential diagnosis of atopic dermatitis

WORKUP

Diagnosis is based on the presence of three of the following major features and three minor features.

MAJOR FEATURES:

- Pruritus
- Personal or family history of atopy: Asthma, allergic rhinitis, atopic dermatitis
- Facial and extensor involvement in infants and children
- Flexural lichenification in adults

MINOR FEATURES:

- Elevated IgE
- Eczema-perifollicular accentuation
- Recurrent conjunctivitis
- Ichthyosis
- Nipple dermatitis
- Wool intolerance
- Cutaneous *S. aureus* infections or herpes simplex infections
- Food intolerance
- Hand dermatitis (nonallergic irritant)
- Facial pallor, facial erythema
- Cheilitis
- White dermographism
- Early age of onset (after 2 mo of age)

LABORATORY TESTS

- Laboratory tests are generally not helpful, though 80% to 90% of patients have elevated IgE levels.
- Consider skin biopsy only in cases unresponsive to treatment.

TABLE 2 Differential Diagnosis of Atopic Dermatitis (AD)

	Main Age Group Affected	Frequency*	Characteristics and Clinical Features
Other Types of Dermatitis			
Seborrheic dermatitis	Infants	Common	Salmon-red greasy scaly lesions, often on the scalp (cradle cap) and napkin area; generally presents in the first 6 wk of life; typically clears within weeks
Seborrheic dermatitis	Adults	Common	Erythematous patches with yellow, white, or grayish scales in seborrheic areas, particularly the scalp, central face, and anterior chest
Nummular dermatitis	Children and adults	Common	Coin-shaped scaly patches, mostly on legs and buttocks; usually no itch
Irritant contact dermatitis	Children and adults	Common	Acute to chronic eczematous lesions, mostly confined to the site of exposure; history of locally applied irritants is a risk factor; might coexist with AD
Allergic contact dermatitis	Children and adults	Common	Eczematous rash with maximum expression at sites of direct exposure but might spread; history of locally applied irritants is a risk factor; might coexist with AD
Lichen simplex chronicus	Adults	Uncommon	One or more localized, circumscribed, lichenified plaques that result from repetitive scratching or rubbing because of intense itch
Asteatotic eczema	Adults	Common	Scaly, fissured patches of dermatitis overlying dry skin, most often on lower legs
Infectious Skin Diseases			
Dermatophyte infection	Children and adults	Common	One or more demarcated scaly plaques with central clearing and slightly raised reddened edge; variable itch
Impetigo	Children	Common	Demarcated erythematous patches with blisters or honey-yellow crusting
Scabies	Children	Common†	Itchy superficial burrows and pustules on palms and soles, between fingers, and on genitalia; might produce secondary eczematous changes
HIV	Children and adults	Uncommon	Seborrhea-like rash
Keratinization Disorders			
Ichthyosis vulgaris	Infants and adults	Uncommon	Dry skin with fine scaling, particularly on the lower abdomen and extensor areas; perifollicular skin roughening; palmar hyperlinearity; full form (i.e., 2 *FLG* mutations) is uncommon; often coexists with AD
Nutritional Deficiency–Metabolic Disorders			
Zinc deficiency (acrodermatitis lenteropathica)	Children	Uncommon	Erythematous scaly patches and plaques, most often around the mouth and anus; rare congenital form accompanied by diarrhea and alopecia
Biotin deficiency (nutritional or biotinidase deficiency)	Infants	Uncommon	Scaly periorofacial dermatitis, alopecia, conjunctivitis, lethargy, hypotonia
Pellagra (niacin deficiency)	All ages	Uncommon	Scaly crusted epidermis, desquamation, sun-exposed areas, diarrhea
Kwashiorkor	Infants and children	Geographic dependent	Flaky scaly dermatitis, swollen limbs with cracked peeling patches
Phenylketonuria	Infants	Uncommon	Eczematous rash, hypopigmentation, blonde hair, developmental delay
Neoplastic Disease			
Cutaneous T-cell lymphoma	Adults	Uncommon	Erythematous pink-brown macules and plaques with a fine scale; poorly responsive to topical corticosteroids; variable itch (in early stages)
Langerhans cell histiocytosis	Infants	Uncommon	Scaly and purpuric dermatosis, hepatosplenomegaly, cytopenias

FLG, Filaggrin gene; *HIV*, human immunodeficiency virus.
*Common = approximately 1 in 10 to 1 in 100; uncommon = 1 in 100 to 1 in 1000; rare = 1 in 1000 to 1 in 10,000; very rare ≤1 in 10,000.
†Especially in developing countries.
From Kliegman RM: *Nelson textbook of pediatrics,* ed 21, Philadelphia, 2020, Elsevier.

Rx TREATMENT

NONPHARMACOLOGIC THERAPY

- Proactive skin care:
  1. Clip nails to decrease abrasion of skin.
  2. Moisturize daily with emollients or ceramides, ideally immediately after bathing when the skin is still damp. Severely affected skin can be further hydrated by occlusion with wet dressings.
  3. Limit showers to 5 to 10 minutes with warm water.
  4. Utilize fragrance-free soaps and detergents.
- Bleach baths may be helpful for certain patients.
- Avoidance of triggering factors:
  1. Sudden temperature changes, sweating, low humidity in the winter
  2. Contact with irritating substance (e.g., wool, cosmetics, some soaps and detergents, tobacco)
  3. Foods that provoke exacerbations (e.g., eggs, peanuts, fish, soy, wheat, milk)
  4. Stressful situations
  5. Allergens and dust
  6. Excessive hand washing
  7. Very hot, long showers
- Phototherapy in moderation may be effective in resistant cases and typically requires dermatology referral.

ACUTE GENERAL Rx

- Low-potency topical corticosteroids (e.g., 1% to 2.5% hydrocortisone) may be helpful and are generally considered first-line therapy. Use intermediate-potency steroids (e.g., triamcinolone, fluocinolone) for more severe cases and limit potent corticosteroids (e.g., betamethasone, desoximetasone, clobetasol) to severe cases. Table 3 summarizes relative potencies of topical corticosteroids.
- Crisaborole 2% ointment is a phosphodiesterase type-4 (PDE4) inhibitor modestly effective for short-term treatment of mild to moderate atopic dermatitis, but use can be limited by patient report of discomfort. Cost is also a limiting factor.
- Oral antihistamines (e.g., hydroxyzine, diphenhydramine) have not been shown to be effective and are generally not recommended but may be useful in controlling pruritus and inducing sedation, restful sleep, and prevention of scratching during sleep. Doxepin and other tricyclic antidepressants also have antihistamine effect, induce sleep, and reduce pruritus.
- The topical immunomodulators pimecrolimus and tacrolimus can be used in conjunction with topical corticosteroids and are useful for the face and intertriginous sites, where steroid-induced atrophy may occur. The FDA recommends limiting their use for short periods in a specific subset of patients, given concerns about the potential for rare, carcinogenic effects. Pimecrolimus cream 1% has anti-inflammatory effects secondary to blockage of activated T-cell cytokine production. Tacrolimus ointment (0.03% or 0.1%) suppresses humoral and cell-mediated immune responses.
- Oral prednisone, intramuscular triamcinolone, psoralen, ultraviolet A light therapy, and Goeckerman regimen are generally reserved for severe cases.
- Cyclosporine, azathioprine, and methotrexate are sometimes tried for recalcitrant disease in adults by physicians who specialize in severe inflammatory skin conditions.
- The monoclonal antibody dupilumab has been shown to be effective in children and adults with moderate to severe atopic dermatitis. It can be used with or without topical steroids and is injected subcutaneously. Cost is a limiting factor.

TABLE 3 Relative Potencies of Topical Corticosteroids (from Most Potent to Weakest)

Class	Drug	Dosage Form(s)	Strength (%)
I. Very high potency			
	Augmented betamethasone dipropionate	Ointment	0.05
	Clobetasol propionate	Cream, ointment, foam	0.05
	Diflorasone diacetate	Ointment	0.05
	Halobetasol propionate	Cream, ointment	0.05
II. High potency			
	Amcinonide	Cream, lotion, ointment	0.1
	Augmented betamethasone dipropionate	Cream	0.05
	Betamethasone dipropionate	Cream, ointment, foam, solution	0.05
	Desoximetasone	Cream, ointment	0.25
	Desoximetasone	Gel	0.05
	Diflorasone diacetate	Cream	0.05
	Fluocinonide	Cream, ointment, gel, solution	0.05
	Halcinonide	Cream, ointment	0.1
	Mometasone furoate	Ointment	0.1
	Triamcinolone acetonide	Cream, ointment	0.5
III-IV. Medium potency			
	Betamethasone valerate	Cream, ointment, lotion, foam	0.1
	Clocortolone pivalate	Cream	0.1
	Desoximetasone	Cream	0.05
	Fluocinolone acetonide	Cream, ointment	0.025
	Flurandrenolide	Cream, ointment	0.05
	Fluticasone propionate	Cream	0.05
	Fluticasone propionate	Ointment	0.005
	Mometasone furoate	Cream	0.1
	Triamcinolone acetonide	Cream, ointment	0.1
V. Lower-medium potency			
	Hydrocortisone butyrate	Cream, ointment, solution	0.1
	Hydrocortisone probutate	Cream	0.1
	Hydrocortisone valerate	Cream, ointment	0.2
	Prednicarbate	Cream	0.1
VI. Low potency			
	Alclometasone dipropionate	Cream, ointment	0.05
	Desonide	Cream, gel, foam, ointment	0.05
	Fluocinolone acetonide	Cream, solution, oil	0.01
VII. Lowest potency			
	Dexamethasone	Cream	0.1
	Hydrocortisone	Cream, ointment, lotion, solution	0.25, 0.5, 1
	Hydrocortisone acetate	Cream, ointment	0.5-1

From Paller AS, Mancini AJ: *Hurwitz clinical pediatric dermatology, a textbook of skin disorders of childhood and adolescence*, ed 5, 2016, Elsevier.

TABLE 4 Management of Mild, Moderate, and Severe Forms of Atopic Dermatitis

Mild	Moderate	Severe
Bathing and barrier repair* Avoidance of irritant and allergic triggers Intermittent, short-term use of class VI or VII topical steroids ± topical calcineurin inhibitors Treatment of superinfection	Bathing and barrier repair* Avoidance of irritant and allergic triggers Intermittent, short-term use of class III-V topical steroids ± topical calcineurin inhibitors Treatment of superinfection Oral antihistamines	Bathing and barrier repair* Avoidance of irritant and allergic triggers Class II topical steroids for flares; class III-V topical steroids ± tacrolimus ointment for maintenance Treatment of superinfection Oral antihistamines Systemic antiinflammatory agents, ultraviolet light therapy

*Barrier repair may be accomplished by application of effective emollients or from barrier-repair agents.
From Paller AS, Mancini AJ: *Hurwitz clinical pediatric dermatology, a textbook of skin disorders of childhood and adolescence*, ed 5, 2016, Elsevier.

- Antistaphylococcal antibiotics are effective in treating secondary skin infections.
- Table 4 summarizes the management of atopic dermatitis.

DISPOSITION

- Resolution occurs in approximately 70% of patients by adulthood.
- Most patients have a course characterized by remissions and intermittent flares.

SUGGESTED READINGS

Available at ExpertConsult.com

RELATED CONTENT

Dermatitis (Patient Information)
Eczema (Patient Information)

AUTHORS: **Sonia A. Havele, MD,** and **Anna-Marie Tierney, MD**

Atrial Fibrillation (ALG) (PTG)

DEFINITION

Atrial fibrillation (AF) is a supraventricular tachyarrhythmia characterized by disorganized and rapid atrial activation and uncoordinated atrial contraction. AF occurs when structural and/or electrophysiologic abnormalities alter atrial tissue to promote abnormal impulse formation and/or propagation. The ventricular rate is dependent on the conduction properties of the atrioventricular (AV) node, which can be influenced by vagal/sympathetic tone, medications, or disease of the AV node.

Multiple classification schemes have been used in the past to characterize AF. The current classification scheme (divided into three major types) used by the American College of Cardiology (ACC)/American Heart Association (AHA) guideline committee is as follows:

- Paroxysmal AF: More than one episode of AF that terminate spontaneously or with intervention within 7 days
- Persistent AF: Episodes of AF that last longer than 7 days
  1. Early-persistent AF: AF that has been continuous for longer than 7 days but fewer than 3 mo
  2. Long-standing persistent AF: AF that has persisted for longer than 1 yr, either because cardioversion has failed or because cardioversion has not been attempted
- Permanent AF: When patient and physician decide to stop pursuing restoring sinus rhythm
- In addition to the previous AF categories, which are mainly defined by episode timing and termination, the ACC/AHA/European Society of Cardiology (ESC) guidelines describe additional AF categories in terms of other characteristics of the patient:
  1. Lone atrial fibrillation (LAF): Generally refers to AF in younger patients without clinical or echocardiographic evidence of cardiopulmonary disease, diabetes, or hypertension
  2. Nonvalvular AF: Atrial fibrillation in the absence of moderate-to-severe mitral stenosis or in the presence of a mechanical heart valve
  3. Secondary AF: Occurs in the setting of a primary condition that may be the cause of the AF, such as acute myocardial infarction, cardiac surgery, pericarditis, myocarditis, hyperthyroidism, pulmonary embolism, pneumonia, or other acute disease. It is considered separately because AF is less likely to recur once the precipitating condition has resolved
  4. Silent AF: Asymptomatic AF diagnosed by an ECG or rhythm strip

SYNONYMS

AF
Paroxysmal atrial fibrillation (PAF)
AFib

ICD-10CM CODES

I48.0	Paroxysmal atrial fibrillation
I48.1	Persistent atrial fibrillation
I48.2	Chronic atrial fibrillation
I48.91	Unspecified atrial fibrillation

EPIDEMIOLOGY & DEMOGRAPHICS

- The prevalence of AF increases with age, from 2% in adults <65 yr to 9% of those >65 yr.
- AF affects over 3 million people in the United States. AF is uncommon in infants and children and, when present, almost always occurs in association with structural heart disease.
- The incidence of AF is significantly higher in men than in women in all age groups (1.1% versus 0.8%). AF appears to be more common in whites than in blacks, who may have lower awareness of the disease.
- Stroke due to thromboembolism is the most common and dreaded complication of AF. The rate of ischemic stroke in patients with nonrheumatic AF averages 5% a yr, which is somewhere between 2 and 7× the rate of stroke in patients without AF. The risk of stroke is not due solely to AF; changes in the endothelium and elevated markers of inflammation that may contribute to thrombosis are found in patients with AF, regardless of their rhythm at the time. The attributable risk of stroke from AF is estimated to be 1.5% for those aged 50 to 59 yr, and it approaches 36% for those aged 80 to 89 yr.
- Table 1 summarizes the thromboembolic risk score.

PHYSICAL FINDINGS & CLINICAL PRESENTATION

Clinical presentation is variable:

- Palpitations, dizziness, or light-headedness
- Fatigue, weakness, or impaired exercise tolerance
- Angina
- Dyspnea
- Some patients are asymptomatic
- Cardiac auscultation revealing irregularly irregular rhythm
- Thromboembolic phenomenon such as stroke

TABLE 1 Thromboembolic Risk Score

CHA_2DS_2-VASc Risk Factors	Score
Congestive heart failure	1
Hypertension	1
Age ≥75	2
Diabetes	1
Previous stroke, TIA, or thromboembolism	2
Vascular disease	1
Age 65-75	1
Female	1

European Society of Cardiology (ESC), American Heart Association (AHA), and American College of Cardiology (ACC) Guidelines recommend to use CHA2DS2-VASc Score to assess the risk of stroke in patients with atrial fibrillation. ESC Guidelines recommend patients with risk factor(s) ≥1 to receive effective stroke prevention therapy. Antithrombotic therapy is not recommended in patients with AF (irrespective of gender) who are aged <65 and with lone AF as they have very low absolute event rates. AHA/ACC Guidelines recommend oral anticoagulation for patients with CHA2DS2-VASc ≥2; for patients with nonvalvular AF and a CHA_2DS_2-VASc score of 1, no antithrombotic therapy or treatment with an oral anticoagulant or aspirin may be considered.

CHA2DS2-VASc, Congestive heart failure, hypertension, age, diabetes, stroke/TIA, and vascular disease; *TIA,* transient ischemic attack.

From Ronco C et al: *Critical care nephrology,* ed 3, Philadelphia, 2019, Elsevier.

ETIOLOGY

- The most frequent change in AF is the loss of atrial muscle mass and atrial fibrosis
- Fibrillation is presumed to be caused by multiple wandering wavelets, usually originating from the pulmonary veins. Both reentrant and focal mechanisms have been proposed. See Fig. 1 for mechanisms of atrial fibrillation. Fig. 2 illustrates an approach to selecting drug therapy for ventricular rate control
- Vascular causes: Hypertensive heart disease
- Valvular heart disease
- Pulmonary causes: Pulmonary embolism, chronic obstructive pulmonary disease, obstructive sleep apnea, carbon monoxide poisoning
- Structural cardiac disease: Hypertrophic cardiomyopathy, congestive heart failure, coronary artery disease, myocardial infarction, congenital heart disease (especially those that lead to atrial enlargement such as atrial septal defect)
- Pericarditis and myocarditis
- Arrhythmias: Atrial tachycardias and atrial flutters have been associated with atrial fibrillation, as has Wolff-Parkinson-White syndrome
- Endocrine: Thyrotoxicosis, hyperthyroidism or subclinical hyperthyroidism, pheochromocytoma, obesity
- Surgery: Both cardiac and noncardiac
- Electrolytes: Hypokalemia, hypomagnesemia
- Systemic stress: Fever, anemia, hypoxia, sepsis, infections (e.g., pneumonia)
- Medications/toxins: Digitalis, adenosine, theophylline, amphetamines, cocaine, antihistamines, alcohol abuse and/or withdrawal, caffeine, steroidal antiinflammatory drugs (SAIDs), nonsteroidal antiinflammatory drugs (NSAIDs)
- Frequency of vigorous exercise is associated with an increased risk of developing AF in young men and joggers
- Porphyrias have been associated with autonomic dysfunction and increased risk of AF
- Patients with metabolic syndrome, excessive vitamin D intake, or excessive niacin intake have a higher risk of AF

Dx DIAGNOSIS

DIFFERENTIAL DIAGNOSIS

- Multifocal atrial tachycardia
- Atrial flutter
- Frequent atrial premature beats
- Atrial tachycardia
- AV nodal reentry tachycardia (AVNRT)
- Wolff-Parkinson-White syndrome

WORKUP

The evaluation of atrial fibrillation involves diagnosis, determination of the etiology, and

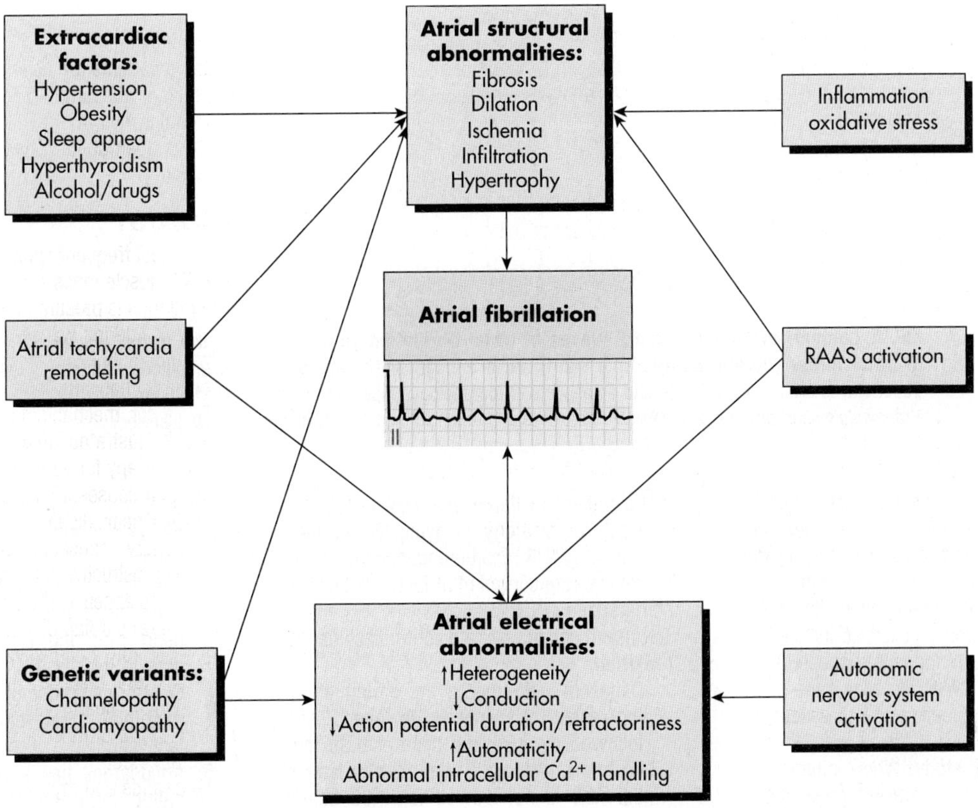

FIG. 1 Mechanisms of atrial fibrillation. *Ca^{2+},* Ionized calcium; *RAAS,* renin-angiotensin-aldosterone system. (From Parrillo JE, Dellinger RP: *Critical care medicine, principles of diagnosis and management in the adult,* ed 5, Philadelphia, 2019, Elsevier.)

classification of the arrhythmia. A minimal evaluation includes a history and physical examination, ECG, transthoracic echocardiogram, and case-specific laboratory work to rule out secondary AF.

LABORATORY TESTS

- Thyroid-stimulating hormone, free T_4
- Serum electrolytes
- Toxicity screen
- CBC count (looking for anemia, infection)
- Renal and hepatic function tests
- D-dimer/CT scan of chest pulmonary embolism protocol (if the patient has risk factors to merit a pulmonary embolism workup)

IMAGING STUDIES

- ECG (Fig. E3)
- Absence of P waves
- Fibrillatory or F waves at the isoelectric baseline with varying amplitude, morphology, and intervals (Fig. 4)
- Irregular ventricular rate
- Echocardiography to rule out structural heart disease (evaluate ventricular size, thickness, and function, atrial size, pericardial disease, and valve function)
- Chest radiography (if pulmonary disease or congestive heart failure [CHF] is suspected)
- Transesophageal echocardiography (TEE): Helpful to evaluate for left atrial thrombus (particularly in the left atrium appendage) to guide cardioversion or ablation (if thrombus is seen, cardioversion should be delayed)

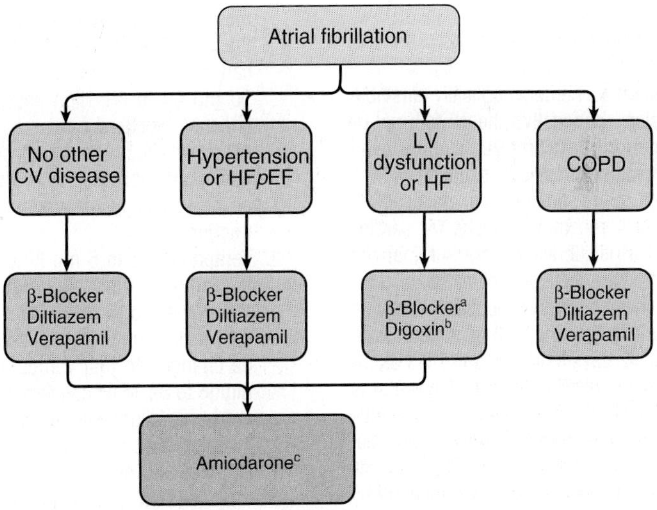

FIG. 2 Approach to selecting drug therapy for ventricular rate control. Drugs are listed alphabetically.
[A]β-Blockers should be instituted after stabilization of patients with decompensated heart failure (HF). The choice of β-blocker (e.g., cardioselective) depends on the patient's clinical condition.
[B]Digoxin is not usually first-line therapy. It may be combined with a β-blocker and/or a nondihydropyridine calcium channel blocker when ventricular rate control is insufficient and may be useful in patients with heart failure.
[C]In part because of concern over its side effect profile, use of amiodarone for chronic control of ventricular rate should be reserved for patients who do not respond to or are intolerant of β-blockers or nondihydropyridine calcium antagonists.
COPD, Chronic obstructive pulmonary disease; *CV,* cardiovascular; *HF,* heart failure; *HFpEF,* heart failure with preserved ejection fraction; *LV,* left ventricular. (From Parrillo JE, Dellinger RP: *Critical care medicine, principles of diagnosis and management in the adult,* ed 5, Philadelphia, 2019, Elsevier.)

- CT and MRI: In patients with a positive D-dimer result, chest CT angiogram may be necessary to rule out pulmonary embolus. 3D imaging technologies (CT scan or MRI) are often helpful to evaluate atrial anatomy if AF ablation is planned

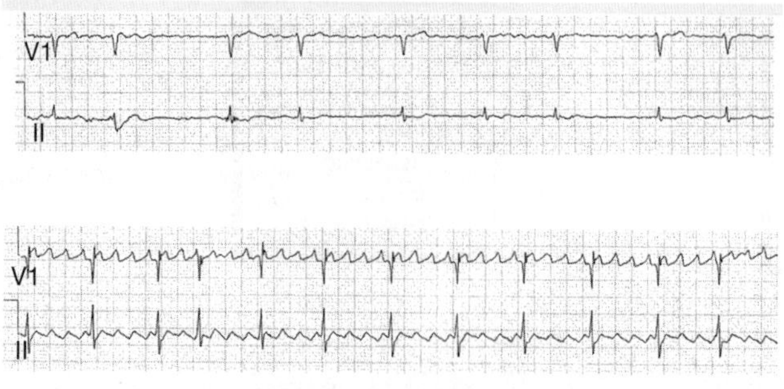

FIG. 4 Comparison between the F waves of atrial fibrillation *(top panel)* and the flutter waves of atrial flutter *(bottom panel)*. Note that F waves are variable in rate, shape, and amplitude, whereas flutter waves are constant in rate and all aspects of morphology. Shown are leads V1 and II. (From Zipes DP: *Braunwald's heart disease, a textbook of cardiovascular medicine,* ed 11, Philadelphia, 2019, Elsevier.)

- 6-minute walk test or exercise test: 6-minute walk or exercise testing can help assess the adequacy of rate control. Exercise testing can also exclude ischemia prior to treatment of patients with class Ic antiarrhythmic drugs and can be used to reproduce exercise-induced AF
- Sleep study (if sleep apnea is suspected)
- Holter monitor or event recorder if the diagnosis of AF is in question and to assess AF burden
- Electrophysiologic study: When initiation of AF is secondary to a supraventricular tachycardia, such as AVNRT or Wolff-Parkinson-White syndrome

Rx TREATMENT

ACUTE GENERAL Rx

New-onset AF:

- If the patient is hemodynamically unstable (hypotension, congestive heart failure, or angina), perform synchronized cardioversion after immediate conscious sedation with a rapid short-acting sedative (e.g., midazolam). The ACC/AHA recommendations for cardioversion of atrial fibrillation are summarized in Table 2. The likelihood of cardioversion-related clinical thromboembolism is low in patients with AF lasting <48 hr. Patients with AF lasting >2 days have a 5% to 7% risk for clinical thromboembolism if cardioversion is not preceded by several weeks of anticoagulation therapy. However, if transesophageal echocardiography reveals no atrial thrombus, cardioversion may be performed safely after therapeutic anticoagulation has been achieved. Alternatively, patients can be safely anticoagulated for approximately 1 mo and then undergo cardioversion without transesophageal echocardiogram. Anticoagulant therapy should be continued for at least 1 mo after cardioversion to minimize the incidence of adverse thromboembolic events. It can be stopped after 1 mo as long as AF has not recurred if the patient is deemed low risk of stroke using the congestive heart failure, hypertension, age, diabetes, stroke/TIA, and vascular disease (CHA2DS2-VASc) scoring system (Table 1).
- If the patient is hemodynamically stable, a rate-control strategy is typically pursued initially. ACC/AHA recommendations for pharmacologic rate control of atrial fibrillation are summarized in Table 3.
- Treatment options for rate control include the following:
  1. Diltiazem 0.25 mg/kg (maximum of 25 mg) given intravenously (IV) over 2 min followed by a second dose of 0.35 mg/kg (maximum of 25 mg) 15 min later if the rate is not slowed to <100 beats/min. May then follow with IV infusion 10 mg/hr (range, 5 to 15 mg/hr) to achieve a resting heart rate of <100 beats/min. Onset of action after IV administration is usually within 3 min, with peak effect most often occurring within 10 min. After the ventricular rate is slowed, the patient can be changed to oral diltiazem 60 to 90 mg q4 to 6h. High doses of calcium channel blockers can exacerbate heart failure and thus should be used with caution in patients presenting with symptoms of heart failure or depressed ejection fraction.
  2. Verapamil 2.5 to 5 mg IV initially, then 5 to 10 mg IV 10 min later if the rate is still not slowed to <100 beats/min. After the ventricular rate is slowed, the patient can be changed to oral verapamil 80 to 120 mg q6 to 8h. Main concern is hypotension and heart failure with this medication, and it should not be used in patients with CHF.
  3. Esmolol and metoprolol are beta-blockers available in IV preparations that can be used. High doses of beta-blockers can have negative inotropic effects in heart failure and should be used with caution.
  4. Digoxin is not a potent AV nodal blocking agent and has a potential for toxicity and therefore cannot be relied on for acute control of the ventricular response, but it may be used in conjunction with beta-blockers and calcium channel blockers. It may be a useful adjunct to a beta-blocker in the hypotensive or heart failure patient, which is not infrequent. When used, give 0.5 mg IV loading dose (slow) and then 0.25 mg IV 6 hr later. A third dose may be needed after 6 to 8 hr; the daily dose varies from 0.125 to 0.25 mg (decrease dosage in patients with renal insufficiency and elderly patients) depending on the heart rate and signs or symptoms of digoxin toxicity. Toxicity is manifested by GI and visual complaints, atrial tachyarrhythmias, heart block, and ventricular tachycardia.
  5. Amiodarone has a class IIa recommendation from the ACC/AHA/ESC for use as a rate-controlling agent for patients who are intolerant of or unresponsive to other agents, such as patients with heart failure who may otherwise not tolerate diltiazem or metoprolol. Caution should be exercised in those who are not receiving anticoagulation because amiodarone can promote cardioversion, thereby posing a thromboembolic risk.
- AV nodal blocking agents, particularly calcium channel blockers and digoxin, should be avoided in patients with Wolff-Parkinson-White syndrome and AF because, by blocking the AV node, AF impulses may be transmitted exclusively down the accessory pathway, which can result in ventricular fibrillation. If this happens, the patient will require immediate defibrillation. Procainamide, flecainide, or amiodarone can be used instead if Wolff-Parkinson-White syndrome is suspected.
- In the acute setting, pharmacologic cardioversion (e.g., ibutilide, dofetilide) is less commonly used than electrical cardioversion. A major disadvantage with pharmacologic cardioversion is the risk of development of ventricular tachycardia and other serious arrhythmias, especially due to acute prolongation of the QT interval.
- ACC/AHA recommendations for maintenance of sinus rhythm in patients with atrial fibrillation are summarized in Table 4.

CHRONIC THERAPY

- Avoidance of alcohol in patients with suspected excessive alcohol use.
- Treatment of underlying source or cause, if any found.

TABLE 2 ACC/AHA Recommendations for Cardioversion of Atrial Fibrillation

Class	Indication	Level of Evidence
Pharmacologic Cardioversion		
Class I (indicated)	Administration of flecainide, dofetilide, propafenone, or ibutilide is recommended for pharmacologic cardioversion of AF.	A
Class IIa (reasonable)	Administration of amiodarone is a reasonable option for pharmacologic cardioversion of AF.	A
	A single oral bolus dose of propafenone or flecainide ("pill-in-the-pocket") can be administered to terminate persistent AF outside the hospital once treatment has proved safe in the hospital for selected patients without sinus or AV node dysfunction, bundle branch block, QT interval prolongation, the Brugada syndrome, or structural heart disease. Before antiarrhythmic medication is initiated, a beta-blocker or nondihydropyridine calcium channel antagonist should be given to prevent rapid AV conduction in the event atrial flutter occurs.	C
	Administration of amiodarone can be beneficial on an outpatient basis in patients with paroxysmal or persistent AF when rapid restoration of sinus rhythm is not deemed necessary.	C
Class IIb (may be considered)	Administration of quinidine or procainamide might be considered for pharmacologic cardioversion of AF, but the usefulness of these agents is not well established.	C
Class III (not indicated)	Digoxin and sotalol may be harmful when used for pharmacologic cardioversion of AF and are not recommended.	A
	Quinidine, procainamide, disopyramide, and dofetilide should not be started out of the hospital for conversion of AF to sinus rhythm.	B
Direct-Current Cardioversion		
Class I (indicated)	When a rapid ventricular response does not respond promptly to pharmacologic measures for patients with AF with ongoing myocardial ischemia, symptomatic hypotension, angina, or heart failure, immediate R wave–synchronized direct-current cardioversion is recommended.	C
	Immediate direct-current cardioversion is recommended for patients with AF involving preexcitation when very rapid tachycardia or hemodynamic instability occurs.	B
	Cardioversion is recommended in patients without hemodynamic instability when symptoms of AF are unacceptable to the patient. In case of early relapse of AF after cardioversion, repeated direct-current cardioversion attempts may be made after administration of antiarrhythmic medication.	C
Class IIa (reasonable)	Direct-current cardioversion can be useful to restore sinus rhythm as part of a long-term management strategy for patients with AF.	B
	The patient's preference is a reasonable consideration in the selection of infrequently repeated cardioversions for the management of symptomatic or recurrent AF.	C
Class III (not indicated)	Frequent repetition of direct-current cardioversion is not recommended for patients who have relatively short periods of sinus rhythm between relapses of AF after multiple cardioversion procedures despite prophylactic antiarrhythmic drug therapy.	C
	Electrical cardioversion is contraindicated in patients with digitalis toxicity or hypokalemia.	C
Pharmacologic Enhancement of Direct-Current Cardioversion		
Class IIa (reasonable)	Pretreatment with amiodarone, flecainide, ibutilide, propafenone, or sotalol can be useful to enhance the success of direct-current cardioversion and to prevent recurrent AF.	B
	In patients who relapse to AF after successful cardioversion, it can be useful to repeat the procedure after prophylactic administration of antiarrhythmic medication.	C
Class IIb (may be considered)	For patients with persistent AF, administration of beta-blockers, disopyramide, diltiazem, dofetilide, procainamide, or verapamil may be considered, although the efficacy of these agents to enhance the success of direct-current cardioversion or to prevent early recurrence of AF is uncertain.	C
	Out-of-hospital initiation of antiarrhythmic medications may be considered in patients without heart disease to enhance the success of cardioversion of AF.	C
	Out-of-hospital administration of antiarrhythmic medications may be considered to enhance the success of cardioversion of AF in patients with certain forms of heart disease once the safety of the drug has been verified for the patient.	C
Prevention of Thromboembolism in Patients with Atrial Fibrillation Undergoing Cardioversion		
Class I (indicated)	For patients with AF of 48-hr duration or longer, or when the duration of AF is unknown, anticoagulation (INR 2.0-3.0) is recommended for at least 3 wk before and 4 wk after cardioversion, regardless of the method (electrical or pharmacologic) used to restore sinus rhythm.	B
	For patients with AF of more than 48-hr duration requiring immediate cardioversion because of hemodynamic instability, heparin should be administered concurrently (unless contraindicated) by an initial intravenous bolus injection, followed by a continuous infusion in a dose adjusted to prolong the activated partial thromboplastin time to 1.5-2× the reference control value. Thereafter, oral anticoagulation (INR, 2.0-3.0) should be provided for at least 4 wk, as for patients undergoing elective cardioversion. Limited data support subcutaneous administration of low-molecular-weight heparin in this indication.	C
	For patients with AF of less than 48-hr duration associated with hemodynamic instability (angina pectoris, myocardial infarction, shock, or pulmonary edema), cardioversion should be performed immediately, without delay, for prior initiation of anticoagulation.	C

TABLE 2 ACC/AHA Recommendations for Cardioversion of Atrial Fibrillation—cont'd

Class	Indication	Level of Evidence
Class IIa (reasonable)	During the 48 hr after onset of AF, the need for anticoagulation before and after cardioversion may be based on the patient's risk of thromboembolism.	C
	As an alternative to anticoagulation before cardioversion of AF, it is reasonable to perform transesophageal echocardiography in search of thrombus in the left atrium or left atrial appendage.	B
	a. For patients with no identifiable thrombus, cardioversion is reasonable immediately after anticoagulation with unfractionated heparin (e.g., initiated by intravenous bolus injection and an infusion continued at a dose adjusted to prolong the activated partial thromboplastin time to 1.5-2× the control value until oral anticoagulation has been established with an oral vitamin K antagonist [e.g., warfarin] as evidenced by an INR ≥2.0).	B
	Thereafter, continuation of oral anticoagulation (INR, 2.0-3.0) is reasonable for a total anticoagulation period of at least 4 wk, as for patients undergoing elective cardioversion.	B
	Limited data are available to support the subcutaneous administration of a low-molecular-weight heparin in this indication.	C
	b. For patients in whom thrombus is identified by transesophageal echocardiography, oral anticoagulation (INR, 2.0-3.0) is reasonable for at least 3 wk before and 4 wk after restoration of sinus rhythm, and a longer period of anticoagulation may be appropriate even after apparently successful cardioversion because the risk of thromboembolism often remains elevated in such cases.	C
	For patients with atrial flutter undergoing cardioversion, anticoagulation can be beneficial according to the recommendations as for patients with AF.	C

ACC, American College of Cardiology; *AF,* atrial fibrillation; *AHA,* American Heart Association; *AV,* atrioventricular; *INR,* international normalized ratio.
From Zipes DP: *Braunwald's heart disease, a textbook of cardiovascular medicine,* ed 11, Philadelphia, 2019, Elsevier.

TABLE 3 ACC/AHA Recommendations for Pharmacologic Rate Control of Atrial Fibrillation

Class	Indication	Level of Evidence
Class I (indicated)	Measurement of the heart rate at rest and control of the rate with pharmacologic agents (either a beta-blocker or nondihydropyridine calcium channel antagonist, in most cases) are recommended for patients with persistent or permanent AF.	B
	In the absence of preexcitation, intravenous administration of beta-blockers (esmolol, metoprolol, or propranolol) or nondihydropyridine calcium channel antagonists (verapamil, diltiazem) is recommended to slow the ventricular response to AF in the acute setting, exercising caution in patients with hypotension or heart failure.	B
	Intravenous administration of digoxin or amiodarone is recommended to control heart rate in patients with AF and heart failure who do not have an accessory pathway.	B
	In patients who experience symptoms related to AF during activity, the adequacy of heart rate control should be assessed during exercise, adjusting pharmacologic treatment as necessary to keep the rate in the physiologic range.	C
	Digoxin is effective after oral administration to control the heart rate at rest in patients with AF and is indicated for patients with heart failure or left ventricular dysfunction and for sedentary individuals.	C
Class IIa (reasonable)	A combination of digoxin and either a beta-blocker or nondihydropyridine calcium channel antagonist is reasonable to control the heart rate both at rest and during exercise in patients with AF. The choice of medication should be individualized and the dose modulated to avoid bradycardia.	B
	It is reasonable to use ablation of the AV node or accessory pathway to control heart rate when pharmacologic therapy is insufficient or associated with side effects.	B
	Intravenous amiodarone can be useful to control heart rate in patients with AF when other measures are unsuccessful or contraindicated.	C
	When electrical cardioversion is not necessary in patients with AF and an accessory pathway, intravenous procainamide or ibutilide is a reasonable alternative.	C
Class IIb (may be considered)	When the ventricular rate cannot be adequately controlled both at rest and during exercise in patients with AF by a beta-blocker, nondihydropyridine calcium channel antagonist, or digoxin, alone or in combination, oral amiodarone may be administered to control the heart rate.	C
	Intravenous procainamide, disopyramide, ibutilide, or amiodarone may be considered for hemodynamically stable patients with AF involving conduction over an accessory pathway	B
	When the rate cannot be controlled with pharmacologic agents or tachycardia-mediated cardiomyopathy is suspected, catheter-directed ablation of the AV node may be considered in patients with AF to control the heart rate.	C
Class III (not indicated)	Strict rate control (<80 beats/min at rest or <110 beats/min during 6-minute walk) is not beneficial compared to a resting rate <110 beats/min in asymptomatic patients with persistent AF and an ejection fraction >40%, although uncontrolled tachycardia can lead to reversible left ventricular dysfunction over time.	B
	Digitalis should not be used as the sole agent to control the rate of ventricular response in patients with paroxysmal AF.	B
	Catheter ablation of the AV node should not be attempted without a prior trial of medication to control the ventricular rate in patients with AF.	C
	In patients with decompensated heart failure and AF, intravenous administration of a nondihydropyridine calcium channel antagonist may exacerbate hemodynamic compromise and is not recommended.	C
	Intravenous administration of digitalis glycosides or nondihydropyridine calcium channel antagonists to patients with AF and a preexcitation syndrome may paradoxically accelerate the ventricular response and is not recommended.	C

ACC, American College of Cardiology; *AF,* atrial fibrillation; *AHA,* American Heart Association; *AV,* atrioventricular.
From Zipes DP: *Braunwald's heart disease, a textbook of cardiovascular medicine,* ed 11, Philadelphia, 2019, Elsevier.

TABLE 4 ACC/AHA Recommendations for Maintenance of Sinus Rhythm in Patients with Atrial Fibrillation

Class	Indication	Level of Evidence
Class I (indicated)	Before initiation of antiarrhythmic drug therapy, treatment of precipitating or reversible causes of AF is recommended.	C
	Catheter ablation by an experienced operator is useful in selected patients with symptomatic paroxysmal AF who have failed treatment with an antiarrhythmic drug and have a normal or mildly dilated left atrium and normal or mildly reduced left ventricular function.	A
Class IIa (reasonable)	Pharmacologic therapy can be useful in patients with AF to maintain sinus rhythm and to prevent tachycardia-induced cardiomyopathy.	C
	Infrequent, well-tolerated recurrence of AF is reasonable as a successful outcome of antiarrhythmic drug therapy.	C
	Outpatient initiation of antiarrhythmic drug therapy is reasonable in patients with AF who have no associated heart disease when the agent is well tolerated.	C
	In patients with lone AF without structural heart disease, initiation of propafenone or flecainide can be beneficial on an outpatient basis in patients with paroxysmal AF who are in sinus rhythm at the time of drug initiation.	B
	Sotalol can be beneficial in outpatients in sinus rhythm with little or no heart disease, prone to paroxysmal AF, if the baseline uncorrected QT interval is shorter than 460 milliseconds, serum electrolyte values are normal, and risk factors associated with class III drug–related proarrhythmia are not present.	C
	Catheter ablation is a reasonable for treatment of symptomatic persistent AF.	A
Class IIb (may be considered)	Catheter ablation may be reasonable for patients with symptomatic paroxysmal AF and significant left atrial dilation or significant left ventricular dysfunction.	A
Class III (not indicated)	Antiarrhythmic therapy with a particular drug is not recommended for maintenance of sinus rhythm in patients with AF who have well-defined risk factors for proarrhythmia with that agent.	A
	Pharmacologic therapy is not recommended for maintenance of sinus rhythm in patients with advanced sinus node disease or AV node dysfunction unless they have a functioning electronic cardiac pacemaker.	C

ACC, American College of Cardiology; *AF,* atrial fibrillation; *AHA,* American Heart Association.
From Zipes DP: *Braunwald's heart disease, a textbook of cardiovascular medicine,* ed 11, Philadelphia, 2019, Elsevier.

- Treatment of modifiable risk factors such as obstructive sleep apnea, hypertension, and obesity have been shown to decrease AF burden in patients.
- Per the Atrial Fibrillation Follow-up Investigation of Rhythm Management (AFFIRM) and Rate Control versus Electrical Cardioversion (RACE) trials, either rate control or rhythm control strategies show no difference in composite cardiovascular end points of death, CHF, bleeding, drug side effects, or thromboembolism. However, the more recent EAST-AFNET 4 trial suggested that an initial rhythm control strategy may result in lower risk of the combined cardiovascular endpoint of death, stroke, or hospitalization. Both approaches require appropriate anticoagulation to reduce stroke risk.
- For patients without symptomatic AF, a rate-control strategy with calcium channel blockers, beta-blockers, or digoxin may be a reasonable option. The RACE 2 trial indicates that a lenient rate control strategy, with a target resting heart rate of <110 beats/min, is noninferior to a strict control strategy, with a target resting heart rate of <80 beats/min and an exercise heart rate of <110 beats/min. Most recent ACC/AHA guidelines, however, recommend targeting a heart rate <80 beats/min over a target of <110 beats/min.
- In patients with symptomatic AF, younger patients, or those with difficult to control heart rate, an attempt should be made to maintain sinus rhythm with antiarrhythmic agents. Options of antiarrhythmic agents include amiodarone, dronedarone, (paroxysmal atrial fibrillation only without heart failure), dofetilide, flecainide, propafenone (contraindicated with structural heart disease), or sotalol. The decision of which strategy to follow should be best made in consultation with a cardiologist. Use of dronedarone should be avoided in patients with persistent or permanent atrial fibrillation because of worsened cardiovascular outcomes, especially in those with concomitant symptomatic heart failure (see Fig. 5 for a proposed algorithm to guide maintenance of sinus rhythm).

NONPHARMACOLOGIC THERAPY

- Catheter ablation of AF has become a common procedure for symptomatic drug-refractory or drug-intolerant patients. Sinus rhythm can be maintained long term in the majority of patients with paroxysmal atrial fibrillation (PAF) by circumferential pulmonary vein ablation performed in experienced centers. Established centers have reported success rates of 70% to 85% in patients with paroxysmal AF, but up to 50% of patients may require more than one ablation to achieve success. Complication rates are 4.5% in the largest international survey of hospitals performing this procedure. Success with persistent AF is much lower, with long-term success rates of 40% to 50% in many studies, and such patients often require more than one procedure. The most common techniques used to isolate the pulmonary veins are radiofrequency ablation and cryoballoon ablation, which have shown similar results for patients with PAF.
- Pulmonary vein isolation is being increasingly used to treat AF in patients with heart failure. Trials have shown that pulmonary vein isolation is superior to AV node ablation with biventricular pacing in patients with heart failure who have drug-refractory AF.
- AV nodal ablation with permanent pacemaker implantation may become necessary in some patients in whom rate and rhythm are difficult to control despite drugs and cardioversion, although it is generally used as a therapy of last resort.
- The Cox-Maze III surgical procedure, with its modifications creating electrical barriers to the macroreentrant circuits that are believed to underlie AF, is being performed with good results in some medical centers (preservation of sinus rhythm in 70% to 95% of patients without the use of long-term antiarrhythmic medication). Success rates are higher in paroxysmal than in persistent or permanent atrial fibrillation. Surgical ablation is often used for patients undergoing aortic or mitral valve surgery. As a stand-alone procedure, it is a Class IIb recommendation per ACC/AHA Guidelines in 2017. Some centers perform surgical pulmonary vein isolation similar to this procedure using a mini-thoracotomy or video thoracoscopic "Mini-Maze" approach. Another surgical method is a pericardioscopic approach that allows extensive posterior wall ablation and, when combined with catheter ablation in a "hybrid" approach, has shown promising results for patients with persistent AF.
- It is important to understand that ablation therapy will not eliminate the need to take anticoagulant drugs. Even after ablation, patients with AF face increased risk of thromboembolic events and most electrophysiologists suggest lifelong anticoagulation for patients with elevated stroke risk score. Due to the increasing success rate of ablation, catheter-based therapy is considered the first-line treatment for paroxysmal AF patients intolerant or refractory to one

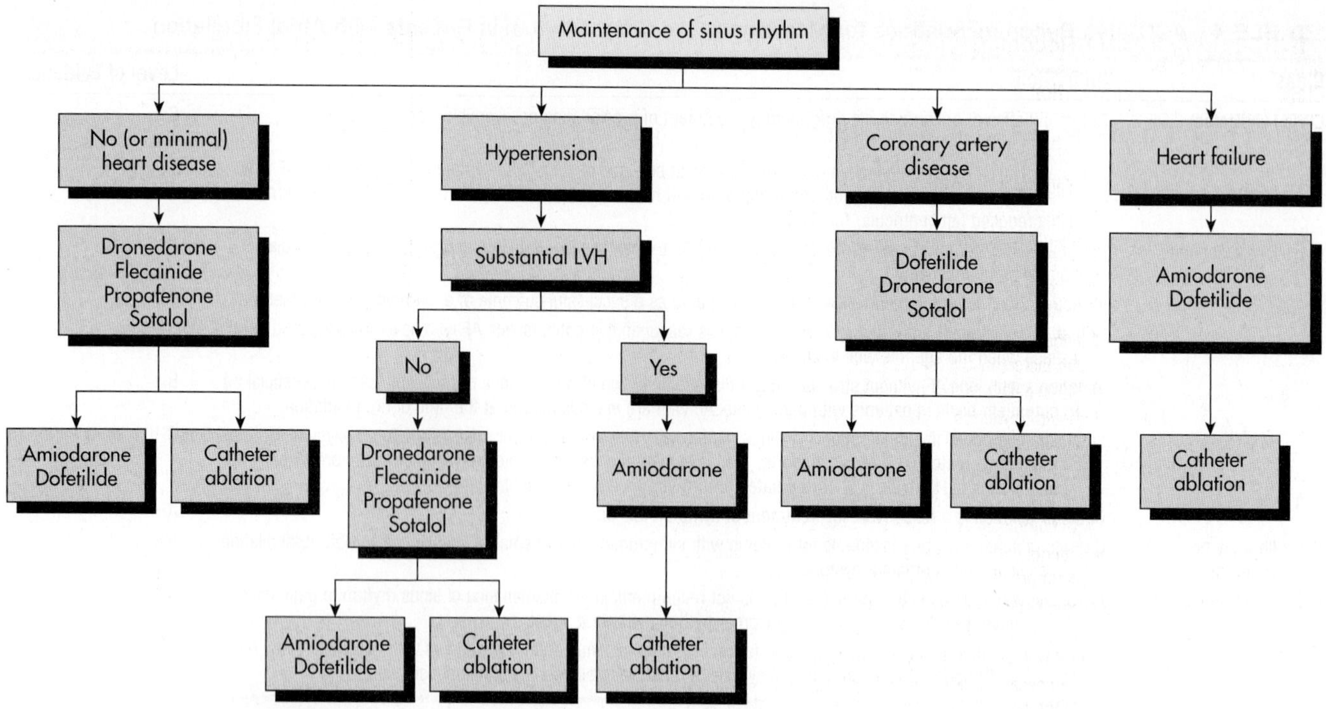

FIG. 5 Therapy to maintain sinus rhythm in patients with recurrent paroxysmal or persistent atrial fibrillation. Drugs are listed alphabetically and not in order of suggested use. The seriousness of heart disease progresses from left to right, and selection of therapy in patients with multiple conditions depends on the most serious condition present. *LVH,* Left ventricular hypertrophy. (From Wann LS et al: 2011 ACCF/AHA/HRS Focused update on the management of patients with atrial fibrillation [updating the 2006 guideline]: a report of the American College of Cardiology Foundation/American Heart Association Task Force on Practice Guidelines, *J Am Coll Cardiol* 57[2]:223-242, 2011.)

medication or IIa for persistent patients in the ACC/AHA AF Ablation Guidelines in 2017. It remains a IIb indication for patients in longstanding persistent atrial fibrillation.

STROKE PREVENTION

- The decision whether to pursue long-term anticoagulation must be made in light of the patient's risk for a cardioembolic event versus risk for a bleeding event. ACC/AHA recommendations for prevention of thromboembolism in atrial fibrillation are summarized in Table 5. In nonvalvular AF, CHA2DS2-VASc has superseded the CHADS2 scoring system (C = congestive heart failure; H = hypertension; A = age [>75 yr is 2 points]; D = diabetes; S = stroke, transient ischemic attack, or thromboembolic disease [2 points]; V = vascular disease, A = age 65 to 74 yr; and Sc = sex category, with females getting 1 extra point). Patients with a CHA2DS2-VASc score of 0 are considered low risk, 1 to 2 are considered moderate risk, and >2 are considered high risk. Per guidelines, patients with a score of 0 do not merit anticoagulation. Patients with a score of 1 can be treated at the discretion of the physician with either aspirin or an oral anticoagulant (warfarin or a novel oral anticoagulant). Anticoagulation with either warfarin or a novel oral anticoagulant is recommended for all men with a CHADS2-VASc score of 2 or above and women with a CHADS2-VASc score of 3 or above. The available direct-acting oral anticoagulants (DOACs) are recommended over warfarin in DOAC-eligible patients with atrial fibrillation in the new 2019 AHA/ACC/Heart Rhythm Society (HRS) Focused Update of the 2014 AHA/ACC/HRS Guidelines.
- Increasing amounts of evidence now show that aspirin likely does not protect a person from stroke in AF and has recently been dropped from most of the ACC/AHA and European Atrial Fibrillation guidelines. Target INR for patients on warfarin with an indication for anticoagulation is 2 to 3 and should be diligently monitored to avoid risk of stroke versus bleeding. Patients with hypertrophic cardiomyopathy or thyrotoxicosis with AF also have a high risk of stroke and should be anticoagulated irrespective of their CHADS2-VASc score.
- The DOACs include several factor Xa inhibitors (Table 6) and a direct thrombin inhibitor.
  1. Dabigatran is a direct thrombin inhibitor indicated to reduce the risk of stroke and systemic embolism in patients with nonvalvular atrial fibrillation. In the RE-LY trial of 18,113 patients with mean CHADS2 score of 2.1, dabigatran 110 mg bid was noninferior to warfarin, and 150 mg bid was superior to warfarin in prevention of thromboembolic events. Bleeding risk was similar to that of warfarin for both doses. Idarucizumab has been approved as a dabigatran reversal agent. Onset is immediate, and it provides full reversal for at least 24 hr in most patients.
  2. Factor Xa inhibitors (apixaban, rivaroxaban, edoxaban) are also effective in reducing stroke and systemic embolism in patients with atrial fibrillation. The Apixaban for Reduction in Stroke and Other Thromboembolic Events in Atrial Fibrillation (ARISTOTLE) trial in patients at high risk for stroke (mean CHADS2 score 2.1) using apixaban, the Rivaroxaban Once Daily Oral Direct Factor Xa Inhibition Compared with Vitamin K Antagonism for Prevention of Stroke and Embolism Trial in Atrial Fibrillation (ROCKET AF) trial using rivaroxaban in patients with CHADS2 score 3.5, and the Effective Anticoagulation with Factor Xa Next Generation in Atrial Fibrillation (ENGAGE-AF) trial using edoxaban in patients with a CHADS2 score of at least 2, showed that these anticoagulants reduce the risk of stroke, systemic embolism, and serious bleeding compared with warfarin. Rivaroxaban showed noninferior efficacy to warfarin in prevention of thromboembolism. Apixaban showed superior stroke reduction, reduced bleeding events, and an overall mortality benefit when compared with warfarin. Edoxaban showed noninferiority to warfarin with respect to stroke and systemic embolism prevention, with lower rates of bleeding and death from cardiovascular causes, but benefit was limited to patients with moderately impaired renal function.

TABLE 5 ACC/AHA Recommendations for Prevention of Thromboembolism in Atrial Fibrillation

Class	Indication	Level of Evidence
Class I (indicated)	Antithrombotic therapy to prevent thromboembolism is recommended for all patients with AF, except those with lone AF or contraindications.	A
	The selection of the antithrombotic agent should be based on the absolute risks of stroke and bleeding and the relative risk and benefit for a given patient.	A
	For patients without mechanical heart valves at high risk of stroke, chronic oral anticoagulant therapy with a vitamin K antagonist is recommended in a dose adjusted to achieve the target intensity international normalized ratio (INR) of 2.0-3.0 unless contraindicated. Factors associated with highest risk for stroke in patients with AF are prior thromboembolism (stroke, transient ischemic attack, or systemic embolism) and rheumatic mitral stenosis.	A
	Anticoagulation with a vitamin K antagonist is recommended for patients with more than one moderate risk factor. Such factors include age ≥75 yr, hypertension, heart failure, impaired left ventricular systolic function (ejection fraction ≤35% or fractional shortening <25%), and diabetes mellitus.	A
	INR should be determined at least weekly during initiation of therapy and monthly when anticoagulation is stable.	A
	Dabigatran is a useful alternative to warfarin in patients with AF and risk factors for stroke who do not have a prosthetic heart valve or significant valve disease, a creatinine clearance <15 ml/min, or advanced liver disease.	B
	Aspirin, 81-325 mg daily, is recommended as an alternative to vitamin K antagonists in low-risk patients or in those with contraindications to oral anticoagulation.	A
	For patients with AF who have mechanical heart valves, the target intensity of anticoagulation should be based on the type of prosthesis, maintaining an INR of at least 2.5.	B
	Antithrombotic therapy is recommended for patients with atrial flutter as for those with AF.	C
Class IIa (reasonable)	For primary prevention of thromboembolism in patients with nonvalvular AF who have just one of the following validated risk factors, antithrombotic therapy with either aspirin or a vitamin K antagonist is reasonable, based on an assessment of the risk of bleeding complications, ability to safely sustain adjusted chronic anticoagulation, and the patient's preferences: Age ≥75 yr (especially in female patients), hypertension, heart failure, impaired left ventricular function, or diabetes mellitus	A
	For patients with nonvalvular AF who have one or more of the following less well-validated risk factors, antithrombotic therapy with either aspirin or a vitamin K antagonist is reasonable for prevention of thromboembolism: Age 65-74 yr, female gender, or coronary artery disease. The choice of agent should be based on the risk of bleeding complications, ability to sustain adjusted chronic anticoagulation, and the patient's preferences.	B
	It is reasonable to select antithrombotic therapy by the same criteria irrespective of the pattern (i.e., paroxysmal, persistent, or permanent) of AF.	B
	In patients with AF who do not have mechanical prosthetic heart valves, it is reasonable to interrupt anticoagulation for up to 1 wk without substituting heparin for surgical or diagnostic procedures that carry a risk of bleeding.	C
	It is reasonable to reevaluate the need for anticoagulation at regular intervals.	C
Class IIb (may be considered)	In patients ≥75 yr at increased risk of bleeding but without frank contraindications to oral anticoagulant therapy, and in other patients with moderate risk factors for thromboembolism who are unable to safely tolerate anticoagulation at the standard intensity of INR 2.0-3.0, a lower INR target of 2.0 (range, 1.6-2.5) may be considered for prevention of ischemic stroke and systemic embolism.	C
	When surgical procedures require interruption of oral anticoagulant therapy for longer than 1 wk in high-risk patients, unfractionated heparin may be administered or low-molecular-weight heparin given by subcutaneous injection, although the efficacy of these alternatives in this situation is uncertain.	C
	After percutaneous coronary intervention or revascularization surgery in patients with AF, low-dose aspirin (<100 mg/day) and/or clopidogrel (75 mg/day) may be given concurrently with anticoagulation to prevent myocardial ischemic events, but these strategies have not been thoroughly evaluated and are associated with an increased risk of bleeding.	C
	In patients undergoing percutaneous coronary intervention, anticoagulation may be interrupted to prevent bleeding at the site of peripheral arterial puncture, but the vitamin K antagonist should be resumed as soon as possible after the procedure and the dose adjusted to achieve an INR in the therapeutic range. Aspirin may be given temporarily during the hiatus, but the maintenance regimen should then consist of the combination of clopidogrel, 75 mg daily, plus warfarin (INR, 2.0-3.0). Clopidogrel should be given for a minimum of 1 mo after implantation of a bare-metal stent, at least 3 mo for a sirolimus-eluting stent, at least 6 mo for a paclitaxel-eluting stent, and 12 mo or longer in selected patients, following which warfarin may be continued as monotherapy in the absence of a subsequent coronary event. When warfarin is given in combination with clopidogrel or low-dose aspirin, the dose intensity must be carefully regulated.	C
	In patients with AF younger than 60 yr without heart disease or risk factors for thromboembolism (lone AF), the risk of thromboembolism is low without treatment, and the effectiveness of aspirin for primary prevention of stroke relative to the risk of bleeding has not been established.	C
	In patients with AF who sustain ischemic stroke or systemic embolism during treatment with low-intensity anticoagulation (INR, 2.0-3.0), rather than add an antiplatelet agent, it may be reasonable to raise the intensity of the anticoagulation to a maximum target INR of 3.0-3.5.	C
	Clopidogrel plus aspirin may be considered in patients who cannot tolerate or who refuse an oral anticoagulant.	B
Class III (not indicated)	Long-term anticoagulation with a vitamin K antagonist is not recommended for primary prevention of stroke in patients younger than 60 yr without heart disease (lone AF) or any risk factors for thromboembolism.	C

ACC, American College of Cardiology; *AF*, atrial fibrillation; *AHA*, American Heart Association.
From Zipes DP: *Braunwald's heart disease, a textbook of cardiovascular medicine*, ed 11, Philadelphia, 2019, Elsevier.

TABLE 6 Comparison of the Features of the Direct Oral Anticoagulants

	Dabigatran	Rivaroxaban	Apixaban	Edoxaban
Target	Thrombin (IIa)	Factor Xa	Factor Xa	Factor Xa
Active Drug	No	Yes	Yes	Yes
Onset Time (h)	0.5-2	2-4	3-4	1-3
Half-Life (h)	12-17	5-13	~12	9-11
Renal Excretion (%)	80	33	27	50
Reversal Agent	Idarucizumab 5 g IV bolus	Andexanet alfa or PCC	Andexanet alfa or PCC	Andexanet alfa or PCC

IV, Intravenous; *PCC,* prothrombin complex concentrate.
From Hoffman R et al: *Hematology, basic principles and practice*, ed 7, Philadelphia, 2018, Elsevier.

TABLE 7 Bleeding Risk Score

HAS-BLED Risk Factors	Score
Hypertension	1
Abnormal liver function	1
Abnormal renal function	1
Stroke	1
Bleeding	1
Labile INRs	1
Elderly (age >65)	1
Drugs	1
Alcohol	1

HAS-BLED is the most validated bleeding score for patients with AF in whom antithrombotic therapy is indicated. When HAS-BLED score ≥3, caution and regular review are appropriate, as well as efforts to correct the potentially reversible risk factors for bleeding. *INRs,* International normalized ratio.
From Ronco C et al: *Critical care nephrology*, ed 3, Philadelphia, 2019, Elsevier.

Rivaroxaban and edoxaban are dosed once a day, and apixaban is dosed twice a day. A factor Xa reversal agent, andexanet alfa, has received FDA approval as a reversal for the anticoagulant effect of these agents.

- The decision to anticoagulate should be made irrespective of whether the atrial fibrillation is paroxysmal, persistent, or permanent.
- For patients in whom anticoagulation with warfarin or other anticoagulants is contraindicated due to high bleeding risk (Table 7), left atrial appendage exclusion is an alternative. Several methods can be used, including the Lariat procedure and the AtriClip, but these are still considered unproven for stroke prevention in AF. The Watchman device is a left atrial appendage occlusion device and is the only device approved by the FDA for stroke prevention specifically for patients with AF that require anticoagulation but have an appropriate reason to seek an alternative. Patients with surgical ligation of the left atrial appendage still have an indication for anticoagulation due to lack of clinical trials showing a stroke risk reduction and inconsistent techniques.
- Perioperative bridging anticoagulation in patients with AF: Current guidelines advise perioperative continuation of warfarin in low-risk patients (CHADS2 score 0 to 2) and bridging anticoagulation only in those at highest risk of thromboembolism (CHADS2 score 5 to 6). The recent Bridging Anticoagulation in Patients who Require Temporary Interruption of Warfarin Therapy for an Elective Invasive Procedure or Surgery (BRIDGE) Study found that for patients who require procedure-related warfarin interruption, forgoing bridging anticoagulation was noninferior to perioperative bridging with low-molecular-weight heparin and decrease the risk of major bleeding. Based on this study, a no-bridging strategy is appropriate for lower-risk AF and minor procedures, but in high-risk patients having major surgery the answer remains debatable.

PROGNOSIS

- AF is associated with a 1.5- to 1.9-fold higher risk of death, which is in part due to the strong association between AF and thromboembolic events.
- AF is also independently associated with an increased risk of incident myocardial infarction, especially in women and blacks.
- Development of AF predicts heart failure and is associated with a worse New York Heart Association Heart Failure classification. AF may also worsen heart failure in individuals who are dependent on the atrial component of the cardiac output.
- AF in the setting of acute myocardial infarction was associated with a 40% increase in mortality compared to patients in sinus rhythm.
- ACC/AHA recommendations for special considerations in atrial fibrillation are summarized in Table 8.

DISPOSITION

Factors associated with maintenance of sinus rhythm after cardioversion include:

- Left atrium diameter <60 mm
- Absence of mitral valve disease
- Short duration of AF

REFERRAL

Refer to a cardiologist those patients in whom antiarrhythmic therapy or catheter-based/surgical intervention is being considered.

PEARLS & CONSIDERATIONS

COMMENTS

The number of patients anticoagulated in the United States is approximately half the number that should be anticoagulated for AF, resulting in a large burden of stroke. The exact burden of AF needed to trigger the need for anticoagulation is not known, though recent pacemaker trials have suggested that as little as 6 min confers significant stroke risk. Reversal agents for the new class of anticoagulation are now available: Idarucizumab for reversal of dabigatran; andexanet alfa for reversal of apixaban and rivaroxaban (pending FDA approval).

The American Academy of Family Physicians and the American College of Physicians provide the following recommendations for the management of newly detected AF:

- Rate control with chronic anticoagulation is the recommended strategy for the majority of asymptomatic patients with chronic AF. Rhythm control has not been shown to be superior to rate control (with chronic anticoagulation) in reducing morbidity and mortality and may be inferior in some patient subgroups to rate control. Rhythm control is appropriate when based on other special considerations, such as patient symptoms, exercise tolerance, and patient preference.
- Patients with AF should receive chronic anticoagulation, unless they are at low risk for stroke as stated earlier or have specific contraindications.
- For patients with AF, the following drugs are recommended for their demonstrated efficacy in rate control during exercise and while at rest: Atenolol, metoprolol, diltiazem, and verapamil (drugs listed alphabetically by class). Digoxin is effective only for rate control at rest and, therefore, should be used only as a second-line agent for rate control in AF.
- For patients who elect to undergo acute cardioversion to achieve sinus rhythm in AF, both direct-current cardioversion and pharmacologic conversion are appropriate options in an otherwise healthy patient.
- Both transesophageal echocardiography with short-term prior anticoagulation followed by early acute cardioversion (in absence of

TABLE 8 ACC/AHA Recommendations for Special Considerations in Atrial Fibrillation

Class	Indication	Level of Evidence
Postoperative Atrial Fibrillation		
Class I (indicated)	Unless contraindicated, treatment with an oral beta-blocker to prevent postoperative AF is recommended for patients undergoing cardiac surgery.	A
	Administration of AV nodal blocking agents is recommended to achieve rate control in patients who develop postoperative AF.	B
Class IIa (reasonable)	Preoperative administration of amiodarone reduces the incidence of AF in patients undergoing cardiac surgery and represents appropriate prophylactic therapy for patients at high risk for postoperative AF.	A
	It is reasonable to restore sinus rhythm by pharmacologic cardioversion with ibutilide or direct-current cardioversion in patients who develop postoperative AF, as advised for nonsurgical patients.	B
	It is reasonable to administer antiarrhythmic medications in an attempt to maintain sinus rhythm in patients with recurrent or refractory postoperative AF, as recommended for other patients who develop AF.	B
	It is reasonable to administer antithrombotic medication in patients who develop postoperative AF, as recommended for nonsurgical patients.	B
Class IIb (may be considered)	Prophylactic administration of sotalol may be considered for patients at risk for development of AF after cardiac surgery.	B
Acute Myocardial Infarction		
Class I (indicated)	Direct-current cardioversion is recommended for patients with severe hemodynamic compromise or intractable ischemia, or when adequate rate control cannot be achieved with pharmacologic agents in patients with acute myocardial infarction and AF.	C
	Intravenous administration of amiodarone is recommended to slow a rapid ventricular response to AF and to improve left ventricular function in patients with acute myocardial infarction.	C
	Intravenous beta-blockers and nondihydropyridine calcium antagonists are recommended to slow a rapid ventricular response to AF in patients with acute myocardial infarction who do not display clinical left ventricular dysfunction, bronchospasm, or AV block.	C
	For patients with AF and acute myocardial infarction, administration of unfractionated heparin by either continuous intravenous infusion or intermittent subcutaneous injection is recommended in a dose sufficient to prolong the activated partial thromboplastin time to 1.5-2× the control value, unless contraindications to anticoagulation exist.	C
Class IIa (reasonable)	Intravenous administration of digitalis is reasonable to slow a rapid ventricular response and to improve left ventricular function in patients with acute myocardial infarction and AF associated with severe left ventricular dysfunction and heart failure.	C
Class III (not indicated)	The administration of class IC antiarrhythmic drugs is not recommended in patients with AF in the setting of acute myocardial infarction.	C
Management of Atrial Fibrillation Associated with Wolff-Parkinson-White (WPW) Preexcitation Syndrome		
Class I (indicated)	Catheter ablation of the accessory pathway is recommended for symptomatic patients with AF who have WPW syndrome, particularly those with syncope due to rapid heart rate or those with a short bypass tract refractory period.	B
	Immediate direct-current cardioversion is recommended to prevent ventricular fibrillation in patients with a short anterograde bypass tract refractory period in whom AF occurs with a rapid ventricular response associated with hemodynamic instability.	B
	Intravenous procainamide or ibutilide is recommended to restore sinus rhythm in patients with WPW in whom AF occurs without hemodynamic instability in association with a wide QRS complex on the electrocardiogram (≥120-msec duration) or with a rapid preexcited ventricular response.	C
Class IIa (reasonable)	Intravenous flecainide or direct-current cardioversion is reasonable when very rapid ventricular rates occur in patients with AF involving conduction over an accessory pathway.	B
Class IIb (may be considered)	It may be reasonable to administer intravenous quinidine, procainamide, disopyramide, ibutilide, or amiodarone to hemodynamically stable patients with AF involving conduction over an accessory pathway.	B
Class III (not indicated)	Intravenous administration of digitalis glycosides or nondihydropyridine calcium channel antagonists is not recommended in patients with WPW syndrome who have preexcited ventricular activation during AF.	B
Hyperthyroidism		
Class I (indicated)	Administration of a beta-blocker is recommended to control the rate of ventricular response in patients with AF complicating thyrotoxicosis, unless contraindicated.	B
	In circumstances when a beta-blocker cannot be used, administration of a nondihydropyridine calcium channel antagonist (diltiazem or verapamil) is recommended to control the ventricular rate in patients with AF and thyrotoxicosis.	B
	In patients with AF associated with thyrotoxicosis, oral anticoagulation (INR, 2.0-3.0) is recommended to prevent thromboembolism, as recommended for AF patients with other risk factors for stroke.	C
	Once a euthyroid state is restored, recommendations for antithrombotic prophylaxis are the same as for patients without hyperthyroidism.	C
Management of Atrial Fibrillation during Pregnancy		
Class I (indicated)	Digoxin, a beta-blocker, or a nondihydropyridine calcium channel antagonist is recommended to control the rate of ventricular response in pregnant patients with AF.	C
	Direct-current cardioversion is recommended in pregnant patients who become hemodynamically unstable because of AF.	C
	Protection against thromboembolism is recommended throughout pregnancy for all patients with AF (except those with lone AF and/or low thromboembolic risk). Therapy (anticoagulant or aspirin) should be chosen according to the stage of pregnancy.	C

TABLE 8 ACC/AHA Recommendations for Special Considerations in Atrial Fibrillation—cont'd

Class	Indication	Level of Evidence
Class IIb (may be considered)	Administration of heparin may be considered during the first trimester and last month of pregnancy for patients with AF and risk factors for thromboembolism. Unfractionated heparin may be administered either by continuous intravenous infusion in a dose sufficient to prolong the activated partial thromboplastin time to 1.5-2× the control value or by intermittent subcutaneous injection in a dose of 10,000-20,000 units every 12 hr, adjusted to prolong the midinterval (6 hr after injection) activated partial thromboplastin time to 1.5× control.	B
	Despite the limited data available, subcutaneous administration of low-molecular-weight heparin may be considered during the first trimester and last month of pregnancy for patients with AF and risk factors for thromboembolism.	C
	Administration of an oral anticoagulant may be considered during the second trimester for pregnant patients with AF at high thromboembolic risk.	C
	Administration of quinidine or procainamide may be considered to achieve pharmacologic cardioversion in hemodynamically stable patients who develop AF during pregnancy.	C
Management of Atrial Fibrillation in Patients with Hypertrophic Cardiomyopathy (HCM)		
Class I (indicated)	Oral anticoagulation (INR, 2.0-3.0) is recommended in patients with HCM who develop AF, as for other patients at high risk of thromboembolism.	B
Class IIa (may be considered)	Antiarrhythmic medications can be useful to prevent recurrent AF in patients with HCM. Available data are insufficient to recommend one agent over another in this situation, but (a) disopyramide combined with a beta-blocker or nondihydropyridine calcium channel antagonist or (b) amiodarone alone is generally preferred.	C
Management of Atrial Fibrillation in Patients with Pulmonary Disease		
Class I (indicated)	Correction of hypoxemia and acidosis is the recommended primary therapeutic measure for patients who develop AF during an acute pulmonary illness or exacerbation of chronic pulmonary disease.	C
	A nondihydropyridine calcium channel antagonist (diltiazem or verapamil) is recommended to control the ventricular rate in patients with obstructive pulmonary disease who develop AF.	C
	Direct-current cardioversion should be attempted in patients with pulmonary disease who become hemodynamically unstable as a consequence of AF.	C
Class III (not indicated)	Theophylline and beta-adrenergic agonist agents are not recommended for patients with bronchospastic lung disease who develop AF.	C
	Beta-blockers, sotalol, propafenone, and adenosine are not recommended in patients with obstructive lung disease who develop AF.	C

ACC, American College of Cardiology; *AF,* atrial fibrillation; *AHA,* American Heart Association; *AV,* atrioventricular; *INR,* international normalized ratio.
From Zipes DP: *Braunwald's heart disease, a textbook of cardiovascular medicine,* ed 11, Philadelphia, 2019, Elsevier.

intracardiac thrombus) with postcardioversion anticoagulation vs. delayed cardioversion with preanticoagulation and postanticoagulation are appropriate management strategies for patients who elect to undergo cardioversion.

- Among patients with paroxysmal AF without previous antiarrhythmic drug treatment, ablation compared with antiarrhythmic drugs resulted in a lower rate of recurrent atrial tachyarrhythmias at 2 yr. However, recurrence was frequent in both groups.
- Among patients with atrial fibrillation who undergo packed cell volume, the risk of bleeding is lower among those who receive dual therapy with dabigatran and a $P2Y_{12}$ inhibitor (clopidogrel or ticagrelor) than among those who receive triple therapy with warfarin, a $P2Y_{12}$ inhibitor, and aspirin. Dual therapy has been shown to be noninferior to triple therapy with respect to the risk of thromboembolic events.[1]
- In patients with atrial fibrillation and stable coronary artery disease, rivaroxaban monotherapy is noninferior to combination therapy with rivaroxaban plus a single antiplatelet agent for efficacy and superior for safety.[2]
- In patients presenting to the ED with recent-onset, symptomatic atrial fibrillation, a wait-and-see approach is noninferior to early cardioversion in achieving a return to sinus rhythm at 4 wk.[3]

[1] Cannon CP et al: Dual antithrombotic therapy with dabigatran after PCV in atrial fibrillation, *N Engl J Med* 377:1513-1524, 2017.

[2] Yasuda S et al: Antithrombotic therapy for atrial fibrillation with stable coronary disease, *N Engl J Med* 381:1103-1113, 2019.

SUGGESTED READINGS

Available at ExpertConsult.com

RELATED CONTENT

Atrial Fibrillation (Patient Information)

AUTHOR: **Tania B. Babar, MD**

[3] Pluymaekers N et al: Early or delayed cardioversion in recent-onset atrial fibrillation, *N Engl J Med* 380:1499-1508, 2019.

BASIC INFORMATION

DEFINITION

Typical atrial flutter is the term commonly applied to the atrial macroreentrant circuit that circulates around the tricuspid annulus in the right atrium. The critical isthmus of the circuit is the tissue between the inferior vena cava and the tricuspid annulus, and a more precise name for this arrhythmia is *cavotricuspid isthmus-dependent atrial flutter,* or CTI flutter. Because of its anatomic and physiologic stability, the result is regular atrial depolarizations, typically at a rate of 250 to 350 beats/min. Regular, macroreentrant atrial arrhythmias at this rate that do not use the CTI are referred to as *atypical atrial flutter.* Because of its anatomic and physiologic stability, the result is regular atrial depolarizations, typically at an atrial rate of 250 to 350 beats/min. Regular, supraventricular arrhythmias at this atrial rate that do not use the CTI are referred to as *atypical atrial flutter.* Because of the stability of atrial flutter, conduction through the atrioventricular node (AVN) is often predictable at a common mathematical denominator. For example, when the flutter rate is 300 beats/min, 2:1 conduction results in a ventricular rate of 150 beats/min. By extension, 3:1 conduction results in a ventricular rate of 100 beats/min, 4:1 in a rate of 75 beats/min, and 5:1 in a rate of 60 beats/min. If the regular atrial impulses conduct at a variable rate through the AVN, the result may be an irregular QRS pattern. However, a common denominator atrial interval is often present.

Table 1 summarizes the different types of atrial flutter and distinguishing features on scalar electrocardiography.

ICD-10CM CODE

I48.3 Typical atrial flutter
I48.4 Atypical atrial flutter
I48.92 Unspecified atrial flutter

EPIDEMIOLOGY & DEMOGRAPHICS

- Atrial flutter is the second most common atrial tachyarrhythmia after atrial fibrillation, with an estimated 200,000 new cases annually in the U.S.
- Atrial flutter is common in patients with congestive heart failure, chronic obstructive pulmonary disease (COPD), pulmonary vascular disorders such as pulmonary embolism, or during the first week after open heart surgery.
- Atrial flutter occurs more frequently with advancing age (5/100,000 age <50 vs. 587/100,000 age >80 yr) and 2.5 times more frequently in men than in women.
- Patients taking antiarrhythmics for chronic suppression of atrial fibrillation may present with atrial flutter.
- Atrial flutter is typically seen in patients with underlying structural heart disease and is uncommon in children or young adults without congenital heart disease.
- More than 50% of patients with atrial flutter will develop atrial fibrillation in 3 yr, and more than 80% will develop atrial fibrillation within 5 yr. This is important when considering treatment options for atrial flutter, especially anticoagulation.

CLASSIFICATION

Historically, the Wells classification designated atrial flutter as type I and type II. However, it is now recognized that tachycardias satisfying either of the definitions for type I or type II can be caused by reentrant circuits or by rapid focal atrial tachycardia, and this classification is infrequently used. Designating atrial flutter based on whether or not it is CTI dependent is more useful because of the management options (i.e., ablation). Type I CTI-dependent atrial flutter, also known as common atrial flutter or typical atrial flutter, has an atrial rate of 240 to 350 beats/min. The reentrant loop circles the right atrium, passing through the CTI, a body of fibrous tissue in the lower atrium between the inferior vena cava and the tricuspid valve. CTI flutter can revolve around the tricuspid annulus in either direction (counterclockwise or clockwise) when viewing the tricuspid annulus *en face.*

- Counterclockwise atrial flutter is the more common type (~75%). The flutter waves are "sawtooth" and negative on the surface ECG leads II, III, and aVF; positive in V1; and negative in V6. (Fig. E1)
- Clockwise atrial flutter is less common (~25%): The reentry loop cycles in the opposite direction; thus, the flutter waves are upright in leads II, III, and aVF; negative in V1; and positive in V6. (Fig. 2)
- Atypical atrial flutter is defined by absence of CTI dependence and may occur in patients with prior cardiac surgery, congenital heart disease, or prior radiofrequency ablation (especially left atrial ablation for atrial fibrillation) or may be idiopathic. One ECG feature is the lack of discordance of the flutter wave polarity between the inferior leads (leads II, III, and aVF) and V1. Flutter circuits in the left atrium often have upright flutter waves in all precordial leads.

PHYSICAL FINDINGS & CLINICAL PRESENTATION

- Palpitations
- Dizziness, lightheadedness, syncope, or near syncope
- Angina
- Congestive heart failure
- Embolic phenomena from intracardiac thrombus

TABLE 1 Characteristics of Different Types of Atrial Flutter and Distinguishing Features on Scalar Electrocardiography

Type	Reentrant Circuit	ECG Pattern	Lead V1/V6
Typical counterclockwise	Tricuspid annulus dependent on the CTI	Sawtooth flutter wave; negative in II, III, and aVF	Positive V1 Negative V6
Typical clockwise	Tricuspid annulus dependent on the CTI	"Inverse sawtooth"; positive and often notched in II, III, and aVF	Broad and negative in V1 (often notched) Positive in V6
Lower loop reentry	CTI	Usually similar to typical counterclockwise CTI flutter except subtle loss of terminal positive deflection in leads II, III, and aVF	Usually similar to typical counterclockwise
Upper loop reentry	Superior vena cava and upper crista terminalis	Similar to typical clockwise flutter	Similar to typical clockwise flutter
Right atrial free wall	Around areas of scar in lateral or posterior right atrium (caused by previous atrial surgery or spontaneously)	Variable	Typically negative or biphasic with terminal negative deflection in V1
Septal atrial flutter	Atrial septum, typically after previous surgery	Variable	Usually biphasic or isoelectric in V1
Mitral annular flutter	Around mitral annulus, often slow zone of block around PV interval; frequently occurs in setting of left atrial surgery or ablation	Variable; I, III, and aVF, often positive but low amplitude	Usually positive in V1 (or rarely isoelectric) and often broad
Postatrial fibrillation ablation/maze flutter	Variable; circuit involves previous ablations or scar in left atrium	Variable	Variable

aVF, Augmented vector foot; *CTI,* cavotricuspid isthmus; *PV,* pulmonary vein.
From Zipes DP: *Braunwald's heart disease, a textbook of cardiovascular medicine,* ed 11, Philadelphia, 2019, Elsevier.

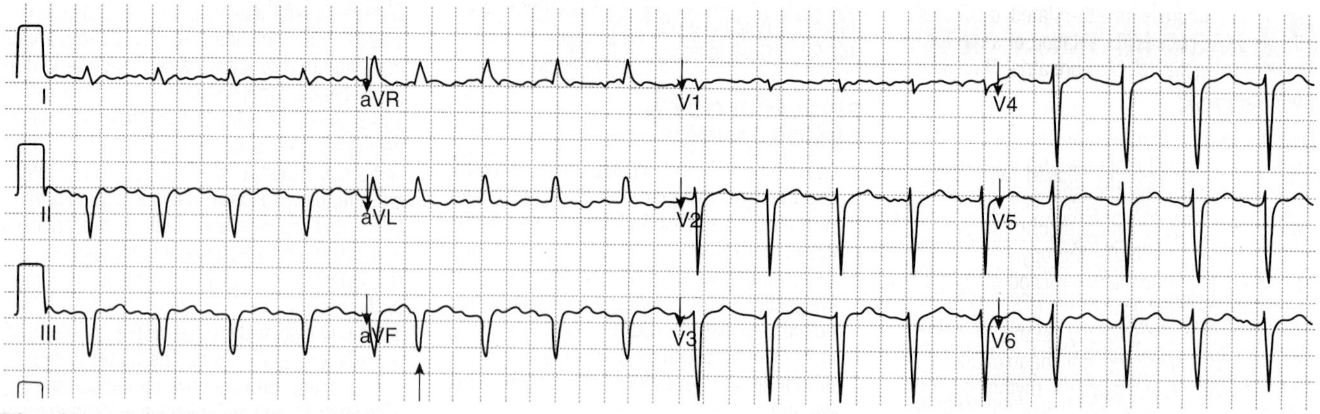

FIG. 2 Clockwise atrial flutter with predominant 2:1 atrioventricular conduction. Note the positive flutter waves in leads II, III, and F, negative in V1 and positive in V6. The overall ventricular rate is slower than in Fig. 1 due to a slow flutter rate of approximately 200 bpm. One beat is conducted 1:1 *(arrow)*. *aVF,* Augmented vector foot; *aVL,* augmented vector left; *aVR,* augmented vector right.

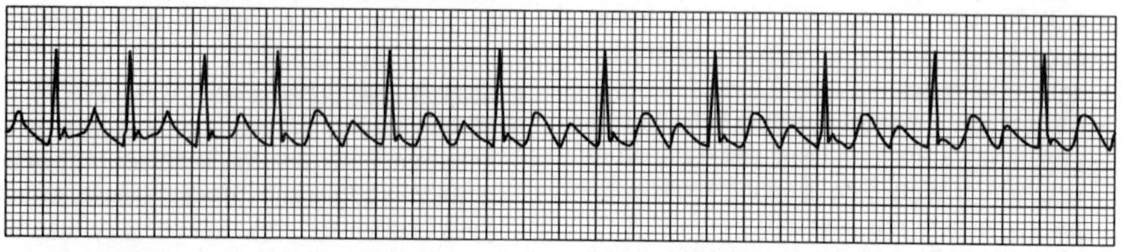

FIG. 3 Rhythm strip of atrial flutter. (From Cameron P: *Textbook of adult emergency medicine,* ed 5, Philadelphia, 2020, Elsevier.)

ETIOLOGY

- Age-related degenerative changes
- Rheumatic heart disease
- Congenital heart disease
- Left ventricular dysfunction or congestive heart failure
- Acute myocardial infarction (rarely)
- Thyrotoxicosis
- Pulmonary embolism
- Mitral valve disease
- Cardiac surgery
- Chronic obstructive pulmonary disease
- Obesity
- Pericarditis
- Pulmonary hypertension
- Antiarrhythmic therapy use in patients with atrial fibrillation

Dx DIAGNOSIS

DIFFERENTIAL DIAGNOSIS

- Atrial fibrillation
- Atrial tachycardia
- Supraventricular tachycardia:
  1. Atrioventricular node reentry
  2. Orthodromic reciprocating tachycardia (using a concealed bypass tract)
  3. Junctional ectopic tachycardia
  4. Wolff-Parkinson-White syndrome
- Sinus tachycardia

WORKUP

- ECG (Fig. 3)
- Laboratory evaluation
- Assessment of CHA_2DS_2-VaSc score

LABORATORY TESTS

- Thyroid function studies
- Serum electrolytes, including renal and hepatic tests (anticipating antiarrhythmic therapy use)
- CBC and PT/INR values (anticipating anticoagulation therapy)

IMAGING STUDIES

- ECG:
  1. Absence of P waves.
  2. Regular, "sawtooth," or "F" (flutter) wave pattern without an isoelectric baseline in leads II, III, and aVF (seen most commonly with counterclockwise typical CTI-flutter). The discordance of the polarity of the flutter waves between the inferior leads and V1 is a constant finding.
  3. There is rarely 1:1 atrioventricular (AV) conduction in atrial flutter (unless preexcitation is present). Rather, AV conduction is usually in a 2:1 (see Fig. E1), 3:1, or 4:1 fashion, with corresponding usual ventricular rates of 150, 100, or 75 beats/min, respectively (assuming an atrial rate of 300 beats/min). With high vagal tone or AV block, ventricular rates may be slow in atrial flutter.
- Echocardiography (for new diagnoses) to evaluate for structural heart disease (ventricular size, thickness, and function; atrial size, and valve function).
- Transesophageal echocardiography: Consider in patients with associated structural or functional heart disease to ascertain the presence of intracardiac (e.g., left atrial appendage) thrombi, in the absence of an appropriate duration of anticoagulation.
- Holter monitoring or event recorder to assess for paroxysmal atrial flutter or rate control or to identify the arrhythmia if symptoms are nonspecific or to identify triggering events.
- Electrophysiologic studies: Required for a precise diagnosis and for ablation.

Rx TREATMENT

NONPHARMACOLOGIC THERAPY

- Vagal maneuvers (e.g., the Valsalva maneuver or carotid sinus massage) may transiently slow the ventricular rate (by increasing AV block) and may make flutter waves more evident. Adenosine may be similarly helpful for diagnostic purposes, allowing the unmasking of the atrial rhythm in the absence of ventricular activity. Maneuvers that affect AV conduction are unlikely to terminate atrial flutter.
- Direct current cardioversion is the treatment of choice for acute management of atrial flutter associated with hemodynamic instability or debilitating symptoms such as angina, congestive heart failure, or hypotension. Electrical cardioversion may be successful with energies as low as 25 joules, but because 100 joules is virtually always successful, this may be a reasonable initial shock strength. If the electrical shock results in atrial fibrillation, a second shock at a higher energy level is used to restore normal sinus rhythm. Sedation of a conscious patient is highly recommended before cardioversion is performed. Patients should be therapeutically anticoagulated for at least a mo or longer depending on their stroke risk (CHA_2DS_2-VASc score; Table 2).
- Overdrive pacing in the atrium may also terminate atrial flutter. This method is especially useful in patients who have recently undergone cardiac surgery and still have temporary atrial pacing wires and in patients who have an implanted pacemaker or defibrillator with an atrial lead.
- Radiofrequency ablation to terminate the atrial flutter and prevent recurrence is highly effective for patients with chronic or recurring atrial flutter and is generally considered first-line therapy in those with recurrent episodes of atrial flutter and may be offered for a first-ever episode of atrial flutter. It has been

shown to improve health-related quality of life. Despite successful ablation of atrial flutter, however, the risk of future atrial fibrillation remains.

ACUTE Rx

- Treatment choices are based on clinical circumstances. Fig. 4 describes an acute treatment of atrial flutter algorithm. Table 3 summarizes atrial flutter therapy.
- If the patient is unstable, proceed directly to electrical cardioversion.
- In the hemodynamically stable patient, assess the need for anticoagulation and proceed with rate control or rhythm control strategy.
- AV blocking agents such as calcium channel blockers, beta-blockers, and digitalis (second-line treatment) may all be used for rate control. Atrial flutter may spontaneously convert to normal sinus rhythm with this strategy.

TABLE 2 CHA_2DS_2-VASc Risk Score for Prediction of Stroke Risk in Atrial Fibrillation

Risk Factor	Points
CHF/LV dysfunction	1
Hypertension	1
Age ≥75 yr	2
Diabetes mellitus	1
Stroke/TIA/embolism	2
Vascular disease	1
Age 64-74 yr	1
Sex category (female)	1
Maximum score	9

CHF, Congestive heart failure; *LV,* left ventricular; *TIA,* transient ischemic attack.

- In general, atrial flutter is more difficult to rate-control than atrial fibrillation.
- The rate of recurrence of atrial flutter with cardioversion alone is difficult to determine because most published data combine atrial flutter with atrial fibrillation. However, the recurrence rate is substantial, perhaps 50% at 1 yr.
- Intravenous ibutilide is a first-line medication for pharmacologic cardioversion of atrial flutter in patients with normal systolic function and QT intervals. The success rate is approximately 60%, and it is more effective than procainamide, sotalol, or amiodarone.

CHRONIC Rx

- Few data exist to decide on the choice of rate control versus rhythm control in patients with atrial flutter. However, rate control may be difficult in atrial flutter, and ablation success exceeds 90%. Although ablation results in more durable freedom from atrial flutter recurrence, there are several pharmacologic options to help maintain sinus rhythm after cardioversion of atrial flutter, such as dofetilide, amiodarone, flecainide, propafenone, or sotalol. The choice of antiarrhythmic therapy is, in part, dictated by the presence or absence of underlying structural heart disease.
- Elective outpatient cardioversion or ablation can be performed either immediately preceded by transesophageal echocardiography (TEE) to evaluate the left atrium and the left atrial appendage for thrombus or after a period of at least 3 wk of documented therapeutic anticoagulation before cardioversion. At least 4 wk of anticoagulation should be administered after cardioversion, if not longer, depending on the overall thromboembolic risk of the patient as determined by the CHA_2DS_2-VASc score.

DISPOSITION

More than 85% of patients convert to regular sinus rhythm after cardioversion. Ablation success rates exceed 90%.

REFERRAL

Refer patients who are considered for rhythm control of atrial flutter to a cardiac electrophysiologist, especially patients who are candidates for radiofrequency ablation.

PEARLS & CONSIDERATIONS

COMMENTS

- The surface ECG is the best tool for recognizing atrial flutter and distinguishing atrial flutter from atrial fibrillation.
- Ablation for typical atrial flutter is highly effective, straightforward, and relatively safe. It should be considered for patients with recurrent episodes and even for a first-ever episode.
- Patients with atrial flutter carry a significant risk for subsequent development of atrial fibrillation.
- Anticoagulation should be considered for all patients whose CHA_2DS_2-VaSc score is ≥2. Anticoagulation is generally not recommended in patients with a CHA_2DS_2-VaSc score of zero. For patients with a CHA_2DS_2-VaSc score of 1, low-dose aspirin or oral anticoagulants (warfarin, dabigatran, rivaroxaban, apixaban, or edoxaban) are appropriate options.
- Although anticoagulation recommendations for atrial flutter are identical to those for atrial fibrillation, studies suggest that the absolute risk of stroke is lower from atrial flutter than from fibrillation.

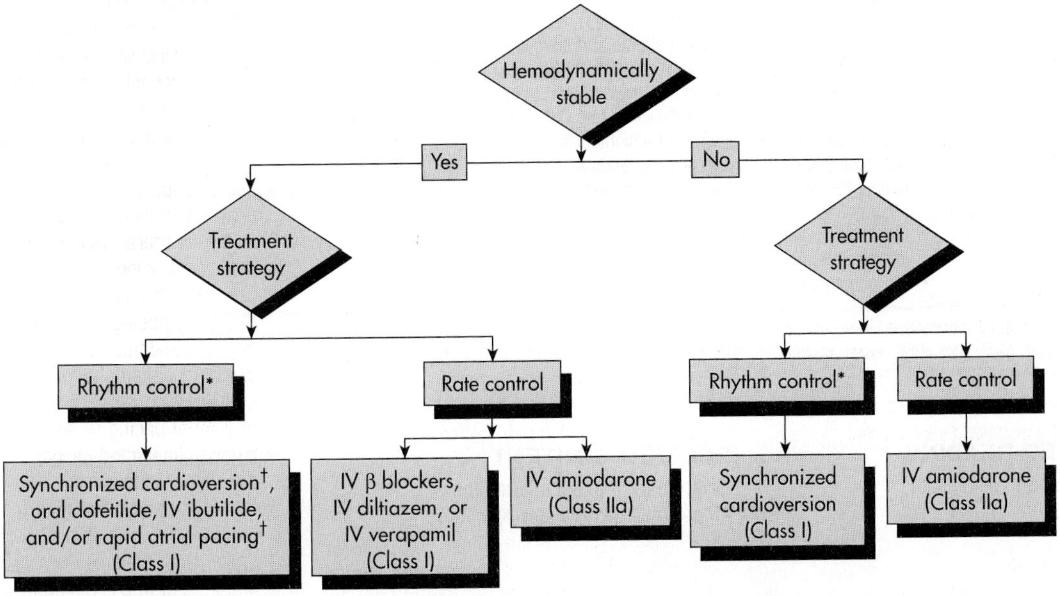

FIG. 4 Acute treatment of atrial flutter. *Anticoagulation as per guideline is mandatory. †For rhythms that break or recur spontaneously, synchronized cardioversion, or rapid atrial pacing is not appropriate. *IV,* Intravenous. (Reproduced with permission from Page RL et al: 2015 ACC/AHA/HRS Guideline for the management of adult patients with supraventricular tachycardia, *JACC* 67[13]:e27-e115, 2016. In Olshansky B et al: *Arrhythmia essentials,* ed 2, Philadelphia, 2017, Elsevier.)

TABLE 3 Atrial Flutter Therapy

Acute therapy for poorly tolerated AFL or continuous rapid ventricular rate	• If prolonged (i.e., >48-72 hr), anticoagulation is required as cardioversion may be associated with thromboembolic risk. Anticoagulation guidelines for cardioversion are the same as for atrial fibrillation and may indicate need for a TEE for prolonged episodes. Adenosine and carotid massage can be used to help diagnose AFL masquerading as sinus rhythm. • **First line:** Electrical cardioversion under sedation with anticoagulation as necessary. Consider the length of the episode. • **Second line:** Ibutilide or procainamide may be attempted for conversion before electrical cardioversion attempts. Ibutilide may be 60%-70% effective if AFL has been present for <48 hr. • **Alternate:** Rapid atrial pacing (esophageal, epicardial, or endocardial, depending on the situation). To pace terminate, pace for 10-15 sec at a rate of 10%-20% faster than rate of flutter. If ineffective, burst pace 10 beats/min faster at a time for 10-15 sec at a time until conversion to AF or sinus rhythm. When AF occurs, it is usually short lived and terminates spontaneously within 24 hr. If persistent, electrical cardioversion can be attempted with or without antiarrhythmic drugs. Atrial fibrillation cannot be pace terminated. However, slower AFL (rate <350) of any flutter wave morphology can often be pace terminated. • Oral drug loading alone to terminate AFL is rarely useful. • If recurrent episodes, use class IC or III antiarrhythmic drugs until steady state is achieved, then attempt cardioversion. These drugs (particularly 1C drugs) may stabilize the flutter circuit. It may also create another form of AFL—"1C" AFL—from AF. Ablation remains first-line therapy, especially if AFL is isthmus dependent. • Consider ablation for cases of AFL. However, despite AFL ablation, AF may occur, especially in individuals with underlying structural heart disease. • AV nodal ablation, although not preferable, could be considered when ventricular rate control cannot be achieved and flutter cannot be ablated (e.g., in the presence of a left atrial appendage clot), or if symptomatic, refractory, and/or if associated with tachycardia-induced cardiomyopathy. This option may be considered in cases where individuals have multiple forms of nonablatable AFL or AF and especially for those who do have non–isthmus-dependent AFL.
Chronic prevention	• If structural heart disease without CHF: Sotalol (often initiated in the hospital), dofetilide, amiodarone. • If structural heart disease with CHF: Amiodarone, dofetilide. • If no structural heart disease: Propafenone, flecainide, sotalol, dofetilide, or amiodarone, but propafenone or flecainide may need concomitant AV nodal blocking drugs to prevent 1:1 conduction. • If class I or III drugs are used, first control the ventricular response rate with an AV nodal blocking drug. Otherwise, the vagolytic effects of class IA drugs can enhance AV nodal conduction, and both 1A and 1C drugs can lead to AFL with 1:1 AV conduction. • Drug therapy alone for pure AFL flutter is usually not effective. • Consider radiofrequency catheter ablation early; it has become first-line therapy.
Nonresponders with severe symptoms	• If typical AFL, radiofrequency ablation within the cavotricuspid isthmus is highly effective. • Atypical AFL is more difficult to ablate and depends on the location of reentrant circuit. Success rates are lower than that for typical AFL. It is more difficult when there is congenital heart disease, valve disease, or prior surgery in which significant areas of scar are present. • Ventricular rate control, antiarrhythmic drugs, or AV node ablation (less preferable) can be performed for atypical, nonablatable AFL. • If AV node ablation and pacing is performed and AFL is intermittent, mode-switching function should be programmed "ON."
MI	• If hemodynamic intolerance or ongoing refractory myocardial ischemia, emergent cardioversion. AFL may increase MVO_2 due to rapid ventricular rate, causing further ischemia, diastolic dysfunction, and pulmonary congestion and edema. • If recurrent, IV amiodarone or procainamide. • Consider temporary antitachycardia pacing if recurrent and poorly tolerated.
Preoperative	• For cardiac surgery, convert AFL to NSR if adequate anticoagulation has been achieved, or ensure that ventricular response is well controlled. • If surgery is elective and AFL is chronic, antiarrhythmic drugs or catheter ablation may be considered. However, anticoagulation should be continued at least 4 wk after conversion of longer-term (>48 hr) AFL prior to elective surgery. • For more urgent surgery in which anticoagulation cannot be used, consider rate control without cardioversion. • For short-duration (<48 hr) AFL, DCC can be performed (may consider therapeutic anticoagulation before electrical cardioversion with surgical consultation as to risk).
Postoperative	• AFL occurs in 10%-20% of all patients after cardiac surgery; it typically occurs with AF. Incidence peaks at days 2-3. It is more common in older patients. It rarely occurs after other types of surgery. The AFL may resolve spontaneously; however, the rhythm can increase the length of hospital stay, exacerbate heart failure, slow the recovery process, and cause symptoms. • Control rate with β-adrenergic blocker if no CHF or bronchospastic disease and LVEF >40%. Diltiazem is often successful as a second-line drug, but use with caution in patients with a reduced LVEF. Digoxin for rate control is less effective but may be considered, particularly in patients with poor LV function. • IV amiodarone may be useful for persistent and poorly tolerated AFL; amiodarone or other antiarrhythmic drugs may be helpful for recurrent episodes. • Electrical cardioversion or atrial pace termination (if atrial pacing leads are present) is often successful, especially when employed early after the AFL onset. • Discontinue inotropic drugs, if possible.

AF, Atrial fibrillation; *AFL,* atrial flutter; *AV,* atrioventricular; *CHF,* congestive heart failure; *DCC,* direct current cardioversion; *IV,* intravenous; *LV,* left ventricle; *LVEF,* left ventricular ejection fraction; *MI,* myocardial infarction; *MVO_2,* myocardial oxygen consumption; *NSR,* normal sinus rhythm; *TEE,* transesophageal echocardiography.
From Olshansky B et al: *Arrhythmia essentials,* ed 2, Philadelphia, 2017, Elsevier.

SUGGESTED READING

Available at ExpertConsult.com

RELATED CONTENT

Atrial Flutter (Patient Information)
Atrial Fibrillation (Related Key Topic)

AUTHOR: **Daniel R. Frisch, MD**

BASIC INFORMATION

DEFINITION

An atrial septal defect (ASD) is a true defect in the interatrial septum that allows blood flow between the atria. Fig. 1 illustrates the physiology of ASD. The five forms of ASD are described below and illustrated in Fig. 2.

- Primum: This type of ASD occurs when the anterior and posterior endocardial cushions do not fuse with the septum primum creating a deficiency in the inferior portion of the septum primum. This defect is frequently associated with a cleft anterior mitral leaflet.
- Secundum: This is the most common form of ASD. It is caused by failure of the septum primum to fuse with the septum secundum. This defect can form anywhere along the septum, but it is most commonly found near the fossa ovalis.
- Sinus venosus defect: This defect is located at the junction of the right atrium and the superior vena cava or inferior vena cava. In a sinus venosus defect, a left-to-right shunt develops through an opening in the wall between the pulmonary veins and the right atrium. Most commonly this defect involves an anterior wall deficiency in the right upper pulmonary vein, which allows it to drain into the right atrium while remaining anatomically connected to the left atrium. Less commonly, the right lower pulmonary vein is involved. The left pulmonary veins can also drain into a vertical vein that communicates with the superior vena cava.
- Coronary sinus septal defect (unroofed coronary sinus): This is a defect between the wall of the coronary sinus and the left atrium that results in a left-to-right shunt. This defect is often associated with a persistent left superior vena cava.
- Iatrogenic atrial septal defect (iASD) is a complication of electrophysiology and structural interventional procedures that require transseptal puncture.

ASD should be distinguished from a patent foramen ovale (PFO), a flap-like opening between the two atria, caused by failure of the septum primum to fuse to the superior limb of the septum secundum in postnatal life. Whereas ASDs represent a congenital defect established in utero due to failure of normal atrial septal development, a persistent PFO in postnatal life represents the failure of an anatomically necessary defect to close. PFO occurs in approximately 20% to 25% of the normal adult population.

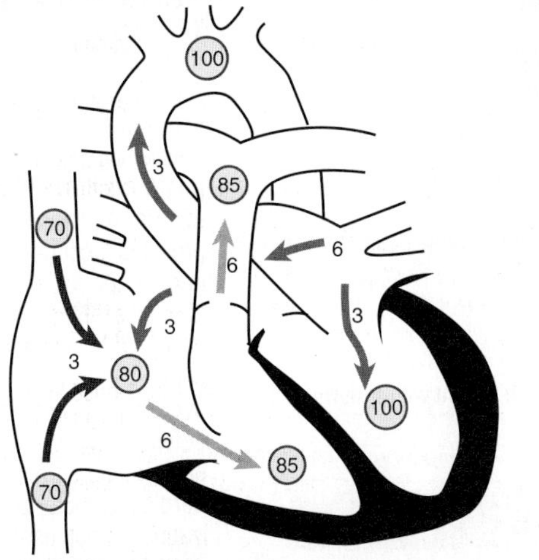

FIG. 1 Physiology of atrial septal defect (ASD). Circled numbers represent oxygen saturation values. The numbers next to the arrows represent volumes of blood flow (in L/min/m^2). This illustration shows a hypothetical patient with a pulmonary-to-systemic blood flow ratio (Qp/Qs) of 2:1. Desaturated blood enters the right atrium from the venae cavae at a volume of 3 L/min/m^2 and mixes with an additional 3 L of fully saturated blood shunting left to right across the ASD; the result is an increase in oxygen saturation in the right atrium. Six liters of blood flow through the tricuspid valve causing a mid-diastolic flow rumble. Oxygen saturation may be slightly higher in the RV because of incomplete mixing at the atrial level. The full 6 L of blood flows across the RV outflow tract and causes a systolic ejection flow murmur. Six liters return to the left atrium, with 3 L shunting left to right across the defect and 3 L crossing the mitral valve to be ejected by the left ventricle into the ascending aorta (normal cardiac output). (From Kliegman RM et al: *Nelson textbook of pediatrics,* ed 19, Philadelphia, 2011, Saunders.)

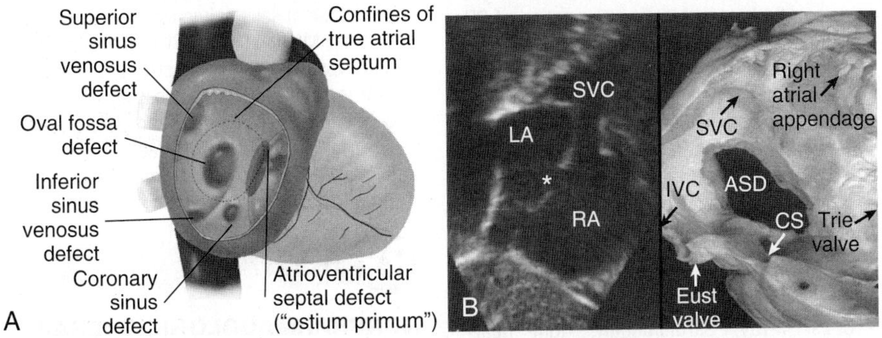

FIG. 2 A, Schematic diagram outlining the different types of interatrial shunting that can be encountered. Note that only the central defect is suitable for device closure. **B,** Subcostal right anterior oblique view of a secundum atrial septal defect *(ASD) (asterisk)* that is suitable for device closure. The right panel is a specimen as seen in a similar view, outlining the landmarks of defect. *CS,* Coronary sinus; *IVC,* inferior vena cava; *LA,* left atrium; *RA,* right atrium; *SVC,* superior vena cava. (From Zipes DP et al [eds]: *Braunwald's heart disease,* ed 7, Philadelphia, 2005, Saunders.)

SYNONYMS

ASD
Interatrial septal defect

ICD-10CM CODES

Q21.1	Atrial septal defect
I23.1	Atrial septal defect as current complication following acute myocardial infarction

EPIDEMIOLOGY & DEMOGRAPHICS

- Secundum, 75%; primum, 15% to 20%; sinus venosus, 5% to 10%; coronary sinus, <1%
- Incidence of ASD is greater in females and in patients with Down syndrome
- Accounts for 8% to 10% of congenital heart abnormalities
- Prevalence is 1.6 per 1000 live births
- Holt-Oram syndrome is an autosomal dominant disorder that involves skeletal anomalies, ASD, and cardiac conduction disease (most commonly atrioventricular [AV] blocks)
- Secundum defects are associated with multiple genetic syndromes including Noonan syndrome, Treacher Collins syndrome, thrombocytopenia–absent radii syndrome, and Down syndrome (trisomy 21)
- ASD may occur as an isolated defect or as part of other congenital cardiac syndromes such as Ebstein anomaly, Lutembacher syndrome, or fetal alcohol syndrome

PHYSICAL FINDINGS & CLINICAL PRESENTATION

- Small ASDs or PFOs may close spontaneously during infancy whereas infants with large ASDs may develop heart failure, recurrent respiratory infections, or failure to thrive. The majority of ASDs are small and do not cause any symptoms during infancy. Patients with small ASDs are usually diagnosed by the presence of a cardiac murmur auscultated during routine physical examination.
- Exertional fatigue and dyspnea are usually the main presenting symptoms.

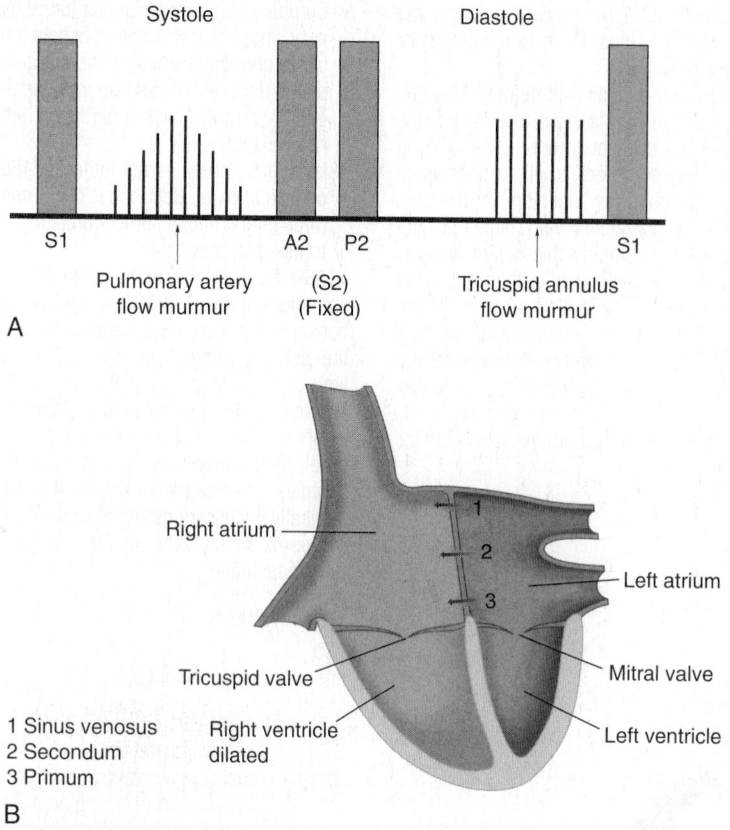

FIG. 3 Atrial septal defect. A, Murmur at the left sternal edge. **B,** Anatomy. (From The patient with a murmur. In Baker T et al [eds]: *Practical cardiology,* Philadelphia, 2008, Elsevier.)

- On rare occasions, young adults may present with ischemic stroke caused by paradoxical embolism through the ASD or PFO.
- Platypnea-orthodeoxia (characterized by dyspnea and deoxygenation when changing from a recumbent position to sitting or standing).
- Patients with ASDs caused by congenital syndromes may present with clinical features to the underlying syndrome.
- Atrial arrhythmias such as atrial fibrillation and atrial flutter are significantly increased in patients with ASDs.

CLINICAL FEATURES

- Cyanosis and clubbing (due to right-to-left shunting)
- Increased jugular venous pressure (may be due to RV failure from left-to-right shunting through a small ASD, or elevated left atrial pressures when a large ASD is present)
- Prominent RV impulse
- Visible and palpable pulmonary artery pulsations
- Wide fixed splitting of S_2
- An accentuated pulmonic component of S_2 (if the patient has pulmonary hypertension)
- Pansystolic murmur best heard at the apex (secondary to mitral regurgitation associated with the ostium primum defect)
- Ejection systolic flow murmur (pulmonary valve flow murmur; Fig. 3
- Diastolic rumble (atrioventricular valve flow murmur)

Dx DIAGNOSIS

DIFFERENTIAL DIAGNOSIS

- Primary pulmonary hypertension
- Pulmonary stenosis
- Rheumatic heart disease
- Mitral valve prolapse
- Cor pulmonale
- Anomalous pulmonary venous connection

WORKUP

- ECG:
  1. Ostium primum defect: Extreme left axis deviation, incomplete or total right bundle branch block, prolongation of PR interval
  2. Sinus venosus defect: Right axis deviation, abnormal P axis (suggesting an absent or deficient sinus node)
  3. Ostium secundum defect: Right axis deviation, incomplete or total right bundle branch block, right atrial enlargement

IMAGING STUDIES

- Chest x-ray: Cardiomegaly, right heart enlargement, increased pulmonary vascular pattern.
- Echocardiography: Transthoracic echocardiography (TTE) has a high degree of sensitivity for diagnosing secundum and primum ASDs when a complete examination is performed by a trained sonographer. Findings suspicious of a secundum or primum defect include abrupt dropout out of the interatrial septum. One must note that the interatrial septum is best visualized in the subcostal view and not the apical 4-chamber view as the alignment of the ultrasound beam is perpendicular and not parallel to the septum. The use of color flow Doppler on TTE can help identify or confirm the presence of an ASD and indicate the overall direction of the flow across the atrial septum. Reducing the Nyquist limit helps identifying lower flow with lower velocities across the defect. Sinus venosus and coronary sinus ASDs, due to their unusual locations, should be sought after when no ASD is readily identified on regular TTE imaging as these can be frequently missed.
- Transesophageal echocardiography (TEE): TEE nearly has a 100% sensitivity and more than 98% specificity in identifying all forms of ASD. It is specifically useful in locating sinus venosus ASDs. TEE is usually required when device closure is contemplated for appropriate sizing of the rims (Fig. 4). Addition of three-dimensional (3D) echocardiography provides accurate visualization of the size and shape of the defect and its rims on unique en-face views. Proper ASD sizing is essential in selecting the device size to avoid complications from using an undersized or oversized closure device (such as incomplete defect closure, device embolization, or disc erosion into surrounding cardiac structures).
- Cardiac catheterization: Left heart catheterization is not used to diagnose ASDs; it is used to assess the coronary arteries before ASD repair. Right-sided heart catheterization is used to assess the severity of the shunt, the extent of pulmonary hypertension, pulmonary vascular resistance (PVR), and pulmonary artery vasoreactivity to vasodilators. In ASD, right-sided heart catheterization will often reveal a "step-up" in arterial oxygen saturation in the right atrium compared with the superior vena cava due to left-to-right shunting from primum or secundum defects. This may not be the case in patients with ASDs from sinus venous defects who develop only partial anomalous pulmonary venous return.
- Cardiac MRI and CT: MRI is the gold standard for assessing RV size and function. MRI is also useful for assessing anomalous pulmonary venous return and persistent left superior vena cava. Cardiac CT can offer similar information. This imaging is useful when echocardiography is not diagnostic.

Rx TREATMENT

NONPHARMACOLOGIC THERAPY

- Asymptomatic patients with small defects, shunts with a pulmonary to systemic flow ratio (Qp/Qs) of <1.5:1, normal RV size, and without pulmonary artery hypertension (PAH) do not require closure with the exception of preventing paradoxical emboli in older

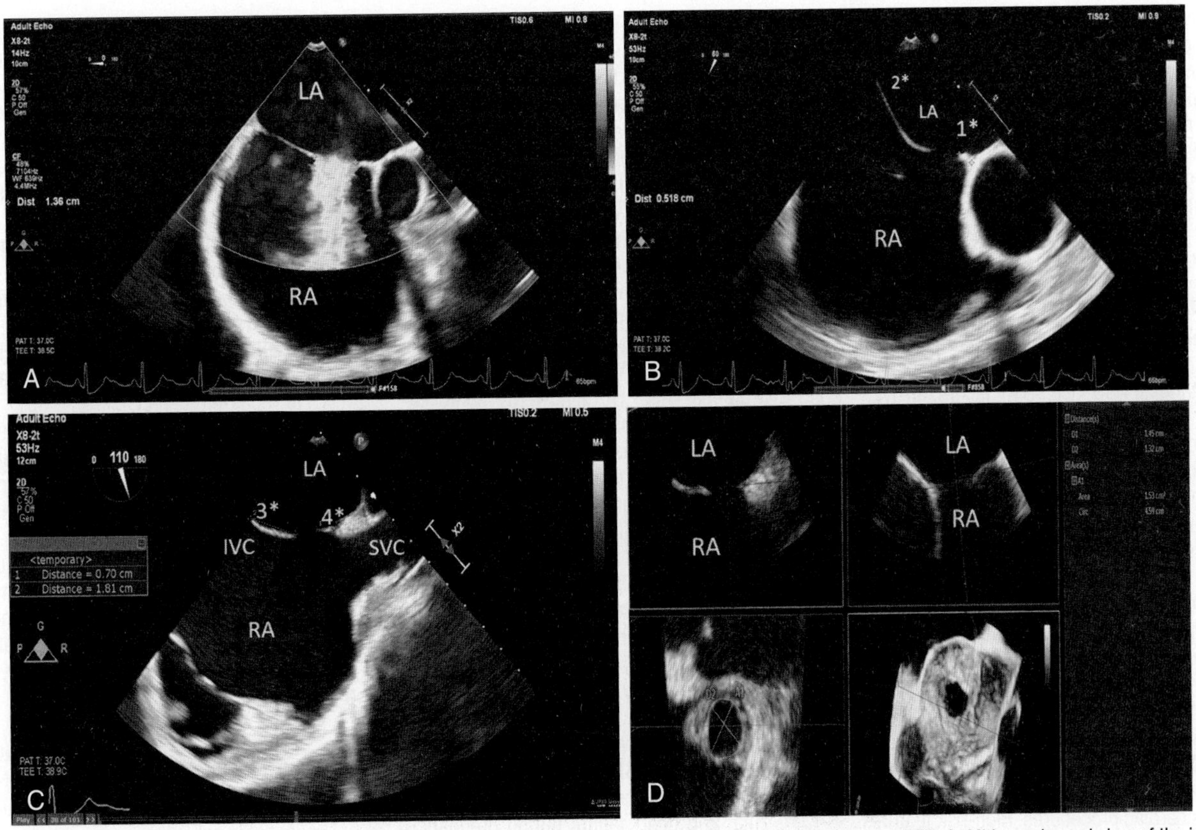

FIG. 4 TEE images for a 56-yr-old female lab with shortness of breath and enlarged right sided chambers on TTE. A, Mid-esophageal view of the interatrial septum identifying a secundum ASD with linear anteroposterior diameter of 1.35 cm. Color flow Doppler imaging demonstrates a left to right shunt. Note the RA appears to be enlarged. **B,** Secundum ASD noted at 60 degrees in the mid-esophageal aortic short axis view. Aortic (1*) and the posteroinferior (2*) rims are seen here. **C,** Bicaval view at 110 degrees demonstrate the diagnostic view for a secundum ASD with their IVC (3*) and SVC (4*) rims. **D,** 3D TEE imaging measuring the ASD defect with two orthogonal views on 2D TEE. Note the defect size is 1.53 cm^2. *LA,* Left atrium; *RA,* right atrium; *IVC,* inferior vena cava; *SVC,* superior vena cava.

patients after a stroke. However, they should be routinely assessed and monitored for development of clinical symptoms, arrhythmias, embolic events, and progression of structural disease (right-sided dysfunction) with serial echocardiography.
- Patients should undergo echocardiography every 2 to 3 yr.
- To monitor RV size and function and pulmonary pressure. Left-to-right shunting is expected to increase with age due to progressive noncompliance of the left ventricle and age-acquired heart disease.

GENERAL Rx

- Children and infants: ASD closure is indicated before age 10 if Qp/Qs is >2:1 (many experts advocate closure for Qp/Qs >1.5:1), if ASD size is >5 mm, or if there is evidence of RV dilation.
  1. ASDs with a diameter of <5 mm and no evidence of RV volume overload do not require closure unless associated with paradoxical embolism.
  2. ASD closure (either percutaneously or surgically) is indicated for either right atrial or right ventricular enlargement even if the patient is asymptomatic.
  3. Sinus venosus, coronary sinus, or primum variant ASDs should be repaired surgically rather than by percutaneous closure.
  4. Surgical closure of a secundum variant ASD is appropriate when other defects exist that require surgical intervention, or when the anatomy of the defect precludes the use of a percutaneous device.
- Adults: ASD closure should be considered if any of the following are present: Left-to-right shunting with Qp/Qs >1.5:1, right-sided chamber enlargement, clinical symptoms, pulmonary hypertension with pulmonary artery pressure less than two-thirds systemic levels, PVR less than two-thirds systemic vascular resistance, or pulmonary hypertension that responds to vasodilation therapy. These patients should be managed by specialists in adult congenital heart disease and pulmonary hypertension.
- Patients with severe, irreversible PAH and no evidence of a left-to-right shunt should not undergo ASD closure.
- ASD closure is reasonable in the presence of:
  1. Paradoxical embolism (Class IIa indication).
  2. Documented Platypnea-orthodeoxia (Class IIa indication).
- The majority of iASDs close spontaneously. However, ASD closure should be actively pursued if high risk features are present such as iASD >8 mm, right-to-left shunting, large left-to-right shunt, a predisposition to thromboembolism, or right ventricular dysfunction.
- Percutaneous catheter device closure has >95% success rate in appropriate candidates. Early complications include device thrombus formation, atrial arrhythmias, erosion, and device dislodgement. Potential mid- and long-term complications include late device erosion into the aortic root or pericardium, atrial dysrhythmias, and infective endocarditis. A combination of low-dose aspirin and clopidogrel is required for 3 to 6 mo after the procedure to prevent thrombus formation. Close clinical follow-up that includes echocardiogram is recommended before discharge, then at 1 wk, 6 mo, and 12 mo postintervention.
- Percutaneous closure is contraindicated in patients with sinus venosus, primum, or unroofed coronary sinus variant ASDs. Successful percutaneous ASD closure in patients with secundum defects depends on the anatomy of the defect. Percutaneous closure is not indicated for secundum defects if the defect is too large; too close to the coronary sinus, AV valves, or pulmonary veins; or if there are inadequate rims. Percutaneous closure of secundum ASD may be successful if the stretched diameter is <41 mm with adequate rims. The procedure should not be performed in the presence of sepsis, bleeding disorder, or intracardiac thrombi.
- Surgical closure involves the placement of a pericardial or Dacron patch through a

minimally invasive approach (with or without robotic assistance). Surgical closure of ASD improves function status, exercise capacity, and patient survival; however, it does not prevent atrial fibrillation or stroke, especially if patients pursue ASD repair after age 40.

- Cox maze procedure should be considered for patients with intermittent or chronic atrial fibrillation when they undergo ASD closure.

DISPOSITION

- Mortality rate increases in patients with large ASDs that go untreated. Complications of longstanding ASD include RV failure, arrhythmias, paradoxical embolism, and PAH leading to right-to-left shunting (Eisenmenger syndrome).
- Patients with small shunts (<1.5:1) have a normal life expectancy.
- Spontaneous closure or size reduction is more likely in younger patients with defects <10 mm in diameter.
- A basic assessment for adults with congenital heart disease should include systemic arterial oximetry, ECG, chest radiograph, transthoracic echocardiography, and blood tests for complete blood count and coagulation screen.
- Intracardiac shunts constitute moderate risk for noncardiac procedures. High-risk features include severe systolic dysfunction (ejection fraction <35%), severe pulmonary hypertension, cyanotic heart disease, and severe left-side outlet obstruction.
- Annual postoperative clinical follow-up is recommended for patients who pursue ASD repair as adults in order to monitor for PAH, atrial arrhythmias, RV or LV dysfunction, and coexisting valvular lesions.
- Preoperative atrial fibrillation is a risk factor for both postoperative and long-term atrial fibrillation. The older the patient undergoing ASD repair, the more likely that patient is to develop atrial fibrillation, even after the ASD is repaired.
  1. The benefits of ASD repair include improved functional status and exercise capacity, improved survival (if closed in childhood), improved quality of life, prevention of right-sided heart failure, and prevention of PAH.
  2. Potential mid- to long-term complications of ASD closure in adulthood include tachyarrhythmias (atrial fibrillation or atrial flutter), bradyarrhythmias (sinus node dysfunction or heart block), stroke (greater risk in older patients), residual ASDs (due to incomplete initial closure or patch dehiscence), right-sided heart failure, PAH (risk is correlated with the size of the original defect and inversely related to age at time of closure), mitral valve regurgitation or subaortic stenosis (associated with primum ASDs), device migration/erosion, and pulmonary venous congestion.
  3. Women with ASD have an increased risk of paradoxical embolus, stroke, arrhythmia, and heart failure during pregnancy. ASD repair before pregnancy reduces these risks. However, if ASD is undiagnosed before pregnancy, close monitoring for the duration of pregnancy is sufficient. The only contraindication to pregnancy in women with ASD is severe PAH.
  4. Scuba diving is contraindicated in patients with unrepaired ASDs because the pressure from deep sea diving increases the risk of paradoxical emboli. In addition, high-altitude climbing should be avoided because it can lead to right-to-left shunting and oxygen desaturation.
- In regard to infective endocarditis prophylaxis for dental procedures:
  1. Prophylaxis is not indicated for an unrepaired ASD.
  2. Prophylaxis is indicated for 6 mo following ASD repair if prosthetic material was used to repair the defect.
  3. Prophylaxis is indicated for a repaired ASD (or any congenital heart defect) if residual defects remain either at or near the site of the prosthetic material or device used for repair.

The estrogen-containing oral contraceptive pill is not recommended in acute congenital heart disease patients at risk for thromboembolism. This includes patients with atrial fibrillation, severe PAH, Fontan repair, or cyanosis related to an intracardiac shunt.

SUGGESTED READINGS

Available at ExpertConsult.com

RELATED CONTENT

Atrial Septal Defect (ASD) (Patient Information)

AUTHORS: **Zain Kassam, MD,** and **Craig L. Basman, MD**

BASIC INFORMATION

DEFINITION

Attention-deficit/hyperactivity disorder (ADHD) is a chronic disorder of inattention and/or hyperactivity or impulsivity. Symptoms must be present before 12 yr of age, last at least 6 mo, and cause functional impairment in multiple settings (e.g., school, home, with friends). The diagnostic keys for ADHD are described in Table 1.

SYNONYMS

Hyperactivity
Attention deficit disorder (ADD)
ADHD

ICD-10CM CODES

F90.0	Attention-deficit/hyperactivity disorder, predominantly inattentive type
F90.1	Attention-deficit/hyperactivity disorder, predominantly hyperactive/impulsive type
F90.2	Attention-deficit/hyperactivity disorder, combined type
F90.8	Attention-deficit/hyperactivity disorder, other type
F90.9	Attention-deficit/hyperactivity disorder, unspecified type

DSM-5 CODES

314.00	Predominantly inattentive presentation
314.01	Predominantly hyperactive-impulsive presentation

EPIDEMIOLOGY & DEMOGRAPHICS

PREVALENCE: 8% to 12% of school-aged children (most prevalent neurodevelopmental disorder among children); up to 14% of adolescents and 3% to 5% of adults. Children from families with low socioeconomic status and children with public insurance are diagnosed with ADHD at higher rates than their peers.

PREDOMINANT SEX: Among children, male predominance with ratio of 2:1 to 4:1. Among adults, ratio is closer to 1:1 (sex difference may reflect referral bias).

PREDOMINANT AGE: Some symptoms must occur before age 12 yr. Symptoms (especially hyperactivity symptoms) tend to diminish with age. Up to 80% continue to meet criteria in adolescence, and an estimated 35% to 65% have some symptoms in adulthood.

PEAK INCIDENCE: Diagnosis is usually first made in school-aged children (6 to 9 yr).

RISK FACTORS: Possible risk factors include in utero tobacco/alcohol/illicit substance exposure or hypoxia, low birth weight, prematurity, genetics, lead exposure (though most children with elevated lead levels do not develop ADHD), head trauma in young children, family dysfunction, low socioeconomic status. Evidence supports possible association between dietary factors (e.g., refined sugar, food additives) and ADHD in a small percentage of patients. A causal link between environmental toxins and ADHD has not been clearly established.

GENETICS: Strong polygenetic component. First-degree relatives of ADHD patients have 2-6 times greater risk of ADHD relative to controls. Studies suggest potential involvement of several genes, including those associated with serotonin and glutamate transporters as well as dopamine metabolism in addition to neuronal development.

TABLE 1 Diagnostic Keys for Attention Deficit Hyperactivity Disorder

1. Inattention
   a. Careless mistakes in schoolwork, work, or other activities
   b. Seems not to listen when spoken to directly
   c. Poor follow-through on schoolwork or chores
   d. Difficulty organizing
   e. Easily distracted by extraneous stimuli and is forgetful
2. Hyperactivity
   a. Trouble sitting still
   b. May act as if "driven by a motor"
   c. May talk excessively
3. Impulsivity
   a. Trouble holding back in class
   b. Trouble taking turns
   c. Interrupts

PHYSICAL FINDINGS & CLINICAL PRESENTATION

- Three types:
  1. Predominantly inattentive: Difficulty organizing, planning, remembering, concentrating, starting/completing tasks; symptoms may not be present during preferred activities
  2. Predominantly hyperactive/impulsive: Edgy/restless, talkative, disruptive/intrusive, disinhibited, impatient
  3. Combined
- Usually diagnosed in elementary school when achievement is compromised and behavioral problems are not tolerated. Children with academic underproductivity, problems with peer and family relations, or discipline issues are often referred for evaluation. Of the more than six million children in the U.S. who have ADHD, most have comorbid conditions (see the following) and nearly half use special education and mental health services.
- Up to 64% may have associated disorders such as psychiatric diagnoses (oppositional defiant disorder, autism spectrum disorder, depression, anxiety), learning disabilities, or substance abuse disorders.
- In adults, motoric hyperactivity is less common, but restlessness, edginess, and difficulty relaxing are often seen. Disorganization and difficulty completing tasks are other common complaints.

ETIOLOGY

Strongest evidence exists for genetic inheritance. Other theories include abnormal metabolism of brain catecholamines, delayed maturation of cerebral cortex, altered reward processing, and disrupted default mode network, as well as environmental factors (see earlier).

Dx DIAGNOSIS

DIFFERENTIAL DIAGNOSIS

- Medical: Visual/hearing impairment, seizure disorder, head injury, sleep disorder, medication interactions, intellectual disability, specific learning disorder, autism spectrum disorder/development delay, thyroid abnormalities, lead toxicity, movement disorders
- Psychiatric: Depression, bipolar disorder, disruptive mood dysregulation disorder, anxiety, obsessive-compulsive disorder, oppositional defiant disorder, intermittent explosive disorder, conduct disorder, posttraumatic stress disorder, reactive attachment disorder, and substance abuse disorder
- Psychosocial: Mismatch of learning environment with ability, family dysfunction, abuse/neglect

WORKUP

- Clinical interview should include assessment of symptoms and impact on work/school and relationships; developmental history; personal and family psychiatric history, including substance abuse; social history, including family dysfunction; medical history, including personal or family history of cardiac conditions.
- Physical examination should be performed to investigate medical causes for symptoms, coexisting conditions, and contraindications to treatment. Special focus should be paid to evaluation of dysmorphic features; neurologic examination, including assessment for neurocutaneous findings; and assessment of hearing and vision.
- Information from collateral sources (parents, partners, teachers) is crucial to diagnosis. Many patients will not display symptoms during an office visit and may underreport or overreport symptoms.
- Self-rating scales and standardized symptom-specific questionnaires from collateral sources can help diagnose and assess response to treatment. The use of ADHD-specific rating scales over broader behavioral rating scales is associated with improved sensitivity and specificity.
- Laboratory or imaging studies should be undertaken only if indicated by history or physical examination.
- The FDA has approved a quantitative electroencephalogram test to aid in the diagnosis of ADHD in children, but sufficient evidence to support its routine use is lacking.
- Ancillary testing (e.g., neuropsychological testing including verbal and performance IQ/achievement testing and language evaluation, and mental health assessment) may be indicated based on clinical findings and may require referral.

Rx TREATMENT

NONPHARMACOLOGIC THERAPY

- The majority of studies comparing the efficacy of pharmacologic vs. nonpharmacologic interventions demonstrate the superiority of pharmacologic treatments. Proposed interventions have included restrictive or elimination diets, artificial food color exclusions, free fatty acid supplementation, cognitive training, neurofeedback, and focused behavioral interventions.
- Studies on combined treatments have not shown significant improvements in core ADHD symptoms when behavioral treatments are added to stimulant medications. However, improvements in related areas such as parent-child relations, aggressiveness, teacher-rated social skills, and reaching achievement have been seen in combined treatment groups.
- Prevailing opinion favors a multimodal approach in which nonpharmacologic behavioral therapies including parent-child behavioral therapy and social skills training can be used to target comorbid conditions or behaviors that have not responded to medication.
- Behavioral therapy/interventions alone are often considered when children are under 6 yr, symptoms and impairment are mild, if parents are opposed to or patients cannot tolerate medications, or if there is uncertainty or disagreement about the diagnosis (e.g., between parents and teachers).
- Educational interventions are recommended. Children with ADHD are entitled to reasonable educational accommodations under a 504 Plan or the Individuals with Disabilities Education Act.
- Behavioral interventions (e.g., goal setting and rewards systems) show short-term efficacy and are endorsed by most national organizations. Time management and organizational skills appear useful. Social skills training may also be useful.
- Psychotherapy such as cognitive therapy, play therapy, or insight-oriented therapy are unlikely to be useful in addressing the core symptoms of ADHD.
- Digital therapeutics are emerging for the treatment of ADHD. One digital therapeutic, delivered through a video game format, has been approved by the FDA for treatment of ADHD.
- Elimination diets are not routinely recommended.
- Many support and advocacy groups provide education and other resources (e.g., Children and Adolescents with ADHD, National ADD Association, American Academy of Child and Adolescent Psychiatry).

ACUTE GENERAL Rx

- Most studies on treatment of ADHD are performed in children; less data available on adults.
- Mainstay of treatment is stimulant medication. Second-line therapies include antidepressants and alpha-agonists. Table 2 summarizes FDA-approved treatments for ADHD.
- Stimulants:
    1. Release or block uptake of dopamine and norepinephrine
    2. Include short- and long-acting methylphenidate, dextroamphetamine, and dextroamphetamine/amphetamine combinations (mixed amphetamine salts). A methylphenidate patch (Daytrana) is available, as is a pro-drug form of dextroamphetamine, lisdexamfetamine (Vyvanse), which is designed to limit the abuse potential. A long-acting oral suspension of methylphenidate (Quillivant XR), a long-acting chewable tablet of methylphenidate (QuilliChew ER), a long-acting orally disintegrating tablet of mixed amphetamine preparation (Adzenys XR-ODT), and a long-acting liquid amphetamine preparation (Dyanavel XR) are also available.
    3. All stimulants equally effective; however, not all patients improve with stimulants. Patients who do not respond well to one stimulant may respond to another.
    4. Do not cause euphoria or lead to addiction when taken as directed.
    5. Improve cognition, inattention, impulsiveness/hyperactivity, and driving skills. Limited impact on academic performance, learning, and emotional problems.
    6. Side effects are usually mild, reversible, and dose dependent, including anorexia, weight loss, sleep disturbances, increased heart rate and blood pressure, irritability, moodiness, headache, onset or worsening of motor tics, reduction of growth velocity (but not adult height). Do not worsen seizures in patients on adequate anticonvulsant therapy. Rebound of symptoms can occur with withdrawal of medication.
    7. Stimulants are associated with an increased risk of cardiovascular events and death. Patients should be carefully evaluated for cardiovascular disease before beginning therapy and be periodically monitored, including blood pressure checks, while they are treated. However, despite concerns regarding cardiovascular risk, these medications are generally safe. Recent studies have shown that among young and middle-aged adults, current or new use of ADHD medications, compared with nonuse or remote use, is not associated with an increased risk of serious cardiovascular events. Routine, pre-treatment screening with ECGs is not currently recommended by the American Academy of Pediatrics or the American Academy of Child and Adolescent Psychiatry.
    8. There are reports of psychotic or manic symptoms (particularly hallucinations) associated with stimulant use in children and adolescents, emerging in <1% of treated children (1 in 400 to 1 in 600).
- Atomoxetine (Strattera):
    1. Selective norepinephrine reuptake inhibitor
    2. Generally felt to be less effective than stimulants, but a useful alternative in patients who have not tolerated or responded to stimulants or in the setting of patient or family substance abuse.
    3. Efficacy and safety of use beyond 2 yr of treatment have not been studied. There have been reports of behavioral abnormalities and increased suicidality in children and adolescents.
    4. Side effects: Gastrointestinal upset, sleep disturbance, decreased appetite, dizziness, sexual side effects in men. Cardiovascular side effects have also been reported.
    5. There have been rare reports of severe liver injury in adults and children.
- Antidepressants (bupropion, imipramine, desipramine, nortriptyline):
    1. May be useful in patients with coexisting psychiatric disorders.
    2. Studies comparing efficacy versus stimulants are inconclusive.
    3. Side effects: Arrhythmias, anticholinergic effects, lowering of seizure threshold, insomnia.
- Alpha-2-adrenergic agonists (clonidine, guanfacine):
    1. Appear to be less effective than stimulants, but may be particularly useful as an adjunctive treatment to stimulants, particularly in patients with a partial stimulant response or who experience side effects such as sleep disturbance or concurrent symptoms of overarousal, irritability, or aggression.
    2. Extended-release formulations of guanfacine (Intuniv) and clonidine (Kapvay) have been approved by the FDA for treatment of ADHD in children ages 6 to 17r. A transdermal clonidine patch is also available.
    3. Potential side effects include sedation, fatigue, headache, bradycardia, hypotension, rebound hypertension, and depression.
- Use of medications, particularly stimulants (which are monitored under the Controlled Substance Act), requires frequent monitoring.

DISPOSITION

- Although symptoms may change over time, for many patients ADHD represents a chronic condition that requires lifelong management.
- Patients are at higher risk for academic underachievement, lower socioeconomic status, work and relationship difficulties, high-risk behavior, and psychiatric comorbidities.

REFERRAL

- Diagnosis complicated by difficult-to-treat comorbid psychiatric conditions, developmental disorders, or mental retardation
- Lack of adequate response to stimulants/atomoxetine/alpha-adrenergic agents

TABLE 2 Select FDA-Approved Treatments for Attention Deficit Hyperactivity Disorder

Generic Name	Brand Name	Formulations and Strengths	Duration of Behavioral Effect (hr)	Comments
Amphetamines				
D-amphetamine	Dexedrine	Tablets: 5, 10 mg	3-6	
	Dexedrine Spansule	Spansules: 5, 10, 15 mg		
	ProCentra	Oral solution: 5 mg/5 ml		
Mixed amphetamine/dextroamphetamine	Adderall	Tablets: 5, 7.5, 10, 12.5, 15, 20, 30 mg	4-6	
	Adderall XR	Capsules: 5, 10, 15, 20, 25, 30 mg	8-10	Capsule with 1:1 ratio of IR to DR beads
	Evekeo	Tablets: 5, 10 mg	10	Racemic amphetamine sulfate, 1:1 D-amphetamine and L-amphetamine
	Dyanavel	Oral suspension: 2.5 mg/ml	8-13	Shake the bottle before administering the dose
Lisdexamfetamine dimesylate	Vyvanse	Capsules: 20, 30, 40, 50, 60, 70 mg	8-12	Inactive prodrug in which L-lysine is chemically bonded to D-amphetamine
Methylphenidates				
Methylphenidate	Ritalin	Tablets: 5, 10, 20 mg	3-4	
	Methylin	Tablets, chewable: 2.5, 5, 10 mg	3-4	
		Oral solution: 5 mg/5 ml, 10 mg/5 ml (500 ml)	3-4	
	Ritalin LA	Capsules: 10, 20, 30, 40 mg	8-9	Capsule with 1:1 ratio of IR beads to DR beads
	Metadate ER	Tablets: 10, 20 mg	5-8	
	Metadate CD	Capsules: 10, 20, 30 mg	8-9	Capsule with 3:7 ratio of IR beads to DR beads
	Concerta	Tablets: 18, 27, 36, 54 mg	8-12	Ascending profile, OROS technology
	Daytrana	Transdermal patch: 10, 15, 20, 30 mg/9 hr	9	Delivery rate of 1.1, 1.6, 2.2, 3.3 mg/hr for the patches, respectively, based on 9-hr wear times in patients ages 6-12 yr
	Quillivant XR	Oral suspension: 25 mg/ 5 ml	8-12	Shake the bottle before administering the dose
	QuilliChew ER	Chewable tablets: 20, 30, 40 mg	8	
	Aptensio XR	Capsules: 10, 15, 20, 30, 40, 50, 60 mg	9-12	May be swallowed or opened and contents mixed into food.
	Adhansia XR	Capsules: 25, 35, 45, 55, 70, 85 mg	IR portion: 1.5-2.5 DR portion: 8.5-16	IR layer with 20% of dose, controlled release layer with 80%
Dexmethylphenidate	Focalin	Tablets: 2.5, 5, 10 mg	IR: 0.5-4	*d-threo*-enantiomer of methylphenidate, twice as potent as racemic methylphenidate; XR capsule contains IR component
	Focalin XR	Capsules: 5, 10, 20 mg	XR: 6.5-12	
Nonstimulant Medications				
Atomoxetine	Strattera	Capsules: 10, 18, 25, 40, 60, 80, 100 mg		Steady state requires 4-6 wk to see effect
Guanfacine	Intuniv	Tablets: 1, 2, 3, 4 mg	8	
Clonidine	Kapvay	Tablets: 0.1, 0.2 mg	12-24	
Digital Therapeutics				
Digital Attention Treatment	EndeavorRx			Video game platform, improves attention

DR, Delayed-release; *IR,* immediate-release; *OROS,* osmotic-controlled release oral delivery system.
Adapted from Stern TA et al: *Massachusetts General Hospital handbook of general hospital psychiatry,* ed 7, Philadelphia, 2018, Elsevier.

PEARLS & CONSIDERATIONS

- The World Health Organization's Adult Self-Report Scale (ASRS) v1.1 has good sensitivity and adaptability to the primary care setting.
- Among adults with persistent ADHD symptoms treated with medication, trials have shown that the use of cognitive behavioral therapy compared with relaxation with educational support resulted in improved ADHD symptoms, which were maintained at 12 mo.
- ADHD has been associated with criminal behavior in some studies. Data analysis has shown that among patients with ADHD, rates of criminality are lower during periods when they receive ADHD medication.
- Recommendations for the diagnosis and management of ADHD have been published by the Centers for Disease Control and Prevention (www.cdc.gov/ncbddd/adhd/guidelines.html).

SUGGESTED READINGS

Available at ExpertConsult.com

RELATED CONTENT

Attention Deficit Hyperactivity Disorder (ADHD) (Patient Information)

AUTHORS: **Nicole M. Benson, MD,** and **Judith A. Restrepo, MD**

Autism Spectrum Disorder (PTG)

BASIC INFORMATION

DEFINITION

Autism spectrum disorder (ASD) encompasses a continuum of developmental disabilities characterized by marked social and behavioral impairment. Box 1 describes the diagnostic keys and case determination criteria under *Diagnostic and Statistical Manual of Mental Disorders* (DSM-5). There is usually impairment in several domains integral to social functioning, including language, nonverbal communication, and social interactions. Restricted/repetitive interests and behaviors, as well as sensory issues (e.g., hypersensitivity), also are prominent. Comorbid intellectual disability, neurological and medical problems, and an increased risk of psychiatric disorders are frequently present in ASD. Both core and associated features can vary dramatically among individuals. In addition, timing of onset can differ, as about one quarter of children with ASD are noted to lose skills after developing normally for as long as 2 yr, whereas others present with delays across most developmental domains within the first yr of life. The majority of children with ASD are identified through primary care screening by age 2, generally for having failed to achieve developmental milestones for communication. However, gender and cognitive, linguistic, and adaptive functioning impact ASD presentation and can affect age of diagnosis. DSM-5 criteria no longer differentiate separate disorders. Instead, an overarching diagnosis of ASD is given; severity levels (1, 2, or 3) have been introduced to identify the magnitude of social and behavioral impairment and the support required to ensure the safety and well-being of the individual. Specifiers have been added to capture associated features (e.g., intellectual disability, language impairment, medical or genetic conditions, and catatonia).

SYNONYMS

ASD
Autism
Autistic disorder
Early infantile autism
Childhood autism
Kanner autism
Asperger disorder
Pervasive developmental disorder
Pervasive developmental disorder–not otherwise specified (PDD-NOS)

ICD-10CM CODE
F84.0 Autism spectrum disorder
DSM-5 CODE
299.00 Autism spectrum disorder

EPIDEMIOLOGY & DEMOGRAPHICS

INCIDENCE (IN U.S.): Autism spectrum disorder afflicts an estimated 1% to 3% of children in the United States.

PREVALENCE (IN U.S.): Approximately 1:54 (1:34 for boys, 1:145 for girls). Prevalence has increased over the past few decades. It is unclear whether this increase reflects an expansion of the diagnosis to include subthreshold cases, increased awareness of the disorder, improvement in diagnostic accuracy, changes in public policy related to service eligibility, or a true increase in the frequency of autism spectrum disorder.

PREDOMINANT SEX AND AGE: Male:female ratio of 3 to 4:1; Lifelong.

PEAK INCIDENCE: Before age 3 yr.

RISK FACTORS: Prenatal and perinatal risk factors identified include hypoxia-related obstetric complications, prenatal infections, maternal use of certain medications (e.g., valproic acid) during pregnancy, maternal health conditions such as diabetes and hypertension, advanced parental age, multiple birth, preterm birth, congenital sensory deficits, and significant exposure to air pollution (during pregnancy and in the postnatal period). However, it is not established whether any of these are causal factors.

GENETICS:
- Autism spectrum disorder is highly inheritable with an estimated heritability index of about 83%.
- The concordance rate for ASD varies across studies and ranges from 36% to 95% for monozygotic twins; the concordance rate is estimated between 20% and 40% for dizygotic twins and between 10% and 20% for nontwin siblings.
- A variety of genetic variations, including copy number and single nucleotide variants, have been identified, but each is rare (accounting for no more than 1% of cases). Genetic variations have been identified in up to 25% of cases, in aggregate.
- The general consensus is that ASD arises from a combination of genetic susceptibility, epigenetic factors, and environmental influences.

PHYSICAL FINDINGS & CLINICAL PRESENTATION

- Common triad of marked impairment in social interactions (poor social-emotional reciprocity), impaired and atypical verbal and nonverbal communication, and repetitive and unusual behavior or play
- Marked impairment in the understanding and use of both verbal and nonverbal communication,

BOX 1 Autism Spectrum Disorder (ASD) Case Determination Criteria under DSM-5

DSM-5 Behavioral Criteria	
A. Persistent deficits in social communication and social interaction	A1: Deficits in social emotional reciprocity A2. Deficits in nonverbal communicative behaviors A3. Deficits in developing, maintaining, and understanding relationships
A. Restricted, repetitive patterns of behavior, interests, or activities, currently or by history	B1: Stereotyped or repetitive motor movements, use of objects or speech B2. Insistence on sameness, inflexible adherence to routines, or ritualized patterns of verbal or nonverbal behavior B3. Highly restricted interests that are abnormal in intensity or focus B4. Hyper- or hyporeactivity to sensory input or unusual interest in sensory aspects of the environment
Historical PDD diagnosis	Any ASD diagnosis documented in a comprehensive evaluation, including a DSM-IV diagnosis of autistic disorder, Asperger disorder, or pervasive developmental disorder–not otherwise specified (PDD-NOS)
DSM-5 case determination	All three behavioral criteria coded under part A, and at least two behavioral criteria coded under part B OR Any ASD diagnosis documented in a comprehensive evaluation, whether based on DSM-IV-TR or DSM-5 diagnostic criteria NOTE: A child might be disqualified from meeting the DSM-5 surveillance case definition for ASD if, based on the clinical judgment of one or more reviewers, there is insufficient or conflicting information in support of ASD, sufficient information to rule out ASD, or if one or more other diagnosed conditions better account for the child's symptoms.

DSM-IV, *Diagnostic and Statistical Manual of Mental Disorders, Fourth Edition*; DSM-IV-TR, *Diagnostic and Statistical Manual of Mental Disorders, Fourth Edition, Text Revision*; DSM-5, *Diagnostic and Statistical Manual of Mental Disorders, Fifth Edition*; *PDD*, pervasive developmental disorder

From Baio J et al: Prevalence of autism spectrum disorder among children aged 8 years—Autism and Developmental Disabilities Monitoring Network, 11 Sites, United States, 2014. MMWR Surveill Summ 67(No. SS-6):1-23, 2018. https://dx.doi.org/10.15585/mmwr.ss6706a1.

BOX 2 Red Flags for Social Communication Development

Prompt evaluation should occur for any of the following: **No vocalizations by 6 mo:** *A parent should be able to have a reciprocal "conversation" by this age, consisting of at least several volleys back and forth.* **No polysyllabic consonant babbling by 12 mo:** *At least some of these vocalizations should be directed at someone with communicative intent.* **No gestures by 12 mo:** *The earliest gesture an infant learns is to raise his/her arms to request to be picked up, usually once sitting independently. Pointing should be with an isolated index finger, not the whole hand, and should be used "to request" or "to show," not just pointing at pictures in a book or pointing to have an adult label items. Any use of hand-over-hand by the child (e.g., putting a parent's hand on the cabinet door where the cookies are kept or using the parent's hand to point at pictures in a book) is a hallmark of ASD.* **No spontaneous (not echoed) single words by 16 mo other than mama or dada:** *Spontaneous words must be beyond those used to simply label items and must be used by the child to communicate, to request, to show, or to share.* **No spontaneous (not echoed) phrases by 24 mo or sentences by 36 mo:** *Spontaneous phrases and sentences must be used by the child to communicate, to request, to show, or to share.* **Any loss of social communication abilities, including babbling, single words, phrases, response to name, social engagement, or gestures:** *If a parent reports their infant has decreased or stopped any social communication milestones, this is usually the hallmark of the onset of regression.*

From Swaiman KF et al: *Swaiman's pediatric neurology, principles and practice*, ed 6, Philadelphia, 2017, Elsevier.

including unchanging facial expression and lack of gestures during interactions
- Stereotypic behavior (e.g., hand flapping, body rocking) or language (e.g., echolalia)
- Perceptual hypersensitivity (i.e., auditory, tactile, olfactory, gustatory) and avoidance of novel stimuli; or perceptual hyposensitivity (e.g., abnormally high threshold for pain)
- Brain abnormalities have been identified at anatomical and functional levels; abnormalities are detected as early as the first yr of life and are accompanied by atypical brain maturation trajectories
- No biomarkers have been identified

ETIOLOGY

- Majority of cases are not associated with a comorbid medical condition
- High prevalence of comorbid seizure disorder and intellectual disability
- Sometimes present in the context of medical conditions (e.g., encephalitis, cytomegalovirus, toxoplasmosis, phenylketonuria [PKU], fragile X syndrome, tuberous sclerosis complex, neurofibromatosis)
- Numerous studies have shown **no** association between immunizations (specifically MMR vaccine) or thimerosal-containing vaccines (i.e., diphtheria, pertussis, and tetanus) and autism spectrum disorder

Dx DIAGNOSIS

DIFFERENTIAL DIAGNOSIS

- Several genetic syndromes manifest with a phenotype similar to ASD (e.g., 22q11.2 deletion syndrome, Angelman syndrome, Aicardi syndrome, Cornelia de Lange syndrome, Christianson syndrome, fragile X syndrome, Landau-Kleffner syndrome, Klinefelter syndrome, neurofibromatosis, Prader-Willi syndrome, Rett syndrome, tuberous sclerosis complex, Williams syndrome).
- Several psychiatric or neurodevelopmental disorders present with some symptoms similar to ASD (e.g., ADHD, Tourette syndrome, selective mutism, catatonia, social phobia, obsessive/compulsive disorder, expressive language disorder, mixed receptive-expressive language disorder, stereotypic movement disorder, intellectual disability). Notable differences are present in age of onset and developmental trajectories.
- Social (pragmatic) communication disorder: Introduced in DSM-5 and characterized by significant difficulties with verbal and nonverbal communication (but without restricted/repetitive interests and behaviors).
- Attachment disorders: Individuals with these disorders can present with language delays, cognitive delays, social difficulties, and stereotypies, often in the context of early childhood neglect.

WORKUP

- Rule out underlying medical condition, including genetic syndromes.
- "Red flags" for critical delays in social communication development should be recognized or queried and should initiate evaluation for an ASD (Box 2). Validated autism spectrum disorder–specific screening tools are available for children age ≥18 mo. All children should be screened specifically for ASD at 18 and 24 mo. General developmental screening tools are currently used in children 9 to 18 mo.
- Gold standard assessment includes detailed developmental and family history, assessment of developmental/intellectual functioning, assessment of ASD symptomatology, and assessment of adaptive behaviors.
- Additional workup may include assessment of language functioning, neuropsychological functioning, and psychiatric presentation.

LABORATORY TESTS

- PKU screen (usually done at birth in the United States)
- Lead exposure screening
- Audiology testing for young children with ASD; school-based hearing screening may be sufficient in older children with autism spectrum disorders and without significant language or learning deficits
- Karyotype, chromosome microarray analysis, and DNA testing for fragile X syndrome in both boys and girls, as well as for different de novo copy number variants or mutations in specific genes associated with the disorder

IMAGING STUDIES

- Electroencephalogram to diagnose coexisting seizure disorder if seizures are suspected or if language regression is present (i.e., Landau-Kleffner syndrome).
- Brain MRI if tuberous sclerosis complex or Aicardi syndrome (callosal agenesis) is suspected.

Rx TREATMENT

NONPHARMACOLOGIC THERAPY

- Consistent behavioral training program in both the home and school environments
- A number of treatment programs have been developed; many are based on applied behavioral analysis (ABA) (e.g., Discrete Trial Training); others combine ABA procedures with social-emotional development (e.g., Pivotal Response Training, Floortime, Early Start Denver Model)
- Special educational program focused on language and communication skills, social and life skills development (e.g., TEACCH)
- Cognitive-Behavioral Therapy (CBT) has proven effective to ameliorate symptoms of anxiety in higher functioning individuals with ASD
- Highly structured home and school environments
- Education for families and teachers; the Autism Speaks™ website may be helpful in this regard: www.autismspeaks.org

ACUTE GENERAL Rx

- Obsessive or ritualistic behaviors: Selective serotonin reuptake inhibitors (SSRIs), atypical antipsychotics, valproic acid
- Aggression, irritability, self-injury: Atypical antipsychotics (e.g., risperidone, aripiprazole), alpha-2 agonists (e.g., clonidine), anticonvulsant mood stabilizers, opiate antagonist (self-injury only)
- Hyperactivity, impulsivity, inattention: Stimulants, alpha-2 agonists (e.g., clonidine), atypical antipsychotics
- Anxiety: SSRIs, buspirone, mirtazapine
- Mood lability: Valproic acid, carbamazepine, lithium, aripiprazole
- Depression: SSRIs, mirtazapine
- Catatonia: Avoid antipsychotics, which make catatonia worse and potentially malignant, and use lorazepam; if unsuccessful, electroconvulsive therapy may be indicated
- Only risperidone and aripiprazole are FDA-approved for the management of symptoms associated with ASD
- Medications used to decrease specific symptoms associated with Autism Spectrum Disorder are summarized in Table 1

TABLE 1 Medications Used to Decrease Specific Symptoms Associated with Autism Spectrum Disorder*

Drug	Dose	Age†	N	Efficacy	Side Effects
Neuroleptic Agents					
Risperidone	0.25-2.5 mg/d <20 kg 0.5-2.5 mg/d 20-45 kg 0.5-3.5 mg/d >45 kg Mean = 2.4 mg/d	5-17	101	Decreased tantrums, aggression, self-injury, hyperactivity	Weight gain, increased appetite, transient sedation
Risperidone	1.2-2.9 mg/d child Mean = 2.0 mg/d 2.4-5.3 mg/d adult Mean = 3.6 mg/d	8-56	36	Decreased irritability, hyperactivity	Increased appetite, weight gain, sedation
Risperidone	0.125-0.175 vs. 1.25-1.75 vs. placebo	5-17	96	Higher dose improves global function and irritability	Somnolence sedation increased appetite
Risperidone	0.01-0.06 mg/kg/d Mean = 1.17 mg/d	5-12	79	Decreased irritability, hyperactivity, noncompliance, conduct problems	Weight gain, transient somnolence, mildly increased heart rate and blood pressure
Risperidone	0.5-1.5 mg/d Mean = 1.14 mg/d	2.5-6	24	Minimal improvement in global autism severity scores	Weight gain, increased prolactin levels
Risperidone	1.0-10.0 mg/d	18-43	n =?	Reduced repetitive behavior, aggression, self-injury, property destruction	Transient sedation
Aripiprazole	5 mg/d, 10 mg/d, or 15 mg/d	6-17	218	Reduced irritability, hyperactivity, stereotypy at all doses	Sedation, EPS, weight gain
Aripiprazole	2-15 mg/d	6-17	98	Reduced irritability, hyperactivity, stereotypy, inappropriate speech, global improvement	Decreased prolactin level, weight gain, EPS
Aripiprazole	2-15 mg/d continuation active tx vs. placebo	6-17	85	No difference in time to relapse	
Opiate Antagonists					
Naltrexone	1.0 mg/kg/d	3-8	41	No improvement over placebo in behavior and learning; improved hyperactivity	None greater than placebo
Naltrexone	1.0 mg/kg/d 2 wk only	3-8	24	No improvement in communication skills	Transient sedation
Naltrexone	40 mg/d Single dose	3-7	23	Decreased hyperactivity, improved attention	Not reported
Naltrexone	1 mg/kg/dose	3-7	23	Decreased hyperactivity and improved attention by teacher, but not parent, report	No side effects
Serotonin Reuptake Inhibitors					
Fluvoxamine	Mean dose = 276.7 mg/d	18-53	n = 30	Reduced repetitive thoughts and behavior, and aggression; improved social communication	Transient nausea and sedation
Buspirone	2.5 mg or 5 mg/d	2-6	166	Improvement in repetitive behaviors not total ADOS	
Clomipramine	5-10 mg/d	8-17	34	No improvement executive function	Diarrhea, headache, fatigue
Fluoxetine	4.8-20 mg/d Mean = 10.6 mg/d; 0.38 mg/kg/d	5-17	39	Modest reduction in repetitive behaviors, but no improvement in global functioning	Agitation requiring dose reduction
Citalopram	2.5-20 mg/d Mean = 16.5 mg/d	5-17	149	No improvement in repetitive behavior or global functioning	Increased energy, inattention, impulsivity, hyperactivity, stereotypy, diarrhea, insomnia, dry skin
Stimulants					
Methylphenidate	0.125, 0.25, or 0.5 t.i.d. mg/kg/day	5-14	72	Reduced inattention, distractibility, hyperactivity, and impulsivity	Irritability, decreased appetite, difficulty falling asleep, emotional outbursts
Methylphenidate	0.25, 0.5 mg/kg/dose	5-13	33	Positive efforts on social behavior	None discussed
Methylphenidate	10-40 LA AM, 2.5-10 mg afternoon	7-13	24	Decreased hyperactive and impulsive behavior	Loss of appetite, insomnia
Atomoxetine	20-100 mg/d Mean = 44.2 mg/d	5-15	16	Reduced hyperactivity, impulsivity, social withdrawal	Transient nausea and fatigue
Antiseizure Drugs					
Lamotrigine	Mean = 5.0 mg/kg/d	3-11	28	No improvement greater than placebo in disruptive behavior and autism symptoms	Aggression, insomnia, echolalia
Levetiracetam	20-30 mg/kg/d	5-17	20	No improvement in disruptive behavior or irritability	Aggression, agitation
Divalproex sodium	500-1500 mg/d	5-17	13	Reduction in compulsive-type repetitive behavior	Irritability, weight gain, aggression
Divalproex sodium	125 mg QD titrated up to 500 bid	5-17	27	Reduction in irritability	Irritability
Bumetanide	0.5 mg bid	3-11	60	Improved autistic behaviors and global function	Diarrhea, increased irritability

ADOS, Autism Diagnostic Observation Schedule; *EPS*, extrapyramidal symptoms; *LA AM*, L-alpha-acetylmethadol; *QD*, every day; *t.i.d.*, three times per day; *tx*, treatment.
*Includes only double-blind, randomized, placebo-controlled trials.
†Age in years.
From Swaiman KF et al: *Swaiman's pediatric neurology, principles and practice*, ed 6, Philadelphia, 2017, Elsevier.

CHRONIC Rx

- Extended use of medications for acute management of comorbid psychiatric disorder
- Use of medications for comorbid medical conditions, including sleep problems and gastrointestinal problems
- Pharmacotherapy is palliative, not curative, of autism spectrum disorder

COMPLEMENTARY & ALTERNATIVE MEDICINE

- Preliminary evidence is available for effectiveness of melatonin in ameliorating sleep problems.
- Very limited rigorous evidence is available on the effectiveness of complementary and alternative medicine, including nutritional interventions.

DISPOSITION

- Most children will require some degree of assistance as adults.
- DSM-5 identifies three severity levels based on social communication and restricted, repetitive behaviors: Level 1 (requiring support), Level 2 (requiring substantial support), and Level 3 (requiring very substantial support).
- With early diagnosis and proper treatment/support, the prognosis for children without language and intellectual impairment is fair to very good despite lifelong symptoms.
- Poorer outcomes include a lack of joint attention by age 4 yr, a lack of functional speech by age 5 yr, intellectual disability, seizures, comorbid medical or psychiatric syndromes, and a pervasive lack of social relatedness.
- Best outcomes are associated with early identification and treatment, the development of oral communication skills, and the cognitive and behavioral capacity for inclusion in regular education settings with typically developing peers.

REFERRAL

Assistance may be needed in diagnosis (child psychiatrist, clinical psychologist, geneticist, pediatric neurologist, developmental pediatrician), symptom management (speech language pathologist, occupational therapist, behavioral therapist, clinical psychologist), parental teaching (clinical psychologist, psychiatric social worker), and intervention with the school system (educational advocate, attorney).

PEARLS & CONSIDERATIONS

- There is no scientific evidence of a relationship between childhood vaccination and the development of autism spectrum disorder.
- Evidence suggests that a disproportionate number of children with autism spectrum disorder suffer from a variety of medical problems including sleep difficulties, gastrointestinal problems, and oral health problems.
- Psychiatric comorbidities are very prominent across the life span, with estimated prevalence ranging from 30% to 70%.
- The new U.S. Preventive Services Task Force (USPSTF) recommendation on screening for ASD in young children concludes that the current evidence is insufficient to assess the balance of benefits and harms of screening for ASD in young children for whom no concerns of ASD have been raised by their parents or a clinician.
- The American Academy of Pediatrics (AAP) in contrast to the USPSTF recommends screening for ASD at 18 and 24 mo of age with the modified checklist for autism in toddlers (M-CHAT) for initial screening in children up to 30 mo of age.[1]

SUGGESTED READINGS

Available at ExpertConsult.com

RELATED CONTENT

Autism (Patient Information)

AUTHORS: **Kristin Bevington, MD, MEd,** and **Giulia Righi, PhD**

[1]Sanchack KE: Autism spectrum disorder: updated guidelines from the American Academy of Pediatrics, Am Fam Phys 102: 629-631, 2020.

Autoimmune Hepatitis (ALG) (PTG)

BASIC INFORMATION

DEFINITION

Autoimmune hepatitis (AIH) is an immune-mediated, inflammatory liver disease characterized by elevated serum globulin levels (IgG), the presence of circulating characteristic autoantibodies, and the typical histology of interface hepatitis, plasma cell rich infiltration, and lobular hepatitis. Three types have been described:

- Type 1, or "classic," autoimmune hepatitis is the most predominant form in the U.S. and worldwide (80%) and has a bimodal age distribution with peaks between 10 and 20 and 45 and 70 yr of age. Patients are positive for antinuclear antibodies (ANA) and/or anti-smooth muscle antibodies (ASMA) and have specific associated human leukocyte antigen (HLA) haplotypes: DR3, DR4, DR13. Usually excellent treatment response, but variable relapse rates after drug withdrawal; usually need for long-term maintenance therapy.
- Type 2, up to 10% of AIH cases, primarily affects young children between 2 and 14 yr of age, and is characterized by the presence of antibodies to liver/kidney microsomes (anti-LKM-1) or liver cytosol 1. Patients have associated HLA haplotypes: DR3 and DR7. This form is generally more advanced at presentation and is more difficult to treat; need for long-term maintenance therapy is very common.
- Type 3 is seen in up to 10% of AIH cases and is only soluble liver antigen/liver pancreas antigen (SLA/LP) positive. Otherwise, it is very similar to AIH-1. Often, patients are also Ro52-antibody positive. Lifelong immunosuppression in most, if not all patients.

SYNONYMS

Autoimmune chronic active hepatitis
AIH
Chronic active hepatitis
Lupoid hepatitis
Plasma cell hepatitis

ICD-10CM CODES

K75.4 Autoimmune hepatitis
K73.2 Chronic active hepatitis, not elsewhere classified

EPIDEMIOLOGY & DEMOGRAPHICS

- Due to paucity of epidemiological data, the exact incidence and prevalence in the United States is unknown.
- Approximately 100,000 to 200,000 persons affected in the U.S.
- Based on European studies, the incidence of AIH 0.9 to 2/100,000 populations per year, with a prevalence of 11 to 25/100,000 per year.
- Type 1: Age of onset has a bimodal distribution with peaks between 10 and 20 and 45 and 70 yr.
- Type 2: More common in young children 2 to 14 yr of age.
- Occurs predominantly in women.
  1. Type 1 has a female:male ratio of 4:1.
  2. Type 2 has a ratio of 10:1.
- Accounts for 4% to 6% of liver transplants in the U.S.
- Associated with HLA-DRB1*0301 and HLA-DRB1*0401 alleles.

PHYSICAL FINDINGS & CLINICAL PRESENTATION

- The spectrum of AIH presentation is broad and may range anywhere from asymptomatic elevations of liver enzymes to advanced cirrhosis or fulminant liver failure. One third of adults and one half of child patients with AIH have cirrhosis at presentation.
- Symptoms may include fatigue, anorexia, nausea, abdominal pain, pruritus, and arthralgia.
- Autoimmune findings may include arthritis, xerostomia, keratoconjunctivitis, cutaneous vasculitis, and erythema nodosum.
- Patients with advanced disease can show hepatosplenomegaly, ascites, peripheral edema, abnormal bleeding, and jaundice.

ETIOLOGY

- Exact etiology is unknown; liver histology demonstrates T-cell mediated immune attack against hepatocytes.
- Presence of a variety of autoantibodies suggests an autoimmune mechanism.
- Observational studies have supported the idea of the main inflammatory activity being driven by T cells recognizing antigens expressed in the liver.
- There are likely two components involved: Genetic predisposition and an inciting environmental trigger.
- Potential triggering agents such as viruses (hepatitis A, B, C) or drugs (minocycline, nitrofurantoin, biological agents, tumor necrosis factor [TNF] blockade) likely possess some homology similar to liver-specific antigens.

Dx DIAGNOSIS

- A simplified diagnostic criteria for routine clinical practice has been developed by the International Autoimmune Hepatitis Group (see Table 1).
- Suggestive findings on histology: Lymphoplasmacytic infiltrate invading the hepatocyte boundary surrounding the portal triad (limiting plate). Also, a periportal infiltrate may be seen (interface hepatitis). Pericentric necrosis may be present in acute-onset AIH, indistinguishable from drug-induced liver injury (DILI).
- If coexistent findings of cholestatic liver disease on histology, rule out PSC and PBC, consider magnetic resonance cholangiography.
- The European Association for the Study of the Liver guidelines require liver biopsy as part of the diagnostic evaluation.
- The American Association for the Study of Liver Disease (AASLD) approach is to obtain a liver biopsy if the diagnosis is unclear or to assess disease activity prior to initiating treatment.

DIFFERENTIAL DIAGNOSIS

AIH should be considered in any patient with acute or chronic liver disease.

- Acute viral hepatitis (A, B, C, D, E, cytomegalovirus, Epstein-Barr, herpes)
- Chronic viral hepatitis (B, C)
- Toxic hepatitis (alcohol, drugs)
- Primary biliary cirrhosis
- Primary sclerosing cholangitis
- Hemochromatosis
- Nonalcoholic steatohepatitis
- Systemic lupus erythematosus
- Wilson disease
- Alpha-1 antitrypsin deficiency

WORKUP

- History and physical examination with attention to the presence of autoimmune abnormalities such as autoimmune thyroiditis, Graves disease, inflammatory bowel disease, celiac sprue, and rheumatoid arthritis. Fig. 1 illustrates a diagnostic algorithm for autoimmune hepatitis
- Liver function tests and serum gamma-globulins
- Tests for autoantibodies: ANA, ASMA, anti-LKM, SLA/LP
- Liver biopsy for establishing diagnosis and disease severity

LABORATORY TESTS

- Aminotransferases generally elevated and may fluctuate, generally alanine aminotransferase (ALT) > aspartate aminotransferase (AST)
- Bilirubin and alkaline phosphatase moderately elevated or normal
- Elevation of gamma globulin (>2.0 g/dl [20 g/L]) and immunoglobulin G seen in 90% of patients, seen as markers of activity

TABLE 1 Simplified Diagnostic Criteria for Autoimmune Hepatitis

Variable	Cutoff	Points	Cutoff	Points
ANA or SMA	≥1:40	1	≥1:80	2
LKM	N/A	N/A	≥1:40	2
SLA	N/A	N/A	Positive	2
IgG	≥ULN	1	≥1.1 × ULN	2
Histology	Compatible with AIH	1	Typical of AIH	2
Absence of viral hepatitis	N/A	N/A	Yes	2

Maximum number of points for all antibodies = 2, total = 8. Probable AIH ≥6 points, definite AIH ≥7 points. 88% sensitivity and 97% specificity. *AIH,* Autoimmune hepatitis; *ANA,* antinuclear antibody; *IgG,* immunoglobulin G; *LKM,* liver/kidney microsomes; *SLA,* soluble liver antigen; *SMA,* smooth muscle antibody; *ULN,* upper limit of normal.

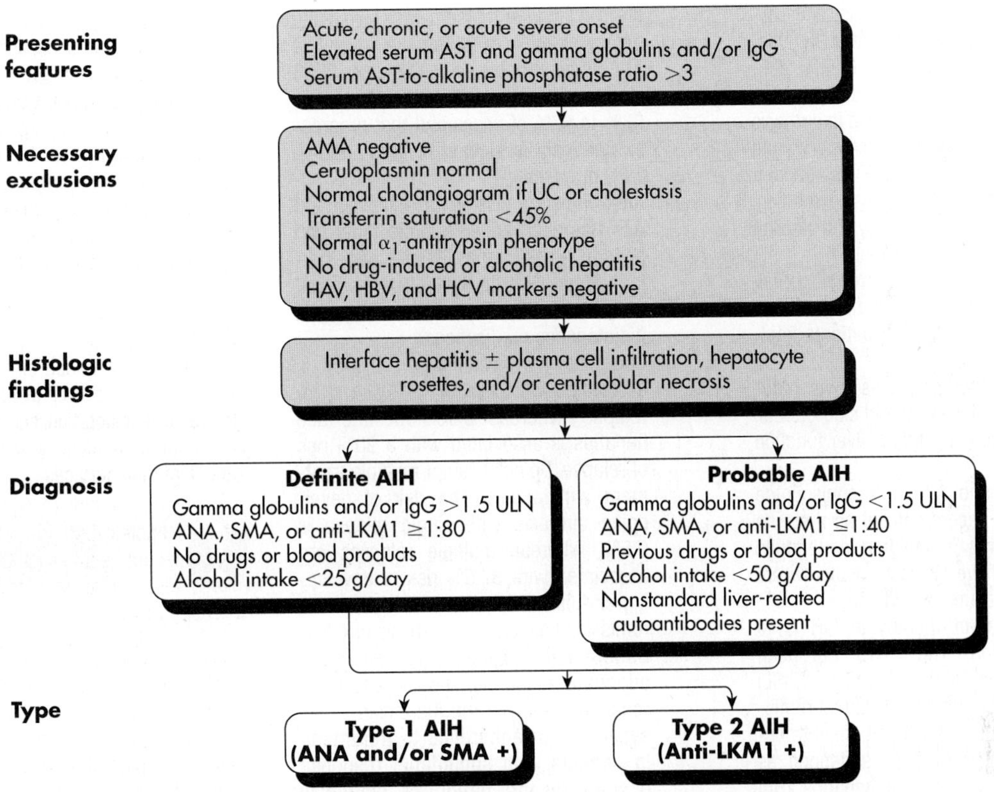

FIG. 1 Diagnostic algorithm for autoimmune hepatitis *(AIH)*. The diagnosis requires exclusion of other hepatic diseases (especially primary biliary cirrhosis, primary sclerosing cholangitis, Wilson disease, hemochromatosis, α1-antitrypsin deficiency, drug-induced or alcoholic hepatitis, and viral hepatitis). Antimitochondrial antibodies *(AMA)* should be absent; cholangiography should be negative in patients with concurrent UC or cholestasis; and the serologic markers of HAV, HBV, and HCV should be negative. Interface hepatitis should be present on histologic examination, and laboratory manifestations of immune reactivity should be evident by abnormal elevation of the serum gamma globulin and/or immunoglobulin G *(IgG)* level and the presence of antinuclear antibodies *(ANA)*, smooth muscle antibodies *(SMA)*, or antibodies to liver kidney microsome type 1 *(anti-LKM1)*. The degree of immune reactivity and the presence of confounding etiologic factors, such as alcohol and drug or blood product exposure, distinguish definite from probable AIH. Classification as type 1 AIH or type 2 AIH is based on the type of autoantibodies that predominate in the disease. *AST*, Aspartate aminotransferase; *HAV*, hepatitis A virus; *HBV*, hepatitis B virus; *HCV*, hepatitis C virus; *UC*, ulcerative cholitis; *ULN*, upper limit of normal. (From Feldman M et al: *Sleisenger and Fortran's gastrointestinal and liver disease*, ed 10, Philadelphia, 2016, Elsevier.)

- Circulating autoantibodies (Table E2) often present:
  1. Rheumatoid factor
  2. ANA:
     a. Present in two thirds of patients
     b. Typical pattern is homogeneous or speckled
     c. Titer does not correlate with the stage, activity, or prognosis
  3. AntiSMA (ASMA):
     a. Found in many but not all patients with AIH
     b. Nonspecific: Found in 4% of patients with elevated liver enzymes and 4% of patients with nonalcoholic steatohepatitis (NASH)
     c. Titer does not correlate with course or prognosis
  4. Anti-LKM antibodies:
     a. Typically found in patients who are ANA negative and SMA negative
     b. Characterizes type 2 AIH
     c. Present in pediatric population and up to 20% of adults in Europe; also present in patients with drug-induced hepatitis
  5. Autoantibodies against soluble liver antigen and liver-pancreas antigen (anti-SLA/LP):
     a. Present in 10% to 30% of patients
     b. Associated with higher rate of relapse after corticosteroid therapy
     c. Several studies suggest that patients with anti-SLA/LP have a more severe course

Serum perinuclear anti-neutrophil cytoplasmic antibodies levels are useful for diagnosis of the 10% to 15% of patients with negative ASMA, negative ANA, and low gamma globulin levels.

- Hypoalbuminemia and prolonged prothrombin time with advanced disease
- There is a well-described overlap syndrome with primary biliary cirrhosis (7%), primary sclerosing cholangitis (6%), and autoimmune cholangitis (11%). In patients who do not respond to therapy after 3 mo, consider cholangiographic studies to evaluate for primary sclerosing cholangitis

IMAGING STUDIES

- Ultrasound of liver and biliary tree to rule out obstruction or hepatic mass
- MR cholangiography if signs of concurrent cholestatic liver disease
- Cirrhosis secondary to AIH is a risk factor for development of hepatocellular carcinoma (although less so than viral hepatitis). Patients with cirrhosis should get ultrasonography and AFP every 6 mo

Rx TREATMENT

NONPHARMACOLOGIC THERAPY

- Avoid alcohol and hepatotoxic medications.
- Liver transplantation is an option for end-stage disease or fulminant hepatic failure.

PHARMACOLOGIC THERAPY

- Initial treatment:
  1. Predniso(lo)ne 0.5 to 1 mg/kg/day followed by addition of azathioprine (AZA) when bilirubin levels are <6 mg/dl, ideally 2 wk after initiation of steroid treatment. Initial dose 50 mg/day, increase depending on toxicity and response up to 1 to 2 mg/kg. A combination of oral budesonide (6 to 9 mg/day) and AZA (1-2 mg/kg/day) can be used to induce and maintain remission in patients with noncirrhotic AIH, with a lower rate of steroid-specific side effects. Treatment of AIH should be response-guided, and regimens should be individualized. Steroids are contraindicated in brittle diabetes mellitus, uncontrolled hypertension, prior steroid

intolerance, severe osteopenia, and psychosis. AZA is contraindicated by thiopurine S-methyltransferase (TPMT) deficiency, leukopenia, or thrombocytopenia. Budesonide is contraindicated in cirrhosis because portal systemic shunting and abnormal hepatic metabolism prevent complete hepatic first-pass extraction, reducing therapeutic efficacy and causing systemic steroid side effects.
2. The AZA metabolite, 6-mercaptopurine, has shown promise in small studies in maintaining remission for patients intolerant of azathioprine.
3. Combination therapy allows lower prednisone doses, fewer steroid side effects, and faster normalization of liver function tests.
4. Budesonide and AZA or predniso(lo)ne and AZA are recommended as first-line AIH treatments in children and adults who do not have cirrhosis, acute severe hepatitis, or acute liver failure.

- The primary goal of therapy in AIH is to achieve remission. The 2015 European Association for the Study of the Liver (EASL) Practice Guideline define biochemical remission as normalization of IgG and aminotransferases. Histologic remission is defined as normal histology or minimal hepatitis (HAI <4 or equivalent) based on the hepatic activity index (HAI). Secondary goals of therapy are the prevention of progression of fibrosis to cirrhosis and reversion of cirrhosis to a lower stage of fibrosis, which has been documented.
- Indications for treatment:
  1. Advanced fibrosis/cirrhosis.
  2. Active disease (HAI >4) on histology.
- Treatment not indicated:
  1. Mild disease with ALT <3× ULN; HAI <4 and no advanced fibrosis (in these cases treatment is optional).
  2. Patients can be monitored every 3 mo with laboratory tests (ALT, IgG).
- Evaluation of treatment response:
  1. Goals are the absence of symptoms, normalization of liver function tests, and absence of inflammatory activity on liver biopsy. Generally, this is a steroid-responsive condition, but up to 20% do not respond.
  2. Patients whose transaminase levels normalize may continue to have ongoing active hepatitis involving inflammation and fibrosis.
  3. Histologic improvement may lag behind clinical and laboratory improvement by as much as 6 mo. Because of this, repeat liver biopsy should be considered after normalization of transaminase levels and before stopping treatment. A review of AIH studies between 1972 and 2013 shows that hepatic fibrosis improves in 53% to 57% of cases and that progressive fibrosis is slowed or prevented in 79% of patients.
  4. After initial remission is achieved and AZA has been added, steroid taper can be initiated as long as liver tests are normal. About 50% to 86% of patients will relapse after this and require long-term maintenance medications.
  5. Complete normalization on biopsy is associated with a 15% to 20% risk of relapse, whereas persistent interface hepatitis is associated with a 90% risk of relapse. Do not attempt multiple treatment withdrawals. The risk of developing cirrhosis with single relapse is 9.5%, whereas multiple relapses are associated with 37.5% risk of developing cirrhosis. The patient with sustained remission has a risk of cirrhosis of 4.5%.
  6. Suboptimal response: A failure to adequate response should lead to a reconsideration of the diagnosis or re-evaluation of adherence to treatment. In patients with suboptimal response despite reconfirmation of diagnosis and adherence, doses of prednisolone and azathioprine should be increased, or alternative medications should be used.
  7. According to AASLD 2019 guidelines, patients with acute severe AIH should be treated with predniso(lon)ne followed by liver transplantation if no improvement is seen within 2 wk. Patients with AIH and acute liver failure should be evaluated directly for liver transplantation.

DISPOSITION

- Long-term treatment may be necessary for sustained remission in individuals who relapse after initial immunosuppression withdrawal and in partial responders.
- 65% of patients achieve remission by 18 mo; 80% achieve remission by 3 yr.
- Approximately 10% to 15% of patients do not respond to conventional therapy. The risk factors for nonresponse include presence of underlying cirrhosis, younger age, or longer duration of disease, HLA-B8 or DR3. High-dose therapy can achieve remission in 70%: Prednisone 60 mg or dual therapy with prednisone 30 mg and AZA 150 mg. Other alternatives such as mycophenolate, the calcineurin inhibitors (CNIs), tacrolimus (TAC) and cyclosporine (CSA), sirolimus (SIR), everolimus (EVR), rituximab, and infliximab, have been used successfully. However, none of the alternative therapies has been studied in multicenter, randomized, controlled trials.
- Orthotopic liver transplantation (OLT) is a life-saving option for AIH patients with acute liver failure, decompensated cirrhosis, or HCC. Allograft and patient survival are excellent; however, AIH recurs in the allograft in a minority (25% probability in first 5 yr, 50% in 10 yr).

REFERRAL

Patients with advanced cirrhosis or who progress to end-stage liver disease are candidates for liver transplantation and should be referred to appropriate medical centers that provide liver transplantation services.

PEARLS & CONSIDERATIONS

COMMENTS

- ANA and SMA are observed together in 60% of cases. Serum titers >1:40 suggest autoimmune hepatitis.
- A variety of autoimmune conditions can be seen in association with autoimmune hepatitis, including thyroiditis, Graves disease, ulcerative colitis, rheumatoid arthritis, uveitis, pernicious anemia, Sjögren syndrome, mixed connective tissue disease, CREST syndrome, and vitiligo.
- Variant forms of autoimmune hepatitis (overlap syndrome) have clinical and serologic findings of autoimmune hepatitis plus features of other forms of chronic liver disease such as PBC or PSC.

PATIENT & FAMILY EDUCATION

- American Liver Foundation (ALF): Phone: 800-GO-LIVER (465-4837); www.liverfoundation.org
- National Institute of Diabetes and Digestive and Kidney Diseases (NIDDK). National Digestive Diseases Information Clearinghouse: www.niddk.nih.gov/health-information/digestive-diseases

SUGGESTED READINGS

Available at ExpertConsult.com

RELATED CONTENT

Autoimmune Hepatitis (Patient Information)

AUTHORS: **Aruj Choudhry, MD** and **Andreea M. Catana, MD**

BASIC INFORMATION

DEFINITION

Autosomal dominant polycystic kidney disease (ADPKD) is the most common inherited kidney disease. ADPKD is a systemic, inherited disorder due to mutations in the majority (approximately 93%) in either the *PKD1* or *PKD2* genes. These mutations lead to fluid-filled cyst formation, proliferation, and growth in multiple organs including the kidneys, liver, and pancreas. ADPKD is also associated with multiple gastrointestinal, connective tissue, and cardiovascular abnormalities.

SYNONYMS

Polycystic Kidney Disease
ADPKD
PKD
Hereditary Polycystic Kidney Disease

ICD-10CM CODES

Q61.3	Polycystic kidney, unspecified
Q61.2	Polycystic kidney, adult type
Q61.19	Other polycystic kidney, infantile type
Z82.71	Family history of polycystic kidney

EPIDEMIOLOGY & DEMOGRAPHICS

- Most common genetic cause of chronic kidney disease (CKD) and end-stage renal disease (ESRD)
- Mendelian autosomal dominant disorder
- Each child of an affected parent has a 50% chance of inheriting the mutated gene
- Affects all ethnic groups equally worldwide
- Autosomal dominant polycystic kidney disease type 1: Approximately 78% of affected individuals with genetically resolved cases have a gene mutation on chromosome 16 (*PKD1* gene)
- Autosomal dominant polycystic kidney disease type 2: Approximately 15% of affected individuals with genetically resolved cases have a gene mutation located on chromosome 4 (*PKD2* gene)
- Autosomal dominant polycystic kidney disease type 3: Increasing number of cases (nearly 7%) linked to mutations of the alpha glucosidase II gene (*GANAB*) located on chromosome 11q12.3
- Disease has 100% penetrance and does not skip generations

INCIDENCE: ADPKD prevalence has been reported to be between 1 in 400 and 1 in 1000 live births, based on earlier studies from Denmark. The U.S. ADPKD prevalence has been reported in subsequent studies from Europe and Japan between 1 in 2525 and 1 in 4000.

GENETICS: The majority of ADPKD cases stem from a mutation in the *PKD1* gene, located on the short arm of chromosome 16. The gene encoding polycystin-1 (PC1) plays a vital role in cell-cell and cell-matrix interactions and primary ciliary function. Mutations in the *PKD1* gene lead to altered differentiation of epithelial cells and the abnormal phenotypic expression that characterizes ADPKD. ADPKD is less commonly (approximately 17%) caused by a mutation in the *PKD2* gene, located on chromosome 4. The *PKD2* gene encodes the protein polycystin-2 (PC2) that is involved in intracellular calcium signaling. *PKD2* patients typically have milder disease with later onset of hypertension, ESRD, and death. PC1 and PC2 form a single functional protein complex via interactions of their intracellular carboxy termini. Consequently, mutation of either the *PKD1* or *PKD2* gene produces a similar phenotype that cannot be distinguished clinically.

ADPKD is also caused by mutations in the *GANAB* gene, which is located on chromosome 11q12.3 and expressed in kidney and liver. The gene product plays an important role in PC1 maturation. Typically, ADPKD patients with *GANAB* gene mutations have mild PKD and mild-to-severe polycystic liver disease.

CLINICAL PRESENTATION

ADPKD is a systemic disorder, and symptoms relate primarily to kidney cyst burden or total kidney volume (TKV) and extrarenal involvement, including polycystic liver disease and vascular complications (Fig. E1). TKV and kidney cyst volume increases exponentially with time and follow a patient-specific curvilinear increase.

RENAL MANIFESTATIONS

Most patients with ADPKD are relatively asymptomatic, particularly in the first three decades of life. A diagnosis of ADPKD is typically established by identification of an affected family member with asymptomatic screening (approximately 40% of cases), or renal imaging performed for clinical indications. Patients may present with gross hematuria, flank mass/pain, polyuria/nocturia, fever due to a kidney or lower urinary tract infection, nephrolithiasis, or blood pressure elevation. Typically, more than half of patients will experience one of these complications by age 30. All of these complications represent manifestations of increased cyst burden or TKV.

Acute flank pain can be caused by a kidney stone, kidney or liver cyst rupture, or hemorrhage. Chronic pain is typically due to enlarged kidneys, unilaterally or bilaterally. Gross hematuria occurs in 35% to 50% of patients and associates with greater TKV. Gross hematuria may also result from spontaneous or traumatic cyst rupture into the collecting system. Less often microscopic hematuria secondary to nephrolithiasis occurs. Nephrolithiasis occurs in approximately 27% of ADPKD patients, due in part to low levels of urinary citrate, increased serum uric acid concentrations, and alterations in calcium oxalate and calcium phosphate supersaturation. Nephrolithiasis may present with acute flank pain with radiation to the groin, often with fever and hematuria, which is often microscopic.

Polyuria, nocturia, and increased thirst in ADPKD are manifestations of impaired urinary concentrating ability. Proteinuria is not a common feature of ADPKD (approximately 18% of adults and 27% of children) and is usually less than 1 gram per day. However, detectable proteinuria and microalbuminuria correlate with increased TKV and more severe kidney disease.

Lower urinary tract infections are common in ADPKD and may not occur more frequently than in the general population. Renal cyst infections are specific to ADPKD, and patients typically present with localized flank pain, fevers, and nausea and vomiting, similar to pyelonephritis.

CARDIAC MANIFESTATIONS

Hypertension occurs in 60% of patients with ADPKD before any substantial decline in kidney function, and it appears earlier in men than in women. Hypertension in ADPKD is due primarily to upregulation of the renin-angiotensin-aldosterone system (RAAS). Hypertension strongly associates with increased cyst burden or TKV. Hypertension is a predictor of worse renal outcomes and is associated with cardiovascular morbidity and mortality. Cardiac valvular abnormalities occur in 25% to 30% of ADPKD patients and include mitral valve prolapse and aortic regurgitation.

EXTRARENAL MANIFESTATIONS

- The prevalence of intracranial aneurysms (ICAs) in ADPKD is approximately 5% and increases to as high as 20% in patients who have a first-degree relative with a known intracranial aneurysm rupture.
- ICA rupture is a serious complication and may produce significant permanent morbidity or death. Routine ICA screening is recommended for patients with a family history of ICA or intracerebral bleed. Recently, smoking exposure and concurrent hypertension have been shown to associate with ICA in ADPKD. Screening is also recommended for ADPKD patients before major elective surgery, patients employed in high-risk occupations that would potentially place the lives of others at risk from a ruptured aneurysm (e.g., pilots, heavy machine operators), or patients with warning symptoms such as a sentinel headache.
- In addition to kidney cysts, cysts can develop in the liver, pancreas, and seminal vesicles. Hepatic cysts are the most common extrarenal manifestation and occur in nearly 85% of ADPKD patients by age 30. Liver cystic disease is typically asymptomatic and develops slightly later than kidney cysts in ADPKD. However, hepatic cysts can cause serious complications including pain, infection, bleeding, and biliary obstruction. Liver cysts continue to grow and expand even after ESRD occurs.
- Colonic diverticula and abdominal or inguinal hernias occur more frequently in ADPKD patients.
- Seminal vesical cysts have been reported to occur in up to 40% of men with ADPKD, but are not associated with reduced fertility.
- Patients with ADPKD may be at an increased risk of developing liver, colon, and kidney cancer. However, there is sparse evidence on which to recommend any change

in current cancer-screening guidelines for ADPKD patients.

NATURAL HISTORY

- Patients with *PKD1* gene mutations typically have more severe disease progression than patients with *PKD2* gene mutations. The median age of onset of ESRD is 54 yr in *PKD1* gene patients and 74 yr in *PKD2* patients.
- Patients with truncating *PKD1* gene mutations experience more severe disease progression than patients with nontruncating *PKD1* gene mutations. The median age of onset of ESRD is 55 yr in *PKD1* patients with truncating mutations and 67 yr with nontruncating mutations.
- Other clinical risk factors associated with progressive kidney disease in ADPKD include male gender, onset of hypertension before 35 yr of age, gross hematuria before age 40 yr, proteinuria or microalbuminuria, increased urinary sodium excretion, and increased circulatory low-density lipoprotein cholesterol levels. However, all of these risk factors are mediated through cyst burden or TKV.
- Data from the Consortium of Radiologic Imaging Studies of Polycystic Kidney Disease (CRISP) indicate that a decline in renal blood flow and increases of TKV and cyst volume are strong predictors of future renal functional decline and progression to CKD stage 3. A baseline height-adjusted TKV (htTKV) of 600 ml/min predicts the risk of developing CKD stage 3 within 8 yr. Patients with ADPKD may be classified as 1A-1E based on the Mayo Clinic Imaging Classification of ADPKD that helps physicians identify patients with severe disease (www.mayo.edu/research/documents/pkd-center-adpkd-classification/doc-20094754). This classification is based on annual growth rates estimated from age-based htTKV (<1.5% (1A), 1.5% to 3% (1B), 3% to 4.5% (1C), 4.5% to 6% (1D), >6%/year (1E)). This classification should only be applied in cases of ADPKD classified as typical ADPKD (i.e., large kidneys with extensive cysts scattered throughout both kidneys at ages 15 to 80 yr). Patients in class 1A are at a low risk for renal function decline. Patients in classes 1C-1E are at a high risk for progressive disease.

Dx DIAGNOSIS

- Ultrasound of the kidneys is the most commonly used imaging modality for screening and diagnosis. It is inexpensive, readily available, noninvasive, and free of radiation. CT and MRI are also used, but typically in the setting of acute complications. CT scans (Fig. E2) and MRI are more sensitive than ultrasound, with cyst detection at <1 cm in size.
- The following diagnostic criteria are used for diagnosis of ADPKD in asymptomatic individuals at risk for development of disease (i.e., positive family history of ADPKD):
  - Individuals 15 to 39 yr of age: At least three unilateral or bilateral kidney cysts.
  - Individuals 40 to 59 yr of age: At least two cysts in each kidney.
  - Individuals older than 60 yr of age: At least four cysts in each kidney.
- With no family history of ADPKD, there is no definitive number of cysts and/or cyst location that provides an unequivocal diagnosis. The diagnosis is strongly suspected when multiple and bilateral kidney cysts are present along with hepatic cysts. Currently, more than 20 cysts distributed bilaterally with a consistent phenotype is considered reliable for making a diagnosis.
- Genetic testing can be done to diagnose ADPKD when imaging results are equivocal and when a definitive diagnosis is required in a young at-risk individual, e.g., potential living kidney donor or family planning.

DIFFERENTIAL DIAGNOSIS

- Multiple benign simple cysts
- Autosomal recessive PKD
- Familial juvenile nephronophthisis
- Medullary cystic or UMOD (uromodulin) disease
- Medullary sponge kidney
- Tuberous sclerosis
- von Hippel-Lindau syndrome
- Acquired cystic kidney disease (Fig. E3)
- Table 1 compares clinical features of cystic kidney diseases

LABORATORY TESTS

- Hemoglobin and hematocrit may be elevated because of increased erythropoietin production; however, these levels are usually similar to levels in other CKD patients.
- Urinalysis can show microscopic hematuria and proteinuria (rarely >1 g per day).
- With decreased kidney function, blood urea nitrogen and creatinine are elevated.
- Platelet counts can be mildly reduced in patients with extensive polycystic liver disease from splenic sequestration.
- Metabolic acidosis, hyperparathyroidism, and hyperphosphatemia are associated with CKD in ADPKD.

Rx TREATMENT

NONPHARMACOLOGIC THERAPY

Dietary intervention is prescribed to all ADPKD patients.

- Restriction of dietary salt (<2 grams sodium per day) and calories is recommended. Post hoc analysis of the HALT-PKD trial in which all patients were instructed to follow a sodium-restricted diet (2.4 g per day) showed that greater urine sodium excretion was associated with kidney growth or increase in htTKV and more rapid renal function decline.
- Intracellular cyclic adenosine monophosphate (cAMP) contributes to cyst formation and growth in ADPKD. Circulating vasopressin stimulates renal cAMP production. Increasing water intake to greater than 3 L per day can suppress circulating vasopressin levels. Consequently, increasing water intake is recommended for all ADPKD patients with preserved kidney function. However, serum sodium should be monitored carefully in advanced CKD because patients are vulnerable for development of hyponatremia.

CHRONIC GENERAL Rx

- In young individuals with preserved kidney function, the HALT-PKD trial showed that strict BP control of <110/75 mm Hg was associated with a slower increase of TKV (15% slower over 5 yr), reduced urinary albumin excretion, and greater reduction of left ventricular mass index.
- For ADPKD patients over the age of 35 yr or with renal dysfunction, the goal BP is <130/80 mm Hg. For young, healthy patients with ADPKD and with intact kidney function, the goal BP target can be <110/75 mm Hg.
- Angiotensin–converting-enzyme inhibitors or angiotensin II type 1 receptor blockers are the drug of choice as first-line treatment for hypertension.
- Hyperlipidemia should be aggressively treated, and the LDL-cholesterol target is <80 mg/dl.
- Pravastatin has been found to have a beneficial effect on htTKV, left ventricular mass index, and urinary albumin excretion in a randomized, double-blind, placebo-controlled phase 2 trial involving 91 children and young adults with ADPKD. Over a 3-year period, a 23% increase in htTKV was observed in the pravastatin group compared to 31% in the placebo group.
- Statin therapy did not show any benefit in a post hoc analysis of the HALT-PKD trials. However, this study was not randomized, different statin drugs and doses were used, and only a small number of statin users were in this study.
- Currently, statin use in the management of ADPKD is by physician choice. A larger, randomized controlled trial is required to study the effect of statins on cyst growth.
- Patients who progress to ESRD require renal replacement therapy. Both peritoneal dialysis and hemodialysis can be used as a bridge to kidney transplantation, but preemptive transplantation is preferred.

The complication rates after nephrectomy are higher with pre-kidney transplant nephrectomy compared with posttransplant nephrectomy. Blood transfusion during pre-kidney transplant nephrectomy may cause allosensitization and delay transplantation evaluation. Consequently, routine pre-kidney transplant nephrectomy is not recommended. Pre-kidney transplant unilateral or bilateral nephrectomy is recommended only in select patients with recurrent infections, recurrent or severe bleeding, renal cell carcinoma, and significant kidney enlargement causing limitation of daily activities, and malnutrition.

ACUTE GENERAL Rx

- The treatment of gross hematuria is typically supportive with bed rest (compress

TABLE 1 Comparison of Clinical Features of Cystic Kidney Diseases

Disease	Inheritance	Frequency	Gene Product	Age of Onset	Cyst Origin	Renomegaly	Cause of ESRD	Other Manifestations
ADPKD	AD	1 : 400-1000	Polycystin-1(PC1); Polycystin-2(PC2); Glucosidase II alpha subunit (GIIα); DnaJB11	20s and 30s	Anywhere (including Bowman capsule)	Yes	Yes (for PC1, PC2, or DnaJB11) No (for GIIα)	Liver cysts Cerebral aneurysms Hypertension Mitral valve prolapse Kidney stones UTIs
ARPKD	AR	1 : 10,000-40,000	Fibrocystin/polyductin	First year of life	Distal nephron, CD	Yes	Yes	Hepatic fibrosis Pulmonary hypoplasia
ACKD	No	90% of ESRD patients at 8 yr	None*	Years after onset of ESRD	Proximal and distal tubules	Rarely	No	None
Simple cysts	No	50% in those older than 40 yr	None*	Adulthood	Anywhere (usually cortical)	No	No	None
NPHP	AR	1 : 80,000	Nephrocystins (NPHP1–20)	Childhood or adolescence	Medullary DCT	No	Yes	Retinal degeneration; neurologic, skeletal, hepatic, cardiac malformations
ADTKD-UMOD	AD	Rare	Uromodulin	Adults	Corticomedullary	No	Yes	Gout
ADTKD-MUC1	AD	Rare	Mucin-1	Adults	Corticomedullary	No	Yes	None
ADTKD-REN	AD	Rare	Renin	Childhood	Corticomedullary	No	Yes	Anemia, gout, hyperkalemia
ADTKD-HNF1B	AD; spontaneous	Rare	HNF1β	Childhood or adulthood	Corticomedullary	Rarely	Variable	Early-onset diabetes, pancreatic hypoplasia, hypomagnesemia, hyperthyroidism, liver function abnormalities, gout, renal and urogenital anomalies, mental retardation, risk of renal cell carcinoma
MSK	No	1 : 5000-20,000	None*	30s	Medullary CD	No	No	Kidney stones
Tuberous sclerosis	AD	1 : 10,000	Hamartin (TSC1), tuberin (TSC2)	Childhood	Loop of Henle, DCT	Rarely	Rarely	Renal cell carcinoma, tubers, seizures, angiomyolipoma, hypertension
VHL syndrome	AD	1 : 40,000	VHL protein	20s	Cortical nephrons	Rarely	Rarely	Retinal angioma, CNS hemangioblastoma, renal cell carcinoma, pheochromocytoma
Oral-facial-digital syndrome-1	XD	1 : 250,000	OFD1 protein	Childhood or adulthood	Renal glomeruli	Rarely	Yes	Malformation of the face, oral cavity, and digits; liver cysts; mental retardation
HIPKD	AR	Rare	Phosphomannomutase 2	Childhood	Renal glomeruli	Yes	Yes	Hypoglycemic seizures; occasional liver cysts
BBS	AR	1 : 65,000-160,000	BBS 1-18	Adulthood	Renal calyces	Rarely	Yes	Syndactyly and polydactyly, obesity, retinal dystrophy, male hypogenitalism, hypertension, mental retardation

ACKD, acquired cystic kidney disease; *AD*, autosomal dominant; *ADPKD*, autosomal dominant polycystic kidney disease; *DnaJB11*, DnaJ homolog subfamily B member 11; *AR*, autosomal recessive; *ARPKD*, autosomal recessive polycystic kidney disease; *BBS*, Bardet-Biedl syndrome; *CD*, collecting duct; *CNS*, central nervous system; *DCT*, distal convoluted tubule; *ESRD*, end-stage renal disease; *ADTKD*, autosomal dominant tubulointerstitial kidney disease; *UMOD*, uromodulin; *MUC1*, mucin-1; *REN*, renin; *HNF1β*, hepatocyte nuclear factor 1 β; *MSK*, medullary sponge kidney; *HIPKD*, PKD with hyperinsulinemic hypoglycemia; *NPHP*, nephronophthisis; *UTI*, urinary tract infection; *VHL*, von Hippel-Lindau; *XD*, X-linked dominant.

*No known genetic susceptibility.

From Goldman L, Shafer AI: *Goldman-Cecil medicine*, ed 26, Philadelphia, 2020, Elsevier.

bleeding cyst), hydration, and analgesics without nonsteroidal antiinflammatory drugs. Antihypertensive medications should be stopped during this time.
- Extracorporeal shock wave lithotripsy (ESWL) has been used in patients with small obstructing kidney stones (<2 cm diameter) in the renal pelvis or calyces. There is some concern that residual stone fragments cause renal dysfunction. Percutaneous nephrolithotomy is a potentially safer option in certain cases.
- Infections are treated with antibiotics that penetrate cysts, including fluoroquinolones, trimethoprim/sulfamethoxazole, vancomycin, and rarely, chloramphenicol.
- New therapies affecting cyst growth.

TOLVAPTAN

- In a phase 3, double-blind, placebo-controlled, randomized trial (TEMPO 3:4 trial) involving 1450 patients with PKD and preserved kidney function, the vasopressin-receptor 2 antagonist, tolvaptan, significantly decreased kidney volume and slowed the decline in kidney function. The benefits of tolvaptan on TKV rate of increase and decline of kidney function are greater in patients with increased albuminuria. The benefits of tolvaptan on TKV were seen across CKD stages 1 to 3.
- The effect of tolvaptan on delaying renal function decline was maintained for an additional 2 yr in the extension study, TEMPO 4:4 trial, in which all participants were offered tolvaptan treatment for an additional 2 yr.
- A second tolvaptan trial (REPRISE) examined the safety and efficacy of tolvaptan in more advanced ADPKD. This was a 12-month, phase III, randomized withdrawal, multicenter, placebo-controlled, and double-blind trial that included 1370 patients with eGFRs between 25 and 65 ml/min/1.73 m^2. Tolvaptan-treated patients demonstrated a reduction in eGFR decline of 35% compared to placebo. Those receiving placebo lost 3.61 ml/min per 1.73 m^2 per year. Tolvaptan-treated patients demonstrated an eGFR decline of 2.34 ml/min per 1.73 m^2 per year, a statistically significant difference of 1.27 ml/min per 1.73 m^2 per year. The beneficial effect of tolvaptan on renal function decline was established in all subgroups (<55 yr age, men and women, and patients with CKD stages 3A, 3B, and 4). Beneficial effects were not present in subjects older than 55 yr. Firm conclusions cannot be made in this subgroup due to relatively smaller numbers.
- Based on the above studies, on April 24, 2018, the FDA approved tolvaptan for treatment of ADPKD in adult patients at risk for rapidly progressing ADPKD.
- Patients at Mayo classes 1C-1E levels of cyst burden (faster rates of cyst growth) likely have rapidly progressive disease and should be considered for treatment with tolvaptan. Treated individuals may experience polyuria, nocturia, abnormally frequent urination, and polydipsia. Post-hoc analyses of TEMPO 3:4 and TEMPO 4:4 trials suggest that drug effects are more pronounced early on following drug initiation and in subjects with better kidney function. Appropriate hydration is essential to prevent thirst, dehydration, and hypernatremia.
- A minor eGFR reduction of 5% to 10% is anticipated after initiation of tolvaptan and reversible upon drug discontinuation. Tolvaptan dose reduction or withholding of the agent is recommended if a significant decline of eGFR of >20% is observed. Renal function testing should be carried out 2 and 4 wk after initiation of therapy, then monthly for the next 18 mo, and every 3 mo afterward. To ensure that patients are maintaining hydration while on tolvaptan, plasma sodium concentration measurements must be obtained. Urinary osmolality can be used to assess treatment response and target drug dosing.
- Another important adverse event associated with tolvaptan is liver toxicity. Two patients in the TEMPO 3:4 trial (https://pubmed.ncbi.nlm.nih.gov/23121377/) and 1 patient in the TEMPO 4:4 trial (https://pubmed.ncbi.nlm.nih.gov/28379536/) developed serious drug-induced liver injury. In the REPRISE trial, liver adverse effects were greater in the tolvaptan group compared to placebo (5.6% vs. 1.2%). Because of the risks of serious liver injury, tolvaptan prescriptions are only available through a restricted distribution program called the Risk Evaluation and Mitigation Strategy (REMS). Under this program, liver function testing is done before initiation of treatment, at 2 wk and 4 wk after initiation, then monthly for the first 18 mo and every 3 mo afterward.

OTHER THERAPIES AFFECTING CYST GROWTH

A small trial involving the somatostatin analogue, octreotide long-acting repeatable depot, showed that there was significantly less increase in TKV in the octreotide group compared to placebo. Another randomized phase III trial involving 100 ADPKD patients with eGFRs between 15 and 40 ml/min per 1.73 m^2 demonstrated that a 3-year treatment with octreotide long-acting release (octreotide LAR) significantly slowed kidney volume growth. Octreotide LAR did not affect GFR decline compared with placebo. However, fewer patients in the octreotide group progressed to the combined end point of doubling of serum creatinine or ESRD compared to placebo (19% vs. 43%). A 1-year, randomized, placebo-controlled study of another somatostatin analogue, pasireotide long-acting release, demonstrated slow rates of increase of total liver and volumes.

- In a phase 2, randomized, double-blind, placebo-controlled study, the oral tyrosine kinase inhibitor bosutinib reduced kidney growth and preserved kidney function. However, medication-related adverse events (diarrhea, rash, and pancreatitis) and acute declines in kidney function have limited development of this agent. A phase II trial of another tyrosine kinase inhibitor, tesevatinib is ongoing.
- Two randomized, double-blind trials investigating mammalian target of rapamycin inhibitors, sirolimus and everolimus, did not show any effect on renal function in ADPKD subjects. The shorter duration of these trials and inadequate dosing of the medications may have affected the outcome.
- Renal cyst formation and growth over time results in increased interstitial inflammation, oxidative stress, and fibrosis. Bardoxolone has antiinflammatory and antioxidant properties and is undergoing investigation as treatment of ADPKD in a phase III randomized trial.

REFERRAL

- Patients with ADPKD should be referred at time of diagnosis to a nephrologist for ongoing care. Urology can also be consulted in patients with nephrolithiasis for recurrent episodes of gross hematuria or consideration of nephrectomy pre-kidney transplantation.
- Genetic counseling should be offered if patients plan to start a family or are considering kidney screening examinations for children. Individuals at risk for ADPKD should undergo pretest and posttest counseling if ADPKD is discovered.

PEARLS & CONSIDERATIONS

- ADPKD is the most common, single, genetic cause of CKD.
- TKV increases exponentially over time, and the increase of TKV is a strong predictor of future kidney functional decline.
- Increasing water intake to >3 L per day is recommended in patients with ADPKD and preserved kidney function.
- Tolvaptan is recommended for patients with rapidly progressing ADPKD.
- Strict blood pressure control is recommended for all ADPKD patients.

SUGGESTED READINGS

Available at ExpertConsult.com

RELATED CONTENT

Polycystic Kidney Disease (Patient Information)

AUTHORS: **Bharathi V. Reddy, MD,** and **Arlene B. Chapman, MD**

BASIC INFORMATION

DEFINITION

Cerebral arteriovenous malformations (AVMs) are congenital vascular lesions that are characterized by blood flow from high-pressure arterial vessels directly into thin-walled veins without passing through an intervening capillary/venule system (Fig. 1).

SYNONYMS

Arteriovenous malformations of the brain
AVM
Brain AVM
Cerebral AV malformations

ICD-10CM CODE
Q28.2 Arteriovenous malformations of cerebral vessels

EPIDEMIOLOGY & DEMOGRAPHICS

INCIDENCE:
- Detection rates in large prospective studies range from 1.1 to 1.4 per 100,000 person-yr.
- Incidence of hemorrhage, the most common and often most clinically dangerous presentation, is estimated to be 2% to 4% per yr.

PREVALENCE: Estimated about 1.3 per 100,000

PREDOMINANT SEX AND AGE:
- There is a slight male preponderance; studies of varying populations show 1.04:1 to 1.2:1 male:female ratio.
- Peak age at time of hemorrhage occurrence is about 20 yr, but it can occur in younger and older patients.

RISK FACTORS:
- Male sex and presence of HHT are risk factors for AVM.
- The risk of hemorrhage is increased with prior hemorrhage, presence of a single draining vein, and diffuse nidus morphology.

GENETICS:
- Cerebral AVMs are sporadic in most cases.
- AVMs are present in about 20% of cases of Osler-Weber-Rendu syndrome (also known as hereditary hemorrhagic telangiectasia [HHT]), an autosomal dominant disorder that results in abnormal blood vessel formation in the skin, lungs, liver, brain, and other organs.

PHYSICAL FINDINGS & CLINICAL PRESENTATION

- The most common presentation is hemorrhage; symptoms vary based on location and magnitude of hemorrhage.
- Patients may present with seizures or neurologic deficits related to mass effect of the AVM nidus.
- Headache and pulsatile tinnitus may be present.
- In infants, AVM may present as cyanotic heart failure, macrocephaly, or hydrocephalus.
- A bruit may be auscultated through the scalp or orbit.
- AVMs may also present with associated intracranial aneurysms that occur on distant, unrelated vessels, on a proximal artery that feeds the aneurysm (flow-related aneurysm), or within the AVM nidus itself (intranidal aneurysm). Patients may present with a subarachnoid hemorrhage related to the aneurysm rather than to the AVM.

ETIOLOGY

In most cases, AVMs are congenital abnormalities caused by failure of formation of a capillary bed between embryonic arterial and venous vascular plexuses during the first trimester of gestation; however, de novo sporadic AVMs have been reported.

DIAGNOSIS

DIFFERENTIAL DIAGNOSIS

The differential diagnosis of cerebral AVMs includes other vascular lesions such as cavernous malformations, dural arteriovenous fistulas, and intracranial aneurysms. Table E1 compares vascular malformations, and Table E2 describes major differences between hemangiomas and vascular malformations.

LABORATORY TESTS

- CBC and basic metabolic panel (BMP) with renal function panel prior to contrast dye administration with CT angiography/cerebral angiogram.
- Prothrombin time/international normalized ratio/partial thromboplastin time (PT/INR/PTT) should be drawn and corrected in the case of bleeding diathesis.

IMAGING STUDIES

- In the acute setting, a CT scan of the head to check for hemorrhage and a CT angiogram of the head for characterization of the lesion may be helpful (although calcification may be present and potentially pose as small acute blood).
- MRI of the brain delineates the nidus and its relationship to surrounding soft tissue structures better than a CT scan; however, in the setting of an acute hemorrhage these details will be obscured.
- Four-vessel cerebral angiogram (arteriogram) is the best study to evaluate AVM. Angiography in multiple projections helps identify the number and location of feeding and draining vessels for treatment planning (Fig. 2). High-resolution images of the nidus may also reveal other irregularities such as aneurysms that often arise given the abnormal histology of the vessel walls and the high-pressure blood flow traversing them.

TREATMENT

Pharmacologic management of seizures with antiseizure drugs and of headaches with oral analgesics can provide symptomatic relief.

NONPHARMACOLOGIC THERAPY

- Observation: The advisability of intervention for unruptured AVMs remains controversial. A randomized trial comparing medical management with specific interventions to obliterate AVMs (neurosurgery, embolization, radiotherapy, or a combination) and prospective follow-up data showed that the rates of neurological disability were higher in the intervention group than with conservative treatment in the form of observation. Whereas patients with unruptured asymptomatic brain AVMs should be observed, treatment may be considered to reduce epileptic seizures or neurologic deficits caused by the AVMs.
- Nonemergent outpatient setting: Cerebral angiogram provides characterization of the lesion. Based on angiographic characteristics, the Spetzler-Martin AVM grading system may be used to help guide treatment. In general, grade 5 AVMs are considered unresectable; they are not treated because the risks of treatment likely outweigh the risk of hemorrhage. Current tools for the treatment of AVMs include surgical resection,

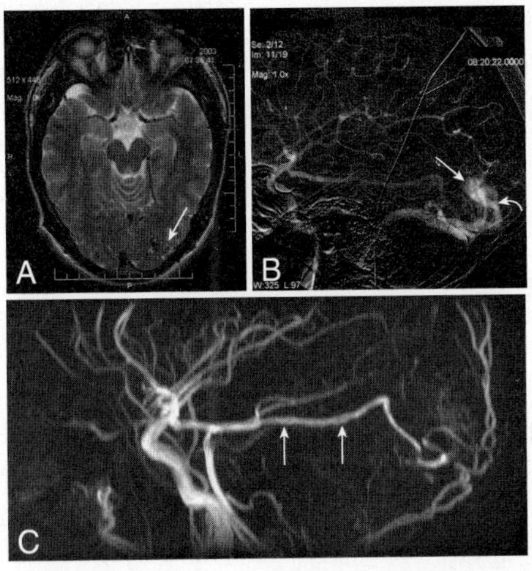

FIG. 1 A 14-year-old child with a left occipital arteriovenous malformation (AVM). A, Magnetic resonance image shows multiple flow voids in the left occipital lobe *(arrow).* **B,** Lateral view from catheter angiogram confirms the presence of an AVM *(arrow)* and early draining veins *(curved arrow).* **C,** Lateral maximum intensity projection image from a magnetic resonance angiogram shows an enlarged posterior cerebral artery branch *(arrows),* which feeds the tangle of abnormal vessels. (From Fuhrman BP et al: *Pediatric critical care,* ed 4, Philadelphia, 2011, Saunders.)

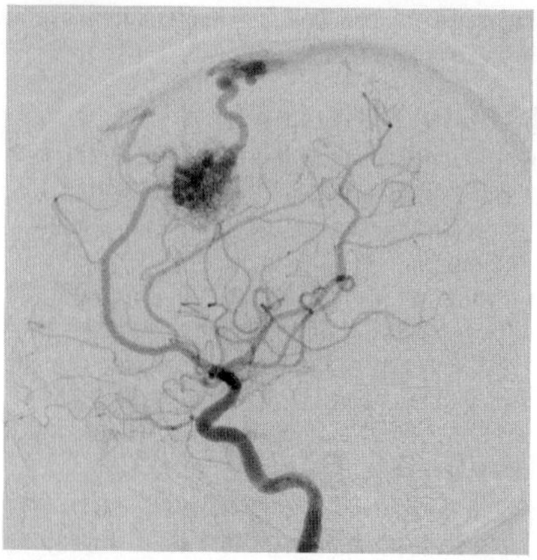

FIG. 2 Arteriovenous malformation of the frontal lobe. The anterior cerebral artery provides primary arterial supply with venous drainage superficially into the superior sagittal sinus.

radiosurgery, and endovascular embolization (with liquid glues or embolic agents).

- Surgical resection: In low-grade lesions by an experienced neurosurgeon yields a high cure rate (~95% in published studies). Resection should include removal of all of the nidus of the AVM; failure to remove the complete nidus may increase the risk of recurrence. An increasing Spetzler-Martin grading scale increases risk of neurologic complications. Intraoperative imaging techniques such as indocyanine-green in-field angiography and conventional digital subtraction angiography are used to verify complete resection.
- Radiosurgery: Alternative definitive treatment for AVMs. Traditionally employed to treat AVMs in eloquent areas (e.g., brainstem); stereotactic radiosurgery is increasingly used for higher Spetzler-Martin grade AVM. Reported rates of confirmed radiographic obliteration after AVM radiosurgery range from 47% to 90%.
- Endovascular embolization involves transarterial superselective blockage of the AVM. It has become an important adjunctive tool. Currently recommended and approved for use before resection, preoperative embolization can reduce arterial flow and pressure within the AVM, assisting in speed and safety of surgical resection. In addition, embolization may often be used to treat intranidal or flow-related aneurysms in coordination with either resection or radiosurgery. Embolization alone in obliterating an AVM is not routinely recommended.
- Treatment decisions should take into consideration the morbidity associated with the treatment modality versus the risk of future hemorrhage or neurologic deterioration. Disability stemming from intractable seizures or severe headaches may make invasive definitive treatment a more attractive option.
- Acute cerebral hemorrhage: In the case of an acute hemorrhage, airway and breathing must be maintained, with intubation if necessary. Acute neurosurgical intervention for clot evacuation may be warranted. Microsurgical resection of the AVM may or may not be feasible in the acute setting and is controversial.

DISPOSITION

Whether the patient is receiving elective treatment of a known lesion or presenting with an acute hemorrhage, the patient should receive care in a progressive or intensive care unit with experience dealing with cerebrovascular disease. Once the patient is stabilized, appropriate rehabilitation should be arranged.

REFERRAL

- Cerebral AVMs should be managed by a qualified neurosurgeon.
- Referral to radiation medicine for adjuvant radiosurgery should be made when indicated.
- Referral to an interventional radiologist for endovascular treatment may be warranted.
- Treatment in a primary stroke center or other specialized center that offers all treatment modalities is recommended.

PEARLS & CONSIDERATIONS

COMMENTS

- No two AVMs are exactly the same; individualization of treatment decisions is the mainstay. Additionally, many AVMs could be effectively treated through one of several modalities or a combination thereof. Factors such as patient age, overall health status, radiographic characteristics, route of surgical access, and potential morbidities of each treatment modality are vital variables in consideration for treatment. Unruptured, asymptomatic AVMs should be observed rather than treated.
- The annual risk of hemorrhage from a cerebral AVM is approximately 3%. However, depending on the clinical and anatomical features of the malformations, the risk may be as low as 1% or as high as 33%. The risk of bleeding is increased if the patient has had previous episodes of bleeding, if there is a berry aneurysm on an artery feeding the AVM, and if there is a restriction of venous drainage from the AVM.[1]

PATIENT & FAMILY EDUCATION

If a patient with a known AVM suffers from acute-onset neurologic deficits or stroke-like symptoms, emergency medical attention is warranted for potential hemorrhage. Presence of AVMs, cerebral or otherwise, in family members should be disclosed to the patient's primary care physician because the presence of a genetic condition predisposing to cerebral AVMs should be considered.

SUGGESTED READINGS

Available at ExpertConsult.com

AUTHOR: **Joseph S. Kass, MD, JD, FAAN**

[1]Solomon RA, Connolly ES: Arteriovenous malformations of the brain, *N Engl J Med* 376:1859-1866, 2017.

BASIC INFORMATION

DEFINITION

Babesiosis is a tick-transmitted protozoan disease of animals, caused by intraerythrocytic parasites of the genus *Babesia.* Humans are incidentally infected, resulting in a nonspecific febrile illness. The disease can be severe in immunocompromised hosts.

ICD-10CM CODE
B60.0 Babesiosis

EPIDEMIOLOGY & DEMOGRAPHICS

INCIDENCE (IN U.S.): From 2011 to 2015 the CDC was notified of 7612 cases of babesiosis. Cases were reported in 27 states, with 94.5% of cases occurring in 7 states (Fig. E1). In 2017, there were 2350 reported cases in the U.S.

PREVALENCE (IN U.S.):
- In areas of high endemicity, seropositivity ranging from 9% (Rhode Island) to 21% (Connecticut)
- Highest number of reported cases in New York

PREDOMINANT SEX: Males (most likely through increased exposure to vectors during recreational or occupational activities)

PREDOMINANT AGE: Severity apparently increasing with age greater than 50 yr or neonate

PEAK INCIDENCE: Spring and summer months, May through September

GENETICS: None known

CONGENITAL INFECTION: Definite evidence of vertical transmission

NEONATAL INFECTION: Many cases of perinatal transmission

BLOOD TRANSFUSION: Many instances. Blood donation screening for antibodies to and DNA from *B. microti* has been shown to significantly decrease the risk of transfusion-transmitted babesiosis

PHYSICAL FINDINGS & CLINICAL PRESENTATION

- Incubation period is 1 to 4 wk; 6 to 9 wk, occasionally longer in transfusion-associated disease.
- Gradual onset of irregular fever, chills, diaphoresis, headache, myalgia, arthralgia, fatigue, and dark urine. Symptoms usually begin within 1 mo after tick bite and within 6 mo after transfusion of infected blood products. Fever is the most frequently reported clinical manifestation.
- On physical examination: Petechiae, frank or mild hepatosplenomegaly, and jaundice. Most patients have a normal physical examination.
- Infection with *B. divergens* (Europe) produces a more severe illness with a rapid onset of symptoms and increasing parasitemia progressing to massive intravascular hemolysis and renal failure.

ETIOLOGY

- Vector: Deer tick, *Ixodes scapularis* (also known as *I. dammini*).
  1. Feeds on rodents during the spring and summer while in its larval and nymphal stages and on deer as an adult
  2. Requires a blood meal to mature to each stage, hence human infection
  3. During the warmer months in endemic areas, humans are readily infected while engaging in outdoor activities
  4. Tick must attach for 36 to 72 hours to transmit infection
  5. Babesia life cycle is illustrated in Fig. 2.
- *B. microti* and *B. divergens* account for most human infections. Table 1 compares causal agents and clinical manifestations of babesiosis.
- In the U.S., cases caused by *B. microti* are acquired on offshore islands of the northeastern coast, including Nantucket Island, Cape Cod, and Martha's Vineyard in Massachusetts; Block Island in Rhode Island; and Long Island, Fire Island, and Shelter Island in New York; as well as the nearby mainland including Connecticut, Rhode Island, Massachusetts, New York, and New Jersey.
- Sporadic cases reported from California, Georgia, Maryland, Minnesota, Virginia,

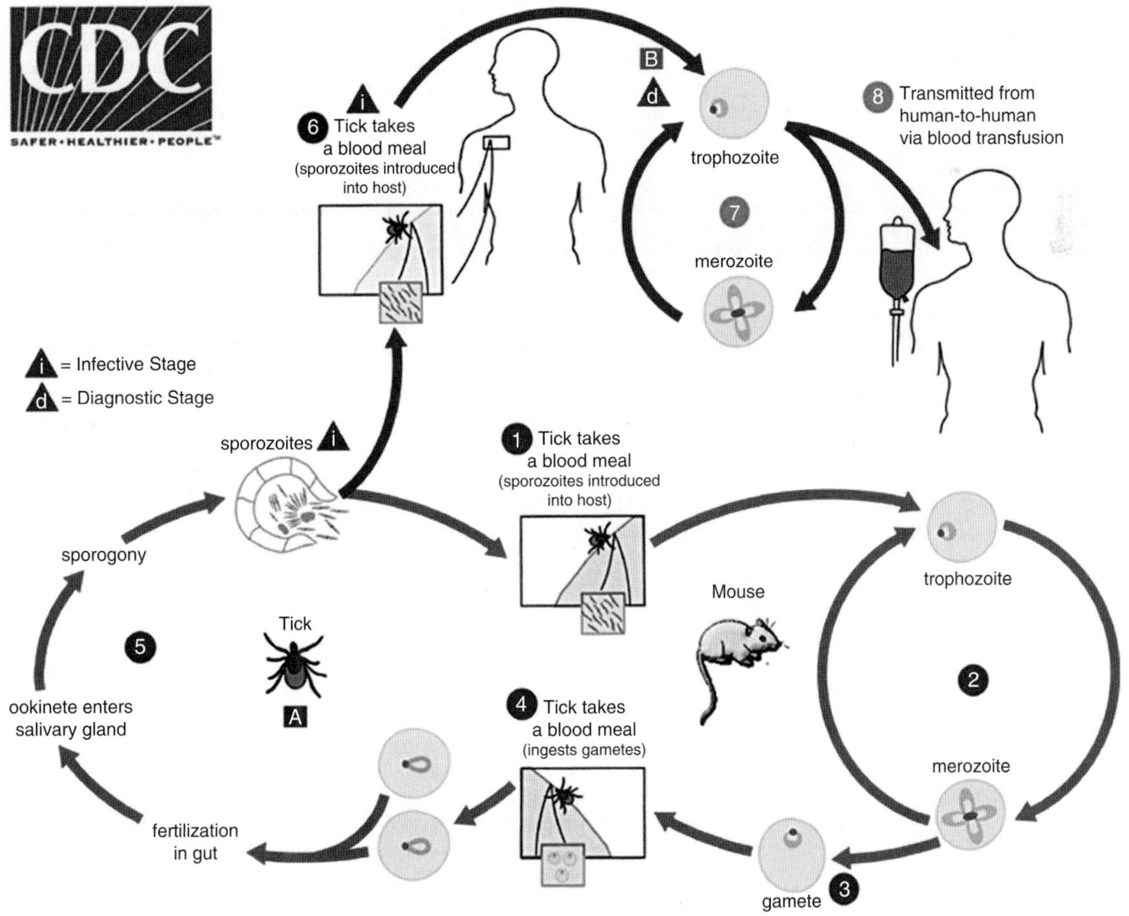

FIG. 2 Babesia life cycle. (From Rifai N et al (eds): *Tietz textbook of clinical chemistry and molecular diagnostics*, ed 6, 2018, Elsevier; In Spec A et al: *Comprehensive review of infectious diseases*, 2020, Elsevier. Courtesy of the CDC DPDx: http://www.cdc.gov/dpdx/.)

TABLE 1 Causal Agents and Clinical Manifestations of Babesiosis

Babesia Species	Geographic Distribution	Tick Vectors	Animal Reservoirs	Epidemiology	Clinical Manifestations
B. divergens	United Kingdom, Western Europe, Eastern Europe, Sweden, Russia; not reported in United States	*Ixodes ricinus*	Cattle, reindeer	Incubation, 1-4 wk. Occurs during summer months in cattle-raising regions Targets splenectomized or immunocompromised patients primarily	Fulminant course with high case-fatality rate Fever, rigors, headache, myalgia, jaundice, hemoglobinuria, hemolytic anemia, acute renal failure, multiorgan failure
B. microti	Parallels the U.S. Northeast endemic regions for *Borrelia burgdorferi*, especially the islands off New York, Massachusetts, Connecticut, and Rhode Island and focal areas in Connecticut, New Jersey, Wisconsin, and Minnesota	Deer ticks: *Ixodes dammini* and *Ixodes scapularis*	White-footed mouse *(Peromyscus leucopus)*	Incubation, 1-4 wk after tick bites or 4-9 wk after blood transfusions Transmission primarily by nymphal ticks Targets older, not necessarily immunocompromised patients, particularly severe in those immunocompromised by HIV infection, advanced age, coinfections with *B. burgdorferi* Seasonality parallels tick nymph activity; 80% of cases occur from May to August	Often asymptomatic in young, healthy patients Self-limited influenza-like febrile illness with onset of anorexia, malaise, and lethargy followed in 1 wk by high fever, diaphoresis, myalgias; mild splenomegaly and rarely hepatomegaly Later hemolysis, hemolytic anemia, thrombocytopenia, jaundice, acute renal failure, especially in the splenectomized, older adults, or the immunocompromised Complications include ARDS and DIC Case-fatality rate, 5%
MO-1 (a relative or subspecies of *B. divergens*)	Rural Missouri and Kentucky	*Ixodes dentatus* (rabbit tick)	Rabbits, birds	Incubation, 1-4 wk after tick bites Spring to autumn seasonality Targets the splenectomized, like *B. divergens*	Same as above—often asymptomatic, except in the splenectomized, who will develop high parasitemia and multiorgan failure
WA-1 (a relative or subspecies of *B. gibsoni*)	Rural Washington state	Ixodid ticks, including *Ixodes dentatus*	Unknown—wild canids and ungulates suspected	Incubation, 1-4 wk Targets the splenectomized, older adults, immunocompromised, premature infants May be transmitted by blood transfusion	Same as above—often asymptomatic, except in the splenectomized, who will develop high parasitemia and multiorgan failure
CA-1, CA-2, etc. subspecies (relatives or subspecies of mule deer and bighorn sheep *Babesia* species)	U.S. Pacific coast, primarily rural and semirural areas of California	Ixodid ticks	Unknown—mule deer and bighorn sheep suspected	Incubation, 1-4 wk Targets the splenectomized, elderly, immunocompromised, and premature infants	Same as above—often asymptomatic, except in the splenectomized, who will develop high parasitemia and multiorgan failure

ARDS, Acute respiratory distress syndrome; *DIC,* disseminated intravascular coagulation; *HIV,* human immunodeficiency virus.
From Bennett JE et al: Mandell, Douglas, and Bennett's principles and practice of infectious diseases, ed 8, Philadelphia, 2015, Saunders.

Wisconsin, and most recently the WA-1 strain from Washington State and the MO-1 strain from Missouri.

- *B. divergens* is implicated in human disease in Europe, where the disease remains rare and predominantly associated with asplenia.
- *B. venatorum* is emerging as an important pathogen in mainland China.
- Majority of cases of *B. microti* are asymptomatic.
- Is transmissible by transfusion of erythrocytes, or through red cell-contaminated platelets.
- Mixed infections (*B. microti* and *Borrelia burgdorferi,* the causative agent of Lyme disease) are estimated to occur in 30% (Rhode Island and Connecticut) to 60% (New York) of cases.

Dx DIAGNOSIS

DIFFERENTIAL DIAGNOSIS

- Malaria
- Ehrlichiosis
- Leptospirosis
- Salmonellosis, including typhoid fever
- Acute viral hepatitis
- Hemorrhagic fevers
- Subacute bacterial endocarditis

WORKUP

Babesiosis should be suspected in any febrile patient living or traveling in an endemic area, irrespective of exposure history to ticks or tick bites, especially if asplenic. The hallmark of babesiosis is hemolysis with resulting anemia. Elevated liver enzymes, thrombocytopenia, and acute kidney injury may occur.

LABORATORY TESTS

- The preferred method for diagnosing babesiosis is polymerase chain reaction (PCR) using whole blood specimens.
- In experienced hands, sequential examination of Giemsa stained thin smears is equally effective.
- Babesial DNA by PCR has comparable sensitivity and specificity to microscopic analysis of thin blood smears. PCR is more sensitive than smears at the onset of infection when parasite load may be minimal.
- Diagnosis is achieved serologically by indirect immunofluorescence assay (IFA) specific for *B. microti.*
  1. Assay is hampered by the inability to distinguish between exposed patients and those who are actively infected.
  2. Immunoglobulin G titer of ≥1:64 is indicative of seropositivity, whereas one ≥1:1024 is considered diagnostic of acute infection. Immunoglobulin M (IgM) titer of 1:64 is considered indicative of acute infection.
  3. IgM indirect immunofluorescent-antibody test may be highly sensitive and specific for diagnosis. IgM titer of 1:64 is considered indicative of acute infection.
- CBC may reveal mild to moderate thrombocytopenia and anemia. The white blood cell (WBC) count may be normal, elevated, or low. Abnormally elevated serum chemistries, including creatinine, liver function profile,

lactate dehydrogenase, and indirect and total bilirubin levels; haptoglobin is low.
- Urinalysis may reveal proteinuria and hemoglobinuria.
- Examination of Giemsa- or Wright-stained thin blood films for intraerythrocytic parasites (Fig. 3):
  1. In its classic, though infrequently seen, form a "tetrad" or "Maltese cross" composed of four daughter cells attached by cytoplasmic strands is observed.
  2. More commonly, smaller forms composed of a single chromatin dot are eccentrically located within bluish cytoplasm.
  3. Parasitized erythrocytes may be multiply infected but not enlarged.
  4. Extra-erythrocytic forms may be seen.
  5. Gametocytes are *not* seen; this is a characteristic of malaria.

Rx TREATMENT

NONPHARMACOLOGIC THERAPY

Supportive care with adequate hydration

ACUTE GENERAL Rx

- In patients with intact spleens: Predominantly asymptomatic or if symptomatic, generally self-limited
- Therapy may be offered to any symptomatic patient. Table 2 summarizes treatment recommendations.
- Therapy is mandatory for the severely ill patient, especially if asplenic, elderly, or immunosuppressed. Combination of atovaquone 750 mg q12h and azithromycin 500 mg on day 1 and 250 mg per day thereafter for 7 to 10 days appears to be as effective as a regimen of clindamycin and quinine with fewer adverse reactions. This is the preferred regimen for mild disease.
- Combination of quinine sulfate 650 mg PO tid plus clindamycin 600 mg PO tid (600 mg parenterally qid) taken for 7 to 10 days. Severely ill patients are hospitalized and treated with clindamycin and quinine or azithromycin plus atovaquone.
- Exchange transfusions in addition to antimicrobial therapy: Successful treatment for severe infections in asplenic patients associated with high levels of *B. microti* or *B. divergens* parasitemia. Exchange transfusion is recommended for patients with >10% parasitemia, but may be considered for any severely ill patient.
- Relapsed and immunocompromised patients may require a longer duration of therapy.

DISPOSITION

Prognosis is usually good and fatal outcomes are rare.

REFERRAL

- For prompt consultation with an infectious disease specialist if the diagnosis is acutely suspected, especially in the asplenic, elderly, or immunocompromised patient
- For hospitalization for the severely ill patient who may require exchange transfusions in addition to antibiotic therapy

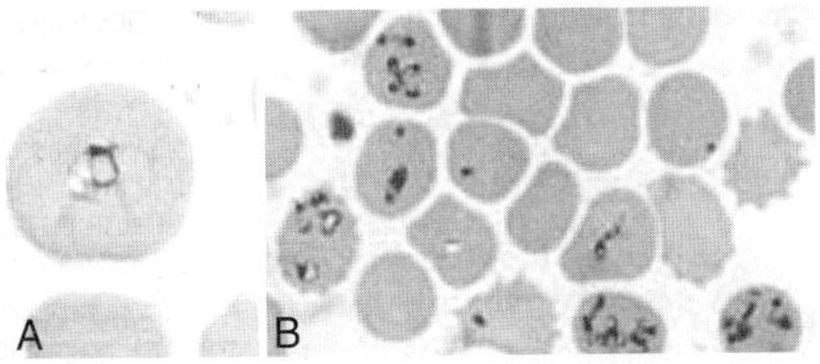

FIG. 3 Babesia parasites. Human infection with species of piroplasm transmitted by the bite of the tick *Ixodes ricinus* infected from cattle is a rare occurrence. Infection in normal people with this piroplasm may give rise to a self-limiting fever and parasitemia, as in the case of infection with the rodent parasite *Babesia microti* on the northeastern seaboard of the United States via the tick *Ixodes scapularis* **(A).** Heavy red-cell infection may develop, however, in splenectomized patients, leading to fatal hemolytic anemia. This patient died as a result of an infection acquired from the cattle parasite *Babesia divergens* in Scotland **(B).** Other species of *Babesia* that occasionally infect humans, for example, the WA-1, CA-1, and MO-1 isolates from the United States, are distinguished by molecular means. (From Hoffman R et al: *Hematology, basic principles and practice*, ed 7, Philadelphia, 2018, Elsevier.)

TABLE 2 Treatment of Human Babesiosis

Organism	Severity	Adults	Children
*Babesia microti**	Mild†	Atovaquone 750 mg q12h PO plus azithromycin 500 mg PO on day 1 and 250 mg/day PO from day 2 on	Atovaquone 20 mg/kg q12h PO (maximum 750 mg/dose) plus azithromycin 10 mg/kg PO on day 1 (maximum 500 mg/dose) and 5 mg/kg/day PO from day 2 on (maximum 250 mg/dose)
	Severe‡,§	Clindamycin 300-600 mg q6h IV or 600 mg q8h PO plus quinine 650 mg q8h PO	Clindamycin 7-10 mg/kg q6-8h IV or 7-10 mg/kg q6-8h PO (maximum 600 mg/dose) plus quinine 8 mg/kg q8h PO (maximum 650 mg/dose)
*Babesia divergens**		Immediate complete RBC exchange transfusion plus clindamycin 600 mg q6-8h IV plus quinine 650 mg q8h PO	Immediate complete RBC exchange transfusion plus clindamycin 7-10 mg/kg q6-8h IV (maximum 600 mg/dose) plus quinine 8 mg/kg q8h PO (maximum 650 mg/dose)

IV, Intravenously; *PO*, orally; *RBC*, red blood cell.
NOTE: Monitor patients on quinine with electrocardiography; monitor quinine serum levels in the setting of hepatic or renal disease.
*Treatment for 7-10 days, but duration may vary.
†Atovaquone (750 mg twice daily) combined with higher doses of azithromycin (600-1000 mg/day) has been used in immunocompromised patients. With this regimen, symptoms and parasitemia resolve faster.
‡Consider partial or complete RBC exchange transfusion in cases of high-grade parasitemia (≥10%), severe anemia (<10 g/dl), or pulmonary, renal, or hepatic compromise. Even when parasitemia is less than 10%, consider exchange transfusion if acute respiratory distress syndrome or syndrome resembling a systemic inflammatory response syndrome is present.
§In asplenic individuals and in immunocompromised patients, persistent or relapsing babesiosis should be treated for at least 6 wk, including 2 wk during which parasites are no longer detected.
From Bennet et al: *Principles and practice of infectious diseases*, ed 8, Philadelphia, 2015, Elsevier.

PEARLS & CONSIDERATIONS

COMMENTS

- Prevention of babesiosis in asplenic or immunocompromised hosts is best achieved by avoidance of areas where the vector is endemic, especially May through September.
- If residence or travel in endemic areas is unavoidable, advise patients to perform daily cutaneous self-examination, wear light-colored clothing (to facilitate removal of ticks), tuck pants into socks, and apply tick repellent (diethyltoluamide and dimethyl phthalate) to skin or clothing.
- Advise a daily inspection for ticks in family pets (e.g., cats and dogs).
- Infection with *B. divergens,* especially in the asplenic patient, is often fatal.
- Concurrent cases of babesiosis and Lyme disease, anaplasma, *Borrelia miyamotoi*, and Powassan virus have been documented—check for combined infection in severely ill patients.
- A combination of clindamycin and quinine has been successfully used to treat babesiosis during the third trimester of pregnancy without incurring apparent adverse effect on the fetus.

- In 2011 the CDC added babesiosis to the list of nationally notifiable diseases.
- Tick avoidance is paramount in prevention of babesiosis.

SUGGESTED READINGS

Available at ExpertConsult.com

RELATED CONTENT

Babesiosis (Patient Information)

AUTHOR: **Patricia Cristofaro, MD**

BASIC INFORMATION

DEFINITION

Barrett esophagus occurs when the squamocolumnar junction is displaced ≥1 cm proximal to the gastroesophageal junction and the squamous lining of the lower esophagus is replaced by metaplastic columnar epithelium, which predisposes to the development of esophageal adenocarcinoma.[1] While cardia-type epithelium has been shown to predispose to esophageal cancer, the presence of intestinalized epithelium is still considered essential for the diagnosis. Recent data show that the absolute annual risk for esophageal carcinoma in Barrett esophagus is 0.12%, which is much lower than the assumed risk of 0.5% that is the basis for current surveillance guidelines.

SYNONYMS

Esophagus, Barrett
Esophagus, columnar-lined
Ulcer, Barrett

ICD-10CM CODES	
K22.70	Barrett esophagus without dysplasia
K22.710	Barrett esophagus with low grade dysplasia
K22.711	Barrett esophagus with high grade dysplasia
K22.719	Barrett esophagus with dysplasia, unspecified

EPIDEMIOLOGY & DEMOGRAPHICS

- Male/female ratio of 4:1.
- Mean age of onset is 40 yr, with a mean age range of diagnosis of 55 to 60 yr.
- Occurs more frequently in white and Hispanic individuals than in African American individuals, with a ratio of 10 to 20:1.
- Mean prevalence of 5% to 15% in patients undergoing endoscopy (EGD) for symptoms of gastroesophageal reflux disease (GERD). It is estimated that 5.6% of adults in the U.S. have Barrett esophagus. The prevalence rate may be as low as ~1% in patients without risk factors and varies based on patient location (Western vs. non-Western countries) and number of risk factors.
- Independent risk factors include chronic reflux (>5 yr), hiatal hernia, age >50 yr, male gender, white ethnicity, smoking history, and intraabdominal obesity. A family history with at least one first-degree relative with Barrett esophagus or adenocarcinoma of the esophagus is a significant risk factor.

PHYSICAL FINDINGS & CLINICAL PRESENTATION

SYMPTOMS:

- Chronic heartburn
- Dysphagia with solid food
- Less frequent: Chest pain, hematemesis, melena
- Patients may be asymptomatic
- May be an incidental finding on EGD in patients without reflux symptoms

PHYSICAL FINDINGS:

- Nonspecific; can be completely normal
- Epigastric tenderness on palpation

ETIOLOGY

- Metaplasia is thought to result from reepithelialization of esophageal tissue injured as a result of chronic GERD. Activation of proliferative and inflammatory pathways likely induces a molecular phenotypic reprogramming of progenitor cells to form intestinal epithelium. Several candidate cells have been identified, including migrating gastric epithelial cells, residual embryonic cells, transitional columnar epithelium, or submucosal glands or ducts.
- Patients with Barrett esophagus tend to have more severe esophageal motility disturbances (decreased lower esophageal sphincter pressure, ineffective peristalsis) and greater esophageal acid exposure on 24-hr pH monitoring. Table 1 lists some physiologic abnormalities that have been reported in Barrett patients and suggests how these abnormalities may contribute to GERD severity.
- Bile salts in the presence of acid may produce oxidative stress, induce reactive oxygen species, and alter transcriptional factor activity, all of which may induce the formation of Barrett epithelium, DNA damage, and dysplastic progression.
- Familial clustering of GERD and Barrett esophagus suggests a genetic predisposition, but no gene has yet been identified. Early data suggest that patients who develop Barrett are genetically predisposed to a severe inflammatory response to GERD. Candidate susceptibility loci include *CRTC1*, *BARX1*, and *FOXP1*.
- Progression from metaplasia to dysplasia to carcinoma is associated with accumulating changes in gene structure and expression, including the caudal-related homeobox family of transcription factors *(CDX1* and *CDX2),* the embryonic transcription factor SOX2, and the tumor suppressors p16 *(CDKN2A)* and *TP53.*
- One meta-analysis of genome-wide association studies identified eight risk loci associated with Barrett esophagus and esophageal adenocarcinoma.
- Transcriptionally active high-risk human papillomavirus has been described in cohorts of patients with Barrett esophagus with dysplasia and esophageal adenocarcinoma.
- Patients with Barrett esophagus and esophageal adenocarcinoma may have a shift in the esophageal microbiome toward a gram-negative population, which may play a role in oncogenesis through the release of proinflammatory cytokines and activation of oncogenic transcriptional regulators such as nuclear factor-κB (NF-κB).

DIAGNOSIS

DIFFERENTIAL DIAGNOSIS

- GERD, uncomplicated
- Erosive esophagitis
- Gastritis
- Peptic ulcer disease
- Angina
- Malignancy
- Stricture or Schatzki ring

WORKUP

- The American Gastroenterological Association Medical Position Panel gave a weak recommendation for screening patients with multiple risk factors, including age over 50, male sex, white race, chronic GERD, hiatal hernia, elevated body mass index, and intraabdominal distribution of body fat.

TABLE 1 Proposed Physiologic Abnormalities Contributing to Gastroesophageal Reflux Disease in Patients with Barrett Esophagus

Abnormality	Potential Consequences
Extreme hypotension of the lower esophageal sphincter	Gastroesophageal reflux
Ineffective esophageal motility	Defective clearance of refluxed material
Gastric acid hypersecretion	Reflux of highly acidic gastric juice
Duodenogastric reflux	Esophageal injury caused by reflux of bile acids and pancreatic enzymes
Decreased salivary secretion of EGF	Delayed healing of reflux-damaged esophageal mucosa
Decreased esophageal pain sensitivity to refluxed caustic material	Failure to initiate therapy

EGF, Epidermal growth factor.
From Feldman M et al: *Sleisenger and Fordtran's gastrointestinal and liver disease*, ed 10, Philadelphia, 2016, Saunders.

[1]The reason for this 1-cm threshold is based on the original work describing the Prague classification, which shows excellent concordance for length thresholds >1 cm but poor concordance for length thresholds <1 cm. Currently, there is alignment of the ACG, BSG, and ESGE not to biopsy an irregular Z line in the absence of a visible abnormality due to the low risk of progression to esophageal adenocarcinoma in these patients as recently shown by Thota et al.
Thota PN et al. Low risk of high-grade dysplasia or esophageal adenocarcinoma among patients with Barrett's esophagus less than 1 cm (irregular Z Line) within 5 years of index endoscopy. *Gastroenterology.* 2017;152:987-992.

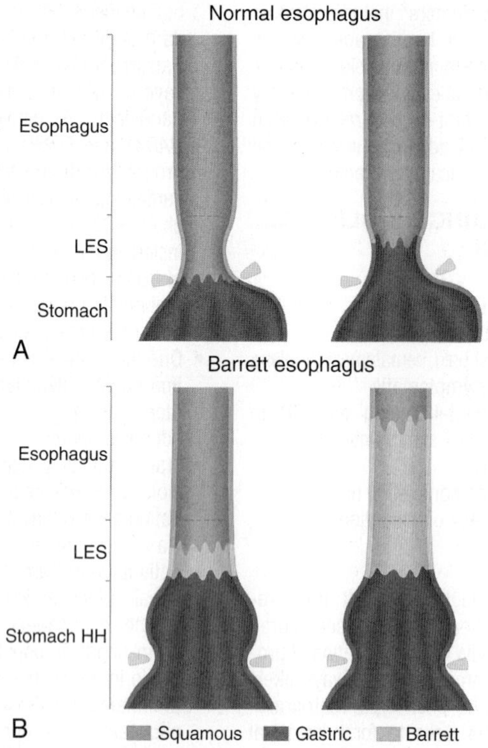

FIG. 1 Anatomic landmarks of the normal LES region **(A)** and of Barrett esophagus **(B).** Note that gastric mucosa is very common and normal in the LES region and that in Barrett esophagus, the squamocolumnar junction is not only proximally displaced within the tubular esophagus, but that the intervening mucosa is composed of intestinalized Barrett metaplastic epithelium. *HH,* Hiatal hernia; *LES,* lower esophageal sphincter.

An international consensus group suggested screening men over 60 with GERD symptoms for more than 10 yr. An American College of Gastroenterology (ACG) Clinical Guideline suggested screening men with >5 yr and/or frequent symptoms of GERD and two or more risk factors including age >50, Caucasian race, presence of central obesity, current or past history of smoking, and a confirmed family history of Barrett or esophageal adenocarcinoma. An American Society for Gastrointestinal Endoscopy (ASGE) guideline stated that although there was insufficient evidence on the effectiveness of screening, if done, it should be performed for high-risk individuals, who were defined as patients with a family history of esophageal adenocarcinoma or Barrett esophagus, or moderate-risk patients with GERD and one of the earlier-defined risk factors. General population screening is not currently recommended. Although screening has become standard of practice in some communities, the effectiveness of screening using current techniques is controversial because it may not improve mortality rates from adenocarcinoma.

- EGD with biopsy is necessary for diagnosis. Ideally, this should be done via high-resolution white-light endoscopy with at least four biopsies for every 2-cm segment. If erosive esophagitis is present, patients should be treated to heal esophagitis with repeat endoscopy and biopsies 8 to 12 wk later to determine if underlying Barrett esophagus is present. ASGE recommends concurrent use of chromoendoscopy or virtual chromoendoscopy if available.
- Unsedated transnasal endoscopy and an esophageal cytology device (Cytosponge) may be acceptable alternatives to conventional endoscopy. Wireless esophageal capsule endoscopy may detect Barrett esophagus but with too low a sensitivity and specificity to be recommended. Imaging studies are not useful.
- Diagnosis requires the presence of metaplastic columnar epithelium at least 1 cm proximal to the gastroesophageal junction (Figs. 1 and E2). Longer-segment (≥3 cm) Barrett esophagus is more readily diagnosed. Barrett esophagus may be described using the Prague criteria, documenting the circumferential and maximal length via a C and M score. The Paris classification may be used to report associated visible lesions. At least two expert gastrointestinal pathologists should concur if any grade of dysplasia is diagnosed.
- Intestinal metaplasia of the gastric cardia is not Barrett esophagus and does not have the same risk for malignancy.
- Biomarkers using tissue samples and, more recently, blood tests involving whole genome sequencing and even breath tests for volatile organic compounds, and advanced imaging techniques, such as mutational load, fluorescence in situ hybridization, autofluorescence imaging, white light postprocessing algorithms, confocal laser endomicroscopy, and optical coherence tomography (recently incorporated into volumetric laser endomicroscopy), are being evaluated to assist with diagnosis and to better understand progression of disease, prediction of response to therapy, or prognosis.
- Screening for *Helicobacter pylori* infection in patients with GERD and Barrett esophagus is not recommended.

Rx TREATMENT

The goal is to control GERD symptoms and maintain healed mucosa.

NONPHARMACOLOGIC THERAPY

Nonpharmacologic therapy includes lifestyle modifications; elevating head of bed; and avoiding chocolate, tobacco, caffeine, mints, and certain drugs (see "Gastroesophageal Reflux Disease").

ACUTE GENERAL Rx

- Proton pump inhibitors are the most effective treatment for GERD. Therapy should be titrated to control symptoms and/or to promote healing of endoscopic signs of disease.
- If patient is asymptomatic and incidentally found to have Barrett esophagus, once-daily proton pump inhibitors should be prescribed, as they may reduce the risk of neoplastic progression. Increasing dosage to twice daily is only recommended if breakthrough symptoms arise.

CHRONIC Rx

- Chronic acid suppression is recommended to control symptoms, maintain healing, and reduce neoplastic progression. For patients with Barrett esophagus, the benefits of the use of proton-pump inhibitors is thought to outweigh the potential risks.
- Antireflux surgery may be considered for management of GERD and associated sequelae, but it has not been proven to be superior to medical therapy. Patients continue to require endoscopic surveillance of their esophagus.
- When GERD is controlled by either medical or surgical therapy, ablation of metaplastic epithelium usually leads to replacement by normal squamous epithelium. Because only a minority of patients with Barrett esophagus progress to high-grade dysplasia or carcinoma, endoscopic eradication therapy is not recommended for the general population of patients with nondysplastic Barrett esophagus.
- Endoscopic eradication therapy is becoming the treatment of choice for low-grade dysplasia and is the treatment of choice for high-grade dysplasia. Radiofrequency ablation or photodynamic therapy, combined with endoscopic mucosal resection (EMR) or endoscopic submucosal dissection (ESD) of visible mucosal irregularities, should be performed in conjunction with aggressive surveillance and eradication of all remaining Barrett epithelium. Endoscopic therapy is preferred over surgical treatment in properly staged individuals, given lower morbidity and mortality rates and similar long-term

survival rates. These therapies may even be considered for patients with focal intramucosal carcinoma, if properly staged (T1 SM1 or lower). Cryotherapy is being evaluated for the complete eradication of both dysplasia and intestinal metaplasia and reduced risk for disease progression. All these options run the risk for residual or buried metaplasia. Ultimate goals of therapy include both complete eradication of dysplasia (CE-D) and complete eradication of intestinal metaplasia (CE-IM). Even with CE-IM, recurrence has been documented in 5% to 39.5% of patients. Modalities for endoscopic treatment of Barrett esophagus are summarized in Table 2.

- Surgical resection is definitive therapy and may be offered for multifocal high-grade dysplasia, carcinoma that has extended into the submucosa (T1 SM2 or 3), or patients with poorly differentiated carcinomas or with evidence of lymphovascular invasion. Surgery may also be considered in patients with resistant, progressive, or recurrent disease in the face of endoscopic therapy. Mortality appears to be lower with experienced surgeons operating in high-volume centers.
- Patients with cardiovascular risk factors may be considered for low-dose aspirin therapy for chemoprevention of esophageal adenocarcinoma. NSAIDs or NSAIDs combined with statins are potentially effective at reducing the risk of esophageal adenocarcinoma but are not currently recommended for use because of the risk of adverse effects.

DISPOSITION

- The relative risk of developing esophageal adenocarcinoma for a patient with Barrett esophagus, as compared with the general population, is 11.3, a substantial drop from the relative risk of 30 or 40 estimated in earlier reports. The risk is greater in men and in patients with longer (≥8 cm) columnar-lined segments.
- The risk of progression to esophageal adenocarcinoma from untreated Barrett with low-grade dysplasia is 0.5% per yr, and with high-grade dysplasia ranges from 6% to 19% per yr.
- Frequency of monitoring is controversial. No prospective studies have proved that endoscopic surveillance is cost effective or increases life expectancy. Although some studies have suggested that close adherence to surveillance protocols is associated with higher rates of detection of dysplasia and cancer, a recent case-control study showed no reduction in mortality.
- Patients with Barrett esophagus currently undergo surveillance EGD and systematic four-quadrant biopsy ("Seattle protocol") at intervals determined by the presence and grade of dysplasia. Wide-area transepithelial sampling with computer-assisted 3D analysis (WATS-3D) may increase the detection of dysplasia. All visible mucosal abnormalities should undergo biopsy.
  1. Patients without dysplasia should have follow-up every 3 to 5 yr. Patients with low-grade dysplasia should have aggressive antisecretory (proton pump inhibitor) therapy, repeat endoscopy within 2 to 6 mo, and endoscopic ablation therapy or extensive mucosal sampling every 12 mo or until dysplasia is no longer present. They then revert to a 3- to 5-yr interval.
  2. Patients with high-grade dysplasia should have expert confirmation and extensive mucosal sampling. Advanced imaging techniques should be used to localize all neoplastic lesions. This includes virtual chromoendoscopy, narrow-band imaging (NBI), blue laser imaging (BLI), and i-scan. A simple and inexpensive technique is the use of acetic acid spray, which turns Barrett epithelium white, before turning neoplastic lesions red after 30 to 40 sec. High-grade dysplasia with visible mucosal irregularities should be removed by EMR or ESD, followed by mucosal ablation. Consider intensive surveillance every 3 mo for at least a yr; the optimal timing and duration of surveillance over the long term is unknown. Indefinite dysplasia requires aggressive medical therapy and close follow-up and resampling. Endoscopic treatment is preferred over intensive surveillance in patients with high-grade dysplasia.
- Patients should be treated aggressively for GERD before surveillance.

REFERRAL

- Consider EGD with biopsy in male or selected female patients with multiple risk factors who have not had previous EGD.
- Refer patients with GERD for evaluation if "red flag" symptoms are present (dysphagia, odynophagia, weight loss, vomiting, early satiety, GI bleeding, iron deficiency).
- Refer patients with biopsy-proved Barrett esophagus for surveillance.
- For those with low-grade or high-grade dysplasia, refer for ablative therapy with EMR or ESD if appropriate, followed by intensive surveillance. Esophageal resection may be considered.

SUGGESTED READINGS

Available at ExpertConsult.com

RELATED CONTENT

Barrett Esophagus (Patient Information)
Esophageal Tumors (Related Key Topic)
Gastroesophageal Reflux Disease (Related Key Topic)

AUTHORS: **Harlan G. Rich, MD, FACP, AGAF,** and **Rei Mitsuyama, MD**

TABLE 2 Modalities for Endoscopic Treatment of Barrett Esophagus

Modality	HGD Resolved	BE Resolved	Recurrence Rate	Subsquamous BE Rate	Stricture Rate	Complication Rate	Advantages	Disadvantages
APC	67%-98.6%	38%-98%	33%-68% low power	25%-45% low power 0-30% high power	4%-10%	24% low power 40%-60% high power	Noncontact, technically simple	Requires several treatment sessions
MPEC	–	25%-88%	7%	7%	2%	41%-43%	Noncontact, technically simple, relatively inexpensive, readily available	Requires several treatment sessions
PDT	77%-88%	13%	5%-11%	2%-24%	4.8%-53%	4.8%-53%	Easy to perform; only FDA-approved ablation method for treatment of precancerous lesions in BE	Photosensitivity, relatively high stricture rate
EMR	59%-97%	53%	4%-30%	–	3%-30%	12%-60%	Histologic assessment; complete removal of circumferential short-segment BE; 1-2 sessions	Difficulty treating long-segment BE

APC, Argon plasma coagulation; *BE,* Barrett esophagus; *EMR,* endoscopic mucosal resection; *FDA,* U.S. Food and Drug Administration; *HGD,* high-grade dysplasia; *MPEC,* multipolar electrocoagulation; *PDT,* photodynamic therapy.
From Cameron JL, Cameron AM: *Current surgical therapy,* ed 12, Philadelphia, 2017, Elsevier.

Bedbug Bite (PTG)

BASIC INFORMATION

DEFINITION

A bedbug's bite is a wound caused by the penetration of the bedbug mouthpiece into the skin as the insect feeds on blood from vessels or extravasated blood from the damaged surrounding tissue. The saliva of the bedbug contains pharmacologically active substances responsible for a spectrum of undesirable skin reactions depending on the individual. The bugs typically feed during times when an individual is at rest and may feed without being detected. Typically feedings take 5 to 10 min.

SYNONYMS

Insect bite
Bedbug *Cimex lectularius* bite

ICD-10CM CODE
T00.9 Multiple superficial (insect bite) injuries, unspecified

EPIDEMIOLOGY & DEMOGRAPHICS

- Traditionally, bedbugs were considered more common in poorer areas, but they are now increasingly found in areas of frequent travel.
- Bedbug infestations may spread among multifamily and institutional facilities with shared walls and are consequently difficult to eradicate.
- Reports of bedbug infestations have increased dramatically in the U.S., as well as worldwide, likely because of the decreased use of pesticides and increased international travel.
- Bedbugs are attracted to carbon dioxide gas and warm bodies.
- Bedbugs do not have a preference for specific age groups, ethnicity, or sex.
- Persons at higher risk include those who have recently stayed overnight in a hotel, dorm room, hospital, or new home.
- Studies have shown increased sensitivity of cutaneous reaction in previous bite victims.

PHYSICAL FINDINGS & CLINICAL PRESENTATION

- Bites typically occur at night on exposed areas of skin, most often the face, neck, arms, and legs.
- The bites are painless and so do not awaken the individual.
- Onset of signs and symptoms of bites can be immediately on awakening or up to 10 days after the bite.
- Firm, purpuric or erythematous macules, urticaria, papules (Fig. 1), or bullae may be present. Bites are often inflammatory and pruritic, although bedbug-naive individuals may be asymptomatic to their first bites.
- Bite may have a central hemorrhagic punctum.
- Victim may observe a linear series often consisting of three bites ("breakfast, lunch, and dinner").
- Bites are typically pruritic.
- The size, degree of itching, and propensity toward vesiculation all increase with repeated bedbug bites.
- Fig. 2 illustrates symptoms and behaviors resulting from bed bug bites.

ETIOLOGY

- The *Cimex lectularius* species, also known as the common bedbug (Fig. 3), have flat, oval bodies and retroverted mouth parts used for taking blood meals. It feeds on mammals and birds. *Cimex hemipterus* is a tropical species that bites mostly humans, and hybrid species of the two insects exist. Both generally feed nocturnally on the blood of sleeping humans. They hide in beds, the floor, or furniture crevices during the day and emerge at night. They go through a larva stage (Fig. 4) and have a life span from 4 mo up to 1 yr. The adult bedbug is about 5 to 7 mm in length. It has a modified mouthpart for piercing and sucking that usually leaves a bite mark of papular urticarial presentation to exposed areas of skin. Bedbugs have weak appendages for latching on to their hosts and are not usually transported from person to person. They have no wings and cannot fly or jump, but they can move 3 to 4 feet per minute. Adult bed bugs that have a food source live up to 5 mo. Starved beg bugs (at any life stage) at room temperature will die within 70 days.[1]
- The saliva of the bedbug contains nitrophorin that enables vasodilation, an anticoagulant that interferes with production of coagulation factor Xa, a salivary apyrase that inhibits platelet aggregation, and an anesthetic. Consequently, the host often does not feel the bite until the effects have worn off.

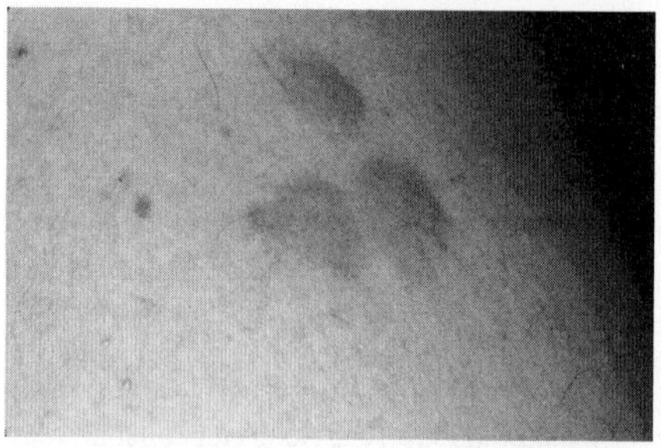

FIG. 1 Pruritic papules after bedbug bites. (From Kliegman RM et al: *Nelson textbook of pediatrics*, ed 19, Philadelphia, 2011, Saunders.)

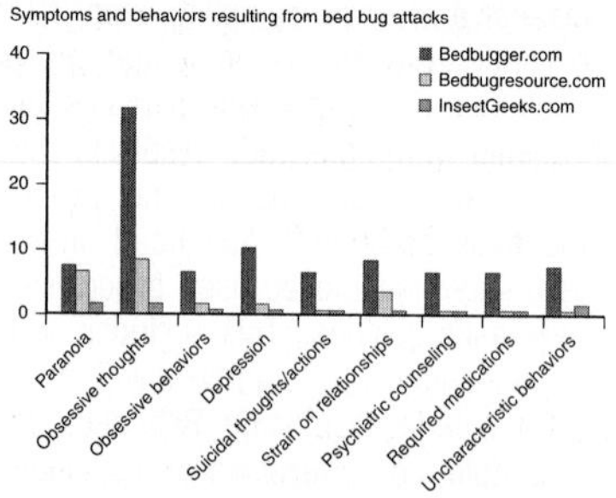

FIG. 2 Distribution of symptoms in 135 Internet reports describing effects of bed bug bites. (From Goddard J, de Shazo R: Psychological effects of bed bug attacks *[Cimex lectularius]*, *Am J Med* 125:101-103, 2012.)

DIAGNOSIS

DIFFERENTIAL DIAGNOSIS

- Scabies
- Flea and mite bites
- Delusional parasitosis

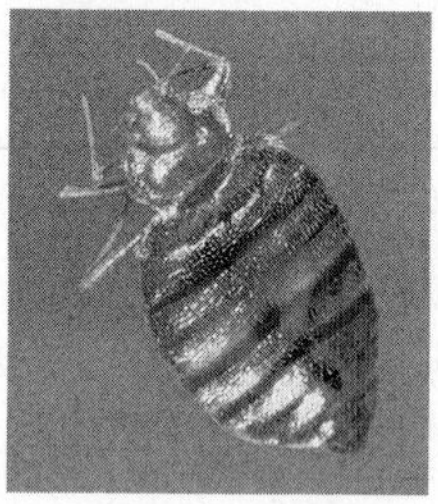

FIG. 3 Bedbug. (From James WD et al: *Andrews' diseases of the skin*, ed 12, Philadelphia, 2016, Saunders.)

[1]Parola P, Izri A: Bedbugs, *N Engl J Med* 382:2230-2237, 2020.

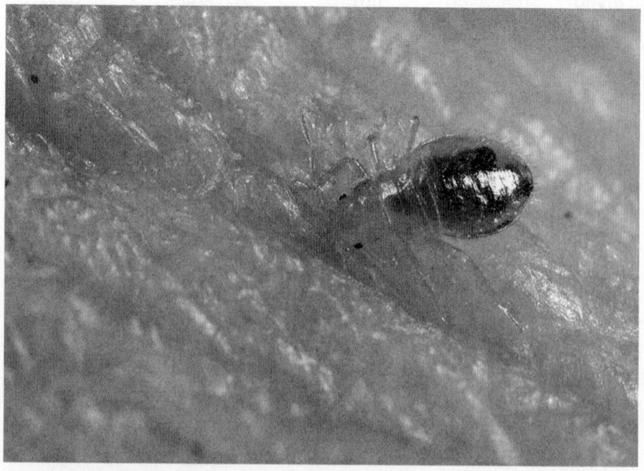

FIG. 4 Bedbug—second-stage larva. (From Habif TP: *Clinical dermatology: a color guide to diagnosis and therapy*, ed 6, Philadelphia, 2016, Elsevier.)

- Vesicular disorders, pemphigus herpetiformis
- Ecthyma
- Drug eruption

WORKUP

- Workup begins with history and physical for clinical symptoms and environmental findings suggestive of insect bites.
- Victims should carefully scrutinize the bedroom for signs of bedbug infestation. One may encounter fecal smears or flecks of blood on bed linens, inside furniture cracks and crevices, and behind peeling wallpaper. Bedbugs may travel as far as 20 feet for a meal. Densely infested rooms may also have a distinctive, pungent, soda syrup–like odor.

LABORATORY TESTS

- No specific tests recommended except for identification of the insect.
- The histology of bedbug bites is similar to other insect bites. Perivascular infiltrate of lymphocytes, histiocytes, eosinophils, and mast cells is seen within the upper dermis. One may also observe collagen bundles with interstitial eosinophils, dermal edema, and extravasated erythrocytes.
- Hypersensitivity to bedbug salivary proteins may be tested via intradermal allergy skin testing.
- Skin biopsy results are nonspecific and are not helpful in making the diagnosis.

Rx TREATMENT

- Specific treatment of bedbug bites is often not necessary. Bites may self-resolve within a week for milder cases and a few weeks for more severe cases. Treatment regimens are based on resolving symptoms of the bites, mainly pruritus.
- To prevent infection, avoid scratching the area.
- Topical glucocorticoids or systemic antihistamines are appropriate in patients with severe pruritus from the bedbug bite.
  1. Triamcinolone cream 0.1%; apply thin film to affected areas bid.
  2. Chlorpheniramine 4 mg PO at bedtime (adults), 2 mg PO at bedtime (children).
- Insecticides may be effective in eradicating the bedbug, but growing resistance has been seen and multi-insecticide therapy is recommended.
  1. Use permethrin spray for clothing and bedsheets or bed nets.
  2. Diethyltoluamide (DEET): Be wary of toxic levels in children when used at high concentrations.
  3. Deltamethrin and chlorfenapyr are two common insecticides used.
  4. Please consult a pest control professional for safe eradication.

NONPHARMACOLOGIC THERAPY

Vacuuming is effective in removing bedbugs but does not remove the eggs. Wash bedsheets and clothing in hot water with detergent with at least 20 min in a dryer. Bedbugs have a high thermal death point of 45° C (113° F) and also may survive at temperatures as low as 7° C (44.6° F). Some companies perform a treatment in which the room is heated above 50° C (122° F), which is a lethal temperature for all stages of a bedbug's life cycle. Coating bedposts with antifriction or adhesive substances such as petrolatum or duct tape may hinder bedbugs from gaining access to the bed.

ACUTE GENERAL Rx

Immunologic response is dependent on immunocompetence and individual sensitivity to the salivary components of the bedbug bite. Often, patients with papular urticaria have IgG antibodies to specific bedbug proteins. IgE antibodies may also mediate bullae formation. Anaphylaxis and death from bites is rare but documented in literature.

DISPOSITION

Patient may resume normal activity and lifestyle. Travelers should inspect their clothing and suitcases before returning home.

BEDBUGS AS POTENTIAL VECTORS

The bedbug has been studied extensively as a potential vector for human pathogens such as HIV, hepatitis B, hepatitis C, and Chagas disease. To date, there is no evidence of transmission from an infected bedbug to a human.

PEARLS & CONSIDERATIONS

COMMENTS

- Bedbugs are an increasing source of anguish and frustration for humans, and clinicians should evaluate for signs of stress and depression. Sleep deprivation, insomnia, nightmares, phobias, hypervigilance, and personal dysfunction with people worrying that they are being bitten at night are often underestimated.
- A combination of chemical and physical intervention is often necessary for complete eradication. All hiding areas must be carefully inspected and cleaned. Treatment may include pesticides, laundering, heat, freezing, vacuuming, and hiring a professional service to eradicate bedbugs.

SUGGESTED READINGS

Available at ExpertConsult.com

RELATED CONTENT

Bedbugs (Patient Information)
Bites and Stings, Insect (Related Key Topic)

AUTHOR: **Fred F. Ferri, MD**

BASIC INFORMATION

DEFINITION

Acute peripheral facial nerve (cranial nerve VII) palsy

SYNONYMS

Idiopathic facial paralysis
Facial nerve palsy

ICD-10CM CODE
G51.0 Bell palsy

EPIDEMIOLOGY & DEMOGRAPHICS

INCIDENCE: 20 to 30 cases per 100,000
PREDOMINANT SEX AND AGE: Sexes are equally affected. The median age is 40.
PEAK INCIDENCE: Patients younger than 70 yr and pregnant females, especially during the third trimester and first postpartum wk
RISK FACTORS: Diabetes and pregnancy

PHYSICAL FINDINGS & CLINICAL PRESENTATION

- Patients present with acute or subacute (hours to days) onset of unilateral facial paralysis with maximal weakness at 3 wk. Clinical findings are dependent on the location of facial nerve injury and involvement of associated branches (Fig. 1). One third of patients demonstrate incomplete paralysis, and the remaining two thirds have complete paralysis. Recovery usually occurs within the first 6 mo.
- Patients may also present with variable involvement of taste over the anterior two thirds of the tongue and/or altered secretion of the lacrimal and salivary glands.

ETIOLOGY

Most cases of Bell palsy are thought to be secondary to either a viral inflammatory or immune injury. Herpes simplex virus is thought to be the most common viral pathogen followed by herpes zoster. Other infectious causes include Epstein-Barr virus, cytomegalovirus, adenovirus, rubella, and mumps.

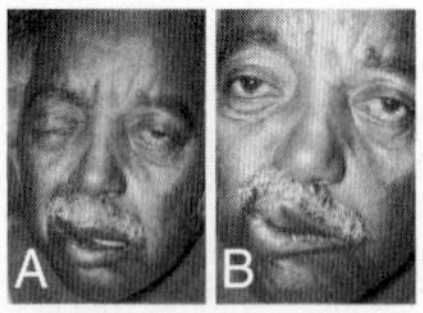

FIG. 1 A patient with a lesion of the facial nerve. A, The patient has difficulty in closing his left eye, and the left corner of his mouth droops. **B,** The latter defect is especially evident when the patient attempts to purse his lips. (From Haines DE: *Fundamental neuroscience for basic and clinical applications,* ed 3, Philadelphia, 2006, Churchill Livingstone.)

DIAGNOSIS

DIFFERENTIAL DIAGNOSIS

- Cortical stroke: Forehead and periorbital muscles are spared in stroke patients because of bilateral innervation of the upper face
- Brain stem stroke: Ipsilateral weakness in the upper and lower muscles of facial expression due to a stroke affecting the nucleus or fascicle of the seventh nerve
- Lyme disease: Facial nerve palsy is the most common cranial neuropathy associated with Lyme disease. In Lyme meningitis, facial nerve palsy may be unilateral or bilateral
- HIV
- Ramsay Hunt syndrome: Facial nerve paralysis associated with ipsilateral zoster oticus
- Parotid gland tumors
- Trauma/temporal bone fracture
- Meningeal processes:
  1. Infectious: Lyme disease, HIV, syphilis, leprosy, tuberculosis meningitis, fungal meningitis
  2. Inflammatory: Sarcoidosis, Sjögren syndrome, and Guillain-Barré syndrome and its variants
  3. Leptomeningeal carcinomatosis or lymphomatosis: Breast cancer, lung cancer, and lymphoma are most common
- Möbius syndrome
- Melkersson-Rosenthal syndrome

WORKUP

- Bell palsy is a clinical diagnosis.
- Additional workup may be necessary in patients with an uncertain diagnosis, complete seventh nerve injury, evidence of neurologic dysfunction in addition to seventh nerve injury, and lack of recovery.

LABORATORY TESTS

Laboratory tests are not typically recommended. However, if the diagnosis of Bell palsy is in question (e.g., bilateral facial nerve palsy, concern for a secondary etiology), then it is reasonable to pursue the following tests:

- Lyme antibody followed by Western blot for positive cases for confirmation. Consider lumbar puncture for CSF analysis for Lyme serologies. In areas with endemic Lyme disease routine testing for Lyme disease may be indicated in all patients with Bell palsy (16% prevalence of Lime disease)[2]
- ACE level
- Glycosylated hemoglobin (HgA1C)
- HIV
- RPR and VDRL in CSF
- ESR

[2] Pacheco A et al: Positive tests for Lyme disease and emergency department visits for Bell palsy patients, *J Emerg Med* 59(6):820-827, 2020.

ELECTRODIAGNOSTIC TESTING

Electrodiagnostic testing may be performed 2 wk after the onset of symptoms to assess the integrity of a motor unit and the degree of nerve damage. Facial motor response remains normal for the first 3 days following an injury and then rapidly decreases depending on the severity of the lesion. A facial motor study may be performed at 10 days and compared to the contralateral side. A motor response that is 10% the amplitude of the unaffected side on electrodiagnostic testing corresponds with 90% motor axon degeneration. One study found that patient recovery was poor when this critical value was reached.

IMAGING STUDIES

Imaging studies are not usually indicated.

- Brain MRI is indicated in certain cases, such as an upper motor neuron pattern (able to wrinkle forehead) where the temporalis branch of the facial nerve is spared.
- Brain MRI with gadolinium is indicated either when other cranial nerve palsies are present or when a meningeal process is suspected.
- CT temporal bone is indicated in cases of either trauma or complete facial paralysis in which the surgeon is considering decompression.

TREATMENT

NONPHARMACOLOGIC THERAPY

- Reassurance that most patients will have a full recovery and that the patient did not sustain a stroke.
- Eye patch to prevent corneal drying/abrasion and subsequent ulceration. Patients may protect their eyes with Lacri-Lube at night and artificial tears during the day.
- Acupuncture with needle manipulation and strong stimulation has been shown to improve recovery after Bell palsy when compared to acupuncture without needle manipulation.[1]

ACUTE GENERAL Rx

- Corticosteroids started within 72 hr will expedite speed and rate of recovery in most patients. Antiviral therapy alone has no benefit.
  1. Two high-quality randomized trials assessed efficacy of early (<72 hr) treatment with glucocorticoids alone, antiviral therapy alone, and combination therapy in the treatment of Bell palsy. Glucocorticoids alone were effective, while antiviral therapy showed no benefit when given either alone or with concomitant glucocorticoid therapy.
  2. The largest study compared groups receiving the following treatments: (a)

[1] Xu SB et al: Effectiveness of strengthened stimulation during acupuncture for the treatment of Bell palsy: a randomized controlled trial, *CMAJ* 185:473-479, 2013.

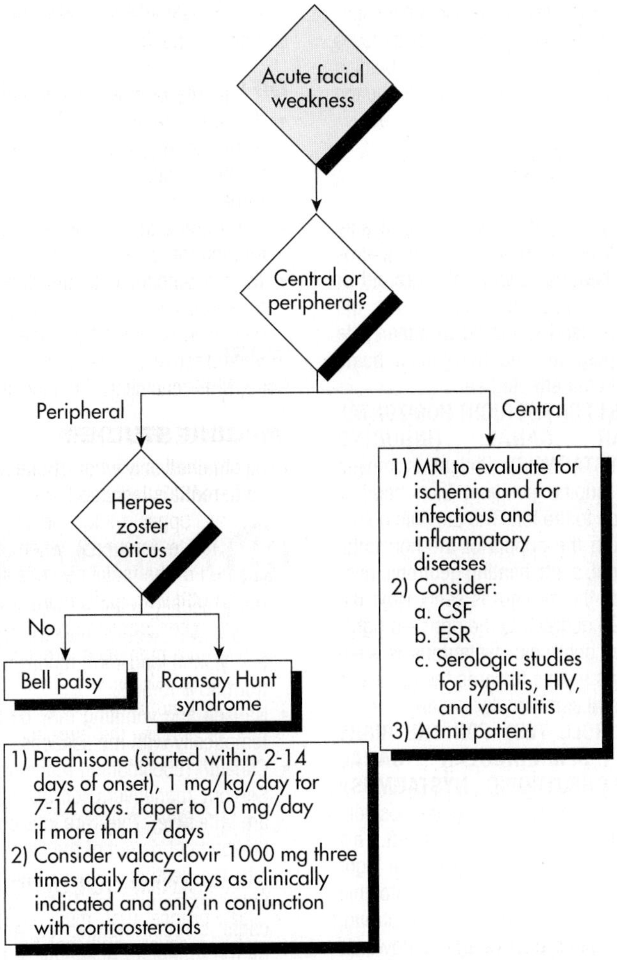

FIG. 2 Algorithm outlining the treatment of patients with Bell palsy. *CSF,* Cerebrospinal fluid; *ESR,* erythrocyte sedimentation rate; *HIV,* human immunodeficiency virus; *MRI,* magnetic resonance imaging. (Modified from Adams JG et al: *Emergency medicine, clinical essentials,* ed 2, St Louis, 2013, Elsevier.)

60 mg prednisolone daily, (b) 1000 mg valacyclovir three times daily for 1 wk, (c) combination therapy, and (d) placebo. All interventions were administered within 72 hr of presentation.

3. Time to recovery, determined at a 1-yr follow-up appointment, was shortest in the group treated with prednisolone monotherapy. The efficacy of valacyclovir monotherapy did not differ from placebo, and no added benefit was seen with combination therapy.

- Treatment guidelines recommend prednisone 60 to 80 mg daily for 1 wk.
  1. Despite the lack of strong clinical evidence, some authors still recommend treatment with valacyclovir (1000 mg 3 times daily for 1 wk) in severe cases (i.e., level IV or greater on the House-Brackmann grading system).
- Surgical decompression is not currently recommended.
  1. The 2001 American Academy of Neurology Practice Parameter concluded there was insufficient evidence to make any recommendation regarding surgical decompression for Bell palsy.
  2. This conclusion was further substantiated by a 2011 Cochrane systematic review, which looked at two additional studies, again citing insufficient evidence regarding surgical decompression for Bell palsy.
- Fig. 2 describes an algorithm for the treatment of patients with Bell palsy.

CHRONIC Rx

Botulinum toxin may be used in cases of hemifacial spasm that may follow recovery from Bell palsy.

DISPOSITION

- Between 70% and 90% of patients with Bell palsy have a complete recovery within a few weeks.

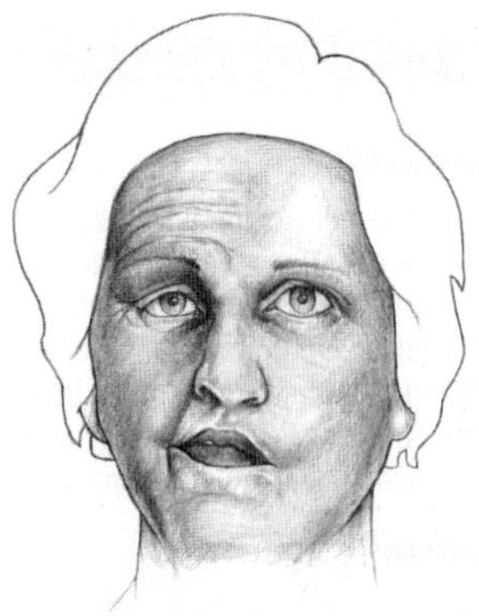

FIG. 3 Bell palsy. The patient with Bell palsy (facial nerve palsy) will demonstrate an unwrinkled forehead, widely opened eyes (with weakness of eyelid closure), flattening of the nasolabial fold, and a droop of the corner of the mouth. (From Remmel KS et al: *Handbook of symptom-oriented neurology,* ed 3, St Louis, 2002, Mosby.)

- 85% show recovery after 3 wk. Prognosis is favorable if recovery is seen during this timeframe.
- 13% have slight sequelae, and 16% have residual weakness, synkinesis, or contracture.
- Recurrence rate is 7%, and the average time to recurrence is 10 yr.

REFERRAL

- Neurologist if clinical diagnosis is in question
- Ophthalmologist if concern for corneal abrasion or ulceration

PEARLS & CONSIDERATIONS

COMMENTS

- Assess wrinkling of forehead (Fig. 3). If present on affected side, ensure that the facial weakness is not central.
- Assess for strength of eye closure. A patient with Bell palsy will have difficulty with ipsilateral eye closure, whereas a patient with a central lesion with have equal eye closure strength bilaterally.
- Assess for other cranial nerve deficits or long-tract signs because brain stem fascicular lesions of the seventh nerve can show peripheral facial pattern of weakness.

SUGGESTED READINGS

Available at ExpertConsult.com

RELATED CONTENT

Bell Palsy (Facial Palsy) (Patient Information)

AUTHOR: **Joseph S. Kass, MD, JD, FAAN**

Benign Paroxysmal Positional Vertigo

BASIC INFORMATION

DEFINITION

Benign paroxysmal positional vertigo (BPPV) is a labyrinthine disorder and is the most common cause of vertigo. It is characterized by paroxysms of brief spinning sensation accompanied by nystagmus that usually last less than a minute. These paroxysms are generally induced by changes in head position with respect to gravity.

SYNONYM

BPPV

ICD-10CM CODE
H81.1 Benign paroxysmal vertigo

EPIDEMIOLOGY & DEMOGRAPHICS

Higher prevalence seen in elderly and women.

INCIDENCE: Incidence increases with advancing age. Unrecognized BPPV can be found in about 10% of certain geriatric populations, and there is a cumulative incidence of nearly 10% by age 80 yr.

PREVALENCE: Lifetime prevalence is 2.4%. Reported prevalence is 10.7% and 64 cases per 100,000 population. BPPV is by far the most common type of vertigo.

PREDOMINANT SEX & AGE: Female (2:1 to 3:1 ratio); peak onset: 50 to 60 yr.

RISK FACTORS: Head trauma, inner ear surgery, viral labyrinthitis, Ménière disease, migraine. The majority are idiopathic.

GENETICS: Unknown

PHYSICAL FINDINGS & CLINICAL PRESENTATION

- Brief paroxysms of vertigo and nystagmus with certain head positions are seen in 70%.
- Episodes are typically triggered by head position changes such as getting in or out of bed, rolling over in bed, tilting the head forward, or bending forward.
- Episodes are brief, usually lasting 30 to 40 seconds but can recur for several days or months.
- Usually no hearing abnormalities are present.
- Direction of nystagmus depends on the canal affected with reversal of direction being seen while sitting up, and fatigability with repeated testing.
- Rarely persistent vertigo and disequilibrium may be seen.

POSTERIOR SEMICIRCULAR CANAL (PSC)

While posterior, horizontal, or superior semicircular canal can be affected as isolated or in different combinations, PSC involvement is most common (60%-90%) and will be discussed in the following sections. Nystagmus is up-beating and torsional and can be elicited by the Dix-Hallpike maneuver.

DIX-HALLPIKE MANEUVER

With head turned to one side at an angle of 45 degrees, patient is moved rapidly from sitting to supine position with head hanging below the end of the table at an angle of 15 to 20 degrees. The posterior semicircular canal comes into the sagittal plane and the free-floating otolith debris moves down and away from the ampulla. An up-beating and torsional nystagmus will be seen with the top poles of the eye beating towards the lower ear.

HORIZONTAL SEMICIRCULAR CANAL

Involvement may be underestimated as it may remit spontaneously. It produces either geotropic nystagmus beating towards the ground or apogeotropic nystagmus beating towards the ceiling when the head is turned to either side in the supine position. The nystagmus beats stronger towards the affected ear.

HEAD ROLL TEST FOR THE RIGHT HORIZONTAL SEMICIRCULAR CANAL (INDUCING GEOTROPIC NYSTAGMUS): Patient is moved from sitting to supine position, then head is rolled 90 degrees to the left. The otolithic debris moves away from the cupula of the horizontal semicircular canal, a left-beating geotropic nystagmus (towards the ground) is seen. Next the head is turned 90 degrees to the right—a right-beating stronger geotropic nystagmus is seen as otolithic debris moves towards the cupula of the right horizontal semicircular canal.

SUPINE HEAD ROLL TEST FOR THE RIGHT HORIZONTAL SEMICIRCULAR CANAL (INDUCING APOGEOTROPIC NYSTAGMUS): Patient is moved from sitting to supine position, then head is rolled 90 degrees to the left. This induces deflection of the cupula of the right horizontal semicircular canal due to otolithic debris near or attached to the cupula. A strong, right-beating apogeotropic nystagmus (towards the ceiling) is induced. Next, the head is turned 90 degrees in the opposite direction. Now the right horizontal semicircular canal cupula is deflected in the opposite direction and a weak, left-beating apogeotropic nystagmus results.

ANTERIOR SEMICIRCULAR CANAL

Involvement is rare as it is located uppermost in the labyrinth and so otolithic debris is unlikely to become trapped. A downbeat and torsional nystagmus where the top poles of the eye beat towards the lower ear is seen. Evaluating for central lesions is a must in these cases.

ETIOLOGY

The fundamental pathologic process is believed to be the movement of otolithic debris in the endolymph of the inner ear. The debris may be present in the cupula (cupulolithiasis) or free floating within the semicircular canal near the cupula (canalithiasis). Static head position changes with respect to gravity, causing the debris to move within the semicircular canal and creating a false sense of rotation.

DIAGNOSIS

Elicitation of a typical nystagmus with Dix-Hallpike is the standard for diagnosing posterior canal BPPV. However, 25% of symptomatic patients may not exhibit nystagmus. Appropriate referral to a neurologist or neuro-otologist should be considered in these cases.

Fig. E1 shows a diagnostic algorithm for vertigo and dizziness.

DIFFERENTIAL DIAGNOSIS

- Vestibular neuritis
- Vestibular migraine
- Ménière disease
- Stroke
- Box 1 lists causes of vertigo with and without hearing loss
- Table 1 describes the differential diagnosis of true vertigo

WORKUP

None; BPPV is a clinical diagnosis.

IMAGING STUDIES

To be obtained only when stroke remains high in the differential diagnosis

TREATMENT

- BPPV usually resolves without treatment in 2 to 4 wk. Recurrences are common in the first yr, and long-term recurrence rates range from 30% to 50%.
- Nausea and vomiting may be treated symptomatically with medications.
- Canalith repositioning maneuvers (Epley and Semont maneuvers for the posterior canal) are effective. They are designed to "flush" otolithic debris out of the semicircular canals into the vestibule where they are resorbed. Epley maneuver for BPPV of the posterior canal is recommended as standard of care by the American Academy of Neurology and American Academy of Otolaryngology-Head and Neck Surgery. When patients do not respond, it may be related to the technique, or they may be refractory. There is no clear

BOX 1 Causes of Vertigo with and without Hearing Loss

Hearing Loss
Conductive
- Otitis media with effusion
- Chronic suppurative otitis media or cholesteatoma should be considered

Sensorineural
- Perilymphatic fistula
- Tumor
- Ménière disease
- Migraine headache
- Genetic syndromes
- Temporal bone fracture
- Vestibular concussion

No Hearing Loss
Acute Vertigo
- Perilymphatic fistula
- Benign positional vertigo
- Seizure
- Labyrinthitis

Recurrent or Chronic Vertigo
- Acoustic neuroma
- Multiple sclerosis

From Marx JA et al: *Rosen's emergency medicine: concepts and clinical practice,* ed 7, Philadelphia, 2010, Elsevier.

TABLE 1 Differential Diagnosis of Patients with True Vertigo

Cause	History	Associated Symptoms	Physical
Peripheral			
1. Benign paroxysmal positional vertigo	Short-lived, positional, fatigable episodes	Nausea, vomiting	Single position can precipitate vertigo. Horizontorotary nystagmus often can be induced at bedside
2. Labyrinthitis			
• Serous	Mild to severe positional symptoms. Usually coexisting or antecedent infection of ear, nose, throat, or meninges	Mild to severe hearing loss can occur	Usually nontoxic patient with minimal fever elevation
• Acute suppurative	Coexisting acute exudative infection of the inner ear. Severe symptoms	Usually severe hearing loss, nausea, vomiting	Febrile patient showing signs of toxicity. Acute otitis media
• Toxic	Gradually progressive symptoms: Patients on medication causing toxicity	Hearing loss that may become rapid and severe, nausea, vomiting	Hearing loss. Ataxia common feature in chronic phase
3. Ménière disease	Recurrent episodes of severe rotational vertigo usually lasting hours. Onset usually abrupt. Attacks may occur in clusters. Long symptom-free remissions	Nausea, vomiting, tinnitus, hearing loss	Positional nystagmus not present
4. Vestibular neuronitis	Sudden onset of severe vertigo, increasing in intensity for hours, then gradually subsiding over several days. Mild positional vertigo often lasts weeks to months. Sometimes history of infection or toxic exposure that precedes initial attack. Highest incidence is found in third and fifth decades	Nausea, vomiting. Auditory symptoms do not occur	Spontaneous nystagmus toward the involved ear may be present
5. Acoustic neuroma	Gradual onset and increase in symptoms. Neurologic signs in later stages. Most occur in women between 30 and 60	Hearing loss, tinnitus. True ataxia and neurologic signs as tumor enlarges	Unilateral decreased hearing. True truncal ataxia and other neurologic signs when tumor enlarges. May have diminution or absence of corneal reflex. Eighth cranial nerve deficit may be present
Central			
1. Vascular disorders			
• Vertebrobasilar insufficiency	Should be considered in any patient of advanced age with isolated new-onset vertigo without an obvious cause. More likely with history of atherosclerosis. Initial episode usually seconds to minutes	Often headache. Usually neurologic symptoms including dysarthria, ataxia, weakness, numbness, double vision. Tinnitus and deafness uncommon	Neurologic deficits usually present, but initially neurologic examination can be normal
• Cerebellar hemorrhage	Sudden onset of severe symptoms	Headache, vomiting, ataxia	Signs of toxicity. Dysmetria, true ataxia. Ipsilateral sixth cranial nerve palsy may be present
• Occlusion of posterior inferior cerebellar artery (Wallenberg syndrome)	Vertigo associated with significant neurologic complaints	Nausea, vomiting, loss of pain and temperature sensation, ataxia, hoarseness	Loss of pain and temperature sensation on the side of the face ipsilateral to the lesion and on the opposite side of the body, paralysis of the palate, pharynx, and larynx. Horner syndrome (ipsilateral ptosis, miosis, and decreased facial sweating)
• Subclavian steal syndrome	Classic picture is syncopal attacks during exercise, but most cases present with more subtle symptoms	Arm fatigue, cramps, mild lightheadedness may be only other symptoms than vertigo	Diminished or absent radial pulses in affected side or systolic blood pressure differentials between the two areas occur in most patients
2. Head trauma	Symptoms begin with or shortly after head trauma. Positional symptoms most common type after trauma. Self-limited symptoms that can persist weeks to months	Usually mild nausea	Occasionally, basilar skull fracture
3. Neck trauma	Usual onset 7-10 days after whiplash injury. Symptoms may last weeks to months. Episodes seconds to minutes when turning head	Neck pain	Neck tenderness, pain on movement, and positional nystagmus and vertigo when head is turned to side of the whiplash
4. Vertebrobasilar migraine	Vertigo almost always followed by headache. Patient has usually had similar episodes in past. Most patients have a family history of migraine. Syndrome usually begins in adolescence	Dysarthria, ataxia, visual disturbances, or paresthesias usually precede headache	No residual neurologic or otologic signs are present after attack

Continued

TABLE 1 Differential Diagnosis of Patients with True Vertigo—cont'd

Cause	History	Associated Symptoms	Physical
5. Multiple sclerosis	Vertigo presenting symptoms in 7%-10% and appears in the course of the disease in a third. Onset may be severe and suggest labyrinth disease. Disease onset usually between ages 20 and 40. Often history of other attacks with varying neurologic signs or symptoms	Nausea and vomiting, which may be severe	May have horizontal, rotary, or vertical nystagmus. Nystagmus may persist after the vertiginous symptoms have subsided. Bilateral internuclear ophthalmoplegia and ataxic eye movements suggest multiple sclerosis
6. Temporal lobe epilepsy	Can be initial or prominent symptom in some patients with the disorder	Memory impairment, hallucinations, trancelike states, seizures	May have aphasia or convulsions
7. Hypoglycemia	Should be considered in diabetics and any other patient with unexplained symptoms	Sweating, anxiety	Tachycardia, mental status change may be present

From Marx JA et al: *Rosen's emergency medicine: concepts and clinical practice,* ed 7, Philadelphia, 2010, Elsevier.

consensus on how many times the maneuver should be performed at a single visit. Many prefer to do it two or three times if nystagmus is still present with the second maneuver. Other maneuvers such as Barbecue, Vannucchi, and Gufoni are used to reposition debris in the horizontal semicircular canal and will not be discussed here.

EPLEY MANEUVER:

- Head is turned 90 degrees towards unaffected side. The head and trunk are then turned an additional 90 degrees in the same direction, so that the patient lies on the unaffected side with head pointing towards the floor. The otolithic debris moves in the same direction, producing a brief nystagmus. The patient is then moved to a sitting position, which allows the debris to fall out of the canal into the utricle through the common crus.
- Each position should be maintained for 30 seconds or until the nystagmus or vertigo resolves. Sometimes nystagmus in the opposite direction is seen. It is prudent for patients to sit still in the upright position for about 15 minutes and then to walk cautiously.

NONPHARMACOLOGIC THERAPY

Transection of the ampullary nerve (singular nerve) and plugging of the involved canal are rarely performed for intractable and treatment-resistant cases.

ACUTE GENERAL Rx

Canalith repositioning

CHRONIC Rx

If multiple treatments are needed, patients should be instructed to perform the maneuvers at home.

REFERRAL

To a neuro-otologist, otolaryngologist, neurologist

PEARLS & CONSIDERATIONS

- BPPV is a benign and self-limiting condition but can be disabling.
- Diagnosis is clinical and canalith repositioning maneuvers are effective.

PATIENT & FAMILY EDUCATION

- Reassurance
- Fall precautions

SUGGESTED READINGS

Available at ExpertConsult.com

RELATED CONTENT

Ménière Disease (Related Key Topic)
Vestibular Neuronitis (Related Key Topic)

AUTHOR: **Joseph S. Kass, MD, JD, FAAN**

BASIC INFORMATION

DEFINITION

Benign prostatic hyperplasia (BPH) is the benign growth of the prostate, generally originating in the periureteral and transition zones, with subsequent obstructive and irritative voiding symptoms. Histologically, BPH refers to the proliferation of smooth muscle, epithelium, and stromal cells within the transition zone of the prostate that surrounds the proximal urethra.

SYNONYMS

Benign prostatic hypertrophy
BPH
Prostatic hypertrophy

ICD-10CM CODES
- N40.1 Enlarged prostate with lower urinary tract symptoms
- N40.0 Enlarged prostate without lower urinary tract symptoms
- N40.3 Nodular prostate with lower urinary tract symptoms
- N40.2 Nodular prostate without lower urinary tract symptoms

EPIDEMIOLOGY & DEMOGRAPHICS

- 80% of men have evidence of BPH by age 80 yr.
- Medical and surgical intervention for problems caused by BPH is required in <20% of males by age 75 yr.
- Transurethral resection of the prostate (TURP) is the tenth most common operative procedure (<400,000/yr in U.S.).
- 10% to 30% of men with BPH have occult prostate cancer.

PHYSICAL FINDINGS & CLINICAL PRESENTATION

- Digital rectal examination (DRE) reveals enlargement of the prostate.
- Focal enlargement may be indicative of malignancy.
- There is poor correlation between size of prostate and symptoms (BPH may be asymptomatic if it does not encroach on the urethral lumen).
- Most patients with BPH report difficulty in initiating urination (hesitancy), decrease in caliber and force of stream, incomplete emptying of bladder often resulting in double voiding (need to urinate again a few minutes after voiding), postvoid "dribbling," and nocturia.

ETIOLOGY

Multifactorial (Fig. E1); a functioning testicle is necessary for development of BPH (as evidenced by the absence in males who were castrated before puberty).

DIAGNOSIS

DIFFERENTIAL DIAGNOSIS

- Prostatitis
- Prostate cancer
- Strictures (urethral)
- Medications interfering with the muscle fibers in the prostate and also with bladder function:
  1. Opiates: Impaired autonomic function
  2. Decongestants: Increased sphincter tone
  3. Antihistamines: Decreased parasympathetic tone
  4. Tricyclic antidepressants: Anticholinergic effects
- Neurogenic bladder
- Bladder cancer

WORKUP

Symptom assessment (use of American Urological Association [AUA] Symptom Index for BPH [Table 1]), laboratory tests, and imaging studies. Fig. E2 describes a diagnostic approach to patients with BPH.

LABORATORY TESTS

- Prostate-specific antigen (PSA): Protease secreted by epithelial cells of the prostate; elevated in 30% to 50% of patients with BPH. Testing for PSA increases detection rate for prostate cancer and tends to detect cancer at an earlier stage. However, the PSA test does not discriminate well between patients with symptomatic BPH and those with prostate cancer, particularly if the cancer is pathologically localized and curable. The test may also trigger additional evaluation, including ultrasound biopsy of the prostate. Asymptomatic men with PSA levels >2 ng/ml do not need annual testing. According to the AUA, PSA testing and DRE should be offered to any asymptomatic man <50 yr with a life expectancy of 10 yr. PSA testing can also be offered at an earlier age in men at higher risk of prostatic cancer (e.g., first-degree relatives with prostate cancer; African American race).
- Measurement of "free" PSA is useful to assess the probability of prostate cancer in patients with normal DRE and total PSA between 4 and 10 ng/ml. In these patients the global risk of prostate cancer is 25%.

TABLE 1 International Prostate Symptom Score (I-PSS)

Symptom	SCORE: Not at All	Less Than 1 Time in 5	Less Than Half the Time	About Half the Time	More Than Half the Time	Almost Always	Total Score
Incomplete emptying: Over the past month, how often have you had a sensation of not emptying your bladder completely after you finished urinating?	0	1	2	3	4	5	
Frequency: Over the past month, how often have you had to urinate again <2 hr after you finished urinating?	0	1	2	3	4	5	
Intermittency: Over the past month, how often have you found you stopped and started again several times when you urinated?	0	1	2	3	4	5	
Urgency: Over the past month, how often have you found it difficult to postpone urination?	0	1	2	3	4	5	
Weak stream: Over the past month, how often have you had a weak urinary stream?	0	1	2	3	4	5	
Straining: Over the past month, how often have you had to push or strain to begin urination?	0	1	2	3	4	5	
	None	1 Time	2 Times	3 Times	4 Times	5 or More Times	
Nocturia: Over the past month, how many times did you most typically get up to urinate from the time you went to bed at night until the time you got up in the morning?	0	1	2	3	4	5	
Total I-PSS score =							

However, if the free PSA is >25%, the risk of prostate cancer decreases to 8%, whereas if the free PSA is <10%, the risk of cancer increases to 56%. Free PSA is also useful to evaluate the aggressiveness of prostate cancer. A low free PSA percentage generally indicates a high-grade cancer, whereas a high free PSA percentage is generally associated with a slower-growing tumor.

- Elevated measurement of prostate cancer gene 3 (*PCA3*) in urine specimens collected after digital exam is helpful in deciding about prostate biopsy in men with elevated PSA (increased *PCA3* = increased likelihood of prostate cancer).
- Urinalysis, urine culture, and sensitivity to rule out infection (if suspected).
- Blood urea nitrogen and creatinine to rule out postrenal insufficiency.

IMAGING STUDIES

- Transrectal ultrasound may be indicated in patients with palpable nodules or significant elevation of PSA. It is also useful to estimate prostate size. BPH may also be evident in suprapubic ultrasound and MRI (Fig. E3).
- Uroflowmetry may be used to determine relative impact of obstruction on urine flow. Urethral pressure profile is useful to predict prostatic hypertrophy within the urethral lumen.
- Pressure flow studies, although invasive, are particularly helpful in patients whose history and/or examination suggest primary bladder dysfunction as a cause of symptoms of prostatism. They are also useful in patients for whom a distinction between prostatic obstruction and impaired detrusor contractility may affect the choice of therapy. However, pressure flow studies may not be useful in the workup of the usual patient with symptoms of prostatism.
- Postvoid residual urine measurement has not been proved useful in predicting the need for or response to treatment; it may be useful in monitoring the course of the disease in patients who elect nonsurgical treatment.
- Urethral cystoscopy is an option during later evaluation if invasive treatment is being planned.

Rx TREATMENT

NONPHARMACOLOGIC THERAPY

- Avoidance of caffeine or any other foods that may exacerbate symptoms
- Avoidance of medications that may exacerbate symptoms (e.g., most cold and allergy remedies)

GENERAL Rx

- Asymptomatic patients with prostate enlargement caused by BPH generally do not require treatment. Patients with mild to moderate symptoms are candidates for pharmacologic treatment (see the following). For patients who have specific complications from BPH, prostate surgery is usually the most appropriate form of treatment. However, surgery may result in significant complications (e.g., incontinence, infection).
- Alpha-blockers (e.g., tamsulosin, alfuzosin, doxazosin, prazosin, terazosin) relax smooth muscle of the bladder neck and prostate and can increase peak urinary flow rate. They have no effect on the size of the prostate. Alpha-1 blockers are useful in symptomatic patients to relieve symptoms of obstruction by causing relaxation of smooth muscle tone in the prostatic capsule, urethra, and bladder neck.
- Hormonal manipulation with finasteride, a 5-alpha-reductase inhibitor that blocks conversion of testosterone to dihydrotestosterone, can reduce the size of the prostate. Usual dose is 5 mg qd. Treatment requires ≥6 mo for maximal effect.
- Dutasteride is also a 5-alpha-reductase inhibitor useful to decrease prostate size and improve urinary flow. In addition to inhibiting the isoform of 5-alpha-reductase located in the prostate, the medication inhibits a second isoform and reduces dihydrotestosterone formation in the skin and liver. Usual dose is 0.5 mg qd.
- Tadalafil 2.5 to 5 mg qd has been FDA-approved to treat patients with signs and symptoms of BPH and patients with both ED and signs and symptoms of BPH. Tadalafil can potentiate the hypotensive effect of alpha-blockers and should not be used in combination with alpha-blockers.
- The dietary supplement saw palmetto is commonly used for relief of symptoms of BPH. Recent trials using 160 mg of saw palmetto bid did not improve symptoms of BPH. This contrasts with the positive findings of many previous studies. Trials with higher dose-ranging protocols are currently in progress.
- Prostatic urethral lift (PUL) is an outpatient treatment option for BPH.
- The prostatic urethral lift implant (UroLift) is an increasingly popular minimally invasive procedure for BPH. It is placed transurethrally at the site of obstruction to open the urethra by compressing the obstructing prostatic lobes and holding them permanently retracted with suture-based implants. Advantages are low risk for ejaculatory or erectile disfunction and use of local anesthesia or propofol sedation. Major disadvantage is 6% annual reintervention rate.[1]
- TURP is the most commonly used surgical procedure for BPH. It is recommended for patients unresponsive to medical therapy who have renal insufficiency, recurrent UTIs, bladder stones, or gross hematuria. Transurethral incision of the prostate (TUIP), a procedure almost equivalent in efficacy, is limited to patients whose estimated resection tissue weight would be 30 g or less. TUIP can be performed in an ambulatory setting or during a 1-day hospitalization. Open prostatectomy is typically performed on patients with very large prostates.
- Laser therapy for BPH is a less invasive alternative to TURP; YAG laser enucleation has minimal effect on potency, libido, or patient satisfaction with his sex life and is associated with retrograde ejaculation. However, recent studies indicate that at least in the initial 7 mo after surgery, TURP is moderately more effective than laser therapy in relieving symptoms of BPH.
- Transurethral needle ablation with radiofrequency to remove periurethral prostate tissue is being increasingly used in patients with prostate volume >60 ml and moderate symptoms. It has a low morbidity rate, but treatment failure is approximately 25% at 5 yr and <80% at 10 yr.
- Balloon dilation of the prostatic urethra is less effective than surgery for relieving symptoms but is associated with fewer complications. It is a reasonable treatment option for patients with smaller prostates and no middle lobe enlargement.
- Surgery need not be the treatment of last resort for most patients; that is, patients need not undergo other treatments for BPH before they can have surgery. However, recommending surgery on the grounds that a patient's surgical risk will "only increase with age" is generally inappropriate.

[1]Miller L et al: Surgical reintervention rate after prostatic urethral lift: systemic review and meta-analysis involving over 2000 patients, *J Urol* 204:1019-1026, 2020.

DISPOSITION

With appropriate therapy, symptoms improve or stabilize in <70% of patients with BPH.

REFERRAL

Urology referral for patients with severe or intolerable symptoms and for any patient suspected of having prostate cancer (10%-30% of men with BPH)

PEARLS & CONSIDERATIONS

COMMENTS

- Emerging technologies for treating BPH, including prostatic artery embolization, transurethral holmium laser enucleation, transurethral electrovaporization, and transurethral microwave thermotherapy of the prostate, appear promising; however, long-term effectiveness has not yet been demonstrated.
- The increase in the use of pharmacologic management has resulted in <30% reduction in the total number of TURP procedures.
- Combined drug therapy for BPH with an alpha-blocker and a 5-alpha-reductase inhibitor is superior to monotherapy with either agent. After 1 yr of combination therapy, withdrawal of the alpha-blocker will usually not exacerbate symptoms.
- Treatment with 5-alpha-reductase inhibitors (finasteride, dutasteride) is associated with approximately 30% higher risk for developing type 2 diabetes.

SUGGESTED READINGS

Available at ExpertConsult.com

RELATED CONTENT

Enlarged Prostate (Patient Information)

AUTHOR: **Fred F. Ferri, MD**

BASIC INFORMATION

DEFINITION

Bicuspid aortic valves (BAVs) are the most common congenital disorder of the heart. It is a result of partial or complete fusion of two of the aortic valve leaflets. Most commonly, fusion of leaflets forms a central raphe, and right and left coronary cusps fuse together. BAV aortopathy results in aortic root and ascending aorta dilation. Aortopathy of the BAV is probably related to rheologic force and shear stress on the aortic wall. It results in cystic medial degeneration of the aortic wall.

SYNONYMS

Bicommissural aortic valve
BAV

ICD-10CM CODE

Q23.1 Bicuspid aortic valve

EPIDEMIOLOGY & DEMOGRAPHICS

PREVALENCE:

- Approximately 1% to 2% of the general population has BAV.
- BAV is the most common cause for valvular aortic stenosis in persons ≤65 yr of age.

PREDOMINANT SEX & AGE: Predominant in males with 2:1 male-to-female ratio.

RISK FACTORS: BAV can be sporadic (more common) and familial. No clear risk factors have been defined. However, multiple clinical conditions are associated with it.

- Coarctation of the aorta
- Turner syndrome
- Shone complex (supravalvular mitral ring, subvalvular aortic membrane, parachute mitral valve, coarctation of the aorta)
- Supravalvular aortic stenosis
- Sinus of Valsalva aneurysm
- Ventricular septal defect

PHYSICAL FINDINGS & CLINICAL PRESENTATION

Symptoms and signs:

- Usually asymptomatic in the young. However, the bicuspid valve degenerates more rapidly than the native tricuspid aortic valve due to rheologic force and shear stress, and causes rapid progression of aortic stenosis. Similar forces on the aortic wall cause aortic root and ascending aorta dilation, which results in aortic aneurysm formation and aortic regurgitation
- Ejection click
- Early peaking ejection systolic murmur
- Early diastolic murmur if aortic root dilated and aortic regurgitation present

ETIOLOGY

It is a common congenital disorder. Embryologically, aortic valve cusps fail to separate, which results in a larger and a smaller cusp.

Dx DIAGNOSIS

DIFFERENTIAL DIAGNOSIS

- Subvalvular aortic membrane
- Aortic valvular stenosis
- Supravalvular stenosis

LABORATORY TESTS

No laboratory tests are recommended for diagnosing BAV.

IMAGING STUDIES

- Transthoracic echocardiogram
- Transesophageal echocardiogram
- Cardiac computed tomography angiogram (CCTA)
- Cardiac magnetic resonance angiogram

Rx TREATMENT

- Echocardiographic surveillance is needed to assess progression of bicuspid valve aortic stenosis, regurgitation, and aortic root dilation. If echocardiogram is not optimal to measure aortic root and ascending aorta diameters, consider aortic magnetic resonance angiography or CT angiography. Surveillance interval is determined by the degree and rate of progression of aortic dilation and by family history. Annual surveillance is needed if the aortic diameter is greater than 4.5 cm.
- Surgical aortic valve replacement (SAVR) is indicated for symptomatic BAV disease without aortopathy in low- to intermediate-risk patients.
- Surgical aortic root and/or ascending aorta repair is recommended in patients with BAV disease and aortic aneurysm diameter ≥5.5 cm. SAVR can be considered for moderate to severe BAV stenosis.
- Surgical aortic root and/or ascending aorta repair with valve replacement is recommended in patients with BAV disease and aortic aneurysm diameter of 5.0 cm if there is a family history of dissection or rapid aortic growth (3 to 5 mm/yr) or aortic coarctation, or small stature. SAVR can be considered for moderate to severe BAV stenosis.
- It is reasonable to surgically repair a 4.5-cm aortic root and/or ascending aorta if patient is undergoing SAVR for moderate to severe BAV disease.
- Transcatheter aortic valve replacement (TAVR) is a reasonable option for symptomatic BAV stenosis with reasonable anatomy (no aortopathy) in intermediate and high surgical risk patients. However, Transcatheter Valve Registry data showed higher rates of stroke, annular rupture, and need for permanent pacemakers with TAVR in BAV stenosis compared with tricuspid aortic valve stenosis.
- In 2019 the PARTNER III trial showed significantly lower risk of annual mortality, stroke, or rehospitalization with TAVR compared with SAVR. However, this trial excluded BAV stenosis patients.
- STS/ACC TVT registry analysis, which included 932 bicuspid aortic valve stenosis patients who underwent TAVR, showed similar mortality, stroke, coronary obstruction, pacemaker implantation, vascular complications, and postprocedural length of stay as compared to tricuspid valve TAVR.

REFERRAL

- If BAV disease present, refer to general cardiologist for surveillance
- Heart team approach for management of BAV aortopathy with BAV disease

PEARLS & CONSIDERATIONS

- Most common congenital cardiac abnormality in general population
- Most commonly associated with aortic root and ascending aorta aneurysm
- Close surveillance needed for early diagnosis of disease progression and referral to a cardiac surgeon or formal heart valve team if regurgitation or stenosis becomes severe or symptomatic

PREVENTION

- No clear data on prevention of BAV
- PROCAS and ASTRONOMER trials showed no effect of statin on delay in progression of aortic valve degeneration

PATIENT & FAMILY EDUCATION

Close follow-up with PCP and cardiologist

SUGGESTED READINGS

Available at ExpertConsult.com

RELATED CONTENT

Aortic Stenosis (Related Key Topic)

AUTHOR: **Maheswara Satya Gangadhara Rao Golla, MD**

BASIC INFORMATION

DEFINITION

Bipolar disorder is an episodic, recurrent, and frequently progressive condition in which the afflicted individual experiences at least one episode of mania, characterized by at least 1 wk of continuous symptoms of elevated, expansive, or irritable mood, in association with three or more of the following symptoms (four if irritability is the presenting mood):

- Decreased need for sleep
- Grandiosity or inflated self-esteem
- Pressured speech
- Flight of ideas or subjective sense of racing thoughts
- Distractibility
- Increased level of goal-directed activity
- Problematic behavior with a high potential for painful consequences

Most individuals with bipolar disorder also experience one or more episodes of major depression over their lifetimes or have symptoms of a depressive episode commingled with those of mania (mixed episode). Hypomanic episodes may also occur.

SYNONYMS

Manic-depression
Cycloid psychosis

ICD-10CM CODES	
F42.0	Bipolar affective disorder, current episode hypomanic
F31.1	Bipolar affective disorder, current episode manic without psychotic symptoms
F31.2	Bipolar affective disorder, current episode manic with psychotic symptoms
F31.3	Bipolar affective disorder, current episode mild or moderate depression
F31.4	Bipolar affective disorder, current episode severe depression without psychotic symptoms
F31.5	Bipolar affective disorder, current episode severe depression with psychotic symptoms
F31.6	Bipolar affective disorder, current episode mixed
F31.8	Bipolar II disorder
DSM-5 CODES	
296.41-296.80	Depends on specific diagnosis

EPIDEMIOLOGY & DEMOGRAPHICS

INCIDENCE: 0.016% to 0.021%

PREVALENCE (IN U.S.): 0.4% to 1.6% (lifetime); bipolar spectrum disorders: 2.8%; approximately 25% attempt suicide (6% to 7% successfully) and suicide deaths occur 20× more frequently than in the general population

PREDOMINANT SEX: The prevalence of bipolar I disorder is similar for males and females, whereas bipolar II disorder occurs more frequently in females[1]

PREDOMINANT AGE: Lifelong condition with usual age of onset 14 to 30 yr; childhood onset can occur.

PEAK INCIDENCE: Onset in 20s

GENETICS:

- Concordance rates for monozygotic twins: 0.7 to 0.8; for dizygotic twins: 0.2
- Risk of affective disorder in offspring with one affected parent with bipolar disorder: 27% to 29%; with two affected parents: 50% to 74%
- Heritability estimate of 0.85
- No specific causal mutations have been identified, but cross-disorder studies indicate an overlap with genes associated with a risk for autism or schizophrenia for BPI, whereas BPII appears genetically closer to major depressive disorder. Large-scale genome-wide association analyses and exome sequencing have identified at least 30 gene loci, and have implicated ion channelopathies, immune and neuronal signaling, insulin regulation, endocannabinoid signaling, and histone methylation in the pathogenesis of bipolar disorder. It is hypothesized that heritability derives from the additive effect of a number of common risk alleles in association with a few higher-risk deleterious variants, but identified genes thus far only account for 25% of heritability

PHYSICAL FINDINGS & CLINICAL PRESENTATION

- Mania associated with:
  1. Psychomotor activation that is usually goal directed but not necessarily productive
  2. Increase in goal-directed activity and excessive involvement in activities leading to unexpected adverse outcomes
  3. Elevated, euphoric, and frequently labile mood
  4. Decreased need for sleep
  5. Flight of ideas with rapid, loud, pressured speech
- Psychosis often occurs (75%), with delusions, hallucinations, and/or formal thought disorder
- Depressive episodes resembling major depressive disorder (see "Depression, Major"), although usually of shorter duration and more frequent; atypical features (hypersomnia, prominent anxiety, weight gain) may be present
- Mixed states, characterized by activation, irritability, and dysphoria also possible

KEY DIAGNOSTIC CRITERIA DISTINGUISHING BIPOLAR I DISORDER FROM BIPOLAR II DISORDER:

Manic episode (Bipolar I Disorder)[2]

- Distinct period during which there is an abnormally and persistently elevated, expansive, or irritable mood and abnormally and persistently increased goal-directed activity or energy lasting at least 1 wk (or less if hospitalization is required).
- Must be accompanied by at least three of the following symptoms (four if mood is only irritable): Inflated self-esteem or grandiosity, decreased need for sleep, pressured speech, racing thoughts, distractibility, increased involvement in goal-directed activity or psychomotor agitation, excessive involvement in pleasurable activities with a high potential for painful consequences.
- Symptoms do not meet criteria for a mixed episode.
- Disturbance must be sufficiently severe to cause marked impairment in social or occupational functioning or to require hospitalization, or it is characterized by the presence of psychotic features.
- Symptoms not due to direct physiologic effect of medication, general medication condition, or substance abuse, although if they persist after a direct condition is addressed, a primary bipolar condition should be considered.

Hypomanic episode (Bipolar II Disorder)

- Distinct period during which there is an abnormally and persistently elevated, expansive, or irritable mood and abnormally and persistently elevated activity or energy lasting at least 4 consecutive days.
- Must be accompanied by at least three of the following symptoms (four if mood is only irritable): Inflated self-esteem or grandiosity, decreased need for sleep, pressured speech, racing thoughts, distractibility, increased involvement in goal-directed activity or psychomotor agitation, excessive involvement in pleasurable activities with a high potential for painful consequences.
- Hypomanic episodes must be clearly different from the person's usual nondepressed mood, and there must be a clear change in functioning that is not characteristic of the person's usual functioning; consider using checklist (HCL-32) for accuracy.
- Changes in mood and functioning must be observable by others. In contrast to a manic episode, a hypomanic episode is not severe enough to cause marked impairment in social or occupational functioning or to require hospitalization, and there are no psychotic features.
- Symptoms not due to direct physiologic effect of medication, general medication condition, or substance abuse.

ETIOLOGY

Hypotheses:

- Abnormalities of GABAA and G protein–coupled receptor and membrane function, calcium dysregulation
- Alteration of cAMP, MAP kinase, protein kinase C, arachidonic acid cascade, and glycogen synthase kinase-3 signal transduction pathways; mitochondrial dysfunction
- Alteration in cell survival pathways, glial and neuronal death and loss of neuroplasticity; proposed biomarkers include BDNF and measures of inflammation, oxidative stress, and endothelial function

Dx DIAGNOSIS

DIFFERENTIAL DIAGNOSIS

- Secondary manias caused by medical disorders (e.g., hyperthyroidism, AIDS, early

[1] Carvalho AF et al: Bipolar disorder. *N Engl J Med*, 383:58-66, 2020.

[2] Criteria are from the American Psychiatric Association: *Diagnostic and statistical manual of mental disorders, fifth edition,* Washington, DC, 2013, American Psychiatric Association.

dementia [particularly frontotemporal dementia]), stroke and nondominant frontal lobe lesions, Cushing syndrome), or pharmacologic treatment (e.g., steroids, stimulants)
- First onset of mania after age 50 yr suggestive of secondary mania
- Less severe, and possibly distinct, conditions of bipolar type II and cyclothymia
- Comorbid substance abuse or dependency occurs in 60% to 75% of patients and may confound diagnosis and treatment
- Presentation can be confused with schizophrenia or paranoid psychosis

WORKUP

- History
- Physical examination
- Mental status examination
- Mood Disorder Questionnaire (MDQ); Composite International Diagnostic Interview (CIDI) (3.0)

LABORATORY TESTS

Because of high rate of secondary manias, initial evaluation to confirm health of all major organ systems (routine chemistries, thyroid panel, complete blood count, urinalysis, sedimentation rate)

IMAGING STUDIES

- Consider brain imaging if late onset or if neurologic examination is abnormal.
- Neuroimaging may show evidence of ventricular enlargement or increased white matter hyperintensities; decrements in prefrontal and temporal lobe cortical thickness also reported. Corresponding changes in neurocognition, including changes in executive function, verbal memory, and processing speed, may occur.

Rx TREATMENT

NONPHARMACOLOGIC THERAPY

- Cognitive-behavioral and family-focused psychoeducational psychotherapy to help patients cope with consequences of the disease, improve adherence with medications, and identify possible environmental triggers; consider life charting
- Bright light therapy in the northern latitudes in individuals exhibiting a seasonal pattern of winter depression
- Lifestyle "regularization"; effective sleep hygiene; interpersonal and social rhythm therapy; integrated care management for chronic conditions
- Many smartphone mobile apps for bipolar disorder are available to provide information, help monitor symptoms, and deliver interventions

ACUTE GENERAL Rx

- First-line agents for acute mania and mixed states: Lithium 1500 to 1800 mg/day (0.8 to 1.2 mEq/L), valproate 1000 to 1500 mg/day (50 to 125 ng/ml), carbamazepine 600 to 800 mg/day (4 to 12 micrograms/ml), oxcarbazepine 900 to 2400 mg/day, olanzapine 10 to 20 mg/day, risperidone 2 to 4 mg/day, quetiapine 350 to 800 mg/day, ziprasidone 80 to 120 mg/day, asenapine 10 to 20 mg/day, cariprazine (3 to 6 mg/day)or aripiprazole 10 to 30 mg/day. Treatment-resistant cases may respond to varying combinations of these agents or to the addition of clozapine. Long-acting injectable forms of antipsychotic agents may be useful in enhancing adherence and improved outcomes.
- Useful adjuncts to acute treatment of mania: Benzodiazepines: Lorazepam 1 to 2 mg q4h, clonazepam 1 to 2 mg q4h.
- Traditional antidepressants can induce manic episodes and exacerbate mania in mixed episodes and may be less effective than in treatment of unipolar depression.
- First-line options for bipolar depression include lithium, lurasidone, quetiapine, lamotrigine, and olanzapine/fluoxetine combination. Bupropion may have a lower risk for triggering mania, and monoamine oxidase inhibitors or electroconvulsive therapy may be efficacious in treatment-resistant cases. Off-label agents with possible efficacy include modafinil, pramipexole, and intravenous ketamine.

CHRONIC Rx

- Goal of long-term treatment: Prevention of relapse or episode recurrence
- Best agents for prophylaxis of mania: Lithium, quetiapine, aripiprazole, and olanzapine (valproate, carbamazepine/oxcarbazepine possibly beneficial)
- Best agents for prophylaxis of depression: Lamotrigine and lithium
- Risk/benefit of atypical antipsychotics versus traditional mood stabilizers in maintenance unclear
- Long-term use of antidepressants: Frequently destabilizes patient and leads to more frequent relapses; depression outweighs mania as the most debilitating dimension over the life span; bipolar disorder accounts for 7% of all disease-related disability-adjusted life yr

DISPOSITION

- Course is variable.
- More than 90% of patients having a single manic episode are likely to experience others.
- Uncontrolled manic or depressive episodes can lead to additional episodes.
- Lithium, in comparison to other mood stabilizers or atypical antipsychotic agents, has been shown to specifically decrease suicidal risk.
- Socioeconomic consequences of both mania and depression can be severe and disabling.
- Mortality rate from all causes is double that of the general population, secondary to suicide and increased comorbidity with physical illnesses.

REFERRAL

- If use of antidepressant contemplated or in cases of pediatric bipolar disorder
- If patient is severely manic, rapid cycling, pregnant, or suicidal or is in a bipolar, mixed episode

! PEARLS & CONSIDERATIONS

COMMENTS

- All patients presenting with depression should be asked about past personal and family history of mania and hypomania; 70% of bipolar patients have previously been misdiagnosed. Onset before age 25, postpartum onset, and poor prior response to antidepressants are additional clues.
- Prompt recognition of the earliest signs of mania in a given individual (e.g., decreased need for sleep, increased rate of speech) allows earlier intervention and a better likelihood of preventing a full episode.
- Bipolar disorder in children frequently manifests as episodic behavioral disinhibition, affective lability, and temper dysregulation, but current consensus indicates that the condition is overdiagnosed in this age group. Disruptive mood dysregulation disorder (DMDD) describes children who exhibit persistent irritability and severe temper outbursts on a frequent basis (at least three times/wk for a yr or more).
- Rapid cycling (greater than three episodes/yr) and mixed states are associated with a poorer prognosis, including a longer course, more treatment resistance, more substance use comorbidity, and increased suicidal risk.
- Patients treated with atypical antipsychotic agents should be carefully monitored for development of metabolic syndrome. Independent of medication effect, there is a higher prevalence of metabolic syndrome and abdominal obesity in those with bipolar disorder.
- Despite some variation in prevalence, the severity, impact, and patterns of comorbidity of bipolar disorder are similar in different countries in world health surveys.
- Bipolar disorder often co-occurs with anxiety disorders and attention deficit hyperactivity disorder (ADHD), making attribution of specific symptoms difficult.
- Patients receiving anticonvulsants or antidepressants should be monitored for a possible increase in suicidal thoughts or behavior.
- There is preliminary evidence that nutraceutical agents like omega-3 fatty acids and *N*-acetyl cysteine (NAC) may have efficacy in the treatment of bipolar disorder.
- Multiple studies show a correlation between bipolar disorder and heightened creativity.
- Patients with bipolar disorder are at risk for catatonic syndrome including manic delirium.
- Early intervention and adjustment of treatment according to stage of illness may result in improved lifetime prognosis.

PATIENT & FAMILY EDUCATION

Information available at www.NMHA.org/ and www.dbsalliance.org/.

SUGGESTED READINGS

Available at ExpertConsult.com

RELATED CONTENT

Bipolar Disorder (Patient Information)
Depression, Major (Related Key Topic)

AUTHOR: **Victor I. Reus MD**

BASIC INFORMATION

DEFINITION

A bite wound can be animal or human, accidental, or intentional.

ICD-10CM CODES

S41.159A	Open bite of unspecified upper arm, initial encounter
T14.1	Open wound of unspecified body region
T01.9	Multiple open wounds, unspecified
S31.000A	Unspecified open wound of lower back and pelvis without penetration into retroperitoneum, initial encounter

EPIDEMIOLOGY & DEMOGRAPHICS

- Bite wounds account for 1% of emergency department visits, and about 2% of patients need hospitalization.
- More than 1 million bites occur in human beings annually in the U.S.
- Dog bites account for 85%-90% of all bites and result in 10 to 20 fatalities yearly in the U.S.; most dog bite victims are children. Cat bites account for 10% to 20%. The animal typically is owned by the victim.
- Infection rates are highest for cat bites (30%-50%), followed by human bites (15%-30%) and dog bites (5%).
- The extremities are involved in 75% of bites.

PHYSICAL FINDINGS & CLINICAL PRESENTATION

- The appearance of the bite wound is variable (e.g., puncture wound, tear, avulsion).
- Cellulitis, lymphangitis, and focal adenopathy may be present in infected bite wounds.
- Patient may have fever and chills.

ETIOLOGY

- Increased risk of infection: Human and cat bites, closed-fist injuries, wounds involving joints, puncture wounds, face and lip bites, bites with skull penetration, bites in immunocompromised hosts
- Mixed aerobes and anaerobes typically compose the bacteria in bite wounds. Most frequent infecting organisms:
    1. *Pasteurella* spp.: Responsible for majority of infections within 24 hr of dog (*P. canis*) and cat (*P. multocida, P. septica*) bites
    2. *Capnocytophaga canimorsus* (formerly DF-2 bacillus): A gram-negative organism responsible for late infection, usually after dog bites
    3. Gram-negative organisms *(Pseudomonas, Haemophilus)*: Often found in human bites
    4. *Streptococcus* spp., *Staphylococcus aureus*
    5. *Eikenella corrodens* in human bites

DIAGNOSIS

DIFFERENTIAL DIAGNOSIS

- Bite from a rabid animal (often the attack is unprovoked)
- Factitious injury

WORKUP

- Determination of the time elapsed since the patient was bitten, status of rabies immunization of the animal, and underlying medical conditions that might predispose the patient to infection (e.g., DM, immunodeficiency).
- Documentation of bite site, notification of appropriate authorities (e.g., police department, animal officer).
- Box 1 summarizes management procedures for bite wounds.

LABORATORY TESTS

- Generally not necessary
- Hematocrit if there has been significant blood loss
- Wound cultures (aerobic and anaerobic) if there is evidence of sepsis or victim is immunocompromised; cultures should be obtained before irrigation of the wound but after superficial cleaning

IMAGING STUDIES

Radiographs are indicated when bony penetration is suspected or if there is suspicion of fracture or significant trauma; they are also useful for detecting foreign bodies (when suspected).

BOX 1 Management Procedures for Bite Wounds

Obtain history from patient:
- Situation leading to injury
- Place of occurrence
- Patient allergies
- Other medications (potential interactions)

Perform evaluation of patient:
- Nerve function
- Tendon function
- Vascular integrity
- Range of motion
- Potential bone and joint involvement

Diagram or photograph wound
Mark leading edge of cellulitis
Culture wound (if infected)
Irrigate wound (do not irrigate puncture wounds)
Débride wound cautiously
Obtain diagnostic imaging for penetrating injuries overlying bones or joints, if fracture suspected or foreign body suspected
Drain abscesses
Operative débridement (for removal of devitalized tissue and for severe bites, as indicated)
Administer antimicrobial agents (prophylactic therapy, 3-5 days; longer duration for established infection)
Elevate injured area
Close the wound (see text)
Immobilize wound area (3 days for hands)
Have the patient exercise the injured area (if previously immobilized)
Administer tetanus toxoid
Submit health department report (if required)

From Cherry JD et al: *Feigin and Cherry's textbook of pediatric infectious diseases*, ed 8, Philadelphia, 2019, Elsevier.

TREATMENT

NONPHARMACOLOGIC THERAPY

- Local care with débridement, vigorous cleansing, and saline irrigation of the wound; débridement of devitalized tissue
- High-pressure irrigation to clean bite wound and ensure removal of contaminants (e.g., use saline solution with a 30- to 35-ml syringe equipped with a 20-gauge needle or catheter with tip of syringe placed 2 to 3 cm above the wound)
- Avoid blunt probing of wounds (increased risk of infection)
- If the animal is suspected to be rabid: Infiltrate wound edges with 1% procaine hydrochloride, swab wound surface vigorously with cotton swabs and 1% benzalkonium solution or other soap, and rinse wound with normal saline

ACUTE GENERAL Rx

- Avoid suturing of hand wounds and any wounds that appear infected.
- Clenched fist injuries that develop after a punch to another's mouth usually require hospitalization, IV antibiotics, and evaluation by a hand specialist.
- Puncture wounds should be left open.
- Give antirabies therapy and tetanus immune globulin (250-500 units IM in limb contralateral to toxoid) and toxoid (adult or child older than 5 yr: 0.5 ml DT given IM, child <5 yr 0.5 ml DPT IM) as needed.
- Use empiric antibiotic therapy in high-risk wounds (e.g., cat bite, hand bites, face bites, genital area bites, bites with joint or bone penetration, human bites, immunocompromised host): Amoxicillin-clavulanate 875 to 1000 mg bid for 7 days or cefuroxime 500 mg bid for 7 days.
- In hospitalized patients, IV antibiotics of choice are cefoxitin 1 to 2 g q6h, ampicillin-sulbactam 1.5 to 3 g q6h, ticarcillin-clavulanate 3 g q6h, cefoxitin 2 g IV q8h, or ceftriaxone 1 to 2 g q24h.
- Penicillin allergy: Animal bite (doxycycline or moxifloxacin or trimethoprim/sulfamethoxazole with either clindamycin or metronidazole); human bite (moxifloxacin plus clindamycin, trimethoprim/sulfamethoxazole plus metronidazole).
- Prophylactic therapy for persons bitten by others with HIV and hepatitis B (see "Section V").
- Table 1 summarizes the treatment of mammalian bites. The comparative in vitro antimicrobial activity of selected oral antimicrobial agents against common bite wound pathogens is summarized in Table 2.

DISPOSITION

- Prognosis is favorable with proper treatment.
- Important prognostic factors are type and depth of wound, which compartments are

TABLE 1 Treatment of Mammalian Bites

Type	Wound Care	Antibiotic PR	Tetanus PR	Rabies PR	HIV PR	Hepatitis PR
Human	High-pressure irrigation of the wound with normal saline or dilute (<1%) povidone-iodine solution; débride devitalized tissue or ragged edges	Amoxicillin-clavulanate, second-generation cephalosporin with anaerobic activity, penicillin plus dicloxacillin, clindamycin plus ciprofloxacin or trimethoprim-sulfamethoxazole	Tetanus immunoglobulin (250 units IM) and tetanus toxoid (0.5 mg IM) if never had a tetanus vaccine or have not had 3 doses of tetanus toxoid; tetanus toxoid (0.5 mg IM) if >5 yr since previous tetanus booster	None	ART therapy started within the first 48-72 hr and continued for 28 days or bite source tested HIV negative; refer to the hospital for the specific drugs used in ART therapy	HBIG (0.06 ml/kg IM); HBV given at separate site from HBIG
Cat	High-pressure irrigation of the wound with normal saline or dilute (<1%) povidone-iodine solution; débride devitalized tissue or ragged edges	Amoxicillin-clavulanate, second-generation cephalosporin with anaerobic activity, penicillin plus a first-generation cephalosporin, clindamycin plus a fluoroquinolone or trimethoprim-sulfamethoxazole	Tetanus immune globulin (250 units IM) and tetanus toxoid (0.5 mg IM) if never had a tetanus vaccine or have not had 3 doses of tetanus toxoid; tetanus toxoid (0.5 mg IM) if >5 yr since previous tetanus booster	HRIG (20 IU/kg) injected IM and/or around the bite site; rabies vaccine (1 ml IM) given in the deltoid in adults and in the thigh in children, on days 0, 3, 7, 14, and 28	None	None
Dog	High-pressure irrigation of the wound with normal saline or dilute (<1%) povidone-iodine solution; débride devitalized tissue or ragged edges	Amoxicillin-clavulanate, second-generation cephalosporin with anaerobic activity, penicillin plus a first-generation cephalosporin, clindamycin plus a fluoroquinolone or trimethoprim-sulfamethoxazole	Tetanus immune globulin (250 units IM) and tetanus toxoid (0.5 mg IM) if never had a tetanus vaccine or have not had 3 doses of tetanus toxoid; tetanus toxoid (0.5 mg IM) if >5 yr since previous tetanus booster	HRIG (20 IU/kg) injected IM and/or around the bite site; rabies vaccine (1 ml IM) given in the deltoid in adults and in the thigh in children, on days 0, 3, 7, 14, and 28	None	None

ART, Antiretroviral therapy; *HBIG*, hepatitis B immune globulin; *HBV*, hepatitis B vaccine; *HIV*, human immunodeficiency virus; *HRIG*, human rabies immune globulin; *IM*, intramuscularly; *PR*, prophylaxis.
From Adams JG et al: *Emergency medicine: clinical essentials*, ed 2, Philadelphia, 2013, Elsevier.

TABLE 2 Comparative in Vitro Antimicrobial Activity of Selected Oral Antimicrobial Agents against Common Bite Wound Pathogens

	Staphylococcus aureus[a]	*Eikenella corrodens*	*Streptococcus*	*Haemophilus*	*Pasteurella*	Anaerobes
Amoxicillin	–	+	V	V	V	V
Amoxicillin–clavulanic acid	V	+	+	+	+	+
Cephalexin	V	–	V	–	V	–
Cefaclor	V	–	V	V	V	–
Cefuroxime	V	V	V	V	V	–
Meropenem	V	+	+	+	+	+
Dicloxacillin	V	–	V	–	–	–
Erythromycin	V	–	V	–	V	–
Azithromycin	V	V	V	–	V	V
Clarithromycin	V	V	V	–	V	–
Trimethoprim-sulfamethoxazole	+	+	V	+	+	–
Moxifloxacin	+	+	+	+	+	+
Clindamycin	+	–	+	–	–	+

+, Active; –, poorly active or inactive; *v*, variable.
[a]Methicillin-resistant *S. aureus* can be a pathogen in bite wounds.
From Cherry JD et al: *Feigin and Cherry's textbook of pediatric infectious diseases*, ed 8, Philadelphia, 2019, Elsevier.

BOX 2 Advice for Avoiding the Bites and Attacks of Common Pets

Dogs

- Do not leave a young child alone with a dog.
- Never approach or try to pet an unfamiliar dog, especially if it is tied up or confined.
- Always ask the dog's owners if you can pet the dog.
- Do not lean over a dog or pet it directly on the head.
- Do not kiss a dog.
- Avoid quick or sudden movements that may startle a dog.
- Never pet or step over a sleeping dog.
- Never try to take a bone or toy away from a dog (other than your own dog).
- Know the appearance of an angry dog: Barking, growling, snarling with teeth showing, ears laid flat, legs stiff, tail up, and hair on the back standing up.
- Never step between two fighting dogs; if you need to separate them, use a bucket of water or a hose.
- Do not approach a female dog that is nursing her pups.
- Teach injury prevention advice to children from an early age.

Cats

- Be aware that some cats do not like prolonged petting.
- Know warning signs of an impending bite: Twitching of the tail, restlessness, and "intention" bites (i.e., the cat moves to bite but does not bite).

Ferrets

- Do not sell or adopt a ferret that is known to bite.
- Do not push your fingers through the wires of a ferret cage.
- Reach for a ferret from the side with the palm upward rather than from above.
- Do not handle food and then handle young ferrets without washing your hands first.
- Do not poke a ferret or pull on its tail or ears.
- Never leave a ferret alone with a child or infant.
- If a ferret bites and locks on very tightly, pour cold and fast-running water over its face.

From Auerbach P: *Wilderness medicine, expert consult,* premium edition—enhanced online features and print, Philadelphia, 2012, Elsevier.

entered, and pathogenicity of inoculated bacteria.

- Punctures that are difficult to irrigate adequately, carnivore bites over vital structures (arteries, nerves, joints), and tissue crushing that cannot be débrided have a worse prognosis.
- In general, human bites have a higher complication and infection rate than do animal bites.
- Nearly 50% of the anaerobic gram-negative bacilli isolated from human bite wounds may be penicillin resistant and beta-lactamase positive.

PREVENTION

Box 2 provides advice for avoiding the bites and attacks of common pets.

REFERRAL

- Hospitalization and IV antibiotic therapy for infected human bites; bites with injury to joints, nerves, or tendons; or any animal bites unresponsive to oral therapy.
- Human bites with tendon involvement should go to operating room for washout.
- In the outpatient setting, bite wounds should be reevaluated within 48 hr to assess for signs of infection.

SUGGESTED READING

Available at ExpertConsult.com

RELATED CONTENT

Animal and Human Bites (Patient Information)

AUTHOR: **Fred F. Ferri, MD**

BASIC INFORMATION

DEFINITION

Most stinging insects belong to the Hymenoptera order and include the winged: Honey bees, hornets, bumblebees, sweat bees, wasps (including yellow jackets), and the unwinged: Harvester ants, fire ants, and the Africanized honey bee ("killer bee"). Thousands of species can sting or bite. Wasps cause 70% of all reactions to stings. Spiders, which are arachnids, not insects, are another cause of bites (see "Bites and Stings, Arachnids"). The venom of the Hymenoptera order (Fig. 1) contains vasoactive and proinflammatory mediators that can cause local reactions. A small number of those stung can develop a systemic hypersensitivity reaction. Bites differ from stings due to the injection of venom. The usual local effect of a sting is intense pain, immediate erythema, edema, and pruritus from the injecting venom. Allergic reactions can be either local or generalized. Generalized reactions can lead to anaphylactic shock. This is a rapid-onset event and can cause death. The majority of reactions occur within the first 6 hr after the sting or bite, but a delayed reaction may occur up to 24 hr after the sting. Delayed reactions are rare and include serum sickness (fever, malaise, urticaria, and arthralgias). A biphasic reaction can occur.

SYNONYM

Venom allergy

ICD-10CM CODES

T63.424	Toxic effect of venom of ants, undetermined, initial encounter
T63.444	Toxic effect of venom of bees, undetermined, initial encounter
T63.464	Toxic effect of venom of wasps, undetermined, initial encounter

EPIDEMIOLOGY & DEMOGRAPHICS

INCIDENCE (IN U.S.): 40 to 100 people die each yr from insect sting anaphylaxis; anaphylaxis occurs most often within 10 to 30 min of a sting. Delayed reactions are rare, occurring only in <0.3% of stings.

PHYSICAL FINDINGS & CLINICAL PRESENTATION

- Stings:
  1. Local reactions:
     a. Cutaneous: The skin is the most common site of a local allergic reaction. Manifestations include flushing, urticaria, pruritus, and angioedema. Local reactions may last several days. Location of sting does not increase risk of a systemic reaction.
  2. Systemic reactions:
     a. Local swelling greater than 10 cm is associated with increased risk of a systemic reaction with repeat exposure.
     b. Respiratory: This is the leading cause of anaphylactic death. Anaphylaxis as defined by consensus of the National Institutes of Health (NIH) 2006 is a severe life-threatening hypersensitivity reaction. Symptoms of upper or lower airway obstruction including hoarseness, choking, throat tightness or tingling that may progress to stridor, laryngeal edema, laryngospasm, and bronchoconstriction.
     c. Cardiovascular: Cardiac manifestations are the second leading cause of death from anaphylaxis; the most common reaction is hypotension that can progress to profound hypovolemic shock. Tachycardia and arrhythmia may occur. Myocardial infarction is rare.
     d. General symptoms: Abdominal pain, nausea, vomiting, lightheadedness, and diarrhea.
- Fire ant bites:
  1. Initial wheal and flare response
  2. Subsequent development of circularly arrayed blisters within 24 hr (Fig. E3)
  3. Blisters may develop the appearance of pustules, but they are not infected
- Flea bites:
  1. Classic linear configuration (Fig. E4)
  2. Multiple excoriated, clustered red papules (Fig. E5)

PREVALENCE (OF BEE STINGS AND INSECT BITES):

- Unknown prevalence, very underreported; can be cause of outdoor sudden death; 56% to 94% of the population has been stung at least once.
- Account for 2.3% of ED visits; 5% to 7.5% of the population is hypersensitive, with large local or systemic reactions to the venom of one or more stinging insects.
- Insect bites are the most common cause of anaphylaxis reactions and account for 20% of all anaphylaxis-related deaths.
- Most anaphylactic reactions occur during summer months in those most likely to be exposed, including children, males, and outdoor workers. There are no tests to predict reaction accurately; the reaction to a prior sting is still the best predictor. Anaphylaxis can occur after a number of uneventful stings.
- Approximately half of fatal reactions occur without prior allergic response.
- Bites by fire ants (Fig. 2) are less likely to cause systemic disease.
- Spider bites are rare; only a few of the thousands of spider species cause a reaction in humans. Observation and collection of the spider inflicting the bite is necessary (see "Bites and Stings, Arachnids").
- Well syndrome, a rare eosinophilic inflammatory skin disorder, can be triggered by a bite or sting.

ETIOLOGY

Stings:

- Most systemic reactions to insect stings are classic immunoglobulin E (IgE)–mediated reactions. Anaphylaxis can be the presenting sign of indolent mastocytosis.
- Reactions occur in previously sensitized patients who have produced high titers of IgE antibody to insect venom antigens.
- Sensitization to wasp venom can occur after a single sting but is more common after a few stings.
- Sensitization to bee venom occurs mainly in people who have been stung frequently by bees.

Bites:

- Fire ant venom contains proteins toxic to the skin.

DIAGNOSIS

DIFFERENTIAL DIAGNOSIS

- Stings: Cellulitis, bites, rash
- Bites: Stings, cellulitis

WORKUP

The history is essential for accurate diagnosis including timing of sting or bite and type of insect (bee, wasp, spider, or ant) if known.

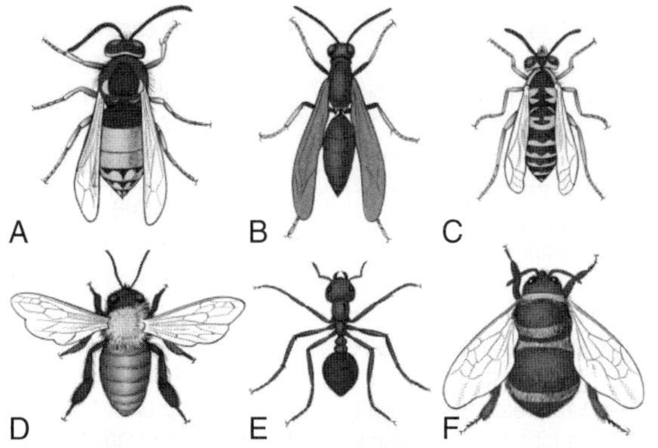

FIG. 1 Representative venomous Hymenoptera. A, Hornet (*Vespula maculata*). **B,** Wasp (*Chlorion ichneumerea*). **C,** Yellowjacket (*Vespula maculiforma*). **D,** Honeybee (*Apis mellifera*). **E,** Fire ant (*Solenopsis invicta*). **F,** Bumblebee (*Bombus* species). (From Erickson TB, Marquez A: Arthropod envenomation and parasitism. In Auerbach PS et al (eds): *Auerbach's wilderness medicine,* ed 7, Philadelphia, 2017, Elsevier, Fig 41-1, p 937. In Kliegman RM: *Nelson textbook of pediatrics,* ed 21, Philadelphia, 2020, Elsevier.)

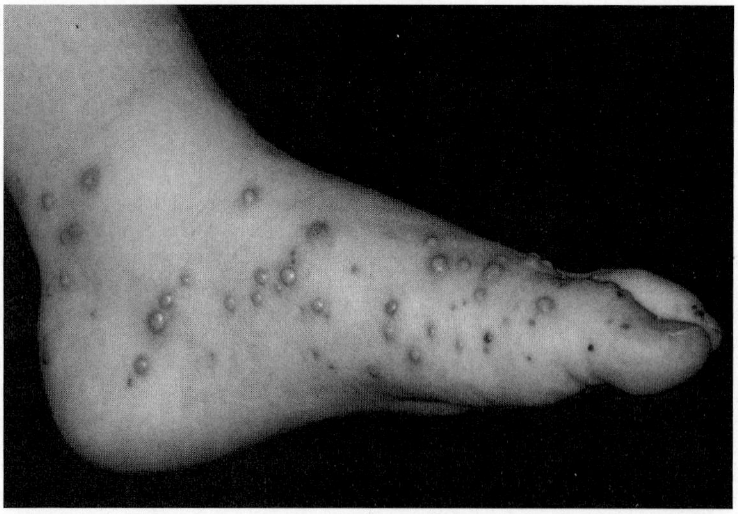

FIG. 2 Fire ant bites presenting as clusters of sterile pustules on the foot. (From Bolognia JL et al: *Dermatology*, ed 4, 2018, Elsevier.)

LABORATORY TESTS (FOR HYPERSENSITIVITY REACTION)

- Skin test: Either skin prick test or intradermal method with fire ant or hymenoptera venom
- Venom skin tests and occasionally radioallergosorbent tests (RAST) to provide additional information, only for those with history of a systemic reaction
- Venom-specific IgE tests
- Basophil activation tests and mast cell mediator testing are being developed to identify those with allergy and predict those who will have more severe reactions
- Measuring baseline serum tryptase can identify patients as high risk for anaphylaxis and those with mastocytosis

Rx TREATMENT

ACUTE GENERAL Rx

Sting:

- Local Poison Control Center can be contacted.
- Removal of the stinger most easily performed with a flat tool such as a credit card within 30 seconds of the sting, followed by cleansing and application of ice.
- Venom may all be released within 20 seconds of bite or sting.
- Avoid squeezing, which may push venom out of the venom sac and into the tissue.
- Supportive care with oral antihistamines, nonsteroidal antiinflammatory medications/pain medications, topical corticosteroids for 5 to 7 days, and cold compresses for limited reactions.
- Large local reactions (LLR>10 cm) may benefit from oral steroids. 50 mg/day prednisone for 5 to 7 days. Oral second-generation antihistamine can treat and prevent this reaction as well as high potency topical steroids. Unknown if future reactions will be severe.
- Patients with previous reactions or multiple stings to the mouth or neck should be evaluated in an emergency department.
- Unusual reactions to multiple stings include cerebrovascular accident or acute kidney injury due to many causes, including hypotension or direct toxicity from venom.
- Systemic reactions = Anaphylaxis: Treat quickly with intramuscular epinephrine (no contraindication for use). Increased risk of death if epinephrine delayed. The patient should be supine with 0.30 mg IM in anterior/lateral thigh. Patient should be observed for 4 to 8 hr. Adults with preexisting cardiovascular (CV) disease are at greater risk due to challenges handling the stress.
  1. H1- and H2-blockers, oxygen, IV glucocorticoids, beta-agonists, pressors, and IV fluids may also be beneficial for anaphylaxis. No data that glucocorticoids improve clinical outcomes.
  2. Patients should be given 2 units of self-injectable epinephrine pens for home use and referral to allergist indicated after a systemic reaction. Patients should be transported to ED if epinephrine is used, due to 20% risk of recurrence of symptoms.
- Tetanus not needed.

Bite:

- Supportive care—wash with soap and water
- Application of ice or cooling. Calamine lotion may be helpful
- Surveillance for secondary cellulitis—more common with yellow jacket bites

DISPOSITION

Sting:

- Prognosis for a limited reaction is excellent.
- Subsequent anaphylaxis may occur in up to 65% of patients stung again with history of prior systemic reaction. Large local reaction does not predict a systemic reaction.
- There is no evidence that the next sting will necessarily cause a more severe reaction. Variable outcome is due to the patient's age, comorbidities, time elapsed since prior exposure, dose of venom injected, and site of sting.
- Watch for secondary cellulitis.
- Patients who have a history of a severe systemic reaction should:
  1. Be educated to avoid stinging insects.
  2. Carry two syringes preloaded with epinephrine for self-administration.
  3. Undergo testing for serum levels of venom-specific IgE.
  4. Be referred to allergist for venom immunotherapy (VIT), which reduces chance of serious allergic reaction from 60% to <5%. VIT is typically needed for 3 to 5 yr.
  5. Carry medical identification for stinging insect hypersensitivity.
  6. Have a baseline tryptase level checked if an anaphylactic reaction to a sting has been experienced in the past to evaluate the possibility of an underlying mast cell disorder. Patients with levels >20 ng/ml need further evaluation. VIT may benefit those with mastocytosis and wasp venom allergy.
  7. Strategies to avoid bites and stings: No food outside, no garbage or open doors/windows near home, no fragrances or use of public outdoor toilets.

Bite:

- Prognosis for fire ant bite is excellent.
- Large lesions from brown recluse spider bites may take months to heal.
- Watch for secondary cellulitis. Some wasp species feed on rotting meat.

REFERRAL

- Consider referral to an allergist for VIT. All patients with severe systemic reactions should be referred for testing and, if positive, should receive VIT for 5 yr.
- Risk of subsequent anaphylaxis with immunotherapy falls to <5%.
- VIT for 5 yr induces long-term protection in most patients. Protects for 2 to 5 yr in some patients.

PEARLS & CONSIDERATIONS

Hypersensitivity to stings is common. Reactions range from local nonallergic reaction to venom to life-threatening systemic reaction with anaphylaxis. This could indicate underlying mast cell disorder; tryptase level is indicated. Venom-specific immunotherapy is highly effective in decreasing subsequent anaphylaxis. Venom immunotherapy is currently indicated for systemic reactions, and there is efficacy for prevention of large local reactions, which can result in significant morbidity.

SUGGESTED READINGS

Available at ExpertConsult.com

RELATED CONTENT

Bites and Stings (Patient Information)
Bites and Stings, Arachnids (Related Key Topic)

AUTHOR: **Lynn A. Bowlby, MD**

BASIC INFORMATION

DEFINITION

Bladder cancer is a field change disease in which the entire urothelium from the renal pelvis to the urethra is susceptible to malignant transformation. The disease stages include non–muscle-invasive bladder cancer, muscle-invasive bladder cancer, and metastatic urothelial carcinoma.

ICD-10CM CODES	
C67.9	Malignant neoplasm of bladder, unspecified
C79.11	Secondary malignant neoplasm of bladder
D09.0	Carcinoma in situ of bladder
D30.3	Benign neoplasm of bladder
D41.4	Neoplasm of uncertain behavior of bladder
D49.4	Neoplasm of unspecified behavior of bladder

EPIDEMIOLOGY & DEMOGRAPHICS

In 2020, 81,400 new cases and 17,980 deaths in the U.S. were estimated to occur due to bladder cancer. It is the sixth commonest malignancy in the U.S., with a median age of diagnosis of 69 yr in men and 71 yr in women. Globally, there are 430,000 new cases and 170,000 deaths reported annually.

PREDOMINANT SEX: It is 3 to 4 times more common in men than in women; lifetime risks are 1 in 26 for men and 1 in 88 for women.

PEAK INCIDENCE: Incidence increases with age: Higher after age 60 yr, uncommon in those younger than 40 yr.

RISK FACTORS:

Smoking:
- More than half of bladder cancers are related to smoking.
- Smoking risk is based on consumption; there is a two- to threefold increase for subjects smoking >10 cigarettes per day.
- Smokers of low-tar and low-nicotine cigarettes have a lower risk when compared with higher tar and nicotine cigarettes.
- Those who smoke unfiltered cigarettes have a 50% increased risk of bladder cancer compared with those who smoke filtered cigarettes.
- Pipe smokers have a lower risk of bladder cancer compared with cigarette smokers.
- Cigars, snuff, and chewing tobacco, although implicated in nonurologic cancers, are not thought to influence bladder cancer risk.

Diet:
- Diets rich in beef, pork, and animal fat increase risk of bladder cancer.
- Beer consumption has been linked to bladder cancer development as a result of the presence of nitrosamines in the beer. Drinking coffee is not thought to contribute to bladder cancer risk.
- Medications: Long-term (>1 yr) use of pioglitazone and rosiglitazone.

GENETICS: It is thought to be multifactorial in etiology, involving both genetic and environmental interactions. Overall, approximately 20% to 25% of the male population in the U.S. with bladder cancer is estimated to have the disease as a result of occupational exposure.

DISTRIBUTION: The three types of bladder cancer are transitional cell carcinoma (93%), squamous cell carcinoma (6%), and adenocarcinoma (1%).

PATHOGENESIS:

Two pathways exist for bladder cancer (TCC):
- Papillary superficial disease occasionally leading to invasive cancer (75%)
- Carcinoma in situ (CIS) and solid invasive cancer with high risk of disease progression (25%)

Two distinct forms of "superficial cancer" exist:
- T_a: Papillary low-grade tumor with a high rate of recurrence; disease progression occurs in 5%
- T_1: Higher-grade papillary tumor that infiltrates the lamina propria; often associated with flat CIS that may involve the urothelium diffusely. Disease progression occurs in 30% to 50%. This is subdivided into:
  1. T_{1a}: Penetration up to the muscularis mucosa; disease progression in 5%
  2. T_{1b}: Penetration through the muscularis mucosa; disease progression in 53%

Flat CIS:
- Entirely different and separate pathway of cancer development whose mechanism is manifested by dysplasia, which leads to the occurrence of poorly differentiated malignant cells that replace or undermine the normal urothelium and extend along the plane of the bladder wall. It penetrates the basement membrane and lamina propria in 20% to 30% of cases and is associated with the development of solid tumor growth. A p53 defect occurs in 50% of these cases.

At presentation, 50% to 51% of cancers are in situ, 34% to 35% are localized to the bladder, 17% are regionally spread to the lymph nodes, and 4% to 5% present with distant metastases. Eighty percent of superficial TCC recur, with up to 30% progressing to a higher stage or grade. Younger patients most commonly develop low-grade papillary noninvasive TCC and are less likely to have recurrences when compared with older patients with similar lesions. Involvement of the upper tracts with tumor occurs in 25% to 50% of cases (see Table E1).

MOLECULAR EPIDEMIOLOGY: TCC is usually a field change disease with tumors arising at different times and sites in the urothelium, suggesting a polyclonal etiology of bladder cancer. Non–muscle-invasive bladder cancer (NMIBC) and muscle-invasive bladder cancer (MIBC) are genetically different. NMIBC is characterized by a high frequency of mutations in the *FGFR* oncogene, leading to constitutive activation of the RAS/MAPK pathway. In MIBC, mutations in the *TP53* gene prevail. In general, mutations in *FGFR* and *TP53* are mutually exclusive, suggesting that NMIBC and MIBC develop along different oncogenetic pathways. However, these mutations often occur simultaneously in stage pT_1 tumors that invade the connective tissue layer underlying the urothelium. Recently, somatic mutations in the *PIK3CA* oncogene, which encodes the catalytic subunit p110α of class-IA PI3 kinase, were described in 13% to 27% of bladder tumors. These mutations often coincided with *FGFR3* mutations. Mutations in the *RAS* oncogenes (*HRAS*, *KRAS*, and *NRAS*) have also been found in 13% of bladder tumors and in all stages and grades; they are mutually exclusive with *FGFR3* mutations.

PHYSICAL FINDINGS & CLINICAL PRESENTATION

- Gross, painless hematuria
- Microhematuria
- Frequency, urgency, occasional dysuria
- With locally invasive to distant metastatic disease, the presentation can include:
  1. Abdominal pain
  2. Flank pain
  3. Lymphedema
  4. Renal failure
  5. Anorexia
  6. Bone pain

ETIOLOGY

Bladder cancer is a potentially preventable disease associated with specific etiologic factors:
- Cigarette smoking is associated with 45% to 65% of cases. The risk of developing a TCC is two to four times higher in smokers, and that risk persists for many yrs, being equal to nonsmokers only after 12 to 15 yr of smoking abstinence. Smoking is associated with higher histologic grade and stage, increase in the numbers of tumors, and increased size
- Occupational exposures: Dye workers, textile workers, tire and rubber workers, petroleum workers
- Chemical exposure: O-toluidine, 2-naphthylamine, benzidine, 4-amino-biphenyl, and nitrosamines
- Exposure to herpes papilloma virus type 16

Squamous carcinomas are associated with:
- Schistosomiasis
- Urinary calculi
- Indwelling catheters
- Bladder diverticula

Miscellaneous causes:
- Phenacetin abuse
- Cyclophosphamide
- Pelvic irradiation
- Tuberculosis

Adenocarcinomas are associated with:
- Exstrophy
- Endometriosis
- Neurogenic bladder
- Urachal abnormalities
- As a secondary site for distant metastases from other organs (e.g., colon cancer)

Dx DIAGNOSIS

- History and physical examination
- Urinalysis

- Cystoscopy with bladder barbotage and biopsy. Fluorescence cystoscopy offers improvement in the detection of flat neoplastic lesions such as carcinoma in situ.
- Transurethral resection of bladder tumor (TURBT).
- There is insufficient evidence to determine whether a decrease in mortality rate from bladder cancer occurs with hematuria testing, urinary cytology, or a variety of other tests on exfoliated urinary cells or other substances.
- In addition to urinary cytology and bladder barbotage, BTA, NMP22, and fibrin degradation products have been approved by the FDA as bladder cancer tumor markers. No marker has general, widespread acceptance because the results are affected by the presence of stents, recent urologic manipulation, stones, infection, bowel interposition, and prostatitis, creating false-positive results.
- Urinary biomarkers: Six urinary biomarkers have been approved by the FDA for diagnosis on surveillance of bladder cancer.
  1. Quantitative nuclear matrix protein 22 (Alere NMP22)
  2. Qualitative NMP22 (BladderChek)
  3. Qualitative bladder tumor antigen (BTA stat)
  4. Quantitative BTA (BTA TRAK)
  5. Fluorescence in situ hybridization (FISH)
  6. Fluorescent immunohistochemistry (ImmunoCyt)
- Generally, urinary biomarkers miss a substantial proportion of patients with bladder cancer and are subject to false-positive results in others. Accuracy is poor for low-stage and low-grade tumors.[1]

DIFFERENTIAL DIAGNOSIS

- Urinary tract infection
- Frequency-urgency syndrome
- Interstitial cystitis
- Stone disease
- Endometriosis
- Neurogenic bladder

WORKUP

Fig. 1 illustrates a diagnostic and treatment algorithm for bladder cancer. Staging is summarized in Table E1.

LABORATORY TESTS

- Urine cytology.
- Urine telomerase: Telomerase activity in voided urine or bladder washings determined by the telomeric repeat amplification protocol (TRAP) assay. This test has been reported to accurately detect the presence of bladder tumors in men. It represents a potentially useful noninvasive diagnostic innovation for bladder cancer detection in high-risk groups such as habitual smokers or in symptomatic patients.

[1]Chou R et al: Urinary biomarkers for diagnosis of bladder cancer: A systematic review and meta-analysis, *Ann Intern Med* 163:922-931, 2015.

RADIOLOGIC TESTS

- Renal ultrasound, retrograde pyelography, CT scan, and MRI.
- One or a combination of studies can be used. In the absence of skeletal symptoms, bone scan is not recommended.

Rx TREATMENT

SURGICAL APPROACHES

- The goal of any resection should be the visual eradication of any tumor burden and the assurance of an adequate depth of resection
- Initially, transurethral resection of bladder tumor (TURBT). Using cutting current, a loop electrode is used to resect the tumor inclusive of muscularis propria (Fig. E2). Histologically, bladder tumors frequently exhibit growth beyond the visible edge, and, as such, resection should include an approximate 2-cm margin of normal-appearing tissue. Wide resection of tumors will ensure completeness, whether the tumor has a broad base or a tentacular growth pattern (Fig. E3)
- Loop biopsy of the prostatic urethra if high-grade TCC is suspected
- If superficial disease, follow-up protocol with repeat TURBT and/or the use of intravesical agents is recommended
- For advanced bladder cancer, radical cystectomy with urethrectomy (unless orthotopic diversion is planned), and either ileal loop conduit or orthotopic diversion

BLADDER PRESERVATION APPROACHES: After cystectomy for muscle-invasive disease, 50% or more of the patients will develop metastases. Most patients develop metastases at distant sites; a third relapse locally. Bladder preservation management is offered in individuals who refuse surgery or who might not be suitable radical cystectomy patients. Bladder-sparing protocols include extensive TURBT or partial cystectomy with external-beam or interstitial radiotherapy and systemic chemotherapy. Radiotherapy as a single treatment modality is not effective. The best predictor of successful bladder preservation is a complete response after the combination of initial TURBT and neoadjuvant chemotherapy with stages T_2 to T_{3a}.

INDICATIONS FOR PARTIAL CYSTECTOMY:
- Tumor within a bladder diverticulum
- Solitary, primary, and muscle-invasive or high-grade lesion of a region of the bladder that allows complete excision with adequate surgical margins
- Inability to adequately resect tumor by TURBT alone because of size or location
- Tumor overlying a ureteral orifice requiring ureteral reimplantation
- Biopsy of a radiation-induced ulceration
- Palliation of severe local symptoms
- Patient refusal of urinary diversion
- Poor-risk patient who is not a diversion candidate

CONTRAINDICATIONS:
- Multiple tumors
- CIS
- Cellular atypia on biopsy
- Prostatic invasion
- Invasion of the trigone
- Inability to achieve adequate surgical margins
- Prior radiotherapy
- Inability to maintain adequate bladder volume after resection
- Evidence of extravesical tumor extension
- Poor surgical risk

ACUTE GENERAL Rx

INDICATIONS FOR INTRAVESICAL CHEMOTHERAPY:
- High-grade tumor
- Tumor size <5 cm
- Multiple tumors
- Presence of CIS
- Positive urinary cytologic findings after a resection
- Incomplete tumor resection

Intravesical agents: Thiotepa, doxorubicin, mitomycin C, BCG, interferon, interleukin-2, keyhole-limpet hemocyanin, and gemcitabine. Photodynamic therapy with hematoporphyrin derivatives has also been used.

INDICATIONS FOR CYSTECTOMY:
- Large tumors not amenable to complete TURBT
- High-grade tumor
- Multiple tumors with frequent recurrences
- Diffuse CIS not responsive to intravesical chemotherapy
- Prostatic urethra involvement
- Irritative bladder symptoms with upper tract deterioration
- Muscle-invasive disease
- Disease outside the bladder

SYSTEMIC THERAPY:
- Nonmetastatic cancers:
  1. Cisplatin-based chemotherapy is used concurrently with radiotherapy in bladder preservation therapy approaches for resectable cases.
  2. Combination chemotherapy regimens are used as perioperative (neoadjuvant and adjuvant) therapy for locally advanced disease in conjunction with bladder resection. Neoadjuvant chemotherapy is preferable given the low rates of completion seen in the postoperative setting in this mostly elderly group of patients.
  3. Neoadjuvant immunotherapy has been associated with high rates of pathologic complete responses in early trials.
- Metastatic or relapsed cancers:
  1. Combination cisplatin-based chemotherapy regimens are used as palliative therapy in fit patients. The most effective combination regimens include MVAC (cisplatin, methotrexate, vinblastine, doxorubicin) and

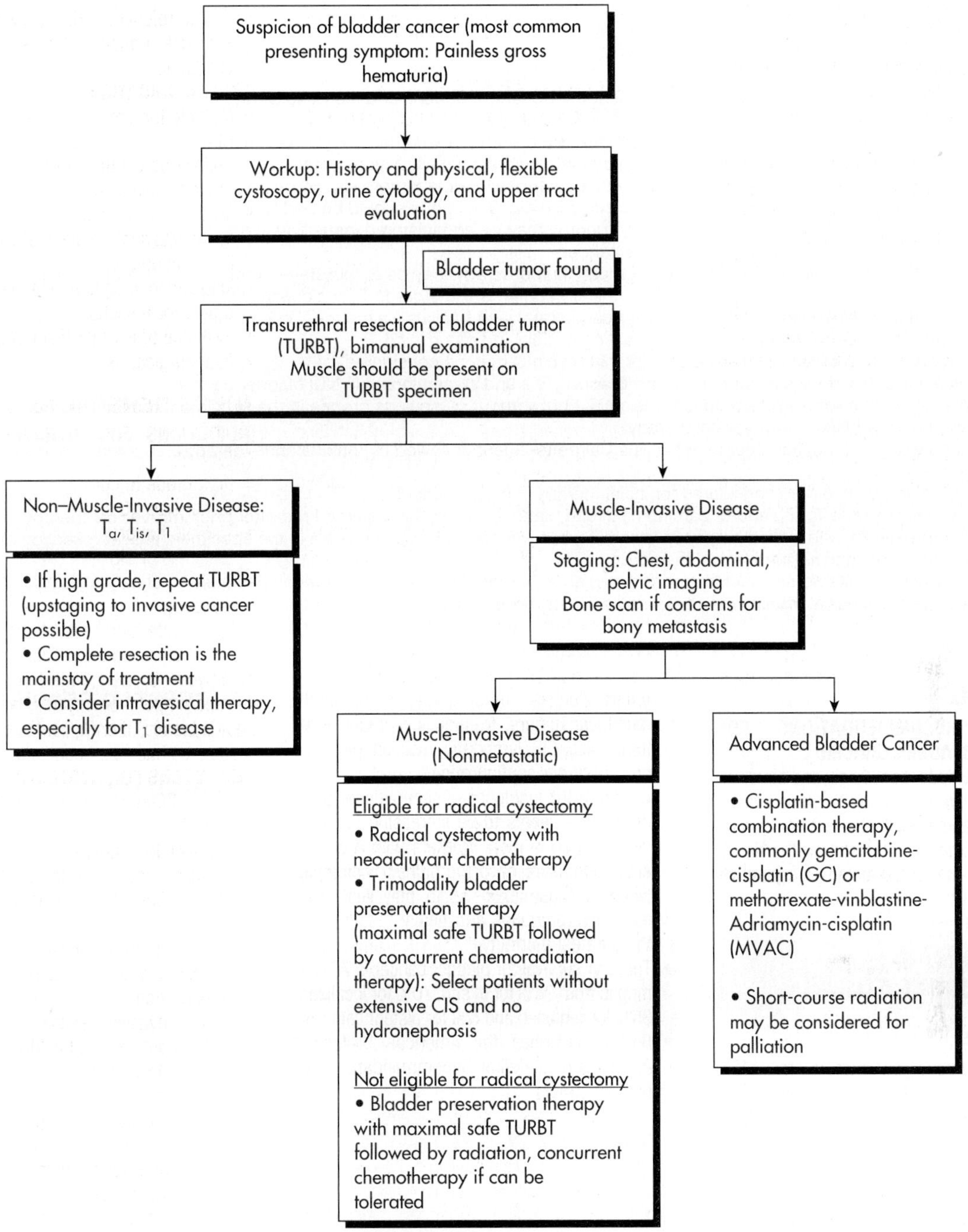

FIG. 1 Diagnostic and treatment algorithm for bladder cancer. *CIS*, Carcinoma in situ. (From Niederhuber JE: *Abeloff's clinical oncology*, ed 6, Philadelphia, 2020, Elsevier.)

GC (gemcitabine, cisplatin), which provide palliation and overall survival benefit.

2. In patients who are unfit to receive cisplatin-based chemotherapy regimens, the use of immune checkpoint inhibitors is the preferred first-line therapy option in patients with PD-L1–expressing tumors. Available agents include the PD-1 inhibitors (nivolumab, pembrolizumab) and PDL-1 inhibitors (atezolizumab, durvalumab, avelumab). These are also used as salvage therapy in patients who have failed prior chemotherapy approaches.
3. Alterations in the gene encoding fibroblast growth factor receptor (FGFR) are detected in 15% to 20% of cases of locally advanced or metastatic urothelial carcinoma. Erdafitinib, a tyrosine kinase inhibitor of FGFR1-4, has shown response rates of 40% in previously treated patients with FGFR alterations, and median survival of approximately 14 mo.
4. Enfortumab vedotin, an antibody drug conjugate consisting of a monoclonal antibody targeting nectin-4 conjugated to monomethyl auristatin E, has been approved for patients who do not respond to both chemotherapy and immune-checkpoint inhibitors.

RADIOTHERAPY: Conflicting reports suggest that superficial bladder cancer is more sensitive to radiotherapy. Only 20% to 30% of patients with invasive bladder cancer can be cured by external-beam radiation therapy alone. It is used in combination with surgery or with systemic agents to treat bladder cancer primarily in patients who are not surgical candidates or who refuse surgery. Combination chemotherapy (cisplatin) given concurrently with radiotherapy has shown significant improved locoregional control of bladder cancer in bladder-preservation strategies.

BOX 1 American Urological Association Guideline Recommendations

For all index patients:
- Standard: Physicians should discuss with the patient the treatment options and the benefits and harms, including side effects, of intravesical treatment.

For a patient who presents with an abnormal growth on the urothelium but who has not yet been diagnosed with bladder cancer:
- Standard: If the patient does not have an established histologic diagnosis, a biopsy should be obtained for pathologic analysis.
- Standard: Under most circumstances, complete eradication of all visible tumors should be performed.
- Standard: If bladder cancer is confirmed, periodic surveillance cystoscopy should be performed.
- Option: An initial single dose of intravesical chemotherapy may be administered immediately postoperatively.

For a patient with small volume, low-grade T_a bladder cancer:
- Recommendation: An initial single dose of intravesical chemotherapy may be administered immediately postoperatively.

For a patient with multifocal and/or large volume, histologically confirmed, low-grade T_a or a patient with recurrent low-grade T_a bladder cancer:
- Recommendation: An induction course of intravesical therapy with bacillus Calmette-Guérin or mitomycin C is recommended for the treatment of these patients with the goal of preventing or delaying recurrence.
- Option: Maintenance bacillus Calmette-Guérin or mitomycin C may be considered.

For a patient with initial histologically confirmed high-grade T_a, T_1, and/or carcinoma in situ bladder cancer:
- Standard: For patients with lamina propria invasion (T_1) but without muscularis propria in the specimen, repeat resection should be performed prior to additional intravesical therapy.
- Recommendation: An induction course of bacillus Calmette-Guérin followed by maintenance therapy is recommended for treatment of these patients.
- Option: Cystectomy should be considered for initial therapy in select patients.

For a patient with high-grade T_a, T_1, and/or carcinoma in situ bladder cancer that has recurred after prior intravesical therapy:
- Standard: For patients with lamina propria invasion (T_1) but without muscularis propria in the specimen, repeat resection should be performed prior to additional intravesical therapy.
- Recommendation: Cystectomy should be considered as a therapeutic alternative for these patients.
- Option: Further intravesical therapy may be considered for these patients.

CHRONIC Rx

FOLLOW-UP RECOMMENDATIONS FOR SUPERFICIAL BLADDER CANCER:
- Cystoscopy, bladder barbotage, and bimanual examination every 3 mo for 2 yr, then every 6 mo for 2 yr, and annually thereafter.
- Upper tract studies are based on the risk of upper tract tumor development, generally every 2 to 5 yr.

PEARLS & CONSIDERATIONS

COMMENTS
- Useful prognostic parameters for bladder tumor recurrence and subsequent progression are tumor grade, tumor depth, multifocal tumors, frequency of recurrence, tumor size, CIS, lymphatic invasion, papillary or solid tumor configuration.
- Currently, the incidence of occupational bladder cancer seems to be increasing faster in women than in men. Workers with aromatic amine exposure have the highest incidence, whereas those exposed to polycyclic aromatic hydrocarbons and heavy metals have the greatest mortality.
- The 5-yr survival for bladder cancer is 76%; it ranges from 96% for in situ, 70% for localized, 35% for regional, and 5% for distant cancers.
- Box 1 describes the American Urological Association Guideline Recommendations for bladder cancer.

SUGGESTED READINGS
Available at ExpertConsult.com

RELATED CONTENT
Bladder Cancer (Patient Information)

AUTHOR: **Bharti Rathore, MD**

BASIC INFORMATION

DEFINITION

The International Continence Society defines bladder pain syndrome, otherwise known as interstitial cystitis (IC), as a clinical syndrome consisting of suprapubic pain related to bladder filling and accompanied by other symptoms, such as increased daytime and nighttime frequency in the absence of proven infection or other obvious pathology. The American Urological Association defines interstitial cystitis/bladder pain syndrome (IC/BPS) as an unpleasant sensation perceived to be related to the urinary bladder that is associated with lower urinary tract symptoms >6 wk duration, in the absence of infection or other unidentifiable causes.

SYNONYMS

Interstitial cystitis
Interstitial cystitis/bladder pain syndrome (IC/BPS)
Painful bladder syndrome
Tic douloureux of bladder

ICD-10CM CODES

N30.1	Interstitial cystitis (chronic)
N30.9	Cystitis, unspecified
N30.10	Interstitial cystitis (chronic) without hematuria
N30.11	Interstitial cystitis (chronic) with hematuria

EPIDEMIOLOGY & DEMOGRAPHICS

INCIDENCE: 21 cases per 100,000 women and 4 cases per 100,000 men annually

PREVALENCE:
- 197 per 100,000 women and 41 per 100,000 men in the U.S.
- Because the disease is substantially underdiagnosed, it may actually affect one in five women and 1 in 20 men.
- More than 81% of women diagnosed with chronic pelvic pain and up to 84% of men initially diagnosed with chronic prostatitis actually have IC.
- More than 90% of patients diagnosed with overactive bladder who do not respond to anticholinergics are subsequently diagnosed with IC.

PREDOMINANT SEX AND AGE:
- White women constitute 95% of patients with IC
- Female:male ratio of 5 to 10:1
- Most prevalent in fourth and fifth decades of life

PHYSICAL FINDINGS & CLINICAL PRESENTATION

- Urinary urgency, frequency (>8 in daytime), nocturia (>2 at night), and suprapubic pain are the most common symptoms
- Suprapubic pain is worse with bladder filling or urinating and relieved after emptying
- Dyspareunia
- Symptoms lasting longer than 6 mo
- Intensity of symptoms waxes and wanes
- Insidious onset and worsens to the final stage within 5 to 15 yr
- Exercise, stress, sexual activity, ejaculation, certain foods with high potassium and acids (beer, spices, bananas, tomatoes, chocolate, strawberries, artificial sweeteners, oranges, cranberries, caffeine), menstruation, prolonged sitting, and activation of allergies exacerbate the symptoms
- Often associated with irritable bowel syndrome, migraine, endometriosis, skin sensitivities, multiple drug allergies, other allergies, vulvodynia, fibromyalgia, chronic fatigue syndrome, systemic lupus erythematosus, and mood disorders
- Dysphoric mood
- Lower abdominal tenderness
- Tender prostate in digital rectal examination
- Levator ani tenderness in female
- Tenderness of anterior vaginal wall/bladder neck in female

ETIOLOGY

Unknown. Fig. 1 illustrates a hypothesis for etiologic cascade of painful bladder syndrome/interstitial cystitis.

DIAGNOSIS

DIFFERENTIAL DIAGNOSIS

- Chronic pelvic pain
- Overactive bladder
- Recurrent urinary tract infection
- Endometriosis
- Pelvic adhesions
- Vulvar vestibulitis
- Vulvodynia
- Urethral pain syndrome
- Chronic nonbacterial prostatitis
- Frequent vaginitis
- Benign prostatic hyperplasia

WORKUP

- IC can be considered a diagnosis of exclusion when no known cause of painful bladder can be identified.
- There is no definite diagnostic test.

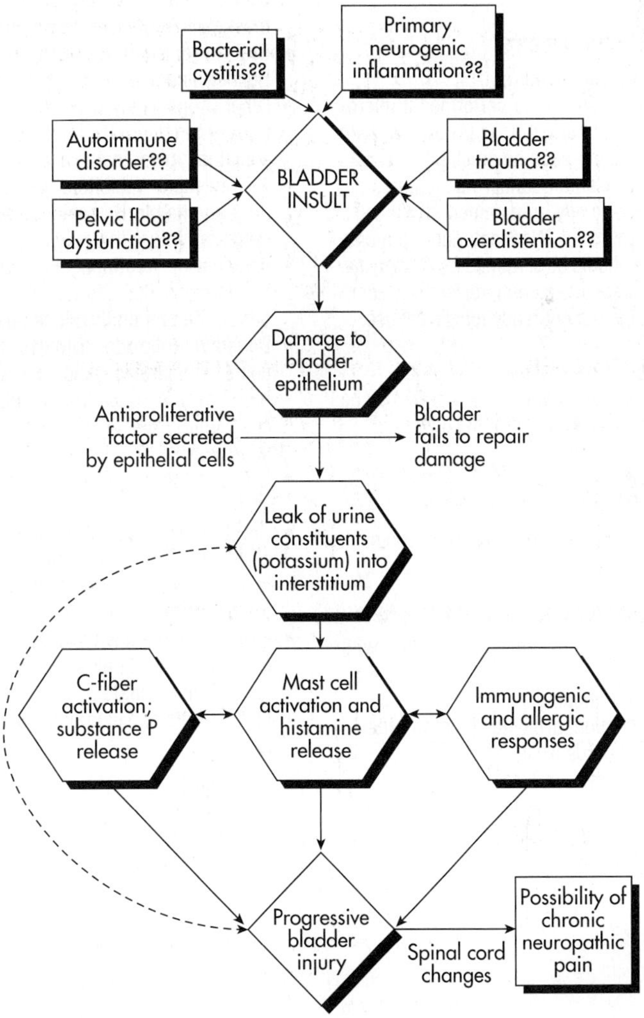

FIG. 1 Hypothesis for etiologic cascade of painful bladder syndrome/interstitial cystitis. (From Wein AJ: Painful bladder syndrome/interstitial cystitis and related disorders. In Wein AJ et al [eds]: *Campbell-Walsh urology*, ed 11, Philadelphia, 2007, Elsevier.)

- Validated questionnaires such as Pelvic Pain and Urgency/Frequency scale (PUF), O'Leary-Sant symptoms and problem index, and Wisconsin IC scale. PUF is the most commonly used.
- Voiding diary shows low-volume (<100 ml) and high-frequency voiding pattern.
- National Institute of Diabetes and Diseases of the Kidney diagnostic criteria misses 60% of IC patients and is not clinically used anymore.
- Anesthetic bladder challenge: With this test the symptoms dissipate on instillation of an anesthetic cocktail into the bladder.
- Cystoscopy and hydrodistention under general anesthesia may show terminal hematuria (Fig. E2), glomerulation, Hunner ulcers (Fig. E3), and small bladder capacity of less than 350 ml. Cystoscopy and/or urodynamic testing should be considered when the diagnosis is in doubt, but the tests are not necessary to confirm an IC/BPS diagnosis in uncomplicated cases.
- Bladder biopsy is not essential for diagnosis of IC.
- Parson potassium sensitivity test (PST).
- Urodynamics are unnecessary in diagnosis of IC.

LABORATORY TESTS

- Urine analysis and culture.
- Urine cytology should be performed if microscopic or gross hematuria is present, or with other risk factors such as smoking, age >40 yr, and other bladder cancer risk factors.
- Culture of sexually transmitted diseases if clinically indicated. Nonbacteriuric patients with pyuria should be screened for *Chlamydia*.
- Urine biomarkers (e.g., antiproliferative factor) are promising but not ready for clinical use.

IMAGING STUDIES

CT or ultrasound of abdomen and pelvis may be considered to rule out other pathology.

Rx TREATMENT

- There is no consensus for optimal management.
- There is no cure for this disease.

NONPHARMACOLOGIC THERAPY

- Avoidance of activities associated with flare-ups
- Avoidance of smoking
- Dietary restriction, avoiding common irritants (e.g., coffee, citrus fruits)
- Physical therapy
- Exercise
- Behavioral therapy
- Bladder retraining
- Biofeedback
- Warm sitz bath, ice, heating pad
- Thiele massage (transrectal and transvaginal manual therapy of pelvic floor muscle) in presence of pelvic floor muscle tenderness and spasm
- Hydrodistention only gives temporary relief, so it is not commonly used anymore

ACUTE AND CHRONIC Rx

- A course of empiric antibiotics if not tried yet. Long-term oral antibiotics are not recommended.
- Oral therapy is tried first.
- Pentosan polysulfate sodium (Elmiron) is the only FDA-approved and most effective oral therapy.
- Most treatment takes 3 to 6 mo before maximum benefit is seen.
- Adjunct oral therapy includes tricyclic antidepressants (amitriptyline), cimetidine, antihistaminics (hydroxyzine, montelukast), neuroleptics (gabapentin, topiramate), analgesics (NSAIDs, opioid analgesics), and occasionally antimuscarinics.
- Oral therapies can be used in combination.
- Antihistaminics are preferred for patients with an allergy history or those who show mast cells in bladder biopsy.
- Oral prednisone is used in presence of Hunner ulcers.
- Other drugs rarely used for IC are cyclosporin A, interleukin-10, imatinib, methotrexate, suplatast, misoprostol, and quercetin.
- Growth factor inhibitors, gene therapy, RDP 58, and vitamin B_3 analogue (BXL 628) may represent future therapies.
- Intravesical treatment is used when oral medications fail, for acute flare-ups, or before the oral medications take full effect.
- Dimethyl sulfoxide (DMSO), heparin, lidocaine, hyaluronic acid, capsaicin, botulinum toxin A, chondroitin sulfate, steroids, and Elmiron are drugs used for intravesical treatment.
- DMSO is the only FDA-approved intravesical treatment.
- DMSO is used less often now because of its side effects, specifically a garlic-like odor or taste on breath or skin that lasts 72 hr after treatment.
- Intravesical therapy typically involves mixture of heparin or Elmiron with lidocaine and sodium bicarbonate.
- Silver nitrate and clorpactin have fallen out of favor.

SURGERY

- Major surgical intervention is not the mainstay of treatment.
- Patients whose condition is extreme and who are miserable may consider surgery if medications fail.
- Sacral neuromodulation (InterStim) is the current preferred surgical intervention.
- Laser ablation, fulguration, or resection is offered when Hunner ulcers are seen in cystoscopy.
- Augmentation cystoplasty is not recommended.
- Cystourethrectomy with urinary diversion is rarely done.

COMPLEMENTARY & ALTERNATIVE MEDICINE

- Transcutaneous electric nerve stimulation
- Intravaginal electric nerve stimulation
- Acupuncture
- Urinary chelating agents such as Polycitra-K crystals, Urocit-K
- Prelief, an over-the-counter food additive
- Herbal remedies such as Algonot Plus, CystoProtek, Cysta-Q, aloe vera

DISPOSITION

Voiding diary and symptom questionnaire are helpful to monitor response to treatment.

REFERRAL

- Urologist
- Pain specialist
- Physical therapist

PEARLS & CONSIDERATIONS

COMMENTS

- On average, these patients see five physicians and endure irritating voiding symptoms for 5 yr before the disease is identified.
- Besides symptom questionnaire and urine analysis, all other diagnostic tests are optional.
- PST is well tolerated.
- Negative cystoscopy does not rule out IC.

PREVENTION

Early identification and timely intervention improve patient outcome.

PATIENT & FAMILY EDUCATION

- IC support groups
- Interstitial Cystitis Association
- Interstitial Cystitis Network

SUGGESTED READINGS

Available at ExpertConsult.com

AUTHOR: **Fred F. Ferri, MD**

BASIC INFORMATION

DEFINITION

A brain abscess is a focal intracerebral infection that can arise as a complication of a bacterial, mycobacterial, fungal, or parasitic infection, or as a sequelae after surgery or trauma.

ICD-10CM CODE
G06.0 Intracranial abscess and granuloma

EPIDEMIOLOGY & DEMOGRAPHICS

INCIDENCE: Uncommon (reported incidence 0.4 to 0.9 cases per 100,000 population; occurs about 2% as commonly as brain tumors)
PREDOMINANT SEX: Men affected more than women (ratio 2:1 to 3:1)
PREDOMINANT AGE: Occurs at any age
PEAK INCIDENCE: Preadolescence and middle age (and depends on predisposing condition); increased rates in the immunocompromised host

PHYSICAL FINDINGS & CLINICAL PRESENTATION

- Classic triad: Fever, headache, and focal neurologic deficit (only present in approximately 20% of cases).
- Clinical presentation is often due to the manifestations of the space-occupying lesion rather than to signs of systemic infection.
- Fever is present in only 32% to 79% of patients.
- Headache is usually localized to the side of the abscess; onset can be gradual or severe; present in an average of 70% to 75% of cases.
- Focal neurologic findings (e.g., seizures, hemiparesis, aphasia, ataxia) depend on the location of the abscess and are seen in 23% to 66% of cases.
- Papilledema is present in 9% to 51% of cases.
- Presence of adjacent infections (dental abscess, otitis media, sinusitis, or postneurosurgical infection) may be a clue to the underlying diagnosis or source and should be sought in any suspected case.
- Time course from symptom onset to presentation ranges from hours in fulminant cases to more than 1 mo; 75% present in the first 2 wk.
- The nonspecific presentation of a brain abscess warrants that clinicians maintain a high index of suspicion. Table 1 describes common initial features of brain abscess.

ETIOLOGY

- Brain abscesses are classified based on the likely portal of entry and can arise from:
  1. Contiguous infection (e.g., dental abscess, otitis media, sinusitis, or post neurosurgical infection)
  2. Hematogenous spread from a remote site (e.g., endocarditis, bacteremia), which typically causes multiple lesions

TABLE 1 Brain Abscess: Initial Features in 123 Cases

Headache	55%
Disturbed consciousness	48%
Fever	58%
Nuchal rigidity	29%
Nausea, vomiting	32%
Seizures	19%
Visual disturbance	15%
Dysarthria	20%
Hemiparesis	48%
Sepsis	17%

From Goldman L, Schafer AI: *Goldman's Cecil medicine*, ed 24, Philadelphia, 2012, Saunders.

- Likely source of abscess and common organisms involved:
  1. Contiguous focus or primary infection (55% of all brain abscesses):
     a. Paranasal sinus: Occur in frontal lobe; streptococci (especially microaerophilic and anaerobic streptococci), *Bacteroides*, *Haemophilus*, and *Fusobacterium* spp.
     b. Otitis media/mastoiditis: Occur in temporal lobe and cerebellum; aerobic and anaerobic streptococci, *Enterobacteriaceae*, *Bacteroides*, and *Pseudomonas* spp.
     c. Dental infection: Occur in frontal lobe; mixed *Fusobacterium*, *Bacteroides*, and *Streptococcus* spp. (especially *S. viridans* and anaerobic streptococci)
     d. Penetrating head injury: Site of abscess depends on site of wound; *Staphylococcus aureus*, aerobic streptococci, *Clostridium* spp., *Enterobacteriaceae*
     e. Postoperative: *Staphylococcus epidermidis* and *S. aureus, Enterobacteriaceae,* and *Pseudomonas aeruginosa*
  2. Hematogenous spread from a distant site of infection (25% of all brain abscesses): Abscesses most commonly multiple, especially in middle cerebral artery distribution; infecting organism(s) depend on source
     a. Congenital heart disease: Streptococci, *Haemophilus* spp.
     b. Endocarditis: *S. aureus*, viridans streptococci
     c. Urinary tract: Enterobacteriaceae, Pseudomonadaceae
     d. Intraabdominal: Streptococci, *Enterobacteriaceae*, anaerobes
     e. Lung: Streptococci, *Actinomyces* spp., *Fusobacterium* spp.
     f. Immunocompromised host: *Toxoplasma* spp., *Enterobacteriaceae*, *Nocardia* spp., listeriosisi, other fungi, tuberculosis
     g. Fungi are responsible for up to 90% of cerebral abscesses in solid organ transplant recipients
  3. Cryptogenic (unknown source): 20% of all brain abscesses

Dx DIAGNOSIS

DIFFERENTIAL DIAGNOSIS

- Other parameningeal infections: Subdural empyema, epidural abscess, thrombophlebitis of the major dural venous sinuses and cortical veins
- Embolic strokes in patients with bacterial endocarditis
- Mycotic aneurysms with leakage
- Acute hemorrhagic leukoencephalitis
- Parasitic infections: Toxoplasmosis, echinococcosis, cysticercosis
- Metastatic or primary brain tumors
- Cerebral infarction
- CNS vasculitis
- Chronic subdural hematoma

WORKUP

Physical examination, laboratory tests, and imaging studies

LABORATORY TESTS

- White blood cell counts are elevated in 60% of patients.
- Erythrocyte sedimentation rate is usually elevated but may be normal.
- Lumbar puncture is contraindicated because of the potential for increased intracranial pressure and the risk for herniation due to the space-occupying abscess. Lumbar puncture may be helpful only in those with suspicion for meningitis or abscess rupture into the ventricular system; however, the risk of herniation must be considered.
- The yield of Gram stain and culture of material aspirated at time of surgical drainage is very high.
- Cultures of contiguous sites of infection should be considered (e.g., paranasal sinus, otitis, skin site abscess from a neurosurgical procedure). These sites of infection may need surgical drainage in order to control the infection.
- Blood cultures and cerebrospinal fluid cultures may identify the causative organism in up to 25% of patients.
- Based on the appearance of lesions on imaging, then antitoxoplasma IgG antibodies from the blood and anticysticercal antibodies in the CSF can aid in the diagnosis of CNS toxoplasma and neurocysticercosis infections, respectively.

IMAGING STUDIES

- CT scan with contrast enhancement or MRI with gadolinium can be used to detect brain abscess. CT is rapid and available in most medical settings. An MRI with gadolinium (Fig. E1) is able to provide more detailed images in order to differentiate between abscess and tumor or other mass.
- CT scan (Fig. 2) with intravenous contrast enhancement is still an excellent test (sensitivity 95% to 99%).
- Serial CT or MRI scanning is recommended to follow the response to therapy.

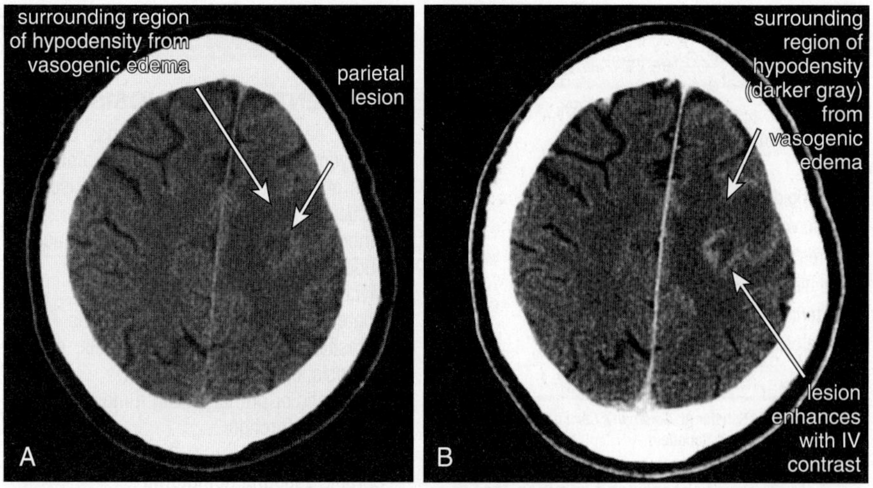

FIG. 2 Brain abscess. This 48-yr-old male presented with status epilepticus. Computed tomography (CT) of the brain showed a parietal mass, which at brain biopsy was found to be an abscess. Cultures grew mixed gram-positive and gram-negative organisms and anaerobes. The patient was subsequently found to be human immunodeficiency virus positive. **A,** Noncontrast head CT, brain windows. **B,** CT with intravenous (IV) contrast moments later, brain windows. Abscesses and other infectious, inflammatory, or neoplastic lesions typically have surrounding hypodense regions representing vasogenic edema. When IV contrast is administered **(B),** the lesion may enhance peripherally, often referred to as ring enhancement. (From Broder JS: *Diagnostic imaging for the emergency physician*, Philadelphia, 2011, Saunders.)

Rx TREATMENT

ACUTE GENERAL Rx

- Effective treatment involves a combination of empiric antibiotic therapy and timely excision or aspiration of the abscess for diagnosis and/or source control. Common pathogens and empirical therapy for brain abscess is summarized in Table E2.
- If evidence of edema or mass effect, treatment of elevated intracranial pressure is paramount.
  1. Hyperventilation of mechanically ventilated patient.
  2. Dexamethasone initially in a dosage of 10 mg IV followed by 4 mg IV q6h until symptoms of cerebral edema subside. Steroids should be discontinued as soon as possible.
  3. Mannitol 0.25 to 1 g/kg IV over 20 to 30 min q6 to 8h; maximum of 6 g/kg in 24 hr.
- Medical therapy is never a substitute for surgical intervention to relieve increased intracranial pressure. Neurologic deterioration usually mandates surgical intervention.
- Steroids should be limited to patients with severe cerebral edema or midline shift.

MEDICAL Rx

If abscess <2.5 cm and patient is neurologically stable and conscious, may start empiric antibiotics and observe. Empiric antibiotic therapy guided by:
- Abscess location
- Suspicion of primary source
- Presence of single or multiple abscesses
- Patient's underlying medical conditions (e.g., HIV, immunocompromised)

Selection of empiric antibiotic therapy:
- Primary infection or contiguous source:
  1. Otitis media/mastoiditis, sinusitis: Third-generation cephalosporin (cefotaxime 2 g q4h IV or ceftriaxone 2 g q12h IV) plus metronidazole 15 mg/kg IV as a loading dose, then 7.5 mg/kg q8h IV, not to exceed 4 g per day
  2. Dental infection: Penicillin G (20 million to 24 million units per day IV in six divided doses) plus metronidazole (dose as above)
  3. Head trauma: Third- or fourth-generation cephalosporin (cefotaxime 2 g IV q4h or ceftriaxone 2 g IV q12h or cefepime 2 g IV q8h) plus vancomycin (30 mg/kg IV in two divided doses adjusted for renal function)
  4. Postoperative neurosurgery: Vancomycin (dose as above) plus ceftazidime (2 g IV q8h) or cefepime (2 g IV q8h), or meropenem (1 g IV q8h). Replace vancomycin with nafcillin (2g IV q4h) if susceptibility testing reveals methicillin-sensitive *S. aureus*
- Hematogenous spread (congenital heart disease, endocarditis, urinary tract, lung, intraabdominal): Vancomycin (empiric therapy, dose as above) or nafcillin (if susceptibility testing reveals methicillin-sensitive *S. aureus*, dose as above) plus metronidazole plus third-generation cephalosporin (cefotaxime 2 g IV q4h or ceftriaxone 2 g IV q12h). Antibiotic therapy can be adjusted based on the etiology of the underlying infection, if known. Depending on the source, many experts advocate for anaerobic coverage, even with no documentation given suboptimal sensitivity of current techniques.
- HIV-infected or immunocompromised patient: Metronidazole plus a third-generation cephalosporin, antifungal, or antiparasitic agent. Duration of antibiotic therapy is guided by the clinical course and by whether the abscess was surgically aspirated or excised; it is usually prolonged. Most recommend parenteral treatment for at least 4 to 8 wk, with serial neuroimaging to ensure adequate resolution. (Imaging weekly could be considered for first 2 wk of therapy, then every 2 wk until resolution.) Surgical therapy may be required for clinical failure (i.e., increasing size of abscess on imaging despite antibiotic therapy).

SURGICAL Rx

- Three indications for surgical intervention:
  1. Collect specimens for culture and sensitivity to guide antibiotic therapy
  2. Reduce mass effect
  3. Clinical failure with antibiotic therapy alone
- Stereotactic biopsy or aspirate of the abscess if surgically feasible
- Essential to selection of targeted antimicrobial coverage
- Timing and choice of surgery depend on:
  1. Primary infection source
  2. Number and location of the abscesses
  3. Whether the procedure is diagnostic or therapeutic
  4. Neurologic status of the patient

DISPOSITION

- Prompt diagnostic consideration, early institution of appropriate antimicrobial therapy, and advanced neuroradiologic imaging have reduced the mortality rate from brain abscesses from 40% to 80% in the preantibiotic era to 10% to 20% at present.
- Morbidity is usually manifest as persistent neurologic sequelae (seizures, intellectual or behavioral impairment, motor deficits).

REFERRAL

Consultation with infectious disease and neurosurgery

! PEARLS & CONSIDERATIONS

COMMENTS

- It is important to maintain a high index of suspicion because a brain abscess often presents with nonspecific symptoms.
- Rapid imaging and early institution of appropriate antimicrobial therapy improve patient morbidity and mortality.
- Neurosurgical consultation is mandatory.

PREVENTION

Because brain abscesses arise from either contiguous infections or hematogenously from a remote site, early and appropriate treatment of predisposing infections is paramount to prevent brain abscess.

SUGGESTED READINGS

Available at ExpertConsult.com

RELATED CONTENT

Brain Abscess (Patient Information)

AUTHOR: **Erica Hardy, MD, MMS**

BASIC INFORMATION

DEFINITION

Brain metastases result from a spread of cancers originating in other organs to the brain and are devastating complications of cancer. Brain metastases are the most common intracranial tumors in adults and account for more than one half of brain tumors.

ICD-10CM CODES	
C79.89	Secondary malignant neoplasm of other specified sites
C80.0	Disseminated malignant neoplasm, unspecified
C80.9	Malignant neoplasm, unspecified

EPIDEMIOLOGY & DEMOGRAPHICS

INCIDENCE:

- The precise incidence and prevalence of brain metastases is unknown. Population studies based on review of historic epidemiological data show an overall incidence of 8.3 to 14.3 per 100,000 population per yr. However, these studies underestimate the true incidence of brain metastases because they rely on data from times when diagnostic imaging was poor. Reported incidence of metastatic brain malignancy is rising, likely due to improved detection and better control of extracerebral disease.
- In the U.S., an estimated 200,000 new cases occur each yr, representing approximately 30% of all cancer patients.

PREDOMINANT SEX & AGE:

- In patients with systemic malignancies, brain metastases occur in 10% to 30% of adults and 6% to 13% of children. Of these, about 60% of patients are between the ages of 50 and 70.
- There is no definite gender predilection. Some data indicate that metastatic brain malignancy has a higher incidence in men because men have a higher incidence of primary lung cancer.

RISK FACTORS:

- In adults, the most common primary cancers for brain metastases are lung (39% to 56%), breast (13% to 30%), melanoma (6% to 11%), renal (5% to 10%), and colon (2% to 8%). In general, almost all malignancies have the potential to metastasize to the brain. The majority (80%) of patients with brain metastases have multiple lesions and also have synchronous extracranial metastases. The cancers with the highest association of intracranial hemorrhage include renal cell carcinoma, melanoma, thyroid carcinoma, choriocarcinoma, and testicular cancer.
- The most common primary pediatric solid tumors associated with brain metastases include sarcomas, neuroblastoma, Wilms, and germ cell tumors. Leukemias are well known to seed the CNS. Metastatic disease is usually never seen when a child first presents with malignancy, with the occasional exception of leukemia. For solid tumors, metastatic disease is seen at the time of disease recurrence. Neuroblastoma CNS lesions have a high propensity to hemorrhage.

PHYSICAL FINDINGS & CLINICAL PRESENTATION

- Clinical presentations vary depending on where the lesion is located. Brain metastases should be suspected in any cancer patient developing acute neurologic signs or symptoms. Neurologic symptoms, however, are nonspecific for brain metastases in patients with systemic cancer. In an analysis of more than 800 patients with neurologic symptoms, brain metastases were found in only 16%.
- Symptoms:
  1. Headache occurs in 40% to 50% of patients with brain metastases. Frequency is higher with metastases located in the posterior fossa, which may result in obstructive hydrocephalus. The headache can be accompanied by nausea, vomiting, focal neurologic signs, and postural variation.
  2. Focal neurologic signs/symptoms are the presenting symptom in 20% to 40% of patients. Hemiparesis is the most frequent complaint. However, the specific neurologic dysfunction depends on the location of the brain metastasis.
  3. Cognitive dysfunction, including memory problems or mood or personality changes, is the presenting problem in 30% to 45% of patients.
  4. Seizures are the presenting symptom for 10% to 20% of patients with metastatic brain tumors and indicate supratentorial metastases.
  5. Acute stroke secondary to hemorrhage into a metastasis, hypercoagulability, or local vascular invasion occurs in 5% to 10% of patients.

ETIOLOGY

The most common mechanism of metastasis to the brain is by hematogenous spread. The most common locations are the cerebral hemispheres (80%), followed by the cerebellum (15%) and brain stem (5%). In the hemispheres, most lesions localize to the gray and white matter junction. Blood vessels decrease in diameter in these regions, which is thought to act like a trap for clusters of tumor cells. Different tumor types have a tendency to metastasize to different regions of the brain. For example, metastases of small cell lung carcinoma are equally distributed in all regions, whereas pelvic (prostate and uterine) and gastrointestinal tumors more commonly metastasize to the posterior fossa.

Dx DIAGNOSIS

DIFFERENTIAL DIAGNOSIS

- Primary brain tumor
- Infection: Bacterial abscess or fungal disease
- Progressive multifocal leukoencephalopathy
- Demyelinating disease: Multiple sclerosis, post-infectious encephalomyelitis
- Cerebral infarction or bleeding
- Effects of treatment, such as radiation necrosis

LABORATORY TESTS

- Routine laboratory studies are not typically helpful.
- Lumbar puncture is generally contraindicated due to increased intracranial pressure and risk of herniation. However, it may be necessary to diagnose metastases to the leptomeninges if suspected.
- Brain biopsy is necessary in some cases for a definitive diagnosis, particularly in the case of unknown primary tumor. Illustrating this situation is a study of cancer patients with solitary brain lesions that were presumed to be metastatic disease; in about 10% of study participants, the lesions were proved to be a different pathology.

IMAGING STUDIES

- MRI (Fig. E1) with and without contrast is the imaging study of choice. Important features on MRI suggesting brain metastases include: Presence of multiple lesions, localization at the junction of the gray and white matter, circumscribed margins, ring enhancement, or large amounts of vasogenic edema. CT of the head with contrast (Fig. E2) can be used when MRI is contraindicated. Noncontrast CT is appropriate for initial presentation with neurological symptoms to rule out intracranial hemorrhage.
- MR spectroscopy and PET may be useful for differentiating tumor from either other space-occupying lesions or radiation necrosis. However, PET has lower resolution than MRI and do not reliably distinguish metastases from high grade gliomas. MRI remains the gold standard, particularly in detection of small metastases (<1 cm).
- In about 80% of patients, brain metastases develop after the diagnosis of systemic cancer. In the remaining patients, brain metastases are diagnosed either simultaneously or before the primary tumor is found. In patients without a known primary tumor, the lung should be the initial focus of evaluation. PET scan may be useful in these patients not only to help identify the primary tumor but also other sites of metastatic disease, which may be more amenable to biopsy.

SCREENING

- There has been debate as to the utility of screening for brain metastases via MRI for high-risk primary tumors in the asymptomatic patient. Currently, the U.S. National Comprehensive Cancer Network (NCCN) guidelines recommend screening only for newly diagnosed small cell lung cancer, stage II-IV non–small cell lung cancer, and stage IV melanoma.

PROGNOSTIC FACTORS

- The Graded Prognostic Assessment (GPA) is used to predict median survival and is based on age, Karnofsky performance score (KPS), number of CNS metastases (>3 being poor prognosis), and presence of extracranial metastases. More recently, a multi-institutional retrospective cohort analysis produced a diagnosis-specific GPA, which is more accurate.

Rx TREATMENT

- Management of patients with brain metastases is influenced by the overall prognosis and are geared toward either treatment targeted at the malignancy or symptomatic management (e.g. edema, seizures).
- Typical treatment of metastatic lesions involves a combination of surgery, whole-brain radiation (WBRT), SRS (stereotactic radiosurgery), and systemic therapy.

SYMPTOMATIC MANAGEMENT

- Steroids are used to reduce peritumoral vasogenic edema, and intracranial pressure in the acute setting. Dexamethasone is the preferred agent. A taper is recommended following symptomatic resolution.
- Antiepileptics are started for patients who present with seizures. Prophylactic treatment for seizures is not indicated in patients without a prior history of seizure.

NONPHARMACOLOGIC THERAPY

- Radiation therapy remains the cornerstone of treatment for brain metastases. Approaches include whole-brain radiation therapy (WBRT) and stereotactic radiosurgery (SRS). WBRT is widely used but primarily provides symptom palliation and local disease control. A meta-analysis of five randomized controlled trials found that WBRT decreased the relative risk of intracranial disease progression at 1 yr by 53% but did not improve survival. SRS is gaining favor over WBRT due to notable adverse effects of WBRT, including cognitive impairment. Emerging data show that in the oligometastatic setting (4-15 metastases), SRS is noninferior to WBRT with regard to median survival and is less associated with neurocognitive decline. Notably, for patients with good prognosis and up to three lesions, addition of SRS to WBRT (vs. WBRT alone) increases overall survival. Therefore, patient involvement in decision-making is important with consideration of quality of life versus survival. In patients with poor prognosis, treatment focuses on WBRT and symptom control.
- Surgery is indicated for large lesions (>3 cm), fewer than three resectable lesions, KPS >70, limited systemic disease, and when tissue diagnosis is needed. A stereotactic approach is standard. Adjuvant radiation therapy is recommended, as most trials demonstrate improvement in overall survival.

PHARMACOLOGIC THERAPY

- The role of systemic therapies and targeted small-molecule therapies is regularly evolving.
- For highly chemosensitive tumors, chemotherapy has been integrated into the primary management of patients with disseminated disease. In most cases, systemic chemotherapies have not demonstrated significant survival benefit and are aimed at palliation. Certain agents have shown efficacy as monotherapies, such as temozolomide for brain metastases from breast cancer.
- Many targeted small-molecule therapies are showing promising results. One of the traditional limitations for small molecules has been penetrating the blood-brain barrier (BBB). Many new targeted therapies have good CNS penetration, including new generation tyrosine kinase inhibitors (TKIs) against EGFR and ALK (for lung cancer primary) that have demonstrated CNS efficacy in phase II/III trials. The combination of lapatinib (which targets both EGFR and HER2/Neu) and capecitabine (an antimetabolite prodrug that is converted to 5-fluorouracil) has also shown efficacy in treating brain metastases in HER2-positive breast cancer patients in phase II studies. For patients with brain metastases from melanoma primary with a *BRAF* mutation, dabrafenib (a TKI against BRAF) has had encouraging response rates, which were improved (to >50%) with combinatorial therapy with trametinib (a MAPK pathway inhibitor). In particular for melanoma, a combination of the immune checkpoint inhibitors ipilimumab (anti-CTLA4 antibody) and nivolumab (anti-PD-1 antibody) resulted in intracranial response rates of nearly 60% as well as 70% overall survival (OS) at 2 yrs, a dramatic improvement over typical median OS of 4 to 5 mo. Whether these targeted therapies synergize with radiation therapy is an area of active investigation.

DISPOSITION

- The median survival of patients who receive supportive care and are treated with corticosteroids only is approximately 1 to 2 mo. With current treatment modalities, median survival is now approximately 7 mo, depending on site of primary.
- Key prognostic factors are performance status, extent of systemic disease, number of CNS lesions, and age. Most favorable outcome is found in patients with Karnofsky performance score ≥90, age <50 yr, no systemic disease or local control of primary tumor without extracranial metastases, and a solitary CNS metastasis. In this group, median survival is estimated at 11.0 mo.

REFERRAL

Treatment involves a multispecialty team. Consultations from oncology, neurosurgery, neurology, radiation oncology, psychiatry, and physical therapy are all warranted.

PEARLS & CONSIDERATIONS

COMMENTS

- Brain metastases are the most common intracranial tumors in adults, accounting for more than half of all brain tumors.
- Lung cancer, melanoma, renal cell carcinoma, and breast cancer are the most common primary tumors that metastasize to the brain.
- MRI of the brain with and without contrast is the most reliable imaging study.
- Treatment (surgery and/or radiation therapy) depends on the patient's overall prognosis, with stereotactic radiosurgery gaining favor over whole-brain radiation therapy.
- New targeted therapies are changing the outlook for brain metastases from specific tumor types.

PATIENT & FAMILY EDUCATION

- American Brain Tumor Association (http://www.abta.org)
- National Brain Tumor Society (http://www.braintumor.org)

RELATED CONTENT

Brain Cancer (Patient Information)

AUTHORS: **Jaray H. Wang, MD, PhD,** and **Lily C. Pham, MD**

BASIC INFORMATION

DEFINITION

Brain neoplasms are a diverse group of primary (predominantly nonmetastatic) tumors arising from one of many different cell types within the central nervous system (CNS). Specific tumor subtypes and prognosis depend on the tumor cell of origin, certain genetic markers, and pattern of growth. The diffuse low-grade gliomas (LGGs) currently include World Health Organization grade II astrocytomas, oligodendrogliomas, and oligoastrocytomas. However, the histologic classification oligoastrocytoma is falling out of favor in lieu of molecular markers specific for either astrocytomas or oligodendrogliomas.

SYNONYMS

Low-grade glioma (LGG)
Glioneuronal tumor
Meningioma
Primary brain tumor

ICD-10CM CODE

D33.2 Benign neoplasm of brain, unspecified

EPIDEMIOLOGY & DEMOGRAPHICS

INCIDENCE: U.S. incidence rate of a new brain tumor is approximately 6.4/100,000 persons per yr for all primary brain tumors (Table 1). One third of these are considered malignant and the remainder benign or borderline malignant. The incidence rate in children aged 0 to 19 yr is lower (5.6 per 100,000 children). Primary brain neoplasms account for ~2% of all cancers, with a disproportionate share of cancer morbidity and mortality. It is the most common cause of cancer death in children up to 15 yr.

PREDOMINANT SEX & AGE: Slight male predominance of malignant brain tumors (8.0 vs. 5.5/100,000 person/yr). Men account for slightly less than half of cases of both benign and malignant brain tumors, as meningiomas have a higher incidence in women.

PEAK INCIDENCE: Depends on histology, though highest peak at ~age 50 yr.

RISK FACTORS: Exposure to ionizing radiation has been implicated in meningiomas, gliomas, and nerve sheath tumors. No convincing evidence has shown a link with trauma, occupation, cellular phone use, diet, or electromagnetic fields.

GENETICS: Most primary CNS neoplasms are sporadic; 5% are associated with hereditary syndromes that predispose to neoplasia. The most common of these include:

- Li-Fraumeni syndrome: *p53* mutation on chromosome 17q13, gliomas
- Von Hippel-Lindau: VHL, chromosome 3p25, hemangioblastoma
- Tuberous sclerosis: *TSC1/TSC2* (chromosome 9q34/16p13), subependymal giant cell astrocytoma
- Neurofibromatosis type 1: NF1, chromosome 17q11, neurofibroma, optic nerve glioma, low-grade glioma
- Neurofibromatosis type 2: NF2, chromosome 22q12, schwannoma, meningioma, ependymoma
- Retinoblastoma: pRB, chromosome 13q, retinoblastoma
- Gorlin syndrome: PTCH, chromosome 9q31, desmoplastic medulloblastoma
- Hereditary nonpolyposis colorectal cancer (HNPCC): Mismatch repair deficiency, high-grade gliomas

PHYSICAL FINDINGS & CLINICAL PRESENTATION

- In general, the location, size, and rate of growth will determine the symptoms and signs of a brain tumor.
- Headache is common and is the worst symptom in nearly half of all patients. The headaches are usually a dull, constant pain that is often worse at night. Symptoms of increased intracranial pressure may also be present, including nausea and vomiting, and may worsen with changes in body position that increase thoracic pressure (coughing, sneezing, Valsalva maneuver). Papilledema is suggestive of obstructive hydrocephalus.
- Seizures occur in 33% of patients and are among the most common symptoms, particularly with brain metastases and low-grade gliomas. The type of seizure and clinical presentation depend on the location of the brain tumor. Tumor-related seizures are typically repetitive and have similar presentation patterns (semiology). It is thought that patients with seizures typically have smaller tumors at the time of diagnosis compared with those with other symptoms, because the onset of seizures prompts an imaging study, leading to an earlier diagnosis.
- Focal neurologic signs and symptoms, including muscle weakness, sensory changes, or visual disturbances are also quite frequent. In addition, cognitive dysfunction, accompanied by changes in memory or personality change, may be recounted, often in retrospect.

ETIOLOGY

Most cases are idiopathic, though specific chromosomal abnormalities have been implicated in some tumor types.

TABLE 1 Frequency of Primary Central Nervous System Tumors

CHILDREN (0-14 YR)		ADULTS (≥15 YR)	
Type	**Percentage**	**Type**	**Percentage**
Glioblastoma	20	Glioblastoma	50
Astrocytoma	21	Astrocytoma	10
Ependymoma	7	Ependymoma	2
Oligodendroglioma	1	Oligodendroglioma	3
Medulloblastoma	24	Medulloblastoma	2
Neuroblastoma	3	Neurilemmoma	2
Neurilemmoma	1	Pituitary adenoma	4
Craniopharyngioma	5	Craniopharyngioma	1
Meningioma	5	Meningioma	17
Teratoma	2	Pinealoma	1
Pinealoma	2	Hemangioma	2
Hemangioma	3	Sarcoma	1
Sarcoma	1	Others	5
Others	5	Total	100
Total	100		

From Goetz CG, Pappert EJ: *Textbook of clinical neurology,* Philadelphia, 1999, Saunders.

DIAGNOSIS

- Diagnosis is typically based on clinical presentation and imaging characteristics. Specifically, neuroimaging is critical for preoperative planning and tumor etiology.
- Tumors are best seen on brain MRI with and without contrast; calcifications are sometimes present. However, most low-grade gliomas are often nonenhancing with contrast. Contrast enhancement is concerning for a higher grade glioma.
- Benign and low-grade tumors, typically in the glioma family, are heterogeneous and are generally seen as an infiltrating hemispheric lesion.

DIFFERENTIAL DIAGNOSIS

- Stroke/cerebral hemorrhage
- Abscess/parasitic cyst
- Demyelinating disease: Multiple sclerosis, postinfectious encephalomyelitis
- Metastatic tumors
- Primary CNS lymphoma

WORKUP

Neuroimaging studies and pathologic sampling are the most important diagnostic modalities in evaluation of brain tumors and may be critical for preoperative planning.

LABORATORY TESTS

- Classically, histologic examination can provide the exact diagnosis. Additional features such as proliferative index, immunohistochemical stains, and electron microscopy can also be used to aid in diagnosis. However, the most recent diagnostic criteria now also demand molecular and genetic classifications (e.g., 1p19q codeletion for the diagnosis of oligodendrogliomas).

- The current classification schema for gliomas is based on molecular genetics and histologic criteria. Tumor histology/histologic diagnosis (World Health Organization [WHO] grading system) includes number of mitoses, capillary endothelial proliferation, and necrosis.
- Molecular genetic analysis of tumors is critical to classification of tumor type, stratification of treatments, and prognosis. Low-grade gliomas are divided into three categories based on molecular genetic findings based on the presence of an isocitrate dehydrogenase (IDH) mutation or 1p/19q codeletion. The presence of both a 1p/19q codeletion and an IDH mutation indicates an oligodendroglioma. The presence of an IDH mutation (without a 1p/19q codeletion) with *TP53* and *ATRX* mutations indicates an astrocytoma. The other category of glioma lacks both an IDH mutation and a 1p/19q codeletion.
- A codeletion of 1p/19q bestows a favorable prognosis. Low-grade gliomas lacking an IDH mutation have a poorer prognosis, one comparable to glioblastoma.
- The presence of the following mutations can upgrade a histologically low-grade glioma to a high-grade glioma: *TERT* promoter mutation, *EGFR* mutation, gain of chromosome 7/loss of chromosome 10, CDKN2A/B homozygous loss.
- However, even tumors with benign histology can cause significant morbidity due to their location and effect on surrounding structures.

IMAGING STUDIES

- MRI with gadolinium enhancement is highly sensitive and permits visualization of the tumor with relation to the surrounding tissue. Specifically, enhancing tumor can be distinguished from surrounding edema. Low-grade tumors often present as an infiltrating lesion without mass effect. MRI is superior to CT scanning for evaluating the meninges, subarachnoid space, and posterior fossa, and for defining relation to major intracranial vessels, although CT scanning is useful if calcification or hemorrhage is suspected (Fig. E1). Fig. E2 shows the appearance of astrocytoma in imaging studies.
- Magnetic resonance spectroscopy can be used as a tool to help differentiate intracranial tumors from other intracranial processes using different chemical markers, usually in the setting of differentiating recurrence vs. radiation necrosis. For example, *N*-acetylaspartate is often decreased in brain tumors, whereas choline, a component of cell membranes, is often increased in brain tumors because of high cellular turnover.
- PET scan is helpful to distinguish neoplastic lesions (with high rate of metabolism) from other lesions such as demyelination or radiation necrosis (with a much lower metabolic rate). Such lesions take up greater amounts of glucose than surrounding tissues or tumors with slower metabolic rates. PET may be useful to help map functional areas of the brain before surgery or radiation.
- Functional MRI is now used as an adjunct in perioperative planning for patients whose lesion is in vital regions, such as those responsible for speech, language, and motor control.

Rx TREATMENT

NONPHARMACOLOGIC THERAPY

- Maximal surgical removal or debulking is the initial treatment of choice and provides tissue for diagnosis and molecular characterization. Maximal safe resection is often favored with a trend toward improved survival with this approach.
- Biopsy alone is performed if the tumor is located in eloquent regions of brain or is inaccessible; this is essential for histopathologic diagnosis. Biopsy can be performed under CT or MRI guidance using stereotactic localization.
- If the tumor is benign (e.g., meningioma, acoustic neuroma), often no further therapy is required.

ACUTE GENERAL Rx

Antiseizure medications have been used perioperatively and to control seizures resulting from focal lesions. Prophylactic use of anticonvulsants is not typically recommended without clear history of seizures.

CHRONIC Rx

- The decision to use chemotherapy and its timing (before, during, or after radiation therapy or surgery) is highly dependent on the age of the patient, grade of the tumor, and the amount of residual following surgery. In children, chemotherapy is often used to delay radiation therapy. In a recent trial in patients with grade 2 glioma who were younger than 40 yr of age and had undergone subtotal tumor resection or who were 40 yr of age or older, progression-free survival and overall survival were longer among those who received combination chemotherapy in addition to radiation therapy than among those who received radiation therapy alone.[1]
- Radiation is useful for certain types of tumors and is often used if there is residual tumor after surgery; conventional radiation uses external beams over a period of weeks, whereas stereotactic radiosurgery delivers a single, high dose of radiation to a well-defined area (usually <1 cm). Long-term effects of radiation therapy include radiation necrosis (particularly of white matter), blood vessel hyalinization, secondary tumors (usually meningiomas, sarcomas, and malignant astrocytomas), and cognitive changes. Radiosensitizers (most often an alkylating agent) may help increase the therapeutic effect of radiation therapy.
- Experimental therapies are continually in development and target molecular characteristics of tumors and signal transduction cascades involved in tumor growth. Some of these therapies involve antisense molecules, biologic agents, immunotherapies, or angiogenesis inhibitors. Intratumoral drug infusions and convection-enhanced delivery of novel agents are currently under study.

DISPOSITION

In general, younger age, high performance status, lower pathologic grade, the presence of an IDH mutation, and a 1p/19q codeletion have more favorable prognosis. For all histologic subtypes of brain tumors, pediatric and young adult patients have a better survival rate.

REFERRAL

- All cases warrant evaluation by a neurooncologist and neurosurgeon. Referral to a neurologist is indicated for management of seizures and headaches related to the tumor if there are no neurooncologists available.
- Patients should be evaluated for physical and occupational therapy.
- Children should undergo neuropsychologic evaluations and screening for learning disabilities.

PEARLS & CONSIDERATIONS

COMMENTS

Molecular genetic characterization is important for diagnosis, therapeutic approach, and prognosis, for which mutations in IDH and the presence of a 1p/19q codeletion represented some of the critical genetic determinations. In general, younger age, high performance status, and lower pathologic grade have more favorable prognosis. For all histologic subtypes of brain tumors, pediatric and young adult patients have a better survival.

PATIENT & FAMILY EDUCATION

American Brain Tumor Association (www.abta.org)
National Brain Tumor Society (www.braintumor.org)
Pediatric Low Grade Astrocytoma (PLGA) (https://akidsbraintumorcure.org)

SUGGESTED READINGS

Available at ExpertConsult.com

RELATED CONTENT

Brain Cancer (Patient Information)
Astrocytoma (Related Key Topic)
Meningioma (Related Key Topic)

AUTHORS: **Lily C. Pham, MD** and **Jaray H. Wang, MD, PhD**

[1] Buckner JC et al: Radiation plus procarbazine, CCNU, and vincristine in low-grade glioma, *N Engl J Med* 374:1344-1355, 2016.

BASIC INFORMATION

DEFINITION

- Glioblastoma (GBM) is the most aggressive primary brain tumor and is classified as WHO Grade IV in the World Health Organization's (WHO) classification system. GBM is diffusely infiltrative and has an astrocytic lineage. GBM is the most common brain and central nervous system (CNS) malignancy, accounting for 48.3% of malignant primary brain and CNS tumors, 54% of all gliomas, and 14.6% of all primary brain and CNS tumors.
- GBM represents a molecularly heterogeneous disease with numerous subclassifications. GBMs comprise primary and secondary subtypes that evolve through different genetic pathways, affect patients at different ages, and have differences in outcomes. Primary (*de novo*) GBMs account for 80% of GBMs and occur in older patients (mean age 65 yr). Secondary GBMs develop from lower-grade astrocytomas or oligodendrogliomas and occur in younger patients (mean age 45 yr).
- Overall prognosis for GBM is poor with median survival being 11 to 16 mo and 5-yr overall survival at 6.8%.

ICD-10CM CODE
C71.9 Malignant neoplasm of brain, unspecified

EPIDEMIOLOGY & DEMOGRAPHICS

INCIDENCE: Based on the 2019 Central Brain Tumor Registry of the United States (CBTRUS) report, the average annual age-adjusted incidence rate (IR) of GBM is 3.22/100,000 population.

PREDOMINANT SEX & AGE: GBM is primarily diagnosed at older ages, with the median age of diagnosis at 65 yr. It is uncommon in children, accounting for ~3% of all brain and CNS tumors reported among infants to 19-yr-olds. A higher incidence of GBM has been reported in men compared with women; the incidence rate is 1.58 times higher in males [3.97 vs. 2.53]. Whites have the highest incidence rates for GBM compared with any other race in the U.S.

RISK FACTORS: Many genetic and environmental factors have been studied in GBM, but no risk factor that accounts for a large proportion of GBM has been identified. Like many cancers, the causes are sporadic. Factors associated with GBM risk are prior therapeutic radiation, decreased susceptibility to allergy, immune factors and immune genes, and some single nucleotide polymorphisms (SNPs) detected by genome-wide association studies (GWAS). There is no substantial evidence of GBM association with lifestyle characteristics such as cigarette smoking, alcohol consumption, drugs, or dietary exposure to N-nitroso compounds (cured or smoked meat or fish). Inconsistent and nondefinitive results have been published regarding the risk of glioma with use of mobile phones.

PHYSICAL FINDINGS & CLINICAL PRESENTATION

Patients present with a variety of symptoms dependent of tumor location, including headache, seizures, symptoms of increased intracranial pressure, weakness, sensory deficits, and cognitive disturbances.

DIAGNOSIS

IMAGING STUDIES

Initial workup includes imaging studies. Brain MRI with and without contrast is the study of choice and demonstrates a contrast-enhancing tumor (Fig. 1). Functional MRI is now used as an adjunct modality in perioperative planning for patients whose lesion is in vital regions (eloquent regions), such as those responsible for speech, language, and motor control.

HISTOLOGY

- Pathologically, GBM is a high-grade astrocytoma characterized by hypercellularity, mitotic activity, nuclear atypia, pseudopalisading necrosis, and microvascular proliferation. Various molecular markers have been identified distinguishing GBM from other lower grade astrocytomas, as well as differentiating primary and secondary subtypes of GBM.
- Recent C-IMPACT-NOW criteria also include various molecular markers for GBM that can predict a more GBM-like prognosis for lower grade gliomas, necessitating treatment similar to histologic GBMs. These markers include: *TERT* promoter mutations, *EGFR* amplification, gain of chromosome 7/loss of chromosome 10, and *CDNK2A/B* homozygous loss.

TREATMENT

- GBM is an aggressive neoplasm with a median survival of 3 mo if untreated.
- Combined modality therapy with surgery, RT, and chemotherapy has significantly improved

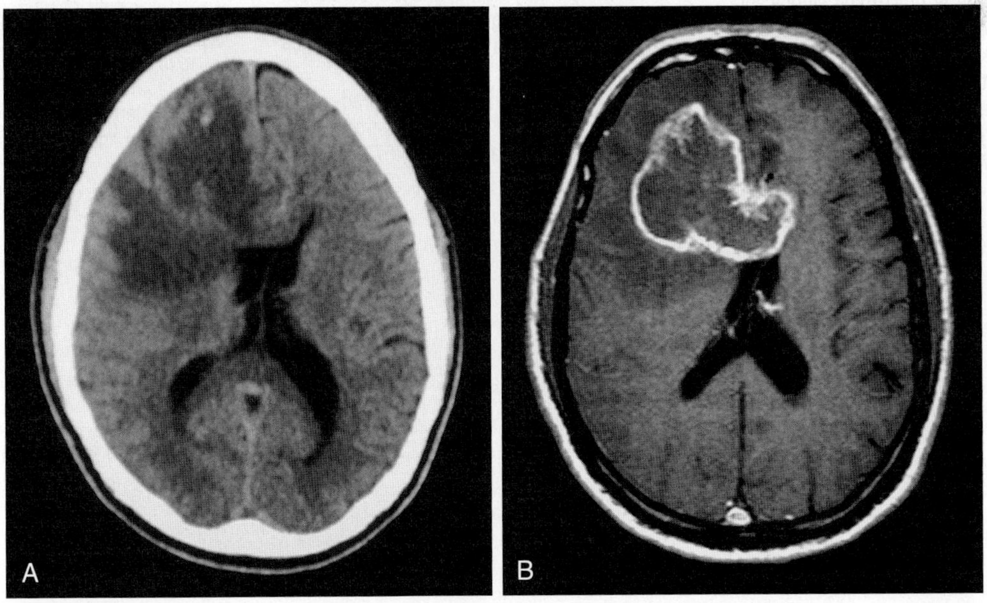

FIG. 1 Glioblastoma multiforme (astrocytoma World Health Organization grade IV/IV). A, On noncontrast computed tomography the mass cannot be clearly separated from the edema. **B,** A postgadolinium T1-weighted image shows an irregular rim of enhancement of this mass that crosses the midline via the corpus callosum. This 50-yr-old man presented with altered mental status. (From Soto JA, Lucey BC: *Emergency radiology: the requisites*, ed 2, Philadelphia, 2017, Elsevier.)

survival of GBM patients. Treatment is complex and initially consists of maximal-safe surgical resection followed by RT with concurrent temozolomide (TMZ) chemotherapy followed by six cycles of maintenance TMZ with tumor-treating fields.

- Surgical intervention has decompressive and cytoreductive effects, and there is increasing evidence of a significant survival advantage with complete resection.
- Various emerging treatment modalities under investigation seem promising, including immunotherapy. Regression of glioblastoma after chimeric antigen receptor T-cell therapy has been reported (see "Brown CE et al," in "Suggested Readings"). Intratumoral infusion of recombinant nonpathogenic polio-rhinovirus chimera (PVSRIPO) has improved survival rate in advanced stage glioblastoma (see "Desjardins et al" in "Suggested Readings").
- Symptomatic treatment includes corticosteroids to reduce cerebral edema, antiepileptic drugs for seizures, and painkillers for headache.

DISPOSITION

Survival: GBM has a poor prognosis with a low relative survival estimate; only a few patients reach long-term survival status of 2.5 yr, and 6.8% of patients survive 5 yr postdiagnosis. The relative survival for the first yr after diagnosis is 35%, falls in the second yr postdiagnosis to 13.7%, and continues to fall thereafter. Median survival of GBM postdiagnosis is 15 mo following standard therapy. Several variables affect the prognosis of GBM patients, including age, preoperative performance status, tumor location, preoperative imaging characteristics of the tumor, and the extent of resection.

Prognostic molecular markers in GBM: All GBMs are WHO grade IV but exhibit significant genetic heterogeneity. Tumor subtypes, based on genetic alterations, exist within this larger homogeneous histologic category and carry prognostic significance. These markers include methylation status of the gene promoter for O^6-methylguanine-DNA methyltransferase (MGMT), isocitrate dehydrogenase enzyme 1/2 *(IDH1/2)* mutation, epidermal growth factor receptor (EGFR) overexpression and amplification, tumor protein *(TP53)* mutation, *ATRX* mutation and genetic losses of chromosomes.

- Primary GBMs show EGFR amplification, phosphatase and tensin homolog gene (*PTEN*) mutations, and loss of heterozygosity (LOH) 10q, p16 deletions; less frequently shown are mouse double-minute 2 (MDM2) amplification, high frequency of telomerase reverse transcriptase (hTERT) promoter mutations, and absence of *IDH1* mutation.
- The hallmark of secondary GBMs is *TP53,* alpha thalassemia/mental retardation syndrome X-linked *(ATRX)* and *IDH1* mutations, and LOH 10q.
- The MGMT promoter is methylated in approximately 50% of newly diagnosed GBMs. MGMT methylation is more common in secondary than primary GBM (75% vs. 36%, respectively) and has prognostic and predictive significance of better overall survival in patients with GBM, irrespective of treatment choices.
- *IDH1/2* mutations are far more common in grades II and III astrocytomas and oligodendrogliomas compared with GBMs, and more than 90% of the mutations involve *IDH1. IDH1/2* mutations are a selective molecular marker of secondary GBMs, help distinguish them from primary GBMs, and are a marker of more favorable prognosis in high-grade gliomas.
- In GBMs, EGFR signaling promotes cell division, tumor invasiveness, and resistance to radiation therapy (RT) and chemotherapy. About 40% of all GBMs have EGFR amplification, and it is more common in primary as compared with secondary GBMs.
- Mutation of the *TP53* gene has been found in 60% to 70% of secondary GBMs and 25% to 30% of primary GBMs, and it occurs more frequently in younger patients. Studies of *TP53* mutations as a prognostic marker have not been definitive.
- *ATRX* is frequently mutated in grade II to III astrocytomas (71%), oligoastrocytomas (68%), and secondary GBMs (57%), but is infrequent in primary (4%) and pediatric GBMs (20%) as well as pure oligodendroglial tumors (14%). In a prospective cohort of patients with astrocytic tumors, those harboring *ATRX* loss had a significantly better prognosis than the ones that expressed *ATRX* and had IDH mutation.
- *TERT* mutation is one of the most frequent genetic alterations in primary adult GBMs and is significantly higher in these tumors as compared with secondary adult or any pediatric GBMs. GBMs with *TERT* mutation have a shorter survival than those without *TERT* mutations. However, when adjusted for GBM subtype (primary and secondary), they do not have a significant impact on survival.

REFERRAL

Treatment involves a multidisciplinary team approach including oncology, neurosurgery, neurology, and radiation oncology.

PEARLS & CONSIDERATIONS

COMMENTS

- Glioblastoma is an aggressive, infiltrative, primary brain cancer with a generally poor prognosis. The median survival is 15 mo with therapy.
- The mainstay of treatment for glioblastoma includes maximum surgical resection, radiation, and chemotherapy. Extent of resection is a prognostic factor in overall survival.
- To date, there are only two FDA-approved medications for the treatment of glioblastoma: Temozolomide and bevacizumab. Newer targeted therapies based on molecular mutations are under investigation in clinical trials.

SUGGESTED READING

Available at ExpertConsult.com

AUTHORS: **Lily C. Pham, MD,** and **Jaray H. Wang, MD, PhD**

BASIC INFORMATION

DEFINITION

Breast abscess is an acute inflammatory process resulting in the formation of a collection of purulent material (pus) in breast tissue. Characterized by a painful, erythematous mass formation in the breast, occasionally draining through the overlying skin or nipple duct.

SYNONYMS

Subareolar abscess
Lactational or puerperal abscess

ICD-10CM CODES

091.111	Abscess of breast associated with pregnancy, first trimester
091.112	Abscess of breast associated with pregnancy, second trimester
091.113	Abscess of breast associated with pregnancy, third trimester
091.119	Abscess of breast associated with pregnancy, unspecified trimester
091.12	Abscess of breast associated with the puerperium
091.13	Abscess of breast associated with lactation

EPIDEMIOLOGY & DEMOGRAPHICS

INCIDENCE: 10% to 30% of all breast abscesses are lactational; acute mastitis occurs in up to 10% of nursing mothers, with one in 15 of these women developing abscess. A recent Cochrane review, however, found that as many as 30% of nursing mothers may have evidence of mastitis. Smoking, obesity, and diabetes may be risk factors for nonpuerperal mastitis with abscess. More recently, nipple piercing may also be associated with infection. Puerperal mastitis is more common in the initial breastfeeding months.

PHYSICAL FINDINGS & CLINICAL PRESENTATION

- Painful, erythematous induration involving breast and leading to fluctuant, possibly palpable abscess
- Systemic symptoms: Fever and malaise
- Note that mastitis and abscess can occur either sequentially or concurrently

ETIOLOGY

- Lactational abscess: Milk stasis (from blockage, fewer feedings, excess supply, weaning, etc.) and bacterial infection leading to mastitis and then abscess, with *Staphylococcus aureus* (commonly MRSA) the most common causative agent. Group A and Group B *Streptococci* also commonly encountered
- Subareolar abscess:
  1. Central ducts involved, with obstructive nipple duct changes leading to bacterial infection
  2. Cultured organisms mixed, including anaerobes, staphylococci, streptococci, and others

DIAGNOSIS

DIFFERENTIAL DIAGNOSIS

- Galactocele
- Inflammatory carcinoma
- Advanced carcinoma with erythema, edema, and/or ulceration
- Tuberculous abscess (rare in the U.S.)
- Hidradenitis of breast skin
- Sebaceous cyst with infection
- Plugged milk duct

WORKUP

- Clinical examination. Fig. E1 illustrates the various areas where breast abscesses can develop
- Ultrasound to identify fluid collection, which can be used to guide treatment options such as facilitating aspiration
- If abscess suspected, referral to surgeon for incision, drainage, and biopsy

LABORATORY TESTS

- Perform culture and sensitivity test of abscess contents.
- If mammogram or ultrasound is required but prevented by discomfort, perform after treatment and subsequent resolution of abscess.

TREATMENT

NONPHARMACOLOGIC THERAPY

- Established abscess: Incision and drainage vs. needle aspiration (latter usually with ultrasound guidance; typically requires multiple procedures for resolution)
  1. High likelihood of patients treated with aspiration subsequently requiring I&D
- Biopsy of abscess cavity wall to exclude carcinoma

ACUTE GENERAL Rx

- Antibiotics: Generally targeting staphylococci (*S. aureus)* for lactational abscess. Recommended initial antibiotic therapy is nafcillin or oxacillin 2 g q4h IV or cefazolin 1 g q8h IV for 10 to 14 days. Alternative includes vancomycin 1 g IV q12h.
- Outpatient management with dicloxacillin 500 mg q6h PO or cephalexin 500 mg q6h PO is reasonable for uncomplicated cases without suspicion for MRSA.
- If acute mastitis is identified and treated early without the development of an abscess, resolution without drainage is possible.
- Subareolar abscess: Broad-spectrum antibiotic treatment (e.g., cephalexin 500 mg PO qid or cefazolin 1 g q8h IV for 10 to 14 days for more severe infection) and drainage (Fig. E1) are needed to control acute phase. If abscess is odoriferous, consider anaerobes as most likely etiology and add metronidazole 500 mg PO/IV tid. Augmentin and clindamycin are reasonable alternatives in this situation.

CHRONIC Rx

Further surgical treatment for recurrences or fistula

DISPOSITION

- Lactational abscess: Possible to continue breastfeeding without risk of infection to the infant
- Subareolar abscess:
  1. High risk for recurrence or complication of fistula formation
  2. I&D often associated with poor cosmetic outcome
  3. Patient informed and referred to General Surgery for evaluation and treatment

REFERRAL

- If abscess drainage required
- If subareolar abscess involved, refer to surgery

RELATED CONTENT

Breast Abscess (Patient Information)
Breast Cancer (Related Key Topic)
Mastodynia (Related Key Topic)

AUTHORS: **Anthony Sciscione, DO** and **Scott J. Merrill, MD**

BASIC INFORMATION

DEFINITION

Breast cancer refers to both in situ and invasive carcinoma of the breast. It can be of either ductal or lobular types.

SYNONYM

Carcinoma of the breast

ICD-10CM CODES

C50.911	Malignant neoplasm of unspecified site of right female breast
C50.912	Malignant neoplasm of unspecified site of left female breast
C50.919	Malignant neoplasm of unspecified site of unspecified female breast
C50.921	Malignant neoplasm of unspecified site of right male breast
C50.922	Malignant neoplasm of unspecified site of left male breast
C50.929	Malignant neoplasm of unspecified site of unspecified male breast

EPIDEMIOLOGY & DEMOGRAPHICS

- In the U.S., there was an estimated 279,100 new patients and an estimated 42,690 deaths in 2020.
- The most common form of breast cancer is hormone-receptor positive; its incidence has increased particularly among young women. Only 1% of breast cancers occur in males.
- Table 1 enumerates risk factors for breast cancer.
- Genetically defined group of women with *BRCA1* or *BRCA2* genes identified to carry lifetime risk as high as 85%.
- Breast cancers that are positive for estrogen receptor (ER) and negative for human epidermal growth factor receptor 2 *(HER2)* are the most common of breast cancers, accounting for 65% of cases of breast cancer among women less than 50 yr of age and 75% of cases among older women.[1]

PHYSICAL FINDINGS & CLINICAL PRESENTATION

- Increasing number of small breast cancers are found by mammograms, in which case patients are usually completely free of symptoms or physical findings.
- Palpable lump or mass which can be self- or physician-detected.
- Skin and/or nipple retraction and skin edema, erythema, ulcer, satellite nodule.
- Nodal enlargement in axilla and supraclavicular areas.
- Nipple discharge may be serous or bloody.
- Generalized symptoms and signs, including fatigue, weight loss, jaundice, and anorexia, may be present in metastatic cases.

[1]Burstein HJ: Systemic therapy for estrogen receptor-positive, *HER2*-negative breast cancer, *N Engl J Med* 383: 2557-2570, 2020.

ETIOLOGY

- The precise mechanism of carcinogenesis is not understood. Endogenous and exogenous estrogen exposure is key to the development of receptor-positive breast cancer
- Breast cancer is no longer perceived as a single disease. Molecular classification based on gene expression profiling has shown breast cancer to be of the following types:
  1. Luminal A type: Endocrine responsive with favorable prognosis
  2. Luminal B type: Endocrine responsive with less favorable prognosis
  3. Normal type: Resemble normal epithelium and prognosis similar to luminal B type
  4. *HER2* amplified type: *HER2* gene amplification. *HER2* is overexpressed in about 15% to 20% of breast cancers
  5. Basal type: Hormone receptor and *HER2* negative cancers with poor prognosis
- Approximately 10% of all women with breast cancer have a germline mutation of *BRCA1, BRCA2, P53*, or other mutations
- Possibly interaction of ovarian estrogen, nonovarian estrogen, estrogens of exogenous origin with breast tissue of varied carcinogenic susceptibility to develop cancer
- Other known or suspected variables: Childbearing, breastfeeding practice, diet, physical activity, body mass, alcohol intake

TABLE 1 Risk Factors for Breast Cancer

Risk Factor	Relative Risk
Any benign breast disease	1.5
Postmenopausal hormone replacement	1.5
Menarche at <12 yr	1.1-1.9
Moderate alcohol intake (2-3 drinks/day)	1.1-1.9
Menopause at >55 yr	1.1-1.9
Increased bone density	1.1-1.9
Sedentary lifestyle and lack of exercise	1.1-1.9
Proliferative breast disease without atypia	2
Age at first birth >30 yr or nulliparous	2-4
First-degree relative with breast cancer	2-4
Postmenopausal obesity	2-4
Upper socioeconomic class	2-4
Personal history of endometrial or ovarian cancer	2-4
Significant radiation to chest	2-4
Increased breast density on mammogram	2-4
Older age	>4
Personal history of breast cancer (in situ or invasive)	>4
Proliferative breast disease with atypia	>4
Two first-degree relatives with breast cancer	5
Atypical hyperplasia and first-degree relative with breast cancer	10

From Goldman L, Schafer AI: *Goldman's Cecil medicine*, ed 24, Philadelphia, 2012, Saunders.

DIAGNOSIS

DIFFERENTIAL DIAGNOSIS

Benign disease is summarized in Table 2. The following nonmalignant breast lesions can simulate breast cancer on both physical and mammogram examinations:

- Fibrocystic changes
- Fibroadenoma
- Hamartoma

WORKUP

- Initial workup:
  1. Mass assessment by medical professional.
  2. Diagnostic mammogram followed by breast ultrasound for suspicious lesions.
  3. MRI (Fig. 1) may detect suspicious lesions better than mammography alone in women with dense breasts or inherited predisposition to breast cancer.
  4. Table 3 summarizes guidelines for evaluation and treatment of nonpalpable ductal carcinoma in situ.
- Diagnosis:
  1. Positive aspiration cytology on a clinically and mammographically suspicious mass is highly accurate, but it requires open biopsy confirmation.
  2. Stereotactic, ultrasound-guided core-needle biopsy procedures are accurate and have low complication rates. Indications for stereotactic core biopsy are summarized in

TABLE 2 American Board of Pathology Histologic Classification of Benign Disease

Histopathologic Findings	Approximate Relative Risk
Nonproliferative	No added risk
Cysts	
Duct ectasia	
Calcification	
Fibroadenoma	
Milk ductal epithelial hyperplasia	
Sclerosing adenosis	No added risk
Papillomatosis	Slight added risk
Radial scars	
Complex sclerosing lesions	?
Moderate florid hyperplasia	1.5:1-2:1
Atypical hyperplasia (ductal and lobular)	4:1
Extensive ductal involvement of atypical hyperplasia	7:1
Lobular carcinoma in situ	10:1
Ductal carcinoma in situ	10:1

From Niederhuber JE: *Abeloff's clinical oncology*, ed 6, Philadelphia, 2020, Elsevier.

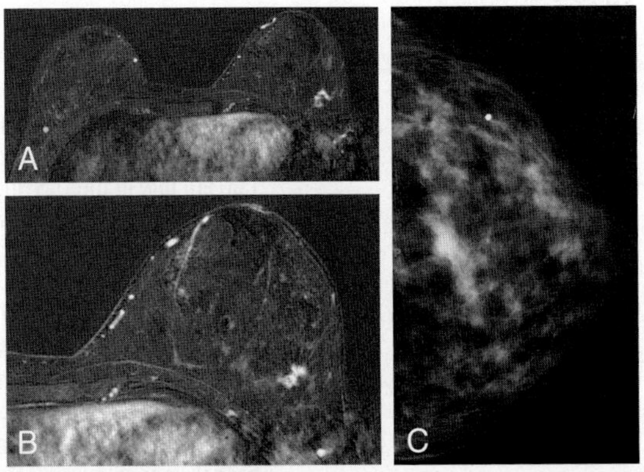

FIG. 1 A 42-yr-old woman with *BRCA2* mutation. Magnetic resonance imaging (MRI) screening showed a 1.2-cm invasive ductal cancer in the lower outer left breast seen only on MRI **(A** and **B)** and subsequently on second-look ultrasound. **C,** The mammogram showed only dense breast tissue. (From Cameron JL, Cameron AM: *Current surgical therapy*, ed 12, Philadelphia, 2017, Elsevier.)

TABLE 3 Guidelines for Evaluation and Treatment of Nonpalpable Ductal Carcinoma In Situ

1. Careful multiview mammography with or without ultrasound and including magnification views
   - Document extent of disease
   - Identify other areas of microcalcification
1. Suspicious microcalcifications and densities cleared with needle localization biopsy
2. Specimen radiography with magnification techniques
3. Radiograph-directed histopathologic evaluation with orientation of specimen by surgeon using multicolored inked margins
4. Complete pathologic description to include:
   - Type of DCIS and size of tumor
   - Relation to microcalcifications
   - Distance of lesion from inked margins
   - Presence of multifocality
   - Presence or risk of microinvasion
1. Repeat mammography with magnification to confirm successful clearing of suspicious areas
2. Repeat breast excision if:
   - Residual microcalcifications are found
   - Margins are unacceptable

DCIS, Ductal carcinoma in situ.
From Niederhuber JE: *Abeloff's clinical oncology*, ed 6, Philadelphia, 2020, Elsevier.

BOX 1 Indications for Stereotactic Core Biopsy

- Certain probably benign lesions, BI-RADS 3, depending on clinical suspicion, patient or physician preference, or when short-term follow-up is not practical
- Lesions suspicious, BI-RADS 4
- Lesions highly suspicious, BI-RADS 5
- New suspicious microcalcifications, developing asymmetries, or architectural distortions
- Nonpalpable asymmetry, focal asymmetry, or solid mass on mammogram not seen on ultrasound
- Mammographic lesions corresponding to suspicious areas of enhancement on MRI

BI-RADS, Breast Imaging-Reporting and Data System; *MRI*, magnetic resonance imaging.
From Cameron JL, Cameron AM: *Current surgical therapy*, ed 12, Philadelphia, 2017, Elsevier.

BOX 2 Contraindications to Stereotactic Core Biopsy

- Patient unable to lie prone or cooperate
- Patient's weight
- Lesion location near nipple, too superficial to skin, or too posterior to chest wall
- Lesion mammographically occult
- Patient has severe kyphosis or movement disorders
- Lack of breast tissue thickness for adequate compression

From Cameron JL, Cameron AM: *Current surgical therapy*, ed 12, Philadelphia, 2017, Elsevier.

Box 1. Box 2 describes contraindications to stereotactic core biopsy.
3. Excisional surgical biopsy establishes diagnosis.
- Breast radiologic evaluation and an algorithm for breast cancer screening and evaluation are described in Section III. The differential diagnosis of breast lumps is described in Section II.

STAGING

Table 4 describes the pathologic staging of breast cancer.

IMAGING STUDIES

Mammograms (Fig. E2, Fig. E3): 30% to 50% of breast cancers are detected by screening mammograms as a spiculated mass, a mass with or without microcalcifications, or a cluster of microcalcifications. MRI is particularly useful in patients with breast implants and when there is a strong family history of breast cancer. MRI is better for assessing response to neoadjuvant chemotherapy and for identifying the primary tumor in patients presenting with axillary adenopathy.

Rx TREATMENT

NONPHARMACOLOGIC THERAPY

- These approaches include various types of surgical resection and reconstruction as well as adjuvant radiotherapy.
- For early breast cancer, the primary therapy is typically surgical. The choice is between modified radical mastectomy and breast-conserving treatment, which consists of lumpectomy, axillary staging with sentinel node biopsy, or axillary dissection.
- Table 5 compares ductal versus lobular carcinoma in situ. Adjuvant treatment guidelines for patients with early-stage invasive breast cancer are described in Table 6.
- Among patients with limited sentinel lymph nodes (SLN) who are treated with breast conservation and systemic therapy, sentinel lymph node dissection (SLND) alone compared with axillary lymph node dissection (ALND) did not result in inferior survival.
- DCIS: Local breast-conserving therapy (lumpectomy plus radiation therapy) or mastectomy followed by endocrine therapy in estrogen receptor-positive cases.
- Invasive breast cancer: Mastectomy or lumpectomy, along with sentinel lymph node evaluation followed by radiation therapy for large tumors.
- Invasive breast cancer may require adjuvant endocrine therapy and chemotherapy. Endocrine therapy is recommended alone or after chemotherapy in patients with hormone-receptor positive tumors. Breast cancer intrinsic subtypes are summarized in Table 7. Treatment according to breast cancer subtypes is described in Table 8. Adjuvant hormone therapy with antiestrogen drugs reduces disease recurrence and mortality in women with breast cancer. Aromatase inhibitors (anastrozole, letrozole, exemestane, fulvestrant) decrease the

TABLE 4 Pathological Staging of Breast Cancer

T_X	Primary tumor cannot be assessed
T_0	No evidence of primary tumor
T_{is}	Carcinoma in situ
T_{is} (DCIS)	Ductal carcinoma in situ
T_{is} (LCIS)	Lobular carcinoma in situ
T_{is} (Paget)	Paget disease of the nipple NOT associated with invasive carcinoma and/or carcinoma in situ (DCIS and/or LCIS) in the underlying breast parenchyma. Carcinomas in the breast parenchyma associated with Paget disease are categorized based on the size and characteristics of the parenchymal disease, although the presence of Paget disease should still be noted
T_1	Tumor ≤20 mm in greatest dimension
T_{1mi}	Tumor ≤1 mm in greatest dimension
T_{1a}	Tumor >1 mm but ≤5 mm in greatest dimension
T_{1b}	Tumor >5 mm but ≤10 mm in greatest dimension
T_{1c}	Tumor >10 mm but ≤20 mm in greatest dimension
T_2	Tumor >20 mm but ≤50 mm in greatest dimension
T_3	Tumor >50 mm in greatest dimension
T_4	Tumor of any size with direct extension to the chest wall and/or to the skin (ulceration or skin nodules)
T_{4a}	Extension to chest wall, not including only pectoralis muscle adherence/invasion
T_{4b}	Ulceration and/or ipsilateral satellite nodules and/or edema (including peau d'orange) of the skin, which do not meet the criteria for inflammatory carcinoma
T_{4c}	Both T_{4a} and T_{4b}
T_{4d}	Inflammatory carcinoma
N_X	Regional lymph nodes cannot be assessed (e.g., previously removed)
N_0	No regional lymph node metastasis
N_1	Metastasis to movable ipsilateral level I, II axillary lymph node(s)
N_2	Metastases in ipsilateral level I, II axillary lymph nodes that are clinically fixed or matted or in clinically detected ipsilateral internal mammary nodes in the *absence* of clinically evident axillary lymph node metastasis
N_{2a}	Metastases in ipsilateral level I, II axillary lymph nodes fixed to one another (matted) or to other structures
N_{2b}	Metastases only in clinically detected ipsilateral internal mammary nodes and in the *absence* of clinically evident level I, II axillary lymph node metastases
N_3	Metastases in ipsilateral infraclavicular (level III axillary) lymph node(s), with or without level I, II axillary node involvement, or in clinically detected ipsilateral internal mammary lymph node(s) and in the *presence* of clinically evident level I, II axillary lymph node metastasis; or metastasis in ipsilateral supraclavicular lymph node(s), with or without axillary or internal mammary lymph node involvement
N_{3a}	Metastasis in ipsilateral infraclavicular lymph node(s)
N_{3b}	Metastasis in ipsilateral internal mammary lymph node(s) and axillary lymph node(s)
N_{3c}	Metastasis in ipsilateral supraclavicular lymph node(s)
M_0	No clinical or radiographic evidence of distant metastasis
$cM_{0(i+)}$	No clinical or radiographic evidence of distant metastases, but deposits of molecularly or microscopically detected tumor cells in circulating blood, bone marrow, or other nonregional nodal tissue that are no larger than 0.2 mm in a patient without symptoms or signs of metastases
M_1	Distant detectable metastases as determined by classic clinical and radiographic means and/or histologically proven >0.2 mm
G_X	Grade cannot be assessed
G_1	Low combined histologic grade (favorable)
G_2	Intermediate combined histologic grade (moderately favorable)
G_3	High combined histologic grade (unfavorable)

Stage Groupings in Breast Cancer

Stage	T	N	M
0	T_{is}	N_0	M_0
I_A	T_1	N_0	M_0
I_B	T_0-T_1	N_{1mi}	M_0
II_A	T_0-T_1	N_1	M_0
	T_2	N_0	M_0
II_B	T_2	N_1	M_0
	T_3	N_0	M_0
III_A	T_0-T_2	N_2	M_0
	T_3	N_1-N_2	M_0
III_B	T_4	N_0-N_2	M_0
III_C	Any T	N_3	M_0
IV	Any T	Any N	M_1

From Goldman L, Schafer AI: *Goldman's Cecil medicine*, ed 24, Philadelphia, 2012, Saunders; AJCC 8th ed., 2018.

agonist effect of estrogen by inhibiting estrogen synthesis and have become preferred first-line hormonal treatment agents over the selective estrogen receptor modulator tamoxifen.

- Standard *adjuvant chemotherapy* regimens in current use in the U.S. include AC (cyclophosphamide plus doxorubicin), AC-T (doxorubicin and cyclophosphamide followed by a taxane), and TC (docetaxel and cyclophosphamide). In patients with *HER2* expressing breast cancers, standard adjuvant regimens also include the addition of trastuzumab and pertuzumab for 1-yr duration. Fig. E4 illustrates considerations for adjuvant chemotherapy in breast cancer.
- *Neoadjuvant chemotherapy* (same regimens as used in the adjuvant setting) results in pathologic complete responses in significant number of cases, causes downstaging, provides an assessment of chemosensitivity, and provides no deleterious effect on survival.
- The benefit of adjuvant chemotherapy or hormone therapy can be assessed by commercially available *multigene assays* (OncotypeDx, Mammaprint) that have demonstrated utility in determining prognostic and predictive benefit with both hormonal therapy and chemotherapy in breast cancer. Results from the prospective TAILORx trial support the routine use of multigene assays so as to identify intermediate-risk score patients in which chemotherapy can be safely omitted.
- *Metastatic breast cancer* is approached based on the extent of bone-only or visceral disease sites as well as the rate of symptomatic progression.
  1. Typically, bone-only metastatic disease is approached with upfront, sequential hormonal therapy. The combination of mTOR inhibitors (everolimus) or CDK4/CDK6 inhibitors (palbociclib, ribociclib, abemaciclib) with aromatase inhibitors has been associated with improved overall survival.
  2. Among patients with *PIK3CA*-mutated, hormone-receptor-positive, *HER2*-negative advanced breast cancer who had received endocrine therapy previously, treatment with the combination of alpelisib plus fulvestrant prolonged progression-free survival, leading to the approval of this combination approach. Commonly used cytotoxic chemotherapy and anti-*HER2* therapy drugs in metastatic breast cancer are summarized in Table 9.
- Patients with progressive bone disease or those with visceral disease are treated with typically single-agent chemotherapy and occasionally with combination chemotherapy regimens. The chemotherapy agents are the same as those used in early stages of disease. Sequential chemotherapy with different classes of chemotherapy agents are usually used to provide palliation with improvement in survival and symptoms.
- Patients whose tumors have germline *BRCA1/2* mutations can be treated with the PARP inhibitors olaparib or talazoparib.
- Patients with triple-negative breast cancer whose tumors express the program death ligand-1 receptor derive a survival benefit with the use of the combination of albumin-bound paclitaxel and the immune inhibitor atezolizumab.

TABLE 5 Carcinoma In Situ: Lobular Versus Ductal

Feature	Lobular Carcinoma In Situ	Ductal Carcinoma In Situ
Age	Younger	Older
Palpable mass	No	Uncommon
Mammographic appearance	Not detected on mammography	Microcalcifications, mass
Immunophenotype	E-cadherin negative	E-cadherin positive
Usual manifestation	Incidental finding on breast biopsy	Microcalcifications on mammography or breast mass
Bilateral involvement	Common	Uncertain
Risk and site of subsequent breast cancer	25% risk for invasive breast cancer in either breast over remaining lifespan	At site of initial lesion; 0.5% risk/yr of invasive breast cancer in opposite breast
Prevention	Consider tamoxifen or raloxifene	Consider tamoxifen or raloxifene if estrogen-receptor positive
Treatment	Yearly mammography and breast examination	Lumpectomy ± radiation; mastectomy for large or multifocal lesions

From Goldman L, Schafer AI: *Goldman's Cecil medicine*, ed 24, Philadelphia, 2012, Saunders.

TABLE 6 Adjuvant Treatment Guidelines for Patients with Early-Stage Invasive Breast Cancer

Patient Group	Treatment
Hormone Receptor-Positive and *HER2* Positive Breast Cancer	
<0.5 cm	Consider adjuvant endocrine therapy
0.6-1 cm	Adjuvant endocrine therapy Consider adjuvant chemotherapy and trastuzumab
>1 cm	Adjuvant endocrine therapy Adjuvant chemotherapy and trastuzumab
Node positive	Adjuvant endocrine therapy Adjuvant chemotherapy with pertuzumab and trastuzumab
Hormone Receptor-Positive and *HER2* Negative Breast Cancer	
<0.5 cm	No adjuvant therapy
>0.5 cm	Adjuvant hormonal therapy Consider adjuvant chemotherapy based on 21-gene recurrence score
Node-positive	Adjuvant hormonal therapy + adjuvant chemotherapy
Hormone Receptor-Negative and *HER2* Positive Breast Cancer	
<0.5 cm	Consider adjuvant chemotherapy and trastuzumab
0.6-1 cm	Consider adjuvant chemotherapy and trastuzumab
>1 cm	Adjuvant chemotherapy and trastuzumab
Node positive	Adjuvant endocrine therapy Adjuvant chemotherapy with pertuzumab and trastuzumab
Hormone Receptor-Negative and *HER2* Negative Breast Cancer	
≤0.5 cm	No adjuvant therapy
0.6-1.0 cm	Consider adjuvant chemotherapy
>1 cm or node positive	Adjuvant chemotherapy

HER2, human epidermal growth factor receptor 2.
Modified from National Comprehensive Cancer Network Guidelines. Available at www.nccn.org.

- In patients with metastatic *HER2*/neu-positive breast cancer, the addition of the monoclonal antibody pertuzumab to the standard regimen of trastuzumab and docetaxel significantly improves the median overall survival. Also, the antibody-drug conjugates TDM-1 and trastuzumab dexrutecan improve survival in this group of patients. In addition, oral *HER2*-directed inhibitors such as neratinib and tucatinib are active in previously treated patients with metastatic disease.

CHRONIC Rx

Follow-up after treatment of early breast cancer stages includes:

- Regular clinical evaluations as delineated by medical oncologist or surgeon.
- Annual mammograms and breast MRI as indicated.
- Laboratory tests as indicated.
- Tumor markers and CT scans for surveillance are not recommended.
- Patient instruction in monthly breast self-examination.
- Systemic adjuvant therapy: Improves prognosis significantly. Women who take tamoxifen for 10 yr lower their recurrence risk by 25% and their dying of breast cancer risk by 27% compared with those who took it for just 5 yr. Adjuvant therapy with an aromatase inhibitor improves survival outcomes, compared with tamoxifen, in postmenopausal women with hormone receptor–positive breast cancer. Recent trials have shown that in premenopausal women with hormone receptor–positive early breast cancer, adjuvant treatment with the aromatase inhibitor exemestane plus ovarian suppression, compared with tamoxifen plus ovarian suppression, significantly reduced recurrence.
- Isolated tumor cells or micrometastases in regional lymph nodes are associated with a reduced 5-yr rate of disease-free survival among women with favorable early-stage breast cancer who do not receive adjuvant therapy. Survival is improved in patients with isolated tumor cells or micrometastases who received adjuvant therapy.
- Retrospective analyses suggest that occult lymph-node metastases are an important prognostic factor for disease recurrence or survival among patients with breast cancer; however, recent trials indicate that the magnitude of the difference in outcome at 5 yr is small (1.2 percentage points). These data do not favor a clinical benefit of additional evaluation (including immunohistochemical analysis) of initially negative sentinel nodes in patients with breast cancer.
- The addition of zoledronic acid to adjuvant endocrine therapy improves disease-free survival in premenopausal patients with estrogen-responsive early breast cancer.

REFERRAL

Referral to a multidisciplinary team consisting of a breast surgeon, reconstructive surgeon, medical oncologist, and radiation oncologist is necessary as soon as breast cancer is suspected.

PEARLS & CONSIDERATIONS

BREAST CANCER IN PREGNANCY AND LACTATION

- Frequency in women 40 yr or younger reported to be 15%
- May carry worse prognosis because disease discovery delayed by engorged and nodular breast changes and/or because disease progression more rapid in pregnancy
- Survival rates similar to those for nonpregnant early-stage patients in same age group
- Expedient workup recommended, including mammography and sonography
- Choice of mastectomy or lumpectomy with axillary dissection for treatment
- Adjuvant chemotherapy delayed until third trimester or after delivery
- Irradiation to breast after lumpectomy delayed until after delivery

DUCTAL CARCINOMA IN SITU (DCIS, INTRADUCTAL CARCINOMA) (SEE TABLE 5)

- Discovered by mammogram as cluster of microcalcifications and/or density
- Presents less often as a palpable mass or nipple discharge

TABLE 7 Breast Cancer Intrinsic Subtypes

Subtype	Characteristics	Markers
Luminal A	Low grade. High ER ~40% of all breast cancer Good prognosis	ER+, PR+, *HER2*– Low Ki-67 (<14%)
Luminal B	Higher grade. Lower ER ~20% of all breast cancer Poorer prognosis than luminal A	ER+, PR+/–, *HER2*+/– High Ki-67 (>14%)
HER2-enriched	High grade. Often node positive *P53* mutations ~10%-15% of all breast cancer	ER–, PR–, *HER2*+
Basal-like	High proliferation. *BRCA* dysfunction ~15%-20% of all breast cancer Poor prognosis	ER–, PR–, *HER2*– CK5/6 Or EGFR+

CK, Cytokeratin; *EGFR*, epidermal growth factor receptor; *ER*, estrogen receptor; *HER2*, human epidermal growth factor receptor 2; *PR*, progesterone receptor.
From Cameron JL, Cameron AM: *Current surgical therapy*, ed 12, Philadelphia, 2017, Elsevier.

TABLE 8 Treatment According to Breast Cancer Subtype

Subtype	Treatment Response and Prognosis
Luminal A	Respond to endocrine therapy • Premenopausal: SERMs (tamoxifen) • Postmenopausal: AIs (exemestane, anastrozole, letrozole)
Luminal B	Response to endocrine therapy lower. Response to chemotherapy greater than luminal A
HER2-enriched	Respond to anti-*HER2* agents (trastuzumab, pertuzumab, lapatinib)
Basal-like	No response to endocrine therapy or anti-*HER2* agents. Chemotherapy only treatment outside of a clinical trial

AIs, Aromatase inhibitors; *HER2*, human epidermal growth factor receptor 2; *SERMs*, selective estrogen receptor modulators.
From Cameron JL, Cameron AM: *Current surgical therapy*, ed 12, Philadelphia, 2017, Elsevier.

TABLE 9 Commonly Used Cytotoxic Chemotherapy and Anti-*HER2* Therapy Drugs in Metastatic Breast Cancer

Cytotoxic Chemotherapy
Albumin-bound paclitaxel
Capecitabine
Cisplatin
Carboplatin
Docetaxel
Doxorubicin
Epirubicin
Eribulin
Gemcitabine
Ixabepilone
Vinorelbine
Anti-*HER2* Therapy
Ado-trastuzumab emtansine
Lapatinib
Pertuzumab
Trastuzumab

HER2, Human epidermal growth factor receptor 2.
From Niederhuber JE: *Abeloff's clinical oncology*, ed 6, Philadelphia, 2020, Elsevier.

- Before mammogram screening, DCIS accounted for 1% of all breast cancers
- Now 15% to 20% or even higher proportion have DCIS
- Treated with lumpectomy with cure rates 98% to 99%
- Higher-risk cases require breast radiation and adjuvant hormone therapy
- Mastectomy possibly required with multifocal and/or high-grade DCIS

INFLAMMATORY CARCINOMA

- Rare, rapidly progressive and often lethal form of breast cancer
- Presents as erythematous and edematous breast resembling mastitis
- Biopsy required, including that of the skin
- Treatment with upfront combination chemotherapy followed by surgery and radiotherapy
- Prognosis once dismal; now 5-yr disease-free survival approaches 50% (Fig. E5)

COMMENTS

- The U.S. Preventive Services Task Force (USPSTF) now recommends against automatic "routine" screening of younger women (age range 40 to 49). The task force recommends biennial screening mammography for all middle-aged women (age range 50 to 74). It also states that current evidence is insufficient to assess the benefits and harms of screening mammography in older women (aged 75 and older). The task force also discourages women from performing breast self-examination. Several other U.S. organizations, such as the American Congress of Obstetricians and Gynecologists, however, still recommend annual screening beginning at age 40 yr. Breast cancer screening recommendations by organization are summarized in Table 10.
- The American Cancer Society guidelines for breast cancer screening are summarized in the following:
  1. Women with an *average risk* of breast cancer should undergo regular screening mammography as below:
     a. Women should have the opportunity to begin annual screening between the ages of 40 and 44 yr. (Qualified recommendation)
     b. Women aged 45 to 54 yr should be screened annually. (Qualified recommendation)
     c. Women 55 yr and older should transition to biennial screening or have the opportunity to continue screening annually. (Qualified recommendation)
  2. Women should continue screening mammography as long as their overall health is good and they have a life expectancy of 10 yr or longer. (Qualified recommendation)
  3. Women who are at *high risk* for breast cancer based on certain factors should get an MRI and a mammogram every yr, typically starting at age 30 yr. This includes women who:
     a. Have a lifetime risk of breast cancer of about 20% to 25% or greater, according to risk assessment tools that are based mainly on family history.
     b. Have a known *BRCA1* or *BRCA2* gene mutation (based on genetic testing).
     c. Have a first-degree relative (parent, brother, sister, or child) with a *BRCA1* or *BRCA2* gene mutation and have not had genetic testing themselves.
     d. Had radiation therapy to the chest between the ages of 10 and 30 yr.
     e. Have Li-Fraumeni syndrome, Cowden syndrome, or Bannayan-Riley-Ruvalcaba syndrome, or have first-degree relatives with one of these syndromes.
- Physicians should be familiar with the risks and benefits of various competing recommendations in order to better counsel patients.
- Breast radiologic evaluation, evaluation of nipple discharge, and evaluation of palpable mass are described in Section III.
- Exposure of the heart to ionizing radiation during breast cancer radiotherapy increases risk of ischemic heart disease. The increased rate of ischemic heart disease begins within a few yrs of exposure and continues for at least 20 yr. The increase is proportional to the mean radiation dose to the heart.

RISK REDUCTION STRATEGIES

- Prophylactic bilateral mastectomy reduces the risk for invasive breast cancer by >90%.
- Counseling points for women with average risk interested in contralateral prophylactic mastectomy (CPM) are summarized in Box 3.
- Selective estrogen receptor modulators (SERM) reduce the incidence of hormone receptor-positive invasive breast cancer by 50%.
- Ovarian failure is a common toxic effect of chemotherapy. Administration of the gonadotropin-releasing hormone (GnRH) agonist goserelin appears to protect against ovarian failure, reducing the risk of early menopause and improving prospects for fertility.

TABLE 10 Breast Cancer Screening Recommendations by Organization

Organization	When to Initiate Screening	Frequency of Screening	When to Stop Screening
American Academy of Family Physicians (AAFP)	Follow U.S. Preventive Services Task Force (USPSTF) recommendations	Follow USPSTF recommendations	Follow USPSTF recommendations
American Cancer Society (ACS)	Opportunity to begin screening at ages 40-44 Regular screening starting at age 45	Annually from age 45-54 Biennially starting at age 55 with opportunity to continue annually	Continue screening mammography as long as overall health is good, and life expectancy is 10 yr or longer
American College of Obstetricians and Gynecologists (ACOG)	Annual screening starting at age 40	Annually	Not specified
American College of Physicians (ACP)	Individualized for women ages 40-49 Regular screening starting at age 50	Biennially	Age 75 yr or older Women of any age with life expectancy <10 yr
American College of Radiology (ACR)	Annual screening starting at age 40	Annually	Should be considered as long as the patient is in good health and is willing to undergo additional testing if an abnormality is detected
National Comprehensive Cancer Network (NCCN)	Annual screening starting at age 40	Annually	Upper age limit is not yet established Consider comorbid conditions limiting life expectancy (e.g., ≤10 yr) and whether therapeutic interventions are planned
U.S. Preventive Services Task Force (USPSTF)	Individualized for women ages 40-49 Regular screening beginning at age 50	Biennially	Insufficient evidence to recommend for or against screening at age 75 or older

From Niederhuber JE: *Abeloff's clinical oncology*, ed 6, Philadelphia, 2020, Elsevier.

BOX 3 Counseling Points for Women with Average Risk Interested in Contralateral Prophylactic Mastectomy (CPM)

- There is a low annual contralateral breast cancer risk in women with average risk factors.
- Risk of contralateral breast cancer is decreasing with use of adjuvant therapy.
- Removing the contralateral breast does not decrease the risk for developing distant metastases.
- Breast cancer does not commonly metastasize from one breast to the other.
- CPM does not improve breast cancer–specific survival.
- CPM does not decrease local recurrence.
- Contralateral breast cancers tend to be at a lower stage than the initial primary cancer.
- CPM increases the surgical complication risk.
- Choice of CPM may influence reconstruction options.
- There are alternatives to CPM, including chemoprevention and surveillance.

From Cameron JL, Cameron AM: *Current surgical therapy*, ed 12, Philadelphia, 2017, Elsevier.

SUGGESTED READINGS

Available at ExpertConsult.com

RELATED CONTENT

Breast Cancer (Patient Information)
Breast Cancer: For Men (Patient Information)
Breast Abscess (Related Key Topic)
Fibrocystic Breast Disease (Related Key Topic)

AUTHOR: **Bharti Rathore, MD**

BASIC INFORMATION

DEFINITION

Bronchiectasis is dilatation of the bronchi or bronchioles resulting from a variety of causes and propagated through an interplay of host factors, environment, and respiratory pathogens. The clinical syndrome of bronchiectasis consists of cough, sputum production, and recurrent respiratory infections. It is often confirmed radiographically by a lack of bronchial tapering and a bronchus-to-arterial ratio greater than 1.5. It can be further divided into cylindrical, varicose, and cystic classes, which often overlap and coexist, but may aid in diagnosis and overall prognosis.

ICD-10CM CODES

J47.0	Bronchiectasis with acute lower respiratory infection
J47.1	Bronchiectasis with (acute) exacerbation
J47.9	Bronchiectasis, uncomplicated
Q33.4	Congenital bronchiectasis

EPIDEMIOLOGY & DEMOGRAPHICS

- The exact prevalence of bronchiectasis is unknown but is rising in the U.S. and Europe.
- Effective childhood immunizations have led to a significant decrease in the incidence of bronchiectasis resulting from pertussis.
- In developed countries, an increasing proportion of patients with an identifiable cause of bronchiectasis is being seen, although idiopathic remains the most frequent worldwide.
- Identified etiologies vary greatly worldwide, and there are growing attempts at global registries to elucidate true prevalence and etiologies across geographic barriers.

PHYSICAL FINDINGS & CLINICAL PRESENTATION

- Chronic cough, typically with expectoration of large amount of purulent sputum
- Fever, night sweats, generalized malaise, weight loss
- Hemoptysis
- Crackles, wheezing, or squeaks on lung exam
- Halitosis, skin pallor
- Clubbing (infrequent)

ETIOLOGY

- Postinfectious (e.g. previous pneumonia, lung abscess, tuberculosis, nontuberculous mycobacterial infections, fungal infections, viral infections)
- Cystic fibrosis
- Ciliary dysfunction (primary ciliary dyskinesia, Kartagener syndrome)
- Chronic obstructive pulmonary diseases (e.g., COPD, asthma)
- Impaired host defense (hypogammaglobulinemia, AIDS, chemotherapy)
- Localized airway obstruction (aspiration, esophageal reflux, congenital structural defects, foreign bodies, neoplasms)
- Inflammation (inflammatory pneumonitis, granulomatous lung disease, allergic aspergillosis)
- Congenital disorders such as tracheobronchomegaly (Mounier Kuhn syndrome), cartilage deficiency (Williams-Campbell syndrome, Marfan syndrome), alpha-1 antitrypsin deficiency
- Connective tissue and autoimmune diseases (Sjogren disease, ulcerative colitis, rheumatoid arthritis)

Dx DIAGNOSIS

DIFFERENTIAL DIAGNOSIS

- Chronic bronchitis or chronic rhinosinusitis
- COPD
- Asthma
- Tuberculosis
- Interstitial fibrosis
- Chronic lung abscess
- Foreign body aspiration
- Cystic fibrosis
- Lung carcinoma
- GERD

LABORATORY TESTS

- Pulmonary function tests with bronchodilators
- Sputum for Gram stain, culture and susceptibilities, and acid-fast bacteria
- Serum immunoglobulins (total IgA, IgM, IgG and subclasses)
- Testing for allergic bronchopulmonary aspergillosis
- Complete blood count with differential (leukocytosis with left shift, anemia)
- Sweat test in patients with suspected cystic fibrosis
- Primary ciliary dyskinesia workup when suspected
- Alpha-1 antitrypsin levels, ANA, RF, SSA/SSB when driven by history or exam
- Serum anti-*Pseudomonas aeruginosa* (PA) IgG antibody testing is highly accurate to detect chronic PA colonization in bronchiectasis patients

IMAGING STUDIES

- Chest x-ray (Fig. 1 and Fig. E2) may be normal or have crowded lung markings, "tram-track" sign of dilated bronchi, or small cystic spaces at the base of the lungs.
- High-resolution CT scan of the chest (Figs. 3 to E6) is the modern gold standard of diagnosis. The CT study should be noncontrast with the use of a 1- to 1.5-mm window every 1 cm with acquisition time of 1 sec. Findings include enlarged bronchoarterial ratio of >1.5 (normal 0.7), lack of tapering of an airway toward periphery, ballooned cysts at the end of bronchi, and airway mucus impaction.
- Bronchoscopy may be helpful to evaluate hemoptysis, rule out obstructive lesions, remove mucus plugs, and obtain microbiologic data on respiratory pathogens.
- Table 1 summarizes diagnostic studies for the classification and management of patients with bronchiectasis.

Rx TREATMENT

NONPHARMACOLOGIC THERAPY

- Mucus clearance is essential: Low risk and shown to improve chronic symptoms of cough, breathlessness, and may reduce frequency of exacerbations. Techniques include positive expiratory pressure (e.g., Acapella, Aerobika), chest wall oscillation (i.e., vest therapy), and postural drainage (reclining prone on a bed with the head down on the side)
- Supplemental oxygen for hypoxemia
- Exercise

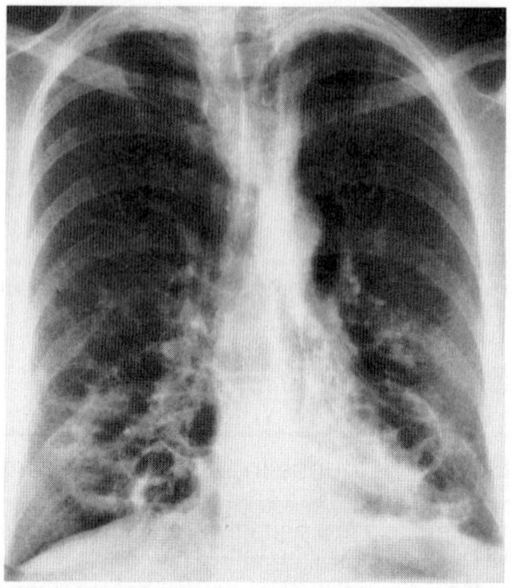

FIG. 1 Bronchiectasis. Multiple ring shadows, many containing air-fluid levels, are present throughout the lower zones of this patient with cystic bronchiectasis. (From Grant LA: *Grainger & Allison's diagnostic radiology essentials,* ed 2, 2019, Elsevier.)

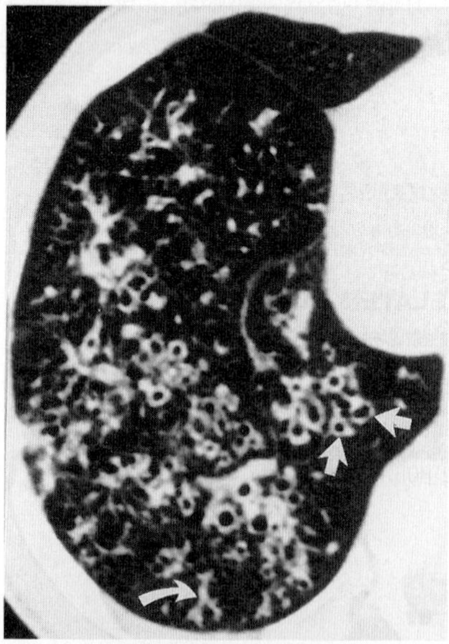

FIG. 3 Bronchiectasis. CT demonstrating dilated subsegmental bronchi. The bronchi are larger than the accompanying vessels with some demonstrating the "signet ring" sign *(arrows).* Plugging of peripheral bronchi is also evident *(curved arrow).* (From Grant LA: *Grainger & Allison's diagnostic radiology essentials,* ed 2, 2019, Elsevier.)

TABLE 1 Diagnostic Studies for the Classification and Management of Patients with Bronchiectasis

Test	Comments
Routine, Universal Studies	
Computed tomography lung scan (CTLS)	If bronchiectasis (BXSIS) is suspected, CTLS is the definitive test. Thin-section, high-resolution images may help detect subtle airway dilation before bronchial walls are grossly thickened. Contrast is generally not helpful and may, in fact, compromise the overall resolution of the study. CTLS may also identify esophageal abnormalities.
Pulmonary function tests (PFTs)	For patients with significant bronchiectasis, comprehensive PFTs, including spirometry, bronchodilator responsiveness, lung volumes, and diffusion capacity, are important studies that aid in management and prognosis. PFTs may also provide useful hints regarding predisposing conditions.
Complete blood count	Anemia may reflect effects of chronic infection or blood loss (consider inflammatory bowel disorders). Leukocytosis may mark severity of infection. Eosinophilia may suggest ABPA/M.
ESR, C-reactive protein	Nonspecific markers of inflammation; very high levels may suggest underlying connective tissue disease or vasculitis.
Routine sputum culture	Antibiotic therapy in bronchiectasis should generally be directed against specific pathogens and guided by in vitro susceptibility. The presence of mucoid strains of *Pseudomonas aeruginosa* and *Staphylococcus aureus* may raise suspicions for CF. *Stenotrophomonas maltophilia, Alcaligenes xylosoxidans,* and *Burkholderia cepacia* are gram-negative bacilli that may prove problematic pathogens in patients with long-standing bronchiectasis. Isolation of *B. cepacia* and *Helicobacter pylori* requires special laboratory techniques.
Mycobacterial sputum culture	Environmental mycobacteria such as *Mycobacterium avium* complex, *M. chelonae,* and *M. abscessus* appear to be increasingly common in contemporary bronchiectasis. May be commensal but often are pathogenic.
Fungal sputum culture	In patients with an asthmatic component, the presence of *Aspergillus* species (or other molds including *Pseudallescheria* or *Penicillium*) may be suggestive of etiology.
CT scan of sinuses	Many patients with bronchiectasis also suffer chronic rhinosinusitis. The presence of extensive sinus involvement suggests possible CF, immunoglobulin deficiencies, or ciliary disorders. Also, optimal management often entails aggressive sinus care.
Specific, Directed Studies	
Sweat chloride, CF genotyping, and nasal potential differences	For bronchiectasis patients with bilateral disease, recurrent sinusitis, and no other identified risk factor, mild variants of CF appear to be relatively common. Sweat chloride is regarded as the primary screening test for CF, but a considerable portion of adults with CF have borderline or normal results. Nasal potential difference may be useful for identifying CF in equivocal cases.
Alpha-1 antitrypsin (AAT) levels and phenotype	AAT anomalies appear to be a substantial risk factor for bronchiectasis, especially with white females. Abnormal proteinase inhibitor (Pi) phenotypes, even heterozygous patterns such as MS, appear to confer risk even with normal levels of AAT. Repletion of AAT may enhance resistance to lower respiratory tract infections.
Immunoglobulin (Ig) levels	Deficiencies of IgG or IgA may promote bronchiectasis; IgG subclass deficiencies may also be a factor. Elevated levels of IgE may suggest ABPA/M or Job syndrome. Hyper-IgM may be associated, as well, with chronic infections.
Ciliary morphology or function	For individuals with suggestive stories, a nasal ciliated epithelium biopsy with transmission electron microscopy may identify primary ciliary dyskinesia. Other studies including ex vivo ciliary activity, the saccharine test, or spermatozoa analysis may aid in this diagnosis.
Nasal nitric oxide (NNO) levels	Patients with documented PCD have significantly lower levels of NNO than normal or patients with CF. Although not universally available, such testing may prove highly useful in identifying PCD. Paradoxically, exhaled NO levels have been elevated in bronchiectasis of diverse etiologies except CF.
Barium swallow (BaS)	The BaS may detect disturbed deglutition, esophageal diverticula, obstructing lesions (tumors or strictures), hypomotility, achalasia, hiatal hernias, or lower esophageal sphincter (LES) incompetence with reflux. The absence of reflux on a BaS, however, does not exclude this problem (see "pH probe").
pH probe	For patients suspected of gastroesophageal reflux, an 18- to 24-hr study with a transnasal pH probe may identify, quantitate, and characterize reflux. Medications that inhibit acid production must be stopped before such tests.
Esophageal manometry	For patients being considered for surgical repair of the LES, manometry should be performed to determine that the esophagus generates sufficient pressure to propel food and liquids through the tightened sphincter.
Tailored hypopharyngography (TH)	TH is useful in detecting abnormalities of the initial phase of swallowing, deglutition. Persons particularly prone to problems include those with prior strokes, Parkinson disease, bulbar disorders including postpolio syndrome, and those with prior laryngeal or pharyngeal surgery. Note that some patients have gross aspiration without clinical manifestations (choking, coughing); this may occur in individuals with none of the above risk factors.
Less Common, Exotic Studies	
Collagen vascular disease (CVD) serologies	Various CVDs may contribute to the risk for bronchiectasis, including RA, ankylosing spondylitis, and systemic lupus erythematosus. Thus, for patients with compatible histories or physical findings, assays for rheumatoid factor, HLA-B27, and ANA may provide insight into predisposing conditions. CVD serologies may also suggest the diagnosis of Sjögren syndrome, particularly SSA/Ro and/or SSB/La.
Schirmer test	For patients with histories suggestive of "sicca syndrome" (dry eyes, dry mouth, oral ulcers), a positive Schirmer test may indicate the presence of either primary or secondary (associated with a CVD) Sjögren syndrome.

ABPA/M, Allergic bronchopulmonary aspergillosis/other mycoses; *ANA,* antinuclear antibody; *CF,* cystic fibrosis; *CT,* computed tomography; *ESR,* erythrocyte sedimentation rate; *HLA,* human leukocyte antigen; *MS,* multiple sclerosis; *NO,* nitric oxide; *PCD,* primary ciliary dyskinesia; *RA,* rheumatoid arthritis.
From Mason RJ: *Murray & Nadel's textbook of respiratory medicine,* ed 5, Philadelphia, 2010, Saunders.

ACUTE GENERAL Rx

- Antibiotic therapy should be based on the results of sputum Gram stain, culture, and susceptibility testing for 14 days of therapy. In those with inadequate or inconclusive sputum test results, empiric therapy with amoxicillin/clavulanate twice a day or a fluoroquinolone daily are reasonable options to ensure broad coverage in patients with complex flora.
- Use intravenous antibiotics in patients who require hospitalizations for acute exacerbation with signs of respiratory distress.
- Bronchodilators are useful in patients with demonstrable airflow obstruction.

COMPLEMENTARY & ALTERNATIVE MEDICINE

- Avoidance of tobacco
- Maintenance of proper nutrition and hydration

CHRONIC Rx

- Infections should be promptly identified and treated.
- Adults with bronchiectasis with a new isolation of *P. aeruginosa* should be offered eradication antibiotic treatment. This should not be offered to adults with bronchiectasis following new isolation of pathogens other than *P. aeruginosa*.
- Bronchodilators should be used before physiotherapy, including inhaled mucoactive drugs and inhaled antibiotics, in those with evidence of obstructive ventilatory defect or bronchospasm as this increases tolerability and optimizes delivery of medications in diseased areas of the lungs.
- Inhaled corticosteroids should not be offered to adults with isolated bronchiectasis. However, the diagnosis of bronchiectasis should not affect the use of inhaled corticosteroid in patients with comorbid asthma of chronic obstructive pulmonary disease.
- Inhaled hyperosmolar agents (e.g., hypertonic saline) should be considered in conjunction with airway clearance in patients who have difficulty expectorating sputum.
- Inhaled mucolytics can be considered in those with difficulty expectorating sputum, poor quality of life, or where standard airway clearance has failed to control symptoms. However, rhDNase should not be offered to patients with bronchiectasis not related to cystic fibrosis.
- Macrolide thrice weekly should be offered for adults with bronchiectasis who have three or more exacerbations per yr.
- Immunoglobulin replacement should be considered in patients with selective immunoglobulin deficiency.

DISPOSITION

- Prognosis is variable with severity of the disease and underlying etiology of bronchiectasis. The bronchiectasis severity index is one helpful scoring system.
- Pulmonary function declines at a faster rate in those with *Pseudomonas* colonization or frequent exacerbations.
- Concomitant rheumatoid arthritis or COPD is associated with worse prognosis.

REFERRAL

- Surgical partial lung resection may be an option in patients with localized, severe disease unresponsive to medical therapy or in patients with massive hemoptysis. Surgical resection of localized bronchiectasis is safe and improves quality of life.
- Referral for lung transplant should be considered similar to patients with cystic fibrosis.

PEARLS & CONSIDERATIONS

COMMENTS

The activity and quantity of neutrophil serine proteases are increased in the sputum of patients with bronchiectasis at baseline and increase further during exacerbations. A recent phase 2 trial revealed a reduction of neutrophil serine protease activity with brensocatib, an oral reversible inhibitor of dipeptidyl peptidase 1 (DPP-1), an enzyme responsible for the activation of neutrophil serine proteases.[1]

SUGGESTED READINGS

Available at ExpertConsult.com

RELATED CONTENT

Bronchiectasis (Patient Information)

AUTHOR: **B. Shoshana Zia, MD, PhD**

[1]Chalmers JD et al: Phase 2 trial of the DPP-1 inhibitor brensocatib in bronchiectasis, *N Engl J Med* 383:2127-2137, 2020.

BASIC INFORMATION

DEFINITION

Brugada syndrome (BRS) is an inherited disorder involving cardiac sodium channels characterized by typical electrocardiographic abnormalities. Patients with a Brugada pattern on ECG and symptoms such as palpitations, syncope, or sudden death are deemed to have BRS. BRS predisposes one to sudden cardiac death (SCD) secondary to polymorphic ventricular tachycardia (PVT) or ventricular fibrillation (VF) in the absence of structural heart disease.

SYNONYMS

BRS
Sudden unexpected nocturnal death syndrome (SUNDS)

ICD-10CM CODES	
I49.9	Cardiac arrhythmia, unspecified
I47.2	Ventricular tachycardia

EPIDEMIOLOGY & DEMOGRAPHICS

INCIDENCE: The incidence ranges from 1 to 5:10,000 people in Europe to 12:10,000 in Southeast Asia.

PREVALENCE: It comprises 4% of SCD and 20% of SCD in structurally normal hearts. Although found in every population, the prevalence is much higher in Asian and Southeast Asian countries; in some Southeast Asian countries, such as Laos and Thailand, it may be the most common form of natural death in younger males.

PREDOMINANT SEX & AGE: BRS is more common in males (58%-80% of patients). Mean age at presentation is 40 to 45.

RISK FACTORS: First-degree relatives with sudden death or known BRS

GENETICS: The disease is autosomal dominant with variable expression

- *SCN5A,* the gene that encodes for the alpha subunit of the cardiac sodium channel, accounts for about 20% to 30% of cases of BRS.
- *SCN10a,* the gene that encodes the Nav1.8 subunit of the sodium channel, has been found in 17% of BRS patients, making it the second most-common-known mutation.
- Known genetic abnormalities are only found in half of patients; thus the impact of genetic testing is limited. When available, it may be useful in identifying silent carriers.
- In all genotypes, the basic abnormality is either a decrease in the inward sodium or calcium current or an increase in the outward potassium current.

PHYSICAL FINDINGS & CLINICAL PRESENTATION

- Physical exam is usually benign
- Classic ECG finding is a pattern of atypical right bundle branch block (RBBB) with persistent ST elevation of cove-like morphology and T-wave inversion in the anterior leads (V1 to V2)
- Often an incidental finding diagnosed from a typical ECG pattern
- Palpitations
- Nocturnal agonal respirations
- Syncope
- Sudden cardiac arrest (SCA)/SCD secondary to rapid PVT that frequently degenerates into VF more often at night
- Fig. 1 illustrates Brugada ECG patterns. Type 1 is the most common and characteristic (Fig. 2)
- Type 1 ECG pattern is defined as an elevated ST segment ≥2 mm that descends in a coved pattern to an inverted T wave. This finding can be transient and may be provoked (sodium channel blockers, vagal maneuvers, increased alpha-adrenergic tone, beta-blockers, tricyclic or tetracyclic antidepressants, fever, hypokalemia, hyperkalemia, hypercalcemia, and alcohol and cocaine toxicity)
- Type 2 ECG pattern (Fig. 3) is not diagnostic of BRS but may be suggestive and warrant further testing. This pattern is a "saddle back" ST-T wave morphology with an upright or biphasic T wave. Type 2 (formerly known as types 2 and 3) can change to a type 1 pattern with the triggers noted above. Table 1 describes drugs used to unmask Brugada ECG pattern

ETIOLOGY

Autosomal dominant inheritance with variable penetration

DIAGNOSIS

Diagnosis is made by the presence of a type 1 ECG *and* symptoms.

- ST segment elevation with type 1 morphology ≥2 mm in one or more right-sided leads ($V_{1\ to}\ V_2$), occurring either spontaneously or after provocative drug testing
- Type 2 ECG that converts into type 1 following sodium channel blocker (procainamide/flecainide/ajmaline) challenge (Fig. 2)

DIFFERENTIAL DIAGNOSIS

A number of diseases can lead to a BRS-like abnormality on the surface ECG, including the following:

- Atypical RBBB
- Early repolarization
- Acute pericarditis
- Acute myocardial infarction or ischemia
- Pulmonary embolism
- Various central and autonomic system abnormalities
- Duchenne muscular dystrophy
- Electrolyte abnormalities such as hyperkalemia and hypercalcemia
- Arrhythmogenic right ventricular cardiomyopathy
- Pectus excavatum

WORKUP

- Clinical history with special emphasis on syncope, palpitations, nocturnal agonal respirations, and family history.
- Echocardiography to rule out structural heart disease. While no structural heart disease is usually apparent, mild abnormalities in the right ventricle and left ventricle and particularly in the right ventricular outflow tract may be seen.
- MRI, especially to rule out ARVC (arrhythmogenic right ventricular cardiomyopathy).

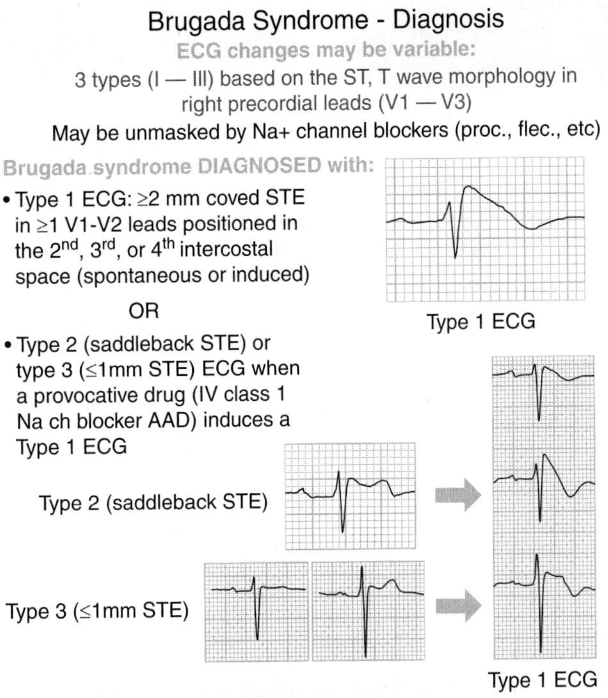

FIG. 1 Brugada electrocardiogram *(ECG)* patterns. A type 1 ECG pattern supports diagnosis of Brugada syndrome. Brugada syndrome can be considered for type 2 or 3 ECG patterns if ECG pattern converts to a type 1 pattern after challenge with a sodium channel *(Na ch)* blocker. *AAD,* Antiarrhythmic drug; *STE,* ST elevation. (From Olshansky B et al: *Arrhythmia essentials,* ed 2, Philadelphia, 2017, Elsevier.)

- Electrophysiology study. No consensus exists on the value of arrhythmia induction in predicting future clinical events in individual patients. However, findings such as HV (His ventricular) conduction interval >60 ms and VERP (ventricular effective refractory period) <200 ms during electrophysiology study can help in supporting a diagnosis. Repeated trials have failed to show a predictive power of electrophysiology study, and it still exists as a IIb recommendation. A recent meta-analysis has suggested it may have some utility in predicting risk of sudden death, and its use in risk stratification remains controversial.
- Laboratory tests are unhelpful. Genetic testing may be helpful for prognosis and family evaluation, but it is not necessary for diagnostic purposes.
- First-degree relatives should obtain ECG and be evaluated for symptoms.
- The following are considered indicators of high risk in an asymptomatic patient:
  1. Spontaneous type 1 ECG at baseline
  2. Presence of fragmented QRS on ECG
  3. RVERP (right ventricular effective refractory period) <200 ms on EPS
  4. Male sex
  5. Spontaneous atrial fibrillation

  Note that family history of sudden death is not considered a high-risk feature in BRS.

Rx TREATMENT

NONPHARMACOLOGIC THERAPY

- The only effective strategy that prevents sudden cardiac death in BRS is implantable cardioverter-defibrillator (ICD). Currently there are no class I recommendations for primary prevention because clinical events are extremely rare, even in high-risk patients. Fig. 4 depicts the algorithm for clinical decision making regarding recommendation of an ICD.
- Definitive candidates for ICD (class I) are patients who survived SCD or have had sustained VT (secondary prevention).
- ICD can be useful (class IIa) for patients who have type 1 ECG pattern (either spontaneous or after class IC drug test) associated with history of syncope.
- ICD may be considered (class IIb) if there is inducible VF on electrophysiologic (EP) study, but this remains controversial.
- Patients with spontaneous type 1 ECG without syncope or inducible VF on EP study or asymptomatic patients with drug-induced type 1 ECG pattern are considered a lower risk group for SCD, and ICD is not indicated in these patients.
- Radiofrequency catheter ablation of the RV epicardium may be performed for patients with recurrent ventricular arrhythmias and may eliminate the Brugada ECG phenotype. It has also been associated with very low recurrence of arrhythmia. This has become an accepted therapy for patients with ICD shocks and requires referral to specialized centers.

ACUTE GENERAL Rx

- Isoproterenol (class IIa) may be used for electrical storm.
- Quinidine, which blocks both Ito and IKr currents in the RV epicardium, is used in patients with a history of multiple appropriate ICD shocks, as well as for electrical storms and treatment of supraventricular tachycardia (SVT) in these patients. It is also useful in cases where the patient refuses an ICD implant or when an ICD implant is contraindicated.

REFERRAL

Consultation with a cardiac electrophysiologist is strongly recommended if BRS is suspected.

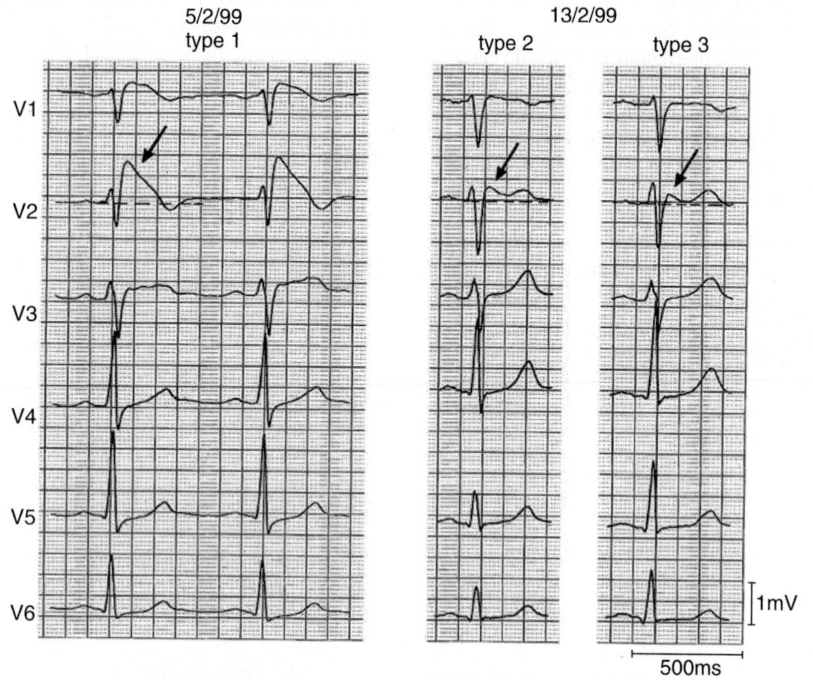

FIG. 2 Electrocardiogram (ECG) changes in Brugada syndrome. ST elevation occurs in the anterior precordial leads, leads V1 and V2. Type 1 (coved) ECGs with 1 mV of ST elevation have the most prognostic significance. (From Strickberger SA et al: AHA/ACCF scientific statement on the evaluation of syncope, *J Am Coll Cardiol* 47:473-484, 2006.)

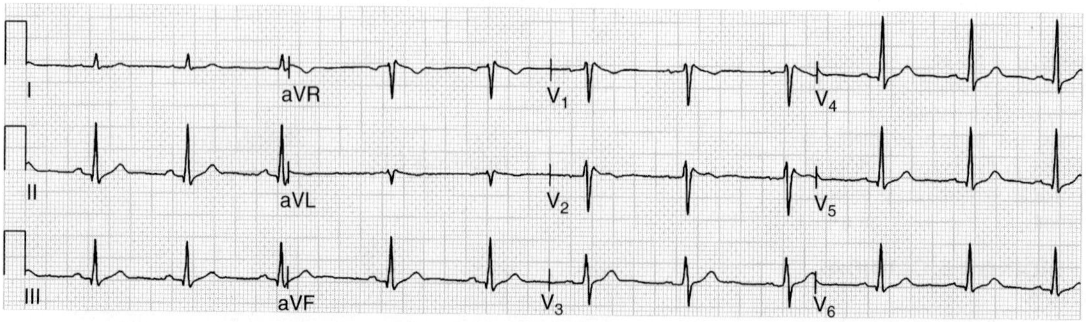

FIG. 3 Type II Brugada pattern electrocardiogram (ECG). This 12-lead ECG shows a type II Brugada pattern in leads V1 and V2. Whereas a type I ECG pattern supports a diagnosis of Brugada syndrome, Brugada syndrome can be considered for type 2 or 3 ECG patterns (see Fig. 1) if the ECG pattern converts to a type 1 pattern after challenge with a sodium channel blocker. *aVF,* Augmented vector foot; *aVL,* augmented vector left; *aVR,* augmented vector right. (From Olshansky B et al: *Arrhythmia essentials*, ed 2, Philadelphia, 2017, Elsevier.)

TABLE 1 Drugs Used to Unmask Brugada ECG Pattern

Drug	Dose
Ajmaline	1-mg/kg IV infusion over 5 min
Flecainide	2-mg/kg IV infusion over 10 min, maximum 150 mg; or 400 mg PO
Procainamide	10-mg/kg IV infusion over 10 min
Pilsicainide	1-mg/kg IV infusion over 10 min

IV, Intravenous.

PEARLS & CONSIDERATIONS

COMMENTS

- The clinical manifestations, such as syncope and SCD, are rare in the pediatric group, but fever can acutely predispose to cardiac arrest. Mean age of presentation is 40 to 45 yr.
- Cardiac events may occur during sleep, at rest, or after a large meal.
- BRS patients should be advised to avoid all drugs that may induce a type 1 ECG pattern and/or be known to trigger ventricular arrhythmias and avoid unnecessary use of drugs (a drug that is not yet identified as potentially dangerous for these patients does not make its use safe). For up-to-date information on this matter, a full list can be found at www.brugadadrugs.org.
- Fever may induce the appearance of a type 1 BRS ECG pattern and may trigger episodes of PVT/VF in BRS patients. In the case of fever, close ECG monitoring is appropriate in combination with lowering of the body temperature.
- The classic ECG changes in BRS can be transient with patients having normal ECGs in between highly abnormal ones.
- The appearance of syncope, seizures, or nocturnal agonal respiration must lead to prompt medical evaluation.
- Family screening for BRS in first-degree relatives is strongly recommended.
- Although participation in sports is not strictly prohibited, competitive training can lead to development of strong vagal tone and subsequent higher risk of clinical events. Hence, participation in sports at a competitive or professional level is not advised.
- Once diagnosed initially by an ECG pattern, all patients must be followed up on a regular basis by an electrophysiologist.

PREVENTION

Identification of patients with BRS, risk stratification, and appropriate screening of family members are paramount to the prevention of SCD. Patients with known BRS should have fevers aggressively treated with antipyretics and avoid drugs associated with drugs that induce a type 1 pattern.

PATIENT & FAMILY EDUCATION

Immediate family members should be notified and be screened for BRS.

SUGGESTED READINGS

Available at ExpertConsult.com

AUTHOR: **John Wylie, MD, FACC**

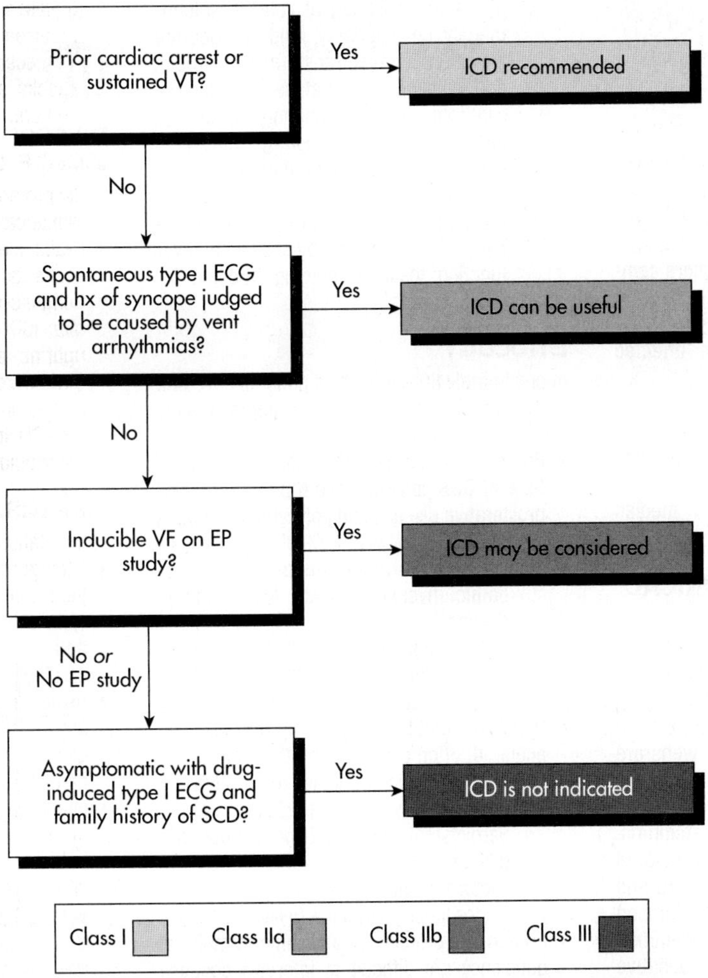

FIG. 4 Consensus recommendations for ICDs in patients diagnosed with Brugada syndrome. (*hx,* History; *ECG,* electrocardiogram; *EP,* electrophysiological; *ICD,* implantable cardioverter-defibrillator; *SCD,* sequential compression device; *VF,* ventricular fibrillation; *VT,* ventricular tachycardia.) (From Priori SG et al: HRS/EHRA/APHRS expert consensus statement on the diagnosis and management of patients with inherited primary arrhythmia syndromes, *Heart Rhythm* 10:1932-1963, 2013.)

Budd-Chiari Syndrome (PTG) (ALG)

BASIC INFORMATION

DEFINITION

Budd-Chiari syndrome (BCS) is a rare disorder defined by the obstruction of hepatic venous outflow anywhere from the small hepatic veins to the junction of the inferior vena cava (IVC) and the right atrium. Primary BCS is defined by endoluminal obstruction as seen in thromboses, phlebitis, or webs. Secondary BCS occurs when the obstruction is caused by compression or invasion by a lesion originating outside of the veins (tumor, abscess, cyst, etc.). It can also be a postoperative complication of orthotopic liver transplantation (OLT).

SYNONYMS

BCS
Hepatic vein thrombosis
Obliterative endophlebitis of the hepatic veins
IVC thrombosis
Chiari-Budd syndrome
Budd syndrome
Chiari disease
Rokitansky disease

ICD-10CM CODE

I82.0 Budd-Chiari syndrome

EPIDEMIOLOGY & DEMOGRAPHICS

INCIDENCE:

- Males: 2.0/1 million persons per yr
- Females: 2.2/1 million persons per yr

PREDOMINANT SEX:

- In Western countries, women are more commonly affected (approximately two thirds of cases).
- In Asia, men are slightly more affected (approximately 1.5/1).

PREDOMINANT AGE:

- In Western countries, presentation is usually in the third and fourth decades of life, with the median age being 35 to 50 yr.
- In Asia, presentation is usually at a median age of 36 yr.

PHYSICAL FINDINGS & CLINICAL PRESENTATION

Clinical presentation and characteristics vary with geography. The classic presentation of Budd-Chiari syndrome includes hepatomegaly, ascites, and right upper quadrant pain. In Africa and South Asia, intravascular webs are more often associated with IVC thrombosis with a stronger association with subsequent liver cirrhosis and hepatocellular carcinoma. In the U.S., BCS is more commonly associated with primary myeloproliferative disorders and underlying hypercoagulable states. Underlying factors that contribute to BCS can be identified in more than 80% of cases; multiple causative factors are identified in up to 50% of cases.

- Clinical manifestations can be caused by complete or partial occlusion of any or all of the three major hepatic veins or the inferior vena cava.
- Presentation is variable according to the degree, location, acuity of obstruction, and presence of collateral circulation:
  1. Fulminant/acute (25%): Severe right upper quadrant abdominal pain, fever, nausea, vomiting, mild jaundice, hepatomegaly, transudative and intractable ascites, marked elevation in serum aminotransferases (AST/ALT >5 times the upper limit of normal), elevation of alkaline phosphatase to 300 to 400 IU/L, serum-ascites albumin gradient ≥1.1 with total protein >2.5 g/dl, coagulopathy (usually international normalized ratio [INR] >1.5), variceal bleeding, encephalopathy within 8 wk of onset of jaundice, renal failure. Biopsy, if performed, would reveal hepatic necrosis. Early recognition and treatment are essential for survival; a slow decrease in ALT is associated with poor survival.
  2. Subacute/chronic (60%): Vague abdominal discomfort, gradual progression to caudate lobe hypertrophy with atrophy of the rest of the liver, portal hypertension with or without cirrhosis and its sequelae, transudative ascites, lower-extremity edema, esophageal varices, splenomegaly, coagulopathy, mild to moderate elevation in aminotransferases, bilirubin, and alkaline phosphatase, hepatorenal syndrome, hepatopulmonary syndrome, and rarely, encephalopathy; biopsy, if performed, could reveal minimal hepatic necrosis.
  3. Asymptomatic (up to 20%): Usually discovered incidentally by abnormal liver function tests or imaging attained for other reasons.

ETIOLOGY

Approximately 80% to 87% of patients have one prothrombotic risk factor, and approximately 50% have multiple.

- Primary myeloproliferative diseases: Up to 53% of BCS patients have a primary myeloproliferative disease and polycythemia vera is responsible for 10% to 40% of these cases.
  1. Essential thrombocythemia and idiopathic myelofibrosis are less common causes.
  2. *JAK2* mutations are implicated in cases of idiopathic BCS (identified in 25% to 60% of cases).
- Hypercoagulable states (inherited and acquired) often coexist with other causes.
  1. Anticardiolipin antibodies (up to 25%)
  2. Hyperhomocysteinemia (22%)
  3. Paroxysmal nocturnal hemoglobinuria (5% to 19%)
  4. Factor V Leiden (25%)
  5. Factor II gene mutation (5%)
- Protein C, protein S, and antithrombin III deficiency are difficult to interpret because the presence of liver disease may confound results. However, they account for 4.0%, 3.0%, and 3.0% of BCS, respectively.
- Heterozygosity for *G20210A* prothrombin gene mutation, methylenetetrahydrofolate reductase (MTHFR) mutation, Tet methylcytosine dioxygenase 2 mutation, and calreticulin mutation may be seen in BCS.
- Pregnancy and oral contraceptive pills are also predisposing factors to develop BCS.
- Malignancy causing external compression or invasion of vascular structures (up to 10% of cases).
  1. Most commonly due to hepatocellular carcinoma but also can be due to neoplasms of the kidney, adrenal gland, pancreas, stomach, lung and sarcomas of the right atrium, inferior vena cava, and hepatic veins.
- Rare but reported: Sickle cell anemia, infections with liver abscess, hydatid cyst (echinococcosis), schistosomiasis, sarcoidosis, Behçet disease, membranous webs of IVC or hepatic veins (more common in Africa and South Asia, can be congenital or acquired secondary to underlying myeloproliferative disorder), abdominal trauma, liver torsion, granulomatous venulitis, ulcerative colitis, celiac disease, systemic lupus erythematous, minimal change nephrotic syndrome, neurofibromatosis, α-1 antitrypsin deficiency, hypereosinophilic syndrome, idiopathic (10% to 25%).

Dx DIAGNOSIS

DIFFERENTIAL DIAGNOSIS

- Hepatitis from ischemia, viral infection, toxin, alcohol
- Cholecystitis
- Hepatic venoocclusive disease (sinusoidal obstruction syndrome)
- Congestive hepatopathy, also known as *cardiac cirrhosis*, from tricuspid regurgitation, right atrial myxoma, constrictive pericarditis
- Cirrhosis from any etiology

LABORATORY TESTS

- Assessment of liver injury and function: Serum aminotransferases, alkaline phosphatase, prothrombin time (PT), albumin, bilirubin.
- Exclusion of another form of liver disease: Viral hepatitis panel, autoantibodies (antinuclear antibody, anti–smooth muscle antibody, anti-mitochondrial antibody), iron studies, ceruloplasmin, and α-1 antitrypsin.
- Ascites protein content ≥2.5 g/dl and serum ascites albumin gradient >1.1 g/dl are suggestive of transudative ascites from BCS or cardiac ascites.
- Evaluation for underlying myeloproliferative disorder and hypercoagulable state: CBC, bone marrow biopsy, tests for hypercoagulable states (Factor V Leiden, prothrombin gene *G20210A* mutation, protein C, protein S, antithrombin deficiencies, antiphospholipid syndrome, and paroxysmal nocturnal hemoglobinuria). Protein C, protein S, and antithrombin deficiencies may be difficult to interpret in the setting of liver dysfunction, but levels <20% of normal are suggestive of a true deficiency; thrombophilia screening for

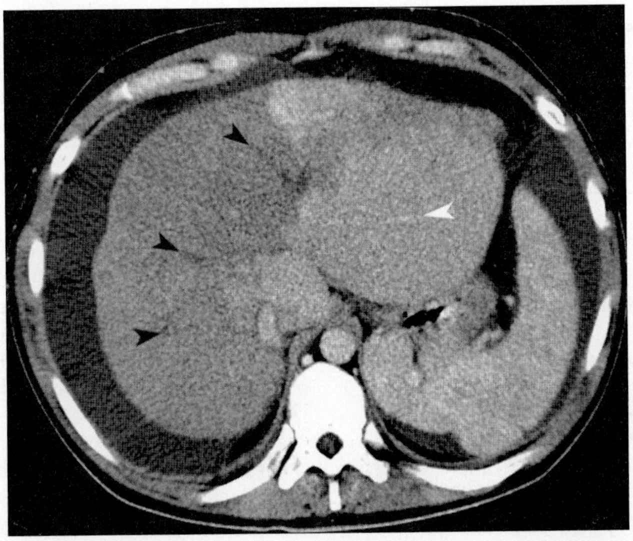

FIG. 2 Acute Budd-Chiari syndrome. On portal phase CT, most of the caudate and left lobe of the liver has enhanced normally and the left hepatic vein can just be seen *(white arrowhead)*, but the right lobe has abnormally low attenuation, and the middle and right hepatic vein branches are attenuated and have failed to opacify *(black arrowheads)*. Ascites is present. (From Grant LA: *Grainger & Allison's diagnostic radiology essentials*, ed 2, Philadelphia, 2019, Elsevier.)

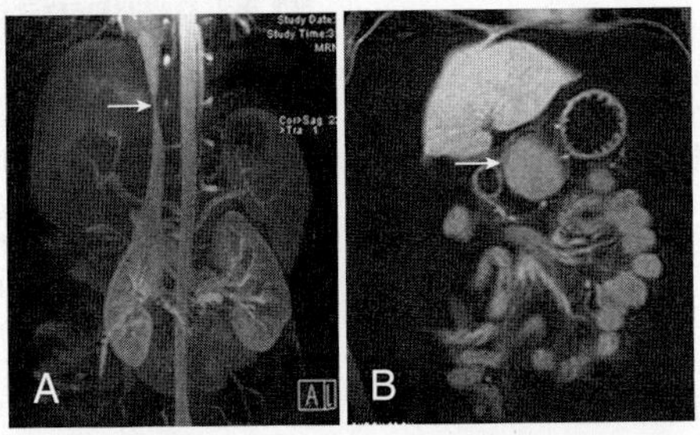

FIG. 5 Magnetic resonance venogram. A, Intravenous cholangiography (IVC) obstruction *(arrow)* at the level of the caudate. **B,** Hypertrophic caudate lobe *(arrow)*. (From Cameron JL, Cameron AM: *Current surgical therapy*, ed 10, Philadelphia, 2011, Saunders.)

the JAK2 V617F mutation, hyperhomocysteinemia, and MTHFR C677T mutation may be useful if no other cause for myeloproliferative disorders or hypercoagulable states are identified.

IMAGING STUDIES

- Diagnosis of BCS is made by radiographic imaging (Figs. E1, 2, and E3).
- Doppler ultrasonography is the first-line test. Diagnostic sensitivity and specificity are 85% to 90%. Findings include large hepatic vein with an absent flow signal, or with reversed or turbulent flow; large intrahepatic or subcapsular collateral vessels; enlarged, stenotic, thickened, or tortuous hepatic veins; spider web pattern near hepatic vein ostia and associated absent flow in that region; caudate lobe hypertrophy (as the caudate lobe has an alternate blood supply through anastomoses); flattened or absent hepatic venous waveform without fluttering; hyperechoic cord replacing a normal vein.
- MRI with gadolinium contrast is the second-line test. It is superior to contrast-enhanced CT (Fig. E4) with a sensitivity and specificity of approximately 90%, and it is preferred in younger patients due to the lack of radiation. Findings include obstructed hepatic veins or IVC, large intrahepatic or subcapsular collaterals, and caudate lobe hypertrophy. MRI is beneficial to visualize the entire length of the IVC and distinguish between acute, subacute, and chronic BCS. Three-dimensional contrast-enhanced magnetic resonance angiography (MRA; see Fig. 5) rivals hepatic venography in sensitivity.
- Contrast-enhanced CT may reveal similar findings as Doppler ultrasound as well as delayed or absent filling of the hepatic veins, parenchymal opacification of the liver, narrowing and/or compression of the inferior vena cava, and caudate lobe hypertrophy. Contrast enhancement localizes more centrally than peripherally and has a patchy and flea-bitten appearance. The use of CT is limited given that in almost 50% of patients, the test is indeterminate or a false-positive. Ultrasonography is more accurate than CT for detecting lesions in the hepatic veins and IVC.
- CT image reconstruction of vasculature is becoming more available.
- Venography: Although it is the gold standard, it is not essential for diagnosis, and it should be performed when other noninvasive imaging tests are nondiagnostic in the setting of strong clinical suspicion for BCS. Measurement of pressure gradients can help predict success of percutaneous or surgical shunt intervention. Confirms the pathognomonic web pattern caused by collateral venous flow.
- Liver biopsy: Not necessary to diagnose BCS but may be helpful in patients with cirrhosis in whom the diagnosis remains uncertain and is critical for differentiating from hepatic venoocclusive disease or congestive hepatopathy. Findings include hepatic congestion, hepatocyte necrosis and fibrosis in centrilobular areas, and compensatory nodular regenerative hyperplasia with progression to fibrosis and cirrhosis. In advanced BCS, infarction caused by concomitant thrombosis of the intrahepatic, extrahepatic, and portal veins may be seen. There are conflicting studies regarding the association of histologic findings and prognosis.

Rx TREATMENT

NONPHARMACOLOGIC THERAPY

- Goal of therapy is decompression of hepatic congestion.
- In general, therapeutic procedures should be introduced by order of increasing invasiveness based on response/failure to therapy rather than disease severity. Fig. 6 illustrates a treatment algorithm for patients with Budd-Chiari syndrome.
- Hypercoagulable states should be investigated in all patients.

ACUTE GENERAL Rx

- Anticoagulation, first with low-molecular-weight heparin (LMWH), followed by warfarin, even in the absence of an underlying hypercoagulable disorder. Recent research also suggests that using direct-acting oral anticoagulants in BCS is safe and effective.
- In situ thrombolysis: Can be successful when performed in patients with recently thrombosed veins (within 2 to 3 wk after symptom onset) that are well defined on venography. Mature clots are nonresponsive to thrombolysis, and bleeding risk is high if portal hypertension has developed.
- Balloon angioplasty: Complicated by 50% restenosis rate within 2 yr; effective when membranous webs or short segment hepatic vein stenosis are the etiology.
- Stenting: May improve long-term patency rates to 90%, but if placed above the intrahepatic IVC, may complicate future liver transplantation.
- Transjugular intrahepatic portosystemic shunt (TIPS) (Fig. 7): Indicated with diffuse hepatic vein thrombosis, refractory ascites, recurrent variceal bleeding and progressive liver failure. Polytetrafluoroethylene (ePTFE)-coated stents have improved TIPS-patency rates, especially in patients with underlying

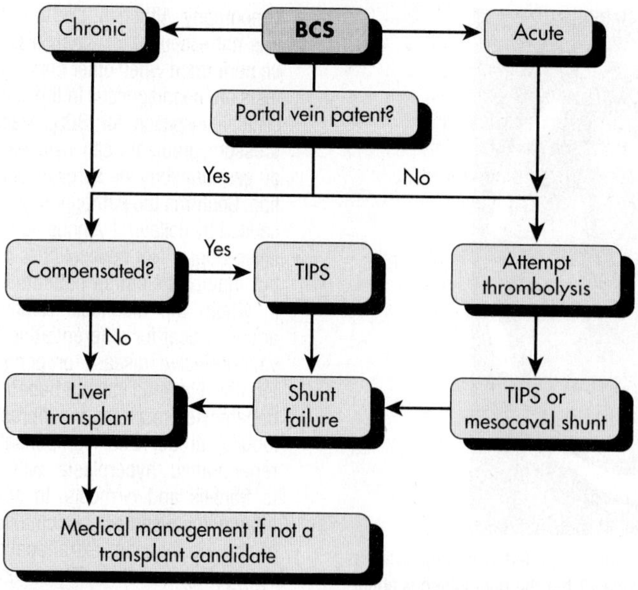

FIG. 6 Treatment algorithm for patients with Budd-Chiari syndrome (BCS). *TIPS,* Transjugular intrahepatic portosystemic shunt. (From Cameron JL, Cameron AM: *Current surgical therapy*, ed 12, Philadelphia, 2017, Elsevier.)

hypercoagulable defects with a 76% 10-yr survival rate.
- Surgical portal systemic shunts: Indicated when angioplasty and stenting have failed and when complications from portal hypertension are also present. This option is no longer common practice and provides no survival benefit.
- Liver transplant may be indicated in patients with cirrhosis or fulminant hepatic failure and in patients who fail to respond to TIPS; 10-yr survival is reported to range between 69% and 84%.
- Supportive measures.

CHRONIC Rx

- Lifelong anticoagulation: Warfarin therapy, with a target INR of 2 to 3 or low-molecular-weight heparin, lessens, but does not completely prevent, recurrence. Anticoagulation should be continued permanently unless the patient has an adverse event to anticoagulation, the obstruction is because of an anatomic cause that has been corrected, or anticoagulation is contraindicated.
- In patients with an underlying myeloproliferative disorder, first-line treatment is with hydroxyurea and aspirin.
- Treat liver dysfunction and complications related to portal hypertension such as ascites and variceal bleeding.
- Invasive interventions should be reserved for symptomatic patients who do not improve with medical therapy.
- Manage shunt thrombosis; which is a common complication.
- Liver transplantation is another treatment option with a 71% to 89% survival rate at 5 yr; up to 27% recurrence of BCS after transplant has been recognized.
- Monitor for development of hepatocellular carcinoma and transformation of myeloproliferative disease in patients with long-standing, well-controlled BCS and posttransplant lymphoma in orthotopic liver transplantation (OLT) recipients.

DISPOSITION

Prognosis is variable and depends on multiple factors, including time to recognition and treatment, etiology, acuity, the type of intervention, and the condition of the patient at the time of treatment. Overall mortality rates are decreasing with the use of anticoagulation and early diagnosis of asymptomatic cases. Given numerous therapeutic options, the survival rate is 90%, 83%, and 72% at 1, 5, and 10 yr from diagnosis.

- A prognostic index called the *Rotterdam BCS Index* has been described: 1.27 × Encephalopathy + 1.04 × Ascites + 0.72 × PT + 0.004 × Bilirubin.
  1. Encephalopathy and ascites are scored as 1 for present or 0 as absent, and PT is scored as greater (1) or less than (0) an INR of 2.3.
  2. An index of <1.1 correlates to low risk (5-yr survival rate, 89%), 1.1 to 1.5 with intermediate risk (5-yr survival rate, 74%), and >1.5 with high risk (5-yr survival rate, 42%).
- There is also the *BCS-TIPS PI score*, which is a prognostic index for survival 1 yr after TIPS: Age (yr) × 0.08 + bilirubin × 0.16 + INR × 0.63.
  1. Seven is the most specific discriminative factor, with those scoring above 7 necessitating emergent OLT as the first-line treatment.

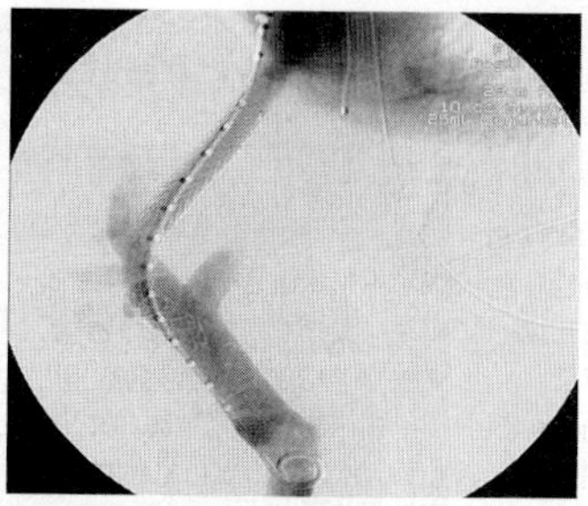

FIG. 7 Transjugular intrahepatic portosystemic shunt extending from the right portal vein into the right atrium. (From Cameron JL, Cameron AM: *Current surgical therapy*, ed 12, Philadelphia, 2017, Elsevier.)

REFERRAL

Fulminant presentations should immediately be referred to a center capable of liver transplantation. All cases benefit from referral to a hepatologist, a hematologist, an interventional radiologist, and a surgeon specializing in hepatobiliary disease.

PEARLS & CONSIDERATIONS

COMMENTS

- Look for one or more underlying causes, especially hypercoagulable or hematologic disorders, and malignancies or space-occupying lesions that may compress or invade the hepatic outflow tract.
- Myeloproliferative disorders are most common.
- Diagnosis relies on imaging; beginning with Doppler ultrasound.
- Treatment with anticoagulation comes first; followed by invasive interventions as needed. Prophylaxis of portal hypertension can reduce the risk of major bleeding associated with anticoagulation therapy.
- Referral for liver transplantation may be necessary.
- Prognostic indices can assist in management and estimate survival rates.

PREVENTION

In the setting of known risk factors, such as a hypercoagulable state or myeloproliferative disorder, any additional risks, such as smoking or oral contraceptive therapy, should be avoided.

SUGGESTED READINGS

Available at ExpertConsult.com

RELATED CONTENT

Budd-Chiari Syndrome (Patient Information)
Hypercoagulable State (Related Key Topic)

AUTHORS: **Jeanette G. Smith, MD,** and **Dina A. Ibrahim, MD**

BASIC INFORMATION

DEFINITION

- Delayed conduction in the His-Purkinje system that meets criteria for right bundle branch block (RBBB), left bundle branch block (LBBB), or hemifascicular block. The latter can be either left anterior fascicular block (LAFB) or left posterior fascicular block (LPFB). Bifascicular block is a combination of RBBB and either LAFB or LPFB. All of these are categories of bundle branch block. Any delayed conduction that does not meet these criteria is not considered bundle branch block and instead categorized as intraventricular conduction delay (IVCD) (see also topic "Intraventricular Conduction Delay"). Repolarization abnormalities may be seen in multiple leads with LBBB and in leads V1 to V3 in RBBB. These include T wave inversion and ST segment depression in the opposite direction from the QRS complex. Fig. 1 illustrates a diagrammatic representation of fascicular blocks in the left ventricle. Table 1 and Table 2 summarize common diagnostic criteria for fascicular blocks and bundle branch blocks.
- The bundle branch block can be persistent or intermittent. Tachycardia-related aberrancy as well as bradycardia-related aberrancy has been described.

SYNONYMS

- Fascicular block
- Aberrancy
- Conduction disturbance
- Conduction delay
- Conduction defect

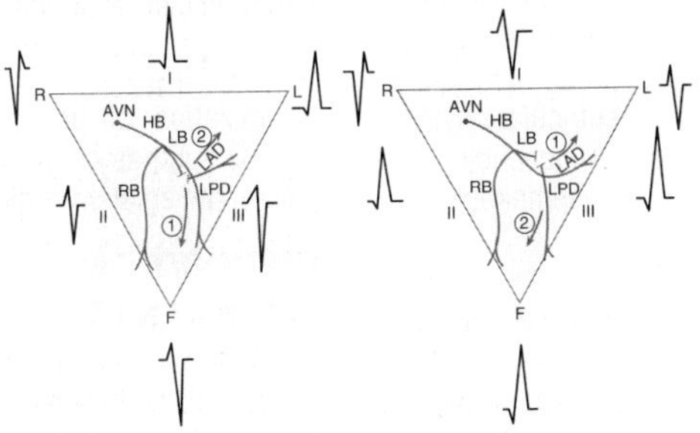

FIG. 1 Diagrammatic representation of fascicular blocks in the left ventricle. *Left,* Interruption of the left anterior fascicle or division (here labeled LAD) results in an initial inferior (1) followed by a dominant superior (2) direction of activation. *Right,* Interruption of the left posterior fascicle or division (here labeled LPD) results in an initial superior (1) followed by a dominant inferior (2) direction of activation. *AVN,* Atrioventricular node; *HB,* His bundle; *LB,* left bundle; *RB,* right bundle. (Courtesy Dr. C. Fisch. From Mann DL et al: *Braunwald's heart disease,* ed 10, Philadelphia, 2015, Elsevier.)

TABLE 1 Common Diagnostic Criteria for Fascicular Blocks

Left Anterior Fascicular Block
Frontal plane mean QRS axis between −45 and −90 degrees
qR pattern in lead aVL
QRS duration <120 msec
Time to peak R wave in aVL ≥45 msec
Left Posterior Fascicular Block
Frontal plane mean QRS axis between +90 and +180 degrees
rS pattern in leads I and aVL with qR patterns in leads III and aVF
QRS duration <120 msec
Exclusion of other factors causing right axis deviation (e.g., right ventricular overload patterns, lateral infarction)

aVF, Augmented vector foot; *aVL,* augmented vector left.
From Mann DL et al: *Braunwald's heart disease,* ed 10, Philadelphia, 2015, Elsevier.

TABLE 2 Common Diagnostic Criteria for Bundle Branch Blocks

Complete Left Bundle Branch Block
QRS duration ≥120 msec
Broad, notched, or slurred R waves in leads I, aVL, V5, and V6
Small or absent initial r waves in right precordial leads (V1 and V2) followed by deep S waves
Absent septal q waves in leads I, V5, and V6
Prolonged time to peak R wave (>60 msec) in V5 and V6
Complete Right Bundle Branch Block
QRS duration ≥120 msec rsr′, rsR′, or rSR′, patterns in leads V1 and V2
S waves in leads I and V6 ≥40 msec wide
Normal time to peak R wave in leads V5 and V6 but >50 msec in V1

aVF, Augmented vector foot; *aVL,* augmented vector left.
From Mann DL et al: *Braunwald's heart disease,* ed 10, Philadelphia, 2015, Elsevier.

ICD-10CM CODES
Bundle branch block (fascicular block):

I44.4	Anterior
I44.5	Posterior
I44.60	Hemiblock (hemifascicular block)
I44.7	Left
I45.10	Right
I45.2	Bilateral (bifascicular)

EPIDEMIOLOGY & DEMOGRAPHICS

INCIDENCE: The cumulative incidence of any type of bundle branch block increases with age (1.5% at age 50, 18% at age 80)

PREVALENCE: The estimated prevalence in the general population for any type of bundle branch block ranges between 0.2% and 3.4% and increases with age.

- Complete LBBB: 0.4% men age 50, 5.7% men age 80, 1.1% women age 50 to 80
- Complete RBBB: 0.2% men before age 30, 0.8% men age 50, 1.3% men age 80, 1.3% women age 50 to 80, 2.3% in men and women age 60
- Incomplete RBBB: 13.5% age 20, 3.4% age 50

PREDOMINANT SEX & AGE: More common in men, incidence increases with age

PEAK INCIDENCE: Cumulative incidence of 18% at age 80 for any type of bundle branch block

RISK FACTORS: Male gender, elder age, structural heart disease, cardiomyopathy, hypertension

GENETICS: Most cases of bundle branch block are not hereditary. The Brugada syndrome is an autosomal dominant genetic disorder with pseudo-RBBB but is not a true bundle branch block (see section on "Brugada Syndrome"). The hereditary bundle branch defect is an autosomal dominant genetic disease that has been described in Lebanon and was mapped to the long arm of chromosome 19.

PHYSICAL FINDINGS & CLINICAL PRESENTATION

- RBBB can cause wide splitting of the second heart sound (S_2). Either LBBB or RBBB can cause continuous splitting of S2 during respiration.
- Isolated bundle branch block is asymptomatic but might reflect heart disease, either in the conduction system or the surrounding cardiac tissues, and its existence can aggravate the clinical picture of the causal entity.
- In patients with heart failure, the presence of LBBB can cause ventricular dyssynchrony and worsen heart failure. LBBB or RBBB, when coexistent with coronary artery disease, diabetes, or heart failure, are markers for increased mortality.
- RBBB can be seen in pulmonary hypertension or acute pulmonary embolism; entities that increase the right ventricular afterload. The presence of bundle branch block can be associated with other conduction defects such as second or third degree AV block.

- Intermittent bundle branch block is predominantly rate-related, usually RBBB, during tachycardia or acute reduction of the R-R interval, which is common during atrial fibrillation.
- Bradycardia-dependent aberrancy has been described. For more, see below on "Etiology" section.
- Alternating bundle branch block between RBBB and LBBB is a sign of conduction system disease and will often progress to complete heart block.

ETIOLOGY

- Bundle branch block can be a result of disease in the His-Purkinje conduction system but can also result from disease or fibrosis surrounding the conduction system (i.e., myocardial infarction), antiarrhythmic drugs, or hyperkalemia. Selected causes of bundle branch block are the following: intracardiac catheter manipulation, myocardial ischemia or infarction, myocarditis, cardiomyopathy, and Lenegre or Lev disease. RBBB in particular is associated with pulmonary hypertension and pulmonary embolism, whereas LBBB can be caused by an anterior myocardial infarction.
- Rate-related branch block in normal hearts is usually seen in tachycardia or in atrial fibrillation where a long R-R interval is followed by a shorter one. This is due to the Ashman phenomenon, where a long cycle length interval causes prolongation in the refractory period resulting in bundle branch block on the subsequent early beat. This is a common property of all cardiac tissues but more evident in the conduction system. The rate-related bundle block is usually RBBB since the right bundle has a longer refractory period than the left bundle for the same heart rate.
- Another phenomenon is bradycardia-dependent aberrancy. This may be due to automaticity in a bundle branch block during diastole leading to BBB on a subsequent beat. Other explanations include vagal tone inhibition or phase 4 block. In phase 4 block the cells have depleted sodium reserves resulting in low resting membrane potentials that impose difficulty in cell excitability, causing conduction block.
- In patients with LBBB, detailed mapping has demonstrated that the site of block is in the proximal left conduction system in 64% of cases.

Dx DIAGNOSIS

DIFFERENTIAL DIAGNOSIS

- Refer to Table 3.
- An accessory pathway can cause an appearance of RBBB or LBBB. If lead V1 is placed higher than the fourth intercostal space or more right than the parasternal area, the EKG can resemble incomplete RBBB.
- An inferior myocardial infarction can resemble left anterior fascicular block.In the inferior myocardial infarction, the inferior leads (II, III, aVF) will have qR or QS morphology, whereas in the left anterior fascicular block they will have rS morphology Left posterior fascicular block can resemble lateral myocardial infarction, right ventricular hypertrophy, dextrocardia, or lateral accessory pathway. Accelerated idioventricular rhythm can resemble LBBB or RBBB, depending on the origin of the ventricular pacemaker site.

WORKUP

- Resting, ambulatory, and exercise electrocardiogram
- Investigation of coexistent comorbidities such as heart failure, myocardial infarction, and cardiomyopathies
- Acute LBBB should prompt investigation for anterior myocardial infarction (Fig. 2) whereas acute RBBB for pulmonary hypertension, or pulmonary embolism (Fig. 3)
- Figs. 2 and 3 illustrate diagnostic evaluations for bundle branch block

LABORATORY TESTS

- Standard laboratory testing appropriate for age, gender, and metabolic abnormalities
- Electrolyte abnormalities and especially hyperkalemia should be excluded

IMAGING STUDIES

Electrocardiogram (Figs. E4 and E5)

Rx TREATMENT

- Treat the underlying cause (Tables 4 and 5).
- In asymptomatic patients with an isolated bundle branch block, no therapy is required.

NONPHARMACOLOGIC THERAPY

Cardiac resynchronization therapy (CRT) with biventricular or His-bundle devices can benefit selected patients with LBBB and depressed EF, if heart failure is present. Permanent pacemaker is appropriate for patients with cardiac syncope or coexisting third degree, or Mobitz type II second degree AV block, when not due to a reversible cause.

ACUTE GENERAL Rx

In acutely established bundle branch block, investigate the cause. In acute LBBB, anterior myocardial infarction should be investigated whereas in acute RBBB investigation should target pulmonary embolism.

CHRONIC Rx

Optimization of potential coexisting comorbidities such as coronary artery disease, heart failure, hyperkalemia, diabetes

DISPOSITION

There is no specific disposition plan for isolated bundle branch block. Entities such as myocardial ischemia or infarction, myocarditis, and cardiomyopathy should be investigated prior to disposition in a new bundle branch block with associated symptoms. Pulmonary embolism should also be investigated in a new RBBB with suspecting symptoms.

REFERRAL

In selected patients at risk for sudden cardiac death such as Brugada syndrome, or in cases of new bundle branch block associated with acute symptoms, referral is indicated.

! PEARLS & CONSIDERATIONS

COMMENTS

Acute LBBB can be caused by anterior myocardial infarction. Acute RBBB can be due to pulmonary

TABLE 3 Differential Diagnosis of Bundle Branch Block

	Right Bundle Branch Block		Left Bundle Branch Block		Hemifascicular Block	
	Incomplete	**Complete**	**Incomplete**	**Complete**	**Left Anterior Fascicular Block**	**Left Posterior Fascicular Block**
QRS Axis	Normal	Normal	Normal or left	Normal or left	Left and >−45°	Right and >+90°
QRS Duration	<120 msec	>120 msec	<120 msec	>130 msec	<120 msec	<120 msec
I	qRs	Deep S	No q wave	Tall R wave, no q wave, no S wave	Positive QRS	rS
aVL	qRs	Deep S		Tall R wave, no q wave, no S wave	qR	rS
II, III, aVF					rS	qR
Precordial Leads	rSR' in V1-V2, qRs in V5-V6	RsR' in V1-V2, deep S in V5-V6	No q wave in V5-V6	QS or rS in V1-V2, tall R wave and no q wave or S wave in V5-V6	Poor R wave progression in V1-V3	
aVR	rsR'				Often tall R wave	

aVF, Augmented vector foot; *aVL*, augmented vector left; *aVR*, augmented vector right.

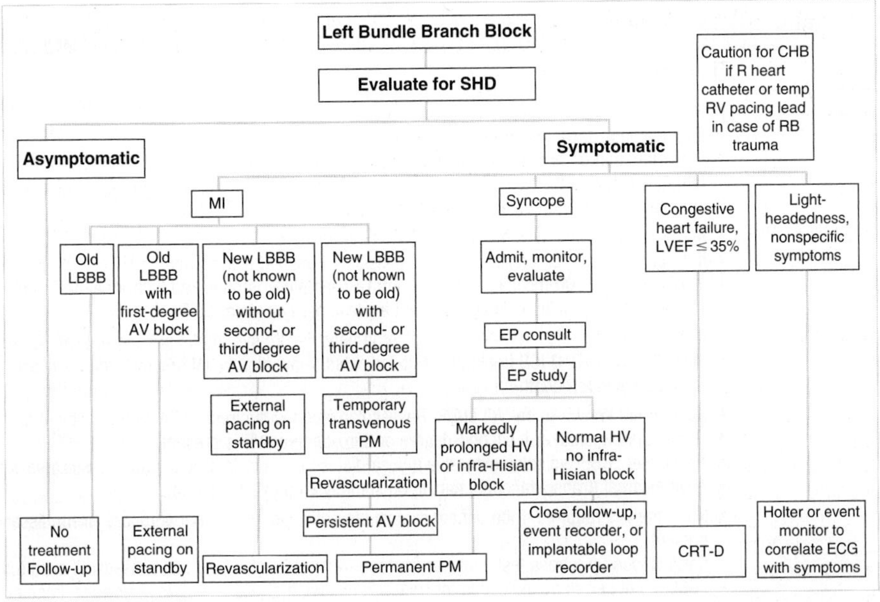

FIG. 2 Left bundle branch block. *AV,* Atrioventricular; *CHB,* complete heart block; *CRT-D,* cardiac resynchronization therapy combined with a defibrillator; *ECG,* electrocardiogram; *EP,* electrophysiology; *HV,* histoventricular; *LBBB,* left bundle branch block; *LVEF,* left ventricular ejection fraction; *MI,* myocardial infarction; *PM,* pacemaker; *RB,* right bundle; *RV,* right ventricular; *SHD,* structural heart disease (no overt evidence of myocardial, valvular, congenital, or coronary heart disease). (From Olshansky B et al: *Arrhythmia essentials,* ed 2, Philadelphia, 2017, Elsevier.)

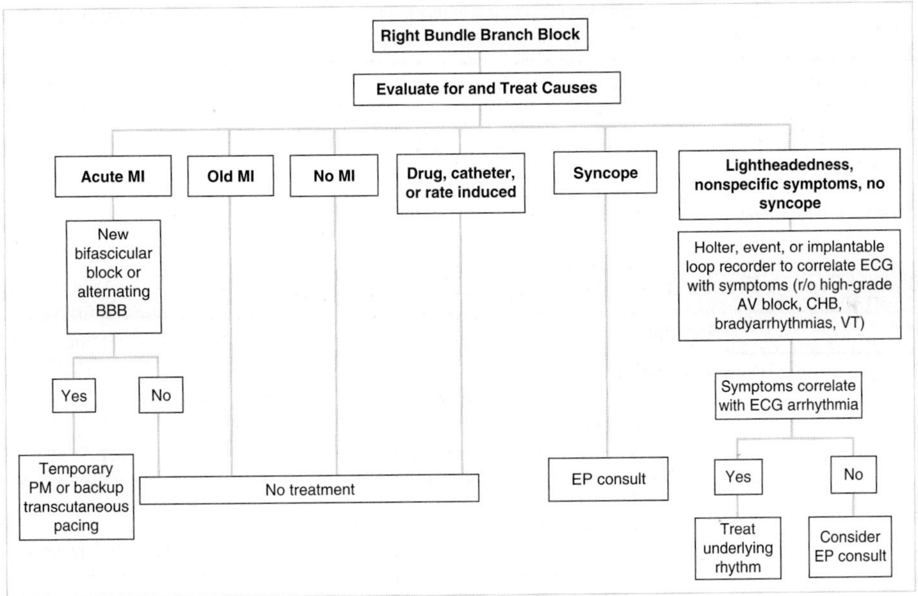

FIG. 3 Right bundle branch block. *AV,* Atrioventricular; *BBB,* bundle branch block; *CHB,* complete heart block; *ECG,* electrocardiogram; *EP,* electrophysiology; *MI,* myocardial infarction; *PM,* pacemaker; *VT,* ventricular tachycardia. (From Olshansky B et al: *Arrhythmia essentials,* ed 2, Philadelphia, 2017, Elsevier.)

embolism. Bundle branch block is a normal variant, especially in young individuals. History and physical exam are needed to identify associated cardiac abnormalities. In patients with heart failure and depressed ejection fraction, cardiac resynchronization is beneficial in the presence of LBBB but not in the presence of RBBB.

PREVENTION

Modification of associated comorbidities such as optimization of heart failure, coronary artery disease, hypertension, and diabetes.

PATIENT & FAMILY EDUCATION

Bundle branch block is a problem in the heart's electrical system. There are several types, but clinically the most important is the left bundle branch block in which one of the two main "wires" in the heart is not functioning correctly. As a result, the heart's pumping chambers are squeezing out of sync and can worsen the heart's ability to pump in people with heart failure. It is more common in older adults and people with serious heart disease.

SUGGESTED READINGS

Available at ExpertConsult.com

RELATED CONTENT

Atrioventricular Dissociation (Related Key Topic)
Brugada Syndrome (Related Key Topic)
Heart Failure (Related Key Topic)
Intraventricular Conduction Delay (Related Key Topic)
Myocardial Infarction (Related Key Topic)
Pulmonary Embolism (Related Key Topic)

AUTHORS: **Ioannis Koulouridis, MD, MS,** and **John Wylie, MD, FACC**

TABLE 4 Left Bundle Branch Block Management

Setting	Therapy
Asymptomatic normal LV function	• No therapy—rule out structural heart disease, ischemic heart disease. • Requires long-term follow-up. • If instrumentation of the right ventricle is planned, be ready to temporarily pace (preferably externally or via a temporary pacemaker wire) if transient traumatic RBBB with resultant complete AVB is induced. • Trauma to the right bundle can last from minutes to more than 24 hours.
Symptomatic (syncope, lightheadedness)	• Admit, monitor, and evaluate for structural heart disease. • If syncope occurs, EP consultation and possible EP testing is indicated. • If HV interval is 100 msec or more or if infra-Hisian block is provoked with atrial pacing at rates of <160 bpm with or without procainamide challenge, implant a permanent pacemaker.
Symptomatic cardiomyopathy (CHF)	• If LVEF is 35% or less, NYHA class II, III, or IV heart failure symptoms are present with LBBB with QRS duration of more than 130 ms: CRT-D ICD implantation is indicated (may improve LV function, reduce heart failure symptoms, and reduce the risk of sudden death).
Myocardial infarction	• New (or not known to be old) LBBB: Revascularization with direct PTCA with or without stent. • Temporary pacemaker if second-degree or third-degree AVB is present. • New onset LBBB indicates extensive myocardial ischemia or infarction and is associated with worse prognosis. • Have external (transcutaneous) pacing on standby if no AVB is present.
Preoperative	• No therapy is required if the patient is asymptomatic, whether or not coronary artery disease or systolic dysfunction is present. • Cardiac workup (stress test, echocardiogram) to exclude structural heart disease if symptomatic. • LBBB is not per se an indication for treadmill testing. If stress testing is performed, imaging must accompany the test if the aim is to document the presence of obstructive coronary artery disease; imaging is not required if the aim of the stress test is the assessment of effort tolerance.
Postoperative	• No therapy if asymptomatic. • Common after aortic valve replacement (usually persistent) and after CABG (transient due to cardioplegia).
Alternating LBBB and RBBB	• Alternating BBB may be due to trifascicular disease • Because of the high rate of progression to CHB, permanent pacemaker implantation is advised. • Alternating BBB may also be seen as a digitalis toxic rhythm, although in current practice this occurs only rarely.

AVB, Atrioventricular block; *BBB,* bundle branch block; *CABG,* coronary artery bypass graft; *CHB,* complete atrioventricular block; *CHF,* congestive heart failure; *CRT-D,* cardiac resynchronization and defibrillation therapy; *EP,* electrophysiology; *HV,* histoventricular; *ICD,* implantable cardioverter defibrillator; *LBBB,* left bundle branch block; *LV,* left ventricular; *LVEF,* left ventricular ejection fraction; *NYHA,* New York Heart Association; *PTCA,* percutaneous transluminal coronary angioplasty; *RBBB,* right bundle branch block.
From Olshansky B et al: *Arrhythmia essentials,* ed 2, Philadelphia, 2017, Elsevier.

TABLE 5 Right Bundle Branch Block Management

Setting	Therapy
Outpatient asymptomatic	• No therapy • May occur with instrumentation of the right ventricle (e.g., Swan-Ganz catheter) and trauma to the right bundle • Can last up to 24 h
Symptomatic (syncope)	• Admit the patient with RBBB who has syncope • If symptoms of syncope occur (may be related to AVB or VT), attempt to correlate symptoms with rhythm by Holter or event monitoring • Evaluate for underlying structural cardiac disease • Consider EP testing to assess AV conduction and the presence of inducible VT (present in up to 30% of symptomatic RBBB patients) if the patient is syncopal

MI	• Isolated RBBB: No therapy
	• RBBB with LAFB or LPFB (that is new or not known to be old) or alternating BBB:
	  • Temporary pacemaker
	  • Alternatively, placement of a transcutaneous pacing system
	• RBBB occurs in 3%-7% of MIs, often with LAFB, and usually because of anterior or anteroseptal infarction
	• The combination is less common in the current era of early revascularization via percutaneous techniques

Preoperative	• No therapy—temporary pacemaker not required • Perform cardiac evaluation to exclude other cardiovascular disease
Postoperative	• No treatment • Most common conduction disturbance in this setting
Alternating LBBB and RBBB	• Permanent pacemaker if not due to reversible cause

AV, Atrioventricular; *AVB,* atrioventricular block; *BBB,* bundle branch block; *EP,* electrophysiology; *LAFB,* left anterior fascicular block; *LBBB,* left bundle branch block; *LPFB,* left posterior fascicular block; *MI,* myocardial infarction; *RBBB,* right bundle branch block; *VT,* ventricular tachycardia.
From Olshansky B et al: *Arrhythmia essentials,* ed 2, Philadelphia, 2017, Elsevier.

BASIC INFORMATION

DEFINITION

- Cutaneous burns can be classified by type of injury (e.g., thermal vs. chemical), burn depth (e.g., first, second, third degree), extent of burn (total burn surface area [TBSA]), and burn severity (e.g., minor vs. major). Types of burn injury include thermal (flames, scalds, hot contactants), chemical, electrical, and radiation burns. This chapter will focus on thermal and electrical burns.
- Burns can affect skin and respiratory, ocular, oral, and genital mucosa.

SYNONYMS

Thermal injury
Chemical injury
Electrical injury
Radiation injury

ICD-10CM CODES

T29.0	Burns of multiple regions, unspecified degree
T30.0	Burn of unspecified body region, unspecified degree
T30.1	Burn of first degree, body region unspecified
T30.2	Burn of second degree, body region unspecified
T30.3	Burn of third degree, body region unspecified
T31.0	Burns involving less than 10% of body surface
T31.1	Burns involving 10%-19% of body surface
T31.2	Burns involving 20%-29% of body surface
T31.3	Burns involving 30%-39% of body surface
T31.4	Burns involving 40%-49% of body surface
T31.5	Burns involving 50%-59% of body surface

EPIDEMIOLOGY & DEMOGRAPHICS

PREVALENCE (IN U.S.):

- More than 1.2 million individuals experience burns in the U.S., and burn injuries account for approximately 500,000 emergency department visits, with 9% (45,000) requiring hospitalization and 0.8% (4000) resulting in death annually.
- Of thermal injury, scald burn from liquid is most common—followed by flame, flash burn, and then contact burn.

PREDOMINANT AGE & SEX: Children ages 2 to 4 yr have the greatest frequency of burns (most commonly scald burns), with male adolescent and young adults ages 17 to 25 with second greatest frequency (most commonly from flammable liquids).

PHYSICAL FINDINGS & CLINICAL PRESENTATION

- It is important to note that burns occur unevenly, often with various depths (Table 1)
- First-degree (superficial) burns: Penetrate epidermis only (minimal barrier loss)
  1. Very painful, intact, erythematous skin with minimal to no edema and no blistering
- Second-degree (partial-thickness) burns: Epidermis and part of dermis is affected
  1. Moist, very painful skin with edema and blistering/blebs
  2. Superficial partial-thickness burns: Cherry red with two-point discrimination intact, incredibly painful
  3. Deep partial-thickness burns: Mottled white and cherry red; only the sensation of pressure is intact in these areas
- Third-degree (full-thickness) burns: Entire epidermis and dermis are affected, with destruction of hair follicles and sweat glands
  1. The skin is dry, charred, pale, painless, and leathery; charred vessels may be visible beneath, little or no pain, and hair pulls out easily

Dx DIAGNOSIS

DIFFERENTIAL DIAGNOSIS

Cultural practices leading to burnlike lesions in distinctive patterns (e.g., cupping, coining, moxibustion), cellulitis, Stevens-Johnson syndrome/toxic epidermolytic necrolysis

CLASSIFICATION

- Burns are classified by (1) depth of injury, (2) extent of injury, and (3) severity, according to the American Burn Association.
- Depth of injury (see Table 1):
  1. Indicates how the wound will heal and whether grafting will be needed.
- Extent of TBSA:
  1. The TBSA is best classified by using age-specific burn charts and the "rule of nines" (Fig. 1).
  2. For scattered burns, utilizing patient's palm including fingers to equate 1% body surface area can be helpful.
  3. TBSA indicates how aggressively the patient will need to be resuscitated.
- Severity: Determined by burn depth, TBSA, age, location, type of injury, and presence/absence of coexisting conditions. Severity classification helps triage patients to outpatient, inpatient, or burn unit care (see Table 2).
  1. Minor burns: Outpatient management
  2. Moderate burns: Admission to hospital with experience managing burns or burn center referral
  3. Major burns: Referral to burn center

LABORATORY STUDIES (MODERATE OR MAJOR BURNS)

- CBC, electrolytes, BUN, creatinine, glucose, liver function tests, venous blood gas, blood coagulation, and type and screen in anticipation of blood transfusion
- *If smoke inhalation expected:* Serial ABG carboxyhemoglobin and continuous ECG
- *If electrical burn or if concern for rhabdomyolysis:* Urinalysis, urine myoglobin, and CPK levels

TABLE 1 Categorization of Burn by Depth

Burn Type	Histologic Depth	Clinical Presentation	Treatment	Healing Time/Prognosis
1st degree	Epidermis	Erythematous but intact skin, no blisters, pain may range in severity	Topical salves, cold compresses, NSAIDs for pain control	2-5 days with no scarring
Superficial 2nd degree (partial thickness)	Papillary dermis	Erythematous with superficial blisters, intense pain	Topical antimicrobials with gauze dressing or biosynthetic dressing (if widespread), pain control	5-21 days with no grafting
Deep 2nd degree (partial thickness)	Reticular dermis	Erythematous with superficial/deep blisters, range of pain depending on nerve involvement	Same	21-35 days with no infection; if infected, converts to full-thickness burn
3rd degree (full thickness)	Through dermis to subcutaneous tissue. Can involve fascia, muscle, and bone	White or black, possible eschar, may or may not be painful depending on nerve damage	Usually requires grafting, may require resuscitation depending on TBSA affected, pain control	Large areas require grafting, but small areas may heal from the edges after wks

NSAID, Nonsteroidal antiinflammatory drug; *TBSA,* total body surface area.
From Kliegman RM et al: *Nelson textbook of pediatrics,* ed 19, Philadelphia, 2011, Saunders; and Kessides MC, Skelsey MK: Management of acute partial-thickness burns, *Cutis* 86:249-257, 2010.

- *If severe lactic acidosis:* Consider checking cyanide level

IMAGING STUDIES

- If smoke inhalation suspected: Chest radiograph and bronchoscopy
- If high-voltage electrical burn: Cardiac monitoring first 24 hours

Rx TREATMENT

ACUTE GENERAL Rx

MINOR BURNS (FIRST-DEGREE BURNS AND SECOND/THIRD-DEGREE BURNS OF LIMITED TBSA):

- Outpatient management: "6 Cs"
  1. Clothing: Remove hot or burned clothing.
  2. Cooling: Cool (approximately 54° F [12.22° C]) for 10 to 30 min (under faucet or compress) to reduce edema/pain by conducting heat away from skin. Not recommended with extensive burns due to theoretical risk of hypothermia and shock. No ice packs.
  3. Cleaning: Wash gently with mild alcohol-free soap, then normal saline daily. Remove all old ointment and any loose skin. Blot dry. No evidence supports vigorous cleansing with antiseptic solutions. Embedded materials should be removed by copious irrigation using a large-gauge syringe.
  4. Chemoprophylaxis: Tetanus immunization (all deep second- and third-degree burns). Routine skin cultures are NOT recommended except when wound infection suspected, and prophylactic systemic antibiotics are NOT recommended. All second- and third-degree burns are treated with a topical antimicrobial agent. This may include silver sulfadiazine, bacitracin, bismuth-impregnated Vaseline gauze, or silver-impregnated synthetic dressings.
  5. Covering: All second- and third-degree burns should be covered with sterile dressing. If financial resources are limited, instead of gauze, can purchase cotton gloves, T-shirts, or similar at discount stores, wash, and reuse.
  6. Comfort: Analgesics (Tylenol and NSAIDs—alone or in combination with opioids) around the clock are recommended. Additional "rescue" analgesics before dressing changes and physical activity recommended.

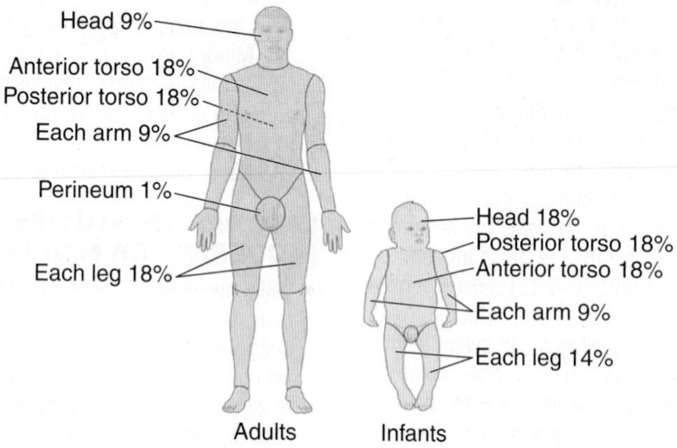

FIG. 1 The "rule of nines" for estimating second-degree and third-degree burns. Because infants have significantly larger heads and smaller legs than do adults, different rules must be used in evaluating these patients. A simple, practical rule is that the palm of the patient's hand, with fingers, equals 1% of the total body area. (From Ferri F: *Practical guide to the care of the medical patient,* ed 9, St Louis, 2014, Elsevier.)

MODERATE AND MAJOR BURNS (SECOND/THIRD-DEGREE BURNS OF EXTENSIVE TBSA):

- Patients with moderate/major burns (Fig. 1) should be admitted to the hospital or referred to a burn center. Indications for hospitalization for burns are described in Table 2. Burn care can be compartmentalized into four main phases: Initial assessment and triage (phase I), resuscitation (phase II), burn wound coverage and critical care (phase III), and rehabilitation (phase IV) (Fig. 2).
  1. Assessment of ABCs: Establish airway and assess breathing (inspect for inhalation injury and intubate for suspected airway edema, often seen 12 to 24 hours later); O_2; establish circulation (place two large-bore peripheral IV lines, ECG).
  2. IV fluid resuscitation: Various fluid resuscitation formulas have been proposed and used to guide burn providers. These formulas each estimate the amount each patient may require during the course of a 24- to 48-hour postburn resuscitation period. The goal is to maintain optimal end-organ perfusion during this time with volume replacement at the lowest physiologic cost. Parkland formula (Ringer lactate at 2 to 4 ml/kg per % TBSA per 24 hours with half the calculated fluid given in the first 8 hours) is an effective modality in severe burns (Fig. 3) and has been commonly used. Once fluid resuscitation is initiated, the crystalloid rate should be titrated up or down on a regular basis while maintaining a urine output of around 0.5 to 1.0 ml/kg/h in adults. Various algorithms and clinical protocols have been proposed. One such algorithm is depicted in Fig. 4. The goal of burn resuscitation is to provide adequate fluid necessary to avoid end-organ failure while avoiding "fluid creep." Rescue therapy in the form of colloid infusion with albumin has been described as "colloid rescue." The military's Joint Trauma System Clinical Practice Guidelines recommend that 5%

TABLE 2 Classification of Burns by Severity and Indications for Hospitalization or Burn Center Referral

Criteria	Minor Burn	Moderate Burn	Major Burn
Total body surface area (%)	All 1st degree burns <10% adults <5% children or elderly <2% for 3rd degree	2nd degree burns 10%-20% adults, 5%-10% in children or elderly 2%-5% 3rd degree	All 1st degree burns >20% adults, >10% children and elderly >5% 3rd degree
Type of burn injury		Low-voltage burn Suspected inhalation injury	High-voltage burn Chemical burn Known
Location		Circumferential burn	Clinically significant burn to face, eyes, ears, genitalia, over joints
Coexisting conditions		Concomitant medical problem predisposing to infection (e.g., diabetes, sickle cell anemia)	Significant associated injuries (e.g., fracture, other major trauma)
	Outpatient management	Inpatient management—consider referral to burn center*	Referral to burn center

*Per the American Burn Association (ABA), any partial-thickness burn >10% total body surface area or any factors listed in moderate or major burn category warrant referral to burn center. Additional factors per the ABA include burned children in a hospital without qualified personnel or equipment for the care of children and burn injury in a patient who will require special social, emotional, or rehabilitative intervention (including suspected child abuse).

Modified from Singer AJ, Dagum AB: Current management of acute cutaneous wounds, *N Engl J Med* 359 (10):1037-1046, 2008.

albumin should be initiated as early as 8 hours after a burn if certain conditions are met. These conditions include that the hourly IV fluid rate exceeds 1500 ml/h or the projected 24-hour total fluid volume approaches 250 ml/kg.

3. Baseline neurologic and vascular assessment.
4. Foley catheter and NG tube (20% of patients develop an ileus): Urine output 30 ml/h.
5. Optimize nutritional support: Mayes equations to calculate energy requirements after burn (Box 1).

- Frequent reassessment in the first 24 to 72 hours, as wound depth can change significantly.

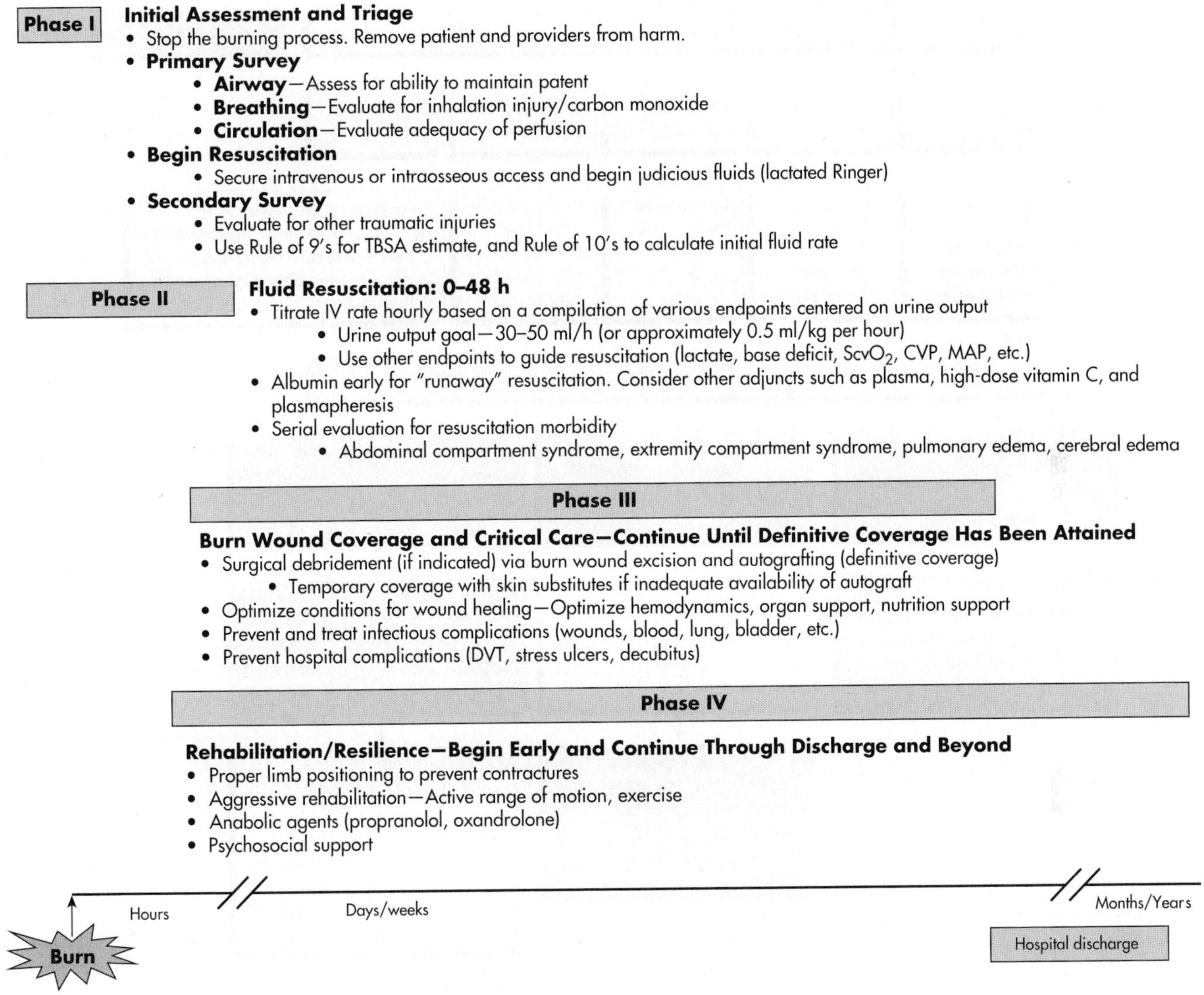

FIG. 2 The four major phases of burn care. Initial assessment and triage (phase I), resuscitation (phase II), burn wound coverage and critical care (phase III), and rehabilitation (phase IV). *CVP,* Central venous pressure; *DVT,* deep vein thromboses; *IV,* intravenous; *MAP,* mean arterial pressure; *ScvO2,* central venous oxygen saturation; *TBSA,* total body surface area. (From Parrillo JE, Dellinger RP: *Critical care medicine, principles of diagnosis and management in the adult,* ed 5, Philadelphia, 2019, Elsevier.)

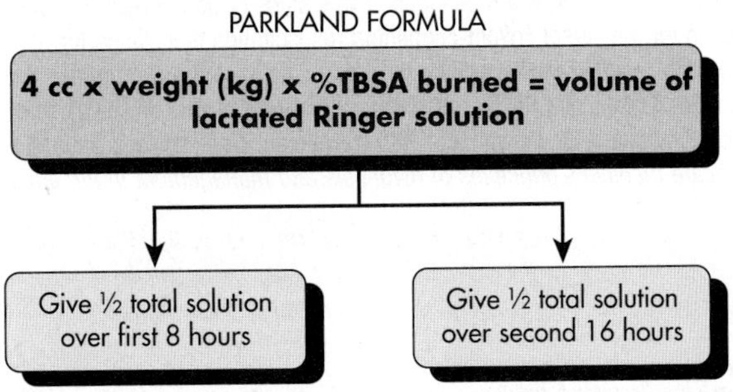

FIG. 3 Parkland formula. *TBSA,* Total body surface area. (From Cameron JL, Cameron AM: *Current surgical therapy,* ed 12, Philadelphia, 2017, Elsevier.)

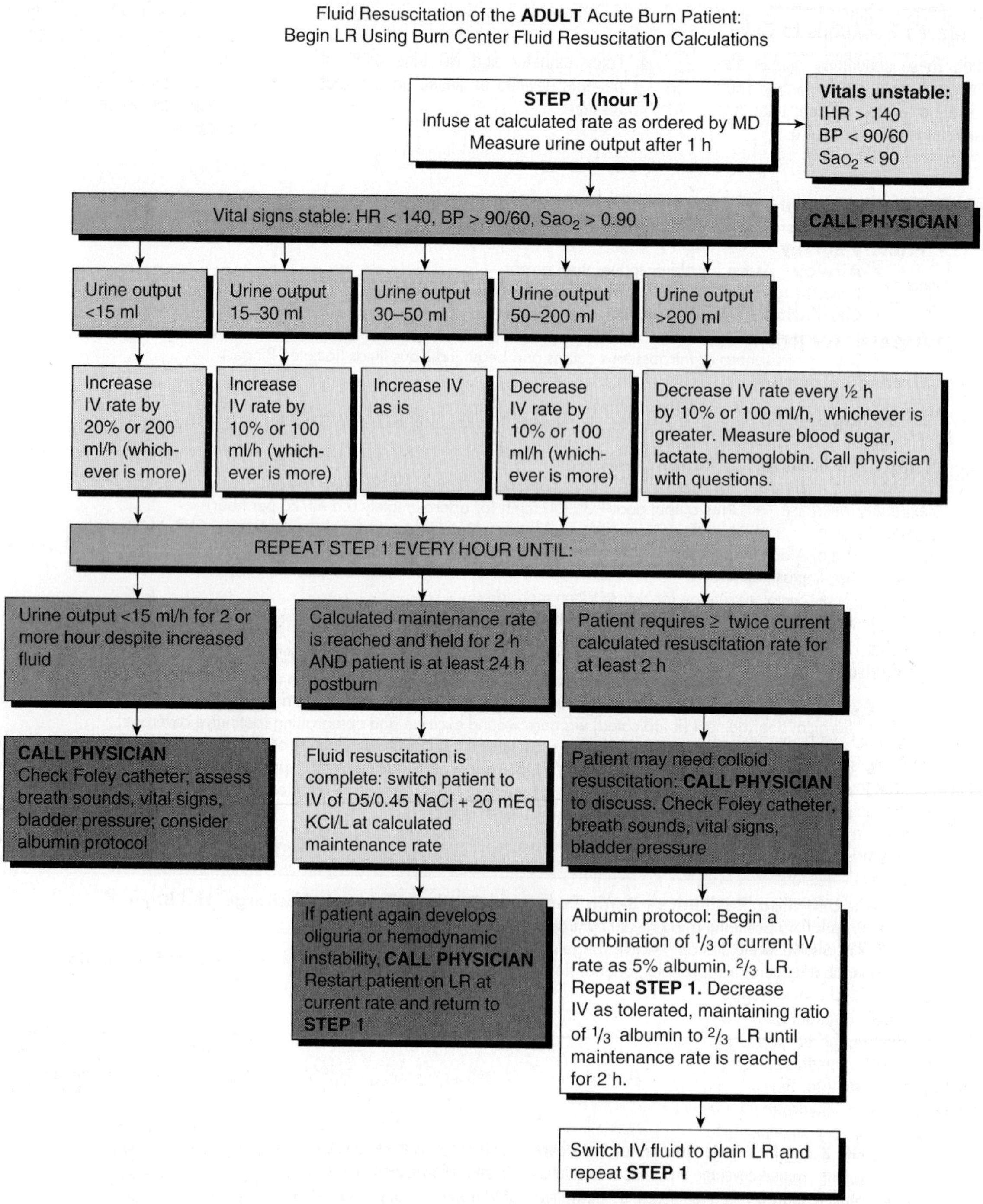

FIG. 4 Burn fluid resuscitation protocol used at the University of Utah. Physicians order an initial infusion rate of lactated Ringer solution based on Parkland formula calculations and indicate the target maintenance rate. The nursing staff measures hourly urine output and increases or decreases fluids based on this response. If patients experience unexpected changes in vital signs or do not respond appropriately, physicians are contacted. An option for the use of colloid-containing resuscitation is included for patients whose requirements fail to decline. This regimen permits close titration of fluids without requiring hourly physician input. *BP,* Blood pressure; *D5/0.45,* glucose 5.0% and sodium chloride 0.45%; *HR,* heart rate; *IHR,* intrinsic heart rate; *IV,* intravenous; *LR,* lactated Ringer solution; *MD,* physician; *Sao₂,* oxygen saturation. (From Parrillo JE, Dellinger RP: *Critical care medicine, principles of diagnosis and management in the adult,* ed 5, Philadelphia, 2019, Elsevier.)

BOX 1 Mayes Equations to Calculate Energy Requirement After a Burn

Mayes equation for a 5- to 10-yr-old burn patient with injury <50% TBSA:

$$818 + 37.4\,(\text{weight in kilograms}) + 9.3 \times \text{TBSA burn}$$

Mayes equation for a 5.5-yr-old patient with a 45% TBSA scald burn weighing 20 kg:

$$818 + 37.4\,(20\text{ kg}) + 9.3 \times 45\text{ TBSA scald}$$

$$818 + 748 + 481.5 = 2047.5\text{ calories / day}$$

TBSA, Total body surface area.
From Fuhrman BP et al: *Pediatric critical care,* ed 4, Philadelphia, 2011, Saunders.

BURN WOUND CARE BY BURN DEPTH Rx

GENERAL:

- Vigilant wound care with dressings to prevent evaporation and minimize threat of wound colonization and infection of nonintact skin
- Daily activity necessary to maintain function of burned extremity, decrease pain and swelling, and promote healing
- First-degree burns (skin intact):
  1. *Dressing:* None required (except to protect from injury); topical antibacterial agents NOT recommended
  2. *Other:* Emollients, cool compresses (avoid ice), if pruritic, trial of antihistamines
  3. *Prognosis:* Heals within 1 wk without scarring; may heal with pigmentary changes (limit by sunscreen and sun avoidance of area for 1 yr)
- Second-degree (superficial partial-thickness) burns without adherent exudate or eschar:
  1. *Blisters:* Sharp debridement of ruptured blisters; leave intact blisters. Quicker healing and reduced infections when intact blisters are not disturbed. Consider unroofing blisters that show no sign of resorption over several wks or contain cloudy fluid.
  2. *Dressing:* Topical antimicrobial ointment (e.g., Bactroban) or petrolatum A&D ointment with nonadherent dressing twice a day. Alternate: Biosynthetic dressing (alginates, hydrofibers, or foam dressings)—many with silver as antimicrobial (absorb exudates, maintain moist environment, require fewer dressing changes, which reduces pain/anxiety).
  3. *Prognosis:* Heals with minimal scarring in 10 to 14 days. May heal with pigmentary changes (reduced with sunscreen and sun avoidance of area for 1 yr).
- Second-degree (deep partial-thickness) burns with adherent exudates; localized third-degree burns; cellulitic wounds:
  1. *Dressing:* Silver sulfadiazine 1%: Broader spectrum, better penetration of necrotic tissue than Bactroban, but inhibits epithelialization and promotes hypertrophic scarring in studies. Must stop use once exudates and eschar have separated from wound. Alternative: Enzymatic debrider (e.g., Santyl or Accuzyme)—chemically debrides devitalized tissue without harming healthy tissue.
  2. *Referral:* Burn specialist for consultation regarding need for excision and grafting.
  3. *Prognosis:* Deep second-degree burns heal with significant scarring, often take 3 to 4 wk to heal. If infected, convert to third-degree burns. Third-degree burns typically require skin graft, but small areas may heal from edges after wks.

DISPOSITION/FOLLOW-UP CARE

- Outpatient: Evaluate next day to assess level of injury, level of pain, and ability to manage dressing changes on own. If insufficient, daily evaluation until complete wound epithelialization recommended. Epithelialization: Tiny islands of epithelialization throughout wound. If no epithelialization after 2 wk, or subsequent evaluation reveals third-degree burn, referral to burn surgeon recommended. Box E2 describes common complications in burn patients.
- Following re-epithelialization, visits every 4 to 6 wk to monitor for hypertrophic scar formation (early referral to burn/scar specialist if occurs).
- Mortality rates higher in patients >60 yr of age, with burns >40% TBSA, or with inhalation injury. Long-term risk of developing squamous cell carcinoma of the skin within burn injury. Long-term skin monitoring necessary.

REFERRAL

Consultation of dermatology and burn specialist or burn center referral per Table 2.

PEARLS & CONSIDERATIONS

COMMENTS

- In circumferential skin burns, look for compartment syndrome of limbs (e.g., tightening, progressive deterioration of peripheral motor and sensory exam findings, severe pain, and loss of arterial Doppler signals). Escharotomy may be necessary.
- If child abuse is suspected, social services at the hospital or child protective services must be contacted.
- Fig. E5 describes an algorithm for the treatment of chemical burns.

SUGGESTED READINGS

Available at ExpertConsult.com

RELATED CONTENT

Burns (Patient Information)
Electrical and Lightning Injury (Related Key Topic)

AUTHOR: **Lisa Pappas-Taffer, MD**

Calcium Pyrophosphate Deposition Disease (Pseudogout) PTG ALG

BASIC INFORMATION

DEFINITION

Calcium pyrophosphate dihydrate crystal deposition (CPPD) disease refers to the precipitation of calcium pyrophosphate dihydrate (CPP) in connective tissues that may be asymptomatic or may be associated with several clinical syndromes, including acute and chronic arthritis. CPP was formerly abbreviated and commonly referred to as "CPPD," but the abbreviation is now reserved for "CPP deposition." Alternative names (Table 1) representing specific clinical or radiographic features of CPPD disease include pseudogout, chondrocalcinosis, and pyrophosphate arthropathy.

Pseudogout/acute CPP crystal arthritis is used to describe acute attacks of CPP crystal-induced arthritis that clinically resembles the arthritis that is commonly encountered in gout. The term *acute CPP crystal arthritis* is now preferred in place of *pseudogout.*

Chondrocalcinosis (CC) refers to radiographic calcification in hyaline cartilage and/or fibrocartilage and does not confirm the diagnosis of CPP-related arthritis as it can be present in other types of crystal deposition diseases or be asymptomatic.

Pyrophosphate arthropathy is the term used for a chronic structural arthropathy related to CPP deposition.

SYNONYMS

Calcium pyrophosphate dihydrate crystal deposition disease
CPP crystal deposition disease
CPPD
Chondrocalcinosis (CC)
Pseudogout
Pyrophosphate arthropathy

ICD-10CM CODES
M11.2 Other chondrocalcinosis
M11.9 Crystal arthropathy, unspecified
M11.8 Other specified crystal arthropathies
M11.1 Familial chondrocalcinosis

EPIDEMIOLOGY & DEMOGRAPHICS

PREVALENCE:
- The epidemiology of CPPD crystal deposition is described in Table 2.
- Most linked with advancing age (average age of 72).

GENETICS: Familial forms
- Associated with *ANKH* (ankylosis human) gene, which functions to transport inorganic pyrophosphate (PPi) out of cells, or the osteoprotegerin gene (TNFRSF11B).
- Familial mutations can increase extracellular PPi levels and lead to onset of CPPD disease in the third or fourth decade of life.

PHYSICAL FINDINGS & CLINICAL PRESENTATION

- *Acute CPP crystal arthritis/pseudogout:* Monoarticular attacks most commonly involve the knee and wrist but can be polyarticular (Fig. E1). Patients, especially the elderly, can have systemic manifestations such as fever and altered mental status. Situations that may trigger acute CPPD crystal arthritis are described in Box E1
- Asymptomatic disease ("asymptomatic CPPD")
- Pseudogout (acute CPP crystal arthritis)
- Pseudo-RA (chronic CPP crystal inflammatory arthritis): Symmetric polyarthritis
- Pseudo-OA, with or without superimposed acute attacks (OA with CPPD)
- Pseudo-neuropathic joint disease
- Crowned-dens syndrome caused by crystal deposition in the ligamentum flavum of the cervical spine, either asymptomatic or causing acute neck pain
- Pseudo-polymyalgia rheumatica (pseudo-PMR): Pain and stiffness in the neck and shoulder girdle mimicking PMR

ETIOLOGY

- Idiopathic
- Familial
- Trauma
- Metabolic and endocrine disorders (Table 3): Hyperparathyroidism, hypophosphatasia, hemochromatosis, hypomagnesemia, Gitelman syndrome, Bartter syndrome, gout, ochronosis, acromegaly, Wilson disease, familial hypocalciuric hypercalcemia, X-linked hypophosphatemic rickets

Dx DIAGNOSIS

DIFFERENTIAL DIAGNOSIS

- Gouty arthritis (Table 4)
- Septic arthritis
- RA
- Spondyloarthritis (ReA, PsA)
- PMR

Table 5 describes metabolic diseases predisposing to CPPD disposition. Section II describes the differential diagnosis of acute monoarticular and oligoarticular arthritis and crystal-induced arthritides. An algorithm for evaluation and treatment of CPPD is shown in Fig. 2.

LABORATORY TESTS

- Arthrocentesis with presence of weakly positive birefringent rhomboid-shaped crystals by compensated polarized light microscopy (Fig. E3).
- Synovial fluid should always be analyzed for cell count with differential, crystals, Gram stain, and culture because acute CPP crystal arthritis/pseudogout and septic arthritis can co-exist.
- Evaluate for possible metabolic causes, especially in younger patients aged <55 yr or patients with florid polyarticular disease. Box 2 describes screening blood tests for metabolic diseases associated with CPPD crystal deposition.

IMAGING STUDIES

- Plain radiographs (Figs. E4, E5, and E6) often reveal CC located parallel to subchondral bone.
  1. Classic locations for CC (Fig. E1) include knee menisci (Fig. E7), wrist triangular fibrocartilage, symphysis pubis, and glenoid and acetabular labra.
- Musculoskeletal ultrasound can detect deposition of CPP crystals within the hyaline

TABLE 1 Nomenclature of Calcium Pyrophosphate and Associated Syndromes

Definition	Old Terms	EULAR Recommendations	Preferred Term (Abbreviation)
Radiographic correlate of CPPD	Chondrocalcinosis, chondrocalcinosis articularis	Chondrocalcinosis	Chondrocalcinosis (CC)
Acute inflammatory arthritis caused by CPP crystals	Pseudogout	Acute CPP crystal arthritis	Acute CPP crystal arthritis
Calcium pyrophosphate dihydrate crystals	Calcium pyrophosphate dehydrate; calcium pyrophosphate dihydrate	Calcium pyrophosphate crystals	Calcium pyrophosphate crystals (CPP crystals)
All clinical syndromes associated with CPP crystals	Calcium pyrophosphate dihydrate deposition disease	None	Calcium pyrophosphate deposition disease (CPPD)
Chronic arthritis caused by CPP crystals ± inflammation	Calcium pyrophosphate dihydrate deposition disease: Pyrophosphate arthropathy; pseudorheumatoid arthritis; pseudoosteoarthritis	Chronic CPP crystal arthritis, OA with CPPD	Chronic CPP crystal arthritis, OA with CPPD
Deposition of calcium pyrophosphate crystals in joints or tissue with or without clinical symptoms	Calcium pyrophosphate dihydrate deposition	CPPD	Calcium pyrophosphate deposition (CPPD)

CPP, Calcium pyrophosphate; *CPPD,* calcium pyrophosphate dihydrate crystal deposition disease; *EULAR,* European League Against Rheumatism; *OA,* osteoarthritis.
From Hochberg MC: *Rheumatology*, ed 7, Philadelphia, 2019, Elsevier.

TABLE 2 Epidemiology of Calcium Pyrophosphate Dihydrate Crystal Deposition

Age Association	Rises with Age
Sex distribution	(F:M) 1:1
Chondrocalcinosis prevalence	8.1% (age range 63-93)
Pyrophosphate arthropathy prevalence	3.4% (age range 40-89)
Geography	Appears ubiquitous
Genetic associations	Mutations of *ANKH* gene on chromosome 5p (CCAL2) and unknown genes on chromosome 8q (CCAL1)

From Hochberg MC et al: *Rheumatology,* ed 5, St Louis, 2011, Mosby.

cartilage and/or fibrocartilage. In contrast to urate crystal deposits in gout, CPP crystals often deposit within the substance of the hyaline cartilage and fibrocartilage, providing a means to distinguish CPP from urate deposition that occurs on the surface of the hyaline cartilage as seen in gout (Fig. E8).

- Early studies suggest that dual-energy CT scan can differentiate mineral deposits through color-coded images and may aid in the diagnosis of CPPD from other crystal arthropathies.

Rx TREATMENT

NONPHARMACOLOGIC THERAPY

General measures such as immobilization of inflamed joint

ACUTE GENERAL Rx

- Monoarticular pseudogout:
  1. Aspiration followed by intraarticular corticosteroid injection (often superior to systemic treatment in the elderly)
- Polyarticular pseudogout:
  1. Oral corticosteroids, colchicine, or NSAIDs, if not contraindicated

CHRONIC GENERAL Rx

Prophylaxis: Colchicine 0.6 mg twice daily or once daily as tolerated

- Pseudo-RA or refractory disease: Hydroxychloroquine or methotrexate
- Anakinra (Interleukin-1 receptor antagonist): Treatment and prophylaxis of polyarticular acute CPP crystal arthritis unresponsive to oral corticosteroids
- Treat underlying metabolic disease
- Management options for CPPD are summarized in Boxes E3 and E4

DISPOSITION

Structural joint damage may occasionally occur, requiring arthroplasty in rare cases.

REFERRAL

Rheumatology

PEARLS & CONSIDERATIONS

COMMENTS

Acute CPP crystal arthritis/pseudogout attacks have been reported to occur in the setting of surgical procedures, diuresis, bisphosphonate administration, and hyaluronate joint injections.

SUGGESTED READINGS

Available at ExpertConsult.com

RELATED CONTENT

Pseudogout (Patient Information)
Gout (Related Key Topic)

AUTHORS: **Nicole B. Yang, MD,** and **Anthony M. Reginato, PhD, MD**

TABLE 3 Diseases Associated with Calcium Pyrophosphate Dihydrate Crystal Deposition Disease

Disease	Strength of Evidence for a Link with CPPD	Recommended Testing
Hyperparathyroidism	Strong	Calcium, parathyroid hormone level
Hemochromatosis	Strong	Fe, TIBC, ferritin, C282Y
Hypophosphatasia	Strong	Alkaline phosphatase
Hypomagnesemia	Strong	Magnesium
Gout	Strong	Synovianalysis
Rheumatoid arthritis	Moderate	Clinical judgement
Osteoporosis	Moderate	Bone density if warranted

CPPD, Calcium pyrophosphate dihydrate crystal deposition disease; *TIBC,* total iron-binding capacity.
From Hochberg MC: *Rheumatology,* ed 7, Philadelphia, 2019, Elsevier.

TABLE 4 Differences Between Acute Gouty Arthritis and Acute Calcium Pyrophosphate Crystal Arthritis

Symptom or Sign	Acute Gout	Acute CPP Crystal Arthritis
Pattern of joint involvement	First MCP joint, other lower extremity joints	Knee, wrist, ankle, spine
Response to colchicine	Excellent in early attack	Variable
Blood in joint fluid	Unusual	Not unusual
Duration of attack	7-10 days	Days to weeks

CPP, Calcium pyrophosphate dihydrate; *MCP,* metacarpophalangeal.
From Hochberg MC: *Rheumatology,* ed 7, Philadelphia, 2019, Elsevier.

TABLE 5 Metabolic Diseases Predisposing to Calcium Pyrophosphate Dihydrate Crystal Deposition

	CC	Pseudogout	Chronic PA
Hemochromatosis	Yes	Yes	Yes
Hyperparathyroidism	Yes	Yes	No
Hypophosphatasia	Yes	Yes	No
Hypomagnesemia	Yes	Yes	No
Gout	Possibly	Possibly	No
Acromegaly	Possibly	No	No
Ochronosis	Yes	Yes	No
Familial hypocalciuric hypercalcemia	Possibly	No	No
X-linked hypophosphatemic rickets	Possibly	Possibly	Possibly

CC, Chondrocalcinosis; *PA,* pyrophosphate arthropathy.

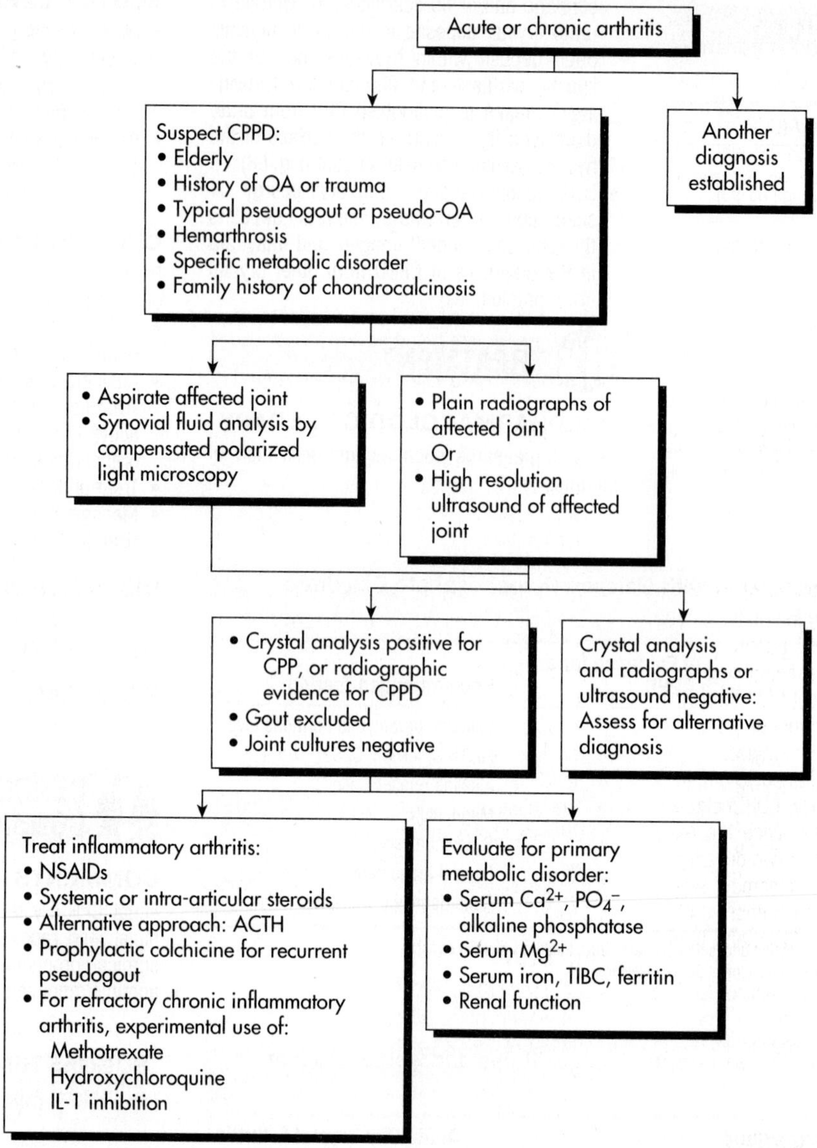

FIG. 2 Algorithm for evaluation and treatment of calcium pyrophosphate dihydrate disease. *ACTH,* Adrenocorticotropic hormone; *CPP,* calcium pyrophosphate dihydrate; *CPPD,* calcium pyrophosphate dihydrate crystal deposition; *IL,* interleukin; *NSAIDs,* nonsteroidal antiinflammatory drugs; *OA,* osteoarthritis; *TIBC,* total iron-binding capacity. (From Firestein GS et al: *Kelley and Firestein's textbook of rheumatology,* ed 10, Philadelphia, 2017, Elsevier.)

BOX 2 Screening Blood Tests for Metabolic Diseases Associated with Calcium Pyrophosphate Dihydrate Crystal Deposition

Calcium
Alkaline phosphatase
Magnesium
Ferritin, iron, transferrin
Liver function
Thyroid-stimulating hormone

From Hochberg MC et al: *Rheumatology,* ed 5, St Louis, 2011, Mosby.

Rx BASIC INFORMATION

DEFINITION

Carcinoma of unknown primary (CUP) refers to a diverse group of malignancies for which the anatomic site of origin cannot be determined despite extensive investigations.

SYNONYMS

Cancer NOS
Cancer unspecified site
Malignancy unspecified site
CUP

ICD-10CM CODE

C80.1 Malignant (primary) neoplasm, unspecified

EPIDEMIOLOGY & DEMOGRAPHICS

- CUP accounts for about 4% of all cancers, and the annual incidence in the United States is 7 to 12 cases per 100,000 persons.
- It is the seventh most frequent common cause of cancer and the fourth most common cause of cancer death. It predominantly occurs in adults and is more common in males.
- In the United States, an estimated 30,000 new cases are expected annually. CUP incidence rates have been decreasing since the early 1980s, 3.6% per yr in the last two decades.
- Most cases of CUP are carcinomas, which are divided into adenocarcinomas (90%), squamous cell carcinomas (5%), and undifferentiated carcinomas (5%).
- Recent data suggest that the risk of CUP is substantially increased in heavy smokers and to a lesser degree increased in obese patients.
- There is a variable rate of mutations detected in CUP (18% to 30%). The tumor suppressor gene *p-53* has overexpression rates (40%-50%) or mutation rates (25%-40%) that are comparable to that seen in other solid tumors. The evaluation of VEGF-A (vascular endothelial growth factor-A, angiogenesis factor) and matrix metalloproteinases (enzymes that degrade stroma) showed that these are universally expressed and active angiogenesis is present in CUP.

PHYSICAL FINDINGS & CLINICAL PRESENTATION

- Physical findings can be variable and include generalized and organ-specific findings.
- General findings can include cachexia, pallor, edema, icterus, edema, skin rash, and muscle wasting, among others.
- Organ-specific findings are related to the dysfunction of the underlying organ(s) involved with CUP.
- The clinical course is often highlighted by a short presentation history, with symptoms and signs associated with metastatic sites, early dissemination, aggressive clinical course, and occasionally an unpredictable metastatic pattern.
- Multiple organs are involved at diagnosis in up to half of patients.
- The clinicopathologic subsets comprising CUP are shown in Table 1.

Dx DIAGNOSIS

WORKUP

- Comprehensive medical history
- Complete physical examination with particular attention to skin, lymph node sites, organ enlargement, and testes; also rectal examination and pelvic examination (in women) (Table 2)
- Histopathology review of biopsy specimens

LABORATORY TESTS

- Complete blood count.
- Comprehensive chemistry panel.
- Urine analysis.
- Stool for occult blood.
- Tumor markers (in selected cases): Prostate-specific antigen (PSA), β-human chorionic gonadotrophin, α-fetoprotein.
- Adequate tissue biopsy with immunohistochemical (IHC) staining is done to guide broad diagnostic category assignments—carcinoma, melanoma, sarcoma, or lymphoma. Commonly used immunoperoxidase stains to assist in the differential diagnosis of carcinoma of unknown primary cancer are summarized in Table 3.
- Subtyping with IHC panels helps further classifying into adenocarcinoma, squamous carcinoma, germ cell tumor, neuroendocrine, thyroid, hepatocellular, or renal origin.
- Stepwise approach for IHC-derived diagnosis of likely site of origin is depicted in Table 4.
- In up to 25% of cases, a single site of origin can be narrowed down by IHC staining (e.g., TTF-1 positive and CK-1 positive lung cancer profile).
- Molecular diagnosis is carried out by commercially available multi-gene assays that utilize micro-array or polymerase chain reaction assays and can assist in finalizing diagnosis in up to 80% to 90% of cases in which initial IHC staining has been inconclusive.

IMAGING STUDIES

- CT scans of the chest, abdomen, and pelvis; also CT of the neck in case of neck lymphadenopathy
- For selected cases
  1. PET scan
  2. Mammography and/or breast MRI
  3. Testicular ultrasonography

Rx TREATMENT

- CUP patients often require early supportive care for their advanced cancer; also there is elevated psychosocial distress with the uncertainties of diagnosis and treatment options. Anxiety and depression are more common in CUP patients compared to patients with known primaries.
- Treatment is based according to the most likely site of origin for the cancer, with systemic chemotherapy typically being the mainstay of therapy.
- Treatment is typically palliative, and standard chemotherapy consists of platinum plus taxane combinations. In addition, gemcitabine-based regimens can be used.
- Next-generation gene sequencing and in situ hybridization techniques in a large study of 1806 CUP cases were able to identify potential biomarkers predictive of therapeutic efficacy in 96% of cases. Additionally, biomarkers associated with a potential lack of benefit were identified in numerous cases, which could further refine the management of patients with CUP.

TABLE 1 Clinicopathologic Subsets of Patients with CUP

	Median Age (Yr)	Sex of Patients (M/F)	Histopathology
Lymph Nodes			
Mediastinal retroperitoneal	<50	70%/30%	UDF or PDF
Axillary	52	0%/100%	Adenocarcinoma (WDF, MDF, or PDF)
Cervical	57-60	80%/20%	SCC
Inguinal	58	50%/50%	UDF, SCC, mixed SCC and adenocarcinoma
Peritoneal Cavity			
Primary peritoneal in women	55-65	0%/100%	Adenocarcinoma (serous papillary)
Ascites of other unknown origin	–	–	Adenocarcinoma (MDF or PDF; mucin; with or without signet ring cells)
Neuroendocrine tumors	63	60%/40%	PDF with neuroendocrine features; low-grade neuroendocrine cancers; small-cell anaplastic cancers
Liver (mainly) or other organs, or both	62	61%/39%	Adenocarcinoma (MDF or PDF)
Lungs			
Pulmonary metastases	–	–	Adenocarcinoma (WDF, MDF, or PDF)
Pleural effusions	–	–	Adenocarcinoma (MDF or PDF)
Bones (one or more)	–	–	Adenocarcinoma (WDF, MDF, or PDF)
Brain (one or more)	51-55	M>F	Adenocarcinoma (WDF, UDF, or PDF); SCC

CUP, Cancer of unknown primary; *F,* women; *M,* men; *MDF,* moderately differentiated; *PDF,* poorly differentiated; *SCC,* squamous cell carcinoma; *UDF,* undifferentiated; *WDF,* well differentiated.
From Pavlidis N, Pentheroudakis G: Cancer of unknown primary site, *Lancet* 379(9824):1428-1435, 2012.

TABLE 2 Recommended Evaluation Following Initial Light Microscopic Diagnosis

Diagnosis	Clinical Evaluation*	Special Pathologic Studies
Adenocarcinoma (or poorly differentiated adenocarcinoma)	PET CT of chest, abdomen; men: Serum PSA; women: Mammogram; additional directed radiologic or endoscopic studies to evaluate abnormal symptoms, signs, laboratory values	Men: PSA stain; women: Estrogen and progesterone receptor stains (if clinical features suggest metastatic breast cancer)
Poorly differentiated carcinoma	PET CT of chest, abdomen; serum hCG, AFP; additional directed radiologic or endoscopic studies to evaluate abnormal symptoms, signs, laboratory values	Immunoperoxidase staining; electron microscopy (if immunoperoxidase stains indeterminate)
Squamous carcinoma, cervical nodes	PET direct laryngoscopy with visualization; biopsy of nasopharynx, pharynx, hypopharynx, larynx; fiberoptic bronchoscopy (if laryngoscopy is negative)	—
Squamous carcinoma, inguinal nodes	PET complete examination of perineal area (including pelvic examination); anoscopy, cystoscopy	—

AFP, α-Fetoprotein; *CT*, computed tomography; *hCG*, human chorionic gonadotropin; *PET*, positron emission tomography; *PSA*, prostate-specific antigen.
*In addition to a history, physical examination, complete blood cell counts, chemistry profile, and chest radiograph.
From Goldman L, Schafer AI: *Goldman's Cecil medicine*, ed 25, Philadelphia, 2016, Saunders.

TABLE 3 Commonly Used Immunoperoxidase Stains to Assist in the Differential Diagnosis of Carcinoma of Unknown Primary Cancers

Primary Tissue Stain	Immunoperoxidase Stain
Lung cancer	Thyroid transcription factor (TTF-1), surfactant protein A precursor (SP-A1)
Breast cancer	Estrogen receptor (ER), gross cystic disease fibrous protein-15 (GCDFP-15), mammaglobin, Her-2/neu, GATA3
Lymphoma	Leukocyte common antigen (LCA), CD3, CD4, CD5, CD20, CD45
Gastrointestinal cancers	CK7, CK20, CDX-2, carcinoembryonic antigen (CEA)
Müllerian or ovarian	CK7, estrogen receptor (ER), WT-1, PAX-8, PAX2
Prostate cancer	PSA, alpha-methylacyl CoA racemase/P504S (AMACR/P504S), P501S (prostein), and prostate-specific membrane antigen (PSMA), NKX3-1
Germ cell tumor	β-hCG, αFP, OCT3/4, CKIT, CD30 (embryonal), SALL4
Hepatocellular cancers	Hep Par-1, arginase-1 (Arg-1), Glypican-3
Sarcoma	Desmin1, factor VIII, CD31, smooth muscle actin for leiomyosarcoma, MyoD1 for rhabdomyosarcoma
Renal cell cancer	RCC, CD10, PAX-8
Neuroendocrine tumor	Chromogranin, synaptophysin, CD56
Melanoma	S100, vimentin, HMB-45, tyrosinase and Melan-A, SOX-10
Urothelial	CK7, CK20, thrombomodulin, uroplakin III
Mesothelioma	Calretinin, WT-1, D2-40, mesothelin

From Niederhuber JE: *Abeloff's clinical oncology*, ed 6, Philadelphia, 2020, Elsevier.

- In another study of 442 patients with CUP, the use of targeted clinical-grade, next-generation sequencing resulted in the detection of alterations in circulating tumor DNA in 80% of patients. Among the patients harboring characterized alterations, distinct genomic profiles were observed in the majority of cases exhibiting potentially targetable alterations with currently available biologic therapies.
- In a recent systematic review of data from 11 studies evaluating genomic profiling of CUPs through NGS technology, 85% of patients demonstrated at least one molecular alteration. The most frequently detected alterations involved *TP53, KRAS, CDKN2A*, and *PIK3CA* genes. A mean of 47.3% of patients harbored a potentially targetable alteration for which approved/off-label/in clinical trials drugs were available.
- Favorable and unfavorable CUP subsets are shown in Table 5.
- ***Favorable CUP:***
  1. Women with peritoneal adenocarcinoma when treated as advanced ovarian cancer with surgical cytoreduction and adjuvant systemic chemotherapy can have median survivals in the 36-mo range.
  2. Patients with a midline tumor characteristically treated as germ cell tumors have median survivals of 12 mo.
  3. Patients with poorly differentiated neuroendocrine cancers are treated with combination platinum-containing chemotherapy and median survivals are in the 15-mo range.
  4. Women with axillary nodal adenocarcinoma are approached as breast cancers with treatment plans incorporating axillary and breast surgery followed by adjuvant chemotherapy, hormone therapy, and radiotherapy; survival rates are comparable to similarly staged breast cancers.
  5. Patients with metastatic squamous neck nodal cancer are treated as head–neck cancers with chemoradiotherapy and/or neck dissection.
  6. Patients with a colon adenocarcinoma profile are treated with systemic regimens as in metastatic colorectal cancers with median survivals in the 24-mo range.
  7. Men with blastic bone metastases and elevated prostate specific antigen are treated with initial androgen deprivation therapy and later on with systemic chemotherapy.

Unfavorable CUP:

- Account for 75% to 80% of all CUP patients.
- The most common presentation is advanced visceral disease, often with liver metastases; median survivals with systemic platinum and taxane-containing chemotherapy are typically in the range of 6 to 7 mo.

DISPOSITION

Newer clinical practice guidelines recommend that gene panel testing be routinely undertaken to support diagnosis based on the findings of genomic mutations and to select a therapeutic drug that is likely to be effective.

SUGGESTED READINGS

Available at ExpertConsult.com

AUTHOR: **Ritesh Rathore, MD**

TABLE 4 Immunohistochemical Approaches for Diagnosis of CUP

	Diagnosis
Step One	
AE1 or AE3 pan-cytokeratin	Carcinoma
Common leukocyte antigen	Lymphoma
S100; HMB-45	Melanoma
S100; vimentin	Sarcoma
Step Two	
CK7 or CK20; PSA	Adenocarcinoma
PLAP; OCT4; AFP; human chorionic gonadotropin	Germ cell tumors
Hepatocyte paraffin1; canalicular pCEA, CD10, or CD13	Hepatocellular carcinoma
RCC; CD10	Renal cell carcinoma
TTF1; thyroglobulin	Thyroid carcinoma
Chromogranin; synaptophysin, PGP9.5; CD56	Neuroendocrine carcinoma
CK5 or CK6; p63	Squamous cell carcinoma
Step Three	
PSA; PAP	Prostate
TTF1	Lung
GCDFP-15; mammaglobin; ER	Breast
CDX2; CK20	Colon
CDX2 (intestinal epithelium); CK20; CK7	Pancreas or biliary
ER; CA-125; mesothelin; WT1	Ovary

Step one detects broad type of cancer. Step two detects subtype. Step three detects origin of adenocarcinoma. Positive results with any of these stains indicates a tumor is present, but without absolute certainty.

AFP, α-Fetoprotein; *CA-125,* cancer antigen 125; *ER,* estrogen receptor; *GCDFP-15,* gross cystic disease fluid protein 15; *OCT4,* octamer-binding transcription factor 4; *PAP,* prostatic acid phosphatase; *pCEA,* polyclonal carcinoembryonic antigen; *PLAP,* placental alkaline phosphatase; *PSA,* prostate-specific antigen; *RCC,* renal cell carcinoma antigen; *TTF1,* thyroid transcription factor 1; *WT1,* Wilms tumor 1.

From Pavlidis N, Pentheroudakis G: Cancer of unknown primary site, *Lancet* 379:1428-1435, 2012.

TABLE 5 Prognostic Classification of CUP Patients

Favorable Subset
Women with papillary adenocarcinoma of the peritoneal cavity
Women with adenocarcinoma involving the axillary lymph nodes
Poorly differentiated carcinoma with midline distribution
Poorly differentiated neuroendocrine carcinoma
Squamous cell carcinoma involving cervical lymph nodes
Adenocarcinoma with a colon-cancer profile (CK20+, CK7−, CDX2+)
Men with blastic bone metastases and elevated prostate-specific antigen (adenocarcinoma)
Isolated inguinal adenopathy (squamous carcinoma)
Patients with one small, potentially resectable tumor
Unfavorable Subset
Adenocarcinoma metastatic to the liver or other organs
Nonpapillary malignant ascites (adenocarcinoma)
Multiple cerebral metastases (adenocarcinoma or squamous carcinoma)
Several lung or pleural metastases (adenocarcinoma)
Multiple metastatic lytic bone disease (adenocarcinoma)
Squamous cell carcinoma of the abdominopelvic cavity

From Pavlidis N, Pentheroudakis G: Cancer of unknown primary site, *Lancet* 379:1428-1435, 2012.

BASIC INFORMATION

DEFINITION

Infection caused by the species of the genus *Candida.* All the different *Candida* species can cause disease, but infections caused by *Candida albicans* are the most common. *Candida* species are ubiquitous and are the most common fungal pathogens affecting mankind. Cutaneous candidiasis comprises superficial *Candida* infections of the skin and mucosal membranes.

Cutaneous candidiasis can be classified into two subgroups: Cutaneous candidiasis syndromes and chronic mucocutaneous syndromes. Cutaneous candidiasis syndromes include:

- Generalized cutaneous candidiasis
- Intertrigo
- *Candida* folliculitis
- Paronychia/onychomycosis
- Perianal candidiasis
- Erosio interdigitalis blastomycetica
- Balanitis

Chronic mucocutaneous syndromes include:

- Oropharyngeal candidiasis
- Esophageal candidiasis
- Vulvovaginal candidiasis
- GI candidiasis (gastric/intestines/perianal)
- *Candida* cystitis

SYNONYMS

Yeast infection
Candidosis
Moniliasis
Oidiomycosis

ICD-10CM CODES	
B37.2	Candidiasis of skin and nail
B37.8	Candidiasis, unspecified
B37.89	Other sites of candidiasis

EPIDEMIOLOGY & DEMOGRAPHICS

- *Candida* species: It is the most common fungal infection in immunocompromised people.
- Most females (75%) experience an episode of vulvovaginal candidiasis in their lifetime.

INCIDENCE: Estimated to be 50 cases per 100,000 persons

PREVALENCE: Colonizes more than 50% of U.S. population

PREDOMINANT SEX AND AGE:

- Female > male
- No predominant age, but neonates and the elderly (adults >65 yr) are susceptible to *Candida* colonization and to getting mucocutaneous candidiasis

RISK FACTORS: Risk factors that allow *Candida* infection include:

- Age >65 yr
- Females in the third trimester
- Defects in the mucocutaneous barrier (e.g., wounds, burns, ulcerations)
- Decreased/defective granulocytes/monocytes
- Diseases of white blood cells (e.g., chronic granulomatous disease)
- Complement deficiency
- Certain diseases associated with cell-mediated immunity (e.g., HIV, DM)
- Use of certain medications (e.g., broad-spectrum antibiotics, high doses of corticosteroids)
- Increased skin pH due to panty liners and occlusive attire
- Chronic mucocutaneous candidiasis: (CMC) is characterized by susceptibility to *Candida* infection of skin, nails (Fig. E1), and mucous membranes. Patients with recessive CMC and autoimmunity have mutations in the autoimmune regulator *AIRE.* Mutations in the CC domain of *STAT1* underlie autosomal-dominant CMC and lead to defective Th1 and Th17 responses, which may explain the increased susceptibility to fungal infections (van de Veerdonk et al). Some patients have autosomal recessive polyglandular autoimmune syndrome type 1 (also autoimmune polyendocrinopathy-candidiasis-ectodermal dystrophy [APECED] syndrome)

Anatomical sites predisposed to *Candida* infection include:

- Axilla
- Beneath the breast, abdominal fold, intertriginous areas
- Periungual creases
- Inguinal creases
- Back and buttocks of bedridden persons

PHYSICAL FINDINGS & CLINICAL PRESENTATION

There are several clinical presentations of cutaneous candidiasis. A few are presented here.

- Cutaneous candidiasis
  1. Presents as erythematous, sometimes shiny with flakes and fluid lesions at the edge of the redness (satellite pustules). It is itchy, and the skin becomes inflamed. Pustules may be present in candidiasis of the scrotal and perineal skin.
- Gastrointestinal tract candidiasis
  1. Oropharyngeal candidiasis [thrush]
     a. Usually seen in diabetics, after exposure to inhaled steroids, broad-spectrum antibiotics, chemotherapy, radiation to head and neck, and in immunosuppressed individuals (e.g., patients with a history of HIV infection). It is also seen in some patients who wear dentures. Symptoms include:
        (1) White, thick patches on the oral mucosa (Fig. E2), tongue, palate, or oropharynx or under dentures
        (2) Dysphagia, mouth soreness, and pain on eating and swallowing
        (3) Tongue burning
        (4) Loss of taste
     b. Physical examination shows:
        (1) Erythema of the buccal mucosa
        (2) White patches on buccal cavity surfaces (described previously)
        (3) Transverse fissuring
  2. Esophageal candidiasis:
     a. Most common in patients with:
        (1) Hematologic cancers
        (2) HIV/AIDS (it is an AIDS-defining illness)
     b. History of oropharyngeal candidiasis. Symptoms include:
        (1) Odynophagia (pain on swallowing), hallmark of the disease
        (2) Dysphagia
        (3) Epigastric pain
        (4) Retrosternal pain
     c. Physical examination shows:
        (1) Affects mainly the distal one third of the esophagus. Endoscopy shows areas of the erythema and edema; scattered white patches or ulcers
  3. Perianal candidiasis:
     a. Skin maceration
     b. Itching
     c. Frequently extends to the perineum
- Paronychia/onychomycosis
  1. Fungal infection of the nail and surrounding tissues
  2. Associated with diabetes mellitus and immersion of hands or feet in water
  3. History: Pain and redness around and beneath the nail and nail bed
  4. Physical exam: Inflammation around the toe nail. There may also be nail thickening and discoloration (dystrophic nails). Nail loss may also occur
- Respiratory tract candidiasis
  1. Usually seen in hospitalized patients.
  2. About 25% of outpatients have their respiratory tract colonized by *Candida* species.
- Genitourinary tract candidiasis
  1. Vulvovaginal candidiasis
     a. Most common form of mucosal candidiasis.
     b. Risk factors include increased estrogen level (e.g., contraceptive pill), steroid or antibiotic use, diabetes, HIV infection, IUD, and diaphragm use.
     c. It causes itching, curdy white discharge, and occasionally dysuria, dyspareunia, and vaginal irritation.
     d. On examination the mucosa may be inflamed with vulvar and vaginal erythema, and vaginal discharge, classically described as white and curdy.
     e. Painful erythema or itchy penile inflammation may occur in male sexual partners of affected females.
  2. *Candida* balanitis
     a. Usually acquired through sexual contact with a partner who has vulvovaginal candidiasis. Common in diabetic patients and uncircumcised individuals. The dominant species is *C. albicans.*
     b. Symptoms include penile pruritus and white patches on penis. There could be severe burning and itching. Infection could also spread to the perineum.
     c. Physical exam: Dry, erythematous, and scaly patches on penis and sometimes on the thighs, scrotum, gluteal folds, and buttocks. Papules, vesicles or pustules and ulceration may also be present.

- **Others**
  1. Erosio interdigitalis blastomycetica: Denudating/macerating area commonly seen in third web space.
  2. Mastitis: Injured nipples in lactating women can lead to infections, including *Candida* infections.
  3. *Candida* folliculitis: Pustulous nodules in hairy areas.
  4. Intertrigo: This occurs in folds of the skin and creases (Fig. E3). It is characterized by erosions, exudation, oozing, and maceration.

ETIOLOGY

The most common cause of cutaneous candidiasis is *Candida albicans*.

Dx DIAGNOSIS

DIFFERENTIAL DIAGNOSIS

- Intertrigo
- Seborrheic dermatitis
- Psoriasis
- Bacterial vaginosis
- Contact dermatitis

WORKUP

- Mucocutaneous and cutaneous candidiasis:
  1. Obtain scrapings from the skin, oral, and vaginal mucosa or nails.
  2. The presence of hyphae/pseudohyphae or budding yeast cells on wet smear, as well as confirmation by culture, is the recommended procedure to diagnose cutaneous candidiasis.
  3. KOH smears are helpful.
- Respiratory candidiasis:
  1. Sputum Gram stain: Shows yeast cells
  2. Sputum cultures
  3. Lung biopsy: Establishes the diagnosis
- Gastrointestinal candidiasis:
  1. Upper endoscopy with or without biopsy (Fig. E4)

Rx TREATMENT

PHARMACOLOGIC THERAPY (TABLE 1)

- Cutaneous candidiasis:
  1. Decrease/prevent moisture in area
  2. Apply antifungal agents (nystatin powder or cream with an azole or ciclopirox [e.g., clotrimazole, econazole, miconazole])
- Gastrointestinal candidiasis:
  1. Oropharyngeal candidiasis
     a. Treat with either
        (1) Oral topical antifungal agent (e.g., nystatin 1:100,000 U/ml, 5 ml swish and swallow qid) OR
        (2) Systemic oral azoles (e.g., fluconazole 100 mg qd ×14 days)
  2. In HIV-positive patients, use high doses of fluconazole (100 to 200 mg PO qd for 7 to 14 days), itraconazole, or posaconazole
- *Candida* esophagitis:
  1. Treat with systemic fluconazole for 2 to 3 wk
  2. Treat with IV fluconazole if patient is unable to take oral medication
- Genitourinary tract candidiasis:
  1. Vulvovaginal candidiasis: Treatment options for acute cases include:
     a. A single dose of oral fluconazole (fluconazole 150 mg PO × 1 dose) OR
     b. Topical antifungal agent
  2. For chronic or recurrent cases, treat with fluconazole 150 mg qd × 3 doses and then 150 mg/wk for 6 mo
- Chronic mucocutaneous candidiasis:
  1. Treatment with azoles is effective (e.g., fluconazole 100 to 400 mg daily)
  2. When patient improves, follow with maintenance treatment with same azole for life

FOLLOW-UP CARE

- Mucocutaneous candidiasis:
  1. Patient should be instructed to call or follow up if symptoms persist, recur, or worsen.
  2. For recurrent infections:
     a. Check HIV antibodies.
     b. Check FBS, HbA_{1c}.
     c. Rule out hematologic malignancy or solid organ malignancy.
     d. Refer to infectious disease specialist if no etiology is found.

PREVENTION

- Maintaining dry environment (e.g., by wearing cotton underwear)
- Decreased use of antibiotic
- No douching

SUGGESTED READING

Available at ExpertConsult.com

RELATED CONTENT

Candidiasis (Patient Information)

AUTHOR: **Daniel K. Asiedu, MD, PhD, FACP**

TABLE 1 Treatment of Mucocutaneous *Candida* Infections
Candidal onychomycosis can be treated with the oral fluconazole or itraconazole regimens for tinea unguium.

Type of Infection	Treatment Regimen (adult doses unless otherwise indicated)
Oropharyngeal candidiasis	**Nystatin*** 100,000 units/ml suspension: • Children and adults—4-6 ml swish and swallow four times daily • Infants—2 ml (1 ml inside each cheek) four times daily **Clotrimazole*** 10 mg troche five times daily **Fluconazole**† 200 mg po on day 1, then 100-200 mg po daily Continue treatment for 7-14 days after clinical resolution
Esophageal candidiasis	**Fluconazole*** 200-400 mg po on day 1, then 100-400 mg daily **Itraconazole** 200 mg po daily **Voriconazole** 200 mg po or iv BID **Posaconazole** 400 mg po BID **Caspofungin** 50 mg po iv daily Continue treatment for 7-14 days following resolution of symptoms, for a minimum of 21 days total
Candidal vulvovaginitis§	**Fluconazole*** 150 mg po single dose or (for severe disease or an immunosuppressed patient) three doses at 3-day intervals **Butoconazole** 2% vaginal cream, 5 g daily for 1-3 days **Clotrimazole***,‡ • 1% vaginal cream (or other topical formulation), 5 g daily for 7-14 days • Vaginal suppositories: 100 mg daily for 7 days or 200 mg daily for 3 days **Miconazole***,‡ • 2% cream, 5 g daily for 7 days • Vaginal suppositories: 100 mg daily for 7 days, 200 mg daily for 3 days, or 1200 mg single dose **Tioconazole*** 6.5% cream, 5 g single dose **Terconazole*** • 0.4% or 0.8% cream, 5 g daily for 7 or 3 days, respectively • 80 mg vaginal suppository daily for 3 days **Nystatin** 100,000 units vaginal suppository daily for 14 days *For suppression in patients with recurrent infections:* **Fluconazole** 150 mg weekly for 6 mo **Clotrimazole** vaginal suppository, 200 mg twice weekly or 500 mg weekly for 6 mo
Chronic mucocutaneous candidiasis	**Fluconazole** • *Eradication:* 400-800 mg po daily for 4-6 mo • *Suppressive therapy*: 200 mg po daily
Candidal intertrigo or balanitis§	Topical **imidazole** or **ciclopirox** cream or lotion twice daily for 1-2 wk or until resolved¶ *Systemic agents for recalcitrant or severe cases:* **Fluconazole** • 50-100 mg po daily for 14 days • 150 mg po weekly for 2-4 wk **Itraconazole** 200 mg po twice daily for 14 days

BID, twice daily; *iv*, intravenously; *po*, orally.
*Recommended as first-line treatment for immunocompetent individuals.
†Recommended as first-line treatment for HIV-infected patients (or other immunosuppressed individuals) with moderate to severe disease, recurrent infection, or a CD4 count of <200 cells/mcl.
‡Preferred treatments (with 7-day regimens) for pregnant patients.
§In cases of recurrent vulvovaginitis, treatment of the patient's sexual partner is controversial; in contrast, for recurrent balanitis, eradication of *Candida* from the sexual partner's genital tract is generally recommended.
¶After clinical resolution, topical treatments may be continued twice weekly to prevent recurrence.
From Bolognia J: *Dermatology*, ed 4, 2018, Elsevier.

BASIC INFORMATION

DEFINITION

Severe and invasive diseases are caused by *Candida* infection. More than 15 different *Candida* species cause disease in humans, but at least 95% of invasive disease is caused by *C. albicans, C. glabrata, C. tropicalis, C. parapsilocis,* and *C. krusei.* These organisms cause serious disease referred to as invasive candidiasis. Invasive candidiasis embodies a variety of diseases caused by hematogenous spread of *Candida* to multiple viscera (e.g., kidney, brain, heart). These diseases include candidemia, disseminated candidiasis, meningitis, and endophthalmitis. Invasive candidiasis is a significant cause of morbidity and mortality for certain groups of patients.

SYNONYM

Systemic candidiasis

ICD-10CM CODES	
B37.89	Other sites of candidiasis
B37.1	Pulmonary candidiasis
B37.2	Candidiasis of skin and nail
B37.5	Candidal meningitis
B37.6	Candidal endocarditis
B37.7	Candidal sepsis
B37.9	Candidiasis unspecified

EPIDEMIOLOGY & DEMOGRAPHICS

INCIDENCE:

- Invasive candidiasis is the most common fungal disease among hospitalized patients in the developed world. It is an important nosocomial infection. It affects over 250,000 people worldwide each yr and causes more than 50,000 deaths.
- In the U.S., *Candida* species cause 8% to 10% of nosocomial bloodstream infections (fourth most common bloodstream infection). *C. albicans* is the most common cause of candidemia, but other non-*albicans* species have been implicated in recent yrs. These include *C. glabrata, C. parapsilosis, C. tropicalis,* and *C. krusei.* Incidence rates of candidemia are between 2 and 14 cases/100,000 persons.

PREVALENCE: No data available

PREDOMINANT SEX AND AGE: Equal between males and females; all ages are susceptible.

RISK FACTORS: Prolonged hospitalization and ICU stay, use of broad-spectrum antibiotics, prolonged indwelling of catheters (especially central venous catheters), acute and chronic renal failure, surgery requiring general anesthesia, cancer (e.g., solid neoplasms), transplantation (bone marrow or solid organ), recent chemotherapy/radiation therapy, use of immunosuppressive drugs, parenteral alimentation, use of internal prosthetic devices, organ transplant, hemodialysis, mechanical, surgical procedures

PHYSICAL FINDINGS & CLINICAL PRESENTATION

- History
  1. Fever unresponsive to broad-spectrum antibiotics
  2. History of prolonged indwelling IV catheter
  3. A personal history of any of the risk factors listed earlier
- Physical findings (general)
  1. Fever
  2. Hypotension
  3. Generalized malaise
  4. Tachycardia
  5. Change in mental status
  6. Signs of multiorgan system failure
- Specific diseases
  1. Candidemia
     a. A positive blood culture is the gold standard for the diagnosis of candidemia. Obtain blood cultures in patients suspected to have candidemia. *Candida* species must be isolated from at least one blood culture. A positive culture for *Candida* should be investigated thoroughly because of the increased risk of morbidity and mortality. Attributable mortality to candidemia in adults is 15% to 20%.
     b. Most common manifestation of invasive candidiasis.
     c. Physical exam may include fever, macronodular skin lesions, septic shock, *Candida* endophthalmitis
  2. Disseminated candidiasis
     a. Seen in patients with neutropenia who have undergone cytotoxic chemotherapy for a hematologic malignancy
     b. Associated with multiple deep-organ infections or failure
     c. Blood culture positive
     d. Fever not responding to broad-spectrum antibiotics
     e. Physical exam: Discrete erythematous or palpable rash, sepsis/septic shock
  3. Endophthalmitis
     a. Iatrogenic/accidental or traumatic fungal infection of the eye (exogenous) or hematogenous seeding of the eye (endogenous); *C. albicans* accounts for about 90% of cases of endogenous endophthalmitis
     b. Starts as choroidal lesion, progresses to vitreitis and endophthalmitis and eventually blindness
     c. Physical exam shows fever. An early funduscopic exam by an ophthalmologist should be performed in all patients with candidemia. Funduscopic examination may show large and off-white cotton ball–like lesions with indistinct borders. Patients usually present with decreased visual acuity and occasional pain
  4. *Candida* infection of the CNS
     a. Meningitis: Candida can spread hematogenously to the meninges during craniotomy or through ventriculoatrial/peritoneal shunts. Culture CSF to establish diagnosis
     b. Commonly found in long-term ICU patients
     c. May present as meningitis, mycotic aneurysms, change in mental status
     d. Physical examination reveals fever, neck rigidity, confusion, headache, and coma
  5. Candidal musculoskeletal infections
     a. Candida infect the skeletal system, especially the joints as a result of trauma, joint injections, and other surgical interventions, such as IV drug use (hematogenous seeding)
     b. Previously uncommon; now relatively common probably due to increased frequency of candidemia and disseminated candidiasis
     c. Knee and vertebral column (especially lumbosacral vertebral disks and vertebral bodies, which can lead to vertebral osteomyelitis, with or without discitis) are involved
     d. Physical exam is usually unremarkable but may show tenderness over involved area, fever, erythema, bone deformity, weight loss, and sometimes a draining fistulous tract
  6. Candidal infections of the heart
     a. Usually found in patients with artificial heart valves, IV drug users, and patients with an indwelling central venous catheter
     b. May present as infective endocarditis, myocarditis, or pericarditis
     c. Physical examination reveals fever, hypotension, tachycardia, new or changing murmur, and signs and symptoms of heart failure
  7. Hepatosplenic candidiasis (chronic systemic candidiasis)
     a. Seen in patients with hematologic malignancy and neutropenia; usually develops during recovery from a neutropenic state (normally after undergoing myeloablative chemotherapy)
     b. On examination, patients have low-grade fever, right upper quadrant pain, palpable/tender liver, splenomegaly, and rarely jaundice
     c. MRI/CT/US may reveal multiple focal abnormalities in the liver, spleen, and kidneys
  8. *Candida* peritonitis
     a. Associated with GI surgery: Perforations, acute necrotizing pancreatitis, peritoneal dialysis. Pancreatic abscess, gangrenous cholecystitis, and common bile duct obstruction are other GI manifestations of *Candida* infection. *C. albicans* is the commonly isolated species in intra-abdominal candida infection
     b. Clinical manifestations include fever, chills, abdominal pain; nausea, vomiting, constipation
     c. Physical examination reveals abdominal distention, abdominal pain, absent bowel sounds
  9. Other forms of invasive candidiasis
     a. *Candida* splenic abscess
     b. *Candida* cholecystitis
     c. Renal candidiasis
     d. Mediastinitis: Usually occurs after thoracic surgery. Clinical manifestations include chest wall erythema, sternal instability, and fever

e. Empyema: Common in patients with malignancies
f. Pneumonia (rare)
g. Septic arthritis

ETIOLOGY

- Several species of *Candida* exist in nature
- Medically significant include:
  1. *C. albicans*: Together with *C. glabrata*, they account for 70% to 80% of *Candida* in invasive candidiasis
  2. *C. glabrata*: Together with *C. albicans*, they account for 70% to 80% of *Candida* in invasive candidiasis
  3. *C. parapsilosis*: Associated with indwelling vascular catheters and prosthetic devices
  4. *C. tropicalis*: Especially in leukemic patients
  5. *C. krusei*: Resistant to fluconazole and ketoconazole

Dx DIAGNOSIS

DIFFERENTIAL DIAGNOSIS

- Sepsis (bacterial)
- Septic shock
- Cryptococcosis
- Aspergillosis

LABORATORY TESTS

- Laboratory studies are nonspecific. It is often necessary to perform several diagnostic tests to achieve maximum accuracy.
- High index of suspicion is needed.
- Candidemia/disseminated candidiasis: Candidemia represents the tip of the iceberg with respect to the more invasive forms of candidiasis. Central lines often contribute to the propagation of candidemia. From the blood, infection can spread to almost any organ.
  1. Blood culture is the gold standard of diagnosis. They are helpful but have low positive yield. Only 40% to 60% of patients with infection have positive culture. 95% of blood cultures that are positive for *Candida* species become positive within 96 hours. Candida in a blood culture is NOT a contamination, and the source of the infection should be sought.
  2. Diagnosis can also be made from normally sterile sites. Specific species identification is necessary since only 10% of known *Candida* species produce disease in humans.
  3. The T2 magnetic resonance assay of whole blood can be performed on blood samples even after initiation of antifungal therapy.
  4. Serum (1,3) beta-D-glucan detection assay: High specificity and high positive predictive value. It can also be used for diagnosing invasive candidiasis when blood cultures are negative.
  5. New techniques allow for quick identification of *Candida* species in blood. These include:
     a. Peptide nucleic acid fluorescence in-situ hybridization (PAN-FISH).
     b. Matrix-assisted laser desorption ionization-time of flight mass spectrometry (MALDI-TOF MS).
- Hepatosplenic candidiasis (focal):
  1. Elevated serum alkaline phosphatase.

IMAGING STUDIES

- Imaging studies are generally not required or useful.
- Ultrasound is useful for diagnosing hepatosplenic abscess. "Bull's eye or target lesions" are observed in the liver and spleen.
- CT scanning may be used to diagnose hepatosplenic candidiasis, as well as intraabdominal/renal abscesses.
- ECHO is useful to rule in or rule out *Candida* endocarditis.

Rx TREATMENT

- To successfully treat invasive *Candida* infection, it is important to start antifungal medication as early as possible. A small delay (approximately 12-24 hr) in starting treatment may result in a significantly excessive mortality rate.
  1. Do not dismiss *Candida* spp. as a contaminant when it is isolated in blood cultures or other sterile sites.
  2. Before treatment, also consider removal of an intravenous catheter.
- Antifungals available include:
  1. Azoles (e.g., fluconazole, posaconazole, itraconazole, voriconazole). They inhibit the synthesis of ergosterol, a fungal cell component.
  2. Echinocandins (e.g., caspofungin, micafungin, anidulafungin). These are glucan synthesis inhibitors. Glucan is an important component of fungal cell walls. Most studies have provided reasonable support for echinocandins as treatment of choice for the majority of patients with invasive candidiasis.
  3. Polyenes (e.g., amphotericin B, lipid formulation of amphotericin, nystatin). Broad spectrum. Their mechanism of action is to increase cytoplasmic permeability.
  4. Antimetabolites (e.g., flucytosine). Flucytosine is deaminated to 5-fluorouracil in fungal cell. 5-Fluorouracil inhibits RNA and protein synthesis.

TREATMENT PLANS

CANDIDEMIA: General principles:

- For documented candidemia, 2 wk of antifungal treatment after the first negative blood culture is recommended.
- In nonneutropenic patients, a dilated funduscopic examination in the first week of treatment is recommended.
- In neutropenic patients, delay (b) above until neutrophil recovery because characteristic ocular findings may be delayed.
- Treatment depends on whether the patient is neutropenic or not.
  1. **Nonneutropenic adult patients:** The initial treatment is with an Echinocandin, e.g., caspofungin 70 mg loading dose, then 50 mg IV daily *or* micafungin 100 mg IV daily. Alternatives include fluconazole 800 mg as loading dose, then 400 mg/day for at least 2 wk after clinical improvement or negative blood culture. Amphotericin B is equally efficacious.
  2. **Neutropenic adult patients:** An echinocandin is the drug of choice (e.g., caspofungin) 70 mg IV loading dose then 50 mg/day IV or micafungin 100 mg/day IV or anidulafungin 200 mg IV loading dose then 100 mg IV all for at least 2 wk after clear blood culture and after clinical improvement. An alternative is fluconazole.
  3. **Preferred oral step-down therapy:** Neutropenic and nonneutropenic clinically stable patients who have:
     a. *Candida*-susceptible fluconazole, and
     b. Negative blood cultures can be transitioned to oral fluconazole (400 mg [6 mg/kg] daily) after about 5 to 7 days.

DISSEMINATED CANDIDIASIS: Fluconazole is the drug of choice.

DISSEMINATED CANDIDIASIS WITH END-ORGAN INFECTION:

- Treatment is the same as for candidemia of nonneutropenic patients. In most cases, therapy is prolonged for at least 4 to 6 wk.
- The echinocandins are the first-line therapy.

OSTEOMYELITIS OR SEPTIC ARTHRITIS:

- Fluconazole 400 mg IV or PO *or*
- Caspofungin 50 mg IV daily *or*
- Micafungin 100 mg IV daily

ENDOCARDITIS:

- Caspofungin 50 to 150 mg/day *or*
- Micafungin 100 to 150 mg/day *or*
- Anidulafungin 100 to 200 mg/day

MYOCARDITIS:

- Lipid-based amphotericin B 3 to 5 mg/kg daily *or*
- Caspofungin 150 mg/d *or* micafungin 100 mg/d

ESOPHAGITIS:

- Caspofungin 50 mg IV daily
- Fluconazole 200 to 400 mg/day

PERICARDITIS: Lipid-based amphotericin B 3 to 5 mg/kg daily

SURGICAL CARE: Includes:

- Drainage
- Removal of any foreign bodies
- Surgical débridement
- Organ-specific care (e.g., valve replacement for endocarditis, splenectomy for splenic abscess, or vitrectomy for fungal endophthalmitis)

DISPOSITION

- Several factors affect prognosis: Infection site, degree of immune suppression, and how quickly diagnosis and therapy are initiated
- Overall mortality rate: 30% to 40%

REFERRAL

- Always involve an infectious disease specialist.

- Referral to specialist will depend on the organ involved. For example:
  1. Endocarditis will require a cardiothoracic surgeon.
  2. Endophthalmitis will require an ophthalmologist.

FOLLOW-UP CARE

- Prolonged periods, mainly in the hospital, of antifungal treatment may be necessary.
- Closely monitor patients on amphotericin B because of the high incidence of side effects. Check basic metabolic panel, magnesium, and CBC at least twice a week.

PEARLS & CONSIDERATIONS

PREVENTION

Basic preventive measures are similar to those used for nosocomial infections. This includes:

- Maximizing hand hygiene recommendations:
  1. Hand washing
  2. Using alcohol/chlorhexidine solution
- Adhering strictly to recommendations for placement and care of central lines and catheters
- Judicious use of antimicrobials
  1. Notes on *C. auris*:
     a. CDC issued warnings in 2016 about the emergence of *C. auris*, a multidrug-resistant *Candida* species. It is resistant to fluconazole and amphotericin B in 93% and 35% of patients, respectively
     b. It has caused invasive health care–associated infections in many countries and has high mortality rates
     c. Initial treatment is with echinocandin. Patient should be closely followed with cultures
     d. Special infection control precautions should be followed for patients infected with or colonized by *C. auris*

PROPHYLAXIS

Antifungal prophylaxis should be limited to patients in whom it has proved beneficial: Patients with gastrointestinal anastomotic leakage, patients undergoing transplantation of the pancreas or small bowel, selected patients undergoing liver transplantation who are at high risk for candidiasis, and extremely low-birth-weight neonates in settings with a high incidence of neonatal candidiasis.

PATIENT & FAMILY EDUCATION

- Inform them about the risk factors for invasive candidiasis.
- Inform them of the seriousness of the disease and the associated high morbidity/mortality rates, thus requiring aggressive treatment.
- Side effects and toxicities associated with treatment.

SUGGESTED READINGS

Available at ExpertConsult.com

RELATED CONTENT

Candidiasis (Patient Information)
Candidiasis, Cutaneous (Related Key Topic)

AUTHOR: **Daniel K. Asiedu, MD, PhD, FACP**

Carbon Monoxide Poisoning (PTG)

BASIC INFORMATION

DEFINITION

Carbon monoxide (CO) is a colorless, odorless, tasteless, nonirritating gas. When inhaled, it produces toxicity by causing cellular hypoxia and damage.

ICD-10CM CODES

T68	Toxic effect of carbon monoxide
T58.01	Toxic effect of carbon monoxide from motor vehicle exhaust, accidental (unintentional), initial encounter

EPIDEMIOLOGY & DEMOGRAPHICS

- A leading cause of accidental and intentional poisoning in the U.S.
- Can occur because of acute toxicity or chronic exposure.
- Associated with poorly ventilated heaters, stoves, and generators or exposure to vehicles in poorly ventilated areas.
- CO poisoning is seen more frequently during the fall and winter months in cold climates. Frequently seen after storm-related power outages, mostly due to the use of portable gasoline-powered electrical generators.
- Most fatal cases of CO poisoning occur in the home.

PHYSICAL FINDINGS & CLINICAL PRESENTATION

- Depends on the severity and duration of exposure. The brain and heart are most sensitive to CO poisoning. Table 1 summarizes carboxyhemoglobin concentration and related symptoms.
- Presentation is often nonspecific and may be mistaken for a flulike illness.
- Severity of poisoning does not correlate with carboxyhemoglobin (COHb) levels.
- Mild to moderate poisoning may present with headache, malaise, dizziness, nausea, dyspnea, difficulty concentrating, confusion, and blurred vision. Patients may have tachypnea and tachycardia.
- Severe poisoning may present with hypotension, arrhythmias, myocardial ischemia, pulmonary edema, lethargy, ataxia, loss of consciousness, seizure, coma, or, rarely, cherry-red skin.
- Delayed neurologic sequelae may develop days to weeks after apparent recovery from acute poisoning. Patients may present with neurologic or psychiatric symptoms (cognitive deficits, memory loss, personality changes, movement disorders, Parkinson, psychosis, neurologic deficits).

ETIOLOGY

- CO results from the incomplete combustion of carbon-containing compounds. CO poisoning occurs from inhaling smoke from fires, motor vehicle/motor boat exhaust, or the burning of fuel (oil, wood, coal, gasoline, natural gas) in poorly functioning or improperly ventilated devices (heating systems, stoves/grills, portable generators, etc.). Methylene chloride (paint stripper) fumes are converted to CO by the liver.
- CO toxicity results from tissue hypoxia and direct CO-mediated damage at the cellular level. This may explain why COHb levels alone are not predictive of clinical toxicity. The mechanisms of CO toxicity are not completely understood.
- CO impairs oxygen delivery. CO reversibly binds hemoglobin with an affinity 250 times greater than oxygen, displacing oxygen from hemoglobin and decreasing the oxygen-carrying capacity of blood. By binding to hemoglobin, CO changes the structure of the hemoglobin molecule and decreases oxygen release to tissue.
- CO may also interfere with peripheral oxygen utilization by binding to other heme-containing proteins including cytochromes and myoglobin. Cellular respiration may be depressed by inhibition of mitochondrial function.
- Neurologic toxicity is not explained by hypoxia alone and is related to the complex intracellular actions of CO. CO precipitates an inflammatory cascade that results in oxidative damage and brain lipid peroxidation.

DIAGNOSIS

DIFFERENTIAL DIAGNOSIS

- Viral syndromes
- Cyanide, hydrogen sulfide
- Methemoglobinemia
- Amphetamines and derivatives
- Cocaine, phencyclidine (PCP)
- Cyclic antidepressants
- Phenothiazines
- Theophylline

WORKUP

History (duration and source of CO exposure, loss of consciousness), physical examination (detailed neurologic examination), laboratory and imaging tests

LABORATORY TESTS

- COHb level measured by CO-oximetry on arterial or venous blood. COHb level >3% in nonsmokers confirms exposure. Heavy smokers may have baseline levels up to 10% to 15%. Levels may be low if the patient has already received supplemental oxygen or if delays occur between exposure and testing.
  - Note: Pulse oximetry and arterial blood gas (ABG) may be falsely normal because neither measures oxygen saturation of hemoglobin directly. Pulse oximetry is inaccurate because of the similar absorption characteristics of oxyhemoglobin and COHb. An ABG is inaccurate because it measures oxygen dissolved in plasma (which is not affected by CO) and then calculates oxygen saturation of hemoglobin.
- Electrolytes, glucose, BUN, creatinine, cardiac biomarkers, ABG (lactic acidosis and rhabdomyolysis may develop), CBC (polycythemia from hypoxia in chronic CO poisoning).
- ECG (ischemia, arrhythmia).
- Pregnancy test (fetus at high risk).
- Consider toxicology screen.
- Table 2 summarizes treatment strategies for acute smoke inhalation.

IMAGING STUDIES

- Chest x-ray (noncardiogenic edema)
- Brain CT, MRI if neurologic abnormalities are present, to exclude other causes

TREATMENT

ACUTE GENERAL Rx

- Remove from site of CO exposure
- Ensure adequate airway
- Continuous ECG monitor
- Fetal monitoring if pregnant
- 100% oxygen by nonrebreather mask, high-flow nasal cannula, or endotracheal tube (decreases half-life of COHb from 4-6 hr to 60-90 min) until COHb level is <5% and patient is asymptomatic. Table 3 describes the half-life of COHb
- Consider hyperbaric oxygen
  1. Disparate findings in various studies: Some suggest hyperbaric oxygen treatment reduces the incidence of neurologic sequelae, and others have found it worsens neurologic outcomes compared to normobaric oxygen treatment. A large retrospective study suggests it may

TABLE 1 Carboxyhemoglobin Concentration and Related Symptoms

COHb (%)	Symptoms
<20	Slight headache and dilation of peripheral blood vessels
21-40	Severe headache and pulsating in temporal blood vessels, vertigo, dizziness, nausea and vomiting, circulatory collapse
41-60	Symptoms as above, syncope, tachycardia, hyperventilation, intermittent seizures, cyanosis, coma, shock, Cheyne-Stokes respiration
61-80	Coma, intermittent seizures, impaired heart and lung function, weak pulses, slow breathing, death within hours
>81	Death occurs within minutes

COHb, Carboxyhemoglobin.
From Parrillo JE, Dellinger RP: *Critical care medicine, principles of diagnosis and management in the adult,* ed 5, Philadelphia, 2019, Elsevier.

TABLE 2 Treatment Strategies for Acute Smoke Inhalation

Current	Under Investigation
Rescue victim from source	Activated protein C
High-flow 100% O_2	Antiinflammatory drugs: • Methylprednisolone • Phenytoin
Body check	Nitric oxide synthase inhibitors
Intravenous access	Antioxidants: • Gamma-tocopherol • 21-aminosteroid
± Intubation	Endothelin-I-receptor antagonist tezosentan
If upper airway edema: • Nebulized adrenaline • Nebulized corticosteroids	P-selectin blockade
If bronchospasm: • Nebulized alpha$_2$-agonists	Nebulized deferoxamine-pentastarch complex
If elevated COHb: • High-flow 100% O_2 • Hyperbaric oxygen	Mechanical ventilation: • High-frequency percussive ventilation • Airway pressure release ventilation • Volumetric diffuse ventilator
If cyanide intoxication: • Amyl nitrate • Sodium thiosulfate • Hydroxocobalamin (Cyanokit)	Extracorporeal membrane oxygenation
Mechanical ventilation, low tidal volume	Arteriovenous carbon dioxide removal
Nebulized heparin	Pulmonary decontamination with nebulized amphoteric chelating agents
Nebulized *N*-acetylcysteine	

COHb, Carboxyhemoglobin.
From Parrillo JE, Dellinger RP: *Critical care medicine, principles of diagnosis and management in the adult,* ed 4, Philadelphia, 2014, Elsevier.

TABLE 3 Half-Life of COHb

Oxygen Concentration	Half-Life
21% (room air)	4-5 hr
100% (mask or endotracheal)	60-90 min
100% (hyperbaric molecular oxygen)	20-30 min

COHb, Carboxyhemoglobin.
From Fuhrman BP et al: *Pediatric critical care,* ed 4, Philadelphia, 2011, Saunders.

decrease short-term and long-term mortality, especially in individuals <20 yr old and those with acute respiratory failure. Multiple sessions were associated with lower mortality than a single session.

2. Decreases half-life of COHb to 20 to 30 min; increases amount of oxygen dissolved in plasma. It also reduces CO binding to other heme-containing proteins
3. Consider for:
   a. Severe intoxication (COHb >25%, history of loss of consciousness, neurologic symptoms or signs, cardiovascular compromise, severe metabolic acidosis)
   b. Pregnant women with COHb >20% or signs of fetal distress. CO elimination is slower in fetus than mother, fetal Hgb has greater affinity for CO than adult Hgb
   c. Should be instituted quickly if deemed necessary

- Consider concomitant poisoning with other toxic/irritant gases that may be present in smoke (e.g., cyanide) or thermal injury to airway. Toxic effects of CO and cyanide are synergistic
- Identify source of exposure and determine if poisoning was accidental

DISPOSITION

- Patients with mild accidental poisoning can be treated in an ambulatory setting. Those with moderate to severe poisoning or coexisting illness require hospitalization.
- About 35% of patients with moderate to severe poisoning have cardiac dysfunction (arrhythmia, LV systolic dysfunction, ischemia).
- Survivors of severe poisoning are at 14% to 40% risk for neurologic sequelae.
  1. Deficits are usually apparent within 3 wk of poisoning but may present months later.
  2. Risk of developing sequelae is greater if patient lost consciousness during acute poisoning and with older age.
  3. Brain MRI and functional CT may reveal changes; damage is seen most often in the globus pallidus and deep white matter.
  4. Recovery may occur over months to years.
- Severe CO poisoning is associated with increased long-term morbidity and mortality.
- High risk of fetal demise.

REFERRAL

- American Association of Poison Control Centers: 800-222-1222
- Hyperbaric unit; accredited facilities are listed on the Undersea & Hyperbaric Medical Society website (www.uhms.org)
- Psychiatric evaluation if intentional poisoning

PEARLS & CONSIDERATIONS

- Hookah smoking is increasingly being recognized as a cause of CO poisoning, especially among young adults.
- Severity of poisoning and prognosis do not correlate with COHb levels because hypoxia represents only a component of CO's toxic effect. New therapies to address CO toxicity are being proposed.
- Neuropsychometric testing is an objective measure of cognitive function but is not universally used.
- Imaging techniques and biomarkers to define severity of CO poisoning, early prediction of CNS damage and prognosis are being studied, but are not ready for application.
- Pulse CO-oximetry measurement of CO saturation has limited clinical use.
- Treatment with hydroxocobalamin (for cyanide toxicity) may make subsequent COHb testing unreliable.
- Contact local fire department to assess environment and identify source of CO.

SUGGESTED READINGS

Available at ExpertConsult.com

RELATED CONTENT

Carbon Monoxide Poisoning (Patient Information)

AUTHOR: **Sudeep K. Aulakh, MD**

BASIC INFORMATION

DEFINITION

Cardiac tamponade is a life-threatening condition in which an accumulation of fluid within the pericardial space causes impaired diastolic filling and cardiac output as well as arterial hypotension due to elevated pericardial pressure.

ICD-10CM CODE
I31.4 Cardiac tamponade

PHYSICAL FINDINGS & CLINICAL PRESENTATION

- Tachypnea/dyspnea
- Chest pain may be present
- Beck triad:
  1. Absolute or relative hypotension
  2. Elevated jugular venous pressure (with prominent *x* descent and blunted *y* descent)
  3. Muffled heart sounds
- Tachycardia
- Pulsus paradoxus (decrease in systolic blood pressure of 10 mm Hg or more during normal inspiration while in normal sinus rhythm). It carries a sensitivity of 80% and a specificity of 40%. Tamponade settings in which pulsus paradoxus may not be present are summarized in Box 1
- Pericardial friction rub may be heard in patients with cardiac tamponade due to inflammatory pericarditis
- Reduced or absent apical cardiac impulse
- Signs of hypoperfusion from reduced cardiac output (diaphoresis, cool extremities, altered mental status, syncope or presyncope)

ETIOLOGY

- Acute (rapidly accumulating pericardial effusion leading to cardiac tamponade): Does not need a large amount of effusion to cause tamponade; rather, it is the rapidity of fluid accumulation that leads to clinical tamponade. It requires urgent reduction of pericardial pressure. Causes for acute cardiac tamponade include:
  1. Penetrating chest trauma
  2. Aortic dissection (more commonly in Type A)
  3. Postinfarction complications such as free wall rupture, immune mediated pericarditis (Dressler syndrome)
  4. Iatrogenic (right ventricular perforation during central line and pacemaker insertions, endomyocardial biopsy, arrhythmia ablation)
- Subacute or chronic: Occurs over days to weeks, and the effusion is usually moderate to large in size; causes include the following:
  1. Malignancy (e.g., lung, breast, lymphoma)
  2. Viral pericarditis (e.g., Coxsackie, human immunodeficiency virus, enterovirus, HSV 6, parvovirus, etc.)
  3. Bacterial, fungal, or tuberculous pericarditis
  4. Uremia
  5. Hypothyroidism/myxedema (rare)
  6. Collagen vascular disease (e.g., lupus, rheumatoid arthritis, scleroderma)
  7. Radiation
  8. Postmyocardial infarction or postcardiac ablation inflammation
  9. Idiopathic (most common)
- Regional cardiac tamponade occurs when the localized or loculated hematoma compresses only selected cardiac chambers

BOX 1 Tamponade Settings in Which Pulsus Paradoxus May Not Be Present

- Nonrestrictive (large) atrial septal defect
- Severe aortic insufficiency
- Loculated effusion
- LV hypertrophy and other causes of elevated LV diastolic pressure
- Shock caused by hypovolemia, or profound circulatory collapse with tamponade
- Severe left ventricular dysfunction
- Low-pressure tamponade
- RV hypertrophy or other cause of impaired RV filling
- Positive-pressure ventilation
- Arrhythmias

LV, Left ventricular; *RV*, right ventricular.

From Parrillo JE, Dellinger RP: *Critical care medicine, principles of diagnosis and management in the adult,* ed 5, Philadelphia, 2019, Elsevier.

DIAGNOSIS

Cardiac tamponade is a clinical diagnosis made at the bedside using patient history and physical examination. The transthoracic echocardiogram can help confirm the clinical diagnosis. Tamponade can also be confirmed invasively by the measurement of elevated intrapericardial pressures with an intrapericardial catheter and right heart catheterization. Typical findings are diastolic equalization of pressures, usually ranging from 10 to 30 mm Hg (diastolic pulmonary artery pressure = right ventricular diastolic pressure = right atrial pressure = intrapericardial pressure), and lowering of the intrapericardial pressure with fluid drainage. Thereafter, the underlying etiology must be determined with specific laboratory work (see "Laboratory Tests").

DIFFERENTIAL DIAGNOSIS

Other conditions that can also lead to elevated jugular venous pressure, decreased systemic pressure, and pulsus paradoxus include:

- Chronic obstructive pulmonary disease and asthma exacerbations
- Constrictive pericarditis (Table 1)
- Effusive-constrictive pericarditis
- Right ventricular infarction
- Pulmonary embolism
- Chronic biventricular heart failure

LABORATORY TESTS

- Electrolytes, blood urea nitrogen, creatinine, erythrocyte sedimentation rate, thyroid function tests, antinuclear antibody, rheumatoid factor, PPD, blood cultures, viral titers, and pericardial fluid analysis including cytology and cultures
- Possible 12-lead ECG findings:
  1. Sinus tachycardia
  2. PR depression and/or diffuse ST elevations if acute pericarditis is present
  3. Electrical alternans (beat to beat alternations in the QRS complex heights), which suggests the presence of a large pericardial effusion with or without tamponade. (Fig. 1)
  4. Low QRS voltage in patients with a pericardial effusion may be a specific manifestation of cardiac tamponade, not of the effusion (QRS complex <0.5 mV in the limb leads and <1.0 mV in precordial leads)

IMAGING STUDIES

- Chest radiograph (enlarged cardiac silhouette with clear lung fields) (Fig. 2).
- Chest CT (may overestimate size of the effusion) (Fig. 3).
- Cardiac MRI (as an adjunct to echocardiography) is usually not required.
- Echocardiogram findings (Fig. 4):
  1. Presence of pericardial effusion. Normally 10 to 50 cc of fluid is present in pericardial sac, and 100 cc of fluid can cause a circumferential effusion.
  2. Right atrial inversion for greater than one third of systole has a sensitivity of 94% and a specificity of 100% for the diagnosis of tamponade.

TABLE 1 Hemodynamics in Cardiac Tamponade and Constrictive Pericarditis

	Tamponade	Constrictive Pericarditis
Paradoxical pulse	Usually present	Present in ~1/3
Equalization left- and right-sided filling pressures	Present	Present
Systemic venous wave morphology	Absent *y* descent	Prominent *y* descent (M or W shape)
Inspiratory change in systemic venous pressure	Decrease (normal)	Increase or no change (Kussmaul sign)
"Square root" sign in ventricular pressure	Absent	Present

From Fuhrman BP et al: *Pediatric critical care,* ed 4, Philadelphia, 2011, Saunders.

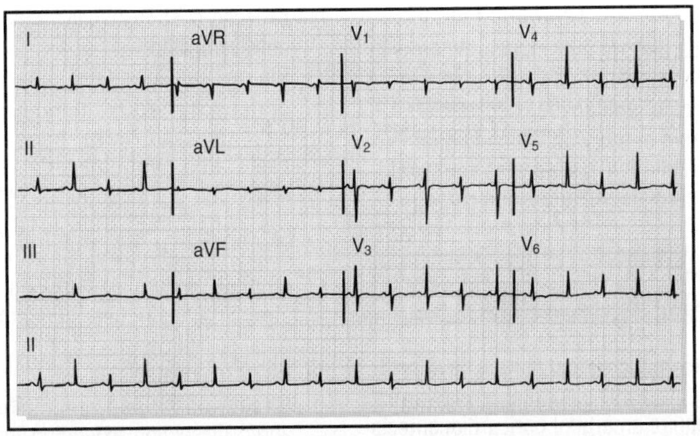

FIG. 1 Total electrical alternans (P-QRS-T) caused by pericardial effusion with tamponade. This finding, particularly in concert with sinus tachycardia and relatively low voltage, is a highly specific, although not sensitive, marker of cardiac tamponade. *aVF,* Augmented vector foot; *aVL,* augmented vector left; *aVR,* augmented vector right. (From Bonow RO: *Heart disease,* ed 9, Philadelphia, 2012, Saunders.)

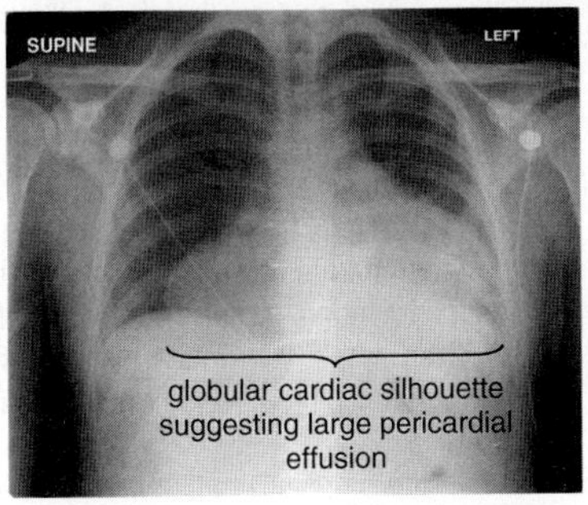

FIG. 2 Massive pericardial effusion and tamponade. This 23-yr-old male has a history of aortic valve replacement for infective endocarditis. He presented with increased chest pain and dyspnea. His chest x-ray shows a globular cardiac silhouette, suggesting a large pericardial effusion. The lung fields and right costophrenic angle appear clear, although the left costophrenic angle is hidden behind the heart and cannot be assessed. The patient underwent chest computed tomography to evaluate his aorta, as he complained of severe interscapular pain as well (see Fig. 3). (From Broder JS: *Diagnostic imaging for the emergency physician,* Philadelphia, 2011, Saunders.)

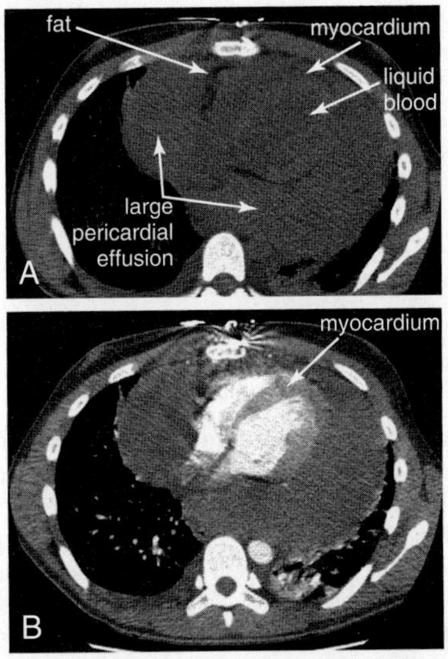

FIG. 3 Massive pericardial effusion. Same patient as Fig. 2. The patient underwent chest computed tomography (CT) without **(A)** and then with **(B)** intravenous contrast to evaluate his aorta, which was normal. However, the CT confirmed a massive pericardial effusion surrounding a normal-appearing heart. Without contrast, note that fluid blood within the chambers of the heart has a slightly lower density than the pericardial effusion, which has a density more similar to that of myocardium. When contrast is administered, the ventricular chambers fill completely, and the myocardium enhances and becomes somewhat brighter than the surrounding pericardial effusion. The heart itself is outlined by a thin stripe of fat, which appears nearly black on soft tissue windows. The patient developed hypotension, suggesting cardiac tamponade, and pericardial window was performed for drainage of the effusion. In the operating room, the effusion was found to be coagulated blood. (From Broder JS: *Diagnostic imaging for the emergency physician,* Philadelphia, 2011, Saunders.)

3. Diastolic collapse of the right ventricle (early diastole) is pathognomonic and 100% specific for the presence of cardiac tamponade.
4. >25% mitral and >40% tricuspid valve inflow variation on the first beat of inspiration and expiration, respectively.
5. Plethoric inferior vena cava (IVC dilation and <50% decrease in the diameter of the IVC during inspiration).
6. Left atrial and ventricular collapse have been noted most commonly in the setting of loculated effusions following cardiac surgery. They can also occur in the setting of tamponade with severe pulmonary hypertension.
7. An inspiratory septal "bounce" toward the left ventricle is commonly noted during inspiration due to phenomenon of ventricular interdependence, but this finding is not specific for tamponade. It is also present in constrictive pericarditis.

- Cardiac catheterization may demonstrate equalization of intracardiac diastolic pressures and increase of right-sided pressures and reduction of left-sided pressures, which causes pulsus paradoxus (the pathognomonic finding on physical examination).

Rx TREATMENT

NONPHARMACOLOGIC THERAPY

- Cardiac tamponade should be treated emergently with removal of the pericardial fluid (Fig. 5).
- Avoid drugs that reduce preload (e.g., nitrates, diuretics).
- Large pericardial effusions (>20 mm) without hemodynamic compromise (tamponade) can be managed conservatively with careful monitoring, IV fluids, and treatment of the underlying cause, clinical follow-up, and frequent serial surveillance echocardiography.

ACUTE GENERAL Rx

- Aggressive intravascular volume expansion (saline or blood)
- Emergency pericardial fluid removal by pericardiocentesis or surgical pericardiotomy by way of the subxiphoid pericardial window
- Pericardiocentesis should be performed under echocardiographic and fluoroscopic guidance when available
- Pericardiocentesis is contraindicated if the etiology of the pericardial effusion is aortic dissection, wherein emergent surgical management is indicated
- Inotropic or vasopressor support if above measures cannot be performed immediately

CHRONIC Rx

- Depends on etiology. Patients with inflammatory causes of pericarditis leading to effusion should be treated with antiinflammatory therapy (NSAIDs) as well as an extended 3-mo course of colchicine
- Pericardiocentesis with draining catheter: The catheter can be left inside the pericardium to allow continued drainage for 24 to 48 hr. If residual fluid still persists with hemodynamic compromise, surgical drainage should be considered. In the absence of significant residual fluid (output <50 ml in 24-hr period), discontinuation of the draining catheter can be done with periodic postprocedure echocardiographic monitoring for reaccumulation (e.g., 24 hr, 7 days, 30 days, 3 mo, 6 mo, 12 mo) depending on the etiology and the rate of reaccumulation
- Other surgical drainage procedures include:
  1. Subxiphoid pericardiotomy drainage
  2. Pericardial window; draining the pericardial fluid into the left hemithorax
  3. Limited pericardiectomy
  4. Complete pericardiectomy, especially in patients with effusive-constrictive pericarditis, bacterial pericarditis, or tuberculous pericarditis (see "Pearls & Considerations")

DISPOSITION

The prognosis of cardiac tamponade depends on the underlying cause.

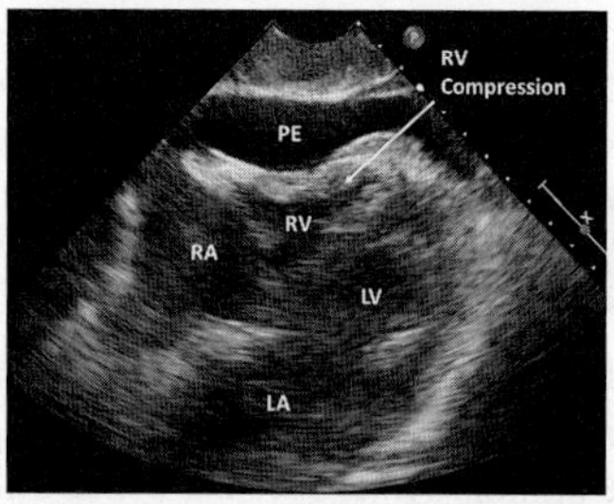

FIG. 4 Cardiac tamponade on echocardiography. Echo shows large pericardial effusion which is compressing the right ventricle. *LA,* Left atrium; *LV,* left ventricle; *PE,* pericardial effusion; *RA,* right atrium; *RV,* right ventricle. (From Parrillo JE, Dellinger RP: *Critical care medicine, principles of diagnosis and management in the adult,* ed 5, Philadelphia, 2019, Elsevier.)

REFERRAL

- Emergent cardiology consultation along with thorough echocardiographic exam should be made if cardiac tamponade is suspected.
- Cardiothoracic surgery or interventional cardiology consultation should also be considered if pericardial drainage is indicated.

PEARLS & CONSIDERATIONS

- Cardiac tamponade should always be considered during pulseless electrical activity arrest and may require emergent pericardiocentesis at the bedside.
- Evaluation for pulsus paradoxus should always be performed during normal respiration because deep inspiration may render a false-positive finding.
- Strong consideration should be given to performing early pericardiocentesis in patients who have pericardial effusion associated with bacterial pneumonia or empyema because the incidence of bacterial pericarditis is especially high in this clinical situation and the subsequent development of cardiac tamponade and severe chronic constrictive pericarditis are ominous complications.
- Pericardiocentesis is contraindicated if the etiology of the pericardial effusion is due to aortic dissection extending into the pericardial sac.
- As little as 100 ml of fluid can lead to acute cardiac tamponade if the rate of accumulation is rapid, whereas with gradual accumulation, the pericardial sac can hold up to a liter of fluid or more before tamponade occurs.
- With effusions that are small, organized, and/or loculated, needle aspiration should generally be avoided. An exception is acute cardiac tamponade complicating a cardiac procedure (e.g., percutaneous coronary intervention) with anticoagulation. In this setting, the effusion is often small, but pericardial pressure rises very quickly, resulting in hemodynamic compromise.

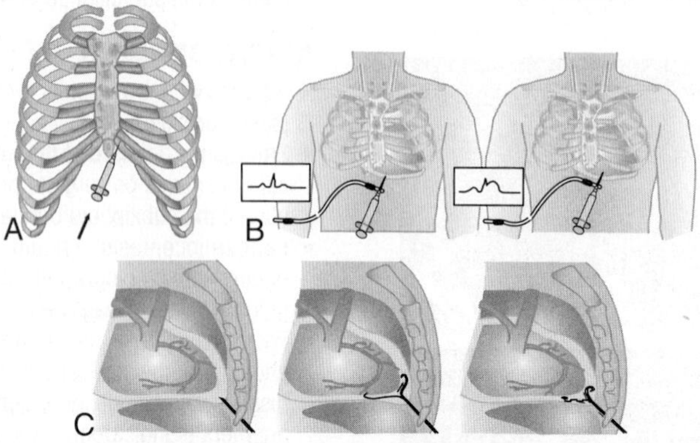

FIG. 5 Diagrammatic representation of a pericardiocentesis procedure via the subxiphoid approach. A, A subxiphoid approach is used. **B,** A pericardial needle is connected to an ECG lead and is advanced left, lateral to the subxiphoid area, aiming toward the left shoulder. ST-segment elevation is seen on the ECG lead tracing when the needle touches the epicardium. The needle should be retracted slightly until the ST-segment elevation disappears. **C,** After the pericardial space is entered with the pericardial needle, a guidewire is introduced in the pericardial space through the needle. The needle is removed, and a catheter is inserted in the pericardial sac over the guidewire (either anteriorly or inferiorly in the pericardial sac). (From Parrillo JE, Dellinger RP: *Critical care medicine, principles of diagnosis and management in the adult,* ed 5, Philadelphia, 2019, Elsevier.)

SUGGESTED READINGS

Available at ExpertConsult.com

RELATED CONTENT

Cardiac Tamponade (Patient Information)
Pericarditis (Related Key Topic)

AUTHORS: **Vrinda Trivedi, MBBS** and **Aravind Rao Kokkirala, MD, FACC**

BASIC INFORMATION

DEFINITION

Cardiomyopathy, chemical-induced (CMc), is a change in myocardial structure and/or function caused by chemical compounds. Many chemicals, including environmental toxins, prescription drugs, and illicit drugs, are associated with cardiomyopathy (CM). These include (but are not limited to) alcohol, cocaine, amphetamines, chloroquine, anabolic steroids, anthracyclines, 5-fluorouracil (5-FU), zidovudine, tyrosine kinase inhibitors, and trastuzumab.

SYNONYMS

Alcoholic cardiomyopathy (ACM)
Cocaine-induced CM
Anabolic steroid-induced CM
Anthracycline-induced CM
Chemotherapy-induced CM
CMc

ICD-10CM CODE
I42.7 Cardiomyopathy due to drug and external agent

EPIDEMIOLOGY & DEMOGRAPHICS

- ACM occurs in about 5% to 10% of alcoholics and accounts for 21% to 36% of dilated cardiomyopathy in high-income countries. Most patients in whom alcoholic cardiomyopathy develops have been drinking more than 80 to 90 g of ethanol per day for more than 5 yr. A key factor for diagnosing ACM is a history of heavy alcohol consumption in the absence of coronary artery disease.
- The risk of doxorubicin-induced cardiotoxicity is dose dependent: 3% to 5% with 400 mg/m^2, 7% to 26% at 550 mg/m^2, and 18% to 48% at 700 mg/m^2.
- The addition of trastuzumab to an anthracycline-based chemotherapy regimen markedly increases the incidence of heart failure (28% vs. 1.7%-21% with trastuzumab alone). Introducing a drug-free interval between the agents can significantly reduce the incidence of heart failure. Long-term follow-up data regarding trastuzumab cardiotoxicity are favorable, as the cardiotoxic effects generally manifest during treatment and are reversible.
- Other chemotherapeutic agents known to cause cardiomyopathy include idarubicin (>90 mg/m^2, 5%-18%), epirubicin (>900 mg/m^2, 0.9%-11.4%), docetaxel (2.3%-13%), cyclophosphamide (7%-28%), bortezomib (2%-5%), sunitinib (2.7%-19%), 5-fluorouracil [5-FU] (6%-7%), and carfilzomib (11% to 25%). Table 1 summarizes chemotherapeutic agents implicated in clinical syndromes of cardiotoxicity.

PREDOMINANT SEX & AGE: The prevalence of ACM appears to be similar among alcoholic men and women, with women developing left ventricular (LV) dysfunction at a lower ethanol dose than men. Significant racial differences exist, with blacks having higher mortality rates than non-Hispanic whites. Anthracycline- and trastuzumab-induced cardiomyopathy is more common in those aged >50 yr.

RISK FACTORS:
- Consumption of more than 80 to 100 g/day of alcohol for more than 10 yr significantly increases the risk of ACM.
- The occurrence of chronic anthracycline-induced CM is correlated to cumulative dose, age, preexisting heart disease, concomitant chemotherapy, and history of mediastinal radiation therapy. Children are more susceptible to anthracycline-induced CM.
- Additional risk factors for anthracycline-induced CM include radiation therapy involving the cardiac silhouette as well as concomitant use of trastuzumab.
- Continuous infusion dosing may reduce the risk for cardiotoxicity compared to bolus regimens.

GENETICS:
- In patients with ACM, the deletion (DD) genotype of angiotensin-converting-enzyme (ACE) is more common than insertion (II) and deletion, insertion (DI) genotypes. The underlying mechanism involves direct toxicity of ethanol to the myocardium through uncoupling of adenosine triphosphate.
- Anthracycline-induced CM is linked to an increase in cardiac oxidative stress via the pathways of mitochondrial nitric oxide synthesis, and nicotinamide adenine dinucleotide phosphate reduction.
- One study suggests that polymorphisms in the carbonyl reductase genes could be related to anthracycline-induced CM.

PHYSICAL FINDINGS & CLINICAL PRESENTATION

The majority of clinical characteristics of CMc are similar to dilated cardiomyopathy of other etiologies. Symptoms may be insidious or acute in onset.
- ACM typically occurs after years of heavy drinking. Concurrent cirrhosis may be present. The presentation is typically heart failure with or without arrhythmia. Atrial fibrillation is the most common arrhythmia associated with chronic alcohol abuse and can also be seen with acute intoxication (holiday heart syndrome).
- Acute anthracycline-induced CM can start at any time after the first dose and may present with arrhythmias (most commonly supraventricular tachycardia), left ventricular (LV) dysfunction, or pericardial disease. Typically the first manifestation of anthracycline-induced cardiotoxicity is subtle diastolic dysfunction noted on tissue Doppler echocardiography. The subacute and chronic symptoms may occur 3 mo to 10 yr after the last dose. Patients usually present with heart failure. More recently, mortality has improved as a result of medical therapy with ACE inhibitors and beta-blockers. In fact, recent trials, including the OVERCOME trial, have demonstrated a benefit in preemptively treating low-cardiac-risk patients undergoing anthracycline therapy with beta-blockers and ACE-inhibitors to prevent the development of CM.
- Cardiac symptoms after 5-FU treatment include angina (most common), myocardial infarction, arrhythmia, acute pulmonary edema, cardiac arrest, and pericarditis. The mechanism of angina and myocardial infarction is coronary vasospasm and endothelial injury. The overall incidence of angina is approximately 10%.
- Patients with cocaine-induced CM may present with adrenergic symptoms (palpitations, pallor, diaphoresis, and anxiety), hypertension, angina, atrial and ventricular arrhythmias, and heart failure.
- Anabolic steroids harm the myocardium in a dose-related manner and can cause left ventricular (LV) hypertrophy and dilation, and lead to heart failure, arrhythmia, myocardial infarction, hypertension, and sudden death.

ETIOLOGY

- Table 2 describes mechanisms of ethanol-induced myocardial injury. Table 3 summarizes the effects of light-to-moderate and heavier alcohol intake on cardiovascular risk factors and outcomes.
- Nutritional deficiencies, such as thiamine deficiency, also play a role in ACM.
- The underlying mechanism of chemotherapy-induced cardiotoxicity is not well established. Several pathways have been proposed (Fig. 1), including an increase in oxidative stress; free radical production; apoptosis; disturbance of DNA, RNA, and protein synthesis; and vasospasm.
- Cocaine-induced LV dysfunction is largely secondary to myocardial scarring, but cocaine also induces adrenergic surge and can cause LV dilation and an acute elevation in LV pressures, even in the absence of ischemic heart disease.
- Chloroquine/hydroxychloroquine-induced cardiomyopathy is caused by inhibition of lysosomal enzymes, leading to lysosomal dysfunction and subsequent toxic accumulation of metabolic products.

Dx DIAGNOSIS

DIFFERENTIAL DIAGNOSIS

- Infectious cardiomyopathy: Viral, HIV-related, Lyme disease, Chagas disease
- Ischemic cardiomyopathy
- Dilated cardiomyopathy, related to valvular disease or hypertension
- Cirrhotic cardiomyopathy
- Tachycardia-induced cardiomyopathy
- Stress-related (takotsubo) cardiomyopathy
- Peripartum cardiomyopathy
- Genetic causes of dilated cardiomyopathy

WORKUP

- Chemical exposure history
- Electrocardiogram, serum electrolytes, renal function, and hepatic function
- Serum troponin and brain natriuretic peptide (BNP) levels

TABLE 1 Chemotherapeutic Agents Implicated in Clinical Syndromes of Cardiotoxicity

Agent	Frequency of Cardiotoxicity*	Comments
Left Ventricular Dysfunction–Heart Failure Chemotherapeutics		
Anthracyclines		
Doxorubicin	+++	Highly dose-dependent
Epirubicin	+	Risk factors include age (old and young), prior mediastinal radiation, history of heart disease, decreased ejection fraction; drop in ejection fraction on drug therapy, female sex (for children), and other agents (especially trastuzumab)
Idarubicin	++	Risk decreased by liposomal encapsulation or dexrazoxane
Alkylating agents		
Cyclophosphamide	+++	Primarily seen with high-dose "conditioning" regimens
Ifosfamide	+++	Risk factors are previous mediastinal irradiation and anthracycline drug therapy Also can have myocarditis, pericarditis, myocardial necrosis
Taxanes		
Paclitaxel	+/++	Also employed in paclitaxel-eluting stent
Docetaxel	+	
Proteasome inhibitor		
Bortezomib	+/++	Moderately high rates of HF seen in trials (5%), but rates only minimally higher than in patients receiving dexamethasone
Targeted Therapeutics		
Monoclonal antibodies		
Trastuzumab	++	Not common as single agent Increased risk with anthracyclines, paclitaxel, cyclophosphamide
Pertuzumab	+/++	Targets HER2 Rates of LV dysfunction as high as ~25% in one series
Bevacizumab	+/++	Targets VEGF-A (ligand for VEGFRs) and serves as a trap, preventing interaction with its receptor HF can be seen in setting of severe hypertension, which occurs in 10%-25% of patients, depending on dose; anthracyclines may increase HF risk
Tyrosine kinase inhibitors		
Imatinib, nilotinib	+	Can cause severe fluid retention with peripheral edema, pleural and pericardial effusion not secondary to LV dysfunction
Dasatinib	++	Same as above regarding fluid retention Can cause severe pulmonary hypertension; mechanism unclear
Sunitinib	+++	LV dysfunction common; hypertension likely plays role
Sorafenib	++	Rate of cardiotoxicity not clear as of yet
Ischemic Syndromes		
Fluorouracil, capecitabine	++	ACS; patients with CAD at increased risk Recurs with rechallenge; multiple mechanisms proposed; etiology remains unknown
Cisplatin, carboplatin	+	ACS caused by vasospasm or vascular injury Hypertension common; thromboembolism more common (see below)
Interferon-α	+	Risk of ischemia increased in patients with CAD; hypertension common
Paclitaxel	+	Myocardial ischemia in 1%-5%; serious ischemic cardiac events not common
Docetaxel	+	Limited data, but rate probably ~1%
Bevacizumab	++	Arterial thrombotic events including MI and stroke
Vinca alkaloids	+	~1% risk of cardiac events; ischemia possibly caused by coronary spasm
Sorafenib	+/++	~2.5% risk of ACS
Erlotinib, nilotinib	+/++	Limited data, but rate ~2%; concern over possible increase in peripheral vascular events
Hypertension		
Cisplatin	++++	
Bevacizumab	++++	Extremely common with all anti-VEGF therapeutics to date
Sunitinib	++++	Intrinsic in mechanism of action of these agents
Sorafenib	+++	
Venous Thrombosis		
Cisplatin	+++	Deep vein thrombosis or pulmonary embolism in 8.5%; most occur early in treatment Additional risk factors for deep vein thrombosis often present
Thalidomide	++++	Uncommon with monotherapy, but risk rises with concurrent chemotherapy
Lenalidomide	+++	See comments for thalidomide
Erlotinib	++	Rate with erlotinib plus gemcitabine ~2% over that with gemcitabine alone

ACS, Acute coronary syndrome; *CAD,* coronary artery disease; *HER2,* human epidermal growth factor receptor 2; *HF,* heart failure; *LV,* left ventricular; *MI,* myocardial infarction; *VEGF,* vascular endothelial cell growth factor; *VEGFR,* vascular endothelial cell growth factor receptor.

*Relative frequency of cardiotoxicity is scored as follows: + = ≤1%; ++ = 1% to 5%; +++ = 6% to 10%; ++++ = >10%.

From Mann DL et al: *Braunwald's heart disease*, ed 10, Philadelphia, 2015, Elsevier.

TABLE 2 Mechanisms of Ethanol-Induced Myocardial Injury

Direct Toxic Effects
Uncoupling of the excitation/contraction system
Reduced calcium sequestration in the sarcoplasmic reticulum
Inhibition of the sarcolemmal adenosine triphosphate–dependent Na^+/K^+ pump
Reduction in the mitochondrial respiratory ratio
Altered substrate uptake
Increased interstitial/extracellular protein synthesis
Toxic Effect of Metabolites
Acetaldehyde
Ethyl esters
Nutritional or Trace Metal Deficiencies
Thiamine
Selenium
Electrolyte Disturbances
Hypomagnesemia
Hypokalemia
Hypophosphatemia
Toxic Additives
Cobalt
Lead
Arsenic

K, Potassium; *Na*, sodium.
From Mann DL et al: *Braunwald's heart disease*, ed 10, Philadelphia, 2015, Elsevier.

TABLE 3 Qualitative Effects of Light-to-Moderate and Heavier Alcohol Intake on Cardiovascular Risk Factors and Outcomes

Cardiovascular Risk Factors and Outcomes	Light-to-Moderate Alcohol Intake (<2 Drinks per Day)	Heavier Alcohol Intake (>2 Drinks per Day)
Blood pressure	↔	↑↑
HDL cholesterol	↑↑	↑↑↑
Triglycerides	↑	↑↑
LDL cholesterol	↔ or ↓	↑
Platelet aggregability/coagulability	↓	↓↓
Systemic inflammation	↓	↑
Congestive heart failure	↓	↑↑
Coronary artery disease (angina, nonfatal MI)	↓↓	↓
Atrial fibrillation	↔	↑↑
Stroke	↓	↑↑
Sudden cardiac death	↓↓	↑

HDL, High-density lipoprotein; *LDL*, low-density lipoprotein; *MI*, myocardial infarction.
From Mann DL et al: *Braunwald's heart disease*, ed 10, Philadelphia, 2015, Elsevier.

- Transthoracic echocardiogram for the evaluation of heart structure and function
- Rule out the diagnosis of coronary artery disease by coronary angiography
- Cardiac magnetic resonance (CMR) imaging can be used to evaluate for myocardial scar and fibrosis

LABORATORY TESTS

- There are no specific diagnostic tests to help differentiate CMc from other forms of CM, but the following laboratory tests are generally helpful; serum electrolytes, renal function, hepatic function, thyroid-stimulating hormone, iron profile, and inflammatory markers.
- Recent studies have suggested that early elevation of troponin levels, BNP, and myeloperoxidase following chemotherapy may be a predictor of future development of cardiomyopathy.

IMAGING STUDIES

- ECG
- Nonspecific findings of a cardiomyopathy may be present, including sinus tachycardia, nonspecific ST-T wave changes, decreased QRS voltage, interventricular conduction delay or bundle branch block, and QT interval abnormalities. In 5-FU toxicity, significant ST segment deviations may be present.
- Echocardiogram
  1. Asymptomatic alcoholics may present with mild LV hypertrophy, diastolic dysfunction, LV dilation, and decrease in left ventricular ejection fraction (LVEF).
  2. Baseline LVEF should be performed before initiation of anthracycline-based chemotherapy, preferably with an echocardiogram or multigated acquisition (MUGA) scan.
     a. Anthracycline-based chemotherapy should generally be avoided for patients with an LVEF ≤40%, or LVEF >40% but <50% with prior heart failure.
     b. Total doxorubicin dose should be limited to 450 mg/m².
     c. If baseline LVEF is ≥55%, then subsequent evaluation should be at the end of treatment if the doxorubicin dose is <200 mg/m² or serially at 200, 300, 350, and 400 mg/m² for higher doses. Doxorubicin therapy should be discontinued if there is a >15% absolute drop in LVEF, decease in LVEF to ≤40%, or symptomatic congestive heart failure with an LVEF <50%. There has been no direct causal link between anthracyclines and the development of heart failure with a preserved ejection fraction.
     d. Peak systolic global longitudinal strain imaging (GLS) is an emerging echocardiographic measurement. A 10% to 15% early decrease in GLS by speckle tracking echocardiography during treatment seems to be the most useful parameter for the early detection of cardiotoxicity. Echocardiographic strain and strain rate imaging are sensitive, noninvasive methods for assessment of myocardial function.
  3. Echocardiographic features of chloroquine/hydroxychloroquine-induced cardiomyopathy include biatrial enlargement and biventricular hypertrophy with a restrictive physiology.
- Radionuclide imaging (Fig. E2).
  1. If baseline LVEF is <50% with no prior history of heart failure, the cardiac risks vs. oncological benefits should be discussed with the patient, cardiologist, and oncologist before initiating therapy. Optimization of cardiovascular status, including hypertension control, is recommended. Cardio-protective agents such as ACE inhibitors and beta-blockers should be initiated and serial LVEF measurements done after each dose.
  2. Even after chemotherapy, periodic screening with echocardiography and/or biomarkers should be considered for up to 10 yr for those with high cumulative anthracycline doses or a history of reversible LV dysfunction during treatment.

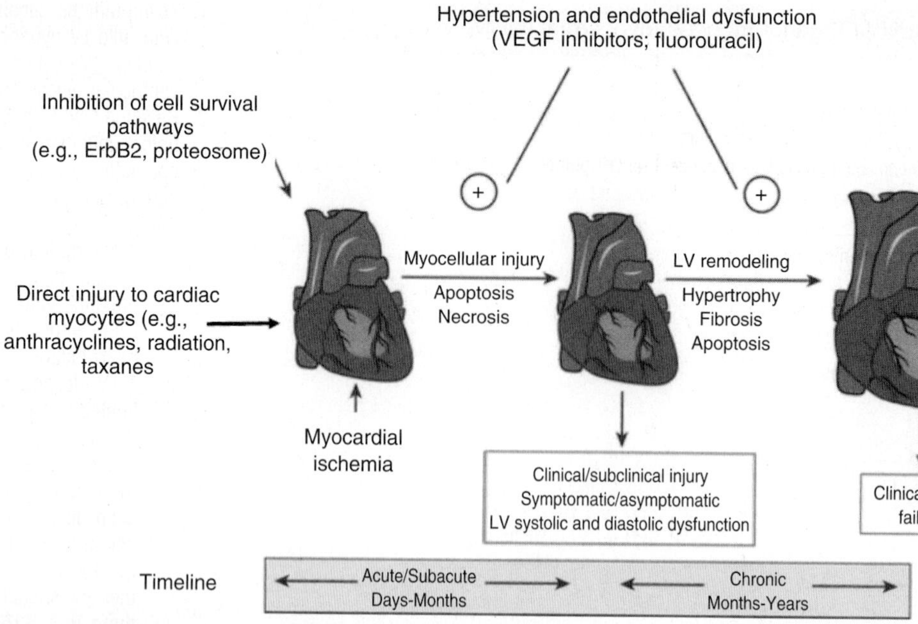

FIG. 1 Pathophysiology of chemotherapy-induced cardiotoxicity. The specific mechanisms and clinical manifestations of cardiac injury may vary according to each chemotherapy class, but the final common pathway linking the initial injury to acute, subacute, and chronic manifestations are often overlapping. Acute and subacute injury are often asymptomatic and may or may not be associated with a measurable change in ejection fraction. Chronic cardiac injury usually is associated with left ventricular *(LV)* remodeling, characterized by LV enlargement, reduced ejection fraction, and eventually symptomatic heart failure. Hypertension associated with inhibitors of the vascular endothelial growth factor *(VEGF)* signaling pathway can exacerbate myocardial injury and cardiac disease progression in the acute, subacute, and chronic settings. (From Niederhuber JE: *Abeloff's clinical oncology,* ed 6, Philadelphia, 2020, Elsevier.)

Rx TREATMENT

ACUTE GENERAL Rx

- Treat decompensated heart failure with diuresis, supplementing with inotropes if there is a low cardiac output state.
- For angina in acute cocaine intoxication or induced by 5-FU, benzodiazepines, nitrites, and calcium channel blockers are first-line therapy. If ECG provides evidence of acute myocardial infarction, patients should proceed to emergent cardiac catheterization and coronary angiography.

CHRONIC Rx

- Thiamine, folic acid, and multivitamins are adjunctive treatments for ACM. Abstinence can usually reverse the cardiomyopathy.
- Dexrazoxane is an ethylenediaminetetraacetic acid-like chelator that acts by binding to iron, which prevents anthracycline cardiotoxicity. Cardiooncology experts suggest a 10:1 ratio of dexrazoxane to anthracycline, given 15 to 30 min before doxorubicin administration. However, its routine use is not currently recommended in adults except in cases of a cumulative doxorubicin dose of 300 mg/m^2 or greater with an ongoing indication to receive doxorubicin-based chemotherapy.
- Those developing anthracycline-induced CM generally should not be rechallenged with the drug, as the cardiac damage is usually irreversible due to cell death.
- Beta-blocker: Carvedilol and nebivolol have been shown to have protective effects on LV systolic function during anthracycline therapy. Larger trials with metoprolol have shown no benefit.
- The following ACE inhibitors and angiotensin receptor blocker (ARB) have been shown to protect against anthracycline cardiotoxicity: Enalapril, ramipril, and telmisartan. Results from the PRADA trial suggest that use of the ARB candesartan mitigates anthracycline-induced decline in LVEF.
- There is growing interest in the use of statins for primary prevention of anthracycline-mediated cardiotoxicity based on their antioxidant and antiinflammatory properties, although a cardioprotective effect has not been established.
- There is an early reversibility of chloroquine-induced cardiomyopathy, and if the offending agent is withdrawn in a timely manner, there may be a partial or complete reversal of cardiomyopathy.

DISPOSITION

Prognosis depends on the dosage of chemicals and the severity of LV dysfunction.

REFERRAL

Close follow-up with a cardiooncologist.

PEARLS & CONSIDERATIONS

The presentation of chemotherapy-induced cardiac toxicity ranges from an asymptomatic decline in LVEF to overt heart failure. The incidence is dose-dependent in the case of anthracyclines and may manifest up to 10 yr after the initial exposure. Therefore, regular clinical follow-up with echocardiographic surveillance is advised.

PREVENTION

- Noninvasive assessment of LV function before, during, and after anthracycline-containing chemotherapy with echocardiography or MUGA scan.
- To reduce the risk of doxorubicin cardiotoxicity, the lifetime cumulative dosage should be limited to <450 mg/m^2 in adults.
- Other approaches include the use of infusion rather than bolus dosing, liposomal encapsulated doxorubicin, less cardiotoxic analogs of doxorubicin such as epirubicin, and coadministration of protective agents such as dexrazoxane.
- 5-FU treatment should be terminated if cardiac symptoms develop. Readministration is not recommended.

SUGGESTED READINGS

Available at ExpertConsult.com

AUTHORS: **Shilpa Vijayakumar, MD,** and **Aravind Rao Kokkirala, MD, FACC**

BASIC INFORMATION

DEFINITION

Dilated cardiomyopathy describes a group of diseases involving the myocardium and characterized by dilation and impaired contraction of one or both ventricles that is not wholly the result of hypertension, coronary atherosclerosis, valvular dysfunction, congenital, or other structural heart disease. As a result, the systolic function of the heart is impaired and may develop overt heart failure, atrial and/or ventricular arrhythmias, and sudden death. The disease is considered idiopathic if primary and secondary causes of heart disease are excluded.

SYNONYMS

Congestive cardiomyopathy
Idiopathic cardiomyopathy

ICD-10CM CODES

B33.24	Viral cardiomyopathy
I11.0	Hypertensive heart disease with heart failure
I42.0	Dilated cardiomyopathy (includes congestive cardiomyopathy)
I42.9	Cardiomyopathy, unspecified (includes cardiomyopathy [primary] [secondary] NOS)
I43	Cardiomyopathy in diseases classified elsewhere
I50.20 to I50.9	(Unspecified, Acute, Chronic, or Acute on Chronic) + (systolic, diastolic, or combined) (congestive) heart failure
O90.3	Peripartum cardiomyopathy

EPIDEMIOLOGY & DEMOGRAPHICS

- The estimated age-adjusted prevalence of dilated cardiomyopathy in the United States general population is approximately 36 per 100,000 and a predilection for men with a male/female ratio of 3:1. The incidence is approximately 6 per 100,000 persons per year, although younger patients (<55 yr) were more frequently affected (incidence up to 18/100,000).
- African Americans have a three-fold increased risk for developing DCM, irrespective of comorbidities or socioeconomic factors, compared with whites.
- DCM is the most common form of cardiomyopathy, comprising approximately 60% of all cardiomyopathies.

PHYSICAL FINDINGS & CLINICAL PRESENTATION

Affected patients may present in a number of ways, and the etiology is most often elucidated with obtaining a focused history. The patient may display common symptoms of congestive heart failure, which may either be insidious or present suddenly. The patient may also be asymptomatic and the diagnosis made only by the incidental finding of cardiomegaly on a chest X-ray. Classical signs of heart failure include:

- Increased jugular venous pressure
- Narrow pulse pressure
- Pulmonary rales, hepatomegaly, peripheral edema
- S3, S4
- Mitral regurgitation, tricuspid regurgitation (less common)
- Pulsus alternans (sign of advanced ventricular dysfunction)

ETIOLOGY

DCM can be attributed to genetic and nongenetic causes, including hypertension, valve disease, inflammatory/infectious causes, and toxins.

- Idiopathic (often a viral infection that cannot be confirmed)
- Infections (viral [human herpesvirus 6, influenza, echovirus, cytomegalovirus, Coxsackie B, adenovirus, parvovirus, HIV], rickettsial, mycobacterial, toxoplasmosis, trichinosis, Chagas' disease)
- Ischemic heart disease
- Alcoholism (15% to 40% of all cases in Western countries)
- Uncontrolled tachyarrhythmia ("tachycardia-mediated")
- Sleep apnea–obstructive or nonobstructive
- Cirrhotic (not necessarily alcohol-induced)
- End-stage renal disease–related
- Nutritional deficiencies (selenium, L-carnitine, thiamine)
- Peripartum (greatest risk from last trimester of pregnancy to 6 mo postpartum)
- Chemotherapeutic (anthracycline, doxorubicin, daunorubicin) or pharmacologic agents (antiretrovirals, phenothiazines) (see "Cardiomyopathy, Chemical-Induced")
- Substance abuse (cocaine, heroin, organic solvents "glue-sniffer's heart")
- Postmyocarditis
- Toxins (cobalt, lead, phosphorus, carbon monoxide, mercury), collagen-vascular disease (systemic lupus, rheumatoid arthritis, polyarteritis, dermatomyositis, sarcoidosis)
- Hereditary familial neuromuscular disorders (e.g., muscular dystrophy, myotonic dystrophy)
- Endocrine dysfunction (acromegaly, osteogenesis imperfecta, myxedema, thyrotoxicosis, diabetes)
- Hematologic (e.g., sickle cell anemia, hereditary sideroblastic anemias and thalassemias, hypereosinophilia, hereditary hemochromatosis)
- Stress-induced (i.e., takotsubo or broken heart syndrome)
- LV noncompaction
- Autoimmunity ("anti-heart antibodies" (AHAs) [beta-1 adrenoceptor, alpha-myosin heavy chain, beta-myosin heavy chain, myosin light chain]) are hypothesized to cause DCM based on animal studies. Appears to be applicable to humans as AHAs can be detected in 38% of patients with an idiopathic DCM.
- *TTN* truncating mutations (mutations in *TTN*, the gene encoding the sarcomere protein titin) are a common cause of dilated cardiomyopathy, occurring in approximately 25% of familial cases of idiopathic dilated cardiomyopathy and in 18% of sporadic cases.

Dx DIAGNOSIS

Dilated cardiomyopathy is a diagnosis of exclusion, made after ruling out other potential causes of myocardial dysfunction.

DIFFERENTIAL DIAGNOSIS

- Coronary atherosclerosis, that is, left ventricular dysfunction secondary to ischemia and/or myocardial infarction
- Valvular dysfunction (especially aortic and mitral regurgitation)
- Other cardiomyopathies (restrictive, hypertrophic)
- Pulmonary disease (embolism, obstructive, restrictive)
- Pericardial abnormalities (constrictive pericarditis, tamponade)
- Hypothyroidism/myxedema
- Athlete's heart

WORKUP

- Medical history: Emphasis on symptoms of dyspnea, orthopnea, paroxysmal nocturnal dyspnea, weight gain, palpitations, fatigue, or signs of systemic and pulmonary embolism, substance abuse history, and possible toxin exposures (especially occupational)
- Physical exam (see "Physical Findings & Clinical Presentation")
- Testing (see "Laboratory Tests" and "Imaging Studies" for more detail): Laboratory, chest X-ray, ECG, echocardiogram, cardiac catheterization; myocardial biopsy is not routinely recommended, unless acute myocarditis requiring immunosuppressive therapy is considered (e.g., giant cell myocarditis)

LABORATORY TESTS

- Chemistries/metabolites (deficiencies), renal function tests (renal dysfunction)
- Cardiac biomarkers (elevation of cardiac troponin or BNP): Persistently increased cardiac troponin T levels are a marker of poor outcome in cardiomyopathy patients
- Endocrine (particularly thyroid)
- Iron studies (hemochromatosis, deficiency)
- Rheumatologic and inflammatory (ANA, ESR, CRP)
- Others as indicated (HIV, Lyme, neurohormonal)

IMAGING STUDIES

Chest x-ray:

- Cardiac silhouette enlargement (particularly left ventricle)
- Pulmonary vascular redistribution and congestion (Kerley B lines, cephalization of vasculature), pleural effusion (may appear as unilateral, most often on the right side)

ECG:

- ECG findings are typically nonspecific, and sinus tachycardia is usually a reflection of underlying heart failure. Large voltage in precordial leads and low voltage in limb leads may be seen in advanced disease.
- Intraventricular conduction defects and left bundle branch block

- Arrhythmias (atrial fibrillation, premature ventricular or atrial contractions, ventricular tachycardia)
- Echocardiogram (Fig. E1): Low ejection fraction with global hypokinesis
- Four-chamber enlargement (LV enlargement usually predominates)
- Mitral or tricuspid regurgitation ("secondary" regurgitation from tethering due to incomplete leaflet closure caused by ventricular dilation)

Cardiac catheterization:
- On initial presentation to exclude obstructive epicardial coronary artery disease

Cardiac magnetic resonance imaging (CMRI):
- Particularly if infiltrative or inflammatory etiology suspected

TABLE 1 Factors Associated with an Adverse Outcome in Dilated Cardiomyopathy

Clinical	Noninvasive	Invasive
NYHA Class III/IV	Low LV ejection fraction	High LV filling pressures
Increasing age	Marked LV dilation	
Low exercise peak oxygen consumption	Low LV mass	
Marked intraventricular conduction delay	≥Moderate mitral regurgitation	
Complex ventricular arrhythmias	Abnormal diastolic function	
Abnormal signal-averaged ECG	Abnormal contractile reserve	
Evidence of excessive sympathetic stimulation	Right ventricular dilation or dysfunction	
Protodiastolic gallop (S_3)		
Elevated serum BNP		
Elevated uric acid		
Decreased serum sodium		

BNP, Brain natriuretic peptide; *ECG*, electrocardiogram; *LV*, left ventricular; *NYHA*, New York Heart Association.
From Hare JM: The dilated, restrictive, and infiltrative cardiomyopathies. In Bonow RO et al (eds): *Braunwald's heart disease—a textbook of cardiovascular medicine*, ed 9, St Louis, 2011, Saunders.

Rx TREATMENT

NONPHARMACOLOGIC THERAPY

- Treatment of underlying disease (systemic lupus, alcoholism)
- Dietary sodium restriction (<2 g/day)
- Exercise training has been shown to be associated with reduced risk for hospitalization and death in patients with history of heart failure in limited trials; enrollment in a formal cardiac rehabilitation program may be beneficial in improving patient's functional status

ACUTE GENERAL Rx

- Identify and treat the etiology of the acute exacerbation, when able. A helpful mnemonic is FAILURE: Failure to take medications, Anemia/Arrhythmia, Ischemia/Infection/Infarction, Lifestyle (dietary indiscretion), Upregulation of cardiac output (hyperthyroidism or pregnancy), Renal failure, Embolus (pulmonary).
- Diuretics are indicated for all patients with current symptoms or history of heart failure and reduced left ventricular ejection fraction (LVEF) with evidence of volume overload (see "Physical Findings and Clinical Presentation") to improve symptoms. Although diuretics are the mainstay for treatment for heart failure exacerbations, it is important to note that diuretics have not been shown to improve mortality rates.
- Patients with associated coronary atherosclerosis (angina, ECG changes, reversible defects on myocardial perfusion imaging) may benefit from percutaneous or surgical revascularization.

CHRONIC Rx

- Diuretics as noted in "Acute General Rx."
- ACE inhibitors (and angiotensin receptor blockers) have been shown to have favorable effects on ventricular remodeling in patients with cardiomyopathy and a demonstrable mortality benefit in these patients. They also reduce afterload and improve cardiac output. Recommended in all patients with reduced LV systolic function (EF ≤40%), regardless of symptoms unless specific contraindications exist.
- Beta-blockers work by inhibiting the adverse effects of the sympathetic nervous system in patients with ventricular systolic dysfunction (EF ≤40%). *Only* carvedilol, long-acting metoprolol succinate, and bisoprolol have shown a mortality benefit in patients with LV systolic dysfunction. Unless specifically contraindicated, they should be started after the acute exacerbation has resolved and titrated to the maximum tolerated dose.
- Aldosterone antagonists (spironolactone and eplerenone) have shown mortality benefit along with a decreased rate of hospitalization for heart failure in patients with symptomatic heart failure and reduced LV systolic function (EF ≤35%). They should be used following label guidelines and with close monitoring of renal function and potassium.
- Hydralazine/nitrates improve both morbidity and mortality, and should be considered in the following populations: African Americans with persistent NYHA class III or IV heart failure with an EF < 40% on optimal medical therapy (beta blocker and ACE or ARB) or for those unable to take an ACE inhibitors or ARBs due to intolerance, hypotension, or renal insufficiency.
- Digoxin is used for its positive inotropic effects in heart failure due to systolic dysfunction. It has no mortality benefit but has been shown to improve patients' quality of life in appropriately selected patients.
- Angiotensin receptor-neprilysin inhibitor (ARNI), sacubitril-valsartan (LCZ696 or Entresto™), approved in the U.S. in 2015, was developed to block harmful effects of renin-angiotensin-aldosterone system (RAAS) activation while raising levels of endogenous vasoactive peptides degraded by neprilysin, such as natriuretic peptides, bradykinin, and adrenomedullin. Used in place of an ACE inhibitor or angiotensin receptor blocker and on top of optimal medical therapy in patients with class II to IV heart failure and an EF of 40% or less was found to significantly reduce multiple heart failure end points, including death, hospitalizations, and CV death in comparison to enalapril.
- Ivabradine was FDA approved in 2015 for patients with stable, symptomatic chronic heart failure with left ventricular ejection fraction ≤35% who are in sinus rhythm with resting heart rates ≥70 beats/min and either of the following: (1) are on maximally tolerated doses of beta-blockers or (2) have a contraindication to beta-blocker use. It acts by blocking the hyperpolarization-activated cyclic nucleotide-gated (HCN) channel responsible for the cardiac pacemaker I_f current, which regulates heart rate.
- Dapagliflozin (Farxiga), a SGLT2 inhibitor, has been found to reduce worsening heart failure and cardiovascular death when added to GDMT in patients with left ventricular ejection fraction <40%, regardless of diabetes status. The FDA approved dapagliflozin in 2020.

DISPOSITION

- Annual mortality rate is 20% in patients with moderate heart failure, and it exceeds 50% in patients with severe heart failure. Once symptomatic, hospitalizations are frequent and readmission rates are high (>50% at 3 mo). A multispecialty treatment approach (e.g., primary care, cardiology, nutrition, and cardiac rehabilitation) is recommended.
- Factors associated with an adverse outcome in dilated cardiomyopathy are described in Table 1.

REFERRAL

- Implantation of a cardiac defibrillator for primary prevention of sudden cardiac death can be considered for patients with LVEF ≤35% and on optimal medical therapy regardless of symptom status.
- Patients with LVEF <35%, left bundle branch block on ECG (QRS ≥0.13 sec) and persistent heart failure symptoms may benefit from cardiac resynchronization therapy via a biventricular pacemaker.
- Consider heart transplantation for relatively young patients (there is no precise age

threshold) free of other significant comorbid conditions who are unresponsive to medical therapy. Dilated cardiomyopathy is the reason for 45% of all heart transplantations in the U.S.

PEARLS & CONSIDERATIONS

COMMENTS

- Patients should be encouraged to restrict or eliminate alcohol and reduce sodium intake (<2 g daily).
- Patients may benefit from daily weight checks as a means of early detection of volume overload and decompensated heart failure.
- Vulnerability to cardiomyopathy among chronic alcohol abusers is partially genetic and related to the presence of the ACE DD genotype.
- Idiopathic dilated cardiomyopathy is often familial, and apparently healthy relatives may have latent, early, or undiagnosed disease. Echocardiographic evaluation of family members is recommended.
- Incorporation of sequencing approaches that detect *TTN* truncations into genetic testing for dilated cardiomyopathy may substantially increase test sensitivity and allow earlier diagnosis of dilated cardiomyopathy.

SUGGESTED READINGS

Available at ExpertConsult.com

RELATED CONTENT

Dilated Cardiomyopathy (Patient Information)
Cardiomyopathy, Chemical Induced (Related Key Topic)

AUTHORS: **Christopher P. Blomberg, DO,** and **Jennifer Bell, MD**

BASIC INFORMATION

DEFINITION

Hypertrophic cardiomyopathy (HCM) is most commonly an autosomal dominant myocardial disorder characterized by disorganized myocyte architecture and marked thickening (hypertrophy) of the left ventricular wall (≥15 mm), without dilation, *not explained by another cardiac or systemic disorder*. The interventricular septum is the most common site of enlargement, though hypertrophy may involve other focal regions or may be concentric. HCM may result in hemodynamically significant obstruction within the left ventricular outflow tract (LVOT) and/or impairment of the diastolic function of the left ventricle. However, about one third of patients have no obstruction at rest or with provocation.

SYNONYMS

HCM
Hypertrophic cardiomyopathy
Idiopathic hypertrophic subaortic stenosis (IHSS)
Hypertrophic obstructive cardiomyopathy (HOCM)
Hypertrophic nonobstructive cardiomyopathy
Asymmetric septal hypertrophy (ASH)
Familial hypertrophic cardiomyopathy

ICD-10CM CODES

I42.1	Obstructive hypertrophic cardiomyopathy (includes hypertrophic subaortic stenosis)
I42.2	Other hypertrophic cardiomyopathy (includes nonobstructive hypertrophic cardiomyopathy)
I42.8	Other cardiomyopathies
I42.9	Cardiomyopathy, unspecified (includes cardiomyopathy [primary] [secondary] not otherwise specified)

EPIDEMIOLOGY & DEMOGRAPHICS

- Prevalence in the general population in the U.S., China, and Japan is estimated to be between 1/500 to 1/200 (the most common genetically transmitted cardiovascular disease).
- HCM is the most common cause of sudden cardiac death in young athletes (more commonly among blacks).
- There is equal prevalence in men and women (probably underdiagnosed in women).
- It occurs across ethnicities, perhaps underdiagnosed among blacks.
- Mortality rate is approximately 1%/yr, as high as to 2%/yr in children.
- The most common form of the disease is familial (60%-70% of cases), and it follows an autosomal dominant inheritance pattern with variable expression.
- Spontaneous mutations can also occur, accounting for approximately 20% of cases. It is otherwise indistinguishable from the familial form.
- A variant form seen in the elderly (5%-10% of cases) has a better prognosis, and it is not typically associated with sudden cardiac death.
- The familial form is usually diagnosed in young patients. It is most often caused by a mutation in one of the contractile protein genes of the cardiac sarcomere. See "Etiology)." for more details.
- Nonsarcomeric genetic mutations that cause storage disease (e.g., Fabry disease) have a very similar clinical presentation.
- Apical HCM is a variant more common among Asians: As many as 41% of Chinese HCM and 15% of Japanese HCM patients. Clinically there is no LVOT obstruction.

PHYSICAL FINDINGS & CLINICAL PRESENTATION

Patients may have subtle symptoms of progressive congestive heart failure (CHF). At the time of diagnosis, most patients are asymptomatic, referred and diagnosed based on family history. HCM may be suspected on the basis of abnormalities found on physical examination. Classic findings include:

- Harsh, systolic, crescendo–decrescendo murmur at the left sternal border or apex. The murmur increases with maneuvers that decrease venous return or LV size (Valsalva, standing), and decreases with those that increase venous return or afterload (squatting, hand grip, post-Valsalva release).
- Paradoxical splitting of S2 (if left ventricular obstruction is present).
- S4 may be present.
- Double or triple LV apical impulse ("triple ripple": Atrial contraction, early rapid ejection, and late slow ejection).
- Pulsus bisferiens (double pulsation on palpation of the carotid pulse).

Increased obstruction can occur with:

- Drugs: Digitalis, β-adrenergic stimulators (isoproterenol, dopamine, epinephrine), nitroglycerin, vasodilators, diuretics, alcohol, inhalation of amyl nitrate
- Hypovolemia
- Tachycardia
- Valsalva maneuver
- Standing position

Decreased obstruction is seen with:

- Drugs: β-adrenergic blockers, calcium channel blockers, disopyramide, α-adrenergic stimulators
- Volume expansion
- Bradycardia
- Hand-grip exercise
- Squatting position
- Release phase of the Valsalva maneuver

Clinical manifestations are as follows:

- Syncope or presyncope (usually seen with exercise)
- Angina
- Palpitations
- Sudden cardiac death
- Heart failure (typically with advanced stages): Dyspnea on exertion, orthopnea, edema, increased jugular venous pressure, paroxysmal nocturnal dyspnea

ETIOLOGY

- Genetic: Autosomal dominant trait with variable penetrance caused by mutations in multiple genes encoding proteins of the cardiac sarcomere and calcium regulation. To date, >1400 mutations have been identified among at least 13 genes, with variable phenotypes, expressivity, and penetrance. The most vigorous evidence indicates that eight genes are known to definitively cause HCM: Beta myosin heavy chain, myosin binding protein C, troponin T, troponin I, tropomyosin alpha-1 chain, actin, regulatory light chain, and essential light chain. HCM may be caused by a single mutation in one of two alleles; however, 5% of patients have at least two mutations. Sarcomeric protein gene mutations account for up to 60% of cases of HCM.
- Metabolic: Most are autosomal recessive, but some are X-linked. Most commonly, they are due to Anderson-Fabry disease (a lysosomal storage disease). Other metabolic etiologies include the glycogen storage diseases Pompe and Danon, AMP-kinase (PRKAG2), and carnitine disorders.
- Mitochondrial: These comprise autosomal dominant, autosomal recessive, X-linked, and maternally inherited traits. Most frequently, they are due to mutations in the respiratory chain protein complexes. The age of onset and severity of involvement are variable.
- Neuromuscular: These are most commonly associated with Friedreich ataxia, but they are also associated with *FHL1*.
- Malformation syndromes: These etiologies include Noonan (formerly referred to as LEOPARD), Costello, and cardiofaciocutaneous.
- Amyloidosis: These include familial ATTR, wild-type TTR (senile), and amyloid light-chain (AL) amyloidosis.
- Drug-induced: Tacrolimus, hydroxychloroquine, and steroids.
- Sporadic occurrence.

Dx DIAGNOSIS

DIFFERENTIAL DIAGNOSIS

- Hypertensive heart disease
- Aortic stenosis
- Subaortic stenosis
- Athlete heart
- Volume depletion

WORKUP

- Medical history: Unexplained clinical manifestations and/or family history of sudden death.
- Physical exam: See "Physical Findings & Clinical Presentation."
- Genetic counseling with or without testing.
- ECG is abnormal in 75% to 95% of patients, although there are no pathognomonic findings. Typical findings include:
  1. Left ventricular (LV) hypertrophy (abnormally tall R waves in the precordial leads) in up to 80% of patients (Fig. E1).

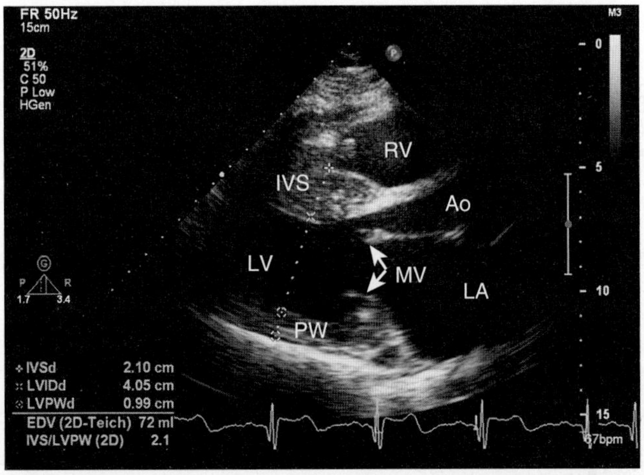

FIG. 2 Echocardiographic appearance of hypertrophic cardiomyopathy. Parasternal long-axis view from a patient with hypertrophic cardiomyopathy demonstrating asymmetrical septal hypertrophy. The interventricular septum (marked by *arrow*) measures 2.1 cm; the posterior wall measures 0.99 cm. *Ao,* Aorta; *IVS,* interventricular septum; *LA,* left atrium; *LV,* left ventricle; *MV,* mitral valve; *PW,* posterior wall; *RV,* right ventricle. (From Issa Z et al: *Clinical arrhythmology and electrophysiology,* ed 2, Philadelphia, 2012, Saunders.)

- Echocardiography (Fig. 2) is usually diagnostic as the majority of patients have significant LV hypertrophy (See "Imaging Studies" for details) and should be repeated every 12 to 24 mo or as clinically needed.
- 24-hr Holter monitor to screen for potentially lethal ventricular arrhythmias (principal cause of syncope or sudden death in obstructive cardiomyopathy) should be performed at the initial diagnosis and in patients that subsequently develop palpitations, lightheadedness, or syncope. The presence of these arrhythmias identifies patients who are candidates for implantable cardioverter-defibrillator (ICD) therapy.
- In the absence of significant LVOT obstruction, exercise testing is indicated at diagnosis and annually thereafter to evaluate for symptoms and response to exercise. A drop in systolic blood pressure by at least 20 mm Hg or failure to augment by at least 20 mm Hg with exercise are markers of poor prognosis and are indicators for referral for myotomy/myomectomy. Cardiopulmonary exercise testing can provide objective evidence for worsening diseases but need only be performed every 2 to 3 yr.
- Biomarkers of myocardial fibrosis in HCM include brain natriuretic peptide and high-sensitivity cardiac troponin T and I. Other labs include complete blood count, basic metabolic panel, liver function test, thyroid stimulating hormone, serum protein electrophoresis, urine protein electrophoresis free light chain ratio (Kappa/Lambda).
- Screening for sarcomere protein gene mutations in family members of patients with HCM can identify a broad subgroup of patients with increased propensity toward long-term impairment of left ventricular function and adverse outcome, irrespective of the myofilament (thick, intermediate, or thin) involvement.
- Specific sarcomere mutation does not predict the prognosis or the risk for sudden death.
- In individuals with pathogenic mutations who do not express the HCM phenotype, it is recommended to perform serial electrocardiogram (ECG), transthoracic echocardiogram (TTE), and clinical assessment at periodic intervals (12-18 mo in children and adolescents and about every 5 yr in adults), based on the patient's age and change in clinical status.
- Endomyocardial biopsy may be helpful to rule out diseases other than HCM if a diagnosis remains inconclusive after extensive testing.

IMAGING STUDIES

- Chest x-ray may be normal or show cardiomegaly.
- Two-dimensional echocardiography is used to establish the diagnosis and assess the severity of obstruction when present. LV wall thickness will usually be ≥15 mm (although some may be genetically positive but phenotype negative), and most patients (up to 95%) will have asymmetric (ratio of septum thickness to left ventricular wall thickness >1.3:1) LV wall hypertrophy. Symmetric LV hypertrophy is less common. The septum is most often affected, followed by the left ventricular mid-cavity and apex. In addition, 25% to 30% of patients will manifest systolic anterior motion (SAM) of the anterior leaflet of the mitral valve, causing obstruction of the LVOT and mitral regurgitation. Two-dimensional strain imaging echocardiography is useful for differentiation of HCM and cardiac amyloidosis from other causes of ventricular wall thickening. Up to 80% of HCM patients will also have diastolic dysfunction as evidenced by pulsed mitral valve inflow pattern and tissue Doppler.
- Cardiac MRI or cardiac CT may be of diagnostic value when echocardiographic studies are technically inadequate. MRI is also useful in identifying unusual segmental hypertrophy undetectable by standard echocardiography and can detect myocardial replacement fibrosis (an independent predictor of adverse cardiac outcomes and ventricular arrhythmias) using late gadolinium enhancement. Cardiac magnetic resonance evaluation may be considered every 5 yr or every 2 to 3 yr in patients with progressive disease.

Rx TREATMENT

NONPHARMACOLOGIC THERAPY

- Avoid volume depletion: An underfilled left ventricle causes closer approximation of the hypertrophic interventricular septum and anterior mitral valve leaflet, worsening the outflow tract obstruction and mitral regurgitation, potentially leading to dizziness, hypotension, and/or syncope.
- Exercise restriction: The risk of sudden cardiac death is increased by exercise in HCM patients and rapid heart rates may cause LV underfilling as described above; therefore, participation in competitive sports and intense physical activity should be avoided. As a part of a healthy lifestyle, low-intensity aerobic exercise is reasonable.
- Avoidance of alcohol: Alcohol use (even in small amounts) may result in increased obstruction of the left ventricular outflow tract. Other stimulants such as cocaine and other sympathomimetic recreational drugs should also be avoided.

ACUTE GENERAL Rx

- Therapy for HCM is directed at blocking the effect of catecholamines and generally avoiding vasodilator or diuretic agents that can exacerbate the dynamic left ventricular outflow tract obstruction.
- Beta-blockers' beneficial effects on symptoms (principally dyspnea and chest pain) and exercise tolerance appear to be largely a result of a decrease in the heart rate with consequent prolongation of diastole and increased passive ventricular filling. By reducing the inotropic response, beta-blockers may also reduce myocardial oxygen demand and decrease the outflow gradient during exercise, when sympathetic tone is increased. Dose titration to a resting heart rate of less than 65 bpm is recommended.
- Nondihydropyridine calcium channel blockers (e.g., verapamil [preferred], diltiazem) can also decrease left ventricular outflow obstruction through a mechanism similar to beta-blockers. However, they are mainly second-line agents used in patients who cannot tolerate beta-blockers as they also theoretically have vasodilatory properties that may worsen severe outflow tract gradients.
- Disopyramide is an antiarrhythmic that is also a negative inotrope, resulting in further

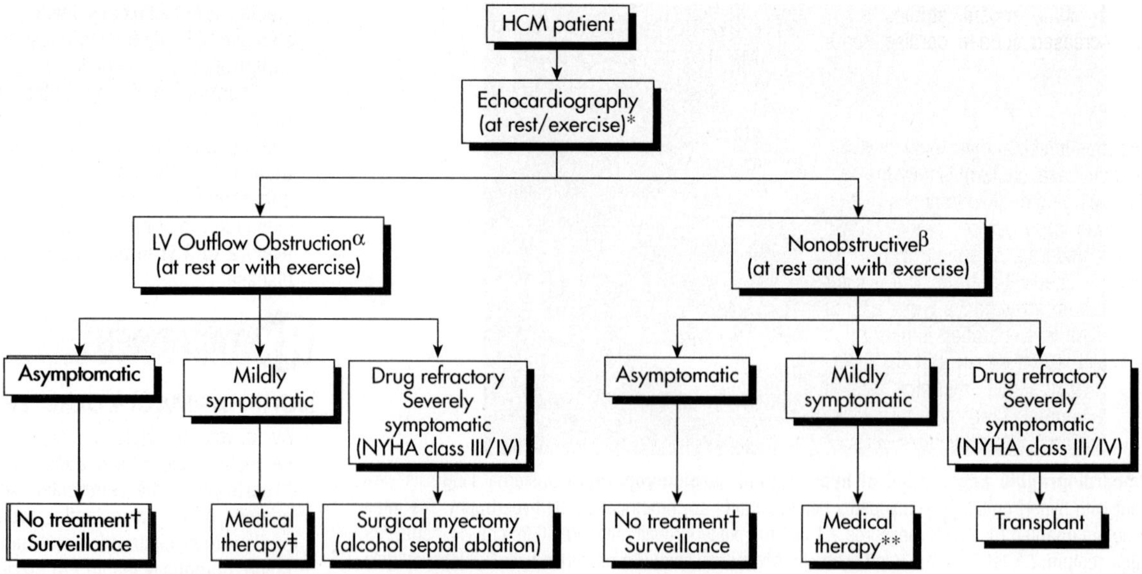

FIG. 3 Heart failure management strategies starting with echocardiography. *Patients without LV outflow tract gradient (<30 mm Hg) at rest should undergo stress (exercise) echocardiography. †No data on benefit of pharmacologic therapy, although beta-blockers often are administered prophylactically in clinical practice. **Beta-blockers, calcium channel antagonists, and possibly diuretics administered judiciously. ‡Usually, beta-blockers or calcium channel antagonists (verapamil), or disopyramide. α, generally regarded, by definition, as ≥30 mm Hg outflow gradient, but ≥50 mm Hg when septal reduction intervention is considered (i.e., septal myectomy; alcohol ablation). β, no or trivial (<30 mm Hg) outflow gradient at rest and with exercise. *HCM,* Hypertrophic cardiomyopathy; *LV,* left ventricle; *NYHA,* New York Heart Association. (From Maron BJ et al: State-of the art review: hypertrophic cardiomyopathy: present and future, with translation into contemporary cardiovascular medicine, *J Am Coll Cardiol* 2014;64:83. In Zipes DP: *Braunwald's heart disease, a textbook of cardiovascular medicine,* ed 11, Philadelphia, 2019, Elsevier.)

decrease in outflow gradient. It is sometimes used in combination with beta-blockers.
- Prophylactic antibiotics before dental, GI, and genitourinary procedures are no longer recommended according to the American Heart Association (AHA) guidelines.
- Avoid use of digitalis, intravenous inotropes, dihydropyridine calcium channel blockers (e.g., nifedipine, amlodipine), nitrates, and vasodilators.
- Diuretics, angiotensin-converting enzyme inhibitors, and angiotensin receptor blockers should be used with caution.
- Intravenous phenylephrine (or another pure vasoconstricting agent) is recommended for the treatment of acute hypotension in patients with obstructive HCM who do not respond to fluid administration.
- ICDs are a safe and effective therapy in HCM patients prone to ventricular arrhythmias. In their practice guidelines, the major cardiology societies (AHA/ACC/HRS) give a strong recommendation (Class I) for ICD implantation in all patients with HCM who have had an episode of sustained ventricular tachycardia or fibrillation. In addition, they endorse the prophylactic placement of an ICD (Class IIa recommendation) for patients with one or more of the major risk factors for sudden cardiac death (outlined in "Disposition"). In patients with New York Heart Association (NYHA) functional class III or IV heart failure symptoms on maximal medical therapy, an ICD also may be considered when ejection fraction (EF) is less than or equal to 50%.
- Dual-chamber pacing may provide symptomatic relief of symptoms attributable to LVOT obstruction and refractory to medical therapy; however, the role is very limited (Class IIb indication (ACC/AHA/HRS guidelines).
- The role of biventricular pacing for treatment of HF in HCM patients remains uncertain and is generally only considered in patients whose EF has dropped to <35%.
- Systolic dysfunction in patients with HCM is defined as an EF of less than or equal to 50%, at which point medical therapy should follow guidelines for heart failure with reduced EF (ACE inhibitors, angiotensin II receptor blockers, beta-blockers, etc.).
- HCM patients are at an increased risk of atrial fibrillation (AF) as well as systemic thromboembolism. AF occurs in over 20% of the HCM population. AF is an important source of symptoms, morbidity, and mortality and correlates to a worse prognosis. Anticoagulation for AF is indicated independent of CHA_2DS_2-VASc score and should aim for thromboembolic risk mitigation with a vitamin K antagonist (unless contraindicated) and symptom alleviation via rhythm (generally preferred due to poor tolerance of AF with HCM) or rate control. If a vitamin K antagonist cannot be used in a patient (due to inability to maintain a therapeutic INR, inability to adequately perform INR monitoring, or other side effects), the 2014 ESC HCM (Class Ib) and 2014 ACC/AHA/HRS AF (Class Ic) guidelines recommend the use of direct thrombin or factor Xa inhibitors, even though there is no data on their use in patients with HCM.
- Cardiac myosin inhibitors (mavacamten) and gene-silencing agents are under investigation as targeted treatment for HCM patients.
- Fig. 3 summarizes heart failure management strategies.

DISPOSITION

HCM is not a static disease. Some adults may experience subtle regression in wall thickness, whereas others (~5%-10%) paradoxically evolve into an end-stage cardiomyopathy resembling dilated cardiomyopathy, characterized by cavity enlargement, left ventricular wall thinning, and systolic dysfunction. Patients with HCM are at increased risk for sudden death, especially if the onset of symptoms began during childhood. Severe left ventricular outflow obstruction at rest is also a strong, independent predictor of severe symptoms of heart failure and death. ICD implantation for primary prevention should be considered if patients (particularly the young) have any of the following high-risk features:
- Personal history of sudden cardiac death or out of hospital cardiac arrest (major risk factor)
- Spontaneous sustained ventricular tachycardia or ventricular fibrillation (major risk factor)
- Family history of premature death in a first-degree relative possibly caused by HCM
- Unexplained syncope
- Nonsustained ventricular tachycardia during Holter monitoring
- Substantial septal hypertrophy (>30 mm)
- LV apical aneurysm
- Abnormal blood pressure response during exercise
- Increased delayed gadolinium enhancement on cardiac magnetic resonance imaging is

suggested in some recent studies as a marker of increased sudden cardiac death risk

REFERRAL

- Surgical treatment (septal myectomy involving resection of the basal septum) is now the gold standard for relieving outflow tract obstruction in patients with large outflow gradient (≥50 mm Hg) and moderate to severe symptoms unresponsive to medical therapy. The risk for sudden death from arrhythmias is not altered by surgery. When this operation is performed by experienced surgeons in tertiary referral centers, the operative mortality rate is <1%, and many patients are able to achieve near-normal exercise capacity after surgery. Mitral valvuloplasty or plication in combination with myectomy may be necessary in <5% of patients. Risks of surgery include AV nodal block, ventricular septal defect, and aortic regurgitation (AR).
- Alcohol septal ablation is a nonsurgical alternative to reduce the size of the interventricular septum. This can be done in patients with HCM refractory to pharmacologic treatment, particularly in those who are not candidates for myectomy due to high surgical risk or patient preference. This technique involves the injection of ethanol in a septal perforator branch of the left anterior descending coronary artery (Fig. E4), producing a controlled myocardial infarction of the interventricular septum, and thereby reducing septal mass and consequently the left ventricular outflow tract gradient. This method may lead to improvement in both subjective and objective measures of exercise capacity, but results are not as effective as surgery because they are associated with a high incidence of heart block, requiring permanent pacing in approximately 25% of patients, and/or recurrence of obstruction and symptoms. This should be done only at centers with experienced operators.
- Refractory end-stage heart failure symptoms can be treated with left ventricular assist device, biventricular assist device, or heart transplant.

TABLE 1 Proposed Clinical Family Screening Strategies with Echocardiography or Cardiovascular Magnetic Resonance (and 12-Lead Electrocardiography) for Detection of HCM with Left Ventricular Hypertrophy*

Age <12 yr
Optional unless:
Malignant family history of premature death from HCM or other adverse complications
Competitive athlete in an intense training program
Onset of symptoms
Other clinical suspicion of early left ventricular hypertrophy
Age 12-21 yr†
Every 12-18 mo
Age >21 yr
Imaging at onset of symptoms, or possibly at 5-yr intervals at least through midlife; more frequent intervals for imaging are appropriate in families with malignant clinical course or history of late-onset HCM

*In family members who had not undergone genetic testing or in whom testing was unresolved or indeterminant.
†Age range takes into consideration individual variability in achieving physical maturity, and in some patients, screening may be justified at an earlier age; initial evaluation should be performed no later than early pubescence.
From Maron BJ et al: Genetics of hypertrophic cardiomyopathy after 20 years: clinical perspectives, *J Am Coll Cardiol* 60:705, 2012. In Zipes DP: *Braunwald's heart disease, a textbook of cardiovascular medicine*, ed 11, Philadelphia, 2019, Elsevier.

PEARLS & CONSIDERATIONS

COMMENTS

- Clinical screening of first-degree relatives with two-dimensional echocardiography and ECG is indicated. Starting at the age of 12, periodic screening at 12- to 18-mo intervals is recommended for children of patients with HCM and in competitive athletes. Periodic screening of first-degree adult family members not in competitive athletics is recommended at 5-yr intervals because hypertrophy may not be detected until the sixth decade of life. If the index patient does not have a definite pathogenic mutation, then genetic testing of relatives is not indicated.
- Genetic counseling and screening (Fig. E5, Table 1) is recommended in first-degree relatives of patients with HCM. Genetic screening of first-degree relatives can refine or eliminate the need for periodic clinical screening. At least 13 genes are known to cause HCM, among them: Cardiac myosin binding protein-C, beta-myosin heavy chain, troponin T, troponin I, alpha tropomyosin, actin regulatory light chain, and essential light chain. Clinical predictors of positive genotype, such as the presence of ventricular arrhythmias, age at diagnosis, degree of left ventricular wall hypertrophy, and family history of HCM, may aid in patient selection for genetic testing and increase the yield of cardiac sarcomere gene screening. Currently a mutation can be identified in 40% to 60% of all cases, sporadic or familial.
- All HCM patients who wish to become pregnant should be given prenatal counseling about the risk of transmission (about 50%) to their offspring and should be followed at a tertiary care center that specializes in high-risk pregnancies. Most patients with HCM tolerate pregnancy well due to the higher circulating blood volume.
- The mortality rate in HCM is approximately 1% to 2% per yr.
- About one third of HCM patients will not have a resting or labile outflow gradient (i.e., nonobstructive form of HCM), but it is important to note that lethal ventricular arrhythmias can occur in the absence of obstruction or symptoms.
- Myocardial fibrosis is a hallmark of hypertrophic cardiomyopathy. (Biomarkers of collagen metabolism such as serum C-terminal propeptide of type I procollagen (PICP) are significantly higher in mutation carriers without left ventricular hypertrophy and in subjects with overt hypertrophic cardiomyopathy than in controls, indicating that a probiotic state precedes the development of hypertrophy of fibrosis identifiable with cardiac MRI.)

SUGGESTED READINGS

Available at ExpertConsult.com

RELATED CONTENT

Hypertrophic Cardiomyopathy (Patient Information)

AUTHOR: **Artem Astsaturov, MD**

BASIC INFORMATION

DEFINITION

Restrictive cardiomyopathy refers to either an idiopathic or a secondary myocardial disorder (in the absence of ischemic, hypertensive, valvular, or congenital heart disease) characterized by restrictive filling (Fig. E1). Other features include normal or reduced left ventricular (LV) and right ventricular (RV) volumes, and normal or near normal systolic LV and RV function. Pathophysiologically, the myocardium is abnormally stiff, resulting in decreased compliance, abnormal relaxation in diastole, and increased filling pressures leading to enlarged left atria.

SYNONYMS

Idiopathic restrictive cardiomyopathy
Infiltrative cardiomyopathy

ICD-10CM CODES	
I43.1	Cardiomyopathy in metabolic diseases
D86.XX	Sarcoidosis-related codes
E83.11X	Hemochromatosis-related codes
E85.X	Amyloidosis-related codes
I42.5	Other restrictive cardiomyopathy
I42.8	Other cardiomyopathies
I42.9	Cardiomyopathy, unspecified

EPIDEMIOLOGY & DEMOGRAPHICS

- A relatively uncommon cardiomyopathy, accounting for 5% of all primary myocardial diseases.
- Most frequently caused by amyloidosis or myocardial fibrosis (following open heart surgery, transplantation, or radiation).
- Patients classified as having "idiopathic" restrictive cardiomyopathy may have mutations in sarcomere components such as troponin T (TNNT2 gene), troponin I (TNNI3), alpha-actin (ACTC), and beta-myosin heavy chain (MYH7). Mostly inherited in an autosomal dominant pattern.
- Restrictive cardiomyopathy may represent an overlap with hypertrophic cardiomyopathy in many familial cases.

PHYSICAL FINDINGS & CLINICAL PRESENTATION

Restrictive cardiomyopathy presents with symptoms of progressive left-sided and right-sided heart failure:

- Fatigue, weakness (caused by low output as patients are unable to augment cardiac output by increasing heart rate without compromising ventricular filling).
- Progressively worsening exercise intolerance and dyspnea.
- Anginal chest pain can be seen (particularly in patients with amyloidosis) from myocardial compression of small coronaries.
- Palpitations (atrial fibrillation is common), dizziness, or syncope (from orthostasis, heart block, or malignant arrhythmia).
- Edema, ascites, hepatomegaly, distended neck veins (from elevated right heart pressures).
- Kussmaul sign may be present (rise, or failure to fall, of the jugular veins on inspiration).
- On auscultation: Murmurs of mitral or tricuspid regurgitation may be heard; an S3 may be present.
- Apical impulse may be palpable (can help distinguish it from constrictive pericarditis) and nondisplaced.

ETIOLOGY

Disease may be classified according to pathophysiologic processes:

- Infiltrative:
  1. Amyloidosis (most common overall): The main types include AA, AL, and ATTR (transthyretin-mutated or wild type [commonly known as senile systemic]). AL amyloidosis is a rare plasma cell disorder with overproduction of monoclonal kappa or lambda light chains that can misfold. Amyloid A amyloidosis (AA) is a rare condition seen in the setting of chronic inflammatory states such as rheumatologic diseases. Wild-type TTR is produced primarily in the liver and is a protein tetramer that breaks into monomers and can deposit into tissues. Mutant TTR is due to a mutation in the gene causing the protein to break down into monomers.
  2. Sarcoidosis (more commonly causing a dilated cardiomyopathy with regional wall motion abnormalities).
- Noninfiltrative:
  1. Idiopathic (familial subtypes may have genetic overlap with hypertrophic cardiomyopathy)
  2. Scleroderma
  3. Diabetic cardiomyopathy
- Storage diseases:
  1. Hemochromatosis (more commonly associated with a dilated cardiomyopathy)
  2. Glycogen or other storage diseases (Gaucher, Hurler, Fabry—all rare)
- Endomyocardial:
  1. Endomyocardial fibrosis
  2. Hypereosinophilic syndrome (Loeffler syndrome)
- Carcinoid heart disease
- Radiation
- Metastatic cancers
- Drug related (anthracyclines, serotonin, ergotamine, busulfan, methysergide)

Dx DIAGNOSIS

The diagnosis of idiopathic or primary restrictive cardiomyopathy is rare and is a diagnosis of exclusion.

DIFFERENTIAL DIAGNOSIS

- Constrictive pericarditis (see Table E1)
- Valvular dysfunction (especially aortic stenosis)
- Hypertrophic cardiomyopathy
- Hypertensive heart disease

WORKUP

- Complete blood count with differential (to identify eosinophilia), iron studies, serum renal function studies, chest x-ray, ECG, echocardiogram
- Right and left heart catheterization, magnetic resonance imaging, and computed tomography (in select cases)
- Aspiration biopsy of subcutaneous fat to detect amyloidosis
- Endomyocardial biopsy if diagnostic confirmation needed
- Brain natriuretic peptide (BNP) serum levels (>400 pg/ml): There are data suggesting that BNP levels are markedly elevated in restrictive cardiomyopathy but near normal in constrictive pericarditis, most likely resulting from the lack of myocardial stretching in constriction that is required for BNP release
- Genetic testing, including testing for transthyretin mutation in amyloidosis

IMAGING STUDIES

- Chest x-ray:
  1. Ranges from normal cardiomediastinal silhouette to moderate cardiomegaly (primarily because of biatrial enlargement).
  2. Evidence of heart failure may be present.
  3. Presence of pericardial calcification favors alternative diagnosis of constrictive pericarditis.
- ECG:
  1. Nonspecific ST-T wave abnormalities are the most common finding. Voltage may be low in infiltrative etiologies such as amyloidosis.
  2. Frequent atrial and ventricular ectopy are often present. Atrial fibrillation may be present.
  3. High-degree atrioventricular block, intraventricular conduction delay may be seen in advanced cases.
- Echocardiogram (Fig. 2):
  1. Biatrial enlargement almost always present.
  2. Wall thickness depends on etiology; often thickened in infiltrative disease.
  3. Myocardial appearance may be altered (speckled pattern with apical sparing suggestive of amyloidosis).
  4. Ventricular chamber sizes and systolic function are often normal or reduced.
  5. Echo Doppler shows evidence of diastolic dysfunction. Tissue Doppler demonstrates low mitral annular velocities.
- Cardiac catheterization:
  1. Characteristic hemodynamic findings are a dip and plateau, or square-root sign, in the left ventricular tracing where a deep and rapid decline in ventricular pressure at the onset of diastole is immediately followed by rapid rise and plateau in early diastolic phase.

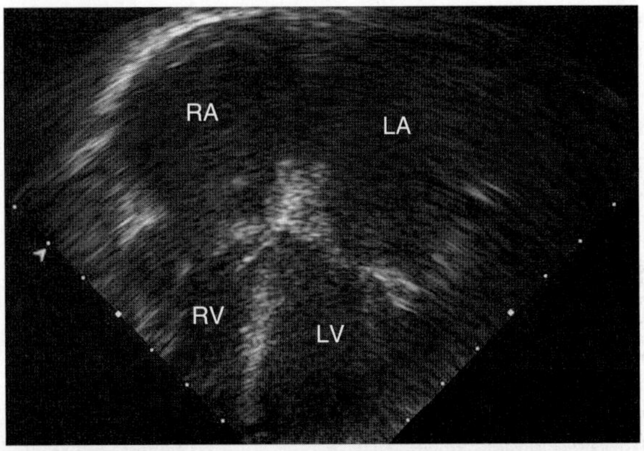

FIG. 2 Echocardiogram of a patient with restrictive cardiomyopathy. The optical four-chamber view shows the markedly enlarged right and left atria, compared to the normal-sized left and right ventricular chambers. *LA,* Left atrium; *LV,* left ventricle; *RA,* right atrium; *RV,* right ventricle. (From Kliegman RM et al: *Nelson textbook of pediatrics,* ed 19, Philadelphia, 2011, Saunders.)

2. To distinguish restrictive cardiomyopathy from constrictive processes (Fig. 3):
   a. Constrictive: Usually involves both ventricles and leads to equalization of diastolic pressures between all four cardiac chambers to within 5 mm Hg. There is discordance in RV and LV pressures generated during inspiration, which is due to increased ventricular interdependence and decreased left atrial filling (caused by a decreased gradient in inspiration between the pulmonary veins, which are outside the constrictive process and the left atrium).
   b. Restrictive cardiomyopathy: Impairs the left ventricle more than the right, often with left-sided end-diastolic pressures of 5 mm Hg greater than the right. The presence of increased pulmonary arterial systolic pressures is also suggestive of restrictive disease. Simultaneous RV and LV pressure tracings demonstrate concordant patterns during the respiratory cycle.

- Cardiac computed tomographic scan may be helpful to identify a thickened and calcified pericardium, consistent with constrictive pericarditis.
- Cardiac magnetic resonance imaging (CMRI) may also be useful to distinguish restrictive cardiomyopathy from constrictive pericarditis (thickness of the pericardium greater than 4 mm in the latter). CMRI is particularly helpful in the diagnosis of the amyloid or sarcoid variants and may have value in other variants as well. Late gadolinium enhancement can be seen with infiltrative diseases.
- Technetium pyrophosphate bone scintigraphy is useful in diagnosis of transthyretin cardiac amyloidosis and differentiates it from light chain amyloidosis.

Rx TREATMENT

NONPHARMACOLOGIC THERAPY

Congestive symptoms may respond to dietary sodium restriction (<2 g/day).

ACUTE GENERAL Rx

Treatment of volume overload and heart failure symptoms with diuretic therapy

CHRONIC Rx

- Treatment involves management of the underlying disease if it exists:
  1. Hemochromatosis may respond to repeated phlebotomy and iron chelators to decrease iron deposition in the heart.
  2. Sarcoidosis may respond to corticosteroid therapy.
  3. Primary amyloidosis may respond to chemotherapy (high-dose melphalan paired with dexamethasone, followed by autologous stem cell therapy or bortezomib-based regimens). ATTR may be treated with liver transplant or other promising novel therapeutic agents that are currently being tested in clinical trials.
  4. Eosinophilic cardiomyopathy may respond to corticosteroid and cytotoxic drugs.
  5. There is no effective therapy for other causes of restrictive cardiomyopathy.
- Overall, the goal of treatment is to reduce symptoms by decreasing filling pressures while preserving cardiac output. Since there is currently no drug available to specifically act on myocardial relaxation, therapy centers on low-dose diuretics to lower the preload.
- Beta-blockers or calcium channel blockers have not been demonstrated to improve symptoms or alter the course of disease. Must be careful not to decrease HR too far, as this will affect cardiac output (CO = HR × stroke volume).
- ACE inhibitors (or angiotensin receptor blockers [ARBs]) and vasodilators should be avoided in patients with amyloidosis as they are poorly tolerated. Even small doses can trigger profound hypotension (probably due to associated autonomic neuropathy). Adequate preload is necessary for LV filling and ultimately cardiac output.
- Atrial fibrillation is common and patients with it or with a history of embolization should be anticoagulated. Tachycardia (of any cause) is poorly tolerated and a common cause of decompensation. Rate control is of paramount importance. Cardioversion in case of rapid atrial fibrillation should be considered. Of note, digoxin should be used with caution as it is potentially arrhythmogenic (particularly in patients with amyloidosis).
- Fibrosis of the cardiac conduction system may result in complete heart block presenting as dizziness or syncope (especially in amyloidosis) and pacemaker implantation may be required. The course of restrictive cardiomyopathy is variable and depends on the underlying etiology. Death usually results from heart failure or arrhythmias, and interventions aimed at addressing these are recommended.
  1. For the amyloid variant, an implantable cardiac defibrillator offers little prophylactic benefit beyond the ability to pace because the cause of sudden cardiac death is usually electromechanical disassociation.

DISPOSITION

Prognosis varies with the etiology of the cardiomyopathy but is poor overall as disease is rarely detected before advanced stages.

REFERRAL

Cardiac transplantation can be considered in patients with refractory symptoms and idiopathic or familial restrictive cardiomyopathies.

SUGGESTED READINGS

Available at ExpertConsult.com

RELATED CONTENT

Restrictive Cardiomyopathy (Patient Information)

AUTHOR: **Nathan Riddell, MD**

DIFFERENTIATION OF RESTRICTIVE CARDIOMYOPATHY FROM CONSTRICTIVE PERICARDITIS

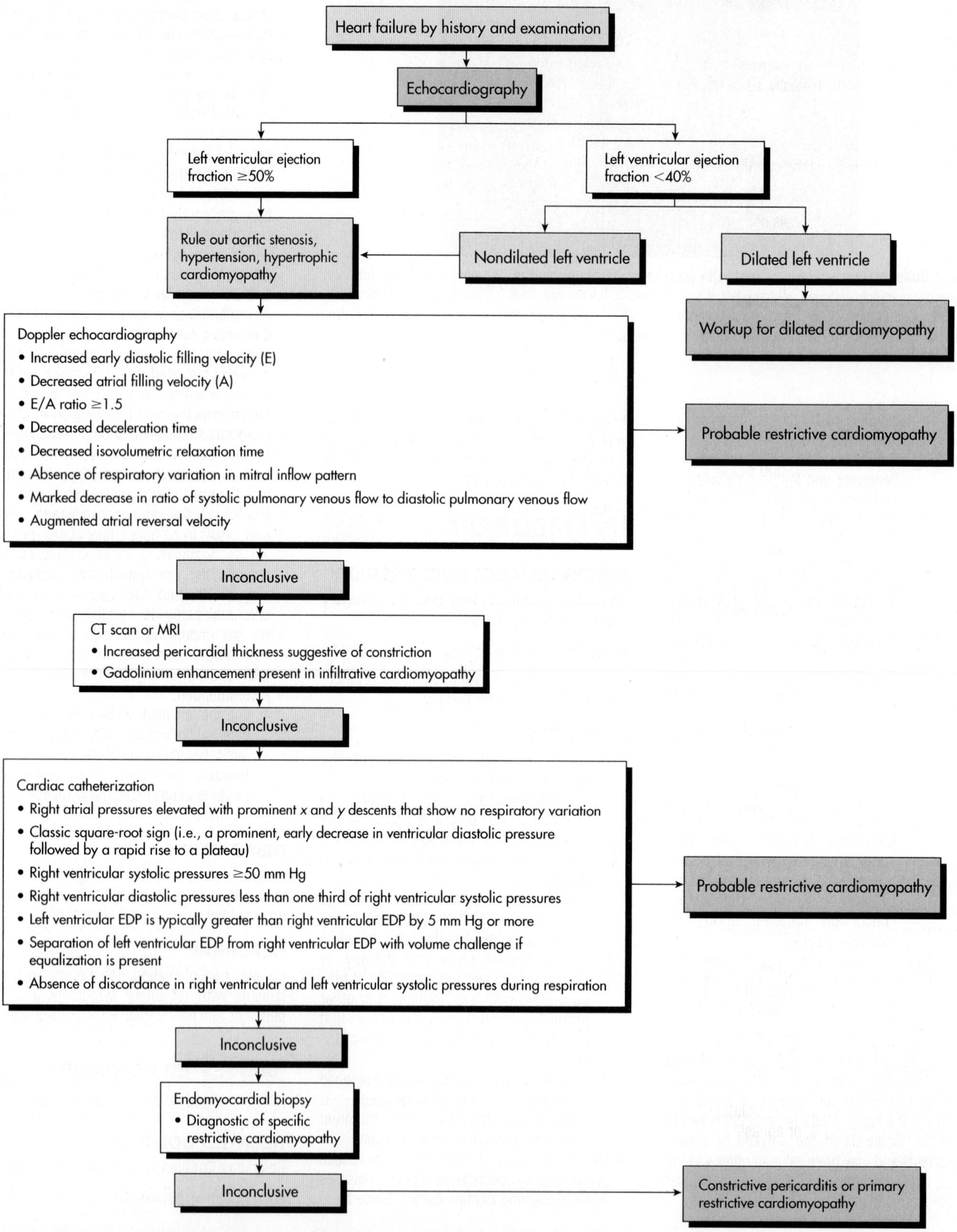

FIG. 3 Differentiation of restrictive cardiomyopathy from constrictive pericarditis. *CT,* Computed tomography; *EDP,* end-diastolic pressure; *MRI,* magnetic resonance image. (From Pereira NL, Dec GW: Restrictive and infiltrative cardiomyopathies. In Crawford MH et al: *Cardiology,* Philadelphia, 2010, Elsevier.)

BASIC INFORMATION

DEFINITION

Carotid artery stenosis is narrowing of the carotid arterial lumen, typically as a result of atherosclerosis.

SYNONYM

Atherosclerotic disease of the carotid artery

ICD-10CM CODES

I65.29	Occlusion and stenosis of unspecified carotid artery
I65.21	Occlusion and stenosis of right carotid artery
I65.22	Occlusion and stenosis of left carotid artery
I65.23	Occlusion and stenosis of bilateral carotid arteries

EPIDEMIOLOGY & DEMOGRAPHICS

INCIDENCE: 2.2 to 8/1000 persons per yr

PREVALENCE: 11 to 77/100,000 persons; it is estimated that 5/1000 persons aged 50 to 60 yr and 100/1000 persons >80 yr have carotid stenosis >50%. (NOTE: The incidence of carotid artery stenosis is unknown as screening is not routine. However, the incidence of transient ischemic attack [TIA], a common presenting symptom of carotid stenosis, is well known.)

PREDOMINANT SEX & AGE: Male:female ratio of 2:1.

PEAK INCIDENCE: Peak incidence is between 50 and 60 yr.

RISK FACTORS: Hypertension, dyslipidemia, diabetes mellitus, and smoking are the four major risk factors.

GENETICS: Multifactorial; twin studies (monozygotic versus dizygotic) suggest a familial influence.

PHYSICAL FINDINGS & CLINICAL PRESENTATION

Patients with carotid artery stenosis are often asymptomatic, but many either have a carotid bruit or experience a TIA.

- Carotid bruit: The presence of a carotid bruit is a better indicator of generalized atherosclerosis and is thus a better predictor of ischemic heart disease than future stroke.
- TIA: Carotid artery stenosis is classically heralded by ipsilateral transient monocular blindness (amaurosis fugax), contralateral numbness or weakness, contralateral homonymous hemianopsia, or aphasia.

ETIOLOGY

- Atherosclerosis (most common by far)
- Aneurysm
- Arteritis
- Carotid dissection
- Fibromuscular dysplasia
- Post-radiation necrosis
- Vasospasm

DIAGNOSIS

DIFFERENTIAL DIAGNOSIS

Aneurysm, arteritis, and carotid dissection

WORKUP

Systematic history, examination, and diagnostic studies to assess for carotid stenosis and other risk factors of TIA and stroke. Carotid artery stenosis is responsible for approximately 10% of all ischemic strokes.

LABORATORY TESTS

CBC, comprehensive metabolic panel, fasting lipid profile, PT/international normalized ratio, APTT, HgA1C

IMAGING STUDIES

- Four imaging modalities are available for the evaluation of carotid artery stenosis (Table 1).
- Patients with transient ischemic attack or stroke should be evaluated for carotid artery stenosis via carotid duplex (Fig. 1), magnetic resonance angiography, or computed tomography angiography. Conventional angiography may be obtained to confirm the degree of stenosis and plan for intervention (Fig. 2).
- The U.S. Preventive Services Task Force recommends against screening for asymptomatic carotid artery stenosis in the general adult population.
- Screening with carotid duplex may be considered in asymptomatic patients with carotid bruit, in those with multiple risk factors for atherosclerosis, or those with known atherosclerotic disease at other sites such as coronary artery disease, peripheral arterial disease, or abdominal aortic aneurysms.
- Patients identified to have >50% stenosis on carotid duplex may be reimaged annually to assess progression and should have intensive medical management of vascular risk factors.

TREATMENT

ACUTE GENERAL Rx

- General medical therapy should be aimed at risk factor reduction. The major risk factors for carotid artery stenosis are hypertension, diabetes mellitus, dyslipidemia, and smoking (see "Stroke, Secondary Prevention").
- Antiplatelet therapy: Three antiplatelet options are available for patients with carotid artery stenosis: ASA, ASA plus dipyridamole, or clopidogrel.

NONPHARMACOLOGIC THERAPY

Carotid endarterectomy (CEA) and carotid angioplasty and stenting (CAS) (Fig. 3) are the two revascularization options available. The decision on which revascularization procedure to favor is dependent upon the presence or absence of symptoms, degree of stenosis, medical comorbidities, operative risk of the patient, and experience and outcomes data of the proceduralist. Factors associated with increased risk from carotid artery surgery are summarized in Table 2.

In a trial involving asymptomatic patients with severe carotid stenosis who were not at high risk for surgical complications, stenting was noninferior to endarterectomy with regard to the rate of the primary composite end point at 1 yr. In analyses that included up to 5 yr of follow-up, there were no significant differences between the study groups in the rates

TABLE 1 Imaging Modalities for Carotid Stenosis

Imaging Modality	Benefit	Drawback
Cerebral angiography	• Gold standard • Assesses plaque morphology • Assesses presence of collaterals	• Invasive • High cost • 4% incidence rate of complications • 1% incidence rate of serious complications or death
Carotid duplex	• Sensitive in detecting high-grade stenosis (>70%) • Less invasive • Lower cost	• Can be limited by body habitus • Technician dependent • Overestimates degree of stenosis • May not distinguish high-grade stenosis from complete occlusion
Magnetic resonance angiography (MRA)	• Sensitive in detecting high-grade stenosis (>70%) • Less operator dependent	• Overestimates degree of stenosis • Cannot be performed in patients who are critically ill, unable to tolerate supine positioning, have pacemaker or other ferromagnetic hardware, or are claustrophobic* • Expensive • Takes much longer to obtain compared with other modalities
Computed tomography angiography (CTA)	• Sensitive for high-grade stenosis	• Contraindicated in patients with serum creatinine concentration >1.5 mg/dl • Uses ionizing radiation

*One study revealed that ~17% of patients are unable to tolerate MRA secondary to claustrophobia or are unable to lie still for procedure.

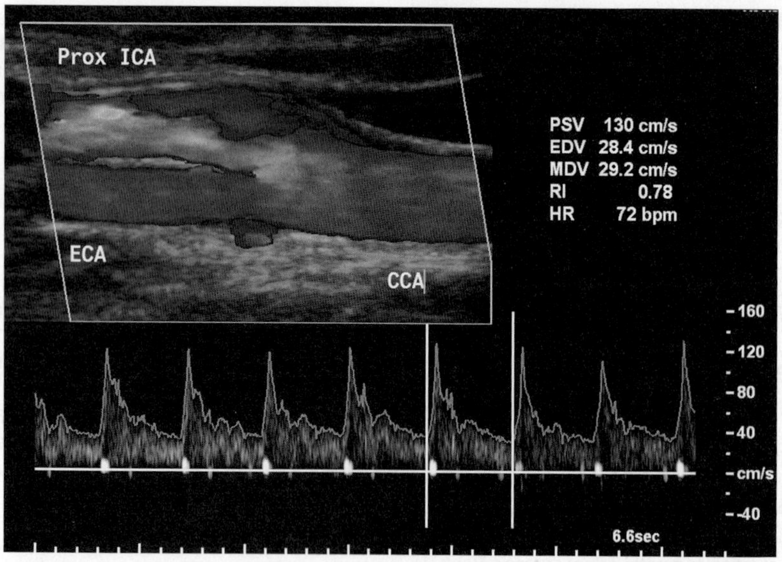

FIG. 1 Duplex ultrasound image of the carotid bifurcation with flow information used to calculate severity of stenosis. (From Fillit HM: *Brocklehurst's textbook of geriatric medicine and gerontology*, ed 8, Philadelphia, 2017, Elsevier.)

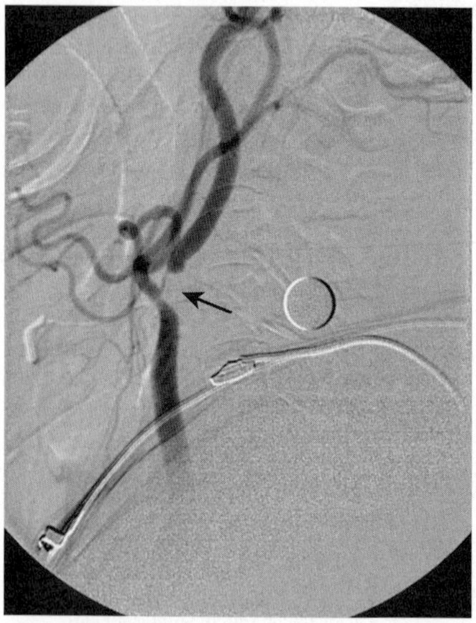

FIG. 2 Conventional angiography demonstrating severe stenosis of the internal carotid artery at the bifurcation.

of nonprocedure-related stroke, all stroke, and survival.[1]

ASYMPTOMATIC CAROTID STENOSIS

The benefit of surgical revascularization of the carotids (CEA or CAS) in asymptomatic patients is not well established. In the U.S., more than 90% of carotid artery interventions are performed in asymptomatic patients, even though evidence suggests that up to 90% of these patients are undergoing an ultimately unnecessary and potentially harmful procedure. In contrast, the percentage of interventions performed for asymptomatic stenosis is approximately 60% in Germany and Italy, 15% in Canada and Australia, and 0% in Denmark.[2]

According to the most recent guidelines, revascularization procedures may be considered in asymptomatic patients with >70% stenosis if the anticipated perioperative risk is less than 3%, but surgery should only be recommended after considering medical comorbidities and life expectancy and after discussing the risks and benefits in detail with the patients. It is important to note that trials of CEA for asymptomatic carotid stenosis were performed prior to the era of aggressive medical management of vascular risk factors. Recently launched studies of asymptomatic carotid stenosis versus aggressive contemporary medical management will answer lingering questions from older studies.

SYMPTOMATIC CAROTID STENOSIS

In patients who have suffered a nondisabling ischemic stroke or TIA in the preceding 6 mo, surgical revascularization by CEA is recommended if the degree of carotid stenosis is severe (70% to 99%) and if the anticipated rate of perioperative stroke or mortality is <6%. The number needed to treat to prevent 1 stroke in 2 yr is 6.

In patients who have suffered a nondisabling ischemic stroke or TIA in the preceding 6 mo, and who have moderate carotid stenosis (50-69%), CEA is recommended based on an assessment of the patient's age, sex, and comorbidities. To prevent 1 stroke in 5 yr, 15 patients with moderate carotid stenosis would have to undergo CEA. Factors to consider in recommending CEA for patients with moderate symptomatic carotid stenosis are age, sex, and comorbidities. The NASCET trial, which studied the efficacy of CEA versus medical management, suggested that women experienced higher complication rates from CEA than men. However, the CREST trial, which compared CEA to carotid stenting, did not find a sex-related outcome difference between the two interventions in terms of primary outcome, which was the composite of stroke, myocardial infarction, or death during the periprocedural period or ipsilateral stroke within 4 yr. However, when periprocedural events are examined alone, CREST data suggest that the periprocedural risk of events seems to be higher in women who have CAS than those who undergo CEA, while men experience no significant difference in periprocedural risk. CREST also found that patients older than 70 did better with CEA than with carotid stenting. All patients undergoing CEA should be started on aspirin (ASA; 81 or 325 mg daily) and a high dose statin before surgery. This therapy, along with blood pressure control and aggressive management of other vascular risk factors, should be continued indefinitely.

CAS can be an alternative to CEA in select patients considered to be at high surgical risk or with unfavorable neck anatomy for surgery.

CEA is preferred over CAS in older patients.

For patients undergoing CAS, dual antiplatelet therapy is recommended for a minimum of 30 days followed by single antiplatlet thereafter.

When feasible, early revascularization within 14 days after incident event should be undertaken unless there are definite contraindications. Data suggest that women with symptomatic lesions lose benefit of intervention of the intervention is delayed beyond 14 days after incident event, and the preferred intervention is CEA. For patients undergoing early intervention, CEA is associated with lower periprocedural complication rate than CAS.

Surgical revascularization is not recommended in <50% stenosis, total occlusion, or in patients with major disabling strokes.

In patients who are considered high surgical risk for either CEA or CAS, the role of medical therapy alone compared with surgical revascularization is not well established.

DISPOSITION

Disposition and prognosis depend on several variables (Table 3): The degree of stenosis, the presence of symptoms, medication compliance, and the type of intervention (if any).

PEARLS & CONSIDERATIONS

The results of ongoing studies concerning the best treatment of patients with carotid artery stenosis may result in guideline changes.

SPECIAL CONSIDERATION

Some studies have shown that in patients with bilateral hemodynamically significant stenosis

[1]Rosenfield K et al, for the ACT I Investigators: Randomized trial of stent versus surgery for asymptomatic carotid stenosis, *N Engl J Med* 374:1011-1020, 2016.

[2]Spence DJ, Naylor AR: Endarterectomy, stenting, or neither for asymptomatic carotid artery stenosis, *N Engl J Med* 374:1087-1088, 2016.

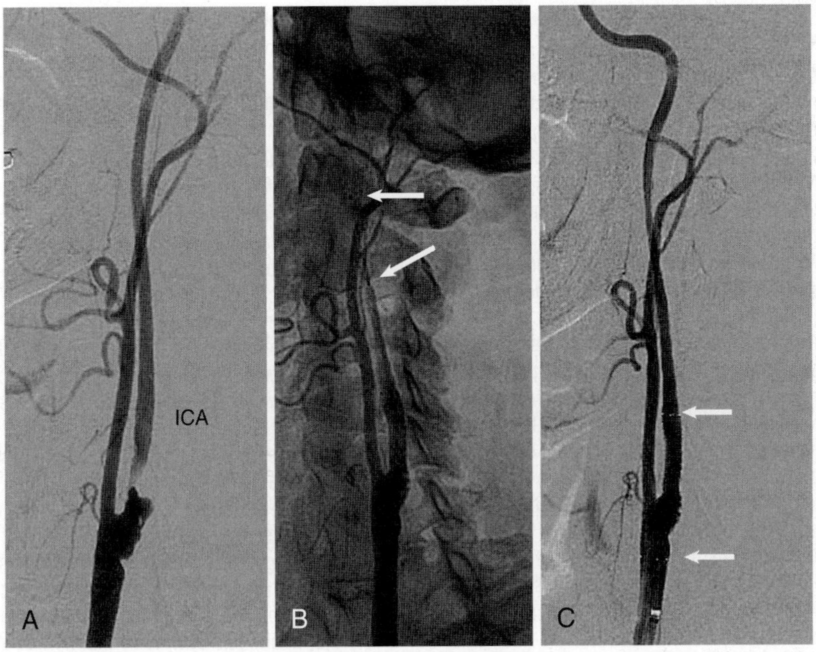

FIG. 3 Carotid stenting for symptomatic carotid stenosis. A, Stenosis at origin of left internal carotid artery. **B,** Stent deployed. Arrows indicate markers of embolic protection filter. **C,** Final angiogram with arrows indicating the margins of the stent. *ICA,* Internal carotid artery. (From Zipes DP: *Braunwald's heart disease, a textbook of cardiovascular medicine*, ed 11, Philadelphia, 2019, Elsevier.)

TABLE 2 Factors Associated with Increased Risk from Carotid Artery Surgery

Anatomic Criteria

High cervical or intrathoracic lesion
Previous neck surgery or radiation therapy
Contralateral carotid artery occlusion
Previous ipsilateral carotid endarterectomy
Contralateral laryngeal nerve palsy
Tracheostomy

Medical Comorbidities

Age >80 yr*
Class III or IV congestive heart failure
Class III or IV angina pectoris
Left main coronary disease
Two- or three-vessel coronary artery disease
Need for open heart surgery
Ejection fraction ≤30%
Recent myocardial infarction
Severe chronic obstructive lung disease

*The risk for a cerebrovascular accident (stroke) with carotid artery stent placement is increased, and the risk for myocardial infarction with carotid endarterectomy is increased.
From Zipes DP: *Braunwald's heart disease, a textbook of cardiovascular medicine*, ed 11, Philadelphia, 2019, Elsevier.

TABLE 3 Carotid Stenosis Management

Degree of Carotid Artery Stenosis	<50%	50%-69%	70%-99%
Asymptomatic	• Medical management	• Medical management • Inconclusive evidence base to favor surgical treatment. May be considered in select patients with >60% stenosis.*	• Medical management • CEA in highly selected patients*
Symptomatic	• Medical management	• CEA • CAS can be an alternative	• CEA • CAS can be an alternative

CAS, Carotid artery stenting; *CEA,* carotid endarterectomy.
*CEA can be considered in asymptomatic patients with >70% stenosis if the anticipated rate of perioperative complications (stroke, myocardial infarction, and death) is <3%, life expectancy is greater than 5 yr, and the risks and benefits (including medical comorbidities) have been discussed thoroughly with the patients and their families.

(>70%), blood pressure reduction resulted in worsened outcomes for stroke. These patients would likely be candidates for CEA.

Symptomatic women with severe carotid stenosis can be managed by CEA provided that the perioperative risk of the operators is low (4%). Although the periprocedural stroke risks may be increased in symptomatic women undergoing CAS, the choice of CAS or CEA should be tailored by subgroups. For example, women with restenosis or severe coronary disease may do best with CAS, whereas those >70 yr of age of having tortuous vessels are best off with CEA.

Both women and men with carotid stenosis should undergo aggressive medical management of cardiovascular risk factors in periprocedural period and beyond for the rest of their lives regardless of whether the patient is undergoing revascularization.

Carotid artery occlusion (100% blockage), for which there is no routine treatment, was reexamined in the national Carotid Occlusion Surgery Study (www.cosstrial.org). Recently published results from the COSS trial demonstrate that superficial temporal artery to middle cerebral artery anastomosis does not provide an overall benefit for ipsilateral 2-yr stroke recurrence when compared to medical therapy alone.

PREVENTION

Prevention of carotid stenosis should include pursuit of a healthy lifestyle and management of risk factors for atherosclerosis.

PATIENT & FAMILY EDUCATION

Patients should be counseled to pursue a healthy lifestyle including exercise and smoking cessation. In addition, patients should take an active role in controlling blood pressure and blood glucose. Further educational materials can be found online at: www.strokecenter.org/education.

SUGGESTED READINGS

Available at ExpertConsult.com

RELATED CONTENT

Carotid Stenosis (Patient Information)
Transient Ischemic Attack (Related Key Topic)

AUTHORS: **Joseph S. Kass, MD, JD, FAAN,** and **Prashanth Krishnamohan, MBBS, MD**

BASIC INFORMATION

DEFINITION

Light-headedness, dizziness, presyncope, or syncope in a patient with carotid sinus hypersensitivity is defined as carotid sinus syndrome (CSS). Carotid sinus hypersensitivity is the exaggerated response to carotid stimulation resulting in bradycardia, hypotension, or both. CSS is often considered a variant of neurocardiogenic syncope. The 2013 European Guidelines (ESC) defines CSS as syncope with reproduction of symptoms during carotid sinus massage of 10-second duration. There are two components of CSS: Cardioinhibitory and vasodepressor.

SYNONYMS

Carotid sinus syncope
CSS
Carotid sinus hypersensitivity

ICD-10CM CODES	
G90.01	Carotid sinus syncope
R55	Syncope and collapse

EPIDEMIOLOGY & DEMOGRAPHICS

- Carotid sinus hypersensitivity accounts for 1% of syncopal episodes (Fig. 1).
- Carotid sinus hypersensitivity is frequently associated with atherosclerosis and diabetes mellitus.
- Incidence increases with age, with an average age of onset at 61 to 74 yr.
- Men are affected more often than women (2:1).
- CSS is rarely found in patients younger than 50 yr.

MECHANISM

- The carotid sinus is located in the internal carotid artery.
- There is a reflex loop between the mechanoreceptors of the carotid sinus and the vagal nucleus in the midbrain.
- There is an exaggerated cardioinhibitory and vasodepressor reaction caused by decreased sympathetic and increased parasympathetic outflow to the heart and vasculature, respectively.

PHYSICAL FINDINGS & CLINICAL PRESENTATION

- Often associated with sudden neck movements, especially rotation, neck palpation, shaving, or tight-fitting collars, but can occur in the absence of clear provocation.
- Mild form has symptoms such as fatigue, light-headedness, nausea, warmth, pallor, or diaphoresis.
- More severe form of the condition has sudden abrupt loss of consciousness without prodrome.

Properly performed carotid sinus massage (CSM) at the bedside is diagnostic. The European Society of Cardiology recommends carotid sinus massage as part of the exam in patients with syncope of unknown etiology and age over 40. This maneuver can elicit three types of responses in patients with carotid sinus hypersensitivity (see "Diagnosis").

- CSM should be performed with the patient in the supine and upright positions while monitoring the patient's blood pressure by cuff and heart rate by ECG.
- CSM should be performed on both the right and left sides but on only one carotid artery at a time.
- Vigorous pressure is applied over the carotid artery, directed posterior to compress the artery against the spinous process of the vertebrae, at the level of the cricoid cartilage for 10 to 30 sec. Repeat on the opposite side if no effect is produced.
- Contraindications to CSM include the presence of carotid artery bruits, documented carotid artery stenosis >70%, history of stroke or transient ischemic attack <3 mo, history of myocardial infarction <6 mo, history of serious ventricular arrhythmia, or prior carotid endarterectomy.
- Complications of CSM are rare (0.1% to 1%) and may include transient visual disturbance, transient paresis, tachyarrhythmias, or bradyarrhythmias.
- False-positive results with carotid sinus massage may be relatively common in the elderly population. Thus alternative explanations for syncope should be investigated prior to attribution of symptoms to carotid sinus hypersensitivity.

ETIOLOGY

- Idiopathic
- Head and neck tumors (e.g., thyroid)
- Significant lymphadenopathy
- Carotid body tumors
- Prior neck surgery

DIAGNOSIS

- The diagnosis of CSS is made in a patient with a history of syncope when carotid sinus hypersensitivity is demonstrated by CSM and no other cause of syncope is identified.
- CSM can elicit three types of responses diagnostic of carotid sinus hypersensitivity:
  1. Cardioinhibitory type: CSM producing (1) asystole for at least 3 sec in the absence of symptoms or (2) reproduction of symptoms occurring with a decline in heart rate of 30% to 40% or asystole of up to 2 sec in duration. Symptoms should not recur when CSM is repeated after atropine infusion.
  2. Vasodepressor type: CSM producing (1) a decrease in systolic blood pressure of 50 mm Hg in the absence of symptoms or 30 mm Hg in the presence of neurologic symptoms; (2) no evidence of asystole; or (3) neurologic symptoms that persist after infusion of atropine.
  3. Mixed type: CSM producing both types of responses.

DIFFERENTIAL DIAGNOSIS

All causes of syncope

WORKUP

- Evaluation for structural heart disease and other arrhythmias
- Exclude other causes of syncope or presyncope: Detailed history, physical examination including orthostatic vital signs, ECG
- Evaluation for vasovagal syncope which may include tilt table testing

TREATMENT

NONPHARMACOLOGIC THERAPY

Reassurance and education are important. Avoid applying neck pressure from tight collars, shaving, or rapid head turning.

ACUTE GENERAL Rx

Treatment will vary according to the type of carotid hypersensitivity response and symptoms present (see "Chronic Rx").

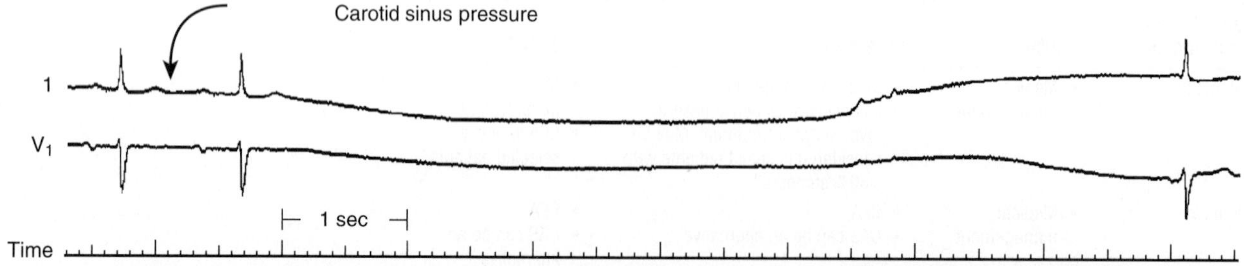

FIG. 1 Carotid sinus hypersensitivity. Two surface electrocardiogram leads are shown during carotid sinus pressure, as indicated. The PR interval is prolonged and followed by a 7.5-second sinus pause ended by a P wave and probable junctional escape complex. The patient was nearly syncopal during this period. (From Issa ZF et al: *Clinical arrhythmology and electrophysiology: a companion to Braunwald's heart disease*, ed 2, Philadelphia, 2012, Saunders.)

CHRONIC Rx

Therapy is divided into three classes: medical, surgical (carotid denervation), and cardiac pacing.

- Surgical therapy has been largely abandoned except in cases of compressing tumors or masses responsible for CSS.
- For infrequent and mildly symptomatic carotid sinus hypersensitivity of either the cardioinhibitory or vasodepressor type, treatment is generally not necessary.
- Cardiac pacing is indicated in patients with recurrent syncope in whom CSM induces ventricular asystole of more than 6 sec and accompanied by syncope. Dual chamber pacing is recommended as there is evidence that single-chamber pacing worsens syncope recurrence.
- Permanent pacing is not indicated for carotid sinus hypersensitivity with no, or only vague, symptoms.

For symptomatic patients with a vasodepressor response to CSM:

- No medical treatment is proven to be effective
- Drugs, such as vasodilators, that would worsen the response should be discontinued or reduced if feasible
- Permissive hypertension
- Increased fluids (≥2 L) and salt intake (>6 g/day)
- Sympathomimetics: Midodrine, titrate from 2.5 to 10 mg tid based on BP and therapeutic response (major side effect in urinary retention in elderly males)
- Serotonin-specific reuptake inhibitors
- Fludrocortisone
- Elastic knee-high or thigh-high stockings
- Carotid sinus denervation

For symptomatic patients with CSS with a mixed response to CSM:

- Combination of dual-chamber permanent pacemaker and agents used to treat vasodepressor response

DISPOSITION

- Up to 50% of the patients have recurrent symptoms.
- No increased mortality rate in patients with idiopathic CSS compared with the general population.

REFERRAL

Cardiology referral is indicated if pacemaker placement is being considered.

PEARLS & CONSIDERATIONS

- The most common type of CSS is cardioinhibitory, followed by mixed and vasodepressor responses.
- Driving restrictions in the 2009 ESC syncope update and 2006 AHA/ACCF consensus document on syncope are stratified according to whether patients have mild or severe syncope.
- Mild carotid sinus syndrome is defined as infrequent mild symptoms (without syncope), with clear precipitating causes (usually standing), warning signs, and infrequent occurrence. For patients with mild sinus hypersensitivity, no driving restrictions are recommended for private or commercial driving.
- Severe carotid sinus syndrome is marked by syncope without warning occurring in any position, without precipitating causes and frequent occurrences. For patients with severe hypersensitivity, all driving is prohibited. If symptoms are controlled, driving is permitted 1 to 6 mo after, based on the modality of treatment.

COMMENTS

Prognosis depends on the underlying cause.

RELATED CONTENT

Syncope (Patient Information)
Orthostatic Hypotension (Related Key Topic)
Syncope (Related Key Topic)

AUTHOR: **John Wylie, MD, FACC**

BASIC INFORMATION

DEFINITION

Carpal tunnel syndrome (CTS) is a compression neuropathy of the median nerve as it passes under the transverse carpal ligament at the wrist (Figs. E1 and E2). It is the most common entrapment neuropathy.

SYNONYM

CTS

ICD-10CM CODES	
G56.0	Carpal tunnel syndrome, unspecified upper limb
G56.01	Carpal tunnel syndrome, right upper limb
G56.02	Carpal tunnel syndrome, left upper limb

EPIDEMIOLOGY & DEMOGRAPHICS

INCIDENCE: 3.8% of the general population (the most common entrapment neuropathy)
PREDOMINANT SEX: Females are affected two to five times as often as males.
PREDOMINANT AGE: 30 to 60 yr

PHYSICAL FINDINGS & CLINICAL PRESENTATION

- Pain, paresthesia in 1st, 2nd, 3rd, and lateral half of 4th fingers, worse at night, with awakenings from sleep due to pain and paresthesias being common.
- ***Tinel sign*** at wrist (Fig. 3): Tapping lightly over the median nerve on the volar surface of the wrist produces a tingling sensation radiating from the wrist to the hand.
- ***Phalen sign*** (Fig. 4): Reproduction of symptoms after 1 min of gentle, unforced wrist flexion.
- Carpal compression (Durkan) test: Direct pressure over the patient's carpal tunnel for 30 sec elicits symptoms.
- Thenar atrophy in long-standing cases with weakness of thumb abduction and opposition.
- Findings may be bilateral in up to 65% of patients.

ETIOLOGY

- Idiopathic in most cases—caused by increased pressure within the carpal tunnel leading to nerve ischemia
- Commonly associated with diabetes, obesity, female gender, advancing age, pregnancy, hypothyroidism, rheumatologic disorders, autoimmune disorders
- Specific occupations with repetitive strain or job-related mechanical overuse
- May also occur due to mass occupying lesions (tenosynovitis, gout, ganglion) or as a result of trauma (distal radius fractures, perilunate and lunate dislocations, etc.)

DIAGNOSIS

DIFFERENTIAL DIAGNOSIS

- Cervical radiculopathy
- Chronic tendinitis
- Pronator teres syndrome
- Anterior interosseous syndrome
- Complex regional pain syndrome
- Brachial plexopathy, thoracic outlet syndrome
- Polyneuropathy
- Other entrapment neuropathies
- Traumatic wrist injuries
- Vascular disorders (Raynaud syndrome)
- Cervical myelopathy

IMAGING STUDIES

Carpal tunnel syndrome is a clinical diagnosis, but imaging may assist workup in uncertain situations. Accumulating evidence suggests that diagnostic ultrasound may be almost as sensitive as nerve conduction velocity tests and may help identify the structural cause of nerve compression. X-ray or MRI may be helpful in ruling out other conditions.

ELECTRODIAGNOSTIC STUDIES

Nerve conduction velocity tests (NCS) demonstrate impaired sensory conduction across the carpal tunnel and may help guide treatment based on the severity of median nerve compression. Electromyography may show active denervation muscle potentials. Specificity of NCS and electromyography for CTS is >95%, and sensitivity is >85%.

TREATMENT

ACUTE GENERAL Rx

- Activity modification and ergonomic optimization (desk, keyboard).
- Nocturnal wrist splint has been shown to be effective.
- No evidence for effectiveness of NSAIDs.
- Corticosteroid injection of carpal canal on ulnar side of palmaris longus tendon proximal to wrist crease (Figs. E5 and E6): Can be done with palpation guidance or under ultrasound guidance. In different clinical studies, injections have increased patient satisfaction and improved clinical symptoms, albeit temporarily.
- Low-dose oral corticosteroids are optional but usually not effective.
- Short-term benefit from ultrasound therapy (physical therapy modality).
- Carpal tunnel release if no response from nonoperative treatment.

DISPOSITION

Clinical course may have remissions and exacerbations. Some may progress from intermittent to persistent sensory complaints (numbness, tingling, paresthesia) and then to motor symptoms. In pregnancy, symptoms usually resolve spontaneously weeks after delivery.

REFERRAL

Surgical referral is needed if conservative treatment fails. Surgery (sectioning of transverse carpal ligament) is performed by open, endoscopic, or minimal incision techniques, with good long-term results. Carpal tunnel release is one of the most common surgeries performed, with approximately 400,000 conducted per yr. Recurrence and complication rates range from 3% to 19% in some series, with revision required in up to 12% of patients.

PEARLS & CONSIDERATIONS

- The sensory changes of carpal tunnel syndrome spare the thenar eminence. This distinctive pattern occurs because the palmar sensory cutaneous branch of the median nerve arises proximal to the wrist, passing superficial to the tunnel.
- Role of repetitive hand or wrist use and workplace factors in the development of carpal tunnel syndrome remains controversial.
- Recent trials from the Mayo Clinic using ultrasound-guided perineural injection therapy (PIT) using 5% dextrose (D_5W) have shown promising results in patients with mild-to-moderate CTS.[1]

SUGGESTED READINGS

Available at ExpertConsult.com

RELATED CONTENT

Carpal Tunnel Syndrome (Patient Information)

AUTHORS: **Shashank Dwivedi, MD,** and **Manuel F. DaSilva, MD**

[1]Wu YT et al: Six-month efficacy of perineural dextrose for carpal tunnel syndrome: a prospective, randomized, double-blind, controlled trial, *Mayo Clin Proc* 92(8):1179-1189, 2017.

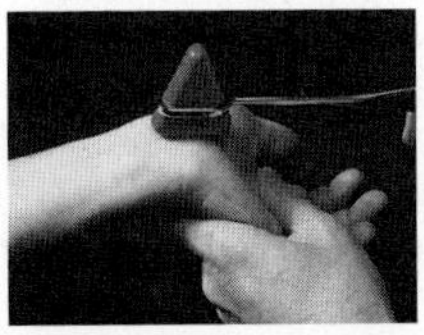

FIG. 3 Tinel sign. The wrist is held in extension while gentle percussion is performed over and just proximal to the transverse carpal ligament. (From Hochberg MC et al: *Rheumatology,* ed 5, St Louis, 2011, Mosby.)

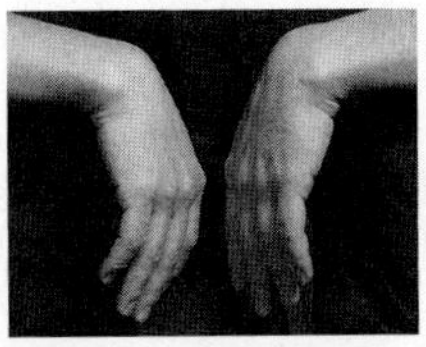

FIG. 4 Phalen (wrist flexion) test. With the wrists held in unforced flexion for 30 to 60 seconds, a positive test reproduces or worsens the patient's symptoms. (From Hochberg MC et al: *Rheumatology,* ed 5, St Louis, 2011, Mosby.)

Cat-Scratch Disease (PTG)

BASIC INFORMATION

DEFINITION

Cat-scratch disease (CSD) is an infectious disease consisting of gradually enlarging regional lymphadenopathy occurring after contact with a feline. Atypical presentations are characterized by a variety of neurologic manifestations as well as granulomatous involvement of the eye, liver, spleen, and bone. The disease is usually self-limiting, and recovery is complete; however, patients with atypical presentations, especially if immunocompromised, may suffer significant morbidity and mortality.

SYNONYMS

CSD
Cat-scratch fever
Benign inoculation lymphoreticulosis
Nonbacterial regional lymphadenitis

ICD-10CM CODE
A28.1 Cat-scratch disease

EPIDEMIOLOGY & DEMOGRAPHICS

INCIDENCE (IN U.S.):
- 9 to 10 cases per 100,000 persons per yr (22,000 cases per yr)
- Majority of reported cases occur in persons <21 yr
- About 500 patients are admitted to the hospital yearly with CSD

PREVALENCE: Unknown
PEAK INCIDENCE: August through January

PHYSICAL FINDINGS & CLINICAL PRESENTATION

- Classic, most common finding: Regional lymphadenopathy occurring within 2 wk of a scratch or contact with felines; usually a new kitten in the household
- Tender, swollen lymph nodes most commonly found in the head and neck (Fig. E1), followed by the axilla and the epitrochlear, inguinal, and femoral areas
- Erythematous overlying skin, showing signs of suppuration from involved lymph nodes
- On careful examination, evidence of cutaneous inoculation in the form of a nonpruritic, slightly tender pustule or papule
- Fever in most patients
- Malaise and headache in fewer than a third of patients
- Atypical presentations in less than 15% of cases
  1. Usually in association with lymphadenopathy and a low-grade or frank fever (>101° F, >38.3° C)
  2. Include granulomatous involvement of the conjunctiva (Parinaud oculoglandular syndrome) and focal masses in the liver, spleen, and mesenteric nodes
- CNS involvement: Neuroretinitis, encephalopathy, encephalitis, transverse myelitis, seizure activity, and coma
- Osteomyelitis in adults and children
- Can be a cause of culture-negative endocarditis
- In HIV-infected and other immunocompromised patients, *Bartonella henselae* is the cause of bacillary angiomatous and peliosis hepatis

ETIOLOGY

- Major cause: *Bartonella henselae*, possibly *Afipia felis* and *Bartonella clarridgeiae*
- Mode of transmission: Predominantly by direct inoculation through the scratch, bite, or lick of a cat, especially a kitten
- Also can be transmitted by flea bite (with the flea obtaining the bacteria from a bacteremic cat); rarely after exposure to a dog, probably secondary to flea bites
- Approximately 2 wk after introduction of the bacteria into the host, regional lymphatic tissues displaying granulomatous infiltration associated with gradual hypertrophy
- Possible dissemination to distant sites (e.g., liver, spleen, and bone), usually characterized by focal masses or discrete parenchymal lesions

DIAGNOSIS

DIFFERENTIAL DIAGNOSIS

Granulomas of this syndrome must be differentiated from those associated with:
- Tularemia
- Tuberculosis or other mycobacterial infections
- Brucellosis
- Sarcoidosis
- Sporotrichosis or other fungal diseases
- Toxoplasmosis
- Lymphogranuloma venereum
- Benign and malignant tumors such as lymphoma

WORKUP

Diagnosis should be considered in patients who present with a predominant complaint of gradually enlarging regional (focal) lymphadenopathy, often with fever and a recent history of having contact with a cat. A primary ulcer at the site of the cat scratch may or may not be present at the time lymphadenopathy becomes manifest.

LABORATORY TESTS

- Serologies: An IFA *Bartonella* serology (titer ≥1:64) is strongly suggestive of infection. An IFA titer >1:256 is diagnostic.
- A PCR assay on tissue, blood, or intraocular fluid is also available but sensitivity is not high.
- Lymph node biopsy: Granulomatous inflammation consistent with CSD.
- Warthin-Starry silver stain on biopsy can identify the bacteria.
- Histopathologically, Warthin-Starry silver stain has been used to identify the bacillus.
- Culture: *B. henselae* is a fastidious, slow-growing, gram-negative rod that requires specific culture techniques for tissue or blood.
- Routine laboratory findings:
  1. Mild leukocytosis or leukopenia
  2. Infrequent eosinophilia
  3. Elevated ESR or CRP
- Abnormalities of bilirubin excretion and elevated hepatic transaminases are usually secondary to hepatic obstruction by granuloma, mass, or lymph node.
- In patients with neurologic manifestations, lumbar puncture usually reveals normal CSF, although there may be a mild pleocytosis and modest elevation in protein.
- CSD skin test is no longer used for clinical purposes.

TREATMENT

NONPHARMACOLOGIC THERAPY

- Warm compresses to the affected nodes
- In cases of encephalitis or coma: Supportive care

ACUTE GENERAL Rx

- This disease is typically self-limited and generally resolves within 2 to 6 mo. Most studies show no additional benefit from antibiotic therapy.
- It would be prudent to treat severely ill patients, especially if immunocompromised, with antibiotic therapy, because these patients tend to suffer dissemination of infection and increased morbidity.
- *Bartonella* is usually sensitive to a 5-day course of azithromycin (500 mg on day 1 followed by 250 mg for 4 days for weight >45.5 kg; 10 mg/kg on day 1 followed by 5 mg/kg for 4 days for weight <45.5 kg) or alternatively tetracycline, sulfa, and the quinolones can be used for 7 to 10 days.
- Hepatosplenic disease, neuroretinitis, and endocarditis require longer courses of therapy.
- Antipyretics and NSAIDs may also be used for lymphadenitis.

DISPOSITION

- Overall prognosis is good.
- Surgical drainage is generally not recommended. Excision of the entire lymph node may be necessary if not responding after prolonged treatment.

REFERRAL

- For diagnostic aspiration or excision in presence of regional lymphadenopathy, bone lesions, and mesenteric lymph nodes and organs
- Infectious diseases specialist for organ involvement including endocarditis
- To ophthalmologist for ocular granulomas

SUGGESTED READING
Available at ExpertConsult.com

RELATED CONTENT

Cat-Scratch Disease (Patient Information)

AUTHOR: **Glenn G. Fort, MD, MPH**

BASIC INFORMATION

DEFINITION

Cavernous sinus thrombosis (CST) is a late complication of either facial or paranasal sinus infection, resulting in thrombosis of the cavernous sinus and inflammation of its surrounding anatomic structures, including cranial nerves III, IV, V (ophthalmic and maxillary branch), and VI, and the internal carotid artery.

SYNONYMS

CST
Intracranial venous sinus thrombosis or thrombophlebitis
Dural sinus thrombosis

ICD-10CM CODE
G08 Intracranial and intraspinal phlebitis and thrombophlebitis

EPIDEMIOLOGY & DEMOGRAPHICS

- CST is rare in the post-antibiotic era.
- Before antibiotics the mortality rate was 80% to 100%.
- With antibiotics and early diagnosis, mortality rates have fallen to ~20%.
- Reported morbidity rates have also declined from between 50% and 70% to about 20% to 30% with advances in imaging modalities and aggressive medical care.

PHYSICAL FINDINGS & CLINICAL PRESENTATION

- Can be either an acute and fulminant disease or an indolent and subacute presentation.
- Septic cases of CST commonly present with high-grade fever (picket fence pattern) and signs of sepsis.
- Headache, although not specific, is the most common presenting symptom and may precede fever and periorbital edema by several days. Elderly patients, however, may only demonstrate alteration in mental status without antecedent headache. The triad of unilateral or bilateral progressive chemosis, periorbital edema, and proptosis with headache is a classical presentation in patients with CST. These signs and symptoms are related to the anatomic structures affected within the cavernous sinus, notably cranial nerves III to VI, as well as impaired venous drainage from the orbit and eye.
  Other common signs and symptoms include:
  - Ptosis.
- Cranial nerve palsies (III, IV, V1, V2, VI).
  1. Ophthalmoplegia caused by involvement of cranial nerves III, IV, and VI is present in most cases. Sixth nerve palsy can occur early in some cases of septic CST, especially when originating from the sphenoid sinus owing to its anatomic proximity.
  2. Hypoesthesia or hyperesthesia of the ophthalmic and maxillary branch of the fifth nerve is common. Periorbital sensory loss and impaired corneal reflex may be noted.
- Papilledema, retinal hemorrhages, and decreased visual acuity progressing to blindness may occur from venous congestion within the retina.
- Pupil may be dilated and sluggishly reactive.
- Headache with nuchal rigidity and changes in mental status may occur if the infection spreads intracranially to the meninges and brain parenchyma.
- Infection can spread to the contralateral cavernous sinus through the intercavernous sinuses within 24 to 48 hr of initial presentation.
- Patients may also develop signs and symptoms of pituitary insufficiency.

ETIOLOGY

- CST most commonly results from contiguous spread of an infection from either the sinuses (sphenoid, ethmoid, or frontal) or the medial third of the face (areas around the eyes and nose that drain to the ophthalmic vein). Nasal furuncles are the most common facial infection to produce this complication. Less-common primary sites of infection include dental abscess, tonsils, soft palate, middle ear, or orbit (orbital cellulitis).
- CST also can result from hematogenous spread of infection to the cavernous sinus by the superior and inferior ophthalmic veins or through the lateral and sigmoid sinuses. Depending on the pressure gradients, infection can spread in a retrograde direction because the dural sinuses are valveless.
- *Staphylococcus aureus* is the most commonly identified pathogen, found in 60% to 70% of the cases.
- *Streptococcus* is the second leading cause.
- Gram-negative rods and anaerobes may also lead to CST.
- Rarely, *Aspergillus fumigatus* and mucormycosis cause CST.
- Risk factors for dural sinus thrombosis include venous hypercoagulable disorders, infections (see previous), trauma, malignancies, systemic inflammatory disorders, pregnancy, and dehydration.

DIAGNOSIS

- The diagnosis of CST is made by clinical suspicion and confirmed by appropriate imaging studies.
- Proptosis, ptosis, chemosis, and cranial nerve palsy beginning in one eye and progressing to the other eye establish the diagnosis.

DIFFERENTIAL DIAGNOSIS

- Orbital or periorbital cellulitis
- Internal carotid artery aneurysm or fistula
- Cerebrovascular disease
- Migraine headache
- Allergic blepharitis
- Thyroid ophthalmopathy
- Orbital neoplasm
- Meningitis
- Epidural and subdural infections
- Epidural and subdural hematoma
- Subarachnoid hemorrhage
- Acute angle-closure glaucoma
- Trauma

WORKUP

CST is a clinical diagnosis, with laboratory tests and imaging studies confirming the clinical impression.

LABORATORY TESTS

- Complete blood count, erythrocyte sedimentation rate, blood cultures, and sinus cultures help establish and identify an infectious primary source. Metabolic panel to look for electrolyte imbalances in cases of suspected pituitary involvement (DI/SIADH).
- Lumbar puncture (LP) helps to distinguish CST from more localized processes (e.g., sinusitis, orbital cellulitis). LP reveals inflammatory cells in 75% of cases. In half of these cases, the cerebrospinal fluid profile is typical for a parameningeal focus (high white blood cells with polymorphonuclear and/or mononuclear cells, normal glucose, normal protein, culture negative), and in one third may be similar to that of bacterial meningitis.

IMAGING STUDIES

- MRI with gadolinium, including magnetic resonance angiography and magnetic resonance venogram (Fig. 1), is more sensitive than CT scan and is the imaging study of choice to diagnose CST. Findings may include deformity of the internal carotid artery within the cavernous sinus and an obvious signal hyperintensity within thrombosed vascular sinuses.
- Noncontrast CT scan of the head and orbits may demonstrate increased density in the region of the cavernous sinus but has relatively low sensitivity. Contrast-enhanced CT scan may reveal underlying sinusitis, thickening of the superior ophthalmic vein, and irregular filling defects within the cavernous sinus; however, findings may be normal early in the disease course.

TREATMENT

NONPHARMACOLOGIC THERAPY

Recognizing the primary source of infection (i.e., facial cellulitis, middle ear, and sinus infections) and treating the primary source expeditiously is the best way to prevent CST.

ACUTE GENERAL Rx

- Appropriate therapy should take into account the primary source of infection as well as possible associated complications such as brain abscess, meningitis, or subdural empyema.
- Broad-spectrum intravenous antibiotics are used as empiric therapy until a definite pathogen is found. Treatment should include vancomycin to cover hospital or community-acquired methicillin-resistant *Staphylococcus aureus* or resistant *Streptococcus pneumoniae* plus a third- or fourth-generation cephalosporin:

1. Vancomycin (1 g q12h with normal renal function) plus either ceftriaxone (2 g q12h) or cefepime (2 g q8-12h).
2. Metronidazole 500 mg IV q6h should be added if anaerobic bacterial infection is suspected (dental or sinus infection).

- Most experts recommend anticoagulation with heparin after the diagnosis is confirmed, unless either surgical intervention is planned or there is evidence of an expanding hematoma. Spontaneous intracranial hemorrhage should first be ruled out before initiating heparin therapy. Early heparinization has been suggested in patients with unilateral CST to prevent clot propagation. Coumadin therapy should be avoided in the acute phase of the illness but should ultimately be instituted to achieve an INR of 2 to 3 and continued until the infection, symptoms, and signs of CST have either resolved or significantly improved. Anticoagulation with warfarin is generally continued for a minimum of 3 to 6 mo. Retrospective case reports and case series have demonstrated a favorable outcome in terms of decreased mortality and morbidity in the anticoagulated patients.
- Steroid therapy is also controversial but may prove helpful in reducing cranial nerve dysfunction or when progression to pituitary insufficiency occurs. Corticosteroids should only be instituted after appropriate antibiotic coverage. Dexamethasone 10 mg q6h is the treatment of choice.
- Emergent surgical drainage with sphenoidotomy is indicated if the primary site of infection is believed to be the sphenoid sinus.

CHRONIC Rx

- Patients with CST are usually treated with prolonged courses (3-4 wk) of IV antibiotics. If there is evidence of complications such as intracranial suppuration, 6 to 8 wk of total therapy may be warranted.
- All patients should be monitored for signs of complicated infection, continued sepsis, or septic emboli while antibiotic therapy is being administered. Relapse of septic CST can occur after an initial improvement weeks after stopping antibiotic treatment.

DISPOSITION

- CST can be a life-threatening, rapidly progressive infectious disease with high morbidity and mortality rates (30%) despite antibiotic use. Morbidity and mortality rates are increased in cases of sphenoid sinus infection.
- Complications of untreated CST include extension of thrombus to other dural sinuses, carotid thrombosis with concomitant strokes, subdural empyema, brain abscess, or meningitis. Septic embolization may also occur to the lungs, resulting in acute respiratory distress syndrome, pulmonary abscess, empyema, and pneumothorax.
- 30% of treated patients develop long-term sequelae, including cranial nerve palsies, blindness, pituitary insufficiency, and hemiparesis.

REFERRAL

If suspected, CST should be considered a medical emergency. Depending on source of infection, appropriate consultation should be made (i.e., ear-nose-throat, ophthalmology, and infectious disease).

PEARLS & CONSIDERATIONS

COMMENTS

CST is a medical emergency and should be suspected with progressing chemosis, proptosis, and cranial neuropathy in a patient with headaches with or without fever.

The anatomy of the cavernous sinus explains the clinical findings: The cavernous sinus lies just above and lateral to the sphenoid sinus and drains the middle portion of the face by the superior and inferior ophthalmic veins; cranial nerves III, IV, V, and VI pass alongside or through the cavernous sinus.

SUGGESTED READINGS

Available at ExpertConsult.com

RELATED CONTENT

Cavernous Sinus Thrombosis (Patient Information)

AUTHOR: **Joseph S. Kass, MD, JD, FAAN**

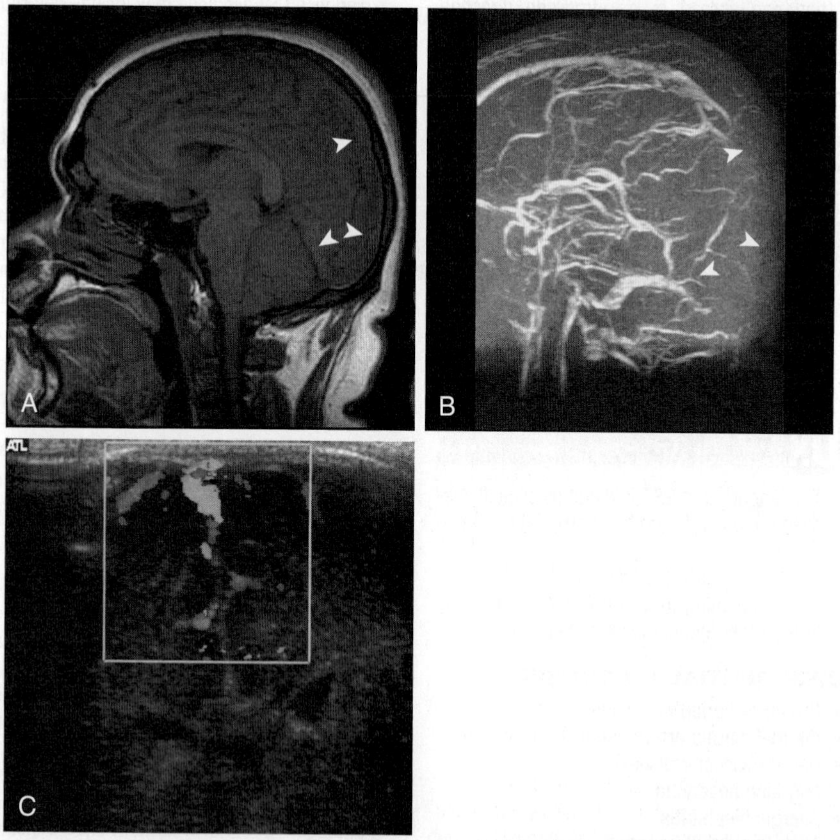

FIG. 1 Superior sagittal sinus (SSS) thrombosis on magnetic resonance venogram (MRV). Sagittal T1 magnetic resonance imaging **(A)** shows intermediate signal intensity in sagittal and straight sinuses *(arrowheads)*. No flow is seen on MRV **(B)** in these vessels *(arrowheads)*, which is consistent with thrombosis. Color Doppler evacuation **(C)** of the SSS in another 6-mo-old patient with suspected thrombosis demonstrated a patent SSS with normal draining cortical veins. (From Fuhrman BP, et al: *Pediatric critical care,* ed 4, Philadelphia, 2011, Saunders.)

BASIC INFORMATION

DEFINITION

Celiac disease is a chronic autoimmune disease characterized by malabsorption and diarrhea precipitated by ingestion of food products containing gluten in genetically susceptible persons. Gluten is a protein complex found in wheat, rye, and barley.

SYNONYMS

Gluten-sensitive enteropathy
Celiac sprue
Nontropical sprue

ICD-10CM CODE
K90.0 Celiac disease

EPIDEMIOLOGY & DEMOGRAPHICS

- The prevalence of celiac disease is 0.5% to 1% in the general population in North America and Western Europe and 5% in high-risk groups such as first-degree relatives of persons with the disease. The prevalence of celiac disease in the U.S. has increased fourfold over the past three decades, but the trend is flattening. The decline in undiagnosed celiac disease may reflect greater public and professional attention to gluten-related issues. Worldwide celiac disease affects 0.6% to 1% of the population. Celiac disease is significantly more common in persons with type 1 diabetes mellitus (DM) and is associated with greater risk of retinopathy and nephropathy in this population.
- Incidence is highest during infancy and the first 36 mo of life (after introduction of foods containing gluten), in the third decade (frequently associated with pregnancy and severe anemia during pregnancy), and in the seventh decade.
- There is a slight female predominance.
- The average age of diagnosis is in the fifth decade of life.
- The risk for celiac disease is 5% to 10% in newborn children of parents with the disease and nearly 20% in siblings.
- It is estimated that only 10% to 15% of persons with celiac disease in the U.S. have been diagnosed.

PHYSICAL FINDINGS & CLINICAL PRESENTATION

- Physical examination may be entirely within normal limits.
- Weight loss, dyspepsia, short stature, and failure to thrive may be noted in children and infants.
- Weight loss, fatigue, and diarrhea are common in adults.
- Abdominal pain, nausea, and vomiting are unusual.
- Pallor as a result of iron-deficiency anemia is common.
- Atypical forms of the disease are being increasingly recognized and include osteoporosis, short stature, anemia, infertility, and neurologic problems. Manifestations of calcium deficiency, such as tetany and seizures, are rare and can be exacerbated by coexistent magnesium deficiency.
- Angular cheilitis, aphthous ulcers, atopic dermatitis, and dermatitis herpetiformis are frequently associated with celiac disease.
- Table 1 summarizes the clinical spectrum of celiac disease.
- Table 2 summarizes extraintestinal manifestations of celiac disease.
- Disorders associated with celiac disease are summarized in Box 1.

ETIOLOGY

- Celiac sprue is considered an autoimmune-type disease, with tissue transglutaminase (tTG) suggested as a major autoantigen. It results from an inappropriate T-cell–mediated immune response against ingested gluten in genetically predisposed individuals who carry either *HLA-DQ2* or *HLA-DQ8* genes. There is sensitivity to gliadin, a protein fraction of gluten found in wheat, rye, and barley. In patients with celiac disease, immune responses to gliadin fractions promote an inflammatory reaction, mainly in the upper small intestine, manifested by infiltration of the lamina propria and the epithelium with chronic inflammatory cells and villous atrophy. The susceptibility to celiac disease may also be related to other environmental factors such as bacterial microbiome and reovirus infection). Table 3 summarizes biomarkers in the diagnosis of celiac disease and monitoring compliance to gluten-free diet.
- Seroconversion to celiac autoimmunity may occur at any time.
- Timing of introduction of gluten into the infant diet in children at risk remains inconclusive. Children initially exposed to gluten in the first 3 mo of life have a fivefold increased risk. Current recommendations are to delay introduction of gluten into the diet of a genetically susceptible infant until 4 to 6 mo of age while the mother continues to breastfeed.
- Trials involving randomized feeding intervention in infants at high risk for celiac disease have shown that as compared to placebo, the introduction of small quantities of gluten at 16 to 24 wk of age did not reduce the risk of celiac disease by 3 yr of age.

DIAGNOSIS

Diagnostic criteria for celiac disease require at least four out of five or three out of four if the *HLA* genotype is not performed:

1. Typical symptoms of celiac disease
2. Positivity of serum celiac disease Immunoglobulin A (IgA) class autoantibodies at high titer
3. *HLA-DQ2* or *HLA-DQ8* genotypes
4. Celiac enteropathy at the small intestinal biopsy
5. Response to gluten-free diet

DIFFERENTIAL DIAGNOSIS

- Inflammatory bowel disease
- Laxative abuse
- Intestinal parasitic infestations
- Lactose intolerance
- Other: Irritable bowel syndrome, tropical sprue, chronic pancreatitis, Zollinger-Ellison syndrome, cystic fibrosis (children), lymphoma, eosinophilic gastroenteritis, short bowel syndrome, Whipple disease
- Intestinal lymphoma, tuberculosis, radiation enteritis, HIV enteropathy

LABORATORY TESTS

- IgA anti-tTG antibody by enzyme-linked immunosorbent assay (tissue transglutaminase [tTG] test) is the best screening serologic test for celiac disease. IgA antiendomysial antibodies (EMA) test is also a good screening test for celiac disease but is best used as a confirmatory test in cases of borderline positive results. In patients with IgA deficiency, the IgG deamidated gliadin peptide (DPG) test (deamidated gliadin peptides) can be used for diagnosis. Screening of close relatives is initially done with polymerase chain reaction (PCR) testing for *HLA-DQ2* or *HLA-DQ8*. Those that are positive should then have serum tTG IgA screening. All diagnostic serologic testing for celiac disease should be performed before a gluten-free diet is initiated. Table 4 summarizes the sensitivity, specificity, and positive and negative predictive values of serologic tests for untreated celiac disease.
- CBC, ferritin level: Iron-deficiency anemia (microcytic anemia, low ferritin level) may be present.
- Celiac disease can lead to malabsorption: Screen for vitamin B_{12} level, folate level, vitamin D level, serum calcium, albumin, magnesium; vitamin B_{12} deficiency, vitamin D deficiency, hypomagnesemia, and hypocalcemia are not uncommon in celiac disease.

TABLE 1 Clinical Spectrum of Celiac Disease

Symptomatic

Frank malabsorption symptoms: Chronic diarrhea, failure to thrive, weight loss

Extraintestinal manifestations: Anemia, fatigue, hypertransaminasemia, neurologic disorders, short stature, dental enamel defects, arthralgia, aphthous stomatitis

Silent

No apparent symptoms in spite of histologic evidence of villous atrophy

In most cases identified by serologic screening in at-risk groups (see "Laboratory Tests")

Latent

Subjects who have a normal histology, but at some other time, before or after, have shown a gluten-dependent enteropathy

Potential

Subjects with positive celiac disease serology but without evidence of altered jejunal histology

It might or might not be symptomatic

From Kliegman RM et al: *Nelson textbook of pediatrics,* ed 19, Philadelphia, 2011, Saunders.

TABLE 2 Extraintestinal Manifestations of Celiac Disease

Manifestation	Probable Cause(s)
Cutaneous	
Ecchymoses and petechiae	Vitamin K deficiency; rarely, thrombocytopenia
Edema	Hypoproteinemia
Dermatitis herpetiformis	Epidermal (type 3) tTG autoimmunity
Follicular hyperkeratosis and dermatitis	Vitamin A malabsorption, vitamin B complex malabsorption
Endocrinologic	
Amenorrhea, infertility, impotence	Malnutrition, hypothalamic-pituitary dysfunction, immune dysfunction
Secondary hyperparathyroidism	Calcium and/or vitamin D malabsorption with hypocalcemia
Hematologic	
Anemia	Iron, folate, vitamin B_{12}, or pyridoxine deficiency
Hemorrhage	Vitamin K deficiency; rarely, thrombocytopenia due to folate deficiency
Thrombocytosis, Howell-Jolly bodies	Hyposplenism
Hepatic	
Elevated liver biochemical test levels	Lymphocytic hepatitis
Autoimmune hepatitis	Autoimmunity
Muscular	
Atrophy	Malnutrition due to malabsorption
Tetany	Calcium, vitamin D, and/or magnesium malabsorption
Weakness	Generalized muscle atrophy, hypokalemia
Neurologic	
Peripheral neuropathy	Deficiencies of vitamin B_{12} and thiamine; immune-based neurologic dysfunction
Ataxia	Cerebellar and posterior column damage
Demyelinating central nervous system lesions	Immune-based neurologic dysfunction
Seizures	Unknown
Skeletal	
Osteopenia, osteomalacia, and osteoporosis	Malabsorption of calcium and vitamin D, secondary hyperparathyroidism, chronic inflammation
Osteoarthropathy	Unknown
Pathologic fractures	Osteopenia and osteoporosis

tTG, Tissue transglutaminase.
From Feldman M et al: *Sleisenger and Fortran's gastrointestinal and liver disease*, ed 10, Philadelphia, 2016, Elsevier.

BOX 1 Disorders Associated with Celiac Disease

Definite Association
Bird-fancier lung
Dermatitis herpetiformis
Diabetes mellitus type 1
Down syndrome
Epilepsy with cerebral calcification
Fibrosing alveolitis
Hypothyroidism or hyperthyroidism
IBD
IgA mesangial nephropathy
Idiopathic pulmonary hemosiderosis
IgA deficiency
Microscopic colitis
Recurrent pericarditis
RA
Sarcoidosis

Negative Association
Diabetes mellitus type 2

Possible Association
Addison disease
Autoimmune hemolytic anemia
Autoimmune liver diseases
Cavitary lung disease
Congenital heart disease
Cystic fibrosis
Immune thrombocytopenic purpura
Iridocyclitis or choroiditis
Macroamylasemia
Myasthenia gravis
Polymyositis
Schizophrenia
Sjögren syndrome
Systemic and cutaneous vasculitides
SLE

IBD, Inflammatory bowel disease; *IgA*, immunoglobulin A; *RA*, rheumatoid arthritis; *SLE*, systemic lupus erythematosus.
Modified from Mulder CJ, Tytgat GN: Coeliac disease and related disorders, *Neth J Med* 31:286-299, 1987. In Feldman M et al: *Sleisenger and Fortran's gastrointestinal and liver disease*, ed 10, Philadelphia, 2016, Elsevier.

- Biopsy of the small bowel, considered the gold standard, has been questioned as a reliable and conclusive test in all cases. It may be reasonable in children with significant elevations of tTG levels (>100 U) to first try a gluten-free diet and consider biopsy in those who do not improve with diet. Repeat small-bowel biopsies are no longer required to show healing when there is a clear response to a gluten-free diet.
- The HLA-DQ2 allele is identified in >90% of patients with celiac disease, and HLA-DQ8 is identified in most of the remaining patients. These genes occur in only 30% to 40% of the general population. Their greatest diagnostic value is in their negative predictive value, making them useful when negative in ruling out the disease.

IMAGING STUDIES

- Consider bone density in newly diagnosed adult patients.
- Capsule endoscopy can be used to evaluate mucosa of the small intestine, especially if future innovations will allow mucosal biopsy.

Rx TREATMENT

NONPHARMACOLOGIC THERAPY

Patients should be instructed on a gluten-free diet (avoidance of wheat, rye, and barley). Safe grains (gluten-free) include rice, corn, oats, buckwheat, millet, amaranth, quinoa, sorghum, and teff (an Ethiopian cereal grain). The lowest amount of daily gluten that causes damage to the celiac intestinal mucosa is 10 to 15 mg/day. One slice of bread contains 1.6 g of gluten. Principles of initial dietary therapy for patients with celiac disease are summarized in Box 2.

GENERAL Rx

- Correct nutritional deficiencies with iron, folic acid, calcium, vitamin D, and vitamin B_{12} as needed.
- Prednisone 20 to 60 mg qd gradually tapered is useful in refractory cases.
- Lifelong gluten-free diet is necessary. A referral to a nutritionist experienced in celiac disease and gluten-free diet is recommended at initial diagnosis.

DISPOSITION

- Prognosis is good with adherence to a gluten-free diet. Rapid improvement is usually seen within a few days of treatment. Healing of the intestinal damage typically occurs within 6 to 24 mo after initiation of the diet. Lack of response to gluten-free diet occurs in 5% of patients and is due to unintentional ingestion of gluten or presence of coexisting GI disorders such as inflammatory bowel disease (IBD), lactose or other carbohydrate intolerance, and pancreatic insufficiency.
- Serial antigliadin or antiendomysial antibody tests can be used to monitor the patient's adherence to a gluten-free diet.
- Repeat small-bowel biopsy after treatment generally reveals significant improvement. It is also useful to evaluate for increased risk of small-bowel T-cell lymphoma in these patients, especially untreated patients. Some experts recommend a repeat biopsy only in selected patients who have an unsatisfactory response to a strict gluten-free diet; however, recent data (Lebwohl et al) show that the risk for lymphoproliferative malignancy (LPM) is affected by the results of follow-up intestinal biopsy performed

TABLE 3 Biomarkers in the Diagnosis of Celiac Disease and Monitoring Compliance to Gluten-Free Diet

Biomarker	Method	Comments
Antireticulin antibodies—IgG/IgA	IFA (rat kidney)	Lack optimal sensitivity and specificity for routine diagnostic use
Total IgA	Quantitative nephelometry	Useful in ruling out IgA deficiency; specific IgG antibodies need to be tested in IgA-deficient individuals
Antigliadin antibodies—IgG/IgA	Quantitative EIA	Low sensitivity and specificity; useful in monitoring dietary compliance
Antideaminated gliadin antibodies—IgG/IgA	Quantitative EIA	Inferior performance relative to other diagnostic assays
Antiendomysial antibodies—IgG/IgA	IFA (rhesus monkey esophagus; human umbilical cord)	High sensitivity and specificity in CD; observer bias limits usefulness
Antitissue glutaminase—IgG/IgA	Quantitative EIA	Assays using purified human or recombinant human tTG are more sensitive than those using guinea pig tTG; useful in both diagnosis and monitoring dietary compliance
HLA-DQ2/HLA-DQ8	PCR-based assays	High negative predictive value; not affected by dietary gluten; found in ≈30% of general population

CD, Celiac disease; *EIA,* enzyme immunoassay; *IFA,* immunofluorescence; *IgA,* immunoglobulin A; *IgG,* immunoglobulin G; *PCR,* polymerase chain reaction; *tTG,* tissue transglutaminase.
From McPherson RA, Pincus MR: *Henry's clinical diagnosis and management by laboratory methods*, ed 23, Philadelphia, 2017, Elsevier.

TABLE 4 Sensitivity, Specificity, and Positive and Negative Predictive Values of Serologic Tests for Untreated Celiac Disease

Serologic Test	Sensitivity* (%)	Specificity* (%)	Positive Predictive Value (%)	Negative Predictive Value (%)
Immunoglobulin A Tissue Transglutaminase				
Endomysial antibody by indirect immunofluorescence assay	85-98	97-100	98-100	80-95
Guinea pig tTG ELISA	95-98	94-95	91-95	96-98
Human tTG ELISA	95-100	97-100	80-95	100
Antigliadin Antibodies (AGAs)				
IgA	75-90	82-95	28-100	65-100
IgG	69-85	73-90	20-95	41-88

AGA, Antigliadin antibodies; *ELISA,* enzyme-linked immunosorbent assay; *IgA,* immunoglobulin A; *IgG,* immunoglobulin G; *tTG,* tissue transglutaminase.
*Wide variations in test sensitivity and specificity rates are reported among different laboratories. (Stern M: Comparative evaluation of serologic tests for celiac disease: a European initiative toward standardization, *J Pediatr Gastroenterol Nutr* 31:513-519, 2000.)
From Feldman M et al: *Sleisenger and Fortran's gastrointestinal and liver disease*, ed 10, Philadelphia, 2016, Elsevier.

to document mucosal healing. Increased risk for LPM in CD is associated with the follow-up biopsy results, with a higher risk among patients with persistent villous atrophy. Follow-up biopsy may effectively stratify patients with CD by risk for subsequent LPM.

PEARLS & CONSIDERATIONS

COMMENTS

- The presence of dermatitis herpetiformis is pathognomonic for celiac disease.
- In close relatives, repeated serum tTG IgA testing may be useful in those with positive *HLA-DQ2* or *HLA-DQ8* tests because celiac disease may not manifest until later in life, and initial negative results do not preclude the possibility of future onset of celiac disease.
- Celiac disease should be considered in patients with unexplained metabolic bone disease, osteoporosis, transaminasemia, or hypocalcemia, because gastrointestinal symptoms are absent or mild. Clinicians should also consider testing children and young adults for celiac disease if unexplained weight loss, abdominal pain or distention, or chronic diarrhea is present.
- Screening for celiac disease is recommended in first-degree relatives. It should also be considered in patients with type 1 diabetes mellitus and in those with certain autoimmune disorders such as primary biliary cirrhosis, primary sclerosing cholangitis, autoimmune hepatitis, IBD, thyroid disease (hypothyroidism occurs in up to 15% of patients with celiac disease), systemic lupus erythematosus, RA, and Sjögren syndrome due to increased risk of celiac disease in these populations. Screening persons with Down syndrome or Turner syndrome has also been recommended.
- The prevalence of celiac disease in patients with dyspepsia is twice that of the general population. Screening for celiac disease should be considered in all patients with persistent dyspepsia.
- Patients with celiac disease have an overall risk of cancer that is almost twice that of the general population. The risk of adenocarcinoma of the small intestine is increased manifold compared with the risk in the general population. Celiac disease is also associated with an increased risk for non-Hodgkin lymphoma, especially of T-cell type and primarily localized in the gut. Lymphoma is 4 to 40 times more common, and death from lymphoma is 11 to 70 times more common in patients with celiac disease. Patients with refractory celiac disease are at greatest risk for T-cell lymphoma.
- Patients with celiac disease who have followed a gluten-free diet for prolonged periods may not experience relapse of symptoms for several months after gluten is reintroduced.

BOX 2 Principles of Initial Dietary Therapy for Patients with Celiac Disease

Avoid all foods containing wheat, rye, and barley gluten (pure oats usually safe).
Avoid malt unless clearly labeled as derived from corn.
Use only rice, corn, maize, buckwheat, millet, amaranth, quinoa, sorghum, potato or potato starch, soybean, tapioca, and teff, bean, and nut flours.
Wheat starch and products containing wheat starch should only be used if they contain less than 20 ppm gluten and are marked "gluten free."
Read all labels and study ingredients of processed foods.
Beware of gluten in medications, supplements, food additives, emulsifiers, or stabilizers.
Limit milk and milk products initially if there is evidence of lactose intolerance.
Avoid all beers, lagers, ales, and stouts (unless labeled gluten free).
Wine, most liqueurs, ciders, and spirits, including whiskey and brandy, are allowed.

ppm, Parts per million.
Modified from Trier JS: Celiac sprue and refractory sprue. In Feldman M et al (eds): *Gastrointestinal and liver disease,* ed 6, Philadelphia, 1997, Saunders, p 1557. In Feldman M et al: *Sleisenger and Fortran's gastrointestinal and liver disease*, ed 10, Philadelphia, 2016, Elsevier.

SUGGESTED READINGS

Available at ExpertConsult.com

RELATED CONTENT

Celiac Disease (Patient Information)
Dermatitis Herpetiformis (Related Key Topic)
Malabsorption (Related Key Topic)

AUTHOR: **Fred F. Ferri, MD**

BASIC INFORMATION

DEFINITION

Cellulitis is an infection of the deep dermis and subcutaneous tissues characterized by erythema, warmth, and tenderness of the involved area. Diagnosis is made on the basis of history and physical examination.

SYNONYMS

Erysipelas (cellulitis generally caused by group A β-hemolytic streptococci [GABHS])
SSSIs (skin and skin structure infections)
ABSSSIs (acute bacterial skin and skin structure infections)

ICD-10CM CODES

H05.011	Cellulitis of right orbit
H05.012	Cellulitis of left orbit
H05.013	Cellulitis of bilateral orbits
H05.019	Cellulitis of unspecified orbit
H60.10	Cellulitis of external ear, unspecified ear
H60.11	Cellulitis of right external ear
H60.12	Cellulitis of left external ear
H60.13	Cellulitis of external ear, bilateral
K12.2	Cellulitis and abscess of mouth
L03.011	Cellulitis of right finger
L03.012	Cellulitis of left finger
L03.019	Cellulitis of unspecified finger
L03.031	Cellulitis of right toe
L03.032	Cellulitis of left toe
L03.039	Cellulitis of unspecified toe
L03.111	Cellulitis of right axilla
L03.112	Cellulitis of left axilla
L03.113	Cellulitis of right upper limb
L03.114	Cellulitis of left upper limb
L03.115	Cellulitis of right lower limb
L03.116	Cellulitis of left lower limb
L03.119	Cellulitis of unspecified part of limb
L03.211	Cellulitis of face
L03.221	Cellulitis of neck
L03.311	Cellulitis of abdominal wall
L03.312	Cellulitis of back [any part except buttock]
L03.313	Cellulitis of chest wall
L03.314	Cellulitis of groin
L03.315	Cellulitis of perineum
L03.316	Cellulitis of umbilicus
L03.317	Cellulitis of buttock
L03.319	Cellulitis of trunk, unspecified
L03.811	Cellulitis of head [any part, except face]
L03.818	Cellulitis of other sites
L03.90	Cellulitis, unspecified

EPIDEMIOLOGY & DEMOGRAPHICS

- Occurs most frequently in diabetics, immunocompromised hosts, and patients with venous and lymphatic compromise.
- Frequently found near skin breaks (trauma, surgical wounds [surgical site infections develop in 2% to 5% of all surgical procedures], ulcerations, tinea infections). Edema, animal or human bites, subadjacent osteomyelitis, and bacteremia are potential sources of cellulitis.
- Skin and soft-tissue infections account for >14 million outpatient visits per yr and $3.7 billion in ambulatory care costs. They also are responsible for more than 650,000 admissions in the U.S./yr.

PHYSICAL FINDINGS & CLINICAL PRESENTATION

Variable with the causative organism:

- Erysipelas (Fig. E1): Superficial-spreading, warm, erythematous lesion distinguished by indurated, elevated margin; lymphatic involvement, vesicle formation common.
- Staphylococcal cellulitis: Area involved is erythematous, hot, and swollen; differentiated from erysipelas by nonelevated, poorly demarcated margin; local tenderness and regional adenopathy are common; up to 85% of cases occur on the legs and feet.
- *Haemophilus influenzae* cellulitis: Area involved is a blue-red/purple-red color; occurs mainly in children; generally involves the face in children and the neck or upper chest in adults.
- *Vibrio vulnificus:* Larger hemorrhagic bullae, cellulitis, lymphadenitis, myositis; often found in critically ill patients in septic shock.
- Table E1 describes anatomic variants of or predispositions to cellulitis. Typically, nonpurulent cellulitis is caused by β-hemolytic streptococci, whereas cellulitis with purulent drainage is caused by MRSA.

ETIOLOGY

- Any disruption of the skin barrier provides a portal for pathogens to enter the skin and soft tissues
- Group A β-hemolytic streptococci (may follow a streptococcal infection of the upper respiratory tract). β-hemolytic streptococci are implicated in most cases of nontraumatic cellulitis
- Staphylococcal cellulitis: Diabetics, athletes, men who have sex with men, people living in public housing, and incarcerated men are at greater risk for methicillin-resistant *Staphylococcus aureus* (MRSA) infection. A community-acquired MRSA strain, USA 300, is replacing nosocomial strains of MRSA in hospitals
- IV drug use: MRSA, *Pseudomonas aeruginosa*
- *V. vulnificus:* Higher incidence in patients with liver disease (75%) and in immunocompromised hosts. *V. vulnificus* infection is the leading cause of death related to seafood consumption in the U.S.
- *Erysipelothrix rhusiopathiae:* Common in people handling poultry, fish, or meat
- *Aeromonas hydrophila:* Generally occurs in contaminated open wounds in fresh water
- Fungi *(Cryptococcus neoformans):* In immunocompromised granulopenic patients
- Gram-negative rods *(Serratia, Enterobacter, Proteus, Pseudomonas):* May be present in immunocompromised or granulopenic patients
- Hot tub exposure: *P. aeruginosa*; fish tank exposure: *Mycobacterium marinum*
- Bites: Human *(Eikenella corrodens)*, dog *(Pasteurella multocida, C. canimorsus)*, cat *(P. multocida)*, rat *(Streptobacillus moniliformis)*

DIAGNOSIS

DIFFERENTIAL DIAGNOSIS

- Necrotizing fasciitis (reddish-purple discoloration of skin, rapid increase in size, woody induration and pale appearance rather than erythema, violaceous bullae, pain out of proportion to appearance, sepsis)
- Deep vein thrombosis
- Peripheral vascular insufficiency (venous stasis dermatitis)
- Paget disease of the breast
- Thrombophlebitis
- Acute gout
- Psoriasis
- *Candida* intertrigo
- Pseudogout
- Osteomyelitis
- Insect bite
- Fixed drug eruption
- Lymphedema
- Contact dermatitis
- Olecranon bursa infection
- Herpetic whitlow, early herpes zoster (before blisters)
- Erythema migrans (Lyme disease)
- Rare: *Vaccinia* vaccination, Kawasaki disease, pyoderma gangrenosum, Sweet syndrome, carcinoma erysipeloides, anaerobic myonecrosis, erythromelalgia, eosinophilic cellulitis (Well syndrome), familial Mediterranean fever

LABORATORY TESTS

- Laboratory testing is generally not required for the evaluation of cellulitis and uncomplicated soft tissue infections in the absence of comorbidities
- CBC with differential: Leukocytosis may be present but is a nonspecific finding
- Gram stain, culture (aerobic and anaerobic):
  1. Aspirated material from:
     a. Advancing edge of cellulitis
     b. Any vesicles
  2. Swab of any drainage material
  3. Punch biopsy (in selected patients)
- Blood cultures in hospitalized patients, patients with cellulitis superimposed on lymphedema, patients with buccal or periorbital cellulitis, and patients suspected of having a salt- or fresh-water source of infection. Bacteremia uncommon in cellulitis (positive blood cultures in 4% of patients)
- Anti-streptolysin O (ASLO) titer (in suspected streptococcal disease)
- The cause of cellulitis remains unidentified in most patients. Patients with recurrent lower-extremity cellulitis should be inspected for tinea pedis. If found, it should be treated

IMAGING STUDIES

- Imaging is generally not necessary but may be helpful in suspected purulent soft tissue infections and osteomyelitis.

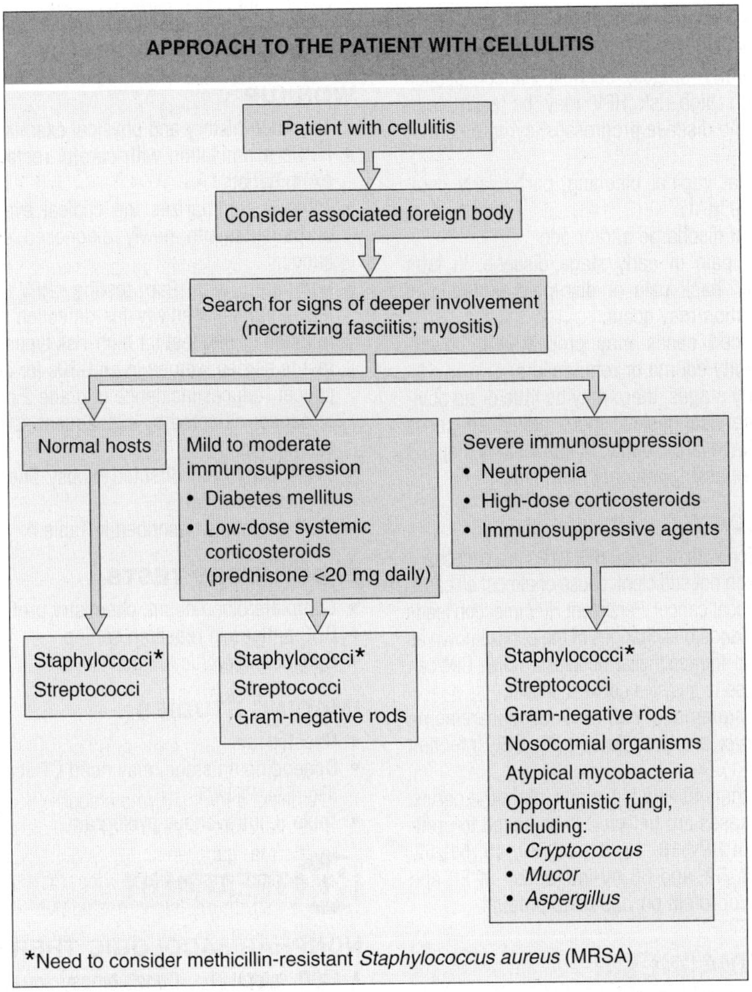

FIG. 2 Approach to the patient with cellulitis. (From Bolognia JL et al: *Dermatology*, ed 4, 2018, Elsevier.)

- CT or MRI in patients with suspected necrotizing fasciitis (deep-seated infection of the subcutaneous tissue that results in the progressive destruction of fascia and fat).

WORKUP

An approach to the patient with cellulitis is illustrated in Fig. 2.

Rx TREATMENT

NONPHARMACOLOGIC THERAPY

Immobilization and elevation of the involved limb. Cool sterile saline dressings to remove purulence from any open lesion. Support stockings in patients with peripheral edema.

ACUTE GENERAL Rx

Treatment should initially cover *Streptococcus* and methicillin-sensitive *S. aureus* and should be expanded for MRSA in patients with risk factors (e.g., IV drug users, residents of long-term care facilities, athletes, children, men who have sex with men, prisoners).

ERYSIPELAS:

- PO: Dicloxacillin 500 mg PO q6h or cephalexin 500 mg qid
- IV: Cefazolin 1 g q6 to 8h or nafcillin 1.0 or 1.5 g IV q4 to 6h

NOTE: Use vancomycin 1 g IV q12h in patients allergic to penicillin.

STAPHYLOCOCCAL CELLULITIS:

- PO: Dicloxacillin 250 to 500 mg qid.
- IV: Nafcillin 1 to 2 g q4 to 6h.
- Cephalosporins (cephalexin 500 mg qid) also provide adequate antistaphylococcal coverage, except for MRSA.
- Trimethoprim-sulfamethoxazole (160 mg/800 mg 1 PO bid) may be appropriate in outpatient mild MRSA infections. Use vancomycin 1.0 to 2.0 g IV qd or linezolid 0.6 g IV q12h in patients with moderate/severe MRSA. Daptomycin (Cubicin), a cyclic lipopeptide, can be used as an alternative to vancomycin for complicated skin and skin structure infections. Usual dose is 4 mg/kg IV given over 30 min every 24 hr. Telavancin is a new glycopeptide derivative of vancomycin effective for gram-positive skin and skin structure infections, including those caused by MRSA. Tedizolid is an oxazolidinone effective in ABSSSI as an alternative to linezolid. Ceftaroline fosamil (Teflaro) is a newer IV cephalosporin also effective against MRSA. Dalbavancin and tedizolid are two new drugs FDA-approved for skin and skin structure infections, including those caused by MRSA.

H. INFLUENZAE CELLULITIS:

- PO: Cefixime or cefuroxime
- IV: Cefuroxime or ceftriaxone

VIBRIO VULNIFICUS:

- Doxycycline 100 mg IV bid + ceftazidime 2 g IV q8h or IV ciprofloxacin 400 mg bid. Mild cases treated with oral antibiotics (doxycycline 100 mg bid + ciprofloxacin 750 mg bid).
- IV support and admission into intensive care unit (mortality rate >50% in septic shock).

E. RHUSIOPATHIAE:

- Penicillin

A. HYDROPHILA:

- Aminoglycosides
- Chloramphenicol
- Complicated skin and skin structure infections in hospitalized patients can be treated with daptomycin (Cubicin) 4 mg/kg IV q24h

PEARLS & CONSIDERATIONS

- 16.6% of acute cellulitis cases are unresponsive to initial treatment mainly due to inappropriate antibiotic selection and dosing (weight-based dosing is preferred).
- Prophylactic antibiotics (e.g., dicloxacillin 500 mg bid or erythromycin 250 mg bid) are controversial but can be considered with patients with ≥4 episodes of cellulitis despite optimized control of risk factors. Recurrent cellulitis with no identifiable cause occurs in 22% of cases despite antibiotic prophylaxis.
- In patients with uncomplicated cellulitis in the outpatient setting, adding trimethoprim-sulfamethoxazole to cephalexin for MRSA coverage is unnecessary and does not increase the likelihood of clinical cure.
- In patients with chronic edema of the leg, daily use of compression garments on the leg can lower the incidence of recurrent cellulitis.[1]

RELATED CONTENT

Cellulitis (Patient Information)
Erysipelas (Related Key Topic)
Necrotizing Fasciitis (Related Key Topic)

SUGGESTED READINGS

Available at ExpertConsult.com

AUTHOR: **Fred F. Ferri, MD**

[1]Webb E et al: Compression therapy to prevent recurrent cellulitis of the leg, *N Engl J Med* 383: 630-639, 2020.

BASIC INFORMATION

DEFINITION

Cervical cancer is the penetration of the basement membrane and infiltration of the stroma of the uterine cervix by malignant cells. The cancer arises from normal cervical epithelium through progressive development of low-grade and high-grade cervical intraepithelial lesions (CINs).

ICD-10CM CODES

C53.8	Malignant neoplasm of overlapping sites of cervix uteri
C53.9	Malignant neoplasm of cervix uteri, unspecified
D06.7	Carcinoma in situ of other parts of cervix
D06.9	Carcinoma in situ of cervix, unspecified

EPIDEMIOLOGY & DEMOGRAPHICS

INCIDENCE: According to the World Health Organization, cervical cancer is the fourth most common malignancy in women. It is reported that nearly 9 out of 10 women who died of cervical cancer were in an underdeveloped region of the world.

PREDOMINANCE: Higher incidence rates occur in developing countries. Among the U.S. population, Hispanics have a higher incidence than African Americans, who likewise have a higher incidence than Caucasians. Compared to Caucasian women, African American and Hispanic women have increased risk of late-stage diagnosis and worse disease progression.

RISK FACTORS: The major risk factor is persistent infection with high-risk human papillomavirus (HPV; types 16 and 18 are the most oncogenic with 31, 33, 35, 45, 52, and 58 also considered high risk). Smoking, early age of coitarche, multiple sexual partners, immunocompromised state, nonbarrier methods of contraception, and multiparity are also risk factors.

PHYSICAL FINDINGS & CLINICAL PRESENTATION

In the early stages, cervical cancer associated with high-risk HPV may be asymptomatic. As the disease progresses, symptoms may include:

- Unusual vaginal bleeding, particularly postcoital (Fig. 1).
- Vaginal discharge and/or odor.
- Pelvic pain in early stage disease. In later stages, back pain or disrupted urination or defecation may occur.
- Advanced cases may present with lower-extremity edema or renal failure.
- In early stages, there may be little or no obvious cervical lesion; more advanced cases may have large, bulky, friable lesions (Fig. E2) encompassing majority of vagina.

ETIOLOGY

- Infection with high-risk HPV types is a necessary, although not sufficient, cause of almost all cases of cervical cancer. Persistent HPV infection leads to precancerous changes of the cervix known as cervical intraepithelial neoplasia (CIN). CIN can progress to invasive cervical cancer.
- Both squamous cell and adenocarcinoma of cervix are associated with HPV infection (Table 1).
- More than 40 HPV types can infect the cervix. Most cases are believed to be linked to presence of HPV 16, 18, 31, 35, 39, 45, 51, 52, 56, 58, 59, and 68 by interaction of E6 and E7 oncoprotein on *p53* gene product.

Dx DIAGNOSIS

DIFFERENTIAL DIAGNOSIS

- Cervical polyp or prolapsed uterine fibroid.
- Neoplasia metastatic from a separate primary neoplasia.
- Box 1 summarizes benign mimics of cervical adenocarcinoma.
- Categories of squamous carcinoma are described in Box 2.
- Table 2 summarizes the differential diagnosis of squamous intraepithelial lesions.

WORKUP

- Thorough history and physical examination
- Pelvic examination with careful rectovaginal examination
- Table 3 summarizes the clinical evaluation of patients with newly diagnosed cervical cancer
- Compared with Pap testing, HPV testing has greater sensitivity for detection of CIN. Addition of HPV test for high-risk types to Pap test to screen women in mid-30s for cervical cancer reduces incidence of grade 2 or 3 CIN or cancer detected by subsequent screening examinations
- Colposcopy with directed biopsy and endocervical curettage
- FIGO staging is described in Table 4

LABORATORY TESTS

- Complete blood count, chemistry profile
- SCC antigen in research setting
- Carcinoembryonic antigen

IMAGING STUDIES

- Chest x-ray
- Depending on stage, may need CT scan, MRI (Fig. E3), PET/CT
- Table 3, intravenous pyelogram

Rx TREATMENT

NONPHARMACOLOGIC THERAPY

- FIGO stage I_A: Cone biopsy or simple hysterectomy
- FIGO stage I_B or II_A: Type III radical hysterectomy and pelvic lymphadenectomy or pelvic radiation therapy. Minimally invasive radical hysterectomy is associated with shorter overall survival than open surgery among women with stage I_{A2} or I_{B2} cervical carcinoma (Melamed A et al, in Suggested Reading *N Engl J Med* 379:1905, 2018.)

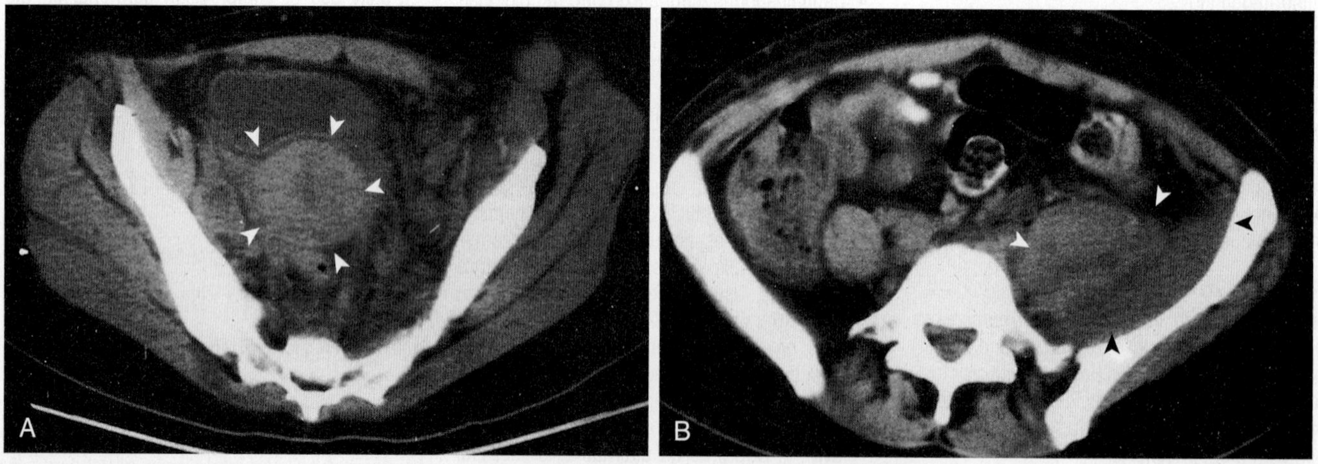

FIG. 1 Stage III_B cervical carcinoma. A 27-yr-old woman presented with increased vaginal bleeding, left leg swelling, and abdominal pain. Examination revealed a large, fixed pelvic mass. Computed tomography scan evaluation **(A)** confirms the mass *(arrowheads)* and **(B)** shows extension into the left psoas and iliacus muscles *(arrowheads)*. She also had hydronephrosis. Pathologic examination showed an adenosquamous carcinoma. (From Skarin AT: *Atlas of diagnostic oncology*, ed 4, Philadelphia, 2010, Mosby.)

TABLE 1 Descriptive Categories of Low-Grade Squamous Intraepithelial Lesion and High-Grade Squamous Intraepithelial Lesion

	Descriptors	Human Papillomavirus	p16 Immunostaining
LSIL	CIN1, flat condyloma, mild dysplasia	HR (70%)	Usually diffuse
	Exophytic condyloma	LR	Negative or patchy
	Immature condyloma (papillary immature metaplasia)	LR	Negative or patchy
	Immature flat metaplastic LSIL	HR	Usually diffuse
HSIL	CIN2 or moderate dysplasia	HR (45% type 16)	Diffuse
	CIN3 or severe dysplasia/carcinoma in situ	HR (60% type 16)	Diffuse
	Keratinizing SIL	HR	Diffuse
	HSIL with immature metaplastic phenotype	HR	Diffuse
	Papillary carcinoma in situ	HR	Diffuse
	Adenosquamous carcinoma in situ	HR	Diffuse

CIN, Cervical intraepithelial lesion; *HR,* high risk; *HSIL,* high-grade squamous intraepithelial lesion; *LR,* low risk; *LSIL,* low-grade squamous intraepithelial lesion; *SIL,* squamous intraepithelial lesion.
From Crum CP et al: *Diagnostic gynecologic and obstetric pathology,* ed 3, Philadelphia, 2018, Elsevier.

BOX 1 Benign Mimics of Cervical Adenocarcinoma

Deep nabothian cysts, florid deep glands
Tunnel clusters
Endocervical gland hyperplasias
  Lobular hyperplasia
  Diffuse laminar hyperplasia
Adenomyoma of the endocervical type
Endocervicosis, florid cystic endosalpingiosis
Müllerian papilloma
Microglandular hyperplasia
Mesonephric hyperplasia
Ectopic prostate
Deep tubal metaplasia

From Crum CP et al: *Diagnostic gynecologic and obstetric pathology*, ed 3, Philadelphia, 2018, Elsevier.

BOX 2 Categories of Squamous Carcinoma

Squamous cell carcinoma
Large cell keratinizing (well-differentiated)
Large cell nonkeratinizing (moderately differentiated)
Small cell nonkeratinizing (poorly differentiated)
Lymphoepithelial-like carcinoma
Spindle cell (sarcomatoid) carcinoma
Verrucopapillary carcinomas
Papillary (squamotransitional) carcinoma
Verrucous carcinoma (rare)[a]
Condylomatous carcinoma[a]
Basaloid carcinomas[b]

[a]In young women, an extensive (giant) condyloma must be excluded.
[b]May be associated with adenoid basal and adenoid cystic carcinomas, as well as carcinosarcomas.
From Crum CP et al: *Diagnostic gynecologic and obstetric pathology,* ed 3, Philadelphia, 2018, Elsevier.

TABLE 2 Differential Diagnosis of Squamous Intraepithelial Lesions

Category	Mimic	Distinguishing Features
LSIL	Mucosal polyp (vaginal)	Minimal acanthosis, no koilocytosis
	Reactive epithelial changes	Mild superficial karyomegaly, occasional binucleated intermediate cells
	Postmenopausal changes	Superficial cell karyomegaly, cytoplasmic halos
HSIL	Immature reactive/repair	Basal hyperchromasia, uniform nuclear spacing and nuclear contour, nucleoli
	Immature metaplasia	Uniform maturation, minimal surface hyperchromasia
	Atrophy	No mitoses, uniform chromasia, nuclear density
	Atypical atrophy	Enlarged nuclei, uncommon
	Implantation site	Uniform and wide nuclear spacing, bizarre nuclei
	Endometrial histiocytes	Small, indented nuclei, granular cytoplasm, lack of polarity

HSIL, High-grade squamous intraepithelial lesion; *LSIL,* low-grade squamous intraepithelial lesion.
From Crum CP et al: *Diagnostic gynecologic and obstetric pathology,* ed 3, Philadelphia, 2018, Elsevier.

- Advanced or bulky disease: Multimodality therapy (radiation, chemotherapy, and/or surgery); platinum use before radiation therapy

ACUTE GENERAL Rx

- Table 4 summarizes treatment according to tumor stage. Fig. 4 describes a treatment algorithm for invasive cervical cancer.
- Chemotherapy is cisplatin-based. In advanced cases, cervical cancer may present with massive and acute vaginal bleeding requiring volume and blood replacement, vaginal packing or other hemostatic modalities, and/or high-dose local radiotherapy.

CHRONIC Rx

- Physical examination with Pap smear every 3 mo for 2 yr, every 6 mo for 3 to 5 yr, annually thereafter. Table 5 summarizes a proposed schedule for interval evaluation of cervical cancer after radiotherapy or surgery in asymptomatic patients
- Chest x-ray annually (optional)
- Other imaging done only as clinically indicated
- Localized pelvic recurrence may be treated and cured with pelvic exenteration

DISPOSITION

Five-yr survival varies by stage:
- Stage I: 90% to 95%
- Stage II: 40% to 80%
- Stage III: <60%
- Stage IV: <15%

Early detection by Pap smear is imperative for long-term improvements in survival. American Cancer Society guidelines for screening by cytology for the early detection of cervical neoplasia and cancer are summarized in Table 6.

REFERRAL

Gynecologic oncologist for all invasive disease

PEARLS & CONSIDERATIONS

- HPV vaccination is indicated in males and females age 9 to 26 yr for the prevention of cervical cancer caused by HPV types 6, 11, 16, and 18. HPV vaccination is over 90% effective in preventing infection and cervical cancer. There are now HPV vaccines that are effective against nine strains of high-risk HPV. Per the Centers for Disease Control and Prevention, those who are between the ages of 27 and 45 may now choose to be vaccinated, if they have not been already, depending on their risk for new HPV infection. However, vaccination among this age range is less effective, as many have already been exposed to HPV.
- Available evidence supports discontinuation of cervical cancer screening among women aged 65 yr or older who have had adequate screening and are not otherwise at high risk.
- Updated recommendations from the American College of Physicians on screening

TABLE 3 Clinical Evaluation of Patients with Newly Diagnosed Cervical Cancer

History	Review of Systems	General Physical Examination
Risk factors (STDs, smoking, OCPs, HIV), prior abnormal Pap tests, previous dysplasia, and treatment	Abnormal vaginal bleeding or discharge, pelvic pain, flank pain, sciatica, hematuria, rectal bleeding, anorexia, weight loss, bone pain	Peripheral lymphadenopathy
Evaluation	Common procedures (FIGO)	Alternative procedures
Invasive cancer	Cervical biopsy	Histologic diagnosis required
	Endocervical curettage	
	Cervical conization	
Tumor size; involvement of the vagina, bladder, rectum, and parametria	Pelvic examination under anesthesia	MRI of pelvis preferred over CT
Anemia	Complete blood count	—
Renal failure	Serum chemistries	—
Hematuria	Urinalysis	—
Bladder involvement	Cystoscopy with biopsy and urine cytology	CT, MRI pelvis
Rectal infiltration	Proctoscopy with biopsy	CT, MRI pelvis; barium enema
Hydronephrosis	IVP	Renal ultrasonography; CT abdomen
Pulmonary metastases	Chest radiography	CT chest; PET scan
Retroperitoneal lymphadenopathy	—	lymphangiogram, CT, MRI, PET scan

CT, Computed tomography; *FIGO,* Federation of International Gynecologists and Obstetricians; *HIV,* human immunodeficiency virus; *IVP,* intravenous pyelography; *MRI,* magnetic resonance imaging; *OCP,* oral contraceptive pill; *PET,* positron emission tomography; *STD,* sexually transmitted disease.
From Disaia PJ et al: *Clinical gynecologic oncology*, ed 9, Philadelphia, 2017, Elsevier.

TABLE 4 Federation of International Obstetrics and Gynecology Staging of Cervical Cancer

Stage	Invasion	Prognosis 5-Yr Survival	Treatment
I_{A1}	Depth of invasion ≤3 mm and width ≤7 mm (includes early stromal invasion of up to 1 mm)	98%-99%	Local excision; if margins of a LLETZ/cone clear (i.e., no residual tumor or CIN) then conization is adequate, with no need for pelvic lymphadenectomy.
I_{A2}	Depth of invasion 3.1-5 mm and width ≤7 mm	95%	Simple hysterectomy and pelvic lymphadenectomy. If fertility sparing required, large cone and lymphadenectomy
I_{B1}	Tumor confined to cervix and diameter <2 cm	90%-95%	Radical hysterectomy (and lymphadenectomy)
I_{B2}	Tumor confined to cervix and diameter ≥ 2 cm to <4 cm	80%	Chemo–radiotherapy
I_{B3}	Tumor confined to cervix and diameter ≥4 cm		Chemo–radiotherapy
II_A	Upper two thirds of vagina	70%-90%	Chemotherapy & radiotherapy
II_B	Upper two thirds of vagina plus parametrial disease but not up to pelvic wall	60%-70%	Chemo–radiotherapy
III_A	Lower third of vagina	30%-50%	Chemotherapy & radiotherapy
III_B	Pelvic sidewall and/or hydronephrosis		Chemo–radiotherapy
IIIc	Involvement of pelvic and/or paraaortic lymph nodes		Chemo-radiotherapy
IV_A	Bladder, rectum	20%	Chemo–radiotherapy
IV_B	Beyond pelvis		

CIN, Cervical intraepithelial neoplasia; *LLETZ,* large loop excision of the transformation zone.
From Magowan BA: *Clinical obstetrics and gynecology*, ed 4, 2019, Elsevier.

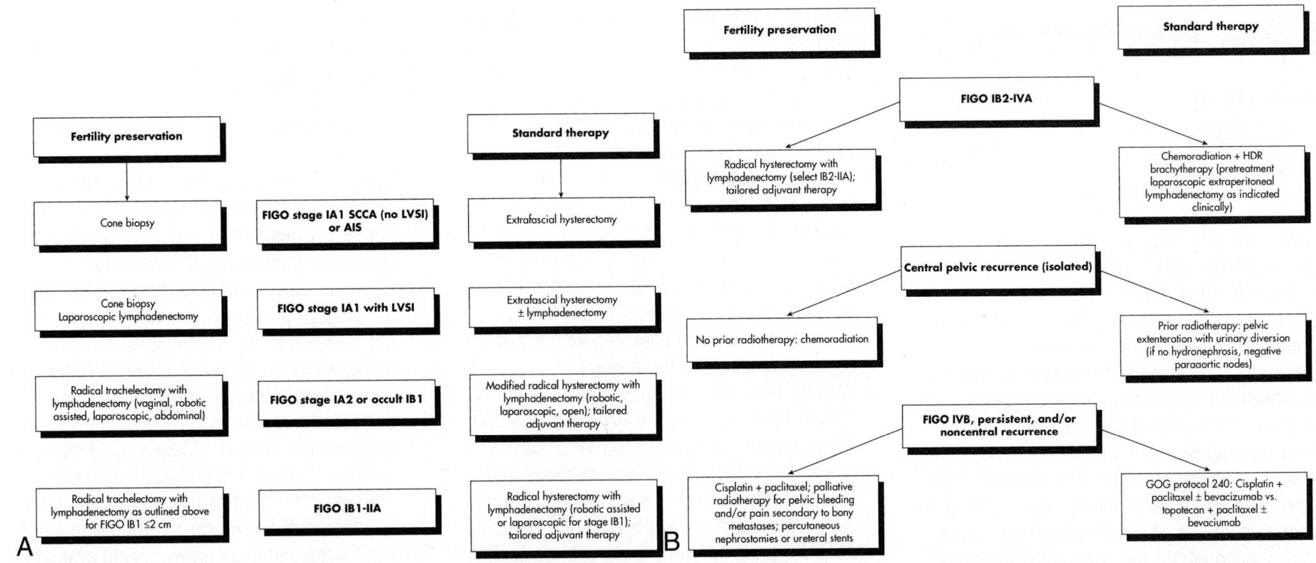

FIG. 4 A and **B,** Algorithm for therapy. *AIS,* Adenocarcinoma *in situ; FIGO,* Federation of International Gynecologists and Obstetricians; *GOG,* gynecologic oncology group; *HDR,* high-dose rate; *LVSI,* lymphovascular space invasion, *SCCA,* squamous cell carcinoma associated antigen. (From Disaia PJ et al: *Clinical gynecologic oncology*, ed 9, Philadelphia, 2017, Elsevier.)

TABLE 5 Proposed Schedule for Interval Evaluation of Cervical Cancer after Radiotherapy or Surgery (Asymptomatic Patient*)

Year	Frequency	Examination
1	3 mo	Pelvic examination, Pap smear
	6 mo	Chest radiography, CBC, BUN, creatinine
	1 yr	IVP or CT scan with contrast
2	4 mo	Pelvic examination, Pap smear
	1 yr	Chest radiography, CBC, BUN, creatinine, IVP or CT scan with contrast
3-5	6 mo	Pelvic examination, Pap smear

BUN, Blood urea nitrogen; *CBC,* complete blood count; *CT,* computed tomography; *IVP,* intravenous pyelogram; *Pap,* Papanicolaou.
*Symptomatic patients should have appropriate examination where indicated.
From Disaia PJ et al: *Clinical gynecologic oncology*, ed 9, Philadelphia, 2017, Elsevier.

TABLE 6 American Cancer Society Guidelines for Screening by Cytology for the Early Detection of Cervical Neoplasia and Cancer

- No screening is recommended regardless of sexual initiation or other risk factors before the age of 21.
- Women between the ages of 21 and 29 yr should have a Pap test every 3 yr. They should not be tested for human papillomavirus (HPV) unless such testing is needed after an abnormal Pap test result.
- Women between the ages of 30 and 65 yr should have both a Pap test and an HPV test every 5 yr. This is the preferred approach, but it is also acceptable to have a Pap test alone every 3 yr.
- Women older than 65 yr who have had regular screenings with normal results should not be screened for cervical cancer. Women who have been diagnosed with cervical precancer should continue to be screened.
- Women who have had their uterus and cervix removed in a hysterectomy and have no history of cervical cancer or precancer should not be screened.
- Women who have had the HPV vaccine should still follow the screening recommendations for their age group.
- Women who are at high risk for cervical cancer may need to be screened more often. Women who are at high risk might include those with human immunodeficiency virus (HIV) infection, organ transplantation, or exposure to the drug diethylstilbestrol (DES). They should talk with a doctor or nurse.

From Niederhuber JE: *Abeloff's clinical oncology*, ed 6, Philadelphia, 2020, Elsevier.

for cervical cancer in average-risk women are as follows.[1]

1. Women should be screened with cervical cytology every 3 yr beginning at age 21 until age 30.
2. After age 30, women can be screened with cytology and HPV testing every 5 yr.
3. Before age 21, women should not be screened unless HIV positive. If HIV positive, they should begin screening within 1 yr of coitarche.
4. Before age 30, women should not be screened with HPV testing.

- At age 65, screening can stop in women with three consecutive negative cytology results or two consecutive negative cytology results combined with a negative HPV test within the last 10 yr (with the most recent test within 5 yr).
- Women without a cervix should not be screened.

SUGGESTED READING

Available at ExpertConsult.com

RELATED CONTENT

Cervical Cancer (Patient Information)
Cervical Dysplasia (Related Key Topic)

AUTHORS: **Shanice Akoto, MD, MPH,** and **Simone Sweeney, MD**

[1]Sawaya GF et al: Cervical cancer screening in average-risk women: best practice advice from the Cervical Guidelines Committee of the American College of Physicians, *Ann Intern Med* 162(12):851-859, 2015.

BASIC INFORMATION

DEFINITION

Cervical dysplasia refers to the atypical development of intraepithelial cells of the cervix that do not cross the basement membrane and is a precursor to cervical cancer. It is caused by persistent infection with human papillomavirus (HPV), most commonly types 16 and 18. Characteristics include increased cellularity, nuclear abnormalities, and increased nuclear/cytoplasmic ratio. A progressive loss of squamous differentiation begins adjacent to the basement membrane and progresses to the most advanced stage (severe dysplasia), which encompasses the entire thickness of the squamous epithelial layer. The revised 2001 Bethesda System terminology was used in a National Institutes of Health consensus conference, sponsored by the American Society for Colposcopy and Cervical Pathology (ASCCP) and its partner professional organizations in 2006. The conference updated therapeutic options for women based on studies such as the **A**SC-US (atypical squamous cells of undetermined significance)/**L**SIL (low-grade squamous intraepithelial lesions) **T**riage **S**tudy (ALTS) that appeared after revision of the Bethesda classification. Fig. 1 provides a comparison of grading systems for cervical squamous dysplasia.

In 2012, the American Cancer Society (ACS), ASCCP, and American Society for Clinical Pathology (ASCP) published a new set of recommendations for lifetime assessment and early diagnosis of cervical dysplasia and cancer. The recommendations attempted to reduce the number of lifetime screenings, thereby reducing the possible morbidity associated with excess testing and also optimizing the co-evaluation with Pap smear and HPV testing. In 2019, the ASCCP published updated consensus guidelines for the management of cervical cancer screening abnormalities, which shifted the focus of management recommendations from test results–based algorithms to risk-based guidelines.

SCREENING PROTOCOL (2012 RECOMMENDATIONS):

- Women younger than 21 yr of age should not have cervical cancer screening unless HIV positive. If HIV positive, screening should start within 1 yr of coitarche.
- Women 21 to 29 yr of age should have testing every 3 yr with cytology only. With negative cytology or HPV-negative ASC-US, patients can repeat every 3 yr. For HPV-positive ASC-US or cytology with LG-SIL or greater, follow-up is as per the 2006 guidelines, typically with a colposcopy as the initial step with follow-up steps depending on the findings.
- Women between the ages of 30 and 65 yr should have co-testing every 5 yr with both Pap cytology and HPV testing. Alternatively, it is also acceptable to perform cytology alone; however, the testing interval should be every 3 yr. With negative cytology or HPV-negative ASC-US, patients can repeat with co-testing every 5 yr. For HPV-positive ASC-US or cytology with LG-SIL, follow-up is as per the 2006 guidelines, as previously documented. For patients with positive HPV but negative cytology, the patient can repeat testing 12 mo later with co-testing. Patients can also specifically test for HPV 16 or HPV 16/18 genotypes and, if positive, should be referred for colposcopy. Patients with positive HPV but negative 16 and/or 18 should be retested in 12 mo with co-testing.
- Women older than the age of 65 and those with a history of hysterectomy (including removal of cervix) should no longer be tested unless they had previous diagnosis of cervical intraepithelial neoplasia (CIN) 2 or greater; these women should be tested for at least 20 yr.
- Women who have been vaccinated for HPV should still use age-specific recommendations for screening.

BETHESDA 2001 UPDATED CLASSIFICATION: The Bethesda 2001 System was the result of a year-long iterative process held to update the original 1991 system and to broaden participation in the consensus process, clarify reporting of abnormalities, and incorporate data that had been collected since the initial system was created.

The reporting system includes the following areas:

- *Specimen adequacy:* The system defines the specimen as either satisfactory for evaluation or unsatisfactory, and then specifies the reason for inadequacy if necessary.
- *General categorization (optional):* This serves to triage the specimen into normal finding (negative for intraepithelial lesion or malignancy) or identifies it as an "epithelial abnormality." The descriptions are meant to be mutually exclusive.
- *Interpretation/result:* Makes a distinction between "interpretation" and "diagnosis" of the specimen so that the interpretation may be incorporated into the overall clinical context for the particular patient being evaluated.
- *Negative for* intraepithelial *lesion or malignancy:* In this screening test, no intraepithelial lesion or malignancy is identified. Nonneoplastic findings such as organisms or reactive cellular findings may be specified but are still considered to be a negative result.
- Epithelial cell abnormalities:
  1. Squamous cell:
     a. Atypical squamous cell (ASC) of undetermined significance (ASC-US) emphasizing the unusual but still possible association with underlying CIN II/III and extremely rare possibility of squamous cell carcinoma.
     b. ASC cannot exclude high-grade squamous intraepithelial lesion (ASC-H), suggesting a risk for CIN II/III that is intermediate between ASC-US and HSIL.
     c. Low-grade squamous intraepithelial lesion (LSIL) suggests a transient viral infection with a greater likelihood for regression, more likely to encompass HPV infection and CIN I histologically.

Histological features	Traditional system	WHO system	British Society for Cervical Cytology	Bethesda system
Atypical squamous cells not meeting the criteria for dysplasia	Mild atypia	Mild atypia	Borderline nuclear abnormality	Atypical squamous cells (ASC)
Koilocytes plus mild atypia	HPV infection	HPV infection	HPV plus borderline change	Low-grade squamous intraepithelial lesion (SIL)
Dysplasia limited to lower third of epithelium	Mild dysplasia	CIN 1	Mild dyskaryosis (low-grade dyskaryosis)	Low-grade SIL
Dysplasia limited to lower two-thirds of epithelium	Moderate dysplasia	CIN 2	Moderate dyskaryosis (high-grade dyskaryosis)	High-grade SIL
Dysplasia extending into upper third of epithelium	Severe dysplasia	CIN 3	Severe dyskaryosis (high-grade dyskaryosis)	High-grade SIL
Dysplasia of full thickness of epithelium	Carcinoma in situ	CIN 3	Severe dyskaryosis (high-grade dyskaryosis)	High-grade SIL

FIG. 1 Comparison of grading systems. *CIN,* Cervical intraepitheial neoplasia; *HPV,* human papilloma virus; *WHO,* World Health Organization. (From Young B et al: Female reproductive system. In *Wheater's basic pathology,* Philadelphia, 2011, Elsevier, pp. 216-315.)

d. High-grade squamous intraepithelial lesion (HSIL) suggestive of a more persistent viral infection and with a greater risk for progressive disease, more likely to encompass CIN II/III and carcinoma in situ (CIS) histologically.
e. Squamous cell carcinoma.
2. Glandular cell:
a. Atypical glandular cells (should specify endocervical, endometrial, or not otherwise specified).
b. Atypical glandular cell, favor neoplasia (should specify endocervical or not otherwise specified).
c. Endocervical adenocarcinoma in situ (AIS).
d. Adenocarcinoma.
3. Other: Because menopausal status is sometimes uncertain, age >40 yr was chosen to discriminate women who might warrant further evaluation with endometrial sampling in those with findings of endometrial cells on cytology.

UPDATED 2019 ASCCP RISK-BASED MANAGEMENT CONSENSUS GUIDELINES:

- Recommendations of colposcopy, treatment, or surveillance will be based on a patient's risk of CIN 3 or greater as determined by a combination of current results and past history.
- Repeat HPV testing or co-testing at 1 yr is recommended for patients with minor screening abnormalities indicating HPV infection with low risk of underlying CIN 3+ (e.g., HPV-positive, low-grade cytologic abnormalities after a documented negative screening HPV test or co-test).
- Expedited treatment was an option for patients with HSIL cytology in the 2012 guidelines; this guidance is now better defined in the 2019 recommendations.
  1. For nonpregnant patients 25 yr or older, expedited treatment, defined as treatment without preceding colposcopic biopsy demonstrating CIN 2+, is preferred when the immediate risk of CIN 3+ is ≥60%, and is acceptable for those with risks between 25% and 60%.
  2. Expedited treatment is preferred for nonpregnant patients 25 yr or older with high-grade squamous intraepithelial lesion (HSIL) cytology and concurrent positive testing for HPV genotype 16 (HPV 16) (i.e., HPV 16–positive HSIL cytology) and never or rarely screened patients with HPV-positive HSIL cytology regardless of HPV genotype.
  3. Shared decision-making should be used when considering expedited treatment, especially for patients with concerns about the potential impact of treatment on pregnancy outcomes.
- Excisional treatment is preferred to ablative treatment for histologic HSIL (CIN 2 or CIN 3) in the U.S. Excision is recommended for adenocarcinoma in situ (AIS).
- For CIN1, observation is preferred to treatment.
- Histopathology reports based on Lower Anogenital Squamous Terminology (LAST)/ World Health Organization (WHO) recommendations for reporting histologic HSIL should include CIN 2 or CIN 3 qualifiers, i.e., HSIL (CIN 2) and HSIL (CIN 3).
- All positive primary HPV screening tests, regardless of genotype, should have additional reflex triage testing performed from the same laboratory specimen (e.g., reflex cytology).
  1. Additional testing from the same laboratory specimen is recommended because the findings may inform colposcopy practice. For example, those HPV-16 positive HSIL cytology qualify for expedited treatment.
  2. HPV 16 or 18 infections have the highest risk for CIN 3 and occult cancer, so additional evaluation (e.g., colposcopy with biopsy) is necessary even when cytology results are negative.
  3. If HPV 16 or 18 testing is positive, and additional laboratory testing of the same sample is not feasible, the patient should proceed directly to colposcopy.
- Continued surveillance with HPV testing or co-testing at 3-yr intervals for at least 25 yr is recommended after treatment and initial post-treatment management of histologic HSIL, CIN 2, CIN 3, or AIS.
- Continued surveillance at 3-yr intervals beyond 25 yr is acceptable for as long as the patient's life expectancy and ability to be screened are not significantly compromised by serious health issues.
  1. The 2012 guidelines recommended return to 5-yr screening intervals and did not specify when screening should cease. New evidence indicates that risk remains elevated for at least 25 yr, with no evidence that treated patients ever return to risk levels compatible with 5-yr intervals.
- Surveillance with cytology alone is acceptable only if testing with HPV or cotesting is not feasible.
- Cytology is less sensitive than HPV testing for detection of precancer and is therefore recommended more often. Cytology is recommended at 6-mo intervals when HPV testing or cotesting is recommended annually. Cytology is recommended annually when 3-yr intervals are recommended for HPV or cotesting.
- Human papillomavirus assays that are Food and Drug Administration (FDA)–approved for screening should be used for management according to their regulatory approval in the U.S. (NOTE: All HPV testing in this document refers to testing for high-risk HPV types only.)
  1. For all management indications, HPV mRNA and HPV DNA tests without FDA approval for primary screening alone should only be used as a co-test with cytology, unless sufficient, rigorous data are available to support use of these particular tests in management.

KEY POINTS:

- The cytologic distinctions of low grade (LSIL) and high grade (HSIL) do not necessarily equate to the histologic classifications CIN I and CIN II/III.
- The 2006 conference noted that one cytologic abnormality can have different histologic risk in different women and highlights "special populations" such as adolescent and young women, and those women who are pregnant. In young women, spontaneous HPV clearance rates are exceptionally high. The testing recommendations essentially removed the possibility of testing women younger than 21 yr of age.
- DNA testing for high-risk HPV types is incorporated into the evaluation and treatment algorithms for women with cytologic cervical abnormalities.

ICD-10CM CODES

N87.9	Dysplasia of cervix uteri, unspecified
R87.610	Atypical squamous cells of undetermined significance on cytologic smear of cervix (ASC-US)
R87.611	Atypical squamous cells cannot exclude high grade squamous intraepithelial lesion on cytologic smear of cervix (ASC-H)
R87.612	Low grade squamous intraepithelial lesion on cytologic smear of cervix (LGSIL)
R87.613	High grade squamous intraepithelial lesion on cytologic smear of cervix (HGSIL)
R87.614	Cytologic evidence of malignancy on smear of cervix
R87.615	Unsatisfactory cytologic smear of cervix
R87.618	Other abnormal cytological findings on specimens from cervix uteri
R87.619	Unspecified abnormal cytological findings in specimens from cervix uteri
Z12.4	Encounter for screening for malignant neoplasm of cervix

EPIDEMIOLOGY & DEMOGRAPHICS

PREDOMINANT AGE:

- Dysplasia: Peak age, 26 yr (3600 cases/100,000 persons)
- CIS: Peak age, 32 yr (1100 cases/100,000 persons)
- Invasive cancer: Peak age <60 yr (800 cases/100,000 persons)

PEAK INCIDENCE:

- Age 35
- Abnormal Pap smear rate revealing dysplasia approximates 2% to 5% depending on population risk factors and false-negative rate variance
- False-negative rate approaching 40%
- Average age-adjusted incidence of severe dysplasia is 35 cases/100,000 persons
- Approximately half of the cases of new cervical cancer had never been screened, and another 10% had not been screened in more than 5 yr. Given that many of these women come from underserved or underresourced communities, reduction of the morbidity and mortality from cervical cancer would necessitate addressing these health disparities.

PHYSICAL FINDINGS & CLINICAL PRESENTATION

- Cervical lesions associated with dysplasia often are not visible to the naked eye;

therefore, physical findings are best viewed by colposcopy of a 3% acetic acid-prepared or Lugol solution–prepared cervix
- Patients evaluated by colposcopy are identified by abnormal cervical cytology screening from Pap smear screening
- Colposcopic findings:
  1. Leukoplakia (white lesion seen by the unaided eye that may represent condyloma, dysplasia, or cancer)
  2. Acetowhite epithelium with or without associated punctation, mosaicism, abnormal vessels
  3. Abnormal transformation zone (abnormal iodine uptake, "cuffed" gland openings)
- Studies have looked at the benefit of taking random biopsies at time of colposcopy and have shown that there may be increased detection of CIN II or greater if biopsies are taken at random rather than only directed toward abnormal appearing lesions

ETIOLOGY

- Strongly associated and initiated by oncogenic HPV infection (high-risk HPV types are 16, 18, 31, 33, 35, 45, 51, 52, 56, and 58; low-risk HPV types are 6, 11, 42, 43, and 44)
- Risk factors:
  1. HPV
  2. Any heterosexual coitus
  3. Coitus during puberty (transformation-zone metaplasia peak)
  4. Diethylstilbestrol exposure
  5. Multiple sexual partners
  6. Lack of prior Pap smear screening
  7. History of STD
  8. Other genital tract neoplasia
  9. HIV
  10. Tuberculosis
  11. Substance abuse
  12. "High-risk" male partner (HPV)
  13. Low socioeconomic status
  14. Early first pregnancy
  15. Tobacco use

Dx DIAGNOSIS

DIFFERENTIAL DIAGNOSIS

- Metaplasia
- Hyperkeratosis
- Condyloma
- Microinvasive carcinoma
- Glandular epithelial abnormalities
- Vulvar intraepithelial neoplasm
- Vaginal intraepithelial neoplasm
- Metastatic tumor involvement of the cervix

WORKUP

- Periodic history and physical examination (including cytologic screening) depending on age, risk factors, and history of preinvasive cervical lesions
- Consider screening for sexually transmitted disease (gonorrhea, *Chlamydia,* herpes, HIV, HPV)
- Abnormal cytology (HSIL/LSIL, initial ASC/ASC-US/ASC-H in high-risk patients, recurrent in low-risk/postmenopausal patients) and grossly evident suspicious lesions should be referred for colposcopy and possible directed biopsy/endocervical curettage (ECC). Examination should include cervix, vagina, vulva, and anus.
- For glandular cell abnormalities (AGCs): Refer for colposcopy and possible directed biopsy/ECC, and consider endometrial sampling
- In pregnancy: Abnormal cytology followed by colposcopy in the first trimester and at 28 to 32 wk; only high-grade lesions suspicious for carcinoma biopsied; ECC is contraindicated

LABORATORY TESTS

- Gonorrhea, chlamydia nucleic-acid amplification tests to rule out STD
- Pap cytology screening (requires appropriate sampling, preparation, cytologist interpretation, and reporting)
- HPV DNA typing
- Colposcopy, directed cervical biopsy, and ECC (for indications see "Workup")
- As compared with Pap testing, HPV testing has greater sensitivity for the detection of intraepithelial neoplasia

IMAGING STUDIES

- Cervicography
- Computer-enhanced Pap cytology screening (e.g., PAPNET)

MANAGEMENT

Refer to the literature for a more comprehensive approach. The following treatment paradigms in Table 1 give a general outline for care.

TABLE 1 Summary of Recommendations

Population	Recommended Screening Method	Management of Screen Results	Comments
<21 yr	No screening		
21-29 yr	Cytology alone every 3 yr	HPV-positive ASC-US or cytology of LSIL or more severe: Refer to ASCCP Guidelines Cytology Negative or HPV-Negative ASC-US; Rescreen with cytology in 3 yr	
30-65 yr	HPV and cytology "co-testing" every 5 yr (preferred)	HPV-positive ASC-US or cytology of LSIL or more severe: Refer to ASCCP guidelines HPV positive, cytology negative: Option 1: Y 12-mo follow-up with co-testing Option 2: Y test for HPV16 or HPV16/18 genotypes. If HPV16 or HPV16/18 positive, refer to colposcopy. If HPV16 or HPV16/18 negative, 12-mo follow-up with co-testing Co-test negative or HPV-negative ASC-US: Rescreen with co-testing in 5 yr	Screening by HPV testing alone is not recommended for most clinical settings.
	Cytology alone every 3 yr (acceptable)	HPV-positive ASC-US or cytology of LSIL or more severe: Refer to ASCCP guidelines Cytology negative or HPV-negative ASC-US: Rescreen with cytology in 3 yr	
>65 yr	No screening following adequate negative prior screening		Women with a history of CIN2 or a more severe diagnosis should continue routine screening for at least 20 yr
After hysterectomy	No screening		Applies to women without a cervix and without a history of CIN2 or a more severe diagnosis in the past 20 yr or cervical cancer ever.
HPV vaccinated	Follow age-specific recommendations (same as unvaccinated women)		

ASCCP, American Society for Colposcopy and Cervical Pathology; *ASC-US,* atypical squamous cells of undetermined significance; *CIN,* cervical intraepithelial neoplasia; *HPV,* human papillomavirus; *LSIL,* low-grade squamous intraepithelial lesions.

Modified from Saslow D et al: American Cancer Society, American Society for Colposcopy and Cervical Pathology, and American Society for Clinical Pathology screening guidelines for the prevention and early detection of cervical cancer, *J Low Gen Tract Dis* 16(3):175-204, 2012.

DISPOSITION

- Because of the large number of women in high-risk groups, the prevalence of HPV, and the high false-negative Pap smear rate, routine Pap smear screening should be strongly encouraged for all women, especially those with a history of cervical dysplasia. Primary HPV testing with reflex cytology and using risk-based guidelines reduces the incidence of CIN II or III, or cancer detected by subsequent screening.
- Success rates for treatment approach 80% to 90%.
- Detection of persistence or recurrence requires careful follow-up.
- Cervical treatment can increase risk for poor obstetric outcomes (cervical incompetence with subsequent miscarriage or preterm birth), which requires careful consideration and discretion for use of loop electrosurgical excision procedure and cone biopsy in women desiring future childbearing.
- Appropriate counseling and informed consent are needed when considering any form of management of cervical dysplasia.

REFERRAL

- Patients with abnormal Pap cytology should be referred to a provider, preferably a trained obstetrician/gynecologist, who can appropriately treat the patient in an age-specific manner and also perform a colposcopy or excisional procedure if indicated as part of the new recommendations. Given the morbidity associated with both under evaluation and treatment, as well as reacting excessively to cytologic findings, a provider who is intimately familiar with ASCCP guidelines should be sought.
- If treatment is required, patient should be referred to a gynecologist or gynecologic oncologist skilled in the diagnosis and treatment of preinvasive cervical disease.

PEARLS & CONSIDERATIONS

COMMENTS

- Testing for human papillomavirus by Hybrid capture 2 DNA test will identify 91% of the small proportion of women with post-treatment residual or recurrent disease, but 30% of all women who are tested will test positive and need colposcopy.
- HPV vaccination is recommended for males and females from ages 9 to 26. As of June 2019, ACIP recommends HPV vaccination based on shared clinical decision-making for individuals ages 27 through 45 yr who are not adequately vaccinated.

RELATED CONTENT

Cervical Cancer (Related Key Topic)
Cervical Dysplasia (Patient Information)
Cervical Polyps (Related Key Topic)
Pap Smear Abnormalities (Patient Information)

SUGGESTED READINGS

Available at ExpertConsult.com

AUTHORS: **Ashlie Sewdass Carter, MD,** and **Kelly McNamara, MD**

BASIC INFORMATION

DEFINITION

Cervicitis is an inflammation of the uterine cervix, primarily affecting the columnar epithelial cells of the endocervical glands. Acute cervicitis results from direct infection of the cervix secondary to a uterine or vaginal infection—most commonly chlamydia or gonorrhea—whereas chronic cervicitis is due to an exposure to a local irritant.

SYNONYMS

Endocervicitis
Ectocervicitis
Mucopurulent cervicitis

ICD-10CM CODES	
N72	Inflammatory disease of cervix uteri
A54.03	Gonococcal cervicitis, unspecified
A74.89	Other chlamydial diseases
A60.03	Herpesviral cervicitis
O86.11	Cervicitis following delivery

EPIDEMIOLOGY & DEMOGRAPHICS

The published prevalence of cervicitis varies greatly, ranging from 8% to as high as 40% of women attending sexually transmitted disease (STD) clinics. Cervicitis is most common in women aged 15 to 24 but it can occur in any sexually active woman. Women who have had sex without condoms or sex with multiple partners are at increased risk of developing cervicitis as well as other STDs.

PHYSICAL FINDINGS & CLINICAL PRESENTATION

- Cervicitis is usually asymptomatic or associated with mild symptoms. Patients may complain of copious purulent or mucopurulent vaginal discharge, pelvic pain, postcoital or intermenstrual bleeding, vulvovaginal irritation, or dyspareunia.
- The CDC emphasizes that the two diagnostic signs of cervicitis are either mucopurulent discharge or sustained cervical bleeding with gentle trauma. On physical exam, the cervix can be erythematous and tender on palpation. The cervix may also bleed easily when obtaining cultures or a Pap smear. Yellow discharge will be seen on a Q-tip inserted into the cervix.

INFECTIOUS ETIOLOGY

- *Chlamydia trachomatis*
- *Neisseria gonorrhoeae*
- *Trichomonas vaginalis*
- Herpes simplex
- Human papillomavirus
- *M. genitalium*
- Bacterial vaginosis

DIAGNOSIS

The diagnosis of acute cervicitis is clinical and based upon the presence of purulent or mucopurulent cervical exudate (Fig. E1) and/or cervical friability—bleeding induced by gently touching the area with a swab.

DIFFERENTIAL DIAGNOSIS

- Carcinoma of the cervix
- Cervical erosion (from tampons or other intravaginal devices)
- Cervical metaplasia
- Cervical ectropion
- Cervical and vaginal irritation due to chemicals or hormonal imbalance

WORKUP

If cervicitis is suspected, testing for infectious causes should be performed and pelvic inflammatory disease (PID) should be excluded.

LABORATORY TESTS

- A finding of leucorrhea (>10 WBC per high-power field on microscopic examination of vaginal fluid) has been associated with chlamydial and gonococcal infection of the cervix.
- Nucleic acid amplification tests (NAAT) should be used for diagnosing *C. trachomatis* and *N. gonorrhoeae* in women with cervicitis; this testing can be performed on vaginal, cervical, or urinary samples.
- Use a wet mount to look for evidence of bacterial vaginitis (BV) and trichomonads, but because the sensitivity of microscopy to detect *T. vaginalis* is relatively low (~50%), symptomatic women with cervicitis and negative microscopy for BV and trichomonads should receive further testing with NAAT or culture if there is concern for resistant infection.
- HIV testing is recommended in all patients with supposed cervicitis.
- Although HSV-2 infection has been associated with cervicitis, the utility of specific testing (i.e., culture or serologic testing) for HSV-2 in this setting is not recommended unless there are clinical findings suggestive of herpes infection.

Rx TREATMENT

NONPHARMACOLOGIC THERAPY

- The patient's history of hygiene habits, which may increase her risk for cervicitis, should be obtained including history of douching, tampon usage, and other potential chemical exposures to vaginal irritants.
- Uncomplicated cervicitis is typically treated as an outpatient.
- Safe sex should be recommended including monogamous relationships and the consistent use of condoms (male and female).
- Sexual partners should be offered treatment in all cases of STD infection proven by culture.

ACUTE GENERAL Rx

- Because *Chlamydia* and *N. gonorrhoeae* cause 50% of cases of infectious cervicitis, if either of these infections is suspected, then treatment should be initiated without waiting for the test results. Administer Ceftriaxone 500 mg IM as a single dose for persons weighing <150 kg (300 lb) or 1 g of IM ceftriaxone for persons weighing ≥150 kg (300 lb) followed by azithromycin 1 g single dose or doxycycline 100 mg PO bid for 7 days. If the patient is pregnant, treat with azithromycin 1 g single dose instead of using doxycycline, which is contraindicated in pregnant or nursing mothers. If *Trichomonas* is the etiologic agent, treat with metronidazole or tinidazole 2 g single dose, which is curative in 95% of cases. An alternative treatment option is metronidazole 500 mg twice daily for 7 days. Alcohol should be avoided during the treatment course.
- For herpes infection, treat with acyclovir, valacyclovir, or famciclovir.
- *M. genitalium* might be considered for cases of clinically significant cervicitis that persist after azithromycin or doxycycline therapy in which reexposure to an infected partner or medical nonadherence is unlikely. If *M. genitalium* infection is confirmed, treatment is with moxifloxacin.

DISPOSITION

Bacterial cervicitis responds well to antibiotics. Possible complications to watch for include subsequent PID and infertility (found in 5% to 10% of patients with increasing rates with repeat episodes of PID). Repeat cervical cultures are recommended after treatment in pregnancy or if there is concern of treatment failure. Screening for reinfection is recommended within 3 mo. Condoms should be recommended and sexual relations should be resumed after negative cultures for both partners.

REFERRAL

If subsequent PID develops, attempt outpatient therapy and consider hospital admission for IV antibiotics for severe or specialty cases as outlined in the CDC guidelines.

PEARLS & CONSIDERATIONS

COMMENTS

- Management of sex partners of women tested for cervicitis should be appropriate for the identified or suspected STD.
- Repeat testing 3 to 6 mo after treatment is recommended for all women diagnosed with chlamydia or gonorrhea, and all sex partners in the preceding 60 days should be evaluated and treated for the STDs for which the index patient received treatment.

SUGGESTED READING

Available at ExpertConsult.com

RELATED CONTENT

Cervicitis (Patient Information)
Chlamydia Genital Infections (Related Key Topic)
Gonorrhea (Related Key Topic)
Urethritis, Nongonococcal (Related Key Topic)

AUTHORS: **Helen B. Gomez, MD,** and **Anthony C. Sciscione, DO**

BASIC INFORMATION

DEFINITION

Chemotherapy-induced nausea and vomiting (CINV) refers to adverse emetic effects associated with the use of systemic therapies used in the treatment of cancer. There are five recognized subtypes:

- Acute-phase CINV: Nausea and vomiting starting within 24 hr after receiving chemotherapy.
- Delayed-phase CINV: Nausea and vomiting beginning or returning > 24 hr after receiving chemotherapy.
- Breakthrough CINV: Nausea and vomiting occurring despite appropriate prophylactic treatment.
- Anticipatory CINV: Nausea and vomiting beginning prior to receiving therapy as a conditioned response in patients who have developed significant emesis during previous chemotherapy administration.
- Refractory CINV: Recurring in subsequent cycles of therapy, excluding anticipatory CINV.

SYNONYMS

Drug-induced nausea and vomiting
Chemotherapy-induced emesis
CINV

ICD-10CM CODES

R11.2	Nausea with vomiting, unspecified
R11.0	Nausea
R11.10	Vomiting, unspecified
Z51.11	Encounter for antineoplastic chemotherapy

EPIDEMIOLOGY & DEMOGRAPHICS

- The patient's risk for development of nausea and vomiting is most strongly dependent on the emetogenicity of the chemotherapy agent(s) being used (Table 1).
- Emetogenicity is classified into four categories: highly emetic (>90%), moderately emetic (>30% to 90%), low emetic (10% to 30%), and minimally emetic (0% to 10%).
- With certain chemotherapy regimens, CINV will occur in the majority of patients. However, patients' tolerance may vary, and symptoms may occur in as low as 10% of patients.
- Symptoms may be dose dependent (the higher the dose, the greater the risk for symptoms).
- CINV is more likely to affect female and younger patients.
- Patients expecting CINV before receiving therapy (anticipatory emesis) are at greater risk of experiencing symptoms.

INCIDENCE: The highest incidence of CINV is before or during the first cycle of chemotherapy.

RISK FACTORS:

- Previous history of CINV
- History of motion sickness or vestibular dysfunction
- Higher levels of anxiety
- History of alcohol use decreases risk

GENETICS: It has been demonstrated that three SNPs in 5-hydroxytryptamine receptor (5- HT3R) genes, two alleles of the cytochrome P450 family 2 subfamily D member 6 (CYP2D6) gene, and three SNPs in ATP binding cassette subfamily B member 1 (ABCB1) gene are associated with the occurrence and severity of CINV.

PHYSICAL FINDINGS & CLINICAL PRESENTATION

- Symptoms may include anxiety and lightheadedness.
- The most common physical findings are increased pulse rate and abnormal blood pressure (elevated if the person is highly anxious, reduced if the patient is dehydrated).
- Symptoms such as diarrhea, fever, headache, and abdominal pain may suggest an alternative diagnosis; physical examination findings such as increased blood pressure, abdominal tenderness, or focal neurologic deficits may suggest symptoms caused by cancer progression or other acute illness such as infection.

TABLE 1 Emetogenic Potential of Commonly Used Oral Antineoplastic Agents

Risk	Frequency of Emesis (%; Without Prophylaxis)	Agent
High	>90	Altretamine
		Procarbazine
Moderate	30-90	Cyclophosphamide
		Crizotinib
		Olaparib
		Temozolomide
Low	10-30	Alectinib
		Axitinib
		Capecitabine
		Ceritinib
		Cobimetinib
		Dasatinib
		Everolimus
		Gefitinib
		Ibrutinib
		Imatinib
		Ixazomib
		Lapatinib
		Lenalidomide
		Nilotinib
		Palbociclib
		Panobinostat
		Pazopanib
		Sorafenib
		Sunitinib
		Thalidomide
		Vemurafenib
Minimal	<10	Alectinib
		Busulfan
		Chlorambucil
		Dabrafenib
		Erlotinib
		Hydroxyurea
		Idelalisib
		Melphalan
		Methotrexate
		Osimertinib
		Ruxolitinib
		6-Thioguanine
		Trametinib
		Vismodegib

Modified from Roila F et al: Guideline update for MASCC and ESMO in the prevention of chemotherapy and radiotherapy-induced nausea and vomiting: results of the Perugia consensus conference, *Ann Oncol* 2010;21(suppl 5):v232-243.

PATHOPHYSIOLOGY

The pathophysiology of nausea and vomiting is illustrated in Fig. E1. CINV is likely the result of chemotherapy acting in two places: Directly in the gastrointestinal tract and in the vomiting center of the brain. In both areas, nausea and vomiting are mediated by the actions of certain neurotransmitters, with serotonin, dopamine, and neurokinin-1 being the most important.

Dx DIAGNOSIS

DIFFERENTIAL DIAGNOSIS

- The two main considerations are progression of cancer and infection
- Intestinal/gastric: Obstruction or partial obstruction of the digestive tract from tumor
- Neurologic: Metastases to the brain causing vomiting; metastatic infiltration of nerves affecting the digestive tract
- Infectious: Acute bacterial, viral, or parasitic infections of the digestive tract causing symptoms (can be associated with diarrhea or pain)
- Renal: Dehydration leading to acute kidney injury and failure, causing worsening of nausea and vomiting

WORKUP

Additional workup is not indicated if patient's symptoms and onset of nausea and vomiting fit the usual presentation for CINV. If other symptoms or unexpected physical examination findings are present, then other likely causes need to be ruled out with a combination of blood work and imaging.

LABORATORY TESTS

- If the onset of symptoms is not typical for CINV, then blood tests such as CBC, liver function tests, electrolytes, and kidney function tests and CNS imaging may be indicated to assess for secondary causes of nausea and/or emesis.
- Stool studies looking for infections from viruses, bacteria, or parasites may be ordered if diarrhea is also present.

IMAGING STUDIES

- Abdominal radiographs may reveal ileus or obstruction of the digestive tract.
- Abdomen and pelvic CT scans may provide more detailed information about local cancer progression/invasion in relation to the digestive tract and whether ileus or obstruction is present.
- CNS imaging with CT or MRI scanning of the brain may provide information about possible brain or leptomeningeal metastases.

BOX 1 Management Approach: Chemotherapy-Induced Nausea and Vomiting (CINV)

Antiemetic therapy for CINV should be based on the emetic potential of the chemotherapy regimen being used and should take into account individual patient factors (e.g., sex, age, history of alcohol use, and previous emesis with chemotherapy). Excellent methods for predicting the likelihood of emesis with single chemotherapeutic agents or combination regimens have been developed.

All patients receiving chemotherapy with moderate or high emetogenic potential should receive antiemetic prophylaxis for acute (day 1) and delayed (days 2-5) nausea and vomiting. Patients receiving highly emetogenic regimens should receive prophylaxis on day 1 with a 5-HT_3 receptor antagonist (preferably palonosetron) plus neurokinin-1 (NK1) receptor antagonist plus dexamethasone, followed on days 2-4 by dexamethasone. Olanzapine should be added in patients judged to be at high risk. For moderately emetogenic regimens, treatment with a 5-HT_3 receptor antagonist (preferably palonosetron) plus dexamethasone on day 1, followed by dexamethasone on days 2 and 3, is recommended.

Patients receiving therapy with low emetic potential should receive dexamethasone (8 mg intravenously or orally); a 5-HT_3 receptor antagonist should be added with subsequent courses only if antiemetic control is inadequate. Routine prophylaxis is not necessary for patients receiving agents or regimens of minimal risk. Patients with inadequate control should have intensification of their antiemetic prophylaxis during subsequent treatment cycles.

5-HT_3, 5-Hydroxytryptamine 3 (serotonin).
From Niederhuber JE: *Abeloff's clinical oncology*, ed 6, Philadelphia, 2020, Elsevier.

TABLE 2 Antiemetic Agents: Recommended Dosing

	Recommended Dose	
Antiemetic Agent	**Acute Emesis (Before Chemotherapy)**	**Delayed Emesis**
5-HT_3 antagonists		
Ondansetron	0.15 mg/kg or 8 mg IV; 12-16 mg PO	8 mg PO twice a day × 2-3 days
Granisetron	1 mg IV or PO; 10 mg subcutaneous (extended release)	
Dolasetron	1.8 mg/kg or 100 mg IV; 100-200 mg PO	
Palonosetron	0.25 mg IV or 0.5 mg PO	
NK1 receptor antagonists		
Aprepitant	125 mg PO	80 mg PO days 2 and 3
Fosaprepitant	150 mg IV	
Rolapitant	180 mg PO	
Combination 5-HT_3/NK1 receptor antagonist		
NEPA (palonosetron 0.5 mg/netupitant 300 mg)	1 tablet PO	
Multireceptor antagonist		
Olanzapine	10 mg PO	10 mg PO days 2-4
Corticosteroids		
Dexamethasone		
With NK1 antagonist	12 mg IV or PO	8 mg PO for 2-3 days
Without NK1 antagonist	8 mg (moderate risk) or 20 mg (high risk) IV or PO	4-8 mg PO twice a day for 2-3 days
Other agents		
Prochlorperazine		10 mg PO or IV every 3-4 hours as needed
Lorazepam	1-2 mg IV (for anticipatory nausea/vomiting)	
Dronabinol		5 mg/m² PO every 3-4h as needed

5-HT_3, 5-Hydroxytryptamine 3; *NK1*, neurokinin 1; *IV*, intravenous; *PO*, by mouth.
From Niederhuber JE: *Abeloff's clinical oncology*, ed 6, Philadelphia, 2020, Elsevier.

Rx TREATMENT

- A management approach to CINV is summarized in Box 1.
- Choice and duration of antiemetic use are dependent on the emesis-potential of the chemotherapy regimen being used. Commonly used antiemetic agents and recommended dosing are described in Table 2. For chemotherapy agents with high emetogenic potential, the use of multidrug antiemetic regimens has proven to be highly effective as prophylaxis.
- The most common treatment combination includes a serotonin-receptor (5-HT3) antagonist (ondansetron, granisetron, dolasetron, or palonosetron), a corticosteroid (dexamethasone), and a neurokinin-1 (NK-1) receptor antagonist (aprepitant, rolapitant, or fosaprepitant).
- A fixed-dose combination of oral palonosetron and netupitant is now available. Table 3 summarizes recommended antiemetic prophylaxis for patients receiving intravenous chemotherapy.

TABLE 3 Summary of Recommended Antiemetic Prophylaxis for Patients Receiving Intravenous Chemotherapy

Risk of Emesis	Day 1 (Prechemotherapy)	After Day 1
High (includes cyclophosphamide and doxorubicin)	$5\text{-}HT_3$ receptor antagonist (palonosetron preferred) + NK1 receptor antagonist + dexamethasone + olanzapine (if patient considered high risk)	Dexamethasone days 2-4 + aprepitant days 2-3 (if used on day 1) + olanzapine days 2-4 (high-risk patients)
Moderate	$5\text{-}HT_3$ receptor antagonist (palonosetron preferred) + dexamethasone	Dexamethasone days 2 and 3
Low	Dexamethasone	None
Minimal	As needed	None

$5\text{-}HT_3$, 5-Hydroxytryptamine 3; *NK1*, neurokinin 1.
From Niederhuber JE: *Abeloff's clinical oncology*, ed 6, Philadelphia, 2020, Elsevier.

- The commonly used antipsychotic drug olanzapine has been demonstrated across multiple clinical trials to be effective and safe at reducing emesis during the delayed and overall phases of CINV prevention.
- Many other adjunct drugs are available, such as prochlorperazine, metoclopramide, haloperidol, and marinol; comparatively, they are less effective and have greater potential for adverse effects.
- Benzodiazepines (usually lorazepam) may help in patients with significant anxiety levels that lead to anticipatory CINV.
- Patients with uncontrolled symptoms may require hospitalization for supportive care including intravenous medications and fluids.

NONPHARMACOLOGIC THERAPY

Patients who have a significant anxiety component to their CINV may benefit from cognitive behavioral therapy.

DISPOSITION

Although CINV is one of the most feared complications of cancer therapy, its treatment has been revolutionized in the last 20 yr, with a significant majority of patients achieving adequate symptom control.

PEARLS & CONSIDERATIONS

COMMENTS

- Aggressive symptom control in the acute phase of CINV is the key initial therapeutic approach. Prevention of the acute phase has led to much improved control of delayed CINV and also decreased the incidence of anticipatory CINV.
- Prevention of symptoms is much easier to achieve than controlling or treating active symptoms.

SUGGESTED READINGS

Available at ExpertConsult.com

AUTHOR: **Ritesh Rathore, MD**

BASIC INFORMATION

DEFINITION

Chikungunya (CHIK) is a disabling and debilitating mosquito-borne disease transmitted by infected *Aedes* spp mosquitos to humans caused by the Chikungunya virus (CHIKV). It is listed as a WHO Blueprint priority pathogen due to the dramatic increase in spread in recent years to more than 100 countries affecting millions of people.

SYNONYMS

Chikungunya Fever
Chikungunya virus disease
CHIK
CHIKV

ICD 10-CM CODE

A92.0 Chikungunya virus disease

EPIDEMIOLOGY & DEMOGRAPHICS

INCIDENCE:

- This disease was first described in West Africa in the 1950s and spread to Thailand and India in the 1960s. The first major epidemic was in 2004 in Kenya and in 2005 on Reunion Island in the Indian Ocean, which had an outbreak of 250,000 cases. In 2007, an outbreak occurred in Italy with autochthonous cases and in France in 2010, 2014, and 2017. In 2013, autochthonous cases started in the Caribbean and the Americas.
- The first cases in the U.S. were reported in Florida in 2014. Most cases in the U.S. (4000 between 2014 and 2016) were from returning travelers.

PREVALENCE: Chikungunya virus is found in tropical and subtropical regions (Fig. 1) and is endemic to parts of West Africa. Human serosurveys can show up to 35% to 50% of the population have antibodies in some areas.

PREDOMINANT SEX & AGE: Affects male and females of all age groups.

PEAK INCIDENCE: Most outbreaks occur during the tropical rainy season with increased amounts of the mosquito vector. The virus is maintained in a complex sylvatic and rural cycle, progressing to an urban cycle every 5 to 20 yr, which leads to outbreaks.

RISK FACTORS: Transmission can occur via three mechanisms:

- Mosquito bites
- Rarely via maternal-fetal transmission
- Rarely via blood products and solid organ transplants and cornea transplants

GENETICS: Maternal-fetal transmission can occur intrapartum, which results in high rates of infant mortality.

PHYSICAL FINDINGS & CLINICAL PRESENTATION

- Incubation period can vary between 1 and 12 days with an average of 2 to 7 days. CHIK infection is symptomatic in 85% of children and adults. Three phases include acute stage, post-acute stage, and chronic stage.
- Acute Phase: Correlates with the viremia and lasts about 7 days. Common signs and symptoms include:
  1. Fever: Sudden onset and often over 39° C (lasts about 48 hrs)
  2. Macular to maculopapular rash (Fig. E2): 2 to 5 days after the fever
     a. Edema of the face and extremities
     b. Benign bleeding in children (gingival and epistaxis)
  3. Pruritus
  4. Myalgia
  5. Arthralgia
  6. Periorbital pain
  7. Headache
  8. Lymphadenopathy

  Less common: Diarrhea, vomiting, abdominal pain, confusion, optic neuritis, conjunctivitis, oral or gingival ulcers
  1. Disabling polyarthralgia is a key symptom for diagnosis. Joint pain involves many joints (often 10 or more joint groups) and is usually symmetric in both arms and legs involving large joints with morning stiffness. Rash affects extremities, palms and soles of the feet, face, and torso.
- Post-acute Phase: From the fourth wk to end of 3 mo
  1. Inflammatory arthralgia, joint stiffness
  2. Arthritis (synovitis with or without effusion)
  3. Tenosynovitis, bursitis
  4. Decompensation of pre-existing degenerative or traumatic arthropathy
  5. Other: Osteoarthritis, entrapment syndromes, neuropathic pain, severe asthenia
- Chronic Stage: 25% to 75% of patients will enter a chronic stage after the third mo that can last several years. It is more likely in patients over 45 yr old and/or with pre-existing arthritis.
  1. Joints: Articular arthritis, synovitis, degenerative osteoarthritis, bursitis
  2. Tendons: Tendinitis, enthesitis, tenosynovitis
  3. Other: Edema, neuropathic pain, stiffness, loss of physical fitness
- Atypical features of infection and complications include encephalopathy and meningitis, optic neuritis, myelopathy and myelitis, heart failure, myocarditis/pericarditis, arrhythmias, hepatic insufficiency, SIADH, and pancreatitis.

ETIOLOGY

- Chikungunya is an alphavirus of the family *Togaviridiae* and consists of a solitary

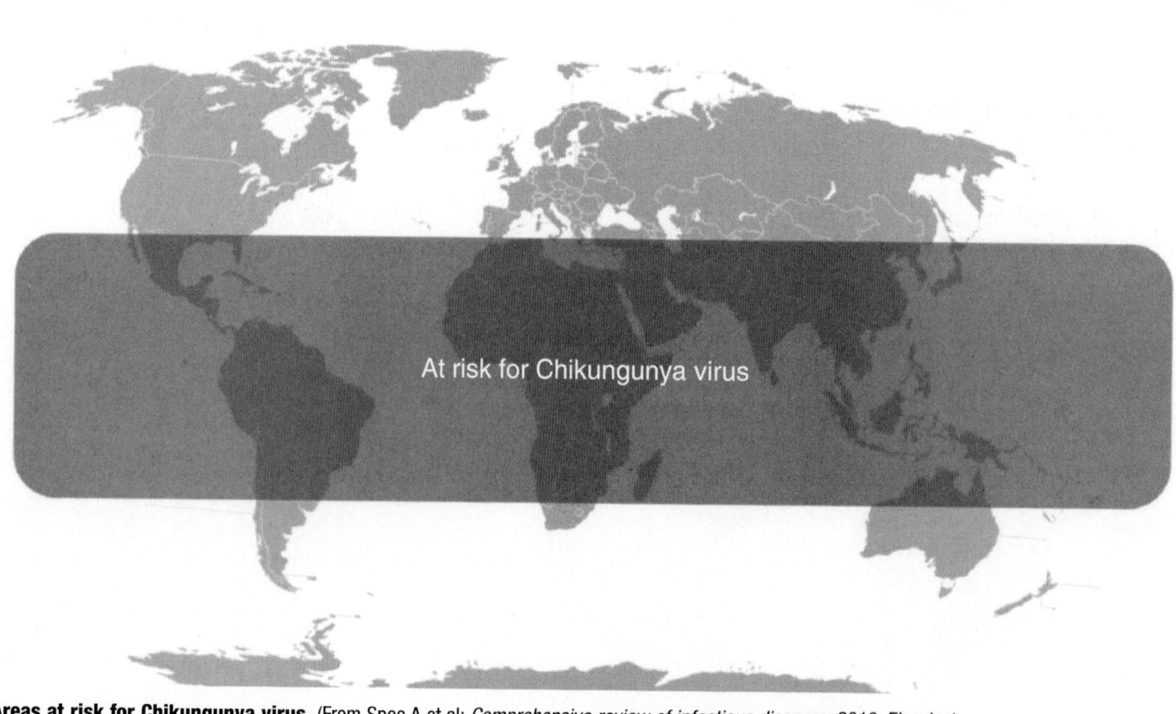

FIG. 1 Areas at risk for Chikungunya virus. (From Spec A et al: *Comprehensive review of infectious diseases,* 2019, Elsevier.)

TABLE 1 Differences Between Dengue, Chikungunya, Yellow Fever, and Leptospirosis

	Dengue	Chikungunya	Yellow Fever	Leptospirosis
Key features	Febrile illness, mosquito exposure Thrombocytopenia Shock	Febrile illness, mosquito exposure Joint pains Milder disease than dengue	Febrile illness, mosquito exposure Transaminitis, jaundice, no vaccine prior to travel	Febrile illness, water exposure Hyperbilirubinemia out of proportion to transaminitis Conjunctival suffusion

From Ryan ET et al: *Hunter's tropical medicine and emerging infectious diseases*, ed 10, 2019, Elsevier.

positive strand of RNA made up of 12,000 nucleotides. There are three major circulating genotypes of CHIKV: East Central South Africa, West Africa, and Asian.

- Mosquito Vector: Major mosquito vectors are *Aedes aegypti*, which is widely distributed in the tropics and subtropics and prefers the human host, and *Aedes albopictus*, which can survive in more temperate climates and has a wider potential distribution, but it bites a range of animal species and thus has a less efficient vector. Both mosquitos prefer to feed on humans more during daylight hours and early evening.

Dx DIAGNOSIS

DIFFERENTIAL DIAGNOSIS

- Dengue Fever (Table 1): Transmitted by same mosquito vector as CHIKV and coinfection can exist
- Zika Virus: Transmitted by the same mosquito vector as CKIKV and coinfection can exist
- Ross River Virus: Fever, rash, and arthritis but limited to Australia
- Other viruses that can cause arthritis include parvovirus, rubella, enterovirus, and adenovirus
- Leptospirosis
- Malaria
- Mimics of chronic arthritis: Seronegative rheumatoid arthritis, Reactive arthritis, SLE

WORKUP

Diagnosis of CHIK should be considered in patients with acute onset of fever and polyarthralgia and consistent epidemiologic exposure (residence or travel where mosquito-borne transmission occurs).

LABORATORY TESTS

- CBC tends to show leukocytopenia but not thrombocytopenia like in Dengue Fever.
- CHIKV IgM ELISA antibodies develop at the end of the first week of illness.
- CHIKV RT-PCR will detect infection 1 to 7 days from onset of symptoms.
- CHIKV IgG will indicate prior infection but will not indicate whether arthritic symptoms are related to prior infection.
- Testing for Zika and Dengue should also be performed.

Rx TREATMENT

There is no specific antiviral therapy and thus consists of supportive therapy.

ACUTE GENERAL Rx

- Acetaminophen is preferred for pain and fever. NSAIDs and salicylates are not recommended in the 14 days after onset of symptoms in case of coinfection with Dengue, which may lead to bleeding complications and risk of Reye syndrome induced by aspirin.
- Use of steroids is not recommended for arthritis symptoms as it may cause rebound of the arthritis and tenosynovitis.
- Experimental treatments include CHIKV IgG-specific monoclonal antibodies; chloroquine and chlorpromazine, which may affect virus entry; ribavirin; interferon alpha; and trigocherriolide A.

DISPOSITION

Chikungunya is self-limiting and not life-threatening with a low mortality rate (about 0.1%) but can have a prolonged recovery; joint pain can persist for months and affects the elderly more seriously.

PEARLS & CONSIDERATIONS

COMMENTS

The term *Chikungunya* is a word from an African language and means "that which bends up" or "to become contorted" due to the stooped bent posture of patients who develop joint pain.

PREVENTION

- Several vaccines have completed phase 2 studies: CHIK VLP (virus-like particle), which had promising results, and live attenuated CHIKV and CHIKV vaccine using measles vector platforms.
- Clothing and insect repellants: Use clothing that reduces skin exposure during daylight hours. Effective mosquito repellants include DEET, IR3535, and icaridin. Permethrin can be used on clothes and bed netting.
  1. *Aedes aegypti* is typically a container-habitat species (Fig. E3) and breeds primarily in artificial containers and receptacles. Therefore, all water tanks, cisterns, barrels, trash containers, etc. need to be covered tightly with a lid. Old tires, tin cans, buckets, drums, and bottles should be removed, as mosquitoes may breed in these containers if they accumulate water. In ornamental garden water tanks, larvivorous fish (e.g., gambusia, guppy) can be introduced. In case water containers cannot be emptied on a daily or weekly basis, larvicidal treatments can be applied.

PATIENT & FAMILY EDUCATION

Part of mosquito vector control in endemic areas includes reducing or eliminating water-filled containers that mosquitos can use to breed.

SUGGESTED READINGS

Available at ExpertConsult.com

RELATED CONTENT

Zika Virus (Related Key Topic)
Dengue Fever (Related Key Topic)

AUTHOR: **Glenn G. Fort, MD, MPH**

Chlamydia Genital Infections

BASIC INFORMATION

DEFINITION

Genital infection with *Chlamydia trachomatis* (CT) is the most prevalent sexually transmitted disease in the U.S. In women, chlamydia infection can result in cervicitis, acute urethral syndrome, endometritis, and pelvic inflammatory disease. These infections can, in turn, lead to ectopic pregnancy, infertility, and chronic pelvic pain (see "Pelvic Inflammatory Disease"). In men, CT infection may cause mucopurulent discharge, urethritis, epididymitis, and prostatitis. Newborns born via an infected birth canal are at risk for conjunctivitis and pneumonia. A majority of the men and women affected with CT are asymptomatic. Thus, screening tests play a very important role in detection of this infection to initiate treatment, impede disease sequelae, and prevent further transmissions.

ICD-10CM CODES

A56.2	Chlamydial infection of genitourinary tract, unspecified
A56	Other sexually transmitted chlamydial diseases
A56.0	Chlamydial infection of lower genitourinary tract
A56.00	Chlamydial infection of lower genitourinary tract, unspecified
A56.01	Chlamydial cystitis and urethritis
A56.02	Chlamydia vulvovaginitis
A56.09	Other chlamydial infection of lower genitourinary tract
A56.1	Chlamydial infection of pelviperitoneum and other genitourinary organs
A56.19	Other chlamydial genitourinary infection
A56.2	Chlamydial infection of genitourinary tract, unspecified
A56.3	Chlamydial infection of anus and rectum
A56.4	Chlamydial infection of pharynx
A56.8	Sexually transmitted chlamydial infection of other sites

EPIDEMIOLOGY & DEMOGRAPHICS

- *C. trachomatis* is the most commonly reported sexually transmitted disease in the U.S., with more than 1.5 million cases reported annually to the Centers for Disease Control and Prevention. However, it is thought that this number is an underestimate, since many cases of CT infection are asymptomatic and likely remain undiagnosed.
- Age is a strong predictor for risk of CT infection. Individuals less than 25 yr old are the largest age group affected by *C. trachomatis.* Chlamydia infections are 10 times more prevalent than gonococcal infections in young women between the ages of 18 and 26 yr.
- The prevalence of chlamydial infection varies according to race; according to a U.S. report in 2017, the rate of reported cases among African Americans was 5.6 times the rate among whites.
- Chlamydia conjunctivitis occurs in 18% to 44% of infants, and chlamydial pneumonia occurs in 3% to 16% of infants who are delivered by mothers with untreated CT infection at the time of delivery.
- Pelvic inflammatory disease develops in 10% to 15% of women with untreated CT infections.
- Untreated CT increases a person's risk of acquiring HIV.
- In men, 15% to 55% of nongonococcal urethritis cases are caused by *C. trachomatis.*
- Table 1 summarizes clinical characteristics of common *C. trachomatis* infections.

PHYSICAL FINDINGS & CLINICAL PRESENTATION

- Clinical manifestations in symptomatic women affected with *C. trachomatis* may include vaginal discharge or irregular vaginal bleeding. Purulent discharge or cervicitis may be visualized on speculum exam. Easily induced endocervical bleeding can be noted on exam and is caused by inflammation of endocervical columnar epithelium. Untreated infection can ascend the reproductive tract, causing pelvic inflammatory disease. Clinical signs of pelvic inflammatory disease are cervical, uterine, or adnexal tenderness on exam. Complications of pelvic disease are ectopic pregnancy, infertility, and chronic pelvic pain.
- Most men are asymptomatic, but when they do experience symptoms, it is usually dysuria or a mucopurulent penile discharge. A complication that can arise from CT infection in men is epididymitis, which manifests as unilateral testicular pain, hydrocele, or swelling of the epididymis. An untreated CT infection can also cause prostatitis in men. Prostatitis may present as urinary dysfunction, pain with ejaculation, and pelvic pain.
- Chlamydial conjunctivitis can be experienced by both men and women and is the result of conjunctiva exposed to infected genital secretions. CT infection can also cause proctitis or infection of the rectum in men and women. This usually presents with rectal pain, discharge, or bleeding. CT infection of the throat is usually asymptomatic in both men and women and not a usual cause of pharyngitis. Less frequent manifestations of CT infection may include perihepatitis (Fitz-Hugh–Curtis syndrome) or reactive arthritis (Reiter syndrome).

ETIOLOGY

- *C. trachomatis* consists of 15 serotypes
- Obligate, intracellular bacteria

DIAGNOSIS

DIFFERENTIAL DIAGNOSIS

Differential diagnosis depends on presenting symptoms. Some of the common differentials are listed in the following:

- Candidiasis
- Conjunctivitis
- Ectopic pregnancy
- Endometriosis
- Gonorrhea
- Mycoplasma infection
- Pelvic inflammatory disease
- Trichomonas
- Urethritis
- Urinary tract infection

WORKUP

Individuals with signs and symptoms mentioned previously should be screened for CT infection. Since the majority of CT infections are asymptomatic, routine screening should be offered to individuals at risk for CT infection. Annual screening is recommended for all sexually active women less than 25 yr of age and women at any age at risk for sexually transmitted infections. Risk factors include a new sexual partner, more than one sexual partner, individuals not in a mutually monogamous relationship, a previous or concurrent sexually transmitted disease, or working in the sex industry for profit. Screening interval is determined by any new risk for exposure since the last negative screening. The CDC recommends CT screening for all pregnant women under the age of 25 and for any pregnant woman over the age of 25 who is at increased risk for acquiring CT. These same pregnant women should be screened again during the third trimester. At a minimum, annual screening is also recommended for men who have sex with men and persons with HIV.

LABORATORY TESTS

- Nucleic acid amplification tests (NAATs) are the gold standard for diagnosis because of their high sensitivity and specificity for the detection of CT infection. The FDA has approved these tests for male and female urine collection and for provider-collected endocervical, vaginal, and male urethral specimens.
- Rectal and pharyngeal collection site specimens may be taken from individuals who engage in receptive anal and oral intercourse, but these collection sites are not FDA approved.
- For best results, urine collection should be completed with a first-void urine sample.
- Self-collected vaginal swab samples for women have the same sensitivity and specificity as provider-collected samples.
- The same specimen can be used to test for chlamydia and gonorrhea.
- Sexual partners of a person testing positive for CT infection should be treated if they had sexual contact with that individual within 60 days prior to onset of symptoms or CT diagnosis.
- Microscopy should not be used for chlamydia diagnosis; however, greater than 10 white blood cells per high-power field with a mucopurulent discharge can be a presumptive diagnosis.

TABLE 1 Clinical Characteristics of Common *Chlamydia trachomatis* Infections

	Infection	Symptoms and Signs	Presumptive Diagnosis	Definitive Diagnosis	Treatment
Men	Nongonococcal urethritis	Urethral discharge, dysuria	Urethral leukocytosis; no gonococci seen	Urine or urethral NAAT	Azithromycin, 1 g PO (single dose) *Or* Doxycycline, 100 mg PO bid, for 7 days
	Epididymitis	Unilateral epididymal tenderness, swelling; pain; fever, presence of NGU	Urine or urethral NAAT	Urethral leukocytosis; pyuria on urinalysis	STI likely: Ceftriaxone 250 mg IM plus doxycycline, 100 mg PO bid, for 10 days *History of insertive anal intercourse:* Ceftriaxone, 250 mg IM, plus levofloxacin, 500 mg bid for 10 days
	Proctitis (non-LGV)	Rectal pain, discharge and bleeding; history of receptive anal intercourse	≥1 PMN/OIF on rectal Gram stain; no gonococci seen	Urine or urethral NAAT; rectal culture or NAAT	Doxycycline, 100 mg PO bid, for 7 days
	LGV	Painful, tender inguinal lymphadenopathy, fever	"Groove sign"	Urine, urethral, lymph node or rectal NAAT; rectal or lymph node culture; LGV-specific testing if available	Doxycycline, 100 mg PO bid, for 21 days
	LGV proctitis	Rectal pain, discharge, and bleeding in MSM; absence of inguinal lymphadenopathy	≥1 PMN/OIF on rectal Gram stain; no gonococci seen	Urine, urethral, or rectal NAAT; rectal culture; LGV-specific testing if available	Doxycycline, 100 mg PO bid, for 21 days
	Conjunctivitis	Ocular pain, redness, discharge; simultaneous genital infection	Gram stain of conjunctival swab negative for bacterial pathogens; PMNs on smear	Rectal culture or NAAT; NAAT of conjunctivae	Azithromycin, 1 g PO (single dose) *Or* Doxycycline, 100 mg PO bid, for 7 days
Women	Cervicitis	Mucopurulent cervical discharge; ectopy, easily induced bleeding	≥20 PMN/OIF on cervical Gram stain	Urine or cervical NAAT	Azithromycin, 1 g PO (single dose) *Or* Doxycycline, 100 mg PO bid, for 7 days
	Urethritis	Dysuria, frequency; no hematuria	Pyuria on UA; negative urine Gram stain and culture	Urine, cervical, or urethral NAAT	Azithromycin, 1 g PO (single dose) *Or* Doxycycline, 100 mg PO bid for 7 days
	Pelvic inflammatory disease	Lower abdominal pain, adnexal pain, cervical motion tenderness	Evidence of mucopurulent cervicitis	Urine or cervical NAAT	Outpatient: Ceftriaxone 250 mg IM as a single dose, plus doxycycline 100 mg PO bid for 14 days, with or without metronidazole, 500 mg PO bid for 14 days
Adults	Conjunctivitis	Ocular pain, redness, discharge; simultaneous genital infection	Gram stain of conjunctival swab negative for bacterial pathogens; PMNs on smear	DFA or NAAT on conjunctival swab	Azithromycin, 1 g PO (single dose) *Or* Doxycycline, 100 mg PO bid for 7 days
Newborns	Conjunctivitis	Ocular pain, redness, discharge; simultaneous genital infection	Gram stain of conjunctival swab negative for bacterial pathogens; PMNs on smear	DFA or NAAT on conjunctival swab; vagina, rectum, pharynx also often positive	Erythromycin base 50 mg/kg/day, orally divided into four doses daily for 14 days; evaluate and treat parents as well
	Pneumonia	Staccato cough, tachypnea, hyperinflation	Diffuse interstitial infiltrate, eosinophilia	Nasopharyngeal NAATs or culture; MIF serology (IgM)	Erythromycin base 50 mg/kg/day, orally divided into four doses daily for 14 days; evaluate and treat parents as well

bid, Twice daily; *DFA,* Direct fluorescent antibody; *IgM,* immunoglobulin M; *IM,* intramuscular; *LGV,* lymphogranuloma venereum; *MIF,* microimmunofluorescence; *MSM,* men who have sex with men; *NAAT,* nucleic acid amplification test; *NGU,* nongonococcal urethritis; *OIF,* oil immersion field; *PMN,* polymorphonuclear neutrophil; *PO,* by mouth; *STI,* sexually transmitted infection; *UA,* urinalysis.
From Bennett JE et al: *Mandell, Douglas, and Bennett's principles and practice of infectious diseases,* ed 8, Philadelphia, 2015, Saunders.

Rx TREATMENT

ACUTE GENERAL Rx

Nongonococcal urethritis, urethritis, cervicitis, conjunctivitis (except for lymphogranuloma venereum):

- Azithromycin 1 g PO × single dose therapy *or*
- Doxycycline 100 mg PO bid for 7 days

Infection in pregnancy:

- Azithromycin 1 gm PO single-dose therapy

Alternatives:

- Erythromycin 500 mg PO qid for 7 days *or*
- Erythromycin ethylsuccinate 800 mg PO qid for 7 days

NOTE: Azithromycin (Pregnancy Risk Category B) is generally considered safe and effective during pregnancy and with lactation. Erythromycin base (Pregnancy Risk Category B) is an acceptable alternate agent for treatment of CT infection in pregnancy. Doxycycline is contraindicated in pregnancy. Erythromycin estolate is contraindicated in pregnancy because of drug-related hepatotoxicity.

FOLLOW-UP

- Observed single-dose therapy should be offered to individuals for whom compliance is a concern.
- To minimize disease transmission to partners, affected persons should be advised to refrain from sexual intercourse for 7 days after single-dose therapy, until completion of 7-day therapy, or until resolution of symptoms.
- To prevent reinfection, affected individuals should refrain from sexual intercourse until all of their partners have been treated.
- Re-collection by NAAT method in less than 3 wk from treatment can yield a false-positive result due to the sensitivity of this testing method.
- Both men and women treated for chlamydia should be retested at approximately 3 mo after treatment to screen for reinfection. If patients do not return to clinical settings within 3 mo, rescreen the patient at the next presentation for clinical care.
- Pregnant women with *Chlamydia trachomatis* infection should have a test of cure 3 to 4 wk after treatment and should then be retested within 3 mo.

Refer partners for evaluation and treatment.

RECURRENT AND PERSISTENT URETHRITIS: Retreat noncompliant patients with the above regimens. If patient was initially compliant, recommended regimens include: Metronidazole 2 g PO in single dose plus erythromycin base 500 mg PO qid for 7 days or erythromycin ethylsuccinate 800 mg PO qid for 7 days.

REFERRAL

Refer to infectious disease specialist if persistent infection or gynecologist if salpingitis is suspected.

SUGGESTED READINGS

Available at ExpertConsult.com

RELATED CONTENT

Cervicitis (Related Key Topic)
Urethritis, Gonococcal (Related Key Topic)
Gonorrhea (Related Key Topic)
Urethritis, Nongonococcal (Related Key Topic)
Pelvic Inflammatory Disease (Related Key Topic)

AUTHORS: **Ruth B. Hennebery, MD,** and **Anthony Sciscione, DO**

BASIC INFORMATION

DEFINITION

Cholangitis refers to an inflammation and/or infection of the hepatic and common bile ducts associated with obstruction of the common bile duct.

SYNONYMS

Biliary sepsis
Ascending cholangitis
Suppurative cholangitis

ICD-10CM CODE
K83.0 Cholangitis

EPIDEMIOLOGY & DEMOGRAPHICS

INCIDENCE (IN U.S.): Complicates approximately 1% of cases of cholelithiasis
PREVALENCE (IN U.S.): 2 cases/1000 hospital admissions
PREDOMINANT SEX:
- Females, for cholangitis secondary to gallstones
- Males, for cholangitis secondary to malignant obstruction and HIV infection

PREDOMINANT AGE: Seventh decade and older; unusual <50 yr of age
PEAK INCIDENCE: Seventh decade

PHYSICAL FINDINGS & CLINICAL PRESENTATION

- Usually acute onset of fever, abdominal pain (RUQ), and jaundice (Charcot triad)
- All signs and symptoms in only 50% to 85% of patients
- Often, dark coloration of the urine resulting from bilirubinuria
- Complications:
  1. Bacteremia (50%) and septic shock
  2. Hepatic abscess and pancreatitis

ETIOLOGY

Obstruction of the common bile duct causing rapid proliferation of bacteria in the biliary tree
- Most common cause of common bile duct obstruction: Stones, usually migrated from the gallbladder
- Other causes: Prior biliary tract surgery with secondary stenosis, tumor (usually arising from the pancreas or biliary tree), and parasitic infections from *Ascaris lumbricoides* or *Fasciola hepatica*
- Iatrogenic after contamination of an obstructed biliary tree by endoscopic retrograde cholangiopancreatoscopy (ERCP) or percutaneous transhepatic cholangiography (PTC)
- Primary sclerosing cholangitis (PSC)
- HIV-associated sclerosing cholangitis: Associated with infection by CMV, *Cryptosporidium,* Microsporidia, and *Mycobacterium avium* complex

DIAGNOSIS

DIFFERENTIAL DIAGNOSIS

- Biliary colic
- Acute cholecystitis
- Liver abscess
- Peptic ulcer disease (PUD)
- Pancreatitis
- Intestinal obstruction
- Right kidney stone
- Hepatitis
- Pyelonephritis

WORKUP

- Blood cultures
- CBC
- Liver function tests
- Procalcitonin

LABORATORY TESTS

- Usually, elevated WBC count with a predominance of polymorphonuclear forms
- Elevated alkaline phosphatase and bilirubin in chronic obstruction
- Elevated transaminases in acute obstruction
- Positive blood cultures in 50% of cases, typically with enteric gram-negative aerobes (e.g., *Escherichia coli*, *Klebsiella pneumoniae*), enterococci, or anaerobes

IMAGING STUDIES

- Ultrasound:
  1. Allows visualization of the gallbladder and bile ducts to differentiate extrahepatic obstruction from intrahepatic cholestasis
  2. Insensitive but specific for visualization of common duct stones
- CT scan:
  1. Less accurate for gallstones
  2. More sensitive than ultrasound for visualization of the distal part of the common bile duct
  3. Also allows better definition of neoplasm
- ERCP:
  1. Confirms obstruction and its level
  2. Allows collection of specimens for culture and cytology
  3. Indicated for diagnosis if ultrasound and CT scan are inconclusive
  4. May be indicated in therapy (see "Treatment")

TREATMENT

NONPHARMACOLOGIC THERAPY

Biliary decompression:
- May be urgent in severely ill patients or those unresponsive to medical therapy within 12 to 24 hr
- May also be performed semielectively in patients who respond
- Options:
  1. ERCP with or without sphincterotomy or placement of a draining stent
  2. Percutaneous transhepatic biliary drainage for the acutely ill patient who is a poor surgical candidate
  3. Recently, endoscopic ultrasound–guided biliary drainage has been proven as an alternative to percutaneous transhepatic biliary drainage in specialized centers when ERCP fails or is not available
  4. Surgical exploration of the common bile duct

ACUTE GENERAL Rx

- Nothing by mouth
- Intravenous hydration
- Broad-spectrum antibiotics directed at gram-negative enteric organisms, anaerobes, and enterococcus such as carbapenems (meropenem: 1 g q8h or imipenem: 500 mg IV q6h if life threatening), piperacillin/tazobactam: 3.375 or 4.5 g IV q6h, or ampicillin-sulbactam, or ticarcillin-clavulanate; if infection is nosocomial, post-ERCP, or the patient is in shock, broaden antibiotic coverage
- Fig 1 illustrates a clinical algorithm for management of acute cholangitis

CHRONIC Rx

Repeated decompression may be necessary, particularly when obstruction is related to neoplasm.

DISPOSITION

Excellent prognosis if obstruction is amenable to definitive surgical therapy; otherwise relapses are common.

REFERRAL

- To biliary endoscopist if obstruction is from stones or a stent needs to be placed
- To interventional radiologist if external drainage is necessary
- To a general surgeon in all other cases
- To an infectious disease specialist if blood cultures are positive or the patient is in shock or otherwise severely ill

PEARLS & CONSIDERATIONS

- Cholangitis is a life-threatening form of intra-abdominal sepsis, though it may appear to be rather innocuous at its onset.
- Antibiotics alone will not resolve cholangitis in the presence of biliary obstruction, because high intrabiliary pressures prevent antibiotic delivery. Decompression and drainage of the biliary tract to alleviate the obstruction with antimicrobial therapy is the therapy of choice.

SUGGESTED READING

Available at ExpertConsult.com

AUTHOR: **Glenn G. Fort, MD, MPH**

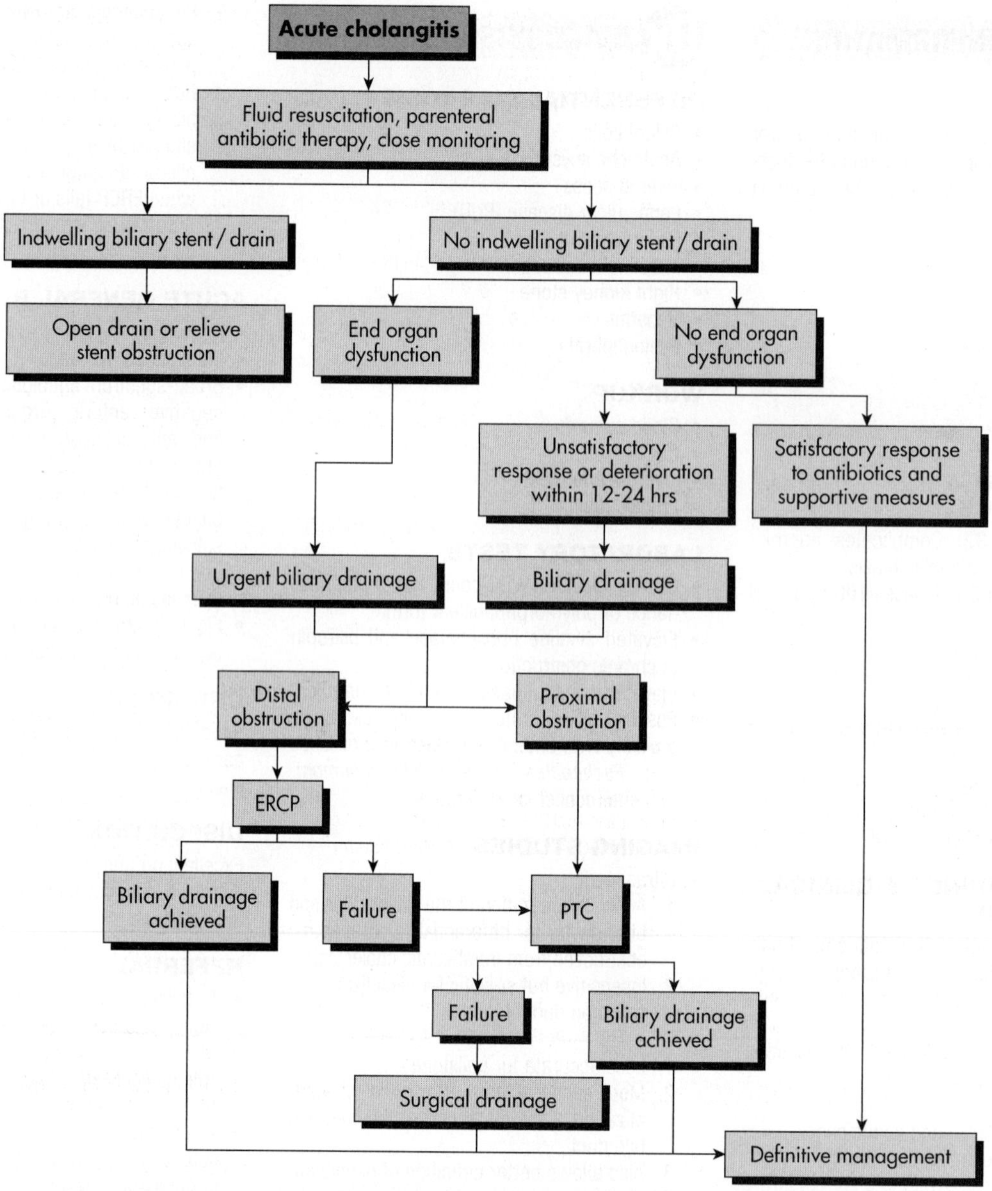

FIG. 1 Management algorithm for patients with acute cholangitis. The priority is prompt biliary drainage, and some patients may require surgical drainage without attempted EUS biliary decompression. *ERCP*, Endoscopic retrograde cholangiopancreatography; *EUS*, endoscopic ultrasound; *PTC*, percutaneous transhepatic cholangiography. (From Cameron JL, Cameron AM: *Surgical therapy*, ed 12, Philadelphia, 2017, Elsevier.)

BASIC INFORMATION

DEFINITION

Cholecystitis is acute or chronic inflammation of the gallbladder generally caused by gallstones (>95% of cases).

SYNONYMS

Gallbladder attack
Biliary colic

ICD-10CM CODES

K81.9	Acute cholecystitis
K80.00	Calculus of gallbladder with acute cholecystitis without obstruction
K81.9	Cholecystitis, unspecified

EPIDEMIOLOGY & DEMOGRAPHICS

- Acute cholecystitis occurs most commonly in women during the fifth and sixth decades. Approximately 120,000 cholecystectomies are performed for acute cholecystitis annually in the U.S.
- The incidence of gallstones is 0.6% in the general population and much higher in certain ethnic groups (>75% of Native Americans by age 60 yr). Most patients with gallstones are asymptomatic. Of such patients, biliary colic develops in 1% to 4% annually.

PHYSICAL FINDINGS & CLINICAL PRESENTATION

- Pain and tenderness in the right hypochondrium or epigastrium; pain possibly radiating to the infrascapular region
- Palpation of the right upper quadrant (RUQ) eliciting marked tenderness and stoppage of inspired breath (Murphy sign)
- Guarding
- Fever (33%)
- Jaundice (25%-50% of patients)
- Palpable gallbladder (20% of cases)
- Nausea and vomiting (>70% of patients)
- Fever and chills (>25% of patients)
- Medical history often revealing ingestion of large, fatty meals before onset of pain in the epigastrium and RUQ

ETIOLOGY

- Gallstones (>95% of cases)
- Ischemic damage to the gallbladder, critically ill patient (acalculous cholecystitis)
- Infectious agents, especially in patients with AIDS (cytomegalovirus, *Cryptosporidium*)
- Strictures of the bile duct
- Neoplasms, primary or metastatic
- Risk factors for cholelithiasis include age, obesity, female sex, rapid weight loss, ethnicity/race (Native American), use of contraceptives, pregnancy, diabetes mellitus, hemolysis, total parenteral nutrition, biliary parasites

DIAGNOSIS

DIFFERENTIAL DIAGNOSIS

- Hepatic: Hepatitis, abscess, hepatic congestion, neoplasm, trauma
- Biliary: Neoplasm, stricture, sphincter of Oddi dysfunction
- Gastric: Pelvic ulcer disease, neoplasm, alcoholic gastritis, hiatal hernia, nonulcer dyspepsia
- Pancreatic: Pancreatitis, neoplasm, stone in the pancreatic duct or ampulla
- Renal: Calculi, infection, inflammation, neoplasm, ruptured kidney
- Pulmonary: Pneumonia, pulmonary infarction, right-sided pleurisy
- Intestinal: Retrocecal appendicitis, intestinal obstruction, high fecal impaction, irritable bowel syndrome (IBS), inflammatory bowel disease (IBD)
- Cardiac: Myocardial ischemia (particularly involving the inferior wall), pericarditis
- Cutaneous: Herpes zoster
- Trauma
- Fitz-Hugh–Curtis syndrome (perihepatitis), ruptured ectopic pregnancy
- Subphrenic abscess
- Dissecting aneurysm
- Nerve root irritation caused by osteoarthritis of the spine

WORKUP

Workup consists of detailed history and physical examination coupled with laboratory evaluation and imaging studies. No single clinical finding or laboratory test is sufficient to establish or exclude cholecystitis without further testing.

LABORATORY TESTS

- Leukocytosis (12,000-20,000) is present in >70% of patients.
- Elevated alkaline phosphatase, ALT, AST, bilirubin; bilirubin elevation >4 mg/dl is unusual and suggests presence of choledocholithiasis.
- Elevated amylase may be present (consider pancreatitis if serum amylase elevation exceeds 500 U).

IMAGING STUDIES

- Ultrasound of the gallbladder (Fig. E1) is the preferred initial test; it will demonstrate the presence of stones and also dilated gallbladder with thickened wall and surrounding edema in patients with acute cholecystitis.
- Nuclear imaging (HIDA scan) (Fig. E2) is useful for diagnosis of cholecystitis when sonogram is inconclusive: Sensitivity and specificity exceed 90% for acute cholecystitis. This test is only reliable when bilirubin is <5 mg/dl. A positive test result (absence of gallbladder filling within 60 min after the administration of tracer) will demonstrate obstruction of the cystic or common hepatic duct; the test will not demonstrate the presence of stones.
- CT scan of abdomen is useful in cases of suspected abscess, neoplasm, or pancreatitis.
- Plain radiograph of the abdomen generally is not useful because <25% of stones are radiopaque.

TREATMENT

NONPHARMACOLOGIC THERAPY

Provide IV hydration; withhold oral feedings.

ACUTE GENERAL Rx

- Laparoscopic (percutaneous) cholecystectomy (PC) is considered the treatment of choice for most patients. The rate of conversion to open cholecystectomy is higher when laparoscopic cholecystectomy (CCY) is performed for acute cholecystitis rather than for uncomplicated cholelithiasis; conservative management with IV fluids and antibiotics (ampicillin-sulbactam 3 g IV q6h or piperacillin-tazobactam 4.5 g IV q8h) may be justified in some high-risk patients to convert an emergency procedure into an elective one with a lower mortality rate.
- Endoscopic retrograde cholangiopancreatography with sphincterectomy and stone extraction can be performed in conjunction with laparoscopic cholecystectomy for patients with choledochal lithiasis; approximately 7% to 15% of patients with cholelithiasis also have stones in the common bile duct.

DISPOSITION

- Prognosis is good; elective laparoscopic cholecystectomy can be performed as outpatient procedure.
- Hospital stay (when necessary) varies from overnight with laparoscopic cholecystectomy to 4 to 7 days with open cholecystectomy.
- Complication rate is approximately 1% (hemorrhage and bile leak) for laparoscopic cholecystectomy and <0.5% (infection) with open cholecystectomy.

REFERRAL

Surgical referral in all patients with acute cholecystitis

PEARLS & CONSIDERATIONS

COMMENTS

- Patients should be instructed that stones may recur in bile ducts.
- Gallbladder aspiration, in which all fluid visualized by ultrasound is aspirated, represents a nonsurgical treatment when patients who are at high operative risk develop acute cholecystitis. Salvage cholecystectomy is reserved for nonresponders.

SUGGESTED READINGS

Available at ExpertConsult.com

RELATED CONTENT

Gallbladder Attack (Cholecystitis) (Patient Information)
Cholangiocarcinoma (Related Key Topic)
Choledocholithiasis (Related Key Topic)
Cholelithiasis (Related Key Topic)
Cholangitis (Related Key Topic)
Functional Gallbladder Disorder (Related Key Topic)

AUTHOR: **Fred F. Ferri, MD**

Choledocholithiasis (ALG)

DEFINITION

Choledocholithiasis is a derivation from the Greek words of *choli* (bile), *docheion* (container), and *lithos* (stone) and refers to the presence of gallstones within the common bile duct (CBD).

SYNONYM

Common bile duct stone(s)

ICD-10CM CODE

K80.50 Calculus of bile duct

EPIDEMIOLOGY & DEMOGRAPHICS

- While the exact incidence and prevalence are unknown, an estimated 10% to 20% of patients are found to have choledocholithiasis at the time of cholecystectomy.
- Passage of gallstones into the CBD occurs in approximately 10% to 15% of those with cholelithiasis, and the incidence is known to increase with age. Approximately 95% of those with choledocholithiasis will also have cholelithiasis.
- Risk factors for gallstone formation include nonmodifiable factors such age, female sex, family history, ethnic background, and genetic predilection, while modifiable factors are centripetal obesity and metabolic syndrome, rapid weight loss, ileal Crohn disease, cirrhosis, total parenteral nutrition, and medications such as estrogen replacement therapy.

PHYSICAL FINDINGS & CLINICAL PRESENTATION

- Uncomplicated choledocholithiasis presents with biliary colic; it is classically described as intense and constant pain in the right upper quadrant or epigastric region, associated with nausea and vomiting.
- Occasionally patients may remain asymptomatic, but resolution of pain more often reflects passage of stone into the bowel.
- Physical examination demonstrates right upper quadrant or epigastric tenderness and occasionally jaundice.
- Courvoisier sign for a palpable gallbladder is more typically associated with malignant obstruction of the CBD, but it has been reported with choledocholithiasis.
- Other clinical findings of fever (Charcot triad), hypotension, and altered mental status (Reynolds pentad) are found only when choledocholithiasis is complicated by acute cholangitis.
- Choledocholithiasis can also be complicated by acute pancreatitis.

ETIOLOGY

- The majority of cases are due to passage of cholesterol stones from the gallbladder into the common bile duct.
- De novo formation of choledocholithiasis (primary choledocholithiasis) is uncommon but is seen among those with increased propensity for pigment stone formation due to chronic recurrent pyogenic cholangitis from trematodes, congenital biliary duct anomalies, dilated or strictured ducts or *MDR3* gene defects causing impairments in biliary phospholipid secretions, or biliary stasis such as from cystic fibrosis.
- Brown pigment stones comprise the majority of pigment stones in the bile duct, often found proximal to biliary stricture and associated with cholangitis.

Dx DIAGNOSIS

DIFFERENTIAL DIAGNOSIS

- Biliary pain
- Acute cholecystitis
- Sphincter of Oddi dysfunction
- Functional gallbladder disorder
- Malignant obstruction
- Choledochal cyst
- Papillary stenosis
- AIDS-associated cholangiopathy

WORKUP

- The constellation of symptomatic cholelithiasis with elevated liver enzymes should prompt a transabdominal ultrasound (US) of the right upper quadrant to evaluate for a stone in the CBD, which is the most reliable predictor of choledocholithiasis.
- Elevated liver enzymes are 94% sensitive in detecting choledocholithiasis.
- Clinical predictors should be utilized to risk-stratify patients and to inform the next step in management.
- High-risk predictors of choledocholithiasis:
  1. CBD stone seen on US or cross-sectional imaging
  2. Elevated serum bilirubin (>4 mg/dl) with evidence of dilated CBD on imaging
  3. Clinical or biochemical evidence of ascending cholangitis
- Intermediate-risk predictors of choledocholithiasis include abnormal liver biochemistries, age >55 yr and/or a dilated CBD seen on imaging.
- See Fig. 1 for a proposed risk stratification model based on American Society for Gastrointestinal Endoscopy guidelines.

LABORATORY TESTS

- Elevations in serum alanine aminotransferase (ALT) and aspartate aminotransferase (AST) reflect early biliary obstruction, followed by a disproportionate increase in serum bilirubin, alkaline phosphatase (ALP), and gamma-glutamyl transpeptidase (GGT), which are independent predictors of a CBD stone.
- Elevation in ALP is rapid and precedes the rise in bilirubin level, the latter being proportional to the degree of obstruction.
- An isolated and transient increase in alanine transaminase or amylase reflects passage of the gallstone.
- In addition, patients with choledocholithiasis complicated by acute pancreatitis and cholangitis have elevated serum amylase or lipase (>3 times upper limit of normal) and leukocytosis, respectively.

IMAGING STUDIES

- Ultrasound of the gallbladder has a relatively poor sensitivity (22%-55%) for stone detection but is relied on for CBD dilation, which is associated with choledocholithiasis.
- The finding of CBD dilation >6 mm in patients with an intact gallbladder or >8 mm in patients with prior cholecystectomy is indicative of biliary obstruction. Multiple small gallbladder stones (<5 mm) portend a fourfold higher risk of passage of stones into the CBD.
- Other imaging modalities such as helical CT (Fig. 2), magnetic resonance cholangiopancreatography (MRCP), CT cholangiography, and endoscopic ultrasound (EUS) have improved performance characteristics for CBD stone detection; however, their use as first-line diagnostic tools is contingent on diagnostic uncertainty, patient factors, and availability.
- Either MRCP or EUS should be used in intermediate-risk patients to confirm the diagnosis of choledocholithiasis and prompt further therapeutic management.
- High-risk patients should proceed directly to endoscopic retrograde cholangiopancreatography (ERCP) for diagnosis and treatment.

Rx TREATMENT

ACUTE GENERAL Rx

- Presence of choledocholithiasis warrants treatment.
- The mainstay is removal of CBD stones via ERCP and papillotomy either before or at the time of laparoscopic or open cholecystectomy.
- Failure of ERCP to clear the biliary duct warrants biliary stenting for drainage as a temporary measure in the event of acute cholangitis.
- Subsequent cholecystectomy should optimally be performed within 2 wk of pre-operative ERCP to reduce the risk of recurrence.
- ERCP without subsequent cholecystectomy may be performed in select high-risk patients, but 10% of these patients will require a subsequent cholecystectomy for recurrence.

CHRONIC Rx

Patients with recurrent choledocholithiasis from cholesterol gallstones after cholecystectomy might be considered for chronic treatment with ursodeoxycholic acid to facilitate reduction of cholesterol saturation of bile.

REFERRAL

- Gastroenterology
- General surgery

SUGGESTED READINGS

Available at ExpertConsult.com

RELATED CONTENT

Cholangiocarcinoma (Related Key Topic)
Cholelithiasis (Related Key Topic)
Cholecystitis (Related Key Topic)

AUTHORS: **Suqing Li, MD,** and **Talia Zenlea, MD**

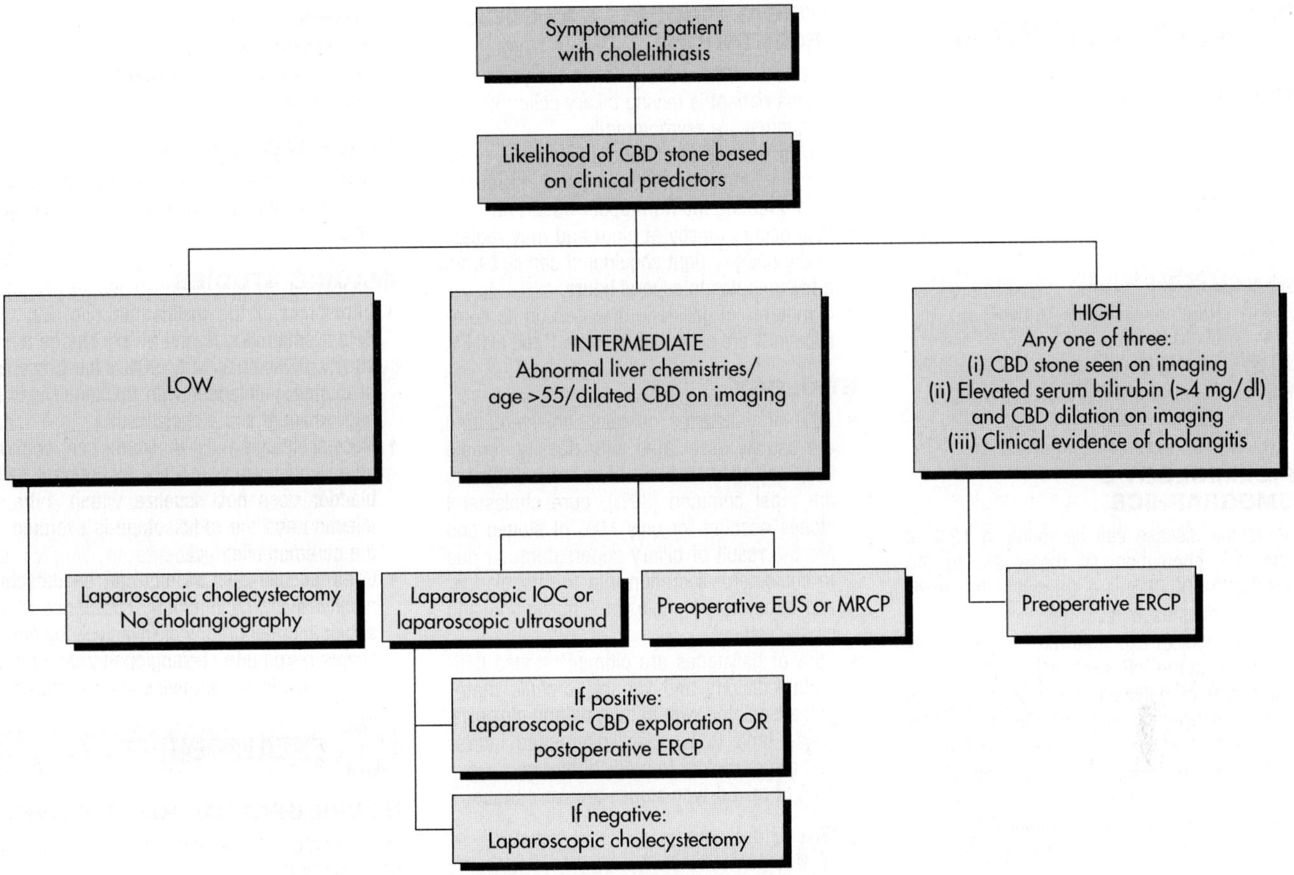

FIG. 1 Algorithm for the management of patients with symptomatic cholelithiasis. *CBD,* Common bile duct; *ERCP,* endoscopic retrograde cholangiopancreatography; *EUS,* endoscopic ultrasound; *IOC,* intraoperative cholangiogram; *MRCP,* magnetic resonance cholangiopancreatography. (Adapted from Feldman M et al: *Sleisenger and Fordtran's gastrointestinal and liver disease,* ed 11, Philadelphia, 2020, Elsevier; and Buxbaum J et al: ASGE guideline on the role of endoscopy in the evaluation and management of choledocholithiasis, *Gastrointest Endosc* 89[6]:1075-1105, 2019.)

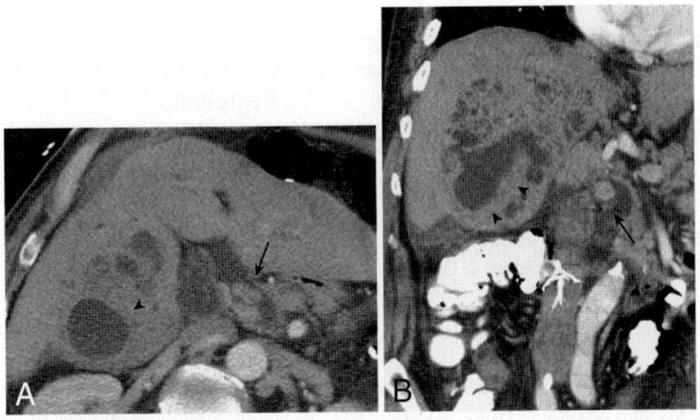

FIG. 2 A 70-yr-old male with choledocholithiasis and a hepatic abscess. Axial **(A)** and coronal **(B)** portal venous phase computed tomography images demonstrate large bile duct stones *(arrows)* with a focal intrahepatic fluid collection *(arrowheads)* consistent with the patient's known pyogenic abscess. (From Soto JA, Lucey BC: *Emergency radiology: the requisites,* ed 2, Philadelphia, 2017, Elsevier.)

Cholelithiasis

BASIC INFORMATION

DEFINITION

Cholelithiasis is the presence of stones in the gallbladder.

SYNONYM

Gallstones

ICD-10CM CODES	
K80.80	Other cholelithiasis without obstruction
K80.81	Other cholelithiasis with obstruction
K91.86	Retained cholelithiasis following cholecystectomy

EPIDEMIOLOGY & DEMOGRAPHICS

- Gallstone disease can be found in 12% of the U.S. population. Of these, 2% to 3% (500,000-600,000) are treated with cholecystectomies each yr.
- Annual medical expenditures for gallbladder surgeries in the U.S. exceed $5 billion.
- Incidence of gallbladder disease increases with age. Highest incidence is in the fifth and sixth decades. Predisposing factors for gallstones are female sex, pregnancy, age >40 yr, family history of gallstones, obesity, ileal disease, oral contraceptives, diabetes mellitus, rapid weight loss, estrogen replacement therapy.
- Patients with gallstones have a 20% chance of developing biliary colic or its complications at the end of a 20-yr period. Significant predictors of gallstone-related events are large stone (>10 mm), presence of multiple stones, and female sex.

PHYSICAL FINDINGS & CLINICAL PRESENTATION

- Physical examination is entirely normal unless patient is having biliary colic; 80% of gallstones are asymptomatic.
- Typical symptoms of obstruction of the cystic duct include intermittent, severe, cramping pain affecting the right upper quadrant.
- Pain occurs mostly at night and may radiate to the back or right shoulder. It can last from a few minutes to several hours.
- Symptoms of gallstone disease and its complications are described in Table 1 and Fig. E1.

ETIOLOGY

- 75% of gallstones contain cholesterol and are usually associated with obesity, female sex, and diabetes mellitus; mixed stones are most common (80%); pure cholesterol stones account for only 10% of stones and are the result of biliary supersaturation due to cholesterol secretion into the gallbladder and accelerated cholesterol nucleation and crystallization.
- 25% of gallstones are pigment stones (bilirubin, calcium, and variable organic material) associated with hemolysis and cirrhosis. These tend to be black-pigmented stones that are refractory to medical therapy.
- 50% of mixed-type stones are radiopaque.

DIAGNOSIS

DIFFERENTIAL DIAGNOSIS

- Peptic ulcer disease
- Gastroesophageal reflux disease
- Irritable bowel disease
- Pancreatitis
- Neoplasms
- Nonnuclear dyspepsia
- Inferior wall myocardial infarction
- Hepatic abscess

LABORATORY TESTS

Generally normal unless patient has biliary obstruction (elevated alkaline phosphatase, bilirubin).

IMAGING STUDIES

- Ultrasound of the gallbladder (Fig. E2) will detect small stones and biliary sludge (sensitivity, 95%; specificity, 90%); the presence of dilated gallbladder with thickened wall is suggestive of acute cholecystitis.
- Nuclear imaging (HIDA scan) can confirm acute cholecystitis (>90% accuracy) if gallbladder does not visualize within 4 hr of injection and the radioisotope is excreted in the common bile duct.
- Common bile duct stones can be detected noninvasively by magnetic resonance cholangiopancreatography or invasively by endoscopic retrograde cholangiopancreatography (ERCP) and intraoperative cholangiography.

TREATMENT

NONPHARMACOLOGIC THERAPY

Lifestyle changes (avoidance of diets high in polyunsaturated fats, weight loss in obese patients; however, avoid rapid weight loss)

ACUTE GENERAL Rx

- The management of gallstones is affected by the clinical presentation.

TABLE 1 Symptoms of Gallstone Disease and Its Complications

Disease	Pathophysiology	Symptoms
Biliary colic	Transient gallstone impaction at the cystic duct or ampulla of Vater	Intermittent RUQ pain associated with nausea or vomiting. Pain in the epigastrium or radiating to the right scapular tip. Episodes last 30 min to several hours with days or months between episodes.
Acute cholecystitis	Inflammation of the gallbladder caused by obstruction of the cystic duct. May occur in the presence or absence of bacterial superinfection	Patients appear ill and cannot take deep breaths. They have constant pain that lasts 30-60 min and worsens with movement. Persistent common bile duct impaction usually promotes vomiting. Physical examination demonstrates RUQ tenderness with voluntary guarding and a positive Murphy sign (arrest of inspiration during deep palpation over the gallbladder).
Emphysematous cholecystitis	Infection with gas-producing bacteria such as *Escherichia coli, Clostridium perfringens*, and anaerobic streptococci	Symptoms are similar to those with acute cholecystitis. Gas may be seen on abdominal plain films or CT. Male diabetics are most commonly affected.
Chronic cholecystitis	Persistent inflammation and fibrosis of the gallbladder with poor motor and absorptive function	Patients are usually asymptomatic but may report multiple previous attacks of colic. Porcelain gallbladder develops from chronic inflammation and may progress to carcinoma.
Acalculous cholecystitis	Probably related to biliary stasis in the setting of critical illness and altered gastrointestinal motility	Seen in patients with traumatic injuries, burns, and critical illness, as well as in those receiving total parenteral nutrition. The mortality for this disorder is twice as high as that for acute calculous cholecystitis.
Gallbladder perforation	Stones erode through an inflamed and necrotic gallbladder wall. Stones may travel into the peritoneal cavity or cause adhesions between nearby structures. Bile peritonitis may develop	More than half of patients with gallbladder perforation have fever and a palpable RUQ mass. Mortality in these patients is 30%.

CT, Computed tomography; *RUQ*, right upper quadrant.
From Adams JG et al: *Emergency medicine, clinical essentials*, ed 2, Philadelphia, 2013, Elsevier.

- Asymptomatic patients do not require therapeutic intervention. Proposed criteria for prophylactic cholecystectomy are described in Table 2.
- Surgical intervention is generally the ideal approach for symptomatic patients. Laparoscopic cholecystectomy is preferred over open cholecystectomy because of the shorter recovery period and lower mortality rate. Between 5% and 26% of patients undergoing elective laparoscopic cholecystectomy will require conversion to an open procedure. Most common reason is the inability to clearly identify the biliary anatomy.
- Laparoscopic cholecystectomy after endoscopic sphincterectomy is recommended for patients with common bile duct stones and residual gallbladder stones. Where possible, single-stage laparoscopic treatments with removal of duct stones and cholecystectomy during the same procedure are preferable. Percutaneous cholecystectomy is an alternative for patients who are critically ill with gallbladder empyema and sepsis.
- Patients who are not appropriate candidates for surgery because of coexisting illness or patients who refuse surgery can be treated with oral bile salts: Ursodiol or chenodiol. Candidates for oral bile salts are patients with cholesterol stones (radiolucent, noncalcified stones), with a diameter of ≤15 mm and having three or fewer stones. Candidates for medical therapy must have a functioning gallbladder and must have absence of calcifications on CT scans.
- Extracorporeal shock wave lithotripsy (ESWL) is another form of medical therapy. It can be used in patients with stone diameter of ≤3 cm and having three or fewer stones.

TABLE 2 Proposed Criteria for Prophylactic Cholecystectomy

Life expectancy >20 yr
Calculi >2 cm in diameter
Calculi >3 mm and patent cystic duct
Radiopaque calculi
Gallbladder polyps >15 mm
Nonfunctioning or calcified gallbladder ("porcelain" gallbladder)
Women <60 yr
Patients in areas with high prevalence of gallbladder cancer

From Cameron JL, Cameron AM: *Current surgical therapy*, ed 10, Philadelphia, 2011, Saunders.

DISPOSITION

- Complicated gallstone events develop in 8% of patients with incidentally discovered gallstones after 17 yr (Shabanzadeh DM et al in Suggested Readings: *Gastroenterology* 150:156, 2016).
- After ESWL, stones recur in approximately 20% of patients after 4 yr.
- Patients with at least one gallstone <5 mm in diameter have a greater than fourfold increased risk of presenting with acute biliary pancreatitis. A policy of watchful waiting in such cases is generally warranted.
- A potential serious complication of gallstones is acute cholangitis. ERCP and endoscopic sphincterectomy followed by interval

TABLE 3 Uncommon Complications of Gallstone Disease

Complication	Pathogenesis	Clinical Features	Diagnosis/Treatment
Emphysematous cholecystitis	Secondary infection of the gallbladder wall with gas-forming organisms (*Clostridium welchii, Escherichia coli,* and anaerobic streptococci) More common in older adult diabetic men; can occur without stones	Symptoms and signs similar to those of severe acute cholecystitis	Plain abdominal films may show gas in the gallbladder fossa US and CT are sensitive for confirming gas Treatment is with IV antibiotics, including anaerobic coverage, and early cholecystectomy High morbidity and mortality rates
Cholecystoenteric fistula	Erosion of a (usually large) stone through the gallbladder wall into the adjacent bowel, most often the duodenum, followed in frequency by the hepatic flexure, stomach, and jejunum	Symptoms and signs similar to those of acute cholecystitis, although sometimes a fistula may be clinically silent Stones >25 mm, especially in older adult women, may produce a bowel obstruction, or "gallstone ileus"; the terminal ileum is the most common site of obstruction Gastric outlet obstruction (Bouveret syndrome) may occur rarely	Plain abdominal films may show gas in the biliary tree and/or a small bowel obstruction in gallstone ileus, as well as a stone in the RLQ if the stone is calcified Contrast upper GI series may demonstrate the fistula A fistula from a solitary stone that passes may close spontaneously Cholecystectomy and bowel closure are curative Gallstone ileus requires emergency laparotomy; the diagnosis is often delayed, with a resulting mortality rate of ≈20%
Mirizzi syndrome	An impacted stone in the gallbladder neck or cystic duct, with extrinsic compression of the common hepatic duct from accompanying inflammation or fistula	Jaundice and RUQ pain	ERCP demonstrates dilated intrahepatic ducts and extrinsic compression of the common hepatic duct and possible fistula Preoperative diagnosis is important to guide surgery and minimize the risk of BD injury
Porcelain gallbladder	Intramural calcification of the gallbladder wall, usually in association with stones	No symptoms attributable to the calcified wall per se, but carcinoma of the gallbladder is a late complication in ≈20%	Plain abdominal films or CT show intramural calcification of the gallbladder wall Prophylactic cholecystectomy is indicated to prevent carcinoma

BD, bile duct; *CT,* computed tomography; *ERCP,* endoscopic retrograde cholangiopancreatography; *GI,* gastrointestinal; *IV,* intravenous; *RLQ,* right lower quadrant; *RUQ,* right upper quadrant; *US,* ultrasound.
From Feldman M et al: *Sleisenger and Fortran's gastrointestinal and liver disease*, ed 10, Philadelphia, 2016, Elsevier.

laparoscopic cholecystectomy are effective in acute cholangitis.

- Uncommon complications of gallstone disease are summarized in Table 3.

SUGGESTED READINGS

Available at ExpertConsult.com

RELATED CONTENT

Gallstones (Patient Information)
Cholecystitis (Related Key Topic)
Choledocholithiasis (Related Key Topic)

AUTHOR: **Fred F. Ferri, MD**

BASIC INFORMATION

DEFINITION

Chronic fatigue syndrome (CFS), also known as myalgic encephalomyelitis/chronic fatigue syndrome (ME/CFS) and systemic exertion intolerance disease (SEID), is characterized by at least three of the following symptoms, present concurrently for at least 6 mo:

- Impaired memory or concentration (cognitive impairment)
- Sore throat
- Tender cervical or axillary lymph nodes
- Muscle pain
- Multijoint pain
- New headaches
- Unrefreshing sleep
- Postexertion malaise for longer than 24 hr
- Orthostatic intolerance

There are currently several sets of clinical criteria to define ME/CFS, yet there is no consensus regarding which set of criteria best identifies patients with this condition. In 2015, the Institute of Medicine (IOM) recommended renaming ME/CSF "systemic exertion intolerance disease (SEID)." Their definition requires that patients have: 1. Substantial reduction or impairment in the ability to engage in premorbid levels of activities persisting for >6 mo and associated with new-onset fatigue not alleviated by rest; 2. Postexertional fatigue; 3. Unrefreshing sleep; and 4. Presence of cognitive impairment and/or orthostatic intolerance.

SYNONYMS

Systemic exertion intolerance disease (SEID)
Yuppie flu
CFS
Chronic Epstein-Barr syndrome
Myalgic encephalomyelitis/chronic fatigue syndrome (ME/CFS)
Neurasthenia

ICD-10CM CODES

R53.82	Chronic fatigue, unspecified
F45.8	Other somatoform disorders

EPIDEMIOLOGY & DEMOGRAPHICS

PREVALENCE IN U.S.: Prevalence rates of CFS in the U.S. range from 0.3% to 2.5%. It is estimated that 800,000 to 2.5 million Americans have CFS

PREDOMINANT SEX: Females affected more often than males

PREDOMINANT AGE: Young adulthood and middle age

ECONOMICS: The estimated annual cost of lost productivity is estimated to be between $17 billion and $24 billion annually

PHYSICAL FINDINGS & CLINICAL PRESENTATION

- There are no physical findings specific for CFS.
- The physical examination may be useful to identify fibromyalgia and other rheumatologic conditions that may coexist with CFS.

ETIOLOGY

- The etiology of CFS is unknown. The pathophysiologic dysregulation of the thalamus, hypothalamus, and amygdala is believed by some to be a potential cause of SEID.
- Some theorize that a viral illness may trigger certain immune responses that lead to the various symptoms. Most patients often report the onset of their symptoms with a flulike illness.
- The presence of numerous psychiatric comorbidities in CFS have led some experts to question the existence of any organic etiology.

DIAGNOSIS

DIFFERENTIAL DIAGNOSIS

- Psychosocial depression, dysthymia, anxiety-related disorders, and other psychiatric diseases
- Sleep apnea
- Infectious diseases (subacute bacterial endocarditis, Lyme disease, fungal diseases, mononucleosis, HIV, chronic hepatitis B or C, tuberculosis [TB], chronic parasitic infections)
- Autoimmune diseases: Systemic lupus erythematosus, myasthenia gravis, multiple sclerosis, thyroiditis, rheumatoid arthritis
- Endocrine abnormalities: Hypothyroidism, hypopituitarism, adrenal insufficiency, Cushing syndrome, diabetes mellitus, hyperparathyroidism, pregnancy, reactive hypoglycemia
- Occult malignant disease
- Substance abuse
- Systemic disorders: Chronic renal failure, chronic obstructive pulmonary disease, cardiovascular disease, anemia, electrolyte abnormalities, liver disease
- Other: Inadequate rest, sleep apnea, narcolepsy, fibromyalgia, sarcoidosis, medications, toxic agent exposure, Wegener granulomatosis, vitamin deficiency

LABORATORY TESTS

- No specific laboratory tests exist for diagnosing CFS. Initial laboratory tests are useful to exclude other conditions that may mimic or may be associated with CFS.
    1. Screening laboratory tests: CBC, ESR, ALT, total protein, albumin, globulin, alkaline phosphatase, calcium, phosphorus, glucose, BUN, creatinine, electrolytes, TSH, and urinalysis are useful.
    2. Serologic tests for Epstein-Barr virus, *Candida albicans,* human herpesvirus 6, and other studies for immune cellular abnormalities are not useful; these tests are expensive and generally not recommended.
- Other tests may be indicated depending on the history and physical examination (e.g., ANA, RF in patients presenting with joint complaints or abnormalities on physical examination, Lyme titer in areas where Lyme disease is endemic).

IMAGING STUDIES

Generally not recommended unless history and physical examination indicate specific abnormalities (e.g., chest radiography in any patient suspected of TB or sarcoidosis)

TREATMENT

NONPHARMACOLOGIC THERAPY

- Patients should be reassured that the illness is not fatal and that most patients improve over time.
- An initially supervised exercise program to preserve and increase strength is beneficial for most patients and can improve symptoms.
- Cognitive-behavioral therapy trials have shown positive effects on fatigue levels, work, depression/anxiety, and social adjustment.

GENERAL Rx

Therapy is generally palliative. The following medications may be helpful; however, evidence is conflicting:

- Antidepressants: The choice of antidepressant varies with the desired side effects. Patients with difficulty sleeping or fibromyalgia-like symptoms may benefit from low-dose trazodone 50 mg hs. When sedation is not desirable, low-dose SSRIs (fluoxetine 20 mg qd) often help alleviate fatigue and associated symptoms.
- NSAIDs can be used to relieve muscle and joint pain and headaches.
- "Alternative" medications (herbs, multivitamins, nutritional supplements) are very popular with many CFS patients but are generally not very helpful.
- B-lymphocyte depletion using rituximab has failed to show any benefit in trials.

PEARLS & CONSIDERATIONS

COMMENTS

- In CFS the symptoms are serious enough to reduce daily activities by >50% in the absence of any other medically identifiable disorders.
- The suicide rate is nearly sevenfold higher in people with CFS.
- Moderate to complete recovery at 1 yr occurs in 22% to 60% of patients with CFS.
- Early trials using an electrical impedance assay have shown promise in identifying CFS patients.

SUGGESTED READINGS

Available at ExpertConsult.com

RELATED CONTENT

Chronic Fatigue Syndrome (Patient Information)

AUTHOR: **Fred F. Ferri, MD**

Chronic Kidney Disease

BASIC INFORMATION

DEFINITION

Chronic kidney disease (CKD) is diagnosed when there is evidence for more than 3 mo of **kidney damage** (urine albumin >30 mg/g creatinine, hematuria, or parenchymal abnormalities) and/or **decreased kidney function** (glomerular filtration rate (GFR) <60 ml/min per 1.73 m^2). Advanced CKD, when GFR is <30 ml/min per 1.73 m^2, is characterized by accumulation of metabolic waste products in blood, electrolyte abnormalities, mineral and bone disorders, and anemia. The pathophysiology of CKD and its manifestations are summarized in Table 1.

CLASSIFICATION

The 2012 Kidney Disease: International Global Outcomes classifies CKD with a C-G-A format: Cause (etiology), GFR (G1 to G5), and Albuminuria (A1 to A3) by urine albumin-to-creatinine ratio. This format now is recommended when documenting and discussing CKD. Fig. E1 depicts how CKD prognosis worsens with either increasing levels of albuminuria or declining GFR.

SYNONYMS

CKD
Chronic renal failure (CRF)
Chronic renal insufficiency (CRI)
Chronic renal disease (CRD)

TABLE 1 Pathophysiology of Chronic Kidney Disease

Manifestation	Mechanisms
Accumulation of nitrogenous waste products	Decrease in glomerular filtration rate
Acidosis	Decreased ammonia synthesis Impaired bicarbonate reabsorption Decreased net acid excretion
Sodium retention	Excessive renin production Oliguria
Sodium wasting	Solute diuresis Tubular damage
Urinary concentrating defect	Solute diuresis Tubular damage
Hyperkalemia	Decrease in glomerular filtration rate Metabolic acidosis Excessive potassium intake Hyporeninemic hypoaldosteronism
Renal osteodystrophy	Impaired renal production of 1,25-dihydroxycholecalciferol Hyperphosphatemia Hypocalcemia Secondary hyperparathyroidism
Growth retardation	Inadequate caloric intake Renal osteodystrophy Metabolic acidosis Anemia Growth hormone resistance
Anemia	Decreased erythropoietin production Iron deficiency Folate deficiency Vitamin B_{12} deficiency Decreased erythrocyte survival
Bleeding tendency	Defective platelet function
Infection	Defective granulocyte function Impaired cellular immune functions Indwelling dialysis catheters
Neurologic symptoms (fatigue, poor concentration, headache, drowsiness, memory loss, seizures, peripheral neuropathy)	Uremic factor(s) Aluminum toxicity Hypertension
Gastrointestinal symptoms (feeding intolerance, abdominal pain)	Gastroesophageal reflux Decreased gastrointestinal motility
Hypertension	Volume overload Excessive renin production
Hyperlipidemia	Decreased plasma lipoprotein lipase activity
Pericarditis, cardiomyopathy	Uremic factor(s) Hypertension Fluid overload
Glucose intolerance	Tissue insulin resistance

From Kliegman RM et al: *Nelson textbook of pediatrics*, ed 19, Philadelphia, 2011, Saunders.

ICD-10CM CODES

N18.1	Chronic kidney disease, stage G1
N18.2	Chronic kidney disease, stage G2
N18.30	Chronic kidney disease, stage G3 NOS
N18.31	Chronic kidney disease, stage G3a
N18.32	Chronic kidney disease, stage G3b
N18.4	Chronic kidney disease, stage G4
N18.5	Chronic kidney disease, stage G5
N18.6	End-stage renal disease
N18.9	Chronic kidney disease, unspecified

EPIDEMIOLOGY & DEMOGRAPHICS

- The point prevalence of CKD is 14%. The prevalence of recognized CKD stage 1 to 5 increased with age from 10.5% at ages 65 to 74 yr to 23.9% at age 85 yr and older in the Medicare database. Males had slightly higher prevalence than females. For end-stage renal disease (ESRD), the crude prevalence was 2203.5 per million population. The incidence of ESRD increased by 1.7% from 2016 to 2017.
- Total Medicare spending on CKD and ESRD patients exceeds $120 billion USD. Accompanying chronic diseases such as diabetes and heart failure compound the cost of caring for these individuals, and CKD is considered a “cost multiplier,” accounting for 25% of Medicare expenditures. Spending per patient-year for those with all three chronic conditions of CKD, DM, and HF was more than twice as high ($40,516) as for beneficiaries with only CKD.
- Kidney transplantation represents the best option for kidney replacement therapy, offering greater longevity and quality of life and at lowest overall cost.

PHYSICAL FINDINGS & CLINICAL PRESENTATION

- Most patients with early CKD have no or few symptoms or physical exam findings.
- Skin pallor, ecchymosis
- Sleep disorder
- Hypertension, edema, jugular venous distension
- Leg cramps, restless legs, peripheral neuropathy
- Emotional lability, depression, decreased cognitive function
- Uremic frost, odor, and fetor in severe cases
- Clinical presentation varies with the degree of kidney disease and its underlying etiology. Common symptoms are generalized fatigue, nausea, anorexia, pruritus, sleep disturbance, smell and taste disturbances, hiccoughs, and seizures

ETIOLOGY

- Diabetes
- Hypertension
- Glomerular disease
- Failed kidney transplant
- Interstitial nephritis (e.g., drug hypersensitivity, analgesic nephropathy)
- Obstructive nephropathies (e.g., nephrolithiasis, prostatic disease)
- Congenital disease (e.g., Alport syndrome, polycystic kidney disease)
- Vascular diseases (renal artery stenosis, hypertensive nephrosclerosis)
- Autoimmune disorders
- Acute kidney injury (AKI)

Dx DIAGNOSIS

GFR is considered the best overall index of kidney function but is not the only measure of kidney health. Although quantitation of albuminuria has been less widely adopted in clinical practice than assessment of estimated GFR (eGFR), its evaluation is critical to determining prognosis. When applying eGFR equations, one must appreciate that CKD is defined over a 3-mo interval. (Table 2)

Therefore, the serum creatinine, which all eGFR equations are based on, must be repeated and trended to establish a diagnosis of CKD. Furthermore, to properly trend the eGFR in a given individual, creatinine must be in a steady state of production. Albuminuria assesses kidney damage and compliments the GFR evaluation. Consequently, the National Kidney Foundation (NKF) and the American Society for Clinical Pathology (ASCP) advocate optimal screening for CKD in the primary care setting using the new "Kidney Profile" test. The "Kidney Profile" combines 1) eGFR (serum creatinine with eGFR: CPT 82565) and 2) urine albumin-to-creatinine ratio (ACR; albumin, urine [e.g., microalbumin], quantitative: CPT 82043 plus urine creatinine: CPT 82570). CKD has an elevated risk for cardiovascular disease, and combining eGFR and ACR testing is a strong predictor of cardiovascular mortality and kidney failure risk.

WORKUP

- Ultrasound: Evaluation for sagittal length, echogenicity, and anatomical abnormalities including causes of obstructive uropathy.
- Kidney biopsy: Greatest diagnostic determination for acute kidney injury of unknown etiology and albuminuric disorders; generally, not performed when kidneys are small (<8.5-9.0 cm in length) or if CKD is advanced.
- Table 3 provides a summary of a practical approach for detection and management of CKD.

LABORATORY TESTS

- Blood urea nitrogen (BUN) and serum creatinine: Serum creatinine is used to determine eGFR via multivariable (creatinine, age, sex, and race) prediction equations normalized to a body surface area of 1.73 m^2. eGFR calculators are available online (www.kidney.org/kls/professionals/gfr_calculator.cfm). The preferred eGFR equation is from the Chronic Kidney Disease Epidemiology Collaboration (CKD–EPI).
- Urinalysis: Biochemical identification of albumin and/or blood. Microscopy may

TABLE 2 Criteria for Definition of Chronic Kidney Disease

KD is defined as abnormalities of kidney structure or function, present for more than 3 mo, with implications for health. These may include the following:

Markers of kidney damage	Albuminuria (AER ≥30 mg/24 h; ACR ≥30 mg/g [≥3 mg/mmol]) Urine sediment abnormalities Electrolyte and other abnormalities caused by tubular disorders Abnormalities detected through histology Structural abnormalities detected through imaging History of kidney transplantation
Decreased GFR	GFR <60 ml/min per 1.73 m^2

ACR, Urine albumin-to-creatinine ratio; *AER,* albumin excretion rate; *GFR,* glomerular filtration rate; *KD,* kidney disease.
From KDIGO 2012 Clinical practice guideline for the evaluation and management of chronic kidney disease, *Kidney Int Suppl* 2013;3:1-150. In Floege J et al: *Comprehensive clinical nephrology,* ed 6, Philadelphia, 2019, Elsevier. Table 80.1

TABLE 3 Management Plan for Patients with Chronic Kidney Disease, According to Stage

Stage & GFR	Action	Clinical Testing	Treatment Considerations
1 **>90 ml/min per 1.73 m^2**	**Establish** risk or etiology of CKD **Diagnose** and treat CVD risk factors and comorbid conditions	***eGFR***: *Every* 12 mo **UA** with microscopic evaluation **UPC** if nondiabetic: *Every* 12 mo **ACR** if diabetic: *Every* 12 mo	**Consult** nephrology if ***eGFR*** declines by ≥4 ml/min per yr **BP:** <130/80 mm Hg **Proteinuria:** UPC <0.2; ACR <30 mg/g with ACEI or ARB
2 **60-89 ml/min per 1.73 m^2**	**Estimate** CKD progression rate **Diagnose** and treat CVD risk factors and comorbid conditions	***eGFR***: *Every* 6-12 mo **CBC**, reticulocyte ct, TSAT, ferritin if Hb 10-12 g/dl: Every 12 mo **Annual** Ca/P/PTH/25(OH)D evaluations **ACR** or UPC: *Every* 6-12 mo	**Avoid** nephrotoxins **Treat** hypertension **Hb:** 10-12 g/dl, TSAT >20%, and ferritin >100 ng/ml **ACR:** <30 mg/g or UPC <0.2 with ACEI or ARB
3A **45-59 ml/min per 1.73 m^2** **3B** **30-44 ml/min per 1.73 m^2**	**Estimate** CKD progression rate **Diagnose** and treat CVD risk factors and comorbid conditions **Kidney** imaging study (e.g., US or CT) **Consider** nephrology **Consultation**	**BP** monitoring: *Every* 3-6 mo ***eGFR***: *Every* 6 mo, if stable every 12 mo **CBC:** Hb <10 g/dl *every* 1-3 mo until Hb 9-12 g/dl; then *every* 3-6 mo **TSAT** and ferritin if Hb <13 g/dl (men) or 12 g/dl (women) and after therapy **Baseline** Ca/P/PTH/Alk Phos/25(OH)D Ca/P/PTH/Alk Phos, depending on baseline and CKD progression **25(OH)D**, depending on baseline and response to treatment **UPC or ACR:** *Every* 6-12 mo	**Avoid** nephrotoxins **Treat** hypertension **Hb:** 9-12 g/dl, TSAT >20%, ferritin >100 ng/ml with p.o. and/or *iv* iron and/or erythropoiesis stimulating agent **Ca & P:** To normal range with P-binders **25(OH)D:** ≥30 ng/ml with vitamin D2/D3 **iPTH:** 130-600 pg/ml with calcitriol or vitamin D analogs If iPTH progressively increases **NaHCO3:** 22-26 mmol/L and titrate $NaHCO_3$ therapy **UPC:** <0.2 or ACR <30 mg/g with ACEI or ARB
4 **15-29 ml/min per 1.73 m^2**	Transition of management and care to Nephrology **Initiate** decisions regarding kidney replacement therapy, vascular access, and kidney transplant **Diagnose** and treat CVD risk factors and comorbid conditions **Adjust** drug dosing for CKD stage	**BP** monitoring: *Every* 3 mo ***eGFR***: *Every* 3 mo **CBC**, TSAT, ferritin: *Every* 3-6 mo **Baseline** Ca/P/PTH/Alk Phos/25(OH)D; then repeat levels every 6-12 mo **UPC or ACR:** *Every* 3-6 mo	**All of the above plus CKD**-specific education: Kidney replacement therapy modality **Immunizations:** Influenza (TIV, QIV but not LAV; PPSV23; and HBV **Reinforce** dietary prescription **Protect** dominant (handwriting) arm **Vascular** access surgery evaluation

ACR, urine albumin-to-creatinine ratio; *ACEI,* Angiotensin converting–enzyme-inhibitors; *Alk* Phos, alkaline phosphatase; *ARB,* angiotensin-receptor blockers; *BP,* blood pressure; *Ca,* serum calcium; *CBC,* complete blood count; *CKD,* chronic kidney disease; *CT,* computed tomography; *ct,* count; *CVD,* cardiovascular disease; *eGFR,* estimated glomerular filtration rate; *GFR,* glomerular filtration rate; *Hb,* hemoglobin; *HBV,* hepatitis B virus; *iPTH,* intact parathyroid hormone; *LAV,* live attenuated virus; *P,* serum phosphorus; *PPSV23,* 23-valent pneumococcal polysaccharide vaccine; *PTH,* parathyroid hormone; *QIV,* quadrivalent influenza vaccine; *TIV,* trivalent influenza vaccine; *TSAT,* transferrin saturation; *UA,* urine analysis; *UPC,* urine protein-to-creatinine ratio; *US,* ultrasonography.
CKD Stage G5 (GFR <15 ml/min per 1.73 m^2) patients require management by a nephrologist.
From Inker LA et al: *Am J Kidney Dis* 63(5);713-735, 2014.

TABLE 4 Recommended Kidney Protective Therapies According to Level of Recommendation

Level 1 Recommendations
- Control blood pressure.
- Administer angiotensin–converting-enzyme inhibitor, angiotensin-receptor blocker, or direct renin inhibitor.
- Avoid dihydropyridine calcium channel blockers (DH-CCBs) unless required for BP control.
- Control protein intake.

Level 2 Recommendations
- Restrict NaCl intake/diuretic therapy.
- Administer nondihydropyridine calcium channel blockers (NDH-CCB) therapy.
- Control each component of the metabolic syndrome.
- Administer mineralocorticoid receptor antagonist therapy.
- Administer β-blocker therapy.
- Control serum phosphorus.
- Instigate smoking cessation.
- Control hyperuricemia.
- Administer alkali therapy.
- Avoid anticoagulant-related nephropathy.
- Monitor serum creatinine in patients receiving proton pump inhibitors.
- Correct vitamin D deficiency.
- Avoid/minimize nonsteroidal antiinflammatory drug use.
- The goal for the chronic kidney disease (CKD) patient is to implement all level 1 recommendations and as many level 2 recommendations as feasible.

BP, Blood pressure; *NaCl,* sodium chloride.
From Floege J et al: *Comprehensive clinical nephrology,* ed 6, Philadelphia, 2019, Elsevier. Box 79.3.

demonstrate formed elements, including red blood cells, white blood cells, casts, and crystals.
- Serum chemistry: Sodium, potassium (elevated), chloride, and total carbon dioxide (primarily bicarbonate; low), calcium (low), phosphorus (elevated), glucose (elevated), and uric acid (elevated).
- Urinary protein excretion. A urine total protein-to-creatinine ratio >1000 mg/g creatinine or albumin-to-creatinine ratio of >500 mg/g creatinine generally indicates glomerular disease, since tubular proteinuria is usually less than this threshold.
- Special studies: Serum and urine immunoelectrophoresis (multiple myeloma), serum free light chains (monoclonal gammopathy of renal significance), antinuclear antibody (i.e., systemic lupus erythematosus), and other serological tests for determination of etiology of glomerular disorders.
- Cystatin C: A small protein biomarker used for determination of glomerular filtration. It is used to estimate GFR when a serum creatinine-based eGFR determination is less accurate, i.e., HIV or malnutrition, or if a more precise eGFR is required.

IMAGING STUDIES

- Ultrasound of kidneys and bladder for kidney length measurements (normal, 10 to 12 cm based on height) and to rule out cause of obstructive uropathy
- Plain radiographs of the aorta and extremities ordered for other reasons may reveal vascular and extraskeletal calcification

Rx TREATMENT

CKD typically progresses slowly. Therefore, even relatively small reductions in GFR loss can delay the onset of ESRD by years. For this reason, an aggressive, multiple risk factor intervention to slow GFR decline is warranted, except in patients with low ESRD risk. CKD treatment plan goals of CKD include reduction of albuminuria to the greatest extent possible and control of hypertension. Albuminuria reduction to less than 500 mg/day or more, often with inhibition of the renin-angiotensin-aldosterone system, and maintenance of blood pressure to <130/<80 mm Hg are the two most important aspects of treatment. Table 4 summarizes recommended kidney protective therapies according to level of recommendation.

NONPHARMACOLOGIC THERAPY

The Kidney Disease: Improving Global Outcomes organization recommends lowering protein intake to 0.8 g/kg per day in adults with CKD and eGFR below 30 ml/min per 1.73 m^2, whereas high protein intake (>1.3 g/kg per day) should be avoided in adults with CKD at risk of progression. Table 5 describes nutritional recommendations in CKD.
- Referral to a dietitian for medical nutritional therapy for patients with eGFR <50 ml/min per 1.73 m^2 is recommended and is a Medicare-covered service.
- Dietary restriction of sodium (~100 mmol/day), potassium (≤60 mmol/day), and phosphorus (<800 mg/day). Potassium restriction is recommended for those with or at risk for hyperkalemia only.
- Blood pressure: Current guidelines from the American College of Cardiology/American Heart Association and the National Kidney Foundation Kidney Disease Outcomes Quality Initiative recommend a goal BP of <130/<80 mm Hg for diabetic and nondiabetic CKD.
- Contrast-enhanced MRI: Gadolinium-based contrast media (GBCM) using group II agents should not be withheld regardless of renal function if MRI is deemed medically necessary.[1]
- Medications: Reviewed for potential toxicity and dosage adjustment based on eGFR.
- Resistance exercise training can preserve lean body mass and improve nutritional status and muscle function in patients with moderate CKD.
- Avoid iodinated radiocontrast media for eGFR <30 ml/min per 1.73 m^2. Prophylactic intravenous volume expansion with sodium chloride or sodium bicarbonate before dye exposure is equally effective usually recommended when eGFR <45 ml/min per 1.73 m^2
- Smoking cessation.
- Nephrology referral: Late or delayed evaluation of patients with CKD is associated with greater burden and severity of comorbid disease and CKD complications, increased risk of hospitalization, reduced access to patient-centric home dialysis and kidney transplant and reduced survival. Criteria for referral are listed in Table 6.
- Referral for kidney transplantation evaluation should be considered for patients with eGFR <20 ml/min per 1.73 m^2, unless absolute contraindications are present, e.g., malignancy within the past year.

ACUTE GENERAL Rx

- Angiotensin–converting-enzyme inhibitors (ACEIs) and angiotensin II type 1 receptor blockers (ARBs) reduce cardiovascular risk and slow progression of CKD. Combining ACEI and ARB agents is not recommended due to increased risks of hyperkalemia and acute kidney injury. Elevations of serum creatinine of 30% or greater than baseline serum creatinine within 3 mo of initiating ACEI or ARB therapy is generally tolerated without complication(s) and does not indicate parenchymal injury or the need to dose adjust or discontinue drug therapy.
- In 2019, the U.S. FDA approved the first novel treatment for type 2 diabetic kidney disease (DKD) in nearly 18 yr, canagliflozin, a sodium-glucose co-transporter (SGLT-2) inhibitor. Canagliflozin was effective in the Evaluation of the Effects of Canagliflozin on Renal and Cardiovascular Outcomes in Participants With Diabetic Nephropathy (CREDENCE) study. CREDENCE achieved its primary end point, compared with placebo, and reduced a composite of progression to end-stage renal disease (ESRD); doubling of serum creatinine; and renal or CV death. Canagliflozin had been previously shown to reduce the decline in eGFR and albuminuria in diabetic kidney disease. Another SGLT-2 inhibitor, dapagliflozin, substantially reduced the rate of progression of CKD and frequency of ESRD in diabetic and nondiabetic patients in A Study

[1]Weinreb JC et al: Use of intravenous gadolinium-based contrast media in patients with kidney disease: consensus statements from the American College of Radiology and the National Kidney Foundation, *Radiology* 298:28-35, 2021.

TABLE 5 Nutritional Recommendations in Chronic Kidney Disease.

Recommendations are for typical patients but always should be individualized on the basis of clinical, biochemical, and anthropometric indices.

Daily Intake	Predialysis CKD	Hemodialysis	Peritoneal Dialysis
Protein (g/kg ideal BW) (see "KDOQI" for estimation of adjusted edema-free BW)	0.6-1.0 Level depends on the view of the nephrologist 1.0 for nephrotic syndrome	min ≥1.1 Recommendations are in conjunction with an adequate energy intake. Requirements may be higher during illness because of multiple comorbidities or during acute periods of infection, including peritonitis.	min 1.0-1.2
Energy (kcal/kg BW)	35 (younger than 60 yr) 30-35 (older than 60 yr)	35 (younger than 60 yr) 30-35 (older than 60 yr) 30-40 kcal/kg ideal BW	35 including dialysate calories (younger than 60 yr) 30-35 including dialysate calories (older than 60 yr)
Sodium (mmol)	<100 (more if salt-wasting)	<100	<100
Potassium	Reduce if hyperkalemic If hyperkalemic, advice will take the form of decreasing certain foods (e.g., some fruits and vegetables) and giving information about cooking methods.	Reduce if hyperkalemic	Reduce if hyperkalemic; potassium restriction is generally not required. May need to increase potassium intake if hypokalemic.
Phosphorus	Reduce because of phosphate retention. Monitor levels. Advice will take the form of reducing certain foods (e.g., dairy, offal, some shellfish) and processed foods with high content of added phosphates, and giving information about the timing of binders with high-phosphorus meals and snacks.		

Recommendations are for typical patients but always should be individualized based on clinical, biochemical, and anthropometric indices. *BW,* Body weight; *CKD,* chronic kidney disease; *KDOQI,* Kidney Disease Outcomes Quality Initiative.
From Floege J et al: *Comprehensive clinical nephrology,* ed 6, Philadelphia, 2019, Elsevier. Table 86.6.

TABLE 6 Suggested Criteria for Referral of Patients with Chronic Kidney Disease to a Nephrologist

	NICE 2008	KDIGO 2012
Advanced CKD	Stage 4 and 5 CKD	Category G4 and G5 CKD
Proteinuria	High proteinuria: ACR ≥70 mg/mmol unless known to be caused by diabetes and appropriately treated	Consistent proteinuria: ACR ≥ 300 mg/g (≥30 mg/mmol)
Hematuria	Proteinuria (ACR ≥30 mg/mmol) together with hematuria	Urinary red cell casts, RBCs >20 per high power field sustained; not readily explained
Progression of CKD	Rapidly declining eGFR: >5 ml/min per 1.73 m^2 in 1 yr >10 ml/min per 1.73 m^2 in 5 yr	Progression of CKD: Sustained decline of eGFR >5 ml/min per 1.73 m^2 per 1 yr Decrease in GFR category with a ≥25% drop in eGFR from baseline
Uncontrolled hypertension	Hypertension that remains poorly controlled despite the use of at least four antihypertensive drugs at therapeutic doses	CKD and hypertension refractory to treatment with four or more antihypertensive agents
Hereditary kidney disease	Known or suspected rare or genetic causes of CKD	Hereditary kidney disease
Other conditions	Suspected renal artery stenosis	Recurrent or extensive nephrolithiasis Persistent abnormalities of serum potassium

ACR, urine albumin-to-creatinine ratio; *CKD,* chronic kidney disease; *eGFR,* estimated glomerular filtration rate; *KDIGO,* Kidney Disease: Improving Global Outcomes; *NICE,* National Institute for Health and Care Excellence; *RBC,* red blood cells.
From Floege J et al: *Comprehensive clinical nephrology,* ed 6, Philadelphia, 2019, Elsevier. (Table 80.3) (Data from KDIGO 2012 Clinical Practice Guideline for the Evaluation and Management of Chronic Kidney Disease, *Kidney Int Suppl* 2013; 3: pp. 1-150; and National Institute for Health and Care Excellence: *Chronic kidney disease in adults: assessment and management.*

to Evaluate the Effect of Dapagliflozin on Renal Outcomes and Cardiovascular Mortality in Patients with Chronic Kidney Disease (DAPA-CKD). Glucagon-like peptide-1 receptor agonists (GLP-1 RA) have shown similar improvements in cardiovascular and kidney outcomes in type 2 diabetes; however, the renal end points were secondary outcomes. The SGLT-2 inhibitor class has been recommended especially for CKD patients with heart failure as salt and water loss occur from glucosuria. GLP-1 RAs are especially recommended for atherosclerotic cardiovascular disease. The addition of chlorthalidone to CKD patients with difficult-to-treat hypertension may reduce blood pressure and proteinuria.

- Erythropoiesis-stimulating agents (ESAs), e.g., epoetins alfa and beta and darbepoetin alfa, are administered to reduce need for transfusions in anemic CKD patients. A target hemoglobin of 9 to 11 g/dl is reasonable to avoid premature and excessive ESA use. Higher hemoglobin values have been associated with adverse cardiovascular events. Iron sufficiency should be present, defined as transferrin saturation >20% and ferritin >100 ng/ml, before ESA therapy is initiated.
- Optimal diuretic therapy should be prescribed for edema or cardiopulmonary congestion.
- ACEIs or ARBs retard progression of CKD and lower blood pressure but cause short-term reductions of GFR and increase serum potassium.
- Treat metabolic acidosis with oral sodium bicarbonate to attain a goal serum HCO3 level of approximately 22 to 26 mmol/L.
- Statin or a combination of statin and ezetimibe is recommended in adults aged ≥50 yr with eGFRs <60 ml/min per 1.73 m^2. Lipid management focuses on absolute risk for coronary events, and there are no target cholesterol levels without any effect on GFR trajectory.
- Therapy of mineral and bone disease in CKD targets normal serum calcium and phosphorus levels. Calcitriol and vitamin D analogs are generally reserved for patients at CKD stages G4 to G5 and severe, progressive hyperparathyroidism (see "CKD–MBD" chapter).
- Dietary phosphate restriction is recommended for nearly all CKD patients. For additional management of hyperphosphatemia, phosphate-binders are recommended. Calcium-based phosphate binders, although

TABLE 7 Factors Affecting Renal Dysfunction in Long-Term Survivors and General Management of Chronic Kidney Disease

Risk Factors	CKD Management
• Pretransplantation HRS • Pretransplantation renal dysfunction • Duration of renal dysfunction in the pretransplant period • Dialysis requirement in the pre- and post-transplantation period • Postoperative AKI • Chronic CNI nephrotoxicity • Use of nephrotoxic drugs • Diabetes mellitus (pre-existing or post-transplantation diabetes mellitus [a.k.a., new onset diabetes after transplantation]) • Hypertension • Hepatitis C infection* (particularly if associated with post-transplant alcohol use) • Older age • Diabetes mellitus and type 2 HRS are associated with CKD progression (limited data)	**KDIGO 2012 Guidelines for CKD** 1. Hypertension • Treat BP to ≤140/90 mm Hg for either diabetic or nondiabetic with CKD and albuminuria <30 mg/24 hr (or equivalent). • Treat BP to ≤130/80 mm Hg for either diabetic or nondiabetic with CKD and albuminuria >30 mg/24 hr (or equivalent). • Use an ACEI or ARB in diabetic adults with CKD and urine albumin excretion (UAE) ≥30 mg/24 hr (or equivalent). • Use an ACEI or ARB in nondiabetic adults with CKD and UAE ≥30 mg/24 hr (or equivalent) in whom treatment with BP-lowering drugs is indicated. 2. Diabetes • Maintain hemoglobin A1C ~7% as safely tolerated 3. Metabolic acidosis • Oral bicarbonate supplement to keep serum HCO_3^- ≥22-27 mEq/L unless contraindicated

ACEI, angiotensin-converting enzyme inhibitor; *AKI,* Acute kidney injury; *ARB,* angiotensin receptor blocker; *BP,* blood pressure; *CKD,* chronic kidney disease; *CNI,* calcineurin inhibitor; *HRS,* hepatorenal syndrome; *KDIGO,* Kidney Disease Improving Global Outcomes.
*Whether successful treatment of chronic hepatitis C with the newer Direct-Acting Antiviral agents alters renal outcome remains to be studied.
From Ronco C: *Critical care nephrology*, ed 3, Elsevier, 2019.

inexpensive, should be restricted if total serum calcium is >10.2 mg/dl or serum phosphorus exceeds 6.0 mg/dl. Sevelamer carbonate and lanthanum carbonate are effective as phosphate binders but more expensive. Two iron-based phosphate-binding agents, sucroferric oxyhydroxide and ferric citrate, are effective phosphate-binders (see "CKD–MBD" chapter).
- Uremic pruritus: Difelikefalin, selective agonist of kappa opioid receptors, reduces itch intensity in hemodialysis patients.
- Recommendations of the current Centers for Disease Control and Prevention's Advisory Committee on Immunization Practices recommend pneumococcal vaccination of individuals >19 yr at time of CKD diagnosis in sequence with both 13-valent strain and 23-valent strain vaccines. An annual influenza vaccination for all persons aged ≥6 mo who do not have a contraindication is recommended. Individuals at high risk of progression of CKD with eGFRs <30 ml/min per 1.73 m^2 should be immunized against hepatitis B to ensure seroconversion.
- Initiation of dialysis: Early initiation of dialysis at eGFR 10 to 15 ml/min per 1.73 m^2 does not enhance survival compared with a symptom-driven strategy for initiation of dialysis at eGFR <8 to 10 ml/min per 1.73 m^2.
  1. Urgent indications: Uremic pericarditis, neuropathy, neuromuscular abnormalities, CHF, hyperkalemia, or seizure.
  2. Other indications: GFR, 10 to 15 ml/min per 1.73 m^2, with progressive anorexia, weight loss, disordered sleep, pruritus, uncontrolled fluid gain with hypertension, and signs of heart failure (see related "ESRD" chapter).

DISPOSITION

- Prognosis is influenced by CKD stage and burden of comorbid illness. Factors affecting renal dysfunction in long-term survivors are summarized in Table 7. Late nephrology referral, or no referral to a nephrologist within 6 to 12 mo before a diagnosis of ESRD is established, is associated with greater morbidity and mortality. Despite recommendations for early referral, nearly two thirds of CKD patients are referred late.
- *Choosing Wisely* is an American Board of Internal Medicine Foundation initiative (https://www.choosingwisely.org/societies/american-society-of-nephrology/) that promotes conversations between clinicians and patients by helping patients choose evidence-base care that avoids wasteful or unnecessary medical tests, treatments, and procedures.
- Genetic susceptibility for CKD is prominent in African Americans. Two high-risk alleles of apolipoprotein L1 predict more rapid CKD progression independent of diabetes, race, and lipid and nonlipid factors. Approximately 14% of African Americans have 2 risk alleles, and 38% have 1 risk allele.
- Kidney transplantation in selected patients improves survival. Whereas the 2-yr kidney graft survival rate for living-related donor transplantations is >80%, the 2-yr graft survival rate for cadaveric donor transplantation is approximately 70%.

SUGGESTED READINGS

Available at ExpertConsult.com

AUTHOR: **Snigdha T. Reddy, MD**

BASIC INFORMATION

DEFINITION

- Chronic kidney disease–mineral bone disease (CKD-MBD) is a comprehensive term that describes the various abnormalities of bone turnover, mineralization, and volume (TMV) that accompany loss of kidney function. These alterations are the result of abnormal hormonal interplay that includes elevated fibroblast growth factor 23 (FGF-23), vitamin D deficiency, and elevated parathyroid hormone (PTH). The bone disorders are frequently accompanied by hypocalcemia, hyperphosphatemia, and vascular calcifications in advanced CKD (i.e., stages 4 and 5). Renal osteodystrophy is histologically identified from a bone biopsy. Four major lesions have been described within the TMV classification (Table 1).
  1. Osteitis fibrosis cystica (OFC): High turnover bone disease with demineralized bone with replacement by fibrotic tissue and characterized by increased porosity and brown tumors of bone (von Recklinghausen's disease).
  2. Osteomalacia: Decreased mineralization with unmineralized osteoid that frequently manifests as bone pain and gait alteration. Osteomalacia has decreased significantly with greatly reduced use of aluminum-based phosphate binders.
  3. Adynamic bone disease (ABD): Bone disorder with reduced osteoblast and osteoclast activities and greatly reduced bone turnover, an essential feature of healthy bone. ABD is more frequently associated with hypercalcemia and vascular calcification.
  4. Mixed uremic osteodystrophy: High turnover disease similar to OFC but with decreased mineralization. Clinical presentation is varied.

SYNONYMS

CKD-MBD
Renal osteodystrophy
Secondary hyperparathyroidism

ICD-10CM CODES

N25.0	Renal osteodystrophy
N25.81	Secondary hyperparathyroidism of renal origin
E83.9	Disorder of mineral metabolism
E83.51	Hypocalcemia
E83.39	Other disorders of phosphorus metabolism

EPIDEMIOLOGY & DEMOGRAPHICS

PREVALENCE: Approximately 26 million American adults have chronic kidney disease (CKD) and are at risk of CKD-MBD. The prevalence of CKD-MBD increases as glomerular filtration rate (GFR) declines (Fig. E1).

RISK FACTORS: Controlling risk factors for CKD and adherence to a low-phosphorus diet may help prevent the development of CKD-MBD.

GENETICS: A number of gene polymorphisms are associated with the development of CKD-MBD, specifically high turnover disease. These include G990R, BSM1, FOK1 C, Q1011E, rs7652589, rs1801725, rs1801725, rs1042636, rs1393199, and rs4300957.

PHYSICAL FINDINGS & CLINICAL PRESENTATION

Examination is typically normal but varies depending on bone pathology. Some patients may complain of bone pain or have signs of fracture. Symptomatic hypocalcemia may manifest as muscle spasm, tetany, or seizure. Some individuals may present instead with sequelae of CKD-MBD such as vascular disease that includes calcification with signs and/or symptoms of vascular insufficiency or calciphylaxis.

ETIOLOGY

- The hormonal cascade that leads to CKD-MBD is multifactorial and can include elevation of FGF-23, klotho deficiency, reduced renal activation of vitamin D, and secondary hyperparathyroidism (SHPT). The interplay of these factors is demonstrated in Fig. 2 and progression in Fig. E1.

DIAGNOSIS

WORKUP

LABORATORY TESTS:

- CKD 3A-B: Measure serum calcium and phosphate levels every 6 to 12 mo and intact-PTH (iPTH) once yearly.
- CKD 4: Measure serum calcium and phosphate levels every 3 to 6 mo and iPTH every 6 to 12 mo.
- CKD 5 and end-stage renal disease (ESRD): Measure calcium and phosphate every 1 to 3 mo and iPTH every 3 to 6 mo.
- For patients with CKD 4-to-ESRD: Measure alkaline phosphatase annually, or more frequently if iPTH is elevated.
- A bone biopsy should be performed if histology will guide therapy.

IMAGING STUDIES:

- Imaging is not performed routinely in the diagnosis of CKD-MBD.
- Computed tomography can show subperiosteal resorption and new bone formation in OFC.
- Reduced mineralization on bone densitometry testing is associated with higher rates of incident fracture. Densitometry is recommended before bone biopsy, if indicated.

TABLE 1 TMV Classification of Common MBD Histologic Phenotypes

Pathology	Turnover	Mineralization	Volume
Osteitis fibrosis cystica	High	Normal	Increased
Osteomalacia	Normal	Abnormal	Increased
Adynamic bone disease	Low	Normal	Normal
Mixed uremic osteodystrophy	High	Abnormal	Decreased

TREATMENT

Treatment, as recommended by the Kidney Disease: Improving Global Outcome (KDIGO) CKD-MBD guideline, begins with monitoring phosphorus, calcium, vitamin D, and iPTH; if derangements are present, all parameters and trends must be analyzed before enacting a therapeutic plan.

If hyperphosphatemia is present (serum phosphorus >4.5 mg/dl), the first intervention is dietary restriction. If no improvement occurs, oral phosphate-binders are added. Calcium- and non–calcium-containing binders are available. The ideal binder is debated; however, non–calcium-based binders are preferable. Treatment of asymptomatic mild hypocalcemia is not required (albumin-corrected calcium <7.5 mg/dl). If there is concurrent hyperphosphatemia or vitamin D deficiency, treatment of associated derangements is advised to elevate the serum calcium level. In the absence of hyperphosphatemia, hypercalcemia, and SHPT, vitamin D deficiency is treated per general population guidelines. When SHPT persists (iPTH consistently >150-200 pg/ml), hyperphosphatemia and vitamin D deficiency are treated. If iPTH elevations persist despite therapy, vitamin D analogs (e.g., calcitriol) or calcimimetics are used to attenuate SHPT. The ideal range of intact parathyroid hormone is unknown; international KDIGO guidelines recommend treatment if marked elevations in iPTH are noted, whereas national Kidney Disease Outcomes Quality Initiative (KDOQI) guidelines suggest iPTH varies by stage of CKD. Frequently encountered pharmacotherapeutics are reviewed in Table 2. Last, if patients have evidence of mineral bone disease (elevated PTH or abnormal bone-specific alkaline phosphatase) or risk factors for osteoporosis, bone mineral density testing is recommended to assess fracture risk if it will affect treatment. Consider bone biopsy to characterize the type of osteodystrophy in cases where its knowledge will alter treatment decisions.

NONPHARMACOLOGIC THERAPY

Dietary phosphorus restriction maybe beneficial in reducing serum phosphorus concentration. Phosphorus intake is limited to 900 mg/day. Dietary counseling by a renal dietitian is advised.

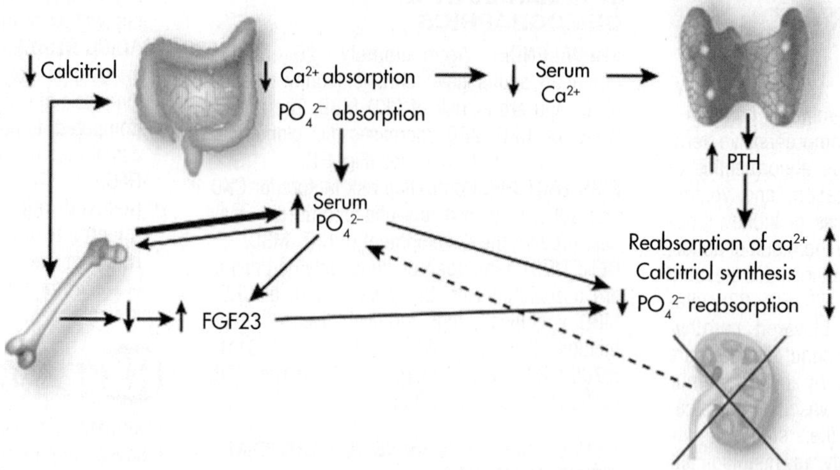

FIG. 2 Interplay of hormones in CKD-MBD. *FGF23,* fibroblastic growth factor-23; *PTH,* parathyroid hormone. (From Hruska KA et al: Hyperphosphatemia of chronic kidney disease. *Kidney Int* 2008;74[2]:148-157.)

TABLE 2 Treatment Options for CKD-MBD

Treatment Options	Examples	Mechanism
Phosphorus binders	• Calcium acetate • Calcium carbonate • Sevelamer carbonate • Lanthanum carbonate • Aluminum hydroxide • Sucroferric oxyhydroxide	• Bind oral phosphorus in the gastrointestinal tract, promoting fecal excretion
Activated vitamin D	• Calcitriol • Doxercalciferol • Paracalcitol	• Activates vitamin D receptor
Calcimimetics	• Cinacalcet • Etelcalcitide	• Activates calcium sensing receptor on parathyroid gland, suppressing PTH secretion

DISPOSITION

The presence of CKD-MBD is associated with increased risk of bone fractures, cardiovascular disease, and mortality. Treatment involves assessment of phosphorus, calcium, vitamin D, and iPTH. Bone density testing and/or bone biopsy may facilitate diagnosis. Importantly, bone lesions may heal, and this reversibility has been demonstrated in kidney transplant patients.

PEARLS & CONSIDERATIONS

- CKD-MBD is a multisystem disorder inversely proportional to reduced GFR and associated with cardiovascular disease and increased mortality, if left untreated.
- CKD-MBD treatment is based on frequent laboratory assessment, management of metabolic derangements, and evaluation and treatment of concurrent bone disease.

SUGGESTED READINGS

Available at ExpertConsult.com

RELATED CONTENT

Chronic Kidney Disease (Key Related Topic)
End-Stage Kidney Disease (Key Related Topic)
Hyperparathyroidism (Key Related Topic)
Hypocalcemia (Key Related Topic)
Hyperphosphatemia (Key Related Topic)

AUTHORS: **Ankur Shah, MD,** and **Natasha Dave, MD**

BASIC INFORMATION

DEFINITION

Chronic lymphocytic leukemia (CLL) is a lymphoproliferative disorder characterized by proliferation and accumulation of mature-appearing neoplastic B cells.

SYNONYM

CLL

ICD-10CM CODES

C91.10	Chronic lymphocytic leukemia of B-cell type not having achieved remission
C91.11	Chronic lymphocytic leukemia of B-cell type in remission
C91.12	Chronic lymphocytic leukemia of B-cell type in relapse

EPIDEMIOLOGY & DEMOGRAPHICS

- Most frequent form of leukemia in Western countries (21,040 new cases and 4060 deaths annually in the U.S.). Incidence rate is 5 per 100,000 person-yr, increasing to 17 cases per 100,000 at age 65. It is more common in patients with a family history of CLL or other lymphoid malignancy.
- Median age at diagnosis in the U.S. is 70 yr with male/female ratio of 2:1.
- CLL accounts for 1% of all cancers and 11% of all hematologic neoplasms. Because of its prolonged clinical course, over 186,000 individuals with CLL are estimated to live in the U.S.
- CLL may be preceded by monoclonal B-cell lymphocytosis—a premalignant, asymptomatic condition with less than 5000 /mm^3 CLL-like cells circulating in the blood.
- CLL confined to the lymph nodes is less common and termed small lymphocytic lymphoma (SLL); SLL is biologically and therapeutically equivalent to CLL.

PHYSICAL FINDINGS & CLINICAL PRESENTATION

- At presentation most patients are asymptomatic. Many are diagnosed on the basis of incidentally discovered lymphocytosis.
- Symptoms include fatigue, recurrent infections (pneumonia, herpes zoster), enlarging lymph nodes.
- B symptoms (fever, weight loss, and drenching night sweats) occur in 10% of patients at presentation.
- Small diffuse lymphadenopathy and splenomegaly are typical findings on clinical examination, but they are absent in most patients at diagnosis.
- A minority of CLL patients (<10%) may develop autoimmune hemolytic anemia or immune thrombocytopenia at diagnosis or during the course of the disease.
- At a rate of 1% per yr, CLL may undergo a histologic transformation into an aggressive lymphoma (Richter transformation), characterized by a rapidly growing nodal mass, elevated LDH, and constitutional symptoms.

ETIOLOGY

Remains largely unknown. Accumulation of genetic defects causing resistance to apoptosis and chronic stimulation of the B-cell receptor by autoantigens or undefined microorganisms have been implicated.

Dx DIAGNOSIS

- The diagnosis of CLL requires presence of >5000/mm^3 clonal B cells, for >3 mo, with a characteristic immunophenotype on flow cytometry, which is essential for diagnosis.
- CLL cells are typically positive for CD5, CD19, CD23 and weakly positive for CD20, while they are negative for CD10, Cyclin D1, and CD103. In some cases, molecular studies for CLL-specific chromosomal alterations (deletion of chromosome 13q, 11q, 17p, or trisomy 12) may be helpful.
- Table 1 describes the evaluation of CLL patients at diagnosis.

DIFFERENTIAL DIAGNOSIS

- Few acute infections with lymphocytosis (mononucleosis, pertussis)
- Other lymphoproliferative disorders that involve blood (can be distinguished using flow cytometry): Follicular lymphoma, mantle cell lymphoma, splenic marginal zone lymphoma, prolymphocytic leukemia, adult T-cell lymphoma/leukemia, hairy cell leukemia (Table 2)
- Acute lymphocytic leukemia can be differentiated by presence of lymphoblasts rather than mature lymphocytes
- Persistent polyclonal B-cell lymphocytosis: A rare, benign condition affecting (predominantly female) middle-aged smokers

LABORATORY TESTS

- Complete blood count demonstrates lymphocytosis with mature lymphocytes and characteristic "smudge cells" on the peripheral smear (Fig. E1); anemia and thrombocytopenia may be present in more advanced cases.
- Bone marrow examination is **not** indicated in most cases, except when differentiation between autoimmune cytopenias and marrow infiltration by CLL is difficult.
- Hypogammaglobulinemia and elevated lactate dehydrogenase may be present at the time of diagnosis.
- Cytogenetic evaluation (using fluorescent *in-situ* hybridization, FISH), mutational status of the immunoglobulin heavy chain variable region (*IGHV*, unmutated gene with >98% homology indicates worse prognosis), and presence of *TP53* mutations are essential for prognostic assessment and optimal treatment selection.
- Other prognostic markers include: High serum beta-2 microglobulin, presence of CD38 or ZAP-70 (also associated with poor prognosis), complex karyotype, and additional somatic mutations associated with worse prognosis (*ATM, NOTCH1, SF3B1,* and *BIRC3* genes).

TABLE 1 Evaluation of Chronic Lymphocytic Leukemia Patients at Diagnosis

History
- B symptom and fatigue assessment
- Infectious history assessment
- Occupational assessment for chemical exposure
- Familial history of CLL and lymphoproliferative disorders
- Preventive interventions for infections and secondary cancers

Physical Examination

Laboratory assessment
- CBC with differential
- Morphology assessment of lymphocytes
- Chemistry, LFT enzymes, LDH
- Flow cytometry assessment to confirm immunophenotype of CLL
- Serum immunoglobulins
- Serum β_2M levels
- Interphase cytogenetics for del(17p13.1), del(11q22.3), del(13q14), del(6q21), and trisomy 12
- *IGHV* mutational analysis
- Stimulated metaphase karyotype (if available)

Selected tests under certain circumstances
- DAT, haptoglobin, reticulocyte count if anemia present
- CT scan if unexplained abdominal pain or enlargement present
- PET scan or biopsy (or both) if large nodal mass present
- BM aspirate and biopsy if cytopenias unexplained by disease burden
- Familial counseling if first-degree relative with CLL

Teaching
- Varicella zoster identification instruction
- Skin cancer identification
- Disease education (Leukemia and Lymphoma Society)

B symptoms, Fever, night sweats, weight loss; *BM,* bone marrow; β_2M, beta-2 microglobulin; *CBC,* complete blood count; *CLL,* chronic lymphocytic leukemia; *CT,* computed tomography; *DAT,* direct antiglobulin test; *IGHV,* immunoglobulin heavy chain variable region; *LDH,* lactate dehydrogenase; *LFT,* liver function test; *PET,* positron emission tomography.
From Hoffman R et al: *Hematology, basic principles and practice,* ed 7, Philadelphia, 2018, Elsevier.

TABLE 2 Diseases that Can Mimic Chronic Lymphocytic Leukemia

- Follicular lymphoma
- Mantle cell lymphoma
- Marginal zone lymphoma (particularly splenic)
- Hairy cell leukemia (particularly variant)
- Acute lymphoblastic leukemia
- T-cell prolymphocytic leukemia
- Large granular natural killer or T-cell leukemia
- Persistent polyclonal B-cell lymphocytosis

From Hoffman R et al: *Hematology, basic principles and practice*, ed 7, Philadelphia, 2018, Elsevier.

TABLE 3 Prognosis of Patients with CLL at the Time of Diagnosis, Stratified by the CLL-International Prognostic Index.

Number of High Risk Factors	Risk Group	Percent of Patients	Median Time to First Chemotherapy	Overall Survival at 5 yr
0-1	Low	38%	5-10 yr	93%
2-3	Intermediate	34%	4-5 yr	79%
4-6	High	23%	1-3 yr	63%
7-10	Very high	5%	<1 yr	23%

Risk factors include age >65 yr (1 point), stage Rai I-IV or Binet B-C (1 point), unmutated *IGVH* (2 points), beta-2-microglobulin >3.5 mg/L (2 points), or deletion 17p/*TP53* mutation (4 points). *CLL,* Chronic lymphocytic leukemia.

STAGING

Staging reflects the clinical burden of disease and aids assessment of prognosis and treatment decision making. The historical staging systems by Rai and Binet remain in clinical use. They use **only** physical examination and the CBC (i.e., no scans). The modified Rai system distinguishes three risk groups:

- Low risk (lymphocytosis alone, or Stage 0)
- Intermediate risk (presence of lymphadenopathy, hepatomegaly, or splenomegaly, formerly Stage I/II)
- High risk (presence of anemia with hemoglobin <11 g/dl, or thrombocytopenia with platelet count <100,000/mm^3, formerly stage III/IV)

The Binet system divides CLL into three stages:

- Stage A: Involvement of <3 nodal areas (counting separately cervical, axillary, or inguinal lymph nodes, spleen, and liver)
- Stage B: Three or more areas involved
- Stage C: Presence of anemia (hemoglobin <10 g/dl) or thrombocytopenia (<100,000/mm^3), independent of the areas involved

Prognosis in CLL can be determined using the CLL-International Prognostic Index (CLL-IPI), which includes five factors: 17p/*TP53* status, *IGVH* mutational status, serum beta-2-microglobulin, Rai/Binet stage (0/A versus others), and age >65 yr. Overall 5-yr survival varies from 93% for the low-risk group to 23% for the very high-risk group (Table 3).

IMAGING STUDIES

Imaging studies (CT or PET/CT scans) are not necessary for asymptomatic patients at diagnosis. They are obtained in case of clinical concerns for bulky internal adenopathy, Richter transformation, or prior to starting therapy.

Rx TREATMENT

- At present, there is no standard curative therapy for CLL, so treatment is only instituted for progressive or symptomatic disease (Table 4) with a goal of symptom relief and prolongation of life. However, novel therapies aim at achieving complete remissions with no detectable "minimal residual disease" (MRD, indicating less than 1:10,000 malignant B-cells in the marrow or blood).
- "Watchful waiting" (i.e., observation without therapy) is the optimal strategy for all early-stage, asymptomatic patients outside of clinical trials because early therapy provides no survival or quality-of-life benefit.
- Chemotherapy is no longer routinely used in CLL.
- Oral Bruton tyrosine kinase (BTK) inhibitors (ibrutinib or acalabrutinib), or the BCL2 inhibitor venetoclax in combination with an anti-CD20 antibody obinutuzumab, are typically initiated for patients with symptoms related to disease, bulky adenopathy, rapidly increasing lymphocyte count, or progressive cytopenias.

ACUTE GENERAL Rx

- Although historically initial treatment was chosen depending on the patient's age, comorbidities, and CLL cytogenetics, BTK inhibitors or venetoclax/obinutuzumab are appropriate for most patients (Fig. 2).
- BTK inhibitors (ibrutinib or acalaburinib) are the most frequently used first-line therapy. Their downsides include lack of complete remissions and need for long-term daily drug therapy. The combination of venetoclax with obinutuzumab offers a time-limited alternative but is associated with a risk of tumor lysis syndrome. Three-drug combinations are currently studied as first-line therapy.
- BTK inhibitors are associated with diarrhea, arthralgias, hypertension, atrial fibrillation, and occasional bleeding (particularly with concurrent anticoagulants).
- Immunochemotherapy with fludarabine, cyclophosphamide, and rituximab (FCR) may provide prolonged (>10 yr) remissions for select fit patients younger than 65 yr with unmutated *IGVH*, but is associated with high rates of toxicity.
- Recurrent CLL is often characterized by acquired deletion or mutation of the *TP53* gene and can be treated with a variety of salvage regimens:
  1. BTK inhibitors for patients who did not receive them as first line of treatment.
  2. Venetoclax alone or in combination with obinutuzumab.
  3. Oral PI3K inhibitors (duvelisib, idelalisib).
  4. Anti-CD20 monoclonal antibodies: Ofatumumab, obinutuzumab, rituximab, alone or in combination with chemotherapy: Purine analogues (fludarabine, pentostatin), alkylating agents (bendamustine, cyclophosphamide, CHOP-like combinations).
  5. Alemtuzumab (anti-CD52 monoclonal antibody).
  6. Palliative radiation therapy to bulky lymph nodes or spleen.
  7. Chimeric antigen receptor (CAR) T cells are currently studied as effective salvage therapy.
- Allogeneic bone marrow transplantation is rarely offered to younger patients with recurrent, refractory disease.

CHRONIC Rx

Treatment of systemic complications:

- Tumor lysis syndrome may occur during initial or subsequent therapy but is extremely unlikely prior to treatment in CLL, even with high lymphocyte counts.
- CLL patients are at increased risk of solid tumors and should adhere to age-appropriate screening modalities; skin cancers, including melanoma, are particularly common.
- Hypogammaglobulinemia is frequent in CLL and may cause recurrent infections, particularly pneumonias. Immunoglobulin supplementation (250 mg/kg IV every 4 wk) may prevent infections but has no effect on the course of CLL.
- Patients who had received chemoimmunotherapy are at risk for opportunistic infections, including herpes zoster and *Pneumocystis jirovecі* pneumonia.
- Specific adverse effects of novel agents are commonly seen in clinical practice. BTK inhibitors may cause hypertension, atrial fibrillation, chronic diarrhea, or hemorrhage, and must be held before surgical procedures. Venetoclax may cause tumor lysis syndrome and neutropenia.
- Autoimmune hemolytic anemia, thrombocytopenia, and (rare) neutropenia may be treated with steroids, immunoglobulin, or immune suppression without CLL-directed therapy.
- CLL is a contraindication to administration of live vaccines (varicella zoster, mumps/measles/rubella, yellow fever, intranasal influenza). Patients should adhere to the recommended schedule of immunization against *Pneumococcus* and influenza.

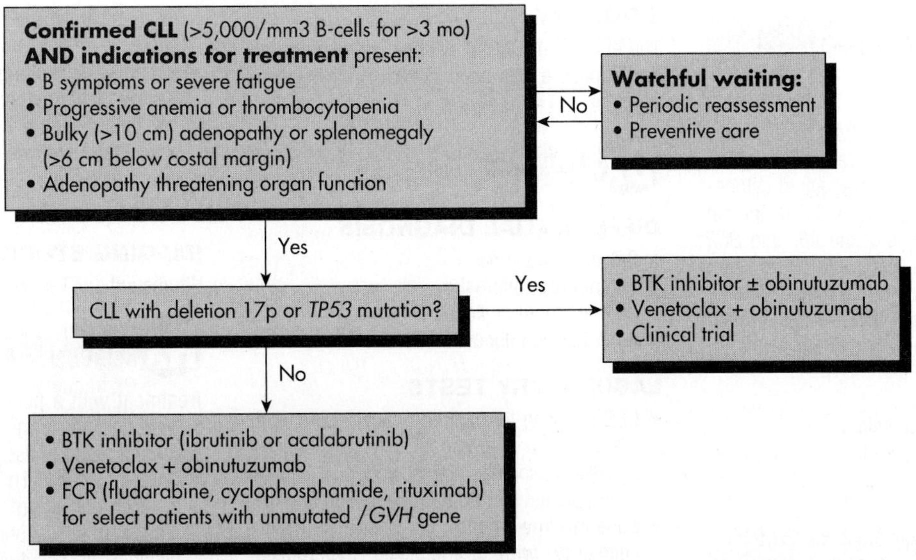

FIG. 2 Initial treatment approach in chronic lymphocytic leukemia. *BTK*, Bruton tyrosine kinase; *CLL*, chronic lymphocytic leukemia. (Courtesy Adam J. Olszewski, MD)

TABLE 4 Modified Indications for Treatment of Chronic Lymphocytic Leukemia

- Grade 2 or greater fatigue limiting life activities
- B symptoms persisting for ≥2 wk
- Lymph nodes >10 cm or progressively enlarging lymph nodes causing symptoms
- Spleen or liver with progressive enlargement or causing symptoms
- Anemia (hemoglobin <11 g/dl) referable to CLL
- Thrombocytopenia (platelets $<100 \times 10^{12}$/L) referable to CLL or ITP poorly responsive to traditional therapy
- Severe paraneoplastic (e.g., insect hypersensitivity, vasculitis, myositis) process related to CLL not responsive to traditional therapies

B symptoms, Fever, night sweats, weight loss; *CLL,* chronic lymphocytic leukemia; *ITP,* idiopathic thrombocytopenic purpura.
From Hoffman R et al: *Hematology, basic principles and practice*, ed 7, Philadelphia, 2018, Elsevier.

- Patients with CLL are at increased risk of complications from COVID-19, although BTK inhibitors may lessen the severity of the coronavirus disease.

DISPOSITION

Most patients have extended survival, though they may die from infectious complications of prior chemotherapy or from Richter's transformation. Palliative treatment should be offered to patients who are no longer benefiting from aggressive therapy to avoid pervasive and futile treatment with distressing complications.

SUGGESTED READINGS

Available at ExpertConsult.com

RELATED CONTENT

Chronic Lymphocytic Leukemia (Patient Information)

AUTHOR: **Adam J. Olszewski, MD**

BASIC INFORMATION

DEFINITION

Chronic myeloid leukemia (CML) is a malignant clonal stem disease characterized by the Philadelphia chromosome, an acquired cytogenetic abnormality arising out of the reciprocal translocation of long arms of the *ABL* and *BCR* genes on chromosomes 9 and 22. The resultant *BCR:ABL* fusion oncogene is associated with the development of abnormal myeloid proliferation and accumulation of immature granulocytes.

SYNONYMS

Chronic granulocytic leukemia
Chronic myelogenous leukemia

ICD-10CM CODES

C92.10	Chronic myeloid leukemia, BCR/ABL-positive, not having achieved remission
C92.11	Chronic myeloid leukemia, BCR/ABL-positive, in remission
C92.12	Chronic myeloid leukemia, BCR/ABL-positive, in relapse

EPIDEMIOLOGY & DEMOGRAPHICS

- CML usually presents in the mid-50s range and accounts for 15% to 20% of adult leukemias.
- Incidence is 1 to 1.5 cases per 100,000 people annually.
- In 2020, nearly 8450 new cases and more than 1130 deaths are estimated to occur in the U.S.

PHYSICAL FINDINGS & CLINICAL PRESENTATION

- Up to 50% patients are asymptomatic, with diagnosis based on abnormal blood counts.
- The initial chronic phase (CP-CML) is marked by a myeloproliferative picture lasting months to years, which evolves into an advanced phase (AP-CML) characterized by poor response to therapy and worsening cytopenias; finally, this phase then evolves into a terminal blast phase (BP-CML), resulting in acute leukemia (70% myeloid and approximately 30% lymphoid subtype). The criteria for accelerated and blast phases of CML are described in Table 1.
- In chronic phase, symptomatic patients have fatigue, weight loss, early satiety, and left abdomen pain, and the examination can reveal splenomegaly. Occasionally, hyperleukocytosis and severe thrombocytosis may lead to hyperviscosity-related symptoms.
- Patients in accelerated phase are usually symptomatic with fevers, sweats, weight loss, abdomen pain, and progressive splenomegaly.
- Patients in blast phase in addition can have bone pain; symptoms of anemia, infectious complications, and bleeding are also present.

ETIOLOGY

The etiology of CML is unclear, although radiation exposure has been linked in its development.

DIAGNOSIS

DIFFERENTIAL DIAGNOSIS

- Splenic lymphoma
- Primary myelofibrosis
- Chronic neutrophilic leukemia
- Essential thrombocythemia

LABORATORY TESTS

- CBC showing left-shifted myeloid cells, with the presence of precursor polymorphonuclear cells, basophils, and eosinophils; can be accompanied by thrombocytosis and anemia.
- Bone marrow biopsy demonstrates hypercellularity with granulocytic hyperplasia, increased ratio of myeloid cells to erythroid cells, and increased megakaryocytes (Fig. E1).
- Bone marrow cytogenetics demonstrated the 9:22 translocation (Philadelphia chromosome) in >95% of patients (Fig. 2).
- Leukocyte alkaline phosphatase is markedly decreased (unlike other myeloproliferative disorders).
- *BCR-ABL* fusion transcripts can be measured using quantitative RT-PCR technology using either peripheral blood or bone marrow; serial peripheral blood monitoring of transcript level is utilized at 3-mo intervals to determine molecular remission status.

RISK STRATIFICATION

- Chronic phase CML patients can be stratified into three categories; low-, intermediate-, or high-risk, using the Sokal, Hasford (EURO) or more recently, the EUTOS long-term (ELTS) score.
- Patients developing secondary mutations have variable response to second- or third-line therapies; the *T315I* mutation is typically associated with resistance and is treated with allogeneic stem cell transplantation (SCT).

IMAGING STUDIES

Ultrasound or CT scan of abdomen can be done.

TREATMENT

Treatment with a potential to either cure CML or prolong long-term survival should be used according to the phase of the disease.

- Chronic phase: The therapeutic approach involves the use of either a first-generation (imatinib) or second-generation (dasatinib, nilotinib, or bosutinib) oral tyrosine kinase inhibitor (TKI). Imatinib mesylate, a 2-phenylaminopyrimidine derivative, binds to the canonic adenosine triphosphate (ATP)–binding site of the Abl kinase domain. It blocks phosphorylation of tyrosine residues on substrate protein. Blocking ATP binding inactivates the Abl kinase because it cannot transfer phosphate to its substrate. Inhibiting phosphorylation prevents activation of signal transduction pathways that cause CML (Fig. E3). Imatinib inhibits several tyrosine kinases, including $p210^{BCR\text{–}ABL1}$, $p190^{BCR\text{–}ABL1}$, v-ABL1, c-ABL1, c-Kit, and platelet-derived growth factor receptor (PDGFR). The decision to select a particular TKI is based on patient comorbidities, age, and often formulary restrictions. The large majority of patients obtain hematologic and cytogenetic remissions; major molecular remissions are observed in 25% to 60% cases. Patients who

TABLE 1 Definitions of the Accelerated and Blastic Phases of Chronic Myeloid Leukemia

Criteria	MD Anderson Cancer Center[a]	International Bone Marrow Transplant Registry	World Health Organization
Accelerated Phase			
Percent blasts	15-29	10-29	10-19
Percent blasts + promyelocytes	≥30	≥20	NA
Percent basophils	≥20	≥20% (basophils + eosinophils)	≥20
Platelets ($\times 10^9$/L)	<100	Unresponsive ↑, persistent ↓	<100 or >1000 unresponsive
Cytogenetics	CE	CE	CE not at diagnosis
WBCs	NA	Difficult to control, or doubling in <5 days	NA
Anemia	NA	Unresponsive	NA
Splenomegaly	NA	Increasing	NA
Other		Chloromas, myelofibrosis	Megakaryocyte proliferation, fibrosis
Blastic Phase			
30% or more blasts; or extramedullary blastic disease, except for the World Health Organization classification, which requires 20% or more			

CE, Clonal evolution; *NA,* not applicable; *WBC,* white blood cell.
[a]These criteria were also used in all the IFN-α and tyrosine kinase inhibitor studies.
From Niederhuber JE: *Abeloff's clinical oncology,* ed 6, Philadelphia, 2020, Elsevier.

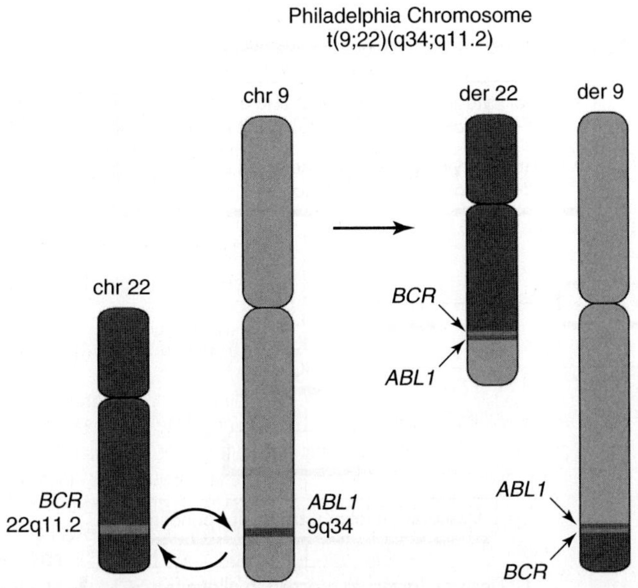

FIG. 2 The Philadelphia chromosome, der(22q), results from the reciprocal translocation of a portion of the ABL1 gene on chromosome 9 at band q34 to the region of the BCR gene on chromosome 22 at band q11.2. In turn, a portion of *BCR* is translocated to chromosome 9 to the region of *ABL1*. In 5%-10% of patients with chronic myeloid leukemia, cryptic or complex rearrangements result in a *BCR-ABL1* fusion gene, even though no Philadelphia chromosome is detected cytogenetically. (From Jaffe ES et al: *Hematopathology*, Philadelphia, 2011, Saunders).

TABLE 2 Approved Indications in Chronic Myeloid Leukemia

	Frontline	Salvage	Accelerated	Blastic
Imatinib	400 mg QD 340 mg/m² per day	400 mg QD (IFN failure)	600 mg QD (IFN failure)	600 mg QD (IFN failure)
Dasatinib	100 mg QD	100 mg QD A	140 mg QD A	140 mg QD A
Nilotinib	300 mg BID	400 mg BID A	400 mg BID A	—
Bosutinib	—	500 mg QD B	500 mg QD B	500 mg QD B
Ponatinib	—	45 mg QD B	45 mg QD B	45 mg QD B
Omacetaxine	—	1.25 mg/m² SC × 14 days every 28 days (induction), then × 7 days every 28 days C	1.25 mg/m² SC × 14 days every 28 days (induction), then × 7 days every 28 days C	—

A, Resistance or intolerance to prior therapies including imatinib; *B,* resistance or intolerance to prior tyrosine kinase inhibitors (TKIs); *BID,* twice daily; *C,* resistance or intolerance to two prior TKIs; *IFN,* interferon; *QD,* daily; *SC,* subcutaneously.
From Niederhuber JE: *Abeloff's clinical oncology*, ed 6, Philadelphia, 2020, Elsevier.

lose their initial response, develop secondary mutations, or develop intolerance to therapy can be treated with newer third-generation TKIs (bosutinib, ponatinib). Omacetaxine, a protein synthesis inhibitor, is also effective in patients who have previously received TKI therapy. The approved indications are summarized in Table 2. An algorithm of the suggested treatment approach in CML is illustrated in Fig. 4.

- Second-generation TKIs (dasatinib, nilotinib, or bosutinib) are preferred for patients with an intermediate- or high-risk Sokal or Hasford score, especially for young women whose goal is to achieve a deep and rapid molecular response and eventual drug discontinuation of TKI therapy for fertility purposes.
- Some patients develop resistance to currently available TKI drugs. The ABL myristoyl pocket (STAMP) inhibitor, asciminib, has recently demonstrated superiority over bosutinib in achieving molecular responses in patients previously treated with >2 other TKIs. Based on these data the drug has been granted fast-track designation by the FDA.
- During therapy for chronic phase CML, treatment efficacy is monitored by the use of serial RT-PCR to measure peripheral blood *BCR-ABL* transcripts every 3 to 6 mo.
- Accelerated phase: Patients are initially treated with second-generation TKIs but ultimately require allogeneic SCT.
- Blast phase: Patients are initially treated with conventional induction chemotherapy as per the type of evolved acute leukemia and then subsequently undergo allogeneic SCT.
- Symptomatic hyperleukocytosis is treated with leukapheresis and hydroxyurea; allopurinol should be started to prevent urate nephropathy after the rapid lysis of the leukemia cells.

DISPOSITION

- Response definition and monitoring are summarized in Table 3.
- Median survival for patients with chronic phase CML undergoing therapy with current TKIs is estimated to last 25+ yr.
- Median survivals for patients with accelerated and blast phase CML are 5 yr and 7 to 11 mo, respectively.
- Discontinuing oral TKI therapy in chronic phase CML patients who have achieved deep, long-term molecular remissions can be considered in select cases but can be associated with molecular relapses in up to half the cases. Criteria for TKI discontinuation include: Age >18 yr, chronic phase CML, prior TKI therapy for at least 3 yr, and stable major molecular response >2 yr as documented on at least four occasions using quantitative RT-PCR assays performed more than 3 mo apart. Nilotinib is currently the only therapy that has been approved by the FDA for treatment-free remission in patients.

REFERRAL

To hematology physician

PEARLS & CONSIDERATIONS

- Chronic-phase CML patients should be risk-stratified at diagnosis to define prognosis upfront; patients achieving complete cytogenetic remission or major molecular remission by 12 mo have consistently superior long-term outcomes.
- Regular monitoring of molecular response using peripheral blood RT-PCR for BCR:ABL transcript levels is done every 3 to 6 mo for disease monitoring.
- Allogeneic stem cell transplantation is a useful modality for advanced CML patients and chronic phase CML patients who develop resistance to standard TKI therapy.

SUGGESTED READINGS

Available at ExpertConsult.com

RELATED CONTENT

Chronic Myeloid Leukemia (Patient Information)

AUTHOR: **Ritesh Rathore, MD**

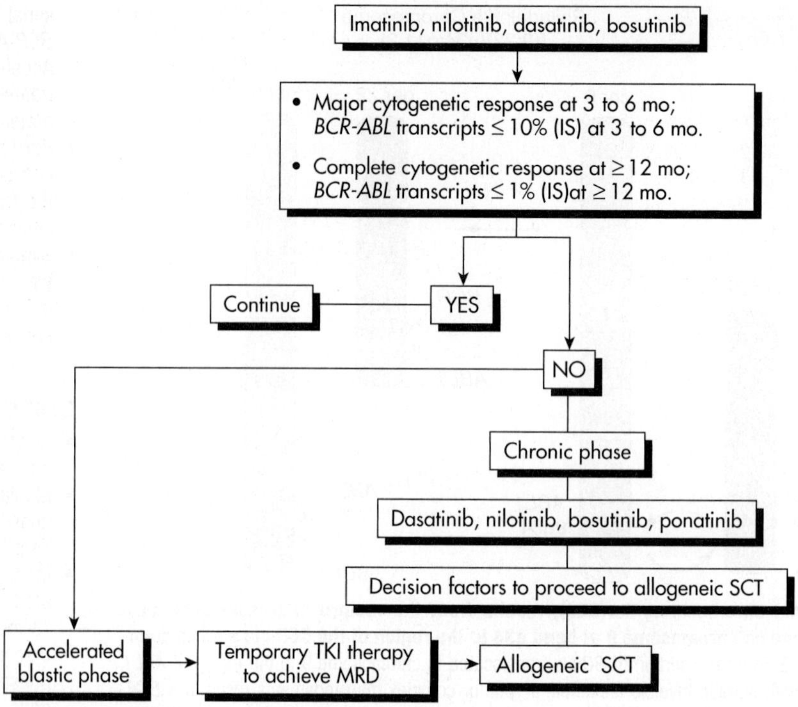

- Choice of salvage (TKI) depends on frontline TKI, and *BCR-ABL* mutation. If *T315I* mutation, only ponatinib is effective; if not available, use hydrea or chemotherapy, and proceed to allogeneic stem cell transplantation (SCT).
- In CML salvage the following are considered:
  - If relapse in accelerated-blastic phase, use TKIs as temporary measure to achieve minimal residual disease (MRD) and proceed to allogeneic SCT.
  - If relapse in chronic phase, choice of TKI based on mutations. Choice to continue on TKI indefinitely depends on presence of absence of clonal evolution, adverse mutations, and response to TKIs.
  - Older patients (≥65 yr) and patients with poor matching donors may decide to continue TKIs in combination with hydroxyurea or other chemotherapy to gain several years of good quality of life, rather than opt for allogeneic SCT.

FIG. 4 Algorithm of the suggested treatment approach in chronic myeloid leukemia (CML). *TKI,* Tyrosine kinase inhibitor. (From Niederhuber JE: *Abeloff's clinical oncology*, ed 6, Philadelphia, 2020, Elsevier.)

TABLE 3 Response Definition and Monitoring

Hematologic Response	Cytogenetic Response	Molecular Response
Complete: Platelet count <450 × 10^9/L; WBC count <10 × 10^9/L; differential without immature granulocytes and with less than 5% basophils; nonpalpable spleen	Complete: Ph+ 0 Major: Ph+ 1-35% Minor: Ph+ 36-65% Minimal: Ph+ 66-95% None: Ph+ <95%	Complete: *BCR-ABL* transcripts nonquantifiable and nondetectable[a] Major: ≤0.10%

BCR-ABL to control gene ratio according to the proposed international scale for measuring molecular response, with a standardized "baseline," as established in the IRIS trial, taken to represent 100% on the international scale, and a 3-log reduction from the standardized baseline (major molecular response) fixed at 0.10%.

ABL, Abelson leukemia virus; *BCR,* breakpoint cluster region; *Ph+,* Philadelphia chromosome positive; *WBC,* white blood cell.

[a]Qualified by the limit of sensitivity of the polymerase chain reaction assay employed.

From Hoffman R et al: *Hematology: basic principles and practice*, ed 7, Philadelphia, 2018, Elsevier.

BASIC INFORMATION

DEFINITION

Chronic obstructive pulmonary disease (COPD) is an inflammatory respiratory disease usually caused by exposure to tobacco smoke. It is an umbrella term for various clinical entities with multiple causes resulting in airflow limitation that is not fully reversible. The pathophysiology of COPD is related to enhanced inflammatory response to noxious particles and gases, chronic airway irritation, mucus production, and pulmonary scarring and changes in pulmonary vasculature.

Acute exacerbations and comorbidities contribute to the overall severity and prognosis of the disease in individual patients.

Traditionally, COPD was described as encompassing *emphysema*, characterized by loss of lung elasticity and destruction of lung parenchyma with enlargement of air spaces, and *chronic bronchitis*, characterized by obstruction of small airways and productive cough >3 mo for more than 2 successive yrs. These terms are no longer included in the formal definition of COPD, although they are still used clinically. Although emphysema and chronic bronchitis are commonly associated with COPD, neither is required to make the diagnosis.

An overlap syndrome known as Asthma-COPD overlap (see Asthma-COPD Overlap chapter), characterized by persistent airflow limitation with several features associated with asthma and several features associated with COPD, has been gaining recognition and may have treatment and mortality implications (Global Initiative for Chronic Obstructive Lung Disease [GOLD] and Global Initiative for Asthma [GINA] consensus statement).

SYNONYMS

COPD
Emphysema
Chronic bronchitis

ICD-10CM CODES

J44.9	Chronic obstructive pulmonary disease, unspecified COPD type
J42	Chronic bronchitis, unspecified chronic bronchitis type
J44.0	Chronic obstructive pulmonary disease with acute lower respiratory infection
J44.1	Chronic obstructive pulmonary disease with acute exacerbation
J43.0	Unilateral emphysema
J43.1	Panlobular emphysema
J43.2	Centrilobular emphysema
J43.8	Other emphysema
J43.9	Pulmonary emphysema, unspecified emphysema type

EPIDEMIOLOGY & DEMOGRAPHICS

- COPD affects 14% of U.S. adults aged 40 to 79 yr
- Between 10% and 20% of COPD in the U.S. is due to occupational or other exposure to chemical vapors, irritants, and fumes; 80% to 90% is due to cigarette smoking.
- COPD is the third leading cause of death in the U.S.
- Highest incidence is in males >40 yr
- 16 million office visits, 500,000 hospitalizations, 126,000 deaths annually, and >$18 billion in direct health care costs annually can be attributed to COPD.
- Patients with COPD living in isolated rural areas of the U.S. are at greater risk for COPD exacerbation-related mortality than those living in urban areas, independent of hospital rurality and volume.

PHYSICAL FINDINGS & CLINICAL PRESENTATION

- Patients with COPD have historically been classically subdivided in two major groups based on their phenotype:
  1. *Blue bloaters* are patients with chronic bronchitis; the name is derived from the bluish tinge of the skin (as a result of chronic hypoxemia and hypercapnia) and from the frequent presence of peripheral edema (from cor pulmonale); chronic cough with production of large amounts of sputum is characteristic.
  2. *Pink puffers* are patients with emphysema; they have a cachectic appearance but pink skin color (adequate oxygen saturation); shortness of breath is manifested by pursed-lip breathing and use of accessory muscles of respiration.
- COPD may present with combinations of the following signs and symptoms:
  1. Cyanosis, chronic cough (usually productive but may be intermittent and may be unproductive), tachypnea, tachycardia.
  2. Dyspnea (persistent, progressive), pursed-lip breathing with use of accessory muscles for respiration, decreased breath sounds, wheezing.
  3. Chronic sputum production.
  4. Chest wall abnormalities (hyperinflation, "barrel chest," protruding abdomen).
  5. Flattening of diaphragm.
- Systemic manifestations and comorbidities of COPD are described in Table 1.
- Acute exacerbation of COPD is mainly a clinical diagnosis and generally manifests with worsening dyspnea, increase in sputum purulence, and increase in sputum volume. Respiratory symptom status, however, is not a reliable indicator of the presence of airflow obstruction. Individuals with normal spirometry values may report respiratory symptoms, whereas individuals who have severe to very severe airflow obstruction by spirometry may report no symptoms. Individuals with sedentary lifestyles may underestimate their symptoms and careful history taking is important to elicit symptoms suggestive of COPD.

ETIOLOGY

- Tobacco exposure (Fig. E1)
- Occupational exposure to pulmonary toxins (e.g., dust, noxious gases, vapors, fumes, cadmium, coal, silica); the industries with the highest exposure risk are plastics, leather, rubber, and textiles
- Atmospheric pollution
- Alpha-1-antitrypsin deficiency (rare; <1% of COPD patients) (see "Alpha-1-Antitrypsin Deficiency" chapter)

DIAGNOSIS

DIFFERENTIAL DIAGNOSIS

- Heart failure (HF)
- Asthma
- Tuberculosis, other respiratory infections
- Bronchiectasis
- Anemia
- Cystic fibrosis
- Neoplasm
- Pulmonary embolism
- Obliterative bronchiolitis
- Diffuse panbronchiolitis
- Sleep apnea, obstructive
- Hypothyroidism <50% predicted
- Neuromuscular disease

DIAGNOSTIC WORKUP

- Chest x-ray is seldom diagnostic but useful to visualize significant hyperinflation and to exclude alternative diagnosis (e.g., CHF, TB).
- Pulmonary function testing (spirometry). Spirometry is the reference standard for diagnosing and assessing the severity of COPD. Measurement of airflow limitation (by forced expiratory volume in 1 second [FEV_1]) is recommended to confirm diagnosis and establish prognosis.
- Oxygen saturation and arterial blood gases (useful in selected patients with FEV_1 <50% predicted, with acute exacerbation or hypoxia by pulse oximetry).
- Alpha-1-antitrypsin: All patients with COPD should be screened one time for alpha-1 antitrypsin deficiency.

LABORATORY TESTS

- CBC: Generally not helpful, may reveal leukocytosis with left shift during acute

TABLE 1 Systemic Manifestations and Comorbidities of COPD

Cardiovascular	Infarction Arrhythmia Congestive heart failure Aortic aneurysm
Hypercoagulability	Stroke Pulmonary embolism Deep vein thrombosis Atrophy
Systemic	Weight loss Osteoporosis Skin wrinkling Anemia Fluid retention
Lung cancer	Depression

From Mason RJ: *Murray & Nadel's textbook of respiratory medicine*, ed 5, Philadelphia, 2010, Saunders.

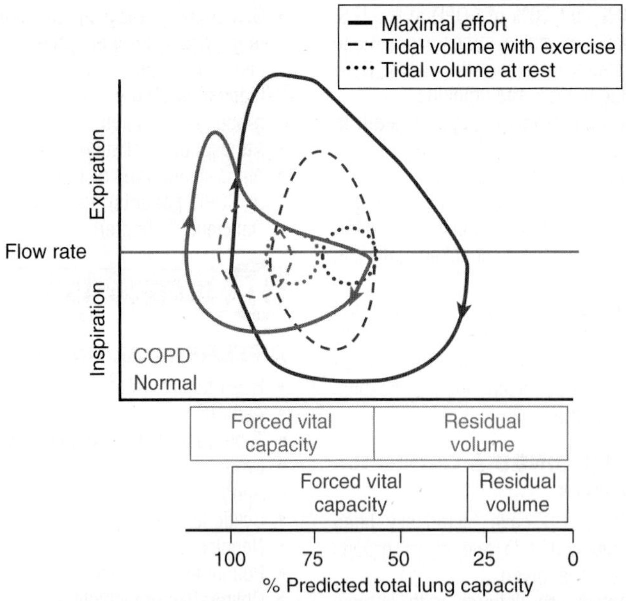

FIG. 2 Representative flow-volume loops in normal subjects (red) and COPD (blue). Flow-volume tracings are shown at rest, with exercise (dashed lines), and with maximal effort. The normal tracings demonstrate that the metabolic demands generated by exercise can be met with increased tidal volumes and frequency without reaching flow limitation, and that lung volumes do not change. In contrast, the patient with COPD has flow limitation during tidal breathing. Increasing tidal volumes and frequency limit expiratory time, and the flow limitation results in a failure to reach resting end-expiratory lung volume. The resulting increases in lung volumes, termed dynamic hyperinflation, are associated with an increased work of breathing and, hence, dyspnea. *COPD,* Chronic obstructive pulmonary disease; *mMRC,* modified Medical Research Council Dyspnea Score; *CAT,* COPD Assessment Test; *FEV_1,* forced expiratory volume in 1 second; *FVC,* forced vital capacity. (From Goldman L, Shafer AI: *Goldman-Cecil medicine*, ed 26, 2019.)

TABLE 2 Stage and Severity of COPD According to Postbronchodilator Spirometry

GOLD Stage and Severity	Definition
I: Mild	FEV_1/FVC <0.70, FEV_1 ≥80% of predicted
II: Moderate	FEV_1/FVC <0.70, 50% ≤ FEV_1 <80% of predicted
III: Severe	FEV_1/FVC <0.70, 30% ≤ FEV_1 <50% of predicted
IV: Very severe	FEV_1/FVC <0.70, FEV_1 <30% of predicted or FEV_1 <50% of predicted plus chronic respiratory failure

COPD, Chronic obstructive pulmonary disease; *FEV_1,* forced expiratory volume in 1 s; *FVC,* forced vital capacity.
Data from the Global Initiative for Chronic Obstructive Lung Disease, 2017 Report.

exacerbation and secondary polycythemia in COPD with significant, chronic hypoxia. Recent trials have shown that eosinophilia in COPD patients predicts response to corticosteroids. Eosinophilia may also be found in an acute exacerbation in Asthma-COPD overlap.

- Sputum may be purulent with bacterial respiratory tract infections. Sputum staining and cultures are usually reserved for cases refractory to antibiotic therapy.
- Arterial blood gases: Normocapnia, mild to moderate hypoxemia may be present. ABGs and pulse oximetry are usually used to determine if a patient is a candidate for long-term oxygen therapy or if hypercapnia is present (ABGs).
- Spirometry pulmonary function testing (PFT) with measurement of forced vital capacity (FVC) and FEV_1. Spirometry should be obtained to diagnose airflow obstruction in clinically stable patients with respiratory symptoms. It should not be used to screen for airflow obstruction in individuals without respiratory symptoms. Spirometry reveals that the primary physiologic abnormality in COPD is an accelerated decline in FEV_1 from the normal rate in adults >30 yr of approximately 30 ml/yr to nearly 60 ml/yr. PFT results in COPD (Fig. 2) reveal abnormal diffusing capacity, increased total lung capacity and/or residual volume, and fixed reduction in FEV_1 in patients with emphysema; normal diffusing capacity and reduced FEV_1 are found in patients with chronic bronchitis. Stage and severity of COPD according to postbronchodilator spirometry are described in Table 2. It is important to note that FEV_1 does not correlate well with individual patients' severity of dyspnea, exercise limitations, or health status. Evaluation of patients should also focus on symptom control and risk for adverse events in addition to FEV_1.
- Patients with COPD can generally be distinguished from asthmatics by their incomplete response to short-acting beta agonist (change in FEV_1 <200 ml and 12%) and absence of an abnormal bronchoconstrictor response to methacholine or other stimuli. Nearly 40% of patients with COPD will, however, respond to bronchodilators. Similarly, patients without a smoking history but with chronic asthmatic bronchitis may have airflow obstruction that is not completely reversible.

ASSESSMENT

The Global Initiative for Chronic Obstructive Lung Disease (GOLD, Fig. 3) assigns patients with COPD into four groups (A, B, C, D) based on (1) the degree of airflow restriction (Table 2), (2) a patient symptom score using one of two symptom questionnaires (CAT or mMRC), or (3) the number of COPD exacerbations in 1 yr.[1]

IMAGING STUDIES

Chest x-ray:

- Hyperinflation with flattened diaphragm, tenting of the diaphragm at the rib, and increased retrosternal chest space (Fig. 4)
- Decreased vascular markings and bullae in patients with emphysema
- Thickened bronchial markings and enlarged right side of the heart in patients with chronic bronchitis
- Computed tomography: Emphysematous lung, tracheobronchomalacia

Rx TREATMENT

NONPHARMACOLOGIC THERAPY

- Smoking cessation and elimination of air pollutants.
- Vaccination (pneumococcal vaccine and annual influenza vaccine).
- Supplemental oxygen, usually through a face mask/nasal cannula, to ensure oxygen saturation >90% as measured by pulse oximetry. Continuous oxygen therapy should be prescribed for patients with COPD who have arterial partial pressure of oxygen 55 mm Hg or less, or oxygen saturation 88% or less as measured by pulse oximetry. In patients with stable COPD and moderate resting desaturation (SpO2 89 to 93%) or moderate exercise-induced moderate desaturation (during the 6-minute walk test, Spo2 ≥80% for ≥5 minutes and <90% for ≥10 seconds), long-term supplemental oxygen did not improve mortality or time to first hospitalization.
- Pulmonary secretion clearance: Careful nasotracheal suction is indicated only in patients with excessive secretions and an inability to expectorate. Mechanical percussion of the chest as applied by a physical or respiratory therapist is ineffective with acute exacerbations of COPD.

[1] Lee H et al: Treatment of stable chronic obstructive pulmonary disease: the GOLD guidelines, *Am Fam Physician* 88(10):655-663, 2013.

- Pulmonary rehabilitation should be considered in COPD patients who remain symptomatic despite optimal medical management. Medicare will cover up to 36 sessions of pulmonary rehabilitation in COPD patients.
- Weight loss in obese patients.
- Identification of depression in patients newly diagnosed with COPD is important, as it may be associated with decreased adherence to maintenance therapy of COPD.
- Use of continuous positive airway pressure (CPAP) in patients with COPD and obstructive sleep apnea, as it improves both survival and reduces hospital admissions.

GENERAL Rx

- Pharmacologic treatment (Table 3) should be administered in a stepwise approach (Fig. 5)

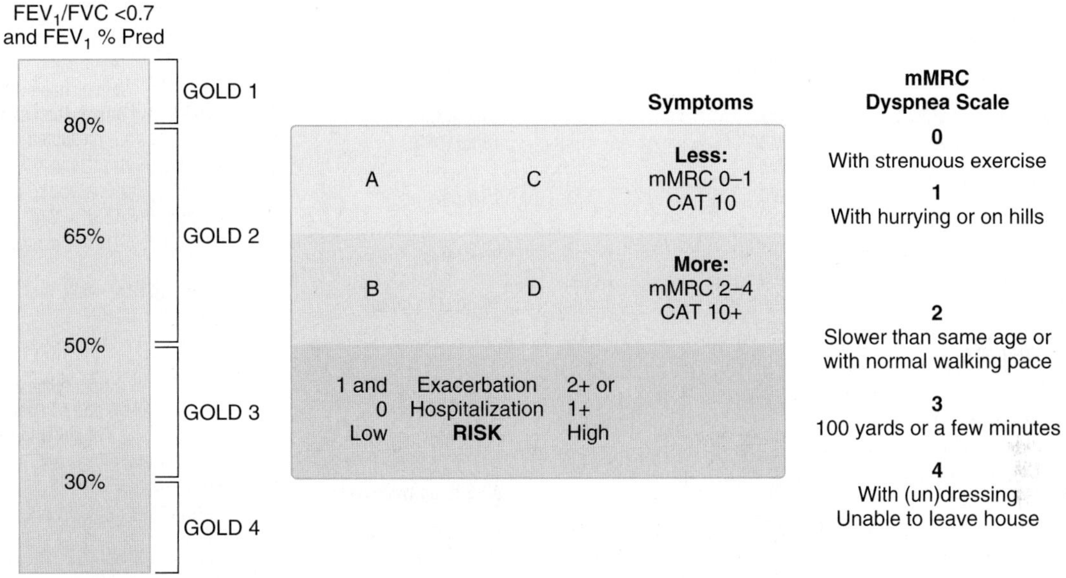

FIG. 3 New GOLD Classification System for COPD. In addition to airflow obstruction (on the left), it incorporates symptoms and risk of exacerbation to create 4 categories: GOLD 1, GOLD 2, GOLD 3, and GOLD 4. These in turn are used to recommend therapy and estimate prognosis. *COPD,* Chronic obstructive pulmonary disease; *mMRC,* modified Medical Research Council Dyspnea Score; *CAT,* COPD Assessment Test; *FEV1,* forced expiratory volume in 1 second; *FVC,* forced vital capacity; *Pred,* predicted. (From Goldman L, Shafer AI: *Goldman-Cecil medicine,* ed 26, 2019.)

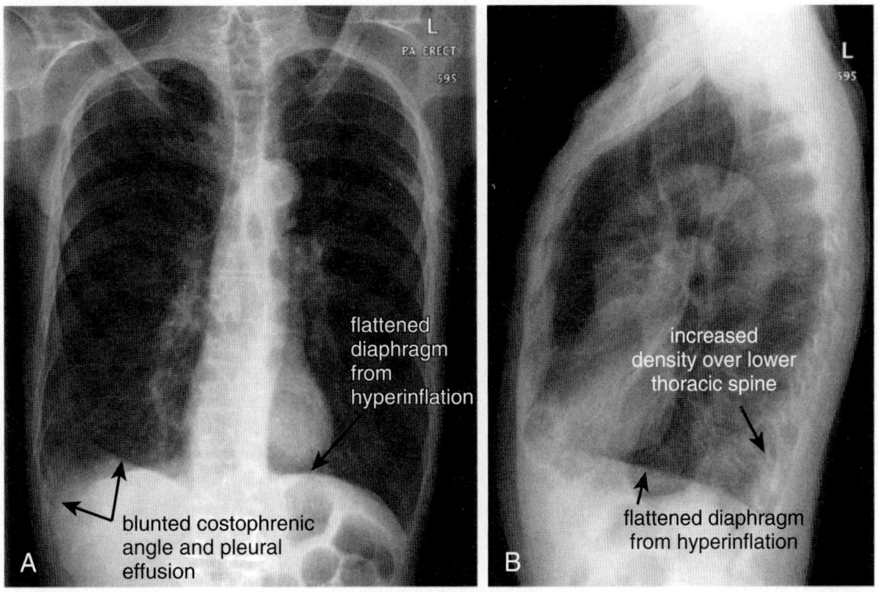

FIG. 4 Chronic obstructive pulmonary disease (COPD). A, Posterior-anterior (PA) upright chest x-ray. **B,** Lateral upright chest x-ray. This 63-yr-old man with a history of COPD presented with 2 wk of worsening cough with yellow sputum and dyspnea. His oxygen saturation was 87% in the emergency room. He has evidence of hyperinflation with flat diaphragm (particularly evident on the lateral x-ray) **(B).** The patient also has a blunted right costophrenic angle with an apparent effusion and increased densities in both the right and the left lung base **(A).** The lateral x-ray also shows increased density overlying the inferior thoracic spine, an abnormal spine sign. (From Broder JS: *Diagnostic imaging for the emergency physician,* Philadelphia, 2011, Saunders.)

TABLE 3 Medications for Chronic Obstructive Pulmonary Diseasen

Drug(s)	Frequency/Formulation	Dosage	Side Effects
β-AGONISTS			
Salmeterol			Palpitations, hypokalemia
Formoterol	BID Nebulizer	20 μg	
Indacaterol			
Olodaterol	QD MDI	5 μg (2.5 μg/puff)	
MUSCARINIC ANTAGONISTS			
Aclidinium bromide	BID DPI	400 μg	Dry mouth Constipation
Tiotropium bromide	QD MDI DPI	5 μg (MDI) 18 μg (DPI)	Aggravation of narrow angle glaucoma
Glycopyrronium	BID DPI	15.6 μg	
Umeclidinium	QD DPI	62.5 μg	
Ipratropium bromide	QID MDI	34 μg (17 μg/puff)	
INHALED CORTICOSTEROIDS			
Fluticasone	BID DPI	88-500 μg	Oropharyngeal candidiasis and hoarseness, and risk of pneumonia
Budesonide	BID or QD Nebulized	0.5-1 mg daily total	
Beclomethasone	BID MDI	40-320 μg twice daily	
Mometasone	QD DPI	220-440 μg	
Flunisolide	BID MDI	220-440 μg twice daily	
PHOSPHODIESTERASE-4 INHIBITORS			
Roflumilast	Pill QD	500 μg	Diarrhea, nausea, and weight loss
COMBINATION INHALERS			
Combination Long-acting β-agonist/Long-acting Muscarinic Antagonist			
Formoterol/glycopyrrolate	BID MDI	9.6 μg formoterol/18 μg glycopyrrolate	Side effects of each constituent
Indacaterol/glycopyrrolate	BID DPI	27.5 μg indacaterol/15.6 μg glycopyrrolate	
Olodaterol/tiotropium	QD MDI	5 μg of each (2 puffs)	
Vilanterol/umeclidinium	QD DPI	25 μg vilanterol/62.5 μg umeclidinium	
Combination Short-acting β Agonist/Short-acting Muscarinic Antagonist			
Albuterol/ipratropium	q4-6 hr	MDI Nebulizer	Side effects of each constituent
Combination Long-acting β Agonist/Inhaled Corticosteroids			
Salmeterol/fluticasone	BID MDI		Side effects of each constituent
Formoterol/budesonide	BID MDI	9 μg formoterol/160-320 μg budesonide (two strengths available)	
Formoterol/mometasone	BID MDI	5 μg formoterol/100 or 200 μg mometasone; 2 inhalations per administration	
Vilanterol/fluticasone	QD DPI	25 μg vilanterol/100 μg fluticasone; one inhalation	
Combination Long-acting β Agonist/Long-acting Muscarinic Antagonist/Inhaled Corticosteroids			
Vilanterol/umeclidinium/fluticasone	QD DPI	25 μg vilanterol/62.5 μg umeclidinium/100 μg fluticasone	Side effects of each constituent

BID, Twice daily; DPI, dry powder inhaler; MDI, metered dose inhaler; QD, once daily.
From Goldman L, Shafer AI. *Goldman-Cecil Medicine*, ed 26, Elsevier, 2020.

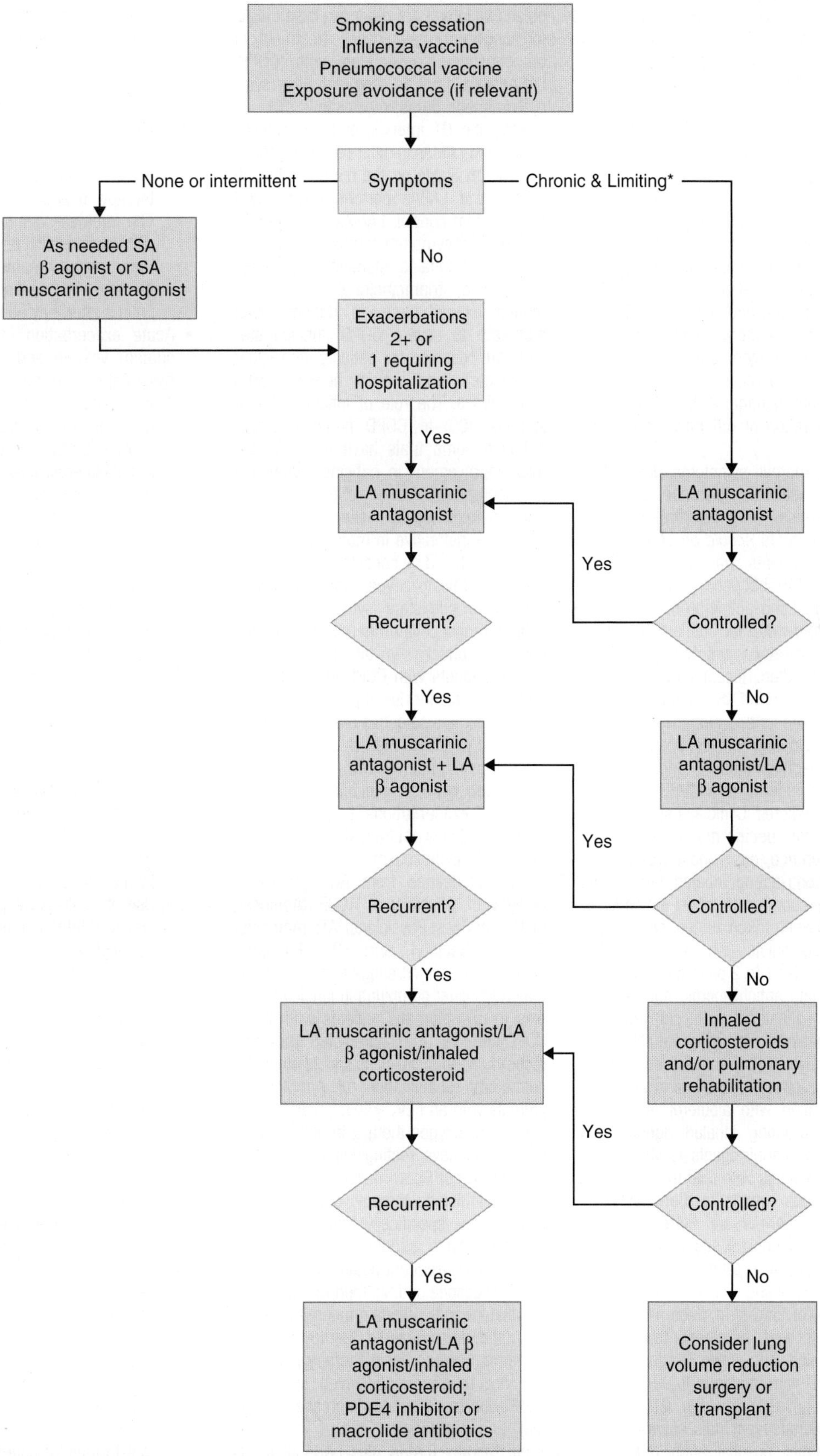

FIG. 5 Approach to the patient with chronic obstructive pulmonary disease. *Dyspnea causes the patient to walk slower than patients of the same age or to stop to catch their breath when walking at their own pace; patient stops for breath after walking 100 yards or less or after a few minutes; or patient is breathless when dressing or housebound due to dyspnea. *COPD*, chronic obstructive pulmonary disease; *LA*, long acting; *PDE*, phosphodiesterase; *SA*, short acting. (From Goldman L, Shafer AI: *Goldman-Cecil medicine*, ed 26, 2019.)

according to the severity of disease and patient's tolerance for specific drugs. When using the GOLD assessment criteria, pulmonary rehabilitation is recommended for patients in groups B, C, and D. Those in group A should receive a short-acting or long-acting anticholinergic or β_2-agonist for mild intermittent symptoms. For patients in group B, long-acting anticholinergics or long-acting β_2-agonists should be added, and both if symptoms persist on one drug. Patients in group C or D are at high risk of exacerbations and should receive a long-acting anticholinergic or a combination of either an inhaled corticosteroid and a long-acting β_2-agonist or a long-acting anticholinergic and long-acting bronchodilator if symptoms persist. Patients in group D are more complicated and require individual management, multiple drugs, and consideration of roflumilast and azithromycin.

1. Bronchodilators improve symptoms, quality of life, and exercise tolerance and decrease incidence of exacerbations. Inhaled bronchodilators *should be offered* for stable COPD patients with respiratory symptoms and FEV[1] between 60% and 80% of predicted. Long-acting bronchodilators are *recommended* for stable COPD patients with respiratory symptoms and FEV_1 <60% of predicted. Recent guidelines from ACP, ACCP, ATS, and ERS recommend that clinicians prescribe monotherapy using either long-acting inhaled anticholinergics or long-acting inhaled β-agonists for symptomatic patients with COPD and FEV_1 <60% of predicted. Clinicians should base the choice of specific monotherapy on patient preference, cost, and adverse effect profile. Long-acting inhaled bronchodilators are superior to short-acting bronchodilators when taken as needed.
2. Short-acting β_2-agonists (e.g., albuterol metered-dose inhaler 1 to 2 puffs q4 to 6h prn) or short-acting anticholinergic agents (e.g., ipratropium inhaler 2 puffs qid) are acceptable in patients with mild, variable symptoms. Anticholinergics (antimuscarinic agents) are also effective and are available in combination with albuterol (e.g., Combivent). Long-acting inhaled agents (long-acting antimuscarinic agents [LAMAs]) are preferred in patients with mild to moderate or continuous symptoms. Currently available inhaled LAMAs are tiotropium (Spiriva), aclidinium (Tudorza), and glycopyrrolate (Seebri Neohaler, Yupelri). Tiotropium is an excellent long-acting bronchodilator. It is very effective for long-term, once-a-day use. It has been shown to be superior to salmeterol, an inhaled long-acting β-agonist (LABA) in patients with moderate to severe COPD and may possibly slow the rate of decline in FEV_1. Some recent trials, however, have shown higher hospitalization rates and mortality with tiotropium compared to LABAs. Indacaterol, umeclidinium, olodaterol, and vilanterol are other available LABAs for long-term maintenance treatment of bronchospasm associated with COPD. LABAs should not be used with other sympathomimetic drugs, medications that can prolong the QT interval, or beta-blockers. LABAs and LAMAs in different combinations are now available on the market. Although LAMAs and LABAs perform equally well for symptom control, LAMAs are generally preferred for symptom control.
3. Addition of inhaled steroids (fluticasone, budesonide, triamcinolone) is used to reduce exacerbations in patients with moderate to severe COPD. Inhaled steroids are reserved for patients with either ≥2 exacerbations annually or FEV_1 <50% of predicted. The role of inhaled corticosteroids (ICS) in COPD is controversial. Although some trials have demonstrated mild improvement in patients' symptoms and decreased frequency of exacerbations, most pulmonologists believe that these drugs are ineffective in most patients with COPD but should be considered for patients with moderate to severe airflow limitation who have persistent symptoms despite optimal bronchodilator therapy. ICS therapy does not affect 1-yr all-cause mortality among patients with COPD and is associated with a higher risk of pneumonia.
4. Roflumilast is a selective oral PDE4 inhibitor useful to reduce the risk of COPD exacerbations in patients with severe COPD associated with chronic bronchitis and a history of exacerbations. It is not a bronchodilator and is not indicated for the relief of acute bronchospasm.
5. Recent guidelines from ACP (American College of Physicians), ACCP (American College of Chest Physicians), ATS (American Thoracic Society), and ERS (European Respiratory Society) suggest that clinicians may administer combination inhaled therapies for symptomatic patients with stable COPD and FEV_1 <60% predicted. They also recommend that clinicians should prescribe pulmonary rehabilitation for symptomatic patients with an FEV_1 <50% predicted and continuous oxygen therapy in patients with COPD who have resting hypoxemia (Pa_{O_2} <55 mm Hg or Sp_{O_2} <88%).
6. Chronic antibiotic therapy: Chronic antibiotic therapy, specifically macrolides such as azithromycin, should be considered in patients with frequent acute exacerbations of COPD despite optimal therapy with bronchodilators and antiinflammatory agents.
7. Systemic glucocorticoid therapy: Chronic systemic glucocorticoid therapy is generally not recommended even in severe COPD due to associated increase in mortality and morbidity.
8. Triple therapy (LAMA plus LABA plus ICS [e.g., vilanterol, umeclidinium, and fluticasone {Trelegy Ellipta}]): Indicated in patients with COPD at high risk for exacerbations. A double-blind, parallel group, RCT (TRINITY) reported that treatment with extrafine fixed triple therapy reduced rates of moderate-to-severe exacerbation and improved baseline FEV_1 at 52 wk as compared with tiotropium in patients with symptomatic COPD, FEV_1 <50%, and a history of exacerbations. Another double-blind RCT (FULFIL) reported similar benefits of single-inhaler triple therapy compared with ICS/LABA therapy in patients with advanced COPD. The greatest benefit occurs in patients with eosinophilia or concomitant asthma. Unfortunately, many patients start triple therapy without clear indications and continue it after they no longer need it.

- Acute exacerbation of COPD (increase in sputum volume and purulence, worsening dyspnea) can be treated with:
  1. Aerosolized β_2-agonists (e.g., metaproterenol nebulizer solution 5% 0.3 ml or albuterol nebulized 5% solution 2.5-5 mg).
  2. Anticholinergic agents, which have equivalent efficacy to inhaled beta-adrenergic agonists. Inhalant solution of ipratropium bromide 0.5 mg can be administered every 4 to 8 hr.
  3. Short courses of systemic corticosteroids have been shown to improve spirometric and clinical outcomes. Treatment failure occurs less often in patients who receive low-dose steroids than in those receiving high-dose parenteral steroids. Oral prednisone 40 mg/day for 5 to 14 days is generally effective. Courses of treatment that are extended for >14 days confer no added benefit and increase the risk of adverse events. Trials have shown that in patients with acute COPD exacerbations, systemic glucocorticoid treatment for 5 days is not inferior to treatment for 14 days.
  4. Use of noninvasive positive pressure ventilation (NIPPV) decreases the risk of endotracheal intubation and decreases intensive care unit admission rates. Contraindications to its use are uncooperative patient, decreased level of consciousness, hemodynamic instability, inadequate mask fit, and severe respiratory acidosis. Increased airway pressure can be delivered by using inspiratory positive airway pressure, continuous positive airway pressure, or bilevel positive airway pressure, which combines the other modalities. When using NIPPV, the nasal mask is usually tolerated the best; however, patients must be instructed to keep their mouths closed while breathing with the nasal apparatus. Oxygen can be delivered at 10 to 15 L/min and started in spontaneous ventilation mode with an initial expiratory positive airway pressure setting of 3 to 5 cm H_2O and an inspiratory positive airway pressure setting of up to 10 cm H_2O. Adjustments in these settings should be made in 2-cm H_2O increments. It is important to monitor patients with frequent vital signs measurements, arterial blood gases, or pulse oximetry. Intubation and mechanical ventilation may be necessary if previous measures fail to provide improvement.

[1] Riley CM, Sciurba FC: Diagnosis and outpatient management of chronic obstructive pulmonary disease: a review, *JAMA* 321(8):786-797, 2019.

5. IV aminophylline administration is controversial and generally not recommended. When used in patients with refractory symptoms, serum levels should be closely monitored (keep level 8-12 mcg/ml) to minimize risks of tachyarrhythmias.

- Approximately 50% of COPD exacerbations are caused by bacterial infection. Antibiotics are indicated in suspected bacterial respiratory infection (e.g., increased purulence and volume of phlegm).
    1. *Haemophilus influenzae* and *Streptococcus pneumoniae* are frequent causes of acute bronchitis.
    2. Oral antibiotics of choice are azithromycin, levofloxacin, amoxicillin-clavulanate, trimethoprim-sulfamethoxazole, doxycycline, and cefuroxime.
    3. The two best predictors of potential benefit from antibiotics are purulent sputum and C-reactive protein (CRP) level >40 mg/L.
    4. Procalcitonin-based protocols to trigger antibiotic use are associated with significantly decreased antibiotic use without affecting clinical outcomes such hospital length of stay, treatment failure, and mortality.
- Guaifenesin may improve cough symptoms and mucus clearance; however, mucolytic medications are generally ineffective. Their benefits may be greatest in patients with more advanced disease.
- Fig. 6 illustrates the management of acute exacerbations of COPD. Guideline recommendations for hospital management of

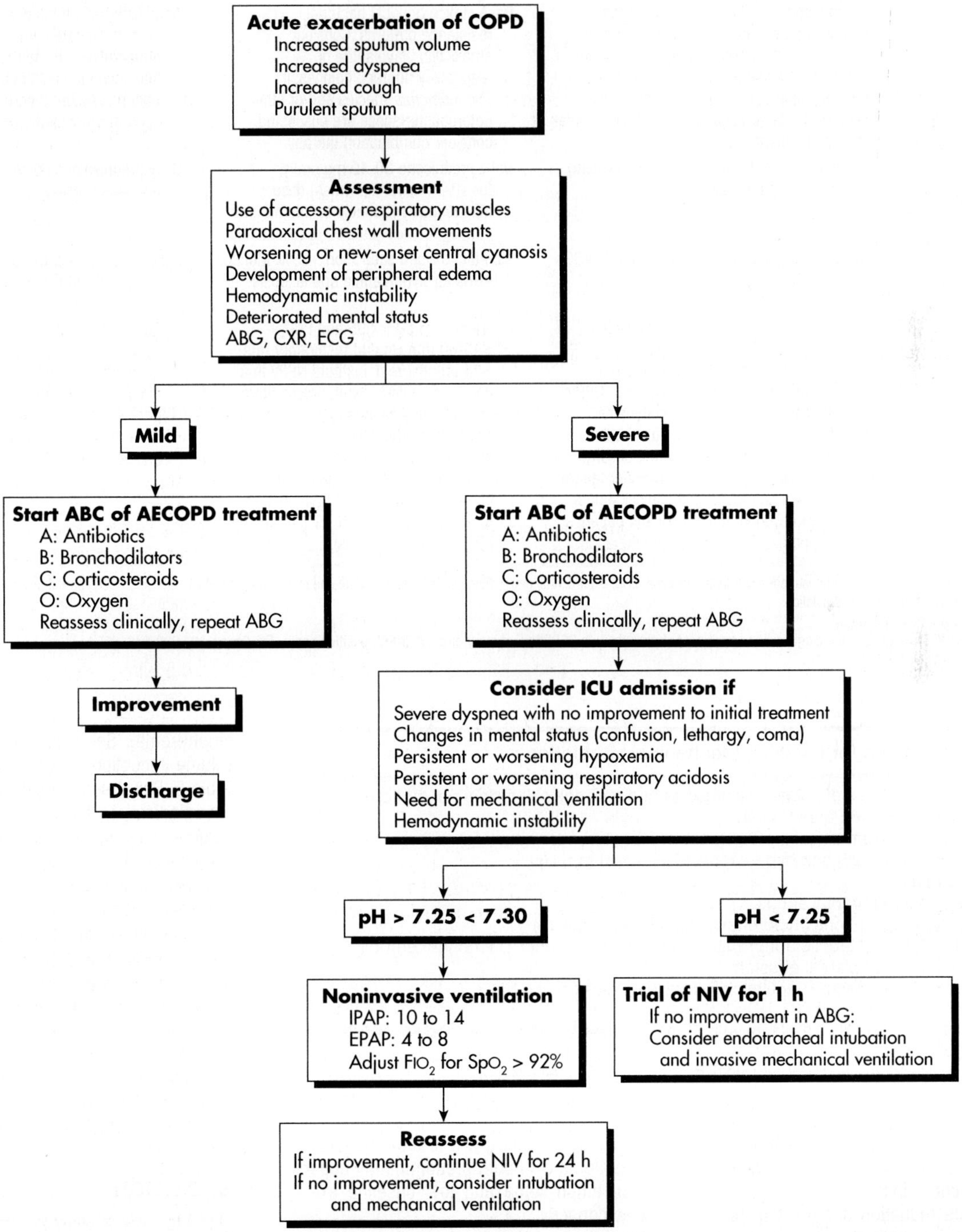

FIG. 6 Management of acute exacerbations of chronic obstructive pulmonary disease. *ABG,* Arterial blood gase; *AECOPD,* acute exacerbations of chronic obstructive pulmonary disease; *COPD,* chronic obstructive pulmonary disease; *CXR,* chest x-ray; *ECG,* electrocardiogram; *EPAP,* expiratory positive airway pressure; *FIO_2,* fraction of inspired oxygen; *ICU,* intensive care unit; *IPAP,* inspiratory positive airway pressure; *NIV,* noninvasive ventilation; *SpO_2,* oxygen saturation measured by pulse oximetry. (From Parrillo JE, Dellinger RP: *Critical care medicine: principles of diagnosis and management in the adult,* ed 5, Philadelphia, 2019, Elsevier.)

TABLE 4 Guideline Recommendations for Hospital Management of COPD Exacerbations

	Global Initiative for Chronic Obstructive Lung Disease*	American Thoracic Society/ European Respiratory Society†	National Institute for Clinical Excellence‡
Date of statement	2017	2017	2010
Diagnostic testing	Chest radiograph, oximetry, ABGs, ECG. Other testing as warranted by clinical indication.	Chest radiograph, oxygen saturation, ABGs, ECG, sputum Gram stain and culture.	Chest radiograph, ABG, ECG, complete blood count, sputum smear and culture, blood cultures if febrile.
Bronchodilator therapy	Inhaled short-acting β_2-agonist is recommended. Consider ipratropium if inadequate clinical response. Methylxanthines are not recommended due to increased side effect profiles.	Inhaled short-acting β_2-agonist and/or ipratropium with spacer or nebulizer, as needed.	Administer inhaled drugs by nebulizer or handheld inhaler. Specific agents and dosing regimens not specified. Consider theophylline if inadequate response to inhaled bronchodilators.
Antibiotics	Recommended if (1) increases in dyspnea, sputum volume, and sputum purulence all are present; (2) increase in sputum purulence along with increase in either dyspnea or sputum volume; or (3) need for assisted ventilation. See original document for complex treatment algorithm.	Base choice on local bacterial resistance patterns. Consider amoxicillin/clavulanate or respiratory fluoroquinolones. If *Pseudomonas* species and/or other Enterobacteriaceae are suspected, consider combination therapy.	Administer only if history of purulent sputum. Initiate with an aminopenicillin, a macrolide, or a tetracycline, taking into account local bacterial resistance patterns. Adjust therapy according to sputum and blood cultures.
Systemic corticosteroids	Daily prednisolone 30-40 mg (or its equivalent) orally for not more than 5-7 days.	Daily prednisone 30-40 mg orally for 10-14 days. Equivalent dose intravenously if unable to tolerate oral intake. Consider inhaled corticosteroids.	Daily prednisolone 30 mg (or its equivalent) orally for 7-14 days.
Supplemental oxygen	Maintain oxygen saturation >90%. Monitor ABGs for hypercapnia and acidosis.	Maintain oxygen saturation >90%. Monitor ABGs for hypercapnia and acidosis.	Maintain oxygen saturation within the individualized target range. Monitor ABGs.
Assisted ventilation	Indications for NPPV include severe dyspnea, acidosis (pH ≤7.35) and/or hypercapnia (PCO_2 >45 mm Hg), and respiratory rate >25 breaths/min. Contraindications to NPPV include respiratory arrest, hemodynamic instability, impaired mental status, copious bronchial secretions, and extreme obesity. Intubate if contraindication to NPPV or failure of NPPV (worsening ABGs or clinical status). Consider likelihood of recovery and patient's wishes and expectations before intubation.	Consider with pH <7.35 and PCO_2 >45-60 mm Hg and respiratory rate >24 breaths/min. Institute NPPV in a controlled environment, unless there are contraindications (e.g., respiratory arrest, hemodynamic instability, impaired mental status, copious bronchial secretions, and extreme obesity). Intubate if contraindication to NPPV or failure of NPPV (worsening ABGs or clinical status).	NPPV treatment of choice for persistent hypercapnic respiratory failure. Consider functional status, body mass index, home oxygen, comorbidities, prior ICU admissions, age, and FEV_1 when assessing suitability for intubation and ventilation.

ABGs, Arterial blood gases; *COPD,* chronic obstructive pulmonary disease; *ECG,* electrocardiogram; *FEV_1,* forced expiratory volume in 1 s; *ICU,* intensive care unit; *PCO2,* partial pressure of carbon dioxide; *NPPV,* noninvasive positive pressure ventilation.
*Data from https://www.goldcopd.org.
†Data from MacNee W: Standards for the diagnosis and treatment of patients with COPD: a summary of the ATS/ERS position paper, *Eur Respir J* 23:932-946, 2004.
‡Data from https://www.nice.org.uk.

BOX 1 Indications for Invasive Mechanical Ventilation

Severe dyspnea, with use of accessory muscles and paradoxical abdominal motion
Respiratory frequency >35 breaths/min
Life-threatening hypoxemia (Pao_2 <40 mm Hg or Pao_2/Fio_2 <200 mm Hg)
Severe acidosis (pH <7.25) and hypercapnia ($Paco_2$ >60 mm Hg)
Respiratory arrest
Somnolence, impaired mental status
Cardiovascular complications (hypotension, shock, heart failure)
Other complications: Metabolic abnormalities, sepsis, pneumonia, pulmonary embolism, barotrauma, massive pleural effusion
Noninvasive positive-pressure ventilation failure (or exclusion criteria)

Fio_2, Inspired oxygen fraction; *$Paco_2$,* partial pressure of carbon dioxide in arterial blood; *Pao_2,* partial pressure of oxygen in arterial blood.
From Vincent JL et al: *Textbook of critical care*, ed 6, Philadelphia, 2011, Saunders.

COPD exacerbations are described in Table 4. Indications for invasive mechanical ventilation are described in Box 1.

- Lung volume reduction surgery has been proposed as a palliative treatment for severe emphysema. Overall it increases the chance of improved exercise capacity but does not confer a survival advantage over medical therapy. It is most beneficial in patients with both predominantly upper-lobe emphysema and low baseline exercise capacity.
- Preliminary trials involving lung volume reduction using bronchoscopic treatment with nitinol coils have shown improved exercise capacity in patients with severe emphysema. Selection criteria for lung volume reduction surgery is described in Table 5. Box 2 summarizes indications and contraindications for lung volume reduction surgery and lung transplantation.
- Endobronchial valve (EBV) placement (Zephyr valve) via bronchoscopy to reduce lung volume with one-way valves that are allowed to leave but not enter a lung segment is now FDA approved since June 2018.
- Single-lung transplantation (Box 2) should be considered a surgical option in patients with end-stage emphysema who have an FEV_1 <25% of predicted normal value after administration of bronchodilator and additional complications such as severe hypoxemia, hypercapnia, and pulmonary hypertension.

DISPOSITION

- After the initial episode of respiratory failure, 5-yr survival is approximately 25%.
- Development of cor pulmonale or hypercapnia and persistent tachycardia are poor prognostic indicators.

TABLE 5 Selection Criteria for Lung Volume Reduction Surgery

Inclusion Criteria	Exclusion Criteria
General	
Disability despite maximal rehabilitation	Inability to participate in rehabilitation
Cessation of tobacco use >6 mo	Continued use of tobacco
Patient's expectation of goals reasonable	Significant comorbidity Previous pleurodesis or thoracotomy
	Underweight, overweight
Anatomic-Radiographic Evaluation	
Marked emphysema	Bronchiectasis
	Minimal radiographic emphysema
Heterogeneously distributed emphysema	Homogeneously distributed emphysema
Target zones of poorly perfused lung	No target zones
Areas with better preserved lung	No preserved lung tissue
Marked thoracic hyperinflation	Chest wall or thoracic cage abnormalities
Physiologic Evaluation	
Marked airflow obstruction	Minimal to moderate airflow obstruction
Marked hyperinflation	Minimal to moderate thoracic hyperinflation
Alveolar gas exchange	Markedly disordered alveolar gas exchange
DL_{co} <50% (steady state)	DL_{co} <10%
	$Paco_2$ >60 mm Hg
Cardiovascular function	Cardiovascular function
Essentially normal ejection fraction	Mean pulmonary artery pressure >35 mm Hg
	Left ventricular ejection fraction <40%
	Significant coronary artery disease

DL_{co}, Diffusing capacity of the lungs for carbon monoxide; *$Paco_2$*, partial pressure of carbon dioxide in arterial blood.
From Sellke FW et al: *Sabiston & Spencer surgery of the chest*, ed 9, Philadelphia, 2016, Elsevier.

BOX 2 Indications and Contraindications for Lung Volume Reduction Surgery and Lung Transplantation

Indications Common to Both Procedures
Emphysema with destruction and hyperinflation
Marked impairment (FEV_1 <35% predicted)
Marked restriction in activities of daily living
Failure of maximal medical treatment to correct symptoms

Contraindications to Both Procedures
Abnormal body weight (<70% or >130% of ideal)
Coexisting major medical problems increasing surgical risk
Inability or unwillingness to participate in pulmonary rehabilitation
Unwillingness to accept the risk of morbidity and mortality of surgery
Tobacco use within the past 6 mo
Recent or current diagnosis of malignant disease
Increasing age (>65 yr for transplantation, >70 yr for volume reduction)
Psychological instability, such as depression or anxiety disorder

Discriminating Conditions Favoring Lung Volume Reduction Surgery
Marked thoracic distention
Heterogeneous disease with obvious apical target areas
FEV_1 >20% predicted
Age between 60 and 70 yr

Discriminating Conditions Favoring Lung Transplantation
Diffuse disease without target areas
FEV_1 <20% predicted
Hypercapnia with $Paco_2$ >55 mm Hg
Pulmonary hypertension
Age younger than 60 yr
α_1-Antitrypsin deficiency

FEV_1, Forced expiratory volume in 1 s.
From Sellke FW et al: *Sabiston & Spencer surgery of the chest*, ed 9, Philadelphia, 2016, Elsevier.

- Supplemental oxygen for patients with resting hypoxemia (defined as SPO_2 <89%) improves survival. The need for oxygen at rest may be the strongest predictor of mortality in chronic respiratory failure from COPD.
- Pulmonary rehabilitation, which includes strength and endurance training and education, nutritional, and psychosocial support, improves symptoms and exercise tolerance but is underutilized.[1]

PEARLS & CONSIDERATIONS

COMMENTS

- All patients with COPD should receive pneumococcal vaccine and yearly influenza vaccine.
- Early antibiotic administration is associated with improved outcomes among patients hospitalized for acute exacerbations of COPD regardless of the risk of treatment failure.
- In assessing the severity of COPD, the FEV_1 is limited by the fact that it does not take into account the systemic manifestations of COPD. The BODE index (body mass index, degree of obstruction, dyspnea, and exercise capacity) has been proposed as a multidimensional scale to better assess the morbidity and mortality associated with COPD. It is better than the FEV_1 alone at predicting the risk of death from any cause and from respiratory causes among patients with COPD. In the BODE index, obstruction is measured by FEV_1 and dyspnea is measured by the modified Medical Research Council (MMRC) dyspnea questionnaire in a 6-minute walk test. A score of 0 on the MMRC indicates that the individual is not troubled with breathlessness except with strenuous exercise, 1 indicates shortness of breath when hurrying or walking up a slight hill, and 2 means the individual walks slower than people of the same age due to breathlessness or has to stop for breath when walking at own pace on level ground. A score of 3 means severe dyspnea because the person has to stop for breath after walking approximately 100 meters or after a few minutes on level ground, and a score of 4 indicates very severe dyspnea and is given when the individual is too breathless to leave the house or is breathless when dressing or undressing.
- Pulmonary artery enlargement as determined by a ratio of the diameter of the pulmonary artery to the diameter of the aorta [PA:A ratio] of >1 detected by CT is associated with severe exacerbations of COPD.
- The average person with COPD has one or two acute exacerbations each yr. Prophylactic use of macrolide antibiotics (azithromycin 250 mg/day) has been shown to decrease the frequency of exacerbations and improve quality of life among selected patients with COPD; however, it leads to hearing decrements in a

small percentage of patients and increased prevalence of macrolide-resistant bacteria colonizing the airway and is therefore not recommended.
- Eosinophilic airway inflammation may contribute to COPD exacerbations. Patients with COPD with eosinophilic phenotype may benefit from mepolizumab, a monoclonal antibody directed against interleukin-5.
- Current and former smokers (within 15 yr) with at least a 30-pack-yr history of smoking should be assessed for lung cancer using low-dose computed tomography.

SUGGESTED READINGS

Available at ExpertConsult.com

RELATED CONTENT

Chronic Obstructive Pulmonary Disease (Patient Information)
Emphysema (Patient Information)
Alpha-1-Antitrypsin Deficiency (Related Key Topic)
Asthma-COPD Overlap (Related Key Topic)

AUTHORS: **Aline N. Zouk, MD**

BASIC INFORMATION

DEFINITION

Chronic pancreatitis is a recurrent or persistent inflammatory process of the pancreas characterized by chronic pain and by pancreatic exocrine and/or endocrine insufficiency. It is classified anatomically as either large-duct disease or small-duct (minimal change) disease.

ICD-10CM CODES
K86.1 Other chronic pancreatitis
K86.0 Alcohol-induced chronic pancreatitis

EPIDEMIOLOGY & DEMOGRAPHICS

- Chronic pancreatitis occurs in approximately five to 10 per 100,000 persons in industrialized countries.
- Average age at diagnosis is 35 to 55 yr; male:female ratio is 5:1.

PHYSICAL FINDINGS & CLINICAL PRESENTATION

- Persistent or recurrent epigastric and left upper quadrant pain that may radiate to the back
- Tenderness over the pancreas, muscle guarding
- Significant weight loss
- Bulky, foul-smelling stools, greasy in appearance
- Epigastric mass (10% of patients)
- Jaundice (5%-10% of patients)

ETIOLOGY

- Chronic alcoholism (most common cause)
- Obstruction (ampullary stenosis, tumor, trauma [with pancreatic duct stricture], pancreas divisum, annular pancreas)
- Tobacco
- Recurrent pancreatitis
- Vascular disease/ischemia
- Hypertriglyceridemia
- Chronic kidney disease
- Hereditary pancreatitis
- Severe malnutrition
- Idiopathic
- Untreated hyperparathyroidism (hypercalcemia)
- Mutations of the cystic fibrosis transmembrane conductance regulator *(CFTR)* gene and the TF genotype
- Other genetic mutations (Cationic trypsinogen gene, chymotrypsinogen C gene, calcium-sensing receptor gene, claudin-2 gene, serine protease inhibitor, Kazal type 1 gene)
- ***Autoimmune pancreatitis (AIP):*** (5% of chronic pancreatitis cases): Presents clinically with jaundice (63% of patients) and abdominal pain (35%). CT may reveal diffusely enlarged pancreas, enhanced peripheral rim of hypoattenuation "halo," and low-attenuation mass in head of pancreas. Laboratory values reveal elevated serum immunoglobulin (Ig) G4, elevated serum Ig or gamma-globulin level, presence of antilactoferrin antibody (ALA), anticarbonic anhydrase (ACA) II level, anti–smooth-muscle antibody (ASMA), or antinuclear antibody (ANA)
- ***Sclerosing pancreatitis:*** A form of chronic pancreatitis characterized by infrequent attacks of abdominal pain, irregular narrowing of the pancreatic duct, and swelling of the pancreatic parenchyma; patients have high levels of serum immunoglobulins (IgG4); chronic sclerosing pancreatitis is also known as *autoimmune pancreatitis*

DIAGNOSIS

DIFFERENTIAL DIAGNOSIS

- Pancreatic cancer
- Peptic ulcer disease
- Cholelithiasis with biliary obstruction
- Malabsorption from other etiologies
- Recurrent acute pancreatitis
- Renal insufficiency
- Intestinal ischemia or infarction
- Other: Crohn disease, gastroparesis, inflammatory bowel disease

WORKUP

Medical history with focus on alcohol use, laboratory tests, diagnostic imaging. Table 1 summarizes available diagnostic tests for chronic pancreatitis.

LABORATORY TESTS

- Serum amylase and lipase may be elevated (normal amylase levels, however, do not exclude the diagnosis).
- Hyperglycemia, glycosuria, hyperbilirubinemia, and elevated serum alkaline phosphatase may also be present.
- 72-hr fecal fat determination (rarely performed) reveals excess fecal fat. Fecal elastase test requires only 20 g of stool.
- Secretin stimulation test is the best test for diagnosing pancreatic exocrine insufficiency. Pancreatic secretory function tests are summarized in Table 2.
- Lipid panel: Significantly elevated triglycerides can cause pancreatitis.
- Serum calcium: Hyperparathyroidism is a rare cause of chronic pancreatitis.
- Elevated levels of serum IgG4 are found in sclerosing pancreatitis and AIP.
- Elevated serum Ig or gamma-globulin level, presence of ALA, ACA II level, ASMA, or ANA in AIP.

IMAGING STUDIES

- Plain abdominal radiographs may reveal pancreatic calcifications (Fig. 1) in 25% of patients (95% specific for chronic pancreatitis).
- Ultrasound of abdomen may reveal duct dilation, pseudocyst, calcification, and presence of ascites.
- Contrast-enhanced CT scan of abdomen is the initial modality of choice. It is useful to detect calcifications (Fig. E2), evaluate for ductal dilation (Fig. E3), AIP, and rule out pancreatic cancer. CT in AIP reveals narrowed main pancreatic duct and a homogenous "sausage-shaped" pancreas.
- Endoscopic retrograde cholangiopancreatography (ERCP) (Fig. E4) had been traditionally used to evaluate for the presence of dilated ducts, strictures, pseudocysts, and intraductal stones. However, for the evaluation of pancreatic parenchyma and duct system newer, less invasive modalities such as magnetic resonance cholangiopancreatography and endoscopic ultrasonography (EUS) are preferred. EUS (Fig. E5) has a sensitivity of 97% and a specificity of 60% for chronic pancreatitis and a very low complication rate. The diagnosis of chronic pancreatitis on EUS is summarized in Table E3. Fine-needle aspiration biopsy combined with EUS is the preferred modality for evaluation of cystic or mass lesions to determine malignancy.

TABLE 1 Available Diagnostic Tests for Chronic Pancreatitis

Tests of Pancreatic Structure	Tests of Pancreatic Function
EUS	Direct hormonal stimulation (with pancreatic stimulation by secretin or CCK or both): Using oroduodenal tube* Using endoscopy*
MRI with MRCP, with or without secretin stimulation	Fecal elastase
CT	Serum trypsinogen (trypsin)
ERCP	Fecal chymotrypsin
Abdominal US	Fecal fat
Plain abdominal film	Blood glucose level

*See text for explanations.
Tests are listed in estimated order of decreasing sensitivity for each category.
CCK, Cholecystokinin; *CT*, computed tomography; *ERCP*, endoscopic retrograde cholangiopancreatography; *EUS*, endoscopic ultrasonography; *MRCP*, magnetic resonance cholangiopancreatography; *MRI*, magnetic resonance imaging.
From Feldman M et al: *Sleisenger and Fordtran's gastrointestinal and liver disease*, ed 10, Philadelphia, 2016, Elsevier.

TREATMENT

NONPHARMACOLOGIC THERAPY

- Avoidance of alcohol and tobacco
- Frequent, small-volume, low-fat meals

ACUTE GENERAL Rx

- Avoidance of narcotics if possible (simple analgesics or NSAIDs can be used). Fig. 6 describes an approach to the patient with painful chronic pancreatitis. Management of chronic pancreatitis focuses on treatment of symptoms.
- Treatment of steatorrhea with pancreatic supplements (e.g., Pancrease, Creon, pancrelipase titrated prn based on the amount

TABLE 2 Pancreatic Secretory Function Tests

Test	Description	Advantages	Disadvantages	Clinical Indications
Direct				
Secretin	Measurements of volume and HCO_3- secretion into the duodenum after IV secretin	Provide the most sensitive and specific measurements of exocrine pancreatic function	Require duodenal intubation and IV administration of hormones; not widely available	Detection of mild, moderate, or severe exocrine pancreatic dysfunction
CCK	Measurements of duodenal outputs of amylase, trypsin, chymotrypsin, and/or lipase after IV CCK			
Secretin and CCK	Measurements of volume, HCO_3-, and enzymes after IV secretin and CCK			
Indirect (Requiring Duodenal Intubation)				
Lundh test meal	Measurement of duodenal trypsin concentration after oral ingestion of a test meal	Does not require IV administration of hormones	Requires duodenal intubation, a test meal, and normal anatomy, including small intestinal mucosa; not widely available	Detection of moderate or severe exocrine pancreatic dysfunction when a direct test cannot be done (e.g., due to limited availability)
Indirect (Tubeless)				
Fecal fat	Measurement of fat in the stool after ingesting meals with a known amount of fat	Provides a quantitative measurement of steatorrhea	Requires sufficient dietary fat intake and collection of stool; only detects severe pancreatic dysfunction	Detection of severe exocrine pancreatic dysfunction and steatorrhea
Fecal chymotrypsin Fecal elastase 1	Measurement of chymotrypsin or elastase 1 in the stool	Do not require IVs, tubes, or administration of oral substrates	Insensitive for detecting mild or moderate dysfunction	Detection of severe exocrine pancreatic dysfunction
NBT-PABA Fluorescein dilaurate	Oral ingestion of NBT-PABA or fluorescein dilaurate with a meal, followed by measurements of PABA or fluorescein in serum or urine	Provide simple measurements for severe pancreatic dysfunction	Do not detect mild or moderate dysfunction; results may be abnormal in patients with small intestinal mucosal disease	Detection of severe exocrine pancreatic dysfunction

CCK, Cholecystokinin; *IV*, intravenous; *NBT-PABA*, *N*-benzoyl-L-tyrosyl-*p*-aminobenzoic acid.
From Feldman M et al: *Sleisenger and Fordtran's gastrointestinal and liver disease*, ed 10, Philadelphia, 2016, Elsevier.

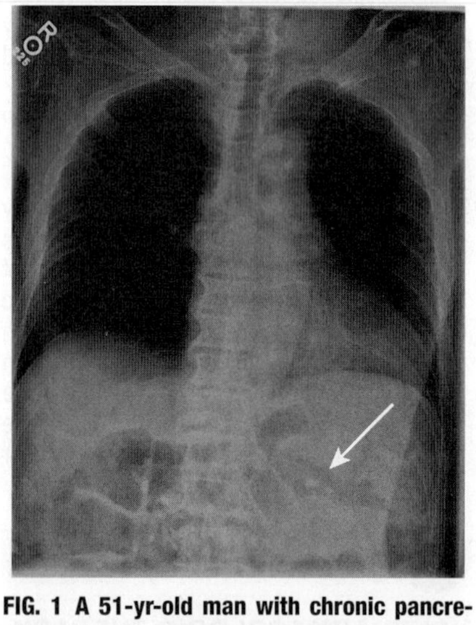

FIG. 1 A 51-yr-old man with chronic pancreatitis. A plain radiograph demonstrates multiple punctate foci of calcification overlying the expected location of the pancreas *(arrow)*, a finding consistent with chronic pancreatitis. (From Soto JA: *Emergency radiology, the requisites*, ed 2, 2017, Elsevier.)

of steatorrhea and patient's weight loss). Enzyme products for the treatment of chronic pancreatitis are summarized in Table 4. All non–enteric-coated enzymes should be used with acid-suppressing medications. Proton pump inhibitors and H_2 blockers reduce inactivation of the enzymes from gastric acid.

- Antioxidants (vitamin A, selenium, vitamin E) may be helpful for pain control in chronic pancreatitis.
- Percutaneous or via EUS celiac plexus blockade with corticosteroids or neurolysis with ethanol may provide temporary pain relief.
- Treatment of complications (e.g., type 1 diabetes mellitus).
- Autoimmune pancreatitis (AIP): Glucocorticoid therapy in patients with AIP and sclerosing pancreatitis can induce clinical remission and significantly decrease serum concentrations of IgG4, immune complexes, and the IgG4 subclass of immune complexes. Starting dose of oral prednisolone is 0.6 to 1.0 mg/kg/day tapered over 3 mo. Recurrent AIP is treated with glucocorticoids and immunomodulators (azathioprine, mycophenolate, mercaptopurine) or rituximab.

CHRONIC Rx

- Surgical intervention (e.g., distal pancreatectomy or pancreaticoduodenectomy) may be necessary in painful chronic pancreatitis to eliminate biliary tract disease and improve flow of bile into the duodenum by eliminating obstruction of pancreatic duct.
- ERCP with endoscopic sphincterectomy and stone extraction and for treatment of pancreatic duct strictures is less invasive and more widely available than surgery and may be preferred as first-line treatment in painful chronic pancreatitis.
- Percutaneous or EUS-guided celiac plexus blockade using glucocorticoids is effective in providing short-term pain relief in nearly half of patients.

DISPOSITION

- Long-term survival is poor (50% of patients die within 10 yr from chronic pancreatitis or malignancy).
- Prognosis is best in patients with recurrent acute pancreatitis resulting from cholelithiasis, hyperparathyroidism, or stenosis of the sphincter of Oddi.

SUGGESTED READINGS

Available at ExpertConsult.com

REFERRAL

Gastrointestinal referral for ERCP, surgical referral in selected patients (see "Chronic Rx")

RELATED CONTENT

Chronic Pancreatitis (Patient Information)
Malabsorption (Related Key Topic)
Pancreatitis, Acute (Related Key Topic)

AUTHOR: **Fred F. Ferri, MD**

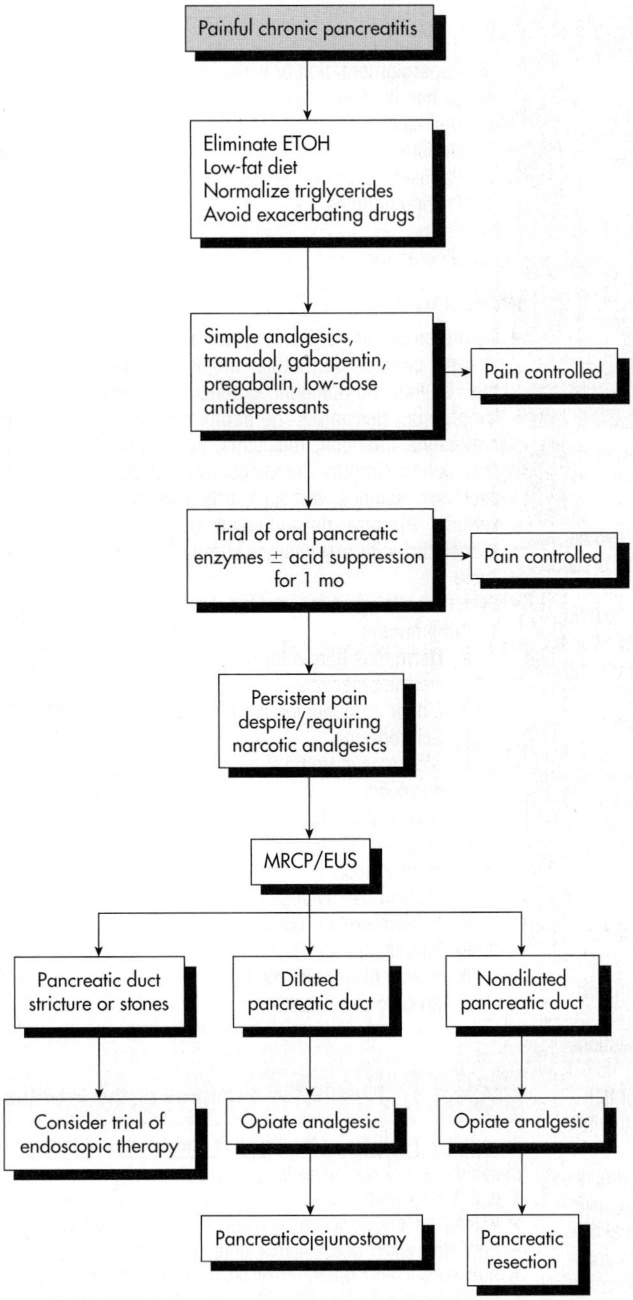

FIG. 6 Approach to the patient with painful chronic pancreatitis. *ETOH,* Alcohol; *EUS,* endoscopic ultrasound; *MRCP,* magnetic resonance cholangiopancreatography. (From Goldman L, Ausiello D [eds]: *Cecil textbook of medicine,* ed 24, Philadelphia, 2012, Saunders.)

TABLE 4 Enzyme Products for the Treatment of Chronic Pancreatitis

Product	Formulation	Lipase Content per Pill or Capsule (USP units)
Creon	Enteric-coated capsule	3000; 6000; 12,000; 24,000; 36,000
Zenpep	Enteric-coated capsule	3000; 5000; 10,000; 15,000; 20,000; 25,000
Pancreaze	Enteric-coated capsule	4200; 10,500; 16,800; 21,000
Ultresa	Enteric-coated capsule	13,800; 20,700; 23,000
Pertzye	Enteric-coated with bicarbonate	8000; 16,000
Viokase	Non–enteric-coated tablet*	10,440; 20,880

The total dose of lipase per meal should be titrated based on response but usually requires at least 60,000 and usually 90,000 USP units (30,000 international units) of lipase per meal and one half that amount with snacks. The dose should be split equally during the meal and immediately after the meal.

*Non–enteric-coated agents require cotreatment with an H2RA or PPI to avoid denaturation of the enzymes by gastric acid.

From Feldman M et al: *Sleisenger and Fordtran's gastrointestinal and liver disease*, ed 10, Philadelphia, 2016, Elsevier.

Chronic Pruritis (ALG)

BASIC INFORMATION

DEFINITION

Chronic pruritus is defined as a generalized itching sensation lasting ≥6 wk in duration.

ICD-10CM CODES

L29	Pruritus
L29.0	Pruritus ani
L29.1	Pruritus scroti
L29.2	Pruritus vulvae
L29.3	Anogenital pruritus, unspecified
L29.8	Other pruritus
L29.9	Pruritus, unspecified

EPIDEMIOLOGY & DEMOGRAPHICS

INCIDENCE: Symptoms of itch are common accounting for about 7 million, or about 1%, of all outpatient office visits in the U.S. per year.

PREVALENCE: Estimates of prevalence within the general population range from 8% to 17%. Reported prevalence between 7% to 60% of geriatric populations.

PREDOMINANT SEX & AGE: More common in women and older adults.

RISK FACTORS: Asthma, xerosis (dry skin), elevated body mass index, anxiety, and liver disease are associated with increased risk for chronic pruritus.

GENETICS: Unknown.

PHYSICAL FINDINGS & CLINICAL PRESENTATION

- Chief concern is typically an itch lasting longer than 6 wk.
- History should be taken including questions about:
  1. Duration, quality, and localization of itch
  2. Presence of skin lesions preceding the itch
  3. Associated skin symptoms
  4. Possible allergies or medication changes
  5. Signs or symptoms of pregnancy, liver disease, gastrointestinal disease, renal disease, neurologic, or psychiatric conditions
  6. Constitutional symptoms indicating underlying systemic illness
  7. Itching or new lesions in family members or close contacts
  8. New sexual contacts
  9. Descriptive features of the pruritus and additional patient history are summarized in Table 1
- Primary skin lesions may be primary due to an underlying skin condition or secondary changes due to persistent scratching.
- Primary lesions may include:
  1. Bullae
  2. Ichthyosis (dry, thickened, scaly skin)
  3. Macular erythema
  4. Papules
  5. Vesicles
  6. Wheals
  7. Xerosis
- Secondary skin changes may include:
  1. Atrophy
  2. Crusting
  3. Excoriation
  4. Hyperpigmentation or hypopigmentation
  5. Lichenification
  6. Necrosis
  7. Nodules
  8. Papules
  9. Prurigo nodules
  10. Scars
  11. Ulcerations

ETIOLOGY

- Dermatologic etiologies for pruritus include allergic contact dermatitis, atopic dermatitis, bullous pemphigoid, cutaneous T-cell lymphoma, dermatitis herpetiformis, dermatophyte infection, folliculitis, lichen planus, lichen simplex chronicus, pediculosis, psoriasis, scabies, sunburn, urticarial, and xerosis. Primary dermatologic conditions associated with pruritus are summarized in Table 2.
- Systemic etiologies for pruritus include:
  1. Autoimmune
     a. Dermatitis herpetiformis
     b. Dermatomyositis
     c. Linear immunoglobulin A disease
     d. Scleroderma
     e. Sjogren syndrome
  2. Hematologic
     a. Hemochromatosis
     b. Iron deficiency anemia
     c. Mastocytosis
     d. Plasma cell dyscrasias
     e. Polycythemia rubra vera
  3. Hepatobiliary
     a. Primry biliary cirrhosis
     b. Chronic pancreatitis
     c. Drug-induced cholestasis
     d. Hepatitis
     e. Sclerosing cholangitis
  4. Infectious disease
     a. Human Immunodeficiency Virus infection
     b. Parasitic disease
     c. Prion disease
  5. Malignancy
     a. Leukemia
     b. Lymphoma
     c. Multiple myeloma
     d. Paraneoplastic syndrome
  6. Endocrine
     a. Carcinoid syndrome
     b. Diabetes mellitus
     c. Hyperthyroidism
     d. Hypothyroidism
     e. Hyperparathyroidism
  7. Neurologic
     a. Cerebral abscess
     b. Cerebral tumor
     c. Peripheral neuropathy

Dx DIAGNOSIS

DIFFERENTIAL DIAGNOSIS

- Liver disease (primary biliary cirrhosis, hepatitis)
- Multiple myeloma
- Lymphoma
- Leukemia
- Xerosis (dry skin)
- Allergic reaction
- Renal disease (uremia)
- Diabetes mellitus
- Medication side effect
- Atopic dermatitis

TABLE 1 Descriptive Features of the Pruritus and Additional Patient History

Descriptive Features of the Pruritus and Additional Patient History

Questions to ask regarding the pruritus

- WHEN did it start? *Duration:* Days, weeks, months, years
- WHERE did it start? WHERE is it now? *Location:* Localized or generalized, unilateral or bilateral
- HOW did it start? *Onset:* Abrupt, gradual, prior history of pruritic episodes
- HOW does it feel? *Nature:* Prickling, crawling, burning, stinging
- HOW intense is it? *Severity:* Mild, moderate, severe; interference with normal activities or sleep
- HOW often do you feel it? *Time course:* Intermittent, continuous, cyclical, nocturnal
- WHAT makes it worse? *Provoking/aggravating factors:* Heat, cold, water, air, exercise, occupation, hobbies
- WHAT makes it better? *Itch relief:* Cold, heat, scratching/rubbing/hurting, cool/hot showering
- WHAT do you think is the cause? *Patient's theory of pruritus etiology*

Additional patient history

- Skin care, bathing habits, exposure to irritants
- Medications (including topical agents): Prescribed, over-the-counter; duration of use and relationship to onset of pruritus
- Use of nicotine, alcohol, and recreational/illicit drugs
- Allergies (known and suspected): Drugs, airborne, food, contact
- Atopic history: Atopic dermatitis, allergic rhinoconjunctivitis, asthma
- Past and present medical history: Thyroid, liver, or renal dysfunction; other systemic diseases; psychologic disease; surgeries or accidents
- Family history: Atopy, skin disease, similar pruritic conditions
- Occupation, hobbies, personal stress
- Household and personal contacts; pets and their care
- Dietary habits
- Sexual history
- Travel history
- Prior diagnoses made by physician or patient

From Bolognia J: *Dermatology*, ed 4, 2018, Elsevier.

TABLE 2 Primary Dermatologic Conditions Associated with Pruritus

PRIMARY DERMATOLOGIC CONDITIONS ASSOCIATED WITH PRURITUS	
Cause	**Dermatologic disease**
Inflammation	• Atopic dermatitis • Allergic or irritant contact dermatitis • Seborrheic dermatitis, especially of the scalp • Stasis dermatitis • Psoriasis • Parapsoriasis • Pityriasis rubra pilaris • Lichen planus • Urticaria, dermographism • Mastocytosis • Papular urticaria, urticarial dermatitis • Drug eruptions, e.g., morbilliform • Polymorphous light eruption, actinic prurigo, chronic actinic dermatitis • Bullous diseases, e.g., DH, BP • Polymorphic eruption of pregnancy (PEP) • Eosinophilic folliculitis • Dermatomyositis • Prurigo pigmentosa • Lichen sclerosis • Graft-versus-host disease
Infestation/bites & stings	• Scabies • Pediculosis • Arthropod bites
Infections	• Bacterial infections, e.g., folliculitis • Viral infections, e.g., varicella • Fungal infections, e.g., inflammatory tinea • Parasitic infections, e.g., schistosomal cercarial dermatitis
Neoplastic	• Cutaneous T-cell lymphoma, e.g., mycosis fungoides, Sézary syndrome
Genetic/nevoid	• Darier disease and Hailey–Hailey disease • Ichthyoses, e.g., Netherton, Sjögren–Larsson, and peeling skin syndromes • Pruriginosa subtype of dominant dystrophic EB • Porphyrias, e.g., porphyria cutanea tarda and erythropoietic protoporphyria • Inflammatory linear verrucous epidermal nevus (ILVEN) • Large/giant congenital melanocytic nevi, occasionally, especially in bulky lesions with neural differentiation
Other	• Xerosis, eczema craquelé • Primary cutaneous amyloidosis (macular, lichenoid) • Postburn pruritus • Scar-associated pruritus • Fiberglass dermatitis

BP, Bullous pemphigoid; *DH*, dermatitis herpetiformis; *EB*, epidermolysis bullosa.
From Bolognia J: *Dermatology*, ed 4, 2018, Elsevier.

- Dermatitis herpetiformis (associated with gluten sensitivity)
- Insect bite and scabies
- Anxiety
- Pregnancy
- Pruritis of elderly skin
- Lichen Simplex Chronicus

WORKUP

Diagnostic testing should be guided by clinical suspicion of underlying causes such as liver disease, HIV, lymphoma, hypothyroidism, renal failure, and polycythemia vera. A simplified approach to the patient with pruritus is illustrated in Fig. 1.

LABORATORY TESTS

- Complete blood count with differential, glucose, creatinine, liver function tests, serum protein electrophoresis, hepatitis serologies, HIV testing, and ferritin can be considered. If diagnosis remains uncertain, skin biopsy should be performed.
- Laboratory and radiographic evaluation in patients with pruritus of unknown etiology are summarized in Table 3.

IMAGING STUDIES

Chest x-ray if diagnosis remains uncertain and concern for underlying pathology.

Rx TREATMENT

Keeping skin cool, using emollients, taking short tepid showers, and avoiding soaking may help symptoms. Moisturizing soaps without fragrance and avoiding antibacterial soaps may help as well.

NONPHARMACOLOGIC THERAPY

- Avoid excessive bathing, frequent use of soap, dry environments, topical irritants or vasodilators such as caffeine, alcohol, and exposure to warm water. Apply emollients liberally after bathing and use fragrance-free soaps. Humidifiers may be used in dry indoor environments, particularly during the winter months. Keeping fingernails short and clean may prevent complications of repetitive scratching.

ACUTE GENERAL Rx

- Antihistamines are usually recommended. H1 blocker diphenhydramine may be sedating. Non-sedating H1 blockers such as cetirizine, fexofenadine, and loratadine are also effective.
- The addition of an H2 blocker (cimetidine, famotidine, ranitidine, nizatidine) should be considered if H1 blockers alone are ineffective.
- Montelukast inhibitors may also be effective when adding to an H1 blocker for symptom control.

CHRONIC Rx

- The management of pruritus should focus on the underlying cause. If patients have pruritus with a systemic cause, itching may slowly improve as the primary disease improves.
- Topical naltrexone and topical or oral doxepin may benefit patients with persistent symptoms.
- Table 4 summarizes drug treatment of pruritus.

COMPLEMENTARY & ALTERNATIVE MEDICINE

Natural supplements for atopic eczema include fish oil, and vitamin D plus vitamin E have demonstrated limited benefit.

DISPOSITION

Overall prognosis depends on the underlying cause of pruritus.

REFERRAL

Patients with psychogenic pruritus may benefit from a referral to a psychologist or psychiatrist.

PEARLS & CONSIDERATIONS

COMMENTS

In patients with an identified underlying cause, the mainstay of treatment is treating the underlying condition.

PREVENTION

Avoid excessive bathing. Avoid frequent use of drying soaps, dry environments, topical irritants, or vasodilators such as caffeine, alcohol, and exposure to warm water. Apply emollients liberally after bathing. Use unscented soaps. A humidifier may be used in dry indoor environments, particularly during the winter months. Keeping fingernails short and clean may prevent complications of repetitive scratching.

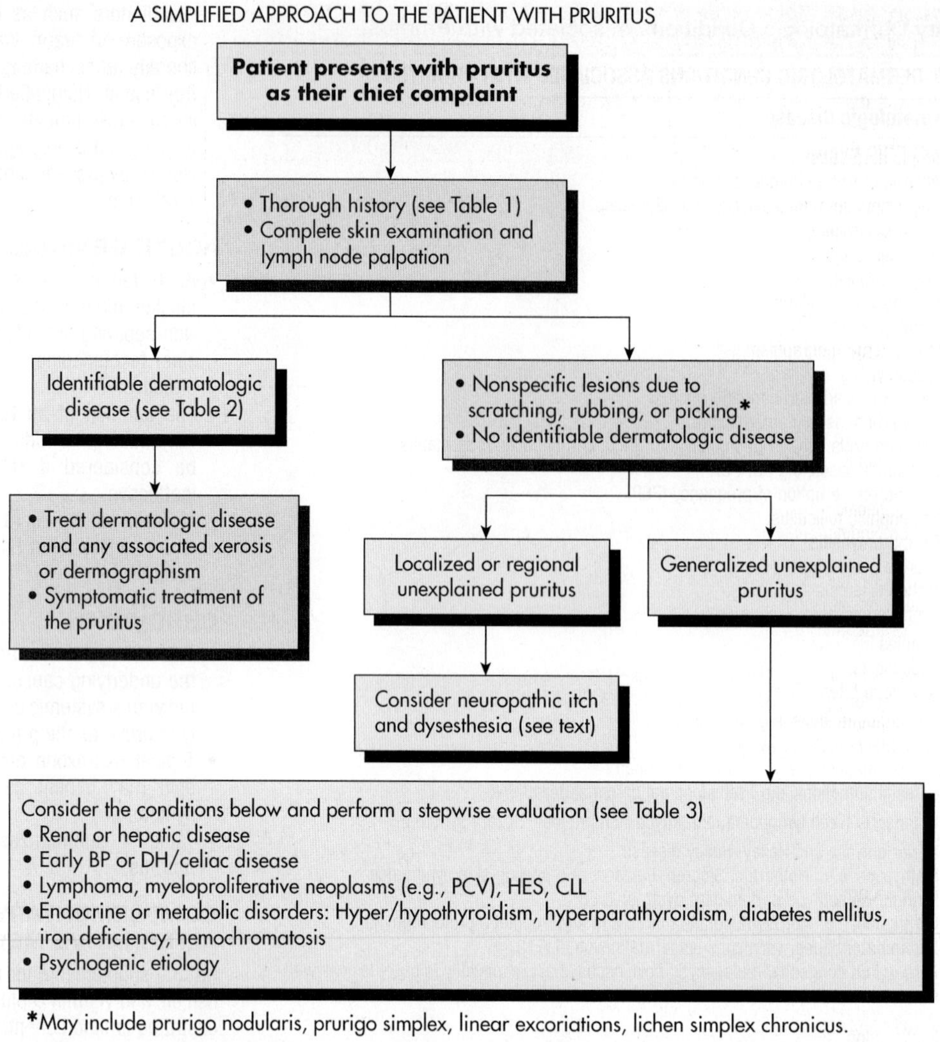

FIG. 1 A simplified approach to the patient with pruritus. *BP*, Bullous pemphigoid; *CLL*, chronic lymphocytic leukemia; *DH*, dermatitis herpetiformis; *HES*, hypereosinophilic syndromes; *PCV*, polycythemia vera. (From Bologna J: *Dermatology*, ed 4, 2018, Elsevier.)

PATIENT & FAMILY EDUCATION

Medline: https://medlineplus.gov/itching.html
American Academy of Family Physicians: https://www.aafp.org/afp/2011/0715/p203.html
DermNetNZ: https://dermnetnz.org/topics/pruritus/

RELATED CONTENT

Primary Biliary Cholangitis (Related Key Topic)
Atopic Dermatitis (Related Key Topic)
Human Immunodeficiency Virus (Related Key Topic)
Hodgkin Lymphoma (Related Key Topic)
Polycythemia Vera (Related Key Topic)

AUTHORS: **Karl T. Clebak, MD, FAAFP,** and **Michael T. Partin, MD**

TABLE 3 Laboratory and Radiographic Evaluation in Patients with Pruritus of Unknown Etiology. A general physical examination should also be performed by the patient's primary care physician. Selection of particular tests beyond the basic initial evaluation is based upon the patient's history, physical examination findings, and pruritus severity. The results of initial testing can also help to direct further evaluation.

Laboratory and Radiographic Evaluation in Patients with Pruritus of Unknown Etiology

Basic initial evaluation

- Complete blood cell count (CBC) with differential and platelet count
- Erythrocyte sedimentation rate (ESR) and C-reactive protein (CRP)
- Creatinine, blood urea nitrogen, electrolytes
- Liver transaminases, alkaline phosphatase, bilirubin
- Lactate dehydrogenase (LDH)
- Fasting glucose
- Thyroid stimulating hormone (TSH) ± free thyroxine

Possible additional evaluation

Skin biopsy

- Routine histology (if skin lesions are present)
- Direct immunofluorescence studies*

Other laboratory tests

- Serum total and/or allergen-specific IgE
- Serum ferritin, iron, total iron binding capacity
- Hemoglobin A1c
- Parathyroid function (calcium, phosphate, and parathyroid hormone levels)
- Stool for ova/parasites and/or occult blood
- Viral hepatitis panel (including hepatitis B and C viruses)
- HIV testing
- Anti-tissue transglutaminase ± epidermal transglutaminase IgA antibodies**
- Anti-BP180 and anti-BP230 bullous pemphigoid IgG antibodies
- Anti-mitochondrial and anti-smooth muscle antibodies
- Serum tryptase, histamine, and/or chromogranin-A levels
- Urinalysis with sediment evaluation
- 24-hour urine collection for 5-hydroxyindoleacetic acid (5-HIAA; a serotonin metabolite) and porphyrins
- Serum protein electrophoresis, serum immunofixation electrophoresis

Radiographic studies

- Chest x-ray or CT scan
- Abdominal and pelvic ultrasonography or CT scan
- Lymph node ultrasonography
- Spinal x-ray or MRI (for regional pruritus)

Other investigations

- Patch testing
- Prick testing for major atopy and relevant occupational allergens
- Age-appropriate cancer screening (in conjunction with primary care physician)
- If hydroxyethyl starch (HES)-induced pruritus is suspected, electron microscopy of a biopsy sample from normal-appearing skin

*Biopsy perilesional skin or normal-appearing skin (in vicinity of lesions if present) to assess for bullous pemphigoid and dermatitis herpetiformis, respectively.
**Often performed in conjunction with serum total IgA; in patients with IgA deficiency, anti-tissue transglutaminase IgG antibodies should be assessed.
From Bolognia J: *Dermatology*, ed 4, 2018, Elsevier.

TABLE 4 Drug Treatment of Pruritus. Topical naltrexone, aspirin, and cannabinoids may also have antipruritic effects, and injections of botulinum toxin type A have been used to treat neuropathic itch. In the future, topical anti-itch medications may target serine proteases (e.g., cathepsin S), nerve growth factor, or neurotrophin 4

DRUG TREATMENT OF PRURITUS

Medication	Mechanism(s) of Action	Uses and Efficacy	Major Adverse Effects
Topical agents			

Capsaicin (active component in hot chili peppers)	• Activates and subsequently desensitizes TRPV1, a vanilloid TRP receptor
	• Causes release from C neurons and (eventually) depleted stores of neuropeptides (e.g., substance P, CGRP, somatostatin)
	• Prolonged use leads to neuronal degeneration at sites of application, which can result in a reversible decrease in epidermal nerve fiber density
		• Used primarily for localized, chronic pruritic disorders, especially those of neuropathic origin
		• Controlled studies support use for:
		  • Notalgia paresthetica
		  • Brachioradial pruritus
		  • Hemodialysis-associated pruritus
		  • Postherpetic neuralgia, with a transdermal patch FDA-approved for this indication
			• Transient burning sensation, which usually resolves after several days of consistent use; application of topical lidocaine or EMLA may be helpful

Doxepin	• Tricyclic compound with potent antihistamine effects (H_1 and H_2); also anticholinergic properties	• Shown to relieve pruritus in patients with atopic dermatitis	• Drowsiness in ~25% of patients due to percutaneous absorption • Allergic contact dermatitis
Menthol	• Activates TRPM8 and TRPA1, producing a cool sensation	• Inconsistent results in controlled studies • May be especially beneficial for patients whose itch is relieved by cold showers	• Skin irritation

Continued

TABLE 4 Drug Treatment of Pruritus. Topical naltrexone, aspirin, and cannabinoids may also have antipruritic effects, and injections of botulinum toxin type A have been used to treat neuropathic itch. In the future, topical anti-itch medications may target serine proteases (e.g. cathepsin S), nerve growth factor, or neurotrophin 4.—cont'd

DRUG TREATMENT OF PRURITUS

Medication	Mechanism(s) of Action	Uses and Efficacy	Major Adverse Effects
Pramoxine	• Anesthetic (blocks transmission of nerve impulses)	• Beneficial for histamine-induced itch and uremic pruritus in end-stage renal disease	• Allergic contact dermatitis (uncommon)
Tacrolimus, pimecrolimus	• Calcineurin inhibitors that block production of multiple proinflammatory cytokines • May initially activate and subsequently desensitize TRPV1	• Can decrease itch related to the inflammation of atopic dermatitis	• Transient burning sensation
"Barrier repair" creams, other emollients and humectants	• Diminish transepidermal water loss and decrease flux between a distended and desiccated state • Minimize microfissures that expose C nerve fibers • Agents that acidify the stratum corneum may reduce itch, as alkaline agents (e.g., bar soaps) can activate proteases and increase lipid rigidity	• Decrease itch in patients with atopic dermatitis	None
Strontium	• Calcimimetic thought to inhibit ion channels in nerve fibers	• Strontium 4% hydrogel was shown to relieve localized cowage-induced itch	None identified
Ketamine-amitriptyline-lidocaine (10%-5%-5% compounded cream)	• Anaesthetic effect; targets ion channels in peripheral nerves and NMDA receptors	• May decrease neuropathic itch and other forms of pruritus, including the itch of prurigo nodularis	• Mild burning sensation • Potential systemic absorption
Systemic agents			
Antihistamines (especially doxepin)	• Doxepin is a tricyclic compound with potent antihistamine effects (H_1 and H_2) and anticholinergic properties; first-generation, sedating antihistamine	• Decrease wheal formation as well as pruritus in patients with urticaria	• Sedation • Anticholinergic effects • Interaction with MAO inhibitors (for doxepin)
Naloxone, naltrexone	• μ-Opioid receptor antagonists*	• Controlled trials show efficacy for cholestatic and renal pruritus • May be of benefit for severe pruritus of other etiologies	• Hepatotoxicity • Nausea/vomiting • Insomnia • Reversal of analgesia
Nalfurafine†	• κ-Opioid receptor agonist*	• Controlled trials show efficacy for renal pruritus	• Insomnia
Butorphanol	• κ-Opioid receptor agonist and μ-opioid receptor antagonist*	• Relieves pruritus associated with morphine with epidural administration of both agents • May reduce severe pruritus associated with systemic disease or inflammatory skin conditions‡	• Nausea/vomiting • Sedation • Dependence (rare)
Mirtazapine	• Serotonin and norepinephrine inverse agonist that reduces central itch perception	• May reduce nocturnal pruritus (at low doses, e.g., 15 mg nightly)	• Sedation • Weight gain
Paroxetine	• Selective serotonin reuptake inhibitor (SSRI)	• A controlled study showed benefit for pruritus related to systemic disease	• Sexual dysfunction • Sedation • Insomnia • Weight gain
Thalidomide	• Blocks neuropathic afferent pathways (peripherally and centrally) • Inhibits TNF synthesis	• May be helpful for prurigo nodularis, actinic prurigo and, pruritus of advanced age	• Teratogenicity • Peripheral neuropathy
Gabapentin, pregabalin	• Structural analogues of the neurotransmitter GABA • Thought to inhibit central itch pathways	• Beneficial for neuropathic itch (e.g., brachioradial pruritus), post-burn pruritus and postherpetic neuralgia	• Peripheral edema • Sedation • Abdominal pain
Aprepitant	• Antagonist of the neurokinin-1 receptor, which is activated by substance P	• Primarily used as an antiemetic in oncology patients; reports of reduced pruritus in patients with atopic dermatitis, Sézary syndrome, and other forms of CTCL as well as decreases in pruritus induced by anti-EGFR antibodies or tyrosine kinase inhibitors	• Fatigue • Hiccups

CGRP, Calcitonin gene-related polypeptide; *EMLA*, eutectic mixture of local anesthetics (lidocaine + prilocaine); *FDA*, U.S. Food and Drug Administration; *MAO*, monoamine oxidase; *TRP*, transient receptor potential ion channel family; *CTCL*, cutaneous T-cell lymphoma; *EGFR*, epidermal growth factor receptor; *GABA*, γ-aminobutyric acid; *NMDA*, N-methyl-D-aspartate; *TNF*, tumor necrosis factor.

*Inhibit itch transmission within the central nervous system.

†Currently not commercially available in the U.S.

‡An intranasal spray is currently available.

From Bolognia J: *Dermatology*, ed 4, 2018, Elsevier.

BASIC INFORMATION

DEFINITION

Chronic rhinosinusitis (CRS) is an inflammatory condition that involves the paranasal passages and linings of the nasal passages that lasts 12 wk or longer despite medical therapy. It can be divided into three categories:
- CRS without nasal polyposis
- CRS with nasal polyposis
- Allergic fungal rhinosinusitis

SYNONYMS

Chronic sinusitis
CRS

ICD-10CM CODE

J32 Chronic sinusitis, unspecified

EPIDEMIOLOGY & DEMOGRAPHICS

INCIDENCE: CRS occurs in children and adults but is most frequently diagnosed in young and middle-aged adults
PREVALENCE: In the U.S. it varies from 1% to 5%
PREDOMINANT SEX & AGE: Some studies suggest women are more affected. In adults, the mean age of diagnosis was 39 yr.
RISK FACTORS:
- Environmental or behavioral risk factors include:
    1. Smoking
    2. Cocaine use
    3. Chemical and air pollutants: Ozone, sulfur dioxide, nitrogen dioxide
- Host-associated risk factors: Allergic rhinitis, atopy, asthma, aspirin-exacerbated respiratory disease
- Innate immunodeficiencies: Cystic fibrosis
- Humoral immunodeficiencies: Common variable immunodeficiency, IgA or IgG subclass deficiencies, types of vasculitis (e.g., Churg-Strauss syndrome), and sarcoidosis
- Allergic fungal sinusitis
- Gastroesophageal reflux disease
- Odontogenic: Infectious agents from maxillary posterior teeth may breech into maxillary sinus

GENETICS: Patients with cystic fibrosis or primary ciliary dyskinesia are more likely to develop CRS.

PHYSICAL FINDINGS & CLINICAL PRESENTATION

- CRS is diagnosed clinically with a physical examination and a detailed sinonasal history. There should be at least two out of the four cardinal symptoms for at least 12 consecutive wk:
    1. Nasal obstruction: 81% to 95% of patients
    2. Nasal drainage: 51% to 83% of patients
    3. Facial pain/pressure: 70% to 85% of patients
    4. Hyposmia/anosmia: 61% to 69% of patients
- Objective evidence on physical examination using anterior rhinoscopy and nasal endoscopy includes mucopurulent drainage, edema, polyps in the middle meatus
- Radiographic evidence includes, preferably, computed tomography (CT) of sinuses.
- Features of specific subtypes:
    1. CRS without nasal polyposis: Most common type (60%-65% of cases) with cardinal clinical symptoms
    2. CRS with nasal polyposis: Characterized with the presence of bilateral nasal polyps in the middle meatus, which are translucent masses composed of gelatinous inflammatory material, as well as cardinal clinical symptoms
    3. Allergic fungal rhinosinusitis:
        a. Type 1 hypersensitivity confirmed by history, skin test, or serology
        b. Nasal polyposis
        c. Positive fungal stain
        d. Eosinophilic mucin showing fungal hyphae without tissue invasion
        e. CT of sinuses showing high-attenuation sinus contents with bony remodeling

ETIOLOGY

- Not fully understood but multifactorial involving host genetics and immunity, as well as environmental and infectious agents that produce chronic inflammation of the upper airways.
- Various cells, including fibroblasts, epithelial cells, endothelial cells, mast cells, eosinophils, antigen-presenting cells (dendritic cells), T cells, and B cells, have been shown to coordinate the immune inflammatory network underlying CRS, by the production of mediators such as cytokines, chemokines, eicosanoids, and antibodies.
- Microbiology: Organisms that may be involved in the pathogenesis of CRX include:
    1. *Staphylococcus aureus:* This is the most common bacterium and contributes to polyp formation. Methicillin-resistant *S. aureus* is isolated in 2% to 20% of patients with CRS.
    2. Coagulase-negative staphylococci: It is not always clear whether they are pathogens or colonizers.
    3. *Pseudomonas aeruginosa:* Occurs especially in patients with cystic fibrosis. Other gram-negative rods include *Klebsiella pneumoniae, Proteus mirabilis, Enterobacter* spp., and *E. Coli.*
    4. Anaerobic bacteria include: *Peptostreptococcus, Fusobacterium, Prevotella* spp., *Porphyromonas* spp.

DIAGNOSIS

DIFFERENTIAL DIAGNOSIS

- Recurrent acute rhinosinusitis: ≥4 episodes a yr but symptom-free in between
- Allergic rhinitis, nonallergic rhinitis, vasomotor rhinitis, and eosinophilic nonallergic rhinitis
- Trigeminal neuralgia
- Tension headache

WORKUP

CRS is diagnosed clinically with a physical examination and focused sinonasal history, including the CRS-associated comorbidities and a pertinent family history

LABORATORY TESTS

Testing should be done to search for chronic conditions that may affect treatment:
- Asthma
- Cystic fibrosis
- Aspirin sensitivity
- Ciliary dyskinesia
- Immunodeficiencies: IgG deficiency, IgG subclass deficiency, IgA deficiency, selective IgA deficiency
- Assessment of patient allergies and immunologic status: IgG, IgA, IgM, and IgE levels; T-cell number; and function evaluation (delayed hypersensitivity skin test and flow cytometric quantification of T cells)
- Bacterial cultures via maxillary tap (maxillary sinus aspirate [MSA]) or endoscopically directed middle meatus culture (EDMM). MSA is the gold standard, with EDMM being considered equivalent

IMAGING STUDIES

- Plain films of sinuses are no longer recommended, with noncontrast-enhanced CT being the study of choice.
- Include all of the forehead and extend to maxillary teeth, also including the ears and nasal tip.
- Maintain a maximum slice of thickness of 1 mm, and obtain scans axially with no gantry tilt.

TREATMENT

The goal of treatment is to manage symptoms and to improve or maintain quality of life. Therapies are targeted to enhancing mucociliary clearance, improving sinus drainage/outflow, eliminating local infection and inflammation, and improving access for topical medications.

NONPHARMACOLOGIC THERAPY

Nasal saline irrigation: Low-pressure, high-volume (240 ml) isotonic or hypertonic saline irrigation can reduce symptoms in 50% of patients and is better than nasal saline spray. Often used in conjunction with intranasal corticosteroid spray.

ACUTE GENERAL Rx

- Topical intranasal corticosteroids: First-generation products include beclomethasone dipropionate (QNASL), flunisolide (Nasalide, Nasarel), budesonide (Rhinocort), and triamcinolone acetonide (Nasacort). Newer agents include fluticasone propionate (Flonase), fluticasone furoate (Veramyst), mometasone furoate (Asmanex), and ciclesonide (Omnaris). Most are used once a day.
- Oral corticosteroids: Oral corticosteroids, such as prednisone, can be used in patients

with severe disease and especially in patients with nasal polyps because they will help reduce the size of polyps. Prednisone will also minimize mucosal inflammation in allergic fungal rhinosinusitis. Dose: 20 mg twice daily for 5 days, then 20 mg daily for 5 days.
- Antibiotics: Often used in conjunction with prednisone. Can be used when evidence of infection present: Facial pain, air–fluid level on sinus CT, or purulent mucus in middle meatus. Use for up to 3 to 4 wk at most. Examples include amoxicillin/clavulanic acid or moxifloxacin.

SURGERY: Endoscopic surgery is appropriate if medical therapy fails. It can provide ventilation and drainage of the paranasal sinuses and enlarge the paranasal sinuses to create better access for topical medications. In general, it does not cure the condition and patients will need continued medical therapies.

CHRONIC Rx

Use of macrolide antibiotics for prolonged periods has been tried, but studies have not shown additional benefit.

COMPLEMENTARY & ALTERNATIVE MEDICINE

Herbal medicines, homeopathy, acupuncture, reflexology, and yoga are used but have not been studied in clinical trials.

REFERRAL

- Otolaryngologist for long-term treatments and possible surgery

PEARLS & CONSIDERATIONS

- Surfactants such as baby shampoo can be added to saline irrigations and may prevent formation of bacterial biofilm on the sinus mucosa.
- Antihistamines such as cetirizine 20 mg used daily are of unproven benefit.

PREVENTION

- Smoking cessation is recommended because it reduces the risk for sinusitis.
- Nasal irrigation can be used as prevention for exacerbations of CRS.

SUGGESTED READINGS

Available at ExpertConsult.com

AUTHOR: **Glenn G. Fort, MD, MPH**

BASIC INFORMATION

DEFINITION

Chronic traumatic encephalopathy (CTE) is a pathologically defined neurogenerative disorder often found in athletes and veterans that is associated with repetitive concussive or subconcussive head injury. CTE presents with cognitive, psychiatric, and sometimes motor symptoms.

SYNONYMS

CTE
Traumatic encephalopathy syndrome (clinical diagnosis)
Dementia pugilistica (older term)
Punch drunk syndrome (older term)

ICD-10CM CODE
G93.49 Other encephalopathy

EPIDEMIOLOGY & DEMOGRAPHICS

PEAK INCIDENCE & PREVALENCE: The incidence and prevalence of CTE are currently unknown. In the largest CTE case series to date, of 202 deceased individuals who had a significant history of repetitive head trauma related to either contact sports or military service, Mez and colleagues reported that CTE was diagnosed in 177 former professional football players (or 87% of the cases) and, more specifically, in 110 out of 111 (99%) of the former National Football League (NFL) players. The authors noted that the study was limited by ascertainment bias since individuals with symptoms consistent with possible CTE were much more likely to participate in the brain donation program, and, therefore, the true frequency of CTE pathology is unknown.

- Among participants with severe CTE pathology, 89% had behavior, mood symptoms, or both, 95% had cognitive symptoms, and 85% had signs of dementia.[1]

PREDOMINANT SEX AND AGE: CTE may present early (20s-30s) or later (50s-60s) in adulthood. The relationship with gender is unknown.

RISK FACTORS: Repetitive head injuries leading to concussions or subconcussive injuries are the strongest risk factor for the development of CTE. Athletes, veterans, and victims of repetitive head trauma are at highest risk. Although repetitive head trauma is required for CTE to develop, head trauma alone is insufficient. The search for genetic and environmental risk factors are underway.

GENETICS: Currently there are no known genetic risk factors that predispose to the development of CTE, although some studies raise the possibility of a relationship to the APOE4 allele and others do not confirm this association.

[1] Mez J et al: Clinicopathological evaluation of chronic traumatic encephalopathy in players of American football, *JAMA* 318(4):360-370, 2017.

PHYSICAL FINDINGS & CLINICAL PRESENTATION

CTE causes progressive cognitive, behavior, and mood changes and may even lead to motor deficits. CTE is a delayed presentation of repetitive concussive or subconcussive injuries and should not be confused with acute or postacute sequelae of traumatic brain injury. The most common cognitive domains affected are memory and executive function. The most common presenting symptoms in patients with autopsy confirmed CTE are found in Table 1. Because CTE is a pathological diagnosis currently made only postmortem, a search for in vivo biomarkers is underway. Patients with a clinical syndrome thought to be the consequence of repetitive blows to the head are considered for research purposes to have traumatic encephalopathy syndrome (TES). Some TES patients are found postmortem to have CTE, whereas others may have other forms of neurodegeneration or even psychiatric conditions lacking specific neurodegenerative pathology. Like CTE, TES does not refer to either the acute or postacute sequelae of TBI such as concussion, postconcussive syndrome, or moderate to severe TBI. TES can take one of four clinical types: (1) behavioral/mood variant, occurring in younger patients; (2) cognitive variant, occurring later in life; (3) a mixed variant; and (4) a dementia variant.

The behavioral/mood variant first presents early in life (later 20s-30s), with primarily psychiatric and behavioral manifestations such as depression, anxiety, paranoia, impulsivity, explosivity, and aggression. Cognitive problems are more common as the disease progresses. The cognitive and dementia forms present later in life (50s-60s), with impairment in episodic memory, attention, and executive function. Currently it is thought that CTE progresses in four stages with increasing severity along each stage. Symptoms progress from headaches, attention problems, and depression to explosivity, aggression, dementia, and suicidality as the disease progresses.

Physical examination findings are not always present in CTE but may include symptoms of parkinsonism and motor dysfunction, such as gait disturbance, tremors, ataxia, and dysarthria. These have been found to be particularly more common in boxers.

Of note, the symptoms of CTE may present similarly to the behavioral variant of frontotemporal dementia (bvFTD), but CTE patents, in addition to their history of repetitive or subconcussive head injury, experience more memory loss than patients with bvFTD. Alzheimer disease (AD) should be in the differential diagnosis for memory loss, but in addition to the apathy or irritability that may be seen in both AD and CTE, CTE patients have explosivity and disinhibition not typically seen in AD. CTE patients with dementia may also develop parkinsonism, raising the possibility of dementia with Lewy bodies (DLB), but parkinsonism is late and rare in CTE. REM behavior disorder is typical of DLB but not a feature of CTE, and disinhibition and explosivity are features of CTE not associated with DLB.

ETIOLOGY

The frequency, severity, and total exposure to head trauma and the exact pathophysiologic mechanism by which repetitive head trauma causes CTE in chronic traumatic encephalopathy are active areas of research.

- Head injury is an important but nonsufficient risk factor in the development of chronic traumatic encephalopathy; other exposure and genetic risk factors are under investigation.
- Currently, no validated clinical diagnostic criteria for chronic traumatic encephalopathy exist, although research diagnostic criteria have been developed.
- Concussion is a clinical syndrome of impaired brain function, typically impacting memory and orientation, with or without loss of consciousness that results from head injury.
- Chronic traumatic encephalopathy is defined by neuropathology: Perivascular aggregation of phosphorylated tau protein within neurons and astrocytes that begins in the depths of sulci and progresses to involve the medial temporal lobes and other parts of the brain.

CTE is believed to occur due to repetitive head injuries. Definitive diagnosis is made only through autopsy, where neurofibrillary tangles and p-tau aggregates may be found around blood vessels and in deep cortical sulci, amygdala, hippocampus, brainstem, and cerebellum depending on the stage of the disease.

DIAGNOSIS

DIFFERENTIAL DIAGNOSIS

- Alzheimer disease
- Frontotemporal dementia

TABLE 1 Clinical Features at Initial Presentation of Patients with Autopsy-Confirmed Chronic Traumatic Encephalopathy

- Memory impairment (85%)
- Executive dysfunction (79%)
- Attention and concentration difficulties (73%)
- Sadness/depression (64%)
- Hopelessness (64%)
- Explosivity (58%)
- Language impairment (58%)
- Visuospatial difficulties (55%)
- "Out of control" (52%)
- Physically violent (52%)
- Verbally violent (49%)
- Impulse and control problems (46%)
- Suicidal ideation/attempts (30%)
- Motor symptoms (30%)

Reprinted with permission from Budson AE, Solomon PR. *Memory loss, Alzheimer's disease, and dementia: a practical guide for clinicians*, ed 2. Edinburgh, UK, 2016, Elsevier Health Sciences, using data from Stern RA et al. Clinical presentation of chronic traumatic encephalopathy, *Neurology* 81(13):1122-1129, 2013. doi:10.1212/ WNL.0b013e3182a55f7f.

- Dementia with Lewy bodies
- Bipolar disorder
- Major depressive disorder

WORKUP

CTE should be suspected in those with a history of repetitive head injuries with or without concussion as a result of contact sports, military service, motor vehicle accidents, domestic abuse, and battery presenting with the symptoms listed in Table 1. The history and progression of symptoms is of most benefit in the diagnostic process. Neuropsychological testing may be helpful in delineating specific cognitive deficits.

LABORATORY TESTS

Tests including complete blood count, comprehensive metabolic panel, thyroid function tests, HIV, syphilis

IMAGING STUDIES

MRI may aid in ruling out other causes of dementia. CTE patients will often have imaging abnormalities such as a cavum septum pellucidum cavum vergae, or fenestrations of the lateral ventricle, evidence of increased cortical thinning consistent with neurodegeneration, cortical atrophy, and a dilated third ventricle.

- The usefulness of advanced imaging such as PET, SPECT, and DTI in CTE is still under investigation. Tau-PET is under investigation for in vivo diagnosis of CTE. The neuropathological diagnosis is based on a specific pattern of Tau deposition with minimal amyloid-beta deposition that differs from other disorders, including Alzheimer disease. An analysis of living former NFL players with cognitive and neuropsychiatric symptoms revealed higher Tau levels measured by PET than controls in brain regions that are affected by CTE and did not have elevated amyloid-beta levels.[1]
- A negative amyloid PET would exclude AD pathology.

Rx TREATMENT

NONPHARMACOLOGIC THERAPY

Cognitive behavioral therapy is helpful for depression and anxiety symptoms.

ACUTE GENERAL Rx

- **SSRIs** may be effective in treating depression symptoms. Close monitoring for suicidality is recommended in all patients with CTE.
- **Acetylcholinesterase inhibitors approved for treating AD may help with memory dysfunction.**
- **Atypical antipsychotics** may be used to control disinhibition and reduce violence, but all antipsychotics carry an FDA boxed warning about an increased mortality in patients with dementia, a risk that should be disclosed to the patient's surrogate decision-maker and weighed on a case-by-case basis.
- **Pain management** to improve quality of life.

DISPOSITION

CTE is chronic and progressive. Emphasis should be placed on improving quality of life through pain management, therapy, and symptom management.

REFERRAL

Patients may benefit from referral to neurology, psychiatry, and psychology.

[1]Stern RA et al: Tau Positron-Emission Tomography in Former National Football League Players, *N Engl J Med* 380;1716-1725, 2019

PEARLS & CONSIDERATIONS

COMMENTS

CTE is a slowly developing illness. Although it should be considered in patients with repetitive head injuries, it is important to conduct a thorough workup to rule out psychiatric illnesses and other forms of dementia that may present with similar symptoms.

PREVENTION

For athletes, wearing proper protective equipment as well as using techniques to avoid direct head impacts when playing sports is important. Furthermore, if a concussion is suspected, the player should not be allowed to resume play without further evaluation.

PATIENT & FAMILY EDUCATION

Concussion foundation—CTE resources
https://concussionfoundation.org/CTE-resources

CDC—HEADS UP: For prevention of concussions
www.cdc.gov/headsup/index.html

SUGGESTED READINGS

Available at ExpertConsult.com

RELATED CONTENT

Concussion (Related Key Topic)
Depression, Major (Related Key Topic)
Postconcussion Syndrome (Related Key Topic)
Suicide (Related Key Topic)

AUTHOR: **Joseph S. Kass, MD, JD, FAAN**

BASIC INFORMATION

DEFINITION

Cirrhosis is defined histologically as the presence of irreversible fibrosis in the liver. It can be classified as micronodular, macronodular, or mixed; however, each form may be seen in the same patient at different stages of the disease, and this classification system has little utility in determining the underlying etiology of cirrhosis. Cirrhosis manifests clinically with portal hypertension, ascites and peripheral edema, hepatic encephalopathy, and variceal bleeding.

ICD-10CM CODES	
K70.30	Alcoholic cirrhosis of liver without ascites
K70.31	Alcoholic cirrhosis of liver with ascites
K71.7	Toxic liver disease with fibrosis and cirrhosis of liver
K74.3	Primary biliary cirrhosis
K74.4	Secondary biliary cirrhosis
K74.5	Biliary cirrhosis, unspecified
K74.60	Unspecified cirrhosis of liver
K74.69	Other cirrhosis of liver
P78.81	Congenital cirrhosis (of liver)

EPIDEMIOLOGY & DEMOGRAPHICS

- Cirrhosis was the fourteenth-leading cause of death in the U.S. in 2015 and the thirteenth-leading cause of death globally. In the U.S., cirrhosis-related deaths increased 3.4% annually between 2009 and 2016.
- Alcohol abuse, hepatitis C, and nonalcoholic steatohepatitis are the major causes of cirrhosis in the U.S.
- Economic burden of cirrhosis in the U.S. exceeds $2 billion in direct costs and over $10 billion in indirect costs.

PHYSICAL FINDINGS & CLINICAL PRESENTATION

GENERAL: Fever (spontaneous bacterial peritonitis)

SKIN: Jaundice, palmar erythema, spider angiomata, ecchymosis (thrombocytopenia or coagulation factor deficiency), increased pigmentation (hemochromatosis), xanthomas (primary biliary cirrhosis), and diffuse pruritus. Cutaneous lesions often accompany cirrhosis and can be found in >40% of people with chronic alcoholism

EYES: Kayser-Fleischer rings (corneal copper deposition seen in Wilson disease; best diagnosed with slit lamp examination), scleral icterus

BREATH: Fetor hepaticus (breath has a sweet musty odor found in cirrhosis with hepatic failure)

CHEST: Possible gynecomastia in men

ABDOMEN: Tender or nontender hepatomegaly (congestive hepatomegaly), small, nodular liver (cirrhosis), palpable, nontender gallbladder (neoplastic extrahepatic biliary obstruction), palpable spleen (portal hypertension), dilated superficial periumbilical vein (caput medusae), venous hum auscultated over periumbilical veins (portal hypertension), ascites (portal hypertension, hypoalbuminemia), diffuse abdominal tenderness (spontaneous bacterial peritonitis)

RECTAL EXAMINATION: Hemorrhoids (portal hypertension), guaiac-positive stools (alcoholic gastritis, bleeding esophageal varices, peptic ulcer disease, bleeding hemorrhoids, portal gastropathy)

GENITALIA: Testicular atrophy in males (chronic liver disease, hemochromatosis)

EXTREMITIES: Pedal edema (hypoalbuminemia, anasarca), arthropathy (hemochromatosis), Dupuytren contractures

NEUROLOGIC: Asterixis (hepatic encephalopathy), choreoathetosis, dysarthria (Wilson disease)

ETIOLOGY

- Chronic hepatitis B virus (HBV) and hepatitis C virus (HCV) infection
- Alcoholism
- Nonalcoholic steatohepatitis
- Primary biliary cholangitis
- Secondary biliary cirrhosis, obstruction of the common bile duct (stone, stricture, pancreatitis, neoplasm, sclerosing cholangitis)
- Autoimmune hepatitis
- Drugs with chronic hepatitis (e.g., acetaminophen, isoniazid, methotrexate, methyldopa)
- Chronic hepatic congestion (e.g., CHF, constrictive pericarditis, tricuspid insufficiency, thrombosis of the hepatic vein, obstruction of the vena cava)
- Hemochromatosis
- Wilson disease
- Alpha-1-antitrypsin deficiency
- Infiltrative diseases (amyloidosis, glycogen storage diseases, nonhepatocellular malignancies)
- Nutritional: Jejunoileal bypass
- Others: Parasitic infections (schistosomiasis), idiopathic portal hypertension, congenital hepatic fibrosis, systemic mastocytosis

Dx DIAGNOSIS

WORKUP

In addition to an assessment of liver function, the evaluation of patients with cirrhosis should also include an assessment of renal and circulatory function. Diagnostic workup is aimed primarily at identifying the most likely cause of cirrhosis. The history is extremely important:

- Alcohol abuse: Alcoholic liver disease
- History of hepatitis B or hepatitis C
- Obesity, type 2 diabetes mellitus, hyperlipidemia (nonalcoholic steatohepatitis)
- History of IBD (primary sclerosing cholangitis)
- History of pruritus, hyperlipoproteinemia, and xanthomas in a middle-aged or elderly woman (primary biliary cholangitis)
- Impotence, diabetes mellitus, hyperpigmentation, arthritis (hemochromatosis)
- Neurologic disturbances (Wilson disease, hepatolenticular degeneration)
- Family history of "liver disease" (hemochromatosis [positive family history in 25% of patients], alpha-1-antitrypsin deficiency)
- History of recurrent episodes of right upper quadrant pain (biliary tract disease)
- History of blood transfusions, IV drug abuse (hepatitis C)
- History of repetitive hepatotoxic drug exposure
- Coexistence of other diseases with immune or autoimmune features (immune thrombocytopenic purpura, myasthenia gravis, thyroiditis, autoimmune hepatitis)
- Biopsy is the gold standard to diagnosis cirrhosis and is helpful when multiple etiologies are possible that might change management (autoimmune hepatitis, small duct primary sclerosing cholangitis, antimitochondrial antibody-negative primary biliary cholangitis, and infiltrative diseases such as lymphoma, amyloidosis, and granulomatous hepatitis). However, it is generally unnecessary if the clinical picture is highly suggestive of cirrhosis and management would not change. Biopsy can be useful in actively drinking patients with cirrhosis to distinguish between decompensated cirrhosis and cirrhosis with alcoholic hepatitis

LABORATORY TESTS

- Decreased hemoglobin and hematocrit, elevated mean corpuscular volume (Fig. E1). Increased blood urea nitrogen (BUN) and creatinine (the BUN may also be "normal" or low if the patient has severely diminished liver function).
- Decreased sodium (dilutional hyponatremia), and decreased potassium (as a result of secondary aldosteronism or urinary losses). Evaluation of renal function should also include measurement of urinary sodium and urinary protein from 24-hr urine collection.
- Decreased glucose in a patient with liver disease indicates severe liver damage.
- Other laboratory abnormalities:
  1. Alcoholic hepatitis and cirrhosis: Possible mild elevation of alanine aminotransferase (ALT) and aspartate aminotransferase (AST), usually <500 IU; AST > ALT (ratio >2:3).
  2. Extrahepatic obstruction: Possible moderate elevations of ALT and AST to levels <500 IU.
  3. Viral, toxic, or ischemic hepatitis: Extreme elevations (>500 IU) of ALT and AST.
  4. Transaminases may be normal despite significant liver disease in patients with jejunoileal bypass operations or hemochromatosis or after methotrexate administration.
  5. Alkaline phosphatase elevation can occur with extrahepatic obstruction, primary biliary cholangitis, and primary sclerosing cholangitis.
  6. Serum lactate dehydrogenase is significantly elevated in metastatic disease of the liver; lesser elevations are seen with hepatitis, cirrhosis, extrahepatic obstruction, and congestive hepatomegaly.

7. Serum gamma-glutamyl transpeptidase is elevated in alcoholic liver disease and may also be elevated with cholestatic disease (primary biliary cholangitis, primary sclerosing cholangitis).
8. Serum bilirubin may be elevated; urinary bilirubin can be present in hepatitis, hepatocellular jaundice, and biliary obstruction.
9. Serum albumin: Significant liver disease results in hypoalbuminemia. Malnutrition occurs in 20% to 60% of patients with cirrhosis.

- Prothrombin time/INR: Elevation in patients with liver disease indicates severe liver damage and poor prognosis. Table 1 summarizes hemostatic balance in liver disease.

1. Presence of hepatitis B surface antigen implies acute or chronic hepatitis B.
2. Presence of antimitochondrial antibody suggests primary biliary cholangitis, chronic hepatitis.
3. Elevated serum copper, decreased serum ceruloplasmin, and elevated 24-hr urine may be diagnostic of Wilson disease.
4. Protein immunoelectrophoresis may reveal decreased α-1 globulins (alpha-1-antitrypsin deficiency), increased IgA (alcoholic cirrhosis), increased IgM (primary biliary cirrhosis), increased IgG (chronic hepatitis, cryptogenic cirrhosis).
5. An elevated serum ferritin and increased iron saturation are suggestive of hemochromatosis.
6. An elevated blood ammonia suggests hepatocellular dysfunction; serial values, however, are generally not useful in monitoring patients with hepatic encephalopathy because there is poor correlation between blood ammonia level and degree of hepatic encephalopathy.
7. Serum cholesterol is elevated in cholestatic disorders.
8. Antinuclear antibodies (ANA) may be found in autoimmune hepatitis.
9. Alpha fetoprotein: Levels >1000 pg/ml are highly suggestive of hepatocellular carcinoma.
10. Hepatitis C viral testing identifies patients with chronic hepatitis C infection.
11. Elevated level of serum globulin (especially gamma-globulins) and positive ANA test may occur with autoimmune hepatitis.
12. End-stage liver disease is characterized by decreased levels of most procoagulant factors with the notable exceptions of factor VIII and von Willebrand factor, which are elevated. Table 2 summarizes hemostatic indices in liver disease.

IMAGING STUDIES

- Ultrasonography is the procedure of choice. It can identify the size and shape of the liver (generally small and nodular in advanced cirrhosis) and can detect gallstones and dilation of bile ducts. The use of sonography on a periodic basis to screen for hepatocellular carcinoma in patients with cirrhosis should be considered.
- CT scan (Figs. 2 and 3) is useful for detecting mass lesions in liver and pancreas, assessing hepatic fat content, identifying idiopathic hemochromatosis, diagnosing Budd-Chiari syndrome early, assessing dilation of intrahepatic bile ducts, and detecting varices and splenomegaly. However, ultrasound is generally the preferred imaging modality of choice.
- MRI can be used to identify hemangiomas, hepatocellular carcinoma.
- Vibration-controlled transient elastography and magnetic resonance elastography are useful to assess advanced fibrosis. These noninvasive tests are less expensive and safer than biopsy and can be repeated over time to monitor disease progression.
- Technetium-99m sulfur colloid scanning is rarely used but can be useful for diagnosing cirrhosis (there is a shift of colloid uptake to the spleen and bone marrow), identifying hepatic adenomas (cold defect is noted), and diagnosing Budd-Chiari syndrome (there is increased uptake by the caudate lobe).
- Endoscopic retrograde cholangiopancreatography can be used for diagnosing periampullary carcinoma and common duct stones; it is also useful in diagnosing primary sclerosing cholangitis.
- Percutaneous transhepatic cholangiography is useful when evaluating patients with cholestatic jaundice and dilated intrahepatic ducts by ultrasonography; presence of intrahepatic strictures and focal dilation is suggestive of primary sclerosing cholangitis.

Rx TREATMENT

NONPHARMACOLOGIC THERAPY

- Avoid any hepatotoxins (e.g., ethanol, acetaminophen), improve nutritional status, vaccinate against hepatitis A and B if not already immune.
- Transjugular intrahepatic portosystemic shunt (TIPS, Fig. E4) in patients with recurrent variceal hemorrhage despite optical

TABLE 1 Hemostatic Balance in Liver Disease

	Promotes Thrombosis	Promotes Bleeding
Primary hemostasis	• Increased vWF • Decreased ADAMTS13	• Thrombocytopenia • Platelet dysfunction
Secondary hemostasis	• Increased factor VIII • Decreased protein C, protein S, antithrombin	• Factor deficiencies: II, V, VII, IX, XI • Vitamin K deficiency • Hypofibrinogenemia • Dysfibrinogenemia
Fibrinolysis	• Reduced plasminogen • Increased PAI-1	• Reduced α2-antiplasmin, TAFI, factor VIII • Increased t-PA

ADAMST13, A disintegrin and metalloproteinase with thrombospondin; *PAI-1,* plasminogen activator inhibitor-1; *TAFI,* thrombin activatable fibrinolysis inhibitor; *t-PA,* tissue plasminogen activator; *vWF,* von Willebrand factor.
From Hoffman R et al: *Hematology: basic principles and practice,* ed 7, Philadelphia, 2018, Elsevier.

TABLE 2 Hemostatic Indices in Liver Disease

Laboratory Changes	PT	PTT	TCT	Fib	Clauss	Plt	Platelet Aggregation	FVII	DD	ELT
Thrombocytopenia	N	N	N	N	N	↓	N	N	N	N
Platelet dysfunction	N	N	N	N	N	N	Abnormal	N	N	N
Vitamin K deficiency[a]	↑	↑	N	N	N	N	N	↓	N	N
Factor deficiency	↑	↑	N	N	N	N	N	↓	N	N
Hypofibrinogenemia	N/↑	N/↑	↑	↓	↓	N	N	N	N	N
Dysfibrinogenemia	N/↑	N/↑	↑	N	↓	N	N	N	N	N
Hyperfibrinolysis	N/↑	N/↑	N/↑	N/↓	N/↓	N	N	↓	↑	↓
DIC	N/↑	N/↑	N/↑	↓	↓	↓	N	N/↓	↑	↓

Clauss, Clauss fibrinogen; *DD,* D-dimer; *DIC,* disseminated intravascular coagulation; *ELT,* euglobulin lysis time (measure of fibrinolysis); *Fib,* fibrinogen; *FVII,* factor VII functional assay; *N,* normal; *Plt,* platelet; *PT,* prothrombin time; *PTT,* partial thromboplastin time; *TCT,* thrombin clotting time.
[a]Differentiating between vitamin K deficiency and liver disease can be challenging with conventional laboratory tests. If available, performing a factor II assay with and without Echis venom (factor II biologic and factor II Echis) may be useful. Ecarin is derived from *Echis carinatus* snake venom and can activate prothrombin irrespective of γ-carboxylation. Factor II activity (biologic) is reduced in both vitamin K deficiency and liver disease. In contrast, the factor II Echis is reduced in liver disease but is normal in vitamin K deficiency.
From Hoffman R et al: *Hematology: basic principles and practice,* ed 7, Philadelphia, 2018, Elsevier.

medical therapy. Early use of TIPS is associated with significant reductions in treatment failure and in mortality in patients with cirrhosis who are hospitalized for acute variceal bleeding and are at high risk for treatment failure.
- Correction of malnutrition: Daily protein intake of 1.0 to 1.5 g per kg of body weight.

ACUTE GENERAL Rx

- Nonselective beta blockers (nadolol, propranolol) in patients with cirrhosis and variceal hemorrhage, and some without hemorrhage but with high-risk bleeding features. Use with caution in patients with severe alcoholic hepatitis and decompensated cirrhosis with refractory ascites. Beta-blockers should be temporarily discontinued in patients with spontaneous bacterial peritonitis due to increased mortality and hepatorenal syndrome incidence.
- Pruritus due to liver disease may be treated with cholestyramine 4 g/day initially. Dose can be increased to 24 g/day as needed.
- Pain management: Avoid opiates (may precipitate or aggravate hepatic encephalopathy) and NSAIDs (increased risk of gastrointestinal bleeding and renal failure). Low-dose tramadol and lidocaine patches are generally well tolerated.
- Sedatives: Benzodiazepines (lorazepam or oxazepam) may be used for alcohol withdrawal but should be avoided in patients with hepatic encephalopathy. Avoid benzodiazepines with liver metabolites (diazepam, chlordiazepoxide).
- Statins: Can be safely started and continued in patients with hyperlipidemia and/or nonalcoholic fatty liver disease.
- Proton pump inhibitors: Not routinely indicated; their use in patients with cirrhosis is associated with excess risk for spontaneous bacterial peritonitis and hepatic encephalopathy; avoid indiscriminate use of PPIs in patients with cirrhosis.
- Antibiotics: Trimethoprim-sulfamethoxazole or ciprofloxacin/norfloxacin for spontaneous bacterial peritonitis prophylaxis in patients with a history of SBP, an ascites protein concentration less than 1 g/dl, or history of variceal hemorrhage.
- Liver transplantation may be indicated in otherwise healthy patients (ages <65 yr) with severe cirrhosis and lack of contraindications. Contraindications to liver transplantation are AIDS, most metastatic malignancies, active substance abuse, uncontrolled sepsis, and uncontrolled cardiac or pulmonary disease.
- Complications of cirrhosis (Fig. 5): Treatment of complications of portal hypertension (ascites, esophagogastric varices, hepatic encephalopathy, spontaneous bacterial peritonitis, and hepatorenal syndrome; refer to these individual topics in Section I).
- Fig. 6 summarizes the management of compensated and decompensated cirrhosis.
- Box 1 summarizes the management of coagulopathy in liver disease.

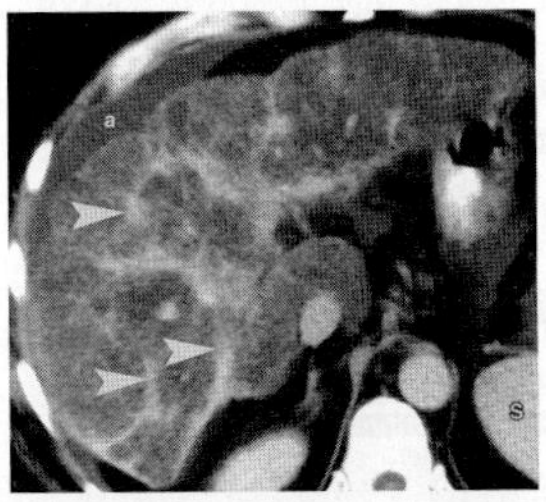

FIG. 2 Advanced cirrhosis with fatty infiltration. Delayed portal venous–phase computed tomography reveals that the liver is misshapen and nodular in contour. Parenchymal density that is significantly lower than that of the spleen *(S)* is indicative of fatty infiltration and continuing liver injury. Prominent scars and bands of fibrosis *(arrowheads)* are seen throughout the liver. Ascites *(a)* is present. (From Webb WR et al: *Fundamentals of body CT*, ed 4, Philadelphia, 2015, Saunders.)

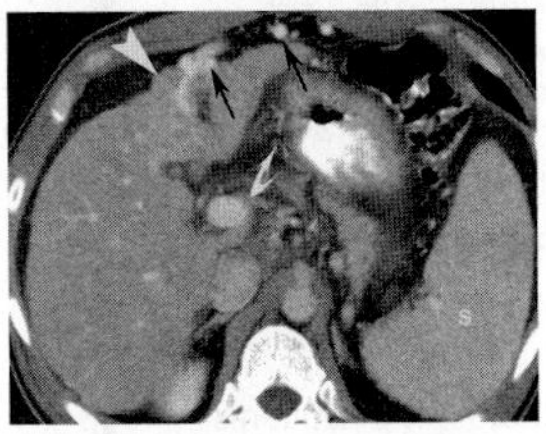

FIG. 3 Cirrhosis with portal hypertension. Postcontrast computed tomography reveals a liver that is nodular in contour *(arrowhead)* with patent enlarged paraumbilical veins *(blue arrows)* and splenomegaly *(S)*, findings indicative of portal hypertension. Mildly enlarged portosystemic collateral vessels *(curved arrow)* are also evident in the gastrohepatic ligament. (From Webb WR et al: *Fundamentals of body CT*, ed 4, Philadelphia, 2015, Saunders.)

TREATMENT BASED ON SPECIFIC CAUSE OF CIRRHOSIS

- Remove excess body iron with phlebotomy and deferoxamine in patients with hemochromatosis.
- Remove copper deposits with D-penicillamine in patients with Wilson disease.
- Long-term ursodiol therapy will slow the progression of primary biliary cholangitis. It is, however, ineffective in primary sclerosing cholangitis.
- Glucocorticoids (prednisone 20 to 30 mg/day initially or combination therapy or prednisone and azathioprine) are useful in autoimmune hepatitis.
- Antivirals in chronic hepatitis C.

PROGNOSIS

- Prognosis varies with the etiology of the patient's cirrhosis and whether there is ongoing hepatic injury. Fig. 7 illustrates the natural history of cirrhosis.
- Patients with compensated cirrhosis (no associated complications or esophageal varices without bleeding) have a good prognosis with median survival over 12 yr.
- In patients with decompensated cirrhosis, the Model of End-stage Liver Disease with sodium (MELDNa) scoring (Table 3) is useful to predict 3-mo mortality and so is the main method of prioritizing patients awaiting liver transplantation. It also has prognostic value following TIPS placement for patients with cirrhosis undergoing nontransplant surgeries. Mortality rate exceeds 80% in patients with hepatorenal syndrome.
- Regression of cirrhosis has been demonstrated after antiviral therapy in some patients with chronic hepatitis C. Regression is associated with decreased disease-related morbidity and improved survival.
- Cirrhosis is associated with an increased risk for hepatocellular carcinoma. However, the risk is low (1% 5-yr cumulative risk in alcoholic cirrhosis).

PEARLS & CONSIDERATIONS

COMMENTS

- Thrombocytopenia and advanced Child-Pugh classes (see Table 3) are associated with the presence of varices. These factors are useful to identify cirrhotic patients who benefit most from referral for endoscopic screening for varices.
- A combination of endoscopic and drug therapy reduces overall and variceal rebleeding in cirrhosis more than either therapy alone.
- PPI use, but not H_2RA use, is associated with risk for serious infections in patients with decompensated cirrhosis.
- In patients with compensated cirrhosis and clinically significant hypertension beta-blockers reduced a composite of decompensation or death.[1]

RELATED CONTENT

Cirrhosis (Patient Information)
Ascites (Related Key Topic)
Esophageal Varices (Related Key Topic)
Hepatic Encephalopathy (Related Key Topic)
Hepatopulmonary Syndrome (Related Key Topic)
Hepatorenal Syndrome (Related Key Topic)
Spontaneous Bacterial Peritonitis (Related Key Topic)
Primary Biliary Cholangitis (Related Key Topic)

SUGGESTED READINGS

Available at ExpertConsult.com

AUTHOR: **David J. Lucier Jr, MD, MBA, MPH**

[1]Villanueva C et al: β blockers to prevent decompensation of cirrhosis in patients with clinically significant portal hypertension (PREDESCI): a randomised, double-blind, placebo-controlled, multicentre trial, *Lancet* 393:1597-1608, 2019.

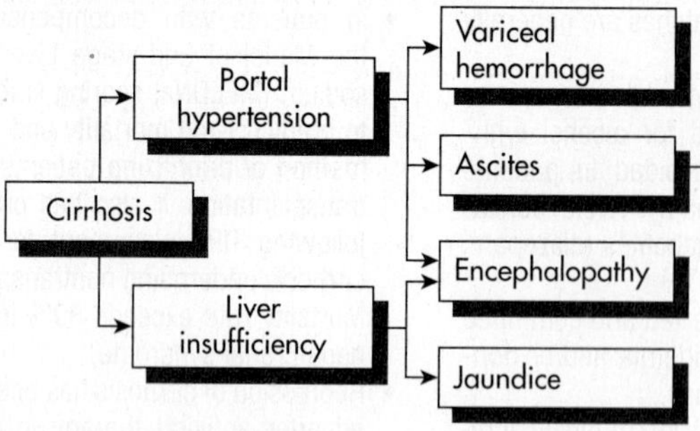

FIG. 5 Complications of cirrhosis result from portal hypertension or liver insufficiency. Varices and variceal hemorrhage are a direct consequence of portal hypertension. Ascites results from sinusoidal portal hypertension and can be complicated by infection (spontaneous bacterial peritonitis [SBP]) or renal dysfunction (hepatorenal syndrome [HRS]). Hepatic encephalopathy results from portosystemic shunting (i.e., portal hypertension) and liver insufficiency. Jaundice results solely from liver insufficiency. (From Goldman L, Schafer AI: *Goldman-Cecil medicine*, ed 26, Philadelphia, 2019, Elsevier.)

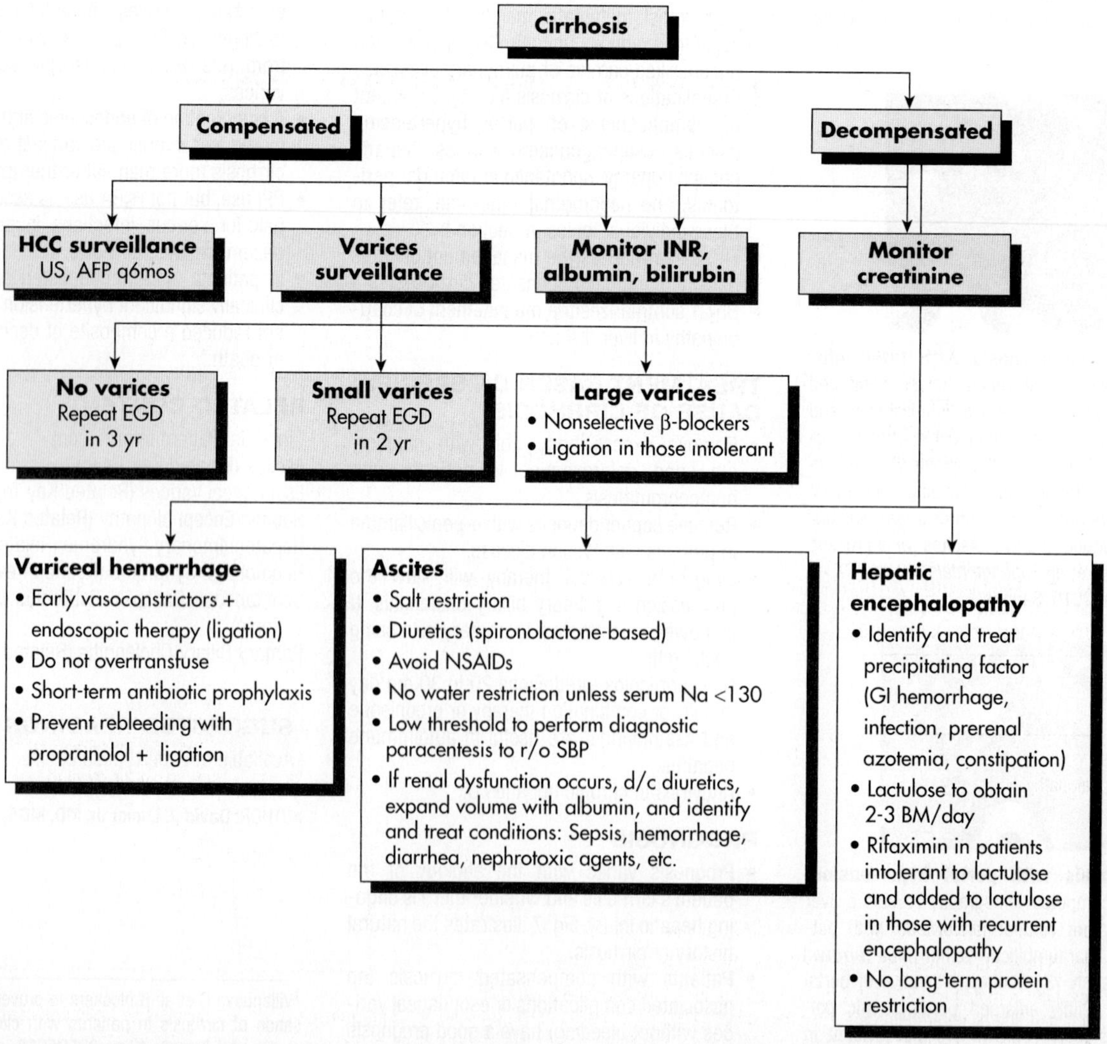

FIG. 6 Summary of the management of compensated and decompensated cirrhosis. *AFP,* α-Fetoprotein; *BM,* bowel movement; *d/c,* discontinue; *EGD,* esophagogastroduodenoscopy; *GI,* gastrointestinal; *HCC,* hepatocellular carcinoma; *INR,* international normalized ratio; *Na,* sodium; *NSAIDs,* nonsteroidal antiinflammatory drugs; *r/o,* rule out; *SBP,* spontaneous bacterial peritonitis; *US,* ultrasound. (From Goldman L, Schafer AI: *Goldman-Cecil medicine*, ed 26, Philadelphia, 2019, Elsevier.)

BOX 1 Management of Coagulopathy in Liver Disease

- Actively bleeding patients should be adequately resuscitated. Admission to the intensive care setting may be appropriate.
- Basic coagulation tests should be ordered to identify the cause of bleeding; these include CBC, PT (INR), PTT, thrombin clotting time, fibrinogen, D-dimer, FDP, and mixing studies. The need for more specialized tests will be dictated by the clinical situation and response to therapy.
- It is important to identify any localized source of bleeding (e.g., varices) amenable to procedural intervention to achieve hemostasis.
- A trial of 5-10 mg of vitamin K is reasonable in asymptomatic patients with prolonged PT and PTT but should be used with other therapies in actively bleeding patients.
- In patients with thrombocytopenia, platelet transfusions can be used, targeting platelet counts greater than 50 × 109 /L.
- In patients who can tolerate volume, FP 4-6 units (1000-1500 ml) given over 1-2 hours can be used to replace coagulation factors. Coagulation parameters should be monitored to document effect and determine the timing and need for additional units.
- Dysfibrinogenemia or hypofibrinogenemia should be suspected if coagulation assays do not correct with FP or fibrinogen levels are low, respectively. Replacement can be attempted with 10-20 units of cryoprecipitate while following laboratory results.
- Patients who are intravascularly overloaded or who do not respond to FP should be considered for rFVIIa. Low doses of rFVIIa (25-50 µg/kg) are generally used, and repeated doses may be required because of the short rfVIIa half-life of 2-3 hours. rFVIIa may be most suitable as a temporizing measure to enable invasive procedures or hemostasis to be achieved by other means. Avoid use in the setting of DIC.

CBC, Complete blood count; *DIC*, disseminated intravascular coagulation; *FDP*, fibrin degradation products; *FP*, frozen plasma; *INR*, international normalized ratio; *PT*, prothrombin time; *PTT*, partial thromboplastin time; *rFVIIa*, recombinant factor VIIa.
From Hoffman R et al: *Hematology: basic principles and practice*, ed 7, Philadelphia, 2018, Elsevier.

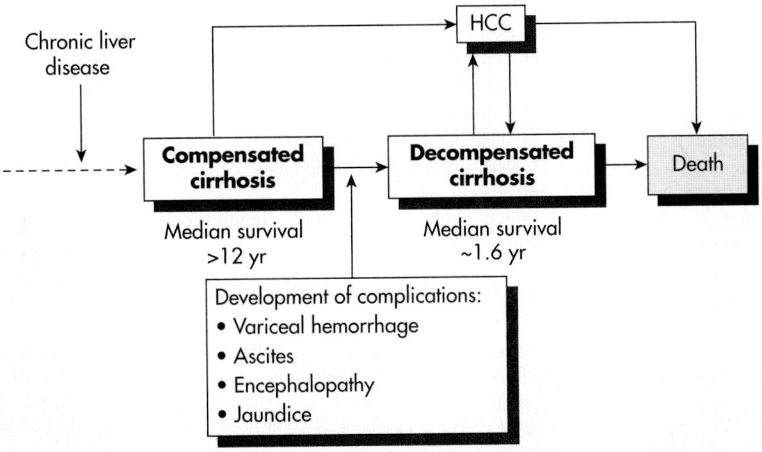

FIG. 7 Natural history of cirrhosis. Any chronic liver disease will lead to cirrhosis. Initially, cirrhosis will be compensated (median survival, >12 yr), but once complications (ascites, variceal hemorrhage, encephalopathy, jaundice) develop, it becomes decompensated (median survival, 1.6 yr). Hepatocellular carcinoma (HCC) can develop at any stage and precipitate decompensation and death. (From Goldman L, Schafer AI: *Goldman-Cecil medicine*, ed 26, Philadelphia, 2019, Elsevier.)

TABLE 3 The Two Most Commonly Used Scoring Systems in Cirrhosis

1. CHILD-TURCOTTE-PUGH (CTP) SCORE (RANGE, 5-15)

	POINTS ASCRIBED		
Parameters	**1**	**2**	**3**
Ascites	None	Grade 1-2 (or easy to treat)	Grade 3-4 (or refractory)
Hepatic encephalopathy	None	Grade 1-2 (or induced by a precipitant)	Grade 3-4 (or spontaneous)
Bilirubin (mg/dl)	<2	2-3	>3
Albumin (g/dl)	>3.5	2.8-3.5	<2.8
Prothrombin time (seconds > control) or INR	<4 <1.7	4-6 1.7-2.3	>6 >2.3

CTP classification: Child A: Score of 5-6; Child B: Score of 7-9; Child C: Score of 10-15

2. MODEL OF END-STAGE LIVER DISEASE (MELD) SCORE (RANGE, 6-40)

[0.957 × LN (creatinine in mg/dl) + 0.378 × LN (bilirubin in mg/dl) + 1.12 × LN (INR) + 0.643] × 10

MELD-Na is calculated first by determining the traditional MELD ($MELD_{(0)}$); if the initial $MELD_{(i)}$ score is 12 or greater, the score is adjusted by incorporating the serum sodium value [$MELD_{(0)}$ + 1.32 × (137-Na) – [0.033 × MELD(i) × (137-Na)]

INR, International normalized ratio; *LN*, natural logarithm.
From Goldman L, Schafer AI: *Goldman-Cecil medicine*, ed 26, Philadelphia, 2019, Elsevier.

BASIC INFORMATION

DEFINITION

Claudication refers to reproducible pain, fatigue, discomfort, or cramping due to vascular origin in a muscle group that is consistently induced by exertion and is relieved with rest. Claudication results from inadequate blood flow to the target muscle group, which is not able to meet increased metabolic demand, resulting in a supply-and-demand mismatch due to peripheral arterial disease (PAD). Intermittent vascular claudication is more common in the lower extremities but can also affect the upper extremities.

SYNONYM

Intermittent claudication

ICD-10CM CODES

I70.211	Atherosclerosis of native arteries of extremities with intermittent claudication, right leg
I70.212	Atherosclerosis of native arteries of extremities with intermittent claudication, left leg
I70.213	Atherosclerosis of native arteries of extremities with intermittent claudication, bilateral legs
I70.219	Atherosclerosis of native arteries of extremities with intermittent claudication, unspecified extremity
I70.311	Atherosclerosis of unspecified type of bypass graft(s) of the extremities with intermittent claudication, right leg
I70.312	Atherosclerosis of unspecified type of bypass graft(s) of the extremities with intermittent claudication, left leg
I70.313	Atherosclerosis of unspecified type of bypass graft(s) of the extremities with intermittent claudication, bilateral legs
I70.319	Atherosclerosis of unspecified type of bypass graft(s) of the extremities with intermittent claudication, unspecified extremity
I70.719	Atherosclerosis of other type of bypass graft(s) of the extremities with intermittent claudication, unspecified extremity

EPIDEMIOLOGY & DEMOGRAPHICS

- Symptomatic claudication in Western countries affects 5% of patients between the ages of 55 and 74.
- PAD, which includes both symptomatic claudication and asymptomatic disease, is estimated to affect approximately 40 to 45 million Americans and over 200 million people around the world.
- At-risk patients include:
  1. All patients age 65 yr or older
  2. Age 50 to 64 yr with risk factors for atherosclerosis, including diabetes mellitus, smoking history, hyperlipidemia, hypertension, or family history of PAD
  3. Age <50 yr, with diabetes mellitus and one additional risk factor for atherosclerosis
  4. Individuals with known atherosclerotic disease in another vascular bed, for example, coronary, carotid, subclavian, renal, mesenteric artery, or abdominal aortic aneurysm (AAA)
- Risk factors associated with development of PAD are similar to coronary atherosclerosis (CAD) (odds ratio 2.6) and include increasing age, cigarette smoking (odds ratio 2.7), hypertension (odds ratio 1.6), diabetes mellitus (odds ratio 1.9), and hypercholesterolemia (odds ratio 1.2). In addition, patients with chronic kidney disease, metabolic syndrome, and elevated levels of C-reactive protein, lipoprotein(a), and homocysteine are at increased risk. Nontraditional risk factors include race/ethnicity, with African American patients being at higher risk. Hispanics also have similar to slightly higher rates of PAD compared to non-Hispanic whites.
- There is a strong correlation among PAD, CAD, carotid artery stenosis, and generalized cerebrovascular disease. Individuals with known atherosclerotic disease in one vascular bed are likely to have disease in another.
- The American College of Cardiology/American Heart Association (ACC/AHA) guidelines suggested the following distribution of clinical presentation of PAD in patients 50 yr of age or older:
  1. Asymptomatic: 20% to 50%
  2. Atypical leg pain: 40% to 50%
  3. Classic intermittent claudication: 10% to 35%
  4. Critical limb ischemia with threatened limb: 1% to 2%

PHYSICAL FINDINGS & CLINICAL PRESENTATION

- The severity of symptoms varies with degree of PAD, collateral blood supply, and exertional demands.
- Classic symptoms include exertional calf pain, which limits the patient's activity and self-resolves with rest within 10 minutes. Claudication can also typically present in the buttock and hip, thigh, calf, or foot, with one or more of the following signs or symptoms, depending on the level and degree of peripheral stenosis:
  1. Diminished or absent pedal pulses
  2. Bruit over the distal aorta, iliac, or femoral arteries
  3. Pallor of the distal extremities and cool to the touch upon elevation
  4. Rubor with prolonged capillary refill upon dependent positioning
  5. Trophic changes, including hair/nail loss and muscle atrophy
  6. Nonhealing ulcers, necrotic tissue, and gangrene
  7. Weakness, numbness, or heaviness in the lower extremities
- True vascular claudication must be distinguished from "pseudoclaudication," which can be caused by severe venous obstruction or insufficiency, chronic compartment syndrome, spinal stenosis, osteoarthritis, and inflammatory muscle diseases. The characteristic features of pseudoclaudication that distinguish it from claudication are summarized in Table 1. Table 2 illustrates the differential diagnosis of intermittent claudication.
- Location of pain usually corresponds to analogous anatomy:
  1. Buttock and hip: Aortic or iliac disease
  2. Thigh: Aorta, iliac, or common femoral artery
  3. Upper two thirds of calf: Superficial femoral artery
  4. Lower one third of calf: Popliteal artery
  5. Foot: Tibial or peroneal artery
- Asymptomatic PAD is typically diagnosed by screening studies (exercise ankle brachial index, lower-extremity ultrasound) or incidentally on physical exam. Patients who are at significant risk for PAD often have multiple comorbidities that can alter their presentation. In the PARTNERS program report, 47% of those with a new diagnosis of PAD had no history of leg symptoms, 47% had atypical symptoms, and only 6% had classic symptoms.
- Symptoms of intermittent claudication classically start distally within a muscle group (below the stenosis) and then ascend with continued activity.
- Rest pain that occurs with leg elevation and is paradoxically relieved by walking may suggest severe PAD.
- Critical limb ischemia may present as tissue ulceration and gangrene, which require prompt intervention.

ETIOLOGY

The primary cause of claudication is peripheral atherosclerosis, resulting in a stenosis that impedes blood flow beyond the level necessary to meet the metabolic demand of limb muscles first with activity and then ultimately at rest.

TABLE 1 Distinguishing Characteristics between Pseudoclaudication and Claudication

	Claudication	Pseudoclaudication
Characteristics	Limb cramping, tightness, fatigue	Similar to claudication with numbness
Location of discomfort	Lower extremity involving buttock, hip, thigh, calf, foot	Similar to claudication
Induced by exercise	Yes	Variable
Reproducible with distance walked	Consistent	Variable
Occurs with standing	No	Yes
Actions which provide relief	Stand	Sit
Time to relief	<5 min	≥30 min

TABLE 2 Differential Diagnosis of Intermittent Claudication

	Intermittent Claudication	Venous Claudication	Neurogenic Claudication
Quality of pain	Cramping	Aching, heaviness, tightness	"Pins and needles" sensation going down the leg, weakness
Onset	Gradual, consistent	Gradual; can, however, be immediate	Can be immediate
Relieved by	Stopping walking	Activity, elevation of leg	Sitting down, stooping, flexion at the waist
Location	Muscle groups (e.g., buttocks, thigh, calf)	Entire leg, worse in calf	Poorly localized, but can affect whole leg
Legs affected	Usually one	Usually one	Often both

From Swartz MH: *Textbook of physical diagnosis,* ed 7, Philadelphia, 2014, Saunders.

Other etiologies include neuropathy, musculoskeletal or degenerative disease, compartment or entrapment syndrome, vasculitis, and embolic events.

Dx DIAGNOSIS

DIFFERENTIAL DIAGNOSIS

- Spinal stenosis (neurogenic or pseudoclaudication)
- Musculoskeletal disorders: Arthritis or myositis
- Degenerative osteoarthritic joint disease, predominantly of the lumbar spine and hips
- Chronic compartment or popliteal artery entrapment syndrome
- Peripheral neuropathy
- Sciatica
- Atheromatous embolization and deep venous thrombosis, superficial thrombophlebitis
- Vasculitis: Thromboangiitis obliterans, Takayasu, or giant cell arteritis
- Symptomatic Baker cyst
- Venous claudication
- Raynaud phenomenon

WORKUP

History and physical findings suggest the diagnosis of claudication and noninvasive studies help confirm the diagnosis.

- Careful physical examinations include:
  1. Measurement of blood pressure in both arms and notation of asymmetry
  2. Palpation and recording of carotid pulses, upstroke, amplitude, and presence of bruits
  3. Auscultation and palpation of abdomen for bruits, aortic pulsation, and diameter
  4. Palpation of brachial, radial, ulnar, femoral, popliteal, dorsalis pedis, and posterior tibial pulses. Pulse intensity should be recorded as follows: 0, absent; 1+, diminished; 2+, normal; 3+, bounding
  5. Auscultation of femoral arteries for the presence of bruits.
  6. Extremities should be inspected for color, temperature, integrity of the skin, hair loss, and hypertrophic nails
- Measurement of resting ankle–brachial index (ABI) should be considered first-line test in patients at risk for PAD.
- An ABI is the ratio of higher ankle systolic pressure (between the dorsalis pedis and posterior tibial arteries) of each leg to the higher systolic pressure of either arm (brachial artery).
- When measuring ABI, brachial pressures in both arms should be taken to avoid underestimating pressure due to subclavian artery stenosis.
- The severity of PAD is based on the resting ABI:
  1. Severe PAD: <0.4
  2. Moderate PAD: 0.4 to 0.69
  3. Mild PAD: 0.70 to 0.90
  4. Borderline: 0.91 to 0.99
  5. Normal: 1.00 to 1.40
  6. Noncompressible: >1.40
- ABI ≤0.90 has 75% sensitivity and 86% specificity in the detection of PAD.
- A low ABI has been shown to be an independent predictor of mortality.
- A high ABI (>1.4) may represent significant PAD caused by arterial wall stiffening. In such cases, measuring a toe–brachial index (TBI) can increase the sensitivity of testing, as highly calcified arteries are incompressible and may have an elevated ABI. A toe–brachial index <0.7 is considered abnormal and diagnostic of PAD.
- Borderline resting ABI (>0.90 and ≤1.40) in patients with exertional leg symptoms should undergo exercise treadmill ABI testing to evaluate for PAD. This can help differentiate claudication from pseudoclaudication. If posttreadmill ABI is normal, alternative causes of leg pain should be considered.
- Progression of PAD is considered to have occurred if a decrease in ABI of 0.15 occurs while the patient is on treatment.
- If a patient has a history concerning for PAD but a normal ABI, and if the clinician is concerned about a potential false-negative finding, performing an exercise stress ABI can potentially demonstrate lower-extremity PAD.
- If after exercise, ABI reading decreases by more than 20% or an ankle pressure decreases by 30 mm Hg, the patient should be considered to have significant PAD.
- Segmental systolic pressures are measured at the level of the thigh, calf, ankle, metatarsal, and toes. Normally, successive segments have <20 mm Hg difference in pressures. If the gradient is >20 mm Hg, a significant stenosis is suspected in the interval vascular segment.

IMAGING STUDIES

- Duplex ultrasound can be used to assess occlusion location, length, and patency of the distal arterial system or prior grafts; it is a good choice for initial imaging and surveillance monitoring after revascularization.
- In patients with prior infrainguinal venous bypass grafts, the long-term patency should be evaluated at regular intervals using a duplex ultrasound approximately 4 to 6 wk postprocedure, 6 and 12 mo after graft placement, and then yearly.
- Magnetic resonance angiography (MRA) and CT angiography (CTA) are effective for imaging of the aorta and peripheral lower-extremity arteries above the knee. MRA has almost replaced catheter-based angiography, with 90% sensitivity and 97% specificity in identification of hemodynamically significant stenosis in the lower extremities.
- MRA and CTA are useful to define the anatomy and assist in planning percutaneous and surgical revascularization; however, the utility of each is decreased by necessity of gadolinium contrast and noniodinated contrast agents, respectively.
- Angiography (Fig. 1) remains the gold standard for diagnosing PAD, particularly below the knee.

Rx TREATMENT

NONPHARMACOLOGIC THERAPY

- Smoking cessation is of paramount importance. Smokers and former smokers should be asked about tobacco use status at every visit and offered pharmacotherapy, counseling, and/or referred to smoking cessation programs (Class I, A).
- Aggressive risk factor modification for hypertension, dyslipidemia, and diabetes mellitus, including diet, weight loss, and lifestyle counseling, is recommended (Fig. 2).
- Supervised exercise training should be performed as a first-line therapy for a minimum of 30 to 45 minutes, in sessions performed at least 3 times per week, for a minimum of 12 wk.
- Supervised exercise training programs under direct supervision in a hospital or outpatient facility and structured exercise are recommended for all patients with PAD. This has been shown to increase maximal walking distance, pain-free walking distance, and the 6-minute walking distance. It typically requires 4 to 6 wk for patients to notice improvement.
- Structured or home-based walking exercise program may be considered as an alternative treatment modality, but it has not been shown to be as efficacious. It can be combined with group-mediated cognitive behavioral intervention that can significantly

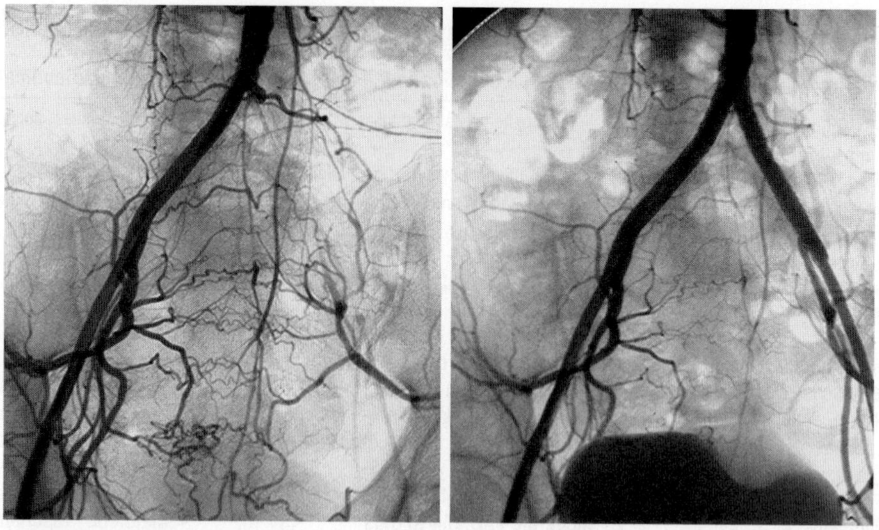

FIG. 1 Angiogram of the distal abdominal aorta and iliac arteries demonstrates an occluded left common iliac artery with extensive collateral circulation from contralateral internal iliac artery (left panel), which resolved after successful stent implantation *(right panel)*. (Images courtesy of Bart Domatch, MD, Radiology Department, University of Texas. Southwestern Medical Center, Dallas, Texas. From Andreoli TE et al: *Andreoli and Carpenter's Cecil essentials of medicine,* ed 8, Philadelphia, 2010, Saunders.)

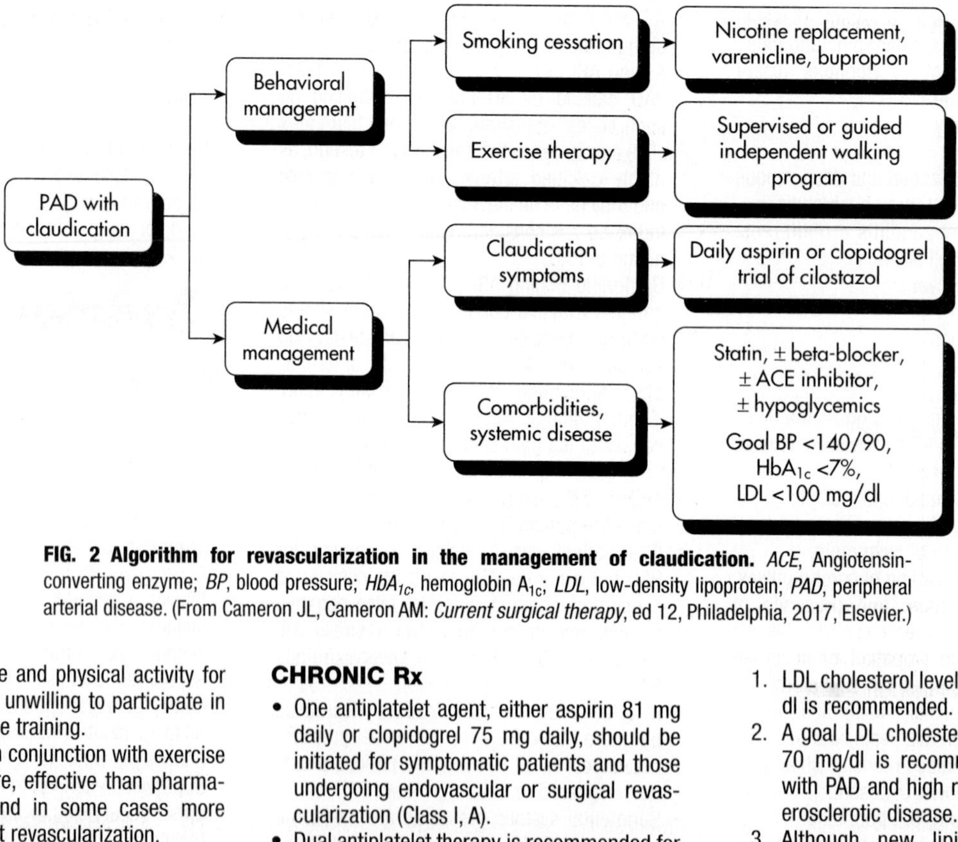

FIG. 2 Algorithm for revascularization in the management of claudication. *ACE,* Angiotensin-converting enzyme; *BP,* blood pressure; *HbA_{1c},* hemoglobin A_{1c}; *LDL,* low-density lipoprotein; *PAD,* peripheral arterial disease. (From Cameron JL, Cameron AM: *Current surgical therapy,* ed 12, Philadelphia, 2017, Elsevier.)

improve endurance and physical activity for patients unable or unwilling to participate in supervised exercise training.

- Lifestyle therapy in conjunction with exercise can be as, or more, effective than pharmacologic therapy and in some cases more effective than stent revascularization.
- Intermittent mechanical compression appears to be an effective noninvasive treatment alternative for patients with intermittent claudication.

ACUTE GENERAL Rx

Revascularization by an endovascular or surgical approach is usually reserved for patients with symptoms refractory to medical therapy or those with impending critical limb ischemia.

CHRONIC Rx

- One antiplatelet agent, either aspirin 81 mg daily or clopidogrel 75 mg daily, should be initiated for symptomatic patients and those undergoing endovascular or surgical revascularization (Class I, A).
- Dual antiplatelet therapy is recommended for after infrainguinal stenting and carotid artery stenting for at least 1 mo (Class IIa, C) and single agent afterward.
- Asymptomatic patients with PAD (ABI ≤0.90) without claudication symptoms may benefit from the addition of an antiplatelet agent (Class IIa, C), either ASA or clopidogrel, as there is an increased cardiovascular risk in this subgroup.
- Statin medications are indicated for all patients with PAD (Class I, A).
    1. LDL cholesterol level of less than 100 mg/dl is recommended.
    2. A goal LDL cholesterol level of less than 70 mg/dl is recommended for patients with PAD and high risk for coronary atherosclerotic disease.
    3. Although new lipid guidelines have been published, the guidelines did not specifically address patients with PAD; therefore, the numerical targets can be considered. In those unable to reach the targets, a reduction in LDL >50% should be approached at a minimum.
- Antihypertensive therapy with beta-adrenergic blocking drugs and/or ACE inhibitors should be administered to all hypertensive patients with PAD to reduce the risk of MI,

stroke, congestive heart failure, and cardiovascular death.

- Cilostazol 100 mg bid may be used in conjunction with aspirin or clopidogrel. It has been shown to increase walking distance by 50% to 67% in symptomatic patients (Class I, A).
- Among patients with intermittent claudication, a single randomized controlled trial has shown a 24-wk treatment with ramipril resulted in significant increases in pain-free and maximum treadmill walking times compared with placebo.
- Pentoxifylline is not effective for treatment of claudication. In a review of 24 studies with over 3000 participants, results remained unclear, and a randomized control trial showed no difference between pentoxifylline and placebo; thus this is not recommended as a treatment for claudication.
- In patients with type II diabetes, a secondary analysis of the BARI 2D trial showed that an insulin-sensitizing approach (metformin, thiazolidinediones) reduces the risk of developing PAD when compared to insulin-providing therapy (glipizide, insulin). These patients also have lower rates of revascularization and amputation.
- Patients who are tobacco smokers should be strongly advised to quit smoking at every visit and offered either varenicline or bupropion along with nicotine replacement therapy in the absence of any contraindications. Patients with PAD should avoid tobacco smoke exposure at work, at home, and in public places.
- Anticoagulation should not be used to reduce the risk of cardiovascular ischemic events in patients with PAD as there is increased morbidity with no mortality benefit. Its use to improve patency after bypass is uncertain (Class III, A).
- Novel agents, such as protease-activated receptor-1 (e.g., vorapaxar), added to existing antiplatelet therapy may have some benefit in decreasing acute limb-related ischemic events; however, its association with a risk of moderate to severe bleeding makes its benefits uncertain at this time.
- Fig. 3 summarizes the nonoperative management of claudication.
- Revascularization through either a percutaneous or surgical approach is indicated in patients with lifestyle-limiting claudication and inadequate response to goal-directed medical therapy. It is also indicated in those with nonhealing ulcers or gangrene and in select patients with functional disability. Before such revascularization, each patient should have:
  1. Participated in a supervised exercise training program and been given goal-directed medical therapy.
  2. Received comprehensive risk factor modification, including smoking cessation and optimal management of comorbidities.
  3. Significant disability with either the inability to perform normal work or a serious impairment of other activities important to the patient.
  4. Lower-extremity PAD lesion anatomy amenable to revascularization defined as low risk with high probability of initial and long-term success.
- Common procedures include:
  1. Percutaneous balloon angioplasty can be used for long lesions or diffuse disease and has initial success rate of 90% but >60% restenosis rate over 12 mo. Balloon angioplasty combined with stenting is primarily used on discrete stenotic lesions in the iliac or femoropopliteal arteries.

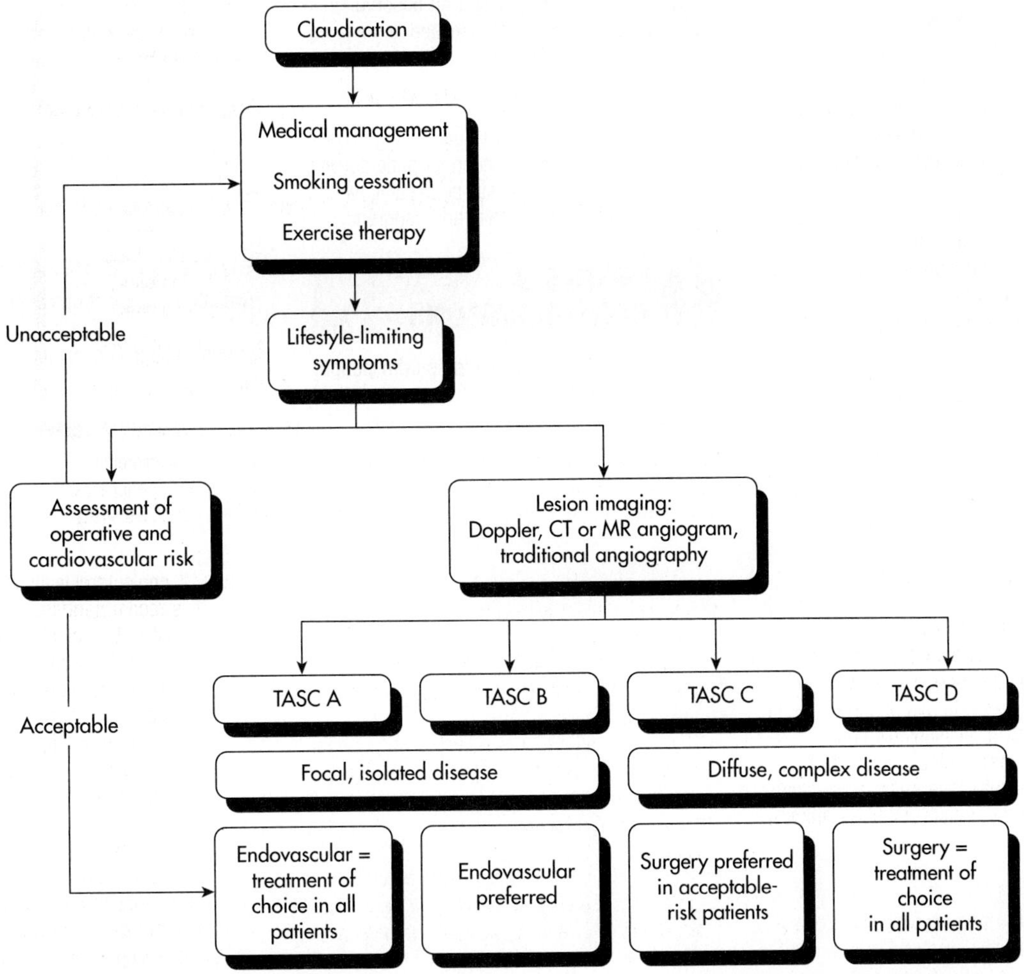

FIG. 3 Nonoperative management of claudication. *CT*, Computed tomographic; *MR*, magnetic resonance; *TASC*, TransAtlantic Inter-Society Consensus class. (From Cameron JL, Cameron AM: *Current surgical therapy*, ed 12, Philadelphia, 2017, Elsevier.)

2. Aortoiliofemoral reconstruction or bypass or infrainguinal bypass (e.g., femoropopliteal, femorotibial).
3. Endovascular intervention is recommended as the preferred revascularization technique for iliac and femoropopliteal arterial lesions. In LEVANT II trial, endovascular stenting had greater primary patency rate than balloon angioplasty in patients with claudication at 12 mo.
4. Stenting is an effective primary therapy for common and external iliac artery stenosis and occlusions. However, it is not recommended in the femoral, popliteal, or tibial arteries due to a low success rate except to salvage suboptimal balloon dilation.
5. In severe, nonreversible cases with gangrene, amputation may be required.

- Endovascular procedures should not be performed in patients with PAD solely to prevent progression to critical limb ischemia, as reported rates of amputation or progression to critical limb ischemia are <10% to 15% over 5 yr or more, and increased mortality rate associated with claudication is usually the result of cardiovascular events rather than limb-related events.

COMPLEMENTARY & ALTERNATIVE MEDICINE

- A meta-analysis found that over 12 to 24 wk, ginkgo biloba increased pain-free walking distance by 34 m compared with placebo, although the benefit is not well established according to ACC/AHA guidelines.
- Naftidrofuryl, a serotonin receptor inhibitor, available in Europe and other parts of the world, has shown some efficacy in improving claudication symptoms.
- Estrogen replacement therapy, propionyl-L-carnitine, L-arginine, oral vasodilators, prostaglandins, and chelation therapy are ineffective in the treatment of intermittent claudication.
- B-complex vitamin supplementation to lower homocysteine levels for prevention of cardiovascular events in patients with PAD is not recommended (HOPE-2 trial).
- Acupuncture has shown some improvement in symptom relief and functional capacity in small studies but mainly in neurogenic claudication or mild peripheral arterial disease.

PROGNOSIS

- It is unusual for intermittent claudication to progress to ischemic leg or limb loss, especially with aggressive use of conservative treatments, risk factor modification, exercise, and smoking cessation.
- Among patients with claudication, 70% to 80% remain with stable claudication, 10% to 20% with worsening symptoms, and critical limb ischemia in 1% to 2% in 5 yr. The risk for nonfatal cardiovascular event is 20% and death is 15% to 30%.
- The 5-yr risk for development of ischemic ulceration in patients treated for diabetes and with ABI <0.5 was 30% compared with only 5% in patients without either characteristic.
- A screening duplex ultrasound for AAA is recommended for patients with symptomatic PAD.
- All patients with PAD should receive annual influenza vaccination based on observational studies that have demonstrated a reduced cardiovascular event rate.

REFERRAL

Consultation with physicians specializing in vascular medicine is recommended for patients with threatened limb loss, rest pain, nonhealing ulcers, functional disability from pain, and gangrene.

PEARLS & CONSIDERATIONS

- Approximately 70% of patients with peripheral vascular disease will have concomitant coronary artery disease.
- Beta-blockers may worsen claudication symptoms in some patients, although their underuse is associated with excess cardiovascular death. Patients with intermittent claudication are less likely to receive beta-blocker therapy after a myocardial infarction. Those who do not receive post-MI beta-blockers have at least a threefold higher mortality.
- Patients with peripheral vascular disease may benefit from secondary cardiovascular prevention with clopidogrel versus aspirin more so than other high-risk patients.
- PAD can be asymptomatic or with atypical symptoms, and a thorough history, physical exam, and clinical suspicion based on medical comorbidities may help guide therapy before lifestyle-limiting claudication or limb ischemia develops.

COMMENTS

- Claudication is a marker for generalized atherosclerosis. Patients have a higher risk of death from cardiovascular events than from limb loss. Patients with PAD experience diminished overall quality of life similar to patients diagnosed coronary artery or cerebrovascular disease.
- The ABI is more closely associated with exercise tolerance and severity of disease in persons with PAD rather than intermittent claudication or other leg symptoms.

RELATED CONTENT

Poor Circulation (Claudication) (Patient Information)
Peripheral Artery Disease (Related Key Topic)

SUGGESTED READINGS

Available at ExpertConsult.com

AUTHORS: **Stephani C. Wang, MD,** and **Pranav M. Patel, MD, FACC, FAHA, FSCAI**

BASIC INFORMATION

DEFINITION

Clostridium difficile infection (CDI) is the occurrence of diarrhea and bowel inflammation associated with antibiotic use caused by *C. difficile*, an anaerobic gram-positive, spore-forming, toxin-producing bacillus transmitted through the fecal–oral route. CDI can manifest clinically in several forms ranging from fulminant diarrhea and leukocytosis associated with pseudomembranous colitis, mild to severe acute diarrhea, short-term colonization seen typically in health care facilities, and recurrent CDI within 60 days after initial treatment occurring in 20% to 30% of cases.

SYNONYMS

Antibiotic-induced colitis
Pseudomembranous colitis
CDI

ICD-10CM CODE

A04.7 Enterocolitis due to *Clostridium difficile*

EPIDEMIOLOGY & DEMOGRAPHICS

- Cephalosporins are the most frequent offending agent in CDI because of their high rates of use.
- The antibiotic with the highest incidence is clindamycin (10% incidence of CDI with its use).
- Since 1996, the incidence of CDI has more than doubled. Severity of CDI has also increased due to the emergence of an epidemic virulent strain (NAP1/BI/027). CDI is the most common infectious cause of health-care–associated diarrhea in adults. In the U.S. *C. difficile* is responsible for nearly half a million infections per year and is associated with approximately 29,000 deaths/yr.
- Nosocomial CDI quadruples the cost of hospitalizations and increases annual expenditures by $4 and $6 billion in the U.S.
- Asymptomatic carriage of *C. difficile* is identified in more than 20% of patients hospitalized without diarrhea.

PHYSICAL FINDINGS & CLINICAL PRESENTATION

- Abdominal tenderness (generalized or lower abdominal)
- Fever
- In patients with prolonged diarrhea, poor skin turgor, dry mucous membranes, and other signs of dehydration may be present

ETIOLOGY

C. difficile colonizes the large intestines and releases two protein exotoxins (TcdA and TcdB) that cause colitis. Infection is transmitted by spores that are resistant to antibiotics, heat, and acid. The NAP1 strain is predominant among patients with *C. difficile* infection, whereas asymptomatic patients are more likely to be colonized with other strains. Risk factors for *C. difficile* (the major identifiable agent of antibiotic-induced diarrhea and colitis):

- Administration of antibiotics: Can occur with any antibiotic, but occurs most frequently with clindamycin, ampicillin, cephalosporins, and fluoroquinolone
- Prolonged hospitalization
- Advanced age
- Abdominal surgery
- Underlying disease (malignancy, renal failure, debilitated status)
- Hospitalized, tube-fed patients are at risk for *C. difficile*–associated diarrhea. Clinicians should consider testing for *C. difficile* in tube-fed patients with diarrhea unrelated to the feeding solution
- Proton pump inhibitor (PPI) and H_2 blocker therapy increases risk of CDI and recurrent CDI. Risk is 1.7-fold higher with PPIs

Dx DIAGNOSIS

The clinical signs of CDI generally include diarrhea, fever, and abdominal cramps after use of antibiotics. Although a history of recent antibiotic use is common, it is not a requirement for diagnosis.

CLASSIFICATION

The American College of Gastroenterology (ACG), the Infectious Diseases Society of America (IDSA), and the European Congress of Clinical Microbiology and Infectious Diseases (ECCMID) classify CDI as:

- Mild/moderate
  1. Diarrhea but no signs or symptoms of severe or fulminant CDI (ACG)
  2. WBC <15 x 10^9/L, serum creat <1.5 mg/dL (IDSA)
  3. Stool frequency <4 times daily, no signs of severe colitis (ECCMID)
- Severe
  1. Serum albumin <3 g/dL and WBC >1.5 x 10^9/dL or abdominal tenderness (ACG)
  2. WBC ≥15 x 10^9/L, serum creatinine > 1.5 mg/dL (IDSA)
  3. Fever >38.5°C, rigors, hemodynamic instability (ECCMID)
- Fulminant
  1. Hypotension or fever ≥38.5, or ileus, mental status change, and organ failure WBC ≥35 x 10^9/L, hypotension, ICU admission (ACG)
  2. Hypotension or shock, ileus, megacolon (IDSA)
  3. Peritoneal signs, ileus WBC >16 x 10^9/L, elevated serum lactate increase in serum creatinine (≥1.5 x baseline) (ECCMID)

DIFFERENTIAL DIAGNOSIS

- Gastrointestinal bacterial infections (e.g., *Salmonella, Shigella, Campylobacter, Yersinia*)
- Enteric parasites (e.g., *Cryptosporidium, Entamoeba histolytica*)
- Inflammatory bowel disease
- Celiac sprue
- Irritable bowel syndrome
- Ischemic colitis
- Antibiotic intolerance

WORKUP

- All patients with diarrhea accompanied by current or recent antibiotic use should be tested for *C. difficile* (see later discussion). *C. difficile* stool tests are positive in 3% of outpatients and up to 29% of inpatients without signs of infection. Testing and treatment for CDI is not recommended in asymptomatic individuals.
- Sigmoidoscopy (without cleansing enema) may be necessary when the clinical and laboratory diagnosis is inconclusive and the diarrhea persists.
- In antibiotic-induced pseudomembranous colitis, the sigmoidoscopy often reveals raised white-yellow exudative plaques adherent to the colonic mucosa pseudomembranes (Fig. E1). These are seen more commonly in severe CDI.

LABORATORY TESTS

- Stool test for *C. difficile* toxin: Enzyme-linked immunosorbent assay for *C. difficile* toxins A and B. The latter is used most widely in the clinical setting. It has a sensitivity of 85% and a specificity of 100%.
- *C. difficile* toxin can be detected by cytotoxin tissue culture assay (cytotoxin assay, gold standard for identifying *C. difficile* toxin in stool specimen). This test is difficult to perform, and results are not available for 24 to 48 hr.
- Fecal leukocytes (assessed by microscopy or lactoferrin assay) are generally present in stool samples.
- Complete blood count usually reveals leukocytosis. A sudden increase in white blood cells to >30,000/mm^3 may be indicative of fulminant colitis.
- Laboratory indicators of **severe CDI** are leukocyte count >15,000/mm^3, serum creatinine ≥1.5 times baseline level, serum albumin <2.5 g/dl.

IMAGING STUDIES

- Abdominal film (flat plate and upright) is useful in patients with abdominal pain or evidence of obstruction on physical examination.
- CT can demonstrate typical findings of colonic wall thickening, dilatation, and the so-called *accordion sign* (thickened haustral folds and trapped contrast material, ascites, or pericolonic stranding [Fig. 2]).

Rx TREATMENT

NONPHARMACOLOGIC THERAPY

- Discontinue offending antibiotic.
- Fluid hydration and correction of electrolyte abnormalities.
- Probiotics to restore natural defense mechanisms may be useful as adjuvant therapy; however, evidence is limited. Probiotic trials have failed to show benefit in preventing *C. difficile*–associated diarrhea.

- Fecal microbiota transplantation (FMT) is an excellent treatment modality for recurrent CDI. It replaces the altered gut flora to allow colonization resistance. Trials have shown that it is more effective than vancomycin and may become standard treatment for recurrent CDI. Recent trials have shown that donor stool administered via colonoscopy are safe and more efficacious than autologous FMT in preventing further CDI episodes.

ACUTE GENERAL Rx

- Vancomycin 125 mg PO qid for 10 days can be used as initial treatment in patients with nonsevere or severe CDI. Patients with fulminant CDI will require 500 mg qid for 10 days.
- Fidaxomicin 200 mg bid for 10 days has shown noninferiority to vancomycin and a lower rate of CDI recurrence (25% with vancomycin vs. 15% with fidaxomicin); however, its higher cost is a limiting factor. Fidaxomicin can be used for initial treatment of nonsevere or severe CDI or for recurrence of CDI if vancomycin was used for initial treatment.
- Metronidazole 500 mg PO qid for 10 days can be used in patients with mild disease if oral vancomycin or fidaxomicin are not available or contraindicated. A significant rise in clinical failure has been seen with metronidazole over the past decade, especially in patients with the BI/NAP/027 strain.
- When parenteral therapy is necessary (e.g., patient with paralytic ileus), IV metronidazole 500 mg qid can be used. It can also be supplemented with vancomycin 500 mg by nasogastric tube with intermittent clamping or retention enema.
- Fecal microbiota transplantation (FMT): When standard treatment has failed, intestinal microbiota transplantation (IMT) is an effective alternative therapy (eradication rate is 94%). It involves infusing intestinal microorganisms (in a suspension of healthy donor stool) into the intestine of a sick patient via enema, oral capsule, gastroscope/colonoscope, or nasojejunal tube to restore the microbiota. In patients with recurrent *C. difficile* infection, FMT by oral capsule has been shown to be noninferior to transplantation by colonoscopy for recurrence at 12 wk. Trials comparing fresh versus frozen fecal microbiota transplantation have shown equal efficacy.
- The human monoclonal antibody bezlotoxumab has been FDA-approved for use with antibacterial drug treatment to reduce recurrence of CDI. Cost is a limiting factor.

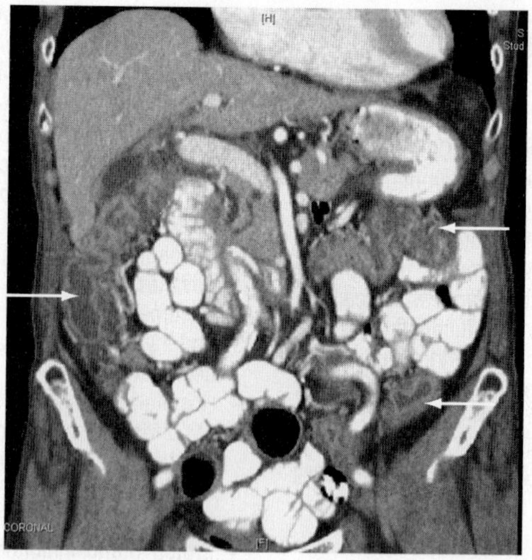

FIG. 2 Computed tomography with oral and intravenous contrast in a patient with Clostridium difficile colitis. Typical findings include colonic wall thickening *(arrows)*, dilation, and accordion sign (thickened haustral fold and trapped contrast material, ascites, and pericolonic stranding). (From Vincent JL et al: *Textbook of critical care*, ed 7, Philadelphia, 2017, Elsevier.)

SURGICAL MANAGEMENT

- Indications: CDI unresponsive to medical therapy, fulminant colitis
- Clinical features: Colonic distention, severe abdominal pain/tenderness, systemic inflammatory response syndrome. Diarrhea may be absent because of ileus
- Surgical approaches:
  1. Traditional (subtotal or total colectomy), high mortality (50%)
  2. Colon-sparing (loop ileostomy with intraoperative colonic lavage using warmed polyethylene glycol solution via the ileostomy and instillations of postoperative vancomycin flushes via the ileostomy); lower mortality compared to traditional approach

CHRONIC Rx

- Judicious future use of antibiotics to prevent recurrences (e.g., avoid prolonged antibiotic therapy).
- Probiotics have been shown mildly effective in reducing the risk for CDI among patients prescribed antibiotics. They should not be used in immunocompromised or severely debilitated patients.
- Alcohol-based hand gels are inadequate for eradication of spores. They are inferior to soap and water for eradication of spores.
- Gastric acid suppression with PPIs increases risk of CDI. Preferential use of H_2RA should be considered in these patients.

DISPOSITION

- Most patients recover completely with appropriate therapy. Fever resolves within 48 hr and diarrhea within 4 to 5 days. Overall mortality rate is 1% to 2.5% but exceeds 10% in untreated patients. CDI recurrence after an initial episode is 20% to 25% regardless of initial treatment with metronidazole or vancomycin. Each recurrence increases risk of repeat episodes (65% chance of recurrence after three CDI episodes). Recurrent CDI usually represents relapse rather than reinfection, no matter how long between episodes (Fig. E3). Recurrent episodes are best treated with a prolonged course of oral vancomycin tapered off over several weeks to months.
- Hospital-acquired CDI is independently associated with an increased risk of in-hospital death. All hospitalized patients with CDI should be placed in contact isolation at least until resolution of diarrhea.

SUGGESTED READINGS

Available at ExpertConsult.com

RELATED CONTENT

Clostridium difficile Infection (Patient Information)

AUTHOR: **Fred F. Ferri, MD**

BASIC INFORMATION

DEFINITION

The term *cluster headache* refers to attacks of severe, unilateral pain that is orbital, supraorbital, temporal, or any combination of these sites, lasting 15 to 180 minutes, and occurring from once every other day to eight times a day over a span of weeks to months. The attacks are associated with one or more ipsilateral signs and symptoms of parasympathetic activation: conjunctival injection, lacrimation (Fig. 1), nasal congestion, rhinorrhea, forehead and facial sweating, miosis, ptosis, or eyelid edema. Most patients are restless or agitated during an attack.

SYNONYMS

Headache, cluster
Ciliary neuralgia
Erythromelalgia of the head
Erythroprosopalgia of Bing
Horton headache

ICD-10CM CODES

G44.001	Cluster headache syndrome, unspecified, intractable
G44.009	Cluster headache syndrome, unspecified, not intractable
G44.011	Episodic cluster headache, intractable
G44.019	Episodic cluster headache, not intractable
G44.021	Chronic cluster headache, intractable
G44.029	Chronic cluster headache, not intractable

EPIDEMIOLOGY & DEMOGRAPHICS

INCIDENCE: Estimated to occur in 0.05% to 1% of the population

PREDOMINANT SEX: Occurs in males at least five times more commonly than in females

PREDOMINANT AGE: Peak age of onset between 20 and 40 yr

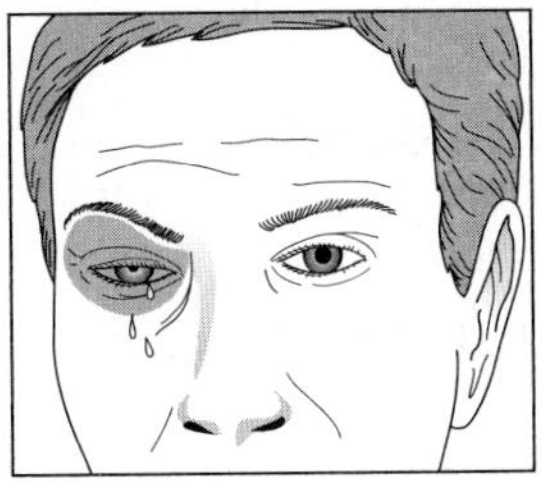

FIG. 1 This 43-yr-old man with cluster headaches suffers from nightly right-sided unrelenting, severe, stabbing unilateral periorbital pain for 45 minutes to 3 hours accompanied by ipsilateral tearing and nasal discharge, along with ptosis and miosis (a partial Horner syndrome). Note that the ptosis prompts compensatory elevation of the eyebrow. (From Kaufman DM et al: *Kaufman's clinical neurology for psychiatrists*, ed 8, Philadelphia, 2017, Elsevier.)

GENETICS: May be inherited in up to 20% of cases, although uncertainty exists over the mode or modes of inheritance.

PHYSICAL FINDINGS & CLINICAL PRESENTATION

- Many of the attacks are nocturnal, and some may be provoked by alcohol ingestion.
- During attack: Conjunctival injection, lacrimation, nasal congestion, rhinorrhea, facial sweating, Horner syndrome.
- In contrast to migraine sufferers, patients are agitated and active during an attack.
- Symptoms associated with an attack remain ipsilateral during the attack but may switch sides from one attack to the next.
- Permanent partial Horner syndrome in 5% of patients; otherwise examination is normal.

ETIOLOGY

Activation of the posterior hypothalamic gray matter resulting in trigeminal activation coupled with parasympathetic activation. The pathophysiology remains controversial.

DIAGNOSIS

Per the *International Classification of Headache Disorders,* 3rd edition, the diagnosis of cluster headache requires all of the following:

- At least five attacks of severe or very severe unilateral orbital, supraorbital, and/or temporal pain lasting 15 to 180 minutes
- Frequency of every other day to eight per day; they may cluster seasonally or at a certain time in a patient's life
- Headache is accompanied by a sense of restlessness or agitation and/or at least one of the following (ipsilateral):
  1. Conjunctival injection and/or lacrimation
  2. Nasal congestion and/or rhinorrhea
  3. Eyelid edema
  4. Forehead and facial sweating
  5. Forehead and facial flushing
  6. Miosis and/or ptosis
  7. Sensation of fullness in the ear
  8. Restlessness or agitation
- A diagnosis of episodic cluster headache requires the above criteria plus attacks that occur in bouts, also called cluster periods. These periods last 1 wk to 1 yr and are separated by attack-free intervals lasting at least 1 mo.
- A diagnosis of chronic cluster headache requires meeting the criteria for cluster headache plus at least 1 yr of attacks without a pain-free interval of at least 1 mo.

DIFFERENTIAL DIAGNOSIS

- Migraine
- Trigeminal neuralgia
- Primary stabbing headache
- Temporal arteritis
- Postherpetic neuralgia
- Venous sinus thrombosis
- Carotid-cavernous fistula or other cavernous sinus lesions
- Other trigeminal autonomic cephalalgias
- Section II describes the differential diagnosis of headaches

WORKUP

Diagnosis is made clinically.

IMAGING STUDIES

- None, unless history or examination suggests focal neurologic deficit or headaches change in character or are of new onset.
- MRI of the brain along with vascular imaging may be necessary to exclude secondary headaches at the time of initial diagnosis.

TREATMENT

NONPHARMACOLOGIC THERAPY

Avoidance of alcohol, histamine, nitroglycerin, and tobacco during clusters

ABORTIVE Rx

- Inhalation of 100% oxygen by face mask at a flow rate of 12 L/min or greater for 15 min aborts the attack in 60% to 80% of patients.
- In approximately 75% of patients, subcutaneous or nasal triptans (e.g., sumatriptan, zolmitriptan) will result in freedom from pain within 20 minutes. Only injectable and nasal formulations achieve a response that is rapid enough to be efficacious.
- Galcanezumab-gnlm is the first FDA-approved medication for episodic cluster headache in adults. First approved for migraine, this injectable medication is a humanized monoclonal antibody to calcitonin gene-related peptide (CGRP), blocking its binding to the CGRP receptor. It reduces the average number of cluster headaches per week from baseline compared to placebo.
- Cafergot, octreotide, intranasal lidocaine, or IV dihydroergotamine may abort an attack or prevent one if given just before a predictable episode. An attack typically resolves before oral analgesics can take effect, although indomethacin and other NSAIDs may be effective in prolonged attacks.

PROPHYLAXIS Rx

For patients with episodic cluster headache, prophylactic treatment should be started at the onset of the cluster period and tapered at its end. Patients with chronic cluster headache should be started on prophylactic treatment at increasing doses until good control is achieved. Preventative therapy should begin with verapamil. Alternative treatment options are also listed below.

- Verapamil: Start at 240 mg/day total dose; increase up to 960 mg/day as tolerated. The total dose should be given as three divided doses per day. Dosing three times per day may be more effective than extended release. First-degree AV block may develop with escalating doses, so ECG should be checked.
- Topiramate: Up to 50 mg bid; can be used as add-on to verapamil.
- Lithium: Typical initial dose is 300 mg once daily, with frequent monitoring and

adjustment to maintain therapeutic serum level of 0.4 to 1 mEq/L. Maintenance dose is usually 900 to 1200 mg/day. Equally effective as verapamil, but with more side effects.
- Galcanezumab: 300 mg monthly during the cluster period.
- Melatonin: 10 mg per night. Evidence is weak and comes from scattered case reports.
- Prednisone: 60 mg PO daily for 1 wk followed by taper; headaches can return during taper.
- Ergotamine tartrate: 3 to 4 mg/day during clusters.
- Greater and lesser occipital nerve blocks (with lidocaine or bupivacaine) and steroid injections (Depo-Medrol, dexamethasone, or triamcinolone) may be used to shorten the duration of the cluster period. Consensus guidelines from the American Headache Society have been published recently.
- There is emerging evidence for benefit of a sphenopalatine ganglion block that may be available at some centers for both treatment and prophylaxis of cluster attacks.
- Treatments under investigation include non-invasive vagus nerve stimulation, deep brain stimulation, and occipital nerve stimulation.

DISPOSITION

Headache-free periods tend to increase with increasing age.

REFERRAL

Refractory cluster headaches may require referral to a headache specialist.

PEARLS & CONSIDERATIONS

COMMENTS

- Cluster headaches are divided into episodic (attacks lasting up to 1 yr with more than 1 mo pain-free periods) and chronic (>1 yr without remission). Episodic cluster headache is six times more common than the chronic form.
- Home oxygen therapy is reasonable for cluster headache sufferers.

SUGGESTED READINGS

Available at ExpertConsult.com

RELATED CONTENT

Cluster Headaches (Patient Information)

AUTHORS: **Marco Pares, MD,** and **Joseph S. Kass, MD, JD, FAAN**

BASIC INFORMATION

DEFINITION

Cocaine is an alkaloid derived from the coca plant *Erythroxylum coca,* native to South America, which contains approximately 0.5% to 1% cocaine. The drug produces physiologic and behavioral effects when administered orally, intranasally, intravenously, or by inhalation after smoking. Cocaine has potent pharmacologic effects on dopamine, norepinephrine, and serotonin neurons in the central nervous system (CNS) involving alteration and blockade of cellular membrane transport and prevention of reuptake. Cocaine's second action involves the blockage of voltage-gated sodium ion membrane channels, which is responsible for its anesthetic effect. Table 1 describes the pharmacokinetics of cocaine according to route of administration. The mechanism by which cocaine alters sympathetic tone is illustrated in Fig. 1.

SYNONYMS

Cocaine hydrochloride: Topical solution (FDA approved as a topical anesthetic)

Crack: This is produced when the hydrochloride molecule is removed by ether extraction, which frees the basic cocaine molecule or "free base." Heating does not destroy the free base; rather, it melts at 98° F and vaporizes at higher temperatures, allowing it to be smoked.

Freebase: Aqueous solution of cocaine hydrochloride converted to a more volatile base state by the addition of alkali, thereby extracting the cocaine base in a residue or precipitate.

Street names include Bernice, Blow, C, Carrie, Cecil, Charlie, Coke, Dust, Dynamite, Flake, Gin, Girl, Gold dust, Green gold, Jet, Powder, Star dust, Paradise, Pimp's drug, Snow, Stardust, White girl, Yay, Yayo

Liquid lady: Alcohol + cocaine

Speedball: Heroin + cocaine

Street measures: Git (2-200 mg), snort, line, dose, spoon (approximately 1 g)

ICD-10CM CODES

T40.5 Poisoning, cocaine

F14.20 Cocaine dependence, uncomplicated

EPIDEMIOLOGY & DEMOGRAPHICS

- The 2019 National Survey on Drug Use and Health (NSDUH) released by the U.S. Substance Abuse and Mental Health Services Administration (SAMHSA) estimates that, in 2019, 1.97 million people aged 12 or older were current users of cocaine. This is unchanged from previous yrs but antedates the impact of the COVID-19 pandemic.
- Table 2 summarizes characteristics of patients with cocaine-induced myocardial infarction.

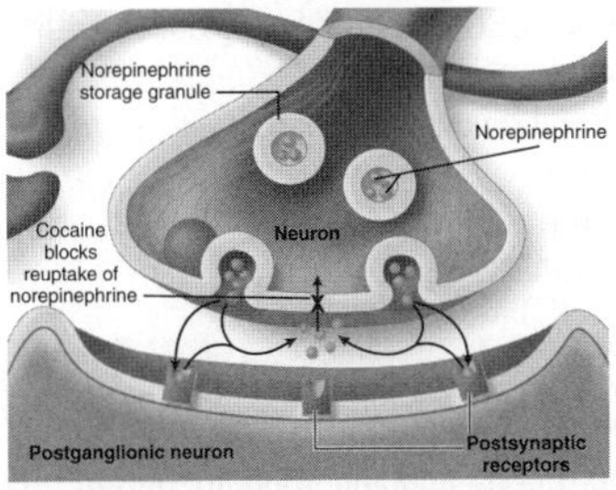

FIG. 1 Mechanism by which cocaine alters sympathetic tone. Cocaine blocks the reuptake of norepinephrine by the preganglionic neuron (X), thereby resulting in excess amounts of this neurotransmitter at postganglionic receptor sites. (From Mann DL et al: *Braunwald's heart disease*, ed 10, Philadelphia, 2015, Elsevier.)

PHYSICAL FINDINGS & CLINICAL PRESENTATION

PHASE I:
- CNS: Euphoria, agitation, headache, vertigo, twitching, bruxism, unintentional tremor
- Nausea, vomiting, fever, hypertension, tachycardia

PHASE II:
- CNS: Lethargy, hyperreactive deep tendon reflexes, seizures (status epilepticus)
- Sympathetic overdrive: Tachycardia, hypertension, hyperthermia
- Incontinence

PHASE III:
- CNS: Flaccid paralysis, coma, fixed dilated pupils, loss of reflexes
- Pulmonary edema
- Cardiopulmonary arrest

Psychological dependence manifests with habituation, paranoia, and hallucinations (cocaine "bugs").

CNS: Cerebral ischemia and infarction, cerebral arterial spasm, cerebral vasculitis, cerebral vascular thrombosis, subarachnoid hemorrhage, intraparenchymal hemorrhage, seizures, cerebral atrophy, movement disorders, and hyperthermia

Cardiac: Acute myocardial ischemia and infarction (Fig. 2), arrhythmias (Table 3), and sudden death, dilated cardiomyopathy and myocarditis, infective endocarditis, aortic rupture, acceleration of coronary atherosclerosis

Pulmonary: Inhalation injuries (secondary to smoking crack cocaine): Cartilage and nasal septal perforation, oropharyngeal ulcers; immunologically mediated diseases: Hypersensitivity pneumonitis, bronchiolitis obliterans; pulmonary vascular lesions and hemorrhage, pulmonary infarction, pulmonary edema secondary to left ventricular failure, pneumomediastinum, and pneumothorax

Gastrointestinal: Gastroduodenal ulceration and perforation; intestinal infarction or perforation, colitis

Renal: Acute renal failure secondary to rhabdomyolysis and myoglobinuria; renal infarction; focal segmental glomerulosclerosis

Obstetric: Placental abruption, low infant weight, prematurity, microcephaly

Psychiatric: Anxiety, depression, paranoia, delirium, psychosis, suicide

Adulterants such as levamisole (an immunomodulator) and clenbuterol (a beta-adrenergic agonist) have been found mixed with cocaine. Levamisole can cause agranulocytosis, leukoencephalopathy, and cutaneous vasculitis leading to necrosis of the skin. Clenbuterol may cause tachycardia, hyperglycemia, and hypokalemia.

ETIOLOGY

Cocaine may be absorbed through different routes with varying degrees of speed:
- Nasal insufflation/snorting: 2.5 min
- Smoking: <30 sec
- Oral: 2 to 5 min
- Mucosal: <20 min
- Intravenous injection: <30 sec

DIAGNOSIS

DIFFERENTIAL DIAGNOSIS

- Methamphetamine ("speed") abuse

TABLE 1 Pharmacokinetics of Cocaine According to Route of Administration

Route of Administration	Onset of Action	Peak Effect	Duration of Action
Inhalation (smoking)	3-5 sec	1-3 min	5-15 min
Intravenous	10-60 sec	3-5 min	20-60 min
Intranasal or other mucosal	1-5 min	15-20 min	60-90 min

From Bonow RO et al: *Heart disease,* ed 9, Philadelphia, 2012, Saunders.

TABLE 2 Characteristics of Patients with Cocaine-Induced Myocardial Infarction

Dose of Cocaine

5-6 lines (150 mg) to as much as 2 g

Serum concentration, 0.01-1.02 mg/L

Frequency of Use

Reported in chronic, recreational, and first-time users

Route of Administration

Occurs with all routes of administration

75% of reported MIs occurred after intranasal use

Age

Mean, 34 (range, 17-71) yr

20% younger than 25 yr

Sex

80%-90% male

Timing

Often within minutes of cocaine use

Reported as late as 5-15 hr after use

MI, Myocardial infarction.

From Mann DL et al: *Braunwald's heart disease*, ed 10, Philadelphia, 2015, Elsevier.

- Methylenedioxyamphetamine ("ecstasy") abuse
- Cathinone ("khat") abuse
- Lysergic acid diethylamide (LSD) abuse

WORKUP

Physical examination and laboratory evaluation

LABORATORY TESTS

- Toxicology screen (urine): Cocaine is metabolized within 2 hr by the liver to major metabolites, benzoylecgonine, and ecgonine methyl ester, which are excreted in the urine. Metabolites can be identified in urine within 5 min of IV use and up to 48 hr after oral ingestion
- Blood: CBC, electrolytes, glucose, BUN, creatinine, calcium
- Arterial blood gas analysis
- ECG
- Serum creatine kinase and troponin concentration
- A suspected "body packer" should have an abdominal radiograph to detect the continued presence of cocaine-containing condoms in the intestinal tract.
  - If present, gentle catharsis with charcoal and mineral oil should be performed with ICU admission and monitoring.

TABLE 3 Cardiac Dysrhythmias and Conduction Disturbances Reported with Cocaine Use

Sinus tachycardia
Sinus bradycardia
Supraventricular tachycardia
Bundle branch block
Complete heart block
Accelerated idioventricular rhythm
Ventricular tachycardia
Ventricular fibrillation
Asystole
Torsades de pointes
Brugada pattern (right bundle branch block with ST-segment elevation in leads V_1, V_2, and V_3)

From Mann DL et al: *Braunwald's heart disease*, ed 10, Philadelphia, 2015, Elsevier.

Rx TREATMENT

- There is no specific antidote, and at present, no drug therapy is uniquely effective in treating cocaine abuse and dependence.
- Modifying cocaine's pharmacokinetic properties by sequestering or hydrolyzing it in serum and limiting its access to its sites of action may prove helpful by using a bacterial cocaine esterase, currently investigational.
- Adulterants (such as levamisole and clenbuterol, discussed earlier), contaminants, and other drugs may be admixed with street cocaine and should be kept in mind with patients presenting with unusual manifestations.
- Amantadine may provide effective treatment for cocaine-dependent patients with severe cocaine withdrawal symptoms, as well as the other dopamine agonist, bromocriptine (1.5 mg PO tid), which may alleviate some of the symptoms of craving associated with acute cocaine withdrawal.

ACUTE GENERAL Rx

- Acute cocaine toxicity requires following advanced poisoning treatment and life support.

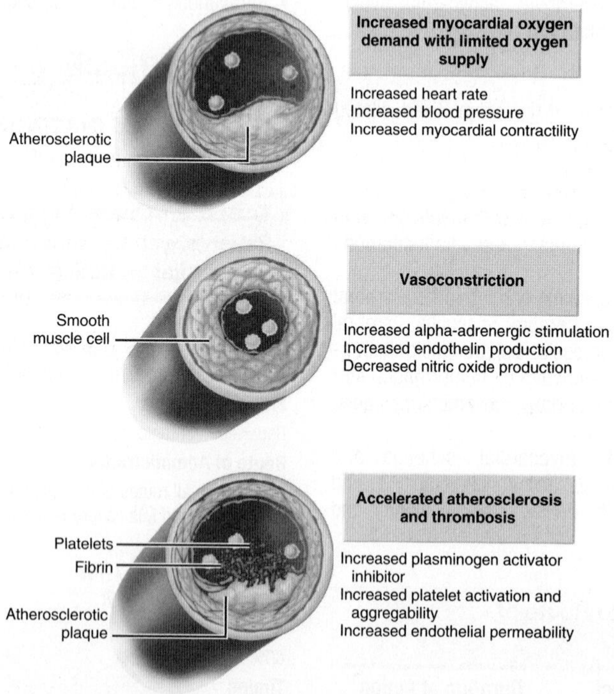

FIG. 2 Mechanisms by which cocaine may induce myocardial ischemia or infarction. Cocaine may induce myocardial ischemia or infarction by increasing the determinants of myocardial oxygen demand in the setting of limited oxygen supply (*top*), thereby causing intense coronary arterial vasoconstriction (*middle*) or inducing accelerated atherosclerosis and thrombosis (*bottom*). (From Mann DL et al: *Braunwald's heart disease*, ed 10, Philadelphia, 2015, Elsevier.)

SPECIFIC TREATMENT

INHALATION: Wash nasal passages

AGITATION:

- Check STAT glucose
- Diazepam 15 to 20 mg PO or 2 to 10 mg IM or IV for severe agitation

HYPERTHERMIA:

- Check rectal temperature, creatine kinase, electrolytes
- Monitor with continuous rectal probe; bring temperature down to 101° F within 30 to 45 min

RHABDOMYOLYSIS:

- Vigorous hydration with urine output at least 2 ml/kg
- Mannitol or bicarbonate for rhabdomyolysis resistant to hydration

SEIZURE MANAGEMENT (STATUS EPILEPTICUS):

- Diazepam 5 to 10 mg IV over 2 to 3 min; may be repeated every 10 to 15 min
- Lorazepam 2 to 3 mg IV over 2 to 3 min; may be repeated
- Phenytoin loading dose 15 to 18 mg/kg IV at a rate not to exceed 25 to 50 mg/min under cardiac monitoring
- Phenobarbital loading dose 10 to 15 mg/kg IV at a rate of 25 mg/min; an additional 5 mg/kg may be given in 30 to 45 min if seizures are not controlled
- For refractory seizures, consider:
  1. Pancuronium 0.1 mg/kg IV
  2. Halothane general anesthesia
  3. Both require EEG monitoring to determine brain seizure activity

HYPERTENSION: Cocaine-induced hypertension usually responds to benzodiazepines. If this fails:

- Consider arterial line for continuous blood pressure monitoring.
- The use of beta-blockers may exacerbate cocaine-induced vasoconstriction and may cause paradoxical hypertension, worsening patient outcomes.
- Phentolamine (unopposed adrenergic effects) or nitroglycerin may be required.
- If diastolic pressure >120 mm Hg: Hydralazine hydrochloride 25 mg IM or IV; may repeat q1h.
- If hypertension is uncontrolled or hypertensive encephalopathy is present: Sodium nitroprusside initially at 0.5 mg/kg/min not to exceed 10 mg/kg/min.

CHEST PAIN:

- Chest radiograph, ECG, cardiac enzymes.
- Benzodiazepines (diazepam 5 mg IV or lorazepam 1 mg IV every 5 min) for agitation until sedation is achieved.
- Acetylsalicylic acid and nitroglycerin for ischemic pain. (Aspirin is contraindicated if dissection is suspected.)

- Percutaneous transluminal coronary angioplasty possibly better than thrombolysis for cocaine-associated myocardial infarction.
- Phentolamine will reverse cocaine-induced vasoconstriction and may be administered 5 to 10 mg every 5 to 10 min.
- Calcium channel blockers (diltiazem 20 mg IV or verapamil 2.5-5 mg IV) are considered safe and may be used in patients with ongoing ischemic pain.
- The use of beta-adrenergic blockers is not generally recommended for reasons highlighted earlier.
- If beta-blockers are to be used, this should be preceded by administration of phentolamine to prevent unopposed alpha-adrenergic stimulation. Many authors recommend not using beta-blockers until the cocaine has been systemically eliminated.

VENTRICULAR ARRHYTHMIAS (CONSIDERATIONS):

- The Advanced Cardiac Life Support (ACLS) protocol should be followed.
- Antiarrhythmic agents should be used with caution during the early period after cocaine exposure as a result of their proarrhythmic and proconvulsant effects.
- Termination of ventricular arrhythmias may be resistant to lidocaine and even cardioversion.
- In a cardiac arrest situation secondary to cocaine toxicity, vasopressin offers a theoretical advantage over epinephrine as it increases coronary blood flow and myocardial oxygen availability. In the 2015 ACLS update, however, vasopressin was removed from the treatment algorithm, so it may not be readily available.

DISPOSITION

Although many patients who use cocaine may not require treatment because of the short half-life of the drug, others may require specific treatment for possible cocaine-related complications. Box 1 summarizes complications associated with cocaine use.

REFERRAL

Consider psychotherapy or behavioral therapy once stable. There is some evidence that topiramate 300 mg orally daily added to cognitive behavioral therapy may be beneficial in patients with severe withdrawal symptoms.

BOX 1 Complications Associated with Cocaine Use

Cardiovascular
Myocardial ischemia, infarction
Arrhythmias
Aortic dissection, rupture
Hypertension
Atherosclerosis
Cardiomyopathy
Vasculitis

Central Nervous System
Seizures
Cerebral infarction
Transient ischemic attack
Intracranial hemorrhage (intraparenchymal, intraventricular, subarachnoid)
Cerebral vasculitis
Cognitive dysfunction

Pulmonary
Bronchospasm
Barotrauma
Noncardiogenic edema
Pulmonary hypertension

Renal
Renal infarction
Renal failure
Scleroderma renal crisis

Gastrointestinal
Mesenteric ischemia, infarction
Gastrointestinal tract perforations

Metabolic
Hyperthermia
Rhabdomyolysis
Weight loss
Multiple organ failure

Other
Deep venous thrombosis
Skin ischemia
Dystonic reactions

From Parrillo JE, Dellinger RP: *Critical care medicine, principles of diagnosis and management in the adult,* ed 4, Philadelphia, 2014, Elsevier.

PEARLS & CONSIDERATIONS

- Cocaine-induced vasoconstriction may be exacerbated by the use of selective and nonselective beta-adrenergic blocking agents.
- The use of lidocaine in treating ventricular arrhythmias may precipitate seizures and further arrhythmias.
- Clinical trials with the SSRI sertraline 200 mg/day have shown that it may help prevent relapse in individuals with some depression symptoms.

SUGGESTED READINGS

Available at ExpertConsult.com

RELATED CONTENT

Cocaine Abuse and Dependence (Patient Information)
Drug Use Disorder (Patient Information)
Drug Use Disorder (Related Key Topic)

AUTHOR: **Sajeev Handa, MD, SFHM**

BASIC INFORMATION

DEFINITION

Colorectal cancer (CRC) is a neoplasm arising from the luminal surface of the large bowel; locations include descending colon (40%-42%), rectosigmoid and rectum (30%-33%), cecum and ascending colon (25%-30%), and transverse colon (10%-13%).

ICD-10CM CODES

C18	Malignant neoplasm of colon
C18.2	Malignant neoplasm of colon, ascending colon
C18.4	Malignant neoplasm of colon, transverse colon
C18.6	Malignant neoplasm of colon, descending colon
C18.7	Malignant neoplasm of colon, sigmoid colon
C19	Malignant neoplasm of rectosigmoid junction

EPIDEMIOLOGY & DEMOGRAPHICS

- Worldwide, CRC accounts for about 1.4 million new cases and 700,000 deaths annually. The highest incidence is in North America, Australasia, Europe, and South Korea
- CRC is the fourth most common cancer and the second leading cause of cancer deaths in the U.S. (147,950 new cases and 53,200 deaths for 2020). Distant metastatic disease is present in 18% to 22% of patients at time of diagnosis
- The peak incidence is in the seventh decade of life. The lifetime risk for development of CRC is 1 in 17, with 90% of cases occurring after age 50 yr
- Risk factors (Table 1):
  1. Hereditary polyposis syndromes
  2. Familial polyposis (high risk)
  3. Gardner syndrome (high risk)
  4. Turcot syndrome (high risk)
  5. Peutz-Jeghers syndrome (low to moderate risk)
  6. Inflammatory bowel disease (IBD), both ulcerative colitis and Crohn disease
  7. Family history of "cancer family syndrome"
  8. Heredofamilial breast cancer and colon carcinoma
  9. Pelvic irradiation history
  10. First-degree relatives with colorectal carcinoma
  11. Age >50 yr
  12. Dietary factors (diet high in fat or red meat, alcohol use, low vegetable intake)
  13. Hereditary nonpolyposis colon cancer (HNPCC): Autosomal dominant disorder characterized by early age of onset (mean age, 44 yr) and right-sided or proximal colon cancers, synchronous and metachronous colon cancers, mucinous and poorly differentiated colon cancers; accounts for 1% to 5% of all cases of CRC; Criteria for diagnosis of HNPCC are summarized in Table 2
  14. Previous endometrial or ovarian cancer, particularly when diagnosed at an early age

PHYSICAL FINDINGS & CLINICAL PRESENTATION

- Physical examination may be completely unremarkable.
- Digital rectal examination can detect approximately 50% of rectal cancers.
- Palpable abdominal masses may indicate metastasis or complications of colorectal carcinoma (abscess, intussusception, volvulus).
- Abdominal distention and tenderness are suggestive of colonic obstruction.
- Hepatomegaly is indicative of hepatic metastasis.

ETIOLOGY

CRC can arise through either of two mutational pathways: Microsatellite instability or chromosomal instability. Germline genetic mutations are the basis of inherited colon cancer syndromes; an accumulation of somatic mutations in a cell is the basis of sporadic colon cancer. Fig. E1 illustrates the molecular carcinogenesis of colon cancer. Approximately 15% of CRC lack one or more mismatch repair enzymes (mismatch repair deficient [dMMR]-CRC).

Dx DIAGNOSIS

DIFFERENTIAL DIAGNOSIS

- Diverticular disease
- Strictures or adhesions
- Inflammatory bowel disease (IBD)
- Infectious or inflammatory lesions
- Arteriovenous malformations
- Metastatic carcinoma
- Extrinsic masses (cysts, abscesses)

WORKUP

The clinical presentation of colorectal malignancies may consist of nonspecific symptoms (weight loss, anorexia, malaise) or of specific symptoms related to mass effect or bleeding. It is useful to divide colon cancer symptoms into those usually associated with the right- or left-sided cancers because the clinical presentation can vary with the location.

- Right side of colon:
  1. Anemia (from chronic blood loss).
  2. Abdominal pain may be present, or the patient may be completely asymptomatic.
  3. Rectal bleeding is often missed because blood is mixed with feces.
  4. Obstruction and constipation are unusual because of large lumen and more liquid stools.
- Left side of colon:
  1. Change in bowel habits (constipation, diarrhea, tenesmus, pencil-thin stools).
  2. Rectal bleeding (bright red blood coating the surface of the stool).
  3. Intestinal obstruction is frequent because of small lumen.

CLASSIFICATION (TABLE 3) AND STAGING

AJCC 8th edition classification for CRC:

A. Confined to the mucosa-submucosa (stage I)
B. Invasion of muscularis propria (stage II)
C. Local node involvement (stage III)
D. Distant metastasis (stage IV)

TNM Classification:

Stage	TNM Classification
I	T_{1-2}, N_0, M_0
II_A	T_3, N_0, M_0
II_B	T_{4a}, N_0, M_0
II_C	T_{4b}, N_0, M_0
III_A	T_{1-2}, N_1, M_0; T_1, N_{2a}, M_0
III_B	T_{3-4a}, N_1, M_0 T_{2-3}, N_{2a}, M_0 T_{1-2}, N_{2b}, M_0
III_C	T_{4a}, N_{2a}, M_0 T_{3-4a}, N_{2b}, M_0 T_{4b}, N_{1-2}, M_0
IV_A	T(any), N(any), M_{1a}
IV_B	T(any), N(any), M_{1b}
IV_C	T(any), N(any), M_{1c}

LABORATORY TESTS

- Positive fecal occult blood test (FOBT): Many primary care physicians use single digital

TABLE 1 Recognized Risk Factors for Colorectal Cancer

Family History
- Colorectal cancer (CRC)
- Inherited syndromes (e.g., familial adenomatous polyposis [FAP])
- Racial and ethnic background (e.g., African American, Ashkenazi Jews)

Personal History
- Age
- Male sex
- Previous colonic polyps or CRC
- History of inflammatory bowel disease
- Diabetes mellitus

Lifestyle
- Obesity
- High consumption of alcohol
- Diet high in red meat and fat, low in fiber

From Niederhuber JE: *Abeloff's clinical oncology*, ed 6, Philadelphia, 2020, Elsevier.

C

TABLE 2 Criteria for Diagnosis of Hereditary Nonpolyposis Colon Cancer (HNPCC)

Amsterdam Criteria[1]
- At least three relatives have colorectal cancer, and all of the following are present:
  - One is a first-degree relative (parent, sibling, or child) of the other two
  - At least two successive generations are involved
  - At least one relative had colorectal cancer when he or she was younger than 50
  - Familial adenomatous polyposis has been excluded

Revised Bethesda Guidelines[2]
(Indicates tumors to select for microsatellite instability testing)
- Colorectal cancer in a patient younger than 50 yr
- A second synchronous or metachronous colorectal cancer or cancer associated with HNPCC
- Presence of high-level microsatellite instability histologically in a patient younger than 60 yr
- One or more first-degree relatives with either colorectal cancer or HNPCC-associated tumor diagnosed at younger than 50 yr
- Colorectal cancer in two or more first- or second-degree relatives with HNPCC-related tumors at any age

Either all of the Amsterdam criteria or one of the Bethesda criteria is used to identify an individual at risk of HNPCC
- HNPCC-associated tumors include endometrial, gastric, ovarian, pancreatic, ureter, renal pelvis, biliary tract, small bowel, and brain

[1]Vasen HF et al: New clinical criteria for hereditary nonpolyposis colorectal cancer (HNPCC, Lynch syndrome) proposed by the International Collaborative group on HNPCC, *Gastroenterology* 116:1453-1456, 1999.
[2]Umar A et al: Revised Bethesda Guidelines for hereditary nonpolyposis colorectal cancer (Lynch syndrome) and microsatellite instability, *J Natl Cancer Inst* 96:261-268, 2004.
From Niederhuber JE: *Abeloff's clinical oncology*, ed 6, Philadelphia, 2020, Elsevier.

TABLE 3 World Health Organization Classification of Colorectal Carcinoma

- Adenocarcinoma
- Cribriform comedo-type adenocarcinoma
- Medullary carcinoma
- Micropapillary carcinoma
- Mucinous adenocarcinoma
- Serrated adenocarcinoma
- Signet ring cell carcinoma
- Adenosquamous carcinoma
- Spindle cell carcinoma
- Squamous cell carcinoma
- Undifferentiated carcinoma
- Neuroendocrine carcinoma (NEC):
  - Large NEC
  - Small NEC
- Mixed adenoneuroendocrine carcinoma

From Niederhuber JE: *Abeloff's clinical oncology*, ed 6, Philadelphia, 2020, Elsevier.

FOBT as their primary screening test for CRC. Single FOBT has low specificity for detecting human hemoglobin, is a poor screening method for CRC (sensitivity, 4.9%), and is inappropriate as the only test because negative results do not decrease the odds of advanced neoplasia. The American College of Gastroenterology recommends the fecal immunochemical test (FIT), which measures intact human globin protein (as opposed to heme) in the stool and detects more advanced adenomas than FOBT.

- Fecal DNA testing is a newer screening method that detects colonic cells shed into the fecal stream that possess specific genetic or epigenetic changes. The technique has a reported sensitivity of 97% and a specificity of 90% for CRC stages I to III. In trials involving asymptomatic persons at average risk for colorectal cancer, multitarget stool DNA testing detects significantly more cancers than FIT but has more false-positive results. High cost and rate of false positives are the main obstacles inhibiting broader adoption of fecal DNA testing.
- Molecular markers (Table 4) including abnormal DNA from cancerous cells can be detected in stool. FIT combined with stool DNA test (FIT-DNA) has been approved by the FDA for colorectal screening. One study showed that one-time FIT-DNA had a higher sensitivity for detection of colorectal cancer than one-time FIT alone (92.3% vs. 73.8%), but specificity was lower (86.6% vs. 94.9%).[1]
- Circulating methylated SEPT9 DNA: Does not reliably detect precancerous neoplasia. Studies showing mortality benefit are lacking.

[1] Inadomi JM: Screening for colorectal neoplasia, *N Engl J Med* 376:149-156, 2017.

- Plasma carcinoembryonic antigen (CEA) level is not useful for screening because it can be increased in nonmalignant conditions (smoking, IBD, alcoholic liver disease). A normal CEA result does not exclude the diagnosis of CRC.

IMAGING STUDIES

- Colonoscopy with biopsy (primary assessment tool): The American College of Physicians (ACP) recommends that patients should be offered a colonoscopy beginning at age 50, and it should be repeated every 10 yr in average-risk patients. Screening is recommended in African Americans beginning at age 45 yr. Persons with only one first-degree relative with CRC or advanced adenomas diagnosed at 60 yr or older may be screened as at average risk. The U.S. Preventive Services Task Force guidelines state that screening should not be routinely recommended in persons older than 75 yr, and it should not be recommended at all in persons older than 85 yr. If persons between the ages of 75 and 85 yr have never undergone screening, the decision about screening should be individualized according to health status. The ACP recommends that clinicians stop screening for colorectal cancer in adults over age 75 yr or in adults with a life expectancy of <10 yr. Table 5 describes CRC screening and surveillance recommendations.
- Computed tomography colonoscopy (CTC) virtual colonoscopy (VC) uses helical (spiral) CT scanning to generate a two- or three-dimensional virtual colorectal image (Fig. E2). CTC does not require sedation, but, like optical colonoscopy, it requires some bowel preparation (either bowel cathartics or ingestion of iodinated contrast medium with meals during the 48 hr before CT) and air insufflation. It also involves substantial exposure to radiation. In addition, patients with lesions detected by VC will require traditional colonoscopy. Compared with colonoscopy, CTC sensitivity for detection of polyps >10 mm ranges from 70% to 96%, and specificity ranges from 72% to 96%. CTC has replaced double-contrast barium enema as the radiographic screening alternative when patients decline colonoscopy.
- Capsule endoscopy allows visualization of the colonic mucosa but is not recommended as a screening procedure because its sensitivity for detecting colonic lesions is low compared with colonoscopy.
- CT scanning of the abdomen (Fig. E3), pelvis, and chest assists in preoperative staging.
- PET scanning (Fig. E4) can display functional information and is accurate in the detection of CRC and its distant metastases. Colonography composed of a combined modality of PET and CT is a newer diagnostic modality that can provide whole-body tumor staging in a single session.

Rx TREATMENT

GENERAL Rx

- Surgical resection is the definitive and curative upfront treatment for stages I to III colon cancers. Selected patients (high-risk stage II, all stage III) are recommended to receive adjuvant chemotherapy. Microsatellite instability can be used alongside clinicopathologic factors in stage II and III colorectal cancer to guide therapy (Fig. 5).
- The standard chemotherapy regimen for adjuvant therapy of resected CRC is the combination of oxaliplatin with a fluoropyrimidine (5-fluorouracil or capecitabine) for a period of 3 to 6 mo. Older patients and patients with significant comorbidities have more toxicity with combination chemotherapy; treatment with single-agent fluoropyrimidine therapy only is recommended in these patients.

- Neoadjuvant chemotherapy and radiation therapy are used to downsize and downstage rectal cancers before definitive resection and improve overall survival and local disease control in stage II and III cancers.
- Adjuvant chemotherapy in stage II disease provides a modest improvement in overall survival by 3% to 4%, with current 5-yr survival rates in the 80% range. As such, current guidelines recommend consideration of adjuvant chemotherapy only in high-risk stage II patients. The magnitude of survival benefit is significantly higher in stage III patients, and combination chemotherapy is associated with 5-yr overall survival rate in the 70% range with wide variation in the subgroups. More recent data have revealed that low-risk stage III colon cancer patients may have equivalent survival with adjuvant multiagent chemotherapy of only 3 mo in duration.
- The outlook for patients with metastatic and relapsed CRC has improved dramatically in the past few yr. Median overall survival in patients with unresectable metastases is now expected in the 30-mo range with modern chemotherapeutic regimens. In patients with limited, resectable metastases in sites such as the liver, the 5-yr median overall survival is in the 50% range.
- Chemotherapy agents used in the metastatic setting include 5-fluorouracil (5-FU), capecitabine, irinotecan, oxaliplatin, and mitomycin. Chemotherapy regimens using a combination of antimetabolite (5-FU or capecitabine) in combination with either oxaliplatin or irinotecan form the backbone of systemic chemotherapy.
- Molecularly targeted therapy against the epidermal growth factor receptor (EGFR) and the angiogenesis pathway are used in combination with the chemotherapy backbone in metastatic CRC. Antiangiogenic agents (bevacizumab, aflibercept, and ramucirumab) and the EGFR receptor blockers (cetuximab and panitumumab) are utilized in combination with standard chemotherapy regimens in metastatic CRC patients. The recent KEYNOTE-177 trial revealed that pembrolizumab led to significantly longer progression-free survival that chemotherapy when received as first-line therapy for MSI-H-dMMR metastatic colorectal cancer with fewer treatment-related adverse events.[1]
- The liver is generally the initial and most common site of CRC metastases. Resection of liver-limited metastases followed by systemic combination chemotherapy is curative in more than 30% of selected patients. Metastasectomy of limited pulmonary metastases can also be considered in selected cases.
- Unresectable multiple liver metastases are often approached by locoregional therapeutic approaches such as transarterial chemoembolization (TACE), selective internal radiation therapy (SIRT) using yttrium-90 brachytherapy, or hepatic arterial infusional chemotherapy.
- The oral multitargeted kinase inhibitor regorafenib and the oral antimetabolite drug TAS-102 provide modest survival benefit in patients who have failed standard chemotherapy approaches.
- Patients with tumors harboring BRAF mutations can now have improved survival with the use of combination molecularly targeted therapy consisting of encorafenib, binimetinib, and cetuximab.
- In patients with pathologically confirmed microsatellite instability in their cancers (Fig. 5), the checkpoint inhibitors (pembrolizumab, nivolumab) are effective options after failure of standard therapies and have been recently approved in this setting. Recent data have shown that upfront treatment with pembrolizumab is superior to conventional chemotherapy and results in doubling of progression-free survival in newly diagnosed patients with microsatellite instability-driven colorectal cancers.
- Reviews of randomized trials in metastatic CRC have demonstrated that right-sided cancers are associated with shorter overall survival when compared with left-sided cancers.

[1]André T et al: Pembrolizumab in microsatellite-instability-high advanced colorectal cancer, *N Engl J Med* 383:2207-2218, 2020.

TABLE 4 Molecular Biomarkers Used in Clinical Standard-of-Care Decision Making in Colorectal Cancer

Biomarker	Purpose
APC mutation detection	Diagnosis of FAP
MMR protein expression *(MSH2, MLH1, MSH6, PMS2)*	Diagnosis of HNPCC
MSI analysis	
MMR mutation detection *(MSH2, MLH1, MSH6, PMS2)*	
BRAF mutation detection	
MYH mutation detection	Diagnosis of MYH-associated polyposis
LKB1, SMAD4, BMPR1A, PTEN mutation detection	Diagnosis of hamartomatous polyp syndromes
KRAS mutation analysis	Molecular stratification for treatment with EGFR inhibitors
BRAF mutation analysis	
Thymidylate synthase protein expression	Identification of response to 5-FU
MSI	Identification of response to 5-FU
Gene expression signature	Prognostication
PD-1	Stratification for response to PD-L1 blockade

EGFR, Epidermal growth factor receptor; *FAP,* familial adenomatous polyposis; *5-FU,* 5-fluorouracil; *HNPCC,* hereditary nonpolyposis colorectal cancer; *MMR,* mismatch repair; *MSI,* microsatellite instability.
From Niederhuber JE: *Abeloff's clinical oncology,* ed 6, Philadelphia, 2020, Elsevier.

TABLE 5 Colorectal Cancer (CRC) Screening and Surveillance Recommendations*

Indication	Recommendations
Average risk	Beginning at age 50 yr: Colonoscopy every 10 yr; computed tomographic colonography every 5 yr; flexible sigmoidoscopy every 5 yr; double-contrast barium enema every 5 yr; stool blood testing annually or stool; DNA testing acceptable but not preferred
One or two first-degree relatives with CRC at any age or adenoma at age <60 yr	Colonoscopy every 5 yr beginning at age 40 yr, or 10 yr younger than earliest diagnosis, whichever comes first
Hereditary nonpolyposis CRC	Genetic counseling and screening† Colonoscopy every 1-2 yr beginning at age 25 yr and then yearly after age 40 yr‡
Familial adenomatous polyposis and variants	Genetic counseling and testing† Flexible sigmoidoscopy yearly beginning at puberty‡
Personal history of CRC	Colonoscopy within 1 yr of curative resection; repeat at 3 yr and then every 5 yr if normal
Personal history of colorectal adenoma	Colonoscopy every 3-5 yr after removal of all index polyps
Inflammatory bowel disease	Colonoscopy every 1-2 yr beginning after 8 yr of pancolitis or after 15 yr if only left-sided disease

*Recommendations proposed by the American Cancer Society and U.S. Multi-Society Task Force on Colorectal Cancer; recommendations for average-risk patients also endorsed by the American College of Radiology.
†Whenever possible, affected relatives should be tested first because of potential false-negative results.
‡Screening recommendation for individuals with positive or indeterminate tests as well as for those who refuse genetic testing.
DNA, Deoxyribonucleic acid.
From Andreoli TE et al: *Andreoli and Carpenter's Cecil essentials of medicine,* ed 8, Philadelphia, 2010, Saunders.

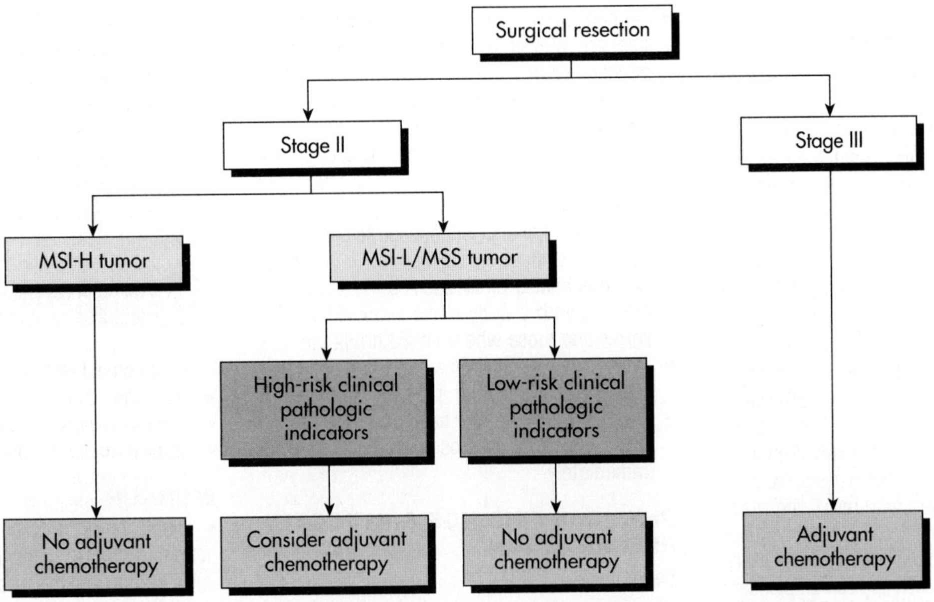

FIG. 5 Proposed algorithm for using microsatellite instability *(MSI)* alongside clinicopathologic factors in stages II and III colorectal cancer. ASCO guidelines: Inadequate samples nodes, T4 lesions, perforation, poorly differentiated histology. *MSI-H,* High-level microsatellite instability; *MSI-L/MSS,* low-level microsatellite instability/microsatellite stability. (From Niederhuber JE: *Abeloff's clinical oncology*, ed 6, Philadelphia, 2020, Elsevier.)

CHRONIC Rx

Follow-up is indicated with:

- Physician visits with a focus on clinical and disease-related history, directed physical examination, coordination of follow-up, and counseling every 3 to 4 mo for the first 3 yr and then every 6 mo for 2 yr.
- Colonoscopy at end of first yr, then after 3 yr, and subsequently every 5 yr.
- Baseline CEA level, if elevated, can be used after surgery as a measure of completeness of tumor resection. It is used to monitor tumor recurrence and is obtained every 3 to 6 mo for up to 5 yr.

DISPOSITION

The 5-yr survival rate varies with the stage of the carcinoma:

TNM Stage	5-yr Survival Rate (%)
I	>90
II_{A-C}	60-85
III_{A-C}	25-65
IV	5-10

- Overall 5-yr disease-free survival rate has increased from 50% to 63% during the past two decades.
- High-frequency microsatellite instability in CRC is independently predictive of a relatively favorable outcome and reduces the likelihood of metastases.
- In patients with high-risk stage II and with stage III CRC, there is improved 5-yr survival among patients treated with adjuvant chemotherapy.
- Expression patterns of microRNA are systemically altered in colon adenocarcinomas. High miR-21 expression is associated with poor survival and poor therapeutic outcome.
- The optimal timing from surgery to initiation of adjuvant chemotherapy is 4 to 8 wk. A longer time to initiation of adjuvant chemotherapy is associated with worse survival rates.
- Regular aspirin use after the diagnosis of CRC has been reported to be associated with lower risk for CRC-specific and overall mortality, especially among individuals with tumors that overexpress cyclooxygenase-2. Regular aspirin use is associated with lower BRAF-wild type colorectal cancer but not with BRAF-mutated cancer risk. All aspirin doses starting with 75 mg daily had similar effects on CRC incidence and mortality.

REFERRAL

Multidisciplinary referral to colorectal surgery or surgical oncology, medical oncology, radiation oncology

PEARLS & CONSIDERATIONS

COMMENTS

- Metastases of tumor cells to regional lymph nodes is the single most important prognostic factor in patients with colon cancer.
- Decreased fat intake to 30% of total energy intake, increased fiber through fruit and vegetable consumption may reduce CRC risk.
- Chemoprophylaxis with aspirin (81 mg/day) reduces the incidence of colorectal adenomas in persons at risk.
- The National Cancer Institute has published consensus guidelines for universal screening for HNPCC in patients with newly diagnosed CRC. Tumors in mutation carriers of HNPCC typically exhibit microsatellite instability, a characteristic phenotype caused by expansion or contraction of short nucleotide repeat sequences. These guidelines (Bethesda Guidelines) are useful for selective patients for microsatellite instability testing. Screening patients with newly diagnosed CRC for HNPCC is cost effective, especially if the benefits to their immediate relatives are considered.
- The use of either annual or biennial FOBT significantly reduces the incidence of CRC.
- The detection of mutations in the *APC* gene from stool samples is a promising new modality for early detection of colorectal neoplasms.

RELATED CONTENT

Colon Cancer (Patient Information)
Familial Adenomatous Polyposis and Gardner Syndrome (Related Key Topic)
Lynch Syndrome (Related Key Topic)
Peutz-Jeghers Syndrome and Other Polyposis Syndromes (Related Key Topic)

SUGGESTED READINGS

Available at ExpertConsult.com

AUTHOR: **Ritesh Rathore, MD**

BASIC INFORMATION

DEFINITION

Concussion is a mild traumatic brain injury manifesting with self-limited symptoms at the less severe end of the brain injury spectrum.

The Fifth International Conference on Concussion in Sport (2016) defines sports-related concussion as *a traumatic brain injury induced by biomechanical forces* caused either by a direct blow to the head, face, neck or elsewhere on the body with an impulsive force transmitted to the head. (However, this definition is also applicable to concussion in general.) This injury results in the rapid onset of short-lived, spontaneously resolving neurological impairment. In some cases, signs and symptoms evolve over a number of minutes to hours. Although neuropathological changes may result, the acute clinical signs and symptoms largely reflect a functional disturbance rather than brain structural injury, and therefore no abnormality is seen on standard structural neuroimaging studies. A range of clinical signs and symptoms may develop that may or may not involve loss of consciousness. Resolution of the clinical and cognitive features typically follows a sequential course, but in some cases symptoms may be prolonged. The clinical signs and symptoms cannot be explained by drug, alcohol or medication use, other injuries (such as cervical injuries, peripheral vestibular dysfunction, etc.), or other comorbidities (e.g., psychological factors or coexisting medical conditions).

SYNONYM

Mild traumatic brain injury (mTBI)

ICD-10CM CODES

S06.0	Concussion
S06.0X0A	Concussion without loss of consciousness, initial encounter
S06.0X0D	Concussion without loss of consciousness, subsequent encounter
S06.0X0S	Concussion without loss of consciousness, sequela
S06.0X1A	Concussion with loss of consciousness of 30 minutes or less, initial encounter
S06.0X9A	Concussion with loss of consciousness of unspecified duration, initial encounter

EPIDEMIOLOGY & DEMOGRAPHICS

INCIDENCE: 3.8 million sports- and recreation-related concussions occur each yr in the U.S. It is estimated that as many as 50% of concussions go unreported.

PREVALENCE: Each yr, U.S. emergency departments treat an estimated 135,000 sports- and recreation-related TBIs, including concussions, among children ages 5 to 18.

PREDOMINANT SEX AND AGE:

- Children and teens are more likely to get a concussion and take longer to recover than adults.
- Limited studies have shown that in sports that are played by both men and women, women are at more risk of sustaining a concussion. In males the incidence is highest in football, followed by hockey, and in females, soccer. Player contact is the most common cause.

RISK FACTORS:

- Participating in high-impact sports and recreational activities
- Previous history of concussion
- Athletes with a body mass index (BMI) >27 kg/m^2 and those who train <3 hr/wk
- Individuals who sustain a sports-related concussion and continue playing immediately after the injury require nearly twice as much time to recover as those who are removed immediately

PHYSICAL FINDINGS & CLINICAL PRESENTATION

See Table 1.

TABLE 1 Symptoms and Signs of Concussion

Mental Status Changes
Amnesia
Confusion
Disorientation
Easily distracted
Excessive drowsiness
Feeling dinged, stunned, or foggy
Impaired level of consciousness
Inappropriate play behaviors
Poor concentration and attention
Seeing stars or flashing lights
Slow to answer questions or to follow directions
Physical or Somatic
Ataxia or loss of balance
Blurry vision
Decreased performance or playing ability
Dizziness
Double vision
Fatigue
Headache
Light-headedness
Nausea, vomiting
Poor coordination
Ringing in the ears
Seizures
Slurred, incoherent speech
Vacant stare/glassy-eyed
Vertigo
Behavior or Psychosomatic
Emotional lability
Irritability
Low frustration tolerance
Personality changes
Nervousness, anxiety
Sadness, depressed mood

From Patel DR et al: Sports concussions in adolescents, *Pediatr Clin N Am* 57:652, 2010.

ETIOLOGY

- Occurs when rotational or angular acceleration forces are applied to the brain, resulting in shear strain of the underlying neural elements, including altered autonomic function and impaired control of cerebral blood flow
- May be associated with a blow to the skull; however, direct impact to the head is not required

Dx DIAGNOSIS

DIFFERENTIAL DIAGNOSIS

- Migraine
- Cervical strain
- Posttraumatic vestibular injury

WORKUP

- There is no definitive diagnostic test for concussion. A standardized protocol (Table 2) can help first responders identify more subtle mental status changes. Physical exam should include smooth pursuits (examiner moves finger horizontally across field of vision), saccades, gaze instability, near point of convergence, accommodation, and balance. Patients with loss of consciousness or posttraumatic convulsive seizures should be transported to the emergency department.
- Sideline assessment:
  1. No athlete with a suspected concussion should return to play that day.
  2. Neurologic assessment using a standardized tool, such as s SCAT-3 (Sports Concussion Assessment Tool), which includes the BESS (Balance Error

TABLE 2 Standardized Assessment of Concussion

Task	Possible Score
Orientation	
Month, date, day of week, year, time (1 point for each correct answer)	0-5
Immediate Memory	
Patient repeats a 5-word list spoken by examiner; 3 trials (1 point for each word correctly remembered)	0-15
Concentration	
Digits backward; 3-, 4-, 5-, and 6-digit strings (1 point for each digit string correctly repeated backward)	0-4
Months of the year in reverse order (1 point for repeating backward in correct sequence)	0-1
Delayed Memory Recall	
Patient repeats the 5 words from Immediate Memory test (1 point for each word correctly recalled)	0-5
TOTAL SCORE	0-30

Goldman L, Shafer AI: *Goldman-Cecil medicine*, ed 26, Philadelphia, 2020, Elsevier.

Scoring System), Maddocks Questions, and SAC (Standardized Assessment of Concussion).
3. Monitor for deterioration; no athlete should be left alone.

- Office assessment:
  1. History focused on current symptoms. Consider using Postconcussion Symptom Checklist. According to the Consensus Statement on Concussion in Sport issued by the Fifth International Conference on Concussion in Sport, the following domains should be investigated when considering a diagnosis of sports-related concussion. A problem in one domain in the proper historical context should raise concern for sports-related concussion.
     a. Symptoms: Somatic (e.g., headache), cognitive (e.g., feeling like in a fog), and/or emotional symptoms (e.g., lability)
     b. Physical signs (e.g., loss of consciousness, amnesia, neurological deficit)
     c. Balance impairment (e.g., gait unsteadiness)
     d. Behavioral changes (e.g., irritability)
     e. Cognitive impairment (e.g., slowed reaction times)
     f. Sleep/wake disturbance (e.g., somnolence, drowsiness)
  2. Neurologic exam
     a. Gait/balance testing. Consider the Balance Error Scoring System (BESS)
     b. Cerebellar coordination: Finger-to-nose testing (tested on SCAT-3 card)
     c. Convergence of Accommodative Sufficiency
- Neurocognitive testing:
  1. Computer-based programs, such as ImPACT, ANAM, CogSport
  2. Neuropsychiatric testing administered by a neuropsychologist
- When used in combination, symptom assessment, balance assessment, and neurocognitive testing provide a sensitivity of >90% for the identification of concussion.
- Consider the Buffalo Concussion Treadmill Test, which identifies physiologic dysfunction in concussion, rules out other diagnoses, and can quantify a safe level of activity in concussion recovery.

IMAGING STUDIES

- CT imaging is not universally indicated and should be considered on an individual basis. It is indicated in any athlete with a rapidly changing or focal neurologic exam or with a suspected intracranial bleed.
- Consider following PECARN guidelines.

Rx TREATMENT

ACUTE GENERAL Rx

- Removal from game
- Physical rest
  1. No return to play until asymptomatic for at least 24 hours.
  2. Follow the return-to-play guidelines (Table 3).
  3. There is no evidence to support prolonged rest in concussed athletes longer than several weeks (see "Postconcussive Syndrome"). Prolonged inactivity after concussion has been linked to negative health effect. Light aerobic activity that avoids risk for reinjury decreases concussion symptoms, suggesting that low-level physical activity postconcussion might be beneficial.
- Cognitive rest to limit symptoms
  1. Limit screen time to less than 2 hours per day.
  2. Academic accommodations at school. Consider return to school for half-days when tolerating 2 hours of work at home.
  3. Encourage good sleep hygiene.

CHRONIC Rx

See "Postconcussive Syndrome."

DISPOSITION

- Physiologic recovery is slower than symptomatic recovery. Protocols involving a symptom-free waiting period before return to play are warranted. Table 3 summarizes the American Academy of Neurology, American Medical Society for Sports Medicine, and International Conference on Concussion recommendations on returning to play after a concussion.
- If concussion symptoms occur with activity at one level, the athlete should stop the activity, rest until symptoms resolve, and then restart his or her progression at the level that did not elicit symptoms.
- There are no evidence-based guidelines for disqualifying or retiring an athlete from sport after a concussion. Each case should be individually considered.

TABLE 3 Graduated Return to Play Protocol

Rehabilitation Stage	Functional Exercise at Each Stage of Rehabilitation	Objective of Each Stage
1. No activity	Complete physical and cognitive rest	Recovery
2. Light aerobic exercise	Walking, swimming, or stationary cycling, keeping intensity <70% maximum predicted heart rate. No resistance training	Increase heart rate
3. Sport-specific exercise	Skating drills in ice hockey, running drills in soccer. No head impact activities	Add movement
4. Noncontact training drills	Progression to more complex training drills, e.g., passing drills in football and ice hockey. May start progressive resistance training	Exercise, coordination, and cognitive load
5. Full contact practice	After medical clearance, participate in normal training activities	Restore confidence and assess functional skills by coaching staff
6. Return to play	Normal game play	

From Putukian M: The acute symptoms of sports-related concussion: diagnosis and on-field management, *Clin Sports Med* 30(58), 2011.

REFERRAL

Referral to sports-medicine physician, neuropsychology, or concussion center is indicated if there is concern about the timing of return to contact or collision sport. Referral is also indicated in patients with preexisting neurologic disorders such as migraines, depression or anxiety, and in those who have had multiple concussions.

PEARLS & CONSIDERATIONS

PREVENTION

- Preparticipation evaluations for all athletes.
- Preparticipation neurocognitive and balance testing to establish a baseline.
- There is currently no evidence to support the use of concussion prevention headbands or mouth guards.
- Spontaneous recovery from acute concussion ranges from 1 to 2 wk in adults and up to 4 wk in adolescents.

PATIENT & FAMILY EDUCATION

Centers for Disease Control and Prevention: www.cdc.gov/TraumaticBrainInjury/get_the_facts.html.

SUGGESTED READINGS

Available at ExpertConsult.com

RELATED CONTENT

Concussion (Patient Information)
Postconcussion Syndrome (Related Key Topic)
Traumatic Brain Injury (Related Key Topic)

AUTHOR: **Joseph S. Kass, MD, JD, FAAN**

Condyloma Acuminatum

BASIC INFORMATION

DEFINITION

Condyloma acuminatum, also known as anogenital warts, is a sexually transmitted viral disease of the penis, vulva, vagina, cervix, perineum, and perianal area caused by the human papillomavirus (HPV). More than 100 subtypes of the HPV virus have been identified, yet 90% of genital warts are caused by HPV types 6 or 11.

SYNONYMS

Genital warts
Venereal warts
Anogenital warts

ICD-10CM CODE

A63.0 Anogenital (venereal) warts

EPIDEMIOLOGY & DEMOGRAPHICS

- The estimated prevalence rate of HPV anogenital infection in the U.S. adult population is 10% to 20% among unvaccinated individuals
- Seen mostly in young adults, with peak age of onset of 16 to 25 yr
- A sexually transmitted disease spread by skin-to-skin contact
- Highly contagious, with 75% of sexually active adults in the U.S. having been infected with at least one genital HPV type at some time
- Virus shed from both macroscopic and microscopic lesions
- Average incubation time is 2 mo (range, 1-8 mo)
- Predisposing conditions: Diabetes, pregnancy, local trauma, and immunosuppression (e.g., transplant recipients, those with HIV infection)

PHYSICAL FINDINGS & CLINICAL PRESENTATION

- Usually found in genital area but can be present elsewhere on the body (larynx, oropharynx, trachea, and extremities)
- Lesions usually in similar positions on both sides of perineum
- Initial lesions are pedunculated, soft papules about 2 to 3 mm in diameter, 10 to 20 mm long; may occur as single papule or in clusters
- Size of lesions varies from pinhead to large cauliflower-like masses (Fig. E1)
- Usually asymptomatic, but if infected can cause pain, odor, or bleeding
- Vulvar condyloma more common than vaginal and cervical
- Four morphologic types: Condylomatous, keratotic, papular, and flat warts
- Intra-anal warts are observed predominantly in persons who have had receptive anal intercourse

ETIOLOGY

- HPV is a group of nonenveloped, double-stranded DNA viruses belonging to the family Papillomaviridae.
- HPV DNA types 6 and 11 usually found in exophytic warts and have no malignant potential. 90% of genital warts are caused by HPV 6 and 11.
- HPV types 16 and 18 usually found in flat warts and are associated with increased risk of malignancy.
- Recurrence associated with persisting viral infection of adjacent normal skin in 25% to 50% of cases.

Dx DIAGNOSIS

DIFFERENTIAL DIAGNOSIS

- Molluscum contagiosum
- Seborrhea keratosis
- Fordyce spots
- Lichen planus
- Lichen nitidus
- Condylomata lata of syphilis
- Malignancy
- Abnormal anatomic variants or skin tags around labia minora and introitus
- Dysplastic warts
- Table 1 summarizes treatment options for anal warts.

WORKUP

- Colposcopic examination of lower genital tract from cervix to perianal skin with 3% to 5% acetic acid
- Biopsy of vulvar lesions that lack the classic appearance of warts and that become ulcerated or do not respond to treatment
- Biopsy of flat, white, or ulcerated cervical lesions

LABORATORY TESTS

- HPV tests are available to detect oncogenic types of HPV infection and are used in the context of cervical cancer screening and management or follow-up of abnormal cervical cytology or histology.
- Cervical cultures for *Neisseria gonorrhoeae* and Chlamydia
- Serologic test for syphilis
- HIV testing offered
- Wet mount or DNA testing for trichomoniasis, *Candida albicans*, and *Gardnerella vaginalis* (if patient has abnormal vaginal discharge)

Rx TREATMENT

NONPHARMACOLOGIC THERAPY

- Cryotherapy with liquid nitrogen
- Surgical removal

ACUTE GENERAL Rx

Factors that influence selection of treatment include wart size, wart number, anatomic site of wart, wart morphology, patient preference, cost of treatment, convenience, adverse effects, and provider experience.

Keratolytic agents:

- Podophyllin (Podofilox 0.5% solution or gel)
  1. Acts by poisoning mitotic spindle and causing intense vasospasm
  2. Applied by patient directly to lesion weekly and washed off in 6 hr
  3. Used in minimal vulvar or anal disease
  4. Applied cautiously to nonkeratinized epithelial surfaces
  5. Contraindicated in pregnancy
  6. Discontinued if lesions do not disappear in 6 wk; switch to other treatment
- Sinecatechins 15% ointment (green tea flavonoid extracts)
  1. Acts by upregulating apoptosis-associated genes
  2. Applied by patient three time daily (0.5 cm strand of ointment to each wart)
  3. Should not be continued longer than 16 wk
- Trichloroacetic acid (30%-80% solution)
  1. Acts by destruction of the warty lesions through precipitation of surface proteins
  2. Applied weekly to lesion by a trained clinician
  3. Indicated for vulvar, anal, and vaginal lesions; can be used for cervical lesions
  4. Less painful and irritating to normal tissue than podophyllin
- 5-Fluorouracil
  1. Acts by causing necrosis and sloughing of growing tissue
  2. Can be used intravaginally or for vulvar, anal, or urethral lesions
  3. Better tolerated; 3 g (two thirds of vaginal applicator) applied weekly for 12 wk
  4. Possible vaginal ulceration and erythema
  5. Patient's vagina examined after four to six applications
  6. 80% cure rate

Physical agents:

- Cryotherapy with liquid nitrogen or cryoprobe
  1. Acts by causing tissue damage by formation of ice crystals, leading to disruption of cell membranes and cell death
  2. Can be used weekly for 3 to 6 wk
  3. 62% to 79% cure rate
  4. Not suitable for large warts
- Laser therapy
  1. Done by physician with necessary expertise and equipment
  2. Painful; requires anesthesia
- Electrocautery or excision
  1. For recurrent, very large lesions
  2. Local anesthesia needed

Immunotherapy:

- Interferon A
  1. Injected intralesionally at a dose of 3 million U/m^2 three times weekly for 8 wk
  2. Side effects: Fever, chills, malaise, headache
- Imiquimod 5% cream: Immunomodulatory drug that increases the immune response to warts
  1. Applied by patient at night, 3× per wk; wash off after 6 to 10 hr
  2. Usage for 16 wk maximum
  3. Increases wart clearance after 3 mo
- 40% to 77% cure rate
- Interferon, topical: Increases wart clearance at 4 wk

C

TABLE 1 Treatment Options for Anal Warts

Treatment	Success Rate	Comments
Podophyllin	20%-50%	May need repeat applications Skin irritation can occur Not used in the anal canal Poorly absorbed by keratinized lesions (most chronic warts are keratinized)
Trichloroacetic or dichloroacetic acid	75%	Can be used in the anal canal Care is required to control the size of the slough
Cryotherapy	75%	Can be used in the anal canal Care is required to limit the size of the wound Fumes from the therapy can contain active HPV*
Topical 5-fluorouracil	50%-75%	Probably better used after surgical excision to decrease the frequency of recurrence
Imiquimod	75% in women 33% in men	Cannot be used in the anal canal; works better in women than in men
Surgical excision (usually combined with cautery)	60%-90%	Fumes from the cautery may contain HPV* May need to be done in more than one session to avoid excising or burning excessive anoderm if a thick carpet of lesions is present
Intralesional interferon-α	>70%	Injected into the base of up to 5 warts 3 times a wk for 3-8 wk Approved by the FDA for refractory condyloma
HspE7	Experimental	Promising treatment involving subcutaneous injections Fusion protein that combines immune-stimulating properties and a target antigen from HPV
External-beam radiation therapy	Variable	Reserved for giant cavitating condyloma (Buschke-Löwenstein lesions) Used as a last resort, usually when bleeding or tissue invasion cannot be controlled

FDA, Food and Drug Administration; *HPV,* human papillomavirus.
*The risk of HPV transmission from such fumes is unknown.
From Feldman M et al: *Sleisenger and Fordtran's gastrointestinal and liver disease,* ed 10, Philadelphia, 2016, Elsevier.

DISPOSITION

- Most genital warts resolve without therapy.
- Follow-up exam every 6 to 12 mo as needed.
- Referral to a specialist experienced in the treatment of anogenital warts (e.g., dermatologist, urologist, or colorectal surgeon) is appropriate for patients who are immunosuppressed or who have treatment-refractory anogenital warts.
- Patients with large, bulky perianal or genital warts that may require extensive surgical removal should be referred to a colorectal surgeon or urologist.

PREVENTION

- Male and female condoms should be used consistently and correctly to lower the risks of acquiring and transmitting HPV. However, because HPV can infect areas not covered by a condom, condoms will not fully protect against HPV.
- Guidelines for the routine vaccination of young adolescents (females and males) ages 9 to 14 are two doses of the HPV vaccine given at a 6- to 12-mo interval, which offers the same protection as the three-dose vaccination.
- Young women from ages 15 to 26 should receive three doses of the HPV vaccine (the 9vHPV, 4vHPV, and 2vHPV are approved for females).
- Young males from ages 15 to 21 should receive three doses of the HPV vaccine. The age limit for male HPV vaccination may be extended up to age 26 (only the 4vHPV and 9vHPV vaccines are approved for males). For men who have sex with men (including young men who identify as gay and bisexual), for young transgender adults, and for young adults who are immunocompromised (secondary to HIV, chronic steroid usage, or prior history of transplant), HPV vaccination is recommended up to age 26. Three-dose HPV vaccination series are administered as IM injections over a 6-mo period, with the second and third doses given 1 to 2 and 6 mo after the first dose, respectively. The same vaccine type should be used for the entire three-dosage series.
- 4vHPV (Gardasil) vaccinates against types 6, 11, 16, and 18, which account for 66% of all cervical cancers.
- 2vHPV (Cervarix) vaccinates against types 16 and 18 (licensed for females only).
- 9vHPV (Gardasil 9) vaccine is available for preventing infection against HPV types 6, 11, 16, 18, 31, 33, 45, 52, and 58. It offers protection against five additional types of HPV accounting for 15% of cervical cancers not covered by Gardasil or Cervarix.
- HPV vaccines are not recommended for use in pregnant women.

Diseases and Disorders

I

SUGGESTED READING

Available at ExpertConsult.com

RELATED CONTENT

Genital Warts (Patient Information)
Warts (Related Key Topic)

AUTHORS: **Helen B. Gomez, MD,** and **Rachel Wright Heinle, MD, FACOG**

BASIC INFORMATION

DEFINITION

The term *conjunctivitis* refers to an inflammation of the conjunctiva resulting from a variety of causes, including allergies and bacterial, viral, and chlamydial infections.

SYNONYMS

Red eye
Pink eye
Acute conjunctivitis
Subacute conjunctivitis
Chronic conjunctivitis
Purulent conjunctivitis
Pseudomembranous conjunctivitis
Papillary conjunctivitis
Follicular conjunctivitis
Newborn conjunctivitis

ICD-10CM CODES

H10.9	Unspecified conjunctivitis
B30	Viral conjunctivitis
H10.0	Mucopurulent conjunctivitis
H10.1	Acute atopic conjunctivitis
H10.4	Chronic conjunctivitis

EPIDEMIOLOGY & DEMOGRAPHICS

INCIDENCE (IN U.S.): 1.6% to 12% in newborns

PREVALENCE (IN U.S.):

- Allergic conjunctivitis (Fig. E1), the most common form of ocular allergy, is usually associated with allergic rhinitis and may be seasonal or perennial.
- Bacterial or viral conjunctivitis is often seasonal and can be extremely contagious.

PREDOMINANT AGE: Occurs at any age. Most cases in adults are due to viral infection. Children are more prone to develop bacterial conjunctivitis than viral forms.

PEAK INCIDENCE: More common in the spring and fall, when viral infections and pollens increase

PHYSICAL FINDINGS & CLINICAL PRESENTATION

- Infection and chemosis of conjunctivae with discharge. Gluing of the eyelids and no itching is more indicative of a bacterial cause (Fig. E2).
- Cornea is clear or can be involved (certain bacteria, such as *Neisseria*, can rapidly develop into corneal infection).
- Vision is often normal but can be blurred. Mucus and watering can cause fluctuating vision.
- Fig. E3 illustrates the difference between papillary and follicular conjunctivitis.

ETIOLOGY

- Bacterial: *Haemophilus influenzae, Streptococcus pneumoniae,* and *Moraxella catarrhalis* in children; *Staphylococcus* species in adults. Gram-negative infections are more common in contact lens wearers. *Gonococcal ophthalmia neonatorum* is caused by *Neisseria gonorrhoeae* acquired by exposure of the neonatal conjunctivae to infected cervicovaginal secretions during delivery
- Viral: Most common overall cause of infectious conjunctivitis
- Chlamydial
- Allergic
- Traumatic (chemical or toxin exposure)
- Chronic eyelid inflammation (blepharitis)

DIAGNOSIS

DIFFERENTIAL DIAGNOSIS

- Acute glaucoma (fixed pupil with headache may indicate acute angle closure)
- Corneal lesions
- Acute iritis (with pain and photophobia, blurred vision)
- Episcleritis
- Scleritis (more severe pain, local globe tenderness, and no drainage)
- Canalicular obstruction (eye watering, inflammation near the tear punctum)
- Table 1 compares allergic diseases of the eye; histologic and laboratory manifestations of allergic ocular disease are described in Table 2

WORKUP

- History and physical examination
- Visual acuity and eye examination
- Reports of itching, pain, and visual changes

LABORATORY TESTS

Cultures are useful if not *successfully* treated with antibiotics; initial culture is usually not necessary, since normal conjunctival flora interferes with helpful culture results.

TREATMENT

NONPHARMACOLOGIC THERAPY

- Warm compresses if infective conjunctivitis
- Cold compresses if allergic conjunctivitis
- Contact lenses should be taken out until an infection is completely resolved. Nondisposable lenses should be cleaned thoroughly as recommended by the manufacturer, and a new lens case should be used. Disposable contact lenses should be thrown away

ACUTE GENERAL Rx

- The majority of cases of bacterial conjunctivitis are self-limiting, and no treatment is necessary in uncomplicated cases.[1] Antibiotic drops (e.g., levofloxacin, ofloxacin, ciprofloxacin, tobramycin, gentamicin ophthalmic solution, 1 or 2 drops q2-4h) are indicated for complicated bacterial conjunctivitis, in conjunctivitis caused by gonorrhea or chlamydia, and in bacterial conjunctivitis in contact lens wearers.
- Caution: Be careful with ophthalmic corticosteroid treatment and avoid unless sure of diagnosis; corticosteroids can exacerbate infections and have been associated with increased intraocular pressure and cataract formation.
- An oral antihistamine (e.g., cetirizine, loratadine, desloratadine, or fexofenadine) is effective in relieving itching.
- Mast cell stabilizers (e.g., ketotifen, olopatadine, azelastine bid) are effective for allergic conjunctivitis. Others include Elestat, Optivar, and Patanol.
- Bepotastine, alcaftadine, azelastine, epinastine, and ketotifen are H_1-antihistamines and mast cell stabilizers effective for topical treatment of itching associated with allergic conjunctivitis. The topical NSAID ketorolac (0.5%, 1 drop qd) is also useful in allergic conjunctivitis. Table 3 describes topical ophthalmic medications for allergic conjunctivitis.
- Antihistamine/decongestant combinations such as pheniramine/naphazoline (Visine A), available over the counter, are more effective than either agent alone but have a short duration and can result in rebound vasodilation with prolonged use. Others include Naphcon-A, Albalon-A, and Opcon-A.

CHRONIC Rx

- Depends on cause.
- If allergic, nonsteroidals such as ketorolac and bromfenac ophthalmic solution; mast cell stabilizers such as Patanol and Zaditor (ketotifen) are useful for improving ocular itching in patients with allergic conjunctivitis.
- If an infection, use antibiotic drops (see "Acute General Rx").
- Dry eyes need artificial tears, topical cyclosporine, or lacrimal duct plugs when indicated.
- Chronic and recurrent conjunctivitis often occurs with blepharitis. Daily warm compresses and lid scrub treatment may help relieve symptoms.

DISPOSITION

Follow carefully for the first 2 wk to ensure secondary complications do not occur. Otitis media can develop in 25% of children with *H. influenzae* conjunctivitis. Bacterial keratitis occurs in 30/1000 contact lens wearers.

REFERRAL

To ophthalmologist if symptoms are refractory to initial treatment. Indications for urgent referral are severe eye pain or headache, photophobia, decreased vision, and contact lens use.

---

[1] Azari AA, Barney NP: Conjunctivitis, a systematic review of diagnosis and treatment, *JAMA* 310(16):1721-1729, 2013.

TABLE 1 Allergic Diseases of the Eye

Disease	Clinical Parameters	Signs and Symptoms	Differential Diagnosis
Seasonal allergic conjunctivitis (SAC)	Occurs in sensitized individuals Both females and males affected Bilateral involvement Seasonal allergens Self-limiting	Ocular itching Tearing (watery discharge) Chemosis, redness Often associated with rhinitis Not sight-threatening	Infective conjunctivitis Preservative toxicity (any eye drop with preservative) Medicamentosa Dry eye Perennial allergic conjunctivitis Vernal keratoconjunctivitis (VKC) Atopic keratoconjunctivitis (AKC)
Perennial allergic conjunctivitis (PAC)	Occurs in sensitized individuals Both females and males affected Bilateral involvement Year-round allergens Self-limiting	Ocular itching Tearing (watery discharge) Chemosis, redness Often associated with rhinitis Not sight-threatening	Infective conjunctivitis Preservative toxicity Dry eye SAC/AKC/VKC
Atopic keratoconjunctivitis (AKC)	Occurs in sensitized individuals Peak incidence: 20-50 yr of age Both females and males affected Bilateral involvement Seasonal or perennial allergens Atopic dermatitis Chronic symptoms	Severe ocular itching Red, flaking periocular skin Mucoid discharge, photophobia Corneal erosions Scarring of conjunctiva Cataract (anterior subcapsular) Sight-threatening	Contact dermatitis Infective conjunctivitis Blepharitis Pemphigoid VKC/SAC/PAC/GPC
Vernal keratoconjunctivitis (VKC)	Occurs in some sensitized individuals Peak incidence: 3-20 yr of age Males predominate (in 3:1 ratio) Bilateral involvement Warm, dry climate Seasonal/perennial allergens Chronic symptoms	Severe ocular itching Severe photophobia Thick, ropy discharge Cobblestone papillae Corneal ulceration and scarring Sight-threatening	Infective conjunctivitis Blepharitis AKC/SAC/PAC/GPC
Giant papillary conjunctivitis (GPC)	Sensitization not necessary Both females and males affected Bilateral involvement Prosthetic and contact lens exposure Occurs anytime Chronic symptoms Nonseasonal occurrence	Mild ocular itching Mild mucoid discharge Giant papillae Contact lens intolerance Foreign body sensation Protein buildup on contact lens Not sight-threatening	Infective conjunctivitis Preservative toxicity SAC/PAC/AKC/VKC

From Adkinson NF et al: *Middleton's allergy principles and practice*, ed 8, Philadelphia, 2014, Saunders.

TABLE 2 Histopathologic and Laboratory Manifestations of Allergic Ocular Disease

Disease	Histopathologic Features	Laboratory Manifestations
Seasonal/perennial allergic conjunctivitis	Mast cell/eosinophil infiltration in conjunctival epithelium and substantia propria Mast cell activation Upregulation of ICAM-1 on epithelial cells	Increased in tears: Specific IgE antibody Histamine Tryptase TNF-α
Atopic keratoconjunctivitis	Increased mast cells, eosinophils in conjunctival epithelium and substantia propria Epithelial cell/goblet cell hypertrophy Increased CD4/CD8 ratio in conjunctival epithelium and substantia propria Increased collagen	Increased specific IgE antibody in tears Depressed cell-mediated immunity Increased IgE antibody and eosinophils in blood Eosinophils found in conjunctival scrapings
Vernal keratoconjunctivitis	Increased mast cells, eosinophils in conjunctival epithelium and substantia propria Eosinophil major basic protein deposition in conjunctiva CD4+ clones from conjunctiva found to have helper function for local production of IgE antibody Increased collagen Increased ICAM-1 on corneal epithelium	Increased specific IgE/IgG antibody in tears Elevated histamine and tryptase in tears Reduced serum histaminase activity Increased serum levels of nerve growth factor and substance P
Giant papillary conjunctivitis	Giant papillae Conjunctival thickening Mast cells in epithelium	No increased histamine in tears Increased tryptase in tears

ICAM-1, Intercellular adhesion molecule 1; *IgE*, immunoglobulin E; *IgG*, immunoglobulin G; *TNF-α*, tumor necrosis factor-α.
From Adkinson NF et al: *Middleton's allergy principles and practice,* ed 8, Philadelphia, 2014, Saunders.

TABLE 3 Topical Ophthalmic Medications for Allergic Conjunctivitis

Drug and Trade Names	Mechanism of Action and Dosing	Cautions and Adverse Events
Azelastine hydrochloride 0.05% Optivar	Antihistamine Children ≥3 yr: 1 gtt bid	Not for treatment of contact lens–related irritation; the preservative may be absorbed by soft contact lenses. Wait at least 10 min after administration before inserting soft contact lenses.
Cetirizine 0.24% (Zerviate) opthalmic solution		
Emedastine difumarate 0.05% Emadine	Antihistamine Children ≥3 yr: 1 gtt qid	Soft contact lenses should not be worn if the eye is red. Wait at least 10 min after administration before inserting soft contact lenses.
Levocabastine hydrochloride 0.05% Livostin	Antihistamine Children ≥12 yr: 1 gtt bid-qid up to 2 wk	Not for use in patients wearing soft contact lenses during treatment.
Pheniramine maleate	Antihistamine/vasoconstrictor	Avoid prolonged use (>3-4 days) to avoid rebound symptoms. Not for use with contact lenses.
0.3% Naphazoline hydrochloride 0.025% Naphcon-A, Opcon-A	Children >6 yr: 1-2 gtt qid	
Cromolyn sodium 4% Crolom, Opticrom	Mast cell stabilizer Children >4 yr: 1-2 gtt q4-6h	Can be used to treat giant papillary conjunctivitis and vernal keratitis. Not for use with contact lenses.
Lodoxamide tromethamine 0.1% Alomide	Mast cell stabilizer Children ≥2 yr: 1-2 gtt qid up to 3 mo	Can be used to treat vernal keratoconjunctivitis. Not for use in patients wearing soft contact lenses during treatment.
Nedocromil sodium 2% Alocril	Mast cell stabilizer Children ≥3 yr: 1-2 gtt bid	Avoid wearing contact lenses while exhibiting the signs and symptoms of allergic conjunctivitis.
Pemirolast potassium 0.1% Alamast	Mast cell stabilizer Children >3 yr: 1-2 gtt qid	Not for treatment of contact lens–related irritation; the preservative may be absorbed by soft contact lenses. Wait at least 10 min after administration before inserting soft contact lenses.
Epinastine hydrochloride 0.05% Elestat	Antihistamine/mast cell stabilizer Children ≥3 yr: 1 gtt bid	Contact lenses should be removed before use. Wait at least 15 min after administration before inserting soft contact lenses. Not for the treatment of contact lens irritation.
Ketotifen fumarate 0.025% Zaditor	Antihistamine/mast cell stabilizer Children ≥3 yr: 1 gtt bid q8-12h	Not for treatment of contact lens–related irritation; the preservative may be absorbed by soft contact lenses. Wait at least 10 min after administration before inserting soft contact lenses.
Olopatadine hydrochloride 0.1%, 0.2%, 0.7% Patanol Pataday Pazeo	Antihistamine/mast cell stabilizer Children ≥3 yr: 1 gtt bid (8 hr apart) Children ≥2 yr: 1 gtt qd	Not for treatment of contact lens–related irritation; the preservative may be absorbed by soft contact lenses. Wait at least 10 min after administration before inserting soft contact lenses.
Alcaftadine, 0.25% Lastacaft	Antihistamine/mast cell stabilizer Children >2 yr: 1 gtt bid q8-12h	Contact lenses should be removed before application; may be inserted after 10 min. Not for the treatment of contact lens irritation.
Bepotastine besilate 1.5% Bepreve	Antihistamine/mast cell stabilizer Children >2 yr: 1 gtt bid q8-12h	Contact lenses should be removed before application, may be inserted after 10 min. Not for the treatment of contact lens irritation.
Ketorolac tromethamine 0.5% Acular	NSAID Children ≥3 yr: 1 gtt qid	Avoid with aspirin or NSAID sensitivity. Use ocular product with caution in patients with complicated ocular surgeries, corneal denervation or epithelial defects, ocular surface diseases (e.g., dry eye syndrome), repeated ocular surgeries within a short period, diabetes mellitus, or rheumatoid arthritis; these patients may be at risk for corneal adverse events that may be sight-threatening. *Do not use while wearing contact lenses.*
Fluorometholone0.1%, 0.25% suspension (0.1%, 0.25%) and ointment (0.1%) FML, FML Forte, Flarex	Fluorinated corticosteroid Children ≥2 yr, 1 gtt into conjunctival sac of affected eye(s) bid-qid. During initial 24-48 hr, dosage may be increased to 1 gtt q4h. Ointment (~1.3 cm in length) into conjunctival sac of affected eye(s) 1-3 times daily. May be applied q4h during initial 24-48 hr of therapy	If improvement does not occur after 2 days, patient should be reevaluated. Patient should remove soft contact lenses before administering (contains benzalkonium chloride) and delay reinsertion of lenses for ≥15 min after administration. Close monitoring for development of glaucoma and cataracts.

bid, Two times daily; *gtt,* drops; *NSAID,* nonsteroidal antiinflammatory drug; *q4-6h,* every 4-6 h; *qd,* every day; *qid,* four times daily.
From Kliegman RM: *Nelson textbook of pediatrics,* ed 21, Philadelphia, 2020, Elsevier.

PEARLS & CONSIDERATIONS

COMMENTS

- Red eyes are not simply conjunctivitis when the patient has significant pain or loss of sight. However, it is usually safe to treat pain-free eyes and the normal-seeing red eye with lid hygiene and topical treatment.
- Use caution with patients wearing soft contact lenses, infants, and the elderly.
- Do not use steroids indiscriminately; use only when the diagnosis is certain.
- Bacterial conjunctivitis is generally self-limiting. More than 60% of persons will improve with placebo within 2 to 5 days.

RELATED CONTENT

Conjunctivitis (Patient Information)

AUTHOR: **R. Scott Hoffman, MD**

BASIC INFORMATION

DEFINITION

Decreased stool frequency (fewer than three bowel movements [BM] per week) with complaints of excessive straining, lower abdominal fullness, hard stools, feeling of incomplete evacuation, commonly associated with hardened feces or another underlying disorder.

Rome IV criteria (see "Diagnosis") are used to classify patients.

ICD-10CM CODES	
K59.0	Constipation
K59.00	Unspecified
K59.01	Slow-transit constipation
K59.02	Outlet dysfunction constipaiton
K59.03	Drug-induced constipation
K59.04	Chronic idiopathic constipation
K59.09	Other constipation
K59.8	Other specified functional intestinal disorders
K59.9	Functional intestinal disorder, unspecified

EPIDEMIOLOGY & DEMOGRAPHICS

PREVALENCE:

- 12% to 19% of adults all ages
- Chronic constipation increases with age
- 33.5% adults 60 to 101 yr of age
- Approximately 26% of men and 34% of women >65 have constipation

RISK FACTORS: More prevalent in patients who are: Women; nonwhites; low income; over 60 yr; sedentary; less educated; or diagnosed with a medical condition predisposing them to constipation (e.g., Parkinson disease)

PHYSICAL FINDINGS & CLINICAL PRESENTATION

- A thorough history includes the duration of constipation, change in BM, medication history, or any comorbidities.
- Clinical presentation varies for every patient as their personal definition of constipation may differ from medical lexicon.
- Constipation can be accompanied by an increased frequency of liquid stools (overflow diarrhea) typically caused by stool impaction.
- Rule out alarm features such as hematochezia or melena, weight loss of greater than 10 lbs, a family history of colon cancer or inflammatory bowel disease (IBD), anemia or acute onset of constipation.
- Physical examination must include a digital rectal exam (DRE). Pain on examination, asymmetric anal opening, impaired sphincter function, masses, strictures, or the presence and character of stool (soft, hard, impacted) can help determine the etiology.

ETIOLOGY

Idiopathic vs. secondary causes of constipation

- Secondary causes include neurologic, metabolic, or endocrine disturbances; psychiatric disorders; gastrointestinal malignancies; and medication-induced.
- Types of anorectal dysfunction causing rectal outlet delay in older people are summarized in Table 1.
- Medication-induced constipation is very common; frequent offenders include:
  1. Anticholinergics
  2. Iron supplements
  3. Antacids
  4. Opiates
  5. Antihypertensive medications (especially calcium channel blockers)
  6. Serotonin antagonists
  7. Ganglionic blockers

Dx DIAGNOSIS

BASED ON ROME IV CRITERIA

- Symptoms present for at least 3 mo out of the previous 6 mo.
- Loose stools are rarely present without the use of laxatives.
- Does not meet criteria for Rome IV irritable bowel syndrome (IBS).
- Presence of two or more of the following symptoms:
  1. Straining during more than 25% of defecations
  2. Lumpy or hard stools in more than 25% of defecations
  3. Sensation of incomplete evacuation for more than 25% of defecations
  4. Sensation of anorectal obstruction/blockage for more than 25% of defecations
  5. Manual maneuvers to facilitate more than 25% of defecations (e.g., digital evacuation, support of the pelvic floor)
  6. Fewer than three spontaneous bowel movements per week
- See Fig. 1 for an algorithmic approach to the diagnosis of constipation.

DIFFERENTIAL DIAGNOSIS

- First delineate between functional and secondary constipation.
- Functional constipation must be differentiated from IBS, IBD, appendicitis, ileus, and Ogilvie syndrome.

WORKUP

- A thorough history should include presence of alarm symptoms, dietary habits, medications, underlying systemic or neurologic disorders, and patient's activity level.
- Physical examination must include a rectal examination as mentioned earlier. The sensitivity and specificity of DRE to diagnose dyssynergic defecation are 75% and 87%, respectively.
- Stool impaction can present as diarrhea and is diagnosed with DRE and physical/radiologic findings of increased stool burden.

LABORATORY TESTS

Routine laboratory tests are not required to diagnose constipation. However, patients with alarm signs should get a complete blood cell count, basic metabolic panel, thyroid-stimulating hormone, and fecal occult blood test.

IMAGING STUDIES

- Not routinely needed but may help rule out secondary causes.

TABLE 1 Types of Anorectal Dysfunction Causing Rectal Outlet Delay in Older People

	Pathophysiology	Clinical Picture
Rectal dysmotility	Reduced rectal motility and contractions Increased rectal compliance Variable degree of rectal dilation Impaired rectal sensation with blunting of urge to pass stool Over time, increasing rectal distention required to reflexively trigger the defecation mechanism	Rectal hard or soft stool retention on digital examination of which patient may be unaware Chronic rectal distention leads to relaxation of the internal sphincter and fecal soiling One postulated cause is diminished parasympathetic outflow as a result of impaired sacral cord function (e.g., from ischemia or spinal stenosis). May also develop through persistent disregard or suppression of the urge to defecate as a result of dementia, depression, immobility, or painful anorectal conditions
Pelvic floor dyssynergia	Paradoxical contraction or failure to relax the pelvic floor and external anal sphincter muscles during defecation Manometric studies show paradoxical increases in anal canal pressure on straining	Severe and long-standing symptoms of rectal outlet delay Parkinson disease More common in younger women
Irritable bowel syndrome	Increased rectal tone and reduced compliance Lower pain threshold on distending the rectum during anorectal function tests	Usually constipation-predominant in older people Rome criteria symptoms: Abdominal distention or pain relieved by defecation, passage of mucus, and feeling of incomplete emptying

From Fillit HM: *Brocklehurst's textbook of geriatric medicine and gerontology,* ed 8, Philadelphia, 2017, Elsevier.

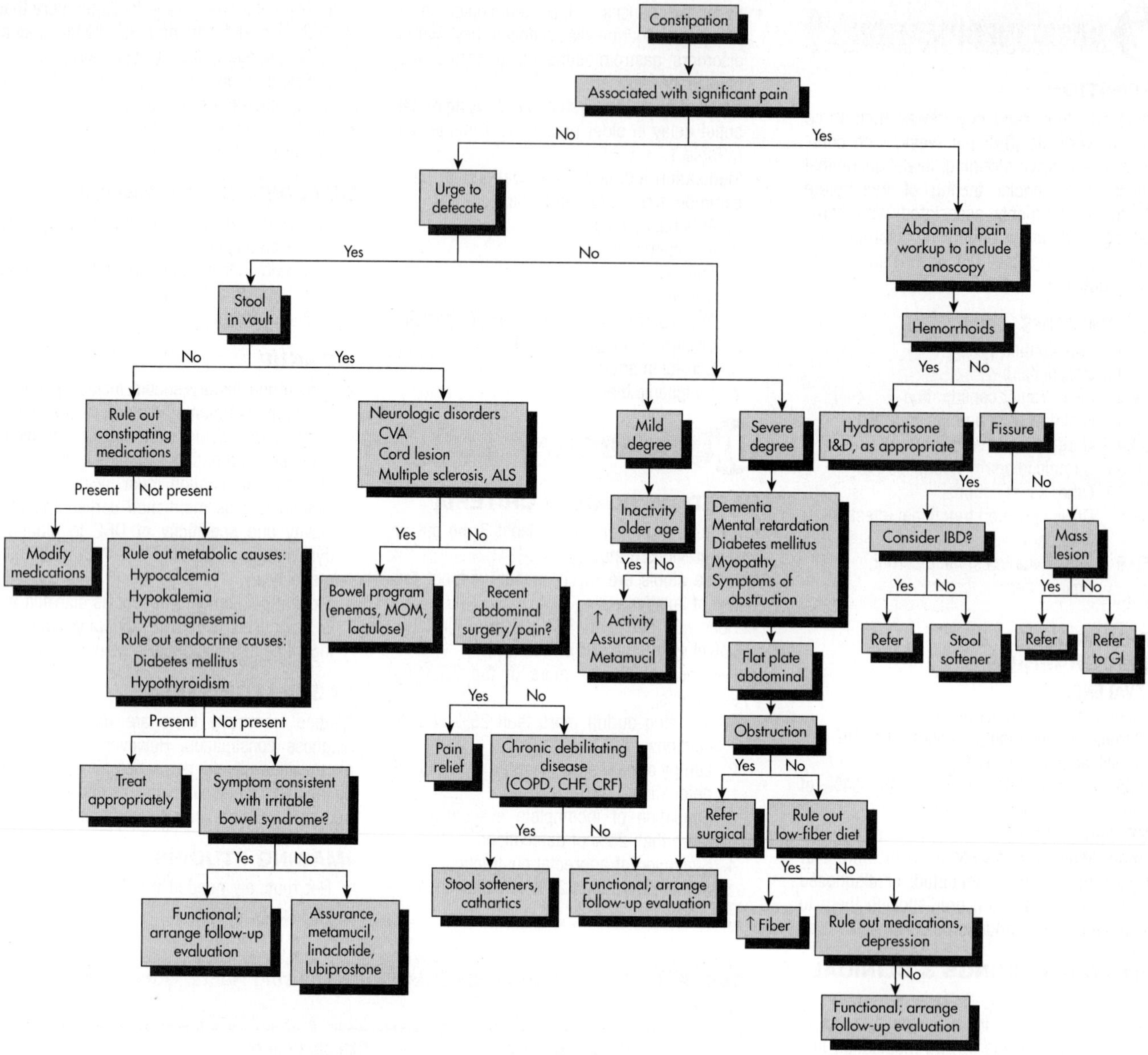

FIG. 1 Algorithmic approach to the diagnosis of constipation. *ALS,* Amyotrophic lateral sclerosis; *CHF,* congestive heart failure; *COPD,* chronic obstructive pulmonary disease; *CRF,* chronic renal failure; *CVA,* cerebrovascular accident; *GI,* gastroenterology; *IBD,* inflammatory bowel disease; *I&D,* incision and drainage; *MOM,* milk of magnesia. (From Marx JA et al: *Rosen's emergency medicine,* ed 8, Philadelphia, 2014, Saunders.)

- Plain films of the abdomen can help diagnose stool retention, which can suggest ileus, obstruction, or possible malignancy.
- Colon transit studies (via wireless motility capsule study) and whole-gut transit times can be useful but are only indicated in patients with chronic constipation that is refractory to laxatives and other conservative measures.
- Defecography is performed when the anorectum has anatomic and functional changes thought to contribute to constipation.
- Motility studies include anorectal manometry, colonic manometry, and balloon expulsion.

Rx TREATMENT

After a thorough history and physical examination, initiate empiric treatment, including patient education, dietary changes, and fiber therapy without further diagnostic workup. If no response occurs, laxative therapy is indicated.

See Box 1 for a general approach to the treatment of constipation.

NONPHARMACOLOGIC THERAPY

- Biofeedback is a behavioral approach to correcting inappropriate contraction of the pelvic floor muscles and external anal sphincter during defecation for patients with pelvic floor dysfunction as the major cause of constipation.
- Manual disimpaction removes hard stool in the rectal vault; occasionally this must be done in the operating room (depending on the volume of impacted stool).
- In patients unresponsive to medical therapy and with favorable manometry studies, subtotal colectomy with ileorectal anastomosis may be considered.

ACUTE GENERAL Rx

- Fiber is the first-line treatment.
- Laxatives, including bulk-forming, osmotic, and stimulant, are the next therapy to utilize.
    1. Suppositories and/or enemas should be used if oral therapy is ineffective.
- Many agents can be used in combination if no alarm signs are present.
- Bowel preparation in older people is summarized in Table 3.

CHRONIC Rx

- Many of the agents used in acute constipation also have a role in chronic constipation.
- Be wary of the chronic use of stimulant laxatives, which can cause colonic epithelial dysfunction.

BOX 1 General Approach to Treatment of Constipation

For specific agents, dosages, and precautions, see Table 2.

I. Core Program for All Patients

- Adequate intake of fluid and fiber is one key to preventing constipation. Fiber is available primarily from grains and bran cereals. Flatulence, bloating, and cramps are common side effects encountered when bran fiber is introduced.
- Another source of bulk is from synthetic bulk agents (e.g., psyllium). Bulk agents require an adequate amount of fluid intake; otherwise, they may worsen constipation.
- Avoid irritant laxatives as part of a core program, because long-term use may decrease bowel motility. Encourage the patient to exercise and respond promptly to the urge to defecate.

II. Individualized Program-Specific Indications and General Comments

Stimulant laxatives (e.g., senna, bisacodyl): Many believe that long-term use of these agents leads to dependency and habituation, but this is not substantiated. When used appropriately, these medications are not harmful and are very effective. Senna is probably the first-line choice among this class of laxatives.

- *Osmotic laxatives (e.g., polyethylene glycol [PEG], lactulose, milk of magnesia, magnesium citrate):* These agents are most commonly used for colonic preparation before bowel procedures. These agents are safe and well tolerated. PEG has been shown to be slightly more effective than lactulose and causes less bloating and flatus.
- *Lubricants and stool softeners:* Oral mineral oil lubricants and stool softeners are particularly helpful in patients who have acute painful perianal lesions. The softening and coating of the stool can make passage much easier and less painful, preventing constipation. Mineral oil is contraindicated in patients with swallowing problems or in those who are particularly debilitated, to prevent aspiration leading to lipid pneumonia.
- *Suppositories and enemas:* These agents may be helpful in patients who tend to have trouble expelling soft stool from the rectum. Glycerin suppositories may have a soothing effect and be helpful in patients with constipation caused by local, painful perianal lesions. Tap-water enemas are helpful when disimpaction is necessary.

From Marx JA et al: *Rosen's emergency medicine*, ed 8, Philadelphia, 2014, Saunders.

TABLE 2 Preparations Used in the Symptomatic Treatment of Constipation

Medication	Maximal Recommended Dose	Onset of Action	Comments
Bulk Laxatives			Indigestible fiber attracts water, which leads to larger, softer fecal mass.
Psyllium (Metamucil)	Titrate up to 20 g	12-72 hr	Natural fiber that undergoes bacterial degradation, which may contribute to bloating and flatus. Should be taken with plenty of water to avoid intestinal obstruction.
Methylcellulose (Citrucel)	Titrate up to 20 g		Semisynthetic cellulose fiber that is relatively resistant to colonic bacterial degradation.
Polycarbophil (Fibercon)	Titrate up to 20 g		Synthetic fiber of polymer of acrylic acid, resistant to bacterial degradation.
Osmotic Laxatives			Draw water into the intestines along osmotic gradient.
Magnesium or Sodium Salts			
Magnesium Hydroxide (Milk of Magnesia)	30-45 ml once daily	1-6 hr	A small percentage of magnesium is absorbed. Use caution in patients with renal insufficiency and in children.
Magnesium Citrate	150-300 ml as needed	3-6 hr	
Sodium Phosphate (Fleet Phospho-soda)	20-45 ml with 12 oz of water as needed		Hyperphosphatemia may result if patient has renal insufficiency. Commonly used before colonoscopy.
Poorly Absorbed Sugars			
Lactulose	15-30 ml once or twice a day	24-48 hr	Synthetic disaccharide not absorbed by the small intestine. Gas and bloating common.
Sorbitol	15-30 ml once or twice a day		Poorly absorbed by small intestine.
Polyethylene Glycol and Electrolytes (GoLYTELY, MiraLax)	17 g two or three times a day	12-24 hr	Organic polymers that are poorly absorbed and not metabolized by bacteria, thus may cause less bloating and cramping. Can be mixed with noncarbonated beverages.
Stimulant Laxatives			Stimulate intestinal motility or secretion.
Senna (Senokot, Ex-Lax)	8-34 mg daily	6-12 hr	Stimulates secretion and motility of small intestine and colon.
Bisacodyl (Dulcolax, Correctol)	5-10 mg daily		
Stool Softeners			Increase water penetration and soften stool.
Docusate Sodium (Colace)	100 mg twice a day; some use higher doses	24-48 hr	In many studies, no better than placebo. Not recommended as first-line or solo therapy.
Mineral Oil (Fleet Mineral Oil)	5-15 ml orally at night		Provides lubrication for the passage of stool. Long-term use is not recommended. Lipid pneumonia can occur in patients predisposed to aspiration.
Newer Agents			
Lubiprostone (Amitiza)	24 μg once or twice per day	1 hr	A chloride channel activator. FDA-approved for treatment of chronic idiopathic constipation in adults. Adverse effects: Headache, nausea, diarrhea.
Methylnaltrexone (Relistor)	8-12 mg SQ		Used in refractory opioid-induced constipation.
Linaclotide (Linzess)	145 mcg daily 30 min prior to meals	2-6 hr	Peptide agonist of the guanylate cyclase 2C. It increases smooth muscle contractions. Useful in IBS with constipation.
Plecanatide (Trulance)	3 mg once/day	<24 hr	Peptide agonist of the guanylate cyclase 2C. It increases smooth muscle contractions. Useful in IBS with constipation.
Naldemedine (Symproic)	0.2 mg once/day	2 h	Opioid receptor antagonist

FDA, U.S. Food and Drug Administration; *IBS*, irritable bowel syndrome; *SQ*, subcutaneously.
Modified from Marx JA et al: *Rosen's emergency medicine*, ed 8, Philadelphia, 2014, Saunders.

TABLE 3 Bowel Preparation in Older People

- Older age, constipation, reported laxative use, tricyclic antidepressants, stroke, diabetes, and dementia are associated with inadequate preparation and thus takes longer to instrument the cecum.
- Even in those who take 75%-100% of their prescribed treatment, bowel preparation is satisfactory in only 50%.

Guidance

- Give regular laxatives (e.g., Movicol two sachets daily) and enemas or suppositories for at least 1 wk before the procedure, with a longer run-up period in patients known to have constipation and in those with comorbidities such as diabetes.
- Individualize the cathartic regimen (e.g., 1-2 L of GoLYTELY daily over 2-3 days in those unable to drink 4 L, or use of alternative preparations such as sodium picosulfate).
- Identify potential nonadherence. ("Can the patient drink 4 L of GoLYTELY in 24 hours?")
- Preempt unpleasant side effects. ("Will the patient be able to reach the toilet in time to avoid fecal leakage?")
- Use oral phospho soda with caution because administration in older people increases serum phosphate, even in patients with normal creatinine clearance.
- Consider preprocedure plain abdominal x-ray for evaluation of persisting fecal loading.
- Where possible, give clear fluid diet before administration of bowel preparation.

From Fillit HM: *Brocklehurst's textbook of geriatric medicine and gerontology*, ed 8, Philadelphia, 2017, Elsevier.

- Less commonly used options for chronic constipation, include:
  1. Linaclotide and plecanatide: Guanylate cyclase-c reactor agonists, stimulate intestinal fluid secretion and transit.
  2. Lubiprostone: Chloride channel activator, enhances chloride-rich intestinal fluid secretion.
  3. Misoprostol: Prostaglandin analog.
  4. Botulinum toxins: Relaxes pelvic floor muscles.
  5. Naldemedine: Opioid receptor antagonist useful for opioid-induced constipation.

COMPLEMENTARY & ALTERNATIVE MEDICINE

Acupuncture may be recommended for chronic idiopathic constipation, but the efficacy of this treatment methodology has not been established.

DISPOSITION

Constipation can be treated in outpatient clinic settings with dietary modifications, medications, and follow-up visits.

- Occasionally, constipation must be addressed in the inpatient setting.

REFERRAL

A referral to a gastroenterologist is essential for refractory patients or those who may need a colonoscopy, sigmoidoscopy, or manometric studies.

- A referral to a surgeon may be required in patients with large volumes of impacted stool, megacolon, megarectum, or chronic slow transit constipation that is nonresponsive to medical treatment.

PEARLS & CONSIDERATIONS

- A thorough history and physical exam including DRE are important in identifying the cause of constipation.
- History that includes a survey of the patient's diet, medications, and psychosocial issues is key to the successful treatment of constipation.
- The presence of weight loss, rectal bleeding, or anemia mandates a colonoscopy or flexible sigmoidoscopy.

SUGGESTED READINGS

Available at ExpertConsult.com

AUTHORS: **Samantha Ni, MD,** and **Amanda Box, MD, MS**

BASIC INFORMATION

DEFINITION

Contraception refers to the various modalities that a sexually active couple uses to prevent pregnancy. These options can be either medical or nonmedical and used by men or women or both. There are numerous options, and this chapter should not be considered to be fully comprehensive of every option. The options are as follows:

- No contraception (unprotected intercourse); failure rate 85% both typical use and perfect use
- Abstinence: Failure rate 0%
- Withdrawal: Failure rate with perfect use, 4%; with typical use, 19%
- Rhythm method (natural family planning)
  1. Failure rate with perfect use, 1%-9%; with typical use, 20%
  2. Lactation amenorrhea method (LAM): 0.5% to 2.0% failure rate in the first 6 mo after delivery when exclusively breastfeeding and amenorrheic
- Barriers
  1. Male condom: Failure rate with perfect use, 3%; with typical use, 12%
  2. Female condom: Failure rate with perfect use, 5.1%; with typical use, 12.4%; FDA labeling states 25% failure rate
  3. Diaphragm and cervical cap: Failure rate 5% to 9% in nulliparous women, 20% in multiparous women
  4. Spermicides (aerosols, foam, jellies, creams, tabs): Failure rate with perfect use, 3%; with typical use, 21%
- Combined hormonal contraceptives
  1. Oral Pill (various estrogen/progestin combinations): Failure rate with perfect use, <1%; with typical use, 3%
  2. Vaginal ring (NuvaRing): Failure rate Pearl index, 0.77
  3. Contraceptive patch: Failure rate, 0.4% to 0.7%
- Progesterone only pill ("Mini pill")
  1. Failure rate with typical use, 1.1% to 13.2%
  2. With perfect use, 5 pregnancies per 1000 women
  3. Requires precise timing of daily use for effectiveness
- Hormonal implants and injectables
  1. Nexplanon (etonogestrel) single rod subdermal implant: Failure rate of 0.05%
  2. Depo-Provera (medroxyprogesterone acetate): Failure rate, 0.3% in first yr of use
- Emergency contraception (EC)
  1. Combined estrogen-progesterone regimen: Decreases pregnancy rate by 74% or more with women treated within 72 hr of coitus
  2. Progestin-only method "Plan B": 2.2% pregnancy rate
  3. Selective progesterone receptor modulator (Ulipristal acetate): 1.4% pregnancy rate
  4. Copper IUD: 0.1% pregnancy rate, most effective option
- Intrauterine device (IUD) or intrauterine system (IUS)
  1. Copper T (380-A): Hormone Free. Failure rate with perfect use, 0.6%; with typical use, 0.8%
  2. Levonorgestrel (LNG) IUD
     a. 52 mg LNG IUD (Mirena and Liletta): 1-yr failure rate, 0.1% to 0.2%, 5-yr cumulative failure rate 0.5% to 1.1%
     b. 19.5 LNG IUD (Kylenna): 5-yr cumulative failure rate, 0.6% to 1.6%
     c. 13.5 LNG IUD (Skyla): First year Pearl index, 0.48
- Female sterilization (tubal ligation): Failure rate with perfect use, 0.2%; with typical use, 3%
- Male sterilization (vasectomy): Failure rate of 0.1% in first yr

SYNONYMS

Birth control
Family planning

ICD-10CM CODES	
Z30	Encounter for contraceptive management
Z30.0	Encounter for general counseling and advice on contraception
Z30.011	Encounter for initial prescription of contraceptive pills
Z30.012	Encounter for prescription of emergency contraception
Z30.013	Encounter for initial prescription of injectable contraceptive
Z30.014	Encounter for initial prescription of intrauterine contraceptive device
Z30.015	Encounter for initial prescription of vaginal ring hormonal contraceptive
Z30.016	Encounter for initial prescription of transdermal patch hormonal contraceptive device
Z30.017	Encounter for initial prescription of implantable subdermal contraceptive
Z30.018	Encounter for initial prescription of other contraceptives
Z30.09	Encounter for other general counseling and advice on contraception
Z30.2	Encounter for sterilization
Z30.4	Encounter for surveillance of contraceptives
Z30.430	Encounter for insertion of intrauterine contraceptive device

DIAGNOSIS

WORKUP

- To help facilitate method selection for the patient, we recommend obtaining the below information and consulting with CDC Medical Eligibility Criteria.
  1. Thorough medical and surgical history
  2. Obstetric history (was fertility desired with conception?)
  3. Gynecologic history, including:
     a. History of previous sexually transmitted diseases
     b. Previous difficulties with contraception
     c. Frequency of intercourse
  4. Family history
- Table E1 summarizes when to start using contraceptive methods.
- Examinations and tests needed before initiation of contraceptive methods described in Table 2.
- Recommendations for routine follow-up after contraceptive initiation summarized in Table E3.

LABORATORY TESTS

- Pap smear should be done as routine and is not required prior to initiation of contraception
- *Chlamydia* and *Gonorrhea* screening when appropriate
- Pregnancy test if suspected pregnancy
- Lipid profile if family history of premature vascular event

TREATMENT

NONPHARMACOLOGIC THERAPY

- Male condoms
  1. 95% latex (rubber), 5% polyurethane, or natural membrane (lamb's intestine does not block transmission of sexually transmitted infections).
  2. Proper use: Place on an erect penis and leave ½-inch empty space at the tip of the condom; use with non–oil-based lubricants.
  3. Effectiveness is increased when used with spermicides.
  4. Main advantage: Condoms are the only method shown to reduce HIV transmission.
- Female condoms
  1. Composed of polyurethane, with one end open and one end closed
  2. Proper use: Place closed end over cervix, open end hanging out of vagina to cover penis and scrotum
  3. Highly effective against HIV
- Spermicides
  1. Types: Nonoxynol, octoxynol
  2. Forms: Jellies, creams, foams, suppositories, tablets, soluble films
  3. Proper use: Put in immediately before intercourse; may be used with other barrier methods
- Diaphragm and cervical cap
  1. Must be fitted by practitioner, used with contraceptive gels, and refitted with weight gain or loss of 4.5 kg. Must also be refitted after pregnancy.
  2. Diaphragm sizes: 50 to 105 mm; cervical cap sizes 26, 28, and 30 mm.
  3. The correct fit allows the woman to remain ambulatory without feeling the device.
  4. Proper use of diaphragm: Put in immediately before intercourse and keep in for 6 hr after intercourse; must not remain in the vagina for longer than 24 hr.
  5. Proper use of cervical cap: Fit over the cervix exactly; must not remain in place for longer than 48 hr.
- Lactation amenorrhea method (LAM)
  1. Three criteria must be met for this method to be effective: Exclusive breastfeeding

TABLE 2 Examinations and Tests Needed before Initiation of Contraceptive Methods

	CONTRACEPTIVE METHOD AND CLASS							
Examination or Test	Cu-IUD and LNG-IUD	Implant	Injectable	CHC	POP	Condom	Diaphragm or Cervical Cap	Spermicide
Examination								
Blood pressure	C	C	C	A*	C	C	C	C
Weight (BMI) (weight [kg]/height [m]²)	—†	—†	—†	—†	—†	C	C	C
Clinical breast examination	C	C	C	C	C	C	C	C
Bimanual examination and cervical inspection	A	C	C	C	C	C	A‡	C
Laboratory Test								
Glucose	C	C	C	C	C	C	C	C
Lipids	C	C	C	C	C	C	C	C
Liver enzymes	C	C	C	C	C	C	C	C
Hemoglobin	C	C	C	C	C	C	C	C
Thrombogenic mutations	C	C	C	C	C	C	C	C
Cervical cytology (Papanicolaou test)	C	C	C	C	C	C	C	C
STD screening with laboratory tests	—¶	C	C	C	C	C	C	C
HIV screening with laboratory tests	C	C	C	C	C	C	C	C

BMI, Body mass index; *CDC*, Centers for Disease Control and Prevention; *CHC*, combined hormonal contraceptive; *Cu-IUD*, copper-containing intrauterine device; *HIV*, human immunodeficiency virus; *LNG-IUD*, levonorgestrel-releasing intrauterine device; *POP*, progestin-only pill; *STD*, sexually transmitted disease; *U.S. MEC*, U.S. Medical Eligibility Criteria for Contraceptive Use.

*In instances in which blood pressure cannot be measured by a provider, blood pressure measured in other settings can be reported by the woman to her provider.

†Weight (BMI) measurement is not needed to determine medical eligibility for any methods of contraception because all methods can be used (U.S. MEC 1) or generally can be used (U.S. MEC 2) among obese women. However, measuring weight and calculating BMI at baseline might be helpful for monitoring any changes and counseling women who might be concerned about weight change perceived to be associated with their contraceptive method.

‡A bimanual examination (not cervical inspection) is needed for diaphragm fitting.

¶Most women do not require additional STD screening at the time of IUD insertion. If a woman with risk factors for STDs has not been screened for gonorrhea and chlamydia according to CDC's *STD Treatment Guidelines* (www.cdc.gov/std/treatment), screening can be performed at the time of IUD insertion, and insertion should not be delayed. Women with current purulent cervicitis or chlamydial infection or gonococcal infection should not undergo IUD insertion (U.S. MEC 4).

From Curtis KM et al: U.S. selected practice recommendations for contraceptive use, 2016, *MMWR Recomm Rep* 65(4):1-66, 2016.

(~every 3 hr), amenorrhea, and must be within 6 mo postpartum.
2. If patient begins supplementing with formula, pumping and feeding by bottle, or has any vaginal bleeding, or once infant is 6 mo old, recommend alternative contraception.
3. Not a common practice in the U.S. but may be used with another method, such as the progesterone-only pill.

- Withdrawal
  1. Withdrawal of the penis from the vagina before ejaculation
  2. Depends on self-control, but there is a high typical use failure rate
- Rhythm method
  1. Symptothermal type: Mucus method and ovulation pain combined with basal body temperature
  2. Ovulation (Billings method): Takes into account mucus quality
  3. Basal body temperature method: Uses biphasic temperature chart
  4. Depends on awareness of physiology of male and female reproductive tracts
     a. Sperm viable in vagina for 2 to 7 days
     b. Ovum lifespan 24 hr
- Sterilization
  1. Male
     a. Vasectomy to interrupt vas deferens and block passage of sperm to seminal ejaculate
     b. Scalpel and nonscalpel techniques available
     c. More easily performed procedure than female sterilization and does not require general anesthesia
  2. Female
     a. Leading method of birth control in U.S. in women older than 30 yr
     b. Interrupts fallopian tubes, blocking passage of ovum proximally and sperm distally through tube
     c. Methods: Bilateral salpingectomy, tubal ligation via removal of segment of fallopian tube, fulguration, application of clips (Filshie, Hulka) or band (Falope Ring)
     d. Essure-tubal occlusion through hysteroscopic placement of micro-inserts into the fallopian tubes. Has been removed from the market

ACUTE GENERAL Rx

- Combination oral contraceptives
  1. Standard administration: Taken daily for 21 to 24 days, placebo or pill-free interval of 4 to 7 days
  2. Alternative regimen: Extended or continuous administration of active pills.
  3. Less than 50 mcg ethinyl estradiol in most common combination oral contraceptives; progestins most commonly used in combination pills are norethindrone, levonorgestrel, norgestrel, norethindrone acetate, ethynodiol diacetate, norgestimate, or desogestrel.
  4. Triphasic combination oral contraceptives (give varying doses of progestin and estrogens throughout cycle), monophasic oral contraceptives (offer same dose of progestin and estrogen throughout cycle), Estrophasic pill (constant progesterone with variation of estrogen throughout the cycle).
  5. If pill taken with antibiotics, efficacy affected by inadequate gastrointestinal absorption in most cases; only rifampin truly reduces pill's effectiveness.
  6. Increased body weight decreases effectiveness.
  7. Table E4 describes oral contraceptive formulations available in the U.S. Guidelines for use of combination estrogen-progestin contraceptives in women 35 yr of age and older are described in Table E5.
  8. Fig. E1 describes recommended actions after late or missed combined oral contraceptives.
  9. Recommended actions after vomiting or diarrhea while using combined oral contraceptives are described in Fig. E2.
- Mini pill
  1. Progestin only; no placebo pills or pill-free intervals
  2. May cause irregular bleeding because of the lack of estrogen effect on the lining of the uterus
  3. Table E6 provides a summary and recommendations for progestin-only oral contraceptive use
- Hormonal implants and injectables
  1. Nexplanon
     a. Single etonogestrel-secreting device that is inserted underneath the skin
     b. The most effective contraceptive available
     c. Approved by FDA in 2006 and effective over 3-yr period

2. Depo-Provera
   a. Medroxyprogesterone acetate given every 3 mo in IM injection form
   b. Major side effect: Irregular bleeding; can also affect bone density
   c. Fertility return possibly delayed up to 1 yr or longer after last injection
   d. Table E7 provides a summary and recommendations for depot medroxyprogesterone acetate (DMPA) use

- Emergency contraception (EC)
  1. Done on emergency basis, if no contraceptive method used or failure of birth control (e.g., condom breakage or missed doses)
  2. Methods:
     a. Hormonal methods:
        (1) Levonorgestrel is available either as two 0.75-mg tablets taken 12 hr apart (next choice) or as a 1.5-mg tablet taken once (Plan B, one step). It is indicated for emergency contraception to be used within 72 hr after unexpected intercourse. It can be obtained OTC by women >15 yr of age and by prescription by younger patients. May be less effective in overweight and obese women.
        (2) Ulipristal (Ella) is a progesterone-receptor agonist/antagonist available by prescription only. It is a 30-mg, single-dose tablet and can be taken up to 5 days after unexpected intercourse. More effective than Plan B. Requires a prescription.
        (3) Combined estrogen-progesterone pills (Yuzpe regimen): In general, involves a first dose of 4 to 6 tablets (to achieve a dose of 100-120 mcg of ethinyl estradiol and 0.5-0.6 mg of levonorgestrel), followed by a second dose of 4 to 6 tablets 12 hr later. Less effective option.
     b. Nonhormonal method: Copper IUD inserted within 5 days of coitus. Requires an office visit and insertion by trained provider.
- IUD
  1. Device inserted into uterus to prevent sperm and ovum from uniting in fallopian tube
  2. Types available in the U.S.:
     a. ParaGard (Copper T/380-A): A polyethylene T wrapped with a fine copper wire effective for 10 yr
     b. Mirena LNG IUD: A T-shaped system with a chamber that contains levonorgestrel. Releases 20 mcg/day. Approved for 5 yr
     c. Liletta LNG IUD: Lower cost. Releases 18.6 mcg/day. Recently approved for 6 yr
     d. Kyleena LNG IUD: Releases 9.8 mcg/day. Approved for 5 yr
     e. Skyla LNG IUD: Slightly smaller device and lowest dose of levonorgestrel (may cause more irregular bleeding). Releases 8 mcg/day. Approved for 3 yr
- Vaginal ring (NuvaRing)
  1. Provides daily dose of 120 mcg of etonogestrel and 15 mcg ethinyl estradiol
  2. Stays in vagina 3 wk and is removed the fourth for a contraceptive-free interval analogous to the placebo pills in combined oral contraceptive pills
  3. Increased body weight decreases effectiveness
  4. Delivers lower total dose of estrogen than the combination oral contraceptive, but may have higher risk of DVT
  5. Recommended actions after delayed insertion or reinsertion with combined vaginal ring are described in Fig. E3
- Contraceptive patch
  1. Each patch contains 6 mg norelgestromin and delivers an estimated continuous systemic dose of 150 mcg norelgestromin and 15 mcg of ethinyl estradiol daily
  2. Worn 3 out of 4 wk
  3. Increased body weight decreases effectiveness
  4. Concern for increased risk of thromboembolic events
  5. Ortho Evra brand discontinued; Xulane (generic) available in the U.S.
  6. Recommended actions after delayed application or detachment with combined hormonal patch are described in Fig. E4

CHRONIC Rx

- With all the previously mentioned types of birth control, patient is followed up at least yearly, or as necessary, if problems arise.
- Pap test should be completed per ASCCP guidelines.
- STI cultures should be performed if indicated.
- Patients with medical problems are followed up approximately every 6 mo when taking hormonal therapy.

DISPOSITION

- Follow yearly or more frequently according to patient's side effects.
- Tailor birth control to patient according to different needs or side effects present at different times in life. Effective counseling also requires an understanding of a woman's preference and medical risks, benefits, side effects, and contraindications of each contraceptive method.

COMMENTS

- With hormonal contraception, if neurologic or cardiac symptoms arise, stop method immediately, evaluate, and refer to internist when appropriate.
- The effectiveness of long-acting reversible contraception (IUDs and implants) is superior to that of contraceptive pills, patch, or ring and is not altered in adolescents and young women.
- Management of women with bleeding irregularities while using contraception is described in Fig. E5.

REFERRAL

- If patient is medically complex, refer to a gynecologist for guidance on safe options.

PEARLS & CONSIDERATIONS

- The most effective option is the one the woman chooses to use, as she is more likely to use her chosen method correctly and consistently.
- Educate all women at risk for pregnancy about the option for emergency contraception if needed.

SUGGESTED READINGS

Available at ExpertConsult.com

RELATED CONTENT

Contraception (Patient Information)
Emergency Contraception (Related Key Topic)

AUTHOR: **Siri M. Holton, MD**

BASIC INFORMATION

DEFINITION

Cor pulmonale is an alteration in the structure and function of the right ventricle (RV) from pulmonary hypertension (PH) caused by diseases of the upper or lower airways, lungs, or pulmonary vasculature. It is the end result of disorders of pulmonary circulation due to chronic lung disease. Cor pulmonale can also occur acutely in the setting of acute pulmonary embolism (PE) or acute respiratory distress syndrome (ARDS) in which the RV is dilated and the muscular wall is stretched thin because of acute increase in RV afterload. This may present with often life-threatening obstructive shock or death, but if the patient survives the initial event, they may experience PH, right ventricular hypertrophy, and subsequent right heart failure. Chronic cor pulmonale is a disorder where RV is dilated and hypertrophied because of PH caused by long-standing lung disease. Right-sided heart failure resulting from primary disease of the left heart and congenital heart disease is not considered in this disorder. There is debate as to whether right-sided heart failure resulting from pulmonary arterial hypertension should be included in this disorder.

SYNONYMS

Acute cor pulmonale
Chronic cor pulmonale

ICD-10CM CODES

I27.81	Cor pulmonale (chronic)
I26.0	Pulmonary embolism with acute cor pulmonale
I26.01	Septic pulmonary embolism with acute cor pulmonale
I26.02	Saddle embolus of pulmonary artery with acute cor pulmonale
I26.09	Other pulmonary embolism with acute cor pulmonale
I26.90	Septic pulmonary embolism without acute cor pulmonale
I26.92	Saddle embolus of pulmonary artery without acute cor pulmonale
I26.99	Other pulmonary embolism without acute cor pulmonale

ETIOLOGY

- Acute cor pulmonale is mainly caused by a massive PE or ARDS.
- Chronic cor pulmonale is the end result of a diverse group of diseases that affect the pulmonary microcirculation. Survivors of acute cor pulmonale may also experience chronic disease over the long term. The pathophysiology of cor pulmonale is outlined in Fig. E1.
- Common conditions that lead to cor pulmonale:
  1. Chronic obstructive pulmonary disease (COPD) – leading cause
  2. Interstitial lung disease (ILD)
  3. Chronic thromboembolic disease
  4. Sleep disordered breathing
  5. Chest wall disease, such as kyphoscoliosis
  6. Chronic mountain sickness

PHYSICAL FINDINGS & CLINICAL PRESENTATION

No symptoms are specific for cor pulmonale. The symptoms are often a result of right ventricular failure as well as the underlying disease process:

- Dyspnea, fatigue, chest pain, or syncope with exertion (from PH, RV ischemia, and impaired cardiac output)
- Right upper quadrant abdominal pain and anorexia (from passive hepatic congestion)
- Cyanosis (late finding, secondary to low cardiac output)
- Hoarseness (caused by compression of the left recurrent laryngeal nerve by dilation of the main pulmonary artery; known as *Ortner syndrome*)
- Signs of right ventricular failure: Jugular venous distention, peripheral edema, hepatic congestion, ascites, and a right ventricular third heart sound
- Signs of associated tricuspid regurgitation: Holosystolic murmur heard best along the left parasternal border (augments during inspiration), prominent V-wave on jugular venous pulse, and pulsatile hepatomegaly (in severe tricuspid regurgitation)
- PH will increase the intensity of the pulmonic component of S2, which may be narrowly split
- Rarely, cough and hemoptysis

Dx DIAGNOSIS

WORKUP

Search for an underlying pulmonary process resulting in PH.

- As left ventricular (LV) dysfunction is the most common cause of PH, an initial echocardiogram (ECG) should be performed to exclude LV systolic or diastolic dysfunction.
- Echocardiography also helps with diagnosis of acute cor pulmonale as the presence of RV dilation, along with a paradoxical interventricular septal motion in systole and diastole, suggesting both RV pressure and volume overload.
- Workup should include complete pulmonary function tests (PFTs) and chest CT since the prevalence of cor pulmonale cases attributable to COPD is around 50%.
- In the majority of cases of COPD and ILD, the PH is usually mild to moderate and rarely severe.
- Consideration of obstructive sleep apnea (OSA), chronic thromboembolic disease, pulmonary arterial hypertension, and musculoskeletal disease should be given in the absence of parenchymal lung disease.
- A multiple gated acquisition right ventricular ejection fraction (MUGA RVEF) <45% is considered abnormal. However, MUGA scan is largely being replaced by cardiac MRI (CMR), which is the gold standard for RV function and size.

LABORATORY TESTS

- Complete blood count may show erythrocytosis from chronic hypoxia.
- Arterial blood gas levels confirm hypoxemia and acidosis or hypercapnia.
- B-type natriuretic peptide (BNP) may be elevated from RV dilation and/or hypoxia.
- Connective tissue disorder workup to exclude scleroderma, lupus, rheumatoid arthritis.
- Stool ova and parasites in suspected cases of schistosomiasis.
- HIV testing.

IMAGING STUDIES

- Chest radiography may show underlying pulmonary disease and evidence of PH (e.g., enlargement of the pulmonary arteries or right atrium and right ventricular dilation or "pruning" of the peripheral vasculature) (Fig. E2).
- ECG (Fig. 3) may reveal right ventricular hypertrophy with R/S ratio >1 in leads V_1 and R/S ratio <1 in leads V_5, V_6, right atrial enlargement (P-pulmonale), right-axis deviation, or the triad of $S_1Q_3T_3$ indicative of RV strain.
- ECG to detect RV enlargement and/or hypertrophy and to estimate systolic pulmonary artery pressure. In acute cor pulmonale, McConnell sign may be seen, which is a relative hyperkinesis of the RV apex relative to mid-free wall. It is caused by an abrupt increase in RV afterload resulting in regional wall stress.
- PFTs, including spirometry, lung volumes, and diffusion capacity, should be performed in all patients to evaluate for restrictive, obstructive, or combined restrictive-obstructive lung disease. Severe reductions in diffusion capacity that are out of proportion to the parenchymal lung disease can be seen.
- Perfusion scintigraphy (VQ scan) to rule out chronic thromboembolic pulmonary hypertension (CTEPH).
- Cardiac MRI can accurately measure right ventricular dimensions and function.
- Right-sided heart catheterization is the gold standard and measures pulmonary artery pressures and pulmonary vascular resistance. Importantly, right heart catheterization allows assessment of pulmonary capillary wedge pressure, allowing right heart failure from pulmonary venous hypertension due to left heart disease to be ruled out.
- Vasoreactivity testing is not indicated in cor pulmonale; however, when pulmonary arterial hypertension is thought to coexist with PH due to lung disease, as in cases of severe PH with only mild lung disease, vasoreactivity testing can be performed.
- High-resolution computed tomography (HRCT) of the chest is useful in the diagnosis of various pulmonary parenchymal diseases and also for the presence of PH. A main pulmonary artery diameter >29 mm has shown to diagnose the presence of PH with 84% sensitivity and 75% specificity.

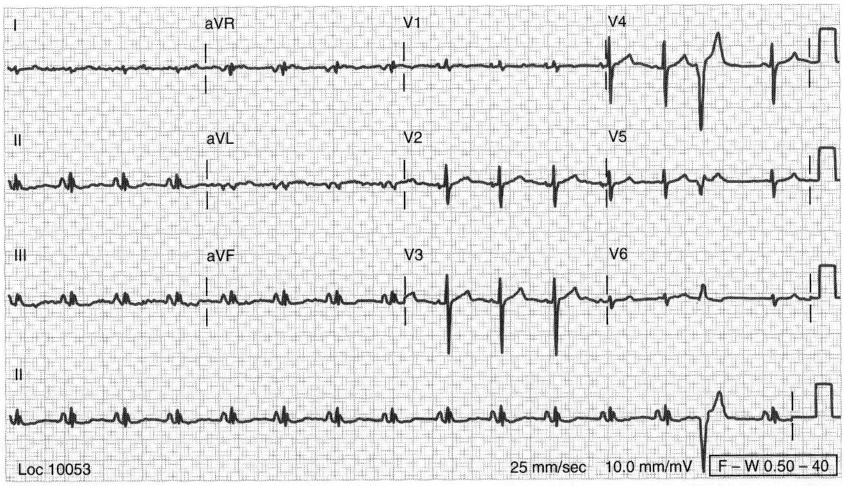

FIG. 3 An electrocardiogram in a patient with chronic cor pulmonale reveals prominent "P pulmonale" and other characteristic features (see text). *aVF,* Augmented vector foot; *aVL,* augmented vector left; *aVR,* augmented vector right. (From Mason RJ: *Murray & Nadel's textbook of respiratory medicine,* ed 5, Philadelphia, 2010, Saunders.)

TABLE 1 Therapeutic Strategies for Cor Pulmonale

Diet and Lifestyle
Smoking cessation
Weight loss
Sodium restriction
Judicious exercise training
Structured rehabilitation and breathing training programs
Avoidance of overexertion
Avoidance of pregnancy
Avoidance of high altitudes
Interventions
Treatment of underlying condition
• COPD (bronchodilators, corticosteroids, antibiotics, oxygen)
• ILD (immunosuppression, oxygen, interferon gamma [investigational])
• Sleep-disordered breathing and alveolar hypoventilation disorders (CPAP, BiPAP, surgery)
• Chronic exposure to high altitudes (return to sea level)
• Chronic thromboembolic disease (anticoagulation, inferior vena cava filters, thromboendarterectomy)
Supplemental oxygen
Pulmonary vasodilators
Anticoagulation
Diuretics
Digitalis glycosides (chronic therapy)
Nonglycoside inotropes (low-dose dobutamine or milrinone in acute severe right heart decompensation with hypoperfusion)
Lung volume reduction surgery
Lung transplantation
Heart-lung transplantation (PAH secondary to complex congenital heart disease)
Percutaneous blade-balloon atrial septostomy (investigational)
• Severe right-sided heart failure
• Recurrent syncope

BiPAP, Bilevel positive airway pressure; *COPD,* chronic obstructive pulmonary disease; *CPAP,* continuous positive airway pressure; *ILD,* interstitial lung disease; *PAH,* pulmonary arterial hypertension.
From Mason RJ: *Murray & Nadel's textbook of respiratory medicine,* ed 5, Philadelphia, 2010, Saunders.

- Additional tests: Several additional tests may be undertaken if the underlying cause of cor pulmonale is not exactly clear or to exclude other etiologies. These tests include:
  1. Overnight oximetry for nocturnal hypoxemia
  2. Polysomnography for OSA
  3. CT angiography to detect pulmonary thromboembolism
  4. Six-minute walk test to determine the WHO functional class

Rx TREATMENT

The treatment of cor pulmonale is directed toward the underlying etiology and also reversing hypoxemia, improving right ventricular contractility, decreasing pulmonary artery vascular resistance, and improving PH. Table 1 summarizes therapeutic strategies for cor pulmonale.

NONPHARMACOLOGIC THERAPY

- Supplemental oxygen to correct hypoxemia is an important management step in the treatment of cor pulmonale related to hypoxemia. Goal O_2 saturation of 90% to 96% is recommended. Oxygen is the only modality that has demonstrated mortality benefit in patients with group 3 PH.
- Continuous positive airway pressure is used in patients with OSA.
- Sodium and fluid restriction in setting of edema from RV failure.
- Low-level aerobic exercise, avoiding heavy physical exercise or isometric exercises that may cause syncope.

ACUTE GENERAL Rx

- PE is the most common cause of acute cor pulmonale (see "Pulmonary Embolism"). The treatment is anticoagulation, hemodynamic support, and consideration of thrombolytics. Thrombolytics are reserved for patients with large PE resulting in hemodynamic instability. Catheter-based thrombectomy or surgical embolectomy are potential salvage therapies in patients who cannot receive anticoagulation or thrombolysis, or whose condition continues to deteriorate despite thrombolytics and anticoagulation.
- Acute cor pulmonale may also be seen in cases of ARDS, related to hypercapnia/acidosis, hypoxic pulmonary vasoconstriction, and the effects of mechanical ventilation. The treatment is supportive care for ARDS with low tidal volume ventilation. Extracorporeal membrane oxygen support (ECMO) while awaiting lung recovery from ARDS may also be helpful in maintaining blood oxygenation.
- In patients with preexisting cor pulmonale, acute pulmonary illnesses or hypoxia can increase PH and worsen right ventricular function. The underlying exacerbating conditions should be treated.
- Careful attention to fluid balance is important in the management of acute decompensated right heart failure. Both overhydration and overdiuresis should be avoided, with careful monitoring of intake and output, electrolytes and creatinine, and hemodynamics.
- Intravenous inotropes may be employed to support right heart contractility in decompensated right heart failure. Dobutamine, milrinone, or epinephrine all have been used in clinical studies with variable success.

CHRONIC Rx

- Primary treatment of cor pulmonale is treating the underlying cause of hypoxemia. Treatment of primary associated conditions, such as COPD, ILD, and OSA, is indicated in all patients.
- The long-term use of oxygen therapy results in decreased clinical right heart failure and improved pulmonary hemodynamics in hypoxic patients. This is because oxygen reduces hypoxic vasoconstriction, RV afterload, and/or pulmonary vascular remodeling.

- Indications for oxygen in chronic obstructive pulmonary disease (COPD) patients with cor pulmonale include the following:
    1. Resting PaO_2 ≤59 mm Hg on arterial blood gas
    2. SpO_2 less than or equal to 89%
    3. EKG evidence of P pulmonale
    4. Hematocrit >55%
    5. Clinical evidence of right heart failure
- Based on the Nocturnal Oxygen Therapy Trial (NOTT), continuous oxygen therapy has a greater mortality benefit over nocturnal oxygen therapy alone.
- Volume overload should be treated with loop diuretics such as furosemide and potassium-sparing diuretics such as spironolactone.
- Anticoagulation with warfarin has been shown to have some benefit in patients with CTEPH, provided that there are no obvious contraindications to long-term anticoagulation. Experience with use of direct oral anticoagulants (DOACs) for this condition is still limited, and hence warfarin remains the drug of choice for anticoagulation.
- Pulmonary endarterectomy may be curative in cor pulmonale due to CTEPH in proximal pulmonary arteries. Before proceeding with surgery, a trial of 3 mo of anticoagulation is required.
- Digoxin, though controversial, may be employed as an oral inotropic agent to improve right heart contractility and control atrial arrhythmias.
- When vasoreactivity testing is indicated and response to vasodilators is established, selective oral or parenteral pulmonary vasodilators such as oral calcium channel blockers (CCBs), prostanoids, phosphodiesterase inhibitors, and endothelin receptor blockers may be used (refer to "Pulmonary Hypertension").
- These drugs may be effective in patients whose parenchymal destruction is mild or mild to moderate and cor pulmonale is clearly linked to changes in the pulmonary artery itself. However, in patients with severe parenchymal damage, these medications need special caution because they may cause ventilation-perfusion mismatch.
- The soluble guanylate cyclase stimulator Riociguat has been shown to improve exercise capacity and WHO functional class in CTEPH and idiopathic PH. It can be used as monotherapy or in combination with endothelin receptor antagonists or prostanoids. In small observational studies, long-term treatment with riociguat has been shown to reduce RV size and improve RV function.
- Lung transplantation or heart-lung transplantation should be considered in patients who progress despite medical management.
- All patients should be encouraged to quit smoking and should be vaccinated against influenza and with two doses of pneumococcal vaccine.

DISPOSITION

Patients with cor pulmonale should have regular assessment of their functional class (i.e., New York Heart Association or World Health Organization [NYHA or WHO] functional class); worse functional class portends a poorer prognosis. Other poor prognostic features include high right atrial pressure, impaired cardiac output, elevated BNP levels, low systemic blood pressure, and poor exercise tolerance as demonstrated by a 6-minute walk test.

REFERRAL

Patients with pulmonary disease who have progressed to cor pulmonale should be followed by a pulmonologist and a tertiary care center that specializes in treatment of advanced PH.

PEARLS & CONSIDERATIONS

- Identification and treatment of the underlying cause of cor pulmonale is key.
- Prognosis and treatment are related to the underlying cause, whereas the presence of cor pulmonale is merely a marker of the underlying disease severity.
- Right heart catheterization is the gold standard to establish diagnosis.

COMMENTS

- There is increasing interest in selective pulmonary vasodilators to improve right ventricular heart function in patients with cor pulmonale outside of the setting of idiopathic PAH, PAH related to connective tissue disease, and PAH related to congenital heart disease. However, more data on the safety and efficacy of these agents, especially in the setting of hypoxemic lung disease, is needed.
- The importance of maintaining or improving right heart function, rather than solely lowering pulmonary pressures, is becoming increasingly apparent in the therapeutic management of patients with PH and right heart failure.
- Long-term survival is related to improved pulmonary artery hemodynamics (lower mean PAP). Improved pulmonary hemodynamics are apparent within the first 6 mo of oxygen therapy.
- Continuous oxygen therapy improves pulmonary hemodynamics with more than 19 hr/day therapy.

SUGGESTED READINGS

Available at ExpertConsult.com

RELATED CONTENT

Pulmonary Embolism (Related Key Topic)
Pulmonary Hypertension (Related Key Topic)
Chronic Obstructive Pulmonary Disease (Related Key Topic)

AUTHOR: **Caroline Zahm, MD**

BASIC INFORMATION

DEFINITION

Coronary artery disease (CAD) is a clinical syndrome that suggests limitation of coronary blood flow to the myocardium as a result of atherosclerotic lesions. Atherosclerosis can be defined as the narrowing of the artery due to plaque formation in the setting of lipid accumulation inside the arterial walls. It is silent in the early stages and characterized by exertional symptoms in later stages as described in the following.

This topic addresses only stable CAD. Acute coronary syndromes (ACS), angina pectoris, and myocardial infarction are addressed as separate topics elsewhere.

SYNONYMS

Atherosclerotic heart disease
CAD
Chronic stable angina
Stable ischemic heart disease
Coronary arteriosclerosis

ICD-10CM CODES	
I25.0	Atherosclerotic cardiovascular disease
I25.1	Atherosclerotic heart disease
I25.10	Atherosclerotic heart disease of native coronary artery without angina pectoris
I25.110	Atherosclerotic heart disease of native coronary artery with unstable angina pectoris
I25.111	Atherosclerotic heart disease of native coronary artery with angina pectoris with documented spasm
I25.118	Atherosclerotic heart disease of native coronary artery with other forms of angina pectoris
I25.119	Atherosclerotic heart disease of native coronary artery with unspecified angina pectoris

EPIDEMIOLOGY & DEMOGRAPHICS

INCIDENCE:

- For persons who are 40 yr old, the lifetime risk of developing CAD is 49% in men and 32% in women. The risk increases with age in both men and women; however, the incidence in women lags behind that seen in men by approximately 10 yr.
- The incidence in premenopausal women is relatively low, while the incidence increases significantly in postmenopausal women.
- The initial presentation in men is more likely to be that of a myocardial infarction, whereas women often present initially with angina.

PREVALENCE: The 2017 Heart Disease and Stroke Statistics update from the American Heart Association estimated that 16.5 million Americans ≥20 yr of age have CAD. There is a slight male predominance at 55%, with incidence increasing with age. CAD prevalence is 7.9% for men and 5.1% for women.

RISK FACTORS: The most prevalent risk factors include age, male sex, hypertension, hyperlipidemia, diabetes mellitus, obesity, tobacco use, family history, and peripheral vascular disease. Coronary plaque, especially noncalcified plaque, is more prevalent and extensive in HIV-infected men, independent of CAD risk factors.

PHYSICAL FINDINGS & CLINICAL PRESENTATION

- Left anterior chest discomfort often described as squeezing, heavy pressure, and burning. Associated symptoms include fatigue, dyspnea, weakness, lightheadedness, nausea, diaphoresis, altered mental status, and syncope.
- Discomfort that radiates to the neck, jaw, shoulder, and arm (left more than right) is common.
- Typical angina is exertional, resolves with rest after 3 to 5 min, and rarely lasts more than 30 min.
- Women and diabetics may not present with classic symptoms but may manifest more frequently with dyspnea or GI complaints.
- Discomfort is elicited by physical exertion, emotional stress, cold exposure, consumption of a large meal, and smoking.
- Early coronary disease is asymptomatic.
- Stigmata of atherosclerosis may include xanthelasma, tendon xanthomata, and evidence of peripheral vascular disease such as claudication and diminished peripheral pulses.

ETIOLOGY

The process of atherosclerosis begins when the endothelium is damaged by a variety of different pathways/disease states: Hypertension, hyperlipidemia, trauma, toxins from drugs or tobacco use, or simple endothelial dysfunction sometime thought to be related to genetics. When the endothelium is dysfunctional, LDL cholesterol circulating in the blood begins to accumulate within the intima. As the cholesterol accumulates within this plaque precursor, it begins to oxidize over time, which subsequently signals monocytes to migrate into the intima and convert to macrophages—this accumulation is known as a fatty streak. The macrophage cells enlarge and engulf cholesterol but can become overwhelmed and subsequently undergo apoptosis, leaving behind foam cells (the remnants of cholesterol-filled macrophages), as well as releasing inflammatory cytokines. Atherogenesis is further propagated by this resultant cellular necrosis within the forming plaque, promoting inflammatory mediator expression, intimal thickening, and migration of more macrophage cells.

Initially atheromatous plaques develop in an outward direction, with enlargement of the external radius of the artery, thereby maintaining the inner luminal diameter and thus blood flow. This positive remodeling is frequently referred to as the "Glagov" phenomenon or remodeling. Luminal obstruction and vascular calcification are both later stages of atherogenesis. As the process continues, a well-defined core of extracellular lipids form—the collection is, at this stage, called an atheroma or fibrous plaque. Signals from the apoptotic macrophages prompt smooth muscle cell migration from the media, accelerating plaque formation by multiple actions, including secretion of collagen and elastin forming a protein fibrous cap, deposition of calcium, and releasing signals for neovascularization. By this time in the formation of the atheroma, the internal elastin membrane has become dysfunctional, allowing the passage of smooth muscle cells and perforations of neovascularization. Due to the previously mentioned changes and thickening of the intimal layer, there can be luminal narrowing, which reduces flow and ultimately can lead to symptoms of ischemia. This process of atherosclerosis typically occurs over many years.

DIAGNOSIS

DIFFERENTIAL DIAGNOSIS OF ACUTE CHEST PAIN

- Cardiovascular causes
  1. Acute coronary syndrome
  2. Aortic dissection
  3. Pericarditis
  4. Coronary arterial vasospasm
- Pulmonary causes
  1. Pulmonary embolism
  2. Pneumonia
  3. Pleuritis
  4. Pneumothorax
- Gastrointestinal causes
  1. Esophageal spasm
  2. Esophagitis
  3. GERD
- Chest wall causes
  1. Rib fracture
  2. Sternoclavicular arthritis
  3. Herpes zoster
  4. Costochondritis
- Psychiatric causes
  1. Anxiety disorders

WORKUP

See Fig. 1. ACCF/HFA guidelines for stress testing and advanced imaging are summarized in Tables 1 to 3.

LABORATORY TESTS

- Focused metabolic studies to rule out noncardiac causes (BMP, liver function tests).
- Complete blood count can help rule out anemia-related chest discomfort.
- Fasting cholesterol panel is important in assessment of lipid-related risk factors.
- Hemoglobin A1c is important to follow glycemic control.
- High-sensitivity C-reactive protein.

IMAGING STUDIES

- When choosing the appropriate imaging study, one must keep in mind the patient's baseline activity levels and baseline EKG findings. In general, an exercise-based stress test yields a better idea of the patient's ischemic burden. Furthermore, each imaging modality focuses on a different element within the ischemia cascade. The ischemia cascade suggests that, with coronary artery luminal narrowing, there is a progression of findings as the demand for oxygen-carrying hemoglobin overwhelms the delivered blood supply. The ischemia cascade: Perfusion defect > diastolic dysfunction >

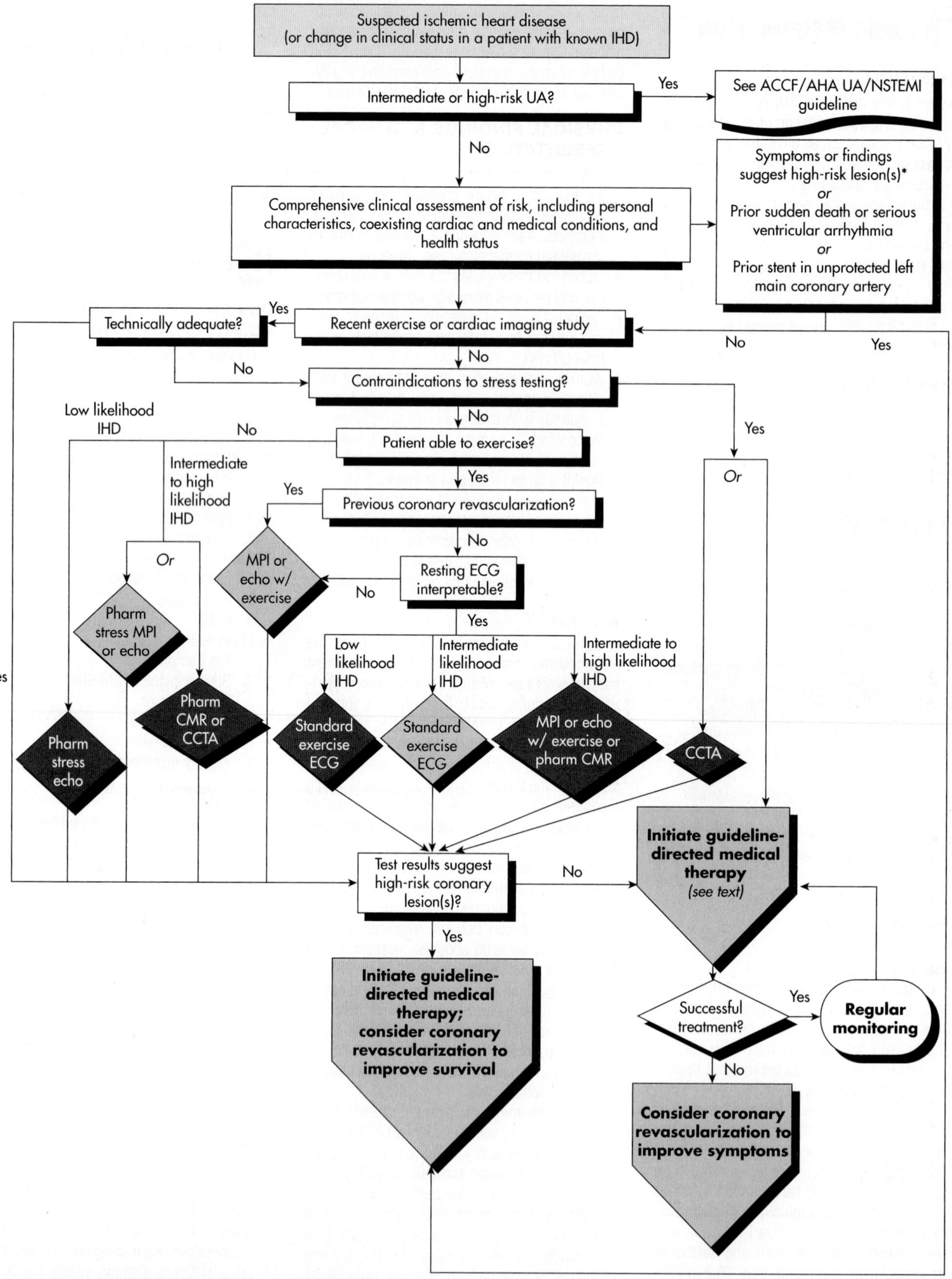

FIG. 1 Diagnosis of patients with suspected ischemic heart disease.

*CCTA is reasonable only for patients with intermediate probability of IHD. *ACCF/AHA,* American College of Cardiology Foundation/American Heart Association; *CCTA,* Computed coronary tomography angiography; *CMR,* cardiac magnetic resonance; *ECG,* electrocardiogram; *Echo,* echocardiography; *IHD,* ischemic heart disease; *MPI,* myocardial perfusion imaging; *Pharm,* pharmacologic; *UA,* unstable angina; *UA/NSTEMI,* unstable angina/non–ST-elevation myocardial infarction. (From 2012 ACCF/AHA/ACP/AATS/PCNA/SCAI/STS Guideline for the Diagnosis and Management of Patients With Stable Ischemic Heart Disease: A report of the American College of Cardiology Foundation/American Heart Association Task Force on Practice Guidelines, and the American College of Physicians, American Association for Thoracic Surgery, Preventive Cardiovascular Nurses Association, Society for Cardiovascular Angiography and Interventions, and Society of Thoracic Surgeons, *J Am Coll Cardiol* 60:e44-e164, 2012.)

TABLE 1 ACCF/AHA Guidelines for Stress Testing and Advanced Imaging for Initial Diagnosis in Patients with Suspected Stable Ischemic Heart Disease Who Require Noninvasive Testing

Test	Exercise Status		ECG Interpretable		Pretest Probability of Ischemic Heart Disease			Recommendation	Level of Evidence
	Able	Unable	Yes	No	Low	Intermediate	High		
Patients Able to Exercise									
Exercise ECG	X		X			X		I	A
Exercise ECG with MPI or Echo	X			X		X	X	I	B
Exercise ECG	X		X		X			IIa	C
Exercise ECG with MPI or Echo	X		X			X	X	IIa	B
Pharmacologic stress CMR	X			X		X	X	IIa	B
CCTA	X		Either			X		IIb	B
Exercise Echo	X		X			X		IIb	C
Pharmacologic stress with nuclear MPI, Echo, or CMR	X		X			Any		III	C
Exercise stress with MPI	X		X		X			III	C
Patients Unable to Exercise									
Pharmacologic stress with nuclear MPI or Echo		X	Either			X	X	I	B
Pharmacologic stress Echo		X	Either		X			IIa	C
CCTA		X	Either		X	X		IIa	B
Pharmacologic stress CMR		X	Either			X	X	IIa	B
Exercise ECG		X		X		Any		III	C
Other Reasons for Cardiac Computed Tomography Angiography									
Continued symptoms after normal test results Inconclusive stress test results Unable to undergo stress test	Either		Either			X		IIa	C
CAC	Either		Either		X			IIb	C

ACCF/AHA, American College of Cardiology Foundation/American Heart Association; *CAC,* coronary artery calcium (imaging); *CCTA,* coronary computed tomography angiography; *CMR,* cardiac magnetic resonance; *ECG,* electrocardiography; *Echo,* echocardiography; *MPI,* myocardial perfusion imaging.
From Zipes DP: *Braunwald's heart disease, a textbook of cardiovascular medicine,* ed 11, Philadelphia, 2019, Elsevier.

TABLE 2 ACCF/AHA Guidelines for Stress Testing and Advanced Imaging for Patients with Known Stable Ischemic Heart Disease Who Require Noninvasive Testing for Risk Assessment

Test	Exercise Status		ECG Interpretable		Additional Considerations	Recommendation	Level of Evidence
	Able	Unable	Yes	No			
Patients Able to Exercise							
Exercise ECG	X		X			I	B
Exercise ECG with MPI or Echo	X			X	Abnormalities other than LBBB or ventricular pacing	I	B
Exercise ECG with MPI or Echo	X		X			IIa	B
Pharmacologic stress CMR	X			X		IIa	B
CCTA	X			X		IIb	B
Pharmacologic stress imaging or CCTA	X		X			III	C
Patients Unable to Exercise							
Pharmacologic stress with nuclear MPI or Echo		X	Either			I	B
Pharmacologic stress CMR		X	Either			IIa	B
CCTA		X	Either		Without previous stress test	IIa	C
Regardless of Ability to Exercise							
Pharmacologic stress with nuclear MPI or Echo	Either			X	LBBB present	I	B
Exercise or pharmacologic stress with nuclear MPI, Echo, or CMR	Either		Either		Known coronary stenosis being considered for revascularization	I	B
CCTA	Either		Either		Indeterminate result of functional testing	IIa	C
	Either		Either		Unable to undergo stress imaging	IIb	C
	Either		Either		Alternative to invasive coronary angiography when functional testing indicates moderate to high risk	IIb	C
Multiple stress tests or cardiac imaging at the same time	Either		Either			III	

ACCF/AHA, American College of Cardiology Foundation/American Heart Association; *CCTA,* coronary computed tomography angiography; *CMR,* cardiac magnetic resonance; *ECG,* electrocardiography; *Echo,* echocardiography; *LBBB,* left bundle branch block; *MPI,* myocardial perfusion imaging.
From Zipes DP: *Braunwald's heart disease, a textbook of cardiovascular medicine,* ed 11, Philadelphia, 2019, Elsevier.

TABLE 3 ACCF/AHA Guidelines for Coronary Angiography to Assess Risk in Patients with Known or Suspected Stable Ischemic Heart Disease

Class	Indication	Level of Evidence
I (indicated)	1. Patients with SIHD who have survived sudden cardiac death or potentially life-threatening ventricular arrhythmia should undergo coronary angiography to assess cardiac risk.	B
	2. Patients with SIHD in whom symptoms and signs of heart failure develop should be evaluated to determine whether coronary angiography should be performed for risk assessment.	B
	3. Coronary arteriography is recommended for patients with SIHD whose clinical characteristics and results of noninvasive testing indicate a high likelihood of severe IHD and when the benefits are deemed to exceed risk.	C
IIa (good supportive evidence)	1. Coronary angiography is reasonable to further assess risk in patients with SIHD who have depressed LV function (EF <50%) and moderate-risk criteria on noninvasive testing with demonstrable ischemia.	C
	2. Coronary angiography is reasonable to further assess risk in patients with SIHD and inconclusive prognostic information after noninvasive testing or in patients for whom noninvasive testing is contraindicated or inadequate.	C
	3. Coronary angiography for risk assessment is reasonable for patients with SIHD who have unsatisfactory quality of life because of angina, have preserved LV function (EF >50%), and have intermediate-risk criteria on noninvasive testing.	C
III (no benefit)	1. Coronary angiography for risk assessment is not recommended in patients with SIHD who elect not to undergo revascularization or who are not candidates for revascularization because of comorbid conditions or individual preferences.	B
	2. Coronary angiography is not recommended to further assess risk in patients with SIHD who have preserved LV function (EF >50%) and low-risk criteria on noninvasive testing.	B
	3. Coronary angiography is not recommended to assess risk in patients who are at low risk according to clinical criteria and who have not undergone noninvasive risk testing.	C
	4. Coronary angiography is not recommended to assess risk in asymptomatic patients with no evidence of ischemia on noninvasive testing.	C

ACCF/AHA, American College of Cardiology Foundation/American Heart Association; *EF*, ejection fraction; *IHD*, ischemic heart disease; *LV*, left ventricle; *SIHD*, stable ischemic heart disease.
From Zipes DP: *Braunwald's heart disease, a textbook of cardiovascular medicine*, ed 11, Philadelphia, 2019, Elsevier.

systolic dysfunction > EKG changes and finally chest pain. See Tables 1 and 2 for further guidance on appropriate stress testing.

- Electrocardiography (ECG) is important for assessing for prior cardiac injury or ischemia.
- Exercise treadmill test (ETT) is the gold standard to assess physiologic cardiac stress response if the patient is able to exercise and has a normal baseline ECG.
- Stress tests combined with imaging (exercise stress echo or exercise myocardial perfusion study) are the next best options if ETT cannot be performed due to physical limitation or if baseline ECG is abnormal.
- Echocardiogram to assess left ventricular ejection fraction (LVEF) and the presence of wall motion abnormalities.
- Although not used in the acute setting, a coronary artery calcium (CAC) score can be used to improve CVD risk classification. The CAC is estimated from noncontrast CT (Fig. E2) images. Normal coronary arteries do not have plaques or calcium, and the normal score is 0. A CAC score of 300 or higher, or 75th percentile or higher for age, sex, and ethnicity is considered a high risk. According to the recent ACC/AHA guidelines, CAC is most appropriate among adults with an estimated 10-yr ASCVD risk <7.5% in whom questions remain about whether statin therapy is indicated. A CAC score >75th percentile for age, sex, and ethnicity is considered high risk and would justify revising a patient's risk upward.
- Those with high-risk features (Box 1) should undergo coronary angiography to assess coronary anatomy for revascularization.
- Cardiac computed tomography angiography is an emerging imaging modality that can be considered as an alternative to stress testing.
- Coronary angiography is useful for both diagnostic and therapeutic interventions if there is evidence of significant ischemia by noninvasive assessment or progressive symptoms despite optimal medical therapy (OMT) (as in the following).

Rx TREATMENT

- See Fig. 3. Table 4 summarizes ACCF/AHA guidelines for risk factor modification. Note that hypertension and cholesterol management guidelines have been revised since release of these CAD guidelines, and these are summarized in the "Hypertension" and "Hypercholesterolemia" chapters in this text.
- Successful treatment of CAD entails minimizing the likelihood of major adverse cardiac events (MACE), which include death, myocardial infarction, need for emergent coronary artery bypass grafting, or target lesion revascularization, while maximizing health and function.

NONPHARMACOLOGIC THERAPY

LIFESTYLE MODIFICATION:

- ≥150 min/wk of moderate-intensity activity or ≥75 min/wk of vigorous-intensity activity or a combination thereof (for adults) as 1 of the 7 components of ideal cardiovascular health.
- Mediterranean diet with a focus on vegetables, fruit, fish, whole grains, and olive oil has proven to reduce cardiovascular events to a degree greater than low-fat diets and equal to or greater than the benefit observed in statin trials.
- Smoking cessation.
- Weight reduction can reduce various risk factors with improved lipid, blood pressure and glycemic control.

THERAPEUTIC INTERVENTIONS: Coronary angiography with percutaneous coronary intervention (PCI) or coronary artery bypass graft (CABG) for patients on optimal medical therapy with persistent symptoms.

ACUTE GENERAL Rx FOR STABLE ANGINA

- Rest
- Sublingual nitroglycerin if rest does not provide adequate relief

CHRONIC Rx

- Antianginal therapy:
  1. Nitrates (isosorbide mononitrate and isosorbide dinitrate). These medications treat ischemia by venodilation to decrease preload, dilate epicardial coronary arteries and recruit coronary collaterals. Furthermore, they attenuate platelet aggregation. Although they do not influence survival or decrease cardiovascular death in patients with chronic CAD, they do lower the rate of angina frequency and increase time to ischemic ECG findings on treadmill testing.
  2. Beta-adrenergic antagonists (metoprolol, atenolol, carvedilol, or any other beta-blockers with the exception of those with intrinsic sympathomimetic activity). These medications work to relieve angina by decreasing myocardial oxygen demand by reducing heart rate, blood pressure, and contractility. Drugs should be titrated to a heart rate of 50 to 60 beats/min at rest and ≤100 beats/min with exercise.
  3. Calcium channel blockers (CCBs; amlodipine or verapamil). The antianginal efficacy of CCBs is comparable to beta-blockers; however, the efficacy of

BOX 1 Noninvasive Risk Stratification

High risk (>3% annual mortality rate)

1. Severe resting left ventricular dysfunction (LVEF <35%).
2. High-risk treadmill score (≤−11).
3. Severe exercise left ventricular dysfunction (exercise LVEF <35%).
4. Stress-induced large perfusion defect (particularly if anterior).
5. Stress-induced multiple perfusion defects of moderate size.
6. Large, fixed perfusion defect with LV dilation or increased lung uptake (thallium-201).
7. Stress-induced moderate perfusion defect with LV dilation or increased lung uptake (thallium-201).
8. Echocardiographic wall motion abnormality (involving >2 segments) developing at low dose of dobutamine (≤10 mg/kg/min) or at a low heart rate (<120 beats/min).
9. Stress echocardiographic evidence of extensive ischemia.

Intermediate risk (1%-3% annual mortality rate)

1. Mild/moderate resting left ventricular dysfunction (LVEF 35%-49%).
2. Intermediate-risk treadmill score (score between −11 and <5).
3. Stress-induced moderate perfusion defect without LV dilation or increased lung intake (thallium-201).
4. Limited stress echocardiographic ischemia with a wall motion abnormality only at doses of dobutamine involving ≤2 segments.

Low risk (<1% annual mortality rate)

1. Low-risk treadmill score (≥5).
2. Normal or small myocardial perfusion defect at rest or with stress.
3. Normal stress echocardiographic wall motion or no change of limited resting wall motion abnormalities during stress.

LV, Left ventricle; *LVEF*, left ventricular ejection fraction.

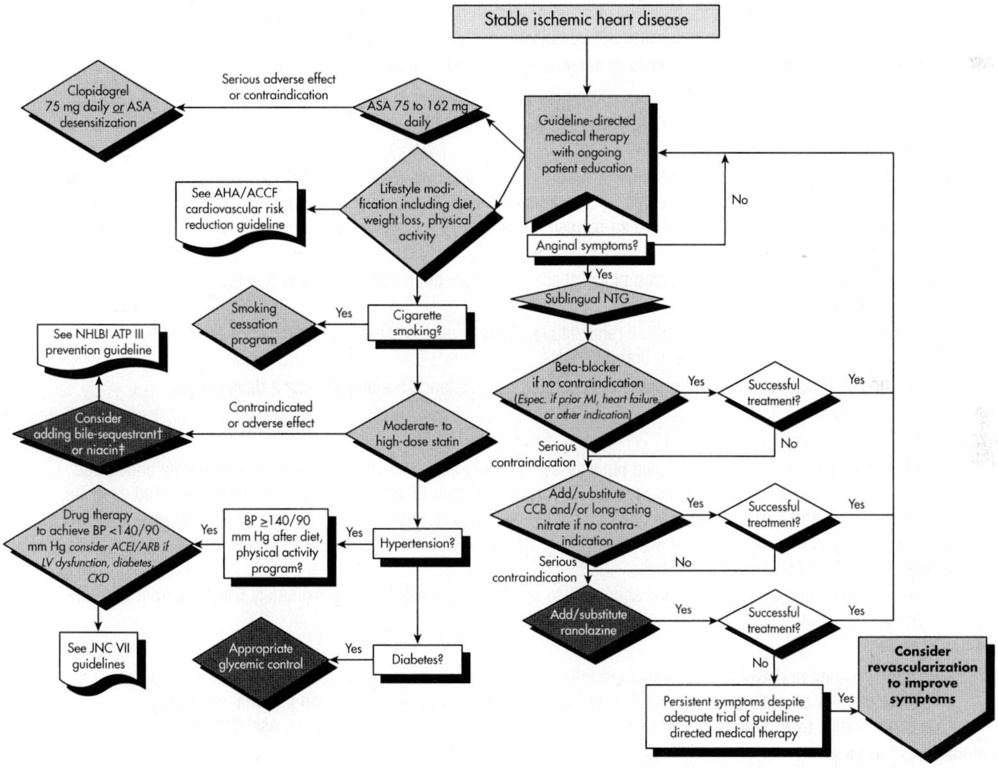

FIG. 3 Algorithm for guideline-directed medical therapy for patients with SIHD.

**The algorithms do not represent a comprehensive list of recommendations (see text for all recommendations). †The use of bile acid sequestrant is relatively contraindicated when triglycerides are ≥200 mg/dl and is contraindicated when triglycerides are ≥500 mg/dl. ‡Dietary supplement niacin must not be used as a substitute for prescription niacin. *ACCF*, American College of Cardiology Foundation; *ACEI*, angiotensin-converting enzyme inhibitor; *AHA*, American Heart Association; *ARB*, angiotensin-receptor blocker; *ASA*, aspirin; *ATP III*, Adult Treatment Panel 3; *BP*, blood pressure; *CCB*, calcium channel blocker; *CKD*, chronic kidney disease; *JNC VII*, Seventh Report of the Joint National Committee on Prevention, Detection, Evaluation, and Treatment of High Blood Pressure; *LV*, left ventricular; *MI*, myocardial infarction; *NHLBI*, National Heart, Lung, and Blood Institute; *NTG*, nitroglycerin; *SIHD*, stable ischemic heart disease. (From Fihn SD et al: 2012 ACCF/AHA/ACP/AATS/PCNA/SCAI/STS Guideline for the diagnosis and management of patients with stable ischemic heart disease: a report of the American College of Cardiology Foundation/American Heart Association Task Force on Practice Guidelines, and the American College of Physicians, American Association for Thoracic Surgery, Preventive Cardiovascular Nurses Association, Society for Cardiovascular Angiography and Interventions, and Society of Thoracic Surgeons, *J Am Coll Cardiol* 60:e44-e164, 2012.)

TABLE 4 ACCF/AHA Guidelines for Risk Factor Modification

Class	Indication	Level of Evidence
Lipid Management		
I (indicated)	1. Lifestyle modifications, including daily physical activity and weight management, are strongly recommended for all patients with SIHD.	B
	2. Dietary therapy for all patients should include reduced intake of saturated fats (to <7% of total calories), trans fatty acids (to <1% of total calories), and cholesterol (to <200 mg/day).	B
	3. In addition to therapeutic lifestyle changes, a moderate or high dose of a statin should be prescribed in the absence of contraindications or documented adverse effects.	A
IIa (good supportive evidence)	For patients who do not tolerate statins, LDL cholesterol–lowering therapy with bile acid sequestrants, niacin, or both is reasonable.	B
Blood Pressure Management		
I (indicated)	1. All patients should be counseled about the need for lifestyle modification: Weight control; increased physical activity; alcohol moderation; sodium reduction; and emphasis on increased consumption of fresh fruits, vegetables, and low-fat dairy products.	B
	2. In patients with SIHD and a BP of 140/90 mm Hg or higher, antihypertensive drug therapy should be instituted in addition to or after a trial of lifestyle modifications.	A
	3. The specific medications used for the treatment of high BP should be based on specific patient characteristics and may include ACE inhibitors and/or beta-blocking agents, as well as the addition of other drugs such as thiazide diuretics or calcium channel blocking agents if needed to achieve a goal BP of less than 140/90 mm Hg.	B
Diabetes Management		
IIa (good supportive evidence)	1. For selected individual patients, such as those with a short duration of diabetes mellitus and a long life expectancy, a goal hemoglobin A1c (HbA1c) of 7% or less is reasonable.	B
	2. A goal HbA1c between 7% and 9% is reasonable for certain patients according to age, history of hypoglycemia, presence of microvascular or macrovascular complications, or presence of coexisting medical conditions.	C
IIb (weak supportive evidence)	Initiation of pharmacotherapy interventions to achieve a target HbA1c might be reasonable.	A
III (not indicated)	Therapy with rosiglitazone should not be initiated in patients with SIHD.	C
Physical Activity		
I (indicated)	1. For all patients, clinicians should encourage 30-60 min of moderate-intensity aerobic activity at least 5 days and preferably 7 days per wk, supplemented by an increase in daily lifestyle activities (e.g., walking breaks at work, gardening, household work) to improve cardiorespiratory fitness and move patients out of the least-fit, least-active, high-risk cohort (bottom 20%).	B
	2. For all patients, risk assessment with a physical activity history and/or an exercise test is recommended to guide prognosis and prescription.	B
	3. Medically supervised programs (cardiac rehabilitation) and physician-directed, home-based programs are recommended for at-risk patients at first diagnosis.	A
IIa (good supportive evidence)	It is reasonable for clinicians to recommend complementary resistance training at least 2 days per wk.	C
Weight Management		
I (indicated)	1. BMI and/or waist circumference should be assessed at every visit, and clinicians should consistently encourage weight maintenance or reduction through an appropriate balance of lifestyle physical activity, structured exercise, caloric intake, and formal behavioral programs when indicated to maintain or achieve a BMI of between 18.5 and 24.9 kg/m^2 and a waist circumference of less than 102 cm (40 inches) in men and less than 88 cm (35 inches) in women (less for certain racial groups)	B
	2. The initial goal of weight loss therapy should be to reduce body weight by approximately 5%-10% from baseline. With success, further weight loss can be attempted if indicated.	C
Smoking Cessation		
I (indicated)	Smoking cessation and avoidance of exposure to environmental tobacco smoke at work and home should be encouraged for all patients with SIHD. Follow-up, referral to special programs, and pharmacotherapy are recommended, as is a stepwise strategy for smoking cessation (Ask, Advise, Assess, Assist, Arrange, Avoid).	B
Management of Psychological Factors		
IIa (good supportive evidence)	It is reasonable to consider screening patients with SIHD for depression and to refer or treat when indicated.	B
IIb (weak supportive evidence)	Treatment of depression has not been shown to improve cardiovascular disease outcomes but might be reasonable for its other clinical benefits.	C
Alcohol Consumption		
IIb (weak supportive evidence)	In patients with SIHD who drink alcohol, it might be reasonable for nonpregnant women to have 1 drink (4 oz of wine, 12 oz of beer, or 1 oz of spirits) a day and for men to have 1 or 2 drinks a day unless alcohol is contraindicated (such as in patients with a history of alcohol abuse or dependence or those with liver disease).	C
Exposure to Air Pollution		
IIa (good supportive evidence)	It is reasonable for patients with SIHD to avoid exposure to increased air pollution to reduce their risk for cardiovascular events.	C

ACE, Angiotensin-converting enzyme; *ACCF/AHA,* American College of Cardiology Foundation/American Heart Association; *BMI,* body mass index; *BP,* blood pressure; *LDL,* low-density lipoprotein; *SIHD,* stable ischemic heart disease.

From Zipes DP: *Braunwald's heart disease, a textbook of cardiovascular medicine,* ed 11, Philadelphia, 2019, Elsevier.

monotherapy for reducing MI or cardiac death has not been demonstrated.

4. Ranolazine. This is a selective inhibitor of late sodium influx into myocytes, which leads to decreased myocardial contractility. It can be used in combination with beta-blockers and significantly reduces frequency of angina and increases exercise duration and time to onset of angina (CARISA trial). Although it rarely may cause QT prolongation, it has not been linked to any clinically important arrhythmias.
5. May benefit from combination therapy of the above.

- Antiplatelet therapy:
  1. Aspirin therapy (81 to 162 mg/day).
  2. Clopidogrel for those intolerant to aspirin therapy.
  3. Combination of aspirin and clopidogrel does not reduce cardiovascular events in stable CAD (CHARISMA trial).
  4. Newer antiplatelet drugs such as Prasugrel and Ticagrelor have been studied and are recommended in ACS.
- Statins:
  1. HMG-CoA reductase inhibitors (statins) (atorvastatin, rosuvastatin) with high-intensity therapy for a target LDL reduction of >50% if safely achieved in high-risk patients; if not a candidate for high-intensity therapy, patient should receive at least moderate-intensity statin therapy that lowers LDL by 30% to 50%. The initiation of a statin can be determined by the ASCVD 10-yr risk calculator. Statins are recommended for primary prevention in patients with LDL >190, patients with type 2 diabetes mellitus (moderate intensity for ASCVD score <7.5% and high intensity for ASCVD risk score >7.5%) and patients with an elevated ASCVD risk score of >7.5%.
- PCSK9 inhibitors:
  1. This is a novel class of monoclonal antibodies that inhibit proprotein convertase subtilisin/kexin type 9. They cause dramatic reductions in LDL cholesterol and have been shown to reduce cardiovascular events. They are generally reserved for patients with familial hypercholesterolemia and patients with established vascular disease with LDL above goal despite maximal tolerated dose of statin. No overall mortality benefit has been demonstrated in studies to date.
- ACE-inhibitors (captopril, enalapril, lisinopril) are a class I recommendation for patients with chronic CAD with LV dysfunction LVEF <40% or diabetes and a class II recommendation for CAD patients without these features.
- Colchicine: In a randomized trial involving patients with chronic coronary disease, the risk of cardiovascular events was 31% lower among those who received 0.5 mg of colchicine once daily than among those who received placebo.[1]

CORONARY ARTERY REVASCULARIZATION

- Patients with symptoms refractory to OMT as above or those with high clinical, stress testing, or an angiographic risk profile and suitable coronary anatomy may benefit from revascularization with either PCI or CABG surgery. ACCF/AHA guidelines for revascularization are summarized in Tables 5 and 6.
- ACC/AHA class I indications for bypass surgery in chronic CAD patients include the following:
  1. High grade (>50%) left main CAD
  2. Left main CAD-equivalent anatomy including >70% luminal stenosis in the left anterior descending artery and left circumflex arteries
  3. Three-vessel disease with LVEF <50%
  4. Single- or two-vessel CAD with a large area of viable myocardium at risk
  5. Severe angina despite medical therapy if CABG can be performed with acceptable risk
- PCI has not been shown to reduce long-term rates of MI and death in patients with stable chronic CAD and therefore has no class I indications in this group. PCI is suitable in patients with suitable anatomy with refractory or lifestyle-limiting angina who have failed optimal medical therapy (OMT). Recent trials such as the COURAGE Trial have demonstrated no significant difference between OMT and PCI in overall survival, MI, and ACS over 5 yr in patients with chronic stable CAD.

[1] Nidorf SM et al: Colchicine in patients with chronic coronary disease, *N Engl J Med* 383: 1838-1847, 2020.

- The SYNTAX trial, which used a numerical score based on qualitative plaque features on angiography, showed that surgical revascularization was associated with a lesser risk of stroke and major cardiac events if the SYNTAX score was high (>33).
- Trials continue to support CABG as superior to PCI in diabetic patients with multivessel CAD and should remain the revascularization strategy of choice in this patient population.

DISPOSITION

CAD is a common chronic condition with which many patients can live for years with good symptom control on optimal medical therapy.

REFERRAL

Cardiovascular disease specialist

PEARLS & CONSIDERATIONS

COMMENTS

- The transition from stable CAD to unstable angina must be carefully monitored. Symptoms of concern include more frequent episodes of chest pain, exertional dyspnea, chest pain that is less responsive to nitroglycerin, or first episode of chest pain. Regarding unstable angina, please refer to section on acute coronary syndromes.
- ACC/AHA guidelines for follow-up noninvasive testing are summarized in Tables 7 and 8.

SUGGESTED READINGS

Available at ExpertConsult.com

RELATED CONTENT

Coronary Artery Disease (Patient Information)
Acute Coronary Syndrome (Related Key Topic)
Angina Pectoris (Related Key Topic)
Hypercholesterolemia (Related Key Topic)
Hyperlipoproteinemia, Primary (Related Key Topic)
Myocardial Infarction (Related Key Topic)

AUTHOR: **Gerhard H. Daly, MD, MSc**

TABLE 5 ACCF/AHA Guidelines for Revascularization to Improve Survival Versus Medical Therapy in Patients with Stable Ischemic Heart Disease

Anatomic Setting	Class	Recommendation	Level of Evidence
Unprotected Left Main or Complex Coronary Artery Disease			
CABG and PCI	I	Heart team approach	C
CABG and PCI	IIa	Calculation of STS and SYNTAX Scores	B
Unprotected Left Main			
CABG	I		B
PCI	IIa	For SIHD when both of the following are present: 1. Anatomic conditions associated with a low risk for PCI procedural complications and a high likelihood of a good long-term outcome 2. Clinical characteristics that predict a significantly increased risk for adverse surgical outcomes	B
	IIb	For SIHD when both of the following are present: 1. Anatomic conditions associated with a low to intermediate risk for PCI procedural complications and an intermediate to high likelihood of a good long-term outcome 2. Clinical characteristics that predict increased risk for adverse surgical outcomes (e.g. STS-predicted operative mortality >2%)	B
	III	For SIHD in patients (versus performing CABG) with unfavorable anatomy for PCI and who are good candidates for CABG	B
Three-Vessel Coronary Artery Disease with or without Proximal Left Anterior Descending Coronary Artery Disease			
CABG	I		B
	IIa	It is reasonable to choose CABG over PCI in patients with complex 3-vessel CAD (e.g., SYNTAX score ≥22) who are good candidates for CABG	B
PCI	IIb		B
Two-Vessel Coronary Artery Disease with Proximal Left Anterior Descending Coronary Artery Disease			
CABG	I		B
PCI	IIb		B
Two-Vessel Coronary Artery Disease without Proximal Left Anterior Descending Coronary Artery Disease			
CABG	IIa	With extensive ischemia	B
	IIb	Without extensive ischemia	C
PCI	IIb		B
One-Vessel Proximal Left Anterior Descending Coronary Artery Disease			
CABG	IIa	With LIMA	B
PCI	IIb		B
One-Vessel Coronary Artery Disease without Proximal Left Anterior Descending Coronary Artery Disease			
CABG	III	Harm	B
PCI	III	Harm	B
Left Ventricular Dysfunction			
CABG	IIa	EF of 35%-50%	B
CABG	IIb	EF <35% without significant left main disease	B
PCI	N/A	Insufficient data	
Survivors of Sudden Cardiac Death with Presumed Ischemia-Mediated Ventricular Tachycardia			
CABG	I		B
PCI	I		C
No Anatomic or Physiologic Criteria for Revascularization			
CABG	III	Harm	B
PCI	III	Harm	B

ACCF/AHA, American College of Cardiology Foundation/American Heart Association; *CABG,* coronary artery bypass graft; *CAD,* coronary artery disease; *EF,* ejection fraction; *LIMA,* left internal mammary artery; *N/A,* not applicable; *PCI,* percutaneous coronary intervention; *SIHD,* stable ischemic heart disease; *STS,* Society of Thoracic Surgery; *SYNTAX,* synergy between PCI with taxus and cardiac surgery.
From Zipes DP: *Braunwald's heart disease, a textbook of cardiovascular medicine*, ed 11, Philadelphia, 2019, Elsevier.

TABLE 6 ACCF/AHA Guidelines for Revascularization to Improve Symptoms in Patients with Significant Anatomic (>50% Left Main or >70% NonLeft Main Coronary Artery Disease) or Physiologic (Fractional Flow Reserve <0.80) Coronary Artery Stenoses

Clinical Setting		Recommendation	Level of Evidence
≥1 significant stenosis amenable to revascularization and unacceptable angina despite GDMT	I	CABG or PCI	A
≥1 significant stenoses and unacceptable angina in whom GDMT cannot be implemented because of medication contraindications, adverse effects, or patient preferences	IIa	CABG or PCI	C
Previous CABG with ≥1 significant stenosis associated with ischemia and unacceptable angina despite GDMT	IIa	PCI	C
	IIb	CABG	C
Complex 3-vessel CAD (e.g., SYNTAX score ≥22) with or without involvement of the proximal LAD artery and a good candidate for CABG	IIa	CABG preferred over PCI	B
Viable ischemic myocardium that is perfused by coronary arteries that are not amenable to grafting	IIb	TMR as an adjunct to CABG	B
No anatomic or physiologic criteria for revascularization	III	CABG or PCI	C

ACCF/AHA, American College of Cardiology Foundation/American Heart Association; *CABG,* coronary artery bypass graft; *GDMT,* guideline-directed medical therapy; *LAD,* left anterior descending; *PCI,* percutaneous coronary intervention; *SYNTAX,* synergy between PCI with taxus and cardiac surgery; *TMR,* transmyocardial revascularization.
From Zipes DP: *Braunwald's heart disease, a textbook of cardiovascular medicine,* ed 11, Philadelphia, 2019, Elsevier.

TABLE 7 ACC/AHA Guidelines for Follow-Up Noninvasive Testing in Patients with Known Stable Ischemic Heart Disease: New, Recurrent, or Worsening Symptoms (Not Consistent with Unstable Angina)

	Exercise Status		ECG Interpretable				
Test	**Able**	**Unable**	**Yes**	**No**	**Additional Considerations**	**Recommendation**	**Level of Evidence**
Patients Able to Exercise							
Exercise ECG	X		X			I	B
Exercise ECG with MPI or Echo	X			X		I	B
Exercise ECG with MPI or Echo	X		Either		Previous requirement for imaging or known to be at high risk for multivessel CAD	IIa	B
Pharmacologic stress MPI, Echo, or CMR	X		X			III	C
Patients Unable to Exercise							
Pharmacologic stress with nuclear MPI or Echo		X	Either			I	B
Pharmacologic stress CMR		X	Either			IIa	B
Exercise ECG		X		X		III	C
Regardless of Ability to Exercise							
CCTA	Either		Either		To assess patency of coronary stent or bypass graft ≥3 mm in diameter	IIb	C
	Either		Either		In absence of known moderate or severe calcification and to assess coronary stent <3 mm in diameter	IIb	C
	Either		Either		Known moderate or severe calcification or assessment of stent <3 mm in diameter	III	C

ACC/AHA, American College of Cardiology/American Heart Association; *CAD,* coronary artery disease; *CCTA,* cardiac computed tomography angiography; *CMR,* cardiac magnetic resonance; *ECG,* electrocardiography; *Echo,* echocardiography; *MPI,* myocardial perfusion imaging.
From Zipes DP: *Braunwald's heart disease, a textbook of cardiovascular medicine,* ed 11, Philadelphia, 2019, Elsevier.

TABLE 8 ACC/AHA Guidelines for Follow-Up Noninvasive Testing in Patients with Known Stable Ischemic Heart Disease: Asymptomatic or Stable Symptoms

	Exercise Status		ECG Interpretable					
Test	**Able**	**Unable**	**Yes**	**No**	**Pretest Probability of Ischemia**	**Additional Considerations**	**Recommendation**	**Level of Evidence**
Exercise or pharmacologic stress with MPI, Echo, or CMR at ≥2-yr intervals		X		X	Previous evidence of silent ischemia or at high risk for recurrent event	Unable to exercise, uninterpretable ECG, or incomplete revascularization	IIa	C
Exercise ECG at ≥1-yr intervals	X		X		Previous silent ischemia or at high risk for recurrent event		IIb	C
Exercise ECG	X		X		No previous silent ischemia and not at high risk for recurrent events		IIb	C
Exercise or pharmacologic stress imaging or CCTA	Either		Either			<5-yr intervals after CABG or <2 yr intervals after PCI	III	C

ACC/AHA, American College of Cardiology/American Heart Association; *CABG,* coronary artery bypass graft; *CCTA,* cardiac computed tomography angiography; *CMR,* cardiac magnetic resonance; *ECG,* electrocardiography; *Echo,* echocardiography; *MPI,* myocardial perfusion imaging; *MPI,* myocardial perfusion imaging; *PCI,* percutaneous coronary intervention.
From Zipes DP: *Braunwald's heart disease, a textbook of cardiovascular medicine,* ed 11, Philadelphia, 2019, Elsevier.

BASIC INFORMATION

DEFINITION

Coronavirus disease–2019 (COVID-19), a viral illness caused by severe acute respiratory syndrome coronavirus 2 (SARS-CoV-2), was declared a global pandemic by the World Health Organization (WHO). Presentations of infection vary widely, ranging from asymptomatic to multiorgan failure and mortality. COVID-19 was originally thought to be a primarily respiratory disorder, although association between COVID-19 and incident cardiovascular disease has been increasingly elucidated.

ICD-10CM CODE
U07.1 COVID-19

EPIDEMIOLOGY & DEMOGRAPHICS

INCIDENCE: The U.S. incidence was 1.83% as of December 2020.

PREVALENCE:

- On December 31, 2019, the WHO was informed of numerous cases of pneumonia of unknown cause in Wuhan City, China. The cause of these pneumonias was subsequently linked to SARS-CoV-2. On March 11, 2020, the WHO declared COVID-19 a global pandemic.
- The prevalence of acute myocardial injury in patients with COVID-19 infection ranges from 5% to 38%, with a weighted pooled prevalence estimate of 20% (Bavishi et al, 2020).

PREDOMINANT SEX AND AGE:

- There are no apparent differences between genders in the prevalence of COVID-19 cases. However, men have higher rates of morbidity and all-cause mortality than women.
- Males diagnosed with COVID-19 infection are also older, are more likely to be hospitalized, and have higher prevalence of comorbid conditions, including hypertension, diabetes mellitus, coronary artery disease, and heart failure. Even after adjusting for age and comorbidities, men face higher rates of death. These sex differences are not yet well understood.
- Age also appears to be a significant risk factor for mortality, with the vast majority of deaths in the U.S. occurring in those over 75 yr of age.

RISK FACTORS:

- Older age, male sex, smoking, and numerous comorbid conditions—including cardiovascular disease, diabetes mellitus, chronic airway and lung disease, hypertension, chronic kidney disease, cancer, immunocompromised state, and obesity—have been reported with increased risk of developing severe COVID-19 illness and cardiovascular complications.
- In a case surveillance of patients in the U.S. with confirmed COVID-19 infection reported to the Centers for Disease Control and Prevention (CDC), hospitalizations were six times greater in patients with underlying preexisting conditions (45.4%) than those without any underlying conditions (7.6%). Rates of death were also 12 times higher in those with underlying conditions (19.5%) than those without any underlying conditions (1.6%).

GENETICS:

Coronaviruses are single-stranded RNA viruses. SARS-CoV-2 is the seventh known coronavirus to infect humans. Its genetic composition is similar to two prior coronaviruses also known to be pathogenic in humans—severe acute respiratory syndrome coronavirus (SARS-CoV) and Middle East respiratory syndrome coronavirus (MERS-CoV). Genomic sequence studies have shown SARS-CoV-2 to share approximately 80% identity with SARS-CoV and 96% with certain bat coronaviruses. Thus, SARS-CoV-2 is believed to have originated in bats with subsequent spread to an intermediate animal host before human transmission.

PHYSICAL FINDINGS & CLINICAL PRESENTATION

- COVID-19 infection can have highly varied clinical presentations, ranging from asymptomatic to critical illness with severe multiorgan dysfunction.
- The most common symptoms in the U.S. reported to the CDC per case surveillance of over 1 million people with confirmed COVID-19 include cough (50%), subjective or objective fever of >100.4° F/38° C (43%), myalgia (36%), headache (34%), dyspnea (29%), sore throat (20%), diarrhea (19%), nausea or vomiting (12%), anosmia or dysgeusia (<10%), abdominal pain (<10%), and rhinorrhea (<10%).
- Multiple cardiovascular complications of COVID-19 infection have been reported and can be categorized into the following (Table 1):
  1. *Myocardial Injury*
     a. Myocardial injury, as defined by elevations in cardiac biomarkers, has been commonly described in COVID-19 and, per early studies in China, reported in nearly one fourth of patients hospitalized with the infection.
     b. There appears to be a direct correlation between higher troponin levels and more severe disease.
     c. In a recent multicenter prospective cohort study (ECHOVID-19) of hospitalized patients with confirmed COVID-19, among 129 patients, 79.1% had evidence of myocardial injury as defined by decreased systolic function by echocardiography and/or elevated cardiac biomarkers; 20 patients (15%) with evidence of myocardial injury developed acute respiratory distress syndrome (ARDS) whereas only 2 patients (1.5%) without any evidence of myocardial injury developed ARDS.
     d. In a prospective observational cohort study of 100 patients recently recovered from COVID-19 illness in Germany, 78 patients (78%) had abnormal cardiac magnetic resonance imaging (MRI) markers, with 60 patients (60%)

TABLE 1 Categorization of the Various Cardiac Manifestations and Complications of COVID-19 Infection

COVID-19 CARDIAC EFFECTS			
Myocardial Injury			
Elevated cardiac biomarkers	Electrocardiographic abnormalities	Echocardiographic abnormalities	Cardiac MRI abnormalities
Acute Coronary Syndrome			
Can present atypically including absence of chest pain	Increased rates of venous and arterial thromboembolic events	Increased risk of coronary stent thrombosis	STEMI mimics including stress cardiomyopathy and myopericarditis
Heart Failure			
Wide spectrum ranging from mild pulmonary edema to cardiogenic shock	Multiple reports of myocarditis/myopericarditis and stress cardiomyopathy	Right ventricular dysfunction and myocardial strain	BNP can be used as a biomarker and prognostic indicator of HF
Arrhythmia			
Both tachyarrhythmias and bradyarrhythmias can be seen	Brugada-like electrocardiogram pattern	Malignant ventricular arrhythmias have been reported, although in-hospital cardiac arrests most likely due to asystole	Investigational drug therapies used for COVID-19 treatment can prolong QT interval and lead to ventricular arrhythmias

BNP, Brain natriuretic peptide; *HF,* heart failure; *MRI,* magnetic resonance imaging; *STEMI,* ST elevation myocardial infarction.

showing cardiac MRI signs of active myocardial inflammation, independent of coexisting medical conditions.

2. *Acute Coronary Syndrome*
   a. As evidenced by prior viruses, including SARS and influenza, viral infection can lead to increased incidence of acute coronary syndrome.
   b. Patients with acute ST elevation myocardial infarction (STEMI) in the setting of COVID-19 infection presented with more atypical symptoms (including symptoms more typical of COVID-19 infection such as fever, cough, and dyspnea) rather than with chest pain.
   c. Multiple case series have shown that the majority of patients who present with concomitant STEMI and COVID-19 required revascularization with percutaneous coronary intervention.
   d. Reports have also suggested increased risk of coronary stent thrombosis in patients with COVID-19 and coronary artery disease.
   e. Increased rates of venous and arterial thromboembolic events have been described in patients diagnosed with COVID-19 infection, including reports of spontaneous thrombosis involving the aorta, peripheral arteries, cerebrovascular arteries, and renal arteries.
   f. STEMI mimickers, including stress cardiomyopathy and myopericarditis, have also been described in patients with COVID-19.
3. *Heart Failure*
   a. Among early cases in China, heart failure (HF) was recognized as a common manifestation of COVID-19, seen in approximately 20% of all patients and 49% of those who died of COVID-19.
   b. The spectrum of heart failure in COVID-19 can range from mild cardiogenic pulmonary edema to cardiogenic shock.
   c. Numerous case reports have documented typical features of myocarditis, ranging from mild to fulminant, in patients with COVID-19. Stress (Takotsubo) cardiomyopathy has also been reported.
   d. Right-sided myocardial strain has also been frequently reported and secondary to submassive or massive pulmonary embolism, pulmonary hypertension secondary to ARDS, sepsis-associated myocardial dysfunction, or HF.
   e. Brain natriuretic peptide (BNP) has been used as a biomarker and prognostic indicator of HF in patients with COVID-19, although patients with COVID-19 infection have been shown to have elevated levels of BNP even in the absence of ventricular dysfunction.
4. *Arrhythmia*
   a. Multiple observational reports have found increased tachycardia in patients hospitalized with COVID-19 infection, even in the absence of hypotension or fever. This tachycardia persisted in up to 40% of patients on discharge.
   b. Both tachyarrhythmias and bradyarrhythmias have been reported in patients with COVID-19 disease, including atrial fibrillation, atrial flutter, supraventricular tachycardia, ventricular tachycardia, ventricular fibrillation, sinus node dysfunction, and atrioventricular node dysfunction, leading to high-grade atrioventricular blocks including complete heart block.
   c. One case report also details a Brugada-like electrocardiogram (ECG) pattern in a patient with confirmed COVID-19 illness.
   d. Early studies from Wuhan, China, analyzing in-hospital cardiac arrests in patients hospitalized with COVID-19 showed that cardiac arrests were mainly secondary to asystole (89.7%), followed by shockable rhythm (5.9%) and pulseless electrical activity (4.4%).
   e. Cardiac arrhythmias and cardiac arrests are likely due to overall systemic illness rather than purely caused by COVID-19 infection.
   f. Investigational drug therapies such as hydroxychloroquine can prolong the QT interval and lead to malignant arrhythmias. Patients with QTc ≥450 msec are at greater risk of developing prolonged QTc interval and subsequent arrhythmias.

ETIOLOGY

- Myocardial injury in COVID-19 illness can be secondary to both direct and indirect mechanisms. Direct mechanisms include acute plaque rupture leading to acute coronary syndrome or direct infiltration of the myocardium by the virus. Indirect mechanisms are due to the increased inflammatory response consequent to cytokine storm, microvascular thrombosis, and myocardial oxygen supply/demand mismatch.
- The etiology of heart failure in COVID-19 has not yet been well studied. Mechanisms proposed have included increased cytokine release and myocardial inflammation as well as direct viral infiltration leading to myocarditis (Clerkin et al, 2020).
- Arrhythmias associated with COVID-19 may be caused by myocardial strain and myocarditis, myocardial ischemia, hypoxia, electrolyte derangements, fluid shifts and volume imbalances, and side effects of medications.

Dx DIAGNOSIS

DIFFERENTIAL DIAGNOSIS

- Other infectious etiologies, including other coronaviruses, influenza, acute HIV
- Myocarditis
- Ischemic cardiomyopathy
- Stress (Takotsubo) cardiomyopathy
- Tachycardia-induced cardiomyopathy
- Pulmonary hypertension/cor pulmonale
- Acute coronary syndrome
- Valvular disease
- Pulmonary embolism
- ARDS

WORKUP

- Exposure history
- ECG
- Serum troponin and BNP levels
- SARS-CoV-2 PCR
- Transthoracic echocardiogram
- Coronary angiography to evaluate for coronary artery disease and acute coronary syndrome
- Cardiac MRI

LABORATORY TESTS

- Laboratory markers, including complete blood count with differential, serum electrolytes, renal function, hepatic function, lactate dehydrogenase, prothrombin time, partial prothrombin time, fibrinogen, ferritin, D-dimer, C-reactive protein, erythrocyte sedimentation rate, troponin, BNP, and inflammatory markers, are useful in the evaluation of suspected COVID-19 infection.
- Common abnormalities found on laboratory testing include lymphopenia, thrombocytopenia, elevated troponin and BNP, elevated aminotransferase and lactate dehydrogenase levels, and elevated inflammatory markers, including D-dimer levels.

IMAGING STUDIES

- Baseline ECG will help evaluate for presence of arrhythmias, signs of myocardial injury or acute coronary syndrome, and baseline QT interval.
- Chest radiographs or chest computed tomography (CT) may show evidence of consolidations, ground-glass opacities, air bronchograms, pleural effusions, or pericardial effusions.
- Transthoracic echocardiography can be used if the results will change the prognosis or significantly affect management. Transthoracic echocardiographic findings in COVID-19 infection may show ventricular dysfunction (both left and right) with and without regional variation, valvular dysfunction, and pericardial effusion.
- Cardiovascular MRI with possible endomyocardial biopsy can be used to diagnose myocarditis and differentiate this from other cardiomyopathies.

Rx TREATMENT

Treatment for the cardiac effects of COVID-19 remains supportive. Therapies to target COVID-19 are limited and investigational. Given the current pandemic, the Food and Drug Administration (FDA) has issued an emergency use authorization for some of these trial therapies in select populations.

NONPHARMACOLOGIC THERAPY

- In patients with severe COVID-19 illness with mixed shock and respiratory failure with unclear extent of cardiac involvement, placement of a pulmonary artery catheter may help guide management.
- Patients with multiorgan dysfunction and mixed or refractory cardiogenic shock may benefit from extracorporeal membrane oxygenation (ECMO) support. A multidisciplinary approach should be taken to determine which patients should be initiated on ECMO. Other temporary mechanical circulatory support devices such as percutaneous left ventricular assist device and intraaortic balloon pump can also be considered.
- Patients with signs and symptoms of acute coronary syndrome and confirmed COVID-19 infection should be managed on a case-by-case basis, although coronary angiography and primary percutaneous coronary intervention are preferred in most cases. A fibrinolytic strategy may be more appropriate for some patients. During intervention, protective measures should be taken to ensure safety of all staff and other patients.

ACUTE GENERAL Rx

- Dexamethasone may be beneficial in patients hospitalized with severe illness on supplemental oxygen or mechanical ventilation.
- Monoclonal antibodies: Bamlanivimab has received FDA Emergency Use Authorization (EUA) for outpatient treatment of recently diagnosed mild to moderate COVID-19 in patients who are older than 12 yr of age, weigh at least 40 kg, and are at high risk for progressing to severe disease and/or hospitalization. The drug is infused over 1 hour in the outpatient setting. It has not been shown to be beneficial in hospitalized patients.
- Remdesivir is an antiviral therapy that prevents RNA replication. It was issued EUA by the FDA in 2020 for patients with severe COVID-19 illness with signs of hypoxia requiring supplemental oxygen, mechanical ventilation, or mechanical circulatory support requirements. The recommended dosage is 200 mg IV on day 1, infused over 30 to 120 min, followed by 100 mg once daily. The recommended treatment duration is 10 days for patients who need mechanical ventilation and/or ECMO and 5 days for those who do not. It should be avoided in patients with an eGFR <30 ml/min. Clinical trials have produced mixed results. The drug has been shown to shorten the time to recovery in hospitalized adults. It appears to be most beneficial when given earlier in the illness.
- Convalescent plasma obtained from patients who recovered from COVID-19 infection may be useful for patients with severe COVID-19 illness. Observational data suggest favorable clinical effects and reduction of mortality. The FDA has approved emergency authorization use in patients with severe COVID-19 illness.
- Chloroquine and hydroxychloroquine prevent entry of SARS-CoV-2 into cells. Initial studies suggested clinical benefit. However, multiple subsequent studies showed no evident clinical benefit of hydroxychloroquine (with or without azithromycin) as well as potential increased risk of harm from side effects. Thus, these agents are not recommended for use in patients with severe COVID-19 illness.
- Inotropic support should be considered in patients with cardiogenic shock or mixed shock with a cardiac component.
- In patients with arrhythmias, secondary causes should be addressed, including correction of electrolyte derangements, treatment of hypoxia, treatment of myocardial injury or ischemia, and withdrawal of any offending medications. Patients with unstable tachyarrhythmias and bradyarrhythmias, including malignant ventricular arrhythmias, should be treated according to standard resuscitation protocols. In patients with Brugada-pattern ECG in the setting of febrile COVID-19 illness, aggressive measures should be taken to reduce fever.

CHRONIC Rx

- There was initial apprehension for using angiotensin-converting enzyme (ACE) inhibitors or angiotensin receptor blockers (ARBs) since SARS-CoV-2 uses the ACE-2 cell receptors for entry. Initially, there was theoretical concern that renin-angiotensin-aldosterone system inhibition may upregulate ACE-2 receptors and thereby render a host more susceptible to infection. However, clinical data do not support this theory, and COVID-19–infected patients on ACE-inhibitor and ARB therapy were found to have lower all-cause mortality compared to those not on ACE inhibitors or ARBs. Therefore, patients receiving ACE inhibitors or ARBs should continue treatment with these agents without discontinuation in the setting of COVID-19 infection (unless there are other reasons for discontinuation such as hypotension).
- Telehealth visits should be used to closely follow up with patients diagnosed with COVID-19.

DISPOSITION

Disposition varies based on signs and symptoms, but in general, those with severe dyspnea, hypoxia, altered mental status, signs or symptoms of acute coronary syndrome including chest pain, and hypotension will likely require emergency department evaluation and possible hospitalization.

REFERRAL

Close follow-up with a cardiologist.

PEARLS & CONSIDERATIONS

COMMENTS

- COVID-19 will remain a pandemic with significant global impact until there is adequate vaccine distribution and vaccination of the general population.
- Cardiovascular manifestations and complications occur commonly in patients with COVID-19 infection and can lead to a worsened prognosis. These manifestations can be categorized as myocardial injury, acute coronary syndrome, heart failure, and arrhythmia.
- Treatment of cardiac effects of COVID-19 illness remains largely supportive. Treatments targeting SARS-CoV-2 and COVID-19 are becoming increasingly available.

PREVENTION

- Vaccinations: Three vaccines (BioNTECH/Fosun Pharma/Pfizer, Moderna, and Johnson & Johnson) are now FDA approved in adults for prevention of COVID-19 illness. Others may be approved by early 2021.
- Preventive measures are of utmost importance to combat the COVID-19 pandemic and reduce the spread of disease. Widespread vaccination of the general population and following basic safety protocols, such as maintaining social distancing (at least 6 ft), practicing proper hand hygiene, quarantining if symptomatic, and wearing masks in public, are strongly recommended during the course of the pandemic.
- Proper mask use reduces the transmission of respiratory viruses, including SARS-CoV-2, by about 40% (fitted filtration efficiency [FFE] 38%-72%). N95 masks are more effective than surgical masks (FFE >95%) and are preferred for prevention of respiratory infection. The CDC recommends use of N95 respirators while caring for patients with confirmed or suspected COVID-19 (especially during aerosol-generating procedures such as intubation).

SUGGESTED READINGS

Available at ExpertConsult.com

RELATED CONTENT

COVID-19 Disease (Related Key Topic)
Pediatric COVID-19 Disease (Related Key Topic)

AUTHORS: **Shilpa Vijayakumar, MD,** and **Aravind Rao Kokkirala, MD, FACC**

BASIC INFORMATION

DEFINITION

COVID-19 disease is a human respiratory illness transmitted person-to-person primarily via respiratory droplets as well as contact with contaminated surfaces caused by a novel coronavirus, SARS-CoV-2, that emerged in December 2019 in Wuhan, China. By March 2020 it was declared a worldwide pandemic by the World Health Organization.

SYNONYM

SARS-CoV-2

ICD-10CM CODES	
U07.1	Confirmed diagnosis
U07.1 and J12.89	COVID-19 with pneumonia, other viral pneumonia
U07.1 and J80	COVID-19 with ARDS, acute respiratory distress syndrome
U07.1 and J98.8	COVID-19 with lower respiratory infection, other specified respiratory disorder

EPIDEMIOLOGY & DEMOGRAPHICS

INCIDENCE: After originating in China, the worst countries/areas affected worldwide include the United States, Europe, Brazil, India, and Russia. Most current information on incidence: www.coronavirus.jhu.edu

PREDOMINANT SEX & AGE: Men are more at risk for worse outcomes and death, independent of age, with COVID-19. Whereas males and females have the same prevalence of COVID-19, male patients have a higher mortality rate. Children also get infected but have milder disease, much better outcomes, and a lower mortality rate of about 0.1% in the United States.

PEAK INCIDENCE: The pandemic started in the winter of 2019. It was hoped that it would be a winter seasonal infection similar to influenza, but by the summer months of 2020 that did not prove to happen, and cases continued unabated with a second spike occurring in the winter months.

RISK FACTORS:

Age:

- Most reported cases are in adults of middle age or older, but pediatric infections in adolescents and children also occur.
- Risk of severe disease increases with age; in the United States, 94% of deaths occur in people older than 50 yr. Percentage of total mortality by age group:
  1. 0 to 49 yr: less than 5%
  2. 50 to 64 yr: 15.7%
  3. 65 to 74 yr: 21.2%
  4. 75 to 84 yr: 26.4%
  5. 85 yr or older: 31.7%

Sex:

- Overall, where sex or gender data are available, it appears that females are more often affected, but disease is more severe in males.

Other Risk Factors/Associations: Various underlying medical conditions have been associated with increased risk for severe disease, especially if they are not well controlled:

- Chronic kidney disease
- Chronic obstructive pulmonary disease
- Immunosuppression because of previous solid organ transplant
- Malignancy
- Obesity (body mass index [BMI] of 30 or higher)
- Serious cardiac conditions (e.g., heart failure, coronary artery disease, cardiomyopathy)
- Sickle cell disease
- Diabetes type 2

Conditions that may be associated with higher risk for severe disease:

- Asthma (moderate to severe)
- Cerebrovascular disease
- Cystic fibrosis
- Hypertension
- Immunodeficiency from various other causes (e.g., bone marrow or hematopoietic stem cell transplant, primary immunodeficiencies, HIV disease, chronic treatment with corticosteroids or other agents with immunosuppressive effects)
- Neurologic dysfunction
- Chronic liver disease
- Pregnancy
- Pulmonary fibrosis
- Smoking
- Thalassemia
- Diabetes type 1
- Children with medically complex conditions (e.g., neurologic, metabolic, genetic, cardiac) are also at higher risk for severe disease.
- Residents of nursing homes and long-term care facilities are at high risk for acquiring infection and for severe disease, probably owing to a combination of heightened transmission in a close-quarters community and prevalence of compromised health status.

GENETICS: Variations in the DNA sequences of the ACE2 and TMPRSS2 genes in humans may affect susceptibility to the infection by altering how the virus attaches to the receptor on human cells.

PHYSICAL FINDINGS & CLINICAL PRESENTATION

- Incubation period: Within 14 days of exposure but most patients exhibit symptoms by day 4 to 5 after exposure
- Spectrum of disease:
  1. Asymptomatic disease: May be as high as 30% to 40%
  2. Mild disease: No or mild pneumonia—about 80% of symptomatic cases
  3. Severe disease: Dyspnea, hypoxia, or >50% lung involvement within 24 to 48 hours—about 14%
  4. Critical disease: Respiratory failure, shock, or multiorgan failure—5%
  5. Overall case fatality rate is about 2.3%
- Initial presentation: Pneumonia manifested by fever, cough, dyspnea, and bilateral infiltrates on chest imaging is the most serious presentation of the infection; however, in a study of 370,00 confirmed cases in the United States, a variety of symptoms were associated with COVID-19 infection:
  1. Cough: 50%
  2. Fever: subjective or >100.4° F: 43%
  3. Myalgia: 36%
  4. Headache: 34%
  5. Dyspnea: 29%
  6. Sore throat: 20%
  7. Diarrhea: 19%
  8. Nausea/vomiting: 12%
  9. Loss of smell or taste, abdominal pain, and rhinorrhea: Less than 10% each
- In some patients gastrointestinal manifestations (nausea and diarrhea) may be how the infection presents.
- Clinicians should be particularly attuned to pulmonary and hemodynamic indicators of severe disease:
  1. Patients with severe disease may appear quite ill, with tachypnea and labored respirations.
  2. Patients in apparent distress require immediate assessment of airway, breathing, and circulation (e.g., pulses, blood pressure).
  3. Clinicians should be aware of the COVID-19–related phenomenon of silent (or "happy") hypoxemia; absence of signs of respiratory distress may be misleading.
  4. Oxygenation should be assessed promptly by peripheral saturation (e.g., pulse oximetry).
- Fever is typical, occasionally exceeding 39° C. Patients in the extremes of age or with immunodeficiency may not develop fever.
- Conjunctival secretions, injection, and chemosis have been reported.
- A variety of skin changes have been described, including erythematous rashes, purpura, petechiae, and vesicles; acral lesions resembling chilblains or Janeway lesions have been seen, particularly in young patients.
- Hypotension, tachycardia, and cool/clammy extremities suggest shock.
- In children, hypotension plus two or more of the following criteria may be indicative of COVID-19-associated multisystem inflammatory syndrome:
  1. Altered mental status
  2. Tachycardia (heart rate more than 160 beats per minute in infants or 150 in older children) or bradycardia (heart rate less than 90 in infants or 70 in older children)
  3. Prolonged capillary refill (more than 2 seconds) or warm vasodilation and bounding pulses
  4. Tachypnea
  5. Mottled skin, petechiae, or purpura
  6. Oliguria
  7. Hyperthermia or hypothermia

COMPLICATIONS

- Respiratory failure:
  1. High-flow nasal cannula (HFNC) is recommended over noninvasive positive pressure ventilation (NIPPV).

2. If hypoxemia persists and intubation is not indicated, it is recommended to use a trial of awake prone positioning to improve oxygenation.
3. If patient requires intubation, use a higher positive end expiratory pressure (PEEP) strategy over a lower PEEP strategy.
4. If still hypoxemic despite intubation, prone ventilation for 12 to 16 hours a day is recommended.

- Cardiac and cardiovascular complications:
  1. Acute coronary syndrome (ACS): There has been an increased coronary artery thrombus burden in patients with COVID-19 and an increased risk of developing an STEMI. This is likely related to the hypercoagulable state produced by COVID-19. The ability to reperfuse the patient with PCI or fibrinolysis will depend on how ill the patient is.
  2. Myocarditis is a known complication and likely results from a combination of direct viral injury and cardiac damage due to the host's immune response. Clinical findings include changes in electrocardiogram or cardiac biomarkers and impaired cardiac function. Cardiac magnetic resonance imaging or cardiac computed tomography (CT) with angiography may help in the diagnosis.
  3. Arrhythmias, congestive heart failure, and cardiac shock can also occur.
- Thromboembolic complications: Severe COVID-19 illness is associated with intense inflammation, leading to high rates of thrombotic complications that lead to higher morbidity and mortality rates. One study showed a 25% incidence of deep vein thrombosis (DVT) in severe COVID-19, and another study found a combined incidence of 31% for DVT, pulmonary embolus, and arterial embolism.
  1. Histopathologic studies show diffuse alveolar damage with profound inflammation, thrombosis, and thrombotic microangiopathy of small vessels and capillaries of the lung.
  2. Measurement of D-dimer, fibrinogen, prothrombin time, INR, and APTT should be obtained every 48 hours.
  3. Prophylaxis against DVT is recommended for all patients with COVID-19 in the hospital using low-molecular-weight heparin, unfractionated heparin for those in renal failure, or fondaparinux for those with heparin-induced thrombocytopenia, as long as platelet count is above 25×10^9/L.
  4. Patients with a D-dimer level of 3.0 μg/ml or higher should undergo screening with point-of-care ultrasound to rule out DVT and receive more intensive prophylaxis.
     a. Elevated levels of D-dimer on presentation are associated with more severe disease.
     b. Levels of 0.5 μg/ml or higher were found in 59.6% of patients with severe disease.
     c. Higher levels correlate with the need for intensive care and increased risk of death.
- Other complications: Stroke
  1. Encephalopathy with agitated delirium (common in the intensive care unit [ICU] setting)
  2. Acute kidney injury
  3. Multisystem inflammatory syndrome seen in children

ETIOLOGY

- The SARS-CoV-2 is a coronavirus, an enveloped positive stranded RNA virus. It is in the same subgenus as the severe acute respiratory virus (SARS) as well as several bat coronaviruses. It is not known if there was direct transmission from bats or some other intermediary host.
- The name coronavirus comes from the Latin word meaning "crown" or "halo" because on two-dimensional electron microscopy the virus has a "crown-like" appearance caused by club-shaped spike peplomers covering the surface.
- The virus enters cells through an endocytosis pathway, using surface spike (S) proteins to bind to angiotensin-converting enzyme 2 (ACE-2) and dipeptidyl peptidase 4 (DPP4) receptors on the ciliated bronchial epithelial cells and type II pneumocytes. Once the virus enters a host cell, viral RNA is exposed and replication occurs.

Dx DIAGNOSIS

DIFFERENTIAL DIAGNOSIS

- Early stages:
  1. Viral: Influenza, parainfluenza, adenovirus, respiratory syncytial virus, human metapneumovirus, other coronaviruses
  2. *Streptococcus pneumoniae* pneumonia
  3. *Haemophilus pneumoniae* pneumonia
  4. *Moraxella catarrhalis* pneumonia
  5. Atypical bacterial pneumonia: *Legionella* or *Mycoplasma pneumoniae*
- Severe acute respiratory syndrome (SARS)
- Middle East respiratory syndrome (MERS)
- Noninfectious: Heart failure, pulmonary embolism, salicylate poisoning, toxic shock

WORKUP

- Consists of a combination of laboratory tests, viral diagnostic tests, radiology, and a compatible clinical course. The Centers for Disease Control and Prevention (CDC) has the following guidelines for COVID-19 diagnostic testing:
  1. High priority:
     a. Hospitalized patients *with symptoms*
     b. Health care facility workers, workers in congregate settings, and first responders *with symptoms*
     c. Residents in long-term care facilities or other congregate living settings, including prisons and shelters, *with symptoms*
  2. Priority:
     a. Persons *with symptoms* of potential COVID-19 infection, including fever, cough, shortness of breath, chills, muscle pain, new loss of taste or smell, vomiting or diarrhea, and/or sore throat
     b. Persons *without symptoms* who are prioritized by health departments or clinicians, for any reason, including but not limited to public health monitoring, sentinel surveillance, or screening of other asymptomatic individuals according to state or local plans

LABORATORY TESTS

Virologic testing for SARS-CoV-2 infection uses a molecular diagnostic or antigen test. Initial tests used a reverse transcriptase polymerase chain reaction (PCR) platform; however, more recent tests use additional platforms such as the antigen rapid tests, including one on saliva and tests that take 15 min. False negatives are unusual but can occur.

- The CDC recommends nasopharynx swab samples, but nasal swabs or oropharyngeal swabs are acceptable alternatives.
- Although lower respiratory tract samples have a higher yield than upper tract samples, they are often not done because of concerns of aerosolization of virus during sample collection procedures.
- Serology testing is not useful in early diagnosis because it may take 21 days to develop IgM/IgG antibodies, plus there is variability in terms of sensitivity and specificity of these tests. In areas of low prevalence of infection, false positives may be quite high.
- It is not recommended to use serology tests to see if a patient is still immune because it is currently unknown how long antibodies persist following infection and whether the presence of antibody confers immunity against future infection.

OTHER LABORATORY TESTS

Laboratory tests associated with worse outcomes include the following:

- Lymphopenia
- Thrombocytopenia
- Elevated liver function tests
- Elevated lactate dehydrogenase (LDH)
- Elevated inflammatory markers: C-reactive protein (CRP), ferritin
- Elevated D-dimer: >1 μg/ml
- Elevated prothrombin time (PT)
- Elevated troponin
- Elevated creatine phosphokinase (CPK)
- Elevated creatinine
- Elevated interleukin-6 (IL-6) levels
- Procalcitonin level initially normal but may become elevated in critically ill patients

IMAGING STUDIES

- Radiologic findings of SARS-CoV-2 pneumonia are variable.
- More than 75% of patients present with bilateral lung involvement, and multilobe involvement is also common (over 70%).

- On CT, ground-glass opacity (GGO) is the most common finding in over 80% of patients, with one-third of patients presenting GGO in the periphery; consolidation is also present in 30% of patients.
- Nodules, cavitation, pleural effusions, and lymphadenopathy are not seen on CT.
- Due to the hypercoagulable state of COVID-19, pulmonary embolism (PE) or DVT is not uncommon and a high D-dimer should prompt consideration for workup with CT.
- CT angiography is used to rule out PE.

Rx TREATMENT

PHARMACOLOGIC THERAPY CURRENTLY IN USE

- Corticosteroids: A large randomized open label trial (RECOVERY trial) in the UK showed that oral or IV dexamethasone at 6 mg/day for 7 to 10 days reduced mortality rates among hospitalized patients.
    1. Overall relative reduction for all patients was 17%.
    2. Relative reduction in mortality in patients intubated or on extracorporeal membrane oxygenation (ECMO) was 35%.
    3. For patients on noninvasive oxygen therapy relative reduction was 18%.
    4. There was not a benefit in patients who either did not require oxygen or were intubated.
- Monoclonal antibodies: Bamlanivimab has received Food and Drug Administration (FDA) Emergency Use Authorization (EUA) for outpatient treatment of recently diagnosed mild to moderate COVID-19 in patients who are older than 12 yr of age, weight at least 40 kg, and are at high risk for progressing to severe disease and/or hospitalization. The drug is infused over 1 hour in the outpatient setting. It has not been shown to be beneficial in hospitalized patients.
- Remdesivir is an antiviral therapy that prevents RNA replication. It was issued emergency use authorization by the FDA in 2020 for patients with severe COVID-19 illness with signs of hypoxia requiring supplemental oxygen, mechanical ventilation, or mechanical circulatory support requirements. The recommended dosage is 200 mg IV on day 1, infused over 30 to 120 min, followed by 100 mg once daily. The recommended treatment duration is 10 days for patients who need mechanical ventilation and/or ECMO and 5 days for those who do not. It should be avoided in patients with an eGFR < 30 ml/min. Clinical trials have produced mixed results. The drug has been shown to shorten the time to recovery in hospitalized adults. It appears to be most beneficial when given earlier in the illness.
- Chloroquine and hydroxychloroquine prevent entry of SARS-CoV-2 into cells. Initial studies suggested clinical benefit. However, multiple subsequent studies showed no evident clinical benefit of hydroxychloroquine (with or without azithromycin) as well as potential increased risk of harm from side effects. Thus, these agents are not recommended for use in patients with severe COVID-19 illness.

NONPHARMACOLOGIC THERAPY

Convalescent plasma: Plasma from donors who have recovered from COVID-19 may contain antibodies to SARS-CoV-2 that may help suppress the virus and modify the inflammatory response. The largest clinical trial was from the Mayo Clinic and enrolled over 70,000 patients in the United States as of August 2020. Side effects were <1% and are the usual side effects of any blood product transfusion. Convalescent plasma received EUA in August 2020.

VACCINES

Two vaccines (BioNTECH/Fosun Pharma/Pfizer and Moderna) are now FDA approved in adults for prevention of COVID-19 illness. Others may be approved by early 2021.

- Messenger RNA (mRNA)–based vaccines: Moderna (mRNA-1273) and BioNTECH/Fosun Pharma/Pfizer (BNT162a1). mRNA is the intermediate step between the translation of DNA and production of proteins in the cytoplasm, and both vaccines use mRNA to encode for the spike protein of the virus.
- Viral vector vaccines use adenovirus as the vector. A gene from the SARS-CoV-2 is inserted into the adenovirus. Johnson & Johnson/Janssen vaccine uses replication-defective human adenovirus 26 vector and the AstraZeneca/University of Oxford uses a replication-defective simian adenovirus vector. Another viral-based vaccine uses recombinant vesicular stomatitis virus vector: Merck Sharp & Dohme/International Aids Vaccine Initiative. The viral vector vaccines also target the spike protein.

REFERRAL

Infectious diseases, pulmonary, and intensivist, if patient requires ICU level of care, should be consulted for hospitalized patients.

! PEARLS & CONSIDERATIONS

MULTISYSTEM INFLAMMATORY SYNDROME IN CHILDREN (MIS-C) ASSOCIATED WITH COVID-19

The clinical presentation includes fever, severe illness, and the involvement of two or more organ systems, in combination with laboratory evidence of inflammation and laboratory or epidemiologic evidence of COVID-19 infection. It appears to be a rare complication with an incidence of 2 per 100,000.

- Organ system involvement can be cardiac, renal, respiratory, dermatologic, hematologic, gastrointestinal, or neurologic.
- Lab evidence: Elevated CRP, erythrocyte sedimentation rate, fibrinogen, procalcitonin, D-dimer, ferritin, LDH, or IL-6; elevated neutrophils or reduced lymphocytes; low albumin.
- Positive SARS-CoV-2 testing by RT-PCR, serology, or antigen *or* COVID-19 exposure within 4 wk before onset of symptoms. There appears to be a lag of several weeks between the peak of COVID-19 cases within a community and the rise of MIS-C cases.
- It appears that the pathogenesis involves a postinfectious immune dysfunction similar to what is seen in Kawasaki disease.
- Treatment options include intravenous immunoglobulin (IVIG), aspirin, and corticosteroids (Solu-Medrol). Clinical trials are ongoing with anakinra (IL-1 blocker) and tocilizumab (IL-6 blocker).

INFECTION CONTROL

- Patients undergoing aerosol-generating procedures should be placed in a negative pressure room. Otherwise patients can go into a well-ventilated single-occupancy room with a closed door and dedicated bathroom. Two COVID-19–positive patients can be placed in a room if necessary.
- Personal protective equipment (PPE): Gowns and gloves and eye protection should be worn.
    1. On COVID-19 units gowns do not need to be routinely changed between patients.
    2. The CDC recommends an N-95 respirator for patient care but acknowledges that a medical mask is acceptable when supplies of respirators are limited.
    3. Goggles or a disposable face shield that covers the front and sides of the face must be used.
    4. Some hospitals require shoe covers, and hair covers may also be used.
    5. Health care workers should pay special attention to appropriate sequence (donning and doffing) of putting on and taking off the PPE. Videos are available to educate health care workers (www.cdc.gov/coronavirus/2019-ncov/hcp/using-ppe.html).

PREVENTION

- Preventive measures are of utmost importance to combat the COVID-19 pandemic and reduce the spread of disease. Widespread vaccination of the general population and following basic safety protocols such as maintaining social distancing (at least 6 feet), practicing proper hand hygiene, quarantining if symptomatic, and wearing masks in public are strongly recommended during the course of the pandemic.
- Proper mask use reduces the transmission of respiratory viruses, including SARS-CoV-2, by about 40% (fitted filtration efficiency [FFE] 38%-72%). N95 masks are more effective than surgical masks (FFE >95%) and are preferred for prevention of respiratory infection. The CDC recommends use of N95 respirators while caring for patients with confirmed or suspected COVID-19 (especially during aerosol-generating procedures such as intubation).

COMMUNITY/FAMILY EDUCATION

- Social distancing: Avoid crowds and stay at least 6 feet (2 meters) from others in public.
- Cover cough or sneeze.
- Hand washing: Especially after touching surfaces in public. Use soap and water for 30 seconds or hand sanitizer of at least 60% alcohol.
- Avoid touching the face, especially eyes, nose, and mouth.
- Wearing masks in the community: The CDC recommends the use of a nonmedical cloth mask in public settings where social distancing may be more difficult. It is thought that this will contain secretions of and prevent transmission from individuals with infection, including those who are asymptomatic or presymptomatic.
- Individuals who develop any of the symptoms of COVID-19 should self-isolate at home away from other people or, if they need to be around others, wear a mask until they can be tested and results known.

REINFECTION

In most cases of persons who became reinfected several months after an initial episode of COVID-19, genetic material of the virus analyzed from each episode suggested that patients had two distinct viral infections of the COVID-19 virus.

RELATED CONTENT

Multisystem inflammatory syndrome in children
SARS (Related Key Topic)
MERS: Middle Eastern respiratory syndrome (Related Key Topic)

SUGGESTED READINGS

Available at ExpertConsult.com

AUTHOR: **Glenn G. Fort, MD, MPH**

BASIC INFORMATION

DEFINITION

Crohn disease (CD) is an inflammatory disease of the bowel of unknown etiology, most commonly involving the terminal ileum and manifesting primarily with diarrhea, abdominal pain, fatigue, and weight loss.

SYNONYMS

CD
Regional enteritis
Inflammatory bowel disease (IBD)

ICD-10CM CODES

K50.00	Crohn disease of small intestine without complications
K50.011	Crohn disease of small intestine with rectal bleeding
K50.012	Crohn disease of small intestine with intestinal obstruction
K50.013	Crohn disease of small intestine with fistula
K50.014	Crohn disease of small intestine with abscess
K50.018	Crohn disease of small intestine with other complication
K50.019	Crohn disease of small intestine with unspecified complications
K50.10	Crohn disease of large intestine without complications
K50.111	Crohn disease of large intestine with rectal bleeding
K50.112	Crohn disease of large intestine with intestinal obstruction
K50.113	Crohn disease of large intestine with fistula
K50.114	Crohn disease of large intestine with abscess
K50.118	Crohn disease of large intestine with other complication
K50.119	Crohn disease of large intestine with unspecified complications
K50.80	Crohn disease of both small and large intestine without complications
K50.811	Crohn disease of both small and large intestine with rectal bleeding
K50.812	Crohn disease of both small and large intestine with intestinal obstruction
K50.813	Crohn disease of both small and large intestine with fistula
K50.814	Crohn disease of both small and large intestine with abscess
K50.818	Crohn disease of both small and large intestine with other complication
K50.819	Crohn disease of both small and large intestine with unspecified complications
K50.90	Crohn disease, unspecified, without complications
K50.911	Crohn disease, unspecified, with rectal bleeding
K50.912	Crohn disease, unspecified, with intestinal obstruction
K50.913	Crohn disease, unspecified, with fistula
K50.914	Crohn disease, unspecified, with abscess
K50.918	Crohn disease, unspecified, with other complication
K50.919	Crohn disease, unspecified, with unspecified complications

EPIDEMIOLOGY & DEMOGRAPHICS

PREVALENCE:

- Annual incidence ranges from 3 to 20 cases per 100,000.
- Median age of onset is 30 yr.
- Crohn disease has two peaks, the first between age 20 and 30 yr and the second a smaller peak around 50 yr.

PHYSICAL FINDINGS & CLINICAL PRESENTATION

- Physical exam findings vary depending on disease location and severity
- Abdominal tenderness, mass, or distention
- Chronic or nocturnal diarrhea
- Weight loss, fever, night sweats
- Hyperactive bowel sounds in patients with partial obstruction, bloody diarrhea
- Delayed growth and failure of normal development in children
- Perianal and rectal abscesses, multiple sinuses and scarring (Fig. E1), mouth ulcers, cobblestone appearance of oral mucosa (Fig. E2), and atrophic glossitis
- Extraintestinal manifestations (Table E1): Joint swelling and tenderness, hepatosplenomegaly, erythema nodosum, clubbing, tenderness to palpation of the sacroiliac joints
- Symptoms may be intermittent, with varying periods of remission
- Overall, 45% to 50% of patients have ileocolonic inflammation, 30% have isolated small bowel disease, 20% have isolated colonic disease, and 5% have isolated upper GI or perianal manifestations

ETIOLOGY

Unknown. Pathophysiologically, Crohn disease involves an immune system dysfunction.

DIAGNOSIS

DIFFERENTIAL DIAGNOSIS

- Ulcerative colitis (see Table 2)
- Infectious diseases (tuberculosis, *Yersinia, Salmonella, Shigella, Campylobacter*)
- Parasitic infections (amebic infection)
- Pseudomembranous colitis
- Ischemic colitis in elderly patients
- Lymphoma
- Colon carcinoma
- Diverticulitis
- Radiation enteritis
- Collagenous colitis
- Fungal infections *(Histoplasma, Actinomyces)*
- Anorectal and colon diseases, formerly referred to as gay bowel syndrome
- Carcinoid tumors
- Celiac sprue
- Mesenteric adenitis

LABORATORY TESTS

- Decreased hemoglobin and hematocrit from chronic blood loss, effect of inflammation on bone marrow, and malabsorption of vitamin B_{12}
- Hypokalemia, hypomagnesemia, hypocalcemia, and low albumin in patients with chronic diarrhea
- Vitamin B_{12} and folate deficiency
- Elevated erythrocyte sedimentation rate and CRP
- Positive anti–*Saccharomyces cerevisiae* antibodies

TABLE 2 Differentiating Features

	Ulcerative Colitis	Crohn Disease
Site of involvement	Only involves colon Rectum almost always involved	Any area of the gastrointestinal tract Rectum usually spared
Pattern of involvement	Continuous	Skip lesions
Diarrhea	Bloody	Usually nonbloody
Severe abdominal pain	Rare	Frequent
Perianal disease	No	In 30% of patients
Fistula	No	Yes
Endoscopic findings	Erythematous and friable Superficial ulceration	Aphthoid and deep ulcers Cobblestoning
Radiologic findings	Tubular appearance resulting from loss of haustral folds	String sign of terminal ileum RLQ mass, fistulas, abscesses
Histologic features	Mucosa only Crypt abscesses	Transmural crypt abscesses, granulomas (about 30%)
Smoking	Protective	Worsens course
Serology	p-ANCA more common	ASCA more common

ASCA, Anti–*Saccharomyces cerevisiae* antibodies; *p-ANCA,* perinuclear antineutrophil cytoplasmic antibody; *RLQ,* right lower quadrant.
From Andreoli TE et al: *Andreoli and Carpenter's Cecil essentials of medicine,* ed 8, Philadelphia, 2010, Saunders.

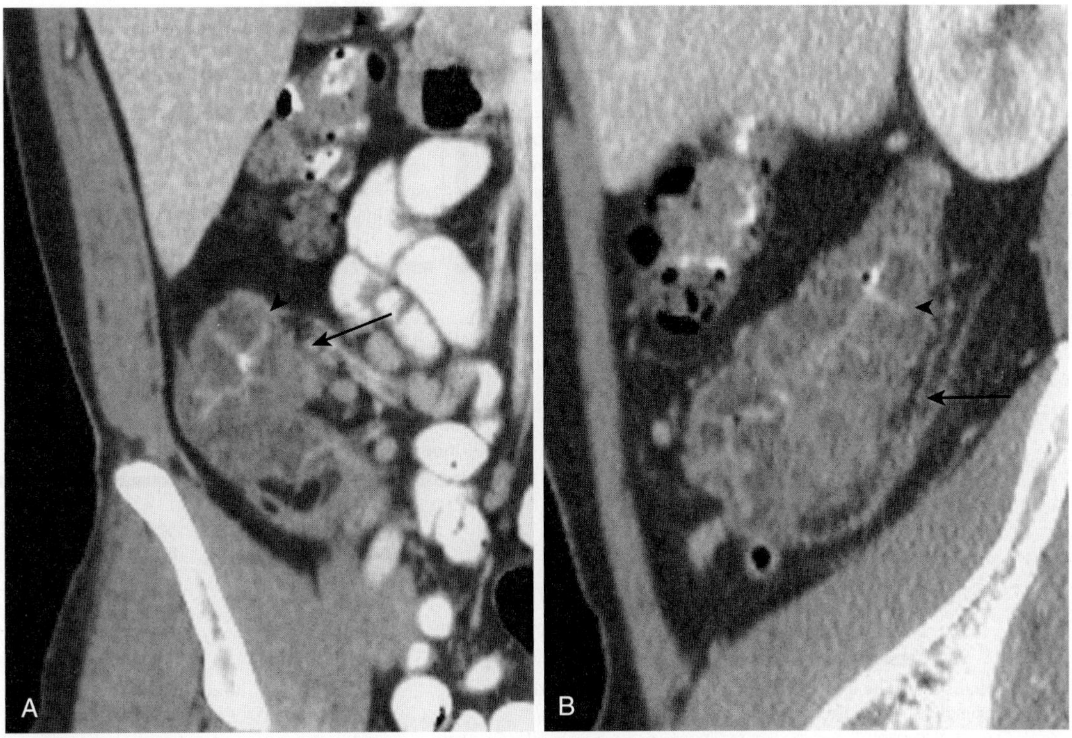

FIG. 4 A 38-yr-old man with Crohn disease. Coronal **(A)** and sagittal **(B)** portal venous phase images demonstrate significant cecal wall thickening *(arrows)*, with oral contrast material identified between the thickened haustra *(arrowheads)*, the so-called "accordion" sign. (From Soto JA, Lucey BC: *Emergency radiology: the requisites*, ed 2, Philadelphia, 2017, Elsevier.)

- Elevated INR (due to vitamin K malabsorption)
- Fecal calprotectin has been reported as useful in screening of patients with suspected IBD. Based on a pretest probability of 32% in adults, an abnormal calprotectin test result increases the posttest probability to 91%, and a normal result reduces the probability of IBD to 3%. False elevations may occur with other gastrointestinal diseases such as bacterial, viral, and protozoal causes of infective diarrhea

ENDOSCOPIC EVALUATION

Endoscopic features of Crohn disease include asymmetric and discontinued disease, deep longitudinal fissures, cobblestone appearance, and presence of strictures (Fig. E3). Crypt distortion and inflammation are also present. Granulomas may be present.

IMAGING STUDIES

- CT of abdomen (Fig. 4) may show thickening of the terminal ileum and is helpful in identifying abscesses, fistulas (Fig. E5), and other complications.
- Magnetic resonance enterography (MRe) is superior to other imaging modalities in its ability to distinguish active from chronic fibrotic disease. It is, however, more expensive.
- In 10% to 15% of patients with IBD, a clear distinction between ulcerative colitis and Crohn disease cannot be made. In general, Crohn disease can be distinguished from ulcerative colitis by the presence of transmural involvement and the frequent presence of noncaseating granulomas and lymphoid aggregates on biopsy.

Rx TREATMENT

- The medical management of Crohn disease is based on disease activity (Fig. 6).
- According to Hanauer and Sanborn, disease activity can be defined as follows:
  1. Mild to moderate disease: The patient is ambulatory and able to take oral alimentation. There is no dehydration, high fever, abdominal tenderness, painful mass, obstruction, or weight loss of >10%.
  2. Moderate to severe disease: Either the patient has not responded to treatment for mild to moderate disease or has more pronounced symptoms, including fever, significant weight loss, abdominal pain or tenderness, intermittent nausea and vomiting, or significant anemia.
  3. Severe fulminant disease: Either the patient has persistent symptoms despite outpatient steroid therapy or has high fever, persistent vomiting, evidence of intestinal obstruction, rebound tenderness, cachexia, or evidence of an abscess.
  4. Remission: The patient is asymptomatic or without inflammatory sequelae, including patients responding to acute medical intervention.

NONPHARMACOLOGIC THERAPY

- Nutritional supplementation is needed in patients with advanced disease. Total parenteral nutrition may be necessary in selected patients.
- Low-residue diet is necessary when obstructive symptoms are present.
- If diarrhea is prominent, increased dietary fiber and decreased fat in the diet are sometimes helpful.
- Psychotherapy is useful for situational adjustment crises. A trusting and mutually understanding relationship and referral to self-help groups are very important because of the chronicity of the disease and the relatively young age of the patients.
- Avoid oral feedings during acute exacerbation to decrease colonic activity: A low-roughage diet may be helpful in early relapse.

ACUTE GENERAL Rx

- Corticosteroids are used to induce remission. They have been the mainstay for treating moderate to severe active Crohn disease. Prednisone 40 to 60 mg/day is useful for acute exacerbation. Steroids are usually tapered over approximately 2 to 3 mo. Some patients require a low dose for a prolonged period of maintenance.
- Steroid analogues are locally active corticosteroids that target specific areas of inflammation in the gastrointestinal tract. Budesonide is available as a controlled-release formulation and is approved for mild to moderate active Crohn disease involving the ileum and/or ascending colon. The adult dose is 9 mg qd for a maximum of 8 wk.

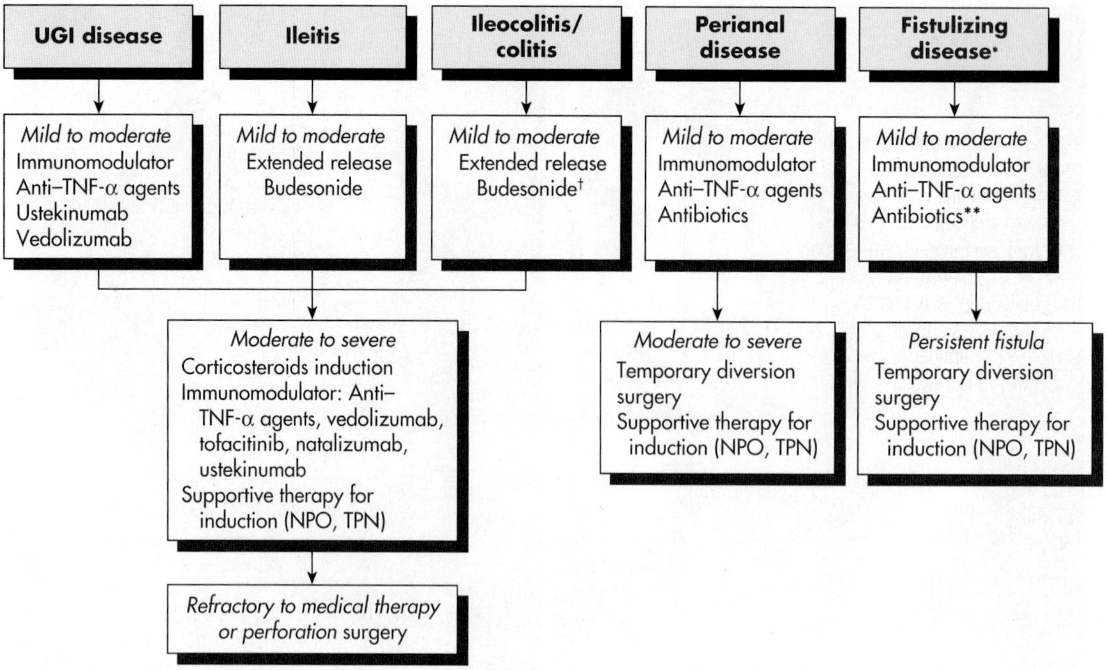

*Abscess should be excluded before initiating medical therapy.
†Proximal colon disease involvement.
**Perianal location.

FIG. 6 Crohn disease treatment algorithm. *NPO*, Nothing by mouth; *TNF-α*, tumor Necrosis factor-α; *TPN*, total parenteral nutrition; *UGI*, upper gastrointestinal. (From Goldman L, Schafer AI: *Goldman-Cecil medicine*, ed 26, Philadelphia, 2020, Elsevier.)

- Patients responding to glucocorticoids are transitioned to immunomodulators as their glucocorticoid is tapered.
- Immunosuppressants such as azathioprine or mercaptopurine are used for maintenance of remission. Methotrexate is an alternative agent.
- Metronidazole 500 mg qid may be useful for colonic fistulas and treatment of mild to moderate active Crohn disease. Ciprofloxacin 1 g qd has also been found to be effective in decreasing disease activity.
- TNF inhibitors are agents useful to induce remission and maintain remission in patients with moderate to severe Crohn disease. Infliximab, a chimeric monoclonal antibody targeting tumor necrosis factor-α, is effective in the treatment of enterocutaneous fistulas. This medication can induce clinical improvement in 80% of patients with Crohn disease refractory to other agents. It can be used in combination with other medications such as azathioprine in patients with severe Crohn disease. A PPD test should be done before using this medication. Adalimumab and certolizumab are other TNF inhibitors also effective in inducing remissions and may be useful in adult patients with Crohn disease who cannot tolerate infliximab or have symptoms despite receiving infliximab therapy. Efficacy is better when an anti-TNF is used together with an immunomodulator.
- Natalizumab, a selective adhesion-molecule inhibitor, has been reported to be effective in increasing the rate of remission and response in patients with active Crohn disease. It is effective for patients in whom anti-TNF therapy has been unsuccessful. Prior to using natalizumab, serologic testing should be done for JC virus, which causes multifocal leukoencephalopathy (PML), and if the patient is seronegative, the risk of PML from natalizumab is low. Vedolizumab is another IV integrin receptor antagonist recently FDA approved for moderate to severe Crohn disease patients who have not responded to or cannot tolerate standard treatment. Vedolizumab use is not associated with high risk of PML. Ustekinumab, a monoclonal antibody to the P_40 subunit of interleukin-12 and interleukin-23, has shown efficacy for induction and maintenance therapy for Crohn disease. It has been FDA-approved for moderate to severely active Crohn disease unresponsive to immunomodulators or corticosteroids or a tumor necrosis factor inhibitor.
- Hydrocortisone enema bid or tid is useful for proctitis.
- Most patients who have anemia associated with Crohn disease respond to iron supplementation. Erythropoietin is useful in patients with anemia refractory to treatment with iron and vitamins.

CHRONIC Rx

- Monitor disease activity with symptom review and laboratory evaluation (complete blood count and sedimentation rate).
- Liver tests and vitamin B_{12} levels monitored on a yearly basis.

DISPOSITION

There is no cure for CD, and most patients require at least one surgical resection. One tenth of patients have prolonged remission, three quarters have a chronic intermittent disease course, and one eighth have an unremitting course. Patients with IBD are at increased risk of colon cancer.

REFERRAL

Surgical referral is needed for complications such as abscess formation, obstruction, fistulas, toxic megacolon, refractory disease, or severe hemorrhage. Approximately 40% to 50% of patients will require some type of bowel surgery within the first 5 yr of Crohn disease. A conservative surgical approach is necessary because surgery is not curative. Multiple surgeries may also result in short bowel syndrome.

SUGGESTED READINGS

Available at ExpertConsult.com

RELATED CONTENT

Crohn Disease (Patient Information)

AUTHOR: **Fred F. Ferri, MD**

BASIC INFORMATION

DEFINITION

Cryoglobulins are serum immunoglobulins that precipitate when cooled and redissolve when heated. A classification of cryoglobulins is described in Table 1 and Fig. 1. Cryoglobulinemia is a clinical syndrome that results from systemic inflammation caused by cryoglobulin-containing immune complexes. Mixed cryoglobulinemia is a vasculitis of small and medium-sized arteries and veins due to the deposition of complexes of antigen, cryoglobulin, and complement in the vessel walls.

SYNONYMS

Cryoglobulinemic vasculitis
Cryoproteinemia
Mixed cryoglobulinemia
Essential cryoglobulinemia

ICD-10CM CODE

D89.1 Cryoglobulinemia

EPIDEMIOLOGY & DEMOGRAPHICS

PREVALENCE:

- Prevalence of mixed cryoglobulinemia is approximately 1:100,000.
- Approximately 50% of patients with HCV are found to have mixed cryoglobulinemia; only 5% to 10% develop vasculitis.
- Three types: I (monoclonal), II (IgM monoclonal and IgG polyclonal), and III (polyclonal).

PREDOMINANT SEX: Female-to-male ratio of 3:1.

PREDOMINANT AGE: Mean age reported is 42 to 52 yr.

RISK FACTORS:

- Hepatitis C virus (HCV) infection
- Connective tissue disorders
- Lymphoproliferative disorders

PHYSICAL FINDINGS & CLINICAL PRESENTATION

- ***Meltzer triad*** of purpura, arthralgias/myalgia, and weakness is seen in one third of patients.
- Other symptoms include dyspnea, cough, numbness, abdominal pain, acrocyanosis.
- Hypertension, hepatosplenomegaly, Raynaud phenomenon, and in severe cases, distal necrosis and ulcerations of lower limbs (Fig. 2).

ETIOLOGY

- Intravascular deposition of cryoglobulins leading to ischemic insults in territory supplied by vasa nervorum
- Necrotizing vasculitis caused by cryoglobulin precipitation in cooler areas (distal extremities) and kidneys (increased concentration due to ultrafiltration)
- Infections: HCV, mycosis fungoides, HBV, HIV, Epstein-Barr virus, cytomegalovirus, *Treponema pallidum,* Mycobacterium leprae, and in post-streptococcal glomerulonephritis
- Lymphoproliferative disorders: Chronic lymphocytic leukemia, Waldenström macroglobulinemia, multiple myeloma

TABLE 1 Classification of Cryoglobulins

Type	Composition	Associated Disease
I	Monoclonal IgG, IgA, or IgM	Multiple myeloma (IgG, IgM) Chronic lymphocytic leukemia Waldenström macroglobulinemia Idiopathic monoclonal gammopathy Lymphoproliferative disorders
II	Polyclonal IgG and monoclonal IgM (with rheumatoid factor activity)	Hepatitis C, hepatitis B, HIV neoplasms: Chronic lymphocytic leukemia, diffuse lymphoma, B lymphocytic neoplasia
III	Polyclonal IgG and polyclonal IgM	Infections: Viral (hepatitis B and C, Epstein-Barr virus, cytomegalovirus), bacterial (endocarditis, leprosy, poststreptococcal glomerulonephritis), parasitic (schistosomiasis, toxoplasmosis, malaria) Autoimmune disorders: Systemic lupus erythematosus, rheumatoid arthritis Lymphoproliferative disorders Chronic liver disease

HIV, Human immunodeficiency virus; *Ig,* immunoglobulin.
From Floege J et al: *Comprehensive clinical nephrology,* ed 4, Philadelphia, 2010, Saunders.

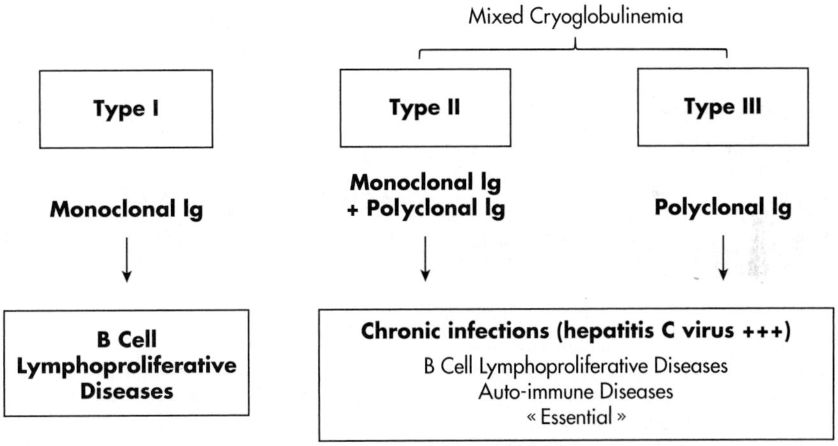

FIG. 1 Cryoglobulin immunotyping and related underlying diseases. *Ig,* Immunoglobulin. (From Cacoub P et al: Cryoglobulinemia vasculitis, *Am J Med* 128[9]:950-955.)

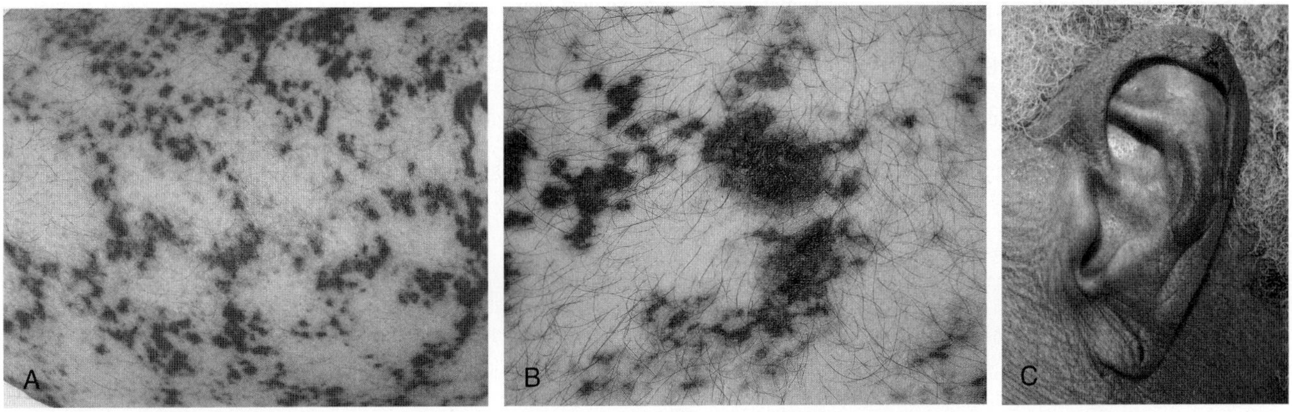

FIG. 2 Cryoglobulinemia. (From Hoffman R et al: *Hematology, basic principles and practice,* ed 6, New York, 2013, Elsevier.)

- Connective tissue disorders: Rheumatoid arthritis, systemic lupus erythematosus (SLE), scleroderma, Sjögren syndrome, vasculitis
- Renal diseases including proliferative glomerulonephritis

Dx DIAGNOSIS

DIFFERENTIAL DIAGNOSIS

- Antiphospholipid syndrome
- SLE
- Churg-Strauss syndrome
- Cirrhosis
- Glomerulonephritis
- Goodpasture syndrome
- Hemolytic uremic syndrome
- Hepatitis
- Lymphoma
- Sarcoidosis
- Waldenström hypergammaglobulinemia

WORKUP

History and physical examination; laboratory tests; imaging tests depending on patient's presentation.

LABORATORY TESTS

- Serum cryoglobulins, rheumatoid factor, serum complement, hepatitis C titer, urinalysis, CBC, ALT, AST, BUN, creatinine
- Electromyogram/nerve conduction studies may demonstrate axonal changes and distal muscle denervation
- Sural nerve and skin biopsy

IMAGING STUDIES

Chest x-ray for pulmonary involvement, CT scan to evaluate for malignancy, and angiography for vasculitis.

Rx TREATMENT

- Management of type I cryoglobulinemia is directed at treating the underlying disorder.
- For noninfectious mixed cryoglobulinemia, treatment is based on disease severity. Low-dose corticosteroids, NSAIDs, and colchicine should be given for mild symptoms. Rituximab, high-dose corticosteroids, cyclophosphamide, and/or plasmapheresis should be given for severe disease.
- In patients with HCV, mild symptoms can be managed by treatment with direct-acting antivirals (DAA). Therapy is aimed at eradicating the HCV infection, suppressing B-cell clonal expansion and cryoglobulin production, and ameliorating symptoms.
- For severe disease in HCV-infected patients, initial immunosuppression with rituximab is warranted, followed by initiation of antiviral therapy.
- Fig. 3 illustrates the treatment of HCV-related mixed cryoglobulinemia vasculitis according to presentation.
- Sustained virologic response due to DAA does not always fully eradicate cryoglobulinemia but can help mitigate its manifestations.

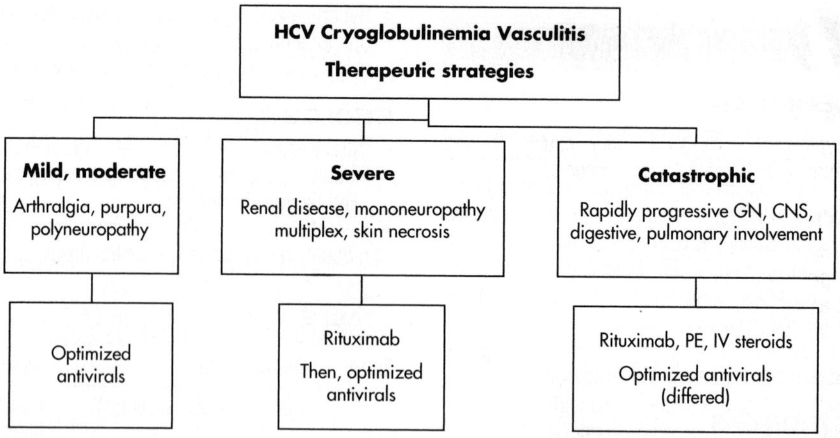

FIG. 3 Treatment of HCV-related mixed cryoglobulinemia vasculitis according to the presentation. *CNS,* Central nervous system; *GN,* glomerulonephritis; *HCV,* hepatitis C virus. (From Cacoub P et al: Cryoglobulinemia vasculitis, *Am J Med* 128[9]:950-955.)

NONPHARMACOLOGIC THERAPY

Avoidance of cold exposure, diabetic food care guidelines

ACUTE GENERAL Rx

NSAIDs in those with general fatigue and arthralgia; see "Treatment" for further management.

DISPOSITION

Overall prognosis is worse with concomitant renal disease. Mean survival rate is ~50% at 10 yr.

REFERRAL

Consider referring to a

- Nephrologist if there is renal involvement
- Hematologist in patients with lymphoproliferative disorders
- Gastroenterologist/hepatologist in patients with hepatitis
- Rheumatologist in patients with connective tissue disease cases
- Clinical immunologist in severe cases

PEARLS & CONSIDERATIONS

COMMENTS

Always look for underlying cause of cryoglobulinemia.

PREVENTION

Avoidance of cold exposure, avoidance of late complications.

PATIENT & FAMILY EDUCATION

Inform patients about early signs/symptoms of cryoglobulinemia so that treatment can be rendered before the development of complications.

SUGGESTED READINGS

Available at ExpertConsult.com

AUTHOR: **Rebecca Soinski, MD**

BASIC INFORMATION

DEFINITION

Cryptococcosis is an infection caused by the encapsulated yeast *Cryptococcus* spp.

SYNONYMS

C. neoformans infection
C. gattii infection
C. albidus infection
C. laurentii infection

ICD-10CM CODES

B45.9	Cryptococcosis, unspecified
B45.09	Pulmonary cryptococcosis
B45.1	Cerebral cryptococcosis
B45.2	Cutaneous cryptococcosis
B45.3	Osseous cryptococcosis
B45.7	Disseminated cryptococcosis

EPIDEMIOLOGY & DEMOGRAPHICS

INCIDENCE (IN U.S.):

- 0.8 cases per million persons/yr; *C. neoformans* is an important opportunistic infection in patients with deficits in cell-mediated immunity.
- 2 to 7 per 1000 persons living with AIDS/yr.

PREDOMINANT SEX: Equal sex distribution when adjusted for HIV status
PREDOMINANT AGE: Less than 2 yr of age; 20 to 40 yr of age
PEAK INCIDENCE: 20 to 40 yr (parallel to HIV/AIDS epidemic)
NEONATAL INFECTION: Very uncommon

PHYSICAL FINDINGS & CLINICAL PRESENTATION

- More than 90% present with meningitis (generally subacute); almost all have fever and headache.
- Meningismus, photophobia, mental status changes are seen in approximately 25%.
- Increased intracranial pressure may be present.
- Most common infections outside the CNS:
  1. In the lungs (fever, cough, dyspnea, and typically with lobar consolidation)
  2. In the skin (cellulitis, papular eruption)
  3. In the lymph nodes (lymphadenitis)
  4. Potential involvement of virtually any organ (e.g., prostate and bone)

ETIOLOGY

- There are four *Cryptococcus spp.* that cause disease in humans, although most laboratories are not able to differentiate between species. *C. neoformans* (Table E1) is the cause of a majority of global disease burden, primarily in immunocompromised patients. *C. gattii* infections are much less common and occur more often in normal hosts, with recent outbreaks in the Pacific Northwest. *C. albidus* and *C. laurentii* are even rarer causes of disease.
- Infection originates by inhalation into the respiratory tract followed by dissemination to the CNS in most cases, usually without recognizable lung involvement.
- Almost always in the setting of AIDS (most with CD4 counts <100) or other disorders of cellular immune function, such as organ transplantation.
- Neutropenia alone poses a much lower risk of significant cryptococcal infection.

Dx DIAGNOSIS

DIFFERENTIAL DIAGNOSIS

- Subacute meningitis (caused by *Listeria monocytogenes,* Mycobacterium tuberculosis, *Histoplasma capsulatum,* viruses)
- Intracranial mass lesion (neoplasms, toxoplasmosis, TB)
- Pulmonary involvement confused with *Pneumocystis jiroveci* pneumonia when diffuse or confused with TB or bacterial pneumonia when focal or involving the pleura
- Skin lesions can take many forms and may be confused with bacterial cellulitis or molluscum contagiosum

WORKUP

- Lumbar puncture to exclude cryptococcal meningitis, with measurement of opening pressure because CSF opening pressure is elevated in 60% to 80% of HIV patients and may require drainage. In cryptococcal meningitis, CSF reveals lymphocytic pleocytosis (although a paucity of WBCs may be found in CSF of HIV patients)
- CT scan of the head when focal lesion or increased intracranial pressure is suspected
- Biopsy of enlarged lymph nodes and skin lesions if feasible

LABORATORY TESTS

- Culture and India ink stain (60%-80% sensitive in culture-proven cases [Fig. E1]); examination of the CSF in all cases when CNS involvement is suspected
- Blood and serum cryptococcal antigen assay (>90% sensitivity and specificity in immunocompromised patients; lower sensitivity in immunocompetent patients)
- Culture and histologic examination of biopsy material
- HIV antibody testing

IMAGING STUDIES

- CT scan or MRI of the head if focal neurologic involvement or cryptococcoma is suspected.
- Chest x-ray examination to exclude pulmonary involvement.

Rx TREATMENT

ACUTE GENERAL Rx

- Treatment of cryptococcosis consists of three stages: Induction, consolidation, and maintenance. Induction therapy for CNS disease (meningitis) was historically initiated with IV amphotericin B deoxycholate (0.7-1.0 mg/kg/day) with flucytosine 100 mg/kg/day PO in four divided doses; however, there is growing clinical evidence for liposomal amphotericin B (3 to 6 mg/kg/day) plus flucytosine, especially in HIV-infected patients and in those with renal dysfunction. Induction therapy is generally recommended for 2 to 4 wk and until repeat CSF cultures are negative; it is then recommended to transition to consolidation therapy with fluconazole 400 mg PO q24h for 8 wk, followed by ongoing fluconazole 200 mg PO q24h maintenance therapy (up to 2 yr) to reduce relapse rate. Maintenance therapy is indicated in patients with AIDS until these patients have been receiving antifungal therapy for at least 1 yr and they have responded to antiretroviral therapy (CD4 cell count ≥100/microliter for ≥3 mo). In patients without HIV, the duration of maintenance therapy is generally 6 to 12 mo. Lifelong antifungal therapy is needed in organ transplant patients.
- Alternative: IV fluconazole combined with flucytosine for initial therapy in patients unable to tolerate amphotericin B.
- If symptomatic increased intracranial pressure, consider multiple therapeutic lumbar taps or intraventricular shunt.
- Data support increased mortality with early initiation of antiretroviral therapy in the setting of cryptococcal meningitis due to immune reconstitution syndrome; therefore it is generally recommended to wait 2 to 10 wk after starting cryptococcal therapy prior to starting antiretroviral therapy.
- CSF removal with daily lumbar puncture or insertion of a shunt is beneficial in patients with elevated intracranial pressure.

CHRONIC Rx

- Fluconazole (200-400 mg PO qd) is highly effective in preventing a relapse in HIV-infected patients; development of resistance may occur. Itraconazole is an alternative agent, along with growing evidence for voriconazole and posaconazole use.

DISPOSITION

Without maintenance therapy, relapse rate is >50% among AIDS patients.

REFERRAL

- For consultation with infectious diseases specialist in all cases
- For neurologic consultation if level of consciousness is depressed or focal lesion is present

SUGGESTED READINGS

Available at ExpertConsult.com

RELATED CONTENT

Cryptococcosis (Patient Information)

AUTHORS: **Tara C. Bouton, MD, MPH & TM,** and **Philip A. Chan, MD, MS**

Cryptosporidium Infection

BASIC INFORMATION

DEFINITION

The intracellular protozoan parasite *Cryptosporidium parvum* is associated with gastrointestinal disease and diarrhea, especially in patients with AIDS or other immunocompromised hosts. It is also associated with sporadic infections and waterborne outbreaks in immunocompetent hosts. Cryptosporidiosis is a notifiable disease in the U.S.

Other species, including *C. hominis, C. felis, C. muris, C. canis,* and *C. meleagridis,* are now described to be pathogens as well.

SYNONYM

Cryptosporidiosis

ICD-10CM CODE

A07.2 Cryptosporidiosis

EPIDEMIOLOGY & DEMOGRAPHICS

INCIDENCE:
- Approximately 2% of diarrheal illness in industrial countries, 5% to 10% in developing countries.
- Immunocompromised patients, especially those with HIV/AIDS, are particularly susceptible to infection. 10% to 20% of HIV patients in the United States may excrete cyst.
- Cryptosporidiosis is a leading cause of all waterborne outbreaks in the U.S. An estimated 748,000 cryptosporidiosis cases occur annually, although fewer than 2% are reported. In 2011, more than 9000 cases of cryptosporidiosis were reported in the country. The highest overall reporting rates were observed in the Midwest.[1]

PREVALENCE: Worldwide, especially third-world countries; associated with poor hygiene as a waterborne pathogen.

PREDOMINANT SEX: Male = female

TRANSMISSION:
- Person-to-person (day care, family members)
- Animal-to-person (pets, farm animals). Fig. E1 describes the life cycle of *Cryptosporidium*
- Environmental (water-associated outbreaks, including travel associated with swimming in or drinking contaminated water or eating contaminated food)
- May be significant pathogen causing diarrhea in patients with AIDS

PHYSICAL FINDINGS & CLINICAL PRESENTATION

- Spectrum of illness ranging from asymptomatic to severe enteritis (Table 1). Typical cases in immunocompetent hosts result in self-limited diarrhea, whereas immunocompromised hosts are characterized by profuse, watery, nonbloody diarrhea that may lead to dehydration and weight loss
- Usually limited to the gastrointestinal tract; however, in individuals with AIDS, the disease may be fulminant and life-threatening (CD4 counts <50)
- Diarrhea, severe abdominal pain (2-28 days)
- Impaired digestion, dehydration
- Fever, malaise, fatigue, nausea, vomiting
- Pneumonia if aspirated

ETIOLOGY

C. hominis, C. parvum, C. felis, C. muris, C. meleagridis

Dx DIAGNOSIS

Clinical presentation of acute gastrointestinal illness, especially associated with HIV/AIDS or with travel and waterborne outbreaks.

DIFFERENTIAL DIAGNOSIS

- *Campylobacter*
- *Clostridium difficile*
- *Entamoeba histolytica*
- *Giardia lamblia*
- *Salmonella*
- *Shigella*
- Microsporidia
- Cytomegalovirus
- *Mycobacterium avium*
- Disease may cause cholecystitis, reactive arthritis, hepatitis, urethritis, pancreatitis, or pneumonia in immunocompromised or HIV-infected patients.

WORKUP

- Stool evaluation looking for characteristic oocyst by modified acid-fast stain (Fig. E2)
- Direct immunofluorescence using monoclonal antibodies is the gold standard for stool exams
- Rapid antigen detection
- PCR
- HIV antibody testing
- Table 2 summarizes diagnostic tests for diagnosing *Cryptosporidium* infection

Rx TREATMENT

- Handwashing and appropriate decontamination of drinking and recreational water sources.
- May be self-limited in normal host, lasting days to weeks. Antidiarrheal agents Pepto-Bismol, Kaopectate, or loperamide may give symptomatic relief.
- Pharmacologic treatment with antibiotics has been largely unsatisfactory in patients with AIDS. Antiviral therapy is the treatment of choice to restore the immune system. Consider prolonged therapy while awaiting CD4 count recovery and combination therapy in those who fail initial course.
- Oocyst excretion reduction has been shown with nitazoxanide 500 mg PO bid for 3 days in immunocompetent patients. If treatment fails, consider paromomycin, metronidazole, azithromycin, or trimethoprim/sulfamethoxazole. However, these medications have not been approved for treatment of *Cryptosporidium.*
- Nitazoxanide elixir has been approved for the treatment of cryptosporidiosis in children ages 1 to 11 yr.
- Biliary cryptosporidiosis can be treated with antiretroviral therapy in the HIV setting.
- Box 1 outlines a treatment protocol for cryptosporidiosis.

DISPOSITION

- A self-limited disease in immunocompetent patients with complete recovery over 2 to 3 wk.
- In patients with AIDS, chronic infection often clears with initiation and maintenance of antiretroviral therapy.
- Chronic arthralgia, headache, malaise, and weakness may persist after infection, even in immunologically normal people.
- If severe and prolonged disease (>30 days), testing for HIV and other immunocompromised states is appropriate, along with a referral to an infectious diseases specialist or gastroenterologist.

REFERRAL

- To an infectious diseases specialist if symptoms persist and/or HIV infection is found
- To a gastroenterologist if chronic malabsorption, or biliary or pancreatic complications occur

PEARLS & CONSIDERATIONS

- Chronic cryptosporidiosis (>30 days of diarrhea from *Cryptosporidium* spp. infection) in a patient with HIV is an AIDS-qualifying opportunistic infection.
- *Cryptosporidium hominis* has a limited host range (humans), whereas *Cryptosporidium parvum* has a wide host range including humans, horses, cattle, other domesticated animals, and wild animals; both species present similarly in humans.

SUGGESTED READING

Available at ExpertConsult.com

AUTHORS: **Tara C. Bouton, MD, MPH & TM, Philip A. Chan, MD, MS,** and **Glenn G. Fort, MD, MPH**

[1]Cryptosporidiosis surveillance, United States, 2011-2012. MMWR 64 3 (2015).

TABLE 1 Clinical Manifestation of Cryptosporidiosis

Host	Clinical Manifestations	Comments
Normal host	Acute watery diarrhea	Relapses common Persistent diarrhea common
Children in developing countries	Acute watery diarrhea	Diarrhea more severe in children with malnutrition
	Persistent diarrhea	Persistent diarrhea affecting nutritional status, growth, and intellectual function
Immunocompromised host	Acute watery diarrhea	Transient, self-limited, similar to disease in normal host
	Relapsing diarrhea	Very common
	Persistent or chronic diarrhea	Usually found in patients with low CD4 count or malnutrition
	Cholera-like illness	Voluminous watery diarrhea, only with very low CD4 count
	Extraintestinal involvement	Respiratory tract, biliary tract, and pancreas

From Cherry JD et al: *Feigin and Cherry's pediatric infectious diseases*, ed 8, Philadelphia, 2019, Elsevier.

TABLE 2 Diagnosis of *Cryptosporidium* Infection

Test Type	Method	Comments
Microscopic examination of stools	Modified acid-fast stain of stools	Inexpensive and widely available diagnostic test
	Fluorescent stains (auramine O, auramine-rhodamine)	Faster than other acid-fast stains and may improve sensitivity
	Immunofluorescent assays	More sensitive than acid-fast staining but also more expensive
Antigen-detection assays	Enzyme immunoassay and immunochromatographic tests: Direct and indirect immunofluorescence assay	Good sensitivity (66%-100%) and excellent specificity (93%-100%), but occasional lots associated with false-positive test results
Molecular methods	Polymerase chain reaction	Increased sensitivity in contrast to microscopic or antigen-detection studies

From Cherry JD et al: *Feigin and Cherry's pediatric infectious diseases*, ed 8, Philadelphia, 2019, Elsevier.

BOX 1 Treatment of Cryptosporidiosis

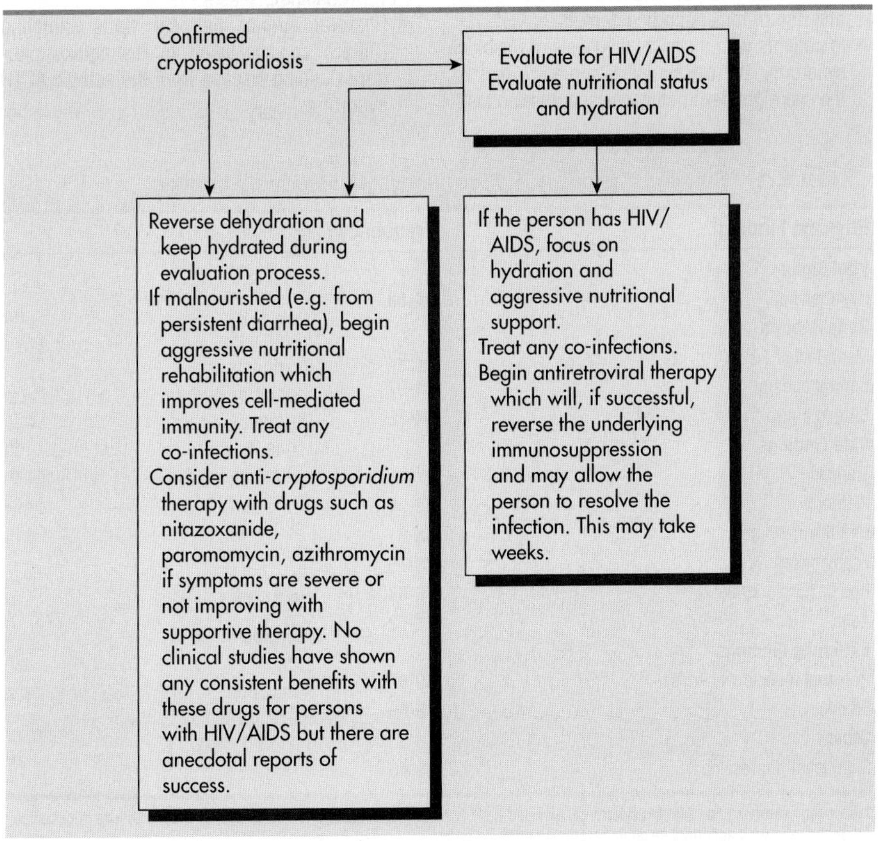

From Ryan ET: *Hunter's tropical medicine and emerging infectious diseases*, ed 10, 2020, Elsevier.

BASIC INFORMATION

DEFINITION

- Cushing syndrome is the occurrence of clinical abnormalities associated with glucocorticoid excess as a result of exaggerated adrenal cortisol production or long-term glucocorticoid therapy.
- Cushing disease is Cushing syndrome caused by pituitary adrenocorticotropic hormone (ACTH) excess.

ICD-10CM CODES

E24	Cushing syndrome
E24.2	Drug-induced Cushing syndrome
E24.3	Ectopic ACTH syndrome
E24.8	Other Cushing syndrome
E24.9	Cushing's syndrome, unspecified
E24.9	Pituitary-dependent Cushing disease

PHYSICAL FINDINGS & CLINICAL PRESENTATION

- Hypertension
- Central obesity with rounding of the facies (moon facies); thin extremities. Fig. 1 illustrates the distribution of adipose tissue in Cushing syndrome
- Hirsutism, menstrual irregularities, hypogonadism
- Skin fragility, ecchymoses, red-purple abdominal striae (Fig. E2), acne, poor wound healing, hair loss, facial plethora, hyperpigmentation (with ACTH excess). The frequency of individual findings in Cushing syndrome is summarized in Table 1
- Psychosis, emotional lability, paranoia
- Muscle wasting with proximal myopathy

NOTE: The previous characteristics are not commonly present in Cushing syndrome caused by ectopic ACTH production. Many of these tumors secrete a biologically inactive ACTH that does not activate adrenal steroid synthesis. These patients may have only weight loss and weakness.

ETIOLOGY

- Iatrogenic from long-term glucocorticoid therapy (common).
- Pituitary ACTH excess (Cushing disease; 60%).
- Adrenal neoplasms (30%).
- Ectopic ACTH production (neoplasms of lung, pancreas, kidney, thyroid, thymus; 10%).
- Table E2 summarizes the incidence of tumors associated with the ectopic adrenocorticotropic hormone syndrome.
- A classification of causes of Cushing syndrome is described in Table E3.

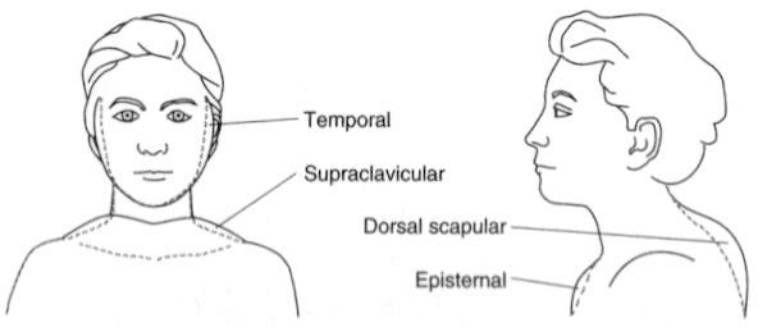

FIG. 1 Distribution of adipose tissue in Cushing syndrome. Rounding of the cheeks and prominent bitemporal fat produce the characteristic moon facies. Fat also may accumulate bilaterally above the clavicles (supraclavicular collar), in front of the sternum (episternal area, or dewlap), and over the back of the neck (dorsal cervical fat pad, or buffalo hump). In these drawings, the dotted line depicts normal contours of patients without Cushing syndrome. (From McGee S: *Evidence-based physical diagnosis*, ed 4, Philadelphia, 2018, Elsevier.)

DIAGNOSIS

DIFFERENTIAL DIAGNOSIS

- Alcoholic pseudo-Cushing syndrome (endogenous cortisol overproduction)
- Obesity associated with diabetes mellitus
- Adrenogenital syndrome

WORKUP

- Initial tests include the overnight low-dose dexamethasone suppression test (LDST), 24-hour urine free cortisol (UFC), and late-night (LN) salivary cortisol. The LN and UFC tend to be more convenient.
- Late-night salivary cortisol: A single midnight serum cortisol level (normal diurnal variation leads to a nadir around midnight) >7.5 mcg/dl has been reported as 96% sensitive and 100% specific for the diagnosis of Cushing syndrome. This test assesses the normal diurnal rhythm of cortisol (lost in Cushing syndrome) and is not useful in patients who have inconsistent sleep patterns or do shift work. It can also be affected by tobacco use and use of topical corticosteroids.
- In patients with a clinical diagnosis of Cushing syndrome, the classic initial screening test is the overnight dexamethasone suppression test:
  1. Dexamethasone 1 mg PO given at 11 pm.
  2. Plasma cortisol level measured 9 hr later (8 am).
  3. Plasma cortisol level <5 mcg/100 ml excludes Cushing syndrome.
- Serial measurements (two or three consecutive measurements) of 24-hr urinary free cortisol and creatinine (to ensure adequacy of collection) are undertaken if overnight dexamethasone test is suggestive of Cushing syndrome. Persistent elevated cortisol excretion (>300 mcg/24 hr) indicates Cushing syndrome.
- The low-dose (2 mg) dexamethasone suppression test is useful to exclude pseudo-Cushing syndrome if the previous results are equivocal. Corticotropic-releasing hormone (CRH) stimulation after low-dose dexamethasone administration (dexamethasone-CRH test) is also used to distinguish patients with suspected Cushing syndrome from those who have mildly elevated urinary free cortisol level and equivocal findings.
- The high-dose (8 mg) dexamethasone test and measurement of ACTH by radioimmunoassay are useful to determine the etiology of Cushing syndrome.
  1. ACTH undetectable or decreased and lack of suppression indicate adrenal cause of Cushing syndrome.
  2. ACTH normal or increased and lack of suppression indicate ectopic ACTH production.
  3. ACTH normal or increased and partial suppression suggest pituitary excess (Cushing disease).
- Bilateral inferior petrosal sinus sampling (BIPSS) can be used to distinguish pituitary Cushing disease from the ectopic ACTH syndrome.

TABLE 1 Cushing Syndrome—Frequency of Individual Findings

Physical Finding[†]	Frequency (%)[‡]
Vital Signs	
Hypertension	64-88
Body Habitus	
Moon facies	67-92
Central obesity	44-97
Buffalo hump	34-75
Skin Findings	
Thin skin	27
Plethora	28-94
Hirsutism, women	48-81
Ecchymoses	23-75
Red or purple striae	46-68
Acne	21-52
Extremity Findings	
Proximal muscle weakness	39-68
Edema	15-66
Other	
Significant depression	12-40

[†]*Diagnostic standard*: For Cushing syndrome, elevated daily cortisol or corticosteroid metabolites, or both, with loss of circadian rhythm and with abnormal dexamethasone suppression tests.
[‡]Results are overall mean frequency or, if statistically heterogeneous, the range of values.
From McGee S: *Evidence-based physical diagnosis*, ed 4, Philadelphia, 2018, Elsevier.

LABORATORY TESTS

- Hypokalemia, hypochloremia, metabolic alkalosis, hyperglycemia, hypercholesterolemia.
- Increased 24-hr urinary free cortisol (>100 mcg/24 hr).
- Table 4 describes the differential diagnosis of hormonal values seen in Cushing syndrome.
- Fig. 3 describes an algorithm for the evaluation of Cushing syndrome.

IMAGING STUDIES

- CT scan or MRI of adrenal glands in suspected adrenal Cushing syndrome (Fig. E4).
- MRI of pituitary gland with gadolinium is the preferred procedure for localizing a pituitary edema in suspected pituitary Cushing syndrome.
- Additional imaging studies to localize neoplasms of the lung, pancreas, kidney, thyroid, or thymus in patients with ectopic ACTH production.

TABLE 4 Differential Diagnosis of Hormonal Values Seen in Cushing Syndrome

Cause	Plasma ACTH	Plasma Cortisol (PM)	High-Dose or Overnight Dexamethasone Suppression
Pituitary-dependent	N—slightly ↑	↑	Yes
Adrenal disease	↓—undetectable	↑	No
Ectopic Cushing*	↑↑↑	↑↑	Usually no
Pseudo-Cushing	N—slightly ↑	N–↑	Usually yes

ACTH, Adrenocorticotropin; *N,* normal.
*ACTH levels may overlap with values seen in pituitary-dependent disease.
From McPherson RA, Pincus MR (eds): *Henry's clinical diagnosis and management by laboratory methods*, ed 23, St Louis, 2017, Elsevier.

Rx TREATMENT

GENERAL Rx

The definitive treatment of Cushing syndrome is surgical removal of the tumor causing excessive production of cortisol:

- Pituitary adenoma: Transsphenoidal microadenomectomy is the therapy of choice in adults. Pituitary irradiation is reserved for patients not cured by transsphenoidal surgery. In children, pituitary irradiation may be considered as initial therapy because 85% of children are cured by radiation. Stereotactic radiotherapy (photon knife or gamma knife) is effective and exposes the surrounding neuronal tissues to less irradiation than does conventional radiotherapy. Total bilateral adrenalectomy is reserved for patients not cured by transsphenoidal surgery or pituitary irradiation
- Adrenal neoplasm:
  1. Surgical resection of the affected adrenal
  2. Glucocorticoid replacement for approximately 9 to 12 mo after the surgery to allow time for the contralateral adrenal gland to recover from its prolonged suppression
  3. In nonsurgical candidates, suppression of adrenal steroid production can be accomplished with ketoconazole. Mifepristone, an antiprogestin, can also be used for control of hyperglycemia secondary to hypercortisolism in adults with endogenous Cushing syndrome. It should be avoided in women who are or who could become pregnant
- Bilateral micronodular or macronodular adrenal hyperplasia: Bilateral total adrenalectomy
- Ectopic ACTH:
  1. Surgical resection of the ACTH-secreting neoplasm
  2. Control of cortisol excess with metyrapone, aminoglutethimide, mifepristone, or ketoconazole
  3. Control of the mineralocorticoid effects of cortisol and 11-deoxycorticosteroid with spironolactone
  4. Bilateral adrenalectomy: A rational approach to patients with indolent, unresectable tumors

DISPOSITION

Prognosis is favorable in patients with surgically amenable disease.

PEARLS & CONSIDERATIONS

COMMENTS

Screening for multiple endocrine neoplasia type I should be considered in patients with Cushing disease.

SUGGESTED READING

Available at ExpertConsult.com

RELATED CONTENT

Cushing Syndrome (Patient Information)

AUTHOR: **Fred F. Ferri, MD**

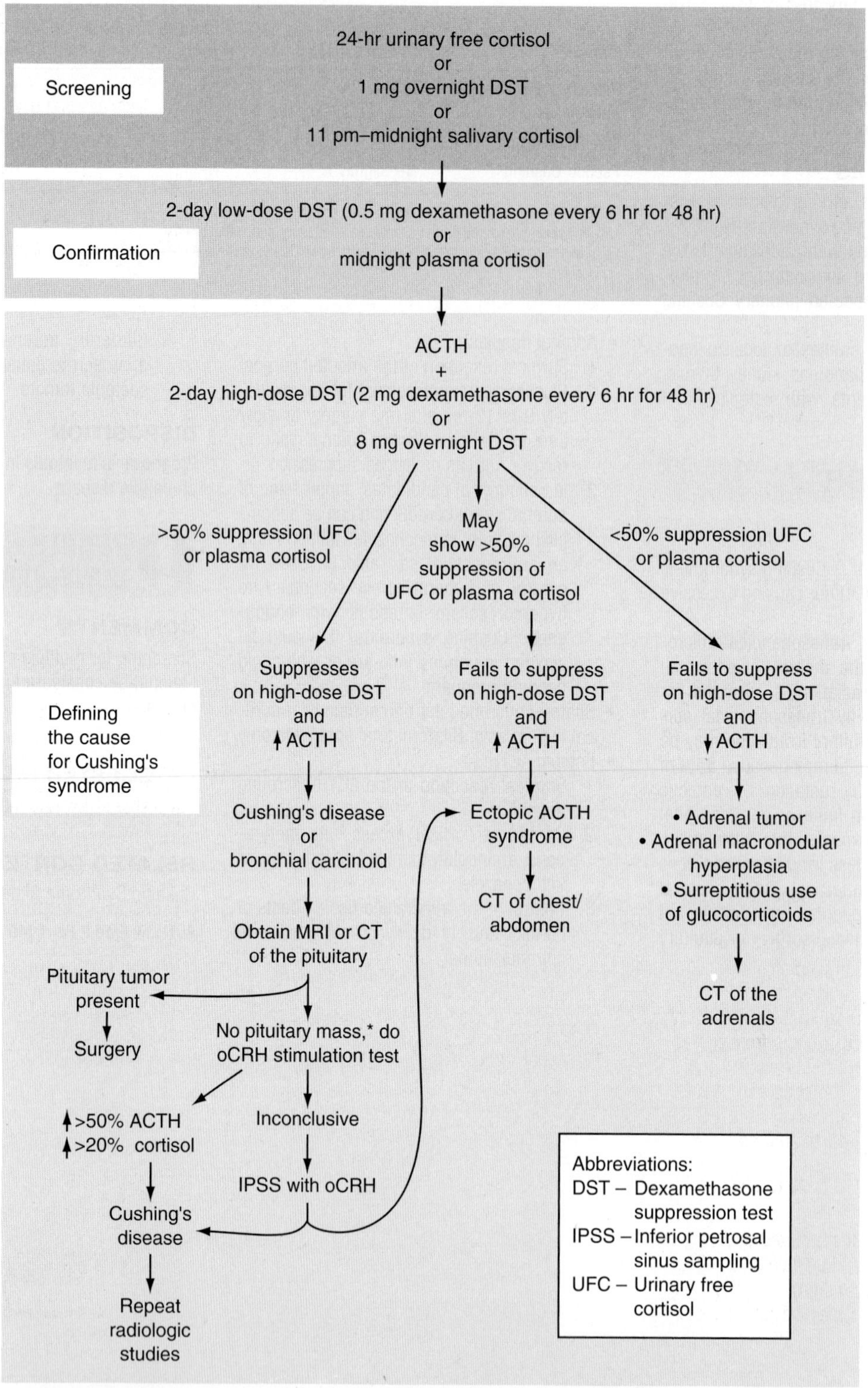

FIG. 3 Algorithm for the evaluation of Cushing syndrome. All screening tests must be followed by a confirmatory test. If there is no pituitary mass, obtain a chest radiograph and chest CT to rule out bronchial carcinoid before proceeding to IPSS. *ACTH,* Adrenocorticotropin; *CT,* computed tomography; *MRI,* magnetic resonance imaging; *oCRH,* ovine corticotropin-releasing hormone. (From McPherson RA, Pincus MR: *Henry's clinical diagnosis and management by laboratory methods,* ed 23, Philadelphia, 2017, Elsevier.)

BASIC INFORMATION

DEFINITION

Venous thromboembolism is any thromboembolic event occurring within the venous system. Deep vein thrombosis (DVT) is the development of thrombi in the deep veins of the extremities or pelvis.

SYNONYMS

DVT
Venous thromboembolism (VTE) (VTE includes DVT and pulmonary embolism [PE])
Deep venous thrombosis
VTE

ICD-10CM CODES

I82.401	Acute embolism and thrombosis of unspecified deep veins of right lower extremity
I82.402	Acute embolism and thrombosis of unspecified deep veins of left lower extremity
I82.403	Acute embolism and thrombosis of unspecified deep veins of lower extremity, bilateral
I82.621	Acute embolism and thrombosis of deep veins of right upper extremity
I82.622	Acute embolism and thrombosis of deep veins of left upper extremity
I82.623	Acute embolism and thrombosis of deep veins of upper extremity, bilateral

EPIDEMIOLOGY & DEMOGRAPHICS

- Annual incidence of VTE is 0.1% to 0.27%, affecting up to 5% of the population during their lifetimes.
- The risk of recurrent thromboembolism is higher among men than women.
- In the U.S., there are approximately 900,000 DVT events annually. About 5% to 15% of persons with untreated DVT die from pulmonary embolism.
- Venous thromboembolism occurs in nearly 2 cases per 1000 pregnancies and is a leading cause of maternal mortality and morbidity.

PHYSICAL FINDINGS & CLINICAL PRESENTATION

- Pain and swelling of the affected extremity
- In lower extremity DVT: Leg pain on dorsiflexion of the foot (***Homan*** **sign**)
- Physical examination may be unremarkable in early DVT

ETIOLOGY

The etiology is often multifactorial (prolonged stasis, coagulation abnormalities, vessel wall trauma (Fig. 1). The following are risk factors for DVT:

- Prolonged immobilization (>3 days)
- Postoperative state
- Trauma to pelvis and lower extremities for lower extremity DVT; central line placement for upper extremity DVT
- Birth control pills, high-dose estrogen therapy; conjugated equine estrogen but not esterified estrogen is associated with increased risk of DVT; estrogen plus progestin is associated with doubling the risk of venous thrombosis. The use of bevacizumab is also significantly associated with an increased risk of developing DVT in cancer patients receiving this drug
- Visceral cancer (lung, pancreas, alimentary tract, genitourinary tract)
- Occult cancer is detected in 1 in 20 patients within a year of receiving a diagnosis of unprovoked VTE
- Age >60 yr
- History of thromboembolic disease
- Hematologic disorders (e.g., factor V Leiden mutation [FVL], antithrombin III deficiency, protein C deficiency, protein S deficiency, heparin cofactor II deficiency, sticky platelet syndrome, G20210A prothrombin mutation, lupus anticoagulant, dysfibrinogenemias, anticardiolipin antibody, hyperhomocysteinemia, concurrent homocystinuria, high levels of factors VIII, XI, and single nucleotide polymorphisms [SNPs] such as CYP4V2). A classification of hypercoagulable states is described in Table 1
- Pregnancy and early puerperium
- Obesity (BMI >30)
- Congestive heart failure
- Surgery, fracture, or injury involving lower leg or pelvis
- Plaster cast immobilization
- Surgery requiring >30 min of anesthesia
- Gynecologic surgery (particularly gynecologic cancer surgery)
- Recent travel (within 2 wk, lasting ≥2 hr). Every 2 hr spent traveling increases VTE risk by 18%
- Smoking and abdominal obesity
- Central venous catheter or pacemaker insertion
- Superficial vein thrombosis (10% risk of DVT within 3 mo), varicose veins
- Collagen vascular disease
- Nephrotic syndrome
- Myeloproliferative disorders
- Testosterone therapy
- Long-term exposure to particulate air pollution is also associated with altered coagulation function and DVT risk
- Varicose veins

DIAGNOSIS

DIFFERENTIAL DIAGNOSIS

- Postphlebitic syndrome
- Superficial thrombophlebitis
- Ruptured Baker cyst
- Cellulitis, lymphangitis, Achilles tendinitis
- Hematoma
- Muscle or soft tissue injury, stress fracture
- Varicose veins, lymphedema
- Arterial insufficiency
- Abscess
- Claudication
- Venous stasis

WORKUP

- The clinical diagnosis of DVT is inaccurate. Pain, tenderness, swelling, or color changes are not specific for DVT.
- Clinical prediction rules can be used to establish pretest probability of DVT. The Wells prediction rules for DVT and for pulmonary embolism are described in Table 2. These rules perform better in younger patients without a history of DVT and in those without comorbidities. In younger patients without associated comorbidities and a low pretest

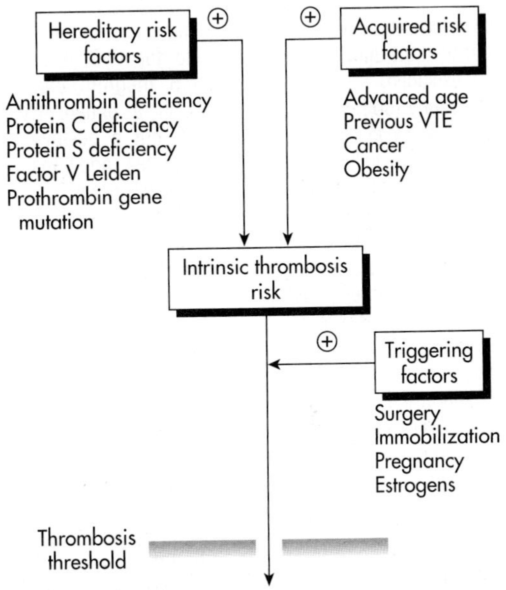

FIG. 1 Thrombosis threshold. Hereditary and acquired risk factors combine to create an intrinsic risk for thrombosis in each individual. This risk is increased by extrinsic triggering factors. If the intrinsic and extrinsic forces exceed a critical threshold at which thrombin generation overwhelms protective mechanisms, thrombosis occurs. *VTE,* Venous thromboembolism. (From Zipes DP: *Braunwald's heart disease, a textbook of cardiovascular medicine,* ed 11, Philadelphia, 2019, Elsevier.)

TABLE 1 Classification of Hypercoagulable States

Hereditary	Mixed	Acquired
Loss of Function		
Antithrombin deficiency	Hyperhomocysteinemia	Advanced age
Protein C deficiency		Previous venous thromboembolism
Protein S deficiency		Surgery
Gain of Function		Immobilization
Factor V Leiden		Obesity
Prothrombin gene mutation		Cancer
Elevated factor VIII, IX, or XI levels		Pregnancy, puerperium
		Drug-induced: L-asparaginase, hormonal therapy

From Zipes DP: *Braunwald's heart disease, a textbook of cardiovascular medicine,* ed 11, Philadelphia, 2019, Elsevier.

TABLE 2 Wells Scoring Scheme for Pre-Test Probability of Deep Vein Thrombosis*

Clinical Feature	Points
Risk Factors	
Active cancer	1
Paralysis, paresis, or recent plaster immobilization of the lower extremities	1
Recently bedridden >3 days or major surgery, within 4 wk	1
Signs	
Localized tenderness along the distribution of the deep venous system	1
Entire leg swollen	1
Asymmetric calf swelling (>3 cm difference, 10 cm below tibial tuberosity)	1
Asymmetric pitting edema	1
Collateral superficial veins (nonvaricose)	1
Alternative Diagnosis	
Alternative diagnosis as likely or more likely than deep venous thrombosis	−2

*Interpretation of score: High probability if 3 points or more, moderate probability if 1 or 2 points, and low probability if 0 points or less.

From Wells PS et al: Value of assessment of pretest probability of deep-vein thrombosis in clinical management, *Lancet* 350:1795-1798, 1997. In McGee S: *Evidence-based physical diagnosis*, ed 4, Philadelphia, 2018, Elsevier.

probability using Wells criteria and a negative high-sensitivity D-dimer test, the diagnosis of DVT can be reasonably excluded.

- Compression ultrasonography (CUS; Fig. E2) is preferred as the initial study to diagnose DVT in patients with intermediate to high pretest probability. An initial negative test limited to the proximal leg should be repeated after 5 days (if the clinical suspicion of DVT persists) to exclude DVT that is propagating proximally from the calf. Comprehensive ultrasonography (whole-leg CUS) is a more extensive test that examines the deep veins from the inguinal ligament to the level of the malleolus. Literature reports indicate that it may be safe to withhold anticoagulation after negative results on comprehensive duplex ultrasonography in nonpregnant patients with a suspected first episode of symptomatic DVT of the leg.

LABORATORY TESTS

- Laboratory tests are not specific for DVT.
- Baseline prothrombin time (INR), partial thromboplastin time, and platelet count should be obtained on all patients.
- D-dimer testing is sensitive but not specific for DVT. A negative result (D-dimer <0.5 mcg/ml) can exclude the diagnosis in a patient with low probability of DVT, but a positive result (≥0.5 mcg/ml) mandates additional testing with venous ultrasonography.
- Laboratory evaluation of young patients with DVT, patients with recurrent thrombosis without obvious causes, and those with a family history of thrombosis should include protein S (both total and free PS), protein C, fibrinogen, antithrombin III level, lupus anticoagulant, anticardiolipin antibodies, anti-b2 glycoprotein1, factor V Leiden, factor VIII, factor IX, and fasting plasma homocysteine levels. It is important to remember that the lupus anticoagulant assay and antithrombin, protein C, protein S, and dysfibrinogenemia testing cannot be properly interpreted if a patient is already on warfarin, whereas anticardiolipin antibody test, prothrombin G20210A, factor VII:C, factor V Leiden, and PT polymorphism can be performed when a patient is on warfarin.

IMAGING STUDIES

- Compression ultrasonography (CUS) is generally preferred as the initial study because it is noninvasive and can be repeated serially (useful to monitor suspected acute DVT); it offers good sensitivity for detecting proximal vein thrombosis (in the popliteal or femoral vein). Its disadvantages are poor visualization of deep iliac and pelvic veins and poor sensitivity in isolated or nonocclusive calf vein thrombi. Whole-leg compression ultrasound can generally exclude proximal and distal DVT in a single evaluation. Withholding anticoagulation following a single negative whole-leg CUS is associated with a relatively low risk of venous thromboembolism (3.5% of inpatients will develop DVT) during a 3-mo follow-up.
- Contrast venography is the gold standard for evaluation of DVT of the lower extremity. It is, however, invasive and painful and rarely used in clinical practice. Additional disadvantages are the increased risk of phlebitis, new thrombosis, renal failure, and hypersensitivity reaction to contrast media; it also gives poor visualization of the deep femoral vein in the thigh and the internal iliac vein and its tributaries.
- Magnetic resonance direct thrombus imaging (MRDTI) is an accurate noninvasive test for diagnosis of DVT. It is particularly useful in suspected DVT patients with leg casts, which prevent CUS, and in pregnant patients with positive D-dimer and negative CUS. Current limitations are its cost and lack of widespread availability.

Rx TREATMENT

NONPHARMACOLOGIC THERAPY

- Gradual resumption of normal activity. Immobility promotes stasis and propagation of DVT. Patients should get up and walk as tolerated. The theoretical risk that ambulation may dislodge thrombi in the legs, precipitating PE, is unfounded.
- Patient education on anticoagulant therapy and associated risks.

ACUTE GENERAL Rx

- Direct oral anticoagulants (DOACs) apixaban or rivaroxaban are preferred as monotherapy for initial treatment of DVT. These new anticoagulants (Table 3) are noninferior to warfarin, do not require periodic lab monitoring, and have a relatively low bleeding risk. They are preferred agents for extended treatment of venous thromboembolism if cost is not a significant issue.
- When apixaban or rivaroxaban are not available or contraindicated, initial treatment of DVT requires therapeutic doses of heparin (low-molecular-weight heparin [LMWH] or unfractionated). LMWH is preferred due to ease of administration, less hemorrhage, and significantly fewer deaths. Unfractionated heparin is preferred in patients with renal insufficiency because LMWH is predominantly excreted in the urine.
- LMWH is generally administered for 5 to 7 days. Recommended dose of enoxaparin is

TABLE 3 Comparison of Dabigatran, Rivaroxaban, Apixaban, and Edoxaban

	Dabigatran	Rivaroxaban	Apixaban	Edoxaban
Target	Thrombin (IIa)	Factor Xa	Factor Xa	Factor Xa
Active drug	No	Yes	Yes	Yes
Onset time (hr)	0.5-2	2-4	3-4	1-3
Half-life (hr)	12-17	5-13	~12	9-11
Renal excretion (%)	80	33	27	50

From Hoffman R et al: *Hematology, basic principles and practice*, ed 7, Philadelphia, 2017, Elsevier.

BOX 1 Contraindications to Outpatient Treatment of Venous Thromboembolism[a]

- Active or high risk of bleeding
- Recent surgery (within 7 days)
- Cardiopulmonary instability
- Severe symptomatic venous obstruction
- High risk of pulmonary embolism
- Thrombocytopenia (platelets <50,000/μL)
- Other medical or surgical condition requiring inpatient management
- Medical noncompliance
- Geographic or telephone inaccessibility
- Poor hepatic function (international normalized ratio ≥1.5)
- Unstable renal function (e.g., rising serum creatinine)
- Poor home health care support environment

[a]Not an all-inclusive list.
From Niederhuber JE: *Abeloff's clinical oncology*, ed 6, Philadelphia, 2020, Elsevier.

1 mg/kg q12h SC. Once-daily fondaparinux, a synthetic analogue of heparin, is also as effective and safe as twice-daily enoxaparin in the initial treatment of patients with symptomatic DVT. Once systemic anticoagulation is initiated, vitamin K antagonist warfarin is initiated. Warfarin is titrated to maintain an INR between 2 and 3. After ≥5 days, heparin is stopped and warfarin is continued as monotherapy. Long-term LMWH may be preferable to warfarin in patients with cancer or those whose INR is difficult to control.

- Outpatient treatment of DVT is appropriate for patients without thrombophilic conditions or substantial comorbidity. Exclusions from outpatient treatment of DVT (Box 1) include patients with potential high complication risk (e.g., active or high risk of bleeding, hemoglobin <7, platelet count <50,000, guaiac-positive stool, recent cerebrovascular accident or noncutaneous surgery, noncompliance).
- Compression stockings are effective in reducing the incidence of postthrombotic syndrome and should be used starting within 1 mo of proximal DVT and continued for at least 1 yr after diagnosis.
- Insertion of an inferior vena cava filter to prevent pulmonary embolism is recommended in patients with contraindications to anticoagulation (e.g., hemorrhagic stroke, active internal bleeding, pregnancy), HIT in a patient with an active VTE/PE, recurrent PE despite adequate anticoagulant therapy, emergent surgery in patient with DVT, presence of free-floating iliofemoral thrombus, lower IVC thrombosis (incipient embolization), and chronic pulmonary (thromboembolic) hypertension with limited pulmonary reserve. Table 4 summarizes indications for IVC filter placement.
- Potential harms associated with IVC filters include migration, vessel penetration, excess DVT risk, fracture.[1]
- Thrombolytic therapy (streptokinase) can be used in rare cases (unless contraindicated) in patients with extensive iliofemoral venous thrombosis and a low risk of bleeding. There are concerns about hemorrhagic complications related to the large doses of thrombolytics required in systemic thrombolysis for DVT (2%-10% risk of major hemorrhagic complications).
- Other treatment modalities for DVT include surgical thrombectomy and catheter-directed thrombolysis (CDT). Thromboreduction by surgical thrombectomy is effective but invasive and expensive. CDT is also invasive, carries a bleeding risk, and will generally require ICU admission.

CHRONIC Rx

- The optimal duration of anticoagulant therapy varies with the cause of DVT and the patient's risk factors. The risk of recurrence is low if VTE is provoked by surgery, intermediate if provoked by a nonsurgical risk factor, and high if unprovoked. These risks should determine whether patients with VTE should undergo short-term vs. indefinite treatment.
- Therapy for 3 mo is generally satisfactory in patients with reversible risk factors (low-risk group). A high D-dimer level measured after 3 mo of anticoagulation in patients with unprovoked DVT should favor a longer duration of therapy. The American College of Chest Physicians Guidelines suggests that patients with first unprovoked VTE receive indefinite anticoagulation unless their bleeding risk is high.
- The risk of recurrence in patients with a first unprovoked VTE who have negative D-dimer results is not low enough to justify stopping anticoagulant therapy in men but may be low enough in some cases to justify stopping therapy in women who were taking estrogen at the time of initial VTE.[2]
- Anticoagulation for 6 mo is recommended for patients with idiopathic venous thrombosis or medical risk factors for DVT (intermediate-risk group). About 20% of patients with unprovoked venous thromboembolism have a recurrence within 2 yr after the withdrawal of oral anticoagulant therapy. Use of daily low-dose aspirin after discontinuation of anticoagulant treatment may provide a modest reduction in DVT risk.
- Indefinite anticoagulation is necessary in patients with DVT associated with active cancer; long-term anticoagulation is also indicated in patients with inherited thrombophilia (e.g., deficiency of antithrombin III, protein C or S antibody), high factor VIII levels, antiphospholipid antibody, and those with recurrent episodes of idiopathic DVT (high-risk group). Long-term anticoagulation should also be considered in the presence of comorbidities such as paroxysmal nocturnal hemoglobinuria (PNH), SLE (especially with nephrotic syndrome), some myeloproliferative disorders, IBD, and Cushing syndrome.
- Measurement of D-dimer after withdrawal of oral anticoagulation may be useful to estimate the risk of recurrence in selected patients. In patients with a first unprovoked DVT, positive D-dimer test results after cessation of anticoagulation predict recurrence, regardless of test timing or patient's age. Patients with a first spontaneous DVT and a D-dimer level <250 mg/ml after withdrawal of oral anticoagulation have a low risk of DVT recurrence. Risk is lower in women than in men. In patients who have completed at least 3 mo of anticoagulation for a first episode of unprovoked DVT and after approximately 2 yr of follow-up, a negative D-dimer result is associated with a 3.5% annual risk of recurrent disease, whereas a positive D-dimer result is associated with an 8.9% annual risk for recurrence. Hence, elevated D-dimer levels would be an indication for prolonged therapy (for 1 or 2 more yr at a minimum).
- The presence of residual thrombosis on ultrasonography when anticoagulant therapy is discontinued is also associated with an increased risk for subsequent recurrent DVT; a recent trial showed that tailoring the duration of anticoagulation on the basis of the persistence of residual thrombi on ultrasonography may

[1] Kaufman JA et al: Society of Interventional Radiology Clinical Practice Guideline for Inferior Vena Cava Filters in the Treatment of Patients with Venous Thromboembolic Disease: Developed in collaboration with the American College of Cardiology, American College of Chest Physicians, American College of Surgeons Committee on Trauma, American Heart Association, Society for Vascular Surgery, and Society for Vascular Medicine, *J Vasc Interv Radiol* 31:1529-1544, 2020.

[2] Kearon C et al: D-dimer testing to select patients with a first unprovoked venous thromboembolism who can stop anticoagulant therapy: a cohort study. *Ann Intern Med* 162:27-34, 2015.

reduce the rate of recurrent DVT. Additional trials are needed before this approach can be adapted for all patients.

- Patients with DVT and pulmonary embolism are at high risk of recurrence whenever anticoagulation is discontinued; therefore, many experts recommend prolonged anticoagulation in this population group, especially if other risk factors for recurrence are present.

PEARLS & CONSIDERATIONS

COMMENTS

- The prevalence of occult cancer is low among patients with a first unprovoked venous embolism. Routine screening with CT of the abdomen and pelvis does not provide a clinically significant benefit.[3]
- When using heparin, there is a risk of heparin-induced thrombocytopenia (HIT) (with unfractionated more so than with LMWH). Platelet count should be obtained initially and repeated every 3 days while on heparin.
- Therapeutic options for cancer-associated venous thromboembolism are summarized in Box 2.
- ISOLATED DEEP VEIN THROMBOSIS OF THE CALF: The American College of Chest Physicians Guidelines suggest (1) anticoagulation in patients with severe symptoms or risk factors for proximal extension, and (2) repeat sonogram in 2 wk in lower risk patients and anticoagulation only in those patients whose DVTs extend proximally.
- Prophylaxis of DVT: Recommended in all patients at risk (e.g., low-molecular-weight heparin [enoxaparin 30 mg SC bid or fondaparinux 2.5 mg SC daily] after major trauma, postsurgery of hip and knee; enoxaparin 40 mg SC qd post–abdominal surgery in patients with moderate to high DVT risk; gradient elastic stockings alone or in combination with intermittent pneumatic compression [IPC] boots following neurosurgery). Graduated compression stockings (GCSs) are effective for preventing air-travel-related DVT and in reducing the risk of DVT in patients hospitalized for conditions other than stroke. The type of GCSs is also important because proximal DVT occurs more often in patients with stroke who wear below-knee stockings than in those who wear high-length stockings. The new oral anticoagulants (rivaroxaban, apixaban, etc.) are effective for thromboprophylaxis after THR and TKR. However, their clinical benefits over LMWH are marginal. Betrixaban is the first FDA-approved once-daily oral direct factor Xa inhibitor for prophylaxis of VTE in adults hospitalized for an acute medical illness with risk factors for VTE and moderately or severely restricted mobility. Apixaban appears to be as effective as LMWH for thromboprophylaxis in cancer patients but poses similar risk of bleeding and should be used with caution in patients with GI malignancies, thrombocytopenia, or renal impairment. Common regimens for venous thromboembolism prevention are summarized in Table 5. Box 3 describes traditional absolute and relative contraindications to pharmacologic and mechanical venous thromboembolism prophylaxis.
- RECURRENT THROMBOEMBOLISM: The risk of recurrent venous thromboembolism in heterozygous carriers of factor V Leiden and a first spontaneous venous thromboembolism is similar to that of noncarriers of factor V Leiden; therefore, heterozygous patients should receive secondary thromboprophylaxis for a similar length of time as patients without factor V Leiden. Management of recurrent venous thromboembolism in patients with cancer is summarized in Table 6.
- POSTTHROMBOTIC SYNDROME: Approximately 20% to 50% of patients with DVT develop postthrombotic syndrome characterized by leg edema, pain, venous ectasia, skin induration, and ulceration. Patients with extensive DVT

[3]Carrier M et al: Screening for occult cancer in unprovoked venous thromboembolism, *N Engl J Med* 373:697-704, 2015.

TABLE 4 Indications for Inferior Vena Cava Filter Placement

	Indications for IVC Filter Placement	Examples
1.	DVT and contraindication to anticoagulation (A)	Hemorrhage while on anticoagulation
2.	DVT and failure of anticoagulation (A)	Recurrent DVT or PE despite anticoagulation, inability to achieve or maintain adequate anticoagulation
3.	DVT and low cardiopulmonary reserve or high mortality risk from possible PE (R)	Severe pulmonary hypertension, right heart failure, known large right-to-left shunt
4.	Populations with very high risk for PE (R)	Some postbariatric, orthopedic, or neurosurgical patients or multitrauma patients. Patients with expected prolonged immobilization
5.	High risk for life-threatening PE (R)	Large, unstable (free-floating) IVC clot
6.	DVT and high fall risk (R)	
7.	Prophylaxis during catheter-directed thrombolysis of DVT (R)	

There are two absolute indications for IVC filter placement: First, if the patient is at risk for PE (i.e., DVT) but for whatever reason he/she is not a candidate for systemic anticoagulation (i.e., hemorrhage); and second, if the patient developed a PE, new DVT, or an extension of DVT while on proper anticoagulation. There are a number of relative indications for filter placement. They are presented in rows 3 through 7. In every case the decision to place a filter compels careful consideration of the risks and benefits and may require multidisciplinary input. *(A)*, Absolute; *DVT*, deep vein thrombosis; *IVC*, inferior vena cava; *PE*, pulmonary embolism; *(R)*, relative.

From Cameron JL, Cameron AM: *Current surgical therapy*, ed 12, Philadelphia, 2017, Elsevier.

BOX 2 Therapeutic Options for Cancer-Associated Venous Thromboembolism (VTE)

Acute VTE Treatment Options

- Unfractionated heparin: 80 units/kg intravenous bolus followed by 18 units/kg/hr infusion adjusted to aPTT ratio
- Dalteparin, 200 units/kg subcutaneously every 24 hr
- Enoxaparin, 1 mg/kg subcutaneously every 12 hr
- Tinzaparin, 175 units/kg subcutaneously every 24 hr
- Fondaparinux, 5-10 mg subcutaneously every 24 hr (5 mg for weight <50 kg, 7.5 mg for weight 50-100 kg, and 10 mg for weight >100 kg)
- Initial rivaroxaban dose 15 mg twice daily; switch to 20 mg once daily after 3 wk
- Dabigatran 150 mg bid after 5 days of parenteral agent
- Apixaban 10 mg bid × 7 days followed by 5 mg bid[a]
- Edoxaban 60 mg once daily after 5 days of parenteral agent
- Vena caval filter

Chronic VTE Treatment Options

- Dalteparin, 200 units/kg subcutaneously every 24 hr for 1 mo then 150 units/kg subcutaneously every 24 hr
- Enoxaparin, 1 mg/kg every 12 hr or 1.5 mg/kg subcutaneously every 24 hr
- Tinzaparin, 175 units/kg subcutaneously every 24 hr
- Vitamin K antagonists (e.g., warfarin) adjusted for an INR of 2-3
- Rivaroxaban 20 mg once daily; consider 10 mg once daily if appropriate
- Dabigatran 150 bid after 5 days of parenteral agent
- Apixaban 10 mg bid initial × 7 days followed by 5 mg bid
- Edoxaban 60 mg once daily after 5 days of parenteral agent
- Vena cava filter

Rivaroxaban should be used with caution in patients with cancer, given the limited information on this medication in patients with cancer.

aPTT, Activated partial thromboplastin time; *bid*, twice daily; *INR*, international normalized ratio.
[a]No data currently available for use in the cancer population.
From Niederhuber JE: *Abeloff's clinical oncology*, ed 6, Philadelphia, 2020, Elsevier.

and those with more severe postthrombotic manifestations 1 mo after DVT have poorer long-term outcomes. Recent trials have shown that compression stockings after DVT do not prevent postthrombotic syndrome.

- Exercise following DVT is reasonable because it improves flexibility of the affected leg and does not increase symptoms in patients with postthrombotic syndrome.
- UPPER EXTREMITY DVT: It is less common than lower extremity DVT and is seen more frequently in patients requiring central venous catheters or wires. It confers risk for mortality, recurrent thromboembolic events, and postthrombotic syndrome similar to that of lower extremity DVT. It is classified as primary upper extremity DVT (Paget-Schroetter syndrome), defined as a thrombus in the axillary and subclavian veins in absence of identifiable thrombosis risk factors. It accounts for 20% of upper extremity DVT cases and may be due to an underlying anatomic abnormality at the thoracic outlet in combination with local hypercoagulability due to venous stretching or perivascular fibrosis from recurrent venous compression. Secondary upper extremity DVT is defined as any DVT related to a predisposing factor (e.g., insertion of central venous catheter, wires, or other devices; malignancy). In patients with secondary upper extremity DVT, removal of the catheter is not routinely recommended but is warranted if there is a catheter malfunction or infection, if anticoagulation therapy is contraindicated or has failed, or if the catheter is no longer needed. Anticoagulation therapy in upper extremity DVT consists of use of vitamin K antagonists, except in patients with cancer, for whom LMWH is preferred. Optimal duration of anticoagulation treatment in upper extremity DVT is 3 to 6 mo (including in those in whom a central catheter has been removed).
- DVT THERAPY IN PREGNANCY: Vitamin K antagonists such as warfarin are contraindicated in pregnancy. Low-molecular-weight heparins are safe and effective. Typical agents used in pregnancy include dalteparin (200 IU per kg of body weight daily or 100 IU per kg twice daily) or enoxaparin (1.5 mg per kg daily or 1 mg per kg twice daily).
- REVERSAL OF ANTICOAGULATION: Vitamin K (1 mg PO or 2 mg IV) can be used to reverse elevated INR (3-6) from warfarin when elective or urgent procedures are needed. The administration of vitamin K can take more than 24 hr to fully restore vitamin K-dependent coagulation factors II, VII, IX, and X. The American College of Chest Physicians recommends the following guidelines for managing elevated INRs or bleeding in patients receiving vitamin A antagonist therapy:
  1. INR between 4.5 and 10 and no significant bleeding: Omit dose and monitor the next day, routine use of vitamin K is not recommended.
  2. INR >10 and no significant bleeding: Hold vitamin K antagonist, give 5 to 10 mg

TABLE 5 Common Regimens for Venous Thromboembolism Prevention

Condition	Prophylaxis
Hospitalization with medical illness	Unfractionated heparin 5000 units SC bid or tid *or* Enoxaparin 40 mg SC qd *or* Dalteparin 2500 units or 5000 units SC qd *or* Fondaparinux 2.5 mg SC qd with normal renal function (in patients with a heparin allergy such as heparin-induced thrombocytopenia) *or* Graduated compression stockings or intermittent pneumatic compression for patients with contraindications to anticoagulation Consider combination pharmacologic and mechanical prophylaxis for high-risk patients
General surgery	Unfractionated heparin 5000 units SC bid or tid *or* Enoxaparin 40 mg SC qd *or* Dalteparin 2500 or 5000 units SC qd
Major orthopedic surgery	Warfarin (target INR 2-3) *or* Enoxaparin 30 mg SC bid *or* Enoxaparin 40 mg SC qd *or* Dalteparin 2500 or 5000 units SC qd *or* Fondaparinux 2.5 mg SC qd *or* Rivaroxaban 10 mg qd *or* Aspirin 81 mg qd *or* Dabigatran 220 mg qd *or* Apixaban 2.5 mg twice daily *or* Intermittent pneumatic compression (with or without pharmacologic prophylaxis)

bid, Twice daily; *INR,* international normalized ratio; *qd,* every day; *SC,* subcutaneous; *tid,* three times a day.
From Zipes DP: *Braunwald's heart disease, a textbook of cardiovascular medicine*, ed 11, Philadelphia, 2019, Elsevier.

BOX 3 Traditional Absolute and Relative Contraindications to Pharmacologic and Mechanical Venous Thromboembolism Prophylaxis[a]

Contraindications to Pharmacologic Prophylaxis
- Active, recent, or high risk of clinically significant bleeding
- Thrombocytopenia (platelet count <50,000/μL)
- Systemic coagulopathy (e.g., disseminated intravascular coagulation, international normalized ratio >1.4, or activated partial thromboplastin time ratio >1.2, excluding lupus inhibitors)
- Known congenital bleeding disorders (e.g., hemophilia A or B and von Willebrand disease)
- Known functional acquired or congenital platelet disorder (e.g., Bernard-Soulier syndrome and uremic platelet dysfunction)
- Heparin-induced thrombocytopenia (for unfractionated or low-molecular-weight heparin)

Contraindications to Mechanical Prophylaxis
- Acute or recent deep venous thrombosis (within 3 mo)
- Arterial insufficiency in target limb
- Open lower extremity wound

[a]List not inclusive.
From Niederhuber JE: *Abeloff's clinical oncology,* ed 6, Philadelphia, 2020, Elsevier.

TABLE 6 Management of Recurrent Venous Thromboembolism in Patients with Cancer

Causes	Management
Extrinsic vascular compression (causes sluggish flow)	Relieve vascular compression due to tumor, nodal masses, or anatomic abnormalities (i.e., May-Thurner syndrome/iliac vein compression, thoracic outlet syndrome) with surgical decompression, vascular stents, or other
Intrinsic vascular obstruction	Remove central venous catheter or devices responsible for sluggish flow
Trousseau syndrome	Switch to LMWH
Heparin-induced thrombocytopenia	Discontinue unfractionated or LMWH and start a direct thrombin inhibitor (preferred) or fondaparinux
Therapeutic resistance	If the patient is taking warfarin, switch to LMWH If the patient is taking LMWH, check to ensure the correct full weight-based dose is being used, switch to twice-daily dosing (if administration is once daily), consider checking LMWH (anti-Xa) level, initiate an empiric 25% dose increase, or switch to fondaparinux

LMWH, Low-molecular-weight heparin.
From Niederhuber JE: *Abeloff's clinical oncology,* ed 6, Philadelphia, 2020, Elsevier.

orally of vitamin K. Monitor the next day and use additional vitamin K if necessary. Resume therapy at lower dose when INR therapeutic.

3. Serious bleeding at any elevation of INR: Hold vitamin K antagonist and supplement with prothrombin complex concentrates (PCC). Give vitamin K (10 mg by slow IV infusion over 30 min to reduce the risk of anaphylaxis). Vitamin K1 can be repeated every 12 hr. PCC composition in the U.S. (3-factor PCC) includes clotting factors II, IX, and X but minimal amounts of factor VII (unlike PCC products available outside of the U.S. [4-factor PCC], which have a significant amount of factor VII). In order to replace the low factor VII, some clinicians in the U.S. will also give fresh frozen plasma (FFP) in addition to vitamin K and PCC in patients with life-threatening warfarin-related bleeding.

- SPECIFIC REVERSAL AGENTS FOR NON–VITAMIN K ANTAGONIST ANTICOAGULANTS (Table 7):
  1. Idarucizumab, an antibody fragment given at a dose of 5 g IV, has been shown to completely reverse the anticoagulant effect of dabigatran within minutes.
  2. The anticoagulant activity of factor Xa inhibitors apixaban, rivaroxaban, and edoxaban can be rapidly reversed with IV administration of andexanet alfa.
  3. These reversal agents are very expensive (over $20,000 for each use).

TABLE 7 Reversal Agents for Direct Oral Anticoagulants

Feature	Idarucizumab	Andexanet Alfa	Ciraparantag
Structure	Humanized antibody fragment	Recombinant human factor Xa variant	Synthetic, small cationic molecule
Mass (Da)	47,776	39,000	573
Mechanism of action	Binds dabigatran with high affinity	Competes with factors Xa (and IIa) for binding	Binds via hydrogen bonding
Target	Dabigatran	Rivaroxaban, apixaban, edoxaban and heparins	Dabigatran, rivaroxaban, apixaban, edoxaban and heparins
Administration	Intravenous bolus	Intravenous bolus followed by a 2-hour infusion	Intravenous bolus
Measurement of reversal	Activated partial thromboplastin time, diluted thrombin time, or ecarin clotting time or chromogenic assay	Calibrated anti-factor Xa assays	Whole-blood clotting time
Elimination	Renal (catabolism)	Not reported	Not reported
Cost	$3500 per dose in the U.S.	Unknown; likely to be at least as much as idarucizumab	Likely to be low

From Zipes DP: *Braunwald's heart disease, a textbook of cardiovascular medicine,* ed 11, Philadelphia, 2019, Elsevier.

RELATED CONTENT

Deep Vein Thrombosis (DVT) (Patient Information)
Antiphospholipid Antibody Syndrome (Related Key Topic)
Hypercoagulable State (Related Key Topic)
Postthrombotic Syndrome (Related Key Topic)
Pulmonary Embolism (Related Key Topic)
Upper Extremity Deep Vein Thrombosis (Related Key Topic)

SUGGESTED READINGS

Available at ExpertConsult.com

AUTHOR: **Fred F. Ferri, MD**

BASIC INFORMATION

DEFINITION

The American Psychiatric Association's *Diagnostic and Statistical Manual*, 5th edition, (DSM-5) defines delirium as:

- Disturbance of consciousness with reduced ability to focus, sustain, or shift attention.
- The disturbance develops over a short period of time (usually hours to days) and tends to fluctuate during the course of a day.
- An additional disturbance in cognition (e.g., memory deficit, disorganization, language, visuospatial ability, or perception).
- A change in cognition or development of a perceptual disturbance that is not better accounted for by a preexisting, established, or evolving dementia.
- There is evidence from history, physical exam, or lab findings that the disturbance is caused by medical condition, substance intoxication or withdrawal (i.e., due to a drug of abuse or to a medication), or exposure to a toxin, or is due to multiple etiologies.

SYNONYMS

Acute confusional state
Toxic or metabolic encephalopathy

THEORIES REGARDING PATHOPHYSIOLOGY

- Neuroinflammation, with increased permeability of the blood-brain barrier
- Acetylcholine deficiency
- Other neurotransmitter imbalances, including excesses of norepinephrine, serotonin, and, most important, dopamine

CLASSIFICATION

Hyperactive, hypoactive, and mixed subtype

ICD-10CM CODES

F05	Delirium, not induced by alcohol and other psychoactive substances
F05.9	Delirium, unspecified
F06.0	Organic hallucinosis
F05.8	Other delirium
F05.0	Delirium not superimposed on dementia
F05.1	Delirium superimposed on dementia

EPIDEMIOLOGY & DEMOGRAPHICS

Nearly 30% of older patients experience delirium at some time during the hospital course. In older surgical patients, the risk varies from 10% to 50%. Hypoactive is more common. Delirium is the most common mental disorder in patients with medical illness. Any age, race, or gender can be affected. Pediatric delirium is often missed but remains important because delirium is associated with longer hospital stays, decreased cognitive performance, and increased mortality. Risk factors include extremes of age, severe pain, illicit substance use, surgery, dementia, and kidney or liver failure (Table 1).

PHYSICAL FINDINGS & CLINICAL PRESENTATION

- One of the earliest symptoms is change in level of awareness and ability to focus, sustain, or shift attention. Symptoms may differ both among patients and within one patient. Family members or caregivers report that the patient "isn't acting quite right." Symptoms may include poor attention, sleepiness, agitation, or psychosis.
- Acuteness of presentation helps in differentiating delirium with dementia. Change in cognition, perceptual problems (such as visual, auditory, or somatosensory hallucination usually with lack of insight), memory loss, disorientation, difficulty with speech and language. It is important to ascertain from family member or caregivers the patient's level of functioning before onset of delirium.
- Elderly patients with delirium often do not look sick, but patients with delirium are sick by definition.
- Hyperactive delirium represents only 25% of cases, with the others having hypoactive (quiet) delirium.
- There is often a prodrome phase that later blends into hypoactive delirium or erupts into an agitated confusional state.
- Physical examination should be performed, focusing on signs of infection, dehydration, or chronic disease that may be exacerbated. Vital signs are key. Consider using the Mini-Mental Status Exam or the Montreal Cognitive Assessment.
- Fig. 1 describes an algorithm for evaluation of mental status changes in an older patient.
- Table 2 summarizes delirium assessment tools.

ETIOLOGY

Can be multifactorial; often falls into one of the following categories:

- Drugs: Benzodiazepines are the worst offenders, but other drugs such as narcotics, anticholinergics, beta-blockers, steroids, nonsteroidal antiinflammatory drugs, digoxin, cimetidine can cause delirium; also, withdrawal states such as alcohol withdrawal or benzodiazepine withdrawal can cause delirium
- Infection or inflammation
- Metabolic: Kidney or liver failure, thyroid, adrenal, or glucose dysregulation, anemia, vitamin deficiency such as Wernicke encephalopathy or vitamin B_{12} deficiency, inborn metabolic errors such as porphyrias or Wilson disease
- Stress: Surgery, sleep problems, pain, fever, hypoxia, anesthesia, environmental changes, fecal or urinary retention, burns
- Fluids, electrolytes, nutrition (FEN): Dysregulation of calcium, magnesium, potassium, or sodium; dehydration; volume overload; altered pH
- Brain disorder: CNS infection, head injury, hypertensive encephalopathy

DIAGNOSIS

DIFFERENTIAL DIAGNOSIS

- Primary psychiatric illness
- Focal syndromes
- Dementia
- Sundowning
- Nonconvulsive status epilepticus

Remember, delirium may coexist with any of the above. Table 3 summarizes the differential diagnosis of delirium. Table 4 describes clinical factors that help differentiate delirium and dementia from psychiatric disease.

LABORATORY TESTS

- Complete blood count, electrolytes, liver function tests, ammonia, drug levels (digoxin, lithium)
- Toxicology screen, urinalysis, urine culture
- Thyroid function tests, vitamin B_{12}, and folate levels
- Rapid plasma reagin for syphilis, blood, urine, and spinal fluid culture
- Arterial blood gas
- Lumbar puncture is mandatory when cause of delirium is not obvious

IMAGING STUDIES

- Consider head CT (to look for bleed, trauma, tumor, atrophy, dementia, stroke)

TABLE 1 Mnemonic for Risk Factors for Delirium and Agitation

I Watch Death	Delirium
Infection	**D**rugs
Withdrawal	**E**lectrolyte and physiologic abnormalities
Acute metabolic	**L**ack of drugs (withdrawal)
Trauma/pain	**I**nfection
Central nervous system pathology	**R**educed sensory input (blindness, deafness)
Hypoxia	**I**ntracranial problems (CVA, meningitis, seizure)
Deficiencies (vitamin B_{12}, thiamine)	**U**rinary retention and fecal impaction
Endocrinopathies (thyroid, adrenal)	**M**yocardial problems (MI, arrhythmia, CHF)
Acute vascular (hypertension, shock)	
Toxins/drugs	
Heavy metals	

CHF, Congestive heart failure; *CVA,* cerebrovascular accident; *MI,* myocardial infarction.
From Vincent JL et al: *Textbook of critical care,* ed 6, Philadelphia, 2011, Saunders.

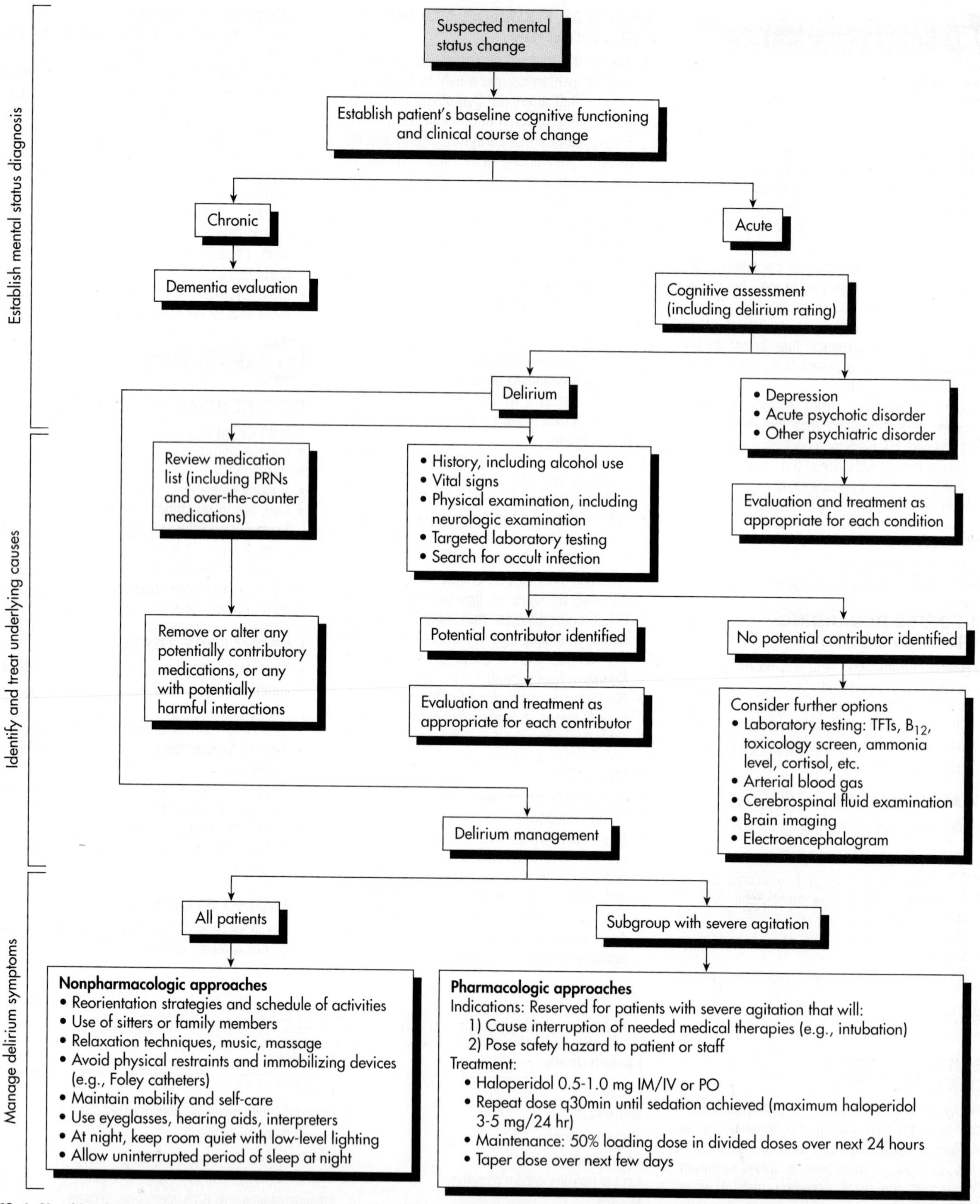

FIG. 1 Algorithm for evaluation of suspected mental status change in an older patient. *IM*, Intramuscular; *IV*, intravenous; *NG*, nasogastric; *PO*, by mouth; *PRN*, as needed; *TFTs*, thyroid function tests. (Modified from Goldman L, Ausiello D [eds]: *Cecil textbook of medicine*, ed 24, Philadelphia, 2012, Saunders.)

TABLE 2 Delirium Assessment Tools

Tool	Structure	Notes
Confusion Assessment Method (CAM)	Full scale of 11 items Abbreviated algorithm targeting four cardinal symptoms	Intended for use by nonpsychiatric clinicians
Confusion Assessment Method for the Intensive Care Unit (CAM-ICU)	Algorithm targeting four cardinal symptoms	Designed for use by nursing staff in the ICU
Intensive Care Delirium Screening Checklist (ICDSC)	8-item screening checklist	Bedside screening tool for use by nonpsychiatric physicians or nurses in the ICU
Delirium Rating Scale (DRS)	Full scale of 10 items Abbreviated 7- or 8-item subscales for repeated administration	Provides data for confirmation of diagnosis and measurement of severity
Delirium Rating Scale—Revised–98 (DRS-R-98)	16-item scale that can be divided into a 3-item diagnostic subscale and a 13-item severity subscale	Revision of DRS is better suited to repeat administration
Memorial Delirium Assessment Scale (MDAS)	10-item severity rating scale	Grades severity of delirium once diagnosis has been made
Neecham Confusion Scale	10-item rating scale	Designed for use by nursing staff and primarily validated for use in elderly populations in acute medical or nursing home setting

ICU, Intensive care unit.
From Stern TA et al: *Massachusetts General Hospital handbook of general hospital psychiatry,* ed 7, Philadelphia, 2017, Elsevier.

- Chest radiograph (to look for tumor, infection)

ELECTROENCEPHALOGRAM

To exclude seizure, confirm diagnosis of metabolic encephalopathy

Rx TREATMENT

NONPHARMACOLOGIC THERAPY

- The most important consideration is to keep the patient safe by using a variety of methods, including frequent reorientation.
- A quiet, restful, simplified environment with cues to time and location such as clock or calendar is helpful, as well as consistent staff providing both personal and medical care. If possible, encourage familiar family members and friends to keep the patient company.
- Early mobilization and minimized use of physical restraints (use of physical restraints if necessary to ensure safety).
- Visual and hearing aids for patients with these impairments.

ACUTE GENERAL Rx

- Reverse any treatable cause, such as volume repletion for patients with dehydration, antibiotics for urinary tract infection.
- Antipsychotic agents should not be used routinely for preventing or treating delirium. Pharmacologic treatment with antipsychotic agents should be initiated only when symptoms are severe, dangerous, or cause significant distress to the patient. In general these agents are similarly effective and the choice among them is usually made on the basis of side effects. Haloperidol is the least sedating but has a high risk of extrapyramidal side effects; quetiapine has the fewest side effects but is highly sedating.
- Haloperidol can be used with caution to control agitation, with doses ranging from 0.25 to 2 mg IM/IV twice daily, repeating the dose every 20 to 30 min until patient has calmed and using lower doses for the elderly.
- Most antipsychotics can prolong the QT interval and increase the risk of torsades de pointes. The effect is greatest with IV haloperidol and least with aripiprazole. Aripiprazole is available in tablets, solution, and injection. Starting dose is 1 mg twice a day.
- Risperidone 0.5 mg twice daily (off-label use, non-FDA approved) can also be used with caution with a slow increase to desired dose, not to exceed 1.0 to 2.0 mg.
- Avoid benzodiazepines and meperidine. Drug toxicity accounts for approximately 30% cases of delirium.

CHRONIC Rx

Delirium is not a chronic condition; if assessing a more long-term mental status change, consider other diagnoses.

DISPOSITION

Requires frequent monitoring often necessitating hospital level of care to ensure safety and assess etiology.

REFERRAL

Consider neurologic or psychiatric consultation if not improved in several days or in complicated cases.

PEARLS & CONSIDERATIONS

COMMENTS

Although benzodiazepines are frequently used in hospitalized patients for sedation and are the mainstay of therapy for alcohol withdrawal, they must be used with caution in the elderly because they can have a paradoxical effect on agitation.

PREVENTION (TABLE 5)

- Avoid polypharmacy as much as possible.
- Optimize chronic medical conditions.
- Provide frequent reorientation and a soothing environment for high-risk patients (e.g., lights on during the day, off at night; open curtains during the day so patient can see the weather).
- In patients over 70 without dementia, regular exercise has been associated with lower risk for developing delirium, and early return to physical activity can improve outcomes in ill patients.

PATIENT & FAMILY EDUCATION

Inform about the above preventive techniques, especially polypharmacy risks.

RELATED CONTENT

Delirium Tremens (Related Key Topic)

SUGGESTED READINGS

Available at ExpertConsult.com

AUTHOR: **Fred F. Ferri, MD**

TABLE 3 Differential Diagnosis of Delirium

General Cause	Specific Cause
Vascular	Hypertensive encephalopathy Cerebral arteriosclerosis Intracranial hemorrhage or thrombosis Emboli from atrial fibrillation, patent foramen ovale, or endocarditic valve Circulatory collapse (shock) Systemic lupus erythematosus Polyarteritis nodosa Thrombotic thrombocytopenic purpura Hyperviscosity syndrome Sarcoid Posterior reversible encephalopathy syndrome (PRES) Cerebral aneurysm
Infectious	Encephalitis Bacterial or viral meningitis, fungal meningitis *(cryptococcal, coccidioidal, histoplasma)* Sepsis General paresis Brain, epidural, or subdural abscess Malaria Human immunodeficiency virus Lyme disease Typhoid fever Parasitic *(toxoplasma, trichinosis, cysticercosis, echinococcosis)* Behçet syndrome Mumps
Neoplastic	Space-occupying lesions, such as gliomas, meningiomas, abscesses Paraneoplastic syndromes Carcinomatous meningitis
Degenerative	Dementias Huntington disease Creutzfeldt–Jakob disease Wilson disease
Intoxication	Chronic intoxication or withdrawal effect of drugs, including sedative-hypnotics, opiates, tranquilizers, anticholinergics, dissociative anesthetics, anticonvulsants
Neurophysiologic	Epilepsy Postictal states Complex partial status epilepticus
Traumatic	Intracranial bleeds Postoperative trauma Heat stroke Fat emboli syndrome
Intraventricular	Normal-pressure hydrocephalus
Vitamin deficiency	Thiamine (Wernicke–Korsakoff syndrome) Niacin (pellagra) B_{12} (pernicious anemia)
Endocrine/metabolic	Diabetic coma and shock Uremia Myxedema Hyperthyroidism Parathyroid dysfunction Hypoglycemia Hepatic or renal failure Porphyria Severe electrolyte or acid/base disturbances Cushing or Addison syndrome Sleep apnea Carcinoid Whipple disease
Autoimmune	Autoimmune encephalitides Steroid-responsive encephalopathy associated with thyroiditis (SREAT)/Hashimoto encephalopathy Systemic lupus erythematosus Multiple sclerosis
Poisoning	Heavy metals (lead, manganese, mercury) Carbon monoxide Anticholinergics Other toxins
Anoxia	Hypoxia and anoxia secondary to pulmonary or cardiac failure, anesthesia, anemia
Psychiatric	Depressive pseudodementia, catatonia, Bell mania

From Stern TA et al: *Massachusetts General Hospital handbook of general hospital psychiatry,* ed 7, Philadelphia, 2017, Elsevier.

TABLE 4 Clinical Factors That Help Differentiate Delirium and Dementia from Psychiatric Disease

Characteristic	Delirium	Dementia	Psychiatric Illness
Symptoms			
Age at onset	<12 or >40 yr	Usually elderly, >50 yr	13-40 yr
Onset	Acute	Gradual or insidious	Gradual
Symptom course	Rapid, fluctuating	Stable and progressive	Stable
Duration	Days to weeks	Months to years	Months to years
Reversibility	Usually	Rarely	Rarely
History			
Past medical history	Substance abuse, medical illness	Comorbid conditions of aging	Previous psychiatric history
Family history	Unusual	History of dementia	History of psychiatric illness
Physical Examination			
Vital signs	Usually abnormal	Usually normal	Usually normal
Involuntary activity	May have tremors, asterixis, etc.	None unless coexistent disease	None
Mental Status			
Affect	Emotional lability	Flat affect with advanced disease	Flat affect
Orientation	Usually impaired	Impaired with advanced disease	Rarely impaired
Attention	Impaired	Slow to focus	Disorganized
Hallucinations	Primarily visual	Rare	Primarily auditory
Speech	Slow, incoherent, dysarthric	Usually coherent	Usually coherent
Consciousness	Decreased to impaired	Normal (clear)	Alert
Intellectual function	Usually impaired	Impaired	Intact

From Adams JG et al: *Emergency medicine, clinical essentials*, ed 2, Philadelphia, 2013, Elsevier.

TABLE 5 Priorities (Consensus, Evidence-Based, and Speculative) for the Prevention, Management, and Advancement of the Treatment of Delirium

Community-Based Prevention	Hospital-Based Prevention	Hospital-Based Management	Postdischarge Management	Clinical Research Opportunities
Hospital avoidance strategies	Implementation of basic standards (e.g., screening for delirium) Minimization of iatrogenesis*	Implementation of basic standards (e.g., review of medications)*	Responsive, proportionate, and holistic follow-up*	Pragmatic research into optimizing care delivery
Identification and management of frailty	Multicomponent interventions to address frailty† Reorientation† Nutrition† Multidisciplinary care* Physiologic correction† Sensory optimization† Minimization of ward transfers* Avoidance of polypharmacy†	Multicomponent interventions to address frailty* Reorientation* Nutrition* Multidisciplinary care* Physiologic correction* Sensory optimization* Minimization of ward transfers* Reduction of drug burden*	Identification and management of frailty Reduction and cessation of antipsychotics	The interaction between frailty, interventions to ameliorate frailty, and delirium Transference from basic science models to trials of newer therapies Validation of delirium models using advanced imaging
Pleiotropic interventions (e.g., exercise/ nutrition)	Monitor and promote early mobilization†	Monitor and promote early mobilization*	Review of the primary triggers for delirium and other state variables (e.g., mobility)	Delirium, mobility, and response to physical therapy
Early diagnosis and management of dementia	Screening for dementia*	Screening for delirium resolution and residual cognitive impairment	Screening for subsyndromal delirium or dementia*	The interaction between dementia, including non-Alzheimer dementia, and delirium
Education of nursing home facilities and staff	Education of nursing and medical staff*	Education of medical and nursing staff*	Caregiver support and education	The role of education of nonmedical staff, families,‡ and general public using multimedia solutions
Integrated geriatric care for planned major surgery	Targeted drug treatments (e.g., melatonin for sleep disturbance)† Family-based screening/ reorientation†	Delirium units Supported early discharge Family-based screening/ reorientation* Management in the nursing home with CGA capability	Adaptive and versatile methods of follow-up such as telemedicine	The role of novel and targeted interventions and models of care supported by assistive technologies
Public health awareness	Audit of care and cycle of care improvement†	Audit of care and cycle of care improvement*	Public health awareness/ NGO engagement	Development of key indicators in the management of delirium

CGA, Comprehensive geriatric assessment; *NGO*, nongovernmental organization.
*Consensus role.
†Evidence-based role.
‡Speculative role.
From Fillit HM: *Brocklehurst's textbook of geriatric medicine and gerontology*, ed 8, 2017, Elsevier.

Delirium Tremens (PTG)

BASIC INFORMATION

DEFINITION

Delirium tremens, also known as withdrawal delirium, is overactivity of the central nervous system after cessation of alcohol intake. The time interval is variable; it usually occurs within 1 wk after reduction or cessation of heavy alcohol intake and persists for 1 to 3 days.

SYNONYMS

Withdrawal delirium
Alcohol withdrawal syndrome
DTs
Alcoholic delirium

ICD-10CM CODE
F10.231 Alcohol dependence with withdrawal delirium

EPIDEMIOLOGY & DEMOGRAPHICS

INCIDENCE (IN U.S.): Up to 500,000 cases annually, 3% to 5% of patients who are hospitalized for alcohol withdrawal meet the criteria for withdrawal delirium
PREDOMINANT SEX: Male
PREDOMINANT AGE: Teenage yrs and older
PEAK INCIDENCE: 30 yr and older
GENETICS: More common with patients who have relatives who are alcoholics

PHYSICAL FINDINGS & CLINICAL PRESENTATION

- Ethanol withdrawal symptoms usually begin within 8 hours after blood alcohol levels decrease, peak at about 72 hr, and are markedly reduced by days 5 to 7 of abstinence
- Initially: Anxiety, insomnia, tremulousness
- Early: Tachycardia, sweating, anorexia, agitation, headache, gastrointestinal distress
- Late: Seizures, visual hallucinations, delirium

ETIOLOGY

Alcoholism

DIAGNOSIS

DIFFERENTIAL DIAGNOSIS

- Coexisting illness
- Trauma
- Drug use

WORKUP

- Frequent rating of symptoms (hallucinations, tremor, sweating, agitation, orientation)
- The Clinical Institute Withdrawal Assessment-Alcohol (CIWA-A) scale can be used to measure the severity of alcohol withdrawal. It consists of the 10 following items:
  1. Nausea
  2. Tremor
  3. Autonomic hyperactivity
  4. Anxiety
  5. Agitation
  6. Tactile disturbances
  7. Visual disturbances
  8. Auditory disturbances
  9. Headache
  10. Disorientation

  The maximum score is 67. Scores <8 indicate mild symptoms; scores 8 to 15 indicate moderate withdrawal symptoms; and scores >15 indicate severe withdrawal symptoms.

LABORATORY TESTS

- Electrolytes (including magnesium, phosphate)
- Close monitoring of glucose levels
- Drug screen (blood and urine)

IMAGING STUDIES

CT scan of head if there is a history of head trauma.

TREATMENT

NONPHARMACOLOGIC THERAPY

Refer to drug rehabilitation program after patient recovers.

ACUTE GENERAL Rx

- Admission to a detoxification unit where patient can be observed closely.
- Vital signs q30min initially (neurologic signs, if necessary).
- Use of lateral decubitus or prone position if restraints are necessary.
- Nothing by mouth: Nasogastric tube for abdominal distention may be necessary but should not be routinely used.
- Vigorous hydration (4-6 L/day): IV with glucose (Na^+, K^+, PO_4^{-3}, and Mg^{2+} replacement). May be necessary in some patients but commonly there is little support for routine administration of magnesium. Use vigorous hydration with caution in patients with CHF.
- Vitamins: Thiamine 500 mg infused IV over the course of 30 minutes daily for 3 days. The initial dose of thiamine should precede the administration of IV dextrose; multivitamins (may be added to the hydrating solution).
- Sedation (sedation can be achieved using fixed-dose regimen or individualized benzodiazepine administration [see CIWA-Ar score] in "Alcohol Abuse" Chapter):
  1. Initially: Lorazepam 8 mg IM/IV every 15 minutes as needed, after the patient has received 16 mg. If delirium is still severe, administer an 8 mg bolus IV, then administer 10 to 30 mg/hr.1
  2. Maintenance (individualized dosage): Chlordiazepoxide, 50 to 100 mg PO q4 to 6h, lorazepam 2 mg PO q4h, or diazepam 5 to 10 mg PO tid; withhold doses or decrease subsequent doses if signs of oversedation are apparent.
  3. Midazolam is also effective for managing DTs. Its rapid onset (sedation within 2 to 4 min of IV injection) and short duration of action (approximately 30 min) make it an ideal agent for titration in continuous infusion.
- In addition to benzodiazepines, administer medications such as the antipsychotic agent haloperidol for uncontrolled agitation or hallucinations (0.5-5 mg IV/IM every 30-60 minutes as needed for severe agitation or hallucinations, not to exceed 20 mg).
- Treatment of seizures: Diazepam 2.5 mg/min IV until seizure is controlled (check for respiratory depression or hypotension) may be beneficial for prolonged seizure activity; IV lorazepam 1 to 2 mg q2h can be used in place of diazepam. In general, withdrawal seizures are self-limited and treatment is not required; the use of phenytoin or other anticonvulsants for short-term treatment of alcohol withdrawal seizures is not recommended.
- Diagnosis and treatment of concomitant medical, surgical, or psychiatric conditions.[1]

CHRONIC Rx

Alcoholics Anonymous has the best record in breaking addiction, but the results are still disappointing.

DISPOSITION

Refer to drug rehabilitation program

REFERRAL

If cardiac arrhythmias are prominent or respiratory distress develops.

PEARLS & CONSIDERATIONS

COMMENTS

This is a potentially lethal disease if not carefully treated. Mortality rate is 15% in untreated patients, and approximately 1% to 6% of hospitalized patients who have withdrawal delirium die.

SUGGESTED READING
Available at ExpertConsult.com

RELATED CONTENT

Delirium Tremens (Patient Information)
Alcohol Abuse (Related Key Topic)
Delirium (Related Key Topic)
Wernicke Syndrome (Related Key Topic)

AUTHOR: **Fred F. Ferri, MD**

[1]Schuckit MA: Recognition and management of withdrawal delirium (delirium tremens), *N Engl J Med* 371:2109-2113, 2014.

BASIC INFORMATION

DEFINITION

Dementia with Lewy bodies (DLB) is a neurodegenerative dementia occurring concurrently with or within 1 yr (either before or after) of the onset of parkinsonism. DLB also has other core features including fluctuations in attention and alertness and recurrent vivid visual hallucinations. Diagnostic criteria for dementia syndrome associated with Lewy body pathology are described in Table 1. Patients generally respond to cholinesterase inhibitors, are very sensitive to the adverse effects of neuroleptics, and are less responsive to levodopa compared with Parkinson disease patients.

SYNONYMS

DLB
Lewy body dementia
Diffuse Lewy body disease
Lewy body type senile dementia
Cortical Lewy body disease

ICD-10CM CODE
G31.83 Dementia with Lewy bodies

EPIDEMIOLOGY & DEMOGRAPHICS

INCIDENCE: Accounts for 10% to 15% of all dementias. DLB is the second most common neurodegenerative cause of dementia after Alzheimer disease.

PREVALENCE: Estimated 0.7% of individuals older than age 65

PREDOMINANT SEX & AGE:
- Sex: Male predominance
- Mean age of onset: 75 yr. On average, 10 yr greater for dementia with Lewy bodies (DLB) than Parkinson disease (PD).

PEAK INCIDENCE: Affects individuals in their sixth decade or older

RISK FACTORS:
- Male sex
- Advanced age

GENETICS:
- Most cases are sporadic with a discordance among monozygotic twins, suggesting that either environmental or other epigenetic factors may play a major role in the incidence of DLB.
- Copy number variation of the alpha-synuclein gene (*SNCA*) has been reported in families with DLB. Rare autosomal dominant variants in *LRRK2* have also been reported. These genes are associated with Parkinson disease and Parkinson disease dementia in addition to DLB, suggesting a common molecular etiology with a spectrum of clinical phenotypes.
- The *APOE* ε4 allele has a higher prevalence in DLB than in control individuals, suggesting heightened disease risk conferred by the allele. Conversely, the *APOE* ε2 allele is enriched in control individuals, suggesting a neuroprotective role, or at least the lack of a deleterious effect, for the allele.
- Other factors include glucocerebrosidase genetic mutations, high prevalence of Lewy bodies with presenilin-1 mutations, and polymorphisms of the coding region for the synuclein genes.

PHYSICAL FINDINGS & CLINICAL PRESENTATION

- Importance of recognizing DLB relates to its pharmacologic management, including responsiveness to cholinesterase inhibitors, sensitivity to the adverse effects of neuroleptics, and relative unresponsiveness to levodopa.
- Onset of dementia is insidious, with core features of fluctuations in cognition, attention, and alertness; recurrent vivid visual hallucinations; and extrapyramidal motor symptoms, along with other features either suggestive or supportive of the clinical diagnosis.
- Syncopal events or unexplained episodes of severe alteration in mentation.
- Repeated falls.
- Detailed neuropsychological assessment demonstrates a characteristic profile of impairments in visuoperceptual, attentional, and executive functions, with relative sparing of episodic memory (in contradistinction to Alzheimer diseases, in which impairment in episodic memory is a hallmark), reflecting a combination of cortical and subcortical damage.

ETIOLOGY

- *SNCA* encodes for a protein normally found at the synapse with a role in vesicle production. In its insoluble form, SNCA aggregates into Lewy bodies found at the cortical and subcortical levels.
- Lewy bodies (Fig. E1) are round, eosinophilic, intracytoplasmic inclusions in the nuclei of neurons.
- Cortical Lewy bodies are found in deep cortical layers of the anterior frontal and temporal lobes, the cingulate gyrus, and insula.
- As in Parkinson disease, Lewy bodies aggregate in the following structures: Substantia nigra, locus ceruleus, raphe nuclei, nucleus basalis of Meynert, and brainstem nuclei.
- Fig. E2 shows the relationships among the subtypes of dementia.
- Many patients with DLB also have evidence of amyloidosis and tauopathy typical of Alzheimer disease. These patients often have a worse cognitive profile than pure DLB, with a cognitive phenotype typical of both Alzheimer disease (episodic memory loss) and DLB (inattention, executive dysfunction, and visuospatial dysfunction).

DIAGNOSIS

DIFFERENTIAL DIAGNOSIS

- Diagnosis of DLB when dementia occurs before or concurrently with extrapyramidal features—arbitrarily set as the "1-yr rule" vs. Parkinson disease with dementia, which occurs in the setting of well-established Parkinson disease.
- Dementia: Alzheimer disease (AD), vascular dementia, frontotemporal dementia. However, some patients have pathological overlap of AD and DLB or DLB and vascular dementia.
- Parkinsonian features: Parkinson disease dementia, progressive supranuclear palsy (PSP), corticobasal syndrome (CBS), and multisystem atrophy (MSA).
- Rapidly progressive form: Creutzfeldt-Jakob disease (CJD). Lack of cerebellar signs and lack of typical MRI may help distinguish DLB from classic CJD (but not variant form of CJD).
- Psychiatric features: Late-onset psychosis or depression with psychotic features.
- Hallucinations with fluctuations in consciousness: Temporal lobe epilepsy (TLE) or delirium due to metabolic or autoimmune derangement.

WORKUP

- MRI of the brain to evaluate for structural causes of dementia and exclude MRI features of vascular dementia or CJD
- Lumbar puncture to rule out underlying chronic infections, especially if there are atypical features
- Electroencephalogram (EEG) if there is concern about TLE. However, both DLB and TLE may show nonspecific slowing or periodic complexes.
- DaTscan [Ioflupane (123I)] imaging is a SPECT scan preceded by injection of a radiopharmaceutical that detects the loss of functional dopaminergic neuron terminals in the striatum, reflecting underlying Parkinson disease or DLB.

LABORATORY TESTS

Rule out other potential reversible causes for dementia including: Complete blood count, complete metabolic panel, thyroid stimulating hormone, and B12. Consider RPR and HIV testing as well.

IMAGING STUDIES

- MRI typically shows a relative preservation of the hippocampi and medial temporal lobe volumes (in contrast to AD) but generalized atrophy and white matter changes.
- Functional imaging including single photon emission computed tomography (SPECT) may demonstrate hypoperfusion of the parietal lobes, and in those with visual hallucinations, occipital region (specific finding but not sensitive).

TREATMENT

Patient and caregiver education about benefits, side effects, and limitations of treatment is very important. Caregivers may be encouraged to avoid neuroleptics unless the psychotic features either trouble or endanger the patient. If neuroleptics must be used, typical neuroleptics must be avoided.

TABLE 1 Revised Criteria for the Clinical Diagnosis of Probable and Possible Dementia with Lewy Bodies (DLB)

Essential for a diagnosis of DLB is dementia, defined as a progressive cognitive decline of sufficient magnitude to interfere with normal social or occupational functions, or with usual daily activities. Prominent or persistent memory impairment may not necessarily occur in the early stages but is usually evident with progression. Deficits on tests of attention, executive function, and visuoperceptual ability may be especially prominent and occur early.

Core clinical features (*The first 3 typically occur early and may persist throughout the course.*)

- Fluctuating cognition with pronounced variations in attention and alertness.
- Recurrent visual hallucinations that are typically well formed and detailed.
- REM sleep behavior disorder, which may precede cognitive decline.
- One or more spontaneous cardinal features of parkinsonism: These are bradykinesia (defined as slowness of movement and decrement in amplitude or speed), rest tremor, or rigidity.

Supportive clinical features

- Severe sensitivity to antipsychotic agents; postural instability, repeated falls, syncope or other transient episodes of unresponsiveness; severe autonomic dysfunction, e.g., constipation, orthostatic hypotension, urinary incontinence; hypersomnia; hyposmia; hallucinations in other modalities; systematized delusions; apathy, anxiety, and depression.

Indicative biomarkers

- Relative preservation of medial temporal lobe structures on CT/MRI scan.
- Generalized low uptake on SPECT/PET perfusion/metabolism scan with reduced occipital activity ± the cingulate island sign on FDG-PET imaging.
- Prominent posterior slow-wave activity on EEG with periodic fluctuations in the pre-alpha/theta range.

Probable DLB can be diagnosed if:

a. Two or more core clinical features of DLB are present, with or without the presence of indicative biomarkers, or

b. Only one core clinical feature is present but with one or more indicative biomarkers.

Probable DLB should not be diagnosed on the basis of biomarkers alone.

Probable DLB can be diagnosed if:

a. Only one core clinical feature of DLB is present, with no indicative biomarkers evidence, or

b. One or more indicative biomarkers is present but there are no clinical features.

DLB is less likely:

a. In the presence of any other physical illness or brain disorder including cerebrovascular disease, sufficient to account in part of in total for the clinical picture, although these do not exclude a DLB diagnosis and may serve to indicate mixed or multiple pathologies contributing to the clinical presentation, or

b. If parkinsonian features are the only core clinical feature and appear for the first time at a state of severe dementia.

DLB should be diagnosed when dementia occurs before or concurrently with parkinsonism. The term Parkinson disease dementia (PDD) should be used to describe dementia that occurs in the context of well-established Parkinson disease. In a practice setting, the term that is most appropriate to the clinical situation should be used, and generic terms such as Lewy body disease are often helpful. In research studies in which distinction need to be made between DLB and PDD, the existing 1-yr-rule between the onset of dementia and parkinsonism continues to be recommended.

CT, Computed tomography; *EEG,* electroencephalogram; *FDG-PET,* fluorodeoxyglucose-positron emission tomography; *MRI,* magnetic resonance imaging; *PET,* positron emission tomography; *REM,* rapid eye movements; *SPECT,* single-photon emission computerized tomography.

From McKeith IG et al: Diagnosis and management of dementia with Lewy bodies: fourth consensus report of the DLB Consortium, *Neurology* 89(1):88-100, 2017.

NONPHARMACOLOGIC THERAPY

- Social interaction and environmental novelty may improve cognitive dysfunction and psychiatric features often exacerbated by low levels of arousal and attention
- Behavioral methods, such as avoiding previously exposed environmental triggers known to cause anxiety, agitation, or aggression
- Physical therapy, mobility aids, and daily exercise

ACUTE GENERAL Rx

Atypical neuroleptic for disabling, persistent, bothersome (to the patient) psychotic features despite initiation of a cholinesterase inhibitor. A very low dose of an atypical antipsychotic (quetiapine 12.5 mg daily) may be started after patient/caregiver education regarding the sensitivity to neuroleptics. However, all neuroleptics do carry a boxed warning from the FDA about the increased mortality risk associated with neuroleptic use in patients with dementia. Patients and/or caregivers should be informed of this risk and allowed to balance the risk against the perceived benefit.

CHRONIC Rx

- Cholinesterase inhibitors for cognitive and behavioral symptoms. Rivastigmine (6-12 mg per day orally or 9.5 mg per day by transdermal patch) has shown in randomized controlled trial (RCT) to significantly reduce anxiety, delusions, and hallucinations, as well as significantly improved performance on neuropsychological testing.
- Parkinson disease medications for disabling parkinsonian features. Carbidopa/levodopa is reported to be more effective with fewer side effects than dopamine agonists. Begin at a low dose—25/100 mg three times a day—and slowly titrate over several weeks as tolerated and according to response.
- Selective serotonin reuptake inhibitors are commonly used for depression.
- If rapid eye movement (REM) sleep disorder remains disabling (or patient has not responded to an atypical antipsychotic initiated for psychosis), a trial of low-dose clonazepam (0.25-0.5 mg) or melatonin (3 mg) at bedtime remains an option.
- Orthostatic hypotension may be aided by nonpharmacologic therapy such as supportive stockings or pharmacologically by midodrine, fludrocortisone, or droxidopa.
- Memantine demonstrated an improvement in clinical global measure and remains well tolerated but may worsen hallucinations or delusions.
- Avoid anticholinergics (including tricyclic antidepressants), benzodiazepines, and typical neuroleptics as they can trigger delirium and worsen symptoms.

DISPOSITION

- Survival resembles the progression of AD, but a minority of cases may have a rapid disease course.
- Progression in cognitive decline, similar to AD, by approximately 10% per yr on cognitive testing.

REFERRAL

DLB requires a multidisciplinary approach including the general practitioner, neurologist, neuropsychologist, and/or neuropsychiatrist.

PEARLS & CONSIDERATIONS

COMMENTS

- Clinical presentation helps differentiate DLB from AD. AD presents with early signs of anterograde episodic memory loss without the benefit of cues on neuropsychological testing due to cortical atrophy at the medial temporal lobe region.
- Vascular dementia may also present with evidence of frontal-subcortical features but typically without the core features listed in the criteria above.
- Bed partners may report that individuals with DLB "act out their dreams," sometimes violently, leading to sleeping in separate beds. This history may indicate REM sleep behavior disorder. A history of REM sleep behavior may precede the diagnosis by many yr. However, REM sleep behavior does not necessarily lead to DLB.

PATIENT & FAMILY EDUCATION

- Visual hallucinations (VH) typically consist of innocuous, well-formed, detailed images of animate figures. These are classically labeled

Lilliputian, as the hallucinatory images are often relatively small. Unless VH lead to a potential threat to self or others, avoid antipsychotics due to the sensitivity of neuroleptics. Family/friends are often more alarmed by the VH than the patient with DLB.

- Apathy is a common clinical feature of DLB and mimics changes in mood, including depression or excessive daytime somnolence. These features are often noticed by family/friends.

SUGGESTED READINGS

Available at ExpertConsult.com

AUTHORS: **Angad Jolly, PhD,** and **Joseph S. Kass, MD, JD, FAAN**

BASIC INFORMATION

DEFINITION

Major depression is an episodic, frequently recurring syndrome. The diagnosis requires that five of nine criteria be present for 2 wk. One of these nine criteria must be either a persistent depressed mood or pervasive anhedonia (loss of interest or pleasure in all, or almost all, usual interests or activities). Other symptoms include sleep disturbance (insomnia, hypersomnia, or interrupted sleep), appetite loss/gain or weight loss/gain, fatigue, psychomotor retardation or agitation, difficulty concentrating or indecisiveness, feelings of guilt or worthlessness, and recurrent thoughts of death or suicidal ideation.

SYNONYMS

Unipolar affective disorder
Clinical depression
Melancholia
Manic-depressive illness, depressed type
Depressive episode

Codes depend on whether the episode is single or recurrent, and also on clinical severity.

ICD-10CM CODES	
F32.9	Depressive episode, unspecified
F33.0	Recurrent depressive episode, current episode mild
F33.1	Recurrent depressive disorder, current episode moderate
F33.2	Recurrent depressive disorder, current episode severe without psychotic symptoms
F33.3	Recurrent depressive disorder, current episode severe with psychotic symptoms
F33.4	Recurrent depressive disorder, currently in remission
F33.9	Recurrent depressive disorder, unspecified
DSM-5 CODES	
296.21	Single episode
296.22	Single episode, moderate
296.23	Single episode, severe
296.24	Single episode, with psychotic features
296.31	Recurrent, mild
296.32	Recurrent, moderate
296.33	Recurrent severe
296.34	Recurrent, with psychotic features

EPIDEMIOLOGY & DEMOGRAPHICS

LIFETIME RISK (IN U.S.): 15% of men, 26% of women

PREVALENCE (IN U.S.): Point prevalence in a community sample is 3% of men, 4.5% to 9.3% of women, and 1% of children. 12-mo prevalence is 7.2% in men and 13% in women. Prevalence is 20% to 40% in patients with comorbid medical conditions.

PREDOMINANT SEX: Lifetime risk female/male ratio 1.7:1.

PREDOMINANT AGE: Mean age of onset of first episode is 29, though prevalent in all ages, and 5% in adolescents.

PEAK INCIDENCE: 25 to 40 yr; 13% of postpartum women.

GENETICS:
- Clear evidence of familial predominance.
- Prevalence is 2 to 3 times greater among first-degree relatives.
- Concordance among monozygotic twins approximately 50%.
- Several studies have documented associations between various genes and increased risk for major depressive disorder (MDD), but there remains no established pattern of inheritance.

PHYSICAL FINDINGS & CLINICAL PRESENTATION

- Clinical evaluation facilitated by organizing the major symptoms into four hallmarks: (1) Depressed mood, (2) anhedonia, (3) physical symptoms (sleep disturbance, appetite problem, fatigue, psychomotor changes), and (4) psychological symptoms (difficulty concentrating or indecisiveness, guilt or worthlessness, and suicidal ideation).
- A stressful life event, typically a serious loss, may trigger a depressive episode. DSM-5 recommends that clinical judgment be used to determine if depression in the context of a loss should be diagnosed as a major depressive episode versus normal grief or adjustment disorder.
- Somatic complaints such as pain, fatigue, insomnia, dizziness, headache, or gastrointestinal problems occur in more than two-thirds of patients presenting to primary care with underlying depression.
- Comorbid psychiatric disorders are often present. Anxiety disorders are the most common comorbid conditions.
- Subtypes of depression include those with psychotic features. May be associated with mood-congruent delusional thinking (paranoid and melancholic themes).
- May be associated with active or passive suicidal ideation.
- May be underdiagnosed in elderly patients, with signs and symptoms attributed to normal aging or cognitive impairment.
- May be underdiagnosed in medically ill patients, with signs and symptoms attributed to medical illness or considered appropriate reaction to medical condition.

ETIOLOGY

- A heterogeneous group of disorders probably arising from various etiologies.
- Genetic and environmental experiences, and their interaction, each contribute.
- Significant psychosocial stressors, including losses, trauma, and ramifications of adverse childhood events, often trigger depression, particularly for first episodes.
- Numerous biologic correlates have been identified, though none is considered causative or diagnostic. Genes that influence the production and reuptake of serotonin, norepinephrine, dopamine, and glutamate, as well as nerve cell growth in brain regions underlying memory and emotional processing, are of greatest interest. Abnormalities in brain regions underlying executive functioning, emotion regulation, and reward processing, as well as irregularities in functional connectivity have been identified. Irregularities in cortisol responding and inflammation also may play a role.
- Cognitive risk factors include a pessimistic style of explaining negative events, a tendency to ruminate, and biases in processing emotional information and events.

Dx DIAGNOSIS

DIFFERENTIAL DIAGNOSIS

- Time-course and symptomatology can distinguish MDD from persistent depressive disorder (dysthymia), premenstrual dysphoric disorder, and substance-induced mood disorder.
- Anxiety disorders, posttraumatic stress disorder [PTSD], obsessive compulsive disorder, substance abuse, and personality disorders often present with depressive symptoms or coexist with major depressive disorder.
- Important to determine if a depressive episode is part of major depression or part of bipolar disorder, which entails carefully screening for a history of manic symptoms.
- Important to distinguish from adjustment disorder. Depression in the context of a stressful life event is diagnosed as major depressive disorder if the symptom criteria are met and adjustment disorder if the symptom criteria are not met. Psychotherapy, rather than medication, is the treatment mainstay for adjustment disorder.
- Approximately 10% to 15% of depression is caused by general medical illnesses, such as Alzheimer disease, Parkinson disease, stroke, end-stage renal failure, cardiac disease, HIV infection, and cancer.
- Some medical conditions can present with depressive symptoms (e.g., hypothyroidism, hyperthyroidism, pancreatic cancer, and neurosyphilis).
- Depression can coexist with dementia, though depression-related cognitive dysfunction (formerly known as "pseudo-dementia") must also be considered in such populations.

WORKUP

- Careful medical history is required to rule out nonprimary psychiatric etiology.
- Physical examination reveals no specific diagnostic signs of depression, though psychomotor changes can be observed.
- Mental status examination.
- Self-report scales can assist in screening.
- Commonly used validated screening tools include the 15-item Geriatric Depression Scale in the elderly and the Patient Health Questionnaire (PHQ)-2 and PHQ-9. The PHQ-2

has a 97% sensitivity and 67% specificity in adults. If it is positive for depression, the PHQ-9 should be administered. The PHQ-9 has a 61% sensitivity and 94% specificity for depression in adults.

LABORATORY TESTS

- Research is underway to identify biomarkers that may be useful in diagnosis, but as of yet no laboratory studies are diagnostic.
- The following can assist in ruling out other confounding issues:
  1. Routine blood chemistry evaluation
  2. CBC with differential
  3. Thyroid function studies
  4. Vitamin B_{12} levels

IMAGING STUDIES

With unusual presentations (e.g., associated with new-onset severe headache, focal neurologic signs, a cognitive or sensory disturbance), the following may be performed:

- Electroencephalogram (EEG) (diffuse slowing indicates metabolic encephalopathy)
- Anatomic brain imaging (CT scan or MRI)

Rx TREATMENT

NONPHARMACOLOGIC THERAPY

- Good evidence exists that cognitive-behavioral therapy is as effective as antidepressant medication in achieving significant reduction or remission (Table 1). Meta-analysis indicates that combining psychotherapy with medication is modestly more effective than either modality alone.
- Problem-solving and interpersonal psychotherapies are comparably efficacious.
- Various forms of cognitive-behavioral therapy (e.g., acceptance and commitment, mindfulness-based [MBCT], and dialectical behavioral [DBT]), as well as traditional CBT, have demonstrated efficacy in numerous studies.
- Growing evidence indicates that internet-based CBT and brief therapy interventions integrated into primary care to expand access to therapy are efficacious, with some studies finding comparable efficacy to standard length interventions.
- By 12 wk or earlier, psychotherapy and medication approaches are equally effective.
- Augmentation of standard depression treatment with CBT to address insomnia (CBT-I) was found to significantly improve response rates.
- Official treatment guidelines recommend that medication be used as the first-line treatment for patients with severe depression, although some studies have found equal efficacy of medication and psychotherapy in the treatment of severe depression.
- Factors, including history of adverse childhood events, presence of precipitant stressful life events, family psychiatric history, the presence of anhedonia, and depression severity may affect treatment response and risk of recurrence. Numerous genetic and neurobiologic variables that predict treatment response have been identified, particularly in combination with one another or with clinical characteristics. However, at present, there are no universally accepted markers that can aid clinicians in matching individuals to particular medications or interventions.

TABLE 1 Treatments of Depression

Name of Psychotherapy	Approach
Cognitive psychotherapy	Identify and correct negativistic patterns of thinking.
Interpersonal psychotherapy	Identify and work through role transitions or interpersonal losses, conflicts, or deficits.
Problem-solving therapy	Identify and prioritize situational problems; plan and implement strategies to deal with top-priority problems.
Psychodynamic psychotherapy	Use therapeutic relationship to maximize use of the healthiest defense mechanisms and coping strategies.

From Goldman L et al: *Goldman's Cecil medicine,* ed 24, Philadelphia, 2012, Saunders.

ACUTE GENERAL Rx

- Concurrent medical or psychiatric illnesses, history of prior response, cost, patient preference, and side effects should be considered when selecting initial treatment.
- Antidepressants are helpful in approximately 60% to 70% of cases, though sustained remission rates are lower.
- Selective serotonin reuptake inhibitors (SSRIs) are generally first line. According to the Sequenced Treatment Alternatives to Relieve Depression (STAR-D) trial, approximately 30% achieve remission with the first prescribed medication after 3 mo of treatment. Another 25% to 30% respond to treatment but do not achieve remission. Treatment-refractory patients may be switched to another SSRI or another class of medication may be more helpful, offered adjunctive medication such as bupropion, or referred for evidence-based counseling. Approximately 25% more patients will achieve remission with this secondary intervention.
- According to a network meta-analysis of 21 antidepressants, escitalopram, mirtazapine, paroxetine, and sertraline had higher response and lower dropout rates than other antidepressants, and all antidepressants were more effective than placebo.
- Response to antidepressants for many patients is seen as early as 2 wk, and among patients showing little to no response, the odds of later response decrease the longer patients remain unimproved. Conversely, rapid response to treatment predicted improved outcomes in multiple studies.
- Antidepressants may transiently increase suicidality and aggression in patients under 25, an important side effect to discuss prior to treatment initiation.
- To date, there are no data to support combining antidepressants as first-line treatment. There is also no clear advantage to switching medications within vs. across different classes, or to switching vs. augmentation. The Veterans Affairs (VA) Augmentation and Switching Treatments for Improving Depression Outcomes (VAST-D) trial found that switching to the antipsychotic aripiprazole resulted in statistically significant, though modest, improvement in remission rates compared with switching or augmenting with an antidepressant, although greater side effects resulted. More research is needed.
- Therapy should be continued for 4 to 9 mo after the full remission of symptoms.
- Electroconvulsive therapy (ECT) is the most effective means available for the treatment of severe, refractory depression. Transcranial magnetic stimulation (TMS) has also shown evidence of efficacy, though the magnitude of effects is more variable and overall smaller than ECT. Research is underway to investigate mechanisms to increase the efficacy of TMS.
- Antipsychotic medication should be added for psychotic depression. Antipsychotic medication has also been shown to be helpful in augmenting antidepressants for nonpsychotic depression, and it may be beneficial for individuals with mixed manic-depressive features, although more research is needed.
- Ketamine IV has been found to be rapidly effective in treatment-resistant and suicidal depression. Intranasal esketamine (Spravato) is approved for use in treatment-resistant depression. Further research is needed to determine whether positive effects are maintained, as effectiveness appears to fade without repeated use.
- Early data from open-label trials of psilocybin for treatment-resistant depression suggest sustained improvement of depressive symptoms at 3 and 6 mo, though more research is needed.

CHRONIC Rx

Long-term treatment, in some cases lifelong, is recommended for multiple depressive episodes, an episode duration longer than 2 yr, a severe episode or significant suicidality, or a strong family history of severe depression or bipolar disorder.

DISPOSITION

- Major depression is often a relapsing and remitting illness.

- Additional episodes are experienced by >50% of patients after one episode, with each additional episode linked to increased risk for subsequent episodes.
- Without treatment, episodes last an average of 6 to 12 mo; risk of recurrence higher without treatment.
- For many depressed individuals, subthreshold residual symptoms are present between episodes and define the majority of an individual's course of depression. Such symptoms may lead to impairment and warrant prolonged treatment.

REFERRAL

- If treatment-refractory
- If patient is suicidal or psychotic
- For suspected bipolar depression

PEARLS & CONSIDERATIONS

COMMENTS

- All threats of suicide should be taken very seriously. Clinicians can use the mnemonic SAL: Is the method specific? Is it available? Is it lethal?
- Rule out bipolar affective disorder before initiating antidepressant medication. Screening scales for bipolar disorder can be helpful in primary care settings to identify patients at increased risk for bipolar disorder. Antidepressants can induce mania in susceptible patients.
- Comorbid or diagnostically-related entities such as OCD, generalized anxiety, and PTSD, while sometimes difficult to differentiate from MDD, share similar pharmacologic and therapy-based treatment principles.
- A two-question screener (PHQ2) is as effective as longer instruments. A positive answer to either question warrants a full assessment.
  1. Over the past 2 wk, have you ever felt down, depressed, or hopeless?
  2. Over the past 2 wk, have you felt little interest or pleasure in doing things?
- Depression screening programs without treatment programs are unlikely to improve depression outcomes.
- Strict monitoring of patients who initiate antidepressant therapy is necessary both for safety and to ensure optimal treatment. Use of self-report scales to measure symptom severity is helpful in monitoring outcome and may result in improved outcomes.
- St. John's wort *(Hypericum perforatum)* is sold as a dietary supplement in the United States and is used for depression in the community. It is not consistently effective and should not be used in combination with antidepressants given the possibility of severe serotonin-related side effects, as well as effects on the metabolism of other drugs.

SUGGESTED READINGS

Available at ExpertConsult.com

RELATED CONTENT

Depression (Patient Information)
Bipolar Disorder (Related Key Topic)

AUTHORS: **Rachel L. MacLean, MD,** and **Mark Zimmerman, MD**

BASIC INFORMATION

DEFINITION

Dermatitis herpetiformis (DH) is an autoimmune blistering disease that is considered to be a cutaneous manifestation of celiac disease (CD). It is associated with gluten-sensitive enteropathy in nearly all cases, although only 20% of patients have gastrointestinal symptoms. 15% to 25% of patients with CD will have DH.

SYNONYMS

DH
Duhring disease

ICD-10CM CODE
L13.0 Dermatitis herpetiformis

EPIDEMIOLOGY & DEMOGRAPHICS

PREVALENCE (IN U.S.): 11 cases per 100,000 persons per yr; prevalence for CD is one in 133 adults
PREDOMINANT SEX: Male predominance (2:1); however, female predominance in children
PREDOMINANT AGE: Fourth decade of life, but can occur at any age
PREDOMINANT RACE: Most common in Caucasians of northern European ancestry
GENETICS: Both CD and DH have a strong genetic component. 10% to 15% of patients with DH have a first-degree relative with either DH or CD. Specific HLA genes (involved in processing gliadin antigen in genetically susceptible individuals) have also been shown to predispose to developing DH (HLA-DQ2 in 90%, DQ8 in the remaining 10%). However, less than 50% of genetic predisposition is attributed to HLA genes. Autoimmune disorders associated with dermatitis herpetiformis are summarized in Table E1.

PHYSICAL FINDINGS & CLINICAL PRESENTATION

- Classically, the lesions of DH are small, grouped, "herpetiform" vesicles that are distributed symmetrically on extensor surfaces (elbows, knees [Fig. E1], scalp, back, and buttocks). However, due to intense pruritus and scratching, pinpoint erosions and excoriations in the above distribution are often the most prominent findings on examination, with intact vesicles rarely seen.
- Spontaneous improvement with cyclic exacerbations is common.
- Celiac-type enamel defects to permanent teeth, oral vesicles, or palmoplantar purpura have been reported as potential associated findings.

PATHOGENESIS

CD and DH are both autoimmune-mediated by immunoglobulin A (IgA) class autoantibodies. Dietary gluten is central to the pathogenesis in both. In genetically predisposed individuals, it is hypothesized that the gluten by-product, gliadin, complexes with tissue transglutaminase (tTG) in the gut, binding as an antigen to HLA-DQ2 on T cells, creating an immune response that results in anti-tTG IgA antibodies (i.e., antiendomysial antibodies) in the blood. tTG cross-reacts with epidermal TG (eTG). The blood of CD patients with and without skin disease is found to have both skin and gut anti-TG IgA antibodies. Yet, it is thought that the high-affinity IgA against eTG form complexes that are responsible for DH. The deposition of IgA-eTG complexes in the papillary dermis triggers an immunologic cascade resulting in neutrophil recruitment and complement activation.

DIAGNOSIS

Physical examination and routine histopathology are often suggestive of DH; however, direct immunofluorescence (DIF) of a perilesional skin biopsy has pathognomonic findings and is the gold standard for diagnosis. Fig. 2 describes an approach to the patient with suspected dermatitis herpetiformis.

DIFFERENTIAL DIAGNOSIS

- Clinically and histologically, the differential diagnosis includes:
  1. Linear IgA dermatosis
  2. Bullous pemphigoid
  3. Bullous lupus

  These diagnoses can be differentiated by DIF on perilesional skin biopsy.
- Other clinical diagnoses to consider:
  1. Scabies (check for interdigital burrows and involvement of genitalia)
  2. Arthropod bite (urticarial papules, often in groups of 3, over-exposed areas)
  3. Eczematous dermatitis (ill-defined, erythematous and xerotic plaques or deep seeded vesicles on hands)
  4. Herpes simplex or zoster infection (painful, not symmetric)
  5. Generalized pruritus (no blister history, not limited to extensor surfaces)

WORKUP AND LABORATORY TESTS

- Evaluation for gastrointestinal symptoms, family history of DH or CD, and pruritus should be sought in patients with suspected DH.
- **Lesional skin biopsy:** Will demonstrate a neutrophil-rich subepidermal bulla and rule out many conditions.
- **DIF of normal-appearing perilesional skin biopsy:** Will demonstrate pathognomonic IgA deposits localized to the dermal papillae and dermal-epidermal junction in a granular pattern.
- Serology (enzyme-linked immunosorbent assay [ELISA]) for IgA tissue transglutaminase, ELISA for IgA epidermal transglutaminase, if available, and indirect immunofluorescence for IgA endomysial antibodies (total IgA) can be used to aid in the diagnosis of DH in cases where the DIF is negative or equivocal, or for monitoring disease activity response to treatment. Although these circulating antibodies in the blood exist, there is a high false-negative rate for antitissue TG and for antiendomysial antibodies (one third of DH patients are negative for antiendomysial antibodies), and their absence does not exclude the diagnosis. Also, IgA-deficient DH patients may also have negative serologic results. Those with the presence of circulating antibodies will have a reduction in levels in response to treatment adherence.

TREATMENT

A gluten-free diet (GFD) and dapsone are considered first-line therapy and are often started in conjunction.

- GFD improves symptoms of both GI and skin disease, with GI responding quicker (skin responds after 2 mo). A retrospective study showed remission (2 yr without symptoms) in 12%.
- Dapsone results in improvement of skin manifestations within days but does not treat GI manifestations. Dapsone is typically tapered over time, while lifelong gluten avoidance is often necessary.
- One study demonstrated GFD alone was comparable to GFD plus dapsone in the treatment of DH; hence GFD is an essential component in the treatment of DH.

NONPHARMACOLOGIC THERAPY

- First line: GFD:
  1. Avoid barley, rye, wheat (can consume rice, corn, and oats).
  2. Consultation with a dietitian is recommended.
  3. Most patients need to follow diet indefinitely; however, cases of spontaneous remission have been reported.
- Second line: Elemental diet (controversial):
  1. Can consider elemental diet (avoidance of whole proteins) in those patients who do not adequately respond to a strict GFD; however, data are limited.

ACUTE GENERAL Rx

- First line: Dapsone:
  1. Initial dose 25 to 50 mg PO daily with gradual increase to an average maintenance dose of 0.5 to 1 mg/kg daily (often maintenance dose of 100 mg daily).
  2. Clinical monitoring weekly is recommended to optimize dose (optimal dose is when 1-2 new lesions/wk).
  3. Caution: Dapsone may produce hemolysis (especially if G6PD deficiency), agranulocytosis, methemoglobinemia, systemic drug hypersensitivity reaction (DRESS), and long-term, a peripheral neuropathy.
  4. Baseline labs: CBC, LFTs, G6PD levels. After the initiation of therapy, monitor CBC every wk ×1 mo, then every other wk ×2 mo, monthly ×3 mo, then every 3 to 4 mo. Monitor LFTs every 3 to 4 mo.
- Second-line alternatives:
  1. Sulfapyridine (500-1500 mg/day, compounded medication) or sulfasalazine (500-1000 mg bid) may be substituted in cases of dapsone intolerance or in

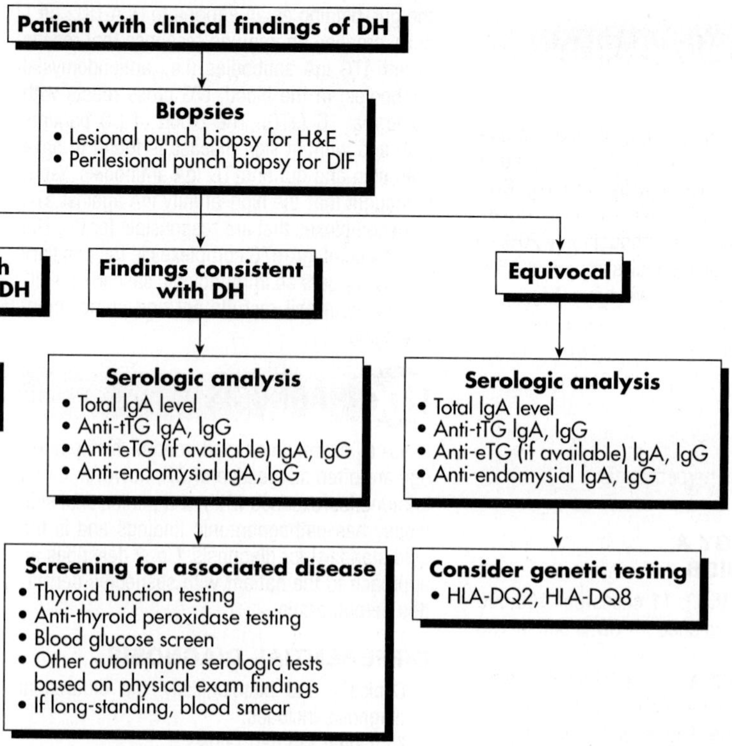

FIG. 2 Approach to the patient with suspected dermatitis herpetiformis. *DH,* Dermatitis herpetiformis; *DIF,* direct immunofluorescence; *eTG,* epidermal transglutaminase; *H&E,* hematoxylin and eosin; *HLA-DQ2,* histocompatibility locus antigen haplotype DQ2; *HLA-DQ8,* histocompatibility locus antigen haplotype DQ8; *Ig,* immunoglobulin; *tIG,* tetanus immune globulin. (From Bolotin D, Petronic-Rosic V: Dermatitis herpetiformis: part II. Diagnosis, management, and prognosis, *J Am Acad Dermatol* 64:1027-1033, 2011.)

the rare case that neuropathy develops. Sulfapyridine must be compounded.

2. Case reports of efficacy using topical dapsone 5% twice daily in patients who do not tolerate oral dapsone; also reported to be efficacious as an adjuvant to oral dapsone.
3. Uncontrolled studies and case reports have suggested efficacy with tetracyclines, nicotinamide, cyclosporine, colchicine, and heparin.

- Symptomatic relief for pruritus:
  1. Potent and superpotent topical corticosteroids (atrophy with prolonged use, limit to 14 days per mo), nonsedating antihistamines twice daily, sedating antihistamines at bedtime, mentholated lotion

CHRONIC Rx

- As DH is considered to represent the cutaneous manifestations of CD, lifelong avoidance of gluten is typically recommended. Information about educational resources, such as national and local support groups, should be provided (www.celiac.org).
- Patients with DH and CD have an increased risk of developing Hashimoto thyroiditis (50% with thyroid disease), non-Hodgkin lymphoma, and GI lymphomas. An increased incidence of other autoimmune disorders (type 1 diabetes mellitus, pernicious anemia, Addison disease, vitiligo, systemic lupus erythematosus, rheumatoid arthritis, and Sjögren syndrome) and osteoporosis have also been reported.
  1. Screening for thyroid disease (TSH, antithyroid peroxidase antibody titers) is typically recommended.
  2. Screening for autoimmune connective tissue diseases should be considered if there are suspicious signs or symptoms.
  3. Routine screening for GI lymphomas is controversial.

REFERRAL

- Dermatologist for skin biopsy and management of cutaneous disease
- Gastroenterologist for evaluation of CD
- Nutritionist to educate patients about gluten-free diet
- National support groups (www.celiac.org) and local support groups

PEARLS & CONSIDERATIONS

- Classic areas involved are those that are exposed if in a "fetal position."
- Lesions may be worsened by iodides and certain NSAIDs; systemic steroids ineffective.
- Location of biopsies is IMPORTANT: False-negative DIF can result if biopsies are taken from lesional skin (should be taken from normal-appearing skin adjacent to lesion) as diagnostic IgA deposits are usually destroyed by the blistering process.
- GFD results in reduced IgA in skin on DIF (with eventual disappearance) and reduced antiendomysial antibodies in the blood. Hence, serologies (e.g., antiendomysial antibodies) can be used to monitor degree of compliance to dietary gluten restriction.
- Some studies have suggested a possible protective effect of GFD against intestinal lymphoma. First-degree relatives do not appear to be at increased risk for GI or systemic lymphomas in the absence of DH or CD.

SUGGESTED READINGS

Available at ExpertConsult.com

RELATED CONTENT

Celiac Disease (Related Key Topic)

AUTHOR: **Lisa Pappas-Taffer, MD**

BASIC INFORMATION

DEFINITION

- Diabetes mellitus (DM) refers to a syndrome of hyperglycemia resulting from many different causes (see "Etiology"). It is broadly classified into type 1 (T1DM) and type 2 DM (T2DM). The terms *insulin-dependent* and *non–insulin-dependent* diabetes are obsolete because when a person with type 2 diabetes needs insulin, he or she remains labeled as type 2 and is not reclassified as type 1. Immune-mediated type 1 DM (type 1A) represents 5% to 10% of newly diagnosed diabetics. Tables 1 and 2 provide a general comparison of the two types of DM. One difference is that type 1 has usually complete or near-total knockout of insulin reserves mediated solely by immunogenic responses from carriers of certain genotypes, whereas type 2 is of polygenetic origin and may have patients who may start with hyperinsulinemia but have insulin resistance and through environmental factors such as diet and sedentary lifestyle leads to an imbalance between glucagon and insulin levels, resulting in combination of causes toward hyperglycemia.
- Some type 1 diabetics also may exhibit high levels of glucagon and not all type 1 diabetics have complete islet cell destruction.
- The classification of diabetes also includes:
  1. **LADA**: Latent autoimmune diabetes of adult onset (sometimes called type 1.5 DM). These individuals are typically not insulin dependent initially and are often misclassified as having type 2 DM.
  2. **MODY**: Maturity onset diabetes of youth. These have various genetic expressions and can be classified into various subtypes:
     a. MODY 1, 2, 3, 4, and 5 (with 3 being most prevalent: 70% incidence with HNF-1-alpha [12q24] genetic expression)
     b. MODY 7 and 8 (rare)
  3. Ketosis-prone diabetes: Relapsing/remitting beta cell function with slow deterioration over time. It presents with ketoacidosis requiring insulin, then regains beta cell function and patient is able to discontinue insulin. This form is most common under age 40, in those of African or Afro-Caribbean origin, and in obese or overweight patients.
  4. Secondary diabetes:
     a. Pancreatic disease or resection (e.g., cystic fibrosis)
     b. Chronic excessive corticosteroid exposure or Cushing syndrome
     c. Glucagonoma
     d. Acromegaly
     e. Other rare genetic disorders (e.g., mitochondrial diabetes MELAS syndrome)
  5. Rare autoimmune (e.g., type A and B insulin resistance syndrome)
- A classification of diabetes mellitus is shown in Box 1.
- Diabetes mellitus can be diagnosed by the following tests:
  1. A hemoglobin A_{1c} (HbA_{1c}) value ≥6.5% is considered diagnostic for diabetes. This test is preferred because of ease of administration and reliability.
  2. A fasting plasma glucose (FPG) ≥126 mg/dl, which should be confirmed with repeat testing on a different day. Fasting is defined as no caloric intake for at least 8 hr.
  3. An oral glucose tolerance test (OGTT) with a plasma glucose ≥200 mg/dl 2 hr after a 75 g (100 g for pregnant women) glucose load.
  4. Symptoms of hyperglycemia and a casual (random) plasma glucose ≥200 mg/dl are also indicative of DM. Classic symptoms of hyperglycemia include polyuria, polydipsia, and unexplained weight loss. At the time of diagnosis as a diabetic, B-cell function is at 25% to 30%.
- Individuals with glucose levels higher than normal but not high enough to meet the criteria for diagnosis of DM are considered to have "prediabetes," the diagnosis of which is made as follows:
  1. A fasting plasma glucose 100 to 125 mg/dl; this is referred to as ***impaired fasting glucose.***
  2. After OGTT, a 2-hr plasma glucose of 140 to 199; this is referred to as ***impaired glucose tolerance.*** Patients with impaired glucose tolerance or prediabetes have B-cell function at 50% of normal.
  3. A hemoglobin A_{1c} value of 5.7% to 6.4%.
- Table 3 describes diagnostic categories for DM and at-risk states.

SYNONYMS

IDDM (insulin-dependent diabetes mellitus)
NIDDM (non–insulin-dependent diabetes mellitus)
Type 1 diabetes mellitus (insulin-dependent diabetes mellitus)
Type 2 diabetes mellitus (non–insulin-dependent diabetes mellitus)
LADA (latent autoimmune diabetes of adult)
MODY (mature onset diabetes of youth)

ICD-10CM CODES

E11.5	Type 2 diabetes mellitus with peripheral circulatory complications
E11.7	Type 2 diabetes mellitus with multiple complications

TABLE 1 Characteristic Comparison of Type 1 Versus Type 2 Diabetes Mellitus

Characteristic	Type 1	Type 2
Nature *Very different*	Autoimmune disorder marked by destruction of insulin-producing beta cells and loss of insulin production	A disorder of insulin deficiency involving an interplay between both pancreatic and extrapancreatic contributions to disease
Symptoms *Partial overlap*	Rapid onset; very high to extremely high blood glucose levels; polyphagia; polydipsia, polyuria; ketoacidosis	Mild to moderate onset; modest to high elevations in blood glucose; mild polydipsia/polyuria; fatigue; visual changes/headache
Onset *Very different*	Sudden (symptoms for days to weeks)	Slower onset (symptoms for months to years)
Risk factors *Typically different but overlap*	Family history of autoimmune disease but particularly type 1 diabetes mellitus (10-fold increased risk vs. general population)	Overweight/obese; poor diet; sedentary lifestyle; ethnicity (higher in African Americans, Hispanics); family history of type 2 diabetes mellitus; history of gestational diabetes
Onset age *Typically different but overlap*	Typically early life through adolescence but can occur at any age	Typically adults but trending toward earlier age of onset
Treatment strategy *Typically different*	Absolute requirement for insulin (multiple daily injections or insulin pump); self-management lifestyle modification (monitor food types, exercise, etc.)	Dietary modifications and exercise alongside oral agents (for most); increasingly greater percentage of patients require insulin over time
Can it be prevented? *Very different*	Not at present (subject of major research efforts); future cases can be predicted by autoantibodies and genetics	Yes, for more than half of potential cases, with dietary modifications and exercise
Can it be reversed? *Very different*	Not at present (subject of major research efforts)	No, but for a limited few; patients can see disease managed and risk for complications reduced through diet modifications, exercise; growing evidence for disease improvements through combination therapies
Complications *Mostly similar, but some variation*	Acute emergencies of hypoglycemia and ketoacidosis leading to hypoglycemic unawareness; chronic effects of hyperglycemia can lead to retinopathy, nephropathy, neuropathy, cardiovascular disease, etc.	Acute emergencies of hypoglycemia and ketoacidosis leading to hypoglycemic unawareness; chronic effects of hyperglycemia can lead to retinopathy, nephropathy, neuropathy, cardiovascular disease, etc.

From Melmed S et al: *Williams textbook of endocrinology*, ed 14, Philadelphia, 2020, Elsevier.

E11.8 Type 2 diabetes mellitus with unspecified complications
E11.9 Type 2 diabetes mellitus without complications
E10.69 Type 1 diabetes mellitus with other specified complication
E10.8 Type 1 diabetes mellitus with unspecified complications
E10.9 Type 1 diabetes mellitus without complications
E11.69 Type 2 diabetes mellitus with other specified complication
E11.8 Type 2 diabetes mellitus with unspecified complications
E11.9 Type 2 diabetes mellitus without complications

EPIDEMIOLOGY & DEMOGRAPHICS

- DM affects 9% to 10% of the U.S. population. Prevalence rates vary considerably by race/ethnicity. T1DM accounts for approximately 5% of diagnosed diabetes cases and is defined by the presence of one or more autoimmune markers. Risk factors for type 1 DM are summarized in Table 4. While incidence of diabetes in adolescents is mostly type 1, the rate of type 2 being diagnosed in adolescents has increased by 1.5 times in certain given areas. This seems to correlate with the epidemic of pediatric obesity. Table 5 summarizes epidemiological determinants of and risk factors for type 2 DM.
- Incidence rate increases with age, varying from 2% in persons age 20 to 44 yr to 18% in persons 65 to 74 yr. T2DM can have a long presymptomatic phase, leading to a 4- to 7-yr delay in diagnosis. In the U.S. 1.2 million new cases of diabetes are diagnosed each yr, and 86 million have prediabetes. Currently, 30 million Americans have diabetes; with this current trend, it is predicted that by 2050 1 out of 3 Americans will be diabetic.
- Diabetes accounts for 8% of all legal blindness in the U.S. and is the leading cause of end-stage renal disease (ESRD). Approximately 40% of patients in a given dialysis center are diabetic.
- Patients with diabetes are 2 to 4 times more likely than nondiabetic patients to experience development of cardiovascular disease (CVD).

PHYSICAL FINDINGS & CLINICAL PRESENTATION

- Physical examination varies with the presence of complications and may be normal in early stages.
- Diabetic retinopathy:
  1. Nonproliferative (background diabetic retinopathy):
     a. Initially: Microaneurysms, capillary dilation, waxy or hard exudates, dot and flame hemorrhages, arteriovenous shunts
     b. Advanced stage: Microinfarcts with cotton wool exudates, macular edema

TABLE 2 Characteristics of Type 1 and Type 2 Diabetes Mellitus

	Type 1 Diabetes	Type 2 Diabetes
Frequency	5%-10%	90%-95%
Age of onset	Any, but most common in children and young adults	More common with advancing age, but can occur in children and adolescents
Risk factors	Genetic, autoimmune, environmental	Genetic, obesity, sedentary lifestyle, race/ethnicity, hypertension, dyslipidemia, polycystic ovarian syndrome
Pathogenesis	Destruction of pancreatic beta cells, usually autoimmune	No autoimmunity Insulin resistance and progressive insulin deficiency
C-peptide levels	Very low or undetectable	Detectable
Prediabetes	Autoantibodies (GAD65, IA-2, IAA, ZnT8) may be present.	Autoantibodies absent
Medication therapy	Insulin absolutely necessary; multiple daily injections or insulin pump	Oral agents and/or noninsulin injectable hypoglycemic drugs Insulin commonly needed
Therapy to prevent or delay onset of diabetes	None known Clinical trials in progress	Lifestyle (weight loss and increased physical activity) Oral medications (metformin, acarbose) may be helpful.

From McPherson RA, Pincus MR: *Henry's clinical diagnosis and management by laboratory method*, ed 23, St. Louis, 2017, Elsevier.

BOX 1 Classification of Diabetes Mellitus

I. Type 1 diabetes (beta cell destruction, usually leading to absolute insulin deficiency)
   A. Immune mediated
   B. Idiopathic
II. Type 2 diabetes (may range from predominantly insulin resistance with relative insulin deficiency to a predominantly secretory defect with insulin resistance)
III. Other specific types
   A. Genetic defects of beta cell function
      1. Chromosome 12, HNF-1α (MODY3)
      2. Chromosome 7, glucokinase (MODY2)
      3. Chromosome 20, HNF-4α (MODY1)
      4. Chromosome 13, insulin promoter factor-1 (IPF-1; MODY4)
      5. Chromosome 17, HNF-1β (MODY5)
      6. Chromosome 2, NeuroD1 (MODY6)
      7. Mitochondrial DNA
      8. Others
   B. Genetic defects in insulin action
      1. Type A insulin resistance
      2. Leprechaunism
      3. Rabson-Mendenhall syndrome
      4. Lipoatrophic diabetes
      5. Others
   C. Diseases of the exocrine pancreas
      1. Pancreatitis
      2. Trauma/pancreatectomy
      3. Neoplasia
      4. Cystic fibrosis
      5. Hemochromatosis
      6. Fibrocalculous pancreatopathy
      7. Others
   D. Endocrinopathies
      1. Acromegaly
      2. Cushing syndrome
      3. Glucagonoma
      4. Pheochromocytoma
      5. Hyperthyroidism
      6. Somatostatinoma
      7. Aldosteronoma
      8. Others
   E. Drug or chemical induced
      1. Vacor
      2. Pentamidine
      3. Nicotinic acid
      4. Glucocorticoids
      5. Thyroid hormone
      6. Diazoxide
      7. β-Adrenergic agonists
      8. Thiazides
      9. Dilantin
      10. γ-Interferon
      11. Others
   F. Infections
      1. Congenital rubella
      2. Cytomegalovirus
      3. Others
   G. Uncommon forms of immune-mediated diabetes
      1. "Stiff-man" syndrome
      2. Anti-insulin receptor antibodies
      3. Others
   H. Other genetic syndromes sometimes associated with diabetes
      1. Down syndrome
      2. Klinefelter syndrome
      3. Turner syndrome
      4. Wolfram syndrome
      5. Friedreich ataxia
      6. Huntington chorea
      7. Laurence-Moon-Biedl syndrome
      8. Myotonic dystrophy
      9. Porphyria
      10. Prader-Willi syndrome
      11. Others
IV. Gestational diabetes mellitus

From McPherson RA, Pincus MR: *Henry's clinical diagnosis and management by laboratory method*, ed 23, St. Louis, 2017, Elsevier.

TABLE 3 Diagnostic Categories*: Diabetes Mellitus and At-Risk States

Fasting Plasma Glucose Level	2-hr (75-g) OGTT Result		
	<140 mg/dl	140-199 mg/dl	≥200 mg/dl
<100 mg/dl	Normal	IGT†	DM
100-125 mg/dl	IFG†	IGT† *and* IFG†	DM
≥126 mg/dl	DM	DM	DM
HbA_{1C} Level	**<5.7%**	**5.7-6.4%**	**≥6.5%**
	Normal	High-risk†	DM

DM, Diabetes mellitus; *HbA_{1c},* glycosylated hemoglobin; *IFG,* impaired fasting glucose; *IGT,* impaired glucose tolerance; *OGTT,* oral glucose tolerance test.

*These diagnostic categories are based on the combined fasting plasma glucose level and a 2-hr, 75-g oral glucose tolerance test (OGTT) result. Note that a confirmed random plasma glucose level of 200 mg/dl or higher in the appropriate clinical setting is diagnostic of diabetes and precludes the need for further testing.

†May be referred to as prediabetes.

From Goldman L, Schafer Al: *Goldman's Cecil medicine,* ed 24, Philadelphia, 2012, Saunders.

TABLE 4 Risk of Type 1 Diabetes Mellitus

Group	Childhood Annual Incidence
US general population	0.3% (15-25/100,000)
Offspring	1%
Sibling	3.2% (through adolescence); 6% lifetime
Dizygotic twin	6%
Mother	2%
Father	4.6%
Both parents	~10%
Monozygotic twin	50%, but incidence varies with age of index twin

From Melmed S et al: *Williams textbook of endocrinology,* ed 14, Philadelphia, 2020, Elsevier.

TABLE 5 Epidemiologic Determinants of and Risk Factors for Type 2 Diabetes Mellitus

Genetic Factors
Genetic markers
Family history

Demographic Characteristics
Age
Ethnicity

Behavioral and Lifestyle-Related Risk Factors
Obesity (including distribution of obesity and duration)
Physical inactivity
Diet
Stress
Westernization, urbanization, modernization
Medications
Shift work

Metabolic Determinants and Intermediate-Risk Categories of Type 2 Diabetes
Impaired glucose tolerance
Insulin resistance
Gestational diabetes
Offspring of women with diabetes during pregnancy
Intrauterine malnutrition or overnutrition
Microbiome composition

From Melmed S et al: *Williams textbook of endocrinology,* ed 14, Philadelphia, 2020, Elsevier.

2. Proliferative retinopathy: Characterized by formation of new vessels, vitreous hemorrhages, fibrous scarring, and retinal detachment
- Cataracts and glaucoma occur with increased frequency in patients with diabetes.
- Diabetic macular edema: Swelling of the macula leading to loss of sharp vision in this part of the eye. People with this disorder usually already have retinopathy but may present separately as well.
- Diabetic neuropathy:
  1. Distal sensorimotor polyneuropathy:
     a. Symptoms include paresthesia, hyperesthesia, or burning pain involving bilateral distal extremities in a "stocking glove" distribution. This can progress to motor weakness and ataxia.
     b. Physical examination may reveal decreased pinprick sensation, decreased sensation to light touch, decreased vibration sense, and loss of proprioception. Motor disturbances such as decreased deep tendon reflexes and atrophy of interosseous muscles can also be seen.
  2. Autonomic neuropathy:
     a. GI disturbances: Esophageal motility abnormalities, gastroparesis, diarrhea (usually nocturnal):
        (1) Increased gastric emptying seen in type 2.
        (2) Decreased gastric emptying seen in type 1.
     b. Genitourinary (GU) disturbances: Neurogenic bladder (hesitancy, weak stream, and dribbling), impotence
     c. Cardiovascular (CV) disturbances: Orthostatic hypotension, tachycardia, decreased heart rate variability (HRV). Decreased heart rate variability is associated with increased cardiac mortality, independent of ejection fraction.
  3. Polyradiculopathy: Painful weakness and atrophy in the distribution of ≥1 contiguous nerve root.
  4. Mononeuropathy involving cranial nerves III, IV, or VI or peripheral nerves can also occur.
- Diabetic nephropathy: Pedal edema, pallor, weakness, uremic appearance
- Nephrotic syndrome: Proteinuria, hypertriglyceridemia, edema
- Nephritis: Progressive degeneration of nephrons focal glomerulosclerosis

Type IV renal tubular acidosis, hyperkalemic nephropathy, interstitial nephritis, causing hyporeninemic hypoaldosteronism. It is important to keep in mind that NSAIDs, ACE inhibitors, trimethoprim, and heparin can all reduce aldosterone and can cause or exacerbate the condition. 50% of patients on dialysis have diabetes as primary diagnosis; whereas glycemia is important to prevent nephropathy, the most significant contributing factor is hypertension.

- Foot ulcers: Occur in 15% of individuals with diabetes (annual incidence rate 2%) and are the leading causes of hospitalization; they are usually secondary to a combination of factors, including peripheral vascular insufficiency, repeated trauma (unrecognized because of sensory loss), and superimposed infection.
  1. Patient symptoms are usually less than would be expected from clinical findings, due to loss of sensation related to peripheral neuropathy.
  2. Comprehensive foot exams include visual inspection, assessment of pedal pulses, and assessment of protective sensation using a 10-g monofilament to test sensation.
  3. Prevention of foot ulcers in an individual with diabetes includes strict glucose control, patient education, prescription

BOX 2 Some Cutaneous Associations with Diabetes Mellitus

Established or Probable Association
- Necrobiosis lipoidica (NL) diabeticorum
- Diabetic dermopathy
- Diabetic bullae
- Acanthosis nigricans
- Acrochordons (skin tags)
- Scleroderma diabeticorum
- Limited joint mobility and waxy skin syndrome
- Partial lipodystrophy
- Malignant otitis externa
- Neuropathic leg ulcers
- Perforating disorders
- Eruptive xanthomas
- Hemochromatosis
- Carotenemia
- Pruritus
- Xerosis and anhidrosis
- Yellow nails, koilonychia

Increased susceptibility to infections:
- *Candida albicans*
- *Staphylococcus aureus*
- Group A β-hemolytic streptococcus
- *Pseudomonas aeruginosa*
- Dermatophytes (tinea pedis, onychomycosis)
- *Corynebacterium minutissimum* (erythrasma)

Possible Association
- Disseminated granuloma annulare
- Vitiligo

From Paller AS, Mancini AJ: *Hurwitz clinical pediatric dermatology: a textbook of skin disorders of childhood and adolescence,* ed 5, Philadelphia, 2016, Elsevier.

footwear, intensive podiatric care, and evaluation for surgical interventions.
4. Foot examination should be done annually on all diabetics.

- Neuropathic arthropathy (Charcot joints): Bone or joint deformities from repeated trauma (secondary to peripheral neuropathy; Fig. E1).
- Necrobiosis lipoidica diabeticorum: Plaque-like reddened areas with a central area that fades to white-yellow, found on the anterior surfaces of the legs (Fig. E2); in these areas, the skin becomes very thin and can ulcerate easily.
- Other diabetic skin manifestations with diabetes include:
  1. Scleroderma diabeticorum: Thickening of skin and epidermis giving skin a "leather-like texture"; typically affects type 2, mainly on upper back and neck.
  2. Dermatitis herpetiformis: Diffuse petechial rash associated with gluten insensitivity.
  3. Vitiligo: Associated with type 1 and type 2, and affects skin coloration due to autoimmune reaction to pigmentation (at times may be associated with adrenal insufficiency, especially in type 1 patients). Patients should use SPF 30 sunscreen to prevent sunburn.
  4. Acanthosis nigricans: Darkening of skin folds in neck and axilla, at times raised and velvety, thought to be associated with insulin resistance; other conditions such as Cushing and acromegaly can have this as well.
  5. Diabetic dermopathy: Appears as shiny round or oval lesions on thin skin of the lower extremity, also known as "shin spots"; these are usually not painful and do not require treatment.
  6. Eruptive xanthomatosis: Associated with uncontrolled blood sugars and extremely high triglycerides. There is a high risk for pancreatitis in patients with this finding; treatment is aimed at lowering blood sugars with insulin and fibrates.
  7. Digital sclerosis: Skin on toes fingers and hands become waxy, thick, and tight, with joint stiffness; treatment is aimed at lowering blood sugars and encouraging use of lotions and moisturizers.
  8. Bullosis diabeticorum: Rare disorder manifesting with blisters on hands, forearms, toes, and feet, usually painless. Lesions generally heal on their own.
  9. Box 2 summarizes cutaneous associations with diabetes mellitus.

ETIOLOGY

IDIOPATHIC DIABETES: Type 1 DM: Results from autoimmune beta-cell destruction, usually leading to absolute insulin deficiency.
- Hereditary factors:
  1. Islet cell antibodies (found in 90% of patients within the first yr of diagnosis)
  2. Higher incidence of human leukocyte antigen (HLA) types DR3, DR4
  3. 50% concordance rate in identical twins
- Environmental factors: Viral infection (possibly coxsackievirus, mumps virus)

Type 2 DM: Results from insulin resistance and a progressive defect in insulin secretion.
- Hereditary factors: 90% concordance rate in identical twins
- Environmental factors: Obesity, sedentary lifestyle, high carbohydrate content in food

DIABETES SECONDARY TO OTHER FACTORS:
- Hormonal excess: Cushing syndrome, acromegaly, glucagonoma, pheochromocytoma
- Drugs: Glucocorticoids, diuretics, oral contraceptives
- Insulin receptor unavailability (with or without circulating antibodies)
- Pancreatic disease: Pancreatitis, pancreatectomy, hemochromatosis, cystic fibrosis
- Genetic syndromes: Maturity onset diabetes of the young (MODY, monogenetic diabetes accounting for 2% to 5% of diabetes), familial hyperlipidemias, myotonic dystrophy, lipoatrophy
- Gestational diabetes (GDM): Diabetes diagnosed during pregnancy that is due to pregnancy-related insulin resistance

Dx DIAGNOSIS

DIFFERENTIAL DIAGNOSIS

- Diabetes insipidus
- Stress hyperglycemia
- Diabetes secondary to hormonal excess, drugs, pancreatic disease

LABORATORY TESTS

- Diagnosis of DM is made on the basis of the following tests:
  1. Fasting glucose ≥126 mg/dl on two occasions.
  2. Non-FPG ≥200 mg/dl and symptoms of DM.
  3. OGTT (75 g glucose load for nonpregnant individuals) with 2-hr value >200 mg/dl.
  4. Glycosylated hemoglobin (HbA_{1c}) ≥6.5%. HbA_{1c} level reflects average glycemia over previous 3 mo or longer. In known diabetics, this test should be performed at least twice yearly in stable patients and more frequently when therapy changes or patients are not meeting glycemic goals. HbA_{1c} alone does not provide a measure of glycemic variability or hypoglycemia and is affected by the presence of hemoglobin variants, hemolysis, or blood loss.
- Measurement of autoantibodies glutamic acid decarboxylase (GAD65) and tyrosine phosphatase IA-2 are useful in suspected immune mediated type 1 DM (strong association).
- Screening for prediabetes and diabetes in asymptomatic patients (see Table 6):
  1. Should be considered in adults of any age who are overweight (body mass index [BMI] >25 kg/m^2) or obese (BMI >30) and who have one or more additional risk factors for diabetes.
  2. In those who are without these risk factors, testing should begin at age 45 yr.
  3. If screen is normal, repeat testing should be carried out at least at 3-yr intervals.
  4. ADA recommends screening all Asian Americans with BMI 23 or higher every 2 yr.
- Detection and diagnosis of gestational diabetes mellitus (GDM):
  1. Screen for GDM using risk factor analysis and use of an OGTT. Pregnant women who are not known to have diabetes should be screened for gestational diabetes at 24 to 28 wks' gestation with a "1-step" strategy with 75 g oral glucose tolerance test or a "2-step" approach with a 50-g (nonfasting) screen followed by a 100-g oral glucose tolerance test for those who screen positive. A diagnosis of GDM is made if any of the following levels of plasma glucose are exceeded: ≥92 mg/dl (5.1 mmol/L) when fasting, ≥80 mg/dl (10 mmol/L) at 1 hr, or ≥153 mg/dl (8.5 mmol/L) at 2 hr.
  2. Women with GDM should be screened for diabetes 6 to 12 wk postpartum and should be followed with subsequent screening for the development of diabetes or prediabetes at least every 3 yr. A woman who had GDM during pregnancy has 50% risk of developing diabetes later in life; this is dependent on ethnicity (e.g., Pima Indians, Hispanic, African American).
- Screening for diabetic nephropathy:
  1. Screening should be done at diagnosis and then yearly for type 2 diabetes and

5 yr after diagnosis then yearly in type 1 diabetes. 18% of type 1 DM may have early kidney changes, and future guidelines may change screening to 1 yr after diagnosis if poorly controlled then annually for both type 1 and type 2.

2. Screening can be performed using an albumin:creatinine ratio (microalbumin) in a random spot urine collection or by measurement of a 24-hr urine collection for albumin and creatinine clearance. The urine albumin to creatinine ratio (ACR) is independently associated with mortality at all levels of estimated glomerular filtration rate (eGFR) in older adults with diabetes.
3. The diagnosis of microalbuminuria (ACR 30 to 299 mg/24 hr) should be based on 2 to 3 elevated levels within a 3- to 6-mo period because there is a marked variability in day-to-day albumin excretion. Patients with overt macroalbuminuria (>300 mg albumin/24 hr or albumin:creatinine ratio >300) should be followed by urine protein:creatinine ratio.

- A fasting serum lipid panel, serum creatinine, and electrolytes should be obtained yearly on all adult patients with diabetes.
- Self-monitoring of blood glucose (SMBG) is crucial for assessing the effectiveness of the management plan. The frequency and timing of SMBG varies with the needs and goals of each patient. In most patients with type 1 DM and pregnant women taking insulin, SMBG is recommended at least 3 times/day. In patients with type 2 DM not on insulin, recommendations are unclear for SMBG, but testing once or twice/day is acceptable in most patients. Glycemic control is best evaluated when SMBG is combined with HbA_{1c} testing.
- Continuous glucose monitoring (CGM) is now starting to play a more prominent role in reducing the number of fingersticks. Dexcom CGM has been approved by FDA for use by patients to adjust insulin based on CGM readings.
- The use of insulin pump and CGM readings and computer software can adjust insulin automatically (known as the "artificial pancreas").
- CGM can also be used in patients with type 2 on multiple daily injections.
- Limitations of CGM are that it cannot predict accuracy of blood glucose when <70 mg/dl.
- Screening for thyroid dysfunction (TSH level), vitamin B_{12} deficiency, and celiac disease should be considered in type 1 diabetes due to the increased frequency of other autoimmune diseases in these individuals.
- Consider screening for autoimmune polyendocrine syndromes (APS-2):
  1. APS-2: Most commonly known as Schmidt syndrome, heterogeneous not linked to one gene (HDLA-DQ2, HDLA-DQ8, AND HLA-DR4). Patients can have IDDM, hyperthyroidism, other autoimmune conditions, B_{12} deficiency, and myasthenia.

TABLE 6 Criteria for Diabetes Screening in Asymptomatic Individuals

1. Testing should be considered in all adults who are overweight (BMI >25 kg/m²*) and have additional risk factors:
   1. Physical inactivity
   2. A first-degree relative with diabetes
   3. High-risk ethnic population (e.g., African American, Hispanic American, Native American, Asian American, Pacific Islander)
   4. Delivered a baby weighing more than 9 lb or diagnosed with gestational diabetes mellitus
   5. Systemic hypertension (blood pressure >140/90 mm Hg or on antihypertensive therapy)
   6. High-density lipoprotein cholesterol level <35 mg/dl or triglyceride level >250 mg/dl
   7. Polycystic ovary syndrome
   8. Hemoglobin A_{1c} ≥5.7%, impaired glucose tolerance or impaired fasting glucose on prior testing
   9. Other clinical conditions associated with insulin resistance (e.g., severe obesity, acanthosis nigricans)
   10. History of cardiovascular disease
2. If none of the above criteria are present, screening for diabetes should begin at age 45 yr.
3. If the results are normal, screening should be repeated at least every 3 yr. Depending on initial results and risk status, more frequent testing may need to be considered.

*In some ethnic groups, such as Asians, at-risk body mass index (BMI) may be lower.
Modified from American Diabetes Association: Diagnosis and classification of diabetes mellitus, *Diabetes Care* 33(Suppl 1):S14, 2010; and from Goldman L, Schafer AI: *Goldman's Cecil medicine,* ed 24, Philadelphia, 2012, Saunders.

TABLE 7 Glycemic Goals in Adults*

	Preprandial Glucose		Postprandial Glucose**		
Hemoglobin A_{1c} (%)	mg/dl	mmol/L	mg/dl	mmol/L	
ADA†: Adults	<7.0‡	80-130	4.4-7.2	<180	<10.0
Pregnant adults	<6.0	60-99	3.3-5.5	100-129	5.6-7.2
Older adults:					
Healthy	<7.5	90-130	5.0-7.2	90-150	5.0-8.3
Intermediate	<8.0	90-150	5.0-8.3	100-180	5.6-10.0
Poor health	<8.5	100-180	5.6-10.0	110-200	6.1-11.1
AACE§,¶	≤6.5	≤110	≤6.1	≤140	<7.8

*Youth <18 yr of age: Goal hemoglobin A_{1c}<7.5%.
**1 to 2 hr after beginning a meal for adults, except bedtime for older adults.
†ADA, American Diabetes Association (2015); Chiang et al (2014).
‡Lower goals may be appropriate for selected individuals if this can be accomplished safely (without significant hypoglycemia). Higher goals may be appropriate in some individuals (e.g., with a history of severe hypoglycemia, limited life expectancy, advanced complications, extensive comorbid conditions, or long-standing diabetes in whom the goal is difficult to achieve with appropriate education, monitoring, and therapies, including insulin).
§AACE, American Association of Clinical Endocrinologists, 2015.
¶For patients without concurrent serious illness and at low hypoglycemia risk.
From McPherson RA, Pincus MR: *Henry's clinical diagnosis and management by laboratory method,* ed 23, St. Louis, 2017, Elsevier.

Rx TREATMENT

- Glycemic goals in adult diabetics are summarized in Table 7.
- Type 1 diabetes requires immediate initiation of insulin therapy.
- In type 1 diabetes, intensive glycemic control (HbA_{1c} <7) has been shown in randomized controlled trials (RCT) to reduce the risk of microvascular (neuropathy, retinopathy, nephropathy) and macrovascular (cardiovascular events) complications.
- Type 2 DM: The ADA and European Association for the Study of Diabetes recommend lifestyle intervention (diet and exercise) and metformin initiation (unless contraindications exist such as serum creatinine levels ≥1.5 mg/dl in males or ≥1.4 mg/dl in females or patients ≥30 yr of age with reduced renal function as measured by creatinine clearance) at the time of diagnosis of type 2 diabetes. Therapy should then be augmented with additional agents (including early initiation of insulin therapy) to achieve adequate glycemic control.
- In type 2 diabetes, intensive glycemic control (HbA_{1c} <7) has been shown in RCT to reduce the risk of microvascular complications. While intensive glucose control reduced the risk of some CVD outcomes (such as nonfatal MI), it did not reduce the risk of cardiovascular death or all-cause mortality and increased the risk of severe hypoglycemia.
- Table 8 summarizes American College of Cardiology/American Heart Association (ACC/AHA) recommendations for primary prevention of CVD in patients with diabetes. Recommendations for secondary prevention of CVD are described in Table 9.
- It is important to remember that tight glycemic control may burden patients with complex treatment programs, hypoglycemia, weight gain, and costs. Clinicians should individualize HbA_{1c} targets so that they are reasonable and reflect patients' personal and clinical contexts and their informed values and preferences. A target HbA_{1c} <7 is reasonable for motivated new diabetic patients with long life expectancies, whereas less stringent controls (HbA_{1c} 7.5 or higher) may

TABLE 8 American College of Cardiology Foundation/American Heart Association Recommendations for Primary Prevention of Cardiovascular Disease in People with Diabetes

Lifestyle Management

Weight

Structured programs that emphasize lifestyle changes such as reduced fat (<30%-35% of daily energy) and total energy intake and increased regular physical activity, along with regular participant contact, can produce long-term weight loss on the order of 5% to 7% of starting weight, with improvement in BP.

For persons with elevated plasma triglycerides and reduced HDL-C, improved glycemic control, moderate weight loss (5%-7% of starting weight), dietary saturated fat restriction, increased physical activity, and modest replacement of dietary carbohydrate (5%-7%) by either monounsaturated or polyunsaturated fats may be beneficial.

Medical Nutrition Therapy

To achieve reductions in LDL-C:

Saturated fats should be less than 7% of energy intake.

Dietary cholesterol intake should be less than 200 mg/day. Intake of *trans* unsaturated fatty acids should be less than 1% of energy intake.

Total energy intake should be adjusted to achieve body weight goals.

Total dietary fat intake should be moderated (<30%-35% of total calories) and should consist mainly of monounsaturated or polyunsaturated fat.

Ample intake of dietary fiber (≥14 g/1000 calories consumed) may be of benefit.

If individuals choose to drink alcohol, daily intake should be limited to one drink for adult women and two drinks for adult men. One drink is defined as 12 ounces (oz) of beer, 4 oz of wine, or 1.5 oz of distilled spirits. Alcohol ingestion increases caloric intake and should be minimized when weight loss is the goal.

Individuals with elevated plasma triglyceride levels should limit intake of alcohol because it may exacerbate hypertriglyceridemia.

In both normotensive and hypertensive persons, a reduction in sodium intake may lower BP. The goal should be to reduce sodium intake to 1200-2300 mg/day (50-100 mmol/day), equivalent to 3000-6000 mg/day sodium chloride.

Physical Activity

To improve glycemic control, assist with weight loss or maintenance, and reduce risk for CVD, at least 150 min of moderate-intensity aerobic physical activity or at least 90 min of vigorous aerobic exercise per wk is recommended. The physical activity should be distributed over at least 3 days per wk, with no more than 2 consecutive days without physical activity.

For long-term maintenance of major weight loss, a larger amount of exercise (7 hr of moderate or vigorous aerobic physical activity per wk) may be helpful.

Blood Pressure

BP should be measured at every routine diabetes visit. Patients found to have SBP ≥130 mm Hg or DBP ≥80 mm Hg should have BP confirmed on a separate day.

Patients with diabetes should be treated to achieve SBP at least <140 mm Hg and DBP <90 mm Hg, and for patients who can tolerate without adverse symptoms, targets can be as low as SBP <130 mm Hg and DBP <80-85 mm Hg. Patients with SBP of 130-139 mm Hg or DBP of 80-89 mm Hg should initiate lifestyle modification alone (weight control, increased physical activity, alcohol moderation, sodium reduction, and emphasis on increased consumption of fresh fruits, vegetables, and low-fat dairy products) for a maximum of 3 mo. If, after these efforts, targets are not achieved, treatment with pharmacologic agents should be initiated.

Patients with hypertension (SBP ≥140 mm Hg or DBP ≥90 mm Hg) should receive drug therapy in addition to lifestyle and behavioral therapy.

All patients with diabetes and hypertension should be treated with a regimen that includes either an ACE inhibitor, or if intolerant to an ACE inhibitor, an ARB. If one class is not tolerated, the other should be substituted. Other drug classes demonstrated to reduce CVD events in patients with diabetes—dihydropyridine calcium channel blockers, thiazide diuretics (chlorthalidone and indapamide), and beta-blockers—should be added, in listed order of preference, as needed to achieve BP targets.

If ACE inhibitors, ARBs, or diuretics are used, kidney function and serum potassium levels should be monitored within the first 3 mo. If BP is stable, follow-up could occur every 6 mo thereafter.

Multidrug therapy generally is required to achieve BP targets.

In elderly hypertensive patients, BP should be lowered gradually to avoid complications.

Orthostatic measurement of BP should be performed in people with diabetes and hypertension when clinically indicated.

Patients not achieving target BP despite multidrug therapy should be referred to a physician specializing in the care of patients with hypertension.

Lipids

In adult patients with diabetes, lipid levels should be measured at least annually and more often if needed to achieve goals. In adults with diabetes who are younger than 40 with low-risk lipid values (LDL-C <100 mg/dl, HDL-C >50 mg/dl, triglycerides <150 mg/dl), lipid assessments may be repeated every 2 yr.

Lifestyle modification deserves primary emphasis in all individuals with diabetes. Patients should focus on the reduction of saturated fat and cholesterol intake, weight loss (if indicated), and increases in dietary fiber and physical activity. These lifestyle changes have been shown to improve the lipid profile in patients with diabetes. In persons with diabetes who are older than 40 yr, without overt CVD, statin therapy should be considered for primary prevention with recommendation to use at least moderate-dose and ideally intense-dose statins, independent of baseline LDL-C levels. On maximally tolerated statin, the goal is an LDL-C level <100 mg/dl (2.6 mmol/L), and ideally <70 mg/dl (1.8 mmol/L) for those at highest CVD risk. If LDL-lowering drugs are used, a reduction of at least 50% in LDL-C levels should be obtained.

If baseline LDL-C is <100 mg/dl, statin therapy should be initiated based on risk factor assessment and clinical judgment. Major risk factors in this category include age, sex, race/ethnicity, cigarette smoking, hypertension (BP >140/90 mm Hg or use of antihypertensive medication), high total cholesterol and low HDL-C (<40 mg/dl), and family history of premature CHD (CHD in male first-degree relatives ≤55 yr of age; CHD in female first-degree relatives ≤65 yr of age).

In people with diabetes who are younger than 40, without overt CVD, but who are estimated to be at increased risk for CVD either by clinical judgment or by risk calculator, at least moderate-intensity statin therapy is recommended, with an LDL-C goal of <100 mg/dl.

Combination therapy with LDL-lowering drugs (e.g., statins, ezetimibe, PCSK9 inhibitors) and fibrates or niacin may be necessary to achieve lipid targets, but to date, only the addition of ezetimibe to statin therapy has proven incremental CV outcomes benefit.

Beyond the consensus of therapeutic lifestyle intervention, the ADA and AHA guidelines have evolved significantly over recent years, no longer recommending pharmacologic treatment of low HDL-C or high triglyceride levels, except for those with extremely high fasting triglyceride levels, to consider fish oil or a fibrate to mitigate pancreatitis risk.

Tobacco

All patients with diabetes should be asked about tobacco use status at every visit.

Every tobacco user should be advised to quit.

The tobacco user's willingness to quit should be assessed.

The patient can be assisted by counseling and by developing a plan to quit.

Follow-up, referral to special programs, or pharmacotherapy (including nicotine replacement and bupropion) should be incorporated as needed.

TABLE 8 American College of Cardiology Foundation/American Heart Association Recommendations for Primary Prevention of Cardiovascular Disease in People with Diabetes–cont'd

Antiplatelet Agents

The ADA and AHA recommend aspirin therapy (75-162 mg/day) for primary prevention in patients with diabetes at increased CV risk (e.g., estimated 10-yr risk >10%), including most age ≥50 yr who have additional risk factors (e.g., family history of CVD, hypertension, smoking, dyslipidemia, albuminuria). In contrast, the ESC/EASD guidelines discourage aspirin for primary prevention in patients with diabetes, except for those estimated to be at the very highest CV risk, in whom such use may be considered.

People with aspirin allergy, bleeding tendency, existing anticoagulant therapy, recent gastrointestinal bleeding, and clinically active hepatic disease are poor candidates for aspirin, especially for primary prevention. Other antiplatelet agents may be a reasonable alternative for patients with high risk.

Glycemic Control

The HbA_{1c} goal for most patients with diabetes in general is less than 7% in the absence of CVD, with higher targets such as 8% (or higher) endorsed for patients with moderate to severe CVD or other serious comorbidities.

Type 1 Diabetes Mellitus

At present, all of the recommendations listed above for patients with type 2 DM appear to be appropriate for those with type 1 DM as well.

ACE, Angiotensin-converting enzyme; *ADA,* American Diabetes Association; *AHA,* American Heart Association; *ARB,* angiotensin receptor blocker; *BP,* blood pressure; *CHD,* coronary heart disease; *CV,* cardiovascular; *CVD,* cardiovascular disease; *DBP,* diastolic blood pressure; *DM,* diabetes mellitus; *EASD,* European Association for the Study of Diabetes; *ESC,* European Society of Cardiology; *HbA_{1c},* glycosylated hemoglobin; *HDL-C,* high-density lipoprotein cholesterol; *LDL-C,* low-density lipoprotein cholesterol; *SBP,* systolic blood pressure.

Data are from Fox CS et al: Update on prevention of cardiovascular disease in adults with type 2 diabetes mellitus in light of recent evidence: a scientific statement from the American Heart Association and the American Diabetes Association, *Circulation* 132:691-718, 2015; Ryden L et al: ESC guidelines on diabetes, pre-diabetes, and cardiovascular diseases developed in collaboration with the EASD. The Task Force on Diabetes, Pre-diabetes, and Cardiovascular Diseases of the European Society of Cardiology (ESC) and developed in collaboration with the European Association for the Study of Diabetes (EASD), *Eur Heart J* 34:3035-3087, 2013; ADA Standards of Medical Care in Diabetes—2016: abridged for primary care providers, *Diabetes Care* 34:3-21, 2016; Inzucchi SE et al: Management of hyperglycemia in type 2 diabetes, 2015: a patient-centered approach—update to a position statement of the American Diabetes Association and the European Association for the Study of Diabetes, *Diabetes Care* 38:140-149, 2013; and Stone NJ et al: 2013 ACC/AHA guideline on the treatment of blood cholesterol to reduce atherosclerotic cardiovascular risk in adults: a report of the American College of Cardiology/American Heart Association Task Force on Practice Guidelines, *Circulation* 129(Suppl 2):S1-S45, 2014; in Zipes DP: *Braunwald's heart disease: a textbook of cardiovascular medicine,* ed 11, Philadelphia, 2019, Elsevier.

TABLE 9 American College of Cardiology Foundation/American Heart Association Recommendations for Secondary Prevention of Cardiovascular Disease Specific to Patients with Diabetes

Class	Indication	Level of Evidence
I	Care for diabetes should be coordinated with the patient's primary care physician and/or endocrinologist.	C
	Lifestyle modifications including daily physical activity, weight management, blood pressure control, and LDL cholesterol management are recommended for all patients with diabetes.	B
	ACE inhibitors (or ARBs for those with ACE inhibitor intolerance) should be started and continued indefinitely in patients with diabetes, unless contraindicated.	A
	Use of aldosterone blockade in post-MI patients without significant kidney dysfunction or hyperkalemia is recommended in patients who are already receiving therapeutic doses of an ACE inhibitor and beta-blocker, who have a left ventricular ejection fraction ≤40% and diabetes.	A
IIa	Metformin is an effective first-line pharmacotherapy and can be useful if not contraindicated.	A
	Individualizing the intensity of blood glucose–lowering interventions based on the individual patient's risk for hypoglycemia during treatment is reasonable.	C
IIb	Initiation of pharmacotherapy interventions to achieve target HbA_{1c} may be reasonable.	A
	A target HbA_{1c} of ≤7% may be considered, whereas the ADA/EASD endorse a target ≥8% for those with moderate to severe CVD.	C
	Less stringent HbA_{1c} goals may be considered for other patients with a history of severe hypoglycemia, limited life expectancy, advanced microvascular complications, or extensive comorbidity, or those in whom the goal is difficult to attain despite intensive therapeutic interventions.	C

ACE, Angiotensin-converting enzyme; *ADA,* American Diabetes Association; *ARB,* angiotensin receptor blocker; *CVD,* cardiovascular disease; *EASD,* European Association for the Study of Diabetes; *HbA_{1c},* glycosylated hemoglobin; *LDL,* low-density lipoprotein; *MI,* myocardial infarction.

Data are from Fox CS et al: Update on prevention of cardiovascular disease in adults with type 2 diabetes mellitus in light of recent evidence: a scientific statement from the American Heart Association and the American Diabetes Association, *Circulation* 132:691-718, 2015; Ryden L et al: ESC guidelines on diabetes, pre-diabetes, and cardiovascular diseases developed in collaboration with the EASD. The Task Force on Diabetes, Pre-diabetes, and Cardiovascular Diseases of the European Society of Cardiology (ESC) and developed in collaboration with the European Association for the Study of Diabetes (EASD), *Eur Heart J* 34:3035-3087, 2013; ADA Standards of Medical Care in Diabetes—2016: abridged for primary care providers, *Diabetes Care* 34:3-21, 2016; Inzucchi SE et al: Management of hyperglycemia in type 2 diabetes, 2015: a patient-centered approach—update to a position statement of the American Diabetes Association and the European Association for the Study of Diabetes, *Diabetes Care* 38:140-149, 2015; and Stone NJ et al: 2013 ACC/AHA guideline on the treatment of blood cholesterol to reduce atherosclerotic cardiovascular risk in adults: a report of the American College of Cardiology/American Heart Association Task Force on Practice Guidelines, *Circulation* 129(Suppl 2):S1-S45, 2014; in Zipes DP: *Braunwald's heart disease: a textbook of cardiovascular medicine,* ed 11, Philadelphia, 2019, Elsevier.

be reasonable in elderly patients with limited life expectancy and elevated risk of hypoglycemia. The American Geriatrics Society recommends a general goal for glycated hemoglobin in older adults of 7.5% to 8.0%. Higher HbA_{1c} targets (8% to 9%) are appropriate for older adults with multiple comorbidities, poor health, and limited life expectancy.[1]

[1]Huang ES, Davis AM: Glycemic control in older adults with diabetes mellitus, *JAMA* 314:1509-1510, 2015.

NONPHARMACOLOGIC THERAPY

- Diet: The ADA does not recommend a special diet. However, newly diagnosed diabetics who are overweight or obese should be counseled to lose at least 5% of their body weight. Consultation with a registered dietitian is recommended.
  1. Calories:
     a. The patient with diabetes can be started on 15 calories/lb of ideal body weight; this number can be increased to 20 calories/lb for an active person and 25 calories/lb if the patient does heavy physical labor.
     b. The calories should be distributed as 45% to 65% carbohydrates, <30% fat, with saturated fat limited to <7% of total calories, and 10% to 30% protein. Daily cholesterol intake should not exceed 300 mg.

c. The emphasis should be on complex carbohydrates rather than simple and refined starches, and on polyunsaturated instead of saturated fats in a ratio of 2:1.
d. The glycemic index compares the increase in blood sugar after the ingestion of simple sugars and complex carbohydrates with the increase that occurs after the absorption of glucose; equal amounts of starches do not give the same increase in plasma glucose (pasta equal in calories to a baked potato causes less of an increase than the potato); thus, it is helpful to know the glycemic index of a particular food product.

2. Fiber: Insoluble fiber (bran, celery) and soluble globular fiber (pectin in fruit) delay glucose absorption and attenuate the postprandial serum glucose peak.
   a. They also appear to reduce the increased triglyceride level often present in patients with uncontrolled diabetes. A diet high in fiber should be emphasized (20 to 35 g/day of soluble and insoluble fiber).
   b. Diet programs: In 2015, a meta-analysis review of all research revealed that weight loss was equal no matter which diet program patients were involved in.
   c. However, the only data to show evidence-based prevention of diabetes in prediabetics was the "Mediterranean diet."
   d. The Mediterranean diet also showed a significant decrease in the percentage of established diabetics from needing insulin in the future and significant benefit in reducing cardiovascular events.
3. Other principles:
   a. Modest sodium restriction to 2400 to 3000 mg/day. If hypertension is present, restrict to <2400 mg/day; if nephropathy and hypertension are present, restrict to <2000 mg/day.
   b. Moderation of alcohol intake recommended (≤2 drinks/day in men, ≤1 drink/day in women).
   c. Nonnutritive artificial sweeteners are acceptable in moderate amounts.
      (1) However, it has been shown that artificial sweeteners may actually increase insulin resistance by affecting the action of insulin at receptor level.

- Exercise: Increases the cellular glucose uptake by increasing the number of insulin receptors. The following points must be considered:
  1. Exercise program must be individualized and built up slowly. Consider beginning with 15 min of low-impact aerobic exercise 3 times per wk and increasing the frequency and duration to 30 to 45 min of moderate aerobic activity (50% to 70% of maximum age predicted heart rate) to 3 to 5 days/wk.
     a. In the absence of contraindications, resistance training three times per wk should be encouraged.
  2. Insulin is more rapidly absorbed when injected into a limb that is then exercised, and this can result in hypoglycemia.
  3. Physical activity can result in hypoglycemia if medication dose or carbohydrate consumption is not modified. Ingestion of additional carbohydrates is recommended if pre-exercise glucose levels are <100 mg/dl.
  4. Diabetes prevention program: Low-fat diet with exercise reduced diabetes by 58%. This encompassed diet of 1200 to 1800 kcal/day <30% from fat, exercise unsupervised and supervised, akin to brisk walking >150 min/wk of moderately intensity physical activity.
- Weight loss: To ideal body weight if the patient is overweight. Recent trials have shown that although weight loss has many positive health benefits for people with type 2 DM, such as slower decline in mobility, it does not reduce the number of cardiovascular events.
- Screening for nephropathy, neuropathy, and retinopathy: Annual serum creatinine and urine albumin excretion; initial comprehensive eye examination and at least annually thereafter.
- Diabetes self-management education: Could also address psychosocial issues.
- Self-monitoring of blood glucose should occur three to four times per day for patients using multiple insulin injections or on insulin pump therapy.
- Perform HbA_{1c} at least two times a yr in patients who are meeting treatment goals and who have stable glycemic control.
  1. HbA_{1c} quarterly in patients whose therapy has changed or who are not meeting glycemic goals.
  2. The HbA_{1c} goal for nonpregnant adults in general is <7%.
  3. In the elderly, those with comorbidities, or those at risk for complications from hypoglycemia, a more moderate glycemic target (HbA_{1c} 7 to 8) may be appropriate.
  4. In elderly patients (>80 yr of age) with average life expectancy of 5 yr, a target HbA_{1c} <8.0 is reasonable. In patients >80 yr with comorbidities and life expectancy of 3 yr, a target HbA_{1c} of <9.0 may be appropriate.

TABLE 10 Examples of Insulin Regimens Used in Type 1 Diabetes

Intensive Insulin Regimens

Multiple Daily Injections

- Long-acting insulin given once daily, and rapid-acting insulin given at meals, snacks, and periodically to correct high blood sugars

Continuous Subcutaneous Insulin Infusion via Insulin Pump

- Rapid-acting insulin given at basal rate (rate can vary throughout the day) and as a bolus at meals, snacks, and as needed to correct high blood sugars
- Rapid-acting insulin given via pump according to automated insulin delivery algorithm and based on continuous glucose monitoring

Simplified Insulin Regimens

Multiple Daily Injections

- Long-acting insulin given once daily, NPH given at breakfast, and rapid-acting insulin given at breakfast and dinner (may be used when lunchtime insulin dosing is logistically difficult; lunch carbohydrate intake must be consistent)
- NPH given twice daily (breakfast and bedtime), and rapid-acting insulin given at meals
- NPH and rapid- or short-acting insulin given twice daily (breakfast and dinner)
- Premixed insulin (70/30, 75/25, 50/50) given twice daily (breakfast and dinner)

From Melmed S et al: *Williams Textbook of Endocrinology*, ed 14, Philadelphia, 2020, Elsevier.

GENERAL Rx

- Type 1 DM: Lifelong insulin therapy is required for persons with type 1 DM. It should consist of basal coverage, prandial coverage, and supplemental insulin for correction of hyperglycemia. Initial total insulin dosing ranges from 0.4 to 1.0 U/kg/day, 50% of which is basal insulin and 50% prandial insulin. Examples of insulin regimens used in type 1 DM are described in Table 10.
- Type 2 DM: When the previous measures fail to normalize the serum glucose, oral hypoglycemic agents should be added to the regimen in T2DM. Treatment options in patient with type 2 diabetes should be tailored to try to target core diabetic defects and apply therapies that lower HbA_{1c} in a weight-neutral or weight-lowering fashion if possible; of course, cost of therapies needs to be considered as well. Clinical features of commonly used oral antihyperglycemic agents are summarized in Table 11. Commonly used injectable agents other than insulin are described in Table 12.
- **Metformin:** The primary mechanism of metformin is to decrease hepatic glucose production and improve insulin sensitivity. Because metformin does not produce hypoglycemia when used as a monotherapy, it is preferred initially for most patients. Metformin reduces mean HbA_{1c} level by 1.1%. It is contraindicated in patients with severe renal insufficiency with an estimated glomerular filtrate rate <30 ml/min, serum creatinine level of 1.5 per dl or greater in men or 1.4 per dl or greater in women, heart failure, or other clinical states of hypoperfusion, and in patients with

TABLE 11 Clinical Features of Commonly Used Oral Antihyperglycemic Agents

Classes and Specific Agents (Commercial Names)	Commonly Used Dosages	Contraindications	Side Effects	%HbA$_{1c}$ Reduction as First or Second Therapy
Biguanide				
Metformin (Glucophage)	500-1000 mg bid	T1D, DKA eGFR <30	Nausea, diarrhea, abdominal pain	1-2
Metformin-ER	500-1000 mg bid	Severe cardiac, hepatic disease	Vitamin B_{12} deficiency	
Secretagogue				
Glipizide (Glucotrol)	5-20 mg bid	T1D, DKA	Hypoglycemia	1-2
Glipizide-ER	2.5-10 mg qd		Weight gain	
Gliclazide (Diamicron)	80-160 bid			
Gliclazide-MR	30-120 qd			
Glimepiride (Amaryl)	0.5-4 mg qd			
Glyburide (Micronase et al)	2.5-10 mg bid			
Repaglinide (Prandin)	0.5-2 mg tid			
Nateglinide (Starlix)	60-120 mg tid			
Thiazolidinedione				
Pioglitazone (Actos)	15-30 mg qd	T1D, DKA	Weight gain	0.75-1.5
Rosiglitazone (Avandia)	4-8 mg qd	Symptomatic heart failure	Edema	
			Fractures	
DPP4 inhibitor[a]				
Sitagliptin (Januvia)	25-100 mg qd	T1D, DKA	Hypersensitivity	0.5-1
Vildagliptin (Galvus)	50 mg qd or bid			
Saxagliptin (Onglyza)	2.5-5 mg qd			
Linagliptin (Tradjenta)	5 mg qd			
Alogliptin (Nesina)	6.25-25 mg qd			
α-Glucosidase inhibitor[b]				
Acarbose (Precose)	25-50 mg tid	T1D, DKA	Flatulence, diarrhea, abdominal discomfort	0.5-1
Miglitol (Glyset)	25-50 mg tid			
SGLT inhibitor				
Canagliflozin (Invokana)	100-300 mg qd	TID, DKA eGFR <30	Urinary frequency	0.5-1
Dapagliflozin (Farxiga)	5-10 mg qd		Urogenital infections	
Empagliflozin (Jardiance)	10-25 mg qd		Nausea, diarrhea	
Ertugliflozin (Steglatro)	5-15 mg qd		Hypotension	
Bile-acid sequestrant				
Colesevelam (Welchol)	Six 625-mg tabs qd	T1D, DKA Pancreatitis, intestinal disease, hypertriglyceridemia	Constipation	0.5-1
Dopamine agonist				
Bromocriptine (Cycloset)	1.6-4.8 mg qd	T1D, DKA	Somnolence, dizziness, hypotension	0.5-1

bid, Twice daily; *DKA,* diabetic ketoacidosis; *eGFR,* estimated glomerular filtration rate; *ER,* extended release; *HbA$_{1c}$,* glycosylated hemoglobin; *MR,* modified release; *qd,* once daily; *tid,* three times daily.

[a]The DPP4 inhibitors listed here are approved in the U.S. and/or the European Union. Other DPP4 inhibitors are available in certain countries, including anagliptin (Suiny), evogliptin (Suganon), gemigliptin (Zemiglo), gosogliptin (SatRx), omarigliptin (Marizef), teneligliptin (Tenelia), trelagliptin (Zafatek), and vildagliptin (Galvus).

[b]Acarbose and miglitol are available in the United States and the European Union. Voglibose (Basen et al) is available in other countries.

From Melmed S et al: *Williams textbook of endocrinology*, ed 14, Philadelphia, 2020, Elsevier.

TABLE 12 Clinical Features of Commonly Used Injectable Agents Other Than Insulin

Types and Generic Names (Commercial Names)	Administration	Main Effects	Contraindications	Side Effects
Short-acting GLP1 agonist				
Exenatide (Byetta)	5-10 μg bid before breakfast and dinner	Postprandial glucose control and weight loss	T1D DKA Pancreatitis History medullary carcinoma	Nausea, diarrhea, abdominal pain Pancreatitis?
Lixisenatide (Adlyxin)	10-20 μg qd before breakfast			
Long-acting GLP1 agonist				
Liraglutide (Victoza)	0.6-1.8 mg daily	Basal glucose control and weight loss	T1D DKA Pancreatitis History medullary carcinoma	Nausea, diarrhea, abdominal pain Pancreatitis?
Dulaglutide (Trulicity)	0.75 or 1.5 mg weekly			
Extended-release exenatide (Bydureon)	2 mg weekly			
Semaglutide (Ozempic)	0.5 or 1 mg weekly			
Fixed-dose GLP1/insulin combination				
Liraglutide/degludec (Xultophy)	Daily, titrated	Glucose and weight control	T1D DKA Pancreatitis History medullary carcinoma	Hypoglycemia Nausea, diarrhea, abdominal pain Pancreatitis?
Lixisenatide/glargine (Soliqua)	Daily before breakfast, titrated			
Amylin agonist				
Pramlintide (Symlin)	tid before meals in T1D or T2D requiring prandial insulin	Postprandial glucose control and weight loss	Confirmed gastroparesis	Nausea Abdominal pain Hypoglycemia

DKA, Diabetic ketoacidosis.

From Melmed S et al: *Williams textbook of endocrinology*, ed 14, Philadelphia, 2020, Elsevier.

significant liver disease. Starting metformin in patients with GFR between 30 and 45 ml/min is also not recommended. Renal dosing of metformin is preferred, based on GFR levels rather than creatinine levels. The excess risk for lactic acidosis is however negligible in patients with mild to moderate reductions in kidney function.[2] When metformin alone does not achieve the desired A_{1C} goal, the choice of a second drug is dictated by the comorbidities or cost. For example, an SLGT2 inhibitor is preferred in patients with heart failure or cardiovascular disease.

1. When the HbA_{1c} level is 9% or greater, initial dual-regimen combination therapy should be considered. It is important to consider that some drug classes provide benefit in cardiovascular and renal outcomes that may be independent of glucose control. Clinicians should consider adding either a GLP-1 agonist or an SGLT-2 inhibitor to metformin to improve glycemic control when a dual regimen is considered.

- **GLP-1 agonists:** Exenatide, dulaglutide, semaglutide, lixisenatide, and liraglutide are glucagon-like peptide-1 (GLP-1) agonists. These injectable agents are incretin mimetics that stimulate release of insulin from pancreatic beta cells and can be used as adjunctive therapy for patients with T2DM. GLP-1 agonists are not indicated in T1DM and are contraindicated in patients with severe renal impairment. Advantages are weight loss, no hypoglycemia when used as monotherapy and reduced incidence of cardiovascular events and nephropathy. Side effects include injection site reactions, GI side effects (nausea, diarrhea, vomiting), increased risk of pancreatitis and thyroid C-cell carcinoma. Cost is a barrier to their use.
- **Sodium-glucose co-transporter 2 ($SGLT_2$) inhibitors** (e.g., canagliflozin, dapagliflozin, sotagliflozin, empagliflozin) are useful for oral treatment of type 2 DM. By inhibiting $SGLT_2$, these medications decrease glucose reabsorption, increase urinary glucose excretion, and lower blood glucose levels (decrease HbA_{1c} by 0.7%). Empagliflozin has been shown to slow progression of renal disease in type 2 diabetics with CVD. $SGLT_2$ inhibitors reduce the risk of hospitalization for heart failure or death from cardiovascular disease among patients with stable heart failure. Sotagliflozin therapy initiated before or shortly after discharge in patients with diabetes and recent worsening heart failure resulted in a significantly lower total number of deaths from cardiovascular causes and hospitalizations and urgent visits for heart failure versus placebo in a recent trial.[3] Potential advantages include weight loss (up to 3.5% of BMI) and mild lowering of blood pressure (2 to 4 mm Hg). Side effects include increased risk of genital mycotic infections, UTIs, and volume depletion. Renal function should be evaluated before starting $SGLT_2$ inhibitors and periodically thereafter. Temporary discontinuation of these meds is recommended in cases of reduced oral intake or fluid loss. Higher cost and limited drug formulary availability are limiting factors.
- **DPP-4 inhibitors:** Sitagliptin, saxagliptin, vildagliptin, alogliptin, and linagliptin inhibit the enzyme DPP-4, responsible for inactivation and degradation of glucagon-like peptide-1 (GLP-1) and glucose-dependent insulinotropic polypeptide (GIP). These drugs, known as "DPP-4 inhibitors" or "gliptins," raise blood incretin levels, thereby inhibiting glucagon release and lowering blood glucose levels. When used with metformin, they do not cause hypoglycemia. They have modest efficacy (hemoglobin A_{1C} reductions of 0.5% to 1%, neutral effect on weight). Linagliptin does not require a dosage adjustment in renal insufficiency. Cost is a major barrier to their use. Sitagliptin can be used in any degree of kidney disease but needs to be dosed based on GFR and creatinine levels.
- **Sulfonylureas:** Sulfonylureas increase insulin secretion and work best when given before meals. All sulfonylureas are contraindicated in patients who are allergic to sulfa. Use of sulfonylureas confers a greater risk of hypoglycemia than the other agents. These agents are now being considered to be used as last or later resort or when cost is of major concern for the patient and when other therapies cannot be incorporated or are contraindicated.
- **Acarbose and miglitol:** These agonists inhibit pancreatic amylase and small intestinal glucosidases, thereby delaying carbohydrate absorption in the gut and reducing associated postprandial hyperglycemia. The major side effects are flatulence, diarrhea, and abdominal cramps.
- **The meglitinides nateglinide and repaglinide and the bile acid sequestrant colesevelam** can also be used to lower glucose levels but are expensive and generally poorly tolerated.
- **Pramlintide** is a synthetic analog of human amylin, which is synthesized by pancreatic beta cells and cosecreted with insulin in response to food intake. It suppresses glucagon secretion and slows stomach emptying and can be used as an adjunctive treatment for patients with T1DM or T2DM who inject insulin at mealtime. Nausea is its major side effect. This therapy has been largely replaced with use of GLP-1 analogs.
- **Thiazolidinediones (pioglitazone and rosiglitazone)** increase insulin sensitivity and have been used in the therapy of type 2 diabetes. Serum transaminase levels should be obtained before starting therapy and monitored periodically. Thiazolidinediones, in general, result in moderate weight gain and increase the risk for heart failure and osteoporosis/fractures. Rosiglitazone has an FDA black box warning for heart failure exacerbations and myocardial ischemia. Pioglitazone and rosiglitazone cause increased incidence of bladder cancer. Use thiazolidinediones with caution with calcium channel blockers, especially amlodipine (can cause fluid retention and edema).
- Combination therapy of various hypoglycemic agents is commonly used when dual therapy results in inadequate glycemic control.

1. **Insulin** is indicated for the treatment of all T1DM and for T2DM patients whose condition cannot be adequately controlled with diet and oral agents. The American College of Endocrinology and the American Association of Clinical Endocrinologists recommend initiation of insulin therapy in patients with type 2 diabetes and an initial HbA_{1c} level >9%, or if the diabetes is uncontrolled despite optimal oral glycemic therapy. Insulin therapy may be initiated as augmentation, starting at 0.1 to 0.2 unit/kg of body weight, or as replacement, starting at 0.6 to 1.0 unit/kg. Tables 13 and 14 summarize onset, peak, and duration of action of currently available insulin preparations. The risks of insulin therapy include weight gain, hypoglycemia, and in rare cases, allergic or cutaneous reactions.
2. Replacement insulin therapy should mimic normal release patterns.
   a. Approximately 50% to 60% of daily insulin can be given as a long-acting insulin (NPH, Ultralente, glargine, detemir) injected once or twice daily.
   b. The remaining 40% to 50% can be short-acting (regular) or rapid-acting (lispro, aspart, glulisine) to cover mealtime carbohydrates and correct increased current glucose levels.
   c. NPH and older basal insulins can be mixed with rapid-acting insulins like Humalog and regular; all newer basal insulins cannot be mixed in one syringe.
   d. Basal-bolus regimens are now preferred on injection of long-acting basal at bedtime or in AM to target fasting glycemia between 80 and 130, and rapid-acting mealtime insulins to target lower postprandial blood glucose <140 mg/dl.
   e. New combinations of basal insulins with GLP-1 analogs are now available:
      (1) Soliqua: Combines glargine insulin and lixisenatide in one pen. Patients taking <30 units start at 15 units and patient taking >30 units start at 30 units and are titrated every 3 to 4 days until fasting blood glucose levels are between 80 and 130 mg/dl. One should not exceed 60 units of glargine insulin.
      (2) Xultophy 100/3.6 is degludec insulin and liraglutide combination in one pen. Dosing is based on Tresiba dose. Patients start at 16 units and increase by 2 units every 5 to 7 days

[2] Chu PY et al: Hospitalization for lactic acidosis among patients with reduced kidney function treated with metformin or sulfonylureas, *Diabetes Care* 43:1462-1470, 2020.

[3] Bhatt DL et al: Sotagliflozin in patients with diabetes and recent worsening heart failure, *N Engl J Med* 384:117-128, 2020.

TABLE 13 Insulin Types and Action Profiles

Product	Onset of Action	Peak Action	Duration	
Rapid acting	Aspart (*Novolog* [Novo Nordisk, Princeton, NJ]) Lispro (*Humalog U-100* [Eli Lilly, Indianapolis, IN], *Humalog U-200* [Eli Lilly, Indianapolis, IN], *Admelog* [Sanofi, Bridgewater, NJ]) Glulisine (*Apidra* [Sanofi, Bridgewater, NJ])	10-30 min	30-180 min	3-5 hr
	Aspart (*Fiasp* [Novo Nordisk, Princeton, NJ])	2.5 min	40-50 min	
	Insulin human (*Afrezza* [MannKind, Westlake Village, CA]) inhalation powder	12 min	35-45 min	1.5-3 hr
Short acting	Regular U-100 (Humulin R U-100 [Eli Lilly, Indianapolis, IN]) Regular U-100 (Novolin R [Novo Nordisk, Princeton, NJ]) Regular U-500 (Humulin U-500)	30-60 min	2-4 hr	U-100: Up to 10 hr U-500: Up to 24 hr
Intermediate acting	NPH (Humulin N) NPH (Novolin N)	2-4 hr	4-8 hr	12-18 hr
Long acting	Detemir (*Levemir* [Novo Nordisk, Princeton, NJ]) Glargine (*Lantus* [Sanofi, Bridgewater, NJ], *Basaglar* [Eli Lilly, Indianapolis, IN], Toujeo U-300 [Sanofi, Bridgewater, NJ]) Degludec (*Tresiba U-100* [Novo Nordisk, Princeton, NJ], *Tresiba U-200*)	2-4 hr	Minimal	Detemir: 12-24 hr Glargine: Up to 24 hr Degludec: Up to 48 hr
Premixed	70/30 (NPH/Aspart) (*Novolog 70/30*) 70/30 NPH/Regular (*Humulin 70/30*) 75/25 (NPH/Lispro) (*Humalog 75/25*) 50/50 (NPH/Lispro) (*Humalog 50/50*) [Other combinations may be available in Europe.]	5-60 min	Dual	12-18 hr

TABLE 14 Clinical Features of Commonly Used Insulins

Types and Generic Names (Commercial Names)	Onset of Action (Min)	Time to Peak (hr)	Duration (hr)	Administration
Rapid Acting				
Aspart (Fiasp)	<5	0.5-1.5	3-5	Just before or just after meals
Aspart (Novolog)	10-20	0.5-1.5	3-5	
Lispro (Humalog)	10-20	0.5-1.5	3-5	0-15 min before or just after meals
Glulisine (Apidra)	10-20	0.5-1.5	3-5	
Short Acting				
Regular human (Humulin R, Novolin R)	30-45	2-4	4-8	15-30 min before meals
Intermediate Acting				
NPH (Humulin N, Novolin N)	60-120	4-8	12-20	Once or twice daily
Long Acting				
Detemir (Levemir)	60-120	6-10	16-24	Usually once daily
Glargine (Lantus, Basaglar)	60-120	No pronounced peak	~24	
Degludec (Tresiba)	60-120	No pronounced peak	Up to 72	
Premixed				
70/30 NPH/R (Humulin 70/30, Novolin 70/30)	30-40	4-8	12-20	Usually twice daily, 0-30 min before meals
75/25 Protamine-lispro/lispro (Humalog Mix 70/30)	10-20	4-8	12-20	
70/30 Protamine-aspart/aspart (Novolog Mix 70/30)	10-20	4-8	12-20	
50/50 Protamine-lispro/lispro (Humalog Mix 50/50)	10-20	4-8	12-20	
50/50 Protamine-aspart/aspart (Novolog Mix 50/50)	15-60	4-8	12-20	
Concentrated				
U-500 human regular (Humulin U-500)	30-45	6-12	12-24	Twice daily
U-200 degludec (Tresiba U-200)	60-120	No pronounced peak	>24	Once daily
U-300 glargine (Toujeo 300 U/ml)	60-120	No pronounced peak	Up to 72	Once daily

From Melmed S et al: *Williams textbook of endocrinology*, ed 14, Philadelphia, 2020, Elsevier.

to target fasting glycemia between 80 and 130 mg/dl, and dose cannot exceed 50 units. The use of this combination may eliminate or reduce prandial insulin needs and limits weight gain caused by insulin.

- Continuous subcutaneous insulin infusion (CSII, or insulin pump [Fig. 3]) provides comparable or slightly better control than multiple daily injections. It should be considered for diabetes presenting in childhood or adolescence and during pregnancy. The guidelines for insulin pump therapy from the American Association of Diabetes Educators include "frequent and unpredictable fluctuations in blood glucose" and "patient perceptions that diabetes management impedes the pursuit of personal or professional goals." Use of insulin pumps are today coupled with CGM monitoring and with software in which the computer is making the automatic adjustments to glucose levels, constituting what is referred to as an "artificial pancreas." This allows for fewer fluctuations of glycemia.
- Antiplatelet therapy: Low-dose aspirin (ASA; 81 mg/day) has been proven to lower the risk of subsequent myocardial infarction, stroke, or vascular death in secondary prevention studies. The ADA recommends low-dose aspirin for primary prevention in diabetic patients with one additional cardiovascular risk factor, including age older than 50 yr, cigarette smoking, hypertension, obesity, albuminuria, hyperlipidemia, and family history of coronary artery disease. Clopidogrel can be used in patients with atherosclerotic cardiovascular disease (ASCVD) and a documented aspirin allergy. The ADA does not recommend aspirin therapy in diabetics younger than 50 yr of age at low risk for coronary artery disease.
- Lipid management: Measure fasting lipid profile at least annually in adults.
  1. All patients with diabetes with one or more additional risk factors for CVD should be on statin therapy together with lifestyle

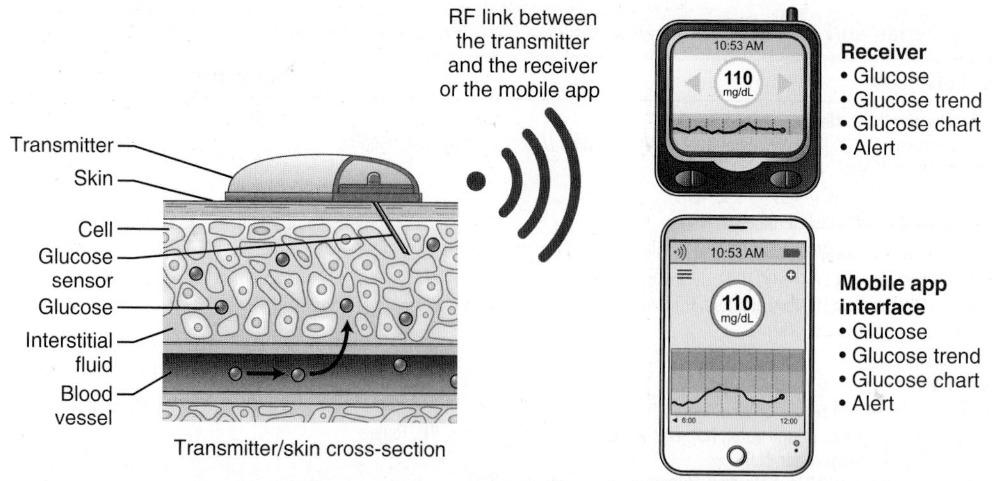

FIG. 3 The components of a continuous glucose monitoring system, which include the glucose sensor that resides in the subcutaneous tissue along with the transmitter that wirelessly transmits the glucose data to a separate receiver that can be a stand-alone device or an application on a mobile device. Wireless transmission occurs via radio frequency (RF) and Bluetooth. Both glucose concentrations and trends can be displayed. Alerts can notify the user when glucose levels are rising or falling. (From Melmed S et al: *Williams textbook of endocrinology*, ed 14, Philadelphia, 2020, Elsevier.)

TABLE 15 Classification of Hypoglycemia in Diabetes

Clinical Classification	Definition
Severe hypoglycemia	An event requiring the assistance of another person to actively administer carbohydrate, glucagon, or other resuscitative actions. Plasma glucose measurements may not be available during such an event, but neurologic recovery attributable to the restoration of plasma glucose to a normal level is considered sufficient evidence that the event was induced by a low plasma glucose concentration.
Documented symptomatic hypoglycemia	An event during which typical symptoms of hypoglycemia are accompanied by a measured plasma glucose concentration of ≤70 mg/dl (3.9 mmol/L).
Asymptomatic hypoglycemia	An event not accompanied by typical symptoms of hypoglycemia but with a measured plasma glucose concentration of ≤70 mg/dl (3.9 mmol/L).
Probable symptomatic hypoglycemia	An event during which symptoms typical of hypoglycemia are not accompanied by a plasma glucose determination but were presumably caused by a plasma glucose concentration of ≤70 mg/dl (3.9 mmol/L).
Pseudohypoglycemia	An event during which the person with diabetes reports any of the typical symptoms of hypoglycemia and interprets those as indicative of hypoglycemia, with a measured plasma glucose concentration that is >70 mg/dl (3.9 mmol/L) but is approaching that level.

From Melmed S et al: *Williams textbook of endocrinology*, ed 14, Philadelphia, 2020, Elsevier.

modification regardless of baseline lipid levels.

2. Diabetic patients aged 40 to 75 with LDL cholesterol of 70 to 189 mg/dl and without clinical ASCVD should receive at least moderate-intensity statin therapy and consider high-intensity statin therapy if 10-yr ASCVD risk is ≥7.5%.
3. Ezetimibe can be added to moderate-intensity statin therapy in those who cannot tolerate high-intensity statin therapy.
4. Combination therapy with statin and fenofibrate is not recommended but may be considered in those with triglyceride levels equal or greater than 204 mg/dl. If triglycerides are not at goal with combination of statin and fibrate, then prescription fish oil is advised if triglyceride levels still exceed 300 mg/dl.
5. PCK-9 inhibitors may be considered in diabetics with CAD risk when statins are insufficient and in those who cannot tolerate statins, have had cardiovascular events, and cannot achieve A_{1c} to target goal.

- Hypertension: Antihypertensive therapy is recommended to keep systolic blood pressure (BP) <140 and diastolic BP <90 mm Hg. Use of angiotensin-converting enzyme (ACE) inhibitors or angiotensin receptor blockers (ARBs) to decrease albuminuria and for prevention of progression of kidney disease should be considered regardless of presence of hypertension. Combination therapy with an ACE inhibitor and an ARB should be avoided due to increased risk of adverse effects among patients with diabetic nephropathy. In older adults a treatment goal of <130/70 mm Hg is not recommended due to higher mortality and morbidity.
- Bariatric surgery should be considered in adults with BMI >35 kg/m^2 and type 2 diabetes, especially if the diabetes is difficult to control with lifestyle and pharmacologic therapy. Five-yr outcome data showed that, among patients with type 2 DM and a BMR of 27 to 43, bariatric surgery plus intensive medical therapy was more effective than intensive medical therapy alone in decreasing, or in some cases resolving, hyperglycemia.[4]

[4]Schauer PR et al: Bariatric surgery versus intensive medical therapy for diabetes—5-year outcomes, *N Engl J Med* 376(7):641-651, 2017.

- Hypoglycemia—a plasma glucose concentration low enough to cause symptoms or signs—is a rare occurrence in individuals without diabetes but is common in sulfonylurea-, glinide-, or insulin-treated diabetes.
- The plasma glucose concentration is normally maintained in a relatively narrow range, 72 to 144 mg/dl (4.0 to 8.0 mmol/L), owing to a fine balance between glucose influx (exogenous glucose delivery and endogenous glucose production) and glucose efflux (glucose utilization by insulin-sensitive tissues, such as the skeletal muscle, and insulin-insensitive tissues, particularly the brain).
- A classification of hypoglycemia in diabetics is shown in Table 15. Hypoglycemia results from an imbalance between glucose influx and glucose efflux due to either excessive glucose removal from the circulation, deficient glucose delivery into the circulation, or both.
- Hypoglycemia in diabetes is typically the result of the interplay of therapeutic hyperinsulinemia and compromised defenses against falling glucose levels resulting in hypoglycemia-associated autonomic failure (HAAF), including defective glucose

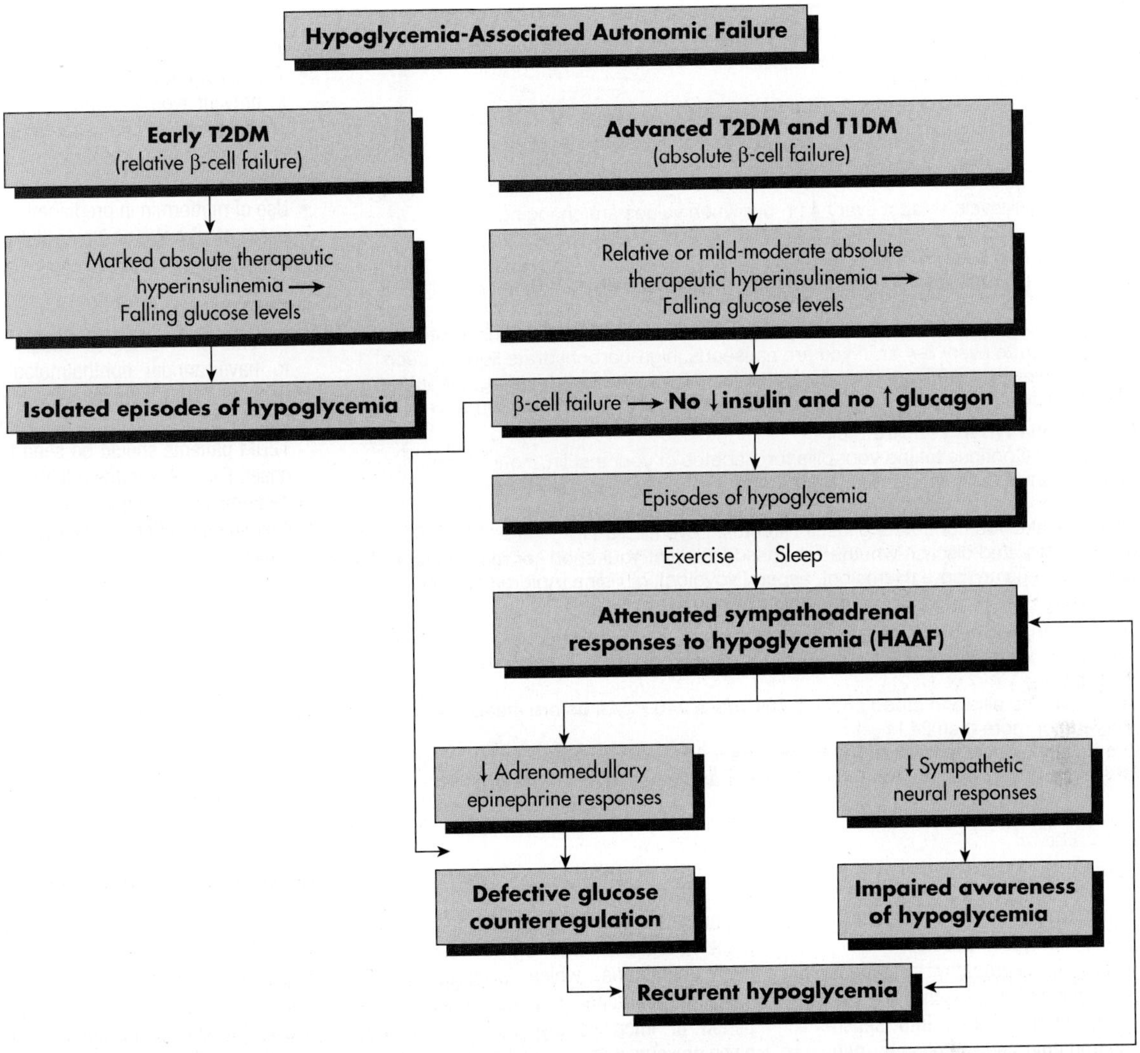

FIG. 4 Schematic representation of the concept of hypoglycemia-associated autonomic failure (HAAF) in diabetes and the pathogenesis of iatrogenic hypoglycemia including the clinical syndromes of defective glucose counterregulation and impaired awareness of hypoglycemia. *β-cell,* Pancreatic islet beta cell; *T1DM,* type 1 diabetes mellitus; *T2DM,* type 2 diabetes mellitus. (From Melmed S et al: *Williams textbook of endocrinology*, ed 14, Philadelphia, 2020, Elsevier.)

TABLE 16 Risk Factors for Hypoglycemia in Diabetes

Conventional Risk Factors: Absolute or Relative Insulin Excess
Insulin or insulin secretagogue doses are excessive, ill timed, or of the wrong type
Exogenous glucose delivery is decreased (e.g., after missed meals, during the overnight fast)
Glucose utilization is increased (e.g., during exercise)
Endogenous glucose production is decreased (e.g., after alcohol ingestion)
Sensitivity to insulin is increased (e.g., after weight loss, with improved fitness or improved glycemic control, in the middle of the night)
Insulin clearance is decreased (e.g., with renal failure)
Risk Factors for Hypoglycemia-Associated Autonomic Failure
Absolute endogenous insulin deficiency
A history of severe hypoglycemia, impaired awareness of hypoglycemia, or both, and recent antecedent hypoglycemia, prior exercise, or sleep
Aggressive glycemic therapy per se (lower HbA_{1c} levels, lower glycemic goals, or both)

HbA_{1c}, Glycosylated hemoglobin.
From Melmed S et al: *Williams textbook of endocrinology*, ed 14, Philadelphia, 2020, Elsevier.

counterregulation and impaired awareness of hypoglycemia (Fig. 4).

- An attenuated sympathoadrenal response to falling glucose levels, the key feature of HAAF, is induced by recent antecedent hypoglycemia, sleep, or prior exercise, and is reversible by short-term scrupulous avoidance of hypoglycemia.
- Iatrogenic hypoglycemia is associated with both morbidity and fatality in type 1 and type 2 diabetes mellitus. Risk factors for hypoglycemia are summarized in Table 16. Treat hypoglycemia in a conscious person with glucose tab or gel 15 to 20 g, and intramuscular injection of glucagon if unconscious. Patient and family members should be instructed on the administration of glucagon for individuals at significant risk for severe hypoglycemia. A sick day management protocol for diabetic patients is described in Box 3.

DISPOSITION

- Diabetic retinopathy occurs in nearly 15% of patients with diabetes after 15 yr of diagnosis and increases 1%/yr after diagnosis. Glycemic, lipid, and blood pressure controls are essential to reduce the risk and progression of diabetic retinopathy. An annual comprehensive eye exam by an ophthalmologist or optometrist should begin at the time of diagnosis for those with T2DM and after 5 yr in those with T1DM. Retinal laser photocoagulation and vitrectomy are effective treatment modalities. Prevention is best accomplished by strict glucose and BP control. Early blockade of the renin-angiotensin system has

BOX 3 Sick Day Management Protocol for Diabetic Patients

Examples of "Sick Day" Scenarios
- Feeling sick or presence of fever for 2 days or longer without getting better
- Vomiting or diarrhea for more than 6 hr

Management
General Measures
- Check blood sugar levels at least every 4 hr, but when values are changing quickly, check more often.
- Check urine or blood ketones.
- Modify usual insulin regimen according to a plan developed by the diabetes physician or team.
- Maintain adequate food and fluid intake. If your appetite is poor, aim for consumption of 50 g of carbohydrate every 3-4 hr. If you are nauseous, high-carbohydrate liquids, such as regular (not diet) soft drinks or juice, or frozen juice bars, sherbet, pudding, creamed soups, or fruit-flavored yogurt usually are tolerated. Broth also is a good alternative.

Taking Medications When You Are Sick
- If you are eating: Continue taking your pills for diabetes or your insulin. Your blood sugar may continue to rise because of your illness.
- If you are nauseous or vomiting or otherwise cannot take your medicines:
  - Continue to take your long-acting insulin (Lantus, Levemir, NPH).
  - Call your doctor and discuss whether you need to adjust your short- or rapid-acting insulin dose (regular, lispro [Humalog], aspart [Novolog], glulisine [Apidra]) or your other diabetes medicines.

Examples of When to Call Physician or Diabetes Team
- If glucose levels are higher than 240 mg/dl despite taking extra insulin according to a sick day plan
- If you take diabetes pills and blood sugar is still above 240 mg/dl before meals and remains there for more than 24 hr
- If symptoms/signs develop that might signal diabetic ketoacidosis or dehydration, such as dizziness, trouble breathing, fruity breath, or dry and cracked lips or tongue

From Parrillo JE, Dellinger RP: *Critical care medicine: principles of diagnosis and management in the adult,* ed 5, Philadelphia, 2019, Elsevier.

been shown to slow progression of retinopathy in patients with type 1 diabetes.
- The frequency of neuropathy in patients with type 2 diabetes approaches 70% to 80%. It can be subdivided into sensorimotor neuropathy and autonomic neuropathy. Duloxetine, a selective serotonin and norepinephrine reuptake inhibitor, is effective and FDA approved for relief of diabetic peripheral neuropathy. Pregabalin and gabapentin (900 to 3600 mg/day) are also effective for the symptomatic treatment of peripheral neuropathic pain. Topical capsaicin, 5% lidocaine transdermal patches, amitriptyline, and carbamazepine are also modestly effective. Use of high-dose vitamin combination of B_{12}, B_6 with alpha lipoic acid may help with nerve preservation and worsening of neuropathy, but will have no immediate effect on pain.
- Diabetic gastroparesis is most often seen in patients who have had diabetes for at least 10 yr and typically have retinopathy, neuropathy, and nephropathy. Major manifestations are postprandial fullness, nausea, vomiting, and bloating. Pharmacologic therapy involves prokinetic agents (metoclopramide). Endoscopic injection of botulinum toxin into the pylorus and gastric electrical stimulation (using f electrodes placed laparoscopically in the muscle wall of the stomach antrum and connected to a neurostimulator) represent newer approaches to nonpharmacologic therapy.
- Nephropathy: The first sign of renal involvement in patients with DM is most often microalbuminuria, which is classified as incipient nephropathy. Before the current period of intensive glycemic control and blood pressure with ACE inhibitors and angiotensin receptor blockade, it was suggested that 25% to 45% of diabetic patients would develop clinically evident renal disease (proteinuria) and 4% to 17% would progress to end-stage renal disease. In the current era of intensive glycemic and blood pressure control and ACE/ARB use, clinically evident diabetic nephropathy has declined to 9% and end-stage renal disease 2% to 7%. Use of ACE inhibitor or ARB is not recommended in diabetics with normal blood pressure, no microalbuminuria (urine albumin to creatinine ratio less than 30 mg/g creatinine) and normal renal function (eGFR >60 ml/min/1.73 m^2).
- Infections are generally more common in patients with diabetes because of multiple factors, such as impaired leukocyte function, decreased tissue perfusion secondary to vascular disease, repeated trauma because of loss of sensation, and urinary retention secondary to neuropathy.
- Prevention/delay of type 2 diabetes: Patients with prediabetes should achieve weight loss of 5% to 10% of body weight and increase physical activity to at least 150 min/wk of moderate activity such as walking. Metformin therapy may be considered in those at high risk, especially if they have hyperglycemia (HbA_{1c} ≥6) despite lifestyle interventions.
- The Mediterranean diet has been shown to prevent type 2 diabetes in patients with prediabetes and can delay the need of insulin use in type 2 diabetes in up to 50% of patients.
- Use of metformin in prediabetics can prevent onset of diabetes in up to 30% of patients, independent of diet.

REFERRAL

- Patients with diabetes should be advised to have annual ophthalmologic examinations. In T1DM, ophthalmologic visits should usually begin 5 yr after diagnosis, whereas T2DM patients should be seen from disease onset. Fig. 5 illustrates a flow chart useful in determining the timing of initial ophthalmic examination after a diagnosis of diabetes mellitus.
- Podiatric care can significantly reduce the rate of foot infections and amputations in patients with DM. Noninfected neuropathic foot ulcers require debridement and reduction of pressure.
- Nephrology consultation in all cases of proteinuria, hyperkalemia, uncontrolled BP, and when GFR has decreased to <30 ml/min/1.73 m^2.

PEARLS & CONSIDERATIONS

COMMENTS

- Because normalization of serum glucose level is the ultimate goal, every patient with diabetes should measure his or her blood glucose with commercially available glucometers unless contraindicated by senility or blindness.
- Continuous glucose monitoring is now commercially available for all types of diabetics on multiple daily injections of insulin. In the near future there will be weekly disposable sensors that can replace fingersticks. The advantage of CGM is that it not only gives a patient a value, but it shows a rate of change at that moment and predicts impending hyperglycemia or hypoglycemia, allowing a patient to react appropriately.
- Underinsured children and those with psychiatric illness are at greater risk for acute complications in T1DM and require frequent monitoring and aggressive risk management with diet, exercise, and periodic laboratory evaluation.
- Significant sustained weight loss using bariatric surgery has been reported as effective in achieving remission of type 2 diabetes in morbidly obese patients. Bariatric surgery may be considered for adults with BMI >35 kg/m^2 and T2DM, especially if diabetes or associated comorbidities are difficult to control with lifestyle and pharmacologic therapy.
- Cigarette smoking predicts incident type 2 diabetes. For a smoker at risk for diabetes, smoking cessation should be coupled with

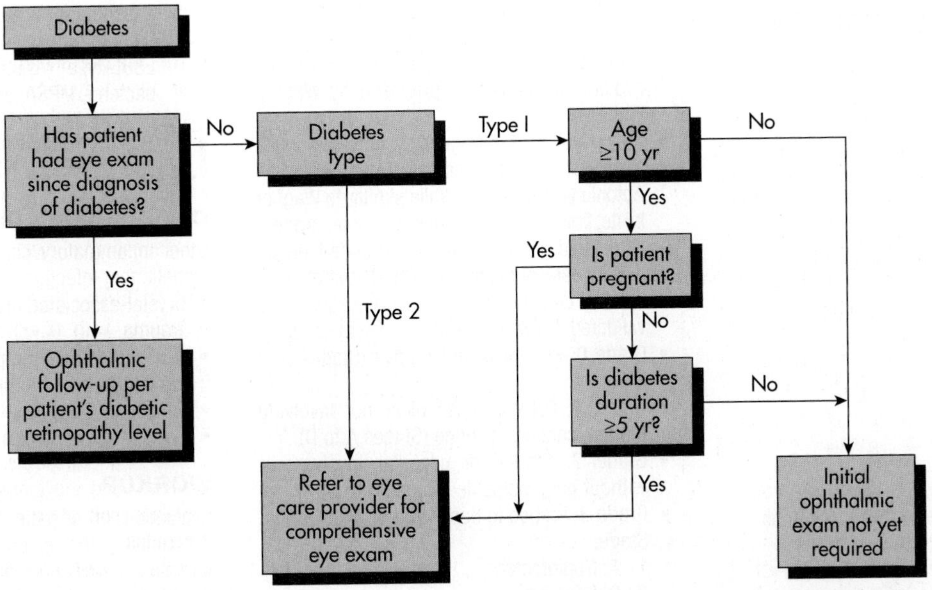

FIG. 5 Schematic flow chart of major principles involved in determining the timing of initial ophthalmic examination after a diagnosis of diabetes mellitus. These are minimal recommended times. Ocular symptoms, complaints, or other associated medical issues can necessitate earlier evaluation. Guidelines are regularly reevaluated based on new study results. (From Melmed S et al: *Williams textbook of endocrinology*, ed 14, Philadelphia, 2020, Elsevier.)

strategies for diabetes prevention and early detection.

- Glycemic control in hospitalized patients: The American College of Physicians (ACP) recommends against using intensive insulin therapy to strictly control blood glucose in nonsurgical intensive care unit (SICU)/medical intensive care unit (MICU) in patients with or without DM. The ACP recommends a target blood glucose level of 130 to 180 mg/dl if insulin therapy is used.
- Studies have shown that tight glycemic control in SICU patients can reduce infection rates and ICU stay. This was not seen in MICU patients. However, there is evidence showing that patients using continuous IV insulin infusions to keep tight glycemic control after open heart surgery reduces sternal wound infection rates.
- Now many institutions are incorporating automated log adjustment, such as Glucommander, which reduces workload of staff in maintaining smooth glycemic control.

SUGGESTED READINGS

Available at ExpertConsult.com

RELATED CONTENT

Diabetes Mellitus Type 1 (Patient Information)
Diabetes Mellitus Type 2 (Patient Information)
Diabetic Foot (Related Key Topic)
Diabetic Gastroparesis (Related Key Topic)
Diabetic Ketoacidosis (Related Key Topic)
Diabetic Polyneuropathy (Related Key Topic)
Diabetic Retinopathy (Related Key Topic)
Gestational Diabetes Mellitus (Related Key Topic)
Hyperglycemic Hyperosmolar Syndrome (Related Key Topic)

AUTHORS: **David J. Domenichini, MD,** and **Fred F. Ferri, MD**

BASIC INFORMATION

DEFINITION

Diabetic foot infections (DFIs) are a common and potentially serious problem in persons with diabetes. They usually arise from either a skin ulceration that occurs secondarily to peripheral neuropathy or in a wound caused by some form of trauma. The infection usually involves one or more bacteria and can spread to contiguous tissues including bone, causing an osteomyelitis.

SYNONYMS

Diabetic foot ulcer
Diabetic foot infection
DFI

ICD-10CM CODES

E11.621	Type 2 diabetes mellitus with foot ulcer
E10.5	Diabetes mellitus with peripheral circulatory complications
E10.6D	Diabetes mellitus with other specific complications

EPIDEMIOLOGY & DEMOGRAPHICS

INCIDENCE: DFIs are the most common cause of hospitalizations for diabetic patients. They account for 20% of all hospital admissions. Nearly one in six patients will die within 1 yr of their infection.

PREVALENCE: 25 million people in the U.S. have diabetes, of which 19% to 34% will develop a foot ulcer in their lifetime and more than 50% of these will become infected.

PREDOMINANT SEX & AGE: Females greater than males

PEAK INCIDENCE: More common in Hispanics, African Americans, and Native Americans due to increased rates of diabetes in those populations

RISK FACTORS:
- Diabetes greater than 10 yr
- Poor glucose control
- Peripheral neuropathy: Altered protective sensation and altered pain response
- Diabetic angiopathy: Atherosclerotic obstruction of larger vessels leading to peripheral vascular disease
- Evidence of increased local pressure: Callus or erythema

PHYSICAL FINDINGS & CLINICAL PRESENTATION

- Based on guidelines by Infectious Diseases Society of America, infection is present if obvious purulent drainage and/or the presence of two or more signs of inflammation:
  1. Erythema
  2. Pain
  3. Tenderness
  4. Warmth
  5. Induration
- Systemic signs of infection include:
  1. Anorexia, nausea/vomiting
  2. Fever, chills, night sweats
  3. Change in mental status and recent worsening of glycemic control
- An earlier and commonly used classification system was originally proposed by Wagner (Table 1).
- An update to the Wagner system was introduced at the University of Texas (UT), San Antonio (Table 2), U.S. While similar to Wagner in its first three categories, this later system eliminated grades 4 and 5 and added stages A-D for each of the grades. The UT system was the first diabetic foot ulcer classification to be validated. University of Texas system Grade:
- Grade 0: Pre- or postulcerative (Stages A to D)
- Grade 1: Full-thickness ulcer not involving tendon, capsule, or bone (Stages A to D)
- Grade 2: Tendon or capsular involvement without bone palpable (Stages A to D)
- Grade 3: Probes to bone (Stages A to D)
  Stage:
  1. A: Noninfected
  2. B: Infected
  3. C: Ischemic
  4. D: Infected and ischemic

ETIOLOGY

- Most diabetic foot infections are polymicrobial (can involve 5 to 7 different bacteria) and depend on the extent of involvement.
- Superficial infections are likely due to gram-positive skin bacteria:
  1. *Staphylococcus aureus*, includes methicillin-resistant *S. aureus* (MRSA)
  2. *Streptococcus agalactiae* (group B streptococcus) and *Streptococcus pyogenes* (group A streptococcus)
  3. Coagulase-negative *Staphylococcus*
- Infections that are deep, chronically infected, or previously treated are likely to be polymicrobial:
  1. Include above bacteria plus enterococci, gram-negative rods including *Pseudomonas aeruginosa* and anaerobes
  2. With gangrene can expect more anaerobic bacteria such as *Clostridia* and *Bacteroides* species
  3. Patients with multiple admissions can have more resistant bacteria such as ESBL-type resistant gram-negative rod bacteria, MRSA, and *Acinetobacter*

TABLE 1 Wagner Diabetic Foot Ulcer Classification System

Grade	Description
0	No ulcer, but high-risk foot (e.g., deformity, callus, insensitivity)
1	Superficial full-thickness ulcer
2	Deeper ulcer, penetrating tendons, no bone involvement
3	Deeper ulcer with bone involvement, osteitis
4	Partial gangrene (e.g., toes, forefoot)
5	Gangrene of whole foot

Modified from Oyibo S et al: A comparison of two diabetic foot ulcer classification systems: the Wagner and the University of Texas wound classification systems, *Diabetes Care* 24:84-88, 2001. In Melmed S et al: *Williams textbook of endocrinology*, ed 14, Philadelphia, 2020, Elsevier.

DIAGNOSIS

DIFFERENTIAL DIAGNOSIS

Other inflammatory conditions that can mimic diabetic foot infections include:
- Crystal-associated arthritis such as gout
- Trauma
- Acute Charcot arthropathy from long-standing diabetes
- Venous stasis ulcers
- Deep vein thrombosis

WORKUP

Evaluation of a patient with a DFI involves determining the extent and severity of the infection, identifying the underlying factors that predispose to the infection, and determining the microbiologic etiology. An algorithm for risk screening in the diabetic foot is illustrated in Fig. 1.

PHYSICAL EXAMINATION

- Vital signs: Fever, chills, hypotension, tachycardia can be present.
- Detailed wound description: Length, width, and depth of wound, consistency of drainage, character of wound base: Granular fibrous necrotic.
- Determination of osteomyelitis: Highly likely if bone visible. A positive probe test to bone has a sensitivity of 66% and specificity of 85% in diagnosing bone infection.
- Necrotizing infections may present with cutaneous bullae, soft tissue gas, foul odor, and skin discoloration (Fig. E2).
- Severe infections may present with gangrene, tissue necrosis, and evidence of tissue ischemia (Fig. E3), all of which may be limb threatening.

LABORATORY TESTS

Important to obtain at baseline and to assess response to therapy:
- Fewer than 50% of patients have an elevated WBC.
- Determine BUN/Cr, acidosis, hemoglobin A_{1C}, and blood sugar.
- Acute phase reactants: Sed rate and CRP are markers for inflammation.
  1. Sed rate >70 increases probability of bone infection.
- Serum prealbumin and albumin are markers for nutritional status and ability to heal.
- An ulcer size larger than 2 cm^2 is indicative of osteomyelitis.
- Gram stains and cultures: Superficial cultures should not be obtained as they may contain colonizing bacteria; instead deep tissue cultures (aerobic and anaerobic) should be obtained.

TABLE 2 University of Texas Wound Classification System

Stage	Grade 0	Grade 1	Grade 2	Grade 3
A	Preulcer or postulcer lesion; no skin break	Superficial ulcer	Deep ulcer to tendon or capsule	Wound penetrating bone or joint
B	+ Infection	+ Infection	+ Infection	+ Infection
C	+ Ischemia	+ Ischemia	+ Ischemia	+ Ischemia
D	+ Infection and ischemia	+ Infection and ischemia	+ Infection and ischemia	+ Infection and ischemia

Modified from Armstrong DG et al: Validation of a diabetic wound classification system. The contribution of depth, infection, and ischemia to risk of amputation, *Diabetes Care* 12:855-859, 1998. In Melmed S et al: *Williams textbook of endocrinology*, ed 14, Philadelphia, 2020, Elsevier.

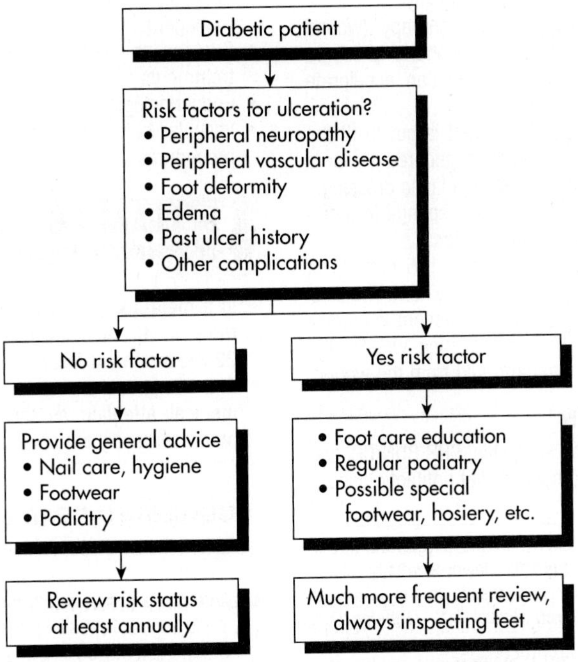

FIG. 1 Simple algorithm for risk screening in the diabetic foot. (From Melmed S et al: *Williams textbook of endocrinology*, ed 14, Philadelphia, 2020, Elsevier.)

IMAGING STUDIES

- Plain film x-ray evaluates bones and soft tissues and can detect presence of tissue gas, which would represent an emergent situation (Fig. 4).
- Osteomyelitis appears as radiolucencies, periosteal reaction, and destructive changes. Plain films are 67% specific and 60% sensitive for osteomyelitis.
- Bone scan: Indium-111 or technetium-99 can distinguish acute and chronic infections.
- CT and MRI: MRI is the most sensitive and specific test to detect osteomyelitis and abscess formation.

OTHER DIAGNOSTIC TESTS

- Annual noninvasive vascular studies: Ankle brachial index (ABI): <0.90 or >1.30 indicates peripheral arterial disease
- Transcutaneous oxygen (TcPO2) tension measurements: Predictive of wound healing failure at levels below 25 mm Hg

Rx TREATMENT

Empiric antibiotic regimen should be started based on likely pathogens suspected and severity of disease. Wound management and debridement including surgical consultation are important as well.

NONPHARMACOLOGIC THERAPY

- Good nutrition will promote wound healing.
- Glycemic control will promote healing.
- Fluid and electrolyte balance will improve healing.

ACUTE GENERAL TREATMENT

WOUND MANAGEMENT:

- Debridement of callus and necrotic tissues by wound care specialist or surgeon and at times may require multiple debridements.
- Wound dressing: To absorb exudates and promote healing. Many products are available but none has been proven superior and include:
  1. Enzymes
  2. Gels
  3. Hydrocolloids
  4. Antiseptics containing iodine or silver salts
  5. Honey
- Relieve pressure on the foot: Casts or special shoes.
- Amputation or revascularization procedures such as angioplasty or bypass grafting may be necessary.

ANTIBIOTIC MANAGEMENT:

- Prior to receiving culture results an empiric antibiotic regimen should be started as soon as possible to cover skin bacteria, gram-negative rods, and anaerobes. Options for intravenous therapy include:
  1. Piperacillin-tazobactam: 3.375 g IV q6h with normal kidney function. Will cover gram-negative rods including *Pseudomonas aeruginosa,* streptococci, anaerobes, and *Staphylococcus aureus.* Adjust dose based on CrCl.
  2. Meropenem: 1 g IV q8h with normal kidney function has comparable coverage as piperacillin-tazobactam. Similar agents include imipenem and doripenem.
  3. Third-generation cephalosporin such as cefepime, 2 g IV q8h, or ceftriaxone, 2 g IV qd, have excellent gram-negative coverage, and for anaerobic coverage add metronidazole, 500 mg IV q8h, or clindamycin 900 mg IV q8h. Cefepime will cover *Pseudomonas aeruginosa* but ceftriaxone will not.
  4. For penicillin-allergic patients a combination of ciprofloxacin, 400 mg IV q12h, plus metronidazole or clindamycin is an option. Aztreonam is another option for gram-negative rod coverage, 2 g IV q8h.
  5. If MRSA is suspected, need to add IV vancomycin, 15 to 20 mg/kg IV q8 to 12h, depending on age and CrCL and follow trough levels to keep above 15. Other options include daptomycin, 4 mg/kg IV qd, which does not have to be adjusted for CrCL, or linezolid, 400 to 600 mg IV q12h.
  6. If VRE is suspected, options include tigecycline, 100-mg IV load dose, then 50-mg IV q12h, which also covers MRSA and gram-negative rods but not *Pseudomonas aeruginosa,* or can use daptomycin or linezolid.
  7. If ESBL gram-negative bacteria are suspected, then options include meropenem or ertapenem, 1 g IV qd, or tigecycline.
  8. Once culture results are known can tailor antibiotics to more specific agent.
- Oral antibiotics used for milder infections include amoxicillin-clavulanate, 875 mg PO q12h, which will cover gram-negative rods, streptococci, and anaerobes, or ciprofloxacin plus metronidazole or clindamycin. Bactrim will cover MRSA and MSSA and some gram-negative rods.

The expert panel on diabetic foot infection (DFI) of the International Working Group on the Diabetic Foot conducted a systematic review.

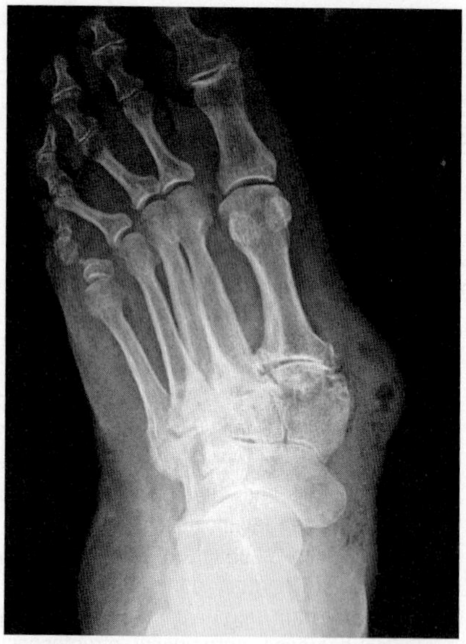

FIG. 4 X-ray. Significant soft tissue swelling in midfoot with numerous gas bubbles seen in the soft tissues.

Results of comparisons of different antibiotic regimens generally demonstrated that newly introduced antibiotic regimens appeared to be as effective as conventional therapy.

CHRONIC TREATMENT

- Length of therapy: Highly variable depending on the severity of the infection. In general, 2 to 4 wk of antibiotics is sufficient. If bone infection suspected or documented, may need 4 to 8 wk of antibiotics, preferably intravenous via a peripherally inserted central line (PICC line).
- Surgical debridement may also be necessary for several weeks.

COMPLEMENTARY MEDICINE

- Hyperbaric oxygen (HBO): Used as an adjunct to antibiotics, debridement, and revascularization in the therapy of chronic, nonhealing wounds associated with diabetes. Evidence of effectiveness is conflicting.[1,2] HBO acts by:
  1. Inducing vasoconstriction and reducing vasogenic edema
  2. Facilitating fibroblast activity, angiogenesis, and wound healing
  3. Killing anaerobic bacteria and augmenting neutrophil bactericidal activity
- Negative pressure wound therapy (wound vac): Controlled, subatmospheric pressure applied to an open wound can accelerate healing and closure.
  1. An open cell foam insert is cut to fit the open wound and then secured under a clear, vapor-permeable, plastic dressing.
  2. Tubing extends from the sponge to a disposable collection canister.
  3. A portable pump applies 125 mm Hg of controlled suction to the system. The subatmospheric pressure (suction) is equally distributed across the open wound and evacuates stagnant fluid from the wound.

DISPOSITION

- Following up on sed rates, CRP, BUN/CR, and levels of vancomycin if that antibiotic used.
- Surgical or wound center care follow-up.
- HBO usually involves multiple sessions over several weeks.
- Wound vac is applied for weeks and requires periodic nursing follow-up.
- The risk of death at 5 yr for a patient with a diabetic foot ulcer is 2 to 5 times as high as the risk for a patient with diabetes without a foot ulcer.

REFERRAL

- Infectious disease consultant for antibiotic management
- Surgeon or wound care center for surgical treatments
- Endocrinologist for good diabetes care
- Vascular surgeon for angioplasty or bypass procedures

PEARLS & CONSIDERATIONS

- In a meta-analysis of randomized controlled trials on the outcome of DFIs, there was a 22.7% treatment failure rate.
- Patients should be advised to seek prompt medical attention as these infections can progress rapidly to gangrene.

SUGGESTED READINGS

Available at ExpertConsult.com

AUTHOR: **Glenn G. Fort, MD, MPH**

[1] Santema KTB et al: Hyperbaric oxygen therapy in the treatment of ischemic lower-extremity ulcers in patients with diabetes: results of the Damocles multicenter randomized clinical trial, *Diabetes Care* 41:112, 2018.

[2] Frykberg RG et al: A multinational, multicenter, randomized, double-blinded, placebo-controlled trial to evaluate the efficacy of cyclical topical wound oxygen therapy (TWO2) in the treatment of chronic diabetic foot ulcers: the TWO2 study, *Diabetes Care* 43(3), 616-624, 2020.

BASIC INFORMATION

DEFINITION

Gastroparesis is a syndrome characterized by delayed gastric emptying in the absence of a mechanical obstruction of the stomach. It is associated with the cardinal symptoms of nausea, vomiting, early satiety, belching, bloating, and/or upper abdominal pain. It is commonly associated with longstanding, poorly controlled diabetes.

SYNONYMS

Gastroparesis diabeticorum
Gastrointestinal autonomic neuropathy
Delayed gastric emptying

ICD-10CM CODE

K31.84 Diabetic gastroparesis

EPIDEMIOLOGY & DEMOGRAPHICS

- Age-adjusted incidence of gastroparesis is 2.4 per 100,000 person-yr for men and 9.8 per 100,000 person-yr for women. The age-adjusted prevalence of definite gastroparesis is 9.6 per 100,000 persons for men and 38 per 100,000 persons for women
- Gastroparesis is seen more commonly in women, and there is no known genetic predisposition to the disease
- There are certain risk factors for development of gastroparesis, and diabetes is the most frequently recognized systemic disease. However, the most common form is idiopathic, where no detectable primary underlying abnormality is found. The idiopathic form accounts for approximately 50% of the patients with delayed gastric emptying
- Other risk factors include:
  1. Postviral, especially rotavirus and Norwalk virus
  2. Medications including narcotics, calcium channel blockers, and tricyclic antidepressants
  3. Postsurgical
  4. Neurologic illnesses, such as multiple sclerosis, brain stem stroke, or tumor, etc.
  5. Autoimmune gastrointestinal dysmotility
  6. Others such as mesenteric ischemia, scleroderma

PHYSICAL FINDINGS & CLINICAL PRESENTATION

- Patients with gastroparesis present with nausea, vomiting (vomitus may contain food ingested a few hours earlier), abdominal pain, early satiety, postprandial fullness, bloating, and in severe cases, weight loss. Although abdominal pain is a frequent symptom in patients with gastroparesis, it is rarely the predominant symptom.
- Interestingly, in patients with diabetes as the cause for gastroparesis, severe retching and vomiting are more commonly reported.
- Symptoms of gastroparesis are more pronounced in patients with type 1 diabetes, as compared with patients with type 2 diabetes.
- Physical examination findings may include epigastric distention or tenderness, but not guarding or rigidity. A succussion splash may be heard on auscultation by gently rocking the patient.

ETIOLOGY

- Diabetic gastroparesis is thought to result from impairment of neural control of gastric function. Various mechanisms of nerve injury include inflammatory changes to the autonomic ganglia or dropout of myelinated fibers involving the vagus nerve.
- Acute hyperglycemia has been found to have effects on the gastric sensory and motor functions by causing altered gastric electrical activity. It can also result in relaxation of the proximal stomach and decreased pressure in the antrum and pylorus. All of these processes can contribute to the retardation of gastric emptying.
- Achieving euglycemia can correct the gastric emptying delay.
- The effect of chronic hyperglycemia on the stomach is less clear, but there is some evidence that gastric emptying of meals is slower in patients with high glycated hemoglobin levels.

DIAGNOSIS

DIFFERENTIAL DIAGNOSIS

- Gastric outlet obstruction
- Cyclic vomiting syndrome
- Chronic use of cannabinoids
- Functional dyspepsia
- Irritable bowel syndrome
- Rumination syndrome
- Eating disorders such as anorexia nervosa and bulimia

WORKUP

- Thorough history and physical examination.
  1. An associated history of poorly controlled blood sugars may be present.
  2. A history of retinopathy, nephropathy, and neuropathy may be present in association with diabetes.
- All medications that can delay gastric emptying should be stopped before formal workup.

LABORATORY TESTS

No specific labs are needed to confirm the diagnosis, but the following can help to arrive at diagnosis:

- Hemoglobin A_{1c} (HbA_{1c})
- TSH
- Total protein/albumin
- Hemoglobin
- Vitamin B_{12}
- Antinuclear antibody titers

IMAGING STUDIES

- Initial imaging should be done to rule out a mass causing mechanical obstruction.
  1. Upper GI endoscopy is first line.
  2. Computed tomography (CT) enterography vs. magnetic resonance (MR) enterography may also be done to rule out mechanical obstruction from a small-bowel mass.
  3. Barium follow-through if CT or MR enterography unavailable.
- Food retained after overnight fasting may be suggestive of gastroparesis.
- After a mechanical obstruction has been ruled out, scintigraphic gastric emptying should be done as a confirmatory test.
  1. It is the simplest and most cost-effective test.
  2. Documenting the presence of delayed gastric emptying and assessing its severity is best done by measuring the delay in gastric emptying of solids.
  3. Patient is asked to ingest a standard, low-fat meal.
  4. Abnormal gastric emptying is defined as >10% gastric retention of solid food at 4 h and/or >60% at 2 h.
- ^{13}C breath test can also be used to measure gastric emptying.
  1. Not as sensitive as the scintigraphy method
- An alternative testing modality, called the *wireless motility capsule,* is as sensitive and specific as scintigraphy, but it is rather expensive and has not been shown to offer any added clinical information that scintigraphy has already provided.
  1. It is an ingestible, wireless capsule that measures pH, pressure, and temperature as it traverses the GI tract. Gastric emptying of the capsule occurs with phase III of the migrating motor complex, signifying completion of the postprandial phase.

TREATMENT

- Diabetic gastroparesis is not progressive, and treatment is mainly directed toward alleviating patient symptoms. Exacerbating factors must be corrected as well.
- Patients can have a calorie-deficient diet, along with deficiencies in minerals and vitamins.

NONPHARMACOLOGIC THERAPY

- Nonpharmacologic therapy includes provision of nutritional support along with dietary modifications.
  1. Oral nutrition is preferred in mild disease. Diet should include small meals that are low in fiber (low-residue) and fat.
  2. Avoidance of carbonated beverages is recommended because these can lead to symptoms of bloating.
  3. Alcohol and tobacco smoking should also be stopped because these also delay gastric emptying.
  4. For patients with severe disease, a feeding jejunostomy tube may be considered. A successful trial of a nasojejunal feeding tube should precede placement.
  5. Optimize glucose and electrolyte levels.

ACUTE GENERAL Rx

- Prokinetic agents can be used to improve gastric motility.

1. Metoclopramide and erythromycin are both available in intravenous and liquid form, which makes medication administration, tolerance, and efficacy more acceptable if patient symptoms are severe.
2. The FDA has approved a nasal spray formulation of metoclopramide called Gimoti for diabetic gastroparesis in adults. Cost is a limiting factor.
3. Domperidone is only available in the U.S. through investigational drug application due to increased risk of QT interval prolongation and arrhythmias.

- Antiemetic agents may also be needed for symptom relief in the acute setting.
  1. Phenothiazines, such as promethazine.
  2. 5-HT3 antagonists, such as ondansetron.
  3. Neurokinin receptor antagonist, such as aprepitant.
  4. Scopolamine patch
- Intravenous fluid resuscitation may be required if signs or symptoms of dehydration are present due to persistent nausea and vomiting.
- Correct hyperglycemia even in the acute setting, because delayed gastric emptying can be quickly corrected in the immediate setting.
- Discontinue medications that may delay gastric emptying.
  1. Pain medications.
     a. Avoid opioids.
     b. Tramadol may be used; however, one study showed that although gastric emptying was improved, colonic transit time was delayed.
  2. Incretin-based therapies and glucagon-like peptide 1 (GLP-1) analogues have been shown to retard gastric emptying.

CHRONIC Rx

- Metoclopramide should not be used for more than 12 wk unless the benefits outweigh the risks. Side effects include restlessness, anxiety, QT prolongation, and extrapyramidal effects such as dystonia and tardive dyskinesia.
- Erythromycin use is limited to 4 wk because longer use leads to tachyphylaxis. Similar effect is seen with the higher dose (250 mg) vs. a lower dose (40 mg).
- Pain management may need to be addressed for patients receiving chronic opioids.
  1. Low-dose tricyclic antidepressants (TCAs), selective serotonin reuptake inhibitors (SSRIs), and pregabalin can be used as alternatives for long-term pain control.
- Endoscopic intrapyloric injection of botulinum toxin may be considered.
  1. Not shown to improve symptoms associated with diabetic gastroparesis but does have a modest effect on improving gastric emptying.
  2. Not approved as a mainstay treatment modality.
- Gastric electrical stimulation via a gastric electrical neurostimulator can be offered to patients with diabetic gastroparesis.
  1. Shown to improve symptom severity and gastric emptying.
  2. Approved as a humanitarian exemption device for patients with refractory symptoms.
- Surgical intervention.
  1. Venting gastrostomy, gastrojejunostomy, pyloroplasty, and gastrectomy are available.
  2. Rarely employed and is reserved for patients with severe, debilitating disease.

COMPLEMENTARY & ALTERNATIVE MEDICINE

- Dietary modifications as described earlier
- Acupuncture
- Autonomic retraining

PEARLS & CONSIDERATIONS

COMMENTS

- Gastroparesis can be one of the consequences of chronic, poorly controlled diabetes.
- Symptoms of nausea, vomiting, bloating, early satiety, and abdominal pain in a patient with chronic, poorly controlled diabetes should prompt the possibility of gastroparesis.
- The diagnostic study of choice is gastric scintigraphy, performed by the nuclear medicine department.
- Discontinue all medications that can slow gastric emptying, especially opioids.
- Improve blood sugar control and avoid hyperglycemia.
- Antiemetics with prokinetic properties, such as metoclopramide, are most helpful in relieving nausea and vomiting, in both the acute and chronic presentations.
- Refer to gastroenterology for consideration of botulinum toxin injection or gastric neurostimulator placement if patients have poorly controlled and refractory disease.

PREVENTION

Focus on improved glycemic control in the long term.

PATIENT & FAMILY EDUCATION

- Gastroparesis Patient Association for Cures and Treatments (G-PACT)
- Association of Gastrointestinal Motility Disorders, Inc. (AGMD)

RELATED CONTENT

Diabetes Mellitus (Key Related Topic)
Diabetic Polyneuropathy (Key Related Topic)

SUGGESTED READINGS

Available at ExpertConsultcom

AUTHOR: **Hussain R. Khawaja, MD, FACP**

BASIC INFORMATION

DEFINITION

Diabetic ketoacidosis (DKA) is a life-threatening complication of diabetes mellitus (DM). It results from an absolute or relative insulin deficiency that results in insulin resistance when paired with counterregulatory hormone and free fatty acid excess. DKA is characterized by the presence of an anion gap metabolic acidosis, ketonemia, and hyperglycemia.

ICD-10CM CODES	
E13.10	Diabetic ketoacidosis
E10.10	Type 2 diabetes mellitus with other specified complication
E10.11	Diabetic ketoacidosis with coma associated with type 1 diabetes mellitus
E08.10	Diabetes mellitus due to underlying condition with ketoacidosis without coma
E08.11	Diabetes mellitus due to underlying condition with ketoacidosis with coma
E13.11	Diabetic ketoacidosis with coma

EPIDEMIOLOGY & DEMOGRAPHICS

DKA is the most common hyperglycemic emergency among patients with type 1 (T1D) and type 2 diabetes (T2D). In the past decade, the frequency of DKA has increased in the U.S., with more than 160,000 hospital admissions in 2017. DKA most commonly occurs in T1D, with one third in T2D. Those with ketosis-prone T2D are especially vulnerable. Overall, DKA prevalence has increased, yet mortality has decreased to <5%, significantly less than from hyperglycemic hyperosmolar syndrome (HHS). Mortality from DKA in children and adolescents is most commonly due to cerebral edema, whereas in adults it is usually related to the precipitating illness (i.e., sepsis, cardiac or CNS ischemia, pneumonia). Elderly patients present with multiple comorbidities that can complicate DKA even further. The most common precipitating factor for DKA in the elderly is related to insulin noncompliance and their underlying comorbidities. They often present with sepsis, and frequently with atrial fibrillation (AF). The combination of atrial fibrillation and diabetes increases morbidity and mortality associated with AF. In addition, elderly patients may be prescribed antipsychotic medications for underlying dementia, which have been associated with higher incidence of DKA admissions.

PHYSICAL FINDINGS & CLINICAL PRESENTATION

- Polyuria, polydipsia, polyphagia, weight loss, weakness
- Signs of dehydration (tachycardia, hypotension, dry mucous membranes, sunken eyes, poor skin turgor)
- Nausea, vomiting, abdominal tenderness, ileus
- Mental obtundation (can range from full alertness to coma)
- Tachypnea with air hunger (Kussmaul respirations)
- Fruity breath (caused by acetone)
- Evidence of precipitating factors (i.e., ischemia or infection)

ETIOLOGY

Hyperglycemia occurs from relative insulinopenia for the degree of transient insulin resistance plus an increase in counterregulatory hormones, which leads to increased hepatic gluconeogenesis and glycogenolysis. The resulting lipolysis and fatty oxidation produce ketonemia and metabolic acidosis. Both hyperglycemia and ketonemia result in an osmotic diuresis, which can lead to hypovolemia and subsequent decline in renal function.

DKA can be precipitated by various conditions:

- Infection (commonly of the respiratory or urinary tract, or dermatological).
- Insulin deficiency (undiagnosed diabetes, medication nonadherence/inadequacy, insulin pump malfunction/disconnect, diabulimia)
- Inflammatory conditions (i.e., acute pancreatitis)
- Ischemia/infarction (i.e., myocardial infarction, stroke, bowel ischemia)
- Severe extracellular fluid volume depletion
- Drugs (i.e., steroids, thiazides, atypical antipsychotics, SGLT2 inhibitors, alcohol, sympathomimetics including cocaine, cancer immunotherapy [such as antiprogrammed death 1 {PD-1} antibody treatment])

DIAGNOSIS

DIFFERENTIAL DIAGNOSIS

- Hyperosmolar nonketotic state
- Alcoholic/starvation ketoacidosis
- Lactic acidosis
- Acute kidney injury/chronic kidney disease
- Metabolic acidosis caused by exogenous poisons, e.g., methanol, ethylene glycol, paraldehyde
- Salicylate poisoning
- Hypovolemic or septic shock

WORKUP

After initial history is obtained, perform physical examination, including evaluation of airway, breathing, circulation, mental status, volume status, and signs suggestive of precipitating event(s).

LABORATORY TESTS

- Serum glucose level: Generally >250 mg/dl. However, "euglycemic DKA" can occur in 10% of the DKA population [i.e., exogenous insulin injection en route to hospital, food restriction, administration of an SGLT inhibitor (SGLTi)].
- Arterial blood gas (demonstrating metabolic acidosis): Arterial pH <7.30 (<7.00 in severe cases).
- Serum beta hydroxybutyrate and urine ketones: Positive (beta hydroxybutyrate >3 mmol/L, ≥2+ urine ketones).
- Serum electrolytes:
  1. Serum bicarbonate concentration: <15 mmol/L (mild DKA may reduce levels to <18 mmol/L).
  2. Serum potassium concentration: Levels may initially measure as normal or high from extracellular shift with insulin deficiency and hyperosmolality. However, overall total body potassium depletion occurs from urinary losses and vomiting.
  3. Serum sodium concentration: May be low, normal, or high. Hyperglycemia increases plasma osmolality, which attracts intracellular water to the extracellular compartment and decreases the sodium level. Correct the serum sodium concentration: Add 1.6 mmol/L to the measured serum sodium level for every 100 mg/dl increase of serum glucose >100 mg/dl and <400 mg/dl, and then increase the sodium level by 4 mmol/L for each glucose increment of 100 mg/dl above 400 mg/dl.
  4. Serum calcium, magnesium, and phosphorus: May be significantly low and may decrease further with DKA treatment.
  5. Anion gap (AG): Na − (Cl + HCO_3). AG is increased (>10 mmol/L) from elevated ketones.
  6. Blood urea nitrogen (BUN) and creatinine: Generally reveals acute kidney injury.
- Hemoglobin A1c if not performed within the preceding 3 mo.
- Complete blood count with differential: May indicate underlying infection (leukocytosis >25,000/mm^3), inflammatory condition, or hemoconcentration. A leukocytosis of 10,000 to 15,000/mm^3 is expected from the stress of illness alone.
- Urinalysis, urine/blood cultures: As indicated based on exam findings.
- Pregnancy test: Perform in all female patients of reproductive age. DKA in pregnancy bodes significant fetal morbidity and mortality.
- Lipase/liver enzymes: Obtain if abdominal pain present. Elevated lipase can occur without underlying pancreatitis.

IMAGING STUDIES

ECG, chest x-ray, and other imaging studies as indicated to evaluate the precipitating cause(s).

TREATMENT

NONPHARMACOLOGIC THERAPY

- Monitor mental status, vital signs, and urine output hourly until improved.
- Monitor serum glucose hourly and serum electrolytes, BUN, and creatinine every 2 to 4 hr until DKA resolves.

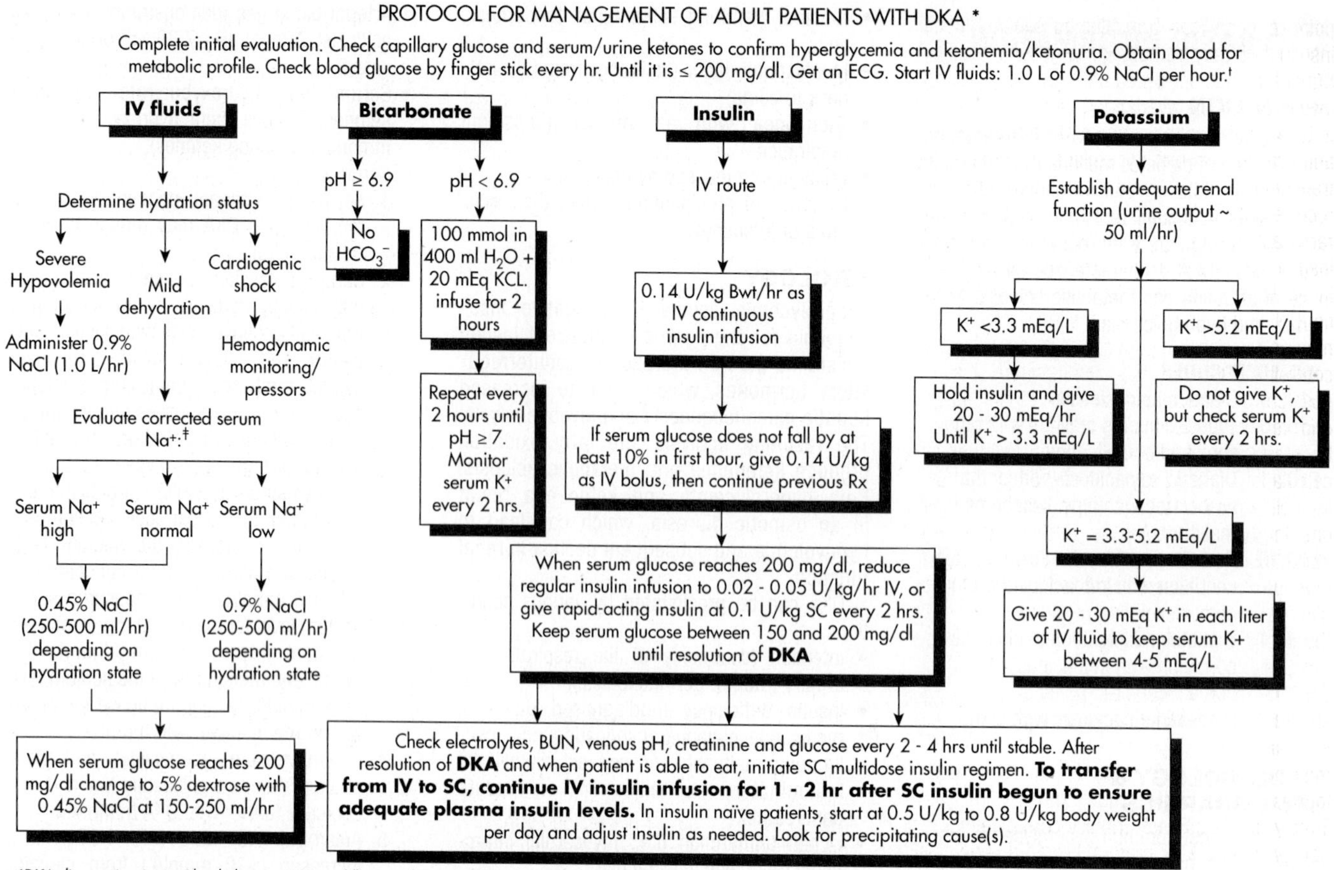

*DKA diagnostic criteria: Blood glucose >250 mg/dl, arterial pH <7.3, bicarbonate <15, mEq/l, and moderate ketonuria or ketonemia.
†Serum Na+ should be corrected for hyperglycemia (for each 200 mg/dl glucose, add 1.6 mEq to sodium value for corrected serum value)

FIG. 1 Management of diabetic ketoacidosis. *BUN,* Blood urea nitrogen; *DKA,* diabetic ketoacidosis; *ECG,* electrocardiogram; *IV,* intravenous; *Rx,* prescription; *SC,* subcutaneous. (From Nyenwe EA et al: The evolution of diabetic ketoacidosis: an update of its etiology, pathogenesis, and management, *Metabolism* 65[4]:507-521, 2016.)

ACUTE GENERAL Rx (FIG. 1)

FLUID REPLACEMENT: Fluid therapy is initiated to expand volume and restore renal perfusion for a typical total body water deficit of 8 to 10 L. In the absence of cardiac compromise or severe kidney impairment, infuse 0.9% normal saline (NS) at an initial rate of 1 to 1.5 L/hr (alternatively, use 15-20 ml/kg per hour) for the first 1 to 2 hr. The subsequent fluid choice depends on patient hemodynamics, electrolytes, and urinary output. If corrected serum sodium is normal or high, infuse 0.45% NS at 250 to 500 ml/hr. If corrected serum sodium is low, continue 0.9% NS at a similar rate. Once serum glucose decreases to 200 mg/dl, add 5% dextrose to the IV fluid. The recommended sodium decline is 0.5 mmol/L per hr and should not surpass 10 to 12 mmol/L per day. Hyperglycemia (>250 mg/dl) resolves sooner than ketoacidosis (6 versus 12 hr, respectively).

INSULIN ADMINISTRATION: Insulin should not be started until after initiation of IV fluid resuscitation and correction of hypokalemia. Once these are addressed, administer initial bolus of IV regular insulin 0.1 units/kg followed by 0.1 units/kg per hour infusion or a continuous infusion of 0.14 units/kg per hour without initial bolus. If the serum glucose declines by less than 50 to 75 mg/dl in the first hr, increase insulin infusion rate hourly until a steady glucose decline is seen. After the serum glucose reaches 200 mg/dl and until DKA resolves, maintain the serum glucose concentration between 150 and 200 mg/dl by decreasing the insulin infusion to 0.02 to 0.05 units/kg per hr or deliver subcutaneous rapid-acting insulin at 0.1 units/kg every 2 hr. Alternative to IV insulin includes use of subcutaneous (SQ) rapid-acting insulin for those presenting with mild-to-moderate DKA. Potential candidates for SQ insulin include those patients who are alert, do not require admission to a critical care area, have a pH >7.0, are able to tolerate oral intake, and have a bicarbonate level of at least 10mEq/L. SQ rapid-acting insulin can be given as an initial bolus of 0.3 units/kg bolus, followed by maintenance doses of 0.2 units/kg every 2 hr. Once blood glucose is <250 mg/dL, administer 0.05 to 0.1 units/kg every 2 hr until DKA resolves. If anion gap is not closed within 12 hr, the patient should be switched to an IV insulin infusion.

POTASSIUM REPLACEMENT: Insulin therapy shifts potassium intracellularly, frequently causing hypokalemia. If the serum potassium concentration at presentation is between 3.3 and 5.2 mmol/L, infuse 20 to 30 mmol of potassium chloride (KCl) with each liter of IV fluid to maintain serum potassium at 4 to 5 mmol/L. If serum potassium is <3.3 mmol/L, withhold insulin until the serum potassium level is >3.3 mmol/L, and replace potassium by administering KCl infusion at 20 to 30 mmol/hr. If the serum potassium level at presentation is >5.2 mmol/L, monitor the level every 2 hr without replacement.

BICARBONATE REPLACEMENT: The administration of bicarbonate in DKA is generally not recommended. Bicarbonate does not improve time to resolution of acidosis or discharge, although adverse effects are associated with severe metabolic acidosis (decreased cardiac contractility, cerebral vasodilation). In adult patients with pH <6.9, administer 100 mmol (2 ampules) of sodium bicarbonate in 800 ml of sterile water (isotonic solution) with 20 mmol KCl at 200 ml/hr for 2 hr until venous pH is >7.0. If pH is still <7 after infusion, repeat infusion every 2 hr until pH is >7.

PHOSPHATE REPLACEMENT: Phosphate replacement is not routinely recommended, although phosphorus concentrations decrease with insulin administration. In patients with cardiac dysfunction, respiratory depression, or anemia and serum phosphorus <1 mg/dl, add 20 to 30 mmol/L of potassium phosphate to IV fluids to prevent diaphragmatic muscle weakness.

TRANSITION TO SUBCUTANEOUS INSULIN: Resolution of DKA occurs when blood glucose is <200 mg/dl and two of the following occur: Venous pH >7.3, serum bicarbonate >15 mmol/L, anion gap ≤12 mmol/L. At this point, patients can transition to subcutaneous insulin but may remain on IV insulin if NPO. Subcutaneous intermediate- or long-acting insulin should be overlapped with IV insulin by 2 to 4 hr to maintain adequate insulin levels and prevent rebound hyperglycemia. When this transition occurs before a meal, the patient may receive a dose of prandial insulin with short- or rapid-acting analogs together with the basal insulin, and the IB insulin may be discontinued in an hr. In patients with a known history of controlled diabetes, their home insulin regimens may be resumed. In patients with known poorly controlled diabetes, the subcutaneous insulin dose can be determined based on stable insulin drip requirements. Insulin-naïve patients may be started on basal-bolus insulin therapy by calculation of total daily dose of 0.5 to 0.8 units/kg (split as half-basal and half-bolus; administer one third of total bolus for each meal) or by stable insulin drip requirements. Further subcutaneous insulin dose titration is based on blood glucose results. Resolution of glucotoxicity and the inciting condition(s) will decrease insulin requirements.

DISPOSITION: In general, patients with DKA should be admitted to an intensive care unit with an insulin infusion. Those with mild DKA may be treated with rapid-acting insulin analogues under observation and discharged. Timely follow-up with primary care or endocrinology is important, preferably with an appointment made before discharge, as over 40% of patients may be readmitted within 2 wk of hospital discharge.

PEARLS & CONSIDERATIONS

COMMENTS

- DKA is the initial presentation of diabetes in 15% to 20% of adults and 30% to 40% of children. This underscores the importance of educating patients, families, and school administrators regarding early symptoms of diabetes with the aim of earlier diagnosis.
- Ketosis-prone diabetes, also referred to as Flatbush diabetes, is found more often in certain ethnic populations, including African Americans and Asians, among others. Initial therapy with insulin is required for acute management; however, diet alone or oral hypoglycemic agents can be used to achieve glycemic control without the need of insulin.
- The development of euglycemic DKA is characterized by normal or modestly elevated blood sugars with anion gap metabolic acidosis, ketonemia, and ketonuria. Management is similar to DKA management. Mainstays of treatment involve correction of electrolytes and dehydration with IV fluids. However, higher percentages of dextrose (10% or 20%) are used to allow for concomitant high-dose insulin, required to correct the acidosis. If patient is taking an SGLTi, stop immediately. Patient may resume SGLTi only after resolution of DKA, feeling well, and discusses with primary outpatient managing physician.
- DKA in end-stage renal disease (ESRD) patients is relatively uncommon secondary to decreased insulin clearance. In fact, low GFR increases the risk for hypoglycemia. However, when ESRD patients develop DKA, special management considerations are needed. These patients are usually anuric and do not produce an osmotic diuresis, negating the need for aggressive volume repletion. Vigorous volume resuscitation may lead an ESRD patient to volume overload, pulmonary edema, and respiratory distress. Anuric ESRD patients do not have urinary potassium loss, thus making potassium replacement unnecessary. Similarly, phosphorus supplementation is not required. In fact, in severe acidosis, transcellular potassium shifts for hydrogen may produce hyperkalemia, prompting some providers to request immediate dialysis. Insulin therapy alone for hyperglycemia may also correct hyperkalemia without the need for dialysis. During DKA in ESRD patients, dialysis is generally only recommended if there are hyperkalemia-induced electrocardiographic manifestations. A precipitous drop in serum glucose from an insulin infusion and hemodialysis may result in rapid tonicity shifts, predisposing to cerebral edema. Thus, hemodialysis is typically delayed until the serum glucose is corrected. Due to increased risk for hypoglycemia, ESRD patients require careful and preemptive insulin reduction from the hospital DKA protocol.
- Address affordability of insulin before discharge. Consider use of NPH and Regular insulin for as little as $25 per vial.
- Proper instructions for insulin storage, dosing, timing of mealtime insulin before meals, preparation of insulin before injection (i.e., resuspend NPH), and use of syringe/vial or pen are essential.

PREVENTION

Many cases of DKA can be prevented by effective patient education and communication. Education of patients regarding sick day management includes early communication with the health care provider, continuing insulin during illness, checking ketones, and continuing an easily digestible liquid diet that contains carbohydrates.

SUGGESTED READINGS

Available at ExpertConsult.com

RELATED CONTENT

Diabetes Mellitus (Related Key Topic)
Hyperglycemic Hyperosmolar Syndrome (Related Key Topic)

AUTHORS: **Jaspreet K. Hehar, DO,** and **Jessica E. Shill, MD**

BASIC INFORMATION

DEFINITION

Diabetic nephropathy (DN) is chronic kidney disease defined by structural and functional changes that develop as a result of microvascular complications associated with long-standing or poorly controlled diabetes mellitus (DM). The clinical presentation includes albuminuria, hypertension (HTN), and progressive reduction in renal function. This is demonstrated histologically as glomerular basement membrane thickening, mesangial matrix expansion, foot process effacement, arteriolar hyalinosis, microaneurysms, nodular glomerulosclerosis (Kimmelstiel-Wilson lesion), and tubulointerstitial fibrosis.

SYNONYMS

Diabetic kidney disease
DN

ICD-10CM CODES	
E10.21	Type 1 diabetes mellitus with diabetic nephropathy
E11.21	Type 2 diabetes mellitus with diabetic nephropathy

EPIDEMIOLOGY & DEMOGRAPHICS

INCIDENCE: Diabetes is present in 10% of the U.S. population. DN occurs in approximately 40% of patients who have diabetes for more than 10 yr.

PREVALENCE: DN develops in approximately 30% of patients with type 1 diabetes mellitus (T1DM) and 40% of patients with type 2 diabetes mellitus (T2DM). DN is the leading cause of chronic kidney disease (CKD) and end-stage renal disease (ESRD) worldwide. Among U.S. ESRD patients, approximately 47% have DN as the primary cause for ESRD.

PREDOMINANT SEX & AGE: Male patients and older age

RISK FACTORS:

- Male
- Older age
- Race: People of African descent, American Indian, Hispanic, Asian/Pacific Islander
- Family history of diabetic nephropathy
- Hyperglycemia
- Hypertension
- Obesity
- Diabetic retinopathy
- Smoking
- Hyperlipidemia
- Early onset T2DM
- Low socioeconomic status

GENETICS: Polygenetic. Patients with first-degree relative with DN are at increased risk.

PHYSICAL FINDINGS & CLINICAL PRESENTATION

- Peripheral edema
- Foamy urine
- Weight gain or weight loss
- Hypertension
- Diabetic retinopathy
- Microalbuminuria/proteinuria
- Decline in estimated glomerular filtration rate (eGFR)

ETIOLOGY

- DN develops as a result of microvascular complications associated with long-standing DM.
- DN is characterized by histologic changes (Fig. E1) including glomerular basement membrane thickening, mesangial matrix expansion, foot process effacement, arteriolar hyalinosis, microaneurysms, nodular glomerulosclerosis (Kimmelstiel-Wilson nodules) and tubulointerstitial fibrosis. These changes lead to urine albumin/protein excretion and decreased eGFR.
- The pathophysiology leading to DN (Fig. 2) includes the generation of advance glycation end products, elaboration of growth factors, hemodynamic changes, and hormonal changes resulting in the release of reactive oxygen species and inflammatory mediators such as TNF-A, IL-1, and IL-6. These changes lead to glomerular hyperfiltration, glomerular hypertension, renal hypertrophy, and altered glomerular composition, which manifest as albuminuria, HTN, and progressive decline in renal function.

DIAGNOSIS

DIFFERENTIAL DIAGNOSIS

- Hypertensive nephrosclerosis
- Focal segmental glomerulosclerosis
- Amyloidosis and light chain deposition disease
- IgA nephropathy
- Membranous nephropathy

WORKUP

- Workup should include thorough history and physical with focus on duration of DM, degree of hyperglycemia, and presence of complications (including retinopathy) and appropriate laboratory testing (Fig. E3). Stages of diabetic nephropathy are illustrated in Fig. 4.

LABORATORY TESTS

- Urine albumin-to-creatinine ratio (UACR)
  1. Microalbuminuria ("moderately increased albuminuria") is defined as 30 to 299 mg/g and macroalbuminuria ("severely increased albuminuria") is defined as >300 mg/g
  2. Screening should be performed annually in patients with T1DM with >5-yr duration and annually for T2DM from its onset
  3. Confirm microalbuminuria with 2 to 3 elevated levels within a 3- to 6-mo period
  4. Early morning urine sample is recommended to identify albuminuria. Prolonged standing, heavy exercise, UTI, uncontrolled hyperglycemia, and acute illness can cause transient albuminuria
  5. In T1DM, microalbuminuria occurs 5 to 10 yr from onset
  6. In T2DM, up to 25% of patients with DN may have little or no proteinuria
- eGFR <60 ml/min per 1.73 m^2
- Other tests
  1. Electrolytes
  2. Lipid profile

IMAGING STUDIES

- Renal ultrasound may help identify disease since kidney volume increases by an average of 15% with the onset of diabetes mellitus.
- Renal biopsy is confirmatory but is only reserved for patients with atypical features. Atypical features include rapid decline in eGFR (>5 ml/min per 1.73 m^2 per year), overt proteinuria without prior microalbuminuria, active urine sediment, or features to suggest other systemic disease. Microscopic hematuria with isomorphic erythrocyturia may be seen with DN. In T2DM, DN can be present from the onset whereas in T1DM it typically

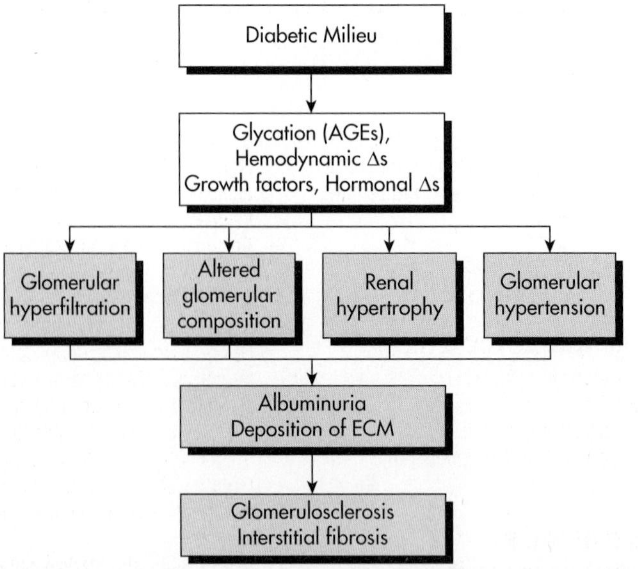

FIG. 2 Pathophysiology. *AGEs,* Advanced glycation end products; *ECM,* extracellular matrix. (From Umanath K et al: Update on diabetic nephropathy, *Am J Kidney Dis* 71:884, 2018.)

	Stage I	Stage II	Stage III	Stage IV
Median year of onset	0	10	15-17	18-20
Patients with diabetes (%)	100	30-35	30	30

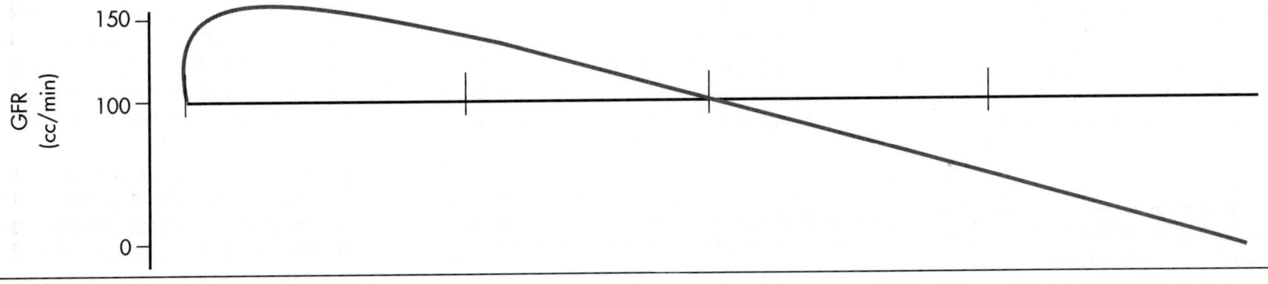

Urinary protein	Occasional and transient microalbuminuria	Fixed microalbuminuria	Proteinuria (>500 mg/24 hr) and microalbuminuria (200 mg/24 hr)	Nephrotic-range proteinuria (<3.5 g/24 hr)
Systemic manifestations	Hypertension: absent in type 1; often present in type 2		Hypertension: absent in type 1 and worsening in type 2	Manifestations of chronic renal insufficiency
Renal morphology and history	Kidney hypertrophy	Glomerular basement membrane thickening and mesangial matrix expansion	Focal glomerulosclerosis (± nodular or Kimmelstiel-Wilson lesions) Microvascular hyalinosis and tubulointerstitial fibrosis	Kidney may still be inappropriately large for level of renal insufficiency Global glomerulosclerosis and tubulointerstitial fibrosis

FIG. 4 Stages of diabetic nephropathy. *GFR*, Glomerular filtration rate. (From Goldman L, Schafer AI: *Goldman-Cecil medicine*, ed 26, Philadelphia, 2020, Elsevier.)

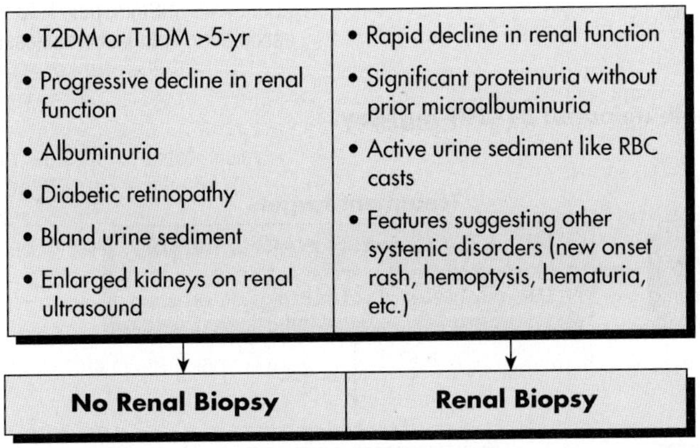

FIG. 5 Role of renal biopsy. *RBC*, Red blood cell; *T1DM*, type 1 diabetes mellitus; *T2DM*, type 2 diabetes mellitus.

develops after 5 yr. In general, patients with albuminuria, retinopathy, and progressive decline of kidney function do not require kidney biopsy (Fig. 5).

Rx TREATMENT (Table 1)

NONPHARMACOLOGIC THERAPY

- Smoking cessation
- Weight loss
- Dietary modification, including a low-carbohydrate, low-fat, and reduced-potassium diet

ACUTE GENERAL Rx

- Early identification and an aggressive multiprong approach of treatment of DN is key to slowing progressive disease (Table E2). Figure 6 illustrates the management of diabetic nephropathy before the onset of renal failure.
- Glycemic control with a goal A1C <7% is recommended as per Kidney Disease Outcomes Quality Initiative (KDOQI) guidelines, with modification for patients at risk for hypoglycemia. Glycemic control delays microvascular complications and progression of DN.
- The ideal blood pressure goal is debatable. The current KDOQI guideline recommends a goal BP <130/80 mm Hg; however, the Eighth Joint National Committee (JNC 8) guidelines recommend a goal BP <140/90 mm Hg.
- Use of renin-angiotensin-aldosterone system (RAAS) blockers should be the cornerstone of HTN management. Angiotensin type 1 receptor blockers (ARBs) and angiotensin–converting-enzyme inhibitors (ACE-Is) reduce proteinuria, lower blood pressure, and slow progression of DN. Combination therapy of ARB and ACE-I is not recommended due to greater risk of hyperkalemia and acute kidney injury.
- Cardiovascular events, including death, occur more frequently than ESRD; therefore lipid-lowering therapy with a goal of cardiovascular risk reduction is recommended.

CHRONIC Rx

- Identify anemia in CKD. Patients with DN are twice as likely to develop anemia compared to nondiabetic CKD and may need treatment with erythropoiesis-stimulating agents.
- Identify CKD-bone and mineral disorder, especially adynamic bone disease, which develops more often with DN.
- Figure 7 illustrates the management of diabetic nephropathy after the onset of renal failure.
- Patients with DN should have timely referral for kidney transplantation and vascular access evaluation as eGFR declines to 20 ml/min per 1.73 m^2.
- Type IV renal tubular acidosis from hyporeninemic hypoaldosteronism and hyperkalemia is common in DN, especially with RAAS blockade. Treatment with low-potassium diet, diuretics, and/or potassium binders may be required.
- Figure 8 illustrates the management of diabetic nephropathy after the onset of clinical proteinuria.

- Treatment options for end-stage renal disease in diabetic patients are summarized in Table 3.

DISPOSITION

- DN should ideally be monitored every 3 to 6 mo with assessment of BP, eGFR, potassium, and UACR.
- Patients with DN with severe albuminuria and decreased eGFR have poor prognosis and are at higher risk of cardiovascular events and deaths.
- The 5-yr survival rate of patients with diabetes and ESRD is approximately 30%.

REFERRAL

- Nephrology for CKD management
- Endocrinology for glycemic control
- Podiatry for foot care in the setting of neuropathy/peripheral vascular disease
- Ophthalmology for retinopathy management
- Dietician for specific dietary counseling

TABLE 1 Treatment of Diabetic Nephropathy

Stage 1	Tight glucose control BP control—consider use of ACEI or ARB
Stage II	Tight glucose control ACEI or ARB BP control Smoking cessation Weight reduction Exercise Annual eye examination
Stage III	ACEI or ARB BP control Restriction of dietary protein (to 0.8 g/kg/day of ideal body weight) Antihyperlipidemic medications
Stage IV	Treat manifestations of nephrotic syndrome and chronic renal insufficiency Prepare for renal replacement therapy, including prevention of abnormalities in calcium and phosphorus metabolism and prevention of anemia by early use of erythropoietin

ACEI, Angiotensin-converting enzyme inhibitor; *ARB*, angiotensin-receptor blocker; *BP*, blood pressure.
From Goldman L, Schafer AI: *Goldman-Cecil medicine*, ed 26, Philadelphia, 2020, Elsevier.

PEARLS & CONSIDERATIONS

- DN is the leading cause of CKD and ESRD worldwide. Early identification and an aggressive multiprong approach toward treatment of DN are key to slow its progression. Timely referral for renal transplant and access evaluation as they progress to ESRD are essential.
- DN is characterized by specific histologic findings; however, the diagnosis usually is made without renal biopsy with the presence of clinical indicators including long duration of disease (usually >5 yr) and presence of other complications of the disease (albuminuria, retinopathy).
- RAAS blockage is a vital component of DN treatment. After initiation of RAAS blockage, chemistry panel should be monitored in 1 to 2 wk to identify hyperkalemia or AKI. DN should ideally be monitored every 3 to 6 mo with assessment of BP, eGFR, potassium, and UACR.
- Insulin and many oral diabetic mediations are metabolized and cleared by kidneys and need dose adjustment with decline in renal function. Metformin is contraindicated with eGFR <30 ml/min per 1.73 m^2 and should be limited to <1000 mg/day in patients with eGFR <45 ml/min per 1.73 m^2 due to its association with lactic acidosis.

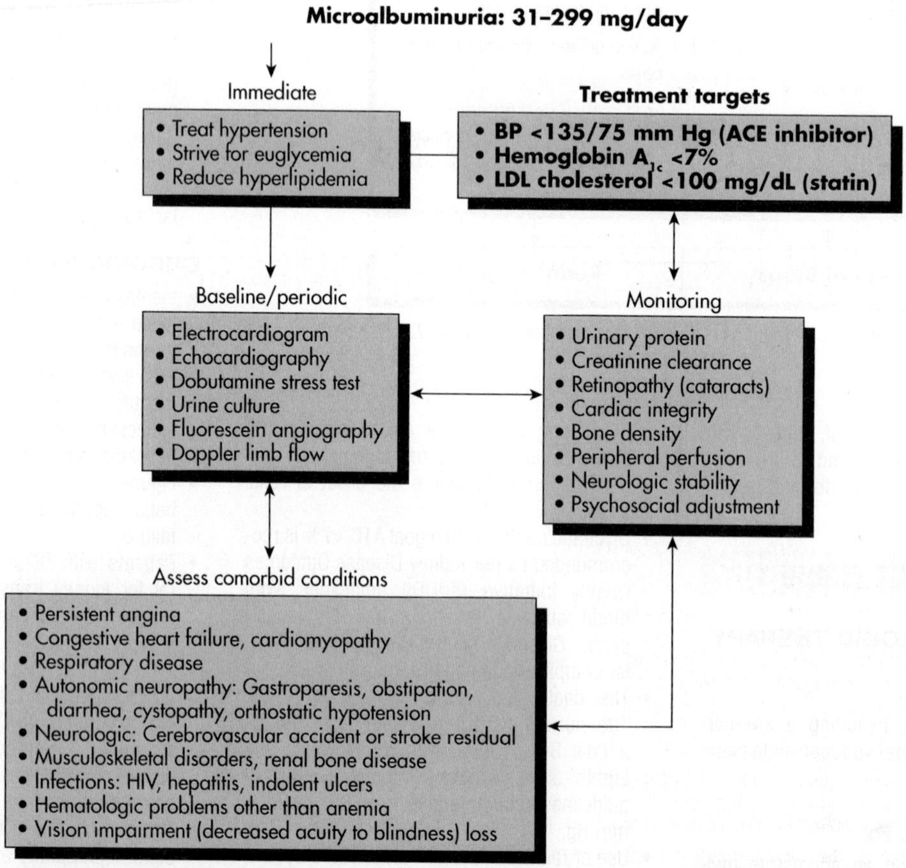

FIG. 6 Flow chart illustrating the management of diabetic nephropathy before the onset of renal failure. *ACE*, Angiotensin-converting enzyme; *BP*, blood pressure; *HIV*, human immunodeficiency virus; *LDL*, low-density lipoprotein. (From Melmed S et al: *Williams textbook of endocrinology*, ed 14, Philadelphia, 2020, Elsevier.)

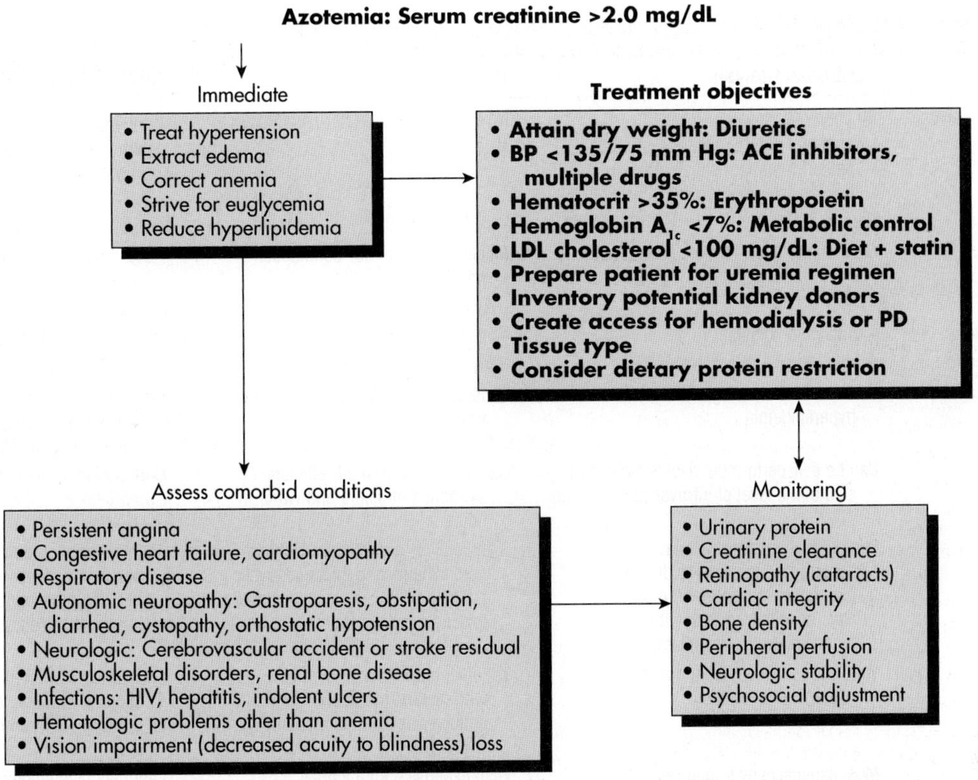

FIG. 7 Flow chart illustrating the management of diabetic nephropathy after onset of renal failure. *ACE,* Angiotensin-converting enzyme; *BP,* blood pressure; *HIV,* human immunodeficiency virus; *LDL,* low-density lipoprotein; *PD,* peritoneal dialysis. (From Melmed S et al: *Williams textbook of endocrinology,* ed 14, Philadelphia, 2020, Elsevier.)

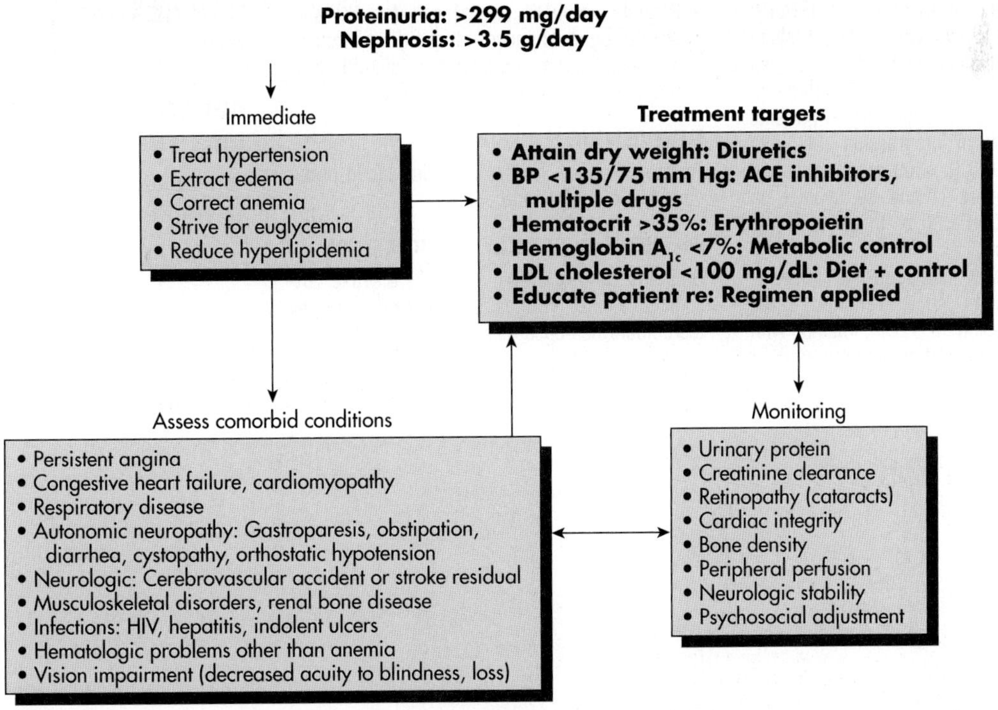

FIG. 8 Flow chart illustrating the management of diabetic nephropathy after the onset of clinical proteinuria. *ACE,* Angiotensin-converting enzyme; *BP,* blood pressure; *HIV,* human immunodeficiency virus; *LDL,* low-density lipoprotein. (From Melmed S et al: *Williams textbook of endocrinology,* ed 14, Philadelphia, 2020, Elsevier.)

TABLE 3 Options in Therapy for End-Stage Renal Disease in Diabetic Patients

Variable	Peritoneal Dialysis	Hemodialysis	Kidney Transplantation
Extensive extrarenal disease	No limitation	No limitation except for hypotension	Excluded in cardiovascular insufficiency
Geriatric patients	Limited by frailty, cognitive dysfunction; patient treatment satisfaction greater with assisted peritoneal dialysis	No limitation	Arbitrary exclusion as determined by program
Complete rehabilitation	Rare, if ever	Very few patients	Common as long as graft functions
Death rate	Much higher than for nondiabetic patients	Much higher than for nondiabetic patients	About the same as for nondiabetic patients
First-year survival rate	~75%	~75%	>90%
Morbidity during first year	~15 days in hospital	~12 days in hospital	Weeks to months hospitalized
Survival to second decade	Almost never	<5%	~1 in 5
Progression of complications	Usual and unremitting; hyperglycemia and hyperlipidemia	Usual and unremitting; might benefit from metabolic control	Interdicted by functioning pancreas plus kidney; partially ameliorated by correction of azotemia
Special advantage	Can be self-performed; avoids swings in solute and level of intravascular volume	Can be self-performed; efficient extraction of solute and water in hours	Cures uremia; freedom to travel
Disadvantages	Peritonitis; hyperinsulinemia; hyperglycemia, hyperlipidemia; long hours of treatment; more days hospitalized than with either hemodialysis or transplantation	Blood access a hazard for clotting, hemorrhage, and infection; cyclic hypotension, weakness, aluminum toxicity, amyloidosis	Cosmetic disfigurement, hypertension, personal expense for cytotoxic drugs; induced malignancy; HIV (human immunodeficiency virus) transmission
Patient acceptance	Variable, usual compliance with passive tolerance for regimen	Variable; often noncompliant with dietary, metabolic, or antihypertensive components of regimen	Enthusiastic during periods of good renal allograft function; exalted when pancreas proffers euglycemia
Relative cost	Most expensive over long run	Less expensive than kidney transplantation in the first year; subsequent years more expensive	Pancreas plus kidney engraftment most expensive uremia therapy for diabetics; after first year, kidney transplantation alone is lowest cost option

From Melmed S et al: *Williams textbook of endocrinology*, ed 14, Philadelphia, 2020, Elsevier.

- Sodium-glucose cotransporter 2 (SGLT2) inhibitors have been shown in recent trials to improve renal and cardiovascular outcomes in patients with T2DM. SGLT2 inhibitors should be considered, especially in patients with higher risk of progression (DN with eGFR <60 and UACR >300 mg/g). Initiation of SGLT2 inhibitors should be avoided in patients with eGFR <30 or those at risk of limb amputation.
- Recent trials with glucagon-like peptide-1(GLP-1) agonists show reduced renal disease progression in T2DM, mainly with reduction in the onset of albuminuria.
- Patients with DN are at risk for AKI and should be counselled to avoid nephrotoxins such as nonsteroidal anti-inflammatory drugs (NSAIDs) and contrast studies.

PREVENTION

Treatment of risk factors including blood pressure, blood sugars, and obesity.

PATIENT & FAMILY EDUCATION

Diabetes and Chronic Kidney disease by National Kidney Foundation www.kidney.org/sites/default/files/docs/diabckd_stg5.pdf

SUGGESTED READINGS

Available at ExpertConsult.com

RELATED CONTENT

Diabetes Mellitus (Related Key Topic)

AUTHORS: **Jyothsna I. Herek, MD,** and **Yuvraj Sharma, MD**

BASIC INFORMATION

DEFINITION

Diabetic polyneuropathy is a distal symmetric polyneuropathy (DSPN) characterized by numbness, tingling, pain, or weakness that affects the nerves in a stocking-and-glove pattern, beginning in the distal extremities. DSPN leads to substantial pain, morbidity, and impaired quality of life. A number of different classification schemes exist for diabetic neuropathy; a common one is outlined in Box 1.

SYNONYMS

Distal symmetric polyneuropathy
Diabetic peripheral neuropathy
DSPN

ICD-10CM CODES

E11.40	Type 2 diabetes mellitus with neurological complications
E11.40	Type 2 diabetes mellitus with diabetic neuropathy, unspecified
E11.41	Type 2 diabetes mellitus with diabetic mononeuropathy
E11.42	Type 2 diabetes mellitus with diabetic polyneuropathy
E11.43	Type 2 diabetes mellitus with diabetic autonomic (poly)neuropathy
E11.44	Type 2 diabetes mellitus with diabetic amyotrophy
E11.49	Type 2 diabetes mellitus with other diabetic neurological complication

EPIDEMIOLOGY & DEMOGRAPHICS

PREVALENCE: The prevalence of diabetic polyneuropathy varies from 10% to 100% in patients with diabetes mellitus in population-based studies. It is the most common form of peripheral neuropathy in the Western world.

RISK FACTORS: Patients with poor glycemic control, diabetic nephropathy, or retinopathy are at increased risk.

PHYSICAL FINDINGS & CLINICAL PRESENTATION

- Patients most commonly experience numbness and tingling, but they may also experience either feelings of tightness or a sensation of heat or cold.
- Pain is common, is often worst at night, and can be burning, aching, shooting, or lancinating in nature.
- Sensory symptoms begin in the feet and may slowly ascend over months to years. Symptoms in the hands do not generally occur until symptoms in the lower extremities have reached the level of the knees. In more severe cases, the symptoms can spread to the trunk and head.
- Neurologic examination reveals early loss of small-fiber modalities resulting in decreased pinprick and temperature sensation and later involvement of large-fiber modalities leading to a reduction in vibratory and proprioceptive sensation. Ankle reflexes are usually reduced or absent, and more proximal reflexes may also become involved as the neuropathy progresses. Strength is usually normal, but there can be some motor involvement leading to mild weakness and atrophy, which is usually limited to intrinsic foot muscles and ankle dorsiflexors.

BOX 1 Clinical Classification of Diabetic Neuropathies

Symmetric
- Diabetic polyneuropathy
- Diabetic autonomic neuropathy
- Painful diabetic neuropathy

Asymmetric
- Diabetic radiculoplexopathy
- Diabetic thoracic radiculoneuropathy
- Mononeuropathies
- Carpal tunnel syndrome
- Ulnar neuropathy at the elbow
- Peroneal neuropathy at fibular head
- Cranial neuropathies

From Fillit HM: *Brocklehurst's textbook of geriatric medicine and gerontology,* ed 8, Philadelphia, 2017, Elsevier.

ETIOLOGY

The precise etiology is unknown but most likely involves a complex interaction of metabolic derangements and microvascular insults occurring in the setting of diabetes.

DIAGNOSIS

DIFFERENTIAL DIAGNOSIS

Although diabetes is the leading cause of peripheral neuropathy in developed countries, there are numerous other causes requiring further investigation(s).

WORKUP

- A thorough history and neurologic examination are essential to confirm features consistent with a diabetic polyneuropathy and exclude other features suggesting alternative diagnoses.
- For some patients, neuropathy may be the presenting feature of previously undiagnosed diabetes.
- Electrodiagnostic evaluation to include nerve conduction studies and electromyography can be helpful in confirming the presence, extent, and severity of a neuropathy.
- Patients with DSPN typically have a reduction of amplitudes and slowing of conduction velocities involving sensory and possibly motor nerves in a length-dependent and symmetric fashion.
- Electromyographic examination of distal muscles may reveal fibrillation potentials, positive sharp waves, and large motor unit action potentials, all suggestive of denervation and reinnervation.
- Electrodiagnostic testing may be negative if the neuropathy is limited to small fiber involvement.
- Neither skin biopsy nor nerve biopsy is necessary in the vast majority of cases.
- Fig. 1 describes a diagnosis and treatment algorithm of diabetic autonomic neuropathy.

LABORATORY TESTS

- Fasting blood sugar, hemoglobin A1c, and 2-hr oral glucose tolerance tests should all be considered in patients with peripheral neuropathy without a known history of diabetes.
- A focused laboratory evaluation for other common or potentially treatable causes of neuropathy is also indicated: Complete blood cell count, comprehensive metabolic panel to include electrolytes and liver function tests, vitamin B_{12} and folate levels, thyroid function tests, serum protein electrophoresis with immunofixation.
- Additional laboratory tests can be considered, based on either history or exam findings suggesting other underlying diagnoses, such as antinuclear antibodies, extractable nuclear antigens, ANCAs, rheumatoid factor, HIV, hepatitis B and C, and cryoglobulins.

IMAGING STUDIES

Imaging is not necessary unless there is concern for an alternate or coexisting process based on the history and examination.

TREATMENT

CHRONIC Rx

- Table 1 summarizes clinical features, diagnosis, and treatment of diabetic autonomic neuropathy.
- Glycemic control: The primary treatment for diabetic polyneuropathy is effective glycemic control, as this may either improve or at least slow progression of the neuropathy.
- Symptomatic management: Another aspect of treatment is the symptomatic management of pain and paresthesias. The American Academy of Neurology, the American Association of Neuromuscular and Electrodiagnostic Medicine, and the American Academy of Physical Medicine and Rehabilitation have together developed an evidence-based guideline for the treatment of painful diabetic neuropathy. Pregabalin, an anticonvulsant, is the only agent in the guideline that has been established as effective for painful diabetic neuropathy. Other probably effective agents are listed in the following:
  1. Topical agents: Lidocaine 5% patch can be applied to painful areas for 12 hr a day, capsaicin 0.075% applied qid.
  2. Anticonvulsants: Gabapentin (100-1200 mg tid), pregabalin (50-100 mg tid), carbamazepine (100 mg bid).
  3. Antidepressants: Amitriptyline (10-100 mg qhs), nortriptyline (25-150 mg qhs), duloxetine (60-120 mg daily).
  4. Tramadol (50 mg qid as needed) can be a useful adjunctive analgesic.
- Fig. 2 describes a treatment algorithm for neuropathic pain after exclusion of nondiabetic etiologies and stabilization of glycemic control.

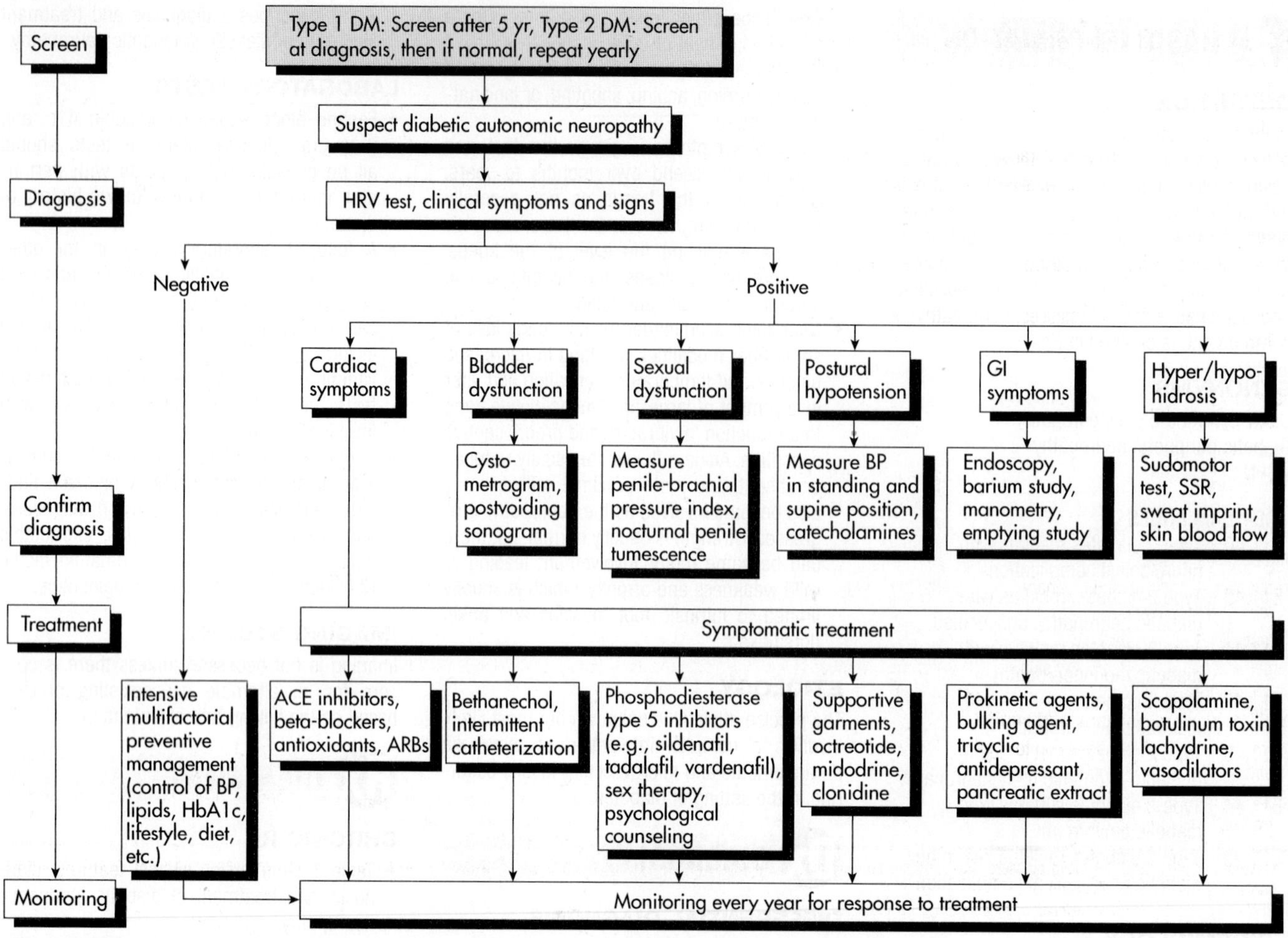

FIG. 1 Diagnosis and treatment algorithm of diabetic autonomic neuropathy. *ACE*, Angiotensin-converting enzyme; *ARBs*, angiotensin receptor blockers; *BP*, blood pressure; *DM*, diabetes mellitus; *GI*, gastrointestinal; *HbA1c*, glycohemoglobin; *HRV*, heart rate variability; *SSR*, sympathetic skin response. (Modified from Larsen PR et al [eds]: *Williams textbook of endocrinology*, ed 11, Philadelphia, 2008, Saunders.)

DISPOSITION

The distal sensory loss of diabetic polyneuropathy places patients at increased risk of trauma to the extremities, with the potential for ulceration and infection that could ultimately require amputation if not attended to in a timely fashion.

REFERRAL

- A neurologist can assist in the diagnosis and management of diabetic polyneuropathy.
- Patients with diabetic polyneuropathy should also be evaluated at least annually by a podiatrist and ophthalmologist.
- Progression of diabetic polyneuropathy can be minimized by paying close attention to strict glycemic control as well as other risk factors such as hypertension and obesity.

PEARLS & CONSIDERATIONS

COMMENTS

- For many patients, either DSPN or another form of diabetic neuropathy may be the initial presentation of previously undiagnosed diabetes.
- In addition to regular visits with podiatry, patients with diabetic polyneuropathy should be educated on aggressive foot hygiene and the importance of examining their own feet.

PATIENT & FAMILY EDUCATION

The following website is recommended:
www.mayoclinic.com/health/diabetic-neuropathy/DS01045

SUGGESTED READINGS

Available at ExpertConsult.com

AUTHOR: **Lydia Sharp, MD**

TABLE 1 Clinical Features, Diagnosis, and Treatment of Diabetic Autonomic Neuropathy

Symptoms	Tests	Treatments
Cardiac		
Resting tachycardia, exercise intolerance	HRV, MUGA thallium scan, MIBG scan	Graded supervised exercise, ACE inhibitors, β-blockers
Postural hypotension, dizziness, weakness, fatigue, syncope	HRV, supine and standing BP, catecholamines	Mechanical measures, clonidine, midodrine, octreotide, erythropoietin
Gastrointestinal		
Gastroparesis, erratic glucose control	Gastric emptying study, barium study	Frequent small meals, prokinetic agents (metoclopramide, domperidone, erythromycin)
Abdominal pain, early satiety, nausea, vomiting, bloating, belching	Endoscopy, manometry, electrogastrogram	Antibiotics, antiemetics, bulking agents, tricyclic antidepressants, pyloric botulinum toxin, gastric pacing
Constipation	Endoscopy	High-fiber diet, bulking agents, osmotic laxatives, lubricating agents
Diarrhea (often nocturnal alternating with constipation)		Soluble fiber, gluten and lactose restriction, anticholinergic agents, cholestyramine, antibiotics, somatostatin, pancreatic enzyme supplements
Sexual Dysfunction		
Erectile dysfunction	H&P, HRV, penile-brachial pressure index, nocturnal penile tumescence	Sex therapy, psychological counseling, phosphodiesterase inhibitors, PGE_1 injections, devices or prostheses
Vaginal dryness		Vaginal lubricants
Bladder Dysfunction		
Frequency, urgency, nocturia, urinary retention, incontinence	Cystometrogram, postvoid sonography	Bethanechol, intermittent catheterization
Sudomotor Dysfunction		
Anhidrosis, heat intolerance, dry skin, hyperhidrosis	Quantitative sudomotor axon reflex, sweat test, skin blood flow	Emollients and skin lubricants, scopolamine, glycopyrrolate, botulinum toxin, vasodilators
Pupillomotor and Visceral Dysfunction		
Blurred vision, impaired adaptation to ambient light, Argyll-Robertson pupil	Pupillometry, HRV	Care with driving at night
Impaired visceral sensation: Silent MI, hypoglycemia unawareness		Recognition of unusual presentation of MI, control of risk factors, control of plasma glucose levels

ACE, Acetylcholinesterase; *BP*, blood pressure; *H&P*, history and physical examination; *HRV*, heart rate variability; *MI*, myocardial infarction; *MIBG*, metaiodobenzylguanidine; *MUGA*, multigated angiography; PGE_1, prostaglandin E_1.
From Melmed S et al: *Williams textbook of endocrinology*, ed 12, Philadelphia, 2011, Saunders.

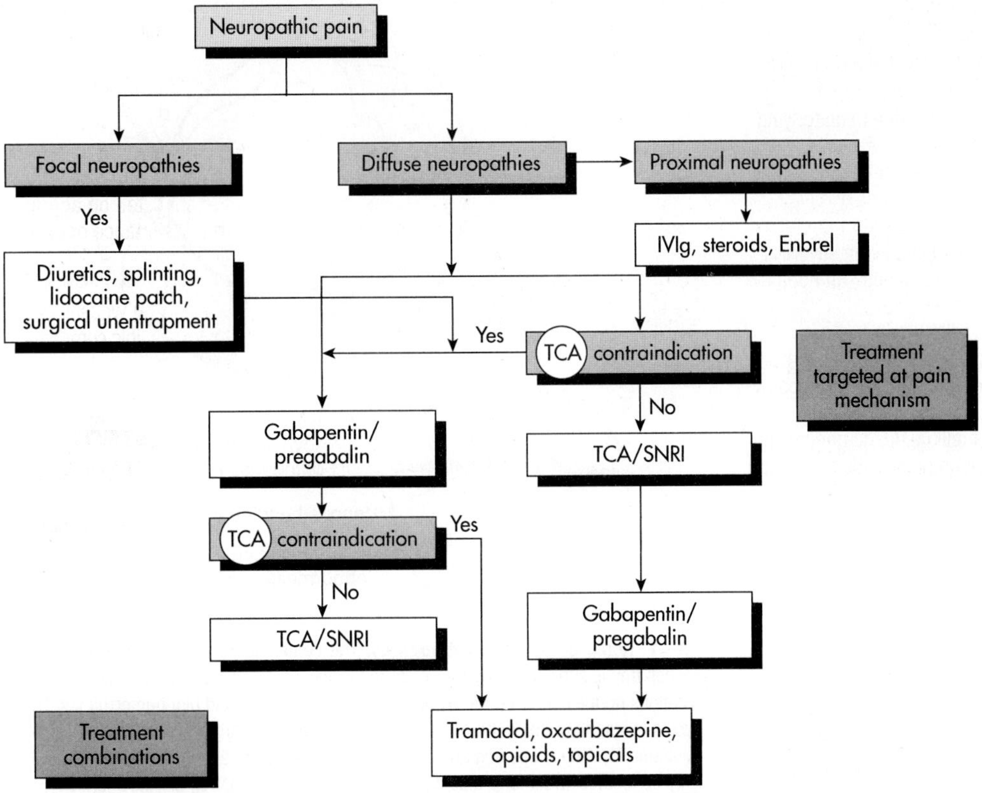

FIG. 2 Treatment algorithm for neuropathic pain after exclusion of nondiabetic etiologies and stabilization of glycemic control. *IVIg*, Intravenous immune globulin; *SNRI*, serotonin-norepinephrine reuptake inhibitors; *TCA*, tricyclic antidepressants. (From Melmed S et al: *Williams textbook of endocrinology*, ed 12, Philadelphia, 2011, Saunders.)

Diabetic Retinopathy

BASIC INFORMATION

DEFINITION

Diabetic retinopathy (Fig. 1) is a microvascular abnormality of the retina resulting in microaneurysms (Fig. E2), retinal hemorrhages, lipid exudates (Fig. E3), macular edema, and neovascular vessel growth (Fig. E4) and can ultimately end in blindness. Diabetic retinopathy can be classified into two stages: Nonproliferative (mild, moderate, and severe) and proliferative. A glossary and abbreviations pertinent to diabetic eye disease are described in Table E1.

SYNONYMS

Nonproliferative diabetic retinopathy (NPDR)
Proliferative diabetic retinopathy (PDR)
Diabetic macular edema (DME)

ICD-10CM CODES

E08.311	Diabetes mellitus due to underlying condition with unspecified diabetic retinopathy with macular edema
E08.319	Diabetes mellitus due to underlying condition with unspecified diabetic retinopathy without macular edema
E08.321	Diabetes mellitus due to underlying condition with mild nonproliferative diabetic retinopathy with macular edema
E08.329	Diabetes mellitus due to underlying condition with mild nonproliferative diabetic retinopathy without macular edema
E08.331	Diabetes mellitus due to underlying condition with moderate nonproliferative diabetic retinopathy with macular edema
E08.339	Diabetes mellitus due to underlying condition with moderate nonproliferative diabetic retinopathy without macular edema
E08.341	Diabetes mellitus due to underlying condition with severe nonproliferative diabetic retinopathy with macular edema
E08.349	Diabetes mellitus due to underlying condition with severe nonproliferative diabetic retinopathy without macular edema
E08.351	Diabetes mellitus due to underlying condition with proliferative diabetic retinopathy with macular edema
E08.359	Diabetes mellitus due to underlying condition with proliferative diabetic retinopathy without macular edema

EPIDEMIOLOGY & DEMOGRAPHICS

INCIDENCE (IN U.S.):

- After 20 yr of diabetes mellitus, nearly 99% of patients with type 1 and 60% with type 2 disease demonstrate some degree of diabetic retinopathy.
- A leading preventable cause of blindness in the U.S. between the ages of 20 and 74 yr.
- There are approximately 8000 new cases of diabetic retinopathy–induced blindness each year in the U.S.

PREVALENCE (IN U.S.):

- Prevalence of retinopathy increases with duration of diabetes. Found in 18% of people diagnosed with diabetes for 3- to 4-yr duration and in up to 80% of diabetics with a diagnosis of ≥15 yr.
- In the U.S., the prevalence of diabetic macular edema (the most common cause of vision impairment) is 4%, or approximately 750,000 people.
- CDC data reveal that 4 million Americans were visually impaired due to diabetic retinopathy in 2011.
- The number of Americans with diabetic retinopathy is expected to nearly double, from 7.7 million to 14.6 million between 2010 and 2050. Expected to triple in the Hispanic population.

PREDOMINANT SEX: Males and females affected equally

PREDOMINANT AGE: ≥30 yr

GENETICS:

- The development of diabetes involves the interaction of genetic and nongenetic factors.
- Type 1 has an autoimmune basis, resulting in destruction of beta islet cells and has strong HLA associations.
- Type 2 has genetic predisposition, but the specific genes are not yet well characterized.

PHYSICAL FINDINGS & CLINICAL PRESENTATION

- Microaneurysms
- Hemorrhages
- Cotton-wool spots
- Lipid exudates
- Macular edema
- Neovascularization
- Retinal detachment (in advanced cases)
- Vitreous hemorrhage
- In early cases, patient may not report a visual disturbance

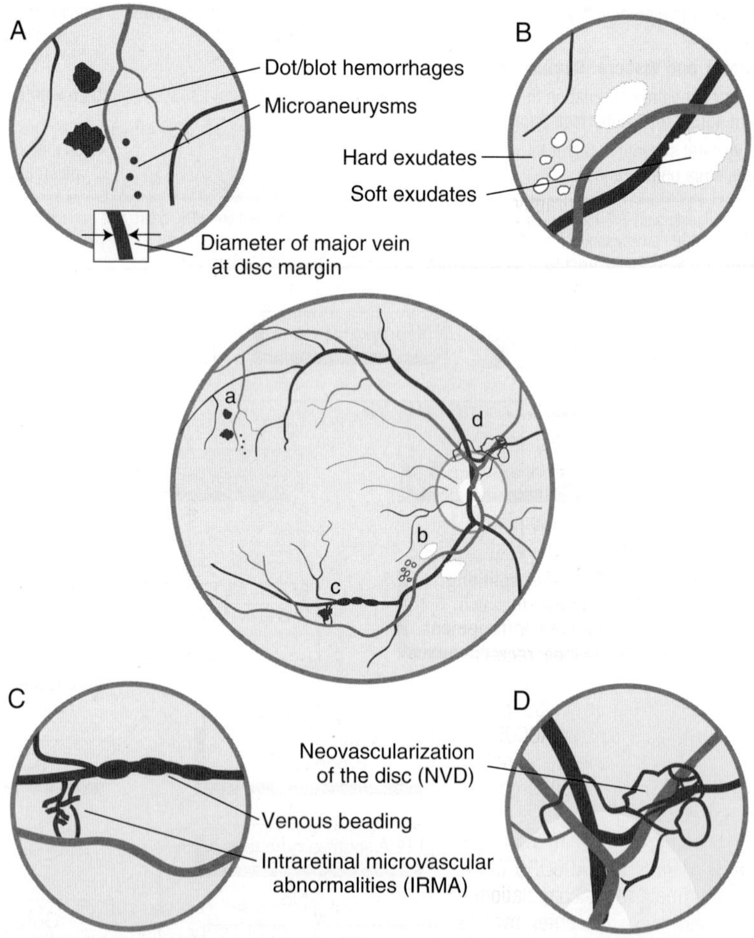

FIG. 1 Types of diabetic retinopathy. The center figure depicting the fundus of a patient with diabetic retinopathy is surrounded by four enlarged views, each labeled with a letter (a to d) corresponding to specific locations on the center figure. **A,** Microaneurysms and dot and blot hemorrhages. The diameter of microaneurysms is less than the width of a major vein at the disc margin (reproduced in square inset). **B,** Hard and soft exudates. **C,** Venous beading and intraretinal microvascular abnormalities (IRMA). **D,** Neovascularization, which may be located within one disc diameter of the optic disc (NVD) or elsewhere (NVE). Although both IRMA and neovascularization represent the formation of new blood vessels, IRMA are confined to the layers of the retina, whereas neovascularization is on the inner surface of the retina or vitreous. (From McGee S: *Evidence-based physical diagnosis,* ed 4, Philadelphia, 2018, Elsevier.)

ETIOLOGY

Prolonged hyperglycemia results in basement membrane thickening in retinal capillaries with subsequent loss of pericytes and endothelial decompensation resulting in breakdown of the blood–retina barrier and capillary occlusion, ischemia, and serum leakage (Fig. 5). This leads to the clinical findings of dot hemorrhages, microaneurysms, lipid exudate, and edema. Upregulation of vascular endothelial growth factor (VEGF) and other cytokines contributes to vascular incompetence and promotes growth of neovascular tissue.

Dx DIAGNOSIS

DIFFERENTIAL DIAGNOSIS

- Branch or central retinal vein occlusion
- Hypertensive retinopathy
- Ocular ischemic syndrome (carotid occlusion)
- Radiation retinopathy
- Retinal macroaneurysm
- Sickle cell retinopathy
- Valsalva retinopathy
- Lupus
- Retinal vasculitis
- Terson syndrome

WORKUP

- Fundus photography
- Optical coherence tomography
- Optical coherence angiography
- Fluorescein angiogram (Fig. E6)
- Laboratory workup if indicated based on DDx

Rx TREATMENT

NONPHARMACOLOGIC THERAPY

- Tight glycemic control remains the cornerstone in the primary prevention of diabetic retinopathy, particularly in type 1 as seen in the Diabetes Control and Complications Trial (DCCT) and less so in type 2 as seen in the United Kingdom Prospective Diabetes Study (UKPDS) and more recently in the Action to Control Cardiovascular Risk in Diabetes Trial (ACCORD). ADA guidelines recommend A1c <7.0.
- Intensive lowering of blood pressure was shown in UKPDS but not ACCORD to reduce progression of diabetic retinopathy. ADA guidelines recommend BP target of <140/90 mm Hg.
- Lipid lowering results in reduction of retinopathy progression (ACCORD Trial).
- Laser treatment (photocoagulation) for proliferative disease or noncenter involving macular edema. The International Classification of Diabetic Macular Edema (DME) is described in Table E2.

TABLE 3 Abbreviated Early Treatment Diabetic Retinopathy Study (ETDRS) Classification of Diabetic Retinopathy

Category/Description	Management
Nonproliferative diabetic retinopathy (NPDR)	
No DR	Review in 12 mo
Very mild NPDR Microaneurysms only	Review most patients in 12 mo
Mild NPDR Any or all of: Microaneurysms, retinal hemorrhages, exudates, cotton wool spots, up to the level of moderate NPDR. No intraretinal microvascular anomalies (IRMA) or significant beading	Review range 6-12 mo, depending on severity of signs, stability, systemic factors, and patient's personal circumstances
Moderate NPDR • Severe retinal hemorrhages (more than ETDRS standard photograph 2A: About 20 medium to large per quadrant) in 1-3 quadrants or mild IRMA • Significant venous beading can be present in no more than 1 quadrant • Cotton wool spots commonly present	Review in approximately 6 mo Proliferative diabetic retinopathy (PDR) in up to 26%, high-risk PDR in up to 8% within a year
Severe NPDR The 4–2–1 rule; one or more of: • Severe hemorrhages in all 4 quadrants • Significant venous beading in 2 or more quadrants • Moderate IRMA in 1 or more quadrants	Review in 4 mo PDR in up to 50%, high-risk PDR in up to 15% within a year Consider panretinal photocoagulation
Very severe NPDR Two or more of the criteria for severe NPDR	Review in 2-3 mo High-risk PDR in up to 45% within a year
Proliferative diabetic retinopathy (PDR)	
Mild–moderate PDR New vessels on the disc (NVD) or new vessels elsewhere (NVE), but extent insufficient to meet the high-risk criteria	Treatment considered according to severity of signs, stability, systemic factors, and patient's personal circumstances such as reliability of attendance for review. If not treated, review in up to 2 mo
High-risk PDR • New vessels on the disc (NVD) greater than ETDRS standard photograph 10A (about ⅓ disc area) • Any NVD with vitreous hemorrhage • NVE greater than ½ disc area with vitreous hemorrhage	Treatment advised (see text) Should be performed immediately when possible, and certainly same day if symptomatic presentation with good retinal view

DR, Diabetic retinopathy.
From Bowling B: *Kanski's clinical ophthalmology, a systematic approach*, ed 8, Philadelphia, 2016, Elsevier.

- Table 3 summarizes classification and management of diabetic retinopathy. A diabetic retinopathy and macular edema examination and treatment flow chart for nonpregnant patients is illustrated in Fig. E7 and Fig. E8 for pregnant patients.

ACUTE GENERAL Rx

- Intravitreal pharmacotherapy with anti-VEGF agents (e.g., bevacizumab, ranibizumab, aflibercept) and/or corticosteroids is the standard of care for patients with center-involved diabetic macular edema.
- Laser therapy: Panretinal laser photocoagulation (Fig. E9) reduces the risk of severe visual loss in patients with proliferative retinopathy.
- Focal laser reduces risk of moderate visual loss by 50% in patients with clinically significant macular edema.
- Vitrectomy for traction retinal detachment or vitreous hemorrhage.

CHRONIC Rx

- Monthly anti-VEGF injections until macular edema has resolved with surveillance at regular intervals for additional treatment
- Both ranibizumab (Lucentis) and aflibercept (Eylea) have been FDA-approved for treatment of diabetic retinopathy in patients with macular edema
- Repeated laser treatments may be necessary
- Diet and exercise; good medical control of disease, blood pressure, and cholesterol

DISPOSITION

- Retinal examination should be performed on all routine medical visits. Referral if abnormality seen.
- Routine annual eye examination in all patients with diabetes.
- Prognosis is improved with early diagnosis and treatment.

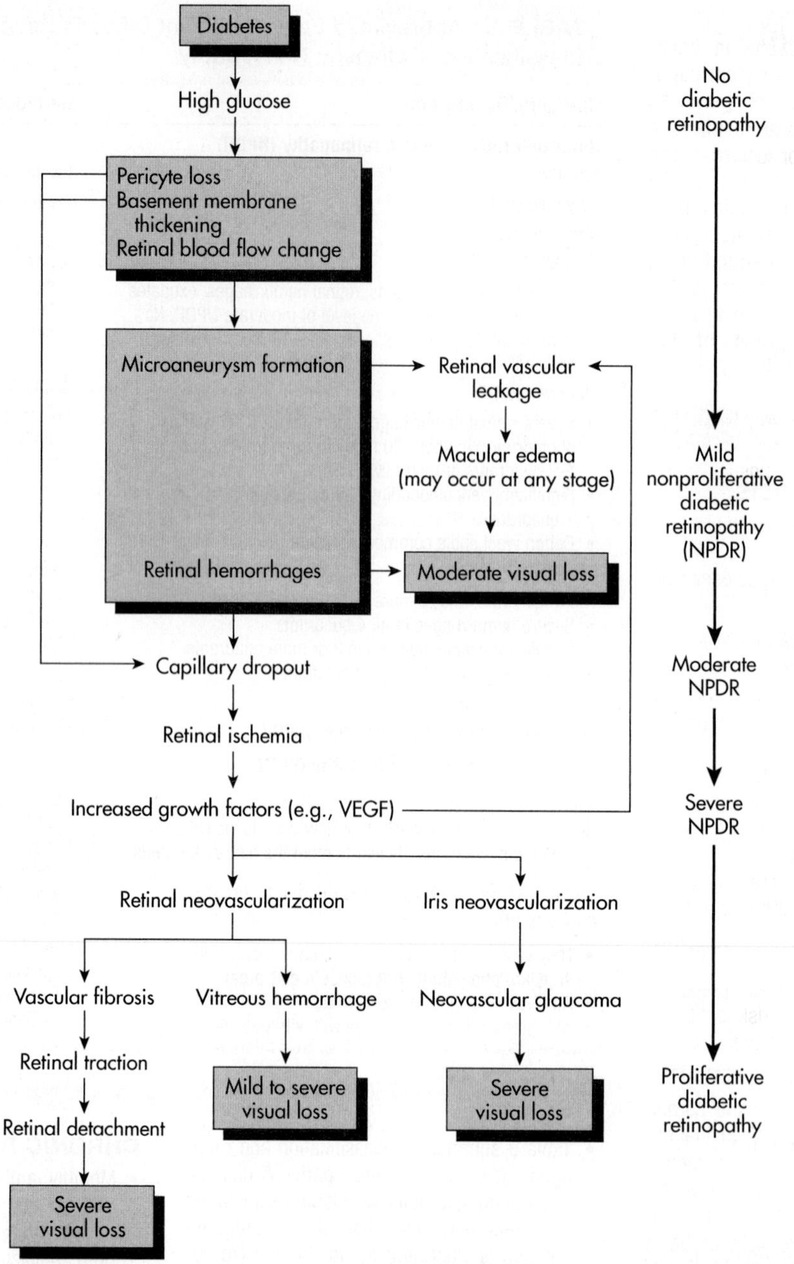

FIG. 5 Pathogenesis of diabetic retinopathy. This schematic flow chart represents the major preclinical and clinical findings associated with the full spectrum of diabetic retinopathy and macular edema. *VEGF,* Vascular endothelial growth factor. (From Melmed S et al: *Williams textbook of endocrinology,* ed 14, Philadelphia, 2020, Elsevier.)

REFERRAL

Refer to ophthalmologist immediately on finding retinal abnormality to institute early treatment.

PEARLS & CONSIDERATIONS

COMMENTS

- Early treatment of severe nonproliferative and proliferative retinopathy may minimize complications and visual loss.
- Tight blood sugar control in type 1 patients significantly reduces the probability of developing new-onset retinopathy as well as progression of existing retinopathy.
- Retinopathy is an independent risk marker for cardiovascular disease in patients with type 2 DM.

RELATED CONTENT

Diabetic Retinopathy (Patient Information)
Diabetes Mellitus (Related Key Topic)

SUGGESTED READINGS

Available at ExpertConsult.com

AUTHOR: **Robert H. Janigian Jr, MD**

BASIC INFORMATION

DEFINITION

Persistent diarrhea is defined as an increase in stool frequency (>3 per day) or loose consistency for ≥4 wk.

SYNONYM

Chronic diarrhea

ICD-10CM CODES

R19.7	Diarrhea, unspecified
K52.9	Noninfective gastroenteritis and colitis, unspecified
K58.0	Irritable bowel syndrome with diarrhea
K59.1	Functional diarrhea
K90.9	Intestinal malabsorption, unspecified

EPIDEMIOLOGY & DEMOGRAPHICS

PREVALENCE: Chronic diarrhea affects 3% to 5% of the U.S. population.

PREDOMINANT SEX & AGE, RISK FACTORS, & GENETICS: Dependent on etiology:

- Irritable bowel syndrome (IBS) has a female:male ratio of 2:1, with peak prevalence from 20 to 39 yr of age.
- Celiac disease has a female predominance, with highest incidence during infancy. Genetic risk factors include homozygosity for HLA DR3-DQ2 and DR4-DQ8.
- Crohn disease has female predominance, with highest incidence during the second decade. Smoking is associated with increased incidence.
- Ulcerative colitis (UC) has male predominance. Smoking *cessation* is a risk factor.
- Lactose intolerance incidence increases with age, with a lower prevalence in European Americans.

PHYSICAL FINDINGS & CLINICAL PRESENTATION

History:

- Age of onset: Varies
- Duration and nature of onset: Abrupt (infectious) or gradual
- Timing: Nocturnal (suggests secretory)
- Change in bowel movements: Loose, frequent, urgent, incontinent
- Stool characteristics: Watery, bloody, fatty, malodorous
- Stool volume: Watery, voluminous (disorder of small bowel or proximal colon), frequent and small (disorder of left colon or rectum)
- Aggravating and alleviating factors: Diet
- Abdominal pain: Location, relation to meals or bowel movements (inflammatory bowel disease [IBD], IBS, ischemia)
- Associated symptoms: Excessive flatus, bloating (carbohydrate malabsorption)
- Systemic symptoms: Weight loss, fever (malabsorption, malignancy, IBD)
- Medical history: Immunologic, endocrine, neoplastic, human immunodeficiency virus (HIV), diabetes, radiation
- Psychiatric history: Stress, depression
- Surgical history: Prior GI operations
- Travel history: Areas with infectious sources
- Medications: All medications and supplements; see Box 1
- Dietary history: Recent changes, "sugar-free" foods; fiber intake; raw seafood, shellfish, milk; impure drinking water; alcohol
- Family history: Lactose intolerance, IBD, celiac disease, IBS, cancer
- Social history: HIV risk factors, receptive anal intercourse

Physical:

- General: Volume and nutritional status
- Skin: Flushing (carcinoid syndrome), dermatitis herpetiformis (celiac disease), erythema nodosum or pyoderma gangrenosum (IBD), migratory necrotizing erythema (glucagonoma)
- Mouth: Ulcers (Crohn disease)
- Neck: Thyroid mass or nodule (hyperthyroidism), lymphadenopathy (malignancy, infection)
- Abdomen
  1. Hepatomegaly (endocrine tumor)
  2. Splenomegaly (Whipple disease, lymphoma, mastocytosis)
  3. Scars (prior operation)
  4. Tenderness (inflammation)
  5. Mass (cancer)
  6. Bruit (chronic mesenteric ischemia)
- Rectal: Sphincter weakness, anal fistula, fecal impaction

ETIOLOGY

Cause-specific etiology: Steatorrheal; inflammatory; watery; secretory; factitial; iatrogenic

Dx DIAGNOSIS

DIFFERENTIAL DIAGNOSIS (Box 2)

- Steatorrheal (fatty) diarrhea
  1. Malabsorption syndromes
     a. Mesenteric ischemia
     b. Mucosal diseases (celiac, Whipple disease)
     c. Small intestinal bacterial overgrowth
     d. Short bowel syndrome
     e. Drug-induced enteropathy
  2. Maldigestion
     a. Inadequate luminal bile acid
     b. Pancreatic exocrine insufficiency
     c. Liver disease
     d. Bariatric surgery
     e. Lactose intolerance
- Inflammatory diarrhea (Table 1)
  1. Diverticulitis
  2. IBD
  3. Infectious diseases
     a. Bacterial (tuberculosis, yersiniosis, *Salmonella, Shigella, Campylobacter*)
     b. Parasitic (amebiasis, strongyloidiasis)
     c. Pseudomembranous colitis (*C. difficile*)
     d. Ulcerating viral (CMV, HSV)
     e. Toxin mediated (*E. coli* 0157:H7)
  4. Ischemic colitis
  5. Neoplasia (colon cancer, lymphoma)
  6. Radiation colitis
- Watery diarrhea (Table 2)
  1. Osmotic diarrhea
     a. Carbohydrate (lactose) malabsorption
     b. Osmotic laxatives (magnesium, phosphate, sulfate, sorbitol)
  2. Gluten and FODMAP intolerance
- Secretory diarrhea
  1. Infectious (cholera, rotavirus, *Cryptosporidium*)
  2. Congenital syndromes (chloridorrhea, Hirschsprung)
  3. Disordered motility
     a. Diabetic neuropathy
     b. Post-sympathectomy
     c. Post-vagotomy
  4. Endocrinopathies
     a. Addison disease
     b. Carcinoid syndrome
     c. Hyperthyroidism
     d. Mastocytosis
     e. Medullary carcinoma of the thyroid
     f. Gastrinoma, pheochromocytoma, somatostatinoma, VIPoma
  5. Idiopathic secretory diarrhea
  6. Alcoholism
  7. Laxative abuse
  8. Lymphocytic colitis
  9. Neoplasia

BOX 1 Medications and Toxins Associated with Diarrhea

Acid-reducing agents (e.g., H_2RAs, PPIs)
Antacids (e.g., containing magnesium)
Antiarrhythmics (e.g., quinidine)
Antibiotics (most)
Antinflammatory agents (e.g., 5-aminosalicylates, NSAIDs)
Antihypertensives (e.g., β-adrenergic receptor blocking drugs)
Antineoplastic agents
Antiretroviral agents
Colchicine
Heavy metals
Herbal products
Prostaglandin analogs (e.g., misoprostol)
Theophylline
Vitamin and mineral supplements

H_2RA, Histamine-2 receptor agonist; *NSAID*, nonsteroidal anti-inflammatory drug; *PPI*, proton pump inhibitor.
From Feldman M et al: *Sleisenger and Fordtran's gastrointestinal and liver disease*, ed 10, Philadelphia, 2016, Elsevier.

BOX 2 Differential Diagnosis of Diarrhea

Acute Diarrhea
- Infection
  - Bacteria
  - Parasites
  - Protozoa
  - Viruses
- Food allergies
- Food poisoning
- Medications
- Initial presentation of chronic diarrhea

Chronic Diarrhea
- Steatorrheal diarrhea
  - Malabsorption syndromes
    - Mesenteric ischemia
    - Mucosal diseases (Celiac, Whipple disease)
    - Short bowel syndrome
    - SIBO
  - Maldigestion
    - Inadequate luminal bile acid
    - Pancreatic exocrine insufficiency
    - Lactose intolerance
- Inflammatory Diarrhea
  - Diverticulitis
  - Infectious diseases
    - Invasive bacterial infections (tuberculosis, yersiniosis)
    - Invasive parasitic infections (amebiasis, strongyloidiasis)
    - Pseudomembranous colitis (*C. difficile* infection)
    - Ulcerating viral infections (CMV, HSV)
  - Inflammatory bowel diseases
    - Crohn disease
    - Ulcerative colitis
    - Microscopic colitis
  - Ischemic colitis
  - Neoplasia
  - Radiation colitis
- Watery Diarrhea
  - Osmotic diarrhea
    - Carbohydrate malabsorption
    - Osmotic laxatives (Mg^{2+}, PO_4^{3-}, SO_4^{2-})
  - Secretory diarrhea
    - Bacterial toxins
    - Congenital syndromes (chloridorrhea)
    - Diabetic autonomic neuropathy
    - IBS
    - Post-sympathectomy
    - Post-vagotomy
    - Endocrinopathies
      - Addison disease
      - Carcinoid syndrome
      - Hyperthyroidism
      - Mastocytosis
      - Medullary carcinoma of the thyroid
      - Gastrinoma, pheochromocytoma, somatostatinoma, VIPoma
    - Idiopathic secretory diarrhea
    - Ileal bile acid malabsorption
    - Laxative abuse
    - Medications and toxins (Box 1)
    - Neoplasia
    - Vasculitis

CMV, Cytomegalovirus; *HSV*, herpes simplex virus; *IBS*, inflammatory bowel syndrome; *SIBO*, small intestine bacterial overgrowth

From Feldman M et al: *Sleisenger and Fordtran's gastrointestinal and liver disease*, ed 10, Philadelphia, 2016, Elsevier.

TABLE 1 Clinical Findings Suggesting the Causative Organisms for Some Inflammatory Diarrheas

Finding	Causative Organisms
Hemolytic-uremic syndrome/thrombotic thrombocytopenic purpura	Shiga toxin-producing *Escherichia coli*; most common with *Shigella dysenteriae*, but *S. dysenteriae* is not found in the U.S.
Reactive arthritis*	*Salmonella* spp., *Shigella* spp., *Campylobacter* spp., *Yersinia* spp.
Bone-marrow suppression	*Salmonella* serovars Typhi and Paratyphi
Guillain-Barré syndrome	*Campylobacter jejuni*
Toxic megacolon	*Shigella* spp., *Clostridium difficile, Salmonella*
Aortitis/endovascular infection	Nontyphoidal *Salmonellae*
Intestinal hemorrhage/perforation	*Salmonella* serovars Typhi and Paratyphi, TB enteritis
Right lower quadrant tenderness	*Yersinia* spp.
Cellulitis	*Vibrio vulnificus* and *alginolyticus*
Postinfection IBS	All, including viral gastroenteritis; viruses typically yield less severe symptoms
Small-bowel lymphoproliferative disease	*Campylobacter jejuni*

IBS, Inflammatory bowel syndrome; *TB,* tuberculosis; *spp.*, species.
*Can occur with any enteric pathogen.
From Feldman M et al: *Sleisenger and Fordtran's gastrointestinal and liver disease*, ed 10, Philadelphia, 2016, Elsevier.

- Factitial causes (Munchausen)
- Iatrogenic causes
  1. Cholecystectomy
  2. Ileal resection
  3. Bariatric surgery
  4. Medications and toxins

WORKUP

- Using the same tests on every patient is impractical. Obtain a good history and physical examination and tailor the workup accordingly.
- First determine the type of diarrhea (watery, fatty, or inflammatory) based on the history and physical. Next obtain further testing to differentiate the subtype of diarrhea.
- Basic laboratory testing may include complete blood count (anemia, leukocytosis), electrolytes, liver function tests, albumin, inflammatory markers, and thyroid-stimulating hormone.
- Initial stool studies may include fecal leukocyte and occult blood testing.
- Further testing is indicated by clinical suspicion:
  1. IBD: Fecal calprotectin, terminal ileum biopsy
  2. Diarrhea after hospitalization or antibiotics: *C. difficile* stool toxin
  3. Laxative abuse: Stool laxative screen
  4. Malabsorption: Fecal fat, Sudan stain
  5. Celiac: Tissue transglutaminase immunoglobulin A, small bowel biopsy
  6. Watery diarrhea
     a. Fecal osmotic gap
        (1) >125 mOsm/kg: Osmotic diarrhea
        (2) <50 mOsm/kg: Secretory diarrhea
     b. Fecal pH <5.3: Carbohydrate malabsorption
  7. If no other etiology is determined: Hormone studies

Rx TREATMENT

NONPHARMACOLOGIC THERAPY

- Eliminate offending substances if the etiology can be managed with diet modification.
- Consider trials of reduced lactose, alcohol, and caffeine intake.
- Fiber supplementation can thicken stool consistency but may increase stool output.
- Patients with stool output greater than 1000 g per day often need intravenous or oral rehydration solutions.

CHRONIC Rx

- General principles:
  1. Opiates are the most effective nonspecific antidiarrheal but should be avoided in acute infection, massive intestinal resection, or presence of secretagogues.
  2. Attempt low-potency opiates first, escalating treatment if these fail.
  3. Avoid high-potency agents if concerned for narcotic abuse and/or dependence.
  4. Prescribe opiates as scheduled rather than as needed.
- Low-potency opiates
  1. Diphenoxylate with atropine (Lomotil) 2.5 to 5 mg 4 times daily
  2. Loperamide (Imodium) 2 to 4 mg 4 times daily
- More potent opiates
  1. Codeine 15 to 60 mg 4 times daily
  2. Morphine 2 to 20 mg 4 times daily
- Alpha-2 agonist
  1. Affects colonic motility and secretion.
  2. Clonidine 0.1 to 0.3 mg 3 times daily.

TABLE 2 Secretory versus Osmotic Diarrhea

Type of Diarrhea	Causes	Examples
Secretory	Exogenous secretagogues	Enterotoxins (e.g., cholera)
	Endogenous secretagogues	Neuroendocrine tumors (e.g., carcinoid syndrome)
	Absence of ion transporter	Congenital chloridorrhea
	Loss of intestinal surface area	Intestinal resection, diffuse intestinal mucosal disease
	Intestinal ischemia	Diffuse mesenteric atherosclerosis
	Rapid intestinal transit	Intestinal hurry following vagotomy
Osmotic	Ingestion of poorly absorbed agent	Magnesium ingestion
	Reduced nutrient transport	Lactase deficiency

From Feldman M et al: *Sleisenger and Fordtran's gastrointestinal and liver disease*, ed 10, Philadelphia, 2016, Elsevier.

3. Utility limited by hypotension. Attempt opiate agents first.

- Intraluminal agents
  1. Bind toxins and change stool consistency
  2. Usually ineffective as monotherapy
  3. Fibers: Psyllium, calcium polycarbophil, methylcellulose
  4. Bismuth
  5. Clays: Attapulgite, kaolin
  6. Bile acid–binding resins: Cholestyramine, colestipol

COMPLEMENTARY & ALTERNATIVE MEDICINE

Growing evidence suggests some benefit of probiotics in the treatment of infectious diarrhea, IBS, *C. difficile* disease, and antibiotic-associated diarrhea.

DISPOSITION

Typically treat outpatient unless signs of sepsis or dehydration are present.

REFERRAL

Gastroenterology referral is warranted depending on the severity of symptoms and need for endoscopic procedures and/or long-term disease management.

PEARLS & CONSIDERATIONS

COMMENTS

- A good history is crucial in the evaluation of persistent diarrhea. Attempt to classify diarrhea as watery, secretory, steatorrheal, or inflammatory.
- Patients often describe fecal incontinence as diarrhea, and many are reluctant to share this information unless specifically asked.
- IBS is one of the most common causes of chronic diarrhea and requires minimal workup. Screen patients appropriately.

PATIENT & FAMILY EDUCATION

- Disease-specific education
- Hygiene information

SUGGESTED READINGS

Available at ExpertConsult.com

RELATED CONTENT

Amebiasis (Related Key Topic)
Celiac Disease (Related Key Topic)
Colorectal Cancer (Related Key Topic)
Crohn Disease (Related Key Topic)
Gastroenteritis (Related Key Topic)
Giardiasis (Related Key Topic)
Hyperthyroidism (Related Key Topic)
Incontinence, Bowel, Elderly Patient (Related Key Topic)
Irritable Bowel Syndrome (Related Key Topic)
Lactose Intolerance (Related Key Topic)
Malabsorption (Related Key Topic)
Small Bowel Intestinal Bacterial Overgrowth (Related Key Topic)
Traveler's Diarrhea (Related Key Topic)
Tropical Sprue (Related Key Topic)
Ulcerative Colitis (Related Key Topic)
Whipple Disease (Related Key Topic)

AUTHORS: **Diana Zhou, MD,** and **Amanda Box, MD, MS**

BASIC INFORMATION

DEFINITION

Disseminated intravascular coagulation (DIC) is an acquired thromboembolic disorder characterized by generalized activation of the clotting pathways, which results in the intravascular formation of fibrin and ultimately thrombotic occlusion of small and midsize vessels, followed by end-organ damage.

SYNONYMS

Consumptive coagulopathy
DIC
Defibrination syndrome

ICD-10CM CODE

D65 Disseminated intravascular coagulation [defibrination syndrome]

EPIDEMIOLOGY & DEMOGRAPHICS

About 1% of hospitalized patients may have evidence of DIC. There is no predilection for age or gender. More than 50% of cases are associated with gram-negative sepsis or other septicemic infections, and up to 35% of patients with severe sepsis have DIC.

PHYSICAL FINDINGS & CLINICAL PRESENTATION

DIC occurs in both acute and chronic forms and can present with bleeding, thrombosis, or laboratory evidence of clotting cascade activation and fibrinolysis without evident clinical sequelae. Acute DIC is more common and predominantly manifests as bleeding complications. The risk of bleeding increases with worsening thrombocytopenia and is fivefold higher when platelet count is below $<50 \times 10^9$/liter. Sudden exposure to procoagulants may extensively activate a coagulation cascade and platelet consumption, resulting in thrombosis. In contrast, chronic DIC more frequently causes thrombotic complications. The diagnosis of chronic DIC can be challenging, as the PT and PTT are frequently normal. Multiple pathways are involved simultaneously in DIC to create the clinical presentation. These include: (1) thrombin generation due to release of tissue factor, (2) suppression of physiologic anticoagulant (e.g., protein C or antithrombin insufficiency), (3) impaired fibrinolysis characterized by increased level of plasminogen activator inhibitor type 1 (PAI-1), and (4) activation of inflammatory pathways.

With DIC, multiple organs may be involved, and clinical presentations may vary. They can include:

- Central nervous system: Altered mental status, transient neurologic deficits
- Cardiovascular: Hypotension, tachycardia
- Respiratory: Hypoxia, dyspnea, localized rales, and acute respiratory syndrome
- Gastrointestinal: Intestinal bleeding, bowel infarction
- Genitourinary: Oliguria, anuria, uremia, acidosis, metrorrhagia
- Skin: Wound site bleeding, epistaxis, gingival bleeding, hemorrhagic bullae, petechiae, ecchymosis, purpura

ETIOLOGY

DIC results from the aberrant and generalized activation of the clotting system, resulting in simultaneous formulation of coagulation and fibrinolysis. Clotting factors are consumed at a rate in excess of the capacity of the liver to synthesize them, and platelets are consumed in excess of the capacity of the bone marrow megakaryocytes to release them. It frequently occurs in the setting of severe infection; common triggers are listed below:

- Infections (e.g., gram-negative sepsis, Rocky Mountain spotted fever, malaria, viral or fungal infection)
- Obstetric complications (e.g., fetal demise, amniotic fluid embolism, toxemia, abruptio placentae, septic abortion, eclampsia, placenta previa, uterine atony)
- Tissue trauma (e.g., burns, hypothermia rewarming)
- Malignancy (e.g., adenocarcinomas [gastrointestinal, prostate, lung, breast], lymphoproliferative/myeloproliferative; DIC is a hallmark of acute promyelocytic leukemia and a main cause of mortality)
- Quinine, cocaine-induced rhabdomyolysis
- Liver failure
- Acute pancreatitis
- Transfusion reactions
- Respiratory distress syndrome
- Toxins (snake bites, amphetamine overdose)
- Other: Systemic lupus erythematosus (SLE), vasculitis, aneurysms, polyarteritis, hemangiomas with thrombocytopenia, and consumptive coagulopathy (Kasabach-Merritt syndrome)

Dx DIAGNOSIS

DIFFERENTIAL DIAGNOSIS

- Hepatic necrosis: Normal or elevated factor VIII concentrations
- Vitamin K deficiency: Normal platelet count
- Hemolytic uremic syndrome: Coagulation assays are usually normal
- Thrombotic thrombocytopenic purpura: Low ADAMTS13 activity
- Renal failure, SLE, sickle cell crisis, dysfibrinogenemias
- HELLP syndrome (**h**emolysis, **e**levated **l**iver function tests, and **l**ow **p**latelets)

WORKUP

The diagnostic workup includes laboratory testing to characterize the coagulopathy and its severity and exclude conditions noted in the differential diagnosis (Tables 1 and 2, Box 1). Additional workup is guided by the clinical scenario and may include distinguishing DIC progression (acute vs. chronic), chief manifestations (thrombotic or hemorrhagic), and extent (localized or systemic).

LABORATORY TESTS

- Peripheral blood smear generally shows red blood cell fragments (schistocytes) and low platelet counts.
- Coagulation testing: Diagnostic characteristics of DIC are decreased fibrinogen level; thrombocytopenia; and increased prothrombin time (PT), partial thromboplastin time (PTT), thrombin time (TT), fibrin split products, and D-dimer.
- Coagulopathy secondary to DIC must be differentiated from other coagulopathies that result from underproduction of clotting

TABLE 1 Differential Diagnosis of Thrombocytopenia in Suspected Disseminated Intravascular Coagulation

Differential Diagnosis	Additional Diagnostic Clues
DIC	Prolonged aPTT and PT, increased FDP, low levels of antithrombin or protein C
Sepsis without DIC	Positive (blood) cultures, positive sepsis criteria, hemophagocytosis in bone marrow
Massive blood loss	Major bleeding, low hemoglobin, prolonged aPTT and PT
Thrombotic microangiopathy	Schistocytes evident on blood smear, Coombs-negative hemolysis, fever, neurologic symptoms, renal insufficiency, coagulation tests usually normal, ADAMTS13 levels decreased
Heparin-induced thrombocytopenia	Use of heparin, venous or arterial thrombosis, positive HIT test (usually immunoassay for heparin-platelet factor 4 antibodies), increase in platelet count after cessation of heparin; coagulation tests usually normal
Immune thrombocytopenia	Antiplatelet antibodies, normal or increased number of megakaryocytes in bone marrow aspirate, normal levels of TPO (TPO levels are usually normal or slightly increased in ITP); coagulation tests usually normal
Drug-induced thrombocytopenia	Decreased number of megakaryocytes in bone marrow aspirate or detection of drug-induced antiplatelet antibodies, increase in platelet count after cessation of drug; coagulation tests usually normal

ADAMTS13, A disintegrin and metalloproteinase with thrombospondin 13; *aPTT,* activated partial thromboplastin time; *DIC,* disseminated intravascular coagulation; *FDP,* fibrin degradation products; *HIT,* heparin-induced thrombocytopenia; *PT,* prothrombin time; *ITP,* immune thrombocytopenia; *TPO,* thrombopoietin.
From Hoffman R et al: *Hematology, basic principles and practice,* ed 7, Philadelphia, 2018, Elsevier.

TABLE 2 Differential Diagnosis of Prolonged aPTT and/or PT in Suspected Disseminated Intravascular Coagulation

Test Result	Cause
PT prolonged, aPTT normal	Factor VII deficiency Mild vitamin K deficiency Mild liver insufficiency Low doses of vitamin K antagonists
PT normal, aPTT prolonged	Factor VIII, IX, or XI deficiency Unfractionated heparin Inhibitory antibody and/or antiphospholipid antibody Factor XII or prekallikrein deficiency
Both PT and aPTT prolonged	Factor X, V, II, or fibrinogen deficiency Severe vitamin K deficiency Vitamin K antagonists Global clotting factor deficiency • Decreased synthesis: Liver failure • Increased loss: Massive bleeding, DIC

aPTT, Activated partial thromboplastin time; *PT,* prothrombin time.
From Hoffman R et al: *Hematology, basic principles and practice,* ed 7, Philadelphia, 2018, Elsevier.

BOX 1 Diagnostic Algorithm for the Diagnosis of Overt Disseminated Intravascular Coagulation[a]

- Presence of an underlying disorder known to be associated with disseminated intravascular coagulation (DIC) (Table 2) (no = 0, yes = 2)
- Score global coagulation test results
  1. Platelet count (>100 = score 0; <100 = score 1; <50 = score 2)
  2. Level of fibrin markers (e.g., D-dimer, fibrin degradation products) (no increase = score 0; moderate increase = score 2; strong increase = score 3)[b]
  3. Prolonged prothrombin time (<3 s = score 0; >3 s but <6 s = score 1; >6 s = score 2)
  4. Fibrinogen level (>1.0 g/L = score 0; <1.0 g/L = score 1)
- Calculate score
- If ≥5: Compatible with overt DIC; repeat scoring daily if <5: Suggestive (not affirmative) for nonovert DIC; repeat next 1-2 days.

[a]According to the Scientific Standardization Committee of the International Society of Thrombosis and Haemostasis.
[b]Strong increase, greater than 5× upper limit of normal; moderate increase, greater than upper limit of normal but less than 5× upper limit of normal.
From Hoffman R et al: *Hematology, basic principles and practice,* ed 7, Philadelphia, 2018, Elsevier.

factors, including liver disease or vitamin K deficiency.
1. Vitamin K deficiency manifests with prolonged PT but normal PTT, TT, platelet, and fibrinogen levels; PTT may be elevated in severe cases.
2. Patients with liver disease have abnormal PT and PTT; TT and fibrinogen are usually normal unless severe disease is present; platelets are usually normal unless splenomegaly is present.
3. Factor VIII is not synthesized exclusively by the liver. It can differentiate between DIC, where it is low, and coagulopathy of liver disease, where it is normal.

IMAGING STUDIES

Imaging studies are generally not useful. Imaging may be helpful for identifying sequelae of DIC, including chest radiographs to exclude infectious processes in patients with pulmonary symptoms such as dyspnea, cough, or hemoptysis.

Rx TREATMENT

ACUTE GENERAL Rx

- Correcting and eliminating the underlying cause is often sufficient to halt DIC (e.g., antimicrobial therapy for infection, removal of necrotic bowel, evacuation of uterus in obstetric emergencies).
- Patients with bleeding should be given replacement therapy with fresh frozen plasma (FFP) and platelets:
  1. FFP 10 to 15 ml/kg can be given with a goal of normalizing international normalized ratio.
  2. Platelet transfusions are given when platelet count is <10,000 (or higher if major bleeding is present).
  3. Cryoprecipitate 1 U/5 kg is given for low fibrinogen. It also can be given for prevention of bleeding in patients with fibrinogen level <100 mg/dl.
- Patients with extensive thrombosis (e.g., in acute promyelocytic leukemia, purpura fulminans, acral ischemia) require anticoagulation, despite thrombocytopenia and abnormal coagulation parameters. Heparin therapy using unfractionated heparin at lower doses than those used in venous thrombosis may be useful with a view to increase neutralization of thrombin. Low-molecular-weight heparin also may be used in this scenario.
- The mainstays of supportive treatment of DIC are summarized in Box E2.

DISPOSITION

Mortality rate in severe DIC exceeds 75%. The high mortality rate is often due to the severity of the underlying trigger and complications including acute renal failure, intracerebral bleeding, shock, or cardiac tamponade.

REFERRAL

Hematology consultation is recommended in all cases of severe DIC and DIC with hemorrhagic or thrombotic complications.

PEARLS & CONSIDERATIONS

COMMENTS

The treatment of chronic DIC is controversial. Low-dose SC heparin and/or combination antiplatelet agents such as aspirin and dipyridamole may be useful.

SUGGESTED READINGS

Available at ExpertConsult.com

RELATED CONTENT

Disseminated Intravascular Coagulation (Patient Information)

AUTHORS: **Zachary Cohn, MD,** and **Patan Gultawatvichai, MD**

Diverticular Disease (Diverticulosis, Diverticulitis, Diverticular Hemorrhage) ALG PTG

BASIC INFORMATION

DEFINITION

- Colonic diverticula are herniations of mucosa and submucosa (Figs. 1 and 2) through the muscularis. They are generally found along the colon's mesenteric border at the site where the vasa recta penetrates the muscle wall (anatomic weak point).
- *Diverticulosis* is the asymptomatic presence of multiple colonic diverticula.
- *Diverticulitis* is an inflammatory process or localized perforation of diverticulum.

ICD-10CM CODES

K57.30	Diverticulosis of large intestine without perforation or abscess without bleeding
K57.32	Diverticulitis of large intestine without perforation or abscess without bleeding
K57.31	Diverticulosis of large intestine without perforation or abscess with bleeding

EPIDEMIOLOGY & DEMOGRAPHICS

- Incidence of diverticulosis in the general population is 35% to 50%. Prevalence of diverticulosis increases with ages (<10% under age 40 to over 50% in those >85).
- Diverticulosis is more common in Western countries, affecting >30% of people >40 yr and >50% of people >70 yr.
- Approximately 20% of patients with diverticula have an episode of diverticulitis.

PHYSICAL FINDINGS & CLINICAL PRESENTATION

- Physical examination in patients with diverticulosis is generally normal.
- Painful diverticular disease can present with left lower quadrant (LLQ) pain, often relieved by defecation; location of pain may be anywhere in the lower abdomen because of the redundancy of the sigmoid colon.
- An estimated 10% to 16% of patients with acute diverticulitis present with complicated disease (i.e., abscess or fistula formulation, perforation, or hemorrhage).[1]
- Diverticulitis can cause muscle spasm, guarding, and rebound tenderness predominantly affecting the LLQ. Factors associated with diverticulitis are pain localized to left lower quadrant and exacerbated by movement, left-lower-quadrant tenderness on examination, fever 38.5°C or higher, absence of vomiting, age >50 yr, and history of one or more episodes of diverticulitis.

ETIOLOGY

- Diverticular disease is believed to be secondary to low intake of dietary fiber.
- There are reports of a pathogenetic role for inflammation in diverticulitis that may be similar to that of IBS, IBD, or both, based on common histologic findings such as granulomas, infiltrating lymphocytes, TNF, histamine, and matrix metalloproteinases.[2]

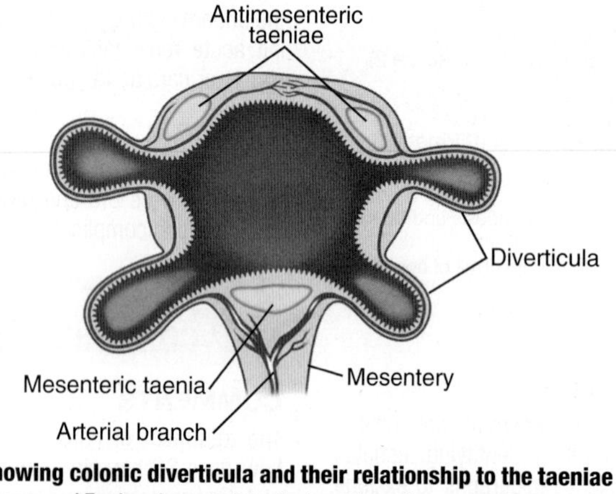

FIG. 1 Diagram showing colonic diverticula and their relationship to the taeniae coli. (From Feldman M et al [eds.]: *Sleisenger and Fordtran's gastrointestinal and liver disease*, ed 10, Philadelphia, 2016, Saunders.)

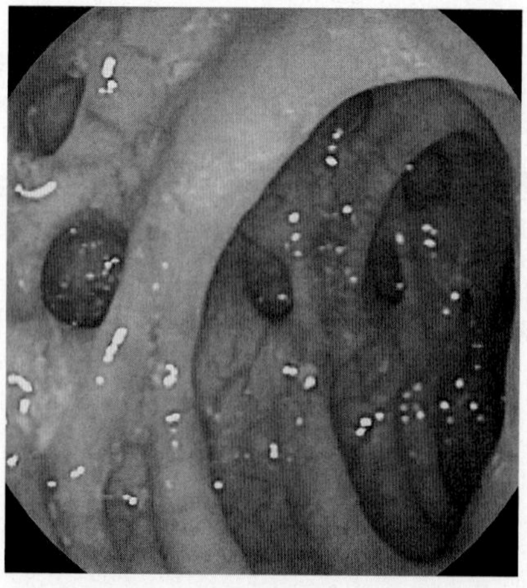

FIG. 2 Colonoscopic view of sigmoid diverticulosis. (From Feldman M et al [eds.]: *Sleisenger and Fordtran's gastrointestinal and liver disease*, ed 10, Philadelphia, 2016, Saunders.)

DIAGNOSIS

DIFFERENTIAL DIAGNOSIS

- IBS
- IBD
- Colorectal cancer
- Endometriosis
- Ischemic colitis
- Bowel obstruction/volvulus
- Urinary tract disorders (urolithiasis, hydronephrosis)
- Infections (pseudomembranous colitis, appendicitis, pyelonephritis, PID)
- Lactose intolerance
- Celiac disease
- Epiploic appendagitis
- Gynecologic disorders (ectopic pregnancy, menstrual irregularities, dyspareunia, endometriosis)
- Cholecystitis, biliary disease

LABORATORY TESTS

- WBC count in diverticulitis reveals leukocytosis with left shift.
- Microcytic anemia can be present in patients with chronic bleeding from diverticular disease. MCV may be elevated in acute bleeding secondary to reticulocytosis.
- Urinalysis is useful to exclude urinary causes of pain.
- Pregnancy test is indicated in women of child-bearing age.
- Electrolytes and liver enzymes are useful in ruling out biliary causes of pain.
- CRP levels of 50 mg/L or greater is common in acute diverticulitis.

[1] von Strauss Und Torney M et al: Risk of emergency surgery or death after initial nonoperative management of complicated diverticulitis in Scotland and Switzerland, *JAMA Surg* 155:600-606, 2020.
[2] Morris AM et al: Sigmoid diverticulitis: a systematic review, *JAMA* 311(3):287-297, 2014.

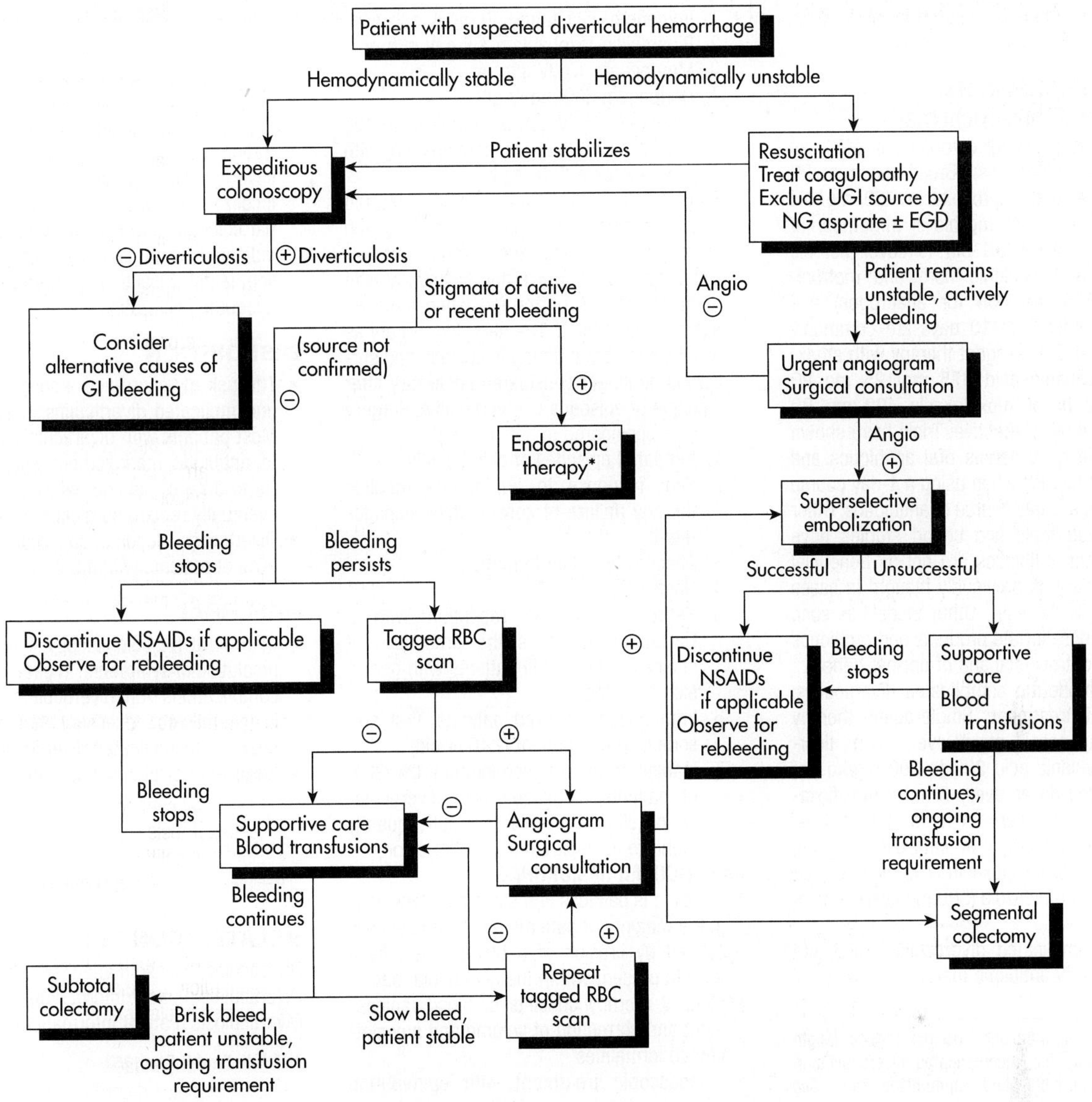

FIG. 4 Algorithm for the management of patients with suspected diverticular hemorrhage. *Angio,* Angiogram; *EGD,* esophagogastroduodenoscopy; *GI,* gastrointestinal; *NG,* nasogastric; *NSAID,* nonsteroidal antiinflammatory drug; *RBC,* red blood cell; *UGI,* upper GI. *Endoscopic therapy may consist of epinephrine injection alone or in combination with other therapies, such as heater probe coagulation, bipolar coagulation, endoclips, fibrin sealant, and band ligation. (From Feldman M et al [eds.]: *Sleisenger and Fordtran's gastrointestinal and liver disease,* ed 10, Philadelphia, 2016, Saunders.)

PROCEDURES: Colonoscopy should be avoided during acute diverticulitis due to the risk of perforation. It can generally be performed after 6 wk to rule out the presence of cancer and IBD.

IMAGING STUDIES

- If clinical features are highly suggestive of diverticulitis, imaging studies are generally not necessary.
- A CT scan of the abdomen (Fig. E3) with IV and luminal contrast is the preferred radiologic examination to diagnose acute diverticulitis. It can also diagnose diverticulosis. It has a sensitivity of 93% to 97% and a specificity approaching 100% for diverticulitis. Typical findings are thickening of the bowel wall, fistulas, or abscess formation. CT may also reveal other disease processes (e.g., appendicitis, tuboovarian abscess, Crohn disease) accounting for lower abdominal pain. In the Hinchey classification scheme based on CT results, stages 0 and Ia indicate uncomplicated diverticulitis, whereas stages Ib (pericolic or mesenteric abscess in proximity to the primary inflammatory process), II (intraabdominal abscess distant from primary inflammatory process or pelvic/retroperitoneal abscess), III (generalized purulent peritonitis), and IV (generalized fecal peritonitis) indicate complicated diverticulitis. Ultrasonography and MRI can also be used. Abdominal ultrasonography has a 90% sensitivity and specificity for acute diverticulitis. MRI is also highly sensitive and specific for acute diverticulitis.
- Evaluation of suspected diverticular bleeding (Fig. 4):
  1. Arteriography if the bleeding is faster than 1 ml/min (advantage: The possible infusion of vasopressin directly into the arteries supplying the bleeding, as well as selective arterial embolization; disadvantages: Its cost and invasive nature)
  2. Technetium-99m sulfa colloid
  3. Technetium-99m labeled RBC (can detect bleeding rates as low as 0.12-5 ml/min)

Rx TREATMENT

NONPHARMACOLOGIC THERAPY

- Increase in dietary fiber intake and regular exercise to improve bowel function. However, recent studies have challenged the common view that fiber intake protects against diverticulosis.
- Oral diet of clear liquids is recommended until pain resolves in cases of mild uncomplicated diverticulitis.
- NPO and IV hydration in severe diverticulitis; NG suction if ileus or small bowel obstruction is present.

- Emergent surgery is required for perforation, peritonitis, or uncontrolled sepsis.

ACUTE GENERAL Rx

TREATMENT OF DIVERTICULITIS:

- Mild uncomplicated diverticulitis (75% of cases of diverticulitis): Broad-spectrum PO antibiotics (e.g., ciprofloxacin 750 mg bid or levofloxacin 750 mg bid or trimethoprim/sulfamethoxazole DS bid to cover aerobic component of colonic flora *and* metronidazole 500 mg q6h for anaerobes) and liquid diet for 7 to 10 days are commonly prescribed. Single-agent therapy with amoxicillin-clavulanic acid 875 mg/125 mg PO every 12 hr or moxifloxacin 400 mg PO every hr is also effective. Trials have shown no benefit of IV versus oral antibiotics and similar outcomes when using a 4-day course instead of a 7-day course of antibiotics. Other randomized trials and cohort studies have shown that antibiotics are not as beneficial or necessary as previously thought in cases of mild diverticulitis.[3] Other modalities such as 5-aminosalicylate products and probiotics remain controversial and of unclear benefit.
- Mild to moderate complicated diverticulitis, in-patient treatment: Single-agent therapy with ertapenem 1 mg IV every 24 hr, ticarcillin-clavulanic acid 200 to 300 mg/kg per day divided doses every 6 hr, or moxifloxacin 400 mg IV every 24 hr for 4 to 7 days. Combination therapy of cefazolin (1-2 mg every 8 hr) or levofloxacin (750 mg every 24 hr) plus metronidazole (500 mg every 8 hr) is also effective.
- Severe complicated diverticulitis: NPO and aggressive IV antibiotic therapy
  1. Imipenem- cilastatin 500 mg IV q6h *or*
  2. Piperacillin-tazobactam 4.5 g IV q8h *or*
  3. Meropenem 1 g IV q8h *or*
  4. Doripenem 500 mg IV q8h
  5. Cefepime 2 g IV q8h or ciprofloxacin 400 mg IV q12h each in combination with metronidazole 500 mg IV q8h
- Surgical treatment (laparoscopic preferred over open colectomy) consisting of resection of involved areas and reanastomosis (if feasible); otherwise, a diverting colostomy with reanastomosis is performed when infection has been controlled. The need for surgery as well as its optimal timing is unclear, and surgery is no longer considered necessary after a couple of episodes of diverticulitis. Surgery may be considered in patients with:
  1. Repeated episodes of diverticulitis
  2. Poor response to appropriate medical therapy (failure of conservative management)
  3. Abscess or fistula formation
  4. Obstruction
  5. Peritonitis: Colonic resection with a Hartmann pouch is the procedure of choice in critically ill patients with generalized peritonitis
  6. Immunocompromised patients, first episode in young patient (<40 yr old)
  7. Inability to exclude carcinoma (10%-20% of patients diagnosed with diverticulosis on clinical grounds are subsequently found to have carcinoma of the colon)

DIVERTICULAR HEMORRHAGE:

- Bleeding is painless and stops spontaneously in the majority of patients (60%); it is usually caused by erosion of a blood vessel by a fecalith present within the diverticular sac.
- Medical therapy consists of blood replacement and correction of volume and any clotting abnormalities.
- Colonoscopic treatment with epinephrine injections, bipolar coagulation, or both may prevent recurrent bleeding and decrease the need for surgery. Endoclips (Fig. E5) can also be used to stop the bleeding.
- Surgical resection is necessary if bleeding does not stop spontaneously after administration of 4 to 5 U of PRBCs or recurs with severity within a few days; if attempts at localization are unsuccessful, total abdominal colectomy with ileoproctostomy may be indicated (high incidence of rebleeding if segmental resection is performed without adequate localization).

DISPOSITION

- The risk of recurrence among patients with uncomplicated diverticulitis is 32% to 36%. Most patients with diverticulitis respond well to antibiotic management and bowel rest. Up to 30% of patients with diverticulitis will eventually require surgical management.
- Diverticular bleeding can recur in 15% to 20% of patients within 5 yr.

REFERRAL

- GI referral for colonoscopy 4 to 6 wk after resolution of symptoms. In patients who have complications from diverticulitis, colonoscopy is generally not necessary after radiologically proven uncomplicated diverticulitis.
- Surgical referral when considering resection.

SUGGESTED READINGS

Available at ExpertConsult.com

RELATED CONTENT

Diverticular Disease (Patient Information)
Diverticulitis (Patient Information)
Diverticulosis (Patient Information)

AUTHOR: **Fred F. Ferri, MD**

[3] Jaung R et al: antibiotics do not reduce length of hospital stay for uncomplicated diverticulitis in a pragmatic double-blind randomized trial, *Clin Gastroenterol Hepatol* 19:503-510, 2021.

BASIC INFORMATION

DEFINITION

Drug use disorder is a recurring pattern of harmful use of a substance despite adverse consequences to work, school, relationships, the legal system, or physical health. This may occur concurrently with or independently from *substance dependence,* in which the impairment or distress is more pervasive and often (though not necessarily) includes physical dependence and withdrawal symptoms (Table 1).

SYNONYMS

Substance use disorder
Substance abuse
Substance dependence
Addiction

ICD-10CM CODES

F19.129	Other psychoactive substance abuse, with intoxication, unspecified
F10-F19	Defined by specific substance; abuse and dependence specifiers
Z71.51	Drug abuse counseling and surveillance of drug abuser

DSM-5 CODE

Defined by specific substance; mild, moderate, severe specifiers

EPIDEMIOLOGY & DEMOGRAPHICS

INCIDENCE (IN U.S.): Alcohol or other drug dependence: 5% to 10% of population. Peak incidence for most substances: Ages 15 to 30.

PREVALENCE (IN U.S.): Approximately 15% of patients in primary care practice have an at-risk pattern of drug and/or alcohol use. Lifetime prevalence of alcohol use disorder is 30% in the U.S., compared to 8.6% worldwide. Rates of prescription pain reliever misuse have decreased, with 3.6% past-year prevalence; past-year prevalence of stimulant and sedative/tranquilizer use are 1.9% and 2.4%, respectively. Among the U.S. population >12 yr, 19.4% (or nearly 1 in 5) have used an illicit drug (including marijuana) in the past year and 3.0% meet the classification for an illicit drug use disorder (2018 National Survey on Drug Use and Health).

TABLE 1 Key Features of Substance Abuse

1. The substance is often taken in larger amounts over a longer period than intended
2. Unsuccessful efforts to cut down
3. A great deal of time spent obtaining the substance or recovering from its effects
4. Craving
5. Social, occupational, or recreational
6. Recurrent despite hazards
7. Tolerance or withdrawal

From Goldman L, Bennett JC (eds): *Cecil textbook of medicine,* ed 22, Philadelphia, 2004, Saunders.

PREDOMINANT SEX: Alcohol and other drug use are more prevalent among males than females. However, drug use rates in the U.S. show an increase in female consumption of alcohol and alcohol use disorders in recent years.

PREDOMINANT AGE:

- Problematic use of substances may begin in early life (8-10 yr).
- Mean age of onset of problem drinking is approximately 25 yr for men and 30 yr for women.
- Rates of binge alcohol use among the baby boomer generation and older adults (ages 65+) are on the rise.

DURATION OF CONDITION:

- Men: Average >20 yr of heavy drinking
- Women: Average 15 yr of heavy drinking
- In general, substance use disorders are chronic, relapsing, and often progressive. Younger onset of use tends to be correlated with worse prognosis

GENETICS: There is evidence of nonspecific genetic factors. Addiction may result in part from underlying, inherited abnormalities in brain structure that impair behavior control and encourage impulsive behavior.

PHYSICAL FINDINGS & CLINICAL PRESENTATION

- Polysubstance use and comorbidity with psychiatric disorders are common.
- History often reveals recurring behavioral and psychosocial problems, such as relationship, work, financial, housing, or legal problems; violence and traumatic injuries; and anxiety, depression, insomnia, and cognitive and memory dysfunction.
- Repeated requests for early refills of controlled substances and obtaining prescriptions from multiple providers should raise concern for prescription drug use disorder (Table 2).
- Physical findings may include injection marks (Figs. E1 and E2), nasal lesions or recurrent epistaxis (Table E3), poor dentition, scars or bruises from falls or trauma, sudden weight change, and poor nutritional status. Signs/symptoms of intoxication (e.g., dilated or constricted pupils, involuntary head nodding) or withdrawal are highly suggestive of substance use disorder. Infectious complications of drug abuse are summarized in Table E4.

ETIOLOGY

Several models of addiction have been proposed, with consensus that addiction likely results from a combination of both biologic/genetic and social/environmental factors.

- Disease model: Addiction is a chronic brain disease, which occurs as a result of the impairment of healthy neurochemical or behavioral processes.
- Genetic model: Genetic predisposition is often a factor in dependency and certain addictive behaviors.
- Social model: Person–environment interactions (i.e., socialization, imitation of observable behavior, and the influence of modeling) shape addictive behavior.

DIAGNOSIS

DIFFERENTIAL DIAGNOSIS

- Psychiatric disorders and symptoms such as depression, mania, psychosis, insomnia, posttraumatic stress disorder, and anxiety disorders may coexist or occur as a consequence of substance use.
- Rule out seizure disorder and underlying medical illness.

WORKUP

- A thorough history is crucial for diagnosis.
- The physician's history-taking style and techniques strongly affect patient's willingness to report use and to participate in future treatment activities. Common trade and "street names" of opioids available in the U.S. are summarized in Box E1.

TABLE 2 "Red Flags" for Abuse Behavior and Opioid Addiction

Potential Abuse/Addiction Behaviors*

1. Patient displays an overwhelming focus on opioid issues during clinic visits that occupies a significant proportion of the clinic visit and impedes progress with other pain issues or medical problems.
2. Patient has a pattern of early refills (three or more) or escalating drug use in the absence of acute change or progression of his or her medical condition.
3. Patient generates multiple telephone calls or unscheduled visits to request more opioids, early refills, or problems associated with the opioid prescription that often creates a disturbance of the clinic staff.
4. There is a pattern of prescription problems with reports of medications lost, spilled, or stolen.
5. Patient has supplemental sources of opioids from multiple providers, emergency departments, or illegal sources.

Additional "Red Flag" Abuse Behavior

1. Selling prescribed medications
2. Prescription forgery
3. Stealing another patient's medications
4. Injecting or snorting oral medication
5. Concurrent use of illicit drug(s)
6. Appearing intoxicated or oversedated
7. Insisting on obtaining a specific opioid medication

*Adapted from Chabal criteria for opioid abuse.
From Hochberg MC et al: *Rheumatology,* ed 5, St Louis, 2011, Mosby.

- A structured, nonjudgmental approach is generally preferable:
  1. Ask about quantity and frequency of alcohol or drug use, as well as method of administration (e.g., IV, smoke). The National Institute on Alcohol Abuse and Alcoholism (NIAAA) declares that *problem drinking* is defined as more than two drinks per day for men and more than one drink per day for women or anyone older than age 65.
  2. Use a short screening instrument such as the CAGE questionnaire ("1. Have you ever felt you need to **C**ut down on your alcohol or drug use? 2. Have people **A**nnoyed you by criticizing your alcohol or drug use? 3. Have you ever felt **G**uilty about alcohol or drug use? 4. Have you ever felt you need to drink first thing in the morning [**E**ye opener] to stop shakiness?").
- Problematic behavior during intoxication or withdrawal is diagnostic.
- Because self-report of substance use and its consequences can be unreliable, laboratory tests and obtaining corroborating information, such as from family members, past detoxifications, or drug rehabilitations, is often helpful.
- Adolescent drug use disorder detection and treatment is extremely challenging. Stages of adolescent substance use are described in Table E5. An assessment for evaluating the seriousness of adolescent drug use disorder is described in Table E6.

LABORATORY TESTS

- Blood alcohol content (BAC) measured on the breath is practical to define intoxication and provides a rough measure of impairment. In general, two standard drinks may cause BAC 0.08% or higher, which is considered legally impaired.
- Obtain toxicology screen in urine, oral swab, or blood samples. Oral swabs are more resistant to tampering than are urine screens.
- Biologic markers such as elevated mean corpuscular volume (MCV), γ-glutamyltransferase (GGT), liver function tests (AST and ALT; AST:ALT ratio of 2:1 or greater is suggestive of alcoholic liver disease), and carbohydrate deficient transferrin (CDT) may also be used to diagnose and monitor.

IMAGING STUDIES

Not helpful in routine diagnosis and management of substance misuse, but possibly useful in the management of sequelae of substance misuse (e.g., brain imaging to evaluate the alcohol abuse–associated increased risk of subdural hematomas or increased evidence of cerebral atrophy). Imaging studies have also revealed adaptations within the brain's reward circuit following repeated alcohol and drug use; these adaptations reduce the impact of dopamine, often resulting in depressed mood and anhedonia among persons who misuse substances.

Rx TREATMENT

NONPHARMACOLOGIC THERAPY

- Motivational interviewing (MI) is an evidence-based approach that preserves patient autonomy in defining treatment goals and working toward change. For patients who express lack of readiness/commitment to change, it can be helpful to discuss the functions of their use and advantages/disadvantages the patient has personally experienced. Use an Elicit-Provide-Elicit format to counsel about risks of use and benefits of abstinence; in other words, elicit a patient's consent and feedback before and after providing information.
- Nonpharmacologic strategies have the greatest documented efficacy: Education, feedback, goal setting, problem solving, and additional contacts for further assistance.
- Opiate contracts, prohibiting a patient from getting early refills, or obtaining opiates from multiple prescribers should be considered for all patients with chronic pain receiving opioid painkillers, especially for patients with a history of substance misuse or misuse of prescribed medication.
- Behavioral relapse prevention approaches teach patients how to avoid trigger stimuli or uncouple trigger stimuli from substance ingestion.
- Self-help and 12-step support groups such as Alcoholics Anonymous and Narcotics Anonymous are helpful in achieving and maintaining sobriety. Alternative self-help and peer groups include SMART Recovery, Dharma Recovery, Refuge Recovery, and Recovery Coach services.
- Consider psychotherapy/psychiatry referrals to address co-occurring psychiatric conditions, as well as case management referrals to address common barriers to recovery (e.g., safe housing).
- Residential or inpatient treatment programs should be a consideration for any individual with continued or escalating use despite outpatient treatment.

ACUTE GENERAL Rx

- Detoxification is an important first step. Seizure risk is greatest within the first 48 hours of alcohol abstinence. Detoxification goals are to facilitate withdrawal and initiate abstinence safely, prevent withdrawal seizures and reduce symptoms, and refer the patient to ongoing treatment.
- Benzodiazepines are effective in acute alcohol withdrawal for the management of symptoms as well as the prevention of seizures. One strategy is to give the patient a loading dose of a long-acting benzodiazepine (e.g., 20 mg of diazepam) and then continue the benzodiazepine as scheduled while tapering down the dose gradually. An example would be chlordiazepoxide 25 to 50 mg every 6 hr on day 1, 25 to 50 mg every 8 hr on day 2, 25 to 50 mg every 12 hr on day 3, and 25 to 50 mg at hour of sleep on day 4 and day 5 and then discontinue. An alternative "symptom-driven" strategy is to follow the patient closely with serial assessments, such as the Clinical Institute Withdrawal Assessment for Alcohol (CIWA) scale, and to dose with 1 to 2 mg of lorazepam as needed to treat specified withdrawal symptoms.
- The prophylactic administration of thiamine and folic acid (first intravenously or intramuscularly followed by supplemental oral doses) in alcohol withdrawal is recommended before starting any carbohydrate-containing fluids or food to prevent Wernicke-Korsakoff syndrome (alcoholic encephalopathy and psychosis). Magnesium appears to be effective in the treatment of alcohol withdrawal–related cardiac arrhythmias, but not other symptoms of alcohol withdrawal.
- Beta-blockers and clonidine generally should be avoided in alcohol withdrawal; they may mask markers of the severity of the withdrawal (blood pressure and pulse rate).
- Unlike withdrawal from alcohol or benzodiazepines, opioid withdrawal is not life threatening.
- Clonidine alleviates the discomfort of opiate withdrawal. Clonidine tablets, 0.1 mg q4-6h as needed, can be used while monitoring patient's blood pressure. Clonidine transdermal patch, 0.1 mg/24 hr, can be used to treat autonomic hyperactivity symptoms; however, it has a very slow onset and may take 2 to 3 days to achieve therapeutic levels. Antidiarrheals, ibuprofen, and dicyclomine can be used as adjuncts to treat opiate withdrawal symptoms.
- Methadone taper is an effective approach for detoxification in opioid dependence.
- Buprenorphine is a partial μ-opioid receptor agonist that may be used for detoxification and maintenance in treatment of opioid dependence (see dosing in next section).

LONG-TERM Rx

- Naltrexone helps reduce craving for alcohol. Naltrexone 50 mg once daily for 12 wk can be a useful adjunct to substance abuse counseling or rehabilitation programs. Randomized treatment studies are equivocal for long-term outcomes. Naltrexone reduces relapse and the intensity or frequency of any drinking that does occur. It can be hepatotoxic and is contraindicated in opiate users. Intramuscular naltrexone (380 mg monthly) may be considered if adherence is an issue.
- Acamprosate also helps reduce craving for alcohol. Acamprosate 666 mg three times daily may be an effective adjunct to counseling. A recent meta-analysis showed overall benefit with increase in the number of abstinent days.
- Disulfiram provokes acetaldehyde accumulation after alcohol ingestion, producing a toxic state manifested by nausea, headache, flushing, and respiratory distress. Studies have shown limited efficacy mostly due to noncompliance.

- Topiramate may be an alternative treatment for alcoholism. In a 12-wk randomized trial, topiramate up to 300 mg daily significantly reduced the number of heavy drinking days.
- Methadone maintenance for opiate addiction is effective and involves once-daily dosing of methadone in a controlled setting via methadone clinics.
- Buprenorphine is as effective as low-dose methadone and may be prescribed by physicians who have completed approved training. For induction, initiate 12 to 24 hr after short-acting opioid use and 24 to 48 hr after long-acting opioid use. Use buprenorphine/naloxone (Suboxone) tablets in most patients, since buprenorphine-only tablets have risk of abuse. Maximum first-day dosage is 4 to 8 mg of buprenorphine. Titrate buprenorphine dose up to 12 mg on day 2 for signs of withdrawal. Then adjust dosage in frequent outpatient visits (weekly) to minimum needed for maintenance (up to 32 mg daily).
- Naltrexone (oral or injectable) may also be used for maintenance in opioid dependence treatment, though evidence of effectiveness is limited.
- Always combine pharmacotherapy with counseling. There is good evidence that this combination improves outcome.
- Treatment of comorbid psychiatric disorders improves outcomes.

COCAINE: Health effects of cocaine use include:

- Constricted blood vessels
- Dilated pupils
- Nausea
- Raised body temperature and blood pressure
- Fast or irregular heartbeat
- Tremors and muscle twitches
- Restlessness

Long-term effects of cocaine use include vulnerability to HIV and hepatitis C infections; malnourishment because cocaine decreases appetite; and movement disorders, including Parkinson disease, irritability and restlessness from cocaine binges, and severe paranoia and perceptual changes such as auditory hallucinations. Cocaine abuse can cause cardiomyopathy, myocardial infarction and arrhythmias, cerebrovascular accidents, and lower the threshold for seizures.

During cocaine withdrawal, patients can experience:

- Depression
- Suicidal ideation
- Agitation
- Intense cravings
- Need for higher doses
- Apathy
- Exhaustion
- Long periods of sleep

Behavioral therapy may be used to treat cocaine addiction. Examples include:

- Cognitive-behavioral therapy (CBT)
- Contingency management or motivational incentives—providing rewards to patients who remain substance free
- Therapeutic communities
- Community-based recovery groups, such as 12-step programs

Most pharmacotherapies have been ineffective for treating cocaine use disorder. Bupropion, psychostimulants, and topiramate may improve abstinence. While no government-approved medicines are currently available to treat cocaine addiction, researchers are testing some treatments that have been used to treat other disorders, including:

- Disulfiram (used to treat alcoholism)
- Modafinil (used to treat *narcolepsy*—a disorder characterized by uncontrollable episodes of deep sleep)
- Lorcaserin (used to treat obesity)
- Buprenorphine (used to treat opioid addiction)

Observational studies suggest that cannabidiol may reduce problems related with crack-cocaine addiction, such as withdrawal symptoms, craving, impulsivity, and paranoia.

METHAMPHETAMINE: Even small amounts of methamphetamine can result in many of the same health effects as those of other stimulants, such as cocaine or amphetamines. These include:

- Increased wakefulness and physical activity
- Decreased appetite
- Faster breathing
- Rapid and/or irregular heartbeat
- Increased blood pressure and body temperature

Injecting methamphetamine increases risk of contracting HIV and hepatitis B and C. Methamphetamine use can also alter judgment and decision making leading to risky behaviors, such as unprotected sex, which also increases risk for infection. Methamphetamine may worsen the progression of HIV/AIDS and its consequences. Long-term methamphetamine use has many other negative consequences, including:

- Extreme weight loss
- Addiction
- Severe dental problems ("meth mouth")
- Intense itching, leading to skin sores from scratching
- Anxiety
- Changes in brain structure and function
- Confusion
- Memory loss
- Sleeping problems
- Violent behavior
- Delusions
- Hallucinations

There are no approved medications for methamphetamine treatment, although medications are used for symptoms such as psychotic symptoms. Behavior therapies such as CBT and contingency management or motivational incentives as noted above for cocaine treatment are also used for methamphetamine treatment.

DISPOSITION

- Drug use disorders are chronic relapsing illnesses, so relapses are best approached as part of the course of the illness, as opposed to treatment failure.
- The goal of treatment is often abstinence, but success of treatment is measured by return of function, increasing duration between relapses, and prevention of sequelae of use.

REFERRAL

Physicians should refer patients who do not make progress on changing substance use patterns to addiction specialists and/or specialized substance use disorder or dual-diagnosis (mental health and addiction) programs. Patients with comorbid psychiatric illness should be referred for mental health care.

PEARLS & CONSIDERATIONS

- The opioid crisis, which has led to an epidemic of overdose deaths in the U.S., was partially fueled by the use of oral narcotics in the treatment of chronic pain and this has prompted a revision of chronic pain management with strict guidelines for the use of opiate medications for this condition.
- Fentanyl involvement in opioid overdose deaths rose from 14.3% in 2010 to 46% in 2016 (National Vital Statistics System data). In 2018, fentanyl was found in 73.9% of opioid overdose deaths (Morbidity and Mortality Weekly Report, 2020). In many deaths, more than one drug is involved, and combining fentanyl with heroin may enhance its lethality.
- Between 2012 and 2018, the rate of drug overdose deaths from cocaine use have more than tripled and the rates of overdose deaths involving psychostimulants with abuse potential (e.g., methamphetamine) have increased nearly fivefold (National Vital Statistics System data).
- Racial disparities have long been an issue in the diagnosis and treatment of drug use disorders. Purposeful reflection on implicit biases and their impact on treatment practice is critical when addressing substance misuse.
- Acute withdrawal from alcohol and benzodiazepines can become life threatening.
- Withdrawal from opioids can resemble a severe case of the flu.
- A brief intervention (providing information and advising the patient to reduce consumption of alcohol) by the primary care doctor has been demonstrated in randomized trials to reduce drinking in at-risk patients.
- Treatment rates for alcohol use disorders remain low despite available effective treatments.

SUGGESTED READINGS

Available at ExpertConsult.com

RELATED CONTENT

Drug Use Disorder (Patient Information)
Substance Use Disorder (Related Key Topic)
Alcohol Use Disorder (Related Key Topic)
Opioid Use Disorder (Related Key Topic)

AUTHORS: **René Lento, PhD,** and **Tahir Tellioglu, MD**

BASIC INFORMATION

DEFINITION

Dysmenorrhea is painful menstrual cramps of uterine origin. Prevalence is estimated to vary between 45% and 95%. Dysmenorrhea is the most common gynecologic condition in women, regardless of age and nationality.

Types of dysmenorrhea:

- Primary dysmenorrhea is menstrual pain without organic disease.
- Secondary dysmenorrhea is menstrual pain associated with an identifiable disease.

SYNONYMS

Menstrual cramps
Painful periods

ICD-10CM CODES
N94.3 Primary dysmenorrhea
N94.5 Secondary dysmenorrhea
N94.6 Dysmenorrhea, unspecified

EPIDEMIOLOGY & DEMOGRAPHICS

- Approximately 50% of menstruating women are affected by dysmenorrhea, with approximately 10% of them having severe dysmenorrhea with incapacitation for 1 to 3 days/mo.
- Dysmenorrhea is most common in the age group from 20 to 24 yr.
- Primary dysmenorrhea may appear 6 to 12 mo after ovulatory menstrual cycles begin.
- Secondary dysmenorrhea may occur at any time after menarche, but it may arise in a woman's 30s to 40s due to a causative underlying condition. The woman may also complain of dyspareunia, menorrhagia, intermenstrual bleeding, or postcoital bleeding.

PHYSICAL FINDINGS & CLINICAL PRESENTATION

- Sharp, crampy, midline, lower abdominal pain without a lower quadrant or adnexal component but possible radiation to the lower back and upper thighs
- Unremarkable pelvic examination in nonmenstruating patient
- Accompanying symptoms: Nausea, vomiting, headaches, anxiety, fatigue, diarrhea, fainting, and abdominal bloating
- Cramps usually lasting <24 hr and seldom lasting >2 to 3 days
- Secondary dysmenorrhea: Dyspareunia is a common complaint, and bimanual pelvic-abdominal examination may demonstrate uterine or adnexal tenderness, fixed uterine retroflexion, uterosacral nodularity, a pelvic mass, or an enlarged, irregular uterus

ETIOLOGY

Prostaglandin $F_2\alpha$ is the agent responsible for dysmenorrhea. It stimulates uterine contractions and cervical stenosis (narrowing) and increases vasopressin release. Behavior and psychological factors have also been implicated in the etiology of primary dysmenorrhea. Primary dysmenorrhea only occurs in ovulatory cycles. Secondary dysmenorrhea is usually caused by endometriosis, adenomyosis, leiomyomas, and, less commonly, intrauterine device (IUD) use, or congenital or acquired outflow tract obstruction, including cervical stenosis.

DIAGNOSIS

DIFFERENTIAL DIAGNOSIS: SECONDARY DYSMENORRHEA

- Adenomyosis
- Adhesions
- Cervical structures or stenosis
- Congenital malformation of Müllerian system
- Ectopic pregnancy
- Endometriosis
- Imperforate hymen
- IUD use
- Leiomyomas
- Ovarian cysts
- Pelvic congestion syndrome
- Pelvic inflammatory disease
- Polyps
- Transverse vaginal septum
- Table 1 summarizes the differential diagnosis of dysmenorrhea in adolescents

WORKUP AND EVALUATION

- Primary dysmenorrhea: Characteristic history, physical examination and ultrasound normal with the absence of an identifiable cause of pelvic pain
- Secondary dysmenorrhea: Physical examination and ultrasound may reveal vaginal/uterine abnormalities, fibroids, adenomyosis, polyps, endometriomas

LABORATORY TESTS

- No specific tests diagnostic for dysmenorrhea
- Elevated white blood cell count in the presence of infection
- Human chorionic gonadotropin to rule out ectopic pregnancy

IMAGING STUDIES

- Ultrasound scan of the pelvis to evaluate the presence of leiomyomas, adenomyosis, ovarian cysts
- Saline ultrasonography to assess the uterine cavity to rule out endometrial polyps or submucosal or intraluminal leiomyomas

TREATMENT

NONPHARMACOLOGIC THERAPY

- Applying heat to the lower abdomen with hot compresses, heating pads, or hot water bottles seems to offer some relief.
- Offer reassurance that this is a treatable condition.

TABLE 1 Differential Diagnosis of Dysmenorrhea in Adolescents

	Presentation	Diagnosis
Primary	Crampy pelvic pain may be accompanied by aching/heaviness in lower back and upper thighs, nausea, emesis, diarrhea, headache, mastalgia, fatigue, and dizziness; symptoms begin at or shortly before onset of menstrual flow and last 1-3 days.	Normal physical exam; internal exam only for sexually active adolescents. Ultrasound can be reserved for those patients with atypical presentations (e.g., onset at menarche) or those whose pain does not respond to NSAIDs and hormonal therapy.
Endometriosis and adenomyosis*	**Increasingly severe dysmenorrhea despite adequate therapy;** pain exacerbated during menses can occur acyclically as well.	Increased risk in patients with obstructive anomalies and possibly bleeding disorders; however, most teenagers with endometriosis have normal anatomy and bleeding indices; diagnosis is made visually during surgery. *Found in up to 69% of adolescents who underwent laparoscopy for persistent pelvic pain.*
Müllerian anomalies with partial outflow obstruction	**Pain begins at or shortly after menarche** and occurs with bleeding; presence of **known renal tract anomaly** (often coexists with Müllerian anomaly).	Pelvic ultrasound will demonstrate uterine anomalies (e.g., rudimentary uterine horn); MRI may be required to identify some lesions (e.g., obstructed hemivagina). *Found in 8% of adolescents who underwent laparoscopy for persistent pelvic pain.*
Pelvic inflammatory disease	Abrupt onset of dysmenorrhea more severe than baseline in a sexually active adolescent; presentation can range from mild discomfort to acute abdomen.	Clinical diagnosis made by findings of uterine or adnexal tenderness on bimanual pelvic examination; supporting features include dysuria, dyspareunia, **vaginal discharge,** fever, and increased white blood cell count.
Pregnancy complication	Coincident pain and bleeding may be misdiagnosed as dysmenorrhea.	Urine test positive for human chorionic gonadotropin.

MRI, Magnetic resonance imaging; *NSAID,* nonsteroidal antiinflammatory drug.
Bold entries indicate "red flags" for diagnosis.
*Adenomyosis is the presence of endometrial tissue within the uterine myometrium.
From Kliegman RM: *Nelson Textbook of Pediatrics,* ed 21, Philadelphia, 2020, Elsevier.

TABLE 2 Treatment for Dysmenorrhea

	Medication	Regimen	Comments
NSAIDs for up to 5 days	Ibuprofen, 200 mg	2 tablets PO q4-6h	Over-the-counter
	Naproxen sodium, 275 mg	550 mg loading dose, then 275 mg PO q6h	Patients may prefer the equivalent 550 mg PO q12h dosing regimen
	Celecoxib (cyclooxygenase [COX]-2 inhibitor)*	400 mg, then 200 mg PO q12h prn pain	Can be used for patients with von Willebrand disease
Hormonal contraception	Combined oral contraceptive pills or vaginal ring	Continuous hormone regimens (vs standard 21 hormone days followed by 7 placebo days) may offer better relief but may increase the risk of unexpected intermenstrual bleeding	The data favoring rings and pills over the combined hormone patch for this indication are sparse; treatment can be based on patient preference.
	Progestin-only methods	DMPA 150 mg IM or 104 mg SC q3 mo; levonorgestrel intrauterine device for up to 5 yr; etonogestrel implant for up to 3 yr	DMPA has potential side effects of weight gain and interference with expected bone density increase during adolescence, as well as a higher discontinuation rate than LARC methods.
Gonadotropin-releasing hormone agonist	Depot leuprolide	11.25 mg IM q3 mo	Consider for patients with presumed endometriosis not responsive to hormonal methods; add-back hormones are recommended to prevent bone loss.

DMPA, Depot medroxyprogesterone acetate; *IM*, intramuscular; *LARC*, long-acting reversible contraceptive; *NSAIDs*, nonsteroidal antiinflammatory drugs; *PO*, by mouth; *prn*, as needed; *SC*, subcutaneous.

*This medication may cause serious cardiovascular and gastrointestinal events. Use with caution in patients with impaired renal or liver function, heart failure, or a history of GI bleeding or ulcer. Full prescribing information can be found at: www.accessdata.fda.gov/drugsatfda_docs/label/2011/020998s033,021156s003lbl.pdf.

From Kliegman RM: *Nelson textbook of pediatrics*, ed 21, Philadelphia, 2020, Elsevier.

ACUTE GENERAL Rx

- Treatment of dysmenorrhea is summarized in Table 2
- Nonsteroidal antiinflammatory drugs such as ibuprofen 400 to 600 mg q4 to 6h or naproxen sodium 500 mg q12h
- Oral contraceptives cyclically or continuously (taking only active pills), primarily in women with primary dysmenorrhea
- The levonorgestrel-containing IUD is increasingly being used to ameliorate symptoms of dysmenorrhea. Pain improvement has been shown in many cases to be even better than oral contraceptive pills
- Magnesium supplements (research ongoing)
- Thiamine supplements (research ongoing)
- Fish oil supplements (research ongoing)
- Secondary dysmenorrhea: Treatment directed to the specific underlying condition

CHRONIC Rx

Acupuncture and transcutaneous electrical nerve stimulation may be tried. However, there is not enough evidence to support the use of yoga, acupuncture, or massage. In cases in which medical therapy has not worked, laparoscopy or other surgical treatments should be considered depending on the secondary cause of the dysmenorrhea. A directed physical examination looking for gynecologic masses or nodularity should be performed. Nontraditional approaches such as acupuncture have been tried with relief in some patients. The levonorgestrel IUD has been shown to effectively reduce pain in women with primary dysmenorrhea.

DISPOSITION

The majority of patients are satisfactorily treated with good outcomes. Possible chronic complications with primary dysmenorrhea that has not been adequately treated can lead to anxiety and depression. With certain causes of secondary dysmenorrhea, infertility can become a problem.

REFERRAL

If a secondary cause of dysmenorrhea is revealed, refer to the appropriate specialist for further medical or surgical treatment (e.g., gynecologist, urogynecologist, reproductive endocrinologist, pain management center).

RELATED CONTENT

Dysmenorrhea (Patient Information)
Dyspareunia (Related Key Topic)
Endometriosis (Related Key Topic)
Premenstrual Dysphoric Disorder (Related Key Topic)
Premenstrual Syndrome (Related Key Topic)

AUTHOR: **Barbara McGuirk, MD**

BASIC INFORMATION

DEFINITION

Dyspepsia is a constellation of symptoms referable to the gastroduodenal region of the upper GI tract. *Nonulcerative dyspepsia* is a term used to describe signs and symptoms of persistent or recurrent dyspepsia that have no identifiable organic cause.

- Functional dyspepsia (FD) is defined as discomfort or pain in the upper abdomen.
- Postprandial distress syndrome is characterized by postprandial fullness and early satiation. It is the most common subtype of functional dyspepsia.

SYNONYMS

Nonulcer dyspepsia
Functional dyspepsia
Idiopathic dyspepsia
Postprandial distress syndrome (PDS)

ICD-10CM CODE
K30 Functional dyspepsia

EPIDEMIOLOGY & DEMOGRAPHICS

Up to 25% of the general population will experience dyspepsia each yr. Of these, 75% will have no evident causative agent. Functional dyspepsia is a common disorder, with an estimated prevalence of 8% to 12% based on Rome IV criteria and up to 40% when less restrictive criteria are used. Data suggest that less than 15% of patients with functional dyspepsia are actually given the correct diagnosis. In the U.S., the diagnosis, treatment, and work absenteeism related to functional dyspepsia have been estimated to cost $18.4 billion per year.

PHYSICAL FINDINGS & CLINICAL PRESENTATION

Typical clinical presentation is dyspepsia without findings on physical examination to explain the symptoms.

ETIOLOGY

The etiology and pathophysiology are still unclear. Box 1 summarizes causes of dyspepsia. Research is focused on abnormalities of gastric motor function and visceral hypersensitivity, as well as:

- *Helicobacter pylori* infection
- Psychosocial factors—associated with anxiety and depression

RISK FACTORS

Risk factors include the following:

- Genetic predisposition: Homozygous *GNB3* gene
- Dietary habits such as caffeine, alcohol, or smoking
- Medications such as NSAIDs, calcium channel blockers, methylxanthines, alendronate, orlistat, acarbose, and potassium supplements
- Psychological disorders such as anxiety, depression, somatization, or personal history of childhood sexual or physical abuse

DIAGNOSIS

DIFFERENTIAL DIAGNOSIS

Nonulcerative dyspepsia is diagnosed when all other organic causes have been excluded, including:

- Peptic ulcer disease (PUD)
- Gastroesophageal reflux
- Gastric/esophageal/other abdominal cancers
- Biliary tract disease
- Gastroparesis, including diabetic gastroparesis
- Pancreatitis
- Medications (i.e., NSAIDs, erythromycin)
- Metabolic disturbances (i.e., hypercalcemia, heavy metals, or hyperkalemia)
- Ischemic bowel disease
- Systemic disorders (i.e., eosinophilic gastritis, Crohn disease, sarcoidosis, celiac disease, thyroid disorders)

DIAGNOSIS

The Rome IV criteria (Table 1) lists the following factors, which must be present at least 3 mo and first noticed within 6 mo of diagnosis:

- At least one of the following:
  1. Postprandial fullness, *or*
  2. Early satiety, *or*
  3. Epigastric pain, *or*
  4. Epigastric burning
  5. *And* no evidence of structural disease likely to explain the symptoms

WORKUP

The American Gastroenterological Association, as well as the Maastricht III and the IV European consensus, suggest the following:

- The pattern of symptoms overlaps considerably for all types of dyspepsia; therefore, the history and physical should focus on finding specific symptoms that help exclude other causes of dyspepsia.
- Endoscopy should be performed only in patients >55 yr old and in younger patients with alarming symptoms (e.g., weight loss, progressive dysphagia, recurrent vomiting, evidence of gastrointestinal bleeding, or

BOX 1 Causes of Dyspepsia

Luminal GI Tract
Functional dyspepsia
Chronic gastric volvulus
Chronic gastric or intestinal (mesenteric) ischemia
Food intolerance
Gastric or esophageal neoplasm
Gastric infections (cytomegalovirus, fungus, tuberculosis, syphilis)
Gastroparesis (diabetes mellitus, postvagotomy, scleroderma, chronic intestinal pseudo-obstruction, postviral, idiopathic)
GERD
Infiltrative gastric disorders (Ménétrier disease, Crohn disease, eosinophilic gastroenteritis, sarcoidosis, amyloidosis)
IBS
Parasites (*Giardia lamblia, Strongyloides stercoralis*)
PUD

Systemic Conditions
Adrenal insufficiency
Diabetes mellitus
Heart failure, myocardial ischemia
Intraabdominal malignancy
Pregnancy
Renal insufficiency
Thyroid disease, hyperparathyroidism

Medications
Acarbose
Aspirin and other NSAIDs (including COX-2 selective agents)
Colchicine
Digitalis preparations
Estrogens
Ethanol
Gemfibrozil
Glucocorticoids
Iron
Levodopa
Narcotics
Niacin
Nitrates
Orlistat
Potassium chloride
Quinidine
Sildenafil
Theophylline

Pancreaticobiliary Disorders
Biliary pain: Cholelithiasis, choledocholithiasis, sphincter of Oddi dysfunction
Chronic pancreatitis
Pancreatic neoplasms

COX-2, Cyclooxygenase-2; *GERD*, gastroesophageal reflux disease; *IBS*, irritable bowel syndrome; *NSAID*, nonsteroidal antiinflammatory drug; *PUD*, peptic ulcer disease.
From Feldman M et al (eds): *Sleisenger and Fordtran's gastrointestinal and liver disease,* ed 10, Philadelphia, 2016, Elsevier.

TABLE 1 Rome IV Diagnostic Criteria for Functional Dyspepsia*

1. One or more of the following bothersome symptoms:
   Postprandial fullness
   Early satiation
   Epigastric pain
   Epigastric burning *and*
2. No evidence of structural disease (including at upper endoscopy) that is likely to explain the symptoms

*The criteria must be fulfilled for the last 3 mo with onset of symptoms at least 6 mo before diagnosis.
From Goldman L, Shafer AI: *Goldman-Cecil medicine*, ed 26, 2020, Elsevier.

family history of cancer) presenting with new-onset dyspepsia. Findings consistent with diagnosis of nonulcerative dyspepsia are not conclusive, no presence of *H. pylori*, no signs of gastroesophageal reflux disease, no mucosal inflammation. NOTE: Patients <55 yr old and without any alarming symptoms can be treated without endoscopy.

LABORATORY TESTS

H. pylori: Laboratory methods include serologic tests,[1] monoclonal stool antigen, or urea breath test.

Rx TREATMENT

ACUTE GENERAL Rx

PHARMACOLOGIC THERAPY: Primary treatment is usually initiated with proton pump inhibitors (PPIs), which can be started without performing endoscopy, especially if the patient comes from a population with low prevalence of *H. pylori* infection. If symptoms persist, a trial of antidepressants can be started. An algorithm for the management of patients with dyspepsia is described in Fig. E1.

Treatment of accompanying symptoms includes:

Predominant Symptom	Possible Etiology	Medication Recommended
Nausea	Motility dysfunction	Prokinetic agent
Bloating	Motility dysfunction	Simethicone and/ or prokinetic agent
Pain	Mucosal disease or *H. pylori* infection	Antibiotic trial
Somatic complaints	Psychosocial	Psychotropic medication trial

Medication categories:
- Antacids (i.e., aluminum hydroxide, calcium carbonate)
- Gas-reducing agents, such as those containing simethicone
- H_2-receptor antagonists (i.e., cimetidine)
- PPIs (i.e., omeprazole)
- Prokinetic agents (i.e., metoclopramide, domperidone)
- Antidepressants (i.e., selective serotonin receptor inhibitors, tricyclics)
- *H. pylori* therapy/antibiotic therapy (various antibiotic regimens, usually 1 PPI) if *H. pylori* present

CHRONIC Rx

Controversy currently exists around the long-term use of PPIs. Due to the high association with psychological factors, patients with functional dyspepsia should undergo psychological intervention, even if there is good response to pharmacotherapeutic approaches.

COMPLEMENTARY & ALTERNATIVE THERAPIES

Peppermint and caraway oil may be helpful; however, no definitive trials have been performed.
- In a recent trial among patients with PDS, acupuncture resulted in increased response rate and elimination rate of postprandial fullness, upper abdominal bloating, and early satiation after 4 wk of treatment.[2]

REFERRAL

- Referral to gastroenterology if patient has alarming symptoms (such as GI bleeding, dysphagia, odynophagia, unexplained anemia, change in appetite, and weight loss) or when endoscopy is indicated—although controversy exists about the workup of younger patients
- Referral to cardiology if cardiac etiology suspected

PEARLS & CONSIDERATIONS

PREVENTION

Avoid excessive amounts of caffeine, alcohol, smoking, or long-term use of steroids and NSAIDs.

PATIENT & FAMILY EDUCATION

www.mayoclinic.org/diseases-conditions/functional-dyspepsia/symptoms-causes/syc-20375709

SUGGESTED READINGS

Available at ExpertConsult.com

RELATED CONTENT

Approach to the patient with dyspepsia (Algorithm, Section III)

AUTHORS: **Alvaro M. Rivera, MD,** and **Nadine Mbuyi, MD**

[1] Serologic testing for *H. pylori* has a low predictive value because colonization is lifelong; it can therefore determine prevalence better than incidence.

[2] Yang JW et al: Effect of acupuncture for postprandial distress syndrome: a randomized clinical trial, *Ann Intern Med* 172:777-785, 2020

BASIC INFORMATION

DEFINITION

The term "dysphagia" is derived from the Greek words *dys* (with difficulty) and *phagia* (to eat). It is characterized by abnormal transfer of food from mouth to the stomach, which may involve the oral, pharyngeal, or esophageal stages of swallowing.

ICD-10CM CODES	
D50.1	Sideropenic dysphagia
I69.091	Dysphagia following nontraumatic subarachnoid hemorrhage
I69.191	Dysphagia following nontraumatic intracerebral hemorrhage
I69.291	Dysphagia following other nontraumatic intracranial hemorrhage
I69.391	Dysphagia following cerebral infarction
I69.891	Dysphagia following other cerebrovascular disease
I69.991	Dysphagia following unspecified cerebrovascular disease
R13.10	Dysphagia, unspecified
R13.11	Dysphagia, oral phase
R13.12	Dysphagia, oropharyngeal phase
R13.13	Dysphagia, pharyngeal phase
R13.14	Dysphagia, pharyngoesophageal phase
R13.19	Other dysphagia

EPIDEMIOLOGY & DEMOGRAPHICS

- This is seen in 10% of individuals above the age of 50 yr. Its prevalence increases with advancing age.
- Nearly 12% of hospitalized patients have symptoms of dysphagia.
- Up to 30% to 60% of nursing home patients have some form of dysphagia.
- Special populations, including patients with head injury, stroke, or Parkinson disease, have 30% to 50% prevalence of oropharyngeal dysphagia.

ETIOLOGY

- Oropharyngeal:
  1. Neuromuscular causes:
     a. Stroke
     b. Parkinson disease
     c. Multiple sclerosis
     d. Myasthenia gravis
     e. Amyotrophic lateral sclerosis
     f. CNS tumors
     g. Muscular dystrophy
     h. Thyroid dysfunction
     i. Polymyositis and dermatomyositis
     j. Sarcoidosis
     k. Cerebral palsy
     l. Head trauma
     m. Metabolic encephalopathy
     n. Dementia
     o. Bell palsy
  2. Structural causes:
     a. Oropharyngeal tumors
     b. Zenker diverticulum
     c. Infection of pharynx or neck (mucositis from *Candida,* herpes, and CMV)
     d. Thyromegaly
     e. Prior surgery or radiotherapy
     f. Osteophytes and other spinal disorders
     g. Proximal esophageal webs
     h. Congenital anomalies (e.g., cleft palate)
     i. Poor dentition
- Esophageal:
  1. Neuromuscular disorders:
     a. Achalasia
     b. Diffuse esophageal spasm
     c. Nutcracker esophagus
     d. Hypertensive lower esophageal sphincter
     e. Ineffective esophageal motility
     f. Scleroderma
     g. Reflex-associated dysmotility
  2. Structural disorder:
     a. Peptic stricture
     b. Esophageal rings and webs
     c. Diverticuli
     d. Carcinoma and benign tumors
     e. Foreign bodies
     f. Vascular compression
     g. Mediastinal masses
     h. Spinal osteophytes
     i. Mucosal injury (from pills, infection, gastroesophageal reflux disease [GERD], etc.)

PATHOGENESIS

The inability to swallow is caused either by a problem in strength or coordination of the muscles required to move material from the mouth to stomach or by a fixed obstruction somewhere between the mouth and the stomach.

CLINICAL FEATURES

Oropharyngeal dysphagia (transfer dysphagia):

- The patient is unable to transfer the food bolus from the mouth to the upper esophagus. Problem arises within 2 sec of initiating the voluntary phase of swallowing.
- Typical symptoms include drooling, spillage of food, postnasal regurgitation, difficulty in initiation of swallowing, sialorrhea, sensation of food stuck in the neck, coughing or choking during swallowing, the need to swallow repeatedly to clear food or fluid from the pharynx, dysphonia, nasal speech, hoarseness of voice, and dysarthria.
- A thorough physical examination including that of the nervous system, oral cavity, and the head/neck is very important in patients with oropharyngeal dysphagia.

Esophageal dysphagia:

- Problem usually arises several seconds after swallowing.
- Patients often complain of food being stuck in lower substernal area.
- Dysphagia to solids suggests mechanical obstruction whereas dysphagia with liquids or combination of solids and liquids favors a motility disorder.
- Neuromuscular causes result in dysphagia to both solids and liquids. Particularly, patients with achalasia tend to drink a lot of fluids while eating or apply maneuvers such as straightening the back, raising their arms over their heads, or standing to increase intraesophageal pressure to facilitate the emptying of food into the stomach.
- Oftentimes, ingestion of very cold or very hot foods precipitates the dysphagia associated with neuromuscular disorder.
- Delayed regurgitation of food, heartburn, and chest pain are usually present.
- Weight loss is usually associated with malignancy or achalasia.
- Symptoms are intermittent in patients with esophageal dysphagia from benign causes of structural obstruction or diffuse esophageal spasm. However, it is progressive in patients with peptic stricture, esophageal carcinoma, scleroderma, and achalasia.
- In patients with structural obstruction, when the luminal diameter is more than 18 to 20 mm, they are rarely symptomatic, whereas those with a diameter of less than 13 mm are nearly always symptomatic.
- These patients with esophageal dysphagia usually do not have any characteristic physical findings.

Dx DIAGNOSIS

Laboratory Evaluation:

- CBC
- Thyroid studies
- Nutritional assessment by checking serum protein and albumin levels
- Other studies based on specific clinical conditions

Special studies:

- Oropharyngeal dysphagia
  1. Videofluoroscopy is the first test often ordered in evaluation of patients with oropharyngeal dysphagia.
  2. Double contrast modified barium swallow study (Fig. 1).
  3. Fiberoptic flexible nasopharyngeal laryngoscopy is mandatory in all cases when a structural lesion, particularly malignancy, is suspected.
  4. Pharyngeal and upper esophageal manometry (Fig. 2) is occasionally of value to predict which patients will have a favorable outcome from cricopharyngeal myotomy or dilation.
  5. Radiography of head and neck when indicated.
- Esophageal dysphagia
  1. Barium esophagography should precede upper endoscopies to identify patients at risk from potential perforation with an endoscopy and to help plan fluoroscopically guided dilation. It is often the first step in evaluating patients with dysphagia, especially if an obstructive lesion is suspected
  2. EGD
  3. Esophageal manometry is indicated if no abnormality is identified by barium study or EGD

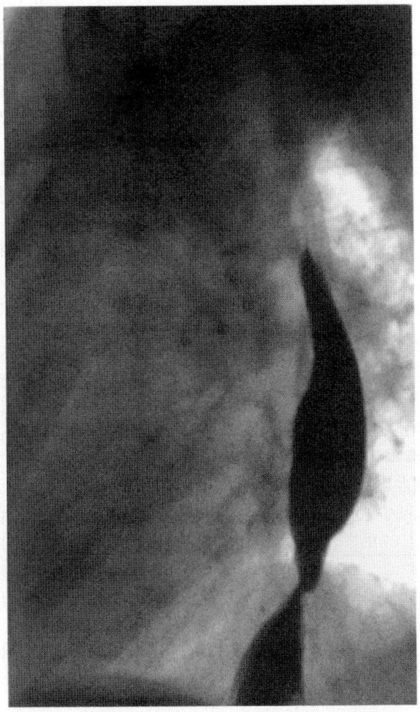

FIG. 1 Barium swallow demonstrating a benign peptic stricture in a patient with gastroesophageal reflux disease and dysphagia. (From Talley NJ, Martin C: *Clinical gastroenterology: a practical problem-based approach,* ed 2, Sydney, 2006, Churchill Livingstone.)

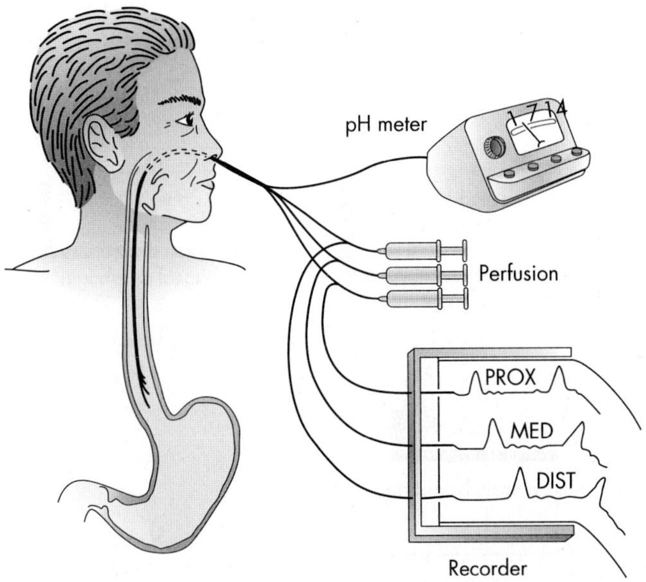

FIG. 2 Combined manometric-pH recording system used in the evaluation of esophageal function. The triple-lumen perfused recording catheter measures intraluminal pressures from three levels in the esophagus. Measurements are made in terms of centimeters from the nostrils to the proximal opening of the recording catheter *(PROX).* The medial catheter *(MED)* records pressures 5 cm distal to the proximal opening and the distal catheter *(DIST)* 5 cm below this. The intraesophageal pH electrode is used to document gastroesophageal reflux. (From Townsend CM et al: *Sabiston textbook of surgery,* ed 17, Philadelphia, 2004, Saunders.)

4. Esophageal pH monitoring in patients with suspected reflux disease
5. Endoscopic ultrasonography
6. Radiograph, CT, and MRI of chest

DIFFERENTIAL DIAGNOSIS (FIG. 3)

- Globus pharyngeus
- Odynophagia
- Phagophobia
- GERD

Rx TREATMENT

- Treatment should be approached with the help of specialists of multiple disciplines (ENT, head and neck surgeon, radiologist, speech pathologist, physical therapist, dietitian, gastroenterologist, physical medicine and rehabilitation specialist, dentist, neurologist, etc.).
- Goal of therapy is airway protection and maintenance of nutrition.
- Alteration of food consistency, volume, and delivery rate plays a major role.
- The goal of direct therapy is to change swallowing physiology with medical treatment of primary disease, maxillofacial prosthesis, and cricopharyngeal myotomy.
- Indirect therapies include exercise programs for tongue coordination and chewing under the guidance of a speech therapist.
- Maintenance of oral feeding often requires compensatory techniques such as chin-tuck position, rotation of head to the affected side, tilting of head to the strong side, and lying on one's back or on one's side during swallowing.
- Some of the voluntary maneuvers applied include supraglottic swallow, effortful swallow, Mendelson maneuver, Shaker exercise, and the Heimlich maneuver.
- Placement of nasogastric tube, jejunostomy tube, or percutaneous endoscopic gastrotomy (PEG) tube is considered for enteral feeding when other measures fail and the patient remains at significant risk for aspiration or nutrition becomes compromised.
- Treatment of associated GERD should not be forgotten.
- Surgery for chronic aspiration may involve tracheostomy, medialization, laryngeal suspension, laryngeal closure, and/or laryngotracheal separation-diversion.
- Other measures include esophageal dilation removal of foreign body, esophageal resection, chemotherapy, radiotherapy, endoscopic ablation of tumor, photodynamic therapy, esophageal prosthesis/stents, diverticulectomy, intrasphincteric injection of botulinum toxin, surgical myotomy, and others. Smooth muscle relaxants such as nitrates and calcium channel blockers have been used to effectively treat patients with diffuse esophageal spasm and nutcracker esophagus.
- Several scales have been suggested to determine patients' functional outcome. One of them is the "Swallowing Rating Scale."

COMPLICATIONS

- Dehydration
- Malnutrition
- Aspiration pneumonia
- Airway obstruction
- Death resulting from pulmonary complications

PROGNOSIS

- Depends on the etiology.
- Nursing home patients with oropharyngeal dysphagia and a history of aspiration have an approximately 45% mortality rate over 1 yr.
- All patients, especially the elderly, should take their medications with a full glass of water while in upright position well before bedtime.
- Dysphagia should be considered an alarm symptom, indicating the need for immediate evaluation.

PATIENT EDUCATION

Elderly patients with dysphagia should not attribute their symptoms to aging.

SUGGESTED READING

Available at ExpertConsult.com

RELATED CONTENT

Achalasia (Related Key Topic)
Dyspepsia, Nonulcerative (Related Key Topic)
Esophageal Tumors (Related Key Topic)
Gastroesophageal Reflux Disease (Related Key Topic)

AUTHOR: **Fred F. Ferri, MD**

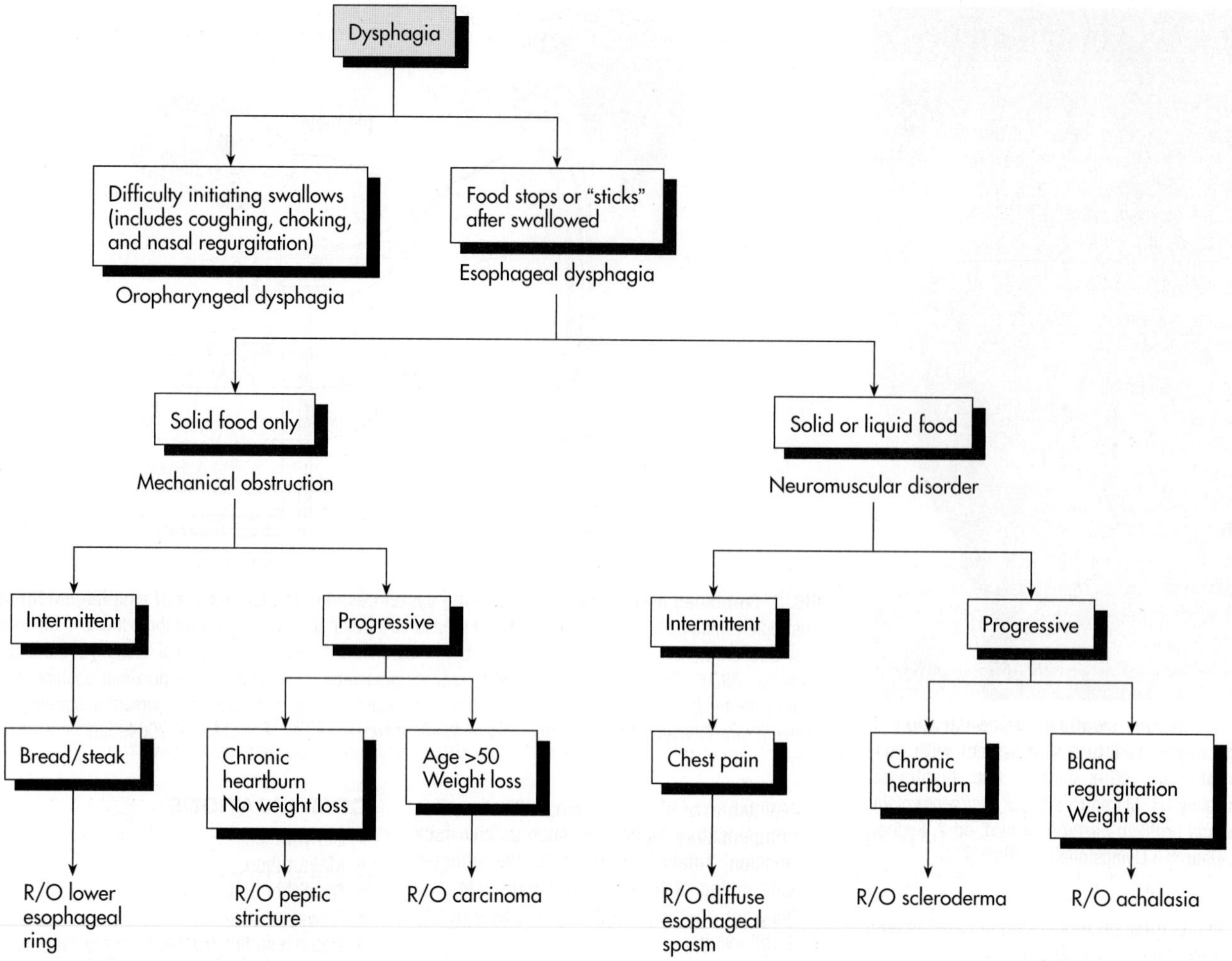

FIG. 3 Differential diagnosis of dysphagia. *R/O,* Rule out. (Modified from Andreoli TE [ed]: *Cecil essentials of medicine,* ed 7, Philadelphia, 2008, Saunders.)

BASIC INFORMATION

DEFINITION

Early pregnancy loss is an intrauterine pregnancy that is determined to be nonviable via an empty gestational sac or a sac containing an embryo or fetus without fetal heart activity before 13 wk of pregnancy.

SYNONYMS

Spontaneous abortion
Miscarriage

ICD-10CM CODE
O03.9 Complete or unspecified spontaneous abortion without complication

EPIDEMIOLOGY & DEMOGRAPHICS

INCIDENCE: Approximately 10% to 15% of all pregnancies. Approximately 80% of pregnancy losses overall are early and occur in the first trimester.

PREDOMINANT SEX & AGE: Affects females postmenarche and premenopause.

RISK FACTORS: The most common risk factors of early pregnancy loss are advanced maternal age (with a positive correlation between age and risk) and a prior early pregnancy loss. The incidence of clinically known early pregnancy loss for women ages 20 to 30 yr is 9% to 17%, with an increase in rate from 20% at age 35 yr to 40% at age 40 yr and 80% at age 45 yr.

GENETICS: Over two thirds of early pregnancy losses before 12 wk of estimated gestational age are associated with chromosomal abnormalities. The most frequent are autosomal trisomies.

PHYSICAL FINDINGS & CLINICAL PRESENTATION

Common symptoms include vaginal bleeding and uterine cramping; however, these symptoms are also common in normal gestation, ectopic pregnancy, and molar pregnancy.

DIAGNOSIS

DIFFERENTIAL DIAGNOSIS

- Viable intrauterine pregnancy
- Ectopic pregnancy
- Molar pregnancy
- Vaginal trauma

WORKUP

- Thorough history and physical examination.
  1. Timing, quantity, and quality of symptoms
  2. Abdominal and pelvic examinations
- Serum beta–human chorionic gonadotropin (β-hCG), with serial values to determine true resolution of the pregnancy.
- Ultrasonography is the preferred modality to verify the presence of a viable intrauterine gestation.
- Depending on the specific clinical circumstances and how much diagnostic certainty the patient desires, a single serum β-hCG test or ultrasound examination may not be sufficient to confirm the diagnosis of early pregnancy loss.

LABORATORY TESTS

- Serial serum β-hCG measurements in addition to serial ultrasound can be helpful in differentiating possible ectopic, molar, resolution of spontaneous abortion, or viable intrauterine gestation.

IMAGING STUDIES

Ultrasound is indicated in determining the status of an intrauterine pregnancy.

- Crown–rump length (CRL) of 5 mm without cardiac activity and an empty gestational sac measuring 16 mm in mean gestational sac diameter have been used as diagnostic criteria to confirm early pregnancy loss.
- A fetal heart rate of under 100 beats per minute at 5 to 7 wk of gestation and subchorionic hemorrhage are suggestive of an early pregnancy loss, but are not regarded as diagnostic alone.

TREATMENT

NONPHARMACOLOGIC THERAPY

- Expectant management with adequate follow-up
- Surgical evacuation with adequate follow-up

PHARMACOLOGIC THERAPY

- To be considered only in women without infection, hemorrhage, severe anemia, or a history of bleeding disorders
- Decreases time of expulsion and increases rate of complete expulsion without surgical intervention when compared with expectant management

ACUTE GENERAL Rx

- 800 μg of vaginal misoprostol is recommended, with a repeat dose as needed within 7 days if there is no response to the first dose.
- Women who are Rh(D) negative and unsensitized should receive Rh(D) immune globulin within 72 hr of the first misoprostol administration.
- The addition of 200-mg oral mifepristone 24 hr before misoprostol administration may significantly improve treatment efficacy.

COMPLEMENTARY & ALTERNATIVE MEDICINE

No evidence-based recommendations

DISPOSITION

- Complete passage of tissue may be noted via follow-up ultrasound in 7 to 14 days.
- If fetal tissue is not visible on ultrasonography or ultrasonography is unavailable, serial serum β-hCG measurements may be used instead.

REFERRAL

No further workup generally is recommended until after the second consecutive clinical early pregnancy loss; however, patients should follow up with their routine OB/GYN.

PEARLS & CONSIDERATIONS

COMMENTS

It is imperative to differentiate early pregnancy loss from other etiologies of symptoms before initiating treatment at the risk of disruption of a normal viable intrauterine pregnancy, pregnancy complications, or birth defects.

PREVENTION

No evidence-based interventions have been proven to prevent early pregnancy loss. Women who have experienced at least three prior pregnancy losses, however, may benefit from progesterone therapy in the first trimester.

PATIENT & FAMILY EDUCATION

Patient education material can be obtained from local women's health clinics and also from the American College of Obstetricians and Gynecologists. Patients should follow up with their primary OB/GYN after pregnancy loss.

RELATED TOPICS

Miscarriage (Patient Information)
Ectopic Pregnancy (Key Related Topic)
Molar Pregnancy (Key Related Topic)
Vaginal Bleeding During Pregnancy (Key Related Topic)

SUGGESTED READINGS
Available at ExpertConsult.com

AUTHORS: **Lauren Davis Rivera, MD MSEd, Helen B. Gomez, MD,** and **Anthony Sciscione, DO**

BASIC INFORMATION

DEFINITION

Eclampsia is the occurrence of new-onset tonic-clonic, focal, or multifocal seizures in the absence of other causative conditions in pregnant or postpartum women often, but not always, associated with other signs and symptoms of preeclampsia. Atypical eclampsia occurs at <20 wk of gestation or as much as 23 days postpartum.

SYNONYMS

Toxemia
Seizures of pregnancy

ICD-10CM CODES	
015.00	Eclampsia in pregnancy, unspecified trimester
015.02	Eclampsia in pregnancy, second trimester
015.03	Eclampsia in pregnancy, third trimester
015.1	Eclampsia in labor
015.2	Eclampsia in the puerperium
015.9	Eclampsia, unspecified as to time period

EPIDEMIOLOGY & DEMOGRAPHICS

INCIDENCE: Based on a World Health Organization multicountry survey, the global prevalence of eclampsia is reported to be 0.3%. And although preeclampsia is a known risk factor for eclampsia, studies have shown that only 1.9% and 3.2% of patients with preeclampsia and severe preeclampsia, respectively, went on to develop eclampsia.

RISK FACTORS: Multifetal gestation (3.6% in twin gestation), molar pregnancy, nonimmune hydrops fetalis, uncontrolled hypertension, preexisting hypertension, renal disease, systemic lupus, and existing heart disease.

GENETICS: Increased incidence with a first-degree relative (sister or mother) having had eclampsia.

PHYSICAL FINDINGS & CLINICAL PRESENTATION

- Seizure often begins as facial twitching, then spreads to generalized tonic-clonic state, with cessation of respiration followed by a postictal period of amnesia, agitation, and confusion.
- The most common symptoms preceding eclampsia are headache (80%), visual disturbance (45%), and epigastric pain (20%). Seventeen percent are completely asymptomatic prior to seizure.
- Forty percent have severe hypertension, 40% have mild to moderate hypertension, and 20% are normotensive.
- Generalized edema with rapid weight gain (>2 lb/wk) may precede eclampsia.

ETIOLOGY

Common pathway relates to abnormalities in autoregulation of cerebral blood flow. This may involve transient vasospasm, ischemia, cerebral hemorrhage, and edema occurring by a mechanism involving hypertensive encephalopathy, decreased colloid osmotic pressure, and prostaglandin imbalance.

Dx DIAGNOSIS

DIFFERENTIAL DIAGNOSIS

- Preexisting seizure disorder
- Metabolic abnormalities (hypoglycemia, hyponatremia, hypocalcemia)
- Substance abuse
- Head trauma, infection (meningitis, encephalitis)
- Intracerebral bleeding or thrombosis
- Amniotic fluid embolism
- Space-occupying brain lesions or neoplasms
- Pseudoseizure
- Postdural puncture syndrome
- Hypertensive encephalopathy
- Venous or arterial thrombosis, arterial embolism
- Posterior reversible encephalopathy syndrome (often seen in eclampsia)
- Vasculitis, angiopathy
- Thrombotic thrombocytopenic purpura

WORKUP

- Rule out other causes of seizures during pregnancy.
- Atypical presentations such as prolonged postictal state; status epilepticus; gestational age <20 wk or >48 hr postpartum; or signs of meningitis, substance abuse, or severe uncontrolled hypertension should prompt a search for other seizure etiologies.

LABORATORY TESTS

- Proteinuria: Severe (49%), mild to moderate (29%), absent (22%)
- HCT: Elevated as a result of hemoconcentration
- Platelet count: Decreased; LFTs elevated in HELLP syndrome (hemolysis, elevated liver enzymes, and low platelet count)
- BUN and creatinine: Elevated with renal involvement
- Serum electrolytes, glucose, calcium, toxicology profile: Rule out other causes of seizures
- ABG: Maternal acidemia and hypoxia

IMAGING STUDIES

- CT scan or MRI indicated in atypical presentation, suspected intracerebral bleeding, or focal neurologic deficit.
- Over 90% of patients will have findings consistent with posterior reversible encephalopathy syndrome on MRI.
- There are other abnormal findings, including cerebral edema, hemorrhage, and infarction, in 50% of patients.

Rx TREATMENT

ACUTE GENERAL Rx

- Elevate bed side rails, place patient in the lateral decubitus position (physical restraints may be necessary), suction oropharyngeal secretions and vomitus.
- Maintain airway, adequate oxygenation, and IV access.
- Fetal resuscitation involving maternal oxygenation, left lateral positioning, and continuous fetal heart rate monitoring is needed.
- Magnesium sulfate is the drug of choice. Give magnesium sulfate 6 g IV load over 20 min, then 2 g/hr maintenance, for treatment and recurrent seizure prophylaxis. Adjust maintenance dose for renal insufficiency. If there is no IV access, may give 10 g IM (5 g to each buttock). If repeated convulsions, may give an additional 2 g IV over 3 to 5 min. Approximately 10% to 15% of patients will have a second seizure after initial loading dose. Clinical signs of progressive Mg2+ toxicity, such as loss of reflexes, should also be followed. If magnesium toxicity is suspected, check magnesium level (therapeutic range 4-7 mEq/L). If serum level >9.6 mg/dl, stop infusion. Respiratory and cardiac arrest occur at extremely high magnesium levels. Antidote for toxicity is calcium gluconate 10 ml of 10% solution. Phenytoin has been used as an alternative in patients in whom magnesium sulfate is contraindicated (e.g., heart block, myasthenia gravis).
- Give sodium amobarbital 250 mg IV over 3 min for persistent seizures not responsive to magnesium sulfate.
- Treat BP >160 mm Hg systolic or BP >110 mm Hg diastolic with either hydralazine 5 to 10 mg IV, then 10 mg, then 10 mg every 20 minutes to a maximum of 20 mg; or labetalol hydrochloride 20, 40, 80 mg IV, escalating the dose every 10 minutes to maximum total dose of 300 mg; or nifedipine 10 to 20 mg orally every 20 minutes can be used for acute blood pressure control, if no IV access, to a total dose of 180 mg/day. If maximum dose of one medication is reached, add an additional medication to reach goal of BP 140 to 150/90 to 100 mm Hg.
- Evaluate patient for delivery.

CHRONIC Rx

- The first priority is stabilization of the mother in terms of adequate oxygenation, hemodynamics, and laboratory abnormalities, such as associated coagulopathies.
- Cervical status and gestational age should be assessed. If unfavorable cervix and <30 wk of gestation, consider C-section; otherwise consider induction.
- Give antenatal corticosteroids if 24 to 34 wk gestation. Consider antenatal corticosteroids if 34 to 36-6/7 wk gestation or 23-0/7 to 24 wk gestation.
- Controlled epidural is the anesthesia of choice for labor or C-section.
- Avoid general anesthesia in uncontrolled hypertension to minimize risk of catastrophic cerebral events.
- Continue magnesium sulfate through delivery process and for 24 hr postpartum or for at least 24 hr after the last convulsion.

DISPOSITION

- The maternal mortality rate for eclampsia averages 5% to 6%. Morbidity rate is 25%, including placental abruption (10%), disseminated intravascular coagulation, maternal apnea with fetal asphyxia, aspiration pneumonia, pulmonary edema (4%), renal failure, cardiopulmonary arrest, and coma.
- There is an increased risk of fetal death, neonatal death, preterm birth, and small-for-gestational-age birth.
- In patients with eclampsia, the risk of recurrence of eclampsia in a subsequent pregnancy is about 2% and the risk of preeclampsia is about 25%. The use of daily low-dose aspirin starting at 12 to 16 (28) wk may decrease that risk.

REFERRAL

Because of the potential for serious permanent maternal and fetal sequelae, all cases should be managed by a team approach of obstetrician, maternal and fetal medicine, neonatologist, and intensivist.

SUGGESTED READINGS

Available at ExpertConsult.com

RELATED CONTENT

Eclampsia (Patient Information)
HELLP Syndrome (Related Key Topic)
Preeclampsia (Related Key Topic)

AUTHORS: **Emily E. Nuss, MD,** and **Philip A. Shlossman, MD**

Ectopic Pregnancy (PTG) (ALG)

BASIC INFORMATION

DEFINITION

An ectopic pregnancy (EP) occurs when a fertilized ovum implants outside the endometrial cavity.

SYNONYMS

Tubal pregnancy (97%)
Interstitial (cornual) pregnancy (1% to 2%)
Ovarian pregnancy (1% to 3%)
Abdominal pregnancy (0.03% to 1%)
Cervical pregnancy (0.5%)
Cesarean scar pregnancy (1% to 3%, 6% of all EP in women with prior cesarean)
Heterotopic pregnancy (1/4000 to 1/30,000)

ICD-10CM CODES	
000.9	Ectopic pregnancy, unspecified
000.0	Abdominal pregnancy
000.1	Tubal ectopic pregnancy
000.2	Ovarian ectopic pregnancy
000.8	Other ectopic pregnancy

EPIDEMIOLOGY & DEMOGRAPHICS

- 1.5% to 2% of pregnancies
- 2.7% of maternal deaths

PREVALENCE (IN U.S.): Accounts for up to 18% of women presenting to the emergency room with vaginal bleeding or abdominal pain. Currently over 100,000 reported cases/year.

RISK FACTORS: Previous EP, previous pelvic infection (pelvic inflammatory disease, tubo-ovarian abscess, salpingitis), previous tubal ligation, previous tuboplasty, previous cesarean section, intrauterine device use, assisted reproductive techniques, infertility, cigarette use, age >35, multiple lifetime sexual partners, DES exposure in utero

PHYSICAL FINDINGS & CLINICAL PRESENTATION

- Abdominal tenderness: 95%
- Adnexal tenderness: 87% to 99%
- Amenorrhea or abnormal vaginal bleeding: 75%
- Peritoneal signs: 71% to 76%
- Adnexal mass: 33% to 53%
- Enlarged uterus: 6% to 30%
- Shoulder pain: 10%
- Tissue passage: 6% to 7%
- Shock: 2% to 17%

ETIOLOGY

- Anatomic obstruction to zygote passage
- Abnormalities in tubal motility
- Transperitoneal migration of the zygote

Dx DIAGNOSIS

DIFFERENTIAL DIAGNOSIS

- Corpus luteum cyst
- Rupture or torsion of ovarian cyst, especially hemorrhagic
- Threatened or incomplete abortion
- Pelvic inflammatory disease/tubo-ovarian abscess
- Appendicitis
- Gastroenteritis
- Dysfunctional uterine bleeding
- Degenerating uterine fibroids
- Endometriosis

WORKUP

- The classic presentation of EP includes the triad of abnormal vaginal bleeding, pelvic pain, and an adnexal mass.
    1. Fig. 1 describes a diagnostic approach to suspected EP.
    2. Fig. 2 *(top)* describes potential sites of ectopic implantations.
- Consider in all women with abdominopelvic pain and a positive pregnancy test.
- Transvaginal ultrasound (Fig. 2 [bottom]).
- Quantitative serum human chorionic gonadotropin level.
    1. Consider progesterone level if ultrasound and sonographic findings are inconclusive
- Type and screen if presents with vaginal bleeding
    1. give Rhogam if Rh-negative status on initial presentation of vaginal bleeding with positive pregnancy test.
- Laparoscopy (Fig. E3) in equivocal situations and possibly for treatment.

LABORATORY TESTS

- Quantitative human chorionic gonadotropin (qhCG): Check on initial presentation. qhCG allows one to interpret initial ultrasound. If qhCG >6000 mIU/ml, should see intrauterine pregnancy (IUP) on abdominal scan; qhCG >1500 mIU/ml for transvaginal scan. The ability to visualize an early pregnancy is dependent on the gestational age and expertise of the ultrasonographer; therefore, some may use up to qhCG >3500 mIU/ml as the discriminatory threshold for transvaginal ultrasonography.
    1. Approximately 25% to 50% of women with an EP present with a pregnancy of unknown location (PUL), meaning that the initial ultrasound does not show a pregnancy in the uterus or the fallopian tube. Therefore, serial measurement of qhCG, typically obtained every 2 days, can help distinguish between an IUP, resolving miscarriage, or EP. The expected rate of qhCG increase varies by the initial starting hCG. For an initial hCG level <1500 mIU/ml, the expected rate of increase is 49%, compared to 40% for an initial hCG level between 1500 and 3000 mIU/ml, and a 33% increase for an initial hCG >3000 mIU/ml.
- Serum progesterone level between 5 and 10 wk of gestation varies minimally. A single progesterone level <5 ng/ml has 99% specificity to predict nonviable pregnancy in women with inconclusive sonographic findings. However, this may not be able to distinguish between EP and failed IUP.
- Dropping hematocrit may be associated with tubal rupture or possible abnormal intrauterine pregnancy.

IMAGING STUDIES

- Ultrasound: Presence of an intrauterine yolk sac makes EP extremely unlikely. However, if the patient used assisted reproductive technologies, a heterotopic pregnancy (an EP with concurrent IUP) is a possibility. A repeat ultrasonographic examination within 7 days after presentation may identify the location of a pregnancy that was not identified on initial ultrasonographic examination.
- Findings on ultrasound in EP include:
    1. Empty uterus (i.e., no yolk sac or fetal pole; a pseudosac in uterus may appear similar to a gestational sac)
    2. Adnexal mass (typically separate from adjacent ovary, commonly seen with "ring of fire" appearance)
    3. Enlarged hysterotomy scar, may bulge beyond contour of the uterus
    4. Fluid in cul-de-sac
    5. Yolk sac and/or fetal pole in tube
    6. Fetal cardiac activity in adnexa

Rx TREATMENT

NONPHARMACOLOGIC THERAPY

Surgery performed via laparoscopy is preferred; however, laparotomy is appropriate if patient is very unstable or if visualization of the pelvis is poor at the time of laparoscopy.

- Salpingostomy, or resecting EP with conservation of tube, has the potential benefit of higher rates of subsequent IUP; however, recent randomized controlled trials suggest there is no difference in fecundity rate between salpingostomy and salpingectomy. The procedure requires postoperative serial monitoring of qhCG.
- Salpingectomy, or removal of affected fallopian tube, is considered the standard surgical procedure and is preferred in the following circumstances:
    1. Ruptured tube
    2. Future fertility not desired
    3. Recurrent EP in the same tube
    4. Uncontrolled hemorrhage
- Direct injection of chemotherapy into the EP by laparoscopy, transvaginal ultrasound, or hysteroscopy. Direct injection of methotrexate, and possibly KCl if there is active cardiac activity, may be performed when the pregnancy is in a location where there is high morbidity, such as the cervix, cesarean section scar, or cornua.
- Cervical and cesarean scar pregnancies may be managed with a combination of methotrexate administration, laparoscopic and/or hysteroscopic techniques, uterine artery embolization, laparotomy, and possible hysterectomy.

ACUTE GENERAL Rx

- Medical management with methotrexate, a folic acid antagonist, is a safe alternative if the patient is stable. Check labs prior to administration (CBC, creatinine, LFTs).

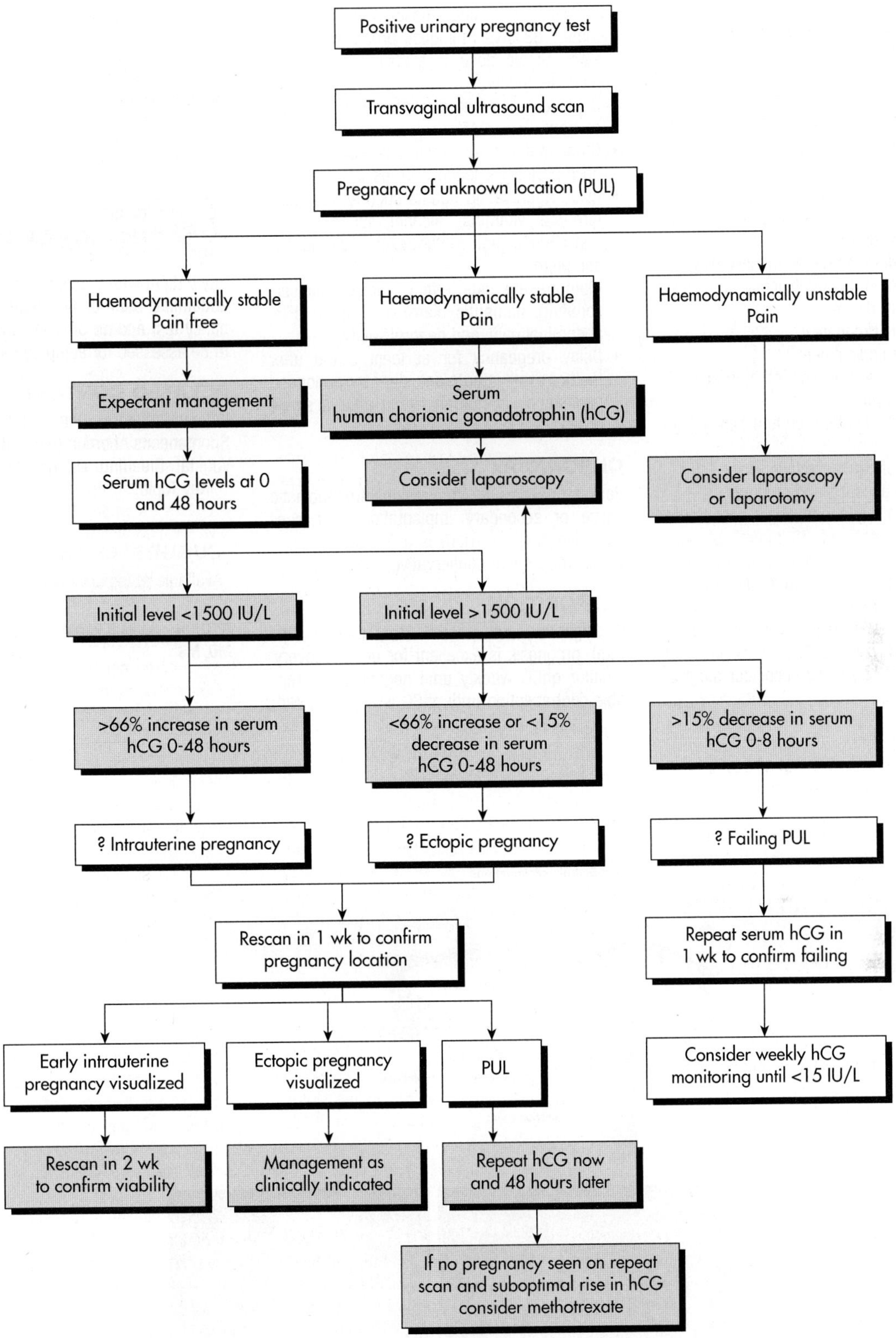

FIG. 1 Algorithm for managing suspected ectopic pregnancy. (From Magowan BA: *Clinical obstetrics & gynecology,* ed 4, 2019, Elsevier.)

- Contraindications:
  1. Allergy or sensitivity to methotrexate
  2. Hemodynamically unstable; ruptured EP
  3. Patient unable to comply with follow-up
  4. Medical contraindication to methotrexate including the following: Clinically relevant hepatic or renal disease, preexisting blood dyscrasias (thrombocytopenia, leukopenia, or significant anemia), as it is directly toxic to hepatocytes and renally excreted.
  5. Breastfeeding, active pulmonary disease, evidence of immunodeficiency, and active peptic ulcer disease
  6. Intrauterine pregnancy
- Relative contraindications:
  1. EP >4 cm mass as imaged by transvaginal ultrasound
  2. qhCG >5000 mIU/ml (up to a 14% failure rate)
  3. Presence of cardiac activity in the fetus
  4. Refusal to accept blood products
- Most common regimen is single-dose methotrexate at a dose of 50 mg/m^2 of body surface area and is administered intramuscularly on day 1. May require second dose or surgical intervention if qhCG increases or plateaus (<15% drop) when comparing values from day 4 and 7. If qhCG does not decrease after two doses, consider surgical management.
- Success rate of single-dose protocol approximately 88% vs multidose protocol which is 92%. Single dose is associated with less adverse effects.
- Rupture during methotrexate treatment ranges from 7% to 14%.
- Other methotrexate regimens include multidose protocol ± leucovorin rescue.
- Avoid aggravating agents such as folic acid (prenatal vitamins), alcohol, sun exposure, and NSAIDs until methotrexate treatment is complete.
- Methotrexate side effects include nausea, vomiting, stomatitis, diarrhea, elevated LFTs, abdominal pain, and nephrotoxicity.
- Delay pregnancy for at least 3 mo after methotrexate treatment due to prolonged persistence in human tissue after a single dose.

CHRONIC Rx

Persistent EP results from residual trophoblastic tissue or secondary implantation after conservative surgery. There is a 5% incidence of persistent EP with conservative treatment.

DISPOSITION

If diagnosed and treated early (before rupture), prognosis is excellent for good recovery. Monitor qhCG weekly until negative. Use reliable contraception until qhCG is negative. With subsequent pregnancies, follow qhCG and perform early ultrasound to confirm IUP. There is a 10% recurrence rate for EP.

REFERRAL

Should obtain gynecologic consultation if EP is suspected.

PEARLS & CONSIDERATIONS

Any patient who presents with vaginal bleeding, abdominal pain, or both with a positive pregnancy test and no prior documented IUP needs to be assessed for ectopic pregnancy.

RELATED CONTENT

Ectopic Pregnancy (Patient Information)
Spontaneous Abortion (Related Key Topic)
Vaginal Bleeding During Pregnancy (Related Key Topic)

SUGGESTED READINGS

Available at ExpertConsult.com

AUTHORS: **Shivani Parikh, MD,** and **Nima R. Patel, MD, MS**

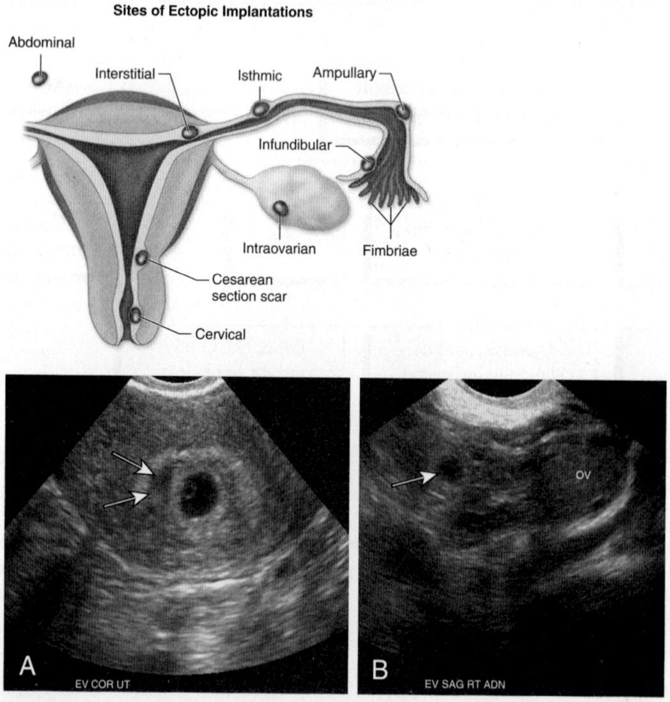

FIG. 2 ***Top*, Schematic drawing depicting implantation sites of ectopic pregnancies. A** and **B,** Heterotopic pregnancy. This pregnant patient presented with vaginal bleeding at 5 to 6 wk of gestational age. **A,** Transverse transvaginal ultrasound (TVUS) image of the uterus reveals an intrauterine gestational sac containing a yolk sac. Note small subchorionic hemorrhage *(arrows)*, most likely accounting for the vaginal bleeding. **B,** Sagittal TVUS image of the right adnexa reveals an echogenic tubal ring *(arrow)* clearly separate from the right ovary *(OV)*, which was surgically confirmed to be an ectopic pregnancy. (From Fielding JR et al: *Gynecologic imaging*, Philadelphia, 2011, Saunders.)

BASIC INFORMATION

DEFINITION

Human monocytic ehrlichiosis (HME) and human granulocytic anaplasmosis (HGA) are tick-borne rickettsial diseases. Ehrlichiosis is the generic name for infections caused by both *Ehrlichia* and *Anaplasma* genera. Table 1 describes the agent, vector, and geographic prevalence of these diseases.

SYNONYMS

Human granulocytic ehrlichiosis (HGE)
Ehrlichiosis
Human monocytic ehrlichiosis (HME)
Human monocytotropic ehrlichiosis
Human granulocytic anaplasmosis (HGA)
Human granulocytotropic ehrlichiosis
Anaplasmosis
Human granulocytropic anaplasmosis
HGE
HGA
HME

ICD-10CM CODES

A77.40	Ehrlichiosis, unspecified
A77.41	Ehrlichiosis chaffeensis [*E. chaffeensis*]
A77.49	Other ehrlichiosis

EPIDEMIOLOGY & DEMOGRAPHICS

INCIDENCE (IN U.S.): Highest overall incidence in Rhode Island (36.5 per 1 million), New York, New Jersey, Connecticut, Wisconsin, Minnesota, and northern California; >3000 cases identified in the United States since 2006.
PREDOMINANT SEX: Males outnumber females by 2 to 1.
PREDOMINANT AGE: Most severe disease 50 to 70 yr
PEAK INCIDENCE: Occurs throughout the yr, with peak incidence between May and July and again in September

PHYSICAL FINDINGS & CLINICAL PRESENTATION

- Symptoms of ehrlichiosis typically appear after a median of 9 days (range 5-14 days) after a tick bite
- Most common initial symptoms
  1. Fever (96%)
  2. Chills, rigor
  3. Headache (72%)
  4. Myalgia
- Subsequent symptoms
  1. Anorexia, nausea
  2. Arthralgia
  3. Cough
  4. Confusion (meningoencephalitis in 20% of patients with HME)
  5. Abdominal pain
  6. Rash (erythematous to pustular) <30% in HME, uncommon in HGA
- Complications
  1. Hepatitis
  2. Interstitial pneumonitis; acute respiratory distress syndrome
  3. Renal and respiratory failure
  4. Demyelinating polyneuropathy
  5. Toxic shock–like syndrome
  6. Life-threatening opportunistic infections, usually HGA

ETIOLOGY

- The causative agents are *Ehrlichia chaffeensis* for human monocytic ehrlichiosis (HME), *Anaplasma phagocytophilum* for human granulocytic anaplasmosis (HGA), and *Ehrlichia ewingii* for human granulocytic ehrlichiosis (HGE).
- Vector:
  1. Almost certainly tick-borne, recently confirmed to be rarely transmitted by infected blood (including nosocomial infection). Perinatal and transplant transmission have been documented.
  2. Transmitted by *Ixodes scapularis* in the northeastern states and *Amblyomma americanum* in the south central, southeastern, and mid-Atlantic states. Fig. 1 illustrates the life cycles of human monocytic ehrlichiosis (HME, with *Ehrlichia chaffeensis*) and human granulocytic ehrlichiosis (anaplasmosis).
  3. Tick exposure reported in >90% of patients, with ~60% reporting tick bite.
- Mammalian host: Deer, horses, dogs, white-footed mice, cattle, sheep, goats, bison.
- Host inflammatory and immune responses define final spectrum of disease beyond granulocytes, including hepatitis, interstitial pneumonitis, and nephritis with mild azotemia.
- Between 6% and 21% of patients with HGA also have serologic evidence of other *Ixodes* spp. tick-borne diseases: Lyme disease or babesiosis.
- Recovery is usual outcome; fatality rate of HGE is about 1%.
- ICU care required: 7%.

DIAGNOSIS

DIFFERENTIAL DIAGNOSIS

- Rocky Mountain spotted fever
- Colorado tick fever
- Q fever
- Relapsing fever
- Babesiosis
- Leptospirosis
- Lyme disease
- Tularemia
- Typhoid fever, paratyphoid fever
- Brucellosis
- Viral hepatitis
- Meningococcemia
- Infectious mononucleosis
- COVID-19
- Hematologic malignancy
- TTP (thrombotic thrombocytopenic purpura)
- Table 2 describes clinical clues suggesting a diagnosis of a tick-borne illness manifesting as a nonspecific febrile illness

WORKUP

- Acute blood samples for Giemsa-stained smears
- CBC (leukopenia, thrombocytopenia), liver function (elevated), blood urea nitrogen (BUN)/creatinine
- Acute serum samples for serology: Antibodies are seldom detected at time of acute infection (they usually appear 2 to 4 wk following clinical illness)
- Chest radiograph examination
- Bone marrow rarely needed

LABORATORY TESTS

- Polymerase chain reaction (PCR) to facilitate early diagnosis: Detection of *Ehrlichia/Anaplasma* DNA in blood or cerebrospinal fluid (CSF) by PCR (Table E3)
- Giemsa-stained smear demonstrating morulae of the organism within granulocytes or monocytes (sensitivity 20%-75%) (Fig. E2)
- CBC: Progressive leukopenia and thrombocytopenia with nadir near day 7
- C-reactive protein concentration is generally elevated
- Liver function tests (LFTs): Increase in hepatic transaminases, lactate dehydrogenase, and alkaline phosphatase
- Elevated plasma creatinine concentration may be seen
- Serologic titer (IFA) >80 or fourfold increase in titer to antigen

IMAGING STUDIES

- Chest radiograph examination may show interstitial pneumonitis (unusual)
- MRI of the brain in cases of encephalitis

TREATMENT

ACUTE GENERAL Rx

- Immediate therapy in order to limit extent of acute illness and complication
- Doxycycline: 100 mg twice a day for 7 to 14 days is therapy of choice for adults and children >8 yr (4 mg/kg/day in 2 divided doses)
- Doxycycline is now recommended as well for children aged <8 yr (Redbook 2018)
- Rifampin: 300 mg twice a day for 7 to 10 days; can be used in pregnancy and for children <8 yr at 10 mg/kg twice per day
- Most patients defervesce within 24 to 48 hr given appropriate treatment

PROGNOSIS

Poor prognostic indicators include:
- Advanced age or immunosuppression
- Concomitant chronic illness (such as diabetes mellitus, collagen-vascular disease)
- Diagnostic delay
- Delayed onset of specific antibiotic therapy
- Concomitant HIV or organ transplant status

DISPOSITION

Repeat CBC every 2 to 4 wk until normal.

REFERRAL

For consultation with infectious diseases specialist in suspected cases

PEARLS & CONSIDERATIONS

- A new pathogenic *Ehrlichia* species, closely related to *E. muris,* has been identified in Minnesota and Wisconsin. Organism-specific PCR and serologic testing can be used for identification.
- Duration of time tick must be attached to produce illness as few as 4 hr.
- Delay in antibiotic treatment results in poorer outcome. Antibiotic treatment should be initiated as soon as infection is suspected.

SUGGESTED READINGS

Available at ExpertConsult.com

RELATED CONTENT

Anaplasmosis (Patient Information)

AUTHOR: **Patricia Cristofaro, MD**

TABLE 1 Human Ehrlichioses and Anaplasmosis

	Human Monocytotropic Ehrlichiosis	Human Granulocytotropic Ehrlichiosis	Human Granulocytotropic Anaplasmosis
Former disease nomenclature	Human monocytic ehrlichiosis	Human granulocytic ehrlichiosis	Human granulocytic ehrlichiosis
Causative agent(s)	*Ehrlichia chaffeensis*	*Ehrlichia ewingii, Ehrlichia cani*—one asymptomatic human case reported in Venezuela	*Anaplasma phagocytophilum*
Leukocyte targets	Monocytic cell phagosomes	Neutrophil phagosomes	Granulocyte-neutrophil phagosomes
Tick vectors	*Amblyomma americanum* (lone star ticks)	*Amblyomma americanum* (lone star ticks), *Dermacentor variabilis* (American dog ticks)	*Ixodes persulcatus* complex (American deer ticks)—*I. scapularis, I. ricinus, I. pacificus*
Animal reservoirs	White-tailed deer, coyotes, dogs	White-tailed deer, dogs	Rodents, deer, ruminants, horses
U.S. regional distribution	Southeastern and south central United States	South central United States	Northeastern United States, upper Midwest, northern California
U.S. regional prevalence	2-5 cases/100,000	≤10% of presumed HME cases have *E. ewingii* infections in south central United States	50-60 cases/100,000; high seroprevalence rates in children (>20%) who have had subclinical infections
Seasonal occurrences	April-September, peaking in July	Spring-fall	May-July
Incubation periods (wk)	1-4	1-4	1-4
Modes of transmission	Tick bite, blood product transfusion	Tick bite, blood product transfusion	Tick bite, blood product transfusion, nosocomial
Frequently presenting clinical manifestations	Fever, malaise, headache, myalgias, rash in <40%	Same initial manifestations, but much milder, except in immunocompromised individuals	Fever, malaise, headache, myalgias; rarely rash
Laboratory abnormalities	Leukopenia, thrombocytopenia, transaminitis	Leukopenia, thrombocytopenia, transaminitis	More pronounced and prolonged leukopenia, thrombocytopenia, transaminitis
Potential complications, especially in immunocompromised individuals	Meningoencephalitis, acute renal and respiratory failure, hepatitis, myocarditis	Milder and less likely, except in patients immunocompromised by HIV/AIDS, organ transplantation, prolonged corticosteroid therapy	May be significant in immunocompromised patients with high fevers, seizures, confusion, hemorrhagic diathesis, rhabdomyolysis, shock, acute tubular necrosis, adult respiratory distress syndrome; some specific CNS complications may include eighth nerve palsy, brachial plexopathy, demyelinating polyneuropathy
Case-fatality rate (CFR)	3%, higher in immunocompromised individuals	No deaths reported	0.5%, higher CFR in immunocompromised individuals
Recommended confirmatory diagnostic tests	Wright-stained peripheral blood smears with characteristic intracytoplasmic morulae in monocytes, DNA detection by PCR assay, culture	Wright-stained peripheral blood smears with characteristic intracytoplasmic morulae in neutrophils, DNA detection by PCR	Wright-stained peripheral blood smears with characteristic intracytoplasmic aggregates in neutrophils, DNA detection by PCR assay, increased immunofluorescent antibodies in initial and paired serum samples
Current antibiotic resistance	Fluoroquinolones	Fluoroquinolones	Fluoroquinolones
Currently recommended antibiotic therapy, adults	Doxycycline, 100 mg PO bid, or tetracycline, 250-500 mg PO qid, for minimum of 3 days after defervescence to maximum of 14-21 days	Doxycycline, 100 mg PO bid, or tetracycline, 250-500 mg PO qid, for minimum of 3 days after defervescence to maximum of 14-21 days	Doxycycline, 100 mg PO bid, or tetracycline, 250-500 mg PO qid for minimum of 3 days after defervescence to maximum of 14-21 days
Currently recommended antibiotic therapy, children	Doxycycline, 4.4 mg/kg PO bid, or tetracycline, 25-50 mg/kg PO qid, for minimum of 3 days after defervescence to maximum of 14-21 days	Doxycycline, 4.4 mg/kg PO bid, or tetracycline, 25-50 mg/kg PO qid, for minimum of 3 days after defervescence to maximum of 14-21 days	Doxycycline, 4.4 mg/kg PO bid, or tetracycline, 25-50 mg/kg PO qid, for minimum of 3 days after defervescence to maximum of 14-21 days

bid, Twice daily; *CNS,* central nervous system; *DNA,* deoxyribonucleic acid; *HME,* human monocytotropic ehrlichiosis; *HIV/AIDS,* human immunodeficiency virus infection/acquired immunodeficiency syndrome; *PCR,* polymerase chain reaction; *PO,* by mouth; *qid,* four times a day.
From Bennett JE et al: *Mandell, Douglas, and Bennett's principles and practice of infectious diseases,* ed 8, Philadelphia, 2015, Saunders.

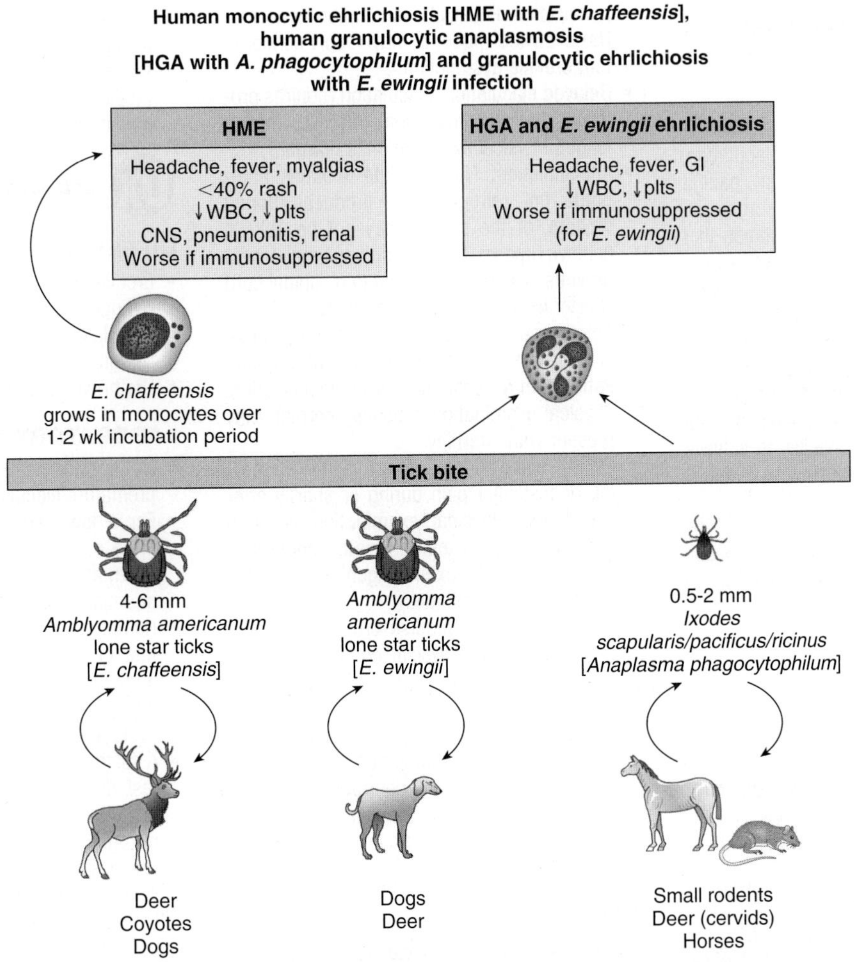

FIG. 1 Life cycles of human monocytic ehrlichiosis *(HME,* with *Ehrlichia chaffeensis)* and human granulocytic ehrlichiosis (anaplasmosis, *HGA* with *Anaplasma phagocytophilum*) or infection with *E. ewingii*. *CNS*, Central nervous system; *GI*, gastrointestinal; *WBC*, white blood cell count. (From Dumler JS: Ehrlichiosis and anaplasmosis. In Guerrant RL et al [eds]: *Tropical infectious diseases: principles, pathogens and practice*, ed 3, Philadelphia, 2011, Elsevier, pp. 339-343.)

TABLE 2 Clinical Clues (History, Physical Examination, or Laboratory) Suggesting the Diagnosis of a Tick-Borne Illness Manifesting as a Nonspecific Febrile Illness*

Disease	Clues
Anaplasmosis	Faint rash possible Low white blood cell or platelet count Elevated hepatic transaminases
Babesiosis	Findings of hemolysis History of splenectomy Presence of faint rash, hepatomegaly, or splenomegaly
Lyme disease	Careful skin examination for any rash consistent with erythema migrans Bradycardia from heart block Associated seventh nerve palsy or lymphocytic meningitis
Colorado tick fever	Saddle-back fever curve
Rocky Mountain spotted fever	Maculopapular or petechial rash Normal white blood cell count or low platelet count Hyponatremia Peripheral edema
Relapsing fever	Recurring episodes of fever with afebrile intervals
Tularemia	Acrally located ulcer Regional lymphadenopathy Possible associated pneumonia

*Apart from an epidemiologic context suggesting a tick-borne disease.

BASIC INFORMATION

DEFINITION

Disorders of ejaculation and orgasm include premature ejaculation, delayed ejaculation, anejaculation, retrograde ejaculation, painful ejaculation, hematospermia, and anorgasmia. Premature ejaculation refers to ejaculation that occurs sooner than desired, while delayed ejaculation refers to ejaculation that occurs after prolonged sexual stimulation. Anejaculation is the absence of semen propulsion from the urethra, with or without orgasm. Retrograde ejaculation is the backward flow of semen into the bladder. Hematospermia is the appearance of blood in the ejaculate. Anorgasmia is the inability to achieve orgasm despite sexual stimulation.

SYNONYMS

Ejaculatory dysfunction
Anejaculation
Anorgasmia
Aspermia
Dry orgasm
Dry ejaculate
Failure of emission

ICD-10CM CODES	
R36.1	Hematospermia; Bloody ejaculation
F52.4	Premature ejaculation
F52.32	Male orgasmic disorder; Inhibited male orgasm; Anorgasmia
N53.11	Delayed ejaculation; Retarded ejaculation
N53.12	Painful ejaculation
N53.13	Anejaculatory orgasm; Anejaculation
N53.14	Retrograde ejaculation
N53.19	Other ejaculatory dysfunction

EPIDEMIOLOGY & DEMOGRAPHICS

INCIDENCE: Not well understood, due to variability in definitions and reporting.
PREVALENCE: Premature ejaculation ranks among the most prevalent male sexual complaints, affecting up to 30% of men in self-reported studies. Delayed ejaculation is least commonly reported and studied, with a prevalence rate of 1% to 5% according to some studies.
PREDOMINANT SEX & AGE: These disorders have been reported among men aged 18 to 70 yr.
PEAK INCIDENCE: Not well understood. Ejaculatory and orgasmic disorders may be primary (lifelong) if the condition has always been present, or secondary (acquired) if the condition developed after a period of normal function.
RISK FACTORS: Men with ejaculatory dysfunction of any type usually indicate higher levels of relationship stress, sexual dissatisfaction, anxiety about sexual performance, and general health issues, compared to sexually functional men.
GENETICS: No known genetic predisposition.

PHYSICAL FINDINGS & CLINICAL PRESENTATION

- Premature ejaculation: Ejaculation occurs sooner than desired, often within 2 min of penetration. Physical examination is normal. Up to 30% of patients may report concomitant erectile dysfunction.
- Delayed ejaculation: Ejaculation requires prolonged sexual stimulation, often 25 min or longer. Physical examination is normal.
- Anejaculation: No ejaculate (neither antegrade nor retrograde) is produced during orgasm, or the patient may not be able to achieve orgasm. Physical findings may reveal nervous system dysfunction (e.g., spinal cord injury); may present with infertility.
- Retrograde ejaculation: Little or no ejaculate is expelled out of the urethra at orgasm. Patients may report cloudy postcoital urine. Physical examination is usually normal; may present with infertility.
- Painful ejaculation: Urethral, perineal, scrotal, or testicular pain during or shortly after ejaculation. Physical examination is often normal but may demonstrate tenderness with palpation of external genitalia, or with digital rectal examination.
- Hematospermia: Reddish-brown ejaculate, usually painless. Physical findings are usually unremarkable; not associated with malignancy.
- Anorgasmia: The inability to achieve orgasm, despite adequate stimulation. Patients will not experience perineal contractions nor the pleasurable sensation associated with normal orgasm. Physical findings are usually unremarkable.

ETIOLOGY

- Premature and delayed ejaculation represent opposite ends of the spectrum of ejaculatory disorders. The underlying etiology is complex and multifactorial, and includes organic and psychogenic contributions. Box E1 summarizes the recommended and optional questions to establish the diagnosis of delayed ejaculation and to direct treatment.
- Anejaculation may result from pelvic surgery, trauma, or radiation; from neurologic sequalae of Parkinson disease, multiple sclerosis, spinal cord injury, or diabetes mellitus; from bilateral ejaculatory duct obstruction; or from psychological stress and anxiety.
- Retrograde ejaculation is most commonly caused by the use of medications (e.g., alpha-blockers) or surgical procedures (e.g., transurethral resection of prostate) that relax or disrupt the bladder neck. It can also result from retroperitoneal surgery, diabetes mellitus, and the previously mentioned neurologic diseases. Box 2 summarizes the causes of retrograde ejaculation, delayed ejaculation, anejaculation, and anorgasmia.
- Causes of painful ejaculation may be infectious (e.g., epididymo-orchitis, urethritis, prostatitis), obstructive (e.g., vasectomy, prostatectomy, hernia repair), nervous/musculoskeletal, or psychological.
- Hematospermia is usually idiopathic and self-resolving, but may be secondary to prolonged abstinence, or due to infection or inflammation of the genitourinary tract; it is not commonly linked to malignancy.
- Anorgasmia may be caused by spinal cord injury, hormonal dysfunction, psychological factors, dysfunctional sexual techniques, or medications, particularly serotonin reuptake inhibitors.

DIAGNOSIS

DIFFERENTIAL DIAGNOSIS

- Erectile dysfunction
- Hypogonadism
- Ejaculatory duct obstruction
- Urethral stricture disease
- Urethritis or sexually transmitted infection

LABORATORY TESTS

- No specific testing is needed for lifelong premature ejaculation.
- For a low-volume ejaculate, post-ejaculate urine may be evaluated for the presence of spermatozoa to differentiate between failure of emission and retrograde ejaculation.
- Hematuria, in the setting of hematospermia or painful ejaculation, may signal an underlying inflammatory disorder or a malignancy and should prompt a complete urologic evaluation.
- A fasting blood glucose or hemoglobin A1c test may be considered if diabetes is suspected as a cause of lack of emission or retrograde ejaculation.
- Urinalysis, urine culture, and screening for sexually transmitted diseases, when indicated, can rule out an infectious etiology of painful ejaculation.

IMAGING STUDIES

Transrectal ultrasonography or pelvic MRI may detect an ejaculatory duct obstruction or absence of the seminal vesicles. While not routinely used in the evaluation of ejaculatory and orgasmic disorders, they may be useful for the evaluation of persistently painful ejaculation.

TREATMENT

NONPHARMACOLOGIC THERAPY

- Premature ejaculation can improve with psychotherapy and behavioral interventions (e.g., "coronal squeeze" or "start-and-stop" technique) and effective partner communication. These approaches may be more effective when combined with pharmacologic therapy.
- Delayed ejaculation may likewise be improved with counseling and sexual therapy to address psychological issues and explore sexual positions or techniques that may enhance arousal.
- Retrograde ejaculation and anejaculation do not require treatment unless fertility is desired.
  1. In the setting of retrograde ejaculation, viable sperm can be recovered from the post-ejaculate urine and used for intrauterine insemination or in vitro fertilization.

BOX 2 Causes of Retrograde Ejaculation, Delayed Ejaculation, Anejaculation, and Anorgasmia

Aging Male
Degeneration of penile afferent nerves

Psychogenic
Inhibited ejaculation

Congenital
Müllerian duct cyst
Wolffian duct abnormality
Prune belly syndrome

Anatomic Causes
Transurethral resection of prostate
Bladder neck incision

Neurogenic Causes
Diabetic autonomic neuropathy
Multiple sclerosis
Spinal cord injury
Radical prostatectomy
Retroperitoneal lymph node dissection
Proctocolectomy
Bilateral sympathectomy
Abdominal aortic aneurysmectomy
Para-aortic lymphadenectomy

Infectious
Urethritis
Genitourinary tuberculosis
Schistosomiasis

Endocrine
Hypogonadism
Hypothyroidism

Medication
α-Methyldopa
Alpha blockers
Thiazide diuretics
Tricyclic and SSRI antidepressants
Phenothiazine
Alcohol abuse

SSRI, Selective serotonin reuptake inhibitor.
From Wein AJ et al: *Campbell-Walsh urology*, ed 11, Philadelphia, 2016, Elsevier.

2. Vibratory or electrical stimulation of emission is helpful in selected cases of anejaculation.

- Idiopathic hematospermia may be followed expectantly and is usually self-limited to 10 or 15 ejaculations.
- Painful ejaculation that is myofascial rather than infectious in origin may benefit from pelvic floor physical therapy.

ACUTE GENERAL Rx

- Premature ejaculation: Selective serotonin reuptake inhibitors (SSRI) (e.g., sertraline, fluoxetine) and the tricyclic antidepressant clomipramine can successfully delay ejaculation when taken daily. Dapoxetine, a short-acting SSRI, may be used as an "on-demand" treatment for premature ejaculation (not available in the U.S.). Topical anesthetics such as lidocaine cream and topical sprays have been used with variable success. Patients who have failed SSRIs or topical anesthetics may consider on-demand tramadol or daily α1-adrenoceptor antagonists. The use of phosphodiesterase inhibitors (PDE5i) (e.g., sildenafil, vardenafil, tadalafil) with SSRIs may be beneficial in men with concomitant erectile dysfunction and premature ejaculation. Fig. E1 illustrates an algorithm for the office management of premature ejaculation; Table E1 summarizes drug therapy for premature ejaculation.
- Delayed ejaculation or anorgasmia caused by serotonin reuptake inhibitors usually improves with withdrawal of the medication. Fig. E2 illustrates an algorithm for the management of delayed ejaculation, anejaculation, and anorgasmia. Drug therapy for delayed ejaculation and anejaculation is summarized in Table E2.
- Retrograde ejaculation: Pharmacologic therapy is only effective in patients without an anatomic disturbance of the bladder neck. Sympathomimetic medications (phenylpropanolamine, ephedrine, pseudoephedrine) and imipramine may be useful in converting retrograde ejaculation to antegrade ejaculation.
- Antimicrobial treatment for infections, NSAIDs, and muscle relaxants may help decrease discomfort associated with painful ejaculation.
- The use of the pharmacologic therapies listed above for the treatment of various disorders of ejaculation is strictly off label in the U.S. and does not carry FDA approval.

CHRONIC Rx

Rarely, painful ejaculation due to long-standing obstructive causes may show improvement with surgical intervention (e.g., vasectomy reversal). The pharmacologic therapies listed above can also be used for the chronic treatment of disorders of ejaculation and orgasm.

COMPLEMENTARY & ALTERNATIVE MEDICINE

- A variety of nutritional supplements and herbs have been used for the treatment of erectile dysfunction, but their benefit for the specific treatment of ejaculation and orgasm disorders is unknown.
- Acupuncture and traditional Chinese medicine may be helpful in treating underlying hormonal imbalances.
- Yoga and meditation can reduce the effects of stress and relieve anxiety about sexual dysfunction.
- Therapeutic massage can decrease stress.

DISPOSITION

Prognosis varies with etiology. Ejaculatory dysfunction attributable to sexual techniques, psychological issues, or pelvic floor musculature can improve with psychotherapy or physiotherapy. Pharmacologic treatment may be helpful in treating premature, retrograde, or painful ejaculation.

REFERRAL

All male infertility issues and suspected anatomic problems should be referred to a urologist. Professional psychotherapy should be considered for appropriate patients.

PEARLS & CONSIDERATIONS

COMMENTS

Ejaculatory and orgasmic disorders are common male sexual dysfunctions and include premature ejaculation, delayed ejaculation, anejaculation, retrograde ejaculation, painful ejaculation, hematospermia, and anorgasmia. Physical exam is usually normal.

PREVENTION

Preventing sexually transmitted infections and treating other inflammatory disorders of the genitourinary tract may be of some benefit in reducing the incidence of these sexual disorders.

PATIENT & FAMILY EDUCATION

These sexual disorders can exert a significant psychological burden on affected men and their partners. A combination of pharmacologic and nonpharmacologic therapies, including a urologic and psychologic evaluation, when indicated, may be helpful in the treatment of these complaints.

SUGGESTED READINGS

Available at ExpertConsult.com

RELATED CONTENT

Erectile Dysfunction (Patient Information)
Premature Ejaculation (Patient Information)
Erectile Dysfunction (Related Key Topic)

AUTHORS: **David Guo, MD**, and **Mark Sigman, MD**

BASIC INFORMATION

DEFINITION

Electronic cigarette (e-cigarette) or vaping-associated lung injury (EVALI) refers to an acute lung injury due to inhalation of vaporized liquid, which contains nicotine or cannabis products, with or without added flavorings. The syndrome is heterogenous, with variable severity, presentation, and duration.

SYNONYMS

E-cigarette or vaping product use–associated lung injury
(E-cigarette or) vaping–associated pulmonary injury; (E)VAPI
Vaping (product use)–associated lung injury; VALI
"Popcorn lung"—referring specifically to lung injury caused by diacetyl-containing flavor additives
EVALI

ICD-10CM CODES

J68.0	Bronchitis and pneumonitis due to chemicals, gases, fumes, and vapors; includes chemical pneumonitis
J69.1	Pneumonitis due to inhalation of oils and essences; includes lipoid pneumonia
J80	Acute respiratory distress syndrome
J82	Pulmonary eosinophilia, not elsewhere classified
J84.114	Acute interstitial pneumonitis
J84.89	Other specified interstitial pulmonary disease
J68.9	Unspecified respiratory condition due to chemicals, gases, fumes, and vapors

EPIDEMIOLOGY & DEMOGRAPHICS

INCIDENCE & PREVALENCE: Because of the relatively recent discovery of EVALI, as well as the subsequent COVID-19 pandemic, exact incidence rates of EVALI are difficult to ascertain. As of February 18, 2020, a total of 2,807 hospitalized EVALI cases or deaths had been reported to the Centers for Disease Control and Prevention.

PREDOMINANT SEX & AGE: EVALI primarily affects young men; the median age of individuals with EVALI is 24. Males compose 66% of EVALI cases.

PEAK INCIDENCE: The incidence of known EVALI cases increased significantly in August 2019 and peaked during September 2019. The subsequent COVID-19 pandemic has made identification of EVALI cases more challenging, but there have been no signs of a second rise in EVALI incidence.

RISK FACTORS:

- Vaping products that contain tetrahydrocannabinol (THC) are associated with increased risk of EVALI compared with those that contain nicotine.
- A history of prior EVALI markedly increases the risk of subsequent EVALI if a patient is reexposed to vaping products.

GENETICS: Ethnic and racial minorities appear to be at greater risk. Although the majority of EVALI patients have been non-Hispanic white individuals, ethnic minorities are overrepresented compared with their baseline frequencies of vaping-product use.

PHYSICAL FINDINGS & CLINICAL PRESENTATION

- Patients with EVALI may present with symptoms ranging from mild dyspnea to immediately life-threatening respiratory failure. Milder cases generally present with cough, shortness of breath, and dyspnea on exertion. Chest pain and fever are frequently encountered complaints. Patients may also report chills and gastrointestinal symptoms (diarrhea, nausea, and vomiting). Sputum production is less frequent (36% in one case series) and hemoptysis relatively uncommon. More severe cases are marked by profound dyspnea, tachycardia, tachypnea, and hypoxemia.
- Laboratory abnormalities are nonspecific, with elevated leukocyte count, C-reactive protein, erythrocyte sedimentation rate, and procalcitonin. Peripheral eosinophilia is not generally found in EVALI cases.
- Chest imaging findings are also nonspecific, but generally consist of patchy, ground glass opacities, occasionally with subpleural sparing seen on CT scans.
- Although EVALI generally presents with a diffuse alveolar damage phenotype, cases have been reported with more varied presentations, including hypersensitivity pneumonitis, acute eosinophilic pneumonia, organizing pneumonia, and lipoid pneumonia.

ETIOLOGY

- The etiology of EVALI is not fully understood; several mechanisms have been proposed, including direct toxicity of e-liquid components causing lung epithelial necrosis and alteration of the inflammatory state of the lung by increasing pro-inflammatory cytokine release by macrophages.
- Vitamin E (tocopherol acetate) is the causative compound most consistently found in bronchoalveolar lavage (BAL) fluid of patients with EVALI and in the vaping products they used. The vitamin E is thought to have a direct toxic effect on pulmonary epithelium.

DIAGNOSIS

DIFFERENTIAL DIAGNOSIS

Because of the nonspecific nature of the history, physical, laboratory, and radiologic findings in EVALI, it is considered a diagnosis of exclusion (in the setting of known or suspected vaping-product use). The differential diagnosis is broad, including the following:

- Infection
  1. Bacterial
     a. Atypical bacterial pneumonia (including *Chlamydophila, Mycoplasma, Legionella,* and others)
     b. Severe or diffuse typical bacterial pneumonia
  2. Viral
     a. Seasonal influenza infection
     b. COVID-19 infection
     c. Other respiratory viral infections (including common strains of parainfluenza, respiratory syncytial virus, coronavirus, adenovirus, rhinovirus, enterovirus, and metapneumovirus)
  3. Fungal, parasitic, or mycobacterial infection
     a. Including but not limited to *Pneumocystis jirovecii* pneumonia, strongyloidiasis, miliary tuberculosis, disseminated histoplasmosis, coccidioidomycosis, or blastomycosis
     b. More commonly (but not exclusively) a consideration in immunocompromised patients, severe cases can closely mimic EVALI and should be excluded with appropriate laboratory evaluation in the correct setting
- Autoimmune/idiopathic inflammatory conditions
  1. Vasculitis (including granulomatosis with polyangiitis or eosinophilic granulomatosis with polyangiitis)—generally associated with additional extrapulmonary manifestations or a preexisting history of pulmonary disease
  2. Diffuse alveolar hemorrhage
     a. Characterized by increasingly bloody BAL fluid return
- Other inhalational exposures/toxins
  1. Chemical pneumonitis—it is important to question patients and families regarding any other potentially toxic inhalational exposures
  2. Aspiration pneumonitis—due to gastric contents aspiration; of particular concern in patients with a history of dysphagia, reflux, or alcoholism
- Malignancy
  1. Generally excluded by the rapid onset of symptoms; however, some hematologic malignancies may cause leukemic infiltrates that can mimic clinical findings of EVALI
- Cardiogenic pulmonary edema
  1. A transthoracic echocardiogram should be obtained on all patients presenting with severe suspected EVALI to evaluate for cardiac causes of pulmonary edema

WORKUP

- Because there is no specific diagnostic test for EVALI, the majority of the workup is directed at excluding other potential etiologies.
- If the patient is sufficiently stable, bronchoscopy should be strongly considered to rule out infection in cases of suspected EVALI.
  1. Bronchoscopy should be done with BAL fluid sent for cell count and differential; bacterial, acid-fast bacteria (AFB), and fungal culture.
  2. Mycobacterial polymerase chain reaction (PCR), respiratory viral PCR, and galactomannan of the BAL fluid can be helpful to exclude tuberculous infection, respiratory

viral infection, and disseminated aspergillosis, respectively.
3. If diffuse alveolar hemorrhage is suspected, serial lavage should also be performed, observing for increasingly bloody return.

LABORATORY TESTS

- In addition to basic lab work (complete blood count, basic metabolic panel, liver function tests, and coagulation tests), we suggest the following for patients hospitalized with suspected EVALI:
  1. Blood culture and sputum culture
  2. Erythrocyte sedimentation rate, C-reactive protein
  3. *Legionella* antigen
  4. Respiratory viral panel (including assays for COVID-19 and influenza)
  5. Testing for endemic fungal infection (if locally prevalent or patient has had recent travel)
- In addition, we also recommend the following for immunocompromised hosts with suspected EVALI:
  1. Sputum culture (fungal and AFB), as well as TB PCR; recommend induced sputum or bronchoscopy if patient is unable to produce sputum
  2. Silver stain for *Pneumocytis jirovecii* of induced sputum, tracheal aspirate, or BAL

IMAGING STUDIES

- Chest x-rays are recommended in all suspected cases of EVALI. Typical findings include diffuse opacities in a central distribution.
- CT scans can assist in the diagnosis of EVALI by elucidating parenchymal abnormalities seen on chest x-ray. Findings are also nonspecific, but frequently include diffuse ground glass opacities, with subpleural sparing.

Rx TREATMENT

NONPHARMACOLOGIC THERAPY

The primary treatment of EVALI, regardless of severity, is supportive, and includes supplemental oxygen (via endotracheal intubation if necessary) and close monitoring in the hospital setting.

ACUTE GENERAL Rx

- No EVALI-specific therapies have been shown to improve outcomes. Therapy is generally supportive, as described earlier. Glucocorticoids have been suggested as a possible treatment for severe cases of EVALI, but data concerning their efficacy are limited. No consensus exists on the appropriate dose of steroids, but methylprednisolone 0.5 to 1 mg/kg daily, tapered over 5 to 10 days, is a reasonable approach.
- Empiric, broad-spectrum antimicrobial therapy should also be initiated for suspected EVALI cases, pending results of cultures.

CHRONIC Rx

- To our knowledge, no cases of "chronic" EVALI exist; patients either recover or succumb to the effects of the disease. Patients may also be left with residual pulmonary dysfunction due to scarring.
- Patients with persistent cough or dyspnea after EVALI should be managed as described later under "Disposition."

COMPLEMENTARY & ALTERNATIVE MEDICINE

- No evidence-based complementary/alternative medicine approaches to EVALI exist.

DISPOSITION

- Patients with suspected EVALI requiring supplemental oxygen should be managed in a hospital (rather than an outpatient setting).
- Once patients with EVALI are clinically improving and stable for discharge, short-interval follow-up with a primary care provider and pulmonologist should be arranged.
- Older patients with comorbidities are at higher risk of rehospitalization or death.
- Patients with persistent dyspnea should be evaluated with pulmonary function testing.
- Persistent cough can be treated symptomatically with an antitussive.

REFERRAL

- We recommend follow-up with a pulmonologist for all diagnosed cases of EVALI.
- Patients admitted to the intensive care unit (ICU) may also benefit from evaluation in an ICU Recovery Clinic (if available), to evaluate for symptoms of post-ICU syndrome (including posttraumatic stress disorder, anxiety, weakness, or cognitive dysfunction).

PEARLS & CONSIDERATIONS

COMMENTS

- EVALI emerged as a cause of severe respiratory failure in early 2019, with cases peaking in the fall of 2019.
- Diagnosis of EVALI is based on excluding other potential causes of respiratory failure, including infection or autoimmune disease.
- Treatment is primarily supportive, though glucocorticoids may also be beneficial.
- Reducing the incidence of EVALI depends on decreasing e-cigarette use, particularly among teens and children.

PREVENTION

- Primary care and pulmonary clinicians should regularly screen for e-cigarette or vaping product use.
- In particular, patients with a personal history of EVALI should be cautioned that they are at high risk of recurrent (and more severe) disease if they again use vaping products.
- Public health efforts to discourage underage use of e-cigarettes show promise in preventing future cases of EVALI.

PATIENT & FAMILY EDUCATION

- Any patient reporting e-cigarette or vaping use should be counseled on the risks, including the risk of EVALI.
- In particular, all patients with a personal history of EVALI should be cautioned that they are at high risk of recurrent (and more severe) disease if they again use vaping products.

SUGGESTED READINGS

Available at ExpertConsult.com

RELATED CONTENT

Acute Respiratory Distress Syndrome (Key Related Topic)

AUTHORS: **Amy L. Bellinghausen, MD,** and **Angela Wang, MD**

Empyema

BASIC INFORMATION

DEFINITION

Infection of the pleural space, most often bacterial, as identified by aspiration of pus, positive pleural cultures, or a positive Gram stain on pleural fluid smear.

SYNONYMS

Infected pleural effusion
Purulent pleural effusion
Pleural sepsis

ICD-10CM CODES	
A16.5	Empyema due to tuberculosis
J86	Pyothorax

EPIDEMIOLOGY & DEMOGRAPHICS

- Empyema is most commonly a complication of bacterial pneumonia, especially in association with pneumococcal or anaerobic infection (40%-60% of cases of empyema)
- Iatrogenic complications from thoracic surgery or indwelling pleural catheters occur less frequently (<20% of cases)
- Penetrating chest trauma may also lead to empyema (4%-10% of cases)

PHYSICAL FINDINGS & CLINICAL PRESENTATION

- Presentation may vary from mild pleuritic chest pain and low-grade fever to more severe symptoms with malaise, dyspnea, and a productive cough.
- Rarely empyemas can present as slowly enlarging chest wall masses or form a fistula (e.g., empyema necessitans).
- Physical findings of empyema are those of pleural effusion: Decreased breath sounds and dullness to percussion over the involved part of the thorax. Systemic signs include fever, tachycardia, leukocytosis, and warmth and erythema over the involved area.

ETIOLOGY

Pleural bacteriology differs based on setting:
Community acquired:
- *Streptococcus* spp. (e.g., *S. milleri, S. pneumonia*)
- *Staphylococcus aureus*
- *Haemophilus influenzae*
- Oral anaerobic bacteria (e.g., *Bacteroides fragilis, Prevotella* spp., *Fusobacterium nucleatum,* and *Peptostreptococcus*)
- *Legionella* spp.
- *Mycobacterium tuberculosis*
- *Actinomyces* spp.

Hospital acquired:
- Methicillin-resistant *Staphylococcus aureus* (MRSA)
- Methicillin-susceptible *Staphylococcus aureus* (MSSA)
- Gram-negative anaerobes

DIAGNOSIS

- Differential Diagnosis (see section on pleural effusion)
- Uninfected parapneumonic effusion
- Lung abscess (see Fig. 1)
- Heart failure
- Malignancy
- Tuberculous pleurisy
- Collagen vascular disease (particularly rheumatoid lung and systemic lupus erythematosus)

LABORATORY TESTS

- Blood and pleural fluid cultures: Pleural fluid cultures identify pathogens in only 60% of cases (yield increases when sent in culture medium bottles).
- Pleural fluid analysis in the acute phase of empyema is a neutrophilic-predominant exudate (pleural to serum protein ratio >0.5 or pleural to serum LDH >0.6).
- Complete blood count
- C-reactive protein
- BUN and albumin: 3-mo survival prognostic calculators incorporating BUN, age, purulence, infection source, serum albumin have been developed.

IMAGING STUDIES

- Chest x-ray (Fig. E2*A*)
- Lateral decubitus view to establish the presence of free fluid in the pleural space
- Computed tomography (Fig. E2*B*) to establish the presence of fluid loculation, underlying mass lesions, and other intrathoracic pathology
- Ultrasound to evaluate effusion complexity, procedure planning, and effusion surveillance (Fig. E3)

TREATMENT

NONPHARMACOLOGIC THERAPY

- Pleural glucose <50 mg/dl or pH <7.2 warrants immediate drainage by chest tube, given the high risk of progressive loculation.

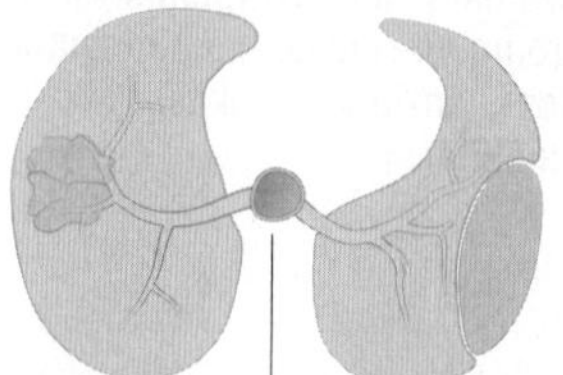

FIG. 1 Empyema versus lung abscess. (From Webb WR et al: *Fundamentals of body CT*, ed 4, Philadelphia, 2015, Saunders.)

- Early instillation of thrombolytic agents (tPA and DNAse) has been shown to improve radiographic appearance, decrease duration of hospital stay, and reduce surgical consults.
- Open decortication or video-assisted thoracoscopic surgery (VATS) may be required in cases where the lung remains unexpandable or source control is not obtained through conservative measures.

ACUTE GENERAL Rx

- Maintenance of drainage until infection controlled.
- Antibiotics directed at suspected or proven bacterial or fungal pathogens. Initial regimens include cefotaxime or ceftriaxone for suspected *S. pneumoniae* or group A *Streptococcus,* nafcillin or oxacillin for suspected methicillin-sensitive *S. aureus,* vancomycin or linezolid for suspected MRSA, ceftriaxone for suspected *H. influenzae,* and clindamycin plus ceftriaxone when suspecting anaerobes. Other agents with excellent anaerobic coverage include carbapenem antibiotics such as meropenem and ertapenem and piperacillin/tazobactam. These agents also have excellent gram-negative coverage.

CHRONIC Rx

- Pleural decortication may be indicated if sufficient pleural drainage cannot be accomplished using nonsurgical methods or if lung re-expansion is limited due to a pleural rind.
- Lung function should be monitored following completion of therapy.

DISPOSITION

Hospitalization with supplemental oxygen with ventilatory support if necessary

REFERRAL

Consultation by infectious diseases, pulmonary, or thoracic surgery specialists as needed

PEARLS & CONSIDERATIONS

- Chest tube sizes (large vs. small bore) are of equal efficacy for empyema drainage

SUGGESTED READINGS

Available at ExpertConsult.com

AUTHOR: **Yaron B. Gesthalter, MD**

BASIC INFORMATION

DEFINITION

Acute viral encephalitis is an acute febrile syndrome with evidence of meningeal involvement and of derangement of the function of the cerebrum, cerebellum, or brain stem.

SYNONYMS

Arboviral encephalitis
Brain stem encephalitis
Acute necrotizing encephalitis
Rasmussen encephalitis
Encephalitis lethargica

ICD-10CM CODES	
A86	Unspecified viral encephalitis
A83.0	Japanese encephalitis
A83.1	Western equine encephalitis
A83.2	Eastern equine encephalitis
A83.3	St Louis encephalitis
A83.4	Australian encephalitis
A83.5	California encephalitis
A83.8	Other mosquito-borne viral encephalitis
A83.9	Mosquito-borne viral encephalitis, unspecified
A84.8	Other tick-borne viral encephalitis
A84.9	Tick-borne viral encephalitis, unspecified
A85.0	Enteroviral encephalitis
A85.1	Adenoviral encephalitis
A85.2	Arthropod-borne viral encephalitis, unspecified
A85.8	Other specified viral encephalitis
A92.31	West Nile virus infection with encephalitis
B00.4	Herpesviral encephalitis
B01.11	Varicella encephalitis and encephalomyelitis
B02.0	Zoster encephalitis
B05.0	Measles complicated by encephalitis
B06.01	Rubella encephalitis
B10.01	Human herpesvirus 6 encephalitis
B10.09	Other human herpesvirus encephalitis
B26.2	Mumps encephalitis
B94.1	Sequelae of viral encephalitis
G04.00	Acute disseminated encephalitis and encephalomyelitis, unspecified
G04.81	Other encephalitis and encephalomyelitis
G04.90	Encephalitis and encephalomyelitis, unspecified
G05.3	Encephalitis and encephalomyelitis in diseases classified elsewhere

EPIDEMIOLOGY & DEMOGRAPHICS

INCIDENCE (IN U.S.): About 20,000 cases/yr are reported to the CDC. In 2019, there were 958 cases of West Nile virus with 54 deaths. Each yr in the U.S. approximately 7 patients are hospitalized for encephalitis per 100,000 population.

PREVALENCE (IN U.S.):
- Arbovirus infections are transmitted by mosquitoes and thus cause infection when mosquitoes are active, especially summer and fall. Herpes simplex infections can occur at any time.
- Geography also plays a role (Fig. 1): Whereas Eastern equine encephalitis is more likely on the East Coast of U.S., West Nile virus has spread to 48 states. Powassan virus is more common in northern New England and Canada. La Crosse virus is more common in the upper Midwestern and mid-Atlantic and southeastern states.

PREDOMINANT SEX: Male = female
PREDOMINANT AGE: Any age
PEAK INCIDENCE: Any age, but children and older adults are more likely to have significant morbidity
GENETICS: No specific genetic or congenital predisposition

ETIOLOGY

- Can be caused by a host of viruses (Table E1), with herpes simplex the most common virus identified.
- Arboviruses transmitted by mosquitoes include Eastern equine encephalitis, Western equine encephalitis, St. Louis encephalitis, Venezuelan equine encephalitis, California virus encephalitis, Japanese B encephalitis, La Crosse encephalitis, Murray Valley and West Nile encephalitis. Tick-borne diseases include Russian spring-summer encephalitis, Powassan encephalitis, and other lesser known agents.
- Also implicated: Rabies-causing agents, CMV, Epstein-Barr, varicella-zoster, echo virus, mumps, adenovirus, coxsackie, rubeola, and herpes viruses.
- Meningoencephalitis: Acute retroviral infection from HIV.
- In the U.S., the most commonly identified etiologies are herpes simplex virus, West Nile virus, and the enteroviruses.

PHYSICAL FINDINGS & CLINICAL PRESENTATION

- Initially, fever and evidence of meningeal irritation
- Headache and stiff neck
- Later, development of signs of cortical dysfunction: Lethargy, coma, stupor, weakness, seizures, facial weakness, as well as brainstem findings
- Cerebellar findings: Ataxia, nystagmus, hypotonia, myoclonus, cranial nerve palsies, and abnormal tendon reflexes
- Patients with rabies: Hydrophobia, anxiety, facial numbness, psychosis, coma, or dysarthria
- Rarely, movement disorders, such as chorea, hemiballismus, or dystonia
- Recall of a prodromal viral-like illness (this finding is not at all uniform)

Dx DIAGNOSIS

DIFFERENTIAL DIAGNOSIS

- Bacterial infections: Brain abscess, toxic encephalopathies, TB
- Protozoal infections
- Behçet syndrome
- Lupus encephalitis
- Sjögren syndrome
- Multiple sclerosis
- Syphilis
- Cryptococcus
- Toxoplasmosis
- Brucellosis
- Leukemic or lymphomatous meningitis
- Other metastatic tumors
- Lyme disease
- Cat-scratch disease
- Vogt-Koyanagi-Harada syndrome
- Mollaret meningitis

WORKUP (BOX 1)

- Lumbar puncture to reveal pleocytosis, usually lymphocytic, although neutrophils may be seen early on.
- Usually, elevated CSF protein.
- Normal or low CSF glucose
- In herpes simplex encephalitis: RBCs and xanthochromia.
- Selected tests on CSF fluid in viral encephalitis are described in Table 2.
- EEG changes showing periodic high-voltage sharp waves in the temporal regions and slow wave complexes suggestive of herpes encephalitis (Fig. E2).
- CT scan and MRI (Fig. 3) to reveal edema and hemorrhage in the frontal and temporal lobes.
- Temporal lobe involvement suggests herpes simplex encephalitis (Fig. E4).
- Basal ganglia and thalami are areas involved as generally seen in Eastern equine encephalitis.
- With West Nile infection, MRI changes have shown changes in basal ganglia, thalami, mesial temporal structures, brain stem, and cerebellum.
- Arboviral infections suspected during outbreaks in specific areas.
- Rising titers of neutralizing antibodies from the acute to the convalescent stage demonstrated but often not helpful in the acutely ill patient.
- Polymerase chain reaction (PCR) that amplifies DNA from the CSF for herpes simplex encephalitis.
- Rarely, brain biopsy to assist in the diagnosis; viral culture of cerebral tissue obtained if biopsy done.
- Classic herpetic skin lesions suggestive of herpes encephalitis.
- In diagnosing arboviral encephalitis:
  1. Presence of antiviral IgM within the first few days of symptomatic disease; detected and quantified by ELISA
  2. Unusual to recover an arbovirus from the blood or CSF

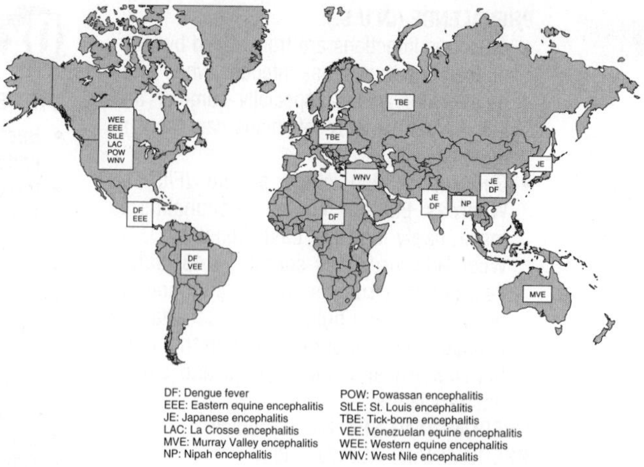

FIG. 1 Map showing the worldwide geographic distribution of encephalitis caused by arthropod-borne viruses (the "arboviruses"). (From Swaiman KF et al: *Swaiman's pediatric neurology, principles and practice*, ed 6, Philadelphia, 2017, Elsevier.)

BOX 1 Diagnostic Algorithm

All Cases

CSF
- WBC count with differential, RBC count, protein, glucose
- Gram stain and bacterial culture
- Herpes simplex virus-1/2 PCR (if test available, consider HSV CSF IgG and IgM in addition)
- VZV PCR (sensitivity may be low; if test available, consider VZV CSF IgG and IgM in addition)
- Enterovirus PCR

Blood/Serum
- Routine blood culture
- Epstein-Barr virus (EBV) antibodies (if positive for acute infection, check CSF EBV PCR)
- Hold acute serum and collect convalescent serum 10-14 days later for paired antibody testing

Respiratory, Stool
- Enterovirus PCR (respiratory, stool)
- Enterovirus (stool)

Conditional

Host Factors
- Neonate: Herpes simplex virus-2 PCR (CSF), swabs of skin vesicles, mouth, nasopharynx, conjunctivae, and rectum (viral culture)
- ≤3 yr: Parechovirus PCR (CSF and respiratory)
- Immunocompromised: Cytomegalovirus, human herpesvirus-6/7, JC virus, human immunodeficiency virus PCR (CSF)

Season and Exposure
- Summer/fall: West Nile virus (WNV) IgM (CSF, serum), WNV IgG (paired serum), and other appropriate arboviruses as geographically relevant
- Cat (particularly if with seizures and paucicellular CSF): *Bartonella* antibody (serum)
- Animal bite exposure: Rabies test[a]
- Rodent exposure: LCM antibody (serum)
- Tick and/or camping exposure: *Rickettsia* spp., antibody (serum), *Anaplasma* phagocytophila antibody (serum)
- Swimming or diving in brackish water: *Naegleria fowleri* (wet mount)[a]
- If history of sexual activity: Herpes simplex virus-2 (CSF PCR)

Signs and Symptoms
- Psychotic component or movement disorder: Anti-NMDAR antibody (CSF and serum), and abdominal ultrasound evaluation for teratoma
- Vesicular rash: Varicella zoster virus PCR (CSF)
- Rapid decompensation (especially with bite history or foreign travel): Rabies test[a]
- Respiratory (during influenza season): Influenza PCR (respiratory)
- Diarrhea and seizure (especially young child): Rotavirus (check stool for antigen), if positive then rotavirus PCR (CSF)

Laboratory Features
- CSF protein >100 mg/dl or CSF glucose less than two-thirds peripheral glucose and/or lymphocytic pleocytosis:
  1. Mycobacterial tuberculosis: Culture (CSF, respiratory), place PPD, and check IGRA, chest radiograph, fungal culture (CSF)
  2. Fungal (specific types depend on geographic residence and/ or travel to endemic areas): Culture CSF *and* check antibody and antigen
  3. *Balamuthia mandrillaris:* Contact health department/CDC for assistance with testing
- CSF eosinophilia: *Baylisascaris procyonis* antibody

Travel
- Consider consultation with public health department concerning specific diseases such as arboviruses, rabies, and other diseases

CDC, Centers for Disease Control and Prevention; *CSF*, cerebrospinal fluid; *HSV*, herpes simplex virus; *Ig*, immunoglobulin; *IGRA*, interferon gamma release assay; *LCM*, lymphocytic choriomeningitis; *NMDAR*, N-methyl-d-aspartate receptor; *PCR*, polymerase chain reaction; *PPD*, purified protein derivative; *RBC*, red blood cell; *VZV*, varicella zoster virus; *WBC,* white blood cell.

[a]Contact health department for assistance with testing.

From Cherry JD et al: *Feigin and Cherry's pediatric infectious diseases,* ed 8, Philadelphia, 2019, Elsevier.

TABLE 2 Selected Tests for Viral Encephalitis

Organism/Syndrome	Test	Comment
West Nile Virus		
West Nile encephalitis	IgM in CSF	Diagnostic of CNS invasive disease or acute flaccid paralysis
Herpes Simplex Virus Type 1		
Herpes simplex encephalitis	PCR in CSF	Sensitive and specific in the acute phase
	CSF–serum antibody ratio	Useful 2 wk to 3 mo after onset
Herpes Simplex Virus Type 2		
Neonatal encephalitis	PCR in CSF	Confirmatory, high sensitivity
Relapsing meningitis	PCR in CSF	Sensitive and specific in first 3 days of illness
Varicella-Zoster Virus		
Meningoencephalitis	PCR in CSF	Confirmatory when used with clinical and spinal fluid findings; sensitivity unclear
Epstein-Barr Virus		
EBV encephalitis	PCR in CSF	Suggests CNS invasion by virus
JC virus		
Progressive multifocal leukoencephalopathy	PCR in CSF	Diagnostic but incompletely (70%) sensitive
Cytomegalovirus		
CMV ventriculitis	PCR in CSF	Sensitive and specific

CMV, Cytomegalovirus; *CNS,* central nervous system; *CSF,* cerebrospinal fluid; *EBV,* Epstein-Barr virus; *IgM,* immunoglobulin M; *PCR,* polymerase chain reaction.
From Goldman L, Schafer AI: *Goldman's Cecil medicine,* ed 24, Philadelphia, 2011, Saunders.

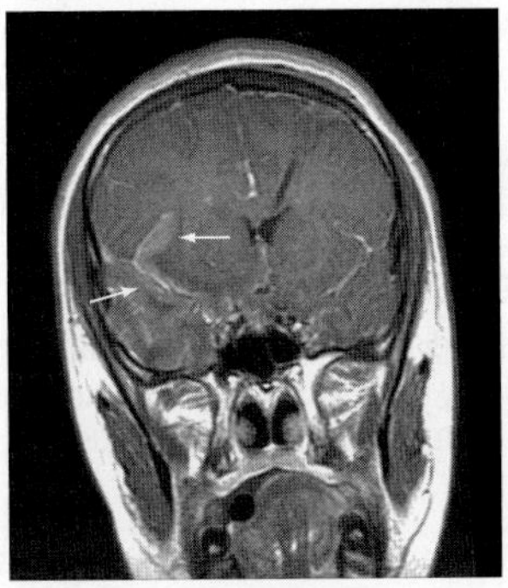

FIG. 3 Gadolinium-enhanced, T1-weighted brain magnetic resonance imaging in a teenager with herpes simplex virus encephalitis. The scan shows gadolinium enhancement in the right insular cortex *(arrows).* (From Swaiman KF et al: *Swaiman's pediatric neurology, principles and practice,* ed 6, Philadelphia, 2017, Elsevier.)

LABORATORY TESTS

- Aside from the lumbar puncture, most other laboratory studies are nonspecific.
- Skin lesions and urine may be cultured for herpes simplex and CMV.

Rx TREATMENT

ACUTE GENERAL Rx

- Supportive care, frequent evaluation, and neurologic examination
- Ventilatory assistance for patients who are moribund or at risk for aspiration
- Avoidance of infusion of hypotonic fluids to minimize the risk of hyponatremia
- For patients who develop seizures: Anticonvulsant therapy and follow-up in a critical care setting
- For comatose patients:
  1. Aggressive care to avoid decubitus ulcers, contractures, and DVT
  2. Close attention to weights, input/output, and serum electrolytes
- Acyclovir 30 mg/kg/day IV total dose divided in q8h intervals for 14 days for herpes simplex encephalitis
- Short courses of corticosteroids to control brain edema and prevent herniation
- In patients with suspected rabies:
  1. Human rabies immune globulin (HRIG) should be given at a dose of 20 U/kg
  2. Active immunization may be stimulated by rabies vaccine, which is grown on a human diploid cell line (HDCV) and has reduced the number of doses needed to five
  3. If suspect animal is a dog or cat and can be found, observe closely for 10 days to detect rabid behavior; any significant illness in the animal should promptly initiate humane sacrifice of the animal with the brain submitted to local or state health departments for pathology and immunologic testing for rabies. Any wild animal suspected of rabies should be humanely sacrificed, if possible, and submitted for rabies testing immediately
  4. If signs are seen, animal should be euthanized and its brain examined for signs of rabies
- No specific pharmacologic therapy for most other viral pathogens

CHRONIC Rx

Some patients may develop permanent neurologic sequelae; these patients will benefit from intensive rehabilitation programs, including physical, occupational, and speech therapy.

DISPOSITION

- Patients with suspected encephalitis of any cause should generally be admitted for initial diagnostic workup and specific treatment (if available).
- Long-term management of patients with significant neurologic sequelae from encephalitis (e.g., memory defects, depression, difficulty with organization of thoughts, movement disorders) may benefit from rehabilitation services, home care, or nursing home placement.

REFERRAL

- To a neurologist for initial workup and management
- To an infectious disease specialist for diagnostic and therapeutic plan
- To a rehabilitation service for long-term evaluation and convalescent services

PEARLS & CONSIDERATIONS

- West Nile virus encephalitis occurs primarily in elderly patients >65 yr of age.
- Rabies may occur months after contact with the rabid animal, and the exposure (especially bat rabies) may have been seemingly insignificant and even inapparent.
- Experimental therapies are worthy of consideration for some forms of viral encephalitis (e.g., immune plasma, ribavirin, interferons), and expert consultation should be obtained early on for possible treatment interventions with promising experimental therapies.

SUGGESTED READINGS

Available at ExpertConsult.com

RELATED CONTENT

Herpes Encephalitis (Patient Information)
Rabies (Related Key Topic)
West Nile Virus Infection (Related Key Topic)

AUTHOR: **Glenn G. Fort, MD, MPH**

BASIC INFORMATION

DEFINITION

Encephalopathy is a clinical syndrome of global cognitive impairment characterized by impaired arousal, inattention, and disorientation.

SYNONYMS

Acute confusional state
Altered mental status

ICD-10CM CODES

G93.40	Encephalopathy, unspecified
G93.41	Metabolic encephalopathy
G93.49	Other encephalopathy
G92	Toxic encephalopathy
E51.2	Wernicke encephalopathy
G04.30	Acute necrotizing hemorrhagic encephalopathy, unspecified
G04.31	Postinfectious acute necrotizing hemorrhagic encephalopathy
G04.32	Postimmunization acute necrotizing hemorrhagic encephalopathy
G04.39	Other acute necrotizing hemorrhagic encephalopathy
G93.49	Other encephalopathy
I67.4	Hypertensive encephalopathy
I67.83	Posterior reversible encephalopathy syndrome
J10.81	Influenza due to other identified influenza virus with encephalopathy
J11.81	Influenza due to unidentified influenza virus with encephalopathy
P91.60	Hypoxic ischemic encephalopathy [HIE], unspecified
P91.61	Mild hypoxic ischemic encephalopathy [HIE]
P91.62	Moderate hypoxic ischemic encephalopathy [HIE]
P91.63	Severe hypoxic ischemic encephalopathy [HIE]

EPIDEMIOLOGY & DEMOGRAPHICS

POINT PREVALENCE: 1.1% of adults in the general population >55 yr, 10% to 40% of hospitalized elderly, and 60% of nursing home patients >75 yr; 100,000 to 200,000 cases annually with anoxic encephalopathy

RISK FACTORS: Advanced age; cancer; AIDS; terminal illness; bone marrow transplant; postoperative state; poor nutritional status; acute or chronic cardiac, pulmonary, renal, or hepatic dysfunction; history of previous insult to the brain; epilepsy; drug abuse; alcoholism; overtreatment and undertreatment of pain; use of anticholinergics, benzodiazepines, narcotics, barbiturates, and neuroleptics

PHYSICAL FINDINGS & CLINICAL PRESENTATION

- Common to all encephalopathies is a fluctuating level of arousal, poor attention, and dysfunction of other cognitive domains Table 1 summarizes stages of encephalopathy in chronic liver disease.
- Some patients may appear agitated and others lethargic.
- Delusions (fixed false beliefs) and hallucinations are common.
- Asterixis (negative myoclonus) is common.
- Other physical findings, such as fever, ascites, jaundice, or tachycardia, may vary depending on the underlying cause of encephalopathy.
- Because toxins and metabolic disturbances are common causes of encephalopathy, the history should focus on exposure to toxins, especially medications, and symptoms suggesting a concurrent illness such as a urinary tract infection, pneumonia, sepsis, meningitis, or encephalitis. Clinical events precipitating hepatic encephalopathy in patients with cirrhosis are summarized in Box 1.

ETIOLOGY

The final common pathway of all causes of encephalopathy is widespread neuronal dysfunction from either a structural or functional cause. Many conditions are reversible and carry a good prognosis if treated in a timely manner.

- Organ failure (e.g., hepatic encephalopathy [Fig. 1], hypoxia, hypercapnia, uremia)
- Infection: Systemic (e.g., urinary tract, pneumonia, sepsis) or involving the central nervous system (e.g., meningitis, encephalitis)
- Toxin ingestion or withdrawal: Special consideration should be paid to alcohol, benzodiazepines, anticholinergics, neuroleptics, antibiotics (such as fluoroquinolones), and recreational drugs
- Metabolic disturbance: Hyperosmolar states, hypernatremia, hyponatremia, hyperglycemia, hypoglycemia, hypercalcemia, hypophosphatemia, acidosis, alkalosis, inborn errors of metabolism
- Endocrinopathy: Hyperthyroidism, hypothyroidism, Cushing syndrome, adrenal insufficiency, pituitary failure
- Neoplasm: Tumors of the central nervous system, primary or metastatic; effects of distant tumors (e.g., paraneoplastic limbic encephalitis)
- Nutritional deficiency, mostly in alcoholics and chronically ill patients, such as vitamin B_1 deficiency (Wernicke encephalopathy)
- Seizures: Postictal state, nonconvulsive status epilepticus, complex partial seizures, absence seizures
- Trauma: Concussion, contusion, subdural hematoma, epidural hematoma, diffuse axonal injury
- Vascular: Ischemic and hemorrhagic strokes, vasculitis, venous thrombosis
- Post-anoxic encephalopathy
- Psychiatric disease: Acute psychosis, depression with psychiatric features
- Acute demyelinating disease: Acute disseminating encephalomyelitis, tumefactive multiple sclerosis
- Other autoimmune diseases: Autoimmune encephalitis (e.g., anti-NMDA receptor encephalitis), lupus cerebritis, cerebral vasculitis (primary angiitis of the central nervous system or a secondary cerebral vasculitis)
- Other: Posterior reversible encephalopathy syndrome (PRES), hypertensive encephalopathy, postoperative status, sleep deprivation

DIAGNOSIS

DIFFERENTIAL DIAGNOSIS

Differential diagnosis for encephalopathy is broad. It is typically helpful to distinguish toxic/metabolic causes from primary neurologic causes.

TABLE 1 Stages of Encephalopathy in Chronic Liver Disease (West Haven Criteria)

Stage	Clinical Signs
Stage I	Mental slowness, euphoria or anxiety, shortened attention span, impaired calculating ability
Stage II	Lethargy or apathy, inappropriate behavior, personality change, more obvious problems with calculations
Stage III	Lethargic, somnolent, marked confusion and disorientation, but responds to verbal stimuli
Stage IV	Coma, patient may or may not respond to noxious stimuli

Patients with chronic liver disease rarely, if ever, demonstrate cerebral edema, regardless of the stage of encephalopathy.
From Vincent JL et al: *Textbook of critical care*, ed 7, Philadelphia, 2017, Elsevier.

BOX 1 Clinical Events Precipitating Hepatic Encephalopathy in Patients with Cirrhosis

Gastrointestinal hemorrhage
Infection (including spontaneous bacterial peritonitis)
Sepsis
Dehydration
Imbalance of electrolytes or acid-base
Renal failure
Drugs, toxins, medications (especially sedative-hypnotics or narcotics)
Illicit substances
Alcohol
Dietary indiscretion (excessive protein intake)

From Vincent JL et al: *Textbook of critical care*, ed 7, Philadelphia, 2017, Elsevier.

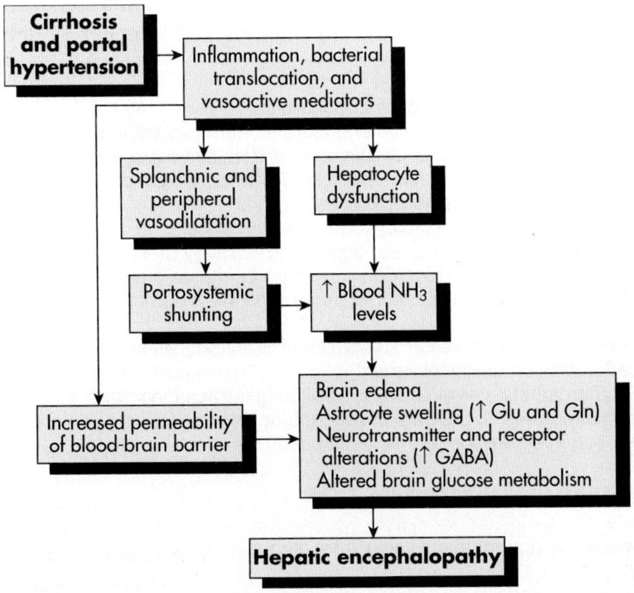

FIG. 1 Proposed pathophysiology of hepatic encephalopathy. *GABA*, Gamma-aminobutyric acid; *Gln*, glutamine; *Glu*, glutamate; *NH_3*, ammonia. (From Feldman M et al [eds]: *Sleisenger and Fordtran's gastrointestinal and liver disease*, ed 10, Philadelphia, 2016, Saunders.)

- Dementia: Distinguished from encephalopathy by a history of slowly progressive cognitive decline over time (fluctuating cognitive function is rare except in dementia with Lewy bodies)
- Hypersomnia
- Aphasia: Distinguished from encephalopathy by virtue of its representing a specific disorder of language rather than a global disturbance of cognitive function
- Depression
- Psychosis: Some overlap with encephalopathy because delusions and hallucinations may be common to both
- Mania
- Vegetative state from cerebral injury; these patients appear awake (eyes are open) but there is no content to their consciousness
- Akinetic mutism: These patients do not talk and do not move; there is little fluctuation in their state, and there is no asterixis or other focal deficit
- Locked-in syndrome: May be distinguished from encephalopathy by the presence of fixed neurologic deficits (e.g., paralysis of all four limbs); however, the patient is aware of his or her environment

WORKUP

The best tool in the evaluation of encephalopathy is a good history and physical exam, which will help tailor the remainder of the diagnostic workup. Interview family members and other providers to identify preceding events, medication changes, and medical history. Evaluate focal deficits.

LABORATORY TESTS

- Comprehensive metabolic panel, amylase, lipase, ammonia, TSH, B_{12}
- Complete blood count with differential
- Drug screen and alcohol level (must order ethylene glycol separately if suspected)
- Lumbar puncture if meningitis, encephalitis, autoimmune process, or subarachnoid hemorrhage with negative imaging is suspected
- HIV, RPR
- Urinalysis and microscopy, urine culture, blood cultures
- Arterial blood gases

IMAGING STUDIES

The following imaging and diagnostic studies may be indicated depending on history and physical examination:

- Chest radiograph to rule out pneumonia
- Head CT to rule out intracranial hemorrhage, hydrocephalus, tumors
- Brain MRI with and without contrast and with diffusion-weighted images for suspected encephalitis, tumors, acute strokes, or acute autoimmune processes
- Magnetic resonance angiography/venography for strokes, arterial dissection, venous thrombosis
- Conventional angiography for CNS vasculitis and aneurysms
- EEG: Evaluate for subclinical status epilepticus

Rx TREATMENT

The encephalopathy itself is a symptom of these underlying problems. In general, it is best to avoid treating the symptom of encephalopathy with antipsychotics or sedatives. The best approach is to treat the underlying toxic or metabolic disturbance.

- Thiamine supplementation.
- Glucose for hypoglycemia.
- Antibiotics in cases of infections (choose an agent with good CNS penetration in cases of primary CNS infections; to prevent exacerbation of underlying problem, ensure also that the agent is not associated with causing encephalopathy, if possible).
- Insulin in hyperglycemic conditions (e.g., diabetic ketoacidosis, hyperosmolar nonketosis, and sepsis).
- Correct electrolyte disturbances properly.
- Treat organ failure and its sequelae; for example, implement appropriate therapy for hyperammonemia and uremia.
- Ensure hemodynamic stability (blood pressure and heart rate).
- Eliminate medications that can cause or exacerbate encephalopathy: Anticholinergic drugs, benzodiazepines and other sedative-hypnotics, neuroleptics, and narcotics.
- Consider acute intoxication with, or withdrawal from, drugs or alcohol and treat withdrawal appropriately.
- Consider serotonin syndrome and neuroleptic malignant syndrome in the appropriate clinical setting.

RELATED CONTENT

Delirium (Related Key Topic)
Encephalitis, Acute Viral (Related Key Topic)
Hepatic Encephalopathy (Related Key Topic)

SUGGESTED READINGS

Available at ExpertConsult.com

AUTHOR: **Joseph S. Kass, MD, JD, FAAN**

BASIC INFORMATION

DEFINITION

Infective endocarditis is an infection of the endocardial surface of the heart or mural endocardium. Box 1 describes the modified Duke criteria for the diagnosis of infective endocarditis.

ACUTE ENDOCARDITIS: Usually caused by *Staphylococcus aureus, Streptococcus pyogenes, S. pneumoniae,* and *Neisseria* organisms; classic clinical presentation of high fever, positive blood cultures, vascular and immunologic phenomenon

SUBACUTE ENDOCARDITIS: Usually caused by *Viridans streptococci* in the presence of valvular pathology; less toxic, often indolent presentation with lower fevers, night sweats, fatigue

ENDOCARDITIS IN INJECTION DRUG USERS: Often involving *S. aureus* or *Pseudomonas aeruginosa* with variation that may be geographically influenced; tricuspid or multiple valvular involvement; high mortality rate of 50% to 60%

PROSTHETIC VALVE ENDOCARDITIS (EARLY): Usually caused by *S. aureus* (leading cause of PVE) within 2 mo of valve replacement; other organisms include *S. epidermidis*, gram-negative bacilli, diphtheroids, *Candida* organisms

PROSTHETIC VALVE ENDOCARDITIS (LATE): Typically develops >60 days after valvular replacement; involved organisms similar to early prosthetic valve endocarditis, including *Viridans streptococci,* enterococci, and group D streptococci

NOSOCOMIAL ENDOCARDITIS
- Secondary to intravenous catheters, TPN lines, pacemakers; coagulase-negative staphylococci, *S. aureus,* and streptococci most common
- Non-HACEK gram-negative bacillus endocarditis is not primarily a disease of injection drug users. More than half of all cases are associated with health care contact

SYNONYMS

Bacterial endocarditis
Subacute bacterial endocarditis (SBE)
Endocarditis

ICD-10CM CODES

I33.0	Acute and subacute infective endocarditis
I33.9	Acute endocarditis, unspecified

BOX 1 Modified Duke Criteria for the Diagnosis of Infective Endocarditis*

Major Criteria
- Positive blood cultures for infective endocarditis.
- Typical microorganism for infective endocarditis from two separate blood cultures in the absence of a primary focus: *Streptococcus viridans, Streptococcus bovis*
- HACEK group: *Haemophilus* species, *Actinobacillus actinomycetemcomitans, Cardiobacterium hominis, Eikenella corrodens,* and *Kingella kingae*
- Community-acquired *Staphylococcus aureus* or enterococci
- Persistently positive blood cultures, defined as recovery of a microorganism consistent with infective endocarditis from blood cultures drawn more than 12 hr apart or all of three or the majority of four or more separate blood cultures, with first and last drawn at least 1 hr apart
- Single positive blood culture for *Coxiella burnetii* or antiphase IgG antibody titer >1:800
- Evidence for endocardial involvement
- TTE (TEE in prosthetic valve) showing oscillating intracardiac mass on a valve or supporting structures, in the path of regurgitant jet or on implanted material, in the absence of an alternative anatomic explanation, or
- Abscess, or
- New partial dehiscence of prosthetic valve.

Minor Criteria
- Predisposition (e.g., prosthetic valve, intravenous drug use).
- Fever: 38° C (100.4° F).
- Vascular phenomena.
- Immunologic phenomena.
- Microbiologic evidence: Positive blood culture but not meeting major criteria.

*Adapted from Li JS et al: Proposed modifications to the Duke criteria for the diagnosis of infective endocarditis, *Clin Infect Dis* 30:633-638, 2000.
Ig, Immunoglobulin; *TEE,* transesophageal echocardiogram; *TTE,* transthoracic echocardiogram.
From Ballinger A: *Kumar & Clark's essentials of clinical medicine,* ed 6, Edinburgh, 2012, Saunders.

EPIDEMIOLOGY & DEMOGRAPHICS

INCIDENCE (IN U.S.): Yearly incidence is 15 cases/100,000 persons and is increasing due to medical interventions in the elderly and an increase in implanted cardiac devices.

NOSOCOMIAL ENDOCARDITIS: 14% to 28% of cases

PREVALENCE (IN U.S.): 0.3 to 3 cases/1000 hospital admissions. 40,000 to 50,000 new cases a yr in the U.S.

PREDOMINANT SEX: Male < female

PREDOMINANT AGE: 45 to 65 yr

PEAK INCIDENCE: Females: Often <35 yr old; males: 45 to 65 yr old

ENDOCARDITIS TRENDS: From 1998 through 2013 the population of patients with prosthetic valve endocarditis increased from 2% to 13.8%, as did cardiac device-related endocarditis, from 1.3% to 4.1%, whereas native valve endocarditis decreased from 74.5% to 68.4%.

PHYSICAL FINDINGS & CLINICAL PRESENTATION

- Clinical manifestations of infective endocarditis are described in Table 1 and Table 2.
- Fever may be variable in presentation; may be high, hectic, or absent.
- Fever, chills, fatigue, and rigors occur in 25% to 80% of patients.
- Heart murmur may be absent in right-sided endocarditis.
- Embolic phenomenon with peripheral manifestations is found in 50% of patients.
- Skin manifestations include petechiae, Osler nodes (Fig. E1), splinter hemorrhages, Janeway lesions (Fig. E2).
- Splenomegaly is more common with subacute course.

ETIOLOGY

Staphylococcal infection is now the leading cause of native or prosthetic valve infection. Variation in incidence may occur that is influenced by the patient's risk for developing infection. Table 3 summarizes the microbiology of infective endocarditis. Risk factors include hemodialysis (8%), IV drug use (10%), mitral regurgitation (43%), aortic regurgitation (26%), and rheumatic heart disease (3.3%).

ACUTE ENDOCARDITIS:
- *Staphylococcus aureus* (MSSA and MRSA)
- *Staphylococcus lugdunensis*

TABLE 1 Symptoms in Infective Endocarditis

Symptom	Patients Affected (%)
Fever	80-95
Chills	40-70
Weakness	40-50
Malaise	20-40
Sweats	20-40
Anorexia	20-40
Headache	20-40
Dyspnea	20-40
Cough	20-30
Weight loss	20-30
Myalgia/arthralgia	10-30
Stroke	10-20
Confusion/delirium	10-20
Nausea/vomiting	10-20
Edema	5-15
Chest pain	5-15
Abdominal pain	5-15
Hemoptysis	5-10
Back pain	5-10

From Zipes DP: *Braunwald's heart disease, a textbook of cardiovascular medicine,* ed 11, Philadelphia, 2019, Elsevier.

- *Streptococcus pneumoniae*
- Streptococcal species and groups A through G
- *Haemophilus influenzae*

SUBACUTE ENDOCARDITIS:
- *Viridans streptococci* (alpha-hemolytic) including nutritionally variant species:
  1. *Abiotrophia* spp. and *Granulicatella* spp.

TABLE 2 Physical Findings in Infective Endocarditis

Finding	Patients Affected (%)
Fever	80-90
Heart murmur	75-85
New murmur	10-50
Changing murmur	5-20
Central neurologic abnormality	20-40
Splenomegaly	10-40
Petechiae/ conjunctival hemorrhage	10-40
Splinter hemorrhages	5-15
Janeway lesions	5-10
Osler nodes	3-10
Retinal lesion or Roth spot	2-10

From Zipes DP: *Braunwald's heart disease, a textbook of cardiovascular medicine*, ed 11, Philadelphia, 2019, Elsevier.

- *S. bovis* (now called *S. gallollyticus*)
- Enterococci
- *S. aureus*

ENDOCARDITIS IN INJECTION DRUG USERS:
- *S. aureus*
- *P. aeruginosa*
- *Candida* spp.
- Enterococci

PROSTHETIC VALVE ENDOCARDITIS (EARLY):
- *S. epidermidis*
- *S. aureus*
- Gram-negative bacilli
- Group D streptococci

PROSTHETIC VALVE ENDOCARDITIS (LATE):
- *S. epidermidis*
- *Viridans streptococci*
- *S. aureus*
- Enterococci and group D streptococci

NOSOCOMIAL ENDOCARDITIS:
- Coagulase-negative staphylococci
- *S. aureus*
- Streptococci: Viridans, group B, enterococcus

HACEK ORGANISMS:
- Fastidious gram-negative bacilli
- ***H.** parainfluenzae*
- ***H.** aphrophilus*
- ***A.** actinomycetemcomitans*
- ***C**ardiobacterium hominis*
- ***E**ikenella corrodens*
- ***K**ingella kingae*

Other unusual pathogens:
- Q fever: *Coxiella burnetii*
- *Bartonella henselae* (etiologic agent of cat scratch disease)
- *Tropheryma whippelii* (Whipple disease)

RISK FACTORS

- Poor dental hygiene
- Long-term hemodialysis
- Diabetes mellitus
- HIV infection
- Mitral valve prolapse

Dx DIAGNOSIS

DIFFERENTIAL DIAGNOSIS

- Brain abscess
- FUO
- Pericarditis
- Meningitis
- Rheumatic fever
- Osteomyelitis
- Salmonella
- TB
- Bacteremia
- Pericarditis
- Glomerulonephritis

WORKUP

Physical examination to evaluate for the previous physical findings followed by laboratory testing (see "Laboratory Tests"). Fig. 3 describes a diagnostic evaluation of suspected endocarditis. The modified Duke criteria for diagnosis of endocarditis defines "major criteria" as persistently positive blood cultures of organisms typical of endocarditis or endocardial involvement (new valvular regurgitation or positive echocardiogram). "Minor criteria" are defined as presence of predisposing condition or injection drug use, fever, embolic vascular pneumonia (e.g., glomerulonephritis, rheumatoid factor), or positive blood cultures not meeting major criteria. Definite endocarditis is two major criteria or one major criteria and three minor criteria or five minor criteria or presence of organisms by culture or histologic examination of a vegetation.

LABORATORY TESTS

- Blood cultures: Three sets in first 24 hr. Table 4 describes causes of culture-negative endocarditis.
- More culturing if patient has received prior antibiotic
- CBC (anemia possibly present, subacute)
- WBC (leukocytosis is higher in acute endocarditis)
- ESR and C-reactive protein (elevated)
- Positive rheumatoid factor (subacute endocarditis)
- Proteinuria, hematuria, RBC casts
- Serologies or PCR for more unusual pathogens (*B. henselae, C. burnetii*, etc.)

IMAGING STUDIES

- Echocardiogram: Two-dimensional. Transthoracic echocardiography (TTE) (Fig. E4) is noninvasive and more easily available but has less-than-optimal sensitivity (50%-80%) for endocarditis.
- Transesophageal echocardiography (TEE): More sensitive in detecting vegetations and preferred diagnostic modality. It is especially helpful with prosthetic valves or in detecting perivalvular disease (Fig. E5). Echocardiographic features that suggest potential need for surgical intervention are summarized in Table 5.
- Electrocardiogram: Look for cardiac conduction abnormalities, injury pattern, or evidence of pericarditis—any such new findings are suggestive of myocardial abscess.

Rx TREATMENT

Initial IV antibiotic therapy (before culture results) is aimed at the most likely organism. The American Heart Association has developed guidelines based on the most frequently encountered bacteria. Tables 6 through 10 summarize treatment recommendations.

- **Native valve endocarditis** caused by penicillin-susceptible *S. viridians, S. gallolyticus* (previously called *S. bovis*), and other streptococci (MIC of penicillin ≤0.12 mcg/ml): Pen G 12 to 18 million U IV q24h continuous or divided q4h for 4 wk **or** ceftriaxone 2 g IV or IM q day for 4 wk for penicillin-allergic patients. Vancomycin at 30 mg/kg per 24 hr in two equally divided doses assuming normal kidney function, for 4 wk.
- **Native valve endocarditis** caused by strains of viridians streptococci and *S. gallolyticus (S. bovis)* relatively resistant to penicillin (MIC >0.12 mcg/ml): Pen G: 24 million units per 24 hr IV either continuously or in 4 or 6 equally divided doses for 4 wk **or** ceftriaxone 2 g per 24 hr IV or IM for 4 wk **plus** gentamicin 3 mg/kg per 24 hr IV or IM in one dose or in 2 to 3 equally divided doses for 2 wk or monotherapy with vancomycin 30 mg/kg per 24 hr IV in 2 equally divided doses for 4 wk not to exceed 2 g per 24 hr unless concentrations in serum too low.
- **Native valve endocarditis** due to *Staphylococcus:*
  1. **MSSA:** Nafcillin (or oxacillin) 12 per 24 hr IV in 4 or 6 equally divided doses for 6 wk **plus** optional addition of gentamicin 3 mg/kg per 24 hr IV or IM in 2 or 3 equally divided doses for 3 to 5 days **or** cefazolin 6 g per 24 hr IV in 3 equally divided doses for 6 wk, **plus** optional addition of gentamicin 3 mg/kg per 24 hr IV or IM in 2 or 3 equally divided doses for 3 to 5 days. A newer antibiotic daptomycin has an indication for right-sided endocarditis with MSSA at 6 mg/kg IV q24h.
  2. **MRSA:** Vancomycin 30 mg/kg per 24 hr in 2 equally divided doses for 6 wk; not to exceed 2 g per 24 hr unless concentrations in serum are low.
- For culture-negative native valve endocarditis one of the following regimens is suggested: Ampicillin-sulbactam: 12 g per 24 hr IV in 4 equally divided doses for 4 to 6 wk **plus** gentamicin 3 mg/kg per 24 hr IV or IM in 3 equally divided doses for 4 to 6 wk **or** vancomycin 30 mg/kg per 24 hr IV in 2 equally divided doses for 4 to 6 wk; not to exceed 2 g per 24 hr unless concentrations in serum low **plus** gentamicin 3 mg/kg per 24 hr IV or IM in 3 equally divided doses for 4 to 6 wk **plus** ciprofloxacin 1000 mg per 24 hr orally or 800 mg per 24 hr IV in 2 equally divided doses for 4 to 6 wk.

TABLE 3 Microbiology of Infective Endocarditis (IE)

	Native Valve				Prosthetic Valve	
	Health Care-Associated IE (%)					
Organism	**Community-Acquired IE (%) (*n* = 1201)[19,26]**	**Nosocomial (*n* = 370)[18,26]**	**Nonnosocomial (*n* = 254)[18]**	**Intravenous Drug Users with IE (%) (*n* = 237)[7]**	**Early IE (%) (*n* = 140)[27-29]**	**Late IE (%) (*n* = 390)[27,29]**
Staphylococcus aureus	21	45	42	68	34	19
Coagulase-negative staphylococci	6	12	15	3	28	20
Enterococcus species	10	14	16	5	10	13
Viridans group streptococci	26	10	6	10	1	11
Streptococcus gallolyticus	10	3	3	1	1	7
HACEK	3	0	0	0	0	2
Fungi	0	2	2	1	6	3
Other	13	7	10	7	6	15
Negative blood culture	11	7	6	5	14	10

HACEK, Haemophilus spp., *Aggregatibacter* spp., *Cardiobacterium hominis, Eikenella corrodens,* and *Kingella* spp.
From Zipes DP: *Braunwald's heart disease, a textbook of cardiovascular medicine*, ed 11, Philadelphia, 2019, Elsevier.

- For treatment of native valve endocarditis due to HACEK organisms: Ceftriaxone 2 g per 24 hr IV or IM in 1 dose for 4 wk **or** ampicillin-sulbactam 12 g per 24 hr IV in 4 equally divided doses for 4 wk **or** ciprofloxacin 1000 mg per 24 hr orally or 800 mg per 24 hr IV in 2 equally divided doses for 4 wk.
- **Patients with prosthetic valves** endocarditis:
- Methicillin-susceptible strains: Nafcillin or oxacillin 12 g per 24 hr IV in 6 equally divided doses for at least 6 wk **plus** rifampin 900 mg per 24 hr IV or orally in 3 equally divided doses for at least 6 wk **plus** gentamicin 3 mg/kg IV or IM in 2 or 3 equally divided doses for 2 wk.
- Methicillin-resistant strains: Vancomycin 30 mg/kg per 24 hr in two equally divided doses for at least 6 wk **plus** rifampin 900 mg per 24 hr IV or orally in three equally divided doses for at least 6 wk **plus** gentamicin 3 mg/kg per 24 hr IV or IM in two or three equally divided doses for 2 wk.

Antibiotic therapy after identification of the organism should be guided by susceptibility testing, preferably by formal testing by MIC (minimum inhibitory concentration).

DISPOSITION

- The patient may need outpatient IV antibiotic therapy, and arrangements need to be made to ensure safe vascular access and continuity of care with outpatient IV therapy team.
- Long-term follow-up is essential after therapy has ended; relapse of endocarditis may occur.
- Prophylaxis with antibiotics will be needed before dental procedures as a previous episode of endocarditis increases the risk of recurrent endocarditis associated with transient bacteremia from dental procedures.

REFERRAL

- To an infectious disease specialist.
- To a cardiologist or a cardiac surgeon if evidence of heart failure, refractory infection, myocardial abscess, valve disruption, or major embolic events occur.
- The timing and indications for surgical intervention to prevent systemic embolism in infective endocarditis remain controversial. Trials have shown that early surgery in patients with infective endocarditis and large vegetations significantly reduced death and embolic events by decreasing the risk of systemic embolism.

PEARLS & CONSIDERATIONS

- Serologies and/or PCR exist for more unusual zoonotic causes of endocarditis such as *Bartonella henselae* (cat exposure), *Coxiella burnetii* (farm animals), *Brucella* spp. (unpasteurized milk or cheese), and *Tropheryma whiplei* (soil and farm animals).
- 1-yr mortality has not improved and remains at 30%.

COMMENTS

- For endocarditis prophylaxis refer to Section V.
- In regards to antibiotic prophylaxis before dental procedures in patients with orthopedic implants, the 2013 guidelines from the American Academy of Orthopedic Surgeons (AAOS) and the American Dental Association (ADA) advises clinicians to consider discontinuing the practice of routinely prescribing prophylactic antibiotics for patients with hip and knee prosthetic joint implants undergoing dental procedures.
- *Streptococcus viridians* are a large group of commensal bacteria that are either alpha hemolytic on blood agar plates or nonhemolytic. Common members of this family include *S. mutans*, *S. anginosus*, *S. mitis*, *S. sanguis*, *S. oralis,* and *S. salivarius.* These tend to be oral/dental flora and most highly penicillin susceptible.
- Trials have shown that in patients with endocarditis in the left side of the heart who were in stable condition, changing to oral antibiotic treatment was noninferior to continued intravenous antibiotic treatment.[1,2] Additional trials will be necessary before changing current parenteral antibiotic guidelines to include oral antibiotic regimens.

SUGGESTED READINGS

Available at ExpertConsult.com

RELATED CONTENT

Endocarditis (Patient Information)

AUTHOR: **Glenn G. Fort, MD, MPH**

[1] Iverson K et al: Partial oral versus intravenous antibiotic treatment of endocarditis, *N Engl J Med* 380:415-424, 2019.
[2] Spellberg B et al: Evaluation of a paradigm shift from intravenous antibiotics to oral step-down therapy for the treatment of infective endocarditis: a narrative review, *JAMA Intern Med*, 2020 March.

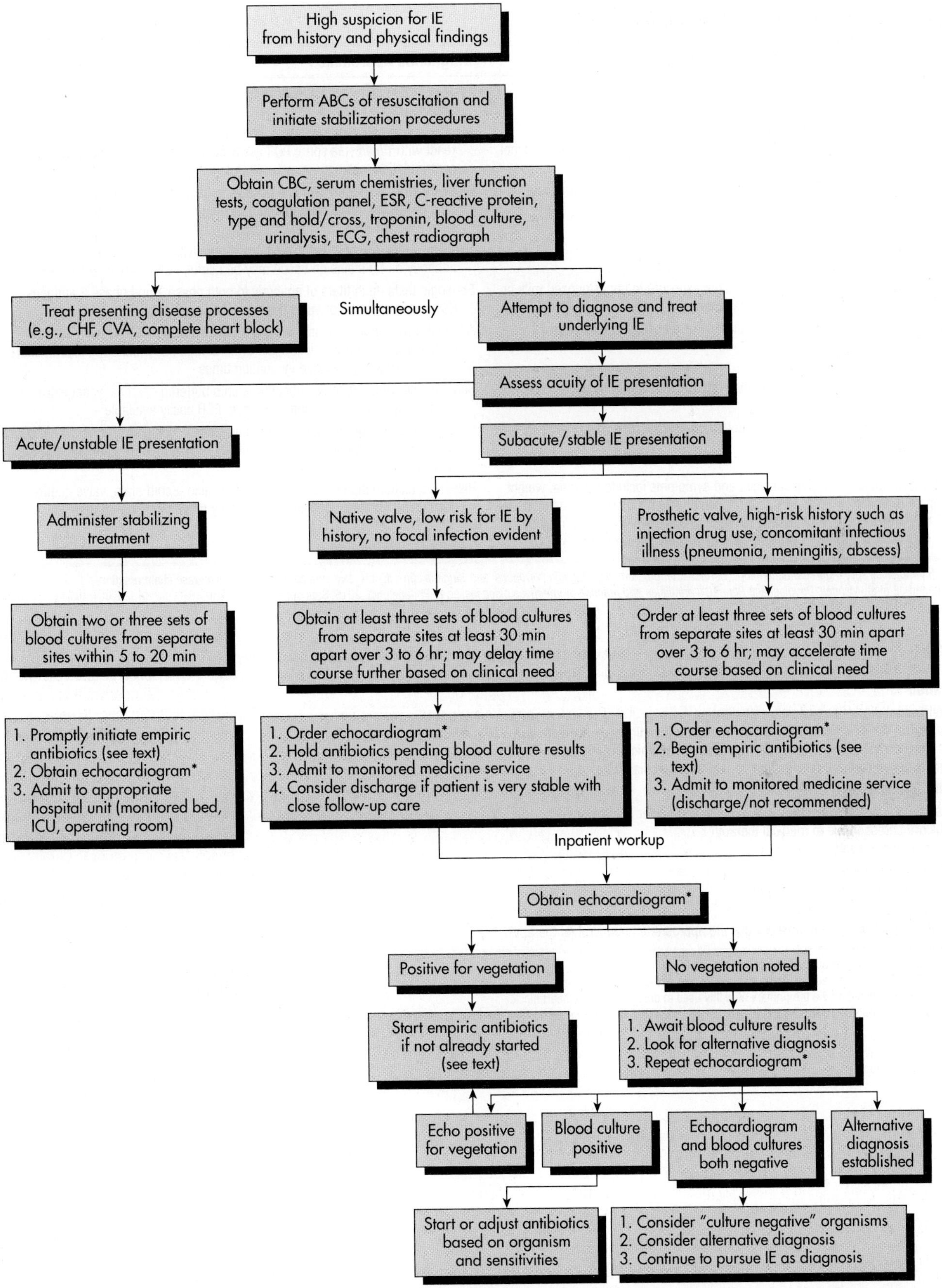

FIG. 3 Diagnostic algorithm for the emergency department management of patients in whom infective endocarditis *(IE)* is suspected. *Echocardiography can be performed via either the transthoracic *(TTE)* or transesophageal *(TEE)* technique. TEE is more invasive but is more sensitive for detecting vegetations and complications of IE, such as perivalvular abscesses; it is recommended for prosthetic valves; for situations in which optimal visualization by TTE will be difficult, such as emphysema and morbid obesity; for high suspicion of IE but normal TTE findings; and for high suspicion of a complication of IE, such as perivalvular abscess. Normal findings with either technique do not exclude IE if clinical suspicion is high. Echocardiograms can be repeated in an attempt to identify problems such as vegetations and abscesses that may not be noted initially. *ABCs,* Airway, breathing, and circulation; *CBC,* complete blood count; *CHF,* congestive heart failure; *CVA,* cerebrovascular accident; *ECG,* electrocardiogram; *ESR,* erythrocyte sedimentation rate; *ICU,* intensive care unit. (From Adams JG et al: *Emergency medicine, clinical essentials,* ed 2, Philadelphia, 2013, Elsevier.)

TABLE 4 Causes of Culture-Negative Endocarditis

Organism	Epidemiology and Exposures	Diagnostic Approaches
Aspergillus and other noncandidal fungi	Prosthetic valve	Lysis-centrifugation technique; also culture and histopathologic examination of any emboli
Bartonella spp.	*B. henselae:* Exposure to cats or cat fleas *B. quintana:* Louse infestation; homelessness, alcohol abuse	Most common cause of culture-negative IE in U.S.; serologic testing (may cross-react with *Chlamydia* spp.); PCR assay of valve or emboli is best test; lysis-centrifugation technique may be useful
Brucella spp.	Ingestion of unpasteurized milk or dairy products; livestock contact	Blood cultures ultimately become positive in 80% of cases with extended incubation time of 4-6 wk; lysis-centrifugation technique may expedite growth; serologic tests are available
Chlamydia psittaci	Bird exposure	Serologic tests available but exhibit cross-reactivity with *Bartonella;* monoclonal antibody direct stains on tissue may be useful; PCR assay now available
Coxiella burnetii (Q fever)	Global distribution; exposure to unpasteurized milk or agricultural areas	Serologic tests (high titers of antibody to both phase 1 and phase 2 antigens); also PCR assay on blood or valve tissue
HACEK spp.	Periodontal disease or preceding dental work	Although traditionally a cause of culture-negative IE, HACEK species are now routinely isolated from most liquid broth continuous monitoring blood culture systems without prolonged incubation times
Legionella spp.	Contaminated water distribution systems; prosthetic valves	Serology available; periodic subcultures onto buffered charcoal yeast extract medium; lysis-centrifugation technique; PCR assay available
Nutritionally variant streptococci	Slow and indolent course	Supplemented culture media or growth as satellite colonies around *Staphylococcus aureus* streak; antimicrobial susceptibility testing often requires processing specialized microbiology laboratory
Tropheryma whipplei (Whipple disease)	Typical signs and symptoms include diarrhea, weight loss, arthralgias, abdominal pain, lymphadenopathy, central nervous system involvement; IE may be present without systemic symptoms	Histologic examination of valve with periodic acid–Schiff stain; valve cultures may be done using fibroblast cell lines; PCR assay on vegetation material

HACEK, Haemophilus spp., *Aggregatibacter* spp., *Cardiobacterium hominis, Eikenella corrodens,* and *Kingella* spp.; *IE,* infective endocarditis; *PCR,* polymerase chain reaction.
From Bennett JE et al: *Mandell, Douglas, and Bennett's principles and practice of infectious diseases,* ed 8, Philadelphia, 2015, Saunders.

TABLE 5 Echocardiographic Features That Suggest Potential Need for Surgical Intervention

Vegetation

Persistent vegetation after systemic embolization
Anterior mitral valve leaflet vegetation, particularly if it is highly mobile with size >10 mm*
One or more embolic events during the first 2 wk of antimicrobial therapy*
Increase in vegetation size despite appropriate antimicrobial therapy*,†

Valvular Dysfunction

Acute aortic or mitral insufficiency with signs of ventricular failure†
Heart failure unresponsive to medical therapy†
Valve perforation or rupture†

Perivalvular Extension

Valvular dehiscence, rupture, or fistula†
New heart block†,‡
Large abscess or extension of abscess despite appropriate antimicrobial therapy†

*Surgery may be required because of risk of embolization.
†Surgery may be required because of heart failure or failure of medical therapy.
‡Echocardiography should not be the primary modality used to detect or monitor heart block.
From Zipes DP: *Braunwald's heart disease, a textbook of cardiovascular medicine,* ed 11, Philadelphia, 2019, Elsevier.

TABLE 6 Therapy of Native Valve Endocarditis Caused by Highly Penicillin-Susceptible Viridans Group Streptococci and *Streptococcus gallolyticus*

Regimen	Dosage* and Route	Duration (wk)	Class	LOE	Comments
Aqueous crystalline penicillin G sodium	12-18 million U/24 hr IV either continuously or in four or six equally divided doses	4	IIa	B	Preferred in most patients >65 yr of age or patients with impairment of 8th cranial nerve function or renal function
Or					
Ceftriaxone sodium	2 g/24 hr IV/IM in one dose	4	IIa	B	
Aqueous crystalline penicillin G sodium	12-18 million U/24 hr IV either continuously or in six equally divided doses	2	IIa	B	2-wk regimen not intended for patients with known cardiac or extracardiac abscess or for those with creatinine clearance of <20 ml/min, impaired 8th cranial nerve function, or *Abiotrophia, Granulicatella*, or *Gemella* spp. infection; gentamicin dosage should be adjusted to achieve peak serum concentration of 3-4 μg/ml and trough serum concentration of <1 μg/ml when three divided doses are used; there are no optimal drug concentrations for single daily dosing‡
Or					
Ceftriaxone sodium	2 g/24 hr IV/IM in one dose	2	IIa	B	
Plus					
Gentamicin sulfate†	3 mg/kg/24 hr IV/IM in one dose	2			
Vancomycin hydrochloride§	30 mg/kg/24 hr IV in two equally divided doses, not to exceed 2 g/24 hr unless concentrations in serum are inappropriately low	4	IIa	B	Vancomycin recommended only for patients unable to tolerate penicillin or ceftriaxone; vancomycin dosage should be adjusted to a trough concentration range of 10-15 μg/ml

MIC ≤0.12 μg/ml.
IM, Intramuscular; *IV*, intravenous; *LOE*, level of evidence; *MIC*, minimum inhibitory concentration.
§Vancomycin dosages should be infused over at least 1 hr to reduce the risk of histamine-release "red man" syndrome.
*Dosages recommended are for patients with normal renal function.
†Other potentially nephrotoxic drugs (e.g., nonsteroidal antiinflammatory drugs) should be used with caution in patients receiving gentamicin therapy.
‡Data for once-daily dosing of aminoglycosides for children exist, but no data for treatment of IE are available.
From Mann DL et al: *Braunwald's heart disease*, ed 10, Philadelphia, 2015, Elsevier.

TABLE 7 Therapy of Native Valve Endocarditis Caused by Strains of Viridans Group Streptococci and *Streptococcus gallolyticus* Relatively Resistant to Penicillin

Regimen	Dosage* and Route	Duration (wk)	Class	LOE	Comments
Aqueous crystalline penicillin G sodium	24 million U/24 hr IV either continuously or in four to six equally divided doses	4	IIa	B	Patients with endocarditis caused by penicillin-resistant (MIC ≥0.5 μg/ml) strains should be treated with regimen recommended for enterococcal
or					
Ceftriaxone sodium	2 g/24 hr IV/IM in one dose	4	IIa	B	
plus					
Gentamicin sulfate†	3 mg/kg/24 hr IV/IM in one dose	2			
Vancomycin hydrochloride	30 mg/kg/24 hr IV in two equally divided doses, not to exceed 2 g/24 hr, unless serum concentrations are inappropriately low	4	IIb	C	Vancomycin‡ therapy recommended only for patients unable to tolerate penicillin or ceftriaxone therapy

Minimum inhibitory concentration (MIC) >0.12 μg/ml to <0.5 μg/ml.
IM, Intramuscular; *IV*, intravenous; *LOE*, level of evidence.
*Dosages recommended are for patients with normal renal function.
†See Table 6 for appropriate dosage of gentamicin.
‡See Table 6 for appropriate dosage of vancomycin.
From Mann DL et al: *Braunwald's heart disease*, ed 10, Philadelphia, 2015, Elsevier.

TABLE 8 Therapy for Endocarditis of Prosthetic Valves or Other Prosthetic Material Caused by Viridans Group Streptococci and *Streptococcus gallolyticus*

Regimen	Dosage* and Route	Duration (wk)	Class	LOE	Comments
Penicillin-Susceptible Strain (MIC ≤0.12 μg/ml)					
Aqueous crystalline penicillin G sodium	24 million U/24 hr IV either continuously or in four to six equally divided doses	6	IIa	B	Penicillin or ceftriaxone together with gentamicin has not demonstrated cure rates superior to those for monotherapy with penicillin or ceftriaxone for patients with highly susceptible strain; gentamicin should not be administered to patients with creatinine clearance of <30 ml/min.
or					
Ceftriaxone	2 g/24 hr IV/IM in one dose	6	IIa	B	
with or without					
Gentamicin sulfate†	3 mg/kg/24 hr IV/IM in one dose	2			
Vancomycin hydrochloride‡	30 mg/kg per 24 h IV in two equally divided doses	6	IIa	B	Vancomycin therapy recommended only for patients unable to tolerate penicillin or ceftriaxone.
Penicillin–Relatively or Fully Resistant Strain (MIC >0.12 μg/ml)					
Aqueous crystalline penicillin sodium	24 million U/24 hr IV either continuously or in four to six equally divided doses	6	IIa	B	
or					
Ceftriaxone	2 g/24 hr IV/IM in one dose	6	IIa	B	
plus					
Gentamicin sulfate	3 mg/kg/24 hr IV/IM in one dose	6			
Vancomycin hydrochloride	30 mg/kg/24 hr IV in two equally divided doses	6	IIb	C	Vancomycin therapy is recommended only for patients unable to tolerate penicillin or ceftriaxone.

IM, Intramuscular; *IV,* intravenous; *LOE,* level of evidence; *MIC,* minimum inhibitory concentration.
*Dosages recommended are for patients with normal renal function.
†See Table 6 for appropriate dosage of gentamicin.
‡See text and Table 6 for appropriate dosage of vancomycin.
From Mann DL et al: *Braunwald's heart disease*, ed 10, Philadelphia, 2015, Elsevier.

TABLE 9 Therapy for Endocarditis Caused by Staphylococci in the Absence of Prosthetic Materials

Regimen	Dosage* and Route	Duration (wk)	Class	LOE	Comments
Oxacillin-Susceptible Strains					
Nafcillin or oxacillin†	12 g/24 hr IV in four to six equally divided doses	6	IIa	B	For complicated right-sided IE and for left-sided IE; for uncomplicated right-sided IE, 2 wk (see text)
For penicillin-allergic (nonanaphylactoid type) patients:					Consider skin testing for oxacillin-susceptible staphylococci and questionable history of immediate-type hypersensitivity to penicillin
Cefazolin	6 g/24 hr IV in three equally divided doses	6	IIa	B	Cephalosporins should be avoided in patients with anaphylactoid-type hypersensitivity to β-lactams; vancomycin should be used in these cases‡
Oxacillin-Resistant Strains					
Vancomycin‡	30 mg/kg/24 hr IV in two equally divided doses	6	IIa	B	Adjust vancomycin dosage to a trough serum concentration of 10-15 μg/ml (see text for vancomycin alternatives)

IE, Infective endocarditis; *IV,* intravenous; *LOE,* Level of evidence.
*Dosages recommended are for patients with normal renal function.
†Penicillin G 24 million U/24 hr IV in four to six equally divided doses may be used in place of nafcillin or oxacillin if strain is penicillin-susceptible (MIC ≤0.1 μg/ml) and does not produce beta-lactamase.
‡For specific dosing adjustment and issues concerning vancomycin, see Table 6 footnotes.
From Mann DL et al: *Braunwald's heart disease*, ed 10, Philadelphia, 2015, Elsevier.

TABLE 10 Therapy for Endocarditis of Prosthetic Valves or Other Prosthetic Material Caused by Staphylococci

Regimen	Dosage* and Route	Duration (wk)	Class	LOE	Comments
Oxacillin-Susceptible Strains					
Nafcillin or oxacillin	12 g/24 hr IV in six equally divided doses	≥6	IIa	B	Penicillin G 24 million U/24 hr IV in four to six equally divided doses may be used in place of nafcillin or oxacillin if strain is penicillin susceptible (MIC ≤0.1 μg/ml) and does not produce beta-lactamase; vancomycin should be used in patients with immediate-type hypersensitivity reactions to beta-lactam antibiotics (see Table 6 for dosing guidelines); cefazolin may be substituted for nafcillin or oxacillin in patients with nonimmediate hypersensitivity reactions to penicillins
Plus					
Rifampin	900 mg/24 hr IV/PO in three equally divided doses	≥6			
Plus					
Gentamicin†	3 mg/kg/24 hr IV/IM in two or three equally divided doses	2			
Oxacillin-Resistant Strains					
Vancomycin	30 mg/kg/24 hr in two equally divided doses	≥6	IIa	B	Adjust vancomycin to achieve a trough serum concentration of 10-15 μg/ml (see text for gentamicin alternatives)
plus					
Rifampin	900 mg/24 hr IV/PO in three equally divided doses	≥6			
plus					
Gentamicin	3 mg/kg/24 hr IV/IM in two or three equally divided doses	2			

IM, Intramuscular; *IV,* intravenous; *LOE,* level of evidence; *MIC,* minimum inhibitory concentration; *PO,* oral.
*Dosages recommended are for patients with normal renal function.
†Gentamicin should be administered in close proximity to vancomycin, nafcillin, or oxacillin dosing.
From Mann DL et al: *Braunwald's heart disease*, ed 10, Philadelphia, 2015, Elsevier.

BASIC INFORMATION

DEFINITION

Endometrial carcinoma (EC) is the malignant transformation of endometrial glands with stromal invasion. The changes are typified by irregular nuclear membranes, nuclear atypia, mitotic activity, loss of glandular pattern, loss of intervening stroma, and irregular cell size. The two main histologic subcategories of EC (Table 1), low-grade endometrioid (type 1) and high-grade endometrioid and nonendometrioid EC (type 2), show unique molecular aberrations and differing clinical behaviors.

SYNONYMS

Uterine cancer (some forms)
Carcinoma of the endometrium
EC

ICD-10CM CODES

C54.1	Malignant neoplasm of endometrium
C54.9	Malignant neoplasm of corpus uteri, unspecified
C55	Malignant neoplasm of uterus, part unspecified

EPIDEMIOLOGY & DEMOGRAPHICS

INCIDENCE:

- In 2015, 53,911 new cases of uterine cancer were diagnosed. This corresponds to an incidence of 27 cases per 100,000 women. Incidence was greater among white and black women compared with American Indian/Alaska Native, Hispanic, and Asian Pacific Islander women. It is the most common gynecologic malignancy in the U.S. A woman's lifetime risk for development of endometrial cancer is between 2% and 3%.
- Unlike most cancers in the U.S., endometrial cancer is rising in both incidence and associated mortality.[1]

PREDOMINANT SEX & AGE: Median age at diagnosis: 62 yr; only 5% occur in women <40 yr; 5-yr survival >80%

RISK FACTORS: Obesity, diabetes, nulliparity, early menarche and late menopause, unopposed estrogen therapy, tamoxifen use, oligoovulation with chronic unopposed estrogen exposure such as with polycystic ovary syndrome (PCOS), endometrial atypical hyperplasia, endometrial polyps (malignancy is found in 3.6% of endometrial polyps), family history. Other risk factors include a personal history of ovarian, breast, or colonic cancer, as well as certain genetic syndromes, such as Lynch syndrome and Cowden syndrome. The relative risk for endometrial cancer is summarized in Table 2.

PHYSICAL FINDINGS & CLINICAL PRESENTATION

- Abnormal uterine bleeding or postmenopausal bleeding in 90%
- Pyometra or hematometra
- Abnormal Pap smear: Endometrial cells, atypical glandular cells, or adenocarcinoma
- Incidental finding at hysterectomy

ETIOLOGY

Endogenous or exogenous chronic unopposed estrogen stimulation of the endometrium

Dx DIAGNOSIS

DIFFERENTIAL DIAGNOSIS

- Endometrial atypical hyperplasia
- Other genital tract malignancy
- Uterine polyps
- Atrophic vaginitis
- Granulosa cell tumor
- Fibroid uterus
- Adenomyosis

WORKUP

- Complete history and physical examination
- Endometrial biopsy or dilation and curettage (Table 3)

TABLE 1 Pathogenetic Subsets of Endometrial Carcinoma

Parameter	Type I	Type II
Age	50s-60s	60s-70s
Obesity	Common	Uncommon
Estrogenic stimuli	Common	Uncommon
Endometrium	Anovulatory	Atrophic
Precursor	Endometrial intraepithelial neoplasia	Presumed EmGD
Transition	Slow	Unknown
Type	Endometrioid	Papillary serous or mixed
Molecular genetics	MSI, *PTEN* mutation; loss of PAX2	p53 mutation, 1p deletions; loss of PAX2
Familial	Hereditary nonpolyposis colonic cancer syndrome	
Spread	Lymph nodes	Peritoneum
Concurrent ovarian	Common	Uncommon
Prognosis	Good	Poor

EmGD, Endometrial glandular dysplasia; *MSI*, microsatellite instability.
From Crum CP et al: *Diagnostic gynecologic and obstetric pathology*, ed 3, Philadelphia, 2018, Elsevier.

TABLE 2 Risk Factors for Endometrial Cancer

Factor	Relative Risk
Overweight (lb):	
• 20-50	3.0
• 50+	10.0
Nulliparous:	
• vs. one child	2.0
• vs. five children	5.0
Late menopause (>52 vs. 49 yr)	2.4
Diabetes mellitus	2.7
Unopposed estrogen therapy	6.0
Tamoxifen therapy	2.0
Sequential oral contraceptives	7.0
Combination oral contraceptives	0.5
Cowden syndrome (*PTEN* mutation)	Three- to fivefold increased risk
Hereditary nonpolyposis colonic cancer syndrome	40%-60% lifetime risk
Family member with endometrial cancer	3.4

From Crum CP et al: *Diagnostic gynecologic and obstetric pathology*, ed 3, Philadelphia, 2018, Elsevier.

TABLE 3 Differential Diagnosis of Endometrial Carcinoma (Curettings)

Parameter	Mimicking	Differential Diagnosis
Gland architecture	Cancer	Telescoping artifact; stromal collapse breakdown; sectioning artifacts
	Benign	Microglandular mucinous carcinoma; surface endometrioid carcinoma
Nuclear atypia	Cancer	Surface or glandular repair; Arias-Stella changes (hormonal therapy); radiation effect
Papillary changes	Cancer	Exfoliation artifact; stromal breakdown with papillary changes; papillary syncytial changes
	Benign	Papillary mucinous carcinoma

From Crum CP et al: *Diagnostic gynecologic and obstetric pathology*, ed 3, Philadelphia, 2018, Elsevier.

[1]Henley SJ et al: Annual report to the nation on the status of cancer, part I: National cancer statistics, *Cancer* 126:2225-2249, 2020.

TABLE 4 National Comprehensive Cancer Network Treatment Guidelines for Endometrial Carcinoma after Comprehensive Surgical Staging

Stage I_A	
Grade 1 without ARF	Observe
Grade 1 with ARF	Observe or VBT
Grade 2 or 3 without ARF	Observe or VBT
Grade 2 or 3 with ARF	Observe or VBT and/or pelvic RT
Stage I_B	
Grade 1 without ARF	Observe
Grade 1 with ARF	Observe or VBT
Grade 2 without ARF	Observe or VBT
Grade 2 with ARF	Observe or VBT and/or pelvic RT
Grade 3 without ARF	Observe or VBT and/or pelvic RT
Grade 3 with ARF	Observe or VBT and/or pelvic RT ± chemotherapy
Stage II	
Grade 1	VBT and/or pelvic RT
Grade 2	Pelvic RT and VBT
Grade 3	Pelvic RT and VBT ± chemotherapy
Stage III_A	Chemotherapy ± pelvic RT or tumor-directed RT ± chemotherapy or pelvic RT ± VBT
Stage III_B-III_C	Chemotherapy and/or tumor-directed RT
Stage IV_A-IV_B	Chemotherapy ± RT

ARF, Adverse risk factors (age, positive lymphovascular space invasion, tumor size, lower uterine or cervical involvement); *RT,* radiation therapy; *VBT,* vaginal brachytherapy.
From Niederhuber JE: *Abeloff's clinical oncology,* ed 6, Philadelphia, 2020, Elsevier.

TABLE 5 Revised FIGO Staging for Endometrial Cancer (adopted 2009)

Stages*	Characteristic
I	Tumor confined to the corpus uteri
I_A	No or less than half myometrial invasion
I_B	Invasion equal to or more than half of the myometrium
II	Tumor invades cervical stroma but does not extend beyond the uterus†
III	Local or regional spread of the tumor
III_A	Tumor invades serosa of the corpus uteri or the adnexa‡
III_B	Vaginal or parametrial involvement‡
III_C	Metastases to pelvic or paraaortic lymph nodes‡
III_{C1}	Positive pelvic nodes
III_{C2}	Positive paraaortic lymph nodes with or without positive pelvic lymph nodes
IV	Tumor invades bladder or bowel mucosa, or distant metastasis
IV_A*	Tumor invasion of bladder or bowel mucosa
IV_B	Distant metastases, including intraabdominal or inguinal lymph nodes

*G1, G2, or G3.
†Endocervical glandular involvement should be considered only as stage I and no longer as stage II.
‡Positive cytology has to be reported separately without changing the stage.
FIGO, Fédération Internationale de Gynécologie et d'Obstétrique (International Federation of Gynecology and Obstetrics).
From Lobo RA et al: *Comprehensive gynecology,* ed 7, Philadelphia, 2017, Elsevier.

- Assessment of operative risk
- Staging (Tables 4, 5, and 6)
- Fig. 1 is a diagnostic algorithm for diagnosing endometrial carcinoma for women with abnormal uterine bleeding.

LABORATORY TESTS

- Complete blood count
- Prothrombin time and partial thromboplastin time if bleeding is heavy
- Chemistry profile including liver function tests
- Consider CA-125 level

IMAGING STUDIES

- Chest x-ray
- CT scan if concern for metastatic disease, and/or pelvic ultrasound (Fig. E2)
- Transvaginal ultrasound (Fig. E3) in postmenopausal women with vaginal bleeding

Rx TREATMENT

NONPHARMACOLOGIC THERAPY

- Surgery is the mainstay of treatment, with or without adjuvant radiation and/or chemotherapy, depending on tumor histology, stage, and grade. Laparoscopic surgery for early-stage EC is as safe and effective as laparotomy. Robotic laparoscopy procedures have increased significantly in recent yrs for this indication.
- Surgery generally consists of pelvic washings, total hysterectomy and bilateral salpingo-oophorectomy, selective pelvic and periaortic lymphadenectomy, and omental biopsy depending on stage, grade, and histology.
- Brachytherapy and/or teletherapy are added in an advanced stage.
- Chemotherapy (carboplatin, paclitaxel) may be used for patients with high-risk endometrial cancer. Hormonal therapy (progestins alone or in combination with tamoxifen, selective estrogen-receptor modulators, aromatase inhibitors, synthetic steroid derivatives, and gonadotropin-releasing hormone analogues) may also be considered in cases where palliation, rather than cure, is the main intent of treatment, or in patients with multiple coexisting medical conditions who may not be surgical candidates.
- Hormonal therapy, commonly a levonorgestrel intrauterine device, is an option for some young women with early-stage, low-grade EC who wish to preserve fertility. This choice should be discussed with a gynecologic oncologist.

ACUTE GENERAL Rx

- A thorough workup should be completed before any therapy for EC.
- Surgery hysterectomy with bilateral salpingo-oophorectomy is the treatment of choice.

CHRONIC Rx

- Physical and pelvic examination every 3 mo for 2 yr, then every 6 mo for 2 yr, and annually thereafter with imaging as clinically indicated
- Hormone replacement (combination) a consideration in low-risk patients (stage I or early stage II)

DISPOSITION

- Survival is generally defined by the stage of the disease and histology.
- The majority of cases present early, and the 5-yr survival is generally good (Fig. E4).
- Some histologic types (clear cell, papillary serous) have worse survival rates, as they tend to be more aggressive with higher rates of metastatic disease at the time of diagnosis.

PEARLS & CONSIDERATIONS

Any woman with postmenopausal bleeding or abnormal uterine bleeding with risk factors for endometrial cancer needs evaluation by a gynecologist and either endometrial biopsy and/or pelvic ultrasound. When endometrial cancer is diagnosed, the patient should be cared for by a gynecologic oncologist and undergo surgical staging in a minimally invasive procedure when possible.

TABLE 6 Carcinoma of the Corpus Uteri: Patients Treated in 1990-1992: Survival by 1988 FIGO Surgical Stage, $N = 5562$

Stage	5-Yr Survival Rate
I_A	90.9%
I_B	88.2%
I_C	81.0%
II	71.6%
III	51.4%
IV	8.9%

FIGO, Fédération Internationale de Gynécologie et d'Obstétrique (International Federation of Gynecology and Obstetrics).
From Lobo RA et al: *Comprehensive gynecology*, ed 7, Philadelphia, 2017, Elsevier.

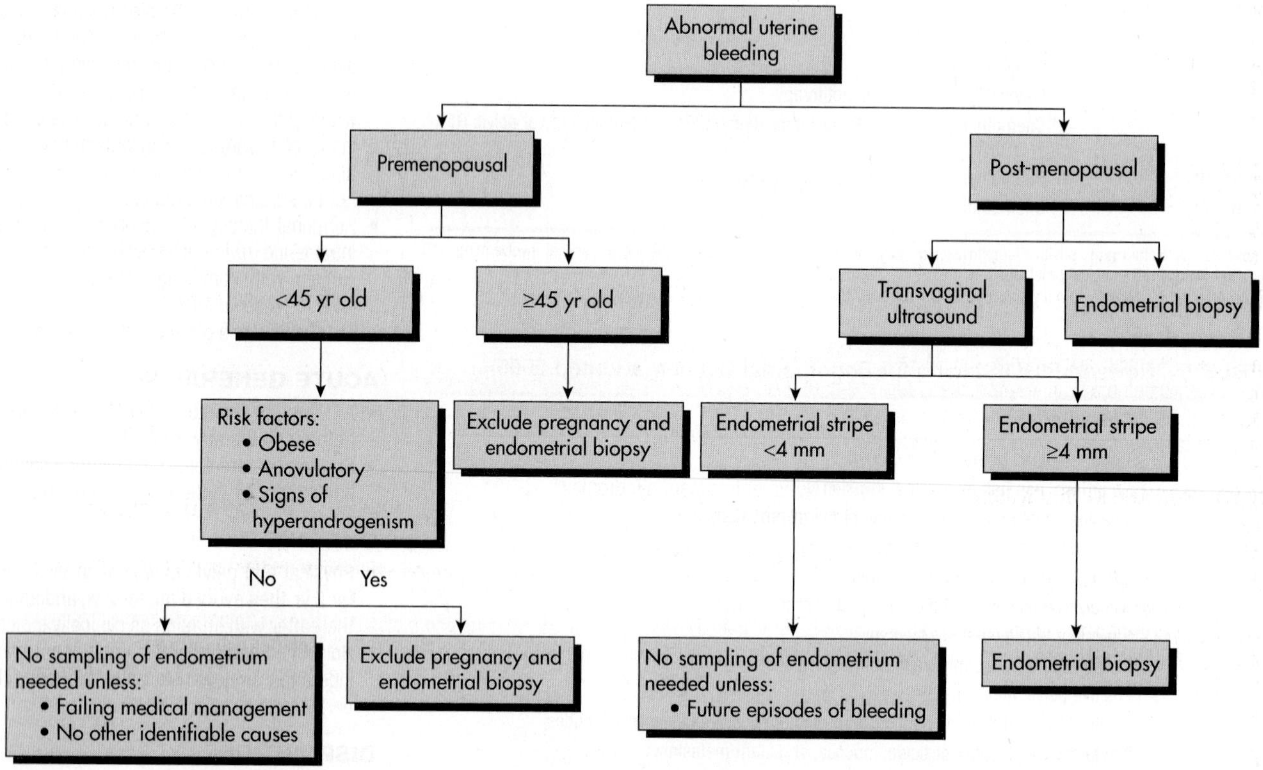

FIG. 1 Diagnostic algorithm to diagnose endometrial carcinoma for women with abnormal uterine bleeding. (From Niederhuber JE: *Abeloff's clinical oncology,* ed 6, Philadelphia, 2020, Elsevier.)

SUGGESTED READINGS

Available at ExpertConsult.com

RELATED CONTENT

Endometrial Cancer (Patient Information)
Abnormal Uterine Bleeding (Related Key Topic)
Uterine Malignancy (Related Key Topic)

AUTHORS: **Emily Sauck, DO, MBA,** and **Anthony Sciscione, DO**

BASIC INFORMATION

DEFINITION

Endometriosis is defined as the presence of functioning endometrial glands and stroma outside the uterine cavity. It is a chronic, estrogen-dependent condition that causes dysmenorrhea and pelvic pain.

ICD-10CM CODES

N80.9	Endometriosis, unspecified
N80.0	Endometriosis of uterus
N80.1	Endometriosis of ovary
N80.2	Endometriosis of fallopian tube
N80.3	Endometriosis of pelvic peritoneum
N80.4	Endometriosis of rectovaginal septum and vagina
N80.5	Endometriosis of intestine
N80.6	Endometriosis in cutaneous scar
N80.8	Other endometriosis

EPIDEMIOLOGY & DEMOGRAPHICS

PREVALENCE:

- Endometriosis affects 10% of reproductive-aged women.
- Women with dysmenorrhea: 40% to 60%.
- Subfertile women: 28% to 50%.
- Among symptomatic adolescents, the prevalence of endometriosis ranges from 49% for those with chronic pain to 75% for those with pain that is unresponsive to medical treatment.[1]
- Incidence peaks at approximately 40 yr.

MOST COMMON AGE AT DIAGNOSIS:

25 to 29 yr.

GENETICS:

- Familial association: If first-degree relative is affected, the patient has a seven- to tenfold increased risk of having the disease.
- Polygenic-multifactorial inheritance pattern.
- 6.9% occurrence rate in first-degree female relatives.

PHYSICAL FINDINGS & CLINICAL PRESENTATION

- Classic triad is dysmenorrhea, dyspareunia, and infertility.
- Presence of pelvic pain does not correlate with the total area of endometriosis (stage of disease), type of lesion, or volume of disease but is correlated with the depth of infiltration.
- Other symptoms include abnormal bleeding (premenstrual spotting, menorrhagia), cyclic abdominal pain, intermittent constipation/diarrhea, dyschezia, dysuria, hematuria, and urinary frequency.
- Rare manifestations: Catamenial hemothorax, bloody pleural effusion, massive ascites occurring during menses.
- Most severe discomfort is associated with lesions >1 cm in depth.
- Bimanual examination may reveal tender uterosacral ligaments, cul-de-sac nodularity, induration of the rectovaginal septum, fixed retroversion of the uterus, adnexal mass, and generalized or localized tenderness.

[1]Shafrir AL et al: Risk for and consequences of endometriosis: A critical epidemiologic review, *Best Pract Res Clin Obstet Gynaecol* 51:1-15, 2018.

ETIOLOGY

- Reflux and direct implantation theory: Retrograde menstruation with implantation of viable endometrial cells to surrounding pelvic structures (Sampson theory)
- Coelomic metaplasia theory: Transformation of multipotential cells of the coelomic epithelium into endometrium-like cells
- Vascular dissemination theory: Transport of endometrial cells to distant sites by the uterine vascular and lymphatic systems
- Autoimmune disease theory: Disorder of immune surveillance allows growth of endometrial implants
- Molecular mechanisms in endometriosis are illustrated in Fig. E1

Dx DIAGNOSIS

DIFFERENTIAL DIAGNOSIS

- Ectopic pregnancy
- Acute appendicitis
- Chronic appendicitis
- Pelvic inflammatory disease (PID)
- Pelvic adhesions
- Hemorrhagic cyst
- Hernia
- Irritable bowel syndrome
- Uterine leiomyomata
- Adenomyosis
- Nerve entrapment syndrome
- Interstitial cystitis

WORKUP

- Thorough history and physical examination including ultrasound.
- Definitive diagnosis of endometriosis can be made only by histologic confirmation during surgery (gold standard).
- Fig. 2 illustrates a diagnostic and management algorithm for endometriosis.

SURGICAL STAGING

- American Society for Reproductive Medicine classification system for endometriosis (ASRM revised 1996) is the most widely accepted staging system.
- Value: Uniform recording of operative findings.
- Limitations
  1. Not a good predictor of successful pregnancy after treatment.
  2. Does not correlate well with the symptoms of pain, dyspareunia, or infertility.

Stage I	Minimal
Stage II	Mild
Stage III	Moderate
Stage IV	Severe

LABORATORY TESTS

Cancer antigen 125 (CA125): Limited overall value in the diagnosis of endometriosis

- Also elevated in ovarian epithelial neoplasm, myomas, adenomyosis, acute PID, ovarian cysts, pancreatitis, chronic liver disease, menstruation, and pregnancy.
- CA125 value >35 U/ml: Positive predictive value of 0.58 and a negative predictive value of 0.96 for the presence of endometriosis.

IMAGING STUDIES

- Ultrasound: For evaluating adnexal mass; ultrasound characteristics may suggest endometriomas versus other benign or malignant ovarian conditions but persistent solid or cystic-solid ovarian masses require definitive tissue diagnosis with laparoscopy.
- MRI:
  1. Highly accurate in detecting endometriomas.
  2. Limited sensitivity in detecting diffuse pelvic endometriosis, especially if sessile lesions.
- CT scan may show adnexal masses of varying density (Fig. 3).

Rx TREATMENT

NONPHARMACOLOGIC THERAPY

Expectant management (observation for 5-12 mo) for stage I or stage II endometriosis-associated infertility. Evaluation should take place if the couple meets the diagnostic criteria for infertility.

ACUTE GENERAL Rx

Nonsteroidal antiinflammatory drugs for symptomatic relief of dysmenorrhea.

CHRONIC Rx

PHARMACOLOGIC MANAGEMENT:

Estrogen-progesterone:

- State of "pseudopregnancy" created by continuous (discarding pill pack when placebo pills remaining and starting active pills from new pill pack) use of combination oral contraceptives for minimum of 6 mo and continuing indefinitely.

Progestins:

- Medroxyprogesterone acetate 10 to 30 mg orally qd and occasionally up to 100 mg orally qd.
- Alternatively, 100 mg IM q2wk for four doses, followed by 200 mg IM monthly for 4 mo.
- Comparison with danazol: Progestins cost less, have a more tolerable side-effect profile, and have comparable efficacy with regard to pain relief and so are often the first-line drug. Very little justification for the use of danazol.

Gonadotropin-releasing hormone (GnRH) agonists:

- Induces medical menopause.
- Use usually limited to 6 to 12 mo due to hypoestrogenic effects such as osteopenia or osteoporosis but can be given longer in certain circumstances, particularly when paired with estrogen add-back therapy. Referral to specialist strongly advised.
- Elagolix is an oral GnRH antagonist that provides partial to nearly full estrogen suppression. Dosage is 150 mg once daily or 200 mg twice daily. It is effective in improving dysmenorrhea and nonmenstrual pain, but is associated with

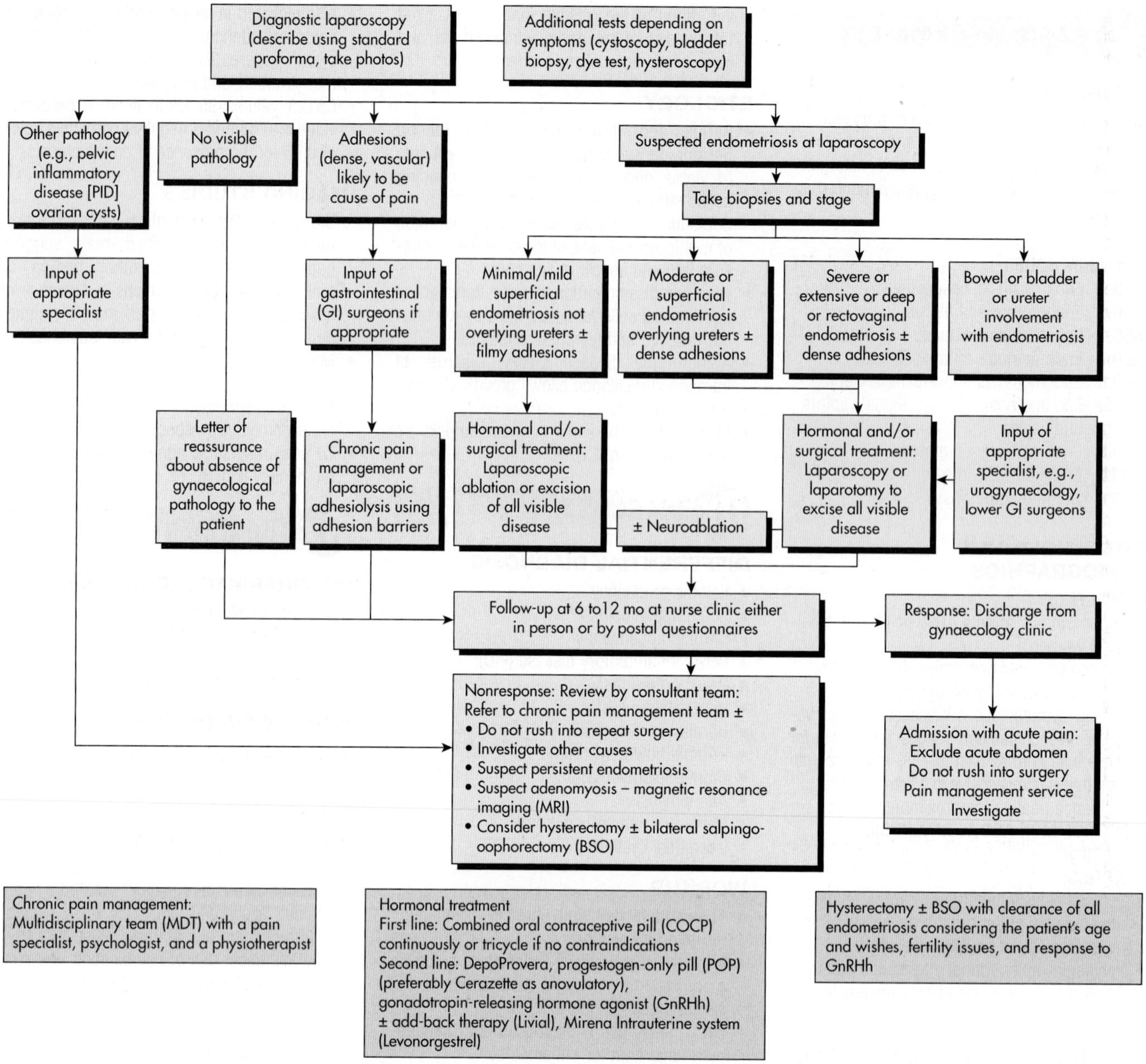

FIG. 2 An example of a management pathway for patients with endometriosis after laparoscopy. (From Magowan BA: *Clinical obstetrics and gynecology*, ed 4, Philadelphia, 2019, Elsevier.)

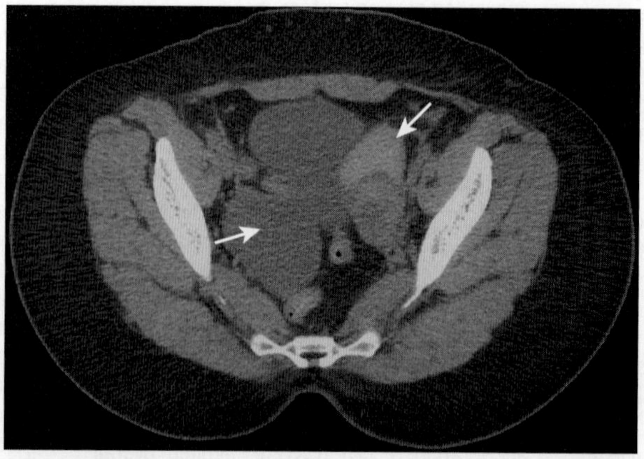

FIG. 3 Computed tomography scan demonstrates adnexal masses of varying density, subsequently proven to be endometriomas. (From Fielding JR et al: *Gynecologic imaging*, Philadelphia, 2011, Saunders.)

hypoestrogenic side effects (hot flashes, hyperlipidemia, decreased bone density).

- Leuprolide acetate depot 3.75 mg IM monthly or 11.25 mg IM q3mo or nafarelin 400 mcg nasal puffs bid or goserelin 3.6 mg SC monthly.
- Add-back therapy for protection against vasomotor symptoms and bone loss: Norethindrone acetate 5 mg PO qd alone or in combination with conjugated estrogen 0.625 mg orally qd.
- Add-back therapy allows gonadotropin-releasing hormone (GnRH) agonist use to be extended to 1 yr based on limited studies available.

Alternative therapies for inhibition of estrogen action currently under investigation are:

- Aromatase inhibitors: Anastrozole, letrozole
- SERM: Raloxifene
- Agents enhancing cell-mediated immunity are cytokines (interleukin-12 and interferon-α2b)
- Immunomodulators (loxoribine, levamisole)
- Antiinflammatory: Pentoxifylline

SURGICAL MANAGEMENT:

Conservative:

- Directed at enhancing fertility or treating pain unresponsive to first-line medical treatment.
- Usually accomplished through laparoscopy.
- Removal or destruction of endometriotic implants by excision, electrocautery, or laser.
- Cystectomy for endometrioma; must remove cyst wall to be effective long-term.
- Laparoscopic uterosacral nerve ablation (LUNA) for midline pain such as dysmenorrhea or dyspareunia (evidence does not support its use).
- Unless pregnancy is desired, patient is usually started on GnRH agonist therapy or continuous OCP immediately after surgery.
- For those desiring pregnancy, surgery alone results in significant increase in fertility.

Definitive:

- Directed at relieving endometriosis-associated pain.
- Total abdominal hysterectomy with bilateral salpingo-oophorectomy and complete excision or ablation of endometriosis.
- Thorough abdominal exploration to ensure removal of all disease.
- Must be prepared to manage possible gastrointestinal and urinary tract endometriosis.
- 90% effective in pain relief; patient must be counseled that pain relief is not guaranteed.
- Estrogen replacement therapy (ERT) to be considered in all women undergoing definitive surgical management; after ERT, recurrence rate is 0% to 5% in women with endometriosis confined to the pelvis but 18% in women with bowel involvement.
- Concern for malignant degeneration exists in implants if unopposed estrogen is used after definitive surgical therapy.

MANAGEMENT OF ENDOMETRIOSIS-ASSOCIATED INFERTILITY:

Conservative surgery:

- Yields significantly higher pregnancy rate than does expectant management, in part because of correction of mechanical factors such as adhesions.

Assisted reproductive technologies:

- Can be used to circumvent unknown mechanism of endometriosis-associated infertility.
- Superovulation with clomiphene citrate or human menopausal gonadotropins; clomiphene citrate results in threefold pregnancy rate over expectant management.
- Further improvement with intrauterine insemination combined with superovulation.
- In vitro fertilization if above procedures are unsuccessful.

DISPOSITION

Tends to recur unless definitive surgery is performed, and should be considered a chronic condition.

REFERRAL

To a reproductive endocrinologist for advanced surgical management or infertility management

PEARLS & CONSIDERATIONS

COMMENTS

Patient information can be obtained through the following organizations: Endometriosis Association, 8585 North 76th Place, Milwaukee, WI 53223, 414-355-2200 or 800-992-ENDO; Women's Reproductive Health Network, P.O. Box 30167, Portland, OR 97230-9067 or 503-667-7757.

SUGGESTED READINGS

Available at ExpertConsult.com

RELATED CONTENT

Endometriosis (Patient Information)
Dysmenorrhea (Related Key Topic)
Dyspareunia (Related Key Topic)

AUTHOR: **Barbara McGuirk, MD**

BASIC INFORMATION

DEFINITION

Per the Centers for Medicare and Medicaid Services, end-stage renal disease (ESRD) is a medical condition in which a person's kidneys cease functioning on a permanent basis leading to the need for a regular course of long-term dialysis or a kidney transplant to maintain life. Briefly, ESRD is chronic kidney disease (CKD) that requires long-term renal replacement therapy (RRT). Increasingly, the term end-stage kidney disease (ESKD) is used instead of ESRD because the word "kidney" is more recognizable than "renal" to the lay public.

SYNONYMS

Dialysis dependency
Renal replacement therapy
Chronic irreversible renal failure

ICD-10CM CODES

N18.6	End-stage renal disease
Z99.2	Dependence on renal dialysis
Z94.0	Kidney transplant status

EPIDEMIOLOGY & DEMOGRAPHICS

INCIDENCE: According to the U.S. Renal Data System (USRDS), there were approximately 124,500 incident cases of ESRD in the U.S. in 2017.

- 86.9% of incident individuals began RRT with hemodialysis (HD)
- 10.1% of incident individuals began RRT peritoneal dialysis (PD)
- 2.9% of incident individuals began RRT with a preemptive kidney transplant
- More recently, there has been an increase in incident PD cases
- There is a significant cost difference among modalities, with average Medicare spending for HD at $91,795 per patient-yr versus PD at $78,159 per patient-yr

The incidence of ESKD differs among countries; the highest frequencies are in Taiwan, U.S., and the Jalisco region of Mexico.

PREVALENCE: Per USRDS, there were 726,331 prevalent cases of ESKD in 2017. The number of prevalent cases has increased by approximately 20,000 annually.

- 62.7% of all prevalent ESKD patients in the U.S. were treated by HD (98% dialyzing at an in-center facility and 2% dialyzing at home).
- 7.1% of all prevalent ESKD patients were treated by PD.
- 29.9% of all prevalent ESKD patients had a functioning kidney transplant.

ESKD prevalence varies greatly by country, with Hong Kong, the Jalisco region of Mexico, and Guatemala having >50% PD utilization. Home HD use is highest in New Zealand and Australia.

PREDOMINANT SEX & AGE: The incidence and prevalence of ESKD increases with age, but individuals can experience ESKD at any age. Older patients are more likely to be dialyzed with HD than PD. Males constitute 57% of prevalent ESKD patients.

RISK FACTORS: Risk factors for the development of ESKD include proteinuria, higher body mass index, diabetes mellitus, high blood pressure, higher serum creatinine, male gender, lower educational status, and African American descent.

GENETICS: Genome-wide association studies (GWAS) have shown several genes that are associated with the development of CKD and progression to ESKD. The *APOL1* gene is most strongly implicated. Single-nucleotide polymorphisms of the following genes are associated with greater risk for the development of ESKD: *UMOD, PRKAG2, ANXA9, DAB2,* and *SHROOM3.*

PHYSICAL FINDINGS & CLINICAL PRESENTATION

Clinical presentations of uremia are myriad. Signs and symptoms may include hypertension, edema, uremic frost, asterixis, ankle clonus, altered mentation, pallor, peripheral neuropathy, coma, and pericardial friction rub. Classic uremic symptoms include anorexia, dysgeusia, aversion to meat, nausea or vomiting, hiccups, pruritus, weight loss, reversal of sleep cycles, restless legs, and loss of energy.

ETIOLOGY

The most common causes of ESKD in the U.S. are, in order of frequency, diabetes, hypertension, glomerulonephritis, and cystic diseases.

DIAGNOSIS

WORKUP

The diagnosis of ESKD is made in the setting of CKD, manifested by an elevated serum creatinine concentration and decreased glomerular filtration rate, typically <10 ml/min per 1.73 m^2. RRT is initiated when uremia, volume overload refractory to diuretic therapy, or electrolyte abnormalities refractory to medical therapy is present. The workup of CKD is discussed elsewhere (see "Chronic Kidney Disease"). The ongoing workup of the consequences of ESKD include measures of anemia, iron metabolism, metabolic acidosis, and mineral and bone disease.

LABORATORY TESTS

Laboratory tests that warrant monitoring in ESKD include electrolytes, blood urea nitrogen, creatinine, glucose, calcium, phosphorus, intact parathyroid hormone, 25-hydroxyvitamin D, complete blood count with reticulocyte count, serum iron, transferrin saturation, and ferritin.

TREATMENT

- A patient with HD will require vascular access for dialysis that is typically a hemodialysis catheter or arteriovenous fistula or graft (Table 1).
  1. A subcutaneously tunneled dialysis catheter is ideally placed in the right internal jugular vein.
  2. An arteriovenous graft or fistula should be palpated regularly to ensure flow, which is noted by the presence of bruit and thrill. If the thrill is decreased or absent, the vascular access is clotting, which prompts vascular access intervention.
  3. The most common arteriovenous fistulas are radiocephalic, brachiocephalic, and brachiobasilic. It is important in patients with CKD and ESKD to preserve veins in nondominant upper extremities by avoiding unnecessary venipunctures and intravenous lines, including central venous catheters and peripherally inserted central catheters.
- Patients who require dialysis have two primary options for RRT: HD and PD.
  1. In HD, the bloodstream is cannulated and diverted through a hemodialyzer that filters the plasma phase of blood running countercurrent to a dialysate enriched in bicarbonate and that contains other minerals and glucose (Table 2).
     a. Dialysis is effective only for the clearance of non–protein-bound molecules.
     b. Typical blood flow rate varies from 300 to 500 ml/min. Dialysate flow rate ranges from 500 to 800 ml/min.
     c. Small solutes such as potassium will equilibrate quickly, whereas larger solutes such as beta 2-microglobulin take longer to equilibrate.
     d. The volume of ultrafiltrate, or plasma without protein, that is removed is determined clinically.

TABLE 1 Hemodialysis Vascular Access

Vascular Access	Description	Benefits	Drawbacks
Tunneled catheter	Subcutaneously tunneled under skin to reduce contamination by skin flora	Immediate use	High infection risk High thrombosis risk
Arteriovenous graft	Synthetic tube connecting artery to vein	Ready to use when swelling resolves (~2 wk) Able to use in most patients	High stenosis/thrombosis rate Moderate infectious risk
Arteriovenous fistula	Vein cross-cut attached end-to-side to artery High-pressure flow dilates and thickens vein	Lowest infectious risk Longest lasting with lowest thrombosis risk	Maturation time Primary patency

TABLE 2 Composition of Typical Hemodialysis and Peritoneal Dialysis Solutions

Component	Concentration in Hemodialysis Solutions	Concentration in Peritoneal Dialysis Solutions
Sodium	135-145 mEq/L	132 mEq/L
Potassium	1-3 mEq/L	0 mEq/L
Calcium	2.5-3.5 mEq/L	2.5-3.5 mEq/L
Chloride	95-110 mEq/L	95-105 mEq/L
Magnesium	0.5-1 mEq/L	0.5 mEq/L
Bicarbonate	32-40 mEq/L	
Lactate		35-40 mEq/L
Acetate	2.5-5 mEq/L	
Glucose	200 mg/dl	1500-4250 mg/dl

2. In PD, the blood flow originates from the vascular parietal and visceral peritoneum, with the peritoneal membrane representing the "dialysis" membrane. Peritoneal dialysate is dextrose-based and hypertonic. The hypertonicity produces ultrafiltration. The concentration of dextrose is varied to increase or decrease ultrafiltration according to the clinical requirements.
   a. A tunneled catheter is placed through the abdominal wall. Peritoneal dialysate is infused into the peritoneum and left to "dwell" as solute transfer occurs via convection or diffusion across concentration gradients.
   b. PD can be performed manually throughout the day or overnight via an automated cycler device.

- In patients who require RRT, withholding treatment has substantial risk.
  1. Patients with late-stage CKD are hypertensive in nearly 90% of cases. If hypertension is untreated, the risks for accelerated heart disease and/or stroke increase.
  2. Hyperkalemic patients have increased risk of sudden cardiac death. Metabolic acidosis may increase risk for cardiovascular failure and bone demineralization.
  3. Patients with untreated uremia may manifest neuromuscular irritability, including seizures, or confusion, altered mentation, and coma.
  4. Uremia may cause platelet dysfunction and increased risk for bleeding.
- In addition to RRT, patient management of ESKD patients involves treatment of anemia in CKD, disorders of bone and mineral metabolism, and cardiovascular disease.
  1. Patients receiving dialysis experience anemia for several reasons, including erythropoietin deficiency, gastrointestinal bleeding, functional and absolute iron deficiency, increased red blood cell fragility, and blood loss from HD.
     a. Management of anemia in CKD depends on the primary causative factor.
     b. Iron utilization is estimated using ferritin (>100 ng/ml) and transferrin saturation (>20%). Patients who do not meet these parameters are first managed with intravenous iron or a trial of oral iron. Intravenous iron may be administered without a trial of oral iron. In patients who are iron replete, erythropoiesis-stimulating agents are used to increase hemoglobin. Large randomized controlled trials demonstrate an association between increased cancer death and stroke with attainment of hemoglobin levels >11 g/dl. The target hemoglobin range for a dialysis patient is 9.0 to 11.0 g/dl, and these are not absolute criteria.
- Patients with ESKD are at risk for several different metabolic bone disorders.
  1. Secondary hyperparathyroidism of renal origin occurs in the majority of individuals who require RRT. This disorder is aggravated by concurrent metabolic acidosis. The intact PTH level is characteristically elevated in these individuals, with an entry level of nearly 500 pg/ml at initiation of RRT.
  2. The gold-standard diagnosis for establishing a histologic diagnosis is bone biopsy. Bone lesion parameters are reported as turnover, mineralization, and volume.
  3. Patients who do not undergo bone biopsy are managed by serologic markers, calcium, phosphate, and intact parathyroid hormone.
  4. Adynamic bone disease occurs more frequently in diabetic ESKD patients. Typically, the intact PTH level is low (<150 pg/ml). PD has a greater risk for adynamic bone disease. Patients undergoing HD are at greatest risk for osteitis fibrosis cystica and mixed lesions.
  5. Mixed uremic osteodystrophy that has histological characteristics of hyperdynamic and adynamic bone remodeling.
  6. Osteopenia.
- ESKD is considered a coronary heart disease equivalent with enhanced risk of mortality from cardiovascular causes. However, data are lacking regarding the efficacy of cardiovascular risk modification.
  1. Studies of statin therapy in patients with ESKD have not shown a reduction in cardiovascular mortality. Initiation of statin therapy after beginning RRT is not recommended.
  2. Levels of cardiac biomarkers such as troponin-I and N-terminal pro-B-type natriuretic peptide (NT-proBNP) are frequently and chronically elevated in ESKD. Interpretation of these biomarkers must be considered in the context of clinical findings.
  3. Hemoglobin A1c levels are reduced in ESKD patients due to shortened red blood cell lifespan. Add approximately 0.3% to the A1c level of an ESKD patient.
- Because multiple medications are renally excreted or nephrotoxic, careful attention must be paid to choice and dosing of medications. Commonly used medications that should be used with caution in ESKD include low-molecular-weight heparin, morphine, oxycodone, gabapentin, pregabalin, digoxin, bisphosphonates, sodium glucose contransport inhibitors, metformin, and electrolyte-containing solutions, including milk of magnesium, magnesium citrate, aluminum hydroxide, and magnesium hydroxide.
- Management of ESKD patients in the Intensive Care Unit is summarized in Table E3.

DISPOSITION

Morbidity and mortality remain exceptionally high for patients who require RRT.

- Dialysis patients in 2017 had a mortality rate of 165 deaths per 1000 patient-yr.
- This rate has been improving, with net reductions in mortality from 2001 to 2017 of 27% for HD patients and 43% for PD patients.
- HD patients have greater earlier mortality, and PD patients have greater delayed mortality.
- 5-yr survival probability rates are 42% for HD patients and 52.1% for PD patients. The difference in survival rates is likely related to patient-selection factors rather than differences between modalities.

SUGGESTED READINGS

Available at ExpertConsult.com

RELATED CONTENT

Chronic Kidney Disease (Related Key Topic)

AUTHORS: **Ankur Shah, MD**

BASIC INFORMATION

DEFINITION

Enteropathic arthritis (EA) is an inflammatory joint disease associated with inflammatory bowel diseases (IBD) such as Crohn disease (CD), ulcerative colitis (UC), and microscopic colitis. Less frequently, EA is associated with other gastrointestinal disorders, including Whipple disease, celiac disease, and bowel-associated dermatitis-arthritis syndrome related to bypass surgery or intestinal disease. EA is included in the family of spondyloarthropathies (SpA), which have features of peripheral inflammatory arthritis, axial spondylitis and sacroiliitis, enthesitis, dactylitis, uveitis, and rashes. Arthritis is the most common extraintestinal manifestation of IBD.

SYNONYMS

IBD-related spondyloarthropathy
Enteroarthritis
Arthritis associated with gastrointestinal disease

ICD-10CM CODES	
M07.60	Enteropathic arthropathies, unspecified sites
M07.68	Enteropathic arthropathies, vertebra
M07.69	Enteropathic arthropathies, multiple sites
M07.611	Enteropathic arthropathies, right shoulder
M07.612	Enteropathic arthropathies, left shoulder
M07.619	Enteropathic arthropathies, unspecified shoulder
M07.621	Enteropathic arthropathies, right elbow
M07.622	Enteropathic arthropathies, left elbow
M07.629	Enteropathic arthropathies, unspecified elbow
M07.631	Enteropathic arthropathies, right wrist
M07.632	Enteropathic arthropathies, left wrist
M07.639	Enteropathic arthropathies, unspecified wrist
M07.641	Enteropathic arthropathies, right hand
M07.642	Enteropathic arthropathies, left hand
M07.649	Enteropathic arthropathies, unspecified hand
M07.651	Enteropathic arthropathies, right hip
M07.652	Enteropathic arthropathies, left hip
M07.659	Enteropathic arthropathies, unspecified hip
M07.661	Enteropathic arthropathies, right knee
M07.662	Enteropathic arthropathies, left knee
M07.669	Enteropathic arthropathies, unspecified knee
M07.671	Enteropathic arthropathies, right ankle and foot
M07.672	Enteropathic arthropathies, left ankle and foot
M07.679	Enteropathic arthropathies, unspecified ankle and foot
M07.68	Enteropathic arthropathies, vertebrae
M07.69	Enteropathic arthropathies, multiple sites

EPIDEMIOLOGY & DEMOGRAPHICS

Peripheral arthritis occurs in 5% to 15% of patients with IBD in most studies and is slightly more common in CD than in UC. Spinal involvement occurs in 10% to 20% of cases and may be the only articular manifestation or be accompanied by peripheral arthritis.

PREDOMINANT SEX & AGE: Males and females equally affected. Inflammatory back pain usually presents before the age of 45 yr. Onset of peripheral arthritis is usually between 25 and 45 yr of age.

RISK FACTORS:

- Active large bowel disease
- Family history of IBD
- Cigarette smoking
- Genetics
- Complicating intestinal manifestations such as abscesses and perianal disease

GENETICS: The presence of *HLA-B27* is the strongest association with SpA. Recent genome-wide association studies demonstrated a genetic overlap between IBD and SpA, implicating *NOD2 (CARD15)* and interleukin 23 receptor *(IL23R)* as susceptibility genes.

PHYSICAL FINDINGS & CLINICAL PRESENTATION

- Two types of joint involvement in IBD: Peripheral and/or axial. Peripheral: Affects peripheral joints, predominantly lower limb joints. Axial: Affects the spine in the form of sacroiliitis with or without spondylitis; can be similar to ankylosing spondylitis or other idiopathic SpA (e.g., psoriatic arthritis, reactive arthritis, undifferentiated SpA).
- Axial involvement is found more commonly in CD than in UC. Axial disease is independent of IBD activity. Can have asymptomatic sacroiliitis.
- Peripheral arthritis is the most frequent extraintestinal finding in both CD and UC. Peripheral and spinal disease equally affects both sexes (Table 1).
- Type 1 peripheral arthropathy (pauciarticular, fewer than five joints): Usually acute and self-limited asymmetric inflammatory arthritis; commonly affects large joints of legs such as the knee; occurs early in the course of IBD and commonly parallels the disease activity or flares of IBD, generally self-limiting.
- Type 2 peripheral arthropathy (polyarticular, five or more joints): Affects mainly the metacarpophalangeal, proximal interphalangeal, knee and ankle joints; bilateral and symmetric; may be migratory, nonerosive. Symptoms may take a more chronic course, independent of IBD activity.
- Main complaints are inflammatory back pain, buttock pain, joint pain, and swelling (with prolonged morning stiffness and fatigue); symptoms worse with rest or inactivity and improve with exercise.
- Examination reveals evidence of synovitis, progressive limitation of spinal mobility.
- Periarticular and other extraintestinal manifestations include enthesitis (inflammation of tendon insertion sites into bone such as Achilles or plantar fascia), dactylitis (flexor tenosynovitis of a finger or toe causing sausage like swelling of digit), uveitis, and psoriasis.
- Uveitis in IBD is more often bilateral and more prone to chronicity.

TABLE 1 Enteropathic Arthritis

Feature	Peripheral Arthritis	Sacroiliitis, Spondylitis
Crohn Disease		
Frequency in CD	10%-20%	2%-7%
HLA-B27 associated	No	Yes
Pattern	Transient, symmetrical	Chronic
Course	Related to activity of CD	Unrelated to activity of CD
Effect of surgery	Remission of arthritis uncommon	No effect
Effect of anti-TNF therapy	Effective	Effective
Ulcerative Colitis		
Frequency in UC	5%-10%	2%-7%
HLA-B27 associated	No	Yes
Pattern	Transient	Chronic
Course	More common in pancolitis than proctitis; related to activity of UC	Unrelated
Effect of surgery	Remission of arthritis	No effect

CD, Crohn disease; *HLA,* human leukocyte antigen; *TNF,* tumor necrosis factor; *UC,* ulcerative colitis.
From Goldman L, Schafer AI: *Goldman's Cecil medicine,* ed 24, Philadelphia, 2012, Saunders.

- Erythema nodosum, pyoderma gangrenosum can be skin lesions seen in IBD.

ETIOLOGY

In genetically predisposed individuals with intestinal disease, the co-occurrence of joint inflammation provides important support to the theory that dysbiosis in the gut microbiome can link colitis to the development of EA.

Dx DIAGNOSIS

DIFFERENTIAL DIAGNOSIS

- Hypertrophic osteoarthropathy
- Osteonecrosis (avascular necrosis)
- Septic arthritis
- Other idiopathic seronegative spondyloarthropathies (e.g., reactive arthritis, psoriatic arthritis, ankylosing spondylitis)
- Behçet syndrome
- Rheumatoid arthritis

WORKUP

Diagnosis mainly relies on clinical features and imaging data. There is no gold standard for diagnosis.

LABORATORY TESTS

- Laboratory testing: Markers of inflammation such as sedimentation rate and C-reactive protein (CRP) may reflect underlying disease activity of bowel disease and thus may not be useful to track for EA activity. CBC can reveal leukocytosis, anemia, thrombocytosis suggestive of inflammatory response.
- Synovial fluid is nonspecific; shows mild to marked inflammation: WBC 1500-50,000/mm^3.
- Serologic tests for rheumatoid arthritis are negative (rheumatoid factor, cyclic-citrullinated peptide antibodies), and lupus-related antinuclear antibodies are usually absent.
- Tests for other intestinal diseases based on clinical suspicion: Whipple diagnosis is based on histology with Periodic acid–Schiff (PAS)-positive cells, serology for *T. whipplei*, and culture; celiac disease immunoglobulin A (IgA) antitissue transglutaminase and antiendomysial antibodies along with diagnostic villous atrophy on small bowel biopsy; microscopic colitis diagnosed only through histology from colonoscopy showing collagenous colitis or lymphocytic colitis.
- Calprotectin measured in the serum or in the stools has been used to identify subclinical bowel inflammation in patients with SpA. Individuals who had both CRP and calprotectin elevated had an increased frequency of bowel inflammation compared to patients who had low levels of these proteins.

IMAGING STUDIES

- Plain x-ray of the spine and pelvis may appear normal in early disease but with progression may show evidence of sacroiliitis, spondylitis, ankyloses.
- X-ray of peripheral joints may show soft tissue swelling, periostitis, or joint effusion.
- MRI may be used to assess early changes of spondyloarthritis when plain x-rays are negative. MRI is the most sensitive method of detecting sacroiliitis in IBD patients.
- Musculoskeletal ultrasonography is a noninvasive, safe, and easily reproducible means of detecting early pathologic changes in SpA patients. It can identify characteristic features of enthesitis, bone erosions, synovitis, bursitis, and tenosynovitis.

Rx TREATMENT

- Effective treatment of underlying IBD is helpful in controlling the peripheral arthritis. The goal of treatment of EA is reducing inflammation to relieve suffering and prevent joint deformity and disability.
- When IBD and SpA coexist, treatment strategy should also address extraintestinal and extraarticular features such as enthesitis, dactylitis, uveitis, and psoriasis, with need for tailored consideration of certain limited biologic options.
- Avoidance of NSAIDs due to controversial increased risk of exacerbation of intestinal disease.

NONPHARMACOLOGIC THERAPY

Rest, physical therapy, and exercise such as swimming

ACUTE GENERAL Rx

- There has been concern that NSAIDs exacerbate IBD and that NSAID-related adverse events such as ulcers and GI bleeding may mimic IBD flares. COX-2 inhibitors may be preferred to traditional NSAIDs, but similar concerns and cautions apply.
- Intraarticular steroid injections may help treat joint synovitis.
- Systemic steroids can help reduce polyarticular joint and IBD activity but should be used at the lowest effective dose and ideally for only short courses.

CHRONIC Rx

- Immunomodulatory agents such as sulfasalazine, azathioprine, 6-mercaptopurine, methotrexate, and cyclosporine can be used to treat active IBD, peripheral arthritis, and associated skin conditions. Peripheral joint disease responds better to these agents than axial disease. Tumor necrosis factor (TNF) inhibitors, particularly infliximab, adalimumab, and certolizumab, are useful to treat both arthritis (axial or peripheral) and severe, refractory IBD. Golimumab is also in use for refractory IBD and is used for arthritis. Etanercept is not effective to control IBD.
- The axial disease associated with IBD is treated similar to other SpA. Medications approved for other SpAs, such as ustekinumab (anti-IL12/23), secukinumab (anti-IL17A), ixekizumab (anti-IL17), and Janus kinase (JAK) inhibitors, may be effective therapies for EA, though not all have clear efficacy in IBD. Anti-IL17 is usually avoided with IBD, given possible worsening of IBD. Ustekinumab is approved to treat Crohn disease. Tofacitinib (JAKi) is approved to treat UC.
- The choice of biologic requires the consideration of extraarticular and extraintestinal features such as skin disease or uveitis. The latter can be treated with infliximab or adalimumab, both of which also treat IBD.
- For highly active IBD, particularly UC, colectomy has been found to ameliorate peripheral joint inflammatory disease but does not influence axial involvement.
- Interdisciplinary approach and active cooperation between rheumatologist and gastroenterologist through combined clinics, for example, are essential.

REFERRAL

Rheumatology and gastroenterology

PEARLS & CONSIDERATIONS

- When a single joint is affected, consider joint aspiration to rule out septic arthritis. Signs of infection may be atypical in those receiving antiinflammatory or immunosuppressive medications.
- Other extraintestinal manifestations of enteropathic arthritis include skin and mucous membrane involvement, anterior uveitis, Hashimoto thyroiditis, genitourinary involvement (nephrolithiasis), aortic insufficiency, and cardiac conduction abnormalities. These are often seen in patients with prolonged disease activity and positive *HLA-B27.*

SUGGESTED READINGS

Available at ExpertConsult.com

RELATED TOPICS

Ankylosing Spondylitis (Related Key Topic)
Crohn Disease (Related Key Topic)
Psoriatic Arthritis (Related Key Topic)
Spondyloarthropathies (Related Key Topic)
Ulcerative Colitis (Related Key Topic)

AUTHORS: **Candice Reyes, MD, RhMSUS,** and **Amani A. Elghafri, MD, MSc, MEd**

BASIC INFORMATION

DEFINITION

Eosinophilic esophagitis is a chronic, antigen- and immune-mediated disease, which requires these inclusion criteria after secondary causes of esophageal eosinophilia are excluded:

1. Inflammation secondary to eosinophilic infiltration within the esophagus (confirmed with at least 15 eosinophils per high power field [HPF] detected on biopsy of mucosa taken at proximal and distal esophagus)
2. Symptoms related to esophageal dysfunction

Mucosal eosinophilia is isolated to the esophagus and persists after a proton pump inhibitor (PPI) trial.

SYNONYMS

Esophageal eosinophilia
EoE
EE

ICD-10CM CODE

K20.0 Eosinophilic esophagitis

EPIDEMIOLOGY & DEMOGRAPHICS

INCIDENCE (IN U.S.): 1 to 20 new cases per 100,000 inhabitants per yr, increased from last year

PREVALENCE: Between 13 and 49 cases per 100,000 inhabitants

PREDOMINANT SEX: Male predominance (ratio ~3:1)

PREDOMINANT AGE: Peak of disease activity at age 35 to 39

PEAK INCIDENCE: Older children; in adults, ages 30 to 50

RISK FACTORS/ETIOLOGY: Genetic (see below), host immune, and environmental. Allergy plays a significant role in the pathophysiology of EoE. Elimination of food antigens with an elemental diet leads to resolution of esophageal eosinophilia in over 90% of patients.

GENETICS:

- Association between thymic stromal lymphopoietin *(TSL)* gene mutation and risk for EoE
- Higher risk in those with homozygous pattern for the mutation
- *TSL* gene found on Yp11.3 chromosome
- Association with polymorphism on eotaxin-3 (CCL-26)

PHYSICAL FINDINGS & CLINICAL PRESENTATION

- Adults: Dysphagia to solid foods, food impaction, heartburn, noncardiac chest pain, increased time to consume meals, concurrent atopic diseases (asthma, eczema, rhinitis, atopic dermatitis, seasonal/food allergies)
- Children: Vomiting, regurgitation, nausea, epigastric/abdominal pain, chest pain, water brash, globus, decreased appetite, gagging, choking, refusal of food, possible atopy, failure to thrive
- Often associated with asthma, rhinitis, dermatitis, and other atopic conditions

DIAGNOSIS

DIFFERENTIAL DIAGNOSIS

- Gastroesophageal reflux disease
- PPI-responsive esophageal eosinophilia (PPI-REE)—see "Acute General Rx"
- Celiac disease
- Eosinophilic gastroenteritis
- Crohn disease
- Hypereosinophilic syndrome
- Achalasia
- Vasculitis/pemphigus/connective tissue diseases
- Infectious (fungal/viral)
- Graft-versus-host disease
- Pemphigus
- Connective tissue disease

WORKUP

- Esophagogastroduodenoscopy (EGD) with at least two to four biopsies from distal and mid/proximal esophagus after a PPI trial
- Confirmation: Persistence of symptoms *and* ≥15 eosinophils/HPF on pathology (Fig. 1) although esophagus is normal in ~5% to 10% of patients.
- Other histological findings can include basal zone hyperplasia, dilated intracellular spaces, and subepithelial fibrosis.
- Endoscopic findings can include white mucosal papules, which represent eosinophilic microabscesses, linear furrows, esophageal narrowing with stricture, mucosal tearing, and esophageal trachealization (Fig. 2), esophageal rings, felinization of esophagus. Felinization of the esophagus is a radiologic term used to describe 1- to 2-mm transverse folds found circumferentially along the entire lumen of the esophagus that appear transiently on EGD and barium studies, possibly attributed to thickened and contracted muscularis mucosae.

LABORATORY TESTS

- 40% to 50% have elevated peripheral eosinophilia
- 50% to 60% have elevated serum immunoglobulin E (IgE) levels

IMAGING STUDIES

Esophagram can reveal rings and strictures. In one study 26% of esophageal strictures less than 15 mm in diameter were detected on esophogram but missed on endoscopy.[1]

[1] Gentile N et al: Oesophageal narrowing is common and frequently under-appreciated at endoscopy in patients with oesophageal eosinophilia, *Aliment Pharmacol Ther* 40:1333-1340, 2014.

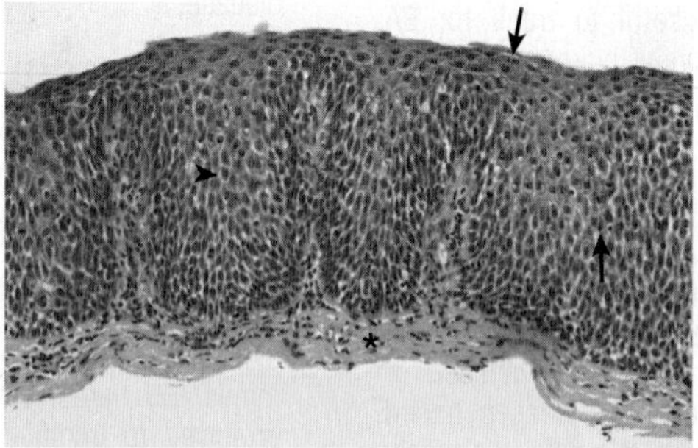

FIG. 1 H&E staining of an esophageal specimen from a patient with eosinophilic esophagitis. *Arrows* point to eosinophils, including some at the surface. *Arrowhead* points to dilated intercellular spaces. *Asterisk* marks the lamina propria, showing inflammation and fibrosis. *Green arrow* points to elongated papillae. There is also marked basal layer hyperplasia, with the basal layer reaching almost to the luminal surface. *H&E*, hematoxylin and eosin. (From Feldman M et al: *Sleisenger and Fordtran's gastrointestinal and liver disease*, ed 10, Philadelphia, 2016, Elsevier.)

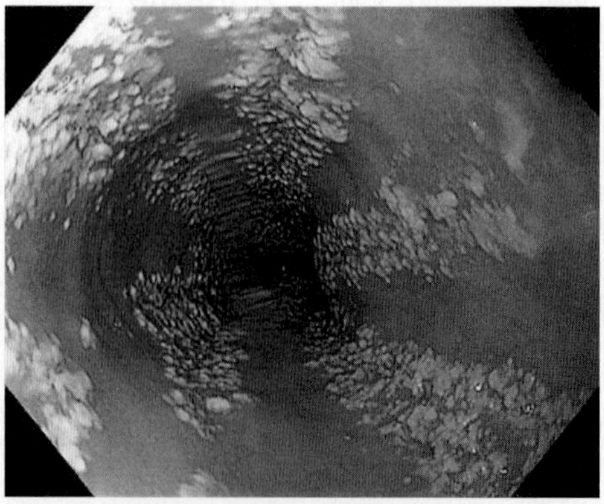

FIG. 2 Endoscopic view of eosinophilic esophagitis with furrowing and exudates. (From Feldman M et al: *Sleisenger and Fordtran's gastrointestinal and liver disease*, ed 10, Philadelphia, 2016, Elsevier.)

Rx TREATMENT

NONPHARMACOLOGIC THERAPY

Three strategies of dietary therapy:

- Empiric six-food elimination diet (eliminates milk, soy, egg, wheat, nuts, and seafood)
  For patients with response, foods can be reintroduced one at a time for 6 wk
- Total elimination of all food allergens with elemental or amino acid–based formula
- Targeted elimination diet guided by allergy testing, typically skin prick testing or patch testing
- Dilation if stricture is present and/or patient is refractory to therapy with the goal of creating a tear in the mucosa

ACUTE GENERAL Rx

- An 8-wk trial of PPI therapy to exclude PPI-responsive esophageal eosinophilia should be initiated after an initial EGD with biopsy based on clinical symptoms with subsequent EGD (with biopsies).
  1. If eosinophilia persists on biopsy despite PPI use, diagnosis is EoE.
  2. If eosinophilia is reduced on repeat biopsies, patient is considered to have proton pump inhibitor-responsive esophageal eosinophilia (PPI-REE), not EoE.
- An EGD (with biopsies) should be performed initially if a critical stricture is present (e.g., patient presents with food impaction).
- If EoE is confirmed, patient should be tried on aerosolized topical glucocorticoids (fluticasone or budesonide) and/or dietary elimination.
  1. Topical steroids shown to be most effective:
     a. Swallowed fluticasone 880 to 1760 mcg/day in a divided dose bid (adult dosing)
        (1) Delivered by meter-dosed inhaler without a spacer.
        (2) Medication is sprayed into the patient's mouth and then swallowed.
        (3) Patient should **not** inhale when the medication is being delivered.
        (4) Patient should not eat or drink for 30 to 60 min following administration.
     b. Swallowed budesonide 2 mg daily, typically in divided doses
        (1) Administered using a nebulizer: Patient then instructed to swallow accumulated liquid
        (2) Administered as viscous slurry: Mixing 1 mg/2 ml nebulizer ampules with sucralose (five 1-g packets per 1 mg of budesonide)
        (3) Patient should not eat or drink for 30 to 60 min after taking the budesonide suspension

CHRONIC Rx

- If patient is responsive to PPI therapy, EoE has been excluded and patient can be continued on PPI therapy with surveillance of symptoms.
- If patient is responsive to aerosolized topical steroids and/or dietary modification, continue steroids at lowest dose and/or continue dietary elimination.
- If lack of response to initial therapy:
  1. Assess compliance
  2. Restrict diet further
  3. Increase steroid dose or consider alternative steroid
  4. Switch from dietary modification to steroid therapy and vice versa
  5. Consider second-line agents or clinical trials
  6. Reevaluate diagnosis and secondary causes of esophageal eosinophilia (see "Differential Diagnosis" earlier)
- Chronic histologic and symptomatic surveillance is recommended
- If dysphagia persists, endoscopic dilation is recommended for amelioration of symptoms.

DISPOSITION

Follow-up by gastroenterologist is important to gauge progression or regression of disease.

REFERRAL

Referrals to gastroenterologists, allergists, and dieticians allow for a multidisciplinary approach to diagnosis and management of EoE.

PEARLS & CONSIDERATIONS

COMMENTS

- EoE can be confused with PPI-REE, and patients should undergo a PPI trial before confirmation of EoE and utilization of topical steroids, step-up elimination diet, or esophageal dilation.
- Endoscopic surveillance of disease with or without symptoms is important.
- While esophageal dilation is the mainstay of therapy in patients with esophageal strictures, narrowing of esophagus, and esophageal rings, dilation will not reduce the risk of recurrence as eosinophilic burden is unaffected.

SUGGESTED READINGS

Available at ExpertConsult.com

RELATED CONTENT

Gastroesophageal Reflux Disease (Related Key Topic)

AUTHOR: **Zilla Hussain, MD**

BASIC INFORMATION

DEFINITION

- Epididymitis is an inflammatory reaction of the epididymis caused by either an infectious agent or local trauma. In most cases of acute epididymitis, the testis is also involved (orchitis).
- Epididymitis is considered chronic if lasting ≥6 wk. Chronic epididymitis has been subcategorized into inflammatory chronic epididymitis, obstructive chronic epididymitis, and chronic epididymalgia.

SYNONYMS

Nonspecific bacterial epididymitis
Sexually transmitted epididymitis

ICD-10CM CODES	
N45.1	Epididymitis
A54.00	Gonococcal infection of lower genitourinary tract, unspecified

EPIDEMIOLOGY & DEMOGRAPHICS

INCIDENCE (IN U.S.): Cause of >600,000 visits to physicians per yr
PREDOMINANT SEX: Exclusive to males
PREDOMINANT AGE: All ages affected but usually in sexually active men or older males
CONGENITAL: Congenital urologic structural disorders possibly predisposing to infections
PEAK INCIDENCE: Sexually active years

PHYSICAL FINDINGS & CLINICAL PRESENTATION

- Tender swelling of the scrotum with erythema, usually unilateral testicular pain and tenderness
- Dysuria and/or urethral discharge
- Fever and signs of systemic illness (less common)
- Pain and redness on scrotal examination
- Hydrocele or even epididymo-orchitis, especially late
- Chronic draining scrotal sinuses with a "beadlike" enlargement of the vas deferens in tuberculous disease

ETIOLOGY

- In young, sexually active men (<35 yr of age), the most common causes of infections are *Neisseria gonorrhoeae* and *Chlamydia trachomatis.*
- In older men (>35 yr of age) or those with underlying urologic disease:
  1. Gram-negative aerobic rods are predominant (i.e., *Escherichia coli*).
  2. Similar organisms are found in men following invasive urologic procedures.
  3. Gram-positive cocci are rarely seen in these groups.
  4. *Mycobacterium tuberculosis* (TB) may also be a cause of epididymitis.
- Acute epididymitis caused by sexually transmitted enteric organisms (e.g., *Escherichia coli*) also occurs among men who are the insertive partner during anal intercourse.
- Young, prepubertal boys may present with epididymitis caused by coliform bacteria; almost always a complication of underlying urologic disease such as reflux.
- In AIDS patients, CMV and *Salmonella* epididymitis have been described. CMV may have a negative urine culture. Toxoplasmosis and *Cryptococcus* should also be considered as a cause of epididymitis in AIDS patients.
- Chronic infectious epididymitis is most frequently seen in conditions associated with granulomatous reaction; TB is the most common granulomatous disease affecting the epididymis.

Dx DIAGNOSIS

DIFFERENTIAL DIAGNOSIS

- Orchitis
- Testicular torsion, trauma, or tumor
- Epididymal cyst
- Hydrocele
- Varicocele
- Spermatocele
- Testicular torsion should be considered in all cases (Table E1).

WORKUP

- Consideration of a full assessment of the urologic tract in patients with bacterial infection, especially if recurrent
- If discharge is present, cultures and Gram stain smear of urethral exudate. Gram stain should demonstrate ≥2 WBC per oil immersion field
- If testicular torsion a consideration: Radionuclear imaging
- Examination of first void uncentrifuged urine for leukocytes if the urethral Gram stain is negative. Positive leukocyte esterase test on first-void urine or microscopic examination of first-void urine sediment will demonstrate ≥2 WBC per high power field. A culture and Gram-stained smear of this urine specimen should be obtained along with nucleic acid amplification testing (NAAT) from urine samples for gonorrhea and chlamydia. *Mycoplasma genitalium* should also be considered. Rectal and oropharyngeal NAAT for gonorrhea and chlamydia may also be helpful in diagnosis if indicated.
- Imaging with sonogram (Fig. E1)

LABORATORY TESTS

- All suspected cases of acute epididymitis should be tested for *C. trachomatis* and for *N. gonorrhoeae* by NAAT. Urine is the preferred specimen for NAAT testing.
- Urinalysis and urine culture if dysuria is present or if urinary tract infection is suspected.
- HIV testing and counseling.
- PPD placed and chest x-ray viewed if TB suspected (rare cases).
- Rarely, biopsy to ensure the diagnosis of tuberculous epididymitis.

Rx TREATMENT

ACUTE GENERAL Rx

- Ice packs and scrotal elevation for relief of pain
- Analgesia with acetaminophen with or without codeine or NSAIDs
- Antibiotics to cover suspected pathogens. Empiric therapy is indicated before laboratory test results are available, but treatment should be guided by culture and susceptibility data.
- Recommended empiric regimens include ceftriaxone 250 mg IM in a single dose plus doxycycline 100 mg bid for 10 days. For acute epididymitis most likely caused by enteric organisms, levofloxacin 500 mg qd × 10 days could be considered.
- Best treatment for older men with gram-negative bacteriuria: Ofloxacin 300 mg PO bid for 10 days or levofloxacin 500 mg PO qd for 10 days
- *Pseudomonas* treatment should be based on antimicrobial susceptibilities, but could be covered by ciprofloxacin PO or IV or cefepime (2 g IV q8h)
- Consider ampicillin-sulbactam, third-generation cephalosporin, ticarcillin-clavulanate, or piperacillin-tazobactam in toxic-appearing patients
- Surgical aspiration of local abscesses or even open surgical drainage
- Diabetics: Especially prone to develop more extensive scrotal infections, including Fournier gangrene
- Reinforcement of compliance with antibiotics to avoid partial treatment

CHRONIC Rx

- Repair of underlying structural defects is considered especially if infections are severe or recur.
- Surgical repair of reflux in young boys should be undertaken promptly and at a young age when possible.
- Sex partners of patient should be referred for evaluation and treatment.

REFERRAL

- If abscess or chronic structural problems suspected
- If another diagnosis, such as testicular torsion, is suspected

PEARLS & CONSIDERATIONS

- Recurrent epididymitis in sexually active men is usually related to failure to simultaneously treat sexual partners for STDs.
- Recurrent epididymitis in nonsexually active men is generally related to structural-anatomic defects in the genitourinary system or relapsing disease from inadequate initial treatment or antimicrobial resistance.
- Tuberculous epididymitis fails to respond to seemingly adequate antimicrobial therapy even without characteristic radiographic changes on chest films.

RELATED CONTENT

Epididymitis (Patient Information)
Orchitis (Related Key Topic)
Testicular Torsion (Related Key Topic)

AUTHORS: **Philip A. Chan, MD, MS,** and **Glenn G. Fort, MD, MPH**

BASIC INFORMATION

DEFINITION

Epidural abscess is a suppurative infection of the central nervous system localized between the dura mater and the overlying skull or vertebral column. There are two types of epidural abscess: Spinal epidural abscess (SEA) and intracranial epidural abscess (IEA), depending on the location within the central nervous system.

SYNONYMS

SEA
Spinal epidural abscess
IEA
Intraspinal abscess

ICD-10CM CODE
G06.2 Extradural and subdural abscess, unspecified

EPIDEMIOLOGY & DEMOGRAPHICS

INCIDENCE: Spinal epidural abscess: 2 to 25 patients per 100,000 admissions; spinal epidural abscess is 9 times more common than intracranial abscess
PREVALENCE: Greatest between 50 and 70 yr of age
PREDOMINANT SEX: More common in men
PEAK INCIDENCE: Median age at onset of spinal epidural abscess: 50 yr old
RISK FACTORS: Bacteremia, secondary to distant infection; epidural catheter placement (0.5% 3% risk), paraspinal injections of glucocorticoids or for pain management, contiguous bone or soft tissue infection, intravenous drug abuse, diabetes, immunosuppressive therapy, HIV

PHYSICAL FINDINGS & CLINICAL PRESENTATION

- Initially nonspecific, such as fever and malaise
- Classic triad: Fever, spinal pain, and neurologic deficits are not common
- More commonly:
  1. Localized and significant back pain is present.
  2. Nerve root pain is present ("shooting" or "electrical" from involved nerve root).
  3. Motor weakness, sensory changes, and even paralysis can occur.
  4. Fever may not be a prominent sign.

ETIOLOGY

- Bacteria enter the epidural space most often secondary to hematogenous spread from foci elsewhere in the body (25%-50% of cases) or by direct extension from nearby infected tissues such as vertebral body or psoas muscle. A local intervention such as injection can also cause infection.
- Hematogenous foci include furuncles, cellulitis, urinary tract infection, pharyngitis, and pneumonia.
- Microbiology:
  1. *Staphylococcus aureus*, including methicillin-resistant S. *aureus* (MRSA), accounts for 50% to 90% of cases.
  2. Aerobic and anaerobic streptococci account for 8% to 17% of cases.
  3. Aerobic gram-negative rods *(Escherichia coli* and *Pseudomonas)* account for 10% to 17% of cases.
  4. Coagulase-negative staphylococci can be seen with spinal procedures.

DIAGNOSIS

DIFFERENTIAL DIAGNOSIS

- Disc and degenerative bone disease
- Metastatic tumors
- Vertebral discitis and osteomyelitis

WORKUP

Includes a combination of physical exam with neurologic evaluation, blood work, and radiographic studies

LABORATORY TESTS

- Blood cultures
- Culture of fluid or pus for bacteria aerobically and anaerobically by CT-guided aspiration if possible. Fungal stain and cultures and AFB stain and culture should also be obtained to exclude more unusual pathogens.
- Erythrocyte sedimentation rate and/or C-reactive protein
- CBC with differential

IMAGING STUDIES

- MRI with gadolinium is the diagnostic test of choice (Fig. E1) and imperative if diagnosis is considered.
- CT is an alternative but not as good as MRI for visualizing spinal cord and epidural space.
- CT myelography can be performed if MRI is not available.

TREATMENT

NONPHARMACOLOGIC THERAPY

- Immediate surgery is required if neurologic deficits occur or the patient worsens with medical therapy.
- CT-guided aspiration of abscess with antimicrobial therapy is an alternative treatment to surgery for patients without neurologic deficits.

ACUTE GENERAL Rx

- Empiric antibiotic regimen should include antibiotics effective against staphylococci (including MRSA), streptococci, and gram-negative rods.
- Examples are vancomycin: 30 to 60 mg/kg daily divided in q12h doses adjusted for creatinine clearance *plus* metronidazole (500 mg IV q8h) *plus* ceftriaxone (2 g IV q12h) or ceftazidime (2 g IV q8h) if *Pseudomonas* is suspected. Meropenem: 1 g IV q8h with vancomycin as an alternative, especially if penicillin allergic.
- If cultures reveal methicillin-sensitive *S. aureus*, use nafcillin 2 g IV q4h.

CHRONIC Rx

Antimicrobial therapy tailored to culture results may have to be continued for 4 to 6 wk depending on whether or not there was surgical or CT-guided drainage. If osteomyelitis is suspected, treat for 6 to 8 wk.

DISPOSITION

- Mortality rates vary from 5% to 32%. Irreversible paralysis can affect 4% to 22% of patients.
- Complete recovery is more likely if neurologic signs are present less than 24 hr before the start of treatment.
- Final functional capacity may continue to improve for up to 1 yr after the end of treatment.

REFERRAL

- Neurosurgery should be involved early when this diagnosis is considered.
- Refer to an interventional radiologist for possible aspiration.
- An infectious diseases evaluation is needed for antimicrobial therapy.

PEARLS & CONSIDERATIONS

COMMENTS

It is important to think of spinal epidural abscess early to permit early treatment and prevent permanent neurologic deficits.

SUGGESTED READINGS
Available at ExpertConsult.com

RELATED CONTENT

Brain Abscess (Related Key Topic)

AUTHOR: **Glenn G. Fort, MD, MPH**

BASIC INFORMATION

DEFINITION

Epidural hematoma (EDH) is the accumulation of blood in the potential space surrounding the brain, between the dura mater and the inner surface of the skull.

SYNONYMS

Extradural hematoma/hemorrhage
EDH

ICD-10CM CODES	
S06.4	Epidural hemorrhage
I62.1	Non-traumatic extradural hemorrhage
S06.4X0A	Epidural hemorrhage without loss of consciousness, initial encounter
S06.4X1A	Epidural hemorrhage with loss of consciousness of 30 minutes or less, initial encounter
S06.4X9A	Epidural hemorrhage with loss of consciousness of unspecified duration, initial encounter

EPIDEMIOLOGY & DEMOGRAPHICS

INCIDENCE: Exact incidence is unknown; however, it is found in 1% to 4% of traumatic head injury cases and 5% to 15% of autopsy series.
PREDOMINANT SEX & AGE: Male > female
PEAK INCIDENCE: Peak incidence is among adolescents and young adults. It is rarely found in patients older than 50 to 60 yr old.
RISK FACTORS: Head trauma, especially in cases involving skull fracture
GENETICS: There is a role for genetics in spontaneous (nontraumatic) EDH caused by coagulopathies and vascular malformations.

PHYSICAL FINDINGS & CLINICAL PRESENTATION

- History of head trauma is present.
- Signs and symptoms vary depending on severity.
- Symptoms: Altered mental status, nuchal rigidity, headache, vomiting, drowsiness, confusion, aphasia, photophobia, and paralysis.
- Signs: Transient loss of consciousness, followed by a "lucid interval" in 47% of cases, in which the patient is free of any neurologic signs or symptoms. This is followed by clinical deterioration including vomiting, lethargy, confusion, or seizures. Other signs may include focal neurologic deficits such as paralysis of limbs, unequal pupils, and coma. Signs of increased intracranial pressure could be found including the Cushing reflex of hypertension, bradycardia, and respiratory distress. External signs of skull fracture—lacerations, ecchymoses, cerebrospinal fluid (CSF) rhinorrhea or otorrhea—may be observed. Skull fractures can be found in 75% to 95% of EDH patients.
- Coma or stupor with ipsilateral cranial nerve III palsy and contralateral hemiparesis may indicate transtentorial (uncal) herniation.

ETIOLOGY

- Traumatic: Commonly caused by arterial injury (the middle meningeal artery) from a temporal bone fracture (Fig. 1) but may also be injury of the anterior meningeal artery, a dural arteriovenous (AV) fistula at the vertex, or from venous bleeding
- Nontraumatic: Caused by an infection/eroding abscess, coagulopathy, hemorrhagic tumors, vascular malformations, postsurgical procedures, and in special populations (e.g., pregnant women, patients receiving hemodialysis)

DIAGNOSIS

DIFFERENTIAL DIAGNOSIS

In the setting of head trauma: Subdural hematoma, subarachnoid hemorrhage, cerebral contusion, brain laceration, diffuse brain swelling

WORKUP

- Imaging is the mainstay of diagnosis.
- Serial head CT is the test most commonly used due to its simplicity, widespread use, and availability. Typical appearance is a "lens shaped," or "lentiform" hyperdensity (Fig. 2). Box 1 describes CT findings of EDH.
- Note: Head CT is not conclusive in 8% of cases possibly due to severe anemia, early scanning (before blood has time to accumulate), and severe hypotension.
- Brain MRI: More sensitive. Indicated in situations in which there is a strong clinical suspicion but no evidence of EDH on head CT (Fig. 3).
- Angiography: Rarely necessary but may be used to evaluate an underlying vascular lesion.
- Note: Lumbar puncture (LP) is contraindicated in EDH due to risk of brain stem herniation.

LABORATORY TESTS

- Laboratory tests are helpful as adjunct to diagnosis but are not the mainstay of diagnosis or treatment.
- CBC may be helpful to evaluate for anemia, although in an acute onset of bleeding hemoglobin levels can be normal.
- Other tests: Renal functions, electrolytes, liver functions, INR may be helpful depending on the case scenario.

TREATMENT

Acute symptomatic EDH is a neurologic emergency that requires surgical treatment to prevent permanent brain injury.

NONPHARMACOLOGIC THERAPY

- Immediate surgical decompression, ideally within 1 to 2 hr after traumatic event

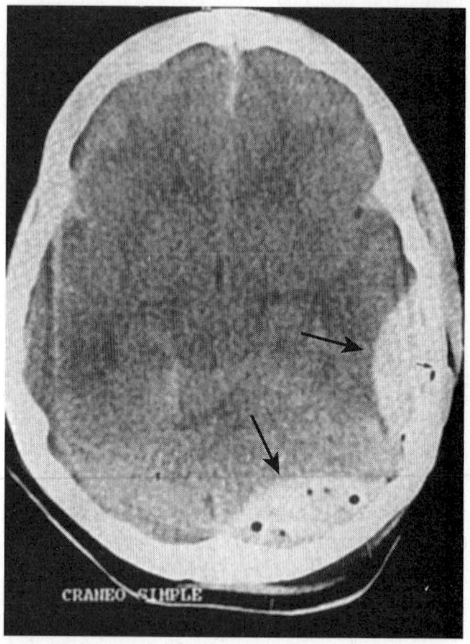

FIG. 2 Head computed tomography showing two epidural hematomas in a 23-yr-old involved in a motor vehicle accident. Note air bubbles that are a result of linear fracture in the left temporal bone *(short arrow)*.

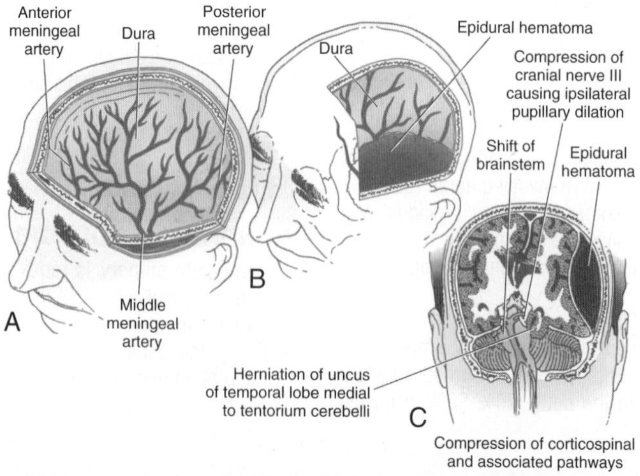

FIG. 1 Epidural hematoma is typically caused by trauma resulting in laceration of the middle meningeal artery. A, The middle meningeal artery. The typical traumatic epidural hematoma is caused by a laceration of this vessel. **B and C,** A linear fracture of the squamous portion of the temporal bone has torn the middle meningeal artery, which has resulted in an epidural hematoma. (From Rothrock JC: Neurosurgery. In Rothrock JC [ed.]: *Alexander's care of the patient in surgery,* ed 13, Philadelphia, 2007, Elsevier.)

BOX 1 Computed Tomography (CT) Findings of Epidural Hematoma

- CT appearance: Variable white to gray on brain windows
- Location: Peripheral to brain, variable but usually temporal region
- Shape: Biconvex disc or lens
- Pearl: Does not cross suture lines
- White swirl sign means active bleeding
- Significance: May cause mass effect and herniation
- Look for midline shift
- Look for effacement of ventricles and sulci
- Surgical indications: 15-mm thickness or 5-mm midline shift

From Broder JS: *Diagnostic imaging for the emergency physician,* Philadelphia, 2011, Saunders.

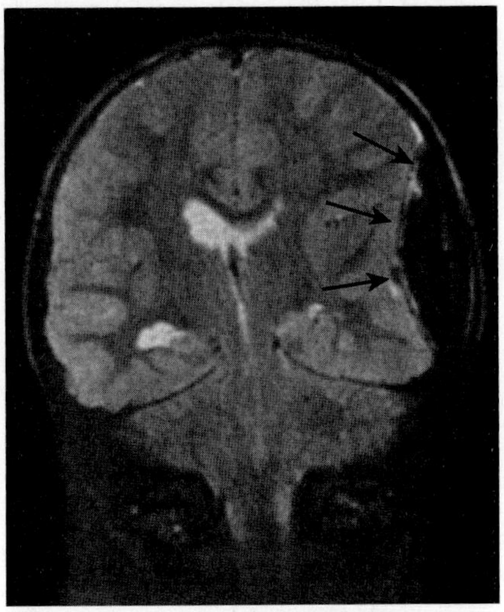

FIG. 3 Epidural hematoma on magnetic resonance image. Coronal T2-weighted images show hypointense biconvex extraaxial collection in the left temporal region.

- Craniotomy and hematoma evacuation is the treatment of choice. When indicated, identify and ligate the bleeding vessel.
- Burr hole evacuation: This involves drilling a hole in the skull to evacuate the hematoma. It is a lifesaving procedure that is indicated if surgical expertise is limited.

ACUTE GENERAL Rx

- Cardiopulmonary resuscitation and assessment for disability.
- Medical resuscitation maneuvers: Head elevation, hyperventilation, monitoring of vital signs and avoidance of hypotension and hyperthermia, sedation if necessary.
- Medications: Osmotic diuresis with IV mannitol, cerebrosedating medications, antiepileptics may be used to treat or, in some situations, prevent seizures. The patient should also be started on a proton pump inhibitor to decrease risks of developing an upper gastrointestinal bleed.
- Reversing anticoagulation should be weighed in terms of advantages versus disadvantages.
- NOTE: Glucocorticoid therapy is *not* indicated following head injury and may be related to increased mortality.
- Evaluation for surgery: The best available evidence points toward advantages of decompression procedures. Nonoperative treatment may only be indicated if the patient has no symptoms, no focal neurologic deficit, no coma (Glasgow coma score >8), and EDH volume is less than 30 ml by CT scan, with clot thickness <15 mm and midline shift of less than 5 mm.
- Nonoperative treatment involves close monitoring, hourly neurologic checks, and serial head CT scans.

CHRONIC Rx

- There is a risk of permanent brain damage whether the disorder is treated or not. Most recovery occurs in the first 6 mo with some improvement over 2 yr.
- Children have a tendency to recover more quickly.
- Patients should be educated on rehabilitative exercises and to alert medical professionals in the event of new neurologic symptoms.
- Support and encouragement to patient and family should always be provided.

REFERRAL

Neurosurgery should be the first service consulted. If not available, then general surgery needs to be called. Clinical nurse practitioners, pastoral care staff, and social workers to help patients and families are also appropriate.

PEARLS & CONSIDERATIONS

- Acute symptomatic EDH is a neurologic emergency. Urgent surgical evacuation is necessary in patients with Glasgow coma score less than 9, hematoma greater than 30 ml in volume, or presence of anisocoria.
- EDH should be suspected in any patient with a history of blow to the head leading to a period of loss of consciousness.
- Initial resuscitation is extremely important, but surgery is the mainstay of treatment for acute symptomatic EDH.

PREVENTION

Should be directed toward preventing head trauma: Use of appropriate safety equipment (e.g., helmets, hard hats, safe driving, avoiding diving into unknown depths).

PATIENT & FAMILY EDUCATION

Online head injury support groups are helpful: www.headinjury.com/linktbisup.htm, www.headinjury.com/, www.dailystrengthorg/c/Brain-Injury/support-group.

AUTHOR: **Fred F. Ferri, MD**

BASIC INFORMATION

DEFINITION

Epiglottitis is a rapidly progressive cellulitis of the epiglottis and adjacent soft tissue structures with the potential to cause abrupt airway obstruction, which can be life-threatening.

SYNONYMS

Supraglottitis
Cherry-red epiglottitis

ICD-10CM CODE
J05.1 Acute epiglottitis

EPIDEMIOLOGY & DEMOGRAPHICS

INCIDENCE (IN U.S.): Due to vaccination against *Haemophilus influenzae* type B, this is a rare infection in children estimated at between 0.6 to 0.8 per 100,000 in one study and for adults at 1.6 per 100,000.
PREDOMINANT SEX: Males
PEAK INCIDENCE: Now highest in children ages 6 to 12 yr old

PHYSICAL FINDINGS & CLINICAL PRESENTATION

- Irritability, fever, dysphonia, and dysphagia
- Respiratory distress with "tripoding" (child sitting up, leaning forward, and bracing upper body)
- Drooling or increased oral secretions
- Tachycardia and tachypnea are common
- Edematous and cherry-red epiglottis
- Absence of cough
- Anxiety
- Possibly fulminant course (especially in children), leading to complete airway obstruction

ETIOLOGY

- *Haemophilus influenzae* type b, while rare due to vaccination, remains a causative agent in children. Other bacterial pathogens include *Streptococcus pyogenes,* (group A Streptococcus) *Streptococcus pneumoniae, and Staphylococcus aureus* (includes MRSA).
- In adults, *Streptococcus pyogenes* (group A Streptococcus) and *H. influenzae* are most common (isolated from blood and/or epiglottis in 26% of cases).
- Pneumococci, streptococci, and staphylococci are also implicated.
- The role of viruses in epiglottitis is unclear.

DIAGNOSIS

DIFFERENTIAL DIAGNOSIS

- Croup (Table 1)
- Angioedema
- Retropharyngeal or peritonsillar abscess
- Diphtheria
- Foreign body aspiration causing obstruction
- Lingual tonsillitis
- Bacterial tracheitis

WORKUP

- Minimize causes of stress and anxiety if high suspicion for epiglottitis.
- Attempt to visualize epiglottis with oral exam.
- Cultures of blood, urine, and epiglottis.
- Lateral neck radiograph to show an enlarged epiglottis, ballooning of the hypopharynx, and normal subglottic structures (Fig. 1).
  1. Radiographs are of only moderate sensitivity and specificity and take time to perform.
  2. Visualization of the epiglottis may be safer in adults than in children.

LABORATORY TESTS

- CBC: May reveal a leukocytosis with a shift to the left.
- Chest radiograph examination: May reveal evidence of pneumonia in close to 25% of cases.
- Cultures of blood, urine, and the epiglottis, as noted previously.

TREATMENT

ACUTE GENERAL Rx

- Maintenance of adequate airway is critical. Fig. E2 describes the optimal assessment and management of upper airway obstruction caused by epiglottitis or severe croup. It is crucial to have a tracheostomy set "at bedside."
- With high concern for epiglottitis, early placement of an endotracheal or nasotracheal tube in a child is advised.
- Prepare for intubation utilizing most experienced staff and advanced technology possible.
- Minimize intubation attempts and time to intubation if there is concern for obstruction due to epiglottitis.
- Visualization and intubation are best done in the most controlled environment.
- Closely follow the adult patient, if no signs of airway obstruction, defer intubation.

Empiric antibiotics (two-drug regimens):

- **In children:** Use cefotaxime 50 mg/kg IV q8h (max daily dose 10 g) or ceftriaxone 50 to 100 mg/kg IV q24h (max dose 2 g) *plus* either vancomycin, clindamycin, cefazolin, or nafcillin or oxacillin. If penicillin allergic, use levofloxacin *plus* clindamycin.
- **In adults:** Ceftriaxone 2 g IV q24h or cefotaxime 2 g q4 to 6h *plus* vancomycin, clindamycin, cefazolin, or nafcillin or oxacillin.
- If possible, obtain cultures prior to initiating antibiotics.
- **Prophylaxis:** If a child >4 yr is unvaccinated for *H. influenzae* and resides at home or in day care, treat close family contacts of the patient (including adults) with rifampin 20 mg/kg/day for 4 days (up to 600 mg/day).
- The role of epinephrine or corticosteroids in the management of epiglottitis is not firmly established.

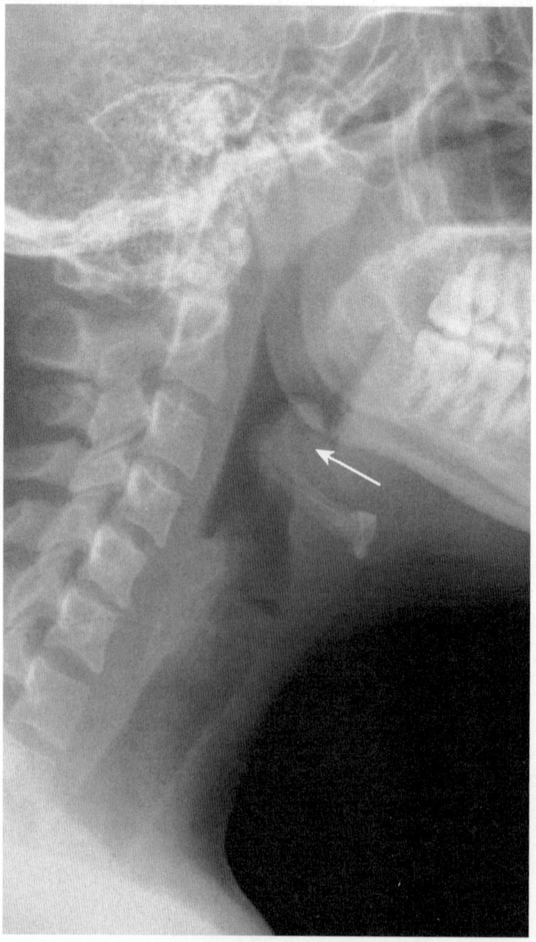

FIG. 1 Epiglottitis. In this young child who presented with difficulty breathing, a lateral neck radiograph demonstrates the classic "thumbprint" sign *(arrow)* of the inflamed epiglottis. (From Soto JA, Lucey BC: *Emergency Radiology: the requisites,* ed 2, Philadelphia, 2017, Elsevier.)

TABLE 1 Comparison of Croup, Epiglottitis, and Bacterial Tracheitis

	Croup	Epiglottitis	Bacterial Tracheitis
Peak age	6 mo-3 yr	5-7 yr, but can be seen throughout childhood	3-5 yr, but seen throughout childhood
Pathologic features	Subglottic inflammation, edema	Inflammation and edema of the epiglottis, aryepiglottic folds	Bacterial superinfection with inflammation of the tracheal mucosa, copious mucopurulent secretions obstructing the trachea
Organisms	Parainfluenza virus, RSV, adenovirus	Group A beta-hemolytic streptococcus, *Staphylococcus aureus, Streptococcus pneumoniae, Haemophilus influenzae*	*Staphylococcus aureus* or mixed flora
Clinical features	Onset follows URI prodrome consisting of croupy cough, hoarse voice, low-grade fever, inspiratory stridor	Rapid progression of high fever, toxicity, drooling, and stridor	Several-day prodrome of croup-like illness progressing to toxicity, inspiratory and expiratory stridor, and marked distress
Laboratory and radiographic findings	Steeple sign on PA view of the neck, or normal	Thumbprint sign on lateral view of the neck, thickened aryepiglottic folds, loss of air in the vallecula	Normal upper airway structures, shaggy tracheal air column
Management	Steroids, aerosolized epinephrine	Intubation, antibiotics	Intubation, antibiotics

PA, Posteroanterior; *RSV,* respiratory syncytial virus; *URI,* upper respiratory infection.
From Marx JA et al: *Rosen's emergency medicine,* ed 8, Philadelphia, 2014, Saunders.

DISPOSITION

Invasive *H. influenzae* infections and epiglottitis are reportable illnesses; recognition of outbreaks in a day care center with unvaccinated children is crucial.

REFERRAL

- Best managed in a critical care setting or ICU.
- Close cooperation between the pediatrician or internist, anesthesiologist, and otorhinolaryngologist, especially when epiglottis is visualized and when the patient requires endotracheal intubation.

PEARLS & CONSIDERATIONS

The incidence of epiglottitis has diminished markedly since the introduction of the protein conjugate vaccine against *H. influenzae* serotype B into routine childhood immunization.

The mortality rate now in children is about 1%, but still remains about 7% in adults.

SUGGESTED READING

Available at ExpertConsult.com

RELATED CONTENT

Epiglottitis (Patient Information)

AUTHORS: **Erin Alpert-Rathhauser, MD,** and **Jon Farkas, MD**

BASIC INFORMATION

DEFINITION

Epstein-Barr virus infection refers to a disease caused by Epstein-Barr virus (EBV), a human herpesvirus.

SYNONYMS

Infectious mononucleosis (IM)
Kissing disease

ICD-10CM CODES

B27.80	Other infectious mononucleosis without complication
B27.81	Other infectious mononucleosis with polyneuropathy
B27.82	Other infectious mononucleosis with meningitis
B27.89	Other infectious mononucleosis with other complication
B27.90	Infectious mononucleosis, unspecified without complication
B27.91	Infectious mononucleosis, unspecified with polyneuropathy
B27.92	Infectious mononucleosis, unspecified with meningitis
B27.99	Infectious mononucleosis, unspecified with other complication

EPIDEMIOLOGY & DEMOGRAPHICS

INCIDENCE (IN U.S.): 5 cases/100,000 persons per yr of IM
PREDOMINANT SEX: Neither, although peak incidence occurs about 2 yr earlier in women
PREDOMINANT AGE:
- Clinical evidence of IM: Occurs most commonly at ages 15 to 24 yr
- EBV infection: Occurs earlier in life in lower socioeconomic groups

PHYSICAL FINDINGS & CLINICAL PRESENTATION

- Most EBV infections either are asymptomatic or cause a nonspecific viral illness.
- Incubation period is 1 to 2 mo, possibly followed by a prodrome of anorexia, low-grade fever, malaise, headache, and chills; after several days, clinical triad of pharyngitis, moderate to high fever, and adenopathy may appear, accompanied by fatigue and malaise.
- Pharyngitis is usually the most severe symptom; white or necrotic exudates are common.
- Symmetrical lymphadenopathy is most prominent in the posterior more than anterior cervical region but may be diffuse.
- Splenomegaly (50% of cases) is possible, most commonly during the second week of illness.
- Maculopapular or morbilliform rash is uncommon but will often occur in patients who receive ampicillin (Fig. E1). Patients may have palatal petechiae, periorbital, or palpebral edema. Mucocutaneous oral hairy leukoplakia (OHL), which is associated with intense EBV replication and the action of EBV-encoded proteins such as latent membrane protein-1, may occur.
- Possible IM presentation: Fever and adenopathy without pharyngitis.
- Nausea, vomiting, and anorexia are frequent in patients with IM, probably reflecting mild hepatitis encountered in 90% of infected individuals.
- Although complications such as spleen rupture, airway obstruction, and malignancy may be severe and fatal, they are uncommon and tend to resolve completely.
- Hematologic involvement includes hemolytic or aplastic anemia, thrombocytopenia, thrombotic thrombocytopenic purpura/hemolytic-uremic syndrome, and disseminated intravascular coagulation (DIC). Pneumonia, myocarditis, pancreatitis, mesenteric adenitis, myositis, and glomerulonephritis may occur as well. Nervous system involvement includes Guillain-Barré syndrome, facial nerve palsy, meningoencephalitis, aseptic meningitis, transverse myelitis, peripheral neuritis, and optic neuritis.
- IM is usually a self-limited illness. Acute symptoms resolve in 1 to 2 wk, but symptoms of malaise and fatigue often persist for months.
- EBV is related to lymphoproliferative syndromes in transplant recipients and in AIDS patients.
- Increasing evidence showing an association between EBV infection and African Burkitt, B-cell or T-cell lymphoma, and nasopharyngeal carcinoma. Table 1 describes EBV-associated disorders.

ETIOLOGY

- EBV is a ubiquitous virus.
- Infection during childhood is much less likely to cause significant illness.
- Frequency of IM in late adolescence is attributed to the onset of social contact between the sexes.
- Close personal contact is usually necessary for transmission, although EBV is occasionally transmitted by blood transfusion; transfer via saliva while kissing may be responsible for many cases.

Dx DIAGNOSIS

DIFFERENTIAL DIAGNOSIS

- Heterophile-negative IM caused by cytomegalovirus (CMV)

TABLE 1 EBV-Associated Disorders

EBV-Associated Disorders
- Infectious mononucleosis
- Gianotti–Crosti syndrome
- Genital ulcers*
- Periodontal disease
- Oral hairy leukoplakia
- Hydroa vacciniforme and related conditions
  1. Typical hydroa vacciniforme
  2. Severe hydroa vacciniforme-like eruptions**
  3. Hydroa vacciniforme-like lymphoproliferative disorder***
- Severe hypersensitivity to mosquito bites*
- Lymphadenitis, including Kikuchi disease
- Lymphoproliferative disorders and lymphomas
  1. Posttransplant lymphoproliferative disorder/lymphoma
  2. Methotrexate-associated lymphoproliferative disorder (usually in patients with rheumatoid arthritis)
  3. Systemic EBV+ T-cell lymphoma of childhood
  4. EBV+ mucocutaneous ulcer
  5. X-linked lymphoproliferative syndrome
  6. Hemophagocytic lymphohistiocytosis (susceptibility to develop)
  7. Lymphomatoid granulomatosis
  8. Burkitt lymphoma, endemic ≫ sporadic
  9. Extranodal NK/T-cell lymphoma, nasal type
  10. EBV+ diffuse large B-cell lymphoma, NOS
  11. Angioimmunoblastic T-cell lymphoma
  12. Other non-Hodgkin lymphomas (including T-cell), particularly in HIV-infected patients
  13. Hodgkin disease
- Other malignancies
  1. Nasopharyngeal carcinoma
  2. Gastric carcinoma
  3. Leiomyosarcoma
- Smooth muscle tumors

*There may or may not be evidence of EBV within the ulcer; reactive non–sexually related acute genital ulcers (formerly referred to as Lipschütz ulcers) can be triggered by EBV and other infections (e.g., cytomegalovirus, influenza, *Mycoplasma pneumoniae*), most often in adolescent girls; this is thought to represent a form of aphthosis, which may be recurrent and associated with a history of oral aphthous ulcers.
**Present with bullous, necrotic, and ulcerative skin lesions together with fever, lymphadenopathy, hepatosplenomegaly, and natural killer (NK)–cell lymphocytosis.
***Can progress to a T- or NK-cell lymphoma or hemophagocytic lymphohistiocytosis.
EBV, Epstein-Barr virus; *NOS*, not otherwise specified.
From Bolognia J: *Dermatology*, ed 4, 2018, Elsevier.

TABLE 2 Frequently Determined EBV-Specific Antibodies

Antibody Specificity	Positive in IM (%)	Time of Appearance in IM	Persistence	Comments
Viral Capsid Antigen				
VCA-IgM	100	At clinical presentation	4-8 wk	Highly sensitive and specific; of major diagnostic utility
VCA-IgG	100	At clinical presentation	Lifelong	Useful for documentation of past EBV infection
Early Antigen				
Anti-D	70	Peaks 3-4 wk after onset	3-6 mo	Correlates with disease severity; seen in NPC patients
Anti-R	Low	2 wk to several months after onset	2 mo to >3 yr	Occasionally seen with unusually severe cases; seen in African Burkitt lymphoma patients
EBNA	100	3-4 wk after onset	Lifelong	Presence excludes primary EBV infection

EBNA, EBV nuclear antigen; *EBV,* Epstein-Barr virus; *Ig,* immunoglobulin; *IM,* infectious mononucleosis; *NPC,* nasopharyngeal carcinoma; *VCA,* viral capsid antigen.
Adapted from Schooley RT: Epstein-Barr virus (infectious mononucleosis). In Mandell GL et al (eds): *Principles and practice of infectious diseases,* Philadelphia, 2010, Churchill Livingstone.

- Although clinical presentation similar, CMV more frequently follows transfusion
- Bacterial and viral causes of pharyngitis
- Toxoplasmosis
- Acute retroviral syndrome of HIV
- Lymphoma
- Lyme disease

WORKUP

Heterophile antibody and CBC with blood smear. Table 2 describes frequently determined EBV-specific antibodies.

LABORATORY TESTS

- Increased WBC common, with a relative lymphocytosis of more than 50% and neutropenia identified.
- Hallmark of IM: Atypical lymphocytes of more than 10% (not pathognomonic) are found.
- Mild thrombocytopenia is present.
- Falling hematocrit signals the possibility of splenic rupture or immune hemolytic anemia.
- Elevated hepatocellular enzymes and cryoglobulins are found in most cases.
- Heterophile antibody:
  1. As measured by the monospot test, may be positive at presentation or may appear later in the course of illness. Its accuracy is 71% to 90% but has a 25% false-negative rate in the first week of illness.
  2. A negative test should be repeated in 1 wk if clinical suspicion is high.
  3. A false-positive test has been reported with primary HIV infection.
- Viral capsid antigen (VCA) IgG and IgM are rarely used for diagnosis, but better value in children because heterophile antibody is negative in most children younger than 8 yr.
- PCR DNA for CMV is the test of choice in transplant recipients who develop lymphoproliferative syndromes.

IMAGING STUDIES

Chest radiograph examination:
- May rarely show infiltrates
- Possible elevated left hemidiaphragm with splenic rupture

Rx TREATMENT

NONPHARMACOLOGIC THERAPY

- Supportive including rest
- Splenectomy if rupture occurs
- Transfusions for severe anemia or thrombocytopenia

ACUTE GENERAL Rx

- Pharmacologic therapy is not indicated in uncomplicated illness.
- Avoid aspirin due to the risk of Reye syndrome.
- Avoid ampicillin and amoxicillin as their use can frequently precipitate a nonallergic rash. Azithromycin has also been implicated.
- Use of steroids is suggested in patients who have severe thrombocytopenia, hemolytic anemia, impending airway obstruction resulting from enlarged tonsils, or fulminant liver failure. Prednisone 60 to 80 mg PO qd for 3 days, then tapered over 1 to 2 wk.
- Although it may reduce initial viral shedding, there is little evidence to support the use of antiviral agents such as acyclovir in the management of IM.

CHRONIC Rx

An extremely rare, chronic form of IM with persistent fevers and fatigue has been described and should be differentiated from chronic fatigue syndrome, which is not related to EBV.

DISPOSITION

Eventual resolution of all symptoms

REFERRAL

If more than mild illness

PEARLS & CONSIDERATIONS

- Epstein-Barr infection will occur in 95% of the world population at some point in life.
- It is felt the antibiotic-induced rash in IM is a transient virus-mediated immune alteration that sets the stage for loss of antigenic tolerance and the development of a reversible, delayed-type hypersensitivity reaction to the antibiotic

COMMENTS

Avoidance of contact sports during the first month of illness because splenic rupture can occur even in the absence of clinically detectable splenomegaly in 0.1% to 0.5% of patients.

SUGGESTED READINGS

Available at ExpertConsult.com

RELATED CONTENT

Epstein-Barr Virus Infection (Patient Information)
Mononucleosis (Related Key Topic)

AUTHOR: **Glenn G. Fort, MD, MPH**

BASIC INFORMATION

DEFINITION

Erectile dysfunction (ED) is the persistent inability to achieve or sustain a penile erection of adequate rigidity to make sexual penetration possible or satisfactory.

SYNONYMS

ED
Impotence
Male erectile disorder
Sexual dysfunction (a nonspecific term)

ICD-10CM CODES

N48.4	Impotence of organic origin
F52.2	Failure of genital response
F52.9	Unspecified sexual dysfunction, not caused by organic disorder or disease
N52.01	Erectile dysfunction due to arterial insufficiency
N52.02	Corporo-venous occlusive erectile dysfunction
N52.03	Combined arterial insufficiency and corporo-venous occlusive erectile dysfunction
N52.1	Erectile dysfunction due to diseases classified elsewhere
N52.2	Drug-induced erectile dysfunction
N52.31	Erectile dysfunction following radical prostatectomy
N52.32	Erectile dysfunction following radical cystectomy
N52.33	Erectile dysfunction following urethral surgery
N52.34	Erectile dysfunction following simple prostatectomy
N52.39	Other post-surgical erectile dysfunction
N52.8	Other male erectile dysfunction
N52.9	Male erectile dysfunction, unspecified

DSM-5 CODE

302.72	Failure of genital response

EPIDEMIOLOGY & DEMOGRAPHICS

PREVALENCE (IN U.S.):
- Prevalence increases with age and presence of specific medical comorbidities
- Approximately 8% in the 20s to 30s, 18% in the 50s, 25% in the 60s, 37% in the 70s, 80% in the 80s

PREDOMINANT SEX: By definition, only in males

PREDOMINANT AGE: Increases with age

RISK FACTORS: Age, coronary artery disease, peripheral vascular disease, hypertension, hypogonadism, diabetes mellitus, hypercholesterolemia, prostate surgery, neurologic injury, numerous medications, alcohol, tobacco or drug use, obesity, obstructive sleep apnea, systemic sclerosis; psychological distress, partner-related stress, performance anxiety

ETIOLOGY (TABLE 1)

- A classification of male erectile dysfunction is described in Box 1.
- Most cases involving men older than 50 yr are caused by organic problems related to neurologic, hormonal, or vascular abnormalities and prescription or recreational drugs. In organic ED, nocturnal penile tumescence is generally diminished or absent. ED is also experienced during private masturbation and across partners.
- Psychogenic ED results from psychological stress, depression, stressful partner relationship, a partner's sexual and mental health problems, and performance anxiety. Performance anxiety is extremely common and is characterized by a focus on the performance outcome of sex (i.e., obtaining and maintaining an erection) rather than a focus on the process and enjoyment of sex. Psychogenic ED is characterized by normal nocturnal penile tumescence and/or erections associated with erotic material or other

TABLE 1 Causes of Hypoactive Sexual Desire Disorder and Erectile Dysfunction

Cause	Examples
Brain Disorders	
Psychogenic disorders	Stress or preoccupation, performance anxiety, depression, major psychiatric illness
Chronic systemic illness	Heart, respiratory, kidney, or liver failure; cancer
CNS-active drugs	Alcohol; antihypertensive, narcotic, sedative-hypnotic, anticonvulsant, antidepressant, antipsychotic medications
Structural brain disease	Temporal lobe or limbic system disorders, Parkinson or other neurodegenerative brain disease, vascular brain disorders
Androgen deficiency	Primary and secondary hypogonadism
Other endocrine disorders	Hyperprolactinemia, Cushing syndrome, hyperthyroidism, hypothyroidism
Spinal Cord and Peripheral Disorders	
Spinal cord disorders	Trauma, vascular compromise, spinal stenosis, epidural abscess, tumor, transverse myelitis, multiple sclerosis, other spinal cord lesions
Peripheral nerve disorders	Diabetes mellitus; pelvic, prostate, or retroperitoneal surgery or damage; other causes of peripheral neuropathy
PNS-active drugs	Anticholinergic, antihistamine, antidepressant, sympathomimetic, α-adrenergic agonist, β-adrenergic antagonist medications
Peripheral vascular disease	Aortoiliac atherosclerosis, diabetes mellitus, trauma, surgery, vasculitis, venous incompetence (venous leakage), smoking
Antihypertensive drugs	Diuretics, β-adrenergic antagonists, calcium channel antagonists
Penile abnormalities	Peyronie disease, chordee, trauma, priapism, phimosis

CNS, Central nervous system; *PNS,* peripheral nervous system.
From Melmed S et al: *Williams textbook of endocrinology*, ed 14, Philadelphia, 2020, Elsevier.

BOX 1 Classification of Male Erectile Dysfunction

Organic
- I. Vasculogenic
  - A. Arteriogenic
  - B. Cavernosal
  - C. Mixed
- II. Neurogenic
- III. Anatomic
- IV. Endocrinologic

Psychogenic
- I. Generalized
  - A. Generalized unresponsiveness
    1. Primary lack of sexual arousability
    2. Aging-related decline in sexual arousability
  - B. Generalized inhibition
    1. Chronic disorder of sexual intimacy
- II. Situational
  - A. Partner-related
    1. Lack of arousability in specific relationship
    2. Lack of arousability owing to sexual object preference
    3. High central inhibition owing to partner conflict or threat
  - B. Performance-related
    1. Associated with other sexual dysfunction (e.g., rapid ejaculation)
    2. Situational performance anxiety (e.g., fear of failure)
  - C. Psychological distress or adjustment related
    1. Associated with negative mood state (e.g., depression) or major life stress (e.g., death of partner)

From Wein AJ et al: *Campbell-Walsh urology,* ed 11, Philadelphia, 2016, Elsevier.

TABLE 2 Drug-Induced Erectile Dysfunction and Suggested Alternatives

Class	Known to Cause Erectile Dysfunction	Suggested Alternatives
Antihypertensives	Thiazide diuretics General β blockers	α-Blockers Calcium channel blockers Specific β-blockers Angiotensin-converting enzyme inhibitors Angiotensin II receptor antagonists
Psychotropics	Antipsychotics Antidepressants Anxiolytics	Anxiolytic (buspirone); antidepressant (bupropion)
Antiandrogen	Androgen receptor antagonists Luteinizing hormone–releasing hormone agonists 5α-Reductase inhibitors	
Opiates		
Antiretroviral agents		
Tobacco		Quit smoking
Alcohol	Large amount	Small amount

From Wein AJ et al: *Campbell-Walsh urology,* ed 11, Philadelphia, 2016, Elsevier.

partners, and by otherwise negative medical test results.

- Vascular disease: History of hypertension (HTN), peripheral vascular disease, ischemic heart disease, diabetes, smoking. In approximately 40% of men >50 yr, the primary cause of ED is related to atherosclerotic disease, diabetes mellitus (DM), neuropathy, or vascular disease.
- Obesity and metabolic syndrome.
- Medication side effects: Antihypertensives such as thiazides and clonidine, guanethidine or methyldopa; antiandrogens such as spironolactone, finasteride, ketoconazole; cimetidine (but not ranitidine or famotidine); antidepressants such as selective serotonin reuptake inhibitors [SSRIs]; and antipsychotics. Table 2 summarizes drug-induced erectile dysfunction and suggested alternatives.
- Excessive alcohol and nicotine use.
- Recreational drugs, including cocaine, heroin, amphetamines, and marijuana. These may increase libido but impair performance.
- Hormonal dysfunction such as testosterone deficiency (decreases libido and erection), hypothyroidism or hyperthyroidism, hyperprolactinemia, and adrenal insufficiency.
- Neurogenic causes including spinal cord lesions, cortical lesions, and peripheral neuropathies.
- Trauma or pelvic surgeries such as radical prostatectomy or cystectomy.

Dx DIAGNOSIS

DIFFERENTIAL DIAGNOSIS

- A useful tool to diagnose/evaluate ED severity is the Sexual Health Inventory for Men (SHIM).
- Distinguish psychogenic and organic contributions to ED.
- Evaluate for underlying etiology of organic ED and comorbid psychiatric condition.

WORKUP

- A diagnostic directed evaluation of ED is summarized in Table 3. Clinical history should include time course (abrupt onset may correlate with reversible causes such as medications, psychosocial stress, psychiatric concerns, trauma; gradual onset may correlate with vascular or neurologic issues), cause (psychogenic vs. organic), and change in libido. Box 2 describes symptoms suggesting neurologic sexual impairment.
- Report of spontaneous nocturnal or morning erections indicate intact neurologic reflexes and penile blood flow.
- Decreased libido may indicate endocrinologic or psychogenic cause.
- If possible, interview partner regarding partner's sexual function, relationship satisfaction, and mental health history.
- Medical and social history should address cardiac disease symptoms and risk factors (HTN, DM, hyperlipidemia, smoking, and substance abuse), pelvic surgery, medications, and mental health. Coronary artery calcium score (CAC) is best indicator of subclinical coronary artery disease.
- Physical examination to check blood pressure; visual field defects to evaluate for pituitary tumors, thyroid examination; femoral and peripheral pulses, femoral bruits; gynecomastia; neuronal damage (genital sensation, cremasteric reflex); direct penile damage (e.g., plaque formation such as Peyronie disease); prostate examination; or testicular atrophy and other secondary sexual characteristics. Signs of neurologic sexual impairment are summarized in Box 3.

LABORATORY TESTS

Screen for diabetes mellitus with fasting glucose. Consider lipid panel, thyroid-stimulating hormone, morning serum testosterone (free and total). If decreased testosterone, check prolactin, follicle-stimulating hormone, and luteinizing hormone.

IMAGING STUDIES

Imaging studies are rarely performed except in situations of pelvic trauma or surgery.

OTHER STUDIES

- Nocturnal penile tumescence testing is very specific for distinguishing psychogenic versus organic causes.
- Neurogenic etiologies examined by the cremasteric reflex (inner-thigh touch elicits scrotal contraction), the bulbocavernosus reflex, or the pudendal-evoked response.
- Intracorporeal injection of prostaglandin E_1 to distinguish vascular and nonvascular etiologies (erection is achieved in patients with normal vascular systems). If no erection with direct injection of vasoactive substance, consider duplex ultrasound of penile vasculature.
- In patients without an obvious cause of ED, consider screening for cardiovascular disease prior to starting treatment.

Rx TREATMENT (FIG. 1)

NONPHARMACOLOGIC THERAPY

- Various psychotherapeutic approaches: Cognitive-behavioral therapy preferred; success rates decrease with advancing age and duration of symptoms.
- Psychosexual therapy is first line for psychogenic ED. Psychosexual therapy may be used as adjunctive therapy in ED from any cause to address contributing factors, including performance anxiety, relationship issues, and other psychosocial factors.
- Performance anxiety is best addressed by sensate focus in which a couple is asked to focus on touch and refrain from behavior centered around the genitals, including sexual penetration.
- Mechanical vacuum devices (function by drawing blood into corpus cavernosum) are 70% to 90% effective but are difficult to use and subject to nonadherence.
- Incorporate vascular risk factor reduction including education on diet, exercise, smoking cessation, ETOH intake and screening/treatment for HTN, insulin resistance, and hypercholesterolemia as appropriate. Trials have shown that lifestyle modification and pharmacotherapy for cardiovascular risk factors are effective in improving sexual function in men with ED.

ACUTE GENERAL Rx

- First-line treatment: In setting of sexual stimulation, four selective phosphodiesterase type 5 (PDE5) inhibitors (Table 4) prolong nitric oxide–induced vasodilation by increase of intracavernosal cyclic guanosine monophosphate levels. Sildenafil (Viagra) and vardenafil (Levitra, Staxyn) can be taken 30 to 60 min before sexual activity, and both are effective for about 4 hr. Avanafil

TABLE 3 Directed Diagnostic Evaluation of ED

History

Ascertain Psychosexual History

- Nature of sexual dysfunction: Whether the primary problem is decreased desire, erectile dysfunction, premature or delayed ejaculation, or difficulty in achieving orgasms
- Strength of marital relationship and marital discord
- Depression
- Stress
- Sexual performance anxiety
- Knowledge and beliefs about sexuality

Ascertain Risk Factors

- Presence of diabetes mellitus, hypertension, hyperlipidemia, coronary artery disease, end-stage renal disease, and peripheral vascular disease
- History of spinal cord injury, stroke, Alzheimer disease, or other neurologic disorder
- Prostate or pelvic surgery
- Pelvic injury
- Medications such as antihypertensives, antidepressants, antipsychotics, opioid analgesics, and inhibitors of androgen production or action
- Use of recreational drugs such as alcohol, cocaine, opiates, and tobacco

Ascertain Factors That Might Affect Choice of Therapy and the Patient's Response to It

- Coexisting coronary artery disease and its symptoms and severity
- Exercise tolerance
- Use of nitrates or nitrate donors
- Use of α-adrenergic blockers
- Use of vasodilators for hypertension or congestive heart failure
- Use of foods (e.g., cranberry juice) or drugs (e.g., erythromycin, protease inhibitors, ketoconazole, and itraconazole) that might affect metabolism of PDE5 inhibitors

Physical Examination

- Ascertain signs of androgen deficiency, such as loss of body hair, eunuchoidal proportions, small testicular volume, or breast enlargement
- Genital and perineal sensation to evaluate neurologic deficit from spinal cord lesion, previous stroke, peripheral neuropathy, or other neurologic disorder
- Blood pressure and postural change in blood pressure
- Evaluate femoral and pedal pulses and evidence of lower extremity ischemia
- Penile examination to exclude Peyronie disease or other penile deformities

Basic Laboratory Evaluation That Should Be Performed in All Men With ED

- Fasting blood glucose
- Plasma lipids
- Serum total and free testosterone level using reliable assays

ED, Erectile dysfunction; *PDE5,* phosphodiesterase 5.
From Melmed S et al: *Williams textbook of endocrinology*, ed 14, Philadelphia, 2020, Elsevier.

BOX 2 Symptoms Suggesting Neurologic Sexual Impairment

Continual erectile dysfunction
- Absence of morning erections
- No erection or orgasm during masturbation or sex with different partners

Related somatic complaints
Sensory loss in genitals, pelvis, or legs
Urinary incontinence
Certain neurologic conditions
- Spinal cord injury
- Diabetic neuropathy
- Multiple sclerosis
- Herniated intervertebral disk

Use of many medications

From Kaufman DM et al: *Kaufman's clinical neurology for psychiatrists*, ed 8, Philadelphia, 2017, Elsevier.

BOX 3 Signs of Neurologic Sexual Impairment

Signs of spinal cord injury
- Paraparesis or quadriparesis
- Leg spasticity
- Urinary incontinence

Signs of autonomic nervous system injury
- Orthostatic hypotension or lightheadedness
- Anhidrosis in groin and legs
- Urinary incontinence
- Retrograde ejaculation

Signs of peripheral nervous system injury
- Loss of sensation in the genitals, "saddle area," and legs
- Paresis and areflexia in legs
- Scrotal, cremasteric, and anal reflex loss

From Kaufman DM et al: *Kaufman's clinical neurology for psychiatrists*, ed 8, Philadelphia, 2017, Elsevier.

(Stendra) can be taken 15 to 30 min before sexual activity and is effective for about 6 hr. Tadalafil (Cialis) can be taken several hours before sexual activity (although 50% respond within 30 min) and lasts up to 36 hr. All four PDE5 inhibitors have similar efficacy and tolerability, but tadalafil has a longer duration of action and is less affected by high-fat meals and alcohol. Counsel patients to avoid high-fat meals and excessive alcohol when taking PDE5 inhibitors, as they may impede effectiveness.

- With PDE5 inhibitors, avoid concomitant use of nitrates (absolute contraindication), drugs that inhibit or induce cytochrome P450 CYP3A4, and drugs that prolong the QT interval. Caution in men on alpha-adrenergic blocker therapy because of concern for hypotension; start the lowest dose of PDE5 inhibitor. Caution in men who have had myocardial infarction in the past 6 mo, resting hypotension or uncontrolled hypertension, unstable angina, positive exercise stress test or poor exercise tolerance. Counsel on side effects of headache, flushing, dyspepsia, nasal congestion, changes in color perception (including blue vision for sildenafil and vardenafil but not tadalafil), sudden hearing loss, and priapism (rare). Nonarteritic anterior ischemic optic neuropathy is also a rare association with sildenafil and tadalafil. Consider counseling on safe sexual practices when prescribing PDE5 inhibitors.
- Second-line treatment if PDE5 inhibitors fail: Self-injection with intraurethral alprostadil (prostaglandin E_1 [medicated urethral suppository]) applied into meatus of penis before intercourse; or intracavernosal injections of vasodilators (e.g., papaverine or prostaglandin E_1). Consider combining intraurethral alprostadil with PDE5 inhibitor. Relatively high success with self-injection, but attrition is high (Table 5).
- Second-line treatment alternative: Vacuum constriction pump; has variable satisfaction rate.

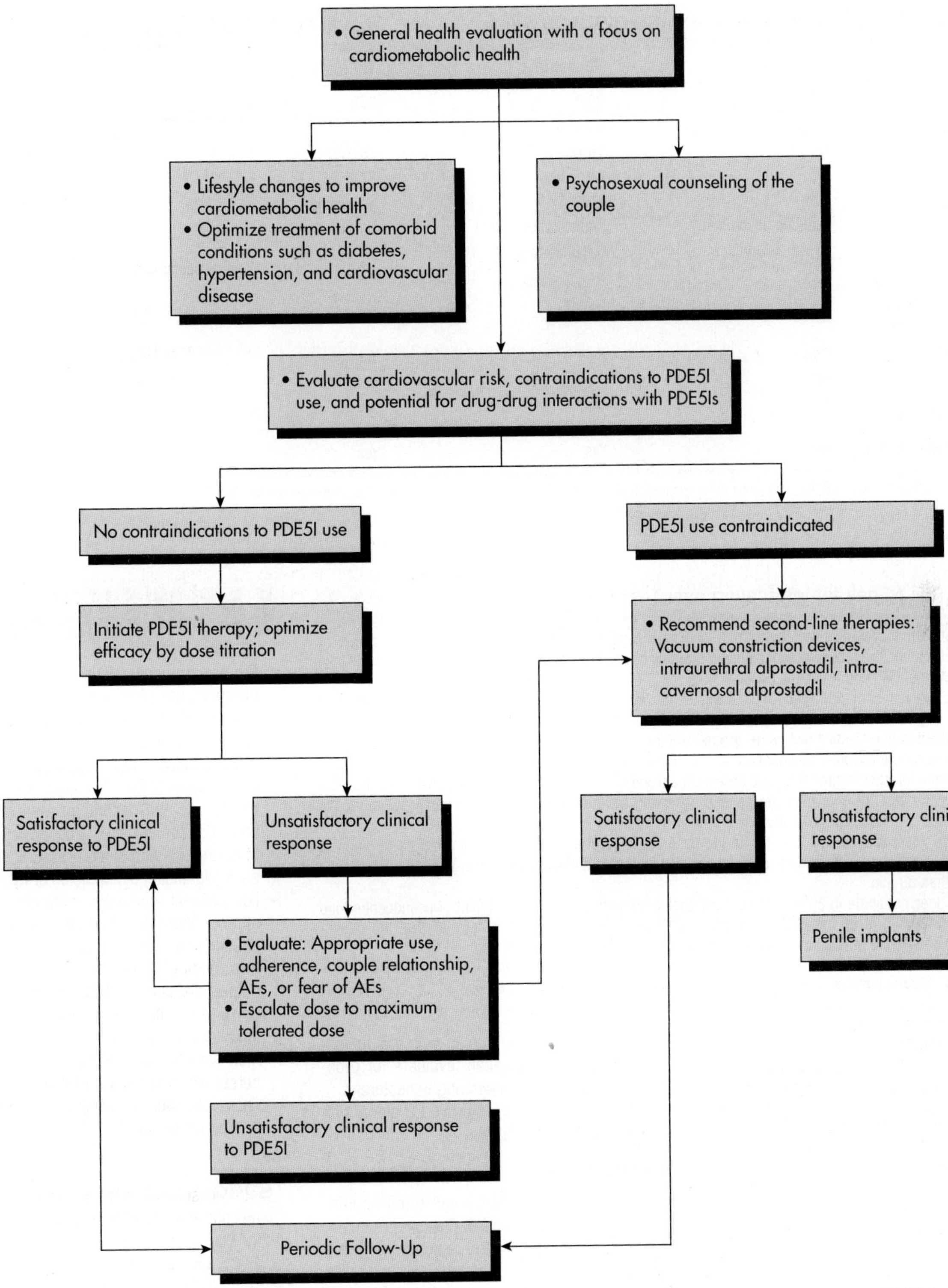

FIG. 1 An algorithmic approach to the treatment of men with erectile dysfunction. *AE*, adverse event; *PDE5I*, phosphodiesterase 5 inhibitor. (From Melmed S et al: *Williams textbook of endocrinology*, ed 14, Philadelphia, 2020, Elsevier.)

TABLE 4 Comparison of Four Phosphodiesterase Type 5 Inhibitors Currently Available in the United States

	Sildenafil	Vardenafil	Tadalafil	Avanafil
C_{max} (ng/ml)	450	20.9	378	2153
T_{max} (hr)	0.8	0.7-0.9	2	0.3-0.5
Onset of action (min)	15-60	15-60	15-120	15-60
Half-life (hr)	3-5	4-5	17.5	3-5
Bioavailability	40%	15%	Not tested	30%
Fatty food	Reduced absorption	Reduced absorption	No effect	Reduced absorption
Recommended dosage	25, 50, 100 mg	5, 10, 20 mg	5, 10, 20 mg	50, 100, 200 mg
Side effects				
Headache, dyspepsia, facial flushing	Yes	Yes	Yes	Yes
Backache, myalgia	Rare	Rare	Yes	Rare
Blurred/blue vision	Yes	Rare	Rare	No
Precaution with antiarrhythmics	No	Yes	No	No
Contraindication with nitrates	Yes	Yes	Yes	Yes

C_{max}, Maximal plasma concentration; *half-life,* time required for elimination of one half of the medication from plasma; *T_{max},* time required to attain C_{max}.
From Wein AJ et al: *Campbell-Walsh urology,* ed 11, Philadelphia, 2016, Elsevier.

TABLE 5 Guidelines for Intracavernosal Therapy

1. Do not prescribe intracavernosal therapy to men who have psychiatric disorders, hypercoagulable states, or sickle cell disease; who are receiving anticoagulant therapy; or who are unable to comprehend the risks or take appropriate action should complications occur.
2. Designate a physician or a urologist to be available to handle emergencies related to complications of intracavernosal injections, such as prolonged erection and priapism.
3. Instruct the patient in the injection technique, the risks of intracavernosal therapy, and the steps to be taken in the event of prolonged erection or priapism.
4. Administer the first injection in the office, and observe the blood pressure and heart rate response. This provides an excellent opportunity for educating the patient, observing adverse effects, and determining whether the patient will respond to intracavernosal therapy.
5. Start with a low dose of alprostadil and titrate the dose based on the erectile response and the duration of erection. Adjust the dose of alprostadil to achieve an erection that is sufficient for sexual intercourse but does not last more than 30 min.
6. If the erection does not abate in 30 min, the patient should be instructed to take a tablet of pseudoephedrine or terbutaline (Brethine) or an intracavernosal injection of phenylephrine. If this is not effective, the patient should call the designated physician or urologist and go to the emergency department.

From Melmed S et al: *Williams textbook of endocrinology,* ed 12, Philadelphia, 2011, Saunders, Elsevier.

CHRONIC RX

- Psychosexual therapy is helpful as an adjunctive treatment regardless of cause of ED.
- Psychogenic impotence: PDE5 inhibitors are effective in patients with depression because tissues, nerves, hormones, and vasculature are normal. PDE5 inhibitors are also effective as a way of providing positive experiences and building sexual confidence. Full psychological evaluation is recommended before starting treatment.
- For men not responding to other approaches: Surgical implantation of penile prosthesis may be considered. Full psychological evaluation is recommended to evaluate the possibility of unrealistic expectations or partner problems contributing to ED.
- Testosterone therapy in men with low testosterone (i.e., hypogonadal); evaluate for prostate cancer before prescribing testosterone.
- Aerobic exercise may improve ED along with pharmacologic treatment.

DISPOSITION

- Psychogenic-acquired ED will remit spontaneously in 15% to 30% of cases.
- Lifelong ED is usually a chronic and unremitting condition.
- Situational ED may remit with changes in social environment and reducing performance anxiety.

REFERRAL

- Refer if psychotherapy, sexual focused therapy, or invasive organic treatment required
- Refer to urology if PDE5 inhibitors fail or sudden onset occurs after penile trauma

PEARLS & CONSIDERATIONS

- ED is commonly evaluated and treated by primary care physician; refer to urologist if oral therapy fails, history of penile trauma, or surgery is required.
- PDE5 inhibitors are treatment of choice for most causes of ED. Main contraindications are nitrate use and decompensated cardiac disease. Caution in patients on alpha-adrenergic blockers and with blood pressures at extreme ends (significant hypotension or hypertension).
- For optimal response, patients should be appropriately informed of proper use, precautions, and adverse effects of PDE5 inhibitors. Try six to eight times at optimal doses before declaring PDE5 inhibitors a failure. Consider switching among the four PDE5 inhibitors if one fails.
- Men with ED have higher rates of coronary, cerebrovascular, and peripheral vascular diseases. Screen for cardiovascular risk factors in these patients.

SUGGESTED READINGS

Available at ExpertConsult.com

RELATED CONTENT

Erectile Dysfunction (Patient Information)
Ejaculation and Orgasm Disorders (Related Key Topic)
Hypogonadism, Male (Related Key Topic)

AUTHORS: **Mackenzie Davis, MD,** and **John P. Wincze, PhD**

BASIC INFORMATION

DEFINITION

Erysipelas is an infection of the superficial dermal layers of the skin; the infection may also extend to the cutaneous lymphatics. Erysipelas is characterized by redness, induration, lymphangitis, lymphadenopathy, and a sharply demarcated, raised border. It can affect any part of the body but is most commonly seen on the face and lower extremities.

SYNONYM

St. Anthony's Fire

ICD-10CM CODE

A46 Erysipelas

EPIDEMIOLOGY & DEMOGRAPHICS

PREDOMINANT AGE: Occurs most often in the young or old

RISK FACTORS: Breaks in the skin lead to introduction of bacteria. This can occur due to trauma, surgical incisions, ulceration, or insect bites. Athlete's foot is another common portal of entry.

Patients with impaired lymphatic or venous drainage (mastectomy, saphenous vein harvesting) and immunocompromised patients.

RECURRENCE RATE: Relatively common and often occurs at the same site.

PHYSICAL FINDINGS & CLINICAL PRESENTATION

- Distinctive red, warm, tender skin lesion with induration and a sharply defined, advancing, raised border (Fig. E1).
- Most common sites are lower extremities and face.
- Systemic signs of infection (fever and chills) are often present and may occur before the skin lesion appears.
- Vesicles or bullae may develop in severe disease.
- After several days, lesions may appear ecchymotic, and desquamation of the affected area may occur.

ETIOLOGY

- Most commonly caused by group A β-hemolytic streptococci (GABHS)
- Less often group B, C, or G streptococci
- Rarely *Staphylococcus aureus*

COMPLICATIONS

- Abscess
- Necrotizing fasciitis
- Thrombophlebitis
- Gangrene
- Metastatic infection

Dx DIAGNOSIS

DIFFERENTIAL DIAGNOSIS

- Cellulitis
- Necrotizing fasciitis
- Deep vein thrombosis
- Stasis dermatitis
- Erythema nodosum
- Contact dermatitis
- Erythema migrans (Lyme disease)
- Insect bite
- Herpes zoster
- Erysipeloid
- Acute gout
- Pseudogout

WORKUP

- Diagnosis is mainly clinical, which stresses the importance of a careful history and physical examination.
- Laboratory evaluation is not required as it will likely not change management in healthy patients. However, laboratory studies should be performed in ill-appearing or immunocompromised individuals.

LABORATORY TESTS

- Leukocytosis
- Increased ESR/CRP
- Blood cultures are positive in 5% of patients
- Gram stain and culture of any drainage from skin lesions has low yield

IMAGING STUDIES

- Not routinely indicated
- Duplex ultrasound for patients suspected of having deep vein thrombosis
- CT scan or MRI for patients with suspected necrotizing fasciitis

Rx TREATMENT

NONPHARMACOLOGIC THERAPY

- Elevation of the affected limb
- Warm compresses

ACUTE GENERAL Rx

Typical erysipelas of extremity in nondiabetic patient:

- PO: Penicillin V 500 mg q6h. Use clindamycin in patients who are allergic to penicillin.
- IV: Penicillin G (aqueous) 1 to 2 million units q6h. Use vancomycin 15 mg/kg IV q12h in penicillin-allergic patients.

Facial erysipelas (include coverage for *Staphylococcus aureus*):

- Dicloxacillin 500 mg PO q6h
- Nafcillin or oxacillin 2 g IV q4h
- Vancomycin 1 g IV q12h
- Daptomycin 4 mg/kg IV q24h
- Linezolid 600 mg IV q12h

DISPOSITION

Prognosis is good with antibiotic treatment but recurrence is common.

REFERRAL

Surgical consultation for debridement for patients with necrotizing fasciitis or for drainage of abscess.

PEARLS & CONSIDERATIONS

- Consider early surgical referral when necrotizing fasciitis suspected. Consider skin biopsy when not responding to appropriate antibiotics.
- Look for tinea pedis as portal of entry in erysipelas of lower extremities, and treat if present.

SUGGESTED READINGS

Available at ExpertConsult.com

RELATED CONTENT

Erysipelas (Patient Information)
Cellulitis (Related Key Topic)

AUTHOR: **Christina M. Bortz, MD**

BASIC INFORMATION

DEFINITION

Erythema nodosum (EN) is an acute, tender, erythematous, nodular skin eruption resulting from inflammation of subcutaneous fat, often associated with bruising. It is the most common form of panniculitis.

SYNONYM

EN

ICD-10CM CODE
L52 Erythema nodosum

EPIDEMIOLOGY & DEMOGRAPHICS

INCIDENCE: It is the most common form of panniculitis. Two to three cases/100,000 persons per yr.
PREDOMINANT SEX: Female:male ratio of 3 to 4:1
PREDOMINANT AGE: 25 to 40 yr

PHYSICAL FINDINGS & CLINICAL PRESENTATION

- Prodromal symptoms of fatigue, malaise, upper respiratory infection symptoms may precede eruption by 1 to 2 wk.
- Acute onset of tender nodules typically located on the shins and occasionally seen on the thighs and forearms (Fig. E1).
- The nodules are usually 1/8 to 1 inch in diameter but can be as large as 4 inches; they begin as light red lesions, then become darker and often ecchymotic. The nodules heal within 8 wk without ulceration.
- Associated findings:
  1. Fever (60%)
  2. Lymphadenopathy (<50%)
  3. Arthralgia (64%)
  4. Signs of the underlying illness

ETIOLOGY

Cell-mediated hypersensitivity reaction is seen more frequently in persons with human leukocyte antigen (HLA) B8. The lesion results from an exaggerated interaction between an antigen and cell-mediated immune mechanisms leading to granuloma formation. Up to 55% of cases of EN are idiopathic.
Infections:
- Bacteria:
  1. Campylobacter
  2. Streptococcal pharyngitis (28%-48%)
  3. *Salmonella* enteritis
  4. *Yersinia* enteritis
  5. Psittacosis
  6. *Chlamydia pneumoniae* infection
  7. *Mycoplasma* pneumonia
  8. Meningococcal infection
  9. Gonorrhea
  10. Syphilis
  11. Lymphogranuloma venereum
  12. Tularemia
  13. Cat-scratch disease
  14. Leprosy
  15. Tuberculosis
- Fungi:
  1. Histoplasmosis
  2. Coccidioidomycosis
  3. Blastomycosis
  4. *Trichophyton verrucosum*
- Viruses:
  1. Cytomegalovirus
  2. Hepatitis B
  3. Epstein-Barr virus
- Drugs (3%-10%):
  1. Sulfonylureas
  2. Sulfonamides
  3. Penicillins
  4. Oral contraceptives
  5. Gold salts
  6. Prazosin
  7. Aspirin
  8. Bromides
- Sarcoidosis (11%-25%)
- Inflammatory bowel disease
- Hodgkin disease, non-Hodgkin lymphoma
- Ankylosing spondylosis and reactive arthropathies (e.g., associated with inflammatory bowel disease)
- Behçet disease
- Löfgren syndrome
- Acute myelogenous leukemia

DIAGNOSIS

DIFFERENTIAL DIAGNOSIS

- Insect bites
- Posttraumatic ecchymoses
- Vasculitis
- Weber-Christian disease
- Fat necrosis associated with pancreatitis
- Necrobiosis lipoidica
- Scleroderma
- Lupus panniculitis
- Subcutaneous granuloma

WORKUP

- Physical examination
- Diagnosis of underlying illness by history, physical examination, and laboratory tests as indicated

LABORATORY TESTS

- Erythrocyte sedimentation rate
- Throat culture and antistreptolysin O titer
- Purified protein derivative
- Others depending on index of suspicion (e.g., stool culture and evaluation for ova and parasites in patients with diarrhea and gastrointestinal symptoms)
- Skin biopsy in doubtful cases:
  1. Early lesion: Inflammation and hemorrhage in subcutaneous tissue
  2. Late lesion: Giant cells and granulomata

IMAGING STUDIES

Chest radiograph to rule out sarcoidosis and tuberculosis

TREATMENT

- Treatment recommendations are summarized in Table E1.
- The disease is self-limited and treatment is symptomatic. EN nodules develop in pretibial locations and resolve spontaneously over several weeks without scarring or ulceration.
- Treatment of underlying disorders.
- Avoidance of contact irritation of affected areas.
- Nonsteroidal antiinflammatory drugs for pain.
- Systemic steroids (prednisone 1 mg/kg of body weight/day, tapered over several days) may be useful in severe cases if underlying risk of sepsis and malignancy have been excluded.
- Potassium iodide given as tablet 300 mg tid or as a supersaturated solution (five drops three times/day in orange juice) has been reported as effective for symptom control.
- Intralesional corticosteroid injections for persistent lesions.

PROGNOSIS

Typical case:
- Pain for 2 wk
- Resolution within 8 wk

RELATED CONTENT

Erythema Nodosum (Patient Information)
Sarcoidosis (Related Key Topic)

AUTHOR: **Fred F. Ferri, MD**

BASIC INFORMATION

DEFINITION

Esophageal tumors include benign and malignant neoplasms of the esophageal mucosa and wall. Carcinomas of the esophageal epithelium, both squamous cell carcinoma and adenocarcinoma (including adenoacanthoma, mucoepidermoid, and adenoid cystic), are the most common tumors of the esophagus. Rare esophageal tumors include both malignant (spindle cell, small cell, sarcoma, lymphoma, melanoma, and choriocarcinoma) and benign neoplasms (leiomyoma, papilloma, and fibrovascular polyps). One can also develop metastatic disease from a cancer that originated in another organ, but this is very rare. Breast cancer, lung cancer, and melanoma would be the most likely culprits. Other cancers can directly extend to the esophagus from the larynx, pharynx, lung, thyroid, or stomach. Approximately 15% of esophageal tumors arise in the proximal esophagus, 50% in the middle third of the esophagus, and 35% in the lower third. Tumors involving the esophageal-gastric junction are usually staged and treated as esophageal cancers if the tumor epicenter is no more than 2 cm into the proximal stomach. Tumors in the upper two thirds are usually squamous cell cancers, and tumors in the lower third are usually adenocarcinomas. The incidence of superficial esophageal cancers is increasing. These invade no deeper than the submucosa.

ICD-10CM CODES

C15.X	Malignant neoplasm of the esophagus (X defines location)
C15.3	Malignant neoplasm of upper third of esophagus
C15.4	Malignant neoplasm of middle third of esophagus
C15.5	Malignant neoplasm of lower third of esophagus
D00.2	Carcinoma of esophagus, in situ

EPIDEMIOLOGY & DEMOGRAPHICS

INCIDENCE: It is the eighth most common cancer worldwide and the seventh leading cause of cancer deaths. Rates are increasing every decade and are highest in the Asian esophageal cancer belt, extending from the Caspian Sea to northern China, with certain high-incidence pockets in Finland, Ireland, southeast Africa, and northwest France. Incidence has increased sixfold since 1975. Foods including cured meats and spicy regional fare likely play a role in certain areas. Increasing substance abuse with tobacco and alcohol also coincides with a rise in esophageal cancers. Rates of squamous cell carcinoma are decreasing while those of adenocarcinomas are dramatically increasing. The direct causes of squamous cell carcinoma most commonly include tobacco and alcohol abuse. Epithelial dysplasia usually occurs, which progresses to carcinoma in situ. Adenocarcinomas are usually the result of GERD and obesity. The mucosa of the esophagus undergoes intestinal metaplasia. Genetic alterations occur and perpetuate during proliferation.

PREVALENCE: In the U.S., there was an estimated 16,000 new cases and 15,000 deaths are reported yearly, making it the seventh leading cause of death by cancer among men. The majority of cases are diagnosed at an advanced stage (unresectable or metastatic disease).

RACE, AGE, & SEX PREDOMINANCE: In the U.S., squamous cell esophageal cancer more common among African Americans compared to whites, whereas adenocarcinoma more common in whites. The overall male:female ratio is 3 to 4:1; the highest male/female ratio is in the Hispanic population. Usually develops in fifth to seventh decades and associated with lower socioeconomic status.

GENETICS: Increasing evidence shows that genetics may play a role by increasing susceptibility to esophageal cancer. One well-identified disease associated with esophageal cancer is tylosis (focal nonepidermolytic palmoplantar keratoderma), linked to loss of heterozygosity on chromosome 17q. Familiar clustering of Barrett esophagus and the recent identification of germline mutations in affected sibling pairs support a genetic link to esophageal adenocarcinoma. Also, up to 35% of esophageal adenocarcinomas can have overexpression of HER2, which can lead to the use of targeted therapy (trastuzumab) in the treatment plan.

CLINICAL PRESENTATION

Symptoms and signs:

- Dysphagia (74%): Initially with solid foods, gradually progresses to semisolids and liquids; latter signs usually indicate incurable disease with tumor involving more than 60% of the esophageal circumference. It may be felt as chest pain
- Unintentional weight loss of short duration. Loss >10% body mass predicts poor outcome
- Hoarseness: Suggests recurrent laryngeal nerve involvement
- Odynophagia and halitosis: Unusual symptoms
- Cervical adenopathy: Usually involving supraclavicular lymph nodes
- Dry cough: Suggests tracheal involvement
- Aspiration pneumonia: Caused by fistula between the esophagus and trachea
- Iron deficiency anemia: Related to chronic GI blood loss
- Massive hemoptysis or hematemesis from the invasion of vascular structures
- Advanced disease spreads to lymph nodes, liver, lungs, peritoneum, and pleura
- Hypercalcemia: Associated with squamous cell carcinoma from secretion of a parathyroid-like tumor peptide

Clinical findings:

- 50% to 60% of patients present with inoperative disease (locally advanced/metastatic).

ETIOLOGY

The pathogenesis of esophageal cancers is attributable to chronic recurrent oxidative damage from any of the following etiologic agents, which cause inflammation, and esophagitis, increased cell turnover, and, ultimately, initiation of the carcinogenic process.

ETIOLOGIC AGENTS: Squamous cell carcinoma

- Excess alcohol consumption is strongly associated with squamous cell esophageal cancer in the U.S.; hard liquor is associated with a higher incidence than wine or beer.
- Tobacco and alcohol synergistically increase risk for squamous cell cancer
- Other ingested carcinogens:
  1. Nitrates (converted to nitrites): South Asia, China
  2. Smoked opiates: Northern Iran
  3. Fungal toxins in pickled vegetables
  4. Betel nut chewing
- Mucosal damage:
  1. Long-term exposure to extremely hot tea (>70 °C [158 °F])
  2. Ingestion of lye or extremely acidic solutions, including reflux of stomach acid
- Radiation-induced strictures
- Achalasia: Incidence of esophageal cancer is seven times greater in this population
- Host susceptibility as a result of precancerous lesions:
  1. Plummer-Vinson syndrome (Paterson-Kelly): Glossitis with iron deficiency
  2. Congenital hyperkeratosis and pitting of palms and soles (tylosis)
- HPV infection (types 16 and 18) has been detected in squamous cell carcinoma of the esophagus, sometimes associated with p53 tumor suppressor gene mutations
- Possible relationship with prolonged bisphosphonates (≥10 prescriptions, or >3 yr use)
- Possible association with celiac sprue or dietary deficiencies molybdenum, selenium, zinc, vitamin A

ADENOCARCINOMA:

- The incidence of adenocarcinoma is continually rising.
- Smoking increases risk of adenocarcinoma, particularly in patients with Barrett.
- Obesity, hiatal hernia, and diets lacking in fresh fruit and vegetables and high in fat (particularly from red meat and processed foods) increase risk.
- Chronic GERD leading to Barrett metaplasia and adenocarcinoma via immune cell infiltration and production of inflammatory mediators and reactive oxygen species. The annual rate of transformation from Barrett to adenocarcinoma is <0.5%.
- *H. pylori* infection may reduce risk of adenocarcinoma but can increase risk of lymphoma.

Dx DIAGNOSIS

DIFFERENTIAL DIAGNOSIS

- Achalasia
- Scleroderma of the esophagus
- Diffuse esophageal spasm
- Esophageal rings and webs

LABORATORY TESTS

Complete blood cell count, blood chemistry, and liver enzymes should be obtained at diagnosis. No biomarkers are currently recommended to diagnose, monitor, or predict outcomes. While both the CEA and CA-19-9 can be elevated in patients with esophageal cancer (up to 70%), the sensitivity is low (18%-35%) and there is no proven predictive value.

IMAGING STUDIES

Imaging studies are important not only for diagnosis but for accurate staging:

- Esophagogastroduodenoscopy (EGD) (Fig. E1) should be performed initially to visualize all tumors and allow histopathologic confirmation.
- Endoscopic inspection of the larynx, trachea, and bronchi may identify concomitant cancers of head, neck, and lung ("triple endoscopy").
- Endoscopic ultrasound (EUS) (Fig. E1) appears to be the most accurate method for locoregional staging: To determine the depth of tumor invasion and to assess for and possibly obtain fine needle aspiration biopsies of suspicious lymph nodes.
- PET CT has become the standard of care along with EUS, for the most accurate staging. These modalities can determine tumor spread for preoperative staging. CT scans of the chest (Fig. E2) and abdomen are more useful for restaging patients after initial therapy.

STAGING

Table 1 describes the TNM staging system for cancer of the esophagus from the American Joint Committee on Cancer Criteria. Fig. 3 illustrates an algorithm for staging thoracic esophageal cancer.

TABLE 1 TNM Staging System for Cancer of the Esophagus (American Joint Committee on Cancer Criteria)

Primary Tumor (T)*	
T_X	Primary tumor cannot be assessed
T_0	No evidence of primary tumor
T_{is}	High-grade dysplasia†
T_1	Tumor invades lamina propria, muscularis mucosae, or submucosa
T_{1a}	Tumor invades lamina propria or muscularis mucosae
T_{1b}	Tumor invades submucosa
T_2	Tumor invades muscularis propria
T_3	Tumor invades adventitia
T_4	Tumor invades adjacent structures
T_{4a}	Resectable tumor invading pleura, pericardium, or diaphragm
T_{4b}	Unresectable tumor invading other adjacent structures, such as aorta, vertebral body, trachea, etc.
Lymph Node (N)‡	
N_X	Regional lymph nodes cannot be assessed
N_0	No regional lymph node metastasis
N_1	Metastasis in 1-2 regional lymph nodes
N_2	Metastasis in 3-6 regional lymph nodes
N_3	Metastasis in 7 or more regional lymph nodes
Distant Metastasis (M)	
M_X	Metastasis cannot be assessed
M_0	No distant metastasis
M_1	Distant metastasis

TNM, tumor, node, metastases.
*(1) At least maximal dimension of the tumor must be recorded and (2) multiple tumors require the T(m) suffix.
†High-grade dysplasia includes all noninvasive neoplastic epithelia that was formerly called carcinoma in situ.
‡Number must be recorded for total number of regional nodes sampled and total number of reported nodes with metastasis.
From Edge S et al (eds): *AJCC cancer staging manual,* ed 7, New York, 2010, Springer.

Rx TREATMENT

ALL STAGES OF ESOPHAGEAL CANCER

Although the histology of esophageal cancer can differ, most studies have combined tissue types in exploring treatment options. The histology develops secondary to differing pathogenesis and causative agents with tumor biology likely playing a role through varying mutations. The likelihood of response and prognosis can differ as well. However, as there is a lack of data on how histology should dictate the treatment approach, we generally attack this cancer in a uniform manner as most studies have suggested the optimum benefit be obtained through a neoadjuvant chemoradiation approach followed by surgery when applicable in up to stage III disease.

COMBINATION THERAPY: CHEMORADIOTHERAPY FOLLOWED BY SURGICAL RESECTION: Induction chemotherapy, given before chemoradiation for patients with locally advanced but still possibly resectable disease, has been administered with good results. However, no studies have shown this approach superior to chemoradiation alone. Standard fractionation 3D-RT is utilized in chemoradiotherapy.

- Chemotherapy is most often given with concurrent radiotherapy. Chemotherapy acts as a radiosensitizer and makes tumor cells more vulnerable to the effects of ionizing radiation, thus improving tumoricidal effects on cancer. Neoadjuvant chemoradiotherapy followed by surgery is the most common approach for patients with resectable disease but is employed primarily for patients with stage IIA or higher disease. Five-yr survival is improved with a neoadjuvant approach (39%) versus surgery alone (16%). Several trials have now shown that preoperative therapy improves survival among patients with potentially curable esophageal or esophagogastric junction cancer. Neoadjuvant chemotherapy alone is another option for locally advanced disease, but results are not as good as with neoadjuvant chemoradiotherapy.
- Chemoradiotherapy followed by surgery should be offered to late stage I ($T_{1b}N_0$ or higher), stage II, and stage III esophageal cancer patients as the current standard of care. In several studies, this approach significantly improved local control, reduced recurrence, and reduced mortality compared with surgery alone in patients with resectable esophageal cancer. This also increases the chance of an R0 resection. Trimodality therapy is the preferred treatment for most esophageal cancers.
- Chemoradiotherapy alone may be offered as definitive treatment for patients who are not surgical candidates, and some of these patients may be cured.
- Combination chemotherapy using a platinum doublet (platinum agent plus second agent) can achieve significant tumor reduction in 30% to 60% of patients. Cisplatin, oxaliplatin, or carboplatin is usually given with 5-FU (5-fluorouracil) or paclitaxel to obtain the desired tumoricidal effects. Other chemotherapeutic agents with activity in esophageal cancer include docetaxel, irinotecan, and epirubicin. The latter two are not used with concurrent radiotherapy secondary to increased toxicities.
- Capecitabine in combination with either cisplatin or oxaliplatin is as effective as 5FU in the neoadjuvant or definitive treatment setting.
- Complications of chemoradiotherapy primarily include mucositis, nausea, vomiting, diarrhea, myelosuppression, nephrotoxicity, ototoxicity, neurotoxicity with peripheral neuropathy, esophageal stricture, esophageal rupture, trachea-esophageal fistula (6%), and radiation pneumonitis. These can occur to varying degrees and are certainly more significant in the elderly and those with significant comorbidities.
- Postoperative adjuvant chemoradiotherapy should be offered to node-positive patients who underwent surgical resection without neoadjuvant chemoradiotherapy.

SURGICAL RESECTION:

- Surgical resection of both squamous cell and adenocarcinoma of the middle esophagus and lower third of the esophagus is an acceptable initial modality for local and resectable disease in the absence of widespread metastases detected by CT-PET and transesophageal ultrasound (T_1 and T_2 tumors). Gastric pull-through or colonic interposition typically is used to provide luminal continuity.
- Endoscopic mucosal resection may replace radical surgical resection in patients with dysplasia and some small early tumors with no lymph node involvement (T_{is} or T_{1a}), but a recent Cochrane review found no studies comparing endoscopic resection vs. surgery. Endoscopic mucosal resection may be beneficial for patients who are poor surgical candidates. It may be performed in conjunction with ablative therapies, including radiofrequency ablation, thermal ablation techniques, laser ablation, argon plasma coagulation,

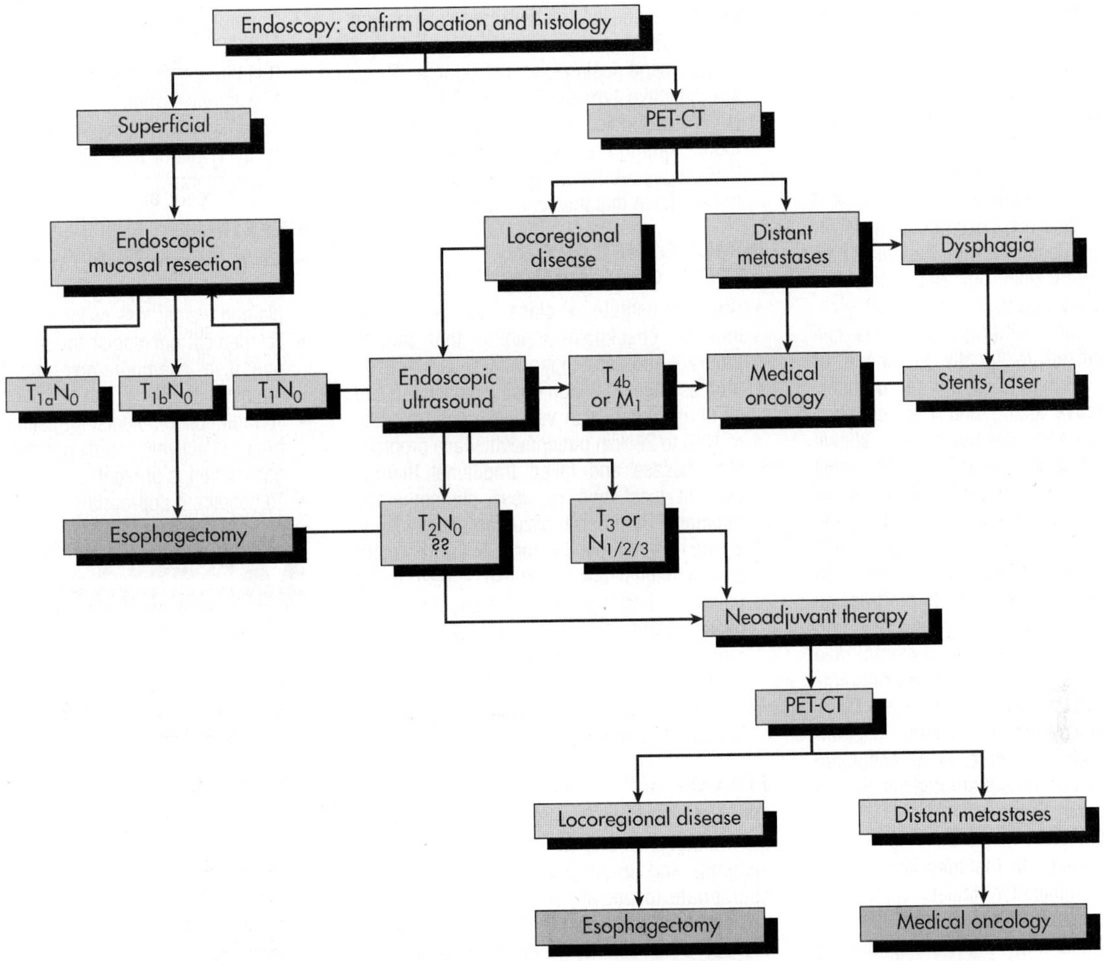

FIG. 3 An algorithm for staging a thoracic esophageal cancer patient. Metastatic disease must always be confirmed by pathologic evaluation of the tissue in question. *PET-CT,* Positron emission tomography–computed tomography. (From Sellke FW et al: *Sabiston & Spencer surgery of the chest,* ed 9, Philadelphia, 2016, Elsevier.)

or photodynamic therapy. Electrocoagulation (electrofulguration) is also being used and may aid in the relief of esophageal blockage.

- Complications of surgery, including endoscopic resection and local therapy:
  1. Esophageal rupture
  2. Anatomic fistula (usually with colon interposition, subphrenic abscesses).
  3. Respiratory complications.
  4. Cardiovascular complications are most common, including MI, CVA, and PE.
  5. Mortality is lower and clinical outcomes are better at high-volume hospitals and with minimally invasive surgery.
  6. Hybrid minimally invasive esophagectomy has been reported to have a lower incidence of intraoperative and postoperative major complications, specifically pulmonary complications, than open esophagectomy, without compromising overall and disease-free survival over a 3-yr period (Mariette et al, 2019).

Despite adequate preoperative staging, 25% of patients initially treated with surgical resection will have microscopically positive resection margins and are upstaged at the time of surgery. This has led to the majority of patients receiving neoadjuvant chemoradiotherapy as demonstrated in the CROSS Trial. The median disease-free survival for this group of patients was significantly prolonged as compared with the surgery-alone group. Death from recurrent cancer was decreased by 9% in the neoadjuvant group as well. The benefit of neoadjuvant therapy on survival was consistent regardless of histologic subtype.

PRETREATMENT PATIENT PREPARATION

The patient needs to stop smoking and drinking alcohol if at all possible. Before neoadjuvant or definitive chemoradiotherapy, the patient should have placement of an intravenous access device and a feeding tube (J-tube is preferable before surgical resection).

RADIATION THERAPY:

- Squamous cell carcinoma is more radiosensitive than adenocarcinoma. Radiotherapy achieves good local control but is generally only used as monotherapy in a palliative mode for obstructive symptoms in patients with unresectable or advanced cancer or those with multiple comorbidities that limit treatment. It is best used for cervical esophageal tumors, but response rates are best when combined with chemotherapy.
- Radiotherapy in the preoperative/neoadjuvant setting is taken to a total dose of 40 to 50 Gy. For definitive therapy, the dose range is 50 to 55 Gy.
- Palliative radiotherapy for bone metastasis is also effective.
- Complications of radiotherapy: Can best be avoided by 3D conformal therapy.
  1. Esophageal stricture, fistula formation, radiation-induced pulmonary fibrosis, and transverse myelitis are the most common adverse events.
  2. Radiotherapy-induced cardiomyopathy and skin changes are rare but can occur. It is difficult to shield the heart from radiation as these organs are positioned so close.
- IMRT can also be used for the treatment of esophageal cancers. It is associated with a more favorable toxicity profile. Very few studies have been completed to date using chemotherapy with IMRT and is therefore not considered a standard approach at this time for neoadjuvant therapy.
- Brachytherapy: This is also an option for patients in a palliative mode. It provides high-dose radiation to a localized area and may prevent the need for a stent in patients

with dysphagia. Its use is very limited in prior irradiated tissue for fear of fistula and perforation of the esophagus.

TREATMENT OF UNRESECTABLE, LOCALLY ADVANCED, OR METASTATIC DISEASE

- Combination chemotherapy regimens as a rule have a higher response rate than single-agent therapy. Response rates can be as high as 50% but that does not always translate into prolonged survival.
- Neoadjuvant chemotherapy regimens can also be utilized in locally advanced or metastatic settings. Cisplatin is probably the most active agent, and this combined with 5FU can yield response rates shown in several studies of up to 50%. The most widely used regimen in both squamous cell and adenocarcinoma is FOLFOX. If a taxane is added to this regimen in the metastatic setting, the triple drug regimen can lead to a prolongation in disease progression by about 2 mo, which may translate into prolonged survival. However, patients have to be carefully chosen for a triple drug regimen because of increased toxicity. Other active doublet regimens combine cisplatin with irinotecan, etoposide, or gemcitabine. Capecitabine can be substituted for 5FU in these regimens.
- Trifluridine/tipiracil is another option for metastatic disease in the third-line setting. Fixed-dose combination tablets comprising trifluridine, an antineoplastic nucleoside analog, and tipiracil, a thymidine phosphorylase inhibitor, are available. In the TAGS trial, this combination improved both PFS and OS compared to best supportive care. However, OS was improved by only 2 mo, not a major breakthrough.

TARGETED MOLECULAR THERAPY

Two drugs have been approved for adenocarcinoma of the esophagus. Ramucirumab is a VEGF inhibitor and trastuzumab is effective in cancers with overexpression of HER2. There is no apparent role for either drug in squamous cell carcinoma.

- Ramucirumab is a recombinant monoclonal IgG1 antibody that is a vascular endothelial growth factor receptor 2 (VEGFR-2) antagonist approved in 2014. It inhibits ligand proliferation and migration of endothelial cells and ultimately inhibits angiogenesis. Indicated for second-line therapy in with paclitaxel or as third line monotherapy.
- Trastuzumab, in combination with oxaliplatin and 5FU (FOLFOX), is considered the standard of care as first-line therapy for metastatic esophageal cancer in patients with HER-2 overexpressing adenocarcinoma. This was approved based on the results of the ToGA trial (2010). Approximately 22% of adenocarcinomas will overexpress the type II epidermal growth factor receptor HER2. The overall response rate is 47%.
- Entrectinib and larotrectinib are also approved for neurotrophic-tropomyosin receptor kinase (NTRK) gene fusion–positive tumors. These are selective tyrosine kinase inhibitors. The NTRK gene fusion and amplification is much more common in adenocarcinoma, but in both types of histology, less than 1% of tumors have this molecular marker.

IMMUNOTHERAPY IN ESOPHAGEAL CANCER

- Drugs constitute a class that act as an immune checkpoint inhibitor that targets programmed death ligand 1 (PD-1).
- Studies have been done using nivolumab and pembrolizumab with varying response rates of 10% to 25% in patients who have progressive disease and failed traditional therapy with at least two previous chemotherapy regimens. Both pembrolizumab and nivolumab are now approved in the U.S. for treatment of esophageal cancer. These appear to be most effective in patients with squamous cell histology, but adenocarcinomas also respond regardless of PD-L1 status, as noted in the KEYNOTE-181 study.
- Patients with MSI-H and dMMR positive tumors also are more likely to respond.

FOLLOW-UP CARE

The majority of recurrences develop within 12 mo of diagnosis. Clinical monitoring, lab tests, imaging, and endoscopic evaluation where appropriate (especially in Barrett esophagus), are performed for postoperative surveillance, without clear benefit of earlier detection or decreased mortality. For patients who have undergone definitive therapy, endoscopic surveillance should be performed every 3 mo for the first yr, and then at least annually. Palliative procedures such as endoscopic dilation, endoscopic ablation, endoscopic mucosal resection, photodynamic therapy, brachytherapy, feeding tube insertion, or placement of expandable metal stents or polyvinyl prostheses to bypass tumors have all been used for unresectable patients. The morbidity and mortality associated with resection in patients with advanced disease and/or for palliation argues against offering surgery to most of these patients.

SURVIVORSHIP

- Overall 5-yr survival for all stages at presentation is 15% (39% for localized disease, 21% for regional disease, and 4% for distant disease).
- Endoscopic therapy for highly selected stage 0 or stage I patients with disease limited to the submucosa may have 5-yr survival rates of 70% to 90%.
- Surgical resection without neoadjuvant treatment: 5 to yr survival rate is 5% to 30%, with higher survival (45%-50%) in early-stage cancers.
- Radiation therapy without chemotherapy or surgery: 5-yr survival rate of 6% to 20%.
- Chemoradiotherapy without surgery: 5-yr survival up to 30%.
- Combined trimodality treatment: 45% to 50% 5-yr survival rates (all stages of disease).
- Patients with metastatic disease have median survivals of less than 1 yr with palliative chemotherapy.

REFERRAL

- To gastroenterologist for endoscopy for patients with dysphagia, odynophagia, unexplained weight loss or for palliative care
- To medical oncologist for evaluation of preoperative chemotherapy and care of the metastatic patient
- To radiation oncologist for palliative therapy if tumor is actively bleeding, unresectable, or if obstruction is present
- To hospice if appropriate

PEARLS & CONSIDERATIONS

COMMENTS

More than 50% of patients with esophageal cancer are diagnosed when the disease is metastatic or unresectable.

PREVENTION

- A diet high in fruits, vegetables, and antioxidants may be associated with lower risk of esophageal cancer.
- Avoid tobacco and excessive alcohol use.
- Avoid ingested toxins known to cause esophageal cancers.
- Aspirin may have a chemopreventive role in Barrett esophagus, but is only currently recommended for patients with other (e.g., cardiac) indications.
- No evidence that vitamins, Chinese herbs, or green tea prevents esophageal cancer.
- Screening the general population is not recommended. If Barrett esophagus is detected, regularly scheduled surveillance endoscopies are necessary, with consideration for radiofrequency or other ablation therapy if dysplasia is detected.

PATIENT & FAMILY EDUCATION

Provide education and support about the likely prognosis because most esophageal cancers are diagnosed at an advanced stage.

SUGGESTED READINGS

Available at ExpertConsult.com

RELATED CONTENT

Esophageal Cancer (Patient Information)
Barrett Esophagus (Related Key Topic)

AUTHOR: **Anthony G. Thomas, DO, FACP**

BASIC INFORMATION

DEFINITION

Esophageal varices are dilated submucosal veins that occur in patients with underlying portal hypertension, function as a shunt between the portal venous and systemic venous circulation, and can result in severe upper GI hemorrhage.

ICD-10CM CODES	
I85.00	Esophageal varices without bleeding
I85.01	Esophageal varices with bleeding

EPIDEMIOLOGY & DEMOGRAPHICS

INCIDENCE:
- Esophageal varices: 5% to 15% per yr in patients with cirrhosis
- Hemorrhage:
  1. One third of all patients with varices will develop hemorrhage.
  2. Variceal hemorrhage occurs in 25% to 40% of patients with cirrhosis.
  3. The risk of bleeding from varices is approximately 15% at 1 yr.
  4. Survivors of an episode of active bleeding have a 70% risk of recurrent hemorrhage within 1 yr.

PREVALENCE: Approximately 50% of patients with cirrhosis have varices at the time of diagnosis.

RISK FACTORS: Cirrhosis, low platelet count and advanced Child-Pugh class, hepatitis C with advanced fibrosis

PHYSICAL FINDINGS & CLINICAL PRESENTATION

- Often asymptomatic until acute upper GI hemorrhage: Hematemesis, hypovolemia
- No physical findings specific for esophageal varices
- Stigmata of cirrhosis and portal hypertension may be evident: Palmar erythema, telangiectasias, gynecomastia, testicular atrophy, jaundice, caput medusae, lower extremity edema, ascites, splenomegaly, hemorrhoids, asterixis

ETIOLOGY

- Portal hypertension results from obstruction to portal venous outflow, and varices subsequently develop in order to decompress the hypertensive portal vein and return blood to the systemic circulation.
- Varices may appear when portal vein pressures rise above 10 to 12 mm Hg.
- Cirrhosis is the most common cause of portal hypertension.

DIAGNOSIS

DIFFERENTIAL DIAGNOSIS

- Budd-Chiari syndrome, cirrhosis, portal vein thrombosis, schistosomiasis, Wilson disease
- Other causes of upper GI bleeding: Duodenal or gastric ulcers, gastric cancer, Mallory-Weiss tear

WORKUP

Upper endoscopy, laboratory tests, and imaging

LABORATORY TESTS

- CBC:
  1. Anemia (blood loss, nutritional deficiencies, alcohol myelosuppression)
  2. Thrombocytopenia (hypersplenism, alcohol myelosuppression)
- Renal function panel:
  1. BUN: Often increased in setting of upper GI bleeding
  2. Creatinine: Often elevated by hypovolemia, monitor for hepatorenal syndrome
  3. Sodium: Dilutional hyponatremia
- Heme-positive stools
- Type and crossmatch: In preparation for blood transfusion
- INR/PT and PTT: Coagulation factors produced in liver and may be prolonged in liver disease or impairment
- Liver function tests: ALT/AST may be normal in cirrhotic patients due to longstanding fibrosis; elevated alkaline phosphatase and a direct hyperbilirubinemia may be present if cholestatic liver disease is present
- Serum albumin: Severe liver disease results in hypoalbuminemia

IMAGING STUDIES

Invasive:
- Esophagogastroduodenoscopy (EGD) (upper endoscopy):
  1. In all patients with cirrhosis, screen for the presence or absence of varices and determine subsequent risk for variceal hemorrhage.
  2. In patients with small varices (<5 mm) repeat EGD in 2 yr (unless decompensation occurs).
  3. In patients with compensated cirrhosis who do not have varices, screening is repeated every 2 to 3 yr.
  4. In patients with decompensated cirrhosis (ascites, hepatic encephalopathy, variceal hemorrhage, or jaundice), it is repeated every yr or at the time of first decompensation.
  5. Emergently performed if there is evidence of acute upper GI bleeding to diagnose and treat variceal hemorrhage.

Noninvasive:
- Esophagography with barium can diagnose esophageal varices (Fig. E1).
- Capsule endoscopy can also diagnose esophageal varices, although sensitivity is not yet established.
- CT scan (Fig. E2).

TREATMENT

NONPHARMACOLOGIC THERAPY

- Endoscopic variceal ligation (Fig. E3) is an alternative to nonselective beta-blockers for primary prophylaxis against variceal hemorrhage. It is also used in patients unable to tolerate beta-blockers.
  1. Typically for patients with medium or large varices at highest risk for hemorrhage (Child-Pugh B/C or red wale markings viewed on endoscopy)
  2. Usually two to four sessions
  3. May not be a permanent solution because varices can recur after initial eradication
  4. Associated with significant complications, including hemorrhage from banding-induced ulcerations
     a. Therefore should be performed by endoscopists with expertise in prophylactic banding
     b. First surveillance endoscopy 1 to 3 mo after obliteration, then every 6 to 12 mo indefinitely

ACUTE GENERAL Rx

- Variceal hemorrhage: Acute hemodynamic resuscitation with packed red blood cell transfusion, correct coagulopathy and thrombocytopenia, airway protection and intubation as necessary, antibiotics (ceftriaxone or norfloxacin) for SBP prophylaxis, octreotide maintained for 2 to 5 days in conjunction with endoscopic therapy. The use of balloon tamponade in the control of active variceal bleeding should be a last resort when other forms of therapy are not available or fail to achieve hemostasis. Balloon tamponade (Fig. E4) should be used only as a temporary means of stabilization and a bridge to a more definitive form of therapy.
- EGD to treat bleeding esophageal varices by esophageal band ligation or sclerotherapy (Fig. 5).

CHRONIC Rx

Primary prophylaxis (Fig. 6):
- Nonselective beta-blockers such as propranolol (20 mg twice daily), nadolol (40 mg once daily) or carvedilol (6.25 mg twice daily)
  1. Increase as tolerated for goal heart rate of approximately 55 beats/min
  2. Blocks the adrenergic dilatory tone in mesenteric arterioles, resulting in unopposed alpha-adrenergic mediated vasoconstriction and therefore a decrease in portal inflow

Secondary prophylaxis (Fig. E7):
- All patients with compensated cirrhosis who have bled from esophageal varices should receive esophageal band ligation and beta-blockers, unless beta-blockers are contraindicated.
  1. Transjugular intrahepatic portosystemic shunt or surgical shunt may be performed if bleeding from esophageal varices continues or recurs despite this dual therapy.
- For patients with decompensated cirrhosis there is evidence, although limited, against the use of prophylactic beta-blockers due to the risk for increased mortality.

REFERRAL

Consultation with a gastroenterologist is recommended in all patients with cirrhosis or portal hypertension in order to screen for esophageal varices.

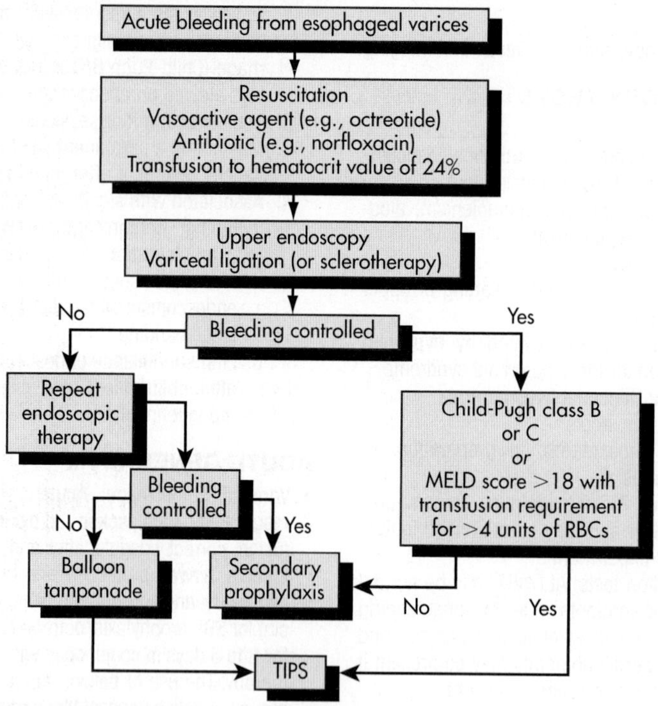

FIG. 5 Algorithm for the management of bleeding esophageal varices. *RBC,* Red blood cell; *MELD,* model end state liver disease; *TIPS,* transjugular intrahepatic portosystemic shunt. (From Feldman M et al: *Sleisenger and Fordtran's gastrointestinal and liver disease*, ed 10, Philadelphia, 2016, Elsevier.)

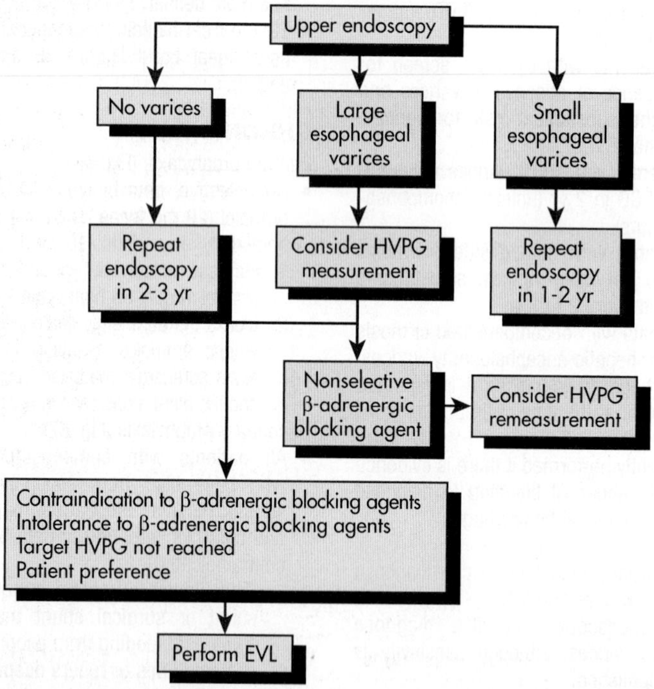

FIG. 6 Algorithm for the primary prophylaxis of esophageal variceal hemorrhage in patients with cirrhosis. The hepatic vein pressure gradient *(HVPG)* may be measured in patients with large varices before a nonselective β-adrenergic blocking agent is started and remeasured 1 mo after the maximum tolerated dose of the beta-blocker is reached. The goal of treatment is to reduce the HVPG to <12 mm Hg or by ≥20%. *EVL,* Endoscopic variceal ligation. (From Feldman M et al: *Sleisenger and Fordtran's gastrointestinal and liver disease*, ed 10, Philadelphia, 2016, Elsevier.)

PEARLS & CONSIDERATIONS

Besides variceal size, risk factors for variceal hemorrhage include Child-Pugh class B/C or variceal red wale markings on endoscopy.

RELATED CONTENT

Cirrhosis (Related Key Topic)
Portal Hypertension (Related Key Topic)

AUTHOR: **Fred F. Ferri, MD**

BASIC INFORMATION

DEFINITION

A tremor is an oscillatory movement of a body part. Essential tremor is a predominantly postural and action tremor that is bilateral and tends to progress slowly over the years in the absence of other neurologic abnormalities.

SYNONYMS

Benign essential tremor
Familial tremor

ICD-10CM CODE
G25.0 Essential tremor

EPIDEMIOLOGY & DEMOGRAPHICS

Essential tremor is one of the most prevalent neurologic diseases. It affects nearly 7 million persons in the U.S. It is the most common movement disorder.

PREDOMINANT AGE: Can begin at any age, but incidence increases after age 40 yr. Prevalence is 6% to 9% for those >60 yr of age.

GENETICS: Positive family history is found in 50% of patients. No gender or racial predominance.

PHYSICAL FINDINGS & CLINICAL PRESENTATION

- Essential tremor is characterized by a bilateral action tremor of 6 to 12 Hz that tends to be more prominent one side of the body than the other. In approximately 50% of patients, the tremor also worsens with intention, specifically at the termination of a goal-directed movement. This can be seen at the very end of the finger-to-nose maneuver or while drinking from a glass. The tremor can be found in the upper extremities (90%-95%), head (30%), legs (10%-15%), or voice (20%), and is usually absent when the affected body part is at rest.
- In addition to the action tremor, a postural tremor may be seen when the patient holds the body part against gravity. The postural tremor is usually most noticeable at the wrist and is usually of lower amplitude than the action tremor.
- Patients with essential tremor may also have gait ataxia on tandem walk and may report a history of increased falls or near falls.
- No other neurologic abnormalities are found on examination.
- Symptoms worsen with emotional distress, fatigue, or the use of caffeine or other stimulants and improve with intake of small amounts of alcohol.

ETIOLOGY

Often an inherited disease in an autosomal dominant pattern. Sporadic cases without a family history can occur.

DIAGNOSIS

DIFFERENTIAL DIAGNOSIS (SEE TABLE 1)

- Parkinson disease: The tremor is usually asymmetric, especially early on in the disease, and is predominantly a resting tremor. Patients with Parkinson disease will also have increased tone, decreased facial expression, slowness of movement, and shuffling gait.
- Cerebellar tremor: This is an intention tremor that increases steadily right before arriving at the target during a goal-directed movement (such as finger to nose testing). Other associated neurologic abnormalities include ataxia, dysarthria, dysmetria, wide-based gait, and difficulty with tandem gait.
- Drug-induced: Many drugs enhance normal, physiologic tremor. These include caffeine, nicotine, lithium, levothyroxine, β-adrenergic bronchodilators, amiodarone, valproate, and SSRIs.
- Wilson disease: This is often characterized by a wing-beating tremor that is most pronounced with shoulders abducted, elbows flexed, and fingers pointing toward each other. Usually there are other neurologic abnormalities including dysarthria, dystonia, and Kayser-Fleischer rings on ophthalmologic examination.
- Physiologic tremor.

WORKUP

- Essential tremor is a clinical diagnosis. Review of medications is essential.
- All imaging studies (MRI, CT) are unnecessary unless other neurologic abnormalities are present.
- Obtain TSH to rule out hyperthyroidism and ionized calcium to rule out calcium abnormalities.
- In patients younger than 40 yr old with other neurologic abnormalities, send ceruloplasmin, serum copper, and 24-hr urine copper to evaluate for Wilson disease.

TREATMENT

Treat essential tremor when it is functionally impairing. Treatments are up to 75% effective.

NONPHARMACOLOGIC THERAPY

- Stress management.
- Minimization of caffeine use if consumption is correlated with worsened symptoms.
- Wrist weights and use of weighted utensils may be helpful in reducing tremor amplitude during feeding.
- Consumption of small quantities of alcohol at social functions, although the symptom relief may be short in duration and may be followed by tremor rebound.
- A recent trial using MRI-guided focus ultrasound thalamotomy found it effective in reducing hand tremor in patients with essential tremor. Side effects included sensory and gait disturbances.

ACUTE GENERAL Rx

Propranolol (20-40 mg) may be used in preparation for specific event.

CHRONIC Rx

First-line agents:

- Propranolol: Typical starting dose of 40 mg BID titrating to 60 mg BID.
- Propranolol LA: Typical starting dose is 30 mg/day. The usual therapeutic dose is 160 mg/day. Although not contraindicated, this medication must be used with caution in those with asthma, depression, cardiac disease, and diabetes. Atenolol or sotalol are also effective.
- Primidone: Typical starting dose is 12.5 to 25 mg qhs. Increase by 12.5 to 25 mg/day every week. Usual therapeutic dose is between 62.5 and 750 mg daily (assuming side effects are tolerated). Sedation and nausea are common at treatment initiation.
- Topiramate: 25 mg qhs, may titrate up to by 25 mg per week in BID dosing to maximum of 400 mg (200 mg BID).

Other (second-line) agents:

- Gabapentin: Typical starting dose is 300 mg tid. Usual therapeutic dose is 1200 to 3600 mg daily in three divided doses
- Benzodiazepines (i.e., alprazolam): 0.125 to 3 mg daily in divided doses
- Focal botulinum toxin injections

SURGICAL Rx

Thalamic deep brain stimulation (or possibly thalamotomy) contralateral to side of tremor is

TABLE 1 Overlapping Features of Various Types of Tremor

Feature	Parkinson Syndrome	Cerebellar Tremor	Essential Tremor
Present at rest	Yes	No	No
Increased tone	Yes	No	No
Decreased tone	No	Yes	No
Postural abnormality	Yes	Yes	No
Head involvement	Yes	Yes	Yes
Intentional component	No	Yes	Yes
Incoordination	No	Yes	No

From Remmel KS et al: *Handbook of symptom-oriented neurology,* ed 3, St Louis, 2002, Mosby.

reserved for resistant tremor or for patients who do not tolerate drug therapy. Surgical ablation of the neutral intermediate nucleus or the thalamus with use of magnetic resonance-guided focused ultrasound was recently FDA approved.

DISPOSITION

Patients should be reassured that the condition is not associated with other neurologic disabilities; however, it can become quite functionally disabling over time.

REFERRAL

This is a condition that usually can be treated by the primary care physician; however, if patient fails first-line therapies, the patient should be referred to a neurologist for other drug trials and discussion of possible surgical options.

PEARLS & CONSIDERATIONS

- Essential tremor is the most common of all movement disorders. It is characterized by an action tremor that increases at the end of goal-directed movement.
- In addition to motor dysfunction, essential tremor can cause significant psychological impact on patients in social situations.

SUGGESTED READINGS

Available at ExpertConsult.com

AUTHORS: **Marco Pares, MD,** and **Joseph S. Kass, MD, JD, FAAN**

BASIC INFORMATION

DEFINITION

Exocrine pancreatic insufficiency (EPI) is a serious condition characterized by a deficiency in pancreatic digestive enzymes resulting in inadequate digestion of fats, carbohydrates, and proteins. The most common cause of EPI is chronic pancreatitis (CP) in adults and cystic fibrosis (CF) in children. Clinically, EPI commonly results in fat malabsorption and is characterized by steatorrhea, weight loss, and maldigestion. In mild cases, it may be asymptomatic or result in mild abdominal discomfort with normal appearing bowel movements.

SYNONYMS

Pancreatic insufficiency
EPI
Fat malabsorption

ICD-10CM CODE

K86.81 Exocrine pancreatic insufficiency

EPIDEMIOLOGY & DEMOGRAPHICS

PREVALENCE: Approximately 40% in patients with CP and 90% in patients with CF

PREDOMINANT SEX & AGE: More common in males than females

RISK FACTORS:

- Excessive alcohol consumption, leading to recurrent pancreatitis and CP
- Cystic fibrosis
- Smoking
- Ductal obstruction (congenital or acquired-pancreatic malignancy, stones)
- Pancreatitis
- Genetic predisposition
- Pancreatic resection
- History of inflammatory bowel disease
- History of celiac disease
- Type 1 and type 2 diabetes mellitus

PHYSICAL FINDINGS & CLINICAL PRESENTATION

EPI manifests as a malabsorption syndrome. The clinical features may mimic and coexist with common gastrointestinal conditions (i.e., irritable bowel syndrome [IBS], small-intestinal bacterial overgrowth [SIBO], celiac disease), which may delay diagnosis. Patients often limit dietary fat intake to avoid or reduce steatorrhea. Severity depends on the degree of pancreatic loss and can be categorized into mild or moderate-to-severe disease as follows:

- *Mild disease*
  1. Asymptomatic
  2. Normal bowel movements
  3. Mild abdominal discomfort
  4. Bloating
- *Moderate-to-severe disease*
  1. Chronic diarrhea
  2. Excessive weight loss
  3. Excessive flatulence
  4. Abdominal pain/bloating
  5. Voluminous and foul-smelling stools
  6. Fatty food intolerance
  7. Failure to thrive in children
  8. Steatorrhea (stool fat >6 g/day) when >90% of pancreatic glandular function is lost
- Edema (as a result of protein malnutrition and hypoalbuminemia)
- Fat-soluble vitamins deficiencies (rare):
  1. Vitamin A (impaired night vision)
  2. Vitamin D (osteoporosis, metabolic bone disease, hyperparathyroidism, hypocalcemia)
  3. Vitamin E (neuropathy, anemia)
  4. Vitamin K (ecchymosis)

ETIOLOGY (TABLE 1)

EPI usually results from CP in adults or CF in children. Pancreatic exocrine insufficiency is also a common occurrence in patients recovering from severe acute pancreatitis, with the severity of symptoms correlating with the degree of pancreatic necrosis. Causative factors can generally be classified into pancreatic and extrapancreatic conditions.

DIAGNOSIS

The diagnosis of EPI is challenging because patients often present with nonspecific signs and symptoms, and reliable diagnostic tests are lacking.

DIFFERENTIAL DIAGNOSIS

With the exception of voluminous and foul-smelling stools, the following conditions may present in a manner similar to EPI:

- Celiac disease
- IBS
- Inflammatory bowel disease
- SIBO
- Short bowel syndrome

WORKUP

- A complete history, physical examination, and laboratory evaluation are essential to making the diagnosis and excluding other common causes of diarrhea and weight loss.
- Complete electrolyte panel to detect hypokalemia, hypocalcemia (in setting of vitamin D deficiency), hypomagnesemia, and metabolic acidosis from malabsorption and gastrointestinal losses. In children, genetic testing for cystic fibrosis transmembrane conductance regulator (CFTR) mutations should be carried out.
- Complete blood count (CBC) may reveal anemia from iron, vitamin B_{12}, or folate deficiencies.
- Prolonged prothrombin times may be elevated because of vitamin K malabsorption.
- Alternative causes of maldigestion should be investigated, such as infection with *Giardia lamblia,* celiac serology, liver disease, and SIBO tests.

LABORATORY TESTS

Direct and indirect pancreatic function tests are available to diagnose EPI.

- **Indirect:** Measures the level of pancreatic enzymes or the consequences of exocrine insufficiency. Used to monitor the effectiveness of pancreatic enzyme replacement therapy (PERT).
  1. **Fecal fat quantification:** Considered the gold standard for evaluating fat digestion. However, it does not distinguish between maldigestion and malabsorption.
  2. **Fecal elastase-1 (FE-1):** The most sensitive and specific test of pancreatic function. This enzyme is minimally degraded during intestinal transit. The test measures enzymatic production of FE-1 and can be used to screen for moderate-to-severe EPI with high sensitivity. FE-1 levels >200 μg/g are normal, levels of 100 to 200 μg/g are considered mild, and levels <100 μg/g are severe for EPI. Liquid stool can lead to falsely low results because of dilution.
  3. **Fecal chymotrypsin:** Sensitive and specific test of pancreatic function. Variably degraded during transit in the intestinal lumen. Accurate levels require an interruption of PERT, generally for 2 days before testing.
  4. **Serum trypsinogen:** Reflects pancreatic acinar cell mass. Highly sensitive for severe EPI when levels <20 ng/ml. This test is not commonly employed in clinical practice.
  5. **^{13}C-Triglyceride breath test:** Monitors the digestion of isotope-labeled fat meal to reflect absorption and metabolization of

TABLE 1 Etiologies of Exocrine Pancreatic Insufficiencies

Pancreatic	Extrapancreatic
Acute/chronic pancreatitis (alcohol abuse, trauma, hereditary, idiopathic)	Celiac disease
Pancreatic cancer	Inflammatory bowel disease
Pancreatic, ampullary, and duct obstruction	Autoimmune pancreatitis
Cystic fibrosis	Zollinger-Ellison syndrome
Diabetes mellitus type 1 or 2	Gastrointestinal surgeries (gastrectomy, gastric bypass, extensive small-bowel surgery)
Shwachman-Diamond syndrome (EPI with anemia, neutropenia, and bony abnormalities)	
Hemochromatosis	

EPI, Exocrine pancreatic insufficiency.

TABLE 2 Enzyme Products for the Treatment of Chronic Pancreatitis

Product	Formulation	Lipase Content per Pill or Capsule (USP units)
Creon	Enteric-coated capsule	3000; 6000; 12,000; 24,000; 36,000
Zenpep	Enteric-coated capsule	3000; 5000; 10,000; 15,000; 20,000; 25,000
Pancreaze	Enteric-coated capsule	4200; 10,500; 16,800; 21,000
Ultresa	Enteric-coated capsule	13,800; 20,700; 23,000
Pertzye	Enteric-coated with bicarbonate	8000; 16,000
Viokase	Non–enteric-coated tablet*	10,440; 20,880

The total dose of lipase per meal should be titrated based on response but usually requires at least 60,000 and usually 90,000 USP units (30,000 IU) of lipase per meal and half that amount with snacks. The dose should be split equally during the meal and immediately after the meal.

*Non–enteric-coated agents require cotreatment with an H_2 receptor antagonist or proton pump inhibitor to avoid denaturation of the enzymes by gastric acid.

USP, United States Pharmacopeia.

From Feldman M et al: *Sleisenger and Fordtran's gastrointestinal and liver disease*, ed 10, Philadelphia, 2016, Elsevier.

product. It is used to measure the efficacy of PERT.

- **Direct:** Most sensitive and specific diagnostic tests for the diagnosis of EPI. Tests use hormonal secretagogues to stimulate the pancreas and then collect duodenal fluid to measure secretory content. Tests use CCK, secretin, and CCK-secretin.
  1. Endoscopic pancreatic function test: Requires fluoroscopic placement of an oro-duodenal collection tube with topical anesthesia. Gastric and duodenal ports sample duodenal fluid for serial measurements of bicarbonate over one hour. Severe EPI is reflected by a peak bicarbonate concentration of <50 mEq/L
  2. Traditional direct pancreatic function test: Endoscopic procedure performed under sedation for the collection of duodenal fluid. Generally, better tolerated by patients. A peak bicarbonate concentration <80mEq/L is considered abnormal for one hour testing.

IMAGING STUDIES

- Computed tomography (CT): First-line imaging study of choice. Permits visualization of calcifications, cysts, deformation/obstruction of bile ducts, pancreatic/peripancreatic tumors, fibrosis, and parenchyma loss.
- Magnetic resonance cholangiopancreatography: Provides 3D-imaging of the pancreatic-biliary ductal system

Rx TREATMENT

The management of EPI includes dietary and lifestyle modifications, as well as PERT and vitamin supplementation, to relieve maldigestion-related symptoms and restore normal nutritional health. Underlying diseases leading to EPI should also be treated.

NONPHARMACOLOGIC THERAPY

Nutritional therapy aims to relieve maldigestion-related symptoms and ensure normal nutritional status. Patients should be encouraged to consume small and frequent meals. In addition, patients should abstain from consuming alcohol and smoking. Limiting dietary fat has not been shown to improve outcomes.

PHARMACOLOGIC THERAPY

Oral administration of pancreatic enzyme replacements (Table 2) is the method of choice for treatment of EPI. It is indicated for patients with weight loss, symptomatic steatorrhea, or steatorrhea of >15 g/day. The aim of PERT is to compensate for the deficiencies of normal pancreatic enzyme secretion and increase fat absorption. Doses are individually tailored and depend upon residual pancreatic function and fat content of the meal, but usually start at 25,000 to 40,000 IU of lipase in the form of enteric-coated mini-microspheres per main meal. PERT improves malabsorption of fat and protein and helps to relieve symptoms of abdominal pain, steatorrhea, and flatulence. Inadequate responses can be managed by either dose escalation or the addition of proton pump inhibitors or H_2 antagonists to prevent acid inactivation of lipase.

DISPOSITION

- Consider further evaluation in patients with persistent weight loss and steatorrhea.

REFERRAL

- Consultation with a gastroenterologist can help expedite diagnosis and rule out alternate diagnoses.
- Referral to a nutritionist can aid the patient with malnutrition and alleviate symptoms.

PEARLS & CONSIDERATIONS

- The pancreas has an important role in the digestion of all nutrients, but fats in particular.
- EPI is a condition related to decreased pancreatic enzyme release resulting from loss of pancreatic parenchyma, inadequate pancreatic stimulation, pancreatic duct obstruction, or pancreatic enzyme inactivation.
- Common symptoms of EPI include weight loss, steatorrhea, and abdominal bloating.
- Timely diagnosis and adequate treatment with PERT therapy by the clinician is crucial because delay may impair growth in children, and lead to adverse outcomes of malnutrition, and increased morbidity and mortality in patients of all ages.
- Individualized dietary advice together with the appropriate PERT are the cornerstones of EPI therapy.

SUGGESTED READINGS

Available at ExpertConsult.com

RELATED TOPICS

Chronic Pancreatitis (Related Key Topic)
Pancreatitis, Acute (Related Key Topic)
Cystic Fibrosis (Related Key Topic)
Celiac Disease (Related Key Topic)
Crohn Disease (Related Key Topic)
Ulcerative Colitis (Related Key Topic)

AUTHORS: **Ethan Pearlstein, MD,** and **Dominick Tammaro, MD**

BASIC INFORMATION

DEFINITION

A fall is an "event which results in a person coming to rest inadvertently on the ground and other than a consequence of the following: Loss of consciousness, sudden onset of paralysis, or epileptic seizure."

SYNONYMS

Syncope
Collapse

ICD-10CM CODES

E880-E888.9	Accidental fall
R29.6	Repeated falls

EPIDEMIOLOGY & DEMOGRAPHICS

INCIDENCE:

- Trauma is the fifth leading cause of death in persons >65 yr of age, and falls are responsible for 70% of accidental deaths in persons ≥75 yr.
- The incidence of falls among community-dwelling older adults is 30% to 40%. Two thirds of falls in the community are preventable; 6% to 7% of these falls result in fracture.
- The incidence of falls for nursing home and hospitalized older adults is three times the rate of community-dwelling older adults. Over 50% of nursing home residents fall during their stay.
- 20% to 30% of older adults who fall suffer significant injury leading to immobility, dependence, and an increased risk of early death.

HEALTH CARE COST: In 2006, patients ≥65 had over 2.1 million visits to the ED for injurious falls, which was 10.5% of all ED visits among the elderly and 29.6% of these visits required hospital admission. In those that were admitted, the mean length of stay was 5.5 days with a mean cost of $10,800. The aggregate hospital cost for those requiring admission in 2006 was $6.8 billion. (Source: Healthcare Cost and Utilization Project.)

PREDOMINANT SEX & AGE:

- Fall-related mortality is highest among older white men followed by white women, African American men, and African American women.
- The incidence rates of falls increase with advancing age.
- Older adults ≥85 yr are 10 to 15 times more likely to have a fracture compared with those aged 60 to 65 yr.

RISK FACTORS: Four groups of risk factors for falls have been identified (Table 1):

- Intrinsic factors inherent in the older adult who falls.
- Extrinsic factors circumstantial to the older adult who falls.
- Falls in nursing homes.
- Situational or the activity in which the older adult is engaged in when a fall occurs.

CLINICAL PRESENTATION

- Older adults who fall may present with minor soft tissue injuries, such as lacerations or bruising, hip fracture, or head trauma; however, most falls are not reported unless an injury has occurred.
- If an older adult presents for medical attention for a fall or reports recurrent falls in the past year or difficulties in walking or balance, a multifactorial fall risk assessment should be completed.
- The multifactorial fall risk assessment should include:
  1. Focused history: A detailed history of events and circumstances surrounding fall, relevant risk factors including review of medications, acute and chronic medical problems (e.g., osteoporosis, urinary incontinence, and cardiovascular disease), and whether the fall was witnessed
  2. Physical examination:
     a. Vital signs including orthostatics.
     b. Cardiovascular examination assessing for arrhythmias, carotid bruits, or new murmurs.
     c. Neurologic examination including vision assessment, evaluation of lower-extremity strength, peripheral nerves, proprioception, and testing of cortical, extrapyramidal, and cerebellar function.
     d. Gait and balance assessment: Multiple screening tools are available for fall risk screening and balance assessment (Tables 2 and 3). "Get up and go test" is a rapid assessment that will quickly tell you if the patient needs rehabilitation and what to work on. (Ask patient to stand from a seated position without use of hands, walk 10 feet forward, turn around, and return to chair and sit).
     e. Musculoskeletal exam with attention to joints of lower extremity, feet, and footwear.
  3. Functional assessment including the older adult's activities of daily living skills, use of adaptive equipment, and fear of falling
  4. Environmental assessment of home safety

TABLE 1 Risk Factors for Falls in the Elderly

Intrinsic

Aging

Age-related decline in vestibular function might lead to loss of balance, dizziness, and falls. Aging of the vision system (e.g., glaucoma, cataracts, retinopathy) may result in decreased visual acuity, inability to discriminate dark/light, and decreased spatial perception.

Cardiac

Cardiac arrhythmias, carotid sinus hypersensitivity, neurocardiogenic syncope.

Neurologic

Parkinson disease, normal pressure hydrocephalus (NPH), sensory neuropathy, dementia/impaired cognition, cervical myelopathy, senile gait disorder, prior stroke. (One third of the elderly have abnormal position sense.)

Musculoskeletal

Lower extremity weakness, impaired knee extension and ankle plantar flexion strength contribute to abnormalities in gait velocity and step length, deconditioning, arthritis, foot abnormalities (such as bunions, calluses, or nail abnormalities).

Vascular

Vertebrobasilar insufficiency, postural hypotension, postprandial hypotension.

Metabolic

Hypoglycemia, hypothyroidism, hyponatremia.

Psychiatric

Depression.

Medications

Use of more than four medications may be associated with an increased risk of falls. Medications that may increase fall risk include benzodiazepines, sleeping medications, neuroleptics, antidepressants, anticonvulsants, class I antiarrhythmics, and antihypertensives.

Extrinsic

Environmental

Environmental hazards cause >50% of falls in the elderly (cords, furniture, small objects, ill-fitting shoes, slippery surfaces, loose rugs, uneven steps, optical patterns on escalators). Majority occurs with mild-moderate activity (walking, stepping up/down, changing position); 70% occur at home and 10% on stairs (descending > ascending).

Nursing Home Falls

20% have a cardiovascular cause (hypotension: Drug induced, postprandial, postural, or bradycardia). 5% are the result of an acute illness such as PNA, febrile illness, UTI, CHF. 3% are from an overwhelming intrinsic event such as syncope, seizure, stroke, psychoactive drugs.

Situational

Tripping over obstacles, carrying heavy items, descending/ascending stairs, rapid turning, reaching overhead, climbing ladders, ill-fitting shoes, lack of assistive devices.

CHF, Congestive heart failure; *PNA,* pneumonia; *UTI,* urinary tract infection.

TABLE 2 Scales Used for Fall Risk Screening and Balance Assessment

Instrument	Items	Setting: Community	Setting: Acute	Setting: Chronic
Multifactorial Reports				
STRATIFY	Five items—history of falls, agitation, visual impairment, frequent toileting, able to stand but needs assistance with moving		X	X
Morse Fall Scale	Six items—history of falls, secondary diagnoses, parenteral therapy, use of ambulation aids, gait, mental status		X	X
FROP-Com	13 risk factors in 26 items—fall and fall injury history, medications, medical conditions, sensory loss, feet, cognitive status, toileting, nutrition, environment, function, behavior, balance, gait; total score, 0-60; fall risk high with score >24	X		
Fall risk for residential care	Among persons who can stand without assistance—poor balance or two of three the following: Fall history, nursing home residence, urinary incontinence Among persons who cannot stand without assistance—one of three of the following: Fall history, hostel residence, use of nine or more medications			X
Functional Mobility				
Berg Balance test	14 tasks scored 0-4; total range 0-56; fall risk increases as score decreases	X	X	X
Functional reach	Distance reached in inches without moving the feet; fall risk <7 inches	X	X	X
Performance-oriented mobility and balance	Balance subscale score 0-16, gait subscale 0-12, summary score 0-28; summary score <19 indicates high fall risk	X		X
Timed up and go	Time in seconds to rise from a chair, walk 3 m, turn, walk back, and sit down; <10 sec normal; fall risk increases with time >13.5 sec	X		X
Dynamic gait index	Eight walking tasks scored 0-3, total score 0-24; <18 or 19 indicates fall risk	X		
Functional mobility tests	Time to complete eight step ups (alternate step test) >10 sec, timed sit to stand five times >12 sec, 6-m walk time >6 sec increased fall risk	X		
Physiologic profile assessment	Performance in five domains: Sway, reaction time, strength, proprioception, contrast sensitivity; total score 0 to >3; fall risk increased with score ≥2	X		

FROP-Com, Falls Risk for Older People in the Community; *STRATIFY,* St. Thomas Risk Assessment Tool in Falling elderly inpatients.
From Fillit HM et al: *Brocklehurst's textbook of geriatric medicine and gerontology,* ed 8, Philadelphia, 2017, Elsevier.

TABLE 3 Clinical Assessment Based on Components of Postural Control

Organ System	Impairment	Clinical Evaluation	Potential Cause
Eye	Decreased acuity	Vision chart	Presbyopia, macular degeneration, cataracts
	Reduced visual fields	Confrontation, perimetry	Glaucoma, posterior circulation stroke
	Decreased depth perception	Stereo or depth testing	Monocular vision
	Decreased dark adaptation	Self-report—inability to dilate pupil in low light	Aging, miotic agents for glaucoma
Vestibular apparatus	Otoliths	Ability to detect true vertical, Hallpike maneuver	Benign positional vertigo
	Semicircular canals	Ability to detect position during rotation with eyes closed, nystagmus, visual acuity during head motion	Meniere disease, vestibular hypofunction
Peripheral nerve	Peripheral neuropathy	Light touch, filaments, two-point discrimination, vibratory sense	Diabetes, peripheral vascular disease, vitamin B_{12} deficiency
Circulation	Reduced cerebral perfusion	Low blood pressure, altered level of consciousness, light-headedness	Medications, arrhythmias, postprandial hypotension
	Orthostatic hypotension	Positional change in blood pressure	Medications, autonomic dysfunction, dehydration
Brain	Reduced attention	Ability to perform dual tasks like timed up and go with cup of water, executive function tasks	Mild cognitive impairment, dementia, medications
	Psychomotor slowing	Timed tapping, timed finger to nose test, trails A test (connect the dots)	Medications, degenerative and vascular brain diseases
	Altered postural reflexes	Absent or slowed righting reflexes	Parkinson disease, other extrapyramidal and degenerative brain diseases
Muscle	Reduced strength	Manual muscle testing, strength-based functional performance (chair rise, squat)	Generalized—inactivity, sarcopenia, vitamin D deficiency, myopathies Focal deficits, spinal cord and peripheral motor nerve conditions
Musculoskeletal pain	Loss of flexibility	Contractures, decreased range of motion	Arthritis, inactivity
	Bone and joint deficits	Weight-bearing pain	Arthritis, fractures, periarticular conditions, foot problems
	Disturbance of spinal cord, roots, nerves	Leg and back pain with activity	Spinal stenosis, radiculopathies, peripheral neuropathies

From Fillit HM et al: *Brocklehurst's textbook of geriatric medicine and gerontology,* ed 8, Philadelphia, 2017, Elsevier.

ETIOLOGY

- Falls are a multifactorial syndrome resulting from the cumulative effects of impaired gait and balance, aging, polypharmacy, depression, cognitive impairment, acute medical illness, or environmental factors (Fig. E1).
- Most falls among community-dwelling older adults are due to environmental factors, whereas falls among nursing home residents are a result of confusion, gait impairment, or postural hypotension.

Dx DIAGNOSIS

DIFFERENTIAL DIAGNOSIS

Falls are often a nonspecific symptom of an acute illness (such as delirium, urinary tract infection, acute anemia, or pneumonia) or an exacerbation of a chronic disease (chronic heart failure [CHF] or chronic obstructive pulmonary disease [COPD]). The mnemonic "DELIRIUMS" can be used to assess the differential diagnosis in acute delirium. (**D**rugs, **E**motional [depression], **L**ow PaO_2 [CHF, COPD], **I**nfection, **R**etention [urinary, fecal], **I**ctal status, **U**nder nutrition/hydration, **M**etabolic, **S**ubdural/ Sensory [all neurologic causes] workup).

WORKUP

- Older adults presenting with a noninjurious fall need a detailed history and physical exam to identify acute medical illnesses and potential modifiable risk factors. Laboratory and neuroimaging studies may be necessary if the history and physical exam indicate a specific problem. ECG and Holter monitoring may be considered if cardiac arrhythmia is suspected.
- See Fig. E1.

LABORATORY TESTS

CBC, stool guaiac, blood chemistries, thyroid function, liver function, vitamin B_{12} level, folate level, erythrocyte sedimentation rate, vitamin D level, drug levels, and urinalysis depending on physical/historical findings.

IMAGING STUDIES

- CT or MRI of the brain or cervical spine films in the presence of neurologic or gait impairment.
- Chest x-ray if pulmonary pathology (pneumonia, pulmonary edema) is suspected.
- Consider ECG, echocardiography, or Holter monitor if suspicious for structural cardiac abnormality or syncope.

Rx TREATMENT

NONPHARMACOLOGIC THERAPY

- Physical therapy evaluation for gait and balance training, evaluation of appropriate assisted devices (e.g., cane, walker), the use of fall prevention equipment (e.g., low beds, bed alarms).
- Home safety assessment: Studies show that 50% of recurrent fallers fell doing the same activity that caused them to fall the first time. This can be prevented by creating a home safety evaluation checklist (preferably done by family member to improve compliance) or arranging for a home safety inspection by a visiting nurse or occupational therapist.
- Minimization or discontinuation of certain medications associated with falls (psychotropics).
- Customized exercise program to improve strength, gait, and balance.
- Evaluation of proper footwear, hard sole, and low heel height.

ACUTE GENERAL Rx

Hospitalization may be necessary for treatment of hip fracture, subdural hematoma, lacerations, or trauma as well as the treatment of underlying cause of the fall such as infection, metabolic disturbances, cardiovascular (e.g., carotid sinus hypersensitivity, vasovagal syndrome, bradyarrhythmias, and tachyarrhythmias) or neurologic abnormality.

CHRONIC Rx

- Screen and treat for osteoporosis as low bone density increases the risk of hip or other fractures.
- Optimize treatment of chronic illnesses such as CHF, COPD, osteoarthritis, Parkinson disease, dementia, postural hypotension, and visual problems.
- The effect of vitamin D supplementation on fall risk in the elderly is controversial. A recent randomized clinical trial of vitamin D supplementation at doses of 1000 IU or higher did not prevent prevent falls, and fall risk increased at higher doses.[1]
- Table 4 summarizes the management of impairments that contribute to instability and falls.

DISPOSITION

Falls increase the older adult's risk of hospitalization, institutionalization, and mortality.

COMPLEMENTARY & ALTERNATIVE MEDICINE

T'ai chi has been shown to reduce the risk of falls in community-dwelling study participants.

REFERRAL

- Referral may be appropriate to cardiologist, ophthalmologist, neurologist, or podiatrist depending on the presence of a specific condition.
- Consider referral to physical therapist for gait and balance training, evaluation for assisted device, or strengthening program.

[1]Appel LJ et al: The effects of four doses of vitamin D supplements on falls in older adults: a response-adaptive, randomized clinical trial, *Ann Intern Med*, 2020 Dec.

PEARLS & CONSIDERATIONS

COMMENTS

- Fear of falling may lead to restriction of activities, social isolation, and dependence.
- Older adults with four or more risk factors have a 78% chance of falling.
- Mortality from falls has increased by 42% over the past decade.

PREVENTION

The U.S. Preventive Services Task Force recommends exercise or physical therapy and vitamin D supplementation to prevent falls in community-dwelling adults aged ≥65 who are at increased risk for falls. It does not recommend automatically performing an in-depth multifactorial risk assessment in conjunction with comprehensive management of identified risks to prevent falls in community-dwelling adults aged 65 or older because the likelihood of benefit is small. In determining whether this service is appropriate in individual cases, patients and clinicians should consider the balance of benefits and harms on the basis of the circumstances of prior falls, comorbid medical conditions, and patient values.

SCREENING

The "get up and go test" is a quick assessment of balance and gait. A more in-depth screening tool for falls is the Tinetti gait and balance assessment, which evaluates normal and adaptive ability to maintain balance when rising from a chair, standing with eyes closed, turning, and receiving a sternal nudge. It also evaluates several components of gait (step height, postural sway, path deviation). The test is scored on the patient's ability to perform specific tasks. Scoring is done on a 3-point scale with a range of 0 to 2. Individual scores are combined to form three measures: An overall gait assessment score (maximum score = 12), an overall balance assessment score (maximum score = 16), and a gait and balance score (maximum score = 28). In general, patients who score below 19 are at high risk for falls, and those who score 19 to 24 are at risk for falls.

PATIENT & FAMILY EDUCATION

Providing education and information for the patient and caregiver regarding fall prevention strategies in addition to multifactorial risk reduction strategies

SUGGESTED READINGS

Available at ExpertConsult.com

AUTHORS: **Sean H. Uiterwyk, MD, Alicia J. Curtin, PhD,** and **Keith Brennan, MD**

TABLE 4 Management of Impairments That Contribute to Instability and Falls

Organ System	Impairment	Medical Management	Restorative Services	Environmental Modifications
Eye	Decreased acuity	Corrective lenses	Low vision rehabilitation	Lighting
	Reduced visual fields	Prisms in spectacles	Low vision rehabilitation, teach to scan using head rotation	
	Loss of depth perception	Cataract removal, if indicated	Teach to use shadows to detect depth	Lighting to accent shadows, contrast
	Poor dark adaptation	Switching to glaucoma medications that do not cause miosis		Lighting
Vestibular system	Benign paroxysmal positional vertigo (BPPV)	Epley maneuver	Vestibular rehabilitation	
	Meniere disease	Cautious use of meclizine, diuretics; rarely, surgery	Vestibular rehabilitation	
Peripheral nerve	Neuropathy	Footwear to protect foot and maximize sensation	Assistive devices for haptic enhancement	Hand holds, railings
Central circulation	Reduced brain perfusion	Treatment varies by cause Arrhythmias—medications to control rate and rhythm, pacemakers Postprandial hypotension—frequent small meals		
	Orthostatic hypotension	Treatment varies by cause Adjust offending medications Autonomic neuropathy—salt loading, fluorinated corticosteroids Dehydration—hydration, reduce diuretic dose	Compression hose, calf muscle contractions	
Brain	Reduced attention	Medication adjustment	Practice dual tasks	
	Psychomotor slowing	Medication adjustment	Practice movement speed	
	Abnormal righting reflexes	Antiparkinsonian medication helps bradykinesia more than balance	Assistive devices, practice getting up after a fall	Protective clothing
Effector muscle	Weakness	Reduced activity—treat contributing causes (e.g., CHF, anemia, COPD, arthritis) Focal motor deficit due to spinal stenosis—sometimes surgery Myopathy—adjust offending medications, possibly steroids for myositis	Strength-training exercises Orthotics, exercise, assistive devices	Raise chair height
Musculoskeletal	Decreased range of motion		Active and passive range of motion exercise, orthotics	
Pain	Bone and joint	Analgesics, injections	Physical modalities (e.g., heat, massage, assistive devices, orthoses, adaptive equipment)	Place items within easy reach
	Spinal cord, roots, nerves	Injections, surgery, analgesics	Orthoses, assistive devices	Place items within easy reach

CHF, Congestive heart failure; *COPD,* chronic obstructive pulmonary disease.
From Fillit HM et al: *Brocklehurst's textbook of geriatric medicine and gerontology,* ed 8, Philadelphia, 2017, Elsevier.

BASIC INFORMATION

DEFINITION

Familial adenomatous polyposis (FAP) is a highly penetrant, autosomal-dominant condition characterized by hundreds of colorectal adenomatous polyps that inevitably progress to cancer (Fig. E1). ***Gardner syndrome*** is a subset of FAP, with prominent extraintestinal manifestations including dental abnormalities, soft tissue lesions, desmoid tumors, and osteomas.

ICD-10CM CODES

D12.2	Benign neoplasm of ascending colon
D12.3	Benign neoplasm of transverse colon
D12.4	Benign neoplasm of descending colon
D12.5	Benign neoplasm of sigmoid colon
D12.6	Benign neoplasm of colon, unspecified

EPIDEMIOLOGY & DEMOGRAPHICS

- FAP occurs in approximately 1 in 10,000 births worldwide.
- FAP accounts for <1% of all colorectal cancers.
- Individuals develop hundreds to thousands of adenomatous colorectal polyps.
- Polyps usually present in adolescence.
- 100% lifetime risk for colorectal cancer; most diagnosed by 40 yr of age.
- Gastric, duodenal, periampullary, and small bowel polyps occur but have lower malignant potential.
- Increased risk for other tumors: Desmoid (15%), duodenal/periampullary (7%), thyroid (2%), brain (1%), childhood hepatoblastoma (1%), nasopharyngeal angiofibroma (benign), pancreatic (2%), adrenal adenoma (10%), and gastric (1%).

PHYSICAL FINDINGS & CLINICAL PRESENTATION

Phenotypic variability is seen in individuals and families with the same mutation. Extraintestinal manifestations may precede intestinal disease. These findings are reported in at least 20% of individuals with FAP.

- Congenital hypertrophy of the retinal pigment epithelium (CHRPE): Benign fundus lesions, usually present at birth
- Dental abnormalities: Supernumerary or unerupted teeth
- Soft tissue lesions: Epidermal or sebaceous cysts, fibromas, lipomas, desmoid tumors (benign, locally invasive, aggressive connective tissue tumor)
- Osteomas (benign bone growths): Skull, mandible, long bone
- Anemia, occult blood in stool, bowel obstruction, weight loss

ETIOLOGY

- FAP is caused by mutations of the tumor suppressor gene adenomatous polyposis coli *(APC)* on chromosome 5q21 to q22; more than 1000 disease-causing mutations identified. The site of the mutation often correlates with the extraintestinal findings.
- De novo mutations are responsible for approximately 20% of FAP cases. These may be due to germline mutations or somatic cell mosaicism, which is seen when a new mutation occurs in the *APC* gene post-fertilization and is present in only a subset of cell types or tissues.
- Table E1 summarizes the genetics of colonic polyposis.

DIAGNOSIS

In individuals with a family history, more than 100 adenomatous colorectal polyps, CHRPE lesions, or positive genetic testing confirms diagnosis. In those without a family history, more than 100 adenomatous colorectal polyps suggest the diagnosis, and genetic testing confirms it. The diagnosis should be considered in individuals with ≥10 adenomatous colorectal polyps or fewer polyps in the presence of extraintestinal findings.

DIFFERENTIAL DIAGNOSIS

- Turcot syndrome
- Attenuated FAP (also *APC* gene mutation, but presents with fewer polyps [<100], at a later age, and has lower cancer risk than FAP [~80% lifetime risk])
- MUTYH-associated polyposis
- Peutz-Jeghers syndrome
- Juvenile polyposis syndrome
- Cowden disease
- Lynch syndrome
- Hereditary mixed polyposis syndrome
- Polymerase proofreading-associated polyposis
- Hyperplastic polyposis
- Table 2 compares various adenomatous polyposis syndromes

WORKUP

History, physical examination, laboratory tests, imaging studies

DIAGNOSTIC SCREENING OPTIONS

GENETIC TESTING: NOTE: Genetic counseling should be performed, and written informed consent obtained before testing. Refer to a specialized center for counseling and evaluation.

- Should be offered to first-degree relatives of affected individuals (with an identified mutation) at age 10 to 12 yr and clinically suspected individuals.
- Able to identify a mutation in approximately 80% of families. To ensure that the family has a detectable mutation, test an affected family member first.
- If positive in the affected individual, the test can differentiate with 100% accuracy affected and unaffected family members. If negative in the affected individual, screening family members will not be useful in determining disease status.
- If no known family history exists, screening the clinically suspected individual is reasonable. A positive test rules in FAP but a negative test does not rule it out.
- Numerous testing techniques available; may require multiple tests to identify the mutation.

SIGMOIDOSCOPY:

- Individuals with a positive genetic test: Annual flexible sigmoidoscopy or colonoscopy beginning at 10 to 12 yr of age.
- Untested at-risk family members or individuals from families with an unidentified *APC* mutation: Annual flexible sigmoidoscopy or colonoscopy beginning at 10 to 12 yr of age. Screening frequency can decrease at 24 yr of age if no polyps detected.
- Once adenomatous polyps are detected, patients should undergo colonoscopy and evaluation for colectomy.
- Negative genetic test in patients from families with an identified mutation: Average risk screening.

CHRPE: Lesions occur in up to 80% of families and are a reliable indicator of affected status in these families.

TREATMENT

- Prophylactic colectomy or proctocolectomy: Timing determined by polyp number, size, and degree of dysplasia. Postsurgical endoscopic surveillance annually.
- Additional screening:
  1. Annual physical examination: History, examination (including thyroid), and blood tests
  2. Upper endoscopy to screen for gastric/duodenal polyps (include visualization of duodenal papilla): Baseline at age 25 yr (earlier if colon polyps detected) and repeated every 3 mo to 4 yr based on findings
  3. Annual thyroid ultrasound: Begin in teenage yrs
  4. Other possible cancer sites imaged if symptoms occur or if these cancers have occurred in relatives
- Treat soft tissue lesions and osteomas for symptoms or cosmetic concerns. Treat desmoid tumors if they pose a risk to adjacent structures.

DISPOSITION

- 100% chance of colorectal cancer in untreated individuals. Many other neoplasms occur at higher rates.
- Metastatic colorectal cancer is the leading cause of death (58%), followed by desmoid tumors (11%), and duodenal/periampullary adenocarcinoma (8%).

REFERRAL

- Patients should be managed at centers with expertise in FAP, including a gastroenterologist, medical geneticist, and surgeon.
- Genetic counselors can be found at www.nsgc.org.
- Genetic clinics and laboratories can be found at www.ncbi.nlm.nih.gov/gtr.

TABLE 2 Adenomatous Polyposis Syndromes

Syndrome	Gene Mutation	Polyps	Extraintestinal Abnormalities
Classic FAP	*APC* (usually truncated protein)	Colonic adenomas (thousands) Duodenal, periampullary adenomas Gastric fundic gland polyps Jejunal and ileal adenomas Ileal lymphoid polyps	Mandibular osteomas Dental abnormalities
Gardner variant of FAP	*APC*	Same as FAP	Osteomas (mandible, skull, long bones) CHRPE Desmoid tumors Epidermoid and sebaceous cysts Fibromas, lipomas Thyroid, adrenal tumors
Turcot variant of FAP	*APC* DNA MMR*	Colonic adenomas (sometimes fewer than in classic FAP)	Medulloblastoma Glioblastoma multiforme CHRPE
Attenuated FAP	*APC* 5′ and 3′ regions	Colonic adenomas (<100; proximal colon) Duodenal, periampullary adenomas Gastric fundic gland polyps	Mandibular osteomas (rare)
Familial tooth agenesis	*Axin2* (APC pathway)	Colonic adenomas Hyperplastic polyps	Agenesis of teeth
Bloom syndrome	*BLM*	Colonic adenomas	Small stature Facial erythema/telangiectasia Male sterility Adenocarcinomas, leukemia, lymphoma
MUTYH polyposis	*MUTYH (MYH)*	Colonic adenomas (5-100) Duodenal polyposis Gastric cancer	CHRPE Osteomas

*May be more appropriately classified under hereditary nonpolyposis colon cancer.
APC, Adenomatous polyposis coli; *CHRPE*, congenital hypertrophy of the retinal pigment epithelium; *DNA*, deoxyribonucleic acid; *FAP*, familial adenomatous polyposis; *MMR*, mismatch repair.
From Feldman M et al (eds): *Sleisenger and Fordtran's gastrointestinal and liver disease*, ed 10, Philadelphia, 2016, Saunders.

PEARLS & CONSIDERATIONS

- Management should be individualized based on genotype, phenotype, and individual preferences.
- Sulindac (NSAID) and celecoxib (COX-2 inhibitor) can cause duodenal and colorectal polyp regression in individuals with FAP. Preliminary studies with other agents also show polyp regression. Their ability to reduce cancer risk remains unknown; they do not replace colon resection for cancer prevention.
- Desmoid tumors usually present in the 30s, frequently occur in the abdomen, and are difficult to treat with high rates of recurrence. Growth and recurrence are stimulated by surgery.
- Screen children of affected parents (from infancy to age 7 yr) biannually with alpha-fetoprotein level and liver ultrasound to rule out hepatoblastoma.
- Preimplantation and prenatal genetic testing is available.
- Attenuated FAP: Screening colonoscopy every 1 to 2 yr starting at 20 yr of age.

SUGGESTED READINGS

Available at ExpertConsult.com

RELATED CONTENT

Familial Adenomatous Polyposis and Polyposis Syndromes (Patient Information)
Colorectal Cancer (Related Key Topic)
Lynch Syndrome (Related Key Topic)
Peutz-Jeghers Syndrome and Other Polyposis Syndromes (Related Key Topic)

AUTHOR: **Sudeep K. Aulakh, MD**

BASIC INFORMATION

DEFINITION

Acute fatty liver of pregnancy (AFLP) is characterized histologically by microvesicular fatty cytoplasmic infiltration of hepatocytes with minimal hepatocellular necrosis.

SYNONYMS

Acute fatty metamorphosis
Acute yellow atrophy
AFLP
Acute fatty liver of pregnancy

ICD-10CM CODES

026.611	Liver and biliary tract disorders in pregnancy, first trimester
026.612	Liver and biliary tract disorders in pregnancy, second trimester
026.613	Liver and biliary tract disorders in pregnancy, third trimester
026.619	Liver and biliary tract disorders in pregnancy, unspecified trimester

EPIDEMIOLOGY & DEMOGRAPHICS

INCIDENCE:
- Rare: 1 in 10,000 to 1 in 20,000 pregnancies
- Equal frequencies in all races and at all maternal ages

AVERAGE GESTATIONAL AGE: 37 wk (range 28-42 wk)
- 20% present postnatally

RISK FACTORS:
- Primiparity
- Multiple gestation
- Male fetus
- History of type 2 diabetes mellitus
- Preeclampsia

GENETICS: Some with a familial deficiency of long-chain 3-hydroxyacyl-coenzyme A dehydrogenase (LCHAD)

PHYSICAL FINDINGS & CLINICAL PRESENTATION

- Initial manifestations:
  1. Nausea and vomiting (70%)
  2. Pain in right upper quadrant or epigastrium (50%-80%)
  3. Malaise and anorexia
- Jaundice often in 1 to 2 wk
- Hypoglycemia
- Late manifestations:
  1. Fulminant hepatic failure
  2. Encephalopathy
  3. Renal failure
  4. Pancreatitis
  5. Gastrointestinal and uterine bleeding
  6. Disseminated intravascular coagulation (10%)
  7. Seizures
  8. Coma
- Liver:
  1. Usually small
  2. Normal or enlarged in preeclampsia, eclampsia, HELLP syndrome (hemolysis, elevated liver enzymes, and low platelets), and acute hepatitis
  3. Coexistent preeclampsia in up to 46% of patients

ETIOLOGY

- Fetal long-chain L-3 hydroxyacyl-CoA dehydrogenase deficiency (LCHAD) deficiency results in transplacental passage of excess fetal fatty acids and subsequent accumulation in the maternal liver.
- Postulated that inhibition of mitochondrial oxidation of fatty acids may lead to microvesicular fatty infiltration of liver.
- Fatty metamorphosis of preeclamptic liver disease believed to be of different etiology.

DIAGNOSIS

DIFFERENTIAL DIAGNOSIS

- Acute gastroenteritis
- Preeclampsia or eclampsia with liver involvement
- HELLP syndrome
- Acute viral hepatitis
- Fulminant hepatitis
- Drug-induced hepatitis caused by halothane, phenytoin, methyldopa, isoniazid, hydrochlorothiazide, or tetracycline
- Intrahepatic cholestasis of pregnancy
- Gallbladder disease
- Reye syndrome
- Hemolytic-uremic syndrome
- Budd-Chiari syndrome
- Systemic lupus erythematosus

WORKUP

- A clinical diagnosis is based predominantly on physical and laboratory findings (Swansea criteria).
- Most definitive diagnosis is through liver biopsy with oil red O staining and electron microscopy.
- Liver biopsy is reserved for atypical cases only and only after any existing coagulopathy is corrected with fresh frozen plasma because of concerns for excessive bleeding.

LABORATORY TESTS

Tests to determine the following:
- Hypoglycemia (often profound <60 mg/dl)
- Hyperammonemia
- Elevated aminotransferases (usually <500 U/ml)
- Thrombocytopenia
- Leukocytosis (white blood cell count >15,000)
- Hyperbilirubinemia (usually <10 mg/dl)
- Low albumin
- Hypofibrinogenemia (<300 mg/dl)
- Disseminated intravascular coagulation (DIC) (in 75%)

IMAGING STUDIES

- Ultrasound: Best used to rule out other diseases in the differential diagnosis such as gallbladder disease
- CT scan: Plays minimal role because of a high false-negative rate

TREATMENT

NONPHARMACOLOGIC THERAPY

- Patient is admitted to intensive care unit for stabilization.
- Fetus is delivered; spontaneous resolution usually follows delivery.
- Mode of delivery is based on obstetric indications and clinical assessment of disease severity.

ACUTE GENERAL Rx

- Decrease in endogenous ammonia through dietary protein restriction; neomycin 6 to 12 g/day PO to decrease presence of ammonia-producing bacteria; magnesium citrate 30 to 50 ml PO or enema to evacuate nitrogenous wastes from colon.
- Administration of IV fluids with glucose to keep glucose levels >60 mg/dl.
- Coagulopathy corrected with fresh frozen plasma.
- Avoidance of drugs metabolized by liver.
- Aggressive avoidance and treatment for nosocomial infections; consideration of prophylactic antibiotics.
- Monitor closely for development of complications such as hepatic encephalopathy, pulmonary edema, DIC, and respiratory arrest.
- Plasma exchange after delivery may result in a lower maternal mortality.

CHRONIC Rx

Orthotopic liver transplantation is the only treatment for irreversible liver failure.

DISPOSITION

- Before 1980, both maternal and fetal mortality rates were approximately 85%.
- Since 2008, maternal mortality rates have been less than 10%.
- Usually rapid return of liver function to normal after delivery.
- Minimal risk of recurrence with future pregnancies.

REFERRAL

- To tertiary health care facility as soon as diagnosis is suspected.
- Twenty percent of infants born to mothers with AFLP have LCHAD; after birth, all infants should be evaluated for the deficiency.

RELATED CONTENT

Eclampsia (Related Key Topic)
Preeclampsia (Related Key Topic)
HELLP Syndrome (Related Key Topic)

SUGGESTED READINGS
Available at ExpertConsult.com

AUTHOR: **Kelly Ruhstaller, MD**

BASIC INFORMATION

DEFINITION

Febrile seizures are seizures that occur in febrile children (fever of at least 100.4° F [38° C]) between the ages of 6 mo and 5 yr in the absence of infection of the central nervous system (CNS), metabolic disturbance, or history of neonatal seizures or a previous unprovoked seizure. Febrile seizures are subdivided into two categories: Simple and complex. Simple febrile seizures last <15 min, are generalized (without a focal component), and occur once in a 24-hr period, whereas complex febrile seizures are prolonged (>15 min), show focal neurologic signs, or occur more than once in 24 hr.

SYNONYMS

Febrile convulsions
Seizures, febrile

ICD-10CM CODE

R56.0 Febrile convulsions

EPIDEMIOLOGY & DEMOGRAPHICS

INCIDENCE: Febrile seizures are the most common seizures of childhood. 2% to 5% of children will have a febrile seizure by age 5 yr. Simple febrile seizures represent 65% to 90% of febrile seizures.
PREVALENCE: Represents up to 18% of all pediatric epilepsy syndromes
PREDOMINANT SEX & AGE: Slightly more common in boys than girls
PEAK INCIDENCE: 6 mo to 5 yr

PHYSICAL FINDINGS & CLINICAL PRESENTATION

- Children with febrile seizures have normal physical and neurologic examinations.

ETIOLOGY

- Viral infections are a common cause of a fever that triggers febrile seizures.
- Febrile seizures tend to occur in families. Although clear evidence exists for a genetic basis of febrile seizures, the mode of inheritance is unknown.
- Febrile seizures are likely multifactorial with genetic and environmental factors.

Dx DIAGNOSIS

DIFFERENTIAL DIAGNOSIS

- CNS infection (i.e., meningitis)
- Epilepsy

WORKUP

- It is important to first investigate whether an underlying infection exists. Fig. 1 describes guidelines for febrile seizure evaluation.
- In patients with simple self-limited febrile seizures with rapid return to consciousness and a normal neurologic examination, further workup is not routinely recommended.
- In patients with complex febrile seizures, laboratory workup and brain imaging are recommended.
- Electroencephalogram (EEG) is not routinely recommended in the evaluation of a neurologically healthy child with simple febrile seizures.

LABORATORY TESTS

- Routine blood workup (CBC with differential, complete metabolic panel (CMP), electrolytes), blood and urine cultures are often performed, but there is no evidence that these tests are necessary for identifying the cause of a simple febrile seizure.
- Lumbar puncture should be performed in children with febrile seizures and signs and symptoms of meningitis (e.g., neck stiffness, Kernig sign, Brudzinski sign), or if the patient history or examination suggests the presence of meningitis or other intracranial infection.
- In infants 6 to 12 mo of age with febrile seizures, lumbar puncture is an option if they have not received the recommended *Haemophilus influenza* type b (Hib) or pneumococcal vaccinations, or if their immunization status is unknown.
- Lumbar puncture is also considered an option in children with febrile seizures pretreated with antibiotics.

IMAGING STUDIES

- MRI of the brain is not required in the routine evaluation of patients with simple febrile seizures.
- Imaging of the brain should be considered in children with complex febrile seizures and in children with focal neurologic deficits.
- CT scans of the head should be avoided in children, if possible, due to exposure to radiation and the relative low yield of the test compared with MRI. CT scans of the head are reserved for neurologic emergencies and are dose-adjusted for weight in children.

Rx TREATMENT

Febrile seizures do not usually require antiepileptic drug treatment.

NONPHARMACOLOGIC THERAPY

Not applicable

GENERAL Rx

Symptomatic treatment of fever

CHRONIC Rx

No chronic treatment for febrile seizures is recommended.

COMPLEMENTARY & ALTERNATIVE MEDICINE

Not applicable

DISPOSITION

- Treatment is not recommended.
- Febrile seizures should stop by age 5.
- Risk of recurrence in the first 2 yr after an initial febrile seizure is 15% to 70%.

REFERRAL

Patients with recurrent febrile seizures need to be referred for a consultation by a pediatric neurologist.

PEARLS & CONSIDERATIONS

COMMENTS

- It is crucial to find out the etiology of the fever and to treat it appropriately.
- Patient with seizures and fever after age 5 are not classified as febrile seizures.

PREVENTION

Antipyretics do not reduce the recurrence risk of febrile seizures. However, fever should be treated and worked up independently of the diagnosis of febrile seizures.

PATIENT & FAMILY EDUCATION

- Children with febrile seizures do not need antiepileptic drug treatment.
- Patient education and information can be obtained at the Epilepsy Foundation: www.epilepsyfoundation.org. Parents should be reassured that children without underlying developmental problems will usually not have lasting neurologic effects from febrile seizures.

RELATED CONTENT

Fever Seizures (Patient Information)

SUGGESTED READINGS

Available at ExpertConsult.com

AUTHOR: **Patricio Sebastian Espinosa, MD, MPH, FAAN**

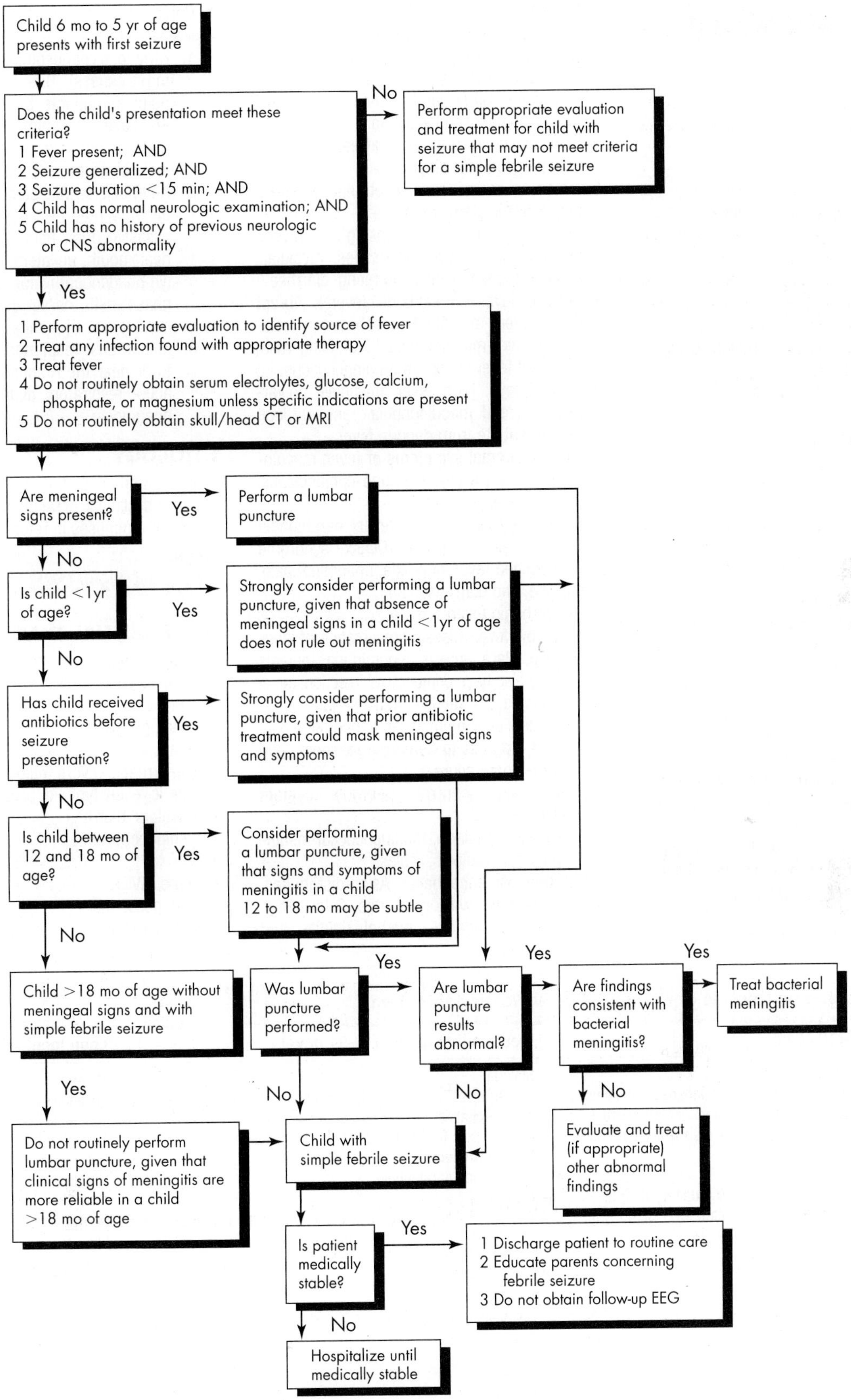

FIG. 1 Guidelines for febrile seizure evaluation. *CNS,* Central nervous system; *CT,* computed tomography; *EEG,* electroencephalogram; *MRI,* magnetic resonance imaging. (From Custer JW, Rau RE: *The Harriet Lane handbook,* ed 18, St Louis, 2009, Mosby.)

Fever in the Returning Traveler

BASIC INFORMATION

DEFINITION

A traveler who returns from a foreign country with a fever or develops a fever within a month of returning.

ICD10-CM CODES	
A01	Typhoid and paratyphoid fever
A50	Fever of other and unknown origin
A90	Dengue fever
A92	Chikungunya fever
A92.5	Zika virus disease
A95	Yellow fever
A98.8	Other specified viral hemorrhagic fever
B54	Malaria, malarial fever
B56	African trypanosomiasis

EPIDEMIOLOGY & DEMOGRAPHICS

INCIDENCE: Fever was the chief complaint in 28% of travelers who presented to a travel clinic. Mortality is between 0.2% and 0.5%. The specific cause of fever may not be diagnosed in up to 25%.

PEAK INCIDENCE: Incidence dependent on location and timing of travel.

RISK FACTORS: Extremes of age, immunocompromised

PHYSICAL FINDINGS & CLINICAL PRESENTATION

- A detailed history of the travel must be obtained, including areas of travel, activities, sleeping arrangements, pre-trip immunizations, comorbidities, and use of malaria prophylaxis.
- If fever develops in less than 21 days, the most common diseases include malaria, typhoid fever, and dengue. Also consider Japanese encephalitis, plague, typhus, yellow fever, and viral hemorrhagic fevers.
- If fever develops after 21 days, the most common diseases include malaria, tuberculosis (TB), and hepatitis A. Consider acute HIV infection, acute systemic schistosomiasis, borreliosis, other viral hepatitis, and West African trypanosomiasis (Table 1).
- Skin lesions in returned travelers (Table 2) may be useful for diagnosis

Common causes of fever in returning travelers and their associated symptoms:

- Malaria: Abrupt rigors, relapsing high fevers, diaphoresis, malaise, headaches, myalgias, abdominal pain, nausea, vomiting, diarrhea.
- Dengue fever ("breakbone fever"): Abrupt fever, severe myalgia, headaches with retro-orbital pain, maculopapular blanching rash, petechial fever similar to meningococcus.
- Chikungunya: High fever, myalgias, polyarthralgias, and maculopapular rash. Difficult to differentiate from dengue fever.
- Zika: Prodromal symptoms of fever, maculopapular rash, arthralgias, and conjunctivitis. Up to 80% asymptomatic.
- Enteric fevers (typhoid fever, paratyphoid fever, travelers' diarrhea): Clinical syndrome of sustained fever, anorexia, abdominal pain, malaise, and diarrhea.
- Hemorrhagic fevers:
  1. Yellow fever: Classic presentation of jaundice, black emesis, albuminuria. Patients may also have conjunctival injection, facial flushing, and relative bradycardia.
  2. Ebola: Fever, myalgia, and abdominal pain that progress to hemorrhage, shock, and end-organ failure.
- Fever with central nervous system involvement:
  1. Consider malaria, meningococcal meningitis, tuberculosis, rabies.
  2. Japanese encephalitis: Asian distribution, associated with rural rice fields. High fevers, headache, nuchal rigidity, and seizures.
- Chronic fevers: Relapsing or constant fever >3 wk:
  1. African trypanosomiasis (African sleeping sickness): Bite from the tsetse fly, painless chancre that grows for 2 to 3 wk. Fever unresponsive to antimalarials, malaise, wasting, behavioral and neurologic changes, encephalitis, coma occur.
  2. American trypanosomiasis (Chagas disease): Spread by reduviid bug (kissing or assassin bug). Painful edema at wound near mouth, unilateral periorbital edema, lymphadenopathy for 2 to 4 wk. Latent phase with nerve destruction causing cardiac and GI manifestations.
  3. Middle East respiratory syndrome (travel to or near the Arabian Peninsula): Fever, acute respiratory distress syndrome, or pneumonia.

ETIOLOGY

Table 3 summarizes the constellations of exposures and clinical presentations suggestive of particular diagnoses in returning travelers.

DIAGNOSIS

DIFFERENTIAL DIAGNOSIS

- Malaria (most common cause of fever after travel to endemic areas)
- Dengue
- Chikungunya
- Zika
- Hemorrhagic fevers: Yellow fever, Ebola
- Enteric fever: Typhoid, paratyphoid
- Travelers' diarrhea
- Meningococcemia
- TB
- Acute HIV
- Trypanosomiasis
- Viral hepatitis

TABLE 1 Incubation Periods of Common Travel-Related Infections*

Short Incubation (<10 days)	Medium Incubation (10-21 days)	Long Incubation (>21 days)
Malaria	Malaria	Malaria
Arboviruses including dengue, yellow fever, Japanese encephalitis	Flaviviruses: Tick-borne encephalitis and Japanese encephalitis	Schistosomiasis
Hemorrhagic fevers: Lassa, ebola, South American arenaviruses	Hemorrhagic fevers: Lassa, ebola, Crimean-Congo	Tuberculosis
Respiratory viruses including severe acute respiratory syndrome	Acute HIV infection	Acute HIV infection
Typhoid and paratyphoid	Typhoid and paratyphoid	Viral hepatitis
Bacterial enteritis	*Giardia*	Filariasis
Rickettsia: Spotted fever group—Rocky Mountain spotted fever, African tick typhus, Mediterranean spotted fever, scrub typhus, Q fever	*Rickettsia*: Flea-borne, louse-borne, and scrub typhus, Q fever, spotted fevers (rare)	*Rickettsia:* Q fever
Bacterial pneumonia including *Legionella*	Cytomegalovirus	Secondary syphilis
Relapsing fever	*Toxoplasma*	Epstein-Barr virus including mononucleosis
Amebic dysentery	Amebic dysentery	Amebic liver disease
Meningococcemia	Histoplasmosis	Leishmaniasis
Brucella (rarely)	*Brucella*	*Brucella*
Leptospirosis	Leptospirosis	Bartonellosis (chronic)
Fascioliasis	Babesiosis	Babesiosis
Rabies (rarely)	Rabies	Rabies
African trypanosomiasis (acute), East African (rarely)	East African trypanosomiasis (acute)	West African trypanosomiasis (chronic)
	Hepatitis A (rarely)	Cytomegalovirus
	Measles	

HIV, Human immunodeficiency virus.

*Diseases that commonly have variable incubation periods are shown more than once. However, most diseases may rarely have an atypical incubation period, and this is not shown here.

From Bennet et al: *Mandell, Douglas, and Bennett's principles and practice of infectious diseases,* ed 8, Philadelphia, 2015, Elsevier.

TABLE 2 Skin Lesions in Returned Travelers

Linear	Cutaneous larva migrans (*Ancylostoma* spp.)	Pruritic serpiginous lesions that advance slowly
	Larva currens	Urticarial linear lesions moving faster due to cutaneous migration of *Strongyloides stercoralis* filariform larvae
	Phytophotodermatitis	Noninfectious lesion due to interaction of natural psoralens (in lime juice spilled on skin) that interacts with UV radiation
Macular	Generalized	Consider drug reactions
	Localized	Consider tinea corporis or tinea versicolor
	Leprosy	Hypopigmented macular lesions with hypoesthesia or peripheral nerve enlargement
Maculopapular	With fever	Arbovirus: Dengue, chikungunya, measles, rubella, parvovirus, EBV, CMV, HIV, syphilis
		VHF
		Rickettsial infection
Nodular	Bacterial skin infection (staphylococcal/streptococcal)	May follow bug bites; pyoderma, impetigo, abscess formation, erysipelas, cellulitis, lymphangitis, or ulceration
	Gnathostomiasis	Migratory panniculitis common in Southeast Asia, less in Africa and Latin America
	Myiasis	Painful "boil"-like lesions in Africa (*Cordylobia anthropophaga)*; or Latin America (*Dermatobia hominis*)
	Tungiasis (*Tunga penetrans*)	Nodular pale subcutaneous lesion with central dark spot
Papular	Bug bites = most common	Grouped papules due to bed bug and flea bites
	Endemic mycoses	Histoplasmosis, penicilliosis
	Onchocerciasis (sub-Saharan Africa)	Generalized pruritic papular dermatitis
	Scabies	Regional or generalized pruritic papular rash
Ulcerative	Anthrax	Necrotic ulcer surrounded by edema
	Buruli ulcer (*Mycobacterium ulcerans*)	Destructive ulcer with undermining edges
	Chancre	*Trypanosoma brucei rhodesiense*: Occurs 48 hours after tsetse fly bite; itchy, painful red/purple nodule, 2-5 cm diameter which ulcerates, with surrounding edema and associated lymphadenopathy
	Cutaneous leishmaniasis	Chronic, usually painless ulcer unless superinfected, with heaped-up margins on exposed skin surfaces, in travelers from high-risk areas, including Latin America, Mediterranean, Middle East, Asia, and parts of Africa
	Rickettsial infection such as African tick-bite fever or scrub typhus	Eschar: Dark, scabbed lesion at site of insect bite
	Ulceroglandular tularemia	Papule develops at site of inoculation with fever onset; becomes vesicular and pustular, then ulcerates. Tender, associated with painful lymphadenitis

CMV, cytomegalovirus; *EBV*, Epstein–Barr virus; *HIV*, human immunodeficiency virus; *UV*, ultraviolet; *VHF*, viral hemorrhagic fever.
From Spec A et al: *Comprehensive review of infectious diseases,* Philadelphia, 2019, Elsevier.

- Common nontravel causes of fever: Urinary tract infection, upper and lower respiratory tract infections, sepsis

Table 4 is from the CDC, with clinical findings and infections to consider. Table 5 is also from the CDC, pairing regions with common tropical diseases that may be causing fever.

WORKUP

Must consider travel location, activities, endemic diseases

LABORATORY TESTS

Consider:
- CBC
- Comprehensive metabolic panel
- Prothrombin time/international normalized ratio, partial thromboplastin time
- Urinalysis
- Blood, urine stool cultures
- Cerebrospinal fluid analysis, Gram stain, culture
- Rapid HIV screen
- Serial blood smears q8 to 12h over 2 days
- Specific serology for suspected infections

IMAGING STUDIES

Not usually required, but consider as clinically indicated:
- Chest x-ray
- Upright abdominal x-ray
- CT: Head
- CT: Abdomen and pelvis

Rx TREATMENT

Pretravel prevention should focus on proper vaccinations and prophylactic antimalarial antibiotics. Posttravel treatment is dependent on the specific disease. Treatment ranges from supportive care to IV antibiotics. Treatment for the more common causes of fever in travelers is listed below, with an emphasis on malaria, given its prevalence:
- Malaria, uncomplicated *Plasmodium falciparum* or species not identified:
  1. Artemether-lumefantrine (Coartem) 1 tab is 20 mg artemether/120 mg lumefantrine
     3 day treatment schedule, 6 doses total
     Day 1: 1 dose and the second dose 8 hr later
     Days 2 and 3: 1 dose PO bid
     5 to <15 kg: 1 tab per dose
     15 to <25 kg: 2 tabs per dose
     25 to <35 kg: 3 tabs per dose
     35 kg and up: 4 tabs per dose
  2. Malarone (atovaquone/proguanil): 250 mg atovaquone/100 mg proguanil
     Malarone 4 tabs PO qd for 3 days
  3. Quinine sulfate 542 mg base (650 mg salt) PO q8h for 3 to 7 days *plus*
     Doxycycline 100 mg PO q12h for 7 days *or*
     Tetracycline: 250 mg PO qid for 7 days *or*
     Clindamycin: 20 mg base/kg/day PO divided tid for 7 days
  4. Mefloquine (not suggested unless the others cannot be taken because of high incidence of neuropsychiatric side effects, high resistance in Southeast Asia): 684 mg base (750 mg salt) PO initial dose, 456 mg base (500 mg salt) PO 6 to 12 hr after the first dose; total dose: 1250 mg salt
  5. For pediatric dosing, refer to CDC treatment table
- Severe malaria:
  1. IV artesunate: Give 2.4 mg/kg per dose; administer 1 dose at 0, 12, 24, and 48 hr for a total of 4 doses

TABLE 3 Constellations of Exposures and Clinical Presentations Suggestive of Particular Diagnoses in Returned Travelers*

Exposure Scenario	Distinctive Findings	Diagnosis
Any exposure in any area with documented malaria transmission	Fever with or without any other finding	Malaria
Most tropical countries	Fever and altered mental status	Malaria, meningococcal meningitis, rabies, West Nile virus
Budget travel to India, Nepal, Pakistan, or Bangladesh	Insidious onset, high unremitting fever, toxic patient, paucity of physical findings	Enteric fever due to *Salmonella typhi* or *Salmonella paratyphi*
Freshwater recreational exposure in Africa	Fever, eosinophilia, hepatomegaly, negative malaria smear	Acute schistosomiasis (Katayama fever)
Bitten by *Aedes aegypti* in Central America, Southeast Asia, or the South Pacific	Fever, headache, myalgia, diffuse macular rash, mild to moderate thrombocytopenia	Dengue
Bitten by *A. aegypti* or *Aedes albopictus* in India, Malaysia, Singapore, the Caribbean, or an island in the Indian Ocean	Fever, headache, myalgia, diffuse macular rash, arthralgia, tenosynovitis often followed by chronic polyarthritis after the fever resolves	Chikungunya fever
Hunting or visiting game reserves in southern Africa	Fever, eschar, diffuse petechial rash	African tick typhus due to *Rickettsia africae*
Travel to Southeast Asia	Fever, eschar, diffuse petechial rash	Scrub typhus due to *Orientia tsutsugamushi*
Hiking, biking, swimming, rafting with exposure to fresh surface water	Fever, myalgia, conjunctival suffusion, mild to severe jaundice, variable rash	Leptospirosis
Cruise, elderly traveler	Influenza-like illness	Influenza A or B
Outdoor exposure anywhere in the Americas	Large, single furuncular lesion anywhere on body, with sense of movement inside	Myiasis due to *Dermatobia hominis* (botfly)
Clothing washed or dried out of doors in Africa	Multiple furuncular lesions around clothing contact points with skin	Myiasis due to *Cordylobia anthropophaga* (tumbu fly)
New sexual partner during travel	Fever, rash, mononucleosis-like illness	Acute human immunodeficiency virus infection
Travel to any developing country or to Western Europe	Coryza, conjunctivitis, Koplik spots, rash	Measles
Longer visit to humid areas of Africa, the Americas, or Southeast Asia	Asymptomatic eosinophilia or with periodic cough or wheezing	Strongyloidiasis
Sand fly bite in tropical areas	Painless skin ulcer with clean, moist base in exposed area	Cutaneous leishmaniasis
Resort hotel in southern Europe, ± exposure to whirlpool spas	Pneumonia	Legionnaires' disease
Explored a cave in the Americas	Fever, cough, retrosternal chest pain, hilar adenopathy	Histoplasmosis
Ingestion of unpasteurized goat cheese	Chronic fever, fatigue	*Brucella melitensis*
Long trip to West/Central Africa	Afebrile, intensely pruritic, evanescent truncal maculopapular rash	Onchocerciasis
Long trip to West/Central Africa	Migratory localized angioedema or swellings over large joints, eosinophilia	Loiasis
Safari to game parks of East Africa	Fever, nongenital chancre, fine macular rash	East African trypanosomiasis
Travel to Australia	Fever, fatigue, polyarthritis	Ross River virus
Farming areas of India and Southeast Asia	Fever, altered mental status, paralysis	Japanese encephalitis
Forested areas of central and eastern Europe and across Russia	Fever, altered mental status, paralysis	Tick-borne encephalitis
Rodent exposure in West Africa	Fever, sore throat, jaundice, hemorrhagic manifestations	Lassa fever
Ingestion of sushi, ceviche, or raw freshwater fish	Migratory nodules in truncal areas with overlying erythema or mild hemorrhage	Gnathostomiasis
Returning Hajj pilgrim or family contact	Fever, meningitis	Meningococcal meningitis
Ingestion of snails, fish, or shellfish in Asia or Australia	Eosinophilic meningitis	Angiostrongyliasis, gnathostomiasis
Diabetic or compromised host with exposure to moist terrain in Asia or Australia	Fever, sepsis, pneumonia or multifocal abscesses	Melioidosis
Summertime exposure to rodent droppings in Scandinavia	Fever with decreased renal function	Puumala virus
Ingestion of undercooked meat of any animal in any country	Fever, facial edema, myositis, increased creatine phosphokinase, massive eosinophilia, normal erythrocyte sedimentation rate	Trichinosis
Unvaccinated, returning from sub-Saharan Africa or forested areas of Amazonia	Fever, jaundice, proteinuria, hemorrhage	Yellow fever
Exposure to farm animals	Pneumonia, mild hepatitis	Q fever
Possible tick exposure almost anywhere	Fever, headache, rash, conjunctival injection, hepatosplenomegaly	Tick-borne relapsing fever
Poor hygienic conditions with possible body louse exposure in Ethiopia or Sudan	Fever, headache, rash, conjunctival injection, hepatosplenomegaly	Louse-borne relapsing fever

*The table includes illnesses of travelers (listed first) as well as less common diseases with presentations that should suggest the possibility of the appropriate diagnosis. Many diseases have a spectrum of presentation, and the table describes the most common presentations of these diseases. Many diseases have a spectrum of geographic origins, and the table describes the most common exposures seen in daily practice.

From Bennet et al: *Mandell, Douglas, and Bennett's principles and practice of infectious diseases*, ed 8, Philadelphia, 2015, Elsevier.

TABLE 4 CDC: Clinical Findings and Select Associated Infectious Diseases

Common Clinical Findings	Infections to Consider after Tropical Travel
Fever and rash	Dengue, chikungunya, Zika, measles, spotted fever or typhus group rickettsioses, enteric fever (skin lesions may be there or not), meningococcemia, acute HIV infection, varicella
Fever and abdominal pain	Enteric fever, amebic or pyogenic liver abscess
Fever and normal or low WBC count	Dengue, malaria, rickettsial infection, enteric fever, chikungunya, Zika, acute HIV
Fever and hemorrhage	Viral hemorrhagic fevers (e.g., dengue, yellow, ebola, Lassa fever), meningococcemia, leptospirosis, spotted fever group rickettsial infections)
Fever and arthralgia or myalgia (sometimes persistent)	Chikungunya, dengue, Zika, Ross River virus, muscular sarcocystosis, trichinellosis
Fever and eosinophilia	Acute schistosomiasis, drug hypersensitivity reaction, fascioliasis, sarcocystosis, trichinellosis, angiostrongyliasis, and other parasitic infections
Fever and respiratory symptoms / pulmonary infiltrates	Influenza and other common bacterial and viral pathogens, legionellosis, tuberculosis, acute schistosomiasis, Q fever, leptospirosis, Middle East respiratory syndrome, acute histoplasmosis, or coccidioidomycosis, psittacosis, melioidosis, pneumonic plague
Fever and altered mental status / CNS involvement	Cerebral malaria, arboviral encephalitides (Jap. Encephalitis, West Nile virus), meningococcal meningitis, rabies, African trypanosomiasis, scrub typhus, angiostrongyliasis, tickborne encephalitis, rabies
Fever and jaundice	Acute viral hepatitis (A, B, C, E), yellow fever and other viral hemorrhagic fevers, severe malaria, leptospirosis
Mononucleosis syndrome	EBV, CMV, toxoplasmosis, acute HIV
Fever persisting >2 wk	Malaria, enteric fever, EBV, CMV, toxoplasmosis, acute HIV, acute schistosomiasis, brucellosis, tuberculosis, Q fever, visceral leishmaniasis
Fever with onset >6 wk after travel	Plasmodium vivax or ovale malaria, acute hepatitis (B, C, E), tuberculosis, amebic liver abscess, melioidosis, African trypanosomiasis

CMV, Cytomegalovirus; *CNS,* central nervous system; *EBV,* Epstein-Barr virus; *HIV,* human immunodeficiency virus; *WBC,* white blood cells.

TABLE 5 Regions with Common Tropical Disease

Geographic Area	Common Tropical Disease Causing Fever	Other Infections Causing Outbreaks or Clusters in Travelers
Caribbean	Chikungunya, dengue, malaria, Zika	Acute histoplasmosis, leptospirosis
Central America	Chikungunya, dengue, malaria (primarily Plasmodium vivax), Zika, enteric fever	Leptospirosis, histoplasmosis, coccidioidomycosis, leishmaniasis
South America	Chikungunya, dengue, malaria (primarily *P. vivax*), Zika	Bartonellosis, leptospirosis, enteric fever, histoplasmosis
South Central Asia	Dengue, enteric fever, malaria (primarily non-falciparum)	Chikungunya, scrub typhus
Southeast Asia	Dengue, malaria (primarily nonfalciparum)	Chikungunya, leptospirosis
Sub-Saharan Africa	Malaria (primarily P. falciparum), tickborne rickettsiae, acute schistosomiasis, dengue fever	African trypanosomiasis, chikungunya enteric fever, meningococcal meningitis

CDC, last update 6/2019.

Followed by 1 of the following:
a. Coartem: reatment as above
b. Doxycycline (clindamycin in pregnant patients): Treatment as above if patient can tolerate PO, otherwise give 100 mg IV q12h and then switch to oral doxycycline as soon as patient can take oral medication; for IV use, avoid rapid administration; treatment course = 7 days
c. Clindamycin: Treatment as above, unless patient cannot tolerate PO, 10 mg base/kg loading dose IV followed by 5 mg base/kg IV q8h; switch to PO clindamycin as soon as possible; avoid rapid administration for IV use; treatment course is 7 days
d. Mefloquine if there is no other option

- Dengue: Supportive care, fever and pain control, prevent dehydration
  1. NSAIDs and aspirin contraindicated due to increased bleeding risk
  2. Acetaminophen or paracetamol q6h
  3. Cool compresses, ice compresses, bath if necessary
- Chikungunya: Supportive care similar to dengue.
- Typhoid fever: Fluoroquinolone (ciprofloxacin), third-generation cephalosporins (cefixime or ceftriaxone), azithromycin. Duration varies based on severity.
- Travelers' diarrhea: Ciprofloxacin, azithromycin.
- Hemorrhagic viruses: Typically only supportive care

DISPOSITION

- Depends on the specific disease, severity of disease, and possibility of transmission.
- Can range from outpatient treatment to ICU level of care.

REFERRAL

- Infectious disease consultation
- Contact the CDC for recommendations pertaining to endemic diseases and treatment
- Some medical treatments and diagnostic testing must be sent from the CDC
- Mandatory reporting of some diseases to the CDC

PEARLS & CONSIDERATIONS

COMMENTS

- The differential depends on the geography and the patient's individual risk factors (pretravel immunizations, comorbidities, activities, etc.)
- Until demonstrated otherwise, some travel medicine experts recommend assuming that all febrile travelers coming from malaria endemic regions have malaria.
- However, keep a broad differential of other common sources of fever (UTIs, respiratory tract infections, hyperthyroid, sepsis, etc.) until a specific diagnosis is made.

PREVENTION

Check the CDC website and the Yellow Book for pretravel vaccinations.

PATIENT & FAMILY EDUCATION

Visit www.cdc.gov for further information.

RELATED CONTENT

Brucellosis (Related Key Topic)
Dengue Fever (Related Key Topic)
Histoplasmosis (Related Key Topic)
Human Immunodeficiency Virus (Related Key Topic)
Leishmaniasis (Related Key Topic)
Malaria (Related Key Topic)
Measles (Rubeola) (Related Key Topic)
Q Fever (Related Key Topic)
Rabies (Related Key Topic)
Salmonellosis (Related Key Topic)
Trichinellosis (Related Key Topic)
West Nile Virus Infection (Related Key Topic)
Yellow Fever (Related Key Topic)
Zika Virus (Related Key Topic)

SUGGESTED READINGS

Available at ExpertConsult.com

AUTHORS: **Nicholas J. Inman, MD,** and **J. Richard Walker III, MD, MS, FACEP**

BASIC INFORMATION

DEFINITION

Fever of undetermined origin (FUO) was first defined by Petersdorf and Beeson in 1961 as an illness characterized by temperatures >38.3° C (101° F) on several occasions for >3 wk with an uncertain diagnosis after 1 wk of evaluation in the hospital. With the increased availability of outpatient evaluation, the requirement of hospitalization for diagnosis was removed. As of 2017, the widely accepted definition of FUO is:

- Temperature ≥38.3° C (101° F) on at least two occasions
- Duration of illness ≥3 wk or multiple febrile episodes in ≥3 wk
- Not immunocompromised
  1. Neutropenic >1 wk in last 3 mo
  2. Known HIV
  3. Hypogammaglobulinemia
  4. 10 mg prednisone or equivalent for at least 2 wk

FUO can be classified into classic, nosocomial (health care associated), neutropenic (immune deficient), and HIV-associated. Table 1 provides a summary of definitions and major features of subtypes of FUO.

SYNONYMS

Fever of unknown origin
Pyrexia of unknown origin

ICD-10CM CODE
R50.9 Fever, unspecified

EPIDEMIOLOGY & DEMOGRAPHICS

- Due to advances in medical knowledge and technology, the distribution of causes of FUO has changed.
- Improved imaging and culture techniques have led to decreased diagnosis secondary to malignancy or infection.
- In recent yrs, more FUOs have no identified cause and eluded diagnosis:
  1. In prospective study of 73 immunocompetent patients with FUO, 51% had no identified cause.

CLINICAL PRESENTATION

Significant fever (≥38.3° C [101° F]) that has persisted for longer than an acute self-limiting illness would be expected to and without identified etiology despite reasonable investigations in whatever setting is appropriate.

ETIOLOGY

FUO can be divided into four categories:

- Infectious (17%-35%)
  1. Localized:
     a. Abscess (intraabdominal, pelvic, renal, dental, intracranial)
     b. Endocarditis (including subacute and culture negative)
     c. Infected peripheral vessels
     d. Osteomyelitis
     e. Urinary tract infection
     f. Sinusitis
     g. *Clostridium difficile* colitis
  2. Generalized:
     a. Bacterial: Typhoid fever, bartonellosis, brucellosis, Q fever
     b. Viral: HIV, cytomegalovirus (CMV), Epstein-Barr virus (EBV), multicentric Castleman disease
     c. Fungal: Histoplasmosis, blastomycosis, cryptococcosis, coccidioidomycosis
     d. Mycobacterial: Tuberculosis (extrapulmonary, military)
     e. Parasitic: Malaria, toxoplasmosis, visceral leishmaniosis, amoebic abscess
- Noninfectious inflammatory (24%-36%)
  1. Adult Still disease
  2. Giant cell arteritis, temporal arteritis, polymyalgia rheumatics
  3. Other vasculitides: Polyarteritis nodosa, Takayasu arteritis, granulomatosis with polyangiitis, mixed cryoglobulinemia
  4. Other rheumatologic disorders: Systemic lupus erythematous, rheumatoid arthritis
- Malignancy (10%-20%)
  1. Lymphoma
  2. Leukemia
  3. Myelodysplastic syndrome
  4. Solid tumors: Renal cell carcinoma, hepatocellular carcinoma, metastatic disease

TABLE 1 Summary of Definitions and Major Features of the Four Subtypes of Fever of Undetermined Origin

Feature	Classic FUO	Health Care–Associated FUO	Immune-Deficient FUO	HIV-Related FUO
Definition	>38.0° C (100.4° F), >3 wk, >2 visits or 1 wk in hospital	≥38.0° C (100.4° F), >1 wk, not present or incubating on admission	≥38.0° C (100.4° F), >1 wk, negative cultures after 48 hr	≥38.0° C (100.4° F), >3 wk for outpatients, >1 wk for inpatients, HIV infection confirmed
Patient location	Community, clinic, or hospital	Acute care hospital	Hospital or clinic	Community, clinic, or hospital
Leading causes	Cancer, infections, inflammatory conditions, undiagnosed, habitual hyperthermia	Health care–associated infections, postoperative complications, drug fever	Majority due to infections, but cause documented in only 40%-60%	HIV (primary infection), typical and atypical mycobacteria, CMV, lymphomas, toxoplasmosis, cryptococcosis, immune reconstitution inflammatory syndrome (IRIS)
History emphasis	Travel, contacts, animal and insect exposure, medications, immunizations, family history, cardiac valve disorder	Operations and procedures, devices, anatomic considerations, drug treatment	Stage of chemotherapy, drugs administered, underlying immunosuppressive disorder	Drugs, exposures, risk factors, travel, contacts, stage of HIV infection
Examination emphasis	Fundi, oropharynx, temporal artery, abdomen, lymph nodes, spleen, joints, skin, nails, genitalia, rectum or prostate, lower limb deep veins	Wounds, drains, devices, sinuses, urine	Skinfolds, IV sites, lungs, perianal area	Mouth, sinuses, skin, lymph nodes, eyes, lungs, perianal area
Investigation emphasis	Imaging, biopsies, sedimentation rate, skin tests	Imaging, bacterial cultures	CXR, bacterial cultures	Blood and lymphocyte count; serologic tests; CXR; stool examination; biopsies of lung, bone marrow, and liver for cultures and cytologic tests; brain imaging
Management	Observation, outpatient temperature chart, investigations, avoidance of empirical drug treatments	Depends on situation	Antimicrobial treatment protocols	Antiviral and antimicrobial protocols, vaccines, revision of treatment regimens, good nutrition
Time course of disease	Months	Weeks	Days	Weeks to months
Tempo of investigation	Weeks	Days	Hours	Days to weeks

CMV, Cytomegalovirus; *CXR,* chest radiograph; *FUO,* fever of undetermined origin; *HIV,* human immunodeficiency virus; *IV,* intravenous.
Adapted from Mandell GL et al (eds): *Mandell, Douglas, and Bennett's principles and practice of infectious diseases,* ed 7, Philadelphia, 2010, Churchill Livingstone. Borrowed from Kliegman RM et al: *Nelson textbook of pediatrics,* ed 19, Philadelphia, 2011, Saunders.

- Miscellaneous (3%-15%)
  1. Drug-induced fever
  2. Inflammatory bowel disease
  3. Sarcoidosis
  4. Pulmonary embolism/deep vein thrombosis
  5. Alcoholic hepatitis
  6. Familial Mediterranean fever
  7. Factitious fever
- No diagnosis in 16% to 39% of cases

Dx DIAGNOSIS

DIFFERENTIAL DIAGNOSIS

Over 200 possible diagnoses for FUO

WORKUP

- By definition, FUO is a diagnostic challenge. As the list of possible causes is extensive, there is no useful, clear-cut algorithmic approach.
- Accurate history and careful physical examination are essential. Table E2 describes an approach to the patient with FUO based on history and physical findings.
- Laboratory tests and imaging dependent on medical history clues and physical findings.
- When in doubt, perform another complete history and physical examination. Examples of subtle physical findings in patients with FUO are described in Table 3.

MEDICAL HISTORY CLUES

- Duration, accompanying symptoms (rigor, drenching sweats)
  1. Degree of fever, nature of fever curve, apparent toxicity, and response to antipyretic have not been found to be helpful.
- Unintentional weight loss
- Drenching night sweats
- Rash
- Myalgias
- Joint pain
- Unilateral retro-orbital headache or jaw claudication
- History of immunosuppression
- Thromboembolic risk factors (previous episodes, prolonged immobility, oral contraceptive pills recent surgeries)
- Medications
- Sick contacts
- Social history:
  1. Alcohol intake
  2. Occupational exposures
  3. Animal exposures
  4. Insect bites
  5. Sexual exposures
  6. Travel history
- Family history:
  1. Autoimmune disorders
  2. Malignancies
  3. Familial Mediterranean fever

PHYSICAL FINDINGS

- HEENT (head, ears, eyes, nose, throat): Sinus tenderness, dental abscesses, funduscopic lesions
- Neck: Adenopathy, palpable thyroid
- Lungs: Auscultate for rales
- Heart: Murmur
- Abdomen: Organomegaly
- Rectal: Prostate tenderness
- Pelvic: Cervical motion tenderness, fundal or adnexal masses or pain, inguinal adenopathy
- Extremities: Clubbing, splinter hemorrhages, tenderness or fluctuance at IV access site
- Musculoskeletal: Joint effusions
- Skin: Rashes, wounds

LABORATORY TESTS

- Initial laboratory testing:
  1. Complete blood count with differential
  2. Comprehensive metabolic panel
  3. Inflammatory markers (erythrocyte sedimentation rate [ESR], C-reactive protein)
  4. Urinalysis
  5. Lactate dehydrogenase
  6. Blood cultures
  7. Thyroid-stimulating hormone
  8. HIV antibody testing
- Consider:
  1. HIV viral load
  2. Hepatitis serologies
  3. TB testing (purified protein derivative or interferon gamma release assay)
  4. Testing for endemic fungal infections (based on geographic location and exposure)
  5. Peripheral smear (thick and thin)
  6. Creatine kinase
  7. Ferritin
  8. Antinuclear antibody testing
  9. Rheumatoid factor
  10. Serum protein electrophoresis
  11. Lumbar puncture
  12. Biopsy (based on clinical and laboratory findings)
- May need to repeat tests at regular intervals until diagnosis is established

IMAGING STUDIES

- Initial:
  1. CXR
  2. Abdominal imaging (CT or ultrasound [US])
- Consider:
  1. Venous duplex imaging
  2. Fluorodeoxyglucose (FDG)-PET
     a. Anatomic localization of focally increased FDG uptake
     b. Consider when initial workup negative and no clear diagnostic clues

TABLE 3 Examples of Subtle Physical Findings Having Special Significance in Patients with Fever of Undetermined Origin

Body Site	Physical Finding	Diagnosis
Head	Sinus tenderness	Sinusitis
Temporal artery	Nodules, reduced pulsations	Temporal arteritis
Oropharynx	Ulceration	Disseminated histoplasmosis
	Tender tooth	Periapical abscess
Fundi or conjunctivae	Choroid tubercle	Disseminated granulomatosis*
	Petechiae, Roth spot	Endocarditis
Thyroid	Enlargement, tenderness	Thyroiditis
Heart	Murmur	Infective or marantic endocarditis
Abdomen	Enlarged iliac crest lymph nodes, splenomegaly	Lymphoma, endocarditis, disseminated granulomatosis*
Rectum	Perirectal fluctuance, tenderness	Abscess
	Prostatic tenderness, fluctuance	Abscess
Genitalia	Testicular nodule	Periarteritis nodosa
	Epididymal nodule	Disseminated granulomatosis
Lower extremities	Deep venous tenderness	Thrombosis or thrombophlebitis
Skin and nails	Petechiae, splinter hemorrhages, subcutaneous nodules, clubbing	Vasculitis, endocarditis

*Includes tuberculosis, histoplasmosis, coccidioidomycosis, sarcoidosis, and syphilis.
From Mandell GL et al (eds): *Mandell, Douglas, and Bennett's principles and practice of infectious diseases*, ed 7, Philadelphia, 2010, Churchill Livingstone.

Rx TREATMENT

- Therapy should be tailored once etiology of FUO has been established.
- When the cause of FUO remains unknown, empiric treatment with broad spectrum antibiotics should be reserved for patients who are severely ill.

DISPOSITION

- Prognosis is determined primarily by the underlying disease.
- FUO patients who remain undiagnosed after an extensive evaluation generally have a favorable outcome.

REFERRAL

To an infectious disease specialist, hematologist, or rheumatologist if no diagnosis after thoughtful workup

RELATED CONTENT

Fever of Unknown Origin (Patient Information)

SUGGESTED READINGS

Available at ExpertConsult.com

AUTHORS: **Alexandra Abrams-Downey, MD,** and **Erna Milunka Kojic, MD**

Fibrocystic Breast Disease (PTG)

BASIC INFORMATION

DEFINITION

Fibrocystic breast disease (FBD), now called "fibrocystic breast changes" (FBC), is a category of benign breast lesions that includes:

- Microcystic and macrocystic changes
- Fibrosis
- Mild and moderate hyperplasia
- Sclerosing adenosis
- Apocrine metaplasia
- Fibroadenoma
- Papilloma
- Papillomatosis
- Radial scar

Nonmalignant breast lesions can be divided into nonproliferative, proliferative without atypia, and atypical hyperplasia. Nonproliferative lesions such as simple breast cysts are considered not to be at increased risk for breast cancer (RR = 1.17). Proliferative lesions, including ductal hyperplasia, intraductal papillomas, sclerosing adenosis, radial scars, and fibroadenomas, are considered markers for a small increase in risk of progressing to breast cancer (proliferation without atypia RR = 1.76, with hyperplastic atypia RR = 3.93), and patients should be counseled on risk reduction.

SYNONYMS

Cystic changes
Chronic cystic mastitis
Fibrocystic breast changes
Mammary dysplasia
Fibrocystic mastopathy
Diffuse cystic mastopathy

ICD-10CM CODES

N60.01	Solitary cyst of right breast
N60.02	Solitary cyst of left breast
N60.09	Solitary cyst of unspecified breast
N60.11	Diffuse cystic mastopathy of right breast
N60.12	Diffuse cystic mastopathy of left breast
N60.19	Diffuse cystic mastopathy of unspecified breast
N60.3	Fibrosclerosis

EPIDEMIOLOGY & DEMOGRAPHICS

- FBC affects 30% to 60% of reproductive-age women.
- Most commonly seen in women ages 30 to 50 yr.

ETIOLOGY

The cause of FBC is unknown but is thought to be influenced by reproductive hormones, estrogen in particular. Because the majority of FBC is found in healthy breasts, it is regarded as a nonpathologic process.

DIAGNOSIS

DIFFERENTIAL DIAGNOSIS

See Table E1.

PHYSICAL FINDINGS & CLINICAL PRESENTATION

- Lumpy or ropey breast texture
- Nodular areas
- Tenderness of breasts and/or nipples
- Dominant mass more often in the upper outer quadrants
- Symptoms tend to be affected by changes in the menstrual cycle
- Symptoms can be aggravated in postmenopausal women who initiate hormone therapy
- Nipple discharge

For differentiation of breast masses, see Table 2. Characteristics of breast masses suspect for cancer (90% sensitivity, 40%-60% specificity) are:

- Fixed mass
- Poorly defined mass
- Hard (scirrhous) mass

WORKUP

- Rule out breast carcinoma if breast mass, thickening, discharge, and/or pain are present.
- Perform biopsy of suspected area for histologic confirmation.

IMAGING STUDIES

Mammography and ultrasound studies required:

- For mammographic changes (suspicious densities, microcalcifications [Fig. E1], architectural distortion): Careful evaluation, including possibly biopsy to exclude breast cancer
- Ultrasound study (Fig. E2): To evaluate the presence of a solid vs. cystic mass
- MRI is not recommended for routine evaluation of breast pain or fibrocystic changes

TREATMENT

NONPHARMACOLOGIC THERAPY

Treatment is symptomatic:

- Reassurance
- Supportive bra
- OTC pain medications including NSAIDs and Tylenol
- Reduced intake of methylxanthines (coffee, chocolate), although this is not as effective as previously thought
- Decreasing vitamin E or salt has not proved to be effective
- Periodic physician examination to monitor patients with FBC who have pronounced nodular features
- Aspiration for palpable or symptomatic cysts (NOTE: Cysts often recur; repeat aspiration is not always required unless pain is a problem)

PHARMACOLOGIC TREATMENT

For breast pain:

- Danocrine (Danazol): This is the only FDA-approved drug for breast pain. Moderate success has been reported, but the side effect profile is significant due to androgenic effects.
- Bromocriptine: This inhibits prolactin, and its effects are better than a placebo, but side effects such as lightheadedness and gastrointestinal symptoms limit its use.
- Tamoxifen: This has been found to reduce breast pain in 70% of affected women with cyclic breast pain, but the side effects of hot flashes and vaginal dryness interfere with compliance.
- Pharmacologic therapy is usually tapered down after 3 to 6 mo of treatment.

FOLLOW-UP

- Evaluate carefully to exclude breast cancer; then offer reassurance and periodic reevaluation as required.
- For all women, ACOG recommends breast self-awareness, regular clinical breast exams (every 1-3 yr for women ages 25-39, annually for women over 40), and mammograms every 1 to 2 yr starting at age 40.

REFERRAL TO BREAST SURGEON

- If suspicious changes are associated with FBC (including progression of dominant mass or thickening, persistent or bloody nipple discharge, or suspicious mammographic changes or lesions), refer for further evaluation and/or biopsy.
- Refer to alleviate anxiety associated with breast symptoms or changes.

SUGGESTED READINGS

Available at ExpertConsult.com

RELATED CONTENT

Fibrocystic Breast Changes (Patient Information)
Breast Cancer (Related Key Topic)
Mastodynia (Related Key Topic)
Mastitis (Related Key Topic)

AUTHORS: **Kathryn G. Vollum, MD,** and **Kelly McNamara, MD**

TABLE 2 Differentiation of Breast Masses

Characteristic	Cystic Disease	Benign Adenoma	Malignant Tumor
Patient age	25-60 yr	10-55 yr	25-85 yr
Number	One or more	One	One
Shape	Round	Round	Irregular
Consistency	Elastic, soft to hard	Firm	Stony hard
Delimitation	Well delimited	Well delimited	Poorly delimited
Mobility	Mobile	Mobile	Fixed
Tenderness	Present	Absent	Absent
Skin retraction	Absent	Absent	Present

From Swartz MH: *Textbook of physical diagnosis,* ed 7, Philadelphia, 2014, Saunders.

BASIC INFORMATION

DEFINITION

Fibromyalgia (FM) is a syndrome characterized by chronic, widespread musculoskeletal pain without evidence of soft tissue inflammation. Key features include fatigue, sleep disruption, cognitive disturbance, and psychiatric and somatic symptoms. Research suggests that FM is a disorder of pain regulation, which is often classified as a form of central sensitization.

SYNONYMS

"Fibrositis" is a term that is no longer used, because there is no evidence of connective tissue inflammation in FM.

ICD-10CM CODE
M79.7 Fibromyalgia

EPIDEMIOLOGY & DEMOGRAPHICS

Worldwide, the prevalence of FM is estimated to be between 2% and 8%, and it increases with age. In the U.S., FM is the most common cause of musculoskeletal pain in women between 20 and 55 yr of age. Using the 2010 American College of Rheumatology (ACR) diagnostic criteria for FM, the female:male ratio is approximately 2:1.

PHYSICAL FINDINGS & CLINICAL PRESENTATION

Patients with FM often report the following symptoms:

- Chronic (>3 mo) widespread (affecting both sides of the body, above and below the waist, and involving the axial spine) musculoskeletal pain
- Cognitive disturbances
- Fatigue and sleep disturbances (e.g., unrefreshed sleep, easy fatigability)
- Psychiatric symptoms (e.g., anxiety, depression)
- Headache (present in more than half of patients with FM; this includes migraine and tension-type headaches)
- Paresthesias
- Associated disorders: Irritable bowel syndrome, interstitial cystitis/painful bladder syndrome

On physical examination, patients with FM can have tenderness, in particular soft tissue locations called tender points. Examination of tender points requires that the examiner be familiar with the areas to palpate and that they apply enough pressure (4 kg/cm^2 or enough pressure to whiten the nail bed of the fingertips of the examiner).

ETIOLOGY

Although the exact cause of FM is unknown, its etiology is thought to be multifactorial:

- Genetic and environmental factors may play a role. Evidence suggests that both the ascending and descending pain pathways operate abnormally, resulting in central amplification of pain signals. Familial associations of FM provide strongest evidence that reflect both these factors.
- In those predisposed, FM may be precipitated by stressful events such as abuse, injury from accidents, illnesses (including autoimmune disorders), infections, surgical procedures, and psychologic stressors.
- Psychosocial, neuroendocrine, hormonal, and sociocultural factors also influence symptom expression.

PATHOGENESIS

Much remains to be discovered about the pathogenesis of FM, even though significant advances have been made in our understanding of this syndrome over the past few decades. Researchers have shown that biochemical, metabolic, and immunoregulatory abnormalities exist in patients with FM. Hence, this condition is now believed to be neurosensory in nature.

- Augmented pain and sensory processing is a hallmark, resulting in diffuse pain, allodynia (pain brought on by nonpainful stimuli), and hyperalgesia (more intense and prolonged pain perception).
- Afflicted persons show altered physiologic responses to painful stimulation at spinal and supraspinal levels.
- Brain neuroimaging studies found differences in brain structure, neurochemical concentrations, and functional brain networks in FM compared with control subjects. PET scans have revealed widespread activation of glial cells in the cortex, particularly in the frontal and parietal lobes.
- Pain augmentation may also result from a loss of tonic inhibition by descending inhibitory pathways from the brain to the spinal cord.

DIAGNOSIS

DIFFERENTIAL DIAGNOSIS

The presence of any of the disorders mentioned below does not necessarily exclude a diagnosis of FM because it can coexist with many conditions:

- Other functional somatic or "central sensitivity" syndromes: Myofascial pain, chronic fatigue syndrome, irritable bowel syndrome, headache/migraines, chronic pelvic and bladder pain disorders, and temporomandibular disorder
- Disorders that can mimic FM and must be ruled out include metabolic (e.g., hypothyroidism), infectious, and neurologic disorders. Arthritis and rheumatic diseases (e.g., rheumatoid arthritis, systemic lupus erythematosus, osteoarthritis, Sjögren's syndrome)
- Myalgias and other muscle disease (e.g., inflammatory and metabolic myopathies)
- Mood and anxiety disorders
- Sleep disorders (e.g., sleep apnea, restless leg syndrome)
- Neurologic disorders
- Medications: Statin-induced muscle pain, opioid-induced hyperalgesia

WORKUP

A thorough history, physical examination, and appropriately selected laboratory or imaging studies can usually differentiate FM from connective tissue or other systemic diseases.

- Chronic (>3 mo) widespread pain is the hallmark symptom of FM, but fatigue, tenderness, depression/anxiety, nonrestorative sleep, cognitive difficulties (the so-called "fibrofog"), and functional impairment are other key symptoms.
- The 1990 ACR FM Classification Criteria were used for clinical studies:
  1. Chronic, widespread pain in all four quadrants of the body and the axial skeleton
  2. Pain on digital palpation of at least 11 of 18 tender points
- The 2010 ACR diagnostic criteria for FM do not require a tender point examination; other disorders that would otherwise explain the musculoskeletal pain must be excluded (Table 1).
- A diagnostic screening tool (Fibromyalgia Diagnostic Screen) developed by Arnold and colleagues was found to accurately screen for FM. This tool includes a patient self-reported questionnaire and an abbreviated physical examination with targeted lab tests.
- The most recent FM diagnostic criteria are by ACTION-APS Pain Taxonomy (AAPT), an international working group. To fulfill AAPT criteria for FM, a patient is required to have a history of at least 3 mo of widespread pain in at least 6 of 9 possible pain sites, and moderate to severe sleep disturbance or fatigue.

LABORATORY TESTS

- Selective use of ancillary tests complements the history and physical examination in the diagnosis of FM. Testing should be highly focused on the exclusion of FM mimickers or suspected concurrent diseases.
- Complete blood cell count, routine chemistries, thyroid-stimulating hormone (TSH), 25-hydroxy vitamin D level (low levels can cause muscle pain), vitamin B^{12} level (low levels can cause fatigue and pain), iron studies (low levels can cause fatigue and depressive symptoms), and magnesium levels (low levels can cause muscle spasms).
- Erythrocyte sedimentation rate (ESR) and C-reactive protein (CRP) are generally normal.
- Routine testing for antinuclear antibody (ANA) and/or rheumatoid factor should be avoided unless history and physical examination suggest an autoimmune disease.

TREATMENT

GENERAL Rx

The goal in treating patients with fibromyalgia is to reduce the main symptoms of the syndrome (musculoskeletal pain, fatigue, depression, anxiety, poor sleep).

- Challenging to treat; best approach may be combination of drug and nondrug therapies.

TABLE 1 2010 Fibromyalgia Diagnostic Criteria

Criteria

A patient satisfies diagnostic criteria for fibromyalgia if the following three conditions are met:
1. Widespread pain index (WPI) 7 and symptom severity (SS) scale score of 5 or WPI 3-6 and SS scale score of 9.
2. Symptoms have been present at a similar level for at least 3 mo.
3. The patient does not have a disorder that would otherwise explain the pain.

Ascertainment

1. WPI: Note the number of areas in which the patient has had pain over the past week. In how many areas has the patient had pain?
   Score will be between 0 and 19.

Shoulder girdle, left	Hip (buttock, trochanter), left	Jaw, left	Upper back
Shoulder girdle, right	Hip (buttock, trochanter), right	Jaw, right	Lower back
Upper arm, left	Upper leg, left	Chest	Neck
Upper arm, right	Upper leg, right	Abdomen	
Lower arm, left	Lower leg, left		
Lower arm, right	Lower leg, right		

2. SS scale score:
   Fatigue
   Waking unrefreshed
   Cognitive symptoms

For the each of the three symptoms above, indicate the level of severity over the past week using the following scale:
- 0, No problem
- 1, Slight or mild problems, generally mild or intermittent
- 2, Moderate, considerable problems, often present at a moderate level
- 3, Severe: Pervasive, continuous, life-disturbing problems

Considering somatic symptoms in general, indicate whether the patient has:*
- 0, No symptoms
- 1, Few symptoms
- 2, A moderate number of symptoms
- 3, A great deal of symptoms

The SS scale score is the sum of the severity of the three symptoms (fatigue, waking unrefreshed, cognitive symptoms) plus the extent (severity) of somatic symptoms in general. The final score is between 0 and 12.

*Somatic symptoms that might be considered include muscle pain, irritable bowel syndrome, fatigue or tiredness, thinking or remembering problem, muscle weakness, headache, pain or cramps in the abdomen, numbness or tingling, dizziness, insomnia, depression, constipation, pain in the upper abdomen, nausea, nervousness, chest pain, blurred vision, fever, diarrhea, dry mouth, itching, wheezing, Raynaud phenomenon, hives or welts, ringing in ears, vomiting, heartburn, oral ulcers, loss of or change in taste, seizures, dry eyes, shortness of breath, loss of appetite, rash, sun sensitivity, hearing difficulties, easy bruising, hair loss, frequent urination, painful urination, and bladder spasms.

Adapted from Wolfe F et al: The American College of Rheumatology preliminary diagnostic criteria for fibromyalgia and measurement of symptom severity, *Arthritis Care Res* 62:600-610, 2010.

- Nonpharmacologic (Table E2): Strong evidence to support exercise (aerobic, strengthening, and stretching exercises; tai chi; yoga), cognitive behavioral therapy, physical therapy, and patient education (e.g., regarding the disease, importance of good sleep and hygiene).
- FM can be due to abnormalities in many different neurotransmitter systems; thus, approaches and treatment responses may vary.
- Pharmacologic therapies for fibromyalgia are summarized in Table 3.
- Best evidence for tricyclics (low-dose amitriptyline, cyclobenzaprine), serotonin-norepinephrine reuptake inhibitors (milnacipran, duloxetine), gabapentinoids (gabapentin, pregabalin).
- Second-tier drug classes include SSRIs.
- "Start low, go slow" approach is best to avoid side effects, which are common. Medication adherence is generally poor.
- There is no evidence that acetaminophen, NSAIDs, or corticosteroids are effective in FM.
- The only analgesic that has demonstrated some efficacy in FM has been tramadol; can consider for treatment-resistant cases.
- Avoid narcotic use. Opioid use and abuse may aggravate chronic widespread pain.

DISPOSITION

- The pain and symptoms of FM can wax and wane, vary in physical location and in intensity day-to-day; many patients continue to have chronic pain and fatigue regardless of therapy.
- Disability rates vary from 10% to 30%.

REFERRAL

Referral to rheumatology, neurology, mental health professionals, physical medicine and rehabilitation, including PT. Multidisciplinary team approach is generally most helpful.

PEARLS & CONSIDERATIONS

- Fibromyalgia is a neurosensory disorder whereby affected individuals have abnormal central nociceptive processing.
- Diagnosis is based on the presence of chronic musculoskeletal pain in the absence of physical or laboratory evidence of inflammation and in the absence of any other condition that would explain the symptoms.
- Treatment options are varied, but a combination of drug and nondrug options is likely to provide optimal results.
- Myofascial pain syndrome may represent a localized form of FM. It is associated with trigger points (rather than tender points as seen in FM). Some patients with myofascial pain syndrome may progress to FM.

COMMENTS

FM occurs frequently in patients with some rheumatic diseases, such as rheumatoid arthritis, ankylosing spondylitis, and systemic lupus erythematosus, in which prevalence of FM may reach 20%.

SUGGESTED READINGS

Available at ExpertConsult.com

RELATED CONTENT

Fibromyalgia (Patient Information)

AUTHOR: **Nadine Mbuyi, MD**

TABLE 3 Pharmacologic Therapies for Fibromyalgia

Treatment	Cost	Specifics	Evidence level	Side Effects	Suggestions
Pharmacologic therapies		Pharmacologic therapy is best chosen based on the predominant symptoms and initiated in low dose with slow dose escalation.	5, Consensus		• Some practitioners find that getting patients on a drug regimen that helps improve symptoms before initiating nonpharmacologic therapies can help improve compliance.
Tricyclic compounds		• Amitriptyline 10-70 mg qhs • Cyclobenzaprine 5-20 mg qhs	1, A	Dry mouth, weight gain, constipation, "groggy" or drugged feeling	• When effective, can improve a wide range of symptoms, including pain, sleep, bowel, and bladder symptoms. • Taking these drugs several hours before bedtime improves side effect profile.
Serotonin norepinephrine reuptake inhibitors	Duloxetine is generic, milnacipran not	• Duloxetine, 30-120 mg/day • Milnacipran, 100-200 mg/day	1, A	Nausea, palpitations, headache, fatigue, tachycardia, hypertension	• Warning patients about transient nausea, taking with food, and slowly increasing dose can increase tolerability. • Milnacipran might be slightly more noradrenergic than duloxetine and thus potentially more helpful for fatigue and memory problems, but it is also more likely to cause HTN.
Gabapentinoids	Gabapentin is generic, pregabalin not	Gabapentin 800-2400 mg/day in divided doses Pregabalin up to 600 mg/day in divided doses	1, A	Sedation, weight gain, dizziness	Giving most or all of the dose at bedtime can increase tolerability.
γ-Hydroxybutyrate	Available for treating narcolepsy, cataplexy	GHB 4.5-6.0 g per night in divided doses	1, A	Sedation, respiratory depression, and death	Shown to be efficacious but not approved by U.S. FDA because of safety concerns.
Low-dose naltrexone	Low	4.5 mg/day	Two small single center RCTs		
Cannabinoids	NA	Nabilone 0.5 mg PO qhs-1.0 mg bid	1, A	Sedation, dizziness, dry mouth	No synthetic cannabinoid is approved in the U.S. for treatment of pain.
Selective serotonin reuptake inhibitors (SSRIs)	SSRIs that should be used in FM (see Suggestions) are all generic	Fluoxetine, sertraline, paroxetine	1, A	Nausea, sexual dysfunction, weight gain, sleep disturbance	Older, less selective SSRIs may have some efficacy in improving pain, especially at higher doses that have more prominent noradrenergic effects. Newer SSRIs (citalopram, escitalopram, desvenlafaxine) are less effective or ineffective as analgesics.
NSAIDs		No evidence of efficacy Can be helpful to treat comorbid "peripheral pain generators"	5, D	GI, renal, and cardiac side effects	Use the lowest dose for the shortest period of time to reduce side effects.
Opioids		Tramadol with or without acetaminophen, 50-100 mg every 6 hours No evidence of efficacy for stronger opioids	5, D	Sedation, addiction, tolerance, opioid-induced hyperalgesia	There is increasing evidence that opioids are less effective for treating chronic pain than previously thought, and their risk-benefit profile is worse than other classes of analgesics.

bid, Twice a day; *FDA,* U.S. Food and Drug Administration; *FM,* fibromyalgia; *GHB,* gammahydroxybutyrate; *GI,* gastrointestinal; *HTN,* hypertension; *NSAIDs,* nonsteroidal antiinflammatory drugs; *PO,* oral; *qhs,* at bedtime; *RCT,* randomized controlled trial.
From Hochberg MC: *Rheumatology,* ed 7, Philadelphia, 2019, Elsevier.

First-Degree Atrioventricular Block

BASIC INFORMATION

DEFINITION

First-degree atrioventricular (AV) block is defined as a PR interval exceeding 200 msec with preserved 1:1 AV conduction relationship. AV block is actually a misnomer because every atrial impulse is conducted to ventricles, and some refer to this finding as *first-degree AV delay.*

SYNONYMS

First-degree heart block
Atrioventricular conduction delay
First-degree AV delay

ICD-10CM CODE
I44.0 Atrioventricular block, first degree; heart block, first degree

EPIDEMIOLOGY & DEMOGRAPHICS

INCIDENCE: Based on studies conducted in healthy volunteers, the incidence varies between 5 and 10 in 1000.

PREVALENCE: Overall prevalence between 1% and 2% has been reported. It increases with age from ~1% in young (20- to 30-yr-old) adults to ~3% to 4% by age 60. In a cohort over age 60, prevalence is ~6%.

PREDOMINANT SEX & AGE: More common in older male patients.

RISK FACTORS: Age (more common with advanced age), male sex (men on average have longer PR intervals), race (African Americans tend to have longer PR intervals), family history, and comorbid conditions (e.g., hypertension, diabetes) are major risk factors.

GENETICS: Genome-wide association studies identified genes (e.g., SCN5A and more recently SCN10A, encoding voltage-gated sodium channel) that can determine PR interval duration.

PHYSICAL FINDINGS & CLINICAL PRESENTATION

- Clinical presentation of a first-degree AV block depends on the duration of PR interval. Insignificant prolongation has no hemodynamic consequences and hence is asymptomatic. Progressive prolongation causes decrease in intensity of the S1 heart sound and sometimes its complete disappearance. This is due to premature partial or complete closure of atrioventricular valves caused by reverse diastolic ventriculoatrial pressure gradient, especially with decreased ventricular compliance.
- In some patients, diastolic mitral regurgitation can be demonstrated. Further lengthening of AV conduction time (particularly beyond 300 msec, termed *marked first-degree AV block*) causes "pseudo-pacemaker syndrome" when atria contract against closed atrioventricular valves due to encroachment of atrial systole on the previous ventricular systole. This leads to increased pressure in both atria, inferior vena cava, superior vena cava, and pulmonary veins, and loss of "atrial kick" with ensuing drop in end-diastolic volume, stroke volume, and cardiac output. Typical symptoms of the pseudo-pacemaker syndrome include malaise, poor exercise tolerance, dyspnea, orthopnea, cough, atypical chest discomfort, sensation of throat fullness, and occasionally presyncope or syncope.
- Physical examination may reveal hypotension, rales, increased jugular venous pressure with cannon A waves, peripheral edema, and murmurs of tricuspid and/or mitral regurgitation.

ETIOLOGY

Causes of AV block are numerous. They can be broadly divided into congenital and acquired. Acquired causes can in turn be broken down into infectious, inflammatory, degenerative, ischemic, vagotonic, metabolic, and iatrogenic. Congenital causes include conditions where a heart block is a part of a syndrome (such as myotonic dystrophy type 1, Emery-Dreifuss, limb-girdle type 1B) or a primary abnormality (as in familial Lev-Lenègre disease due to mutation of the SCN5A gene). A number of infections (Lyme disease, Chagas disease, toxoplasmosis), metabolic disorders (hyperkalemia, hypothyroidism), inflammatory conditions (systemic lupus erythematosus, rheumatoid arthritis, sarcoidosis), therapeutic interventions (beta-blockers, nondihydropyridine calcium channel blockers, valve surgeries, digoxin, etc.), toxins (CO, cyanide, mercury), degenerative processes (senile idiopathic fibrosis of the conduction system, aortic valve calcification), ischemia (acute myocardial infarction, chronic stable coronary artery disease), and increased vagal tone (in athletes or patients with sleep apnea) can be responsible for acquired AV block.

DIAGNOSIS

DIFFERENTIAL DIAGNOSIS

Diagnosis of first-degree AV block is typically straightforward (see definition) and made on a 12-lead electrocardiogram (ECG) or rhythm strip (Fig. 1). In rare cases of extreme AV delay, the P wave may be buried in preceding T wave or QRS complex, causing apparent AV dissociation.

WORKUP

The goal of workup is to establish the level of AV delay, its etiology, and its relationship to symptoms (if present). Workup is also indicated in asymptomatic patients who are at risk for progression to higher degrees of AV block (e.g., when certain hereditary conduction system disorders are suspected). It includes full history, physical examination, laboratory tests, and imaging studies.

LABORATORY TESTS

Selection of a particular test(s) is dictated by preliminary diagnosis(es), considered most likely based on the history and physical findings. Examples include thyroid function studies, basic metabolic panel, Lyme serology, endocardial biopsy, and genetic testing.

IMAGING STUDIES

- Can be divided into three broad categories:
  1. Studies that help establish relationship between AV delay and symptoms (outpatient electrocardiographic monitoring, treadmill stress test)
  2. Studies that help diagnose underlying cause of AV conduction delay (cardiac magnetic resonance imaging, echocardiogram, cardiac computed tomography, left-sided heart catheterization)
  3. Studies that help determine a level of AV conduction delay (surface ECG and/or intracardiac electrogram recording during various pharmacologic and physiologic maneuvers)

However, an electrophysiology study is not generally performed in the evaluation of AV conduction delay.

TREATMENT

Treatment (Fig. 2) is indicated in patients with symptoms that correlate with the first-degree AV block or in patients without symptoms, but who are at risk for progression to higher degrees of AV block. The management of first-degree AV block is summarized in Table 1.

NONPHARMACOLOGIC THERAPY

In asymptomatic patients without high risk of progression to advanced AV block, treatment includes observation, reassurance, and education. Cardiac pacing is a nonpharmacologic treatment modality for appropriately selected patients (see below).

ACUTE GENERAL Rx

Patients with symptoms due to reversible causes of AV conduction delay should receive appropriate treatment (e.g., correction of electrolyte abnormalities, antimicrobial therapy of infections associated with AV block, withdrawal of offending medications) of underlying conditions responsible for AV block.

CHRONIC Rx

Permanent cardiac pacing may be indicated in patients with symptoms that correlate with the first-degree AV block and persist after correction of reversible causes (class IIA). Patients without symptoms but at risk for progression to higher degrees of AV block also benefit from permanent cardiac pacing (Lamin A/C mutations with PR >240 msec and left bundle branch block class IIA), certain neurodegenerative disorders (including myotonic dystrophy type 1) with PR >240 msec and QRS>120 msec, or fascicular block (class IIB).

DISPOSITION

AV conduction delay has been shown to be associated with increased risk of all-cause mortality, heart failure, and atrial fibrillation.

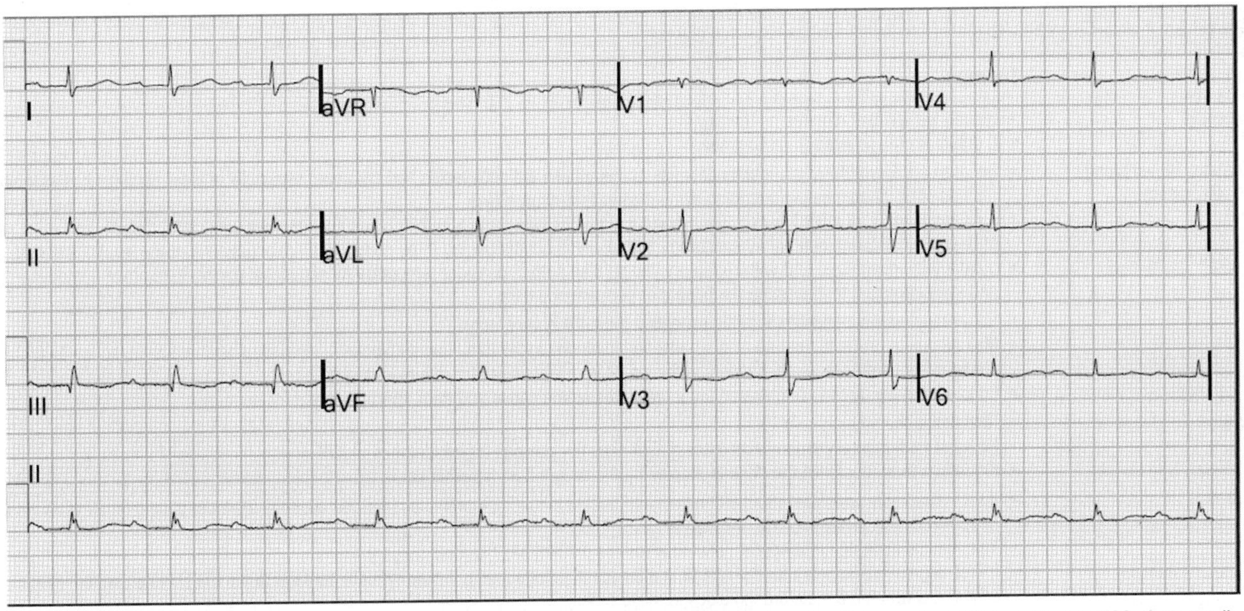

FIG. 1 76-yr-old man with marked first-degree AV conduction delay on 12-lead ECG (PR interval = 393 msec). *AV,* Atrioventricular; *ECG,* electrocardiogram.

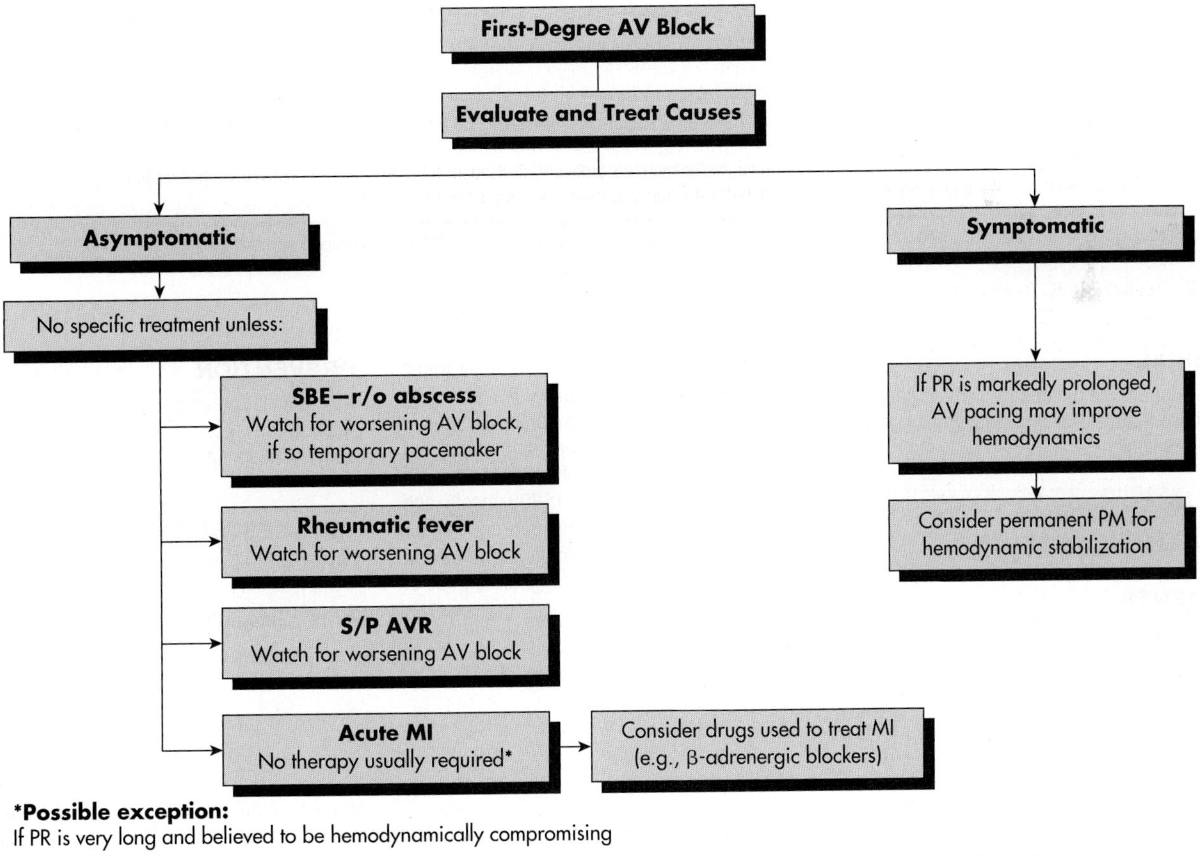

FIG. 2 First-degree atrioventricular (AV) block. *AVR,* Aortic valve replacement; *MI,* myocardial infarction; *PM,* pacemaker. (From Olshansky B et al: *Arrhythmia essentials,* ed 2, Philadelphia, 2017, Elsevier.)

TABLE 1 First-Degree Atrioventricular Block Management

Setting	Therapy
Asymptomatic	• Usually benign and requires no therapy. • If due to drugs, no need to discontinue.
Symptomatic, PR very long (300-400 msec)	• Because such symptoms as lightheadedness and dizziness are nonspecific and common, especially in older persons, it is essential to exclude other causes before ascribing symptoms to first-degree AVB. • A rare indication for a DDD pacemaker. Shortening the PR interval to 150-200 msec may improve weakness, fatigue, and shortness of breath by restoring optimal AV synchrony. Consider His bundle pacing if the conduction prolongation is at the level of the AVN. • If patient is hospitalized and with refractory low cardiac output, consider temporary AV sequential pacing to improve hemodynamics and symptoms and to determine the benefit of permanent pacing.
MI	• No therapy usually required (possible exception if the PR is very long). • May be due to drugs to treat MI (e.g., β-adrenergic blockers, calcium channel blockers, digoxin). If asymptomatic, no medication changes are usually required. If symptomatic or PR very long, consider reducing dosage. • Consider atrial infarction or elevated atrial pressures as the cause and treat appropriately.
Preoperative	• No specific therapy. • No need for temporary prophylactic pacing as it does not presage higher degrees of AVB. • If due to a drug, decrease the dose or stop using the drug if it is not essential.
Postoperative	• If PR is markedly prolonged (300-400 msec) and hemodynamic compromise is suspected, dual-chamber pacing (at PV or AV interval of 150-200 msec) may improve hemodynamics. • This may be instituted if temporary pacing wires are present after cardiac surgery. • If first-degree AVB appears for the first time after aortic valve surgery, it may indicate damage to the His-Purkinje system (usually associated with left bundle branch block in these cases). • Prolonged PR intervals can cause hemodynamic problems after cardiac surgery since the timing of the "atrial kick" may be more important during this time in which diastolic dysfunction is possible.
Endocarditis	• Carefully evaluate for the presence of aortic insufficiency; consider TEE. • Acute development of first-degree AVB, especially if it occurs with a new bundle branch block (transient or persistent), is highly suspicious for the presence of a valve ring abscess. • Requires surgical treatment. • Consider TEE. • Transfer patient to a unit with cardiac telemetry (if not already there), as progression to higher levels of AVB can occur.
Rheumatic fever	• First-degree AVB is a sign of rheumatic carditis and may presage the development of higher levels of AVB, including complete heart block. • May be an indication for steroids.
Infiltrative and restrictive cardiomyopathies	• If PR is markedly prolonged (> 300 msec), dual-chamber pacing (at PV or AV interval of 150-200 msec) may improve hemodynamics and symptoms. • Ventricles with severe diastolic dysfunction are especially dependent on atrial kick to maximize cardiac output. • If prolongation is at the level of the AV node, consider His bundle pacing.

AV, Atrioventricular; *AVB,* atrioventricular block; *AVN,* atrioventricular node; *DDD,* dual-chamber; *MI,* myocardial infarction; *TEE,* transesophageal echocardiography.
From Olshansky B et al: *Arrhythmia essentials,* ed 2, Philadelphia, 2017, Elsevier.

REFERRAL

Patients who are candidates for cardiac pacing should be referred to a cardiologist or cardiac electrophysiologist.

PEARLS & CONSIDERATIONS

COMMENTS

- First-degree AV block can be caused by slowing of electrical impulse conduction at any of the following levels: Atria, AV node (most often), His-Purkinje system.
- Typically it is a benign condition (if caused by increased vagal tone) and does not require treatment except in patients with marked PR prolongation (≥300 msec) and associated symptoms (pseudo-pacemaker syndrome) or in asymptomatic individuals at high risk of progression to higher degrees of AV block.

PREVENTION

No specific preventive measures exist other than those recommended for prevention of underlying conditions.

SUGGESTED READINGS

Available at ExpertConsult.com

AUTHOR: **Danylo Zorin, MD**

BASIC INFORMATION

DEFINITION

In 2017, the International League Against Epilepsy (ILAE) revised its classification of seizures. This article uses this updated nomenclature for focal seizures. Focal seizures (previously known as partial seizures) are caused by electrical discharges that originate in one hemisphere of the brain and cause symptoms based on the neuronal area they affect. There are two subtypes of focal seizure, categorized based on whether or not the seizures affect consciousness. Focal aware seizures (previously known as simple partial seizures) do not cause impairment of consciousness. Patients with this subtype of focal seizure will be able to accurately state who they are and what is going on in their surroundings during a seizure. However, the patient may not be aware that a seizure is occurring. The other subtype of focal seizure, focal impaired awareness seizures (previously known as complex partial seizures), refers to a seizure that impairs a patient's awareness for any part of the seizure.

These two subtypes of focal seizure can be further classified by whether they initially cause motor or nonmotor symptoms, as well as if they evolve into bilateral tonic-clonic seizures (previously known as secondary generalized tonic-clonic seizures).

SYNONYMS

Simple partial seizures
Seizures, partial
Partial seizures

ICD-10CM CODES	
G40.0	Localization-related (focal) (partial) idiopathic epilepsy and epileptic syndromes with seizures of localized onset
G40.109	Localization-related (focal) (partial) symptomatic epilepsy and epileptic syndromes with simple partial seizures, not intractable, without status epilepticus

EPIDEMIOLOGY & DEMOGRAPHICS

INCIDENCE: 30 to 50 cases per 100,000 persons per year
PREVALENCE: 5 to 8 cases per 1000 persons
PREDOMINANT SEX AND AGE: No gender preference

PHYSICAL FINDINGS & CLINICAL PRESENTATION

- Patients with focal seizures usually have normal physical and neurologic examinations when in a nonseizure state; however, if their seizures are secondary to a structural abnormality, such as a stroke, they will have a neurologic exam consistent with the area of CNS structural damage.
- During focal aware seizures, patients are conscious. They will be able to correctly state their name and accurately describe their surroundings. Patients with focal impaired awareness seizures will not be able to correctly state this information.
- Both of these focal seizure types can be further classified by their initial presenting symptoms.
- Focal seizures with initial motor symptoms include clonic (regularly spaced, rhythmic jerking), myoclonic (irregular jerking), hyperkinetic (thrashing or pedaling), tonic (increased tone), and atonic (loss of tone) seizures, as well as automatisms (lip smacking, fumbling of fingers). To avoid confusion, automatisms can also be seen in absence seizures, a type of nonmotor generalized seizure that will not be discussed here.
- Focal seizures with initial nonmotor symptoms include autonomic (e.g., changes in heart rate, blood pressure, sweating), sensory (e.g., changes in taste, smell, hearing, tactile sensation), emotional (sudden onset of emotions such as fear, anxiety, pleasure, etc.), or cognitive (e.g., change in language ability, thinking, feelings of déjà vu) changes and behavioral arrest (cessation of movement or talking) seizures.
- All focal seizures have the possibility of evolving into bilateral tonic-clonic seizures. These are distinct from generalized seizures, which are not discussed in this article.
- Patients with focal seizures can experience postictal weakness/paralysis that usually resolves within 24 hr (Todd paralysis). However, persistent focal neurologic deficits may also be indicative of a new structural brain lesion.

ETIOLOGY

- The etiology of focal seizures can be either genetic or due to a neurologic injury.
- Frequent causes of focal seizures are tumors, stroke, CNS infections (neurocysticercosis among others), arteriovenous malformations (AVMs), cavernous malformations, traumatic brain injury, cortical dysplasia, and structural abnormalities.

DIAGNOSIS

DIFFERENTIAL DIAGNOSIS

- Transient ischemic attack
- Movement disorders
- Psychogenic nonepileptic spells
- Migraines
- The differential diagnosis of nonepileptic events is summarized in Table 1. Table 2 summarizes clinical characteristics that help distinguish epileptic from nonepileptic events

WORKUP

EEG. Ambulatory EEG and/or video EEG recommended for patients with diagnostic uncertainty.

LABORATORY TESTS

Routine blood workup (CMP, CBC, glucose, electrolytes, TSH) and urine toxicology may be considered in appropriate clinical situations.

IMAGING STUDIES

- In the absence of contraindications, MRI with defined epilepsy protocol is preferred over CT due to its increased sensitivity to both acute and remote causes of seizure.
- However, in the setting of acute trauma, acute focal deficit, or if there is concern for a space-occupying lesion, a noncontrast CT may be obtained first, followed later by an MRI.

TREATMENT

- Almost all antiepileptic drugs are approved for focal seizures, either in monotherapy or in adjunct. Carbamazepine traditionally has been the standard initial drug treatment for focal seizures. However, newer antiepileptic drugs have better side effect profiles.
- Lamotrigine, levetiracetam, and oxcarbazepine are effective and well-tolerated antiepileptic drugs for treating focal seizures.
- Eslicarbazepine is indicated for the treatment of focal-onset seizures as monotherapy or adjunctive therapy. The recommended initial

TABLE 1 Differential Diagnosis of Nonepileptic Events

General Medical Conditions
- Transient ischemic attack (TIA)
- Complicated migraine
- Syncope
- Hypoglycemia
- Parasomnia (e.g., rapid eye movement [REM], behavior disorder, or night terrors)
- Narcolepsy
- Myoclonus (from metabolic disturbance)

Psychiatric Causes
- Conversion disorder
- Somatic symptom disorder
- Dissociative disorder
- Panic disorder (simulating focal seizures)

Volitional Deception
- Factitious disorder (goal is to maintain the sick role)
- Malingering (goal is to obtain secondary gain, e.g., disability income)

From Stern TA et al: *Massachusetts General Hospital handbook of general hospital psychiatry*, ed 7, Philadelphia, 2018, Elsevier.

TABLE 2 Clinical Characteristics that Help Distinguish Epileptic from Nonepileptic Events

	Epileptic Seizures	Nonepileptic Seizures/Events
Onset	Sudden onset and offset	Often gradual
Duration	Often <3 min	Variable
Perception	May experience olfactory, gustatory, visual hallucination; déjà vu; derealization	May experience auditory hallucinations; paranoia
Eyes during event	Open	Closed
Incontinence	Common	Rare
Awareness	Often impaired; can stay aware during some focal seizures	Variable; may be responsive during parts of the event
Recall of event	None or limited (e.g., aura)	Usually intact
Ictal EEG	Almost always abnormal	Unchanged from baseline
Interictal EEG	Normal or abnormal	Often normal
Tongue bite	Lateral tongue	None or tip of tongue
Injury	May be present	Rarely present (suggestive of serious psychopathology)
Incontinence	May be present	Rare
Postictal state	Confusion or drowsiness is common	Rare
Prolactin	Elevated; or normal	Normal; rarely elevated from baseline

EEG, Electroencephalogram.
From Stern TA et al: *Massachusetts General Hospital handbook of general hospital psychiatry,* ed 7, Philadelphia, 2018, Elsevier.

dose of eslicarbazepine is 400 mg once daily. Increase the dose in weekly increments of 200 mg, based on clinical response and tolerability, to a recommended maintenance dose of 800 to 1600 mg once daily.
- Lacosamide is indicated as monotherapy or adjunctive therapy in patients with focal-onset seizures. The initial recommended dose is 50 mg twice daily; increase at weekly intervals by 50 mg twice daily, up to a recommended maintenance dose of 100 to 200 mg twice daily.
- Patients who continue to have seizures despite a trial of two antiepileptic drugs and adequate doses should be referred for evaluation for epilepsy surgery. Surgical treatments (e.g., temporal lobectomy in mesial temporal sclerosis) may be indicated in refractory cases of focal seizures.

GENERAL Rx

- Several considerations should be taken into account when deciding if a patient should receive antiepileptic drug therapy after a first-time unprovoked seizure. An unprovoked seizure is one that was not caused by a toxic or metabolic disturbance, head trauma, or an acute stroke.
- According to evidence-based guidelines and several randomized trials, the greatest risk for seizure recurrence is in the first 2 yr after the first unprovoked seizure. Clinical factors that increase this risk include epileptiform discharges on EEG, a history of brain injury, a significant abnormality found on brain imaging (e.g., tumor, scarring), and the initial seizure having occurred at night.
- Immediate initiation of antiseizure medications after a first-time unprovoked seizure reduces the 2-yr risk of seizure recurrence by approximately 35%. However, it does not significantly impact long-term outcomes, as patients who were started on antiepileptic medication after their first seizure and those started after their second seizure had similar rates of long-term seizure remission.
- Thus, if a patient has their first unprovoked seizure and is subsequently found to have risk factors for developing seizure recurrence, such as EEG or neuroimaging abnormalities, it is reasonable to start them on an antiepileptic medication.
- However, if a patient has a normal neurological exam and does not have the above risk factors, drug therapy may be deferred until after a second unprovoked seizure.
- Recurrent seizures and seizures with abnormal studies may require treatment in the form of other medications, consideration of surgery, or with approved medical devices.

DISPOSITION

- Response to treatment often depends on the etiology of the focal seizures.
- 47% of patients become seizure free with monotherapy and 67% with polytherapy.
- Patients who do not respond to two drugs should be referred to an epilepsy center for consideration of surgical treatment.
- Patients should not drive until seizure free in accordance with local laws and regulations.
- Patients should avoid situations that may cause injuries or accidents in the event of a seizure, such as climbing ladders, swimming unsupervised, or taking baths (rather than showers).
- Many antiepileptic drugs also affect vitamin D absorption or metabolism, prompting attention to patients' bone health.
- All patients with epilepsy are at higher risk for depression and should be screened.

REFERRAL

Patients with epilepsy and seizures should be referred for a consultation by a neurologist, preferably one with a special interest in epilepsy.

PEARLS & CONSIDERATIONS

- Focal seizures can be divided into those that impair awareness and those that do not. In both categories, seizures will initially have either motor or nonmotor symptoms. Sometimes, focal seizures can evolve into bilateral tonic-clonic seizures.
- Initial workup should include EEG, MRI (if possible), CMP, and CBC. Other lab tests may be ordered based on clinical suspicion in order to rule out systemic or provoked causes of seizures.
- Drug therapy after a patient's first unprovoked seizure is recommended for those who have EEG or MRI abnormalities, or a history of brain trauma or surgery.
- Carbamazepine has traditionally been the initial drug treatment for focal seizures. However, lamotrigine, levetiracetam, oxcarbazepine, and many other antiepileptic medications are equally useful for treatment. The patient's comorbidities and gender should be taken into account when prescribing antiepileptic medication.

PREVENTION

- Sleep deprivation and alcohol consumption should be avoided.
- Drug compliance is compulsory to prevent seizure recurrence.

PATIENT & FAMILY EDUCATION

- Patient education and information can be obtained at the Epilepsy Foundation: www.epilepsyfoundation.org.
- Patients should be counseled on general seizure precautions such as swimming, bathing, and heights.

SUGGESTED READINGS

Available at ExpertConsult.com

RELATED CONTENT

Focal Motor Seizures (Patient Information)

AUTHORS: **Marco Pares, MD,** and **Joseph S. Kass, MD, JD, FAAN**

BASIC INFORMATION

DEFINITION

Food allergies are divided into IgE-mediated and immunologically mediated non-IgE reactions. They include a spectrum of disorders that involve adverse immunologic responses to dietary antigens.

ICD-10CM CODES	
T78.0	Adverse food reaction (including anaphylactic shock)
T78.1	Other adverse food reactions, not elsewhere classified
L27.2	Dermatitis due to ingested food
Z91.010	Allergy to peanuts
Z91.011	Allergy to milk products
Z91.012	Allergy to eggs
Z91.013	Allergy to seafood
Z91.018	Allergy to other foods
Z91.02	Food additives allergy status

EPIDEMIOLOGY & DEMOGRAPHICS

INCIDENCE: Food allergies have a cumulative incidence of 6% to 8% for the first 3 yr of life.

PREVALENCE:

- Overall prevalence is 1% to 2% in general population, ~3.9% to 8% in children.
- Patient self-reported food allergies have a prevalence of 12% to 13%, demonstrating the importance of objective measures in assessing food allergies.
- Nearly 40% of children with food allergy have a history of severe reactions that, if not treated immediately with proper medication, can lead to hospitalization or even death.[1]
- There is insufficient evidence to conclude a racial predilection (Greenhawt, 2013).

GENETICS: Children with parents or close relatives with allergies may have a tendency to become allergic to foods.

PHYSICAL FINDINGS & CLINICAL PRESENTATION

- IgE-mediated reactions: (Within minutes to a few hours): Pruritus, urticaria or angioedema, atopic dermatitis, GI symptoms, conjunctival injection, sneezing, nasal congestion, rhinorrhea, bronchospasm, and anaphylaxis.
- Non–IgE-mediated reactions: Food-induced enterocolitis, celiac disease, Crohn disease, dermatitis herpetiformis, and pulmonary reactions such as Heiner syndrome. These illnesses are discussed separately.
- Signs, symptoms, and presentation reflect specific allergic manifestation, but in food allergies there is a reproducible temporal relationship to ingested food allergens.

ETIOLOGY

Failure to establish tolerance to food antigens. IL-33 mediated epithelial permeability and Th2 skewing result in sensitization to food proteins which are presented to primed T cells. Food processing conditions that may affect allergenic activity are described in Table 1.

DIAGNOSIS

- Thorough history (to identify specific food[s], quantity consumed, timing, and nature of reaction) and physical exam should be performed.
- The temporal relationship and reproducibility of the symptoms are most important to establishing the diagnosis.
- A review of ingredient labels may be helpful.
- Confirmatory testing can include skin testing or in vitro testing.
- Skin prick testing (SPT): Positive predictive value <50%, but negative predictive value >95%. Thus a negative skin test effectively rules out an IgE-mediated process.
- In vitro testing: RAST testing: Historically it is less sensitive than skin testing, but sensitivity has improved with cut off points indicating a positive predictive value of 95% for allergies to eggs, milk, peanuts, wheat, and fish.
- Atopy patch test: Used in conjunction with RAST and skin testing in multiallergic children to plan widening the elimination diet. However, it is not recommended in the routine evaluation of food allergies.
- Double-blind, placebo-controlled food challenges are the gold standard test for determining food allergies. These need to be done in a supervised and controlled setting.
- In summary, if the history and lab tests are suggestive of a specific food allergy, that food should be confirmed by SPT, RAST, or food challenge and, once confirmed, eliminated from the diet.

DIFFERENTIAL DIAGNOSIS

- Gastrointestinal disorders
- Irritable bowel syndrome
- Carcinoid syndrome
- Giardiasis
- Structural abnormalities like hiatal hernia, pyloric stenosis, Hirschsprung disease, tracheoesophageal fistula
- Disaccharidase deficiencies: Lactase, sucrase-isomaltase complex, glucose-galactose complex
- Pancreatic insufficiency: Cystic fibrosis
- Gallbladder disease
- Peptic ulcer disease
- Malignancy
- Metabolic disorders
- Galactosemia
- Phenylketonuria
- Pharmacologic-related conditions
- Gustatory rhinitis
- Auriculotemporal syndrome (facial flush from tart food)

TREATMENT

NONPHARMACOLOGIC THERAPY

- Elimination diet should be used in conjunction with nutritional counseling. Fig. 1 illustrates an algorithm for the management of food allergy.
- Formula-fed infants: Brief trial of hydrolyzed milk formula as most children with milk allergy–induced skin symptoms will respond to the change of formula. Nonresponders may require amino acid–based formula.
- In older children: Elimination of one to two suspected foods is appropriate for 2 wk or longer and then reintroducing the foods to determine if symptoms recur.

ACUTE GENERAL Rx

- Antihistamines (both H1 and H2 antihistamines), albuterol if wheezing, epinephrine and glucocorticoids in patients with anaphylaxis.
- Patients with documented IgE-mediated reactions should receive and be counseled on the use of epinephrine autoinjector.

NEW TREATMENTS FOR FOOD ALLERGIES

- Oral and sublingual immunotherapy may play a role in management of food allergies, but this is currently under investigation.
- Recombinant vaccines and other immunomodulatory strategies are under development, although monoclonal anti-IgE antibody has shown benefit in adults with peanut allergy.

PEARLS & CONSIDERATIONS

- Eczema that develops in first 6 to 12 mo of life is usually the first manifestation of atopy.
- Egg allergy or sensitization is the strongest recognized predictor of respiratory allergies in children and asthma in adults.
- Consultation with trained dietitian is critical to avoid potentially adverse nutritional consequences in children with multiple food allergies.
- Skin testing is the preferred method for identifying food-specific IgE. RAST is useful if there is chance of severe food reaction causing risk to the patient.
- American Academy of Pediatrics no longer recommends avoiding the influenza and MMR vaccines in patients with severe systemic allergic reactions to egg.

COMMENTS

- Milk allergy usually resolves by age 5. Risk factors for persistence are early cutaneous manifestations following milk ingestion, development of other atopic conditions, and persistence of milk-specific high IgE titers. Soy milk is recommended for these children, keeping in mind that about 15% of these children can develop soy allergy.
- Egg allergy has been thought to resolve in 66% of children by 5 yr of age and in 75% of children by 7 yr of age. Trials have shown that oral immunotherapy can desensitize a high proportion of children with egg allergy and induce sustained unresponsiveness in a clinically significant subset.

[1]Gupta RS et al: The prevalence, severity, and distribution of childhood food allergy in the United States, *Pediatrics* 128(l):e9-e17, 2011.

TABLE 1 Food Processing Conditions that May Affect Allergenic Activity

Processing Stage	Nature of Processing	Impact of Processing on Allergens	Food-Level Evidence	Clinical Implications
Post-harvest treatments	Modified atmosphere for storage of fruit and vegetables	Expression of Bet v 1 homologs is upregulated during storage; levels are higher in fruit stored for 4-5 mo compared with fresh fruit. Expression of LTP allergens is downregulated during storage; levels are higher in fresh fruit and decrease during storage.	Apple	Individuals with birch pollen–related fruit allergies may tolerate freshly picked but not stored fruit. LTP-allergic individuals may experience reverse symptoms, although severity of LTP allergies may completely preclude consumption of problem fruit.
Primary processing	Removal of outer layers by physical or chemical peeling	Loss of allergens such as LTPs located in the outer layers.	Peach	Peeling fruits can make them safe for consumption by certain individuals with LTP allergies.
Secondary processing	Fruit purees and fresh juices	Labile Bet v 1 homologs are modified. Prolamin superfamily fruit LTPs retain a native-like structure.	Peach, apple	Individuals with Bet v 1–related fruit allergies usually can consume pureed fruit products. These foods can still trigger reactions in individuals with LTP fruit allergies.
	Preparation of pasteurized, UHT fruit juices and milk	Labile Bet v 1 homologs are modified. Prolamin superfamily fruit LTPs retain a native-like structure. Milk allergens retain much of their native structure.	Peach, apple, milk	Individuals with Bet v 1–related fruit allergies usually can consume UHT-processed fruit products. Processing is insufficient to make UHT juices safe for individuals with LTP fruit allergies. The allergenic potential of UHT milk resembles that of pasteurized and raw milk.
	Boiling	The prolamin superfamily LTPs and 2S albumin retain a native-like structure after boiling, although when seeds are boiled, much of the protein is lost into cooking water. Boiling alters the structure of milk, egg, and fish allergens. Boiling alters the structure of cupin allergens (7S and 11S seed storage proteins) and can render them insoluble.	Maize, wheat, peanut, lentil, fish, milk, egg	Boiling seeds (e.g., peanuts) and milk reduces their allergenicity but does not abolish it. For some foods (e.g., polenta), the extent of cooking affects the residual level of allergenic activity.
	Roasting and frying	Thermostable allergens, notably the prolamin superfamily 2S albumin allergens, retain their native structure and solubility after roasting and frying. Some cupin allergens (7S and 11S seed storage proteins) are altered by roasting and become insoluble. Maillard modification of allergens may take place under these processing conditions.	Peanut	The major peanut 2S albumin allergens retain their allergenic activity, explaining why roasted peanuts possess significant allergenic activity. Allergenic activity of the 7S and 11S globulins is retained to some extent after roasting. Maillard modifications may further contribute to the allergenic activity of roasted peanuts.
	Preparation of powdered ingredients, such as celery spice, skimmed milk, and pasteurized egg white powder	Major allergens retain their three-dimensional structure and activity in dry-processed goods. Maillard modifications take place under these processing conditions when residual sugars are present (e.g., lactose in skimmed milk powder).	Celery spice, milk	Powdered food ingredients have allergenic activity similar to unprocessed foods and can promote trigger reactions when included in recipes or through cross-contact in other foods (e.g., residual milk powder in foods otherwise free from milk).
	Deamidation	Acidic conditions are used to treat food ingredients (notably gluten) to improve their food functional properties through deamidation.	Gluten	Induces formation of novel IgE epitopes through glutamine deamidation, which results in individuals reacting to foods prepared with deamidated gluten ingredients who can otherwise safely consume wheat flour–containing foods.

TABLE 1 Food Processing Conditions that May Affect Allergenic Activity—cont'd

Processing Stage	Nature of Processing	Impact of Processing on Allergens	Food-Level Evidence	Clinical Implications
	Hydrolyzed food ingredients	Enzymatic (usually microbial proteases) and chemical treatments are used to hydrolyze protein ingredients to change their functional properties. Ingredients may originate from soy, milk (e.g., caseinates, whey protein), gluten, and other sources.	Milk, egg, gluten	Hydrolysis reduces IgE reactivity but does not abolish it completely, which may in part result from the presence of residual intact protein. Evidence is largely limited to in vitro IgE binding studies and animal models with little direct in vivo evidence for allergic humans.
	Oil refining	Proteins are removed during the refining process, and residual protein levels in highly refined oils are very low.	Soybean, peanut	In the EU, highly refined soybean oils are considered safe for consumption by individuals with soy allergies. Highly refined peanut oils do not appear to cause adverse reactions in peanut-allergic individuals, but these oils do not have an EU labeling derogation.
Complex foods	Fining agents added to alcoholic beverages	Certain beverages contain residual levels of fining agents based on isinglass, fish gelatin, milk casein, egg albumin, or lysozyme. Fining agents and their residues in beverages usually are highly modified compared with the raw, unprocessed foods.	Beer, wine, and spirits	Individuals with allergies to fish triggered by collagen or egg can react to alcoholic beverages when they are used as fining agents, although this depends on the nature of the individual's allergy and whether fining agents are used in conjunction with other agents, such as bentonite. Reactions to fining agents are rare, and many individuals with egg, milk, or fish allergy can safely consume these beverages.
	Fermented foods	Lactic acid fermentations can cause proteins to unfold and precipitate or form gelled networks due to the reduced pH. Fermentative organisms secrete proteases that can hydrolyze proteins.	Milk, soybean	Although fermented milk and yogurt may retain some allergenic activity, other highly modified foods, such as soy sauce, may have substantially reduced allergenic activity and may not present a hazard to certain allergic patients.
	Baked foods	Food ingredients may be included that are raw or have already been processed (e.g., skimmed milk powder, pasteurized egg white). Complex interactions between different food ingredients coupled with further cooking modify allergens and result in their becoming part of the insoluble food matrix, but data are limited because of the poor solubility of allergens in physiologic buffers.	Milk	Evidence from oral food challenge studies indicates that baking reduces the allergenic activity of milk, and foods with baked milk may be given to children whose infantile cow's milk allergy is beginning to resolve.

EU, European Union; *Ig*, immunoglobulin; *LTP*, lipid transfer protein; *UHT*, ultrahigh temperature.
From Adkinson NF et al: *Middleton's allergy principles and practice*, ed 8, Philadelphia, 2014, Saunders.

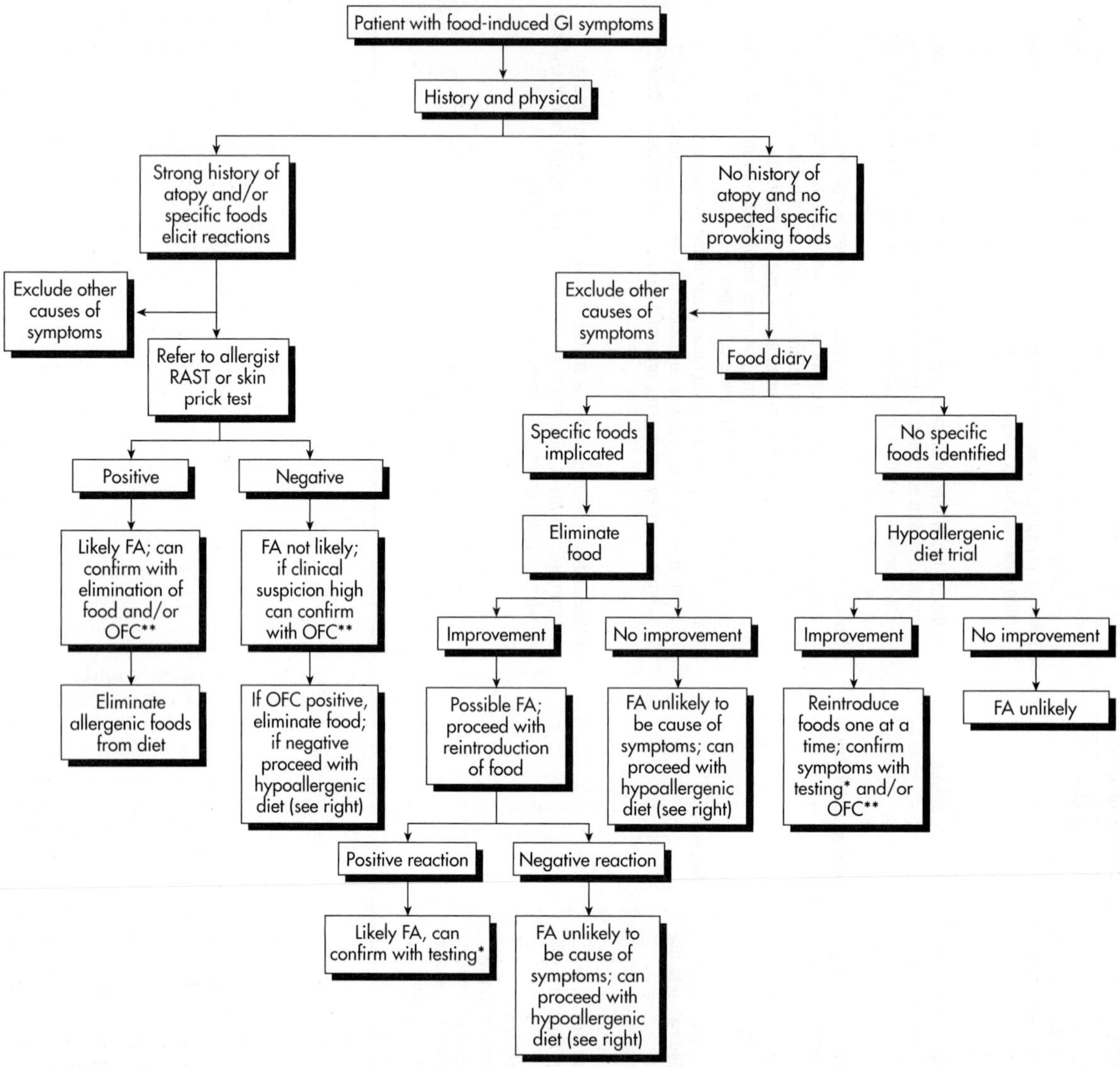

FIG. 1 Algorithm for the management of food allergy. *Testing indicates skin-prick testing, radioallergosorbent tests *(RAST)*, IgG_4 assay, and/or patch testing. Note that clinical symptoms must be associated with the food(s) that test positive before the food(s) should be eliminated from the diet. **Oral food challenge *(OFC)* involves reintroducing the food and observing for signs/symptoms of food allergy *(FA)*. Treatment of food allergy involves elimination of the causative food(s) from the diet. *GI,* Gastrointestinal.

- Wheat allergy found to resolve by 5 yr of age and soybean allergy by 2 yr of age.

PREVENTION

- There is conflicting evidence regarding the protective effect of breastfeeding on food allergies.
- There is no evidence to suggest that exclusive breastfeeding for 6 mo or more is superior to exclusive breastfeeding for 4 to 6 mo in terms of developing food allergies.
- In high-risk infants who are not exclusively breastfed, there is limited evidence to suggest that feeding with hydrolyzed formula compared to cow's milk formula reduces allergies.
- Currently, there is no evidence to support the use of prebiotics and/or probiotics for the prevention of allergic diseases.
- No current evidence exists to support delaying the introduction of solid foods beyond 4 to 6 mo.
- The early introduction of peanuts significantly decreases the frequency of the development of peanut allergy among children at high risk for this allergy and modulated immune responses to peanuts.[2] Early peanut introduction (ages 4-11 mo) lowers the risk of developing peanut allergy by 80% compared with peanut introduction after age 5 yr.
- In recent phase 3 trials of oral immunotherapy in children and adolescents who were highly allergic to peanut, treatment with AR101 resulted in higher doses of peanut protein that could be ingested without dose-limiting symptoms.

[2] Gupta RS et al: The prevalence, severity, and distribution of childhood food allergy in the United States, *Pediatrics* 128(l):e9-e17, 2011.

PATIENT & FAMILY EDUCATION

Information can be found on American Academy of Allergy, Asthma and Immunology (www.aaaai.org), the Food Allergy and Anaphylaxis Network (www.foodallergy.org), and the Anaphylaxis Campaign (www.anaphylaxis.org.uk).

REFERRAL

Patients may be referred to an allergy/immunology specialist when the diagnosis is uncertain or if avoidance measures are not successful.

SUGGESTED READINGS

Available at ExpertConsult.com

RELATED CONTENT

Food Allergies (Patient Information)

AUTHOR: **Fred F. Ferri, MD**

BASIC INFORMATION

DEFINITION

Food poisoning is an illness caused by ingestion of food contaminated by bacteria and/or bacterial toxins. A foodborne disease outbreak is defined as two or more cases of a similar illness resulting from ingestion of a common food.

SYNONYMS

Enterotoxin-poisoning
Epidemic vomiting disease

ICD-10CM CODE
A05.9 Bacterial foodborne intoxication, unspecified

EPIDEMIOLOGY & DEMOGRAPHICS

INCIDENCE (IN U.S.):

- CDC estimates that each year one in six Americans will experience a foodborne illness.
- Approximately 800 foodborne disease outbreaks are reported in the U.S. each year, accounting for approximately 15,000 illnesses, 800 hospitalizations, and 20 deaths. Outbreak-associated foodborne illnesses are only a small subset of the estimated 9.4 million foodborne illnesses that occur annually in the U.S.[1]
- Majority of identifiable causes are bacterial, although more than 250 known diseases can be transmitted through food.

PREDOMINANT AGE: Varies with specific agent
PEAK INCIDENCE: Varies with specific organism

- Summer: *Staphylococcus aureus, Salmonella, Shigella* spp.
- Summer and fall: *Clostridium botulinum, Vibrio parahaemolyticus*
- Spring and fall: *Campylobacter jejuni*
- Winter: *Clostridium perfringens, Yersinia enterocolitica*

NEONATAL INFECTION: Rare but severe with *Shigella* and *Salmonella* spp.

PHYSICAL FINDINGS & CLINICAL PRESENTATION

- Any combination of GI symptoms and fever. Orthostatic pulse and blood pressure changes should be noted
- Specific organisms suspected on the basis of the incubation period and predominant symptoms (Table 1), although a great deal of overlap exists
  1. Short incubation period (1-6 hr): Involve the ingestion of preformed toxin; noninvasive.
     a. *S. aureus:* Nausea, profuse vomiting, and abdominal cramps common; diarrhea possible, but fever uncommon; usually resolves within 24 hr; foods implicated in outbreaks include meats, mayonnaise, and cream pastries.
     b. *B. cereus:* Two forms, a short incubation (emetic) form (characterized by vomiting and abdominal cramps in virtually all patients, diarrhea in one third of patients, fever uncommon) and a long incubation (diarrheal) form; illness usually mild, resolves within 12 hr; unrefrigerated rice most often implicated as vehicle. Other sources include gravy, meats, stews, vanilla, and sauces.
  2. Moderate incubation period (8-16 hr): Involves the in vivo production of toxin; noninvasive.
     a. *C. perfringens:* Severe crampy abdominal pain and watery diarrhea common; fever and vomiting unlikely; symptoms usually resolving within 24 hr; outbreaks invariably related to cooked meat or poultry that is allowed to cool without refrigeration; most cases in the fall and winter months. *C. perfringens* is the third most common cause of foodborne illness in the United States.
     b. *B. cereus:* Diarrheal (or long incubation) form most commonly beginning with diarrhea, abdominal cramps, and occasionally vomiting; fever uncommon; usually resolves within 24 hr; the responsible food is usually fried rice.
  3. Long incubation period (>16 hr): Some toxin-mediated, some invasive.
- Toxin-producing organisms include
  1. *C. botulinum:* Should be considered when a diarrheal illness coincides with or precedes paralysis; severity of illness related to the quantity of toxin ingested; characteristic cranial nerve palsies progressing to a descending paralysis; fever usually absent; usually associated with home-canned foods.
  2. Enterotoxigenic *E. coli* (ETEC): Most common cause of travelers' diarrhea; after 1- to 2-day incubation period, abdominal cramps and copious diarrhea occur; vomiting and fever uncommon; usually resolves after 3 to 4 days; vehicle usually unbottled water or contaminated salad or ice.
  3. Enterohemorrhagic *E. coli* (EHEC): Can cause severe abdominal cramps and watery diarrhea, which may eventually become bloody; bacteria (strain O157:H7) are noninvasive; no fever; illness may be complicated by hemolytic-uremic syndrome; associated with contaminated beef (especially hamburger), unpasteurized milk or juice. Table 2 summarizes the various strains of diarrheagenic *E. coli.*
  4. *V. cholerae:* Varies from a mild, self-limited illness to life-threatening cholera; diarrhea, nausea and vomiting, abdominal cramps, and muscle cramps; no fever; severe cases may progress to shock and death within hours of onset; survivors usually have resolution of symptoms in 1 wk; U.S. cases are either imported or result from ingestion of imported food.
- Invasive organisms include
  1. *Salmonella:* Associated most often with nontyphoidal strains; incubation period generally 12 to 48 hr; nausea, vomiting, diarrhea, and abdominal cramps typical; fever possible; outbreaks of gastroenteritis related to contaminated poultry, meat, and dairy products.
  2. *Shigella:* Asymptomatic infection possible, but some with fever and watery diarrhea that may progress to bloody diarrhea and dysentery; with mild illness, usually self-limited, resolves in a few days; with severe illness, may develop complications; transmission usually from person to person but can occur via contaminated food or water.
  3. *C. jejuni:* The most common foodborne bacterial pathogen; incubation period is about 1 day, then a prodrome of fever, headache, and myalgias; intestinal phase marked by diarrhea associated with fever, malaise, and abdominal pain; diarrhea mild to profuse and bloody; usually resolves in about 7 days, but relapse is possible; associated with undercooked meats and poultry, unpasteurized dairy products, and drinking from freshwater streams.
  4. *Y. enterocolitica* and *Y. pseudotuberculosis:* Infrequent causes of enteritis in the United States; children affected more often than adults; fever, diarrhea, and abdominal pain lasting 1 to 3 wk; some with mesenteric adenitis that mimics acute appendicitis; contaminated food or water is usually responsible.
  5. *V. parahaemolyticus:* In the United States, most outbreaks in coastal states or on cruise ships during the summer months; incubation period usually >1 day, followed by explosive watery diarrhea in the majority of cases; nausea, vomiting, abdominal cramps, and headache also common; fever less common; usually resolves by 1 wk; related to ingestion of seafood.
  6. Enteroinvasive *E. coli* (EIEC): A rare cause of disease in the United States; high incidence of fever and bloody diarrhea; may resemble bacillary dysentery.
  7. *V. vulnificus:* May cause serious, often fatal illness in persons with chronic liver disease; GI symptoms usually absent, but fever, chills, hypotension, and hemorrhagic skin lesions possible; patients with liver disease or at increased risk of developing liver disease should avoid eating raw oysters.

ETIOLOGY

- Table 3 describes pathogenic mechanisms in bacterial foodborne disease.
- Classically categorized as either inflammatory (invasive) or noninflammatory.

[1] Dewey-Mattia D et al: Surveillance for foodborne disease outbreaks–United States 2009-2015, *MMWR Surveill Summ* 67(10):1-11, 2018.

TABLE 1 Foodborne Disease Agents and Clinical Presentation

Usual Incubation Periods	Causative Agent	Clinical Illness: Fever	Diarrhea	Vomiting	Epidemiologic and Laboratory Diagnosis
5 min-6 hr (usually <3 hr)	Chemical or toxin	Rare	Occasional	Common	Demonstration of toxin or chemical from food or epidemiologic incrimination of food
1-6 hr (usually <1 hr)	*Staphylococcus aureus* enterotoxin	Rare	Occasional	Profuse	Isolation of organisms in food (>10^5/g)/vomitus/stool; detection of enterotoxin in food
	Bacillus cereus emetic toxin	Rare	Occasional	Profuse	Isolation of organisms in food (>10^5/g)/vomitus/stool
6-24 hr	*Clostridium perfringens* enterotoxin	Rare	Typical	Occasional	Isolation of organisms or toxin from food (10^5/g) or stools of ill persons, epidemiologic incrimination of food; detection of enterotoxin in food
	B. cereus enterotoxin	Rare	Typical	Occasional	
12-72 hr	*Clostridium botulinum*	Clinical sydrome compatible with botulism	Constipation more common		Isolation of organism or toxin from food (10^5/g) or stools; demonstration of toxin in serum or food
16-96 hr	*Shigella*	Common	Typical, often bloody	Occasional	Isolation of organism from clinical specimens from two or more ill persons; isolation of organism from epidemiologically implicated food
	Nontyphoidal *Salmonella*	Common	Typical	Occasional	
	Enteroinvasive *E. coli* (EIEC)	Common	Typical, may be bloody	Occasional	
	Enteropathogenic *E. coli* (EPEC)	Occasional	Typical	Occasional	
	Enterotoxigenic *E. coli* (ETEC)	Rare	Typical	Rare	
	Vibrio parahaemolyticus; V. cholerae enterotoxin	Occasional	Typical	Occasional	
1-3 days	Caliciviruses (noroviruses) Rotavirus	Occasional	Typical	Common	Antigen detection (enzyme immunoassay) in stool; immune electron microscopy of stool; detection of viral RNA in stool or vomitus by PCR
1-10 days	*Yersinia*	Uncommon	Typical, severe abdominal pain	Uncommon	Isolation of organisms from food or clinical specimens of ill persons
2-10 days	*Campylobacter jejuni*	Common	Typical, often bloody	Uncommon	Isolation of organisms from food or clinical specimens of ill persons
1-11 days	*Cryptosporidium*	Occasional	Common	Occasional	Demonstration of oocysts in stool or in small bowel biopsy of ill persons; demonstration of organism in epidemiologically implicated food
	Cyclospora	Occasional	Common	Occasional	Demonstration of parasite in stool or in small bowel biopsy of ill persons; demonstration of organism in epidemiologically implicated food
	Giardia intestinalis	Occasional	Common	Occasional	Demonstration of parasite in stool or in small bowel biopsy of ill persons; demonstration of organism in epidemiologically implicated food
2 days-weeks	*Bacillus anthracis*	Common	Typical	Frequent	Isolation of organism from blood or contaminated meat
1-7 days	*E. coli* 0157:H7 and other Shiga toxin–producing *E. coli*	Uncommon	Typical	Frequent	Isolation of organism from food or stool or identification of toxin in stools of ill persons
3-60 days, usually 7-14	*Salmonella typhi*	Common	Diarrhea or constipation	Uncommon	Isolation of organisms from food or clinical specimens of ill persons
7-21 days	*Brucella* spp.	Common	Common	Rare	Isolation of organisms from blood or bone marrow culture of ill persons; fourfold increase in standard agglutination titer overall several weeks or single titer 1:160 in person with compatible clinical syndrome
1-4 wk	*Giardia lamblia*	Rare	Common	Rare	Stool for ova and parasite examination enzyme immunoassay
2 days-8 wk	*Trichinella spiralis*	Common	Common	Common	Serology, muscle biopsy

PCR, Polymerase chain reaction; *RNA*, ribonucleic acid.
From Cherry JD et al: Feigin and Cherry's *pediatric infectious diseases*, ed 8, Philadelphia, 2019, Elsevier.

TABLE 2 Diarrheagenic *Escherichia coli*

Strains	Pathogenic Mechanisms	Persons Affected	Clinical Features
DAEC	Diffuse adherence to Hep-2 cells	Children in developing countries	Watery diarrhea (acute) and persistent diarrhea
EAEC	Aggregative adherence to Hep-2 cells	Children in developing countries	Watery diarrhea (acute) and persistent diarrhea
STEC 0157:H7 Non-0157:H7 0104:H4*	Shiga toxins 1 and 2	Children and adults Persons who ingest contaminated food, especially hamburger (outbreaks)	Watery diarrhea Bloody diarrhea (classic)
EIEC	Epithelial cell invasion	Children and adults	Watery diarrhea Dysentery
EPEC Typical Atypical	Attaching and effacing Bundle-forming pilus, attachment and effacement lesions or atypical adherence pattern	Children	Watery diarrhea (acute) Persistent diarrhea
ETEC	Heat-labile and/or heat-stable toxin Adherence	Children in developing countries; travelers	Watery diarrhea

DAEC, Diffusely adhering *Escherichia coli; EAEC,* enteroaggregative *E. coli; EIEC,* enteroinvasive *E. coli; EPEC,* enteropathogenic *E. coli; ETEC,* enterotoxigenic *E. coli; STEC,* Shiga toxin–producing *E. coli.*
From Feldman M et al: *Sleisenger and Fordtran's gastrointestinal and liver disease,* ed 10, Philadelphia, 2016, Elsevier.

TABLE 3 Pathogenic Mechanisms in Bacterial Foodborne Disease

Preformed Toxin	Toxin Production in Vivo	Tissue Invasion	Toxin Production and/or Tissue Invasion
Staphylococcus aureus *Bacillus cereus* (short incubation) *Clostridium botulinum*	*Clostridium perfringens* *B. cereus* (long incubation) *C. botulinum* (infant botulism) Enterotoxigenic *Escherichia coli* *Vibrio cholerae* 01 or 0139 *V. cholerae* non-01 Shiga toxin–producing *E. coli*	*Campylobacter jejuni* *Salmonella* *Shigella* Invasive *E. coli*	*Vibrio parahaemolyticus* *Yersinia enterocolitica*

From Mandell GL et al: *Principles and practice of infectious diseases,* ed 6, Philadelphia, 2005, Churchill Livingstone.

1. Noninflammatory: *B. cereus, S. aureus, C. botulinum, C. perfringens, V. cholerae,* enterotoxigenic *E. coli* (ETEC), and enterohemorrhagic *E. coli* (EHEC); toxin-producing organisms that are noninvasive; fecal leukocytes are not seen.
2. Inflammatory: *Campylobacter,* enteroinvasive *E. coli* (EIEC), *Salmonella, Shigella, V. parahaemolyticus,* and *Yersinia;* cause disease by invasion of intestinal tissue; fecal leukocytes are seen.

Dx DIAGNOSIS

DIFFERENTIAL DIAGNOSIS

Gastroenteritis caused by viruses (Norwalk, Noro, or rotavirus), parasites *(Amoeba histolytica, Giardia lamblia),* or toxins (ciguatoxins, mushrooms, heavy metals).

LABORATORY TESTS

- Watchful waiting is often the most appropriate option and ancillary testing is usually not necessary.
- In severe or persistent cases, stool test for fecal leukocytes may help narrow the differential diagnosis.
  1. Send stool for culture and for ova and parasites.
  2. Send stool for *C. difficile* toxin in patients with current or recent antibiotic use.
  3. Note: Some pathogens are not identified on routine stool culture; laboratory should be advised if *Yersinia, C. botulinum, Vibrio,* or enterohemorrhagic *E. coli* (0157:H7) are suspected.
  4. Finding *B. cereus, C. perfringens,* or *E. coli* in stool is of little value, because these may be part of the normal bowel flora.
  5. Stool cultures are positive in less than 40% of cases.
  6. Newer techniques such as polymerase chain reaction (PCR) testing provide a more rapid and reliable determination of specific pathogens.
- If botulism suspected, send food, serum, and stool for toxin assay.
- Blood cultures should be considered for all febrile patients.
- Consider toxic megacolon (identified on plain abdominal sonography).
- Consider sigmoidoscopy to obtain tissue and histology in hospitalized patients with bloody diarrhea.
- Consider lactoferrin measurement if an inflammatory etiology is suspected.

Rx TREATMENT

NONPHARMACOLOGIC THERAPY

Adequate rehydration is the mainstay of therapy.

ACUTE GENERAL Rx

- Most cases of acute infectious diarrhea are viral and antibiotics are not indicated.
- Gastroenteritis caused by the following bacterial organisms requires no antimicrobial treatment: *B. cereus, S. aureus, C. perfringens, V. parahaemolyticus, Yersinia,* and enterohemorrhagic and enteroinvasive *E. coli.*
- The usual cause of travelers' diarrhea is enterotoxigenic *E. coli.* Although usually a self-limited illness, antibiotics can shorten the course in patients with fever or dysentery.
  1. Azithromycin 1000 mg in a single oral dose or
  2. SMX/TMP one DS tab bid for 3 days or
  3. Ciprofloxacin 500 mg PO bid for 3 days
- The mainstay of therapy for cholera is fluid replacement. Antibiotics should be given to decrease shedding and duration of illness.
  1. Doxycycline 300 mg in a single dose or 100 mg PO bid for 3 days
  2. SMX/TMP 1 DS tab bid for 3 days
- Treatment is not indicated for *Salmonella* gastroenteritis. Patients who are at high risk of developing bacteremia may be treated for 48 to 72 hr (see "Salmonellosis").
- Although shigellosis tends to be a self-limited illness, antibiotics shorten the course of illness and may limit transmission of the illness (see "Shigellosis").
- Those with moderate or severe *Campylobacter* diarrhea may benefit from treatment.

TABLE 4 Antibiotic Therapy for Nonsevere Infections with Common Bacterial Enteropathogens in Immunocompetent Adults

Organism	Recommended Antibiotic(s)	Alternative Antibiotic(s)
***Shigella* Species**		
Shigella infection (non-*dysenteriae;* for *Shigella dysenteriae* type 1, see text)	Ciprofloxacin 500 mg twice daily (or levofloxacin 500 mg daily) × 3 days	Azithromycin 500 mg-1 g daily × 3-5 days TMP/SMX 160 mg/800 mg twice daily, if sensitive, × 3 days
***Salmonella* Species**		
Enterocolitis, uncomplicated	Not usually recommended (see text)	Can consider in areas of high fluoroquinolone quinolone resistance; azithromycin 1 g daily × 5 days
Typhoid and enteric fevers*	Ciprofloxacin 500 mg twice daily (or ofloxacin 400 mg twice daily) × 7-14 days Ceftriaxone 2-3 g IV daily × 7-14 days	
***Campylobacter* Species**		
Campylobacter jejuni	Not usually required Ciprofloxacin 500 mg twice daily × 3 days	Azithromycin 500 mg-1 g × 3-5 days
Yersinia enterocolitica		
Enterocolitis, uncomplicated	Not usually required	An aminoglycoside (parenteral) Tetracycline 500 mg 4 times daily × 5 days TMP/SMX 160 mg/800 mg twice daily × 5 days Ciprofloxacin 500 mg twice daily × 5 days Doxycycline 100 mg twice daily × 5 days
Escherichia coli†		
Enterotoxigenic	Endemic disease; usually self-limited, supportive care (see text). Travelers' diarrhea: Ciprofloxacin 500 mg twice daily × 3 days Rifaximin 200 mg 3 times daily × 3 days	Azithromycin 500 mg-1 g daily × 3-5 days TMP/SMX 160 mg/800 mg twice daily, if sensitive, × 3 days
Shiga toxin–producing	Unclear if antibiotics are effective; may be harmful	
***Vibrio* Species**		
Vibrio cholera	Doxycycline 300 mg × 1 dose	Ciprofloxacin 1 g × 1 dose Azithromycin 1 g × 1 dose Tetracycline 500 mg every 6 hr × 3 days
Vibrio parahaemolyticus	Usually not required; no controlled trials	As for *V. cholerae*

TMP/SMX, Trimethoprim/sulfamethoxazole.

NOTE: All antibiotics are administered orally unless otherwise indicated. Recommendations are given for treatment of mild/moderate infections only. Treatments for complicated infections or severely ill, bacteremic, or immunocompromised patients are not listed above and may differ from treatments for mild disease.

*For severe typhoid fever, consider the addition of glucocorticoids (dexamethasone 3 mg/kg × 1, then 1 mg/kg every 6 hr × 48 hr) to parenteral antimicrobial therapy. Antimicrobial sensitivity testing is required. Fluoroquinolones (e.g., ciprofloxacin) should not be used as empiric therapy in Asia or other areas with high fluoroquinolone resistance.

†Enteropathogenic, enteroaggregative, and diffusely enteroadherent *E. coli* are omitted from this table because these types are defined in research laboratories and are not diagnosed in routine clinical practice. Enteroinvasive *E. coli* presenting as inflammatory diarrhea should be treated empirically as for *Shigella* spp.

From Feldman M et al: *Sleisenger and Fordtran's gastrointestinal and liver disease,* ed 10, Philadelphia, 2016, Elsevier.

1. Azithromycin 500 mg qd for 3 days or
2. Erythromycin 500 mg PO qid for 5 days or
3. Ciprofloxacin 500 mg PO bid for 5 days

- *V. vulnificus* sepsis should be treated with
  1. Doxycycline 100 mg IV bid for 2 wk
  2. Ceftazidime 2 g IV q8h for 2 wk
- For suspected botulism, antitoxin should be administered early (see "Botulism").
- Table 4 summarizes antibiotic therapy for nonsevere infections with common bacterial enteropathogens in immunocompetent adults.

CHRONIC Rx

Patients with *Salmonella* infections may become carriers and may require treatment (see "Salmonellosis").

DISPOSITION

- Most infections are self-limited and do not require therapy.
- In immunocompromised host or patient with underlying disease, serious complications are possible.
- Postinfectious syndromes are important with some infections.
  1. Reiter syndrome: *Salmonella, Shigella, Campylobacter, Yersinia* spp.; more common in genetically susceptible host (HLA-B27+)
  2. Guillain-Barré syndrome: *Campylobacter* spp

REFERRAL

If more than a mild illness

PEARLS & CONSIDERATIONS

COMMENTS

- Grossly underreported and undiagnosed
- All cases to be reported to the local health department
- Table 5 summarizes control and prevention measures of foodborne diseases

SUGGESTED READINGS

Available at ExpertConsult.com

RELATED CONTENT

Bacterial Food Poisoning (Patient Information)
Salmonellosis (Related Key Topic)
Botulism (Related Key Topic)
Shigellosis (Related Key Topic)

AUTHOR: **Glenn G. Fort, MD, MPH**

TABLE 5 Control and Prevention of Foodborne Diseases

General Recommendations for All Persons

- Thoroughly cook raw food from animal sources, such as beef, pork, poultry, fish, and eggs, to temperatures that eliminate most pathogens.*
- Wash raw fruits and vegetables before eating.
- Keep uncooked meats separate from fruits, vegetables, cooked foods, and ready-to-eat foods.
- Do not thaw meat, poultry, or fish on the counter (instead, thaw in a refrigerator, in cold water, or in a microwave oven).
- Wash hands before, during, and after preparing food and before eating food.
- Wash knives, other utensils, and cutting boards after handling uncooked foods.
- Keep refrigerators set to below 40° F and freezers set to 0° F or lower and verify with a thermometer.
- Refrigerate perishable foods within 2 hr (or within 1 hr if left out at temperatures >90°F).
- Read and follow all cooking and storage instructions on food product packaging. This is especially important for foods prepared in microwave ovens because these ovens heat foods unevenly. Even foods that may appear ready to eat may require thorough cooking.
- Persons with diarrhea or vomiting possibly caused by an infectious agent should not prepare foods for others.
- Keep all animals, including reptiles and amphibians, away from surfaces where foods or drinks are prepared.
- Do not drink unpasteurized (raw) milk or eat foods made from unpasteurized milk. (Exception: Hard cheeses made from raw milk that have been aged >60 days are generally safe to eat.)
- Do not eat home-canned foods that were not known to be adequately heat processed during canning.

Recommendations for Persons at High Risk, Such as Pregnant Women and People with Weakened Immune Systems, in Addition to the Recommendations Listed Above

Measures to Prevent a Variety of Bacterial Infections

- Do not eat uncooked sprouts.
- Do not drink prepackaged juice or juice-containing beverages that have not been processed to reduce or eliminate microbial contamination (e.g., by pasteurization).

Listeriosis Prevention Measures

- Do not eat soft cheeses, such as feta, Brie, and Camembert; blue-veined cheeses; and Mexican-style cheeses, such as queso blanco, queso fresco, and panela, unless the package has a label that clearly states that the cheese is made from pasteurized milk.
- Do not eat refrigerated pâtés or meat spreads. Canned or shelf-stable pâtés and meat spreads are safe to eat.
- Do not eat refrigerated smoked seafood unless it is contained in a cooked dish, such as a casserole. Refrigerated smoked seafood, such as salmon, trout, whitefish, cod, tuna, and mackerel, is most often labeled as "nova-style," "lox," "kippered," "smoked," or "jerky." The fish is found in the refrigerator section or sold at delicatessen counters of grocery stores and delicatessens. Canned or shelf-stable smoked seafood is safe to eat.
- Do not eat hot dogs, luncheon meats, or delicatessen meats unless they are reheated until steaming hot.
- Avoid getting fluid from hot dog packages on other foods, utensils, and food preparation surfaces, and wash hands after handling hot dogs, luncheon meats, and delicatessen meats.

Salmonellosis Prevention Measures

- Choose pasteurized eggs.

Vibriosis, Toxoplasmosis, and Norovirus Prevention Measures

- Do not eat raw or lightly steamed oysters, clams, or other raw shellfish (especially important for patients with liver disease).

More food safety information can be found at www.foodsafety.gov/keep/index.html.

*Poultry: 165° F (73.9° C); ground meats: 160° F (71.1° C); intact cuts of beef, pork, ham, veal, and lamb: 145° F (62.8° C) and allow to rest for at least 3 minutes before eating; fish and shellfish: 145° F (62.8° C); egg dishes: 160° F (71.1° C).

From Bennett JE et al: *Mandell, Douglas, and Bennett's principles and practice of infectious diseases,* ed 8, Philadelphia, 2015, Saunders.

BASIC INFORMATION

DEFINITION

Frontotemporal dementia (FTD) is an umbrella term that encompasses three distinct syndromes: Behavioral variant FTD (bvFTD), semantic dementia (SD), and progressive nonfluent aphasia (PNFA). All three syndromes are marked by frontal and/or temporal lobe atrophy; however, they manifest with different clinical presentations. The most common subtype is bvFTD, which is marked by changes in behavior and personality with disinhibition and the breaking of social norms. SD is characterized by a loss of word comprehension and meaning, and PNFA presents with agrammatic, nonfluent speech.

SYNONYMS

- FTD
- FTLD
- Frontotemporal lobar degeneration (FTLD) is the term used for the neuropathologic findings seen in the different FTD syndromes.
- Pick disease: This term was historically used to refer to FTD. However, it is now strictly a neuropathologic diagnosis for patients found to have Pick bodies at autopsy, as very few diagnoses of FTD are associated with these neuropathologic findings.

ICD-10CM CODES

G31.0	Frontotemporal dementia
G31.01	Pick disease
G31.09	Other frontotemporal dementia

EPIDEMIOLOGY & DEMOGRAPHICS

The current data on epidemiology of FTD are variable due to misdiagnosis and underreporting. The following data are estimations obtained through systematic reviews.

INCIDENCE: The estimated annual incidence is 2.7 to 4.1 per 100,000 persons.

PREVALENCE: The estimated point prevalence is 15 to 22 per 100,000 persons.

PREDOMINANT SEX AND AGE: There is a nearly equal distribution by sex, and the average age of presentation is 58 yr.

GENETICS: Approximately 40% of FTD cases have a positive family history, and several genes (Table 1) have been associated with the development of familial FTD. The most common are mutations in *C9ORF72, MAPT,* and *GRN* (Table 2).

PHYSICAL FINDINGS & CLINICAL PRESENTATION

- The early stage of bvFTD is characterized by changes in behavior and personality. Patients display a lack of insight into these changes, and family members may initially think they are suffering a midlife crisis or a new-onset psychiatric disorder. Therefore, careful history-taking is required.
- Behavioral changes include disinhibition, impulsivity, distractibility, violation of social norms (such as offensive, insensitive, or inappropriate sexual remarks; inappropriate behaviors; inappropriately explicit or personal conversations; or encroachment on the personal space of others), as well as increased irritability and impulsive criminal behavior (such as shoplifting or violating traffic laws).
- Patients also display decreased ability to empathize with others, insensitivity to the needs and emotions of their loved ones, and distance/detachment in their personal relationships.
- Apathy and inertia are also common symptoms, with possible development of immobility as the disorder progresses.
- Other associated symptoms that may develop are changes in language and speech (verbal aspontaneity, stereotyped phrases, mutism in late stages), repetitive motor movements, or hyperphagia, especially for sweet foods.
- Physical exam findings for bvFTD can include upper and/or lower motor neuron signs, dysarthria, dysphagia, and pseudobulbar affect. Some patients meet criteria for both FTD and amyotrophic lateral sclerosis. This overlap is typically related to a C9orf72 mutation.
- Although behavioral changes can also occur in the other FTD syndromes SD and PNFA, these two primarily have language deficits that precede the behavioral changes.
    1. SD is characterized by a gradual loss of the knowledge of words, objects, and concepts, with preservation of speech fluency and syntax.
    2. PNFA is characterized by effortful, nonfluent speech, word-finding difficulties, and agrammatism, with preservation of single-word comprehension.

DIAGNOSIS

Diagnosis of bvFTD is primarily clinical, with neuroimaging and pathology/genetics required for further confirmation. In 2011, the International Behavioral Variant FTD Consortium (FTDC) developed revised criteria for the diagnosis of bvFTD (Table 3).

- In summary, six core symptoms that can be seen in bvFTD were identified. The presence of any three is sufficient to diagnose *possible* bvFTD.
- Diagnosis of *probable* bvFTD requires meeting the following three conditions: (1) patient has diagnosed possible bvFTD, (2) significant functional decline, and (3) frontal and/or anterior temporal atrophy/hypoperfusion seen on imaging.
- Diagnosis of *definitive* bvFTD can be made only when the patient has possible or probable bvFTD, plus either (1) pathologic evidence of FTLD on biopsy or postmortem, or (2) presence of a known causal genetic mutation.

DIFFERENTIAL DIAGNOSIS

- Other neurodegenerative disorders, including Alzheimer disease (AD), Parkinson disease, dementia with Lewy bodies, corticobasal

TABLE 1 Clinical, Genetic, and Pathologic Correlations in Frontotemporal Lobar Degeneration

Clinical Presentation	% of FTLD	Associated Genes		Comorbidities: Parkinsonism	Comorbidities: MND	Comorbidities: IBM PDB	Neuropathologic Subtypes: FTLD-tau	Neuropathologic Subtypes: FTLD-TDP	Neuropathologic Subtypes: FTLD-FUS	Neuropathologic Subtypes: FTLD-UPS	Neuropathologic Subtypes: FTLD-ni
bvFTD	57%			+	+	+/–	++	++	+	+/–	+/–
		C9orf72	++	+	++			Type B > A		+/–	
		GRN	+	+				Type A			
		MAPT	+	+			+				
		VCP	+/–		+/–	+		Type D			
		CHMP2B	+/–	+/–	+/–					+	
nfvPPA	24%			+	+/–		++	+			
		C9orf72	+								
		GRN	++	+				Type A			
		MAPT	+	+			+				
svPPA	19%			+/–	+/–		+/–	++ (Type C)			
		Rarely genetic									

Number of plus signs (+) signifies relative frequency of the observation; +/– indicates rare observation.

bv, Behavioral variant; *FTD,* frontotemporal dementia; *FTLD,* frontotemporal lobar degeneration; *FUS,* fused in sarcoma; *IBM,* inclusion body myopathy; *MND,* motor neuron disease; *nfv,* agrammatic or nonfluent variant; *ni,* no inclusions; *PDB,* Paget disease of the bone; *PPA,* primary progressive aphasia; *sv,* semantic variant; *TDP,* TAR DNA-binding protein; *UPS,* ubiquitin-proteasome system.

From Fillit HM: *Brocklehurst's textbook of geriatric medicine and gerontology,* ed 8, Philadelphia, 2017, Elsevier.

TABLE 2 Gene Mutations Associated with Frontotemporal Dementia

Gene	Chromosome	Protein	Protein Function	Mode of Inheritance	Mutation Frequency in Familial FTD	Mutation Frequency in Sporadic FTD	Age of Onset (Mean, Range)
C9ORF72	9p21.2	Unknown	Unknown	AD	21%	6%	50s (mid 20-80s)
MAPT	17q21.31	Microtubule-associated tau protein	Microtubule stabilization and assembly	AD	6.3%	1.5%	Mid-50s (20-80s)
GRN	17q21.31	Progranulin	Activates signaling cascades for development, inflammation, and wound repair	AD	5%-15%	5%	60s (mid 30-80s)

AD, Autosomal dominant; *FTD,* frontotemporal dementia.
From Deleon J, Miller BL: Frontotemporal dementia. In Daniel CK et al (eds), *Handbook of clinical neurology,* ed 148, Philadelphia, 2018, Elsevier, pp 409-430.

TABLE 3 International Consensus Criteria for Behavioral Variant FTD

Must be present for any FTD clinical syndrome:
- Shows progressive deterioration of behavior and/or cognition by observation or history

Possible bvFTD
- Three of the features (A-F) must be present; symptoms should occur repeatedly, not just as a single instance:
  - A. Early (3 yr) behavioral disinhibition
  - B. Early (3 yr) apathy or inertia
  - C. Early (3 yr) loss of sympathy or empathy
  - D. Early (3 yr) perseverative, stereotyped, or compulsive/ritualistic behavior
  - E. Hyperorality and dietary changes
  - F. Neuropsychologic profile: Executive function deficits with relative sparing of memory and visuospatial functions

Probable bvFTD
- All the following criteria must be present to meet diagnosis:
  - A. Meets criteria for possible bvFTD
  - B. Significant functional decline
  - C. Imaging results consistent with bvFTD (frontal and/or anterior temporal atrophy on CT or MRI or frontal hypoperfusion or hypometabolism on SPECT or PET)

Definite bvFTD
- Criteria A and either B or C must be present to meet diagnosis:
  - A. Meets criteria for possible or probable bvFTD
  - B. Histopathologic evidence of FTLD on biopsy at post mortem
  - C. Presence of a known pathogenic mutation

Exclusion criteria for bvFTD
- Criteria A and B must both be answered negatively; criterion C can be positive for possible bvFTD but must be negative for probable bvFTD:
  - A. Pattern of deficits is better accounted for by other non degenerative nervous system or medical disorders
  - B. Behavioral disturbance is better accounted for by a psychiatric diagnosis
  - C. Biomarkers strongly indicative of Alzheimer disease or other neurodegenerative process

Additional features
- Presence of motor neuron findings suggestive of motor neuron disease
- Motor symptoms and signs similar to corticobasal degeneration and progressive supranuclear palsy
- Impaired word and object knowledge
- Motor speech deficits
- Substantial grammatical deficits

bvFTD, Behavioral variant frontotemporal dementia; *CT,* computed tomography; *FTD,* frontotemporal dementia; *FTLD,* frontotemporal lobar degeneration; *MRI,* magnetic resonance imaging; *PET,* positron emission tomography; *SPECT,* single-photon emission computed tomography.
From Rascovsky K et al: Sensitivity of revised diagnostic criteria for the behavioural variant of frontotemporal dementia TT, *Brain* 2011;134:1-22.

syndrome, progressive supranuclear palsy, and chronic traumatic encephalopathy
- Psychiatric disorders (bipolar disorder, schizophrenia, obsessive-compulsive disorder, depression, personality disorders)
- Spontaneous low intracranial pressure with sagging of the front lobes
- Subdural hematomas, especially frontal
- CNS tumors in the prefrontal cortex or compressing the prefrontal cortex
- Metabolic disturbances or nutritional deficiencies (hypothyroidism, B_{12} deficiency)
- Substance abuse/toxicities (ethanol, drugs of abuse, heavy metal poisoning)
- Infections (chronic meningitis, HIV-associated dementia, neurosyphilis)
- Cerebrovascular disease (stroke, vascular dementia, lacunar infarctions)
- Autoimmune encephalitis, sarcoidosis

WORKUP

- Careful history-taking with specific attention paid to initial symptoms, time course, progression of symptoms, family history, psychiatric history, and other medical history
- Comprehensive neurologic physical exam to help rule out other CNS etiologies
- Use of the International Behavioral Variant FTD Criteria for diagnosis (Table 3)
- Genetic testing for causal mutations of FTD *(C9ORF72, MAPT,* and *GRN)*
- Medication review (especially drugs that may alter mental status, such as anticholinergics, opiates, benzodiazepines, barbiturates, and neuroleptics)
- Neuropsychologic tests of executive function, memory, and social cognition to rule out other neurodegenerative disorders
- Psychiatric evaluation to rule out psychiatric disorders

LABORATORY TESTS

- CBC, serum electrolytes, glucose, BUN/creatinine, liver function tests
- Cerebrospinal fluid (CSF) analysis for infection and measurement of CSF tau and amyloid (which can help differentiate between FTD and AD—not typically measured in clinical practice)
- Vitamin B_{12}, thyroid function tests, HIV, and syphilis screening
- Urine toxicity screen
- In vivo histopathology:
  1. Almost all cases of FTLD have one of the following protein inclusions found on pathologic examination: TAR DNA-binding protein with molecular weight 43 kDa (TDP-43), microtubule-associated protein tau (MAPT), or fused-in-sarcoma protein (FUS). If feasible and as medical technology advances, in vivo histopathologic testing can confirm the diagnosis.

IMAGING STUDIES

- In general, structural MRI and CT will show gray matter atrophy in the frontal and/or temporal lobes, anterior cingulate cortex, and insula with variation in distribution between the different FTD subtypes.
  1. Patients with bvFTD specifically will usually show atrophy in the orbitofrontal, anterior cingulate, anterior insular, and anterior temporal cortices.
  2. SD is associated with atrophy in the temporal poles, and PNFA with atrophy in the left perisylvian region.
- A normal MRI scan does not exclude FTD, however, because changes may not be seen

in early stages of the disorder. In these cases, PET or SPECT can be used to visualize areas of hypoperfusion/hypometabolism.

Rx TREATMENT

- No disease-modifying drugs currently exist for the treatment of FTD. With advances in the understanding of FTD pathophysiology and genetics, however, new therapies such as antisense oligonucleotides and tau-specific antibodies are being investigated for their efficacy in treating or altering the progression of the syndrome and may see eventual clinical application.
- Current management of FTD is aimed at management of behavioral symptoms through both pharmacologic and nonpharmacologic means.

NONPHARMACOLOGIC THERAPY

- Due to the impulsivity and the risk for injury seen in bvFTD, discussions with family members about driving, the patient's access to finances, and safety of the physical environment should be conducted early in management.
- For patients with motor symptoms, regular exercise and physical therapy are helpful.
- Speech therapy is helpful for patients with language deficits.
- Diet counseling can aid in prevention of weight gain in patients with hyperphagia.

ACUTE GENERAL Rx

None

CHRONIC Rx

- There are conflicting reports of the efficacy of several medications in the symptomatic treatment of FTD. These include selective serotonin reuptake inhibitors (SSRIs), serotonin and norepinephrine reuptake inhibitors, and antipsychotics.
- SSRIs have the most consensus on their benefit in the management of FTD. They have been shown to help decrease the severity of disinhibition, impulsivity, eating disorders, and repetitive behaviors.
- The use of antipsychotics is controversial, but they are sometimes given to control symptoms of aggression, agitation, and psychosis. However, patients with FTD are also at an increased risk for extrapyramidal side effects due to poorly functioning dopaminergic pathways, and thus are usually used only when SSRIs are not successful.

DISPOSITION

- Patients with FTD benefit from having the social support and specialized care offered in dementia-focused care homes and skilled nursing facilities.
- The range and severity of behaviors seen in FTD can put great burden on family and friends. Education, counseling, and connection with social support or referral to a dementia-focused care home can help reduce caregiver stress.

REFERRAL

Patients who have severe or complex presentations should be referred to a neurologist with expertise in dementia or neurodegenerative disorders.

PEARLS & CONSIDERATIONS

FTD is a complex neurologic disorder with a wide variety of presenting symptoms. The most common syndrome seen is bvFTD; therefore, patients with gradual-onset changes in personality, disinhibition, and increased impulsivity should be investigated for FTD. Therapy is aimed at management of the behavioral symptoms, most commonly through the use of SSRIs. Social support and dementia-specific care facilities are helpful for both patients and family members.

PATIENT & FAMILY EDUCATION

The Association for Frontotemporal Degeneration (www.theaftd.org; 866-507-7222)

SUGGESTED READINGS

Available at ExpertConsult.com

RELATED CONTENT

Alzheimer Disease (Related Key Topic)
Parkinson Disease (Related Key Topic)
Dementia with Lewy Bodies (Related Key Topic)

AUTHORS: **Marco Pares, MD,** and **Joseph S. Kass, MD, JD, FAAN**

BASIC INFORMATION

DEFINITION

Frostbite represents tissue injury (or death) from freezing and vasoconstriction induced by severe environmental cold exposure.

SYNONYM

Cold-induced tissue injury

ICD-10CM CODES

T35.0	Superficial frostbite involving multiple body regions
T34	Frostbite with tissue necrosis
T345	Frostbite with tissue necrosis of wrist and hand
T34.8	Frostbite with tissue necrosis of ankle and foot
T34.9	Frostbite with tissue necrosis of other and unspecified sites
T35.4	Superficial frostbite involving multiple body regions
T33.9	Superficial frostbite of unspecified sites, initial encounter

EPIDEMIOLOGY & DEMOGRAPHICS

- Environmental factors include windchill factor, temperature, duration of exposure, altitude, and degree of wetness. Hands and feet account for >90% of injuries; nose, cheeks, ears, and male genitalia are also more susceptible.
- Host factors include psychiatric illness and neuroleptic and sedative drugs (especially alcohol, which, in addition to impairing judgment, inhibits shivering and causes cutaneous vasodilation). Other risk factors include immobility, previous frostbite, malnutrition, tobacco use, peripheral neuropathy, peripheral vascular disease, diabetes, exhaustion, and constricting clothing and footwear.
- Patients at the extremes of age are at greatest risk, but frostbite is more common in adults between 30 and 49 yrs of age with a strong male predominance (10:1)

PHYSICAL FINDINGS & CLINICAL PRESENTATION

- Frostbite may be classified into four degrees of injury severity or, more practically, into *superficial* (corresponding to first and second degree) and *deep* (corresponding to third and fourth degree) groups. In both cases, the degree of frostbite can only be accurately determined after rewarming as initially most frostbite injuries appear similar.
- *Superficial* frostbite involves the skin and subcutaneous tissue. The frozen part is waxy, white (or mottled), and firm but soft and resilient below the surface when gently depressed. After rewarming, there is an initial hyperemia that may be followed by swelling and formation of superficial blisters with clear or milky fluid within 6 to 24 hr. There is no ultimate tissue loss.
- *Deep* frostbite extends into the dermis and may involve muscles, nerves, tendons, or bones. The skin may be hard or wooden, without tissue resilience. Nonblanching cyanosis, hemorrhagic blisters, tissue necrosis (Fig. E1), and gangrene may develop. Affected tissue has a poor prognosis and débridement or amputation is generally required.
- Patients initially feel numbness, prickling, and itching. More severe injury can produce paresthesias and stiffness, with burning or throbbing pain upon thawing.

PATHOPHYSIOLOGY

Two phases of tissue injury:

1. The actual freezing of the tissues, during which cellular damage is caused by the formation of extracellular ice crystals, which cause osmotic shifts, cellular dehydration, cell membrane lysis, and cell death.
2. The reperfusion injury, during which the thawing of damaged endothelial cells releases a cascade of inflammatory mediators (e.g., prostaglandin F, thromboxane A2, bradykinins, histamine), resulting in capillary compression, vascular stasis, progressive ischemic injury, and thrombus formation. These conditions ultimately lead to the destruction of the microcirculation and to cell death.

DIAGNOSIS

DIFFERENTIAL DIAGNOSIS

- Frostnip: A superficial nonfreezing cold injury associated with intense vasoconstriction and characterized by frost forming on the surface of the skin. Transient numbness, tingling, and pallor resolve quickly with warming
- Pernio (chilblains): Self-limited, cold-induced vasculitis associated with purple plaques or nodules, often affecting dorsum of hands and feet; seen with prolonged cold exposure to above-freezing temperatures
- Cold immersion (trench foot): Caused by ischemic injury resulting from sustained, severe vasoconstriction in appendages exposed to wet cold at temperatures above freezing

WORKUP

- Laboratory workup is not indicated unless the patient has systemic hypothermia.
- Early presentation (<24 hr from thawing): If there is deep frostbite with potential significant morbidity, perfusion evaluation with Tc-99 triple phase scanning or MRA should be done emergently in anticipation of potential thrombolysis treatment.
- Late presentation (>24 hr from thawing): Noninvasive imaging with MRA or multiphase bone scintigraphy (ideally with SPECT/CT) can be used to predict the likely levels of tissue viability for future reconstruction after amputation.

TREATMENT (3 PHASES)

1. FIELD MANAGEMENT

- Prioritize treatment of hypothermia (core body temperature <35° C; 95° F) with systemic and adjunctive rewarming measures if available (e.g., warmed, humidified oxygen, heated IV saline [45° C; 113° F], and warming blankets) before thawing frostbitten extremities.
  1. Shelter patient out of wind and give warm fluids.
- Remove constricting or wet clothing and jewelry from affected digits.
  1. Place cold extremity in a companion's axilla or groin for 10 min, then replace dry gloves/boots.
- Insulate, splint, and elevate affected areas if practical to do so.
  1. Never rub or massage the affected area. Avoid dry heat (e.g., fires and heaters).
- Avoid thawing if there is any risk of refreezing and if possible avoid ambulation on thawed lower extremities (unless only distal toes affected).
- Box 1 describes the Alaska State Guidelines for prehospital treatment of frostbite.

2. REWARMING

- Rapid rewarming (with warm water) limits the freezing injury and yields better outcomes than slow rewarming (e.g., moving to a warmer location).
- Rapid rewarming is achieved by immersing the affected area in a circulating warm water bath with or without a mild antibacterial agent (e.g., chlorhexidine or povidone-iodine) maintained at 37° to 39° C for at least 15 to 30 min up to 1 hour, until all tissues are thoroughly rewarmed and pliable with a red-purple color. Active motion during rewarming is advisable; massage is not.
- Administer analgesics during rewarming (ibuprofen and possibly narcotics).

3. POST-THAW TREATMENT

- Tetanus prophylaxis and topical antibiotics if potentially contaminated skin wound.
- Consider systemic antibiotics for patients with significant trauma or signs of infection.
- Débride broken clear vesicles and avoid disrupting intact blisters (especially hemorrhagic ones) unless they interfere with mobility.
- Topical aloe vera (a potent anti-prostaglandin agent) q6h and ibuprofen (a thromboxane inhibitor) 400 to 600 mg bid to tid (or daily aspirin) can be given until wounds are healed or surgery occurs.
- Thrombolytic therapy: May consider if <24 hr from thawing in a patient with severe frostbite and poor prognostic indicators (e.g., cool skin after rewarming, numb, dusky or blue digits, hemorrhagic blisters). First, evaluate perfusion with angiography (or possibly MRA) to assess for arterial compromise. Next,

BOX 1 Alaska State Guidelines for Prehospital Treatment of Frostbite

First Responder/Emergency Medical Technician—I, II, III/Paramedic/Small Bush Clinic
Evaluation and Treatment

A. Anticipate, assess, and treat the patient for hypothermia, if present.
B. Assess the frostbitten area carefully because the loss of sensation may cause the patient to be unaware of soft tissue injuries in that area.
C. Obtain a complete set of vital signs and the patient's temperature.
D. Remove jewelry and clothing, if present, from the affected area.
E. Obtain a patient history, including the date of the patient's last tetanus immunization.
F. If there is frostbite distal to a fracture, attempt to align the limb unless there is resistance. Splint the fracture in a manner that does not compromise distal circulation.
G. Determine whether rewarming the frostbitten tissue can be accomplished in a medical facility. If it can, transport the patient while protecting the tissue from further injury from cold or impacts.
H. If the decision is made to rewarm frostbitten tissue in the field, you should prepare a warm water bath in a container large enough to accommodate the frostbitten tissues without them touching the sides or bottom of the container. The temperature of the water bath should be 99°-102° F (37°-39° C).
   1. Generally, patients with frostbite do not require opiates for pain relief; they occasionally need nonopiate pain medication or anxiolytics. If possible, consult a physician regarding the administration of oral analgesics, such as acetaminophen, ibuprofen or aspirin. Aspirin or ibuprofen may help improve outcomes by blocking the arachidonic acid pathway.
   2. Immersion injury or frostbite with other associated injuries may produce significant edema and high pain levels. These patients may need opiate pain medications for initial treatment. In this case, advanced life support personnel should administer morphine or other analgesics in accordance with physician-signed standing orders or online medical control.
I. A source of additional warm water must be available.
J. Water should be maintained at approximately at 99°-102° F (37°-39° C) and gently circulated around the frostbitten tissue until the distal tip of the frostbitten part becomes flushed.
K. Pain after rewarming usually indicates that viable tissue has been successfully rewarmed.
L. After rewarming, let the frostbitten tissues dry in the warm air. Do **not** towel dry.
M. After thawing, tissues that were deeply frostbitten may develop blisters or appear cyanotic. Blisters should not be broken and must be protected from injury.
N. Pad between affected digits and bandage affected tissues loosely with a soft, sterile dressing. Avoid putting undue pressure on the affected parts.
O. Rewarmed extremities should be kept at a level above the heart, if possible.
P. Protect the rewarmed area from refreezing and other trauma during transport. A frame around the frostbitten area should be constructed to prevent blankets from pressing directly on the injured area.
Q. Do not allow an individual who has frostbitten feet to walk except when the life of the patient or rescuer is in danger. Once frostbitten feet are rewarmed, the patient becomes nonambulatory.

administer intraarterial (or intravenous) tPA if perfusion defects are demonstrated and there is no contraindication to thrombolysis. Tissue salvage rate appears to correlate with elapsed time to treatment from time of rewarming, and best outcomes are seen within the first 12 hours. Although the use of early thrombolytic therapy appears to limit reperfusion injury and reduce subsequent digit amputation significantly, high-quality studies are lacking, and this treatment is not yet U.S. FDA-approved.

- Some protocols include heparin or prostacyclin in addition to tPA to prevent recurrent thrombosis.
- Vasodilator therapy: Various vasodilators (NTG, pentoxifylline, phenoxybenzamine, nifedipine, reserpine, and buflomedil) have been tried, with the best evidence favoring prostacyclines (e.g., iloprost, an injectable available in Europe that has vasodilatory, fibrinolytic-enhancing, and antiplatelet activity). If iloprost is available, at least one study has shown superior efficacy to tPA, and it is easier to administer, has a better safety profile, has fewer contraindications, and can be managed on a general ward. A small study of Himalayan climbers suggested that it can be beneficial even after the standard 48-hour window and perhaps for up to 72 hours.
- Daily dressing changes with dry, sterile, noncompressive, and nonadherent dressings. Splint and elevate hands and feet to reduce edema and separate digits with cotton gauze. Avoid any abrasion to limit risk of infection.
- Whirlpool hydrotherapy: 1 to 2 times per day for 30 min with warm water (37°-39° C), with or without an antiseptic solution if severe edema is present, until there is a clear demarcation of necrotic tissues or evidence of tissue healing.
- Gentle, progressive physical therapy after edema resolves.
- Keep site warm, and avoid all vasoconstrictors, including nicotine.
- Adjunctive treatments including dextran, warfarin, sympathectomy, and hyperbaric oxygen are of potential but unproven benefit.

DISPOSITION

A majority of patients have long-term residual symptoms, including cold hypersensitivity, neuropathic pain, sensory deficits, hyperhidrosis, secondary Raynaud disease, localized osteoporosis, edema, hair or nail deformities, and (rarely) arthritis. Treatment with tricyclics, gabapentin, calcium channel blockers, and careful protection from further cold exposure may be helpful.

REFERRAL

- Hospitalize for hypothermia or deep frostbite; a burn unit is best.
- Surgical decisions regarding amputation should be deferred until demarcation of viable tissue is clear. Traditionally, this can take 6 to 12 wk by clinical examination. Triple phase Tc-99m bone scan with SPECT/CT in the days after injury can be used to predict level of amputation accurately. Early surgical intervention is indicated if refractory pain, sepsis, or gangrene occurs.

SUGGESTED READINGS

Available at ExpertConsult.com

RELATED CONTENT

Frostbite (Patient Information)

AUTHOR: **Michael P. Johnson, MD**

BASIC INFORMATION

DEFINITION

Biliary pain caused by gallbladder dysmotility in the absence of gallstones, sludge, or microlithiasis. It is a diagnosis of exclusion with no evidence of structural disease seen with normal hepatobiliary and pancreatic laboratory and diagnostic imaging modalities.

SYNONYMS

Biliary dyskinesia
Gallbladder dyskinesia
Gallbladder spasm
Acalculous biliary disease
Chronic acalculous cholecystitis
Chronic acalculous
Gallbladder dysfunction
Cystic duct syndrome

ICD-10CM CODE
K82.9 Disease of gallbladder, unspecified

EPIDEMIOLOGY & DEMOGRAPHICS

INCIDENCE: Biliary dyspepsia has an incidence rate of 1% to 6%.
PREVALENCE: 10% to 45% of total population report dyspepsia.
PREDOMINANT SEX AND AGE: There is a 3:1 female-to-male predominance.
RISK FACTORS: There is no consistent relationship to meals or fatty meal intake.

PHYSICAL FINDINGS & CLINICAL PRESENTATION

These patients present with typical biliary pain that fulfills the Rome III criteria:

- Patients present with sporadic epigastric or right upper quadrant pain lasting for 30 min but less than 6 hr.
- Episodes are recurrent and occur in sporadic intervals (but not daily).
- The pain is not relieved by bowel movements.
- The pain is not relieved by postural movements.
- The pain is not relieved by antacids.
- The pain builds up to a steady level.
- The pain is severe enough it impedes daily activities and may even require an emergency department visit.

DIAGNOSIS

DIFFERENTIAL DIAGNOSIS

- Primary gallbladder disorders: Gallstones, cholecystitis
- Pancreatobiliary disorders: Cholelithiasis, choledocholithiasis, pancreatitis, pancreatic neoplasm
- Gastrointestinal disorders: Gastroesophageal reflux disorder, peptic ulcer disease, inflammatory bowel disease, irritable bowel syndrome, gastric or esophageal neoplasm
- Metabolic disorders: Obesity, diabetes mellitus
- Cholecystokinin deficiency: Celiac disease

WORKUP

This is a diagnosis of exclusion in a patient with biliary pain. Patients will have normal blood test results and hepatobiliary and pancreatic enzymes, including aspartate aminotransferase (AST), alanine aminotransferase (ALT), alkaline phosphatase (ALP), bilirubin, amylase, and lipase. Imaging, including abdominal ultrasound, is essentially normal without evidence of gallstone or gallbladder sludge pathology.

LABORATORY TESTS

Laboratory tests, including serum AST, ALT, ALP, bilirubin, gamma-glutamyl transferase, amylase, and lipase, are within normal limits.

IMAGING STUDIES

- To exclude gallstone pathology, a transabdominal ultrasound is initial choice for imaging. Transabdominal ultrasound is capable of detecting gallstones up to 3 to 5 mm in size. Patients should fast for at least 8 hr before ultrasound to optimize visualization of the gallbladder.
- If gallstones or gallbladder are not found on ultrasound but still suspected, endoscopic ultrasound (EUS) may be used to detect microlithiasis or gallstones smaller than 3 mm.
- Assessing gallbladder emptying through cholecystokinin (CCK)–stimulated cholescintigraphy is essential in the diagnosis. CCK-stimulated cholescintigraphy allows for the calculation of gallbladder ejection fraction (GBEF). Normal GBEF is >38%. Patients with a GBEF <35% to 40% with reproducible pain on CCK stimulation is suggestive of functional gallbladder disorder.

TREATMENT

In patients with appropriate evaluation for suspected functional gallbladder disorder, surgical management with cholecystectomy is the preferred method of treatment.

NONPHARMACOLOGIC THERAPY

Surgical cholecystectomy is the preferred method of treatment. Studies have shown symptomatic relief in up to 98% of patients postcholecystectomy.

ACUTE GENERAL Rx

- Initial management should include adequate analgesic control for abdominal pain.
- Opioid analgesics should be avoided because they may exacerbate symptoms involved in a hypofunctioning gallbladder.

COMPLEMENTARY & ALTERNATIVE MEDICINE

Turmeric (Curcuma) has been known to alleviate biliary dyspepsia by stimulating gallbladder contractions.

DISPOSITION

Patients with functional gallbladder disorder are often misdiagnosed. These patients require appropriate evaluation to exclude other hepatobiliary etiology. After they are properly diagnosed, these patients have a favorable prognosis after surgical intervention.

REFERRAL

- Gastroenterology consultation may be considered to rule out microlithiasis via EUS.
- Surgical consultation should be considered for possible cholecystectomy in select patients.

PEARLS & CONSIDERATIONS

COMMENTS

Functional gallbladder disorder is a diagnosis of exclusion. It is essential that other hepatobiliary pathology be ruled out first. CCK-stimulation scintigraphy showing a reduced GBEF without any other pathology is suggestive of this disorder. Patients fare well with surgical intervention.

RELATED TOPICS

Cholangiocarcinoma (Related Key Topic)
Cholecystitis (Related Key Topic)
Choledocholithiasis (Related Key Topic)
Cholelithiasis (Related Key Topic)

AUTHORS: **Rosann Cholankeril, MD,** and **George Cholankeril, MD**

BASIC INFORMATION

DEFINITION

The *Diagnostic and Statistical Manual of Mental Disorders, Fifth Edition* (DSM-5) states that Internet gaming disorder (IGD) applies to excessive gaming through Internet and non-Internet sources such as playing on personal computers, consoles, or handheld devices. The DSM-5 Workgroup concluded that insufficient data exist to confirm it as a mental disorder. No diagnostic criteria are universally accepted.

SYNONYMS

Internet use disorder
Internet addiction

ICD-10CM CODES
F63.0 Pathological Gambling
Z72.6 Gambling and Betting

ICD-11 CODES
6C51.0 Gaming disorder, predominantly online
6C51.1 Gaming disorder, predominantly offline; bipolar disorder must not be present

EPIDEMIOLOGY & DEMOGRAPHICS

INCIDENCE:

- Estimates range from 0.8% to 11.8% in Western samples and over 10% in some Asian samples.
- Some evidence that rates of "smartphone addiction" or social media addiction can exceed 30% in some samples.

PREVALENCE:

- Prevalence rates are not well established.
- Surveys suggest prevalence rates of 10% to 15% among young people in Asian countries and 1% to 10% of youth in Western countries.
- In children and adolescents, IGD is estimated at 2% on average.
- The mean prevalence rate approaches 5.5%.
- Using stringent criteria, IGD prevalence ranged between 0.5% and 6%; actual prevalence probably falls within this range.

PREDOMINANT SEX & AGE:

- Male gender is a risk factor; IGD was reported in 11.9% of boys but only 2.9% of girls.
- Rates appear to decrease slightly over time. Studies suggest that 50% to 86% of adolescents with IGD persist with their problems over 1 to 2 yr, whereas 14% to 50% recover.

RISK FACTORS:

- Relatively little research has looked at potential race or ethnicity or cross-cultural differences.
- IGD subjects have higher rates of depressive symptoms, and greater depression predicted more gaming as well as reduced time spent in other activities.
- Excessive amounts of playing time at the start may predict risk for persistent IGD and depressive symptoms.
- Low sociability or reduced social competence may confer a risk.
- Impulsivity and attention problems are associated with IGD.
- Some IGD may be associated with illicit drug use and cigarette smoking.

GENETICS:

- The study of IGD genetics is in its infancy.
- The rs2229910 of neurotrophic tyrosine kinase receptor, type 3 (NTRK3), was the only single nucleotide polymorphism (SNP) that showed a significant minor allele frequency difference and may have a protective effect against IGD. Subjects with this SNP spent less time on Internet gaming.
- The *del*-genotype of the *-141C* of the dopamine D2 receptor (*DRD2*) was associated with IGD and use of gaming to avoid negative feelings.
- In a transcriptomic study, persons with more frequent positive Internet gaming-related experiences were less likely to show the elevated conserved transcriptional response to adversity (CTRA) genomic profile of the elevated gene expression of NF-kB innate immune response that leads to chronic inflammation.

PHYSICAL FINDINGS & CLINICAL PRESENTATION

- DSM-5 lists nine criteria. Many are drawn from gambling and substance use disorders.
  1. Preoccupation relates to being all-absorbed by gaming thoughts and should be present not only while playing but throughout the day when engaged in other activities as well.
  2. Withdrawal refers to distressing symptoms emerging when the person does not have the opportunity to play or attempts to stop.
  3. Tolerance involves an increase in time spent playing due to a growing desire to play or need for more exciting games.
  4. Desire to reduce playing accompanied by unsuccessful attempts to control or stop playing, often reflecting a tendency to relapse.
  5. Loss of previously enjoyable interests with constriction of behaviors in favor of game playing.
  6. Continued excessive play despite knowledge of clinically significant problems caused by the excessive gaming.
  7. Concealment or overtly lying about the extent of playing.
  8. Playing to forget about real-life problems or to relieve negative mood states.
  9. Risking or losing a relationship or opportunity at school or work because of excessive game playing.
- DSM-5 suggests endorsing at least five of nine criteria in the past 12 mo.
- Sequelae include parental conflict, poor school performance, and worsening of mood, anxiety, and social phobia symptoms over time.

ETIOLOGY

- Etiology and course of IGD are not well understood, and the neurobiologic basis of IGD is in the early stages of investigation.
- A systematic review by Kuss et al (2018) of 27 studies meeting inclusion criteria found that IGD subjects have poorer response-inhibition and emotion regulation, impaired medial prefrontal cortex (mPFC) functioning and cognitive control, poorer working memory and decision-making capabilities, decreased visual and auditory functioning, and a deficiency in their brain reward system, similar to those found in individuals with substance-related addictions.
- A review by Park et al (2017) of 84 neuroimaging and neurophysiologic studies found associations with structural or functional impairment in regions associated with the brain reward and motivation circuitries, memory, and cognitive control, including the orbitofrontal cortex (OFC), dorsolateral prefrontal cortex (DLPFC), anterior cingulate cortex (ACC), and posterior cingulate cortex.
- IGD is associated with impaired dopamine D2 receptor function, which is associated with mPFC dysregulation.
- While these results suggest that IGD and substance use disorder (SUD) share neurobiologic mechanisms, some recent studies directly report differences in biologic and psychologic markers.

Dx DIAGNOSIS

DIFFERENTIAL DIAGNOSIS

- Significant correlations exist between IGD and other mental health problems including disorders that are part of the differential diagnosis.
  1. 92% correlation with anxiety
  2. 89% correlation with depression
  3. 85% correlation with attention deficit hyperactivity disorder (ADHD)
  4. 75% correlation with social phobia/anxiety and obsessive-compulsive symptoms
- At present, due to lack of quality longitudinal studies, directionality is not discoverable and is further complicated by the complex interrelationship among phenomenologies.

WORKUP

- Screening instruments have been developed.
- Greater gaming time, loneliness, aggression, and poorer prosocial behaviors correlated with higher IGD scores.
- Life satisfaction and self-esteem negatively correlated.
- Endorsement of five or more DSM-5 criteria had high classification accuracy. The threshold of five appears appropriate for distinguishing clinically significant levels of gaming.

IMAGING STUDIES

- Voxel-based morphometry demonstrates decreased gray matter in brain areas involved in cognitive control, error processing, decision-making, and reward in persons with IGD relative to controls.
- Functional magnetic resonance imaging (fMRI) using the cue-induced craving paradigm in IGD show reactivity in the ACC, DLPFC, and parahippocampus.

- Other fMRI results using the Go/No Go task suggest there is altered response inhibition in IGD that resembles that in SUD.
- Conclusions regarding IGD brain mechanisms are premature due to self-report–based diagnoses and small sample sizes. The large number of different regions identified and inconsistencies are problematic.

Rx TREATMENT

- Little is known about the effective treatment. There are few randomized controlled studies.
- Treatment camps for adolescents have generated anecdotal reports of effectiveness.
- There are inpatient and residential programs for Internet addiction in the United States.
- Individual, group, and family therapy are used to strengthen motivation to change and improve social and cognitive-behavioral skills to better control Internet use urges.
- Clinicians also promote alternative activities, including work and exercise.
- Psychiatric assessments are made and medications are prescribed for comorbid mental disorders.
- IGD symptoms are reported to decline but studies are uncontrolled and not randomized. In one of the few randomized trials, Internet use decreased similarly in both the active treatment group and the control group, but those assigned to cognitive-behavioral therapy (CBT) displayed improvements in time management skills and reductions in psychosocial symptoms.

PHARMACOLOGIC TREATMENT

- Screening for and treating comorbid psychiatric conditions in the context of addressing IGD is critical.
- As patients with IGD tend to have other psychiatric conditions, effective treatment for the comorbid condition, which may be delivered concurrently, may have pronounced effects on gaming problems.
- Medication trials for IGD have examined psychotropic drugs typically used for treating depression or ADHD.
- A methylphenidate pre–post trial involved a sample with comorbid IGD and ADHD and found that improvements in IGD improvements were positively correlated with ADHD improvements.
- A bupropion pre–post trial showed that it was superior to both a no medication control group and a placebo condition in reducing IGD symptoms in young adult subjects.
- An escitalopram trial showed it to be superior to no medication, but inferior to bupropion in reducing IGD.
- A 12-wk randomized controlled trial (RCT) found that adolescents receiving either atomoxetine or methylphenidate (but no placebo group) showed reductions in IGD symptoms with an advantage for methylphenidate over atomoxetine in improving ADHD symptoms.

NONPHARMACOLOGIC THERAPY

- CBT has been associated with significantly fewer weekly gaming hours and IGD symptoms compared with no-intervention control groups.
- In a randomized study, both CBT and basic supportive counseling produced significant reductions in IGD symptoms, with no significant difference between groups.
- In another randomized study, CBT plus bupropion was superior to bupropion alone in adolescents with comorbid IGD and major depression.
- CBT for IGD may be an effective short-term intervention for reducing IGD with and without depressive symptoms, but there is need for rigorous studies to determine potential long-term benefits of CBT given the scarcity and limitations of the evidence.
- Family therapy has been tried in IGD, but more research is needed to evaluate results.
- A 2017 systematic treatment review by Zajac et al (2017) summarized 26 psychotherapy studies that met criteria. The conclusion was that well-designed treatment outcome studies were limited by methodological flaws, small sample sizes, lack of control groups, and little information on treatment adherence with lack of evidence for the effectiveness of any treatment modality. Additional treatment for IGD is sorely needed.

COMPLEMENTARY & ALTERNATIVE MEDICINE

- Recreational therapies, music therapy using drumming activity, and art therapy are being considered as complementary treatments for IGD, though no real evidence base exists.
- Exercise rehabilitation using systematic and comprehensive activities to aid in healthy living is being tried in connection with family and outdoor activities, but research is not yet available.
- Parental engagement in the course of shared daily routines and participation is encouraged, with the goal of encouraging a positive attitude toward leisure and the skills to reduce overdependence on online gaming behaviors.
- Mindfulness programs based on yoga or tai chi combine physical activity with meditation and can be embedded in an exercise rehabilitation approach to IGD.

CONCLUSIONS

The inclusion of IGD as a research category in the DSM-5 is helpful as it allows researchers and clinicians a process for studying and treating this condition. Evidence of the clinical morbidity associated with IGD suggests it may have important public health consequences. Achieving clarity of the clinical definition will enhance research and treatment, and an important related issue will be to clarify the comorbid association of IGD with other mental disorders.

! PEARLS & CONSIDERATIONS

PREVENTION

- Pediatricians and child mental health clinicians are in a position to educate parents and patients about the potential harmful effects of Internet gaming. They can help parents feel they have the agency to make guidelines and set limits around gaming.
- Clinicians can help parents understand when use becomes excessive and help them halt a slide into dysfunctional use. A timer can be set before starting play, for example.
- Electronic media should not be located in the child's bedroom, and video game use before bedtime is to be discouraged.
- Regular media-free and rewarding family time can be encouraged.
- Recommendations can be made to use rating systems for video games, and parents can limit use to age- and content-appropriate games (e.g., www.esrb.org/ratings/search.aspx).

PATIENT & FAMILY EDUCATION

PARENTS CAN LEARN TO SPOT THE SIGNS OF IGD:

- Talking incessantly about their game.
- Playing for hours on end and getting defensive or even angry and aggressive when made to stop.
- Neglecting other activities including their daily needs such as food and sleep.
- Developing physical symptoms such as dry or red eyes; soreness in the fingers, back, or neck; or complaints of headaches.
- Appearing preoccupied or depressed.
- Becoming socially isolated.

PARENTS CAN TAKE STEPS TO PREVENT IGD:

- Establish limits when it comes to how long children are allowed to play.
- Do not allow children to have tech in their room after lights out.
- Provide opportunities for rewarding activities such as sports or clubs that provide social engagement with their peers.
- If still concerned about overuse, they should seek the help of a mental health clinician.

However, it should be noted that one recent RCT found no evidence for the effectiveness of the psychoeducational parental guidelines on preventing problematic video gaming in children.

WILDERNESS THERAPY

- Unplugged @ Outback (https://www.outbacktreatment.com/unplugged-internet-addiction-therapy/)
- Pacific Quest (https://pacificquest.org/whom-we-serve/adolescent-profile/video-game-addiction/)
- Trails Carolina (https://trailscarolina.com/video-game-addiction-help-struggling-teens/)
- Camp Pocono Trails (https://www.summerlandcamps.com/gaming-addiction/summer-camp-video-game-addiction/ • https://trailsmomentum.com/video-game-addiction-fortnite-league-of-legends-call-of-duty/)

FAMILY & INDIVIDUAL THERAPY

- Perspectives Counseling (https://perspectivesoftroy.com/michigan/gaming-addiction-treatment/)
- Rise Gaming Recovery (https://www.risegamingrecovery.com/)

- Tech Addiction (http://www.techaddiction.ca/video_game_addiction_books.html)
- Book: *Overcoming Video Game Addiction* (Author: Simon Somlai)
- Book: *Gaming Addiction, Online Addiction, Internet Addiction* (Author: Ace McCloud)

SCHOOL-BASED SCREENING & PREVENTION

- School-based education: Schools should include education about IGD and expand the infrastructure they have in place for other potentially problematic behaviors (drugs, alcohol, risky sex, gambling, etc.) to include problems with electronic media.
- School-based screening: Because of links between IGD and poor school performance, schools may be an effective place for screening for IGD and for providing referrals for services when problems are discovered.
- School-based parental training: Schools should provide training to parents to recognize potential problems.
- School-based activities: Schools and community centers can aid parents in identifying nongaming creative opportunities.

SUGGESTED READINGS

Available at ExpertConsult.com

AUTHOR: **Gregory L. Fricchione, MD**

BASIC INFORMATION

DEFINITION

Gastric cancer is an adenocarcinoma arising from the stomach. Cancers in the cardia arising within 5 cm of the gastroesophageal junction (GEJ) are typically classified as GEJ cancers. It is subdivided into intestinal and diffuse histology. The diffuse form of gastric cancer is more common in women and young patients, whereas the intestinal type is predominantly related to environmental factors (smoking, diet high in smoked, salted, and pickled food, nitrates and nitrites) and ethnicity (Asian and Pacific descent). The classification of gastric adenocarcinoma by depth of invasion is illustrated in Fig. 1.

SYNONYMS

Gastric adenocarcinoma
Stomach cancer
Linitis plastica

ICD-10CM CODES

C16	Malignant neoplasm of stomach
C16.0	Malignant neoplasm of cardia of stomach
C16.1	Malignant neoplasm of stomach
C16.2	Malignant neoplasm of body of stomach
C16.3	Malignant neoplasm of pyloric antrum
C16.5	Malignant neoplasm of lesser curvature of stomach, unspecified
C16.6	Malignant neoplasm of greater curvature of stomach, unspecified
C16.8	Malignant neoplasm of overlapping sites of stomach

EPIDEMIOLOGY & DEMOGRAPHICS

- Gastric cancer is the sixth most common cancer worldwide, with an estimated 1,033,000 new cases diagnosed in 2018. It is the second-leading cause of cancer-related deaths worldwide, with an estimated 782,000 deaths from gastric cancer in 2018. Seventy percent of new cases occur in developing countries, and Asia accounts for the highest incidence.
- In the U.S., an estimated 27,600 new cases and 11,010 deaths were predicted in 2020.
- The incidence and mortality rate of gastric cancer is 6.7 and 3.4, respectively, per 100,000 persons in the U.S. Although the incidence of distal stomach tumors has greatly declined over the past 30 yr, incidences of proximal tumors of the cardia and fundus is increasing.
- Gastric cancer is more common in male patients >65 yr (70% of patients are >50 yr).
- Male:female ratio of 3:2.
- Hereditary diffuse gastric cancer (HDGC) has an autosomal-dominant inheritance, and cancer develops at a young age (average age 37 yr). Germline truncating mutations in the tumor-suppressor E-cadherin gene *(CDH1)* are found in up to 50% of these families. It is associated with an 80% lifetime risk of gastric cancer.
- Increased risk of gastric cancer is also seen with Lynch syndrome, FAP, Peutz-Jeghers, juvenile polyposis syndrome, and hyperplastic gastric polyps.

PHYSICAL FINDINGS & CLINICAL PRESENTATION

- Medical history may reveal complaints of postprandial fullness with significant weight loss (70% to 80%), nausea/vomiting (20% to 40%), dysphagia (20%), and dyspepsia, usually unrelieved by antacids; epigastric discomfort, usually lessened by fasting and exacerbated by food intake, is also common.
- Epigastric or abdominal mass (30% to 50%), epigastric pain.
- Iron deficiency anemia is typically seen from tumor bleeding, and hemoccult-positive stools are detected.
- Hard, nodular liver: May indicate metastatic disease to the liver.
- Ascites, lymphadenopathy, or pleural effusions: May indicate metastases.

ETIOLOGY

RISK FACTORS:

- Chronic *Helicobacter pylori* gastritis. Gastric cancer develops in persons infected with *H. pylori* but not in uninfected persons. Those with histologic findings of severe gastric atrophy, corpus-predominant gastritis, or intestinal metaplasia are at increased risk. Persons with *H. pylori* infection and duodenal ulcer are not at risk, whereas those with gastric ulcers, nonulcer dyspepsia, and gastric hyperplastic polyps are. Eradication of *H. pylori* reduces gastric cancer risk
- Tobacco abuse, heavy alcohol consumption
- Food additives (nitrosamines), smoked foods, occupational exposure to heavy metals, rubber, asbestos
- Chronic atrophic gastritis with intestinal metaplasia, hypertrophic gastritis, and pernicious anemia
- Box 1 summarizes risk factors for gastric adenocarcinoma

Dx DIAGNOSIS

DIFFERENTIAL DIAGNOSIS

- Gastric lymphoma (5% of gastric malignancies)
- Hypertrophic gastritis
- Peptic ulcer
- Reflux esophagitis

WORKUP

Upper endoscopy (Fig. E2) with biopsy will confirm diagnosis. Endoscopic ultrasonography in combination with PET/CT scanning and operative lymph node dissection can be used in staging of the tumor. Table 1 and Fig. 1 describe staging systems for gastric carcinoma.

LABORATORY TESTS

- Complete blood count reveals microcytic anemia.
- Hemoccult-positive stools are detected.
- Chemistry tests can reveal hypoalbuminemia or abnormal liver enzymes in patients with metastasis to the liver.

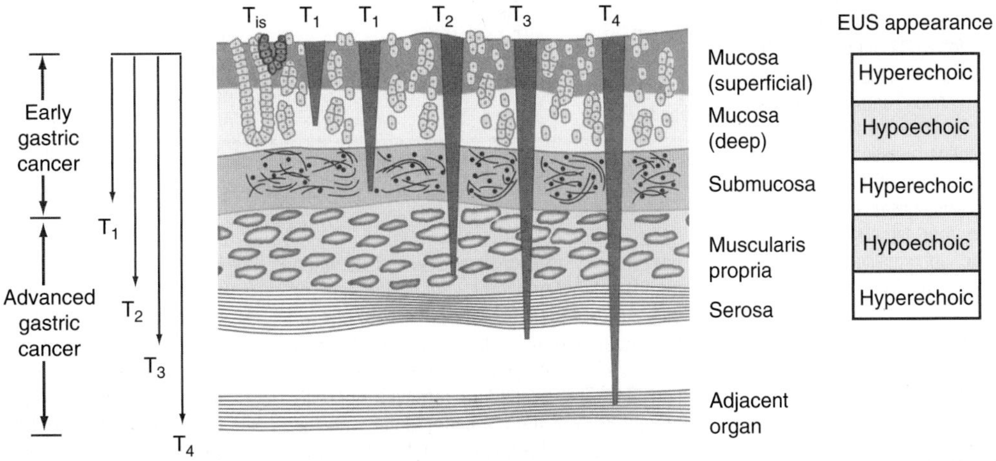

FIG. 1 Classification of gastric adenocarcinoma by depth of invasion (T classification). In the TNM classification, T denotes depth of invasion: T_{is} designates carcinoma in situ; T_1 tumors are confined to the mucosa (T_{1a}) and submucosa (T_{1b}); T_2 tumors invade the muscularis propria but not the serosa; T_3 tumors penetrate the subserosal connective tissue without involving the visceral peritoneum or contiguous structures; and T_4 tumors invade the serosa (visceral peritoneum) and may involve adjacent organs and tissues. In early gastric cancer, the disease is confined to the mucosa and submucosa (T_1), regardless of nodal involvement. (From Feldman M et al [eds]: *Sleisenger and Fordtran's gastrointestinal and liver disease,* ed 10, Philadelphia, 2016, Saunders.)

BOX 1 Risk Factors for Gastric Adenocarcinoma

Definite
H. pylori infection
Chronic atrophic gastritis
Intestinal metaplasia
Dysplasia*
Adenomatous gastric polyps
Cigarette smoking
History of gastric surgery (especially Billroth II)
Genetic factors:
- Family history of gastric cancer (first-degree relative)
- Familial adenomatous polyposis (with fundic gland polyps)
- Hereditary nonpolyposis colorectal cancer
- Peutz-Jeghers syndrome
- Juvenile polyposis

Probable
High salt intake
Obesity (adenocarcinoma of the cardia only)
Snuff tobacco use
History of gastric ulcer
Pernicious anemia
Regular aspirin or other NSAID use (protective)

Possible
Statin use (protective)
Heavy alcohol use
Low socioeconomic status
Ménétrier disease
High intake of fresh fruits and vegetables (protective)
High ascorbate intake (protective)

Questionable
Hyperplastic and fundic gland polyps
Diet high in nitrates
High green tea consumption (protective)

*Surveillance for cancer is recommended in patients with this risk factor.
NSAID, Nonsteroidal antiinflammatory drug.
From Feldman M et al (eds): *Sleisenger and Fordtran's gastrointestinal and liver disease,* ed 10, Philadelphia, 2016, Saunders.

TABLE 1 TNM Staging Criteria and Stages for Gastric Carcinoma Based on AJCC 8th Edition

T Category	T Criteria
T_X	Primary tumor cannot be assessed
T_0	No evidence of primary tumor
T_{is}	Carcinoma *in situ*: Intraepithelial tumor without invasion of the lamina propria, high-grade dysplasia
T_1	Tumor invades the lamina propria, muscularis mucosae, or submucosa
T_{1a}	Tumor invades the lamina propria or muscularis mucosae
T_{1b}	Tumor invades the submucosa
T_2	Tumor invades the muscularis propria
T_3	Tumor penetrates the subserosal connective tissue without invasion of the visceral peritoneum or adjacent structures
T_4	Tumor invades the serosa (visceral peritoneum) or adjacent structures
T_{4a}	Tumor invades the serosa (visceral peritoneum)
N Category	**N Criteria**
N_X	Regional lymph node(s) cannot be assessed
N_0	No regional lymph node metastasis
N_1	Metastasis in one or two regional lymph nodes
N_2	Metastasis in three to six regional lymph nodes
N_3	Metastasis in seven or more regional lymph nodes
N_{3a}	Metastasis in 7 to 15 regional lymph nodes
M Category	**M Criteria**
M_0	No distant metastasis
M_1	Distant metastasis

Stage	pT	pN	M
Stage 0	T_{is}	N_0	M_0
Stage IA	T_1	N_0	M_0
Stage IB	T_1	N_1	M_0
	T_2	N_0	M_0
Stage IIA	T_1	N_2	M_0
	T_2	N_1	M_0
	T_3	N_0	M_0
Stage IIB	T_1	N_{3a}	M_0
	T_2	N_2	M_0
	T_3	N_1	M_0
	T_{4a}	N_0	M_0
Stage IIIA	T_2	N_{3a}	M_0
	T_3	N_2	M_0
	T_{4a}	N_1 or N_2	M_0
	T_{4b}	N_0	M_0
Stage IIIB	T_1	N_{3b}	M_0
	T_2	N_{3b}	M_0
	T_3	N_{3a}	M_0
	T_{4a}	N_{3a}	M_0
	T_{4b}	N_1 or N_2	M_0
Stage IIIC	T_3	N_{3b}	M_0
	T_{4a}	N_{3b}	M_0
	T_{4b}	N_{3a} or N_{3b}	M_0
Stage IV	Any T	Any N	M_1

AJCC, American Joint Committee on Cancer; *TNM,* tumor, node, metastasis.

- Up to 25% of gastric cancers overexpress the HER2/neu growth factor receptor, and it is now standard practice to evaluate gastroesophageal tumors for HER2 overexpression.
- Mutation-specific predictive genetic testing by polymerase chain reaction amplification followed by restriction: Enzyme digestion and DNA sequencing for truncating mutations in *CDH1* is recommended in families of patients with familial diffuse cancer because gastric cancer develops in three of every four carriers of a mutant *CDH1* gene. Genetic abnormalities in gastric adenocarcinoma are summarized in Table E2.

IMAGING STUDIES

Chest and abdomen PET/CT scan (Fig. E3) to evaluate for metastases

Rx TREATMENT

ACUTE GENERAL Rx

- Gastrectomy: Most curable tumors can be removed with adequate margins by subtotal gastrectomy; total gastrectomy is used when mandated by proximal cancer location or disease extent. The preferred treatment for lesions arising in the body or antrum of the stomach is a radical distal subtotal resection (Fig. E4). This procedure removes approximately 80% of the stomach, along with the first portion of the duodenum, the gastrohepatic and gastrocolic omenta, and the nodal tissue adjacent to the three branches of the celiac axis. Extensive or proximal cancers require a total gastrectomy to achieve an adequate proximal gastric margin (Fig. E5). If total gastrectomy is necessary, a splenectomy is sometimes performed, particularly in gastric cancers of the proximal third of the stomach and tumors of the body near the greater curvature. These cancers are more apt to metastasize to lymph nodes in the splenic hilum that cannot be completely excised without a splenectomy. Routine splenectomy is no longer practiced because of the increased complications. A splenectomy should be performed when worrisome, palpable nodes are present in the splenic hilum.

- Finding from recent data indicate that laparoscopic distal gastrectomy with extended D2 lymphadenectomy is comparable to open surgery in terms of relapse-free survival for patients with locally advanced gastric cancer. This approach could become a potential standard treatment option for locally advanced gastric cancer.
- In advanced cases, palliative gastrectomy (bleeding, obstruction) can be performed. Outlet obstruction can be addressed by performing a gastrojejunostomy.
- In patients with operable gastric cancer, the perioperative chemotherapy regimen can decrease tumor size and stage while improving progression-free and overall survival. The current standard neoadjuvant regimen in use is the FLOT (5-fluorouracil [5-FU], leucovorin, oxaliplatin, docetaxel) regimen.
- Postoperative adjuvant chemoradiotherapy using the older 5-FU and leucovorin regimen is an option for stage II to III patients. Alternatively, the modern approach is combination chemotherapy with FOLFOX (5-FU, leucovorin, oxaliplatin) or CAPOX (capecitabine, oxaliplatin) regimens with radiotherapy reserved for high-risk patients only.
- In metastatic gastric cancer, the use of combination chemotherapy regimens results in improved overall survival. Patients progressing after first-line chemotherapy can derive a survival benefit with the use of chemotherapy in combination with antivascular endothelial growth factor receptor-2 antibody ramucirumab. The oral antimetabolite, trifluridine/tipiracil, has been shown to significantly improve overall survival compared with placebo in heavily pretreated patients with advanced gastric cancer.
- In the subset of patients with gastric cancer expressing *HER2-2/neu* oncogene (20% to 25% of patients), the addition of trastuzumab to systemic chemotherapy prolongs overall survival. Recent data have indicated improved survival rates in patients when treated with trastuzumab deruxtecan (an antibody drug conjugate [ADC]) when compared to conventional salvage chemotherapy approaches.
- Immunotherapy with program death receptor-1 antibodies (nivolumab, pembrolizumab) has been shown to improve survival in previously treated patients with high-MSI tumors.
- Treatment algorithms for newly diagnosed gastric or gastroesophageal junction cancer are illustrated in Figs. E6 and E7.

DISPOSITION

- Median survival rate of metastatic or recurrent gastric carcinoma is 10 to 15 mo overall.
- The 5-yr survival rate for early gastric cancers is >35%.

PEARLS & CONSIDERATIONS

COMMENTS

- Gastrectomy patients will need vitamin B_{12} replacement. They are also at risk for dumping syndrome and should be advised to ingest frequent, small meals.
- Prophylactic gastrectomy should be considered in young, asymptomatic carriers of germ-line truncating *CDH1* mutations who belong to families with highly penetrant heredity diffuse gastric cancer.
- Gastric cancer screening for average-risk patients is not recommended in the U.S.

SUGGESTED READINGS

Available at ExpertConsult.com

RELATED CONTENT

Stomach Cancer (Patient Information)

AUTHOR: **Ritesh Rathore, MD**

BASIC INFORMATION

DEFINITION

Gastric outlet obstruction (GOO) is a mechanical obstruction involving the distal stomach or proximal duodenum resulting in delayed gastric emptying. It is not a single entity but rather can be the result of a variety of causes.

SYNONYMS

Pyloric obstruction
Stenosis of the pylorus
GOO

ICD-10CM CODE

K31.5 Obstruction of the duodenum

EPIDEMIOLOGY & DEMOGRAPHICS

INCIDENCE: Accurate statistics on incidence are not available. It is postulated that GOO has decreased over the past several decades due to improved treatment options for peptic ulcer disease, which is historically the leading cause for GOO. More recent data suggest that up to 50% to 80% of new cases are cancer related.

RISK FACTORS:
- History of pancreatic or gastric malignancy
- Untreated peptic ulcer disease
- Chronic NSAID use
- *Helicobacter pylori* infection

PHYSICAL FINDINGS & CLINICAL PRESENTATION

- Signs of dehydration (tachycardia, hypotension, dry mucous membranes) are often present.
- Malnutrition may be evident depending on the chronicity of the obstruction.
- Epigastric tenderness may be present.
- Abdominal distention/tympanic mass in epigastric area or left upper quadrant (LUQ).
- Succession splash may be heard with a stethoscope placed on the abdomen while the patient rocks side to side. It has a low sensitivity and is positive if present 3 hours after a meal, which suggests retained gastric contents.
- Sister Mary Joseph nodule (a periumbilical node) or Virchow's node (a left supraclavicular node) may be palpated in the setting of metastatic gastric cancer.

Patients with GOO often present with postprandial nonbilious vomiting, epigastric pain, nausea, easy satiety, and weight loss, though the presentation may differ depending on the cause of the obstruction. Patients with malignancy as the underlying cause often present with a more acute onset of symptoms, whereas those with peptic ulcer disease have more chronic symptoms. Physical examination findings most commonly include signs of dehydration and malnutrition, as well as abdominal tympanic distention and epigastric tenderness.

ETIOLOGY

- Historically, the most common cause of GOO was peptic ulcer disease; however, with the availability of proton pump inhibitors and treatment to eradicate *H. pylori* infection, this has been drastically reduced. Malignancy now accounts for the majority of cases, most frequently pancreatic adenocarcinoma with spread to the duodenum or stomach, or gastric cancer. Other rarer malignant causes include advanced gallbladder carcinoma or cholangiocarcinoma, gastric lymphoma, malignancy of the duodenum, ampullary cancer, and gastric carcinoid.
- Benign causes include peptic ulcer disease, caustic ingestion, stricture and scarring from NSAIDs or postsurgery, acute or chronic pancreatitis, and pancreatic pseudocysts. Rare causes include gastric obstructing polyps, bezoars or volvulus, Bouveret syndrome (gallstone in the proximal duodenum), congenital annular pancreas, or infiltrative disease from Crohn, amyloid, or tuberculosis. See Table 1.

DIAGNOSIS

Diagnosis is based on clinical presentation, imaging, and often endoscopy with biopsy.

DIFFERENTIAL DIAGNOSIS

It is important to exclude motility causes such as gastroparesis from diabetes, medications, or viral infections. The primary differential diagnosis to be considered in GOO is in determining the causes of the obstruction. See Table 1.

TABLE 1 Causes of Gastric Outlet Obstruction

Benign	Malignant
Peptic ulcer disease	Pancreatic cancer
Gastric polyps	Gastric cancer
Caustic ingestion	Gallbladder carcinoma
Stricture/scarring from NSAIDs, radiation, postsurgical	Cholangiocarcinoma Gastric lymphoma
Acute or chronic pancreatitis	Ampullary cancer
Pancreatic pseudocyst	Duodenum cancer
Bouveret syndrome (gallstone in the proximal duodenum)	Gastric carcinoid
Congenital annular pancreas	
Infiltrative disease (Crohn, amyloid, tuberculosis)	
Bezoars	

NSAID, Nonsteroidal antiinflammatory drug.

WORKUP

During the initial work up of GOO, it is important assess hydration and nutrition status and to determine the underlying cause. Consider the following:
- Complete blood count, electrolytes, abdominal CT scan, and upper endoscopy

LABORATORY TESTS

Laboratory tests are not diagnostic but should include a complete blood count and electrolytes.
- Electrolytes may reveal evidence of contraction alkalosis and hypokalemia, especially in the setting of repeated vomiting.
- The complete blood count may show evidence of anemia in a patient with underlying malignancy that may become more apparent after fluid replacement.

IMAGING STUDIES

- Abdominal x-rays are often not diagnostic but may reveal a significant gastric bubble.
- CT scan of abdomen may reveal gastric distention, mass, and evidence of malignant spread. This should be ordered without oral contrast if upper endoscopy is anticipated.
- Upper endoscopy is usually needed for both diagnostic and therapeutic purposes. This should occur after nasogastric tube placement and suction to remove gastric contents to reduce the chance of aspiration during the procedure. Endoscopy can determine the location and extension of the obstruction and may offer a diagnosis through biopsy.

TREATMENT

The general management of gastric outlet obstruction consists of hydration, correcting metabolic abnormalities, pain management, and alleviating the obstruction.

NONPHARMACOLOGIC THERAPY

- Nothing by mouth (NPO) and nasogastric tube for gastric decompression
- Intravenous fluids using isotonic saline with potassium replacement
- Nutritional support

BENIGN CAUSES

- Management of the obstruction depends on the underlying cause. The following recommendations are for GOO from peptic ulcer disease, the most common benign cause of GOO. Patients with rarer, benign causes of GOO may benefit from some of the following interventions as well but treatment will be more specifically tailored to the underlying cause and decided with consultations from gastroenterology and surgery.
- GOO can be initially managed with 48 to 72 hours of gastric decompression, fluid replacement, correction of metabolic abnormalities, and acid suppression. *H. pylori* infection should be treated if appropriate. If this approach is unsuccessful endoscopic dilation or surgery should be considered.

ENDOSCOPIC BALLOON DILATION

Endoscopic balloon dilation (EBD) is most commonly indicated in patients with GOO from peptic ulcer disease. It results in a lasting response in 70% to 80% of patients; however, narrow strictures often need gradual dilations performed in a stepwise fashion over several sessions. Recurrent stenosis requiring two or more dilations is an indication for surgery.

SURGICAL INTERVENTIONS

- The goals of surgery include alleviating the obstruction and suppressing acid secretion.
- Surgical inventions such as laparoscopic antrectomy or distal gastrectomy with vagotomy, vagotomy with drainage via pyloroplasty, and laparoscopic gastrojejunostomy are potential options.

ENDOSCOPIC ULTRASOUND-GUIDED GASTROENTEROSTOMY

Endoscopic ultrasound-guided gastroenterostomy (EUS-GE) is emerging as an potential treatment option for benign (and malignant) GOO and might be associated with fewer adverse effects, fewer recurring symptoms, and decreased need for subsequent interventions compared with other techniques. However, further research is necessary to determine optimal technique and to directly compare the efficacy of EUS-GE with other endoscopic procedures and surgical options.

MALIGNANT CAUSES

Management of malignant GOO depends on the type and extent of the underlying malignancy. General therapeutic options include endoscopic stenting, surgical resection or bypass, gastrostomy with possible feeding tube placement, and EUS-GE. Surgery is the treatment of choice when resection can be potentially curative. Consultation with gastroenterology, surgery, oncology, and palliative care can guide treatment decisions.

ACUTE GENERAL Rx

- Proton pump inhibitors to decrease gastric secretions
- Antiemetics to treat nausea
- Pain management
- Eradication of *H. pylori* infection, if applicable

CHRONIC Rx

- Avoidance of nonsteroidal antiinflammatory medications
- Proton pump inhibitors

DISPOSITION

Prognosis depends on the underlying cause of the GOO.

REFERRAL

Gastroenterology should be consulted for initial diagnostic and therapeutic options with consultations from surgery, oncology, and palliative care as needed.

PEARLS & CONSIDERATIONS

COMMENTS

- Malignancy should be considered as the primary cause until proven otherwise.
- All patients, regardless of cause, benefit from a proton pump inhibitor.

RELATED CONTENT

Pancreatic Cancer (Related Key Topic)
Gastric Cancer (Related Key Topic)
Peptic Ulcer Disease (Related Key Topic)
Gallbladder Cancer (Related Key Topic)

SUGGESTED READINGS

Available at ExpertConsult.com

AUTHOR: **Dana Ricci Chofay, MD**

BASIC INFORMATION

DEFINITION

Histologically, *gastritis* refers to inflammation in the stomach. Endoscopically, gastritis refers to several abnormal features such as erythema, erosions, and subepithelial hemorrhages. Gastritis can also be subdivided into erosive, nonerosive, and specific types of gastritis with distinctive features both endoscopically and histologically.

SYNONYMS

Erosive gastritis
Hemorrhagic gastritis
Helicobacter pylori gastritis

ICD-10CM CODES

K29.00	Acute gastritis without bleeding
K29.01	Acute gastritis with bleeding
K29.20	Alcoholic gastritis without bleeding
K29.21	Alcoholic gastritis with bleeding
K29.30	Chronic superficial gastritis without bleeding
K29.31	Chronic superficial gastritis with bleeding
K29.40	Chronic atrophic gastritis without bleeding
K29.41	Chronic atrophic gastritis with bleeding
K29.50	Unspecified chronic gastritis without bleeding
K29.51	Unspecified chronic gastritis with bleeding
K29.60	Other gastritis without bleeding
K29.61	Other gastritis with bleeding
K29.70	Gastritis, unspecified, without bleeding
K29.71	Gastritis, unspecified, with bleeding
K52.81	Eosinophilic gastritis or gastroenteritis

EPIDEMIOLOGY & DEMOGRAPHICS

- Erosive and hemorrhagic gastritis is most commonly seen in patients taking nonsteroidal antiinflammatory drugs (NSAIDs), alcoholics, and critically ill patients (usually on ventilator support).
- *H. pylori* infection with gastritis is believed to be present in 30% to 50% of the population; however, the majority of cases are asymptomatic.
- The prevalence of *H. pylori* infection increases with age from <10% in patients <40 yr to >50% in patients >50 yr.

PHYSICAL FINDINGS & CLINICAL PRESENTATION

- Patients with gastritis generally present with nonspecific clinical signs and symptoms (e.g., epigastric pain, abdominal tenderness, bloating, anorexia, nausea [with or without vomiting]). Symptoms may be aggravated by eating.
- Epigastric tenderness in acute alcoholic gastritis (may be absent in chronic gastritis).
- Foul-smelling breath.
- Hematemesis ("coffee grounds" emesis).

ETIOLOGY

- Alcohol, NSAIDs, stress (critically ill patients usually on mechanical respiration), hepatic or renal failure, multiorgan failure
- *H. pylori* infection
- Bile reflux, pancreatic enzyme reflux
- Gastric mucosal atrophy, portal hypertension gastropathy
- Irradiation

DIAGNOSIS

DIFFERENTIAL DIAGNOSIS

- Peptic ulcer disease
- Gastroesophageal reflux disease
- Nonulcer dyspepsia
- Gastric lymphoma or carcinoma
- Pancreatitis
- Gastroparesis

WORKUP

Diagnostic workup includes a comprehensive history and endoscopy with biopsy.

LABORATORY TESTS

- *H. pylori* testing by urea breath test, stool antigen test (*H. pylori* stool antigen), endoscopic biopsy, or specific antibody test is recommended.
  1. The urea breath test documents active infection (sensitivity and specificity >90%). It uses a flat breath card read by a small analyzer.
  2. The stool antigen test is an enzyme-linked immunoassay (ELISA) that identifies *H. pylori* antigen in a stool specimen with a polyclonal anti–*H. pylori* antibody. It is as accurate as the urea breath test for diagnosis of active infection and follow-up evaluation of patients treated for *H. pylori.* A negative result on the stool antigen test 8 wk after completion of therapy identifies patients in whom eradication of *H. pylori* was successful.
  3. Histologic evaluation of endoscopic biopsy samples is considered by many to be the gold standard for accurate diagnosis of *H. pylori* infection. However, detection of *H. pylori* depends on the site and number of biopsy samples, the method of staining, and experience of the pathologist.
  4. Serologic testing for antibodies to *H. pylori* is easy and inexpensive; however, the presence of antibodies demonstrates previous but not necessarily current infection. Antibodies to *H. pylori* can remain elevated for mo to yr after infection has cleared; therefore, antibody levels must be interpreted in light of patient's symptoms and other test results (e.g., peptic ulcer disease [PUD] seen on upper gastrointestinal series).
- Vitamin B_{12} level in patients with atrophic gastritis.
- Hematocrit (low if significant bleeding has occurred).

TREATMENT

NONPHARMACOLOGIC THERAPY

- Avoidance of mucosal irritants such as alcohol and NSAIDs
- Lifestyle modifications with avoidance of tobacco and foods that trigger symptoms

ACUTE GENERAL Rx

- Eradication of *H. pylori,* when present, can be accomplished with various regimens:
  1. Quadruple therapy: Proton pump inhibitor (PPI) (omeprazole 20 mg, lansoprazole 30 mg, pantoprazole 40 mg, rabeprazole 20 mg) bid *plus* clarithromycin 500 mg bid plus amoxicillin 1000 mg bid *plus* metronidazole 500 mg bid for 14 days.
  2. Triple therapy: PPI bid *plus* clarithromycin 500 mg bid *and* metronidazole 500 mg bid for 14 days. This regimen is useful in those with penicillin allergy.
  3. Triple therapy: Clarithromycin 500 mg bid plus amoxicillin 1 g bid plus PPI bid for 14 days. Useful only in areas with clarithromycin resistance <15%.
  4. Bismuth quadruple therapy: Bismuth subsalicylate (e.g., Pepto-Bismol) 525 mg qid plus metronidazole 500 mg qid plus tetracycline 500 mg qid plus PPI bid for 14 days.
- Prophylaxis and treatment of stress gastritis with sucralfate suspension 1 g orally q4 to 6h, H_2-receptor antagonists, or PPIs in patients on ventilator support.

CHRONIC Rx

- Omeprazole, H2RB, or sucralfate in patients receiving long-term NSAIDs.
- Avoidance of alcohol, tobacco, and prolonged NSAID or corticosteroid use.

DISPOSITION

- Patients should be tested for eradication ≥4 wk after completion of therapy. Undetectable stool antigen tested at least 4 wk after therapy accurately confirms cure of *H. pylori* infection in initially seropositive healthy subjects with reasonable sensitivity. PPI therapy should be stopped at least 2 wk prior to testing.
- Surveillance gastroscopy in patients with atrophic gastritis (increased risk of gastric cancer).

RELATED CONTENT

Gastritis (Patient Information)
Helicobacter pylori Infection (Related Key Topic)
Peptic Ulcer Disease (Related Key Topic)

AUTHOR: **Fred F. Ferri, MD**

BASIC INFORMATION

DEFINITION

- Gastroenteritis is a broad term used for various gastrointestinal pathologic states. The main manifestation is diarrhea, defined as daily stool of at least 200 g or at least 3 times a day of rapid onset that lasts less than 2 wk and often accompanied by nausea (93% of cases), vomiting (81%), malaise, anorexia, fever, abdominal pain, and dehydration. Gastroenteritis is usually self-limited, but if it is not managed properly, it can lead to a prolonged course. It usually lasts less than 7 days and not longer than 2 wk. Diarrhea lasting more than 14 days is chronic or persistent.
- May be caused by viruses, bacteria, or parasites. Viruses are responsible for acute gastroenteritis in most patients.
- Gastroenteritis is a common cause of morbidity/mortality around the world. In the developing world, it is a leading cause of death.

ICD-10CM CODES

K52.9	Non-infective gastroenteritis and colitis
558.3	Allergic gastroenteritis and colitis
K52.1	Infectious gastroenteritis and colitis
K52.0	Gastroenteritis and colitis due to radiation

EPIDEMIOLOGY & DEMOGRAPHICS

- Frequency is difficult to determine. Gastroenteritis is underreported in adults. It accounts for about 250,000 hospitalizations each yr.
- Statistics on sporadic cases of adult viral gastroenteritis are not known. Norovirus is the leading cause of medically attended acute gastroenteritis in U.S. children and is associated with nearly 1 million health care visits annually.
- It is estimated that there are 1.5 billion cases a year worldwide.
- It is the leading cause of death in many developing countries. Children under the age of 5 yr are most vulnerable.
- Viral gastroenteritis may be transmitted by the fecal-oral route, by asymptomatic carriers, or by symptomatic patients before the symptoms start.
- Traveler diarrhea affects 20% to 50% of residents of industrialized countries who travel to developing countries.

PREDOMINANT SEX:

- No sexual predilection
- Higher mortality seen in women
- Females have a higher incidence of *Campylobacter* infections

PREDOMINANT AGE:

- May occur at any age
- High morbidity and mortality in the very young (younger than 5 yr), the elderly (people aged 65 or older), and the immunosuppressed

RISK FACTORS

Use of proton pump inhibitors (PPI) may increase the risk of developing gastroenteritis.

PHYSICAL FINDINGS & CLINICAL PRESENTATION

- Diagnosis is made clinically. Laboratory studies are not routinely necessary.
- A well-taken history is important. The onset, duration, and frequency of diarrhea should be noted. The aim of the physical examination is to assess the patient's degree of hydration. This also helps to identify the cause of diarrhea and identify patients at risk of complications.
- Viral gastroenteritis has a short prodrome with vomiting, mild fever, and nonbloody and watery diarrhea, usually for 1 to 4 days.
- Bacterial gastroenteritis presents with high fever, bloody diarrhea, severe abdominal pain, and at least six stools in a 24-hour period.
- Patients usually present with
  1. Diarrhea: Usually more than six stools a day indicates bacterial cause of gastroenteritis.
  2. Vomiting.
  3. Abdominal pain (mild, diffuse abdominal tenderness on palpation).
  4. Mucus and/or blood in stool: Indicating bacterial or parasitic infection.
  5. Fever (101° F-102° F).
  6. Dehydration: This is the main cause of morbidity and mortality. Check for lethargy, dry mucous membrane, decreased skin turgor, hypotension, sunken eyes as signs of moderate to severe dehydration.
  7. Malnutrition: This occurs when diarrhea is chronic. There is reduced muscle and fat mass.
  8. Borborygmi: There is significantly increased peristaltic activity, which may cause audible or palpable bowel activity.
  9. Perianal erythema: Secondary to constantly wet area. Wet buttock and perianal area may result in redness and skin breakdown.

ETIOLOGY

- Viral gastroenteritis (in adults): The caliciviruses, such as *Norovirus* genogroup I (e.g., Norwalk), *Norovirus* (Fig. E1) genogroup II (e.g., South Hampton), *Sapovirus* (e.g., Sapporo)
- Nongroup A *Rotavirus*
- *Astrovirus*
- Adenovirus
- Table 1 describes the characteristics of the major gastroenteritis viruses
- Bacterial gastroenteritis: The top three leading causes of bacterial diarrhea worldwide are *Salmonella, Shigella,* and *Campylobacter* spp.
  1. *Salmonella* (eggs, dairy)
  2. *Shigella*
  3. *Campylobacter* (dairy, poultry)
  4. *Aeromonas species* (seafood, oysters)
  5. *Yersinia* (pork)
  6. Enterohemorrhagic *Escherichia coli* (ground beef)
  7. E. coli
  8. *Clostridium perfringens* (pork, vegetables)
- Parasitic gastroenteritis
  1. Giardia
  2. Cryptosporidium
  3. Microsporidia
  4. Cyclospora
- Traveler diarrhea
  1. Usually caused by Enterotoxigenic *E. coli,* but other organisms implicated include *Salmonella, Shigella,* and *Campylobacter.*
  2. Risk is highest in travelers to Africa, but it is also common in travelers to Portugal, Spain, and some Eastern European countries.

Dx DIAGNOSIS

DIFFERENTIAL DIAGNOSIS

- Amebiasis
- Appendicitis
- Celiac disease
- Inflammatory bowel disease (ulcerative colitis, Crohn disease)
- Colon cancer
- Bowel obstruction
- Botulism
- Hemolytic uremic syndrome
- Food poisoning
- Intraabdominal abscess
- Cholera
- Table 2 summarizes the differential diagnosis for gastroenteritis in adults

WORKUP

- Take a thorough history (see "Physical Findings & Clinical Presentation").
- In most cases, laboratory tests are not indicated.
- Further workup is indicated in patients who
  1. Have persistent diarrhea
  2. Are extremely dehydrated
  3. Appear seriously ill
  4. Have high fever
  5. Present with severe abdominal pain
  6. Have bloody diarrhea
  7. Have persistent nausea

LABORATORY TESTS

- Routine laboratory tests
  1. Tests such as CBC and BMP may not be indicated in making a diagnosis. However, electrolytes and BUN are indicated in patients with severe diarrhea or dehydration.
  2. CBC is indicated with severe diarrhea or toxicity. WBC is increased in *Salmonella* infection; eosinophilia is present in parasitic infections.
- Stool studies
  1. Presence of blood/leukocytes in stool may indicate inflammatory diarrhea.
  2. In *Salmonella* or *Shigella* infections there is an increased fecal leukocyte.

TABLE 1 Characteristics of the Major Gastroenteritis Viruses

Virus	Virus Characteristics	Methods of Detection	Epidemiologic Features
Rotavirus (species *Rotavirus A*, genus Rotavirus, family Reoviridae)	Nonenveloped, characteristic wheel-like, triple-layered capsid, 70-80 nm in diameter, double-stranded RNA genome	EM, ELISA LFI, PAGE, PCR	The most important cause of severe acute gastroenteritis in infants and young children. Vaccines are available for infants.
Norovirus (family Caliciviridae)	Indistinct substructure of virion surface, nonenveloped, 27-35 nm in diameter, single-stranded (+) RNA	EM, ELISA, LFI, PCR	Causes gastroenteritis in all age groups. Endemic in children and associated with outbreaks across the age groups. It can lead to severe disease among elderly and immunodeficient patients. Major cause of food-borne gastroenteritis.
Sapovirus (family Caliciviridae)	Characteristic cup-like depression on the surface, 27-35 nm in diameter, single-stranded (+) RNA	EM, PCR	Causes sporadic cases of gastroenteritis in all age groups. Rarely associated with outbreaks.
Enteric adenovirus (family Adenoviridae)	Nonenveloped, characteristic icosahedrons, 70 nm in diameter, double-stranded DNA	EM, ELISA, LFI, PCR	Serotypes 40/41. Causes sporadic cases of acute gastroenteritis mostly in children <5 yr of age.
Astrovirus (family Astroviridae)	Nonenveloped, characteristic star-like structure on the surface, 27-35 nm in diameter, single-stranded (+) RNA	EM, ELISA, PCR	Causes sporadic cases of acute gastroenteritis primarily in children and occasional outbreaks.

ELISA, Enzyme-linked immunosorbent assay; *EM*, electron microscopy; *DNA*, deoxyribonucleic acid; *LFI*, lateral flow immunoassay; *PAGE*, polyacrylamide gel electrophoresis; *PCR*, polymerase chain reaction; *RNA*, ribonucleic acid.
From Ryan ET: *Hunter's tropical medicine and emerging infectious diseases*, ed 10, 2020, Elsevier.

TABLE 2 Differential Diagnosis for Gastroenteritis in Adults

Incubation Period	Pathogen	Duration of Illness	Food Risk Factors	Type of Diarrhea
1-6 hr	*Staphylococcal aureus* *Bacillus cereus*	24-48 hr	Preformed toxin in unrefrigerated foods	Watery diarrhea; prominent vomiting
24-48 hr	Norovirus, rotavirus	48-72 hr	Molluscs and shellfish, leafy vegetables, fruit such as melon and raspberries, sandwiches, seasonal vomiting virus	Watery diarrhea; prominent vomiting; may have fever
8-16 hr	*Clostridium perfringens*	24-48 hr	Meat, poultry, canned foods	Watery diarrhea
10-16 hr	Enteric viruses (rotavirus, enteric adenovirus, astrovirus, sapovirus)	2-9 days	Fecally contaminated food or water	Watery diarrhea
24 hr	*Listeria monocytogenes*	Variable	Processed/delicatessen meats, hot dogs, soft cheese, pâtés, and fruit	Watery diarrhea
1-3 days	Enterotoxigenic *Escherichia coli*	2-3 days	Fecally contaminated food or water	Watery diarrhea
1-3 days	Nontyphoidal *Salmonella*	1-7 days	Poultry, eggs and egg products, fresh produce, meat, fish, unpasteurized milk or juice	Inflammatory diarrhea with fever, mucus, or bloody stools
1-3 days	*Campylobacter* spp.	5-14 days	Poultry, meat, unpasteurized milk	Inflammatory diarrhea with fever, mucus, or bloody stools
1-3 days	*Shigella* spp.	2-3 days	Raw vegetables, MSM activity	Inflammatory diarrhea with fever, mucus, or bloody stools
1-3 days	*Vibrio parahaemolyticus*	3 days	Raw seafood and shellfish	Inflammatory diarrhea with fever, mucus, or bloody stools
1-8 days	Enterohemorrhagic *E. coli*	1 wk	Ground beef and other meat, fresh produce, unpasteurized milk and juice	Inflammatory diarrhea with fever, mucus, or bloody stools
4-6 days	*Yersinia* spp.	1-3 wk	Pork or pork products, untreated water	Inflammatory diarrhea with fever, mucus, or bloody stools
7-14 days	*Giardia lamblia*	Days to weeks	Fecally contaminated food or water	Watery diarrhea
1-11 days	*Cyclospora cayetanensis*	May remit and relapse over a few weeks	Herbs and berries	Watery diarrhea
2-28 days	*Cryptosporidium parvum*	May remit and relapse over a few weeks	Vegetables, fruit, unpasteurized milk	Watery diarrhea
N/A	*Clostridioides difficile*	Varies but can be up to 10-14 days or longer	Antibiotic associated colitis, proton pump inhibitors	Watery or inflammatory diarrhea with fever, mucus, or bloody stools

From Spec A et al: *Comprehensive review of infectious diseases*, 2020, Elsevier

3. Stool leukocytes are absent in viral diarrhea.

- Stool culture:
  1. Are only useful when positive
  2. Usually not necessary in most cases of diarrhea
  3. Indications for stool cultures include: Bloody stools; prolonged, untreated diarrhea; fever; leukocytes in stool; immunosuppressed patients; immunocompromised patients; and patients who have traveled to remote, exotic, or developing nations. It should also be considered in patients with concurrent or very recent use of antibiotics to rule out *Clostridium difficile* infection as a cause of the diarrhea
- Examination for ova and parasites (O&P) is indicated in immunosuppressed patients; immunocompromised patients; and patients who have traveled to remote, exotic, or developing nations.

IMAGING STUDIES

- In patients with suspected bowel obstruction, perforation, or toxic megacolon, abdominal series is warranted.
- Consider CT scan of the abdomen in older patients with severe abdominal pain.

Rx TREATMENT

GENERAL CONSIDERATIONS

- Most infectious diarrhea is self-limited. Medical care is mainly supportive. Fig. E2 describes an approach to the management of gastroenteritis.
- It is important to assess the degree of dehydration by checking BP, pulse, HR, skin turgor, mucous membrane, thirst, urine output, and mental status change.
- Oral rehydration therapy is very important in diarrhea treatment.
- Consider intravenous rehydration when oral rehydration fails. Watch out for potassium depletion.
- Early re-feeding decreases recovery time.

Principles of treatment include

- Rehydration: Orally or intravenously, PRN
- Treatment of symptoms such as fever, abdominal pain, nausea, vomiting as needed
- Identify and treat complications

REHYDRATION:

- Oral hydration with sports drinks and broth in patients without signs of volume depletion. Oral rehydration solutions are preferred to sports drinks in patients with mild and moderate hypovolemia. These solutions provide hydration and electrolytes. Avoid soft drinks and fruit juices that have high sugar content.
  1. Indications for IV hydration include intractable vomiting/unable to tolerate oral hydration, severe dehydration/hypovolemia, change in mental status or consciousness, and ileus.
  2. Oral hydration is not appropriate due to environmental conditions.
- Intravenous solutions used include dextrose 5% in 0.5 isotonic NaCl with 50 mEq $NaHCO_3$ and 10 to 20 mEq KCl.

TREATMENT OF SYMPTOMS:

- Infectious diarrhea sometimes requires empiric treatment with antibiotics. Foodborne toxigenic diarrhea usually does not.
- Traveler diarrhea: Patients without fever or dysentery may be treated with rifaximin 200 mg thrice daily for 3 days, or ciprofloxacin 500 mg twice daily or 750 mg daily for 1 to 3 days; patients with fever or dysentery can be treated with azithromycin 1000 mg in a single dose.
- *C. difficile* diarrhea and parasitic infestations with *Giardia* or *Entamoeba* are treated with metronidazole or vancomycin. For *C. difficile,* it is important to discontinue the causative antibiotic.
- Treat severe nausea and vomiting with antiemetics.
- Antidiarrheal agents may be useful for systemic relief in mild to moderate diarrhea.
- Loperamide (Imodium) or bismuth subsalicylate (Pepto-Bismol) may provide limited relief in traveler or nonbloody diarrhea.

Dietary measures:

- Patient should eat as tolerated
- No restriction to diet
- Smaller meals, as well as bland, low-residue foods

As early as possible introduce lean meats and clear liquid

- Note that the evidence for banana, rice, applesauce, toast diet (BRAT diet), or eliminating milk and dairy products during a diarrheal episode is weak.

In recent years the use of probiotics (nonpathogenic live microorganism) has increased; however, recent multicenter trials of combination probiotic (combined *L. rhamnosus-L. helveticus* given twice/day) for children with gastroenteritis did not show any significant benefit and should not be recommended in young children with acute gastroenteritis.[1]

REFERRAL

Referral to infectious disease or gastroenterologist specialist may be indicated in patients

- With diarrhea lasting more than 7 days
- Hypernatremia
- Severe dehydration associated with cardiovascular symptoms
- In whom a parasitic etiology is suspected
- With *C. difficile* resistant to treatment with metronidazole and vancomycin
- With HIV/AIDS, immunocompromised
- With clinical features indicating extraintestinal involvement (e.g., meningitis, sepsis, pneumonia) or another etiology (e.g., hemolytic uremic syndrome)
- Who relapse

[1]Freedman SB et al: Multicenter trial of a combination probiotic for children with gastroenteritis, *N Engl J Med* 379:2015-2026, 2018.

PEARLS AND CONSIDERATIONS

PREVENTION

- Perform proper hand washing before and after eating and after each bowel movement to prevent spread to family members.
- Avoid (raw) shellfish served in certain unregulated places.
- Avoid raw or undercooked eggs and/or poultry.
- Wash all produce before consumption.
- For travelers to high-risk areas
  1. Eat only cooked foods.
  2. Drink hot or carbonated beverages.
  3. Avoid water, raw peeled fruits/vegetables, green leafy vegetables, and street food sold by street vendors.
  4. Vaccines are available for *Salmonella typhi* and *Vibrio cholerae* (the latter provides about 50% protection for 3-6 mo).

PATIENT & FAMILY EDUCATION

- Stress the importance of oral rehydration.
- Stress the need for early appropriate feeding.
- Relapse occurs due to dietary noncompliance.
- Travelers to developing areas should be educated on proper avoidance measures and treatment.
- Also stress the importance of good hygiene, hand washing, safe food preparation, and access to clean water as key in preventing gastroenteritis.

SUGGESTED READINGS

Available at ExpertConsult.com

RELATED CONTENT

Clostridium difficile Infection (Related Key Topic)
Gastroenteritis (Patient Information)
Giardiasis (Related Key Topic)
Traveler Diarrhea (Related Key Topic)

AUTHOR: **Daniel K. Asiedu, MD, PhD, FACP**

Gastroesophageal Reflux Disease (GERD) PTG

BASIC INFORMATION

DEFINITION

Gastroesophageal reflux disease (GERD) is a motility disorder characterized primarily by heartburn and caused by the reflux of gastric contents into the esophagus. A current definition is a condition that develops when the reflux of stomach contents causes at least two heartburn episodes per week and/or complications. Table 1 describes a classification system for esophagitis.

SYNONYMS

Peptic esophagitis
Reflux esophagitis
GERD

ICD-10CM CODES

K21.9 Gastroesophageal reflux disease without esophagitis
R12 Heartburn

EPIDEMIOLOGY & DEMOGRAPHICS

- GERD is one of the most prevalent gastrointestinal disorders. It is the most common GI diagnosis recorded during visits to outpatient clinics. From 18% to 28% of adults are affected.
- Nearly 7% of persons in the United States have heartburn daily, 20% have it monthly, and 60% have it intermittently. Incidence in pregnant women exceeds 80%.
- Nearly 20% of adults use antacids or over-the-counter H_2 blockers at least once a week for relief of heartburn.

PHYSICAL FINDINGS & CLINICAL PRESENTATION

- Physical examination: Generally unremarkable
- Clinical signs and symptoms: Heartburn, dysphagia, sour taste, regurgitation of gastric contents into the mouth
- Chronic cough and bronchospasm
- Chest pain, laryngitis, early satiety, abdominal fullness, and bloating with belching
- Dental erosions in children

ETIOLOGY

- Incompetent lower esophageal sphincter (LES) (see Fig. E1)
- Medications that lower LES pressure (calcium channel blockers, alpha-adrenergic antagonists, nitrates, theophylline, anticholinergics, sedatives, prostaglandins).
- Foods that lower LES pressure (chocolate, yellow onions, peppermint). Table 2 summarizes modulators of lower esophageal sphincter (LES) pressure
- Tobacco abuse, alcohol, coffee
- Pregnancy
- Gastric acid hypersecretion
- Hiatal hernia (controversial) present in >70% of patients with GERD; however, most patients with hiatal hernia are asymptomatic
- Obesity is associated with a statistically significant increase in the risk for GERD symptoms, erosive esophagitis, and esophageal carcinoma

Dx DIAGNOSIS

DIFFERENTIAL DIAGNOSIS

- Peptic ulcer disease
- Unstable angina
- Esophagitis (from infections such as herpes, *Candida*), medication induced (doxycycline, potassium chloride), eosinophilic esophagitis
- Esophageal spasm (nutcracker esophagus)
- Cancer of esophagus

WORKUP

- Aimed at eliminating the conditions noted in the differential diagnosis and documenting the type and extent of tissue damage. Generally, when symptoms of GERD are typical and the patient responds to therapy, there is no need for further diagnostic tests to verify the diagnosis.
- Upper GI endoscopy (Fig. E2) is useful to document the type and extent of tissue damage in persistent GERD and to exclude eosinophilic esophagitis and potentially malignant conditions such as Barrett esophagus. The American College of Physicians recommends endoscopy in the setting of GERD in people with heartburn and alarm symptoms (dysphagia, bleeding, anemia, weight loss, and recurrent vomiting). It is also indicated in people with GERD symptoms that persist despite a therapeutic trial of 4 to 8 wk of bid proton pump inhibitor (PPI) therapy in patients with severe erosive esophagus after a 2-mo course of PPI therapy to assess healing and rule out Barrett esophagus.

LABORATORY TESTS

- 24-hr esophageal pH monitoring with transnasal catheter or a 48-hr wireless capsule are sensitive diagnostic tests to assess the degree of acid exposure in the esophagus in patients not responding to acid-reducing therapy; however, they are not practical and generally not done. They are useful in patients with atypical manifestations of GERD, such as chest pain or chronic cough.
- High-resolution esophageal manometry (HRM) is indicated in patients with refractory reflux in whom surgical therapy is planned.
- *Helicobacter pylori* testing is not indicated in GERD.

IMAGING STUDIES

An upper GI series is useful in patients unwilling to have endoscopy or with medical contraindications to the procedure. It can identify ulcerations and strictures; however, it may miss mucosal abnormalities. Only one third of

TABLE 1 Los Angeles Endoscopic Classification System for Esophagitis

Grade A	**One or more mucosal breaks confined to folds, ≤5 mm**
Grade B	One or more mucosal breaks >5 mm confined to folds but not continuous between the tops of mucosal folds
Grade C	Mucosal breaks continuous between tops of two or more mucosal folds but not the circumferential
Grade D	Circumferential mucosal break

From Feldman M et al: *Sleisenger and Fordtran's gastrointestinal and liver disease,* ed 10, Philadelphia, 2016, Elsevier.

TABLE 2 Modulators of Lower Esophageal Sphincter (LES) Pressure

	Increase LES Pressure	Decrease LES Pressure
Hormones/peptides	Gastrin	CCK
	Motilin	Secretin
	Substance P	Somatostatin
		Vasoactive intestinal peptide
Neural agents	α-Adrenergic agonists	α-Adrenergic antagonists
	β-Adrenergic antagonists	β-Adrenergic agonists
	Cholinergic agonists	Cholinergic antagonists
Foods and nutrients	Protein	Chocolate
		Fat
		Peppermint
Other factors	Antacids	Barbiturates
	Baclofen	Calcium channel blockers
	Cisapride	Diazepam
	Domperidone	Dopamine
	Histamine	Meperidine
	Metoclopramide	Morphine
	Prostaglandin $F_{2}\alpha$	Prostaglandins E_2 and I_2
		Serotonin
		Theophylline

CCK, Cholecystokinin.
From Feldman M et al: *Sleisenger and Fordtran's gastrointestinal and liver disease,* ed 10, Philadelphia, 2016, Elsevier.

patients with GERD have radiographic signs of esophagitis on an upper GI series.

Rx TREATMENT

NONPHARMACOLOGIC THERAPY

- Lifestyle modifications with avoidance of foods (e.g., citrus- and tomato-based products, onions, spicy foods, carbonated beverages, mint, chocolate, fried foods) and drugs that exacerbate reflux (e.g., caffeine, β-blockers, calcium channel blockers, α-adrenergic agonists, theophylline)
- Avoidance of tobacco and alcohol use
- Elevation of head of bed (4 to 8 in) with blocks
- Avoidance of lying down directly after late or large evening meals, consumption of smaller and more frequent meals
- Weight reduction to BMI <25, decreased fat intake
- Avoidance of clothing that is tight around the waist

GENERAL Rx

- PPIs (esomeprazole 40 mg qd, omeprazole 20 mg qd, lansoprazole 30 mg qd, rabeprazole 20 mg qd, or pantoprazole 40 mg qd, or dexlansoprazole 30 mg) are generally safe, tolerated, and highly effective in most patients (Table E3). Omeprazole and esomeprazole are inhibitors of CYP2C19 and can increase serum concentrations of phenytoin and diazepam. Concomitant use of clopidogrel should also be avoided with omeprazole and esomeprazole. Increased risk of pneumonia has been documented in hospitalized patients. Long-term use of PPIs has been associated with increased risk of osteoporosis and patients should be warned about an increased risk of fractures with long-term use. Use of PPIs in patients with cirrhosis increases risk of spontaneous bacterial peritonitis and hepatic encephalopathy. Rare side effects of PPIs include acute interstitial nephritis, hypomagnesemia, and QT prolongation.
- H_2 blocker (famotidine 40 mg qhs) can be used but is generally much less effective than PPIs.
- Antacids (may be useful for relief of mild symptoms; however, they are generally ineffective in severe cases of reflux).
- Prokinetic agents (metoclopramide) are indicated only when PPIs are not fully effective. They can be used in combination therapy; however, side effects limit their use.
- Combination of PPE with an agent that reduces esophageal sphincter relaxation (baclofen) plus a neuromodulator (desipramine) may be tried in patients with refractory heartburn before considering surgery.
- For refractory cases: Think first, cut last. Surgery with Nissen fundoplication (Fig. E3). Potential surgical candidates should have reflux esophagitis documented by esophagogastroduodenoscopy and normal esophageal motility as evaluated by manometry. Surgery generally consists of reduction of hiatal hernia when present and placement of a gastric wrap around the gastroesophageal (GE) junction (fundoplication). Although laparoscopic fundoplication is now widely used, long-term medical therapy is a better choice for most patients who are willing to remain on daily acid-reduction medication. In patients preferring surgical intervention, surgery should not be advised with the expectation that patients with GERD will no longer need to take antisecretory medications or that the procedure will prevent esophageal cancer among those with GERD and Barrett esophagus. Approximately 17.7% of patients who undergo primary laparoscopic antireflux surgery will experience recurrent gastroesophageal reflux requiring long-term medication use or secondary antireflux surgery. Risk factors for recurrence are older age, female sex, and comorbidity.
- Endoscopic radiofrequency heating of the GE junction (Stretta procedure) is a treatment modality for GERD patients unresponsive to traditional therapy. Its mechanism of action remains unclear. Endoscopic gastroplasty (EndoCinch procedure) is also aimed at treating GERD. Initial results appear encouraging; however, long-term studies are needed before recommending these procedures.
- Lifestyle modification must be followed for life because GERD is generally an irreversible condition in most patients.

DISPOSITION

- Recurrence of reflux is common if treatment is discontinued. Preliminary trials have shown that in patients with severe reflux esophagitis successfully treated with PPI therapy, stopping PPI medication was associated with T lymphocyte–predominant esophageal inflammation and basal cell and papillary hyperplasia without loss of surface cells.
- The majority of patients respond well to therapy. In patients with chronic GERD, long-term outcomes are similar between medical therapy with PPIs and antireflux surgery. Prolonged use of PPIs is associated with increased risk of fractures of hip, wrist, and spine; increased risk of diarrhea from *Clostridium difficile;* pneumonia; and possible iron deficiency from impaired iron absorption. PPIs also block the effects of clopidogrel by inhibiting cytochrome P450 2C19 isozyme. Therefore all PPIs (other than pantoprazole) should be avoided in patients using clopidogrel. H_2 blockers can be used for patients with GERD taking clopidogrel.
- Postsurgical complications occur in nearly 20% of patients (dysphagia, gas, bloating, diarrhea, nausea). Long-term follow-up studies also reveal that within 3 to 5 yr, 52% of patients who had undergone antireflux surgery are taking antireflux medications again.

REFERRAL

- There is a strong and probably causal relation between symptomatic prolonged and untreated GERD, Barrett esophagus, and esophageal adenocarcinoma. GI referral for upper endoscopy is needed when there are concerns about associated peptic ulcer disease, Barrett esophagus, or esophageal cancer.
- Patients with Barrett esophagus should undergo surveillance endoscopy with mucosal biopsy every 2 yr or less because the risk of developing adenocarcinoma of esophagus is at least 30 times greater than that of the general population.
- Testing and treating for *Helicobacter pylori* in patients with GERD has not been shown to improve symptoms.
- All children with dental erosions should be evaluated for GERD.

RELATED CONTENT

Gastroesophageal Reflux Disease (GERD) (Patient Information)
Achalasia (Related Key Topic)
Dysphagia (Related Key Topic)

SUGGESTED READINGS

Available at ExpertConsult.com

AUTHOR: **Fred F. Ferri, MD**

Gestational Diabetes Mellitus (GDM)

BASIC INFORMATION

DEFINITION

Gestational diabetes mellitus (GDM) is hyperglycemia occurring during the second or third trimester in absence of a prepregnancy diagnosis of type 1 or type 2 diabetes.

Screening for gestational diabetes mellitus in asymptomatic pregnant women after 24 wk' gestation is a grade B recommendation by the U.S. Preventive Services Task Force (USPSTF). In the U.S., a two-step approach to screening is commonly used and is currently endorsed by the American College of Obstetricians and Gynecologists (ACOG) and the National Institutes of Health (NIH). The International Association of Diabetes in Pregnancy Study Group has recommended a simplified, one-step approach for screening and diagnosing GDM, which has been endorsed by the American Diabetes Association since 2011, with the acknowledgment that the one-step approach increases the prevalence of GDM without clear evidence of benefit. Pregnant women with diabetes mellitus (DM) (gestational or preexisting) are classified according to White classification (Table 1).

SYNONYMS

Gestational diabetes
Diet-controlled gestational diabetes (A1)
Medication-treated gestational diabetes (A2)

ICD-10CM CODES

O24.410	Gestational diabetes mellitus in pregnancy, diet controlled
O24.414	Gestational diabetes mellitus in pregnancy, insulin controlled
O24.419	Gestational diabetes mellitus in pregnancy, unspecified control
O99.810	Abnormal glucose complicating pregnancy

EPIDEMIOLOGY & DEMOGRAPHICS

INCIDENCE: Approximately 5% of pregnant women in the U.S. will be diagnosed with GDM using the two-step approach and 18% using the one-step approach.

PREDOMINANT SEX AND AGE: Women of childbearing age; increased risk is observed in women >35 yr.

RISK FACTORS:
- Overweight or obesity
- Family history of GDM or type 2 diabetes, particularly in first-degree relatives
- Polycystic ovarian syndrome
- Multiple gestation
- Hypertensive disorder of pregnancy or chronic hypertension
- Chronic systemic steroid use
- History of macrosomia in prior pregnancy
- Personal history of abnormal glucose tolerance or GDM in previous pregnancy
- Hispanic, Native American, African American, Asian, or Pacific Islander ethnicity
- Advanced maternal age (over age 35)
- Unexplained perinatal loss or malformation in previous or current pregnancy may be suggestive of preexisting diabetes

GENETICS: Higher rate in women with a family history of GDM or type 2 diabetes in a first-degree relative; specific human leukocyte antigen (HLA) alleles (DR3 or DR4) predispose to the development of DM type 2 after pregnancy.

PHYSICAL FINDINGS & CLINICAL PRESENTATION

Suspect GDM if:
- Fetal size greater than dates on Leopold or increased fundal height measurement
- Ultrasound findings of fetal macrosomia (especially enlarged abdominal circumference) or polyhydramnios
- Marked maternal obesity or weight gain above expected range
- Acanthosis nigricans (as underlying insulin resistance increases risk)
- Symptoms of diabetes
- Glucosuria
- Hemoglobin A1c greater than or equal to 5.7 in the first trimester

ETIOLOGY

During normal pregnancy several mechanisms contribute to increased insulin resistance. Placental secretion of human placental lactogen (hPL) decreases maternal insulin sensitivity, decreases maternal glucose utilization, and increases lipolysis, all to ensure adequate glucose availability to the growing fetus. Maternal pancreatic beta cells are increased in order to secrete additional insulin to compensate for the increased circulating blood glucose. Insulin resistance is also exacerbated by an increase in maternal adipose deposition, decreased exercise, and increased caloric intake. GDM occurs when maternal insulin secretion cannot meet the increased glucose burden, resulting in carbohydrate intolerance and hyperglycemia.

Dx DIAGNOSIS

DIFFERENTIAL DIAGNOSIS

Preexisting type 1 or 2 DM not previously diagnosed

WORKUP

- History with focus on personal medical history, prior pregnancy history, and family history
- Routine prenatal examination
- Laboratory evaluation (see the following)

LABORATORY TESTS

- Exclude preexisting diabetes.
- For women with risk factors (see above), order a 1-hr glucose tolerance test at the first prenatal visit, then repeat at 24 to 28 wk if initial screen was normal. If abnormal at intake, consider the probability of undiagnosed preexisting DM or underlying insulin resistance and check hemoglobin A1c. A diagnosis of diabetes is made if a woman meets any of the following criteria: Fasting plasma glucose >126 mg/dl, A1c >6.5%, random plasma glucose >200 mg/dl. The authors consider a first-trimester A1c of ≥5.7 suggestive of preexisting insulin resistance and would be inclined to monitor closely for hyperglycemia.
- Two-step approach:
  1. For screening without risk factors, a 1-hr, nonfasting 50-g oral glucose tolerance test (OGTT) is appropriate. If the result is abnormal (≥130 mg/dl, as defined by Carpenter and Coustan), a 3-hr, 100-g oral glucose tolerance test is performed. The diagnosis of GDM is made if two or more of the following glucose values are met or exceeded:
     a. Fasting: 95 mg/dl
     b. 1-hr plasma glucose: 180 mg/dl
     c. 2-hr plasma glucose: 155 mg/dl
     d. 3-hr plasma glucose: 140 mg/dl
  2. If one of four values on 3-hr glucose tolerance test is abnormal, consider repeat testing in 1 mo and recommend a low-carbohydrate diet immediately and consultation with a nutritionist. At least one study has demonstrated increased perinatal risk in women with only one of four abnormal values on 3-hr OGTT.
- One-step approach:
  1. Like the two-step, a one-step screening is performed at 24 to 28 wk on all pregnant patients who have not already been diagnosed with diabetes. This is a 2-hr, 75-g oral glucose tolerance test performed after an overnight, 8-hr fast. A diagnosis of GDM is made if one or more of the following values are met or exceeded:

TABLE 1 White Classification for Pregnant Women with Diabetes (Gestational or Preexisting)

Class	Description
A1	DM diagnosed during pregnancy and controlled by diet
A2	DM diagnosed during pregnancy and requiring medication
B	Insulin-requiring DM diagnosed before pregnancy, age >20 yr, lasting <10 yr
C	Insulin-requiring DM, onset at age 10 to 19 yr, with a duration 10 to 19 yr
D	Onset >10 yr or duration >20 yr, or associated with hypertension or background retinopathy
F	DM with renal disease
H	DM with coronary artery disease
R	DM with proliferative retinopathy
T	DM with renal transplant

DM, Diabetes mellitus.

a. Fasting: ≥92 mg/dl
b. 1-hr plasma glucose ≥180 mg/dl
c. 2-hr plasma glucose ≥153 mg/dl

- After pregnancy, women with GDM have an increased risk of developing diabetes during their lifetime. Women with GDM should be screened at or after 6 wk postpartum with a 75-g, 2-hr GTT to diagnose type 2 diabetes using the same criteria as nonpregnant patients. Alternatively, an HgbA1c can be performed at or after 12 wk postpartum.

IMAGING STUDIES

Ultrasound for fetal size is performed in women with GDM. It may be initiated at the time of diagnosis and repeated every 3 to 4 wk if macrosomia is suspected. Clinicians should consider local standards of care.

Rx TREATMENT

NONPHARMACOLOGIC THERAPY

- Glucose monitoring:
  1. Four times daily: Fasting and 2-hr postprandial (defined as 2 hr after the start of each meal)
  2. Goals: Fasting <95 mg/dl; 2-hr postprandial <120 mg/dl
  3. Can also use 1-hr postprandial goal of <140 mg/dl
- Dietary modifications for glycemic control:
  1. Follow a low-carbohydrate diet; avoid sugar and concentrated sweets; and eat small, frequent meals (three meals with two snacks is often recommended).
  2. Complex carbohydrates should be consumed over simple carbohydrates to prevent glucose fluctuations.
  3. Diet should adequately meet the needs of pregnancy (below) while restricting carbohydrates to 33% to 40% of daily calories. Caloric needs in pregnancy:
     a. BMI <30: 30 kcal/kg/day
     b. BMI >30: 25 kcal/kg/day
     c. BMI >40: 12 to 14 kcal/kg/day
  4. Regular moderate exercise, defined as 30 min five times per week.
  5. Ongoing nutrition counseling throughout pregnancy.

PHARMACOLOGIC Rx

Initiate if >20% of glucose values are elevated after trial of diet control:

- Insulin: Considered the gold standard in GDM management.
  1. There are no randomized controlled trials on insulin regimens, and therapy is largely guided by expert opinion.
  2. Insulin is the only FDA-approved medication for GDM (Pregnancy Class B) and does not cross placenta.
  3. Insulin may be started first line or added when oral medications have failed to achieve glycemic control. The authors consider factors such as the degree of hyperglycemia, obstacles to medication adherence, and gestational age at time of diagnosis (with early-onset diagnosis more likely to progress and require insulin) when initiating therapy. The ADA recommends insulin as first-line pharmacotherapy for GDM, and ACOG (2017) mirrors this recommendation (Level A).
  4. Regardless of insulin regimen initiated, blood glucose values should be reviewed frequently, and the regimen adjusted and customized to optimize each woman's blood glucose levels, using a single agent or combination of long, intermediate and/or short-acting insulins.
  5. One commonly used regimen:
     a. Insulin 0.7 to 1.0 U/kg/day SQ (based on current pregnant weight), with two thirds of the total daily dose given in the morning and one third of the total daily dose given in the evening.
     b. One third of each dose is given as short-acting insulin and the remaining two thirds as long-acting insulin.
- Oral hypoglycemics:
  1. Oral antidiabetic agents continue to be used in the management of GDM, despite a lack of FDA approval for this indication.
  2. Several recent studies have examined the potential benefits and harms of metformin and glyburide, comparing them with the gold-standard insulin and with each other. Metformin (compared with insulin) has been demonstrated to decrease maternal glucose levels, maternal weight gain, and the risk of gestational hypertension. Evidence grows that it may decrease the risk of preeclampsia as well. Although known to cross the placenta, concerns about the long-term risk in exposed offspring have been mitigated by at least one recent study showing no neurodevelopmental differences with intrauterine exposure to metformin versus insulin. Meanwhile, recent meta-analyses have demonstrated worse neonatal outcomes with the use of glyburide compared with insulin. With both metformin and glyburide, many women go on to require insulin therapy.
  3. As of 2017, ACOG recommends "in women who decline insulin therapy or for those women whom the obstetrician or obstetric care provider believes the patient will be unable to safely administer insulin, metformin is a reasonable second-line choice" (Level B); while suggesting that glyburide should not be recommended as a first-line agent due to a failure to achieve equivalent outcomes to insulin in most studies (also Level B).
  4. Metformin: Begin at 500 mg PO nightly or bid, and titrate up to a maximum of 2500 mg daily in divided doses.
  5. Glyburide: Begin at 2.5 mg qd, and titrate up to a maximum of 20 mg qd (10 mg bid). Increase dose as needed by 2.5 to 5 mg/wk.

ANTENATAL TESTING

Antepartum testing is recommended for women with pregestational diabetes and gestational diabetes. There is no consensus regarding initiation, frequency, or modality of antepartum testing in gestational diabetes, and this should be guided by local standards.

ONE COMMONLY USED REGIMEN

- Weekly NST/AFI beginning at 32 wk or when medications are initiated in women with GDMA2. Less frequent testing or delayed initiation of testing may be considered in women who maintain glycemic control with diet alone (GDMA1), as increased rates of stillbirth have not been observed in these women before 40 wk of gestation.
- Preexisting or poorly controlled diabetes, vascular complications, or concomitant hypertension: Twice weekly NST/AFI beginning at 28 wk. Consider hospital admission to obtain glycemic control.

TIMING AND ROUTE OF DELIVERY

- Women with preexisting diabetes should be induced at 39 wk.
- Women with GDMA2 may also be induced at 39 wk unless otherwise indicated, with decisions regarding induction guided by local standards of care.
- In women with GDMA1, ACOG supports expectant management of up to 40 and 6/7 wk with appropriate antepartum testing.
- Counsel regarding elective cesarean section at or after 39 wk if estimated fetal weight is over 4500 g.
- Consider delivery earlier than 39 wk if poor glycemic control or other medical indications such as growth restriction or preeclampsia.

INTRAPARTUM MANAGEMENT

- Goal is normoglycemia (80 to 120 mg/dl) using insulin and D5 lactated Ringer IV fluid if needed.
- Monitor glucose every 1 to 2 hr in active labor.
- Preparation for shoulder dystocia.
- If on glyburide, discontinue in labor or 12 hr before a scheduled induction.
- If on insulin, consider decreased long-acting insulin by one third to one half before scheduled induction. Most experts recommend holding insulin entirely the morning of a scheduled cesarean delivery.

POSTPARTUM MANAGEMENT

- Class A2: Check fasting blood glucose level before discharge; if abnormal, continue checking at home and schedule early follow-up with primary care physician to confirm diagnosis of DM.
- 6-wk postpartum visit: Screen for impaired glucose tolerance and diabetes with a 75-g, 2-hr glucose tolerance test. Alternatively, an HgbA1c may be performed at or after 12 wk postpartum.

- If no evidence of DM, screen annually for DM and counsel on risk factor modification.

REFERRAL

- Nutritionist
- Maternal-fetal medicine
- Diabetes educator
- Nurse care manager, when available

COMPLICATIONS

- Maternal: Preeclampsia, future type 2 DM or GDM, operative delivery
- Fetal: Polyhydramnios, macrosomia, congenital malformations, shoulder dystocia, birth trauma, IUFD
- Neonatal: Hypoglycemia, hypocalcemia, hyperbilirubinemia, polycythemia, perinatal death, respiratory distress, future obesity, and DM

PEARLS & CONSIDERATIONS

- Trials have shown that although treatment of mild gestational DM did not significantly reduce the frequency of a composite outcome that included stillbirth or perinatal death and several neonatal complications, it did reduce the risks of fetal overgrowth, shoulder dystocia, cesarean delivery, and hypertensive disorders.
- Lactation improves maternal glucose metabolism and may prevent or delay the development of type 2 DM following GDM. Higher lactation intensity and longer duration are independently associated with lower 2-yr incidences of DM after a GDM-affected pregnancy.

PREVENTION

Regular exercise, maintenance of ideal body weight, and high-fiber low-glycemic diet

SUGGESTED READINGS

Available at ExpertConsult.com

RELATED CONTENT

Gestational Diabetes (Patient Information)
Diabetes Mellitus (Related Key Topic)

AUTHORS: **Helen B. Gomez, MD,** and **Anthony Sciscione, DO**

BASIC INFORMATION

DEFINITION

Gestational trophoblastic disease (GTD) refers to a spectrum of neoplastic conditions that arise from abnormal proliferation of trophoblastic cells (cells that ultimately form the placenta). Gestational trophoblastic neoplasia (GTN) specifically refers to GTD with the potential for tissue invasion and metastases. GTN is a clinical and laboratory diagnosis and is characterized by a plateaued, rising, or prolonged persistence of elevated human chorionic gonadotropin (HCG) levels after evacuation of a mole; histologic diagnosis of choriocarcinoma, invasive mole, placental site trophoblastic tumor (PSTT), or epithelioid trophoblastic tumor (ETT); or evidence of metastatic disease after evacuation of a mole.

SYNONYM

Gestational trophoblastic neoplasia

ICD-10CM CODE

C58 Malignant neoplasm of placenta

TABLE 1 Risk Factors for Trophoblastic Neoplasia

Factor	Qualifier	Relative Risk
Maternal age	<20 yr	1.5
	>40	5.2
Prior SAB	1.9-3.3	
Parity	>1	0.4
Vitamin A	Median consumption	0.6
		Incidence
Race	Indonesia	1:85
	Japan	1:522
	Sweden	1:1560
	United States	1:1724
Socioeconomic status	Philippines (wealthy)	1:2000
	Philippines (poor)	1:200
Prior molar pregnancy	1	1:100
	>1	1:6 to 1:4
		Trend
Smoking	>15 cigarettes/day	Increasing
Infertility		Increasing
Theca-lutein cyst	>6 cm by ultrasound	Increasing (GTD subsequently develops in up to 50%)

GTD, Gestational trophoblastic disease; *SAB*, spontaneous abortion.
From Crum CP: *Diagnostic gynecologic and obstetric pathology*, ed 3, Philadelphia, 2018, Elsevier.

EPIDEMIOLOGY & DEMOGRAPHICS

INCIDENCE: In North America and Europe the incidence of GTD is approximately 1 to 2 per 1000 deliveries. The incidence of molar pregnancies in the United States is 1 in 1500 pregnancies. On a global scale, the incidence is thought to be less than 1 in 1000 pregnancies. From 15% to 20% of patients develop GTN after complete mole (CM) evacuation and 1% to 5% after partial mole (PM).

PREDOMINANT SEX AND AGE: There appears to be bimodal distribution in the incidence of molar pregnancy with a significantly higher incidence in women younger than 15 yr and older than 40 yr of age.

RISK FACTORS (TABLE 1):
- Extremes of reproductive age (younger than 15 and older than 40 yr of age)
- Personal history of GTD increases the risk of a subsequent molar pregnancy 10-fold
- A history of prior unsuccessful pregnancies increases the risk of GTD
- High HCG levels before evacuation, uterine size larger than dates, and theca-lutein cysts increase the risk of developing postmolar GTN

PHYSICAL FINDINGS & CLINICAL PRESENTATION

- Vaginal bleeding is typically the hallmark symptom of hydatidiform mole. Patients usually have delayed or irregular menses.
- Patients usually present with vaginal bleeding in the first trimester that spans from spotting to hemorrhage potentially requiring blood transfusion.
- Other clinical manifestation of GTD can vary depending on whether the molar pregnancy is complete or partial.
- CM may present with excessive uterine size for dates, theca-lutein cysts, preeclampsia, hyperthyroidism, or respiratory problems.
- Presentation of patients with GTN is highly variable (Table 2). Many are asymptomatic. If metastatic, GTN most commonly spreads to the lungs, vagina, pelvis, liver, and brain (Table 3). Therefore patients may present with symptoms related to the site of spread.

ETIOLOGY

- Complete moles have a diploid karyotype; 85% to 90% of cases are 46,XX. The chromosomes, however, are entirely of paternal origin. In 46,XX cases a haploid sperm duplicates its own chromosomes after meiosis. Dispermic fertilization of an ovum is possible and produces a 46,XY karyotype.
- Partial moles have a triploid karyotype, 69,XXX, 69,XXY, or less commonly 69,XYY. Composed of one maternal and two paternal haploid sets of chromosomes.

DIAGNOSIS

DIFFERENTIAL DIAGNOSIS

- Vaginal bleeding in women of reproductive age includes gynecologic causes as well as complications of first-trimester pregnancy.
- Malignant GTN should be considered in a woman of reproductive age who presents with metastatic disease from an unknown primary site or cerebral hemorrhage.

WORKUP

- Full patient history
- Past pregnancy history specifically asking about miscarriages, terminations, prior molar pregnancies
- Physical exam
- Blood work (Table 4)
- Imaging (Table 4)
- Staging if GTN is diagnosed (Table 5)
- FIGO score if GTN is diagnosed (Table 6)

LABORATORY TESTS

- Urine β-HCG
- Serum β-HCG levels
- CBC
- CMP
- Type and Rh
- Thyroid function tests
- Histopathologic evaluation of any products of conception, uterine curettings, etc.

IMAGING STUDIES

- Transvaginal ultrasound
- If there is concern for GTN, chest radiograph (CXR) should be obtained to look for metastasis
- Chest computed tomography (CT) and magnetic resonance (MR) imaging of the brain should be performed if lesions are seen in CXR

TREATMENT

- Suction dilation and evacuation (D&E) is the preferred treatment, especially when future fertility is desired. Hysterectomy in selected patients, however, may be considered.
- Chemotherapy is the mainstay of treatment for malignant GTN.
- Table 7 summarizes the management and outcome of trophoblastic neoplasia.

NONPHARMACOLOGIC THERAPY

- Following serial dilation of the cervix, the largest cannula that can be introduced through

TABLE 2 Clinico-Radiologic and Gross Pathologic Presentation of Trophoblastic Neoplasia

Disorder	Clinico-Radiologic Features	Beta–Human Chorionic Gonadotropin	Endometrial Curettings/ Hysterectomy (Gross)	Exclude
PHM	11-25 wk gestation ± fetal cardiac activity Vaginal bleeding Missed/incomplete pregnancy loss	Variable	Moderate amount of tissue Hydropic and normal villi Sac/membranes ± fetal parts (esp. syndactyly)	SAB CHM Aneuploid gestation (e.g., trisomy 13)
CHM	"Snowstorm" U/S Vaginal bleeding Toxemia Hyperemesis Thyrotoxicosis[a]	High (>100K mIU/mL)	Voluminous grapelike, transparent vesicles Ectopic pregnancy Mild diffuse swelling under dissecting microscope (early CHM)	SAB PHM
Persistent GTD/ invasive mole	Vaginal bleeding Prior CHM or PHM	Plateau (<10% drop in 14 days) or rising (>10% increase × 3 wk)	Minimal residual villous tissue Subtle, sometimes hemorrhagic myometrial nodule	Choriocarcinoma Unsuspected degenerating IUP
Choriocarcinoma	Irregular/severe bleeding Recent CHM or normal pregnancy Pulmonary, neurologic, or gastrointestinal symptoms	Rising, 2 wk after delivery After CHM: Plateau (<10% drop in 14 days) or rising (>10% incr. × 3 wk)	Hemorrhagic tumor nodules in endomyometrium	Persistent mole PSTT Unsuspected degenerating IUP
PSTT	Irregular vaginal bleeding Pregnancy months to years earlier	Persistent, low (50 mU/mL)	Discrete or infiltrative, polypoid or endophytic, tan, fleshy mass in endomyometrium	Exaggerated implantation site Placental site nodule Ectopic pregnancy Unsuspected IUP
ETT	Irregular vaginal bleeding Pregnancy months to years earlier	Persistent low (<150 mU/ mL)	Expansile mass, may be centered in cervix or lower uterine segment	Squamous cell carcinoma Placental site nodule Ectopic pregnancy PSTT
Spontaneous pregnancy loss/SAB	Vaginal bleeding, first/second trimester	Declining	Minimal villous edema (not typically grossly evident; by dissecting microscope or histology usually)	CHM PHM Ectopic pregnancy

[a]With first-trimester ultrasound screening and quantitative β-hCG, complete hydatidiform moles are most often diagnosed before clinical manifestations are evident.
β-hCG, Beta–human chorionic gonadotropin; *CHM*, complete hydatidiform mole; *ETT*, epithelioid trophoblastic tumor; *GTD*, gestational trophoblastic disease; *IUP*, intrauterine pregnancy; *PHM*, partial hydatidiform mole; *PSTT*, placental site trophoblastic tumor; *SAB*, spontaneous abortion; *U/S*, ultrasound.
From Crum CP: *Diagnostic gynecologic and obstetric pathology*, ed 3, Philadelphia, 2018, Elsevier.

TABLE 3 Clinical Classification System for Patients with Malignant Gestational Trophoblastic Neoplasia

Category	Criteria
Nonmetastatic GTN	No evidence of metastases; not assigned to prognostic category
Metastatic GTN	Any extrauterine metastases
Good-prognosis metastatic GTN	Short duration (<4 mo) No brain or liver metastases Pretherapy hCG <40,000 mIU/mL No antecedent term pregnancy No prior chemotherapy
Poor-prognosis metastatic GTN	Any one risk factor: Long duration (>4 mo) Pretherapy hCG >40,000 mIU/mL Brain or liver metastases Antecedent term pregnancy Prior chemotherapy

GTN, Gestational trophoblastic neoplasia; *hCG*, human chorionic gonadotropin.
From Disaia PJ et al: *Clinical gynecologic oncology*, ed 9, Philadelphia, 2018, Elsevier.

the cervix should be used. After complete suction D&E, gentle sharp curettage may be performed. Significant hemorrhage may occur at the time of D&E, therefore various uterotonics should be available at the time of procedure (oxytocin, methylergonovine, misoprostol). Rh immune globulin should be administered to nonsensitized RhD-negative women given the possibility of a partial mole and concomitant fetal tissue. Rh immune globulin can be withheld if complete mole is certain, but a diagnosis is often not known at the time of the procedure.

- Medical induction of labor with oxytocin or prostaglandin is not recommended given the risk of increased blood loss as well as an

TABLE 4 Diagnosis and Evaluation of Gestational Trophoblastic Neoplasia

Diagnosis of GTN	
After molar evacuation: Four values or more of plateaued hCG (±10%) over at least 3 wk: Days 1, 7, 14, and 21	
After molar evacuation: A rise of hCG of 10% or greater for three values or more over at least 2 wk: Days 1, 7, and 14	
After molar evacuation: Persistence of hCG beyond 6 mo	
The histologic diagnosis of choriocarcinoma, invasive mole, or PSTT	
Metastatic disease without established primary site with elevated hCG (pregnancy has been excluded)	
Evaluation of GTN	
Complete physical and pelvic examination; baseline hematologic, renal, and hepatic functions	
Baseline quantitative hCG level	
Chest radiograph or CT scan of chest	
Brain MRI	
CT or MRI scan of abdomen and pelvis	

CT, Computed tomography; *GTN*, gestational trophoblastic neoplasia; *hCG*, human chorionic gonadotropin; *MRI*, magnetic resonance imaging; *PSTT*, placental site trophoblastic tumor.
From Disaia PJ et al: *Clinical gynecologic oncology*, ed 9, Philadelphia, 2018, Elsevier.

TABLE 5 FIGO staging for Gestational Trophoblastic Neoplasia

Stage	Criteria
I	Disease confined to the uterus
II	Disease outside of the uterus but is limited to the genital structures
III	Disease extends to the lungs with or without known genital tract involvement
IV	All other metastatic sites

FIGO, International Federation of Gynecology and Obstetrics.
Modified from Kohorn EI: The new FIGO 2000 staging and risk factor scoring system for gestational trophoblastic disease: description and critical assessment, *Int J Gynecol Cancer* 2000;11:73. In Disaia PJ et al: *Clinical gynecologic oncology*, ed 9, Philadelphia, 2018, Elsevier.

increased risk of malignant sequelae when compared with suction D&E.

- If a patient does not desire future fertility, hysterectomy is an alternative to suction D&E. However, this also increases blood loss and does not eliminate the risk of malignant postmolar GTN sequelae.

PHARMACOLOGIC THERAPY

Various chemotherapeutic agents including methotrexate, dactinomycin, etoposide, actinomycin, chlorambucil, cyclophosphamide, and vincristine are used in the treatment of malignant GTN. Single- versus multiple-agent treatment depends on the staging of disease. Specifics of chemotherapy treatment are beyond the scope of this chapter, and patients diagnosed with malignant GTN should be referred to a gynecologic oncologist.

ACUTE GENERAL Rx

- Expeditious evacuation of suspected molar pregnancy should be performed.
- Effective contraception during postmolar surveillance is important because an early pregnancy may mask an elevation in HCG caused by GTN.
- Duration of chemotherapy depends on decrease in β-HCG to normal levels.

CHRONIC Rx

- Following D&E for a mole, close surveillance is necessary to monitor for the development of GTN. HCG levels are obtained every 1 to 2 wk until there are 3 consecutive normal levels and then at monthly intervals until 6 mo after the initial normal value.
- After 6 mo of surveillance, documenting remission, pregnancy can be recommended and β-HCG monitoring discontinued.
- No long-term therapy after successful treatment of GTN is needed.
- Surveillance of remission of GTN is necessary. HCG levels should be obtained every 2 wk for 3 mo, then every month to complete a year of follow-up. Physical exam every 6 to 12 mo for 3 to 5 yr should be performed.

DISPOSITION

- Cure rates for women with low-risk, nonmetastatic GTN approach 100%.
- Overall survival for patients with high-risk GTN is 86% to 92%.

TABLE 6 Scoring system for Gestational Trophoblastic Neoplasia

FIGO Score	0	1	2	4
Age (years)	<40	≥40		
Antecedent pregnancy	Hydatidiform mole	Abortion	Term pregnancy	
Interval from index pregnancy (months)	<4	4-6	7-12	≥13
Pretreatment HCG	<1000	1000-<10,000	10,000-100,000	≥100,000
Largest tumor size including uterus (cm)	<3	3-5	≥5	
Site of metastases	Lung	Spleen, kidney	Gastrointestinal	Brain, liver
Number of metastases		1-4	5-8	>8
Previous failed chemotherapy			Single drug	≥2 drugs

FIGO, International Federation of Gynecology and Obstetrics; *HCG*, human chorionic gonadotropin.
*Total score for a patient is obtained by adding the individual scores for each prognostic factor. Total score 0-6= low risk; >7= high risk.
From Kohorn EI: The new FIGO 2000 staging and risk factor scoring system for gestational trophoblastic disease: description and critical assessment, *Int J Gynecol Cancer* 2000;11:73.In Disaia PJ et al: *Clinical gynecologic oncology*, ed 9, Philadelphia, 2018, Elsevier.

TABLE 7 Management and Outcome of Trophoblastic Neoplasia

Disorder	Therapy	Risk of Progression	Comments/Caveats
PHM	1. Suction curettage 2. Follow β-hCG every week until <5 mIU/mL × 3 wk, then every month × 6 mo, then every year × 1-3 yr 3. Contraception × 1 yr	Persistent GTD = 4%-15% (often as retained products of conception with no or minimal proliferation) ChorioCa = essentially 0%	Confusion with a twin complete and normal gestation (rare)
CHM	Low-risk; same as PHM High-risk; chemoprophylaxis	Persistent GTD = 10%-30% Invasive mole = 15% ChorioCa: 2%-3%	If persistently elevated β-hCG: 75% have persistent GTD; 25% risk of ChorioCa
Persistent invasive mole	1. Evaluate for metastatic disease 2. Single-agent chemo until β-hCG <5 mIU/mL 3. Contraception for 1 yr 4. Hysterectomy for local control (optional) or bleeding complications		"Persistent GTD" is a clinical diagnosis applied to persistently elevated serum β-hCG following molar pregnancy and often treated empirically without pathologic sampling to distinguish persistent/invasive mole versus ChorioCa
Choriocarcinoma	1. Evaluate for metastatic disease 2. Single-agent chemo if low risk 3. Multiagent chemo if high risk 4. Hysterectomy for local control (optional)	Based on FIGO staging and WHO score Remission: No metastases = 80% Metastases = 67% Overall disease-free survival with single-agent chemo = 87%	
PSTT and ETT	1. Hysterectomy (therapy of choice) 2. Evaluate for metastatic disease 3. Multiagent chemo	Nonmetastatic disease: Cured by surgery Metastases = >30% at diagnosis Recurrence = 30% Mortality: 21%-36%	Poor prognosis: >5 mitoses/10 HPFs (recurrence), pulmonary metastases, antecedent pregnancy >4 yr prior

β-hCG, Beta–human chorionic gonadotropin; chemo, chemotherapy; *CHM*, complete hydatidiform mole; *ChorioCa*, choriocarcinoma; *ETT*, epithelioid trophoblastic tumor; *FIGO*, International Federation of Gynecology and Obstetrics; *GTD*, gestational trophoblast disease; *HPF*, high-power field; *PHM*, partial hydatidiform mole; *PSTT*, placental site trophoblastic tumor; *WHO*, World Health Organization.
From Crum CP: *Diagnostic gynecologic and obstetric pathology*, ed 3, Philadelphia, 2018, Elsevier.

TABLE 8 Surveillance during and after Therapy of Gestational Trophoblastic Neoplasia

Monitor serum quantitative hCG levels every week during chemotherapy:
1. Response: >10% decline in hCG during 1 cycle
2. Plateau: ±10% change in hCG during 1 cycle
3. Resistance: >10% rise in hCG during 1 cycle or plateau for 2 cycles of chemotherapy
   - Evaluate for new metastases
   - Consider alternative chemotherapy (see text)
   - Consider extirpation of drug-resistant sites of disease

Remission: Three consecutive normal weekly hCG values
1. Maintenance chemotherapy (see text)

Surveillance of remission:
1. hCG values every 2 wk × 3 mo
2. hCG values every month to complete 1 yr of follow-up
3. Physical examination every 6-12 mo for at least 3-5 yr

hCG, Human chorionic gonadotropin.
From Disaia PJ et al: *Clinical gynecologic oncology*, ed 9, Philadelphia, 2018, Elsevier.

- Overall, pregnancy outcomes in women with a history of molar gestations are similar to those without such a history.
- Surveillance during and after therapy of gestational trophoblastic neoplasia is summarized in Table 8.

REFERRAL

- Treatment of molar pregnancy and postmolar surveillance can safely be performed by a general OB/GYN.
- Patients diagnosed with malignant GTN should be referred to a gynecologic oncologist.

SUGGESTED READING

Available at ExpertConsult.com

AUTHORS: **Helen Toma, MD, MSPH, Kellie C. Forbes, MD,** and **Anthony Sciscione, DO**

BASIC INFORMATION

DEFINITION

Giant cell arteritis (GCA) is a segmental systemic granulomatous arteritis affecting medium and large arteries in individuals >50 yr. Inflammation primarily targets branches of the extracranial head and neck blood vessels (external carotids, temporal arteries, ciliary and ophthalmic arteries). The aorta and subclavian and brachial arteries can also be affected. Intracranial arteritis is rare.

SYNONYMS

Temporal arteritis
Cranial arteritis
GCA
Horton disease

ICD-10CM CODES	
M31.5	Giant cell arteritis with polymyalgia rheumatica
M31.6	Other giant cell arteritis

EPIDEMIOLOGY & DEMOGRAPHICS

INCIDENCE: Approximately 20 new cases per 100,000 persons >50 yr; peak incidence is in patients ages 60 to 80 yr.

PREVALENCE: 200 cases per 100,000 persons; it is the most common primary vasculitis; female/male predominance of twofold to fourfold; more common in Caucasians.

PHYSICAL FINDINGS & CLINICAL PRESENTATION

GCA can present with the following clinical manifestations:

BOX 1 Atypical Manifestations of Giant Cell Arteritis

Fever of unknown origin
Respiratory symptoms (especially cough)
Otolaryngeal manifestations
- Glossitis
- Lingual infarction
- Throat pain
- Hearing loss

Large-artery disease
- Aortic aneurysm
- Aortic dissection
- Limb claudication
- Raynaud phenomenon

Neurologic manifestations
- Peripheral neuropathy
- Transient ischemic attack (TIA) or stroke
- Dementia
- Delirium

Myocardial infarction
Tumorlike lesions
- Breast mass
- Ovarian and uterine mass

Syndrome of inappropriate antidiuretic hormone secretion (SIADH)
Microangiopathic hemolytic anemia

From Harris ED et al: *Kelly's textbook of rheumatology*, ed 7, Philadelphia, 2005, Saunders.

- Headache, often associated with marked scalp tenderness—noticed while brushing hair (hair comb allodynia)
- Constitutional symptoms (fever, weight loss, anorexia, fatigue)
- Polymyalgia rheumatica (aching and stiffness of the trunk and proximal muscle groups)
- Visual disturbances (transient or permanent monocular or binocular visual loss)
- Intermittent claudication of jaw and tongue on mastication that is especially prominent when solid food such as steak is chewed
- Box 1 describes atypical manifestations of GCA

Important physical findings in GCA:

- Vascular examination: The temporal artery demonstrates tenderness, decreased pulsation, and nodularity (ropy) (Fig. E1); diminished or absent pulses in upper extremities may be seen.

ETIOLOGY

Vasculitis of unknown etiology. An association with HLA-DRB*04 has been identified. Recent demonstration of varicella zoster virus virion, antigen, and DNA within the vessel walls of the temporal arteries on histopathologic specimens of giant cell arteritis suggest an association.

DIAGNOSIS

Clinical history and vascular examination remain cornerstones of diagnosis. An algorithm for diagnosing GCA is described in Fig. 2. The American College of Rheumatology has proposed classification criteria to aid in the diagnosis of GCA. Presence of three or more of these criteria in a patient with suspected vasculitis is considered suggestive of GCA:

- Age of onset of symptoms >50 yr
- New onset of or new type of localized headache
- Temporal artery abnormalities including tenderness or decreased pulsation
- Westergren erythrocyte sedimentation rate (ESR) elevated (typically >50 mm/hr)
- Temporal artery biopsy with vasculitis and mononuclear cell infiltrate or granulomatous changes

DIFFERENTIAL DIAGNOSIS

- Other vasculitis syndromes
- Nonarteritic anterior ischemic optic neuropathy (NAION)
- Pituitary apoplexy
- Primary amyloidosis
- Transient ischemic attack, stroke
- Infections
- Occult neoplasm, multiple myeloma

LABORATORY TESTS

- ESR elevated, although up to 22% of patients with GCA have normal ESR before treatment.
- C-reactive protein (CRP) is typically included in laboratory investigation; it may have greater sensitivity than ESR. CRP typically rises before the ESR.
- Mild to moderate normochromic normocytic anemia, elevated platelet count.

IMAGING STUDIES

Imaging studies do not play a major role in diagnosing GCA and are rarely indicated:

- Color duplex ultrasonography (CDUS) of temporal artery produces three characteristic features—periluminal "halo" over the temporal artery involved, segmental arterial stenosis, and arterial luminal occlusion in severe cases. CDUS of the temporal artery has 40% to 75% sensitivity and 79% to 83% specificity for diagnosis of GCA. Clinical utility is not superior to clinical examination with biopsy.
- Contrasted MRI of temporal artery may be performed in patients with contraindications to surgical biopsy of the superficial

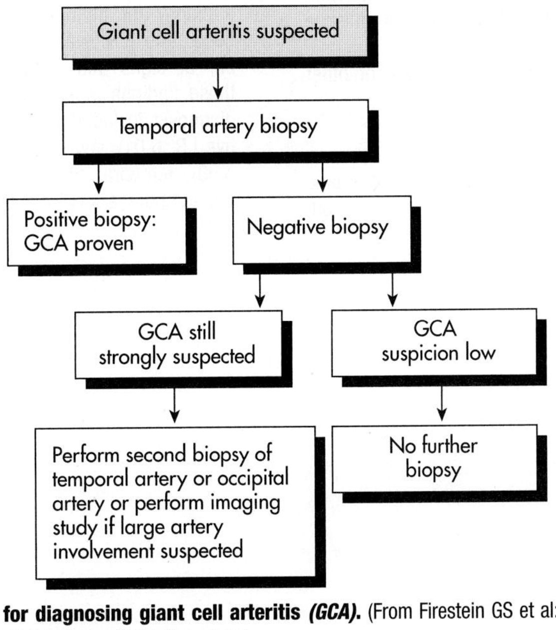

FIG. 2 Algorithm for diagnosing giant cell arteritis *(GCA)*. (From Firestein GS et al: *Kelly's textbook of rheumatology*, ed 9, Philadelphia, 2013, Saunders.)

temporal artery if treatment with steroids has not been initiated. MRI has a 78.4% sensitivity and 90.4% specificity in detecting temporal artery involvement in patients with a clinical diagnosis of GCA.
- Angiography of the arms is indicated in patients with peripheral vascular insufficiency.
- Fluorine-18-fluorodeoxyglucose (18F-FDG) positron emission tomography/computed tomography (18F-FDG PET/CT) imaging may be used to detect large-vessel inflammation in GCA. Sensitivity is 64% in the maxillary or temporal arteries and increases to 82% if vertebral arteries and increases specificity is 100%.

Rx TREATMENT

ACUTE GENERAL Rx

- If there is clinical suspicion of GCA, treatment should be initiated without waiting for results of laboratory or imaging studies.
- IV methylprednisolone (250-1000 mg for 1-3 days) is considered standard of care in patients with severe clinical manifestations such as visual loss from ischemic optic neuropathy.
- Oral prednisone (1 mg/kg/day): High-dose oral regimen should be continued at least until symptoms resolve and ESR returns to normal; usually 3 to 4 wk after treatment initiation. Steroid taper is very slow (10%-20% per mo) with monitoring of clinical features as well as ESR and CRP. When dose <10 mg/day, taper by 1 mg/mo. Treatment may last up to 2 yr or more.
- Although corticosteroids have traditionally been the treatment of choice, tocilizumab, an IL-6 receptor blocker, was recently approved by the FDA for the treatment of GCA. Patients treated with tocilizumab and prednisone achieved remission faster, had a greater reduction in steroid dosage, and had prolonged maintenance of remission when compared with those treated with prednisone alone.
- There is no evidence for the role of other steroid-sparing agents.

DISPOSITION

- With steroid therapy there is a dramatic improvement of systemic symptoms, but not vision in patients with ischemic optic neuropathy. In one study only 4% of eyes improved in both visual acuity and central visual field.
- Management of flares: Repeat prednisone induction if patient experiences severe flare. If mild flare, increase prednisone by 10% to 20% and slow down prednisone taper.

REFERRAL

- Surgical or ophthalmologic referral for biopsy of temporal artery
- Rheumatology referral for long-term immunosuppressive treatment management

PEARLS & CONSIDERATIONS

- Treatment of GCA should be started if there is clinical suspicion of the disease. This usually includes patients above the age of 50 presenting with a severe headache and systemic features that suggest GCA as well. Physicians should not wait for laboratory or pathologic confirmation before starting treatment as the risk of visual loss increases. Blindness from untreated GCA is permanent.
- Temporal artery biopsy should be performed as soon as possible, but within 2 wk of initiating treatment with steroids. The biopsy may remain positive for 2 to 6 wk after initiation of corticosteroids.
- Treatment should not be withheld pending temporal artery biopsy.
- A 2020 review and meta-analysis of 68 unique studies involving >14,000 patients with suspected GCA (approximately two thirds of which were women) set out to determine the clinical and laboratory features that were most helpful in supporting or refuting the diagnosis of biopsy-proven GCA. No single feature has strong enough positive or negative predictive value for the diagnosis, supporting the requirement of a biopsy for definitive diagnosis. A likelihood ratio (LR) was calculated for a number of signs and symptoms of GCA, and those findings most associated with a GCA diagnosis included limb claudication (positive LR, 6.01), jaw claudication (positive LR, 4.90), temporal artery thickening (positive LR), temporal artery loss of pulse (positive LR, 3.25), platelet count >400,000/μL (positive LR, 3.75), temporal tenderness (positive LR, 3.14), and ESR greater than 100 mm/h (positive LR, 3.11). Findings associated with an absence of GCA included the absence of ESR >40 mm/h (negative LR, 0.18), absence of C-reactive protein level of 2.5 mg/dl or more (negative LR, 0.38), and absence of age >70 yr (negative LR, 0.48).[1]

COMMENTS

- The relation between polymyalgia rheumatica and GCA is unclear, but the two frequently coexist. They are considered to be different points along the gradient or spectrum of the same disease.
- Clinical picture rather than ESR should be the prime yardstick for continuing prednisone therapy. A rising ESR in a clinically asymptomatic patient with normal hematocrit should raise suspicion for alternate explanations (e.g., infections, neoplasms).
- GCA is associated with a markedly increased risk for the development of aortic aneurysm, which is often a late complication and may cause death. Annual chest radiograph in chronic CGA patients has been suggested, as well as emergent chest CT or MRI for clinical suspicion.
- GCA is also associated with increased risk of myocardial infarction, stroke, and peripheral vascular disease.
- Coadministration of low dose aspirin (81 mg/day) has been reported by some as effective for further reduction of risk of blindness. Additional trials may be needed before it can be recommended as standard therapy.

SUGGESTED READINGS

Available at ExpertConsult.com

RELATED CONTENT

Giant Cell Arteritis (Patient Information)
Vasculitis, Systemic (Related Key Topic)

AUTHOR: **Joseph S. Kass, MD, JD, FAAN**

[1]van der Geest KSM et al: Diagnostic accuracy of symptoms, physical signs, and laboratory tests for giant cell arteritis: a systematic review and meta-analysis, *JAMA Intern Med* 180(10):1295-1304, 2020, https://doi.org/10.1001/jamainternmed.2020.3050.

BASIC INFORMATION

DEFINITION

Giardiasis is an intestinal and/or biliary tract infection caused by the noninvasive protozoal parasite *Giardia intestinalis* (also known as *G. lamblia* or *G. duodenalis*). The organism is a widespread zoonotic parasite and frequently contaminates fresh water sources worldwide.

SYNONYMS

Giardiasis
Giardia duodenalis (accepted species name by the CDC)
Giardia intestinalis

ICD-10CM CODE

A07.1 Giardiasis [lambliasis]

EPIDEMIOLOGY & DEMOGRAPHICS

INCIDENCE (IN U.S.):

- Exact incidence unknown. CDC estimates 20,000 cases a yr in the U.S.
- Frequently occurs as waterborne outbreaks in international adoptees, travelers, immunocompromised patients, and those with cystic fibrosis.
- *G. lamblia* has been demonstrated in 4% to 7% of submitted stool specimens, making it the most commonly identified intestinal parasite.

PREVALENCE (IN U.S.): 4%

PREDOMINANT SEX: Male = female

PREDOMINANT AGE:

- Preschool children, especially if in day care
- 20 to 40 yr of age, especially among sexually active homosexual men (oral-anal contact)

PEAK INCIDENCE:

- Varies with risk factors, outbreaks, but peak onset from early summer through early fall
- All age groups affected

GENETICS: Familial disposition: Patients with common variable immunodeficiency or X-linked agammaglobulinemia are at increased risk of infection.

PHYSICAL FINDINGS & CLINICAL PRESENTATION

- More than 70% with one or more intestinal symptoms (diarrhea, flatulence, cramps, bloating, nausea). Table 1 summarizes clinical signs and symptoms of giardiasis
- Incubation period averages 7 to 21 days
- Fever in <30%
- Chronic diarrhea, malabsorption, and weight loss, which can be up to 10% of body weight, are common
- GI bleeding is unusual
- Continuous or intermittent symptoms, lasting for 2 to 4 wk
- Of infected patients, 20% to 25% are asymptomatic and can shed cysts for months

TABLE 1 Symptoms of Giardiasis

Symptom	Frequency (%)
Flatulence	56-74
Anorexia	40-64
Abdominal cramps	55-80
Foul-smelling stool	57-72
Abdominal distention	31
Bloating	55-69
Nausea	58-68
Malaise	84
Diarrhea	89
Belching	30
Weight loss	48-64
Fever	17-28

From Cherry JD et al: *Feigin and Cherry's pediatric infectious diseases*, ed 8, Philadelphia, 2019, Elsevier.

ETIOLOGY

Infection is acquired by ingestion of viable cysts of the organism (Fig. 1), typically in contaminated water or food or by fecal-oral contact. *Giardia* cysts are resistant to chlorination and survive well in cold mountain streams. Fig. E2 illustrates the life cycle of *Giardia duodenalis.*

DIAGNOSIS

DIFFERENTIAL DIAGNOSIS

- Other agents of infective diarrhea (amebae, *Salmonella* sp., *Shigella* sp., *Staphylococcus aureus, Cryptosporidium,* etc.)
- Noninfectious causes of malabsorption

WORKUP

- Stool specimen (three specimens yield 90% sensitivity) as a saline suspension or duodenal aspirate for microscopic examination to establish diagnosis and exclude other pathogens.
- Immunoassays for *Giardia* sp. Antigens in stool samples such as the DFA or ELISA are now routinely used in most clinical laboratories. These assays are 85% to 98% sensitive and 90% to 100% specific. They are more sensitive than stool microscopy for confirming the diagnosis. They also have a faster turnaround time.

LABORATORY TESTS

Serum albumin, vitamin B_{12} levels, and stool fat test to exclude malabsorption

IMAGING STUDIES

- Not necessary unless biliary obstruction is suspected
- In detection of organism, possible interference by barium in stool from radiographic studies

TREATMENT

NONPHARMACOLOGIC THERAPY

Avoidance of milk products to reduce symptoms of transient lactase deficiency that occur in many patients and can last for weeks to months.

GENERAL Rx

Adult and pediatric (see Table E2):

- Metronidazole: 250 mg PO tid for 5 to 10 days. Pediatric dose: 5 mg/kg tid × 7 days (metronidazole should be avoided in pregnancy)
- Alternative regimen: Tinidazole: 2-g single dose (50 mg/kg in children over 3 yr of age)
- Nitazoxanide: In children aged 12 to 47 mo: 100 mg bid × 3 days. Aged 4 to 11 yr: 200 mg bid × 3 days
- Quinacrine: 100 mg PO tid × 5 to 7 days
- Albendazole: 400 mg PO qd × 5 days
- Paromomycin: 25 to 35 mg/kg/day in three doses for 5 to 10 days. Safe for pregnancy

DISPOSITION

Re-infection is possible. Postinfection lactose intolerance is common and is frequently mistaken for recurrent infection.

PEARLS & CONSIDERATIONS

COMMENTS

Travelers to endemic areas (developing world, wilderness areas) should be cautioned to boil drinking water or use water purification tablets (for iodine-containing products, chlorination is not effective). Chronic giardiasis as seen in developing nations can cause delays in growth and development in children due to malabsorption and diarrhea.

SUGGESTED READINGS

Available at ExpertConsult.com

RELATED CONTENT

Giardiasis (Patient Information)

AUTHOR: **Glenn G. Fort, MD, MPH**

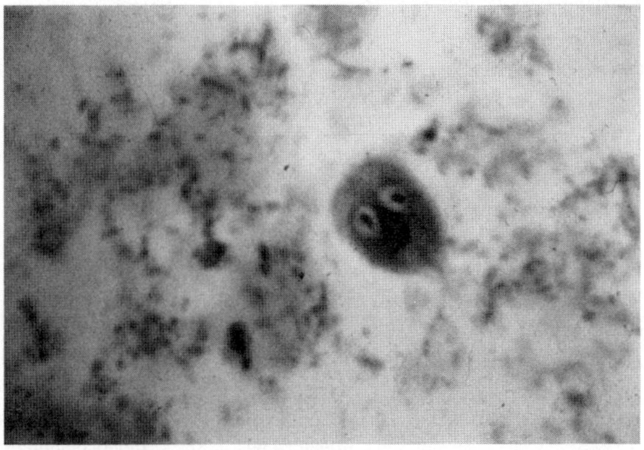

FIG. 1 ***Giardia lamblia*** **trophozoite demonstrated in a trichrome stain of fecal material.** Note the prominent nuclei in the trophozoite. (From Bennett JE et al: *Mandell, Douglas, and Bennett's principles and practice of infectious diseases*, ed 8, Philadelphia, 2015, Saunders.)

Gilbert Syndrome ALG

BASIC INFORMATION

DEFINITION

Gilbert syndrome is an autosomal-dominant disorder characterized by indirect hyperbilirubinemia caused by impaired glucuronyl transferase activity.

SYNONYM

Gilbert disease

ICD-10CM CODE

E80.4 Gilbert syndrome

EPIDEMIOLOGY & DEMOGRAPHICS

INCIDENCE (IN U.S.): Probable autosomal-dominant disease affecting >5% of the U.S. population

PREDOMINANT SEX: Male:female ratio of 3:1

GENETICS: Most common hereditary hyperbilirubinemia (genotypic prevalence 12%)

PHYSICAL FINDINGS & CLINICAL PRESENTATION

- No abnormalities on physical examination other than mild jaundice when bilirubin exceeds 3 mg/dl.
- A family history of unconjugated hyperbilirubinemia may be present.

ETIOLOGY

- Decreased elimination of bilirubin in bile is caused by inadequate conjugation of bilirubin.
- Alcohol consumption and starvation diet can increase bilirubin level.
- The pathogenesis of Gilbert syndrome has been linked to a reduction in the bilirubin UGT-1 gene *(HUG-Brl)* transcription, resulting from a mutation in the promoter region.

DIAGNOSIS

DIFFERENTIAL DIAGNOSIS

- Hemolytic anemia
- Liver disease (chronic hepatitis, cirrhosis)
- Crigler-Najjar syndrome
- Table 1 summarizes principal features of hereditary disorders of bilirubin metabolism

WORKUP

- Most patients are diagnosed during or after adolescence, when isolated hyperbilirubinemia is detected as an incidental finding on routine biochemical testing.
- Laboratory evaluation to exclude hemolysis and liver diseases as a cause of the elevated bilirubin level (Table 2 and Fig. 1).

LABORATORY TESTS

Elevated indirect (unconjugated) bilirubin (rarely exceeds 5 mg/dl)

TREATMENT

ACUTE GENERAL Rx

Treatment is generally unnecessary. Phenobarbital (if clinical jaundice is present) can rapidly decrease serum indirect bilirubin level.

DISPOSITION

Prognosis is excellent. Treatment is generally unnecessary.

REFERRAL

Referral is generally not necessary.

PEARLS & CONSIDERATIONS

COMMENTS

- Patients should be reassured about the benign nature of the condition.
- Fasting for 2 days or significant dehydration may raise the bilirubin level and result in the clinical recognition of jaundice.

AUTHOR: **Fred F. Ferri, MD**

TABLE 1 Principal Features of the Hereditary Disorders of Bilirubin Metabolism

Feature	Crigler-Najjar Syndrome Type I	Crigler-Najjar Syndrome Type II	Gilbert Syndrome	Dubin-Johnson Syndrome	Rotor Syndrome
Incidence	Very rare	Uncommon	Up to 12% of population	Uncommon	Rare
Total serum bilirubin (mg/dl)	18-45 (usually >20), unconjugated	6-25 (usually ≤20), unconjugated	Typically ≤4 in absence of fasting or overt hemolysis; mostly unconjugated	Typically 2-5, less often ≤25; approximately 60% direct reacting	Usually 3-7, occasionally ≤20; approximately 60% direct reacting
Defect(s) in bilirubin metabolism*	Bilirubin UGT1A1 conjugating activity markedly reduced: Trace to absent	Bilirubin UGT1A1 conjugating activity reduced: ≤10% of normal	Complex haplotype Bilirubin UGT1A1 conjugating activity typically reduced to 10%-33% of normal; reduced bilirubin uptake in some cases; mild hemolysis in up to 50% of patients	Impaired canalicular secretion of conjugated bilirubin owing to MRP2/cMOAT mutation	Impaired hepatic secretion or storage of conjugated bilirubin owing to impaired reuptake of bilirubin conjugates resulting from simultaneous OATP1B1 and OATP1B3 mutations
Routine liver tests	Normal	Normal	Normal	Normal	Normal
Serum bile acids	Normal	Normal	Normal	Usually normal	Normal
Pharmacologic responses/special features†	No response to phenobarbital	Phenobarbital reduces bilirubin by ≤75%	Phenobarbital reduces bilirubin, often to normal	Increased bilirubin concentration with estrogens; diagnostic urine coproporphyrin isomer pattern (total is normal, with isomer I increased to ≥80% of total)	Characteristic urine coproporphyrin excretion pattern (total is increased ≤2.5-fold in ≈65% of cases but isomer I always <80% of total)
Major clinical features	Kernicterus in infancy if untreated; may occur later despite therapy	Rare late-onset kernicterus with fasting	None	Occasional hepatosplenomegaly	None
Hepatic morphology/histology	Normal	Normal	Normal; occasionally increased lipofuscin pigment	Liver grossly black; coarse, dark centrilobular pigment	Normal
Bile bilirubin fractions‡	>90% unconjugated	Largest fraction (mean 57%) monoconjugates	Mainly diconjugates but monoconjugates are increased (mean 23%)	Mixed conjugates, reported increase in diconjugates	Increased conjugates

Continued

TABLE 1 Principal Features of the Hereditary Disorders of Bilirubin Metabolism—cont'd

Feature	Crigler-Najjar Syndrome Type I	Crigler-Najjar Syndrome Type II	Gilbert Syndrome	Dubin-Johnson Syndrome	Rotor Syndrome
Inheritance (all autosomal)	Recessive	Recessive	Promoter mutation is recessive; missense mutation often dominant	Recessive; rare kindred appears dominant	Recessive
Diagnosis	Clinical and laboratory findings, lack of response to phenobarbital	Clinical and laboratory findings, response to phenobarbital	Clinical and laboratory findings; promoter genotyping; liver biopsy rarely necessary	Clinical and laboratory findings; liver biopsy unnecessary if coproporphyrin studies available	Clinical and laboratory findings; urine coproporphyrin analysis
Treatment	Phototherapy or tin protoporphyrin as short-term therapy; liver transplantation definitive	Consider phenobarbital if baseline bilirubin ≥8 mg/dl	None necessary	Avoid estrogens; no other therapy necessary	No treatment necessary

*UGT1A1 = bilirubin specific isoform of the UGT1 family of uridine diphosphate glucuronosyltransferases.
†Sulfobromophthalein (BSP) was historically used to distinguish between Dubin-Johnson and Rotor syndromes based on the rate of removal of the dye from the circulation.
‡Bilirubin in normal bile: <5% unconjugated bilirubin, with an average of 7% bilirubin monoconjugates and 90% bilirubin diconjugates.
From Goldman L, Shafer AI: *Goldman-Cecil medicine,* ed 26, 2020, Elsevier.

TABLE 2 Characteristic Patterns of Liver Function Tests

Disorder	Bilirubin	Alkaline Phosphatase	AST	ALT	Prothrombin Time	Albumin
Gilbert syndrome (abnormal bilirubin metabolism)	↑	NL	NL	NL	NL	NL
Bile duct obstruction (pancreatic cancer)	↑↑↑	↑↑↑	↑	↑	↑-↑↑	NL
Acute hepatocellular damage (toxic, viral hepatitis)	↑-↑↑↑	↑-↑↑	↑↑↑	↑↑↑	NL-↑↑↑	NL-↓↓
Cirrhosis	NL-↑	NL-↑	NL-↑	NL-↑	NL-↑↑	NL-↓↓

ALT, Alanine aminotransferase; *AST,* aspartate aminotransferase; *NL,* normal; *↑,* increase; *↓,* decrease (arrows indicate extent of change: ↑-↑↑↑, slight to large).
From Andreoli TE (ed): *Cecil essentials of medicine,* ed 6, Philadelphia, 2005, WB Saunders.

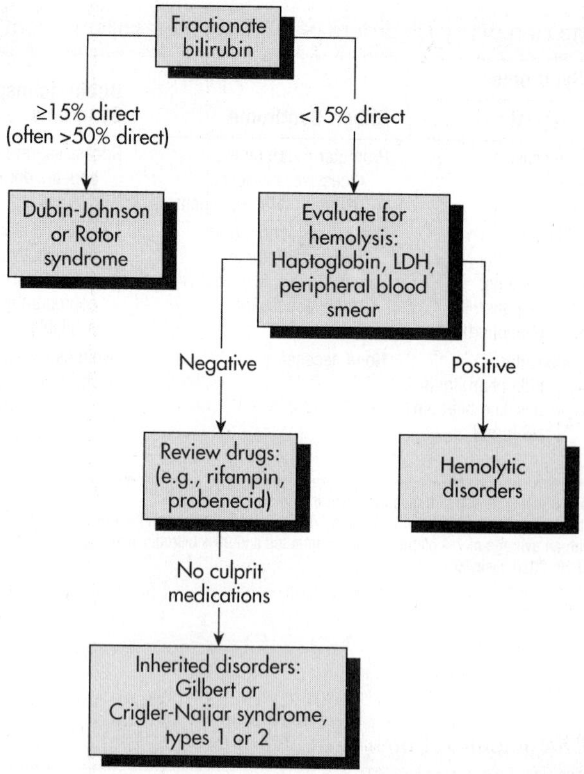

FIG. 1 Evaluation of an isolated elevation of the serum bilirubin level. *LDH,* Lactic dehydrogenase. (From Feldman M et al [eds]: *Sleisenger and Fordtran's gastrointestinal and liver disease,* ed 10, Philadelphia, 2016, WB Saunders.)

BASIC INFORMATION

DEFINITION

Glaucoma is a chronic degenerative optic neuropathy (or the high potential for such degeneration due to risk factors) in which the neuro-retinal rim of the optic nerve becomes progressively thinner, thereby enlarging the optic-nerve cup. The classification of glaucoma is based on the appearance of the iridocorneal angle (open angle vs. narrow or closed angle) and is further subdivided into primary and secondary types. Fig. 1 and Table 1 illustrate the difference between open-angle and narrow-angle glaucoma. Primary open-angle glaucoma can occur with or without elevated intraocular pressure (IOP). Normal tension glaucoma refers to primary open-angle glaucoma without elevated intraocular pressure.

SYNONYMS

Primary open-angle glaucoma (POAG)
Open-angle glaucoma or chronic open-angle glaucoma (OAG, COAG)
Secondary open-angle glaucoma (e.g., pseudoexfoliation, pigment dispersion, trauma, inflammatory)
Ocular hypertension (elevated intraocular pressure with no evidence of optic nerve damage)
Optic nerve cupping, glaucoma suspect

ICD-10CM CODES	
H40.10X0	Unspecified open-angle glaucoma, stage unspecified
H40.10X1	Unspecified open-angle glaucoma, mild stage
H40.10X2	Unspecified open-angle glaucoma, moderate stage
H40.10X3	Unspecified open-angle glaucoma, severe stage
H40.10X4	Unspecified open-angle glaucoma, indeterminate stage
H40.11X0	Primary open-angle glaucoma, stage unspecified
H40.11X1	Primary open-angle glaucoma, mild stage
H40.11X2	Primary open-angle glaucoma, moderate stage
H40.11X3	Primary open-angle glaucoma, severe stage
H40.11X4	Primary open-angle glaucoma, indeterminate stage

EPIDEMIOLOGY & DEMOGRAPHICS

INCIDENCE (IN U.S.): Third most common cause of vision loss (75%-95% of all forms of glaucoma are open angle)

PREVALENCE (IN U.S.):
- Overall prevalence in U.S. population aged >40 yr is estimated to be 1.86%.
- Prevalence is higher in people with diabetes, those with high myopia, and older persons.
- More common in African American population (three times the age-adjusted prevalence than whites). There is a genetic tendency to OAG; multiple genes have been isolated that are associated with development of high IOP and optic nerve damage.

PREDOMINANT AGE:
- Persons >50 yr
- Can occur in third and fourth decades, and juvenile forms are rare

PEAK INCIDENCE:
- Increases after age 40 yr
- Three million cases in 2019, rising with the rapid increase in aging population

PHYSICAL FINDINGS & CLINICAL PRESENTATION

- High intraocular pressures and/or large optic nerve cup (Fig. E2). Ocular Hypertension Treatment Study results help to delineate important risk factors, including high eye pressure, thin corneal central thickness, age, and visual field results.
- Abnormal visual fields (with advanced glaucoma damage to the optic nerve).
- Open anterior chamber angle—evaluated with gonioscopy at slit lamp.
- Figs. E3 and E4 illustrate stages of open-angle glaucoma.
- Because early treatable stages of OAG normally have no symptoms, routine eye exams are imperative, especially for patients with family history and patients over age 60 yr.
- Secondary forms of OAG may exhibit ocular findings such as pseudoexfoliation, pigment dispersion, blood in anterior chamber, inflammation.

ETIOLOGY

- Uncertain hereditary tendency (multifactorial genetics)
- Topical steroids can induce high IOP and cause glaucoma
- Trauma
- Inflammatory (e.g., history of uveitis)
- High-dose oral corticosteroids taken for prolonged periods

Dx DIAGNOSIS

DIFFERENTIAL DIAGNOSIS

- Other optic neuropathies (previous retinal vascular disorders, optic nerve pits, or coloboma).
- Physiologic cupping of the optic nerve: The optic nerve may appear similar to glaucoma damage but does not progress. This is followed for any signs of progression.
- Ocular hypertension: IOP is chronically elevated, but not causing optic nerve damage, must monitor closely.
- Secondary glaucoma from inflammation and steroid therapy.
- Trauma

WORKUP

- Comprehensive eye examination
- Intraocular pressure
- Slit lamp examination
- Visual fields
- Gonioscopy: To determine the type of glaucoma (narrow, open, or closed angles)
- Nerve fiber analysis (e.g., optical coherence topography [OCT] and Heidelberg Retinal tomography [HRT])

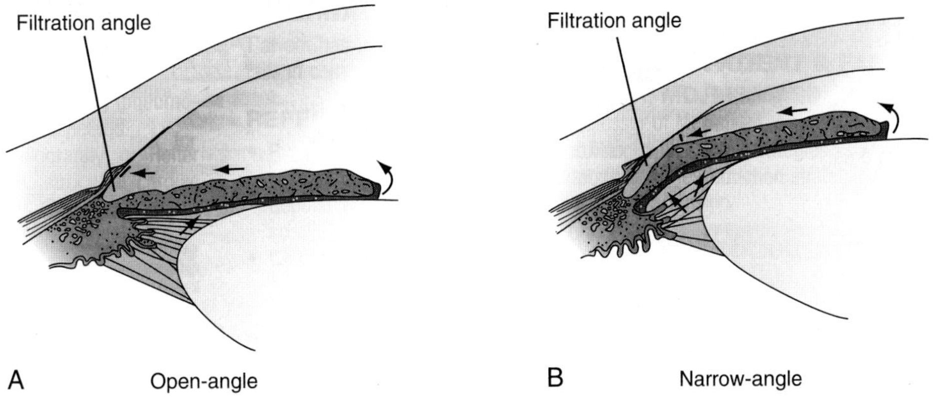

FIG. 1 **A,** Open-angle glaucoma: Drainage of the aqueous humor becomes obstructed, and impaired flow from the eye leads to gradually increased intraocular pressure. **B,** Narrow-angle glaucoma: When the iris moves forward, as may occur during pupil dilation, the angle is narrowed or even closed. Obstruction of aqueous humor flow leads to angle-closure glaucoma. (From Kaufman DM et al: *Kaufman's clinical neurology for psychiatrists*, ed 8, Philadelphia, 2017, Elsevier.)

TABLE 1 Characteristics of Glaucoma

Feature	Primary Open-Angle Glaucoma	Narrow-Angle Glaucoma
Occurrence	85% of all glaucoma cases	15% of all glaucoma cases
Cause	Unclear*	Closed angle prevents aqueous drainage
Age at onset	Variable	50 to 85 yr
Anterior chamber	Usually normal	Shallow
Chamber angle	Normal	Narrow
Symptoms	Usually none Decreased vision, late	Headache Seeing halos around lights Sudden onset of severe eye pain Vomiting during attack
Cupping of disc	Progressive if not treated	After one or more untreated attacks
Visual fields	Peripheral fields are involved early Central involvement is a very late sign	Involvement is a late sign
Ocular pressure	Progressively higher if not medically controlled Late: High	Early: Detected with provocative tests only
Other signs		Fixed, partially dilated pupil Conjunctival injection "Steamy" cornea†
Treatment	Medical Laser surgery	Surgical
Prognosis	Good if recognized early Very dependent on patient compliance	Good

*Thought to be a defect in the trabecular network ultrastructure.
†Like looking through a steamy window.
From Swartz MH: *Textbook of physical diagnosis, history and examination,* ed 7, Philadelphia, 2014, Elsevier.

- Corneal thickness (thick central cornea will result in possible overestimation of the true physiologic IOP, and vice versa, so this is important information in diagnosis and treatment of OAG)

LABORATORY TESTS

Blood sugar

IMAGING STUDIES

- Optic nerve photography—stereo photographs
- Visual field testing
- Laser scan of nerve fiber layer, OCT, HRT. Rarely, MRI of orbits if the glaucoma findings are atypical or suspicious of other causes of optic nerve atrophy.

Rx TREATMENT

ACUTE GENERAL Rx

- β-Blockers (e.g., timolol) qd to bid depending on individual response to drug.
- Carbonic anhydrase inhibitors (e.g., Diamox 250 mg qid or 500 mg bid).
- Prostaglandin analogues (latanoprost, bimatoprost, travoprost, tafluprost) are commonly used as first-line treatment. They lower intraocular pressure by 25% to 30% by increasing uveoscleral outflow and reducing aqueous production. These products are available as opthalmic solutions and emulsions. Bimatoprost is also available as an intracameral implant.
- Alpha-2 agonists and cholinergic agonists.
- Hyperosmotic agents (mannitol) in acute treatment (IV).
- Selective laser trabeculoplasty (SLT) may delay or forestall need for second eye drop. The effect may be temporary, but the laser can be repeated.

CHRONIC Rx

- At least biannual checks of intraocular pressure and adjustment of medication.
- Surgical trabeculectomy and filter valve surgeries can be considered for glaucoma that progresses (optic nerve changes or visual field progression) despite maximal tolerated medical therapies. Recently, minimally invasive glaucoma surgeries (MIGS) have been advocated for IOP control. Some are performed at the time of cataract procedures and some are independent procedures. The effort is to reduce the risks associated with traditional trabeculectomy.

DISPOSITION

Must be followed by ophthalmologist

REFERRAL

Immediately to ophthalmologist

PEARLS & CONSIDERATIONS

COMMENTS

- Glaucoma is a serious blinding disease that must be monitored professionally by an ophthalmologist. It is mostly asymptomatic until late in the disease when visual problems arise. Even in developed countries half of glaucoma cases are undiagnosed.
- Risk factors that should prompt referral to an ophthalmologist for evaluation of glaucoma are high intraocular pressure, family history of glaucoma, use of systemic or topical corticosteroids, older age, and black race.
- Vision loss from glaucoma cannot be recovered. Early diagnosis and treatment may minimize visual loss.
- Glaucoma is not solely caused by increased intraocular pressure because approximately 20% of patients with glaucoma have normal intraocular pressure. However, high pressure is definitely a risk factor to be considered.

SUGGESTED READINGS

Available at ExpertConsult.com

RELATED CONTENT

Glaucoma (Patient Information)

AUTHOR: **R. Scott Hoffman, MD**

BASIC INFORMATION

DEFINITION

Primary angle-closure glaucoma occurs when elevated intraocular pressure is associated with closure of the filtration angle or obstruction in the circulating pathway of the aqueous humor.

SYNONYMS

Acute glaucoma, angle-closure glaucoma (ACG)
Pupillary block glaucoma
Narrow-angle glaucoma
Angle-closure glaucoma
alt2

ICD-10CM CODES

H40.061	Primary angle closure without glaucoma damage, right eye
H40.062	Primary angle closure without glaucoma damage, left eye
H40.063	Primary angle closure without glaucoma damage, bilateral
H40.069	Primary angle closure without glaucoma damage, unspecified eye

EPIDEMIOLOGY & DEMOGRAPHICS

INCIDENCE (IN U.S.):

- 2% to 8% of all patients with glaucoma.
- Higher incidence among those with hyperopia, small eyes, dense cataracts, shallow anterior chambers.

PREDOMINANT SEX: Females are affected more often than males.

PREDOMINANT AGE: 50 to 60 yr.

PEAK INCIDENCE: >50 yr of age; high association with hyperopia and cataracts.

GENETICS: Family history is not particularly helpful; far-sighted (hyperopes) individuals with thickening lenses (i.e., cataracts) are often those with angle-closure attacks.

PHYSICAL FINDINGS & CLINICAL PRESENTATION

- Although angle-closure glaucoma can present with an acute painful crisis associated with blurred vision, more than 75% of patients present with an asymptomatic course with progressive loss of the visual field (similar to that in patients with primary open-angle glaucoma; referred to as intermittent, subacute, or chronic angle closure)
- Hazy cornea
- Narrow angle
- Pain may be present (supraorbital headache is typical)
- Injection of conjunctiva, red eye (often severe limbal conjunctival injection with very high intraocular pressure [IOP])
- Shallow anterior chamber (one can shine a light from the side to perceive the forward position of the iris with narrow AC angles)
- Thick cataract
- Pupil may be mid-dilated and nonreactive to light
- Figs. E1 and Fig. E2 illustrate gonioscopy in primary angle-closure glaucoma

ETIOLOGY

- Narrow angles with acute closure: Blockage of circulatory path of the aqueous humor (Fig. E3) causing increase in IOP. ACG (primary angle-closure glaucoma) occurs more commonly in eyes with shorter axial length (farsightedness), shallower anterior chamber, and a relatively larger lens (enlarging cataract).
- Secondary angle-closure glaucoma (more rare) resulting from neovascularization of iris, iris tumors, lens induced, iris scarring, trauma, chronic inflammation with scarring, malignant glaucoma with aqueous misdirection.

DIAGNOSIS

DIFFERENTIAL DIAGNOSIS

- Open-angle glaucoma: Angle-closure glaucoma is distinguished from open-angle glaucoma by the closure of the angle between the iris and cornea, obstructing outflow of aqueous humor
- High intraocular pressure (normal IOP is usually 8 to 21 mm Hg)
- Optic nerve cupping
- Shallow chamber
- Open-angle glaucoma
- Conjunctivitis
- Corneal disease, keratitis
- Uveitis
- Scleritis
- Allergies
- Contact lens wearing with irritation

WORKUP

Comprehensive eye examination: If one suspects narrow angle or angle closure, avoid pupil dilation, as this may exacerbate the attack.

- Intraocular pressure (with ACG, IOP can be extremely high, >60 mm Hg)
- Gonioscopy for direct visualization of the chamber angle
- Slit lamp examination
- Visual field examination
- Laser scan of nerve fiber layer and optic nerve, optical coherence tomography (OCT)
- Optic nerve evaluation
- Anterior chamber depth

LABORATORY TESTS

- Blood sugar and complete blood count (if diabetes or inflammatory disease is suspected)
- Visual field
- Nerve fiber analysis, OCT, Heidelberg retinal tomography

IMAGING STUDIES

- Fundus photography (optic nerve photos): Very helpful for comparing changes in shape of optic nerve
- Fluorescein angiography for neovascular disease such as diabetic retinopathy, retinal vein occlusions
- Ultrasound biomicroscopy and anterior OCT can show relationships of anterior eye structures

TREATMENT

The goal of treatment is to acutely lower pressure on the eye and keep it down.

NONPHARMACOLOGIC THERAPY

Laser iridotomy early in disease process

ACUTE GENERAL Rx

- IV mannitol
- Pilocarpine
- β-Blockers
- Diamox
- Laser iridotomy
- Anterior chamber paracentesis (as emergency treatment)

CHRONIC Rx

- Iridotomy: When there is an adequate peripheral hole in the iris, the chance for future angle closure is usually eliminated unless there are rare other angle anomalies (i.e., plateau iris or peripheral synechiae).
- Lens removal (cataract extraction) can also eliminate the possibility of ACG.
- Trabeculectomy and filter valve procedures for nonresponsive cases.
- Other laser procedures, such as gonioplasty, for atypical angle closures.

DISPOSITION

Refer to ophthalmologist immediately.

REFERRAL

If acute angle-closure episode is suspected, should refer emergently to ophthalmologist.

PEARLS & CONSIDERATIONS

COMMENTS

- Do not use antihistamines or vasodilators with narrow-angle glaucoma.
- Iridotomy cures the majority of patients, and they will need no further medication and have no visual loss.
- Lower socioeconomic status and higher levels of social deprivation are risk factors for delayed detection and probable worse outcomes in glaucoma.

- Risk factors that should prompt referral to an ophthalmologist for evaluation of glaucoma are high intraocular pressure, family history of glaucoma, use of systemic or topical corticosteroids, older age, and black race.
- Glaucoma is undiagnosed in 9 out of 10 affected people worldwide and is undiagnosed in 50% of those in developed countries.
- Angle closure has become rarer because most people have cataract extractions at an earlier stage than in the past.

RELATED CONTENT

Glaucoma (Patient Information)
Glaucoma, Open Angle (Related Key Topic)

SUGGESTED READINGS

Available at ExpertConsult.com

AUTHOR: **R. Scott Hoffman, MD**

BASIC INFORMATION

DEFINITION

Gonorrhea is a sexually transmitted bacterial infection with a predilection for columnar and transitional epithelial cells. It commonly manifests as urethritis, cervicitis, or salpingitis. Infection may be asymptomatic. It differs between males and females in course, severity, and ease of recognition.

SYNONYMS

Gonococcal urethritis
Gonococcal vulvovaginitis
Gonococcal cervicitis
Gonococcal bartholinitis
GC

ICD-10CM CODES

A54.9	Gonococcal infection, unspecified
098.211	Gonorrhea complicating pregnancy, first trimester
098.212	Gonorrhea complicating pregnancy, second trimester
098.213	Gonorrhea complicating pregnancy, third trimester
098.219	Gonorrhea complicating pregnancy, unspecified trimester
098.22	Gonorrhea complicating childbirth
098.23	Gonorrhea complicating the puerperium
A54.03	Gonococcal cervicitis, unspecified
A54.00	Gonococcal infection of lower genitourinary tract, unspecified

EPIDEMIOLOGY & DEMOGRAPHICS

- The disease is common worldwide, affects both sexes and all ages, especially younger adults; highest incidence is in inner-city areas. Per CDC reports, approximately 470,000 new cases were found in the U.S. in 2016, with more than 60% found in metropolitan statistical centers. Gonorrhea is the second most-commonly reported communicable disease.
- Asymptomatic anterior urethral carriage may occur in 12% to 50% of cases in men.
- Asymptomatic in 50% to 80% of cases in women. Most common dissemination is by mucosal passage to fallopian tubes, resulting in pelvic inflammatory disease (PID) in 10% to 15% of infected women. Hematogenous spread may result in septic arthritis and skin lesions. Conjunctivitis rarely occurs but may result in blindness if not rapidly treated. Infection can occur in both men and women in oropharynx and anorectally.
- The World Health Organization (WHO) reported 78 million new cases of gonorrhea worldwide among adults in 2012.

PHYSICAL FINDINGS & CLINICAL PRESENTATION

- Males: Purulent discharge from anterior urethra (Fig. E1), with dysuria appearing 2 to 7 days after infecting exposure. May have rectal infection causing pruritus, tenesmus, and discharge, or may be asymptomatic.
- Females: Initial urethritis or cervicitis may occur a few days after exposure, frequently mild. Infections may be asymptomatic or may not produce recognizable symptoms until complications have occurred. In approximately 20% of cases, uterine invasion occurs after menstrual period with signs and symptoms of endometritis, salpingitis, or pelvic peritonitis. The patient may have purulent discharge or inflamed Skene or Bartholin glands.
- Classic presentation of acute gonococcal PID is fever, abdominal and adnexal tenderness, and, often, absence of purulent discharge. Physical examination may be normal if asymptomatic. Disseminated gonococcal infection (DGI) may manifest with petechial or pustular acral skin lesions (Fig. E2), asymmetric polyarthralgia, tenosynovitis, or oligoarticular septic arthritis. The infection is occasionally complicated by perihepatitis and, rarely, endocarditis or meningitis.

ETIOLOGY

- *Neisseria gonorrhoeae* is also known as gonococcus. Plasmids coding for β-lactamase render some strains resistant to penicillin or tetracycline. There is an increasing frequency of chromosomally mediated resistance to penicillin, tetracycline, fluoroquinolones, and cefoxitin. In the Far East, high-level resistance to spectinomycin is endemic.
- There are a rising number of cases of quinolone-resistant *N. gonorrhoeae* worldwide, with the expected number to rise in the U.S. from importation.
- Men who have sex with men are vulnerable to the emerging threat of antimicrobial-resistant *N. gonorrhoeae.*

Dx DIAGNOSIS

DIFFERENTIAL DIAGNOSIS

- Nongonococcal urethritis (NGU)
- Nongonococcal mucopurulent cervicitis
- *Chlamydia trachomatis*
- *Trichomonas vaginalis*

WORKUP

Diagnosis depends on bacteriologic investigation. Culture and nucleic acid amplification tests (NAAT) are available for the detection of genitourinary infection with *N. gonorrhoeae.*

- NAATs are preferred testing modalities for the detection of genitourinary infection with *N. gonorrhoeae.* The performance of NAATs with respect to overall sensitivity, specificity, and ease of specimen transport is better than that of any other tests available for the diagnosis of gonococcal infections. NAATs should be used to detect gonorrhea except in cases of child sexual assault involving boys and rectal and oropharyngeal infections in prepubescent girls. When evaluating a potential gonorrhea treatment failure, case culture and susceptibility testing might be required. NAATs allow testing of the widest variety of specimen types, including endocervical swabs, vaginal swabs, urethral swabs (men), and urine (from both men and women).
- Culture: Gonorrhea culture on Thayer-Martin medium (organism is fastidious; requires aerobic conditions with increased carbon dioxide atmosphere; incubate ASAP). Culture has a sensitivity of 95% or more for urethral specimens from men with symptomatic urethritis and 80% to 90% for endocervical infection in women. Gram-negative intracellular diplococci are diagnostic in male urethral smears (Fig. E3). There is a false-negative rate of 60% to 70% in female cervical or urethral smears.
  1. Concomitant serologic testing for syphilis for all patients
  2. Concomitant *Chlamydia* testing for all patients
  3. Offer of HIV testing and counseling to all patients

LABORATORY TESTS

- First-catch urine (or genital swab) sample NAAT is the preferred screening and diagnostic test for gonorrhea. These tests have largely replaced collecting culture in many settings where persons are screened for asymptomatic genital infection. These tests are not more sensitive than culture for detecting *N. gonorrhoeae* in cervical or urethral specimen; however, they have specificities >99% and retain sensitivity when used to test voided urine or self-collected vaginal swabs.
- Gonorrhea culture on Thayer-Martin medium (organism is fastidious; requires aerobic conditions with increased carbon dioxide atmosphere; incubate ASAP). Culture has a sensitivity of 95% or more for urethral specimens from men with symptomatic urethritis and 80% to 90% for endocervical infection in women.
- Nonamplified DNA probe tests are less sensitive than culture or NAATs and are not useful in the diagnosis of rectal or pharyngeal infection or for testing urine; however, they are inexpensive, readily available, and offered in many laboratories in combination assays for *C. trachomatis.*
- Concomitant serologic testing for syphilis on all patients.
- Concomitant *Chlamydia* testing on all patients.
- Offer of HIV testing and counseling to all patients.

Rx TREATMENT

ACUTE GENERAL Rx

For treatment of uncomplicated urogenital, rectal, or pharyngeal gonorrhea, the CDC[1] recommends a single 500-mg IM dose of ceftriaxone.

[1]St. Cyr S, Barbee L, Workowski KA et al: Update to CDC's treatment guidelines for gonococcal infection, *MMWR Morb Mortal Wkly Rep* 69:1911-1916, 2020, https://doi.org/10.15585/mmwr.mm6950a6external icon. 2020.

For persons weighing ≥150 kg (300 lbs), a single 1-g IM dose of ceftriaxone should be administered. If chlamydial infection has not been excluded, doxycycline 100 mg orally twice a day for 7 days is recommended. When ceftriaxone cannot be used for treating urogenital or rectal gonorrhea because of cephalosporin allergy, a single 240-mg IM dose of gentamicin, plus a single 2-g oral dose of azithromycin is an option. Gastrointestinal symptoms, primarily vomiting within 1 hr of dosing, have been reported among 3% to 4% of treated persons. If administration of IM ceftriaxone is not available, a single 800-mg oral dose of cefixime is an alternative regimen. However, cefixime does not provide as high or sustained bactericidal blood levels as does ceftriaxone, and demonstrates limited treatment efficacy for pharyngeal gonorrhea.

When gonococcal expedited partner therapy (provision of prescriptions or medications for the patient to give to a sex partner without the health care provider first examining the partner) is permissible by state law and the partner is unable or unlikely to seek timely treatment, the partner may be treated with a single 800-mg oral dose of cefixime, provided that concurrent chlamydial infection in the patient has been excluded. Otherwise, the partner may be treated with a single 800-mg oral dose of cefixime plus oral doxycycline 100 mg twice daily for 7 days.

In cases of suspected cephalosporin treatment failure, clinicians should obtain relevant clinical specimens for culture and antimicrobial susceptibility testing, consult an infectious disease specialist or STD clinical expert (https://www.stdccn.org/external icon) for guidance in clinical management, and report the case to the CDC through state and local public health authorities within 24 hr. Health departments should prioritize notification and culture evaluation for the patient's sex partner(s) from the preceding 60 days for those with suspected cephalosporin treatment failure or persons whose gonococcal isolates demonstrate reduced susceptibility to cephalosporins.

A test-of-cure is unnecessary for persons with uncomplicated urogenital or rectal gonorrhea who are treated with any of the recommended or alternative regimens. However, for persons with pharyngeal gonorrhea, a test-of-cure is recommended, using culture or nucleic acid amplification tests 7 to 14 days after initial treatment, regardless of the treatment regimen. Because re-infection within 12 mo ranges from 7% to 12% among persons previously treated for gonorrhea, those who have been treated should be retested 3 mo after treatment, regardless of whether they believe their sex partners were treated. If retesting at 3 mo is not possible, clinicians should retest within 12 mo after initial treatment.

Treatment of arthritis and arthritis-dermatitis syndrome:

- Recommended regimen: Ceftriaxone 1 g IM or IV every 24 hr plus azithromycin 1 g orally as a single dose.
- Alternative regimens: Cefotaxime 1 g IV every 8 hr or ceftizoxime 1 g IV every 8 hr *plus* azithromycin 1 g orally in a single dose.

Pregnancy

- Pregnant women infected with *N. gonorrhoeae* should be treated with dual therapy consisting of ceftriaxone 500 mg IM as a single dose for persons weighing <150 kg (300 lbs), 1 g of IM ceftriaxone for persons weighing ≥150 kg (300 lbs) and azithromycin 1 g PO as a single dose. When cephalosporin allergy or other considerations preclude treatment and spectinomycin is not available, consultation with an ID specialist is recommended.

DISPOSITION

- All sexual partners should be identified, examined, tested, and receive presumptive treatment.
- Patients should be counseled to avoid unprotected intercourse with partners for 1 wk after all partners have completed treatment.
- Men or women who have been treated for gonorrhea should be retested in 3 mo because of risk of re-infection. If they are unable to be retested in 3 mo, then they should be retested when they next present to care within 12 mo of their care.

REFERRAL

PID requiring hospitalization, disseminated gonococcal infection

PEARLS & CONSIDERATIONS

COMMENTS

- This is a reportable disease.
- The proportion of gonorrhea cases in heterosexual men who are fluoroquinolone resistant (QRNG) has reached 6.7%, an elevenfold increase from 0.6% in 2001. Fluoroquinolone antibiotics are no longer recommended to treat gonorrhea in the U.S.
- The use of azithromycin as the second antimicrobial is preferred over doxycycline in areas of high prevalence of tetracycline resistance.
- The U.S. Preventive Services Task Force (USPSTF) recommends screening for gonorrhea in sexually active females younger than 25 yr and in older women who are at increased risk for infection (multiple partners, new partner, partner who has concurrent partners). The USPSTF also concludes that the current evidence is insufficient to assess the balance of benefits and harms of screening for gonorrhea in men.
- High-intensity counseling on sexual risk reduction has been shown to reduce sexually transmitted infections (STIs) in primary care and related settings.

SUGGESTED READINGS

Available at www.expertconsult.com

RELATED CONTENT

Gonorrhea (Patient Information)
Cervicitis (Related Key Topic)
Chlamydia Genital Infections (Related Key Topic)
Pelvic Inflammatory Disease (Related Key Topic)
Urethritis, gonococcal (Related Key Topic)

AUTHORS: **Anthony Sciscione, DO,** and **Ella Stern, MD**

BASIC INFORMATION

DEFINITION

Gout is a term used to refer to a group of disease states caused by tissue deposition of monosodium urate resulting from prolonged hyperuricemia. Clinical manifestations of gout include acute and chronic arthritis, soft tissue inflammation, tophus formation, gouty nephropathy, and nephrolithiasis. Untreated hyperuricemia in patients with gout may lead to chronic destructive deforming arthritis.

ICD-10CM CODES	
M10	Gout
M10.0	Idiopathic gout
M10.1	Lead-induced gout
M10.2	Drug-induced gout
M10.3	Gout due to impairment of renal function
M10.4	Other secondary gout
M10.9	Gout, unspecified

EPIDEMIOLOGY & DEMOGRAPHICS

PREVALENCE: Self-reported prevalence in the U.S. is estimated at 3.9% of adults.

PREDOMINANT SEX: Male:female ratio ~4:1

PREDOMINANT AGE: 30 to 50 yr in men; older than 60 yr in women

ETIOLOGY

- Gout is induced by inflammation from monosodium urate (MSU) crystal deposition. The primary risk factor for MSU deposition is hyperuricemia, although local factors such as temperature, pH, and mechanical stress may play a role. Fig. E1 illustrates the pathophysiology of gout.
- Hyperuricemia and gout develop from excessive uric acid production, a decrease in the renal excretion of uric acid, or both.
- Primary hyperuricemia results from an inborn error of metabolism and may be attributed to several biochemical defects.
- Secondary hyperuricemia may develop as a complication of acquired disorders (e.g., leukemia) or as a result of the use of certain drugs (e.g., diuretics). Consumption of alcohol, especially beer, increases the risk of gout, and fructose-rich beverage intake is associated with hyperuricemia. Gout promoters and inhibitors are summarized in Table 1.

PHYSICAL FINDINGS & CLINICAL PRESENTAITON

ACUTE GOUT:

- Rapid onset of pain and swelling and erythema of a distal joint and/or periarticular soft tissue. Box 1 summarizes clinical pearls in acute gout attacks.
- May present as monoarthritis of any joint. Acute gout of the first metatarsophalangeal (MTP) joint is known as *podagra.*
- 10% to 15% of attacks are polyarticular.
- Spontaneous resolution occurs over days to weeks.

CHRONIC TOPHACEOUS GOUT (Fig. E2):

- Insidious onset of painless arthritis and soft tissue swelling
- Distal small joints characteristic
- May be confused with nodal osteoarthritis
- Box 2 summarizes clinical pearls in chronic gout

DIAGNOSIS

DIFFERNTIAL DIAGNOSIS OF ACUTE GOUT

- Septic arthritis, cellulitis
- Pseudogout, calcium pyrophosphate crystal deposition disease
- Trauma

DIFFERENTIAL DIAGNOSIS OF CHRONIC GOUT

- Osteoarthritis (especially nodal OA in women)
- Rheumatoid arthritis
- Psoriatic arthritis

Section II describes the differential diagnosis of acute monoarticular and oligoarticular arthritis.

WORKUP

Arthrocentesis and examination of synovial fluid

LABORATORY TESTS

- Uric acid: All patients with gout are hyperuricemic at some time, but during an acute attack the serum uric acid may be normal or low.
- Synovial aspirate: Usually cloudy and markedly inflammatory in nature (elevated WBC). Urate crystals in fluid are needle shaped and strongly negatively birefringent under polarized microscopy (Fig. E3).
- CBC: Neutrophilic leukocytosis often present.
- Inflammatory markers: ESR and CRP often elevated.

IMAGING STUDIES

- Plain radiography for diagnosis and evaluation. No typical findings in early gouty arthritis, but late disease is associated with characteristic punched-out marginal erosions (Fig. E4) and overhanging edges.
- Musculoskeletal ultrasound has been shown to be an effective means of detecting monosodium urate crystal deposition. Ultrasound can differentiate urate crystals that are found on the surface of articular cartilage from CPPD crystals that are seen within the substance of the cartilage (Fig. E5). Double contour sign can be seen.
- Dual-energy computed tomography (DECT) allows for color-coded images and detection of gout deposits, and may be beneficial if there is difficulty in establishing the diagnosis.

TREATMENT

TREATMENT OPTIONS FOR ACUTE GOUT (Table 2)

- Nonsteroidal antiinflammatory medication (see Table 3).
  1. Indomethacin 75 mg bid
  2. Ibuprofen 800 mg tid
  3. Naproxen 500 mg bid
  4. Celecoxib 200 mg bid
- Low-dose colchicine (less toxic, as effective as traditional high-dose colchicine): 1.2 mg PO, followed by 0.6 mg PO 1 hr later, then 0.6 mg daily or bid. Dose for renal function.
- Intraarticular corticosteroid injection (treatment of choice for monoarticular large joint attack): Triamcinolone acetonide 40 mg or equivalent for knee.

TABLE 1 Gout Promoters and Inhibitors*

Crystal formation	Seed nucleus (particulate) Immunoglobulin Phagocytes Low temperature Low pH Cation concentration Intraarticular dehydration Other (unknown) macromolecules
Triggering the acute flare (local factors)	Rapid change in urate level Microcrystal release IgG coat (apolipoproteins B, E inhibitory) Complement activation (classical, alternate, MAC) Inflammasome activation Cytokine and chemokine release Endothelial activation (e-selectin, ICAM-1, VCAM-1) Local trauma?
Presence of susceptible phagocytes, mast cells (systemic events)	Surgery, trauma Infections, other intercurrent systemic illness Alcohol, dietary intake Drugs that raise or lower circulating urate level

From Hochberg MC: *Rheumatology,* ed 7, Philadelphia, 2019, Elsevier.

*A diverse array of proteins and other mediators have been identified on the surfaces of urate crystals. In addition to their proinflammatory effect through opsonizing existing crystals, immunoglobulin M (IgM) and immunoglobulin G (IgG) antibodies may promote crystal formation by providing a stable molecular platform for crystal nucleation and growth. Apolipoproteins are the best characterized of the antiinflammatory molecules that coat crystals. The characteristics of the phagocytes encountering the crystals may be crucial; macrophages that are more differentiated are less likely to elicit proinflammatory cytokines.

ICAM-1, Intercellular adhesion molecule 1; *Ig,* immunoglobulin; *MAC,* membrane attack complex; *VCAM-1,* vascular cell adhesion molecule 1.

BOX 1 Acute Gout: Clinical Pearls

- Abrupt and rapid onset
- Maximal symptom intensity at 8-12 hr
- Attacks often come on at night or early morning
- Most commonly monoarticular in men during first attack
- Metatarsophalangeal joint is first affected in 50% of cases; other commonly affected joints: Ankle, heel, knee, wrists, and hands
- Joints are red, hot, swollen, and exquisitely tender
- Attacks resolve within days to weeks without treatment

From Hochberg MC: *Rheumatology,* ed 7, Philadelphia, 2019, Elsevier.

BOX 2 Chronic Gout: Clinical Pearls

- Pattern of symptom changes: Time between attacks shortens; more joints may be involved
- Tophaceous disease may result in a destructive arthropathy
- Tophaceous deposits may be bothersome and cause marked reduction in quality of life
- Increased risk for nephrolithiasis
- Associated with comorbidities such as metabolic syndrome, diabetes mellitus, chronic kidney disease, cardiovascular disease, hyperlipidemia, and obesity

From Hochberg MC: *Rheumatology,* ed 7, Philadelphia, 2019, Elsevier.

- Systemic corticosteroid therapy: Prednisone 40 mg PO for 3 days, then taper over 10 days (effective and safe, but evidence is lacking).

TREATMENT OF HYPERURICEMIA IN PATIENTS WITH GOUT

The American College of Rheumatology and most international rheumatology guidelines recommend that every patient with gout who has tophi, more than two attacks of gout per year, chronic kidney disease, or nephrolithiasis be treated with pharmacologic urate-lowering therapy. Serum uric acid should be monitored on a regular basis and urate-lowering therapy intensified until a target of less than 6 mg/dl is reached. In most cases, urate-lowering therapy should be continued for life. Fig. 6 summarizes pharmacologic serum urate–lowering treatment.

The American College of Physicians Guidelines recommends a more conservative approach based on recurrence of symptoms. These guidelines have been criticized as ignoring the progressive nature of gout and perpetuating the well-documented underutilization and under-dosing of urate-lowering therapy.

NONPHARMACOLOGIC THERAPY

Lifestyle and dietary modification should always be a component of therapy for patients with gout, but this is rarely effective without concomitant pharmacologic urate-lowering therapy, as dietary modification can lower uric acid only about 1 mg/dl. Recommendations include reducing ingestion of red meat, kidney, liver, yeast extract, shellfish, and overall protein along with restricting alcohol intake. Discontinuation of diuretic therapy may help lower serum uric acid.

PHARMACOLOGIC TREATMENT OF SYMPTOMATIC HYPERURICEMIA

ALLOPURINOL: Allopurinol is very effective and safe when used properly. Correct dosing and patient compliance are essential elements in the prevention of erosive and tophaceous gout. Patients with renal insufficiency are at increased risk for allopurinol hypersensitivity, which manifests as fever, rash, and hepatitis occurring most commonly in the first 3 mo of therapy. The rash may progress to life-threatening toxic epidermal necrolysis if not recognized early.

Traditionally, therapy with allopurinol is initiated several weeks after the acute attack has resolved. However, initiation of allopurinol at presentation may improve long-term compliance without reducing the efficacy of acute treatment. The initial dose should be low (≤100 mg/day depending on creatinine clearance) in patients with renal insufficiency and those with very high uric acid levels. High initial doses are associated with increased incidence of allopurinol hypersensitivity. The serum uric acid should be reevaluated after 4 to 6 wk of therapy, and the allopurinol dose adjusted to reduce the serum uric acid to less than 6 mg/dl. The most common therapeutic dosage of allopurinol is 300 mg/day, but dose may be increased by 50 to 100 mg every 2 to 3 wk until the target serum uric acid level is achieved. There is evidence that increasing allopurinol doses in patients with renal insufficiency does not result in significant toxicity, but concurrent use with statins and colchicine is associated with a higher incidence of adverse effects. Some authors have reported using doses as high as 800 mg daily without excess toxicity. It is recommended that patients of Han Chinese, Thai, and Korean ancestry be tested for HLA-B*5801 before initiating allopurinol as these individuals are at high risk of allopurinol hypersensitivity if this allele is present.

FEBUXOSTAT: Febuxostat is a xanthine oxidase inhibitor that has been shown to be more potent than allopurinol 300 mg daily for reducing serum uric acid. The chemical structure of febuxostat is different from allopurinol, making cross-reactive allergy unlikely. The metabolism of febuxostat is primarily hepatic, which obviates the need for dose adjustments due to renal insufficiency. Some cases of hepatic toxicity have been reported, and it is recommended that liver function tests be monitored. Febuxostat may help preserve renal function in patients with chronic kidney disease (CKD) but has not been tested in patients with severe renal failure.

The primary indication for febuxostat is demonstrated allergy to allopurinol. The cost of febuxostat may be as much as 40 times that of allopurinol, and there is some evidence suggesting that febuxostat may be associated with higher cardiovascular and all-cause mortality than allopurinol in patients with cardiovascular risk factors. In 2019, the FDA added a boxed warning for increased risk of death with febuxostat.

PROBENECID: Uricosuric agents may be used in patients with good renal function and urinary uric acid less than 600 mg in a 24-hr collection. Probenecid can be used in patients with intolerance to xanthene-oxidase inhibitors. Compliance is poor due to the necessity of taking the drug more often than once daily.

LESINURAD: Lesinurad is a URAT1 and OAT4 inhibitor approved by the FDA in 2015 for gout-associated hyperuricemia unresponsive to xanthine oxidase inhibitor monotherapy, to be taken in combination with a xanthene oxidase inhibitor. This drug was withdrawn in 2019 because of business-related reasons without safety concerns noted.

PEGLOTICASE: Intravenous PEGylated uricase is FDA approved for treatment of severe refractory tophaceous gout. It is a PEGylated recombinant mammalian uricase that rapidly degrades urate when given intravenously. Use is limited by very high cost and potential toxicities, including frequent gout flares and anaphylaxis. Rasburicase is a nonpegylated uricase used in tumor lysis syndrome and is not indicated for gout treatment.

PATIENT & FAMILY EDUCATION

It is essential that patients, families, physicians, and other members of the health care team appreciate the importance of compliance with a daily allopurinol regimen if recurrent flares and progression to chronic arthritis and tophi are to be avoided. Allopurinol should be discontinued only for symptoms suggesting hypersensitivity; otherwise, it should be continued during flares, medical illnesses, and surgical procedures.

REFERRAL

- Rheumatologist if diagnosis is not clear or therapy is complicated
- Podiatrist for management of pedal complications

PEARLS & CONSIDERATIONS

- The interleukin-1 receptor antagonist anakinra (Kineret) is an effective off-label agent for treatment of gout in complex patients with contraindications to standard therapies.
- Do not stop allopurinol during hospitalizations, surgery, or acute attacks unless there is evidence of drug allergy. The dosage of allopurinol should be adjusted in patients with acute kidney injury.

SUGGESTED READINGS

Available at ExpertConsult.com

RELATED CONTENT

Gout (Patient Information)
Hyperuricemia (Related Key Topic)

AUTHOR: **Kevin V. Plumley, MD, MPH**

TABLE 2 Therapeutic Options for Acute Gouty Inflammation

Drug Option	Level of Evidence	Typical Regimens
COX-nonselective NSAIDs	Grade A evidence for each regimen listed	Naproxen, 750-1000 mg PO daily in divided doses for 3 days; then 500-750 mg total daily for 4-7 days Sulindac, 300-400 mg/day in divided doses for 7-10 days Indomethacin, 150-200 mg PO daily in divided doses for 3 days; then 100 mg PO daily in divided doses for 4-7 days
COX-2–selective NSAIDs	Grade A	For example: Celecoxib, 800 mg; then 400 mg on day 1, followed by 400 mg bid for 7 days
Systemic corticosteroids	Grade A evidence for oral prednisolone, 35 mg/day for five or six doses; lower evidence grades for other regimens	Prednisone, 30-60 mg/day for 3 days; then taper every 3 days by 10-15 mg less as a daily dose until discontinuation Oral prednisolone, 35 mg/day for 5-7 days Medrol dose pack (for less severe flares) or to initiate therapy In an NPO patient: • Triamcinolone, 60 mg IM once with additional corticosteroid treatment as needed • Methylprednisolone, 100-150 mg IV for 1-2 days
Intraarticular corticosteroids	Grade C evidence	Particularly useful for flares in a single large joint Triamcinolone acetonide preparations are especially useful Dose titrated to the size of the joint
ACTH	Grade C evidence	25 USP units of synthetic ACTH SC for less severe flares; 40 USP units IM or IV once for more severe flares (including larger joint flares and polyarticular gout) One or two repeated doses of synthetic ACTH at intervals of 12 hr are often required with each of these regimens
Oral colchicine	Grade A evidence for FDA-approved regimen	In the U.S: To treat an early acute gout flare: 1.2 mg once followed by 0.6 mg in 1 hr and then 12 hr later; oral low-dose colchicine at prophylaxis doses until the acute gout flare resolves Outside the U.S: 0.5 mg tid for several days is the EULAR-recommended dosing regimen Oral colchicine treatment of acute gout should be limited to once every 2 wk in those already taking a maintenance low dose of colchicine
Off-label use in U.S: IL-1 antagonism	Grade C for anakinra; grade A for canakinumab	Use of anakinra (e.g., 100 mg SC daily for 3 days) or canakinumab (150 mg SC as single dose) for acute gout flare is not approved by the FDA, but canakinumab is approved by the EMA for this indication

ACTH, Adrenocorticotropic hormone; *bid,* twice a day; *COX,* cyclooxygenase; *EMA,* European Medicines Agency; *EULAR,* European League Against Rheumatism; *FDA,* U.S. Food and Drug Administration; *IL-1,* interleukin-1; *IM,* intramuscularly; *IV,* intravenously; *NPO,* nothing by mouth; *NSAID,* nonsteroidal antiinflammatory drug; *PO,* by mouth; *SC,* subcutaneously; *tid,* three times a day; *USP,* U.S. Pharmacopeia.
From Hochberg MC: *Rheumatology,* ed 7, Philadelphia, 2019, Elsevier.

TABLE 3 Treatment of Gout

Acute Gout	Interval Gout	Treatment of Hyperuricemia
NSAIDs (preferred): Indomethacin 50 mg qid or ibuprofen 800 mg tid (or other NSAID in full doses). Contraindicated in patients with renal insufficiency and gastrointestinal disorders. *Or* **Colchicine, oral:** 1.2 mg followed by a second dose of 0.6 mg 1 hr later. Contraindicated in patients with renal insufficiency and gastrointestinal disorders *Or* **Intraarticular steroids** (Treatment of choice for large joint monoarthritis): Triamcinolone 40 mg or equivalent for knee *Or* Systemic steroid therapy (for patients in whom NSAIDs and colchicine are contraindicated) Prednisone 30-50 mg PO daily or in divided doses. May use lower dose in diabetic or postsurgical patients.	**Colchicine, oral:** 0.6-1.2 mg/day as prophylaxis against recurrent attacks. **NSAIDs may also be used for prophylaxis.** **Hypouricemic agent:** Indicated for patients with recurrent attacks despite prophylaxis, severe hyperuricemia, presence of tophi, urolithiasis, or gouty arthritis **Other:** Weight loss, reduce alcohol (especially beer), diet low in seafood, red meat, organ meat, and fructose	**Colchicine, oral:** 0.6-1.2 mg/day for 4-6 wk before initiating hypouricemic therapy and for several mo afterward to prevent recurrent attacks during initiation of hypouricemic therapy. *And* **Allopurinol:** Initial dose 100 mg/day in patients with renal insufficiency or very high uric acid levels. Increase dose as needed to attain uric acid less than 6 mg/dl. *Or* **Uricosuric agent** (Use only in patients with good renal function and <600 mg uric acid in a 24-hr collection): probenecid, 0.5-1 g bid, or sulfinpyrazone 100 mg tid or qid. **Other:** Consider febuxostat for patients allergic to allopurinol and the addition of lesinurad in patients resistant to xanthine oxidase inhibitors. Pegloticase may be useful for selected patients with severe tophaceous gout.

bid, Twice a day; *NSAID,* nonsteroidal antiinflammatory drug; *PO,* by mouth; *qid,* four times a day; *tid,* three times a day.

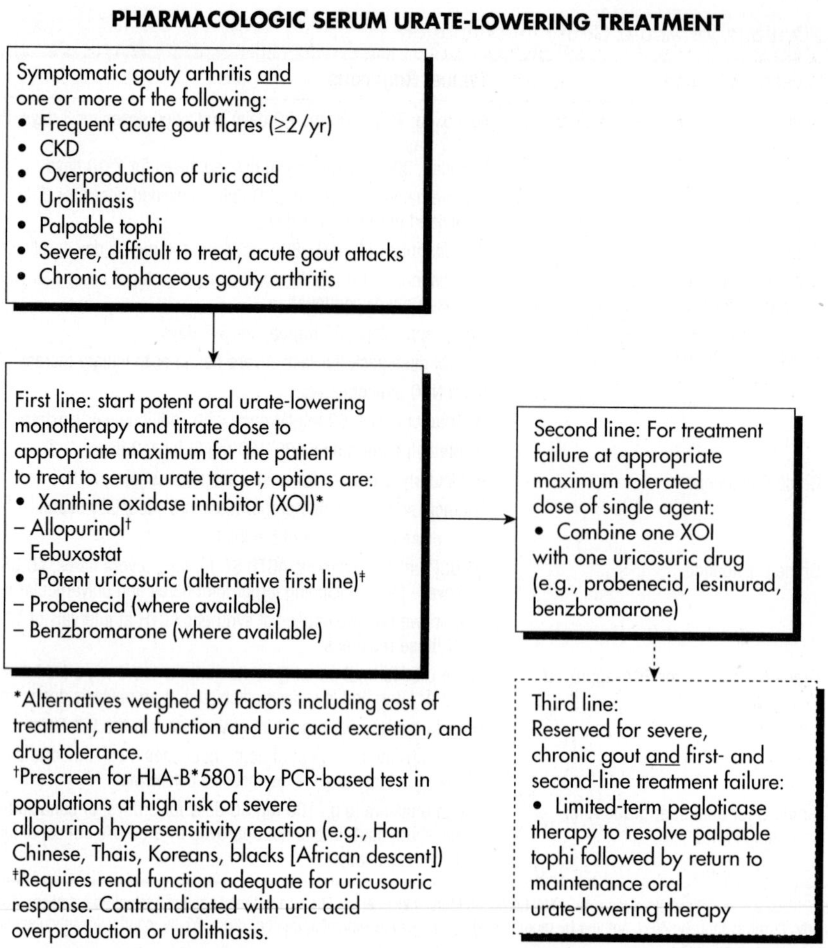

FIG. 6 Algorithm for pharmacologic serum urate–lowering treatment of hyperuricemia in patients with a confirmed diagnosis of gout. The algorithm, discussed in the text, summarizes the first-, second-, and third-line approaches to pharmacologic urate-lowering therapy, including management of refractory hyperuricemia in difficult gout. *CKD,* Chronic kidney disease; *PCR,* polymerase chain reaction. (From Hochberg MC: *Rheumatology,* ed 7, Philadelphia, 2019, Elsevier.)

BASIC INFORMATION

DEFINITION

Graves disease is a hypermetabolic state caused by circulating immunoglobulin G (IgG) antibodies that bind to and activate the G-protein–coupled thyrotropin receptor. This activation stimulates follicular hypertrophy and hyperplasia, causing thyroid enlargement as well as increases in thyroid hormone production. It affects the thyroid, ocular muscles and shin. It is characterized by thyrotoxicosis, diffuse goiter, and infiltrative ophthalmopathy (edema and inflammation of the extraocular muscles and an increase in orbital connective tissue and fat); infiltrative dermopathy characterized by lymphocytic infiltration of the dermis; accumulation of glycosaminoglycans; and occasionally edema.

SYNONYM

Thyrotoxicosis

ICD-10CM CODES	
E05.00	Thyrotoxicosis with diffuse goiter without thyrotoxic crisis or storm
E05.01	Thyrotoxicosis with diffuse goiter with thyrotoxic crisis or storm

EPIDEMIOLOGY & DEMOGRAPHICS

INCIDENCE & PREVALENCE: Graves disease is the most common cause of hyperthyroidism. It affects 3% of women and 0.5% of men during their lifetime. There is a slight increased incidence among young African Americans. The annual incidence of Graves disease–associated ophthalmopathy is 16 cases per 100,000 women and 3 cases per 100,000 men. It is more common in whites than Asians. Cigarette smoking is a risk factor.

PREDOMINANT AGE: Peak incidence is between 30 and 60 yr.

GENETICS: Patients often report a family history of Hashimoto thyroiditis, Graves disease, or other autoimmune conditions. Increased prevalence of *HLA-B8* and *HLA-DR3* in whites with Graves disease. Concordance rate is 20% among monozygotic twins.

PHYSICAL FINDINGS & CLINICAL PRESENTATION

- Diffusely enlarged thyroid. Thyroid bruit may be present. Cervical lymphadenopathy may also be present
- Elevated systolic blood pressure with a widened pulse pressure
- Tachycardia, palpitations, tremor, hyperreflexia
- Exophthalmos (50% of patients) (Fig. E1), lid retraction (lid lag), in which contraction of the levator palpebrae muscles of the eyelids show immobility of the upper eyelid with downward rotation of the eye
- Nervousness, weight loss (weight gain in 10% of patients), heat intolerance, pruritus, muscle weakness, atrial fibrillation
- Increased sweating, brittle nails, clubbing of fingers
- Localized infiltrative dermopathy (1% to 2% of patients) is most frequent over the anterolateral aspects of the legs, commonly over the pretibial area (pretibial myxedema) but can be found at other sites (especially after trauma). It is nonpitting and indurated. It is typically patchy with a peau d'orange appearance to the skin
- Men may have gynecomastia, reduced libido, and erectile dysfunction. Women often have irregular menses

ETIOLOGY

Autoimmune etiology: Thyrotropin receptor antibodies (TRAb) mediated activation of thyroid-stimulating hormone receptor (TSHR). The activity of the thyroid gland is stimulated by the action of T cells, which induce specific B cells to synthesize antibodies against TSHRs in the follicular cell membrane.

DIAGNOSIS

DIFFERENTIAL DIAGNOSIS

- Anxiety disorder
- Premenopausal state
- Thyroiditis
- Other causes of hyperthyroidism (e.g., toxic multinodular goiter, toxic adenoma)
- Other: Metastatic neoplasm, diabetes mellitus, pheochromocytoma

WORKUP

- The diagnosis is made clinically on most instances. The clinical assessment of the patient with Graves orbitopathy is summarized in Table 1.
- The diagnostic workup includes a detailed medical history followed by laboratory and imaging studies and ECG. Patients often present with anxiety, heat intolerance, menstrual dysfunction, increased appetite, and weight loss. Elderly patients can have an atypical presentation (apathetic hyperparathyroidism). For additional information, refer to the topic "Hyperthyroidism."

LABORATORY TESTS

- Increased free thyroxine (T_4) and free triiodothyronine (T_3)
- Decreased TSH
- Measurement of thyroid-stimulating antibodies (TSI) and TRAb
- Table 2 summarizes assays of TSHR antibody nomenclature and indications.

IMAGING STUDIES

- 24-hr radioactive iodine uptake (RAIU): Increased homogeneous uptake.
- CT (Fig. E2) or MRI of the orbits (Fig. E3) is useful if there is uncertainty about the cause of ophthalmopathy.

TREATMENT

NONPHARMACOLOGIC THERAPY

- Patient education and discussion of therapeutic options.
- Smoking cessation: Smoking is associated with an increased risk of progression of Graves ophthalmopathy.

ACUTE GENERAL Rx

- Advantages and disadvantages of treatment options for Graves hyperthyroidism are summarized in Table 3.
- Antithyroid drugs (thionamides, ATDs) to inhibit thyroid hormone synthesis or peripheral conversion of T_4 to T_3:
  1. Methimazole or propylthiouracil (PTU) are available. Methimazole is generally preferred because it has a longer half-life, allowing for once-daily dosing. PTU is preferred during pregnancy.
  2. Side effects: Skin rash (3% to 5%), arthralgias, myalgias, granulocytopenia (0.5%); rare side effects: Aplastic anemia, hepatic necrosis (PTU), cholestatic jaundice.
  3. Thionamide antithyroid drug therapy results in a remission in 40% to 50% of patients treated for 12 to 18 mo.
- Radioactive iodine (RAI):
  1. Treatment of choice for patients >21 yr and younger patients who have not achieved remission after 1 yr of ATD therapy
  2. Contraindicated during pregnancy and lactation
  3. After radioactive therapy there may be an acute elevation of thyroid antibody titers and exacerbation of ocular symptoms in 15% to 20% of patients
- Surgery: Near-total thyroidectomy. Indications: Obstructing goiters despite RAI and ATD therapy, patients who refuse RAI and cannot be adequately managed with ATDs, and pregnant women inadequately managed with ATDs. Complications of surgery include hypoparathyroidism (4%) and vocal cord paralysis (1%).
- Adjunctive therapy: Beta-adrenergic receptor blockers (e.g., atenolol 50 to 100 mg/day) to alleviate the beta-adrenergic symptoms of hyperthyroidism (tachycardia, tremor); contraindicated in patients with bronchospasm.
- Graves ophthalmopathy: Methylcellulose eye drops to protect against excessive dryness, sunglasses to decrease photophobia, intraocular and systemic high-dose corticosteroids for severe exophthalmos. Worsening of ophthalmopathy after RAI therapy is often transient and can be prevented by the administration of prednisone. Other treatment options include antiinflammatory and immunosuppressive agents, radiation, and corrective surgical procedures. The administration of the antioxidant selenium (100 μg PO bid) has been recently reported as effective in improving quality of life, reducing ocular involvement, and slowing progression of the disease in patients with mild Graves orbitopathy. Its mechanism of action is believed to be an effect on the oxygen free radicals and cytokines that play a pathogenic role in Graves orbitopathy. Inhibition of the insulin-like growth factor I receptor (IGF-IR)

TABLE 1 Clinical Assessment of Patient with Graves Orbitopathy

SEVERITY MEASURES (USING THE MNEMONIC NO SPECS)		
NO SPECS Class	**Item**	**Method**
0. **N**o signs or symptoms		
1. **O**nly signs, no symptoms	Lid aperture	With ruler in midline in mm
2. **S**oft tissue involvement	Eyelid and conjunctiva swelling and redness	Inspection, color pictures[a]
3. **P**roptosis	Exophthalmos	Hertel in mm
4. **E**xtraocular muscle involvement	Eye muscle motility Diplopia	Impaired elevation, abduction Subjective grading[b]
5. **C**orneal involvement	Keratitis, ulcer	Fluoresceine
6. **S**ight loss caused by optic nerve involvement	Dysthyroid optic neuropathy (DON)	Visual acuity, color vision, visual fields, optic disc

ACTIVITY MEASURES (USING THE CLINICAL ACTIVITY SCORE [CAS])		
Inflammatory Sign	**Item**	**Score**
Pain	Spontaneous retrobulbar pain Pain on up gaze, side gaze, or down gaze	1 1
Redness	Redness of the eyelids Redness of the conjunctiva	1 1
Swelling	Swelling of the eyelids Swelling of the caruncle and/or plica Chemosis	1 1 1
Maximum CAS score (assessed momently)		*7*
Impaired function	Increase in proptosis ≥2 mm in 1-3 mo Decrease of ≥8° in eye muscle motility in any direction in 1-3 mo Decrease in visual acuity of more than one line on the Snellen chart (using pinhole) in 1-3 mo	1 1 1
Maximum CAS score (assessed over time)		*10*

CAS, Clinical activity score.
[a]Color atlas in Dickinson AJ, Perros P: Controversies in the clinical evaluation of active thyroid-associated orbitopathy: Use of a detailed protocol with comparative photographs for objective assessment, *Clin Endocrinol (Oxf)*, 55:283–303, 2001.
[b]Intermittent diplopia = at awakening or when tired; inconstant diplopia = at extremes of gaze; constant diplopia = in primary or reading position.
From Melmed S et al: *Williams textbook of endocrinology*, ed 14, Philadelphia, 2020, Elsevier.

TABLE 2 Assays of Thyroid-Stimulating Hormone Receptor Antibodies: Nomenclature and Indications

Nomenclature of TSHRAb Assays	
TBII (TSH-binding inhibitory immunoglobulins)	Measurement of inhibition of labelled TSH (or labelled thyroid-stimulating monoclonal antibody) binding to recombinant TSHR by serum antibodies
TSAb or TSI (thyroid-stimulating antibodies)	Measurement of cAMP production by thyroid cell lines transfected with TSHR
TBAb (thyroid-blocking antibodies)	Measurement of inhibition of cAMP production after TSH-mediated stimulation of thyroid cells or TSHR-transfected cells
Indications for Assay of TSHRAb	
Diagnosis	Graves hyperthyroidism Graves orbitopathy and Graves dermopathy Fetal and neonatal thyrotoxicosis
Treatment	Chance of remission of hyperthyroidism at baseline, and during treatment with antithyroid drugs.

cAMP, Cyclic adenosine monophosphate; *TSH*, thyroid-stimulating hormone; *TSHR*, thyroid-stimulating hormone receptor; *TSHRAb*, thyroid-stimulating hormone receptor antibodies.
From Melmed S et al: *Williams textbook of endocrinology*, ed 14, Philadelphia, 2020, Elsevier.

TABLE 3 Advantages and Disadvantages of Treatment Options for Graves Hyperthyroidism

Treatment Option	Advantages	Disadvantages
Antithyroid drugs	Chance of permanent remission (~35%)	Side effects of ATDs Long duration (12-18 mo) High recurrence risk
Radioactive iodine	Simplicity Low recurrence risk	Risk of orbitopathy Lifelong LT_4 needed Possible small increase in cancer risk
Thyroidectomy	Rapidity Almost no recurrences	Low but unavoidable morbidity Lifelong LT_4 needed

ATDs, Antithyroid drugs; *LT_4*, l-thyroxine.
From Melmed S et al: *Williams textbook of endocrinology*, ed 14, Philadelphia, 2020, Elsevier.

is a new therapeutic strategy to combat the underlying autoimmune etiology of ophthalmopathy. Trials with teprotumumab, a human monoclonal antibody inhibitor of IGF-IR, in patients with active, moderate-to-severe ophthalmopathy have shown effectiveness in reducing proptosis.[1]

- Dermopathy and acropachy: Topical corticosteroids are often used but are generally ineffective. Trials using rituximab infusion for dermopathy have shown striking improvement.

[1] Douglas RS et al: Teprotumumab for the treatment of active thyroid eye disease, *N Engl J Med* 382(4):341-352, 2020.

CHRONIC Rx

Patients undergoing treatment with ATDs should be seen every 1 to 3 mo until euthyroidism is achieved and every 3 to 4 mo while they are receiving ATDs.

DISPOSITION

- ATDs induce sustained remission in <60% of cases.
- The incidence of hypothyroidism after RAI is >50% within the first yr and 2% per yr thereafter.
- Complications of surgery include hypothyroidism (28% to 43% after 10 yr), hypoparathyroidism (4%), and vocal cord paralysis (1%).
- Successful treatment of hyperthyroidism requires lifelong monitoring for the onset of hypothyroidism or the recurrence of thyrotoxicosis.
- RAI therapy is followed by the appearance or worsening of ophthalmopathy more often than is therapy with methimazole, particularly in patients who are cigarette smokers. It can be prevented with the administration of prednisone 0.5 mg/kg body weight per day starting 2 to 3 days after RAI, continued for 1 mo, then tapered off over 2 mo.
- Mild to moderate ophthalmopathy often improves spontaneously. Severe cases can be treated with high-dose glucocorticoids, orbital irradiation, or both. Orbital decompression may be used in patients with optic neuropathy and exophthalmos (see "Hyperthyroidism").

SUGGESTED READINGS

Available at ExpertConsult.com

RELATED CONTENT

Graves Disease (Patient Information)
Hyperthyroidism (Related Key Topic)

AUTHOR: **Fred F. Ferri, MD**

BASIC INFORMATION

DEFINITION

Guillain-Barré syndrome (GBS) is an acute immune-mediated polyradiculoneuropathy (affects nerve roots and peripheral nerves), with predominant motor involvement. It is the most common cause of acute flaccid paralysis in the Western hemisphere and probably worldwide. By definition, maximal clinical weakness, the clinical nadir, occurs within 4 wk of disease onset.

SYNONYMS

AIDP (acute inflammatory demyelinating polyradiculoneuropathy)
Acute polyneuropathy
Ascending paralysis
GBS
Postinfectious polyneuritis

ICD-10CM CODE
G61.0 Guillain-Barré syndrome

EPIDEMIOLOGY & DEMOGRAPHICS

INCIDENCE: 0.6 to 1.9 cases/100,000 persons annually without geographic variation. Incidence increases with age. A slight peak in incidence occurs between late adolescence and early adulthood. A slight male preponderance (1.25:1) also exists.

PREDISPOSING FACTORS: Viral (HIV, CMV, EBV, influenza) and bacterial *(Campylobacter jejuni, Mycoplasma pneumoniae)* infections; systemic illness (Hodgkin lymphoma, immunizations). Major antecedents of GBS are described in Box E1.

PHYSICAL FINDINGS & CLINICAL PRESENTATION

- Symmetric weakness, most commonly involving proximal muscles initially, subsequently involving both proximal and distal muscles; difficulty in ambulating, getting up from a chair, or climbing stairs (Box E2)
- Depressed or absent reflexes bilaterally
- Minimal to moderate glove and stocking paresthesias/dysesthesia/anesthesia or back pain
- Pain (caused by involvement of posterior nerve roots) may be prominent
- Autonomic abnormalities (bradyarrhythmias or tachyarrhythmias, hypotension or hypertension, constipation, urinary retention)
- Respiratory insufficiency (caused by weakness of bulbar/intercostal muscles)
- Facial paresis, ophthalmoparesis, dysphagia (secondary to cranial nerve involvement)
- GBS consists of several clinical variants based on the pattern of clinical involvement and electrophysiologic findings. These include:
  1. AIDP (most common form in Europe and North America)
  2. Acute motor axonal neuropathy (AMAN; most prevalent form in China and Japan)
  3. Acute motor and sensory axonal neuropathy (AMSAN; has more severe sensory involvement and is associated with more severe clinical course and poorer prognosis)
  4. Miller Fisher syndrome (MFS; triad of ophthalmoplegia, ataxia, and areflexia)
  5. Acute pandysautonomia (rapid onset of parasympathetic and sympathetic failure without motor or sensory involvement)
  6. Regional variants (e.g., pharyngeal-cervical-brachial GBS, pure ataxic GBS)

ETIOLOGY

- Unknown, but believed to be caused by infection-induced aberrant immune response.
- Preceding infectious illness 1 to 4 wk before disease onset has been noted. The most frequent antecedent infection is *C. jejuni* (associated with 30% of cases of GBS and 20% of cases of Miller Fisher syndrome).
- Humoral and cell-mediated immune attack of peripheral nerve myelin, Schwann cells; sometimes with primary axonal involvement.

DIAGNOSIS

DIFFERENTIAL DIAGNOSIS

- Toxic peripheral neuropathies: Heavy metal poisoning (lead [microcytic anemia], thallium [alopecia], arsenic [typically accompanied by acute GI illness]), medications (vincristine, disulfiram), organophosphate poisoning, hexacarbon (glue sniffer's neuropathy)
- Nontoxic peripheral neuropathies: Acute intermittent porphyria, fulminant vasculitic polyneuropathy, infectious (poliomyelitis, diphtheria, Lyme disease, West Nile virus), tick paralysis
- Neuromuscular junction disorders: Myasthenia gravis, botulism, snake envenomation
- Polymyositis and acute necrotizing myopathies
- Metabolic derangements such as hypermagnesemia, hypokalemia, hypophosphatemia
- Acute CNS disorders such as basilar artery thrombosis with brain stem infarction, brain stem encephalomyelitis, transverse myelitis, or spinal cord compression
- Conversion disorder
- Malingering
- Table 1 differentiates clinical patterns of acute neuromuscular weakness

WORKUP

- Exclude other causes based on clinical history, examination, and laboratory tests.
- Lumbar puncture (may be normal in the first 1 to 2 wk of the illness). Typical findings include elevated CSF protein with few mononuclear leukocytes (albuminocytologic dissociation) in 80% to 90% of patients. Elevated CSF cell counts is an expected characteristic in cases associated with HIV seroconversion.
- EMG/nerve conduction study (NCS) may be normal in the first 10 to 14 days of the disease. The earliest electrodiagnostic abnormality is prolongation or absence of H-reflexes. NCS evidence of demyelination (prolonged distal latency, conduction velocity slowing, conduction block, temporal dispersion, and prolonged F-waves) in two or more motor nerves confirms diagnosis of AIDP in the appropriate clinical context.

LABORATORY TESTS

- CBC may reveal early leukocytosis with left shift. Electrolytes are tested to exclude metabolic causes of weakness.
- Heavy metal testing; urine porphyria screen; creatine kinase; HIV testing, including tests for HIV seroconversion, especially if CSF demonstrates lymphocytic pleocytosis. MRI of brain and spinal cord with and without contrast may be indicated if diagnosis is uncertain. In GBS, a gadolinium-enhanced MRI of the lumbosacral spine may reveal nerve root enhancement.
- Antibodies against ganglioside GQ1b may be present in up to 90% of patients with MFS. IgG antibodies against ganglioside GM1 may be associated with AMAN. There are no anti-ganglioside antibodies commonly associated with AIDP.
- In equivocal cases, especially if peripheral nerve vasculitis is a concern, nerve biopsy may aid in confirming a diagnosis of GBS. Sensory nerve biopsy demonstrates segmental demyelination with infiltration of monocytes and T cells into the endoneurium. Axonal loss is commonly seen in sensory nerve biopsy specimens in GBS.

TREATMENT

NONPHARMACOLOGIC THERAPY

- Close monitoring of respiratory function (frequent measurements of vital capacity, negative inspiratory force, and tidal volume) and pulmonary toilet should be done because respiratory failure is the major complication in GBS
- Frequent repositioning of patient to minimize formation of pressure sores
- Prevention of venous thromboembolism with antithrombotic stockings as a supplement to pharmacologic venous thromboembolism prevention
- Emotional support and social counseling for patient and family
- Pain control
- Cardiac monitoring to detect arrhythmias
- Physical and occupational therapy once patient is medically stable and able to participate

ACUTE GENERAL Rx

- Option 1: Infusion of IV immunoglobulins (IVIG; 0.4 g/kg/day for 5 days). Always check serum IgA levels before infusion to prevent anaphylaxis in IgA-deficient patients.
- Option 2: Early therapeutic plasma exchange (TPE or plasmapheresis: 200 to 250 ml/kg over five sessions every other day), started within 7 days of onset of symptoms, is

TABLE 1 Clinical Patterns of Acute Neuromuscular Weakness

Cause	Cranial Nerve Involvement	Limb Weakness	Reflexes	Sensory	Autonomic Changes
Guillain-Barré syndrome	Common, facial diplegia	Distal (ascending)	Absent	Common	Possible (20%)
Miller Fisher syndrome	Hallmark: Ophthalmoplegia	Variable hallmark: Ataxia	Absent	Rare	Rare
Myasthenia gravis	Common, ptosis, facial, oculomotor	Proximal (shoulders and thighs)	Normal	Present	Present
Botulism	Symmetric diplopia, ptosis, dysarthria, dysphagia	Descending	Absent or decreased	No	Yes (e.g., ileus, mydriasis, reduced salivation, urinary retention)
Organophosphate poisoning	Bulbar dysfunction, dysarthria, dysphagia	Diffuse	Decreased	Late	Yes (e.g., bradycardia, sialorrhea, bronchorrhea, lacrimation, diarrhea, miosis causing blurry vision)
Brain stem	Common, ocular movement	Crossed findings (face/ limbs)	Increased	Common	Rare
Spinal cord	No	Quadriparesis or paraparesis	Decreased then increased	Loss below level	If above thoracic level

From Parrillo JE, Dellinger RP: *Critical care medicine: principles of diagnosis and management in the adult,* ed 5, Philadelphia, 2019, Elsevier.

beneficial in reducing the need for mechanical ventilation in patients with rapidly progressive disease and results in improved rate of recovery. It is contraindicated in patients with cardiovascular disease (recent MI, unstable angina), active sepsis, and autonomic dysfunction.

- Both therapies are equally effective and may shorten recovery time by 50%. There is no proven benefit from combining IVIG and plasma exchange. Glucocorticoids are contraindicated.
- Mechanical ventilation may be needed if FVC is <12 to 15 ml/kg, vital capacity is rapidly decreasing or is <1000 ml, negative inspiratory force is <20 cm H_2O, PaO_2 is <70, or the patient is having significant difficulty clearing secretions or is aspirating.

CHRONIC Rx

- Ventilatory support may be necessary in 10% to 20% of patients. Adequate fluid/electrolyte support and nutrition are necessary, especially in patients with dysautonomia or bulbar dysfunction.
- Aggressive nursing care to prevent decubitus, infections, fecal impactions, and pressure nerve palsies.
- Monitoring and treatment of autonomic dysfunction (bradyarrhythmias or tachyarrhythmias, orthostatic hypotension, systemic hypertension).
- Treatment of back pain and dysesthesia with neuropathic pain medications such as tricyclic antidepressants or gabapentin. Opiate narcotics can be used cautiously in the short term but may compound dysautonomia.
- Pharmacologic venous thromboembolism prevention with agents such as heparin (5000 U SC q12h) or enoxaparin (40 mg SC daily) in poorly ambulating and nonambulatory patients.
- Stress ulcer prevention in patients receiving ventilator support.
- Physical and occupational therapy rehabilitation, including supportive devices.

DISPOSITION

- Mortality rate is approximately 5% to 10% worldwide. Causes of death include cardiac arrest, pulmonary embolism, and fulminant infections. A recent study showed 62% complete motor recovery, 14% mild weakness, 9% moderate weakness, 4% bed-bound or ventilated, and 8% dead at 1 yr. Another study suggested that approximately 33% of patients were free from sensory symptoms at 1 yr, with residual sensory loss present in the lower extremities in 67% and 36% in the upper extremities. About 32% had to change their work, 30% were unable to function at home as well as they could before the disease, and 52% had to alter their leisure activities 1 yr after GBS onset. Excessive fatigue is a common complaint in patients during the recovery phase of GBS. This may be treated with exercise therapy (e.g., bicycle exercise training).
- Predictors for poor recovery (inability to walk independently at 1 yr): Age >60 yr, preceding diarrheal illness, recent CMV infection, fulminant or rapidly progressing course, ventilatory dependence, reduced motor amplitudes (<20% normal), or unexcitable nerves on NCS. Outcomes may also be influenced by complications of medical therapy.
- GBS is typically a monophasic illness. Recurrence may occur in <5% of patients following full recovery.

REFERRAL

- Neurology to aid in diagnosis and direct treatment
- Pulmonary/critical care for ICU management
- Otolaryngology or general surgery for tracheostomy in patients requiring prolonged ventilatory support
- Gastroenterology for percutaneous endoscopic gastrostomy for patients with prolonged inability to obtain nutrition orally

PEARLS & CONSIDERATIONS

- GBS is the most common cause of acute flaccid paralysis.
- Close monitoring of ventilatory function with respiratory mechanics (FVC and NIF) is of paramount importance in all patients with suspected GBS.
- Glucocorticoids are not indicated in GBS and may even slow recovery.

PATIENT & FAMILY EDUCATION

Patient education information may be obtained from the Guillain-Barré Foundation International, The Holly Building, 104½ Forrest Avenue, Narberth, PA 19072; phone: (610) 667-0131; fax: (610) 667-7036; toll-free: (866) 224-3301; email: info@gbs-cidp.org.

SUGGESTED READINGS

Available at ExpertConsult.com

RELATED CONTENT

Guillain-Barré Syndrome (Patient Information)

AUTHOR: **Lydia Sharp, MD**

BASIC INFORMATION

DEFINITION

Head and neck squamous cell carcinoma is a malignant disease entity that arises from the epithelium of the mucosal surfaces of the upper aerodigestive tract and accounts for nearly 90% of head and neck cancers. This disease results from exposure to carcinogens and from the accumulation of genetic alterations. The workup and management of these patients depends upon the specific subsite of the aerodigestive tract in the head and neck from which the primary tumor arises. These subsites are the oral cavity, oropharynx, nasopharynx, hypopharynx, and larynx. Cutaneous malignancies, thyroid neoplasms, and salivary gland neoplasms also occur in the head and neck but are beyond the scope of this chapter.

SYNONYMS

HNC
Head and neck cancer
HNSCC
Head and neck squamous cell carcinoma

ICD-10CM CODES	
C00-C14	Malignant neoplasms of lip, oral cavity, and pharynx
C30	Malignant neoplasm of nasal cavities, middle ear, and accessory sinuses
C32	Malignant neoplasm of larynx
C77.0	Secondary and unspecified malignant neoplasm of lymph nodes of head, face, and neck

EPIDEMIOLOGY & DEMOGRAPHICS

INCIDENCE:

- U.S. annual incidence of head and neck cancer (90% of which is squamous cell carcinoma) is approximately 62,000 persons per year.
- Annual mortality is approximately 13,000 persons per year.
- Accounts for approximately 3% of all cancers in the U.S. and over 1.5% of all cancer deaths.
- Head and neck cancer was the seventh most common cancer worldwide in 2018.
- Human papilloma virus (HPV)-associated squamous cell carcinoma of the head and neck accounts for 5% to 20% of all HNSCCs, and 40% to 90% of those arise in oropharynx.
- Incidence of all forms of HNSCC is on the decline, except oropharyngeal squamous cell carcinoma, which is increasing in incidence, likely related to the rise in human papilloma virus (HPV) associated HNSCC.

PREDOMINANT SEX & AGE: Male:female ratio is approximately 3:1. Risk increases significantly over the age of 40.

PEAK INCIDENCE: Sixth decade of life

RISK FACTORS: The two most strongly implicated risk factors associated with HNSCC are tobacco and alcohol use. These carcinogens place the entire epithelium of the upper respiratory tract at risk for multiple primary tumors via a process known as field cancerization. More recently, a new subset of HNSCC caused by the HPV has been increasing in prevalence. HPV 16 is the most common genotype detected. Patients are more likely to be white middle-aged men, nonsmokers, with minimal alcohol use and higher socioeconomic status.

GENETICS: Research is ongoing in genetic factors that lead to the development and progression of HNSCC. Tumor-suppressor genes including *p53, NOTCH1,* and *CDKN2A,* among others, have been shown to harbor mutations in patients with HNSCC.

PHYSICAL FINDINGS & CLINICAL PRESENTATION

- Presenting signs and symptoms are related to local effects of the primary tumor, regional spread, metastatic disease, or paraneoplastic phenomena:
  1. Oral cavity, oropharynx, hypopharynx: Painful mass or ulceration (Fig. E1), dysphagia, odynophagia, weight loss
  2. Larynx: Hoarseness, voice change, shortness of breath, stridor
  3. Nasal cavity, paranasal sinus, nasopharynx: Referred otalgia, conductive hearing loss from middle ear effusion, epistaxis, cranial nerve palsies
  4. All sites: Cranial nerve palsies, painless neck mass from regional metastases to cervical lymph nodes. Most common site of distant metastases is the lung, with bone and liver being much less common
- Physical exam: A thorough examination of the head and neck, including cranial nerve exam, otoscopy, inspection and palpation of oral cavity, oropharynx, and neck, and general physical exam:
  1. Concerning exam findings: Unilateral middle ear effusion, ulcerated mass of the oral cavity (Fig. E2) or oropharynx, trismus, painless neck mass

ETIOLOGY

Exposure to carcinogens including tobacco and alcohol causes genetic alterations in the epithelium of mucosal surfaces lining the upper aerodigestive tract, leading to malignant transformation of epithelial cells. HPV-associated HNSCC is a direct result of the carcinogenic effects of the virus and is not related to alcohol and tobacco use. Primary nasopharyngeal carcinoma has a weak association with tobacco and alcohol and is endemic to southern China, Southeast Asia, and northern Africa. There is a strong association between Epstein-Barr virus infection and primary nasopharyngeal carcinoma.

DIAGNOSIS

DIFFERENTIAL DIAGNOSIS

Lymphoma, primary salivary gland malignancy, thyroid malignancy, benign tumors of the upper aerodigestive tract, metastases

WORKUP

- Initial workup includes a full physical examination, indirect and/or direct laryngoscopy, imaging studies of the head and neck as well as the chest and/or body to assess for metastases, laboratory tests as indicated, and referral to a head and neck cancer specialist.
- Additional workup by head and neck cancer specialist:
  1. Flexible fiber-optic laryngoscopy or mirror laryngoscopy
  2. Biopsy of the tumor in office or under anesthesia
  3. Fine-needle aspiration (FNA) and biopsy for patient who presents with a suspicious neck mass
  4. Panendoscopy with biopsy under anesthesia, which may include direct laryngoscopy, esophagoscopy, and/or bronchoscopy

LABORATORY TESTS

Complete blood count (CBC), coagulation studies, electrolytes, ECG, liver function tests (albumin, transaminases, alkaline phosphatase), TSH

IMAGING STUDIES

- CT scan of the neck with contrast: Necessary to evaluate extent of primary tumor and nodal metastases in neck (Fig. E3)
- MRI of head and neck (optional): Useful for nasopharyngeal, infratemporal fossa, temporal bone, parotid, parapharyngeal, skull base, or intracranial involvement
- Chest x-ray or CT chest with contrast: To evaluate for lung metastases
- PET/CT (Fig. E4): Highlights areas in the body with increased metabolic uptake. Useful initially to assess extent of primary tumor, location of unknown primary tumor, cervical metastases, distant metastases, and second primary tumors. Can be used to monitor for recurrence in the posttreatment setting

STAGING

Staging is based on the tumor, node, metastasis (TNM) staging system provided by the AJCC (Table 1). Staging varies depending on the head and neck subsite that is involved. Any nodal metastasis in the neck automatically classifies as advanced disease (Stage III or IV). Distant metastases place patients at Stage IVC. The exception to this is HPV-positive cancer of the oropharynx, in which the most recent staging system allows for a patient to be classified as low as Stage II even with cervical nodal metastases given the excellent response to treatment and prognosis for these tumors.

TREATMENT

- Treatment consists of surgery, radiation, chemotherapy, or a combination of any or all of the three modalities. The goal is to use as few modalities as possible to minimize side effects of treatment without compromising oncologic success.
  1. Surgery (Fig. E5): Complete surgical resection of the primary tumor along with unilateral or bilateral neck dissections to remove involved or potentially involved lymph nodes as clinically indicated.

TABLE 1 TNM Staging System for Cutaneous Squamous Cell Carcinoma of the Head and Neck

T: Primary Tumor

T_X	Primary tumor cannot be assessed
T_{is}	Carcinoma in situ
T_1	Tumor <2 cm in greatest dimension
T_2	Tumor ≥2 cm, but <4 cm in greatest dimension
T_3	Tumor ≥4 cm in maximum dimension or minor bone erosion or perineural invasion*
T_4	Tumor with gross cortical bone/marrow, skull base invasion and/or skull base foramen invasion
T_{4a}	Tumor with gross cortical bone/marrow invasion
T_{4b}	Tumor with skull base invasion and/or skull base foramen involvement

N: Regional Lymph Nodes

Clinical N (cN)

N_X	Regional lymph nodes cannot be assessed
N_0	No regional lymph node metastasis
N_1	Metastasis in single ipsilateral lymph node, ≤3 cm in greatest dimension and ENE(−)
N_2	Metastasis in single ipsilateral lymph node, >3 cm but not >6 cm in greatest dimension and ENE(−); or in multiple ipsilateral lymph nodes, none >6 cm in greatest dimension; or in bilateral or contralateral lymph nodes and ENE(−), none >6 cm in greatest dimension and ENE(−)
N_{2a}	Metastasis in single ipsilateral lymph node, >3 cm but no >6 cm in greatest dimension and ENE(−)
N_{2b}	Metastasis in multiple ipsilateral lymph nodes, none >6 cm in greatest dimension and ENE(−)
N_{2c}	Metastasis in bilateral or contralateral lymph nodes, none >6 cm in greatest dimension and ENE(−)
N_3	Metastasis in lymph node, >6 cm in greatest dimension and ENE(−); *or* metastasis in any node(s) and clinically overt ENE [ENE(+)]
N_{3a}	Metastasis in a lymph node >6 cm in greatest dimension and ENE(−)
N_{3b}	Metastasis in any node(s) and ENE(+)

Pathologic N (pN)

N_X	Regional lymph nodes cannot be assessed
N_0	No regional lymph node metastasis
N_1	Metastasis in single ipsilateral lymph node, ≤3 cm in greatest dimension and ENE(−)
N_2	Metastasis in single ipsilateral lymph node, ≤3 cm in greatest dimension and ENE(+), or >3 cm but not >6 cm in greatest dimension and ENE(−); or metastases in multiple ipsilateral lymph nodes, none >6 cm in greatest dimension and ENE(−); or in bilateral or contralateral lymph nodes, none >6 cm in greatest dimension and ENE(−)
N_{2a}	Metastasis in single ipsilateral lymph node, ≤3 cm in greatest dimension and ENE(+), *or* a single ipsilateral node >3 cm but not >6 cm in greatest dimension and ENE(−)
N_{2b}	Metastasis in multiple ipsilateral lymph nodes, none >6 cm in greatest dimension and ENE(−)
N_{2c}	Metastasis in bilateral or contralateral lymph nodes, none >6 cm in greatest dimension and ENE(−)
N_3	Metastasis in lymph node, >6 cm in greatest dimension and ENE(−); *or* in a single ipsilateral node >3 cm in greatest dimension and ENE(+), *or* multiple ipsilateral, contralateral, or bilateral nodes, any with ENE(+)
N_{3a}	Metastasis in a lymph node >6 cm in greatest dimension and ENE(−)
N_{3b}	Metastasis in a single ipsilateral node >3 cm in greatest dimension and ENE(+), *or* multiple ipsilateral, contralateral, or bilateral nodes, any with ENE(+)

Note: A designation of *U* or *L* may be used for any N category to indicate metastasis above the lower border of the cricoid *(U)* or below the lower border of the cricoid *(L)*. Similarly, clinical and pathologic ENE should be recorded as ENE(−) or ENE(+).

M: Metastasis

M_0	No distant metastasis
M_1	Present distant metastasis

Staging for Cutaneous Squamous Cell Carcinoma

Stage 0	T_{is}	N_0	M_0
Stage I	T_1	N_0	M_0
Stage II	T_2	N_0	M_0
Stage III	T_3	N_0	M_0
Stage III	T_1	N_1	M_0
Stage III	T_2	N_1	M_0
Stage III	T_3	N_1	M_0
Stage IV	T_1	N_2	M_0
Stage IV	T_2	N_2	M_0
Stage IV	T_3	N_2	M_0
Stage IV	Any T	N_3	M_0
Stage IV	T_4	Any N	M_0
Stage IV	Any T	Any N	M_1

*Deep invasion is defined as invasion beyond the subcutaneous fat or >6 mm (as measured from the granular layer of adjacent normal epidermis to the base of the tumor); perineural invasion for T_3 classification is defined as tumor cells within the nerve sheath of a nerve lying deeper than the dermis or measuring ≥0.1 mm in caliper, or manifesting with clinical or radiographic involvement of named nerves without skull base invasion or transgression.

ENE, Extranodal extension; *TNM,* tumor, node, metastasis.

From *American Joint Committee on Cancer staging manual,* ed 8, 2017.

2. Radiation: Allows for easier access to poorly exposed tumors such as those of the larynx, oropharynx, nasopharynx, or hypopharynx. Disadvantages include lengthy, time-intensive treatment course, xerostomia, pain, and higher surgical morbidity if salvage surgery is needed.
3. Chemotherapy: Useful only as an adjuvant to radiation therapy or for palliation. Single-agent cisplatin therapy is widely accepted in the U.S. as a standard for chemoradiation regimens for head and neck cancers of any site. Major toxicities include nausea, vomiting, renal toxicity, ototoxicity, and myelosuppression.
4. Reconstruction: Performed with the goal of optimizing functional and cosmetic outcomes. Options include primary closure, local flaps, regional flaps, skin grafts, and microvascular free flaps from other parts of the body (e.g., radial forearm, fibula, anterolateral thigh, latissimus, etc.).

ACUTE GENERAL Rx

- Early-stage disease (Stage I or II):
  1. Single-modality treatment with surgery or radiation alone may be appropriate for early-stage head and neck cancer. The choice between one or the other depends on the specific subsite of the head and neck that is involved and the side effects profile for each modality.
  2. Treatment of the potentially involved lymph nodes in the neck with either neck dissection or radiation is controversial and depends on the clinical scenario and the judgment of the treatment team.
- Locoregionally advanced disease (Stage III or IV):
  1. In general, these patients have large tumors >4 cm and/or cervical nodal metastases. Treatment typically involves multimodality therapy with either surgery followed by radiation therapy or upfront chemoradiation alone. Depending on the presence of certain adverse pathologic features of the surgical specimen, adjuvant chemoradiation may be necessary. If chemoradiation is the initial treatment modality, surgery may be needed in the adjuvant setting for residual or recurrent disease.
  2. Laryngeal cancers are the exception where select advanced disease with T3 or N1 tumors can be managed with single-modality therapy with surgery or radiation alone.
  3. Nasopharyngeal cancer is also an exception. This is not a surgical disease. Managed primarily by radiation to primary site and neck for early-stage disease. Chemoradiation is primary treatment for advanced disease. Surgery is reserved for recurrent or residual disease of primary site or neck following radiation therapy.
- Metastatic disease (Stage IVC):
  1. Palliation of symptoms is the primary goal of treatment.
- All patients should be counseled on smoking cessation and avoidance of alcohol.

DISPOSITION

- Prognosis depends on the specific subsite of the head and neck that is involved. Overall 5-yr survival rate for head and neck squamous cell carcinoma is about 55%. This varies with 5-yr survival rates for carcinoma of the lip as high as 89.7% and carcinomas of the hypopharynx as low as approximately 30%.
- Patients are followed on a regular basis multiple times a year by a head and neck cancer specialist. After a 5-yr disease-free survival, patients are followed on a yearly basis.

REFERRAL

Referral should be made to an otolaryngologist or oral surgeon who specializes in head and neck cancer.

PEARLS & CONSIDERATIONS

PREVENTION

- Encourage all patients to cease using tobacco and to limit alcohol consumption.
- Examine the oral cavity and palpate the neck during the annual physical examination. Work up any suspicious masses or lesions.

PATIENT & FAMILY EDUCATION

- www.entnet.org/content/head-and-neck-cancer
- www.cancer.gov/types/head-and-neck

SUGGESTED READINGS

Available at ExpertConsult.com

RELATED CONTENT

Laryngeal Carcinoma (Related Key Topic)
Oral Cancer (Related Key Topic)

AUTHOR: **Louis F. Insalaco, MD**

BASIC INFORMATION

DEFINITION

Complete heart block (CHB) is the absence of electrical impulse transmission from the atria to the ventricles when atrioventricular (AV) junction is not physiologically refractory, due to a functional or anatomical impairment of the conduction system, resulting in a bradycardia characterized by AV dissociation. It may be acquired or congenital. CHB can be permanent or reversible. Degenerative changes are the most common cause of CHB.

SYNONYMS

Third-degree AV block
CHB
Complete AV block

ICD-10CM CODE

I44.2 Atrioventricular block, complete

EPIDEMIOLOGY & DEMOGRAPHICS

- The prevalence of CHB is 0.04%.
- The prevalence of CHB increases with age.

PHYSICAL FINDINGS & CLINICAL PRESENTATION

Physical examination may be normal. Cannon A waves may appear in the jugular vein periodically due to the right atrium contracting (against closed tricuspid valve) during ventricular systole. Patients may present with the following clinical manifestations:

- Dizziness, palpitations
- Syncope or presyncope (due to reduced cardiac output)
- Fatigue, shortness of breath, and impaired exercise tolerance
- Mental status changes
- Congestive heart failure
- Angina pectoris
- Some patients may be asymptomatic (e.g., congenital CHB, fast junctional escape rhythm)
- Sudden cardiac arrest

ETIOLOGY

- Fibrosis or sclerosis of the conduction system, Lenègre and Lev diseases
- Acute myocardial infarction—inferior (14%) or anterior (2%) wall of patients, usually within 24 hours
- Drug effect (digitalis, calcium channel blockers, beta-blockers, amiodarone)
- Cardiomyopathy and myocarditis (rheumatic fever, diphtheria, viruses, toxoplasmosis, syphilis)
- Bacterial endocarditis with paravalvular abscess formation (e.g., AV endocarditis)
- Infiltrative processes of the myocardium (amyloidosis, sarcoidosis, scleroderma, tumor)
- Metabolic abnormalities (hyperkalemia, hypoxia, hypothyroidism)
- Lyme carditis, rheumatoid nodules, polymyositis, Chagas disease
- Neuromuscular disorders (Becker muscular dystrophy, myotonic muscular dystrophy)
- Congenital (birth from mothers with systemic lupus, large ASDs, and AV canal defects)
- Familial: SCN5 sodium channel mutations have been associated with CHB
- Iatrogenic (cardiac surgery, catheter ablation of arrhythmias, percutaneous coronary intervention). Transcatheter aortic valve implantation (TAVI) is shown to be frequently associated with new conduction abnormalities; patients with preexisting right bundle branch block are at increased risk of CHB (resolves over time in most patients).
- Paroxysmal due to phase 4 block of the His-Purkinje system

DIAGNOSIS

DIFFERENTIAL DIAGNOSIS

- The differential diagnosis includes lesser degree of AV block, automatic accelerated junctional rhythms, and nonconducted premature atrial contractions.
- The atrial rate must be faster than the ventricular rate (more As than Vs), and the junctional or ventricular rate is regular. Episodes of AV dissociation with an accelerated ventricular or junctional pacemaker overtaking the sinus node can often look like heart block on a single electrocardiogram.

WORKUP

- Workup such as routine labs, cardiac biomarkers, and cardiac imaging should be dictated by the clinical circumstances.
- ECG: Diagnostic of the disease (Figs. 1 and 2):
  1. P waves are present with a regular atrial rate that is faster than the ventricular rate.
  2. P waves are not related to the QRS complexes. The PR intervals are variable.
  3. RR intervals are regular.
  4. QRS complexes may be narrow with a rate of 40 to 60 beats/min (block proximal to His bundle) or wide with a rate of <40 beats/min (block distal to His bundle), depending on the location of the block in the conduction system.
  5. Complete AV block can result from block at the level of AV node, within the His bundle, or distal to it, in the Purkinje system.

TREATMENT

ACUTE GENERAL Rx

- Initial treatment should focus on the hemodynamic stability and symptoms of the patient.
- Fig. 3 illustrates the evaluation and management of third-degree AV block.
- Consider temporary pacemaker insertion if ventricular escape rate is slow (<40 beats/min) and associated with symptoms or hemodynamic compromise as well as wide QRS escape rhythms, which can be unstable, and QT prolongation above 500 ms, increasing the risk of torsade de pointes ventricular tachycardias.
- CHB as a complication of inferior MI usually only requires temporary pacing; however, a CHB as a result of anterior MI often requires permanent pacing (Table 1).
- Acquired CHB usually requires pacing, but patients with congenital CHB often have sufficiently rapid escape rhythm to prevent symptoms and avoid permanent pacemaker implantation.
- Withdraw AV-nodal blocking agents if any.
- Short-term therapy (until adequate pacing therapy is established):
  1. Vagolytic agents such as atropine may be used to increase the rate of the escape rhythm (for AV nodal level blocks).
  2. Catecholamines such as isoproterenol transiently used for a CHB at any site (use with extreme caution or not at all in patients with coronary artery disease or in patients with digitalis toxicity).
  3. Percutaneous external cardiac pacing (uncomfortable for patients and not always reliably capturing the ventricle).
- Drugs cannot be relied on to increase HR for more than several hours or days without side effects; therefore, temporary or permanent pacemaker insertion is indicated.
- Symptomatic CHB in the absence of a condition that is likely to resolve is an ACC/AHA/HRS Class I indication for permanent pacemaker (PPM) placement.
- Class I indications for PPM placement in asymptomatic patients according to the ACC/AHA guidelines include:
  1. Patients in sinus rhythm, with documented asystolic pauses greater than or equal to 3.0 sec or an escape rate <40 beats/min, or with an escape rhythm that is below the AV node
  2. Patients with atrial fibrillation and bradycardia with one or more pauses of at least 5 sec or longer
  3. After catheter ablation of the AV junction
  4. If cardiomegaly or LV dysfunction is present with ventricular rates of 40 beats/min or faster
  5. Postoperative CHB that is not expected to resolve
  6. Symptomatic AV block as a consequence of guideline-directed medical therapy for which there is no alternative treatment with strong evidence of therapy benefit (beta-blockers in CAD or HFrEF)
  7. When it is associated with neuromuscular diseases, such as Erb dystrophy (limb-girdle muscular dystrophy), Kearns-Sayre syndrome, myotonic muscular dystrophy, and peroneal muscular atrophy
  8. CHB present during exercise in the absence of myocardial ischemia
- Therapy is directed toward the underlying etiology if there is a reversible source (i.e., IV antibiotics for Lyme disease).

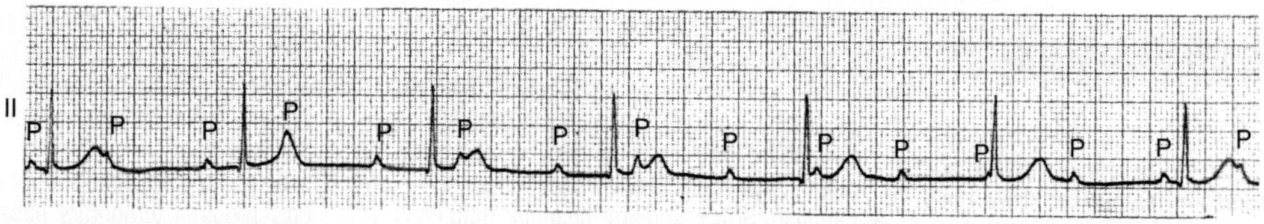

FIG. 1 Third-degree (complete) atrioventricular heart block is characterized by independent atrial (P) and ventricular (QRS) activity. The atrial rate is always faster than the ventricular rate. The PR intervals are completely variable. Some P waves fall on the T wave, distorting its shape. Others may fall in the QRS complex and be "lost." Notice that the QRS complexes are of normal width, indicating that the ventricles are being paced from the atrioventricular junction. (From Goldberger AL, [ed]: *Clinical electrocardiography*, ed 5, St Louis, 1994, Mosby.)

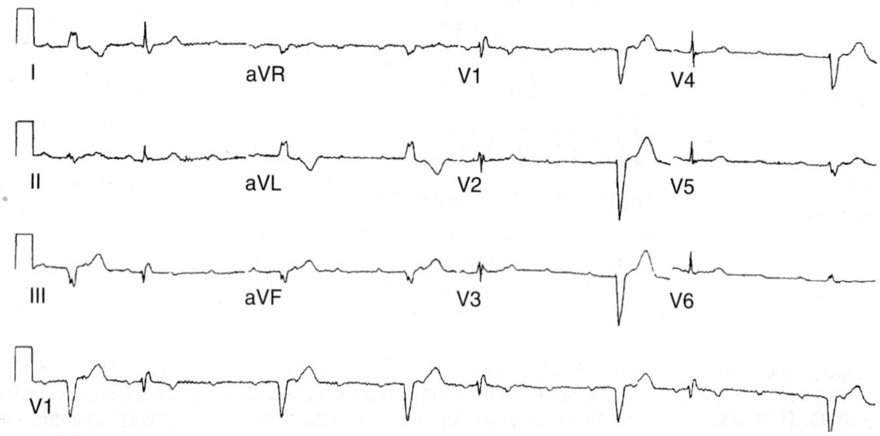

FIG. 2 High-grade atrioventricular block. Note that only three P waves conducted to the ventricle in the whole tracing. Conducted P waves were associated with normal PR intervals and right bundle branch block, a finding suggesting infranodal block. All other P waves were blocked, and ventricular escape rhythm with a left bundle branch block pattern is observed. Note that the block is not caused by retrograde concealment in the atrioventricular node or His-Purkinje system from the ventricular escape complexes because the conducted P waves occurred at a short cycle following the escape complexes. *aVF,* Augmented vector foot; *aVL,* augmented vector left; *aVR,* augmented vector right. (From Issa Z et al: *Clinical arrhythmology and electrophysiology,* ed 2, Philadelphia, 2012, Saunders.)

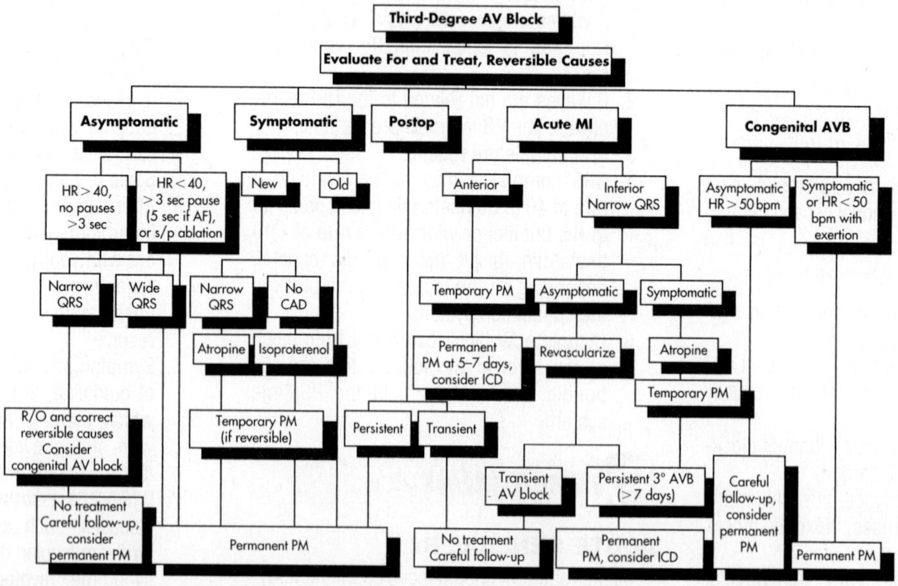

FIG. 3 Evaluation and management of third-degree atrioventricular *(AV)* block. *AF,* Atrial flutter; *AVB,* atrioventricular block; *bpm,* beats per minute; *CAD,* coronary artery disease; *HR,* heart rate; *ICD,* implantable cardioverter defibrillator; *MI,* myocardial infarction; *PM,* pacemaker; *R/O,* rule out; *s/p,* after. (From Olshansky B et al: *Arrhythmia essentials,* ed 2, Philadelphia, 2017, Elsevier.)

TABLE 1 Indications for Pacing in AV Block

Class I

1. Third-degree or advanced second-degree AV block at any anatomic level associated with any one of the following conditions:
   a. Symptoms (including heart failure) attributable to AV block *(Level of Evidence: C)*
   b. Arrhythmias and other medical conditions that require drugs that result in symptomatic bradycardia *(Level of Evidence: C)*
   c. Documented periods of asystole >3.0 seconds, any escape rate <40 beats/min, or any escape rhythm below the AV junction (e.g., a wide QRS morphology) in awake, asymptomatic patients in sinus rhythm *(Level of Evidence: C)*
   d. A documented period of asystole >5 seconds in awake, asymptomatic patients in atrial fibrillation *(Level of Evidence: C)*
   e. After catheter ablation of the AV junction *(Level of Evidence: C)*
   f. Postoperative AV block that is not expected to resolve after cardiac surgery *(Level of Evidence: C)*
   g. Neuromuscular diseases, such as myotonic muscular dystrophy, Kearns–Sayre syndrome, Erb (limb-girdle) dystrophy, and peroneal muscular atrophy, with or without symptoms of bradycardia *(Level of Evidence: B)*
2. Asymptomatic third-degree AV block at any anatomic site with an average awake ventricular rate >40 beats/min in patients with cardiomegaly or left ventricular dysfunction
3. Second-degree or third-degree AV block during exercise in the absence of myocardial ischemia *(Level of Evidence: C)*
4. Symptomatic second-degree AV block regardless of type or site of block *(Level of Evidence: B)*

Class IIa

1. Advanced second-degree or third-degree AV block at any anatomic site with an average ventricular rate >40 beats/min in the absence of cardiomegaly *(Level of Evidence: C)*
2. Asymptomatic second-degree AV block at intra- or infra-His levels found at electrophysiologic study *(Level of Evidence: B)*
3. First-degree or second-degree AV block with symptoms similar to those of pacemaker syndrome *(Level of Evidence: B)*
4. Asymptomatic type II second-degree AV block with a narrow QRS. When type II second-degree AV block occurs with a wide QRS, including isolated right bundle branch block, pacing becomes a Class I recommendation. *(Level of Evidence: B)*

Class IIb

1. AV block due to drug use or toxicity when the block is expected to recur even after withdrawal of the drug *(Level of Evidence: B)*
2. Neuromuscular diseases, such as myotonic muscular dystrophy, Kearns–Sayre syndrome, Erb (limb-girdle) dystrophy, and peroneal muscular atrophy with any degree of AV block (including first-degree AV block), with or without symptoms of bradycardia *(Level of Evidence: B)*

Class III

1. Asymptomatic first-degree AV block *(Level of Evidence: B)*
2. Asymptomatic type I second-degree AV block at a site above the His (i.e., the AV node) level or not known to be intra- or infra-Hisian by electrophysiologic study *(Level of Evidence: B)*
3. AV block expected to resolve and unlikely to recur (e.g., drug toxicity, Lyme disease, nocturnally in sleep apnea, early postoperative status, transient increases in vagal tone) *(Level of Evidence: B)*

AV, Atrioventricular.
From Bonow RO et al: *Braunwald's heart disease: a textbook of cardiovascular medicine,* ed 9, Philadelphia, 2012, Saunders.

- Table 2 summarizes the management of complete heart block.

CHRONIC Rx

Dual-chamber pacemaker implantation. Patients with a pacemaker need regular follow-up and pacemaker monitoring to ensure proper device functioning. Interest has developed recently in placing the ventricular pacing lead in the His bundle region or Left Bundle region, which can result in a narrow-paced QRS and may prevent ventricular dyssynchrony associated with traditional RV pacing.

DISPOSITION

- Mortality is highest in the neonatal period in congenital CHB.
- Prognosis is favorable after insertion of a pacemaker and is related to the underlying etiology of complete AV block (e.g., myocardial infarction, cardiomyopathy).
- Nonrandomized studies have shown that PPM insertion improves survival in patients with CHB.

REFERRAL

All patients with CHB should be referred to a cardiologist for consideration of temporary and/or PPM implantation.

PEARLS & CONSIDERATIONS

COMMENTS

- Patients should be instructed to avoid activities that may damage the pacemaker (e.g., contact sports).
- Pacemaker manufacturers do not recommend any special restrictions regarding proximity to typical household items.
- All pacemaker manufacturers offer pacemakers that are MRI compatible. Older pacemaker models and leads may have a strong relative contraindication for MRI.
- Leadless pacemakers that are implanted directly into the right ventricle using a special delivery system are available for special indications and are primarily used for patients who are at high risk for traditional pacemakers and do not require dual-chamber pacing.
- Some medical procedures, such as lithotripsy, hyperbaric chamber, and electrocautery used during surgery, may require pacemaker programming and testing perioperatively to avoid electromagnetic interference.
- Table 3 describes the five-letter pacemaker code, and Table 4 summarizes common permanent pacemakers.

RELATED CONTENT

Complete Heart Block (Patient Information)

AUTHOR: **Artem Astsaturov, MD**

TABLE 2 Complete Heart Block Management

Setting	Therapy
Asymptomatic–Acquired	• Rule out reversible causes, including: Hyperkalemia Acute inferior MI Digoxin toxicity Excess calcium channel blocker therapy Lyme disease • If HR <40 bpm, first-line therapy is a permanent DDD pacemaker. • Temporary pacing is indicated if heart rate <40 bpm. The patient has impaired hemodynamics, and if permanent, pacing cannot be accomplished expeditiously. The CHB has an identifiable and reversible cause, while awaiting recovery. Temporary transvenous pacing must be used with caution in patients with any escape rhythm, particularly if wide QRS complex and slow. Overdrive suppression can occur rapidly. • If the rate of escape rhythm >40 bpm, permanent pacemaker insertion is controversial. • Temporary pacing is to be avoided in asymptomatic patients whose ventricular rates are >40 bpm, especially if the QRS complex is narrow. • CHB due to radio frequency ablation of the AV junction to control ventricular response rate in atrial fibrillation requires permanent pacing. May occur even if the patient is asymptomatic from a slow ventricular rate (40 bpm) that may be quite stable over time. Acquired CHB is associated with a poor short-term prognosis (>50% mortality in the first 6-12 mo after diagnosis). If irreversible, pacing is indicated.
Symptomatic	• A permanent pacemaker is indicated. • Temporary pacing is indicated if permanent pacing cannot be done expeditiously or if CHB has an identifiable and reversible cause (e.g., drug overdose).
Congenital	• Usually associated with a narrow QRS complex with an escape rhythm arising in the AVN. • Patients are usually asymptomatic. • In patients who are asymptomatic, the indications for a pacemaker are controversial. • Patients will need close follow-up, at least annually, for evaluation of symptoms suggesting chronotropic incompetence. • If symptomatic bradycardia, a permanent pacemaker is indicated. • If rate is consistently <50 bpm and does not increase with exercise (chronotropic incompetence), a permanent pacemaker is indicated.
MI	• If symptomatic bradycardia, a temporary pacemaker is indicated. • If CHB block occurs in the setting of an anterior infarction, permanent pacing is indicated if AVB persists. • CHB in inferior MI is generally in the AVN. There is usually no need for a permanent pacemaker, as it usually resolves. If it does not resolve, a permanent pacemaker may be indicated in some cases.
Preoperative	• Permanent pacemaker first, unless the surgery is emergent. • If surgery is emergent, insert a temporary pacemaker pre-op with the plan for a permanent pacemaker after surgery.
Postoperative	• Transcutaneous or temporary transvenous pacing. • A permanent pacemaker is indicated if there is permanent damage to the AV conduction system (e.g., after aortic valve surgery or VSD repair).

AV, Atrioventricular; *AVB,* atrioventricular block; *AVN,* atrioventricular node; *bpm,* beats per minute; *CHB,* complete atrioventricular block; *DDD,* dual chamber; *HR,* heart rate; *MI,* myocardial infarction; *VSD,* ventricular septal defect.
From Olshansky B et al: *Arrhythmia essentials,* ed 2, Philadelphia, 2017, Elsevier.

TABLE 3 Five-Letter Pacemaker Code

Letter 1 Chamber Paced	Letter 2 Chamber Sensed	Letter 3 Sensing Response	Letter 4 Programmability	Letter 5 Antitachycardia Functions
A = atrium	A = atrium	T = triggered*	P = simple	P = pacing
V = ventricle	V = ventricle	I = inhibited	M = multiprogrammable	S = shock
D = dual	D = dual	D = dual (A and V inhibited)	R = rate adaptive	D = dual (shock pace)
0 = none	0 = none	0 = none	C = communicating	
			0 = none	

*In the triggered response mode, the pacemaker discharges or fires when it recognizes an intrinsic depolarization. As a result, pacemaker spikes occur during inscription of the QRS complex. Because this mode results in high energy consumption and a shortened battery life and because the sensing response can be misinterpreted as pacemaker malfunction, this sensing mode is not used with modern pacemakers.
From Marx JA et al: *Rosen's emergency medicine,* ed 8, Philadelphia, 2014, Saunders.

TABLE 4 Common Permanent Pacemakers

Code	Indication	Advantages	Disadvantages
VVI	Intermittent backup pacing; inactive patient	Simplicity; low cost	Fixed rate; risk of pacemaker syndrome
VVIR	Atrial fibrillation	Rate responsive	Requires advanced programming
DDD	Complete heart block	Atrial tracking restores normal physiology	No rate responsiveness; requires two leads and advanced programming
DDDR	Sinus node dysfunction; for rate responsiveness atrioventricular block and need	Universal pacer; all options available by programming	Complexity, cost, programming, and follow-up evaluation

From Marx JA et al: *Rosen's emergency medicine,* ed 8, Philadelphia, 2014, Saunders.

BASIC INFORMATION

DEFINITION

Second-degree heart block or second-degree atrioventricular (AV) heart block is characterized by a failure of one or more, but not all, atrial impulses to conduct to the ventricles. The block may be at any level of the AV conduction system. In both types of second-degree heart block, the sinus rate will continue at regular intervals, resulting in a constant sinus rate. When more than one atrial impulse is present for each ventricular complex, the rhythm may be described as a ratio of the number of atrial impulses to the number of ventricular complexes. Electrocardiographically there are three types of second-degree block:

- Mobitz I (Wenckebach):
  1. Characterized by a progressive prolongation of the PR interval prior to a blocked nonconducted beat and a shorter PR interval after that blocked beat; the conducted impulse will generally be narrow. The cycle may repeat periodically, leading to "grouped beating."
  2. Site of block is usually AV node (proximal to the His bundle).
- Mobitz type II:
  1. Characterized by fixed PR intervals before and after blocked beats and may be associated with a wide QRS morphology (right bundle branch block [RBBB] or left bundle branch block [LBBB] patterns).
  2. Site of block is usually infranodal, especially when QRS is wide.
  3. It has a greater propensity for progressing to third-degree AV block.
- Pure 2:1 conduction patterns cannot be reliably classified as Mobitz type I or type II because there are not enough P waves to characterize prolongation of the PR interval.

SYNONYMS

Wenckebach block (Mobitz type I block)
Mobitz type II block
AV block

ICD-10CM CODES

I44.1	Atrioventricular block, second degree
I45.5	Other specified heart block
Q24.6	Congenital heart block

EPIDEMIOLOGY & DEMOGRAPHICS

Mobitz type I block is more common and may occur in individuals with heightened vagal tone or as a side effect of medications, such as β-blockers or calcium channel blockers.

PHYSICAL FINDINGS & CLINICAL PRESENTATION

- Patients with Mobitz type I are usually asymptomatic. Patients with either type may feel palpitations or the feeling of "missing a beat." Sudden loss of consciousness without warning (Adams-Stokes attack) can occur in patients with Mobitz type II; however, it is much more common in patients with complete heart block.
- Type I block: There is gradual decrease in the intensity of the first heart sound with widening of the a-c interval in the central venous waveform, ending in a pause, and an a wave not followed by a v wave in the neck along with an irregular pulse.
- Type II block: The first heart sound retains a constant intensity, with intermittent ventricular pauses and a wave not followed by v waves in the neck. There is an irregular pulse for most times with intermittent pauses.

ETIOLOGY

- High vagal tone (young patients, athletes at rest)
- Degenerative changes in the AV conduction system
- Ischemia at the AV nodes (type I with inferior wall myocardial infarction [MI] and type II with anterior wall MI)
- Drugs (digitalis, quinidine, procainamide, adenosine, calcium channel blockers [nondihydropyridines], β-blockers)
- Cardiomyopathies, collagen vascular diseases, infiltrative diseases (amyloidosis, sarcoidosis, hematochromatosis)
- Myocarditis/endocarditis (infectious, e.g., Lyme disease, Chagas disease; and noninfectious, e.g., systemic lupus erythematosus)
- Hyperkalemia, hypermagnesemia
- Hypothyroidism
- Prior cardiac valve surgery
- Catheter trauma, catheter ablation for arrhythmias

DIAGNOSIS

DIFFERENTIAL DIAGNOSIS

The ECG easily and reliably distinguishes Mobitz type I from Mobitz type II block and from other conduction abnormalities. It should be distinguished from the less common phenomenon of second-degree sinoatrial node exit block.

Mobitz type I block with a normal QRS complex tends to be benign and usually does not progress to more advanced forms of AV conduction within a short period of time because the disease is mostly confined to within the AV node. Mobitz type II block often precedes the development of Adams-Stokes syncope, symptoms are frequent, prognosis is compromised, and progression to third-degree AV block is common and sudden. Thus, type II second-degree AV block with a wide QRS typically indicates diffuse conduction system disease involving even the infranodal His-Purkinje system.

WORKUP

ECG, ambulatory monitoring (Holter or external loop recorders) in selected patients

- Mobitz type I (Fig. 1) ECG shows:
  1. Sequential and gradual prolongation of PR interval leading to a nonconducted P wave
  2. Shortened PR interval following the pause as compared with the pre-pause PR interval
  3. Progressive shortening of the R-R interval prior to nonconducted atrial impulse
  4. Usually see "grouped beating" pattern
- Mobitz type II ECG shows (Fig. 2):
  1. Fixed duration of PR interval with constant P-P and R-R intervals
  2. Sudden nonconducted P wave
  3. Abnormal QRS duration or fascicular blocks are common
- In 2:1 AV block (Fig. 3), it cannot be determined based on the 12-lead ECG whether there is Mobitz type I or type II AV block, although a wide QRS complex is suggestive of Mobitz type II.
  1. Administering atropine can improve AV conduction if the AV block is type I or within the AV node; however, if it is infranodal (i.e., type II), the increased sinus rate caused by atropine may worsen the ratio of AV conduction, resulting in worsening bradycardia.
  2. Exercise stress testing may function in the same way as atropine above. If the disease is confined to the AV node, it may improve with exercise, but in cases of Mobitz type II AV block, the degree of AV block will worsen.
  3. Carotid sinus stimulation and other vagal maneuvers may worsen the AV block if it is at the level of the AV node (i.e., Mobitz type I) but will paradoxically improve the ratio of AV conduction by slowing down the sinus rate if it is a Mobitz type II or infranodal AV block.
  4. An algorithm for evaluation of patients with 2:1 AV block is illustrated in Fig. 4.

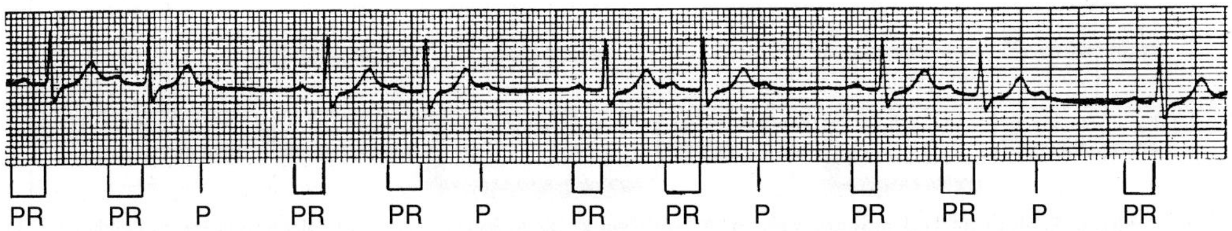

FIG. 1 Wenckebach (Mobitz type I) second-degree atrioventricular block. Notice the progressive increase in PR intervals, with the third P wave in each sequence not followed by a QRS. Wenckebach block produces a characteristically syncopated rhythm with grouping of the QRS complexes (group beating).

Rx TREATMENT

NONPHARMACOLOGIC THERAPY

Elimination of drugs that may induce AV block such as digoxin, beta-blockers, and calcium channel blockers

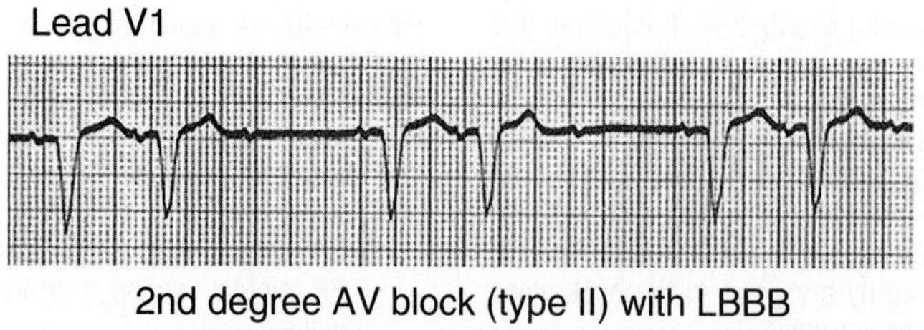

FIG. 2 Mobitz type II atrioventricular (AV) block with left bundle branch block (LBBB). Note the fixed P-P intervals with no change in PR intervals followed by a sudden nonconducted P wave. The LBBB indicates infranodal disease in the His-Purkinje system that is suggestive of Mobitz type II block.

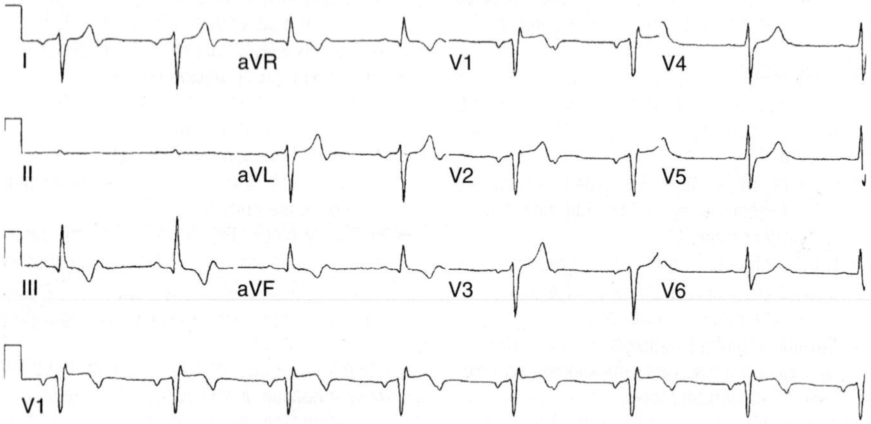

FIG. 3 Second-degree 2:1 atrioventricular block. Notice the short PR interval during conducted complexes and the wide QRS complexes, suggesting block in the His-Purkinje system. (From Issa Z et al: *Clinical arrhythmology and electrophysiology,* ed 2, Philadelphia, 2012, Saunders.)

ACUTE GENERAL Rx

- Treatment is usually not necessary unless the resting heart rate is <40 beats per min (bpm) while awake.
- If symptomatic (e.g., dizziness), atropine 1 mg (may repeat once after 5 min) may be tried to increase AV conduction; if no response, trial of dobutamine or isoproterenol may be helpful prior to insertion of a pacemaker.
- Atropine:
  1. Reduces heart block due to hypervagotonia but not due to AV node ischemia
  2. Does not increase infranodal conduction (third-degree and second-degree AV block that is below the AV node)
  3. Should be used with caution in Mobitz type II AV block due to possible paradoxical decrease in heart rate (as atrial rate increases, AV conduction decreases)
  4. Is ineffective in heart transplantation patients
- If associated with anterior wall MI and wide QRS complex, consider insertion of a temporary pacemaker.
- Indications for permanent pacemaker (PPM) implantation by ACC/AHA/HRS 2008 guidelines:
  1. Second-degree AV block with associated symptomatic bradycardia regardless of the type or site of the block (class I; level of evidence: B)
  2. Second-degree AV block provoked by exercise in the absence of myocardial ischemia (class I; level of evidence: C)
  3. Asymptomatic second-degree AV block at intra- or infra-His levels found at electrophysiologic study (class IIa; level of evidence: B)
  4. First- or second-degree AV block with symptoms similar to those of pacemaker syndrome or hemodynamic compromise (class IIa; level of evidence: B)
  5. Asymptomatic type II second-degree AV block with a wide QRS, including isolated right bundle branch block (class I; level of evidence: B)

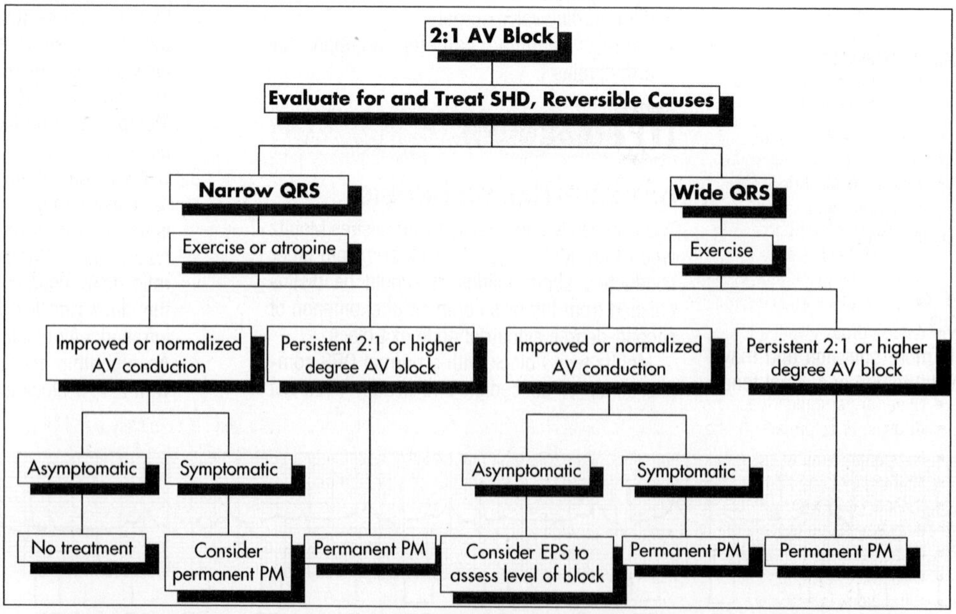

FIG. 4 Evaluation and management of 2:1 AV block. *AV,* Atrioventricular; *EPS,* electrophysiology study; *PM,* pacemaker; *SHD,* structural heart disease (no overt evidence of myocardial, valvular, congenital, or coronary heart disease.) (From Olshansky B et al: *Arrhythmia essentials,* ed 2, Philadelphia, 2017, Elsevier.)

6. PPM is not indicated for asymptomatic type I second-degree AV block at supra-His (AV node) level or that which is not known to be intra- or infra-Hisian (class III; level of evidence: C)

- Table 1 summarizes the management of Mobitz type I second-degree AV block.
- Table 2 summarizes the management of Mobitz type II second-degree AV block.

DISPOSITION

Prognosis is good with insertion of a pacemaker.

REFERRAL

Referral for pacemaker insertion (see "Acute General Rx")

PEARLS & CONSIDERATIONS

COMMENTS

Patients with symptomatic Mobitz type II should be referred for a pacemaker. Asymptomatic patients should be referred if the AV block worsens with exercise and should be followed up routinely for potential development of high-grade AV block.

RELATED CONTENT

Second-Degree Heart Block (Patient Information)

AUTHOR: **Aleem I. Mughal, MD, FHRS**

TABLE 1 Mobitz Type I Second-Degree Atrioventricular Block Management

Setting	Therapy

Outpatient—Asymptomatic	• Treadmill testing will help assess chronotropic competence (if this rhythm is not related to myocardial ischemia), as well as enhance AVN conduction, thereby reducing the degree of Wenckebach block (e.g., from 5:4 to 8:7 or producing first-degree AVB only).
	• Holter monitoring can assess the degree and level of AVB and the persistence of the problem during activities of daily living and any diurnal variation.
	• If the QRS duration is wide and Holter monitoring or stress testing suggests infranodal block, an electrophysiology study may help to confirm the level of AVB.
	• If block is demonstrated to be intra- or infra-Hisian, permanent pacemaker implantation is reasonable, even in an asymptomatic patient. On occasion, intra-Hisian block can be demonstrated in a patient with a narrow, normal-appearing QRS complex by the production of higher degrees of AV block during treadmill testing with the increase in sinus rate.
	• No therapy.
	  • If not due to reversible cause (e.g., drugs or transient damage to the AV node from Lyme disease) and the QRS duration is normal, as more advanced or complete heart block rarely develops.
	  • There may be increased risk of syncope and symptoms in the future.

Outpatient—Symptomatic	• Some AV nodal blocking drugs (digoxin, β-adrenergic blockers, calcium blockers) may be the cause and should be reduced or stopped, if possible, and then only if severe symptomatic bradycardia occurs.
	• If older or at high risk for structural heart disease, consider an echocardiogram to assess LV function (even if no physical findings are present).
	• If due to a correctable cause such as AV nodal blocking drugs, stop the drug, if possible.
	• If there is a wide QRS or bundle branch block, it is possible that Wenckebach can be due to a block below the AV node (in the His-Purkinje system).
	  • In this case, permanent pacemaker implantation is indicated.
	  • Acutely, intravenous atropine or oral theophylline usually increases conduction through the AV node.
	  • These may paradoxically decrease ventricular rate and increase the degree of block if the block is below the bundle of His.
	• Permanent pacemaker implantation is indicated if symptomatic second-degree AVB is not otherwise correctable.

MI	• Is often reversed during thrombolysis or angioplasty.
	• May also appear for the first time concomitantly with these procedures.
	• Transient in nature
	• Temporary DDD pacing for the following:
	  • Persistent low heart rate (<40 bpm)
	  • Low cardiac output
	  • Ischemia
	  • Refractory hypotension
	  • Symptoms of light-headedness and dizziness
	• Atropine or theophylline may reverse the block but can cause unwanted tachycardia during drug administration.
	• These drugs are only rarely indicated except at the time of presentation of the patient.
	• Atypical AV block is more common in inferior-posterior MIs due to the Bezold-Jarisch reflex and the effect of increased vagal tone on the AV node.
	  • This is usually transient, and unless there is hemodynamic collapse, there is no need for a temporary pacemaker.
	  • Rarely is there a need for a permanent pacemaker. This is true even if transient third-degree (complete) AV block occurs, as high degrees of block tend to resolve over 5-7 days.
	  • If the AV block does not resolve but the ventricular rate is >40 bpm, no therapy is required if patient is asymptomatic.
	  • If the block does not resolve after 7 days and/or the ventricular rate is <40 or if patient is symptomatic, a permanent pacemaker is indicated.

Preoperative	• Assess drugs given and their need; stop offending drugs that enhance vagal tone, if possible. • If no symptoms, no therapy. • If symptomatic and no reversible causes, provide temporary pacing before surgery. • Need for permanent pacing can be accomplished in the postoperative setting. • Atropine or isoproterenol may be given to increase AV node conduction if symptomatic or hemodynamically significant.
Postoperative	• Rare after CABG but, if it occurs, consider an offending drug or transient ischemia to the AV node. • No therapy is generally needed. • If associated with wide QRS complex, consider block below the His. • If it persists, consider an EP study to assess the level of the block. • If patient is asymptomatic and block is above His, no need for permanent pacemaker. • If patient is symptomatic or block is below the His, permanent pacemaker is indicated. • If the block is associated with valve (especially aortic) surgery, consider direct damage to the AV node. • If persistent, a pacemaker is indicated for symptoms or persistent slow rate (<40 bpm or no increase in rate with exercise).

AV, Atrioventricular; *AVB,* atrioventricular block; *AVN,* atrioventricular node; *bpm,* beats per minute; *CABG,* coronary artery bypass graft; *DDD,* dual-chamber; *EP,* electrophysiology; *LV,* left ventricular; *MI,* myocardial infarction.

From Olshansky B et al: *Arrhythmia essentials,* ed 2, Philadelphia, 2017, Elsevier.

TABLE 2 Mobitz Type II Second-Degree Atrioventricular Block Management

Setting	Therapy

Outpatient—Asymptomatic	• Risk for complete heart block and death is significant (approximately 50%).
	• A dual-chamber permanent pacemaker is recommended as the pacing system of choice.
	  • Admit the patient for a permanent pacemaker and place on a cardiac monitor.
	  • In the absence of symptoms or progressive (higher-degree AVB), there is no need for a temporary pacemaker before permanent pacemaker implantation.
	  • Avoid atropine.
	  • Evaluate for the presence of underlying cardiac disease, such as infiltrative processes (e.g., amyloid) or MI.

Outpatient—Symptomatic	• Dual-chamber permanent pacemaker implantation is indicated.
	• Admit the patient and place on a cardiac monitor.
	  • If symptomatic or hemodynamically detrimental ventricular bradycardia is present, a temporary pacemaker is indicated if a permanent system cannot be placed expeditiously.
	  • Do not give atropine because this may worsen the AVB and produce a slower ventricular rate.
	  • Exercise, sinus tachycardia, and catecholamines also can worsen the degree of block by enhancing AV nodal conduction and impinging on the refractory period of the His-Purkinje system.

MI	• Place temporary pacemaker.
	  • Mobitz type II second-degree AVB is associated with a high rate of heart failure in this setting.
	  • A permanent pacemaker is indicated if the AVB is persistent because the risk of complete heart block is >50%.
	  • Long-term prognosis may not be improved.
	  • Avoid the use of antiarrhythmic drugs (including lidocaine) in the absence of a pacemaker, unless there is sustained ventricular tachyarrhythmia, as these drugs may worsen the degree of AVB.
	  • Do not give atropine.
	  • Mobitz type II second-degree AVB has a lower (albeit not known with certainty) incidence in the current early revascularization era, but if present or of new onset may improve with time, but this is rare. After being present and persistent, a pacemaker will likely be needed.

Preoperative	• Place permanent pacemaker.
	  • If urgent or emergent surgery, place a temporary pacemaker with the plan for a permanent pacemaker after surgery.
	  • If CABG, epicardial atrial and ventricular wires can be placed, with temporary pacing as standby, until a permanent transvenous pacemaker can be placed.
	  • It is best to place the permanent pacemaker after CABG or other cardiac surgery as leads otherwise tend to dislodge.
	  • If endocarditis, temporary pacemaker until infection resolves and after cardiac surgery.
	  • Avoid antiarrhythmic drugs and atropine.

Postoperative	• If bradycardia, temporary pacing (via epicardial wires, if present, after cardiac surgery).
	• Temporary Mobitz type II AV block may resolve after cardiac surgery.
	  • It may be due to trauma near the His-Purkinje system (e.g., with aortic valve surgery, where left bundle branch block is a not-infrequent accompaniment).
	  • Persistent (e.g., more than 3-5 days) Mobitz type II block will require permanent pacing.
	  • No antiarrhythmic drugs should be given unless an adequate backup ventricular pacing is available.
	  • Endocarditis with abscess near the septum can destroy the His-Purkinje system.
	  • Despite surgical repair, permanent pacing will likely be required.
	  • For patients having tricuspid valve replacement, an endocardial lead can occasionally be placed across a porcine bioprosthesis without producing tricuspid regurgitation but should be avoided if there is a mechanical valve.
	  • Tricuspid valve repair (e.g., annuloplasty) should not pose a problem in positioning a right ventricular lead.

AV, Atrioventricular; *AVB,* atrioventricular block; *CABG,* coronary artery bypass graft; *MI,* myocardial infarction.
From Olshansky B et al: *Arrhythmia essentials*, ed 2, Philadelphia, 2017, Elsevier.

BASIC INFORMATION

DEFINITION

Heart failure (HF) is a complex clinical syndrome that can result from any structural or functional cardiac disorder that impairs the ability of the ventricle to fill with or eject blood. The cardinal manifestations of heart failure are dyspnea, fatigue, and fluid retention. The pathophysiology of HF (Fig. E1) is related to progressive activation of the neuroendocrine system to compensate for decreased effective circulating volume (Table 1), leading to total body volume overload and circulatory insufficiency. These events culminate in the development of pulmonary congestion as well as peripheral edema. Specifically, the renin-angiotensin-aldosterone system (RAAS) is implicated; once activated, it can lead to volume expansion (sodium retention) and cardiac fibrosis (mediated through angiotensin II). Another recognized mechanism is disordered adrenergic stimulation as a key component of progression of disease. The term *congestive heart failure* (CHF) usually denotes a volume-overloaded status as a result of HF. Given that not all patients have volume overload at the time of the evaluation, *congestive heart failure* should be distinguished from the broader term *heart failure*.

CLASSIFICATION: The American College of Cardiology/American Heart Association (ACC/AHA) describes the following four stages of HF. This staging model was designed to emphasize the evolution and progression of HF over a continuum and the preventability of HF in at-risk patients.

- Stage A: Patients at high risk (e.g., with hypertension, atherosclerotic disease, diabetes mellitus, metabolic syndrome, cytotoxin, family history) for HF but without structural heart disease or symptoms of HF
- Stage B: Patients with structural heart disease (e.g., left ventricular [LV] dysfunction) but without symptoms of HF
- Stage C: Patients with structural heart disease with prior or current symptoms of HF
- Stage D: Patients with refractory HF requiring specialized interventions

In addition to the ACC/AHA stages described above, the New York Heart Association (NYHA) defines four functional classes of HF designed to describe the symptoms of stage C and D HF. The functional classes are intended to assess the symptoms of HF and may fluctuate with therapy. It should be noted that current guidelines employ the functional classes to aid in determination of appropriate treatment.

- Asymptomatic or symptomatic only at activity levels that would limit normal individuals
- Symptomatic with ordinary exertion (e.g., 2 city blocks or 1 flight of stairs in a faster than usual pace)
- Symptomatic with less than ordinary exertion (e.g., less than 2 city blocks or 1 flight of stairs)
- Symptomatic at rest

Table 2 compares the ACC/AHA and the NYHA classification. Table 3 describes a simplified classification and common clinical characteristics of patients with acute heart failure.

TERMINOLOGY:

- Although HF has traditionally been classified as systolic vs. diastolic, this was dependent on the imaging modality used. With noted variation in the observed systolic function between studies, the ejection fraction serves as a better marker. HF is now categorized into *HF with reduced ejection fraction* (HFrEF) and HF with *preserved ejection fraction* (HFpEF). Other common classifications include right-sided vs. left-sided and high-output vs. low-output. Systolic HF or HFrEF is defined by the presence of impaired contractility of the LV, as measured by ejection fraction (EF) ≤40% with clinical signs or symptoms of HF. In contrast, HFpEF has been described as evidence (clinical) of HF with an EF ≥50% with or without evidence of diastolic dysfunction. There are two further classifications of HFpEF: HFpEF borderline, used to describe patients with an EF 41% to 49%, and HFpEF improved, used to describe patients who previously had HFrEF with an improvement in their EF.
- Right-sided HF denotes peripheral signs and symptoms of HF without evidence of pulmonary congestion, as opposed to left-sided HF, which typically manifests with pulmonary congestion and subsequent signs and symptoms of right-sided HF. The most common cause of right-sided HF is left-sided HF. High-output HF involves signs and symptoms of HF but features an elevated cardiac output unable to meet the abnormally high metabolic demands of peripheral tissues and is the result of myriad systemic disorders (e.g., systemic arteriovenous fistulas, hyperthyroidism, anemia). The term *acute decompensated HF* (ADHF) refers to worsening of signs or symptoms of HF due to a wide range of causes. Of note, HF is not equivalent to cardiomyopathy or LV dysfunction. These latter terms describe the possible structural or functional reasons for the development of HF, whereas HF is a clinical syndrome characterized by specific symptoms and signs.

SYNONYMS

HF
Congestive heart failure
CHF
Cardiac failure
Cardiogenic shock
Cardiogenic pulmonary edema

ICD-10CM CODES

I50.9	Heart failure, unspecified
I50.20	Unspecified systolic (congestive) heart failure
I50.21	Acute systolic (congestive) heart failure
I50.22	Chronic systolic (congestive) heart failure
I50.23	Acute on chronic systolic (congestive) heart failure
I50.30	Unspecified diastolic (congestive) heart failure
I50.31	Acute diastolic (congestive) heart failure
I50.32	Chronic diastolic (congestive) heart failure
I50.33	Acute on chronic diastolic (congestive) heart failure
I50.40	Unspecified combined systolic (congestive) and diastolic (congestive) heart failure
I50.41	Acute combined systolic (congestive) and diastolic (congestive) heart failure
I50.42	Chronic combined systolic (congestive) and diastolic (congestive) heart failure
I50.43	Acute on chronic combined systolic (congestive) and diastolic (congestive) heart failure

EPIDEMIOLOGY & DEMOGRAPHICS

- There is variability in the reported demographics of HF due to heterogeneous definitions and classifications of HF. Incidence rate is lowest among white women and highest among black men. African Americans have the highest risk for HF of the demographic groups with blacks having a higher 5-yr mortality rate than whites.
- The lifetime risk of developing HF is 20% for Americans ≥40 yr of age.
  1. In the U.S., HF incidence has largely remained stable over the past several decades, with >650,000 new HF cases diagnosed annually.
  2. Based on NHANES data, from 2013 to 2016, an estimated 6.2 million Americans ≥20 yr of age had HF. This represents an increase from an estimated 5.7 million U.S. adults with HF from 2009 to 2012.
  3. Projections show that the prevalence of HF will increase 46% from 2012 to 2030, resulting in >8 million people ≥18 yr of age with HF.
  4. There has been an increase in the prevalence of HF in the population over time. This is primarily due to improved treatment of hypertension and valvular and coronary disease, allowing patients to survive an early death only to later develop HF.
- HF is primarily a condition of the elderly. Approximately 80% of patients hospitalized with HF are older than 65 yr. HF is the most common inpatient diagnosis in the U.S. for patients aged >65 yr.
- HF incidence increases with age, rising from approximately 20 per 1000 individuals 65 to 69 yr to >80 per 1000 individuals among those >85 yr. Before age 75, the incidence of HF is higher in males, but both sexes are equally affected after this age cutoff.
- In the U.S., 809,000 hospital discharges and 2.3 million ED visits/physician visits were associated with HF in 2016, which is a decline compared with 1.02 million hospital discharges in 2006.
- Prevalence: 6.2 million persons in the U.S. and an estimated 26 million persons worldwide. The prevalence of HF is rising, especially in the elderly, particularly due to aging of the population and improved survival from other conditions.
- In 2017, HF was the underlying cause in 80,480 deaths (36,824 males and 43,656 females.

TABLE 1 Compensatory Mechanisms in Heart Failure

Compensatory Response	Stimuli	Beneficial Effects	Adverse Effects	Potential Pharmacologic Interventions
Renin-angiotensin system activation	↓CO/BP ↓Renal blood flow ↑β-adrenergic activity	Maintain vital organ perfusion through vasoconstriction and sodium retention	↑Afterload → worsened LV function Adverse LV remodeling (apoptosis, myocyte hypertrophy)	ACE inhibitors ARBs
Adrenergic activation	↓CO/BP	↑CO through ↑ in heart rate and contractility ↑BP	↑Ischemia ↑Afterload → worsened LV function ↑LVEDP → pulmonary congestion Adverse LV remodeling (apoptosis, myocyte hypertrophy)	β-adrenergic blocking agents
Renal salt and water retention	↑Antidiuretic hormone ↑Norepinephrine ↑Angiotensin II ↑Aldosterone ↓Renal blood flow	↑Preload → ↑Stroke volume and CO	Pulmonary and systemic congestion Adverse LV remodeling	Diuretics Aldosterone inhibitors ACE inhibitors, ARBs β-adrenergic blocking agents
↑Natriuretic peptide secretion	Volume expansion (atrial stretch)	Diuresis Natriuresis Partial inhibition of renin-angiotensin system and norepinephrine	None known	Natriuretic peptides

ACE, Angiotensin-converting enzyme; *ARB,* angiotensin receptor blocker; *BP,* blood pressure; *CO,* cardiac output; *LV,* left ventricular; *LVEDP,* left ventricular end-diastolic pressure.
From Sellke FW et al: *Sabiston & Spencer surgery of the chest,* ed 9, 2016, Elsevier.

TABLE 2 American College of Cardiology/American Heart Association (ACC/AHA) Stages of Heart Failure (HF) Compared to the New York Heart Association (NYHA) Functional Classification

ACC/AHA Stages		NYHA Functional Classification	
A	At high risk for HF but without structural heart disease or symptoms of HF	None	
B	Structural heart disease but without signs or symptoms of HF	I	No limitation of physical activity Ordinary physical activity does not cause symptoms of HF
C	Structural heart disease with prior or current symptoms of HF	I	No limitation of physical activity Ordinary physical activity does not cause symptoms of HF
		II	Slight limitation of physical activity Comfortable at rest, but ordinary physical activity results in symptoms of HF
		III	Marked limitation of physical activity Comfortable at rest, but less than ordinary activity causes symptoms of HF
D	Refractory HF requiring specialized interventions	IV	Unable to carry on any physical activity without symptoms of HF, or symptoms of HF at rest

From Zipes DP: *Braunwald's heart disease, a textbook of cardiovascular medicine,* ed 11, Philadelphia, 2019, Elsevier.

- The estimated (direct and indirect) cost of HF in the U.S. was >$40 billion in 2012, with over half of these costs spent on hospitalizations. The mean cost of HF-related hospitalizations is $23,077 per patient and is higher when HF was a secondary rather than the primary diagnosis.
- HFrEF and HFpEF each make up about half of the overall HF burden.
- Among patients with HF in one large population study, hospitalizations were common after HF diagnosis, with 83% of patients hospitalized at least once and 43% hospitalized at least 4 times. More than half of the hospitalizations were related to noncardiovascular causes.

RISK FACTORS:
Several conditions are associated with an increased risk of developing heart failure. If these are identified and treated appropriately, it may be possible to delay, if not prevent, the onset of HF.
- Hypertension: The incidence of HF is higher in patients with higher blood pressures, older age of the hypertensive patient, and in patients who have been hypertensive for longer.
- Diabetes mellitus: The incidence of HF is increased in patients with diabetes mellitus, independent of the presence of structural heart disease.
- Metabolic syndrome: Appropriately treating hypertension, diabetes mellitus, and dyslipidemia can decrease the incidence of HF.
- Atherosclerotic disease: Patients with atherosclerotic disease are likely to develop HF.

PHYSICAL FINDINGS & CLINICAL PRESENTATION

The clinical and physical exam findings should be given the highest priority when determining the diagnosis of HF. These signs and symptoms are dependent on the severity of disease, precipitant factors, comorbid conditions, and whether the HF symptoms are predominantly right-sided or left-sided. Clues in the patient's history when evaluating HF are summarized in Table 4.

- Common clinical manifestations are:
  1. Dyspnea on exertion, that can progress to dyspnea at rest, caused by increasing pulmonary vascular congestion
  2. Orthopnea, caused by increased venous return in the recumbent position and further elevated pulmonary venous pressure
  3. Paroxysmal nocturnal dyspnea (PND) resulting from multiple factors including increased venous return in the recumbent position, decreased Pa_{O_2}, and decreased adrenergic stimulation of myocardial function during sleep
  4. Nocturnal angina resulting from increased myocardial oxygen demand (secondary to increased venous return in the recumbent position causing increased preload) in patients with concomitant coronary artery disease (CAD)
  5. *Cheyne-Stokes respiration* (alternating phases of apnea and hyperventilation) caused by prolonged circulation time from lungs to brain as a result of impaired cardiac output

TABLE 3 Simplified Classification and Common Clinical Characteristics of Patients with Acute Heart Failure

Clinical Classification	Symptom Onset	Triggers	Signs and Symptoms	Clinical Assessment	Course
Decompensated heart failure	Usually gradual	Noncompliance, ischemia, infections	Peripheral edema, orthopnea, dyspnea on exertion	SBP: Variable CXR: Often clear despite elevated filling pressures	Variable, high rehospitalization rate
Acute hypertensive heart failure	Usually sudden	Hypertension, atrial arrhythmias, ACS	Dyspnea (often severe), tachypnea, tachycardia, rales common	SBP: High (>180/100 mm Hg) CXR with pulmonary edema Hypoxemia common	High acuity, but patient often responds quickly to therapy with vasodilators, noninvasive ventilation Postdischarge mortality is low
Cardiogenic shock	Variable	Progression of advanced HF or major myocardial insult (e.g., large AMI, acute myocarditis)	End-organ hypoperfusion; oliguria, confusion, cool extremities	SBP: Low or low normal LV function usually severely depressed RV dysfunction common Laboratory evidence of end-organ dysfunction (renal, hepatic)	High inpatient mortality Poor prognosis unless readily reversible cause or mechanical support, transplantation

ACS, Acute coronary syndrome; *AMI,* acute myocardial infarction; *CXR,* chest x-ray film; *LV,* left ventricular; *RV,* right ventricular; *SBP,* systolic blood pressure.
From Zipes DP: *Braunwald's heart disease, a textbook of cardiovascular medicine,* ed 11, Philadelphia, 2019, Elsevier.

6. Fatigue, lethargy, and decreased functional capacity resulting from low cardiac output and hypoperfusion of peripheral tissues
7. Table 5 summarizes common presenting symptoms and signs of decompensated heart failure.

- Physical examination (Table 6):
  1. Fine pulmonary crackles, wheezes, tachypnea, hypoxia (due to elevated pulmonary pressures). Crackles may be absent in chronic and longstanding high pulmonary venous pressure because it allows for lymphatic drainage in the lungs to increase.
  2. Tachycardia and narrowed pulse pressure (due to increased sympathetic tone)
  3. S_3 gallop, paradoxical splitting of S_2, jugular venous distention, peripheral edema in dependent tissues, congestive hepatomegaly, ascites, and hepatojugular reflux (due to volume overload)
  4. Perioral and peripheral cyanosis, decreased capillary refill, pulsus alternans, and cool extremities (due to decreased cardiac output)
- Six common clinical presentations identified by European Society of Cardiology of Acute Heart Failure Syndromes:
  1. ADHF presenting with hypertension (SBP >160): The hypertension leads to increased afterload causing pulmonary vascular congestion
  2. Worsening or decompensation of chronic HF
  3. Flash pulmonary edema
  4. Cardiogenic shock
  5. Acute coronary syndrome (ACS) and ADHF
  6. Isolated RV failure
- Each of these scenarios may require different therapies to effectively stabilize and treat the patient.

Acute precipitants of HF decompensation include noncompliance with salt restriction or medications (most common cause), any acute systemic illness, infection, arrhythmias (e.g., atrial fibrillation), ischemia or infarction, uncontrolled hypertension, new medications (e.g., negative inotropic agents such as calcium channel blockers/antiarrhythmic agents), nonsteroidal antiinflammatory drugs (NSAIDs), renal dysfunction, toxins (e.g., ethanol and anthracyclines), surgery, or valvular catastrophe.

TABLE 4 Using the Medical History to Assess the Heart Failure Patient

Symptoms Associated with HF Include:
Fatigue
Shortness of breath at rest or during exercise
Dyspnea
Tachypnea
Cough
Diminished exercise capacity
Orthopnea
Paroxysmal nocturnal dyspnea
Nocturia
Weight gain/weight loss
Edema (of extremities, scrotum, or elsewhere)
Increasing abdominal girth or bloating
Abdominal pain (particularly if confined to right upper quadrant)
Loss of appetite or early satiety
Cheyne-Stokes respirations (often reported by family rather than patient)
Somnolence or diminished mental acuity

Historical Information Helpful in Determining if Symptoms Are Caused by HF
A past history of HF
Cardiac disease (e.g., coronary artery disease, valvular or congenital disease, previous myocardial infarction)
Risk factors for heart failure (e.g., diabetes, hypertension, obesity)
Systemic illnesses that can involve the heart (e.g., amyloidosis, sarcoidosis, inherited neuromuscular diseases)
Recent viral illness or history of HIV infection or Chagas disease
Family history of HF or sudden cardiac death
Environmental and/or medical exposure to cardiotoxic substances
Substance abuse
Noncardiac illnesses that could affect the heart indirectly, including high-output states (e.g., anemia, hyperthyroidism, arteriovenous fistulas)

HIV, Human immunodeficiency virus.
From Zipes DP: *Braunwald's heart disease, a textbook of cardiovascular medicine,* ed 11, Philadelphia, 2019, Elsevier.

ETIOLOGY

LEFT VENTRICULAR FAILURE: The dichotomy of whether HF occurs in the setting of preserved or reduced LV systolic function plays an important role in treatment strategies. Patients with HFpEF may have significant abnormalities in active relaxation and passive stiffness of the LV as well as valvular disease. HFrEF denotes poor pump function.

- Abnormal LV systolic function:
  1. CAD (acute or chronic ischemia, myocardial infarction [MI], LV aneurysm), the most common cause of cardiomyopathy in the U.S., comprising 50% to 75% of HF patients.
  2. Increased afterload or pressure overload (severe hypertension, aortic stenosis)
  3. Increased preload or volume overload (mitral regurgitation, aortic regurgitation)

TABLE 5 Common Presenting Symptoms and Signs of Decompensated Heart Failure

Symptoms	Signs
Predominantly Related to Volume Overload	
Dyspnea (exertional, paroxysmal nocturnal dyspnea, orthopnea, or at rest), cough, wheezing	Rales, pleural effusion
Foot and leg discomfort	Peripheral edema (legs, sacral)
Abdominal discomfort/bloating; early satiety or anorexia	Ascites/increased abdominal girth; right upper quadrant pain or discomfort; hepatomegaly/splenomegaly; scleral icterus
	Increased weight
	Elevated jugular venous pressure, abdominojugular reflux
	Increasing S_3, accentuated P_2
Predominantly Related to Hypoperfusion	
Fatigue	Cool extremities
Altered mental status, daytime drowsiness, confusion, or difficulty concentrating	Pallor, dusky skin discoloration, hypotension
Dizziness, presyncope, or syncope	Pulse pressure (narrow) Proportional pulse pressure (low)
Other Signs/Symptoms of Acute Heart Failure	
Depression	Orthostatic hypotension (hypovolemia)
Sleep disturbances	S_4
Palpitations	Systolic/diastolic cardiac murmurs

From Zipes DP: *Braunwald's heart disease, a textbook of cardiovascular medicine,* ed 11, Philadelphia, 2019, Elsevier.

TABLE 6 Physical Findings of Heart Failure

Tachycardia
Extra beats or irregular rhythm
Narrow pulse pressure or thready pulse*
Pulses alternans*
Tachypnea
Cool and/or mottled extremities*
Elevated jugular venous pressure
Dullness and diminished breath sounds at one or both lung bases
Rales, rhonchi, and/or wheezes
Apical impulse displaced leftward and/or inferiorly
Sustained apical impulse
Parasternal lift
Third and/or fourth heart sound (either palpable and/ or audible)
Tricuspid or mitral regurgitant murmur
Hepatomegaly (often accompanied by right upper quadrant discomfort)
Ascites
Presacral edema
Anasarca*
Pedal edema
Chronic venous stasis changes

*Indicative of more severe disease.

From Zipes DP: *Braunwald's heart disease, a textbook of cardiovascular medicine,* ed 11, Philadelphia, 2019, Elsevier.

4. Cardiomyopathy: Idiopathic, infiltrative (nonischemic)
5. Infectious (Chagas, myocarditis)
6. Infiltrative (amyloidosis, sarcoidosis, hemochromatosis)
7. Toxins (ethanol, cocaine, anthracyclines)
8. Tachycardia induced (e.g., with atrial fibrillation)

- Preserved LV systolic function (Table 7):
  1. Impaired relaxation (myocardial ischemia, diabetes mellitus, metabolic syndrome)
  2. Tachyarrhythmia (featuring reduced diastolic filling time)
  3. Restrictive cardiomyopathy (myocardial stiffness, such as hypereosinophilic syndrome, amyloidosis, hemochromatosis)
  4. High cardiac output (thiamine deficiency, anemia, thyrotoxicosis, arteriovenous malformations)
  5. Increased afterload (uncontrolled hypertension, aortic stenosis, hypertrophic obstructive cardiomyopathy)
  6. Hypervolemia (oliguric renal failure, iatrogenic)

RIGHT VENTRICULAR FAILURE:

- Left-sided HF
- Chronic hypoxemic pulmonary disease
- Valvular heart disease (mitral stenosis or regurgitation)
- Pulmonary embolism
- Primary pulmonary hypertension
- Right-to-left shunts that cause systemic hypoxemia (e.g., large patent foramen ovale and tetralogy of Fallot)
- Left-to-right shunts that cause volume overload (e.g., atrial and ventricular septal defects)
- Bacterial endocarditis (right-sided)
- Right ventricular infarction

Dx DIAGNOSIS

DIFFERENTIAL DIAGNOSIS

- COPD, asthma
- Cirrhosis
- Nephrotic syndrome
- Venous insufficiency
- Pulmonary embolism
- ARDS (adult respiratory distress syndrome)
- Pneumonia, flu, and COVID-19
- Heroin overdose

WORKUP

- ACC/AHAA guidelines for initial and serial evaluation of heart failure are summarized in Table 8.
- Blood work (to diagnose potentially reversible causes, identify comorbidities, and assess disease severity):
  1. CBC (to evaluate for anemia, infections), urinalysis, blood urea nitrogen (BUN), creatinine, electrolytes (worsening hyponatremia is a marker of disease severity and is associated with higher mortality rates), liver enzymes (hepatic congestion), thyroid function (especially in the elderly or patients with comorbid atrial fibrillation or known thyroid disease).
  2. Fig. 2 illustrates the use of biomarkers in HF. B-type natriuretic peptide (BNP) is a cardiac neurohormone secreted from the ventricles in response to elevated LV end-diastolic pressure. While the sensitivity is low in asymptomatic patients, low BNP level has a negative predictive value up to 90% in symptomatic patients. An elevated BNP correlates with severity of disease and parallels closely morbidity and mortality outcome measures. N-terminal-pro-BNP (NT-pro-BNP) is the cleavage remnant of BNP. It has a longer half-life and is renally cleared, making it susceptible to alterations in renal function. A level of <300 pg/ml has an age-independent 98% negative predictive value. There are new data to suggest that BNP screening and early intervention with risk factor modification in patients at risk of developing heart failure may prevent development of left ventricular dysfunction (class IIa recommendation). Natriuretic peptide biomarkers are also useful (class IA recommendation) both for diagnosis in patients presenting with dyspnea and for prognosis in patients with acute decompensated heart failure and chronic heart failure. Measurement of baseline levels of natriuretic peptide biomarkers on admission to the hospital is useful to establish a prognosis in acutely decompensated HF, and predischarge natriuretic peptide level can be useful to establish a postdischarge prognosis. There are insufficient data to recommend natriuretic peptide biomarker–guided therapy or serial measurements for the purpose of reducing hospitalization or deaths. ACC/AHA/HFSA guidelines for the use of biomarkers in HF are summarized in Table 9.
  3. Cardiac biomarkers may be elevated if ischemia is the precipitant factor. However, slight elevations are very common and may not always be due to obstructive coronary artery disease. These elevations could be due to subendocardial ischemia

TABLE 7 Mechanisms/Factors Contributing to the Pathophysiology of Heart Failure with Preserved Ejection Fraction

Cardiovascular

LV Structure

Concentric remodeling, LV hypertrophy

LV Function

Diastolic dysfunction: Abnormal relaxation, decreased recoil, abnormal filling, decreased distensibility, increased diastolic pressure

Systolic dysfunction: Abnormal midwall and long-axis shortening, decreased twist

Hemodynamic load
- Increased afterload and filling load

Heterogeneity
- Dyssynergy, dyssynchrony

Left atrial structure and function
- Increased LA volume and stiffness, decreased LA reservoir function, passive conduit function and active booster pump function

Ischemia
- Subendocardial and microvascular disease, impaired coronary, pulmonary, and peripheral flow reserve

Rate and rhythm abnormalities
- Chronotropic incompetence, atrial fibrillation, supraventricular tachycardia

Vascular dysfunction
- Arterial stiffening, endothelial dysfunction

Cardiomyocyte

Abnormal calcium homeostasis (↑ diastolic calcium or ↓ rate of calcium reuptake → incomplete or impaired relaxation)
- Sarcolemmal calcium channels (Na^+/Ca^{2+} exchanger and calcium pump)
- Sarcoplasmic reticulum Ca^{2+}ATPase (SERCA) abundance and function
- Proteins modifying SERCA activity: Phospholamban, calmodulin, calsequestrin abundance, and phosphorylation state
- Sarcoplasmic reticulum calcium release channels

Energetics (↓ ATP or ↑ ADP slows actin-myosin cross-bridge release)
- ADP/ATP ratio, ADP and P_i concentration, phosphocreatine shuttle function

Proteins regulating cross-bridge formation and calcium sensitivity
- Troponin C: Calcium binding
- Troponin I: Phosphorylation state

Cytoskeletal proteins
- Microtubules (increased density) → ↑ diastolic stiffness
- Titin isoforms (↑ noncompliant isoform and phosphorylation state) → ↑ diastolic stiffness

Extracellular Matrix

Collagen structure, geometry, content, collagen I/III ratio

Collagen homeostasis, synthesis, postsynthetic processing, posttranslational crosslinking, degradation

Basement membrane proteins

Bioactive proteins and peptides: MMP/TIMP, SPARC, TGF-β

Fibroblast structure, function, phenotype

Myofibroblast transdifferentiation

Extra Cardiac

Extrinsic forces (RV-LV interaction and pericardial constraint)

Peripheral muscle and ergoreflex dysfunction

Pulmonary hypertension (secondary to chronic pulmonary venous hypertension)

Neurohormonal activation

Comorbid conditions (renal dysfunction, anemia, chronic lung disease)

ADP, Adenosine diphosphate; *ATP,* adenosine triphosphate; *LA,* left atrium; *LV,* left ventricle; *RV,* right ventricle; *SPARC,* secreted protein, acidic and rich in cysteine [osteonectin]; *TGF,* transforming growth vector.

From Mann DL et al: *Braunwald's heart disease,* ed 10, Philadelphia, 2015, Elsevier.

(due to increased end-diastolic pressure resulting in decreased perfusion) and necrosis, or cardiomyocyte damage from the inflammatory cytokines or oxidative stress. Impaired renal function is very common, and decreased clearance of the biomarkers can contribute to their elevation. Therefore these elevations should be interpreted in the context of the clinical setting. Despite that, in patients with acute decompensated heart failure (ADHF), a positive cardiac troponin test (from whatever mechanism) is associated with worse prognosis.

4. Screening for dyslipidemia and glucose intolerance, which are risk factors for CAD.
5. If hemochromatosis is suspected (specifically in Northern European patients), consider checking a transferrin saturation and ferritin level.
6. Consider HIV testing in high-risk patients and COVID-19 testing in all patients.

- Electrocardiogram (ECG):
  1. Look for signs of prior MI, chamber enlargement, hypertrophy, heart block, arrhythmia, and evidence of pericardial effusion.
  2. More than 25% of patients with HF have some form of intraventricular conduction abnormality that manifests as an increased QRS duration. The most common pattern seen is left bundle-branch block.
- Chest x-ray (Fig. 3):
  1. Evaluate for pulmonary venous congestion, pulmonary edema, pleural effusion, cardiomegaly, chamber dilation, and Kerley B lines.
- Echocardiography:
  1. Plays a critical diagnostic role in patients with HF and is useful in assessment of systolic, diastolic function in addition to assessment of valvular structure and function
- Exercise stress testing:
  1. May be useful in evaluating concomitant ischemic etiologies and assessment of degree of disability in stable compensated patients.
- Cardiac catheterization:
  1. Left heart catheterization can help to identify coronary artery disease as a cause of HF. Right heart catheterization can help to evaluate intracardiac filling pressures, estimates of valvular areas, presence of intracardiac shunts, and calculation of hemodynamic properties such as cardiac output, systemic vascular resistance, and pulmonary artery wedge pressure to further guide management.
- Cardiac MRI:
  1. Useful modality in accurately estimating EF (with less variability than conventional 2D echocardiography). MRI is also useful in excluding pericardial disease, identifying infiltrative disease, and assessing viability in cases of HF caused by underlying ischemic heart disease.

Rx TREATMENT

NONPHARMACOLOGIC GENERAL MEASURES

- Assess the etiology and severity of disease. Educate the patient and family about the nature of the disorder. Assess the home setting and if patient has social support to ensure compliance, especially for patients with dementia.
- Identify and correct precipitating factors (e.g., increased sodium load, medication noncompliance, ischemia, infections, anemia, thyrotoxicosis) and address lifestyle modification (e.g., smoking and alcohol cessation, weight reduction, avoiding use of nonsteroidal anti-inflammatory drugs [NSAIDs]). Anemia is common in patients with HF. In patients with NYHA class II and III symptoms and iron deficiency, IV iron replacement may be reasonable to improve functional status and quality of life (class IIb recommendation). Treatments with erythropoiesis-stimulating agents (ESAs) have not shown improved clinical outcomes in patients with systolic HF

TABLE 8 ACC/AHA Guidelines for Initial and Serial Evaluation of Heart Failure

Class	Indication: History, Physical Examination, and Risk Scoring	Level of Evidence
I	A thorough history and physical examination should be obtained/performed in patients presenting with HF to identify cardiac and noncardiac disorders or behaviors that might cause or accelerate the development or progression of HF.	C
	In patients with idiopathic DCM, a three-generational family history should be obtained to aid in establishing the diagnosis of familial DCM.	C
	Volume status and vital signs should be assessed at each patient encounter. This includes serial assessment of weight, as well as estimates of jugular venous pressure and the presence of peripheral edema or orthopnea.	B
IIa	Validated multivariable risk scores can be useful to estimate subsequent risk of mortality in ambulatory or hospitalized patients with HF.	C
Indication: Diagnostic Tests and Biomarkers (also see below)		
I	Initial laboratory evaluation of patients presenting with HF should include complete blood count, urinalysis, serum electrolytes (including calcium and magnesium), blood urea nitrogen, serum creatinine, glucose, fasting lipid profile, liver function tests, and thyroid-stimulating hormone.	C
	Serial monitoring, when indicated, should include serum electrolytes and renal function.	C
	A 12-lead ECG should be performed initially on all patients presenting with HF.	C
	In ambulatory patients with dyspnea, measurement of BNP or N-terminal pro-B-type natriuretic peptide (NT-proBNP) is useful to support clinical decision making regarding the diagnosis of HF, especially in the setting of clinical uncertainty, and measurement of BNP or NT-proBNP is useful for establishing prognosis or disease severity in chronic HF.	A
IIa	Screening for hemochromatosis or HIV is reasonable in select patients who present with HF.	C
	Diagnostic tests for rheumatologic diseases, amyloidosis, or pheochromocytoma are reasonable in patients presenting with HF in whom there is a clinical suspicion of these diseases.	C
	BNP-guided or NT-proBNP–guided HF therapy can be useful to achieve optimal dosing of GDMT in select, clinically euvolemic patients followed in a well-structured HF disease management program.	B
IIb	The usefulness of serial measurement of BNP or NT-proBNP to reduce hospitalization or mortality in patients with HF is not well established. The measurement of other clinically available tests, such as biomarkers of myocardial injury or "fibrosis," may be considered for additive risk stratification in patients with chronic HF.	B
Indication: Noninvasive Cardiac Imaging		
I	Patients with suspected or new-onset HF, or those presenting with acute decompensated HF, should undergo a chest radiograph to assess heart size and pulmonary congestion and to detect alternative cardiac, pulmonary, and other diseases that may cause or contribute to the patient's symptoms.	C
	A two-dimensional echocardiogram with Doppler should be performed during initial evaluation of patients presenting with HF to assess ventricular function, size, wall thickness, wall motion, and valve function.	C
	Repeat measurement of EF and measurement of the severity of structural remodeling are useful to provide information in patients with HF who have had a significant change in clinical status; who have experienced or recovered from a clinical event; who have received treatment, including GDMT, that might have had a significant effect on cardiac function; or who may be candidates for device therapy.	C
IIa	Noninvasive imaging to detect myocardial ischemia and viability is reasonable in patients presenting with de novo HF who have known CAD and no angina, unless the patient is not eligible for revascularization of any kind.	C
	Viability assessment is reasonable in select situations when planning revascularization in HF patients with CAD.	B
	Radionuclide ventriculography or MRI can be useful to assess LVEF and volume when echocardiography is inadequate.	C
	MRI is reasonable when assessing myocardial infiltrative processes or scar burden.	B
III: No benefit	Routine repeat measurement of LV function assessment in the absence of clinical status change or treatment interventions should not be performed.	B
Indication: Invasive Evaluation		
I	Invasive hemodynamic monitoring with a pulmonary artery catheter should be performed to guide therapy in patients who have respiratory distress or clinical evidence of impaired perfusion in whom the adequacy or excess of intracardiac filling pressures cannot be determined from clinical assessment.	C
IIa	Invasive hemodynamic monitoring can be useful for carefully selected patients with acute HF who have persistent symptoms despite empiric adjustment of standard therapies and (a) whose fluid status, perfusion, or systemic or pulmonary vascular resistance is uncertain; (b) whose systolic pressure remains low, or is associated with symptoms, despite initial therapy; (c) whose renal function is worsening with therapy; (d) who require parenteral vasoactive agents; or (e) who may need consideration for mechanical circulatory support or transplantation.	C
	When ischemia may be contributing to HF, coronary arteriography is reasonable for patients eligible for revascularization.	C
	Endomyocardial biopsy can be useful in patients presenting with HF when a specific diagnosis is suspected that would influence therapy.	C
III: No benefit	Routine use of invasive hemodynamic monitoring is not recommended in normotensive patients with acute decompensated HF and congestion with symptomatic response to diuretics and vasodilators.	B
III: Harm	Endomyocardial biopsy should not be performed in the routine evaluation of patients with HF.	C

ACC, American College of Cardiology; *AHA,* American Heart Association; *BNP,* B-type natriuretic peptide; *CAD,* coronary artery disease; *DCM,* dilated cardiomyopathy, *ECG,* electrocardiogram; *EF,* ejection fraction; *GDMT,* guideline-directed medical therapy; *HIV,* human immunodeficiency virus; *LV,* left ventricle; *LVEF,* left ventricular ejection fraction; *MRI,* magnetic resonance imaging.
From Zipes DP: *Braunwald's heart disease, a textbook of cardiovascular medicine,* ed 11, Philadelphia, 2019, Elsevier.

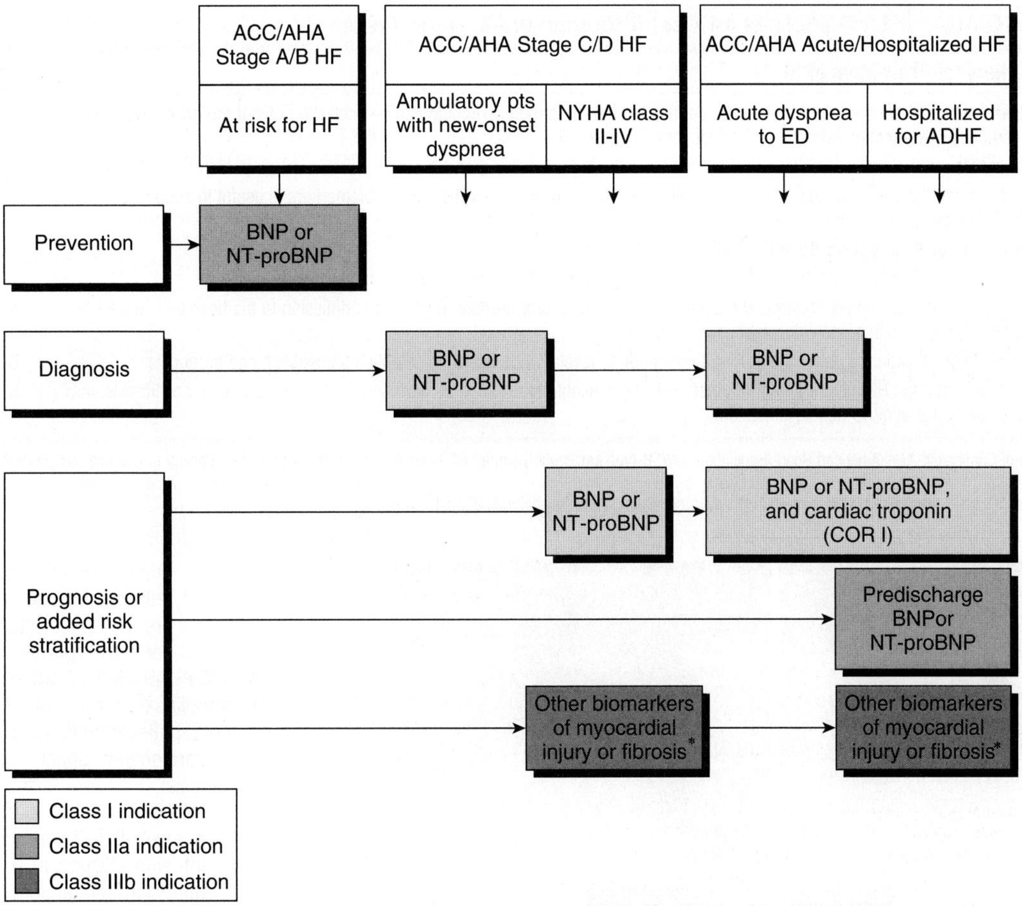

FIG. 2 Indications for the use of biomarkers in heart failure. *Other biomarkers of injury or fibrosis include soluble ST2 receptor, galectin-3, and high-sensitivity troponin. *ACC,* American College of Cardiology; *AHA,* American Heart Association; *ADHF,* acute decompensated heart failure; *BNP,* B-type natriuretic peptide; *COR,* class of recommendation; *ED,* emergency department; *HF,* heart failure; *NT-proBNP,* N-terminal pro-B-type natriuretic peptide; *NYHA,* New York Heart Association; *pts,* patients. (Modified from Yancy CW et al: 2017 ACC/AHA/HFSA focused update of the 2013 ACCF/AHA guideline for the management of heart failure: a report of the American College of Cardiology/American Heart Association Task Force on Clinical Practice Guidelines and the Heart Failure Society of America, *J Am Coll Cardiol* 2017;70[6]:776. In Zipes DP: *Braunwald's heart disease, a textbook of cardiovascular medicine,* ed 11, Philadelphia, 2019, Elsevier.)

and mild-to-moderate anemia and are thus not recommended. Table 10 describes ACC/AHA guidelines for treating patients at high risk for development of heart failure.

- Review list of medications and discontinue the ones that can contribute to HF (e.g., NSAIDs, antiarrhythmic drugs, calcium channel blockers, thiazolidinediones).
- Dietary sodium restriction of <2 g/day is commonly recommended to patients with HF and is endorsed by many guidelines.
- Restrict fluid intake to <2 L/day in patients with hyponatremia.
- Caloric supplementation should be provided to patients with advanced HF with weight loss and muscle wasting due to cardiac cachexia. Weight loss may reflect cachexia caused by the higher total energy expenditure associated with HF compared with that of healthy sedentary subjects. The diagnosis of cardiac cachexia independently predicts a worse prognosis.
- For patients with coexisting obstructive sleep apnea, continuous positive airway pressure (CPAP) may be reasonable after polysomnography (class IIb recommendation).
- Exercise training (or regular physical activity) is recommended as safe and effective for patients with class I to III HF who are able to participate to improve functional status (class I recommendation). Cardiac rehabilitation is unfortunately an underused preventive measure, although it has been shown to reduce morbidity and mortality. Intensive cardiac rehabilitation be useful in clinically stable patients with HF to improve functional capacity, exercise duration, health-related quality of life, and mortality (class IIa recommendation). Home-based cardiac rehabilitation is also an equally effective alternative if patients cannot participate in regular cardiac rehabilitation.
- Pneumococcal vaccination, annual influenza vaccination.
- ACC/AHA guidelines for treatment of asymptomatic left ventricular systolic dysfunction are summarized in Table 11.

TREATMENT OF ADHF

- Four phases in treatment of ADHF:
  1st phase: Initial stabilization and management (Table 12)
  2nd phase: Inpatient hospital care (Table 13)
  3rd phase: Early discharge planning and care
  4th phase: Early postdischarge care
- 1st phase: Initial stabilization and management
  1. Short-term goals: Hemodynamic stabilization, stabilization of respiratory status, symptom relief, optimization of tissue perfusion, and recognition of more immediately life-threatening conditions (e.g., arrhythmias, valvular catastrophe, MI, cardiac tamponade). Initial therapy of ADHF is contingent on appropriate determination of clinical scenario.
  2. Management as per clinical scenario:
     a. ADHF-associated hypertension: Goal is afterload reduction and decrease of systemic hypervolemia. Mode of treatment: Diuresis (IV loop diuretics) and vasodilators (acutely nitrates and

TABLE 9 ACC/AHA/HFSA Guidelines for Use of Biomarkers in Heart Failure

Class	Biomarkers for Prevention of HF	Level of Evidence
IIa	For patients at risk of developing HF, natriuretic peptide biomarker–based screening can be useful to prevent the development of left ventricular dysfunction (systolic or diastolic) or new-onset HF.	B-R
Biomarkers for Diagnosis		
I	In patients presenting with dyspnea (acute or chronic), measurement of natriuretic peptide biomarkers is useful to support a diagnosis or exclusion of HF.	A
Biomarkers for Prognosis or Added Risk Stratification		
I	Measurement of BNP or NT-proBNP is useful for establishing prognosis or disease severity in chronic HF.	A
I	Measurement of baseline levels of natriuretic peptide biomarkers and/or cardiac troponin on admission to the hospital is useful to establish a prognosis in acutely decompensated HF.	A
IIa	During a HF hospitalization, a predischarge natriuretic peptide level can be useful to establish a postdischarge prognosis.	B-NR
IIb	In patients with chronic HF, measurement of other clinically available tests, such as biomarkers of myocardial injury or fibrosis, may be considered for additive risk stratification.	B-NR

ACC, American College of Cardiology; *AHA,* American Heart Association; *BNP,* B-type natriuretic peptide; *HF,* heart failure; *HFSA,* Heart Failure Society of America; *NT-proBNP,* N-terminal pro-B-type natriuretic peptide.
From Zipes DP: *Braunwald's heart disease, a textbook of cardiovascular medicine,* ed 11, Philadelphia, 2019, Elsevier.

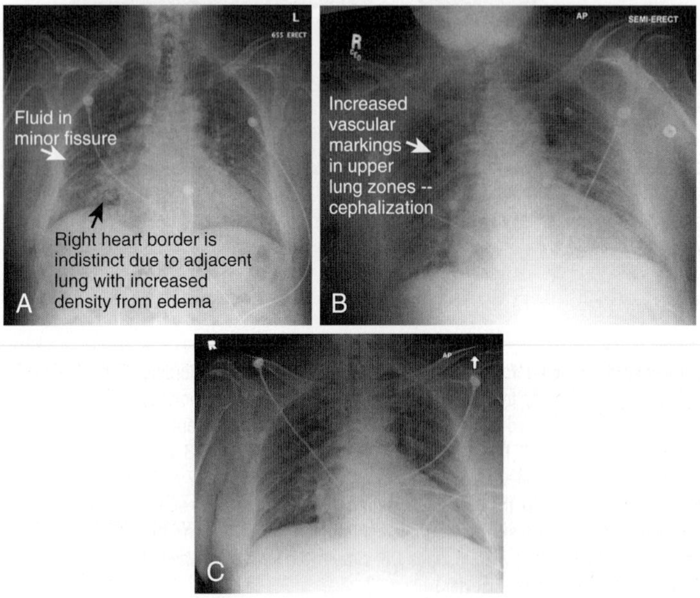

FIG. 3 Congestive heart failure. Mild left ventricular hypertrophy with restricted filling, ejection fraction >55%, and no pericardial effusion. This 63-yr-old man with coronary artery disease, chronic renal insufficiency, and diastolic heart failure (ejection fraction >55%) presented multiple times for dyspnea (**A, B,** and **C,** first through third clinical presentations). Each of these three radiographs shows signs of moderate pulmonary edema. The diaphragms and costophrenic angles are clear, suggesting no pleural effusion. The right heart border in all three images is indistinct because of interstitial edema in these locations. Portions of the left heart border are also indistinct. The upper lung fields have a hazy appearance indicating mild edema. Fluid is visible in the minor fissure on all three images. Does the similarity of these radiographs mean that edema is not the cause of the patient's dyspnea? No, he simply presented with pulmonary edema on all three occasions. (From Broder JS: *Diagnostic imaging for the emergency physician,* Philadelphia, 2011, Saunders.)

morphine followed by treatment with ACE inhibitors or angiotensin receptor blockers [ARBs])

b. Worsening or decompensation of chronic HF (HFrEF or HFpEF): Goal is control of volume status. Treatment is accomplished with vasodilators and diuretics.
c. Flash pulmonary edema: Goal is afterload reduction (vasodilators such as nitrates acutely), respiratory status stabilization, and diuresis (IV loop diuretics). Rate control can be initiated in patients with atrial fibrillation or tachyarrhythmias as it may improve cardiac filling and function.
d. Cardiogenic shock: Goal is hemodynamic stabilization. Treatment consists of inotropes + vasopressors ± mechanical circulatory support ± emergent revascularization if indicated.
e. ACS and ADHF: Goal is hemodynamic stabilization + emergent restoration of coronary perfusion. See "Acute Coronary Syndrome."
f. Isolated RV failure: Goals are identification of etiology: (1) valvular, (2) pulmonary hypertension, and (3) primary RV failure secondary to ischemia. Treatment: Depends on etiology, either corrective surgery vs. treatment of pulmonary hypertension (endothelin antagonists, calcium channel blockers, phosphodiesterase inhibitors) vs. coronary reperfusion therapies.

ACUTE PHARMACOLOGIC TREATMENTS:

- Vasodilators (Table 14) are appropriate in most patients with ADHF (contraindicated in cardiogenic shock and severe aortic stenosis).
  1. Nitroglycerin (0.4 to 0.8 mg sublingually every 3 to 5 min, or by intravenous infusion starting at 0.2 to 0.4 mcg/kg/min with subsequent up titration) may be administered in the emergency setting until relative hypotension ensues. Nitrates are contraindicated after use of phosphodiesterase inhibitors such as sildenafil due to risk of hypotension.
  2. Sodium nitroprusside (0.1 to 0.2 mcg/kg/min as an intravenous infusion) is a potent vasodilator with balanced venous and arteriolar effects that usually requires hemodynamic monitoring with an arterial line and may precipitate coronary steal and thiocyanate toxicity (elevated risk in renal failure).
  3. When given intravenously, loop diuretics have an immediate vasodilator effect that provides clinical relief of symptoms before diuresis begins. Due to gut edema and unpredictable patterns of absorption, oral formulation may become less effective. Therefore intravenous formulation should be used in the acute setting. Studies showed no difference in outcome when using bolus dosing vs. continuous IV infusion. Administration of smaller doses of short-acting loop diuretics multiple times daily is preferable to a single large dose because the kidneys can avidly reabsorb sodium after the initial diuresis. However, if a certain dose is not adequate to force diuresis, the dose, rather than the frequency, should be increased until a single effective dose is reached; more frequent doses can be added as needed. Therefore monitoring of urine output, renal function, and electrolytes is key. The addition of a distal tubule inhibitor such as metolazone

TABLE 10 ACC/AHA Guidelines for Treating Patients at High Risk of Developing Heart Failure (Stage A)

Class	Indication	Level of Evidence
I	Hypertension and lipid disorders should be controlled in accordance with contemporary guidelines to lower the risk of HF.	A
I	In patients at increased risk, stage A, the optimal blood pressure in those with hypertension should be less than 130/80 mm Hg.	B-R
I	Other conditions that may lead to or contribute to HF, such as obesity, diabetes mellitus, tobacco use, and known cardiotoxic agents, should be controlled or avoided.	C
II	For patients at risk of developing HF, natriuretic peptide biomarker–based screening followed by team-based care, including a cardiovascular specialist optimizing GDMT, can be useful to prevent the development of left ventricular dysfunction (systolic or diastolic) or new-onset HF.	B-R

ACC, American College of Cardiology; *AHA,* American Heart Association; *GDMT,* guideline-directed medical therapy; *HF,* heart failure.
From Zipes DP: *Braunwald's heart disease, a textbook of cardiovascular medicine,* ed 11, Philadelphia, 2019, Elsevier.

TABLE 11 ACC/AHA Guidelines for Treatment of Asymptomatic Left Ventricular Systolic Dysfunction (Stage B)

Class	Indication	Level of Evidence
I	In all patients with a recent or remote history of MI or ACS and reduced EF, ACE inhibitors should be used to prevent symptomatic HF and reduce mortality. In patients intolerant of ACE inhibitors, ARBs are appropriate unless contraindicated.	A
	In all patients with a recent or remote history of MI or ACS and reduced EF, evidence-based beta blockers should be used to reduce mortality. Beta blockade and ACE inhibition should be used in all patients with a recent or remote history of MI regardless of EF or presence of HF.	B
	In all patients with a recent or remote history of MI or ACS, statins should be used to prevent symptomatic HF and cardiovascular events.	A
	Blood pressure should be controlled in accordance with clinical practice guidelines for hypertension to prevent symptomatic HF.	A
	ACE inhibitors should be used in all patients with a reduced EF to prevent symptomatic HF.	A
	Beta blockers should be used in all patients with a reduced EF to prevent symptomatic HF.	C
IIa	To prevent sudden death, placement of an ICD is reasonable in patients with asymptomatic ischemic cardiomyopathy who are at least 40 days post-MI, have an LVEF of 30% or less, are on appropriate medical therapy, and have reasonable expectation of survival with a good functional status for more than 1 yr.	B
III: Harm	Nondihydropyridine calcium channel blockers with negative inotropic effects may be harmful in asymptomatic patients with low LVEF and no symptoms of HF after MI.	B

ACC, American College of Cardiology; *ACE,* angiotensin-converting enzyme; *ACS,* acute coronary syndrome; *AHA,* American Heart Association; *ARB,* angiotensin receptor antagonist; *EF,* ejection fraction; *HF,* heart failure; *ICD,* implantable cardioverter-defibrillator; *LVEF,* left ventricular ejection fraction; *MI,* myocardial infarction.
From Zipes DP: *Braunwald's heart disease, a textbook of cardiovascular medicine,* ed 11, Philadelphia, 2019, Elsevier.

30 min prior to loop diuretic dosing has a synergistic effect and often enhances diuresis because it inhibits sodium reabsorption in the distal segment in the face of increased sodium delivery from the loop. Diuretics should be used with caution in patients with aortic stenosis.

- Inotropic agents are used for temporary hemodynamic support in cardiogenic shock, but have not been shown to improve survival. Many of these agents have serious associated adverse events including myocardial necrosis and malignant arrhythmias.
  1. Dobutamine (starting at 2.5 to 5 mcg/kg/min) can be used for inotropic support but is associated with increased myocardial oxygen demand and cardiac arrhythmias and may result in hypotension from decreased systemic vascular resistance.
  2. Milrinone (37.5 to 75 mcg/kg loading dose, followed by 0.375 to 0.75 mcg/kg/min) can be used as a vasodilator and inotropic agent, but is associated with increased oxygen demand and cardiac arrhythmias, and may result in hypotension from decreased systemic vascular resistance.
- Renal replacement therapy or ultrafiltration (can be used as an alternative to pharmacologic diuresis in ADHF when renal function is significantly compromised).
- ACE inhibitors or ARBs, if part of a patient's chronic medication regimen, should be continued in the absence of hypotension, acute renal failure, or hyperkalemia.
- Beta-blockers, if part of a patient's chronic medication regimen, may be continued or reduced in dosage in mild exacerbations of HF but should be discontinued in patients with hypotension or those requiring inotropic support. Beta-blockers should not be initiated in patients who are not on chronic beta-blocker therapy until euvolemia is achieved unless used for rate control.
- Morphine sulfate can cause venodilation and thus reduce cardiac preload. It may be used to reduce patient work of breathing and anxiety, but recent retrospective studies have suggested increased incidence of mechanical ventilation and in-hospital mortality in patients who received morphine.
- If ADHF with preserved EF is suspected, therapy is usually aimed at relief of symptoms and correction of any potential precipitating etiologies (e.g., tachycardia, hypertension, ischemia). Treatment generally involves diuretics to reduce pulmonary congestion with caution to not overdiurese given the need for elevated filling pressures in these patients to ensure adequate stroke volume and cardiac output. Nitrates may be useful in providing symptomatic relief but may precipitate hypotension. Ventricular rate should be controlled in the presence of atrial fibrillation, which, at rapid rates, is poorly tolerated in patients with impaired diastolic filling. Negative inotropic agents such as beta-blockers and calcium channel blockers can be used with caution. ACC/AHA/HSFA guidelines for treatment of patients with stage C HF and preserved left ventricular ejection fraction are summarized in Table 15.
- Nesiritide (recombinant brain natriuretic protein) does not reduce morbidity or mortality (ASCEND-HF trial).
- 2nd phase: Inpatient hospital care.
  1. This phase of treatment includes further diuresis and stabilization of volume status (Table 16). The patient should be carefully brought to euvolemia with daily volume status and electrolyte monitoring. The patient should also be transitioned to oral diuretics when stabilized. While inpatient, the patient should have his/her medical and device management optimized with the therapies discussed later.
- 3rd phase: Early discharge planning and care.
  1. The patient should be transitioned to oral diuretics and be placed on optimum outpatient maintenance therapy. If the patient was on IV inotropic therapy, oral regimens should be adjusted while these infusions are tapered off. Prolonged

TABLE 12 ACC/AHA Guidelines for Treatment of Symptomatic Left Ventricular Systolic Dysfunction (Stage C)

Class	Indication	Level of Evidence
	Nonpharmacologic Interventions	
I	Patients with HF should receive specific education to facilitate HF self-care.	B
	Exercise training (or regular physical activity) is recommended as safe and effective for patients with HF who are able to participate to improve functional status.	A
IIa	Cardiac rehabilitation can be useful in clinically stable patients with HF to improve functional capacity, exercise duration, HRQOL, and mortality.	B
	Sodium restriction is reasonable for patients with symptomatic HF to reduce congestive symptoms.	C
	Continuous positive airway pressure (CPAP) can be beneficial to increase LVEF and improve functional status in patients with HF and sleep apnea.	B
	Pharmacologic Interventions	
I	Measures listed as class I recommendations for patients in stages A and B are recommended where appropriate.	A, B, C
	GDMT should be the mainstay of pharmacologic therapy for HFrEF.	A
	Diuretics	
I	Diuretics are recommended in patients with HFrEF who have evidence of fluid retention, unless contraindicated, to ameliorate symptoms.	C
	Angiotensin-Converting Enzyme Inhibitors/Adrenergic Receptor Blockers	
I	ACE inhibitors are recommended in patients with HFrEF and current or previous symptoms, unless contraindicated, to reduce morbidity and mortality.	A
	ARBs are recommended in patients with HFrEF with current or previous symptoms who are ACE inhibitor–intolerant, unless contraindicated, to reduce morbidity and mortality.	A
IIa	ARBs are a reasonable choice to reduce morbidity and mortality as alternatives to ACE inhibitors for first-line therapy in patients with HFrEF, especially in those already taking ARBs for other indications, unless contraindicated.	A
IIb	Addition of an ARB may be considered in persistently symptomatic patients with HFrEF who are already being treated with an ACE inhibitor and a beta-blocker in whom an aldosterone antagonist is not indicated or tolerated.	A
III: Harm	Routinely combining an ACE inhibitor, an ARB, and an aldosterone antagonist.	C
	Beta-Blockers	
I	Use of one of the three beta-blockers proven to reduce mortality (i.e., bisoprolol, carvedilol, and sustained-release metoprolol succinate) is recommended for all patients with current or previous symptoms of HFrEF, unless contraindicated, to reduce morbidity and mortality.	A
	Aldosterone Receptor Antagonists	
I	Aldosterone receptor antagonists (or mineralocorticoid receptor antagonists) are recommended in patients with NYHA class II-IV and LVEF of ≤35%, unless contraindicated, to reduce morbidity and mortality.	A
I	Aldosterone receptor antagonists are recommended to reduce morbidity and mortality after an acute MI in patients with LVEF of ≤40% who develop symptoms of HF or who have a history of diabetes mellitus, unless contraindicated.	B
III: Harm	Inappropriate use of aldosterone receptor antagonists is potentially harmful because of life-threatening hyperkalemia or renal insufficiency when serum creatinine is >2.5 mg/dl in men or >2.0 mg/dl in women (or estimated glomerular filtration rate <30 ml/min/1.73 m^2), and/or potassium >5.0 mEq/liter.	B
	Hydralazine and Isosorbide Dinitrate	
I	The combination of hydralazine and isosorbide dinitrate is recommended to reduce morbidity and mortality for patients self-described as African Americans with NYHA class III-IV HFrEF receiving optimal therapy with ACE inhibitors and beta-blockers, unless contraindicated.	A
IIa	A combination of hydralazine and isosorbide dinitrate can be useful to reduce morbidity or mortality in patients with current or previous symptomatic HFrEF who cannot be given an ACE inhibitor or ARB because of drug intolerance, hypotension, or renal insufficiency, unless contraindicated.	B
	Digoxin	
IIa	Digoxin can be beneficial in patients with HFrEF, unless contraindicated, to decrease hospitalizations for HF.	B
	Anticoagulation	
I	Patients with chronic HF with permanent/persistent/paroxysmal atrial fibrillation and an additional risk factor for cardioembolic stroke (history of hypertension, diabetes mellitus, previous stroke or transient ischemic attack, or ≥75 yr of age) should receive chronic anticoagulant therapy.	A
I	The selection of an anticoagulant agent (warfarin, dabigatran, apixaban, or rivaroxaban) for permanent/persistent/paroxysmal atrial fibrillation should be individualized on the basis of risk factors, cost, tolerability, patient preference, potential for drug interactions, and other clinical characteristics, including time in the international normalized ratio therapeutic range if the patient has been taking warfarin.	C
IIa	Chronic anticoagulation is reasonable for patients with chronic HF who have permanent/persistent/paroxysmal atrial fibrillation but no additional risk factor for cardioembolic stroke.	B
III: No benefit	Anticoagulation is not recommended in patients with chronic HFrEF without atrial fibrillation, a previous thromboembolic event, or a cardioembolic source.	B
	Statins	
III: No benefit	Statins are not beneficial as adjunctive therapy when prescribed solely for HF.	A
	Omega-3 Fatty Acids	
IIa	Omega-3 PUFA supplementation is reasonable to use as adjunctive therapy in patients with NYHA class II-IV symptoms and HFrEF or HFpEF, unless contraindicated, to reduce mortality and cardiovascular hospitalizations.	B

Continued

TABLE 12 ACC/AHA Guidelines for Treatment of Symptomatic Left Ventricular Systolic Dysfunction (Stage C)—cont'd

Class	Indication	Level of Evidence
	Drugs of Unproven Value or That May Cause Harm	
III: No benefit	Nutritional supplements as treatment for HF are not recommended in patients with current or previous symptoms of HFrEF.	B
	Hormonal therapies other than to correct deficiencies are not recommended for patients with current or previous symptoms of HFrEF.	C
III: Harm	Drugs known to adversely affect the clinical status of patients with current or previous symptoms of HFrEF are potentially harmful and should be avoided or withdrawn whenever possible (e.g., most antiarrhythmic drugs, most calcium channel blocking drugs [except amlodipine], NSAIDs, or thiazolidinediones).	B
	Long-term use of infused positive inotropic drugs is potentially harmful for patients with HFrEF, except as palliation for patients with end-stage disease who cannot be stabilized with standard medical treatment (see recommendations for stage D).	C
	Calcium Channel Blockers	
III: No benefit	Calcium channel blocking drugs are not recommended for routine therapy in patients with HFrEF.	A

ACC, American College of Cardiology; *ACE,* angiotensin-converting-enzyme; *AHA,* American Heart Association; *ARB,* angiotensin-receptor blocker; *GDMT,* guideline-directed medical therapy; *HF,* heart failure; *HFpEF,* heart failure with preserved ejection fraction; *HFrEF,* heart failure with reduced ejection fraction; *HRQOL,* health-related quality of life; *LVEF,* left ventricular ejection fraction; *MI,* myocardial infarction; *NYHA,* New York Heart Association; *NSAID,* nonsteroidal antiinflammatory drug; *PUFA,* polyunsaturated fatty acid.
From Mann DL et al: *Braunwald's heart disease,* ed 10, Philadelphia, 2015, Elsevier.

TABLE 13 ACC/AHA Recommendations for the Hospitalized Patient with Heart Failure (HF)

Class	Indication	Level of Evidence*
I	Thorough history and physical examination to evaluate for adequacy of systemic perfusion, volume status, contribution of precipitating factors and/or comorbidities, and whether HF is associated with preserved ejection fraction.	C
	Concentrations of B-type natriuretic peptide (BNP) or N-terminal pro-B-type natriuretic peptide (NT-proBNP) to evaluate dyspnea if the contribution of heart failure is not known.	A
	Acute coronary syndrome should be promptly identified by electrocardiogram and cardiac troponin testing, and treated, as appropriate to the overall condition and prognosis of patient.	C
	Oxygen therapy should be administered to relieve symptoms related to hypoxemia.	C
	Improve systemic perfusion in patients who present with rapid decompensation and hypoperfusion associated with decreasing urine output and other manifestations of shock.	C
	Treatment of significant fluid overload with intravenous loop diuretics. The diuretic dose should be titrated to relieve symptoms and to reduce extracellular fluid volume excess.	B, C
	Monitor the effects of therapy with careful measurement of fluid intake and output; vital signs; body weight, and symptoms of systemic perfusion and congestion.	C
	Intensify the diuretic regimen when the diuresis is inadequate to relieve congestion.	C
	Intravenous inotropic or vasopressor drugs should be administered to maintain systemic perfusion and preserve end-organ performance in patients with clinical evidence of hypotension associated with hypoperfusion and elevated cardiac filling pressures.	C
	Invasive hemodynamic monitoring to guide therapy in patients who are in respiratory distress or with clinical evidence of impaired perfusion if filling pressures cannot be determined from clinical assessment.	C
	Medications should be reconciled and adjusted as appropriate on admission to and discharge from the hospital.	C
	Maintenance treatment with oral therapies known to improve outcomes (ACE inhibitors or ARBs and beta-blocker therapy) in the absence of hemodynamic instability or contraindications.	C
	Initiation of treatment with oral therapies known to improve outcomes (ACE inhibitors or ARBs and beta-blocker therapy) in stable patients prior to hospital discharge.	B
	During transition from intravenous to oral diuretic therapy, patient should be monitored carefully for supine and upright hypotension, worsening renal function, and HF signs/symptoms.	C
	Comprehensive written discharge instructions for patients and their caregivers is strongly recommended.	C
	Postdischarge systems of care, if available, should be used to facilitate the transition to effective outpatient care.	B
IIa	Urgent cardiac catheterization and revascularization in patients with acute HF with known or suspected acute myocardial ischemia due to occlusive coronary disease when there are signs and symptoms of inadequate systemic perfusion and revascularization is likely to prolong meaningful survival.	C
	Intravenous nitroglycerin, nitroprusside, or nesiritide for patients with evidence of severely symptomatic fluid overload in the absence of systemic hypotension.	C
	Ultrafiltration for patients with refractory congestion not responding to medical therapy.	B
IIb	Intravenous inotropic drugs (dopamine, dobutamine, or milrinone) for patients presenting with documented severe systolic dysfunction, low blood pressure, and evidence of low cardiac output, with or without congestion, to maintain systemic perfusion and preserve end-organ performance.	C
III	Use of parenteral inotropes in normotensive patients with acute decompensated HF without evidence of decreased organ perfusion.	B
	Routine use of invasive hemodynamic monitoring in normotensive patients with acute decompensated HF and congestion with symptomatic response to diuretics and vasodilators.	B

ACC, American College of Cardiology; *ACE,* angiotensin-converting enzyme; *AHA,* American Heart Association; *ARB,* angiotensin-receptor blocker.
*See guidelines text for definition of level of evidence categories.
From Zipes DP: *Braunwald's heart disease, a textbook of cardiovascular medicine,* ed 11, Philadelphia, 2019, Elsevier.

TABLE 14 Intravenous Vasoactive Agents for Treatment of Acute Heart Failure

Intravenous Medication	Initial Dose	Effective Dose Range	Comments
Vasodilators			
Nitroglycerin; glyceryl trinitrate	20 μg/min	40-400 μg/min	Hypotension, headache Tolerance with continuous use after 24 hr
Isosorbide dinitrate	1 mg/hr	2-10 mg/hr	Hypotension, headache Tolerance with continuous use within 24 hr
Nitroprusside	0.3 μg/kg/min	0.3-5 μg/kg/min (usually <4 μg/kg/min)	Caution in patients with active myocardial ischemia Hypotension; cyanide side effects (nausea, dysphoria); thiocyanate toxicity; light sensitive
Nesiritide	2 μg/kg bolus with 0.010-0.030 μg/kg/min infusion*	0.010-0.030 μg/kg/min†	Uptitration: 1 μg/kg bolus, then increase infusion rate by 0.005 μg/kg/min no more frequently than every 3 hr, up to maximum of 0.03 μg/kg/min Hypotension, headache (less than with organic nitrates)
Inotropes			
Dobutamine	1-2 μg/kg/min	2-20 μg/kg/min	For inotropy and vasodilation; hypotension, tachycardia, arrhythmias; ?mortality
Dopamine	1-2 μg/kg/min	2-4 μg/kg/min	For inotropy and vasodilation; hypotension, tachycardia, arrhythmias; ?mortality
	4-5 μg/kg/min	5-20 μg/kg/min	For inotropy and vasoconstriction; tachycardia, arrhythmias; ?mortality
Milrinone	25-75 μg/kg bolus over 10-20 min* followed by infusion	0.10-0.75 μg/kg/min	For vasodilation and inotropy; hypotension, tachycardia, arrhythmias; renal excretion; ?mortality
Enoximone††	0.25-0.75 mg/kg	1.25-7.5 μg/kg/min	For vasodilation and inotropy; hypotension, tachycardia, arrhythmias; ?mortality
Levosimendan††	12-24 μg/kg bolus over 10 min followed by infusion	0.5-2.0 μg/kg/min	For vasodilation and inotropy; active metabolite present for ~84 hr; hypotension, tachycardia, arrhythmias; ?mortality
Epinephrine		0.05-0.5 μg/kg/min	For vasoconstriction and inotropy; tachycardia, arrhythmias, end-organ hypoperfusion; ?mortality
Norepinephrine		0.2-1.0 μg/kg/min	For vasoconstriction and inotropy; tachycardia, arrhythmias, end-organ hypoperfusion; ?mortality

*Some clinicians do not administer a bolus dose to decrease the risk of hypotension. Bolus not recommended in patients with hypotension.
†Lower doses have also been effective in some small studies.
††Not approved for use in all countries.
From Zipes DP: *Braunwald's heart disease, a textbook of cardiovascular medicine,* ed 11, Philadelphia, 2019, Elsevier.

TABLE 15 ACC/AHA/HFSA Guidelines for Treatment of Patients with Stage C Heart Failure and Preserved Left Ventricular Ejection Fraction (HFpEF)

Class	Indication	Level of Evidence
I	Systolic and diastolic blood pressure should be controlled in accordance with published clinical practice guidelines to prevent morbidity.	B
	Diuretics should be used for relief of symptoms due to volume overload.	C
IIa	Coronary revascularization is reasonable in patients with coronary artery disease in whom symptoms (angina) or demonstrable myocardial ischemia is judged to be having an adverse effect on symptomatic heart failure.	C
	Management of atrial fibrillation according to published clinical practice guidelines is reasonable to improve symptomatic heart failure.	C
	The use of beta-blocking agents, ACE inhibitors, and ARBs in patients with hypertension is reasonable to control blood pressure.	C
IIb	In appropriately selected patients with HFpEF (with EF ≥45%, elevated BNP levels or heart failure admission within 1 yr, estimated glomerular filtration rate >30 ml/min, creatinine <2.5 mg/dL, potassium <5.0 mEq/L), aldosterone receptor antagonists might be considered to decrease hospitalizations.	B-R
IIb	The use of ARBs might be considered to decrease hospitalizations.	B
III: No benefit	The routine use of nitrates or phosphodiesterase-5 inhibitors to increase activity or quality of life in patients with HFpEF is ineffective.	B-R
III: No benefit	Routine use of nutritional supplements is not recommended.	C

ACC, American College of Cardiology; *ACE,* angiotensin-converting enzyme; *AHA,* American Heart Association; *ARB,* angiotensin receptor blocker; *BNP,* B-type (brain) natriuretic peptide; *HFSA,* Heart Failure Society of America.
From Zipes DP: *Braunwald's heart disease, a textbook of cardiovascular medicine,* ed 11, Philadelphia, 2019, Elsevier.

physiologic effects of these IV inotropic agents after their discontinuation before discharge may mask the inadequate diuretic regimen and intolerance to the vasodilator doses. This can result in readmission, especially with milrinone due to its long half-life that can be further prolonged by the common coexisting impaired renal function. Therefore it may be recommended that patients who received inotropic infusions remain hospitalized for at least 48 hr after inotropic agents are discontinued and optimize the oral regimen.

- 4th phase: Early postdischarge care
  1. The patient will require reevaluation and constant monitoring in order to avoid another episode of ADHF. Emphasis should be placed on importance of compliance with instructions regarding dietary restrictions and daily body weight monitoring. Early follow-up should be scheduled as well as outpatient electrolyte monitoring if required after medication adjustments.

CHRONIC TREATMENT OF HFrEF: The goals of HF therapy are clinical improvement followed

TABLE 16 Therapeutic Approaches for Volume Management in Acute Heart Failure (AHF)

Severity of Volume Overload	Diuretic	DOSE (mg)	Comments
Moderate	Furosemide, or	20-40, or up to 2.5 times oral dose	IV administration preferable in symptomatic patients
	Bumetanide, or	0.5-1.0	Titrate dose according to clinical response.
	Torsemide	10-20	Monitor Na^+, K^+, creatinine, BP
Severe	Furosemide, or	40-160, or 2.5 times oral dose 5-40 mg/hr infusion	Intravenously
	Bumetanide, or	1-4/0.5-2 mg/hr infusion (max, 2-4 mg/hr, limit 2-4 hr)	Bumetanide and torsemide have higher oral bioavailability than furosemide, but IV administration preferable in AHF.
	Torsemide	20-100/5-20 mg/hr	
	Ultrafiltration	200-500 ml/hr	Adjust ultrafiltration rate to clinical response; monitor for hypotension; consider hematocrit sensor.
Refractory to loop diuretics	Add HCTZ, *or*	25-50 twice daily	Combination with loop diuretic may be better than very high dose of loop diuretics alone.
	Metolazone, *or*	2.5-10 once daily	Metolazone more potent if creatinine clearance <30 ml/min
	Chlorothiazide, *or*	250-500 mg IV 500-1000 mg PO	
	Spironolactone	25-50 once daily	Spironolactone best choice if patient not in renal failure and normal or low serum K^+, although may not be very potent
In case of alkalosis	Acetazolamide	0.5	Intravenously
Refractory to loop diuretics and thiazides	Add dopamine (renal vasodilation), *or* dobutamine or milrinone (inotropic agent) Ultrafiltration, or hemodialysis if coexisting renal failure		

BP, Blood pressure; *IV,* intravenous; *HCTZ,* hydrochlorothiazide; *PO,* by mouth.
From Zipes DP: *Braunwald's heart disease, a textbook of cardiovascular medicine,* ed 11, Philadelphia, 2019, Elsevier.

by stabilizing, slowing, or even reversing deterioration in myocardial function, and ultimately a reduction in risk of morbidity (including hospitalization rates) and mortality.

- ACE inhibitors:
  1. Reduce morbidity and mortality.
  2. Produce both venous and arterial vasodilation acutely, thereby reducing both preload and afterload.
  3. Potential mechanism of long-term benefit is attenuation of RAAS activation and decreased myocardial remodeling and fibrosis.
  4. Used as first-line therapy for asymptomatic LV dysfunction (LVEF <40%) and symptomatic systolic HF (ACC/AHA grades A-D).
  5. Therapy should be initiated at low doses to prevent hypotension and rapidly titrated to higher doses as tolerated.
  6. Contraindications to the use of ACE inhibitors are renal insufficiency (creatinine clearance <30 ml/min), bilateral renal artery stenosis, hyperkalemia, hypotension, or adverse reactions (e.g., angioedema).
- ARBs:
  1. Receptor antagonists to the angiotensin II receptor.
  2. Clinical trials have not shown any superiority compared to ACE inhibitors in patients with systolic HF (LVEF <40%).
  3. Reserved for patients who are ACE inhibitor intolerant.
  4. Combination therapy with ARBs and ACE inhibitors is generally not recommended.
  5. Have a similar contraindication profile to ACE inhibitors. Routine combined use of an ACE inhibitor, ARB, and aldosterone antagonist is potentially harmful for patients with HFrEF.
- Angiotensin receptor–neprilysin inhibitor (ARNI) (valsartan/sacubitril):
  1. Neprilysin is an enzyme that degrades natriuretic peptides, bradykinin, adrenomedullin, and other vasoactive peptides.
  2. In a randomized controlled trial (PARADIGM-HF) that compared valsartan/sacubitril with enalapril in symptomatic patients with HFrEF tolerating an adequate dose of either ACE inhibitor or ARB, the ARNI reduced the composite end point of cardiovascular death or HF hospitalization significantly, by 20%. Additionally, in another randomized controlled trial (PIONEER – HF), in HFrEF patients hospitalized with decompensated HF, initiation of valsartan/sacubitril caused a greater reduction in NT-proBNP concentration than enalapril. Rates of adverse effects did not significantly differ between the two groups.
  3. In patients with chronic symptomatic HFrEF NYHA class II or III who tolerate an ACE inhibitor or ARB, replacement by an ARNI is recommended to further reduce morbidity and mortality (class I).
  4. ARNI should not be administered concomitantly with ACE inhibitors or within 36 hr of the last dose of an ACE inhibitor (class III: Harm).
  5. ARNI should not be administered to patients with a history of angioedema (class III: Harm).
  6. ARNI has not shown additional benefit over ARB in patients with preserved ejection fraction and is not indicated in this group of patients.
- Beta-adrenergic blockers (beta-blockers):
  1. Reduce morbidity and mortality. Such benefits observed with bisoprolol (CIBIS II trial), metoprolol succinate (MERIT-HF trial), and carvedilol (COPERNICUS trial).
  2. Benefit is believed to be conferred by blockade of sympathetic effects of neurohormonal stimulation due to HF.
  3. Are considered first-line therapy for symptomatic patients with systolic HF (NYHA class ≥II and LVEF <35%).
  4. Only carvedilol, bisoprolol, and metoprolol succinate (long acting) have been approved for the medical treatment of chronic HF; these agents are generally started in patients judged to be euvolemic and dosage is to be slowly uptitrated as tolerated.
  5. Adverse effects include worsening HF (due to negative inotropic effects), fatigue, dizziness, bradycardia, hypotension, and bronchospasm.
- Aldosterone receptor antagonists:
  1. Reduce morbidity and mortality.
  2. Indicated in patients with NYHA class II-IV HF, with LVEF ≤35%, already treated with

ACE inhibitors and beta-blockers without significant renal insufficiency or hyperkalemia. Patients with NYHA class II should have a history of prior cardiovascular hospitalization or elevated plasma natriuretic peptide levels to be considered for aldosterone receptor antagonists. Creatinine should be ≤2.5 mg/dl in men or ≤2.0 mg/dl in women (or estimated glomerular filtration rate >30 ml/min/1.73 m2), and potassium should be <5.0 mEq/L. They are also indicated for post-MI patients with EF ≤40% who have either symptomatic HF or diabetes mellitus.
3. Spironolactone may cause gynecomastia, galactorrhea, and hyperkalemia (especially in patients with baseline renal insufficiency or type 4 renal tubular acidosis). It has been best studied in chronic HF with NYHA class III to IV symptoms (RALES study).
4. Eplerenone is associated with fewer endocrine side effects and has especially been studied in postmyocardial infarction left ventricular dysfunction (EPHESUS trial) and in chronic systolic HF with only class II symptoms (EMPHASIS-HF trial).
5. Inappropriate use of aldosterone receptor antagonists is potentially harmful because of life-threatening hyperkalemia or renal insufficiency when serum creatinine is >2.5 mg/dl in men or >2.0 mg/dl in women (or estimated glomerular filtration rate <30 ml/min/1.73 m2), and/or potassium >5.0 mEq/L.

- Diuretics:
  1. They are used to maintain euvolemia and to improve symptoms as discussed previously.
  2. Although data on diuretic efficacy are limited, a meta-analysis of a few small trials found that they were associated with reduction in mortality as well as reduced hospitalization for HF.
  3. Of note, loop diuretics with better bioavailability, such as torsemide and bumetanide, may be used in diuretic-resistant patients but are generally more expensive.
- Combination of isosorbide dinitrate and hydralazine:
  1. Cause venous (nitrates) and arteriolar (hydralazine) vasodilation resulting in decreased preload and afterload.
  2. The combination of hydralazine and isosorbide dinitrate is recommended to reduce morbidity and mortality for patients self-described as African Americans with NYHA class III to IV HFrEF receiving optimal therapy with ACE inhibitors and beta-blockers, unless contraindicated.
  3. A combination of hydralazine and isosorbide dinitrate can be useful to reduce morbidity or mortality in patients with current or prior symptomatic HFrEF who cannot be given an ACE inhibitor or ARB because of drug intolerance, hypotension, or renal insufficiency, unless contraindicated.
  4. Adverse effects of nitrates include hypotension, headaches, and tolerance as well as reflex tachycardia and lupus-like syndrome with hydralazine.
- Digoxin:
  1. Positive inotropic and negative chronotropic drug that works by inhibition of the sodium-potassium transmembrane exchange pump and through its vagomimetic action.
  2. Commonly used in patients with concomitant atrial fibrillation.
  3. Has been shown to reduce HF-related hospitalizations but does not confer any mortality benefit (DIG trial). However, there is evidence suggesting that digoxin may actually have an effect on survival that varies with the serum digoxin level; survival was improved when the level was between 0.5 and 0.8 ng/ml (most often in men) and significantly worsened when it was ≥1.2 ng/ml and >0.9 mg/ml in women.
  4. Caution must be used in patients with abnormal renal function to avoid digoxin toxicity and life-threatening arrhythmia. Avoid hypokalemia because potassium competes with digoxin on the same site of the Na^+-K^+-ATPase pump.
- I_f channel inhibitor (ivabradine):
  1. Ivabradine is a new therapeutic agent that selectively inhibits the I_f current in the sinoatrial node, providing heart rate reduction.
  2. Ivabradine can be beneficial to reduce HF hospitalization for patients with symptomatic (NYHA class II-III) stable chronic HFrEF (LVEF ≤35%) who are receiving guideline-directed therapy, including a beta-blocker at maximum tolerated dose, and who are in sinus rhythm with a heart rate of 70 bpm or greater at rest (class IIa).
- Sodium-Glucose Cotransporter 2 (SGLT2) Inhibitor:
  1. SGLT2 inhibitors, along with its diuretic and related hemodynamic actions, were also proposed to have an effect on myocardial metabolism, ion transporters, fibrosis, adipokines, and vascular function.
  2. Dapagliflozin (a sodium-glucose cotransporter 2 [SGLT2] inhibitor) can be used in patients with HF (LVEF ≤40%) for reduction in cardiovascular deaths and hospitalizations regardless of the presence or absence of diabetes.
  3. Empagliflozin can reduce heart failure hospitalizations and cardiovascular deaths in HF patients (LVEF ≤40%) regardless of diabetes, however dose used in nondiabetics is 10 mg instead of 25 mg as used in diabetics.[1] In patients with diabetes and recent worsening heart failure, sotagliflozin therapy initiated before or shortly after discharge significantly lowers total number of deaths from cardiovascular causes and hospitalizations and urgent visits for heart failure than placebo.[2]
  4. Among patients with HF (EF≤40%), the anticipated aggregate treatment effects of early comprehensive disease-modifying pharmacological therapy are substantial and support the combination use of an ARNI, β blocker, MRA, and SGLT2 inhibitor as a new therapeutic standard.
- Cardiac resynchronization therapy (CRT):
  1. Improves morbidity and mortality rates in selected patients.
  2. The presence of a bundle-branch block or other intraventricular conduction delay (IVCD) can cause ventricular dyssynchrony, which induces regional loading disparities and reduces the efficiency of ventricular contraction, thereby further impairing the systolic function of a failing ventricle.
  3. CRT is indicated for patients who have LVEF ≤35%, sinus rhythm, left bundle-branch block with a QRS duration of 150 ms or greater, and NYHA class II, III, or ambulatory IV symptoms on guideline-directed medical therapy. CRT is NOT indicated in patients whose functional status and life expectancy are limited predominantly by chronic noncardiac conditions. Life expectancy should be >1 yr.
  4. In the appropriate subset of patients, CRT in addition to optimal medical therapy has been shown in numerous clinical trials to improve symptoms by at least one NYHA class, improve 6-min walk distance and quality of life, reduce rate of HF-related hospitalization, and reduce rate of all-cause and cardiovascular mortality.
  5. ACC/AHA guidelines for cardiac resynchronization therapy are summarized in Table 17.
- Implantable cardioverter-defibrillators (ICDs):
  1. Sudden cardiac death (SCD) is a common cause of death in patients with HF in both ischemic and nonischemic cardiomyopathies. Ventricular tachycardia (VT) degenerating into ventricular fibrillation (VF) is the culprit in the majority of patients with SCD, although bradyarrhythmias do also occur with less frequency.
  2. ICD therapy is recommended for primary prevention of SCD to reduce total mortality in selected patients with nonischemic dilated cardiomyopathy or ischemic heart disease at least 40 days post-MI with LVEF ≤35% and NYHA class II or III symptoms on chronic guideline-directed medical therapy, who have reasonable expectation of meaningful survival for >1 yr.
  3. Patients with HF who survive an episode of sudden cardiac arrest or experience sustained VT in the presence of LVEF <35% are at high risk for future arrhythmic events and SCD and obtain a mortality benefit from ICD placement for secondary prevention,

[1] Anker PM et al: Cardiovascular and renal outcomes with empagliflozin in heart failure, *N Engl J Med* 383:1413-1424, 2020.

[2] Bhata DL et al: Sotagliflozin in patients with diabetes and recent worsening heart failure, *N Engl J Med* 384:117-128, 2021.

TABLE 17 ACCF/AHA Guidelines for Cardiac Resynchronization Therapy (CRT)

Class	Indication	Level of Evidence
I	CRT is indicated for patients who have LVEF of 35% or less, sinus rhythm, LBBB with QRS duration of 150 msec or greater, and NYHA Class II, III, or ambulatory IV symptoms on GDMT.	A for NYHA Class III/I B for Class II
IIa	CRT can be useful for patients who have LVEF of 35% or less, sinus rhythm, non-LBBB pattern with QRS duration of 150 msec or greater, and NYHA Class III/ambulatory Class IV symptoms on GDMT.	A
	CRT can be useful for patients who have LVEF of 35% or less, sinus rhythm, LBBB with QRS duration of 120-149 msec, and NYHA Class II, III, or ambulatory IV symptoms on GDMT.	B
	CRT can be useful in patients with atrial fibrillation and LVEF of 35% or less on GDMT if (a) the patient requires ventricular pacing or otherwise meets CRT criteria and (b) atrioventricular nodal ablation or pharmacologic rate control will allow near-100% ventricular pacing with CRT.	B
	CRT can be useful for patients on GDMT who have LVEF of 35% or less and are undergoing placement of new or replacement device with anticipated requirement for significant (>40%) ventricular pacing.	C
IIb	CRT may be considered for patients who have LVEF of 35% or less, sinus rhythm, non-LBBB pattern with QRS duration of 120-149 msec, and NYHA Class III/ambulatory Class IV on GDMT.	B
	CRT may be considered for patients who have LVEF of 35% or less, sinus rhythm, non-LBBB pattern with QRS duration of 150 msec or greater, and NYHA Class II symptoms on GDMT.	B
	CRT may be considered for patients who have LVEF of 30% or less, ischemic etiology of HF, sinus rhythm, LBBB with QRS duration of 150 msec or greater, and NYHA Class I symptoms on GDMT.	C
III: No benefit	CRT is not recommended for patients with NYHA Class I or II symptoms and non-LBBB pattern with QRS duration less than 150 msec.	
	CRT is not indicated for patients whose comorbidities and/or frailty limit survival with good functional capacity to less than 1 yr.	

ACCF, The American College of Cardiology Foundation; *AHA,* American Heart Association; *GDMT,* guideline-directed medical therapy; *LBBB,* left bundle-branch block; *LVEF,* left ventricular ejection fraction; *NYHA,* New York Heart Association.
From Zipes DP: *Braunwald's heart disease, a textbook of cardiovascular medicine,* ed 11, Philadelphia, 2019, Elsevier.

TABLE 18 ACCF/AHA Guidelines for Indications for Implantable Cardioverter-Defibrillators (ICDs)

Class	Indication	Level of Evidence
I	ICD therapy is recommended for primary prevention of SCD in selected patients with HFrEF at least 40 days post-MI with LVEF less than 35% and NYHA Class II or III symptoms receiving chronic GDMT, who are expected to live more than 1 yr.	A
I	ICD therapy is recommended for primary prevention of SCD in selected patients with HFrEF at least 40 days post-MI with LVEF less than 30% and NYHA Class I symptoms receiving GDMT, who are expected to live more than 1 yr.	B
IIa	To prevent SCD, placement of ICD is reasonable in patients with asymptomatic ischemic cardiomyopathy who are at least 40 days post-MI, have an LVEF of 30% or less, are on appropriate medical therapy, and have reasonable expectation of survival with a good functional status for more than 1 yr.	B
IIb	ICD therapy to prevent SCD in patients with nonischemic cardiomyopathy who are at least 40 days post-MI, have LVEF less than 35%, with NYHA Class II or III symptoms while undergoing chronic optimal medical therapy, and have reasonable expectation of survival for more than 1 yr with good functional status.	B
	Usefulness of implantation of ICD is of uncertain benefit to prolong meaningful survival in patients with high risk of non-SCD, as predicted by frequent hospitalizations, advanced frailty, or comorbidities such as systemic malignancy or severe renal dysfunction.	B

HFrEF, Heart failure with reduced ejection fraction; *MI,* myocardial infarction; *SCD,* sudden cardiac death; see Table 17 for other abbreviations.
From Zipes DP: *Braunwald's heart disease, a textbook of cardiovascular medicine,* ed 11, Philadelphia, 2019, Elsevier.

with or without adjunctive therapies such as antiarrhythmic drugs, radiofrequency ablation, surgery, or transplant.

4. ACC/AHA guidelines for indications for implantable cardioverter-defibrillators are summarized in Table 18.

- In the absence of an indication (e.g., atrial fibrillation), routine use of anticoagulation is currently not recommended in patients with HF. Even with the increased risk for LV thrombus formation in dilated cardiomyopathy and subsequent thromboembolization, data are conflicting about benefits of antithrombotic (antiplatelet or anticoagulant) therapy for primary prevention to reduce thromboembolic events or mortality in patients with systolic HF who are in sinus rhythm (SOLVD, V-HeFT, SAVE, HELAS, and WASH trials). It may be reasonable to consider anticoagulation for secondary prevention in patients with HF who had a prior thromboembolic event; however, risks and benefits should be carefully assessed.
- Antiplatelet agents are recommended for patients with concomitant CAD.
- Statins are not beneficial as adjunctive therapy when prescribed solely for the diagnosis of HF in the absence of other indications for their use.
- Calcium channel blocking drugs are not recommended as routine treatment for patients with HFrEF.
- Omega-3 polyunsaturated fatty acid supplementation is reasonable to use as adjunctive therapy in patients with NYHA class II to IV symptoms and HFrEF or HFpEF, unless contraindicated, to reduce mortality and cardiovascular hospitalizations.
- Percutaneous coronary intervention (PCI) or surgical revascularization should be considered in patients with HF and significant CAD who are revascularization candidates.
- In general, the following sequence of drugs is recommended:
  1. Loop diuretics to provide symptom relief and achieve a euvolemic state.
  2. ACE inhibitor or ARB started at low doses, then increased to a moderate dose in 1 to 2 wk. Replace with ARNI in those tolerating ACE inhibitor or ARB.
  3. Beta-blockers after the patient is stable on ACE/ARB treatment. Start a low dose, then uptitrate to goal based on trial data or maximal dose tolerated. Once achieved, uptitration of ACE or ARB to goal doses can be completed.

- The following drugs can be added in selected patients in the absence of contraindications:
  1. Aldosterone antagonists improve survival in NYHA class II with LVEF <30% or NYHA class III-IV with EF <35%. Kidney function should be stable with eGFR ≥30 ml/min and potassium <5 mEq/L.
  2. Combination of hydralazine with a nitrate in patients (particularly African Americans) with a reduced EF.
  3. Digoxin reduces hospitalizations for HF and controls HR in atrial fibrillation. It can also help control symptoms.

CHRONIC TREATMENT OF HFpEF:

- To date, there is a relative dearth of clinical trials examining effective chronic treatment strategies in this subset of patients with HFpEF. Current therapies are mainly for symptomatic relief. ACC/AHA guidelines for treatment of patients with end-stage heart failure are summarized in Table 19.
- Therapy centers on relief of volume overload with judicious diuretic use, treatment of ischemia via coronary revascularization (Table 20), management of atrial fibrillation, controlling heart rate and blood pressure to prevent acute decompensation, and restriction of sodium and fluid to prevent volume overload.
- Diuretics should be used for relief of symptoms due to volume overload in patients with HFpEF.
- The use of beta-blocking agents, ACE inhibitors, and ARBs in patients with hypertension

TABLE 19 ACC/AHA Guidelines for Treatment of Patients with End-Stage Heart Failure (Stage D)

Class	Indication	Level of Evidence
	Nonpharmacologic Interventions	
IIa	Fluid restriction (1.5-2 L/day) is reasonable in stage D, especially in patients with hyponatremia.	B
	Inotropic Support	
I	Until definitive therapy (e.g., coronary revascularization, MCS, heart transplantation) or resolution of the acute precipitating problem, patients with cardiogenic shock should receive temporary IV inotropic support to maintain systemic perfusion and preserve end-organ performance.	C
IIa	Continuous IV inotropic support is reasonable as "bridge therapy" in patients with stage D refractory to GDMT and device therapy who are eligible for and awaiting MCS or cardiac transplantation.	B
IIb	Short-term, continuous IV inotropic support may be reasonable in those hospitalized patients presenting with documented severe systolic dysfunction who present with low blood pressure and significantly depressed cardiac output, to maintain systemic perfusion and preserve end-organ performance.	B
	Long-term, continuous IV inotropic support may be considered as palliative therapy for symptom control in select patients with stage D despite optimal GDMT and device therapy who are not eligible for either MCS or cardiac transplantation.	B
III: Harm	Long-term use of either continuous or intermittent, IV parenteral positive inotropic agents, in the absence of specific indications or for reasons other than palliative care, is potentially harmful in the patient with HF.	B
	Use of parenteral inotropic agents in hospitalized patients without documented severe systolic dysfunction, low blood pressure, or impaired perfusion, and evidence of significantly depressed cardiac output, with or without congestion, is potentially harmful.	B
	Mechanical Circulatory Support (MCS)	
IIa	MCS is beneficial in carefully selected patients with stage D HFrEF in whom definitive management (e.g., cardiac transplantation) or cardiac recovery is anticipated or planned.	B
	Nondurable MCS, including the use of percutaneous and extracorporeal ventricular assist devices (VADs), is reasonable as a "bridge to recovery" or "bridge to decision" for carefully selected patients with HFrEF with acute, profound hemodynamic compromise.	B
	Durable MCS is reasonable to prolong survival for carefully selected patients with stage D HFrEF.	B
	Cardiac Transplantation	
I	Evaluation for cardiac transplantation is indicated for carefully selected patients with stage D HF despite GDMT, device, and surgical management	C

ACC, American College of Cardiology; *AHA,* American Heart Association; *GDMT,* Guideline-directed medical therapy; *HF,* heart failure; *HFrEF,* heart failure with reduced ejection fraction; *IV,* intravenous.
From Zipes DP: *Braunwald's heart disease, a textbook of cardiovascular medicine,* ed 11, Philadelphia, 2019, Elsevier.

TABLE 20 ACC/AHA Guidelines for Surgical/Percutaneous/Transcatheter Interventional Treatments of Heart Failure

Class	Indication	Level of Evidence
I	Coronary artery revascularization via CABG or percutaneous intervention is indicated for patients (HFpEF and HFrEF) on GDMT with angina and suitable coronary artery anatomy, especially for a left main artery stenosis (>50%) or left main–equivalent disease.	C
IIa	CABG to improve survival is reasonable in patients with mild to moderate LV systolic dysfunction (EF 35%-50%) and significant (≥70% diameter stenosis) multivessel CAD or proximal left anterior descending coronary artery stenosis when viable myocardium is present in the region of intended revascularization.	B
	CABG or medical therapy is reasonable to improve morbidity and cardiovascular mortality for patients with severe LV dysfunction (EF <35%), HF, and significant CAD.	B
	Surgical aortic valve replacement is reasonable for patients with critical aortic stenosis and a predicted surgical mortality of no greater than 10%.	B
	Transcatheter aortic valve replacement after careful candidate consideration is reasonable for patients with critical aortic stenosis who are deemed inoperable.	B
IIb	CABG may be considered with the intent of improving survival in patients with ischemic heart disease with severe LV systolic dysfunction (EF <35%) and operable coronary anatomy whether or not viable myocardium is present.	B
	Transcatheter mitral valve repair or mitral valve surgery for functional mitral insufficiency is of uncertain benefit and should only be considered after careful candidate selection and with a background of GDMT.	B
	Surgical reverse remodeling or LV aneurysmectomy may be considered in carefully selected patients with HFrEF for specific indications, including intractable HF and ventricular arrhythmias.	B

ACC, American College of Cardiology; *AHA,* American Heart Association; *CABG,* coronary artery bypass grafting, *CAD,* coronary artery disease; *EF,* ejection fraction; *GDMT,* guideline-directed medical therapy; *HF,* heart failure; *HFpEF,* heart failure with preserved ejection fraction; *HFrEF,* HF with reduced ejection fraction; *LV,* left ventricle.
From Mann DL et al: *Braunwald's heart disease,* ed 10, Philadelphia, 2015, Elsevier.

TABLE 21 Surgery for Management of Heart Failure (HF): Guideline Recommendations

2016 ESC Guidelines for the Diagnosis and Treatment of Acute and Chronic Heart Failure

Recommendations for Myocardial Revascularization in Patients with Chronic HF

- Myocardial revascularization is recommended when angina persists despite antiangina drugs; *class I, level of evidence A.*
  The choice between CABG and PCI should be made by the heart team after careful review.
  CABG is recommended for patients with angina and significant LM or LM-equivalent stenosis to improve prognosis.
  CABG is recommended for patients with HFrEF, significant CAD (LAD or multivessel disease), and LVEF <35%.

2014 ACC/AHA/AATS/PCNA/SCAI/STS Focused Update of the Guideline for the Diagnosis and Management of Patients with Stable Ischemic Heart Disease*

- A heart team approach to revascularization is recommended in patients with diabetes mellitus and complex multivessel CAD; *class 1, level of evidence C.*
- CABG is generally recommended in preference to PCI to improve survival in patients with diabetes mellitus and multivessel CAD for which revascularization is likely to improve survival (3-vessel CAD or complex 2-vessel CAD involving the proximal LAD); *class 1, level of evidence B.*

2014 AHA/ACC Guideline for the Management of Patients with Valvular Heart Disease†

Indications for Aortic Valve Surgery in Aortic Stenosis (as) with Left Ventricular Dysfunction

- AVR is recommended for asymptomatic patients with severe AS and LVEF <50%; *class I, level of evidence B.*
- AVR is reasonable in symptomatic patients with low-flow/low-gradient severe AS with reduced LVEF with a low-dose dobutamine stress study that shows an aortic velocity ≥4.0 m/sec or mean pressure gradient ≥40 mm Hg with a valve area of ≤1.0 cm^2; *class IIa, level of evidence B.*
- AVR is reasonable for patients with moderate AS who are undergoing other cardiac surgery; *class IIa, level of evidence C.*
- TAVR is recommended in patients who meet an indication for AVR for AS and who have a prohibitive surgical risk and post-TAVR survival >12 mo; *class I, level of evidence B.*
- TAVR is a reasonable alternative to surgical AVR in patients who meet an indication for AVR and who have a high surgical risk; *class IIa, level of evidence B.*

Indications for Aortic Valve Surgery in Aortic Regurgitation (AR) with LV Dysfunction

- AVR is recommended for symptomatic patients with severe AR; *class I, level of evidence B.*
- AVR is indicated for patients with severe AR and LV systolic dysfunction; *class I, level of evidence B.*

Indications for Mitral Valve Surgery in Functional Mitral Regurgitation (MR)

- Mitral valve surgery is reasonable for patients with chronic severe functional MR who are undergoing CABG or AVR; *class IIa, level of evidence C.*
- Mitral valve surgery may be considered for severely symptomatic patients (NYHA Class III/IV) with chronic severe functional MR; *class IIb, level of evidence B.*
- Mitral valve repair may be considered for patients with chronic moderate functional MR who are undergoing other cardiac surgery; *class IIb, level of evidence C.*

ESC/EACTS Guidelines on the Management of Valvular Heart Disease (Version 2012)‡

Indications for Mitral Valve Surgery in Chronic Secondary Mitral Regurgitation (MR)

- Surgery is indicated in patients with severe MR undergoing CABG and LVEF >30%; *class I, level of evidence C.*
- Surgery should be considered in patients with moderate MR undergoing CABG; *class IIa, level of evidence C.*
- Surgery should be considered in symptomatic patients with severe MR, LVEF <30%, option for revascularization, and evidence of viability; *class IIa, level of evidence: C.*
- Surgery may be considered in patients with severe MR, LVEF >30%, who remain symptomatic despite optimal medical management (including CRT if indicated) and have low comorbidity, when revascularization is not indicated; *class IIb, level of evidence C.*

AATS, American Association for Thoracic Surgery; *ACC,* American College of Cardiology; *AHA,* American Heart Association; *AS,* aortic stenosis; *AVR,* aortic valve replacement; *CABG,* coronary artery bypass grafting; *CAD,* coronary artery disease; *CRT,* cardiac resynchronization therapy; *EACTS,* European Association for Cardio-Thoracic Surgery; *ESC,* European Society of Cardiology; *HFrEF,* heart failure with reduced ejection fraction; *LAD,* left anterior descending coronary artery; *LM,* left main coronary artery; *LV,* left ventricle; *LVEF,* left ventricular ejection fraction; *NYHA,* New York Heart Association; *PCI,* percutaneous coronary intervention; *PCNA,* Preventive Cardiovascular Nurses Association; *SCAI,* Society for Cardiovascular Angiography and Interventions; *STS,* Society of Thoracic Surgeons; *TAVR,* transcatheter aortic valve replacement.

*Fihn SD et al: 2014 ACC/AHA/AATS/PCNA/SCAI/STS focused update of the guideline for the diagnosis and management of patients with stable ischemic heart disease: a report of the American College of Cardiology/American Heart Association Task Force on Practice Guidelines, and the American Association for Thoracic Surgery, Preventive Cardiovascular Nurses Association, Society for Cardiovascular Angiography and Interventions, and Society of Thoracic Surgeons, *Circulation* 2014;130:1749-67.

†Nishimura RA et al: 2014 AHA/ACC guideline for the management of patients with valvular heart disease, *J Thorac Cardiovasc Surg* 2014;148:E1-E132.

‡Vahanian A et al: Guidelines on the management of valvular heart disease (version 2012), *Eur Heart J* 2012;33:2451-96.

From Zipes DP: *Braunwald's heart disease, a textbook of cardiovascular medicine,* ed 11, Philadelphia, 2019, Elsevier.

TABLE 22 Coordinating Care for Patients with Chronic Heart Failure

Class	Indication	Level of Evidence
I	Effective systems of care coordination with special attention to care transitions should be deployed for every patient with chronic HF that facilitate and ensure effective care that is designed to achieve GDMT and prevent hospitalization.	B
	Every patient with HF should have a clear, detailed, and evidence-based plan of care that ensures the achievement of GDMT goals, effective management of comorbid conditions, timely follow-up with the health care team, appropriate dietary and physical activities, and compliance with secondary prevention guidelines for cardiovascular disease. This plan of care should be updated regularly and made readily available to all members of the patient's health care team.	C
	Palliative and supportive care is effective for patients with symptomatic advanced HF to improve quality of life.	B

GDMT, Guideline directed medical therapy; *HF,* heart failure.
From Mann DL et al: *Braunwald's heart disease,* ed 10, Philadelphia, 2015, Elsevier.

is reasonable to control blood pressure in patients with HFpEF.

- The use of ARBs might be considered to decrease hospitalizations for patients with HFpEF.
- Aldosterone antagonists may be used in appropriate patients with HFpEF (EF >45%, elevated BNP or HF admission in the past yr, potassium <5.0 mEq/L, estimated glomerular filtration rate >30 and creatinine <2.5 mg/dl) to decrease hospitalizations (class IIb recommendation).
- Routine use of nitrates or phosphodiesterase-5 inhibitors to increase activity or quality of life in patients with HFpEF is not recommended as there is no benefit.
- There is no evidence to support routine use of nutritional supplements, and they are not recommended for patients with HFpEF.
- Surgical options (Table 21) for contributing critical aortic stenosis, constrictive pericarditis, and hypertrophic cardiomyopathy (HCM) should be entertained in appropriate patients.
- In patients with comorbidities including anemia, hypertension, and sleep apnea, the following recommendations are made:
  1. Intravenous iron replacement in patients with NYHA class II and III HF and iron deficiency (ferritin <100 ng/ml or 100 to 300 ng/ml with transferrin saturation <20%) to improve functional status and quality of life (class IIb recommendation).
  2. Titration of medical therapy to attain systolic blood pressure <130 mm Hg is

recommended in patients with HFrEF and hypertension, as well as in patients with HFpEF and persistent hypertension after treatment of volume overload (class I recommendation).

3. A formal sleep assessment should be obtained in patients with NYHA class II to IV HF with suspicion of sleep-disordered breathing. Continuous positive airway pressure should be used in patients with HF and obstructive sleep apnea to improve sleep quality and daytime sleepiness (class IIb recommendation).

DISPOSITION

- Coordination of care (Table 22) is essential in patients with chronic heart failure.
- Annual mortality of systolic HF ranges from 10% in stable patients with mild symptoms to 50% in patients with NYHA class IV disease (a mortality rate rivaling some malignancies). The Seattle Heart Failure Model provides an accurate estimate of 1-, 2-, and 3-yr survival before and after different therapies. This model can be useful to assess the need for LV assist device implantation or urgent transplantation. The calculator is available online at http://depts.washington.edu/shfm/.
- Cardiac transplantation has a 5-yr survival rate of ~70% and represents a viable option in selected patients. Fig. E4 describes an algorithm for evaluation of potential heart transplant recipient.
- The use of an LV assist device (LVAD) in patients with advanced HF can result in a clinically meaningful survival benefit and improve quality of life in patients who are not candidates for cardiac transplantation. There are two approved uses of LVADs specifically as a bridge to transplant and as destination therapy. There are two major categories of LVAD pulsatile flow devices vs. continuous flow devices. Continuous flow devices are associated with increased survival as destination therapy as compared to medically managed controls (REMATCH trial).

SUGGESTED READINGS

Available at ExpertConsult.com

RELATED CONTENT

Heart Failure (Patient Information)

AUTHORS: **S. Hammad Jafri, MD, MMSCI,** and **Aravind Rao Kokkirala, MD, FACC**

BASIC INFORMATION

DEFINITION

Heat exhaustion and heat stroke are part of a continuum of heat-related illness, and unless factors leading to heat exhaustion are corrected swiftly, affected patients can progress to heat stroke.

- ***Heat exhaustion:*** An illness resulting from prolonged, heavy activity in a hot environment with subsequent dehydration, electrolyte depletion, and rectal temperature >37.8° C (100° F) but ≤40° C (104° F).
- ***Heat stroke:*** A life-threatening heat illness characterized by extreme hyperthermia (core temperature >40° C [104.0° F]), dehydration, and neurologic manifestations. Heat stroke can be further subdivided into "exertional heat stroke" occurring in generally healthy individuals undergoing strenuous physical activity in warm conditions and "nonexertional heat stroke" often seen in elderly and/or debilitated patients with impaired thermal regulations due to illness or medications (see "Etiology").

SYNONYMS

Heat illness
Hyperthermia

ICD-10CM CODES

T67.5	Heat exhaustion, unspecified
T67.0	Heatstroke and sunstroke
T67.1	Heat syncope
T67.2	Heat cramp
T67.3	Heat exhaustion, anhydrotic
T67.6	Heat fatigue, transient

EPIDEMIOLOGY & DEMOGRAPHICS

INCIDENCE (IN U.S.): Incidence of heat stroke is approximately 20 cases/100,000 population.

PREDOMINANT AGE: Heat exhaustion and stroke occur more frequently in elderly patients, especially those taking diuretics or medications that impair heat dissipation (e.g., phenothiazines, anticholinergics, antihistamines, beta-blockers). Table 1 describes factors predisposing to serious heat illness.

PHYSICAL FINDINGS & CLINICAL PRESENTATION

Heat exhaustion:

- Generalized malaise, weakness, headache, muscle and abdominal cramps, nausea, vomiting, hypotension, tachycardia.
- Rectal temperature is usually normal.
- Sweating is usually present.

Heat stroke:

- Neurologic manifestations (seizures, tremor, hemiplegia, coma, psychosis, other bizarre behavior)
- Evidence of dehydration (poor skin turgor, sunken eyeballs)
- Tachycardia, hyperventilation
- Skin is hot, red, and flushed
- Sweating is often (not always) absent, particularly in elderly patients
- Classic heat stroke generally develops slowly over days and occurs predominantly in older persons and in those with chronic illness. Exertional heat stroke is more common in young, healthy persons; has a more rapid onset; and is associated with higher core temperatures. Table 2 compares classic and exertional heat stroke. Box 1 summarizes organ dysfunction seen in patients with heat stroke

ETIOLOGY

- Exogenous heat gain (increased ambient temperature)
- Increased heat production (exercise, infection, hyperthyroidism, drugs)
- Impaired heat dissipation (high humidity, heavy clothing, neonatal or elderly patients, drugs [phenothiazines, anticholinergics, antihistamines, butyrophenones, amphetamines, cocaine, alcohol, β-blockers])
- Diuretics, laxatives

TABLE 1 Factors Predisposing to Serious Heat Illness

Individual Factors
Lack of acclimatization
Low physical fitness
Excessive body weight
Dehydration
Advanced age
Young age
Health Conditions
Inflammation and fever
Viral infection
Cardiovascular disease
Diabetes mellitus
Gastroenteritis
Rash, sunburn, and previous burns to large areas of skin
Seizures
Thyroid storm
Neuroleptic malignant syndrome
Malignant hyperthermia
Sickle cell trait
Cystic fibrosis
Spinal cord injury
Drugs
Anticholinergic properties (atropine)
Antiepileptic (topiramate)
Antihistamines
Glutethimide (Doriden)
Phenothiazines
Tricyclic antidepressants
Amphetamines, cocaine, "ecstasy"
Ergogenic stimulants (e.g., ephedrine, ephedra)
Lithium
Diuretics
β-Blockers
Ethanol
Environmental Factors
High temperature
High humidity
Little air motion
Lack of shade
Heat wave
Physical exercise
Heavy clothing
Air pollution (nitrogen dioxide)

From Goldman L, Schafer AI: *Goldman's Cecil medicine,* ed 24, Philadelphia, 2012, Saunders.

- Fig. E1 describes an algorithm of the pathophysiology of heat stroke

DIAGNOSIS

DIFFERENTIAL DIAGNOSIS

- Infections (meningitis, encephalitis, sepsis)
- Head trauma
- Epilepsy
- Thyroid storm
- Acute cocaine intoxication
- Malignant hyperthermia
- Heat exhaustion can be differentiated from heat stroke by the following:
    1. Essentially intact mental function and lack of significant fever in heat exhaustion
    2. Mild or absent increases in creatine phosphokinase (CPK), aspartate aminotransferase (AST), lactate dehydrogenase (LDH), and alanine aminotransferase (ALT) in heat exhaustion

WORKUP

- Heat stroke: Comprehensive history, physical examination, and laboratory evaluation.
- Heat exhaustion: In most cases, laboratory tests are not necessary for diagnosis.

LABORATORY TESTS

Laboratory abnormalities may include the following:

- Elevated blood urea nitrogen (BUN), creatinine, hematocrit
- Hyponatremia or hypernatremia, hyperkalemia or hypokalemia
- Elevated LDH, AST, ALT, CPK, bilirubin
- Lactic acidosis, respiratory alkalosis (from hyperventilation)
- Myoglobinuria, hypofibrinogenemia, fibrinolysis, hypocalcemia

TREATMENT

- Treatment of heat exhaustion consists primarily of placing the patient in a cool, shaded area and providing rapid hydration and salt replacement.
    1. Fluid intake should be at least 2 L q4h in patients without history of CHF.
    2. Salt replacement can be accomplished by using one-quarter teaspoon of salt or two 10-grain salt tablets dissolved in 1 L of water.
    3. If IV fluid replacement is necessary, young athletes can be given normal saline IV (3-4 L over 6-8 hr); in elderly patients, consider using D5½NS IV with the rate titrated to cardiovascular status.
- Patients with heat stroke should undergo rapid cooling.
    1. Remove the patient's clothes and place the patient in a cool and well-ventilated room.
    2. If patient is unconscious, position on his or her side and clear the airway. Protect airway and augment oxygenation (e.g.,

TABLE 2 Comparison of Classic and Exertional Heat Stroke

Patient Characteristics	Classic	Exertional
Age	Young children or elderly	15-55 yr
Health	Chronic illness	Usually healthy
Fever	Unusual	Common
Prevailing weather	Frequent in heat waves	Variable
Activity	Sedentary	Strenuous exercise
Drug use	Diuretics, antidepressants, anticholinergics, phenothiazines	Ergogenic stimulants or cocaine
Sweating	Often absent	Common
Acid-base disturbances	Respiratory alkalosis	Lactic acidosis
Acute renal failure	Uncommon	Common (≈15%)
Rhabdomyolysis	Uncommon	Common (≈25%)
CK	Mildly elevated	Markedly elevated (500-1000 U/L)
ALT, AST	Mildly elevated	Markedly elevated
Hyperkalemia	Uncommon	Common
Hypocalcemia	Uncommon	Common
DIC	Mild	Marked
Hypoglycemia	Uncommon	Common

ALT, Alanine aminotransferase; *AST,* aspartate aminotransferase; *CK,* creatine kinase; *DIC,* disseminated intravascular coagulation.
From Goldman L, Schafer AI: *Goldman's Cecil medicine,* ed 24, Philadelphia, 2012, Saunders.

BOX 1 Organ Dysfunction Seen in Patients with Heat Stroke

Encephalopathy
Rhabdomyolysis
Acute renal failure
Acute respiratory distress syndrome
Myocardial injury
Hepatocellular injury
Intestinal ischemia and infarction
Pancreatic injury
Hemorrhagic complication (e.g., disseminated intravascular coagulation)

From Adams JG et al: *Emergency medicine, clinical essentials,* ed 2, Philadelphia, 2013, Elsevier.

nasal O_2 at 4 L/min to keep oxygen saturation >90%).
3. Monitor body temperature every 5 min. Measurement of the patient's core temperature with a rectal probe is recommended. The goal is to reduce the body temperature to 39° C (102.2° F) in 30 to 60 min. Advantages, disadvantages, and efficacy of various cooling methods are described in Table E3.
4. Spray the patient with a cool mist and use fans to enhance airflow over the body (rapid evaporation method).
5. Immersion of the patient in ice water, stomach lavage with iced saline solution, intravenous administration of cooled fluids, and inhalation of cold air are advisable only when the means for rapid evaporation are not available. Immersion in tepid water (15° C, 59° F) is preferred over ice water immersion to minimize risk of shivering.
6. Use of ice packs on axillae, neck, and groin is controversial because they increase peripheral vasoconstriction and may induce shivering.
7. Antipyretics are ineffective because the hypothalamic set point during heat stroke is normal despite the increased body temperature.
8. Intubate a comatose patient, insert a Foley catheter, and start nasal O_2. Continuous ECG monitoring is recommended.
9. Insert at least two large-bore IV lines and begin IV hydration with normal saline (NS) or Ringer lactate.
10. Draw initial laboratory studies: Electrolytes, complete blood count, blood urea nitrogen, creatinine, AST, ALT, CPK, LDH, glucose, PT (INR), PTT, platelet count, Ca^{2+}, lactic acid, and arterial blood gases.
11. Treat complications as follows:
    a. Hypotension: Vigorous hydration with normal saline or Ringer lactate
    b. Convulsions: Diazepam 5 to 10 mg IV (slowly)
    c. Shivering: Chlorpromazine 10 to 50 mg IV
    d. Acidosis: Use bicarbonate judiciously (only in severe acidosis)

- Observe for evidence of rhabdomyolysis and hepatic, renal, or cardiac failure and treat accordingly.

DISPOSITION

Most patients recover completely within 48 hr. Central nervous system injury is permanent in 20% of cases. Mortality rate can exceed 30% in patients with prolonged and severe hyperthermia. Delayed access to cooling is the leading cause of morbidity and mortality in persons with heat stroke.

RELATED CONTENT

Heat Exhaustion and Heat Stroke (Patient Information)
Acute Kidney Injury (Related Key Topic)
Rhabdomyolysis (Related Key Topic)

SUGGESTED READINGS

Available at ExpertConsult.com

AUTHOR: **Fred F. Ferri, MD**

BASIC INFORMATION

DEFINITION

Abnormal uterine bleeding (AUB) is a broad term for variations in normal menses. Normal duration of menstrual flow is 5 days with normal menstrual cycles lasting 21 to 35 days. Heavy menstrual bleeding with normal cycles, called menorrhagia, is a large volume of menstrual blood loss quantified as >80 ml per cycle. Bleeding may also be prolonged, intermenstrual, frequent, and irregular. This language replaces prior terms such as *metrorrhagia* (bleeding between cycles); *polymenorrhea* (menses <21days apart); and *oligomenorrhea* (menses >35 days apart).

The PALM-COEIN classification of abnormal uterine bleeding was adopted in 2011 to standardize terminology and reflect etiology: *P*olyp, *A*denomyosis, *L*eiomyoma, *M*alignancy and hyperplasia, *C*oagulopathy, *O*vulatory dysfunction, *E*ndometrial, *I*atrogenic, and *N*ot yet classified. The PALM-COEIN terminology is used to classify the etiology of the bleeding; for instance, AUB-P would refer to abnormal uterine bleeding due to polyps.

SYNONYMS

Abnormal uterine bleeding
Menometrorrhagia
Dysfunctional uterine bleeding
Irregular menstrual cycle

ICD-10CM CODES	
N92.0	Excessive and frequent menstruation with regular cycle
N92.1	Excessive and frequent menstruation with irregular cycle
N92.2	Excessive menstruation at puberty
N92.4	Excessive bleeding in the premenopausal period
N92.6	Irregular menstruation, unspecified

EPIDEMIOLOGY & DEMOGRAPHICS

INCIDENCE: AUB occurs in 10% to 15% of reproductive-age women, making up 30% of outpatient office visits and 70% of all gynecologic consults.

PREVALENCE: 9% to 14% of all women.

PREDOMINANT SEX & AGE: Females with peak in adolescence and perimenopausal periods ages 13 to 50.

RISK FACTORS: Genetic predisposition, anticoagulation treatment, obesity, endocrinopathies, autoimmune disease, liver disease, renal disease.

GENETICS: Hereditary coagulopathy (most commonly von Willebrand disease or platelet dysfunction disorders), seen in 20% of women with heavy menstrual bleeding, can present in adolescents with prior undiagnosed coagulopathy and can lead to hospitalization in up to 19% of affected women.

PHYSICAL FINDINGS & CLINICAL PRESENTATION

- History: Age, age at menarche or menopause, menstrual bleeding patterns, severity of bleeding, pain, underlying medical conditions, surgical history, medications, family history, hirsutism, acne, symptoms of thyroid dysfunction or other endocrinopathies.
  1. If heavy bleeding since menarche, screen for signs and symptoms of hemostatic disorder, including postpartum hemorrhage, surgery-related bleeding, bleeding from dental work, easy bruising, epistaxis, and frequent gum bleeding.
- Physical exam: Weight, hirsutism, acne, thyroid nodules, signs of insulin resistance (acanthosis nigricans), signs of bleeding disorder (petechiae, ecchymoses, pallor, swollen joints), pelvic examination including external, speculum, and bimanual exam of uterus.

ETIOLOGY

- PALM-COEIN
- Additional etiologies: Pregnancy/miscarriage; AV malformations; cervical/endometrial infections; foreign body, such as IUD malposition; use of hormonal pills; chronic medication use, such as anticoagulation medications; severe kidney or liver disease; endocrine disorder, such as thyroid disorder

DIAGNOSIS

DIFFERENTIAL DIAGNOSIS

In addition to the PALM-COEIN classification, it is also important to consider etiologies as above, including urinary and gastrointestinal tract sources.

Differential diagnosis of AUB can be further narrowed by age. AUB in 13- to 18-yr-olds is most commonly caused by anovulation due to immature or dysregulation of hypothalamic-pituitary-ovarian axis as a function of normal physiology. This can also be when coagulopathy disorders are first identified. AUB in 19- to 39-yr-olds is most commonly due to pregnancy or structural issues such as polyps or fibroids, and cancer is relatively rare in this age range. AUB in women 40 yr old and older commonly is due to ovulation changes with perimenopause, but cancer has increased incidence in this age range.

WORKUP

- History and physical examination
- Laboratory, pathology, and imaging studies

LABORATORY TESTS

- Pregnancy test
- Complete blood count (CBC)
- Thyroid-stimulating hormone (TSH)
- Wet prep and cervical cultures (*Chlamydia trachomatis* and *Neisseria gonorrhoeae*)
- Pap smear if indicated
- Targeted screening for bleeding disorders
- Endometrial sampling by endometrial biopsy or hysteroscopic sampling for women >45 yr or <45 yr with indication such as history of unopposed estrogen (PCOS, obesity), failed medical management, or persistent abnormal bleeding
- Iron studies if anemia is suspected

IMAGING STUDIES

- Pelvic ultrasound, transabdominal and transvaginal. Transvaginal ultrasound provides better assessment than transabdominal and is preferred.
- Sonohysterography or hysteroscopy if ultrasound is not adequate or further evaluation of the cavity is required, especially to assess for intracavitary lesions; superior to ultrasonography in detection of intracavitary lesions.
- MRI if needed for surgical planning or further evaluation of structural abnormality.

TREATMENT

ACUTE GENERAL Rx

Acute severe bleeding may be managed medically with oral progestins, combined oral contraceptive pills, IV estrogen, tranexamic acid, and/or blood transfusion as indicated. Surgical management includes dilation and curettage, endometrial ablation (Fig. 1), uterine artery embolization, or hysterectomy (Table 1).

CHRONIC Rx

- Combined hormonal contraceptives (pill, transdermal patch, vaginal ring) in a cyclic or continuous regimen
- Progesterone intrauterine device
- Oral or injected progesterone
- Gonadotropin-releasing hormone analog
- Nonsteroidal antiinflammatory drugs
- Tranexamic acid, aminocaproic acid
- Danazol (significant side-effect profile requires justification for use; this is rare)
- Selective progesterone receptor modulators (investigational for bleeding related to leiomyomas)
- Replacement of or treatment for any abnormal bleeding factors (i.e., DDAVP)

Recently approved, elagolix (GnRH antagonist with combined estrogen and progestin) was approved in May 2020 for heavy premenstrual bleeding associated with uterine fibroids. Currently it is not recommended for use >24 mo due to concern for bone density loss.

Surgical Management
- Dilation and curettage
- Hysteroscopic resection of uterine pathology including endometrial polyps and submucosal leiomyoma
- Myomectomy
- Endometrial ablation
- Uterine artery embolization
- Hysterectomy

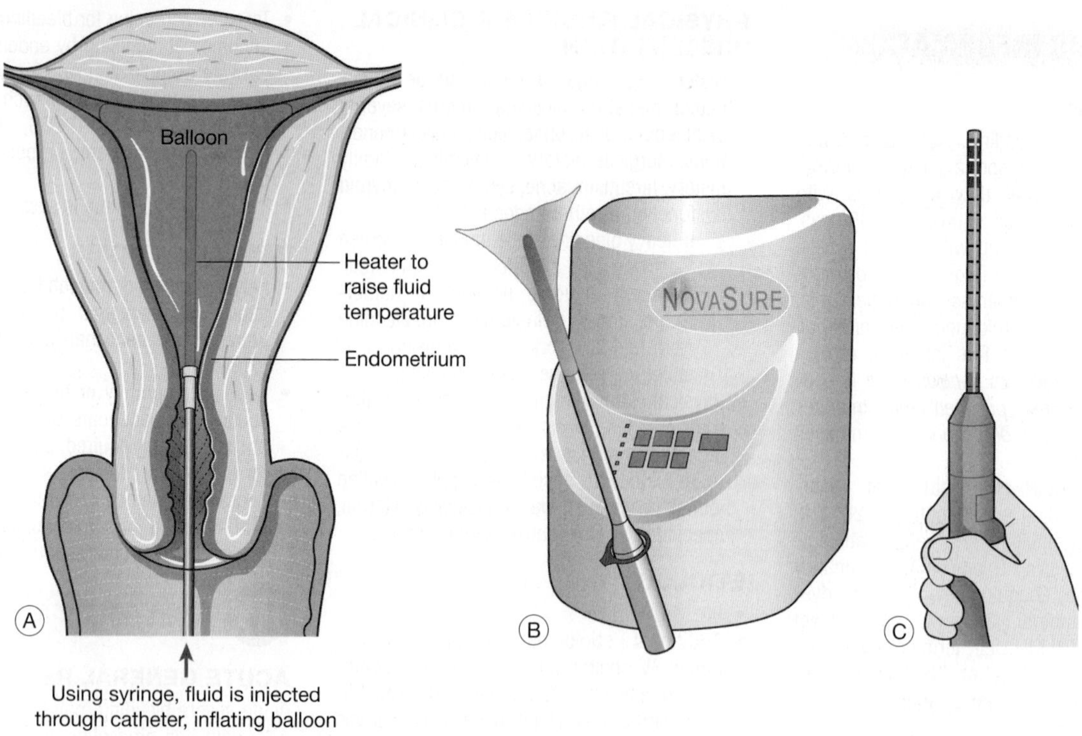

FIG. 1 Conservative surgical treatments for menorrhagia. A, A thermal balloon; B, impedance-controlled ablation; C, microwave endometrial ablation. (From Magowan BA: *Clinical obstetrics and gynecology,* ed 4, Philadelphia, 2019, Elsevier.)

TABLE 1 Pros and Cons of Different Hysterectomy Methods

	Pros	Cons
Total abdominal hysterectomy (TAH)	Cervix is removed, therefore no further need for smears and no further risk of cervical malignancy (thus particularly suitable for those with a history of abnormal cytology) Good access to ovaries	Increased surgical morbidity
Subtotal abdominal hysterectomy	Fewer complications than TAH (↓bleeding, ↓infection, ↓bladder injury, ↓ureteric damage) Good access to ovaries	Risk of cervical cancer remains as before
Vaginal hysterectomy	May be lower incidence of bladder and bowel injury in straightforward cases (compared with abdominal hysterectomy) No painful abdominal wound	Limited ovarian access Contraindicated with: • Large uterus • Restricted uterine mobility • Limited vaginal space • Adnexal pathology • Cervix flush with vagina

From Magowan BA: *Clinical obstetrics and gynecology,* ed 4, Philadelphia, 2019, Elsevier.

REFERRAL

- If unresponsive to initial hormonal management, referral to gynecologist is warranted.
- If concern for a structural etiology or malignancy, referral to a gynecologist for surgical management is indicated.
- If endometrial sampling reveals endometrial hyperplasia or malignancy, referral to a gynecologist or gynecologic oncologist is indicated. Resampling is necessary with progestin therapy for hyperplasia. If endometrial hyperplasia associated with complex glands or atypia, consultation with gynecologic oncologist is warranted due to high degree of progression to malignancy.

SUGGESTED READINGS

Available at ExpertConsult.com

RELATED CONTENT

Heavy Menstrual Bleeding (Menorrhagia) (Patient Information)
Abnormal Uterine Bleeding (Related Key Topic)

AUTHORS: **Leah Saylor, DO,** and **Nima R. Patel, MD, MS**

BASIC INFORMATION

DEFINITION

Infection of the human gastric mucosa with the organism *Helicobacter pylori,* a spiral-shaped gram-negative organism with unique features that allow it to survive in the hostile gastric environment.

SYNONYM

Previously known as *Campylobacter pylori*

ICD-10CM CODE

B96.81 *Helicobacter pylori [H. pylori]* as the cause of diseases classified elsewhere

EPIDEMIOLOGY & DEMOGRAPHICS

H. pylori is the most common chronic bacterial infection in human beings, probably affecting 50% of the Earth's population in all age groups as well as 30% to 40% of the U.S. population. In developing nations, infection is acquired at an earlier age and occurs more frequently.

CLINICAL PRESENTATION

- *H. pylori* causes histologic gastritis in all affected individuals. The majority of cases are asymptomatic and unlikely to proceed to serious consequences.
- *H. pylori* is a causative agent in peptic ulcer disease (PUD), gastric adenocarcinoma, and gastric mucosa-associated lymphoid tissue lymphoma, as well as a risk factor for iron-deficiency anemia and likely chronic idiopathic thrombocytopenic purpura. It may present with the signs and symptoms of these disorders, including abdominal pain, bloating, anorexia, and early satiety. Fig. 1 describes association of *H. pylori* infection and disease states.
- "Alarm symptoms" that should prompt more immediate and aggressive workup include weight loss, dysphagia, protracted nausea or vomiting, anemia, melena, and palpable abdominal mass, particularly in older individuals.

ETIOLOGY

- Route of acquisition is unknown but is presumed to be person to person by fecal-oral or possibly oral-oral transmission.
- The majority of cases are acquired in childhood. Socioeconomic status and living conditions in childhood affect risk of acquisition of infection. These factors include housing density, number of siblings, overcrowding, sharing a bed, and lack of running water.
- Iatrogenic transmission has been documented.
- *H. pylori* does not invade gastroduodenal tissue, but disrupts the mucous layer, causing the underlying mucosa to be more vulnerable to acid peptic damage.
- It is unclear what differentiates the subset of patients with *H. pylori* who go on to develop ulcers or cancer.

DIAGNOSIS

DIFFERENTIAL DIAGNOSIS

- Infection with *H. pylori* should be considered in the face of PUD, gastric cancer, gastritis, and gastric mucosa-associated lymphoid tissue (MALT) lymphoma.
- *H. pylori* should be considered in the differential diagnosis of upper gastrointestinal (GI) tract disease, along with nonulcer dyspepsia, reflux esophagitis, biliary tract disease, gastroparesis, pancreatitis, ischemic bowel, and unexplained iron deficiency anemia.

WORKUP

- Workup is indicated in patients with active PUD, a past history of documented peptic ulcer, or gastric MALT lymphoma, as well as those with immune thrombocytopenic purpura (ITP), and otherwise unexplained iron deficiency. The role of routine screening in high-risk populations is not clear. However, numerous studies suggest that *H. pylori* eradication is protective against progression of premalignant gastric lesions. Consider testing those starting long-term NSAID, low-dose aspirin, or proton pump inhibitor (PPI) therapy. Routine identification and treatment of *H. pylori* in cases of nonulcer dyspepsia, gastroesophageal reflux disease (GERD), and in asymptomatic individuals in populations at high risk for gastric cancer is considered controversial. There is insufficient evidence to advocate screening in asymptomatic first-degree relatives of gastric cancer patients. A test-and-treat strategy may be used in patients younger than 55 with uncomplicated dyspepsia who have no alarm symptoms.
- Results of testing must be interpreted in relation to the individual patient's likelihood of *H. pylori* infection based on demographic risk factors. In the U.S. population, increased probability of infection exists in African Americans, Hispanics/Latinos, immigrants from developing nations, patients with poor socioeconomic status, Native Americans from Alaska, and persons >50 yr.
- Routine screening for *H. pylori* is not indicated in asymptomatic patients who are at low risk of infection.
- Infected patients with functional dyspepsia often benefit from treatment and should be evaluated for *H. pylori.*

LABORATORY TESTS

- Testing may be invasive or noninvasive depending on the need for endoscopy for other indications. There is no indication for endoscopy solely to diagnose *H. pylori.*
- Tests for *H. pylori* are differentiated as active or passive. Active tests provide direct evidence that *H. pylori* infection is currently present and include urea breath testing and stool antigen testing. Passive testing, which includes all serologic testing for *H. pylori,* detects the presence of antibodies to the organism. It is limited by its inability to distinguish between active current infection and prior infection that has resolved.
- Tests that use urease as a marker (urea breath and stool antigen tests and biopsy for urease activity) may result in false-negative results in patients taking antibiotics, bismuth, or antisecretory therapy, as well as those with active ulcer bleeding. Patients should be off antibiotics for 4 wk and off protein pump inhibitors for 2 wk before urea breath or stool antigen testing.

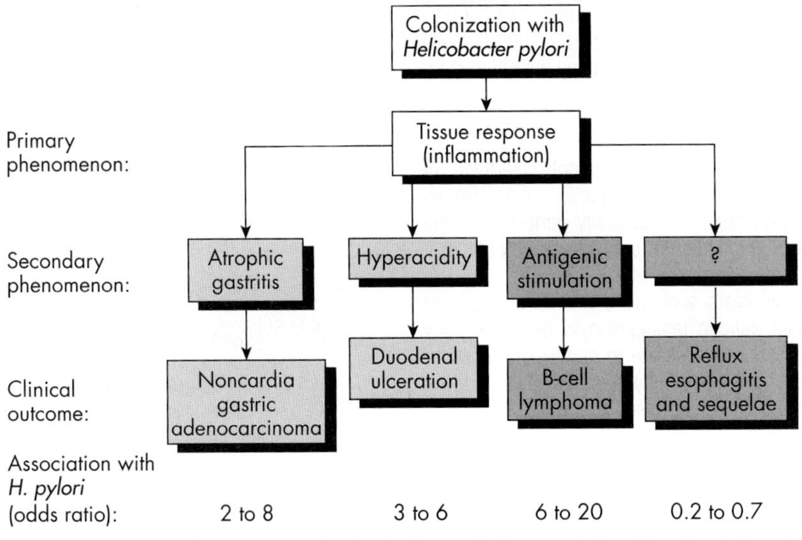

FIG. 1 Association of *Helicobacter pylori* colonization and disease states. After *H. pylori* acquisition, virtually all persons develop persistent colonization that lasts for life. Colonization induces tissue responses termed *chronic gastritis.* This process affects gastric physiology, including glandular structure, acid secretion, and antigen processing, which in turn affect disease risk. Colonization with *H. pylori* increases the risk for certain diseases (duodenal ulcer, gastric ulcer, noncardiac gastric adenocarcinoma, and B-cell lymphomas) but appears to decrease the risk for gastroesophageal reflux disease and its complications, including Barrett esophagus, and adenocarcinoma of the esophagus or gastric cardia. (From Mandell GL et al: *Principles and practice of infectious diseases,* ed 7, Philadelphia, 2010, Churchill Livingstone.)

- When diagnostic endoscopy is indicated (for suspicion or follow-up of PUD or gastric MALT), antral biopsy should be tested for urease activity. If urease testing is likely to show a false-negative result because of recent proton pump inhibitor (PPI), bismuth, or antibiotic use or active ulcer bleeding, the sample should undergo histologic examination.
- In cases in which biopsy is not indicated, urea breath testing or stool antigen testing is indicated to evaluate for active infection. Urea breath testing is slightly more expensive than stool antigen testing, but both costs are in the modest range. Choice can be made based on patient preference and availability. The sensitivities and specificities of these two tests are similar (>90%), but sensitivity may be reduced in the face of active upper GI bleed or recent PPI use.
- Serologic testing should be avoided, although it may be useful in low-risk patients in areas with low prevalence to confirm lack of infection. In this situation, positive results should be confirmed with an active testing method.

Rx TREATMENT

ACUTE GENERAL Rx

- Test only patients whom you intend to treat if positive (see "Workup"). At this time, the value of eradicating *H. pylori* infection has been clearly demonstrated in patients with PUD or gastric MALT lymphoma.
- The optimal antibiotic regimen remains undefined. In addition to efficacy, side effects, cost, and ease of administration must be considered.
- Due to increasing resistance to clarithromycin, decisions regarding appropriate regimens should take into account local rates of clarithromycin resistance, as well as any prior macrolide exposure for the patient. Clarithromycin resistance can be assumed to be >15% in the U.S., unless local resistance information is available.
- The following regimens may be considered for first-line therapy:
  1. Quadruple therapy: PPI (esomeprazole 20 mg, lansoprazole 30 mg, pantoprazole 40 mg, omeprazole 40 mg, or rabeprazole 20 mg, all given bid), with twice-daily clarithromycin (500 mg), amoxicillin (1 g bid), and metronidazole 500 mg bid for 10 to 14 days.
  2. Bismuth quadruple therapy: PPI twice daily (see earlier) combined with bismuth subsalicylate (Pepto-Bismol and others) 262 or 525 mg four times daily, as well as tetracycline (500 mg qid) and metronidazole (250 mg qid or 500 mg tid-qid) for 10 to 14 days. This is now recommended as first-line therapy in areas of high clarithromycin resistance and in patients with penicillin allergy.
- Current guidelines recommend extended treatment of 10 to 14 days. Use of combination capsules may improve compliance but is likely to be more expensive.
- Recent guidelines suggest multiple other regimens that can be considered based on local resistance patterns and patient's allergy profile.
- Prior exposure to a macrolide or metronidazole, for any reason, is associated with increased resistance. A preferable regimen would include medications to which the patient has not been previously exposed.
- Diarrhea and abdominal cramping are commonly observed with many of the regimens. (Probiotics may diminish this effect.) Other side effects may include a metallic taste with metronidazole or clarithromycin, neuropathy, seizures, and disulfiram-like reaction with metronidazole, diarrhea with amoxicillin, photosensitivity with tetracycline, and *Clostridium difficile* infection with any antibiotic exposure. Bismuth may cause black stool and constipation. Tetracycline is contraindicated in pregnant patients.
- 20% of patients may not respond to initial therapy. It is important to reinforce compliance. Second-line therapy should avoid antibiotics used in initial treatment and should include either bismuth-containing quadruple therapy or levofloxacin-containing triple therapy (regardless of local clarithromycin resistance patterns). When possible, management of those who do not respond to two courses of therapy should be guided by antimicrobial sensitivity testing (endoscopy with biopsy for cultures and sensitivity).

CHRONIC Rx

- It is essential to document clearance of infection after the completion of treatment. Repeat testing is generally performed 1 mo after completion of antibiotics and at least 2 wk after cessation of PPI therapy.
- Active tests such as urea breath test and stool antigen testing should be used. They are equally accurate in confirming eradication, and either may be used depending on availability and patient preference.
- Serology does not reliably revert to undetectable levels after treatment and should not be used to determine eradication.

DISPOSITION

Consider further evaluation in patients with recurrent symptoms after appropriate treatment.

REFERRAL

- Patients with gastric MALT lymphoma should be followed by a gastroenterologist and oncologist with expertise in the care of lymphoid neoplasms.
- Patients with dyspepsia who have tested positive for *H. pylori* and failed two courses of treatment should be referred for endoscopy and biopsy for culture and sensitivity.

PEARLS & CONSIDERATIONS

- It remains unclear whether *H. pylori* eradication reduces the risk of progression to gastric cancer.
- Outcomes in PUD and gastric MALT lymphoma are improved with treatment of associated *H. pylori* infection.
- Tests that provide direct evidence of active *H. pylori* infection (urea breath and stool antigen testing) are preferred. These may result in false-negative results in patients taking antibiotics, bismuth, or antisecretory agents, which should be stopped at an appropriate time interval before testing.
- The FDA recently approved a fixed-dose combination of omeprazole, amoxicillin, rifabutin (Talicia) for treatment of *H. pylori* infection in adults. Cost and formulary are significant limiting factors.
- Be aware of high-risk populations in low-prevalence settings, including immigrants from Mexico, South America, Southeast Asia, and Eastern Europe.

RELATED CONTENT

Helicobacter pylori Infection (Patient Information)
Gastritis (Related Key Topic)
Peptic Ulcer Disease (Related Key Topic)

SUGGESTED READINGS

Available at ExpertConsult.com

AUTHOR: **Margaret Tryforos, MD**

BASIC INFORMATION

DEFINITION

Hemochromatosis is an autosomal-recessive disorder that disrupts the body's regulation of iron and is characterized by increased accumulation of iron in various organs (adrenals, liver, pancreas, heart, testes, kidneys, pituitary) and eventual dysfunction of these organs if not treated appropriately.

SYNONYMS

Bronze diabetes
Hereditary hemochromatosis (HH)

ICD-10CM CODES	
E83.110	Hereditary hemochromatosis
E83.111	Hemochromatosis due to repeated red blood cell transfusions
E83.118	Other hemochromatosis
E83.119	Hemochromatosis, unspecified

EPIDEMIOLOGY & DEMOGRAPHICS

INCIDENCE: In whites, approximately 1 in 385 persons

PREDOMINANT SEX & AGE: Generally diagnosed in males in their fifth decade. Diagnosis in females is generally not made until 10 to 20 yr after menopause.

GENETICS: Most common genetic disorder in North European ancestry. Homozygosity for the *C282Y* mutation is now found in approximately 5 of every 1000 persons of European descent.

PHYSICAL FINDINGS & CLINICAL PRESENTATION

- In earlier stages patients completely asymptomatic and diagnosed due to abnormal laboratory tests
- Hepatic dysfunction leading to hepatomegaly, fibrosis, and eventually cirrhosis
- Noninflammatory arthropathy (Fig. E1)
- Gonadal insufficiency leading to loss of libido and testicular atrophy
- Diabetes mellitus: Risk greater in patients with family history
- Iron-induced cardiac disease resulting in cardiomyopathy, heart failure, and arrhythmias
- Skin pigmentation

ETIOLOGY

- The majority of the patients diagnosed with hemochromatosis have mutation in the *HFE* gene and are either homozygous for the *C282Y* mutation *(C282Y/C282Y)* or compound heterozygote for the *C282Y* mutation and either the mutation *H63D (C282Y/H63D)* or less commonly the *S65C (C282Y/S65C)*.
- The remainder of the patients are classified as non–*HFE*-associated hemochromatosis.

DIAGNOSIS

DIFFERENTIAL DIAGNOSIS

- Hereditary anemias with defect of erythropoiesis
- Cirrhosis, chronic liver disease, porphyria cutanea tarda
- Repeated blood transfusions
- Table 1 summarizes hereditary causes of iron overload

WORKUP

Medical history, physical examination, and laboratory evaluation should be focused on affected organ systems (see "Physical Findings & Clinical Presentation"). Fig. E2 outlines evaluation for possible hereditary hemochromatosis in an individual with negative family history. Liver biopsy is the gold standard for diagnosis; it reveals iron deposition in hepatocytes, bile ducts, and supporting tissues.

LABORATORY TESTS

- Transferrin saturation is the best screening test. Values >45% are an indication for further testing.
- Elevated serum ferritin is good evidence of iron overload, but other causes like chronic inflammatory conditions, malignancy, and so forth need to be ruled out as ferritin is also an acute phase reactant.
- Genotypical screening for *C282Y* and *H63D* mutation in *HFE* gene should be done in patients with high transferrin saturation, elevated ferritin, or both.
- Liver biopsy (Fig. E3) is the gold standard but is not needed in somebody who has a persistently elevated transferrin saturation, elevated ferritin, or both.
- Hepatic iron index can help differentiate between various causes of iron overload.
- Elevated aspartate aminotransferase, alanine aminotransferase, and alkaline phosphatase are seen.
- Hyperglycemia is found.
- Endocrine abnormalities (decreased testosterone, luteinizing hormone, follicle-stimulating hormone) are noted.
- Table 2 describes laboratory findings in patients with hereditary hemochromatosis.

IMAGING STUDIES

Routine radiologic imaging is not needed. MRI (Fig. E4) may show low signal intensity in the liver and can be used to estimate hepatic iron concentration.

Rx TREATMENT

The goal of therapy is the removal of excess iron and maintaining it at a normal or near-normal level. Phlebotomy is first line treatment. The goal is to reduce serum ferritin to 50 to 100 mg/ml. Box E1 summarizes the treatment of *HFE*-related hereditary hemochromatosis.

NONPHARMACOLOGIC THERAPY

Phlebotomy is the treatment of choice.

ACUTE GENERAL Rx

- The timing and frequency of phlebotomy needs to be individualized for each patient.
- For patients with heavy iron overload, twice-weekly phlebotomies should be started. In most patients, weekly phlebotomy is adequate.
- The effectiveness of treatment is monitored by periodic ferritin measurement. The goal is to bring ferritin level below 50 ng/ml.
- Patients with iron overload due to transfusion-dependent anemias may not tolerate phlebotomy. For these patients, iron chelation may be needed.
- The chelating agent deferoxamine has to be given daily as a 9- to 12-hr IV or SC infusion, and compliance is difficult.
- The oral chelating agent deferasirox (Exjade) is effective, but should not be used in patients with high-risk myelodysplastic syndrome because it can cause renal impairment, hepatic impairment, or gastrointestinal hemorrhage, which can be fatal.

CHRONIC Rx

After the ferritin has been brought to less than 50 ng/ml, phlebotomy is needed on an as-needed basis to keep the ferritin at that level.

DISPOSITION

- Serum ferritin measurement is the most useful prognostic indicator of disease severity.
- Prognosis is good if phlebotomy is started early (before onset of cirrhosis or diabetes mellitus); women can have the full phenotypic expression of the disease, including cirrhosis, and should also be aggressively treated.

REFERRAL

For liver biopsy if diagnosis is uncertain

PEARLS & CONSIDERATIONS

COMMENTS

- Persons who are homozygous for the *HFE* gene mutation *C282Y* comprise 85% to 90% of phenotypically affected individuals. Patients who are heterozygous for both *C282Y* and *H63D* generally do not have clinically evident disease unless coexisting factors (e.g., excessive alcohol intake) are present.
- Patients with hemochromatosis and serum ferritin levels <1000 ng/ml are unlikely to have cirrhosis. Liver biopsy to screen for cirrhosis may be unnecessary in such patients.
- Cirrhotic patients must be periodically monitored (ultrasound or CT scan) because of their increased risk of hepatocellular carcinoma.
- *HFE* gene testing for *C282Y* mutation is a cost-effective method of screening relatives of patients with hereditary hemochromatosis. The American College of Gastroenterology recommends genotyping persons who have abnormal iron screening tests and first-degree relatives of those identified with *C282Y* homozygosity.
- Established cirrhosis, hypogonadism, destructive arthritis, and insulin-dependent diabetes mellitus secondary to hemochromatosis cannot be reversed with repeated phlebotomy, but their progress can be slowed.

TABLE 1 Hereditary Iron Overload Disorders

Disorder	Gene, Chromosome Location	Inheritance	Plasma Transferrin Saturation	Plasma Ferritin	Iron Deposition Sites	Clinical Manifestations
Hereditary hemochromatosis, *HFE*-associated (type 1; OMIM235200)	*HFE*, 6p21	Autosomal recessive	Early increase; >45%	Later increase after third decade of life	Parenchymal iron overload affecting hepatocytes, heart, pancreas, other organs	Liver and heart disease, diabetes, gonadal failure, arthritis, skin pigmentation
Hereditary hemochromatosis, *TFR2*-associated (type 3; OMIM604250)	*TFR2*, 7q22	Autosomal recessive	Early increase; >45%	Later increase after third decade of life	Parenchymal iron overload affecting hepatocytes, heart, pancreas, other organs	Liver and heart disease, diabetes, gonadal failure, arthritis, skin pigmentation
Juvenile hemochromatosis, hemojuvelin-associated (type 2A; OMIM 602390)	*HJV*, 1q21	Autosomal recessive	Early increase; >45%	Increased by second decade of life	Parenchymal iron overload affecting hepatocytes, heart, pancreas, other organs	As for hereditary hemochromatosis, but liver involvement less prominent
Juvenile hemochromatosis, hepcidin-associated (type 2B; OMIM613313)	*HAMP*, 19q13	Autosomal recessive	Early increase; >45%	Increased by second decade of life	Parenchymal iron overload affecting hepatocytes, heart, pancreas, other organs	As for hereditary hemochromatosis, but liver involvement less prominent
Hemochromatosis, *DMT1*-associated (OMIM 206100)	*SCL11A2*, 12q13	Autosomal recessive	Early increase; >45%	Normal to moderately elevated	Hepatic iron overload, predominantly in hepatocytes	Severe microcytic anemia, liver dysfunction
Atransferrinemia (OMIM 209300)	*TF*, 3q22	Autosomal recessive	No plasma transferrin	Increased	Parenchymal iron overload affecting hepatocytes, heart, pancreas; no iron stores in bone marrow or spleen	Transfusion-dependent iron-deficiency anemia, growth retardation, poor survival
Aceruloplasminemia (OMIM 604290)	*CP*, 3q24-q25	Autosomal recessive	Decreased	Increased	Marked iron accumulation in basal ganglia, liver, pancreas	Diabetes, progressive neurologic disease, retinal degeneration
Hemochromatosis, ferroportin-associated, with impaired iron export (type 4A; OMIM606069)	*SLC40A1*, 2q32	Autosomal dominant	Remains normal or low	Early increase	Predominantly macrophage iron deposition	None
Hemochromatosis, ferroportin-associated, with hepcidin resistance (type 4B; OMIM606069)	*SLC40A1*, 2q32	Autosomal dominant	Early increase; >45%	Early increase	Parenchymal iron overload affecting hepatocytes, heart, pancreas, other organs	Similar to *HFE*-associated hemochromatosis

From Hoffman R et al: *Hematology: basic principles and practice*, ed 7, Philadelphia, 2018, Elsevier.

TABLE 2 Laboratory Findings in Patients with Hereditary Hemochromatosis

Measurements	Normal Subjects	PATIENTS WITH HEREDITARY HEMOCHROMATOSIS: Asymptomatic	Symptomatic
Blood (Fasting)			
Serum iron level (μg/dl)	60-180	150-280	180-300
Serum transferrin level (mg/dl)	220-410	200-280	200-300
Transferrin saturation (%)	20-45	45-100	80-100
Serum ferritin level (ng/ml)			
Men	20-200	150-1000	500-6000
Women	15-150	120-1000	500-6000
Genetic (*HFE* Mutation Analysis)			
C282Y/C282Y	wt/wt‡	*C282Y/C282Y*	*C282Y/C282Y*
*C282Y/H63D**	wt/wt	*C282Y/H63D*	*C282Y/H63D*
Liver			
Hepatic iron concentration			
μg/g dry weight	300-1500	2000-10,000	8000-30,000
μmol/g dry weight	5-27	36-179	140-550
Hepatic iron index†	<1	1 to >1.9	>1.9
Liver histology			
Perls Prussian blue stain	0, 1+	2+ to 4+	3+, 4+

*Compound heterozygote.
†Calculated by dividing the hepatic iron concentration (in μmol/g dry weight) by the age of the patient (in yr). With the increased use of genetic testing in patients with iron overload, the specificity of the hepatic iron index has diminished.
‡wt/wt: Wild type (normal).
From Goldman L, Schafer AI: *Goldman's Cecil medicine*, ed 24, Philadelphia, 2012, Saunders.

- In patients who are heterozygous for *C282Y* or *H63D* mutation, clinically meaningful iron overload does not develop.
- Screening for hepatocellular carcinoma is reserved for those with hereditary hemochromatosis and cirrhosis.

SUGGESTED READINGS

Available at ExpertConsult.com

RELATED CONTENT

Hemochromatosis (Patient Information)

AUTHOR: **Fred F. Ferri, MD**

BASIC INFORMATION

DEFINITION

Hemoptysis is coughing of blood from the lower respiratory tract, ranging from blood-streaked sputum to gross blood. Severity grading is based on quantity (>500 ml/24 hr or bleeding rate is >100 ml/hr is considered massive) and clinical significance.

ICD-10CM CODE

R04.2 Hemoptysis

EPIDEMIOLOGY & DEMOGRAPHICS

INCIDENCE: Unknown, varies based on underlying pathology

RISK FACTORS: Endobronchial cancers are a common cause of hemoptysis. Systemic processes (rheumatologic, renal, hematologic) may contribute to alveolar hemorrhage or vasculitis. Tuberculosis remains the most common infectious etiology for hemoptysis in developing countries where it is widely prevalent. Anticoagulation and bleeding dyscrasias can worsen bleeding.

PHYSICAL FINDINGS & CLINICAL PRESENTATION

- Presentation of hemoptysis can range (Table 1) from minimal blood-tinged sputum to >500 ml of gross blood in 24 hr. Other symptoms depend on the underlying etiology and can include cough, sputum production, fever, shortness of breath, weight loss, night sweats, wheezing, and chest pain.
- There are no specific exam findings, but clues to the etiology may be present, for example, focal wheezing, rhonchi or rales on pulmonary exam, murmur of mitral stenosis on cardiac exam.

ETIOLOGY

Airway disease
- Primary lung cancer or endobronchial metastases
- Inflammatory (chronic bronchitis, bronchiectasis)
- Airway trauma
- Bronchovascular fistula
- Foreign body

Parenchymal disease
- Infections (necrotizing pneumonias, tuberculosis, abscess)
- Inflammatory (granulomatosis with polyangiitis, Goodpasture syndrome, lupus)
- Drugs (cocaine)
- Medications (antiplatelets, anticlotting agents, chemotherapeutics)
- Iatrogenic

Vascular
- Pulmonary embolism
- Cardiac disease (mitral stenosis after rheumatic heart disease, congenital heart disease)
- Arteriovenous malformation
- Iatrogenic

DIAGNOSIS

DIFFERENTIAL DIAGNOSIS

- Various potential causes of lower respiratory tract bleeding
  1. Airway disease (bronchitis, bronchiectasis, bronchovascular fistulas, lung neoplasm)
  2. Infection (necrotizing pneumonia, lung abscess, tuberculosis, fungal infection)
  3. Inflammatory diseases (granulomatosis with polyangiitis, Goodpasture syndrome, lupus)
  4. Cardiac disease (mitral stenosis after rheumatic heart disease, congenital heart diseases)
  5. Pulmonary embolism
  6. Drugs (cocaine use, antiplatelets, anticoagulants)
  7. Foreign body
  8. Arteriovenous malformation
  9. Iatrogenic
- Bleeding from upper respiratory tract
- Pseudohemoptysis: Hematemesis or epistaxis
- Coagulopathy

WORKUP

- Initial history should focus on determining the anatomic origin of the bleeding and on quantifying the volume of the hemoptysis in order to triage appropriately. Attention should be made to exclude causes of pseudohemoptysis and consideration of ENT or GI sources should be considered.
- It is important to ask about duration, frequency, and quantity of hemoptysis and smoking history.
- Complete history and physical exam may suggest a particular etiology. Depending on the results of the initial evaluation and the likely categories of hemoptysis, additional tests can be helpful (Table 2).
- Laboratory testing:
  1. Complete blood count
  2. Coagulation profile
  3. Serum chemistries, including creatinine, urinalysis
  4. If indicated, consider serologic workup (i.e., antinuclear antibody [ANA], antineutrophil cytoplasmic antibodies [ANCA], anti-glomerular basement membrane [anti-GBM])
  5. Arterial blood gas to assess oxygenation
  6. Sputum for bacterial Gram stain and culture, AFB smear and culture, and cytologic studies
  7. Skin test (PPD) or interferon-gamma release assays for tuberculosis

IMAGING STUDIES

- Chest x-ray: All patients with hemoptysis should have a chest x-ray but will likely need additional studies to localize site of bleeding.
- Chest CT: Chest CT scan with contrast combined with flexible bronchoscopy has the highest yield for localizing the site of bleeding.
- Pulmonary angiography with intravenous contrast may increase the sensitivity and specificity of localization for the site of bleeding.

TREATMENT

Varies based on underlying etiology and nonmassive versus massive hemoptysis

TABLE 1 Features of Hemoptysis and Patient Presentation

Hemoptysis Feature	Clinical Presentation
Blood usually bright red	Often dyspneic
Portion of blood usually frothy Alkaline pH	Hypoxemia
Blood usually mixed with sputum	Preceding cough common
Alveolar macrophages may be present in sputum smear	Anemia and melena uncommon

From Parrillo JE, Dellinger RP: *Critical care medicine, principles of diagnosis and management in the adult,* ed 5, Philadelphia, 2019, Elsevier.

TABLE 2 Examples of Special Evaluations for Hemoptysis According to Category of Disease*

Tracheobronchial Disorders
Expectorated sputum for TB, parasites, fungi, and cytology
Bronchoscopy (if not done)
High-resolution chest CT scan
Localized Parenchymal Diseases
Expectorated sputum for TB, parasites, fungi, and cytology
Chest CT scan
Lung biopsy with special stains
Diffuse Parenchymal Diseases
Expectorated sputum for cytology
Blood for BUN, creatinine, ANA, RF, complement, cryoglobulins, ANCA, anti-GBM antibody
High-resolution chest CT scan
Lung or kidney biopsy with special stains
Cardiovascular Disorders
Echocardiogram
Arterial blood gas on 21% and 100% oxygen
Ventilation-perfusion scans
Chest CT with contrast
Aortogram
Hematologic Disorders
Coagulation studies
Bone marrow

ANA, Antinuclear antibody; *ANCA,* antineutrophil cytoplasmic antibody; *BUN,* blood urea nitrogen; *CT,* computed tomography; *GBM,* glomerular basement membrane; *RF,* rheumatoid factor; *TB,* tuberculosis.

*This table is not meant to be all inclusive.

From Goldman L, Shafer AI: *Goldman-Cecil medicine,* ed 26, Philadelphia, 2020, Elsevier.

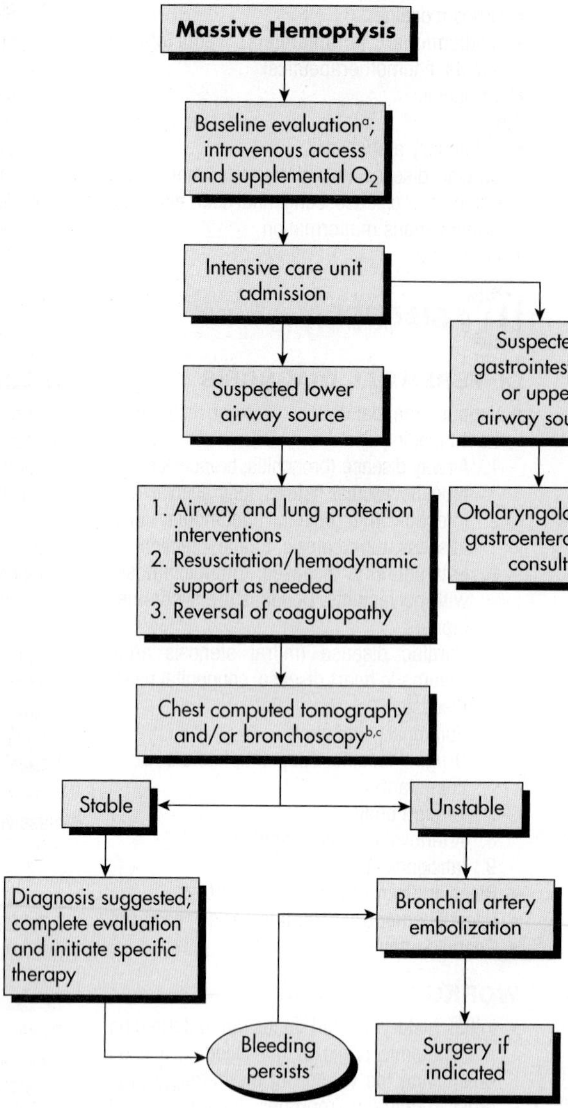

FIG. 1 Massive hemoptysis.
[a]History and physical examination, complete blood cell count, coagulation studies, type and cross-match, chest radiograph, arterial blood gas levels. [b]Local availability and patient stability should guide choice; computed tomography is preferred in initial evaluation in stable patients. [c]Local measures, including topical vasoconstrictors, bronchial blockers, laser photocoagulation, electrocautery, and hemostatic agents, can be used endobronchially. *O_2*, Oxygen. (From Parrillo JE, Dellinger RP: *Critical care medicine, principles of diagnosis and management in the adult*, ed 5, Philadelphia, 2019, Elsevier.)

NONPHARMACOLOGIC THERAPY

Massive hemoptysis:
- Arteriographic embolization of bronchial arteries and/or collateral vessels
- Surgical resection of affected lung

ACUTE GENERAL Rx

Massive hemoptysis (Fig. 1):
- Stabilize hemodynamic status and oxygenation
- Reverse any coagulopathy
- If site of bleeding is known, place patient with bleeding lung in dependent position to prevent blood from spilling into nonaffected lung, and consider selective intubation with large-bore, single-lumen endotracheal tube or double-lumen endotracheal tube.
- Bronchoscopy can be used to identify cause of hemoptysis (e.g., neoplasm), as well as to localize and potentially isolate a site/segment of bleeding.
- Bronchoscopic lavage with iced saline or topical application of epinephrine can be tried as a temporizing measure.
- Bronchoscopic balloon tamponade of bleeding site can be used as temporizing measure.
- Both cold and heat ablative therapies have been used effectively for local and immediate control of bleeding.
- Early consultation with critical care medicine, interventional radiology, interventional pulmonology, and/or thoracic surgery for definitive intervention is recommended.

Nonmassive hemoptysis:
- For nonmassive hemoptysis, identify and treat underlying condition. Refer to pulmonologist or hematologist if indicated.

CHRONIC Rx

For patients requiring anticoagulation or antiplatelet therapy for another disorder, consider risks/benefits of continued anticoagulation or antiplatelet therapy.

DISPOSITION

Generally, patients have a good prognosis after an episode of hemoptysis, but those with massive bleeding and/or malignancy tend to have a poorer prognosis.

RELATED CONTENT

Evaluation of hemoptysis (Algorithm, Section III)

SUGGESTED READING

Available at ExpertConsult.com

AUTHORS: **Hasnain Bawaadam, MD, MPH,** and **Yaron B. Gesthalter, MD**

BASIC INFORMATION

DEFINITION

There are two forms of heparin-induced thrombocytopenia (HIT). Type I HIT is a mild, transient decrease in platelet count that occurs during the first 2 days of heparin exposure due to non–immune-mediated platelet aggregation. This is a benign reaction, and the platelet count will return to normal while heparin is continued. This chapter will address Type II HIT, an antibody-mediated thrombocytopenia with risk of thrombosis.

SYNONYMS

Type II heparin-induced thrombocytopenia
Heparin-induced thrombocytopenia and thrombosis (HITT)
Heparin-associated immune thrombocytopenia

ICD-10CM CODE
D75.82 Heparin-induced thrombocytopenia (HIT)

EPIDEMIOLOGY & DEMOGRAPHICS

INCIDENCE: Occurs in 0.2% to 5% of patients exposed to heparin in various clinical settings. Initially, there was an overwhelming underdiagnosis of HIT; however, since the introduction of HIT antibody ELISA test, there is a propensity to overdiagnose HIT irrespective of the clinical scenario.

PREDOMINANT SEX & AGE: Females are at slightly higher risk than males. More common in adults, but may also occur in children.

RISK FACTORS: Heparin type (unfractionated heparin has up to 10 times greater risk than low–molecular-weight heparin), dose (therapeutic dose may have a greater risk than prophylactic dose, though no dose is considered too low to cause HIT), and duration (longer duration of exposure confers greater risk); type of patient (surgical patients, especially cardiac and orthopedic, are at higher risk than medical patients). Risk factors for HIT are summarized in Table 1.

PHYSICAL FINDINGS & CLINICAL PRESENTATION

Suspect in a patient with:

- Exposure to heparin in prior 3 mo, especially if initiated in the last 5 to 10 days.
- Platelet count decrease to 50% below pretreatment baseline; 5% of patients will not become thrombocytopenic despite this reduction.
- Venous or arterial thrombosis occurs in about 50% of patients without prompt treatment (e.g., DVT, PE, skin necrosis at heparin injection sites, limb gangrene, stroke or cavernous sinus thrombosis, myocardial infarction).
- Bleeding occurred in about 6% of HIT patients, half of which was GI bleed.
- Acute anaphylaxis during administration of heparin bolus.

ETIOLOGY

Occurs when IgG antibodies bind to complexes of heparin and platelet factor 4 (PF4), a prothrombotic cytokine released from platelets during their activation. The resulting immune complexes activate adjacent platelets, leading to further PF4 release, additional antibody production, and eventual platelet aggregation with premature removal from circulation (causing thrombocytopenia). This process also leads to increased thrombin generation, though the full mechanism of thrombosis in HIT is not completely understood.

DIAGNOSIS

DIFFERENTIAL DIAGNOSIS

Thrombocytopenia due to other causes including:

- Sepsis or infection
- Disseminated intravascular coagulation
- Immune thrombocytopenia
- Thrombocytopenic thrombotic purpura
- Hemolytic uremic syndrome
- Drug-induced thrombocytopenia (other than heparin)
- Antiphospholipid antibody syndrome
- Liver failure
- Splenic sequestration
- Intravascular devices

WORKUP

HIT is, first and foremost, a clinical diagnosis that is confirmed with laboratory testing. The 4T score translates clinical findings to pretest probability as outlined in Table 2. If the patient has a low pretest probability score then there is no need for further testing. Moderate or high pretest probability warrants laboratory tests for HIT (Table 3).

LABORATORY TESTS

These can be broadly divided into two categories: Immunoassays (high sensitivity) and functional assays (high specificity).

Immunoassay testing for HIT antibodies with an ELISA is very sensitive, but not specific. The majority of patients with HIT antibodies will not develop clinical HIT. Thus, HIT antibody testing is more effective for ruling out rather than confirming the diagnosis of HIT.

Result of the above immunoassay is reported as HIT antibody optical density (OD), which divides into the following categories: Weakly positive (0.4-1.0), moderately positive (1.0-2.0), and strongly positive (>2.0). A weakly positive OD is rarely associated with functional assay positivity (1%-5%), whereas an OD >2.0 almost always shows functional assay positivity (89%-100%). Of note, the HIT antibody IgG subtype is the pathologic antibody for HIT, therefore the use of IgG-specific ELISA kits increases the test specificity over the polyspecific (IgA/M/G) antibody.

Negative and strongly positive HIT antibody immunoassay results are usually sufficient enough to either exclude or confirm HIT diagnosis, respectively. As for weakly or moderately positive results, however, the functional serotonin release assay (14C-SRA) is often pursued. This test is the gold standard for HIT that measures heparin-dependent platelet activation. Donor platelets are radiolabeled with serotonin and then incubated with patient serum and heparin. If antibodies to the platelet factor 4-heparin complex are present in the patient's serum, the platelets react and release the radiolabeled serotonin, which is then measured. Result of this test ultimately confirms or excludes the diagnosis. Availability and turnaround time of this test is dependent on the institution, and this often limits the test's clinical utility. Heparin-induced platelet aggregation test, flow cytometry, or even combining multiple immunoassays with 4Ts score show promising data to obtain confirmatory data more readily, but their routine utilization is yet premature.

Overall, the diagnosis of HIT is confirmed by (1) a strongly positive ELISA or (2) a positive functional assay. It is excluded by (1) low pretest probability on 4Ts, (2) negative ELISA, or (3) a negative functional assay.

IMAGING STUDIES

DVT screening with bilateral low extremity ultrasound is recommended for all suspected HIT with further imaging (e.g., upper extremity ultrasound) considered for appropriate clinical setting.

TREATMENT

- For patients with a moderate or high pretest probability from 4Ts, discontinue all heparin exposure. Even if the patient does not have a clinically evident thrombosis, there is a significant risk of developing an incident clot within the subsequent 30 days. Thus, the patient must be started on an alternative anticoagulant.

TABLE 1 Risk Factors for Heparin-Induced Thrombocytopenia

Heparin Type	Unfractionated > Low-Molecular-Weight Heparin > Fondaparinux
Patient type	Postoperative (major > minor surgery) > medical > obstetric/pediatric
Dose[a]	Prophylactic dose > therapeutic dose > flushes
Duration	11-14 days[b] > 5-10 days > 4 days or fewer
Sex	Female > male

[a]Importance of heparin dose is uncertain because of compounding effect of patient type (e.g., postoperative patients tend to receive prophylactic-dose heparin whereas medical patients [e.g., with venous thromboembolism] are more likely to receive therapeutic-dose heparin); nevertheless, reported frequencies of heparin-induced thrombocytopenia (HIT) are relatively high in patients given postoperative prophylactic-dose heparin.
[b]Heparin exposure beyond 14 days does not usually increase the risk of HIT beyond that of an 11- to 14-day exposure.
From Hoffman R et al: *Hematology, basic principles and practice,* ed 7, Philadelphia, 2018, Elsevier.

TABLE 2 The 4Ts Score for Estimating the Pretest Probability of Heparin-Induced Thrombocytopenia

	POINTS (0, 1, or 2 for each of the four parameters; maximum points = 8)		
	2	**1**	**0**
Thrombocytopenia (acute)	>50% platelet count fall to nadir ≥20 × 10^9/L	30%-50% platelet count fall; or nadir 10-19 × 10^9/L	<30% platelet count fall; or nadir ≤10 × 10^9/L
Timing of fall in platelet count or other sequelae	Onset day 5-10 or <1 day (if heparin exposure within 30 days)	>Day 10, timing unclear, or <day 1 with recent heparin 31-100 days	Platelet count fall <day 4 (without recent heparin exposure)
Thrombosis or other sequelae	New thrombosis; skin necrosis; post-heparin bolus acute systemic reaction	Progressive or recurrent thrombosis; erythematous skin lesions; suspected thrombosis—not confirmed	None
Other cause for thrombocytopenia	No other cause for platelet count fall is evident	Possible other cause is evident	Definite other cause is present

Pretest probability score: 6-8 = High; 4-5 = Intermediate; 0-3 = Low

From Vincent JL et al: *Textbook of critical care,* ed 7, Philadelphia, 2017, Elsevier.

TABLE 3 Laboratory Assays for Heparin-Induced Thrombocytopenia

Assay	Sensitivity (%)	Specificity (%)	Positive Predictive Value (%)	Negative Predictive Value (%)
Functional assay (e.g., serotonin release assay)	88	~100	~100	81
PF4/heparin enzyme immunoassay (ELISA)	95-98	86	93	95

ELISA, Enzyme-linked immunosorbent assay; *PF4,* platelet factor 4.
From Goldman L, Schafer AI: *Goldman's Cecil medicine,* ed 24, Philadelphia, 2012, Saunders.

TABLE 4 Treatment Schedules for Bivalirudin and Argatroban

Anticoagulant	Dosing Protocol for HIT-Associated Thrombosis	Anticoagulant Monitoring[a]	Clearance	Half-Life (min)	Comment
Bivalirudin	No bolus; initial infusion rate: 0.15-0.20 mg/kg per hour	1.5-2.5 × baseline aPTT	Enzymic (80%); renal (20%)	25	Off-label treatment for HIT (although approved for PCI in patient with HIT); minor prolongation of INR (compared with argatroban)
Argatroban	No bolus; initial infusion rate: 2 μg/kg per minute	1.5-3.0 × baseline aPTT	Hepatobiliary	40-50	Initial dose 0.5 μg/kg per minute in hepatic insufficiency[b]; moderate or marked prolongation of INR, which complicates overlap with warfarin anticoagulation

Dosing protocols shown are appropriate for most patients with strongly suspected or confirmed HIT whether or not complicated by thrombosis. (Dosing for bivalirudin and argatroban is substantially different when given for PCI.) *aPTT,* Activated partial thromboplastin time; *HIT,* heparin-induced thrombocytopenia; *INR,* international normalized ratio; *PCI,* percutaneous coronary intervention.
[a]In general, the patient's baseline aPTT should be used for calculating target range when appropriate; otherwise the mean laboratory normal range can be used.
[b]Reduced initial dosing (e.g., 0.5-1.2 μg/kg per minute) is also appropriate in patients in intensive care units, with cardiac failure, or postcardiac surgery).
Modified from Hoffman R et al: *Hematology, basic principles and practice,* ed 7, Philadelphia, 2018, Elsevier.

- Two agents, both direct thrombin inhibitors, are approved for this indication (Table 4):
  1. Argatroban (preferred agent in renal failure and in hemodialysis patients; avoid in liver dysfunction).
  2. Bivalirudin (approved only for patients with HIT or at risk of HIT who are undergoing PCI; dose adjustment is required in renal failure).
- Note: Lepirudin is no longer available. Outside of the U.S., the factor Xa inhibitor danaparoid may be used.
- Platelet transfusion in the absence of life-threatening hemorrhage or extreme thrombocytopenia should be avoided. Risk of bleeding is low, and platelet transfusions in HIT can increase risk of arterial thrombosis.
- A direct thrombin inhibitor should be continued as a single agent until the platelet count returns to baseline (generally 150 × 109/L, but consider the individual patient's baseline).
- Warfarin can be added after platelet recovery (maximum dose of 5 mg/day to reduce risk of warfarin-induced skin necrosis and venous limb gangrene). This overlap therapy should continue until the platelet count has reached a stable plateau, the INR has reached goal (typically 2-3, though guidelines may vary with argatroban as it artificially elevates the INR), and after a minimum overlap of 5 days with both the direct thrombin inhibitor and warfarin.
- The length of treatment is controversial, but most clinicians agree that at least 1 mo of alternative anticoagulation is required in the absence of thrombosis, while at least 3 to 6 mo of treatment are required in the presence of thrombosis.
- Fondaparinux, a synthetic pentasaccharide that inhibits factor X but not thrombin, is being increasingly used for treatment of HIT despite not yet being FDA approved (Table 5). Observational data suggest it has similar efficacy as direct thrombin inhibitors, with the additional advantages of lower bleeding risk, easier administration (subcutaneous), and lower cost. Rare cases of fondaparinux-induced HIT have been reported, however.
- The use of direct oral anticoagulants (e.g., rivaroxaban, dabigatran, apixaban) is being studied. Retrospective reviews have shown DOACs to be safe and effective for the treatment of HIT, though randomized prospective data remain lacking.
- In patients with confirmed HIT, all heparin products should be avoided for life. A possible exception is in patients who require brief intraoperative anticoagulation such as cardiac bypass surgery.

TABLE 5 Treatment Schedules for Danaparoid and Fondaparinux

Anticoagulant	Therapeutic Dosing Protocol for HIT-Associated Thrombosis[a]	Anticoagulant Monitoring	Clearance	Half-Life (h)	Comment
Danaparoid	Initial bolus, 2250 units[b] IV; accelerated infusion (400 units/hr × 4 hr, 300 units/hr × 4 hr; then 200 units/hr IV, subsequently adjusted by antifactor Xa levels)	Antifactor Xa levels (target, 0.5-0.8 units/ml)	Renal (minor)	25	Widely approved for HIT treatment (although not in the U.S.); not available in the U.S.; low risk for in vivo cross-reactivity; prophylactic-dose therapy[c] may be appropriate when clinical suspicion for HIT is low.
Fondaparinux	7.5 mg[d] subcutaneous once daily	Anti–Xa factor levels (target levels not well established)	Renal (major)	17	Not approved for HIT treatment (although increasingly used as off-label therapy). Prophylactic-dose therapy[e] may be appropriate when clinical suspicion for HIT is low, or if there is renal insufficiency.

HIT, Heparin-induced thrombocytopenia; *IV,* intravenous.
[a]Therapeutic dosing is usually appropriate for strongly suspected or confirmed HIT (including "isolated" HIT, i.e., HIT without apparent thrombosis), or when thrombosis is documented.
[b]Adjust IV danaparoid bolus for body weight: <60 kg, 1500 units; 60-75 kg, 2250 units; 75-90 kg, 3000 units; >90 kg, 3750 units.
[c]Prophylactic-dose regimen, 750 units subcutaneous every 8 hr (for renal failure, reduce to 750 units every 12 hr).
[d]Five milligrams for body weight <50 kg and 10 mg for body weight >100 kg; the author sometimes gives 10 mg as the first and/or second dose (rather than 7.5 mg) for severe HIT. Because HIT treatment is usually started in the afternoon, the author usually gives the second dose (and subsequent doses) at 8 A.M. (i.e., the interval between first and second doses is often only 14-20 hr rather than 24 hr), which helps to achieve steady-state therapy more quickly. Dose reduction and antifactor Xa monitoring (if available) is appropriate if being used in a patient with renal insufficiency.
[e]Prophylactic-dose regimen, 2.5 mg subcutaneous every day (assumes normal renal function).
From Hoffman R et al: *Hematology, basic principles and practice,* ed 7, Philadelphia, 2018, Elsevier.

REFERRAL

Request a hematology consultation.

PEARLS & CONSIDERATIONS

COMMENTS

- HIT paradoxically causes thrombocytopenia and *clotting.* Bleeding is much less common.
- It is unclear whether patients with HIT should be considered heparin allergic lifelong. Risk of recurrent HIT with heparin rechallenge years later is relatively low, about 5% in one small study (though recurrence risk is higher perioperatively). If such a patient requires surgery with heparin (e.g., on-pump cardiac bypass), consider perioperative argatroban.
- Consult the coagulation laboratory and/or hematology when bridging patients on argatroban to warfarin, as argatroban concomitantly raises the INR in most assays. Some clinicians will use a higher target than 2 to 3 during the bridging period for this reason.
- Be alert to heparin exposure in the absence of anticoagulation or DVT prophylaxis: Hospitalized patients are often exposed to heparin lock flushes, heparin-coated catheters, or heparin-coated guidewires—any of which could precipitate HIT.

PREVENTION

Strongly consider the use of low-molecular-weight heparin in place of unfractionated heparin in hospitalized patients with a stable creatinine clearance of 30 ml/min or greater. Such a preventive strategy can reduce the risk of HIT by over 90% and yield cost savings in testing and treatment.

SUGGESTED READINGS

Available at ExpertConsult.com

AUTHORS: **Hyun Lee, MD,** and **John L. Reagan, MD**

BASIC INFORMATION

DEFINITION

Hepatic encephalopathy is a neuropsychiatric syndrome occurring in patients with severe impairment of liver function and consequent accumulation of toxic products not metabolized by the liver. It is characterized by gradual impairment of the ability to perform mental tasks and to react to external stimuli. Fig. 1 illustrates the hepatic encephalopathy grades in acute liver failure. ***Minimal hepatic encephalopathy*** refers to patients with hepatic cirrhosis and mild cognitive impairment, but no history of overt encephalopathy.

SYNONYMS

Hepatic coma
Portal systemic encephalopathy
HE

ICD-10CM CODES

G92	Toxic encephalopathy
G93.40	Encephalopathy, unspecified
G93.41	Metabolic encephalopathy
K70.40	Alcoholic hepatic failure without coma
K70.41	Alcoholic hepatic failure with coma
K72.0	Acute and subacute hepatic failure
K72.00	Acute and subacute hepatic failure without coma
K72.01	Acute and subacute hepatic failure with coma
K72.1	Chronic hepatic failure
K72.10	Chronic hepatic failure without coma
K72.11	Chronic hepatic failure with coma
K72.9	Hepatic failure, unspecified
K72.90	Hepatic failure, unspecified without coma
K72.91	Hepatic failure, unspecified with coma
K91.82	Postprocedural hepatic failure

EPIDEMIOLOGY & DEMOGRAPHICS

INCIDENCE & PREVALENCE: Hepatic encephalopathy occurs in >40% of all cases of cirrhosis.

PHYSICAL FINDINGS & CLINICAL PRESENTATION

Hepatic encephalopathy can be classified by clinical stages described in Table 1. Other widely used scales are the four score criteria and the West Haven criteria. The West Haven criteria for grading hepatic encephalopathy is as follows:

- Grade (0): No abnormalities noted
- Grade (1): Unawareness (mild), euphoria or anxiety, shortened attention span, impairment of calculation ability, lethargy, or apathy
- Grade (2): Disorientation to time, obvious personality change, inappropriate behavior
- Grade (3): Somnolence to stupor, responsiveness to stimuli, gross disorientation, bizarre behavior
- Grade (4): Coma

The physical examination in hepatic encephalopathy varies with the stage and may reveal the following abnormalities:

- Skin: Jaundice, palmar erythema, spider angiomata, ecchymosis, dilated superficial periumbilical veins (caput medusae) in patients with cirrhosis
- Eyes: Scleral icterus, Kayser-Fleischer rings (Wilson disease)
- Breath: Fetor hepaticus
- Chest: Gynecomastia in men with chronic liver disease
- Abdomen: Ascites, small nodular liver (cirrhosis), tender hepatomegaly (congestive hepatomegaly)
- Rectal examination: Hemorrhoids (portal hypertension), guaiac-positive stool (alcoholic gastritis, bleeding esophageal varices, peptic ulcer disease, bleeding hemorrhoids)
- Genitalia: Testicular atrophy in males with chronic liver disease
- Extremities: Pedal edema from hypoalbuminemia
- Neurologic: Flapping tremor (asterixis), obtundation, coma with or without decerebrate posturing

ETIOLOGY

- Hepatic encephalopathy is thought to be caused mainly by accumulation of unmetabolized ammonia. The shunting of ammonia into the systemic circulation results in neuronal dysfunction leading to hepatic encephalopathy
- Precipitating factors in patients with underlying cirrhosis (upper gastrointestinal bleeding, hypokalemia, hypomagnesemia, analgesic and sedative drugs, sepsis, alkalosis, increased dietary protein)
- Acute fulminant viral hepatitis
- Drugs and toxins (e.g., isoniazid, acetaminophen, diclofenac and other NSAIDs, statins, methyldopa, loratadine, propylthiouracil, lisinopril, labetalol, halothane, carbon tetrachloride, erythromycin, nitrofurantoin, troglitazone, herbal products, flavocoxid)
- Reye syndrome
- Shock and/or sepsis
- Fatty liver of pregnancy
- Metastatic carcinoma, hepatocellular carcinoma
- Other: Autoimmune hepatitis, ischemic venoocclusive disease, sclerosing cholangitis, heat stroke, amebic abscesses

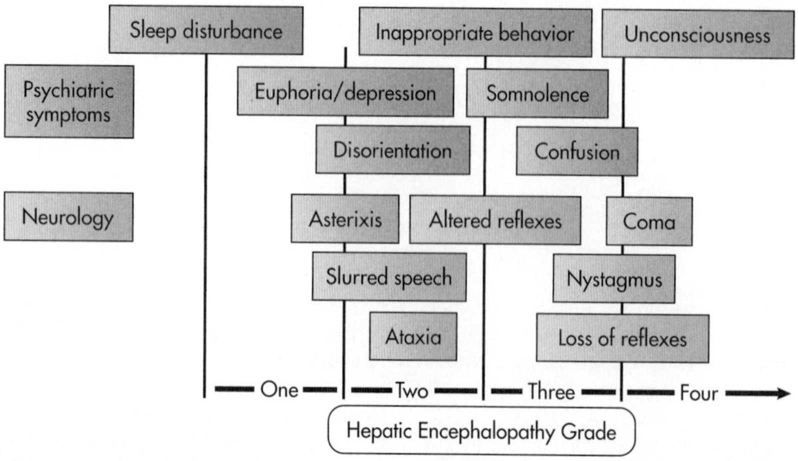

FIG. 1 Hepatic encephalopathy grade in acute liver failure. (From Parrillo JE, Dellinger RP: *Critical care medicine, principles of diagnosis and management in the adult,* ed 4, Philadelphia, 2014, Elsevier.)

DIAGNOSIS

DIFFERENTIAL DIAGNOSIS

- Delirium caused by medications or illicit drugs
- Cerebrovascular accident, subdural hematoma
- Meningitis, encephalitis
- Hypoglycemia
- Uremia
- Cerebral anoxia
- Hypercalcemia
- Metastatic neoplasm to brain
- Alcohol withdrawal syndrome/Wernicke-Korsakoff syndrome
- Hyponatremia
- Postictal state

WORKUP

Hepatic encephalopathy should be considered in any patient with cirrhosis who presents with neuropsychiatric manifestations. Exclude other etiologies with comprehensive history (obtained from patient, relatives, and others), physical examination, and laboratory and imaging studies. A pertinent history should include exposure to hepatitis, ethanol intake, drug history, exposure to toxins, IV drug abuse, measles or influenza with aspirin use (Reye syndrome), and history of carcinoma (primary or metastatic). Minimal hepatic encephalopathy may not be obvious on clinical examination, but can be detected with neurophysiologic and neuropsychiatric testing.

LABORATORY TESTS

- Alanine aminotransferase, aspartate aminotransferase, bilirubin, alkaline phosphatase, glucose, calcium, electrolytes, blood urea nitrogen, creatinine, albumin
- Complete blood count, platelet count, prothrombin time, partial thromboplastin time
- Serum and urine toxicology screen in suspected medication or illegal drug use
- Blood and urine cultures, urinalysis

TABLE 1 Clinical Stages of Hepatic Encephalopathy

Stage	Asterixis	EEG Changes	Clinical Manifestations
I (prodrome)	Slight	Minimal	Mild intellectual impairment, disturbed sleep-wake cycle
II (impending)	Easily elicited	Usually generalized	Drowsiness, confusion, coma/inappropriate behavior, disorientation, mood swings
III (stupor)	Present if patient cooperative	Grossly abnormal slowing of rhythm	Drowsy, unresponsive to verbal commands, markedly confused, delirious, hyperreflexia, positive Babinski sign
IV (coma)	Usually absent	Appearance of delta waves, decreased amplitudes	Unconscious, decerebrate or decorticate response to pain present (stage IVA) or absent (stage IVB)

EEG, Electroencephalogram.
From Fuhrman BP et al: *Pediatric critical care,* ed 4, Philadelphia, 2011, Saunders.

- Venous ammonia level. Measurement of serum ammonia level is useful in the evaluation of acute liver failure because levels correlate with the severity of encephalopathy and elevated levels are predictive of severe encephalopathy and cerebral edema. It is not useful for the evaluation or screening of hepatic encephalopathy in patients with chronic liver disease because it can neither rule in nor rule out hepatic encephalopathy, and levels do not correlate with the degree of encephalopathy
- Arterial blood gases

IMAGING STUDIES

CT scan or MRI of the brain may be useful in selected patients to exclude other etiologies when diagnosis is unclear.

Rx TREATMENT

NONPHARMACOLOGIC THERAPY

- Identification and treatment of precipitating factors.
- Restriction of protein intake is ill-advised and not necessary, since normal protein intake does not appear to exacerbate hepatic encephalopathy.

ACUTE GENERAL Rx

The approach to patients with high grade hepatic encephalopathy is shown in Fig. 2. Table 2 summarizes the management of fulminant hepatic failure.

Reduction of colonic ammonia production:

- Lactulose 25 ml twice daily initially; dose is subsequently adjusted depending on clinical response to achieve production of 3 bowel movements daily. IV ornithine aspartate should be considered for those not responding to lactulose.
- The oral antibiotic rifaximin (550 mg PO bid) is effective in reducing the risk of recurrent hepatic encephalopathy in patients with cirrhosis. It can be taken with lactulose, and the combination of lactulose and rifaximin is superior to lactulose alone in reversing hepatic encephalopathy. Rifaximin has also been shown to be effective in improving psychometric performance and health-related quality of life in patients with minimal hepatic encephalopathy. It is well tolerated but expensive.

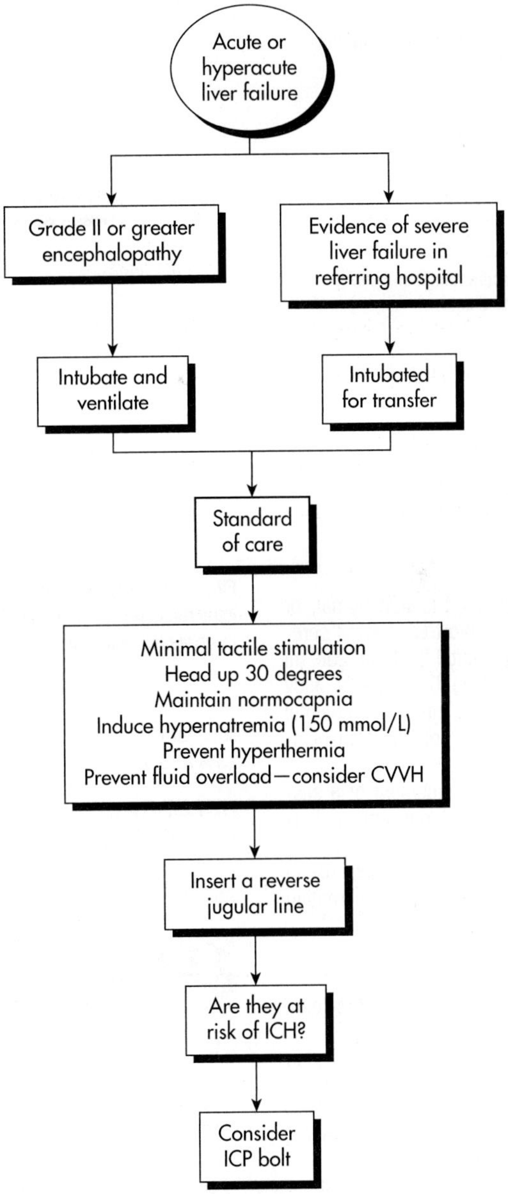

FIG. 2 Initial management of patient with high-grade encephalopathy. *CVVH,* Continuous venovenous hemofiltration; *ICH,* intracranial hypertension; *ICP,* intracranial pressure. (From Parrillo JE, Dellinger RP: *Critical care medicine, principles of diagnosis and management in the adult,* ed 5, Philadelphia, 2019, Elsevier.)

- Probiotics (e.g., 1 capsule containing 112.5 billion viable lyophilized bacteria tid) might also be beneficial in altering gut flora to reduce ammonia production.

Treatment of cerebral edema:

- Cerebral edema is often present in patients with acute liver failure, and it accounts for nearly 50% of deaths. Monitoring intracranial

TABLE 2 Management of Fulminant Hepatic Failure

No sedation except for procedures
Minimal handling
Enteric precautions until infection ruled out
Monitor:
1. Heart and respiratory rate
2. Arterial BP, CVP
3. Core/toe temperature
4. Neurologic observations
5. Gastric pH (>5.0)
6. Blood glucose (>4 mmol/L)
7. Acid-base
8. Electrolytes
9. PT, PTT

Fluid balance:
1. 75% maintenance
2. Dextrose 10%-50% (provide 6-10 mg/kg/min)
3. Sodium (0.5-1 mmol/L)
4. Potassium (2-4 mmol/L)

Maintain circulating volume with colloid/FFP coagulation support only if required
Drugs:
1. Vitamin K
2. H2 antagonist
3. Antacids
4. Lactulose
5. N-acetylcysteine for acetaminophen toxicity
6. Broad-spectrum antibiotics
7. Antifungals

Nutrition:
1. Enteral feeding (1-2 g protein/kg/day)
2. PN if ventilated

BP, Blood pressure; *CVP,* central venous pressure; *FFP,* fresh frozen plasma; *PN,* parenteral nutrition; *PT,* prothrombin time; *PTT,* partial thromboplastin time.
From Fuhrman BP et al: *Pediatric critical care,* ed 4, Philadelphia, 2011, Saunders.

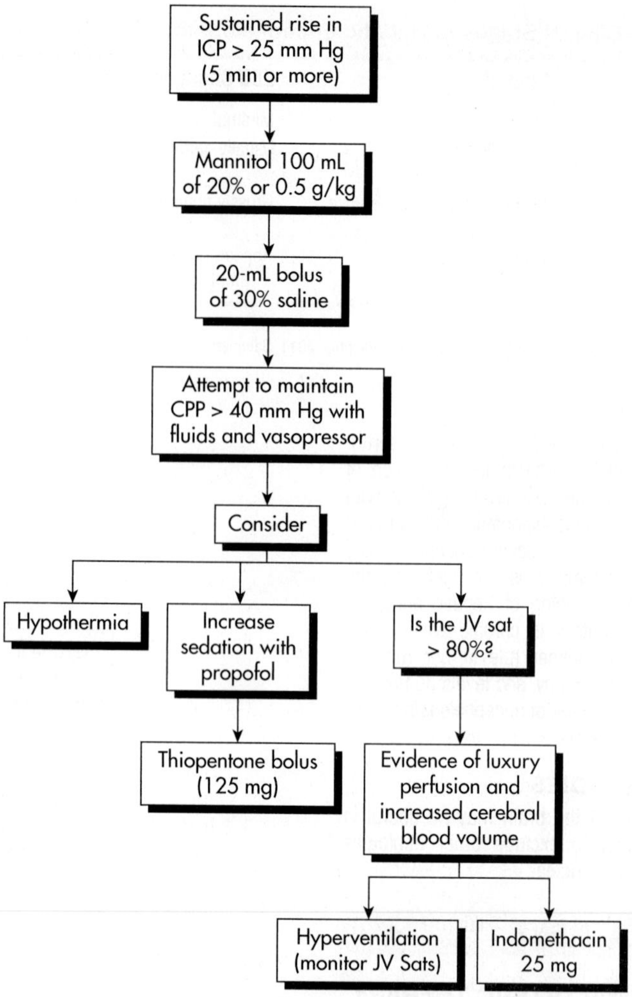

FIG. 3 Management of a sustained rise in intracranial pressure. *CPP,* Cerebral perfusion pressure; *ICP,* intracranial pressure; *JV,* jugular venous; *Sats,* saturation. (From Parrillo JE, Dellinger RP: *Critical care medicine, principles of diagnosis and management in the adult,* ed 5, Philadelphia, 2019, Elsevier.)

pressure by epidural, intraparenchymal, or subdural transducers and treatment of cerebral edema with mannitol (100 to 200 ml of 20% solution [0.3 to 0.4 g/kg of body weight]) given by rapid IV infusion are helpful in selected patients (e.g., potential transplantation patients).
- Fig. 3 illustrates the management of a sustained rise in intracranial pressure in liver failure.
- Dexamethasone and hyperventilation (useful in head injury) are of little value in treating cerebral edema from liver failure.

CHRONIC Rx

- Avoidance of any precipitating factors (e.g., high-protein diet, medications).
- Consideration of liver transplantation in selected patients with progressive or recurrent encephalopathy (Box E1). Liver transplantation remains the only curative therapeutic option.

DISPOSITION

Prognosis varies with the underlying etiology of the liver failure and the grade of encephalopathy (generally good for grades 1 or 2; poor for grades 3 or 4). Without proper therapy, the survival rate at 1 yr is 42% and decreases to 23% at 3 yr.

REFERRAL

The early stages of hepatic encephalopathy can be managed in the outpatient setting, whereas stages III or IV require hospital admission.

PEARLS & CONSIDERATIONS

COMMENTS

- Trials have shown that adding IV albumin to lactulose may improve outcomes in severe hepatic encephalopathy by reducing oxidative stress through reduction of levels of circulating cytokines and endotoxins.
- Long-acting benzodiazepines should not be used to treat anxiety and sleep disorders in patients with cirrhosis, as they may precipitate encephalopathy.
- Patients not responding to supportive therapy should be evaluated for liver transplantation.
- Not all patients with cirrhosis develop hepatic encephalopathy. It has been shown that 40% of persons with cirrhosis and minimal hepatic encephalopathy do not develop overt hepatic encephalopathy in long-term follow-up. There are genetic factors associated with development of hepatic encephalopathy in patients with cirrhosis. Genetic analyses have shown that glutaminase TACC and CACC haplotypes are linked to the risk for overt hepatic encephalopathy.

RELATED CONTENT

Encephalopathy (Patient Information)
Cirrhosis (Related Key Topic)
Hepatic Encephalopathy (Related Key Topic)

SUGGESTED READINGS

Available at ExpertConsult.com

AUTHOR: **Fred F. Ferri, MD**

BASIC INFORMATION

DEFINITION

Hepatitis A is generally an acute self-limiting infection of the liver by an enterically transmitted picornavirus, hepatitis A virus (HAV). Infection may range from asymptomatic to fulminant hepatitis.

SYNONYMS

Infectious hepatitis
Short incubation hepatitis
Type A hepatitis
HAV (hepatitis A virus)

ICD-10CM CODES
B15.9 Hepatitis A without hepatic coma
B15.0 Hepatitis A with hepatic coma

EPIDEMIOLOGY & DEMOGRAPHICS

INCIDENCE:

- Hepatitis A occurs worldwide, affecting 1.4 million people annually and accounting for 20% to 40% of cases of viral hepatitis in the U.S. It is the most common cause of viral hepatitis worldwide.
- The seroprevalence increases with age, ranging from 10% in individuals aged <5 yr to 74% in those aged >50 yr.
- In the U.S., average disease rate was ~15 cases/100,000 persons/yr before routine vaccination of all children in certain states. The incidence after 2005 is about 1 case/100,000. There were 12,474 reported cases in the U.S. in 2018.
- The incidence is relatively higher in some regions in the U.S., including Arizona, Alaska, California, Idaho, Nevada, New Mexico, Oklahoma, Oregon, South Dakota, and Washington.
- At-risk groups include:
  1. Residents and staff of group homes
  2. Children and employees of day care centers
  3. People who engage in oral-anal contact, regardless of sexual orientation
  4. IV drug abusers
  5. Travel to endemic areas
  6. Areas of overcrowding, poor sanitation, inadequate sewage treatment

PREVALENCE:

- Approximately three fourths of the U.S. population has serologic evidence of prior infection.
- Anti-HAV prevalence has an inverse relation to income and household size.

PREDOMINANT SEX: None, except higher infection rates seen in men who have sex with men who engage in oral–anal contact.

PREDOMINANT AGE & PEAK INCIDENCE:

- In areas of high rates of hepatitis A, virtually all children are infected while younger than 10 yr, but disease is rare.
- In areas of moderate rates of hepatitis A, disease occurs in late childhood and young adults.
- In areas of low rates of hepatitis A, most cases occur in young adults.

INCUBATION PERIOD: Averages 30 days (15-50)

PHYSICAL FINDINGS & CLINICAL PRESENTATION

- Infection with HAV may have acute or subacute presentation, icteric or anicteric. Severity of illness seems to increase with age (90% of infection in children aged <5 yr may be subclinical).
- The incubation period of HAV is 2 to 6 wk.
- A preicteric, prodromal phase of approximately 1 to 14 days; 15% no apparent prodrome. Symptoms are usually abrupt in onset and may include anorexia, fatigue, malaise, nausea, vomiting, fever, headache, and mild abdominal pain.
- Less common symptoms are chills, myalgias, arthralgias, upper respiratory symptoms, constipation, diarrhea, pruritus, urticaria.
- Jaundice occurs in >70% of patients. Patients older than 30 yr are more likely than younger individuals to have jaundice.
- The icteric phase is preceded by dark urine.
- Bilirubinuria is typically followed a few days later by clay-colored stools and icterus.

PHYSICAL EXAMINATION

- Jaundice: Peaks in severity 2 wk after onset
- Hepatomegaly
- Splenomegaly
- Cervical lymphadenopathy
- Evanescent rash
- Petechiae
- Cardiac arrhythmias

COMPLICATIONS

- Cholestasis
- Fulminant hepatitis
- Arthritis
- Myocarditis
- Optic neuritis
- Transverse myelitis
- Thrombocytopenic purpura
- Aplastic anemia
- Red cell aplasia
- Henoch-Schönlein purpura
- IgA dominant glomerulonephritis

ETIOLOGY

- Caused by HAV, a 27-nm, nonenveloped, icosahedral, positive-stranded RNA virus.
- Transmission is fecal-oral route, from person to person. Transmission occurs with close contact or with food- or waterborne outbreaks with inadequately purified water or cooked foods. Recent outbreaks have involved green onions and tomatoes.
- Parenteral transmission is considered rare.
- Vertical transmission has also been reported.

Dx DIAGNOSIS

DIFFERENTIAL DIAGNOSIS

- Other hepatitis virus (B, C, D, E): Table 1 summarizes serology and PCR test results
- Infectious mononucleosis
- Cytomegalovirus infection
- Herpes simplex virus infection
- Leptospirosis
- Brucellosis
- Drug-induced liver disease
- Ischemic hepatitis
- Autoimmune hepatitis

WORKUP

- IgM antibody specific for HAV

TABLE 1 Diagnostic Blood Tests: Serology and Viral Polymerase Chain Reaction

HAV	HBV	HCV	HDV	HEV
Acute/Active Infection				
Anti-HAV IgM (+)	Anti-HBc IgM (+)	Anti-HCV (+)	Anti-HDV IgM (+)	Anti-HEV IgM (+)
Blood PCR positive*	HBsAg (+) Anti-HBs (–) HBV DNA (+) (PCR)	HCV RNA (+) (PCR)	Blood PCR positive HBsAg (+) Anti-HBs (–)	Blood PCR positive*
Past Infection (Recovered)				
Anti-HAV IgG (+)	Anti-HBs (+) Anti-HBc IgG (+)†	Anti-HCV (+) Blood PCR (–)	Anti-HDV IgG (+) Blood PCR (–)	Anti-HEV IgG (+) Blood PCR (–)
Chronic Infection				
N/A	Anti-HBc IgG (+) HBsAg (+) Anti-HBs (–) PCR (+) or (–)	Anti-HCV (+) Blood PCR (+)	Anti-HDV IgG (+) Blood PCR (–) HBsAg (+) Anti-HBs (–)	N/A
Vaccine Response				
Anti-HAV IgG (+)	Anti-HBs (+) Anti-HBc (–)	N/A	N/A	N/A

HAV, Hepatitis A virus; *HBc,* hepatitis B core; *HBs,* hepatitis B surface; *HBsAg,* hepatitis B surface antigen; *HBV,* hepatitis B virus; *HCV,* hepatitis C virus; *HDV,* hepatitis D virus; *HEV,* hepatitis E virus; *Ig,* immunoglobulin; *N/A,* not applicable; *PCR,* polymerase chain reaction.
*Research tool.
†Still poses a risk for reactivation.
From Kliegman RM: *Nelson textbook of pediatrics,* ed 21, Philadelphia, 2020, Elsevier.

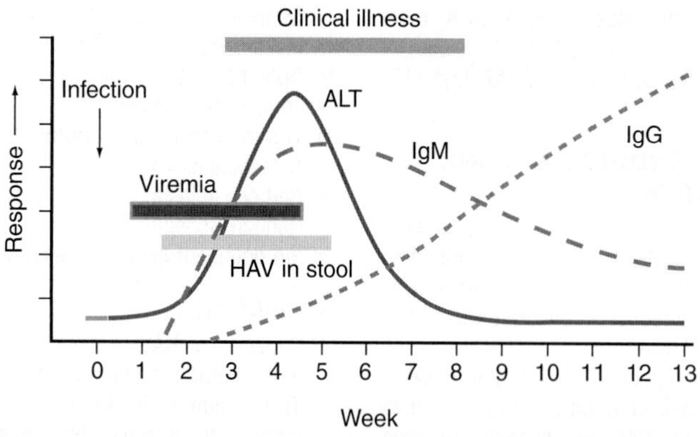

FIG. 1 Immunologic, virologic, and biochemical events during the course of a typical hepatitis A virus (HAV) infection. *ALT,* Alanine transaminase; *HAV,* Hepatitis A virus; *IgG,* immunoglobulin G; *IgM,* immunoglobulin M. (From Cherry JD et al: *Feigin and Cherry's pediatric infectious diseases,* ed 8, Philadelphia, 2019, Elsevier.)

TABLE 2 Recommendations for Routine Preexposure Use of Hepatitis A Virus Vaccine

Group	Comments
Children	Vaccine should be given to all children at age 1 yr (12-23 mo).* Vaccination of children 2-18 yr may also be warranted.†
International travelers‡	IG may be given in addition to or instead of vaccine; children <12 mo should receive IG.
Close contacts of newly arriving international adoptees	All persons who anticipate close personal contact (e.g., household contact or regular babysitter) during the first 60 days after arrival
Men who have sex with men	Includes adolescents
Illicit drug users	Includes adolescents
Persons with chronic liver disease, such as those with hepatitis B or C	Increased risk of fulminant hepatitis A with HAV infection
Persons receiving clotting factor concentrates	
Persons who work with HAV in research laboratory settings	

HAV, Hepatitis A virus; *IG,* immunoglobulin.
*Hepatitis A vaccine is not licensed for children <12 mo.
†States and communities with existing vaccination programs for children aged 2 to 18 yr are encouraged to maintain these programs. Catch-up vaccination for this age group may be warranted elsewhere in the context of ongoing outbreaks among children.
‡Persons traveling to Canada, Western Europe, Japan, Australia, or New Zealand are at no greater risk than in the U.S.
From Bennett JE et al: *Mandell, Douglas, and Bennett's principles and practice of infectious diseases,* ed 8, Philadelphia, 2015, Saunders.

- Liver function tests; ALT and AST elevations are sensitive for liver damage but not specific for HAV
- Elevated ESR
- CBC; may find mild lymphocytosis

LABORATORY TESTS

- Diagnosis confirmed by IgM anti-HAV; it is detectable in almost all infected patients at presentation and remains positive for 3 to 6 mo.
- A fourfold rise in titer of total antibody (IgM and IgG) to HAV confirms acute infection.
- HAV detection in stool and body fluids by electron microscopy.
- HAV RNA detection in stool, body fluids, serum, and liver tissue.
- ALT and AST usually more than 8 times normal in acute infection.
- Bilirubin usually 5 to 15 times normal.
- Alkaline phosphatase minimally elevated, but higher level in cholestasis.
- Albumin and prothrombin time are generally normal; if elevated, they may herald hepatic necrosis.
- Fig. 1 illustrates the typical course of hepatitis A.

IMAGING STUDIES

- Rarely useful
- Sonogram (fulminant hepatitis)

Rx TREATMENT

- Usually self-limited
- Supportive care
- Those with fulminant hepatitis may require hospitalization and treatment of associated complications
- Activity as tolerated
- Advise to avoid alcohol and hepatotoxic drugs
- Patients with fulminant hepatitis should be assessed for liver transplantation

CHRONIC Rx

No chronic HAV and no chronic carrier state. The majority of patients have resolution of symptoms and liver abnormalities within 3 mo.

DISPOSITION

- Follow-up as outpatient.
- Most patients recover within 3 mo of infection, although 5% to 10% of patients will experience a relapse in the first 6 mo.
- HAV is a self-limited infection and does not cause chronic hepatitis.

REFERRAL

- To a hepatologist if severe, fulminant hepatitis develops
- To a transplant surgeon if liver transplant becomes a consideration for fulminant hepatitis and liver failure

PEARLS & CONSIDERATIONS

- All cases of hepatitis A should be reported to the public health authorities because food-borne or water-borne outbreaks may occur, and public health efforts (mass vaccination or immunoglobulin therapy) may prevent secondary cases.
- Hepatitis A is a common illness in internationally traveled and developing countries. Pretravel vaccination is strongly recommended for travelers who are HAV susceptible. Table 2 summarizes recommendations for preexposure use of hepatitis A virus vaccine. Updated dosage recommendations are described in Table 3.
- Handwashing is important because the hepatitis A virus may survive for up to 4 hr on the fingertips.
- There have been significant recent outbreaks of hepatitis A in the U.S. In 2016 to 2018 there was an increase of cases by 294% vs. cases in 2013 to 2015. This was mostly among the homeless, IV drug abusers, men having sex with men, and individuals who consumed certain imported food items.

PREVENTION

- Improvement in hygiene and sanitation
- Heating food
- Avoidance of water and foods from endemic area

PASSIVE IMMUNIZATION

- Immunoglobulin provides protection against HAV through passive transfer of antibody.
- Preexposure prophylaxis indicated for people traveling to endemic areas with immune globulin (Ig 0.02 or 0.06 ml/kg given IM) who have not received or cannot receive the hepatitis A vaccine before departure. The

TABLE 3 Indications and Updated Dosage Recommendations for GamaSTAN S/D Human Immune Globulin for Preexposure and Postexposure Prophylaxis Against Hepatitis A Infection

Indication	Updated Dosage Recommendation
Preexposure prophylaxis	
Up to 1 mo of travel	0.1 ml/kg
Up to 2 mo of travel	0.2 ml/kg
2 mo of travel or longer	0.2 ml/kg (repeat every 2 mo)
Postexposure prophylaxis	0.1 ml/kg

From Kliegman RM: *Nelson textbook of pediatrics,* ed 21, Philadelphia, 2020, Elsevier.

lower dose is effective for up to 3 mo, and the higher dose is effective for up to 5 mo.

- Postexposure prophylaxis (PEP): For individuals with a recent exposure to hepatitis A who have not received the vaccine, post-exposure prophylaxis is warranted with either immunoglobulin (Ig 0.02 ml/kg given IM) or a single dose of the hepatitis A vaccine within 2 wk of the exposure. For healthy persons ages 12 mo to 40 yr of age, a single dose of the hepatitis A vaccine should be given. Children <12 mo, adults >40 yr of age, and persons who have chronic liver disease and who are immunocompromised should receive immunoglobulin.

ACTIVE IMMUNIZATION

- There are several inactivated and attenuated hepatitis vaccines; only the inactivated vaccines are currently available for use and they have been found to be safe and highly immunogenic: HAVRIX or VAQTA. These can be used in adults and children older than 12 mo. They are given as a two-dose regimen 6 mo to 1 yr apart. A combined hepatitis A and hepatitis B vaccine called TWINRX is also available.
- Protective antibody levels were reached in 94% to 100% of adults 1 mo after the first dose; similar results have been found for children and adolescents.
- Theoretic analyses of antibody levels estimate duration of immunity to be 10 to 20 yr.
- Vaccine should be considered for persons who are at risk. Those traveling to or working in endemic areas, men who have sex with men, illegal drug users, persons with chronic liver disease, and children in areas with high rates of hepatitis A infection.
- The Advisory Committee on Immunization Practices recommends routine hepatitis A vaccination for all children beginning at 12 to 23 mo of age. Simultaneous administration of MMR and HCPA vaccines is recommended for infants aged 6 to 11 mo traveling internationally. The travel-related dose for infants aged 6 to 11 mo should not be counted towards the routine 2-dose series.

SUGGESTED READINGS

Available at ExpertConsult.com

RELATED CONTENT

Hepatitis A (Patient Information)

AUTHOR: **Glenn G. Fort, MD, MPH**

BASIC INFORMATION

DEFINITION

Hepatitis B is an acute infection of the liver parenchymal cells caused by the hepatitis B virus (HBV).

SYNONYMS

Serum hepatitis
Long incubation (30 to 180 days) hepatitis HBV
HBV

ICD-10CM CODES

B16	Acute hepatitis B
B16.0	Acute hepatitis B with delta-agent with hepatic coma
B16.1	Acute hepatitis B with delta-agent without hepatic coma
B16.2	Acute hepatitis B without delta-agent with hepatic coma
B16.9	Acute hepatitis B without delta agent and without hepatic coma
B18.0	Chronic viral hepatitis B with delta-agent
B18.1	Chronic viral hepatitis B without delta-agent
B19.1	Unspecified viral hepatitis B
B19.10	Unspecified viral hepatitis B without hepatic coma
B19.11	Unspecified viral hepatitis B with hepatic coma

EPIDEMIOLOGY & DEMOGRAPHICS

INCIDENCE:

- In U.S. overall incidence is approximately 1.1 cases per 100,000.
- Much higher incidence in Europe (~1 million new cases annually) and in areas of high endemicity.
- In the U.S., transmission is mainly horizontal (percutaneous and mucous membrane exposure to infectious blood and other body fluids [e.g., sexual transmission, either homosexual or heterosexual]); also from needle sharing among drug abusers; occupational exposure to contaminated blood and blood products; persons receiving transfusions of blood and blood products; and hemodialysis patients.

  NOTE: Improved screening of blood and blood products has greatly reduced, although not eliminated, the risk of posttransfusion HBV infection.
- In areas of high endemicity, transmission is largely vertical (perinatal): HBV exists in the blood and body fluids. Perinatal transmission from HBsAg-positive mothers is as high as 90% unless immunoprophylaxis is given.

PREVALENCE:

- The WHO estimates that 400 million people worldwide (6% of the population) are chronic HBV carriers. North America, Western Europe, and Australia are areas of low prevalence, <2%. In the U.S. an estimated 800,000 to 2.2 million people have chronic HBV infection. About two thirds of them are unaware that they are infected.
- Africa, Asia, and the Western Pacific region are areas of high prevalence, ≥8%.
- Southern and Eastern Europe have intermediate rates, 2% to 7%.
- Chronically infected persons, those with positive HBsAg for >6 mo, represent the major source of infection.
- As many as 95% of infants and children aged <5, who typically have subclinical acute infection, will become chronic HBV carriers.
- Adults are more likely to have clinically evident acute infection, but only 1% to 5% will develop chronic infection.
- ~0.1% of patients with acute infection will develop fulminant acute hepatitis resulting in death.

PREDOMINANT SEX:

- Predominant in males because of increased IV drug abuse, homosexuality.
- Females more commonly terminate in chronic carrier state.

PREDOMINANT AGE: 20 to 45 yr

PEAK INCIDENCE: 30 to 45 yr of age, at rates of 5% to 20%

GENETICS: Neonatal infection:

- Rare in the U.S.
- High (up to 90%) in areas of high endemicity (only 5% to 10% of perinatal infections occur in utero).

PHYSICAL FINDINGS & CLINICAL PRESENTATION

- The incubation period of HBV infection is 4 to 24 wk. HBV infection presents as acute hepatitis in a minority of patients
- Patients often present with nonspecific symptoms
- Profound malaise (Fig. E1)

Many asymptomatic cases

- Prodrome:
  1. 15% to 20% serum sickness (urticaria, rash, arthralgia) during early HBsAg
  2. HBsAg-Ab complex disease (polyarteritis nodosa–arthritis, arteritis, glomerulonephritis)
- Hepatomegaly (87%) with right upper quadrant (RUQ) tenderness:
  1. Hepatic punch tenderness
  2. Splenomegaly: Rare (10% to 15%)
- Jaundice (30% of patients), dark urine, with occasional pruritus
- Variable fever (when present, generally precedes jaundice and rapidly declines following onset of icteric phase)
- Spider angiomata: Rare; resolves during recovery
- Rare polyarteritis nodosa, cryoglobulinemia

ETIOLOGY

- Caused by HBV (42-nm hepadnavirus with an outer surface coat [HBsAg], inner nucleocapsid core [HBcAg; HBeAg]; DNA polymerase; and partially double-stranded DNA genome). There are eight genotypes (A to H) based on nucleotide sequence. The prevalence of each genotype varies widely.
- Transmission by parenteral route (needle use, tattooing, ear piercing, acupuncture, transfusion of blood and blood products, hemodialysis, sexual contact), perinatal transmission.
- Infection may result from contact of infectious material with mucous membranes and open skin breaks (e.g., HBV is stable and can be transmitted from toothbrushes, utensils, razors, baby toys, assorted medical equipment [respirators, endoscopes]).
- Oral intake of infectious material may result in infection through breaks in the oral mucosa.
- Food or water are virtually never found to be sources of HBV infection.
- Infection occurs primarily in liver, where necrosis probably results from cytotoxic T-cell response, direct cytopathic effect of HBcAg (core antigen), high-level HBsAg (surface antigen) expression, or coinfection with delta (D) hepatitis virus (RNA delta core within HBsAg envelope).
- Recovery (>90%):
  1. Fulminant hepatitis occurring in <1% (especially if coinfected with hepatitis D); 80% fatal
  2. Unusual (5%) prolonged acute disease for 4 to 12 mo, with recovery
  3. Overall fatality increases with age and viral inoculation (e.g., transfusions)
- Chronic hepatitis B (CHB) infection (1% to 2%), four phases:
  1. Immune-tolerant phase: A highly replicative/low-inflammatory phase where HBV DNA levels are high (typically >1 million IU/ml), ALT levels are normal, and biopsies have minimal signs of significant inflammation or fibrosis.
     a. This phase can persist for years, especially in those infected prenatally.
     b. With age there is a likely transformation to an HBeAg-positive immune-active phase.
  2. HBeAg-positive immune-active phase: Elevated ALT and HBV DNA levels in conjunction with liver injury (≥20,000 IU/ml). Median age of onset is 30 yr in those infected at a young age. Biopsy will show moderate to severe inflammation or fibrosis.
  3. Inactive CHB phase: HBV DNA levels are low or undetectable (<2000 IU/ml), ALT levels are normal, and anti-HBe is present. Biopsy shows minimal necroinflammation but variable fibrosis.
  4. HBeAg-negative immune reactivation phase: Elevated ALT and elevated HBV DNA (≥2000 IU/ml). Biopsy will show moderate to severe necroinflammation and fibrosis.
- Table 1 summarizes causes of hepatitis flares in patients with CHB.
- The most feared complications of CHB are cirrhosis and hepatocellular carcinoma (HCC), which kill more than 300,000 people/yr globally. One quarter to one third of patients will go on to develop these complications. The risk of developing HCC appears to be greatest among individuals with the highest serum levels of HBV DNA.

TABLE 1 Causes of Hepatitis Flares in Patients with Chronic Hepatitis B

Cause of Flare	Comment
Spontaneous	Factors that precipitate viral replication are unclear
Immunosuppressive therapy	Flares are often observed during withdrawal of the agent; preemptive antiviral therapy is required
Antiviral therapy for HBV	
Interferon	Flares are often observed during the second to third mo of therapy in 30% of patients; may herald virologic response
Nucleoside analog	
During treatment	Flares are no more common than with placebo
Drug-resistant HBV	Severe consequences can occur in patients with advanced liver disease
On withdrawal	Flares are caused by the rapid reemergence of wild-type HBV; severe consequences can occur in patients with advanced liver disease
HIV treatment	Flares can occur as a result of the direct toxicity of HAART or with immune reconstitution; HBV increases the risk of antiretroviral drug hepatotoxicity
Genotypic variation	
Precore and core promoter mutants	Fluctuations in serum ALT levels are common with precore mutants
Superinfection with other hepatitis viruses	May be associated with suppression of HBV replication

ALT, Alanine aminotransferase; *HAART,* highly active antiretroviral therapy; *HBV,* hepatitis B virus; *HIV,* human immunodeficiency virus.
From Feldman M et al [eds]: *Sleisenger and Fordtran's gastrointestinal and liver disease,* ed 10, Philadelphia, 2016, Saunders.

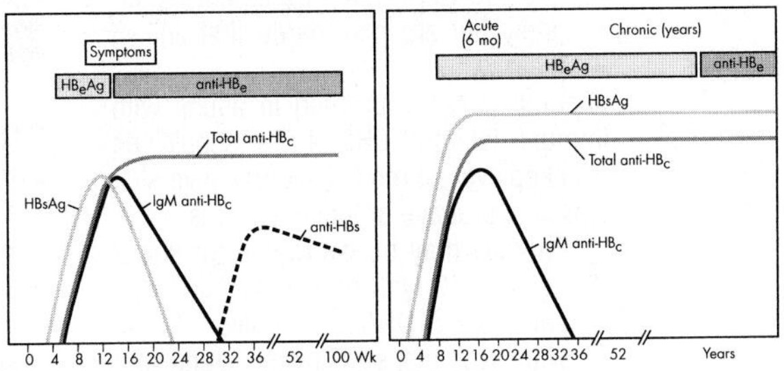

FIG. 2 Typical course of hepatitis B. *Left,* Typical course of acute hepatitis B. *Right,* Chronic hepatitis B. *HBc,* Hepatitis B core; *HBe,* hepatitis B early; *HBeAg,* hepatitis B early antigen; *HBs,* hepatitis B surface; *HBsAg,* hepatitis B surface antigen; *IgM,* immunoglobulin M. (From Mandell GL et al: *Principles and practice of infectious diseases,* ed 7, Philadelphia, 2010, Saunders.)

Dx DIAGNOSIS

DIFFERENTIAL DIAGNOSIS

- Acute disease confused with other viral hepatitis infections (A, C, D, E).
- Any viral illness producing systemic disease and hepatitis (e.g., yellow fever, EBV, CMV, HIV, rubella, rubeola, coxsackie B, adenovirus, herpes simplex or zoster).
- Nonviral causes of hepatitis (e.g., leptospirosis, toxoplasmosis, alcoholic hepatitis, drug-induced [e.g., acetaminophen, INH], toxic hepatitis [carbon tetrachloride, benzene]).

WORKUP

- Acute serum specimen for hepatitis B serology (HBsAg, HBsAb, HBcAb, HBeAg, HBeAb), HBDNA by PCR
- LFTs
- CBC
- Liver biopsy: Rarely indicated for diagnosis of fulminant viral hepatitis, chronic hepatitis, cirrhosis, carcinoma

LABORATORY TESTS

- Diagnosis of acute HBV infection is best confirmed by IgM HBcAb in acute or early convalescent serum or by HBDNA by PCR.
  1. Generally, IgM present during onset of jaundice
  2. Coexisting HBsAg
- HBsAg and IgG-HBcAb during acute jaundice are strongly suggestive of remote HBV infection and another cause for current illness (Fig. 2).
- HBsAb alone is suggestive of immunization response.
- With recovery, HBeAg is rapidly replaced by HBeAb in 2 to 3 mo, and HBsAg is replaced by HBsAb in 5 to 6 mo.
- In chronic HBV hepatitis, HBsAg and HBeAg are persistent without corresponding Ab.
- In chronic carrier state, HBsAg is persistent, but HBeAg is replaced by HBeAb.
- HBcAb develops in all outcomes.
- HBeAg correlation with highest infectivity; appearance of HBeAb heralds recovery.
- LFTs:
  1. ALT and AST: Usually more than eight times normal (often 1000 U/L) at onset of jaundice (minimal acute ALT/AST rises often followed by chronic hepatitis or hepatocellular carcinoma).
  2. Bilirubin: Variably elevated in icteric viral hepatitis.
  3. Alkaline phosphatase: Minimally elevated (one to three times normal) acutely.
- Albumin and prothrombin time:
  1. Generally normal
  2. If abnormal, possible harbinger of impending hepatic necrosis (fulminant hepatitis)
- WBC and ESR: Generally normal.

IMAGING STUDIES

- Sonogram to document rapid reduction in liver size during fulminant hepatitis or mass in hepatocellular carcinoma
- FibroScan (transient elastography): A noninvasive specialized ultrasound test to quantify liver fibrosis without liver biopsy

Rx TREATMENT

NONPHARMACOLOGIC THERAPY

- Symptomatic treatment as necessary
- Activity as tolerated
- High-calorie diet preferred; often best tolerated in morning

ACUTE GENERAL Rx

- In most cases of acute HBV infection, no treatment is necessary; >90% of adults will spontaneously clear infection.
- Hospitalization advisable for any patient in danger from dehydration caused by poor oral intake, whose PT is prolonged, who has rising bilirubin level >15 to 20 μg/dl, or who has any clinical evidence of hepatic failure.

TABLE 2 Indications for Prompt or Urgent Treatment of Hepatitis B

	Indications	Preferred Agent	Principal Supportive Data
Cirrhosis*			
Decompensated	Clinical stabilization; minimizing risk for recurrence after transplant	Entecavir (0.5 mg) or tenofovir (300 mg)†	Open label; multiple large case series
Borderline compensated	Forestalling disease progression; avoidance of transplantation	As above	Undefined
Well compensated	As above	As above	Randomized controlled trials
Acute Liver Failure			
HBV reactivation	Minimizing further liver injury; reducing risk of recurrence after liver transplantation, if needed	Entecavir (0.5 mg) or tenofovir (300 mg)†	Open label with comparison with historical controls
Severe acute hepatitis	Minimizing further liver injury and enhancing full recovery	Consider lamivudine or telbivudine‡	Small case series

HBV, Hepatitis B virus.
*It has been the author's (RP) practice to use maintenance antiviral therapy for all hepatitis B surface antigen (HBsAg)-positive patients with cirrhosis to prevent reactivation of hepatitis B.
†Daily dose should be adjusted according to the patient's renal function, as indicated in the manufacturer's recommendations.
‡Either agent can be used if the anticipated duration of therapy is 6 mo or less.
From Feldman M et al: *Sleisenger and Fordtran's gastrointestinal and liver disease,* ed 10, Philadelphia, 2016, Elsevier.

Table 2 summarizes indications for prompt or urgent treatment of hepatitis B.
- IV therapy needed (rarely) for hydration during severe vomiting.
- Avoid hepatically metabolized drugs.
- No therapeutic measures are beneficial.
- Steroids not shown helpful.

CHRONIC Rx

- Treatment of chronic HBV infection is dependent on which phase the patient is found to be in:
  1. Therapy is warranted for patients in immune-active CHB stage (HBeAg negative or HBeAg positive) to decrease the risk of liver-related complications. Treatment options include:
     a. Pegylated interferon 2a: 180 mcg subcutaneously weekly for 48 wk. This will lead to seroconversion rates of 20% to 30% (HBeAg to anti-HBe), and 65% of patients will have HBV DNA <2000 IU/ml off therapy but cure rates remain low at 3% to 7% and has significant side effects: Bone marrow suppression and exacerbation of existing neuropsychiatric symptoms, including depression. Candidates for interferon therapy should not have significant psychiatric disease, cardiac disease, cytopenia, seizure disorder, autoimmune disease, or pregnancy.
     b. Entecavir: A nucleotide analogue. Dose 0.5 to 1 mg daily, suppresses HBV DNA replication and improves liver inflammation and fibrosis.
     c. Tenofovir disoproxil: 300 mg daily, is another nucleotide analogue. A newer formulation, tenofovir alafenamide (Vemlidy) 25 mg a day, has less renal and bone toxicity in long-term use.
     d. Other nucleotide agents: Lamivudine, telbivudine, and adefovir are less frequently used due to issues of resistance.
     e. Cure rates with nucleotide agents are between 1% and 12%, and thus most patients will require treatment indefinitely but are considered first line of therapy.
  2. Therapy is not warranted in adults with immune-tolerant CHB. LFTs should be checked every 6 mo to look for conversion to immune-active or inactive status.
     a. Therapy may be warranted for select adults >40 with normal ALT and elevated HBV DNA (≥1 million IU/ml) with liver biopsy showing significant necroinflammation or fibrosis.
  3. HBeAg-positive adults without cirrhosis who seroconvert to anti-HBe on therapy with entecavir or tenofovir disoproxil can discontinue treatment after a period of treatment consolidation.
  4. It is recommended that patients receive indefinite therapy with entecavir or tenofovir disoproxil if HBeAg-negative immune-active CHB is present, unless there is a competing rationale for treatment discontinuation.
  5. Adults with compensated cirrhosis and low levels of viremia (<2000 IU/ml) should be treated with entecavir or tenofovir disoproxil to reduce the risk of decompensation, regardless of ALT level.

DISPOSITION

- Follow-up as outpatient
- Acute disease: Infection will resolve (defined as clearance of hepatitis B surface antigen within 6 mo) in 90% of adult patients
- Rare fatalities (fulminant hepatitis)
- Possible chronic carrier state, cirrhosis, hepatocellular carcinoma
- Cure of HBV is an unrealistic goal for most patients with chronic infection since only a few patients will become HBsAb with current treatment modalities

REFERRAL

To infectious disease specialist and gastroenterologist for consultation regarding fulminant hepatitis or prolonged cholestasis, for cases of uncertain etiology, or for treatment of CAH

PEARLS & CONSIDERATIONS

COMMENTS

- Virus and HBsAg in high titers in blood for 1 to 7 wk before jaundice and for a variable time thereafter.
- Screening (HBV surface antigen [HBsAg], HBV core antigen antibody, antibody to HBsAg) should be offered to high-risk groups.
- Transmission is possible during entire period of HBsAg (and especially during HBeAg) in serum.
- Universal precautions should be followed for all contacts with blood or secretions/excretions contaminated with blood.
- Antiviral therapy is recommended in pregnancy to reduce perinatal transmission if HBsAg positive and HBV DNA >200,000 IU/ml. Can use tenofovir disoproxil, lamivudine, or telbivudine. Tenofovir may be preferred because it has a better resistance profile and there are more safety data in pregnant women with hepatitis B. Fig. 3 describes an algorithm for the treatment of hepatitis B surface antigen (HBsAg)-positive mothers during pregnancy.
- Preventing before exposure:
  1. Lifestyle changes.
  2. Meticulous testing of blood supply (although some chronically infected, infectious donors are HBsAg negative).
  3. Sterilization via steam or hypochlorite.
  4. Hepatitis B vaccine for high-risk groups given IM in deltoid to induce HBsAb (response should be confirmed) is protective (>90% effective). Yeast-derived HBsAg vaccines include: Recombivax HB (10 mcg HBsAg/ml) and Engerix-B (20 mcg HBsAg/ml), each as a three-dose series over 6 mo. In 2017, the FDA approved a two-dose hepatitis B virus vaccine (HEPLISAV-B) that uses a novel immunostimulatory adjuvant for use in adults ≥18 yr old, administered at 0 and 1 mo.
  5. Recommendation for universal childhood immunization with doses at birth, 1 mo, and 6 mo.

- Prevention after exposure:
  1. HBV hyperimmune globulin (HBIG) (0.06 ml/kg IM) given immediately after needlestick, within 14 days of sexual exposure, or at birth, followed by HBV vaccination. A second dose of HBIG is given in 28 days for those refusing vaccine or vaccine non-responders.
  2. Standard immune globulin: Nearly as effective as HBIG.
- Preventive therapy with entecavir or tenofovir disoproxil for patients who test positive for HBsAg and are undergoing chemotherapy may reduce the risk for HBV reactivation and HBV-associated morbidity and mortality.
- Hepatitis B prophylaxis is described in Section V.
- Table 3 summarizes interpretation of serologic markers and serum DNA in hepatitis B.
- The U.S. Preventive Services Task Force (USPSTF) recommends screening for hepatitis B infection in adolescents and adults of high risk.[1] Patients at high risk include the following:
  1. People born in countries or area with HBV prevalence ≥ 2%
  2. People who were not vaccinated at birth and were both in the U.S. to parents who were born in countries or areas with prevalence >8%
  3. HIV-positive people
  4. Intravenous-drug users
  5. Men who have sex with men
  6. People who live in households with, or have sex with, HBV-positive people

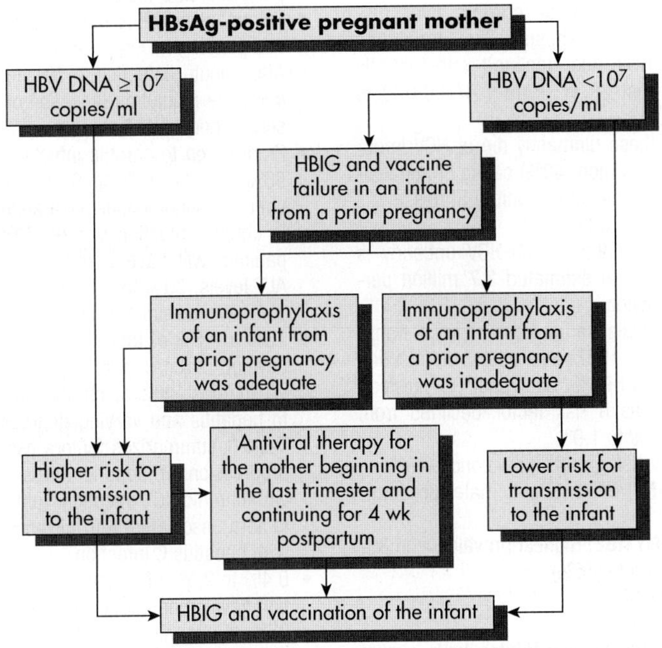

FIG. 3 Algorithm for the treatment of hepatitis B surface antigen (HBsAg)-positive mothers during pregnancy. The goal of treatment in highly viremic mothers is to lower the serum HBV DNA level by several $\log_{10}$ IU/ml by the time of delivery to minimize the chance of newborn infection. The choice of antiviral agent is less important if treatment of the mother is not needed long term. In the event that the treatment needs to be continued after delivery, the patient should be started on a high-genetic-barrier drug initially or switched to one immediately after delivery. See text for further details about drug selection. *DNA,* Deoxyribonucleic acid; *HBIG,* hepatitis B immune globulin; *HBV,* hepatitis B virus. (From Feldman M et al. [eds]: *Sleisenger and Fordtran's gastrointestinal and liver disease,* ed 10, Philadelphia, 2016, Saunders.)

SUGGESTED READINGS

Available at ExpertConsult.com

RELATED CONTENT

Hepatitis B (Patient Information)

AUTHOR: **Glenn G. Fort, MD, MPH**

[1] Krist AR et al: Screening for hepatitis B virus infection in adolescents and adults, U.S. Preventive Task Force recommendation statement, *JAMA* 324:2415-2422, 2020.

TABLE 3 Interpretation of Serologic Markers and Serum DNA in Hepatitis B

	HBsAg	HBeAg	Anti-HBc IgM	Anti-HBc IgG	Anti-HBs	Anti-HBe	HBV DNA*
Acute hepatitis	+	+/−	+				+
Acute hepatitis, window period			+				
Recovery from acute hepatitis			+	+	+	+/−	
Chronic hepatitis	+	+					+
Chronic hepatitis (precore mutant)	+					+	+
Inactive carrier	+					+/−	
Vaccinated					+		

anti-HBc IgG, Hepatitis B core antibody (IgG type); *anti-HBc IgM,* hepatitis B core antibody (IgM type); *anti-HBe,* hepatitis B early antibody; *anti-HBs,* hepatitis B surface antibody; *DNA,* deoxyribonucleic acid; *HBeAg,* hepatitis Be antigen; *HBsAg,* hepatitis B surface antigen; *HBV DNA,* hepatitis B viral DNA.
*HBV DNA >10^5 copies/ml.
From Andreoli TE et al: *Andreoli and Carpenter's Cecil essentials of medicine,* ed 8, Philadelphia, 2010, Saunders.

BASIC INFORMATION

DEFINITION

Hepatitis C is an acute liver parenchymal infection caused by hepatitis C virus (HCV).

SYNONYM

Transfusion-related non-A, non-B hepatitis (incubation period averages 6 wk, intermediate between hepatitis A and B)

ICD-10CM CODES

B17.1	Acute hepatitis C
B18.2	Chronic viral hepatitis C
B17.10	Acute hepatitis C without hepatic coma
B17.11	Acute hepatitis C with hepatic coma
B19.20	Unspecified viral hepatitis C without hepatic coma
B19.21	Unspecified viral hepatitis C with hepatic coma

EPIDEMIOLOGY & DEMOGRAPHICS

Hepatitis C infection is the most common chronic blood-borne infection in the United States. About 3% of baby boomers test positive for the virus. The CDC now recommends[1]

- Hepatitis C screening at least once in a lifetime for all adults ≥18 yr, except in settings where the prevalence of HCV is <0.1%
- Hepatitis C screening for all pregnant women during each pregnancy, except in settings where the prevalence of HCV infection is <0.1%
- Regardless of age or setting prevalence, all persons with risk factors should be tested for hepatitis C with periodic testing while risk factors persist
- Any person who requests hepatitis C testing should receive it, regardless of disclosure risk, because many persons might be reluctant to disclose stigmatizing risk

[1]Schillie S et al: CDC Recommendations for Hepatitis C Screening Among Adults — United States, 2020, *MMWR* 69:1-17, 2020.

The U.S. Preventive Services Task Force (USPSTF) recommends screening of all adults 18 to 79 yr for hepatitis C infection.[2]

INCIDENCE: HCV infects more than 185 million individuals worldwide. Approximately 20% of patients chronically infected with HCV progress to cirrhosis.

- 150,000 new cases/yr (37,500 symptomatic; 93,000 later chronic liver disease; 30,700 cirrhosis). The incidence of acute HCV has declined substantially over the past 30 yr (from 7.4/100,000 to 0.7/100,000).
- ~9000 of these ultimately die of HCV infection; most common (40%) cause of nonalcoholic liver disease in the United States.

PREVALENCE (IN U.S.):

- Overall prevalence of anti-HCV antibody is 1% to 1.2% (an estimated 2.7 million persons nationwide).
- Highest prevalence in hemophiliacs transfused before 1987 and users of injection drugs, 72% to 90%. Over past 30 yr, blood transfusion as a risk factor declined from 15% of cases to 1.9%.
- Among low-risk groups, prevalence 0.6%.

PREDOMINANT SEX: Slight male predominance.

PREDOMINANT AGE: Highest prevalence in 30- to 49-yr age group (65%).

PEAK INCIDENCE:

- 20 to 39 yr of age.
- African Americans and Whites have similar incidence of acute disease; Hispanics have higher rates.
- Prevalence is substantially higher among non-Hispanic Blacks than among non-Hispanic Whites.

GENETICS: Neonatal infection is rare; increased risk with maternal HIV-1 coinfection.

[2]US Preventive Services Task Force; Owens DK et al: Screening for Hepatitis C Virus Infection in Adolescents and Adults: US Preventive Services Task Force Recommendation Statement, *JAMA* [Epub ahead of print]. doi: 10.1001/jama.2020.1123.

TABLE 1 Factors Associated with Progression of Hepatic Fibrosis in Patients with Chronic Hepatitis C Virus Infection

Established	Possible	Not Associated
Age >40 yr	Increased hepatic iron concentration	Viral genotype
Alcohol consumption	Male gender	Viral load
Hepatitis B virus coinfection	Serum ALT level	
HIV coinfection		
Immunosuppressed state		
Insulin resistance		
Marijuana use		
Obesity		
Schistosomiasis		
Severe hepatic necroinflammation		
Smoking		
White race		

ALT, Alanine aminotransferease; *HIV,* human immunodeficiency virus.
From Feldman M et al [eds]: *Sleisenger and Fordtran's gastrointestinal and liver disease,* ed 10, Philadelphia, 2016, Saunders.

PHYSICAL FINDINGS & CLINICAL PRESENTATION

- Symptoms usually develop 7 to 8 wk after infection (range of 2 to 26 wk), but 70% to 80% of cases are subclinical.
- 10% to 20% report acute illness with jaundice and nonspecific symptoms (abdominal pain, anorexia, malaise).
- Fulminant hepatitis may rarely occur during this period.
- After acute infection, 15% to 25% have complete resolution (absence of HCV RNA in serum, normal ALT).
- Progression to chronic infection is common, 50% to 84%. 74% to 86% have persistent viremia; spontaneous clearance of viremia in chronic infection is rare. 60% to 70% of patients will have persistent or fluctuating ALT levels; 30% to 40% with chronic infection have normal ALT levels.
- 15% to 20% of those with chronic HCV will develop cirrhosis over a period of 20 to 30 yr; in most others, chronic infection leads to hepatitis and varying degrees of fibrosis. Table 1 summarizes factors associated with progression of hepatic fibrosis in patients with chronic HCV infection. Table 2 describes factors associated with cirrhosis in persons with hepatitis C infection.
- 0.4% to 2.5% of patients with chronic infection develop hepatocellular carcinoma (HCC).
- 25% of patients with chronic infection continue to have an asymptomatic course with normal LFTs and benign histology.
- In chronic HCV infection, extrahepatic sequelae include a variety of immunologic and lymphoproliferative disorders (e.g., cryoglobulinemia, membranoproliferative glomerulonephritis, and possibly Sjögren syndrome, autoimmune thyroiditis, polyarteritis nodosa, aplastic anemia, lichen planus, porphyria cutanea tarda, B-cell lymphoma, others).
- Fig. 1 illustrates the natural history of HCV infection.

ETIOLOGY

- Caused by HCV (single-stranded RNA flavivirus). HCV genotype 1 accounts for about 75% of HCV in the U.S. Genotypes 2 and 3 account for about 20% to 25% of infections, genotype 4 for 6%, and genotypes 5 and 6 for about 1%.
- Most HCV transmission is parenteral.
- In the United States, advances in screening of blood and blood products have made transfusion-related HCV infection rare (the risk is estimated to be 0.001% per unit transfused).
- Injecting-drug use accounts for most HCV transmission in the United States (60% of newly acquired cases, 20%-50% of chronically infected persons).
- Occupational needlestick exposure from an HCV-positive source has a seroconversion rate of 1.8% (range 0%-7%).
- Nosocomial transmission rates (from surgery and procedures such as colonoscopy and hemodialysis) are extremely low.
- Sexual transmission and maternal-fetal transmission are infrequent (estimated at 5%).

TABLE 2 Factors Associated with Cirrhosis in Persons with Hepatitis C Infection

Factor	Impact	Comment
Environmental		
Alcohol use	+4	The importance of minimal alcohol ingestion (<20 g/day) has not been established
Host		
HIV infection	+4	Increasingly important as HIV-related survival improves; may be masked by competing mortality
HBV infection	+3	Strong effect when HBsAg positive; relatively uncommon
Age	+4	Strong effect; increases as low as 40 yr. Hard to distinguish from infection duration
Body mass index	+2	Associated with metabolic syndrome
Duration of HCV infection	+3	Cirrhosis is rare before 10 yr
HLA type	+1?	HLA B54 is correlated with increased risk of cirrhosis; DRB1*0301 with lack of cirrhosis
Viral		
Quasispecies complexity	+1	Cross-sectional studies cannot assess causality, and complexity may be confounded by duration of infection
HCV genotype 1	+1?	Genotype 1b in some, but not other studies, could be confounded by longer duration of 1b infections
Quantitative measures of viremia (serum or plasma HCV RNA level)	+2	Not always detected or lost in multivariate analysis of age or HIV

HCV, Hepatitis C virus; *HIV,* human immunodeficiency virus; *HLA,* human leukocyte antigen; *RNA,* ribonucleic acid.
From Bennett JE et al: *Mandell, Douglas, and Bennett's principles and practice of infectious diseases,* ed 8, Philadelphia, 2015, Saunders.

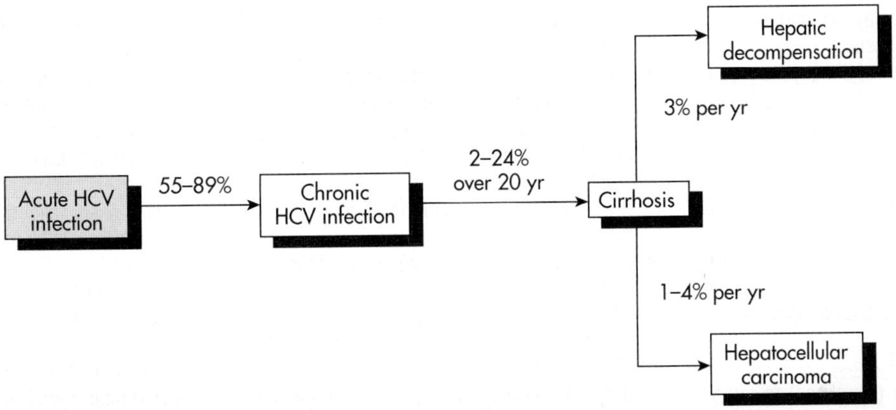

FIG. 1 Natural history of HCV infection. Hepatic decompensation includes ascites, hepatic encephalopathy, variceal hemorrhage, hepatorenal syndrome, or hepatic synthetic dysfunction. *HCV,* Hepatitis C virus. (From Feldman M et al [eds]: *Sleisenger and Fordtran's gastrointestinal and liver disease,* ed 10, Philadelphia, 2016, Saunders.)

- No identifiable risk in 40% to 50% of community-acquired hepatitis C, but snorting of cocaine by shared use of straw or rolled-up paper has been identified as a risk factor because it causes microscopic bleeding of nasal mucosa.
- HCV infection may stimulate production of cytotoxic T lymphocytes and cytokines (INF-γ), which probably mediate hepatic necrosis.

Dx DIAGNOSIS

DIFFERENTIAL DIAGNOSIS

- Other hepatitis viruses (A, B, D, E).
- Other viral illnesses producing systemic disease (e.g., yellow fever, EBV, CMV, HIV, rubella, rubeola, coxsackie B, adenovirus, HSV, HZV).
- Nonviral hepatitis (e.g., leptospirosis, toxoplasmosis, alcoholic hepatitis, drug-induced hepatitis [acetaminophen, INH], toxic hepatitis).

WORKUP

- Acute hepatitis C antibody, viral genotyping, viral titers.
- LFTs; CBC.

NOTE: ALT is an easy and inexpensive test to monitor infection and efficacy of therapy. However, ALT levels may fluctuate or even be normal in active or chronic infection and even with cirrhosis, and ALT may remain elevated even after clearance of viremia.

- Liver biopsy with histologic staging had been the gold standard for assessing the degree of disease activity and the likelihood of disease progression, and also to help rule out other causes of liver disease.
- Transient elastography (FibroScan) is a noninvasive specialized ultrasound assessment that quantifies liver fibrosis and corresponds it to the equivalent in the METAVIR scoring system traditionally used in liver biopsies. It is being increasingly used in place of liver biopsy in many institutions.

LABORATORY TESTS

- Diagnosis is often by exclusion, because it takes 6 wk to 12 mo to develop anti-HCV antibody (70% positive by 6 wk, 90% positive by 6 mo).
- Diagnostic tests include serologic assays for antibodies and molecular tests for viral particles.
  1. Enzyme immunoassay is the test for anti-HCV antibody:
     a. The current version can detect antibody within 4 to 10 wk after infection.
     b. False-negative rate in low-risk populations is 0.5% to 1%.
     c. False negatives also occur in immune-compromised persons, HIV-1, renal failure, HCV-associated essential mixed cryoglobulinemia.
     d. False positives in autoimmune hepatitis, paraproteinemia, and persons with no risk factors.
- The recombinant immunoblot assay that was previously recommended as a follow-up to positive antibody test is no longer available. The CDC now recommends that anyone who tests positive for HCV antibodies receive a follow-up HCV RNA test.
- Qualitative and quantitative HCV RNA tests using PCR: Lower limit of detection is <43 IU/ml.
- Used to confirm viremia and to assess response to treatment.
- Qualitative polymerase chain reaction (PCR) useful in patients with negative enzyme immunoassay in whom infection is suspected.

- Quantitative tests use either branched-chain DNA or reverse transcription PCR; the latter is more sensitive.
- Viral genotyping can distinguish among genotypes 1, 2, 3, 4, 5, and 6, which is helpful in choosing therapy; most of these tests use PCR. Genotypes 1, 2, 3, and 4 predominate in the United States and Europe (genotype 1 is especially common in North America [60%-75% of Hep C infections in the United States]).
- FibroSure score uses a combination of six serum markers of liver function plus age and gender in a patented algorithm to generate a measure of fibrosis and necroinflammatory activity in the liver as a quantitative surrogate marker for the corresponding METAVIR scoring system.
- LFTs: ALT and AST may be elevated to more than eight times normal in acute infection; in chronic infection ALT may be normal or fluctuate.
- Bilirubin may be five to 10 times normal.
- Albumin and prothrombin time generally normal; if abnormal, may be harbinger of impending hepatic necrosis.
- WBC and erythrocyte sedimentation rate (ESR) are generally normal.
- HIV testing. Infection with HCV is seen in 15% to 30% of individuals with HIV infection due to shared risk factors.
- All patients infected with HCV should be tested for Hepatitis B. HBV vaccination is recommended for susceptible individuals, because HBV reactivation may occur during treatment of HCV with direct-acting antiviral therapy.

IMAGING STUDIES

- Transient elastography (FibroScan) to quantify liver fibrosis as an absolute score. Some insurance companies use this score as a basis to determine eligibility for treatment.
- Sonogram: Rapid liver size reduction during fulminant hepatitis or mass in HCC.

Rx TREATMENT

NONPHARMACOLOGIC THERAPY

Activity and diet as tolerated; avoid saw palmetto and green tea leaf herbs.

ACUTE GENERAL Rx

- Supportive care.
- Avoid hepatically metabolized drugs.

CHRONIC Rx

Response to therapy is influenced by HCV genotype. Recommendations for the treatment of hepatitis C in adults are changing constantly as new therapies come to the market. The advent of direct-acting antiviral agents (DAAs) has drastically changed treatment options and improved cure rates to greater than 95%. The most up-to-date guidance is available at the website www.hcvguidelines.org. The following is a brief summary of the guidelines based on genotype. Newer agents containing fixed-dose combinations of direct-acting antiviral (DAA) drugs have been approved for HCV infections caused by any of the six major HCV genotypes in patients without cirrhosis or with compensated cirrhosis. These agents are Mavyret (combination of glecaprevir, an HCV NS3/4A protease inhibitor; and pibrentasvir, an NS5A inhibitor) and Vosevi (combination of the NS5B nucleotide polymerase inhibitor sofosbuvir, the NS5A inhibitor velpatasvir, and the NS3/4A protease inhibitor voxilaprevir). Both agents are approved for use in treatment-experienced patients and Mavyret is also approved for treatment-naïve patients. Currently, these treatment regimens are extremely expensive.

Genotype 1a: Options for treatment-naïve patients without cirrhosis, listed by level of evidence:

- Daily fixed-dose combination of elbasvir (50 mg)/grazoprevir (100 mg) (Zepatier) for 12 wk and in those who do not have baseline NS5A RAVs (amino acid substitutions at 28, 30, 31, or 93 that confer resistance to elbasvir). Rating: Class I, Level A.
- Daily fixed-dose combination of glecaprevir (300 mg)/pibrentasvir (120 mg) (Mavyret) for 8 wk. Rating: Class I, Level A.
- Daily fixed-dose combination of ledipasvir (90 mg)/sofosbuvir (400 mg) (Harvoni) for 12 wk. Rating: Class I, Level A. (Can also use this regimen for only 8 wk for patients who are non-Black, HIV-uninfected, and whose HCV RNA level is <6 million IU/ml. Rating: Class I, Level B.)
- Daily fixed-dose combination of sofosbuvir (400 mg)/velpatasvir (100 mg) (Epclusa) for 12 wk. Rating: Class I, Level A.

Genotype 1a: Options for treatment-naïve patients with compensated cirrhosis:

- Daily fixed-dose combination of elbasvir (50 mg)/grazoprevir (100 mg) [Zepatier] and in those in whom no baseline NS5A RAVs for elbasvir are detected for 12 wk. Rating: Class I, Level A.
- Daily fixed-dose combination of glecaprevir (300 mg)/pibrentasvir (120 mg) [Mavyret] for 12 wk. Rating: Class I, Level A.
- Daily fixed-dose combination of ledipasvir (90 mg)/sofosbuvir (400 mg) [Harvoni] for 12 wk. Rating: Class I, Level A.
- Daily fixed-dose combination of sofosbuvir (400 mg)/velpatasvir (100 mg) [Epclusa] for 12 wk. Rating: Class I, Level A.

Genotype 1b: Treatment-naïve patients without cirrhosis:

- Daily fixed-dose combination of elbasvir (50 mg)/grazoprevir (100 mg) [Zepatier] for 12 wk. Rating: Class I, Level A.
- Daily fixed-dose combination of glecaprevir (300 mg)/pibrentasvir (120 mg) [Mavyret] for 8 wk. Rating: Class I, A.
- Daily fixed-dose combination of ledipasvir (90 mg)/sofosbuvir (400 mg) [Harvoni] for 12 wk. Rating: Class I, Level A. (Can treat for 8 wk in patients who are non-Black, HIV-uninfected, and whose HCV RNA level is <6 million IU/ml. Class I, Level B.)
- Daily fixed-dose combination of sofosbuvir (400 mg)/velpatasvir (100 mg) [Epclusa] for 12 wk. Rating: Class I, Level A.

Genotype 1b: Treatment-naïve patients with compensated cirrhosis:

- Daily fixed-dose combination of elbasvir (50 mg)/grazoprevir (100 mg) [Zepatier] for 12 wk. Rating: Class I, Level A.
- Daily fixed-dose combination of glecaprevir (300 mg)/pibrentasvir (120 mg) [Mavyret] for 12 wk. Rating: Class I, Level A.
- Daily fixed-dose combination of ledipasvir (90 mg)/sofosbuvir [Harvoni] for 12 wk. Rating: Class I, Level A.
- Daily fixed-dose combination of sofosbuvir (400 mg)/velpatasvir (100 mg) [Epclusa] for 12 wk. Rating: Class I, Level A.

Genotype 2: Treatment-naïve regimens without cirrhosis:

- Daily fixed-dose combination of glecaprevir (300 mg)/pibrentasvir (120 mg) [Mavyret] for 8 wk. Rating: Class I, Level A.
- Daily fixed-dose combination of sofosbuvir (400 mg)/velpatasvir (100 mg) [Epclusa] for 12 wk. Rating: Class I, Level A.

Genotype 2: Treatment-naïve patients with compensated cirrhosis:

- Daily fixed-dose combination of sofosbuvir (400 mg)/velpatasvir (100 mg) [Epclusa] for 12 wk. Rating: Class I, Level A.
- Daily fixed-dose combination of glecaprevir (300 mg)/pibrentasvir (120 mg) for 12 wk. Rating: Class I, Level B.

Genotype 3: Treatment-naïve patients without cirrhosis:

- Daily fixed-dose of glecaprevir (300 mg)/pibrentasvir (120 mg) for 8 wk. Rating: Class I, Level A.
- Daily fixed-dose combination of sofosbuvir (400 mg)/velpatasvir (100 mg) [Epclusa] for 12 wk. Rating: Class I, Level A.

Genotype 3: Treatment-naïve patients with compensated cirrhosis:

- Daily fixed-dose combination of glecaprevir (300 mg)/pibrentasvir (120 mg) [Mavyret] for 12 wk. Rating: Class I, Level A.
- Daily fixed-dose combination of sofosbuvir (400 mg)/velpatasvir (100 mg) [Epclusa] for 12 wk. Rating: Class I, Level A.
- Alternative regimens:
  1. Daily fixed-dose combination of sofosbuvir (400 mg)/velpatasvir (100 mg)/voxilaprevir (100 mg) [Vosevi] when Y93H amino acid substitution is present for 12 wk. Rating: IIa, Level B.
  2. Daily fixed-dose combination of sofosbuvir (400 mg)/velpatasvir (100 mg) [Epclusa] with weight-based ribavirin for patients with baseline NS5A RAS Y93H for velatasvir for 12 wk. Rating: Class IIa, Level A.

Genotype 4: Treatment-naïve patients without cirrhosis:

- Daily fixed-dose combination of glecaprevir (300 mg)/pibrentasvir (120 mg) {Mavyret] for 8 wk. Rating: Class I Level A.
- Daily fixed-dose combination of sofosbuvir (400 mg)/velpatasvir (100 mg) [Epclusa] for 12 wk. Rating: Class I, Level A.
- Daily fixed-dose combination of elbasvir (50 mg)/grazoprevir (100 mg) [Zepatier] for 12 wk. Rating: Class IIa, Level B.
- Daily fixed-dose combination of ledipasvir (90 mg)/sofosbuvir (400 mg) [Harvoni] for 12 wk. Rating: Class IIa, Level B.

Genotype 4: Treatment-naïve patients with compensated cirrhosis:

- Daily fixed-dose combination of sofosbuvir (400 mg)/velpatasvir (100 mg) [Epclusa] for 12 wk. Rating: Class I, Level A.
- Daily fixed-dose combination of glecaprevir (300 mg)/pibrentasvir (120 mg) [Mavyret] for 12 wk. Rating: Class I, Level B.
- Daily fixed-dose combination of elbasvir (50 mg)/grazoprevir (100 mg) [Zepatier] for 12 wk. Rating: Class IIa, Level B.
- Daily fixed-dose combination of ledipasvir (90 mg)/sofosbuvir (400 mg) [Harvoni] for 12 wk. Rating: Class IIa, Level B.

Genotypes 5 and 6: Treatment-naïve patients with and without compensated cirrhosis:

- Daily fixed-dose combination of glecaprevir (300 mg)/pibrentasvir (120 mg) for 8 wk Rating: Class I, Level A
- Daily fixed-dose combination of sofosbuvir (400 mg)/velpatasvir (100 mg) [Epclusa] for 12 wk. Rating: Class I, Level B.
- Daily fixed-dose combination of ledipasvir (90 mg)/sofosbuvir (400 mg) [Harvoni] for 12 wk. Rating: Class IIa, Level B.

Drug interactions can be significant with these regimens (www.hep-druginteractions.org/). With DAA regimens, viral loads are measured at 4 wk into the therapy to monitor success and at the end of therapy. A final viral load is measured 12 wk after completing the treatment, and if undetectable, the patient is considered to have a sustained virologic response (SVR), which equates to a cure.

For *treatment-experienced* patients there are guidelines per genotype as well (www.hcvguidelines.org). Treatment is based on genotype and whether the patient is without cirrhosis or with compensated cirrhosis. Regimen will depend on whether the patient had been exposed in the past to interferon/ribavirin-based regimens, NS3 protease inhibitors regimens (telaprevir, boceprevir, simeprevir), or DAA agents.

Determination of Cirrhosis: Liver biopsy is not required. A patient is presumed to have cirrhosis if they have a FIB-4 Score >3.25 or any of the following findings from a previously performed test:

- Transient elastography indicating cirrhosis (e.g., Fibroscan stiffness >12.5 kPA)
- Fibrosure score >0.58 warrants treatment by most insurers. A score of 0.72 to 0.74 equals to a Stage 3 Metavir and >0.74 Stage 4 cirrhosis
- Clinical evidence of cirrhosis (liver nodularity and/or splenomegaly on imaging, platelet <150,000/mm^3
- Prior liver biopsy showing cirrhosis

$$\text{FIB-4 Score} = \frac{\text{Age (Years)} \times \text{AST Level (U/L)}}{\text{Platelet count } (10^9/\text{L}) \times \sqrt{\text{ALT}\left(\frac{\text{U}}{\text{L}}\right)}}$$

In 2017, a new salvage regimen was approved: Once-daily Vosevi (fixed-dose combination of 100-mg voxilaprevir (HCV NS3/4A protease inhibitor) plus 400-mg sofosbuvir and 100-mg velpatasvir. Eligible patients include:

- Genotypes 1, 2, 3, 4, 5, or 6 in patients previously treated with a regimen containing an NS5A inhibitor for 12 wk (NOTE: In clinical trials, prior experience with NS5A inhibitors included daclatasvir, elbasvir, ledipasvir, ombitasvir, or velpatasvir.)
- Genotype 1a or 3 in patients previously treated with sofosbuvir without an NS5A inhibitor for 12 wk. (NOTE: In clinical trials, prior treatment experience included sofosbuvir with or without any of the following: Peginterferon alfa/ribavirin, ribavirin, HCV NS3/4A protease inhibitors: Boceprevir, simeprevir, or telaprevir.)
- Liver transplantation:
  1. Hepatitis C is the main indication for liver transplantation in the United States.
  2. It is the only option for patients with deteriorating HCV-related cirrhosis and for some patients with HCC.
  3. Recurrent infection occurs in almost all patients with progressive fibrosis and cirrhosis; as many as 20% progress to cirrhosis within 5 yr posttransplant.

DISPOSITION

- The absence of HCV RNA in blood 12 wk after completion of treatment is considered a cure. There is no need to check HCV antibodies since they will remain positive indefinitely.
- SVR after treatment among HCV-infected persons at any stage of fibrosis is associated with reduced HCC.
- Periodic abdominal ultrasonography for HCC screening (with or without alpha-feto protein testing) every 6 mo is recommended in patients with cirrhosis even after obtaining virologic cure.

REFERRAL

- To a hepatologist or infectious disease specialist for treatment for hepatitis C in patients who have been previously treated or for treatment failures with DAA agents.
- To a transplant surgeon for consideration of liver transplant if indicated.

PEARLS & CONSIDERATIONS

- More rapid progression of disease in persons who drink alcohol regularly, persons of advanced age at time of infection, and those coinfected with other viruses (HIV, hepatitis B). All persons with identified HCV infection should receive a brief alcohol screening and intervention as clinically indicated.
- Regression of cirrhosis has been demonstrated after antiviral therapy in some patients with chronic hepatitis C. Regression is associated with decreased disease-related morbidity and improved survival.
- The presence of interleukin (IL)-28B and HLA class II is independently associated with spontaneous resolution of HCV infection, and single nucleotide polymorphism IL-28B and DQB1*03:01 may explain approximately 15% of spontaneous resolution of HCV infection.

RELATED CONTENT

Hepatitis C (Patient Information)

SUGGESTED READINGS

Available at ExpertConsult.com

AUTHOR: **Glenn G. Fort, MD, MPH**

BASIC INFORMATION

DEFINITION

Hepatocellular carcinoma (HCC) is a malignant neoplasm of the hepatocytes.

SYNONYMS

Hepatoma
HCC

EPIDEMIOLOGY & DEMOGRAPHICS

HCC is the seventh most common cancer worldwide (~841,000 new cases/yr) and the third most common cause of cancer deaths (~781,000 deaths/yr). Incidence varies worldwide:

- 85% of patients with hepatocellular carcinoma have cirrhosis
- Areas with high rates of hepatitis B and C (East Asia, sub-Saharan Africa) have highest incidence
- Males more affected than females, with ratios between 2:1 and 4:1
- Peak incidence: Fifth and sixth decades in Western countries, earlier in areas with perinatal transmission of hepatitis B
- Incidence has grown in the U.S. due to chronic hepatitis C, increasing nonalcoholic fatty liver disease (NAFLD), metabolic syndrome, obesity, and diabetes mellitus
  1. During the past two decades, the incidence in the U.S. doubled. The incidence in the U.S. is expected to increase to 38,350 cases by 2020 and 56,200 cases by 2030. HCC is the fastest-rising cause of cancer-related deaths in the U.S.
  2. The greatest proportional increase has been among Hispanics and whites between 45 and 60 yr of age.
  3. Mean age of diagnosis approximately 65 yr.
- Risk factors:
  1. Chronic hepatitis B infection accounts for 50% of all cases and most childhood cases
  2. Chronic hepatitis C infection markers are found in 80% to 90% of patients with HCC in Japan and 30% to 50% in the U.S.
  3. Cirrhosis from other causes: Alcoholic liver disease, nonalcoholic steatohepatitis, primary biliary cirrhosis, hemochromatosis, α1-antitrypsin deficiency, and autoimmune hepatitis
  4. Hepatotoxins: Aflatoxin B1
  5. Systemic diseases affecting the liver: Tyrosinemia
  6. Obesity and diabetes mellitus

PHYSICAL FINDINGS & CLINICAL PRESENTATION

- One third of patients are asymptomatic.
- Abdominal pain may be the initial presentation.
- Signs of underlying cirrhosis and portal hypertension are often present.
- Previously compensated cirrhosis with new ascites, encephalopathy, jaundice, or bleeding.
- Paraneoplastic syndromes (hypoglycemia, erythrocytosis, hypercalcemia, severe diarrhea, dermatomyositis) may be present. Box 1 summarizes paraneoplastic syndromes associated with hepatocellular carcinoma.
- Table 1 summarizes symptoms and signs of hepatocellular carcinoma.

Dx DIAGNOSIS

DIFFERENTIAL DIAGNOSIS

- Metastatic cancers to liver
- Intrahepatic cholangiocarcinoma
- Benign liver neoplasms (adenomas, focal nodular hyperplasia, and hemangiomas)
- Focal fatty infiltration

WORKUP

- History regarding risk factors
- Physical examination with attention to signs of chronic liver disease
- Laboratory evaluation and imaging studies
- Imaging studies: Ultrasound for initial testing; 3-phase CT scan or dynamic contrast-enhanced MRI

BOX 1 Paraneoplastic Syndromes Associated with Hepatocellular Carcinoma

Carcinoid syndrome
Hypercalcemia
Hypertension
Hypertrophic osteoarthropathy
Hypoglycemia
Neuropathy
Osteoporosis
Polycythemia (erythrocytosis)
Polymyositis
Porphyria
Sexual changes—isosexual precocity, gynecomastia, feminization
Thyrotoxicosis
Thrombophlebitis migrans
Watery diarrhea syndrome

From Feldman M et al: *Sleisenger and Fordtran's gastrointestinal and liver disease,* ed 10, Philadelphia, 2016, Elsevier.

TABLE 1 Symptoms and Signs of Hepatocellular Carcinoma

Symptom	Frequency (%)
Abdominal pain	59-95
Weight loss	34-71
Weakness	22-53
Abdominal swelling	28-43
Nonspecific GI symptoms	25-28
Jaundice	5-26
Sign	
Hepatomegaly	54-98
Ascites	35-61
Fever	11-54
Splenomegaly	27-42
Wasting	25-41
Jaundice	4-35
Hepatic bruit	6-25

GI, Gastrointestinal.
From Feldman M et al: *Sleisenger and Fordtran's gastrointestinal and liver disease,* ed 10, Philadelphia, 2016, Elsevier.

LABORATORY TESTS

- Liver function tests.
- α-Fetoprotein (AFP) levels can be elevated in 70% of patients. An AFP level >400 ng/ml is highly suggestive of HCC; however, elevations may not be seen in up to 40% of patients with small lesions (1-2 cm).
- Paraneoplastic syndromes associated with HCC may cause hypercalcemia, hypoglycemia, and polycythemia.
- Elevated serum HBV DNA level (≥10,000 copies/ml) is a strong risk predictor of HCC independent of HBeAg, serum aminotransferase level, and liver cirrhosis.

IMAGING STUDIES

Ultrasound (US), CT scan (Fig. E1), or MRI. Ultrasound is most commonly used as a screening test for HCC in high-risk patients every 6 mo. Fig. E2 shows a laparoscopic view of a cirrhotic liver with a nodular hepatoma.

The following imaging modalities are recommended based on US findings:

- Hepatic lesion <1 cm needs to be followed with a repeat US every 3 mo to ensure the lesion does not change in size. If stable for 24 mo, the interval for US can be increased to every 6 mo.
- Hepatic lesion >1 cm needs further confirmatory imaging with either a CT scan or an MRI scan. If the chosen imaging modality shows characteristics typical of HCC (hypervascular in the arterial phase with washout in the portal venous or delayed phase) the diagnosis of HCC is confirmed with no need for additional diagnostic testing or biopsy. If the imaging modality is inconclusive or atypical for HCC, then the alternate imaging test must be performed. If the second imaging modality is also inconclusive, an image-guided biopsy is recommended.

BIOPSY: Percutaneous biopsy under ultrasound or CT scan is obtained in the event that imaging studies are nondiagnostic or atypical for HCC, or if no cirrhosis is present. Negative biopsy results should be followed and the hepatic nodule reassessed every 3 to 6 mo until it is no longer seen, enlarges, or shows diagnostic characteristics.

SCREENING: Screening high-risk patients with US every 6 mo is currently recommended to identify early-stage HCC. The use of AFP in addition to US is debatable; though it does increase detection rate it also increases false-positive results. The use of AFP alone should be discouraged due to limited sensitivity and specificity. Patients on transplant waiting lists should be regularly screened for HCC because in the U.S. the development of HCC gives increased priority for liver transplantation. Screening for HCC is recommended in the following groups:

- Hepatitis B carriers (HBsAg positive): Asian males >40 yr, Asian females >50 yr, all cirrhotic hepatitis B carriers, family history

of HCC and North American blacks/Africans older than age 20 yr
- Cirrhosis (nonhepatitis B): Hepatitis C, alcoholic cirrhosis, hemochromatosis, primary biliary cirrhosis, and possibly α1-antitrypsin deficiency, autoimmune hepatitis, and nonalcoholic steatohepatitis

STAGING: The commonly used Barcelona Clinic Liver Cancer (BCLC) staging system includes patient performance status, cancer symptoms, number and size of nodules, and liver function. The TNM staging classification is described in Table 2.

Treatment is determined according to stage (Fig. 3):
- Early stage (A): Asymptomatic single tumor 5 cm or 3 nodules, each ≤3 cm
- Intermediate stage (B): Patients with tumors that exceed early criteria but do not yet show cancer-related symptoms, vascular invasion, or metastases
- Advanced stage (C): Patients with mild cancer-related symptoms and/or vascular invasion or extrahepatic spread
- End-stage (D): Patients with advanced, symptomatic disease

Rx TREATMENT

- Treatment options for hepatocellular carcinoma are summarized in Table 3. Fig. 4 describes a treatment algorithm for HCC.
- Early stage: Curative treatment (surgical resection or liver transplantation). Patients who have a single lesion can be offered surgical resection if they are noncirrhotic or have cirrhosis with well-preserved liver function, normal bilirubin, and no significant portal hypertension. Liver transplantation is an effective option for patients with HCC corresponding to the Milan criteria (Table 4). Living donor transplantation can be offered for HCC if the waiting time is expected to be long. Local ablation is safe and effective therapy for patients who cannot undergo resection or as a bridge to transplantation. With these options, survival at 5 yr ranges from 50% to 70%. Radiofrequency ablation (RFA) is used in patients with early HCC who are not surgical candidates, and very high local control rates at 2 yr are obtained (>90%), but eventual recurrence rates can approach 70% at 5 yr.
- Intermediate stage: Transarterial chemoembolization (TACE) is recommended as first-line, noncurative therapy for nonsurgical patients with large/multifocal HCC who do not have vascular invasion or extrahepatic spread. More recently, transarterial use of selective internal radiation therapy (SIRT) with yttrium-90 radiolabeled glass microspheres is an alternative to traditional TACE approaches in this setting. Median survivals exceed 2 yr.
- Advanced stage: Multiple options for advanced HCC have been tested and approved in the last few years including targeted therapy, antiangiogenic therapy, and immunotherapy.
- First-line therapy:
  1. Sorafenib and lenvatinib are oral multikinase inhibitors, which are both approved as standard first-line therapy options.
  2. In untreated patients with unresectable hepatocellular carcinoma, the checkpoint inhibitor atezolizumab combined with antiangiogenic antibody bevacizumab resulted in better overall and progression-free survival outcomes than sorafenib.
- Second-line therapy:
  1. In previously treated patients, the oral multikinase inhibitors regorafenib and cabozantinib have shown improved survival.
  2. Also, in previously treated patients, the immune checkpoint inhibitors nivolumab and pembrolizumab have demonstrated improved survival outcomes. In addition, the combination of ipilimumab and nivolumab received accelerated approval in patients previously treated with sorafenib.
  3. The anti-angiogenic antibody ramucirumab has demonstrated improved survival in HCC patients previously treated with sorafenib.

TABLE 2 Hepatocellular Carcinoma TNM Staging Classification and Milan Criteria for Liver Transplantation

T stage	
T_x	The primary tumor is not assessable
T_0	No tumor is present
T_1	A single tumor (of any size) without blood vessel invasion
	T_{1a}: Solitary tumor <2 cm (greatest dimension) without vascular invasion
	T_{1b}: Solitary tumor >2 cm (greatest dimension) without vascular invasion
T_2	A single tumor >2 cm *with* vascular invasion or multiple tumors (none >5 cm)
T_3	Multiple tumors, any more >5 cm
T_4	Tumor(s) invading a major branch of the portal or hepatic vein with direct invasion of adjacent organs including the diaphragm (other than gallbladder) or with perforation of the visceral liver peritoneum
N stage	
N_x	The lymph nodes are not assessable
N_0	There is no regional nodal involvement
N_1	There is regional nodal involvement
M stage	
M_0	There is no distant tumor spread
M_1	There is distant tumor spread
Milan criteria for liver transplantation	
1 tumor ≤5 cm in diameter, or	
Up to 3 tumors ≤3 cm in diameter	
+ No vascular invasion	
+ No extrahepatic disease	
Note	
The tumor/node/metastasis (TNM) staging classification does not consider the background liver function, which is often impaired in cirrhosis and will affect treatment options and prognosis. Other staging systems consider both disease extent and liver function, but have not been compared accurately against one another: • Barcelona Clinic Liver Cancer (BCLC) system • Cancer of the Liver Italian Program (CLIP) system • Okuda system	

From Grant, LA: *Grainger & Allison's diagnostic radiology essentials*, ed 2, Philadelphia, 2019, Elsevier.

DISPOSITION

- For resectable HCC, the 5-yr survival after liver transplantation is 50% to 70% and 30% to 50% with surgical resection. For unresectable HCC, the overall prognosis is poor.
- Tumor size is an independent prognostic factor for resected small HCC (≤50 mm in diameter). Patients with tumors of 0 to 35 mm diameter have a better 60-mo HCC specific survival rate than do those with larger tumors (36-50 mm).[1]
- In the U.S. the 5-yr overall survival rate for HCC is approximately 10%.

REFERRAL

Multidisciplinary gastrointestinal cancer team for treatment planning

PEARLS & CONSIDERATIONS

- Universal hepatitis B vaccination in children in endemic areas has been shown to decrease the incidence of HCC.
- Treatment of patients with chronic hepatitis B–associated cirrhosis with lamivudine

[1]Zhang W et al: Effect of tumor size on cancer-specific survival in small hepatocellular carcinoma, *Mayo Clin Proc* 90(9):1187-1195, 2015.

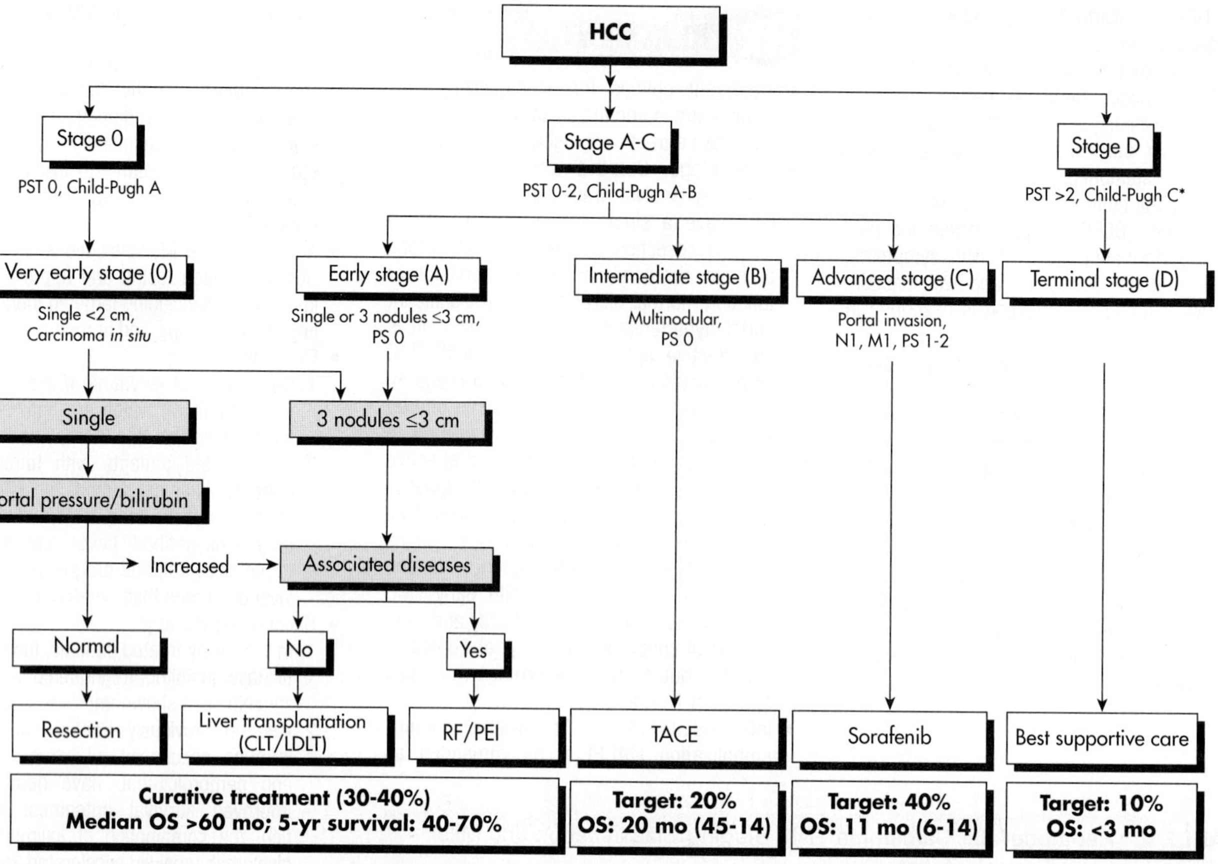

FIG. 3 Updated Barcelona Clinic Liver Cancer staging system and treatment strategy, 2011. *CLT;* Cadaveric liver transplantation; *HCC,* hepatocellular carcinoma; *PEI,* percutaneous ethanol injection; *LDLT,* living donor liver transplant; *RF,* radiofrequency ablation; *TACE,* transarterial chemoembolization. (From Grant, LA: *Grainger & Allison's diagnostic radiology essentials,* ed 2, Philadelphia, 2019, Elsevier.)

TABLE 3 Treatment Options for Hepatocellular Carcinoma

Treatment Modality	Comments
Surgical resection	Curative but limited to noncirrhotic patients and cirrhotic patients without portal hypertension
Liver transplantation	Successful in selected patients with limited disease; requires lifelong immunosuppression
Radiofrequency ablation or ethanol injection	Potentially curative for small tumors, including multiple tumors
Transarterial chemoembolization (TACE)	Prolongs survival in unresectable tumors if hepatic function is preserved; not curative
Immunotherapy	Checkpoint inhibitors improve survival in previously treated patients
Targeted molecular therapies	Sorafenib and lenvatinib improve patient survival in previously untreated patients Regorafenib and cabozantinib improve patient survival in previously treated patients

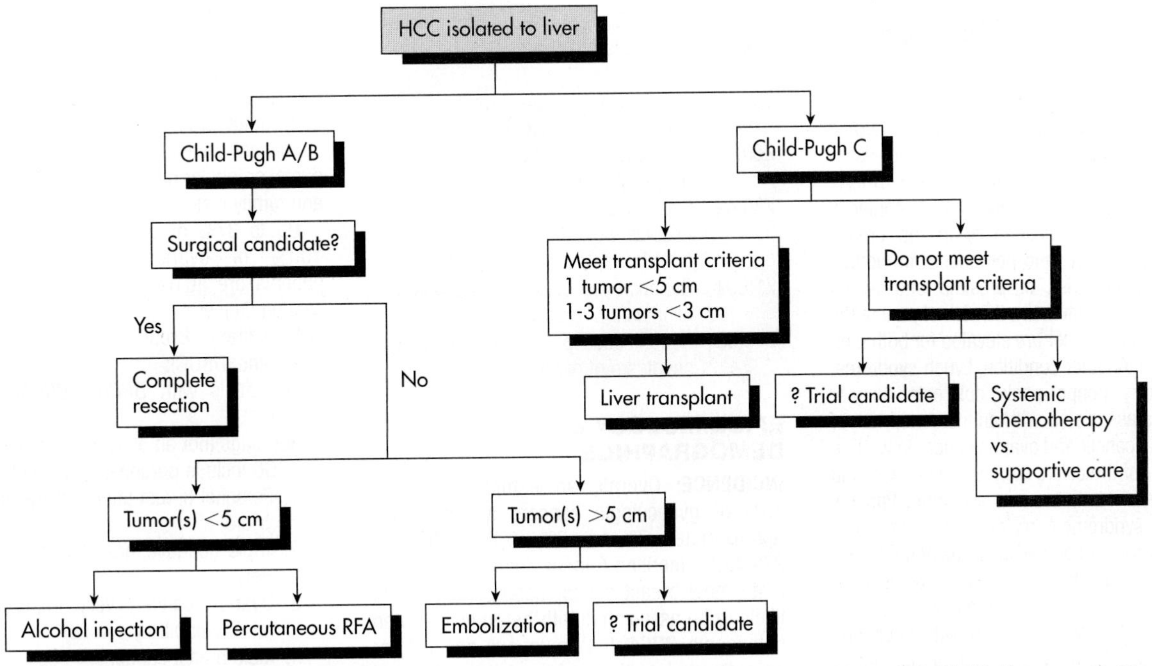

FIG. 4 Treatment algorithm for hepatocellular carcinoma (HCC). *RFA,* Radiofrequency ablation. (From Bruix J, Sherman M: AASLD: Management of hepatocellular carcinoma: an update, *Hepatology* 53(3):1020-1022, 2011.)

TABLE 4 Milan Criteria of Eligibility for Liver Transplantation

Presence of a tumor ≤5 cm in diameter in patients with single hepatocellular carcinomas
Or
≤3 tumor nodules, each 3 cm or less in diameter, in patients with multiple tumors

From Cameron JL, Cameron AM: *Current surgical therapy,* ed 10, Philadelphia, 2011, Saunders.

reduces the incidence of HCC. Treatment with entecavir in chronic hepatitis B-HCC can improve hepatic function and MELD score.

- Treatment with interferon-based therapy in patients with noncirrhotic hepatitis C reduces risk of HCC in patients demonstrating a sustained viral response.
- HCC screening is recommended in high-risk patients because curative therapies are available only for small and early HCC.
- Patients diagnosed with HCC with an AFP >1000 are at increased risk for recurrence after transplantation regardless of tumor size.
- There are numerous ongoing trials with tyrosine kinase inhibitors and monoclonal antibodies for advanced HCC in patients who are intolerant or resistant to sorafenib. The future of therapy for advanced HCC will likely lead to the personalized combination of multiple agents targeting different oncogenic pathways to optimize treatment success.
- Low dose daily aspirin use has been associated with less progression of liver disease in patients with chronic hepatitis B or C and lower HCC risk in those patients.[1]

[1] Simon TG et al: Association of aspirin with hepatocellular carcinoma and liver-related mortality, *N Engl J Med* 382:1018-1028, 2020.

RELATED CONTENT

Liver Cancer (Patient Information)

SUGGESTED READINGS

Available at ExpertConsult.com

AUTHOR: **Bharti Rathore, MD**

Hereditary Breast and Ovarian Cancer

BASIC INFORMATION

DEFINITION

Hereditary breast and ovarian cancer syndrome (HBOC) patients carry a significant cancer-associated alteration in the *BRCA1* and/or *BRCA2* gene. These genetic mutations can confer a heightened risk of malignancy in the breast, ovary, fallopian tube, and peritoneum in women and an elevated risk of prostate and breast cancer in men. Additionally, the risk of pancreatic cancer and skin cancer are elevated for both men and women. Another condition, Lynch syndrome, or hereditary nonpolyposis colorectal cancer (HNPCC), is associated with an increased risk of endometrial cancer and ovarian cancer in women and cancer of the colon, stomach, pancreas, and small bowel in both women and men. Patients with Lynch syndrome carry significant pathogenic alterations in one of five genes, as noted below.

The cancer risk to those who test positive for these genetic mutations is significantly greater than the cancer risk associated with those who test negative: Both in the general population or those with a personal and/or family cancer history. Frequently, a cancer that is associated with a heritable genetic mutation presents at a younger age than that seen in the general population, can be a relatively rarer type of cancer and/or affects multiple same-side family members. Identifying carriers can significantly reduce the morbidity and mortality of the patient and her/his close family members.

SYNONYMS

Hereditary breast and ovarian cancer syndrome (HBOC)

Lynch syndrome/hereditary nonpolyposis colorectal cancer (HNPCC)

Hereditary cancer syndrome

ICD-10CM CODES

Z84.81	Family history of carrier of genetic disease
Z80.3	Family history of malignant neoplasm of breast
Z80.41	Family history of malignant neoplasm of ovary
Z80.49	Family history of malignant neoplasm of other genital organs (uterus, vagina, for example)
Z15.01	Genetic susceptibility to malignant neoplasm of breast
Z15.02	Genetic susceptibility to malignant neoplasm of ovary

EPIDEMIOLOGY & DEMOGRAPHICS

INCIDENCE: Overall, an estimated 6% to 10% of gynecologic cancers are heritable. Approximately 7% to 10% of the estimated 276,480 (American Cancer Society 2020 estimate) new breast cancer cases annually are likely to be associated with heredity. Inherited pathogenic *BRCA 1, 2* mutations account for an estimated 11% to 15% of the estimated 21,750 (American Cancer Society 2020 estimate) annual new ovarian cancer cases. Less than 1% of the general population has a pathogenic mutation in the *BRCA 1* or *2* gene. As noted above, Lynch syndrome–associated mutations increase ovarian and uterine cancer as well as colorectal (up to 5% of colorectal cancers are considered heritable), pancreatic, and gastric cancers. This article will, however, focus on gynecologic disease. Tables 1 and 2 summarize genes associated with hereditary breast and ovarian cancer predisposition.

PREDOMINANT SEX & AGE: Although females are predominantly affected, males who carry deleterious mutations in *BRCA 1, 2* are at a significantly higher risk for cancer. Both sexes can transmit the altered gene to their offspring.

RISK FACTORS: *BRCA1* and *BRCA2* mutations can generate a greater risk of breast cancer than other well-established factors such as increased breast density, history of atypical ductal or lobular hyperplasia, nulliparity, obesity, and family history.

Up to 37% of breast cancer patients and 100% of ovarian/tubal/peritoneal cancer patients are at risk for hereditary breast and ovarian cancer syndrome.

Hereditary Breast and Ovarian Cancer Syndrome (HBOC):

- Individuals with *BRCA1*, *BRCA2* mutations (Fig. 1)
- Red flags (not an exhaustive list) for possible HBOC include personal or family history of:
  1. Personal breast cancer diagnosed at ≤45 yr old
  2. Triple-negative breast cancer (ER-, PR-, Her2-)
  3. Ovarian cancer: Very important factor (mostly papillary serous)
  4. Male breast cancer
  5. Two primary breast cancers
  6. Ashkenazi Jewish ancestry
  7. Breast cancer with ≥2 relatives with an HBOC-associated cancer (breast, ovary, prostate, pancreatic cancers)
  8. A previously identified HBOC mutation
  9. Two or more close relatives with breast cancer, one of whom was diagnosed at age 50 yr or younger
  10. Three or more HBOC-associated cancers at any age

GENETICS: The transmission pattern is autosomal dominant. A child whose father or mother has a *BRCA* mutation has a 50% chance of inheriting that genetic mutation.

NOTE:

TABLE 1 Genes Associated with Hereditary Breast Cancer Predisposition

Gene	Syndrome	Relative Risk of BC	BC Risk by Age 80 Yr	Associated Cancers
High Penetrance				
BRCA1	HBOC	~15-30	70%	Ovarian, other
BRCA2	HBOC	~10-20	70%	Ovarian, pancreatic, prostate, other
p53	Li-Fraumeni syndrome	100	50% by 60 yr	Soft tissue sarcoma, osteosarcoma, brain tumors, adrenocortical carcinoma, leukemia, other
PTEN	Cowden syndrome	No reliable estimate	70%-80%	Thyroid (follicular and rarely papillary) endometrial, genitourinary, other
	Bannayan-Riley-Ruvalcaba syndrome			
	Proteus			
	Proteus-like syndrome			
STK11	Peutz-Jeghers syndrome	No reliable estimate	30% by age 60	Small intestine, colorectal, uterine, testicular and ovarian sex chord tumors, other
CDH1	Hereditary diffuse gastric carcinoma	~3.25	39%	Lobular breast, diffuse gastric, other
Lower or Moderate Penetrance				
ATM (heterozygote)	Ataxia-telangiectasia in homozygotes	~3	30	Undefined in heterozygotes
CHK2 (CHEK2)	Li-Fraumeni variant	1.5-3	20%-30%	Undefined
PALB2	None known	5	~40	Undefined in heterozygotes

BC, Breast cancer; *HBOC,* hereditary breast and ovarian cancer syndrome.
From Niederhuber JE: *Abeloff's clinical oncology,* ed 6, Philadelphia, 2020, Elsevier.

- One half of *BRCA* carriers inherit the mutation from their father.
- Early onset of cancer may be a more important red flag than the number of affected family members, especially if the number of family members is small to begin with.
- Testing criteria (Tables 3 and 4), as per National Comprehensive Cancer Network (NCCN) guidelines, may differ from the red flags noted previously.
- Family history extends to first-, second-, and third-degree relatives.
- Consider Lynch syndrome–associated cancers (e.g., colorectal, gastric, brain, pancreas, small bowel, skin, ureter, renal pelvis, GI polyps), as Lynch syndrome is associated also with ovarian and uterine (endometrial) cancer.
- *BRCA* stands for BReast CAncer.
  1. The majority (84%) of the approximately 7% of breast cancers and 14% of ovarian cancers that result from a heritable mutation are due to a *BRCA1* (52%) and *BRCA2* (32%) gene mutation.
  2. By age 70, in comparison to the 7.3% risk of breast cancer in the general population, or approximately double that risk if one has an affected first-degree relative, *BRCA1* and *BRCA2* mutation carriers have up to an 87% reported risk of developing breast cancer. As opposed to a general-population risk of 2% for developing a second breast primary within 5 yr of the initial diagnosis, women with HBOC mutations have a 12% to 27% risk. This risk climbs to a reported 50% (*BRCA2*) and up to 64% (*BRCA1*) by age 70.
  3. By age 70, in contrast to the 0.7% risk of ovarian cancer in the general population, there is a reported risk of up to 27% to 63% for *BRCA2* and *BRCA1* mutation carriers, respectively. The risk for ovarian cancer within 10 yr of a breast cancer diagnosis is 6.8% (*BRCA2*) to 12.7% (*BRCA1*) as opposed to a general-population risk of less than 1.0%.
  4. Men with HBOC have an up to tenfold increased risk for breast cancer and a more than twofold increase in prostate cancer in comparison to the general-population risk. In men, the *BRCA2* mutation increases the cancer risk more than the *BRCA1* mutation. In fact, the breast cancer risk for a male with a *BRCA2* mutation is up to 80 times the risk seen in the general population.
  5. Both men and women have an elevated risk (up to sevenfold) for pancreatic cancer (*BRCA2* >1) and for melanoma (2.5-fold increase with *BRCA2*).
  6. Ashkenazi Jewish ancestry is associated with founder mutations 187delAG (*BRCA1*), 5382insC (*BRCA1*), and 6174delT (*BRCA2*), which confer a significantly elevated risk for breast and ovarian cancer. As opposed to the 1 in 400 risk in the general population, 1 in 40 individuals of Ashkenazi Jewish descent have a *BRCA 1* or *2* mutation.

Lynch Syndrome (Hereditary Nonpolyposis Colorectal Cancer - HNPCC):

- Individuals with *MLH1, MSH2, MSH6, PMS2, EPCAM* mutations.
- By age 70, Lynch syndrome carriers have—in addition to an increased risk for colorectal, gastric, hepatobiliary, urinary tract, small bowel, brain, skin, and pancreatic cancers—up to an approximately twentyfold increase in ovarian cancer (4% to 12% risk vs. the general-population risk of 0.7%) and up to an approximately fortyfold increase in uterine cancer (25% to 60+% risk vs. the general-population risk of 1.6%).
- The previously listed genes and others (e.g., *PTEN, TP53, CDH1, STK11*) that are found less frequently are considered high-penetrance genes, as they can increase the relative risk of their respective syndromes by greater than four- to fivefold.
- Other, more moderate-penetrant genes (e.g., *CHEK2, ATM, PALB2, BRIP1, RAD51C, RAD51D*), that is, those that are associated with a two- to fourfold increase in the relative risk of cancer, should be considered when assessing risk and ordering genetic tests.
- More than 12 known gene mutations are associated with an elevated risk for breast cancer, and a similar number are associated with an elevated risk for ovarian cancer. As such, screening for *BRCA1, BRCA2* alone will miss these mutations.

TABLE 2 Genes Associated with Hereditary Ovarian Cancer Predisposition

Gene	Syndrome	Relative Risk of OC	OC Risk by Age 80 Yr	Associated Cancers
High Penetrance				
BRCA1	Hereditary breast ovarian cancer syndrome	~50	~40%	Breast, other
BRCA2	Hereditary breast ovarian cancer syndrome	~8	11%-26%	Breast, pancreas, prostate, other
MLH1 *MSH2* *MSH6* *PMS2* *EPCAM*	Lynch syndrome	~4	~20%	Colon Uterine Stomach Small intestine Urinary tract Pancreatic Possible other sites
Lower or Moderate Penetrance				
RAD51C	None	~5	~6%	Undefined Autosomal recessive Fanconi anemia
RAD51D	None	~12	~14%	Undefined Autosomal recessive Fanconi anemia

OC, Ovarian cancer.
From Niederhuber JE: *Abeloff's clinical oncology*, ed 6, Philadelphia, 2020, Elsevier.

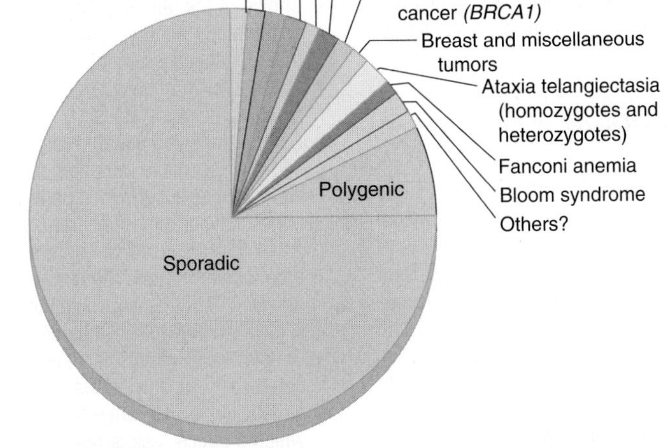

FIG. 1 Schematic depicting heterogeneity in breast cancer. *HBCC*, Hereditary breast and colorectal cancer; *SBLA*, sarcoma, breast and brain tumors, leukemia, laryngeal and lung cancer, and adrenal cortical carcinoma. (From Goldman L, Schafer AI: *Goldman's Cecil medicine,* ed 24, Philadelphia, 2012, Saunders.)

TABLE 3 Testing Criteria for Breast Ovarian Cancer Syndrome*

Individual from a family with a known deleterious *BRCA1* or *BRCA2* gene mutation
Personal history of breast cancer plus one or more of the following:

- Diagnosed at ≤45 yr of age
- Diagnosed at ≤50 yr of age with
  - An additional breast cancer primary
  - At least one close blood relative with breast cancer at any age
  - At least one close relative with pancreatic cancer
  - At least one close relative with prostate cancer
  - An unknown or limited family history
- Diagnosed at age 60 with
  - Triple-negative breast cancer
- Diagnosed at any age with
  - At least one close blood relative with breast cancer before 50 yr of age
  - At least two close blood relatives with breast cancer at any age
  - At least one close blood relative with ovarian cancer
  - At least one close blood relative with pancreatic cancer
  - At least two close blood relatives with prostate cancer
  - A close female blood relative with ovarian cancer
  - An individual of ethnicity associated with a higher mutation frequency
- Personal history of ovarian cancer
- Personal history of male breast cancer
- Personal history of prostate cancer at any age with a close relative with breast, ovarian, or pancreatic cancer at any age
- Personal history of pancreatic cancer and Ashkenazi Jewish ancestry
- Family history meeting any of the above criteria

See NCCN guidelines for the most up-to-date and detailed description for counseling and testing.

*For more detailed information, see the National Comprehensive Cancer Network (NCCN) guidelines.
From Disaia PJ et al: *Clinical gynecologic oncology,* ed 9, Philadelphia, 2017, Elsevier.

TABLE 4 National Comprehensive Cancer Network (NCCN) Guidelines for Recommending Genetic Testing for *BRCA1* or *BRCA2* Mutations*

Personal history of breast cancer and one or more of the following:

- Diagnosed at age ≤45 yr
- Diagnosed with at least two breast cancer primaries (bilateral, separate ipsilateral), the first at age 50 yr
- Diagnosed at age ≤50 yr with one or more close relatives† with breast cancer (prostate or pancreatic) at any age
- Diagnosed with triple-negative breast cancer at age ≤60 yr
- Diagnosed at any age with one or more close relatives with breast cancer at age ≤50 yr
- Diagnosed at any age with two or more close relatives at any age
- Diagnosed at any age with one or more close relatives with invasive ovarian cancer (including fallopian tube and primary peritoneal) at any age
- Diagnosed at any age with two or more close relatives with pancreatic and/or prostate cancer
- Having a close male relative with breast cancer at any age

*Individuals with a limited or unknown family history may have an underestimated probability of a familial gene mutation detection.
†Close relative pertains to first-, second-, or third-degree blood relatives on the same side (either maternal or paternal) of the family.
From Disaia PJ et al: *Clinical gynecologic oncology,* ed 9, Philadelphia, 2017, Elsevier.

- In addition to established deleterious mismatch repair gene mutations, gene alterations that are categorized in the literature as emerging risk mutations are also associated with hereditary gynecologic and other cancers.

PHYSICAL FINDINGS & CLINICAL PRESENTATION

- Present at a younger age
- Bilaterality more likely
- Multiple primaries in one individual

ETIOLOGY

Hereditary cancers are typically due to a tumor suppression gene mutation that interferes with DNA repair thus allowing an otherwise potentially avoidable cancer to develop. This is distinct from familial cancers in which there is no isolated gene mutation. Such cancers appear in the family more than that which would be statistically seen in the general population. Nongenetic factors such as lifestyle habits and environmental influences contribute to cancer risk as well.

Dx DIAGNOSIS

DIFFERENTIAL DIAGNOSIS

- General (sporadic) population or familial basis for the cancer in question.
- Hereditary cancer is more likely to present at a younger age, to span a number of generations, to affect more family members than would be expected (if a large enough family), especially in a suspicious pattern, and to include some rarer (ovary, male breast cancer, pancreatic cancer, for example) presentations.
- In addition to the more common syndromes listed previously, consider Cowden *(PTEN),* Peutz-Jeghers *(STK11),* Li-Fraumeni *(TP53),* and others.

WORKUP

Family history questionnaire, patient and family interviews, genetic counseling/risk assessment (including tools such as Tyrer-Cuzick/Gail/Claus models), and tailored genetic testing. Tablet-based intake questionnaires and computer algorithms are increasingly being used to ferret out at risk patients.

LABORATORY TESTS

- A simple blood or saliva sample drawn in the office or a lab, after informed consent, is needed. This specimen should be sent to a reliable laboratory recognized nationally for its genetic cancer testing accuracy (technologic and interpretative), reporting format, and the support staff ability and availability for consultation, office counseling, and testing integration. Look for a laboratory that has published peer-reviewed data and has an accurate classification methodology that relies on an extensive database. Realize that these labs are not FDA approved and that CLIA certification, while needed, relies on just in-house data. Remember also that most patients get tested only once in their lifetime, and so accuracy is imperative.
- Options include:
  1. Syndrome specific: For example, HBOC-*BRCA* testing (including large rearrangement detection); Lynch syndrome; founder mutation testing (187delAG, 5382insC, 6174delT)—Ashkenazi Jewish population (occasionally recommended as the first test for this population); single-site testing (if a previously identified gene mutation is known in the family); cancer specific, for example, breast cancer panel—*BRCA 1, 2* with/without reflex to broader panel (i.e., sequential testing).
  2. Comprehensive panel testing (can include HBOC syndrome *BRCA1, BRCA2*), Lynch syndrome (*MLH1, MSH2, MSH6, PMS2, EPCAM*), Li-Fraumeni (*TP53*), Cowden (*PTEN*), Peutz-Jeghers (*STK11*), *PALB2, CHEK2, ATM, BRIP1, RAD51C,* and others [upward of 30+ genes]).
- Choice of the test is generally based on personal/family history, although thoroughness of the risk assessment may be limited by attempting to choose a gene test based on history/phenotype alone.
- Comprehensive panel testing has been shown to increase mutation detection. It can aid in test selection when patients qualify for more than one syndrome/cancer-specific test and it can be used to capture a potentially broader view of risk. There may be a concern, however, for detecting mutations that are not clinically actionable, at this time.
- Categories of results include (1) positive or negative for a deleterious mutation or (2) a genetic variant of uncertain significance, in which a cancer risk is not yet established or ruled out. It is critical that the classification of these variants is accurate.

IMAGING STUDIES

Screening transvaginal ultrasonography, annual mammography, annual MRI (when breast cancer risk is 20% or more based on Tyrer-Cuzick or other breast cancer risk screening models)

Rx TREATMENT/RISK REDUCTION

- Heightened surveillance, judicious chemoprevention, and prophylactic surgery have been associated with improved outcomes.
- Surveillance includes patient breast awareness, clinical breast exam, mammography, MRI, transvaginal ultrasonography, and CA-125 blood testing, for example.
- Chemopreventive approaches have been shown to reduce the risk of ovarian cancer by up to 60% (with an oral contraceptive) and risk of contralateral breast cancer by as much as 53% (with tamoxifen).
- In HBOC patients, prophylactic total mastectomy can reduce the risk of breast cancer by 90%, and a bilateral salpingo-oophorectomy, after childbearing or by age 40, can reduce the risk of ovarian cancer by up to 96% and the risk of breast cancer by up to 68%.
- Consider preimplantation genetic diagnosis in conjunction with in vitro fertilization.

REFERRAL

If services are needed beyond one's practice or comfort level, consider consulting with knowledgeable genetic counselors, gynecologists, gynecologic oncologists, breast surgeons, and gastroenterology specialists, among others.

! PEARLS & CONSIDERATIONS

- Be vigilant. Be motivated by the risks: Women with these mutations are approximately 10 times more likely to develop breast cancer and 20 to 30 times more likely to develop ovarian cancer. **Look for red flags during every encounter**, regardless of the patient's chief complaint or scheduled visit type and inquire and regularly update information about the patient's personal and family history of cancer. Consider that approximately 10% of general practice patients have a significant family history. Supply a printed family history questionnaire. Always consider your patient's cancer risk, especially when charting a new treatment course or planning a surgical procedure. Oftentimes, a more comprehensive approach may be taken if a patient proves to be a mutation carrier.
- Adjust the age at which screening/treatment is initiated and the frequency of the visits depending on the age of the youngest affected family member, the at-risk cancer site, and the carrier status of the patient.
- Encourage input from the patient during the screening, workup, follow-up, and treatment.
- Recommend that the patient verify any questionable family history, collect appropriate family documentation/testing, and involve her family in the process; this involvement can include advising, counseling, and testing for close relatives.
- Try to counsel and test (if appropriate) those family member(s) who, if tested, would render testing of progeny/other family members less necessary. Testing an affected family member is oftentimes the most appropriate, efficient, cost-effective, and informative approach.
- Genetic testing can more accurately predict risk and enable a more tailored management approach than relying on one's family history alone. Be mindful that there may be other, although as yet unidentified, mutations at the root of one's patient's personal or family cancer history.
- Refer to your professional societies and the NCCN for screening and surveillance/imaging/treatment guidelines. Don't hesitate to engage the assistance of a genetic counselor, gynecologist, oncologist, breast surgeon, and/or a gastroenterologist during this initial phase.
- Involve other appropriate specialists in the patient's short- and long-term care, depending on the at-risk anatomic systems.
- Remember that *BRCA1*- and *BRCA2*-positive men are at a significantly higher risk for breast and prostate cancer, as well as skin and pancreatic cancer.
- Consider prophylactic bilateral mastectomy and bilateral salpingo-oophorectomy in high-risk patients.
- Encourage high-risk patients to complete childbearing at a younger age and consider, as appropriate, subsequent prophylactic bilateral salpingo-oophorectomy and menopause hormone therapy options.
- Recommend prophylactic bilateral salpingectomy for at-risk pre-menopausal patients during any other surgical procedure—once childbearing is complete. Consider such assistive reproductive options as preimplantation genetic diagnosis.
- Genetic information cannot be used as the basis for a "preexisting condition" with regard to health insurance or employment, according to federal and state laws. However, it may play a role with respect to life insurance, disability insurance, and long-term care insurance.
- While insurance coverage generally is available, panel testing reimbursement may occasionally be challenged. Vocalize and document your support of the appropriate testing and management, with both your patient and her/his insurance company. Enlist the assistance of your local professional society, as needed.
- There may be a medical-legal risk if a failure to identify and/or genetically counsel or test a high-risk patient and/or her family results in a delay in the diagnosis or worsened prognosis of breast or ovarian cancer. The provider, laboratory, and the insurance company/employer may have legal exposure for failing to order testing, for providing inaccurate results, or for denial of coverage, respectively.
- Being aware of a patient's cancer risk facilitates initiation of those preventive screenings and management strategies that have been shown to reduce the likelihood of cancer and improve early cancer detection rates. This can be of tremendous benefit for the patient's family members as well as the patient.

PREVENTION

Consider appropriate screening and surveillance (awareness/physical exam by patient and health care provider, imaging studies, diagnostic procedures/lab studies, counseling, and genetic testing) as well as prophylactic surgery and chemopreventive measures.

PATIENT & FAMILY EDUCATION

Always encourage patients to revisit their personal and family history and to update this information with all of their health care providers and their family members. Recommend that patients initiate discussions with their family members and other health care providers in an ongoing effort to reduce their and their loved ones' risk of heritable cancer.

Refer to NCCN guidelines (www.nccn.org) and national specialty society recommendations.

SUGGESTED READINGS

Available at ExpertConsult.com

RELATED CONTENT

Breast Cancer (Related Key Topic)
Lynch Syndrome (Related Key Topic)
Ovarian Cancer (Related Key Topic)

AUTHOR: **David I. Kurss, MD, FACOG, NCMP**

BASIC INFORMATION

DEFINITION

Herpes simplex is a viral infection caused by the herpes simplex virus (HSV). HSV-1 is associated primarily with oral infections, and HSV-2 causes mainly genital infections. However, either type can infect any site. After the primary infection, the virus enters the nerve endings in the skin directly below the lesions and ascends to the dorsal root ganglia, where it remains in a latent stage until it is reactivated.

SYNONYMS

Genital herpes
Herpes labialis
Herpes gladiatorum
Herpes digitalis
Oral herpes

ICD-10CM CODES

A60	Anogenital herpesviral (herpes simplex) infections
A60.04	Herpesviral vulvovaginitis
B00	Herpesviral (herpes simplex) infections
B00.1	Herpesviral vesicular dermatitis
B00.82	Herpes simplex myelitis
B00.9	Herpesviral infection, unspecified
P35.2	Congenital herpesviral (herpes simplex) infection

EPIDEMIOLOGY & DEMOGRAPHICS

- More than 85% of adults have serologic evidence of HSV-1 infection. The seroprevalence of adults with HSV-2 in the U.S. is 25%; however, only approximately 20% of these persons recall having symptoms of HSV infection.
- Most cases of eye or digital herpetic infections are caused by HSV-1.
- Worldwide, more than 400 million persons have genital herpes caused by HSV-2. In the U.S., 1 in 5 adults is infected with HSV-2, and 1 million new infections occur yearly.
- Frequency of recurrence of HSV-2 genital herpes is higher than HSV-1 oral labial infection.
- The frequency of recurrence is lowest for oral labial HSV-2 infections.
- The incidence of complications from herpes simplex (e.g., herpes encephalitis) is highest in immunocompromised hosts.
- Male circumcision significantly reduces the incidence of HSV-2.

PHYSICAL FINDINGS & CLINICAL PRESENTATION (TABLE 1)

PRIMARY INFECTION:

- Symptoms occur from 3 to 7 days after contact (respiratory droplets, direct contact).
- Constitutional symptoms include low-grade fever, headache and myalgias, regional lymphadenopathy, and localized pain.
- Pain, burning, itching, and tingling last several hours.
- Grouped vesicles, usually with surrounding erythema, appear and generally ulcerate or crust within 48 h (Fig. E1).
- The vesicles are uniform in size (differentiating it from herpes zoster vesicles, which vary in size). Scattered erosions covered with exudate may be noted on genitals (Fig. E2).
- During the acute eruption the patient is uncomfortable; involvement of lips and inside of mouth (Fig. E3) may make it unpleasant for the patient to eat; urinary retention may complicate involvement of the genital area.
- Lesions generally last from 2 to 6 wk and heal without scarring.

RECURRENT INFECTION:

- Generally caused by alteration in the immune system; fatigue, stress, menses, local skin trauma, and exposure to sunlight are contributing factors.
- The prodromal symptoms (fatigue, burning and tingling of the affected area) last 12 to 24 hr.
- A cluster of lesions generally evolves within 24 hr from a macule to a papule and then vesicles surrounded by erythema; the vesicles coalesce and subsequently rupture within 4 days, revealing erosions covered by crusts.
- The crusts are generally shed within 7 to 10 days, revealing a pink surface.
- The most frequent location of the lesions is on the vermilion border of the lips (HSV-1), the penile shaft or glans penis and the labia (HSV-2), buttocks (seen more frequently in women), fingertips (herpetic whitlow), and trunk (may be confused with herpes zoster).
- Rapid onset of diffuse cutaneous herpes simplex (eczema herpeticum) may occur in certain atopic infants and adults. It is a medical emergency, especially in young infants, and should be promptly treated with acyclovir.
- Herpes encephalitis, meningitis, and ocular herpes can occur in patients with immunocompromised status and occasionally in normal hosts.

ETIOLOGY

HSV-1 and HSV-2 are both DNA viruses.

DIAGNOSIS

DIFFERENTIAL DIAGNOSIS

- Impetigo
- Behçet syndrome
- Coxsackie virus infection
- Syphilis
- Stevens-Johnson syndrome
- Herpangina
- Aphthous stomatitis
- Varicella
- Herpes zoster

WORKUP

Diagnosis is based on clinical presentation. Laboratory evaluation confirms diagnosis.

LABORATORY TESTS

- Direct immunofluorescent antibody slide tests provide a rapid diagnosis.
- Viral culture is the most definitive method for diagnosis; results are generally available in 1 or 2 days. The lesions should be sampled during the vesicular or early ulcerative stage; cervical samples should be taken from the endocervix with a swab.
- Pap smear will detect HSV-infected cells in cervical tissue from women without symptoms.
- Serologic tests for HSV: Immunoglobulin (Ig) G and IgM serum antibodies. Antibodies to HSV occur in 50% to 90% of adults. The presence of IgM or a fourfold or greater rise in IgG titers indicates a recent infection (convalescent sample should be drawn 2 to 3 wk after the acute specimen is drawn).
- Tzanck smear is a readily available test that will demonstrate multinucleated giant cells. However, it is not a highly sensitive test.

TREATMENT

- Table 2 summarizes antiviral chemotherapy for HSV infection.
- Topical acyclovir, penciclovir, and docosanol are optional treatments for recurrent herpes labialis, but they are less effective than oral treatments.

DISPOSITION

Most patients recover from the initial episode or recurrences without complications; immunocompromised hosts are at risk for complications (e.g., disseminated herpes simplex infection, herpes encephalitis).

REFERRAL

- Hospital admission in patients with herpes encephalitis or herpes meningitis and in immunocompromised hosts with diffuse herpes simplex infection
- Ophthalmology referral in patients with suspected ocular herpes

PEARLS & CONSIDERATIONS

COMMENTS

- Provide patient education regarding transmission of HSV.
- Condom use offers significant protection against HSV-1 infection in susceptible women.
- Patients should be instructed on the use of condoms for sexual intercourse and on avoiding kissing or sexual intercourse until lesions are crusted. Pericoital application of tenofovir gel, an antiretroviral vaginal gel, has also been shown to reduce the risk of HSV-2 in women. This may be useful in regions of the world where use of condoms is shunned.
- Patients should also avoid contact with immunocompromised hosts or neonates while lesions are present.
- Proper handwashing techniques should be explained.
- Patients with herpes gladiatorum (cutaneous herpes in athletes involved in contact

TABLE 1 Other Clinical Presentations of Herpes Simplex Virus (HSV) Infections

Other Clinical Presentations of Herpes Simplex Virus Infections		
Form of infection	Clinical settings and HSV type(s)	Cutaneous and/or extracutaneous findings
Predominantly mucocutaneous		
Eczema herpeticum (Kaposi varicelliform eruption)	• Affects infants/children > adults with atopic dermatitis; risk is associated with mutations in the gene encoding filaggrin • A similar presentation can occur in patients with an impaired skin barrier due to other conditions such as burns, irritant contact dermatitis, pemphigus (foliaceus, vulgaris), Darier disease, Hailey–Hailey disease, mycosis fungoides, Sézary syndrome, ichthyoses, and rarely Grover disease and pityriasis rubra pilaris with acantholysis, as well as following ablative laser procedures or application of topical 5-fluorouracil • Usually due to HSV-1	• Rapid, widespread cutaneous dissemination of HSV infection in areas of dermatitis/skin barrier disruption • Monomorphic, discrete, 2-3 mm punched-out erosions with hemorrhagic crusts are evident more often than intact vesicles • May have fevers, malaise and lymphadenopathy • Occasionally complicated by bacterial superinfections (e.g., *Staphylococcus aureus* , group A streptococci) or systemic dissemination of HSV infection • Differential diagnosis includes "eczema coxsackium" due to coxsackievirus A6 infection and streptococcal infection
Herpetic whitlow	• Often in young children, usually due to HSV-1 • Increasing frequency in adolescents/adults secondary to digital–genital contact, usually due to HSV-2 • Historically in dental and medical personnel who did not use gloves	• Pain, swelling, and clustered vesicles on a digit; appearance of vesicles may be delayed • Recurrences in the same location can be a clue to the diagnosis • Often misdiagnosed as blistering dactylitis or paronychia
Herpes gladiatorum	• Participation in contact sports such as wrestling • Usually due to HSV-1	• Distribution reflects sites of contact with another athlete's skin lesions and is sometimes widespread
Herpes simplex folliculitis	• Shaving with a blade razor (e.g., *herpetic sycosis*in a man's beard area) • Usually due to HSV-1 • HIV-positive or otherwise immunocompromised individuals	• Rapid development of follicular vesicles and pustules
Severe/chronic HSV infections	• Immunocompromised patients, e.g., hematopoietic stem cell or solid organ transplant recipients, individuals with HIV infection or leukemia/lymphoma	• Most common presentation is chronic, enlarging ulcerations • Cutaneous lesions may affect multiple sites or be disseminated • Skin findings are often atypical, i.e. verrucous, exophytic or pustular lesions • Recurrences can involve oral mucosa, including the tongue and movable areas that do not overlie bone • Involvement of the respiratory tract, esophagus, and remainder of the gastrointestinal tract may also occur
Predominantly extracutaneous		
Ocular HSV infection	• Often due to HSV-2 in newborns (see below) • Usually due to HSV-1 in children and adults	• Primary infection: Unilateral or bilateral keratoconjunctivitis with eyelid edema, tearing, photophobia, chemosis, and preauricular lymphadenopathy • Branching dendritic lesions of the cornea represent a pathognomonic finding • Recurrent episodes are common and typically unilateral • Complications include corneal ulceration and scarring, globe rupture, and blindness
Herpes encephalitis	• Most common cause of fatal sporadic viral encephalitis in the U.S. • Associated with mutations in the genes encoding Toll-like receptor 3 or UNC-93B, which impair interferon-based cellular antiviral responses • Usually due to HSV-1 • Natalizumab, an anti-α4 integrin monoclonal antibody used for the treatment of multiple sclerosis and Crohn disease, increases the risk of encephalitis and meningitis due to HSV and VZV	• Manifestations can include fever, altered mental status, bizarre behavior, and localized neurologic findings • The temporal lobe is often involved • Mortality ≥70% without treatment; residual neurologic defects in most survivors • Herpes labialis may be a coincidental finding
Proctitis	• Most common in men who have sex with men	• Manifestations include diarrhea, anal pain, and a feeling of rectal fullness
Cutaneous and extracutaneous		
Neonatal HSV infection	• Occurs in ~1:10 000 newborns in the U.S.89, usually resulting from exposure to HSV during a vaginal delivery • Risk of transmission is highest (30%-50%) for women who acquire a genital HSV infection (which is often asymptomatic) near the time of delivery • Risk of transmission is low (<1%-3%) for women with recurrent genital herpes • Due to HSV-2 or HSV-1; the latter accounts for 30%-50% of cases	• Onset from birth to 2 wk of age, but usually ≥5 days of age • Localized (favoring the scalp and trunk; or disseminated cutaneous lesions; involvement of the oral mucosa, eye, CNS, and multiple internal organs can occur • Vesicles may progress to bullae and erosions • Encephalitis can present with lethargy, irritability, poor feeding, temperature instability, seizures, and a bulging fontanelle • For CNS or disseminated disease, mortality is >50% without treatment and ~15% with treatment; many survivors have neurologic deficits

From Bolognia JL et al: *Dermatology*, ed 4, 2018, Elsevier.

TABLE 2 Topical and Oral Antiviral Medications Used for Herpes Simplex Virus Infections*

Drug	Formulation	Regimen	Indication/Comment
Topical			
Acyclovir	5% cream (2 g, 5 g)	Apply 5 times/day	Recurrent HL; A: ≥12 yr; 4 days; Rx
	5% ointment (15 g, 30 g)	Apply 6 times/day	Initial GH, localized HSV; A: Adults; 7 days; Rx
Penciclovir	1% cream (1.5 g, 5 g)	Apply q2h (awake)	Recurrent HL; A: ≥12 yr; 4 days; Rx
Docosanol	10% cream (2 g)	Apply 5 times/day	HL; A: ≥12 yr; treat until healed; OTC
Oral (all Rx)			
Acyclovir	200 mg capsule		A: ≥2 yr
	400 mg, 800 mg tablet		
	200 mg/5 ml susp		
		200 mg 5 times/day	Initial GH; 10 days
		200 mg 5 times/day	Recurrent GH; 5 days
		400 mg 2 times/day	Suppression, recurrent GH; up to 12 mo, then reevaluate
Famciclovir	125, 250, 500 mg tablet		A: ≥18 yr
		1500 mg single dose	Recurrent HL
		1000 mg 2 times/day	Recurrent GH; 1 day
		250 mg 2 times/day	Suppression, recurrent GH; up to 12 mo
Valacyclovir	500 mg, 1 g caplet		A: Adults and ≥12 yr for HL
		1 g 2 times/day	Initial GH; 10 days
		500 mg 2 times/day	Recurrent GH; 3 days
		500 mg-1 g once daily	Suppressive GH
		2 g 2 times/day	HL; 1 day; both adults and children ≥12 yr

A, Approved; *GH,* genital herpes; *HL,* herpes labialis; *HSV,* herpes simplex virus; *OTC,* over-the-counter; *Rx,* by prescription.
*Approved indications and regimens listed; often used off-label.
From Paller AS, Mancini AJ: *Hurwitz clinical pediatric dermatology: a textbook of skin disorders of childhood and adolescence*, ed 5, Philadelphia, 2016, Elsevier.

sports) should be excluded from participation in active sports until lesions have resolved.

- Many new HSV-2 infections are asymptomatic. Since HSV-2 antibody tests have become commercially available, an increasing number of persons have learned that they have genital herpes through serologic testing. Persons with asymptomatic HSV-2 infection shed virus in the genital tract less frequently than persons with symptomatic infection, but much of the difference is attributable to less frequent genital lesions because genital lesions are accompanied by frequent viral shedding. The U.S. Preventive Services Task Force (USPSTF) recommends against routine serologic screening for genital HSV infection in asymptomatic adolescents and adults, including those that are pregnant.
- Suppressive treatment of HSV-2 infection lowers the incidence of genital lesions by 70% to 80%, but cuts the rate of HSV-2 transmission to uninfected partners by only 50%.
- Pregnancy: Antiviral prophylaxis with acyclovir is recommended from 36 wk of gestation until delivery in women with a history of genital herpes. Elective cesarean delivery should be performed in laboring patients with active lesions to decrease the risk of neonatal herpes.
- Trials involving investigational herpes simplex vaccine have found it to be effective in preventing HSV-1 genital disease and infection, but not in preventing HSV-2 disease or infection.

RELATED CONTENT

Genital Herpes (Patient Information)
Oral Herpes (Patient Information)

AUTHOR: **Fred F. Ferri, MD**

BASIC INFORMATION

DEFINITION

Herpes zoster is a disease caused by reactivation of the varicella-zoster virus, with spread of the virus alone from the sensory nerve to the dermatome. After the primary infection (chickenpox), the virus becomes latent in the dorsal root ganglia and reemerges when there is a weakening of the immune system (as a result of disease or advanced age). Over 90% of the adult U.S. population is latently infected with varicella zoster virus.

SYNONYMS

Shingles
HZ

ICD-10CM CODES

B02	Herpes zoster
B02.0	Zoster encephalitis
B02.1	Zoster meningitis
B02.30	Zoster ocular disease, unspecified
B02.31	Zoster conjunctivitis
B02.32	Zoster iridocyclitis
B02.33	Zoster keratitis
B02.34	Zoster scleritis
B02.39	Other herpes zoster eye disease
B02.7	Disseminated zoster
B02.8	Zoster with other complications
B02.9	Zoster without complications

EPIDEMIOLOGY & DEMOGRAPHICS

- Herpes zoster occurs during the lifetime of 10% to 20% of the population. There are approximately 1 million cases annually in the U.S. The incidence of herpes zoster has increased fourfold over the past six decades.
- There is an increased incidence in immunocompromised patients (chemotherapy, radiotherapy, immunosuppression due to corticosteroids, AIDS, DM, malignancy), the elderly (most common after age 60) (Fig. E1), and children who acquired chickenpox when younger than 2 mo.

PHYSICAL FINDINGS & CLINICAL PRESENTATION

- Pain generally precedes skin manifestation by 3 to 5 days and is generally localized to the dermatome that will be affected by the skin lesions.
- Constitutional symptoms are often present (malaise, fever, headache).
- The initial rash consists of erythematous maculopapules generally affecting one dermatome (thoracic region in majority of cases [Fig. E2]). Typically, the rash does not cross the midline. Some patients (<30%) may have scattered vesicles outside the affected dermatome. In rare cases the rash can be generalized (Fig. E3).
- The initial maculopapules evolve into vesicles and pustules by the third or the fourth day.
- The vesicles have an erythematous base (Fig. E4), are cloudy, of various sizes (a distinguishing characteristic from herpes simplex, in which the vesicles are of uniform size), and may have a classic appearance of grouped vesicles (Fig. E5).
- The vesicles subsequently become umbilicated and then form crusts that generally fall off within 3 wk; scarring may occur.
- Pain during and after the rash is generally significant. Postherpetic neuralgia occurs after herpes zoster in approximately one third of patients aged 60 yr and older and can persist for mos or yrs.
- Secondary bacterial infection with *Staphylococcus aureus* or *Streptococcus pyogenes* may occur.
- Regional lymphadenopathy may occur.
- Herpes zoster may involve the trigeminal nerve (most frequent cranial nerve involved); involvement of the first division of the trigeminal nerve is known as "herpes zoster ophthalmicus" and can result in blindness. The appearance of blisters on the tip of the nose (Hutchinson sign) is a common manifestation of herpes zoster ophthalmicus. Involvement of the geniculate ganglion can cause facial palsy and a painful ear, with the presence of vesicles on the pinna and external auditory canal (Ramsay Hunt syndrome).
- Pain typical of herpes zoster in the absence of cutaneous lesions, known as "Zoster sine herpete," is rare.

ETIOLOGY

Reactivation of varicella virus (human herpes virus III)

Dx DIAGNOSIS

DIFFERENTIAL DIAGNOSIS

- Rash: Herpes simplex and other viral infections, contact dermatitis
- Pain from herpes zoster: May be confused with acute myocardial infarction, pulmonary embolism, pleuritis, pericarditis, renal colic

WORKUP

The diagnosis of herpes zoster is usually made by the characteristic dermatomal presentation.

LABORATORY TESTS

Laboratory tests are generally not necessary. In cases where the clinical diagnosis is not obvious, PCR testing for varicella zoster virus is has high sensitivity and specificity. It is readily available and results can usually be obtained in less than 24 hr. Other laboratory studies for diagnosis of herpes zoster include viral culture, DFA, and serologic testing.

Rx TREATMENT

NONPHARMACOLOGIC THERAPY

- Wet compresses (using Burow solution or cool tap water) applied for 15 to 30 min five to ten times a day may be useful to break vesicles and remove serum and crust. Then carefully pat dry.
- Care must be taken to prevent any secondary bacterial infection by keeping cutaneous lesions clean and dry.

ACUTE GENERAL Rx

- Oral antiviral agents can shorten the disease course and help prevent post-herpetic neuralgia. They can decrease acute pain, inflammation, and vesicle formation when treatment is begun within 72 hr of onset of rash. Treatment options are:
  1. Valacyclovir 1000 mg tid for 7 days
  2. Famciclovir 500 mg tid for 7 days
  3. Acyclovir 800 mg 5 times daily for 7 to 10 days
- The role of corticosteroids in herpes zoster is controversial. Many physicians prescribe them to improve rash healing and reduce pain severity; however, a Cochrane review failed to show sufficient evidence to support the use of corticosteroids for the prevention of postherpetic neuralgia. Corticosteroids can be considered in older patients within 72 hr of clinical presentation or if new lesions are still appearing if there are no contraindications to their use. Initial dose is prednisone 60 mg/day decreased by 5 mg/day until finished.
- Immunocompromised patients and patients with herpes zoster complicated by CNS involvement should be treated with IV acyclovir 10 to 15 mg/kg q8h in 1-hr infusions for 7 days, with close monitoring of renal function and adequate hydration; vidarabine (continuous 12-hr infusion of 10 mg/kg/day for 7 days) is also effective for treatment of disseminated herpes zoster in immunocompromised hosts.
- Patients with AIDS and transplant recipients may develop acyclovir-resistant varicella-zoster; these patients can be treated with foscarnet (40 mg/kg IV q8h) continued for at least 10 days or until lesions are completely healed.
- Postherpetic neuralgia:
  1. Gabapentin 100 to 600 mg tid is effective in the treatment of pain and sleep interference associated with postherpetic neuralgia. Other effective agents are pregabalin, duloxetine, and tricyclic antidepressants.
  2. Lidocaine patch 5% is also effective in relieving postherpetic neuralgia. Patches are applied to intact skin after resolution of blisters and crusts to cover the most painful area for up to 12 hr within a 24-hr period.
  3. Capsaicin cream can be useful for treatment of postherpetic neuralgia. It is generally applied 3 to 5 times daily for several weeks after the crusts have fallen off. A topical 8% patch formulation of capsaicin is now available by prescription for postherpetic neuralgia.
  4. Sympathetic blocks (stellate ganglion or epidural) with 0.25% bupivacaine and rhizotomy are reserved for severe cases unresponsive to conservative treatment.

DISPOSITION

- The incidence of postherpetic neuralgia (defined as pain that persists more than 90 days after onset of rash) increases with age (<30% by age 40 yr, >70% by age 70 yr); antivirals reduce the risk of postherpetic neuralgia.
- Incidence of disseminated herpes zoster is increased in immunocompromised hosts (e.g., 15% to 50% of patients with active Hodgkin disease).
- Immunocompromised hosts are also more prone to neurologic complications (encephalitis, myelitis, cranial and peripheral nerve palsies, acute retinal necrosis). The mortality rate is 10% to 20% in immunocompromised hosts with disseminated zoster.
- Motor neuropathies occur in 5% of all cases of zoster; complete recovery occurs in >70% of patients.
- Rates of HZ recurrence are more frequent than previously reported and are comparable to rates of first HZ occurrence in immunocompetent individuals.

REFERRAL

- Hospitalization for IV acyclovir in patients with disseminated herpes zoster.
- Patients with herpes zoster ophthalmicus should be referred to an ophthalmologist.
- Consultation with an otolaryngologist is advisable in patients with Ramsey Hunt syndrome.
- Vaccination: In the absence of the herpes zoster vaccine, persons who live to 85 yr of age have a 50% risk of herpes zoster. Immunocompetent adults ≥50 yr (including those who have already received Zostavax) are appropriate candidates for recombinant varicella zoster virus vaccine (Shingrix). It consists of 2 doses 2 to 6 mo apart and is preferred over Zostavax for herpes zoster prevention. Adults who are VZV seronegative (never had varicella) should be immunized against varicella with two doses of varicella vaccine (Varivax). Despite its efficacy and safety, use of this vaccine remains low (<8% of potential recipients).

SUGGESTED READING

Available at ExpertConsult.com

RELATED CONTENT

Shingles (Patient Information)
Postherpetic Neuralgia (Related Key Topic)
Ramsey Hunt Syndrome (Related Key Topic)

AUTHOR: **Fred F. Ferri, MD**

BASIC INFORMATION

DEFINITION

High-altitude illness refers to a spectrum of cerebral and pulmonary syndromes related to hypoxemia occurring during rapid ascent to high altitudes in unacclimatized individuals. Common acute high-altitude illnesses include high-altitude headache (HAH), acute mountain sickness (AMS), high-altitude cerebral edema (HACE), and high-altitude pulmonary edema (HAPE).

SYNONYMS

Altitude sickness
High-altitude headache (HAH)
Acute mountain sickness (AMS)
High-altitude pulmonary edema (HAPE)
High-altitude cerebral edema (HACE)

ICD-10CM CODES

T70.2	Other and unspecified effects of high altitude
W94	Exposure to high and low air pressure and changes in air pressure

EPIDEMIOLOGY & DEMOGRAPHICS

- Millions of people worldwide are at risk of developing altitude sickness annually.
- 80% of people who ascend rapidly to high altitudes develop high-altitude headache (HAH).
- AMS is the most common of the altitude diseases. It affects approximately 40% to 50% of people ascending to 4500 m (14,750 ft) from lowland and 25% of visitors to an altitude of 2000 m (6500 ft).
- The incidence of HACE is reported to be 0.5% to 1% at elevations in excess of 4500 m (14,750 ft).
- HACE is often complicated by concomitant HAPE.
- The incidence of HAPE is reported to be 2% at 3000 m (10,000 ft) and 4% at 4500 m (14,750 ft)
- AMS and HACE affect men and women equally.
- Some studies have suggested that climbers with a prior history of HAPE have a roughly 60% chance of recurrence if they ascend to the same elevation at the same rate.

PHYSICAL FINDINGS & CLINICAL PRESENTATION (TABLE 1)

High Altitude Headache (HAH)
- Headache that develops within 24 hr of ascent.
- Bilateral, frontal or frontotemporal, dull or pressing quality.
- Mild to moderate intensity and aggravated by exertion, movement, straining, coughing, or bending.
- May be worse when lying down.
- Headache resolves within 8 hr of descent.
- HAH should resolve with analgesics and/or 10 to 15 min of supplementary oxygen.
- Difficult to distinguish from headaches secondary to dehydration.

Acute Mountain Sickness (AMS)
- AMS is thought to be a progression of HAH.
- Occurs within 6 to 12 hr after rapid ascent to 2500 m (8000 ft) in 10% to 25% of unacclimatized persons.
- Headache is the most common symptom. Often worse when lying down which may exacerbate sleep disturbance.
- Dizziness and light-headedness.
- Nausea, vomiting, and loss of appetite.
- Fatigue.
- Sleep disturbance from an exaggerated hyperventilatory phase of periodic respiration in response to hypoxemia and alkalosis.
- The Lake Louise AMS Score has been developed to standardize the diagnosis and severity of AMS in research studies.
- AMS can evolve into HAPE and HACE.
- Retinal hemorrhages can be present from increased blood flow or breakdown in the blood-retinal barrier.
- Supplemental oxygen may be used as a temporizing treatment and to support the clinical diagnosis.

High Altitude Cerebral Edema (HACE)
- Usually presents several days after AMS, 24 to 72 after elevation gain.
- Headache, nausea, vomiting, mild fever, confusion, irritability, drowsiness, stupor, hallucinations, seizures, and paralysis.
- Truncal ataxia and encephalopathy.
- Coma and death from brain herniation may develop within hours of the first symptoms.

High Altitude Pulmonary Edema HAPE (Fig. E1)
- Typically occurs 2 to 4 days after ascent to more than 3000 m (10,000 ft); note that HAPE is not always preceded by AMS symptoms.
- It can occur at a lower elevation in patients with pulmonary hypertension.
- Dyspnea out of proportion to the level of exertion, loss of stamina.
- Dry cough or cough with frothy rust- or pink-tinged sputum.
- Chest tightness.
- Tachycardia, tachypnea.
- Rales on auscultation, cyanosis.

ETIOLOGY

- During ascent to altitudes above sea level, the atmospheric pressure and partial pressure of oxygen (PO2) decrease. Although the percentage of oxygen in the air remains the same, the decreased partial pressure reduces the oxygen available in the alveoli and the diffusion gradient across the alveoli into the blood. This causes hypoxemia.
- Competing drives to hyperventilate in response to low oxygen saturation and to hypoventilate due to low pCO2 lead to periodic respiration, which can dramatically disturb sleep exacerbating other symptoms.
- Increased cerebral blood flow and the loss of autoregulation of intracranial pressure may contribute to increased cerebral vascular permeability and subsequent brain edema (HACE).
- Hypobaric hypoxia can trigger elevated pulmonary pressures, resulting in protein-rich, hemorrhagic exudates into the lung alveoli due to a breakdown in the pulmonary blood-gas barrier (HAPE).
- The body responds to low oxygen partial pressures through a process of acclimatization that takes place over days to weeks (see "Comments").

DIAGNOSIS

Made by clinical presentation and physical exam findings.

DIFFERENTIAL DIAGNOSIS

- Dehydration
- Carbon monoxide poisoning
- Hypothermia
- Infection
- Substance abuse
- Congestive heart failure
- Pulmonary embolism
- Cerebrovascular accident
- Box 1 summarizes the differential diagnosis of high-altitude illnesses

WORKUP

Typically, the diagnosis is self-evident after history and physical examination. Subsequent laboratory tests and imaging studies help monitor cardiopulmonary and central nervous system status in patients admitted to the intensive care unit for pulmonary and/or cerebral edema. In patients with HAPE occurring at lower altitudes (< 2500 m [8000 ft]), an evaluation of preexisting pulmonary hypertension or an intracardiac shunt should be considered. Pulse oximetry that does not return to normal on descent can be helpful to evaluate severity of HAPE and follow its resolution.

LABORATORY TESTS

Not useful for initial diagnosis, unless to rule out an alternative diagnosis.

IMAGING STUDIES

- Chest x-ray showing Kerley B-lines and patchy edema. (see Fig. E1)
- CT scan of the head showing diffuse or patchy edema.
- MRI of the head showing characteristic intense T2 signal in the white matter.

TREATMENT

NONPHARMACOLOGIC THERAPY

- Stop the ascent to allow acclimatization or initiate descent until symptoms have resolved.
- Patient with AMS can stay at the same height and may ascend once symptoms resolve.
- If AMS symptoms recur or fail to resolve after 2 to 3 days, descent is indicated.
- Descent is mandatory for all persons with HACE or HAPE and should be initiated immediately with development of symptoms of HACE or HAPE as they may quickly worsen and incapacitate the patient, which can turn

TABLE 1 Clinical Characteristics of High-Altitude Illnesses

	Clinical Classification			
	HAH	**Mild AMS**	**Moderate to Severe AMS**	**HACE**
Symptoms	Headache only	Headache plus one more symptom (nausea/vomiting, fatigue/lassitude, dizziness, or difficulty sleeping) All symptoms of mild severity	Headache plus one or more symptoms (nausea/vomiting, fatigue/lassitude, dizziness, or difficulty sleeping) Symptoms of moderate to severe intensity	±Headache Worsening of symptoms seen in moderate to severe AMS
LL-AMS score*	1-3, headache only	2-4	5-15	
Physical signs	None	Possible peripheral edema	Possible peripheral edema	Ataxia Altered mental status peripheral edema
Findings	None	Possible mild altitude adjusted desaturation	Slightly increased body temperature Slight altitude adjusted desaturation Widened A-a gradient Elevated ICP White matter edema (CT, MRI)	HAPE common: Positive chest radiograph, rales, dyspnea at rest Altitude adjusted desaturation Elevated ICP White matter edema (CT, MRI)

AMS, Acute mountain sickness; *CT,* computed tomography; *HACE,* high-altitude cerebral edema; *HAH,* high-altitude headache; *HAPE,* high-altitude pulmonary edema; *ICP,* intracranial pressure; *LL-AMS,* Lake Louise AMS; *MRI,* magnetic resonance imaging.
*The self-reported Lake Louise AMS score.
From Auerbach P: *Wilderness medicine, expert consult,* premium edition—enhanced online features and print, Philadelphia, 2012, Saunders.

BOX 1 Differential Diagnosis of High-Altitude Illnesses

Acute mountain sickness and high-altitude cerebral edema	Dehydration, exhaustion, viral or bacterial infection, alcohol hangover, hypothermia, carbon monoxide poisoning, migraine, hyponatremia, hypoglycemia, diabetic ketoacidosis, CNS infection, transient ischemic attack, arteriovenous malformation, stroke, seizures, brain tumors, ingestion of toxins or drugs, acute psychosis
High-altitude pulmonary edema	Asthma, bronchitis, pneumonia, mucus plugging (secondary to previous), idiopathic hyperventilation syndrome, pulmonary embolism, heart failure, myocardial infarction

CNS, Central nervous system.
From Auerbach P: *Wilderness medicine, expert consult,* premium edition—enhanced online features and print, Philadelphia, 2012, Saunders.

a relatively easy walk down the mountain into a logistically complicated rescue requiring substantial resources.

- Supplemental oxygen is used for treatment of severe AMS, HAPE, and HACE.
- Portable hyperbaric bags are useful if available at the site and can temporize a difficult situation to allow descent.
- Adequate hydration is key for AMS of any severity.

ACUTE PHARMACOLOGIC PROPHYLAXIS AND THERAPY

- Nonsteroidal antiinflammatory drugs (e.g., ibuprofen 600 mg every 6 hr, beginning 6 hr before ascending) are often used for prophylaxis of traditional altitude sickness and in treating headaches in AMS. However trials have shown that ibuprofen is slightly inferior to acetazolamide for acute mountain sickness prevention, and should not be recommended over acetazolamide for rapid ascent. Headache that does not resolve after treatment with NSAID is concerning, and patients should not ascend further and should consider descent until it improves.
- Acetazolamide 125 to 250 mg PO bid is the preferred agent and has been effective for both prevention and acute therapy in patients with AMS and HACE.
- Dexamethasone is also effective in reducing symptoms of AMS and can be used as an alternative to acetazolamide in individuals who are intolerant to acetazolamide (sulfa allergy). It should be added to acetazolamide in patients with HACE.
- Dexamethasone initial dose of 8 mg PO/IM/IV followed by 4 mg PO every 6 hr is used in patients with severe AMS, HAPE, or HACE.
- Table E2 summarizes recommended medications for the prevention and treatment of altitude sickness.
- Nifedipine 10 mg sublingual followed by long-acting nifedipine 30 mg bid is used for patients with HAPE who cannot descend immediately. Salvage therapy in absence of supplemental oxygen and descent also includes phosphodiesterase-5 inhibitors (sildenafil or tadalafil), which decrease pulmonary artery pressure.

CHRONIC THERAPY

Prevention is the most prudent therapy. Recommendations include:

- Slow, staged ascent to avoid altitude sickness.
- Start the ascent below 2500 meters (8000 ft).
- Ascend 300 m/day (1000 ft/day).
- Spend two nights at the same altitude every 3 days.
- Sleep at lower heights than the altitude climbed ("climb high, sleep low").
- Limiting extreme exertion on arrival at a new higher elevation for 24 hr may also decrease the likelihood of AMS.
- Box 2 summarizes field treatment of high-altitude illness.

DISPOSITION

- AMS typically improves over a period of 2 to 3 days if altitude is unchanged or possibly much quicker if altitude is reduced.
- HAPE is the most common cause of death among patients with altitude illnesses. Aggressive treatment with descent (or hyperbaric therapy if unable to descend) and oxygen are warranted.
- More than 66% of patients with HAPE will have recurrence of symptoms on subsequent climbs.
- In HACE, neurologic deficits may persist for weeks but eventually resolve. If coma occurs, prognosis is poor.

REFERRAL

Cardiology and neurology referrals are made in patients with pulmonary edema and central nervous system findings, respectively.

BOX 2 Field Treatment of High-Altitude Illness

High-Altitude Headache and Mild Acute Mountain Sickness
- Stop ascent, rest, acclimatize at same altitude
- Symptomatic treatment as necessary with analgesics and antiemetics
- Consider acetazolamide, 125 to 250 mg bid, to speed acclimatization
- OR descend 500 m (1640 ft) or more

Moderate to Severe Acute Mountain Sickness
- Low-flow oxygen, if available
- Acetazolamide, 125 to 250 mg bid, with or without dexamethasone, 4 mg PO, IM, or IV q6h
- Hyperbaric therapy
- OR immediate descent

High-Altitude Cerebral Edema
- Immediate descent or evacuation
- Oxygen, 2 to 4 L/min
- Dexamethasone, 8 mg PO, IM, or IV, then 4 mg q6h
- Hyperbaric therapy

High-Altitude Pulmonary Edema
- Minimize exertion and keep warm
- Immediate descent or hyperbaric therapy
- Oxygen, 4 to 6 L/min until improving, then 2 to 4 L/min
  If above unavailable, one of the following:
- Nifedipine, 30 mg extended release q12h
- Sildenafil 50 mg q8h
- Tadalafil 10 mg q12h
- β-agonists may be helpful

Periodic Breathing
- Acetazolamide, 62.5 to 125 mg at bedtime as needed

bid, Twice a day; *IM*, intramuscularly; *IV*, intravenously; *PO*, orally.

From Auerbach P: *Wilderness medicine, expert consult,* premium edition—enhanced online features and print, Philadelphia, 2012, Saunders.

PEARLS & CONSIDERATIONS

COMMENTS

- Acclimatization is the process in which an individual who normally resides at low altitudes adapts to hypobaric hypoxia to improve tolerance and performance at higher altitudes. These mechanisms include:
  1. An increase in respiratory rate and tidal volume. This hyperventilation decreases arterial carbon dioxide improving alveolar oxygenation, even at extreme altitudes.
  2. An early increase in heart rate and stroke volume to improve oxygen delivery via increased cardiac output. After 1 wk, both parameters decrease secondary to diuresis and lower catecholamine levels.
  3. Pulmonary hypertension develops in response to hypoxemia, resulting in improvement of the ventilation-perfusion mismatch (versus response to hypoxemic pulmonary vasoconstriction) but may be maladaptive and lead to the development of HAPE.
  4. Cerebral vasodilation to increase blood flow to the brain.
  5. Rise in hemoglobin. This process can take a week to occur in response to the need for improved oxygen delivery and can take several weeks for a meaningful increase in hemoglobin to occur.
- Adaptation to altitude is different from acclimatization and refers to physiologic differences in permanent residents at high altitude (e.g., an increased oxygen diffusion capacity and very elevated hemoglobin levels).
- Risk factors for the development of altitude sicknesses are:
  1. Rapid ascent
  2. Previous history of altitude sickness
  3. Strenuous exertion on arrival
  4. Obesity
  5. Male gender
  6. Alcohol consumption
- Physical fitness is not protective against nor fully predictive of high-altitude illness.

SUGGESTED READINGS

Available at ExpertConsult.com

RELATED CONTENT

Altitude Sickness (Patient Information)

AUTHORS: **Eugene Carragee, MD, Stephanie Sutter, MD,** and **Jeffrey W. Sall, PhD, MD**

BASIC INFORMATION

DEFINITION

Hodgkin lymphoma is a malignant disorder arising from germinal center B cells and characterized histologically by the presence of multinucleated giant cells (Reed-Sternberg cells) in a mixed inflammatory background.

ICD-10CM CODES	
C81.90	Hodgkin lymphoma, unspecified, unspecified site
C81.00	Nodular lymphocyte predominant Hodgkin lymphoma, unspecified site
C81.10	Nodular sclerosis classical Hodgkin lymphoma, unspecified site
C81.20	Mixed cellularity classical Hodgkin lymphoma, unspecified site
C81.30	Lymphocyte depleted classical Hodgkin lymphoma, unspecified site
C81.79	Other classical Hodgkin lymphoma, extranodal and solid organ sites
C81.90	Hodgkin lymphoma, unspecified, unspecified site
C81.91	Hodgkin lymphoma, unspecified, lymph nodes of head, face, and neck
C81.92	Hodgkin lymphoma, unspecified, intrathoracic lymph nodes
C81.93	Hodgkin lymphoma, unspecified, intra-abdominal lymph nodes
C81.94	Hodgkin lymphoma, unspecified, lymph nodes of axilla and upper limb
C81.95	Hodgkin lymphoma, unspecified, lymph nodes of inguinal region and lower limb
C81.96	Hodgkin lymphoma, unspecified, intrapelvic lymph nodes
C81.97	Hodgkin lymphoma, unspecified, spleen
C81.98	Hodgkin lymphoma, unspecified, lymph nodes of multiple sites
C81.99	Hodgkin lymphoma, unspecified, extranodal and solid organ sites

EPIDEMIOLOGY & DEMOGRAPHICS

- There is a bimodal age distribution (15-34 yr and >50 yr).
- Incidence is 4 in 100,000 cases; >8000 new cases of Hodgkin lymphoma diagnosed annually in the U.S.
- Concordance for Hodgkin lymphoma in identical twins suggests that a genetic susceptibility underlies Hodgkin lymphoma in young adulthood.
- There is association between certain HLA haplotypes, especially HLA-A1.
- The disease is more common in males (in childhood Hodgkin lymphoma, >80% occur in males), whites, and higher socioeconomic groups.
- There is an increased risk in smokers and HIV-infected individuals.

PHYSICAL FINDINGS & CLINICAL PRESENTATION

- Painless palpable lymphadenopathy is the most common presenting symptom.
- The most common site of involvement is the neck region.
- Fever and night sweats: Fever in a cyclical pattern (days or weeks of fever alternating with afebrile periods) is known as Pel-Ebstein fever.
- Unexplained weight loss, generalized malaise.
- Persistent, nonproductive cough.
- Lymph node pain associated with alcohol ingestion often because of heavy eosinophil infiltration of the tumor sites is relatively uncommon.
- Generalized pruritus.
- Hepatosplenomegaly.
- Other: Superior vena cava syndrome, spinal cord compression (rare), erythema nodosum (very rare), ichthyosis (very rare).

ETIOLOGY

- Evidence implicating Epstein-Barr virus remains controversial.
- Cigarette smoking has also been implicated.

DIAGNOSIS

DIFFERENTIAL DIAGNOSIS

- Non-Hodgkin's lymphoma
- Sarcoidosis
- Infections (e.g., cytomegalovirus, Epstein-Barr virus, toxoplasmosis, HIV, tuberculosis)
- Drug reaction

WORKUP

Diagnosis is confirmed by lymph node biopsy. The World Health Organization classifies Hodgkin lymphoma into two groups: Classical Hodgkin lymphoma (92% to 97%) and nodular lymphocyte-predominant Hodgkin lymphoma (3% to 8%). Classical Hodgkin lymphoma has four main histologic subtypes based on the number of lymphocytes, Reed-Sternberg cells, and the presence of fibrous tissue (Table 1):

- Nodular sclerosis (Fig. E1)
- Mixed cellularity (Fig. E2)
- Lymphocyte rich
- Lymphocyte depleted

Nodular sclerosis occurs mainly in young adulthood, whereas the mixed cellularity type is more prevalent after age 50 yr. Table 2 summarizes key features of Hodgkin lymphomas.

Staging: Table 3 describes the Cotswolds staging classification.

Proper staging requires the following:

- Detailed history (with documentation of "B symptoms" and physical examination)
- Excisional biopsy with histologic, immunophenotypic and immunohistochemical analysis
- Laboratory evaluation (complete blood count, erythrocyte sedimentation rate [ESR], blood urea nitrogen, creatinine, liver function tests, albumin, lactate dehydrogenase, HIV test), immunophenotypic markers (see Table 4)
- Positron emission tomography (PET)/computed tomography (CT) scan of the chest, abdomen, and pelvis
- Unilateral bone marrow biopsy in selected patients

Box 1 summarizes recommended staging procedures for Hodgkin lymphoma.

TREATMENT

ACUTE GENERAL Rx

The main therapeutic modality includes chemotherapy with or without radiotherapy depending on stage and other risk factors (Table 5). In general, chemotherapy plus involved-site radiotherapy is standard treatment for Hodgkin lymphoma in the early stages; however, recent data suggest that chemotherapy alone is appropriate for a significant proportion of patients. Chemotherapy (Table 6) is used for advanced stage disease with radiotherapy in selected patients, such as those with bulky disease.

Most oncologists prefer the combination of adriamycin (doxorubicin), bleomycin, vinblastine, and dacarbazine (ABVD). ABVD does not cause infertility or stem cell damage and has also shown to be effective in patients with HIV infection and Hodgkin lymphoma. Table 7 describes characteristics of the ABVD regimen.

Recent trials have shown that in patients with early-stage Hodgkin lymphoma and favorable prognosis, defined by fewer than three nodal sites without bulky or extranodal disease in the absence of ESR >50 without symptoms or 30 with symptoms, treatment with two cycles of ABVD followed by 20 Gy of involved-field radiation therapy may be as effective as, and less toxic than, four cycles of ABVD followed by 30 Gy of involved-field radiation therapy. For patients with early stage disease who do not meet these criteria, options include three or four cycles of ABVD plus involved site radiotherapy to 30 Gy. In addition, chemotherapy alone, in

TABLE 1 Frequency of Histologic Subtypes of Hodgkin Lymphoma According to the 2008 WHO Classification

Classic Hodgkin Lymphoma (cHL)	95%
• Nodular sclerosis classic Hodgkin lymphoma (NSCHL)	70%
• Mixed cellularity classic Hodgkin lymphoma (MCCHL)	20%–25%
• Lymphocyte-rich classic Hodgkin lymphoma (LRCHL)	5%
• Lymphocyte-depleted classic Hodgkin lymphoma (LDCHL)	<1%
Nodular Lymphocyte Predominant Hodgkin Lymphoma (NLPHL)	5%

From Hoffman R et al: *Hematology, basic principles and practice*, ed 7, Philadelphia, 2018, Elsevier.

TABLE 2 Key Features of Hodgkin Lymphomas

Lymphoma	Demographics, Clinical Presentation	Morphology	Cell Surface Markers	Prognosis
Nodular, lymphocyte predominant (NLPHL)	M > F, 30-50 yr, with peripheral lymphadenopathy	Mononuclear cells with convoluted nuclei (popcorn or L&H cells) loosely aggregated in nodules of small B cells	CD45, CD20, bcl-6, J-chain, Oct-2, BOB.1, EBV absent in LP cells	Excellent for stages I, II
Nodular sclerosis	M = F, <30 yr with mediastinal mass, occasional spleen or lung involvement; 40% have B symptoms; most patients present with stage II disease	Broad bands of collagen, nodules of lymphoid tissue with aggregates of HRS cells and lacunar cells, multinucleated variants	CD15, CD30, CD45-EBV in 1%-40%	Good with systemic therapy
Mixed cellularity	M > F; median age, 38 yr; peripheral lymphadenopathy common, spleen, BM; B symptoms common; patients often stage III or IV	Classic HRS cells in mixture of lymphocytes, plasma cells, eosinophils, histiocytes	CD15, CD30, CD45-EBV in 75%	Good with systemic therapy
Lymphocyte depletion	M > F; median age, 30-37 yr; B symptoms, advanced stage common; associated with HIV	Classic HRS cells common with paucity of background lymphocytes; pleomorphic HRS cells mimic sarcoma	CD15, CD30, CD45-EBV positive in HIV-affected patients	Associated with advanced stage
Lymphocyte-rich classical	M > F, older age; peripheral lymphadenopathy; B symptoms rare; most patients with stage I or II disease	Scattered classic HRS cells among numerous small lymphocytes; nodular growth pattern	CD15, CD30; Oct2 and BOB.1 vary; J-chain absent; EBV in 40%-75%	Good, similar to NLPHL

BM, Bone marrow; *CHL,* classical Hodgkin lymphoma; *EBV,* Epstein-Barr virus; *F,* female; *HIV,* human immunodeficiency virus; *HRS,* Hodgkin Reed-Sternberg; *L&H,* lymphocytic and histiocytic; *LP,* lymphoplasmacytic; *M,* male.
From McPherson RA, Pincus MR: *Henry's clinical diagnosis and management by laboratory methods*, ed 23, St Louis, 2017, Elsevier.

TABLE 3 Cotswold-Modified Ann Arbor Staging System for Hodgkin Lymphoma

Stage	Criteria
I	Disease affecting a single lymph node region or lymphoid structure (e.g., spleen, thymus, Waldeyer ring)
II	Disease affecting two or more discrete lymph node regions confined to the same side of the diaphragm
III	Disease affecting two or more discrete lymph node regions or lymphoid structures on both sides of the diaphragm
IV	Disease that has spread to one or more extranodal sites (that do not meet the criteria for E) or extralymphatic structure including involvement of the bone marrow, liver, or lungs
Designation	**Criteria**
A	Absence of B symptoms[a]
B	Presence of B symptoms[a]
S	Involvement of the spleen
E	Single extranodal site or involvement of an extranodal site that is contiguous to an involved nodal region
X	Bulky disease as defined as >1/3 mediastinum at its widest part or a nodal mass >10 cm at its greatest diameter

[a]B symptoms: Constitutional symptoms including night sweats, fevers, or weight loss (>10% over 6 mo).
From Hoffman R et al: *Hematology, basic principles and practice*, ed 7, Philadelphia, 2018, Elsevier.

TABLE 4 Selected Immunophenotypic Markers and Histologic Characteristics of Use in the Differential Diagnosis of Hodgkin Lymphoma and Other Lymphoid Neoplasms

Marker	Classical HL	Nodular Lymphocyte Predominant HL	TCRBCL	ALCL
CD30	+	–	–	+
CD15	+	–	–	–
CD20	–/+*	+	+	–
CD45	–	+	+	+/–
CD79a	–	+	+	–
ALK	–	–	–	+/–
EMA	–	+	+	+
Nodular growth protein	+/–†	+	–	–

+, >90% of cases positive; +/–, majority of cases positive; –/+, minority of cases positive; –, <10% of cases positive; *ALCL,* anaplastic large cell lymphoma; *HL,* Hodgkin lymphoma; *TCRBCL,* T-cell rich B-cell lymphoma.
*CD20 positivity in classical Hodgkin lymphoma is quite heterogeneous, with a wide range in brightness of staining.
†In classical Hodgkin lymphoma, a nodular growth pattern is confined to the nodular sclerosing subtype.
From Abeloff MD: *Clinical oncology*, ed 3, Philadelphia, 2004, Saunders.

the absence of bulky disease, is an alternative approach, especially in women younger than 30 yr given the increased risk of including breast cancer, as well as cardiac and thyroid disease. Although the risk of disease recurrence is slightly higher in patients who receive chemotherapy alone, there is no difference in overall survival.

BEACOPP, an intensified regimen consisting of bleomycin, etoposide, doxorubicin, cyclophosphamide, vincristine, procarbazine, and prednisone, has been advocated by some as the new standard for treatment of advanced Hodgkin lymphoma in place of ABVD. Recent trials have shown that treatment with BEACOPP, as compared with ABVD, results in better initial tumor control, but the long-term clinical outcome does not differ significantly between the two regimens. In addition, with the use of the escalated BEACOPP regimen, the rate of complications is higher (3% treatment-related death, 20% rate of hospitalization, and 3% rate of secondary leukemia, and near-universal infertility). Thus, if the goal is cure with the least overall toxic effects, it is best to favor ABVD therapy, reserving rescue therapy with high-dose chemotherapy and autologous hematopoietic stem-cell transplantation for the small number of patients in whom the primary treatment fails.

In March 2018, the FDA approved the combination of brentuximab vedotin and doxorubicin, vinblastine and dacarbazine (AVD) for previously untreated, stage III or IV Hodgkin lymphoma patients. The combination of brentuximab vedotin and AVD was associated with a longer median modified progression-free survival than ABVD, but also was associated with higher rates of neutropenia and neuropathy.

- Definitions of treatment groups are described in Table 8.
- Recommendations for the primary treatment of Hodgkin lymphoma outside of clinical trials are described in Table 9.
- In 2011, the FDA approved the use of the anti-CD30 antibody drug conjugate brentuximab

BOX 1 Recommended Staging Procedures for Hodgkin Lymphoma

The following staging procedures are recommended for the initial workup of Hodgkin lymphoma:
1. Adequate surgical biopsy reviewed by an experienced hematopathologist
2. Cytologic examination of any effusion in selected cases
3. Detailed history, with attention to the presence or absence of systemic symptoms, and a careful physical examination, emphasizing node chains, size of the liver and spleen, and inspection of Waldeyer ring
4. Routine laboratory tests: Complete blood cell count, erythrocyte sedimentation rate, and liver function tests
5. Neck, chest, and abdominal CT imaging fused with 18-FDG PET scan (Fig. E3)

18-FDG PET, Positron emission tomography with 2-deoxy-2-[fluorine-18]fluoro-D-glucose; *CT;* computed tomography.
From Hoffman R et al: *Hematology: basic principles and practice,* ed 5, Philadelphia, 2009, Churchill Livingstone.

TABLE 5 Standard Treatment Approach According to Prognostic Group

Early-favorable HL	Combined modality therapy • 2-4 cycles of chemotherapy followed by involved-field radiotherapy
Early-unfavorable HL (intermediate-stage)	Combined modality therapy • 4-6 cycles of chemotherapy followed by involved-field radiotherapy
Advanced HL	Extensive chemotherapy • 6-8 cycles of chemotherapy ± consolidation with localized radiotherapy

HL, Hodgkin lymphoma.
From Hoffman R et al: *Hematology, basic principles and practice,* ed 7, Philadelphia, 2018, Elsevier.

TABLE 6 Standard Chemotherapy Regimens for the Treatment of Advanced Hodgkin Lymphoma

Regimen	Drugs	Route	Schedule
ABVD	Adriamycin 25 mg/m^2	IV	Day 1 and 15
	Bleomycin 10 mg/m^2	IV	Day 1 and 15
	Vinblastine 6 mg/m^2	IV	Day 1 and 15
	Dacarbazine 375 mg/m^2	IV	Day 1 and 15
			Every 28 days
BEACOPP (escalated)	Bleomycin 10 mg/m^2	IV	Day 8
	Etoposide 200 mg/m^2	IV	Day 1-3
	Adriamycin 35 mg/m^2	IV	Day 1
	Cyclophosphamide 1250 mg/m^2	IV	Day 1
	Vincristine 1.4 mg/m^2	IV	Day 8
	Procarbazine 100 mg/m^2	PO	Days 1-7
	Prednisolone 40 mg/m^2	PO	Days 1-14
	G-CSF	SC	From day 8
			Every 21 days

ABVD, Adriamycin (doxorubicin), bleomycin, vinblastine, dacarbazine; *BEACOPP,* bleomycin, etoposide, Adriamycin (doxorubicin), cyclophosphamide, Oncovin (vincristine), procarbazine, and prednisone; *G-CSF,* granulocyte colony-stimulating factor; *IV,* intravenous; *PO,* by mouth; *SC,* subcutaneous.
From Hoffman R et al: *Hematology, basic principles and practice,* ed 7, Philadelphia, 2018, Elsevier.

TABLE 7 Characteristics of the ABVD Regimen

Agents: Doxorubicin, bleomycin, vinblastine, dacarbazine
All intravenous, total compliance
80% complete response rate
10% primary refractory disease
60%-65% overall disease-free survival
Most relapses occur within the first 4 yr; however, about 10% of all relapses occur beyond 5 yr
Major side effects are nausea, phlebitis, myelosuppression, less cumulative myelotoxicity than MOPP
No infertility
No leukemia

ABVD, Adriamycin (doxorubicin), bleomycin, vinblastine, dacarbazine; *MOPP,* mechlorethamine, Oncovin (vincristine), procarbazine, prednisone.
From Abeloff MD: *Clinical oncology,* ed 3, Philadelphia, 2004, Saunders.

vedotin for the treatment of patients with Hodgkin lymphoma who have relapsed after autologous stem cell transplant and for patients who have relapsed but are not candidates for transplant. Brentuximab vedotin is associated with an overall response rate of 75%.
- In August 2015, brentuximab vedotin was approved as consolidation therapy after autologous transplant in patients at high risk for relapse. The median progression-free survival with brentuximab vedotin was 43 mo vs. 24 mo in patients who received placebo.
- In May 2016, the FDA approved the anti-PD-1 monoclonal antibody nivolumab for patients with Hodgkin lymphoma who relapsed after autologous stem cell transplant and post-transplant brentuximab vedotin. The overall response rate to nivolumab was 65%, and the complete response rate was 7%.
- In March 2017, the FDA approved the anti-PD-1 monoclonal antibody pembrolizumab in patients with refractory disease or those who have relapsed after three or more lines of therapy. The overall response rate was 69%, and the complete response rate was 22%.

DISPOSITION

- Cure rates as high as 85% to 90% in early stage patients and 75% in stage III/V disease are now possible with appropriate initial therapy.
- Poor prognostic features (Table 10, Table 11) include presence of B symptoms, advanced age, advanced stage at initial presentation, male sex, low albumin, high ESR, lymphocyte depletion histology, and increased number of tumor-associated macrophages.
- Unlike escalated BEACOPP, ABVD is not associated with a risk of leukemia.
- Mediastinal irradiation increases the risk of subsequent cardiac disease, including valvular and pericardial disease, accelerated coronary artery disease, and conduction abnormalities.
- Radiation therapy increases the risk of developing secondary solid tumors, especially breast cancer in women younger than age 30 yr (Table 12).
- Table 13 describes potential late complications of Hodgkin lymphoma treatment and appropriate clinical responses and preventive strategies.

REFERRAL

- To surgery for lymph node biopsy
- Fertility clinic for sperm banking
- Hematology/oncology
- Radiation oncology, in selected cases

PEARLS & CONSIDERATIONS

COMMENTS

- Young male patients should consider sperm banking before the initiation of therapy even though the risk of infertility with ABVD is

TABLE 8 Definition of Treatment Groups According to the EORTC/GELA and GHSG

Treatment Group	EORTC/GELA	GHSG	NCIC/ECOG
Early-stage favorable	CS I-II without risk factors (supradiaphragmatic)	CS I-II without risk factors	Standard risk group: Favorable CSD I-II (without risk factors)
Early-stage unfavorable (intermediate)	CS I-II with ≥1 risk factors (supradiaphragmatic)	CS I, CSIIA ≥1 risk factors; CS IIB with C/D but without A/B	Standard risk group: Unfavorable CS I-II (at least one risk factor)
Advanced stage	CS III-IV	CS IIB with A/B;CS III-IV	High-risk group: CS I or II with bulky disease; intraabdominal disease; CS III, IV
Risk factors (RF)	A large mediastinal mass B age ≥50 yr C elevated ESR* D ≥4 involved regions	A large mediastinal mass B extranodal disease C elevated ESR* D ≥3 involved areas	A ≥40 yr B not NLPHL or NS histology C ESR ≥50 mm/h D ≥4 involved nodal regions

CS, Clinical stage; *ECOG,* Eastern Cooperative Oncology Group; *EORTC,* European Organization for Research and Treatment of Cancer; *GELA,* Groupe d'Etude des Lymphomes de l'Adulte; *GHSG,* German Hodgkin Study Group; *NCIC,* National Cancer Institute of Canada; *NLPHL,* nodular lymphocyte predominant Hodgkin lymphoma.
*Erythrocyte sedimentation rate (ESR) (≥50 mm/h without or ≥30 mm/h with B-symptoms).
From Hoffman R et al: *Hematology, basic principles and practice*, ed 5, New York, 2009, Churchill Livingstone.

TABLE 9 Recommendations for the Primary Treatment of Hodgkin Lymphoma Outside of Clinical Trials

Group	Stage	Recommendation
Early stages (favorable)	CS I-II A/B, no RFs	2 cycles ABVD + ISRT (20 Gy)
	Early stages (unfavorable, intermediate) CS I-II A/B + RFs	4-6 cycles ABVD ±30 Gy for nonbulky disease 4-6 cycles ABVD + 30 Gy for bulky disease
Advanced stages	CS IIB + RFs, CS III A/B, CS IV A/B	6 cycles ABVD; BEACOPP-escalated *or* BEACOPP-14 ± RT, 20-30 Gy for residual tumor (PET positive) and/or bulky disease

ABVD regimen, Adriamycin (doxorubicin), vinblastine, bleomycin, and dacarbazine; *BEACOPP-baseline* regimen, bleomycin, etoposide, Adriamycin (doxorubicin), cyclophosphamide, Oncovin (vincristine), procarbazine, and prednisone; *BEACOPP-escalated* regimen, bleomycin, etoposide, Adriamycin (doxorubicin), cyclophosphamide, Oncovin (vincristine), procarbazine, prednisone, and G-CSF; *BEACOPP-14* regimen, bleomycin, etoposide, Adriamycin (doxorubicin), cyclophosphamide, Oncovin (vincristine), procarbazine, prednisone, and G-CSF; *CS,* clinical stage; *IF,* involved field; *ISRT,* involved-site radiation therapy; *MOPP* regimen, mechlorethamine, Oncovin (vincristine), procarbazine, and prednisone; *PET,* positron emission tomography; *RF,* risk factors; *RT,* radiation therapy; *Stanford V* regimen, nitrogen mustard, doxorubicin, vinblastine, bleomycin, vincristine, etoposide, and prednisone.
From Hoffman R et al: *Hematology, basic principles and practice*, ed 5, New York, 2009, Churchill Livingstone.

TABLE 10 Prognostic Factors in Early and Advanced-Stage Hodgkin Lymphoma

Prognostic Group	EORTC	GHSG	NCCN
Early-favorable	CS I-II without risk factors (supra-diaphragmatic)	CS I-II without risk factors	CS IA-IIA without risk factors
Early-unfavorable (Intermediate)	CS I-II with ≥1 risk factor (supra-diaphragmatic)	CS I-IIA with ≥1 risk factor C/D but not A/B	CS I-II with ≥1 risk factor
Advanced	CS III-IV	CS IIB with risk factors A/B CS III/IV	CS III-IV
Prognostic factors	(A) Bulky mediastinal mass[a] (B) Age ≥50 yr (C) Elevated ESR (>50 mm/h without B symptoms; >30 mm/h with B symptoms)[b] (D) ≥4 nodal areas (out of 5 supra-diaphragmatic EORTC areas)	(A) Bulky mediastinal mass[a] (B) Extranodal disease (>1 lesion) (C) Elevated ESR (>50 mm/h without B symptoms; >30 mm/h with B symptoms)[b] (D) ≥3 nodal areas (out of 11 GHSG areas)	(A) Bulky mediastinal mass[a] (B) Bulk >10 cm (C) Elevated ESR (>50 mm/h without B symptoms) (D) B symptoms (E) ≥4 nodal areas (out of 17 Ann Arbor regions)

CS, Clinical stage; *EORTC,* European Organization for Research and Treatment of Cancer; *ESR,* estimated sedimentation rate; *GHSG,* German Hodgkin Study Group; *NCCN,* National Comprehensive Cancer Network.
[a]Bulky mediastinal mass: Ratio ≥0.035 of the maximum horizontal chest diameter (*EORTC*); ratio ≥1/3 of the maximum horizontal chest diameter (*GHSG*); ratio >1/3 of the maximum horizontal chest diameter (*NCCN*).
[b]B symptoms: Night sweats, fever, weight loss (unexplained, >10% over 6 mo).
From Hoffman R et al: *Hematology, basic principles and practice*, ed 7, Philadelphia, 2018, Elsevier.

TABLE 11 International Prognostic Score (IPS) for Advanced Hodgkin Lymphoma

No. of Prognostic Factors	% of patients	5-yr FFP (%)	5-yr OS (%)
0-1 (low-risk)	29	79	90
2-3 (intermediate-risk)	52	64	80
4-7 (high-risk)	19	47	59

FFP, Freedom from progression; *OS,* overall survival.
From Hoffman R et al: *Hematology, basic principles and practice*, ed 7, Philadelphia, 2018, Elsevier.

TABLE 12 Second Neoplasms Seen with Increased Frequency after Successful Hodgkin Lymphoma Treatment

Acute myelogenous leukemia/myelodysplasia (BEACOPP)
Non-Hodgkin's lymphoma
Melanoma
Soft tissue sarcoma
Adenocarcinoma
Breast
Thyroid
Lung
Stomach and esophagus
Squamous cell carcinoma
Skin
Uterine cervix
Head and neck

BEACOPP, Bleomycin, etoposide, Adriamycin (doxorubicin), cyclophosphamide, Oncovin (vincristine), procarbazine, and prednisone.
From Abeloff MD: *Clinical oncology*, ed 3, Philadelphia, 2004, Saunders.

low. Symptomatic males, particularly with advanced stage Hodgkin lymphoma, may have disease-related oligospermia at diagnosis.

- Chemotherapy with or without involved-field radiotherapy should be the standard treatment for Hodgkin lymphoma with early stage disease. Chemotherapy with radiation in selected cases should be the standard of care for advanced stage.
- After failure of ABVD therapy, more than 60% of patients who have had a relapse and about 30% of patients with initially refractory lymphoma can be reliably cured with high-dose chemotherapy and autologous hematopoietic stem-cell transplantation.

RELATED CONTENT

Hodgkin Lymphoma (Patient Information)

SUGGESTED READINGS

Available at ExpertConsult.com

AUTHORS: **Jorge J. Castillo, MD,** and **Ann S. Lacasce, MD, MMSc**

TABLE 13 Potential Late Complications of Hodgkin Lymphoma Treatment and Appropriate Clinical Responses and Preventive Strategies

Risk/Problem	Incidence/Response
Dental caries	Neck or oropharyngeal irradiation can cause decreased salivation. Patients should have careful dental care follow-up and should make their dentist aware of the previous irradiation.
Hypothyroidism	After external beam irradiation that encompasses the thyroid with doses sufficient to cure Hodgkin lymphoma, at least 50% of patients will eventually become hypothyroid. All patients whose TSH level becomes elevated should be treated with lifelong thyroxine replacement in doses sufficient to suppress TSH levels to low normal. This is also necessary to ensure that the radiation-damaged thyroid is not subjected to long-term stimulation by thyroid-stimulating hormone, which can increase the risk of thyroid neoplasm.
Infertility	ABVD is not known to cause any permanent gonadal toxicity, although oligospermia for 1-2 yr after treatment is common. Direct or scatter radiation to gonadal tissue can cause infertility, amenorrhea, or premature menopause, but this seldom occurs with the current fields used for the treatment of Hodgkin lymphoma. Thus, with the current chemotherapy regimens and radiation fields used, most patients will not develop these problems. In general, after treatment, women who continue menstruating are fertile, but men require semen analysis to provide a specific answer. High-dose chemoradiotherapy and hematopoietic stem cell transplantation almost always cause permanent infertility in both genders, although some young women occasionally recover fertility.
Impaired immunity to infections	Hodgkin lymphoma and its treatment can lead to lifelong impairment of full immunity to infection. All patients should be given annual influenza immunization and pneumococcal immunization every 5 yr. Patients whose spleen has been irradiated or removed should also be immunized against meningococcal types A and C and *Haemophilus influenza* type B. As for all adults, diphtheria and tetanus immunizations should be kept up-to-date.
Secondary neoplasms	Although uncommon, certain secondary neoplasms occur with increased frequency in patients who have been treated for Hodgkin lymphoma. These include acute myelogenous leukemia, thyroid, breast, lung, and upper gastrointestinal carcinoma and melanoma, and cervical carcinoma in situ. It is appropriate to screen for these neoplasms for the rest of the patient's life because they might have lengthy induction periods.

ABVD, Adriamycin, bleomycin, vinblastine, dacarbazine; *TSH*, thyroid-stimulating hormone
From Abeloff MD: *Clinical oncology*, ed 3, Philadelphia, 2004, Saunders.

BASIC INFORMATION

DEFINITION

Hot flashes are sudden onset of intense warmth that begins in the neck or face, or in the chest and progresses to the neck and face; often associated with profuse sweating, flushing, clamminess, anxiety, and palpitations.

SYNONYMS

HFs
Vasomotor symptoms (VMSs)
Hot flushes
Night sweats

ICD-10CM CODES

N95.1	Menopausal and female climacteric states
R23.2	Flushing

EPIDEMIOLOGY & DEMOGRAPHICS

- Hot flashes affect up to 75% of women who are in the menopausal transition.
- Hot flashes typically start during late perimenopause, increase in frequency and severity throughout the menopausal transition, and finally decline over time after the final menstrual period.
- Median total duration of hot flashes is 7 yr, with symptoms lasting for a median of 4.5 yr after the last menstrual period. Women who have hot flashes early in the menopause transition can experience symptoms for more than 12 yr.
- Prevalence of hot flashes differs among racial and ethnic groups in the U.S. with highest frequency among African American women and lowest frequency among Chinese and Japanese women.

PHYSICAL FINDINGS & CLINICAL PRESENTATION

- Profuse sweating and red blotching of skin may be noted during the vasomotor event.
- Palpitations and hyperreflexia may be present during the hot flash.
- Hot flashes typically last 1 to 5 min.
- Each hot flash is associated with increase in temperature, increased pulse rate, and increased blood flow into the hands and face.
- Hot flashes during sleep are common and are referred to as *night sweats.*
- There is considerable variation in the frequency of hot flashes. One third of women report more than 10 flashes per day.

ETIOLOGY

- Dysfunction of central thermoregulatory centers caused by reduction of estrogen levels at the time of menopause
- Tamoxifen use
- Chemotherapy-induced ovarian failure

DIAGNOSIS

DIFFERENTIAL DIAGNOSIS

- Carcinoid syndrome
- Anxiety disorder
- Idiopathic flushing
- Malignancy (lymphoma, solid tumors)
- Hyperthyroidism
- Hyperhidrosis
- Infection

WORKUP

Evaluation of hot flashes is aimed at excluding the conditions listed in the differential diagnosis.

LABORATORY TESTS

- Follicle-stimulating hormone (FSH), luteinizing hormone, estradiol level. The serum FSH levels rather than estradiol levels are associated with greater severity of hot flashes in older postmenopausal women, suggesting that nonestrogen feedback systems may be important in modulating the severity of hot flashes. It is not necessary to obtain an FSH to make the diagnosis of menopausal status, however. An amenorrheic woman over age 50 with vasomotor symptoms is assumed to have made the menopausal transition, and serum markers of menopause are not required to complete the diagnosis.
- Thyroid-stimulating hormone (TSH).

Rx TREATMENT

NONPHARMACOLOGIC THERAPY

- Behavioral interventions such as relaxation training and paced respiration have been reported effective in reducing symptoms in some women.
- Lifestyle changes such as maintaining a healthy body weight, exercising regularly, and avoiding caffeine, alcohol, tobacco, and spicy foods may be beneficial.

ACUTE GENERAL Rx

- Systemic hormone therapy with estrogen alone or in combination with progestin is the most effective way to manage menopausal hot flashes with up to a 75% reduction in weekly episodes. Women receiving hormone therapy are at increased risk of thromboembolic disease and breast cancer; therefore, use should be limited to the shortest duration and smallest possible dose to control symptoms, and only after considering potential risks and benefits for each individual patient.
- While there is some evidence that progestin-only medications may improve hot flashes, it is not considered first-line treatment for vasomotor symptom management.
- The only nonhormonal method that is FDA-approved for management of hot flashes is the SSRI paroxetine (7.5 mg daily). Other antidepressants shown to be effective for treatment of hot flashes include escitalopram (10-20 mg per day), venlafaxine (37.5-75 mg per day), and desvenlafaxine (100-150 mg per day). Caution should be taken in prescribing SSRIs and SNRIs in women taking tamoxifen, as these antidepressants interfere with the cytochrome P-450 metabolism of tamoxifen, reducing its efficacy. Nonhormonal pharmacologic therapy for hot flashes is summarized in Table E1.
- Duavee is a new FDA-approved treatment of moderate to severe vasomotor menopausal symptoms. It consists of a combination of conjugated estrogens and bazedoxifene, a new selective estrogen receptor modulator (SERM).
- The anticonvulsant gabapentin (300-1200 mg/day) represents another nonhormonal alternative in the treatment of hot flashes. It can be used alone or in combination with an antidepressant; however, combining the two medications does not appear to be more effective than just gabapentin alone.
- The antihypertensive clonidine is also somewhat effective in reducing the frequency of hot flashes in mild cases. Adverse effects include dry mouth, sedation, and dizziness.
- Recent trials with the anticholinergic drug oxybutynin have shown effectiveness in reducing the frequency and severity of hot flashes in women with a history of breast cancer.
- Vitamin E (800 IU/day) may be effective in patients with mild symptoms that do not interfere with sleep or daily function.
- Soy protein (use of soy extracts that contain plant-derived estrogens [phytoestrogens]) is often used; however, clinical trials have not shown clear efficacy.
- Several classes of herbal remedies are available to patients and are commonly used, generally without significant benefit. Frequently used agents are *Cimicifuga racemosa* (black cohosh, snakeroot, bugbane), *Angelica sinensis,* and evening primrose (evening star). Recent trials using the isopropanolic extract of black cohosh rootstock (Remifemin) did show some improvement in controlling menopausal symptoms. Such alternative medications may be used to treat mild to moderate symptoms, but it is possible that symptomatic improvements may derive in part from a placebo effect. Acupuncturists are the second most consulted therapists by menopausal women. Evidence of acupuncture efficacy as an HF treatment is conflicting. A recent randomized trial[1] revealed that Chinese medicine acupuncture was not superior to noninsertive sham acupuncture for women with moderately severe menopausal HFs.

SUGGESTED READINGS

Available at ExpertConsult.com

RELATED CONTENT

Hot Flashes (Patient Information)
Menopause (Related Key Topic)

AUTHORS: **Helen Toma, MD, MSPH,** and **Rachel Wright Heinle, MD, FACOG**

[1] Ee C et al: Acupuncture for menopausal hot flashes: a randomized trial, *Ann Intern Med* 164:146-154, 2016.

BASIC INFORMATION

DEFINITION

The human immunodeficiency virus (HIV) is a retrovirus that is responsible for causing acquired immunodeficiency syndrome (AIDS). HIV infection does not necessarily mean a person has AIDS. Table 1 summarizes surveillance case definition for HIV.

SYNONYMS

HIV

AIDS: The result of progressive HIV infection in which a person has a weakened immune system and meets specific diagnostic criteria (See "Acquired Immunodeficiency Syndrome" in Section I and Table 2.)

ICD-10CM CODES

B20 Human immunodeficiency virus (HIV) disease

EPIDEMIOLOGY & DEMOGRAPHICS (IN U.S.)

- An estimated 1.2 million people in the United States are infected with HIV, and approximately 14% of them do not know they are infected.
- There are approximately 38,000 new HIV diagnoses each year, according to the Centers for Disease Control and Prevention (CDC).
- Incidence is highest among gay, bisexual, and other men who have sex with men (MSM) and in minority racial and ethnic populations.

PREDOMINANT RISK GROUPS:

- Gay, bisexual, and other MSM is the group most affected by HIV.
- MSM account for approximately two thirds of all new diagnoses each year, according to the CDC.
- HIV disproportionately affects MSM of younger age and black/African American and Hispanic/Latino background.
- Heterosexual transmission accounts for approximately 25% of new HIV diagnosis. Injection drug use accounts for approximately 6% to 7%.
- Table 3 summarizes risk factors associated with sexual transmission of HIV.

RACIAL DATA:

- African American/black individuals account for over 40% of all new HIV diagnoses despite being 12% of the U.S. population.
- Hispanics/Latinos account for over 25% of all new HIV diagnoses despite being 18% of the U.S. population.

GENETICS:

Familial Disposition:
Individuals with deletions in the *CCR5* gene are immune from infection with macrophage tropic virus (the predominant virus in sexual transmission). Other genetic variants may contribute to rapid progression or long-term control of the virus once infected. One in 300 individuals infected with HIV is an "elite controller," which means they are able to maintain a normal CD4 count and undetectable viral load through immune control.

Congenital Infection:

- Less than 100 children a year younger than 13 yr old receive a diagnosis of perinatally acquired HIV, according to the CDC, which may occur in utero, during delivery, or after delivery via breastfeeding.
- No specific congenital abnormalities are associated with HIV infection, although there is a higher risk of spontaneous abortion and low birth weight.

Neonatal Infection:

- May occur during delivery or via breastfeeding.
- Typically asymptomatic.
- All pregnant women should be tested for HIV and, if positive, take antiretrovirals (ARVs).

PHYSICAL FINDINGS & CLINICAL PRESENTATION

- Signs and symptoms are variable with stage of disease.
- Acute HIV infection (0 to 3 mo, usually within several weeks):
  1. Causes a self-limited mononucleosis-like illness in 50% to 80% of individuals, characterized by fever, sore throat, lymphadenopathy, headache, and a rash resembling roseola. Individuals may also be asymptomatic.
  2. In a minority of acute cases, aseptic meningitis, Bell palsy, or peripheral neuropathy may occur.
  3. Opportunistic infections such as thrush or *Pneumocystis jiroveci* pneumonia (PJP) may occur.
- Chronic HIV infection is usually characterized by a prolonged asymptomatic "latent" phase without symptoms followed by nonspecific symptoms of lymphadenopathy, fatigue, weight loss, diarrhea, and skin changes, including seborrheic dermatitis, localized herpes zoster, and/or fungal infection.

TABLE 1 Surveillance Case Definition for HIV Infection in Adults and Adolescents (Age >13 yr)

Stage	Laboratory Evidence	Clinical Evidence
Stage 1	Laboratory confirmation of HIV infection and CD4+ T-lymphocyte count of ≥500 cells/μL or CD4+ T-lymphocyte percentage of ≥29%[a]	No AIDS-defining condition (see Table 2)
Stage 2	Laboratory confirmation of HIV infection and CD4+ T-lymphocyte count of 200-499 cells/μL or CD4+ T-lymphocyte percentage of 14%-28%[a]	No AIDS-defining condition (see Table 2)
Stage 3	Laboratory confirmation of HIV infection and CD4+ T-lymphocyte count of <200 cells/μL or CD4+ T-lymphocyte percentage of <14%[a]	Documentation of an AIDS-defining condition with laboratory confirmation of HIV infection (see Table 2)
Stage unknown	Laboratory confirmation of HIV infection and no information on CD4+ T-lymphocyte count or percentage	No information on presence of an AIDS-defining condition

[a]The CD4+ T-lymphocyte percentage is a percentage of the total lymphocyte count.
AIDS, Acquired immunodeficiency syndrome.
From Hoffman R et al: *Hematology: basic principles and practice*, ed 7, Philadelphia, 2018, Elsevier.

TABLE 2 Surveillance Definitions of AIDS-Defining Conditions

Opportunistic Infections:

- *Pneumocystis jiroveci (carinii)*
- *Mycobacterium avium* complex
- *Mycobacterium tuberculosis*
- Toxoplasmosis
- Candidiasis: Esophageal and systemic
- Histoplasmosis
- Cryptococcosis
- Cryptosporidiosis and isosporiasis
- Leishmaniasis
- Cytomegalovirus disease
- Recurrent bacterial infections (≥2 episodes/yr)

Lymphomas

Kaposi Sarcoma

Cervical Cancer

AIDS Dementia Syndrome

Wasting Syndrome

AIDS, Acquired immunodeficiency syndrome.
From Hoffman R et al: *Hematology: basic principles and practice*, ed 7, Philadelphia, 2018, Elsevier.

TABLE 3 Risk Factors Associated with Sexual Transmission of HIV

Sexually transmitted infections
- Ulcerative or nonulcerative diseases

Genital tract inflammation

HIV disease
- Higher viral loads
- Lower CD4+ levels
- Acute HIV infection
- Lack of effective antiretroviral therapy
- Lack of heterozygosity or homozygosity for the inactivating 32-base pair deletion in the chemokine receptor gene *(CCR5)*

Anatomic factors
- Lack of circumcision
- Cervical ectopy
- Leukocytospermia
- Hormonal contraception

Sexual practices
- Receptive anal intercourse
- Sexual activity during menses
- Bleeding during intercourse (disruption of vaginal mucosa through trauma)
- Lack of barrier protection

HIV viral features
- Syncytium formation
- Certain viral clades

From Bennett JE et al: *Mandell, Douglas, and Bennett's principles and practice of infectious diseases*, ed 8, Philadelphia, 2015, Saunders.

TABLE 4 Etiology of Anemia in Human Immunodeficiency Virus

HIV Related

HIV Infection

- Anemia of chronic disease
- Blunted production/response to erythropoietin
- Suppression of CFU-GEMM (HIV/inflammatory cytokines)

Neoplasms Infiltrating BM

Non-Hodgkin lymphoma, KS, Hodgkin lymphoma

Infections of the BM

- Parvovirus B19
- Atypical mycobacteria (MAI/MAC)
- M. TB
- Histoplasma
- CMV

Medications Causing Decreased Production	Medications Causing Hemolysis
• RT inhibitors	• Indinavir
• Ganciclovir	• Bactrim and Dapsone in G6PD deficiency
• Bactrim	
• Amphotericin B	

HIV Unrelated

- B_{12} and/or folic acid deficiencies
- Iron deficiency caused by chronic blood loss

BM, Bone marrow; *CFU-GEMM,* colony-forming unit–granulocyte, erythrocyte, macrophage, megakaryocyte; *CMV,* cytomegalovirus; *G6PD,* glucose-6-phosphate dehydrogenase; *KS,* Kaposi sarcoma; *MAC, mycobacterium avium* complex; *MAI, mycobacterium avium-intracellulare; M. TB, Mycobacterium tuberculosis*; *RT,* reverse transcriptase.

From Hoffman R et al: *Hematology: basic principles and practice,* ed 7, Philadelphia, 2018, Elsevier.

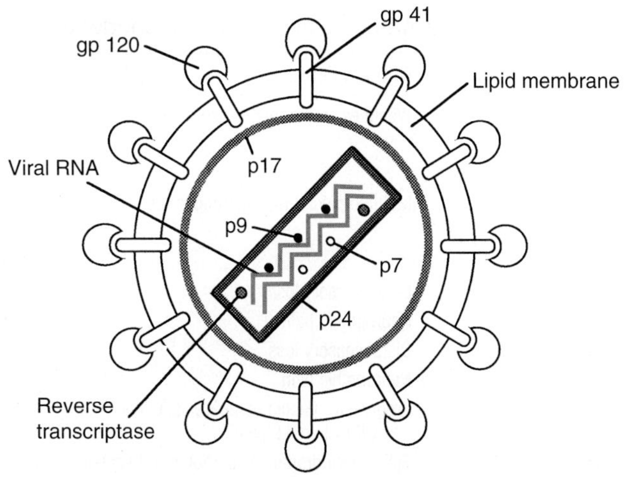

FIG. 1 Structure of the human immunodeficiency virus virion. Two coding strands of genomic ribonucleic acid (RNA) are packaged in the nucleoid core with p7, p9, and p24 proteins and reverse transcriptase. The core is surrounded by the p17 matrix protein lining the inner surface of the envelope. The envelope consists of a lipid bilayer derived from the infected cell and glycoprotein spikes that consist of the outer glycoprotein (GP) 120 molecule, which contains the binding site for CD4, and GP41, which anchors the glycoprotein complex to the envelope and mediates fusion of the viral membrane with the cell membrane during viral penetration. (From Hoffman R et al: *Hematology: basic principles and practice,* ed 7, Philadelphia, 2018, Elsevier.)

- Advanced disease is characterized by AIDS-associated diseases, including infections and malignancies (see specific disorders). Anemia may be multifactorial (Table 4).
- HIV infection in women may be associated with lower levels of viral load at comparable degrees of immunosuppression when compared with men. Furthermore, women may, on average, have higher CD4 counts at the time of HIV diagnosis.
- Another special consideration in women infected with HIV is the high incidence of human papillomavirus (HPV) coinfection and risk for cervical cancer. HIV-positive women should be screened for cervical cancer at time of initial HIV diagnosis and annually thereafter if pap testing is normal. If the results of three consecutive Pap tests are normal, then follow-up testing can occur every 3 yr. HPV vaccination is also recommended in men and women 9- to 26-yr-old who are HIV positive. For adults aged 27- to 45-yr-old, clinicians should discuss and may consider HPV vaccination in persons who are most likely to benefit.
- Coinfection with HIV and hepatitis C virus is common because of similar transmission risk. Hepatitis C is most commonly transmitted by contaminated needles or blood exposure. Hepatitis C can be transmitted sexually, but the risk is low. Patients with HIV and hepatitis C progress faster to cirrhosis. Patients may already have signs of advanced liver disease at the time of diagnosis.

ETIOLOGY

- HIV is a single-stranded RNA retrovirus (Fig. 1) that is categorized as type 1 or 2.
- HIV-1 was derived from transmission of a simian immunodeficiency virus (SIV) from chimpanzees in Central Africa; HIV-2 was derived from an SIV found in sooty mangabey monkeys from West Africa.
- HIV-1 is the predominant pathogenic retrovirus in human populations; HIV-2 has limited distribution (primarily West Africa) and tends to progress less rapidly than HIV-1. HIV-2 should be considered in individuals from West Africa or whose sexual partners are from West Africa.
- HIV is transmitted by sexual contact, shared needles, blood transfusion, or from mother to child during pregnancy, delivery, or breastfeeding.
- Primary target of infection: CD4 lymphocytes.

Dx DIAGNOSIS

DIFFERENTIAL DIAGNOSIS

- Acute HIV infection: Often diagnosed or confused with mononucleosis or other respiratory viral infections.
- Late symptoms: Similar to those produced by other wasting/chronic illnesses such as neoplasms, tuberculosis (TB), disseminated fungal infection (such as *Candida*), malabsorption, or depression.
- HIV-related encephalopathy: Confused with Alzheimer disease or other causes of chronic dementia (cognitive impairment in HIV infection is described in another chapter in Section I); myelopathy and neuropathy possibly resembling other demyelinating diseases such as multiple sclerosis.
- Direct central nervous system (CNS) involvement: Manifests as encephalopathy, myelopathy, or neuropathy in advanced cases. Table 5 summarizes neuromuscular syndromes in HIV infection.
- Renal failure, rheumatologic disorders, thrombocytopenia, or cardiac abnormalities (Table 6) may be seen in association with HIV-1.

WORKUP

Diagnosis is established by testing for HIV antibodies in the blood. The CDC recommends routine testing for patients in all health care settings unless the patient declines (opt-out screening). This includes routine testing of pregnant women. It is also recommended that separate written consent should no longer be required, although by law this is being addressed on a state-by-state basis. Generally, all persons aged 13 to 64 yr should undergo HIV testing at least once, and more frequently (at least once a yr) if sexually active. For individuals who may be at higher risk (e.g., men who are having sex with multiple other men), 3 to 6 mo is recommended.

An FDA-approved at-home rapid HIV screening test is available. It uses swabs of oral fluids from upper and lower gums. A positive test requires confirmatory testing. Clinicians should be aware of the "window period" (i.e., an antibody test may take up to 3 mo to become "reactive" in a person with newly acquired HIV infection).

LABORATORY TESTS

HIV antibodies are detected by a two-step technique:

TABLE 5 Neuromuscular Syndromes in Human Immunodeficiency Virus Type 1 Infection

Diagnosis	Disease Stage	Clinical Features	Diagnostic Studies	Treatment
AIDP CIDP	Early > late	Weakness more than sensory loss	CSF: ↑ WBCs ↑↑ Protein NCS: Demyelination	Early: IVIG, steroids, plasmapheresis Late: Consider ganciclovir/foscarnet
MM	Early or late	Multiple painful mononeuropathies	NCS: Multifocal axonal neuropathy Biopsy: Inflammation/vasculitis CMV	Early: None Late: Steroids/cyclophosphamide Ganciclovir/foscarnet
Nucleoside Neuropathy	Any stage	Distal sensory loss Neuropathic pain	NCS: Distal axonopathy Increased serum lactate	Nucleoside withdrawal
DSPN	Late	Distal sensory loss Neuropathic pain	NCS: Distal axonopathy	NSAIDs, capsaicin AED, tricyclics
PP	Late	Progressive flaccid paraparesis, urinary dysfunction, LS pain	CSF: Increased WBCs (PMNs), CMV PCR+	Ganciclovir/foscarnet Cidofovir
DILS	Late	Sjögren syndrome, distal motor and sensory loss, pain	NCS: Axonal neuropathy Biopsy: $CD8^+$ T cells, HIV-1	Zidovudine/ART Steroids
Zidovudine Myopathy	Any stage	Proximal weakness Myalgias	EMG: ± irritative Biopsy: Ragged red fibers	Zidovudine withdrawal
Polymyositis	Any stage	Proximal weakness Myalgias	EMG: ± irritative Biopsy: Inflammatory infiltrates	Steroids, IVIG Immunosuppressants
ALS-like	Late	Weakness, dysphagia	EMG: Neurogenic	ART

AED, Antiepileptic drug; *AIDP,* acute inflammatory demyelinating polyneuropathy; *ALS,* amyotrophic lateral sclerosis; *ART,* antiretroviral therapy; *CIDP,* chronic inflammatory demyelinating polyneuropathy; *CMV,* cytomegalovirus; *CSF,* cerebrospinal fluid; *DILS,* diffuse infiltrative lymphocytosis syndrome; *DSPN,* distal sensory polyneuropathy; *EMG,* electromyography; *IVIG,* intravenous immunoglobulin; *LS,* lumbosacral; *MM,* mononeuritis multiplex; *NCS,* nerve conduction studies; *NSAID,* nonsteroidal antiinflammatory drug; *PCR,* polymerase chain reaction; *PMNs,* polymorphonuclear leukocytes; *PP,* progressive polyradiculopathy; *WBCs,* white blood cells.

From Bennett JE et al: *Mandell, Douglas, and Bennett's principles and practice of infectious diseases,* ed 8, Philadelphia, 2015, Saunders.

TABLE 6 Summary of HIV-Associated Cardiovascular Diseases

Disease	Possible Causes	Incidence/Prevalence	Diagnosis	Treatment
Accelerated atherosclerosis	Protease inhibitors, atherogenesis with virus-infected macrophages, chronic inflammation, glucose intolerance, dyslipidemia, endothelial dysfunction	Up to 8%	ECG, stress testing, echocardiography, lipid profile, CT angiography, calcium scoring	Smoking cessation, low-fat diet, aerobic exercise, blood pressure control, guideline-based statin use, percutaneous coronary intervention, coronary artery bypass surgery
Dilated cardiomyopathy	Coronary artery disease	Up to 8% of asymptomatic patients	Chest radiographic findings	Diuretics, digoxin, ACE inhibitors, beta blockers
LV systolic dysfunction	Drug related: Cocaine, AZT, IL-2, doxorubicin, interferon Infectious: HIV, *Toxoplasma*, coxsackievirus group B, EBV, CMV, adenovirus Metabolic or endocrine: Selenium or carnitine deficiency, anemia, hypocalcemia, hypophosphatemia, hyponatremia, hypokalemia, hypoalbuminemia, hypothyroidism, growth hormone deficiency, adrenal insufficiency, hyperinsulinemia Cytokines: TNF-β, nitric oxide, TGF-β, endothelin-1, interleukins Immunodeficiency: CD4 count <100 Autoimmune	Up to 25% of autopsy cases	ECG: Nonspecific conduction abnormalities, PVCs, PACs Echocardiographic findings: Low to normal LV wall thickness, increased LV mass, LV dilation, systolic LV dysfunction Possible laboratory studies: Troponin T, brain natriuretic peptide concentration, CD4 count, viral load, viral PCR, *Toxoplasma* serology, thyroid-stimulating hormone, cortisol, carnitine, selenium, serum ACE, stress testing, myocardial biopsy, cardiac catheterization	Adjunctive treatment in HIV patients Treatment of infection Nutritional replacement IVIG Intensify antiretroviral therapy Follow-up serial echocardiograms
LV diastolic dysfunction	TNF, IL-6 Hypertension Chronic viral infection	Up to 37% asymptomatic	Echocardiography Tissue Doppler imaging	Treat hypertension Intensify antiretroviral therapy
Primary pulmonary hypertension	Plexogenic pulmonary arteriopathy	0.5%	ECG, echocardiography, right-heart catheterization	Anticoagulation, vasodilators, prostacyclin analogues Endothelin antagonists PDE-5 inhibitors

Continued

TABLE 6 Summary of HIV-Associated Cardiovascular Diseases

Disease	Possible Causes	Incidence/Prevalence	Diagnosis	Treatment
Pericardial	Bacteria: *Staphylococcus, Streptococcus, Proteus, Klebsiella, Enterococcus, Listeria, Nocardia, Mycobacterium* Viral pathogens: HIV, HSV, CMV, adenovirus, echovirus Other pathogens: *Cryptococcus, Toxoplasma, Histoplasma* Malignancy: Kaposi sarcoma, lymphoma, capillary leak/wasting/malnutrition Hypothyroidism Immunodeficiency Uremia	11%/yr, markedly reduced in post-HAART studies Spontaneous resolution in 42% of affected patients Approximately 30% increase in 6-mo mortality	Pericardial rub on examination Echocardiography Fluid analysis for Gram stain, culture, and cytology ECG—low voltage/PR depression Associated pleural and peritoneal fluid analysis Pericardial biopsy	Treat the cause Follow-up: Serial echocardiograms Intensify antiretroviral therapy Pericardiocentesis or window
Infective endocarditis	Autoimmune Bacteria: *Staphylococcus aureus* or *Staphylococcus epidermidis, Salmonella, Streptococcus, Haemophilus parainfluenzae, Pseudallescheria boydii*, HASEK organisms Fungal: *Aspergillus fumigatus, Candida, Cryptococcus neoformans*	6% increased incidence in IVDAs, regardless of HIV status	Blood cultures; echocardiography	Intravenous antibiotics, valve replacements
Nonbacterial thrombotic endocarditis	Valvular damage, vitamin C deficiency, malnutrition, wasting, DIC, hypercoagulable state, prolonged acquired immunodeficiency	Rare condition, but clinically relevant emboli in 42% of cases	Echocardiography	Anticoagulation Treat vasculitis or underlying illness
Malignancy	Kaposi sarcoma, non-Hodgkin lymphoma, leiomyosarcoma, low CD4 count, prolonged immunodeficiency HHV-8, EBV	Approximately 1% Usually metastatic in HIV-positive patients	Echocardiography, biopsy	Chemotherapy possible
Right ventricular disease	Recurrent pulmonary infections, pulmonary arteritis, microvascular pulmonary emboli, COPD		ECG, echocardiography, right-heart catheterization	Diuretics, treat underlying lung infection or disease, anticoagulation as clinically indicated
Vasculitis	Drug therapy with antibiotics and antivirals	Increasing incidence	Clinical diagnosis	Systemic corticosteroids, withdrawal of drug
Autonomic dysfunction	CNS disease, drug therapy, prolonged immunodeficiency, malnutrition, sedentary lifestyle	Increased in patients with CNS disease	Tilt-table test, Holter or event monitoring	Procedural precautions
Arrhythmias	Drug therapy, pentamidine, autonomic dysfunction, acidosis electrolyte abnormalities		ECG—long QT, Holter monitoring, exercise stress testing	Discontinue drug, procedural precautions, electrolyte replacement
Lipodystrophy	Drug therapy: Protease inhibitors		Echocardiography, lipid profile, cardiac catheterization, coronary calcium score	Lipid therapy (beware of drug interactions), aerobic exercise, altered antiretroviral therapy, cosmetic surgery/fat implantation

ACE, Angiotensin-converting enzyme; *AZT*, zidovudine (azidothymidine); *CMV*, cytomegalovirus; *CNS*, central nervous system; *COPD*, chronic obstructive pulmonary disease; *CT*, computed tomography; *DIC*, disseminated intravascular coagulation; *EBV*, Epstein-Barr virus; *ECG*, electrocardiogram; *HAART*, highly active antiretroviral therapy; *HASEK*, *Haemophilus* species (*Haemophilus parainfluenzae, Haemophilus aphrophilus, Haemophilus paraphrophilus*), *Actinobacillus actinomycetemcomitans, Cardiobacterium hominis, Eikenella corrodens*, and *Kingella* species; *HHV*, human herpesvirus; *HSV*, herpes simplex virus; *IL*, interleukin; *IVDA*, intravenous drug abuser; *IVIG*, intravenous immunoglobulin; *LV*, left ventricle; *PAC*, premature atrial complex; *PCR*, polymerase chain reaction; *PDE*, phosphodiesterase; *PVC*, premature ventricular complex; *TGF*, transforming growth factor; *TNF*, tumor necrosis factor.
From Mann DL et al: *Braunwald's heart disease*, ed 10, Philadelphia, 2015, Elsevier.

- An initial screening test (i.e., enzyme-linked immunosorbent assay [ELISA]).
- Confirmation of an initial positive screening test with more specific assays. The classic confirmatory test is the western blot, but other modalities may be used. Fig. E2 summarizes the laboratory diagnosis of HIV infection.
- Screening antibody tests generally measure HIV-1 and HIV-2 antibodies. Confirmatory tests will generally differentiate between HIV-1 and HIV-2 as well. However, the viral load assays (HIV RNA PCR) are specific only for HIV-1.
- Fourth-generation antibody/antigen tests can detect the "p24" antigen, which is present early in HIV infection and can be used to diagnose HIV earlier than previous generations. An HIV RNA PCR should still be sent if acute HIV is suspected.
- Baseline viral resistance testing (e.g., genotype) is recommended for all newly diagnosed patients with HIV to guide choice of ART.
- The CD4 count and HIV viral load (e.g., HIV RNA PCR) should be measured in all patients.
- The CD4 count is a marker of current immune status. A correlation of CD4 cell count with specific HIV-associated disorders is summarized in Table 7. Table 8 describes the World Health Organization (WHO) immunologic classification for established HIV infection.
- The HIV RNA PCR (viral load) is predictive of disease progression.
- Rapid serologic tests have been increasingly used and are useful in specific settings: Occupational exposures, pregnant women in labor without previous testing, and patients in high seroprevalence areas (for immediate results). Specimens are either blood or saliva and results are given within 1 to 20 min. Although sensitivity is high (99%), false-positive tests are more common in low seroprevalence populations. Thus, all positive results must be confirmed with standard serology.

TABLE 7 Correlation of CD4+ Cell Count with specific HIV-Associated Disorders

Correlation of CD4+ Cell Count with Specific HIV-Associated Disorders				
System*	**>500 CD4+ cells/mm^3**	**<500 CD4+ cells/mm^3**	**<250 CD4+ cells/mm^3**	**<50 CD4+ cells/mm^3**
Dermatologic	• Acute retroviral syndrome • Oral hairy leukoplakia • Vaginal candidiasis • Seborrheic dermatitis	• Oropharyngeal candidiasis (thrush) • Herpes zoster • Psoriasis, severe or refractory • Eruptive atypical melanocytic nevi and melanoma • Kaposi sarcoma	• Eosinophilic folliculitis • Seborrheic dermatitis, refractory • Mollusca, extensive • Bacillary angiomatosis • Miliary/extrapulmonary tuberculosis • Herpes simplex virus infection, disseminated • Cryptococcosis, disseminated • Histoplasmosis, disseminated • Coccidioidomycosis, disseminated • Botryomycosis • Non-Hodgkin lymphoma	• Large, nonhealing mucocutaneous herpes simplex virus infections (e.g., perianal) • Papular pruritic eruption • Giant mollusca • Perianal ulcers due to cytomegalovirus • Aspergillosis • Acquired ichthyosis • *Mycobacterium avium* complex infections • Major aphthae
Respiratory	Bacterial pneumonia and sinusitis	• Pneumococcal pneumonia • Pulmonary tuberculosis • Lymphocytic interstitial pneumonia (pediatric)	*Pneumocystis jiroveci* pneumonia (PCP)	*Pseudomonas* spp. pneumonia
Nervous	• Aseptic meningitis • Guillain–Barré syndrome	Mononeuritis multiplex	• HIV-associated dementia • Cerebral toxoplasmosis • Peripheral neuropathy • Progressive multifocal leukoencephalopathy	Primary CNS lymphoma
Hematologic	Persistent generalized lymphadenopathy	• Anemia • Idiopathic thrombocytopenic purpura	Non-Hodgkin lymphoma	
Other	Myopathy	• Cryptosporidiosis • Cervical/anal intraepithelial neoplasia • Cervical cancer • Anal cancer	• Esophageal candidiasis • Wasting • Microsporidiosis • Vacuolar myelopathy • Cardiomyopathy	• Cryptosporidiosis, refractory • Cytomegalovirus retinitis, extraocular systemic cytomegalovirus infection

*Diseases occur with increasing frequency and severity at lower CD4+ cell counts.
CNS, Central nervous system.
From Bolognia JL et al: *Dermatology*, ed 4, 2018, Elsevier.

TABLE 8 World Health Organization Immunologic Classification for Established HIV Infection

	Age-Related CD4 Values			
HIV-Associated Immunodeficiency	**<11 mo (% CD4+)**	**12-35 mo (% CD4+)**	**36-59 mo (% CD4+)**	**>5 yr (Absolute No./mm^3 or % CD4+)**
None or not significant	>35	>30	>25	>500
Mild	30-35	25-30	20-25	350-500
Advanced	25-29	20-24	15-19	200-349
Severe	<25	<20	<15	<200 or <15%

From Bennett JE et al: *Mandell, Douglas, and Bennett's principles and practice of infectious diseases,* ed 8, Philadelphia, 2015, Saunders.

- Early during infection (i.e., acute HIV infection), standard antibody tests may be negative ("window period"). The fourth-generation antibody/antigen test reduces this window period. The standard for diagnosing HIV during acute infection is by testing for HIV RNA (viral load).
- WHO clinical staging of HIV/AIDS in the setting of confirmed HIV infection is summarized in Table 9. Table 10 compares the WHO and CDC staging systems.

Rx TREATMENT

NONPHARMACOLOGIC THERAPY

Maintenance of adequate nutrition

ACUTE GENERAL Rx

Acute management of opportunistic infections and malignancies (see "AIDS-associated disorders," "Pneumonia, *Pneumocystis jiroveci (carinii);*" "Cryptococcosis;" "Tuberculosis, Pulmonary;" "*Cryptosporidium* Infection;" "Toxoplasmosis;" etc., elsewhere in this text)

CHRONIC Rx

All HIV-infected patients should be considered for ART regardless of CD4 cell count. The benefit of ART is well established in preventing progression to AIDS and associated opportunistic infections. Furthermore, individuals who are on ART and undetectable are highly unlikely to transmit HIV to others. Identifying individuals with HIV as soon as possible and administering ART is the basis of effective public health approaches to addressing HIV (i.e., "Treatment as Prevention").

- Therapy is strongly recommended for all patients with established HIV infection regardless of the CD4 count. Most people with chronic HIV infection are asymptomatic. ART is recommended regardless of CD4 cell counts. The recommendations are due to the safety and benefit of newer antivirals in preventing AIDS and decreasing both morbidity and mortality. Earlier treatment may also help reduce transmission of the virus to others due to reductions in viral loads.
- ART generally consists of using a 3-drug regimen to treat HIV infection. Classes of antiretrovirals include:
  1. Nucleoside/nucleotide reverse transcriptase inhibitor (NRTI): Zidovudine (AZT), lamivudine (3TC), emtricitabine (FTC), tenofovir disoproxil fumarate (TDF), tenofovir alafenamide (TAF), abacavir (ABC), stavudine (D4T), or didanosine (DDI).
  2. Protease inhibitors (PI): Lopinavir/ritonavir, atazanavir, fosamprenavir, darunavir, saquinavir, tipranavir, nelfinavir, and

TABLE 9 WHO Clinical Staging of HIV/AIDS in the Setting of Confirmed HIV infection

All Ages	Adults and Adolescents	Children
Clinical stage 1 – asymptomatic; immunologic correlate*: >500 CD4+ cells/mm^3		
• Asymptomatic • Persistent generalized lymphadenopathy		
Clinical stage 2 – mild; immunologic correlate*: 350-499 CD4+ cells/mm^3		
• **Herpes zoster** • **Fungal nail infection** • **Pruritic papular eruptions** • **Angular cheilitis** • **Recurrent oral ulcerations** • Recurrent/chronic upper respiratory tract infections (sinusitis, otitis media/otorrhea, tonsillitis, pharyngitis)	• **Seborrheic dermatitis** • Moderate unexplained weight loss (<10% of body weight)	• **Extensive warts** • **Extensive molluscum contagiosum** • **Lineal gingival erythema** • Unexplained persistent parotid enlargement • Unexplained persistent hepatosplenomegaly
Clinical stage 3 – advanced; immunologic correlate*: 200-349 CD4+ cells/mm^3		
• **Persistent oral candidiasis (after first 6-8 wk of life)** • **Oral hairy leukoplakia** • **Acute necrotizing ulcerative stomatitis, gingivitis, or periodontitis** • Unexplained chronic diarrhea (>1 mo in adults, >2 wk in children) • Unexplained persistent fever (≥37.6°C intermittent or constant, for >1 mo) • Pulmonary tuberculosis (current) • Unexplained anemia (<8 g/dL), neutropenia (<0.5 × 10^9/L) or chronic thrombocytopenia (<50 × 10^9/L)	• Unexplained severe weight loss (>10% of body weight) • Severe bacterial infections such as pneumonia, empyema, pyomyositis, bone or joint infection, meningitis, bacteremia	• Unexplained moderate malnutrition or wasting not adequately responding to standard therapy • Recurrent severe bacterial pneumonia • Symptomatic lymphoid interstitial pneumonitis • Lymph node tuberculosis • Chronic HIV-associated lung disease including bronchiectasis
Clinical stage 4 – severe/AIDS-defining conditions; immunologic correlate*: <200 CD4+ cells/mm^3		
• **Chronic herpes simplex infection (orolabial, genital, or anorectal of >1 mo duration or visceral at any site)** • **Kaposi sarcoma** • **Extrapulmonary cryptococcosis including meningitis** • **Disseminated endemic mycosis (coccidioidomycosis or histoplasmosis)** • **Disseminated nontuberculous mycobacterial infection** • Unexplained severe wasting, stunting or severe malnutrition not responding to standard therapy (HIV wasting syndrome) • Cytomegalovirus infection (retinitis or infection of other organs; onset at age >1 mo) • HIV encephalopathy • Progressive multifocal leukoencephalopathy • Extrapulmonary tuberculosis • Candidiasis of the esophagus, trachea, bronchi, or lungs • *Pneumocystis* pneumonia • Central nervous system toxoplasmosis (onset at age >1 mo) • Chronic cryptosporidiosis (with diarrhea) • Chronic isosporiasis • Symptomatic HIV-associated nephropathy or symptomatic HIV-associated cardiomyopathy • Cerebral or B-cell non-Hodgkin lymphoma, or other HIV-associated solid tumor	• **Atypical disseminated leishmaniasis** • Recurrent severe bacterial pneumonia • Recurrent nontyphoidal *Salmonella* bacteremia • Invasive cervical carcinoma	• Recurrent severe bacterial infections such as empyema, pyomyositis, bone or joint infection, or meningitis (but excluding pneumonia)

Conditions with mucocutaneous manifestations are in **bold**.
*In individuals ≥6 years of age; corresponding counts in children <6 years of age are available at www.who.int/hiv/pub/guidelines/hivstaging/en/.
AIDS, Acquired immunodeficiency syndrome; *WHO,* World Health Organization.
From Bolognia J: *Dermatology,* ed 4, 2018, Elsevier.

TABLE 10 Comparison of WHO and CDC Staging Systems*

WHO Stage†	WHO T-Lymphocyte Count and Percentage‡	CDC Stage§	CDC T-Lymphocyte Count and Percentage
Stage 1 (HIV infection)	CD4+ T-lymphocyte count of ≥500 cells/mm^3	Stage 1 (HIV infection)	CD4+ T-lymphocyte count of ≥500 cells/mm^3 or CD4+ T-lymphocyte percentage of ≥29
Stage 2 (HIV infection)	CD4+ T-lymphocyte count of 350-499 cells/mm^3	Stage 2 (HIV infection)	CD4+ T-lymphocyte count of 200-499 cells/mm^3 or CD4+ T-lymphocyte percentage of 14-28
Stage 3 (advanced HIV disease [AHD])	CD4+ T-lymphocyte count of 200-349 cells/mm^3	Stage 2 (HIV infection)	CD4+ T-lymphocyte count of 200-499 cells/mm^3 or CD4+ T-lymphocyte percentage of 14-28
Stage 4 (acquired immunodeficiency syndrome [AIDS])	CD4+ T-lymphocyte count of <200 cells/mm^3 or CD4+ T-lymphocyte percentage of <15	Stage 3 (AIDS)	CD4+ T-lymphocyte count of <200 cells/mm^3 or CD4+ T-lymphocyte percentage of <14

CDC, Centers for Disease Control and Prevention; *WHO,* World Health Organization.
*For reporting purposes only.
†Among adults and children aged ≥5 yr.
‡Percentage applicable for stage 4 only.
§Among adults and adolescents (ages ≥13 yr). CDC also includes a fourth stage, stage unknown; laboratory confirmation of HIV infection but no information on CD4+ T-lymphocyte count or percentage and no information on AIDS-defining conditions.
From Bennett JE et al: *Mandell, Douglas, and Bennett's principles and practice of infectious diseases,* ed 8, Philadelphia, 2015, Saunders.

indinavir. These PIs may be "boosted" by ritonavir or cobicistat to increase levels.

3. Nonnucleoside reverse transcriptase inhibitors (NNRTI): Nevirapine, efavirenz, etravirine, doravirine, delavirdine, or rilpivirine.
4. Integrase inhibitors (II): Raltegravir, elvitegravir, bictegravir, and dolutegravir.
5. Fusion inhibitors: Enfuvirtide (T-20). This drug is administered through subcutaneous injections and is only used as part of a salvage regimen for individuals who have failed multiple other regimens.
6. CCR5 inhibitors: Maraviroc. Before using this drug, a viral trophism assay should be checked to determine if the virus uses the CCR5 coreceptor to infect cells. If the virus uses the CXCR4 coreceptor, this drug will not be effective.
7. Postattachment inhibitors: Ibalizumab. Blocks CD4 receptors that HIV needs to enter cells with.

- Adding a fourth drug to the three-drug regimen does not improve viral suppression or outcomes and is not recommended. Treatment interruptions based upon CD4 responses appear harmful in recent comparative studies versus standard continuous treatment protocols and should be avoided. Antiretroviral regimens for initial therapy are summarized in Table 11.
- Typical dosing regimen consists of two NRTIs and either an NNRTI, PI, or II. IIs are now the preferred third drug because of tolerability. Data support inclusion of lamivudine or emtricitabine as one of the two NRTIs.
- Individuals with drug resistant HIV may be on more complex and atypical regimens. Consultation with an HIV specialist is recommended.

Standard NRTIs include:

- Tenofovir disoproxil fumarate/emtricitabine 1 tablet once daily. Individuals with underlying renal dysfunction or requiring other nephrotoxic agents may be at increased risk of renal toxicity while taking tenofovir. TDF may also be associated with reductions in bone mineral density.
- Tenofovir alafenamide/emtricitabine 1 tablet once daily. TAF is a newer formulation of TDF with less nephrotoxicity and bone mineral density effects. Both TDF/FTC, and TAF/FTC are recommended components of the initial regimen (with a "backbone" medication). TDF should be avoided in patients with a creatinine clearance (CrCl) <60 ml/min. TAF should be avoided in patients with a CrCl <30 ml/min.
- Abacavir/lamivudine 1 tablet once daily. Abacavir may be associated with increased risk of myocardial infarction. Before using this drug, individuals should be checked for HLA-B*5701. Individuals with this allele are at higher risk of serious hypersensitivity reactions, and this drug should be avoided.
- Zidovudine/lamivudine 1 tablet twice daily. Once widely prescribed; now rarely used due to lower efficacy compared with tenofovir-emtricitabine; zidovudine is associated with lipoatrophy and anemia, as well as GI and CNS side effects.

Standard backbone regimens include:

- IIs (these are now considered first line):
  1. Bictegravir (50 mg once daily): Fixed-dose combination of bictegravir with the NRTIs TAF and FTC.
  2. Dolutegravir (50 mg once daily): Fixed-dose combination of dolutegravir and the NRTIs abacavir and lamivudine for once-daily treatment of HIV-1 infection. HLA-B*5701 should be checked first.
  3. Elvitegravir: Given with cobicistat (booster) and tenofovir/emtricitabine in a fixed-dose combination.
  4. Raltegravir (400 mg twice a day).
- NNRTIs:
  1. Efavirenz 600 mg daily: Should be used in caution in women in the first trimester or those who are contemplating pregnancy.
  2. Rilpivirine: Given with tenofovir and emtricitabine as part of a fixed-dose combination.
  3. Nevirapine 200 mg two times a day: Avoid with CD4 count >250 in men and >350 cells per cubic millimeter in women because of the risk of hepatitis. Rarely used.
  4. Etravirine 200 mg two times a day: This drug is generally used in patients for whom other regimens have failed. Etravirine retains activity in many patients who have developed resistance against efavirenz and nevirapine.
- PIs (ritonavir boosted):
  1. Darunavir and ritonavir (800 mg and 100 mg a day): This is considered a preferred PI regimen within the U.S.

TABLE 11 Which Antiretroviral Regimen to Choose for Initial Therapy

Preferred Regimens	**Comments**
Integrase inhibitor-based regimen Bictegravir/TAF/FTC Raltegravir + TDF/FTC or TAF/FTC Dolutegravir + TDF/FTC or TAF/FTC Dolutegravir/ABC/3TC	Use abacavir only in individuals who are HLA-B*5701 negative.
PI-based regimen Darunavir/r or Darunavir/c (once daily) + TDF/FTC or TAF/FTC	Use if there is a concern for drug resistance.
Preferred regimen for pregnant women ABC/3TC or TDF/FTC plus Raltegravir or Darunavir/r or Atazanavir/r	TDF should be avoided in renal impairment.
Alternative Regimens	**Comments**
INSTI-based regimens Elvitegravir/cobicistat/TDF/FTC Elvitegravir/cobicistat/TAF/FTC RAL + ABC/3TC	
NNRTI-based regimens (in alphabetical order) DOR/TDF/3TC or DOR + TAF/FTC EFV/TDF/FTC or EFV + TAF/FTC RPV/TDF/FTC or RPV/TAF/FTC	EFV should not be used with caution in the first trimester of pregnancy or in women trying to conceive. NVP should not be used in patients with moderate to severe hepatic impairment (Child-Pugh B or C) Should not be used in women with pretreatment CD4 >250 cells/mm^3 or men with CD4 >400 cells/mm^3.
PI-based regimens (in alphabetical order) ATV/r or ATV/c + TDF/FTC or TAF/FTC DRV/c or DRV/r + ABC/3TC	ABC should not be used in patients who test positive for HLA-B*5701. Use with caution in patients with high risk of cardiovascular disease or with pretreatment HIV RNA >100,000 copies/ml. Once-daily LPV/r is not recommended in pregnant women.

3TC, Lamivudine; *ABC,* abacavir; *ATV,* atazanavir; *DOR,* doravirine; *DRV,* darunavir; *EFV,* efavirenz; *FPV,* fosamprenavir; *FTC,* emtricitabine; *HLA,* human leukocyte antigen; *INSTI,* integrase strand transfer inhibitor; *LPV,* lopinavir; *MRV,* maraviroc; *NNRTI,* nonnucleoside reverse transcriptase inhibitor; *NVP,* nevirapine; *PI,* protease inhibitor; *r,* low dose ritonavir; *RAL,* raltegravir; *RNA,* ribonucleic acid; *RVP,* rilpivirine; *TAF,* tenofovir alafenamide; *TDF,* tenofovir disoproxil fumarate. The following combinations in the recommended list are available as fixed-dose combination formulations: ABC/3TC, EFV/TDF/FTC, LPV/r, TDF/FTC, RPV/TDF/FTC, and ZDV/3TC.

Modified from DHHS Panel on Antiretroviral Guidelines for Adults and Adolescents: Guidelines for the use of antiretroviral agents in adults and adolescents with HIV. Department of Health and Human Services 1-161, 2018. .

Department of Health and Human Services (DHHS) guidelines with either tenofovir disoproxil fumarate or TAF and emtricitabine.
2. Atazanavir and ritonavir (300 mg and 100 mg) 2 tablets a day: Lower pill burden, but use with caution with acid-reducing agents (can alter absorption).
3. Lopinavir and ritonavir (200 mg/50 mg) 2 tablets twice a day (or 4 tablets once a day): Most likely to cause diarrhea and has the greatest negative effect on triglyceride levels; less commonly used.
4. Fosamprenavir and ritonavir (700 mg and 100 mg) 2 tablets twice a day (or 4 tablets once a day): Cannot take fosamprenavir with sulfa allergy; less commonly used.
5. Saquinavir and ritonavir: Saquinavir is no longer recommended for initial treatment of any patient and should be prescribed only in consultation with a specialist.

- All these drugs have their own unique, as well as class-specific, side effects and require careful follow-up to achieve optimal antiviral effects. Compliance with the drug regimen and tolerance of common side effects are critically important to maintain drug efficacy. Antiviral response should be monitored by baseline HIV viral load and CD4 count and repeat measurement at 2 and 4 wk into treatment and then periodically (every 3-6 mo) to ensure viral suppression.
- All patients should have genotypic resistance testing upon entry into medical care and before initiation of ART.
- In experienced patients, an antiretroviral regimen should be constructed based on past antiretroviral use and the results of genotypic or phenotypic testing.
- Patients with a CD4 count $<200/mm^3$ should be given preventive therapy for PJP (Table 12).
- Evaluation of chronic diarrhea in patients with HIV is described in the "Acquired Immunodeficiency Syndrome" topic in Section I.

TABLE 12 Criteria for Discontinuing and Restarting Opportunistic Infection Prophylaxis for Adults and Adolescents with Human Immunodeficiency Virus Infection

Opportunistic Infection	Criteria for Discontinuing Primary Prophylaxis	Criteria for Restarting Primary Prophylaxis	Criteria for Discontinuing Secondary Prophylaxis/Chronic Maintenance Therapy	Criteria for Restarting Secondary Prophylaxis/Chronic Maintenance Therapy
Pneumocystis pneumonia (PJP)	CD4+ count >200 cells/mm^3 for >3 mo in response to ART	CD4+ count <200 cells/mm^3	CD4+ count increased from <200 cells/mm^3 to >200 cells/mm^3 for ≥3 mo in response to ART If PJP is diagnosed when CD4+ count >200 cells/mm^3, prophylaxis should probably be continued for life regardless of CD4+ count rise in response to ART	CD4+ count <200 cells/mm^3, or if PCP recurred at a CD4+ count >200 cells/mm^3
Toxoplasma gondii encephalitis (TE)	CD4+ count >200 cells/mm^3 for >3 mo in response to ART	CD4+ count <100-200 cells/mm^3	Successfully completed initial therapy, remain asymptomatic of signs and symptoms of TE, and CD4+ count >200 cells/mm^3 for >6 mo in response to ART	CD4+ count <100 cells/mm^3
Microsporidiosis	Not applicable	Not applicable	No signs and symptoms of nonocular microsporidiosis and CD4+ count >200 cells/mm^3 for >6 mo in response to ART Patients with ocular microsporidiosis should be on therapy indefinitely regardless of CD4+ count	No recommendation
Disseminated *Mycobacterium avium* complex (MAC) disease	CD4+ count >100 cells/mm^3 for ≥3 mo in response to ART	CD4+ count <50 cells/mm^3	If fulfill the following criteria Completed ≥12 mo therapy, and no signs and symptoms of MAC, and have sustained (≥6 mo) CD4+ count >100 cells/mm^3 in response to ART	CD4+ count <50 cells/mm^3
Bartonellosis	Not applicable	Not applicable	If fulfill the following criteria Received 3-4 mo of treatment CD4+ count >200 cells/mm^3 for ≥6 mo Certain specialists would discontinue therapy only if *Bartonella* titers have also decreased by fourfold	No recommendation
Mucosal candidiasis	Not applicable	Not applicable	If used, reasonable to discontinue when CD4+ count >200 cells/mm^3	No recommendation
Cryptococcal meningitis	Not applicable	Not applicable	If fulfill the following criteria Completed course of initial therapy Remain asymptomatic of cryptococcosis CD4+ count ≥200 cells/mm^3 for >6 mo in response to ART Certain specialists would perform a lumbar puncture to determine if cerebrospinal fluid is culture and antigen negative before stopping therapy	CD4+ count <100 cells/mm^3
Histoplasma capsulatum infection	If used, CD4+ count >150 cells/mm^3 for 6 mo on ART	For patients at high risk for acquiring histoplasmosis, restart at CD4+ count ≤150 cells/mm^3	If fulfill the following criteria received itraconazole for ≥1 yr. Negative blood cultures CD4+ count >150 cells/mm^3 for ≥6 mo in response to ART Serum *Histoplasma* antigen <2 units	CD4+ count ≤150 cells/mm^3
Coccidioidomycosis	If used, CD4+ count ≥250 cells/mm^3 for ≥6 mo	If used, restart at CD4+ count <250 cells/mm^3	**Only for patients with focal coccidioidal pneumonia:** Clinically responded to ≥12 mo of antifungal therapy CD4+ count >250 cells/mm^3 Receiving ART Suppressive therapy should be continued indefinitely, even with increase in CD4+ count on ART for patients with diffuse pulmonary, disseminated, or meningeal diseases	No recommendation

TABLE 12 Criteria for Discontinuing and Restarting Opportunistic Infection Prophylaxis for Adults and Adolescents with Human Immunodeficiency Virus Infection–cont'd

Opportunistic Infection	Criteria for Discontinuing Primary Prophylaxis	Criteria for Restarting Primary Prophylaxis	Criteria for Discontinuing Secondary Prophylaxis/Chronic Maintenance Therapy	Criteria for Restarting Secondary Prophylaxis/Chronic Maintenance Therapy
Cytomegalovirus retinitis	Not applicable	Not applicable	CD4+ count >100 cells/mm^3 for >3-6 mo in response to ART. Therapy should be discontinued only after consultation with an ophthalmologist, taking into account magnitude and duration of CD4+ count increase, anatomic location of the lesions, vision in the contralateral eye, and the feasibility of regular ophthalmologic monitoring. Routine (every 3 mo) ophthalmologic follow-up is recommended for early detection of relapse or immune restoration uveitis	No recommendation
Isospora belli infection	Not applicable	Not applicable	Sustained increase in CD4+ count to >200 cells/mm^3 for >6 mo in response to ART and without evidence of *I. belli* infection	No recommendation

ART, Antiretroviral therapy.
Modified from Centers for Disease Control and Prevention: Guidelines for prevention and treatment of opportunistic infections in HIV-infected adults and adolescents. Recommendations from CDC, the National Institutes of Health, and the HIV Medicine Association of the Infectious Disease Society of America, *MMWR* 58(RR-4), 2009.

TABLE 13 Prophylaxis to Prevent First Episode of HIV-Related Opportunistic Disease

Pathogen	Indication	First Choice	Alternative
Pneumocystis jiroveci pneumonia (PJP, previously referred to as *Pneumocystis carinii,* PCP)	CD4+ count <200 cells/mm^3 or oropharyngeal candidiasis CD4+ <14% or history of AIDS-defining illness CD4+ count >200 but <250 cells/mm^3 if monitoring CD4+ count every 1-3 mo is not possible	Trimethoprim-sulfamethoxazole (TMP-SMX) double-strength PO daily; *or* single-strength daily	TMP-SMX 1 double-strength PO 3 times weekly; *or* dapsone 100 mg PO daily or 50 mg PO bid; *or* aerosolized pentamidine 300 mg via Respirgard II nebulizer every month; *or* atovaquone 1500 mg PO daily
Toxoplasma gondii encephalitis	*Toxoplasma* IgG–positive patients with CD4+ count <100 cells/mm^3 Seronegative patients receiving PCP prophylaxis not active against toxoplasmosis should have *Toxoplasma* serology retested if CD4+ count declines to <100 cells/mm^3 Prophylaxis should be initiated if seroconversion occurred	TMP-SMX, 1 double-strength PO daily	TMP-SMX 1 double-strength PO 3 times weekly; *or* TMP-SMX 1 single-strength PO daily; *or* dapsone 50 mg PO daily + pyrimethamine 50 mg PO weekly + leucovorin 25 mg PO weekly; *or* dapsone 200 mg PO weekly + pyrimethamine 75 mg PO weekly + leucovorin 25 mg PO weekly
Mycobacterium tuberculosis infection (TB) (treatment of latent TB infection or LTBI)	(1) Diagnostic test for LTBI, no evidence of active TB, and no prior history of treatment for active or latent TB (2) Diagnostic test for LTBI, but close contact with a person with infectious pulmonary TB and no evidence of active TB (3) A history of untreated or inadequately treated healed TB (i.e., old fibrotic lesions) regardless of diagnostic tests for LTBI and no evidence of active TB	Isoniazid (INH) 300 mg PO daily or 900 mg PO twice weekly for 9 mo—both plus pyridoxine 25 mg PO daily; *or* for persons exposed to drug-resistant TB, selection of drugs after consultation with public health authorities	Rifampin (RIF) 600 mg PO daily × 4 mo; or rifabutin (dosage depends on ART regimen). Be careful of drug interactions with these medications (PIs and NNRTIs) Isoniazid (15 mg/kg rounded up to the nearest 50 or 100 mg; 900 mg maximum) and rifapentine (10-14.0 kg 300 mg; 14.1-25.0 kg 450 mg; 25.1-32.0 kg 600 mg; 32.1-49.9 kg 750 mg; ≥50.00 kg 900 mg maximum) once weekly for a total of 3 mo
Disseminated *Mycobacterium avium* complex (MAC) disease	CD4+ count <50 cells/mm^3—after ruling out active MAC infection	Azithromycin 1200 mg PO once weekly; *or* clarithromycin 500 mg PO bid; *or* azithromycin 600 mg PO twice weekly	RFB 300 mg PO daily (dosage adjustment based on drug-drug interactions with antiretroviral therapy); rule out active TB before starting RFB
Streptococcus pneumoniae infection	CD4+ count >200 cells/mm^3 and no receipt of pneumococcal vaccine in the past 5 yr. CD4+ count <200 cells/mm^3—vaccination can be offered In patients who received polysaccharide pneumococcal vaccination (PPV) when CD4+ count <200 cells/mm^3 but has increased to >200 cells/mm^3 in response to antiretroviral therapy	A single dose of PCV13 followed by a single dose of PPSV23 at least 8 wk later. A second dose of PPSV23 should be given 5 yr after the initial PPSV23 dose	
Influenza A and B virus infection	All HIV-infected patients	Inactivated influenza vaccine 0.5 ml IM annually	
Histoplasma capsulatum infection	CD4+ count ≤150 cells/mm^3 and at high risk because of occupational exposure or live in a community with a hyperendemic rate of histoplasmosis (>10 cases/100 patient-yr)	Itraconazole 200 mg PO daily	
Coccidioidomycosis	Positive IgM or IgG serologic test result in a patient from a disease-endemic area; and CD4+ count <250 cells/mm^3	Fluconazole 400 mg PO daily itraconazole 200 mg PO bid	

Continued

TABLE 13 Prophylaxis to Prevent First Episode of HIV-Related Opportunistic Disease–cont'd

Pathogen	Indication	First Choice	Alternative
Varicella-zoster virus (VZV) infection	*Preexposure prevention:* Patients with CD4+ count ≥200 cells/mm^3 who have not been vaccinated, have no history of varicella or herpes zoster, or who are seronegative for VZV Note: Routine VZV serologic testing in HIV-infected adults is not recommended. *Postexposure*—close contact with a person who has active varicella or herpes zoster For susceptible patients (those who have no history of vaccination or of either condition, or are known to be VZV seronegative)	*Preexposure prevention:* Primary varicella vaccination (Varivax), 2 doses (0.5 ml SC) administered 3 mo apart. If vaccination results in disease because of vaccine virus, treatment with acyclovir is recommended *Postexposure therapy:* Varicella-zoster immune globulin (VariZIG) 125 IU per 10 kg (maximum of 625 IU) IM, administered within 96 hr after exposure to a person with active varicella or herpes zoster Note: As of June 2007, VariZIG can be obtained only under a treatment IND (1-800-843-7477, FFF Enterprises).	VZV-susceptible household contacts of susceptible HIV-infected persons should be vaccinated to prevent potential transmission of VZV to their HIV-infected contacts. Alternative postexposure therapy: Postexposure varicella vaccine (Varivax) 0.5 ml SC × 2 doses, 3 mo apart if CD4+ count >200 cells/mm^3; *or* preemptive acyclovir 800 mg PO 3×/day for 5 days These two alternatives have not been studied in the HIV population
Human papillomavirus (HPV) infection	Women aged 11-26 yr. Men aged 11-26 yr	HPV quadrivalent vaccine 0.5 ml IM mo 0, 2, and 6	
Hepatitis A virus (HAV) infection	HAV-susceptible patients with chronic liver disease or who are injection-drug users, or men who have sex with men. Certain specialists might delay vaccination until CD4+ count >200 cells/mm^3	Hepatitis A vaccine 1 ml IM × 2 doses—at 0 and 6-12 mo IgG antibody response should be assessed 1 mo after vaccination; nonresponders should be revaccinated	
Hepatitis B virus (HBV) infection	All HIV patients without evidence of prior exposure to HBV should be vaccinated with HBV vaccine, including patients with CD4+ count <200 cells/mm^3. *Patients with isolated anti-HBc:* Consider screening for HBV DNA before vaccination to rule out occult chronic HBV infection	Hepatitis B vaccine IM (Engerix-B 20 μg/ml or Recombivax HB 10 μg/ml) at 0, 1, and 6 mo anti-HBs should be obtained 1 mo after completion of the vaccine series.	Some experts recommend vaccinating with 40-μg doses of either vaccine
	Vaccine nonresponders: Defined as anti-HBs <10 IU/ml 1 mo after a vaccination series For patients with low CD4+ count at the time of first vaccination series, certain specialists might delay revaccination until after a sustained increase in CD4+ count with antiretroviral therapy	Revaccinate with a second vaccine series	Some experts recommend revaccinating with 40-μg doses of either vaccine

AIDS, Acquired immunodeficiency syndrome; *ART,* antiretroviral therapy; *HB,* hepatitis B; *Ig,* immunoglobulin; *IM,* intramuscular; *IND,* investigational new drug; *NNRTI,* nonnucleoside analog reverse transcriptase inhibitor; *PI,* protease inhibitors; *PO,* by mouth; *RFB,* rifabutin.

Modified from Centers for Disease Control and Prevention: Guidelines for prevention and treatment of opportunistic infections in HIV-infected adults and adolescents: recommendations from CDC, the National Institutes of Health, and the HIV Medicine Association of the Infectious Disease Society of America, *MMWR* 58(RR-4), 2009.

- Criteria for discontinuing and restarting opportunistic infection prophylaxis for adults and adolescents with HIV infection is described in Table 13.
- HIV infection in a pregnant woman poses special challenges and considerations. Appropriate and timely ART given to mother and newborn has been shown to dramatically reduce the risk of perinatal transmission of HIV. The goal of therapy is to achieve an undetectable viral load. For HIV-infected pregnant women who are already receiving ART: (1) Continue therapy if suppressing viral replication, but avoid use of efavirenz in the first trimester (substitution is recommended in the first trimester); (2) if viremia on therapy, genotypic testing is recommended. For HIV-infected pregnant women who have never received ART: (1) All women should start on ART as soon as possible. Most antiretrovirals are safe in pregnancy; however, efavirenz should be avoided because of possible teratogenicity (Class D), DDI and D4T should be avoided (potential of lactic acidosis), and some protease inhibitors may be dose-altered in pregnancy. Nevirapine should not be initiated in an antiretroviral-naive pregnant patient with CD4 counts >250 cells/mm^3 because of the risk of hepatotoxicity. (2) Women who do not need ART for their own health should also initiate three-drug therapy, but may do so at the end of the first trimester.
- Preferred ART medications during pregnancy include:
  1. NRTIs: TDF/FTC, TDF/3TC, or ABC/3TC
  2. INSTI: Raltegravir; dolutegravir can be used after the first trimester; limited data with bictegravir. Elvitegravir should not be used in pregnancy because of inadequate drug concentrations.
  3. PIs: ATV/r or DRV/r
- ART should continue through the baby's birth. Zidovudine should also be given intravenously to the woman at the time of labor if the woman has an HIV RNA >1000 copies/ml or there is a concern for poor adherence, regardless of whether it is an existing component of her three-drug regimen. In women with viral loads persistently >1000 copies/ml despite appropriate ART, cesarean section may further lower risk of transmission. For women with HIV RNA <1000 copies/ml zidovudine (AZT) should also be given to the newborn for the first 6 wk of life. If HIV RNA levels are >1000 copies/ml, infants should receive combination ART, which may include zidovudine, lamivudine and nevirapine for 6 wk. Mothers should completely avoid nursing.

DISPOSITION

- Ongoing care consisting of frequent medical evaluations and monitoring of CD4 counts and HIV viral loads.
- Long-term care focused on providing up-to-date ART and prophylaxis of PJP and other opportunistic infections, as well as early detection of complications.

BOX 1 Vaccination in HIV-Positive Adults

Generally Avoid
- BCG
- Oral polio
- Oral typhoid

Avoid if CD4+ Cells <200
- Yellow fever
- Measles
- Varicella-zoster virus (VZV)

Give Routinely
- Tetanus/diphtheria (or Tdap)
- Hepatitis A/B
- *Streptococcus pneumoniae*
- Hib
- Meningococcal
- Influenza, yearly

Give if Indicated for Travel
- Typhoid Vi
- Meningococcal
- Polio, IPV
- Rabies
- Japanese encephalitis
- Tick-borne encephalitis

BCG, Bacillus Calmette-Guerin; *Hib, Haemophilus influenzae* type b; *IPV,* inactivated polio vaccine.
From Auerbach P: *Wilderness medicine, expert consult,* premium edition—enhanced online features and print, Philadelphia, 2012, Saunders.

- Ongoing assessment for cardiovascular risk and other primary prevention interventions.
- Screening for hepatitis A, B, and C. Treatment when indicated. Drugs such as TDF and lamivudine have activity against both HIV and hepatitis B and may be used in patients with coinfection.
- Vaccinations including hepatitis A and B (when susceptible), pneumococcus (PCV13 and PPSV23), tetanus/diphtheria/pertussis, meningococcal, and influenza. Box 1 summarizes vaccinations in HIV-positive adults.
- Yearly screening for other sexually transmitted infections (chlamydia, gonorrhea, and syphilis). This includes trichomonas in women and extragenital testing for chlamydia and gonorrhea (i.e., pharyngeal and rectal) in MSM.
- Consideration of AIDS (lymphomas, HPV) and non-AIDS related (screening for general population, age-specific cancers).

REFERRAL

To a physician knowledgeable and experienced in the management of HIV infection and its complications.

PREVENTION

- TDF/FTC or TAF/FTC may be used as pre-exposure prophylaxis (PrEP). Individuals who are HIV negative may take TDF/FTC or TAF/FTC once a day to prevent HIV infection. TDF/FTC as PrEP has been demonstrated to be effective in MSM, heterosexuals, and injection drug users. Importantly, TAF/FTC as PrEP has been shown to be effective in MSM and transwomen but not for cisgender women. Individuals on PrEP should be monitored every 3 mo for renal dysfunction, HIV status, and adherence.
- Postexposure prophylaxis (PEP) is an effective prevention intervention for individuals exposed to HIV infection, either occupationally or through a sexual exposure. PEP should be taken within 72 hours of an exposure and continued for 28 days. Baseline HIV status, renal function, hepatitis B/C, and liver function should be assessed. The recommended first-line regimen is TDF/FTC or TAF/FTC once daily plus raltegravir 400 mg orally twice daily or dolutegravir 50 mg once daily.

PEARLS & CONSIDERATIONS

COMMENTS

- ART should be initiated in all HIV-infected individuals regardless of CD4 cell counts.
- ART in combination with avoidance of breast-feeding and elective cesarean section in women with viremia reduces risk for mother-to-child transmission.

SUGGESTED READINGS

Available at ExpertConsult.com

RELATED CONTENT

Human Immunodeficiency Virus (HIV) Infection (Patient Information)
Acquired Immunodeficiency Syndrome (Related Key Topic)

AUTHOR: **Philip A. Chan, MD, MS**

BASIC INFORMATION

DEFINITION

Normal pressure hydrocephalus (NPH) is a syndrome of symptomatic hydrocephalus in the setting of normal cerebrospinal fluid (CSF) pressure. The classic clinical triad of NPH includes gait disturbance, cognitive decline, and incontinence.

SYNONYMS

Normal pressure hydrocephalus
NPH
Occult hydrocephalus
Extraventricular obstructive hydrocephalus
Chronic hydrocephalus

ICD-10CM CODES
G91.2 Normal pressure hydrocephalus
G91.8 Other hydrocephalus

EPIDEMIOLOGY & DEMOGRAPHICS

INCIDENCE: The exact incidence is not known. In one study the incidence was found to be 5.5 per 100,000, but it may account for up to 5% of dementia in the U.S. Hospital discharge data suggest approximately 11,500 new cases diagnosed annually (may be overestimated). The prevalence of NPH was found to be 21.9 per 100,000 (~0.22%) in one study but also may be as high as 14% among extended care facility patients.
PREDOMINANT SEX: Males = females
PREDOMINANT AGE: NPH is more common with increasing age. In one study of 1238 patients who had undergone a head CT and neuropsychiatric evaluation, 0.2% of patients between 70 and 79 had probable NPH, and 5.9% of those 80 yr old and older had probable NPH.

PHYSICAL FINDINGS & CLINICAL PRESENTATION

- Gait difficulty: A "magnetic" gait, in which patients have difficulty initiating ambulation. The gait may be broad-based and shuffling, with the appearance that the feet are stuck to the floor. Difficulty with turns may also be seen.
- Cognitive decline: Mental slowing, forgetfulness, and inattention, typically without agnosia, aphasia, or other cortical disturbances.
- Incontinence: Initially may have urinary urgency; incontinence later develops. Fecal incontinence also occasionally occurs. In one prospective study of 55 consecutive patients with idiopathic NPH, nocturia was the most common symptom, urge incontinence was the most bothersome, and 100% had detrusor overactivity on urodynamic studies.
- *Gegenhalten* (paratonia or involuntary resistance with passive movement) or other frontal lobe signs may be seen.

ETIOLOGY

- Approximately 50% of cases are idiopathic; the prevailing thought is that these cases are either due to increased CSF production or reduced absorption.
- The remaining cases are secondary to a variety of causes, including prior subarachnoid hemorrhage, meningitis, head trauma, or intracranial surgery.
- Symptoms are presumed to result from stretching of cortical, limbic, and thalamocortical fibers that lie near the ventricles as dilation occurs.

DIAGNOSIS

DIFFERENTIAL DIAGNOSIS

- Vascular dementia
- Alzheimer disease with extrapyramidal features
- Cognitive impairment in the setting of Parkinson disease or parkinsonism-plus syndromes
- Dementia with Lewy bodies
- Frontotemporal dementia
- Cervical spondylosis with cord compromise in the setting of degenerative dementia
- HIV-associated dementia
- Chronic bifrontal subdural hematomas
- Table 1 differentiates MRI findings between hydrocephalus and atrophy

WORKUP

Large-volume lumbar puncture should be performed with assessment of improvement in gait. Such improvement predicts shunt responsiveness. There are multiple approaches to evaluating for shunt responsiveness using a large-volume lumbar puncture and assessing gait before and after the lumbar puncture. Graff-Radford and colleagues have proposed the following approach: Have the patient walk 30 feet (10 meters), turn 180 degrees, and then return to starting. Videotape and time this action. Count the number of steps the patient takes when turning 180 degrees. Have the patient turn 180 degrees twice and calculate the average the number of steps taken. Count the number of steps the patient takes when turning 360 degrees. Have the patient turn 360 degrees three times and calculate the average number of steps taken. Then, perform a lumbar puncture, removing 30 cc of CSF. Thirty minutes after removing 30 cc, repeat the procedure described above. Videotape the gait and turning as well. If the time to walk 30 feet is reduced or the number of steps taken when turning is reduced, then there is a high probability of shunt response.

- Measurement of CSF outflow resistance by an infusion test or CSF pressure monitoring is sometimes used to help predict surgical outcome. External lumbar drainage (ELD) is being used more commonly and can be done over a period of 1 to 3 days at special centers that specialize in evaluating patients with adult hydrocephalus.

LABORATORY TESTS

- CSF should be sent for routine fluid analysis to exclude other pathologies.
- CSF biomarkers may be useful in excluding Alzheimer disease (e.g., Tau/A-beta 42). However, such biomarker tests are not used in routine clinical practice yet.

IMAGING STUDIES

- CT scan or MRI (Fig. 1) can be used to document ventriculomegaly. The distinguishing feature of NPH is ventricular enlargement out of proportion to sulcal atrophy (Fig. E2), and typically the frontal horn ratio (Evans index) exceeds 0.30. An algorithm for evaluation of patients with enlarged ventricles is described in Fig. 3.
- MRI has advantages over CT, including better ability to visualize structures in the posterior fossa, visualize transependymal CSF flow (seen as periventricular T2 FLAIR hyperintensity), and document extent of white matter lesions. On MRI a flow void in the aqueduct and third ventricle ("jet sign"), thinning and elevation of the corpus callosum on sagittal images, rounding of the frontal horns, and a pattern known as *disproportionately enlarged subarachnoid*

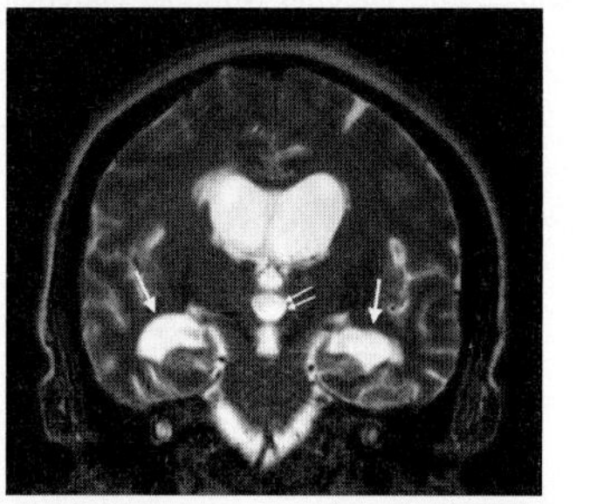

FIG. 1 This MRI study shows a coronal view of the brain of a patient with NPH. It demonstrates the classic findings: Dilation of the lateral ventricles, their temporal horns *(large arrows),* and the third ventricle *(pair of arrows),* and absence of cerebral atrophy. (From Kaufman DM et al: *Kaufman's clinical neurology for psychiatrists,* ed 8, Philadelphia, 2017, Elsevier.)

TABLE 1 Differentiation between Hydrocephalus and Atrophy

	Hydrocephalus	Atrophy
Temporal horns	Enlarged	Normal (except in Alzheimer disease)
Third ventricle	Convex ▸ distended anterior recess	Concave ▸ normal anterior recess
Fourth ventricle	Normal or enlarged	Normal
Transependymal CSF migration	Presents acutely	Absent
Sulci	Flattened	Enlarged out of proportion to age

From Grant LA: *Grainger & Allison's diagnostic radiology essentials,* ed 2, 2019, Elsevier.

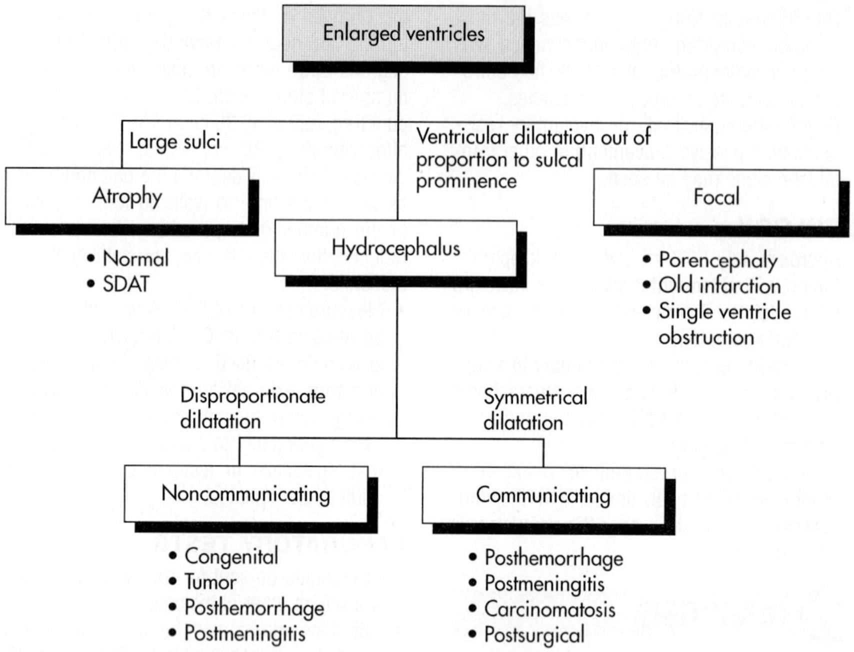

FIG. 3 Radiographic differential diagnosis of enlarged ventricles. *SDAT,* Senile dementia of the Alzheimer type. (From Weissleder R et al: *Primer of diagnostic imaging,* ed 5, St Louis, 2011, Mosby.)

space hydrocephalus (DESH) may be seen. DESH is characterized by narrow CSF space at the high convexity/midline areas and enlarged sylvian fissures and is associated with a good response to CSF shunting. MRI time-resolved 2D phase contrast imaging with velocity encoding can also be used to visualize CSF flow.

- Isotope cisternography and dynamic MRI studies have not been shown to be superior in predicting shunt outcome.

Rx TREATMENT

There is no evidence that NPH can be effectively treated with medications. CSF diversion via a ventriculoperitoneal shunt is a definitive treatment.

NONPHARMACOLOGIC THERAPY

Response to ventriculoperitoneal shunting is variable. Some patients (variable depending on series reported) show significant improvement from shunting; however, effectiveness of shunting has never been demonstrated in a randomized controlled trial. Gait is most likely to improve.

- Factors that may predict positive outcome with surgery:
  1. NPH caused by prior trauma, subarachnoid hemorrhage, or meningitis
  2. History of mild impairment in cognition <2 yr duration
  3. Presence of gait abnormality
  4. Onset of gait abnormality before cognitive decline
  5. Imaging demonstrates hydrocephalus without sulcal enlargement, including normal-size sylvian fissures and cortical sulci, and absent or mild white matter lesions
  6. Transependymal CSF flow visualized on MRI
  7. Large-volume tap or ELD produces dramatic but temporary relief of symptoms
  8. High *normal* opening pressure
- Factors that may predict negative outcome with surgery:
  1. Extensive white matter lesions or diffuse cerebral atrophy on MRI
  2. Moderate to severe cognitive impairment
  3. Onset of cognitive impairment before gait disorder
  4. History of alcohol abuse

ACUTE GENERAL Rx

Shunting in selected patients

DISPOSITION

Symptoms of NPH may progress over time. Prompt diagnosis may improve chances for treatment success.

REFERRAL

Patients should be referred to a neurologist with experience in evaluating NPH followed by a neurosurgeon for shunting in appropriate patients.

PEARLS & CONSIDERATIONS

Each of the cardinal symptoms of NPH is commonly seen in the elderly and occurs in multiple disease processes; therefore, differential diagnoses should always be considered carefully.

CAUTION

Although there has been an increase in positive outcomes after shunting over the last 20 yr, shunt complications, including subdural or intracerebral hematoma, may occur in 30% to 40% of patients. In one retrospective study spanning 10 yr, which included patients with idiopathic as well as other forms of adult hydrocephalus, the shunt failure rate was 32%.

SUGGESTED READINGS

Available at ExpertConsult.com

RELATED CONTENT

Normal Pressure Hydrocephalus (Patient Information)

AUTHORS: **Marco Pares, MD,** and **Joseph S. Kass, MD, JD, FAAN**

BASIC INFORMATION

DEFINITION

Hydronephrosis, Greek for "water inside the kidney," is an anatomic dilation of the collecting system of the kidneys (renal pelvis and/or calyces). When combined with ureteric dilation, the term hydroureteronephrosis is used. Hydronephrosis is a structural finding, not a specific diagnosis, and is *not* synonymous with obstruction. Hydronephrosis can occur with complete, partial, or no obstruction of urine flow.

SYNONYMS

Pelviectasis
Caliectasis
Pelvocaliectasis
Pyelocaliectasis

ICD-10CM CODES

N13.1	Hydronephrosis with ureteral stricture, not elsewhere classified
N13.2	Hydronephrosis with renal and ureteral calculous obstruction
N13.30	Unspecified hydronephrosis
N13.39	Other hydronephrosis
Q62.0	Congenital hydronephrosis
Q62.11	Hydronephrosis with ureteropelvic junction obstruction

EPIDEMIOLOGY & DEMOGRAPHICS

Prevalence from multiple autopsy series ranges from 2% to 4%, with subjects ranging in age from neonates to geriatric patients. Antenatal hydronephrosis is one of the most common findings in prenatal ultrasound scans, affecting up to 5% of pregnancies, with 30% to 40% persisting postnatally. Of these, 40% will resolve spontaneously. Hydronephrosis in children is often caused by congenital and structural abnormalities of the kidneys and ureters, such as ureteropelvic junction obstruction (UPJO) or vesicoureteral reflux (VUR). Hydronephrosis in adults is often a result of obstruction of one or both kidneys, usually caused by stones, tumors, infections, and trauma. Stones are the most common cause overall of upper urinary tract obstruction. In adults 20 to 60 yr in age, hydronephrosis is more common in women, secondary to pregnancy/gynecologic causes. During pregnancy, physiologic hydronephrosis (more commonly on the right) occurs in up to 90% of cases, is often asymptomatic, and typically resolves postpartum. In older patients (age >60 yr), obstruction from prostate enlargement and obstruction from malignancy are the most common causes.

CLINICAL PRESENTATION

Hydronephrosis may present as an asymptomatic, incidental finding during imaging performed for another purpose. Symptoms often indicate an element of obstruction. Presentation depends on degree of obstruction (complete or partial), duration (acute or chronic), and anatomic factors (unilateral, bilateral and intrinsic or extrinsic in the ureter).

HISTORY:

- Pain is usually present along the flank with radiation toward the ipsilateral groin or lower abdominal quadrant. If onset is sudden and severe, consider a ureteral stone. If pain is induced by diuresis (e.g., following consumption of alcohol), consider ureteropelvic junction obstruction ("Dietl crisis"). When obstruction is subacute to chronic, symptoms may be vague, less intense, or absent, and may wax and wane in severity (colic). Extrinsic compression (e.g., malignancy-associated compression of ureters or retroperitoneal fibrosis) usually has a more insidious onset compared with intrinsic obstruction (e.g., ureteral stone or blood clot).
- Nausea and vomiting are typically associated with acute obstruction, usually from an intrinsic process.
- Oliguria/anuria may occur with complete, bilateral obstruction, or with an obstructed solitary kidney.
- Urinary symptoms are often absent, unless there is an associated condition, including urinary tract infection, distal ureteral stone, or urinary retention. These voiding symptoms include dysuria, urinary urgency and frequency, pelvic pressure, and discomfort.
- Hematuria may indicate a stone, urinary tract infection, or malignancy.
- The site of obstruction can relate to the presentation, with upper tract obstruction frequently presenting with flank pain, whereas lower tract obstruction is often associated with obstructive voiding symptoms.

PHYSICAL EXAMINATION: A complete physical examination is warranted, but may not be helpful in the assessment of hydronephrosis. Special attention should be paid to the following:

- Blood pressure.
- Palpable abdominal mass: Rare, except in children or thin patients with massive hydronephrosis. Costovertebral angle tenderness is typically not a helpful finding. An enlarged, often percussible bladder is the most common lower abdominal "mass."
- Complete genitourinary and pelvic exams:
  1. Pelvic exam will assess for pelvic masses or pelvic organ prolapse, which is rarely associated with ureteral obstruction.
  2. Digital rectal exam will assess for prostatic abnormality or rectal mass.
  3. Residual urine volume may demonstrate incomplete emptying of the bladder. Residual urine volume can be evaluated indirectly by bedside ultrasonography or directly by bladder catheterization.

ETIOLOGY

Hydronephrosis can be caused by extrinsic or intrinsic factors relative to the urinary tract (Table 1). Causes may be grouped as congenital or acquired.

DIAGNOSIS

Diagnostic workup depends on age, acuity of presentation, if hydronephrosis was diagnosed incidentally, and associated symptoms.

DIFFERENTIAL DIAGNOSIS

- Extrarenal pelvis: No true obstruction exists
- Urinary stones
- Neoplastic disorders: Kidney, ureter, bladder, urethra, gynecologic, colorectal, metastatic
- Prostatic hyperplasia
- Urethral stricture
- Neurologic disease that produces voiding dysfunction
- Urinary reflux
- Urinary tract infection
- Medication effects

TABLE 1 Causes of Hydronephrosis

Obstructive	
Intrinsic to the Urinary Tract	Ureter: Ureteropelvic junction obstruction, ureterovesical junction obstruction, stricture, tumor, ureterocele, stone, blood clot, sloughed papilla, infection, hyperplastic polyp Bladder: Malignancy, stone, bladder neck obstruction, urine retention Prostate: Benign prostatic enlargement, prostatitis, calculus, abscess, malignancy Urethra: Stricture, stone, diverticulum, malignancy, posterior urethral valves, phimosis
Extrinsic to the Urinary Tract	Reproductive system: Uterus: Pregnancy, prolapse, fibroids, malignancy Ovary: Malignancy, cyst, abscess Vascular system: Aneurysm: Abdominal aorta, iliac vessel Aberrant vessels: Ureteropelvic junction Venous: Retrocaval ureter, ovarian vein syndrome Gastrointestinal system: Inflammatory bowel disease, GI malignancy, abscesses, cysts Diseases of the retroperitoneum: Retroperitoneal fibrosis Retroperitoneal malignancy (primary or metastatic deposits) Hematoma Lymphocele Iatrogenic injury
Nonobstructive	
	Vesicoureteral reflux Extrarenal pelvis Megaureter/megacalycosis Pyelonephritis

GI, Gastrointestinal.

- Trauma
- Congenital abnormality of urinary tract
- Urinary retention
- Retroperitoneal fibrosis
- Urinary trauma
- Iatrogenic injuries

LABORATORY TESTS

- **Evaluation of kidney function:** Blood urea nitrogen and creatinine. If azotemia present, bilateral obstruction or unilateral obstruction of a solitary kidney is present.
- **Electrolyte abnormalities:** Hypo- or hypernatremia, hyperkalemia, and low bicarbonate concentration.
- **Urinalysis and sediment examination:** White blood cells, red blood cells, or bacteria in the appropriate setting (e.g., infection, stones). Urine microscopy facilitates crystal identification, which may suggest urinary stone disease. The sediment may be normal in obstructive renal disease.
- **Urine culture:** Urinalysis or presentation suggests urinary tract infection.
- **Urine cytology:** Suspicion for urothelial cancer.

IMAGING STUDIES

- Ultrasound is an excellent initial screening test, especially for children and pregnant women, with evaluation of the kidneys, portions of the ureters, bladder wall, bladder volume, and contour of the collecting system and ureters. Point-of-care ultrasound provides early, rapid imaging and aids patient triage and justification for additional imaging. Ultrasound is >90% sensitive and specific for hydronephrosis. Although not definitive, the absence of ureteral jets on ultrasound may be an indirect sign of obstruction (Fig. E1).
- Abdominal, plain film, or kidney, ureter, and bladder (KUB) radiographs have limited diagnostic value unless conducted with ultrasound; may demonstrate radiopaque kidney or ureteral stones.
- Abdominal CT scan without intravenous contrast medium localizes sites of obstruction (Figs. E2 and E3), especially if a ureteral calculus is the cause of obstruction. A normal ureteral width by unenhanced CT is 2 to 3 mm wide in adults. If kidney function is normal, CT urography (without and then with contrast, and with delayed images of the ureters), provides anatomic information and is the modality of choice for assessment of upper tract tumors or incidental hydronephrosis.
- MRI is an alternative to CT that provides detail but cannot directly detect a stone. Severely impaired renal function may preclude gadolinium administration. MRI may be used when other tests are inconclusive or contraindicated (e.g., pregnancy, CKD, radiocontrast media allergy).
- Antegrade or retrograde ureterogram/pyelogram is an invasive procedure used when CT or MRI scans with radiocontrast media are contraindicated (e.g., contrast allergy, renal impairment).
- Voiding cystourethrography (VCUG) establishes vesicoureteral reflux and bladder neck or urethral obstruction.
- Radioisotope renography (diuretic renography, Tc-99m MAG3 renogram) is a functional procedure that provides differential renal function and determines presence of functional obstruction.

Rx TREATMENT

ACUTE GENERAL Rx

- Analgesics, antiemetics, and fluids for treatment of pain, nausea, and vomiting
- Antibiotics for urinary tract infection/pyelonephritis

Definitive management:

- Management depends on presence of obstruction, etiology, and location of hydronephrosis. Prompt treatment of infection and relief of obstruction prevent long-term loss of kidney function. Chronic renal obstruction from any cause may produce permanent functional deterioration.
- General principles include the following:
  1. Routine outpatient evaluation for hydronephrosis in asymptomatic or minimally symptomatic patients with no infection, electrolyte derangements, or acute kidney injury.
  2. Surgical treatment is aimed at relieving obstruction when hydronephrosis is associated with urinary tract infection, acute kidney injury, uncontrollable pain, or nausea and vomiting. Surgical treatment is also indicated with complete urinary obstruction from a bilateral obstructing process or unilateral obstruction in a solitary kidney.
  3. Urethral catheter or suprapubic catheter placement is indicated for bladder outlet obstruction. After relief of obstruction, patients should be monitored for postobstructive diuresis.
  4. Ureteral stenting is carried out for decompression of one or both kidneys.
  5. Percutaneous nephrostomy tubes may be required in the setting of extrinsic ureteral compression or when ureteral stenting is not possible or fails.

REFERRAL

Prompt, emergent referral is paramount in the setting of severe symptoms, infection, or impaired renal function.

- Urology for diagnostic and/or therapeutic procedures (pediatric urologist for antenatal or postnatal hydronephrosis)
- Oncology for diagnosed neoplasm
- Gynecology for pregnancy or if female pelvic anatomy is involved
- Nephrology for electrolyte/acid-base disturbances

PEARLS & CONSIDERATIONS

COMMENTS

- Hydronephrosis is not a primary disorder; an underlying etiology must be sought.
- Children often have congenital causes; adults generally have acquired intrinsic or extrinsic causes.
- There are obstructive and nonobstructive causes of hydronephrosis. Further evaluation can be performed without specialty consultation with a computed tomography urogram, magnetic resonance urogram, or diuretic renogram.
- Prompt renal decompression is critical when hydronephrosis is associated with infection, severe kidney injury, and/or electrolyte abnormalities.

PREVENTION

Timely and appropriate management of acute kidney obstruction prevents long-term kidney damage. Hydronephrosis may persist after relief of the obstructing cause.

SUGGESTED READINGS

Available at ExpertConsult.com

AUTHORS: **Natalija Kovacevic, MD,** and **David A. Leavitt, MD**

BASIC INFORMATION

DEFINITION

Hypercholesterolemia refers to a blood cholesterol measurement ≥200 mg/dl.

SYNONYMS

Hyperlipidemia
Hypercholesteremia
Dyslipidemia
Type II familial hyperlipoproteinemia

ICD-10CM CODE

E78.0 Pure hypercholesterolemia

EPIDEMIOLOGY & DEMOGRAPHICS

- More than 105 million (37% of) adults in the U.S. have total blood cholesterol levels higher than 200 mg/dl. Of this group, more than 36 million adults have extremely high-risk cholesterol levels over 240 mg/dl (13%).
- For men over the age of 20 yr, approximately 48% of white men, 45% of black men, and 50% of Hispanic men have high blood cholesterol.
- For women over the age of 20, approximately 50% of white women, 42% of black women, and 50% of Hispanic women have hypercholesterolemia.
- Prevalence of hypercholesterolemia increases with age.
- According to NHANES data for 2009 to 2010, approximately 47% of adults had at least one of three risk factors for cardiovascular disease—uncontrolled high blood pressure, uncontrolled high levels of low-density lipoproteins (LDL) cholesterol, or current smoking.

PHYSICAL FINDINGS & CLINICAL PRESENTATION

- A detailed medication history should be performed because some medications may affect lipid levels (e.g., thiazides, corticosteroids, beta-blockers, and estrogens).
- The physical examination should include measurements of BMI and BP, thyroid and liver assessments, and examining peripheral pulses including carotids for bruits.
- Physical findings, particularly in the familial forms may include:
  1. Tendon xanthomas
  2. Xanthelasma
  3. Arcus corneae
  4. Arterial bruits (young adulthood)

ETIOLOGY

PRIMARY:

- Genetics
- Obesity
- Dietary intake

SECONDARY:

- Hypothyroidism
- Diabetes mellitus
- Nephrotic syndrome
- Obstructive liver disease: Hepatoma, extrahepatic biliary obstruction, primary biliary cirrhosis
- Alcohol or tobacco use
- Dysgammaglobulinemia (multiple myeloma, SLE)
- Drugs: Oral contraceptives, progesterone, corticosteroids, thiazide diuretics, β-blockers, androgenic steroids, retinoic acid derivatives, protease inhibitors

Dx DIAGNOSIS

DIFFERENTIAL DIAGNOSIS

- Always consider underlying secondary causes for the elevated cholesterol.
- Patients with very high LDL cholesterol usually have genetic forms of hypercholesterolemia (see "Hyperlipoproteinemia, Primary"). Early detection of these cases and family testing to identify similarly affected relatives is important.
- Metabolic syndrome:
  1. A constellation of lipid and nonlipid risk factors of a metabolic origin
  2. Diagnosed when three or more of the following are present: abdominal obesity (waist circumference >40 in for men and >35 in for women); fasting triglycerides >150 mg/dl; HDL <40 mg/dl in males and <50 mg/dl in females; systolic BP >130 mm Hg and diastolic BP >85 mm Hg; fasting glucose >110 mg/dl

WHO SHOULD BE SCREENED:

- AACE recommends screening of patients >20 yr of age for elevated cholesterol every 5 yr, males >45 yr and females >55 yr of age every 1 to 2 yr, and >65 yr of age every yr up to 75 yr of age regardless of CAD risk status. Patients above 75 yr of age with multiple CAD risk factors should continue to get screened annually.
- The USPSTF supports routine screening for men aged >35 yr and women aged >45 yr by measurement of nonfasting total and HDL cholesterol alone.
- In 2010 the USPSTF recommended routine screening for overweight and obese persons aged <20 yr.
- In 2011, ACC/AHA recommended screening for hypertriglyceridemia by a nonfasting measurement. A nonfasting level of <200 mg/dl is commensurate with an optimal level of <100 mg/dl and no further testing is required. However, a nonfasting level of >200 mg/dl warrants further testing with a fasting lipid profile.

LABORATORY TESTS

- Obtain a lipid profile. A fasting lipid panel has been traditionally preferred over a nonfasting lipid profile; however, this recommendation has come into question, and expert consensus statements from Canada and Europe recommend nonfasting lipid testing as the new standard for lipid measurement. In nonfasting patients, triglyceride levels ≥175 mg/dl should be considered elevated as compared with <150 mg/dl for fasting panels. Fasting lipid panels are preferred for patients with triglycerides over 400 mg/dl.
- Perform a workup for secondary causes if clinically indicated, such as TSH, metabolic profile, LFTs, and fasting glucose.

Rx TREATMENT

NONPHARMACOLOGIC THERAPY

- First-line treatment: Dietary therapy can result in 5% to 15% reduction in LDL cholesterol level
- Composition of the **TLC diet:**
  1. Total fat 25% to 30% of total calories
  2. Polyunsaturated fat up to 10% of total calories
  3. Monounsaturated fat up to 20% of total calories
  4. Saturated fats <7% of total calories
  5. Carbohydrate 50% to 60% of total calories
  6. Protein 15% of total calories
  7. No more than 200 mg/day of cholesterol
  8. Fiber 20 to 30 g/day
- Increased physical activity: Encourage 30 min of moderately intense physical activity, four to six times a wk (e.g., brisk walking, riding stationary bike, water aerobics)
- Maintenance of a healthy weight
- Avoidance of tobacco products
- Counseling on CAD risk factors (Table 1)
- Plant-based diets (including stanol-containing margarines, oat bran, and nuts) have shown effectiveness in controlling lipids

ACUTE GENERAL Rx

No acute treatment needed

CHRONIC Rx

- Box 1 summarizes the key recommendations for the treatment of blood cholesterol to reduce ASCVD (atherosclerotic cardiovascular disease) risk in adults.
- The guidelines identify four high-risk groups that benefit from statin therapy:
  1. Patients with clinical ASCVD (Table 2, Fig. 1)
  2. LDL ≥190 mg/dl
  3. DM aged 40 to 75 yr and LDL 70 to 189 mg/dl
  4. 10-yr risk for ASCVD ≥7.5% and LDL 70 to 189 mg/dl

TABLE 1 Risk Factors for Heart Disease

1. Cigarette smoking
2. Hypertension (BP ≥140/90 mm Hg or on medications)
3. Low HDL cholesterol (<40 mg/dl)*
4. Family history of premature CHD (<55 yr in first-degree male relative or <65 yr in first-degree female relative)
5. Age (men ≥45 yr, women ≥55 yr)

*HDL cholesterol >60 mg/dl counts as a negative risk factor; its presence removes one risk factor from the total count.
BP, Blood pressure; *CHD,* congenital heart disease; *HDL,* high-density lipoprotein cholesterol.

BOX 1 2013 ACC/AHA Summary of Key Recommendations for the Treatment of Blood Cholesterol to Reduce ASCVD Risk in Adults

A. Heart-healthy lifestyle habits should be encouraged for all individuals
B. The appropriate intensity of statin therapy should be initiated or continued
   1. Clinical ASCVD*
      a. Age 75 yr or less and no safety concerns: High-intensity statin (class I, level A)
      b. Age 75 yr or safety concerns: Moderate-intensity statin (class I, level A)*
   2. Primary prevention: Primary LDL-C 190 mg/dl or greater
      a. Rule out secondary causes of hyperlipidemia (class I, level B)
      b. Age 21 yr or older: High-intensity statin (class I, level B)
      c. Achieve at least a 50% reduction in LDL-C (class IIa, level B)
      d. LDL-C lowering nonstatin therapy may be considered to further reduce LDL-C (class IIb, level C)
   3. Primary prevention: Diabetes, 40 to 75 yr of age, and LDL-C 70 to 189 mg/dl
      a. Moderate-intensity statin (class I, level A)
      b. Consider high-intensity statin when 7.5% or greater 10-yr ASCVD risk using the Pooled Cohort Equations (class IIa, level B)‡
   4. Primary prevention: No diabetes, 40 to 75 yr of age, and LDL-C 70 to 189 mg/dl
      a. Estimate 10-yr ASCVD risk using the Risk Calculator based on the Pooled Cohort Equations in those *not* receiving a statin; estimate risk every 4 to 6 yr (class I, level B)
      b. To determine whether to initiate a statin, engage in a clinician-patient discussion of the potential for ASCVD risk reduction, adverse effects, drug-drug interactions, and patient preferences
      c. Reemphasize heart-healthy lifestyle habits and address other risk factors (class IIa, level C)
         i. 7.5% or greater 10-yr ASCVD risk: Moderate- or high-intensity statin (class I, level A)
         ii. 5% to 7.5% 10-yr ASCVD risk: Consider moderate-intensity statin (class IIa, level B)
         iii. Other factors may be considered: LDL-C 160 mg/dl or greater, family history of premature ASCVD, hs-CRP 2.0 mg/L or greater, CAC score 300 Agatston units or greater, ABI less than 0.9, or lifetime ASCVD risk (class IIb, level C)
   5. Primary prevention when LDL-C is less than 190 mg/dl and age is less than 40 or more than 75 yr, or less than 5% 10-yr ASCVD risk
      a. Statin therapy may be considered in selected individuals (class IIb, level C)
   6. Statin therapy is not routinely recommended for individuals with NYHA class II-IV heart failure or who are receiving maintenance hemodialysis
C. Regularly monitor adherence to lifestyle and drug therapy with lipid and safety assessments
   1. Assess adherence, response to therapy, and adverse effects within 4 to 12 wk following statin initiation or change in therapy (class I, level A)
      a. Measure a fasting lipid panel (class I, level A)
      b. Do not routinely monitor ALT or CK unless symptomatic (class IIa, level C)
      c. Screen and treat type 2 diabetes according to current practice guidelines. Heart-healthy lifestyle habits should be encouraged to prevent progression to diabetes (class I, level B)
      d. Anticipated therapeutic response: Approximately 50% or greater reduction in LDL-C from baseline for high-intensity statin and 30% to 50% for moderate-intensity statin (class IIa, level B)
         i. Insufficient evidence for LDL-C or non–HDL-C treatment targets from RCTs
         ii. For those with unknown baseline LDL-C, an LDL-C less than 100 mg/dl was observed in RCTs of high-intensity statin therapy
      e. Less than anticipated therapeutic response:
         i. Reinforce improved adherence to lifestyle and drug therapy (class I, level A)
         ii. Evaluate for secondary causes of hyperlipidemia if indicated (class I, level A)
         iii. Increase statin intensity, or if on maximally tolerated statin intensity, consider addition of nonstatin therapy in selected high-risk individuals (class IIb, level C)§
      f. Regularly monitor adherence to lifestyle and drug therapy every 3 to 12 mo once adherence has been established. Continue assessment of adherence for optimal ASCVD risk reduction and safety (class I, level A)
D. In individuals intolerant of the recommended intensity of statin therapy, use the maximally tolerated intensity of statin (class I, level B). If there are muscle or other symptoms, establish that they are related to the statin (class IIa, level B)

*Clinical ASCVD includes acute coronary syndromes, history of MI, stable or unstable angina, coronary or other arterial revascularization, stroke, TIA, or peripheral arterial disease presumed to be of atherosclerotic origin.

‡These factors may include primary LDL-C of 160 mg/dl or greater or other evidence of genetic hyperlipidemias; family history of premature ASCVD with onset at less than 55 yr of age in a first-degree male relative or at less than 65 yr of age in a first-degree female relative; hs-CRP 2 mg/L or greater; CAC score 300 Agatston units or greater or 75th percentile or greater for age, sex, and ethnicity; ABI less than 0.9; or lifetime risk of ASCVD. Additional factors that might aid in individual risk assessment could be identified in the future.

§High-risk individuals include those with clinical ASCVD, an untreated LDL-C 190 mg/dl or greater, suggesting genetic hypercholesterolemia, or individuals with diabetes 40 to 75 yr of age and LDL-C 70 to 189 mg/dl.

ABI, Ankle-brachial index; *ACC*, American College of Cardiology; *AHA*, American Heart Association; *ALT*, alanine aminotransferase, a test of hepatic function; *ASCVD*, atherosclerotic cardiovascular disease; *CAC*, coronary artery calcium; *CHD*, coronary heart disease; *CK*, creatine kinase, a test of muscle injury; *HDL-C*, high-density lipoprotein cholesterol; *hs-CRP*, high-sensitivity C-reactive protein; *LDL-C*, low-density lipoprotein cholesterol; *MI*, myocardial infarction; *NYHA*, New York Heart Association; *RCTs*, randomized controlled trials; and *TIA*, transient ischemic attack.

From 2013 ACC/AHA guideline on the treatment of blood cholesterol to reduce atherosclerotic cardiovascular risk in adults: a report of the American College of Cardiology/American Heart Association Task Force on Practice Guidelines, *J Am Coll Cardiol* 63(25 Pt B):2889-2934, 2014.

TABLE 2 Atherosclerotic Cardiovascular Disease

1. Coronary heart disease: Acute coronary syndromes, history of myocardial infarction, stable or unstable angina, coronary or other arterial revascularization
2. Stroke or transient ischemic attack
3. Peripheral arterial disease

- The 10-yr risk of ASCVD is calculated with the risk calculator available at http://my.americanheart.org/cvriskcalculator. Risk enhancing factors favoring statin initiation are summarized in Table 3.
- ASCVD events are reduced by using the maximum tolerated statin intensity in the aforementioned groups shown to benefit the most (Tables 4 and 5).
- Additional factors such as CRP >2 mg/L, primary LDL >160, genetic hyperlipidemias, family history of premature CHD, ABI <0.9, and coronary artery calcium score (CAD) assessed with CT may be used in patients who are not in one of four statin benefit groups and for whom a decision to initiate statin therapy is otherwise unclear. Statins are generally beneficial in patients at

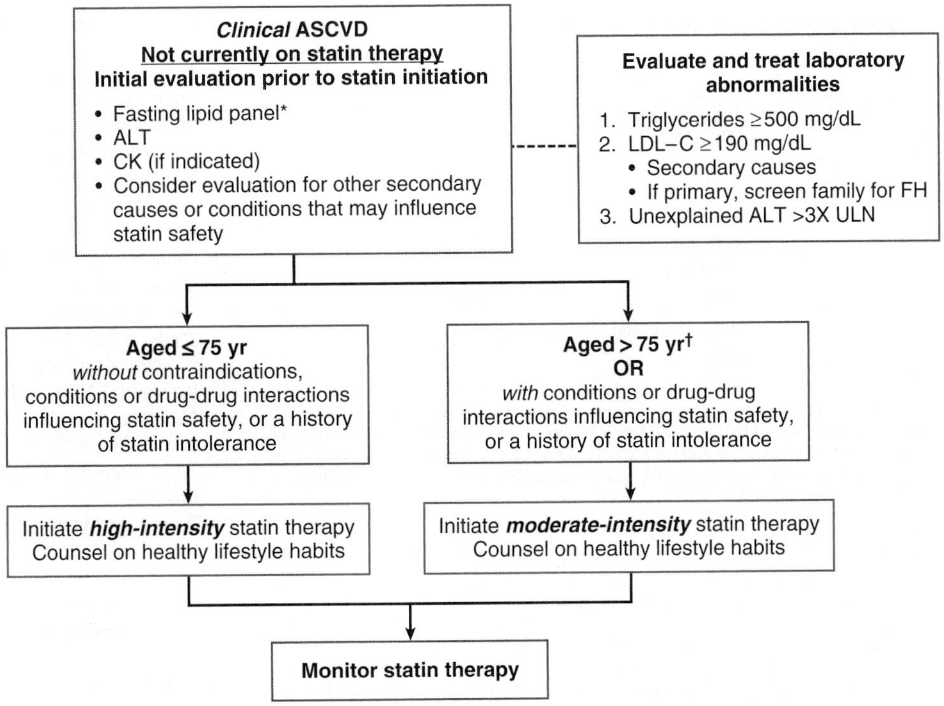

FIG. 1 Initiating statin therapy in individuals with clinical ASCVD. *Fasting lipid panel is preferred. In a nonfasting individual, a nonfasting non–HDL-C >220 mg/dl may indicate genetic hypercholesterolemia that requires further evaluation or a secondary etiology. If nonfasting triglycerides are >500 mg/dl, a fasting lipid panel is required. †It is reasonable to evaluate the potential for ASCVD benefits and for adverse effects and to consider patient preferences in initiating or continuing a moderate- or high-intensity statin in individuals with ASCVD >75 yr of age.

ALT, Alanine transaminase; *ASCVD,* atherosclerotic cardiovascular disease; *CK,* creatine kinase; *FH,* familial hypercholesterolemia; *HDL-C,* high-density lipoprotein cholesterol; *LDL–C,* low-density lipoprotein cholesterol; *ULN,* upper limit of normal. (Modified from Stone NJ et al: 2013 ACC/AHA guideline on the treatment of blood cholesterol to reduce atherosclerotic cardiovascular risk in adults: a report of the American College of Cardiology/American Heart Association Task Force on Practice Guidelines, *J Am Coll Cardiol,* 2013. In Mann DL et al: *Braunwald's heart disease,* ed 10, Philadelphia, 2015, Elsevier.)

TABLE 3 Risk Enhancing Factors Favoring Statin Initiation

These characteristics may confer increased ASCVD risk resulting from genetic or adverse cardiometabolic risk factors:
- Family history of premature ASCVD (males, age < 55 yr; females, age < 65 yr)
- Metabolic syndrome
- CKD (eGFR 15-59 ml/min/1.73 m^2 ± albuminuria; no dialysis or transplantation)
- Chronic inflammatory conditions (e.g., psoriasis, rheumatoid arthritis, HIV/AIDS)
- Premature menopause (before age 40 yr)
- Pregnancy-associated conditions that increase later ASCVD risk (e.g., preeclampsia)
- High-risk race/ethnicities (e.g., South Asian ancestry)
- Ankle-brachial index < 0.9
- LDL-C 160-189 mg/dl (4.1-4.8 mmol/L)
- Non–HDL-C 190-219 mg/dl (4.9-5.6 mmol/L)
- Persistently elevated, primary hypertriglyceridemia (≥175 mg/dl)
- Lp(a) ≥ 50 mg/dl or ≥125 nmol/L
- ApoB ≥ 130 mg/dl
- hs-CRP ≥ 2.0 mg/L

AIDS, Acquired immunodeficiency syndrome; *ASCVD,* atherosclerotic cardiovascular disease; *CKD,* chronic kidney disease; *eGFR,* estimated glomerular filtration rate; *HDL-C,* high-density lipoprotein cholesterol; *HIV,* human immunodeficiency virus; *LDL-C,* low-density lipoprotein cholesterol; *Lp(a),* lipoprotein (a).
2019 AHA/ACC Chol GL.

TABLE 4 Statin Benefit Groups and Recommended Therapy

Statin Benefit Group	High Intensity	Moderate Intensity	Additional Testing
Clinical ASCVD	Yes	Consider†	None
Primary LDL-C >190 mg/dl	Yes	Consider†	None
Diabetes without ASCVD and 10-yr risk ≥7.5%*	Yes	Consider†	None
Diabetes without ASCVD and 10-yr risk <7.5%*	Consider‡	Yes	Case-by-case
Primary prevention and 10-yr risk ≥7.5%*	Consider‡	Yes	Case-by-case
Primary prevention and 10-yr risk <7.5%*	Consider‡	Consider‡	Case-by-case

*Based on Pooled Cohort Risk Equations.
†If age >75 yr or not candidate for high intensity.
‡If abnormal high-sensitivity C-reactive protein, coronary artery calcium, ankle-brachial index, lifetime risk.
ASCVD, Atherosclerotic cardiovascular disease; *LDL-C,* low-density lipoprotein cholesterol.
From Boyden TF et al: Implementing new guidelines in the management of blood cholesterol, *Am J Med* 127:705, 2014.

TABLE 5 High-, Moderate-, and Low-Intensity Statin Therapy*

	DAILY DOSE		
Statin Therapy	**High Intensity† ↓LDL-C ≥50%**	**Moderate Intensity‡ ↓LDL-C 30<50%**	**Low Intensity§ ↓LDL-C <30%**
Atorvastatin	**(40‖)-80 mg**	**10** *(20)* **mg**	
Rosuvastatin	**20** *(40)* **mg**	*(5)* **10 mg**	
Simvastatin		**20-40 mg¶**	*10 mg*
Pravastatin		**40** *(80)* **mg**	**10-20 mg**
Lovastatin		**40 mg**	**20 mg**
Fluvastatin		*80 mg (Fluvastatin XL)*	*20*-**40 mg**
Fluvastatin		**40 mg****	
Pitavastatin		**2-4 mg**	*1 mg*

*Individual responses to statin therapy varied in randomized, controlled trials and vary in clinical practice. A less-than-average response may have a biologic basis. Statins and dosages in bold were reduced in major cardiovascular events in randomized, controlled trials. Statins and doses in italics were approved by the FDA but were not tested in randomized, controlled trials.
†Daily dose decreases LDL-C levels by an average of ≥50%.
‡Daily dose decreases LDL-C levels by an average of 30 to <50%.
§Daily dose decreases LDL-C levels by an average of <30%.
‖Evidence from 1 randomized, controlled trial only; down-titration if patient is unable to tolerate atorvastatin, 80 mg.
¶Although simvastatin, 80 mg, was evaluated in randomized, controlled trials, the FDA recommends against initiation of or titration to 80 mg of simvastatin because of increased risk for myopathy and rhabdomyolysis.
**Twice daily.
FDA, U.S. Food and Drug Administration; *LDL-C,* low-density lipoprotein cholesterol; *XL,* extended-release.
Reprinted with permission of the authors: Stone NJ et al: 2013 ACC/AHA guideline on the treatment of blood cholesterol to reduce atherosclerotic cardiovascular risk in adults: a report of the American College of Cardiology/American Heart Association Task Force on Practice Guidelines, *J Am Coll Cardiol* 63(25, Part B):2889-2934, 2014.

intermediate risk and selected patients with borderline risk who have a calcium score that is 100 or higher or who are in the 75th percentile or higher for their age, sex, and race. Statins should also be considered in persons with scores of 1 to 99, particularly if they are age 55 yr or older.

- Percent reduction in LDL cholesterol is used as a guide to compliance and adherence to therapy in the 2018 AHA/ACC Revised Clinical Practice Guidelines (Fig. 2). Studies have shown that compared with less-intensive LDL-C lowering, more intensive lowering reduces all-cause mortality and cardiovascular mortality; patients with higher baseline LDL-C have greater benefit.
- Moderate-intensity statin therapy should be continued for individuals >75 yr of age for secondary prevention. However, factors such as comorbidities, safety, and priorities of care should be considered before initiating statins for primary prevention of ASCVD.
- Adherence to lifestyle and to statin therapy should be reiterated with patients before the addition of a nonstatin drug.
- High-risk patients with a suboptimal response to statins who are unable to tolerate a recommended intensity or who are completely statin intolerant may benefit from the addition of a nonstatin cholesterol-lowering agent such as ezetimibe. Combination therapies for LDL are summarized in Table 6.
- Table 7 summarizes oral drugs affecting lipoprotein metabolism.
- PCSK9 (proprotein convertase subtilisin/kexin type 9) inhibitors (alirocumab [Praluent], evolocumab [Repatha]) are indicated as adjunct to diet and maximally tolerated statin therapy for the treatment of adults with heterozygous familial hypercholesterolemia or clinical atherosclerotic cardiovascular disease, who require additional lowering of LDL cholesterol. PCSK9 inhibitors lower risk for ischemic cardiovascular events in persons with stable CAD and elevated atherogenic lipoproteins despite statin therapy. These medications are administered by subcutaneous injection and are expensive.
- The management of metabolic syndrome includes weight reduction, increased physical activity, and treatment of hypertension, elevated triglycerides, and low HDL cholesterol.
- According to recent studies, each 40 mg/dl reduction in LDL cholesterol by statin therapy confers a 20% reduction in ASCVD. In other words, a relative risk reduction of 30% in ASCVD by moderate-intensity therapy and 45% by high-intensity therapy has been approximated.
- Recent trials have shown that bempedoic acid, an inhibitor of ATP citrate lyase, reduces LDL cholesterol. The addition of bempedoic acid to maximally tolerated statin therapy did not lead to a higher incidence of overall adverse events than placebo and led to significant lowering of LDL cholesterol.

DISPOSITION & FOLLOW-UP

- Baseline LFT testing should be done before initiation of statin therapy and as clinically indicated thereafter.
- CK level monitoring is not recommended unless a patient reports muscle weakness or myalgias.
- Statin therapy should be monitored by repeating a lipid profile within 4 to 12 wk after initiation of therapy.
- Counseling about behavioral lifestyle changes and risk factors for CHD should be provided at every follow-up visit.
- Adverse effects of statin-associated diabetes vary by statin intensity: 1 excess case of diabetes per 1000 treated individuals with moderate-intensity statin and 3 excess cases of diabetes per 1000 treated individuals with high-intensity statin per yr has been reported. Myopathy and hemorrhagic stroke incidence is around 1 excess case per 10,000 treated individuals.
- Per new guidelines, those who develop diabetes during statin therapy should be advised to continue it to reduce their risk of ASCVD events and should adhere to a heart-healthy diet, engage in physical activity, cease tobacco use, and maintain a healthy body weight (Table 7).
- Maintain patients on simvastatin 80 mg only if they have been taking this dose for 12 or more mo without evidence of muscle toxicity.
- Do not start new patients on simvastatin 80 mg.
- Place patients who do not meet their LDL goal on simvastatin 40 mg on alternative LDL-C-lowering treatment(s) to reach goal.

REFERRAL

Patients with rare lipid disorders, hyperlipoproteinemias, patients resistant to treatment, on complex regimens, and with evidence of disease progression despite treatment should be referred to a lipid specialist.

PEARLS & CONSIDERATIONS

COMMENTS

- New features in the 2018 clinical practice guidelines compared to the 2013 guidelines support the addition of nonstatin medications (ezetimibe or PCSK9 inhibitors) to statin therapy for secondary prevention in patients at very high risk. In primary prevention, a clinical patient risk discussion is strongly recommended before a decision is made about statin treatment. Among intermediate-risk patients, identification of risk-enhancing factors and coronary calcium testing is recommended when considering the use of a statin.
- Familial hypercholesterolemia (FH) is characterized by elevated cholesterol concentrations early in life. Untreated FH is associated with premature cardiovascular disease in adulthood. Screening can detect FH in children, and lipid-lowering treatment in childhood can reduce lipid concentrations in the short term, with little evidence of harm. A 20-yr follow-up study of statin therapy has shown that initiation of statin therapy during childhood in patients with FH slows the progression of carotid intima media thickness and reduces the risk of cardiovascular disease in adulthood.
- The American Academy of Pediatrics (AAP) guideline (*Pediatrics* 122:198, 2008) recommends consideration toward pharmacologic treatment for children with LDL >190 mg/dl or >160 mg/dl if other risk factors are present.

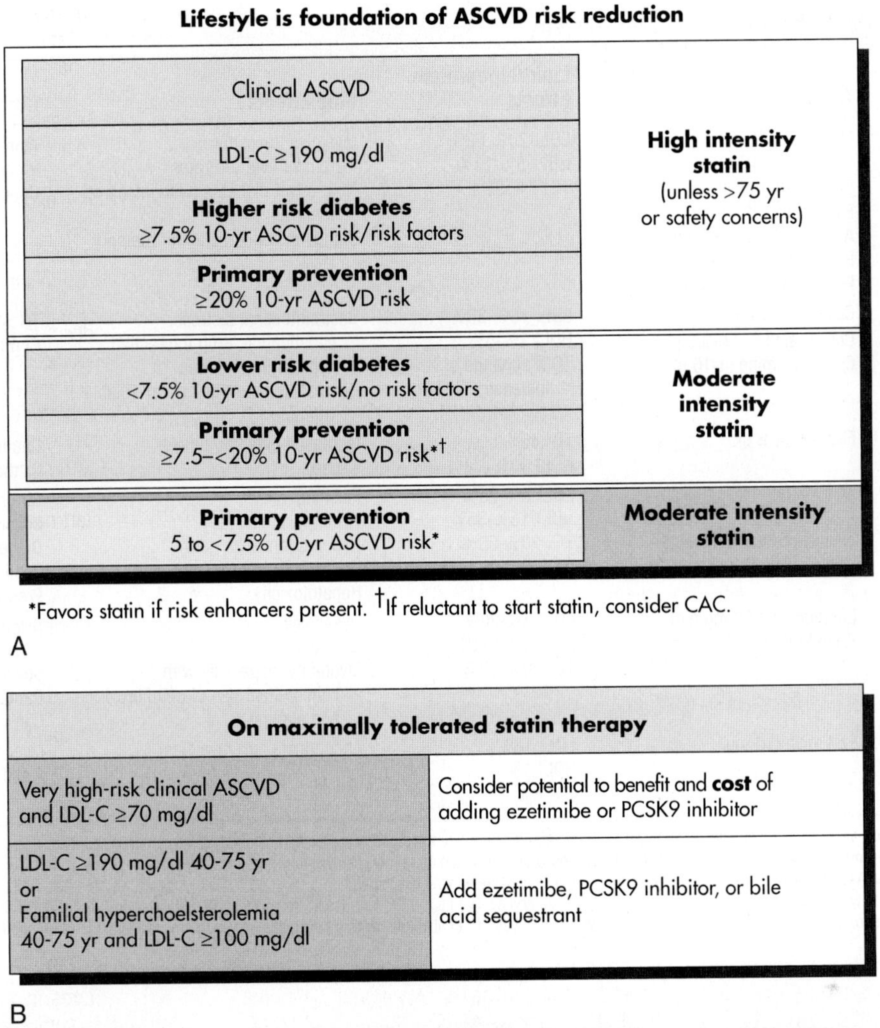

FIG. 2 A and B, Summary of 2018 ACC/AHA cholesterol guideline recommendations for statin and nonstatin therapy. Background color denotes class and level of evidence: Green = Class I (strong) recommendation; yellow = Class IIa (reasonable) recommendation; blue = Grade A (high) level of evidence; orange = Grade B (moderate) level of evidence. *ASCVD,* Atherosclerotic cardiovascular disease; *LDL-C,* low-density lipoprotein cholesterol. (From Goldman L, Shafer AI: *Goldman's Cecil medicine,* ed 26, St Louis, 2019, Elsevier.)

TABLE 6 Combination Therapies for LDL

Statin plus ezetimibe	Ezetimibe added to a statin may further reduce LDL by 20% or more and reduce triglycerides by 7%-13%. The combination provides equivalent LDL reduction to a fourfold increase in statin dose. Daily ezetimibe added to a low-dose statin given 2-3 times/wk can improve tolerance. Combination pills containing statin and ezetimibe are available. Most common side effects reflect those of the individual drugs. Combination ezetimibe and simvastatin has been shown to decrease cardiovascular events in patients with renal disease and acute coronary syndrome.
Statin and PCSK9 inhibitors	This combination is the most effective known treatment for hypercholesterolemia. There are no known negative interactions between these two therapies. This combination reduces CHD events more than statin alone.
Statin plus bile acid sequestrants	Bile acid sequestrants in combination with statins further decrease LDL from 24% to 60%. Cholestyramine and colestipol can interfere with the absorption of statins. Colesevelam does not affect statin absorption. The statin-colesevelam combination is not ideal for patients with high triglycerides but may be useful in those with type 2 diabetes mellitus because colesevelam reduces glycemia.
Statin plus niacin	Adding niacin to a statin can lower LDL by 10% to 20%, in addition to beneficial effects on triglycerides. When used in combination with a statin, the maximum dose of niacin should be 2000 mg/day. This combination in subjects with already low LDL levels did not reduce CHD events.
Bile acid sequestrants plus niacin	Before the availability of statins, bile acid sequestrants plus niacin were used to lower LDL in high-risk patients. The availability of colesevelam and extended-release niacin has made this combination tolerable for many patients who are unable to use statins.
Ezetimibe plus bile acid sequestrants	Ezetimibe inhibits cholesterol absorption, and sequestrants enhance cholesterol excretion through conversion to bile acids. The combination can have additive effects. This combination is useful for patients who cannot take statins.

CHD, Coronary heart disease; *LDL,* low-density lipoprotein; *PCSK9,* proprotein convertase subtilisin/kexin type 9.
From Melmed S et al: *Williams textbook of endocrinology,* ed 14, St Louis, 2019, Elsevier.

TABLE 7 Drugs Affecting Lipoprotein Metabolism

Drug Class	Agents and Daily Doses	Lipid/Lipoprotein Effects	Side Effects	Contraindications
HMG-CoA reductase inhibitors (statins)	Lovastatin (10-40 mg) Pravastatin (10-80 mg) Simvastatin† (5-80 mg) Fluvastatin (20-40 mg) Atorvastatin (10-80 mg) Rosuvastatin (5-40 mg) Pitavastatin (2-4 mg)	LDL↓ 20%-60% HDL↑ 5%-15% TG↓ 7%-30%	Myalgias, myositis Increased liver enzymes New-onset diabetes (with intensive therapy) Unproven concerns about memory loss	Active or chronic liver disease Pregnancy Concomitant use of certain drugs*
Bile acid sequestrants	Colestipol (5-20 g) Colesevelam‡ (2.6-3.8 g) Cholestyramine (4-16 g)	LDL↓ 15%-30% HDL↑ 3%-5% TG No change or increase	Gastrointestinal distress, constipation, drug interaction, hypertriglyceridemia Decreased absorption of fat-soluble vitamins	TG >300 mg/dl GI motility disorder
Omega-3 fatty acids	Fish oils (4-6 g)	TG↓ 45% HDL↑ 13%	Increased bleeding time Nausea	Caution with anticoagulant therapy
Nicotinic acid	Immediate release (niacin) (1.5-3 g) Extended release (Niaspan) (1-2 g)	LDL↓ 5%-25% HDL↑ 15%-35% TG↓ 20%-50%	Flushing Hyperglycemia Hyperuricemia (or gout) Upper GI distress Hepatotoxicity	Chronic liver disease Severe gout Diabetes Peptic ulcer disease Pregnancy/lactation
Fibric acids	Gemfibrozil (600 mg bid) Fenofibrate (45-145 mg)	LDL↓ 5%-20% HDL↑ 10%-20% TG↓ 20%-50%	Dyspepsia Gallstones Myopathy (especially with concomitant use of gemfibrozil and statins)	Severe renal disease (dose adjustment for fenofibrate) Severe hepatic disease Caution with statins Can worsen LDL cholesterol
Ezetimibe (cholesterol absorption inhibitor)	Ezetimibe (10 mg)	LDL↓ 18% HDL↑ 1% TG↓ 8%	Abdominal pain; myalgias	Liver disease Avoid with resins and fibrates

*Cyclosporine, macrolide antibiotics, various antifungal agents, and cytochrome P-450 inhibitors (fibrates and niacin should be used with appropriate caution).
†Dosages of simvastatin 80 mg are no longer recommended. Potential interactions with amlodipine and ranolazine warrant doses ≤2 mg daily.
‡Colesevelam reduces glucose and A1c ~0.5% and has been approved for treatment of diabetes with dyslipidemia.
GI, Gastrointestinal; *HDL,* high-density lipoprotein; *HMG-CoA,* 3-hydroxy-3-methylglutaryl coenzyme A; *LDL,* low-density lipoprotein; *TG,* triglyceride.
Modified from The National Cholesterol Education Program, *JAMA* 285:2486, 2001. In Boyden TF et al: Implementing new guidelines in the management of blood cholesterol, *Am J Med* 127:705, 2014.

- *HDL cholesterol efflux capacity* refers to the ability of HDL to accept cholesterol from macrophages, which is a key step in reverse cholesterol transport. It is inversely associated with the incidence of cardiovascular events and may be a useful biomarker when added to traditional risk factors.

SUGGESTED READINGS

Available at ExpertConsult.com

RELATED CONTENT

High Cholesterol (Patient Information)
Coronary Artery Disease (Related Key Topic)
Hyperlipoproteinemia, Primary (Related Key Topic)
Statin-Induced Muscle Syndrome (Related Key Topic)

AUTHOR: **Fred F. Ferri, MD**

BASIC INFORMATION

DEFINITION

Hypercoagulable state is an inherited or acquired condition associated with an increased risk of thrombosis. A classification of hypercoagulable states is described in Table 1.

SYNONYM

Thrombophilia

ICD-10CM CODES

D68.5 Primary thrombophilia
D68.6 Other thrombophilia
D68.8 Other specified coagulation defects
D68.9 Coagulation defect, unspecified

EPIDEMIOLOGY & DEMOGRAPHICS

INCIDENCE, PREVALENCE, PREDOMINANT SEX AND AGE: See Table 2. Significant variations in the prevalence rates and thrombotic risks for hypercoagulable states are reported. This may reflect geographic variation in the prevalence of genetic defects, different populations, or the presence of other unidentified thrombophilic risk factors. When thrombosis occurs, it is often associated with an acquired risk factor (e.g., surgery, pregnancy, oral contraceptive [OC] use).

RISK FACTORS: Family history of thrombosis, increasing age, tobacco use, immobility, surgery, prior history of deep vein thrombosis (DVT) pregnancy, hormone replacement therapy, trauma, connective tissue disease, underlying malignancy, medications (megestrol acetate, tamoxifen, oral contraceptives). Potential prothrombotic states are summarized in Table 3.

GENETICS:

- Most people with a genetic defect will not have thrombotic disease.
- Approximately half of patients with unprovoked thrombosis have an identifiable inherited thrombophilia. There is a low risk of recurrent thrombosis in patients with a single genetic defect. Multiple genetic defects are not uncommon (1% to 2% prevalence in patients with idiopathic venous thromboembolism [VTE]); a strong synergistic effect occurs when multiple defects are present.

PHYSICAL FINDINGS & CLINICAL PRESENTATION

- Inherited thrombophilia is usually associated with VTE, most commonly DVT.
- Some acquired thrombophilias are associated with arterial thrombosis. Table 2 describes sites of thrombosis according to coagulation defect.
- Pregnancy complications.
- Medical conditions associated with increased risk of thrombosis.

ETIOLOGY

- Thrombosis is often a multifactorial process with genetic, environmental, and acquired factors. Table E4, Table E5, Table E6, and Table E7 describe causes of acquired and inherited deficiencies in antithrombin, protein C, and protein S.
- All thrombotic factors ultimately lead to blood flow stasis, endothelial damage, or change in blood constituents to cause thrombosis. These three components of thrombosis are known as Virchow's triad.
- Thrombotic risk increases with use of OCs or hormone replacement therapy (HRT) and during the pregnancy/postpartum period.
- Adverse pregnancy outcomes may be caused by thrombosis of the uteroplacental circulation.

TABLE 1 Classification of Hypercoagulable States

Hereditary	Mixed	Acquired
Loss of Function		
Antithrombin deficiency	Hyperhomocysteinemia	Previous venous thromboembolism
Protein C deficiency	Obesity	Pregnancy, puerperium
Protein S deficiency	Cancer	
		Drug-induced:
		Heparin-induced thrombocytopenia
		Prothrombin complex concentrates
		L-Asparaginase
		Hormonal therapy
Gain of Function		
Factor V Leiden	Postoperative	
Prothrombin FII G20210A	Myeloproliferative disorders	
Elevated factor VIII, IX, or XI		

Hoffman R et al: *Hematology: basic principles and practice*, ed 7, Philadelphia, 2018, Elsevier.

TABLE 3 Potential Prothrombotic States

Congenital
Deficiency of anticoagulants
AT-III, protein C or protein S, plasminogen
Resistance to cofactor proteolysis
Factor V Leiden
High levels of procoagulants
Prothrombin 20210 mutation
Damage to endothelium

Acquired
Obstruction to flow indwelling lines
Pregnancy
Polycythemia/dehydration
Immobilization
Injury
Trauma, surgery, exercise
Inflammation
IBD, vasculitis, infection, Behçet syndrome
Hypercoagulability
Malignancy
Antiphospholipid syndrome
Nephrotic syndrome
Oral contraceptives
L-Asparaginase

Rare Other Entities
Congenital dysfibrinogenemia
Acquired
Paroxysmal nocturnal hemoglobinuria
Thrombocythemia
Vascular grafts

AT-III, Antithrombin III; *IBD*, inflammatory bowel disease.
From Kliegman RM et al: *Nelson textbook of pediatrics*, ed 19, Philadelphia, 2011, Saunders.

TABLE 2 Hypercoagulable Conditions

	Prevalence in General Population (%)	Prevalence in Population with Thrombosis (%)	A/V Events	Relative Risk of Thrombosis
FVL mutation	5% of whites; rare in nonwhites	12%-40%	V	Heterozygous: 3-7; homozygous: 80
Prothrombin G20210A mutation	3% of whites; rare in nonwhites	6%-18%	V	3
AT deficiency	0.02%	1%-3%	V	20-50
PC deficiency	0.2%-0.4%	3%-5%	V	7-15
PS deficiency	0.03%-0.1%	1%-5%	V	5-11
Antiphospholipid antibody syndrome	1%-2%	5%-21%	V + A	2-11

A, Arterial; *AT*, antithrombin; *FVL*, factor V Leiden; *PC*, protein C; *PS*, protein S; *V*, venous.

Dx DIAGNOSIS

DIFFERENTIAL DIAGNOSIS

INHERITED: Factor V Leiden (FVL) mutation:
- Autosomal-dominant mutation with low penetrance
- Causes activated protein C resistance (APCR); 90% of APCR is caused by FVL mutation
- Most common inherited thrombophilia; accounts for 40% to 50% of cases
- OC use in heterozygous carriers is associated with an eightfold increased risk of VTE compared with noncarriers and a thirty-fivefold increased risk of VTE compared with noncarriers not using OCs
- May be associated with cardiovascular disease in select high-risk subgroups

Prothrombin G20210A mutation:
- Autosomal-dominant mutation with low penetrance
- OC use in heterozygous carriers is associated with a sixteenfold increased risk of VTE compared with noncarriers not using OCs
- May be associated with cardiovascular disease in select high-risk subgroups and young patients with ischemic stroke
- Causes increased mRNA accumulation and protein synthesis, leading to elevated prothrombin plasma concentrations

Protein C, protein S, antithrombin (AT) deficiency:
- Autosomal-dominant inheritance; many mutations identified for each of these conditions
- Decreased level (type I deficiency) or abnormal function (type II deficiency)
- First episode of thrombosis is usually in young adults

Protein C and protein S:
- Homozygous condition is very rare; usually associated with lethal thrombosis in infancy
- Associated with warfarin-induced skin necrosis, which occurs secondary to depletion of vitamin K–dependent anticoagulant factors sooner than procoagulant factors in the first few days of therapy

AT deficiency:
- Most thrombogenic of the inherited thrombophilias; 50% lifetime risk of thrombosis.
- Homozygous condition is very rare, probably not compatible with normal fetal development.
- Arterial thrombosis can occur rarely.
- Can cause heparin resistance.

Other possible causes: Non-O blood group, dysfibrinogenemia, elevated thrombin-activatable fibrinolysis inhibitor, elevated factor IX and factor XI levels

ACQUIRED: Antiphospholipid antibody syndrome (APS):
- Most common cause of acquired thrombophilia
- Can present as arterial or venous thrombosis, recurrent pregnancy loss, and adverse pregnancy outcomes
- Thromboembolic events occur in up to 30% of population; high risk of recurrent thrombosis (up to 70% reported)
- See "Antiphospholipid Antibody Syndrome" for more information

Conditions associated with increased risk of thrombosis:
- Prior thrombosis
- Trauma
- Medical illness: Heart failure, respiratory failure, infection, diabetes mellitus, obesity, nephrotic syndrome, inflammatory bowel disease
- Chronic hemolysis–paroxysmal nocturnal hemoglobinuria, atypical hemolytic uremic syndrome, sickle cell anemia
- Pregnancy (sixfold increased risk of VTE), postpartum, OC use (fourfold increased risk, higher risk with third-generation OCs), transdermal contraceptive patch, HRT (twofold increased risk), tamoxifen, raloxifene
- Immobilization, travel
- Surgery (especially orthopedic), central venous catheters
- Hyperviscosity syndromes
- Myeloproliferative neoplasms
- Malignancy: Disease or treatment related
- Heparin-induced thrombocytopenia and thrombosis
- Smoking

WORKUP

- History (presence of conditions or use of medications predisposing to thrombosis, family history of thrombosis), physical examination, laboratory tests, imaging studies. Routine investigations to evaluate a patient with thrombosis are summarized in Box 1.
- Age-appropriate cancer screening.
- No consensus exists regarding screening for thrombophilia; few cost-effectiveness or outcomes data are available. Thrombophilia screening is probably overused, as results usually do not change management.
- Thrombophilia screening is not recommended for primary prevention of VTE; some advocate testing prior to OC use or pregnancy in women with a strong family history of thrombosis or thrombophilia. Box 2 summarizes recommendations regarding when to perform a thrombophilia screen. Essential tests for thrombophilia screening are described in Box 3.
- Screening not recommended if VTE was associated with an identified risk factor. A possible exception is thrombosis associated with pregnancy, the postpartum period, or with OC use.
- Reasonable to pursue workup for VTE with weak triggers, a strong family history, and female family members of childbearing age; consider testing for FVL, prothrombin *G20210A* mutation, protein C, protein S, and AT deficiency. Consider testing for APS if extensive DVT or pulmonary embolism (PE).
- Unprovoked VTE:
  1. Screen individuals for APCR, prothrombin *G20210A* mutation, protein C, protein S, AT deficiency, and APS if any of the following are present: <50 yr of age at first episode of thrombosis + strong family history of thrombosis or female family member of childbearing age, thrombosis in unusual anatomic location (cerebral veins or splanchnic veins; if splanchnic veins, consider testing as well for myeloproliferative neoplasms [MPN] and paroxysmal nocturnal hemoglobinuria [PNH]).
  2. Screen all others for APS.
- Arterial thrombosis: Screen for APS.
- NOTE: Routine screening for factor VIII level or hyperhomocysteinemia is not recommended.

BOX 1 Routine Investigations to Evaluate a Patient with Thrombosis

Test	Abnormality	Diagnostic Information
Complete blood count	Elevated hematocrit Increased white count Increased platelet count Leukopenia Thrombocytopenia	Myeloproliferative disorder (e.g., essential thrombocythemia, polycythemia vera); may be found in paroxysmal nocturnal hemoglobinuria; if associated with heparin administration, consider heparin-induced thrombocytopenia
Blood film	Leukoerythroblastic changes	Underlying neoplasm invading bone marrow
Liver function tests	Abnormal tests	May point to malignancy
Renal function	Impaired renal function	Assess prior to anticoagulation with heparin, low-molecular-weight heparin or new oral anticoagulants
Urinalysis	Proteinuria	Nephrotic syndrome; may be associated with venous thromboembolism or renal vein thrombosis
PT and aPTT	Prolonged PT and aPTT	To enable safe anticoagulation to proceed if required Need to exclude lupus anticoagulant

aPTT, Activated partial thromboplastin time; *PT*, prothrombin time.
Hoffman R et al: *Hematology: basic principles and practice,* ed 7, Philadelphia, 2018, Elsevier.

BOX 2 When to Perform a Thrombophilia Screen

Clinical Scenario
- First episode of unprovoked venous thromboembolism in individuals younger than 40 yr of age
- Thrombosis in an unusual site (e.g., cerebral or mesenteric thrombosis)
- Two or more first-degree relatives with unprovoked thrombosis
- Three or more early pregnancy losses, or one or more fetal deaths after 10 wk gestation

Hoffman R et al: *Hematology: basic principles and practice,* ed 7, Philadelphia, 2018, Elsevier.

BOX 3 Essential Tests for Thrombophilia Screening

- Basic coagulation screen
  1. International normalized ratio (INR): To exclude warfarin effect—warfarin will lower protein C and S levels
  2. Activated partial thromboplastin time (aPTT): To exclude heparin effect—heparin will lower antithrombin levels
- Functional assay for antithrombin (with heparin to detect type II defects)
- Functional assay for protein C
- Functional assay for protein S (immune assays for total and free protein S)
- APC resistance assay: With genetic test for factor V Leiden for confirmation of abnormal results
- Genetic test for *FIIG 20210A* gene mutation
- Anticardiolipin and β_2 -glycoprotein-1 antibodies (IgG and IgM) and lupus anticoagulant assay

APC, Activated protein C; *Ig,* immunoglobulin.
Hoffman R et al: *Hematology: basic principles and practice,* ed 7, Philadelphia, 2018, Elsevier.

TIMING OF WORKUP:
- Ideally >3 wk after discontinuation of vitamin K antagonists (VKA) and >2 days after discontinuation of direct oral anticoagulant (DOAC) (except for APS, which requires prolonged anticoagulation).
- NOTE: Acute thrombosis, anticoagulation, pregnancy, and many medical conditions can affect the results and must be considered in the timing and interpretation of the workup.

LABORATORY TESTS

- Initial workup: CBC with peripheral smear, electrolytes, calcium, creatinine, blood urea nitrogen (BUN), liver function tests, prothrombin time/partial thromboplastin time, prostate-specific antigen (in men aged >50 yr), urinalysis.
- NOTE: Genetic counseling and written informed consent should be obtained before genetic testing. Abnormal nongenetic tests should be repeated after 6 wk to decrease false-positive results.
- APC-resistance assay tests for factor V Leiden mutation. Presence of lupus anticoagulant causes false positives. Follow-up positive result with a confirmatory genetic test.
- Prothrombin G20210A mutation testing.
- AT, protein C, and protein S deficiency: Functional assays are initial tests, then follow up positive result with antigenic assay to determine the type of deficiency. Note that antigenic assays for protein S should measure free and total levels. The functional assays for protein C and S deficiency testing may be falsely low in the presence of APCR or elevated factor VIII level and falsely high if lupus anticoagulant is present.
- APS: Any one of the following found elevated on two occasions at least 12 wk apart: Lupus anticoagulant, anticardiolipin antibodies, or anti–B_2-glycoprotein-I antibodies.

IMAGING STUDIES

Chest radiograph and other tests as appropriate to diagnose thrombosis and rule out associated conditions

Rx TREATMENT

NONPHARMACOLOGIC THERAPY

OC/HRT use and smoking should be avoided.

PROPHYLAXIS

- Prophylactic anticoagulation in high-risk situations.
- Patients with AT deficiency may benefit from antithrombin concentrates in high-risk situations.
- Pregnancy prophylaxis: Timing and intensity of therapy is based on the patient's risk (genetic or acquired defect and clinical history). Women with thrombophilia and recurrent adverse pregnancy outcomes may benefit from prophylaxis with heparin (low-molecular-weight heparin most commonly used) and low-dose aspirin.

ACUTE GENERAL Rx

Initial therapy is the same as for individuals with and without thrombophilia, with exceptions for protein C, AT, and APS deficiency as detailed in the following.

Venous thrombosis:
- DOACs such as Xa inhibitors (rivaroxaban and apixaban) have been FDA-approved for treatment in acute DVT and are currently recommended as first-line therapy. They have been found to be noninferior to warfarin, appear easier to use with fewer drug interactions, and have a trend toward less major bleeding.
- In patients unable to take DOACs, begin low-molecular-weight heparin (LMWH) and warfarin simultaneously. Continue heparin for at least 5 days and until international normalized ratio (INR) is therapeutic for 2 consecutive days; continue warfarin for at least 3 mo. Aim for INR of 2 to 3. Unfractionated heparin (UH) or fondaparinux (factor Xa inhibitor) may be used as alternatives to LMWH. LMWH is preferred over UH (except in patients with massive pulmonary embolism, increased risk of bleeding, or renal failure) because of equivalent or superior effectiveness and a better safety profile.
- Thrombophilia is not associated with a higher risk of recurrent VTE during warfarin therapy, with the exception of cancer patients in whom LMWH for 3 to 6 mo is associated with lower rates of recurrence than warfarin therapy.
- In pregnancy, anticoagulate with heparin throughout pregnancy and for at least 6 wk postpartum. Minimum duration of anticoagulation should be 6 mo. LMWH is preferred over UH. Warfarin may be used postpartum.
- Consider thrombolysis or thrombectomy in patients with massive pulmonary embolism or large proximal lower extremity DVT.

Protein C deficiency:
- Warfarin-induced skin necrosis: Discontinue warfarin, give vitamin K, and start heparin anticoagulation. Consider protein C replacement with protein C concentrate or fresh frozen plasma. Warfarin may be restarted at a low dose (2 mg daily for 3 days and increase by 2 to 3 mg daily until target INR is reached). Continue heparin for at least 5 days and until warfarin-induced anticoagulation is achieved.

AT deficiency:
- AT concentrates may be used if difficulty achieving anticoagulation (heparin resistance), severe thrombosis, or recurrent thrombosis despite adequate anticoagulation.

APS:
- Warfarin is superior to rivaroxaban in patients with APS. The RAPS trial randomized patients with APS to receive either rivaroxaban or warfarin and found significantly higher rates of thrombosis in the rivaroxaban group. A subsequent trial noted increased endogenous thrombin potential (a marker of less effective anticoagulation) in APS patients switched to rivaroxaban following initial VKA therapy compared to those continued on warfarin. This study was not powered to assess clinical efficacy.

Arterial thrombosis:
- Anticoagulation and evaluation for thrombolysis or surgery

CHRONIC Rx

- Optimal duration of anticoagulation remains unknown. Length of therapy may be individualized by assessing the risk of recurrence. Residual thrombosis (on ultrasonography) or elevated D-dimer levels after completion of anticoagulation are associated with an increased risk of recurrence. With these findings, consider prolonging anticoagulation.

TABLE 8 Management of Women with a History of Venous Thrombosis during Pregnancy and the Puerperium

Clinical History	Thrombophilia	Antepartum	Postpartum[a]
Prior VTE due to a transient risk factor	No	Surveillance	Yes
Prior VTE due to pregnancy or estrogens	Yes or no	Prophylactic LMWH	Yes
Prior idiopathic VTE	Yes or no	Prophylactic LMWH	Yes
Recurrent VTE	Yes or no	Treatment dose LMWH	Resume long-term anticoagulation
No prior VTEPositive family history	Antithrombin deficiency; homozygous FII G20210A; or Factor V Leiden; or dual heterozygosity for both mutations	Prophylactic or intermediate dose LMWH	Yes

LMWH, Low-molecular-weight heparin; *VTE,* venous thromboembolism.
[a]Postpartum prophylaxis involves a 6-wk course of prophylactic doses of LMWH or dose-adjusted warfarin (target INR: 2.0 to 3.0).
Hoffman R et al: *Hematology: basic principles and practice,* ed 7, Philadelphia, 2018, Elsevier.

- Must consider risk and benefit; risk of major bleeding 2% to 3% annually in general population on anticoagulation but higher in the elderly (7% to 9% per yr). Long-term anticoagulation is usually not indicated given the low risk of recurrent thrombosis for most conditions and the bleeding risk associated with anticoagulation.
- Indefinite anticoagulation considered if any of the following:
  1. Life-threatening thrombosis or thrombosis at an unusual site
  2. More than a single genetic defect
  3. Presence of AT deficiency or APS
  4. Unprovoked DVT or PE with low bleeding risk
  5. >1 Provoked DVT or PE with low bleeding risk
- Patients with active cancer may benefit from indefinite anticoagulation.

DISPOSITION

Depends on underlying condition

REFERRAL

Hematology, maternal-fetal medicine, obstetric medicine

PEARLS & CONSIDERATIONS

COMMENTS

- Women with thrombophilic defects but no prior history of venous thromboembolism, or family history of the same, likely do not require antepartum prophylaxis or postpartum treatment, but definitive data are lacking. A summary of these recommendations is provided in Table 8.
- DOACs and warfarin therapy effectively reduce the risk of recurrent VTE; when therapy is discontinued VTE risk increases.
- Warfarin is preferred over DOAC for APS patients based on the data showing rivaroxaban to be inferior to warfarin in this population.
- Previous episode of VTE is a major risk factor for recurrence regardless of the presence of thrombophilia. Risk is greatest in the first 2 yr after thrombosis. 20% of all patients with unprovoked VTE have recurrence within 5 yr.
- Genetic risk factors for thrombosis in non-whites remain largely unknown.
- Interpreting workup: Many medical conditions cause acquired abnormalities.
  1. Acute thrombosis may be associated with lupus anticoagulant, increased anticardiolipin antibodies, and elevated factor VIII levels
     a. Heparin therapy: Antithrombin levels decrease by up to 30%; can affect lupus anticoagulant testing depending on available assay
     b. Warfarin therapy: Cannot measure protein C and protein S (levels and function decrease); antithrombin levels may increase; can affect lupus anticoagulant testing
     c. Acute thrombosis: Antithrombin level, protein C, and protein S levels may be falsely lowered
  2. Protein C, protein S, and antithrombin levels decrease with surgery, liver disease, disseminated intravascular coagulation, and chemotherapy. Protein C level also decreases with severe infection but levels increase with age and hyperlipidemia. Protein S and antithrombin levels also decrease with nephrotic syndrome, pregnancy, and estrogen therapy (HRT, OCs)
  3. APCR is increased with pregnancy, estrogen therapy (HRT, OCs), and certain cancers; elevated factor VIII level and antiphospholipid antibodies can cause APCR

PREVENTION

Risk of postthrombotic syndrome decreases if compression stockings are worn for at least 1 yr, starting in the first month after the DVT.

PATIENT & FAMILY EDUCATION

National Blood Clot Alliance
120 White Plains Road, Suite 100
Tarrytown, NY 10591
www.stoptheclot.org/contact.htm
National Collaborative Outreach Project of the Blood Clot Outreach Program at the Hemophilia and Thrombosis Center University of North Carolina at Chapel Hill
www.clotconnect.org/about-clot-connect/about
Factor V Leiden Resources
www.fvleiden.org/resources/index.html
APS Foundation of America, Inc.
P. O. Box 801
LaCrosse, WI 54602-0801
www.apsfa.org/

RELATED CONTENT

Thrombophilia (Patient Information)
Antiphospholipid Antibody Syndrome (Related Key Topic)
Deep Vein Thrombosis (Related Key Topic)
Pulmonary Embolism (Related Key Topic)

SUGGESTED READINGS

Available at ExpertConsult.com

AUTHORS: **Hyun Lee, MD,** and **John L. Reagan, MD**

BASIC INFORMATION

DEFINITION

Hyperemesis gravidarum refers to a severe and persistent form of nausea and vomiting in pregnancy. While no precise criteria exist to define the severity, it may be characterized by at least a 5% weight loss from prepregnancy weight, dehydration, ketonuria, and electrolyte imbalance. Typical onset occurs at wk 4 to 8 of pregnancy, continuing through wk 14 to 16 of pregnancy.

ICD-10CM CODES

021.0	Mild hyperemesis gravidarum
021.1	Hyperemesis gravidarum with metabolic disturbance

EPIDEMIOLOGY & DEMOGRAPHICS

INCIDENCE: 0.5% to 2% of pregnancies

GENETICS: A genetic predisposition may exist; hyperemesis gravidarum is more common among first-degree relatives of those diagnosed with the condition, and certain placental protein gene variants associated with hyperemesis have been identified.

RISK FACTORS: Women with increased placental mass, including molar pregnancy or multiple gestation, family history or personal history of hyperemesis gravidarum, prior miscarriage, nulliparity, young age, hyperthyroidism, gastrointestinal disorders, vestibular disease, motion sickness, long interpregnancy interval, and supertaster status. Alcohol use, smoking, and anosmia may be protective. A female fetus increases the risk by 1.27-fold.

PHYSICAL FINDINGS & CLINICAL PRESENTATION

- Weight loss of more than 5% from pregravid weight
- Symptoms: Nausea, vomiting, spitting, enhanced olfactory senses, food and/or fluid intolerance, lethargy
- Signs: Poor skin turgor, dry mucous membranes, hypotension, tachycardia
- Complications include inadequate caloric and nutritional intake, dehydration, and electrolyte abnormalities, including hyponatremia, hypocalcemia, hypokalemia, and, in severe cases, hypochloremic metabolic acidosis or Wernicke encephalopathy from thiamine deficiency. Severe hyperemesis gravidarum also has been shown to correlate with higher rates of anxiety and depression

ETIOLOGY

Unknown, but likely multifactorial. Theories include interactions between hCG and the thyroid, gestational hyperestrogenemia, and gastric dysrhythmias.

DIAGNOSIS

DIFFERENTIAL DIAGNOSIS

- Gastrointestinal conditions: Gastroenteritis, gastroparesis, biliary tract disease, hepatitis, intestinal obstruction, peptic ulcer disease, appendicitis, inflammatory bowel disease
- Genitourinary tract conditions: Pyelonephritis, nephrolithiasis
- Metabolic disease: Hyperthyroidism, hyperparathyroidism, diabetic ketoacidosis, cannabinoid hyperemesis syndrome, porphyria, adrenal insufficiency
- Neurologic conditions: Pseudotumor cerebri, vestibular lesions, migraines, tumors of the central nervous system, cyclic vomiting syndrome
- Miscellaneous: Drug toxicity or intolerance, psychogenic
- Pregnancy-related conditions: Acute fatty liver of pregnancy, preeclampsia

WORKUP

Diagnosis is one of exclusion. History and physical examination along with laboratory tests to rule out other causes of vomiting should be performed.

LABORATORY TESTS

- BMP may reveal hyponatremia, hypokalemia, low serum urea.
- Urinalysis may show elevated specific gravity, ketonuria, or proteinuria.
- Liver enzymes (ALT typically more elevated than AST, both usually reaching only two to three times the upper limit of normal).
- Serum bilirubin (<4 mg/dl).
- Serum amylase or lipase (up to 5× greater than normal).
- CBC may show an increase in hematocrit from volume depletion.
- Magnesium and calcium may be low.
- TSH and free T_4 (transient hyperthyroidism occurs in 2/3 of women with hyperemesis gravidarum; this is biochemical hyperthyroidism that usually resolves by 18 wk of gestation; testing and treatment should not be undertaken without additional clinical evidence of intrinsic thyroid disease).

IMAGING STUDIES

- Ultrasound to evaluate for multiple gestation or molar pregnancy
- If the patient is having associated pain, a right upper quadrant ultrasound may be indicated to evaluate biliary tract disease

TREATMENT

NONPHARMACOLOGIC THERAPY

- Avoidance of foods and smells that trigger nausea
- Ginger (200 to 500 mg q8h)
- Protein-heavy meals
- Reassurance and support, in some cases intensive cognitive-behavioral therapy

ACUTE GENERAL Rx

- Pyridoxine (vitamin B_6) 10 to 25 mg PO q8h
- Doxylamine 12.5 to 25 mg qhs
- Pyridoxine (10 mg)/doxylamine (10 mg) combination, starting with 2 tablets qhs and adding an additional 1 tablet q A.M. and 1 tablet q P.M. if needed
- Antiemetics including promethazine, prochlorperazine, metoclopramide, and ondansetron have been shown to be generally safe and effective in improving pregnancy outcome
- Corticosteroids (methylprednisolone, prednisone) may be considered after 10 wk of gestation
- IV fluid and electrolyte administration if evidence of deficiency is found
- Thiamine prior to dextrose administration to avoid Wernicke encephalopathy
- Restart oral intake gradually no less than 48 hr after vomiting has stopped

CHRONIC Rx

- If unable to tolerate oral intake, consider replacing with enteral or parenteral feeding
- Repeated IV fluid and electrolyte replacement can be conducted through outpatient visits

COMPLEMENTARY & ALTERNATIVE MEDICINE

- Supportive psychotherapy
- Acupuncture
- Acupressure with use of a wrist band

DISPOSITION

- Infants born from pregnancies complicated by hyperemesis may have a higher risk of being small for gestational age or low birth weight than those not; however, this may be limited to infants of women who have experienced significant weight loss in the setting of hyperemesis.
- Women with hyperemesis gravidarum should be counseled that they have a higher risk than other women of developing similar symptoms in future pregnancies.

PEARLS & CONSIDERATIONS

COMMENTS

Nausea and vomiting in early pregnancy are associated with psychosocial morbidity.

SUGGESTED READINGS

Available at ExpertConsult.com

RELATED CONTENT

Hyperemesis Gravidarum (Patient Information)

AUTHORS: **T. Caroline Bank, MD,** and **Anthony Sciscione, DO**

BASIC INFORMATION

DEFINITION

Hyperglycemic hyperosmolar syndrome (HHS) is a life-threatening complication of diabetes mellitus characterized by marked hyperglycemia, dehydration, electrolyte derangements, and hyperosmolality with or without mental obtundation, in the absence of significant ketoacidosis.

SYNONYMS

HHS
Hyperosmolar hyperglycemic syndrome
Diabetic hyperosmolar syndrome
Hyperglycemic hyperosmolar nonketotic syndrome
Hyperglycemic hyperosmolar nonketotic coma
Hyperosmolar hyperglycemic state
Nonketotic hyperosmolar syndrome

ICD-10CM CODES

E08.00	Diabetes mellitus due to underlying condition with hyperosmolarity without nonketotic hyperglycemic-hyperosmolar coma (NKHHC)
E08.01	Diabetes mellitus due to underlying condition with hyperosmolarity with coma
E09.00	Drug or chemical induced diabetes mellitus with hyperosmolarity without nonketotic hyperglycemic-hyperosmolar coma (NKHHC)
E09.01	Drug or chemical induced diabetes mellitus with hyperosmolarity with coma
E11.00	Type 2 diabetes mellitus with hyperosmolarity without nonketotic hyperglycemic-hyperosmolar coma (NKHHC)
E11.01	Type 2 diabetes mellitus with hyperosmolarity with coma
E13.00	Other specified diabetes mellitus with hyperosmolarity without nonketotic hyperglycemic-hyperosmolar coma (NKHHC)
E13.01	Other specified diabetes mellitus with hyperosmolarity with coma

EPIDEMIOLOGY & DEMOGRAPHICS

HHS is a rare condition that most commonly affects patients with type 2 diabetes mellitus. Approximately 20% of patients have no history of diabetes. Elderly individuals with new-onset diabetes or those with poorly controlled type 2 diabetes predisposed to extracellular fluid volume depletion (so-called dehydration) are at increased risk for HHS. Mortality from HHS is estimated at 5% to 20%, a greater mortality rate than for diabetic ketoacidosis. Prognosis is determined by several factors, including age, degree of dehydration, and presence of other comorbidities.

PHYSICAL FINDINGS & CLINICAL PRESENTATION

- Polyuria, polydipsia, weight loss, weakness
- Mental status changes that can range from full alertness to coma
- Focal neurologic signs (e.g., hemiplegia, hemianopsia) or seizures (focal or generalized), aphasia, visual hallucinations
- Symptoms of coexisting illnesses or comorbidities that may have precipitated the event
- Signs of extracellular fluid volume depletion, including dry mucous membranes, poor skin turgor, sunken eyes, hypotension, and tachycardia
- Normothermia or hypothermia despite the presence of infection, due to peripheral vasodilation

ETIOLOGY

HHS can be precipitated by various conditions:
- Infection (most common precipitant, especially pneumonia and urinary tract infections)
- Insulin deficiency (undiagnosed diabetes, inadequate insulin, or medication nonadherence)
- Inflammatory conditions (e.g., acute pancreatitis, acute cholecystitis)
- Ischemia/infarction (e.g., myocardial infarction, stroke, bowel ischemia)
- Kidney failure
- Severe dehydration (e.g., burns, heatstroke)
- Drugs (e.g., steroids, thiazides, beta blockers, atypical antipsychotics, sympathomimetics including cocaine, alcohol, pentamidine)

A relative insulin deficiency provides enough insulin to inhibit ketogenesis but is insufficient to inhibit hepatic gluconeogenesis, glycogenolysis, or promote peripheral glucose uptake, with consequent hyperglycemia. With underlying illness, counterregulatory hormone excess leads to further blood glucose elevation. The resultant extreme hyperglycemia leads to osmotic diuresis. If adequate hydration is not maintained, dehydration and worsening renal function ensue. In those with inadequate fluid intake due to altered thirst mechanisms or the inability to access fluids, as may be seen in the elderly population, the risk of severe dehydration further increases. Diminished renal filtration further impairs glucose excretion, thus exacerbating the hyperglycemia, dehydration, and hyperosmolality, and increases the risk for cardiovascular collapse.

Dx DIAGNOSIS

DIFFERENTIAL DIAGNOSIS

- Diabetic ketoacidosis
- Stroke (especially in the elderly with neurologic abnormalities)
- Hypovolemic or septic shock
- Encephalopathy

WORKUP

After the initial history is obtained, perform a physical exam that includes immediate evaluation of airway, breathing, circulation, mental status, volume status, and signs suggestive of precipitating event including infection, myocardial infarction, or stroke.

LABORATORY TESTS

- Hyperglycemia: Blood glucose >600 mg/dl (Box 1)
- Serum osmolality: Usually >320 mOsm/kg
- Complete metabolic panel: Serum creatinine, blood urea nitrogen (BUN), electrolytes, glucose
- Serum sodium: May be low, normal, or high. Hyperglycemia increases plasma osmolality that translocates intracellular water to the extracellular compartment, decreasing serum sodium. Serum sodium can be corrected by adding 1.6 mmol/L to the measured serum sodium for each 100 mg/dl rise in serum glucose above 100 mg/dl. Marked osmotic diuresis induced by hyperglycemia may cause the serum sodium level to be normal or high
- Serum potassium and phosphate: Total body potassium and phosphate deficits typically occur due to urinary losses from osmotic diuresis. However, these levels may be acutely normal or high due to extracellular shift secondary to insulin deficiency and hyperosmolality
- Anion gap and serum lactate: Anion gap may be normal or elevated in the setting of lactic acidosis
- Arterial blood gas: pH >7.30
- Serum and urine ketones: Negative or small
- Serum bicarbonate: >15 mmol/L
- Hemoglobin A1c (if not performed in past 3 mo)
- Complete blood count with differential (may indicate presence of underlying infection [leukocytosis >25,000 mm^3], inflammatory condition, hemoconcentration. A leukocytosis

BOX 1 Diagnostic Testing Criteria for Patients with Hyperglycemic Hyperosmolar State

Glucose higher than 600 mg/dl
Normal pH (classically, however, patients are often mildly acidotic)
No significant ketosis*
Serum osmolarity
- >320 mOsm/L with any mental status changes, *or*
- >350 mOsm/L

*Serum acetoacetate is often present, typically an absent or low β-hydroxybutyrate level.
From Adams JG et al (eds): *Emergency medicine: clinical essentials,* ed 2, Philadelphia, 2013, Saunders.

of 10,000 to 15,000 mm^3 is expected from the stress of illness alone)
- Urinalysis, urine/sputum/blood cultures as indicated based on physical exam findings to evaluate the precipitating illness and other comorbidities

IMAGING STUDIES

ECG, chest radiograph, and other imaging studies as indicated to evaluate the precipitating causes

Rx TREATMENT

ACUTE GENERAL Rx

Aggressive fluid resuscitation, intravenous insulin, and electrolyte correction are the mainstays of treatment. The initial goal of HHS treatment includes restoring the water deficit with intravenous fluids. This will help to normalize the plasma hyperosmolality, improve renal perfusion and insulin resistance, reduce the counterregulatory hormone release, and eventually correct hyperglycemia. Selecting the appropriate type of fluid is important to prevent complications related to dysnatremia. Improper management of plasma sodium concentration and plasma osmolality during treatment of HHS has been associated with the life-threatening complication of cerebral edema.

AGGRESSIVE INTRAVENOUS FLUID REPLACEMENT: Due to trivial ketonemia and the insulin sensitivity of most HHS patients, initial treatment is intravenous fluid alone without insulin. Insulin used prior to intravenous hydration or early in resuscitation risks a precipitous drop in serum osmolality. In the absence of cardiac compromise or end-stage renal disease, infuse 0.9% normal saline (NS) at an initial rate of 1 L/hr for the first hour. This is then followed by adjustments in the rate of infusion based on electrolyte values and hemodynamics. A lower rate of 250 to 500 ml/hr may be adequate in the absence of severe dehydration. If the corrected serum sodium is elevated, 0.45% NS may be infused instead. Reassess corrected sodium needs by frequent checks and calculation. Recommended sodium decline is 0.5 mmol/L/hr and should not surpass 10 to 12 mmol/L per day. Use measured or calculated osmolality to guide the rate of fluid resuscitation for gradual normalization of osmolality. Recommended serum osmolality decline is 3 mOsm/kg per hour. Once serum glucose decreases to 300 mg/dl, change the intravenous fluid to 5% dextrose with 0.45% NS at 150 to 250 ml/hr.

INSULIN: Once glucose is no longer significantly improving with fluids alone, reassess patient's fluid status and initiate intravenous insulin. Administer initial bolus of intravenous regular insulin 0.1 units/kg followed by 0.1 units/kg per hour infusion or a continuous infusion of 0.14 units/kg per hour without initial bolus. If serum glucose declines by less than 50 to 75 mg/dl in the first hour, increase the insulin infusion rate every hour until a decline is noted. Once the serum glucose reaches 300 mg/dl, decrease the insulin infusion rate to 0.02 to 0.05 units/kg per hour to maintain serum glucose between 200 to 300 mg/dl until resolution of HHS.

POTASSIUM REPLACEMENT: Insulin therapy shifts potassium intracellularly, frequently causing hypokalemia. If serum potassium at presentation is between 3.3 and 5.2 mmol/L, infuse 20 to 30 mmol of potassium chloride (KCl) with each liter of intravenous fluid to maintain serum potassium between 4 and 5 mmol/L. If the serum potassium concentration at presentation is <3.3 mmol/L, replace potassium by administering KCl infusion at 20 to 30 mmol/h, and withhold insulin until the serum potassium concentration is >3.3 mmol/L. If the serum potassium at presentation is >5.2 mmol/L, monitor serum potassium level every 2 hours without intravenous potassium supplementation.

PHOSPHORUS AND MAGNESIUM REPLACEMENT:
- Phosphorus and magnesium replacement are not routinely recommended. There are no studies of the utility of phosphate administration during treatment of HHS. Very low phosphorus levels may limit adenosine triphosphate (ATP) generation, thus limiting adequate diaphragm function. In patients with cardiac dysfunction, respiratory depression, or anemia and serum phosphate <1 mg/dl, add 20 to 30 mmol/L potassium phosphate to intravenous fluids.
- Monitor serum glucose hourly and serum electrolytes, BUN, and creatinine every 2 to 4 hours until resolution of HHS.

TRANSITION TO SUBCUTANEOUS INSULIN: Normalization of serum osmolality and mental status indicates resolution of HHS. At this point, a transition to subcutaneous insulin should be performed. Overlap the initiation of subcutaneous intermediate- or long-acting insulin and discontinuation of intravenous insulin by 2 to 4 hours to ensure adequate insulin levels and prevent rebound hyperglycemia. In patients with a known history of diabetes, their home insulin regimen may be initiated if adequate prior to presentation. In patients with poorly controlled diabetes, the subcutaneous insulin dose can be determined based on their stable insulin drip requirement. Insulin-naive patients may be started on basal-bolus insulin therapy either by calculation of total daily dose of 0.5 to 0.8 units/kg (split as half-basal and half-bolus; administer one-third total bolus for each meal) or by their individual stable insulin drip requirements. Further subcutaneous insulin dose titration is based on subsequent blood glucoses. Resolution of glucotoxicity and inciting condition(s) will decrease insulin requirements. The underlying infection/inflammatory condition or precipitating event must be adequately treated.

CHRONIC THERAPY: Most patients will need insulin at discharge, at least short term. Patients whose diabetes was previously well controlled on oral agents may resume oral therapy after blood glucose stabilization by insulin.

DISPOSITION

Most patients require management in an emergency care setting, such as the intensive care unit or in a step-up facility.

PEARLS & CONSIDERATIONS

COMMENTS

- When patients with ESRD experience development of HHS, special management considerations are needed. Aggressive fluid resuscitation is unnecessary in anuric ESRD patients, because most patients cannot produce the osmotic diuresis associated with normal kidney function. Note that urinary potassium and phosphorus losses will not occur, thereby limiting the need for supplementation. Lower continuous insulin infusion rates are required in ESRD patients because of decreased insulin clearance. Hemodialysis is typically delayed until serum glucoses are corrected. Precipitous decreases in serum glucose from insulin administration and hemodialysis may result in rapid shifts in tonicity, predisposing cerebral edema.
- Education of the patient, family, and caregivers at chronic care facilities regarding optimal glycemic control, limiting modifiable risk factors for HHS, and prevention of dehydration is paramount.

SUGGESTED READINGS

Available at ExpertConsult.com

AUTHORS: **Jaspreet K. Hehar, DO,** and **Jessica E. Shill, MD**

BASIC INFORMATION

DEFINITION

- Hyperhidrosis is the excessive production of sweat beyond the body's physiologic need for thermoregulation.
- There are two types of hyperhidrosis: primary and secondary. Primary hyperhidrosis is the idiopathic, bilateral, and symmetric sweating from focal areas. Secondary hyperhidrosis is either generalized or focal excessive sweating resulting from an underlying cause (e.g., diet, medication, or medical condition).
- Primary hyperhidrosis affects many aspects of daily life, which can be detrimental to emotional well-being, self-esteem, and interpersonal relationships, as well as work and productivity. Despite this, only one third of those affected consult a physician about their problem. Primary care physicians are essential in the initial diagnosis and treatment of this condition. Early detection and treatment can significantly improve a patient's quality of life, with treatment efficacy between 90% and 95%.

SYNONYM

Excessive perspiration

ICD-10CM CODES
L74.513 Primary hyperhidrosis
L74.52 Secondary focal hyperhidrosis

EPIDEMIOLOGY & DEMOGRAPHICS

According to recent epidemiologic data, hyperhidrosis affects approximately 4.8% of the U.S. population (15.3 million people), and prevalence in both genders is approximately equal. However, women are more likely to discuss the condition with their physician.

PREVALENCE: The condition is most common among people ages 25 to 64 yr.

PREDOMINANT SEX AND AGE: Equal proportions male and female.

PEAK INCIDENCE: The average age of onset for primary hyperhidrosis is between ages 14 and 25 yr.

RISK FACTORS: None known for primary, but secondary condition has numerous causes (see Table E1).

GENETICS: 35% to 56% of primary hyperhidrosis patients have a positive family history, but a genetic disorder has not been established.

PHYSICAL FINDINGS & CLINICAL PRESENTATION

- History:
  1. Pattern of sweating: Frequency, stress exacerbation, volume, duration, body areas involved, symmetry, triggers, and presence or absence during sleep
  2. Impact on daily life
  3. Family history
  4. Medications that could induce sweating
  5. Excessive intake of coffee or other stimulants
  6. Review of systems to evaluate for systemic disease: Fever; weight loss; anorexia; palpitations; other signs of thyroid, malignant, or neurologic diseases
- Physical examination: Evidence of excessive sweating and location on patient's body

Dx DIAGNOSIS

The initial diagnostic step is to evaluate whether the patient's symptoms represent primary or secondary hyperhidrosis.

- Primary: More than 90% of cases are primary. Criteria for diagnosis include focal and visible excessive sweating for greater than 6 mo without any apparent cause, as well as at least two of the following:
  1. Impairment of daily activities
  2. Bilateral and symmetric sweating (axilla [most common], palms, soles, face, or scalp)
  3. Occurrence at least once per week
  4. Onset younger than 25 yr
  5. No abnormal nocturnal sweating
  6. Positive family history

  NOTE: If four criteria are met, the discrimination between primary and secondary increases (positive predictive value, 0.99; negative predictive value, 0.85)
- Secondary: Less than 10% of cases but with numerous underlying causes, which can be divided between focal and generalized sweating patterns.
  1. Focal:
     a. Neurologic (neuropathy, spinal injury, Horner syndrome, Arnold-Chiari malformation)
     b. Gustatory sweating after eating spicy foods
  2. Generalized:
     a. Medications (cholinergic agents, selective serotonin reuptake inhibitors/serotonin–norepinephrine reuptake inhibitors, selective estrogen receptor modulators, insulin, sulfonylureas, niacin, sildenafil, etc.)
     b. Toxicity (recreational drugs, alcohol, drug/alcohol withdrawal)
     c. Endocrine (hypoglycemia, hyperthyroidism, hyperpituitarism, pheochromocytoma, menopause, pregnancy, acromegaly)
     d. Neurologic (Parkinson disease, cerebrovascular accident)
     e. Malignancy (lymphoma, carcinoid)
     f. Psychiatric (panic attack, social anxiety, generalized anxiety disorder)
     g. Cardiopulmonary (acute respiratory failure, congestive heart failure, chronic obstructive pulmonary disease, myocardial infarction)
     h. Infection and fever
     i. Table E1 summarizes all causes of hyperhidrosis

DIFFERENTIAL DIAGNOSIS

- Primary hyperhidrosis
- Fever
- Anxiety disorder
- Heart attack
- Hyperthyroidism
- Hypoglycemia
- Malignancy
- Menopause
- Heat exposure
- Obesity

WORKUP

No further workup is necessary to diagnose primary hyperhidrosis; secondary hyperhidrosis will require more specific testing to evaluate the underlying cause.

LABORATORY TESTS

There are no specific laboratory tests for primary hyperhidrosis. Underlying causes of secondary hyperhidrosis might dictate further laboratory workup.

IMAGING STUDIES

None

Rx TREATMENT (TABLE 2)

- Primary hyperhidrosis:
  1. Topical:
     a. Aluminum chloride 20% to 25% (first line in mild cases) can produce mild localized burning at application sites.
     b. Glycopyrronium cloth (Qbrexza) is a premoistened cloth containing the long-acting anticholinergic agent glycopyrronium. It is applied once daily for the treatment of excessive underarm sweating (primary axillary hyperhydrosis). It is an expensive alternative first-line treatment useful in severe cases.
     c. Aldehyde agents (formaldehyde, glutaraldehyde) can cause allergic sensitization and localized skin irritation.
  2. Botulinum toxin A injection (first line in severe cases) is safe and effective but expensive; preferred option for axillary hyperhidrosis.
  3. Systemic treatments (oral anticholinergics, beta-blockers, clonazepam).
- Secondary hyperhidrosis:
  1. Diagnose and treat the underlying condition.

NONPHARMACOLOGIC THERAPY

- Electrical current (iontophoresis): Introduction of charged ions into skin to disrupt eccrine gland secretion
- Microwave therapy: Destroys eccrine glands through cellular thermolysis
- Suction curettage: Removes axillary eccrine glands
- Surgery (endoscopic sympathectomy): Destruction of the sympathetic ganglia innervating areas of excessive sweating

DISPOSITION

Hyperhidrosis is a chronic medical condition that will need long-term treatment with either topical medications, oral medications, or surgical intervention. Discuss with patient which treatment option is best for the patient.

REFERRAL

If initial treatments are ineffective, referral to a dermatologist can be considered.

TABLE 2 Treatment of Hyperhidrosis*

TREATMENT OF HYPERHIDROSIS

	Therapy	Frequency & Recommended Dose	Side Effects	Duration	Comments
First line	*Topicals* Aluminum chloride hexahydrate—6.25%-20% Aluminum chloride—12%-20% Aluminum zirconium salts	Use nightly for 3-5 nights, then every few days as needed	Burning Irritant contact dermatitis	Days	Blocks sweat ducts Aluminum zirconium salts may be effective in axillae, but not volar surfaces
	Topical towelette	Single daily application to each axilla	Local: Erythema, burning, pruritus Systemic: Dry mouth > mydriasis > urinary hesitation, blurred vision	Hours	Anticholinergic
Second line	*Acetylcholine release inhibitors (i.e., botulinum toxins)*	Every 4-6 mo	Discomfort during injection Weakness of underlying muscles	Months	Prevents release of acetylcholine
	Iontophoresis	2-3 times a week	Discomfort during procedure	Days	Blocks sweat ducts
	Oral therapy†	As needed		Hours	
	Oxybutynin	1.25-5 mg bid	Dry mouth and urinary retention most common; also confusion and decreased mental status		Anticholinergic
	Glycopyrrolate	1-2 mg bid			Anticholinergic
	Clonidine	0.1-0.3 mg bid	Hypotension, rebound hypertension		α_2-Adrenergic agonist
	Propranolol	10–40 mg bid	Hypotension, bradycardia, hyperhidrosis with long-term use		β-Adrenergic blocker
	Clonazepam	0.25-0.5 mg bid	Sedation		Anxiolytic
	Thermal ablation Nd:YAG laser Microwave	Multiple	Expensive	Years	
Third line	*Liposuction*	Once to more than once‡	Expensive	Semipermanent to permanent	
	Local excision	Once	Scarring	Permanent	Last resort
	Sympathectomy	Once	Compensatory hyperhidrosis Horner syndrome	Usually permanent	

*Examples of commercial products are Xerac® AC, Drysol®, and Driclor® (6.45%, 20%, and 20% aluminum chloride [AlCl] hexahydrate, respectively) and Certain-Dri® (12% AlCl). Contraindications to topical and oral anticholinergics include glaucoma, urinary retention, paralytic ileus or toxic megacolon, and myasthenia gravis.
†Combined with topical therapy.
‡May need to be performed more than once to treat glands that have regenerated or were missed.
bid, Twice daily; *Nd:YAG,* neodymium-doped yttrium aluminum garnet.

SUGGESTED READINGS

Available at ExpertConsult.com

AUTHORS: **Tracy Cherian, BA,** and **Ana Castaneda-Guarderas, MD**

BASIC INFORMATION

DEFINITION

Abnormal elevations of serum potassium concentrations (K^+) in the blood are associated with either normal or altered total body stores of potassium. Normal serum K^+ is 3.5 to 5.0 milliequivalents per liter (mEq/L). Hyperkalemia is defined as mild (5.1 to 6.0 mEq/L), moderate (6.0 to 7.0 mEq/L), and severe (>7.0 mEq/L). K^+ >7 mEq/L can lead to significant hemodynamic and neurologic consequences. Levels >8.5 mEq/L can cause respiratory paralysis or cardiac arrest and are rapidly fatal, if untreated.

SYNONYM

High potassium levels

ICD-10CM CODE

E87.5 Hyperpotassemia

EPIDEMIOLOGY & DEMOGRAPHICS

INCIDENCE & PREVALENCE:

- Overall incidence and prevalence of hyperkalemia is unknown. The rate is low in uncomplicated hypertensive patients taking renin-angiotensin-aldosterone system inhibitors (RAASi), but increases in the setting of other circumstances listed below.
- Rarely detected in the general population, hyperkalemia is encountered in only 2.6% of emergency department visits and 3.5% of hospital admissions.
- Usually multifactorial, associated with various combinations of kidney failure (often oliguric), potassium supplementation, drugs that impair kidney potassium excretion, and movement of potassium out of cells due to hyperglycemia or inorganic metabolic acidosis.
- Chronic kidney disease (CKD) patients are most prevalent at 10%. Increased risk depends on the underlying conditions present, including end-stage kidney disease (ESKD), acute kidney injury (AKI), cardiovascular disease (CVD), diabetes mellitus (DM), metabolic acidosis (especially nonanion gap acidosis), and medications such as renin-angiotensin-aldosterone system inhibitors (RAASi), mineralocorticoid receptor antagonists (MRA), and other potassium-sparing diuretics.
- The prevalence of an ICD-10 diagnosis for hyperkalemia was 14.6%.

PREDOMINANT SEX & AGE:

- More common with increasing age due to increased prevalence of etiological factors such as CKD, DM, CVD, and concomitant use of medications that predispose to hyperkalemia.
- Lower socioeconomic groups also have an increased prevalence, where monitoring of drug therapy and control of DM and hypertension are often inadequate.

GENETIC DISORDERS: Syndromes associated with hyperkalemia include:

- Pseudohypoaldosteronism type 1 (autosomal recessive)
- Pseudohypoaldosteronism type 2 (autosomal dominant; familial hyperkalemic hypertension, i.e., Gordon syndrome):
  1. Rare inherited form of hyperkalemia characterized by hypertension, hyperchloremic metabolic acidosis, and hyperkalemia with normal GFR.
  2. Mutations of several genes that affect renal tubular sodium, potassium, or chloride transport.
  3. All forms respond to treatment with thiazide-like diuretics.
- Hyperkalemic periodic paralysis (autosomal dominant):
  1. Gene mutation resulting in flaccid, generalized weakness and hyperkalemia
- Glomerulopathy with fibronectin deposits (autosomal dominant):
  1. Unknown gene mutation that produces proteinuria, hypertension, and type IV RTA
- Disorders of steroid metabolism and mineralocorticoid receptors:
  1. 21-hydroxylase deficiency with low aldosterone level
  2. Aldosterone synthase deficiency with low aldosterone level
  3. Congenital mineralocorticoid (aldosterone) receptor defect (exceedingly rare)
- Congenital hypoaldosteronism (autosomal recessive):
  1. Gene mutation associated with low aldosterone and salt wasting
  2. Increased serum ratio of 18-hydroxycorticosterone-to-aldosterone
- Nephronophthisis:
  1. Manifestations include bilaterally enlarged kidneys, inflammatory portal fibrosis, and development of ESKD.
- Disorders of chloride homeostasis (autosomal recessive):
  1. Gene mutation causing isolated hyperchlorihidrosis with excessive salt-wasting in sweat resulting in severe hyponatremic dehydration and hyperkalemia

RISK FACTORS: Primary risk factor is CKD, especially if GFR is <15 to 20 ml/min per 1.73 m^2 more commonly associated with diabetes mellitus types 1 or 2, or urinary tract obstruction with nephropathy (especially if there is interstitial nephritis).

Medications associated with hyperkalemia:

- Potassium-sparing diuretics (e.g., spironolactone, triamterene, amiloride, eplerenone)
- Nonsteroidal antiinflammatory drugs (NSAIDs)
- Angiotensin-converting enzyme inhibitors (ACEIs)
- Angiotensin II type 1 receptor blockers (ARBs)
- Direct renin inhibitors
- Calcineurin inhibitors (cyclosporine and tacrolimus)
- Pentamidine
- Digoxin toxicity, particularly in CKD patients
- Trimethoprim-containing medications
- Heparin
- Ketoconazole
- Metyrapone
- Herbs

Clinical risk factors:

- Male sex
- Non-Black
- DM
- CVD
- CHF
- AKI
- CKD
- Metabolic acidosis (hyperchloremic, non-anion gap)
- Urinary obstruction

PHYSICAL FINDINGS & CLINICAL PRESENTATION

Most patients presenting with hyperkalemia are asymptomatic, with the abnormal laboratory parameter discovered inadvertently. Symptoms when present are nonspecific and primarily related to neuromuscular or cardiac dysfunction.

- Muscle paralysis
- Dyspnea
- Palpitations
- Chest pain
- Nausea or vomiting
- Paresthesias

Aside from bradycardia, the physical exam usually does not alert the examiner to a diagnosis of hyperkalemia. Flaccid paralysis and/or depressed or absent deep tendon reflexes may be detected.

ETIOLOGY

- Potassium is maintained in a narrow range of normal (3.8 to 5.0 mEq/L) by redundant and highly efficient homeostatic mechanisms that simultaneously control internal potassium ion redistribution while regulating net potassium excretion. When a defect occurs in one or both of these two processes, a net rise in extracellular potassium occurs, resulting in hyperkalemia. A blunting of insulin-mediated potassium redistribution into muscle cells where the majority of total body potassium resides can produce hyperkalemia. A decrease in aldosterone production or activity, decreased β_2 adrenergic activity, and hyperosmolality from hyperglycemia or another compound can similarly produce redistributional hyperkalemia.
- The kidney is responsible for regulation of potassium reabsorption and excretion (95%). Kidney failure and failure of tubular potassium secretion are the typical reasons for hyperkalemia.
- CKD is the most important condition predisposing hyperkalemia due to a reduction of glomerular filtration. Patients with progressive CKD should consume a potassium-restricted diet. Low sodium intake may be compensated for by an increase in salt-substitute intake that may inadvertently increase potassium intake. AKI is commonly accompanied by hyperkalemia. Hyperkalemia in AKI may be originated from or exacerbated by a potassium load from increased tissue breakdown that may occur with rhabdomyolysis, gastrointestinal bleeding, or blood transfusions with outdated blood. These processes

can often result in the development of severe and life-threatening hyperkalemia.

- DM, with insulin deficiency and/or hypertonicity with hyperglycemia. Cardiovascular disease, especially myocardial infarctions, left ventricular hypertrophy, and congestive heart failure, often associated with various pharmacologic interventions that may induce or worsen hyperkalemia. CVD in association with CKD contributes to the development of hyperkalemia.
- RAASi, potassium-sparing diuretic administration, or digoxin, in association with CKD, may produce hyperkalemia in up to 10% of treated individuals, versus 2% of the non-CKD patients. In patients at risk for hyperkalemia, dual RAASi therapy should generally not be used.
- β_2-receptor blockers, digoxin, heparin: The K^+ elevation is generally small with K^+ increasing mildly, from 0.2 to 0.5 mEq/L.
- Congestive heart failure (CHF). Almost 4 out of 10 CHF patients in a population-based cohort study in Denmark developed hyperkalemia, many with recurrent episodes. Hyperkalemia risk was strongly associated with stage of CKD and use of spironolactone especially in addition to a renin-angiotensin system blocking medication.

Dx DIAGNOSIS

DIFFERENTIAL DIAGNOSIS

Hyperkalemia develops due to three mechanisms: Impaired cellular redistribution, decreased renal potassium secretion, and increased intake. In the presence of normal renal and adrenal function, it is difficult to ingest sufficient potassium to become hyperkalemic. Consequently, hyperkalemia is rarely seen in people without advanced CKD, unless supervening factors are present. The differential diagnosis is listed in Table 1.

TABLE 1 Differential Diagnosis of Hyperkalemia

- Pseudohyperkalemia
- Cellular redistribution from intra- to extracellular space
  1. Mineral acid acidosis (not endogenous organic acidosis)
     a. Hyperkalemia inhibits ammoniagenesis, reducing net acid secretion and compounding metabolic acidosis
  2. Hypertonicity (hyperglycemia, sucrose, mannitol)
  3. DM: Insulin deficiency
  4. Hyperkalemic periodic paralysis
  5. β_2-adrenergic antagonists
  6. α-adrenergic agonists
  7. Drugs
     a. Glucagon
     b. Digoxin overdose
     c. Aminocaproic acid-A
     d. Tetrodotoxin
     e. Succinyl choline
  8. Rebound after labile
  9. Extreme exercise
  10. Crush and tissue injury
     a. Rhabdomyolysis
     b. Hemolysis
     c. Tumor lysis syndrome
- Decreased renal excretion
  1. CKD
     a. Use of nonsteroidal antiinflammatory drugs (NSAIDs)
  2. ESKD
  3. Type 4 renal tubular acidosis
     a. Diabetes mellitus
     b. Obstructive nephropathy
     c. Amiloride
     d. Trimethoprim
     e. Pentamidine
     f. Suxamethonium (muscle depolarizing anesthetic)
     g. Volume depletion
     h. HIV infections
- Excess intake (rare except in advanced CKD or ESKD)
  1. Salt substitute (typically KCl)
  2. Potassium-enriched foods (melons, citrus juice, raw coconut juice [44.3 mmol/L], noni juice [56 mmol/L])
  3. Riverbed clay (red clay) very enriched, with 100 mEq K/100 g clay
- Mineralocorticoid deficiency (Addison disease)
  1. Hypoaldosteronism: Primary or secondary
  2. HIV infection
- Defect of tubular function or voltage defect resulting in hyperkalemia and hypertension:
  1. Genetic
     a. Pseudohyperaldosteronism type 2
- Also known as familial hyperkalemic hypertension or Gordon syndrome
  1. Acquired
     a. Calcineurin inhibitors (tacrolimus and cyclosporine)

CKD, Chronic kidney disease; *DM,* diabetes mellitus; *ESKD,* end-stage kidney disease; *HIV,* human immunodeficiency virus; *KCl,* potassium chloride.

WORKUP

Fig. 1 illustrates a clinical approach to hyperkalemia. The following steps should be followed in the workup of hyperkalemia:

- Rule out pseudohyperkalemia: An in vitro phenomenon caused by mechanical release of potassium from cells during phlebotomy or specimen processing. This may be encountered with severe leukocytosis (>70,000/cm³), thrombocytosis (platelet count >500,000 cm³), prolonged fist-clenching during phlebotomy, and use of a small-bore needle. The diagnosis is made when serum K^+ exceeds the plasma K^+ by >0.5 mEq/L (>0.5 mmol/L). Contamination with potassium-EDTA in some specimen tubes can spuriously increase plasma K^+, and the diagnostic clue is a low plasma calcium concentration.
- If there is no predisposition for hyperkalemia, repeat laboratory testing before treatment is undertaken.
- ECG for electrocardiographic signs of hyperkalemia. ECG changes may not follow a classical progression pattern, described below.
  1. Early ECG changes are seen with serum K^+ of 5.5 to 6.5 mEq/L: Peaked T waves (Fig. 2), especially in precordial leads; shortened QT interval; and variably ST segment depression
  2. Serum K^+ >6.5 mEq/L: Widening QRS complex with intraventricular conduction delay (QRS >120 milliseconds that does not meet the criteria for right or left bundle branch block)
  3. Serum K^+ >7 mEq/L: Decreased P wave amplitude with increased PR interval and development of bradycardia (atrioventricular node block)
  4. Serum K^+ >8.0 mEq/L: Absence of P waves and progressive widening of QRS that merges with T wave (sine wave), followed by ventricular fibrillation or asystole

In hemodialysis patients with hyperkalemia, T wave "tenting" was nonpredictive of serum K^+, especially in the elderly and diabetics. There have even been case reports of severe hyperkalemia with no ECG changes.

- Examine for the symptoms or physical findings of hyperkalemia and order basic studies:
  1. ECG
  2. Complete blood count and platelet count
  3. Basic metabolic profile with a calculated estimated GFR (eGFR) (CKD alone should not develop hyperkalemia until eGFR is <20 to 25 ml/min per 1.73 m²)
  4. Urine potassium and sodium concentrations
  5. Depending on history and results of initial laboratory testing, the following treatments may be indicated:
     a. Serum glucose concentration to rule out hypertonicity
     b. Digoxin level, as applicable
     c. Arterial or venous blood gas, if acidosis is suspected

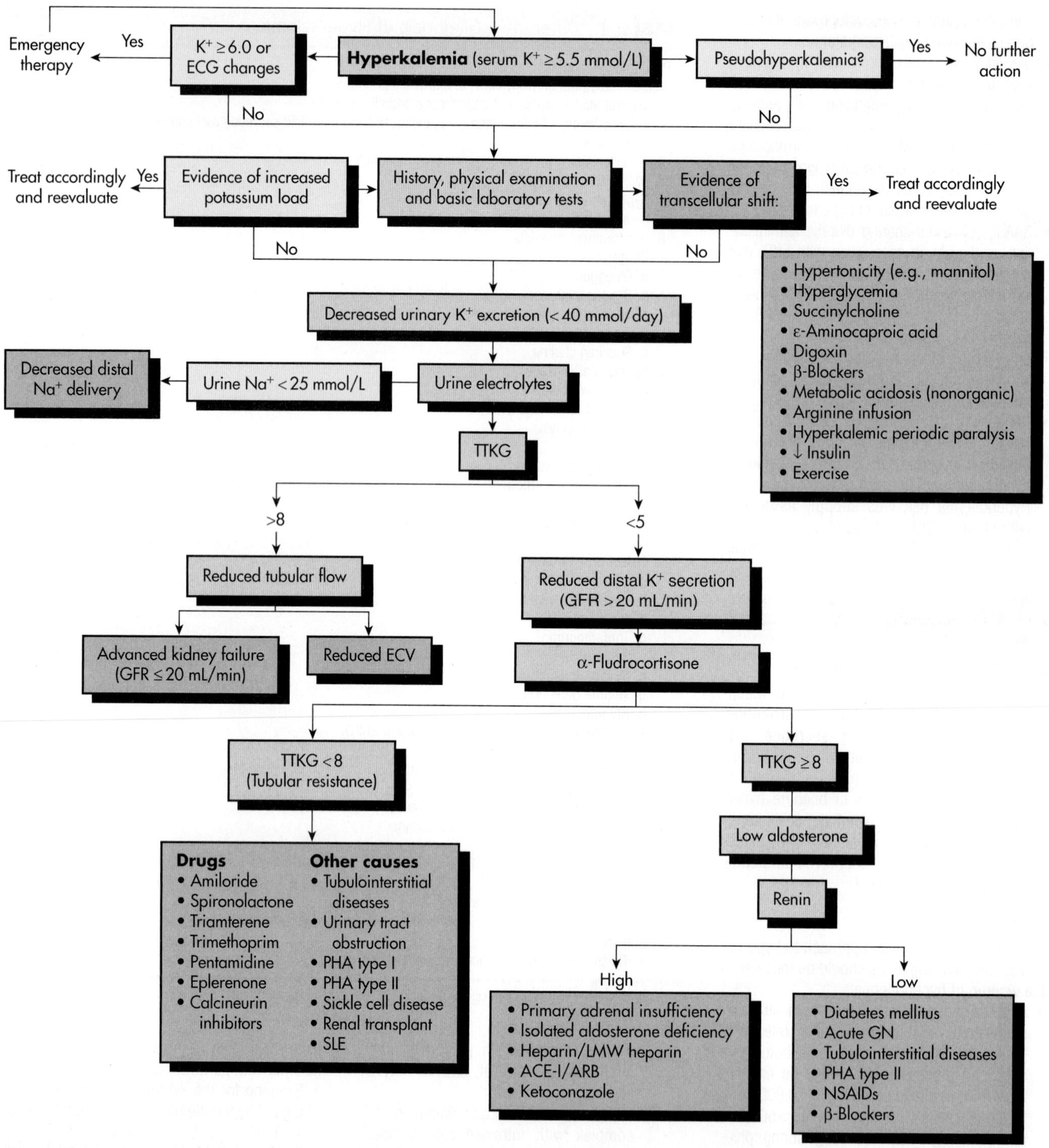

FIG. 1 Clinical approach to hyperkalemia. *ACE-I,* Angiotensin-converting enzyme inhibitor; *ARB,* angiotensin II type 1 receptor blocker; *ECG,* electrocardiogram; *ECV,* effective circulatory volume; *GFR,* glomerular filtration rate; *GN,* glomerulonephritis; *LMW,* low-molecular-weight; *NSAID,* nonsteroidal antiinflammatory drug; *PHA,* pseudohypoaldosteronism; *SLE,* systemic lupus erythematosus; *TTKG,* transtubular potassium gradient. (From Skorecki K et al: *Brenner & Rector's the kidney,* ed 10, Philadelphia, 2016, Elsevier.)

d. Urinalysis with microscopy
e. Serum cortisol and aldosterone levels after other common causes are ruled out
f. Serum uric acid and phosphorus concentration to rule out tumor lysis syndrome
g. Serum creatinine phosphokinase (CPK), calcium, and phosphorus measurements for rhabdomyolysis

- Accurate assessment of kidney function by estimated or calculated GFR to define AKI or CKD stage and risk of hyperkalemia and acid-base status, especially if a hyperchloremic, nonanion gap metabolic acidosis is present.
- Hyperchloremic, nonanion gap metabolic acidosis associated with hyperkalemia is usually a type 4 RTA, with hyporeninemic hypoaldosteronism, which is common with urinary tract outlet obstruction, diabetic kidney disease and acute or chronic kidney disorders involving the tubules.
- Determine presence of a renal origin for hyperkalemia using the urine potassium concentration as renal or endogenous versus exogenous, with nephrology consultation as required.

LABORATORY TESTS

- Serum electrolytes, BUN, and creatinine
- Urinalysis and urine protein–creatinine ratio

- Serum and plasma potassium levels
- Serum and urine creatinine levels
- Cortisol level
- Aldosterone level
- 18-hydroxycorticosterone level

IMAGING STUDIES

- Ultrasound of the kidneys and bladder
- CT scan of the kidneys, ureters, and bladder

Rx TREATMENT

- The treatment of severe hyperkalemia requires three tasks carried out in close succession:
  1. Reverse any electrocardiographic changes caused by the hyperkalemia to prevent a fatal arrhythmia (calcium)
  2. Redistribute potassium into cells (insulin, albuterol, and sodium bicarbonate when there is metabolic acidosis)
  3. Removal of the potassium from the body (sodium polystyrene sulfonate, zirconium cyclosilicate, patiromer, or dialysis)
- Supportive measurements such as fluids, pacing, and pressers do not work in the setting of hyperkalemia. In acute, severe, life-threatening hyperkalemia, the approach is divided into two components. First stabilize the myocardium to prevent a fatal arrhythmia. Giving IV calcium is cardioprotective in the setting of hyperkalemia, commonly reversing all hyperkalemic ECG changes within seconds of administration. However, it does not decrease the potassium levels; therefore, other therapies are needed to reduce the potassium level.
- Before giving calcium, make sure digoxin toxicity is not present, as calcium administration can be fatal in the face of digoxin-induced hyperkalemia.
- Treatment intensity is directly related to rapidity with which hyperkalemia developed, absolute potassium level, and evidence for toxicity by symptoms, neuromuscular examination, and ECG changes. The more rapid the rise in potassium, the higher the level, and the more severe the cardiotoxicity depicted by the ECG changes, the more aggressive the therapy should be.

NONPHARMACOLOGIC THERAPY

- The mainstay of therapy should be educating the patient and the family regarding a low-potassium diet (<3 g/day), as well as providing a list of high-potassium foods to avoid.
- Maintain adequate extracellular fluid volume and prevent volume depletion, which limits potassium excretion by the kidney.

ACUTE GENERAL Rx

In patients with severe hyperkalemia, treatment (Fig. 3) is as follows:

- IV calcium (Fig. 4) to ameliorate cardiac toxicity (if not digoxin toxic).
  1. 10% calcium gluconate or calcium chloride (gluconate preferred)
  2. 10 ml of 10% solution IV over 10 minutes (repeat in 5 minutes if not effective or arrhythmia recurs)
- Identify and remove sources of potassium intake.
- IV glucose and insulin infusion to enhance cellular uptake of potassium.
  1. Make sure to monitor hourly glucose closely for several hours for hypoglycemia, especially in patients with advanced CKD.
- Correct severe acidosis with IV sodium bicarbonate.
- Consider beta-adrenergic agonist therapy (e.g., nebulized albuterol, 10 mg via Venturi mask); preferred over alkali therapy in patients with CKD.
- Increase potassium excretion with administration of loop diuretic IV or cation-exchange medications mentioned previously.
  1. Medications that increase potassium excretion in addition to IV saline and loop diuretics an aldosterone analogue (e.g., 9-alpha fludrocortisone acetate [Florinef]) in patients

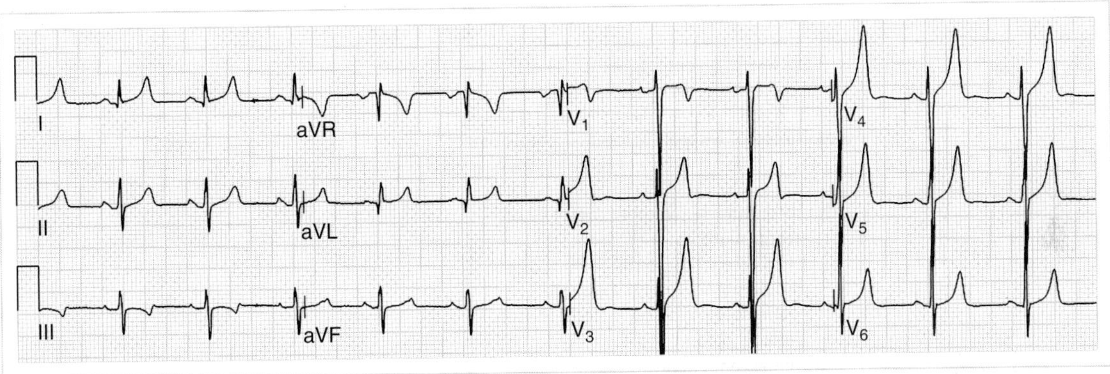

FIG. 2 Tall peaked T waves with hyperkalemia. This 12-lead electrocardiogram shows the tented T waves that are commonly seen in mild to moderate degrees of hyperkalemia. Tented T waves of hyperkalemia need not be tall, although in this case they are. *aVF,* Augmented vector foot; *aVL,* augmented vector left; *aVR,* augmented vector right. (From Olshansky B et al: *Arrhythmia essentials,* ed 2, Philadelphia, 2017, Elsevier.)

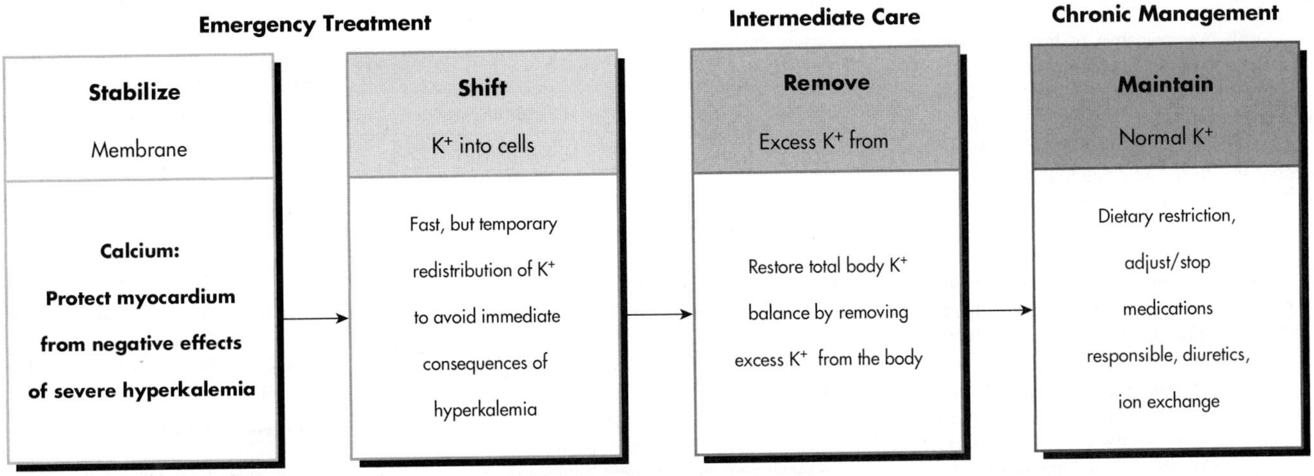

FIG. 3 Management of hyperkalemia.

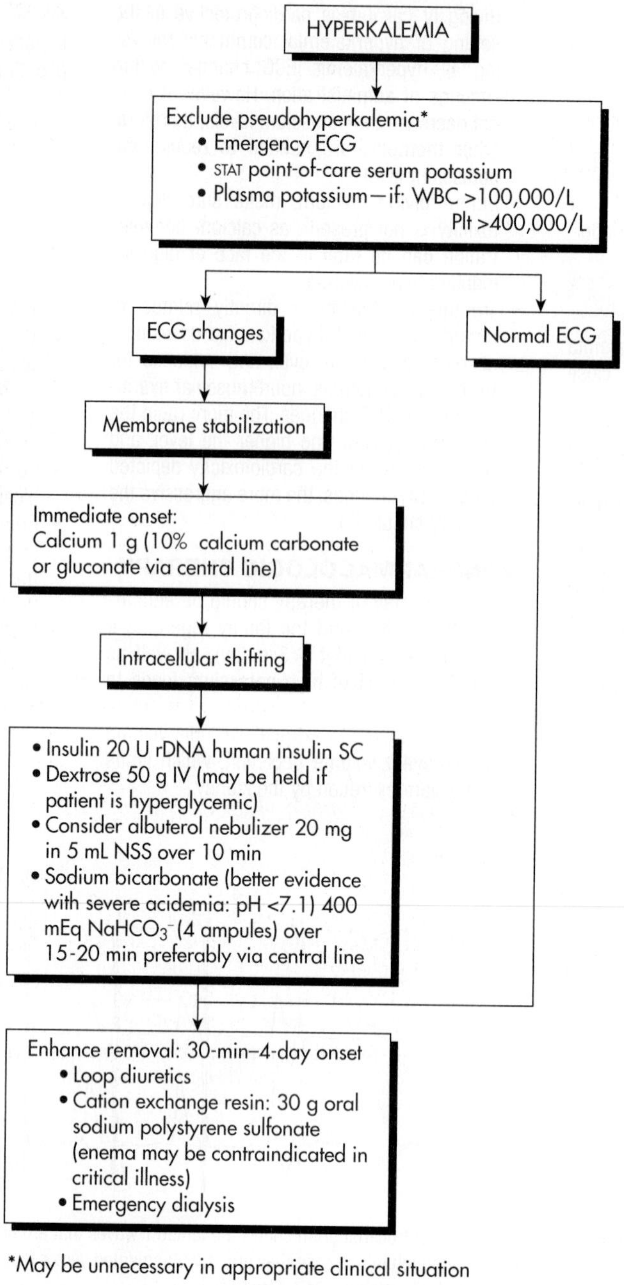

FIG. 4 Algorithm for treatment of hyperkalemia. *ECG,* Electrocardiogram; *IV,* intravenously; *NSS,* normal saline solution; *Plt,* platelet count; *rDNA,* ribosomal deoxyribonucleic acid; *SC,* subcutaneously; *stat,* at once; *WBC,* white blood cell count. (From Ronco C et al: *Critical care nephrology,* ed 3, Philadelphia, 2019, Elsevier.)

with hyporeninemia or hypoaldosteronism or patients with solid organ transplant on calcineurin inhibitor (CNI) and hyperkalemia.

- Emergency dialysis for refractory hyperkalemia, defined as ongoing hyperkalemia unresponsive to conservative measures.
- After correction of hyperkalemia, chronic management should be initiated to maintain a normal potassium. Measures include dietary potassium restriction, adjusting/stopping medications associated with hyperkalemia, and/or administration of newer ion exchange resins sodium zirconium cyclosilicate and patiromer. The use of sodium polystyrene sulfate has greatly decreased due to lack of data demonstrating consistent efficacy and availability of newer agents (i.e., patiromer and zirconium cyclosilicate).

TABLE 2 Available Potassium Ion Exchange Resins

	Patiromer	Sodium Zirconium Cyclosilicate
Dosage	8.4 g, 16.8 g, or 25.2 g Once daily	10 g, 3 times daily for up to 48 hr; then 5 g every other day to 15 g daily
Counterion	Calcium	Sodium
Average daily sodium load	0 mg	400-2400 mg
Concomitant dose separation with other oral medications	3 hours separation	2 hours separation

CHRONIC Rx

In the presence of a moderate elevation of potassium and no ECG abnormalities:

- Correct origin of increased potassium (e.g., inhibited excretion or increased intake)
- Increase potassium excretion (Table 2) with a diuretic:
  1. Patiromer is a nonreabsorbed oral calcium-containing potassium-binding polymer suspension (dose: 8.4 to 25.2 g daily).

a. Shown to lower serum potassium in hyperkalemia associated with diabetic nephropathy and CHF on RAASi.
b. Calcium is the ion exchanger (not sodium), and it can form calcium carbonate in the colon and affect absorption of some medications, especially ciprofloxacin, levothyroxine, and metformin. Administer at least 3 hours before or after all oral medications.
c. Can bind magnesium and may be associated with hypomagnesemia. Magnesium monitoring is recommended with chronic use.

2. Sodium zirconium cyclosilicate is a nonabsorbed inorganic polymer that selectively exchanges potassium for sodium and hydrogen ions. (Initial dose: 10 g three times daily for up to 48 hours: Subsequent dose: 5 g every other day to 15 g daily for chronic use.)
    a. Sodium is the exchanged ion and may be associated with sodium overload if large doses are used for prolonged time.
    b. Agent is taken at least 2 hours before or after all oral medications.

Management of nonurgent hyperkalemia:

- Discontinue or reduce medications that interfere with potassium excretion.
    1. Stop RAASi (special care if in combination)
    2. Stop spironolactone, eplerenone, amiloride, or triamterene
    3. Stop all NSAIDs and COX-2 inhibitors
    4. Herbal medicine: Stop chan su and noni juice
    5. Modify CNI therapy, if feasible
- Prescribe a low-potassium diet (70 mEq/day).
- Administer a loop diuretic or thiazide (CNI-induced hyperkalemia).
- If serum bicarbonate <22 mmol/L, administer sodium bicarbonate tablets (650 mg tablet [7.8 mmol per tablet] or Shohl solution (sodium citrate [1 mmol per ml]) (3 to 60 ml tid).
- Patiromer or sodium zirconium cyclosilicate avoids use of SPS for chronic hyperkalemia.
    1. Neither agent is used for severe/urgent hyperkalemia.
- Continuation of an RAASi may be possible when using patiromer or sodium zirconium cyclosilicate.

DISPOSITION

- Patients with acute symptomatic hyperkalemia with ECG changes should be admitted to a hospital in a monitored bed/intensive care unit.
- Asymptomatic patients with no ECG changes can be treated as outpatients and educated extensively regarding a low-potassium diet with close follow-up including a repeat potassium in 24 to 48 hr, depending on the severity, and a wk later.

REFERRAL

Patients with associated hypertension, proteinuria, CKD, or persistent hyperkalemia should be referred to a nephrologist for evaluation.

PEARLS & CONSIDERATIONS

COMMENTS

- Rule out hemolysis of blood sample.
- If a spurious result is suspected, repeat the test.
- Rule out pseudohyperkalemia, defined as an in vitro phenomenon in which the ex vivo serum potassium level in the specimen tube is elevated, but the in vivo plasma potassium is in the normal range.
- Risk associated with comparable levels of hyperkalemia is higher in individuals with normal kidney function compared with those with chronic kidney disease.
- Do not administer IV calcium or insulin/dextrose if no ECG changes for hyperkalemia.
- Provide education regarding avoidance of rich potassium-containing foodstuffs and encourage dietary restriction of potassium (avoid salt substitutes).
- Evaluate for urinary obstruction, especially in diabetics (neurogenic bladder) and in elderly males (prostatic hypertrophy).

PREVENTION

- Avoid combination therapies of an ARB, ACEI, or direct renin inhibitor.
- In patients with type 4 RTA, provide education regarding rich potassium-containing foodstuffs, avoidance of travel to areas where such foods are common, and avoidance of volume depletion.
- In CKD patients or patients with type 4 RTA, avoid using salt substitutes that contain potassium chloride.

PATIENT & FAMILY EDUCATION

Education regarding potassium content of foods is of practical importance. A certified renal nutritionist should review the patient's medical records for potential dietary interventions and provide necessary education.

SUGGESTED READINGS

Available at ExpertConsult.com

RELATED CONTENT

Chronic Kidney Disease (Related Key Topic)

AUTHORS: **Nelson Kopyt, DO,** and **Jerry Yee, MD**

BASIC INFORMATION

DEFINITION

- Primary hyperlipoproteinemia is a group of genetic disorders of the lipid transport proteins in the blood that manifests as abnormally elevated levels of cholesterol, triglycerides, or both in the serum of affected patients.
- Usually defined as total cholesterol, low-density lipoprotein (LDL), triglycerides, or lipoprotein A levels above 90th percentile or high-density lipoprotein (HDL) or apo A-1 levels below the 10th percentile for the general population. Fig. E1 illustrates the structure of lipoproteins. Plasma lipoprotein composition is described in Table E1.

SYNONYM

Hyperlipidemia

ICD-10CM CODES

E78.0	Pure hypercholesterolemia
E78.2	Mixed hyperlipidemia
E78.1	Pure hyperglyceridemia
E78.4	Other hyperlipidemia
E78.3	Hyperchylomicronemia

EPIDEMIOLOGY & DEMOGRAPHICS

INCIDENCE: The most common types are lipoprotein A excess, hypertriglyceridemia, and combined hyperlipidemia.

- Incidence of heterozygous familial hypercholesterolemia: 1:500
- Incidence of homozygous familial hypercholesterolemia: 1:1 million
- Familial hypercholesterolemia: Autosomal-dominant disorder
- Familial combined hyperlipidemia: Possibly an autosomal-dominant disorder
- Multifactorial predilection: Apparent in majority of affected individuals

GENETICS:

- Familial lipoprotein lipase deficiency: Autosomal recessive, resulting in an elevation in the plasma chylomicrons and triglycerides
- Familial apoprotein CII deficiency: Autosomal recessive, resulting in increased serum chylomicrons, very low-density lipoprotein (VLDL), and hypertriglyceridemia
- Familial type 3 hyperlipoproteinemia: Single-gene defect requiring contributory factors to manifest
- Familial hypercholesterolemia: Autosomal-dominant defect of the LDL receptor, resulting in an elevated serum cholesterol level and normal triglycerides
- Familial hypertriglyceridemia: Common, autosomal-dominant defect resulting in elevated VLDL and triglycerides
- Multiple lipoprotein–type hyperlipidemia: Autosomal dominant, manifesting as isolated hypercholesterolemia, isolated hypertriglyceridemia, or hyperlipidemia
- Polygenic hypercholesterolemia: Multifactorial
- Polygenic hyperalphalipoproteinemia: Autosomal dominant or polygenic, causing an elevated HDL
- A classification of lipoprotein disorders and their clinical findings and management are summarized in Table 2

PHYSICAL FINDINGS & CLINICAL PRESENTATION

- Familial lipoprotein lipase deficiency: Recurrent bouts of abdominal pain in infancy, eruptive xanthomas, hepatomegaly, splenomegaly, lipemia retinalis
- Familial apoprotein CII deficiency: Occasional eruptive xanthomas
- Familial type 3 hyperlipoproteinemia: Xanthoma striata palmaris or tuberoeruptive xanthomas, xanthelasmas, arterial bruits at a young age, gangrene of the lower extremities at a young age
- Familial hypercholesterolemia: Tendon xanthomas, arcus corneae, xanthelasma
- Familial hypertriglyceridemia: Associated obesity; eruptive xanthomas can develop with exacerbations

ETIOLOGY

- Genetic defects causing lipid abnormalities
- Environmental influences, including diet, drugs, and alcohol intake

DIAGNOSIS

DIFFERENTIAL DIAGNOSIS

Secondary causes of hyperlipoproteinemias:

- Hypothyroidism
- Diabetes mellitus
- Pancreatitis
- Autoimmune hyperlipoproteinemia
- Nephrotic syndrome
- Biliary obstruction; Table E3 describes the differential diagnosis of hyperlipidemia and dyslipidemia

WORKUP

- Family history for premature cardiac disease
- Personal history of recurrent pancreatitis
- Detailed physical examination

LABORATORY TESTS

- Standard lipid profile; Table 4 summarizes laboratory findings in lipid disorders
- If normal, further testing with measurement of lipoprotein A, apo B, and apo A-1
- Lipoprotein electrophoresis and ultracentrifugation (for phenotypic classification)
- Workup for secondary causes: Thyroid-stimulating hormone, fasting glucose, liver function, renal function, urinary protein

TREATMENT

NONPHARMACOLOGIC THERAPY

- Cornerstone of treatment: Dietary therapy
  1. TLC diet (**t**herapeutic **l**ifestyle **c**hanges): See "Hypercholesterolemia" topic
- Risk factor reduction includes smoking cessation, treatment of hypertension, exercise
- Familial lipoprotein lipase deficiency and familial apoprotein CII deficiency: Fat-free diet
- Remainder of cases, except those with polygenic hyperalphalipoproteinemia: Fat- and cholesterol-restricted diets

ACUTE GENERAL Rx

No acute treatment is needed.

CHRONIC Rx

- Medications commonly used to treat hyperlipidemias are summarized in Table 5
- Familial lipoprotein lipase deficiency, polygenic hyperalphalipoproteinemia, or familial apoprotein CII deficiency: No chronic drug therapy.
- Familial type 3 hyperlipoproteinemia: Usually responds well to secondary causes being treated and diet therapy; if not, fibric acids may be tried.
- Familial hypercholesterolemia: Statins, bile acid sequestrants, or niacin. Ezetimibe can be added to statins to achieve LDL goals. Alirocumab and evolocumab are subcutaneously injected PCSK9 (protein convertase subtilisin kexin type 9) inhibitors available as an adjunct diet and maximally tolerated statin therapy for adults with heterozygous familial hypercholesterolemia (HeFH). They can be added to statins and ezetimibe. Evinacumab, a monoclonal antibody against the gene encoding angiopoietin-like protein 3 (ANGPTL3) has shown potential benefits in patients with homozygous familial hypercholesterolemia. In a recent phase 3 trial in patients with a homozygous familial hypercholestrolemia receiving maximum doses of lipid-lowering therapy, the reduction from baseline in the LDL cholesterol level in the Evinacumab group, as compared with the subtle increase in the placebo group, resulted in a between-group difference of 49.0 percentage points at 24 weeks.[1]
- Familial hypertriglyceridemia: Fibric acids (fenofibrate), niacin, omega-3 PUFA-containing fish oil capsules. Icosapent ethyl, a highly purified eicosapentaenoic acid ester, has been shown to lower triglyceride levels and cardiovascular risk in patients with hypertriglyceridemia. Icosapent ethyl (Vascepa) is indicated as an adjunct to diet to relieve triglyceride levels in adult patients with severe (≥500 mg/dl) hypertriglyceridemia. It is also indicated as an adjunct to maximally tolerated statin therapy to reduce the risk of myocardial infarction, stroke, coronary revascularization and unstable angina requiring hospitalization in adult patients with elevated triglyceride levels (≥150 mg/dl) and established cardiovascular disease or diabetes mellitus and two or more additional risk factors for cardiovascular disease.
- Multiple lipoprotein–type hyperlipidemia: Drug therapy aimed at the predominant lipid abnormality noted.

[1] Raol FJ et al: Evinacumab for homozygous familial hypercholesterolemia, *N Engl J Med* 383;711-20, 2020

TABLE 2 Disorders of Lipids: Clinical Findings and Management

Disorder	Xanthomas	Cardiovascular	Gastrointestinal	Neurologic	Ophthalmologic	Other Findings	Management
Type I	Eruptive, tendinous, xanthelasmas	None	Acute abdomen, hepatosplenomegaly, pancreatitis	None	Lipemia retinalis, retinal vein occlusion	Diabetes, lipemic plasma	Diet, plasmapheresis
Type II	Planar, especially intertriginous, tendinous, tuberous	Generalized atherosclerosis	None	None	Arcus cornea	None	Type IIa: bile acid sequestrants, statins, niacin, fish oil Type IIb: statins, niacin, fibrate
Type III	Planar, especially palmar, tuberous	Atherosclerosis	None	None	None	Abnormal glucose tolerance, hyperuricemia	Statins, fibrate
Type IV	Eruptive, tuberous	Atherosclerosis	Acute abdomen, hepatosplenomegaly, pancreatitis	None	Lipemia retinalis	Obesity	Statins, fibrate, niacin
Type V	Eruptive, tuberous	Atherosclerosis	Acute abdomen, hepatosplenomegaly, pancreatitis	None	Lipemia retinalis	Obesity, hyperinsulinemia	Niacin, fibrate
Tangier	Macular rash, foam cells in biopsies	Atherosclerosis	Acute abdomen, hepatosplenomegaly	Peripheral neuropathy	Corneal infiltration	Enlarged orange tonsils, lymphadenopathy	
Apolipoprotein A-I and C-III deficiency	Planar and tendon xanthomas, foam cells in biopsies	Atherosclerosis	Normal	Normal	Corneal clouding	None	
HDL deficiency with planar xanthomas	Planar xanthomas, foam cells in biopsies	Atherosclerosis	Hepatomegaly	Normal	Corneal opacity	None	

HDL, High-density lipoprotein.
From Paller AS, Mancini AJ: *Hurwitz clinical pediatric dermatology: a textbook of skin disorders of childhood and adolescence*, ed 5, 2016, Elsevier.

- Recent data suggest in patients with lipoprotein abnormalities that treatment goals should be based on non-HDL cholesterol rather than LDL cholesterol.
- The FDA has approved mipomersen and lomitapide in patients with homozygous familial hypercholesterolemia already taking maximum doses of other lipid-lowering drugs. Both medicines are hepatotoxic and very expensive.
- Recent trials with bempedoic acid, an inhibitor of ATP citrate lyase that lowers LDL cholesterol, have shown to significantly lower LDL when bempedoic acid was added to maximally tolerated statin therapy. The FDA has recently approved bempedoic acid for use alone (Nexletol) and in a fixed-dose combination with ezetimibe (Nexlizet) as an adjunct to diet and maximally tolerated statin therapy in adults with heterozygous familial hypercholesterolemia or established ASCVD who require additional LDL-C lowering.

DISPOSITION

- Those with polygenic hyperalphalipoproteinemia: Excellent prognosis for longevity
- Those with familial hypercholesterolemia, familial type 3 hypercholesterolemia, or multiple lipoprotein–type hyperlipidemia: Even with aggressive treatment, at high risk for accelerated atherosclerosis and coronary artery disease

PEARLS & CONSIDERATIONS

COMMENTS

- Patient information is available through the American Heart Association.
- Lipid-lowering drug therapy is recommended for children ≥10 yr whose LDL-C levels remain extremely elevated after 6 mo to 1 yr of dietary modification. Drug therapy also can be considered for children with LDL-C levels of ≥190 mg/dl.

SUGGESTED READINGS

Available at ExpertConsult.com

RELATED CONTENT

Hypercholesterolemia (Related Key Topic)

AUTHOR: **Fred F. Ferri, MD**

TABLE 4 Laboratory Findings in Lipid Disorders

Disorder	Inheritance	OMIM No.	Prevalence	Cholesterol	Triglycerides	VLDL	Chylomicrons	LDL	HDL	Serum	Cause
Type I	AR		1/million	↑	↑↑↑	↑	↑	↓	↓↓↓	Creamy top	
a: Familial hyperchylomicronemia		239600, 246650, 615947									a. Deficiency from mutations in lipoprotein lipase; *LMF1*; *GPIHBP1*
b: Familial apoprotein C2 or A-V deficiency		207750, 133650									b. Deficient ApoC-2 or ApoA-5 (see Type V)
c: —		118830									c. LP lipase inhibitor in blood
Type II			1 in 500 for heterozygotes	↑	Nl or ↑	↑	Nl	↓	↓	Clear	
a: Familial hypercholesterolemia	AD	143890, 144010, 603776									LDL receptor defect in 60%-80%; *APOB, PCSK9,* each <5%
	AR	603813									*LDLRAP1*
b: Familial combined hyperlipidemia	AD, AR	144250	1 in 100							Clear	Polygenic Decreased LDL receptor and ApoB-100 dysfunction
Type III Familial dysbetalipoproteinemia	AR	107741	1 in 10,000	↑	↑	↑	↑	↓	Nl	Turbid	ApoE-2 synthesis
Type IV Familial hypertriglyceridemia	AD	144600	1 in 100	↑	Nl ↑	↑	Nl	↓	↓↓	Turbid	Renal disease, diabetes
Type V	AR	144650	Very rare	↑	↑↑↑	↑	↑	↓	↓↓↓	Creamy top, turbid bottom	Apo A-V (ApoA-5) deficiency

AD, Autosomal dominant; *Apo,* apolipoprotein; *AR,* autosomal recessive; *HDL,* high-density lipoprotein; *LDL,* low-density lipoprotein; *LP,* lipoprotein; *Nl,* normal; *OMIM,* Online Mendelian Inheritance in Man; *VLDL,* very low-density lipoprotein; ↑, increased; ↓, decreased.

From Paller AS, Mancini AJ: *Hurwitz clinical pediatric dermatology: a textbook of skin disorders of childhood and adolescence*, ed 5, 2016, Elsevier.

TABLE 5 Drugs Used to Treat Hyperlipidemia

Class and Drugs Available	Dosage	Major Lipoprotein Decreased	Mechanism
HMG-CoA Reductase Inhibitors			
Rosuvastatin	5-40 mg qd	LDL	Decrease cholesterol synthesis; increase LDL receptor–mediated removal of LDL
Atorvastatin	10-80 mg qd		
Simvastatin	5-40 mg qd		
Lovastatin	10-80 mg qd		
Pravastatin	10-40 mg qd		
Fluvastatin	20-80 mg qd		
Pitavastatin	1-4 mg qd		
PCSK9 Inhibitors			
Evolocumab	140 mg sc q 2 wk or 420 mg sc q mo	LDL	Prevent degradation of the LDL receptor
Alirocumab	75-150 mg sc q 2 wk		
Intestinal Cholesterol Absorption Inhibitor			
Ezetimibe	10 mg qd	LDL	Inhibits cholesterol absorption
Bile Acid Sequestrants			
Cholestyramine	4-12 g bid	LDL	Increase sterol excretion and LDL clearance
Colestipol	5-15 g bid		
Colesevelam	3.75-4.375 g qd		
Fibric Acid Derivatives			
Gemfibrozil	600 mg bid	VLDL (LDL)	Decrease VLDL production; enhance LPL action
Fenofibrate[a]	30-200 mg qd		
Omega-3 Fatty Acids			
Lovaza (1-g capsule contains EPA and DHA)	4 g qd	VLDL	Inhibit VLDL production
Vascepa (1-g capsule contains EPA)	4 g qd		
Epanova (1-g capsule contains EPA and DHA free fatty acids)	2-4 g qd		
Nicotinic Acid			
Niacin (crystalline)	1-3 g qd	VLDL (LDL)	Decrease VLDL production; enhance LPL action
Niaspan (extended-release niacin)	500-2000 mg qd		
ApoB Antisense Oligonucleotide			
Mipomersen	200 mg once a wk sc injection	VLDL, LDL, Lp(a)	Inhibits synthesis of apolipoprotein B
Microsomal Triglyceride Transfer Protein Inhibitor			
Lomitapide	5-60 mg qd	VLDL, LDL, Lp(a)	Inhibits microsomal triglyceride transfer protein

[a]There are several different preparations of fenofibrate with different doses.
bid, Twice a day; *EPA,* highly concentrated ethyl esters of eicosapentaenoic acid; *DHA,* docosahexaenoic acid; *HMG-CoA,* 3-hydroxy-3-methylglutaryl coenzyme A; *LDL,* low-density lipoproteins; *Lp(a),* lipoprotein(a); *LPL,* lipoprotein lipase; *PCSK9,* proprotein convertase subtilisin/kexin type 9; q, every; *qd,* every day; *sc,* subcutaneously; *VLDL,* very low-density lipoprotein.
From Melmed S et al: *Williams textbook of endocrinology*, ed 14, St Louis, 2019, Elsevier.

BASIC INFORMATION

DEFINITION

Hypernatremia is a clinical disorder that results from net water deficit (i.e., dehydration). It is identified when the serum sodium concentration (S_{Na}) exceeds the upper limit of the normal range (145 mEq/L). Hypernatremia does not reflect the net total body sodium content or extracellular fluid volume status. Consequently, patients with hypernatremia may be hypovolemic, hypervolemic, or normovolemic.

SYNONYMS

Hyperosmolality
Hypertonicity
High serum sodium concentration

ICD-10CM CODES

E87.0	Hyperosmolality and/or hypernatremia
E86.0	Dehydration

EPIDEMIOLOGY & DEMOGRAPHICS

The prevalence of hypernatremia varies based on the defined population and clinical setting. In the outpatient setting, hypernatremia occurs at the extremes of age. Sixty percent of cases develop in hospitalized patients, and approximately 80% of these cases occur in intensive care units.

Among noncritical hospitalized patients, the prevalence rate of hypernatremia is 0.2% to 2.5%. The incidence is greater in critically ill and elderly patients, and the prevalence ranges from 10% to 26% in this population. The severity of hypernatremia correlates with mortality.

RISK FACTORS:
- Age >60 yr
- Acute kidney injury on admission
- Altered mental status
- Mechanical ventilation
- Enteral tube feeding
- Negative fluid balance
- Hyperglycemia
- Hypertonic solution administration (e.g., bicarbonate or mannitol)
- Hypokalemia
- Hypercalcemia
- Underlying polyuric disorders

PHYSICAL FINDINGS & CLINICAL PRESENTATION

- Symptoms generally correlate with severity of hypernatremia, rapidity of development, and underlying cause. In the elderly, symptoms often do not develop until S_{Na} >160 mEq/L.
- In mild hypernatremia, symptoms can include generalized muscle weakness, restlessness, anorexia, nausea, and vomiting.
- With severe hypernatremia, symptoms can begin with lethargy and irritability, with progression to confusion, seizures, and, rarely, coma.
- In extreme scenarios, particularly in infants, hypernatremia-induced brain cell shrinkage can lead to intracranial bleeding from vascular stretching.
- Polydipsia and polyuria may be present in certain types of hypernatremia such as diabetes insipidus (DI).
- Key elements of the history should focus on respective fluid and water intakes and losses, urine output, insensible losses, thirst response, and accessibility to water and fluids.
- Clinicians evaluate the extracellular fluid volume status of patients to facilitate determination of cause and management of hypernatremia (Fig. 1).

ETIOLOGY

- The etiology of hypernatremia is understood through the Edelman equation (refer to "Hyponatremia"). S_{Na} closely approximates the ratio of total exchangeable body cations (sodium and potassium, $TB_{Na} + TB_K$) to total body water (TBW).
- Serum [Na] = $S_{Na} = (TB_{Na} + TB_K)/TBW$.
- Hypernatremia is the result of net water deficit or excessive sodium intake. Renal water regulation and thirst stimuli are the key physiologic components that prevent hypernatremia.
- To prevent hypernatremia, water is retained and urine concentrated by the kidneys under the influence of antidiuretic hormone or arginine vasopressin (AVP). Impairment of AVP

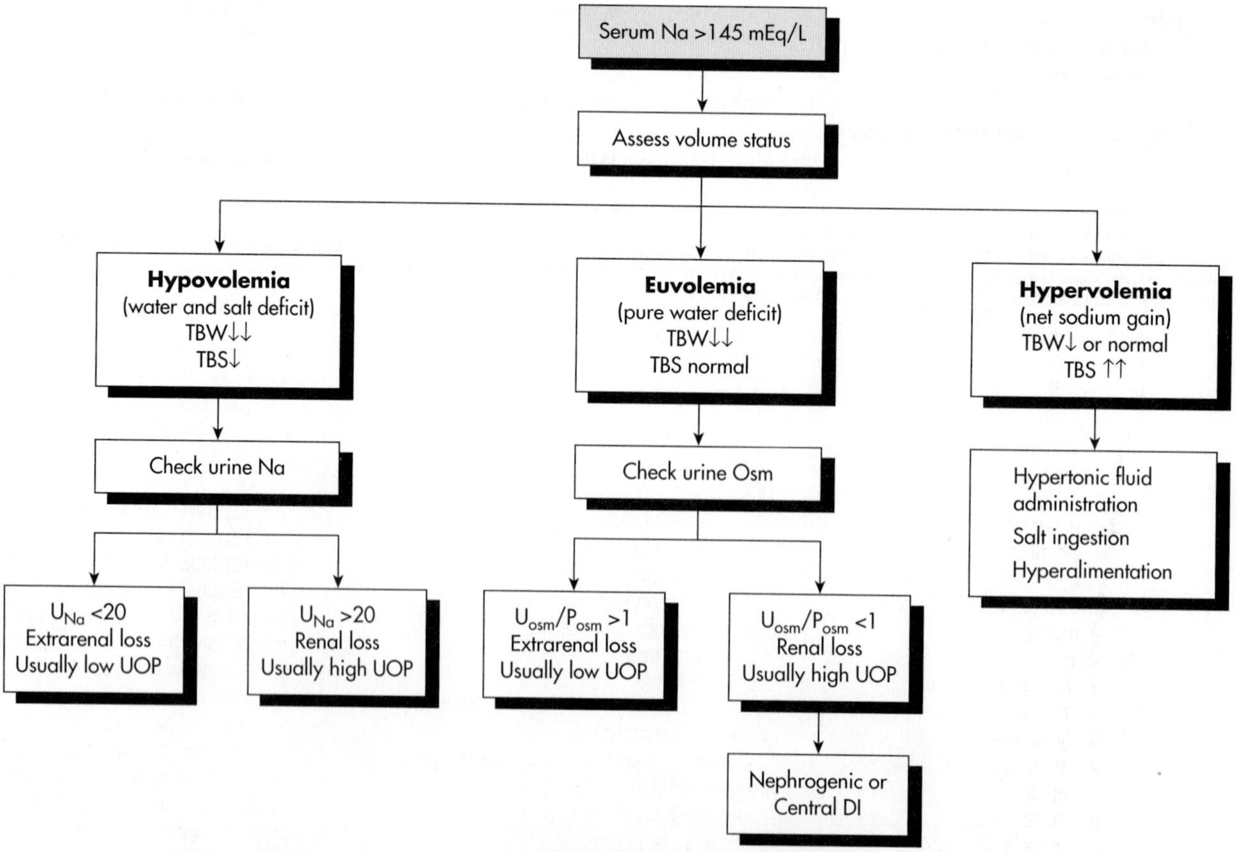

FIG. 1 Diagnostic approach to hypernatremia. *DI,* Diabetes insipidus; *Na,* sodium; *Osm,* osmolality; *TBS,* total body salt; *TBW,* total body water; *UOP,* urine output. (Adapted from Gilbert SJ, Weiner DE: *National Kidney Foundation primer on kidney disease,* ed 6, Philadelphia, 2017, WB Saunders.)

secretion, reduction of the corticomedullary concentration gradient, or inability of AVP to stimulate water reabsorption leads to excessive renal water losses and hypernatremia.

- Elevated plasma osmolality from hypernatremia triggers the hypothalamic thirst response. If water intake exceeds water loss or net solute gain, hypernatremia is avoided. Hypernatremia develops when the thirst response is impaired or when there is a lack of access to water, a common circumstance for mechanically ventilated patients and infants and the elderly resulting from cognitive impairment(s) and physical limitation(s).

Hypernatremia can be classified in the following manner:

- Excessive water loss
  1. Gastrointestinal losses
     a. Vomiting or nasogastric losses
     b. Ileostomy
     c. Pancreaticobiliary fistula
     d. Diarrhea
     e. Laxatives
  2. Renal losses
     a. Osmotic diuresis
        (1). Osmotic diuretics (mannitol, sorbitol, glycine)
        (2). Glucosuria (hyperglycemia, SGLT2 inhibitor administration)
        (3). Urea diuresis (e.g., steroid use, high-protein diet, hypercatabolic state)
        (4). Postobstructive and post–acute tubular necrosis (post-ATN) diuresis
     b. Water diuresis
        (1). Central diabetes insipidus (CDI)
           (a) Genetic
              i. Autosomal dominant
              ii. Autosomal recessive
           (b) Acquired (e.g., post trauma, iatrogenic, craniopharyngioma, metastatic cancers, encephalitis)
           (c) Sarcoidosis
           (d) Langerhans cell histiocytosis
           (e) Eosinophilic granulomatosis
        (2). Nephrogenic diabetes insipidus (NDI)
           (a) Genetic
              i. Arginine vasopressin receptor 2 (AVPR2) or aquaporin 2 (AQP2) gene mutations
              ii. Autosomal dominant polycystic kidney disease
              iii. Familial hypocalciuric hypercalcemia from renal calcium-sensing receptor mutation
           (b) Acquired
              i. Chronic kidney disease
              ii. Post-ATN diuresis
              iii. Hypokalemia
              iv. Hypercalcemia (diverse causes)
              v. Drugs (e.g., lithium, amphotericin, ifosfamide, demeclocycline)
              vi. Gestation (increased placental vasopressinase)
- Impaired water intake
  1. Adipsia or hypodipsia
     a. Septo-optic dysplasia
     b. Craniopharyngioma
  2. Impaired access to water
     a. Mechanical ventilation
     b. Dementia
     c. Cognitive impairment (e.g., dementia)
- Excessive sodium intake
  1. Hypertonic saline or sodium bicarbonate administration
  2. Salt tablet over ingestion
  3. Saltwater drowning

An alternative classification based on extracellular fluid volume status is presented in Table 1.

TABLE 1 Causes of Hypernatremia

Hypovolemic Hypernatremia (Salt Deficit) (U[Na] >20 mEq/dL)

Renal Loss
- Loop diuretics
- Post-AKI diuresis
- Postobstructive diuresis
- Osmotic diuresis (Glucose, mannitol, urea)

Extrarenal Loss
- Gastrointestinal (diarrhea, nasogastric suctioning, vomiting)
- Cutaneous (sweating, burns)

Euvolemic Hypernatremia (Salt Balanced) (Uosm/Posm <1)

Renal Loss
- Diabetes insipidus (ADH-dependent mechanism)
  1. Central DI (complete or partial)
  2. Nephrogenic DI (X-linked recessive with defect in V2 receptor or aquaporin, unresponsive to ADH)
  3. Gestational DI
- Acquired Nephrogenic DI
  1. Electrolyte disturbances (hypercalcemia, hypokalemia)
  2. Drug-induced (amphotericin B, lithium, foscarnet)
  3. Chronic kidney disease (medullary cystic disease, sickle cell anemia, amyloidosis, Sjögren syndrome)
  4. Malnutrition

Extrarenal Loss
- Increased insensible loss (fevers, sweating, tachypnea, burns)
- Decreased intake
  1. Primary hypodipsia
  2. Reset osmostat
  3. Limited access to water (altered mental status, iatrogenic)
- Intracellular shift (seizures, exercise)

Hypervolemic Hypernatremia (Salt Excess)
- Excessive sodium administration (saline or bicarbonate)
- Hyperalimentation
- Salt ingestion
- Mineralocorticoid excess
- Hypertonic dialysis

ADH, Antidiuretic hormone; *AKI,* acute kidney injury; *DI,* diabetes insipidus.

Adapted from Gilbert SJ, Weiner DE: *National Kidney Foundation primer on kidney disease,* ed 7, Philadelphia, 2018, WB Saunders.

Dx DIAGNOSIS

DIFFERENTIAL DIAGNOSIS

Dehydration refers to net water deficit, and its clinical result is hypernatremia. Conversely, volume depletion occurs as a result of net loss of total body sodium and water that reduces the extracellular fluid and intravascular volumes. The combination of dehydration and volume depletion has management implications. For example, normovolemic hypernatremia is caused by pure water loss, and the appropriate volume of water replacement is adequate treatment. This strategy is not appropriate in hypovolemic hypernatremia because volume (sodium and potassium) and water losses also require replacement.

WORKUP

- Workup: Detailed history and physical examination. Historical features that reveal volume depletion and/or dehydration are critical and include a family history of DI and medication or drug use that enhances renal water excretion.
- Hospitalized patients: Frequent monitoring of cumulative fluid intake and fluid losses is mandatory. The most common cause is replacement of total net fluid loss with 0.9% saline.
- Hypernatremia in adults: Usually develops from net water loss and inability to access water (e.g., altered mentation, mechanical ventilation). If access to water is not restricted, etiologies that impair thirst center function should be considered.
- In the presence of polyuria, the underlying etiology should be sought.

LABORATORY TESTS

- Serum chemistry: Serial S_{Na} measurements based on clinical scenario (e.g., 2 to 12 hr). Frequent monitoring maintains the correction rate of S_{Na} at recommended levels. Derangements of other electrolyte and renal parameters frequently accompany hypernatremia.
- Urine osmolality (U_{osm}): With a normal hypothalamic-pituitary-kidney axis, a plasma osmolality (Posm) elevation of 1% or more induces AVP secretion and increases urine concentration (U_{osm} exceeds P_{osm}, typically >600 to 700 mOsm/kg). Accordingly, U_{osm} distinguishes central or nephrogenic the presence of DI from extrarenal water loss.
  1. Low U_{osm} (<300 mOsm/kg) suggests hypernatremia from CDI or NDI. After an initial diagnostic workup is conducted, differentiation between CDI and NDI is required (see "Diabetes Insipidus" chapter).
  2. High U_{osm} typically occurs from extrarenal water losses.
- Urine sodium (U_{Na}) and urine potassium (U_K): U_{Na} assists in the determination of intravascular volume (Fig. 1). The sum of U_{Na} and U_K quantify urine electrolyte-free water clearance to guide therapy as explained later. Electrolyte-free water has no effective osmolality (tonicity) at equilibrium and is water composed of no electrolytes with

- Step 1: Identify rate of correction.
- Step 2: Calculate free water deficit.

$$\text{Water deficit} = \text{TBW}\left[\frac{\text{Current } S_{Na} - \text{Desired } S_{Na}}{\text{Desired } S_{Na}}\right]$$

- Step 3: Choose fluid replacement regimen.

$$\text{Change in } S_{Na} = \frac{\text{Infusate Na} - \text{Current } S_{Na}}{\text{TBW} + 1}$$

- Step 4: Assess ongoing water losses.
  - Urinary water losses estimated by free water clearance

$$C_{\text{electrolyte-free}} = V\left[1 - \frac{U_{Na} + U_K}{S_{Na}}\right]$$

  - Insensible water losses approximately 15-20 mL/kg/day
- Step 5: Determine underlying cause.

FIG. 2 Approach to treatment of hypernatremia. *$C_{electrolyte\text{-}free}$,* Electrolyte-free water clearance; *Na,* sodium; *S_{Na},* serum sodium; *TBW,* total body water; *U_K,* urine potassium; *U_{Na},* urine sodium; *V,* urine volume. (Adapted from Gilbert SJ, Weiner DE: *National Kidney Foundation primer on kidney disease,* ed 6, Philadelphia, 2017, WB Saunders.)

or without urea. Urinary parameters should be monitored every 12 to 24 hr until S_{Na} is adequately corrected.

Rx TREATMENT

- Treatment of hypernatremia requires the replacement of the existing water deficit and ongoing daily electrolyte-free water losses.
- Volume replacement generally precedes replacement of water deficit.
- A stepwise approach to the therapy of hypernatremia is depicted in Fig. 2.
  1. Step 1: Determine rate of S_{Na} correction.
     a. Although the exact risk is unknown, overcorrection of chronic hyponatremia (>48 hr) may induce serious neurologic consequences, namely cerebral edema.
     b. Based on clinical data from infants and critically ill adults, chronic hypernatremia should not be corrected faster than 10 to 12 mEq/L per day or an average of 0.5 mEq/L per hour. This rate would apply to most nonhospitalized elderly patients, because hypernatremia develops over several days.
     c. In rare individuals with acute hypernatremia (e.g., intentional or accidental massive sodium ingestions), the S_{Na} may be rapidly corrected (within 24 hr) to normal S_{Na} levels. The rate of correction should be no less than 0.25 mmol/hr as prolonged hypernatremia is associated with mortality risk.
  2. Step 2: Calculate free water deficit.
     a. Free water deficit is the volume of free water required to correct the current S_{Na} to the target S_{Na}. This is estimated by the Adrogué-Madias formula:
        (1). Water deficit = TBW × [(Current S_{Na}/Target S_{Na}) − 1].
     b. For the preceding formula, TBW is the estimated TBW. TBW estimates are 50% to 60% of lean body weight in men and women. Target S_{Na} is the S_{Na} that should be achieved in a 24-hr period as determined in Step 1.
  3. Step 3: Choose fluid replacement regimen.
     a. With a pure water deficit, the water deficit of Step 2 should be replaced by enteral water or intravenous D_5W.
     b. When possible, the enteral route should is used during hydration therapy to avoid rapid glucose in water infusions that may induce hyperglycemia and produce an osmotic diuresis. This pathophysiologic sequence may occur as D_5W infusion rates are increased to greater than 300 ml/hr.
     c. The rate of water replacement (ml/h) is obtained by dividing the calculated water deficit volume by 24 hr. It is essential that the ongoing rate of water losses must be addressed simultaneously.
     d. Because hypovolemia is present in more than 50% of cases of hypernatremia, concurrent volume replacement with isotonic fluid should be administered (0.9% sodium chloride or Lactated Ringer's solution as required.) An alternative strategy is to use a single infusion of 0.45% saline solution that replaces salt and water along with potassium deficits. For example, 1 L of 0.45% NaCl adds 500 ml of water and 500 ml of 0.9% NaCl to the total body water.
     e. The change in S_{Na} with 1 L of a particular replacement fluid can be predicted by the Adrogué-Madias formula:
        (1). Change in S_{Na} = ($Na_{Infusate}$ − current S_{Na}) / (TBW + 1).
     f. This formula applies to the one-time administration of a 1-L infusate with a sodium concentration ($Na_{Infusate}$). $Na_{Infusate}$ concentrations for 0.45% saline, 0.9% saline, and 3% saline are, respectively, 77, 154, and 513 mEq/L.
  4. Step 4: Assess ongoing water losses.
     a. Ongoing daily water losses (skin, stool, and respiratory tract) must be calculated and treated simultaneously. Failure to account for these losses leads to an undercorrection of hypernatremia.
     b. Urinary losses are estimated by the electrolyte-free water clearance equation shown in Fig. 2.
     c. Insensible water losses can be estimated as 15 to 20 ml/kg per day.

Evaluate for any underlying cause of hypernatremia and treat accordingly. If hypernatremia occurs with hypervolemia, use loop diuretics to remove excess sodium. However, diuretic therapy will also increase water losses that must be accounted for.

Repeat Steps 1 to 4 until S_{Na} is reduced to approximately 140 to 145 mEq/L.

The preceding method represents guidance based on classical estimating equations and periodic monitoring of clinical parameters and is key to achievement of the target S_{Na}.

DISPOSITION

Management of hypernatremia generally warrants inpatient admission because patients have underlying conditions that impair the thirst response.

REFERRAL

Nephrology consultation for management of hypernatremia and evaluation of underlying causes is appropriate. Endocrinology consultation may be warranted if DI is suspected.

PEARLS & CONSIDERATIONS

COMMENTS

- Hypernatremia is a water-deficit problem associated with impaired thirst and/or inability to obtain water.
- Hypernatremia has morbid consequences including mortality.
- Hypernatremia may present with hypovolemia, and the latter is usually treated first.
- The S_{Na} correction rate includes determination of the water deficit plus ongoing water losses.

SUGGESTED READINGS

Available at ExpertConsult.com

RELATED CONTENT

Diabetes Insipidus (Related Key Topic)

AUTHORS: **Lalathaksha Kumbar, MD, Damon Cao, MD,** and **Reem Yusufani, MD**

BASIC INFORMATION

DEFINITION

Hyperparathyroidism is an endocrine disorder caused by excessive secretion of parathyroid hormone (PTH) from the parathyroid glands. Autonomous production of PTH resulting in hypercalcemia defines primary hyperparathyroidism. Secondary hyperparathyroidism occurs when the parathyroid glands appropriately increase PTH production in response to low calcium or vitamin D states. Primary hyperparathyroidism is the focus of this section.

ICD-10CM CODES	
E21.0	Primary hyperparathyroidism
E21.1	Secondary hyperparathyroidism, not elsewhere classified
E21.2	Other hyperparathyroidism
E21.3	Hyperparathyroidism, unspecified
N25.81	Secondary hyperparathyroidism of renal origin

EPIDEMIOLOGY & DEMOGRAPHICS

INCIDENCE: Sixty-six cases per 100,000 person-yr in women and 25 cases per 100,000 person-yr in men in the United States. Although malignancy is the most common cause of hypercalcemia in hospitalized patients, primary hyperparathyroidism is the most common cause of hypercalcemia in the outpatient setting.

PREVALENCE: Varies by country and race with approximately 23 cases per 10,000 women and 8.5 cases per 10,000 men in the United States.

PREDOMINANT SEX & AGE: Higher prevalence in women (female:male ratio 3.5:1) and older age (peaks in the seventh decade of life).

PHYSICAL FINDINGS & CLINICAL PRESENTATION

The majority of patients with primary hyperparathyroidism are asymptomatic. Diagnosis is usually considered in patients after an incidental discovery of elevated calcium or PTH levels on biochemical screening or during the evaluation for decreased bone mass. The development of symptoms varies with severity and rapidity of disease progression and reflects both the hypercalcemia and hyperparathyroid components of the disease process.

- Cardiovascular: Hypertension, shortened QT interval, bradycardia, arrhythmia, valvular calcification, left ventricular hypertrophy, increased mean carotid intima-media thickness
- GI: Anorexia, nausea, vomiting, constipation, abdominal pain, peptic ulcer disease, pancreatitis
- Genitourinary (GU): Nephrolithiasis, nephrocalcinosis, renal insufficiency, polydipsia, polyuria, nocturia, nephrogenic diabetes insipidus, renal tubular acidosis
- Musculoskeletal: Weakness, myopathy, bone pain, osteopenia, osteoporosis, gout, pseudogout, chondrocalcinosis, osteitis fibrosa cystica, subperiosteal bone resorption (Fig. E1)
- CNS: Confusion, anxiety, fatigue, lethargy, obtundation, depression, coma
- Other: Pruritus, metastatic calcifications, band keratopathy

ETIOLOGY

- Most cases of primary hyperparathyroidism are sporadic, but hyperparathyroidism can be associated with rare familial conditions such as multiple endocrine neoplasia (MEN-1 and MEN-2). Mutations in certain genes have been linked to tumor development in both sporadic and familial cases such as hyperparathyroidism-jaw tumor syndrome. Higher prevalence of hyperparathyroidism is noted with head and neck irradiation, chronic low calcium or vitamin D status, and lithium therapy.
- Pathologic characteristics include adenoma (80%), hyperplasia (15% to 20%), or carcinomas (<1%).

DIAGNOSIS

DIFFERENTIAL DIAGNOSIS

- Primary hyperparathyroidism:
  1. Adenoma (80%)
  2. Hyperplasia (15% to 20%)
  3. Carcinomas (<1%)
- Secondary hyperparathyroidism precipitated by conditions that result in hypocalcemia:
  1. Renal calcium loss (i.e., medication: Loop diuretics and hypercalciuria)
  2. Calcium deficiency
  3. Vitamin D deficiency
  4. Malabsorption
  5. Chronic kidney disease (most common)
  6. Pseudohypoparathyroidism (PTH resistance)
  7. Inhibition of bone resorption (i.e., bisphosphonates and denosumab)
- Other causes of hypercalcemia include:
  1. Medications: Thiazide diuretics, lithium therapy
  2. Vitamin D intoxication, milk-alkali syndrome
  3. Familial hypocalciuric hypercalcemia (FHH)
  4. Renal failure (tertiary hyperparathyroidism)
  5. Thyrotoxicosis
  6. Granulomatous disorders (e.g., sarcoidosis)
  7. Malignancy (e.g., lung cancer, lymphoma, multiple myeloma, bone metastasis)
  8. Prolonged immobilization

WORKUP

- Typically, primary hyperparathyroidism is confirmed with an elevated serum calcium and PTH level.
  1. Two measurements of serum calcium are required for the confirmation of hypercalcemia. Total calcium should be corrected for low albumin utilizing the formula: Corrected Calcium = Serum Calcium + 0.8 × 4 − serum albumin. If a reliable laboratory is available, ionized calcium should be considered, especially in conditions associated with acid-base disturbances or low albumin states. Patients with primary hyperparathyroidism can also present with normal calcium levels (normocalcemic primary hyperparathyroidism).
  2. The serum intact PTH (iPTH) level is the best test to evaluate the etiology of hypercalcemia. PTH is elevated or in the high normal range (i.e., inappropriately normal for an elevated calcium state) in primary hyperparathyroidism. PTH is decreased in most other conditions associated with elevated calcium.
- Other causes of hypercalcemia should be ruled out. These are typically associated with low PTH levels. Exceptions include lithium use and FHH.
  1. Review medication history to determine lithium, thiazide, vitamin D, or calcium intake.
  2. Check 24-hour urine calcium:creatinine to rule out FHH. Urine calcium is very low (<100 mg) and calcium clearance/creatinine clearance ratio is <0.01 in FHH. PTH can be normal or high in FHH.
  3. Consider PTH-related peptide (PTHrP) to evaluate hypercalcemia related to malignancies and vitamin D 1,25 to assess hypercalcemia secondary to granulomatous diseases or lymphomas.
  4. Multiple myeloma and bone metastasis can also result in a high calcium state and therefore must be appropriately evaluated.
- Rule out other causes of elevated PTH (i.e., secondary hyperparathyroidism). Serum calcium is typically low or low-normal in secondary hyperparathyroidism.
  1. Check calcium and 25 OH-vitamin D to rule out deficiency states.
  2. Check serum creatinine to assess renal function and 24-hour urine calcium and creatinine to evaluate renal loss.

LABORATORY TESTS

- Serum calcium (ionized or corrected calcium): Normal or elevated in primary hyperparathyroidism
- Serum phosphorus: Low or low-normal in primary hyperparathyroidism
- PTH: Elevated or high-normal in primary hyperparathyroidism
- Serum creatinine and estimated glomerular filtration rate (eGFR)
- 24-hour urine calcium and creatinine
- PTHrP and 1,25 OH-vitamin D levels 25 OH-vitamin D level
- ECG may reveal shortening of the QT interval secondary to severe hypercalcemia (>12 mg/dl)

IMAGING STUDIES

- Parathyroid localization with technetium-99m sestamibi (Fig. E2 and 3) can identify potential adenomas to help with surgical planning.

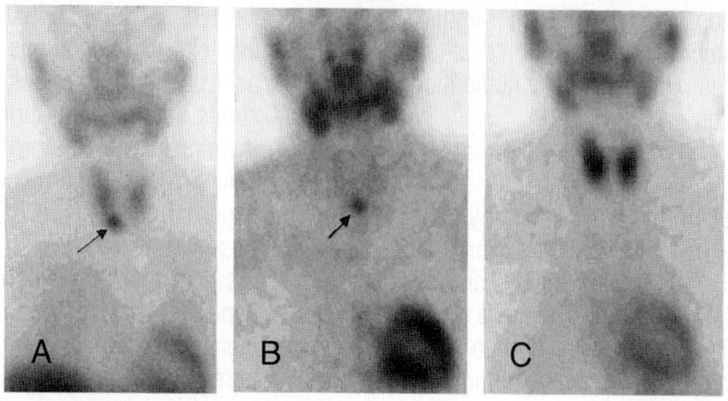

FIG. 3 Parathyroid adenoma. ^{99m}Tc-MIBI images at 10 min **(A)** and 3 hr **(B),** showing a persistent focus of activity inferior to the right lobe of the thyroid; ^{99m}TcO 4 image **(C)** shows normal thyroid uptake but the adenoma is not visualized. (From Grant LA: *Grainger & Allison's diagnostic radiology essentials,* ed 2, Philadelphia, 2019, Elsevier.)

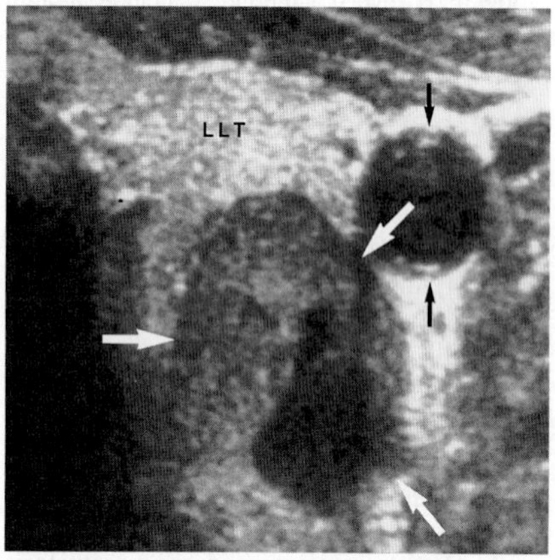

FIG. 4 High-resolution ultrasonography of the left lobe of the thyroid (LLT) anterior to a parathyroid adenoma *(white arrows).* There is a small area of cystic degeneration within the posterior aspect of the adenoma. Carotid artery *(black arrows).* (From Adam A et al: *Grainger & Allison's diagnostic radiology,* ed 5, London, 2007, Churchill Livingstone. In Grant LA: *Grainger & Allison's diagnostic radiology essentials,* ed 2, London, 2019, Elsevier.)

- Parathyroid ultrasound (Fig. 4), dynamic (4D) computed tomography (CT), and magnetic resonance imaging (MRI) are also used to localize the parathyroid adenoma.
- Bone mineral density (BMD) imaging of the spine, hip, and forearm (distal third of radius) is recommended for all patients with hyperparathyroidism to assess the risk for osteoporosis and fragility fractures. Plain radiographic abnormalities are illustrated in Fig. E5 and 6. Cortical bone loss (i.e., forearm) is greater than trabecular bone loss (i.e., hip and spine) in hyperparathyroidism.
- Renal ultrasound can be considered to assess asymptomatic renal stones.

Rx TREATMENT

Modality of treatment depends on disease progression and which patients are more likely to suffer end-organ effects of hyperparathyroidism or benefit the most from surgery. Fig. 7 illustrates an algorithm for managing persistent or recurrent hyperparathyroidism.

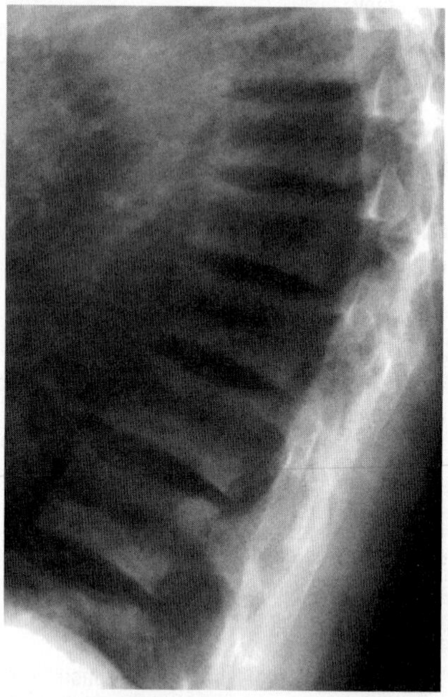

FIG. 6 Secondary hyperparathyroidism. Lateral radiograph of the thoracic spine demonstrating increased sclerosis along the end plates and increased lucency of the central part, giving a "rugger jersey" spine appearance. Also note deformity of the vertebral bodies, with loss of height and increased diameter, in addition to wedge-shaped deformities at the upper thoracic spine related to decreased stability and weakness of the abnormal bone. (From Adam A et al: *Grainger and Allison's diagnostic radiology,* ed 6, London, 2015, Elsevier. In Grant LA: *Grainger & Allison's diagnostic radiology essentials,* ed 2, London, 2019, Elsevier.)

- Surgery is the only definitive treatment for symptomatic primary hyperparathyroidism. Surgery can normalize calcium levels, decrease the risk for kidney stones, improve BMD and fracture risk, and enhance quality-of-life measures.
  1. Indications for parathyroidectomy (Box 1):
     a. All patients younger than 50 yr
     b. Hypercalcemia (Ca >1 mg/dl above upper limit normal)
     c. Creatinine clearance <60 ml/min
     d. 24-hr urine for calcium >400 mg/dl (>10 mmol/dl)
     e. Presence of nephrolithiasis or nephrocalcinosis by x-ray, ultrasound, or CT
     f. Osteoporosis
        (1) BMD by dual-energy x-ray absorptiometry (DXA): T-score ≤2.5 at lumbar spine, total hip, femoral neck, or distal third of radius
        (2) Vertebral fracture by x-ray, CT, MRI, vertebral fracture assessment (VFA) by DXA
  2. Surgical approaches include:
     a. Minimally invasive parathyroidectomy has increased in popularity. The surgeon will identify and remove the abnormal gland that was identified on preoperative imaging. This technique has limited dissection and has improved recovery time. Intraoperative monitoring of PTH level is done to ensure the removal of the abnormal gland. Fall of PTH level by 50% and into the normal range is expected within 10 to 15 min after removal of the abnormal gland.
     b. Bilateral neck exploration under general anesthesia is the traditional surgical approach. All parathyroid glands are identified and compared. An experienced endocrine surgeon cures >95% of patients undergoing bilateral neck exploration. Potential complications include transient and permanent hypocalcemia secondary to hypoparathyroidism and recurrent laryngeal nerve injury.
- Ablation therapy (e.g., ethanol, angiographic, radiofrequency) can be considered in patients who are not surgical candidates. Limited data are available on efficacy and side effects. Repeat ablations may be required if hypercalcemia persists.
- Medical management:
  1. Because inadequate calcium and vitamin D status stimulates PTH, it is not necessary to significantly restrict calcium and vitamin D intake. Vitamin D replacement safely improves vitamin D level and decreases PTH level without significantly increasing serum calcium level and urinary calcium excretion. Repletion of vitamin D is recommended in patients whose levels are <30 mg/dl (75 mmol/L). Dietary calcium intake should be approximately 1000 mg/day.
  2. Encourage physical activity since immobilization increases bone resorption.
  3. Recommend adequate hydration (at least 2 L) to minimize the risk of nephrolithiasis.
     a. For patients who are not surgical candidates or who refuse surgery, pharmacologic options are available. The choice of pharmacologic agents is dependent on the desired goal. Cinacalcet (Sensipar) is an oral calcimimetic agent that activates the calcium-sensing receptor in the parathyroid gland. It decreases PTH production and subsequently normalizes

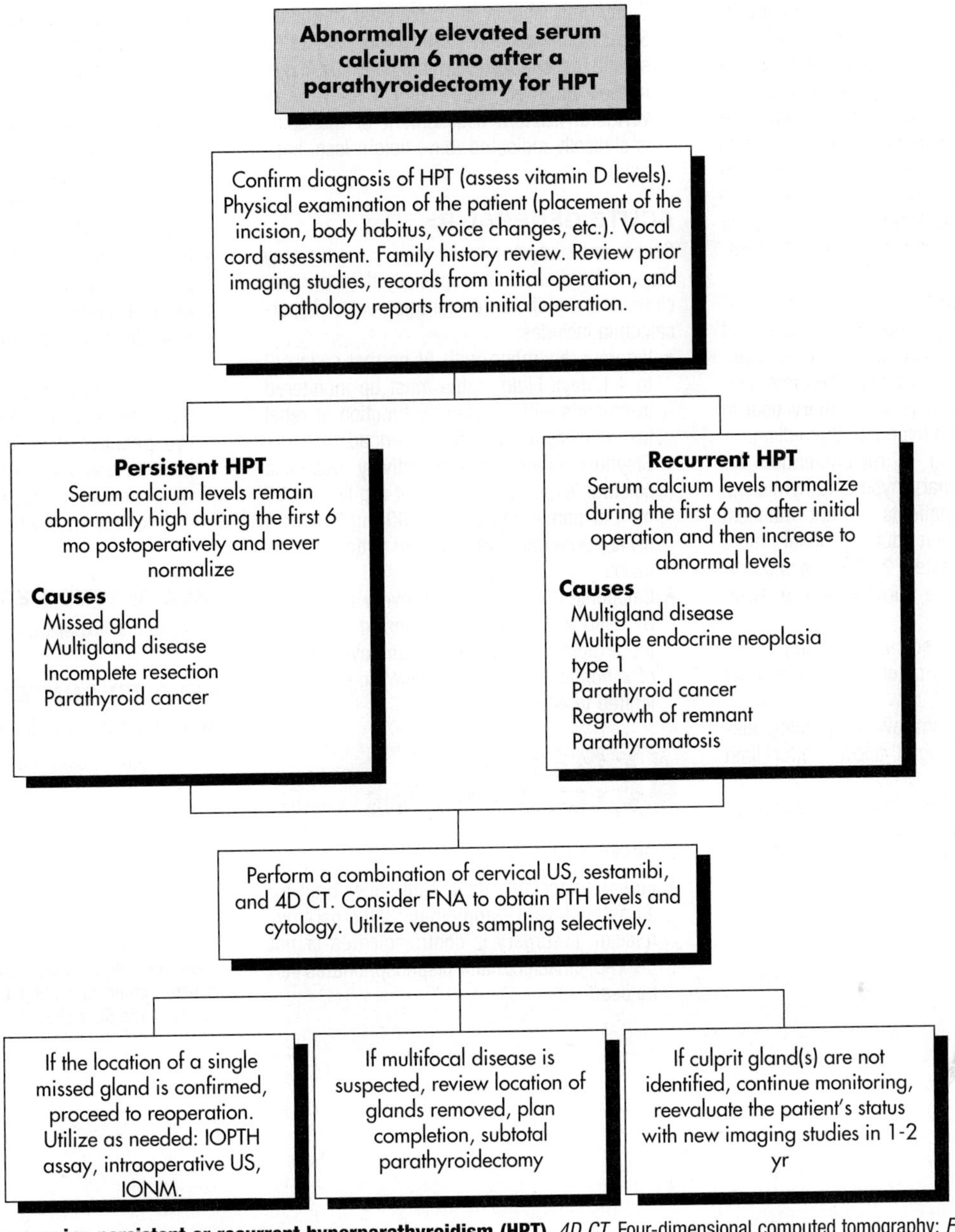

FIG. 7 Algorithm for managing persistent or recurrent hyperparathyroidism (HPT). *4D CT*, Four-dimensional computed tomography; *FNA*, fine-needle aspiration; *IONM*, intraoperative neurophysiologic monitoring; *IOPTH*, intraoperative parathyroid hormone; *PTH*, parathyroid hormone; *sestamibi*, technetium (^{99m}Tc) sestamibi imaging; *US*, ultrasonography. (From Cameron JL, Cameron AM: *Current surgical therapy*, ed 12, Philadelphia, 2017, Elsevier.)

BOX 1 Indications for Parathyroidectomy in Patients with Secondary and Tertiary Hyperparathyroidism

Indications for Parathyroidectomy in Patients with Secondary Hyperparathyroidism (SHPT)

SHPT refractory to medical therapy:
- Parathyroid hormone >1000 pg/ml
- Calcium × Phosphorus product >55

Renal osteodystrophy
Calciphylaxis
Other retractable symptoms, including uremic pruritus, persistent anemia, bone pain, muscle pain, abdominal pain, fatigue, and weakness

Indications for Parathyroidectomy in Patients with Tertiary Hyperparathyroidism

Severe hypercalcemia (calcium >12.5 mg/dl)
Persistent hypercalcemia ≥2 yr after renal transplantation, associated with:
- Decline in renal function, without graft rejection
- Nephrolithiasis
- Progressive bone disease
- Pancreatitis

From Cameron JL, Cameron AM: *Current surgical therapy*, ed 12, Philadelphia, 2017, Elsevier.

or decreases serum calcium levels, without significant BMD changes. It is indicated for the treatment of severe hypercalcemia in patients with primary hyperparathyroidism who are unable to undergo surgery. It is also indicated for the treatment of secondary hyperparathyroidism associated with chronic kidney disease and for hypercalcemia associated with parathyroid carcinoma.

b. Agents such as bisphosphonates (e.g., alendronate, zoledronate) that inhibit bone resorption and increase BMD should be considered when improvement in BMD is the primary goal in patients with hyperparathyroidism.

- Medical monitoring is recommended for asymptomatic primary hyperparathyroidism. The majority of patients do not manifest disease progression during observation. However, approximately 25% of asymptomatic patients require surgery over a 10-yr follow-up period.
  1. Indications for medical monitoring:
     a. Clinically asymptomatic and >50 yr old
     b. Serum calcium level only mildly elevated (<1 mg/dl above upper limit normal)
     c. GFR >60 ml/min and no nephrolithiasis or nephrocalcinosis
     d. No evidence of osteoporosis
     e. Medically unfit for surgery or refusing surgery
- Symptoms should be assessed regularly. Serum calcium, PTH, creatinine, and eGFR should be checked semiannually. DXA performed at three sites every 1 to 2 yr or vertebral fracture assessment of the spine is clinically indicated (e.g., height loss, back pain).

ACUTE GENERAL Rx

Severe and/or symptomatic hypercalcemia may require hospitalization, especially if serum calcium >12 mg/dl. Acute management of hypercalcemia includes:

- Vigorous hydration with IV normal saline (2 to 4 L/day). Fluid status must be monitored in patients with cardiac dysfunction or renal insufficiency to avoid fluid overload.
- Bisphosphonates can effectively decrease calcium levels. Zoledronate (4 mg IV over 15 min) or pamidronate (60 to 90 mg IV over 4 hr) are both effective. Onset of action is 24 to 48 hr.
- Calcitonin (4 units/kg IM/SC every 12 hr) may be used with bisphosphonates to achieve a more rapid reduction of calcium levels. Onset of action is within hours; however, efficacy is limited to 48 hr.

PEARLS & CONSIDERATIONS

COMMENTS

- Parathyroidectomy should be considered for all patients with symptomatic hyperparathyroidism. If surgery is contraindicated or not desired, cinacalcet and bisphosphonates can be used.
- Asymptomatic patients can be monitored with serial calcium, creatinine, eGFR, and BMD measurements. Disease progression may result in surgery.
- Most patients can be managed medically by limiting factors that result in hypercalcemia (e.g., dehydration, immobilization, thiazide diuretics) and maintaining normal calcium and vitamin D intake.
- Patients with osteopenia and high fracture risk may require antiresorptive therapy such as bisphosphonates.
- Patients with nephrolithiasis and and elevated serum calcium should be evaluated for primary hyperparathyroidism. A study of U.S. veterans with kidney stones revealed hypoparathyroidism in 38% of hypercalcemic patients and 26% of these patients underwent parathyroidectomy within 2 yr after their kidney stone episode.[1]

SUGGESTED READINGS

Available at ExpertConsult.com

RELATED CONTENT

Hyperparathyroidism (Patient Information)

AUTHOR: **Vicky Cheng, MD**

[1]Ganesan C et al: Analysis of primary hyperparathyroidism screening among US veterans with kidney stones, *Jama Surg* 155:861-868, 2020

BASIC INFORMATION

DEFINITION

Hypersensitivity pneumonitis (HP) is an inflammatory lung disease caused by the inhalation of an antigen to which the patient is sensitized and hyperresponsive.

SYNONYMS

HP
Extrinsic allergic alveolitis (EAA)
Bird fancier's lung
Farmer's lung
Malt worker's lung
"Ventilation" pneumonitis
Maple bark-stripper's lung
Sauna taker's lung
Hot tub lung

ICD-10CM CODES

J67.x Hypersensitivity pneumonitis due to specific organic dusts
J67.9 Hypersensitivity pneumonitis due to unspecified organic dust

EPIDEMIOLOGY & DEMOGRAPHICS

- Estimates of the prevalence and incidence of HP vary considerably and depend on the definition and methods used to establish the diagnosis.
- Clinical presentation depends on the intensity of exposure, environmental conditions, and genetic risk factors that remain poorly understood.
- More than 300 causative agents have been identified, and the number continues to grow.
- Causative agents in residential and occupational exposures include birds, mold, humidifiers, fountains, steam irons, dry sausage molds, moldy cheese, contaminated wood, biofilm contained within wind instruments (e.g., trombone, saxophone), and organic and inorganic chemicals, including metalworking fluids.
- It is likely that genetic factors are involved that result in an exaggerated lung response to an offending agent. The major histocompatibility complex is the most studied thus far.

PHYSICAL FINDINGS & CLINICAL PRESENTATION

- Presentation is heterogeneous and, until recently, was classified by the clinical presentation as acute, subacute, or chronic HP based on the intensity, frequency, and duration of antigen exposure and symptoms.
  1. Acute HP: Fever, chills, malaise, cough, and dyspnea that occur within 4 to 8 hr of an intense exposure. This flu-like syndrome improves in 24 to 48 hr and can be mistaken for an acute respiratory infection.
  2. Subacute HP: Progressive dyspnea and cough that occurs after weeks or months of sustained low-level exposure or recurrent exposure to an offending antigen.
  3. Chronic HP: Progression of subacute HP, with chronic, progressive dyspnea and cough, fatigue, and weight loss, over months or years of low-level exposure to an offending agent.
- Because these clinical presentations are not consistently associated with outcomes, HP is currently classified as fibrotic or nonfibrotic.
- Physical examination findings include inspiratory crackles and squeaks on lung auscultation, hypoxemia, cyanosis, possibly fever, and clubbing.

ETIOLOGY

- Numerous environmental agents, both at home and in occupational settings.
- Common sources of antigens: "Moldy" hay, silage, grain, or vegetables; bird droppings or feathers (including those found commonly in down pillows, blankets, and upholstered furniture); low–molecular-weight chemicals (e.g., isocyanates); pharmaceutical products.
- Fig. E1 illustrates the pathogenesis of hypersensitivity pneumonitis.

DIAGNOSIS

DIFFERENTIAL DIAGNOSIS

See Table 1 for differential diagnosis at different stages of HP.

TABLE 1 Stages of Hypersensitivity Pneumonitis

Acute Stages	Chronic Stages
Allergic bronchopulmonary aspergillosis	Idiopathic pulmonary fibrosis (IPF)
Pulmonary embolism	Bronchiectasis
Asthma	Chronic bronchitis
Aspiration pneumonia	Nonspecific interstitial pneumonia (NSIP)
Bacterial pneumonia	Connective tissue–related lung disease
Fungal or mycobacterial pneumonia	Sarcoidosis
Bronchiolitis obliterans–organizing pneumonia	
Eosinophilic pneumonia	
Churg-Strauss syndrome	
Wegener granulomatosis	

WORKUP

- Establishing the diagnosis of HP and identifying the offending exposure has treatment and prognostic implications. The diagnosis of HP is based on a combination of exposure history, radiographic findings, bronchoalveolar lavage (BAL), and histologic features.
- Major diagnostic criteria:
  1. **Exposure:** Compatible clinical features (cough and dyspnea) in the setting of an environmental exposure known to cause HP, temporal relation between exposure and disease, clinical improvement with antigen avoidance. Detailed occupational, hobby, and home exposure history is required, along with a high index of suspicion. Questions should address environmental exposure to grain dusts; animal handling; food processing; cooling towers; fountains; metal-working fluids; symptom improvement away from exposure; pets (particularly birds); hobbies involving chemicals, feathers, or fur; organic dusts; presence of humidifiers, dehumidifiers, or hot tubs/saunas; leaking or flooding indoors; visible fungal growth in living or working environment; and feather pillows, bedding, or upholstered furniture. Table 2 describes examples of occupational causes of HP. In up to 50% of patients the specific offending exposure may remain unidentified.

TABLE 2 Examples of Occupational Causes of Hypersensitivity Pneumonitis

Occupation	Cause
Farmer	Thermophilic actinomycetes in moldy hay
Metal worker	Contamination of metal-working fluids with microorganisms such as *Mycobacteria immunogens* or fungi
Worker exposed to humidifiers	Contamination with microorganisms such as protozoa or fungi
Sugarcane worker	Moldy sugarcane (bagassosis)
Maple bark stripper	Fungi
Chicken or turkey worker	Avian proteins
Pharmaceutical worker	Penicillin
Food handler	Soybeans
Office worker	Microorganisms contaminating air conditioners or humidifiers
Swimming pool attendant	Fungal contamination in sprays around pool area
Animal worker	Rat proteins
Mushroom worker	Fungi
Wheat farmer or handler	Weevil-infested flour
Greenhouse worker	Fungi
Workers spraying urethane paint or adhesives/sealants (or less often, other workers using diisocyanate)	Methylene diphenyl diisocyanate, hexamethylene diisocyanate, toluene diisocyanates
Chemical worker using plastics, resins, paints	Trimellitic anhydride

From Goldman L, Schafer AI: *Goldman's Cecil medicine*, ed 24, Philadelphia, 2012, Saunders.

2. **Radiographic:** A typical or compatible HP pattern on high-resolution CT scan (HRCT). Features of small airway disease, including mosaic attenuation, a three-density pattern of normal lung, ground-glass opacity, air trapping, and centrilobular nodules. Findings most often are present with an upper lobe predominance. Fibrosis, including septal thickening, traction bronchiectasis, and honeycombing, may be present and often spares the lower lobes.
3. **BAL:** Lymphocytosis >30%. Bronchoscopy with BAL provides useful supportive data in the diagnosis of HP. Usually reveals intense lymphocytosis (typically T cells >40%) of predominantly CD8+ suppressor cells.
4. **Histological:** A typical or probable HP pattern on transbronchial biopsy or surgical lung biopsy. Poorly formed nonnecrotizing granulomas, giant cells, chronic bronchiolocentric inflammation, airway-centered interstitial fibrosis, absence of alternative diagnosis. In chronic HP, fibrosis can resemble usual interstitial pattern with fibroblastic foci or a nonspecific interstitial pneumonia pattern.

- HP must be suspected in patients presenting with cough, dyspnea, fever, and malaise. A thorough exposure history and an HRCT of the chest are the two most useful tests to make the diagnosis. BAL lymphocytosis supports the diagnosis. Surgical lung biopsy is especially helpful to achieve a confident diagnosis when HRCT shows a usual interstitial pneumonia pattern.

LABORATORY TESTS

- Serum precipitin test for IgG antibodies against offending antigen have a sensitivity and specificity of 83% and 68%, respectively. Asymptomatic patients may have IgG antibodies in serum. HP may occur without a positive precipitin test. When positive, precipitins indicate that the patient has been exposed to the antigen during his or her life. Further exploration to determine if any particular antigen is the cause of the disease is warranted.
- Lactate dehydrogenase (LDH) is increased and tends to decrease with improvement.
- Pulmonary function tests: Restrictive ventilatory pattern is typically seen. Decreased FEV1, decreased forced vital capacity, decreased total lung capacity, decreased diffusing capacity, and decreased static compliance.
- Arterial blood gases show mild hypoxemia (worsens with exercise) and A-a gradient shows slight increase.
- The role for controlled inhalation provocation test using aerosolized materials of the suspected causative agent has not been established.

IMAGING STUDIES

- Chest x-ray: Nonspecific; may be normal in early stages.
- High-resolution chest CT scan (Fig. 2): May vary with stage of disease but often includes features of small airway disease, including mosaic attenuation, a three-density pattern of normal lung, ground-glass opacity, air trapping, and centrilobular nodules. Findings most often are present with an upper lobe predominance. The chronic stage may reveal honeycombing, air trapping, and traction bronchiectasis.

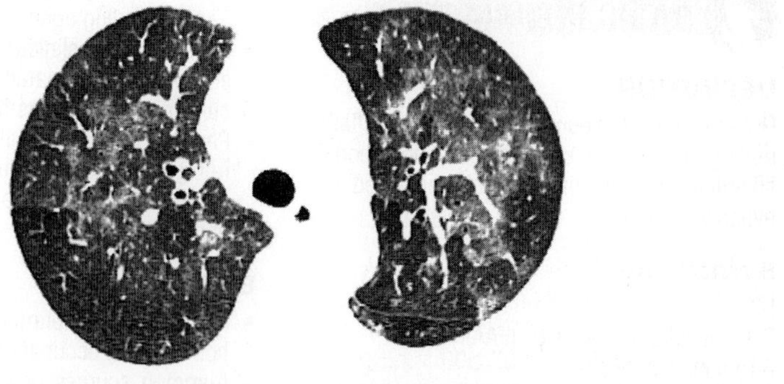

FIG. 2 In this patient with hypersensitivity pneumonitis, patchy ground-glass opacity is visible bilaterally. (From Mason RJ: *Murray & Nadel's textbook of respiratory medicine,* ed 5, Philadelphia, 2010, Saunders.)

Rx TREATMENT

NONPHARMACOLOGIC THERAPY

Identification and complete avoidance of exposure to the offending antigen is the cornerstone of treatment. Avoidance can lead to resolution of acute and subacute HP, as well as to stability and improved survival in chronic HP.

ACUTE GENERAL Rx

- Corticosteroids accelerate initial recovery for acute and subacute HP, but may have no effect long term (from a controlled study in farmer's lung).
- Prednisone 0.5 mg/kg for 1 to 2 wk then tapered over 4 wk.

CHRONIC Rx

- For subacute and chronic HP, steroid-sparing immunosuppression with mofetil mycophenolate or azathioprine, which are better tolerated than prednisone, should be considered for maintenance treatment. Although there are no randomized controlled trials, a retrospective study showed that treatment with either agent was associated with a 4% improvement in DLCO at 1 yr.
- Once the offending antigen exposure has been remediated, and there is improvement or stabilization of symptoms and pulmonary function tests, consider gradual tapering off of immunosuppression.
- For chronic HP with progressive fibrosis despite antigen avoidance and immunosuppression, switching to or adding antifibrotic therapy could be considered. Nintedanib and pirfenidone, medications with antifibrotic and antiinflammatory properties, have been shown to slow the progression of progressive fibrosing interstitial lung disease in randomized clinical trials. Nintedanib has FDA approval.

DISPOSITION/PROGNOSIS

Prognosis is good for patients with acute or subacute HP, especially if the offending antigen is identified. Antigen exposure alone or with immunosuppression can lead to improvement.

Prognosis is worse for patients with chronic HP; approximately 25% die within 5 yr in a cohort of pigeon breeders' lung disease. Chronic HP is associated progressive pulmonary fibrosis, development of pulmonary hypertension, and right heart failure. Honeycombing on HRCT and clubbing indicate advanced disease with poor survival.

REFERRAL

- Pulmonologist: To identify potential exposures and educate patient on its avoidance, establish the diagnosis in multidisciplinary conference and develop a treatment and monitoring strategy.
- Thoracic surgeon for surgical lung biopsy.
- Lung transplant center: To consider lung transplant candidacy. Patients with chronic HP who undergo lung transplant have excellent survival, reported at 89% at 5 yr in a single center series; better than survival after lung transplant for IPF. Can recur in the transplanted lung with exposure to the offending antigen.

PEARLS & CONSIDERATIONS

- HP occurs more frequently in nonsmokers than smokers (likely from an immunosuppressive effect).
- Chronic HP may be difficult to distinguish from IPF. Diagnosis often made in the lung explant at the time of transplant.

RELATED CONTENT

Hypersensitivity Pneumonitis (Patient Information)
Interstitial Lung Disease (Related Key Topic)

SUGGESTED READINGS

Available at ExpertConsult.com

AUTHOR: **Aida Venado, MD, MAS**

BASIC INFORMATION

DEFINITION

Normal blood pressure (BP) in adults can be defined as systolic BP <120 mm Hg and diastolic BP <80 mm Hg. Elevated blood pressure is defined as systolic BP between 120 and 129 mm Hg or diastolic BP <80 mm Hg. Hypertension can be divided into 1) stage 1: systolic BP from 130 to 139 mm Hg or diastolic BP from 80 to 89 mm Hg and 2) stage 2: systolic BP ≥140 mm Hg or diastolic BP ≥90 mm Hg. This definition is based on accurate measurements and average of ≥2 readings on ≥2 occasions.

SYNONYMS

Essential hypertension
Idiopathic hypertension
High BP

ICD-10CM CODES	
I10	Essential (primary) hypertension
I15.0	Renovascular hypertension
I15.1	Hypertension secondary to other renal disorders
I15.2	Hypertension secondary to endocrine disorders
I15.8	Other secondary hypertension
I15.9	Secondary hypertension, unspecified
O10.919	Unspecified pre-existing hypertension complicating pregnancy, unspecified trimester
I67.4	Hypertensive encephalopathy

EPIDEMIOLOGY & DEMOGRAPHICS

- In the U.S., 50% of people age 60 to 69 yr and approximately 75% of people >70 yr of age are affected by hypertension. Worldwide, it is estimated that 41% of people ages 35 to 70 yr have hypertension, and only 46.5% of them are aware of it.
- Peak prevalence increases with age and is highest among non-Hispanic Black adults in the U.S.
- Hypertension is linked with a higher risk of heart attack, stroke, heart failure, and kidney disease.

PHYSICAL FINDINGS & CLINICAL PRESENTATION

Physical examination may be entirely within normal limits, except for the presence of elevated BP. A proper initial physical examination on a hypertensive patient should include the following:

- The BP should be measured with an appropriately sized cuff (bladder of the cuff should cover at least two thirds of the circumference of the arm) and taken in both arms (the higher of the readings being used). Table 1 describes blood pressure cuff size and error in measurement.
- The BP should be measured twice on each visit and separated by at least 1 to 2 min to allow the return of trapped blood.
- The patient should be seated in a calm environment for at least 5 min with the arm in which BP is measured rested on support level with the heart.
- Postural BP change should always be recorded in the elderly to diagnose postural hypotension. This is assessed by taking BP in supine (after 5-min rest) and standing (after 2 min) positions. A drop of ≥20 mm Hg in systolic, a drop of ≥10 mm Hg diastolic BP, or symptoms of cerebral hypoperfusion is suggestive of postural (orthostatic) hypotension.
- A diagnosis of hypertension (HTN) may be established if the BP is markedly elevated (>180/110 mm Hg) or has evidence of end organ damage; otherwise such a diagnosis should wait until BP is found elevated on >2 readings on >2 different occasions.
- Nonoffice (home, workplace, 24-hr ambulatory) BP determination to establish the pattern of HTN (sustained, "white coat," or "masked" HTN) in selected patients.
- Measure heart rate, height, weight, body mass index, and waist circumference.
- Some general clinical clues for when to screen for secondary HTN include:
  1. Severe or resistant HTN
  2. An acute rise in BP developing in a patient with previous stable BP
  3. Age less than 30 yr, nonobese, non-Black with no family history of HTN
  4. Sudden onset or accelerated hypertension
  5. Age of onset before puberty. If above is suspected, additional tests for secondary HTN should be done including renin, aldosterone, cortisol levels, 24-hr urine metanephrines, and serum catecholamines
- Physical examination should include searching for secondary causes, and sequelae of hypertension.
- Examine skin for the presence of café-au-lait spots (neurofibromatosis), uremic appearance (renal failure), and violaceous striae (Cushing syndrome).
- Perform careful funduscopic examination; check for papilledema, retinal exudates, hemorrhages, arterial narrowing, arteriovenous compression.
- Examine neck for carotid bruits, distended neck veins, and enlarged thyroid gland.
- Perform extensive cardiopulmonary examination: Check for a laterally displaced point of maximal intensity, an S3 or S4, and valvular murmurs.
- Palpate abdomen for renal masses (pheochromocytoma, polycystic kidneys), and auscultate for bruit over the aorta and renal arteries.
- Examine arterial pulses (dilated or absent femoral pulses and BP greater in upper extremities than lower extremities suggest aortic coarctation).
- Look for truncal obesity (Cushing syndrome) and pedal edema (congestive heart failure [CHF]).
- Table 2 provides a guide to evaluation of identifiable causes of HTN.
- Table 3 summarizes clinical clues to guide the investigation in young patients with hypertension that has a potentially hereditary cause.

ETIOLOGY

- Essential (primary) HTN (85%)
- Drug induced or drug related (5%)
  1. NSAIDs
  2. Oral contraceptives
  3. Corticosteroids
- Renal HTN (5%)
  1. Renal parenchymal disease (3%)
  2. Renovascular HTN (RVH) (<2%)
- Endocrine (<2%) (Table 4)
  1. Primary aldosteronism (at least 5%)
  2. Pheochromocytoma (0.2%)
  3. Cushing syndrome and long-term steroid therapy (0.2%)
  4. Hyperparathyroidism or thyroid disease (0.2%)
- Coarctation of the aorta (0.2%)

Dx DIAGNOSIS

WORKUP

- The objective for the initial evaluation of HTN is to establish the diagnosis and stage of HTN. Table 5 summarizes initial laboratory evaluation of the hypertensive patient.
- Gather office and nonoffice BP readings, assess presence of target organ damage (TOD), assess the level of global

TABLE 1 Blood Pressure Cuff Size and Error in Measurement*

	Arm Circumference		
Cuff Bladder Size	**28 cm or less**	**29-42 cm**	**43 cm or more**
Regular (12 × 23 cm)	Accurate	Overestimates SBP by 4-8 mm Hg DBP by 3-6 mm Hg	Overestimates SBP by 16-17 mm Hg DBP by 10-11 mm Hg
Large (15 × 33 cm)	Underestimates SBP by 2-3 mm Hg DBP by 1-2 mm Hg	Accurate	Overestimates SBP by 5-7 mm Hg DBP by 2-4 mm Hg
Thigh (18 × 36 cm)	Underestimates SBP by 5-7 mm Hg DBP by 1-3 mm Hg	Underestimates SBP by 5-7 mm Hg DBP by 2-4 mm Hg	Accurate

**Overestimation* means that hypertension may be diagnosed in someone with normal blood pressure; *underestimation* means that the blood pressure reading may be normal in someone who actually has high blood pressure. See text for further discussion.
DBP, Diastolic blood pressure reading; *SBP,* systolic blood pressure reading.
From McGee S: *Evidence-based physical diagnosis,* ed 4, Philadelphia, 2018, Elsevier.

TABLE 2 Guide to Evaluation of Identifiable Causes of Hypertension

Suspected Diagnosis	Clinical Clues	Diagnostic Testing
Chronic kidney disease	Estimated GFR <60 ml/min/1.73 m^2 Urine albumin-to-creatinine ratio ≥30 mg/g	Renal sonography
Renovascular disease	New elevation in serum creatinine, marked elevation in serum creatinine with ACEI or ARB, drug-resistant hypertension, flash pulmonary edema, abdominal, or flank bruit	Renal sonography (atrophic kidney), CT or MR angiography, invasive angiography
Coarctation of the aorta	Arm pulses > leg pulses, arm BP > leg BP, chest bruits, rib notching on chest radiography	MR angiography, TEE, invasive angiography
Primary aldosteronism	Hypokalemia, drug-resistant hypertension	Plasma renin and aldosterone, 24-hr urine aldosterone and potassium after oral salt loading, adrenal vein sampling
Cushing syndrome	Truncal obesity, wide and blanching purple striae, muscle weakness	1 mg dexamethasone-suppression test, urinary cortisol after dexamethasone, adrenal CT
Pheochromocytoma	Paroxysms of hypertension, palpitations, perspiration, and pallor; diabetes	Plasma metanephrines, 24-hr urinary metanephrines and catecholamines, abdominal CT or MR imaging
Obstructive sleep apnea	Loud snoring, large neck, obesity, somnolence	Polysomnography

ACEI, Angiotensin-converting enzyme inhibitor; *ARB,* angiotensin receptor blocker; *BP,* blood pressure; *CT,* computed tomography; *GFR,* glomerular filtration rate; *MR,* magnetic resonance; *TEE,* transesophageal echocardiography.
From Goldman L, Schafer AI: *Goldman's Cecil medicine,* ed 24, Philadelphia, 2012, WB Saunders.

TABLE 3 Clinical Clues to Guide the Investigation in Young Patients with Hypertension That Has a Potentially Hereditary Cause

Specific Conditions	Possible Causes of Familial Hypertension	Clinical Clues
Catecholamine-producing Tumors		
Pheochromocytoma/paraganglioma	Familial cases are responsible for <30% of cases, including MEN2A and MEN2B, von Hippel-Lindau disease, neurofibromatosis, and familial paraganglioma syndromes (SDH complex mutations)	Paroxysmal palpitations, headaches, diaphoresis, pale flushing; syndromic features of any of the associated disorders
Neuroblastomas (adrenal)	1%-2% of neuroblastomas are familial	
Aortic or renovascular lesions		
Coarctation of the aorta	Overrepresented in families but no familial distribution	Asymmetry between upper- and lower-extremity BP, radial-formal pulse delay; associated with Turner syndrome, Williams syndrome, and bicuspid aortic valve
Renal artery stenosis caused by fibromuscular dysplasia or inherited arterial wall lesions	<10% familial with AD pattern	Abnormal renal vascular imaging results; vascular disease in the carotid territory at an early age; common in neurofibromatosis and Williams syndrome; also present in tuberous sclerosis, Ehlers-Danlos syndrome, and Marfan syndrome
Parenchymal kidney disease GN	Alport disease (X-linked, AR, or AD), familial IgA nephropathy (AD with incomplete penetrance)	Proteinuria, hematuria, low eGFR
PKD	ADPKD type 1 or 2, ARPKD	Multiple renal cysts (as few as three in patients under 30 yr)
Adrenocortical disease		
Glucocorticoid-remediable aldosteronism (familial hyperaldosteronism type I)	AD chimeric fusion of the 11β-hydroxylase and aldosterone synthase genes	Cerebral hemorrhages at young age, cerebral aneurysms; mild hypokalemia; high plasma aldosterone, low renin
Familial hyperaldosteronism	AD; unknown defect	Severe type 2 hypertension in early adulthood; high plasma aldosterone, low renin; no response to glucocorticoid treatment
Familial hyperaldosteronism type III	AD; unknown defect	Severe hypertension in childhood with extensive target-organ damage; high plasma aldosterone, low renin; marked bilateral adrenal enlargement
Congenital adrenal hyperplasia	AR mutations in 11β-hydroxylase or 21-hydroxylase	Hirsutism, virilization; hypokalemia and metabolic alkalosis; low plasma aldosterone and renin
Monogenic Primary Renal Tubular Defects		
Gordon syndrome	AD mutations of *KLHL3, CUL3, WNK1,* and *WNK4;* AR mutations of *KLHL3*	Hyperkalemia and metabolic acidosis with normal renal function
Liddle syndrome	AD mutations of the epithelial sodium channel	Hypokalemia and metabolic alkalosis; low plasma aldosterone and renin
Apparent mineralocorticoid excess	AD mutation in 11β-hydroxysteroid dehydrogenase type 2	Hypokalemia and metabolic alkalosis; low plasma aldosterone and renin
Geller syndrome	AD mutation in the mineralocorticoid receptor AD mutations in the phosphodiesterase E3A enzyme	Hypokalemia and metabolic alkalosis; low plasma aldosterone and renin; increased BP during pregnancy or exposure to spironolactone
Hypertension-brachydactyly syndrome		
Unknown mechanisms		
Hypertension-brachydactyly syndrome	AD	Short fingers (small phalanges) and short stature; brain stem compression from vascular tortuosity in the posterior fossa
Essential Hypertension		
	Polygenic	When obesity or metabolic syndrome is present, the likelihood of essential hypertension is higher

AD, Autosomal dominant; *ADPKD,* autosomal dominant polycystic kidney disease; *AR,* autosomal recessive; *ARPKD,* autosomal recessive polycystic kidney disease; *BP,* blood pressure; *eGFR,* estimated glomerular filtration rate; *GN,* glomerulonephritis; *IgA,* immunoglobulin A; *MEN,* multiple endocrine neoplasia; *PKD,* polycystic kidney disease; *SDH,* succinate dehydrogenase.
From Skorecki K et al: *Brenner and Rector's the kidney,* ed 10, Philadelphia, 2016, Elsevier.

TABLE 4 Adrenocortical Causes of Hypertension

Low Renin and High Aldosterone

Primary Aldosteronism

1. Aldosterone-producing adenoma (APA)—30% of cases
2. Bilateral idiopathic hyperplasia (IHA)—60% of cases
3. Primary (unilateral) adrenal hyperplasia—2% of cases
4. Aldosterone-producing adrenocortical carcinoma—<1% of cases
5. Familial hyperaldosteronism (FH)
   a. FH type I (*CYP11B1/CYP11B2* germline chimeric gene)—<1% of cases
   b. FH type II (APA or IHA; germline *CLCN2* mutations—<6% of cases
   c. FH type III (germline *KCNJ5* mutations)—<1% of cases
   d. FH type IV (germline *CACNA1H* mutations)—<0.1% of cases
6. Ectopic aldosterone-producing adenoma or carcinoma—<0.1% of cases

Low Renin and Low Aldosterone

1. Congenital adrenal hyperplasia
   a. 11β-Hydroxylase deficiency
   b. 17α-Hydroxylase deficiency
2. Deoxycorticosterone-producing tumor
3. Primary cortisol resistance
4. Apparent mineralocorticoid excess (AME)/11β-HSD 2 deficiency
   a. Genetic
   b. Type 1 AME
   c. Type 2 AME
5. Acquired
   a. Licorice or carbenoxolone ingestion (type 1 AME)
   b. Cushing syndrome (type 2 AME)

Cushing Syndrome

1. Exogenous glucocorticoid administration—most common cause
2. Endogenous
   a. ACTH-dependent—85% of cases
      1) Pituitary
      2) Ectopic
   b. ACTH-independent—15% of cases
      1) Unilateral adrenal disease (adenoma or carcinoma)
      2) Bilateral adrenal disease
         a) Bilateral adenoma
         b) Macronodular hyperplasia
         c) Primary pigmented nodular adrenal disease (rare)

ACTH, Corticotropin; *HSD,* hydroxysteroid dehydrogenase.
From Melmed S et al: *Williams textbook of endocrinology,* ed 14, 2019, Elsevier.

TABLE 5 Initial Laboratory Evaluation of the Hypertensive Patient to Investigate the Presence of Comorbid Conditions, Secondary Causes, or Established Target-Organ Damage

Test	Clinical Usefulness
Serum creatinine (and estimated glomerular filtration rate)	Assessment of renal function. Identifies parenchymal kidney disease as a possible secondary cause as well as established TOD.
Serum potassium	Low potassium (of renal origin) suggests mineralocorticoid excess (primary or secondary), glucocorticoid excess, Liddle syndrome. High potassium with normal renal function suggests Gordon syndrome. Low levels raise caution about the use of thiazides and loop diuretics. High levels preclude the use of ACEIs, ARBs, renin inhibitors, and potassium-sparing diuretics.
Serum sodium	If high, suggests primary aldosteronism. If low, alerts to the need to avoid thiazide diuretics.
Serum bicarbonate	If high, suggests aldosterone excess (primary or secondary). If low with normal renal function, suggests Gordon syndrome (with high potassium) or primary hyperparathyroidism (with high calcium).
Serum calcium	If high, suggests primary hyperparathyroidism.
Serum glucose	Identifies prediabetes or diabetes. In the appropriate setting, suggests glucocorticoid excess, pheochromocytoma, or acromegaly.
Lipid profile	Identifies hyperlipidemia.
Hemoglobin/hematocrit	If high, in the absence of other hematologic abnormalities or underlying lung disease, suggests sleep apnea.
Urinalysis*	Proteinuria and hematuria identify a possible secondary cause (glomerulonephritis). Proteinuria can also be a marker of TOD.
Electrocardiogram	Identifies left ventricular hypertrophy, old myocardial infarction, or other ischemic changes. Identifies conduction abnormalities that may preclude the use of β-blockers or nondihydropyridine CCBs.

The most recent guidelines do not recommend blood urea nitrogen (BUN) measurement alone.
*Some organizations recommend screening microalbuminuria as a more sensitive tool to identify early renal injury.
ACEI, Angiotensin-converting enzyme inhibitor; *ARB,* angiotensin receptor blocker; *CCB,* calcium channel blocker; *TOD,* target-organ damage.
From Skorecki K et al: *Brenner and Rector's the kidney,* ed 10, Philadelphia, 2016, Elsevier.

cardiovascular disease risk, and produce a plan for individualized monitoring and therapy.
- Patient counseling and education should be prominent features of the initial evaluation.
- Pertinent history:
  1. Age of onset of HTN, previous antihypertensive therapy
  2. Family history of HTN, stroke, cardiovascular disease
- Diet, salt intake, caffeine, alcohol, drugs (e.g., oral contraceptives, NSAIDs, decongestants, steroids).
- Occupation, lifestyle, pain, socioeconomic status, psychologic factors.
- Other cardiovascular risk factors: Hyperlipidemia, obesity, diabetes mellitus.
- Symptoms of secondary HTN:
  1. Headache, palpitations, excessive perspiration (possible pheochromocytoma)
  2. Weakness, polyuria (consider hyperaldosteronism)
  3. Claudication of lower extremities (seen with coarctation of aorta)
  4. Loud snoring, daytime somnolence, morning confusion (may warrant evaluation for sleep apnea)

LABORATORY TESTS

- Routine laboratory tests recommended before initiating therapy include:
  1. Urinalysis with microscopic evaluation; for signs of glomerulopathy
  2. Basic metabolic panel and calcium; for signs of kidney damage, hypokalemia (primary aldosteronism and Cushing syndrome), hypercalcemia (hyperparathyroid)
  3. Complete blood count
  4. Screening for coexisting diseases that may adversely affect prognosis; hemoglobin A1c or fasting glucose level, serum lipid panel
  5. Optional tests include measurement of urinary albumin or albumin/creatinine ratio

IMAGING STUDIES

- ECG: Check for presence of left ventricular hypertrophy (LVH) with strain pattern.
- Renal duplex ultrasonography, CT angiography or magnetic resonance angiography of the renal arteries in suspected renovascular hypertension (renal artery stenosis) may be considered.

Rx TREATMENT

NONPHARMACOLOGIC THERAPY

Lifestyle modifications (the initial treatment of hypertension should focus on lifestyle modifications):
- Weight loss if overweight (target body mass index [BMI] <25).
- Limit alcohol intake to 1 oz of ethanol per day (<2 drinks/day) in men or 0.5 oz (<1 drink/day) in women.
- Regular aerobic exercise (at least 30 min/day on most days).
- Reduce sodium intake to <100 mmol/day (<1.5 g of sodium/day).
- Maintain adequate dietary potassium (>3500 mg/day) intake in patients with normal kidney function.
- Smoking cessation.
- The BP reduction seen ranges from 2 to 20 mm Hg, most significant with substantial weight loss and the implementation of the

Dietary Approaches to Stop Hypertension (DASH) eating plan, which relies on a diet high in fruits and vegetables, moderate in low-fat dairy products, and low in animal protein but with substantial amount of plant protein from legumes and nuts.

ACUTE GENERAL Rx

- Multiple recent consensus documents regarding blood pressure goals and when to initiate treatment have been published.
- According to the 2017 *ACC/AHA/AAPA/ABC/ACPM/AGS/APhA/ASH/ASPC/NMA/PCNA Guideline for the Prevention, Detection, Evaluation, and Management of High Blood Pressure in Adults*, goals of treatment are as follows:
  1. For adults with confirmed hypertension and known cardiovascular disease (CVD) or 10-yr atherosclerotic cardiovascular disease (ASCVD) event risk of 10% or higher, a BP target of less than 130/80 mm Hg is recommended.
  2. For adults with confirmed hypertension without additional markers of increased CVD risk, a BP target of less than 130/80 mm Hg may be reasonable.
- In addition, initiation of therapy recommendations is as follows:
  1. Use of BP-lowering medication is recommended for primary prevention of CVD in adults with no history of CVD and with an estimated 10-yr ASCVD risk <10% and stage 2 hypertension.
  2. Use of BP-lowering medications is recommended for secondary prevention of recurrent CVD events in patients with clinical CVD and for primary prevention in adults with an estimated 10-yr ASCVD risk of 10% or higher and stage 1 hypertension.
  3. Initiate antihypertensive drug therapy with two first-line agents of different classes for adults with stage 2 hypertension and BP more than 20/10 mm Hg higher than their target.
  4. It is reasonable to initiate therapy with a single agent for adults with stage 1 hypertension and a goal less than 130/80 mm Hg.
  5. Patients with diabetes mellitus and chronic kidney disease are considered high risk.
- Additional guidance may be taken from the writers of the JNC 8 guidelines, published in 2014:
  1. In the general non-Black population, preferred initial agents are thiazide-type diuretics, angiotensin-converting enzyme inhibitors (ACEI), calcium channel blockers (CCBs), or angiotensin receptor blockers (ARBs). ACEI or ARBs are preferred initial agents in diabetics and those with chronic kidney disease (CKD) in this population.
  2. Preferred initial agents in the Black population (including diabetics) are thiazide-type diuretics or CCBs.
  3. When selecting drugs, try to give once per day dosages to improve compliance. Also consider the cost of the medication, metabolic and subjective side effects, and drug-drug interactions.
- In a 2020 joint statement by HFSA/ACC/AHA regarding Using RAAS Antagonists in COVID-19:
  1. There is no clinical data demonstrating benefit or adverse outcomes with use of ACEI, ARB, or other RAAS antagonists.
  2. The recommendation is to refrain from adding or removing RAAS agents based on COVID-19 status and to continue standard clinical practice with these agents.
- The major advantages and limitations of each class of drugs are described as follows:
  1. Thiazide diuretics:
     a. Advantages: Inexpensive, once-daily dosing. Useful in edematous states, CHF, chronic renal disease, elderly patients (decreased incidence of hip fractures in elderly patients)
     b. Disadvantages: Significant adverse metabolic effects (hypokalemia), increased risk of cardiac arrhythmias, sexual dysfunction, gout flares, possible adverse effects on lipids and glucose levels
  2. Beta-blockers:
     a. Advantages: Ideal in hypertensive patients with ischemic heart disease or status post myocardial infarction (MI); favored in hyperkinetic, young patients (resting tachycardia, wide pulse pressure, hyperdynamic heart) and stable CHF patients
     b. Disadvantages: Adverse effect on quality of life (increased incidence of fatigue, depression, impotence), bronchospasm, hypoglycemia, peripheral vascular disease, adverse effects on lipids, masking of signs and symptoms of hypoglycemia in diabetics
  3. Calcium antagonists:
     a. Advantages: Helpful in hypertensive patients with ischemic heart disease. Generally favorable effect on quality of life; can be used in patients with bronchospastic disorders, renal disease, peripheral vascular disease, metabolic disorders, and salt sensitivity. CCBs' BP-lowering effect is independent of Na^+ intake.
     b. Disadvantages: Diltiazem and verapamil should be avoided in patients with CHF caused by systolic dysfunction because of their negative inotropic effects; pedal edema may occur with nifedipine and amlodipine; constipation can be severe in elderly patients receiving verapamil. CCB-related edema is positional in nature, but it improves with lying position; additional strategies include switching CCB classes, reducing dosage, giving the medication later in the day, and adding a venodilator (nitrates, an ACE, or an ARB); diuretics may improve edema, but at the expense of a reduction in plasma volume.
  4. ACE inhibitors:
     a. Advantages: First-line therapy for patients with left ventricular dysfunction, helpful in prevention of diabetic renal disease; effective in decreasing LVH, and remodeling.
     b. Disadvantages: Dry cough is a frequent side effect (5% to 20% of patients); hyperkalemia may occur in patients with diabetes or severe renal insufficiency; hypotension may occur in volume-depleted patients; increased risk of renal failure in patients with renal artery stenosis; contraindicated in pregnancy.
  5. ARBs:
     a. Advantages: Well tolerated, favorable impact on quality of life; useful in patients unable to tolerate ACE inhibitors because of persistent cough and in CHF and diabetic patients; single daily dose. An episode of renal insufficiency with ACE inhibitors does not rule out future therapy with an ARB unless high-grade bilateral renal artery stenosis exists.
     b. Disadvantages: Hypotension may occur in volume-depleted patients; hyperkalemia; risk of renal failure in renal artery stenosis; contraindicated in pregnancy.
  6. Alpha-adrenergic blockers:
     a. Advantages: No adverse effect on blood lipids or insulin sensitivity; helpful in benign prostatic hypertrophy.
     b. Disadvantages: Postural hypotension, sedation; syncope can be avoided by giving an initial low dose at bedtime. Generally considered third- or fourth-line agent.
  7. Central alpha-antagonists:
     a. Oral clonidine mainstay of therapy for hypertensive urgencies because of the ease of administration and relative safety.
     b. Transdermal clonidine; useful in management of labile HTN, the hospitalized patient who cannot take medications by mouth, and patients subject to early-morning BP surges. At equivalent doses, transdermal clonidine is more apt to precipitate salt and water retention than is the case with oral clonidine.
     c. Dose beyond 0.4 mg causes fatigue, sedation, dry mouth, salt and water retention, and rebound HTN upon abrupt termination of the medication.
  8. Combined alpha- and beta-adrenergic receptor blockers:
     a. Labetalol, nebivolol, and carvedilol: Use is reserved to treat complicated hypertensive patient when an antihypertensive effect beyond beta-blockade is sought. IV labetalol is used for hypertensive emergencies. Carvedilol is shown to have less adverse effect

TABLE 6 Drugs Used to Treat Hypertension in Pregnancy

Drug	Starting Dose	Maximum Dose	Comments
Acute Treatment of Severe Hypertension			
Hydralazine	5-10 mg IV every 20 min	20 mg*	Avoid in cases of tachycardia and persistent headaches
Labetalol	20-40 mg IV every 10-15 min	220 mg*	Avoid in women with asthma or congestive heart failure
Nifedipine	10-20 mg oral every 30 min	50 mg*	Avoid in case of tachycardia and palpitations
Long-Term Treatment of Hypertension			
Methyldopa	250 mg bid	4 g/day	
Labetalol	100 mg bid	2400 mg/day	
Nifedipine	10 mg bid	120 mg/day	
Thiazide diuretic	12.5 mg bid	50 mg/day	

*If desired blood pressure levels are not achieved, switch to another drug.
bid, Twice daily; *IV,* intravenous.
From Gabbe SG: *Obstetrics,* ed 6, Philadelphia, 2012, Saunders.

on glycemic control than metoprolol and to reduce urinary protein excretion in hypertensive diabetic patients.

9. Direct-acting smooth muscle relaxant: Hydralazine
   a. Advantages: Beneficial in Black patients when used with isosorbide dinitrate.
   b. Disadvantages: May lead to reflex tachycardia, worsening ischemia (best used with nitrates), at higher doses or with renal failure can lead to a reversible drug-induced lupus.
10. Renin inhibitors: Newest class of antihypertensives (Aliskiren):
    a. Advantages: Generally well tolerated; once-daily dosing; can be used alone or in combination with other antihypertensive agents (avoid combining with ACEI or ARBs given increase of hyperkalemia).
    b. Disadvantages: Contraindicated in pregnancy; should not be used in patients with impaired renal function; excessive cost; paucity of cardiovascular outcomes data showing benefit.

TREATMENT OF RENOVASCULAR HYPERTENSION: The therapeutic approach varies with the cause of the renovascular hypertension (RVH) (refer to "Renal Artery Stenosis" for additional information).

- Young patients with fibromuscular dysplasia refractory to medical therapy can be treated with percutaneous transluminal renal angioplasty (PTRA).
- Medical therapy is advisable in elderly patients with atheromatous RVH; useful agents are:
  1. Beta-blockers: Highly effective in patients with elevated plasma renin
  2. ACE inhibitors: Highly effective; however, should be avoided in patients with bilateral renal artery stenosis or with a solitary kidney and renal artery stenosis
  3. Diuretics: Often used in combination with ACE inhibitors
- Surgical revascularization: A recent trial revealed that renal-artery stenting does not confer a significant benefit with respect to the prevention of clinical events when added to comprehensive, multifactorial medical therapy in people with atherosclerotic renal-artery stenosis and hypertension or CKD.

HTN DURING PREGNANCY:

- HTN complicates 5% to 12% of all pregnancies.
- The American Obstetrical Committee defines BP of 130/80 mm Hg as the upper limit of normal at any time during pregnancy.
- A rise of 30 mm Hg systolic or 15 mm Hg diastolic is also considered abnormal regardless of the absolute values obtained.
- Hypertension during pregnancy can be from chronic HTN, gestational HTN, preeclampsia or preeclampsia superimposed on chronic HTN. It is important to distinguish the etiology because the risk to mother and fetus is much greater in preeclampsia.
- Treatment of chronic HTN during pregnancy is as follows:
  a. Initial treatment with conservative measures (proper nutrition, limited physical activity).
  b. When drug therapy is necessary, initiation of methyldopa, hydralazine, labetalol or nifedipine is preferred. Table 6 summarizes drugs used to treat hypertension in pregnancy.
  c. ACE inhibitors can cause fetal and neonatal complications; their use should be avoided in pregnancy.
  d. The safety of CCBs remains unclear.
  e. Diuretics should be used only if there is a specific reason for initiating and maintaining their use (e.g., HTN associated with severe fluid overload or left ventricular dysfunction).

MALIGNANT HTN, HYPERTENSIVE EMERGENCIES, AND HYPERTENSIVE URGENCIES:
Definitions:

- Malignant HTN occurs with HTN when there are grades III and IV retinopathy (exudates, hemorrhages, and papilledema).
  1. The rate of BP rise is a critical factor in the development of malignant HTN.
  2. Complications and mortality rates are much higher in malignant HTN compared with essential HTN.
  3. Requires immediate BP reduction (not necessarily into normal ranges) to prevent or limit target organ disease.
- Hypertensive emergencies occur when the BP elevation is >180 mm Hg systolic and/or >120 mm Hg diastolic without evidence of new or progressive organ dysfunction. It requires rapid lowering of BP to prevent end-organ damage.
- Hypertensive urgencies are BP elevations >180 mm Hg systolic and/or >120 mm Hg diastolic with end-organ damage that should be corrected within 24 hr of presentation.
  1. Most clinicians suggest lowering the BP to <160 mm Hg/<100 mm Hg or to a level no more than 30% lower than the patient's baseline BP.

Therapy: The choice of therapeutic agents varies with the cause. IV medications are preferred in hypertensive emergencies.

- Nitroprusside is the drug of choice in hypertensive encephalopathy, HTN and intracranial bleeding, malignant HTN, HTN and heart failure, dissecting aortic aneurysm (used in combination with propranolol); its onset of action is immediate. Because it is metabolized to cyanide, patients should be carefully monitored for toxicity (mental status changes, acidemia).
- Fenoldopam is a vasodilator agent useful for the short-term (up to 48 hr) management of severe HTN when rapid but quickly reversible reduction of BP is required. It should be avoided in patients with glaucoma.
- Other commonly used agents are the IV CCBs nicardipine and clevidipine (useful for urgent treatment of HTN in the ICU or operating room), the beta-blocker esmolol (useful in aortic dissection or postoperative HTN), labetalol (combined β-adrenergic and α-blocker useful in patients with coronary disease), phentolamine (useful for catecholamine-related emergencies), IV nitroglycerin (used in patients with cardiac ischemia and hypertensive crisis), and hydralazine (used for hypertensive emergencies in pregnancy.
- Table 7 summarizes IV medications useful in hypertensive crisis.

The following are important points to remember when treating hypertensive emergencies:

- Introduce a plan for long-term therapy at the time of the initial emergency treatment.
- Agents that reduce arterial pressure can cause the kidney to retain sodium and water; therefore, the judicious administration of diuretics should accompany their use.
- The initial goal of antihypertensive therapy is not to achieve a normal BP, but rather to gradually reduce the BP; cerebral hypoperfusion may occur if the mean BP is hypertension in patients with CKD.

PEARLS & CONSIDERATIONS

COMMENTS

- "Masked hypertension" refers to the detection of hypertension with home or ambulatory

TABLE 7 Treatment of Hypertensive Crisis: Intravenous Medications

Drug Name and Mechanism of Action	Indications/Advantages/Dose	Disadvantages/Adverse Effects/Metabolism Cautions
Sodium Nitroprusside		
Nitric oxide compound; vasodilation of arteriolar and venous smooth muscle Increases cardiac output by decreasing afterload	Useful in most hypertensive emergencies Onset of action immediate, duration of action 1-2 min Dose: 0.25 μg/kg/min Maximum dose: 8-10 μg/kg/min	Contraindicated in high-output cardiac failure, congenital optic atrophy. Anemia and liver disease at risk of cyanide toxicity: Acidosis, tachycardia, change in mental status, almond smell on breath. Risk of thiocyanate toxicity with renal disease: Psychosis, hyperreflexia, seizure, tinnitus. Cautious use with increased intracranial pressure. Do not use maximum dose for more than 10 min. Crosses the placenta.
Nitroglycerin		
Directly interacts with nitrate receptors on vascular smooth muscle Primarily dilates venous bed Decreases preload	Use with symptoms of cardiac ischemia, perioperative hypertension in cardiac surgery Initial dose: 5 μg/min Maximum dose: 100 μg/min	Contraindicated in angle-closure glaucoma, increased intracranial pressure. Blood pressure decreased secondary to decreased preload, cardiac output—avoid when cerebral or renal perfusion compromised. Caution with right ventricular infarct.
Labetalol		
β- and α-Adrenergic blockade α:β-Blocking ratio is 1:7	Onset of action 2-5 min, duration 3-6 hr Bolus 20 mg, then 20-80 mg every 10 min for maximum dose 300 mg Infuse at 0.5-2 mg/min	Avoid in bronchospasm, bradycardia, congestive heart failure, greater than first-degree heart block, second/third trimester pregnancy. Use caution with hepatic dysfunction, inhalational anesthetics (myocardial depression). Enters breast milk.
Esmolol		
Cardioselective β1-adrenergic blocking agent	Use with aortic dissection Use during intubation, intraoperative, and postoperative hypertension Onset of action 60 sec, duration 10-20 min, 200-500 μg/kg/min for 4 min, then infuse 50-300 μg/kg/min	See labetalol. Not dependent on renal or hepatic function for metabolism (metabolized by hydrolysis in red blood cells).
Fenoldopam		
Postsynaptic dopamine-1 agonist; decreases peripheral vascular resistance; 10 times more potent than dopamine as vasodilator	May be advantageous in kidney disease, increases renal blood flow, increases sodium excretion, no toxic metabolites Initial dose: 0.1 μg/kg/min, with titration every 15 min No bolus	Contraindicated in glaucoma (may increase intraocular pressure) or allergy to sulfites; hypotension, especially with concurrent β-blocker. Check serum potassium every 6 hr. Concurrent acetaminophen may significantly increase blood levels. Dose-related tachycardia.
Hydralazine		
Primarily dilates arteriolar vasculature	Primarily used in pregnancy/eclampsia Dose: 10 mg every 20-130 min; maximum dose 20 mg Decreases blood pressure in 10-20 min Duration of action 2-4 hr	Reflex tachycardia; give β-blocker concurrently. May exacerbate angina. Half-life 3 hr, affects blood pressure for 100 hr. Depends on hepatic acetylation for inactivation.
Phentolamine		
α-Adrenergic blockade	Used primarily to treat hypertension from excessive catecholamine excess (e.g., pheochromocytoma) Dose: 5-15 mg Onset of action 1-2 min, duration 3-10 min	β-Blockade is generally added to control tachycardia or arrhythmias. As in all catecholamine excess states, β-blockers should never be given first, as the loss of β-adrenergically mediated vasodilatation will leave α-adrenergically mediated vasoconstriction unopposed and result in increased pressure.
Nicardipine		
Dihydropyridine calcium channel blocker; inhibits transmembrane influx of calcium ions into cardiac and smooth muscle	Onset of action 10-20 min, duration 1-4 hr Initial dose: 5 mg/hr to maximum of 15 mg/hr	Avoid with congestive heart failure, cardiac ischemia. Adverse effects include tachycardia, flushing, headache.
Clevidipine		
Short-acting dihydropyridine calcium channel antagonist	Initial dose: 1 mg/hr; can be increased to 21 mg/hr	Reduces blood pressure without affecting cardiac filling pressures or causing reflex tachycardia.
Enalaprilat		
Angiotensin-converting enzyme inhibitor	Onset of action 15-20 min, duration 12-24 hr Dose: 1.25-5 mg every 6 hr	Response not predictable, with high renin states may see acute hypotension. Hyperkalemia in setting of reduced glomerular filtration rate. Avoid in pregnancy.
Trimethaphan		
Nondepolarizing ganglionic blocking agent; competes with acetylcholine for postsynaptic receptors	Used in aortic dissection Dose: 0.5-5 mg/min	Does not increase cardiac output. No inotropic cardiac effect. Disadvantages include parasympathetic blockade, resulting in paralytic ileus and bladder atony and development of tachyphylaxis after 24-96 hr of use.

From Vincent JL et al: *Textbook of critical care*, ed 7, Philadelphia, 2017, Elsevier.

monitoring. Up to 40% of patients with BP less than 140/90 mm Hg in the office may have masked hypertension. Automated blood pressure monitors are useful to screen for masked hypertension.

- "White coat hypertension" is defined as an elevated BP during medical office exam, whereas BP is in the normal range while at home. Its prevalence is as high as 30% among patients with an elevated BP in the office. These patients are at increased risk for overt hypertension.
- For patients with hypertension, every 20/10 mm Hg increase in BP doubles the risk of cardiovascular events.
- Most patients will require at least two medications for BP control.
- If BP is greater than 20/10 mm Hg above goal, therapy should be initiated with two drugs.
- Resistant HTN: HTN is considered resistant if the BP cannot be reduced below target levels in patients who are compliant with an optimal triple-drug regimen that includes a diuretic. Terms *refractory* and *resistant* are used interchangeably. Causes include pseudohypertension, measurement artifact, medication nonadherence, volume overload, and secondary HTN.
  1. Pseudohypertension in elderly: Hardened and sclerotic artery is not compressible; hence, falsely elevates BP measurement artifact.
  2. Measurement artifact: BP taken incorrectly (small cuff, improper support).
- Renal sympathetic denervation: A recent blinded trial did not show a significant reduction of systolic blood pressure in patients with resistant hypertension 6 mo after renal artery denervation as compared with a sham control.
- Barriers to BP control: System issues, provider issues; patient issues, and behavior issues. The rate at which physicians adopt recommended changes based on evidence-based findings can be quite slow and has been properly described as "clinical inertia."
- Indications for specialist referral for patients with HTN are described in Table 8.
- New U.S. guidelines for the treatment of hypertension recommend the following:
  1. Use of BP-lowering medication for secondary prevention in patients with cardiovascular disease and average systolic blood pressure (SBP) ≥130 mm Hg or diastolic blood pressure (DBP) ≥80 mm Hg, and for primary prevention in adults with an estimated 10-yr ASCVD risk of >10% and an average SBP ≥130 mm Hg or DBP ≥80 mm Hg.
  2. In patients with no history of cardiovascular disease and an estimated 10-yr ASCVD risk <10%, BP-lowering medication is recommended for those with an average SBP ≥140 mm Hg or an average DBP ≥90 mm Hg.

TABLE 8 Indications for Specialist Referral for Patients with Hypertension

Urgent Treatment Needed
Accelerated hypertension (severe hypertension with grade III-IV retinopathy)
Particularly severe hypertension (>220/120 mm Hg)
Impending complications (e.g., transient ischemic attack, left ventricular failure)
Possible Underlying Cause
Any clue in history or examination of a secondary cause (e.g., hypokalemia with increased or high–normal plasma sodium)
Elevated serum creatinine
Proteinuria or hematuria
Sudden onset or worsening of hypertension
Young age (any hypertension <20 yr; needing treatment <30 yr)
Therapeutic Problems
Multiple drug intolerances
Multiple drug contraindications
Persistent nonadherence or nonconcordance
Special Situations
Unusual blood pressure variability
Possible white coat hypertension
Hypertension in pregnancy

From Floege J et al: *Comprehensive clinical nephrology*, ed 4, Philadelphia, 2010, Saunders.

SUGGESTED READINGS

Available at ExpertConsult.com

RELATED CONTENT

High Blood Pressure (Patient Information)
High Blood Pressure—Child (Patient Information)
Eclampsia (Related Key Topic)
Pheochromocytoma (Related Key Topic)
Preeclampsia (Related Key Topic)
Renal Artery Stenosis (Related Key Topic)

AUTHOR: **Tania B. Babar, MD**

BASIC INFORMATION

DEFINITION

Hyperthyroidism is a hypermetabolic state resulting from excess thyroid hormone. Thyrotoxicosis is a general term for excess circulating and tissue hormone levels.

SYNONYM

Thyrotoxicosis

ICD-10CM CODES	
E05.00	Thyrotoxicosis with diffuse goiter without thyrotoxic crisis or storm
E05.01	Thyrotoxicosis with diffuse goiter with thyrotoxic crisis or storm
E05.10	Thyrotoxicosis with toxic single thyroid nodule without thyrotoxic crisis or storm
E05.11	Thyrotoxicosis with toxic single thyroid nodule with thyrotoxic crisis or storm
E05.20	Thyrotoxicosis with toxic multinodular goiter without thyrotoxic crisis or storm
E05.21	Thyrotoxicosis with toxic multinodular goiter with thyrotoxic crisis or storm
E05.30	Thyrotoxicosis from ectopic thyroid tissue without thyrotoxic crisis or storm
E05.31	Thyrotoxicosis from ectopic thyroid tissue with thyrotoxic crisis or storm
E05.40	Thyrotoxicosis factitia without thyrotoxic crisis or storm
E05.41	Thyrotoxicosis factitia with thyrotoxic crisis or storm
E05.80	Other thyrotoxicosis without thyrotoxic crisis or storm
E05.81	Other thyrotoxicosis with thyrotoxic crisis or storm
E05.90	Thyrotoxicosis, unspecified without thyrotoxic crisis or storm
E05.91	Thyrotoxicosis, unspecified with thyrotoxic crisis or storm
E06.2	Chronic thyroiditis with transient thyrotoxicosis

EPIDEMIOLOGY & DEMOGRAPHICS

INCIDENCE & PREVALENCE:

- Hyperthyroidism affects 2% of women and 0.2% of men in their lifetimes.
- Toxic multinodular goiter usually occurs in women >55 yr and is more common than Graves disease in the elderly.

PHYSICAL FINDINGS & CLINICAL PRESENTATION

- Patients with hyperthyroidism generally present with tachycardia, tremor, hyperreflexia, anxiety, irritability, emotional lability, panic attacks, heat intolerance, sweating, increased appetite, diarrhea, weight loss, menstrual dysfunction (oligomenorrhea, amenorrhea). Presentation may be different in elderly patients (see the following).
- Patients with Graves disease may present with exophthalmos, lid retraction, and lid lag (Graves ophthalmopathy). The following signs and symptoms of ophthalmopathy may be present: blurring of vision, photophobia, increased lacrimation, double vision, and deep orbital pressure. Clubbing of fingers associated with periosteal new bone formation in other skeletal areas (Graves acropachy) and pretibial myxedema may also be noted.
- Clinical signs of hyperthyroidism in the elderly may be masked by manifestations of coexisting disease (e.g., new-onset atrial fibrillation, exacerbation of congestive heart failure).

ETIOLOGY (TABLE 1)

- Graves disease (diffuse toxic goiter): 80% to 90% of all cases of hyperthyroidism
- Toxic multinodular goiter (Plummer disease)
- Toxic adenoma
- Iatrogenic and factitious
- Transient hyperthyroidism (subacute thyroiditis, Hashimoto thyroiditis)
- Rare causes: Hypersecretion of thyroid-stimulating hormone (TSH) (e.g., pituitary neoplasms), struma ovarii, ingestion of large amount of iodine in a patient with preexisting thyroid hyperplasia or adenoma (Jod-Basedow phenomenon), hydatidiform mole, carcinoma of thyroid, amiodarone therapy

DIAGNOSIS

DIFFERENTIAL DIAGNOSIS

- Anxiety disorder
- Pheochromocytoma
- Metastatic neoplasm

TABLE 1 Causes of Hyperthyroidism

I. Excessive TSH-Receptor Stimulation
Graves disease (TRAb)
Pregnancy-associated transient hyperthyroidism (hCG)
Trophoblastic disease (hCG)
Familial gestational hyperthyroidism (mutant TSH receptor)
TSH-producing pituitary adenoma
II. Autonomous Thyroid Hormone Secretion
Multinodular toxic goiter (somatic mutations)
Solitary toxic thyroid adenoma (somatic mutation)
Congenital activating TSH-receptor mutation (genomic mutation)
III. Destruction of Follicles with Release of Hormone
Subacute de Quervain thyroiditis (virus infection)
Painless thyroiditis/postpartum thyroiditis (hashitoxicosis—autoimmune)
Acute thyroiditis (bacterial infection)
Drug-induced thyroiditis (amiodarone, interferon-γ)
IV. Extrathyroidal Sources of Thyroid Hormone
Iatrogenic overreplacement with thyroid hormone
Excessive self-administered thyroid medication
Food and supplements containing excessive thyroid hormone
Functional thyroid cancer metastases
Struma ovarii

hCG, Human chorionic gonadotropin; *TRAb,* thyrotropin-receptor antibodies; *TSH,* thyroid-stimulating hormone (thyrotropin).

From Melmed S et al: *Williams textbook of endocrinology,* ed 14, St Louis, 2019, Elsevier.

- Diabetes mellitus
- Premenopausal state

WORKUP

Suspected hyperthyroidism requires laboratory confirmation and identification of its etiology because treatment varies with cause. A detailed medical history will often provide clues to the diagnosis and etiology of the hyperthyroidism. Fig. E1 describes a diagnostic approach to suspected hyperthyroidism.

LABORATORY TESTS

- Elevated free thyroxine (T_4)
- Elevated free triiodothyronine (T_3): Generally not necessary for diagnosis
- Low TSH (unless hyperthyroidism is a result of the rare hypersecretion of TSH from a pituitary adenoma). Serum TSH is the best test for diagnosis of thyrotoxicosis.
- Thyroid autoantibodies useful in selected cases to differentiate Graves disease from toxic multinodular goiter (absent thyroid antibodies)

IMAGING STUDIES

- 24-hour radioactive iodine uptake (RAIU) is useful to distinguish hyperthyroidism from iatrogenic thyroid hormone synthesis (thyrotoxicosis factitia) and from thyroiditis.
- An overactive thyroid shows increased uptake, whereas a normal underactive thyroid (iatrogenic thyroid ingestion, painless or subacute thyroiditis) shows normal or decreased uptake.
- The RAIU results also vary with the etiology of the hyperthyroidism:
  1. Graves disease: Increased homogeneous uptake
  2. Multinodular goiter: Increased heterogeneous uptake
  3. Hot nodule: Single focus of increased uptake
- RAIU is also generally performed before the therapeutic administration of radioactive iodine to determine the appropriate dose.

TREATMENT

NONPHARMACOLOGIC THERAPY

Patient education regarding thyroid disease and discussion of the therapeutic options. Avoidance of strenuous physical exercise, caffeine, and tobacco in patients with uncontrolled thyrotoxicosis. Patients should be informed that radioiodine, antithyroid drugs, and surgery are all reasonable treatment options for hyperthyroidism. It is crucial for the physician to have a detailed discussion with the patient about the benefits and risks relative to lifestyle, patients' values, and coexisting conditions.

ACUTE GENERAL Rx

ANTITHYROID DRUGS (THIONAMIDES): Propylthiouracil (PTU) and methimazole inhibit thyroid hormone synthesis by blocking production of thyroid peroxidase (PTU and methimazole) or inhibit peripheral conversion of T_4 to T_3 (PTU). Methimazole is favored by most endocrinologists because of the potential for hepatic failure with PTU. PTU is preferred in pregnant women during the first trimester because methimazole has been associated with aplasia cutis and with choanal and esophageal atresia. Complete blood count and differential should be obtained before their use.

- Dosage: Methimazole 15 to 30 mg/day given as a single dose; PTU 50 to 100 mg PO q8h.
- Antithyroid drugs can be used as the primary form of treatment or as adjunctive therapy before radioactive therapy or surgery or afterward if the hyperthyroidism recurs.
- Side effects: Skin rash (3% to 5% of patients), arthralgias, myalgias, granulocytopenia (0.5%). Rare side effects are aplastic anemia, hepatic necrosis from PTU, cholestatic jaundice from methimazole.
- When antithyroid drugs are used as primary therapy, they are usually given for 6 to 18 mo; prolonged therapy may cause hypothyroidism. Monitor thyroid function every 2 mo for 6 mo, then less frequently.
- The use of antithyroid drugs before radioiodine therapy is best reserved for patients in whom exacerbation of hyperthyroidism after radioactive iodine therapy is hazardous (e.g., elderly patients with coronary artery disease or significant coexisting morbidity). In these patients the antithyroid drug can be stopped 2 days before radioactive iodine therapy, resumed 2 days later, and continued for 4 to 6 wk.

RADIOIODINE THERAPY (RADIOACTIVE IODINE [RAI; ^{131}I]):

- RAI is the treatment of choice for patients age >21 yr and younger patients who have not achieved remission after 1 yr of antithyroid drug therapy. RAI is also used in hyperthyroidism caused by toxic adenoma or toxic multinodular goiter.
- Contraindicated during pregnancy (can cause fetal hypothyroidism) and lactation. Pregnancy should be excluded in women of childbearing age before RAI is administered.
- A single dose of RAI is effective in inducing a euthyroid state in nearly 80% of patients.
- There is a high incidence of post-RAI hypothyroidism (>50% within first yr and 2%/yr thereafter); these patients should be frequently evaluated for the onset of hypothyroidism (see "Chronic Rx").

SURGICAL THERAPY (SUBTOTAL THYROIDECTOMY):

- Indicated in obstructing goiters, in any patient who refuses RAI and cannot be adequately managed with antithyroid medications (e.g., patients with toxic adenoma or toxic multinodular goiter), and in pregnant patients who cannot be adequately managed with antithyroid medication or develop side effects to them. Thyroidectomy can also be considered as primary therapy in refractory cases of amiodarone-induced hyperthyroidism. Thyroidectomy is not indicated for low RAIU hyperthyroidism.
- Patients should be rendered euthyroid with antithyroid drugs before surgery.
- Complications of surgery include hypothyroidism (28% to 43% after 10 yr), hypoparathyroidism, and vocal cord paralysis (1%).
- Most patients should be started on replacement doses of levothyroxine (1.7 mcg/kg/day) before discharge from hospital.
- Hyperthyroidism recurs after surgery in 10% to 15% of patients.

ADJUNCTIVE THERAPY: Propranolol alleviates the beta-adrenergic symptoms of hyperthyroidism; initial dose is 20 to 40 mg PO q6h; dosage is gradually increased until symptoms are controlled. Major contraindications to propranolol are congestive heart failure and bronchospasm. Diagnosis and treatment of thyrotoxic storm are also discussed in Section I.

CHRONIC Rx

- Patients undergoing treatment with antithyroid drugs should be seen every 1 to 3 mo until euthyroidism is achieved and every 3 to 4 mo while they remain on antithyroid therapy. After treatment is stopped, periodic monitoring of thyroid function tests with TSH is recommended every 3 mo for 1 yr, then every 6 mo for 1 yr, then annually.
- Orbital decompression surgery can be used to correct Graves orbitopathy (Fig. E2). The administration of the antioxidant selenium (100 mcg PO bid) has been recently reported as effective in improving quality of life, reducing ocular involvement, and slowing progression of the disease in patients with mild Graves orbitopathy. Its mechanism of action is believed to be an effect on the oxygen free radicals and cytokines that play a pathogenic role in Graves orbitopathy.

DISPOSITION

Successful treatment of hyperthyroidism requires lifelong monitoring for the onset of hypothyroidism or the recurrence of thyrotoxicosis.

REFERRAL

- Endocrinology referral is recommended at the time of initial diagnosis and during treatment.
- Surgical referral in selected patients (see "Surgical Therapy").
- Hospitalization of all patients with thyroid storm.

PEARLS & CONSIDERATIONS

COMMENTS

- Elderly hyperthyroid patients may have only subtle signs (weight loss, tachycardia, fine skin, brittle nails). This form is known as ***apathetic hyperthyroidism*** and manifests with lethargy rather than hyperkinetic activity. An enlarged thyroid gland may be absent. Coexisting medical disorders (most commonly cardiac disease) may also mask the symptoms. These patients often have unexplained congestive heart failure, worsening of angina, or new-onset atrial fibrillation resistant to treatment. See the topic "Graves Disease" for additional information on diagnosis and treatment.
- **Subclinical hyperthyroidism** is defined as a normal serum-free thyroxine and free triiodothyronine levels with a TSH level suppressed below the normal range and usually undetectable. Prevalence in the general population is 1% to 2%. These patients usually do not present with signs or symptoms of overt hyperthyroidism. Subclinical hyperthyroidism is associated with an increased risk of atrial fibrillation and heart failure in older adults. Treatment options include observation or a therapeutic trial of low-dose antithyroid agents for 6 mo to attempt to induce remission. The American Thyroid Association and the American Association of Clinical Endocrinologists recommend treatment of patients with TSH levels <0.1 mIU if they are older than 65 or have associated comorbidities (osteoporosis, heart failure).
- ***Thyrotoxic periodic paralysis (TPP)*** is a hyperthyroidism-related hypokalemia and muscle-weakening condition resulting from a sudden shift of potassium into cells. Many patients do not have other symptoms of hyperthyroidism. Typical presentation involves an Asian adult male with acute fatigue and muscle weakness initially presenting in the lower extremities. Physical examination reveals decreased deep tendon reflexes, hypertension, and tachycardia. ECG often reveals U waves, high QRS voltage, and first-degree atrioventricular block. Additional laboratory testing reveals normal acid-base state, hypokalemia with low urinary potassium excretion (spot urinary potassium concentration <20 mEq/L from potassium shift into cells), hypophosphatemia, hypophosphaturia, and hypercalciuria. Electromyography during attacks shows low-amplitude compound muscle action potential of the tested muscle. Therapy consists of cautious potassium supplementation (increased risk of rebound hyperkalemia). Use of nonselective beta-blockers (e.g., propranolol) to counteract hyperadrenergic activity, which may be causing TPP, may also be useful.

RELATED CONTENT

Hyperthyroidism (Patient Information)
Graves Disease (Related Key Topic)
Thyrotoxic Storm (Related Key Topic)

SUGGESTED READINGS

Available at ExpertConsult.com

AUTHOR: **Fred F. Ferri, MD**

BASIC INFORMATION

DEFINITION

Hypertrophic osteoarthropathy (HOA) is a syndrome of abnormal proliferation of the skin and osseous tissues. Clubbing of the digits, periostitis of long bones, and synovial effusions can be seen. Clubbing may be asymptomatic, but patients with periostitis often have deep aching in long bones. HOA may be primary or secondary to other underlying disease processes such as cancer.

SYNONYMS

Primary hypertrophic osteoarthropathy
Pachydermoperiostosis
Idiopathic clubbing
Touraine-Solente-Golé syndrome
Secondary hypertrophic osteoarthropathy
HOA

ICD-10CM CODES

M89.3	Hypertrophy of bone
M89.40	Other hypertrophic osteoarthropathy, unspecified site
M89.411	Other hypertrophic osteoarthropathy, right shoulder
M89.412	Other hypertrophic osteoarthropathy, left shoulder
M89.419	Other hypertrophic osteoarthropathy, unspecified shoulder
M89.421	Other hypertrophic osteoarthropathy, right upper arm
M89.422	Other hypertrophic osteoarthropathy, left upper arm
M89.429	Other hypertrophic osteoarthropathy, unspecified upper arm
M89.431	Other hypertrophic osteoarthropathy, right forearm
M89.432	Other hypertrophic osteoarthropathy, left forearm
M89.439	Other hypertrophic osteoarthropathy, unspecified forearm
M89.441	Other hypertrophic osteoarthropathy, right hand
M89.442	Other hypertrophic osteoarthropathy, left hand
M89.449	Other hypertrophic osteoarthropathy, unspecified hand
M89.451	Other hypertrophic osteoarthropathy, right thigh
M89.452	Other hypertrophic osteoarthropathy, left thigh
M89.459	Other hypertrophic osteoarthropathy, unspecified thigh
M89.461	Other hypertrophic osteoarthropathy, right lower leg
M89.462	Other hypertrophic osteoarthropathy, left lower leg
M89.469	Other hypertrophic osteoarthropathy, unspecified lower leg
M89.471	Other hypertrophic osteoarthropathy, right ankle and foot
M89.472	Other hypertrophic osteoarthropathy, left ankle and foot
M89.479	Other hypertrophic osteoarthropathy, unspecified ankle and foot
M89.48	Other hypertrophic osteoarthropathy, other site
M89.49	Other hypertrophic osteoarthropathy, multiple sites

EPIDEMIOLOGY & DEMOGRAPHICS

- Fig. 1 provides a classification of HOA.
- Primary HOA is a rare familial autosomal-dominant disease affecting the age group between 1 and 20 yr.
- There is a male:female ratio of 9:1.
- Secondary HOA is more common, typically occurs in adults ages 55 to 75 yr. 80% to 90% of secondary HOA is associated with non–small cell lung cancer, most frequently adenocarcinoma; other associated illnesses include:
  1. Pulmonary: Mesothelioma, bronchogenic carcinoma, lung abscesses, empyema, bronchiectasis, cystic fibrosis, pulmonary fibrosis, sarcoidosis, arteriovenous malformations
  2. Gastrointestinal: Carcinoma of esophagus or colon, biliary atresia, peptic ulcer disease, inflammatory bowel disease, hepatocellular carcinoma, liver cirrhosis, amebiasis, laxative abuse, achalasia
  3. Cardiac: Infective endocarditis, right-to-left cardiac shunts, aortic aneurysms, infected aortic bypass graft
  4. Hematologic: Thalassemia, myelofibrosis, Hodgkin lymphoma
  5. Endocrine: Thyroid acropachy, POEMS syndrome (polyneuropathy, organomegaly, endocrinopathy, monoclonal gammopathy, skin abnormalities)
  6. Connective tissue diseases
  7. Thymoma
  8. HIV infection
  9. Osteosarcoma
  10. Nasopharyngeal sarcoma

PHYSICAL FINDINGS & CLINICAL PRESENTATION

- Primary HOA typically presents with the insidious onset of clubbing of the hands and feet, described as "spade-like." Finger clubbing is diagnosed by measurement of the digital index (Fig. 2). Other signs and symptoms of HOA include:
  1. Joint pain and swelling
  2. Sensation of warmth or burning in the hands and feet
  3. Coarsening of facial features with grooves or depressions in the scalp, ptosis of the lids
  4. Thickening of the arms and legs
  5. Oily skin, diaphoresis, gynecomastia, and acne
  6. Thin and shiny appearance of the skin around the nail bed
  7. Nail convexity with nail "floating" sensation within the soft tissue is noticed on palpation of the base of the nail bed
  8. Elephant legs: Nonpitting soft tissue swelling with tenderness can be seen
- Secondary HOA patients may present with clinical symptoms before the underlying disorder can be detected. Signs and symptoms are similar to those seen in primary HOA, but there may be findings related to the underlying disease (e.g., lung carcinoma, infective endocarditis).
- Patients presenting with painful joints prior to developing clubbing can be misdiagnosed as having inflammatory arthritis.

ETIOLOGY

The pathogenesis of HOA (Fig. 3) is not fully understood; current knowledge suggests that HOA results from the activation of one or more growth factors and inflammatory mediators. Levels of vascular endothelial growth factor (VEGF) have been found to be elevated in both primary and secondary HOA. Platelet-derived growth factor secreted by megakaryocytes that normally are inactivated in the lungs and systemic circulation have been implicated in the etiology of HOA in the setting of pulmonary conditions and right-to-left shunts. Primary HOA likely has a genetic basis. Mutations in the HPGD gene that encodes for prostaglandin synthesis have been identified in some patients with this condition. The finding of hyperestrogenism in patients with HOA and simple clubbing led to a new hypothesis on the pathogenesis of HOA involving estrogens, prostaglandin E2, prostaglandin A2, and the inflammatory reflex.

Dx DIAGNOSIS

Diagnosis is primarily clinical; radiographs and bone scans can help confirm the diagnosis.

DIFFERENTIAL DIAGNOSIS

Paget disease, reactive arthritis, psoriatic arthritis, syphilitic periostitis, osteoarthritis, rheumatoid arthritis, osteomyelitis, scleromyxedema, and acromegaly.

WORKUP

HOA warrants an investigation into finding a possible secondary association.

LABORATORY TESTS

- Routine laboratory studies such as blood count, electrolytes, and urine studies are typically normal in primary and secondary HOA.
- Erythrocyte sedimentation rate is usually elevated in secondary HOA.
- Liver function tests may be abnormal in patients with secondary HOA from gastrointestinal pathology.
- Alkaline phosphatase may be elevated as a result of periostitis of long bones.
- Analysis of the synovial fluid from joint effusions reveals a low white blood cell count (<500 WBC) with normal viscosity, color, and complement levels.

CLASSIFICATION OF HYPERTROPHIC OSTEOARTHROPATHY

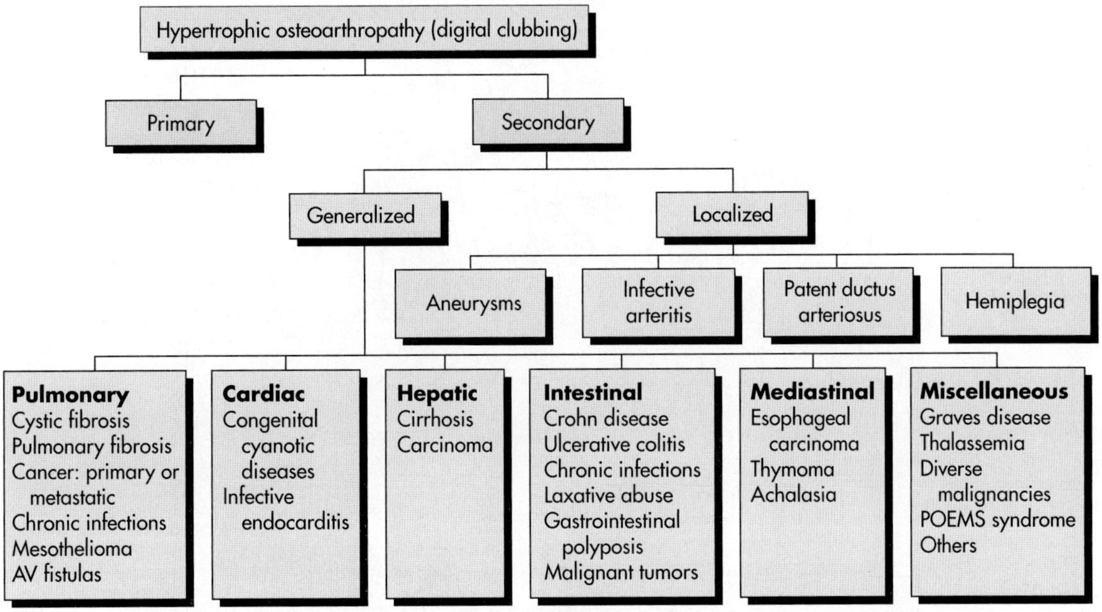

FIG. 1 Various forms of hypertrophic osteoarthropathy (HOA). *AV,* Arteriovenous; *POEMS,* polyneuropathy, organomegaly, endocrinopathy, monoclonal proteins, and skin changes. (From Hochberg MC: *Rheumatology,* ed 7, Philadelphia, 2019, Elsevier.)

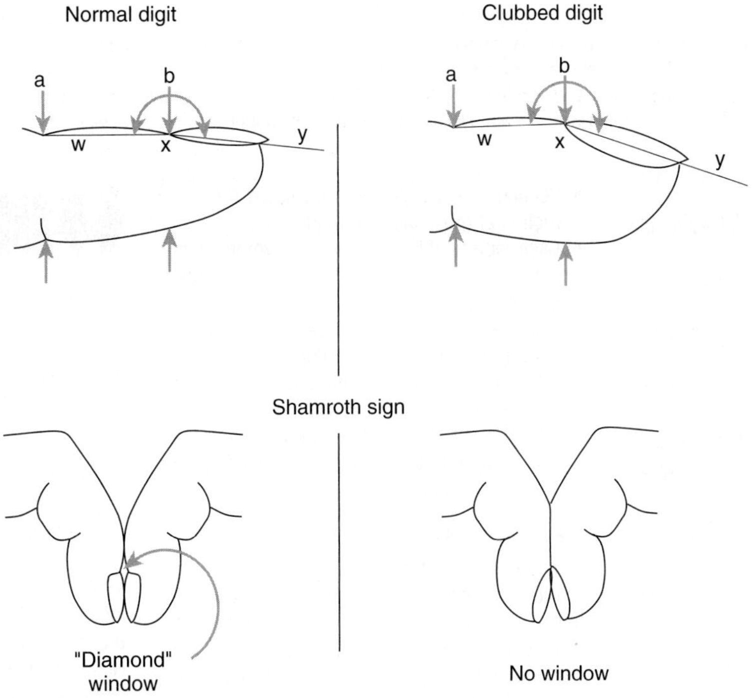

FIG. 2 Clubbing. The normal digit is on the left; the clubbed one, on the right. The distal interphalangeal joint is denoted by **A;** the junction of the nail and skin at the midline is denoted by **B.** The interphalangeal depth ratio is the ratio of the digit's depth measured at **B** divided by that at **A.** The hyponychial angle is the angle *wxy.* In the figure, the depth ratio is 0.9 for the normal digit and 1.2 for the clubbed digit (a ratio >1 indicates clubbing), and the hyponychial angle is 185 degrees for the normal digit and 200 degrees for the clubbed digit (a hyponychial angle >190 degrees indicates clubbing). The Shamroth sign refers to the absence of the diamond-shaped window that normally appears when the terminal phalanges of similar digits are opposed to each other. (From McGee S: *Evidence-based physical diagnosis,* ed 4, Philadelphia, 2018, Elsevier.)

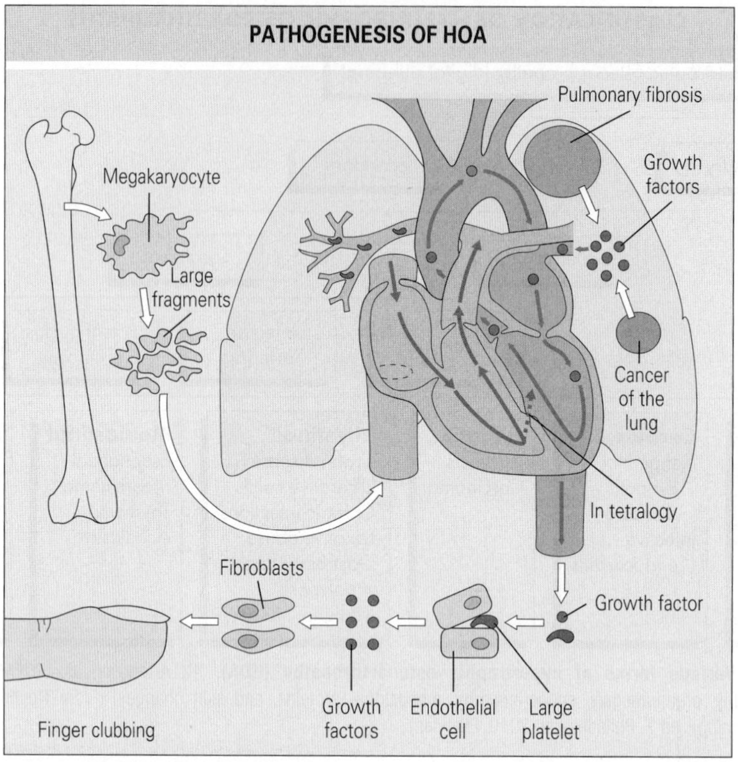

FIG. 3 Theoretic explanation for the development of hypertrophic osteoarthropathy (HOA). Megakaryocytes emerge from the bone marrow and, in normal circumstances, are fragmented in the lung microvasculature. In individuals with cyanotic heart disease (in this case, tetralogy of Fallot), the large fragments would not enter the pulmonary circulation; instead, they would directly enter the systemic circulation, reach its most distal sites, release growth factors, activate endothelial cells, and thus induce finger clubbing. In individuals with lung cancer, a growth factor derived from abnormal tissue would enter the systemic circulation and induce clubbing. (From Hochberg MC: *Rheumatology,* ed 7, Philadelphia, 2019, Elsevier.)

IMAGING STUDIES

- A chest radiograph should be obtained to rule out underlying lung cancer.
- Radiographs of the long bones show periosteal new bone formation (Fig. E4).
- Doppler ultrasound may be useful in identifying periostitis.
- Bone scan with technetium-99m reveals cortical uptake.
- Single photon emission computed tomography (SPECT)/CT can increase specificity by excluding bony metastasis.
- Angiography findings may demonstrate hypervascularization of the finger pads.

Rx TREATMENT

ACUTE GENERAL Rx

- Treatment of primary HOA is symptomatic. NSAIDs, corticosteroids, tamoxifen citrate, or retinoids can be used.
- Asymptomatic patients do not require treatment.
- Colchicine can be helpful for pain resulting from subperiosteal new bone formation.
- Reconstructive surgery is indicated for correction of gross disfigurement.
- Case reports of improvement in symptoms of primary HOA with infliximab and arthroscopic synovectomy.
- Treatment of secondary HOA is to treat the underlying disease. Correction of heart malformation or removal of an underlying tumor can be followed by regression of HOA. Less than 1% of lung cancer patients develop HOA. NSAIDs for symptomatic relief, joint aspiration/injection.

CHRONIC Rx

In patients with secondary HOA refractory to NSAIDs and aspirin, octreotide and bisphosphonates (including pamidronate and zoledronic acid), which inhibit VEGF expression, have been found to be highly effective. Vagotomy has been tried with some success. Definitive treatment remains to treat the underlying disease.

REFERRAL

Referral should be made to rheumatology when the diagnosis of HOA is suspected and the cause remains unclear.

PEARLS & CONSIDERATIONS

- Symptoms of joint pain and swelling in patients with primary HOA often improve with time.
- Prognosis and disease course in patients with secondary HOA will depend on the underlying cause.
- The insidious development of clubbing suggests an infectious process, whereas the rapid progression of clubbing may suggest underlying malignancy.

COMMENTS

Infections and intrathoracic malignancies are the most common causes of secondary HOA. HOA secondary to infection of an arterial graft has been reported.

SUGGESTED READINGS

Available at ExpertConsult.com

AUTHOR: **Long Pham, MD**

BASIC INFORMATION

DEFINITION

Hypoglycemia refers to abnormally low blood glucose levels in circulating plasma. It is defined as a glucose value less than 70 mg/dl (3.9 mmol/L). "Serious hypoglycemia" refers to values <54 mg/dl (3.0 mmol/L). "Severe hypoglycemia" is any glucose value necessitating external assistance to correct it. "Reactive hypoglycemia" refers to symptoms of hypoglycemia with plasma glucose value greater than 70 mg/dl. A multitude of scenarios can lead to this potentially fatal condition.

SYNONYMS

Glycopenia
Low blood glucose
Low blood sugar
HG

ICD-10CM CODES	
E10.641	Type 1 diabetes mellitus with hypoglycemia with coma
E10.649	Type 1 diabetes mellitus with hypoglycemia without coma
E11.641	Type 2 diabetes mellitus with hypoglycemia with coma
E11.649	Type 2 diabetes mellitus with hypoglycemia without coma
E13.641	Other specified diabetes mellitus with hypoglycemia with coma
E13.649	Other specified diabetes mellitus with hypoglycemia without coma
E16.1	Other hypoglycemia
E16.2	Hypoglycemia, unspecified

EPIDEMIOLOGY & DEMOGRAPHICS

- More frequent in type 1 diabetes mellitus (DM). Estimated that glucose levels may be as low as 50 to 60 mg/dl ~10% of the time in type 1 DM.
- Hypoglycemia occurrence 62 to 320 episodes per 100 patient years in type 1 diabetes vs. 35 episodes per 100 patient years in type 2 diabetes.
- Elderly adults with DM are at higher risk of hypoglycemia because of alterations in adaptive physiologic responses to low glucose levels. In addition, this patient population has comorbidities including cognitive and functional decline which interfere with rapid identification and response to hypoglycemic episodes.

PHYSICAL FINDINGS & CLINICAL PRESENTATION

- Symptoms are often nonspecific. Physiologic responses to decreasing plasma glucose concentrations are summarized in Table E1.
- Early symptoms include sweating, pallor, anxiety, palpitations, hunger, and tremor.
- Late symptoms with lower plasma glucose levels include seizures, altered mental status, and coma.
- Profound or prolonged hypoglycemic episodes can cause irreversible brain injury, cardiopulmonary arrest, and death.

ETIOLOGY

- Medications are the most common cause of hypoglycemia. Most common causes include exogenous insulin, insulin secretagogues (sulfonylureas [SU] and meglitinides [MG]), and alcohol
- Critical illness
  1. Organ failure (hepatic, cardiac, or renal)
  2. Sepsis (urinary tract infection and pneumonia common sources in elderly population)
- Hormone deficiency (cortisol, glucagon, and epinephrine)
- Endogenous hyperinsulinism (insulinoma, functional beta-cell disorders, insulin autoimmune hypoglycemia)
- Rare fatal episodes thought to be secondary to ventricular arrhythmias

DIAGNOSIS

Characterized by Whipple triad:
- Symptoms potentially explained by hypoglycemia
- Low blood glucose levels during the symptoms
- Relief of symptoms with administration of glucose or glucagon

DIFFERENTIAL DIAGNOSIS

Hypoglycemic symptoms in the presence of normal plasma glucose levels (>70 mg/dl) point to other etiologies: Postprandial syndrome, stroke, sepsis, seizure/postictal state, cardiac disease, psychiatric disease, metabolic disorders (hyperthyroidism, pheochromocytoma), drug intoxication.

WORKUP

- If Whipple triad is positive, the next step is to consider a patient's medical status.

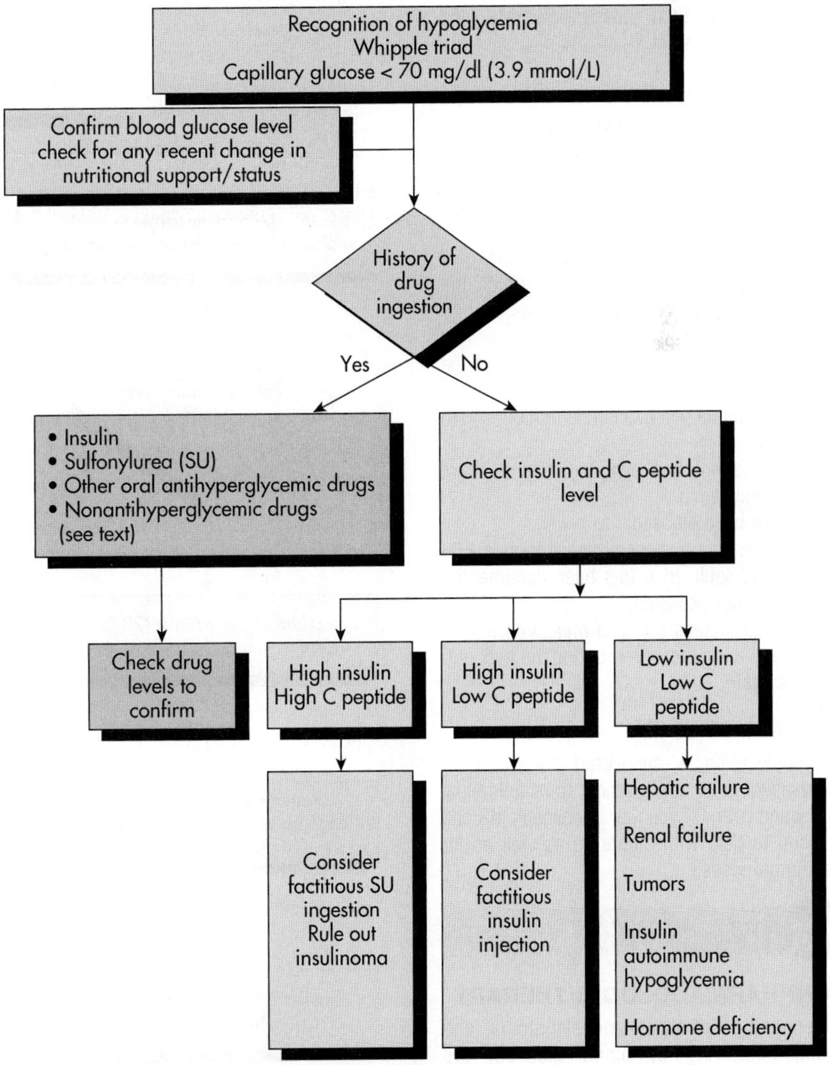

FIG. 1 Recognition and evaluation of hypoglycemia. (From Vincent JL et al: *Textbook of critical care,* ed 7, Philadelphia, 2017, Elsevier.)

- Iatrogenic factors are the most common causes of hypoglycemia in hospitalized patients (review the NPO status, timing of feeding, glucose-lowering medications, and interactions between medications).
- Detailed history, including past medical history, a thorough medication history, and timing of hypoglycemia (in regard to meals and medications).

LABORATORY TESTS

- An algorithm for recognition and evaluation of hypoglycemia is described in Fig. 1.
- If the cause is not apparent after a thorough history, the following is appropriate:

FASTING: If symptoms witnessed when fasting, with verified low blood glucose levels, consider the following labs: Plasma glucose, β-hydroxybutyrate (BHOB), insulin, C-peptide, proinsulin, screen for SU and MG metabolites.

POSTPRANDIAL:

- Plasma glucose, insulin, C-peptide, and proinsulin prior to ingestion of the meal and every 30 min thereafter for 5 hr.
- Only evaluate the samples drawn when glucose levels are <60 mg/dl.
- If a patient has a presentation consistent with Whipple triad, then measure SU, MG, and antibodies to insulin.

72-HR FAST:

- Collect blood specimens for measurement of plasma glucose, insulin, C-peptide, proinsulin, and BHOB every 6 hr until the glucose concentration is <60 mg/dl.
- Increase frequency of sampling to every 1 to 2 hr.
- Insulin, C-peptide, and proinsulin are only relevant in those specimens in which the plasma glucose concentration is <60 mg/dl.
- The fast should be ended when any of the following occurs:
  1. The plasma glucose concentration is <45 mg/dl.
  2. The patient has symptoms or signs of hypoglycemia.
  3. 72 hr have elapsed.
  4. The plasma glucose concentration is <55 and Whipple triad has been documented on a prior occasion.
- Insulin antibodies are also measured but do not need to be measured during the hypoglycemic state.

IMAGING STUDIES

If hypoglycemia is suspected secondary to an insulinoma or malignancy, transabdominal ultrasound (US), CT scan, or endoscopic US can be used to help with diagnosis as well as for staging purposes.

Rx TREATMENT

NONPHARMACOLOGIC THERAPY

- Recognition of signs and symptoms, and self-monitoring of blood glucose, are especially important in insulin-deficient patients.
- Avoiding drugs that can exacerbate condition (e.g., alcohol) if it occurs on repeated occasions.
- Bedtime snacks if hypoglycemia occurs at night.
- In situations caused by tumor etiologies (e.g., islet cell, insulinoma, and non-islet cell), definitive treatment may require surgical removal.

PHARMACOLOGIC THERAPY

- Treating the underlying etiology that exacerbates hypoglycemia (e.g., infection, proper diabetic regimen, proper diabetic diet)
- Fast-acting carbohydrates (e.g., glucose tablets, hard candy, IV dextrose infusion)
- Pure glucose (dextrose) if caused by insulin secretagogue in addition with alpha-glucosidase inhibitor
- In severe hypoglycemia with seizure activity, 25 g of 50% dextrose IV or 0.5 to 1.0 mg IM/subcutaneous glucagon
- Persistent hypoglycemia after IV dextrose therapy think sulfonylurea overdose or insulin pump malfunction. If an insulin pump is present remove it. If sulfonylurea overdose is suspected treat with IV dextrose infusion and octreotide 50 to 100 μg every 6 to 12 hr for adults and 1 to 2 μg/kg every 6 to 12 hr.
- Fig. 2 describes a management algorithm for hypoglycemia

REFERRAL

- Most scenarios of hypoglycemia can be managed by primary care physicians by adjusting medications.
- If the cause is not clear, then endocrinology referral is recommended.
- Severe symptomatic hypoglycemia needs emergent treatment.

PEARLS & CONSIDERATIONS

- Hypoglycemia can cause severe morbidity and death if not dealt with promptly and effectively.
- Hypoglycemia is very common in patients with DM, especially type 1 DM, and most commonly it is a side effect of medications.
- Elderly patients with DM are at higher risk for serious hypoglycemic episodes.
- In patients who are hospitalized, the etiology is often multifactorial.

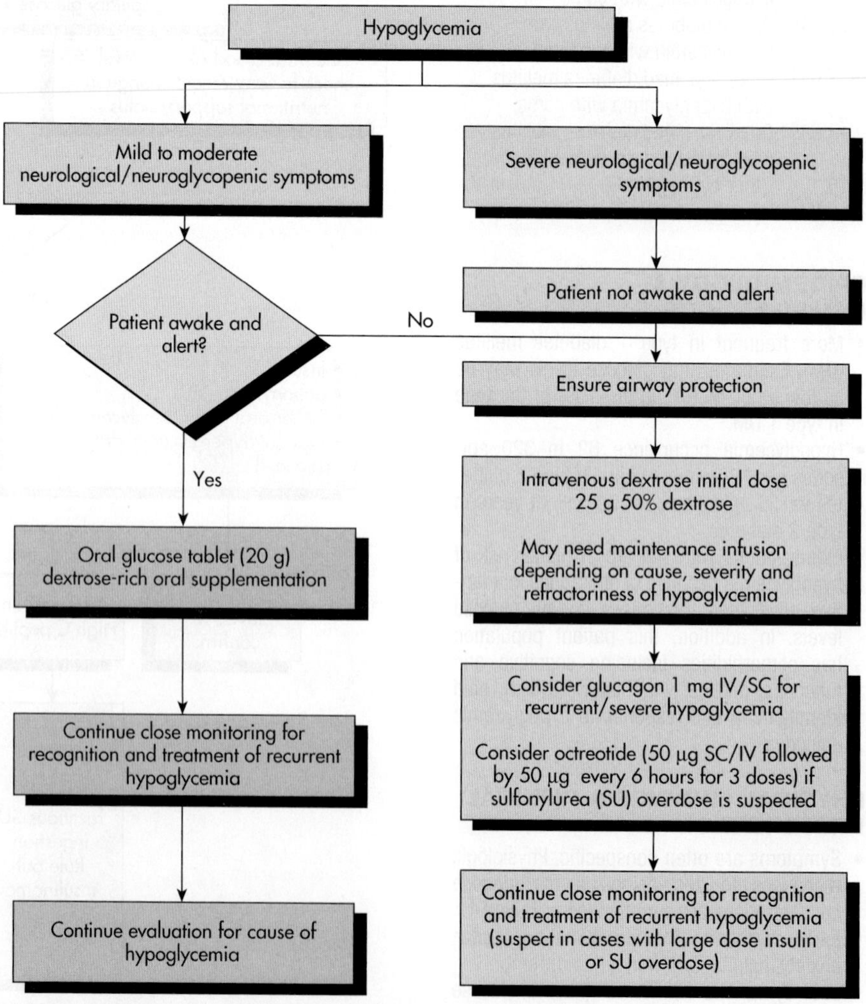

FIG. 2 Management of hypoglycemia. *IV*, Intravenous; *SC*, subcutaneous. (From Vincent JL et al: *Textbook of critical care*, ed 7, dslu, Elsevier.)

- Clinically important hypoglycemia is uncommon in nondiabetic patients, and evaluation for a hypoglycemic disorder in these patients should only occur if the Whipple triad is met.

SUGGESTED READINGS

Available at ExpertConsult.com

RELATED CONTENT

Diabetes Mellitus (Related Key Topic)
Insulinoma (Related Key Topic)

AUTHORS: **Curtis (Trey) Lee Lowery III, PhD, MD, and Thomas M. Triplett, MD**

BASIC INFORMATION

DEFINITION

Male hypogonadism is a clinical syndrome involving subnormal testosterone levels and/or impaired sperm production due to dysfunction at one or both levels of the hypothalamic-pituitary-testicular axis.

SYNONYM

Testicular dysfunction

ICD-10CM CODES

E23.0	Hypopituitarism
E23.1	Drug-induced hypopituitarism
E29	Testicular dysfunction
E29.1	Testicular hypofunction
E29.8	Other testicular dysfunction
E29.9	Testicular dysfunction, unspecified
E89.3	Postprocedural hypopituitarism

EPIDEMIOLOGY & DEMOGRAPHICS

INCIDENCE: Hypogonadism is the most common clinical disorder of the testis. Incidence is unclear due to the many possible underlying factors, nonspecificity of symptoms, and questions relating to the adequacy of a diagnostic serum total testosterone threshold.

PREVALENCE: Prevalence of hypogonadism increases with aging, obesity, diabetes mellitus, and other comorbidities. The average decrease in serum total testosterone levels in aging men is 1% to 2% per yr. Prevalence rises to 23% among men in their 70s. However, in population-based surveys of community-dwelling middle-aged and older males, prevalence of hypogonadism is approximately 6%.

RISK FACTORS: These are many and include genetic abnormalities; the aging process; pituitary and testicular lesions and disorders; medications; drug abuse; HIV disease; acute illnesses; chronic cardiac, hepatic, renal, and pulmonary diseases; cancer; ionizing radiation; chemotherapy; obesity; and malnutrition.

GENETICS: Genetic abnormalities underlie a number of hypogonadal disorders including Klinefelter syndrome, Noonan syndrome, hemochromatosis, Kallmann syndrome, and Prader-Willi syndrome.

PHYSICAL FINDINGS & CLINICAL PRESENTATION

Sexual (specific)

- Decrease in frequency of erections
- Erectile dysfunction
- Decrease in libido
- Decreased fertility
- Small or shrinking testes
- Gynecomastia
- Diminished sexual hair
- Hot flushes and sweats

Neuropsychologic (less specific)

- Depression
- Inability to concentrate
- Diminished motivation and vitality
- Decrease in self-confidence
- Diminished energy and stamina
- Sleep disturbances

Physical features and findings

- Diminished capacity for physical activity
- Decrease in physical endurance and performance
- Diminished muscle mass and strength
- Increase in body fat
- Decrease or loss of axillary and pubic hair and decrease in shaving frequency
- Fine wrinkling over the lateral aspects of the face
- Breast enlargement with or without tenderness
- Change in consistency and decrease in size of testes
- Fragility fractures
- Anemia

ETIOLOGY

- The importance of a careful history and examination cannot be overstated to determine the etiology of possible hypogonadism. Primary hypogonadism is a result of a decrease in testicular testosterone secretion and/or a decrease in spermatogenesis with an associated increase in gonadotropin levels as in Klinefelter syndrome, cryptorchidism, and following orchitis, testicular trauma, chemotherapy, and irradiation. The causes of primary hypogonadism are summarized in Table 1.

TABLE 1 Causes of Primary Hypogonadism

Common Causes	Uncommon Causes
Androgen Deficiency and Impairment of Sperm Production	
Congenital or Developmental Disorders	
Klinefelter syndrome (XXY) and variants	Myotonic dystrophy
	Uncorrected cryptorchidism
	Noonan syndrome
	Bilateral congenital anorchia
	Polyglandular autoimmune syndrome
	Testosterone biosynthetic enzyme defects
	CAH (TART)
	Complex genetic syndromes
	Down syndrome
	LH receptor mutation
Acquired Disorders	
Bilateral surgical castration or trauma	Orchitis
Drugs (spironolactone, ketoconazole, abiraterone, enzalutamide, alcohol, chemotherapy agents)[a]	
Ionizing radiation	
Systemic Disorders	
Chronic liver disease (hepatic cirrhosis)[a,b]	Malignancy (lymphoma, testicular cancer)
Chronic kidney disease[a,b]	Sickle cell disease[b]
Aging[b]	Spinal cord injury
	Vasculitis (polyarteritis)
	Infiltrative disease (amyloidosis, leukemia)
Isolated Impairment of Sperm Production or Function	
Congenital or Developmental Disorders	
Cryptorchidism	Myotonic dystrophy
Varicocele	Sertoli cell–only syndrome
Y chromosome microdeletions	Primary ciliary dyskinesia
	Down syndrome
	FSH receptor mutation
Acquired Disorders	
Orchitis	Environmental toxins
Ionizing radiation	
Chemotherapy agents	
Thermal trauma	
Systemic Disorders	
Acute febrile illness	Spinal cord injury
Malignancy (testicular cancer, Hodgkin disease)[b]	
Idiopathic azoospermia or oligozoospermia	

[a]Functional causes that are potentially reversible with discontinuation of offending medication, or with liver or renal transplantation.

[b]Combined primary and secondary hypogonadism.

CAH, Congenital adrenal hyperplasia; *FSH,* follicle-stimulating hormone; *LH,* luteinizing hormone; *TART,* testicular adrenal rest tumor.

From Melmed S et al: *Williams textbook of endocrinology*, ed 14, Elsevier, 2019.

- Secondary hypogonadism is due to hypothalamic-pituitary dysfunction, which results in a decrease in testosterone levels and/or spermatogenesis with gonadotropin levels that are subnormal or inappropriately within the normal range. Table 2 summarizes causes of secondary hypogonadism.
- Combined primary and secondary hypogonadism is a result of deficits at both the level of the hypothalamic-pituitary axis and testes with variable gonadotropin levels depending upon the predominance of the level of the defect.

TABLE 2 Causes of Secondary Hypogonadism

Common Causes	Uncommon Causes
Androgen Deficiency and Impairment of Sperm Production	
Congenital or Developmental Disorders	
Constitutional delayed puberty	CHH due to genetic mutations
Hemochromatosis	CHH, idiopathic (IHH)
	Kallmann syndrome
	Congenital adrenal hypoplasia
	Isolated LH deficiency, LHβ mutations
	Complex genetic syndromes
Acquired Disorders	
Hyperprolactinemia[a]	Hypopituitarism
Opioids[a]	
Androgenic anabolic steroids, progestins, estrogen excess[a]	
GnRH agonist or antagonist[a]	
	Pituitary or hypothalamic tumor
	Surgical hypophysectomy, pituitary or cranial irradiation
	Vascular compromise, traumatic brain injury
	Granulomatous or infiltrative disease
	Infection
	Pituitary stalk disease
	Lymphocytic or autoimmune hypophysitis
	Acquired IHH
Systemic Disorders	
Glucocorticoid excess (Cushing syndrome)[a,b]	Chronic systemic illness[a,b]
Chronic organ failure[a,b]	Spinal cord injury
Chronic liver disease (hepatic cirrhosis), chronic kidney disease, chronic lung disease, chronic heart failure[a]	Transfusion-related iron overload (β-thalassemia)[a]
Chronic systemic illness[a,b]	Sickle cell disease
Type 2 diabetes mellitus[a]	Cystic fibrosis
Malignancy[a]	
Rheumatic disease (rheumatoid arthritis)[a]	
HIV disease[a]	
Starvation,[b] malnutrition,[b] eating disorders, endurance exercise[a]	
Morbid obesity, obstructive sleep apnea[a]	
Acute and critical illness[a]	
Aging (comorbid illnesses associated with aging)[a,b]	
Isolated Impairment of Sperm Production or Function	
Congenital or Developmental Disorders	
	Congenital adrenal hyperplasia (21-hydroxylase deficiency, 11β-hydroxylase deficiency)
	Isolated FSH deficiency, FSHβ mutations
Acquired Disorders	
Testosterone, androgenic anabolic steroids	Androgen- or hCG-secreting tumors
Malignancy (Hodgkin disease, testicular cancer)[b]	Hyperprolactinemia

CHH, Congenital hypogonadotropic hypogonadism; *FSH,* follicle-stimulating hormone; *GnRH,* gonadotropin-releasing hormone; *hCG,* human chorionic gonadotropin; *HIV,* human immunodeficiency virus; *IHH,* idiopathic hypogonadotropic hypogonadism; *LH,* luteinizing hormone.
[a]Functional causes that are potentially reversible or treatable with discontinuation of offending medication, treatment of underlying cause of gonadotropin suppression or organ transplantation.
[b]Combined primary and secondary hypogonadism.
From Melmed S et al: *Williams textbook of endocrinology*, ed 14, Elsevier, 2019.

Dx DIAGNOSIS (FIG. 1)

DIFFERENTIAL DIAGNOSIS

Hypogonadotropic or secondary hypogonadism
- Pituitary dysfunction: Hypopituitarism, functioning or nonfunctioning pituitary tumor, lymphocytic hypophysitis, infiltrative disease as with sarcoidosis, hemochromatosis, and histiocytosis X
- Hyperprolactinemia: Prolactinoma, medication-related, chronic kidney disease
- Genetic: Kallmann syndrome with anosmia, Prader-Willi syndrome with morbid obesity
- Acute and chronic illnesses, malnutrition, emotional disorders, HIV, sleep apnea, aging, malignancies, obesity, and renal, hepatic, pulmonary, and cardiac diseases
- Opioids, CNS: Active medications, glucocorticoid excess, and GnRH analogues (androgen deprivation therapy)

Hypergonadotropic or primary hypogonadism
- Genetic: Klinefelter syndrome, Noonan syndrome, myotonic dystrophy
- Gonadal damage due to drugs, alcohol, radiation, chemotherapy, trauma
- Congenital anorchia (vanishing testis syndrome)
- Cryptorchidism
- Mumps orchitis, HIV orchitis
- Diabetes mellitus
- Hodgkin disease
- Aging

Combined primary and secondary hypogonadism
- Hemochromatosis, sickle cell disease, thalassemia
- Alcoholism, glucocorticoid therapy, aging
- Chronic cardiac, hepatic, renal, pulmonary diseases, and HIV disease

WORKUP

- Determine the presence or absence of male hypogonadism on the basis of history, clinical manifestations and findings, and documentation of consistently low serum total testosterone levels and/or abnormal seminal fluid analysis.
- Morning serum total testosterone levels should be measured on at least 2 or 3 occasions for confirmation of diagnosis and when necessary followed by measurement of serum free or bioavailable testosterone.
- Serum follicle-stimulating hormone (FSH) and luteinizing hormone (LH) levels are measured to determine whether hypogonadism is primary, secondary, or a result of combined defects of the hypothalamic-pituitary axis and testis. The cause of testosterone deficiency should be definitively determined before initiation of testosterone replacement therapy.
- Hormonal assessment of gonadal status should not be done during an acute or subacute illness.

LABORATORY TESTS

- Serum total testosterone is tightly bound to sex hormone binding globulin (SHBG) and

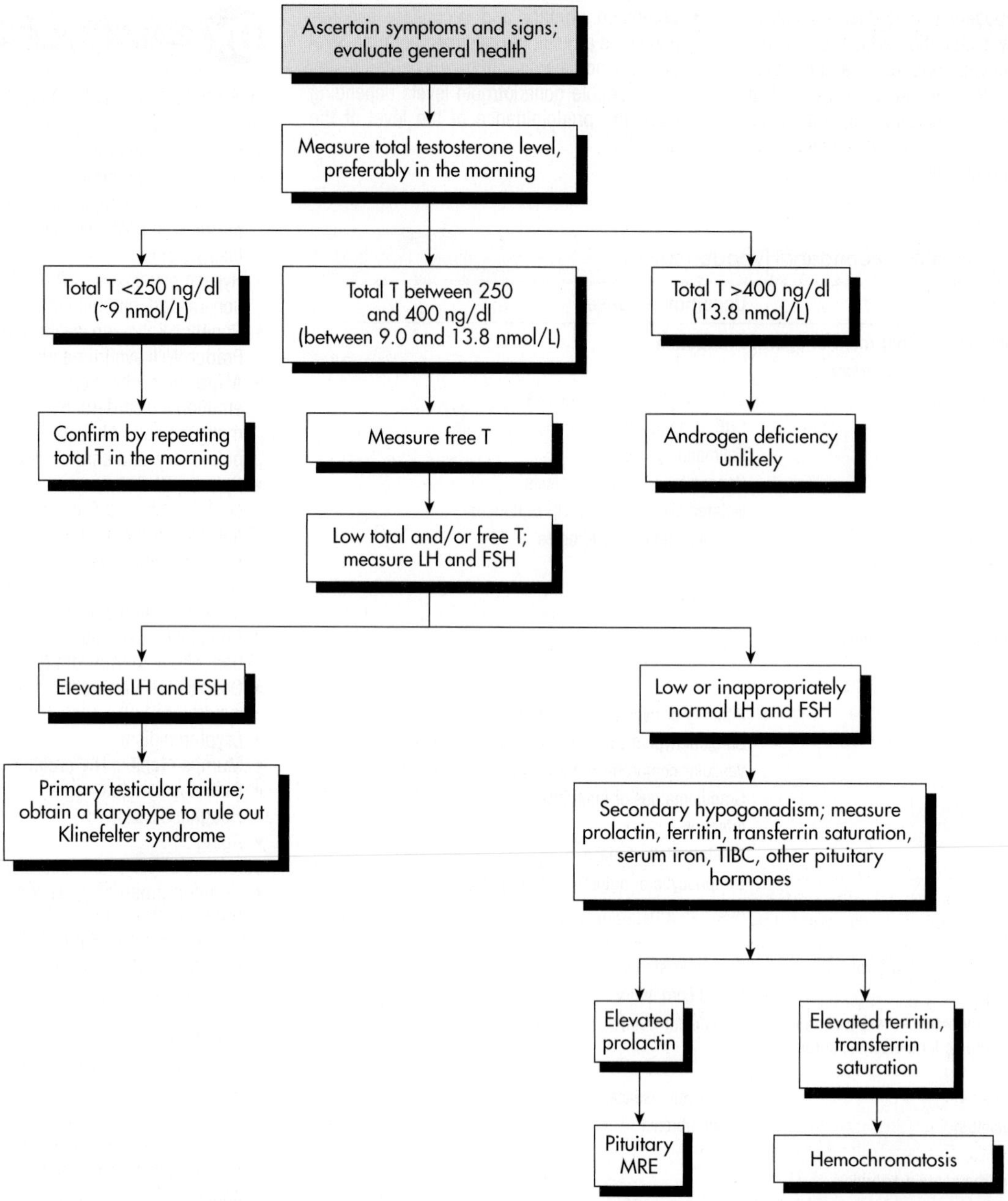

FIG. 1 Algorithm showing an approach for the diagnostic evaluation of adult men suspected of having androgen deficiency. *FSH,* Follicle-stimulating hormone; *LH,* luteinizing hormone; *MRE,* magnetic resonance elastography; *T,* testosterone; *TIBC,* total iron-binding capacity. (From Shalender B, Shehzad B: Diagnosis and treatment of hypogonadism in men, *Best Pract Res Clin Endocrin* 25:251-270, 2011.)

weakly bound to circulating albumin. 0.5% to 3% of serum total testosterone is unbound or free.

- Liquid chromatography tandem mass spectrometry assays for total serum testosterone are more accurate than immunoassays.
- Bioavailable testosterone refers to unbound testosterone plus the testosterone that is loosely bound to albumin.
- Free testosterone, if necessary, is best measured by equilibrium dialysis or centrifugal ultrafiltration.
- An SHBG measurement is helpful in determining the adequacy or normality of a serum total testosterone measurement. Conditions that lower SHBG include obesity, protein-losing states, androgens, hypothyroidism, and familial SHBG deficiency. Increases in SHBG occur in those with hyperthyroidism, hepatitis, cirrhosis, and HIV disease, aging, and by estrogens.
- The lower limit of normal for serum total testosterone in a healthy young male is approximately 240 to 950 ng/dl and a low-normal serum free testosterone in a young normal male is 5 to 20 ng/dl. Serum total testosterone in a healthy young male ranges from 300 to 1000 ng/dl and normal free testosterone ranges from 5 to 20 ng/dl.
- Serum total testosterone levels can vary from day to day, and there is a diurnal rhythm in young normal males with morning levels that are higher by approximately 20% to 25% as compared with levels in the afternoon.
- In elderly males, the diurnal rhythm is diminished with levels approximately 10% lower in the afternoon as compared with morning levels.
- Serum FSH and LH measurements are important in delineating primary, secondary, and combined hypogonadism.
- Hypogonadal symptoms are more likely to be seen in those with total serum testosterone levels of less than 230 ng/dl for young normal males. Serum total testosterone levels of <150 ng/dl are unequivocally low.
- Transient suppression of total serum testosterone may occur during acute illness, in males that are being treated with glucocorticoid, in those taking opiates or CNS-active medications, in those with malnutrition or

poor eating habits, and during excessive physical exercise.

- Quantity and quality of sperm counts and activity can vary in a significant way for a variety of reasons. Therefore, in assessing fertility, seminal fluid analysis should be done on two or more occasions, each separated by 2 or more wk, and on semen collected within an hour of ejaculation after more than 2 days of abstinence.
- Depending on the clinical picture and examination, other studies may be necessary, including a karyotype analysis, for example, for Klinefelter syndrome, or serum prolactin measurement for patients with possible hyperprolactinemia, which may be drug-induced, related to a prolactinoma, or to chronic renal disease.

IMAGING STUDIES

In males with severe androgen deficiency with low serum gonadotropin levels, increased serum prolactin levels, hypopituitarism, severe headaches, and visual defects, an MRI of the pituitary would be appropriate. In males with hypogonadism and a history of fractures, dual energy x-ray absorptiometry (DXA) measurements of spine and hip should be obtained to further delineate the status of the skeletal system.

Rx TREATMENT

Testosterone replacement therapy is indicated when patients have symptoms and signs of hypogonadism and serum testosterone levels that are consistently subnormal with levels of <250 ng/dl. The goal of replacement therapy is to restore serum testosterone levels to within the normal range of values and to have a positive effect on the constellation of hypogonadal symptoms and signs. Subnormal spermatogenesis, if present in such patients, is not affected by testosterone therapy. In patients with hypogonadotropic or secondary hypogonadism, chorionic gonadotropin and/or GnRH therapy can optimize spermatogenesis, whereas, generally in patients with primary hypogonadism, subnormal spermatogenesis and infertility are irreversible. The treatment of adult male hypogonadism is summarized in Table 3.

NONPHARMACOLOGIC THERAPY

- Weight reduction, especially when it appears to be a major factor underlying male hypogonadism
- Discontinuation of anabolic steroids, CNS-active medications, and narcotic abuse
- Surgery or radiation therapy for patients with a pituitary functioning or nonfunctioning tumor with visual field abnormality and headaches who are not candidates for further medical therapy or have been unsuccessfully treated with medication
- Surgery indicated for chronic gynecomastia and, occasionally, in cases with recent-onset gynecomastia that has not responded to testosterone replacement therapy

CHRONIC Rx

Testosterone formulations:

- Parenteral testosterone preparations: Testosterone enanthate (generic) and testosterone cypionate (Depo-Testosterone and generic) 150 to 200 mg are injected intramuscularly every 2 wk. Following injections, there are appreciable fluctuations in serum testosterone, with levels rising within the first several days and a subsequent decrease to normal and in some cases to below normal at the end of the 2 wk. As a result of the varying levels of testosterone, patients may have related symptoms. Adjustments in dose and dosing interval may help to alleviate the serum fluctuations and clinical symptoms. Testosterone undecanoate (AUEFD-ENDO) is an injectable depot formulation FDA-approved for male hypogonadism. The recommended dosage is 750 mg injected IM at 0 and 4 wk, and then every 10 wk thereafter.
- Topical testosterone preparations:
  1. Testosterone adhesive patch (Androderm) delivers 2.5 or 5 mg of testosterone when applied nightly to the back, abdomen, upper arms, or thighs. Serum testosterone levels rise to within normal range in a few hours after application and, thereafter, are relatively stable. Daily doses of up to 10 mg may be necessary.
  2. Testosterone 1% gels (AndroGel and Testim). AndroGel is available in 2.5 g and 5 g gel units that deliver 2.5 mg and 5 mg of testosterone, respectively. The gel is applied daily in the morning by hand over the shoulder, upper arms, or abdomen. Adjustments in dose to 7.5 g or 10 g of gel may be necessary to optimize serum testosterone levels. AndroGel (1.62%) pump is also available for daily application. Testim is available in 5-g and 10-g tubes and with morning applications over the shoulders or arms delivers 5 mg and 10 mg of testosterone, respectively. Both AndroGel and Testim provide relatively stable serum testosterone levels. Two new transdermal formulations, Fortesta and Axiron, are now available and are applied daily by metered dose pumps. With these preparations, care is necessary to avoid skin-to-skin contact exposure with others.
- Testosterone pellets: 3 to 6 pellets of testosterone each containing 75 mg of testosterone are surgically inserted subcutaneously every 3 to 6 mo and provide relatively stable serum testosterone levels.
- Testosterone undecanoate (Jatenzo) is an oral testosterone formulation approved for patients with hypogonadism associated with structural or genetic etiologies and it is not indicated in men with age-related hypogonadism.[1]

RISKS & ADVERSE EFFECTS

- Contraindications to testosterone therapy include prostate cancer, breast cancer, COPD, untreated obstructive sleep apnea, congestive heart failure, and polycythemia. Relative contraindications include severe benign prostatic hyperplasia, hematocrit ≥50% at baseline, sleep apnea, and severe congestive heart failure.
- Patients on chronic testosterone therapy need to be followed carefully with prostate and prostate-specific antigen (PSA) assessments and hematocrit measurements for possible excessive induction of erythrocytosis, initially at 3 to 6 mo and at regular intervals thereafter. Table 4 summarizes monitoring during testosterone treatment.
- Current testosterone use for 6 mo or shorter is associated with 63% higher risk for venous thromboembolism (VTE). VTE risk peaks during the first 6 mo and declines to 25% thereafter.[2]

REFERRAL

Endocrinology for full endocrine and metabolic assessment and therapy. Urology for further assessment and follow-up of the prostate and for evaluation and therapy of erectile dysfunction. Neurosurgery for evaluation and possible surgery for a pituitary lesion. Plastic surgery for chronic gynecomastia. Reproductive endocrinology for those with an infertility problem.

PEARLS & CONSIDERATIONS

COMMENTS

- Do not screen men "routinely" for hypogonadism. Screening men with nonspecific symptoms of hypogonadism (e.g., decreased energy) is also not recommended. Screening should be limited to men with specific signs and symptoms of hypogonadism.
- Male hypogonadism is an important and frequently encountered problem that requires a complete medical history, examination, and hormonal assessment to determine whether a patient has hypogonadism and requires testosterone replacement therapy. Treated patients need to be seen on a regular basis to avoid possible testosterone adverse effects. Patients requiring testosterone replacement should have testosterone, prostate specific antigen, and hematocrit levels monitored.
- Trials to evaluate the effects of testosterone treatment in older men revealed that in symptomatic men 65 yr of age or older, raising testosterone concentrations for 1 yr from moderately low to the mid-normal range had a moderate benefit with respect to sexual function and some benefit with respect to mood and depressive symptoms but no benefit with respect to vitality or walking distance.[3]
- Controversy exists regarding the safety of testosterone replacement therapy following reports of increased risk of cardiovascular

[1] Swerdloff RS et al: A new oral testosterone undecanoate formulation restores testosterone to normal concentrations in hypogonadal men, *J Clin Endocrinol Metab* 105:2515-2531, 2020.

[2] Martinez C et al: Testosterone treatment and risk of venous thromboembolism: population based case-control study, *BMJ* 355:596-598, 2016.

[3] Snyder PJ et al: Effects of testosterone treatment in older men, *N Engl J Med* 374:611-624, 2016.

TABLE 3 Treatment of Adult Male Hypogonadism

Formulation	Dosage	Advantages	Disadvantages
Treatment of Androgen Deficiency			
Formulations Available in the United States			
Parenteral Testosterone Esters			
Testosterone enanthate or cypionate, IM injections	*Adults:* 150-200 mg IM every 2 wk or 75-100 mg IM every wk 50 mg, 75 mg, or 100 mg SC by autoinjector *Prepubertal boys:* 50-100 mg monthly or 25-50 mg every 2 wk, increasing to 50-100 mg every 2 wk and then to adult replacement dosage over 2-4 yr or until spontaneous pubertal development occurs	Extensive clinical use Inexpensive with self-injection Some dose flexibility	IM injections, discomfort Symptomatic fluctuation of T concentrations (supraphysiologic after injection to low normal or low before next injection) Frequent IM injections to reduce fluctuations of T concentrations More erythrocytosis than with transdermal T
Testosterone undecanoate, IM injections	750 mg at 0 and 4 wk, then every 10 wk	Less frequent IM injections Maintenance of normal T concentrations for a longer duration No apparent fluctuations in symptoms	REMS: Slow, deep IM injection in clinic (no self-injection); 30-min observation for potential POME and anaphylaxis IM injections, discomfort Large-volume injection (3 mL) Self-injection not possible Rarely, cough immediately after injection Prolonged maintenance of T level after discontinuation if adverse effects develop
Transdermal Testosterone			
Testosterone patch (nonscrotal)	2 or 4 mg (one patch) or 6 mg (one 2-mg plus one 4-mg patch) applied daily over nonpressure areas	Low- to mid-normal physiologic T concentrations Mimics normal circadian variation when applied nightly No injections Less erythrocytosis than with parenteral T Rapid withdrawal of T replacement if adverse effects occur	Frequent skin irritation Low-normal T concentrations: Two patches may be needed Skin adhesion poor with excessive sweating Daily application More expensive than parenteral T
Testosterone gels and solution	*1% T gel:* 5-10 g of gel (containing 50-100 mg of T) applied daily over shoulders or upper arms; available in foil sachets of 2.5 or 5.0 g (containing 25 or 50 mg of T, respectively), or a tube of 5 g (containing 50 mg of T) *1.62% T gel:* 20.25-81.00 mg (containing 20.25-81.00 mg of T) applied daily to shoulders or upper arms; available in 20.25- and 40.50-mg packets (containing 20.25 and 40.50 mg of T, respectively) or metered-dose pump delivering 12.5 mg per pump depression *2% gel:* 40-70 mg (containing 40-70 mg of T) applied daily to inner thighs; available in a metered-dose pump delivering 10 mg per pump depression *2% solution:* 30-120 mg applied to underarms; available in a metered-dose pump applicator delivering 30 mg per pump depression	Low- to high-normal steady-state physiologic T concentrations No injections Little skin irritation Dose flexibility Rapid withdrawal of T replacement if adverse effects occur For 1.62% or 2% gel: Less gel amount in more concentrated formulations Less gel amount in more concentrated formulations For 2 % solution: Absorption of solution not affected by deodorant or antiperspirant Absorption of solution not affected by deodorant or antiperspirant	Potential for contact transfer of T to women or children Daily application More expensive than parenteral T, especially with higher doses Moderately high DHT concentrations One formulation has a musk odor and another is associated with stickiness or skin dryness Slight skin irritation in some men Solution may drip under arms
Transbuccal testosterone	30-mg tablet applied between cheek and gum two times daily	Mid-normal steady-state physiologic T concentrations No injections, patch or gel application, or their associated disadvantages Rapid withdrawal of T replacement if adverse effects occur	Twice-daily application Gum irritation or inflammation Altered or bitter taste High learning curve for proper application; requires careful instruction or poor acceptability occurs Tablets may be difficult to remove or may fall off prematurely No dose flexibility Moderately high DHT concentrations More expensive than parenteral T

Continued

Formulation	Dosage	Advantages	Disadvantages
Testosterone nasal gel	11 mg (delivering 1.1 mg of T) three times daily (every 6-8 hours) for a total daily dose of 33 mg (delivering 3.3 mg of T) daily Available in a metered-dose pump that delivers 5.5 mg (delivering 0.55 mg of T) per pump depression	No injections No interaction with sympathomimetic nasal decongestants	Thrice-daily administration Learning curve for proper administration Fluctuation in T concentrations from lower- to upper-normal range after administration No nose blowing or sniffing for 1 hour after administration Discontinue with severe rhinitis Nasal irritation Not recommended with other intranasal drugs or chronic nasal conditions
Testosterone pellets	2-6 pellets (each 3.2 mm diameter × 9 mm in length pellet containing 75 mg of T, for a total of 150-450 mg of T delivered) implanted SC every 3-6 mo (usually 3-4 mo)	Maintenance of normal T concentrations for a longer duration	Requires surgical incision Extrusion, bleeding, and infection can occur uncommonly Large number of pellets Not easily removed; fibrosis may occur Lack of ability for rapid withdrawal of T replacement if adverse effects occur Infrequent use
Oral testosterone undecanoate	40-80 mg PO with meals twice a day to three times daily	Oral administration is convenient for many	Twice- or thrice-daily administration Variable T concentrations and clinical responses Requires administration with meal High DHT concentrations
Testosterone Formulations Available Outside the United States			
Testosterone-in-adhesive matrix patch	Two patches (delivering 4.8 mg of T per day) applied every 2 days	Low- to mid-normal physiologic T concentrations Duration 2 days No injections	Some skin irritation Two patches needed
Treatment to Initiate and Maintain Sperm Production in Men with Hypogonadotropic Hypogonadism			
Initially to Stimulate Testosterone and Potentially Sperm Production			
hCG	500-2000 IU given SC two to three times weekly to maintain serum T concentrations within the normal range for 6-12 mo	Effective in stimulating endogenous T production In men with acquired and some men with partial congenital hypogonadotropic hypogonadism, sperm production may be stimulated with hCG treatment alone SC injections easier than IM injections (smaller needle, injection not as deep) Less fluctuation in T concentrations compared with IM T ester injections No injection, patch, or buccal tablet	Injections two to three times weekly Expensive Higher doses needed in men with concomitant primary testicular disease (e.g., cryptorchidism) Breast tenderness or gynecomastia secondary to high estradiol production by testes May require dilution Occasional burning sensation with injection Ineffective in primary hypogonadism
Added to hCG to Stimulate Sperm Production			
FSH Human menopausal gonadotropin, human FSH, or recombinant human FSH	After 6-12 mo of hCG treatment alone resulting in normal T concentrations, add FSH 75-300 IU given SC three times weekly for an additional 6-12 mo or longer	Effective in stimulating sperm production in men with hypogonadotropic hypogonadism	Injections three times weekly Extremely expensive, prohibitive cost for most Breast tenderness or gynecomastia secondary to high estradiol production by testes May require dilution Occasional burning sensation with injection In men with concomitant primary testicular disease (e.g., cryptorchidism), stimulation of spermatogenesis is not likely
To Stimulate Testosterone and Sperm Production			
GnRH	5-25 ng/kg SC every 2 hr by programmable infusion pump for 6-12 mo	Effective in stimulating both endogenous T and sperm production	GnRH not readily available Requires pump use and management, usually in a specialized center Expensive Infrequently used except at certain sites Rarely, local irritation, infection

DHT, Dihydrotestosterone; *FSH,* follicle-stimulating hormone; *GnRH,* gonadotropin-releasing hormone; *hCG,* human chorionic gonadotropin; *IM,* intramuscular; *PO,* orally; *POME,* potential pulmonary oil microembolism; *REMS,* Risk Evaluation and Mitigation Strategy; *SC,* subcutaneous; *T,* testosterone.

From Melmed S et al: *Williams textbook of endocrinology*, ed 14, Elsevier, 2019.

TABLE 4 Monitoring During Testosterone Treatment

Parameter	Timing	Further Management
Measures of Efficacy		
Symptoms and signs of androgen deficiency	At baseline, after 3-12 mo, and then yearly	Continue testosterone treatment in men with clinical improvement and no adverse effects. Consider discontinuing testosterone treatment in men if no clinical improvement.
BMD	For men at high risk for fracture, BMD before treatment; for men with osteoporosis or minimal-trauma fracture, BMD after 1-2 yr	Institute appropriate treatment for men with osteoporosis, including calcium and vitamin D.
Serum testosterone	*Testosterone ester injection:* After 3-6 mo, measured midway between injections or at end of dosing interval (if androgen deficiency symptoms are present at that time) *Testosterone patch:* After 3-4 wk, at 8-10 hr after application *Testosterone gel:* After 2 wk, at any time after application *Buccal testosterone:* After 4-6 wk, at any time after application (preferably in the morning) *Testosterone pellets:* At end of dosing interval *Oral testosterone undecanoate:* After 1 wk, at 3-5 hr after oral dose *Testosterone undecanoate injection:* At end of dosing interval	Adjust dose or dosing interval to achieve serum testosterone concentrations in the mid-normal range.
Adverse Effects		
Hematocrit	At baseline, after 3-6 mo, and then yearly	If hematocrit is >54%, stop or reduce dosage of testosterone until hematocrit declines to normal and reinitiate testosterone at a lower dosage. Investigate for a hypoxic condition such as obstructive sleep apnea or chronic lung disease.
PSA level, with or without DRE (using shared decision making, i.e., if a patient desires prostate cancer screening after discussion of risks and benefits of PSA screening and monitoring), in men >50 yr (>40 if risk factors for prostate cancer)	At baseline, after 3-6 mo, and then according to accepted guidelines	Urologic evaluation with any of the following: • Confirmed PSA >4 ng/mL any time during testosterone treatment • PSA increase >1.4 ng/mL within 12 mo of testosterone treatment • Palpable abnormality (nodule or induration) on DRE • Worsening of lower urinary tract symptoms (e.g., IPSS score >19)
Obstructive sleep apnea (snoring, witnessed apnea, daytime somnolence, unexplained erythrocytosis, worsening hypertension or edema)	At baseline, after 3-12 mo, and then yearly	Evaluate for obstructive sleep apnea or adjustment of CPAP settings. Evaluate for other causes of hypoxia.
Formulation-specific adverse effects	At baseline, after 3-6 mo, and then yearly	Discontinue and switch to another formulation.
Testosterone ester injections	Discomfort, bleeding, or hematoma with IM injections Fluctuations in energy, mood, libido Allergy to oil vehicle (rare)	Reinstruct on the self-injection site technique. Consider shortening the injection interval if the nadir testosterone level is low.
Testosterone patch	Skin irritation Adhesion to skin	Coadministration of corticosteroid cream may reduce skin irritation.
Testosterone gel	Contact transfer to others Skin dryness at site of application	Reinstruct on washing hands and covering application area after gel dries or showering 4-6 hr after application, avoiding prolonged skin-to-skin contact of application site with women and children.
Buccal testosterone tablets	Gum irritation or inflammation Poor adhesion to gums Altered or bitter taste	Reinstruct on proper application and reassure to complete an adequate trial with the correct technique.
SC testosterone pellets	Pellet extrusion Implantation-site infection, bleeding, fibrosis	Reimplant pellets. Treat infection with appropriate drainage and antibiotics.

BMD, Bone mineral density; *CPAP,* continuous positive airway pressure; *DRE,* digital rectal examination; *IM,* intramuscular; *IPSS,* International Prostate Symptom Score; *PSA,* prostate-specific antigen; *SC,* subcutaneous.
From Melmed S et al: *Williams textbook of endocrinology*, ed 14, Elsevier, 2019.

events. However, a recent trial among men with androgen deficiency dispensed testosterone prescriptions revealed lower risk of cardiovascular outcomes over a median follow-up of 3.4 yr.[4]

- Clinical trials have also demonstrated that testosterone replacement in men with low testosterone increases volumetric bone mineral density (vBMD) and estimated bone strength more in trabecular than peripheral bone and more in the spine than the hip.[5]

[4] Cheetham TC et al: Association of testosterone replacement with cardiovascular outcomes among men with androgen deficiency, *JAMA Int Med* 177(4):491-499, 2017.

[5] Synder PJ et al: Effect of testosterone treatment on volumetric bone density and strength in older men with low testosterone, *JAMA Int Med* 177(4):471-479, 2017.

SUGGESTED READINGS

Available at ExpertConsult.com

AUTHOR: **Joseph R. Tucci, MD, FACP, FACE**

BASIC INFORMATION

DEFINITION

Magnesium (Mg), after potassium, is the second most abundant intracellular and fourth most cation in living organisms. This ion plays a vital role in nearly every major metabolic and biochemical process within cells. Magnesium is a critical cofactor of the ubiquitous cellular Na^+-K^+-ATPase and is notable to have coexisting secondary electrolyte disorders when deranged. Serum magnesium concentration is tightly regulated by a dynamic balance among three organ systems: Gut, kidney, and bone. Most of the total body magnesium is found in bone, muscle, and skin. Serum magnesium represents only 0.3% of the total body magnesium. Magnesium has been implicated in and used as treatment for several diseases. Although its importance is widely acknowledged, routine serum magnesium levels are generally not evaluated in clinical medicine.

Magnesium deficiency is defined as a decrease in total body magnesium content. The recommended daily allowance of magnesium is 420 mg for males and 320 mg for females. Fig. 1 illustrates magnesium homeostasis in healthy adults. Magnesium is mainly absorbed through the jejunum and ileum. Poor dietary intake of magnesium usually does not lead to severe magnesium deficiency because normal kidney function prevents magnesium loss through renal conservation of magnesium maintaining homeostasis. Fig. 2 depicts the renal handling of magnesium by the kidney. Hypomagnesemia is typically defined as a total serum magnesium concentration below 1.8 mg/dl and is categorized as mild (1.5 to 1.8 mg/dl), moderate (1 to 1.4 mg/dl), or severe (<1 mg/dl). Serum magnesium levels do not fully correlate with total body magnesium levels given that the different compartments that magnesium is found in do not easily equilibrate like sodium does. Thus, normal magnesium levels in patients where hypomagnesemia would be expected may still need magnesium supplementation, such as in cases of hypocalcemia, hypokalemia, or malnutrition.

SYNONYMS

Magnesium deficiency
Low magnesium

ICD-10CM CODES

E83.42	Hypomagnesemia
E83.40	Disorders of magnesium metabolism, unspecified

EPIDEMIOLOGY & DEMOGRAPHICS

Hypomagnesemia may occur in more than 10% of hospitalized patients. It is especially common among the critically ill, with an incidence as high as 65%. It may be encountered in 25% to 35% of patients with acute pancreatitis. Low magnesium levels frequently are encountered in chronic alcoholics and poorly controlled diabetics. The incidence and prevalence of hypomagnesemia are similar across sexes, races, and ethnicities, but may be greater in the elderly. This observation may be explained by poorer nutritional intake, greater use of certain medications (e.g., diuretics, laxatives, proton pump inhibitors), or comorbidities.

RISK FACTORS

- Alcoholism
- Volume expansion (including pregnancy)
- Poorly controlled diabetes mellitus
- Chronic diuretic use
- Chronic laxative use
- Chronic use of proton pump inhibitors
- Subarachnoid hemorrhage
- Severe sepsis
- Acute phase after liver transplantation
- Large transfusions with citrate-rich blood products
- Postsurgical patients
- Leptospirosis
- Pancreatitis

PHYSICAL FINDINGS & CLINICAL PRESENTATION

- Mild hypomagnesemia is most frequently asymptomatic. Clinical manifestations appear with more severe deficiency.
- Signs and symptoms are not unique and frequently difficult to determine if caused by hypomagnesemia or its complications of hypokalemia or hypocalcemia.
- Symptoms of hypomagnesemia have been reported at modest degrees of depletion, but generally they are more common when serum magnesium levels are <1.2 mg/dl.
- Neuromuscular effects include weakness, cramps, and paresthesias. Manifestations may include Trousseau and Chvostek signs. More severe depletion can cause vertical nystagmus, tetany, and seizures.
- Metabolic effects include hypokalemia from renal potassium wasting that may be refractory to potassium supplementation until magnesium deficiency is repaired. Hypocalcemia is also common in hypomagnesemia, which suppresses release of parathyroid hormone (PTH) and produces end-organ resistance to PTH.
- Cardiovascular effects: Hypomagnesemia is associated with a variety of atrial and ventricular arrhythmias.
- ECG findings: Flattened T-waves, prolonged QT interval, ST depression, and widened QRS complexes, and torsades de pointes.
- The role of magnesium deficiency in the clinical development of seizures and cardiac arrhythmias requires treatment of these conditions with magnesium.

ETIOLOGY

Causes (Table 1)

DIAGNOSIS

WORKUP

- Comprehensive history including medication and dietary history, alcohol use, prior magnesium measurements, and history of disorders associated with hypomagnesemia (e.g., disorders of gastrointestinal tract, vomiting, diarrhea)
- Physical examination and review of vital signs, intake, and output

LABORATORY TESTS

The total serum concentration of magnesium should be measured in hospitalized patients with

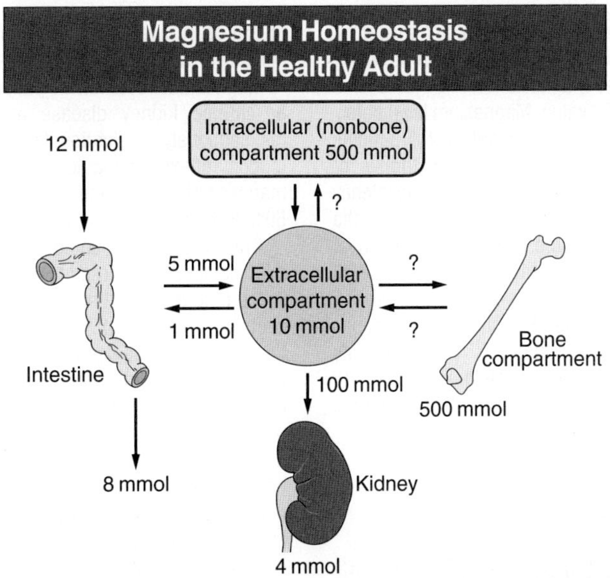

FIG. 1 Magnesium homeostasis in healthy young adults. Net zero balance results from net intestinal uptake (absorption minus secretion) equaling urinary loss. After its passage into the extracellular fluid, Mg^{2+} enters the intracellular space and is deposited in bone or soft tissue or eliminated via the kidneys. Entry and exit fluxes between the extracellular and intracellular spaces (skeletal and nonskeletal compartments) are also of identical magnitude; however, precise values of exchange are still debated. (From Johnson RJ: *Comprehensive clinical nephrology,* ed 6, Philadelphia, 2019, Elsevier.)

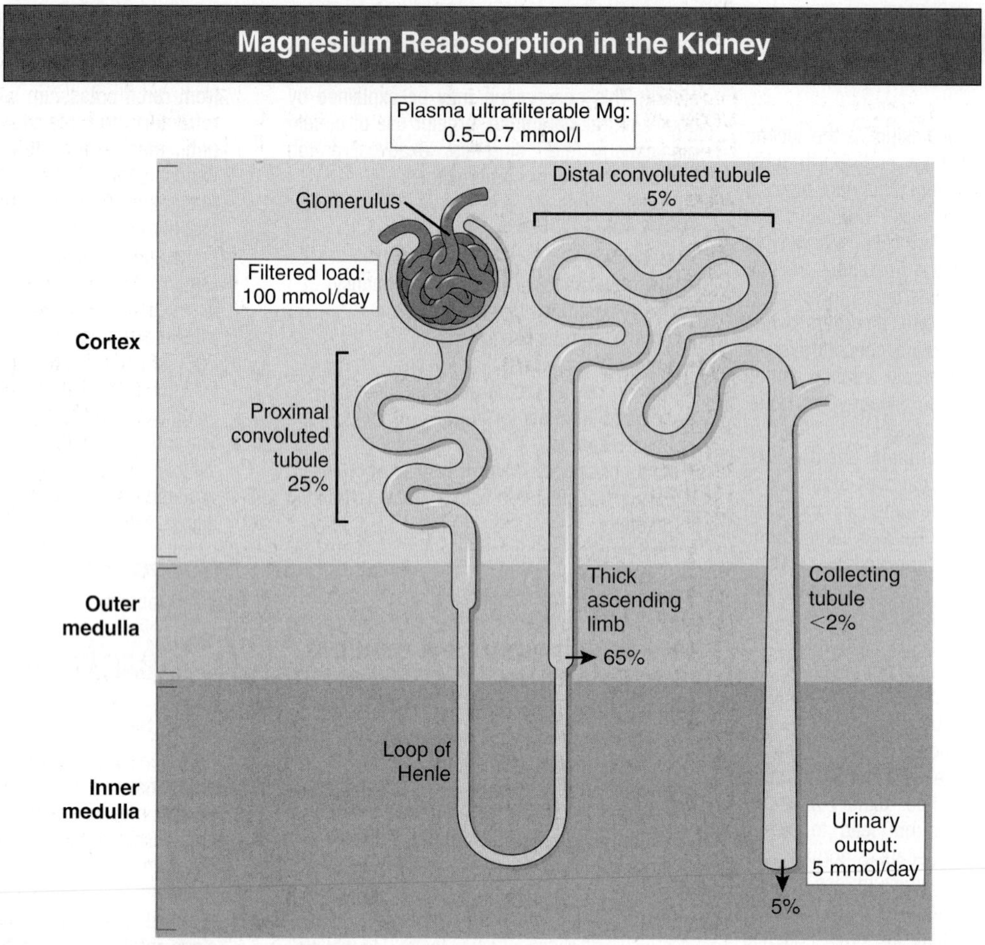

FIG. 2 Sites of magnesium reabsorption in various segments. Percentage absorbed in various segments of the renal tubule from the glomerular ultrafiltrate. (Redrawn from Quamme GA: Control of magnesium transport in the thick ascending limb, *Am J Physiol* 256:F197-F210, 1989. In Johnson RJ: *Comprehensive clinical nephrology,* ed 6, Philadelphia, 2019, Elsevier.)

acute illness to screen for hypomagnesemia. Unlike serum ionized calcium concentrations, obtaining ionized magnesium levels provides no additional clinical value. Magnesium level determinations are indicated for critically ill patients and those at risk for cardiac arrhythmias or seizures. The etiology of magnesium deficiency is often obvious from the history. When the cause is unknown, the fractional excretion of magnesium (FE_{Mg}) may facilitate diagnosis. With extrarenal magnesium loss from malabsorption or laxative abuse, the FE_{Mg} should be appropriately reduced to less than 4%. If FE_{Mg} exceeds 4%, renal magnesium wasting is established and frequently related to surreptitious diuretic use or familial magnesium-wasting disorders.

IMAGING STUDIES

Not routinely recommended

Rx TREATMENT

It is unclear whether mild, asymptomatic hypomagnesemia requires treatment. However, symptomatic hypomagnesemia is treated with intravenous magnesium, typically magnesium sulfate. For treatment of torsades de pointes, 1 to 2 g of intravenous magnesium sulfate as a bolus over 5 minutes is recommended.

Magnesium repletion in patients with acute or chronic kidney disease must be carried out cautiously. Evaluation for depressed deep tendon reflexes, periodic monitoring of serum magnesium levels, and dose reductions from 50% to 75% are recommended.

Oral magnesium supplementation may treat mild cases of hypomagnesemia successfully. In the outpatient setting, oral magnesium salts such as magnesium oxide (250-500 mg 4 times daily) can be used for repletion. However, these agents frequently produce an osmotic diarrhea, particularly at high doses. Patients with gastrointestinal magnesium-wasting who do not achieve normal levels of repletion with one formulation may respond to an alternative formulation. Potassium-sparing diuretics, including triamterene, amiloride, and spironolactone, increase serum magnesium levels. Caution must be exercised to avoid induction of hyperkalemia. Intravenous magnesium supplementation causes an abrupt rise in serum magnesium levels and reduces renal magnesium reabsorption in patients with normal renal function. This limits magnesium repletion. In most cases, oral supplementation of magnesium should suffice.

DISPOSITION

- Potential contributing factors should be evaluated and treated appropriately.
- Patients with symptomatic or severe hypomagnesemia require monitoring in an intensive care setting until the serum magnesium concentration and associated electrolyte abnormalities are corrected and stabilized at safe levels per se >2.0 mg/dl.
- The risk of recurrence depends primarily on the nature of the underlying disorder. Hypomagnesemia has less chance of recurring when the offending medication is discontinued and/or when gastrointestinal and renal losses are not chronic. Inherited disorders may necessitate prolonged supplementation.
- In patients with self-limited reasons for magnesium deficiency, repletion therapy can be accomplished easily. However, in patients with persistent magnesium-wasting, treatment by oral magnesium therapy may not correct the serum level to normal. Nevertheless, most individuals adapt to their chronic hypomagnesemia without sequelae.

TABLE 1 Causes of Magnesium Deficiency

Poor intake	Dietary deprivation or malnutrition Insufficient magnesium in tube-feeding formulas Parenteral nutrition preparations with insufficient magnesium
Redistribution of magnesium from extracellular to intracellular space or bone	Treatment of diabetic ketoacidosis Refeeding syndrome Hungry bone syndrome following parathyroidectomy Correction of metabolic acidosis Acute and chronic pancreatitis (soft tissue sequestration and gastrointestinal loss) Severe burns (sequestration in necrotic tissue) Hyperthyroidism
Poor intestinal absorption/ increased intestinal loss	Diarrhea Inflammatory bowel disease (e.g., Crohn disease, ulcerative colitis) Intestinal fistula Laxative use Nasogastric suction Proton pump inhibitor administration Severe malabsorption Short bowel syndrome Steatorrhea
Excessive renal loss	Diuretics: Loop diuretics (loss of magnesium and calcium) Thiazide-like diuretics (loss of magnesium with calcium retention) Hypercalciuria Metabolic acidosis Osmotic diuretics (hypertonic solutions) Poorly controlled diabetes and diabetic ketoacidosis (especially during recovery phase after phosphorus replacement) Primary hyperaldosteronism Renal tubular acidosis Syndrome of inappropriate antidiuretic hormone secretion (SIADH) Other drugs: Aminoglycosides Amphotericin B Cisplatin, carboplatin Cyclosporine Foscarnet Monoclonal antibodies that target the epidermal growth factor receptor (e.g., cetuximab, panitumumab) Pentamidine Tacrolimus
Inherited causes	Autosomal-dominant hypocalcemia with hypercalciuria (ADHH) Bartter syndrome Familial hypomagnesemia with hypercalciuria and nephrocalcinosis Gitelman syndrome Hypomagnesemia with secondary hypocalcemia (HSH) Isolated dominant hypomagnesemia Isolated recessive hypomagnesemia

REFERRAL

- Outpatient referral to nephrology or endocrinology may be indicated to help manage patients with chronic hypomagnesemia that does not warrant hospital admission.
- Inpatient referral to specialists in nephrology, endocrinology, and/or critical care medicine is recommended in cases of severe or symptomatic hypomagnesemia.
- Consultation with a dietitian can help increase dietary magnesium intake and protein supplementation in malnourished patients.

PEARLS & CONSIDERATIONS

COMMENTS

- Serum magnesium measurement is the most available and most commonly employed test to evaluate magnesium status.
- Routine correction of underlying etiologies and electrolyte and metabolic derangements is recommended for hypomagnesemia while increasing dietary magnesium intake and/or supplementing magnesium. Chronic hypomagnesemia may be associated with various micro- and macrovascular complications.

SUGGESTED READING

Available at ExpertConsult.com

RELATED CONTENT

Hypokalemia (Section II Differential Diagnosis)
Hypoparathyroidism (Related Key Topic)

AUTHOR: **Snigdha T. Reddy, MD**

BASIC INFORMATION

DEFINITION

An osmole is a solute that has the ability displace water. Tonicity or effective osmolality refers to the directionality of water displacement with plasma water as the referent solution. Net water flow into the central nervous system (CNS) from plasma is a hypotonic state, and from the CNS to plasma is a hypertonic state. Solutes that rapidly equilibrate between intracellular and extracellular fluid compartments are ineffective osmoles because no net water movement occurs between the compartments.

Hyponatremia is defined as a measured serum sodium concentration (S_{Na}) less than the lower limit of normal (i.e., <130-135 mmol/L). Since clinical manifestations of hyponatremia are due to hypotonicity, appropriate clinical management depends on distinguishing among the majority of patients with hypotonic hyponatremia from those with hypertonic or isotonic hyponatremia and those with pseudohyponatremia (isotonic hyponatremia: Low measured S_{Na} with normal measured serum osmolality). Hyponatremia will be used synonymously with hypotonic hyponatremia in this chapter. References to pseudohyponatremia and hypertonic/isotonic hyponatremia are specifically identified by these terms.

SYNONYMS

Low serum sodium concentration
Hypo-osmolality

ICD-10CM CODE

E87.1 Hypo-osmolality and hyponatremia

EPIDEMIOLOGY & DEMOGRAPHICS

PREVALENCE: The prevalence of hyponatremia varies widely according to setting and population age. In the general U.S. population dataset of the National Health and Nutrition Examination Survey (NHANES), the overall prevalence was 1.72%. One study of emergency department patients reported a prevalence of 2.3% in patients 16 to 21 yr and 16.9% in patients >80 yr. Following surgery for traumatic hip fracture, the incidence of moderate (<135 mmol/L) and severe (<130 mmol/L) postoperative hyponatremia was 27% (95% CI, 21.7%-32.5%) and 9% (95% CI, 5.7%-12.8%), respectively. The prevalence in stable, older outpatients was reported at approximately 8% and as high as 18% to 20% in sick or frail populations. The overall incidence at or during hospital admission is comparable, with even higher rates in patients admitted for congestive heart failure (CHF), cirrhosis, or elderly patients admitted for fragility fracture.

PREDOMINANT SEX AND AGE: Prevalence of hyponatremia was significantly higher in women in the National Health and Nutrition Examination Survey (NHANES) dataset (2.09%; $P = 0.004$) and increased with age.

RISK FACTORS: In NHANES, hyponatremia was more common in participants with hypertension, diabetes, coronary artery disease, stroke, chronic obstructive pulmonary disease, cancer, and psychiatric disorders, and less common in participants with no comorbidities (1.04%, $P < 0.001$). A significant risk of death was associated with hyponatremia in unadjusted Cox models (hazard ratio [HR], 3.61; $P < 0.001$) and adjusted (HR 2.43; $P < 0.001$). The incidence in outpatients using thiazide diuretics was 15.1%, with an HR of 4.95 (95% CI, 4.12-5.96). Reported frequencies of hyponatremia of outpatients taking selective serotonin reuptake inhibitors or selective norepinephrine reuptake inhibitors varied widely between 0.5% and 32%.

GENETICS: The hyponatremic disorder, nephrogenic syndrome of inappropriate antidiuresis (SIAD), is caused by rare familial gain-of-function mutations of the V2 vasopressin receptor (V2R) gene. Activation of a mutated receptor located in the renal collecting duct produces overt hyponatremia in infancy.

PHYSICAL FINDINGS & CLINICAL PRESENTATION

- Critical history includes detailed documentation of fluid consumption and diet, gastrointestinal and insensible losses of fluid and electrolytes, urine outputs, changes in weight, medication use, changes in behavior or cognition. Recent medical procedures involving irrigation of tissue beds (e.g., transurethral prostatectomy or hysteroscopy with endometrial resection), participation in marathons or other strenuous endurance exercise or attendance at "rave" parties where illicit use of 3,4-methylenedioxy-methamphetamine (MDMA, "Ecstasy") is common should be noted. Comorbid conditions that increase the risk of hyponatremia include malignancy, CNS or pulmonary disease, adrenal insufficiency, congestive heart failure (CHF), liver disease, or nephrotic syndrome.
- The etiology of hyponatremia may affect the clinical presentation directly and/or by its effect on the extracellular fluid volume (ECFV). Hypovolemia and hypervolemia (decreased or increased ECFV, respectively) are identified by conventional clinical criteria. If available, vector bioimpedance analysis has been shown to further increase accuracy. Specific manifestations of the precipitating cause or underlying diseases may be evident (e.g., fever and delirium following the use of MDMA, stigmata of alcoholism or malnutrition, fever and/or localizing symptoms related to pneumonia or other pulmonary disease, or headaches and visual field defects from an intracranial mass).
- Neurologic symptoms predominate as the direct clinical manifestations of hyponatremia due to cerebrocyte swelling. Compensatory processes that reduce cerebral edema by extrusion of electrolytes, amino acids, and carbohydrates from brain cells take 24 hours to become fully active and up to 7 days to reach completion. Therefore, patients who develop hyponatremia over less than 24 to 48 hours have the highest degree of brain swelling, the most severe neurologic symptoms, and greatest risk of permanent or fatal brain injury. Postpubertal, premenopausal women appear to undergo cerebral compensation more slowly, placing them at greater risk from acute hyponatremia.
- Acute hyponatremia may result in nausea and malaise as S_{Na} approaches 130 mmol/L or less. Headache, lethargy, obtundation, neurogenic pulmonary edema, and/or seizures may occur when S_{Na} is <120 mmol/L. In the most severe cases, death from brain stem herniation can occur.
- Chronic hyponatremia rarely presents with life-threatening clinical manifestations. However, subtler neurologic disturbances such as ataxia, short-term memory deficits, fatigue, lethargy, and nausea have been commonly reported. Muscular weakness and elevated creatine kinase and even rhabdomyolysis may occur. Chronic hyponatremia has also been associated with increased risk of falls, fractures, and osteoporosis in elderly patients. In addition, hyponatremia has been associated with increased risk of cardiovascular complications and mortality in a diverse group including elderly outpatients, general hospital admissions, and patients admitted for stroke, subarachnoid hemorrhage, CHF, cirrhosis, pneumonia, hip fracture, and liver transplantation.

ETIOLOGY

- Hypotonic hyponatremia: S_{Na} closely approximates the ratio of total exchangeable body cations (sodium and potassium, $TB_{Na} + TB_K$) to total body water (TBW).
  1. Serum [Na] = $S_{Na} = (TB_{Na} + TB_K)/TBW$
  2. The term *exchangeable* means that sodium or potassium ions can easily enter or exit from their compartment(s), respectively, the ICF and ECF spaces. TB_{Na} is the main determinant of ECF volume and TB_K the principal determinant of ICF volume.
  3. Hypotonic hyponatremia is produced by a decrease of the numerator, increase of the denominator, or both.
- ECFV depletion (disproportionately greater decrease of TB_{Na} and/or TB_K to TBW)
  1. GI losses with intake of hypotonic fluids
  2. Renal losses (diuresis, tubulopathies) with intake of hypotonic fluid
  3. Cerebral salt wasting
- Normovolemic hyponatremia (normal ECFV and TB_{Na})
  1. SIAD (see "Syndrome of Inappropriate Antidiuresis")
  2. Medications (thiazide diuretics, selective and nonselective serotonin reuptake inhibitors, narcotics, Ecstasy, carbamazepine, cyclophosphamide, nicotine, desmopressin, phenothiazines, terlipressin)
  3. Pain, nausea, stress
  4. Marathon running or other endurance exercise
  5. Primary polydipsia

6. Solute-limited water excretion (tea-and-toast diet, beer potomania)
7. Adrenal insufficiency
8. Reset osmostat
9. Severe potassium deficiency with normal total body sodium

- Hypervolemic hyponatremia (disproportionately increased TBW with increased TB_{Na}): Decreased effective arterial blood volume. Hyponatremia results from proportionately greater increase in TBW than TB_{Na} and TB_K.
  1. CHF
  2. Nephrotic syndrome
  3. Cirrhosis

Dx DIAGNOSIS

DIFFERENTIAL DIAGNOSIS

- *Pseudohyponatremia:* This is a laboratory disorder and represents isotonic hyponatremia where no net water movement into the CNS occurs. In pseudohyponatremia, S_{Na} is reported at an abnormal level but measured serum osmolality is normal when serum glucose and blood urea nitrogen (BUN) concentrations are also within normal limits. In pseudohyponatremia, the serum osmolal gap (laboratory-measured serum osmolality [S_{Osm} by freezing point depression] minus calculated S_{Osm}) is informative and usually less than 10 mOsm/kg H_2O.
- Serum Osmolal Gap (mOsm/kg H_2O) = Lab-measured S_{Osm} – Calculated S_{Osm}= S_{Osm} – [(2 × S_{Na} [mmol/l) + (BUN [mg/dl]/2.8 + (Glucose [mg/dl]/18)]. Normally, the lipoprotein phase of plasma occupies approximately 7% of its volume. S_{Na} is an estimated plasma (not plasma water) sodium concentration. Consequently, certain pathologic conditions (severe hypertriglyceridemia, lipoprotein-X, and paraproteinemias) that disproportionately occupy plasma volume may artifactually reduce S_{Na} measurements due to the method of measurement, indirect ion-selective electrode potentiometry. Direct ion-selective electrode potentiometry measurement (blood gas analyzer) of S_{Na} will reveal the presence of hyponatremia and is readily available in clinical laboratories.
- *Hypertonic hyponatremia:* Small solutes such as glucose (in the absence of insulin), mannitol, and sorbitol accumulate in higher concentrations in the ECF than ICF and shift water from the ICF to ECF compartment. Since the ICF is virtually sodium free, the ECF sodium concentration declines producing hyponatremia. In the case of glucose, a decrease in S_{Na} of 1.6 mmol/L occurs for each increment of serum glucose of 100 mg/dl.

WORKUP

- Comprehensive history including medication and drug abuse history, psychiatric history, exercise history, prior serum sodium measurements, dietary history, history of external fluid losses, volume and composition of oral and IV fluid intake, and history suggestive of disorders associated with hyponatremia (e.g., disorders of the lungs, CNS, heart, kidney, liver, or adrenal gland; malignancies; diabetes mellitus; nausea; vomiting; pain; or stress).
- Comprehensive physical examination including careful review of vital signs, weights, intake and outputs; evidence of increased ECFV (e.g., edema, ascites, or pleural effusions) or depletion and evidence of comorbid diseases listed previously (e.g., abnormal pulmonary, neurologic or cardiovascular exam, or hepatomegaly).

LABORATORY TESTS

- Serum glucose to adjust for dilutional effect on S_{Na} (reduced by approximately 1.6 mmol/L for every additional 100 mg/dl increase in serum glucose above 100 mg/dl up to 400 mg/dl and approximately 4 mmol/L for each additional 100 mg/dl above 400 mg/dl)
- Serum potassium: Because S_{Na} = (TB_{Na} + TB_K)/TBW, decreases in TB_K lower S_K and S_{Na}
- Random urine osmolality and 24-hour urine volume: U_{osm} <100 mOsm/kg H_2O usually indicates appropriate suppression of ADH, suggesting diagnoses of solute-limited water excretion, primary polydipsia, or a reset osmostat (if S_{Na} is below the patient's altered setpoint). U_{osm} ≥100 mOsm/kg H_2O generally indicates that ADH is present. However, U_{osm} approximately 300 mOsm/kg is frequently encountered in patients using loop diuretics, and even greater osmolalities can be seen during osmotic diuresis. The latter is characterized by total urine osmolar excretion >900 mOsm/day). However, in both cases urinary ([Na] + [K]) equals approximately 60 to 90 mmol/L
- Random urine sodium (U_{Na}), and urine potassium (U_K). U_{Na} <20 mmol/L: Decreased ECFV or decreased effective arterial blood volume. Urine potassium losses must be monitored and replaced
- Specific testing for comorbid diseases listed previously as clinically indicated (e.g., fasting morning cosyntropin-stimulated serum cortisol level, and brain natriuretic peptide)

IMAGING STUDIES

Not routinely required. Computed tomography or magnetic resonance imaging may be indicated to diagnose associated etiologies or evaluate associated delirium that may be present in acute hyponatremia.

Rx TREATMENT

NONPHARMACOLOGIC THERAPY

Hyponatremic patients excrete less electrolyte-free water (EFW) than input. Moderate fluid restriction (10-15 ml/kg) is indicated while patients are hyponatremic, especially if EFW excretion remains impaired. Diets high in protein, sodium, and potassium increase urine osmolar generation, thereby increasing free water excretion.

ACUTE GENERAL Rx

- Acute (hypotonic) hyponatremia is defined as developing over <24 hours. Acute hyponatremia results in larger increases in brain water than equivalent changes in S_{Na} developing over longer durations due to lack of cellular adaptation to hypotonic stress. Consequently, correction of acute hyponatremia is a medical emergency and mandates an increase in S_{Na} of 4 to 6 mmol/L within the initial 1 to 3 hours of therapy, depending on severity of symptoms and acuity of S_{Na} elevation. Iatrogenic cases, classically children or premenopausal women receiving perioperative hypotonic fluids, are fortunately rare now. These circumstances can present with headache or nausea prior to severe symptoms and require emergent correction. Acute hyponatremia is rare in patients with high ECFV because the increased TB_{Na} partially offsets the decreased (TB_{Na} + TB_K)/TBW ratio, due to the increased TBW.
- Controlled increases of S_{Na} at this rapid rate nearly always require hypertonic (3%) saline: Recommended rate of correction in severe acute hyponatremia is an increase in S_{Na} of 4 to 6 mmol/L in the first hour. In normovolemic patients, furosemide 20 to 40 mg IV may be used with hypertonic saline to prevent expansion of ECFV and increase water excretion.
- Regardless of type of treatment, acute hyponatremia requires monitoring in an intensive care setting with frequent measurements of S_{Na}, urine volume, and U_{osm} until patients are neurologically stable and S_{Na} approaches the lower normal range.

CHRONIC Rx

- Chronic hyponatremia develops over >24 to 48 hours: Prevention of cerebral edema occurs via adaptive loss of intracellular electrolytes and organic osmolytes (i.e., beta taurine, myoinositol, and others). Consequently, the risk for cerebral edema is minimized while the risk of overly rapid correction of the S_{Na} increases. Precipitous increases of the S_{Na} can result in osmotic demyelination syndrome. A recommended target for correction of hyponatremia, in this setting, is 6 to 8 mmol/L per day.
- Hypovolemia with chronic hyponatremia: Usual clinical practice 0.9% saline administration to restore volume status. The saline solution increases S_{Na} minimally. However, suppression of elevated ADH stimulated by hypovolemia can trigger a rapid increase in S_{Na} from rapid water diuresis. Simultaneous application of desmopressin (1-2 mcg IV every 12 hours) is a recommended therapy that prevents overly rapid water excretion. If the rate or magnitude of S_{Na} correction exceeds recommended targets, desmopressin may be re-dosed as needed. Desmopressin may also provide protection against overly rapid elevations of S_{Na} in patients with unrecognized solute-limited water diuresis.

- Overcorrection of S_{Na}: Risk of overly rapid correction is greatest for hyponatremic patients with tea-and-toast diets or beer potomania. These patients have U_{osm} <100 mOsm/kg H_2O with ADH suppression. The preferred treatment of this situation is fluid restriction and dietary supplementation to supply appropriate quantities of protein and electrolytes. Reflex administration of IV saline is contraindicated: 1 L of IV 0.9% saline (308 mOsm/L) supplies enough osmoles to excrete 3 to 6 L of hypotonic urine in the absence of ADH. If saline has already been given, rapid urinary water loss may be blunted by desmopressin to prevent overcorrection of S_{Na}.
- The treatment of normovolemic patients is covered in detail in the "Syndrome of Inappropriate Antidiuresis" and is briefly reviewed here. The goal of therapy in these patients is to reduce TBW in controlled fashion maintaining TB_{Na} and TB_K. Some patients with chronic normovolemic hyponatremia (e.g., drug-induced etiologies or primary polydipsia) have self-limited abnormalities and primarily require monitoring to prevent excessively rapid correction. Active therapy as described below can be started to avoid delays. If required, desmopressin can be administered intermittently to temporarily block further losses of free water to slow the overall rate of correction. If overcorrection has occurred oral and/or IV hypotonic fluids may be quantitatively administered to lower the serum sodium actively. Other disorders may only slowly resolve and require more active therapy as delineated in "Syndrome of Inappropriate Antidiuresis," consisting of either a direct V2R antagonist or a loop diuretic combined with replacement of electrolytes lost during diuresis.

DISPOSITION

- Patients with symptomatic or severe hyponatremia require monitoring in an ICU setting until the S_{Na} has stabilized at a safe level. Frequent monitoring of serum sodium, urine volume, and urine osmolality and electrolytes is required, with adjustments in therapy as outlined previously as needed.
- All potential contributing causes should be evaluated and treated appropriately. Aside from obvious disorders, adrenal insufficiency should be ruled out.
- The risk of recurrence depends primarily on the nature of the underlying disorders present. Hypovolemic hyponatremia (e.g., diarrhea- or diuretic-induced electrolyte and water losses) or drug-induced SIAD generally will not recur, if the offending medication is discontinued or if gastrointestinal losses are not chronic. Elderly patients with solute-limited diuresis due to low electrolyte and protein intake may be resistant to major changes in diet but may agree to oral administration of NaCl tablets and/or protein supplements. Treatment with oral urea powder has recently been used as therapy and should only be done in collaboration with a nephrologist or endocrinologist. In addition to disease-specific management, incurable conditions (e.g., chronic CNS or pulmonary disease, CHF, or cirrhosis) may require lifelong fluid restriction (10-15 ml/kg/day), high protein and electrolyte diets as tolerated, and periodic monitoring of the S_{Na} to reduce the risk of recurrence.

REFERRAL

- Referral to specialists in nephrology, endocrinology, and/or critical care medicine are recommended in cases of severe or symptomatic hyponatremia to aid in setting appropriate rates of correction and to recommend, monitor, and adjust therapeutic regimens to achieve those target rates.
- Outpatient referral to nephrology or endocrinology may be required to facilitate the management of patients with mild hyponatremia or recurrent hyponatremia that does not warrant hospitalization.

PEARLS & CONSIDERATIONS

COMMENTS

PREVENTION: Well-meaning family members, friends, news media, and health care providers often encourage patients with chronic kidney disease or who are taking diuretics to drink large amounts of water. When these patients consume more free water than they can excrete, hyponatremia may develop. Similarly, participants in marathons or other high-intensity endurance activities may ingest enough water that instead of TBW depletion developing, excessive TBW with hyponatremia occurs. Patients at risk for hyponatremia should receive a specific fluid prescription that avoids both extremes. Conversely, patients with diarrheal losses or who develop decreased ECFV from loop diuretics or combination diuretics must be counseled that intake of water or other hypotonic fluids alone will lead to hyponatremia but not effectively restore ECFV. Sodium, potassium, and water catecholaminergic intake are all required for resolution of hyponatremia. Safe, outpatient correction of ECFV requires the consumption of electrolyte-containing solutions such as those marketed for infants. A more recent alternative is the use of commercial electrolyte tablets or packets. Commercially available sports drinks have high sugar content but relatively low quantities of electrolytes and may be inadequate for electrolyte replacement.

SUGGESTED READINGS

Available at ExpertConsult.com

RELATED CONTENT

Syndrome of Inappropriate Antidiuresis (Related Key Topic)

AUTHORS: **Mark D. Faber, MD,** and **Jerry Yee, MD**

BASIC INFORMATION

DEFINITION

A decrease in parathyroid hormone (PTH) secretion or function results in hypoparathyroidism. In **primary hypoparathyroidism,** absence or dysfunction of the parathyroid gland results in inadequate PTH secretion and subsequent hypocalcemia and hyperphosphatemia. Surgical hypoparathyroidism is the most common etiology, followed by autoimmune disorders. Individuals with autoimmune polyglandular syndrome 1 typically present in childhood/adolescence with candidiasis, hypoparathyroidism, and adrenal insufficiency. Impaired function of PTH (i.e., PTH resistance) can also cause hypocalcemia and hyperphosphatemia, but the measured PTH level is elevated in this circumstance. A maternally transmitted mutation in the *GNAS1* gene results in PTH resistance (i.e., pseudohypoparathyroidism). It is associated with characteristic features that include developmental delay, short stature, round facies, and short 4th metacarpal known as Albright hereditary osteodystrophy (AHO). Paternal transmission manifests with AHO without PTH resistance (i.e., pseudopseudohypoparathyroidism; Table 1). **Secondary hypoparathyroidism,** a condition in which PTH levels are low in response to hypercalcemic states, is discussed in Section IV (see hypercalcemia discussion in the "Calcium" topic).

ICD-10CM CODES

E20.0	Idiopathic hypoparathyroidism
E20.1	Pseudohypoparathyroidism
E20.8	Other hypoparathyroidism
E20.9	Hypoparathyroidism, unspecified
E89.2	Postprocedural hypoparathyroidism
P71.4	Transitory neonatal hypoparathyroidism

EPIDEMIOLOGY & DEMOGRAPHICS

The incidence and prevalence of primary hypoparathyroidism depends on the etiology of the condition. Estimated prevalence in the United States is between 23 to 37 cases per 100,000 person-yr. Postoperative hypoparathyroidism is the most common etiology (75%). This occurs in the setting of thyroid or parathyroid surgery as a result of removal of, or vascular compromise of, the parathyroid glands during surgery. Transient hypoparathyroidism (<6 mo) can be as high as 20% postoperatively, but permanent dysfunction (>6 mo) is less common (3%). Autoimmune disorders are the second most common cause of hypoparathyroidism in adults (female/male ratio of 1.4:1.0). Autoimmune polyglandular syndrome type I is reported to have an incidence worldwide of 1:1,000,000. Other etiologies of hypoparathyroidism are very rare.

PHYSICAL FINDINGS & CLINICAL PRESENTATION

The symptoms of hypoparathyroidism are primarily related to hypocalcemia. The presentation of symptoms varies with the severity and duration of illness.

- Cardiovascular: Prolonged QT intervals, QRS and ST segment changes, ventricular arrhythmias
- Musculoskeletal: Muscle cramps, laryngospasm, osteomalacia (adults), rickets (children), weakened tooth enamel, osteosclerosis
- CNS: Tetany (Chvostek sign and Trousseau sign), seizures, paresthesias, visual impairment from cataract formation, altered mental status, papilledema, and basal ganglia calcifications with longstanding disease
- GI: Abdominal pain
- Renal: Hypercalciuria and nephrolithiasis
- Other: Dry scaly skin, brittle nails, dry hair, fatigue, neuropsychiatric issues

In addition to the hypocalcemia-related symptoms, syndromes associated with hypoparathyroidism can have distinct clinical findings. Conditions associated with hypoparathyroidism include:

- Autoimmune polyglandular syndrome type 1: Mucocutaneous candidiasis and adrenal insufficiency
- DiGeorge syndrome: Dysmorphic facies, cleft palate
- Pseudohypoparathyroidism: Developmental delay, short stature, round face, short fourth metacarpal (Albright hereditary osteodystrophy)
- Hypoparathyroidism-retardation-dysmorphism syndrome: Short stature, microcephaly, microphthalmia, small hands and feet, abnormal teeth
- Hypoparathyroidism-deafness-renal dysplasia syndrome: Sensorineural deafness
- Kenny-Caffey syndrome: Short stature
- Kearns-Sayre syndrome: Paralysis of eye muscles and pigmentary retinopathy

ETIOLOGY

There are several etiologies of hypoparathyroidism:

- Postoperative hypoparathyroidism; most common cause (78% of cases)
- Destruction of the parathyroid glands:
  1. Autoimmune polyglandular syndrome type 1
  2. Radiation to the neck
  3. Infiltrative diseases (e.g., metastatic carcinoma, Wilson disease, hemochromatosis, thalassemia, granulomatous disease)
- Developmental defects of the parathyroid glands:
  1. Isolated hypoparathyroidism
  2. Branchial dysembryogenesis (DiGeorge syndrome)
  3. Hypoparathyroidism-retardation-dysmorphism syndrome
  4. Hypoparathyroidism-deafness-renal dysplasia syndrome
  5. Mitochondrial dysfunction associated with hypoparathyroidism
     a. Kearns-Sayre syndrome
     b. Mitochondrial encephalomyopathy with lactic acidosis and strokelike episodes (MELAS) syndrome
     c. Mitochondrial trifunctional protein (MTP) deficiency syndrome
- Functional and secretory defects of the parathyroid glands:
  1. Activating mutation of the calcium-sensing receptor alters the set point of the receptor and decreases PTH secretion
  2. Activating antibodies to calcium-sensing receptor alters the set point of the receptor and decreases PTH secretion
  3. PTH resistance (i.e., target organs unresponsive to PTH action)
     a. Pseudohypoparathyroidism (PHP): Heterogeneous disorder presenting in childhood characterized by hypocalcemia, hyperphosphatemia, and elevated PTH levels. Table 2 summarizes the various types of PHP
     b. Hypermagnesemia and hypomagnesemia

DIAGNOSIS

DIFFERENTIAL DIAGNOSIS

- Secondary hypoparathyroidism as a result of hypercalcemia.
- Other conditions associated with hypocalcemia. These conditions are usually associated with an elevated PTH hormone level.

WORKUP

- Hypoparathyroidism is characterized by hypocalcemia and hyperphosphatemia as a result of inadequate PTH secretion.
  1. Two measurements of serum calcium are required for the confirmation of hypocalcemia. Total calcium should be corrected for low albumin utilizing the

TABLE 1 Types of Hypoparathyroidism

Type	Calcium	PO_4	PTH	Comments
Hypoparathyroidism	↓	↑	↓	Surgical removal (most common cause)
Pseudohypoparathyroidism	↓	↑	Ø↑	End-organ resistance to parathyroid hormone and Albright hereditary osteodystrophy
Pseudo-pseudohypoparathyroidism	Normal	Normal	Normal	Only Albright hereditary osteodystrophy

PO_4, Phosphate; *PTH,* parathyroid hormone.
Adapted from Weissleder R et al: *Primer of diagnostic imaging,* ed 5, St Louis, 2011, Mosby.

TABLE 2 Types of Pseudohypoparathyroidism (PHP)

Disorder	Urinary cAMP Response to PTH	Urinary PO_4 Response to PTH	Other Hormonal Resistance	AHO	Pathophysiology
PHP type 1A	Decreased	Decreased	Yes	Yes	$G_s\alpha$ mutation
Pseudo-PHP	Normal	Normal	No	Yes	$G_s\alpha$ mutation
PHP type 1B	Decreased	Decreased	No	No	*GNAS1* imprinting mutations
PHP type 1C	Decreased	Decreased	Yes	Yes	$G_s\alpha$ activity normal
PHP type 2	Normal	Decreased	No	No	Vitamin D deficiency or myotonic dystrophy in some cases

AHO, Albright hereditary osteodystrophy; *cAMP,* cyclic adenosine monophosphate; *GNAS1,* portion of the *GNAS* complex locus encoding $G_s\alpha$; α-subunit of the stimulatory G protein; *PO_4,* phosphate; *PTH,* parathyroid hormone.
From Melmed S et al: *Williams textbook of endocrinology,* ed 12, Philadelphia, 2011, Saunders.

formula: Corrected calcium = measured calcium + [(4 − albumin) × 0.8]. If a reliable laboratory is available, ionized calcium should be considered especially in conditions associated with acid-base disturbances or low albumin states.

2. Serum phosphorus is usually high-normal or elevated in primary hypoparathyroidism.
3. Serum intact PTH (iPTH) level is the single best test to evaluate the etiology of hypocalcemia. Typically, PTH is low or inappropriately normal in primary hypoparathyroidism and elevated in most other conditions associated with low calcium levels. However, PTH is also elevated in disorders associated with impaired PTH function (i.e., pseudohypoparathyroidism). Genetic studies as indicated if medical or family history is suggestive.

The diagnosis is established by concurrent measurements of ionized calcium or corrected calcium that is within the lower limit of normal range and low or undetectable levels of PTH on two separate occasions at least 2 wk apart.

LABORATORY TESTS

- Total and ionized calcium: Low in hypoparathyroidism
- PTH: Low in hypoparathyroidism and high in PTH resistance states like pseudohypoparathyroidism
- Phosphorus: High-normal or high in hypoparathyroidism
- Magnesium: Both hypomagnesemia and hypermagnesemia can cause hypoparathyroidism
- 24-hr urine calcium and creatinine to evaluate the risk for renal stones
- ECG should be considered. Hypocalcemia is associated with prolonged QT interval, rarely ST-segment elevations

IMAGING

- Renal ultrasonography to detect the presence of nephrocalcinosis
- Soft tissue calcifications may be noted on plain x-rays (Fig.1)

Rx TREATMENT

NONPHARMACOLOGIC THERAPY

Diet:
- Consumption of calcium-enriched food (i.e. dairy)
- Restriction of phosphate intake (i.e. commercially prepared foods)

Parathyroid autotransplantation:
- Hypoparathyroidism and subsequent hypocalcemia are common problems after neck exploration for total or near-total thyroidectomy or parathyroidectomy. In cases where there is concern for postoperative hypoparathyroidism, parathyroid autotransplantation of one or two parathyroid glands into the forearm or sternocleidomastoid muscle should be performed to prevent postoperative hypoparathyroidism.

PHARMACOLOGIC THERAPY

The mainstay of treatment for primary hypoparathyroidism is pharmacologic therapy with calcium and vitamin D supplementation. The goals of therapy are to control symptoms and minimize complications of therapy. The aim should be to achieve a low-normal serum calcium level (8.0 to 8.5 mg/dl), high-normal serum phosphorus level, calcium-phosphorus product <55 mg^2/dl^2, normal magnesium level, 24-hr urinary calcium <300 mg/day, and 25-hydroxyvitamin D > 20 to 30 ng/ml.

- Vitamin D:
  1. There are several vitamin D preparations available on the market, but the treatment of choice for patients with primary hypoparathyroidism is calcitriol. It is an active metabolite that does not require hydroxylation in the liver or kidney and therefore bypasses the PTH-mediated 1-α hydroxylation defect that occurs with hypoparathyroidism.
  2. Dose of 0.25 to 1 μg once or twice daily is usually required to correct hypocalcemia and improve symptoms. Its maximal effect is seen after 10 h and it lasts for 2 to 3 days.
  3. High doses of vitamin D_2 (ergocalciferol) or vitamin D_3 (cholecalciferol) may also be used.
- Calcium:
  1. Calcium carbonate or calcium citrates are common oral agents used for treatment of hypocalcemia associated with hypoparathyroidism. Calcium carbonate contains 40% elemental calcium, and calcium citrate contains 21% elemental calcium. Calcium carbonate requires an acidic environment for effective absorption, and as a result, it must be taken with food. Its effectiveness is decreased with concomitant use of H_2 blockers or proton pump inhibitors. Calcium citrate does not require an acidic environment for effective absorption.
  2. Start with a dose of 500 to 1000 mg of elemental calcium two to three times daily and adjust the dose for a desired calcium in the low-normal range.
- Magnesium:
  1. Hypocalcemia is difficult to correct without normalizing magnesium levels.
  2. Magnesium sulfate IV 2 g over 20 min followed by 1 g/hr infusion can be considered in severe deficiency states. Milder deficiencies can be managed with oral magnesium 100 mg three times a day.
- Thiazide diuretics:
  1. Thiazide diuretics (25 to 100 mg daily) decrease urine calcium excretion and decrease kidney stones. They should be considered in individuals with urine calcium >250 mg/day.
- PTH replacement:
  1. Injectable synthetic human PTH (1-84) decreases urinary calcium excretion and maintains serum calcium in the normal range with reduced requirements for calcium and vitamin D supplementation. It also decreases blood phosphate levels.
  2. PTH (1-84, Natpara, an 84-amino acid single-chain polypeptide identical to native parathyroid hormone) is the first FDA-approved product for use in the treatment of hypoparathyroidism as an adjunct to calcium and vitamin D. PTH (1-84) is recommended for patients who are not well controlled on conventional therapy alone.

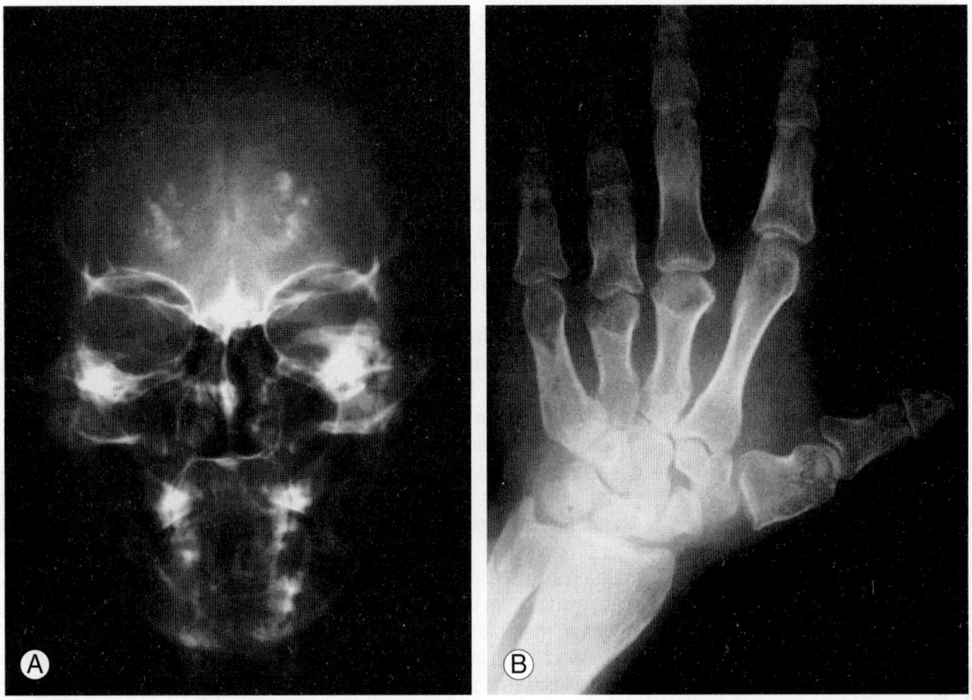

FIG. 1 Hypoparathyroidism. (A) Soft tissue calcification may be present, seen here in the basal ganglia. **(B)** In pseudohypoparathyroidism there are shortened metacarpals, particularly the 4th and 5th. (From Adam A et al: *Grainger & Allison's diagnostic radiology,* ed 5. Churchill Livingstone, 2007. In Grant LA: *Grainger & Allison's diagnostic radiology essentials,* ed 2, 2019, Elsevier.)

ACUTE GENERAL Rx

Severe and/or symptomatic hypocalcemia requires hospitalization. Acute management of hypocalcemia includes:

- Telemetry monitoring for arrhythmias associated with severe hypocalcemia
- IV infusion of 10 ml of a 10% solution of calcium gluconate to receive a bolus of 93 mg of elemental calcium, followed by an infusion of 0.5 to 2 mg/kg/hr until calcium levels are in the low-normal range

PEARLS & CONSIDERATIONS

COMMENTS

- The mainstay of treatment for primary hypoparathyroidism is calcitriol and calcium supplementation to maintain a goal serum calcium level in the low-normal range. IV calcium should be considered if calcium <7.0 mg/dl.
- Treatment of hypothyroidism is commonly associated with hypercalciuria, nephrocalcinosis, nephrolithiasis, and renal insufficiency. It is recommended to target blood calcium levels to the lower end of the normal range in order to reduce hypercalciuria. Urinary calcium levels should also be monitored periodically.
- Hypomagnesemia causes functional, reversible parathyroid hypofunction. Magnesium levels should be assessed and appropriately replaced in all patients with hypocalcemia before a low PTH level is attributed to hypoparathyroidism.
- In patients undergoing neck exploration, consideration should be given to the parathyroid glands. Autotransplantation of one or more parathyroid glands should be considered when appropriate to prevent postoperative hypoparathyroidism.

SUGGESTED READINGS

Available at ExpertConsult.com

AUTHOR: **Vicky Cheng, MD**

BASIC INFORMATION

DEFINITION

Hypopituitarism (from the Latin *pituita,* meaning "phlegm") is the deficiency of one or more of the hormones of the anterior or posterior pituitary gland resulting from diseases of the hypothalamus or pituitary gland. Panhypopituitarism indicates the loss of all the pituitary hormones but is often used in clinical practice to describe patients deficient in growth hormone (GH), gonadotropins, corticotropin, or thyrotropin in whom posterior pituitary function remains intact.

SYNONYMS

Panhypopituitarism
Pituitary insufficiency

ICD-10CM CODES

E23.0 Hypopituitarism
E23.1 Drug-induced hypopituitarism
E89.3 Postprocedural hypopituitarism

EPIDEMIOLOGY & DEMOGRAPHICS

Incidence of 4.2 cases per 100,000 persons

PHYSICAL FINDINGS & CLINICAL PRESENTATION

Symptoms depend on type of onset, number and severity of hormone deficiencies, their target organs, and age of onset.

- Mass effect of a pituitary tumor can cause headaches and visual disturbances (typically as bitemporal hemianopsia).
- Rhinorrhea.
- Corticotropin deficiency:
  1. Fatigue and weakness, no appetite, abdominal pain, nausea, vomiting, failure to thrive in children, and hyponatremia. If the onset is abrupt, hypotension and shock.
- Thyrotropin deficiency:
  1. Fatigue and weakness, weight gain, cold intolerance, anemia, constipation
  2. Bradycardia, hung-up reflexes, pretibial edema, change in voice, and hair loss
- Gonadotropin deficiency:
  1. Loss of libido, erectile dysfunction, amenorrhea, hot flashes, dyspareunia, infertility, gynecomastia, decreased muscle mass, and anemia
- GH deficiency:
  1. Growth retardation in children
  2. Easy fatigue, hypoglycemia
  3. Lean mass is reduced and fat mass is increased, leading to obesity
  4. Decreased bone mineral density, increased low-density lipoprotein cholesterol, obesity, increased inflammatory cardiovascular markers (interleukin-6 and C-reactive protein)
- Hyperprolactinemia:
  1. Galactorrhea, hypogonadism, inability to lactate after delivery
  2. Posterior pituitary (vasopressin; antidiuretic hormone [ADH] deficiency): Diabetes insipidus with polyuria, polydipsia, nocturia, hypotension, and dehydration

ETIOLOGY

It can be congenital or acquired:

- Congenital: Mutations in transcription factors produce multiple hormonal deficiencies. Mutations in genes produce single hormonal deficiency.
- Acquired (Table 1): The result of destruction of pituitary cells caused by:
  1. Pituitary apoplexy: Hemorrhage or infarction of the pituitary gland. Predisposing factors include diabetes mellitus, anticoagulation therapy, head trauma, and radiation therapy. Sheehan syndrome: Postpartum necrosis, a rare complication after pregnancy.
  2. Infiltrative disease, including sarcoidosis, hemochromatosis, histiocytosis X, Wegener granulomatosis, lymphocytic hypophysitis, and infection of the pituitary (tuberculosis, mycosis, syphilis).
  3. Primary empty sella syndrome: Flattening of the pituitary gland caused by extension of the subarachnoid space and filling of cerebrospinal fluid into the sella turcica.
  4. Pituitary tumors: Classified by size (microadenomas, <10 mm; macroadenomas, >10 mm) and function. Prolactin-secreting tumors and nonfunctioning tumors account for the majority of pituitary adenomas.
  5. Suprasellar tumors: Craniopharyngiomas are the most common.

DIAGNOSIS

The diagnosis of hypopituitarism is suspected by clinical history and physical findings and is established by blood tests to confirm the presence of hormone deficiency.

DIFFERENTIAL DIAGNOSIS

The differential diagnosis is as outlined under "Etiology."

WORKUP

Includes baseline determination of each anterior pituitary hormone followed by dynamic provocative stimulation tests, radiograph imaging, and formal visual field testing. Table 2 summarizes testing for assessment of anterior pituitary function.

LABORATORY TESTS

- Corticotropin deficiency:
  1. The presence of a 9:00 A.M. cortisol level >20 mcg/dl or <4 mcg/dl usually confirms sufficiency or deficiency, respectively.
  2. Corticotropin stimulation test using 250 mcg of corticotropin given IV and measuring serum cortisol before and 30 and 60 min after administration. A normal response is an increase in serum cortisol level >20 mcg/dl.
  3. With pituitary disease these test results may be indeterminate, and more dynamic testing such as an insulin-tolerance or metyrapone test may be necessary.
- Thyrotropin deficiency:
  1. Thyroid-stimulating hormone (TSH) and free T_4 measurements
  2. Primary hypothyroidism shows elevated TSH with low free T_4. Secondary hypothyroidism shows normal or low TSH with low free T_4 and low T_3 resin uptake.
- Gonadotropin deficiency:
  1. Follicle-stimulating hormone (FSH), luteinizing hormone (LH), estrogen, and testosterone measurements.
  2. In men, hypogonadotropic hypogonadism is seen with low testosterone levels and normal or low FSH and LH levels (ideally measured at 9:00 A.M. because of diurnal rhythm). Check free testosterone if patient is obese.
  3. In premenopausal women with amenorrhea, low estrogen with normal or low FSH and LH levels is typically seen.
- GH deficiency:
  1. Insulin-induced hypoglycemia stimulation test using 0.1 to 0.15 unit/kg regular insulin given IV and measuring GH 30, 60, and 120 min after administration. A normal response is a GH level >3 mcg/dl. This test is contraindicated in seizure disorder or ischemic heart disease.
  2. Combination of GH-releasing hormone plus arginine is an alternative test, with a diagnostic threshold of 9 mcg/L.
  3. Because the relation between serum insulin-like growth factor (IGF)-1 and GH levels blurs with age, a normal serum IGF-1 does not exclude the diagnosis in older adults.
- Hyperprolactinemia: Prolactin levels may be elevated in prolactin-secreting pituitary adenomas.
- Vasopressin deficiency:
  1. Urinalysis shows low specific gravity.
  2. Urine osmolality is low.
  3. Serum osmolality is high.
  4. Fluid deprivation test over 18 hr with inability to concentrate the urine.
  5. Serum vasopressin level is low.
  6. Electrolytes may show hyponatremia and exclude hyperglycemia.

IMAGING STUDIES

- Imaging is the first step in identifying an underlying cause.
- MRI (Fig. 1) is more sensitive than CT in visualizing the pituitary fossa, sella turcica, optic chiasm, pituitary stalk, and cavernous sinuses. It is also more sensitive in detecting pituitary microadenomas. CT with contrast can be used if MRI is not available.
- Surveillance scan at baseline and 12 mo thereafter depending on protocol and clinical symptoms.

TABLE 1 Causes of Acquired Pituitary Insufficiency

Traumatic
- Surgical resection
- Radiation damage
- Traumatic brain injury

Infiltrative/Inflammatory
- Primary hypophysitis
- Lymphocytic
- Granulomatous
- Xanthomatous
- Secondary hypophysitis
- Sarcoidosis
- Langerhans cell histiocytosis
- Infections
- Granulomatosis with polyangiitis
- Takayasu disease
- Hemochromatosis

Infections
- Tuberculosis
- *Pneumocystis jirovecii* infection
- Fungal (histoplasmosis, aspergillosis)
- Parasites (toxoplasmosis)
- Viral (cytomegalovirus)

Vascular
- Pregnancy related
- Aneurysm
- Apoplexy
- Diabetes
- Hypotension
- Arteritis
- Sickle cell disease

Neoplastic
- Pituitary adenoma
- Parasellar mass
- Rathke cyst
- Dermoid cyst
- Meningioma
- Germinoma
- Ependymoma
- Glioma
- Craniopharyngioma
- Hypothalamic hamartoma, gangliocytoma
- Pituitary metastatic deposits
- Hematologic malignancy
- Leukemia
- Lymphoma

Functional
- Nutritional
- Caloric restriction
- Malnutrition
- Excessive exercise
- Critical illness
- Acute illness
- Chronic renal failure
- Chronic liver failure
- Hormonal
- Hyperprolactinemia
- Hypothyroidism
- Drugs
- Anabolic steroids
- Glucocorticoid excess
- GnRH agonists
- Estrogen
- Dopamine
- Somatostatin analog
- Thyroid hormone excess

GnRH, Gonadotropin-releasing hormone.
Modified from Kaiser U, Ho KKY: Pituitary physiology and diagnostic evaluation. In Melmed S et al (eds): *Williams textbook of endocrinology,* ed 13, Philadelphia, 2016, Elsevier. Table 8.5, p. 193, in Kliegman RM: *Nelson textbook of pediatrics,* ed 21, Philadelphia, 2020, Elsevier.

Rx TREATMENT

Threefold: Removing underlying cause (surgery or radiation), treating hormonal deficiencies, and addressing any other repercussions from deficiency. Table 3 summarizes replacement therapy for adult hypopituitarism.

NONPHARMACOLOGIC THERAPY

- IV fluid resuscitation, correction of electrolyte and metabolic abnormalities with potassium bicarbonate, and oxygen therapy
- Transsphenoidal surgery for tumors causing specific symptoms
- Radiation or stereotactic radiosurgery ("gamma knife") for medically unresponsive, surgically unresectable tumors and tumors for which other modalities are contraindicated. It is both safe and effective for recurrent or residual pituitary adenomas

ACUTE GENERAL Rx

Acute situations such as adrenal crisis or myxedema coma can occur in untreated hypopituitarism and should be treated accordingly with IV corticosteroids (e.g., hydrocortisone 100-250 mg bolus followed by hydrocortisone 100 mg IV q6h for 24 hr) and levothyroxine (e.g., 5-8 mcg/kg IV over 15 min, then 100 mcg IV q24h).

CHRONIC Rx

Treatment is lifelong:
- Adrenocorticotropic hormone (ACTH) deficiency: Hydrocortisone 10 mg PO every morning and 5 mg PO every evening or prednisone 5 mg PO every morning and 2.5 mg PO every evening. Dexamethasone or prednisone is often preferred because of longer duration of action.
- LH and FSH deficiency:
  1. In men, testosterone enanthate or propionate 200 to 300 mg IM every 2 to 3 wk, or transdermal testosterone scrotal patches can be tried.
  2. In women who are not interested in fertility, conjugated estrogen 0.3 to 1.25 mg/day and held the last 5 to 7 days of each mo with the addition of medroxyprogesterone 10 mg/day given during days 15 to 25 of the normal menstrual cycle. In those who have secondary hypogonadism and wish to become pregnant, pulsatile gonadotropic-releasing hormone may be of benefit.
- TSH deficiency: Levothyroxine 0.05 to 0.2 mg/day. Only free thyroxine should be used to monitor appropriate dosing to maintain thyroxine level in the mid to upper half of normal range.
- GH deficiency (Fig. 2):
  1. GH replacement in children is universally accepted.
  2. GH replacement in adults is not generally recommended and requires careful consideration of each individual case. It may have effects on quality of life, body composition, bone density, and cardiovascular risk factors.
  3. Side effects of replacement include peripheral edema, arthralgia, and headaches.
  4. Usual GH dose is between 0.2 and 0.4 mg, determined by the age and gender of a patient and increments of 0.1 mg every 2 to 4 wk until serum IGF-1 is in the upper part of the normal range. Young adults and women taking estrogen require a higher dose.
- ADH deficiency:
  1. Desmopressin (DDAVP) 10 to 20 mcg by intranasal spray or 0.05 to 0.1 mg PO bid is used in patients with diabetes insipidus.
  2. Vasopressin: 5 to 10 U given IM or SC q6h.

DISPOSITION

- Hormone replacement therapy is adjusted according to serum hormone monitoring.
- If untreated can lead to adrenal crisis, severe hyponatremia and hypothyroidism, metabolic abnormalities, and death.
- Complications: Visual deficit, adrenal crisis, susceptibility to infection and other stressors.
- Prognosis: Stable patients have a favorable prognosis with replacement hormone therapy. Patients with acute decompensation are in critical condition with a high mortality rate.

REFERRAL

Consultation with an endocrinologist and neurosurgeon for surgical treatment

PEARLS & CONSIDERATIONS

- All patients sustaining moderate to severe head injury should undergo assessment of anterior pituitary function during the acute phase and at 6 mo.
- IGF-1 can be used as a marker of GH deficiency.
- All tests of GH secretion are more likely to give false-positive results in obese patients.
- The GH axis is the most vulnerable to the effects of radiotherapy; doses as low as 18 Gy in children have caused GH deficiency.
- Sequence of hormonal disruption: GH secretion then gonadotropin secretion. TSH and adrenocorticotropic hormone secretion are somewhat resistant.
- Thyroxine supplementation increases the rate of cortisol metabolism and can lead to adrenal crisis, so corticosteroids should be replaced first.
- All patients receiving glucocorticoid replacement therapy should wear proper identification stating the need for this therapy.
- Stress doses of corticosteroids are indicated before surgery or for any medical emergency (e.g., sepsis, acute myocardial infarction).
- Antidiuretic hormone deficiency may be masked if there is ACTH deficiency with symptoms only appearing when cortisol has been replaced.

TABLE 2 Assessment of Anterior Pituitary Function

Test	Dose	Normal Response	Side Effects
ACTH			
Insulin tolerance	0.1-0.15 U/kg IV	Peak cortisol response >18 μg/dl, or increase by 7 μg/dl	Sweating, palpitation, tremor
Metyrapone	Oral administration of 30 mg/kg at 11 pm	Peak 11-DOC ≥7 μg/dl Peak cortisol ≤7 μg/dl Peak ACTH >75 pg/ml	Nausea, insomnia, adrenal crisis
CRH stimulation	100 μg IV	Peak ACTH ≥ twofold to fourfold Peak cortisol ≥20 μg/dl or ↑ ≥7 μg/dl	Flushing
ACTH stimulation	250 μg IV or IM or 1 μg IV	Peak cortisol ≥20 μg/dl	Rare
TSH			
Serum T_4 (free T_4)			
Total T_3			
TSH—third generation			
TRH stimulation	200-500 μg IV	Peak TSH ≥2.5-fold or ↑ ≥5-6 mU/L (females), ↑ ≥2-3 mU/L (males)	Flushing, nausea, urge to micturate
PRL			
Serum PRL			
TRH stimulation	200-500 μg IV	PRL ≥2.5-fold	Flushing, nausea, urge to micturate
LH/FSH			
Serum LH and FSH		Elevated in menopause and in men with primary testicular failure	
Serum testosterone		300-900 ng/ml (age-adjusted normal ranges)	
GnRH stimulation	100 μg IV	LH ≥ twofold to threefold, or by 10 IU/L FSH 1.5-2-fold, or by 2 IU/L	Rare
GH			
Insulin tolerance	0.1-0.15 U/kg	GH peak >5 μg/L	Sweating, palpitation, tremor
Glucagon	1-1.5 mg IM	GH peak >3 μg/L	Nausea, headaches
L-Arginine plus GHRH	0.5 g/kg (max 30 g) IV over 30 min	Peak GH >9 μg/L	Nausea
GHRH	1 μg/kg		Flushing

ACTH, Adrenocorticotropic hormone; *CRH,* corticotropin-releasing hormone; *11-DOC,* 11-deoxycorticosterone; *FSH,* follicle-stimulating hormone; *GH,* growth hormone; *GHRH,* growth hormone–releasing hormone; *GnRH,* gonadotropin-releasing hormone; *IM,* intramuscular; *IV,* intravenous; *LH,* luteinizing hormone; *PRL,* prolactin; *T_3,* triiodothyronine; *T_4,* thyroxine; *TSH,* thyroid-stimulating hormone; *TRH,* thyrotropin-releasing hormone.
From Melmed S et al: *Williams textbook of endocrinology,* ed 14, Philadelphia, 2019, Elsevier.

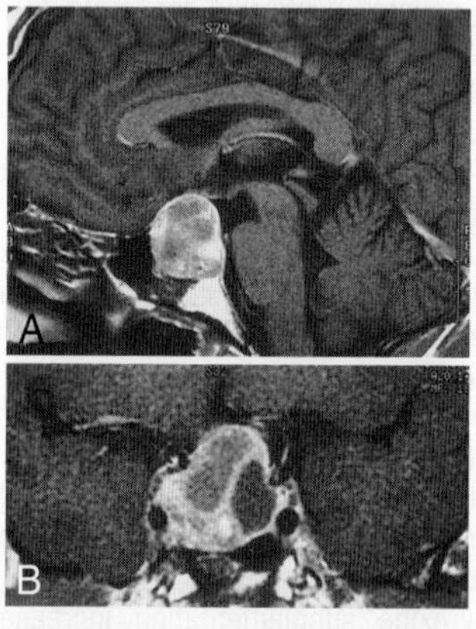

FIG. 1 T1-weighted gadolinium-enhanced MR of a pituitary adenoma. (A) Sagittal and **(B)** coronal images. (Courtesy D. Thomas. From Bowling B: *Kanski's clinical ophthalmology,* ed 8, Philadelphia, 2016, Elsevier.)

COMMENTS

- Mineralocorticoid replacement is not necessary in secondary adrenal insufficiency because the renin-angiotensin-aldosterone system is unaffected by pituitary failure.
- Patients with adult-acquired GH deficiency must meet at least two criteria before replacement therapy: A poor GH response to

TABLE 3 Replacement Therapy for Adult Hypopituitarism[a]

Deficient Hormone	Treatment
ACTH	Hydrocortisone, 10-20 mg daily in divided doses Cortisone acetate, 15-25 mg/day in divided doses
TSH	l-Thyroxine, 0.05-0.2 mg daily according to T_4 levels
FSH/LH	*Males:* Testosterone enanthate, 200 mg IM every 2-3 wk Testosterone undecanoate 1000 mg IM every 3-6 mo Testosterone skin patch, 2.5-5.0 mg/day—can increase dose up to 7.5 mg/day Testosterone gel, 5-10 gm/day (delivering 50-100 mg/day) For fertility: hCG three times weekly, or hCG + FSH or menopausal gonadotropin or GnRH *Females (nonoral route is recommended):* Estradiol skin patch, 4-8 mg, twice weekly Estradiol gel Conjugated estrogen, 0.65 mg daily Micronized estradiol, 1 mg daily Estradiol valerate, 1-2 mg Piperazine estrone sulfate, 1.25 mg All of the estrogens are administered with progesterone or progestin sequentially or in combination if uterus present For fertility: menopausal gonadotropin and hCG or GnRH
GH	*Adults:* Somatotropin, 0.2-1.0 mg SC daily *Children:* Somatotropin, 0.02-0.05 mg/kg/day
Vasopressin	Intranasal desmopressin, via rhinal tube, 5-20 μg twice daily Oral DDAVP, 300-600 μg daily, usually in divided doses

ACTH, Adrenocorticotropic hormone; *DDAVP,* desmopressin acetate; *FSH,* follicle-stimulating hormone; *GH,* growth hormone; *GnRH,* gonadotropin-releasing hormone; *hCG,* human chorionic gonadotropin; *IM,* intramuscularly; *LH,* luteinizing hormone; *SC,* subcutaneously; *T_4,* thyroxine; *TSH,* thyroid-stimulating hormone.
[a]Doses shown should be individualized and reassessed during stress, surgery, or pregnancy.
From Melmed S et al: *Williams textbook of endocrinology,* ed 14, Philadelphia, 2019, Elsevier.

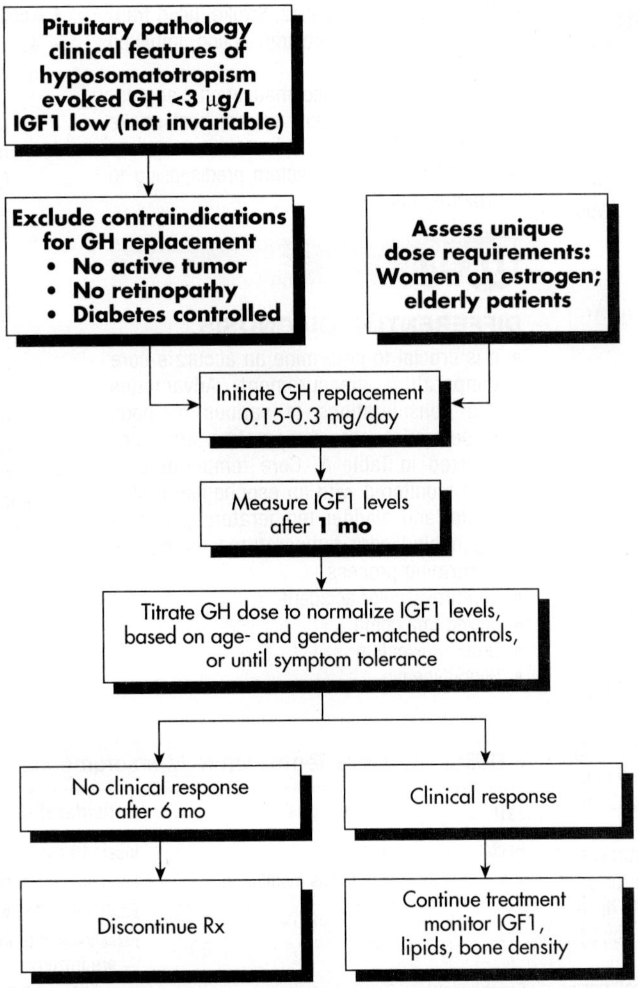

FIG. 2 Management of somatotropin deficiency in adults. Patients older than 60 yr require lower maintenance doses. Women receiving oral estrogen require higher doses than those receiving transdermal estrogen preparations. *GH,* Growth hormone; *IGF1,* insulin-like growth factor 1; *Rx,* treatment. (From Melmed S et al: *Williams textbook of endocrinology,* ed 14, Philadelphia, 2019, Elsevier.)

at least two standard stimuli and hypopituitarism from pituitary or hypothalamic damage. The criteria are different in children in whom GH is required for normal growth.

- Prevention of acute decompensation can be accomplished by reminding patients to increase the dose of hydrocortisone in response to stress.
- Medical therapy should precede surgical therapy.

RELATED CONTENT

Hypopituitarism (Patient Information)

AUTHOR: **Fred F. Ferri, MD**

BASIC INFORMATION

DEFINITION

Hypothermia is a rectal temperature <35° C (95.8° F). "Accidental hypothermia" is an unintentionally induced decrease in core temperature in the absence of preoptic anterior hypothalamic conditions.

ICD-10CM CODES

R68.0	Hypothermia, not associated with low environmental temperature
T68	Hypothermia

EPIDEMIOLOGY & DEMOGRAPHICS

- Hypothermia occurs most frequently in the following groups: Alcoholics; homeless; learning-impaired; patients with cardiovascular, cerebrovascular, or pituitary disorders; those using sedatives or tranquilizers; and elderly patients.
- >700 persons in the U.S. die from hypothermia annually.

PHYSICAL FINDINGS & CLINICAL PRESENTATION

The clinical presentation varies with the severity of hypothermia. Shivering may be absent if body temperature is <33.3° C (92° F) or in patients taking phenothiazines.

Hypothermia may masquerade as cerebrovascular accident, ataxia, or slurred speech, or the patient may appear comatose or clinically dead. Signs of hypothermia are summarized in Box E1. Physiologic stages of hypothermia:

- Stage HT I: Mild hypothermia (typical core temperature 32.2° C to 35 °C [90° F to 95° F]): Arrhythmias, ataxia
- Stage HT II: Moderate hypothermia (core temperature 28° C to 32.2° C [82.4° F to 90° F]):
  1. Progressive decrease of level of consciousness, pulse, cardiac output, and respiration
  2. Fibrillation, dysrhythmias (increased susceptibility to ventricular tachycardia)
  3. Elimination of shivering mechanism for thermogenesis
- Stage HT III: Severe hypothermia (core temperature ≤28° C to 24° C [82.4° F to 75° F]):
  1. Absence of reflexes or response to pain
  2. Decreased cerebral blood flow, decreased CO_2
  3. Increased risk of ventricular fibrillation or asystole
  4. Vital signs present
- Stage IV: No vital signs (core temperature <24° C [75° F])

ETIOLOGY

Exposure to cold temperatures for a prolonged period. Contributing factors include:

- Drugs: Ethanol, phenothiazines, sedative-hypnotics
- Skin disorders: Extensive burns, severe psoriasis, exfoliative dermatitis
- Metabolic disorders: Hypopituitarism, hypothyroidism, hypoadrenalism
- Neurologic abnormalities: Stroke, head trauma, acute spinal cord transection, impaired shivering
- Other: Lack of acclimatization, aggressive fluid resuscitation, sepsis, heat stroke treatment
- Box E2 summarizes factors predisposing to hypothermia

DIAGNOSIS

DIFFERENTIAL DIAGNOSIS

- It is crucial to determine an accurate core temperature measurement. Advantages and considerations of various methods to determine core temperature are summarized in Table 1. Core temperature is best monitored with an esophageal probe. Rectal and bladder temperature generally lag behind core temperatures during the rewarming process
- Cerebrovascular accident
- Myxedema coma
- Drug intoxication
- Hypoglycemia

LABORATORY TESTS

- Metabolic and respiratory acidosis are usually present.
  1. When blood cools, the arterial pH increases, oxygen tension (Po_2) increases, and the pCO_2 falls. Temperature correction factors for arterial blood gas specimens are summarized in Box 3.
  2. Blood gas analyzers warm the blood to 37° C (98.6° F), increasing the partial pressure of dissolved gases, resulting in higher oxygen and carbon dioxide levels and a lower pH than the patient's actual values. A decrease in K^+ initially, then an increase in K^+ with increasing hypothermia; extreme hyperkalemia indicates a poor prognosis.
- Hematocrit increases (caused by hemoconcentration), decreasing leukocytes and platelets (caused by splenic sequestration).
- Blood viscosity, increased clotting time.

IMAGING STUDIES

- Chest x-ray: Generally not helpful; may reveal evidence of aspiration (e.g., intoxicated patient with aspiration pneumonia).

TABLE 1 Core Temperature Measurements

Type	Advantages	Considerations
Rectal	Convenient Continuous monitoring	Insert 15 cm (6 inches) Lags during transition from cooling to rewarming Falsely elevated with peritoneal lavage Falsely low if probe is in cold feces or when lower extremities are frozen
Esophageal	Convenient Continuous monitoring	Insert 24 cm (9.5 in) below larynx Tracheal misplacement Aspiration Falsely elevated with heated inhalation
Tympanic	Approximates hypothalamic temperature via internal carotid artery	Probe: Tympanic membrane perforation; canal hemorrhage Infrared: Unreliable; cerumen effect
Bladder	Convenient Continuous monitoring	Unreliable Falsely elevated with peritoneal lavage Falsely low with cold diuresis

From Auerbach P: *Wilderness medicine, expert consult premium edition—enhanced online features and print,* Philadelphia, 2012, Saunders.

BOX 3 Temperature Correction Factors for Arterial Blood Gas Specimens*

ABG Component Correction Factor

pH + 0.015 (37 − T_c)
Pao_2 − 0.072 (37 − T_c) × Pao_2
$Paco_2$ − 0.044 (37 − T_c) × $Paco_2$

Example

A patient presents with a core temperature of 32° C with the following ABG values: pH 7.12, $Paco_2$ 52 mm Hg, and Pao_2 52 mm Hg. Corrections for temperature are as follows:
pH = 7.12 + [0.015 (37 − 32)] = 7.195
Pao_2 = 52 − [0.072 (37 − 32) × 52] = 33.28 mm Hg
$Paco_2$ = 52 − [0.044 (37 − 32) × 52] = 40.56 mm Hg
These corrections also may be used for hyperthermia.

*Arterial blood gas values not corrected for temperature in significantly hypothermic patients yield falsely low pH and falsely elevated $Paco_2$ and Pao_2 values.

ABG, Arterial blood gas; *Pao_2,* partial pressure of oxygen; *$Paco_2$,* partial pressure of arterial carbon dioxide; *Tc,* core temperature.

From Parrillo JE, Dellinger RP: *Critical care medicine, principles of diagnosis and management in the adult,* ed 5, Philadelphia, 2019, Elsevier.

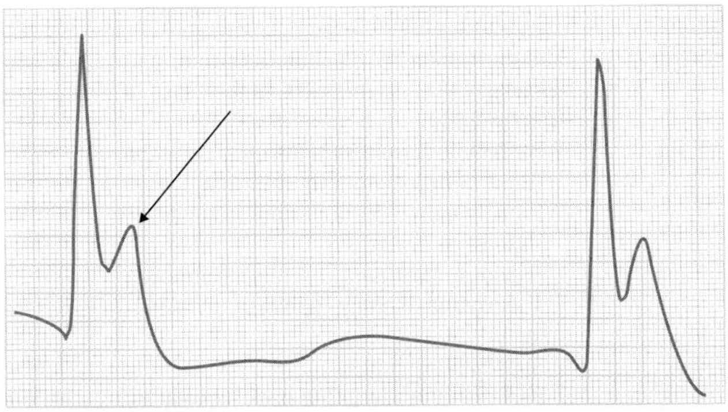

FIG. 1 J (Osborne) wave. (From Goldman L, *Goldman-Cecil medicine*, ed 26, 2020, Elsevier.)

BOX 4 Preparing Hypothermic Patients for Transport

1. The patient must be dry. Gently remove or cut off wet clothing and replace it with dry clothing or a dry insulation system. Keep the patient horizontal, and do not allow exertion or massage of the extremities.
2. Stabilize injuries (i.e., the spine; place fractures in the correct anatomic position). Open wounds should be covered before packaging.
3. Initiate heated intravenous infusions (IVs) if feasible; bags can be placed under the patient's buttocks or in a compressor system. Administer a fluid challenge.
4. Active rewarming should be limited to heated inhalation and truncal heat. Insulate hot water bottles in stockings or mittens, and then place them in the patient's axillae and groin.
5. The patient should be wrapped. Begin building the wrap by placing a large plastic sheet on the available surface (floor, ground), and on it place an insulated sleeping pad. A layer of blankets, a sleeping bag, or bubble wrap insulating material is laid over the sleeping pad. The patient is then placed on the insulation. Heating bottles are put in place along with IVs, and the entire package is wrapped layer over layer, with the plastic as the final closure. The patient's face should be partially covered, but a tunnel should be created to allow access for breathing and monitoring.

From Auerbach P: *Wilderness medicine, expert consult premium edition—enhanced online features and print*, Philadelphia, 2012, Elsevier.

- ECG: Prolonged PR, QT, and QRS segments, depressed ST segments, inverted T waves, atrioventricular block, and hypothermic J waves (Osborne waves) may appear at temperatures less than 33.0° C (91.4° F); characterized by notching of the junction of the QRS complex and ST segments (Fig. 1).

Rx TREATMENT

NONPHARMACOLOGIC THERAPY

- The first critical step in management of accidental hypothermia is initiating passive external rewarming by removing wet clothing and covering the patient with insulating material.
- Specific treatment of hypothermia varies with the following:
  1. Degree of hypothermia
  2. Existence of concomitant diseases (e.g., cardiovascular insufficiency)
  3. Patient's age and medical condition (e.g., elderly, debilitated patients vs. young, healthy patients)
- General measures:
  1. Secure an airway before warming all unconscious patients; precede endotracheal intubation with oxygenation (if possible) to minimize the risk of arrhythmias during the procedure.
  2. Peripheral vasoconstriction may impede placement of a peripheral intravenous catheter; consider femoral venous access as an alternative to the jugular or subclavian sites to avoid ventricular stimulation.
  3. A Foley catheter should be inserted, and urinary output should be monitored and maintained >0.5 to 1 ml/kg/hr with intravascular volume replacement.
  4. Box 4 summarizes measures for preparing hypothermic patients for transport.

ACUTE GENERAL Rx

- Continuous ECG monitoring of patients is recommended. Ventricular arrhythmias can be treated with bretylium; lidocaine is generally ineffective, and procainamide is associated with an increased incidence of ventricular fibrillation in hypothermic patients.
- Correct severe acidosis and electrolyte abnormalities.
- Hypothyroidism, if present, should be promptly treated (see "Myxedema Coma").
- If clinical evidence suggests adrenal insufficiency, administer IV methylprednisolone.

In patients unresponsive to verbal or noxious stimuli or with altered mental status, 100 mg of thiamine, 0.4 mg of naloxone, and 1 ampule of 50% dextrose may be given.

Warm (104° F to 113° F [40° C to 45° C]), humidified oxygen should also be given if available.

- Specific treatment:
  1. Mild hypothermia (rectal temperature <32.3° C [90° F]): Passive external rewarming is indicated. Place the patient in a warm room (temperature >21° C [69.8° F]), and cover with insulating material after gently removing wet clothing; recommended rewarming rates vary between 0.5° C/hr and 20° C/hr (32.9° F/hr and 68° F/hr) but should not exceed 0.55° C/hr (32.99° F/hr) in elderly persons.
  2. Moderate to severe hypothermia:
     a. Active core rewarming
        (1) Delivery of heat by way of fluids: Warm gastrointestinal irrigation (with saline enemas and by nasogastric tube); IV fluids (usually D_5NS without potassium) warmed to 104° F to 107.6° F (40° C to 42° C), peritoneal dialysis with dialysate heated to 40.5° C to 42.5° C (104.9° F/hr to 108.5° F/hr).
        (2) Inhalation of heated, humidified oxygen (warmed to 40° C [104° F]) increases core temperature by 1° C (1.8° F) per hr and decreases evaporative heat loss from respiration.
  3. Active external rewarming: Immersion in a bath of warm water (40° C to 41° C); active external rewarming may produce shock because of excessive peripheral vasodilation. Ideal candidates are previously healthy, young patients with acute immersion hypothermia.
  4. Extracorporeal blood warming with cardiopulmonary bypass appears to be an efficacious rewarming technique in young, otherwise healthy persons.
  5. Patients with cardiac instability and those in cardiac arrest should be transported to a center capable of providing extracorporeal membrane oxygenation (ECMO) unless other conditions (e.g., trauma) require transport to a closer facility.

SUGGESTED READING

Available at ExpertConsult.com

RELATED CONTENT

Hypothermia (Patient Information)

AUTHOR: **Fred F. Ferri, MD**

Hypothyroidism (PTG) (ALG)

BASIC INFORMATION

DEFINITION

Hypothyroidism is a disorder caused by the inadequate secretion of thyroid hormone.

SYNONYM

Myxedema

ICD-10CM CODES

E00.9	Congenital iodine-deficiency syndrome, unspecified
E02	Subclinical iodine-deficiency hypothyroidism
E03.0	Congenital hypothyroidism with diffuse goiter
E03.1	Congenital hypothyroidism without goiter
E03.2	Hypothyroidism due to medicaments and other exogenous substances
E03.3	Postinfectious hypothyroidism
E03.8	Other specified hypothyroidism
E03.9	Hypothyroidism, unspecified
E89.0	Postprocedural hypothyroidism

EPIDEMIOLOGY & DEMOGRAPHICS

INCIDENCE & PREVALENCE: 1.5% to 2% of women and 0.2% of men. Overall, about 1 in 300 persons in the U.S. has hypothyroidism.

PREDOMINANT AGE: Incidence of hypothyroidism increases with age; among persons older than 60 yr, 6% of women and 2.5% of men have laboratory evidence of hypothyroidism (thyroid-stimulating hormone [TSH] more than twice normal level).

PHYSICAL FINDINGS & CLINICAL PRESENTATION

- Hypothyroid patients generally present with the following signs and symptoms: Fatigue, lethargy, weakness, constipation, weight gain, cold intolerance, muscle weakness, slow speech, slow cerebration with poor memory
- Skin: Dry, coarse, thick, cool, sallow (yellow color caused by carotenemia); nonpitting edema in skin of eyelids and hands (myxedema) secondary to infiltration of subcutaneous tissues by a hydrophilic mucopolysaccharide substance (Fig. E1, *A* and *B*)
- Hair: Brittle and coarse; loss of outer third of eyebrows
- Faces: Dulled expression, thickened tongue, thick and slow-moving lips
- Thyroid gland: May or may not be palpable (depending on the cause of the hypothyroidism)
- Heart sounds: Distant, possible pericardial effusion
- Pulse: Bradycardia
- Neurologic: Delayed relaxation phase of the deep tendon reflexes, cerebellar ataxia, hearing impairment, poor memory, peripheral neuropathies with paresthesia
- Musculoskeletal: Carpal tunnel syndrome, muscular stiffness, weakness

ETIOLOGY (TABLE 1)

- Primary hypothyroidism (thyroid gland dysfunction): The cause of >90% of the cases of hypothyroidism
  1. Hashimoto thyroiditis is the most common cause of hypothyroidism after age 8 yr
  2. Idiopathic myxedema (nongoitrous form of Hashimoto thyroiditis)
  3. Previous treatment of hyperthyroidism (radioiodine therapy, subtotal thyroidectomy)
  4. Subacute thyroiditis
  5. Radiation therapy to the neck (usually for malignant disease)
  6. Iodine deficiency or excess
  7. Drugs (lithium, para-aminosalicylate, sulfonamides, phenylbutazone, amiodarone, thiourea)
  8. Congenital (approximately one case per 2000 to 4000 live births)
  9. Prolonged treatment with iodides
- Secondary hypothyroidism: Pituitary dysfunction, postpartum necrosis, neoplasm, infiltrative disease-causing deficiency of TSH
- Tertiary hypothyroidism: Hypothalamic disease (granuloma, neoplasm, or irradiation causing deficiency of thyrotropin-releasing hormone)
- Tissue resistance to thyroid hormone: Rare

Dx DIAGNOSIS

DIFFERENTIAL DIAGNOSIS

- Depression
- Dementia from other causes
- Systemic disorders (e.g., nephrotic syndrome, congestive heart failure, amyloidosis)

LABORATORY TESTS (TABLE 2)

- TSH, free T_4, thyroid peroxidase antibodies (TPOAB).
- Increased TSH: TSH may be normal if patient has secondary or tertiary hypothyroidism, is receiving dopamine or corticosteroids, or the level is obtained after severe illness.
- Decreased free T_4 in hypothyroidism, normal free T_4 in subclinical hypothyroidism.
- Other common laboratory abnormalities: Hyperlipidemia, hyponatremia, and anemia.
- Increased antimicrosomal and antithyroglobulin antibody titers: Useful when autoimmune thyroiditis is suspected as the cause of the hypothyroidism. The American Thyroid Association recommends treatment of pregnant patients with subclinical hypothyroidism and antithyroid peroxidase (anti-TPO) antibody positivity.
- Fig. 2 describes a strategy for the laboratory evaluation of patients with suspected hypothyroidism.

Rx TREATMENT

NONPHARMACOLOGIC THERAPY

Patients should be educated regarding hypothyroidism and its possible complications. Patients should also be instructed about the need for lifelong treatment and monitoring of their thyroid abnormality.

ACUTE GENERAL Rx

Start replacement therapy with levothyroxine (L-thyroxine) 25 to 100 μg/day, depending on the patient's age and the severity of the disease. Physiologic combinations of L-thyroxine plus liothyronine do not offer any objective advantage over L-thyroxine alone. The levothyroxine dose may be increased every 6 to 8 wk, depending on the clinical response and serum TSH level. Elderly patients and patients with coronary artery disease should be started with 12.5 to 25 μg/day (higher doses may precipitate angina). The average maintenance dose of levothyroxine is 1.7 μg/kg/day (100 to 150 μg/day in adults). The elderly may require <1 μg/kg/day, whereas children generally require higher doses (up to 3 to 4 μg/kg/day). Pregnant patients also have increased requirements. Estrogen therapy may also increase the need for thyroxine. Women with hypothyroidism should increase their levothyroxine dose by approximately 30% as soon as pregnancy is confirmed. Close monitoring of serum thyrotropin levels and adjustment of levothyroxine dose to maintain a TSH level of 4.0 mU/L as upper limit is recommended throughout pregnancy. Table E3 summarizes conditions that alter levothyroxine requirements.

CHRONIC Rx

- Periodic monitoring of TSH level is an essential part of treatment. Patients should be evaluated initially with office visit and TSH levels every 6 to 8 wk until the patient is clinically euthyroid and the TSH level is normalized. The frequency of subsequent visits and TSH measurement can then be decreased to every 6 to 12 mo. Pregnant patients should be checked every trimester.
- For monitoring therapy in patients with central hypothyroidism, measurement of serum free thyroxine (free T_4 level) is appropriate and should be maintained in the upper half of the normal range.

REFERRAL

Admission to the hospital intensive care unit is recommended in all patients with myxedema coma. Additional information on the diagnosis and treatment of this life-threatening complication of hypothyroidism is available under "Myxedema Coma" in Section I.

PEARLS & CONSIDERATIONS

COMMENTS

- ***Subclinical hypothyroidism*** occurs in as many as 20% of elderly patients and is characterized by an elevated serum TSH and a normal free T_4 level. Subclinical hypothyroidism can progress to overt hypothyroidism, especially if antithyroid antibodies are present. It is associated with an increased risk of coronary heart disease events and

TABLE 1 Causes of Hypothyroidism

Primary Hypothyroidism

Acquired

- Hashimoto thyroiditis
- Iodine deficiency (endemic goiter)
- Drugs blocking synthesis or release of T_4 (e.g., lithium, ethionamide, sulfonamides, iodide)
- Drug-induced thyroid destruction (e.g., interferon alpha, interleukin 2, tyrosine kinase inhibitors, blockers of CTLA4 or PD1)
- Amiodarone (reversible or permanent)
- Goitrogens in foodstuffs or as endemic substances or pollutants
- Thyroid infiltration (amyloidosis, hemochromatosis, sarcoidosis, Riedel struma, cystinosis, scleroderma)
- Postablative thyroiditis due to ^{131}I, surgery, or therapeutic irradiation for nonthyroidal malignancy
- Transient hypothyroidism following painless thyroiditis (including postpartum) or painful subacute thyroiditis

Congenital

- Iodide transport or utilization defect (NIS or pendrin mutations)
- Iodotyrosine dehalogenase deficiency
- Organification disorders (TPO deficiency or dysfunction)
- Defects in thyroglobulin synthesis or processing
- Thyroid agenesis or dysplasia
- TSH receptor defects
- Thyroidal G_s protein abnormalities (pseudohypoparathyroidism type 1a)
- Idiopathic TSH unresponsiveness

Consumptive Hypothyroidism

- Rapid destruction of thyroid hormone due to D3 expression in large hemangiomas or hemangioendotheliomas

Defects of Thyroxine to Triiodothyronine Conversion

- Selenocysteine insertion sequence–binding protein 2 (SECISBP2) defect

Central Hypothyroidism

Acquired

- Pituitary origin (secondary)
- Hypothalamic disorders (tertiary)
- Bexarotene (retinoid X receptor agonist)
- Dopamine or severe illness

Congenital

- TSH deficiency or structural abnormality
- TSH receptor defect

Resistance to Thyroid Hormone

- Generalized
- "Pituitary" dominant

NIS, Sodium-iodide symporter; *TPO,* thyroid peroxidase; *TSH,* thyroid-stimulating hormone (thyrotropin).
From Melmed S et al: *Williams textbook of endocrinology,* ed 14, Philadelphia, 2019, Elsevier.

TABLE 2 Laboratory Evaluation of Patients with Suspected Hypothyroidism or Thyroid Enlargement[a]

TSH, Free T_4	TPOAb	Diagnosis
TSH >10 mU/L		
Low	+	Primary hypothyroidism due to autoimmune thyroid disease
Low-normal	+	Primary "subclinical" hypothyroidism (autoimmune)
Low or low-normal	–	Recovery from systemic illness
		External irradiation, drug-induced, congenital hypothyroidism
		Iodine deficiency
		Seronegative autoimmune thyroid disease
		Rare thyroid disorders (amyloidosis, sarcoidosis, etc.)
		Recovery from subacute granulomatous thyroiditis
Normal	+, –	Consider TSH or T_4 assay artifacts
Elevated	–	Thyroid hormone resistance
		Blockade of T_4 to T_3 conversion (amiodarone) or a congenital 5′-deiodinase deficiency
		Consider assay artifacts
TSH 5-10 mU/L		
Low, low-normal	+	Early primary autoimmune hypothyroidism
Low, low-normal	–	Milder forms of nonautoimmune hypothyroidism (see earlier)
		Central hypothyroidism with impaired TSH bioactivity
Elevated	– (+)	Consider thyroid hormone resistance
		T_4 to T_3 conversion blockade (e.g., amiodarone)
TSH 0.5-5 mU/L		
Low, low-normal	– (+)	Central hypothyroidism
		Salicylate or phenytoin therapy
		Desiccated thyroid or T_3 replacement
TSH <0.5 μU/L		
Low, low-normal	– (+)	"Post-hyperthyroid" hypothyroidism (^{131}I or surgery)
		Central hypothyroidism
		T_3 or desiccated thyroid excess
		Following excess levothyroxine withdrawal

TgAb, Anti-thyroglobulin antibody; *TPOAb,* thyroid peroxidase autoantibody; *TSH,* thyroid-stimulating hormone (thyrotropin); +, present; –, not present.
[a]Initial tests: serum TSH, serum free T_4, TPO, or TgAb.
From Melmed S et al: *Williams textbook of endocrinology,* ed 14, Philadelphia, 2019, Elsevier.

mortality, particularly in those with a TSH concentration of 10 mU/L or greater. Treatment is individualized and controversial. Some trials have shown that levothyroxine provides no apparent benefit in older persons (≥80 yr of age) with subclinical hypothyroidism. The management of subclinical hypothyroidism should be individualized on the basis of TSH level, comorbid conditions, risk factors, and patient preference. In general, replacement therapy is recommended by most physicians for patients with serum TSH >10 mU/L and with presence of goiter or thyroid autoantibodies or patient has risk factors.

- ***Congenital hypothyroidism*** is a pediatric disorder with an observed prevalence of one in 2000 to 4000 live births in the U.S. Screening is conducted in all newborns in all states and accomplished by measuring TSH from dried whole blood spots collected on a newborn by heel stick within the first 24 to 48 hours of life. Currently 14 states perform a routine second screen at approximately 2 wk of age. A two-screen approach is preferred because retrospective analysis found that 20% of congenital hypothyroidism cases were in infants who had normal TSH on the first screen but elevated TSH concentrations on the second screen.

SUGGESTED READINGS

Available at ExpertConsult.com

RELATED CONTENT

Hypothyroidism (Patient Information)
Myxedema Coma (Related Key Topic)

AUTHOR: **Fred F. Ferri, MD**

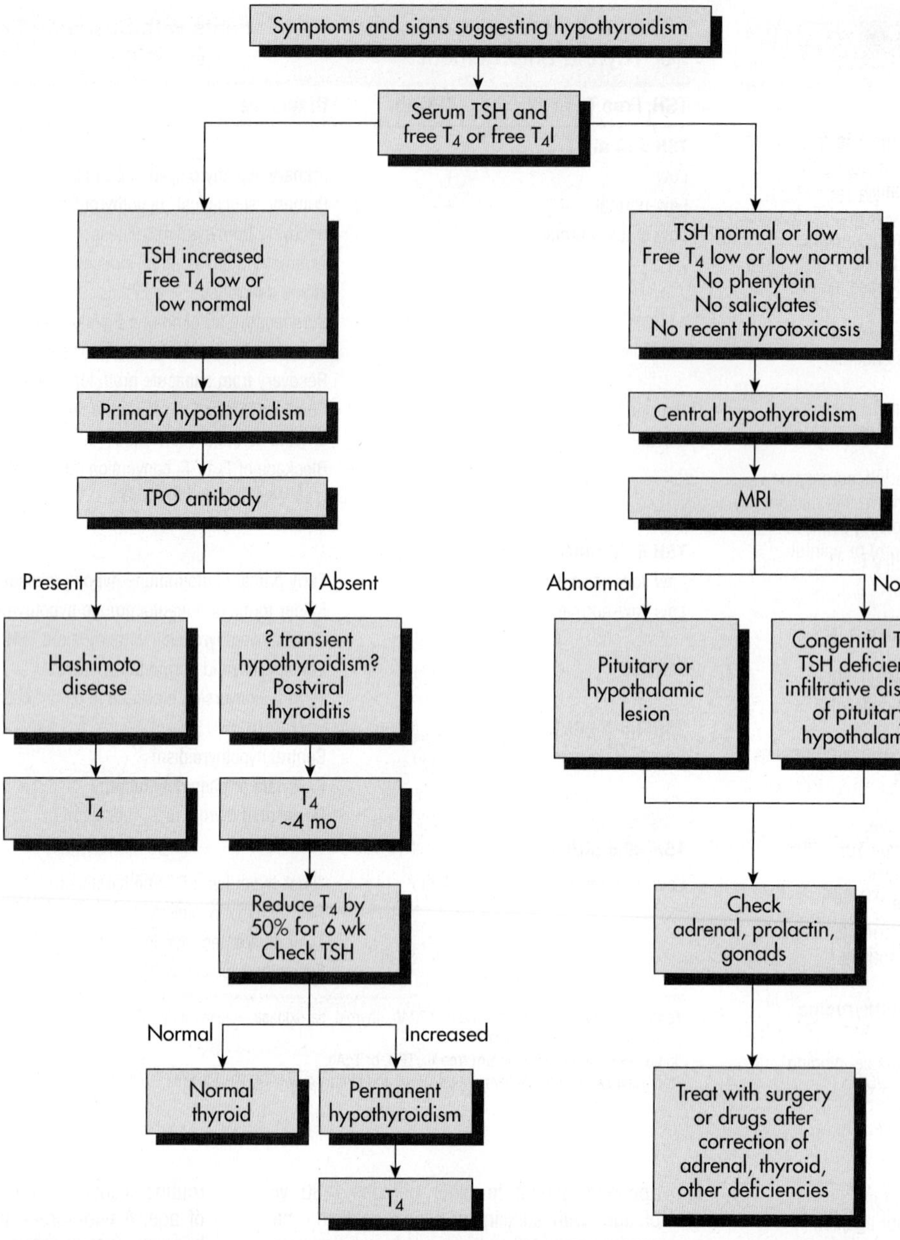

FIG. 2 Strategy for the laboratory evaluation of patients with suspected hypothyroidism. The principal differential diagnosis is between primary and central hypothyroidism. The serum thyrotropin (TSH) concentration is the critical laboratory determination that in general allows recognition of the cause of the disease. An exception is the individual with a recent history of thyrotoxicosis (and suppressed TSH) in whom a low free thyroxine (T_4) level may be associated with a reduced TSH level for several months after relief of the thyrotoxicosis. In patients with primary hypothyroidism, the absence of thyroid peroxidase (TPO) antibodies raises a possible diagnosis of transient hypothyroidism following an undiagnosed episode of subacute or postviral thyroiditis. In such patients, a trial of levothyroxine in reduced dosage after 4 mo may reveal recovery of thyroid function, thus avoiding permanent levothyroxine replacement. *MRI,* Magnetic resonance imaging; *TRH,* thyrotropin-releasing hormone; *T_4I,* thyroxine index. (From Melmed S et al: *Williams textbook of endocrinology,* ed 14, Philadelphia, 2019, Elsevier.)

BASIC INFORMATION

DEFINITION

Idiopathic pulmonary fibrosis (IPF) is a specific form of chronic, progressive, fibrosing interstitial pneumonia with a histologic pattern of usual interstitial pneumonia (UIP) occurring in the absence of an identifiable cause of lung injury. Clinically, it is characterized by progressive parenchymal scarring and loss of pulmonary function.

SYNONYMS

Cryptogenic fibrosing alveolitis
IPF
Pulmonary fibrosis
Usual interstitial pneumonia

ICD-10CM CODE

J84.112 Idiopathic pulmonary fibrosis

EPIDEMIOLOGY & DEMOGRAPHICS

- Incidence: 7 to 16 cases/100,000 person-yr in the United States. Clinically IPF affects >50,000 people in the U.S. and accounts for 20% to 30% of interstitial lung diseases. It is the most common idiopathic interstitial pneumonia
- Most commonly presents in sixth and seventh decades
- More common in men than women
- More common in current and past smokers
- No distinct geographic distribution
- No clear racial predilection
- Familial forms account for 3% to 25% of cases. Genetic variants include mutations in surfactant protein C and telomerase as well as polymorphisms of the *MUC5B* gene

PHYSICAL FINDINGS & CLINICAL PRESENTATION

- Most present with gradual onset (>6 mo) of exertional dyspnea and nonproductive cough. Progressive dyspnea is usually the most prominent symptom. Cough affects up to 80% of patients with IPF and is frequently disabling.
- Fine bibasilar inspiratory crackles, "velcro inspiratory crackles" in >80% of patients, with progression upward as the disease advances.
- Clubbing is found in 25% to 50% of patients.
- Cyanosis and right heart failure (cor pulmonale) may occur late in the disease course.
- There are no extrapulmonary findings beyond clubbing and signs of right heart failure. Fever and wheezing are rare and suggest alternative diagnosis.

ETIOLOGY

- Unknown. Fig. 1 illustrates a proposed pathogenetic sequence in IPF.
- Cigarette smoking, environmental exposures, gastroesophageal reflux, and microaspiration have been associated with IPF.
- Aberrant tissue repair and fibrosis are believed to play a greater role in the pathogenesis than generalized inflammation. Immune system activation and increased vascular permeability contribute to the underlying pathology.

Dx DIAGNOSIS

DIFFERENTIAL DIAGNOSIS

- Occupational exposures (e.g., asbestos) may cause pneumoconiosis with a UIP pattern.
- Connective tissue diseases (e.g., rheumatoid arthritis [RA], systemic sclerosis) can cause a UIP pattern.
- Chronic hypersensitivity pneumonitis (HP)
- Idiopathic fibrotic nonspecific interstitial pneumonia (NSIP)
- Drug-induced interstitial lung disease
- Desquamative interstitial pneumonia (DIP)
- Respiratory bronchitis–interstitial lung disease (RB-ILD)
- Pleuroparenchymal fibroelastosis
- IPF is considered a diagnosis of exclusion

WORKUP

It is critical to establish a confident diagnosis to distinguish IPF from other diseases with better prognosis and different treatment. Multidisciplinary discussion with pulmonology, radiology, and pathology is encouraged as standard of care to decide if a surgical lung biopsy is necessary and to secure the diagnosis.

- Laboratory tests: The are no specific laboratory tests for IPF, however, IPF requires excluding connective tissue disease-associated interstitial lung disease. Thus serologic testing is recommended. Antinuclear antibodies, rheumatoid factor, and anticyclic citrullinated peptide are helpful to exclude rheumatoid arthritis, which often causes UIP.

IMAGING STUDIES

- Chest x-ray shows bilateral reticular opacities most prominent in the periphery and lower lobes. Fig. E2 is a chest x-ray showing diffuse bilateral lower lung predominant reticular opacities in a patient with IPF. High-resolution CT scan (HRCT) of the chest (Fig. 3) is the most useful diagnostic test. HRCT shows one of four radiographic patterns.
  1. UIP: Lower lobe and peripheral predominant honeycombing, reticulation, and traction bronchiectasis. Mild ground-glass opacities (GGO) could be present in areas of fibrosis. It predicts histologic UIP and precludes the need for surgical lung biopsy.
  2. Probable UIP: Same as UIP, but without honeycombing. When the pretest probability is high—severe traction bronchiectasis in a patient of male sex, >60 yr old—it predicts histologic UIP in >90% of cases.
  3. Indeterminate for UIP: Lower-lobe and peripheral predominant subtle reticulation, with or without mild GGO. The pattern does not suggest any specific etiology.
  4. Alternative diagnosis: Findings suggestive of another etiology such as mosaic attenuation, air trapping, predominant GGO, consolidation, nodules, cysts, a peribronchovascular, perilymphatic, or upper/mid lung predominant distribution, pleural plaques, etc.
- Surgical lung biopsy: Obtained by video-assisted thoracoscopy or open thoracotomy in carefully selected patients, when the radiographic pattern does not show UIP and the diagnosis remains unclear. It can show one of four patterns.
  1. UIP: Normal lung with patchy, mostly subpleural or paraseptal, areas of dense

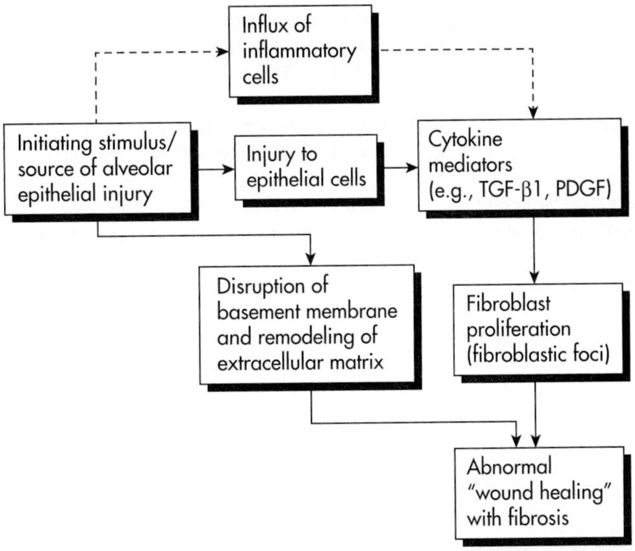

FIG. 1 Proposed pathogenetic sequence in idiopathic pulmonary fibrosis. Dotted lines indicate that although there is an influx of inflammatory cells, this is not thought to be a primary component of pathogenesis. *PDGF*, Platelet-derived growth factor; *TGF-β1*, transforming growth factor-β1. (From Weinberger SE: *Principles of pulmonary medicine,* ed 7, Philadelphia, 2019, Elsevier.)

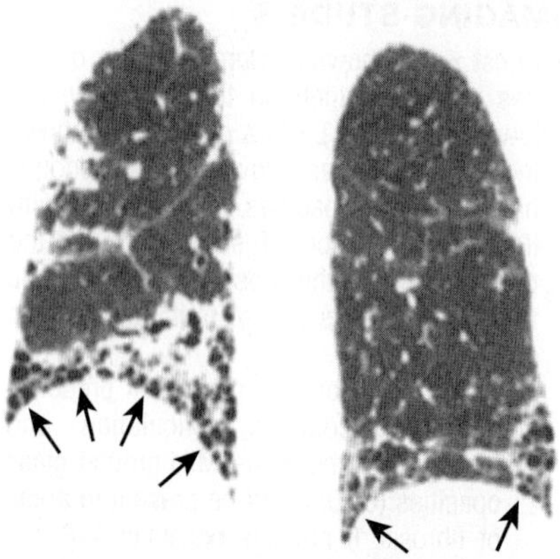

FIG. 3 Pulmonary fibrosis, honeycombing, and a usual interstitial pneumonia (UIP) pattern in idiopathic pulmonary fibrosis (IPF). Coronal high-resolution computed tomography reconstruction shows honeycombing *(arrows)* with a basal and subpleural predominance. This is typical of a UIP pattern. (Webb WR et al: *Fundamentals of body CT*, ed 4, Philadelphia, 2015, Saunders.)

fibrosis with distortion (e.g., microscopic honeycombing), fibroblastic foci, and no features to suggest other diagnosis. Establishes IPF diagnosis in the absence of a radiographic alternative diagnosis.

2. Probable UIP: Same as UIP but the extent is insufficient to exclude other diagnoses. Establishes IPF diagnosis in combination with radiographic probable UIP.
3. Indeterminate for UIP: Some features of UIP but with features suggesting another cause of UIP or an alternative diagnosis. Establishes IPF diagnosis in combination with a radiographic UIP pattern.
4. Alternative diagnosis: Features of other diseases. Excludes IPF. Table 1 summarizes histologic findings for immunologic diseases.

- Pulmonary function tests show a restrictive pattern and reduced diffusing capacity.
- Six-minute walk test may show reduced exercise tolerance and/or exertional hypoxia.

TABLE 1 Summary of Histologic Findings for Immunologic Lung Diseases

Disease	Histology
Granulomatous	
Foreign body, inorganic dust	Simple granuloma
Hypersensitivity pneumonitis	Poorly formed granulomas, peribronchiolar lymphoplasmacytic infiltrate, organizing pneumonia
Infections	
Tuberculosis	Caseating granulomas
Sarcoidosis	Noncaseating granulomas in a lymphangitic pattern
Granulomatous Vasculitides	
Wegener granulomatosis	Necrotizing granulomas involving vasculature
Churg-Strauss syndrome	Necrotizing granulomas involving vasculature
Eosinophilic pneumonias	Granulomas with eosinophilic predominance; interstitial edema
Histiocytosis X	Granulomas with Langerhans cells
Alveolitic	
Drug-associated injury	Interstitial edema with inflammatory cells
Goodpasture syndrome	Linear staining of basement membrane with anti-IgG antibodies typically seen on renal biopsy; interstitial edema with inflammatory cells
Idiopathic Interstitial Pneumonias	
Idiopathic pulmonary fibrosis	Peripheral lobular fibrosis with less involvement of the centrilobular region, and fibroblastic foci in the interface of both
Desquamative interstitial pneumonia	Accumulation of macrophages in the alveolar spaces
Idiopathic nonspecific interstitial pneumonia	Alveolar septa diffusely thickened with inflammation and fibrosis. Preserved architecture
Acute interstitial pneumonia	Diffuse alveolar damage with thickened fibrotic interstitium; proliferating fibroblasts
Respiratory bronchiolitis–associated interstitial lung disease	Macrophages infiltrating distal bronchioles
Organizing pneumonia	Alveolar filling with polypoid plugs of granulation tissue that can contain inflammatory cells.
Lymphocytic interstitial pneumonia	Diffuse thickening of alveolar septa with lymphocytes forming lymphoid aggregates with germinal centers
Idiopathic pleuroparenchymal fibroelastosis	Diffuse alveolar damage with fibrosis

Modified from Sellke FW et al: *Sabiston & Spencer surgery of the chest*, ed 9, 2016, Elsevier; and Jones et al: Histopathologic approach to the surgical lung biopsy in interstitial lung disease. In: Collard HR, Richeldi L. *Interstitial lung disease*. Elsevier, 141-155, 2018.

Rx TREATMENT

- Two FDA-approved oral medications have similar proven efficacy in slowing disease progression, but neither improves quality of life. Both are associated with substantial side effects.
  1. Pirfenidone is an antifibrotic medication without a known mechanism of action. It is taken three times a day with food. Its major side effects are nausea, abdominal discomfort, and photosensitivity. LFTs require periodic surveillance.
  2. Nintedanib is a tyrosine kinase inhibitor taken twice daily. Its major side effect is diarrhea, which often resolves. LFTs also need to be followed.
- Additional new therapies are being investigated and are in phase I, II, and III trials.
- The combination of prednisone, azathioprine, and N-acetylcysteine was associated with increased mortality in a randomized clinical trial and is contraindicated.
- Treatment includes supportive care (pulmonary rehabilitation, supplemental oxygen, influenza and pneumococcal vaccination), referral for lung transplant consideration, and palliative care.
- Gabapentin (up to 1800 mg daily) acts on airway nerves, and is effective for cough, though side effects of sedation and fatigue may limit its use. Other options include benzonatate, guaifenesin with codeine, and menthol lozenges. If post-nasal drip or gastroesophageal reflux could be contributing to cough, it is reasonable to treat them.
- Treatment of asymptomatic gastroesophageal reflux may be reasonable given association between pulmonary fibrosis and reflux or microaspiration.
- Lung transplantation is the only therapy shown to prolong survival in IPF. Guidelines for transplantation by pulmonary disease are summarized in Box 1. Box 2 summarizes absolute contraindications to lung transplantation. Posttransplant 5-yr survival for IPF patients is approximately 50% to 60%. Median survival time is longer after bilateral lung transplantation than single lung transplantation but is associated with more complications during the first year.
- Acute exacerbation of IPF, defined as worsening dyspnea (<1 mo), the presence of new opacities on chest imaging, and the lack of evidence of infection, has a yearly incidence of 10% to 20%. Progressive respiratory failure may require mechanical ventilation; however, a palliative care approach is often chosen instead. Treatment for exacerbations typically includes high-dose corticosteroids and broad-spectrum antibiotics, although the efficacy of this approach is unproven and questionable.

BOX 1 Guidelines for Transplantation by Pulmonary Disease

Chronic Obstructive Pulmonary Disease
Patients with a BODE index* of 7-10 or at least one of the following
- History of hospitalization for exacerbation associated with acute hypercapnia (Pco_2 >50 mm Hg)
- Pulmonary hypertension or cor pulmonale, or both, despite oxygen therapy
- FEV_1 <20% predicted and either DLCO <20% predicted or homogeneous distribution of emphysema

Cystic Fibrosis and Other Causes of Bronchiectasis
Oxygen-dependent respiratory failure
Hypercapnia
Pulmonary hypertension

Idiopathic Pulmonary Fibrosis and NSIP
Histologic or radiographic evidence of usual interstitial pneumonia and any of the following
- DLCO <39% predicted
- 10% or greater decrement in FVC during 6 mo of follow-up
- A decrease in pulse oximetry below 88% during a 6-MWT
- Honeycombing on high-resolution computed tomography (fibrosis score >2)

Histologic evidence of NSIP and any of the following
- DLCO <35% predicted
- 10% or greater decrement in FVC or 15% decrease in DLCO during 6 mo of follow-up

Pulmonary Arterial Hypertension
Persistent New York Heart Association class III or IV on maximal medical therapy
Low (<350 m) or declining 6-MWT
Failing therapy with intravenous epoprostenol or equivalent
Cardiac index <2 L/min/m²
Right atrial pressure >15 mm Hg

*BODE index includes body mass index, degree of airflow obstruction (assessed by percent predicted FEV_1), degree of dyspnea (assessed by the modified Medical Research Council [MMRC] dyspnea scale), and exercise capacity (assessed by the 6-min walk distance). The index increases as body mass index, FEV_1, and distance walked decrease and as the MMRC scale increases.
6-MWT, 6-minute walk test; *DLCO*, diffusing capacity of the lungs for carbon monoxide; *FVC*, forced vital capacity; *NSIP*, nonspecific interstitial pneumonia; Pco_2, partial pressure of carbon dioxide.
From Sellke FW et al: *Sabiston & Spencer surgery of the chest,* ed 9, Philadelphia, 2016, Elsevier.

BOX 2 Absolute Contraindications to Lung Transplantation

- Malignancy within the last 2 yr, with the exception of cutaneous squamous and basal cell carcinomas; the role of lung transplantation in patients with focal pulmonary adenocarcinoma in situ (formerly known as *bronchoalveolar carcinoma*)
- Untreatable advanced dysfunction of another organ system (heart, liver, kidney); coronary artery disease not amenable to percutaneous intervention or bypass grafting, or associated with significant impairment of left ventricular function, is an absolute contraindication to lung transplantation, but heart-lung transplantation could be considered in some cases
- Incurable chronic extrapulmonary infection, including chronic active viral hepatitis B, hepatitis C, and human immunodeficiency virus
- Significant chest-wall or spinal deformity
- Nonadherence or inability to follow through with medical therapy or office follow-up
- Untreatable psychiatric or psychologic condition associated with the inability to cooperate or comply with medical therapy
- Absence of a consistent or reliable social support system
- Substance addiction (alcohol, tobacco, or narcotics) that is either active or has been within the last 6 mo

From Sellke FW et al: *Sabiston & Spencer surgery of the chest,* ed 9, Philadelphia, 2016, Elsevier.

DISPOSITION

- Spontaneous remissions do not occur, although long periods of stability can occur.
- Natural history includes progressive loss of pulmonary function. Predictors of poor outcome include older age, male gender, moderately to severely reduced forced vital capacity (FVC) and diffusion of carbon monoxide (DLCO), and development of pulmonary hypertension.
- There is an increased risk of lung cancer.
- Mean survival after the diagnosis of biopsy-confirmed IPF is 3 to 5 yr, although with new therapies available, survival is less defined.
- Lung transplantation is the only therapy shown to prolong survival.
- Respiratory failure is the most common cause of death.

REFERRAL

- To pulmonologist, with review in multidisciplinary discussion to establish confident diagnosis.
- Referral for participation in clinical trials.
- Early referral to a lung transplant center for evaluation.
- Late stage management should include palliative care referral.

PEARLS & CONSIDERATIONS

- The course is progressive, with a high mortality. The most common cause of death in IPF is respiratory failure.
- Critical to differentiate IPF from other interstitial lung diseases because prognosis and treatment approaches differ.
- Two oral therapies have been shown to slow disease progression are available. Additional novel treatments are being investigated.
- Patients with IPF should be referred early for consideration of lung transplantation.

SUGGESTED READINGS

Available at ExpertConsult.com

RELATED CONTENT

Idiopathic Pulmonary Fibrosis (Patient Information)
Interstitial Lung Disease (Related key topic)

AUTHOR: **Aida Venado, MD, MAS**

BASIC INFORMATION

DEFINITION

Immune thrombocytopenic purpura (ITP) is an autoimmune disorder in which antibody-coated or immune complex-coated platelets are destroyed prematurely, producing defects in cellular immunity that result in peripheral thrombocytopenia. In primary ITP, the thrombocytopenia is isolated, whereas in secondary ITP, the condition is associated with other disorders (e.g., systemic lupus erythematosus [SLE], HIV, chronic lymphocytic leukemia [CLL], lymphomas).

SYNONYM

ITP

ICD-10CM CODE
D69.3 Immune thrombocytopenic purpura

EPIDEMIOLOGY & DEMOGRAPHICS

INCIDENCE: Primary ITP occurs in 10 in 100,000 adults and 5 in 100,000 children.

PREVALENCE: 5 to 10 cases per 100,000 persons.

PREDOMINANT SEX: 72% of patients >10 yr are female; among children, males are more commonly affected.

PREDOMINANT AGE: Children ages 1 to 6 yr and young women (70% are <40 yr). New onset of ITP after age 60 yr is uncommon; comprehensive workup for secondary ITP may be required.

PHYSICAL FINDINGS & CLINICAL PRESENTATION

The presentation of ITP is different in children and adults:

- Children generally present with sudden onset of bruising and petechiae from severe thrombocytopenia.
- In adults, the presentation is insidious; a history of prolonged purpura may be present; many patients are diagnosed incidentally on the basis of automated laboratory tests that now routinely include platelet counts.
- The physical examination may be entirely normal.
- Patients with severe thrombocytopenia may have petechiae, purpura, epistaxis, or heme-positive stool from gastrointestinal bleeding. Life-threatening bleeding is uncommon and generally confined to patients with platelets <10,000/mm^3.
- Splenomegaly is unusual; its presence should alert to the possibility of other etiologies of thrombocytopenia.
- The presence of dysmorphic features (skeletal anomalies, auditory abnormalities) may indicate a congenital disorder as the cause of the thrombocytopenia.

ETIOLOGY

Increased platelet destruction is caused by autoantibody targets to platelet-membrane antigens, in particular, antibodies against platelet GPIIb/IIIa or GPIb/IX. The spleen has a major role in ITP by producing autoantibodies in the white pulp and removing autoantibody-coated platelets in the red pulp. Production of antibodies could be triggered either by immunogenicity of membrane glycoproteins (GPs) on the platelet surface or by external factors such as infections or medications.

DIAGNOSIS

DIFFERENTIAL DIAGNOSIS

- Falsely low platelet count due to aggregation (resulting from EDTA-dependent or cold-dependent agglutinins). Platelet count is corrected by using heparin or citrate anticoagulated tube
- Viral infections (e.g., HIV, hepatitis C, mononucleosis, rubella)
- Drugs commonly implicated are heparin (Heparin induced thrombocytopenia: HIT), quinidine, antibiotics (linezolid, vancomycin, sulfonamides, rifampin), platelet inhibitors (tirofiban, abciximab, eptifibatide), cimetidine, NSAIDs, thiazide diuretics, antirheumatic agents (gold salts, penicillamine), and many chemotherapeutic agents (cyclosporine, fludarabine, carboplatin, oxaliplatin)
- Hypersplenism resulting from liver disease
- Myelodysplastic and lymphoproliferative disorders
- Pregnancy, hypothyroidism
- SLE, thrombotic thrombocytopenic purpura (TTP), hemolytic-uremic syndrome
- Congenital thrombocytopenia (e.g., Fanconi syndrome, May-Hegglin anomaly, Bernard-Soulier syndrome)
- Evan syndrome is a rare autoimmune disorder characterized by autoimmune hemolytic anemia (AIHA) and immune thrombocytopenia (ITP)

LABORATORY TESTS

- Complete blood count, platelet count, and peripheral smear: Platelets are decreased. The peripheral smear should show large platelets and no schistocytes (Fig. E1). Red blood cells and white blood cells have a normal morphology. Unless the patient has been bleeding, the hemoglobin level and leukocyte count should be normal.
- Additional tests may be ordered to exclude other causes of the thrombocytopenia when clinically indicated (e.g. HIV screening test, antinuclear antibody [ANA], thyroid-stimulating hormone [TSH] [hypothyroidism and hyperthyroidism can cause thrombocytopenia], liver enzymes, Hep C Ab).
- Direct assay of platelet-bound antibodies has an estimated positive predictive value of only 80% to 83%. A negative test cannot be used to rule out the diagnosis.
- Bone marrow aspiration and biopsy are recommended in adults older than 60 yr if there is evidence of immature cells on peripheral smear or persistent neutropenia. Biopsy in an ITP patient shows a normal to increased number of megakaryocytes; other hemopoietic lineages are normal.

IMAGING STUDIES

CT scan of abdomen/pelvis in patients with splenomegaly to exclude other disorders causing thrombocytopenia

TREATMENT

NONPHARMACOLOGIC THERAPY

- Minimize activity to prevent injury or bruising (e.g., contact sports should be avoided).
- Stop any potentially offending drugs (see "Etiology"). Avoid medications that increase the risk of bleeding (e.g., aspirin and other NSAIDs).

ACUTE GENERAL Rx

- Treatment varies with the platelet count, patient's age, and bleeding status. For newly diagnosed patients with minimal bleeding, treatment consists of corticosteroids vs. observation when platelet counts are <30,000 /mm^3 and hospital admission when platelet counts are <20,000 /mm^3 (Fig. 2).
- Outpatient observation and frequent monitoring of platelet count are needed in asymptomatic established ITP patients with platelet counts >20,000/mm^3.
- Oral prednisone: 1 mg/kg/day in a tapering course for 4 to 6 wk is the most common initial regimen. Prolonged courses (>6 wk) of prednisone are not recommended. Response rates range from 50% to 75%, and most responses occur within the first 3 wk.
- IV methylprednisolone: 30 mg/kg/day (maximum dose of 1 g/day for 2 or 3 days) infused over 20 to 30 min plus IV immunoglobulin (1 g/kg/day for 2 or 3 days).
- Pulsed-dose oral dexamethasone: Given at a dose of 40 mg/day for 4 consecutive days when given for three to four cycles every 4 wk results in a high response rate (80% to 85%) and has been shown to have fewer side effects when compared to longer courses of prednisone. A meta-analysis of nine randomized trials revealed no major increase in efficacy but confirmed less toxicity and faster increases in platelet counts using high-dose dexamethasone.
- Continuation of corticosteroids is limited by long-term complications associated with its use (osteoporosis, weight gain, opportunistic infections, emotional lability, avascular necrosis).
- Infusion of platelets should only be given to patients with life-threatening hemorrhage or those undergoing emergent surgery.
- IV immunoglobulin (typically 1-2 g/kg in divided doses) is used in two settings: Corticosteroid-refractory patients and pregnant patients. It rapidly increases platelet count in nearly 80% of patients, but its effect is transient.
- Anti-D immunoglobulin, a pooled IgG product derived from the plasma of Rh(D)-negative donors, is also effective. It can be given

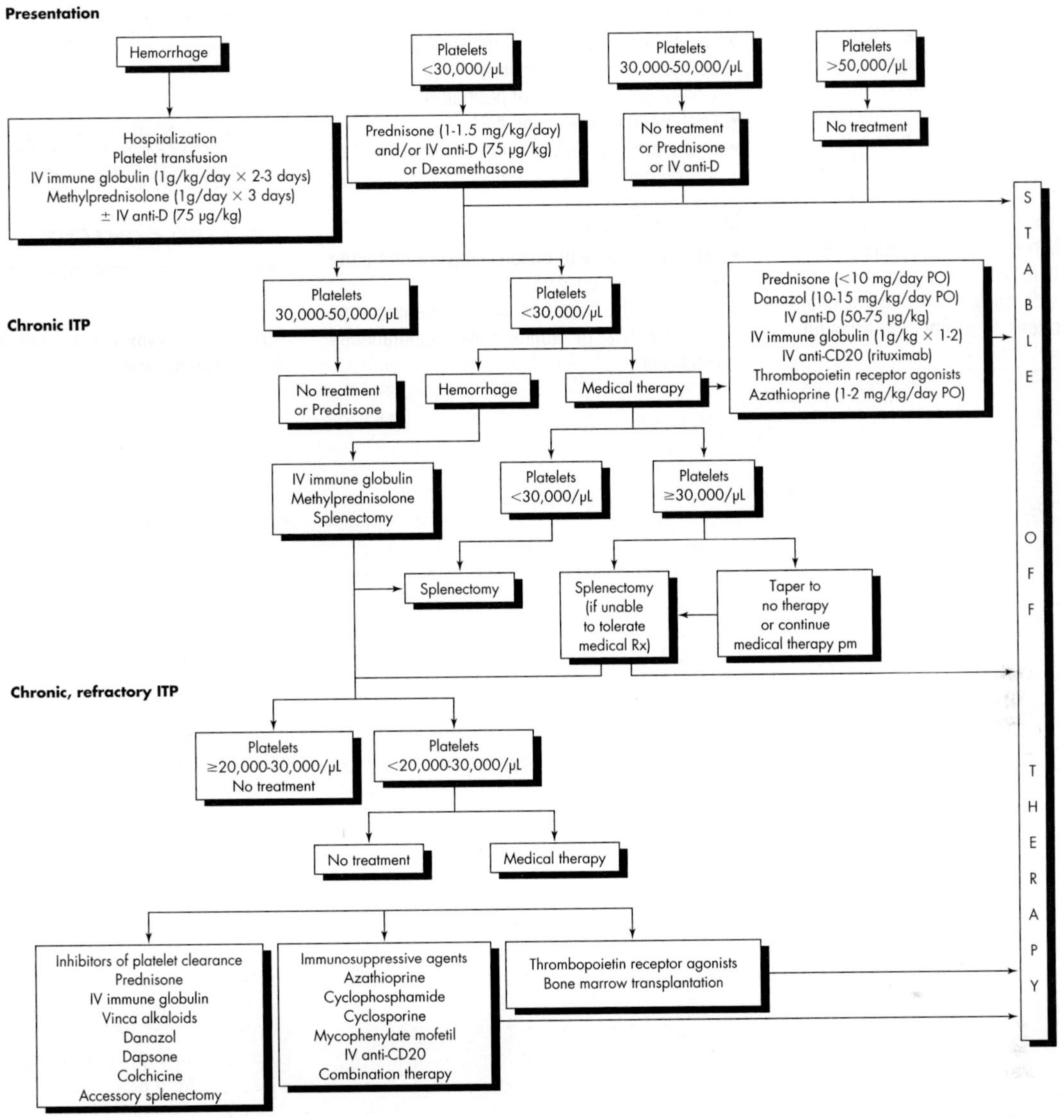

FIG. 2 Treatment algorithm for management of adult-onset immune thrombocytopenic purpura. Some advocate the use of 20,000/mm^3 as a guideline for therapy. The decision to treat patients with platelet counts lower than 50,000/mm^3 is based in part on evidence of bleeding, a history of bleeding, comorbid risk factors, lifestyle, and tolerance of therapy. There is no consensus as to duration of steroid therapy. The use of anti-D as initial therapy is appropriate only for Rh(D)-positive individuals who are not markedly anemic or hemolyzing. The goal of medical therapy is to attain a hemostatic platelet count, generally >20,000-30,000/mm^3. The threshold for treatment depends on comorbid risk factors for bleeding and risk of trauma. Higher platelet counts may be appropriate for surgery or after trauma. Medications can be used individually, but combinations of azathioprine and danazol (or corticosteroids) may provide added benefit and allow lower doses to be used. IVIG and anti-D are generally reserved for severe thrombocytopenia unresponsive to oral agents. The decision to proceed to splenectomy depends on intensity of therapy required, tolerance to side effects, risk of surgery, and patient preference. IVIG and/or methylprednisolone may help to increase the platelet count immediately before splenectomy. Laparoscopic and open splenectomy have comparable outcomes. The decision to treat patients who have platelet counts lower than 20,000-30,000/mm^3 after splenectomy involves an assessment of the risk of hemorrhage versus the side effects of each form of therapy. *ITP,* Immune thrombocytopenic purpura; *IV,* intravenous; *IVIG,* intravenous immunoglobulin; *pm,* precision medicine; *PO,* by mouth; *Rx,* prescription. (Modified from Hoffman R et al: *Hematology, basic principles and practice,* ed 7, Philadelphia, 2018, Churchill Livingstone.)

only to patients who are Rh(D) positive with hemoglobin >8 mg/dL and the usual dose is 50 to 75 mcg/kg.

- Rituximab, a monoclonal antibody directed against the CD20 antigen, is used as a second-line agent. Usual dose is 375 mg/m^2 weekly × 4 wk.
- Splenectomy is considered a subsequent option in case of rituximab failure. Previously, it was considered in adults with platelet count <20,000/mm^3 after 6 wk of medical treatment or after 6 mo if more than 10 to 20 mg of prednisone per day is still required to maintain a platelet count >30,000/mm^3. In children, splenectomy is generally reserved for persistent thrombocytopenia (>1 yr) and clinically significant bleeding. Appropriate immunizations (pneumococcal vaccine in adults and children, *Haemophilus influenzae* vaccine, meningococcal vaccine in children) should be administered earlier than 2 wk before planned splenectomy. Postsplenectomy vaccinations should be performed in all cases.
- Additional second-line agents are thrombopoietin receptor agonists (TPO-RA), azathioprine, cyclosporin A, cyclophosphamide, danazol, dapsone, mycophenolate mofetil, and *Vinca* alkaloids.
- Romiplostim, a recombinant fusion protein, and the oral TPO-RA eltrombopag are effective in increasing platelet count in adult patients with chronic ITP refractory to corticosteroids and/or splenectomy. American Society of Hematology guidelines, revised in 2011, recommend the use of TPO-RA for adult patients with ITP at risk for bleeding who have a contraindication to splenectomy, or who have not responded to at least one other therapy.

- Fostamatinib is an inhibitor of the enzyme spleen tyrosine kinase (Syk). Syk plays an important role in phagocytosis of FcγR-mediated signal transduction and inflammatory propagation. It received FDA approval of chronic ITP in adults who had an insufficient response to previous treatment including corticosteroids, intravenous immunoglobulin (IVIG), splenectomy and/or a TPO-RA. The recommended initial dose is 100 mg oral twice daily. It can be increased to 150 mg twice daily if the platelet count has not responded to at least 50,000/mm^3 at 1 mo.

PREGNANCY Rx

- No treatment is required when platelet count is >30,000/mm^3 or higher until 36 wk gestation, or earlier in case of premature labor.
- Oral corticosteroids and IVIG.
- Refractory ITP may require splenectomy in the second trimester.

DISPOSITION

- More than 80% of children have a complete remission within 8 wk.
- In adults, the course of the disease is chronic; only 5% of adults have spontaneous remission.
- The principal cause of death from ITP is intracranial hemorrhage (1% of children, 5% of adults).

SUGGESTED READINGS

Available at ExpertConsult.com

RELATED CONTENT

Immune Thrombocytopenic Purpura (Patient Information).

AUTHORS: **Sariya Wongsaengsak, MD,** and **Patan Gultawatvichai, MD**

BASIC INFORMATION

DEFINITION

Fecal incontinence is defined as the involuntary loss of gas or liquid stool (minor incontinence) or the involuntary loss of solid stool (major incontinence).

SYNONYMS

Anal or bowel incontinence
Accidental bowel leakage
Fecal incontinence

ICD-10CM CODES

R15.9	Full incontinence of feces
F98.1	Encopresis not due to a substance or known physiological condition

EPIDEMIOLOGY & DEMOGRAPHICS

INCIDENCE: Affects 0.5% to 1.5% of the population younger than age 65, but >10% older than 65. More common in institutionalized patients.

PREVALENCE: Varies widely depending on definition used and population studied; often underreported. In community-based studies, ranges from 1% to 24%. Increases with age and BMI in women.

PREDOMINANT SEX & AGE: Slightly more common in females than males and those of advanced age (older than 65 yr).

RISK FACTORS:

- Cognitive or behavioral dysfunction
- Structural anorectal abnormalities (e.g., rectal prolapse)
- Neurologic disorders, comorbidities (e.g., diabetes mellitus), inflammatory bowel disease (IBD)
- Poor mobility in female gender, advanced age
- Anal sphincter trauma (surgery, obstetrical injury)
- Fecal impaction from constipation or diarrhea

PHYSICAL FINDINGS & CLINICAL PRESENTATION

- Inspect perianal area to evaluate for the presence of fecal material, prolapsing hemorrhoids, chemical dermatitis, scars, fistula, or rectal prolapse.
- Assess for anocutaneous reflex. This may be elicited by stroking skin in each perianal quadrant (normal response is a brisk anal wink). Absent reflex is suggestive of nerve damage.
- Digital rectal examination to assess for impaction, mass, and resting to squeezing anal tone by asking the patient to bear down. Ask patient to bear down to assess for rectal prolapse or excessive perianal descent.

ETIOLOGY

- Usually multifactorial. Table 1 summarizes the mechanisms, causes, and pathophysiology of fecal incontinence. Common types of anorectal dysfunction causing rectal outlet delay in the elderly are summarized in Table 2
- Overflow resulting from fecal impaction
- Anal sphincter weakness:
  1. Trauma (e.g., anorectal surgery, childbirth).
  2. Nontraumatic (e.g., neurologic, spinal cord lesions, diabetes, scleroderma).
- Anorectal inflammation:
  1. Radiation, IBD
- CNS disorders (e.g., dementia, multiple sclerosis, stroke)
- Anatomic disturbance of pelvic floor:
  1. Fistula, prolapse
- Idiopathic

DIAGNOSIS

DIFFERENTIAL DIAGNOSIS

- Fecal encopresis
- Irritable bowel syndrome or IBD

WORKUP

- Requires detailed history taking that includes the onset and precipitating events, duration and severity, stool consistency and urgency.

TABLE 1 Mechanisms, Causes, and Pathophysiology of Fecal Incontinence

Mechanism	Causes	Pathophysiology*
Abnormal Anorectal or Pelvic Floor Structures		
Anal sphincter muscles	Hemorrhoidectomy, neuropathy, obstetric injury	Sphincter weakness, loss of sampling reflex
Puborectalis muscle	Aging, excessive perineal descent, trauma	Obtuse anorectal angle, sphincter weakness
Pudendal nerve	Excessive straining, obstetric or surgical injury, perineal descent	Sphincter weakness, sensory loss, impaired reflexes
Nervous system, spinal cord, autonomic nervous system	Avulsion injury, spine surgery, diabetes mellitus, head injury, multiple sclerosis, spinal cord injury, stroke	Loss of sensation, impaired reflexes, secondary myopathy, loss of accommodation
Rectum	Aging, IBD, IBS, prolapse, radiation	Loss of accommodation, loss of sensation, hypersensitivity
Abnormal Anorectal or Pelvic Floor Function		
Impaired anorectal sensation	Autonomic nervous system disorders, central nervous system disorders, obstetric injury	Loss of stool awareness, rectoanal agnosia
Fecal impaction	Dyssynergic defecation	Fecal retention with overflow, impaired sensation
Altered Stool Characteristics		
Increased volume and loose consistency	Drugs, bile salt malabsorption, infection, IBD, IBS, laxatives, metabolic disorders	Diarrhea and urgency, rapid stool transport, impaired accommodation
Hard stools, retention	Drugs, dyssynergia	Fecal retention with overflow
Miscellaneous		
Physical mobility, cognitive function	Aging, dementia, disability	Multifactorial changes
Psychosis	Willful soiling	Multifactorial changes
Drugs*	Anticholinergics	Constipation
	Antidepressants	Altered sensation, constipation
	Caffeine	Relaxation of sphincter tone
	Laxatives	Diarrhea
	Muscle relaxants	Relaxation of sphincter tone
Food intolerance	Fructose, lactose, or sorbitol malabsorption	Diarrhea, flatus

*Pathophysiology is noted for each class of drugs.
From Feldman M, Friedman LS, Brandt LJ: *Sleisenger and Fordtran's gastrointestinal and liver disease,* ed 10, Philadelphia, 2016, Elsevier.

TABLE 2 Types of Anorectal Dysfunction Causing Rectal Outlet Delay in Older People

Pathophysiology	Clinical Picture	
Rectal dysmotility	Reduced rectal motility and contractions Increased rectal compliance Variable degree of rectal dilation Impaired rectal sensation with blunting of urge to pass stool Over time, increasing rectal distention required to reflexively trigger the defecation mechanism	Rectal hard or soft stool retention on digital examination of which patient may be unaware Chronic rectal distention leads to relaxation of the internal sphincter and fecal soiling One postulated cause is diminished parasympathetic outflow as a result of impaired sacral cord function (e.g., from ischemia or spinal stenosis); may also develop through persistent disregard or suppression of the urge to defecate as a result of dementia, depression, immobility, or painful anorectal conditions
Pelvic floor dyssynergia	Paradoxical contraction or failure to relax the pelvic floor and external anal sphincter muscles during defecation Manometric studies show paradoxical increases in anal canal pressure on straining	Severe and long-standing symptoms of rectal outlet delay Parkinson disease More common in younger women
Irritable bowel syndrome	Increased rectal tone and reduced compliance Lower pain threshold on distending the rectum during anorectal function tests	Constipation usually predominant in older people Rome criteria symptoms: Abdominal distention or pain relieved by defecation, passage of mucus, and feeling of incomplete emptying

From Fillit HM: *Brocklehurst's textbook of geriatric medicine and gerontology*, ed 8, 2017, Elsevier.

Important to evaluate for history of urinary incontinence, anorectal surgery or radiation, neurologic disorders, or prior vaginal deliveries and complete a thorough physical exam. An algorithm for the evaluation and management of patients with fecal incontinence is illustrated in Fig. 1.

- Diagnostic workup may include endoscopy, anorectal manometry, endorectal ultrasound (simple and economical), MRI, defecography, pudendal nerve terminal latency, balloon expulsion test, and anal electromyography (EMG), depending on signs and symptoms. Diagnostic tests for fecal incontinence are summarized in Table 3.

Rx TREATMENT

- Therapy is focused on patient education (Table E4), supportive care, medications, biofeedback, and surgery. Table 5 summarizes bowel preparation in the elderly prior to colonoscopy.
- Medications focus on decreasing stool frequency and improving consistency.
  1. Fiber supplements (e.g., methylcellulose)
  2. Antidiarrheals: Loperamide, diphenoxylate/atropine sulfate, cholestyramine
  3. Topical phenylephrine, oral valproate sodium to increase smooth muscle tone
  4. Injectable anal bulking agent: Dextranomer-hyaluronic acid gel is FDA approved for the treatment of fecal incontinence in adults who fail conservative therapy. Given as four 1-ml injections into the deep submucosal layer of the anal canal. If inadequate response after at least 4 wk, a second course can be attempted.

NONPHARMACOLOGIC THERAPY

- Supportive therapy:
  1. Education, behavioral training, pelvic floor exercises
  2. Dietary modifications (e.g., increased fiber/fluid intake, less caffeine), food diary
  3. Incontinence pads, barrier cream (e.g., zinc oxide)
- Biofeedback therapy
- Electrical stimulation:
  1. Anal electrodes
  2. Sacral nerve stimulation
  3. Posterior tibial nerve stimulation
- Surgery:
  1. Anal sphincteroplasty
  2. Implanted devices (e.g., artificial anal sphincter)
  3. Colostomy (if intractable symptoms and/or failed all other therapies)
  4. Miscellaneous: Radiofrequency ablation, anal sling

REFERRAL

Colorectal surgery

PEARLS & CONSIDERATIONS

COMMENTS

The shame, embarrassment, and stigma associated with fecal and urinary incontinence pose significant barriers to seeking professional treatment, resulting in many people suffering from these conditions without seeking help. Therefore, during routine office visits, asking all patients older than 70 yr about incontinence may be helpful.

PREVENTION

- Reduce constipation and avoid straining during bowel movements.
- Routine episiotomy is the most easily preventable risk factor for fecal incontinence in females.

PATIENT & FAMILY EDUCATION

https://www.niddk.nih.gov/health-information/digestive-diseases/bowel-control-problems-fecal-incontinence

SUGGESTED READINGS

Available at ExpertConsult.com

AUTHOR: **Fred F. Ferri, MD**

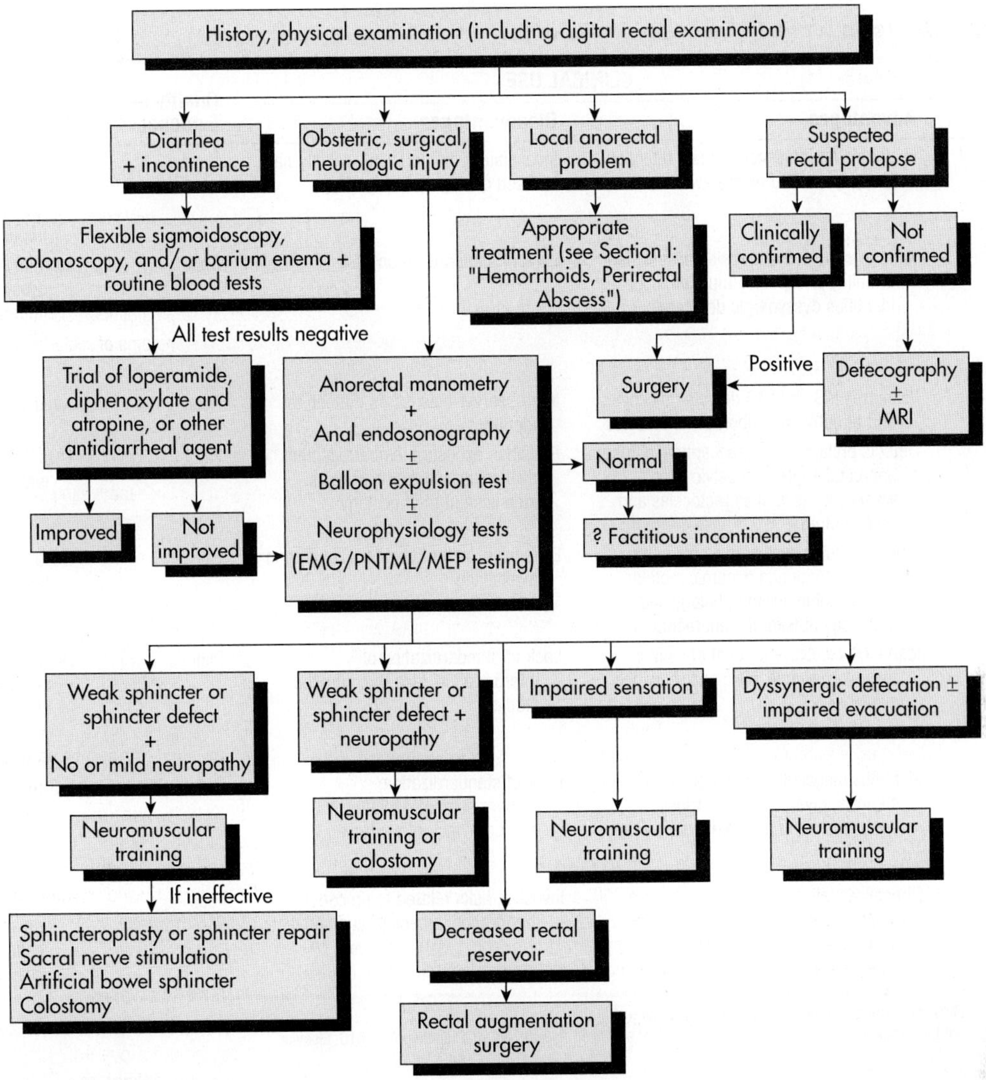

FIG. 1 Algorithm for the evaluation and management of patients with fecal incontinence. *EMG,* Electromyography; *MEP,* motor-evoked potential; *PNTML,* pudendal nerve terminal motor latency. (From Feldman M, Friedman LS, Brandt LJ: *Sleisenger and Fordtran's gastrointestinal and liver disease,* ed 10, Philadelphia, 2016, Elsevier.)

TABLE 3 Diagnostic Tests for Fecal Incontinence

Test	CLINICAL USE: Advantages	CLINICAL USE: Disadvantages	Quality of Evidence	Comments
Physiologic				
Anorectal manometry	Quantifies EAS and IAS pressures; identifies rectal hyposensitivity, rectal hypersensitivity, impaired rectal compliance, dyssynergic defecation	Lack of standardization	Good	Useful for detecting anal sphincter weakness, altered rectal sensation and accommodation, and dyssynergia
Needle EMG	Quantifies spike potentials and re-innervation pattern indicating neuropathy or myopathy	Invasive, painful; not widely available	Fair	Useful but used largely in research laboratories
Surface EMG	Displays EMG activity; can provide information on normal or weak muscle tone	Inaccurate, frequent artifacts	Fair	Used largely for neuromuscular training
Pudendal nerve terminal motor latency (PNTML)	Measures latency of the terminal portion of the pudendal nerve, simple to perform	Minimally invasive, low sensitivity, interobserver differences	Fair	Conflicting data; correlation with other tests and surgical outcome unclear
Translumbar and transsacral motor-evoked potentials	Quantifies the nerve conduction time of the entire spinoanal and spinorectal pathways; minimally invasive	Lack of standardization, training, controlled studies, and availability	Fair	Promising noninvasive test; more objective and higher yield than PNTML

Continued

TABLE 3 Diagnostic Tests for Fecal Incontinence—cont'd

Test	CLINICAL USE: Advantages	CLINICAL USE: Disadvantages	Quality of Evidence	Comments
Colonic transit study with radiopaque markers	Evaluates the presence of fecal retention; inexpensive and widely available	Inconsistent methodology, validity has been questioned	Good	Useful for identifying patients with fecal seepage and older persons with impaction
Balloon expulsion test (BET)	Simple, inexpensive, bedside assessment of ability to expel a simulated stool; identifies dyssynergic defecation	Lack of standardization	Good	Normal BET does not exclude dyssynergia; should be interpreted in the context of other anorectal test results
Imaging				
Anorectal ultrasound	Visualizes IAS and EAS defects, thickness, and atrophy and puborectalis muscles	Interobserver bias; scars difficult to identify	Good	Most widely available
Defecography	Detects prolapse, intussusception, obtuse anorectal angle, and pelvic floor weakness, as well as rectoceles and megarectum	Radiation exposure, embarrassment, availability, interobserver bias, inconsistent methodology	Fair	Useful and complementary with other tests
MRI	Simultaneously evaluates global pelvic floor anatomy and dynamic motion; reveals sphincter morphology and pathology outside the anorectum	Expensive, lack of standardization and availability	Fair	Used as an adjunct to other tests
Plain abdominal film	Identifies excessive amount of stool in the colon; simple, inexpensive, widely available	Lack of standardization of interpretation, lack of controlled studies	Poor	Not recommended for routine evaluation but useful in older adults and children with incontinence and fecal impaction
Barium enema	Identifies megacolon, megarectum, stenosis, diverticulosis, extrinsic compression, and intraluminal masses	Lack of standardization, embarrassment, radiation exposure, lack of controlled studies	Poor	Not recommended as part of routine evaluation
Endoscopy				
Flexible sigmoidoscopy and colonoscopy	Directly visualizes the colon to exclude mucosal lesions (e.g., solitary rectal ulcer syndrome, inflammation, malignancy)	Invasive, risks related to procedure (perforation, bleeding) and sedation	Poor	Indicated in patients with unexplained diarrhea and seepage and patients >age 50

EAS, External anal sphincter; *EMG,* electromyography; *IAS,* internal anal sphincter.
Feldman M, Friedman LS, Brandt LJ: *Sleisenger and Fordtran's gastrointestinal and liver disease,* ed 10, Philadelphia, 2016, Elsevier.

TABLE 5 Bowel Preparation in Older People

- Older age, constipation, reported laxative use, tricyclic antidepressants, stroke, diabetes, and dementia are associated with inadequate preparation and taking longer to perform full colonoscopy.
- Even when patients take 75% to 100% of their prescribed treatments, bowel preparation is satisfactory only 50% of the time.

Guidance

- Give regular laxatives (e.g., Movicol 2 sachets daily) and enemas or suppositories for at least 1 wk before the procedure, with a longer run-up period in patients known to have constipation and those with comorbidities such as diabetes.
- Individualize the cathartic regimen (e.g., 1 to 2 L of GoLYTELY daily over 2 to 3 days in those unable to drink 4 L, or alternative preparations such as sodium picosulfate).
- Identify potential nonadherence. ("Can the patient drink 4 L of GoLYTELY in 24 hours?")
- Preempt unpleasant side effects. ("Will the patient be able to reach the toilet in time to avoid fecal leakage?")
- Use oral phospho soda with caution, as administration in older people increases serum phosphate, even in patients with normal creatinine clearance.
- Consider pre-procedure a plain abdominal x-ray for evaluation of persistent fecal loading.
- Where possible, give a clear fluid diet before administration of bowel preparation.

From Fillit HM: *Brocklehurst's textbook of geriatric medicine and gerontology,* ed 8, 2017, Elsevier.

BASIC INFORMATION

DEFINITION

Urinary incontinence is the involuntary leakage of urine.

SYNONYM

Urinary incontinence

ICD-10CM CODES	
R32	Unspecified urinary incontinence
N39.3	Stress incontinence (female) (male)
N39.41	Urgency urinary incontinence
N39.46	Mixed incontinence
N39.49	Disorder of urinary system, unspecified
R39.81	Functional urinary incontinence

EPIDEMIOLOGY & DEMOGRAPHICS

INCIDENCE/PREVALENCE: In the general population between the ages of 15 and 64 yr, 1.5% to 5% of men and 25% to 57% of women have urinary incontinence. The incidence among young women is 25%, and middle-aged and postmenopausal women is 44% to 57%. In the nursing home population, 75% of the population has some degree of incontinence. Nearly 20% of children through the mid-teenage yr have episodes of urinary incontinence.

CLINICAL, PSYCHOLOGICAL & SOCIAL IMPACT

- Fewer than 50% of women living with incontinence in the U.S. consult health care professionals for care, resulting in significant physical and psychological limitations. Many women choose to turn to home remedies, commercially available absorbent materials, and supportive aids. As the incontinence worsens, many women become depressed, limit social interaction, refrain from sexual intimacy, and become homebound. It is estimated that $19.5 billion in direct costs is spent annually on incontinence in the U.S. Urinary incontinence contributes to approximately 6% of nursing home admissions in the older population, leading to a cost of $3 billion per yr. With aging populations around the world, this cost is dramatically increasing every year.
- The continence mechanisms are complex and include multiple levels of control: Central and peripheral nervous systems, detrusor muscle, urethra, and pelvic floor muscle. Normal function depends on multiple levels of control and dysfunction at any of these levels can lead to incontinence.

MAJOR TYPES OF INCONTINENCE (FIG. 1)

- **Stress urinary incontinence (SUI)** (Table E1) is the complaint of involuntary loss of urine with effort or physical exertion (sporting activities), or on sneezing or coughing (any activity that increases intraabdominal pressure). The most common risk factors are parity and obesity. SUI may be demonstrated with a simple cough stress test during examination. The cotton swab test can determine the degree of urethral mobility, which may be helpful in determining which type of surgical procedure to perform, but this test is not useful for diagnosing SUI.
  1. **Intrinsic sphincter deficiency (ISD)** is the most severe form of SUI and indicates a urethra that cannot remain closed even at rest. Urodynamically, this is diagnosed with a maximal urethral closure pressure <20 cm H_2O and leak point pressure <60 cm H_2O.
- **Urgency urinary incontinence (UUI)** is the complaint of involuntary loss of urine associated with urgency, a sudden compelling desire to pass urine that is difficult to defer. The diagnosis is often made clinically based on patient's report of symptoms but may also be associated with involuntary detrusor contractions on urodynamic investigation. May be idiopathic or neurogenic.
- **Overactive bladder (OAB)** is described as a constellation of symptoms (Fig. E2 and Fig. E3) including urgency, with or without urgency urinary incontinence, usually with urinary frequency and nocturia. It should be distinguished from excessive fluid intake and must exclude urinary tract infection. Can occur in up to 27% of men and up to 43% of women.
- **Mixed urinary incontinence** is the complaint of involuntary leakage of urine associated with urgency and with physical exertion, effort, sneezing or coughing (see Fig. E4).
- **Overflow incontinence** is the leakage of urine resulting from urinary retention with resultant overflow or spilling of the urine. Causes include hypotonic bladder resulting from age, neurologic conditions such as diabetes or spinal cord injury, prior surgery, drug effects (e.g., intravesical Botox), or fecal impaction. It may also be caused by obstruction at the bladder neck and urethra, such as from prior anti-incontinence surgery, pelvic organ prolapse, urethral stenosis, or detrusor-sphincter dyssynergia.
- **Functional urinary incontinence** is the complaint of involuntary leakage of urine resulting from chronic impairments of cognitive, functional, or mobility impairments. This is a diagnosis of exclusion and may be cured by improving the patient's functional status, treating comorbidities, changing medications, and reducing environmental barriers.
- **Extraurethral urinary incontinence** is leakage that bypasses the urethral meatus (i.e., vesicovaginal fistula or ectopic ureter).

DIAGNOSIS

HISTORY

- Because many women are hesitant to bring up symptoms of incontinence, these symptoms should be elicited through simple screening.
- History of present illness, psychosocial factors, congenital disorders, access issues for the physically challenged, neurologic disorders, and medication use are coexistent disorders that may affect the urinary tract.
- Urinary incontinence may be characterized by frequency of incontinence episodes, severity, and extent of bother.
- Voiding diary to assess total voided volume, frequency of micturition, mean volume voided, largest single volume, diurnal distribution, and nature and severity of incontinence.
- Assessments of the severity of symptoms and goals for treatment are important parts of the history.

WORKUP

- General physical examination:
  1. Confounding conditions including mobility issues. Comorbid conditions that can cause or contribute to urinary incontinence in elderly patients are summarized in Table 2. Table 3 describes medications that can cause or contribute to urinary incontinence
  2. Neuromuscular deficits (gait of the patient)

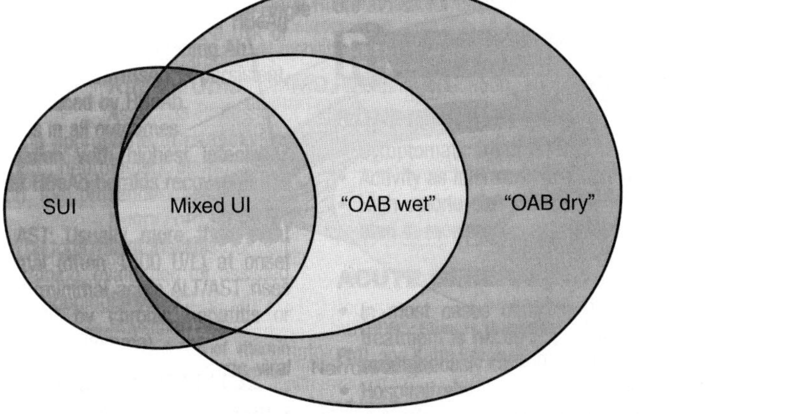

FIG. 1 Incontinence may be stress urinary incontinence *(SUI)*, mixed urinary incontinence *(UI)*, or urgency urinary incontinence ("overactive bladder *[OAB]* wet"), especially in women. SUI can coexist with "OAB dry," giving rise to mixed symptoms of stress incontinence and urgency. (From Wein AJ et al: *Campbell-Walsh urology,* ed 11, Philadelphia, 2016, Elsevier.)

TABLE 2 Comorbid Conditions that Can Cause or Contribute to Urinary Incontinence in Frail Older Adults

Conditions	Comments	Implications for Management
Comorbid Medical Illnesses		
Diabetes mellitus	Poor control can cause polyuria and precipitate or exacerbate incontinence; also associated with increased likelihood of urgency incontinence and diabetic neuropathic bladder	Better control of diabetes can reduce osmotic diuresis and associated polyuria, improve incontinence
Degenerative joint disease	Can impair mobility and precipitate urgency UI	Optimal pharmacologic and nonpharmacologic pain management can improve mobility, toileting ability
Chronic pulmonary disease	Associated cough can worsen stress UI	Cough suppression can reduce stress incontinence and cough-induced urgency UI
Congestive heart failure Lower extremity venous insufficiency	Increased nighttime urine production can contribute to nocturia and UI	Optimizing pharmacologic management of congestive heart failure, sodium restriction, support stockings, leg elevation, and late afternoon dose of rapid-acting diuretic may reduce nocturnal polyuria, associated nocturia, nighttime UI
Sleep apnea	May increase nighttime urine production by increasing production of atrial natriuretic peptide	Diagnosis and treatment of sleep apnea, usually with continuous positive airway pressure devices, may relieve UI, reduce nocturnal polyuria and associated nocturia
Severe constipation and fecal impaction	Associated with "double" incontinence (urine and fecal)	Appropriate use of stool softeners Adequate fluid intake and exercise Dis-impaction if necessary
Neurologic and Psychiatric Conditions		
Stroke	Can precipitate urgency UI and, less often, urinary retention; also impairs mobility	UI after acute stroke often resolves with rehabilitation; persistent UI should be further evaluated. Regular toileting assistance essential for those with persistent mobility impairment
Parkinson disease	Associated with urgency UI; also causes impaired mobility and cognition in late stages	Optimizing management may improve mobility, improve UI. Regular toileting assistance essential for those with mobility and cognitive impairment in late stages
Normal-pressure hydrocephalus	Presents with UI, along with gait and cognitive impairments	Patients presenting with all three symptoms should be considered for brain imaging to rule out this condition; may improve with a ventricular-peritoneal shunt
Dementia (Alzheimer, multi-infarct, others)	Associated with urgency UI; impaired cognition and apraxia interfere with toileting and hygiene	Regular toileting assistance essential for those with mobility and cognitive impairment in late stages
Depression	May impair motivation to be continent; may also be a consequence of incontinence	Optimizing pharmacologic and nonpharmacologic management of depression may improve UI
		Discontinuation or modification of drug regimen
Medications		
Functional Impairments		
Impaired mobility, impaired cognition	Impaired cognition and/or mobility due to a variety of conditions (listed above) and others can interfere with ability to toilet independently and can precipitate UI	Regular toileting assistance essential for those with severe mobility and/or cognitive impairment
Environmental Factors		
Inaccessible toilets Unsafe toilet facilities No contrasting color between toilet and seat Caregivers unavailable for toileting assistance	Frail, functionally impaired persons require accessible and safe toilet facilities and, in many cases, human assistance to be continent	Environmental alterations may be helpful; supportive measures such as pads may be necessary if caregiver assistance not regularly available

UI, Urinary incontinence.
From Fillit HM: *Brocklehurst's textbook of geriatric medicine and gerontology*, ed 8, Philadelphia, 2017, Elsevier.

- Pelvic exam:
    1. Concurrent pelvic organ prolapse
    2. Vaginal discharge
    3. Estrogen status
    4. Pelvic floor strength assessment
    5. Neurologic examination to assess sacral nerves with anal wink and bulbocavernosus reflex
- Rectal examination to assess sphincter tone and stool impaction
- Simple cough stress test
- Urethral hypermobility
- Postvoid residual check with bladder scan or catheter to exclude retention
- 3-day bladder diary to assess frequency, timing, and volume of voids

LABORATORY TESTS

It is important to rule out urinary tract infection and microscopic hematuria with urinalysis and/or culture prior to more invasive testing for other causes for incontinence.

SPECIALIZED STUDIES

- **Urodynamic testing:** Measures different facets of urine storage and evacuation; usually necessary only if basic office evaluation does not elicit the cause of incontinence, if incontinence is persistent despite treatments, or if there are confounding contributors to incontinence including prior surgery
    1. Simple cystometrogram: Graph of bladder and abdominal pressures related to fluid volume during filling/storage/voiding to assess sensation and capacity; also assesses presence of detrusor contractions, whether voluntary or involuntary
    2. Uroflowmetry and pressure-flow studies: Measure the mechanism of bladder emptying and rate of urine flow
    3. Urethral mechanism and pressure studies

TABLE 3 Medications that Can Cause or Contribute to Urinary Incontinence in Frail Older Adults

Medications	Effects on Continence
α-Adrenergic agonists	Increased smooth muscle tone in urethra and prostatic capsule may precipitate obstruction, urinary retention, related symptoms
α-Adrenergic antagonists	Decreased smooth muscle tone in urethra may precipitate stress urinary incontinence in women
Angiotensin-converting enzyme inhibitors	Cause cough that can exacerbate UI
Anticholinergics	May cause impaired emptying, urinary retention, and constipation, which can contribute to UI; may cause cognitive impairment, reduce effective toileting ability
Calcium channel blockers	May cause impaired emptying, urinary retention, and constipation, which can contribute to UI; may cause dependent edema, which can contribute to nocturnal polyuria
Cholinesterase inhibitors	Increase bladder contractility, may precipitate urgency UI
Diuretics	Cause diuresis and precipitate UI
Lithium	Polyuria due to diabetes insipidus
Opioid analgesics	May cause urinary retention, constipation, confusion, immobility, all of which can contribute to UI
Psychotropic drugs Sedatives Hypnotics Antipsychotics Histamine-1 receptor antagonists	May cause confusion and impaired mobility and precipitate UI; anticholinergic effects; confusion
Selective serotonin reuptake inhibitors	Increase cholinergic transmission, may lead to urinary UI
Others—gabapentin, glitazones, nonsteroidal antiinflammatory drugs	Can cause edema, which can lead to nocturnal polyuria and cause nocturia and nighttime UI

UI, Urinary incontinence.
From Fillit HM: *Brocklehurst's textbook of geriatric medicine and gerontology*, ed 8, Philadelphia, 2017, Elsevier.

4. Electromyography: Studies the neuromuscular activity of pelvic muscles and striated urethral sphincter during filling and micturition

- **Cystourethroscopy:** Procedure that can be done in the office or the operating room in which an endoscope is inserted into the urethra to view the inside of the bladder and urethra. This procedure is not routinely used to evaluate incontinence unless hematuria is present or prior pelvic surgery is noted on history

IMAGING STUDIES

- These are usually ordered only if history and/or physical findings suggest other, less common causes of incontinence (i.e., genitourinary fistula) or if microscopic hematuria is present.
- Renal ultrasound may be used to assess for hydronephrosis.
- CT urogram may be used to assess upper tract abnormalities, congenital anomalies, genitourinary fistula, and microscopic hematuria etiologies.

Rx TREATMENT

- The recommended approach to urinary incontinence is a stepped care plan first offering noninvasive behavioral modifications such as bladder training, weight loss, and fluid management. Fig. E5 summarizes the diagnosis and treatment of overactive bladder.
- **Pelvic floor muscle training,** including Kegel exercises and often augmented with biofeedback or electrical stimulation, is an important component of first-line therapy for stress, urge, and mixed incontinence. Women should perform 45 to 50 exercises per day to achieve good results (60% to 85% reduction in incontinence if biofeedback is also used).
- **Estrogen,** oral or vaginal, increases the concentration of alpha-adrenergic receptors in the urethra and bladder, which improves vascularity and subsequently increases thickness of the urethral epithelium in women with urogenital atrophy.
- **Pharmacotherapy** is usually reserved for urgency urinary incontinence:
  1. Antimuscarinic (anticholinergic) medications: Block parasympathetic muscarinic receptors (detrusor M2/M3 receptors) to inhibit involuntary detrusor contractions:
     a. Agents available: Darifenacin, fesoterodine, oxybutynin (available orally and as a transdermal patch), solifenacin, tolterodine, and trospium
     b. Efficacy: Shown to improve symptoms and continence but only modestly compared with placebo
     c. Side effects: High rates of discontinuation due to side effects, most often dry mouth and constipation. May also exacerbate urinary retention, blurred vision, dyspepsia, and impaired cognitive function, with some studies now showing an association with dementia if used for >2 yr; contraindicated in narrow-angle glaucoma
     d. Of note, trospium may have a lower risk of cognitive impairment give the size of the molecule as it is less likely to cross the blood-brain barrier
  2. Beta-agonists: Stimulate β3-adrenergic receptor in the detrusor muscle to cause relaxation and increase bladder capacity
     a. Agent available: Mirabegron
     b. Efficacy: Significant reductions in urgency incontinence in randomized trials
     c. Side effects: Tachycardia, hypertension, headache, and diarrhea (similar to placebo); not recommended in uncontrolled hypertension
  3. OnabotulinumtoxinA (Botox A): Inhibits the presynaptic release of acetylcholine from motor neurons at the neuromuscular junction to paralyze the muscle; given by cystoscopic intravesical injection every 6 to 12 mo:
     a. Efficacy: Similar rates of improvement seen when compared with antimuscarinic medications, but more women reporting complete resolution of urgency urinary incontinence with Botox A (35% to 50% reporting "total continence" in clinical trials); third-line treatment due to adverse effects
     b. Adverse effects: Urinary retention or incomplete bladder emptying (5% requiring catheterization) and urinary tract infections (33%)
- **Peripheral tibial nerve stimulation:** 30-min session of tibial nerve stimulation once per week for 12 wk followed by a customized maintenance plan to treat OAB. Compared with placebo, pooled success rate was 60% in a guideline published by American Urological Association; fewer adverse events noted when compared with antimuscarinic medication.
- **Sacral neuromodulation:** Stimulation of bladder and pelvic floor nerves to treat OAB, UUI, and idiopathic urinary retention. The mechanism is unknown. The procedure occurs in a two-stage process: first the electrode is placed near S3 to determine if symptoms are improved by 50%; if so, then next the pulse generator is implanted. Evidence suggests 70% of women experience significant improvement in their symptoms with sacral neuromodulation.
- **Augmentation cystoplasty:** Older procedure that was used before introduction of sacral neuromodulation in patients with poorly compliant bladders who were at risk for upper tract deterioration, completed by using a gastrointestinal segment.

TABLE 4 Transient Causes of Urinary Incontinence (DIAPPERS)

D	Delirium/AMS state
I	Infection, urinary (symptomatic)
A	Atrophic urethritis/vaginitis
P	Pharmaceuticals (diuretics, and so on)
P	Psychological, especially depression
E	Endocrine (hypercalcemia, hypokalemia, glycosuria)
R	Restricted mobility
S	Stool impaction

AMS, Altered mental status.
From Floege J et al: *Comprehensive clinical nephrology,* ed 4, Philadelphia, 2010, Saunders.

- **Devices:**
  1. Continence pessaries: For women with SUI who wish to defer or avoid surgery; help increase urethral resistance during increased intraabdominal pressure. A large randomized controlled trial demonstrated similar outcomes among women who underwent pessary, behavioral therapy, or a combination of both for incontinence; at 12 mo, approximately 50% of women still using the assigned treatment reported improvement in symptoms.
  2. Over-the-counter vaginal or urethral inserts: Disposable devices used to support the urethra, especially in women with situational stress incontinence (i.e., only when exercising); however, urethral inserts have been associated with a high rate of urinary tract infection.
- **Surgery:** Indicated for women with SUI without symptom control after conservative management or as first-line treatment in appropriately counseled women who decline more conservative treatment:
  1. Synthetic slings are the most common primary surgical treatment for SUI. Cure rates of 62% to 98% have been reported in a recent systematic review:
     a. Transvaginal/retropubic: Trocars are passed through the retropubic space from the midurethra to the abdomen (or vice versa). Short-term cure rates range from 73% to 82%, according to a 2009 Cochrane meta-analysis, with de novo urgency in approximately 6% of patients.
     b. Transobturator: Trocars are passed from the vagina behind the ischium (or vice versa), with similar cure rates as the retropubic slings.
     c. Single-incision slings: Only one vaginal incision is needed beneath the urethra; ends of the sling are secured in the internal obturator muscle.
  2. Autologous fascial slings: Usually considered second line after the failure of synthetic slings due to length and morbidity of the operation. Cure rates estimated to be 50% to 75% depending on definition of cure.
  3. Cadaveric slings: Usually second line; use has declined more recently because of concerns with early failure and declining success rate over time. Cure rates of 74% at 12 to 23 mo and 80% at 48 mo or greater.
  4. Retropubic urethropexy, (i.e., Burch procedure [open abdominal or laparoscopic]): A large meta-analysis estimated cure rates to be 82% at 12 to 23 mo and 73% at 48 mo or longer for open procedures.
- **Bulking Agents:** For treatment of stress incontinence, without hypermobility or in poor surgical candidates:
  1. Available agents: Carbon-coated zirconium beads, calcium hydroxyapatite, cross-linked polydimethylsiloxane
  2. Effectiveness: Relatively noninvasive but less effective than surgical intervention; cure rate at 63% to 80% at 1 yr
- Treatment for urinary retention and overflow incontinence focuses on reversal of modifiable factors and drainage of urine from the bladder:
  1. Clean intermittent self-catheterization
  2. Sacral neuromodulation

PEARLS & CONSIDERATIONS

COMMENTS

- Weight loss and exercise are helpful for urinary incontinence in obese women. Overweight and obese women with urinary incontinence also have a high prevalence of monthly fecal incontinence (16% found to be associated with low dietary fiber intake after adjustment for other known risk factors for fecal incontinence).
- Transient causes of urinary incontinence in the elderly are described in Table 4.
- Other forms of incontinence:
  1. Nocturnal enuresis: Loss of urine occurring during sleep; can occur as idiopathic or neurogenic
  2. Postvoid dribble: A postsphincteric collection of urine seen with urethral diverticulum; can be idiopathic
  3. Extraurethral incontinence: Enterovesical, urethral; also known as *fistula*
- Conditions that predispose to surgical failure: Advanced age, prior failed incontinence surgery, concurrent detrusor instability, abnormal perineal electromyography, pelvic radiation.
- The Women's Preventive Services Initiative (WPSI) recommends screening women for urinary incontinence annually.

RELATED CONTENT

Urinary Incontinence (Patient Information)
Pelvic Organ Prolapse (Related Key Topic)

SUGGESTED READINGS

Available at ExpertConsult.com

AUTHORS: **Shanice Akoto, MD, MPH, Adrienne Werth, MD,** and **Anthony Sciscione, DO**

BASIC INFORMATION

DEFINITION

Infertility in a reproductive-age couple is defined as the inability to conceive after unprotected intercourse for ≥1 yr. When a female is greater than 35 yr of age, an evaluation is recommended after 6 mo without successful pregnancy. Earlier evaluation at any age is warranted with preexisting symptoms or medical conditions.

SYNONYM

Sterility

ICD-10CM CODES	
N46	Male infertility
N46.8	Other male infertility
N46.9	Male infertility, unspecified
N97.0	Female infertility associated with anovulation
N97.1	Female infertility of tubal origin
N97.2	Female infertility of uterine origin
N97.8	Female infertility of other origin
N97.9	Female infertility, unspecified
009.00	Supervision of pregnancy with history of infertility, unspecified trimester
009.01	Supervision of pregnancy with history of infertility, first trimester
009.02	Supervision of pregnancy with history of infertility, second trimester
009.03	Supervision of pregnancy with history of infertility, third trimester
Z31.81	Encounter for male factor infertility in female patient

EPIDEMIOLOGY & DEMOGRAPHICS

PREVALENCE: One in eight reproductive age couples experience infertility. This prevalence is consistent in all developed countries and there is evidence that it is historically stable.

PREDOMINANT SEX & AGE: By definition this is a diagnosis of reproductive age couples. Infertility increases with aging in both males and females, but more dramatically in women. Male factor is responsible in ~40% of couples and the female factor is responsible in ~40% of couples. The remainder of the cases are either combined male and female, or unexplained infertility, meaning a clear cause is not identified.

PEAK INCIDENCE: The incidence of infertility increases with age. Subtle decreases in female fertility start as early as age 30. The rate of infertility increases dramatically after age 37, and unassisted pregnancies become extremely uncommon as women reach the mid-40s. There is also a subtle, but still detectable, decrease in male fertility that may start as early as age 30.

RISK FACTORS: Aging is among the most common risk factors, predominantly among females, although there is evidence that aging affects male fertility as well. Women are increasingly deferring pregnancy due to the lack of a partner or career. Tubal factor infertility can be a result of endometriosis, prior tubal surgery, prior ruptured appendix, or sexually transmitted diseases such as chlamydia and gonorrhea. Ovulatory dysfunction is most commonly caused by polycystic ovarian syndrome (PCOS). Other causes include hypothalamic dysfunction, thyroid disorders, hyperprolactinemia, and extremes of weight, particularly obesity. Male factor infertility may be idiopathic or due to trauma, infection, varicocele, obstruction, hypothalamic dysfunction, or exposure to environmental toxins. Smoking is the most common lifestyle choice that impairs fertility.

PHYSICAL FINDINGS & CLINICAL PRESENTATION

- Age
- Previous fertility, particularly if no pregnancy has occurred in another relationship despite absence of contraception
- Absence of secondary sexual characteristics
- Abnormal uterine bleeding or absent or irregular menstruation
- Clinical signs of androgen excess: Hirsutism, acne, alopecia
- Abnormal pelvic exam: Enlarged uterus, adnexal masses, pelvic/abdominal tenderness
- History of urologic surgery in male or trauma to testes

ETIOLOGY

- Female factor:
  1. Advanced age
  2. Tubal factor: Pelvic inflammatory disease, endometriosis, prior pelvic surgery, history of ruptured appendicitis, prior elective sterilization
  3. Anatomic: Uterine fibroids, polyps, intrauterine adhesions, uterine anomalies
  4. Oligo-/anovulation: Most frequently due to polycystic ovarian syndrome (PCOS), but also due to thyroid abnormalities, hyperprolactinemia, nonclassic congenital adrenal hyperplasia, hypothalamic dysfunction
- Male factor (Table E1):
  1. Abnormal semen analysis
  2. Elective sterilization
- Idiopathic: Both male and female

DIAGNOSIS

WORKUP

- Confirmation of ovulation: History of regular menstrual cycles, mid-luteal serum progesterone, basal body temperature testing, urinary luteinizing hormone predictor kits
- Complete transvaginal pelvic ultrasound
- Ovarian reserve testing: Anti-Müllerian hormone, follicle-stimulating hormone (FSH), and estradiol obtained on cycle day 2, 3, or 4 and antral follicle count
- Fallopian tube evaluation: Hysterosalpingogram (HSG) (Fig. 1) or sonohysterosalpingogram
- Uterine cavity evaluation: HSG, saline infusion sonohysterography, hysteroscopy, or 3D ultrasound of uterus
- Male factor: Semen analysis

LABORATORY TESTS

- Semen analysis, using Kruger strict morphology. Abstain 2 to 5 days prior to test.
- FSH and estradiol collected cycle day 2, 3, or 4 and anti-Müllerian hormone as a measure of ovarian reserve.
- Mid-luteal progesterone (ideally 7 days prior to expected menses). Given variability of serum progesterone measurements throughout the day and absence of a reliable threshold, most practitioners use clinical criteria to diagnose ovulatory dysfunction.
- Thyroid-stimulating hormone (TSH).
- In patients with oligo- or anovulation: Prolactin, testosterone, 17-hydroxyprogesterone.

IMAGING STUDIES

- Day 2 or 3 transvaginal pelvic ultrasound to assess uterine or adnexal abnormalities and to count the number of small antral follicles (2-9 mm) as a measure of ovarian reserve. If oligo- or anovulatory, to assess for polycystic-appearing ovary
- Hysterosalpingogram (early follicular phase after menses complete but before ovulation, typically between days 5 and 12 of the menstrual cycle)
- Also used for imaging of uterine cavity: Saline infusion sonohysterography, 3D ultrasound of uterus, hysteroscopy

TREATMENT

Once the patient presents for evaluation, testing should be completed as quickly as possible, ideally within one menstrual cycle. The couple should follow up with the evaluating provider once all testing is completed and treatment initiated as abnormalities are found.

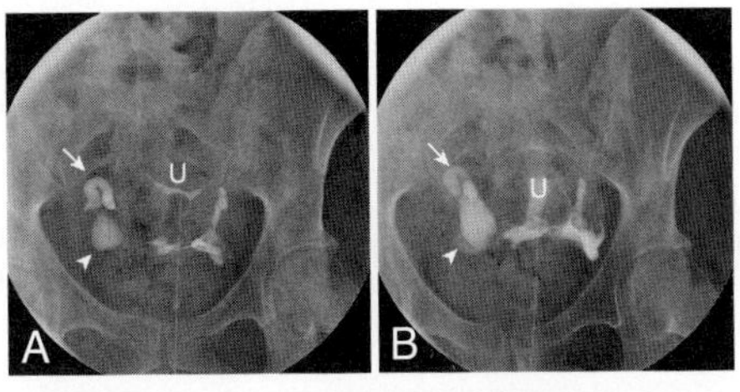

FIG. 1 Hysterosalpingogram spot radiographs early **(A)** and late **(B)** demonstrate a rounded collection of contrast material *(arrowhead)* adjacent to the dilated ampullary portion of the right fallopian tube *(arrow),* caused by peritubal pelvic adhesions related to previous pelvic inflammatory disease. Normal patient left fallopian tube. *U,* Uterus. (From Fielding JR et al: *Gynecologic imaging,* Philadelphia, 2011, Saunders.)

ACUTE GENERAL Rx

- Fertility preservation options among females are summarized in Table E2. Oligo- or anovulation should be treated with ovulation induction agents, such as aromatase inhibitors or clomiphene citrate. A recent multicenter trial found that aromatase inhibitors achieved higher live birth rates than clomiphene citrate. Historically, clomiphene citrate has been used, but a very well done randomized controlled trial convincingly demonstrated that letrozole is superior. Far less commonly, ovulatory dysfunction is the result of hypothalamic dysfunction. In these patients, once hypothalamic or pituitary abnormalities are excluded with MRI, ovulation can be achieved using injectable gonadotropins.
- Tubal factor infertility may be treated surgically if mild, and if the female patient is young and can afford the time to attempt pregnancy over multiple menstrual cycles. If the patient is older or if the tubal pathology is moderate to severe, in vitro fertilization (IVF) is recommended.
- Uterine anatomic abnormalities such as submucosal fibroids, polyps, intrauterine adhesions, or septate uterus should be corrected if they are identified. Fibroids that do not impact the uterine cavity probably do not interfere with fertility. Removal of intramural or subserosal fibroids is reserved for situations in which these cause distortion of the uterine cavity or bothersome symptoms such as excessive vaginal bleeding, pain, or pressure.
- Male infertility: Referral to urologist for complete evaluation. Fertility preservation options for males are summarized in Table E3. If semen analysis is severely abnormal, the following laboratory testing is recommended: Testosterone, FSH, estradiol, luteinizing hormone, TSH and prolactin, karyotype and Y-chromosome microdeletion.
    1. Mild male factor infertility may be treated with intrauterine insemination (IUI), but severe male factor will usually require assisted reproductive technologies (ART) with intracytoplasmic sperm injection (ICSI) in the laboratory, where sperm is injected directly into the oocyte. Some men may require epididymal aspiration or testicular biopsy to obtain sperm for IVF/ICSI. Donor sperm may be necessary in cases of azoospermia due to testicular failure, if male partner has a genetic disorder, or if couple is unable to proceed with IVF/ICSI.
- Unexplained infertility can be treated empirically using superovulation with clomiphene citrate, aromatase inhibitors, or gonadotropins combined with intrauterine insemination with partner's or donor sperm. Most providers recommend using an oral ovulation induction agent with insemination as a first-line superovulatory agent because it is inexpensive. After three cycles, approximately 30% of couples will conceive. After 3 to 4 cycles, few couples will be successful and it is recommended to move forward with IVF. There is evidence suggesting that moving to IVF after 3 mo of clomiphene citrate and intrauterine insemination shortens the time interval to achieving pregnancy. A randomized trial in women with unexplained infertility revealed ovarian stimulation with letrozole resulted in a significantly lower frequency of multiple gestation but also a lower frequency of live birth, as compared with gonadotropin but not as compared with clomiphene.
- Donor egg or embryo may be required in cases of premature ovarian insufficiency or due to age factor. Some couples may elect to pursue adoption.
- For LGBTQ couples, many family building options are available, including IUI or IVF utilizing donor sperm, donor oocytes, and/or gestational carrier, depending on the needs of the couple.

DISPOSITION

- Most couples will achieve a pregnancy, provided that they are willing to proceed with treatment including ovulation induction, superovulation, IUI, IVF, or gamete donation.
- Adoption is also a worthwhile and viable possibility for couples unable to conceive.

COMPLEMENTARY & ALTERNATIVE MEDICINE

Acupuncture is widely used by women being treated for infertility. Limited data suggest some benefit, with possible mechanisms of action including increasing blood flow to the uterus and/or ovaries. Despite these studies, it is unproven whether acupuncture definitely improves IVF outcomes. Patients may additionally benefit from the stress relief that acupuncture provides.

REFERRAL

Couples should be referred to a reproductive endocrinologist once the complexity of treatment exceeds the comfort level of the provider, whether a family physician, internist, or general gynecologist. Complex ovulation and superovulation induction and ART are best managed by a board-certified reproductive endocrinologist.

PEARLS & CONSIDERATIONS

COMMENTS

- The incidence of heterotopic pregnancy in patients who have undergone ART is more common compared with an unassisted conception. Identification of a patient with ultrasound-proved intrauterine pregnancy who used ART to conceive should NOT necessarily exclude the possibility of an ectopic gestation.
- Single-embryo transfer is becoming more common in IVF cycles to reduce the rate of multiple gestation.
- Preimplantation genetic testing for monogenic/single-gene defects (PGT-M) or preimplantation genetic testing for chromosomal structural rearrangement (PGT-SR) is used in selected IVF cycles when one or both parents has one or more known genetic abnormalities or chromosomal rearrangements to test embryos for these specific genetic abnormalities prior to implantation.
- Preimplantation genetic testing for aneuploidy (PGT-A) is used in IVF cycles to screen embryos for aneuploidy prior to implantation.

Prevention

- Techniques that reduce the incidence of pelvic inflammatory disease, such as condom use, can reduce pelvic adhesions that are associated with tubal factor infertility.
- Women should be made aware of the fact that delaying pregnancy into the later reproductive years reduces the likelihood for successful pregnancy. Many women are electing to cryopreserve oocytes or embryos for future use.
- Oocyte, embryo, or sperm cryopreservation is recommended for patients undergoing gonadotoxic chemotherapy or radiation treatment as a means of fertility preservation. Ovarian or testicular tissue cryopreservation may also be performed under a research protocol. All patients should be referred to a reproductive endocrinologist before planned treatment to discuss fertility preservation options.

PATIENT & FAMILY EDUCATION

Patient support groups such as *Resolve* (www.resolve.org) are available to help couples during evaluation and treatment of infertility, which can be extraordinarily stressful.

RELATED CONTENT

Infertility (Patient Information)
Amenorrhea (Related Key Topic)
Pelvic Inflammatory Disease (Related Key Topic)
Polycystic Ovary Syndrome (Related Key Topic)

SUGGESTED READINGS

Available at ExpertConsult.com

AUTHOR: **Emelia Argyropoulos Bachman, MD**

BASIC INFORMATION

DEFINITION

Inflammatory myopathies are idiopathic diseases of muscle characterized clinically by muscle weakness and pathologically by inflammation and muscle fiber breakdown. The four most common are dermatomyositis (DM), necrotizing autoimmune myositis, polymyositis (PM), and inclusion body myositis (IBM). See separate topics on "Inclusion Body Myositis" and "Necrotizing Autoimmune Myopathy" for details regarding these topics.

SYNONYMS

Immune-mediated myopathies
Idiopathic inflammatory myopathies
Myositis syndromes
Polymyositis
Dermatomyositis
IMM

ICD-10CM CODES

M33.02	Juvenile dermatopolymyositis with myopathy
M33.12	Other dermatopolymyositis with myopathy
M33.20	Polymyositis, organ involvement unspecified
M33.22	Polymyositis with myopathy
M33.90	Dermatopolymyositis, unspecified, organ involvement unspecified
M33.92	Dermatopolymyositis, unspecified with myopathy

EPIDEMIOLOGY & DEMOGRAPHICS

Inflammatory myopathies are the largest group of potentially treatable myopathies in children and adults.

DM:

- Occurs in children and in adults (bimodal age peak).
- Average age at diagnosis is 40 yr in adults. Age range in children: 5 to 14 yr.
- More common in females than in males (2:1).
- Incidence 1:100,000.
- Prevalence 1 to 10 cases/million in adults and 1 to 3.2 cases/million in children.
- Up to one third of patients older than 50 with DM have an associated malignancy.

PM:

- Occurs mostly in adults, very rare in children
- Average age at diagnosis >20 yr
- More common in females
- Least common inflammatory myopathy
- Exact incidence unknown

PHYSICAL FINDINGS & CLINICAL PRESENTATION

DM and PM:

- Most patients have a subacute onset over wks to mos.
- Pattern is typically symmetric proximal muscle weakness involving the proximal limbs (shoulder and pelvic girdles).
- Weakness of neck flexion and extension is common.
- Difficulty getting up from a chair, climbing stairs, reaching for objects above head, or combing hair.
- Distal muscle involvement and ocular involvement are uncommon.
- Sensation is preserved.
- Reflexes may be preserved or diminished.
- Dysphagia and dysphonia result from involvement of striated muscle of the pharynx and proximal esophagus.
- Esophageal dysmotility is common in DM.
- Respiratory failure from associated pulmonary fibrosis.
- Cardiac conduction abnormalities can be seen with DM.
- Systemic autoimmune disease occurs frequently in PM, and rarely in DM.
- Skin findings in DM:
  1. Heliotrope rash on the upper eyelids (Fig. E1)
  2. Erythematous rash on the face
  3. May also involve the back and shoulders (shawl sign), neck and chest (V-shape), knees (Fig. E2), and elbows
  4. Photosensitivity
  5. Gottron papules (violaceous papules overlying dorsal interphalangeal or metacarpophalangeal areas, elbow or knee joints [Fig. E3])
  6. Nail cracking, thickening, and irregularity (Fig. E4) with periungual telangiectasia
  7. Mechanic's hand: Fissured, hyperpigmented, scaly, and hyperkeratotic; also associated with increased risk of interstitial lung disease

ETIOLOGY

DM: Complex, immune-mediated microangiopathy. Adaptive immune response via humorally mediated complement attack

PM: Unknown:

- Cell-mediated immune major histocompatibility-I (MHC-1) process directed against muscle fibers is likely, given biopsy features.
- A viral etiology has been proposed secondary to the presence of autoantibodies to histidyl transferase, anti-Jo-1, and signal recognition particle.

DIAGNOSIS

- The diagnosis of each subtype of inflammatory myopathy is based on clinical history, pattern of muscle involvement, electromyographic findings, muscle biopsy (Table E1), and presence of certain antibodies.
- Myopathic pattern of muscle weakness.
- Characteristic rash in DM.
- Electromyography (EMG) shows myopathic (small-amplitude, short-duration, polyphasic) motor potentials with early recruitment.
- Majority of patients have "irritable" features (fibrillations and positive sharp waves) on EMG.
- See "Laboratory Tests."
- Biopsy is required for diagnosis and should confirm inflammation before treatment is started. Table 2 describes histologic features of idiopathic inflammatory myopathies. In idiopathic inflammatory myopathies, myopathic features (variation in fiber size, fiber splitting, fatty replacement of muscle tissue, and increased endomysial connective tissue) should be seen in addition to the following:
  1. DM: Perifascicular atrophy, membrane attack complex (MAC) deposition along capillaries
  2. PM: Endomysial infiltrates composed of CD8+ T cells and macrophages invading nonnecrotic muscle fibers that express MHC-I antigen

DIFFERENTIAL DIAGNOSIS

- IBM
- Muscular dystrophies
- Amyloid myoneuropathy
- Amyotrophic lateral sclerosis
- Myasthenia gravis
- Eaton-Lambert syndrome
- Drug-induced myopathies (e.g., quinidine, NSAIDs, penicillamine, HMG-CoA-reductase inhibitors)
- Diabetic amyotrophy
- Guillain-Barré syndrome
- Hyperthyroidism or hypothyroidism
- Lichen planus
- Amyopathic DM (rash without weakness)
- DM sine rash (weakness with characteristic biopsy, but no rash)
- Systemic lupus erythematosus (SLE)
- Contact atopic or seborrheic dermatitis
- Psoriasis

LABORATORY TESTS

- Creatine kinase (CK) is the most sensitive muscle enzyme test for muscle breakdown. It should be checked at onset, and serially monitored several times during treatment.
- CK is typically elevated (5 to 50× normal) in active PM.
- CK may be normal or only slightly elevated in DM.
- Aldolase, aspartate aminotransferase, alanine aminotransferase, alkaline phosphatase, and lactate dehydrogenase (LDH) may be elevated.
- Anti-Jo-1 antibodies are seen in myositis with associated interstitial lung disease but are not specific for either DM or PM.
- Myositis-specific and myositis-associated autoantibodies in adult polymyositis and dermatomyositis and juvenile dermatomyositis are summarized in Table E3.
- DM: Anti-MDA-5, anti-Mi-2, anti-TIF-1, and anti-NXP2 (implicated in cancer-associated dermatomyositis).
- PM: Antisynthetase antibodies (often seen in overlap myositis) associated with interstitial lung disease, arthritis, fever, and "mechanic's hands."
- Electrolytes, thyroid-stimulating hormone (TSH), Ca, and Mg should be evaluated to exclude other causes of weakness.
- Check ECG for cardiac involvement.

TABLE 2 Histologic Features of Idiopathic Inflammatory Myopathies

Feature	Dermatomyositis	Polymyositis	Inclusion Body Myositis
Necrosis of muscle fibers	+	+	+
Variation in fiber diameter	+	+	+
Regeneration of muscle fibers	+	+	+
Proliferation of connective tissue	+	+	+
Infiltration of mononuclear cells*	+	+	+
Perivascular and perimysial inflammation	+	−/+	−/+
Endomysial inflammation	−/+	+	+
Perifascicular atrophy	+	−	−
Abnormally dilated capillaries	+	−/+	−
Reduced capillary density	+	−/+	−
Deposition of complement on vessel walls	+	−/+	−
Microinfarcts	+	−	−
Invasion of nonnecrotic fibers by cytotoxic T lymphocytes and macrophages	−	+	+
Expression of major histocompatibility complex class I on muscle fibers	−/+	+	+
Rimmed vacuoles with amyloid deposits and tubulofilaments†	−	−	+
Angulated or atrophic and hypertrophic fibers	−	−	+
Ragged red or cytochrome oxidase–negative fibers	−	−	+

*Inflammation is absent in a small proportion of polymyositis and dermatomyositis biopsies.
†Also seen in chronic neurogenic conditions and distal myopathies.
From Firestein GS et al: *Kelley's textbook of rheumatology*, ed 9, Philadelphia, 2013, Saunders, Elsevier.

IMAGING STUDIES

- Chest x-ray is used to rule out pulmonary involvement. If suspicious for pulmonary interstitial disease, a high-resolution CT scan of the chest may be helpful.
- Radiography is an efficient means of identifying and characterizing soft-tissue calcinosis (Fig. E5).
- Although MRI arguably has greater diagnostic value than electromyography or serum enzyme measurements in cases of suspected idiopathic inflammatory myopathy, MRI findings have not been formalized as a diagnostic criterion for idiopathic inflammatory myopathy. The acceptance of MRI as a diagnostic tool in myositis may be inhibited by the high cost and the need for more reliable and validated methods of summarizing the findings of MRI. MRI evaluation before biopsy, however, has become routine at many tertiary care centers. Fascial disease is manifested on MRI by fascial or perifascial hyperintensity on fluid-sensitive sequences. The edema-like signal in the deep subcutis may accompany fasciitis and can indicate associated panniculitis.
- Video fluoroscopy or barium swallow study to look for upper esophageal dysfunction in patients with dysphagia and DM.
- Table E4 summarizes affected organs and their evaluation in inflammatory muscle disease.

Rx TREATMENT

Goal: Maintain function, minimize disease/iatrogenic sequelae

NONPHARMACOLOGIC THERAPY

- Sun-blocking agents with SPF 15 or greater for skin protection in patients with DM
- Physical therapy beneficial for gait training and increasing muscle tone and strength
- Occupational therapy assists with activities of daily living
- Speech therapy to monitor patients with swallowing dysfunction

ACUTE GENERAL Rx

- Corticosteroids are the mainstay of therapy. Start prednisone 1 to 2 mg/kg per day, up to a maximum dose of 100 mg/day. Continue until muscle strength improves or muscle enzymes have normalized for at least 4 wk. Begin tapering by 10 mg/mo until 60 mg/day, then slowly taper by 5 mg/mo. Consider every-other-day prednisone treatment at same dose (may decrease side effects).
- Consider IV immunoglobulin (IVIG) if patient fails to improve on prednisone, or muscle enzymes begin rising when tapering off prednisone. See "Chronic Rx" for specific dosage.
- Hydroxychloroquine can be used to treat the cutaneous lesions of DM.
- A treatment algorithm for adult patients with inflammatory myopathies is illustrated in Fig. 6.

CHRONIC Rx

- Chronic prednisone therapy may be needed for yrs, but other immunosuppressive ("steroid-sparing") agents may be added early to decrease long-term steroid side effects.
- Azathioprine 2 to 3 mg/kg per day tapered to 1 mg/kg per day once steroid is tapered to 15 mg/day. Reduce dosage monthly by 25-mg intervals. Maintenance dosage is 50 mg/day.
- Methotrexate 7.5 to 10 mg PO/wk, increased by 2.5 mg/wk to total of 25 mg/wk; consider IM dosing if PO is ineffective. Use cautiously in patients with interstitial lung disease due to possible pulmonary fibrosis.
- IV immunoglobulin 2 g/kg total dose over 2 to 5 days.
- IV cyclophosphamide 1 g/M^2 monthly for 6 mo is preferred to oral dosing for refractory cases. However, oral dosing of cyclophosphamide is 1 to 3 mg/kg per day PO or 2 to 4 mg/kg per day in conjunction with prednisone.
- Cyclosporine A: Initial dose 2.0 to 2.5 mg/kg bid; long-term maintenance is lowest effective dose.
- Mycophenolate mofetil 500 mg PO bid, titrate to 1500 mg PO bid over 1 to 2 mo.
- Hydroxychloroquine 200 mg PO daily; monitor for visual changes.

DISPOSITION

- 30% to 40% of patients achieve clinical remission with treatment.
- In patients with residual weakness, deficits typically remain stable over long-term follow-up.
- 10% experience recurrent disease.
- Serum CK often returns to normal before symptoms improve.
- During exacerbations, enzymes may rise before clinical symptoms appear.
- Poor prognostic indicators include delay in diagnosis, older age, recalcitrant disease, malignancy, interstitial pulmonary fibrosis, dysphagia, leukocytosis, fever, and anorexia.
- Infection, malignancy, and cardiac and pulmonary dysfunction are the most common causes of death.
- With early treatment, 5- and 8-yr survival rates of 80% and 73%, respectively, have been reported.

REFERRAL

Neurology or rheumatology referral should be made to help establish the diagnosis and implement treatment.

PEARLS & CONSIDERATIONS

- Do not implement treatment before muscle biopsy.
- When assessing response to treatment, clinical muscle strength is more important than muscle enzyme tests.
- The concern for malignancies (ovary, lung, breast, GI) associated with DM is legitimate and merits screening in patients older than

age 40 at time of diagnosis and every 2 to 3 yr thereafter.

- No association exists between juvenile DM and malignancy.
- Overlap syndrome refers to patients with DM who also meet criteria for a connective tissue disorder (e.g., rheumatoid arthritis, scleroderma, SLE).
- In any patient taking steroids, closely monitor for:
  1. Diabetes or glucose intolerance (2-hr oral glucose tolerance test)
  2. Osteopenia/osteoporosis (DEXA scan q6mo)
  3. Cataracts (yearly ophthalmologic appointment)
  4. Hypertension
  5. Psychiatric side effects including depression or psychosis
  6. Poor sleep
  7. Peptic ulcer disease (prescribe H_2 antagonist or proton pump inhibitor)
- Clinical and immune response features can be used for categorizing heterogeneous myositis syndromes and mutually exclusive and stable phenotypes and are useful for predicting clinical signs and symptoms, associated environmental and genetic risk factors, and responses to therapy and prognosis.

SUGGESTED READINGS

Available at ExpertConsult.com

RELATED CONTENT

Dermatomyositis and Polymyositis (Patient Information)
Inclusion Body Myositis (Related Key Topic)
Necrotizing Autoimmune Myopathy (Related Key Topic)

AUTHOR: **Lydia Sharp, MD**

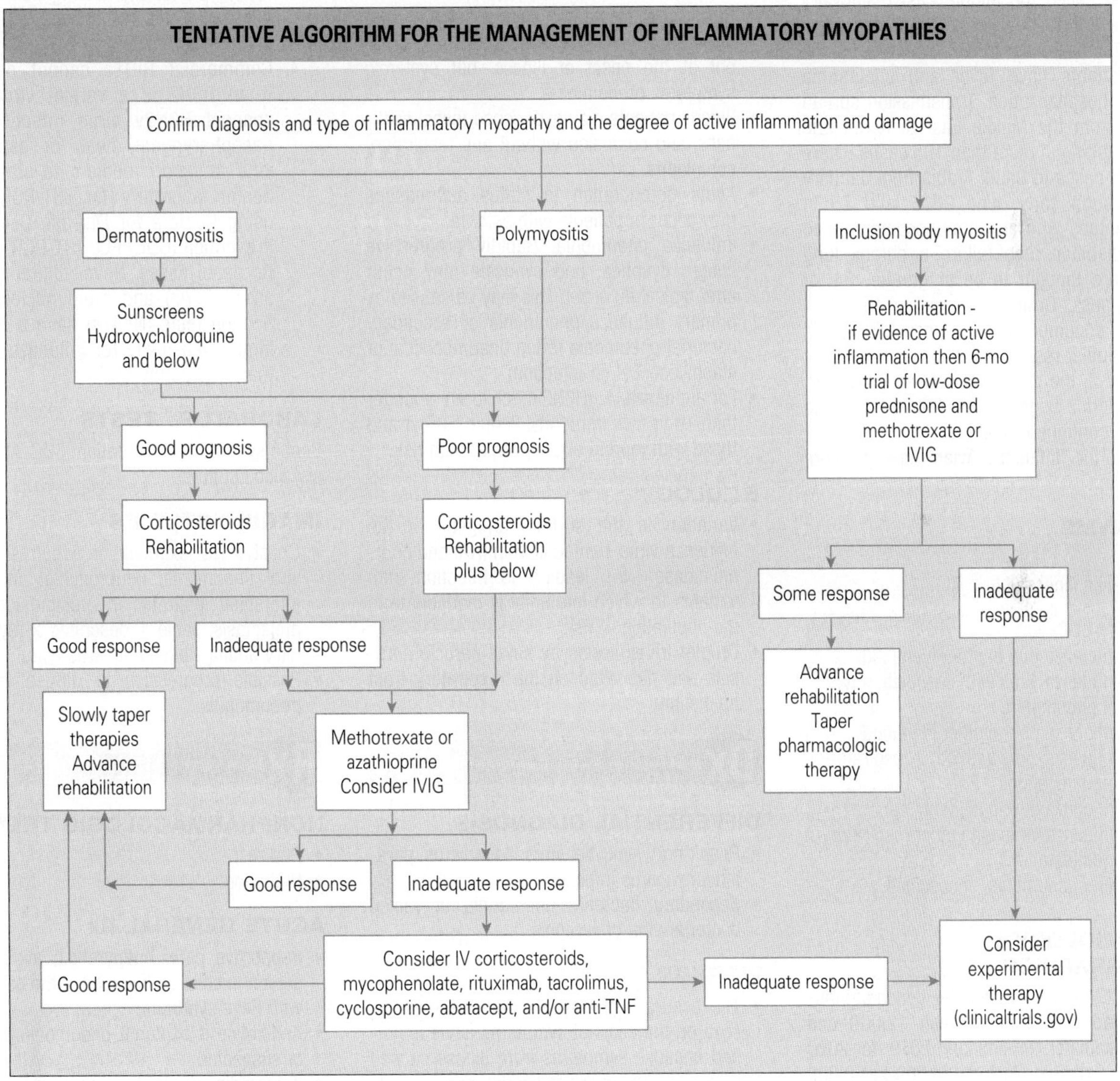

FIG. 6 Tentative algorithm for the management of inflammatory myopathies. *anti-TNF,* Anti–tumor necrosis factor; *IV,* intravenous; *IVIG,* intravenous immunoglobulin. (From Hochberg MC: *Rheumatology,* ed 7, Philadelphia, 2019, Elsevier.)

BASIC INFORMATION

DEFINITION

Influenza is an acute febrile illness caused by infection with influenza type A or B virus. Seasonal influenza can include the H1N1 virus. A similar respiratory illness is severe acute respiratory syndrome (SARS) caused by a coronavirus called SARS-associated coronavirus (SARS-CoV). A new novel coronavirus was recognized in two patients in September 2012. This is a very different virus from the SARS agent; the two patients exhibited acute respiratory distress syndrome, renal failure, consumptive coagulopathy, and/or pericarditis. Now called the Middle East respiratory syndrome (MERS-CoV) virus, it affected more than 2,200 persons in 27 countries since 2012. Patients have fever and pneumonia requiring hospitalization. Transmission spread in 2015 from the Middle East to Korea and China, resulting in more than 185 cases. There were 558 cases in Saudi Arabia from January 2015 through early June 2016, and 75 in 2018. Persons who are immunocompromised or have diabetes, renal failure, or chronic lung disease are thought to be at greater risk of severe illness. Dromedary camels and their milk are documented to harbor MERS-CoV. Another similar respiratory illness is caused by SARS-CoV-2, the virus that causes COVID-19. This pandemic began in the fall of 2019 and will likely continue in 2021.

Refer to the "Influenza, Avian" topic for more information.

SYNONYMS

Flu

Influenza-like illness (ILI)

ICD-10CM CODES

J10.00	Influenza due to other identified influenza virus with unspecified type of pneumonia
J10.1	Influenza due to other identified influenza virus with other respiratory manifestations
J11.1	Influenza due to unidentified influenza virus with other respiratory manifestations
J12.9	Viral pneumonia, unspecified

EPIDEMIOLOGY & DEMOGRAPHICS

INCIDENCE (IN U.S.): Annual incidence of influenza-related deaths is between 12,000 and 51,000 deaths/yr. Preliminary 2019 to 2020 flu season estimates include 24,000 to 62,000 deaths, 39 to 56 million illnesses, and 410,000 to 740,000 hospitalizations.

PREDOMINANT SEX: Male = female

PREDOMINANT AGE: Attack rates are usually higher among children than adults, although children are less prone to pulmonary complications. The severity of the 2017 to 2018 flu season was described by the Centers for Disease Control and Prevention (CDC) as high for all age groups: Children, adults, and older adults. In the 2018 to 2019 season, there were 480 deaths estimated in children; 75% of the 34,000 deaths associated with the flu occurred in older adults.

PEAK INCIDENCE: Winter outbreaks lasting 5 to 6 wk

PHYSICAL FINDINGS & CLINICAL PRESENTATION

- "Classic flu" is characterized by abrupt onset of fever, headache, myalgias, anorexia, and malaise after a 1- to 2-day incubation period.
- Clinical syndromes are similar to those produced by other respiratory viruses, including pharyngitis, common colds, tracheobronchitis, bronchiolitis, and croup.
- Respiratory symptoms such as cough, sore throat, and nasal discharge are usually present at the onset of illness, but systemic symptoms predominate.
- Elderly patients may experience fever, weakness, and confusion without any respiratory complaints.
- Acute deterioration to status asthmaticus may occur in patients with asthma.
- Influenza pneumonia: Rapidly progressive cough, dyspnea, and cyanosis may occur after typical flu onset. This may be caused by primary influenza pneumonia or secondary bacterial pneumonia (often pneumococcal or staphylococcal co-infection).
- For influenza A (H3N2v), children younger than 10 yr lack immunity. People ≥65 yr and those with morbid obesity are at high risk.

ETIOLOGY

- Variation in the surface antigens of the influenza virus, hemagglutinin (HA) and neuraminidase (NA), leading to infection with variants to which immunity is inadequate in the population at risk
- Droplet transmission by small-particle aerosols and deposited on the respiratory tract epithelium

DIAGNOSIS

DIFFERENTIAL DIAGNOSIS

- Respiratory syncytial virus, adenovirus, parainfluenza virus infection
- Secondary bacterial pneumonia or mixed bacterial-viral pneumonia

WORKUP

- The accuracy of clinical diagnosis of influenza on the basis of symptoms alone is limited because symptoms from illness caused by other pathogens can overlap considerably with influenza. Diagnostic tests available for influenza include viral cultures, serology, rapid influenza diagnostic tests (RIDTs), reverse transcription-polymerase chain reaction (RT-PCR), and immunofluorescence assays.
- Virus isolation from nasal or throat swab or sputum specimens is the most rapid diagnostic method in the setting of acute illness.
- Specimens are placed into virus transport medium and processed by a reference laboratory.
- For serologic diagnosis:
  1. Paired serum specimens, acute and convalescent, the latter obtained 10 to 20 days later.
  2. Fourfold rises or falls in the titer of antibodies (various techniques) considered diagnostic of recent infection.
  3. Commercial rapid influenza diagnostic tests (RIDTs) are available. They can detect influenza virus antigens within 15 min of testing. Rapid flu test should be collected as early as possible, ideally within 4 days of onset. False-negative results are common during the flu season. A negative test result does NOT exclude diagnosis of influenza.
  4. Commercial RIDTs cannot determine if an H3N2 is a variant virus; when suspect H3N2v virus infection, send nasopharyngeal swab or aspirate in viral transport medium to state public health laboratory for rRT-PCR testing using Centers for Disease Control and Prevention (CDC) FLU rRT-PCR diagnostic panel assay. Novel digital immunoassay (DIAs) and rapid nucleic amplification tests (NAATs) have a markedly higher sensitivity for influenza A and B than traditional RIDTs.

LABORATORY TESTS

Septic syndrome presentation: CBC, ABG analysis, blood cultures

IMAGING STUDIES

- Chest x-ray examination when suspecting viral pneumonia: Peribronchial and patchy interstitial infiltrates in multiple lobes with atelectasis. Table 1 describes x-ray pulmonary findings based on virus type.
- Possible progression to diffuse interstitial pneumonitis.

TREATMENT

NONPHARMACOLOGIC THERAPY

- Bed rest
- Hydration

ACUTE GENERAL Rx

- Supportive care: Antipyretics; avoid use of aspirin in children because of the association with Reye syndrome.
- Antibiotics if bacterial pneumonia is proved or suspected.
- Amantadine is NOT recommended due to resistant isolates.
- Neuraminidase inhibitors block release of virions from infected cells, resulting in shortened duration of symptoms and decrease in complications; effective against both influenza A and B, including A (H3N2v) for all hospitalized patients, those with severe and progressive illness, and high-risk patients with suspected or confirmed H3N2v.

TABLE 1 Pulmonary Radiographic Findings Based on Virus Type

Virus	Centrilobular Nodules	Lobar Ground-Glass	Diffuse Ground-Glass	Thickened Interlobular Septa	Consolidation
Influenza	+++	+++	+		+
Epstein-Barr	+	+	+		+
Cytomegalovirus	++	++	++	+	+
Varicella-zoster	+++	+	+		
Herpes simplex	+	+++	+		+++
Measles	++	+	+		+
Hantavirus			+++	+	++
Adenovirus	++	+			+++

From Weissleder R et al: *Primer of diagnostic imaging,* ed 5, St Louis, 2011, Mosby.

1. Oseltamivir, administered orally:
   a. For treatment, 75 mg PO twice daily for 5 days
   b. For prevention, 75 mg PO once daily for a minimum of 2 wk in an outbreak setting or 7 days after exposure for an adult
2. Zanamivir, administered via inhaler:
   a. For treatment, 10 mg (2 inhalations of 5 mg each) twice daily for 5 days.
   b. For prevention in households, 10 mg (2 inhalations of 5 mg each) once daily for 7 days. Not recommended in persons with underlying airways disease such as asthma or chronic obstructive pulmonary disease.
   c. Adjust dosing in patients with renal impairment or end-stage renal disease.
3. Baloxavir (Xofluza) was approved by the FDA in 2018 for acute uncomplicated influenza infection in patients ≥ 12 yr of age and in 2020 for post-exposure prophylaxis of influenza. Its mechanism of action is through inhibition of an endonuclease involved in viral RNA replication. It is a single dose drug.

- Placebo-controlled studies have suggested that antiviral therapy with any of the previously mentioned agents must ideally be initiated within 1 to 2 days of the onset of symptoms and reduces the duration of illness by ~1 day.
- Oseltamivir resistance developed on therapy in individuals with avian flu (H5N1) in Asia, and this is associated with poor outcome.
- Amantadine and rimantadine resistance are documented for novel (H1N1) influenza and H3N2 influenza virus.
- Systemic corticosteroids should not be routinely administered to patients with suspected or confirmed influenza, including H3N2v virus infection, except for patients on chronic corticosteroid therapy for COPD, asthma.
- Recent trials[1] have shown that in patients hospitalized with severe influenza infection, triple therapy with clarithromycin 500 mg, naproxen 200 mg, and oseltamivir 75 mg bid for 30 days reduced mortality and did not increase complications compared with oseltamivir (75 mg bid for 5 days) alone.

[1] Hung IFN et al: Efficacy of clarithromycin-naproxen-oseltamivir combination in the treatment of patients hospitalized for influenza (H3N2) infection: an open-lab, randomized, controlled, phase IIb/III trial, *Chest* 151:1069-1080, 2017.

DISPOSITION

Patients are hospitalized if signs of pneumonia are present.

REFERRAL

Infectious disease and/or pulmonary consultation when influenza pneumonia is suspected

PEARLS & CONSIDERATIONS

COMMENTS

- Prevention of influenza in patients at high risk is an important goal of primary care.
- Vaccines reduce the risk of infection and the severity of illness.
  1. Antigenic composition of the vaccine is updated annually. The northern hemisphere's 2020 to 2021 season trivalent egg-based vaccines include an A/Guangdong-Maonan/SWL 1536/2019 (H1N1) pdm09-like virus (updated), an A/Hong Kong/2671/2019 (H3N2)-like virus (updated), and a B/Washingon/02/2019 (B/Victoria lineage)-like virus (updated).
  2. Quadrivalent egg-based vaccines contain these three vaccine viruses, plus a second influenza B vaccine virus strain called B/Phuket/3073/2013-like (Yamagata lineage) virus.
  3. Quadrivalent cell- or recombinant-based vaccines contain: A/Hawaii/70/2019 (H1N1) pdm09-like virus (updated), A/Hong Kong/45/2019 (H3N2)-like virus (updated), B/Washington/02/2019 (B/Victoria lineage)-like virus (updated), and B/Phuket/3073/2013-like (Yamagata lineage) virus.
  4. Revaccination is recommended annually before onset of influenza activity in the community, even for those who received the vaccine in the previous season.
  5. Delaying vaccination to ensure persistence of vaccine-induced protection during flu season could result in missed opportunities to vaccinate.
  6. Seasonal influenza vaccine does not provide protection against the influenza A (H3N2v) virus that is associated with agricultural fairs.
  7. Vaccination should be given at the start of the flu season (September-October) for all persons aged ≥6 mo who do not have contraindications. Vaccination is particularly important for persons who are at high risk and their contacts/caregivers. When vaccine supply is limited, vaccination efforts should focus on the following groups:
     a. All children aged 6 mo to 4 yr (59 mo)
     b. People 50 yr and older
     c. Adults and children with chronic cardiac (except hypertension) or pulmonary (including asthma), renal, hepatic, neurologic, hematologic or metabolic disease (including diabetes mellitus)
     d. Immunocompromised patients (including HIV-infected persons or patients immunosuppressed due to medications)
     e. Women who are or will be pregnant during the influenza season
     f. Children aged 6 mo to 18 yr who are receiving long-term aspirin therapy
     g. Residents of nursing homes and other long-term care facilities
     h. American Indians/Alaska Natives
     i. Persons who are morbidly obese (BMI ≥40)
     j. Health care workers (HCWs)
     k. Household contacts and caregivers of persons in the previous groups
     l. Essential workers during the COVID-19 pandemic
  8. Vaccination precautions include:
     a. Guillain-Barré syndrome within 6 wk following a previous dose of influenza vaccine
     b. Moderate or severe acute illness with or without fever
     c. Asthma in persons >5 yr (LAIV4)
     d. Other underlying medical conditions that might predispose to complications after wild-type influenza infection (e.g., chronic pulmonary, cardiovascular [excluding isolated hypertension], renal, hepatic, neurologic,

TABLE 2 Antiviral Agents for Influenza

	Amantadine	Rimantadine	Zanamivir	Oseltamivir
Protein target	M2	M2	Neuraminidase	Neuraminidase
Activity	A only (H1N1 and H3N2 are resistant)	A only (H1N1 and H3N2 are resistant)	A and B	A and B
Side effects	CNS (13%) GI (3%)	GI (6%)	? Bronchospasm	GI (9%)
Metabolism	None	Multiple (hepatic)	None	Hepatic
Excretion	Renal	Renal, + others	Renal	Renal (tubular secretion)
Drug interactions	Antihistamines, anticholinergics	None	None	Probenecid (increased levels of oseltamivir)
Dose adjustments needed	≥65 yr old CrCl <50 ml/min	≥65 yr old CrCl <10 ml/min	None	CrCl <30 ml/min Severe liver dysfunction
Contraindications	Acute-angle glaucoma	Severe liver dysfunction	Underlying airway disease, asthma	
FDA-Approved Indications				
Therapy	Adults and children ≥1 yr old	Adults only	Adults and children ≥7 yr old	Adults and children ≥1 yr old*
Prophylaxis	Yes	Yes	Adults and children ≥5 yr old	Adults and children ≥13 yr old†

CNS, Central nervous system; *CrCl,* creatinine clearance; *FDA,* U.S. Food and Drug Administration; *GI,* gastrointestinal.
*FDA has authorized treatment of S-OIV (novel H1N1) virus with oseltamivir in children ≥3 mo of age.
†FDA has authorized prophylaxis for S-OIV (novel H1N1) virus with oseltamivir in children ≥1 yr.
From Mandell GL et al: *Principles and practice of infectious diseases,* ed 7, Philadelphia, 2010, Churchill Livingstone.

hematologic, or metabolic disorders [underlying diabetes mellitus]) (LAIV4)
   e. Delay flu vaccination of persons with acute illness from suspected or laboratory-confirmed COVID-19
9. Contraindication to receiving vaccine:
   a. Previous severe allergic reaction to influenza vaccine
   b. For LAIV4: Concomitant aspirin- or salicylate-containing therapy in children and adolescents
   c. For LAIV4: Children 2 to 4 yr with asthma Dx in past 12 mo
   d. For LAIV4: Immunocompromised due to any cause including medications or HIV infection
   e. For LAIV4: Close contacts and caregivers of severely immunosuppressed persons who require a protected environment
   f. For LAIV4: Pregnancy
   g. For LAIV4: Received oseltamivir or zanamivir within past 48 hr, peramivir within past 5 days, or baloxivir within past 17 days
10. Special efforts should be made to vaccinate high-risk patients <65 yr, only 10% to 15% of whom are vaccinated each yr.
11. HCW vaccination minimizes transmission to patients and coworkers. Some states mandate vaccination of HCWs; some healthcare facilities and other states require the wearing of face masks by unvaccinated HCWs during the influenza season, particularly when there is widespread flu.
12. Vaccine efficacy varies by age and by type of circulating virus. Efficacy varies each yr and has ranged from 23% to 60% overall; 2018 to 2019 efficacy varied by age group. Even with low efficacy, hospitalizations are reduced.
13. Alternate vaccine formulations:
   a. Intradermal vaccine for injection via a small needle into skin instead of muscle has not been available for every flu season.
   b. The CDC's Advisory Committee on Immunization Practices (ACIP) found no measurable protective benefit from using nasal spray, live-attenuated influenza vaccine (LAIV) during the 2015 to 2016 flu season. ACIP recently reviewed more data and found LAIV4 effective against influenza B and influenza A (H3N2). Effectiveness of the updated LAIV4 against currently circulating influenza A (H1N1) pdm09-like viruses is unknown. ACIP recommends any licensed, age-appropriate influenza vaccine, including LAIV4. Do not give LAIV4 to patients with cochlear implants, active CSF leaks, and anatomical or functional asplenia.
   c. Give TIV if recipient has egg allergy or asthma or cares for immunosuppressed persons who require a protective environment.
   d. Thimerosal-free vaccine is available.
   e. IIV can be trivalent or quadrivalent, and egg-based or non–egg-based (cell culture or recombinant hemagglutinin).
   f. There is no preference for standard dose IIV or high dose IIV (age 65 or over).
   g. Season 2020-2021 had quadrivalent high-dose vaccine and quadrivalent adjuvanted vaccine for adults age 65 or over.
   h. ACIP guidance for egg allergies:
      (1) If a person with egg allergy experiences only hives, then administer any recommended influenza vaccine (IIV, RIV4, LAIV4) that is otherwise appropriate.
      (2) If person reports past reactions to egg involving symptoms other than urticaria (e.g., angioedema or swelling, respiratory distress, lightheadedness, recurrent emesis) or who required epinephrine or other medical intervention, should be vaccinated in a medical setting with supervision of vaccine administration by health care provider able to recognize and manage severe allergic reactions.
   i. No post-vaccination observation period is recommended for egg-allergic reaction. Consider observing patients for 15 minutes after vaccine administration to decrease risk for injury should syncope occur.

- Storage of vaccines:
   1. Maintain storage temperatures with adequate refrigeration and temperature monitoring.
   2. Do not use beyond expiration date or manufacturer's beyond use date.
   3. Do not access single-dose vial for more than one dose.
- Chemoprophylaxis:
   1. Table 2 describes antiviral agents for influenza. Oseltamivir and zanamivir are recommended in the U.S. during the influenza season. Baloxavir marboxil was FDA approved in 2018 and may eventually replace the other agents as a preferred drug (single-dose treatment for persons 12 yrs and older weighing over 40 kg, low side-effects profile).
   2. Consider (after the current circulating strain of influenza has been shown to be sensitive):
      a. For high-risk patients in whom vaccination is contraindicated
      b. When the available vaccine is known not to include the circulating strain
      c. To provide added protection to immunosuppressed patients likely to have a diminished response to vaccination

d. In the setting of an outbreak, when immediate protection of unvaccinated or recently vaccinated patients at high risk of complications is desired
3. Chemoprophylaxis with antiviral drugs is not recommended for healthy persons exposed to seasonal influenza.
4. Give for 2 wk in the case of late vaccination and for the duration of the flu season in all other patients.
5. Treatment should not wait for laboratory confirmation of influenza.
6. Do not give aspirin or aspirin-containing products to children with influenza-like illness due to the risk of Reye syndrome.

- Other prevention strategies:
  1. Hand hygiene, cough etiquette (cover your cough), respiratory hygiene (use of tissues, facemasks for the ill, and proper disposal).
  2. Seasonal flu personal protective equipment (PPE)—wear gloves and gowns as per universal/standard precautions. Per the CDC, wear a facemask, adhering to Droplet Precautions for 7 days after illness onset or until 24 hr after fever and respiratory symptoms are resolved, whichever is longer. Patient placement in a negative pressure room and N95 respirator for health care workers are recommended when conducting aerosol-generating procedures. During the COVID-19 pandemic, until influenza is confirmed and COVID-19 is definitively ruled out, one needs to take precautions and wear PPE as for COVID-19. Patients can have both influenza and COVID-19 at the same time.
  3. Highly pathogenic Asian avian influenza (HPAI) includes H5N1, H7N9, H5N2, and H5N8. CDC recommends wearing eye protection, N95 respirator, gown, and gloves as for airborne and contact precautions.
  4. Management of ill health care workers—exclude from work until at least 24 hr after they no longer have a fever (without the use of fever-reducing medication). Extended exclusion time period when caring for severely immunocompromised patients.
  5. Standard cleaning and disinfection procedures.
- The Centers for Medicare and Medicaid Services links health care worker vaccine acceptance with payment for performance.

SUGGESTED READINGS

Available at ExpertConsult.com

RELATED CONTENT

Influenza (Flu) (Patient Information)

AUTHOR: **Marlene Fishman Wolpert, MPH, CIC, FAPIC**

BASIC INFORMATION

DEFINITION

Insomnia is a disturbance of initiating or maintaining sleep. Restless, nonrestorative sleep may also be described as another specified insomnia. The disturbance occurs despite adequate circumstances and opportunity for sleep and is accompanied by significant distress or impairment in daytime functioning.

In the DSM-5, the diagnosis of primary insomnia has been replaced with **insomnia disorder** in order to avoid the distinction between primary and secondary forms of the disorder. This paradigm shift relates to widely accepted research in the field suggesting that there is a bidirectional and interactive relationship between insomnia and any coexisting medical and/or mental disorders.

SYNONYMS

Sleeplessness
Sleep disorder, sleep disturbance, dyssomnia (NOTE: The terms *sleep disorder, sleep disturbance,* and *dyssomnia* are generic and can refer to disorders of wakefulness [hypersomnia] or sleep-related behavior disorders [parasomnias])
Insomnia disorder
Chronic insomnia disorder

ICD-10CM CODES

F51.01	Primary insomnia
F51.02	Adjustment insomnia
F51.03	Paradoxical insomnia
F51.04	Psychophysiologic insomnia
F51.05	Insomnia due to other mental disorder
F51.09	Other insomnia not due to a substance or known physiological condition
G47.00	Insomnia, unspecified
G47.01	Insomnia due to medical condition
G47.09	Other insomnia
Z73.810	Behavioral insomnia of childhood, sleep-onset association type
Z73.811	Behavioral insomnia of childhood, limit setting type
Z73.812	Behavioral insomnia of childhood, combined type
Z73.819	Behavioral insomnia of childhood, unspecified type

DSM-5 CODES

Depends on specific diagnosis.

EPIDEMIOLOGY & DEMOGRAPHICS

INCIDENCE (IN U.S.): 20% to 30% of adults experience occasional bouts of acute insomnia.
PREVALENCE (IN U.S.): The prevalence of chronic insomnia disorder ranges from 6% to 10%.
PREDOMINANT SEX: More common in women
PREDOMINANT AGE: Transient insomnia can occur at any age; persistent insomnia can also occur at any age but is more common after age 60 yr.
GENETICS: Can run in families and may be genetically influenced. Circadian rhythm disorders and narcolepsy have been traced to specific genes.

PHYSICAL FINDINGS & CLINICAL PRESENTATION

- Difficulty initiating sleep, inability to maintain sleep, and/or early morning awakening.
- Significant distress or impairment in daytime functioning such as fatigue or low energy, sleepiness, cognitive impairments, mood disturbances, and/or physiologic or behavioral problems.
- Difficulty occurs despite adequate opportunity for sleep.
- Symptoms may be acute and self-limited, chronic but intermittent, or chronic and frequent.

ETIOLOGY

- Transient insomnia:
  1. Any stressful biopsychosocial change in life circumstance (e.g., marriage, divorce, birth of a child, loss of a loved one, illness, retirement, etc.)
  2. Travel (across time zones)
  3. Environmental disruptions (noise, heat, cold, poor bedding, bed partners, unfamiliar surroundings, etc.)
- Persistent insomnia (Fig. 1):
  1. Mood and anxiety disorders (depression, hypomania/mania, PTSD)
  2. Psychophysiologic insomnia (conditioned arousal, extended sleep opportunity, sleep effort, poor sleep hygiene)
  3. Sleep-related breathing disorders (e.g., obstructive apnea and hypopnea, increased upper airway resistance)
  4. Chronobiologic (also known as circadian rhythm) disorder (delayed sleep phase, advanced sleep phase, shift work, non–24-hr sleep-wake disorder secondary to blindness)
  5. Drug and alcohol use disorders.
  6. Restless legs syndrome and periodic leg movements
  7. Neurodegenerative (Alzheimer disease, Parkinson disease, etc.)
  8. Medical (pain, GERD, nocturia, orthopnea, menopause, medications, etc.)

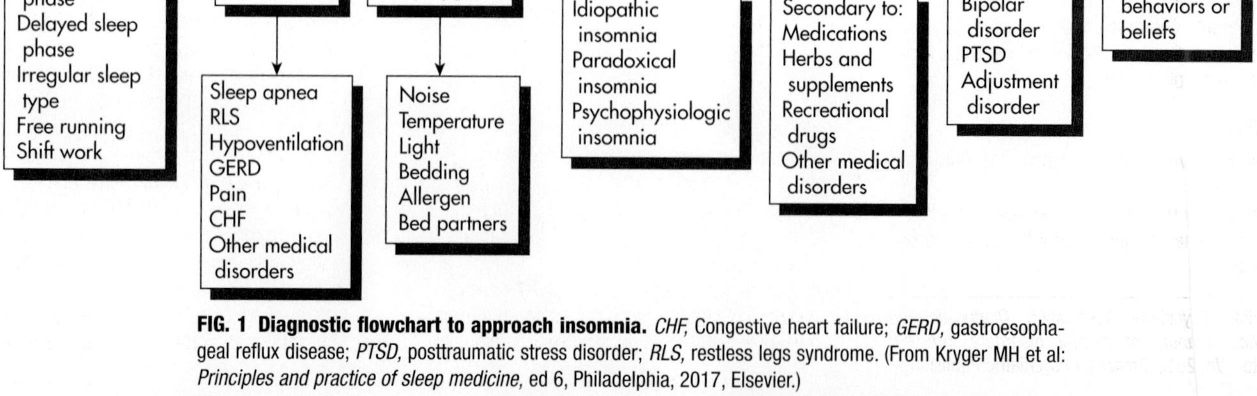

FIG. 1 Diagnostic flowchart to approach insomnia. *CHF,* Congestive heart failure; *GERD,* gastroesophageal reflux disease; *PTSD,* posttraumatic stress disorder; *RLS,* restless legs syndrome. (From Kryger MH et al: *Principles and practice of sleep medicine,* ed 6, Philadelphia, 2017, Elsevier.)

BOX 1 Sleep Habits (Sleep Hygiene Measures) That May Improve Sleep

1. Reduce caffeine, alcohol, or tobacco late in the day or especially evening.
2. Avoid heavy meals at night, but consider a light snack before bed such as toast or a handful of nuts.
3. Increase daytime activity, but avoid exercise within 3-5 hours of bedtime.
4. Increase daytime exposure to natural light.
5. Reduce liquids in the last 4 hours before bedtime.
6. Consider white noise as background sound for the sleep environment.
7. Maintain regular bed and wake times.
8. Go to bed with calm mind; resolve arguments or set a time earlier in the day to review problems and perhaps write down plans, solutions, or things to do.
9. Keep light exposure in the middle of the night to a minimum when awake and attenuate morning light in the bedroom.
10. Avoid pets in the bed.

Dx DIAGNOSIS

Diagnostic and Statistical Manual of Mental Disorders (DSM-5) criteria for the diagnosis of insomnia disorder is as follows[1]:

- Dissatisfaction with sleep quantity or quality, with one or more of the following symptoms:
  1. Difficulty initiating sleep
  2. Difficulty maintaining sleep, characterized by frequent awakenings or trouble returning to sleep after awakenings
  3. Early-morning awakening with inability to return to sleep
- The sleep disturbance causes clinically significant distress or impairment in social, occupational, educational, academic, behavioral, or other important areas of functioning.
- The sleep difficulty occurs at least 3 nights per wk, is present for at least 3 mo, and occurs despite adequate opportunity for sleep

DIFFERENTIAL DIAGNOSIS

- The diagnosis of insomnia disorder should be made only once insomnia related to an underlying medical, substance use, and/or behavioral cause has been ruled out. While insomnia is often precipitated by an underlying cause (e.g., work stress, pain, depression), persistence of symptoms despite treatment of the initial cause should raise concerns for progression to insomnia disorder (see "Etiology"). For medical disorders such as obesity, diabetes mellitus, and renal disease, obstructive sleep apnea is a frequent complication and must be ruled out. Insomnia remains the most resistant symptom following the treatment of depression. Its continued expression complicates the treatment of depression, reduces remission rates, and increases the likelihood of relapse of depression. It is also important to note that sleep dysregulation is a frequent early sign of a manic episode. Restoring sleep will often help reduce manic symptoms.
- Circadian rhythm disturbances such as those seen in shift workers, blind individuals who lack a light-dark cycle to synchronize the body clock, adolescents and young adults with delayed sleep phase syndrome, and people with jet lag can mimic signs and symptoms of insomnia, especially initial and late insomnia. These disorders can be treated with therapies such as chronotherapy, bright light exposure, melatonin, or melatonin agonists. However, the timing of these interventions can be critical to outcome and constitutes therapies that are very different from standard medical and/or behavioral treatment for insomnia.

WORKUP

- History (with bed partner interview, if possible)
- Medication review (e.g., steroids, stimulants, even some antidepressants can disrupt sleep)
- Sleep diary for 1 to 2 wk (Consider the Consensus Sleep Diary [Carney CE et al in Suggested Readings])
- Wrist actigraphy detects gross limb movements and distinguish awake from sleep states. This can be used as an adjunct to self-reported sleep diary data (but not an alternative) and can provide further objective verification of the data reported.
- Validated sleep-quality rating scale (optional).
  1. Insomnia Severity Index
  2. Pittsburgh Sleep Quality Index
  3. Epworth Sleepiness Scale (see Daytime Sleepiness Test at www.sleepfoundation.org)

Other Diagnostic Tests: Evaluate for anemia (especially low ferritin level), uremia (for restless legs), thyroid function (if other signs present), blood glucose, and hemoglobin A1C measurements (for diabetes mellitus).

- Polysomnography (in home or in sleep laboratory) is not required for all cases of insomnia and should be reserved for patients whose history suggests specific sleep-related breathing or movement disorders. It is indicated for symptoms suggestive of daytime somnolence (obstructive sleep apnea, narcolepsy), nonrestorative sleep (periodic leg movements, chronic pain conditions), or sleep behavior suggesting parasomnia (somnambulism, REM sleep behavior).

IMAGING STUDIES

- Not generally helpful
- Brain CT or MRI for severe daytime sleepiness or acute onset

Rx TREATMENT

NONPHARMACOLOGIC THERAPY

- As a monotherapy, sleep hygiene measures (Box 1) may not be fully effective in cases of persistent insomnia. This noted, these simple lifestyle-modification measures should always be reviewed with the patient and used as first treatment modality. Additional treatment modalities (described next) can then be used to augment the effectiveness of sleep hygiene measures.
- Cognitive-behavioral therapy (CBT-I) has been shown to reduce time to fall asleep and time awake during the night, can reduce reliance on sleep medications, and has shown lasting effects after treatment has been discontinued. It should be the initial treatment option in persons with chronic insomnia. A recent study reported improved functional health and psychological well-being with digital CBT (dCBT). Therefore, digital formats may be good alternatives for individuals who cannot participate in one-on-one CBT-I.
- The standard components that comprise CBT-I are as follows:
  1. Stimulus control, which addresses the conditioned cues that create arousal when attempting to sleep by restricting bed activity to sleep and sex, and discouraging activities such as sleep effort, worrying, TV/screen engagement, reading while in bed. Reconditioning of this type can take several days or weeks; patients should be counseled not to expect immediate changes on the first few nights.
  2. Sleep restriction therapy reduces sleep opportunity to the average amount of total sleep time the patient is getting as determined by baseline sleep diary data. Sleep time is increased incrementally, based on improving sleep efficiency. Note that restricted time in bed should never be <5 hr. For the elderly and infirm, average total sleep time plus 30 min is sometimes considered. For patients whose estimated average total sleep time is <4 hr, a diagnosis of paradoxical insomnia should be considered and CBT-I would be contraindicated. Caution should also be exercised when using sleep restriction therapy in bipolar disorder and seizure disorders, as sleep deprivation early in treatment can precipitate a manic episode and lower seizure threshold, respectively.
  3. Cognitive therapy targets unhelpful beliefs and worries about sleep, negative and unwanted thoughts, sleep effort, selective attention bias and monitoring, misperception of sleep and daytime deficits, and counterproductive safety behaviors that are thought to maintain insomnia.
  4. Sleep hygiene is aimed at improving sleep habits (e.g., initiating or maintaining exercise, avoiding heavy meals at night, and altering the timing of or eliminating caffeine, nicotine, and alcohol intake). Environmental factors should

[1] American Psychiatric Association: *Diagnostic and statistical manual of mental disorders,* 5th ed, Arlington, VA, 2013, American Psychiatric Publishing.

also be addressed (e.g., limiting exposure to bright, especially blue, light in the evening; using white noise and/or light-attenuating measures in the bedroom). Caffeine sometimes can prove useful when used judiciously in the morning and early afternoon to combat the increased fatigue and somnolence that are produced early in therapy with sleep restriction and stimulus control. In addition, exercise contingently applied to daytime fatigue can also help to improve alertness during the day and increase sleep pressure at bedtime.

5. Relaxation exercises (e.g., progressive muscle relaxation, diaphragmatic breathing) may be good adjunctive therapy, especially in highly anxious patients, but are not thought to be essential in CBT-I. Increasingly, mindfulness-based practices are being effectively utilized alone and in combination with other elements of CBT-I. Mindfulness may help patients to adopt a more flexible and accepting stance toward insomnia.
6. Nonpharmacologic therapies for insomnia are summarized in Table 1.

TABLE 1 Nonpharmacologic Therapies for Insomnia

COGNITIVE-BEHAVIORAL THERAPY with or without relaxation therapy (Standard)
The combination of multiple modalities noted below
STIMULUS-CONTROL THERAPY (Standard)
Go to bed only when sleepy.
Use the bedroom only for sleeping and sex.
Go to another room when unable to sleep in 15 to 20 minutes, read or engage in other quiet activities, and return to bed only when sleepy; repeat if necessary.
Have a regular wake time regardless of the duration of sleep.
Avoid daytime napping.
SLEEP-RESTRICTION THERAPY (Guideline)
Reduce time in bed to the estimated total sleep time (minimum, 5 hr).
Increase time in bed by 15 minutes every week when the patient estimates the sleep efficiency is at least 85% (ratio of time asleep to time in bed).
RELAXATION THERAPY (Standard)
Physical component: Progressive muscle relaxation, autogenic training
Mental component: Reducing intrusive thoughts through imagery training, meditation, or hypnosis
PARADOXICAL INTENTION (Guideline for sleep-onset difficulties)
Instruct the patient to remain passively awake in bed and avoid any effort to fall asleep.
COGNITIVE THERAPY (Insufficient evidence as a single therapy)
Education to alter maladaptive or unrealistic beliefs and attitudes about sleep, such as that a minimum of 8 hours of sleep per night is required for health.
SLEEP HYGIENE EDUCATION (Insufficient evidence as a single therapy)
Correction of extrinsic factors and behaviors that affect sleep, such as environmental disruption (pets, music, or television); bedroom temperature; fixation on the bedside clock; use of alcohol, nicotine, or caffeine; lack of exercise or exercise too close to bedtime.

From Goldman L, Schafer AI: *Goldman-Cecil medicine*, ed 26, Philadelphia, 2020, Elsevier.

ACUTE GENERAL Rx

- Nonbenzodiazepine benzodiazepine receptor agonists: Zolpidem 5 mg and zaleplon 5 mg for sleep-onset insomnia, and zolpidem continuous-release formulation 6.25 to 12.5 mg and eszopiclone 1 to 3 mg for maintenance insomnia
- Suvorexant is an orexin receptor antagonist FDA approved for insomnia. Signaling of orexin neuropeptides sustains wakefulness. Suvorexant promotes sleep by blocking orexin neuropeptides from binding to their receptors. The initial dose is 10 mg once daily within 30 min of bedtime. Most common side effect (10%) is next-day somnolence.
- Benzodiazepine sedative-hypnotics (e.g., temazepam 7.5-30 mg, triazolam 0.125-0.25 mg). Benzodiazepines should not be used to treat insomnia in older adults due to the increased risk of adverse effects. Benzodiazepines carry a risk of dependence and can be misused. Accordingly, alternatives should always be considered, especially in patients requiring long-term treatment for insomnia. Abrupt discontinuation following protracted treatment with benzodiazepines can be associated with a potentially life-threatening withdrawal and should be avoided whenever possible.
- A low-dose formulation (6 mg) of the tricyclic antidepressant doxepin is also FDA approved for treatment of insomnia associated with sleep maintenance. This dose retains the hypnotic effect of doxepin without the typical tricyclic effects. A generic 10 mg/ml liquid formulation of doxepin is also available. Often tricyclic antidepressants may have adverse cardiovascular effects and thus should be considered with some caution in the elderly and patients with significant cardiovascular illness.
- Atypical neuroleptics, including quetiapine (PO, 12.5-50 mg) and olanzapine (PO/IM/SL, 2.5-5 mg) can be utilized in hospitalized patients, including those in the critical care setting. While less sedating than aforementioned options, haloperidol (IV, 0.5-5 mg) can be used if an intravenous alternative is considered. Benzodiazepines should be avoided whenever possible given risks of propagating delirium. If antipsychotics are utilized, closely monitor QTc given the risk for QTc prolongation with most drugs in the class. Lower doses of the medication should be used in the elderly and in patients deemed to be at higher risk for potential side-effects/complications.
- Melatonin agonist ramelteon 8 mg for sleep-onset insomnia when a mild agent without benzodiazepine side effects is desired.
- Avoid antihistamines except for occasional use.
- Optimize treatment of medical symptoms, especially pain.
- Most prescription and over-the-counter medications carry significant risk of adverse events and drug interactions, especially in the geriatric patient.
- Medications for insomnia are summarized in Table 2.

CHRONIC Rx

- Considerable research supports the efficacy of CBT-I, with acute treatment outcomes equivalent to pharmacotherapy, and better long-term outcomes and maintenance of treatment gains. Although there is limited availability of CBT-I specialists, especially in certain geographic areas, there are now online interactive evidence-based self-help programs that can serve as an effective base for a stepped model of care. Patients who fail these attempts should still be encouraged to seek more tailored treatment with a specialist, especially when the insomnia is comorbid with other conditions.
- When CBT-I is applied to patients with related comorbidities (e.g., depression, chronic pain), evidence suggests that targeted treatment for insomnia not only results in significant improvement of the insomnia but, in many cases, influences the course of the related comorbidities. For example, when CBT-I is applied concurrently with antidepressants, it has the effect of doubling remission rates in depression and reduces suicidal ideation by up to 65%. In a recent study of patients with comorbid depression and insomnia, head-to-head comparison of Internet-based treatments for depression (dCBT-D) and insomnia (dCBT-I) demonstrated that dCBT-I outperformed dCBT-D for insomnia and matched its efficacy in depression.
- Note that the American College of Physicians clinical guidelines for the management of chronic insomnia disorder suggest CBT-I as the first-line treatment for insomnia and recommending that it be attempted before pharmacologic approaches when possible.
- Three sedative-hypnotics—zolpidem continuous release, eszopiclone, and ramelteon—are FDA approved for long-term use.
- Sedating antidepressants (e.g., trazodone 25-150 mg, mirtazapine 7.5-30 mg, amitriptyline 25-50 mg, doxepin 10 mg) are in widespread use, with limited data on safety and efficacy. Amitriptyline should be avoided in older adults.
- Sedating antipsychotics (e.g., quetiapine 25-200 mg, olanzapine 2.5-10 mg at night)

TABLE 2 Medications for Insomnia

Name	Dose	Time of Dose	FDA Indication	Common Side Effects	Half-Life	Mechanism
Zolpidem SL	1.75-10 mg	Bedtime	Yes	Sleepiness, amnesia, falls, parasomnias	1-2 hr	Benzodiazepine receptor agonist (BZRA)
Zolpidem reg	5-10 mg	Bedtime	Yes	Sleepiness amnesia, falls, parasomnias	1-2 hr	BZRA
Zolpidem CR	6.25-12.5 mg	Bedtime	Yes	Sleepiness, amnesia, falls	1-2 hr but continued release	BZRA
Temazepam	7.5-30 mg	Bedtime	Yes	Sleepiness, dizziness	8-10 hr	Benzodiazepine
Zaleplon	5-20 mg	Bedtime	Yes	Sleepiness, dizziness, parasomnias	1 hr	BZRA
Eszopiclone	1-3 mg	Bedtime	Yes	Sleepiness, dizziness	4-8 hr	BZRA
Doxepin	3-6 mg	Bedtime	Yes	Drowsiness, dizziness, nausea	17 hr	Histamine receptor antagonist
Mirtazapine	7.5-15 mg	Bedtime	No	Drowsiness, dizziness, weight gain	20 hr	Histamine receptor antagonist
Ramelteon	4-8 mg	Bedtime	Yes	Sleepiness, headache	1-2 hr	Melatonin receptor agonist
Subvorexant	10-20 mg	Bedtime	Yes	Sleepiness	12 hr	Blocks orexin

CR, Controlled-release; *FDA*, U.S. Food and Drug Administration; *SL*, sublingual.
From Goldman L, Schafer AI: *Goldman-Cecil medicine*, ed 26, Philadelphia, 2020, Elsevier.

can be considered for patients with comorbid mood, anxiety, or thought disorders given adjunct potential for mood stabilization.

COMPLEMENTARY & ALTERNATIVE MEDICINE

- Melatonin 3 to 5 mg has been used for delayed phase insomnia with shortening of sleep initiation time but no real change in sleep efficiency. There can be side effects, especially at higher doses. Melatonin may shorten sleep-onset latency in some individuals. It may have more clinical utility in the management of circadian rhythm disorders. Timing of administration in these types of cases requires careful consideration and would not be often administered at bedtime.
- Cannabinoids: Tetrahydrocannabinol (THC) and cannabidiol (CBD) have been the two main phytocannabinoids recognized as potential regulators of the circadian rhythm. A recent systematic review highlighted the lack of clinical and preclinical evidence supporting cannabinoid-based therapies to treat sleep disorders. Therefore, THC and CBD's efficacy and safety for the treatment of sleep disorders is still unknown.

DISPOSITION

- Transient (acute) insomnia: Usually self-limited. May require follow-up if stress-related or illness-related because of risk of depression or persistence. Prophylactic education regarding maladaptive sleep practices such as extending time in bed, and/or remaining in bed when unable to sleep, might be helpful in avoiding a more protracted course of insomnia.
- Persistent insomnia: Patients who respond well to CBT-I often continue to maintain gains at 1- and 2-yr follow-ups. Patients may need periodic follow-up to reinforce good sleep hygiene and stimulus control and for reevaluation of pharmacologic therapies. There is now a compelling amount of evidence that insomnia, if left untreated, is associated with significant negative mental and health effects over time.

REFERRAL

- A referral to a behavioral medicine specialist may be required for CBT-I or for circadian rhythm disturbances (find a directory at https://www.behavioralsleep.org)
- Excessive daytime sleepiness not obviously caused by insomnia (e.g., narcolepsy, sleep-related breathing disorder)
- Nighttime behavior suggestive of a parasomnia (e.g., somnambulism, REM behavior disorder)
- Severe insomnia not responsive to basic interventions

PEARLS & CONSIDERATIONS

COMMENTS

- CBT-I often results in worse sleep and more fatigue in the short run. Patients often respond to initial worsening of symptoms as a sign of failure; however, they should be encouraged to see this as an important piece of the therapy and to stay the course as new conditioned patterns begin to emerge, sleep efficiency improves, and total sleep time gradually increases.
- Patients should avoid compensating for lost sleep by extending sleep opportunity in the form of going to bed early, sleeping in, or napping. Therefore, early treatment should focus on helping patients to manage daytime fatigue and sleepiness by engaging in activities that help patients stay awake and maintain set bed and wake times.

PREVENTION

It is estimated that 50% to 70% of individuals demonstrating the syndrome of insomnia (e.g., insomnia symptoms more than 3 days per wk for a mo along with deleterious daytime sequelae) are still syndromic 1 to 5 yr later. Therefore, early intervention with medication or education to prevent the development of maladaptive compensatory behaviors (e.g., napping, sleeping late, tossing and turning in bed, avoiding or decreasing daytime activity) may help to reduce the risk of developing persistent insomnia.

PATIENT & FAMILY EDUCATION

The National Sleep Foundation (www.sleepfoundation.org) is a comprehensive resource for health care providers and patients.

SUGGESTED READINGS

Available at ExpertConsult.com

RELATED CONTENT

Fatigue, Chronic (Differential Diagnosis in Section II)
Insomnia (Patient Information)

AUTHORS: **Perla M. Romero Gómez, MD, Mladen Nisavic, MD,** and **John Denninger, MD, PhD**

BASIC INFORMATION

DEFINITION

Interstitial lung disease (ILD) is a heterogenous group of disorders, characterized by varying patterns of lung inflammation and fibrosis. The term "ILD" arises from the histological appearance that the interstitium is abnormal, alhough the alveoli, airways, blood vessels, lymphatic vessels, and pleura are often altered as well. ILDs are classified as either arising from an identified cause or idiopathic. A clinical classification of the interstitial lung diseases is summarized in Table 1.

SYNONYMS

Interstitial pulmonary disease
ILD
Diffuse parenchymal lung disease (DPLD)
Interstitial pneumonia
Pulmonary fibrosis

ICD-10CM CODES

J84.17	Other interstitial pulmonary diseases with fibrosis in diseases classified elsewhere
J84.89	Other specified interstitial pulmonary diseases
J84.9	Interstitial pulmonary disease, unspecified
J84.115	Respiratory bronchiolitis interstitial lung disease
J84.848	Other interstitial lung diseases of childhood

EPIDEMIOLOGY & DEMOGRAPHICS

INCIDENCE AND PREVALENCE: Varies widely with type of ILD. The most common ILDs are sarcoidosis, cryptogenic organizing pneumonia, and idiopathic pulmonary fibrosis. The prevalence of these syndromes varies widely across different populations as defined by age, gender, and race. The overall prevalence of ILD is estimated to be up to 76.0 cases per 100,000 people in Europe and 74.3 cases per 100,000 in the U.S.[1]

PREDOMINANT SEX & AGE: Some ILDs are more common in women, such as those resulting from autoimmune diseases, also known as connective tissue disorders. Lymphangioleiomyomatosis (LAM) occurs exclusively in premenopausal women. ILD caused by occupational exposures are more common in men. Most ILDs occur in people >50 yr; however, sarcoidosis most often presents in younger populations.

RISK FACTORS: Common identifiable risk factors include environmental exposures such as down, mold, silicone, asbestos; reactions to drugs such as chemotherapeutic agents, tyrosine kinase inhibitors, amiodarone, and nitrofurantoin; radiation therapy; connective tissue disease including rheumatoid arthritis, scleroderma, and myositis; and pathologic acid reflux. Both tobacco and drug use can cause ILD. Some individuals have increased genetic susceptibility to developing ILD from impaired cellular repair mechanisms, such as telomere shortening.

[1]Wijsenbeek M, Cottin V: Spectrum of fibrotic lung diseases, *N Engl J Med* 383:(10):958-968, 2020.

TABLE 1 Clinical Classification of the Interstitial Lung Diseases

Connective Tissue Diseases
Scleroderma
Polymyositis-dermatomyositis
Systemic lupus erythematosus
Rheumatoid arthritis
Mixed connective tissue disease
Ankylosing spondylitis
Treatment-Related or Drug-Induced Diseases
Antibiotics (nitrofurantoin, sulfasalazine)
Antiarrhythmics (amiodarone, tocainide, propranolol)
Antiinflammatories (gold, penicillamine)
Anticonvulsants (Dilantin)
Chemotherapeutic agents (mitomycin C, bleomycin, busulfan, cyclophosphamide, chlorambucil, methotrexate, azathioprine, BCNU [carmustine], procarbazine)
Therapeutic radiation
Oxygen toxicity
Narcotics
Primary and Idiopathic Diseases
Sarcoidosis
Primary pulmonary Langerhans cell histiocytosis (eosinophilic granuloma)
Amyloidosis
Pulmonary vasculitis
Gaucher disease
Niemann-Pick disease
Hermansky-Pudlak syndrome
Neurofibromatosis
Lymphangioleiomyomatosis
Tuberous sclerosis
Idiopathic pulmonary fibrosis
Nonspecific interstitial pneumonia
Cryptogenic organizing pneumonia
Respiratory bronchiolitis ILD or desquamative interstitial pneumonia
Acute interstitial pneumonia
Lymphocytic interstitial pneumonia
Pleuroparenchymal fibroelastosis
Bone marrow transplantation
Eosinophilic pneumonia
Alveolar proteinosis
Alveolar microlithiasis
Metastatic calcification
Occupational and Environmental Diseases
Inorganic
Silicosis
Asbestosis
Hard-metal pneumoconiosis
Coal worker's pneumoconiosis
Berylliosis
Talc pneumoconiosis
Siderosis (arc welder)
Stannosis (tin)
Organic (hypersensitivity pneumonitis)
Bird breeder's lung
Farmer's lung

ILD, Interstitial lung disease.
Modified from Mason RJ: *Murray & Nadel's textbook of respiratory medicine*, ed 5, Philadelphia, 2010, Saunders.

PHYSICAL FINDINGS & CLINICAL PRESENTATION

- Shortness of breath (especially with exertion)
- Cough (dry)
- Tachypnea
- Bibasilar end-inspiratory dry crackles
- Pulmonary hypertension
- Cyanosis
- Clubbing

Hallmarks of ILD include restriction of lung volumes and reduced diffusing capacity demonstrated by pulmonary function tests. The restrictive process can result from different abnormalities depending on the type of ILD including acute and subacute inflammatory changes, which are potentially reversible, and fibrosis, which is largely irreversible. Diffusion abnormalities can result from loss of functional capillaries from fibrosis, emphysema, or pulmonary hypertension.

- Specific changes may be seen:
  1. Granulomatous: Accumulation of T lymphocytes, macrophages, and epithelioid cells into granulomas in lung parenchyma
  2. Inflammation and fibrosis: Injury to epithelium causes inflammation; if chronic, inflammation spreads to interstitium and vascular areas

ETIOLOGY

The lungs are constantly exposed to potentially noxious stimuli from environmental and occupational exposures, smoking, drugs, radiation, autoimmune disease, pathologic acid reflux, etc. Lung injury leads to regeneration, repair, or remodeling responses that can result in restoration of normal tissue, inflammation, or fibrosis. Alveolar epithelial damage from repeated injuries promotes migration of inflammatory cells into the lungs. If regeneration or repair of the epithelium fails, remodeling occurs. A fibrotic milieu promotes proliferation of fibroblasts and collagen deposition.

Dx DIAGNOSIS

DIFFERENTIAL DIAGNOSIS

- Heart failure
- Pneumonia: Viral, bacterial, mycobacterial, fungal, and pneumocystis
- Pulmonary embolism
- COPD
- Pulmonary hypertension
- Vasculitis
- Metastatic malignancy manifesting as lymphangitic carcinomatosis

WORKUP

- Establishing a confident ILD diagnosis, as well as the type of ILD, which has treatment and prognostic implications, requires identifying clinical, radiographic, and histologic patterns of lung injury. Multidisciplinary discussion (MDD), which is considered the standard of care to diagnose ILD, includes a pulmonologist, radiologist, and pathologist. Detailed exposure history, exam findings, pulmonary function tests (PFT), laboratory tests, and high-resolution computed tomography (HRCT) scan of the chest are reviewed. If a confident diagnosis remains unclear, surgical lung biopsy should be considered and then reviewed in MDD. Fig. 1 illustrates the approach to ILD diagnosis.

- Pulmonary function tests (PFTs) show restriction, characterized by decreased total lung capacity (TLC) and forced vital capacity (FVC) due to reduced lung compliance caused by alveolar wall thickening or filling of alveolar spaces as a result of inflammation and fibrosis. Inflammation, fibrosis, emphysema, and pulmonary vascular alterations can lead to impaired gas exchange, measured by the diffusing capacity of carbon monoxide (DLCO). FEV_1/FVC is usually normal or increased because lung stiffness keeps small airways open, although some conditions (e.g., sarcoidosis, hypersensitivity pneumonitis) may result in air trapping.
- Bronchoscopy with bronchoalveolar lavage (BAL) can show increased lymphocytes in chronic hypersensitivity pneumonitis and sarcoidosis, increased eosinophils in eosinophilic pneumonia, and can exclude infection.
- Transbronchial biopsy is of limited utility. Criobiopsy may yield sufficient tissue when done by experienced operators. Surgical lung biopsy provides sufficient tissue for diagnosis in >90% of cases. Histologic patterns of lung injury and their ILD associations are summarized in Table 2.

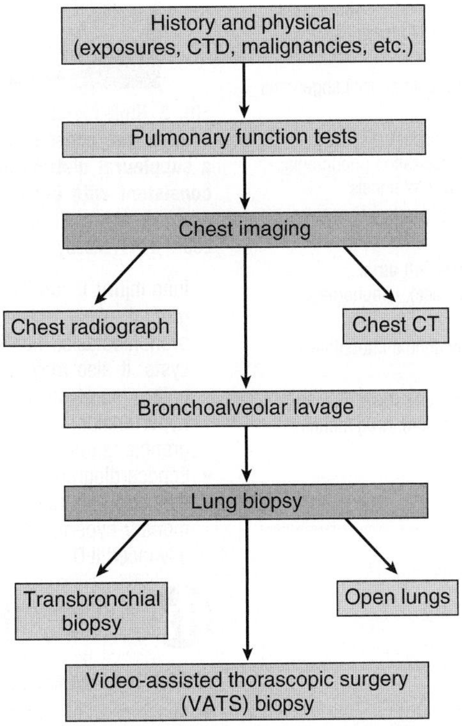

FIG. 1 Algorithm for the approach to a patient with interstitial lung disease. *CT,* computed tomography; *CTD,* connective tissue disease. (From Sellke FW et al: *Sabiston & Spencer surgery of the chest,* ed 9, Philadelphia, 2016, Elsevier.)

LABORATORY TESTS

- ABGs may be normal or show respiratory alkalosis and widened Aa gradient.
- Serologic tests can identify autoimmune features and connective tissue diseases: Antinuclear antibodies, rheumatoid factor, anti-cyclic citrullinated peptide, SS-A, SS-B, Scl-70, RNA pol III, RNP, myositis panel, creatinine kinase, aldolase. Antineutrophil cytoplasmic antibodies or antibasement membrane antibodies should be obtained if vasculitis is suspected.
- Serum precipitins are of limited utility to investigate exposures associated with hypersensitivity pneumonitis.

TABLE 2 Histologic Patterns in the Interstitial Lung Diseases and Their Disease Associations

Histologic Patterns	Clinical Associations
Usual interstitial pneumonia	Idiopathic pulmonary fibrosis; connective tissue diseases (uncommon); asbestosis; chronic hypersensitivity pneumonitis; chronic aspiration pneumonia; chronic radiation pneumonitis; Hermansky-Pudlak syndrome
Nonspecific interstitial pneumonia	Idiopathic; connective tissue diseases; drugs; AIDS
Diffuse alveolar damage	Acute interstitial pneumonia (Hamman-Rich syndrome); acute respiratory distress syndrome (ARDS); drugs (cytotoxic agents, heroin, paraquat, ethchlorvynol, aspirin); toxic gas inhalation; radiation therapy; oxygen toxicity; connective tissue disease; infections
Organizing pneumonia	Cryptogenic organizing pneumonia; organizing stage of diffuse alveolar damage; drugs (amiodarone, cocaine); infections; connective tissue diseases
Desquamative interstitial pneumonia/ respiratory bronchiolitis	Cigarette smoking; idiopathic DIP of childhood
Lymphocytic interstitial pneumonia	Idiopathic; hypogammaglobulinemia; autoimmune diseases, including Hashimoto thyroiditis, lupus erythematosus, primary biliary cirrhosis, Sjögren syndrome, myasthenia gravis, chronic active hepatitis; AIDS; allogeneic bone marrow transplantation
Eosinophilic pneumonia	Idiopathic acute and chronic; tropical filarial eosinophilia; parasitic infections; allergic bronchopulmonary aspergillosis; allergic granulomatosis of Churg and Strauss; hypereosinophilic syndrome; AIDS
Alveolar proteinosis	Pulmonary alveolar proteinosis; acute silicosis; aluminum dust; AIDS; myeloproliferative disorder
Diffuse alveolar hemorrhage	
with capillaritis	Wegener granulomatosis; microscopic polyangiitis; systemic lupus erythematosus; polymyositis; scleroderma; rheumatoid arthritis; mixed connective tissue disease; lung transplantation; drugs (retinoic acid, propylthiouracil, Dilantin); Behçet disease; cryoglobulinemia; Henoch-Schönlein purpura; pauci-immune glomerulonephritis; immune complex glomerulonephritis
without capillaritis	Idiopathic pulmonary hemosiderosis; systemic lupus erythematosus; Goodpasture syndrome; diffuse alveolar damage; pulmonary venoocclusive disease; mitral stenosis; lymphangioleiomyomatosis
Amyloid deposition	Primary amyloidosis; multiple myeloma; lymphocytic interstitial pneumonia
Granuloma	Sarcoidosis; hypersensitivity pneumonitis; pulmonary Langerhans cell histiocytosis; silicosis; intravenous talcosis; berylliosis; lymphocytic interstitial pneumonia; infections

AIDS, Acquired immunodeficiency syndrome; *DIP,* desquamative interstitial pneumonia.
Modified from Mason RJ: *Murray & Nadel's textbook of respiratory medicine,* ed 5, Philadelphia, 2010, Saunders.

TABLE 3 Radiographic Features of the Interstitial Lung Diseases

Feature	Diseases
Upper zone–predominant disease	Radiation pneumonitis; neurofibromatosis; chronic sarcoidosis; pulmonary Langerhans cell histiocytosis; silicosis; chronic hypersensitivity pneumonitis; chronic eosinophilic pneumonia; ankylosing spondylitis; nodular rheumatoid arthritis; berylliosis; drug induced (amiodarone, gold, BCNU [carmustine]); radiation
Increased lung volumes	Lymphangioleiomyomatosis; chronic sarcoidosis; chronic pulmonary Langerhans cell histiocytosis; tuberous sclerosis; neurofibromatosis
Radiographic honeycomb lung	Idiopathic pulmonary fibrosis; connective tissue disease; asbestosis; drug induced; lymphocytic interstitial pneumonia; chronic aspiration pneumonia; hemosiderosis; Hermansky-Pudlak syndrome; alveolar proteinosis
Pneumothorax	Pulmonary Langerhans cell histiocytosis; lymphangioleiomyomatosis; tuberous sclerosis; neurofibromatosis, IPF
Kerley B lines	Lymphangitic carcinomatosis; lymphangioleiomyomatosis; left atrial hypertension (mitral valve disease, venoocclusive disease); lymphoma; amyloidosis
Lymphadenopathy	Sarcoidosis; lymphoma; lymphangitic carcinomatosis; lymphoid interstitial pneumonia; berylliosis; amyloidosis; Gaucher disease
Pleural disease	Lymphangitic carcinomatosis; connective tissue disease; asbestosis (pleural calcification); lymphangioleiomyomatosis (chylous effusion); drug induced (nitrofurantoin, radiation); sarcoidosis
Eggshell calcification of lymph nodes	Silicosis; sarcoidosis; radiation

IPF, Idiopathic pulmonary fibrosis.
From Mason RJ: *Murray & Nadel's textbook of respiratory medicine,* ed 5, Philadelphia, 2010, Saunders.

TABLE 4 Laboratory Findings in the Interstitial Lung Diseases

Finding	Diseases
Leukopenia	Sarcoidosis; connective tissue disease; lymphoma; drug induced
Leukocytosis	Systemic vasculitis; hypersensitivity pneumonitis; lymphoma
Eosinophilia	Eosinophilic pneumonia; sarcoidosis; systemic vasculitis; drug induced (sulfa, methotrexate)
Thrombocytopenia	Sarcoidosis; connective tissue disease; drug induced; Gaucher disease; idiopathic pulmonary fibrosis
Hemolytic anemia	Connective tissue disease; sarcoidosis; lymphoma; drug induced; idiopathic pulmonary fibrosis
Normocytic anemia	Diffuse alveolar hemorrhage syndromes; connective tissue disease; lymphangitic carcinomatosis
Urinary sediment abnormalities	Connective tissue disease; systemic vasculitis; drug induced
Hypogammaglobulinemia	Lymphocytic interstitial pneumonia
Hypergammaglobulinemia	Connective tissue disease; sarcoidosis; systemic vasculitis; idiopathic pulmonary fibrosis; asbestosis; silicosis; lymphocytic interstitial pneumonia; lymphoma
Serum autoantibodies	Rheumatoid arthritis, scleroderma, inflammatory myopathies (dermatomyositis, polymyositis, immune-mediated necrotizing myopathy), mixed connective tissue disease, Sjogren syndrome, systemic lupus erythematosus.
Serum immune complexes	Idiopathic pulmonary fibrosis; lymphocytic interstitial pneumonia; systemic vasculitis; connective tissue disease; pulmonary Langerhans cell histiocytosis
Serum angiotensin-converting enzyme	Sarcoidosis; hypersensitivity pneumonitis; silicosis; acute respiratory distress syndrome; Gaucher disease
Antibasement membrane antibody	Goodpasture syndrome
Antineutrophil cytoplasmic antibody	Systemic vasculitis

Adapted from Mason RJ: *Murray & Nadel's textbook of respiratory medicine,* ed 5, Philadelphia, 2010, Saunders.

- Angiotensin-converting enzyme testing (ACE levels) in sarcoidosis is of unclear value.
- Laboratory findings in the interstitial lung diseases are summarized in Table 3.

IMAGING STUDIES

- Chest x-ray may appear normal or show opacities, often in a reticular pattern.
- High-resolution CT (HRCT) (Fig. 2) is necessary to evaluate the radiographic pattern of lung injury. It can demonstrate consolidation, ground glass opacity, reticulation, traction bronchiectasis, fibrosis, air trapping, and cysts. It also may identify pulmonary artery enlargement in patients with pulmonary hypertension. Table 4 summarizes radiographic features of ILDs.
- Echocardiography is useful to evaluate cardiac size and function, and to screen for pulmonary hypertension, which can complicate advanced ILD.

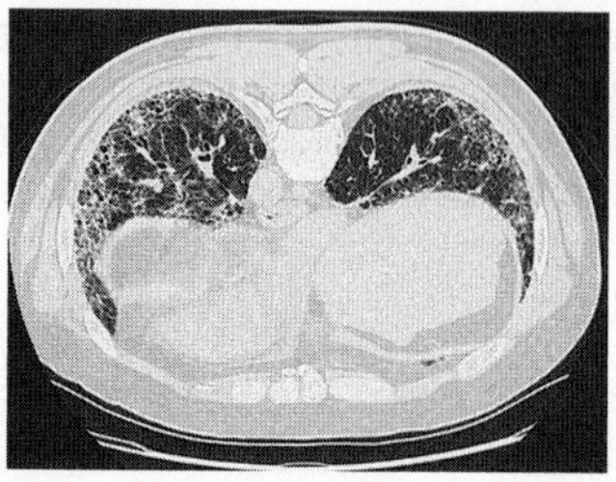

FIG. 2 High-resolution computed tomography scan of the chest shows fibrotic changes in a subpleural distribution with honeycombing consistent with usual interstitial pneumonia. (From Hochberg MC et al: *Rheumatology,* ed 5, St Louis, 2011, Mosby.)

Rx TREATMENT

NONPHARMACOLOGIC THERAPY

- Avoidance of tobacco and occupational exposures
- The mainstay of therapy is to identify the cause of the lung injury and completely avoid it, e.g., discontinue offending drugs or remove environmental exposures. Avoidance alone may be sufficient to reverse acute and subacute inflammation.

ACUTE GENERAL Rx

- Pharmacologic treatment varies significantly depending on the type of ILD, thus it is essential to try to correctly classify the type of ILD. Steroids and immunosuppression should be avoided in idiopathic pulmonary fibrosis; however, they are an important part of the treatment regimen for patients with hypersensitivity pneumonitis. Please see specific chapters on Asbestosis, Cryptogenic Organizing Pneumonia, Eosinophilic Granulomatosis with Polyangiitis, Eosinophilic Pneumonia, Hypersensitivity Pneumonitis, and Idiopathic Pulmonary Fibrosis that discuss specific treatment regimens.
- For patients with acute or subacute inflammation demonstrated by consolidation or ground glass opacity in HRCT, immunosuppression with steroids or steroid-sparing agents, such as mofetil mycophenolate and azathioprine, could expedite improvement. While steroids often cause rapid improvement, their multiple side effects may limit their prolonged use. Patients should be closely monitored with PFT to assess the ILD trajectory. If there is improvement or stabilization after 4 to 12 wk of steroids, the dose should be tapered. If the patient's condition

declines as steroids are weaned, starting mofetil mycophenolate or azathioprine for maintenance may allow steroid tapering. If patients are at high risk for steroid-induced side effects, mofetil mycophenolate or azathioprine monotherapy could be considered from the beginning.

- For patients with scleroderma-associated ILD and those with other progressive fibrosing ILDs, nintedanib added to immunosuppression or monotherapy should be considered. Nintedanib is a tyrosine kinase inhibitor with antifibrotic and antiinflammatory properties that lower the annual rate of decline in FVC in patients using nintedanib rather than placebo.

CHRONIC GENERAL Rx

- Supplemental oxygen in patients with hypoxemia is beneficial to support physical activity and prevent development of pulmonary hypertension. Patients with interstitial disease should receive long-term oxygen therapy (LTOT) for severe resting hypoxemia and ambulatory oxygen for severe exertional desaturation.[2]
- Outpatient pulmonary rehabilitation may be of value.
- Lung transplantation should be considered in appropriate patients in severe stages of the disease.

DISPOSITION

The prognosis is highly variable and depends on the cause, severity of illness, and initial response to treatment.

REFERRAL

- Pulmonary referral for workup and management
- Surgical referral for biopsy
- Referral for lung transplant evaluation

PEARLS & CONSIDERATIONS

COMMENTS

It is very important when working up an ILD to take a thorough history of tobacco and drug use, prior medications, workplace and environmental exposures, and pets, as well as a review of systems, including signs and symptoms that might suggest an underlying connective tissue disease.

PREVENTION

Proper industrial hygiene from a respiratory perspective is important as well as close surveillance when patients are given medications with known pulmonary toxicity. Symptoms of an ILD in the setting of an autoimmune condition need to be evaluated thoroughly.

SUGGESTED READINGS

Available at ExpertConsult.com

RELATED CONTENT

Asbestosis (Related Key Topic)
Cryptogenic Organizing Pneumonia (Related Key Topic)
Eosinophilic Granulomatosis with Polyangiitis (Related Key Topic)
Eosinophilic Pneumonia (Related Key Topic)
Hypersensitivity Pneumonitis (Related Key Topic)
Idiopathic Pulmonary Fibrosis (Related Key Topic)
Interstitial Pulmonary Disease (Patient Information)
Sarcoidosis (Related Key Topic)

AUTHOR: **Aida Venado, MD, MAS**

[2] Jacobs SS et al: Home oxygen therapy for adults with chronic lung disease. An official American Thoracic Society clinical practice guideline, *Am J Respir Crit Care Med* Nov: 202:e121-e141, 2020.

BASIC INFORMATION

DEFINITION

Classified into two broad categories:
1. Acute interstitial nephritis (AIN):
   a. Decrease in kidney function resulting from delayed hypersensitivity immune-mediated injury; most often drug-induced
   b. Characterized on kidney biopsy by edema and leukocyte infiltration of the renal interstitium and tubules *(tubulitis),* which classically spares glomeruli and blood vessels
2. Chronic interstitial nephritis:
   a. Final common pathway of many chronic kidney diseases (CKD) including diabetic kidney disease, hypertensive kidney disease, unresolved AIN, chronic obstruction, high-grade vesicoureteral reflux, and chronic bacterial infections
   b. Characterized on renal biopsy by interstitial fibrosis with mononuclear leukocyte infiltration and tubular atrophy

SYNONYMS

Acute tubulo-interstitial nephritis
Contracted kidney
Cirrhosis of the kidney
Granular kidney
Renal sclerosis

ICD-10CM CODES	
N05.8	Unspecified nephritic syndrome with other morphologic changes
N05.9	Unspecified nephritic syndrome with unspecified morphologic changes
N10	Acute tubulo-interstitial nephritis
N11	Chronic tubulo-interstitial nephritis
N11.8	Other chronic tubulo-interstitial nephritis
N11.9	Chronic tubulo-interstitial nephritis, unspecified
N12	Tubulo-interstitial nephritis, not specified as acute or chronic
N14	Drug- and heavy metal-induced tubulo-interstitial and tubular conditions
N15	Other renal tubulo-interstitial diseases
N16	Renal tubulo-interstitial disorders in diseases classified elsewhere
N17.8	Other acute kidney failure

EPIDEMIOLOGY & DEMOGRAPHICS

PREVALENCE:
- Prevalence is significantly underestimated.
- AIN is found in 0.5% to 2.6% of all kidney biopsies but prevalence may be as high as 12.9% to 18.6% in patients biopsied for acute kidney injury (AKI) of unknown etiology.

DEMOGRAPHICS:
- Increased incidence in elderly, attributed to reduced glomerular filtration rate (GFR), immune-mediated dysfunction, increasing medication use, and comorbidities.
- Median age at presentation is 65 yr.

RISK FACTORS:
- Advanced age (>65 yr)
- Volume depletion
- Underlying kidney disease
- Congestive heart failure
- Diabetes
- HIV infection

PHYSICAL FINDINGS & CLINICAL PRESENTATION

SIGNS AND SYMPTOMS:
- For AIN, the most common presentation is an asymptomatic elevation of serum creatinine and blood urea nitrogen (BUN) levels. When advanced, AIN is associated with nonspecific symptoms of AKI from any cause:
  1. Malaise
  2. Anorexia
  3. Nausea and vomiting
  4. Oliguria or polyuria
  5. Hematuria
  6. Flank pain
- Classic triad (fever, maculopapular rash, and eosinophilia) is present in only 5% of cases:
  1. If present, the rash is usually a truncal maculopapular morbilliform eruption.
  2. Triad is characteristic of methicillin-related AIN; this antibiotic has not been prescribed in the U.S. for 4 decades.
- A small minority present with tubulo-interstitial nephritis and uveitis (TINU) syndrome. The uveitis may be symptomatic or subclinical and may develop before, during, or after kidney injury. Adolescent females are most often affected by TINU.
- For chronic interstitial nephritis, there may be a subacute to protracted rise in serum creatinine without obvious symptomatology that is classified as unspecified CKD.

ETIOLOGY

ACUTE INTERSTITIAL NEPHRITIS:
- **Drug-induced:** Accounts for 70% of cases, and more than 150 agents have been implicated. AKI usually develops 10 to 14 days after exposure to the drug, but may develop earlier when there has been prior drug exposure.
  1. Antibiotics (beta-lactams, sulfonamides, rifampin, fluoroquinolones)
  2. Nonsteroidal antiinflammatory drugs (NSAIDs), including selective cyclo-oxygenase-2 (COX-2) inhibitors
  3. Proton pump inhibitors and H_2 blockers (primarily, cimetidine)
  4. Loop diuretics (furosemide, bumetanide) and thiazide diuretics
  5. Antineoplastic agents
  6. Anticonvulsants
  7. Allopurinol (particularly common cause of drug rash or reaction with eosinophilia and systemic symptoms [DRESS] with AIN)
  8. Immunotherapy with checkpoint pathway inhibitors
  9. 5-aminosalicylates (mesalamine)
- **Infection** (10% to 15%): Systemic or localized to genitourinary system.
  1. Bacteria: *Streptococci, Corynebacterium diphtheria, Legionellae, Yersinia, Mycobacteria, Mycoplasma, Rickettsia, E. coli*
  2. Viruses: *Cytomegalovirus, Epstein–Barr virus, Orthohantavirus,* Hepatitis C Virus, Herpes Simplex Virus-1 and -2, Human Immunodeficiency Virus-1, *Rubulavirus* (mumps), Human Polyomavirus-1 (BK) and -2 (JC), Influenza A Virus
  3. Other: *Treponema pallidum, Toxoplasma gondii, Babesia* species
- **Other Causes** (15% to 20%):
  1. Idiopathic (10%)
  2. Immune disorders: Systemic lupus erythematosus, Sjögren syndrome, small-vessel vasculitides, autoimmune pancreatitis
  3. Neoplastic disorders (multiple myeloma)
  4. DRESS syndrome
  5. IgG4-related disease
  6. Hypocomplementemic tubulointerstitial nephritis

CHRONIC INTERSTITIAL NEPHRITIS:
- Metabolic diseases (urate nephropathy, hypercalcemic nephropathy, hypokalemic nephropathy, oxalate nephropathy)
- Sarcoidosis
- Heavy metals
- Chronic urinary tract obstruction
- Aristolochic acid
- Diabetic kidney disease
- Hypertensive kidney disease
- Chronic pyelonephritis
- Drugs: Indinavir, cisplatin, tacrolimus, cyclosporine, lithium

OVERLAP OF ACUTE AND CHRONIC INTERSTITIAL NEPHRITIS: Some metabolic processes and autoimmune disorders can present either as acute or chronic interstitial nephritis. For example, oxalate nephropathy can present as acute interstitial nephropathy in the setting of ethylene glycol ingestion or chronic interstitial nephritis in cases of bariatric surgery and high oxalate-containing diet.

Dx DIAGNOSIS

DIFFERENTIAL DIAGNOSIS

Other causes of AKI or CKD, including acute tubular necrosis, atheroembolic disease, glomerulonephritis, hypertensive nephrosclerosis, prerenal azotemia, obstructive nephropathy, and renal vascular disease

WORKUP

- Diagnosis is typically recognized by the temporal relationship between onset and resolution of AKI with use and discontinuation of a known culprit drug.
- Gold standard for diagnosis is kidney biopsy. This procedure is reserved for clinical situations with an unclear diagnosis, when removal of the offending agent does not result in improvement or influences medical care, or when steroid initiation is being considered.

LABORATORY TESTS

- No single laboratory test has sufficient positive or negative predictive value to diagnose interstitial nephritis.
- Diagnosis is based on clinical history, urine and serum abnormalities, and clinical course.

URINE TESTS:

- Urine eosinophils: Historical marker of AIN. Eosinophiluria is not sensitive or specific enough to establish AIN and occurs more frequently in noninterstitial kidney disorders.
- Urinalysis: Sterile pyuria, microhematuria, glucosuria, and proteinuria usually <300 mg/dl.
- Nephrogenic diabetes insipidus, especially in chronic tubulointerstitial disease.
- Urine sediment analysis: Leukocytes, leukocyte casts, red cells, and tubular epithelial cells (Fig. E1). However, a bland urine sediment can also be seen in interstitial nephritis, especially if chronic. A lack of pyuria does not exclude AIN. Additionally, granular casts may be noted when tubulitis is present.

BLOOD TESTS

- Serum chemistry profile: Elevated BUN, elevated creatinine, low serum phosphorus, and low serum urate concentrations may be present.
- Complete blood count with differential findings include the following:
  1. Eosinophilia (not sensitive; if present, this finding greatly increases clinical suspicion for a systemic drug reaction. Eosinophilia may also occur in other causes of AKI including cholesterol emboli, vasculitis, and hematologic or solid organ malignancy).
  2. Hemoglobin level that is disproportionately low compared to degree of AKI, attributed to loss of interstitial erythropoietin-producing cells.
- If drug-related AIN is not suspected, laboratory testing for infection, vasculitis, and autoimmune disorders is warranted depending on the clinical context.

IMAGING STUDIES

Gallium scintigraphy (gallium-67 scan), positron emission tomography, and computed tomography have been used to evaluate AIN in patients. These tests may distinguish between AIN and other forms of AKI in patients who are not candidates for kidney biopsy.

KIDNEY BIOPSY

Critical to diagnosis of interstitial nephritis in patients with broad differential diagnosis of AKI. Biopsy findings include the following (Fig. E2):

- Predominant lymphocytic and monocytic infiltrate.
- Eosinophils suggestive of drug-induced AIN.
- Tubulitis (renal tubular invasion by inflammatory cells) compatible with AIN.
- Early inflammation with edema may transition to fibrosis with tubular atrophy as disorder becomes chronic.
- Granuloma formation implies infectious origin of AIN, especially in regions where the infectious etiologies described earlier are endemic. Necrotizing granulomas typically seen in fungal infections and tuberculosis.

Rx TREATMENT

NONPHARMACOLOGIC THERAPY

Largely supportive; removal of offending agent, if known, will resolve 60% of cases.

ACUTE GENERAL Rx

- Maintain adequate hydration and urine output.
- Identify and treat infection(s).
- Avoid nephrotoxins and medications that impair renal blood flow.
- Uveitis in TINU syndrome may be asymptomatic. An ophthalmologic exam is recommended in idiopathic AIN.
- Retrospective studies and anecdotal literature have shown that steroid treatment, initiated within 7 days of diagnosis, may reduce the requirement for long-term dialysis in patients with drug-induced AIN who have not responded to drug withdrawal alone. Steroids are the basis of treatment in idiopathic AIN, AIN associated with systemic disease, and TINU. Regimens vary. Some include an initial steroid pulse of methylprednisolone, 250 to 500 mg for 3 consecutive days, followed by prednisone 1 mg/kg. Alternative regimen: Prednisone 1 mg/kg with no intravenous steroid pulse, with tapering over 4 to 6 wk; prolonged steroid tapering does not improve outcomes. Steroids are not administered to patients with significant kidney fibrosis on histologic examination.
- Cyclophosphamide, cyclosporine, and mycophenolate mofetil are anecdotal therapies for steroid-resistant disease. Mycophenolate mofetil has the most evidence for use as a steroid-sparing agent, if AKI recurs when steroids are tapered or discontinued, or when adverse effects from steroid therapy occur.

CHRONIC Rx

- Limit exposure to known nephrotoxic agents
- Medication dosage adjustments by glomerular filtration rate
- Rigorous control of blood pressure, diabetes, and cholesterol
- Treat causes of chronic obstructive uropathy

DISPOSITION

With AIN:

- Complete recovery with return to baseline creatinine occurs in 60% to 65% of cases
- Partial recovery is seen in 10% to 20%
- Irreversible damage in 5% to 10%
- Relapse is common with repeated exposure to offending agents

REFERRAL

Renal consultation is often required when diagnosis is unclear, biopsy is required, or there is treatment-resistant disease.

PEARLS & CONSIDERATIONS

COMMENTS

Drug-induced acute interstitial nephritis occurs primarily when the offending agent is initiated within the preceding 30 days of diagnosis. The most common drug classes are beta-lactam antibiotics, NSAIDs, and proton pump inhibitors (PPIs). In contrast to acute tubular necrosis, which is often associated with oliguria, early AIN may be associated with polyuria. Therefore, a high index of suspicion in this clinical setting is critical for establishing early diagnosis.

PREVENTION

Use known offending agents with care, especially in the elderly, and persons with known underlying kidney disease.

PATIENT & FAMILY EDUCATION

www.nlm.nih.gov/medlineplus/ency/article/000464.htm

RELATED CONTENT

Interstitial Nephritis (Patient Information)

SUGGESTED READINGS

Available at ExpertConsult.com

AUTHORS: **Vikas Singh, MD,** and **Koyal Jain, MD, MPH**

BASIC INFORMATION

DEFINITION

Intussusception is the invagination (telescoping) of a segment of the intestine into a more distal segment of bowel. The occurrence is idiopathic in most cases. In 25% of pediatric cases, a pathologic lead point is identified. During the invagination of the intestine, its mesentery is dragged into the bowel, causing venous and lymphatic congestion, and intestinal edema. If unrecognized or untreated, intussusception can lead to obstruction, ischemia, and perforation.

ICD-10CM CODE

K56.1 Intussusception

EPIDEMIOLOGY & DEMOGRAPHICS

INCIDENCE: 97 to 126 cases per 100,000 annually

PREDOMINANT SEX AND AGE: M:F ratio 2 to 3:1; most common in children 2 mo to 3 yr.

PEAK INCIDENCE: 5 to 10 mo of age

RISK FACTORS:

- Preceding viral illness
- A small percentage of cases will be due to a lead point. Possible lead points include:
  1. Meckel diverticulum
  2. Polyp syndromes
  3. Duplication cysts
  4. Henoch-Schonlein purpura, causing small bowel wall hematoma
  5. G-J tube
  6. Lymphadenopathy of Peyer patch
  7. Lymphoma
  8. Inspissated stool in cystic fibrosis
- Rotavirus vaccine, although the benefits of decreasing rotavirus infection and hospitalization far outweigh the risk of intussusception

PHYSICAL FINDINGS & CLINICAL PRESENTATION

- Sudden onset intermittent abdominal pain, classically accompanied by the drawing up of legs to the abdomen
- Vomiting, which can become bilious with worsening obstruction
- Bloody or "currant jelly" stools
- Palpable sausage-shaped abdominal mass
- Irritability, lethargy or altered mental status, which may be the only presenting symptom in 10% to 15% of cases
- Episodes of pain may last 15 to 20 min, with the child being relatively normal between episodes

ETIOLOGY

Most commonly, the cecum telescopes into the ileum (ileocolic intussusception). Ileoileal, jejunojejunal, and colonic intussusceptions have also been described.

DIAGNOSIS

DIFFERENTIAL DIAGNOSIS

- Meckel diverticulum
- Malrotation with volvulus
- Gastroenteritis
- Henoch-Schonlein purpura
- Colic
- Appendicitis
- Mesenteric ischemia

WORKUP

If the index of suspicion for intussusception is high, the optimal approach is to proceed directly to ultrasound which can be both diagnostic and therapeutic (using ultrasound-guided reduction).

LABORATORY TESTS

- Fecal occult blood test may be done.

IMAGING STUDIES

- Ultrasound to look for target sign, which is suggestive of layers of intestine within intestine (Fig. E1)
- Abdominal x-ray (Fig. E2) to evaluate for free air
- CT scan to confirm location and presence of a lead point

TREATMENT

Management of intussusception depends on the part of the bowel involved. Most children with ileocolic intussusception who are stable and have no signs of bowel perforation may be treated with nonoperative reduction under fluoroscopy or ultrasound. Small bowel intussusception (jejunojejunal, jejunoileal) with no lead point may resolve spontaneously, and can be observed and managed expectantly.

THERAPY

- Stable patients can have nonoperative reduction under fluoroscopic or ultrasound guidance. Fluoroscopic reduction can be done with air enema (Fig. E3) or a saline/contrast enema. Reduction under ultrasound guidance can only be done with saline enema because air interferes with visualization.
- Surgical reduction is necessary if there are concerns of peritonitis or if the patient is unstable.
  1. Surgical Indications:
     a. Signs of perforation, sepsis, or hemodynamic instability
     b. Failed enema reduction
     c. Presence of a pathologic lead point that requires removal
     d. Signs of bowel necrosis
- If the lead point of the intussusception is the tip of a G-J tube, the G-J tube should be removed or pulled back.
- Recurrence of intussusception is seen in 10% to 20% of children, usually within 72 hr after nonoperative reduction.

ACUTE GENERAL Rx

- Analgesia as needed
- Fluid resuscitation, depending on hydration status
- NPO

CHRONIC Rx

Multiple recurrences of intussusception may be associated with the presence of a pathologic lead point.

DISPOSITION

- Patient may be allowed to eat as soon as fully awake from a successful nonsurgical reduction. Many institutions will observe the patient for 6 to 24 hr further due to risk of recurrence.
- Parental education should be provided prior to discharge regarding return precautions due to risk of recurrence.

REFERRAL

- General surgery follow-up after surgical reduction

PEARLS & CONSIDERATIONS

COMMENTS

- Complications of intussusception include bowel necrosis, perforation, and hemorrhage.
- Intussusception can recur after successful reduction, most commonly within 48 hr.
- For patients with a G-J tube presenting with sudden onset abdomen pain and vomiting, intussusception should be considered in the differential diagnosis.
- Intussusception is uncommon in adults and usually involves a lead point.

RELATED TOPICS

Gastroenteritis (Related Key Topic)
Meckel Diverticulum (Related Key Topic)
Acute Lower Gastrointestinal Bleeding (Related Key Topic)

SUGGESTED READINGS

Available at ExpertConsult.com

AUTHORS: **Brittany Guttadauria, MD,** and **Winona Chua, MD**

BASIC INFORMATION

DEFINITION

Irritable bowel syndrome (IBS) is a chronic functional disorder manifested by alteration in bowel habits and recurrent abdominal pain and bloating. IBS is a symptom complex influenced by a variety of physiologic determinants from gut to brain and back. The ROME IV criteria for diagnosis of IBS are:

- Patient has recurrent abdominal pain ≥1 day per wk, on average, in the previous 3 mo, with an onset ≥6 mo before diagnosis
- Abdominal pain is associated with at least two of the following three symptoms:
  1. Pain related to defecation
  2. Change in frequency of stool
  3. Change in form (appearance) of stool
- Patient has none of the following warning signs:
  1. Age ≥50 yr, no previous colon cancer screening, and presence of symptoms
  2. Recent change in bowel habit
  3. Evidence of overt GI bleeding (e.g., melena or hematochezia)
  4. Nocturnal pain or passage of stool
  5. Unintentional weight loss
  6. Family history of colorectal cancer or inflammatory bowel disease
  7. Palpable abdominal mass or lymphadenopathy
  8. Evidence of iron-deficiency anemia on blood testing
  9. Positive test for fecal occult blood
- The criteria must be fulfilled for at least the past 3 mo with symptom onset at least 6 mo before the diagnosis.
- Table 1 subtypes IBS by predominant stool pattern.

SYNONYMS

Irritable colon
Spastic colon
IBS

ICD-10CM CODES

K58	Irritable bowel syndrome
K58.9	Irritable bowel syndrome without diarrhea
K58.0	Irritable bowel syndrome with diarrhea

EPIDEMIOLOGY & DEMOGRAPHICS

- IBS is the most common functional bowel disorder. An estimated 15 million people in the U.S. have IBS.
- IBS occurs in 7% to 21% of the general population of industrialized countries and is responsible for >50% of gastrointestinal (GI) referrals. Worldwide adult prevalence is 12%. Incidence increases during adolescence and peaks in third and fourth decades of life.
- Female:male ratio is 2:1. Peak prevalence is from 20 to 39 yr of age.
- Nearly 50% of patients have psychiatric abnormalities, with anxiety disorders being most common.

PHYSICAL FINDINGS & CLINICAL PRESENTATION

- The clinical presentation of IBS consists of abdominal pain and abnormalities of defecation, which may include loose stools, usually after meals and in the morning, alternating with episodes of constipation.
- Physical examination is generally normal.
- Nonspecific abdominal tenderness and distention may be present.

ETIOLOGY

- Unknown, believed to be multifactorial. Fig. 1 illustrates a biopsychological model of IBS pathophysiology
- Associated pathophysiology includes altered GI motility, alteration in gut flora, and increased gut sensitivity
- Risk factors: Anxiety, depression, personality disorders, history of childhood sexual abuse, and domestic abuse in women

DIAGNOSIS

DIFFERENTIAL DIAGNOSIS

- Inflammatory bowel disease (IBD)
- Diverticulitis
- Colon malignancy
- Endometriosis
- Peptic ulcer disease
- Biliary liver disease
- Chronic pancreatitis
- Constipation caused by medications (opiates, calcium channel blockers, anticholinergics)
- Diarrhea caused by medications (metformin, colchicine, proton pump inhibitors, antacids, antibiotics)
- Small-bowel overgrowth
- Celiac disease
- Parasites
- Lymphoma of GI tract
- Pelvic floor dyssynergia

TABLE 1 Subtyping Irritable Bowel Syndrome by Predominant Stool Pattern

- IBS with constipation (IBS-C)—hard or lumpy stools* ≥25% and loose (mushy) or watery stools† ≥25% of bowel movements‡
- IBS with diarrhea (IBS-D)—loose (mushy) or watery stools† ≥25% and hard or lumpy stool* ≥25% of bowel movements‡
- Mixed IBS—hard or lumpy stools* ≥25% and loose (mushy) or watery stools† ≥25% of bowel movements‡
- Unsubtyped IBS (IBS unclassified)—insufficient abnormality of stool consistency to meet criteria for IBS with constipation, diarrhea, or mixed‡

IBS, Irritable bowel syndrome.
*Bristol Stool Form Scale 1-2 (separate hard lumps like nuts [difficult to pass] or sausage-shaped but lumpy).
†Bristol Stool Form Scale 6-7 (fluffy pieces with ragged edges, a mushy stool or watery, no solid pieces, entirely liquid).
‡In the absence of use of antidiarrheals or laxatives.
Adapted from Sayuk GS, Gyawali CP: Irritable bowel syndrome: modern concepts and management options, *Am J Med* 128(8):817-827, 2015.

WORKUP

Diagnostic workup (Table 2) is aimed primarily at excluding the conditions listed in the differential diagnoses. A step-wise approach is critical. It is important to identify red flags of other diseases, such as weight loss, rectal bleeding, onset in patients >50 yr, fever, nocturnal pain, and family history of malignancy or IBD. Additional red flags include abnormal examination (e.g., mass, enlarged lymph nodes, stool positive for occult blood, muscle wasting) and abnormal laboratory values (anemia, leukocytosis, abnormal chemistry).

LABORATORY TESTS

- Blood work is generally normal. CBC is reasonable to evaluate for anemia. The presence of anemia should alert to the possibility of a colonic malignancy or IBD.
- Other reasonable tests include C-reactive protein, tissue transglutaminase antibody (rule out celiac disease) and TSH (rule out thyroid abnormalities).
- Fecal calprotectin level is useful to differentiate IBS from inflammatory bowel disease in patients who have IBS with diarrhea or with both diarrhea and constipation. Fecal calprotectin levels less than 40 mcg/g exclude IBD in patients with IBS.
- Testing of stool for ova and parasites should be considered only in patients with chronic diarrhea. Evaluation of stool for *Clostridium difficile* may be helpful in patients with predominant diarrhea symptoms who have recently taken antibiotics.

IMAGING STUDIES

- Imaging studies (e.g., flat and upright abdominal radiograph, small-bowel series, sonogram or CT of abdomen and pelvis) are normal and not necessary for diagnosis.
- Lower endoscopy is generally normal except for the presence of some spasms. Colonoscopic imaging should be performed only in persons who have alarm features to rule out organic disease and in persons older than 50 yr to screen for colorectal cancer.

TREATMENT

NONPHARMACOLOGIC THERAPY

- The patient should be encouraged to maintain an adequate fiber intake and to eliminate foods that aggravate symptoms. Avoidance of caffeine, dairy products, fatty foods, and dietary excesses is also helpful. Several clinical trials have shown that a diet low in fermentable oligosaccharides, disaccharides, monosaccharides, and polyols (FODMAPs) improves symptoms in nearly 70% of patients with IBS.
- Cognitive-behavioral therapy is also recommended, particularly in younger patients because psychosocial stressors are important triggers of IBS. Reassurance that the disorder is benign and education about trigger avoidance and stress management are important.

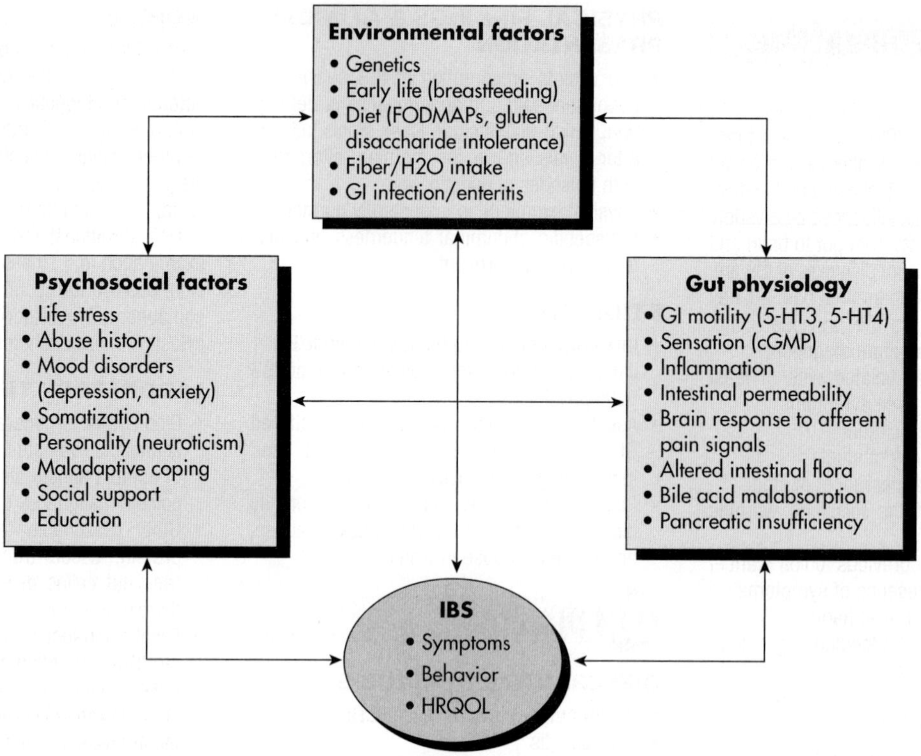

FIG. 1 A biopsychosocial model of irritable bowel syndrome pathophysiology. Irritable bowel syndrome is thought to be a multifactorial disorder, deriving from a potential multitude of etiopathogenic factors, including environmental, psychological, and physiologic factors. This model highlights the complex, often bidirectional interplay of these factors in the experience of irritable bowel syndrome symptoms. *cGMP,* Cyclic guanosine monophosphate; *5-HT3,* serotonin type 3; *5-HT4,* serotonin type 4; *FODMAPS,* fermentable oligosaccharides, disaccharides, monosaccharides, and polyols; *GI,* gastrointestinal; *H20,* water; *HRQOL,* health-related quality of life; *IBS,* irritable bowel syndrome. (Modified from Sayuk GS, Gyawali CP: Irritable bowel syndrome: modern concepts and management options, *Am J Med* 128(8):817-827, 2015.)

- Importance of regular exercise and adequate fluid intake should be stressed.
- Fig. E2 illustrates the management of irritable bowel syndrome.

GENERAL Rx

- The mainstay of treatment of IBS is a high-fiber diet. Fiber is helpful for relief of constipation but not for relief of pain. Because symptoms are chronic, the use of laxatives should generally be avoided.
- Soluble fiber (psyllium) is more effective in symptom relief than insoluble fiber (bran). Fiber supplementation with psyllium 1 tbsp bid or calcium polycarbophil (FiberCon) 2 tablets one to four times daily followed by 8 oz of water may be necessary in some patients.
- Patients should be instructed that there might be some increased bloating on initiation of fiber supplementation, which should resolve within 2 to 3 wk. It is important that patients take these fiber products on a regular basis and not only as needed. Fiber is not effective in patients with diarrhea-predominant IBS and may worsen symptoms in these patients.
- Patients who appear anxious can benefit from use of sedatives or selective serotonin reuptake inhibitors (SSRIs). Tricyclic antidepressants in low doses are also effective in some patients with diarrhea-predominant IBS.
- C-2 chloride channel activators: Lubiprostone (Amitiza) is a chloride channel activator that stimulates chloride-rich intestinal fluid secretion and accelerates small intestine and colonic transmit time. It may be effective in chronic constipation-predominant IBS unresponsive to conventional treatment. Usual dose is 8 to 24 mcg bid with food. Side effects include headache and nausea.
- Linaclotide (Linzess) is a guanylate cyclase-C (GC-C) agonist FDA approved for IBS with constipation. It stimulates secretion of chloride and bicarbonate into the intestinal lumen, mainly through activation of the CFTR ion channel, resulting in increased intestinal fluid and accelerated transit. Usual dose for IBS is 290 mcg 30 min before eating. The most common adverse effects are diarrhea, abdominal pain, flatulence, and abdominal distension.
- Eluxadoline (Viberzi) is a μ-opioid receptor agonist and Δ-opioid receptor antagonist FDA approved for IBS with diarrhea. It decreases muscle contractility, inhibits water and electrolyte secretion, and increases rectal sphincter tone. Usual dose is 100 mg PO bid taken with food.
- Loperamide is effective for diarrhea. Alosetron, a serotonin type-3 receptor antagonist previously withdrawn because of severe constipation and ischemic colitis, has been reintroduced with limited availability. It is indicated only for women with severe chronic diarrhea-predominant IBS unresponsive to conventional therapy and not caused by anatomic or metabolic abnormality. Starting dose is 1 mg qd.
- Alterations in gut flora have been identified as potentially contributing to IBS (84% of IBS patients have an abnormal lactulose breath test, suggesting small-intestinal bacterial overgrowth). Rifaximin, a gut-selective antibiotic, has been used in recent trials to eradicate bacterial overgrowth (70% eradication rate). A dose of 400 mg tid for 10 days was reported effective in improving IBS symptoms up to 10 wk after discontinuation of therapy. Until additional evidence is available, use of rifaximin or other antibiotics in IBS should be reserved for patients with proven bacterial overgrowth.
- Antispasmodics-anticholinergics (e.g., dicyclomine, hyoscyamine) are often used, but efficacy data from clinical trials are inconclusive.
- Probiotics: Bifidobacteria and some combinations of probiotics have shown some limited efficacy. Lactobacilli do not appear to be effective for the treatment of IBS. Additional data showing efficacy is needed before probiotics can be endorsed for treatment of IBS.
- Antidepressants: SSRIs are more effective than placebo for relief of global IBS symptoms.

TABLE 2 Irritable Bowel Syndrome Treatment Strategy: A Way Forward

1. Evaluation
   a. Consider conditions that mimic IBS (e.g., celiac disease, microscopic colitis, bile acid diarrhea, pancreatic insufficiency, carbohydrate intolerances, medication side effects, postsurgical neoanatomy)
   b. Assess for the presence of alarm symptoms
   c. Evaluate for symptom triggers (e.g., stressors, diet)
   d. Explore presence of other functional GI (e.g., functional dyspepsia) and non-GI disorders (e.g., fibromyalgia), psychiatric comorbidity, and drug intolerances
   e. Understand previous IBS treatment experiences
2. Selection of treatment approach
   a. Predicated on symptom severity and dominant symptoms
   b. Symptom severity (intensity, bother, effects on quality of life)
      i. Mild symptoms, intermittent symptoms, low symptom burden: Symptomatic or peripheral therapy
      ii. Moderate symptoms: Centrally acting neuromodulators, especially if symptomatic therapy does not provide adequate benefit
      iii. Severe symptoms and those with comorbidities (non-GI functional disorders, psychiatric): Both centrally acting neuromodulators and peripheral therapy
         a. Concurrent affective disorders need to be managed
         b. Other central therapies (cognitive and behavioral therapy, hypnosis, stress reduction) may need to be considered
   c. Dominant symptoms (diarrhea, constipation, pain, other GI symptoms)
      i. Constipation predominant
         a. Laxatives, fiber
         b. Novel agents (linaclotide, lubiprostone)
      ii. Diarrhea predominant
         a. Antidiarrheals
         b. Alosetron
         c. Address dysbiosis (rifaximin, probiotics)
         d. Diet (low FODMAP)
         e. Bile binders (cholestyramine, colesevelam)
         f. Disaccharidases (lactase)
      iii. Pain predominant
         a. Antidepressants (TCAs and SNRIs preferred)
         b. Linaclotide when constipation present
         c. Avoid narcotics
3. Education and therapeutic alliance
   a. Inform patient about etiopathogenesis
   b. Reaffirm legitimacy of diagnosis; allay concerns about organic disease
   c. Provide information about support organizations (International Foundation for Functional Gastrointestinal Disorders)

FODMAP, Fermentable oligosaccharides, disaccharides, monosaccharides, and polyols; *GI,* gastrointestinal; *IBS,* irritable bowel syndrome; *SNRI,* serotonin-norepinephrine reuptake inhibitor; *TCA,* tricyclic antidepressant.

DISPOSITION

More than 60% of patients respond successfully to treatment over the initial 12 mo; however, IBS is a chronic, relapsing condition and requires prolonged therapy.

REFERRAL

GI referral is recommended in patients with rectal bleeding, fever, nocturnal diarrhea, anemia, weight loss, or onset of symptoms >40 yr. Consultation is also necessary if specialized diagnostic procedures such as endoscopy are necessary.

PEARLS & CONSIDERATIONS

COMMENTS

- Patients should be educated regarding maintenance of a high-fiber diet and elimination of stressors, which can precipitate attacks of IBS. They should be reassured that their condition does not lead to cancer.
- Recent drug efforts (alosetron, tegaserod) are aimed at serotonergic receptors in the gut because most of the serotonin in the body is found in the GI tract and is believed to be involved in the mediation of visceral sensation and motility.
- Cognitive-behavioral therapy is effective in the treatment of patients with IBS and should be considered as part of the armamentarium against this disorder.
- Some patients with IBS but without celiac disease show symptom improvement on a wheat-free diet. A 2- to 3-wk trial of wheat avoidance may be reasonable in patients with treatment-resistant IBS.
- Fecal microbiota transplantation (FMT) delivered via upper endoscopy seems to be efficacious in improving symptoms in all IBS subtypes in early clinical trials.[1]

[1]El-Salhy M et al: Efficacy of faecal microbiota transplantation for patients with irritable bowel syndrome in a randomised, double-blind, placebo-controlled study, *Gut* 69:859-867, 2020.

SUGGESTED READINGS

Available at ExpertConsult.com

RELATED CONTENT

Irritable Bowel Syndrome (Patient Information)

AUTHOR: **Fred F. Ferri, MD**

BASIC INFORMATION

DEFINITION

Ischemic colitis (IC) is tissue damage and inflammation of the large intestine due to a reduction in blood flow.

SYNONYMS

Intestinal ischemia
Colonic ischemia
IC

ICD-10CM CODES

K51.50	Left-sided colitis without complications
K51.51	Left-sided colitis with complications
K51.511	Left-sided colitis with rectal bleeding
K51.512	Left-sided colitis with intestinal obstruction
K51.513	Left-sided colitis with fistula
K51.514	Left-sided colitis with abscess
K51.518	Left-sided colitis with other complication
K51.519	Left-sided colitis with unspecified complications
K52.3	Indeterminate colitis
K55.0	Acute vascular disorders of intestine
K55.031	Focal (segmental) acute (reversible) ischemia of large intestine
K55.032	Diffuse acute (reversible) ischemia of large intestine
K55.039	Acute (reversible) ischemia of large intestine, extent unspecified
K55.9	Vascular disorder of intestine, unspecified

EPIDEMIOLOGY & DEMOGRAPHICS

INCIDENCE: It is the most common type of intestinal ischemia with an annual incidence of 15.6 to 17.7 per 100,000.

PREVALENCE: Unknown

PREDOMINANT SEX AND AGE:
- More common among older patients (60s to 70s)
- Female predominance

PEAK INCIDENCE: Unknown

RISK FACTORS:
- Older age (60s to 70s)
- Atherosclerotic disease
- Hemodialysis
- Hypertension
- Atrial fibrillation
- Diabetes
- Small vessel disease
- Sickle cell disease
- Infection (CMV, *E. coli*)
- Aortic surgery, endovascular intervention, cardiopulmonary bypass surgery
- Long-distance running, extreme exercise
- Hypercoagulable state
- Myocardial ischemia
- Mechanical obstruction
- Hypoalbuminemia
- Pharmacologic
- Shock
- Inflammatory disease

PHYSICAL FINDINGS & CLINICAL PRESENTATION

- Key historical points:
  1. Rapid-onset cramping and abdominal pain (classically thought to involve the left side more often, but newer literature suggests that no one region is affected predominantly). Pain secondary to large bowel ischemia is often not as severe as pain associated with small bowel ischemia
  2. Urge to defecate may accompany developing abdominal pain
  3. Hematochezia (usually within 24 hr). More commonly associated with ischemic colitis of the large bowel compared with small bowel involvement
- Physical exam findings suggestive of ischemic colitis:
  1. Abdominal exam may be normal initially
  2. May have peritoneal signs in severe illness or bowel perforation
  3. Hypotension and tachycardia in severe cases
  4. Guaiac positive stool

ETIOLOGY

GENERAL:
- Caused by a reduction in blood flow, usually sudden, to a segment of the bowel. The resulting blood flow is not enough to provide the oxygen and nutrients necessary for normal cellular metabolism.
- Particularly affected are the watershed regions of the colon (Fig. E1), which have limited collateral circulation (splenic flexure and sigmoid colon).
- Medical and surgical conditions associated with ischemic colitis are summarized in Box 1.

SPECIFIC:
- Nonocclusive disease (20%):
  1. Hypoperfusion: Cardiac failure, septic shock, hemorrhagic shock, hemodialysis, or any other condition that can cause hypotension
  2. Iatrogenic: Drugs (especially constipation-inducing). Medications associated with ischemic colitis are summarized in Box 2
  3. Colonic obstruction: Colon cancer, constipation, volvulus, bowel obstruction
  4. Long-distance running
- Occlusive disease (80%):
  1. Arterial: Thrombus/emboli, cholesterol emboli, small vessel disease (atherosclerosis, diabetes, vasculitis, rheumatoid arthritis, radiation, amyloidosis), trauma
  2. Surgical: Aortic aneurysm repair, cardiac catheterization, cardiopulmonary bypass, colectomy, endoscopy, renal transplant
  3. Venous: Mesenteric venous thrombosis, hypercoagulable state, sickle cell disease, pancreatitis, portal hypertension, lymphocytic phlebitis

DIAGNOSIS

DIFFERENTIAL DIAGNOSIS

- Infectious colitis (e.g., *Clostridium difficile, Salmonella, Shigella*)

BOX 1 Medical and Surgical Conditions Associated with Ischemic Colitis

Cardiovascular/Pulmonary
Atherosclerosis*
Atrial fibrillation
Chronic obstructive pulmonary disease
Hypertension

Gastrointestinal
Constipation
Diarrhea
Irritable bowel syndrome

Low Flow State
Septic shock
Congestive heart failure
Hemorrhagic shock
Hypotension

Surgery
Abdominal surgery
Aortic surgery
Cardiovascular surgery

Invasive Interventions
Postendovascular abdominal manipulations (e.g., chemoembolization)
Postcolonoscopy

Metabolic/Rheumatoid
Diabetes mellitus
Dyslipidemia
Rheumatoid arthritis
Systemic lupus erythematosus

Miscellaneous
Hypercoagulable states†
Sickle cell disease
Long-distance running

*For example, ischemic heart disease, cerebrovascular disease, peripheral vascular disease.
†Antiphospholipid syndrome, factor V Leiden deficiency, protein C and S deficiency.
From Cameron JL, Cameron AM: *Current surgical therapy,* ed 12, Philadelphia, 2017, Elsevier.

BOX 2 Drugs Associated with Ischemic Colitis

Constipation-inducing drugs (opioids and nonopioids)
Immunomodulator drugs (anti-TwNFα, type 1 interferon-α, type 1 interferon-β)
Chemotherapeutic drugs (e.g., Taxanes)
Cocaine and methamphetamines
Female hormones
Oral contraceptive medications
Antibiotics
Pseudoephedrine
Serotoninergic (e.g., Alosetron, Sumatriptan)
Diuretics

TNF, Tumor necrosis factor.
From Cameron JL, Cameron AM: *Current surgical therapy,* ed 12, Philadelphia, 2017, Elsevier.

- Inflammatory bowel disease, inflammatory bowel syndrome, celiac disease
- Small bowel ischemia
- Constipation
- Diverticulitis
- Bowel obstruction
- Pancreatitis
- Malignancy
- Radiation enteritis

WORKUP

The clinical presentation is often vague and can be variable from patient to patient. A high index of suspicion must be maintained in any patient presenting with abdominal pain and bloody stool. In addition to the physical exam, the following are key to confirming the diagnosis:

- Laboratory studies
- Computed tomography
- Lower endoscopy

LABORATORY TESTS

- General:
  1. CBC (may see leukocytosis)
  2. Comprehensive metabolic panel
  3. Liver function panel
- Specific markers: There are no specific laboratory tests for ischemic colitis. However, elevated levels of certain markers suggest inadequate global perfusion:
  1. Lactate
  2. Lactate dehydrogenase
  3. CK
  4. Amylase
- Coagulation studies

IMAGING STUDIES

- Abdominal CT with contrast: Although findings can be nonspecific, the value of CT is in distinguishing ischemic colitis from nonischemic causes of abdominal pain. It also can assess the degree of ischemia and gauge the need for surgical intervention. It may identify arterial emboli or venous obstruction. Specific findings suggestive of ischemic colitis include, but are not limited to, intestinal wall thickening, thumbprinting, pericolonic stranding, and peritoneal free fluid or free air. Pneumatosis (the presence of gas in the colonic wall), portal venous gas, and the presence of megacolon usually indicate severe disease requiring immediate surgical intervention.
- Abdominal radiograph: Should be used in critical patients who are too unstable for a CT scan to look for gas formation in the bowel wall or free air in the abdomen suggestive of perforation.
- Lower endoscopy: This is the gold standard for confirming diagnosis of ischemic colitis in the stable patient. In the absence of peritoneal signs, colonoscopy is the test of choice to evaluate the degree of ischemia. If ischemia is suspected, lower endoscopy should be performed within the first 24 to 48 hr. In most cases, visual inspection of the colonic wall will confirm the diagnosis and dictate the need for conservative versus surgical management. However, endoscopy should not be performed in patients with acute peritonitis or evidence of irreversible ischemic damage on CT.

Rx TREATMENT

- Treatment depends on the severity of disease and the specific etiology of colonic ischemia. However, the mainstay of therapy consists of optimizing blood flow to ischemic regions of bowel and removing any potential exacerbating factors. Initial care consists of aggressive IV crystalloid resuscitation, bowel rest, and broad-spectrum antibiotics with aerobic and anaerobic coverage. A treatment algorithm is illustrated in Fig. 2.
- In mild cases where patients are hemodynamically stable and do not have signs of peritonitis, colonoscopy should be performed. Patients with nonviable bowel seen on endoscopy require immediate operative intervention. However, the remainder of patients should be managed medically with continued IV fluids, bowel rest, and broad-spectrum antibiotics. Consider the use of a nasogastric tube in patients with abdominal distention or signs of ileus or bowel obstruction. Avoid vasoconstrictive medications as these can exacerbate colonic hypoperfusion; however, do not withhold their use in clinically unstable patients. Monitor signs of adequate end organ perfusion (e.g., mental status, abdominal pain, urine output). Management of underlying causes (e.g., heart failure, vascular disease, sepsis) should be considered.
- In severe cases not responding to supportive therapy, where patients are exhibiting acute peritonitis, sepsis, hypotension, or pain out of proportion to clinical exam, surgical abdominal exploration is warranted. Resection of gangrenous segments of bowel may be necessary. Colonoscopy should be avoided in these patients.

NONPHARMACOLOGIC THERAPY

- Open or laparoscopic abdominal exploration to identify necrotic bowel. Box 3 summarizes indications for surgical intervention in patients with ischemic colitis
- NG tube for bowel decompression if ileus or obstruction is present

ACUTE GENERAL Rx

- Supportive care:
  1. IV fluids
  2. Bowel rest
  3. Broad-spectrum antibiotics (aerobic and anaerobic coverage)
  4. Pain control
- Anticoagulation (not indicated in nonocclusive ischemia but may be considered in proven arterial occlusion or mesenteric vein thrombosis)
- Abdominal exploration:
  1. Bowel prep should be given
  2. Bowel resection may be indicated in severe colitis
  3. Repeat surgical exploration normally is performed within 12 to 24 hr, especially after colonic resection, to assess the viability of colonic tissue and state of the anastomosis. Intraoperative infrared angiography based on IV injection of indo cyanine green (Fig. E3) can be used as an adjunct for decisions of whether to resect in determining margins and the integrity of intestinal anastomoses
  4. Primary anastomosis after colonic resection is contraindicated in certain cases (e.g., presence of aortic or iliac grafts; or when tissue is too friable for stable anastomosis)

CHRONIC Rx

- Avoid overly aggressive hypertension treatment.
- Avoid dehydration.
- Avoid extreme exercise.

DISPOSITION

- Most cases of acute ischemic colitis are nongangrenous and resolve completely with medical care in 1 to 2 days. However, the need for surgery in more severe cases portends a worse prognosis and is associated with increased morbidity and mortality. Any risk factors for ischemic colitis should be identified and mitigated as much as possible.

REFERRAL

Prompt general surgery consultation is indicated in patients with the following:

- Hemodynamic instability and peritoneal signs on examination
- CT showing signs of bowel infarction or perforation
- Endoscopy showing nonviable bowel or peritoneal signs

PEARLS & CONSIDERATIONS

COMMENTS

Ischemic colitis typically occurs in older patients who have multiple comorbidities. A high index of suspicion should be maintained for patients with recent endovascular procedures. These patients require close outpatient follow-up and management by a primary care provider.

PREVENTION

Avoid overly aggressive hypertension treatment, dehydration, and extreme exercise.

SUGGESTED READINGS

Available at ExpertConsult.com

RELATED CONTENT

Mesenteric Venous Thrombosis (Related Key Topic)
Acute Mesenteric Ischemia (Related Key Topic)

AUTHORS: **Nicholas J. Inman, MD,** and **Brett Patrick, MD**

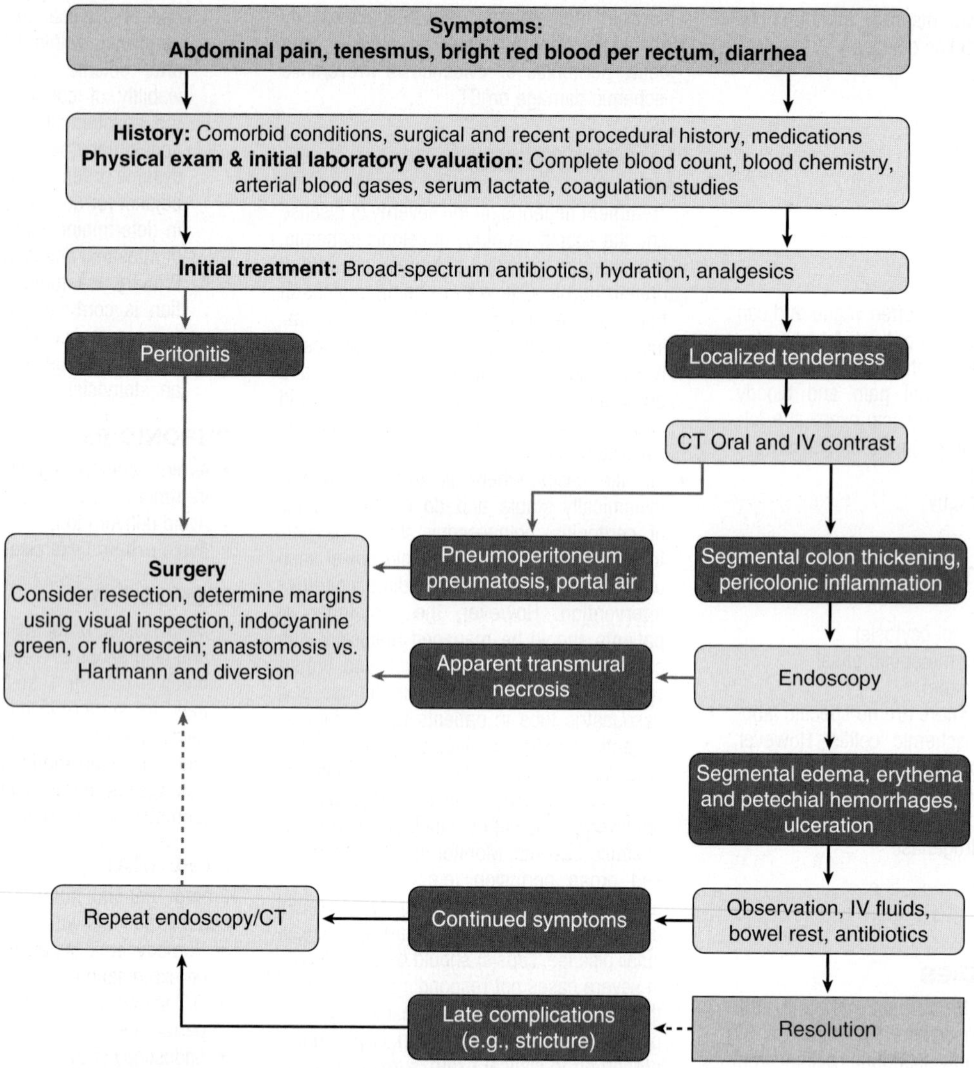

FIG. 2 Treatment algorithm for ischemic colitis. *CT,* Computed tomography; *IV,* intravenous. (From Cameron JL, Cameron AM: *Current surgical therapy,* ed 12, Philadelphia, 2017, Elsevier.)

BOX 3 Indications for Surgical Intervention in Patients with Ischemic Colitis

Acute
Peritonitis
Bowel perforation
Bowel necrosis
Fulminant colitis
Massive hemorrhage
Sepsis

Chronic
Intractable symptoms (abdominal pain, bloody diarrhea, etc.) lasting >2 wk
Recurrent sepsis
Chronic colitis
Ischemic stricture
Malnutrition from protein-losing enteropathy

From Cameron JL, Cameron AM: *Current surgical therapy,* ed 12, Philadelphia, 2017, Elsevier.

BASIC INFORMATION

DEFINITION

- A common form of vascular liver disease
- Occurs when a severe systemic disturbance leads to decreased perfusion to the liver resulting in tissue hypoxia

SYNONYMS

Hypoxic hepatitis
Shock liver
Ischemic hepatopathy
Hepatic necrosis

ICD-10CM CODES	
K76.2	Central hemorrhagic necrosis of liver
K75.89	Other specified inflammatory liver disease

EPIDEMIOLOGY & DEMOGRAPHICS

- Occurs worldwide

INCIDENCE:

- Less than 1% on the inpatient medical wards
- Incidence is higher (2.5%) in intensive care unit

PREVALENCE:

- Recognized as most frequent cause of acute liver injury
- 57% of patients with liver enzymes >1000 IU/L have ischemic hepatitis
- Prevalence up to 10% in the intensive care setting

PREDOMINANT AGE:

- Can occur in all ages
- Most common in elderly

PEAK INCIDENCE: Highest in the cardiac care units

RISK FACTORS:

- Most common is cardiovascular disease
- Chronic heart failure
- Cirrhosis

GENETICS: No genetic predisposition

PHYSICAL FINDINGS & CLINICAL PRESENTATION

- Altered mental status may be present due to decreased cerebral perfusion.
- Other symptoms are often masked by the overall disease state.
- Hepatic synthetic function is usually preserved in ischemic hepatitis.

ETIOLOGY

- Cardiac disease is the most common (Fig. E1)
- This includes myocardial infarction, arrhythmias, cardiac tamponade, and cardiogenic shock
- Majority of patients have markedly increased cardiac filling pressures
- Respiratory failure and sepsis are the second and third most common
- Hypovolemic shock from hemorrhage, dehydration, and heat stroke
- Hypotension (only 1 in 2 patients have documented low blood pressures)
- See Box 1 for a brief summary of the different causes of ischemic hepatitis

DIAGNOSIS

DIFFERENTIAL DIAGNOSIS (BOX 2)

- Acute viral hepatitis
- Autoimmune hepatitis
- Drug-induced liver injury
- Other toxins and medications (i.e., acetaminophen toxicity)

WORKUP

- Diagnosed by laboratory parameters and the clinical context of a hospitalized patient.
- Workup is directed at identifying the predisposing cause.
- Liver biopsy is not required.
- Histology shows centrilobular (zone 3) necrosis with preservation of the hepatic architecture.
- Necrosis can extend to the midzonal hepatocytes in the setting of prolonged ischemia.

LABORATORY TESTS

- Extremely elevated aminotransferase levels, often exceeding 200 times the upper limit of normal.
- Aspartate aminotransferase (AST) and alanine aminotransferase (ALT) rapidly rise after the ischemic insult.
- They peak within 1 to 3 days.
- They usually return to normal within 7 to 10 days if the initial ischemic insult is resolved.
- Lactate dehydrogenase (LDH) level is extremely elevated.
- ALT/LDH ratio of less than 1.5 is suggestive.
- Prothrombin time can be slightly prolonged.
- The serum bilirubin can be mildly increased.
- Serum bilirubin peaks after the aminotransferases peak.
- Increased blood urea nitrogen and creatinine levels from acute tubular necrosis and renal dysfunction.

IMAGING STUDIES

Imaging is not required for the diagnosis.

TREATMENT

NONPHARMACOLOGIC THERAPY

Management is directed at treating the underlying illness causing the systemic disturbance.

ACUTE GENERAL Rx

- Hemodynamic resuscitation
- Inotropic agents for cardiogenic shock
- Intravenous fluid resuscitation with or without vasoconstrictors for septic or hypovolemic shock
- Blood transfusions if hypovolemic shock from blood loss
- These measures optimize hepatic perfusion and resolve tissue hypoxia
- There is no role for *N*-acetylcysteine administration

BOX 1 Causes of Ischemic Hepatitis

Cardiovascular disease (most common): Cardiogenic shock
Respiratory failure
Sepsis/septic shock
Hypovolemic shock: Hemorrhage, volume depletion
Hypotension

BOX 2 Common Differentials of Ischemic Hepatitis

Acute viral hepatitis (e.g., hepatitis A, hepatitis B)
Autoimmune hepatitis
Toxins (e.g., herbal supplements)
Medications (e.g., acetaminophen)

CHRONIC Rx

- Ensure stability of underlying illness
- No specific liver-directed therapy

DISPOSITION

- Most commonly a self-limited and benign condition if promptly managed.
- Occasionally associated with significant mortality.
- Prognosis is determined by the severity of the underlying illness. In-hospital mortality associated with ischemic hepatitis is roughly 50%.
- Patients with underlying chronic heart failure or cirrhosis have worse outcomes.
- Other poor prognostic factors include persistently elevated aminotransferase and multiorgan failure.

REFERRAL

- Referral to a hepatologist is not required once illness is resolved.
- Referral is appropriate if patient has underlying cirrhosis.

PEARLS & CONSIDERATIONS

COMMENTS

- Have a high index of suspicion for this diagnosis in a hospitalized patient with severe systemic illness and significantly elevated AST and ALT.
- Use ALT/LDH ratio to aid in the diagnosis.
- Do not be alarmed if bilirubin continues to rise after AST and ALT peak.
- Hypotension is often not documented or not present at all.
- Patients with significantly elevated liver enzymes should be evaluated for occult heart failure.

PREVENTION

Ensure stability of comorbidities (e.g., cardiac disease)

AUTHOR: **Hirsh D. Trivedi, MD**

BASIC INFORMATION

DEFINITION
Jaundice is a yellowish discoloration of the sclera, skin, and mucous membranes caused by an excessive amount of bilirubin in the bloodstream. Clinically detectable jaundice in adults is a serum bilirubin of 2.5 to 3 mg/dl.

SYNONYM
Icterus

ICD-10CM CODE
R17 Unspecified jaundice

EPIDEMIOLOGY & DEMOGRAPHICS
The prevalent causes of jaundice by age and sex:
- Young adulthood (for either sex): Viral hepatitis, Gilbert disease
- Middle adulthood (for either sex): Drug-induced hepatitis and cirrhosis
- Middle-aged and older men: Alcoholic liver disease, pancreatic cancer, hepatoma, primary hemochromatosis
- Women: Primary biliary cirrhosis, chronic active hepatitis, choledocholithiasis, carcinoma of the gallbladder

PHYSICAL FINDINGS & CLINICAL PRESENTATION
Presentation can vary from an incidental finding to acute and life-threatening. History and physical examination give important clues to the underlying condition.
Key history of present illness findings:
- Duration of jaundice
- Associated symptoms: Abdominal pain, fever, nausea, malaise, pruritus, chills, changes in urine and stool color, anorexia and/or weight loss

Key social history/exposure findings:
- Alcohol use, injection of illicit drugs, use of hepatotoxic medication or herbal products, blood transfusions, unprotected sex, ingestion of shellfish, travel, occupational exposure to toxins

Key medical history findings:
- Prior abdominal/biliary surgery, prior episodes of jaundice, prior diagnosis of hepatitis B or C, inflammatory bowel disease

Key physical findings:
- Vital sign abnormalities: Fever, hypotension, tachycardia
- Signs of acute disease: Abdominal tenderness, splenomegaly, abdominal mass, encephalopathy, Murphy sign
- Signs of chronic liver disease: Palmar erythema, spider angiomas, bruising, gynecomastia, testicular atrophy, ascites, weight loss, Kayser-Fleischer rings (Wilson), caput medusa, internal hemorrhoids, scleral icterus

ETIOLOGY
Disruption in any of the three phases of bilirubin metabolism can lead to jaundice:
- Prehepatic phase: An increase in heme degradation products from red blood cell (RBC) catabolism, ineffective erythropoiesis, or breakdown of muscle myoglobin and cytochromes; leads to indirect (unconjugated) hyperbilirubinemia
- Intrahepatic phase: Destruction of the hepatocytes or disruption of either of the two separate biochemical processes that conjugate bilirubin in the hepatocyte; may lead to indirect (unconjugated) or direct (conjugated) hyperbilirubinemia
- Post-hepatic phase: Blockage of the release of water-soluble bilirubin from the hepatobiliary system, preventing excretion into the stool or urine or recycling within the gut flora; leads to direct (conjugated) hyperbilirubinemia

Dx DIAGNOSIS

DIFFERENTIAL DIAGNOSIS
Prehepatic causes:
- Hemolytic processes (e.g., sickle cell disease, spherocytosis, thalassemia, G6PD, immune hemolysis, HUS), ineffective erythropoiesis (e.g., thalassemia, folate, severe iron deficiency), or large hematoma reabsorption

Intrahepatic causes:
- If unconjugated hyperbilirubinemia: Enzyme metabolism disorders (Gilbert disease, Crigler-Najjar syndrome), drugs that alter the enzymatic pathways such as rifampin, isoniazid, and probenecid
- If conjugated hyperbilirubinemia: Intrahepatic cholestasis caused by:
  1. Viruses: Hepatitis A, B, and C; Epstein-Barr, hemorrhagic viruses (yellow fever, Ebola)
  2. Other infections: Bacteria (leptospirosis, MAI), parasites (schistosomiasis, malaria, amebiasis), fungal *(Blastomyces, Histoplasma)*
  3. Alcohol: Alcoholic hepatitis, alcoholic cirrhosis
  4. Autoimmune: Primary biliary cirrhosis, primary sclerosing cholangitis, autoimmune hepatitis
  5. Hepatotoxic drug-induced: Acetaminophen (most common), penicillins (most commonly Augmentin), chlorpromazine, steroids (estrogenic or anabolic), NSAIDs, valproic acid, some herbals such as kava, ma huang, and off-market weight-loss supplements
  6. Hereditary/metabolic: Sickle cell disease and other RBC dyscrasias, hemochromatosis, Wilson disease, Dubin-Johnson and Rotor syndromes, α-antitrypsin deficiency, glycogen storage disease, NASH (nonalcoholic steatohepatitis), porphyria, benign recurrent intrahepatic cholestasis
  7. Systemic diseases invading liver: Sarcoidosis, amyloidosis, hemochromatosis, tuberculosis, *Mycobacterium avium intracellulare*
  8. Other: Cirrhosis, sepsis, total parenteral nutrition, intrahepatic cholestasis of pregnancy, graft-versus-host disease, environmental toxins, benign postoperative state

Posthepatic causes:
- Intrinsic or extrinsic obstruction of the biliary system:
  1. Blockage within hepatobiliary tree: Strictures, cholangiocarcinoma, gallbladder cancer, carcinoma of ampulla of Vater, infection (e.g., cytomegalovirus, *Cryptosporidium* in patients with AIDS, parasites), choledocholithiasis
  2. Blockage outside of hepatobiliary tree: Pancreatitis, pancreatic carcinoma, pancreatic pseudocyst, lymphoma
- Pseudojaundice: Not related to bilirubin but rather resulting from excessive ingestion of foods containing beta carotene (e.g., carrots, melons, squash)

WORKUP
- History, physical examination, and first-line lab tests can often clarify diagnosis. Fig. 1 describes a clinical approach to jaundice. Table 1 summarizes the differential diagnosis of critical and emergent diagnoses in patients with jaundice.

LABORATORY TESTS
- First-line tests:
  1. Serum total and direct bilirubin
  2. Urinalysis
  3. Liver function tests (AST, ALT, GGTP, alkaline phosphatase), CBC, liver synthetic function (albumin, PT, PTT), pancreatic function (amylase, lipase)
- If serum total bilirubin and direct bilirubin are elevated and urine is positive for bilirubin, consider intrahepatic or posthepatic process. If serum total bilirubin is elevated but direct bilirubin is normal (unconjugated hyperbilirubinemia) and urine is negative for bilirubin, consider prehepatic or intrahepatic processes

Additional tests if diagnosis unclear:
- Screen for hepatitis A, B, and C; if still unclear, then consider following options based on H&P
- Other viruses: EBV, CMV
- Autoimmune disorders: Antimitochondrial antibody (elevated in primary biliary cirrhosis); anti-smooth muscle antibody, ANA (elevated in autoimmune hepatitis); antinuclear cytoplasmic antibody (elevated in primary sclerosing cholangitis)
- Ceruloplasmin (elevated in Wilson disease)
- Alpha-1 antitrypsin deficiency (elevated in cirrhosis and emphysema)
- Ferritin, Fe saturation (elevated in hemochromatosis)
- Blood smear (RBC dyscrasias)
- Diagnosis of exclusion: Gilbert syndrome
- Liver biopsy: Essential in diagnosis of chronic hepatitis. Can be used for diagnosis of liver masses but carries a substantial risk

IMAGING STUDIES
- Abdominal ultrasound: First-line study (Figs. E2 and E3) may be completed bedside, most sensitive for proximal biliary tract disease; presence of dilated ducts hints at an extrahepatic process.

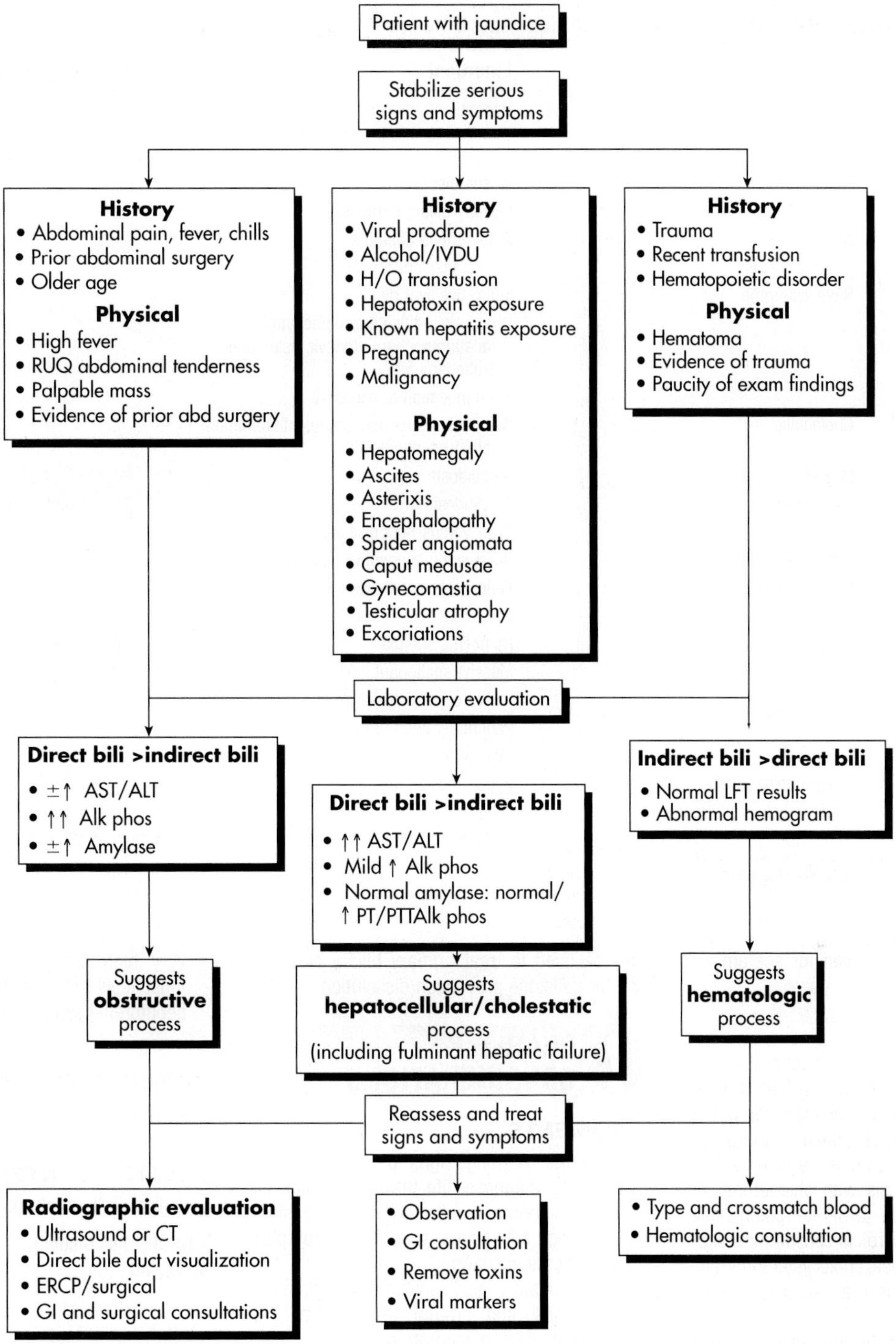

FIG. 1 Management of the patient with jaundice. *Alk phos,* Alkaline phosphatase; *ALT,* alanine aminotransferase; *AST,* aspartate aminotransferase; *bili,* bilirubin; *CT,* computed tomography; *ERCP,* endoscopic retrograde cholangiopancreatography; *GI,* gastrointestinal; *H/O,* history of; *IVDU,* intravenous drug use; *LFT,* liver function test; *PT,* prothrombin time; *PTT,* partial thromboplastin time; *RUQ,* right upper quadrant. (From Marx AJ et al: *Rosen's emergency medicine: concepts and clinical practice,* ed 7, Philadelphia, 2010, Elsevier.)

- Abdominal CT: Often necessary to elucidate more information on liver, pancreas, and distal biliary system.
- Endoscopic retrograde cholangiopancreatography: Rarely necessary for diagnostics. Refer to GI consultant.
- Percutaneous transhepatic cholangiography: Rarely necessary for diagnostics. Refer to GI or surgical consultant.
- Magnetic resonance cholangiopancreatography: Noninvasive visualization of bile and pancreatic ducts. Refer to GI consultant.
- Endoscopic ultrasound: Used for characterization and, if needed, biopsy of any focal lesions found within biliary tree and/or pancreas. Refer to GI consultant.

Rx TREATMENT

NONPHARMACOLOGIC THERAPY

Depends on underlying cause of the jaundice and clinical stability of the patient. Generally, obstructive causes require surgical treatment, while nonobstructive causes require medical treatment.

ACUTE GENERAL Rx

Acute, life-threatening illness (e.g., cholecystitis or ascending cholangitis) requires prompt diagnosis with basic labs and bedside diagnostics, with early surgical and GI consultation in conjunction. Suspicious medications should be stopped. Initiate medical management of symptoms with analgesia, IV fluids, correction of coagulopathies, and consideration of antibiotics.

TABLE 1 Jaundice: Differential Diagnosis of Critical and Emergent Diagnoses

System	Critical	Emergent	Nonemergent
Hepatic	Fulminant hepatic failure	Hepatitis of any cause with confusion, bleeding, or coagulopathy	Hepatitis with normal mental status, normal vital signs, and no active bleeding
	Toxin	Wilson disease	
	Virus	Primary biliary cirrhosis	
	Alcohol	Autoimmune hepatitis	
	Ischemic insult	Liver transplant rejection	
	Reye syndrome	Infiltrative liver disease	
		Drug induced (isoniazid, phenytoin, acetaminophen, ritonavir, halothane, sulfonamides)	
		Toxin ingestion or exposure	
Biliary	Cholangitis	Bile duct obstruction (stone, inflammation, stricture, neoplasm)	
Systemic	Sepsis	Sarcoidosis	Posttraumatic hematoma resorption
	Heatstroke	Amyloidosis	Total parenteral nutrition
		Graft-versus-host disease	
Cardiovascular	Obstructing AAA	Right-sided congestive heart failure	
	Budd-Chiari syndrome	Veno-occlusive disease	
	Severe congestive heart failure		
Hematologic-oncologic	Transfusion reaction	Hemolytic anemia	Gilbert syndrome
		Massive malignant infiltration	Physiologic neonatal jaundice
		Inborn error of metabolism	
		Pancreatic head tumor	
		Metastatic disease	
Reproductive	Preeclampsia or HELLP syndrome	Hyperemesis gravidarum	
	Acute fatty liver of pregnancy		Cholestasis of pregnancy

AAA, Abdominal aortic aneurysm; *HELLP,* hemolysis, elevated liver enzymes, low platelets.
From Marx JA et al: *Rosen's emergency medicine,* ed 8, Philadelphia, 2014, Saunders.

N-Acetylcysteine can be given for acetaminophen overdose.

CHRONIC Rx

Reversible causes must be ruled out first—suspicious medications and EtOH must be discontinued. Consider GI consult for management of many intrahepatic diseases, such as treatment of hepatitis B or C, Wilson disease with penicillamine, hemochromatosis with phlebotomy, or for stent insertion with ERCP for posthepatic obstruction. Consider surgical consult for resection of pancreatic masses, cholecystectomy, etc.

Symptomatic pruritus may be treated with cholestyramine for bilirubin binding or with antihistamines to decrease the itch reflex. Ursodiol may be used to treat primary biliary cirrhosis and for gallstone prevention/dissolution.

PEARLS & CONSIDERATIONS

COMMENTS

- Heed the warning signs of unstable vital signs to diagnose life-threatening illness; early collaboration with surgical and gastroenterology colleagues is helpful in complex patient care scenarios.
- Careful history and physical examination, basic labs, and prompt bedside imaging frequently lead to accurate diagnosis.
- Very high serum bilirubin (>15 mg/dl) is most likely to be seen in cirrhosis. Watch for hepatorenal syndrome in these patients.

SUGGESTED READINGS

Available at ExpertConsult.com

RELATED CONTENT

Jaundice (Patient Information)

AUTHORS: **Alla Goldburt, MD,** and **Paolo G. Pace, MASc, MD**

BASIC INFORMATION

DEFINITION

Junctional rhythm is an abnormal cardiac rhythm originating in the His bundle or atrioventricular (AV) node. This diagnosis includes three distinct entities based on rate:

1. A junctional escape rhythm has a rate of 40 to 60 bpm.
2. Accelerated junctional rhythm has a rate of 60 to 100 bpm.
3. Junctional ectopic tachycardia (JET) has a rate of >100 bpm.

SYNONYMS

Junctional escape rhythm
Accelerated junctional rhythm
Junctional ectopic tachycardia (JET)
Nodal rhythm disorder
Ectopic rhythm disorder
Junctional premature depolarization

ICD-10CM CODE
I49.2 Junctional premature depolarization

EPIDEMIOLOGY & DEMOGRAPHICS

INCIDENCE: Junctional rhythm occurs more commonly in children because of higher vagal tone (13% of 10- to 13-yr-old boys, 45% of 7- to 10-yr-old children, and 19% of infants have junctional rhythm during sleep). Endurance athletes have a 20% incidence of junctional rhythm, for a similar reason.

PREVALENCE: Junctional tachycardia is a rare cause of supraventricular tachycardia. It is rare in the pediatric population and even less common in adults. On the contrary, junctional rhythm is common although the prevalence is not well defined.

RISK FACTORS: Conduction system disease, heart block, digitalis intoxication, heart surgery, endocarditis.

GENETICS: There is no known hereditary component to any of the aforementioned junctional rhythms.

PHYSICAL FINDINGS & CLINICAL PRESENTATION

ESSENTIAL HISTORY:

- Previous history of syncope, presyncope, lightheadedness.
- Drugs, especially digoxin. Amount taken, time of ingestion. The digestion time is especially important because the serum digoxin level ideally should be measured at least 6 hr after ingestion to ensure accuracy. Obtain a thorough medication history to determine if any recent additions or dosing changes were made. Presence of renal failure can result in higher or even toxic serum levels of digoxin. Hypokalemia renders cardiac tissue more susceptible to the effects of digoxin and should be promptly corrected in the event of digoxin toxicity. Other medications such as beta-blockers and nondihydropyridine calcium channel blockers may also result in a junctional escape rhythm primarily by causing AV block.

SYMPTOMS:

- Lightheadedness
- Syncope
- Palpitations
- Symptoms associated with digitalis intoxication: Gastrointestinal symptoms such as anorexia, nausea, vomiting, and abdominal pain. Neurologic manifestation such as lethargy, fatigue, delirium, confusion, weakness. Visual changes: Alteration in color vision, diplopia, photophobia, decreased visual acuity

PHYSICAL EXAMINATION:

- Vital signs
- Look for evidence of hypoperfusion and end organ dysfunction
- Cannon A-waves on examination of the jugular pulse

ETIOLOGY

Junctional tachycardia can occur as a primary arrhythmia (usually in children-JET), secondary to digitalis intoxication or catecholamine intoxication, or in the setting of injury to the His bundle (e.g., after valve surgery, abscess, sarcoidosis, myocarditis, ischemia).

DIAGNOSIS

DIFFERENTIAL DIAGNOSIS

- AVNRT (atrioventricular nodal reentrant tachycardia)
- AVRT (atrioventricular reentrant tachycardia)
- Accelerated idioventricular rhythm, in the case of junctional rhythm with aberrant conduction
- Fig. 1 illustrates arrhythmias originating in the atrioventricular node

WORKUP

- Vital signs
- 12-lead ECG (Figs. 2 and 3). The rhythm is almost perfectly regular and the QRS complex is generally narrow and similar to the complex seen during sinus rhythm. Retrograde P waves with a very short interval from QRS to P wave can be seen
- History of cardiac surgery, fevers, drug ingestion

LABORATORY TESTS

- Serum digoxin concentration
- Serum potassium concentration
- Creatinine and blood urea nitrogen (BUN) to assess renal function
- Troponin
- Serum antibody testing for Lyme disease, if junctional escape rhythm is associated with AV block

IMAGING STUDIES

Echocardiogram

TREATMENT

Junctional tachycardia may be a marker for a serious underlying condition such as digitalis toxicity, post cardiac surgery, endocarditis, hypokalemia, or myocardial ischemia. Underlying conditions should be sought and corrected accordingly.

NONPHARMACOLOGIC THERAPY

- Junctional escape rhythm in the setting of sinus arrest or complete heart block without reversible cause necessitates permanent pacemaker implantation.
- Junctional ectopic tachycardia can be treated with antiarrhythmics or radiofrequency ablation.

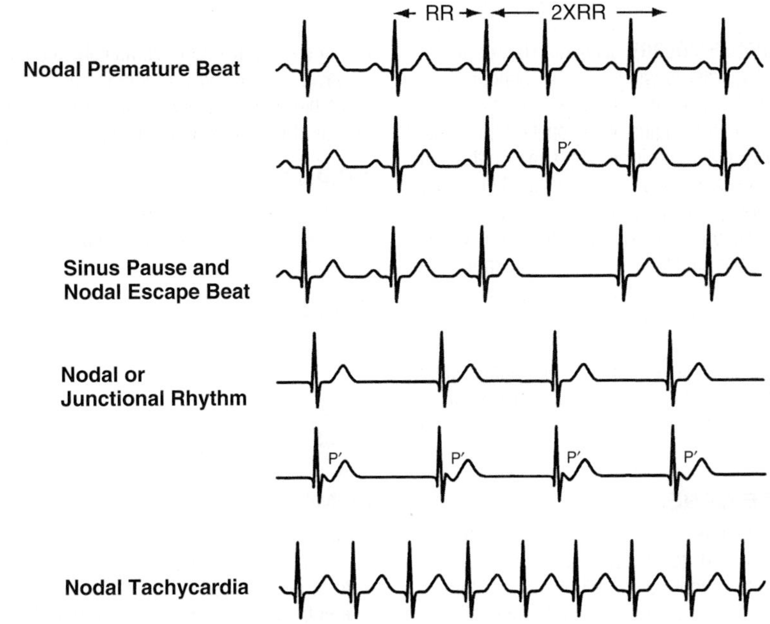

FIG. 1 Arrhythmias originating in the atrioventricular node. (From Park MK: *Park's pediatric cardiology for practitioners,* ed 6, Philadelphia, 2014, Elsevier.)

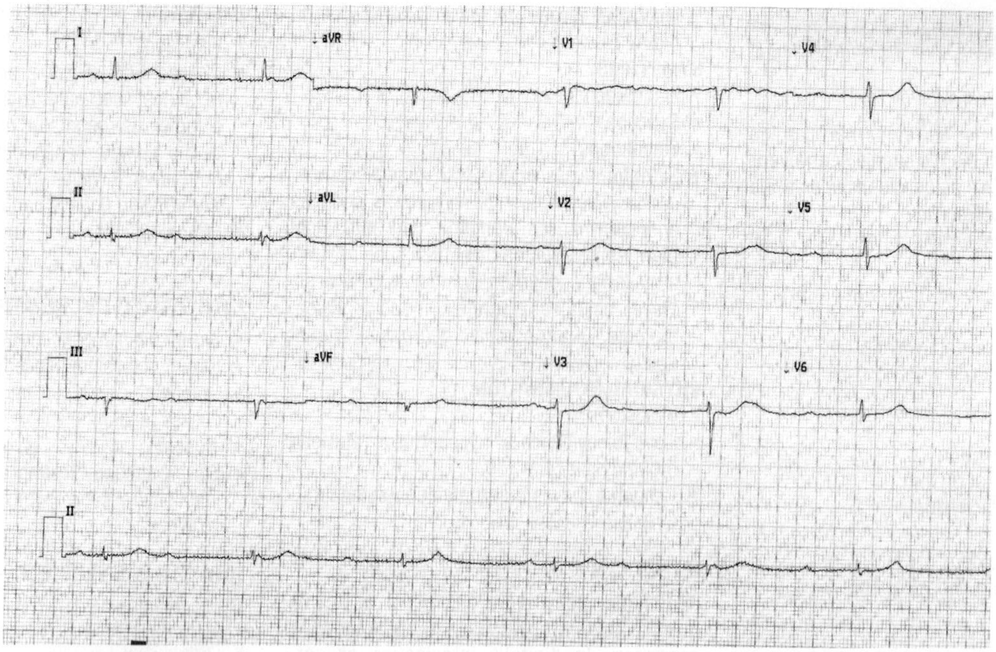

FIG. 2 Electrocardiogram of a patient with junctional rhythm and complete heart block. Note the narrow QRS complex and dissociated P waves. *aVF,* Augmented vector foot; *aVL,* augmented vector left; *aVR,* augmented vector right.

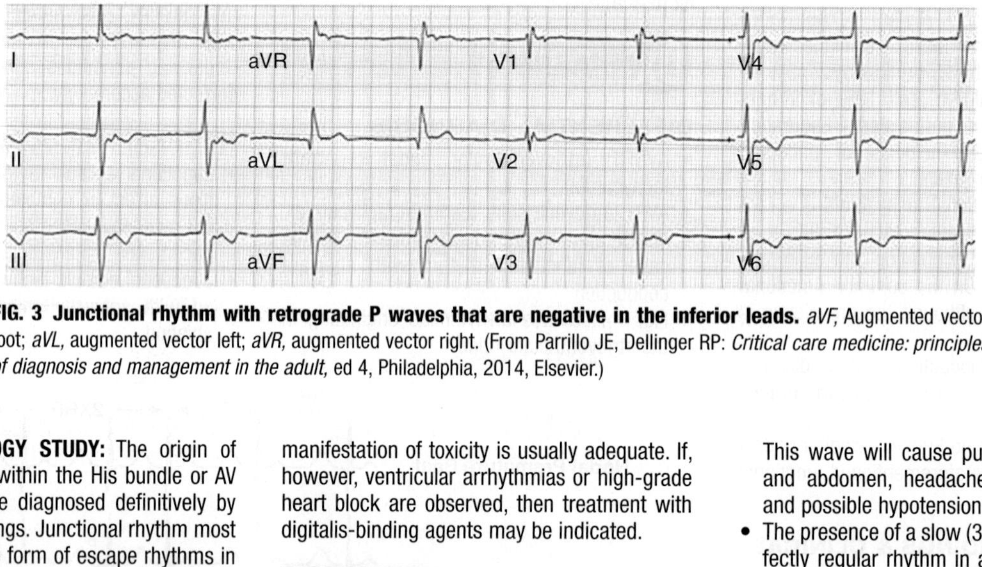

FIG. 3 Junctional rhythm with retrograde P waves that are negative in the inferior leads. *aVF,* Augmented vector foot; *aVL,* augmented vector left; *aVR,* augmented vector right. (From Parrillo JE, Dellinger RP: *Critical care medicine: principles of diagnosis and management in the adult,* ed 4, Philadelphia, 2014, Elsevier.)

ELECTROPHYSIOLOGY STUDY: The origin of this tachycardia is within the His bundle or AV node, and it can be diagnosed definitively by intracardiac recordings. Junctional rhythm most frequently takes the form of escape rhythms in the presence of sinus node dysfunction or AV nodal block, which can be diagnosed on electrophysiology (EP) study. These escape rhythms usually have a QRS morphology identical to that seen during sinus rhythm. In such cases there is no P wave before the QRS complexes. The P waves can occur simultaneously with the QRS complexes; more commonly, they are retrograde. When the junctional rhythm is faster than 100 beats/min, it is called junctional tachycardia.

ACUTE GENERAL Rx

The mainstay of managing nonparoxysmal junctional tachycardia is to correct the underlying abnormality. Withholding digitalis when junctional tachycardia is the only clinical manifestation of toxicity is usually adequate. If, however, ventricular arrhythmias or high-grade heart block are observed, then treatment with digitalis-binding agents may be indicated.

DISPOSITION

Admit to cardiac telemetry if symptomatic. Consider specialty referral to cardiac electrophysiology.

REFERRAL

Refer to cardiologist.

PEARLS & CONSIDERATIONS

COMMENTS

- Junctional rhythm often is observed in patients with AV dissociation, which can lead to atrial contraction against closed atrioventricular valves, resulting in cannon A waves. This wave will cause pulsation in the neck and abdomen, headache, cough, jaw pain and possible hypotension.
- The presence of a slow (30-40 bpm) and perfectly regular rhythm in a patient with atrial fibrillation often indicates junctional rhythm with complete heart block.

PREVENTION

N/A

SUGGESTED READINGS

Available at ExpertConsult.com

RELATED CONTENT

Digoxin Overdose (Related Key Topic)
Sick Sinus Syndrome (Related Key Topic)
Heart Block, Complete (Related Key Topic)
Heart Block, Second-Degree (Related Key Topic)

AUTHOR: **Hrak Chemchirian, MD**

BASIC INFORMATION

DEFINITION

Juvenile idiopathic arthritis (JIA), previously referred to as juvenile rheumatoid arthritis (JRA), is a diverse spectrum of chronic arthritides, involving ≥1 joint for ≥6 wk in a patient ≤16 yr of age. Other causes of arthritis must be excluded.

SYNONYMS

JIA
Juvenile rheumatoid arthritis (JRA)
Still disease (systemic JIA)

ICD-10CM CODES

M08.00	Unspecified juvenile rheumatoid arthritis of unspecified site
M08.09	Unspecified juvenile rheumatoid arthritis, multiple sites
M08.20	Juvenile rheumatoid arthritis with systemic onset, unspecified site
M08.29	Juvenile rheumatoid arthritis with systemic onset, multiple sites
M08.40	Pauciarticular juvenile rheumatoid arthritis, unspecified site

EPIDEMIOLOGY & DEMOGRAPHICS

PREVALENCE: 1 per 1000 children in the U.S.; more common in children of European ancestry

PHYSICAL FINDINGS & CLINICAL PRESENTATION

JIA is subdivided into seven categories based on the International League of Associations for Rheumatology (ILAR) classification criteria (summarized in Table 1). Characteristics of the various categories of JIA are summarized in Table 2.

- Systemic onset JIA (sJIA) (4% to 17%)
  1. Arthritis in ≥1 joint with or preceded by fever (Fig. E1) of at least 2-wk duration that is quotidian (once daily) for at least 3 days and associated with at least one of the following: (1) evanescent erythematous rash (Fig. E2); (2) generalized lymphadenopathy; (3) hepatomegaly, splenomegaly, or both; and (4) serositis
- Oligoarticular JIA (Fig. E3) (27% to 56%)
  1. Arthritis in <4 joints in the first 6 mo of disease. There are two subtypes:
     a. Persistent: ≤4 joints throughout the disease course
     b. Extended: ≤4 joints during the first 6 mo extending to >4 joints after 6 mo
- Polyarthritis, rheumatoid factor (RF) negative (11% to 28%)
  1. Arthritis in >5 joints during first 6 mo of the disease with negative RF
- Polyarthritis, RF positive (2% to 7%)
  1. Arthritis involves ≥5 joints during first 6 mo of the disease with positive RF on >2 tests run 3 mo apart
  2. Anticyclic citrullinated (CCP) antibodies may also be present
  3. Most similar to adult rheumatoid arthritis; most likely to progress
- Psoriatic arthritis (2% to 11%)
  1. Psoriasis and arthritis or psoriasis and ≥2 of the following:
     a. Dactylitis, nail pitting, onycholysis, and psoriasis in a first-degree relative
- Enthesitis-related arthritis (3% to 11%)
  1. Arthritis or enthesitis and ≥2 of the following:
     a. Sacroiliac tenderness, positive HLA-B27 (human leukocyte antigen B27), male age >6 yr, acute anterior uveitis, or first-degree relative with HLA-B27–associated disease
- Undifferentiated arthritis (11% to 21%)
  1. Fulfills criteria in ≥2 categories above, or none of them

ETIOLOGY

Genetically susceptible individuals may develop an inappropriate immune response toward a self-antigen after exposure to an environmental trigger. Variants in HLA, PTPN22, and STAT4 loci may be associated with disease.

Dx DIAGNOSIS

DIFFERENTIAL DIAGNOSIS

- Infection: Viral (parvovirus, toxic synovitis) or bacterial (Lyme, osteomyelitis, septic joints)

TABLE 1 Overview of the Main Features of the Subtypes of Juvenile Idiopathic Arthritis

ILAR Subtype	Peak Age of Onset (yr)	Female:Male; % of All JIA	Arthritis Pattern	Extraarticular Features	Investigations	Notes on Therapy
Systemic arthritis	2-4	1:1; ~10% of JIA cases	Polyarticular, often knees, wrists, and ankles; also fingers, neck, and hips	Daily fever; evanescent rash; pericarditis; pleuritis	Anemia; WBC↑↑; ESR↑↑; CRP↑↑; ferritin↑ platelets↑↑ (normal or ↑ in MAS)	Less responsive to standard treatment with MTX and anti-TNF agents; consider IL-1Ra in resistant cases
Oligoarthritis	>6	4:1; 50%-60% of JIA (but ethnic variation)	Knees ++; ankles, fingers +	Uveitis in ~30%	ANA positive in 60%; other tests usually normal; may have mildly ↑ ESR/CRP	NSAIDs and intraarticular steroids; occasionally require MTX
Polyarthritis, RF negative	6-7	3:1; 30% of JIA cases	Symmetric or asymmetric; small and large joints; cervical spine; TMJ	Uveitis in ~10%	ANA positive in 40%; RF negative; ESR ↑ or; ↑↑ CRP↑/normal; mild anemia	Standard therapy with MTX and NSAIDs, then if nonresponsive, anti-TNF agents or other biologics
Polyarthritis, RF positive	9-12	9:1; >10% of JIA cases	Aggressive symmetric polyarthritis	Rheumatoid nodules in 10%; low-grade fever	RF positive; ESR ↑↑; CRP ↑/normal; mild anemia	Long-term remission unlikely; early aggressive therapy is warranted
Psoriatic arthritis	7-10	2:1; >10% of JIA cases	Asymmetric arthritis of small- or medium-sized joints	Uveitis in 10%; psoriasis in 50%	ANA positive in 50%; ESR ↑; CRP ↑/normal; mild anemia	NSAIDs and intraarticular steroids; second-line agents less commonly
Enthesitis-related arthritis	9-12	1:7; 10% of JIA cases	Predominantly lower limb joints affected; sometimes axial skeleton (but less than adult AS)	Acute anterior uveitis; association with reactive arthritis and IBD	80% HLA-B27	NSAIDs and intraarticular steroids; consider sulfasalazine as alternative to MTX

ANA, Antinuclear antibody; *AS,* ankylosing spondylitis; *CRP,* C-reactive protein; *ESR,* erythrocyte sedimentation rate; *HLA-B27,* human leukocyte antigen B27; *IBD,* inflammatory bowel disease; *ILAR,* International League of Associations for Rheumatology; *IL-1Ra,* interleukin-1 receptor antagonist; *JIA,* juvenile idiopathic arthritis; *MAS,* macrophage activation syndrome; *MTX,* methotrexate; *NSAID,* nonsteroidal antiinflammatory drug; *RF,* rheumatoid factor; *TMJ,* temporomandibular joint; *TNF,* tumor necrosis factor; *WBC,* white blood cell count.
From Firestein G et al: *Kelley's textbook of rheumatology,* ed 9, Philadelphia, 2013, WB Saunders.

TABLE 2 Characteristics of the Various Categories of Juvenile Idiopathic Arthritis

Category	Age at Onset	Affected Joints	Systemic Features	Major Complications
Oligoarticular persistent	Early childhood	Large joints, asymmetric (knee, ankle, wrist, elbow, temporomandibular, cervical spine)	No	Chronic uveitis Local growth disturbances
Oligoarticular extended	Early childhood	Same as above, but more than four joints involved after the first 6 mo of disease	No	Chronic uveitis Local growth disturbances
Polyarticular RF negative	Throughout childhood	Any, often symmetric, often small joints	Malaise (subfebrile)	Chronic uveitis Local growth disturbances
Polyarticular RF positive	Teenage years	Any, usually symmetric and involving small joints	Malaise (subfebrile)	Local growth disturbances and articular damage
Systemic	Throughout childhood	Any (not necessarily at disease onset)	High fever, rash, polyserositis, marked acute-phase response	Acute: Macrophage activation syndrome Chronic: General growth disturbance, amyloidosis
Psoriatic	Late childhood	Spine, lower extremities, distal interphalangeal joints, dactylitis		Psoriasis Local growth disturbances
Enthesitis related	Late childhood	Spine, sacroiliac, lower extremities, thoracic cage joints	Inflammatory bowel disease	Acute symptomatic uveitis

RF, Rheumatoid factor.
From Hochberg MC: *Rheumatology*, ed 7, Philadelphia, 2019, Elsevier.

TABLE 3 Differential Diagnosis of Pediatric Arthralgia/Arthritis

Type of Condition	Examples
Infections	Bacterial arthritis and osteomyelitis Borreliosis (Lyme disease) Viral and mycoplasmal arthritis Tuberculosis
Postinfectious conditions	Rheumatic fever Poststreptococcal arthritis Postenteritis and other reactive arthritis *(Salmonella, Campylobacter, Chlamydia)*
Noninflammatory conditions	Hypermobility and Ehlers-Danlos syndrome Growing pains, trauma, patellofemoral and other overuse syndromes Osgood-Schlatter disease and other juvenile osteochondroses Legg-Calvé-Perthes disease Slipped capital femoral epiphysis Foreign body synovitis Other congenital and genetic disorders of supportive tissue
Hematologic disorders	Sickle cell anemia Hemophilia von Willebrand disease
Systemic inflammatory disorders	Juvenile systemic lupus erythematosus Juvenile dermatomyositis Mixed connective tissue disease Scleroderma Vasculitis (e.g., Henoch-Schönlein purpura, Kawasaki disease, Behçet disease)
Autoinflammatory disorders	Cryopyrin-associated periodic syndrome Familial Mediterranean fever Other monogenic diseases (e.g., mevalonate kinase deficiency [hyperimmunoglobulinemia D], Blau syndrome, tumor necrosis factor receptor–associated periodic syndrome) Chronic recurrent multifocal osteomyelitis Periodic fever, aphthous stomatitis, pharyngitis, and adenitis (PFAPA syndrome)
Malignancies	Leukemia Neuroblastoma Localized bone tumors
Pain	Complex regional pain syndrome Pain amplification syndromes and fibromyalgia Nonspecific musculoskeletal pain
Miscellaneous conditions	Primary immunodeficiencies Sarcoidosis

From Hochberg MC: *Rheumatology*, ed 7, Philadelphia, 2019, Elsevier.

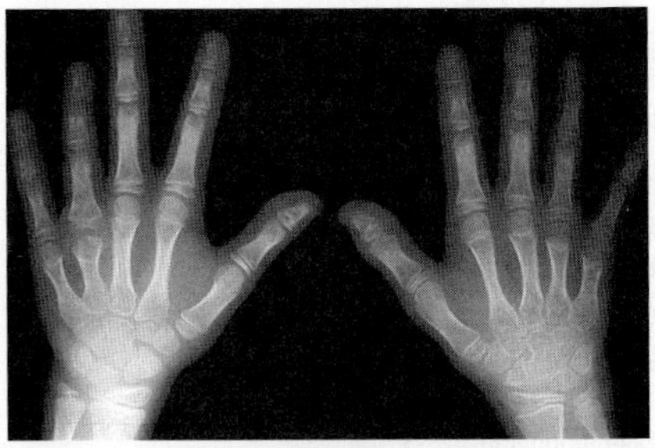

FIG. 4 Juvenile idiopathic arthritis (JIA). Radiograph showing oligoarticular-onset JIA in an 8-yr-old. Epiphyseal destruction and undergrowth of the third metacarpophalangeal joint of the left hand are seen, as well as overgrowth of the carpal bones of the right wrist compared with the left wrist. Also note the widened appearance of the third phalanges caused by periosteal new bone formation. (From Hochberg MC et al: *Rheumatology,* ed 5, St Louis, 2011, Mosby.)

- Inflammation: Lupus, serum sickness, inflammatory bowel disease
- Reactive: Post-streptococcal, rheumatic fever
- Malignancy: Leukemia, bone tumors

Table 3 summarizes conditions with arthralgia/arthritis that might be confused with JIA

LABORATORY TESTS

- No single diagnostic test. Rule out other causes of arthritis
- Elevated sedimentation rate and C-reactive protein; high ferritin
- Mild anemia, leukocytosis
- Rheumatoid factor
- Antinuclear antibodies: Elevation associated with ocular complications
- Pancytopenia, a consumptive coagulopathy, elevated ferritin, and elevated liver enzymes are concerning for macrophage activation syndrome (MAS) in sJIA

IMAGING STUDIES

- Radiographs show soft tissue swelling and periarticular osteopenia early in the disease (Fig. 4).
- Joint destruction (Fig. 5) is less frequent, but bony erosion and cyst formation may be present.

Rx TREATMENT

NONPHARMACOLOGIC THERAPY

Collaboration among the patient's pediatrician, rheumatologist, orthopedist, and physical therapist is essential.

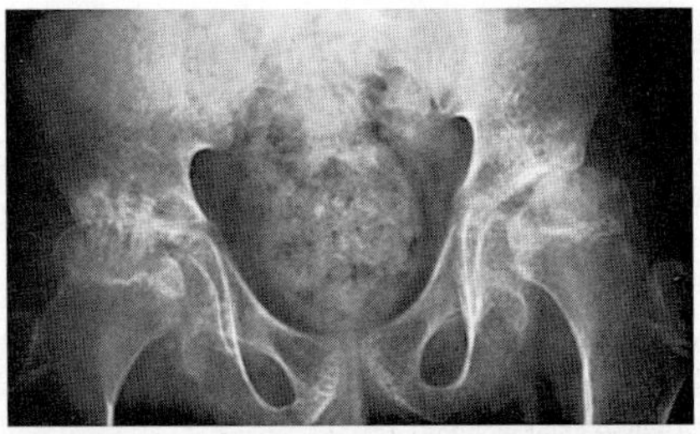

FIG. 5 Severe hip disease in a 13-yr-old boy with active, systemic-onset juvenile idiopathic arthritis. Radiograph shows destruction of the femoral head and acetabula, joint space narrowing, and subluxation of left hip. The patient had received corticosteroids systemically for 9 yr. (From Kliegman RM et al: *Nelson textbook of pediatrics,* ed 19, Philadelphia, 2011, WB Saunders.)

CHRONIC GENERAL Rx

Patients may require combinations of these therapies.

- NSAIDs: Should be used in conjunction with other agents
- DMARDs (disease-modifying antirheumatic drugs): Methotrexate, leflunomide, sulfasalazine
  1. Initial therapy with a DMARD is strongly recommended over NSAID monotherapy
  2. Required by two thirds of children
  3. Axial involvement is less responsive to methotrexate
- Biologics: Improve morbidity associated with JIA. Individual subtypes show different responses to therapy
  1. Tumor necrosis factor antagonists such as etanercept and adalimumab
  2. T-cell modulator, abatacept
  3. IL-1 (anakinra) and IL-6 antagonists (tocilizumab) useful in sJIA

  Meta-analysis of randomized controlled trials did not show statistically significant differences in the efficacy or safety profile of these agents.
- Chronic systemic corticosteroids should be limited when possible.
- Major medications and indications for treatment of JIA are summarized in Table 4. Fig. 6 illustrates an algorithm for medical treatment of oligoarticular-onset JIA. Treatment of polyarticular-onset JIA is illustrated in Fig. 7, and treatment of systemic onset JIA in Fig. 8.

DISPOSITION

- More than 50% continue to have active disease into adulthood.
- Patients with persistent oligoarticular disease are most likely to achieve remission, whereas those who are RF positive are least likely to achieve remission.
- Macrophage activation syndrome is a life-threatening complication of sJIA.
- Asymmetric joint involvement can lead to growth failure and limb length discrepancies.

REFERRAL

- Early rheumatology consultation
- Ophthalmology consultation at diagnosis and at least annually
- Children ages <7 yr, with + ANA are at the highest risk for ocular inflammation (uveitis) and require screening every 3 to 4 mo

PEARLS & CONSIDERATIONS

COMMENTS

JIA is an autoinflammatory disease with a strong genetic component. Children with JIA are at risk of permanent joint damage and decreased health-related quality of life. Normalization of the immune response early in the disease can limit disease progression, and early institution of DMARD therapy is important for optimal outcomes. Immunomodulators have been shown to improve therapy in refractory disease. Children with JIA have an increased rate of malignancy compared with the general population.

SUGGESTED READINGS

Available at ExpertConsult.com

RELATED CONTENT

Juvenile Rheumatoid Arthritis (Patient Information)

AUTHOR: **Michelle C. Maciag, MD**

TABLE 4 Major Medications and Indications for Treatment of Juvenile Idiopathic Arthritis

Medication	Arthritis Subtype	Indication
NSAIDs	All types	Symptomatic: Pain, stiffness, serositis, antiinflammatory in mild cases
Intraarticular corticosteroids	All types, mainly oligoarthritis	Injection of few active joints
Systemic corticosteroids	Systemic, polyarthritis	Fever, serositis, bridging medication, MAS
Methotrexate	All types; less effective for systemic and enthesitis-related axial disease	Disease modifying
Leflunomide	Polyarthritis	Disease modifying
Sulfasalazine	Oligoarthritis, polyarthritis, enthesitis-related peripheral disease	Disease modifying
Cyclosporine	Systemic	MAS
Thalidomide	Systemic	Biologic modifier
Anti-TNF (etanercept infliximab, adalimumab, golimumab, certolizumab)	Polyarthritis, enthesitis-related, uveitis (infliximab, adalimumab), less effective for systemic disease	Biologic modifier
Abatacept	Polyarthritis	Biologic modifier
Anti–IL-1 (anakinra, canakinumab, rilonacept)	Systemic	Biologic modifier, MAS
Anti–IL-6 (tocilizumab)	Systemic, polyarthritis	Biologic modifier
IVIG	Systemic	Steroid sparing, MAS

IL-1, Interleukin-1; *IVIG,* intravenous immune globulin; *MAS,* macrophage activation syndrome; *NSAID,* nonsteroidal antiinflammatory drug; *TNF,* tumor necrosis factor.
From Hochberg MC: *Rheumatology,* ed 7, Philadelphia, 2019, Elsevier.

ALGORITHM FOR MEDICAL TREATMENT OF OLIGOARTICULAR-ONSET JUVENILE IDIOPATHIC ARTHRITIS (JIA)

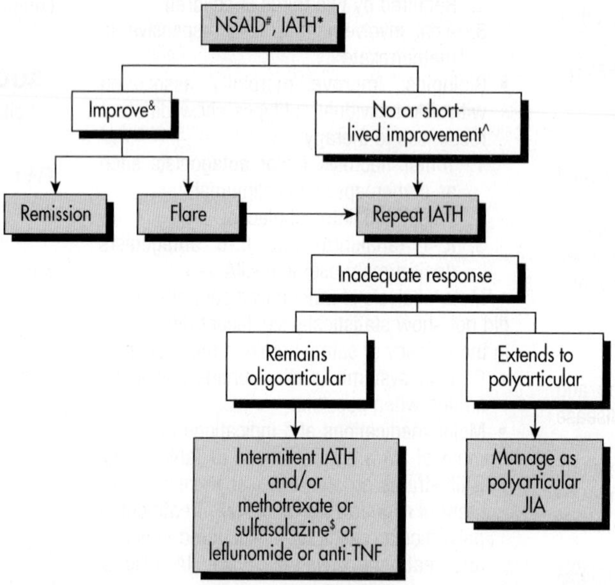

*Prefer early IATH if knee monoarthritis and/or patient has local complications: contractures, leg length discrepancy, significant muscle atrophy
#NSAID trial for 4 to 6 weeks
^ ≤ 4 months
$ Consider sulfasalazine for older boys with enthesitis/peripheral arthritis
& Aim for inactive disease/remission or at least a JADAS score <2

FIG. 6 Medical treatment of the oligoarticular type of juvenile idiopathic arthritis (JIA). *IATH,* Intraarticular triamcinolone hexacetonide; *JADAS,* Juvenile Arthritis Disease Activity Score; *NSAID,* nonsteroidal antiinflammatory drug; *TNF,* tumor necrosis factor. (From Hochberg MC: *Rheumatology,* ed 7, Philadelphia, 2019, Elsevier.)

ALGORITHM FOR MEDICAL TREATMENT OF POLYARTICULAR-ONSET JUVENILE IDIOPATHIC ARTHRITIS (JIA)

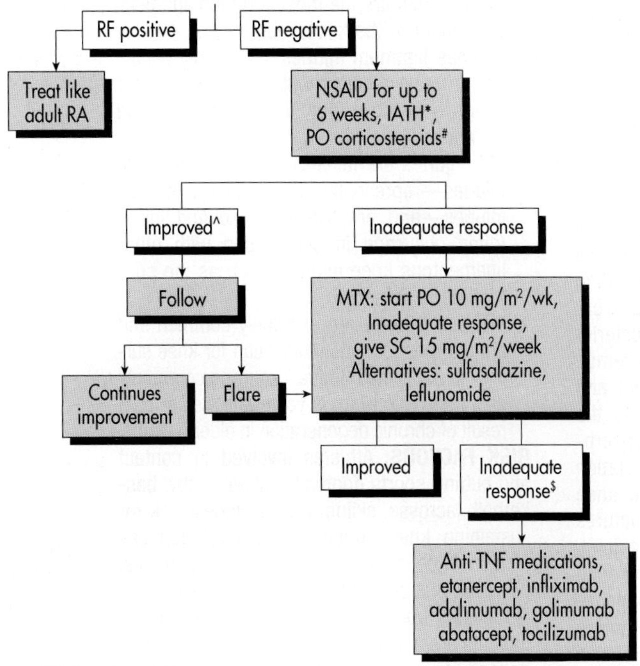

* IATH for selected joints
\# PO steroids can be considered as bridging medicine or during significant flares
$ If fails to respond to one anti-TNF agent, consider changing to another or to abatacept
^ Improved: pediatric ACR 70 response (or JADAS score <3.8)

FIG. 7 Medical treatment of the polyarticular type of juvenile idiopathic arthritis (JIA). *ACR70,* American College of Rheumatology 70% improvement; *IATH,* intraarticular triamcinolone hexacetonide; *JADAS,* Juvenile Arthritis Disease Activity Score; *MTX,* methotrexate; *NSAID,* nonsteroidal antiinflammatory drug; *PO,* oral; *SC,* subcutaneous; *RA,* rheumatoid arthritis; *RF,* rheumatoid factor; *TNF,* tumor necrosis factor. (From Hochberg MC: *Rheumatology,* ed 7, Philadelphia, 2019, Elsevier.)

ALGORITHM FOR MEDICAL TREATMENT OF SYSTEMIC-ONSET JUVENILE IDIOPATHIC ARTHRITIS (JIA)

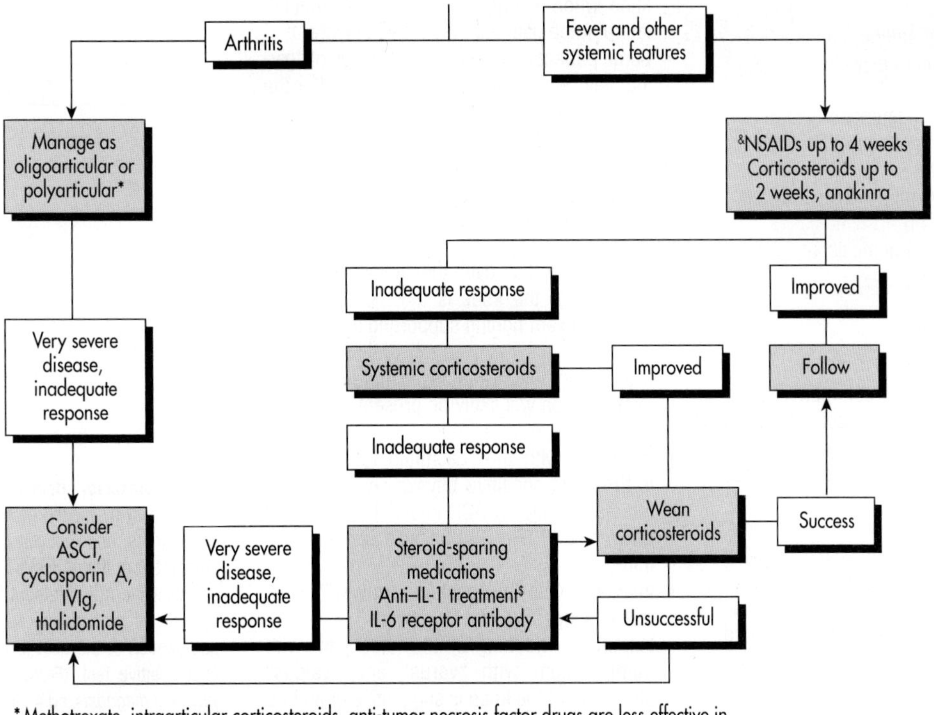

* Methotrexate, intraarticular corticosteroids, anti-tumor necrosis factor drugs are less effective in systemic-onset JIA; anti-IL-1 and IL-6 receptor antibody may be more effective
$ Anti IL-1 treatments include anakinra, rilonacept, canakinumab
& Depends on physician global assessment and number of active joints

FIG. 8 Medical treatment of systemic juvenile idiopathic arthritis (JIA). *ASCT,* Autologous stem cell transplantation; *IL,* interleukin; *IVIG,* intravenous immunoglobulin; *NSAID,* nonsteroidal antiinflammatory drug; *TNF,* tumor necrosis factor. (From Hochberg MC: *Rheumatology,* ed 7, Philadelphia, 2019, Elsevier.)

BASIC INFORMATION

DEFINITION

The topic of "knee sprain" refers to injury sustained to a variety of ligaments and soft tissue supportive structures surrounding the knee, including the anterior and posterior cruciate ligaments (ACL/PCL), the medial and lateral collateral ligaments (MCL/LCL), and the medial and lateral menisci. In addition to providing rotational stability, the ACL and PCL work in concert to prevent anterior and posterior translation of the tibia relative to the femur, while the MCL and LCL prevent medial and lateral translation of the tibia relative to the femur. The menisci function as "shock absorbers" and contribute to the stable articulation of the femur and tibia throughout the knee range of motion. Together, these structures provide static stabilization of the knee joint. Injury to these structures often occur in young athletes who suffer either a twisting, noncontact injury or a direct blow to the knee during sport. Meniscal injuries, however, can also develop as a result of chronic degeneration, and can often present in older individuals as knee pain associated with activity (walking up and down stairs, running, or biking) without a clear traumatic event.

SYNONYMS

Anterior or posterior cruciate ligament tear
Medial or lateral collateral ligament tear
Medial or lateral meniscal tear
Internal derangement of the knee

ICD-10CM CODES	
S83.519 (S83.512A, S83.511A)	Sprain of anterior cruciate ligament of unspecified knee (left, right)
S83.529A (S83.522A, S83.521A)	Sprain of posterior cruciate ligament of unspecified knee (left, right)
S83.242A (S83.241A)	Tear of medial meniscus of left knee (right)
S83.282A (S83.281A)	Tear of lateral meniscus of left knee (right)

EPIDEMIOLOGY & DEMOGRAPHICS

- ACL tears are extremely common injuries, the vast majority of which occur in young athletes, most commonly among female athletes (5:1 female/male ratio in college-aged individuals).
- PCL tears also occur in younger patients, occurring in both the athletic setting (often associated with other ligamentous injuries) and the traumatic setting, such as motor vehicle collisions when the dashboard is driven into a flexed knee ("dashboard injury").
- MCL injuries are the most common ligamentous injury to the knee, representing 40% of all knee ligament injuries, commonly occurring in male athletes with a highest risk for injury in skiing, rugby, football, soccer, and ice hockey.
- LCL injuries are far less common than MCL injuries—representing less than 2% of knee injuries—and are rarely an isolated injury (often occurring in conjunction with other ligamentous knee injuries, such as the posterolateral corner).
- Meniscal injuries are extremely common and are the most common indication for knee surgery in the United States, occurring commonly as a traumatic event in young athletes or as a result of chronic degeneration in older patients.

RISK FACTORS: Athletes involved in contact and cutting sports (football, soccer, rugby, basketball, lacrosse, skiing) are at highest risk for sustaining knee sprains. In general, females sustain knee sprains more often than males, however the discrepancy between sexes varies based upon the injured structure. Older patients are also at increased risk of developing degenerative meniscus tears, often as a result of repetitive activity or in conjunction with other knee pathology (such as osteoarthritis).

PHYSICAL FINDINGS & CLINICAL PRESENTATION

Knee sprains can involve either one or several supporting structures of the knee, and therefore the diagnosis can be challenging:

- Patients may remember an isolated traumatic event (tackled playing football, landing awkwardly when jumping in basketball, twisting knee when skiing) or may endorse medial/lateral knee pain with repetitive activity.
- Some patients may endorse episodes of "giving way" when performing activities after the injury occurred, which is common in injuries to the ACL, PCL, MCL, and LCL.
- Some patients may endorse the feeling of "catching and locking" with range of motion of the knee, which is common in meniscal injuries.
- Point tenderness over the medial or lateral joint line of the knee is the most sensitive physical exam finding supporting a meniscus tear.
- If the injury was traumatic in nature, a knee joint effusion will likely be present on clinical exam.
- Instability with the "Lachman test" (Fig. 1) is the most sensitive physical exam finding for diagnosing an ACL injury. The "anterior drawer test" (Fig. 2) can also suggest ACL injury.
- Instability with the "posterior drawer"(Fig. 3) test is suggestive of a PCL injury.
- Instability (widening of the knee joint with manipulation) with "varus" and "valgus" stress about the knee is suggestive of an LCL

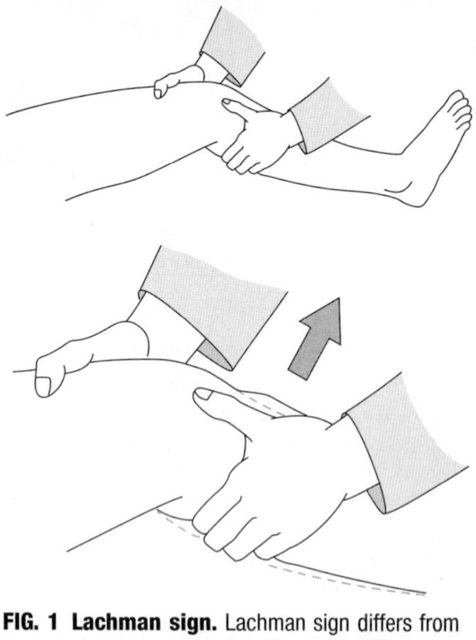

FIG. 1 Lachman sign. Lachman sign differs from the anterior drawer sign (see Fig. 2) by the position of the knee during testing. In Lachman test the hip is extended and the knee flexed at only 20 degrees. The clinician grasps the lower thigh with one hand and the upper calf with the other, pulling forward on the tibia to stress the ligament and reveal the abnormal anterior subluxation of the tibia *(arrow)*. (From McGee S: *Evidence-based physical diagnosis*, ed 4, Philadelphia, 2016, Elsevier.)

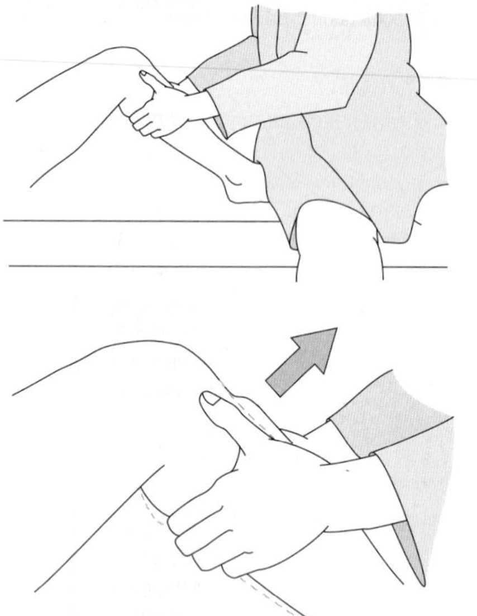

FIG. 2 Anterior drawer sign. The patient lies supine with hip flexed at 45 degrees, knee flexed at 90 degrees, and foot flat on the table. The clinician sits on top of the patient's foot to stabilize it and then stresses the ACL ligament by grasping the patient's upper calf and pulling forward. Abnormal anterior subluxation of the tibia *(arrow)* with a soft end point is a positive test. (From McGee S: *Evidence-based physical diagnosis*, ed 4, Philadelphia, 2016, Elsevier.)

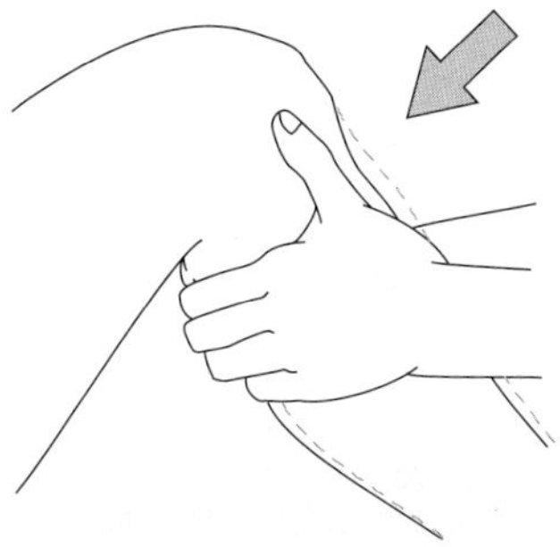

FIG. 3 Posterior drawer sign. With the patient positioned as for the anterior drawer sign (see Fig. 2), the clinician pushes posteriorly on the patient's upper calf. In the posterior cruciate ligament-deficient knee, this force reveals an abnormal posterior tibial movement *(arrow)* with a soft endpoint. (From McGee S: *Evidence-based physical diagnosis,* ed 4, Philadelphia, 2016, Elsevier.)

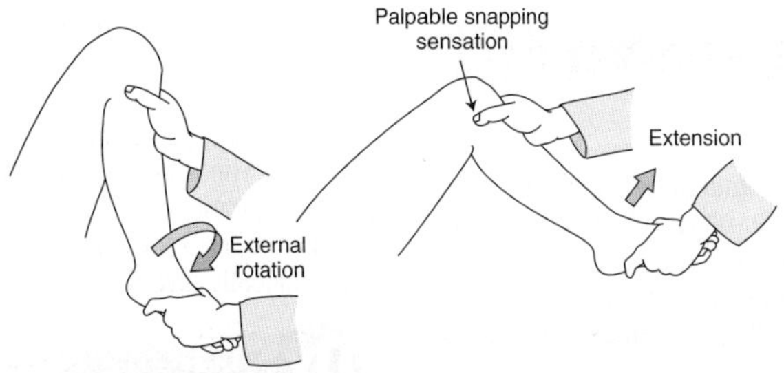

FIG. 4 McMurray test. The clinician flexes the patient's knee fully against the buttock and rotates the tibia (by grasping the patient's foot and ankle). The purpose of rotation is to bring the torn meniscal fragment, located on the posterior half of the meniscus, anterior to the curved surface of the femoral condyle: External rotation brings forward the medial meniscus; internal rotation, the lateral meniscus. Therefore, this figure depicts testing of the medial meniscus: The clinician places a free hand over the medial joint line, fully flexes the patient's knee, and then rotates the tibia externally. The clinician slowly extends the knee while maintaining this rotational force, thereby forcing the medial femoral condyle to glide forward on the tibia and over any torn fragment of meniscus. When the femur passes over the torn fragment, a palpable snapping sensation may be detected at the medial joint line (a positive test). To test the lateral meniscus, the clinician repeats the test while internally rotating the knee and palpating the lateral joint line. (From McGee S: *Evidence-based physical diagnosis,* ed 4, Philadelphia, 2016, Elsevier.)

and MCL injury, respectively. This test performed at various positions of the knee (30 degrees of flexion versus full extension) can also suggest injury to additional ligaments about the knee, such as the ACL and PCL.
- The "McMurray test" (Fig. 4)—palpating the knee joint line on a flexed knee and slowly extending the knee while rotating the leg—a palpable pop/click can correlate with meniscus injury.

ETIOLOGY

- When the traumatic force applied to the knee exceeds the supportive force of any of the surrounding ligaments, these ligaments will tear and result in knee instability.
- Degenerative meniscal injuries occur as a result of wear from repetitive activities accumulating over years (in combination with a less compliant meniscus that develops with age), leading to weakening and eventual tear of the meniscus.

Dx DIAGNOSIS

DIFFERENTIAL DIAGNOSIS

- In a traumatic setting, fracture of the tibia, femur, and patella should always be considered.
- Quadriceps tendon or patellar tendon tear: Can occur in young athletes or older patients after traumatic injury.
- Osteochondral defect: Occurs in young athletes often due to traumatic injury.
- Knee osteoarthritis: Often is present with degenerative meniscus tears in older population and can contribute to symptoms.

WORKUP

Diagnosis of knee sprain may often be suspected from history and physical examination.

IMAGING STUDIES

- X-rays are important in identifying other causes of pain such as fractures and arthritis. Generally, they should be ordered initially when working up knee pain.
- MRI is frequently used to assist in the diagnosis of soft tissue injuries about the knee and often demonstrates both partial and complete tears of the menisci, ACL, PCL, MCL, and LCL. MRI can often reveal bony contusions related to the traumatic injury. MRI is extremely sensitive and specific in diagnosing soft tissue injuries about the knee.
- In the event of continued knee pain suspicious for meniscus or cruciate ligament injury with inconclusive MRI, a diagnostic arthroscopy can be performed to confirm the diagnosis.

Rx TREATMENT

NONSURGICAL THERAPY

Nonsurgical therapy often involves a combination of activity modification (avoiding activities that cause pain), antiinflammatory medications for pain control, and physical therapy for strengthening the muscles about the knee to provide enhanced stability. For meniscal injuries, nonsurgical management is often the first line of treatment, with surgical intervention reserved for patients who do not respond to this management strategy. MCL and LCL tears can often be successfully managed in similar fashion. Patients typically return to their previous level activity as their symptomatic control allows.

SURGICAL TREATMENTS

Surgical management is often reserved for younger patients with traumatic injuries to the ACL, PCL, and various types of meniscal injuries that are unlikely to improve with conservative management (bucket handle tears, meniscal root tears). Due to the poor vascular supply to the ACL, healing of the torn ligament is unlikely, therefore surgical reconstruction of the ligament is often performed. For meniscal injuries, surgical intervention often involves knee arthroscopy with either debridement or repair of the torn portion of the meniscus performed based upon the characteristics of the tear (location, size, orientation).

ACUTE GENERAL Rx

Nonsteroidal antiinflammatory drugs (NSAIDs) are good adjuncts to treatment that expedite the recovery process by decreasing edema, inflammation, and pain.

REFERRAL

With concern for knee sprain, referral to an orthopedic surgeon should be expedited, especially in young athletes with ACL, PCL, and significant meniscal tears, as these often require surgical intervention.

PEARLS & CONSIDERATIONS

COMMENTS

- Knee sprains can be significant injuries to the young athlete, with injuries that require surgical intervention (ACL tears, significant meniscus tears) often requiring up to 6 mo to 1 yr of recovery and rehabilitation before safely returning to sport.
- It should also be noted that with the general population remaining active later into life, knee sprains are becoming more common in the older population and should be considered in the workup of knee pain when encountering older patients.

SUGGESTED READINGS

Available at ExpertConsult.com

AUTHORS: **Stephen E. Maracaccio, MD,** and **Paul Fadale, MD**

BASIC INFORMATION

DEFINITION

Labyrinthitis is a peripheral vestibulopathy characterized by acute onset of vertigo usually associated with nausea and vomiting. It can be associated with hearing loss and gait abnormalities and may be either serous or purulent.

SYNONYMS

Acute labyrinthitis
Acute vestibular neuronopathy
Vestibular neuronitis
Viral neurolabyrinthitis

ICD-10CM CODES

H83.09	Labyrinthitis, unspecified ear
H81.23	Vestibular neuronitis, bilateral
H83.01	Labyrinthitis, right ear
H83.02	Labyrinthitis, left ear
H83.03	Labyrinthitis, bilateral

EPIDEMIOLOGY & DEMOGRAPHICS

INCIDENCE (IN U.S.): Most common cause of prolonged spontaneous vertigo associated with nausea at any age
PREDOMINANT AGE: Any

PHYSICAL FINDINGS & CLINICAL PRESENTATION

CLINICAL PRESENTATION:

- Vertigo, nausea, and vomiting with onset over several hours.
- Symptoms usually peak within 24 hr, then resolve gradually over several weeks.
- During the first day, the patient usually has difficulty focusing the eyes because of spontaneous nystagmus.
- Usually has benign course with complete recovery within 1 to 3 mo, although older patients may have intractable dizziness that persists for many months.

PHYSICAL FINDINGS:

- Nystagmus
- Nausea
- Vomiting
- Vertigo worsening with head movement
- Abnormal caloric ENG tests
- May have hearing loss in the affected ear or ears
- Normal otoscopic exam typically
- Normal neurologic exam; may have signs of vestibular loss, such as a positive head thrust test

ETIOLOGY

Symptoms often preceded for 1 to 2 wk by a viral-like illness. Labyrinthitis may be either bacterial or viral and may be either tympanogenic (i.e., resulting from spread of infection into the inner ear from the middle ear, antrum, or petrous apex), meningogenic, or hematogenic from encephalitis or brain abscess. The round window membrane is considered the most likely pathway of inflammatory mediators from the middle to the inner ear that subsequently give rise to labyrinthitis.

DIAGNOSIS

DIFFERENTIAL DIAGNOSIS

- Acute labyrinthine ischemia (ischemic stroke of the labyrinthine artery)
- Labyrinthine fistula
- Benign paroxysmal positional vertigo
- Ménière disease
- Cholesteatoma
- Drug-induced vestibulocochlear nerve damage
- Vestibulocochlear nerve (cranial nerve VIII) tumor
- Head trauma
- Vertebrobasilar stroke
- Dehiscence of the superior semicircular canal

WORKUP

- Otoscopic examination
- Neurologic examination, with close attention to cranial nerves
- Bedside test of vestibular function, specifically head thrust or head heave test
- Audiogram if symptoms accompanied by hearing loss
- Caloric test if presentation is atypical

LABORATORY TESTS

- Routine laboratory tests are generally not helpful.
- If there is a history of significant emesis, check electrolytes, BUN, and creatinine.

IMAGING STUDIES

- Imaging studies are usually not necessary.
- Gadolinium-enhanced MRI may show enhancement of bony labyrinth. MRI of the brain with and without contrast with fine cuts through the internal auditory canal is indicated if there is an abnormal cranial nerve exam, headache, concern for stroke, or suspicion of cranial nerve VIII nerve tumor.
- Head CT with fine cuts through temporal bones is indicated if there is a history of trauma or suspicion of cholesteatoma.

TREATMENT

NONPHARMACOLOGIC THERAPY

- Reassurance
- Initial bed rest, then encourage increase in activity as tolerated

ACUTE GENERAL Rx

- Treatment is with antiemetics such as promethazine or ondansetron; vestibular suppressants such as the antihistamines meclizine or diphenhydramine; the anticholinergic scopolamine; and the benzodiazepines diazepam or lorazepam. These medications should only be continued for a few days during the acute phase. Some of these medications, especially scopolamine, should be used with caution in the elderly. Methylprednisolone 100 mg per day for 3 days, with slow taper over 3 wk.
- Valacyclovir has not been shown to be helpful.

CHRONIC Rx

- No specific pharmacologic chronic therapy.
- Vestibular rehabilitation is useful for patients with persistent symptoms.

DISPOSITION

Usually does not require hospital admission unless the patient is unable to tolerate oral intake of liquids

REFERRAL

- Refer if symptoms persist or neurologic abnormalities are present.
- Consider vestibular rehabilitation, particularly in the elderly.

PEARLS & CONSIDERATIONS

COMMENTS

Labyrinthitis is a term that usually implies peripheral vestibulopathy associated with hearing loss. The term *vestibular neuronitis* is typically used when hearing is not affected. Despite this technical distinction, many physicians use these terms interchangeably.

RELATED CONTENT

Labyrinthitis (Patient Information)
Benign Paroxysmal Positional Vertigo (Related Key Topic)
Vestibular Neuronitis (Related Key Topic)

AUTHOR: **Joseph S. Kass, MD, JD, FAAN**

BASIC INFORMATION

DEFINITION

Lactose intolerance is the insufficient concentration of lactase enzyme, leading to fermentation of malabsorbed lactose by intestinal bacteria with subsequent production of intestinal gas and various organic acids, manifesting clinically with diarrhea, abdominal pain, flatulence, or bloating after lactose intake. Lactose malabsorption occurs when a substantial amount of lactose is not absorbed in the intestine. Lactase deficiency is defined as brush-border lactase activity that is markedly reduced relative to the activity observed in infants.

SYNONYMS

Lactose malabsorption
Lactase deficiency
Milk intolerance
Carbohydrate malabsorption

ICD-10CM CODES

E73.9	Lactose intolerance, unspecified
E73.8	Other lactose intolerance

EPIDEMIOLOGY & DEMOGRAPHICS

- Nearly 50 million people in the U.S. have partial or complete lactose intolerance. There are racial differences, with <25% of white adults being lactose intolerant but >85% of Asian Americans and >60% of African Americans having some form of lactose intolerance.
- There are geographic variations: Highest in Asians (up to 90%), lowest in northern Europeans (approximately 10%), intermediate in southern Europeans and Middle Eastern populations (up to 40%).

PHYSICAL FINDINGS & CLINICAL PRESENTATION

- Abdominal tenderness and cramping, bloating, flatulence.
- Diarrhea.
- Symptoms are directly related to the osmotic pressure of substrate in the colon and occur approximately 2 hr after ingestion of lactose.
- Physical examination: May be entirely within normal limits.

ETIOLOGY

- Before it can be absorbed, lactose is cleared to glucose and galactose by the enzyme lactase in the brush border of the small intestine. If the amount of lactase is marginal or its expression is left, lactose intolerance will result.
- Congenital lactase deficiency: Common in premature infants; rare in term infants and generally inherited as a chromosomal recessive trait.
- Secondary lactose intolerance: Usually a result of injury of the intestinal mucosa (Crohn disease, viral gastroenteritis, AIDS enteropathy, cryptosporidiosis, Whipple disease, sprue).
- Acquired primary lactase deficiency (adult-type hypolactasia OMIM # 223100) is the most common form of lactase deficiency worldwide. The decline in lactase activity is a multifactorial process that is regulated at the gene transcription level and leads to decreased biosynthesis, retardation of intracellular transport, or maturation of the enzyme lactase-phlorizin hydrolase.

Dx DIAGNOSIS

DIFFERENTIAL DIAGNOSIS

- Inflammatory bowel disease
- Irritable bowel syndrome
- Pancreatic insufficiency
- Nontropical and tropical sprue
- Cystic fibrosis
- Diverticular disease
- Bowel neoplasm
- Laxative abuse
- Celiac disease
- Parasitic disease (e.g., giardiasis)
- Viral or bacterial infections

WORKUP

- A detailed dietary history is essential in the evaluation of patients with suspected carbohydrate malabsorption.
- The diagnosis can usually be made on the basis of the history and improvement with dietary manipulation.
- Diagnostic workup may include confirming the diagnosis with hydrogen breath test and excluding other conditions listed in the differential diagnosis that may also coexist with lactase deficiency.

LABORATORY TESTS

- Laboratory evaluation may not be necessary in patients with significant history.
- Lactose breath hydrogen test: A rise in breath hydrogen >20 ppm within 90 min of ingestion of 50 g of lactose is positive for lactase deficiency. This test is positive in 90% of patients with lactose malabsorption. Common causes of false-negative results are recent use of oral antibiotics or recent high colonic enema. Fig. 1 illustrates the role of symptoms in determining the clinical importance of lactose malabsorption.
- The lactose tolerance test is an older and less accurate testing modality (20% rate of false-positive and false-negative results). The patient is administered an oral dose of 1 to 1.5 g of lactose/kg body weight. Serial measurement of blood glucose level on an hourly basis for 3 hr is then performed. The test is considered positive if the patient develops

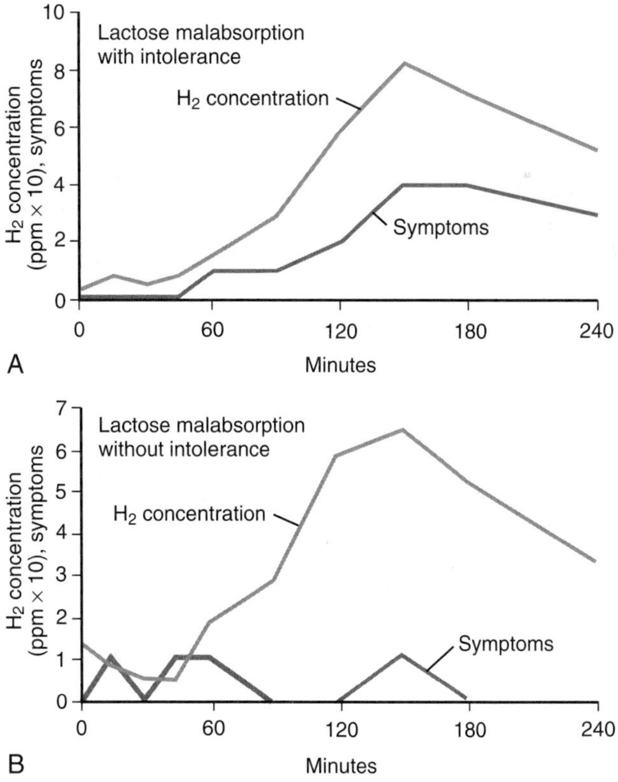

FIG. 1 Graphs illustrating the role of symptoms in determining the clinical importance of lactose malabsorption. Assessment of the clinical relevance of an abnormal lactose hydrogen breath test is made by monitoring abdominal symptoms (bloating, cramps, pain) during the test. Breath hydrogen concentration in parts per million (ppm) and GI symptoms using an arbitrary scoring system for two different patients are plotted on the graphs. **A,** The patient has symptoms associated with an increase in breath hydrogen concentration and therefore can be considered to have lactose intolerance. **B,** The patient has no increase in symptoms, although the breath hydrogen concentration increases considerably, so the patient has lactose malabsorption without lactose intolerance. (From Feldman M et al: *Sleisenger and Fordtran's gastrointestinal and liver disease,* ed 10, Philadelphia, 2016, Elsevier.)

intestinal symptoms and the blood glucose level rises <20 mg/dl above the fasting baseline level.
- Diarrhea associated with lactase deficiency is osmotic in nature with an osmotic gap and a pH <6.5.

IMAGING STUDIES

Imaging studies are generally not indicated. A small bowel series may be useful in patients with significant malabsorption.

Rx TREATMENT

NONPHARMACOLOGIC THERAPY

Management consists of reducing lactose exposure by avoiding milk and milk-containing products or using milk in which the lactose has been prehydrolyzed with lactase. A lactose-free diet generally results in prompt resolution of symptoms. Lactose is primarily found in dairy products but may be present as an ingredient or component of common foods and beverages. Possible sources of lactose include breads, candies, cold cuts, dessert mixes, cream soups, bologna, commercial sauces and gravies, chocolate, drink mixes, salad dressings, and medications. Labels should be read carefully to identify sources of lactose.

ACUTE GENERAL Rx

- Addition of lactase enzyme supplement (Lactaid tablets, Dairy Ease) before the ingestion of milk products may prevent symptoms in some patients. However, it is not effective for all lactose-intolerant patients.
- Lactose-intolerant patients must ensure adequate calcium intake. Calcium supplementation is recommended to prevent osteoporosis.

CHRONIC Rx

Patient education regarding foods high in lactose, such as milk, cottage cheese, or ice cream, is recommended.

DISPOSITION

Clinical improvement with restriction or elimination of milk products

REFERRAL

GI referral for endoscopic procedures if concomitant GI disorders are suspected

PEARLS & CONSIDERATIONS

COMMENTS

- There is great variability in signs and symptoms in patients with lactose intolerance depending on the degree of lactase deficiency. Most individuals with presumed lactose malabsorption can tolerate 12 to 15 g of lactose or up to 12 oz of milk daily without symptoms.
- Nondairy synthetic drinks (e.g., Coffee-Mate) and use of rice milk are generally well tolerated.

SUGGESTED READINGS

Available at ExpertConsult.com

RELATED CONTENT

Lactose Intolerance (Patient Information)

AUTHOR: **Fred F. Ferri, MD**

BASIC INFORMATION

DEFINITION

A mechanical or functional interruption of normal intraluminal flow through the colon

SYNONYM

Colorectal obstruction
LBO

ICD-10CM CODES

K56.609 Unspecified intestinal obstruction
K56.699 Other intestinal obstruction

EPIDEMIOLOGY & DEMOGRAPHICS

PREVALENCE: Approximately 20% to 25% of intestinal obstructions are large bowel obstructions (LBO).

PREDOMINANT SEX AND AGE: Affects males and females equally, more common in the elderly.

PEAK INCIDENCE: Higher in elderly due to increased rates of colorectal cancer. The incidence of large bowel obstruction is approximately 0.15 to 0.29 per 100,000 in patients with colorectal cancer.

RISK FACTORS: Colorectal cancer (usually sigmoid carcinoma), volvulus, fecal impaction, benign strictures related to postoperative changes or inflammatory bowel disease, abscess, radiation, and diverticulitis.

PHYSICAL FINDINGS & CLINICAL PRESENTATION

- History:
  1. Patients commonly present with abdominal pain, abdominal distension, and obstipation.
  2. Patients may have nausea and vomiting, but these can be late-presenting symptoms.
  3. Patients may report a history of bloating or constipation prior to the onset of more severe symptoms.
  4. Inquiries should be made concerning recent weight loss or gain, bowel habits, narcotic use, prior surgery, and malignancy.
- Physical exam:
  1. Patient may be tachycardic or febrile from perforation, strangulation, or ischemia.
  2. Exam should include palpation of the abdomen, investigation for umbilical, inguinal and femoral hernias, as well as a rectal exam.
  3. Physical exam findings may include:
     a. Distended, tympanitic abdomen
     b. Nonspecific tenderness to palpation of the lower abdomen
     c. A palpable hernia
     d. Rectal mass or frank blood on rectal exam
  4. If possible, proctoscopy can be performed to evaluate for rectal or sigmoid mass.

ETIOLOGY

- Most commonly, 50% to 60% of large bowel obstructions are related to colorectal carcinomas. Common sites of malignant obstruction are the descending and rectosigmoid colon. Volvulus accounts for another 10% to 17% of LBO and most often occurs in the sigmoid colon or at the cecum. Diverticular strictures cause 10% of LBO. Acute diverticulitis can also cause colonic obstruction due to abscess compression, stricture, or inflammation.
- Box 1 summarizes causes of adult large bowel obstruction.

DIAGNOSIS

DIFFERENTIAL DIAGNOSIS

- Colorectal cancer
- Volvulus
- Diverticulitis
- Abdominal abscess
- Abdominal adhesions
- Anastomotic stricture
- Hernia
- Fecal impaction
- Crohn disease
- Ischemic colitis
- Intussusception
- Pseudoobstruction (Ogilvie syndrome)
- Constipation
- Toxic megacolon

WORKUP

- Establish IV access with two large-bore IVs.
- Make the patient NPO.
- Flexible sigmoidoscopy or colonoscopy in stable patients.

LABORATORY TESTS

- Complete blood count with differential
- Basic metabolic panel
- Hepatic enzymes
- Lactic acid level

IMAGING STUDIES

- Acute abdominal series should demonstrate dilation of the colon (Fig. E1):
  1. Sensitivity 84%
  2. Specificity 72%
- CT abdomen and pelvis imaging is useful to pinpoint the obstruction and possibly identify the etiology (Fig. E2):
  1. Sensitivity 83%
  2. Specificity 93%
- Water contrast enema is useful for evaluating volvulus or distal obstruction cancer:
  1. Sensitivity 96%
  2. Specificity 98%
  3. Occasionally therapeutic

BOX 1 Causes of Adult Large Bowel Obstruction

Mechanical
- Neoplasm
- Volvulus (sigmoid, cecal, transverse colon)
- Diverticulitis
- Cecal bascule
- Intussusception
- Inflammatory bowel disease
- Incarcerated hernia
- Infection (abscess, inflammation)
- Fecal impaction
- Adhesion-related obstruction
- Foreign body

Functional
- Acute toxic or chronic megacolon
- Colonic pseudoobstruction (Ogilvie syndrome)

From Cameron JL, Cameron AM: *Current surgical therapy,* ed 12, Philadelphia, 2017, Elsevier.

TREATMENT

- IV fluid resuscitation: Consider placing Foley catheter to monitor UOP
- Correction of electrolyte abnormalities
- Pain management
- Antibiotics if concern for gangrene or perforation
- Nasogastric tube to decompress the GI tract
- Cessation of narcotics, antihistamines, and anticholinergics

NONPHARMACOLOGIC THERAPY

- Emergent laparotomy for perforation, closed loop obstruction, peritonitis, or ischemia
- Endoscopic stent placement as a bridge to surgery or palliation compared to emergency laparotomy can be considered
- Rectal cancer: Loop colostomy for cancer, then neoadjuvant chemoradiation
- Pseudo-obstruction and volvulus: Endoscopic decompression
- Diverticular abscess: Percutaneous drainage
- Colon cancer: Depends on location; Hartmann for sigmoid colon cancer, partial or total colectomy for other colon cancers
- Flexible sigmoidoscopy for colonic decompression of volvulus

ACUTE GENERAL Rx

Neostigmine for pseudoobstruction

CHRONIC Rx

Not indicated

DISPOSITION

Immediate referral to general surgery and hospital admission

REFERRAL

- General surgery
- Gastroenterology

RELATED CONTENT

Acute Colonic Pseudo-Obstruction (Ogilvie Syndrome) (Related Key Topic)
Constipation (Related Key Topic)
Colorectal Cancer (Related Key Topic)

SUGGESTED READINGS

Available at ExpertConsult.com

AUTHORS: **Shane Young, MD,** and **Joshua Justice, MD**

BASIC INFORMATION

DEFINITION

Laryngitis is an acute or chronic inflammation of the laryngeal mucous membranes.

SYNONYM

Lower respiratory tract infection

ICD-10CM CODES

J04.0	Acute laryngitis
J37.0	Chronic laryngitis

EPIDEMIOLOGY & DEMOGRAPHICS

It is a common illness worldwide in both genders and all age groups, but the diagnosis is imprecise and, therefore, statistics are not readily available with respect to incidence and prevalence.

PHYSICAL FINDINGS & CLINICAL PRESENTATION

ACUTE LARYNGITIS:

- Clinical syndrome characterized by the onset of hoarseness, voice breaks, or episodes of aphonia; may also have accompanying sore throat, cough, nasal congestion, and rhinorrhea
- Usually associated with viral upper respiratory infection
- Larynx with diffuse erythema, edema, and vascular engorgement of the vocal folds, and occasionally mucosal ulceration
- In young children subglottis is often affected, resulting in airway narrowing with marked hoarseness, inspiratory stridor, dyspnea, and restlessness
- Respiratory compromise rare in adults

CHRONIC LARYNGITIS: Characterized by hoarseness or dysphonia persisting for longer than 2 wk.

ETIOLOGY

ACUTE LARYNGITIS:

- Most often caused by viruses so treatment consists of supportive measures as outlined in "Nonpharmacologic Therapy" section.
- Studies evaluating the use of antibiotics (erythromycin, penicillin) in acute laryngitis failed to show objective clinical benefit over placebo so they are not routinely recommended. Antibiotics and other antimicrobials may be indicated in cases in which specific treatable pathogens are identified.
- Avoid decongestants because of their drying effect.
- Guaifenesin may be a useful adjunct as a mucolytic agent.
- In gastroesophageal reflux disease (GERD)-associated laryngitis use acid-suppressive therapy (H_2 blockers, proton pump inhibitors) and nocturnal antireflux precautions.

CHRONIC LARYNGITIS:

- Results from any of the following: Tuberculosis, usually through bronchogenic spread; leprosy, from nasopharyngeal or oropharyngeal spread; syphilis, in secondary and tertiary stages; rhinoscleroma, extending from the nose and nasopharynx; actinomycosis; cryptococcosis; histoplasmosis; blastomycosis; paracoccidioidomycosis; coccidiosis; candidiasis; aspergillosis; sporotrichosis; rhinosporidiosis; parasitic infections including leishmaniasis and clinostomum infection following raw fresh-water fish ingestion.
- Noninfectious causes of both acute and chronic laryngitis include malignancy, voice abuse (singers), GERD, and chemical or environmental irritants such as cigarettes and allergens. Other causes of inflammatory or granulomatous lesions of the larynx include relapsing polychondritis, Wegener granulomatosis, and sarcoidosis.

Dx DIAGNOSIS

DIFFERENTIAL DIAGNOSIS

- Young children with signs of airway obstruction:
  1. Supraglottitis (epiglottitis)
  2. Laryngotracheobronchitis
  3. Tracheitis
  4. Foreign body aspiration
- In adults with persistent hoarseness, consider noninfectious causes of laryngitis as listed previously.
- Table E1 summarizes the classification and definition of infectious illnesses involving the larynx and supraglottic and infraglottic regions.

WORKUP

- History and physical examination: Diagnosis is usually apparent.
- Laryngoscopy for severe or persistent cases.
- Laryngeal cultures should be performed if a cause other than acute viral infection is suspected.
- Imaging not indicated unless there is evidence of airway compromise. Obtain plain radiographs of neck, anteroposterior and lateral views, to differentiate laryngitis from acute laryngotracheobronchitis or supraglottitis.

Rx TREATMENT

NONPHARMACOLOGIC THERAPY

- Rest the voice.
- Use an air humidifier.
- Ensure adequate hydration. Avoid alcohol and caffeine because of diuretic effect.

ACUTE GENERAL Rx

- Antibiotics and other antimicrobials should generally not be used. They are indicated only when a specific pathogen is isolated; commonly employed antibacterial agents are macrolides; clarithromycin 500 mg by mouth bid for 5 to 7 days or azithromycin 500 mg followed by 250 mg once daily for 4 to 5 days if the cause of laryngitis is found to be *Mycoplasma pneumoniae* or *Chlamydophila pneumoniae* (the new name for what was formerly known as *Chlamydia pneumoniae*).
- Avoid decongestants because of their drying effect.
- Guaifenesin may be a useful adjunct as a mucolytic agent.
- In GERD-associated laryngitis use acid-suppressive therapy (H_2 blockers, proton pump inhibitors) and nocturnal antireflux precautions.

DISPOSITION

Uncomplicated laryngitis is usually benign, with gradual resolution of symptoms.

REFERRAL

- If symptoms persist for >2 wk, refer to otolaryngologist for laryngoscopy.
- Consider referral to gastroenterologist if GERD is suspected.

PEARLS & CONSIDERATIONS

- Most cases of uncomplicated acute laryngitis are viral in origin, and antibacterial agents should not be routinely administered.
- A Cochrane analysis in 2013 found no evidence for the use of empiric antibiotics in adults with laryngitis.
- The most difficult clinical challenge is often convincing patients with acute laryngitis that they do not need and will not benefit from antibacterial agents.

SUGGESTED READING

Available at Expertconsult.com

RELATED CONTENT

Laryngitis (Patient Information)

AUTHOR: **Glenn G. Fort, MD, MPH**

BASIC INFORMATION

DEFINITION

Lead is a potent, pervasive neurotoxicant. Lead poisoning refers to multisystem abnormalities resulting from excessive lead exposure.

SYNONYM

Plumbism

ICD-10CM CODES

T56.0X1A	Toxic effect of lead and its compounds, accidental (unintentional), initial encounter
T56.0X1D	Toxic effect of lead and its compounds, accidental (unintentional), subsequent encounter
T56.0X1S	Toxic effect of lead and its compounds, accidental (unintentional), sequela
T56.0X2A	Toxic effect of lead and its compounds, intentional self-harm, initial encounter
T56.0X2D	Toxic effect of lead and its compounds, intentional self-harm, subsequent encounter
T56.0X2S	Toxic effect of lead and its compounds, intentional self-harm, sequela
T56.0X3A	Toxic effect of lead and its compounds, assault, initial encounter
T56.0X3D	Toxic effect of lead and its compounds, assault, subsequent encounter
T56.0X3S	Toxic effect of lead and its compounds, assault, sequela
T56.0X4A	Toxic effect of lead and its compounds, undetermined, initial encounter
T56.0X4D	Toxic effect of lead and its compounds, undetermined, subsequent encounter
T56.0X4S	Toxic effect of lead and its compounds, undetermined, sequela

EPIDEMIOLOGY & DEMOGRAPHICS

- Lead poisoning is most common in children ages 1 to 5 yr (17,000 cases/100,000 persons). The highest rates are among blacks, those with low income, and urban children.
- In 1991 the Centers for Disease Control and Prevention (CDC) lowered the definition of a safe blood lead level to <10 mcg/dl of whole blood (a blood lead level of 25 mcg/dl was considered acceptable before 1991).
- It is estimated that >15% of preschoolers in the U.S. have a blood lead level >15 mcg/dl.

PHYSICAL FINDINGS & CLINICAL PRESENTATION

- Findings vary with the degree of toxicity (Table 1). Examination may be normal in patients with mild toxicity.
- Myalgias, irritability, headache, and general fatigue may be present initially.
- Abdominal cramping, constipation, weight loss, tremor, paresthesias and peripheral neuritis, seizures, and coma may occur with severe toxicity.
- Motor neuropathy is common in children with lead poisoning; learning disorders are also frequent.

ETIOLOGY

Chronic, repeated exposure to paint containing lead, plumbing, storage of batteries, pottery, or lead soldering. Concentration of lead is generally highest in lead-based paint on exterior surfaces. Among interior surfaces, windows are most likely to have the highest lead content. Table 2 summarizes common sources of lead.

DIAGNOSIS

DIFFERENTIAL DIAGNOSIS

- Polyneuropathies from other sources
- Anxiety disorder, attention deficit disorder
- Malabsorption, acute abdomen
- Iron-deficiency anemia

WORKUP

Laboratory screening: All U.S. children should be considered to be at risk for lead poisoning and should be screened routinely starting at age 1 yr for low-risk children and age 6 mo for high-risk children.

LABORATORY TESTS

- Venous blood lead level: Normal level, <5 mcg/dl; levels of 50 to 70 mcg/dl, indicative of moderate toxicity; levels >70 mcg/dl, associated with severe poisoning
- Mild anemia with basophilic stippling on peripheral smear
- Elevated zinc protoporphyrin levels or free erythrocyte protoporphyrin level
- An increased body burden of lead with previous high-level exposure in patients with occupational lead poisoning can be demonstrated by measuring the excretion of lead in urine after premedication with calcium ethylenediamine tetraacetic acid (EDTA) or another chelating agent

IMAGING STUDIES

- Imaging studies are generally not necessary.
- A plain abdominal film can visualize lead particles in the gut.
- "Lead lines" may be noted on x-ray films of long bones.

TREATMENT

NONPHARMACOLOGIC THERAPY

- Provide adequate amounts of calcium, iron, zinc, and protein in patient's diet.
- Family education on sources of lead exposure and potential adverse health effects.

ACUTE GENERAL Rx

- The use of chelation in cases of acute lead poisoning is guided by the patient's clinical status and the blood lead level (BLL). For children with blood levels of 10 to 19 mcg/dl, the CDC recommends nonpharmacologic interventions (see "Nonpharmacologic Therapy").
- For children with blood levels between 20 and 44 mcg/dl, the CDC recommendations include case management by a qualified social worker, clinical management, environmental assessment, and lead hazard control. Chelation therapy should be considered in children with refractory blood lead levels.
- Chelation therapy (Table 3) is indicated in children with blood lead levels >45 mcg/dl.
- Succimer (DMSA) 10 mg/kg PO q8h for 5 days then q12h for 2 wk can be used in patients with levels between 45 and 70 mcg/dl.

TABLE 1 Serum Lead Levels and Symptoms

	Symptoms	
Level (μg/dl)	Adults	Children
10	None	Decreased IQ Decreased hearing Decreased growth
20	Increased protoporphyrin No symptoms	Decreased nerve conduction velocity Increased protoporphyrin
30	Increased blood pressure Decreased hearing	Decreased vitamin D metabolism
40	Peripheral neuropathies Nephropathy Infertility (men)	Decreased hemoglobin synthesis
50	Decreased hemoglobin synthesis	Lead colic
70	Anemia	Anemia Encephalopathy Nephropathy
100	Encephalopathy	Death

IQ, Intelligence quotient.
From Marx JA et al: *Rosen's emergency medicine*, ed 8, Philadelphia, 2014, Saunders.

- Edetate calcium disodium (EDTA) and dimercaprol (BAL) are effective in patients with severe toxicity.
- Use of both EDTA and DMSA is indicated in children with blood levels >70 mcg/dl.
- d-Penicillamine (Cuprimine) can also be used for lead poisoning, but it is not FDA approved for this condition.

TABLE 2 Sources of Lead

Paint chips
Dust
Soil
Parent's or older child's occupational exposure (auto repair, smelting, construction, remodeling, plumbing, gun/bullet exposure, painting, e-scrap)
Glazed ceramics
Herbal remedies (e.g., Ayurvedic medications)
Home remedies including antiperspirants, deodorants (litargirio)
Jewelry (toys or parents')
Stored battery casings (or living near a battery smelter)
Lead-based gasoline
Moonshine alcohol
Mexican candies; Ecuadorian chocolates
Indoor firing ranges
Retained bullet fragments
Imported spices (*svanuri marili, zafron, kuzhambu*)
Lead-based cosmetics (kohl, surma)
Lead plumbing (water)
Imported foods in lead-containing cans
Imported toys
Home renovations
Antique toys or furniture

From Kliegman RM: *Nelson's textbook of pediatrics,* ed 21, Philadelphia, 2020, Elsevier.

CHRONIC Rx

- Reduce exposure, remove any potential lead sources.
- Correct iron deficiency and any other nutritional deficiencies.
- Recheck blood lead level 7 to 21 days after chelation therapy.

DISPOSITION

Patients with mild to moderate toxicity generally improve without any residual deficits. The presence of encephalopathy at diagnosis is a poor prognostic sign. Residual neurologic deficits may persist in these patients. Chelation therapy seems to slow the progression of renal insufficiency in patients with mildly elevated body lead burden.

REFERRAL

If exposure to lead is work related, it should be reported to the Office of the United States Occupational Safety and Health Administration (OSHA). Follow-up testing is mandatory in all patients after an abnormal screening blood lead level.

PEARLS & CONSIDERATIONS

COMMENTS

- Even blood lead concentrations as low as 5 to 10 mcg/dl are inversely associated with children's IQ scores at age 3 and 5 yr. A recent study evaluating long-term ramifications of childhood lead exposure revealed that childhood lead exposure was associated with lower cognitive function and socioeconomic status at age 38 yr, with declines in IQ, and downward social mobility (Reuben A et al: Association of childhood blood lead levels with cognitive function and socioeconomic status at age 38 and with IQ change and socioeconomic mobility between childhood and adulthood, *JAMA* 317(12):1244-1251, 2017).
- Screening of household members of affected individuals is recommended.
- In children with blood lead levels of >45 mg/dl, treatment with succimer does not improve scores on tests of cognition, behavior, or neuropsychological function.
- Lead toxicity may delay growth and pubertal development in girls.
- Low-level environmental lead exposure may accelerate progressive renal insufficiency in patients without diabetes who have chronic renal disease. Repeated chelation therapy may improve renal function and slow the progression of renal failure.

RELATED CONTENT

Lead Poisoning (Patient Information)

AUTHOR: **Fred F. Ferri, MD**

TABLE 3 Chelators*

Chelator	Dose	Indications	Contraindications
Deferoxamine	15 mg/kg/hr up to 24 hr (titrate up slowly because of hypotension)	Iron level >500 g/dl or systemic symptoms	
Dimercaprol (British anti-Lewisite [BAL])	Lead encephalopathy: 75 mg/m^2 deep IM injection every 4 hr for 5 days in children or 4 mg/kg every 4 hr for adults Arsenic (severe): No established regimen; consider 3 mg/kg IM every 4 hr for 48 hr; then twice daily for 7-10 days Mercury: 5 mg/kg IM first; then 2.5 mg/kg every 12-24 hr	Lead level >70 g/dl or encephalopathy Arsenic: Symptomatic patient with known exposure Mercury: Inorganic	Peanut allergy Organic mercury poisoning
$CaNa_2EDTA$	1500 mg/m^2/day continuous IV infusion 50 mg/kg/day or 1000 mg/m^2/day in 2-4 divided doses for up to 5 days if less severe symptoms	Lead: Given after first dose of BAL for blood lead level above 70 g/dl or encephalopathy	
Succimer (DMSA)	10 mg/kg q8h × 5 days; then q12h for 14 days	Lead level of 45-69 g/dl Arsenic: If tolerated orally for subacute and chronic toxicity Mercury: Acute and chronic	
D-Penicillamine	25 mg/kg q6h × 5 days	Lead level of 45-69 g/dl, succimer not tolerated Arsenic: Only if BAL and DMSA are unavailable Mercury: If BAL and DMSA are unavailable or not tolerated	Penicillin allergy
DMPS (investigational)	5 mg/kg/dose IM q6-8h day 1, q8-12h day 2, q12-24h day 3 and until 24-hr urine is <50 μg/L	Lead (chronic) Arsenic Mercury	

*Indications for chelation and dosing regimens may change. Consult with a toxicologist or poison control center for the most up-to-date recommendations.
DMPS, 2,3-Dimercapto-1-propanesulfonic acid; *EDTA,* edetate calcium disodium; *IM,* intramuscular; *IV,* intravenous; *q,* every.
From Marx JA et al: *Rosen's emergency medicine,* ed 8, Philadelphia, 2014, Saunders.

BASIC INFORMATION

DEFINITION

Pneumonia caused by *Legionella pneumophila*

SYNONYM

Legionella pneumonia

ICD-10CM CODE

A48.1 Legionnaires' disease

EPIDEMIOLOGY & DEMOGRAPHICS

PREVALENCE:

- Accounts for 2% to 5% of cases of community-acquired pneumonia.
- More common in Northeastern U.S. and Mediterranean.
- There are occasional community outbreaks due to contaminated water.
- Nosocomial outbreaks have also been reported.

PREDOMINANT SEX AND AGE:

- Male gender with twofold increased risk
- More common in age >50 yr

RISK FACTORS:

- Chronic heart disease, smoking, end-stage renal disease, immunosuppression, cancer
- No person-to-person transmission

PHYSICAL FINDINGS & CLINICAL PRESENTATION

- Acute respiratory illness similar to other forms of community-acquired pneumonia.
- Hypoxia, cough, physical exam with localizing chest findings including rales, pleural friction rub.
- Febrile prodrome of myalgias, anorexia, and headaches is nonspecific and may be confused with influenza or other viral infections.
- Gastrointestinal symptoms such as diarrhea and abdominal pain are common.

ETIOLOGY

Legionella pneumophila, an aerobic, gram-negative, intracellular bacteria, transmitted from inhalation of aerosols from water or soil. Grows in warm water sources and can cause outbreaks (e.g., cooling towers in the Bronx borough of New York City in 2016).

DIAGNOSIS

DIFFERENTIAL DIAGNOSIS

Clinically indistinguishable from other typical and atypical pneumonias

WORKUP

Similar to other pneumonias. CURB 65 or PSI may be used to stratify patients according to severity.

LABORATORY TESTS

- *Legionella* urinary antigen is highly sensitive for *Legionella* serogroup 1, which causes 70% to 80% of clinical disease but cannot detect other serogroups.
- PCR testing of respiratory samples (sputum or bronchoalveolar lavage) is more sensitive and specific, but many patients cannot produce sputum for testing.
- Culture is gold standard for diagnosis, but many patients cannot produce a sufficient sputum sample to test.
- Additional common lab abnormalities include hyponatremia, elevated creatine kinase, and coagulopathy.

IMAGING STUDIES

Chest x-ray (Fig. E1) with focal or diffuse consolidation, indistinguishable from other pneumonias

TREATMENT

NONPHARMACOLOGIC THERAPY

Supportive therapy: Oxygen, may require intubation for severe hypoxia, fluid management in case of diarrhea.

ACUTE GENERAL Rx

- Antibiotic coverage for atypical pneumonia. Azithromycin or levofloxacin are recommended. Treatment duration similar to other forms of community-acquired pneumonia, with the exception of severely immunosuppressed patients who may require extended courses for up to 21 days.
- Table 1 summarizes preferred therapy for Legionnaire disease.

DISPOSITION

- Mild cases managed as outpatient are likely underdiagnosed, but treated with azithromycin
- Can cause severe illness requiring ICU-level care among admitted patients

REFERRAL

- To pulmonologist and/or infectious disease specialist in severe cases
- To public health authorities for prompt recognition of water source and to contain potential outbreaks

PEARLS & CONSIDERATIONS

COMMENTS

- Pontiac fever is an acute febrile illness also caused by *Legionella* but without pneumonia that resolves spontaneously.
- *Legionella* can also rarely cause cellulitis and other extrapulmonary infections.

PREVENTION

Prompt recognition of clusters to identify water source is pivotal to contain an outbreak.

PATIENT & FAMILY EDUCATION

No risk for transmission to other family members.

SUGGESTED READINGS

Available at ExpertConsult.com

RELATED CONTENT

Pneumonia, Bacterial (Related Key Topic)

AUTHOR: **Brian Block, MD**

TABLE 1 Preferred Therapy for Legionnaires Disease

Clinical Condition	First Choices	Dosage*,†	Second Choices	Dosage*,†
Mild pneumonia inpatient or outpatient, not immunocompromised	Azithromycin *or*	500 mg 1×/day for 3-5 days	Doxycycline	200 mg load, then 100 mg 2×/day for 10-14 days
	Levofloxacin *or*	500 mg 1×/day for 7-10 days	Erythromycin	500 mg 4×/day for 10-14 days
	Ciprofloxacin *or*	500 mg 2×/days for 7-10 days		
	Moxifloxacin *or*	400 mg 1×/day for 7-10 days		
	Clarithromycin	500 mg 2×/day for 10-14 days		
Moderate to severe pneumonia or immunocompromised‡	Azithromycin *or*	500 mg 1×/day for 5-7 days	Ciprofloxacin *or*	750 mg 2×/day for 14 days
			Moxifloxacin *or*	400 mg 1×/day for 14 days
	Levofloxacin	500 mg 1×/day for 7-10 days 750 mg 1×/day for 5-7 days	Erythromycin *or*	750-1000 mg IV 4×/day for 3-7 days, then 500 mg 4×/day for a total course of 21 days
			Clarithromycin	500 mg IV 2×/day for 3-7 days, and then 500 mg 2×/day for a total course of 21 days

IV, Intravenous.

*Dosage adjustments have to be made for renal insufficiency for some of these drugs. Patients with mild disease may be treated entirely with oral therapy, whereas for severely ill patients parenteral therapy is advised until improvement is seen and oral absorption is sufficient.

†Therapy duration may need to be considerably longer for patients with lung abscesses, empyema, endocarditis, or extrathoracic infection.

‡Severely immunocompromised patients may require courses of therapy at the high end of the duration ranges given, or even longer. Close clinical follow-up is required to detect possible relapse after antibiotics have been discontinued.

From Bennett JE et al: *Mandell, Douglas, and Bennett's principles and practice of infectious diseases,* ed 8, Philadelphia, 2015, Elsevier.

Limbic Predominant Age-Related TDP-43 Encephalopathy

BASIC INFORMATION

DEFINITION

- Limbic predominant age-related TDP-43 encephalopathy (LATE) is a form of TDP-43 (TDP-43 or transactive response DNA binding protein 43 kDa) proteinopathy that causes progressive memory loss in older adults in a manner similar to Alzheimer disease (AD).
- TDP-43 intraneuronal cytoplasmic inclusions in the medical temporal lobe are the main pathologic marker and can occur with or without coexisting hippocampal sclerosis (HS). It is often comorbid with other neurodegenerative diseases such as AD.
- LATE typically manifests as an amnestic dementia because of the medial temporal location of the TDP-43 aggregates, and thus in vivo patients are often diagnosed with AD. It is typically a disease of the very old. The clinical picture is also influenced by co-occurring pathology.

SYNONYMS

- LATE encompasses several previously used designations related to TDP-43 proteinopathy that can be associated with cognitive impairment, including hippocampal sclerosis, hippocampal sclerosis of aging, hippocampal sclerosis dementia, cerebral age-related TDP-43 with sclerosis, and TDP-43 pathologies in the elderly
- Limbic-predominant age-related TDP-43 encephalopathy neuropathologic change (LATE-NC)

ICD-10CM CODES

None

EPIDEMIOLOGY & DEMOGRAPHICS

INCIDENCE: LATE-NC is present in >20% (up to 50%) of individuals past 80 yr.

PREVALENCE: Rates of TDP-43 proteinopathy increase at more advanced ages, whereas incidents of severe AD cases become less common as individuals attain such advanced age. TDP-43 pathology in patients with AD is mostly seen in the oldest-old and those with more severe clinical phenotype; between 20% and 50% of AD cases, and 75% of severe cases, exhibit pathophysiologic TDP-43.

PREDOMINANT AGE: Advanced age (>80 yr)

RISK FACTORS: Advanced age

GENETICS: Five alleles have been associated with LATE: GRN, TMEM106B, TARDBP, valosin-containing protein (VCP), and C9ORF72.

PHYSICAL FINDINGS & CLINICAL PRESENTATION

- LATE is associated with progressive memory deficits, in particular episodic memory deficits, but progresses to other cognitive domains as the disease progresses.
- Preliminary evidence suggests that individuals with relatively "pure" LATE (lacking severe comorbid pathologies) decline more gradually compared to those with "pure" AD. Those with comorbid LATE and AD decline faster and have more severe cognitive impairment than those with either LATE or AD alone.
- The concurrent presence of TDP-43 pathology and hippocampal sclerosis is associated with deficits in episodic and semantic memory. However, the occurrence of TDP-43 pathology alone is linked only to poorer episodic memory.
- Pathology is most frequently evident in the medial temporal lobe, correlating with a loss of episodic memory. Other studies have identified TDP-43 deposition in the ventral striatum and basal forebrain, linked to poorer performance on memory, language, and executive tests.
- Individuals with perivascular TDP-43 pathology also frequently exhibit cardiovascular symptoms such as hypertension and cerebral microinfarcts.
- Individuals with pathologic changes in TDP-43 are more likely to show indifference, loss of compassion, stereotyped behavior, and action disorder.

ETIOLOGY

- LATE is caused by TDP-43 proteinopathy. In the pathogenesis of LATE, the normal TDP-43 protein loses its immunoreactivity and begins to accumulate in the nuclei, cytoplasm, and cell processes (neurites) of neurons, oligodendrocytes, and astrocytes.
- As LATE progresses, brain atrophy due to TDP-43 deposition occurs in three stages: Amygdala (stage 1); hippocampus (stage 2); and middle frontal gyrus (MFG) (stage 3).
- In certain cases, TDP-43 aggregation and associated pathology may be a secondary consequence of some upstream neurodegenerative, developmental, or stress-induced influence.

DIAGNOSIS

- As with most other proteinopathies, LATE can only be formally diagnosed on autopsy.
- Symptoms that suggest LATE versus other forms of dementia:
  1. There are no diagnostic tools for the definitive antemortem detection of LATE.
  2. On autopsy, the distinguishing factor of LATE is TDP-43 pathology in medical temporal lobe structures with or without hippocampal sclerosis. The anatomic distribution of TDP-43 proteinopathy is stage 1 in the amygdala only, stage 2 in both amygdala and hippocampus, and stage 3 in amygdala, hippocampus, and middle frontal gyrus.

DIFFERENTIAL DIAGNOSIS

- AD
- Vascular dementia
- Argyrophilic grain disease
- Frontotemporal lobar degeneration associated with TDP-43 inclusions

WORKUP

Neuropsychologic tests similar to those used to diagnose AD can be used, such as the Mini-Mental State Examination (MMSE). However, there are currently no neuropsychologic tests or neuropsychiatric, motor, or autonomic signs that distinguish LATE from other degenerative disorders.

LABORATORY TESTS

There are currently no known biomarkers specific to LATE.

IMAGING STUDIES

MRI may show hippocampal atrophy, especially in LATE with hippocampal sclerosis. Amyloid and tau PET will be negative in pure LATE but may not be in comorbid LATE and AD. There is no TDP-43 fluid marker or PET ligand, but research is ongoing.

TREATMENT

None

REFERRAL

Neurologist with expertise in dementia

PROGNOSIS

Pure LATE has a slower rate of progression than AD. Mixed LATE and AD cases have more rapid progression than AD alone.

- Stage 1
  1. Average age at death: 89.9
  2. % Normal clinical diagnosis: 33.5
  3. % MCI (mild cognitive impairment) or dementia: 66.5
  4. % with comorbid hippocampal sclerosis (HS) pathology: 3.5
- Stage 2
  1. Average age at death: 91.8
  2. % Normal clinical diagnosis: 18.9
  3. % MCI or dementia: 81.1
  4. % with comorbid HS pathology: 13.6
- Stage 3
  1. Average age at death: 91.9
  2. % Normal clinical diagnosis: 7.6
  3. % MCI or dementia: 92.4
  4. % with comorbid HS pathology: 42.9

PREVENTION

Undetermined; possibly similar to AD

SUGGESTED READINGS

Available at ExpertConsult.com

AUTHORS: **Naomi R. Kass, BA,** and **Marco Pares, MD**

BASIC INFORMATION

DEFINITION

Liver abscess is a necrotic infection of the liver usually classified as pyogenic or amebic.

SYNONYMS

Pyogenic hepatic abscess
Amebic hepatic abscess

ICD-10CM CODE
K75.0 Abscess of liver

EPIDEMIOLOGY & DEMOGRAPHICS

INCIDENCE: Incidence of pyogenic liver abscess is 2.3 cases per 100,000 population.
PREVALENCE (WORLDWIDE): Amebic liver abscess is more common than pyogenic liver abscess.
PREVALENCE (IN U.S.): Pyogenic liver abscess is more common than amebic liver abscess.
PREDOMINANT SEX AND AGE: More common in men than women; male/female ratio of 2:1; most common in fourth to sixth decades of life.

PHYSICAL FINDINGS & CLINICAL PRESENTATION

- Fever, chills, and sweats
- Weakness/malaise
- Anorexia with weight loss
- Nausea, vomiting, and diarrhea
- Cough with pleuritic chest pain
- Right upper quadrant abdominal pain
- Hepatomegaly
- Splenomegaly
- Jaundice
- Pleural effusions, rales, and friction rubs may be present
- Most abscesses occur on the right lobe of the liver

ETIOLOGY

- Pyogenic liver abscess is usually polymicrobial (*Klebsiella pneumoniae* [43%], *Escherichia coli* [33%], *Streptococcus* spp. [37%], *Pseudomonas aeruginosa, Proteus* spp., *Bacteroides* spp. [24%], *Fusobacterium* spp., *Actinomyces* spp., gram-positive anaerobes, and *Staphylococcus aureus*).
- Pyogenic liver abscess occurs from:
  1. Biliary disease with cholangitis (accounts for approximately 40% to 60%).
  2. Gallbladder disease with contiguous spread to the liver.
  3. Diverticulitis or appendicitis with spread via the portal circulation.
  4. Hematogenous spread via the hepatic artery, though uncommon; if a solitary organism is isolated, a distant source of hematogenous seeding should be sought.
  5. Penetrating wounds.
  6. Cryptogenic.
  7. Infection by way of portal system (portal pyemia).
  8. No causes found in approximately half of cases.
  9. Incidence increased in patients with diabetes and metastatic cancer.
  10. Table 1 summarizes underlying etiology and bacteriology of liver abscesses.
- Amebic hepatic abscess is caused by the parasite *Entamoeba histolytica.* Amebiasis is usually due to fecal-oral contamination and invades the intestinal mucosa, gaining entry into the portal system to reach the liver. Amebic abscess occurs in 3% to 7% of patients with amebiasis.
- A comparison of pyogenic and amebic liver abscess is summarized in Table 2.

Box 1 describes pearls for amebic liver abscesses. The abscess is usually solitary (85%) and in the right lobe (72%).

DIAGNOSIS

The diagnosis of liver abscess requires a high index of suspicion after a detailed history and physical examination. Imaging studies and microbiologic, serologic, and percutaneous techniques (e.g., aspiration) confirm the presence of a liver abscess.

DIFFERENTIAL DIAGNOSIS

- Cholangitis
- Cholecystitis
- Diverticulitis
- Appendicitis

TABLE 1 Underlying Etiology and Bacteriology

Etiology	Bacteriology
Biliary, benign	*Escherichia coli* *Klebsiella* spp. *Enterococcus*
Biliary, malignant	*Pseudomonas* spp. Multiply resistant GN aerobes VRE Yeast
Diverticulitis/ appendicitis	GN aerobes *Bacteroides fragilis*
Severe cholecystitis	See "Biliary, benign" *Clostridium perfringens* *Bacteroides* spp.
Subcutaneous abscess	*Staphylococcus* spp. MRSA
Endocarditis	*Enterococcus* spp. *Staphylococcus* spp.
Cryptogenic	Anaerobes

GN, Gram-negative; *MRSA,* methicillin-resistant *Staphylococcus aureus; VRE,* Vancomycin-resistant *Enterococcus.*
From Cameron JL, Cameron AM: *Current surgical therapy,* ed 10, Philadelphia, 2011, Saunders.

TABLE 2 Features of Bacterial and Amebic Abscesses

	Demographics	Risk Factors	Symptoms	Laboratory Findings	Radiographic Features	Diagnosis	Treatment
Bacterial liver abscess	50-70 yr Male = female	Recent bacterial infection, biliary obstruction, diabetes mellitus	Fevers, chills, malaise, anorexia, diarrhea, cough, pleuritic chest pain, RUQ pain	Leukocytosis, anemia, elevated alkaline phosphatase and bilirubin, low albumin, positive blood cultures (50%)	Multifocal (50%), usually right lobe, irregular margins	Aspirate (70%-80% positive)	Percutaneous drainage and antibiotics
Amebic liver abscess	18-50 yr Male > female	Alcohol intake, HLA-DR3, oral and anal sex, contaminated enema apparatus, travel to or living in an endemic area	Fever, RUQ pain, hepatic tenderness, anorexia, weight loss, uncommon to have colitis	Leukocytosis, no eosinophilia, mild anemia, elevated alkaline phosphatase, elevated ESR, positive serology	Single abscess (80%), usually right lobe, wall enhancement seen on CT scan with IV contrast	Aspirate (trophozoites rarely seen) can rule out superimposed bacterial infection, positive serology and risk factors	Metronidazole and iodoquinol

CT, Computed tomography; *ESR,* erythrocyte sedimentation rate; *HLA,* human leukocyte antigen; *IV,* intravenous; *RUQ,* right upper quadrant.
From Goldman L, Schafer AI: *Goldman-Cecil medicine,* ed 26, Philadelphia, 2019, Elsevier.

BOX 1 Pearls for Amebic Liver Abscesses

- Only 10%-20% of patients with amebic liver abscess have a history of diarrhea.
- Treat the intestinal infection to prevent relapse of amebic liver abscess. Failure to use luminal amebicidal agents after metronidazole in cases of amebic abscess results in a 10% relapse rate.
- Failure to show response to antiamebic medication requires evaluation for polymicrobial infection with bacteria.
- Amebic abscess usually responds clinically to antimicrobial therapy in 3-7 days, although imaging takes several months to show resolution.
- Percutaneous drainage is rarely required.

From Cameron JL, Cameron AM: *Current surgical therapy*, ed 10, Philadelphia, 2011, Saunders.

- Perforated viscus
- Mesentery ischemia
- Pulmonary embolism
- Pancreatitis

WORKUP

- The workup of a liver abscess should focus on differentiating between amebic and pyogenic causes.
- Features suggesting an amebic cause include travel to an endemic area, single abscess rather than multiple abscesses, subacute onset of symptoms, and absence of conditions predisposing to pyogenic liver abscess, as highlighted under "Etiology."
- Laboratory studies are not specific but are useful as adjunctive tests.
- Imaging studies cannot differentiate between the two, and bacteriologic cultures may be sterile in 50% of the cases.

LABORATORY TESTS

- Complete blood count: Leukocytosis
- Liver function tests: Alkaline phosphatase is most commonly elevated (95% to 100%); aspartate transaminase (AST) and alanine transaminase (ALT) elevated in 50% of cases; elevated bilirubin (28% to 30%); decreased albumin
- Prothrombin time (INR): Prolonged (70%)
- Blood cultures: Positive in 50% of cases
- Aspiration (50% sterile)
- Stool samples for *E. histolytica* trophozoites (positive in 10% to 15% of amebic liver abscess cases)
- Serologic testing for *E. histolytica* should be done on all patients, but it is important to remember that it does not differentiate acute from old infections

IMAGING STUDIES

- Ultrasound (80% to 100% sensitivity in detecting abscesses) shows round or oval hypoechogenic mass (Fig. E1, *A*).
- CT scan is more sensitive in detecting hepatic abscesses and contiguous organ extension and is the imaging study of choice (Fig. E1, *B*, and Fig. E2).
- Chest x-ray: Abnormal in 50% of the cases, may reveal elevated right hemidiaphragm, subdiaphragmatic air-fluid levels, pleural effusions, and consolidating infiltrates.
- Most liver abscesses are single; however, multiple liver abscesses can occur with systemic bacteremia.

Rx TREATMENT

NONPHARMACOLOGIC THERAPY

- The management of pyogenic liver abscess differs from that of amebic liver abscess.
- Medical management is the cornerstone of therapy in amebic liver abscess, whereas early intervention in the form of surgical therapy or catheter drainage and parenteral antibiotics is the rule in pyogenic liver abscess greater than 3 cm. Smaller abscesses (<3 cm) can generally be treated with broad-spectrum antibiotics.

ACUTE GENERAL Rx

- Percutaneous drainage under CT or ultrasound guidance is essential in the treatment of pyogenic liver abscesses.
- Aspiration of hepatic amebic abscesses is not required unless there is no response to treatment or a pyogenic cause is being considered.
- Empiric broad-spectrum antibiotics are recommended initially until culture results are available. Common choices include:
  1. Metronidazole (500 mg IV q8h) plus ceftriaxone or levofloxacin.
  2. Monotherapy with a beta-lactam/beta-lactamase inhibitor, such as piperacillin/tazobactam (4.5 g q6h), ticarcillin-clavulanate (3.1 g q4h), or ampicillin-sulbactam (3 g q6h).
  3. Monotherapy with a carbapenem, such as imipenem (500 mg IV q6h), meropenem (1 g q8h), or ertapenem (1 g daily).
  4. Duration of antibiotic treatment is usually 4 to 6 wk with IV antibiotics used for the first 1 to 2 wk or until a favorable clinical response, followed thereafter with oral antibiotics (e.g., metronidazole 500 mg PO q8h plus ciprofloxacin 500 mg PO q12h).
  5. Third-generation cephalosporins should not be used as single agents for empiric therapy because of risk of the emergence of beta-lactamase–producing bacteria.
- Antibiotic coverage for amebic liver abscesses includes:
  1. Metronidazole 750 mg PO tid for 10 days or tinidazole.
  2. Eradication of the coexistent intestinal infection with paromomycin for 10 days.

CHRONIC Rx

- If fever persists for 2 wk despite percutaneous drainage and antibiotic therapy as outlined under "Acute General Rx," or if there is failure of aspiration or failure of percutaneous drainage, surgery is indicated.
- In patients not responding to intravenous antibiotics and percutaneous drainage, hepatic artery antibiotic infusion can be considered.
- In patients with evidence of metastatic disease that is causing biliary obstruction, a gastroenterology consultation for endoscopic retrograde cholangiopancreatography and stenting should be considered.

DISPOSITION

- Most patients with pyogenic liver abscesses defervesce within 2 wk of treatment with antibiotics and drainage.
- No randomized controlled studies have evaluated the optimal duration of antibiotic therapy for pyogenic liver abscess. Typical duration of antibiotic therapy is at least 4 to 6 wk.
- Pyogenic liver abscess cure rates using percutaneous drainage and antibiotics have been reported to be between 88% and 100%.
- Mortality rate of untreated pyogenic liver abscess is nearly 100%.
- Most patients with amebic liver abscesses defervesce within 4 to 5 days of treatment.
- Amebic liver abscess mortality rate is <1% unless complications occur (see "Comments").
- Follow-up imaging should be used to monitor response to therapy; continue treatment until CT scan shows complete or near-complete resolution of cavity.

REFERRAL

Infectious disease, gastroenterology, interventional radiology, and general surgical consultations are recommended in any patient with hepatic abscess.

PEARLS AND CONSIDERATIONS

COMMENTS

- Complications of pyogenic and amebic liver abscesses include:
  1. Pleuropulmonary extension, resulting in empyema, abscess, and fistula formation
  2. Peritonitis
  3. Purulent pericarditis
  4. Sepsis
- Amebic liver abscesses complicate amebic colitis in nearly 10% of cases.

RELATED CONTENT

Liver Abscess (Patient Information)
Amebiasis (Related Key Topic)

AUTHOR: **Fred F. Ferri, MD**

BASIC INFORMATION

DEFINITION

Long QT syndrome (LQTS) is a disorder of myocardial repolarization characterized by a prolongation of the QT interval on the ECG associated with an increased risk of developing life-threatening ventricular arrhythmias, most commonly torsades de pointes (a specific type of polymorphic ventricular tachycardia), which may lead to ventricular fibrillation and sudden cardiac death (SCD). This syndrome may be either genetic or acquired.

SYNONYMS

LQTS
Congenital forms:
Jervell and Lange-Nielsen syndrome (associated with deafness)
Romano-Ward syndrome (associated with normal hearing)

ICD-10CM CODE

I45.81 Long QT syndrome

EPIDEMIOLOGY & DEMOGRAPHICS

- Congenital LQTS is thought to account for >3000 deaths in childhood per yr in the United States.
- The prevalence of congenital LQTS is at least 1 in 2000 live births and may even be higher because that estimate is based on genetic testing of infants in whom the QTc was in excess of 470 and 460 ms, respectively.
- Incidence of LQTS is thought to be between 1:2500 and 1:10,000 in the general population, although it has been difficult to estimate because of incomplete penetrance. Congenital form associated with deafness is autosomal recessive (Jervell and Lange-Nielsen syndrome) and is less common than the autosomal dominant form as well as more severe.
- Congenital form associated with normal hearing (Romano-Ward syndrome) is autosomal dominant. Although inheritance of LQTS is autosomal dominant, female predominance has often been observed and has been attributed to an increased susceptibility to cardiac arrhythmias in women. LQTS is more likely to express itself before puberty in males and after puberty in females.
- At least 17 different LQTS genes have been identified to date. However, as clinical genetic testing evolves, some previously associated LQTS-susceptibility genes have been reconsidered as unlikely to be causative for congenital LQTS.
- Mortality rate is estimated to be about 1% per yr.
- Multiple mutations causing congenital LQTS have been described. The most common types of LQTS are described in Table 1.

PHYSICAL FINDINGS & CLINICAL PRESENTATION

- Palpitations, presyncope.
- Syncope suggestive of cardiac/arrhythmic origin (not vasovagal syncope).
- Resuscitated sudden cardiac arrest.
- Seizure (often, patients with LQTS are misdiagnosed with epilepsy).
- Family history of LQTS, but a family history of SCD has not been proved to be a risk factor for SCD in patients with LQTS.
- Abnormal ECG (prolonged QT) in asymptomatic relatives of known case.
- Prolonged QTc interval on average among patients with genetically confirmed LQTS is approximately 470 ms. In general the 99th percentile QTc values are 460 ms (prepuberty), 470 ms in postpubertal males, and 480 ms in postpubertal females.
- In case of congenital LQTS the presentation of syncope or SCD is typically triggered by exercise and swimming in LQT1 patients (45% cases); in LQT2 (25%-40% cases) patients by emotion, pregnancy, or noise; and patients with LQT3 (5%-10% cases) are at highest risk of events when at rest or asleep.

ETIOLOGY

- Cardiac repolarization abnormality
- Congenital cause (hundreds of mutations on more than 10 genes have been identified)
- Most of the gene mutations affect function of ion channels leading to prolonged repolarization (i.e., sodium and potassium channels resulting in either increased Na^+ influx or decreased K^+ efflux). These mutations prolong depolarization and predispose the patient to torsades de pointes
- Acquired causes:
  1. Drugs: Dofetilide, ibutilide, bepridil, quinidine, procainamide, sotalol, amiodarone, ranolazine, disopyramide, phenothiazines and antiemetic agents (droperidol, domperidone), tricyclic antidepressants, antipsychotics (quetiapine, ziprasidone, iloperidone), citalopram, antihistamines, quinolones, azithromycin, astemizole or cisapride given with ketoconazole or erythromycin, clarithromycin, and antimalarials, particularly among patients with asthma or those using potassium-lowering medications; also common in patients receiving methadone
  2. Hypokalemia, hypomagnesemia, hypocalcemia (especially in patients with malabsorption syndrome)
  3. Liquid protein diet
  4. Central nervous system lesions
  5. Structural heart disease (heart failure, diastolic dysfunction, myocardial ischemia, and LVH)
  6. Hypothyroidism
  7. Bradyarrhythmias

TABLE 1 Common Types of Long QT (LQT) Syndrome

	LQT1	LQT2	LQT3
Pathophysiology			
Gene	*KCNQ1 (KvLQT1)*	*KCNH2 (formerly "HERG")*	*SCN5A*
Protein	$K_v7.1$	$K_v11.1$	$Na_v1.5$
Ionic current	Decreased I_{Ks}	Decreased I_{Kr}	Increased late I_{Na}
Clinical Presentation			
Incidence of cardiac events	63%	46%	18%
Incidence of SCD	4%	4%	4%
Arrhythmia triggers	Emotional/physical stress (swimming, diving)	Emotional stress, arousal (alarm clock, telephone), rest, postpartum period	Sleep/rest
ECG	Broad-based T wave	Low-amplitude, bifid T wave	Long isoelectric ST segment
QT response to exercise	Attenuated QTc shortening and an exaggerated QTc prolongation during early and peak exercise	Normal QT during exercise but with exaggerated QT hysteresis	Supernormal QT shortening
Management			
Exercise restriction	+++	++	?
Response to beta-blockers	+++	+++	?
Potassium supplement	+	++	+
Left cervicothoracic sympathectomy	++	++	++
Response to mexiletine	+	+	++

From Issa Z et al: *Clinical arrhythmology and electrophysiology*, ed 2, Philadelphia, 2012, Saunders.

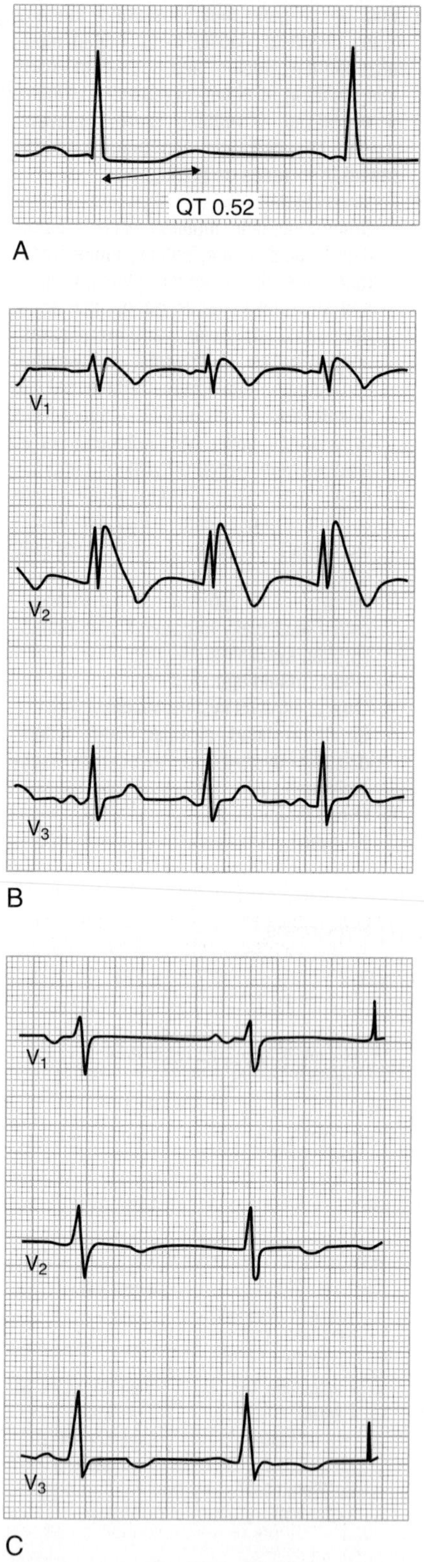

FIG. 1 Sinus rhythm electrocardiogram findings in three genetic sudden death syndromes. A, QT prolongation during sinus rhythm in a patient with long QT syndrome. **B,** ST elevation in V_1 and V_2 in a patient with Brugada syndrome. **C,** T wave inversion in V_1-V_3 in a patient with arrhythmogenic right ventricular dysplasia. (From Goldman L, Schafer AI: *Goldman's Cecil medicine,* ed 24, Philadelphia, 2012, Saunders.)

Dx DIAGNOSIS

DIFFERENTIAL DIAGNOSIS

- See "Syncope."
- Brugada syndrome, arrhythmogenic right ventricular dysplasia, and LQTS are major causes of genetic sudden death syndromes (Fig. 1).

Diagnostic criteria for the congenital LQTS as per 2013 HRS Guidelines:

LQTS is diagnosed:

- In the presence of an LQTS risk score ≥3.5 (Table 2) in the absence of a secondary cause for QT prolongation and/or
- In the presence of an unequivocally pathogenic mutation in one of the LQTS genes or
- In the presence of a QT interval corrected for heart rate using Bazett formula (QTc) ≥500 ms in repeated 12-lead electrocardiogram (ECG) and in the absence of a secondary cause for QT prolongation
- LQTS can be diagnosed in the presence of a QTc between 480 and 499 ms in repeated 12-lead ECGs in a patient with unexplained syncope in the absence of a secondary cause for QT prolongation and in the absence of a pathogenic mutation

WORKUP

Cardiology referral is recommended for all cases.

Genetic analysis is an essential step for risk stratification of patients with congenital prolonged QT and is important for identification of potential mutation carriers within the proband family. There is evidence for gene-specific triggers of events and therapeutic efficacy. Molecular screening should become part of the routine clinical management of LQTS.

In relatives of known patients with LQTS or in young patients with syncope:

- Stress test may prolong the QT interval or cause T-wave alternans.
- Valsalva maneuver: May prolong the QT interval or cause T-wave alternans.
- Prolonged ECG monitoring with various stimulations aimed at increasing catecholamines and assess for QT prolongation (perform in a setting that can provide resuscitation with α- and β-antagonists readily available).
- Epinephrine-induced prolongation of the QT interval (epinephrine infusion QT stress test).
- Genetic analysis:
  1. *LQT1* locus of *KCNQ1* potassium channel gene.
  2. *LQT2* locus of *KCNH2 (formerly "HERG")* potassium channel gene.
  3. *LQT3* locus of *SCN5A* sodium channel gene.
  4. These three variants account for >90% of all genotyped LQTS patients, whereas the remaining genes are responsible for a minority of cases.
- Risk stratification for each genetic variant on the basis of gender and QTc: Groups are defined on the basis of the probability of the first cardiac event (syncope, cardiac arrest, or sudden death) before age 40 yr or before therapy. Specific mutations, depending on type, location, and degree, may confer a high risk even if the ECG abnormalities are mild. Clinically, QT interval duration was the strongest predictor of risk for cardiac events; a QTc exceeding 500 ms identifies patients with the highest risk.
  1. High risk (>50% of cardiac event): QTc ≥500 ms and LQT1 or LQT2, or male with LQT3.
  2. Moderate risk (30%-50%): QTc <500 ms in male with LQT3 or in female with LQT2 or LQT3, and female with LQT3 with QTc ≥500 ms.
  3. Low risk (<30%): QTc <500 ms and LQT1 or male LQT2 with QTc <500 ms.
  4. Prophylactic treatment should be considered in all patients with moderate or high risk for cardiac events based on the above risk stratification scheme (Table 3).

Rx TREATMENT

NONPHARMACOLOGIC THERAPY

- Physical activity and LQTS
  1. *LQT1* patients experience 90% of lethal events under physical and emotional stress. Swimming and diving should be avoided or performed under supervision. In patients with LQT2 and LQT3, children and adolescents can resume participation in physical education classes, and adults should be encouraged to stay physically active.
  2. Regarding competitive athletics for individuals with congenital LQTS, there is a difference of opinion between the 2015 AHA/ACC Scientific Statement on Eligibility and the Disqualification Recommendations for Competitive Athletes, which allows participation in competitive events and training sessions dependent on availability of automated external defibrillator (AED). In contrast, previous European guidelines advise precautionary restriction from competitive sports in these situations.
- Implantation of an implantable cardioverter-defibrillator (ICD) in the vast majority of LQTS patients is not necessary, and most patients with LQTS (90% or more in LQTS expert centers) do not need and should not receive an ICD. Consider ICD placement in following situations (Table 4):
  1. Survivors of sudden cardiac arrest without a reversible cause.
  2. In patients with LQTS-associated sudden cardiac arrest while compliant with beta-blocker therapy.
  3. In patients with recurrent cardiac syncope in spite of beta-blockers and left cardiac sympathetic denervation.
  4. In an asymptomatic patient with either LQT2 or LQT3 whose resting QTc is >550 ms, consider prophylactic ICD.
- ICD is never indicated based solely on the family history, as it is not a personal risk factor for the patient with LQTS.

TABLE 2 Long QT Syndrome Risk Score

ECG CRITERIA	
QTc >480 ms	3 points
QTc 460-480 ms	2 points
QTc 450-460 ms (males)	1 point
QTc 4th minute of recovery from exercise stress test >480 ms	1 point
Torsades de pointes	2 points
T-wave alternans	1 point
Notched T-wave in three leads	1 point
Bradycardia	0.5 point
History	
Syncope with stress	2 points
Syncope without stress	1 point
Congenital deafness	0.5 point
Definite family history of long QT	1 point
Unexplained cardiac death in first-degree relative <30 yr	0.5 point

Total score: 1 point: Low probability of LQTS; 1.5 to 3 points: Intermediate probability of LQTS; ≥3.5 points: High probability of LQTS.
From Schwartz PJ, Crotti L: QTc behavior during exercise and genetic testing for the long-QT syndrome, *Circulation* 124(20):2181-2184, 2011.

TABLE 3 Cardiac Event Risk Stratification Scheme Based on Genes, Gender, and QTc

	QTC <500 MS		QTC ≥550 MS	
Genetic Subtype	**Male**	**Female**	**Male**	**Female**
LQT1	Low	Low	High	High
LQT2	Low	Intermediate	High	High
LQT3	Intermediate	Intermediate	High	Intermediate

Probability of the first cardiac event (syncope, cardiac arrest, or sudden death) before the age of 40 yr or before therapy. High = >50%, Intermediate = 30%-50%, Low = <30%.

TABLE 4 Management of Patients with Long QT Syndrome

Type of Syndrome	Management	Indication
Congenital	Beta-blockers	Asymptomatic patients, symptomatic patients (who do not have bronchospasm)
	Cervicothoracic sympathectomy	Refractory symptoms, especially in pediatric patients
	Cardiac pacing	Refractory symptoms associated with bradycardia, pauses
	Implantable cardioverter-defibrillator	Cardiac arrest, refractory syncope, prophylaxis for moderate- to high-risk patients for cardiac events
Acquired	Elimination of causative drug or condition	All patients
	Magnesium sulfate	Nonsustained ventricular tachycardia, torsades de pointes (even with a normal serum magnesium concentration)
	Administration of potassium (to keep serum K^+ >4.5 mEq/L)	Serum K^+ <4.5 mEq/L
	Maneuvers to increase heart rate (cardiac pacing, isoproterenol)	Bradycardia, arrhythmias refractory to magnesium sulfate

K^+, Potassium.
Adapted from Crawford MH et al [eds]: *Cardiology*, ed 2, St Louis, 2004, Mosby.

PHARMACOLOGIC THERAPY

- All patients with LQTS and a history of syncope, seizures, or resuscitated SCA should be treated with a beta-blocker.
- Beta-blockers, chiefly propranolol and nadolol, are an initial therapy of choice—there are differential responses to β-blocker therapy among different genetic variants; especially effective among LQT1 or LQT2 patients. Studies showed the efficacy of β-blockers with an overall mortality <2% over a mean follow-up exceeding 5 yr.
- In patients with LQT3, mexiletine shortens the QTc and, increasingly, combination therapy with propranolol and mexiletine is utilized in these patients.
- In the 20% to 30% of patients who continue to have symptoms on a β-blocker, the main options are either left cardiac sympathetic denervation (LCSD) or the prophylactic implantation of an ICD.
- In patients with frequent ICD shocks or in those with high risk for SCD where ICD placement cannot be performed, cardiac pacing and/or LCSD may be indicated.
- In patients with recurrent syncope and/or aborted cardiac arrest despite combined ICD and β-blocker, LCSD as adjunctive therapy can be performed.
- For patients with LQTS who continue to receive appropriate ICD shocks or who have a high-risk phenotype but prefer to avoid an ICD, potassium retention strategies are implemented, regardless of the underlying LQTS genotype.
- Correctable factors including electrolyte disorders—hypokalemia and hypomagnesemia—and avoidance of precipitating drugs that may further prolong the QT interval is mandatory. A complete list of drugs that can potentially prolong QT may be found at www.crediblemeds.org.
- For patients with acquired form and torsades de pointes, IV magnesium and atrial or ventricular pacing are initial choices.
- Table 3 summarizes management of patients with LQTS.

PROGNOSIS

- In carefully treated patients, mortality is around 0.5% to 1% over 20 yr.
- The timing and frequency of syncope, QTc prolongation, and gender are predictive of risk for aborted cardiac arrest and SCD during adolescence. Higher risk is present in those with one or two or more episodes of syncope in the last 10 yr compared with those with no syncopal episodes, those with QTc >530 ms, and males ages 10 to 12 yr.

PEARLS & CONSIDERATIONS

COMMENTS

- Family history should be assessed for a history of sudden death and other deaths that may have occurred as manifestations of LQTS (e.g., sudden infant death, drowning, and loss of consciousness while driving).
- ICDs are an important component of therapy, but most LQTS patients do not need and should not receive an ICD based only on LQTS diagnosis.
- Propranolol and nadolol are considered superior to metoprolol for prevention of arrhythmias in LQTS.

SUGGESTED READINGS

Available at ExpertConsult.com

RELATED CONTENT

Long QT Syndrome (Patient Information)
Torsades de Pointes (Related Key Topic)

AUTHOR: **Rizwan Khan, MD**

BASIC INFORMATION

DEFINITION

A lung abscess is an infection of the lung parenchyma resulting in necrosis and cavity formation.

SYNONYM

Pulmonary abscess

ICD-10CM CODES

J85.1 Abscess of lung with pneumonia
J85.2 Abscess of lung without pneumonia
A06.5 Amebic lung abscess

EPIDEMIOLOGY & DEMOGRAPHICS

INCIDENCE:
- The exact incidence is unknown; however, it has significantly decreased with the advent of antibiotics.
- Lung abscess is more common in the elderly because of an increased risk of periodontal disease and dysphagia.

RISK FACTORS (see Table 1):
- Alcohol use disorder
- Seizure disorders
- Cerebrovascular disorders with dysphagia
- Head trauma
- Substance use disorders
- General anesthesia
- Esophageal disorders (e.g., scleroderma, esophageal carcinoma)
- Poor oral hygiene
- Poor cough reflex
- Obstructive lung neoplasm
- Bronchiectasis
- Obstructive foreign body

PHYSICAL FINDINGS & CLINICAL PRESENTATION

Symptoms are generally insidious, occurring over weeks to months.
- Fever
- Cough
- Sputum production (purulent with foul odor)
- Pleuritic chest pain
- Hemoptysis
- Dyspnea
- Malaise, fatigue, and weakness

Physical exam findings
- Tachycardia and tachypnea
- Poor dentition
- Dullness to percussion, whispered pectoriloquy, and bronchophony
- Amphoric breath sounds (low-pitched sound of air moving across a large open cavity)

ETIOLOGY

- Aspiration is the most common cause of lung abscess.
- Periodontal disease is a major predisposing factor.
- Lung abscess is rare in an edentulous person.
- Lung abscesses are most often caused by anaerobic microorganisms (*Peptostreptococci*, microaerophilic streptococci such as *Streptococcus milleri, Bacteroides* species, *Fusobacterium nucleatum, Prevotella, Actinomyces* spp.).
- Frequently are polymicrobial with an anaerobic infection mixed with aerobic or facultative anaerobic organisms *(S. aureus, E. coli, K. pneumoniae, P. aeruginosa).*
- Parasitic organisms including *Paragonimus westermani* and *Entamoeba histolytica.*
- Fungi including *Aspergillus, Cryptococcus, Histoplasma, Blastomyces,* and *Coccidioides* spp.
- Immunocompromised hosts may become infected with *Aspergillus,* mycobacteria, *Nocardia, Legionella micdadei,* and *Rhodococcus equi.*
- Lung necrosis caused by community strains (USA 300 strain) of methicillin-resistant *Staphylococcus aureus* (MRSA) in adolescents and young adults following an acute influenza infection was initially reported in 2002 and can be quite fulminant.
- Multiresistant *Klebsiella pneumoniae* has been isolated from lung abscesses in Taiwan.

Dx DIAGNOSIS

Lung abscess may be classified as primary or secondary.
- *Primary lung abscess* refers to abscess formation in immunocompetent hosts; usually a result of aspiration.
- *Secondary lung abscess* refers to abscess formation in individuals with immunodeficiency or those with a preexisting pulmonary condition (e.g., lung cancer, bronchiectasis).

Lung abscess may be defined as acute or chronic.
- Acute lung abscess denotes symptoms being present for less than 4 to 6 wk.
- Chronic lung abscess denotes symptoms being present for longer than 6 wk.

DIFFERENTIAL DIAGNOSIS

The differential diagnosis for cavitary lung lesions can be separated into infectious and noninfectious causes.

INFECTIOUS:
- Bacterial (anaerobic, aerobic, facultative anaerobes)
- Fungal (histoplasmosis, coccidioidomycosis, blastomycosis, aspergillosis, cryptococcosis, zygomycetes)
- Parasitic (amebiasis, echinococcosis)

NONINFECTIOUS:
- Malignancy (primary lung carcinoma, metastatic lung disease, lymphoma)
- Vasculitis (granulomatosis with polyangiitis)
- Septic emboli
- Bronchiectasis
- Obstructive mass or foreign body

WORKUP

- The workup of a patient with lung abscess attempts to elicit a primary or secondary cause.
- Blood tests are not specific in diagnosing lung abscesses.
- Most diagnoses are made from imaging studies.
- Bacteriologic studies are required to diagnose a specific cause.

LABORATORY TESTS

- CBC with leukocytosis
- Bacteriologic studies:
  1. Sputum Gram stain and culture (commonly contaminated by oral flora).
  2. Fiberoptic bronchoscopy with bronchial brushings and/or bronchoalveolar lavage is commonly performed in those who have failed standard therapy and in immunocompromised individuals to rule out opportunistic infections.
  3. Percutaneous transthoracic aspiration may also be used to identify an organism.
  4. Blood cultures in those with sepsis or septic shock.
  5. If a pleural effusion is present, performing a thoracentesis may provide an uncontaminated specimen to isolate the causative organism of the neighboring abscess.

IMAGING STUDIES

- The diagnosis of lung abscess can be made by chest x-ray demonstrating a cavitary lesion with an air-fluid level.
- Lung abscesses are most commonly found in the posterior segment of the right upper lobe or the superior segment of the lower lobes (the dependent regions of the lung when supine).
- Chest CT scan can help to localize and size the lesion. In addition, it can assist in differentiating lung abscesses from other pathologic processes (e.g., tumor, empyema, infected bulla) (Fig. 1).

TABLE 1 Risk Factors for Aspiration Pneumonia and Lung Abscess

Increased bacterial inoculum	Periodontal disease, gingivitis, tonsillar or dental abscess, drugs that decrease gastric acidity
Impairment of consciousness	Drugs, alcohol, general anesthesia, metabolic encephalopathy, coma, shock, cerebrovascular accident, cardiopulmonary arrest, seizures, surgery, trauma
Impairment of cough and gag reflexes	Vocal cord paralysis, intratracheal anesthesia, endotracheal tube, tracheostomy, myopathy, myelopathy, other neurologic disorders
Impairment of esophageal function	Diverticula, achalasia, strictures, disorders of gastrointestinal motility, neoplasm, tracheoesophageal fistula, pseudobulbar palsy
Emesis	Nasogastric tube, gastric dilation, ileus, intestinal obstruction

From Cohen J, Powderly WG: *Infectious diseases*, ed 2, St Louis, 2004, Mosby.

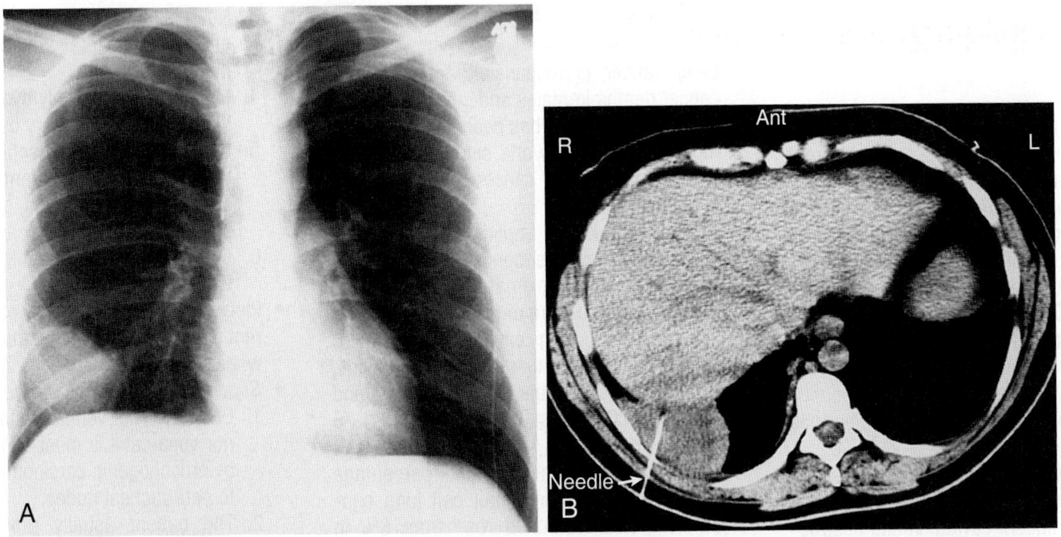

FIG. 1 Lung abscess. On a chest radiograph, a lung abscess may look to be a solid, rounded lesion **(A),** or, if it has a connection with the bronchus, there may be an air-fluid level in a thick-walled cavitary lesion. CT scanning **(B)** can be used to localize the lesion and to place a needle for drainage and aspiration of contents for culture. (From Mettler FA [ed]: *Primary care radiology,* Philadelphia, 2000, Saunders.)

Rx TREATMENT

NONPHARMACOLOGIC THERAPY

- Oxygen therapy
- Airway clearance maneuvers including postural drainage, chest percussion, and deep breathing exercises

ACUTE GENERAL Rx

Antibiotics are the mainstay of treatment and are largely empiric because of the difficulty in isolating anaerobes on culture. Regimens should include combination of a beta-lactam/beta-lactamase inhibitor or a carbapenem.

- Piperacillin/tazobactam 3.375 g IV q6h in aspiration pneumonia with lung abscess.
- Ceftriaxone 1 to 2 g IV q24h plus metronidazole 500 mg IV q8h.
- Clindamycin can be used and is more effective for anaerobic lung abscess than penicillin alone. Dose: 900 mg IV q8h until improved, then 300 to 600 mg PO q6h. We prefer to use other regimens to decrease risk of *C. difficile* infection.
- Penicillin 1 to 2 million units IV q4h until improvement (afebrile, decreased phlegm production, followed by penicillin VK 500 mg PO q6h for 2-3 wk but often up to 6-8 wk) can be given with metronidazole doses of 7.5 mg/kg IV q6h, followed by PO 500 mg bid to qid dosing as an alternative to clindamycin.
- Penicillin should not be used alone because many mouth flora anaerobes now produce penicillinase enzymes.
- Metronidazole should not be used alone because it is not active against microaerophilic streptococci and some anaerobic cocci.
- Other alternatives are ampicillin/sulbactam and carbapenems such as ertapenem and meropenem.

Duration of antibiotic therapy ranges from weeks to months. This largely depends on clinical and radiographic improvement.

CHRONIC Rx

- Bronchoscopy to assist with drainage and/or diagnosis is indicated in patients who fail to respond to antibiotics or if there is suspected underlying malignancy.
- Surgery is indicated on rare occasions (<10%) in patients with complications of lung abscess (see "Comments").

DISPOSITION

- Majority of patients fully recover with the use of antibiotics alone.
- Complications of lung abscesses include:
  1. Empyema
  2. Massive hemoptysis
  3. Pneumothorax
  4. Bronchopleural fistula
  5. Hepatobronchial fistula
  6. Brain abscess
  7. Bronchiectasis
- Mortality from lung abscess is approximately 15% to 20%.
- Despite appropriate therapy, mortality may be as high as 75% in immunocompromised patients, those with bronchial obstruction, or those with large abscesses (>6 cm).

REFERRAL

- Pulmonary and infectious disease consultation is recommended if a lung abscess is present.
- An interventional radiologist may be able to perform drainage and obtain cultures if indicated.

PEARLS & CONSIDERATIONS

COMMENTS

- It is essential to choose antibiotics with good anaerobic coverage.
- Cases refractory to antibiotics are usually the result of:
  1. Large cavity size (>6 cm)
  2. Recurrent aspiration
  3. Thick-walled cavities
  4. Obstructive lesion (e.g., lung mass or foreign body)
  5. Empyema formation
  6. Resistant organisms or other organisms such as mycobacterium, fungi, or parasites that are not covered by current therapy.
- Percutaneous transthoracic tube drainage, endoscopic drainage or surgery may be indicated if the patient is not improving with antibiotic therapy,

SUGGESTED READINGS

Available at ExpertConsult.com

RELATED CONTENT

Lung Abscess (Patient Information)
Aspiration Pneumonia (Related Key Topic)

AUTHOR: **Nisha H. Gidwani, MD**

BASIC INFORMATION

DEFINITION

Primary lung neoplasms are malignancies arising from lung tissue. The two different major subtypes are non–small cell lung cancer (NSCLC, 85% of all lung cancers; squamous cell carcinoma, adenocarcinoma, and large cell carcinoma) and small cell lung cancer (SCLC, 15% of all lung cancers).

ADENOCARCINOMA: Represents 35% to 40% of lung carcinomas; frequently located in mid-lung and periphery; initial metastases are to lymphatics; frequently associated with peripheral scars; adenocarcinoma is described as preinvasive, minimally invasive, or invasive.

SQUAMOUS CELL: Represents 20% to 30% of lung cancers; central location; metastasis by local invasion; frequent cavitation and obstructive phenomena.

SMALL CELL: Represents 15% of lung carcinomas; central location; metastasis through lymphatics; associated with lesion of the short arm of chromosome 3; high cavitation rate.

LARGE CELL: Represents 10% to 15% of lung carcinomas; frequently located in the periphery; metastasis to central nervous system and mediastinum; rapid growth rate with early metastasis.

LEPIDIC-PREDOMINANT PATTERN (BRONCHOALVEOLAR): Represents 5% of lung carcinomas; frequently located in the periphery; may be bilateral; initial metastasis through lymphatic, hematogenous, and local invasion; no correlation with cigarette smoking; cavitation rare.

SYNONYM

Lung cancer

ICD-10CM CODES

C34.10	Malignant neoplasm of upper lobe, unspecified bronchus or lung
C34.11	Malignant neoplasm of upper lobe, right bronchus or lung
C34.12	Malignant neoplasm of upper lobe, left bronchus or lung
C34.2	Malignant neoplasm of middle lobe, bronchus or lung
C34.30	Malignant neoplasm of lower lobe, unspecified bronchus or lung
C34.31	Malignant neoplasm of lower lobe, right bronchus or lung
C34.32	Malignant neoplasm of lower lobe, left bronchus or lung
C34.80	Malignant neoplasm of overlapping sites of unspecified bronchus and lung
C34.81	Malignant neoplasm of overlapping sites of right bronchus and lung
C34.82	Malignant neoplasm of overlapping sites of left bronchus and lung
C34.90	Malignant neoplasm of unspecified part of unspecified bronchus or lung
C34.91	Malignant neoplasm of unspecified part of right bronchus or lung
C34.92	Malignant neoplasm of unspecified part of left bronchus or lung

EPIDEMIOLOGY & DEMOGRAPHICS

- Lung cancer is responsible for >30% of cancer deaths in males and >25% of cancer deaths in females. It has been the most common cancer in the world since 1985 and is the leading cause of cancer-related death in both sexes.
- Tobacco smoke is implicated in 90% of cases; of these, secondhand smoke is responsible for approximately 20% of cases.
- In the U.S., there were an estimated 228,820 new cases of lung cancer and 135,720 deaths from lung cancer in 2020. Worldwide, the estimated number of new cases and deaths in 2018 was 2.01 million and 1.76 million, respectively.
- From 1990 through 2013 the percentage of patients with non–small cell lung cancer who never smoked rose from 8% to 16%, raising concerns about environmental carcinogens.
- Coincident with the decrease in smoking rates, the incidence of new cases and the rate lung cancer deaths in the U.S. continue to decrease. However, death rates among African Americans continue to be disproportionately higher.

PHYSICAL FINDINGS & CLINICAL PRESENTATION

- Weight loss, fatigue, fever, anorexia, dysphagia
- Cough, hemoptysis, dyspnea, wheezing
- Chest, shoulder, and bone pain
- Paraneoplastic syndromes (see Table 1):
  1. Lambert-Eaton myasthenic syndrome: Myopathy involving proximal muscle groups
  2. Endocrine manifestations: Hypercalcemia, ectopic adrenocorticotropic hormone secretion, syndrome of inappropriate excretion of adrenocorticotropic hormone (SIADH)
  3. Neurologic: Subacute cerebellar degeneration, peripheral neuropathy, cortical degeneration
  4. Musculoskeletal: Polymyositis, clubbing, hypertrophic pulmonary osteoarthropathy
  5. Hematologic or vascular: Migratory thrombophlebitis, marantic thrombosis, anemia, thrombocytosis, or thrombocytopenia
  6. Cutaneous: Acanthosis nigricans, dermatomyositis
- Pleural effusion (10% of patients), recurrent pneumonias (from obstruction), localized wheezing
- *Superior vena cava syndrome:*
  1. Obstruction of venous return of the superior vena cava is most commonly caused by bronchogenic carcinoma or metastasis to paratracheal nodes.
  2. The patient usually reports headache, nausea, dizziness, visual changes, syncope, and respiratory distress.
  3. Physical examination reveals distention of thoracic and neck veins, edema of face and upper extremities, facial plethora, and cyanosis.
- *Horner syndrome:* Constricted pupil, ptosis, facial anhidrosis caused by spinal cord damage between C8 and T1 as a result of a superior sulcus tumor (bronchogenic carcinoma of the extreme lung apex)
- *Pancoast tumor:* A superior sulcus tumor (Fig. 1) associated with ipsilateral Horner syndrome and shoulder pain

ETIOLOGY

- Tobacco abuse: The molecular pathology of smoking-related lung cancer is illustrated in Fig. 2. The chance of developing lung cancer for a 40-pack-yr persistent smoker is 20 times that of someone who never smoked.
- Environmental agents (e.g., radon) and industrial agents (e.g., ionizing radiation, asbestos,

TABLE 1 Paraneoplastic Syndromes Associated with Bronchogenic Carcinoma

Syndrome	Cell Type	Mechanism
Hypertrophic pulmonary osteoarthropathy and clubbing	All types	Unknown
Hyponatremia	SCLC most common; may be any type	SIADH, ectopic antidiuretic hormone production by tumor
Hypercalcemia	Usually squamous cell	Bone metastases, osteoclast-activating factor, parathyroid hormone–like hormone, prostaglandins
Cushing syndrome	Usually SCLC	Ectopic ACTH production
Lambert-Eaton myasthenic syndrome	Usually SCLC	Voltage-sensitive calcium channel antibodies in >75%; affects presynaptic neuronal calcium channel activity
Other neuromyopathic disorders	SCLC most common; may be any type	Antineuronal nuclear antibodies, also known as anti-Hu; others unknown
Thrombophlebitis	All types	Unknown

ACTH, Adrenocorticotropic hormone; *SCLC,* small cell lung cancer; *SIADH,* syndrome of inappropriate secretion of antidiuretic hormone.

Adapted from Andreoli TE et al: *Andreoli and Carpenter's Cecil essentials of medicine,* ed 8, Philadelphia, 2010, Saunders.

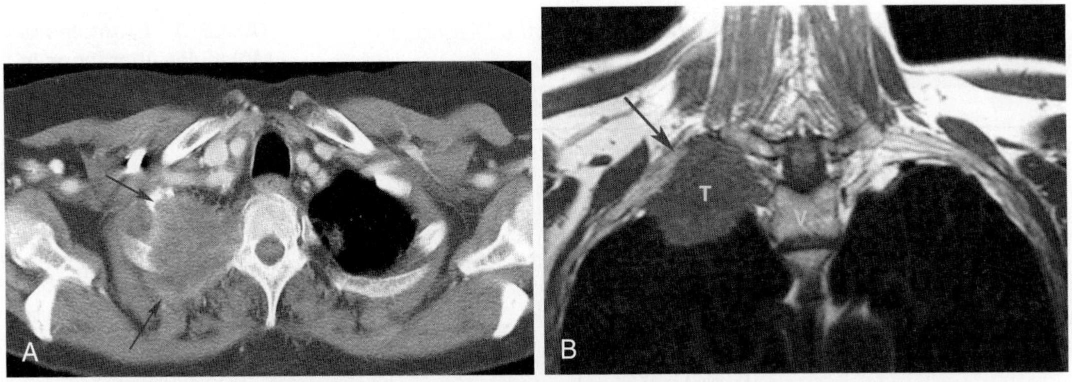

FIG. 1 Pancoast tumor with chest wall invasion. A, On computed tomography, a right apical mass is associated with invasion of the chest wall and rib destruction *(arrows)*. Although the tumor appears to contact the vertebral body, it appears intact. **B,** Coronal magnetic resonance imaging shows the relationship of the tumor (*T*) to the vertebral body (*V*) and the brachial plexus (*arrow*), which appears to be involved. (From Webb WR et al: *Fundamentals of body CT*, ed 4, Philadelphia, 2015, Elsevier.)

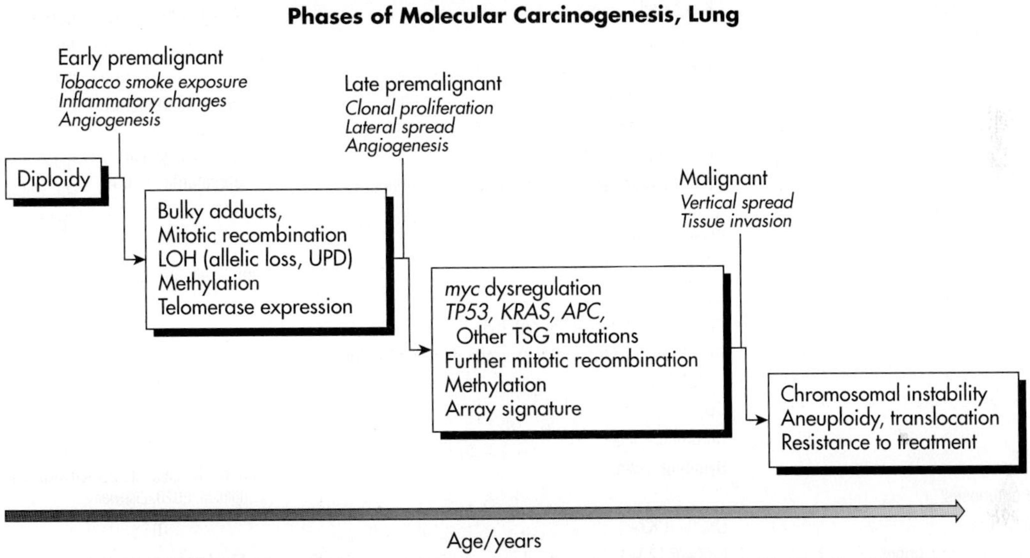

FIG. 2 The molecular pathology of smoking-related lung cancer begins w8ith the direct interaction between metabolites of carcinogenic polyaromatic hydrocarbons in cigarette smoke with host DNA. This creates bulky adducts that affect DNA repair and create transcription errors. The result is a wide range of genomic losses, gains, translocations, and point mutations that account for the high degree of molecular heterogeneity in lung tumors with diverse physiologic effects. *LOH*, Loss of heterozygosity; *TSG*, tumor suppressor gene; *UPD*, uniparental disomy. (From Niederhuber JE: *Abeloff's clinical oncology*, ed 6, Philadelphia, 2020, Elsevier.)

nickel, uranium, vinyl chloride, chromium, arsenic, coal dust).
- Lung cancer susceptibility and risk increased in inherited cancer syndromes caused by germline mutations in p53, retinoblastoma, and epidermal growth factor receptor *(EGFR)* genes.
- Fig. E3 illustrates the multistep cellular carcinogenesis in lung cancer.

Dx DIAGNOSIS

DIFFERENTIAL DIAGNOSIS

- Pneumonia
- Tuberculosis (TB)
- Metastatic carcinoma to the lung
- Lung abscess
- Granulomatous disease
- Carcinoid tumor
- Sarcoidosis
- Benign lesions that simulate thoracic malignancy:
  1. Lobar atelectasis: Pneumonia, chronic inflammatory disease, allergic bronchopulmonary aspergillosis
  2. Multiple pulmonary nodules: Septic emboli, Wegener granulomatosis, sarcoidosis, rheumatoid nodules, fungal disease, multiple pulmonary atrioventricular fistulas
  3. Mediastinal adenopathy: Sarcoidosis, lymphoma, primary TB, fungal disease, silicosis, pneumoconiosis, drug-induced (e.g., phenytoin, trimethadione)
  4. Pleural effusion: Congestive heart failure, pneumonia with parapneumonic effusion, TB, viral pneumonitis, ascites, pancreatitis, collagen-vascular disease

WORKUP

- The workup generally includes chest computed tomography (CT), positron-emission tomographic (PET) scan, and tissue biopsy. Molecular testing for treatable oncogenic alterations should be performed to further classify NSCLC. This includes testing for mutations in the gene encoding epidermal growth factor receptor (EGFR) and in BRAF v600e, searching for translocations in the genes encoding anaplastic lymphoma kinase (ALK) and rat osteosarcoma (ROS1), and assessing expression of programmed death ligand-1 (PD-L1). Common immunohistochemical markers used in the diagnosis of lung tumors are summarized

TABLE 2 Common Immunohistochemical Markers Used in the Diagnosis of Lung Tumors

Diagnosis	Positive Immunohistochemical Markers
Squamous cell carcinoma	Cytokeratin (CK) cocktail (e.g., AE1/AE3) p63 p40 CK5/6 CK7 in up to 30%
Adenocarcinoma, including adenocarcinoma in situ or minimally invasive adenocarcinoma, nonmucinous	CK cocktail CK7 TTF-1 Napsin A
In situ and invasive mucinous adenocarcinoma	CK cocktail CK7 CK20 cdx-2 TTF-1 rare
Large cell neuroendocrine carcinoma	CK cocktail TTF-1 CD56 Chromogranin A Synaptophysin
Carcinoid tumor	CK cocktail TTF-1 (weaker than in high-grade neuroendocrine tumors) CD56 Chromogranin A Synaptophysin
Atypical carcinoid tumor	CK cocktail (tends to be patchy) TTF-1 (weaker than in high-grade neuroendocrine tumors) CD56 Chromogranin A Synaptophysin
Common differential diagnoses:	
• Colonic adenocarcinoma	CK20+/CK7–
• Lung, breast, pancreatobiliary, upper gastrointestinal adenocarcinoma	CK7+/CK20–
• Urothelial carcinoma	CK7+/CK20+
• Prostatic adenocarcinoma	CK7–/CK20–
• Mesothelioma	Calretinin, WT1, CK5/6
• Malignant melanoma	S-100, HMB-45, Melan-A

From Niederhuber JE: *Abeloff's clinical oncology*, ed 6, Philadelphia, 2020, Elsevier.

TABLE 3 Examples of Common Molecular Alterations in Lung Tumors

Diagnosis	Common Molecular Alterations
Squamous preneoplasia	LOH—3p, 9p21, 8p21–23, aneuploidy, methylation
Atypical adenomatous hyperplasia	LOH—3p, 9p, aneuploidy K-ras codon 12 mutation
Adenocarcinoma	p53 mutation p16 mutation/inactivation K-Ras (42%); smokers more common EGFR overexpression (40%) EGFR mutation Her2/neu, COX-2 overexpression
Squamous cell carcinoma	p53 mutation p16 inactivation Allelic loss 3p EGFR overexpression (80%)
Large cell carcinoma	K-Ras, p53, loss p16
Large cell neuroendocrine carcinoma	p53 bcl-2 overexpression Rb mutation 3p21, FHIT, 3p22–24, 5q21,9p21
Small cell carcinoma	Rb mutation (80+%) p53 mutation 50%–80% BCL-2 expression 3p21, FHIT, 3p22–24, 5q21,9p21

COX-2, Cyclooxygenase 2; *EGFR,* epidermal growth factor receptor; *LOH,* loss of heterozygosity.
From Niederhuber JE: *Abeloff's clinical oncology*, ed 6, Philadelphia, 2020, Elsevier.

in Table 2. Table 3 describes common molecular alterations in lung tumors.
- Additional lab tests include CBC, serum chemistry studies.
- Diagnosis and staging of lung cancer should be performed simultaneously to minimize invasive testing.

LABORATORY TESTS

Various modalities are available to obtain a tissue diagnosis:
- Biopsy of any suspicious lymph nodes (e.g., supraclavicular or mediastinal node)
- Flexible fiberoptic bronchoscopy: Brush and biopsy specimens are obtained from any visualized endobronchial lesions. The use of a gene-expression classifier has a high sensitivity across different lesion sizes, locations, stages, and cell type of lung cancer. The combination of the classifier plus bronchoscopy has a sensitivity of >85%. In intermediate-risk patients with a nondiagnostic bronchoscopic examination, a negative classifier score provides support for a more conservative diagnostic approach
- Transbronchial needle aspiration: Done with a special needle passed through the bronchoscope; this technique is useful to sample mediastinal masses or paratracheal lymph nodes
- Transthoracic fine-needle aspiration biopsy with fluoroscopic or CT scan guidance to evaluate peripheral pulmonary nodules
- Endobronchial ultrasound (EBUS) guided biopsy and staging is now routinely used to evaluate suspected mediastinal and hilar nodes
- Mediastinoscopy and anteromedial sternotomy in suspected tumor involvement of the mediastinum
- Pleural biopsy in patients with pleural effusion
- Thoracentesis of pleural effusion and cytologic evaluation of the obtained fluid may confirm diagnosis

IMAGING STUDIES

- Chest x-ray (Fig. 4): The radiographic presentation often varies with the cell type. Presence of pleural effusion, lobar atelectasis, and mediastinal adenopathy can occur in any cell type.
- CT scan of the chest (Fig. 5) can evaluate mediastinal and pleural extension. The chest CT should include liver and adrenal glands (common sites of metastases). CT or MRI of brain should be considered in a patient presenting with neurologic symptoms (e.g., headaches, vision disturbances).
- PET with ^{18}F-fluorodeoxyglucose (^{18}F-FDG) (Fig. E6) is superior to CT in detecting mediastinal and distant metastases in NSCLC. It is useful for preoperative staging of NSCLC.
- The use of PET-CT (Fig. E7) for preoperative staging of NSCLC reduces both the total

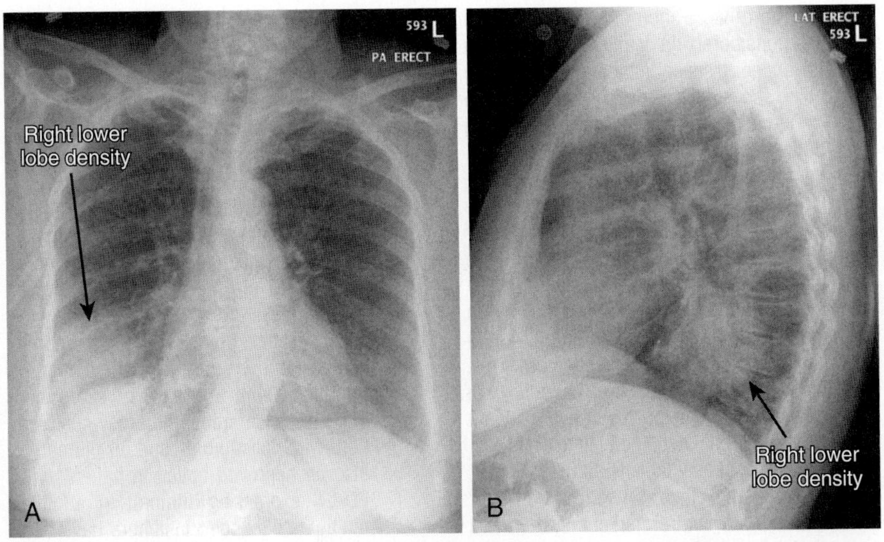

FIG. 4 Lung neoplasm, primary. Lung mass presenting with hemoptysis. **A,** Posterior-anterior (PA) chest x-ray. **B,** Lateral chest x-ray. This 83-yr-old female presented with hemoptysis of a quarter-sized clot. Her posterior-anterior chest x-ray shows a rounded right lower lobe density. On the lateral view, this is visible in the retrocardiac space. This density measures 7.6 cm in diameter. Pneumonia, neoplasm, or abscess could have this appearance on chest x-ray. Computed tomography was performed to further delineate the pathology (see Fig. 5). (From Broder JS: *Diagnostic imaging for the emergency physician,* Philadelphia, 2011, Saunders.)

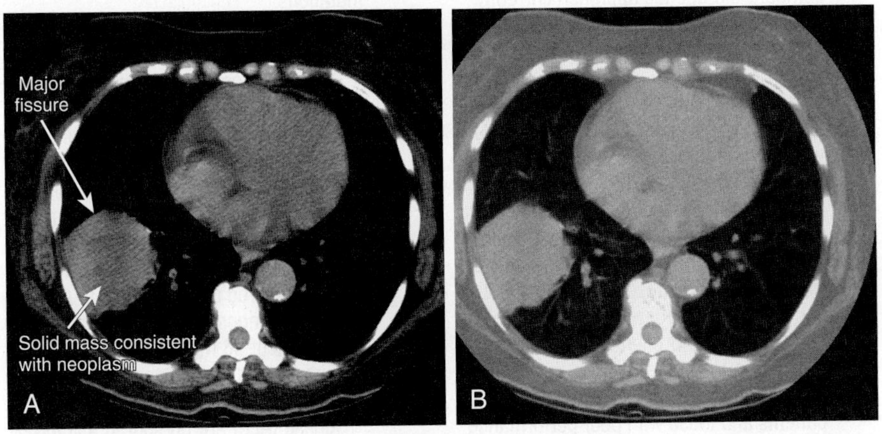

FIG. 5 Lung neoplasm, primary. Lung mass presenting with hemoptysis. Same patient as in Fig. 4. Noncontrast computed tomography was performed (contrast was withheld as a consequence of the patient's renal dysfunction) and shows a 6 x 6 cm round lesion abutting the oblique fissure (also called the major fissure) and lateral chest wall. **A,** Soft tissue windows. **B,** Lung windows. On soft tissue windows the center appears slightly darker, indicating lower density that may represent central necrosis. If IV contrast had been given, an area of necrosis would have failed to enhance. Infection or infarction is technically possible, but a pulmonary neoplasm is the most likely explanation for this lesion. Biopsy showed this to be a moderately differentiated squamous cell carcinoma. (From Broder JS: *Diagnostic imaging for the emergency physician,* Philadelphia, 2011, Saunders.)

number of thoracotomies and the number of futile thoracotomies.

STAGING

After confirmation of diagnosis, patients should undergo staging:

- In NSCLC, the TNM staging system is used. Table 4 summarizes TNM stage groups. Both stage I (no lymph node involvement) and stage II (ipsilateral bronchopulmonary/hilar lymph nodes or T_3 tumor) include localized tumors for which surgical resection is the preferred treatment. Stage III is subdivided into III_A (potentially resectable) and II_B/III_C (unresectable). Stage IV indicates metastatic disease with stage IV_A referring to intrathoracic metastases or pleural involvement or single extra-thoracic metastasis. Stage IV_B includes tumors with multiple extra-thoracic metastases.
- In SCLC, the staging system developed by the Veterans Administration Lung Cancer Study Group is used. It contains two stages:
  1. Limited-stage disease: Confined to the regional lymph nodes and to one hemithorax (excluding pleural surfaces), which can be included in a single radiation portal
  2. Extensive-stage disease: Spread beyond the confines of limited-stage disease
- Pretreatment staging procedures for lung cancer patients, in addition to complete history and physical examination, generally include the following tests:
  1. Chest radiograph (posteroanterior and lateral), ECG
  2. Laboratory evaluation: Complete blood count, complete metabolic panel; arterial blood gases and pulse oximetry in selected cases
  3. Pulmonary function studies
  4. CT scan of chest and PET scan: Trials have shown a reduction in futile thoracotomies for patients with suspected NSCLC who undergo preoperative assessment with PET in addition to conventional workup
  5. Mediastinoscopy or anterior mediastinotomy in patients being considered for possible curative lung resection
  6. Biopsy of any accessible suspect lesions
  7. CT scan to include liver and brain
  8. Bone marrow aspiration and biopsy only in selected patients with small cell carcinoma of the lung. In the absence of an increased lactate dehydrogenase or cytopenias, routine bone marrow examination is not recommended
  9. Newer technologies in preoperative staging include endoscopic bronchial ultrasonography and esophageal ultrasonography to guide biopsies; however, cervical mediastinoscopy is standard criterion in preoperative nodal staging (sensitivity >93%, specificity >95%)

Rx TREATMENT

NONPHARMACOLOGIC THERAPY

- Nutritional support
- Avoidance of tobacco and other substances toxic to the lungs
- Supplemental oxygen

ACUTE GENERAL Rx

NON–SMALL CELL CARCINOMA:

- Surgical resection is standard in patients with operable NSCLC (stage I or II) who are surgical candidates. Lobectomy is the best standard surgical approach. Lesser resections may be necessary in patients with marginal pulmonary reserve. Video-assisted thoracic surgery (VATS) decreases morbidity and shortens the hospital stay.
  1. Surgical resection is indicated in patients with limited disease (not involving mediastinal nodes, ribs, pleura, or distant sites). This represents approximately 15% to 30% of diagnosed cases. Stereotactic ablative radiotherapy is a reasonable option for patients with localized NSCLC who are not surgical candidates. Multimodality treatment guidelines are summarized in Table 5.
  2. Preoperative evaluation includes cardiac status and pulmonary function assessment. Pneumonectomy is possible if the patient has a preoperative FEV_1 = 2 L

or if the maximal voluntary ventilation is >50% of predicted capacity. Individuals with FEV_1 >1.5 L are suitable for lobectomy without further evaluation unless there is evidence of interstitial lung disease or undue dyspnea on exertion. In that case, carbon dioxide diffusion in the lung (DLCO) should be measured. If the DLCO is <80% predicted normal, the individual may not be clearly operable.

3. Conventional radiotherapy fails to durably control the primary lung tumor in nearly 70% of patients and 2-yr survival is less than 40%. Stereotactic body radiation (SBRT) uses several highly focused radiation beams to deliver total higher doses of radiotherapy (in high doses in 3 to 5 fractions) and is much more effective than conventional radiotherapy, with a local control rate equivalent to that with surgery in inoperable early stage lung cancer.

TABLE 4 TNM Stage Groups for Non–Small Cell Lung Cancer

Stage	T	N	M
Stage 0	T_{is}	N_0	M_0
Stage I_{A1}	T_{mi} or T_{1a}	N_0	M_0
Stage I_{A2}	T_{1b}	N_0	M_0
Stage I_{A3}	T_{1c}	N_0	M_0
Stage I_B	T_{2a}	N_0	M_0
Stage II_A	T_{2b}	N_0	M_0
Stage II_B	T_{1a-c}	N_1	M_0
	T_{2a-b}	N_1	M_0
	T_3	N_0	M_0
Stage III_A	T_{1a-c}	N_2	M_0
	T_{2a-b}	N_2	M_0
	T_3	N_1	M_0
	T_4	N_{0-1}	M_0
Stage III_B	T_{1a-c}	N_3	M_0
	T_{2a-b}	N_3	M_0
	T_{3-4}	N_2	M_0
Stage III_C	T_{3-4}	N_3	M_0
Stage IV_A	Any T	Any N	M_{1a-1b}
Stage IV_B	Any T	Any N	M_{1c}

TNM, Tumor, node, metastases.

4. Preoperative chemotherapy should be considered in patients with more advanced disease (stage IIIA) who are being considered for surgery because it increases the median survival time in patients with NSCLC compared with surgery alone.
5. Postoperative adjuvant chemotherapy with doublet regimens significantly increases 5-yr survival (69% vs. 54%) in patients with completely resected stage II-IIIA NSCLC. For stage I NSCLC there may be some patients (tumors >4 cm) who benefit from adjuvant chemotherapy. An algorithm for selecting patients with stage I NSCLC for postoperative adjuvant chemotherapy is outlined in Fig. 8.

- Treatment of unresectable NSCLC:
  1. Radiotherapy alone is used primarily for treatment of central nervous system and skeletal metastases, superior vena cava syndrome.
  2. In unresectable stage 3 disease, concurrent chemotherapy and thoracic radiotherapy, followed by maintenance immunotherapy with checkpoint inhibitor durvalumab (in responding patients), is the standard therapeutic approach currently.
  3. Chemotherapy, targeted therapy, and immune checkpoint therapy are the mainstays of treatment for advanced stage IV or metastatic NSCLC. Initial stratification is done based on pathology (squamous vs. nonsquamous cancers), presence of driver mutations (e.g., *EGFR, ALK, ROS1, BRAF, MET, RET,* and *NTRK* mutations in adenocarcinomas), and expression of programmed death receptor ligand-1 (PDL-1). Table 6 summarizes selected NSCLC oncogenes and targeted therapy.
  4. A platinum-based chemotherapy doublet regimen is recommended for fit patients, and single agents are offered to elderly patients and those with poor performance status. Various combination regimens are available with platinum plus pemetrexed preferred for nonsquamous cancers while other for squamous cancers other doublets such as paclitaxel plus carboplatin, cisplatin plus vinorelbine, gemcitabine plus cisplatin, and cisplatin plus docetaxel are utilized with none being clearly superior to the others. The addition of bevacizumab to paclitaxel plus carboplatin results in significant survival benefit in nonsquamous cancers.
  5. In patients with demonstrated expression of PD-L1 by immunohistochemistry, one standard approach includes combination chemo-immunotherapy regimens (platinum-based chemotherapy plus pembrolizumab or atezolizumab or nivolumab/ipilimumab). Upfront therapy with the immune-checkpoint inhibitor pembrolizumab alone is superior to chemotherapy in patients with >50% PD-L1 expression. The novel dual immunotherapy combination with ipilimumab and nivolumab is also an approved option in patients with PD-L1 expressing tumors. In addition, multiple checkpoint inhibitors have been shown to have superior survival benefit vs. chemotherapy in patients who have previously received chemotherapy.
  6. Tyrosine kinase inhibitors that target activating driver mutations are used as initial and/or subsequent therapy in patients whose adenocarcinomas that harbor such mutations:
     a. EGFR mutations (20%-25% cases) are more commonly detected in never or light smokers and in Asian patients. Gefitinib, erlotinib, afatinib, osimertinib, and dacomitinib are oral EGFR inhibitors that have showed impressive responses and improvements in median overall survival to the range of 30 mo. Currently, first-line therapy with the oral inhibitor osimertinib is the preferred option based on updated data demonstrating median overall survival of 36 mo.
     b. Oncogenic fusion genes consisting of *EML4* and anaplastic lymphoma kinase (ALK) are present in 4% to 5% of cases and can be treated with oral inhibitors crizotinib, ceritinib, alectinib, brigatinib, or lorlatinib.
     c. Approximately 2% of adenocarcinomas have genetic rearrangements involving the ROS1 proto-oncogenic receptor tyrosine kinase (ROS1), and

TABLE 5 Summary of Multimodality Guidelines

Stage	Surgery	Adjuvant Therapy	Radiation	Chemotherapy	Level of Evidence
I	Yes	No	No	No	1B—Surgical resection1B—Against postoperative chemotherapy 1A—Against postoperative radiation therapy
II	Yes	Yes	No	Yes	1B—Surgical resection1A—Postoperative chemotherapy 2A—Against postoperative radiation therapy
IIIA					
(N2-occult)	Yes	Yes	May be considered	Yes	1A—Adjuvant chemo2C—Adjuvant radiation
(N2-discrete)	Yes	No	Yes (Definitive or induction recommended)	Yes	1A—Definite or induction followed by surgery 1C—Against primary resection followed by adjuvant therapy
IIIB (N2, N3)	No	No	Yes (Definitive concurrent)	Yes	1A—Definitive concurrent 1A—Against induction followed by surgery

From Sellke FW et al: *Sabiston & Spencer surgery of the chest*, ed 9, 2016, Philadelphia, Elsevier.

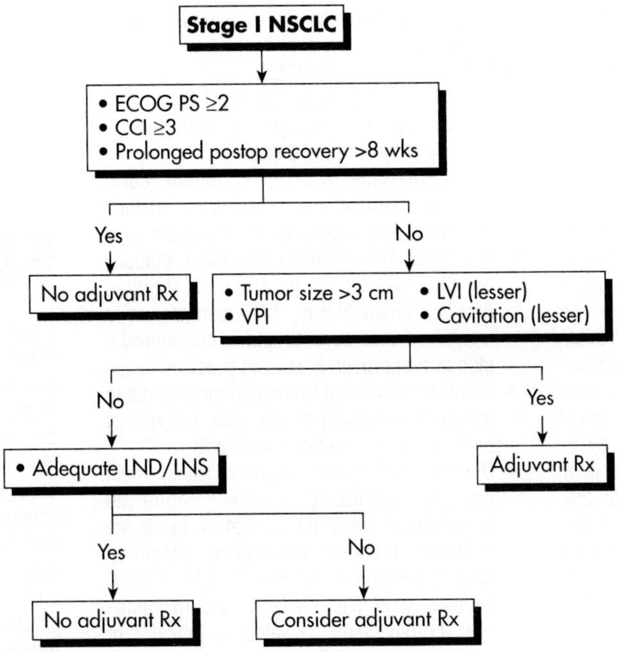

FIG. 8 Algorithm for selecting patients with stage I non–small cell lung cancer *(NSCLC)* for postoperative adjuvant chemotherapy. *CCI,* Charlson Comorbidity Index; *ECOG PS,* Eastern Cooperative Oncology Group Performance Status; *LND,* mediastinal lymph node dissection; *LNS,* systematic mediastinal lymph node sampling; *LVI,* lymphovascular invasion; *Rx,* treatment; *VPI,* visceral pleural invasion. (From Niederhuber JE: *Abeloff's clinical oncology,* ed 6, Philadelphia, 2020, Elsevier.)

TABLE 6 Selected Non–Small Cell Lung Cancer Oncogenes and Targeted Therapy

Oncogene Alteration	Incidence (%)	Clinical Relevance	Treatment
BRAF			
Mutation	1-3	V600E mutation: Most common, equal association with smokers and nonsmokers May be mechanism of acquired EGFR TKI resistance	Dabrafenib plus trametinib
EGFR (ErbB1, HER1)			
Mutation	13-50	Exon 19 deletion and Exon 21-point mutation are the most common Predominantly adenocarcinoma and nonsmokers; up to 50% frequency in Asians	TKI: Gefitinib, erlotinib, afatinib, osimertinib
EML4-ALK			
Fusion	3-7	Most frequent in adenocarcinomas, nonsmokers, men, and younger patients	Nonspecific TKI: Crizotinib, ceritinib, alectinib, brigatinib
Her2/neu (ErbB2)			No approved therapy
Mutation	2-6	Mostly adenocarcinomas and nonsmokers	
Amplification	23	Mechanism of resistance to EGFR TKI	
KRAS			
Mutation	5-30	Mostly adenocarcinomas and smokers May contribute to resistance to ALF, BRAF, and PI3K inhibitors	No approved therapy
MET			No approved therapy
Mutation	<5		
Amplification	21	Mechanism of resistance to EGFR TKI	
PIK3CA			No approved therapy
Mutation	<10	Frequently occurs in association with other mutations; more common in squamous cell	
Amplification	5-43	Mechanism of resistance to EGFR TKI	
PTEN			
Mutation	1.7-10	Associated with PI3K activation, resistance to EGFR TKI, and sensitivity to PI3K inhibitors More frequent in squamous cell	
Loss of function	4-21	Associated with PI3K activation, resistance to EGFR TKI, and sensitivity to PI3K inhibitors More frequent in squamous cell	
RET fusion gene	1-2	Mostly adenocarcinomas and nonsmokers	No approved therapy
ROS1 fusion gene	2	Mostly adenocarcinomas, nonsmokers, and younger patients	TKI: Crizotinib
VEGF			Monoclonal antibodies: Bevacizumab VEGFR TKI

BRAF, v-Raf murine sarcoma viral oncogene homolog B1; *EGFR,* epidermal growth factor receptor; *EML4-ALK,* echinoderm microtubule-associated protein-like 4 anaplastic lymphoma kinase; *ERBB,* avian erythroblastosis oncogene B; *Her2,* human epidermal growth factor receptor 2; *KRAS,* Kirsten Rat sarcoma viral oncogene homolog; *MET,* mesenchymal-epithelial transition; *PIK3CA,* phosphoinositide-3-kinase catalytic alpha polypeptide; *PTEN,* phosphatase and tensin homolog; *RET,* rearranged during transfection; *ROS1,* reactive oxygen species 1; *TKI,* tyrosine kinase inhibitor; *VEGF,* vascular endothelial growth factor; *VEGFR,* vascular endothelial growth factor receptor.
From Sellke FW et al: *Sabiston & Spencer surgery of the chest,* ed 9, 2016, Philadelphia, Elsevier.

these patients can be treated with the oral inhibitors crizotinib and ceritinib.

d. Approximately 2% of adenocarcinomas harbor the BRAF V600E mutation, and these patients can be treated with the combination of oral BRAF/MEK inhibitor (dabrafenib plus trametinib) therapy.
e. Mutations leading to MET exon 14 skipping are found in 3%-4% of patients with advanced non–small cell lung cancer. In 2020 the FDA approved the oral inhibitor capmatinib for the treatment of adult patients with NSCLC harboring this specific MET mutation, which requires confirmatory diagnosis using a companion diagnostic next-generation sequencing (NGS) assay.
f. RET (rearranged during transfection) rearrangements occur in 1% to 2% of unselected NSCLC cases and are commonly found in patients who have never smoked or are minimal smokers. Efficacy of the oral inhibitor selpercatinib in patients with RET fusion-positive NSCLC was 64% in patients who were previously treated with platinum-based chemotherapy and 84% in patients who had never undergone treatment.
g. *NTRK* fusions are clinically targetable and have been identified to be the predominant drivers of growth in <1% of advanced lung cancers. The treatment of patients with NTRK fusion-positive cancers with a first-generation TRK inhibitor, such as larotrectinib or entrectinib, is associated with high response rates but eventual development of resistance.

7. Early initiation of palliative care focusing on management of symptoms, psychosocial support, and assistance with decision making in patients with metastatic NSCLC leads to improved quality of life, longer survival, and less use of aggressive end-of-life care.

SMALL CELL LUNG CANCER:

- Limited-stage disease: Standard treatments include thoracic radiotherapy and chemotherapy (cisplatin and etoposide).
- Extensive-stage disease: Standard combination chemotherapy regimens include platinum plus etoposide or platinum plus irinotecan. The addition of the PD-1 antibody atezolizumab or durvalumab to standard first-line chemotherapy has been proven to improve overall survival and is considered a standard approach in current practice.
- Prophylactic cranial irradiation for patients in complete remission to decrease the risk of central nervous system metastasis.
- Despite high initial response rates, most patients eventually relapse. Topotecan or irinotecan may be an option for these patients. Immune checkpoint inhibitors have demonstrated survival benefit in SCLC patients who have failed standard therapies. Lurbinectedin, a selective inhibitor of oncogenic transcription, is now approved for patients who developed disease progression after first-line therapy.

DISPOSITION

- The 5-yr survival of patients with resectable NSCLC (stages I-III) is approximately 30%. The 5-yr survival for stage 4 patients is increasing, with survival rates in the 25% range reported in current trials with the use of targeted therapy and immunotherapy.
- Median survival time in patients with limited-stage disease SCLC is 15 mo; in patients with extensive-stage SCLC, it is in the range of 12 mo.
- Among patients with metastatic NSCLC, early palliative care results in longer survival and significant improvements in both quality of life and mood.
- Population-level mortality from NSCLC in the United States fell sharply from 2013 to 2016, and survival after diagnosis improved substantially. Reduction in incidence along with modern treatment advances are likely explanations for the reduction in mortality observed.

PEARLS & CONSIDERATIONS

Screening with use of low-dose computed tomography (LDCT) for detection of lung cancer among persons with a heavy history of smoking increases the percentage of lung cancer cases that are diagnosed in stage 1 and reduces mortality from lung cancer. The National Lung Screening Trial (NLST) showed that lung cancer screening with LDCT resulted in a 20% reduction in lung cancer mortality. New guidelines recommend annual LDCT for those who are current or former smokers ages 55 to 74 yr. Screening should be discontinued once a person has not smoked for 15 yr or develops a health problem that substantially limits life expectancy or the ability or willingness to have curative lung surgery.

SUGGESTED READINGS

Available at ExpertConsult.com

RELATED CONTENT

Lung Cancer (Patient Information)
Lung Cancer Screening (Patient Information)
Horner Syndrome (Related Key Topic)
Lambert-Eaton Myasthenic Syndrome (Related Key Topic)
Paraneoplastic Syndromes (Related Key Topic)
Superior Vena Cava Syndrome (Related Key Topic)

AUTHOR: **Ritesh Rathore, MD**

BASIC INFORMATION

DEFINITION

Lyme disease is a multisystem inflammatory disorder caused by the transmission of a spirochete, *Borrelia burgdorferi,* via the bite of infected *Ixodes* ticks, taking 36 to 48 hr for a tick to take a blood meal and transmit the infecting organism to the host. Table E1 summarizes the Centers for Disease Control and Prevention (CDC) Lyme disease surveillance case definition.

SYNONYMS

Bannwarth syndrome (Europe)
Acrodermatitis chronica atrophicans

ICD-10CM CODES	
A69.20	Lyme disease, unspecified
A69.21	Meningitis due to Lyme disease
A69.22	Other neurologic disorders in Lyme disease
A69.23	Arthritis due to Lyme disease
A69.29	Other conditions associated with Lyme disease

EPIDEMIOLOGY & DEMOGRAPHICS

INCIDENCE (IN U.S.): In the U.S., 4.4 cases/100,000 persons; it is the most common vector-borne infection in the U.S., with more than 30,000 new cases reported each year. 90% of cases are found in Massachusetts, Connecticut, Rhode Island, New York, New Jersey, Pennsylvania, Minnesota, Wisconsin, and California. The area of transmission in the U.S. is expanding farther into the South and upper Northeast (Fig. E1). The disease also occurs in Europe and Asia with a different *Ixodes* tick vector. Table E2 summarizes principal vector ticks and spirochetes associated with Lyme borreliosis.
PREDOMINANT SEX: Male = female
PREDOMINANT AGE: Median age of 28 yr
PEAK INCIDENCE: May to November

PHYSICAL FINDINGS & CLINICAL PRESENTATION

Lyme disease may present in the following stages:
- *Early localized stage (incubation period 3 to 30 days):* Early Lyme disease, erythema migrans (EM); skin rash, often at site of tick bite (the CDC has defined EM rash as an expanding red macule or papule that must reach at least 5 cm in size, with or without central clearing); target lesions from ECM can be found in 60% to 80% of localized infections; possible fever, myalgias 3 to 32 days after tick bite
- *Early disseminated stage (incubation period 3 to 6 wk):* Days to weeks later; multiorgan system involvement, including CNS with aseptic meningitis–type picture or Bell palsy, joints (arthritis or arthralgias), cardiac including varying degrees of heart block; related to dissemination of spirochete
- *Late stage (incubation period months to years):* Months to years after tick exposure; affects central and peripheral nervous system, cardiac, joints

Common presenting signs and symptoms include:
- EM (Fig. E2). Most patients with EM (about 80%) have a single lesion but the bacteria can disseminate hematogenously to other sites in the skin and result in often smaller erythema migrans lesions.
- Lymphadenopathy, neck pains, pharyngeal erythema, myalgias, hepatosplenomegaly.
- Patients will complain of malaise, fatigue, lethargy, headache, fever/chills, neck pain, myalgias, back pain.

ETIOLOGY

B. burgdorferi transmitted from bite of an *Ixodes* tick (mostly in the nymph stage, but can also be from adult ticks). Human infection occurs through inoculation of spirochetes in infected saliva and usually requires tick attachment for more than 36 hr.

DIAGNOSIS

Clinical presentation, exposure to ticks in endemic area, and diagnostic testing for antibody response to *B. burgdorferi.* Serologic testing at early stages is usually negative; therefore, in early stage, documentation of erythema migrans lesion with a compatible epidemiologic history is sufficient for diagnosis, and laboratory testing is not indicated.

DIFFERENTIAL DIAGNOSIS

- Chronic fatigue/fibromyalgia
- Acute viral illnesses
- Babesiosis
- Human granulocytic anaplasmosis

WORKUP

Serologic testing is the principal means of laboratory diagnosis of Lyme disease. Current recommendations include using a sensitive enzyme immunoassay (EIA) or immunofluorescence assay, followed by a Western immunoblot assay for specimens yielding positive or equivocal results.

LABORATORY TESTS

- ELISA testing and if positive or equivocal then followed by a Western blot IgM and IgG (Table E3). A Western blot IgM assay is positive if 2 of 3 bands present. The Western blot IgG is positive if 5 of 10 bands present.
- An alternative serologic test is the VlsE C6 ELISA (C6 peptide), which detects an IgG response earlier and may be more sensitive than the ELISA, but its specificity is lower than the two-tier testing method.
- Early disease often is difficult to diagnose serologically, secondary to slow immune response.
- Culturing of skin lesions (EM) and polymerase chain reaction (PCR) of synovial fluid or CSF can also give the diagnosis of active infection.
- Fig. 3 is an algorithm for the diagnosis and treatment of arthritis associated with Lyme disease.

IMAGING STUDIES

- ECG
- Echocardiogram if conduction abnormalities are present with cardiac involvement
- CT scan, MRI of brain in patients with CNS involvement

TREATMENT

Early localized Lyme disease:
- Doxycycline 100 mg bid in adults (children: 2 mg/kg twice daily if ≥8 yr) [doxycycline offers the advantage of treating possible coinfection with the bacterial agents of ehrlichiosis] for 10 to 14 days or amoxicillin 500 mg tid for adults (children: 50 mg/kg per day in three divided doses) for 14 to 21 days.
- Alternative treatments for pregnancy and children ≤8 yr: Cefuroxime axetil 500 mg bid for 14 to 21 days (children: 30 mg/kg per day in two divided doses), azithromycin 500 mg PO for 7 to 10 days but should **not** be used as a first-line agent, as it is less effective than doxycycline and amoxicillin.
- A single dose of 200 mg doxycycline given within 72 hr of removing an engorged *Ixodes* tick can significantly reduce the risk of developing of Lyme disease in endemic areas and is reasonable prophylaxis in nonpregnant adults and children ≥8 yr old.

Early disseminated and late persistent infection:
- 28 days of treatment is often prescribed, although recent evidence supports treating patients with a 14-day course of oral doxycycline for early neurologic Lyme disease in ambulatory patients. Doxycycline and ceftriaxone appear equally effective for acute disseminated Lyme disease.
- Arthritis: 28 days of doxycycline or amoxicillin plus probenecid.
- Neurologic involvement requires parenteral antibiotics. Those who fail to respond should be treated with IV ceftriaxone or cefotaxime.
- Ceftriaxone 2 g/day IV for 21 to 28 days; alternative: Cefotaxime 2 g q8h IV; alternative: Penicillin G 5 million U qid.
- Cardiac involvement: IV ceftriaxone or cefotaxime plus cardiac monitoring.
- Prolonged treatment with IV or PO antibiotic therapy for up to 90 days did not improve symptoms more than placebo.

Post–Lyme disease syndrome:
- Presence of disabling symptoms such as fatigue, malaise, diffuse pains, and poor concentration, which may be due to an exuberant host inflammatory response even in patients who have received proper antibiotic treatment
- Antibiotics are not indicated. Antibiotic treatment of patients with persistent unexplained symptoms despite previous antibiotic treatment of Lyme disease provides little, if any, benefit and carries significant risk
- Supportive care

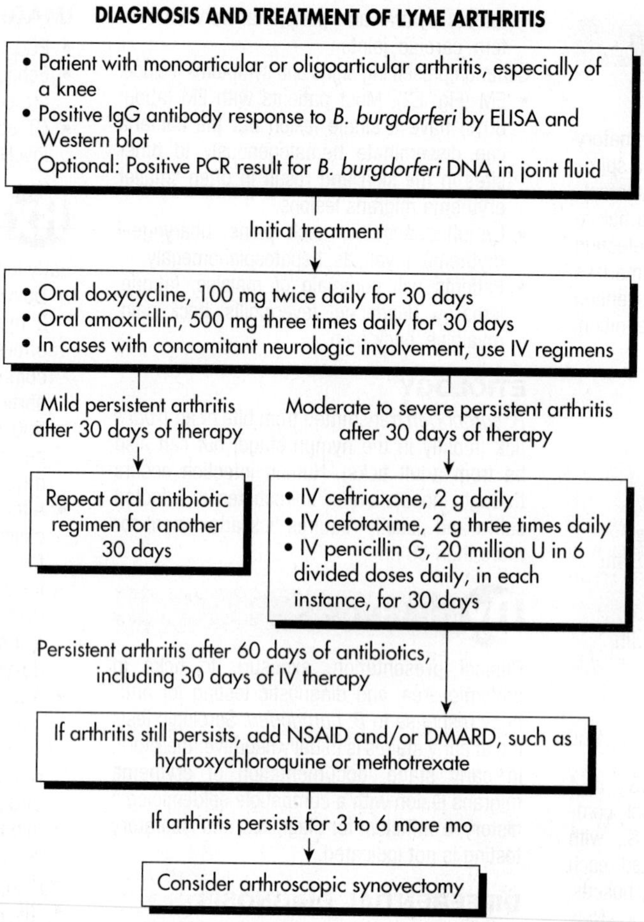

FIG. 3 Algorithm for the diagnosis and treatment of arthritis associated with Lyme disease. *DMARD,* Disease-modifying antirheumatic drug; *DNA,* deoxyribonucleic acid; *ELISA,* enzyme-linked immunosorbent assay; *Ig,* immunoglobulin; *IV,* intravenous; *NSAID,* nonsteroidal antiinflammatory drug; *PCR,* polymerase chain reaction. (From Hochberg MC: *Rheumatology*, ed 7, Philadelphia, 2019, Elsevier.)

DISPOSITION

- The patient often needs careful follow-up and supportive care for the arthralgia-neuritis symptoms.
- 10% to 20% of treated patients may have lingering symptoms of fatigue, disrupted sleep, and musculoskeletal complaints. Repeat episodes of EM in appropriately treated patients are due to reinfection and not to relapse.

REFERRAL

- To a neurologist if significant neurologic complications (meningitis, myelitis, ophthalmoplegia, Bell palsy)
- To a cardiologist if the patient develops evidence of cardiac conduction disturbances or pericarditis

PEARLS & CONSIDERATIONS

- A physician diagnosis of classic EM in an endemic region of Lyme disease is sufficient to make a definitive diagnosis.
- In some patients with Lyme disease, nonspecific complaints such as headache, fatigue, and arthralgia may persist for months after appropriate (and ultimately successful) antibiotic treatment. Long-term antibiotic treatment does not provide additional beneficial effects.
- There is no evidence of current or previous *Borrelia burgdorferi* infection in most patients evaluated at university-based Lyme disease referral centers. Psychiatric comorbidity and other psychologic factors are prominent in the presentation and outcome of some patients who inaccurately ascribe longstanding symptoms to "chronic Lyme disease."
- It is important to realize that one tick bite can transmit Lyme disease *and* the bacterial agents of either ehrlichiosis or babesiosis (protozoan parasite), or even both, and these latter agents require separate serologic testing and possibly therapy. *Ehrlichiosis* is treated with doxycycline, but *Babesia* would require a different therapy. Powassan virus can also be transmitted by the *Ixodes* tick bite and causes an encephalitis seen in eastern Canada and northcentral, northeastern, and upper midwestern United States. Cases have been increasing.
- Tick bite protection: EPA-registered insect repellents containing DEET, picaridin, IR3535, oil of lemon eucalyptus (OLE), para-menthane-3,8-diol (PMD), or 2-undecanone can prevent ticks from attaching when applied, and can last for several hours. OLE and PMD products cannot be used on children under 3 yr of age.

RELATED CONTENT

Lyme Disease (Patient Information)

SUGGESTED READINGS

Available at ExpertConsult.com

AUTHOR: **Glenn G. Fort, MD, MPH**

BASIC INFORMATION

DEFINITION

Lymphangitis refers to the inflammation of lymphatic vessels resulting from infectious or noninfectious causes. Infectious causes include bacteria, mycobacteria, viruses, fungi, and parasites.

SYNONYMS

Nodular lymphangitis
Sporotrichoid lymphangitis

ICD-10CM CODE

I89.1 Lymphangitis

EPIDEMIOLOGY & DEMOGRAPHICS

INCIDENCE (IN U.S.): Several hundred cases/year of sporotrichoid lymphangitis, which is a fungal infection; bacterial lymphangitis more common but not reported.

PHYSICAL FINDINGS & CLINICAL PRESENTATION

ACUTE LYMPHANGITIS:

- Commonly associated with a bacterial cellulitis
- Usually develops after cutaneous inoculation of microorganisms into the lymphatic vessels through disrupted skin or as a result of spread from a distal infection
- May or may not recognize a site of skin trauma (i.e., laceration, puncture, ulcer)
- In hours to days, distal appearance of erythema, edema, and tenderness, with linear erythematous streaks extending proximally to regional lymph nodes
- Possible lymphadenitis and fever
- Predisposition to group A streptococcal infection of the skin in those with uncontrolled diabetes mellitus, chronic lymphedema, and superficial fungal infections (e.g., tinea pedis)
- Nonbacterial causes can include arthropod bites and reaction to medical interventions (e.g., purified protein derivative [PPD] skin testing for tuberculosis)

SPOROTRICHOID OR NODULAR LYMPHANGITIS:

- Includes subcutaneous nodules that develop along the path of involved lymphatics
- Usually preceded by an episode of cutaneous inoculation or trauma to the hand
- Lesions apparent from one to several weeks after inoculation
- Initially, nodular or papular lesion; may ulcerate
- Pain is organism-dependent
- May have frank pus or a serosanguineous discharge
- Systemic complaints uncommon, but infection with certain microorganisms associated with fever, chills, myalgias, and headache

ETIOLOGY

- Acute lymphangitis: Usually associated with *Streptococcus pyogenes* (group A streptococcus), and to a lesser extent staphylococcus species, including community-acquired methicillin-resistant *S. aureus* (CA-MRSA)
- Nodular lymphangitis caused by one of several organisms:
  1. *Sporothrix schenckii* ("Rose gardener's disease," corn cultivation)
     a. Most common recognized cause in the U.S., usually in the Midwest
     b. Fungus found in soil and plant debris
  2. *Nocardia brasiliensis:* Gram-positive rod-shaped bacteria found in soil
  3. *Mycobacterium marinum:* Associated with trauma related to water (e.g., aquariums, swimming pools, fish)
  4. *Leishmania brasiliensis:*
     a. Protozoal parasite transmitted to humans by sand flies, mostly to travelers in endemic areas (Texas, rural Central and South America, Africa, subtropical Asia)
  5. *Francisella tularensis:* Gram-negative bacteria. Also causes lymphadenitis:
     a. Most often in Southern/Midwestern states (Arkansas, Missouri, Oklahoma)
     b. Associated with contact with infected mammals (e.g., rabbits, squirrels, cats), tick bites, and (rarely) water exposure

Dx DIAGNOSIS

DIFFERENTIAL DIAGNOSIS

- Nodular lymphangitis
  1. Blastomyces or Coccidioides, Histoplasma, *Bacillus anthracis,* Mycetoma
- Insect or snake bites
- Filariasis

WORKUP

- Acute lymphangitis: Blood cultures
- Nodular lymphangitis: Various stains and cultures of drainage or biopsy specimens of inoculation sites

LABORATORY TESTS

- WBCs possibly elevated with cellulitis
- Eosinophilia common with helminthic infections
- Skin biopsy and microbiologic cultures may be necessary to confirm diagnosis in nodular lymphangitis

Rx TREATMENT

NONPHARMACOLOGIC THERAPY

Limb elevation

ACUTE GENERAL Rx

- Penicillin possibly sufficient, but 1 wk of dicloxacillin or cephalexin 500 mg PO qid commonly used to ensure antistaphylococcal coverage; if CA-MRSA suspected, then use oral Bactrim DS one PO bid or clindamycin 300 mg PO q6h. Reserve vancomycin 1 g IV every 12 hr for patients requiring IV therapy
- If allergic to penicillin:
  1. Clindamycin 300 mg PO qid for 7 days *or*
  2. Erythromycin 500 mg PO qid for 7 days
  3. Levofloxacin 500 mg PO daily or moxifloxacin 400 mg PO daily for 7 days
- Nodular lymphangitis: Specific therapy directed at etiologic agent
- For superficial fungal infections: Treatment may prevent recurrence of acute lymphangitis

DISPOSITION

- Acute lymphangitis: Usually resolves with therapy
- Recurrent attacks: May lead to chronic lymphedema of limb, rarely resulting in elephantiasis nostras (nonfilarial elephantiasis)
- Nodular lymphangitis: Usually responds to appropriate therapy

REFERRAL

- If acute lymphangitis is more than a mild disease or if it involves the face
- If nodular lymphangitis or filariasis is suspected

PEARLS & CONSIDERATIONS

COMMENTS

- Outside of the U.S., initial episodes of filariasis caused by Brugia malayi resemble acute lymphangitis.
- Chronic lymphedema or elephantiasis results from recurrent episodes.
- For chronic lymphedema, adherence to limb elevation, compression/support stockings, and adequate glycemic control (for patients with diabetes) all can reduce risk of acute lymphangitis.

RELATED CONTENT

Lymphangitis (Patient Information)

SUGGESTED READINGS

Available at www.ExpertConsult.com

AUTHOR: **Russell J. McCulloh, MD**

BASIC INFORMATION

DEFINITION

A primary role of the lymphatic system is to transport proteins from the interstitium to the heart. When the transport capacity of the lymphatic system is reduced, proteins accumulate in the interstitium. Accumulated proteins attract water, which creates a high protein swelling in the subcutaneous tissues called lymphedema.

SYNONYM

Elephantiasis

ICD-10CM CODES	
I89.0	Lymphedema, not elsewhere classified
I97.2	Postmastectomy lymphedema syndrome
Q82.0	Hereditary lymphedema

EPIDEMIOLOGY & DEMOGRAPHICS

PRIMARY LYMPHEDEMA:
- Found in 1.1/100,000 people aged <20 yr
- Females outnumber males 3.5:1
- Incidence peaks between ages 12 and 16 (puberty)

SECONDARY LYMPHEDEMA: See specific etiology in the following.

PHYSICAL FINDINGS & CLINICAL PRESENTATION

Lymphedema is a slow-onset, progressive disease characterized by an asymmetric, inflammatory swelling, traveling distal to proximal, that can affect any body part including limbs, trunk, head/neck, and genitals (Fig. 1). Box 1 summarizes lymphedema staging from the International Society of Lymphology.

STAGE 0: LATENCY:
- Decreased lymphatic system transport capacity due to primary or secondary etiology
- Subjective complaints of affected body part feeling heavy or achy
- No objective findings, no apparent swelling

STAGE I: REVERSIBLE:
- Edema is observable, soft, pitting, and reversible with elevation.
- No secondary skin changes are present.

STAGE II: SPONTANEOUSLY IRREVERSIBLE:
- Skin becomes more firm/fibrotic, therefore less pitting.
- Edema does not reverse to normal with elevation.
- Possibility of infections (cellulitis), wounds, or weeping (lymphorrhea).

STAGE III: ELEPHANTIASIS:
- Skin becomes very firm/fibrotic, therefore nonpitting.
- Evidence of substantial skin changes (e.g., papillomas, lobules, "peau d' orange").

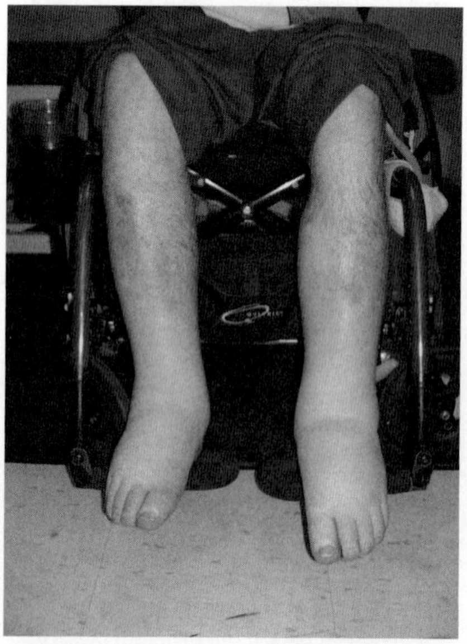

FIG. 1 Lymphedema before treatment.

ETIOLOGY

Lymphedema is caused by a reduction in lymphatic system transport (Table E1) and is classified into primary and secondary forms.

PRIMARY LYMPHEDEMA:
- Occurs when the lymphatic system does not mature properly during fetal development
  1. Aplasia
  2. Hypoplasia
  3. Hyperplasia
- Can be familial, genetic, or hereditary
- Lymphedema congenital: Symptoms present at birth
- Lymphedema praecox: Symptoms onset before the age of 35 (commonly during puberty)
- Lymphedema tardum: Symptoms onset at the age of 35 or after

SECONDARY LYMPHEDEMA:
- Occurs secondary to a disruption or obstruction of the lymphatic system caused by:
  1. Filariasis (number one cause worldwide)
  2. Lymph node surgery/radiation due to cancer (number one cause in the U.S.)
  3. Other: Chronic venous insufficiency (CVI), deep vein thrombosis (DVT), infection, surgery/trauma, lipedema, and obesity

BOX 1 Lymphedema Staging

Stage 0: Latent
- Impaired lymphatic function
- No evident edema; subclinical
- May last months or years before progression

Stage I: Spontaneously Reversible
- Early accumulation of protein-rich fluid
- Pitting edema
- Subsides with elevation

Stage II: Spontaneously Irreversible
- Accumulation of protein-rich fluid
- Pitting edema progresses to fibrosis
- Does not resolve with elevation alone

Stage III: Lymphostatic Elephantiasis
- Nonpitting
- Significant fibrosis
- Trophic skin changes

From International Society of Lymphology: The diagnosis and treatment of peripheral edema: 2009 consensus document of the International Society of Lymphology, *Lymphology* 42(2):51-60, 2009.

DIAGNOSIS

- Lymphedema is primarily a clinical diagnosis made on the basis of past medical history and objective findings that distinguish it from other causes of chronic edema.
- A Stemmer sign is often used to identify lymphedema (inability to pick up or pinch a fold of skin at the base of the second toe or finger).
- When physical examination is inconclusive, other available imaging tests can help make the diagnosis (see "Imaging Studies").

DIFFERENTIAL DIAGNOSIS

Other causes of edema that should be ruled out before treatment for lymphedema include cardiac, renal, hepatic, and thyroid dysfunction.

WORKUP

A detailed history and physical examination should help exclude most of the differential diagnoses.

LABORATORY TESTS

- Blood urea nitrogen, creatinine, liver function tests, albumin, urine analysis, and thyroid function tests are obtained to exclude possible systemic causes of edema.
- Genetic testing may be practical in defining a specific hereditary syndrome with a discrete gene mutation such as lymphedema distichiasis *(FOXC2),* Milroy disease *(VEGFR-3)* (Fig. E2), Meige disease, or Klippel-Trenaunay-Weber syndrome.

IMAGING STUDIES

- Lymphoscintigraphy: Diagnostic image of choice for lymphedema (if needed)
- Indocyanine green (ICG) fluorescent lymphography: Can now be used to identify sentinel nodes, to demonstrate superficial lymph channels and functional lymphatics, to indicate treatment pathways, and to confirm the effectiveness of therapeutic techniques
- Magnetic resonance imaging (MRI): Primarily used in tumor diagnosis
- Duplex ultrasound: Determines venous involvement in the edema
- Computed axial tomography (CAT): Distinguishes between fatty tissue and accumulations of protein-rich fluids
- Lymphography: Phased out in favor of less invasive techniques

TREATMENT

NONPHARMACOLOGIC THERAPY

- Complete decongestive therapy (CDT) is backed by longstanding research and experience as the primary treatment of choice for lymphedema in both children and adults (Fig. 3). It should be delivered by a certified lymphedema therapist (CLT). CDT involves a two-phase treatment program:

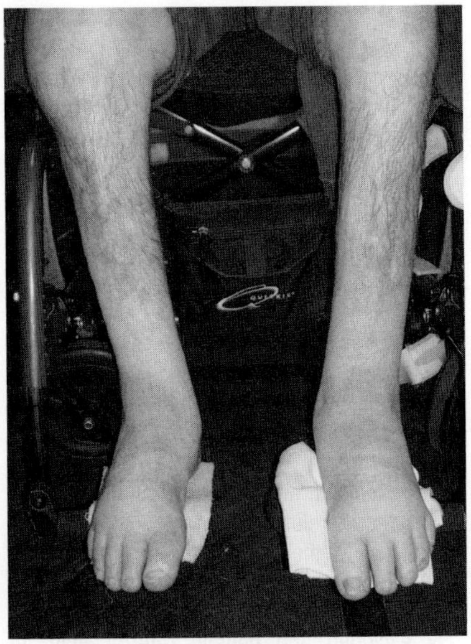

FIG. 3 Lymphedema after treatment.

1. Phase 1—Reduce tissue congestion of affected body part with daily treatments:
   a. Manual lymph drainage
   b. Skin care
   c. Compression wrapping of limb
   d. Decongestive exercises
2. Phase 2—Maintain decongestion with home maintenance program:
   a. Daily use of elastic and inelastic compression garments that are properly fitted according to circumference and length to prevent lymphedema from returning.
   b. Compression is graduated; most of the compression is distal with decreasing compression in the stocking proximally.
   c. Different knits and compression classes are available for different stages of lymphedema.
   d. Choices of garments include below-the-knee stockings, thigh-high stockings, pantyhose, sleeves, bras, and truncal garments.

- Massage (or any modality that increases blood flow) can have negative effects on lymphedema by increasing vasodilation. Therefore it is contraindicated on the lymphedematous quadrants.
- Compression pumps have not been found to be effective in removing proteins from lymphedematous quadrants.
- Nutritional therapy (reducing the amount of proteins ingested) is ineffective in the treatment of lymphedema.

PHARMACOLOGIC THERAPY

No drugs have been shown to be beneficial in the treatment of lymphedema. Diuretics in particular have not been found to be effective in removing proteins from lymphedematous quadrants and may promote the development of volume depletion.

SURGERY

Surgery for lymphedema has been proven largely unsuccessful and should not be considered before CDT. Surgical procedures are divided into two types:

- Physiologic procedures: Those performed to improve lymph node drainage (e.g., anastomoses of the lymph system with the venous system, lymph node transplant).
- Excisional or debulking procedures: Those performed to excise the subcutaneous tissue (e.g., Charles procedure, Thompson procedure, the modified Homans procedure, and liposuction). Liposuction-circumferential suction-assisted lipectomy represents a newly proposed method to reduce morbidity involved in the traditional excisional techniques.

PEARLS & CONSIDERATIONS

- Lymphedema is a chronic, generally incurable but very manageable condition that requires lifelong care and attention along with psychosocial support.
- Children and adolescents (along with parents and adults) should be encouraged to pursue a normal life, participating in school activities and sports (preferably noncontact, such as swimming).
- Infections such as cellulitis should be treated promptly.
- If the etiology is filariasis caused by the parasites *Wuchereria bancrofti* or *Brugia malayi*, treatment is diethylcarbamazine citrate 5 mg/kg in divided doses for 3 wk.
- Patients with lymphedema commonly manifest psychiatric comorbidities as a result of their disease, such as anxiety; depression; adjustment problems; and difficulty in vocational, domestic, or social domains.
- Lymphedema can be complicated in rare cases by development of lymphangiosarcomata or other cutaneous malignancies.
- Gene therapy to develop new lymphangiosis in the affected body parts is a potential clinical remedy in the future.

RELATED CONTENT

Lymphedema (Patient Information)

SUGGESTED READINGS

Available at ExpertConsult.com

AUTHORS: **Frank G. Fort, MD, FACS, RPHS,** and **Kathryn Taylor Anilowski, MS, PT, CLT-LANA**

Lynch Syndrome

BASIC INFORMATION

DEFINITION

Lynch syndrome is a hereditary predisposition to malignancy of the colon that is explained by a germline mutation in a DNA mismatch repair gene. The Lynch syndrome phenotype is characterized by a predominance of cancers on the right side of the colon and a propensity for synchronous and metachronous colorectal cancers.

SYNONYMS

Hereditary nonpolyposis colorectal cancer
HPNCC
Hereditary site-specific colon cancer

ICD-10CM CODE

C18.9 Malignant neoplasm of colon, unspecified

EPIDEMIOLOGY & DEMOGRAPHICS

The lifetime risk for developing colon cancer in the U.S. is approximately 6%. Up to 30% of colon cancer is inherited, and 3% may be attributable to Lynch syndrome. The incidence of Lynch syndrome is estimated to be between 1:660 and 1:2000. Lynch syndrome is the most common form of hereditary colon cancer. The average age of diagnosis for Lynch syndrome is 45 yr, although diagnosis can occur as early as the second decade or as late as the seventh decade.

RISK FACTORS: Family history of colon cancer or other hereditary nonpolyposis colorectal cancer (HNPCC)-related cancers such as endometrial (up to 40% of women with Lynch syndrome may develop endometrial cancer), biliary tract, ovarian, stomach, upper urinary tract, or brain. Table 1 summarizes the risk of Lynch syndrome.

GENETICS: Autosomal-dominant inheritance pattern.

PHYSICAL FINDINGS & CLINICAL PRESENTATION

- Changes in bowel habits (prolonged constipation)
- Melena
- Hematochezia
- Abdominal pain
- Unexplained weight loss
- Decreased appetite
- Right-sided colon cancer (70% to 85% of cases)

ETIOLOGY

Lynch syndrome is thought to be secondary to germline mutations in DNA mismatch repair genes. The predominant genes involved are *MSH2* and *MLH1,* which are tumor suppressor genes, although other genes have documented involvement (*PMS1, PMS2, MSH6,* and *EpCAM*). Mutations in these genes prevent repair of DNA mismatches during DNA replication. This is most prevalent in regions of DNA called microsatellites, causing DNA microsatellite instability and leading to an increased risk for malignancy, especially colon cancer. *MSH6* mutations are associated with a markedly lower cancer risk than *MLH1* or *MSH2* mutations.

DIAGNOSIS

DIFFERENTIAL DIAGNOSIS

- Familial adenomatosis polyposis
- Peutz-Jeghers syndrome
- Juvenile polyposis
- Nonhereditary colorectal cancer. Table 2 compares Lynch syndrome and sporadic colorectal cancer
- Gardner syndrome

WORKUP

If an individual presents with numerous adenomatous polyps or has multiple relatives with cancer at a young age, a family history complete with pedigree must be obtained. Clinical diagnosis of the Lynch syndrome can be made with the Amsterdam or Bethesda criteria (Box 1) as well as newer models such as prediction model for gene mutations 5 (PREMM5).

- Revised Amsterdam (II) criteria (must meet all criteria):
  1. HNPCC-associated carrier diagnosis in at least three individuals in the family
  2. One of the patients is a first-degree family member of two other patients
  3. Involved patients occur in at least two successive generations with diagnosis of HNPCC
  4. At least one diagnosis in family of HNPCC was made before age 50
  5. The diagnoses are histologically confirmed
  6. Familial adenomatous polyposis is excluded
- Bethesda criteria (must meet all criteria):
  1. Colorectal cancer before age 50
  2. Multiple colorectal cancers or other HNPCC-related cancers such as biliary tract, endometrial, stomach, or ovarian
  3. Colorectal cancer with microsatellite instability histology <60 yr of age
  4. Colorectal cancer or HNPCC-related cancer in first-degree relative <50 yr of age
  5. Colorectal cancer or HNPCC-related cancer in at least two first- or second-degree relatives, any age
- If criteria for the Lynch syndrome are not met, no further analysis is necessary (although a genetic syndrome cannot be definitively excluded and genetic referral may be warranted).

LABORATORY TESTS

- If a patient meets criteria for Lynch syndrome, immunohistochemistry can be performed for the presence or absence of mismatch repair genes *MLH1, MSH2, MSH6*, and *PMS2.* Rarely, *MLH3* is identified.
- Microsatellite instability analysis should also be performed if criteria for Lynch syndrome are met.

TREATMENT

- If the mutation has been identified in a family member, screening for this mutation can be performed via genetic testing. Informed consent must be obtained after a thorough explanation has been provided to each individual. Criteria for referral to a genetic counselor for suspected Lynch syndrome is summarized in Box 2.
- Surveillance using colonoscopy can be performed in individuals who screen positive, while those who screen negative can be discharged. The mismatch repair gene that is mutated guides screening.

TABLE 1 Risk of Lynch Syndrome

Condition	Risk (%)
Endometrial cancer at any age	1.8
Endometrial cancer diagnosed before 50 yr of age	9
Endometrial and colon cancer at any age	18
Endometrial and colon cancer before 50 yr of age	43
Endometrial and ovarian cancer	7

From Disaia PJ et al: *Clinical gynecologic oncology*, ed 9, Philadelphia, 2017, Elsevier.

TABLE 2 Comparison of Clinical Features in Lynch Syndrome and Sporadic Colorectal Cancer

Clinical Feature	Lynch Syndrome	Sporadic Colorectal Cancer
Mean age at diagnosis (yr)	45	67
Multiple colon cancers	35%	4%-11%
Synchronous colon cancers	18%	3%-6%
Metachronous colon cancers	24%	1%-5%
Proximal location of the initial cancer*	72%	35%
Increased risk of malignant tumors at other sites	Yes	No
Mucinous and poorly differentiated colon cancers	Common	Infrequent
Prognosis	Favorable†	Variable

*Proximal to the splenic flexure.
†Patients whose tumors demonstrate microsatellite instability have a more favorable prognosis than those with microsatellite-stable tumors.
From Feldman M et al: *Sleisenger and Fordtran's gastrointestinal and liver disease*, ed 10, Philadelphia, 2016, Elsevier.

BOX 1 Amsterdam II Criteria for Hereditary Nonpolyposis Colorectal Cancer (Lynch Syndrome)

Criteria defined by the International Collaborative Group on Hereditary Nonpolyposis Colorectal Cancer
At least three relatives with CRC (one must be a first-degree relative of the other two) or Lynch syndrome–associated cancer*
CRC involving at least two successive generations
One or more cancer cases before age 50 yr
Familial adenomatous polyposis should be excluded
Tumors should be verified by histologic examination

*Endometrium, ovary, stomach, ureter/renal pelvis, pancreas, brain, hepatobiliary tract, small intestine, and multiple sebaceous adenomas and carcinomas and keratoacanthomas in the Muir-Torre variant of Lynch syndrome.
CRC, Colorectal cancer.
From Feldman M et al: *Sleisenger and Fordtran's gastrointestinal and liver disease*, ed 10, Philadelphia, 2016, Elsevier.

BOX 2 Criteria for Referral to a Genetic Counselor for Suspected Lynch Syndrome

Bethesda guidelines
Amsterdam Criteria fulfilled
Persons with two relatives with Lynch syndrome
Colorectal cancer and first-degree relative with a Lynch cancer before 45 yr or a first-degree relative with an adenoma before 40 yr of age
Colorectal cancer or endometrial cancer before 45 yr of age
Right-sided, undifferentiated colon cancer before 45 yr of age
Signet ring colon cancer before 45 yr of age
Adenoma before 40 yr of age

- According to the Netherlands Surveillance Protocol, for example, individuals with mutations in *MLH1, MSH2,* or *MSH6* should have colonoscopies every 1 to 2 yr starting at age 20 to 25 yr; urine cytology every 1 to 2 yr starting at age 30 to 35 yr; esophagogastroduodenoscopy every 1 to 2 yr starting at age 30 to 35 yr; and, in females, ultrasound of endometrium and CA-125 every 1 to 2 yr starting at age 30 to 35 yr.
- *Helicobacter pylori* testing is also indicated in patients with Lynch syndrome or at high risk for it.
- Aspirin may be protective against colorectal cancer in Lynch syndrome patients.

REFERRALS

- To gastroenterology for surveillance colonoscopies
- To genetic counselor if patient satisfies Bethesda criteria
- To psychologist as necessary for psychological support

PEARLS & CONSIDERATIONS

- Before genetic testing is instituted, informed consent must be obtained because consequences of this testing include the necessity of lifelong screenings such as colonoscopies.
- The risk of pancreatic cancer is increased in families with Lynch syndrome compared with the U.S. population.
- **Familial Colorectal Cancer Type X** refers to patients who meet the Amsterdam criteria for HPNCC but have no molecular evidence of a mismatch repair (MMR) deficiency. These patients have a lower risk of colon cancer and no increased risk of extracolonic cancer compared to those with Lynch syndrome.

PATIENT & FAMILY EDUCATION

- For information on local genetic counselors, visit the National Society of Genetic Counselors website at http://www.nsgc.org.
- For information on Lynch syndrome, visit http://www.mayoclinic.com/health/lynch-syndrome/DS00669.

RELATED CONTENT

Colorectal Cancer (Related Key Topic)
Familial Adenomatous Polyposis and Gardner Syndrome (Related Key Topic)
Peutz-Jeghers Syndrome and Other Polyposis Syndromes (Related Key Topic)

SUGGESTED READINGS

Available at ExpertConsult.com

AUTHOR: **Fred F. Ferri, MD**

Malabsorption

BASIC INFORMATION

DEFINITION

Malabsorption is the diminished intestinal absorption of dietary nutrients. The majority of malabsorption is due to either congenital or acquired defects in the membrane transport system, absorption, and brush border processing in the intestinal epithelium.

SYNONYM

Maldigestion

ICD-10CM CODES

K90.4	Malabsorption due to intolerance, not elsewhere classified
K90.89	Other intestinal malabsorption
K90.9	Intestinal malabsorption, unspecified
K91.2	Postsurgical malabsorption, not elsewhere classified

EPIDEMIOLOGY & DEMOGRAPHICS

PREDOMINANT SEX AND AGE: More common in females, with a mean age of 40

RISK FACTORS:
- Excessive alcohol consumption
- History of celiac disease
- History of irritable bowel disease (IBD)
- Intestinal surgery

GENETICS: HLA-DQ2 present in 95% of celiac disease

PHYSICAL FINDINGS & CLINICAL PRESENTATION

- Most commonly nonspecific symptoms such as abdominal flatulence and distention are seen.
- Due to the osmotic load from maldigestion/malabsorption, watery diarrhea may be present. In the case of fat digestive disorder, steatorrhea ensues.
- Weight loss is very common, but many patients are able to compensate by increased caloric load. Diffuse disease often has much more pronounced weight loss.
- Chronic protein malabsorption can cause hypoalbuminemia, leading to edema and ascites.
- Both microcytic and macrocytic anemia can result from micronutrient deficiency (iron/B_{12}). These patients can be pale and present with fatigue.
- Bleeding disorders from vitamin K deficiency can lead to ecchymosis, melena, and hematuria.
- Vitamin D deficiency can lead to bone disorders. Secondary hyperparathyroidism can be a presenting feature.
- Electrolyte and vitamin deficiency can lead to neurologic disorders such as ataxia, weakness, and neuropathy, and may have positive Chvostek or Trousseau sign.
- Autoimmune disease-specific dermatologic findings such as alopecia, pellagra, erythema nodosum, pyoderma gangrenosum, cheilosis, glossitis, and aphthous ulcers may be present.
- Cardinal clinical features of specific malabsorptive disorders are summarized in Table 1.

ETIOLOGY

- Can be congenital or acquired.
- Disease-specific etiology. Mechanisms of malabsorption, malabsorbed substrates, and representative causes are summarized in Table 2.

TABLE 1 Cardinal Clinical Features of Specific Malabsorptive Disorders

Disorder	Cardinal Clinical Features
Adrenal insufficiency	Skin darkening, hyponatremia, hyperkalemia
Amyloidosis	Renal disease, nephrotic syndrome, cardiomyopathy, neuropathy, carpal tunnel syndrome, macroglossia, hepatosplenomegaly
Bile acid deficiency	Ileal resection or disease, liver disease
Carcinoid syndrome	Flushing, cardiac murmur
Celiac disease	Variable symptoms: Dermatitis herpetiformis, alopecia, aphthous mouth ulcers, arthropathy, neurologic symptoms, and (life-threatening) malnutrition; elevated liver biochemical test levels, mild iron deficiency
Crohn disease	Arthritis, aphthous mouth ulcers, episcleritis, uveitis, pyoderma gangrenosum, erythema nodosum, abdominal mass, fistulas, perianal fistulae, primary sclerosing cholangitis (PSC), laboratory signs of inflammation
CF	Chronic sinopulmonary disease, meconium ileus, distal intestinal obstruction syndrome (DIOS), elevated sweat chloride
Cystinuria, Hartnup disease	Kidney stones, dermatosis
Diabetes mellitus	Long history of diabetes and diabetic complications
Disaccharidase deficiency	Bloating and cramping, intermittent diarrhea
GI fistulas	Previous intestinal surgery or trauma, Crohn disease
Glucagonoma	Migratory necrolytic erythema, enlarged gallbladder
Hyperthyroidism, hypothyroidism	Symptoms and signs of thyroid disease
Hypogammaglobulinemia	Recurrent infections
Intestinal ischemia	Other ischemic organ manifestations; abdominal pain with eating (chronic mesenteric ischemia)
Lymphoma	Enlarged mesenteric or retroperitoneal lymph nodes, abdominal mass, abdominal pain, fever
Mastocytosis	Urticaria pigmentosum, peptic ulcer
Mycobacterium avium complex infection	AIDS
Pancreatic insufficiency	History of pancreatitis, abdominal pain, or alcoholism; large-volume fatty, oily stools; passage of orange oil
Parasitic infection	History of travel to endemic areas
PBC	Jaundice, itching
Scleroderma	Dysphagia, inability to open the mouth widely, Raynaud phenomenon, skin tightening
SIBO	Previous intestinal surgery, motility disorder (scleroderma, pseudo-obstruction), small intestinal diverticula, strictures
Tropical sprue	History of travel to endemic area
Tuberculosis	Specific history of exposure, living in or travel to endemic area, immunosuppression, abdominal mass or intestinal obstruction, ascites
Whipple disease	Lymphadenopathy, fever, arthritis, cerebral symptoms, heart murmur (pulmonary valve), oculomasticatory myorhythmia
ZES	Peptic ulcers, diarrhea

AIDS, Acquired immunodeficiency syndrome; *CF,* cystic fibrosis; *GI,* gastrointestinal; *PBC,* primary biliary cholangitis; *SIBO,* small intestinal bacterial overgrowth; *ZES,* Zollinger-Ellison syndrome.
From Feldman M et al: *Sleisenger and Fordtran's gastrointestinal and liver disease*, ed 10, Philadelphia, 2016, Elsevier.

TABLE 2 Mechanisms of Malabsorption, Malabsorbed Substrates, and Representative Causes

Pathophysiologic Mechanism	Malabsorbed Substrate(s)	Representative Causes
Maldigestion		
Conjugated bile acid deficiency	Fat Fat-soluble vitamins Calcium Magnesium	Hepatic parenchymal disease Biliary obstruction SIBO with bile acid deconjugation Ileal bile acid malabsorption CCK deficiency
Pancreatic insufficiency	Fat Protein Carbohydrate Fat-soluble vitamins Vitamin B_{12} (cobalamin)	Congenital defects Chronic pancreatitis Pancreatic tumors Inactivation of pancreatic enzymes (e.g., ZES)
Reduced mucosal digestion	Carbohydrate	Congenital defects Acquired lactase deficiency
	Protein	Generalized mucosal disease (e.g., celiac disease, Crohn disease)
Intraluminal consumption of nutrients	Vitamin B_{12} (cobalamin)	SIBO Helminthic infections (e.g., *Diphyllobothrium latum* infection)
Malabsorption		
Reduced mucosal absorption	Fat Protein Carbohydrate Vitamins Minerals	Congenital transport defects Generalized mucosal diseases (e.g., celiac disease, Crohn disease) Previous intestinal resection or bypass Infections Intestinal lymphoma
Decreased transport from the intestine	Fat Protein	Intestinal lymphangiectasia Primary Secondary (e.g., solid tumors, Whipple disease, lymphomas) Venous stasis (e.g., from heart failure)
Other Mechanisms		
Decreased gastric acid and/or intrinsic factor secretion	Vitamin B_{12}	Pernicious anemia Atrophic gastritis Previous gastric resection
Decreased gastric mixing and/or rapid gastric emptying	Fat Calcium Protein	Previous gastric resection Autonomic neuropathy
Rapid intestinal transit	Fat	Autonomic neuropathy Hyperthyroidism

CCK, Cholecystokinin; *SIBO,* small intestinal bacterial overgrowth; *ZES,* Zollinger-Ellison syndrome.
From Feldman M et al: *Sleisenger and Fordtran's gastrointestinal and liver disease*, ed 10, Philadelphia, 2016, Elsevier.

Dx DIAGNOSIS

DIFFERENTIAL DIAGNOSIS

- Crohn disease
- Celiac disease
- Hartnup disease
- Chronic pancreatitis
- Pancreatic insufficiency
- Cystic fibrosis
- Short bowel syndrome
- Neoplasm
- Abetalipoproteinemia
- Lactose intolerance
- Small intestine bacterial overgrowth
- Chronic atrophic gastritis
- Zollinger-Ellison syndrome
- Chronic cholestasis
- Cirrhosis

WORKUP

- A detailed history including alcohol consumption and surgical history as well as autoimmune disease can help diagnose the underlying disease. It is important to screen for anemia and electrolyte abnormalities due to malabsorption.
- Table E3 summarizes malabsorptive diseases or conditions in which noninvasive tests can establish malabsorption or provide a diagnosis.

LABORATORY TESTS

- CBC, serum iron, Vitamin B_{12}, and folate to detect for anemia.
- **Prothrombin time:** Elevated PT can suggest vitamin K deficiency.
- **Fat malabsorption:** The gold standard is the 72-hour stool elastase or fat collection. More than 6/g day in the stool is pathologic. This test can be cumbersome so other options are available. Sudan III stain and acid steatocrit tests are qualitative measures of steatorrhea. Serologic testing for celiac disease should be considered as well.
- **Carbohydrate malabsorption:** Carbohydrate malabsorption leads to fermentation of the undigested carbohydrates by intestinal bacteria.
- The urinary D-xylose test for carbohydrate absorption in the small intestine. After loading with D-xylose, urinary D-xylose levels are measured. Low levels suggest intestinal malabsorption.
- Lactose intolerance can be tested by the lactose tolerance test or the breath test. The lactose tolerance test measures blood glucose after lactose administration. Development of symptoms or inadequate increase in blood sugar is indicative of lactose intolerance. H_2/CO_2 breath tests using specific forms of carbohydrates can detect malabsorption as well.
- **Protein malabsorption:** Protein malabsorption is likely due to small intestinal bacterial overgrowth or protein gastroenteropathies. Alpha-1 antitrypsin clearance or 99mTc-albumin gamma camera scintigraphy may aid in this diagnosis.
- **Pancreatic insufficiency:** Fecal elastase and chymotrypsin levels can distinguish from pancreatic and intestinal causes.
- **Vitamin deficiency:** It is important to assess serum vitamin B_{12} and methylmalonic acid levels. Schilling test is rarely used but can be useful in some cases.
- **Bile acid malabsorption:** Quantitative stool bile acid measurement is the preferred method of diagnosis. SeHCAT test (selenium homocholic acid taurine test) is another option but less likely used.
- **Bacterial overgrowth:** This can be detected with endoscopic jejunal aspirate culture or a less invasive hydrogen breath test.
- Table 4 summarizes useful laboratory tests for evaluating patients with suspected malabsorption and for establishing possible nutrient deficiencies.

IMAGING STUDIES

- Abdominal ultrasound can identify thickened small bowel wall
- Endoscopy for visualization and biopsy
- Small bowel follow through
- Abdominal CT/MRI
- Endoscopic retrograde cholangiopancreatography/magnetic resonance cholangiopancreatography/endoscopic ultrasound for identification of pancreatic abnormalities
- Capsule endoscopy

Rx TREATMENT

Involves identification and treatment of the underlying illness, treatment of diarrhea, and nutritional repletion

NONPHARMACOLOGIC THERAPY

- A gluten-free diet in patients with celiac disease. Avoidance of lactose-containing product in lactose intolerance.
- Avoidance of caffeine and high sugar containing compounds has been found to decrease diarrhea in some cases.

TABLE 4 Useful Laboratory Tests for Patients with Suspected Malabsorption and for Establishing Possible Nutrient Deficiencies

Test	Comment(s)
Blood Cell Count	
Hematocrit, hemoglobin	Decreased in iron, vitamin B_{12}, and folate malabsorption or with blood loss
Mean corpuscular hemoglobin or mean corpuscular volume	Decreased in iron malabsorption; increased in folate and vitamin B_{12} malabsorption
White blood cells, differential	Decreased in vitamin B_{12} and folate malabsorption; low lymphocyte count in lymphangiectasia
Biochemical Tests (Serum)	
TGs	Decreased in severe fat malabsorption
Cholesterol	Decreased in bile acid malabsorption or severe fat malabsorption
Albumin	Decreased in severe malnutrition, lymphangiectasia, protein-losing enteropathy
Alkaline phosphatase	Increased in calcium and vitamin D malabsorption (severe steatorrhea); decreased in zinc deficiency
Calcium, phosphorus, magnesium	Decreased in extensive small intestinal mucosal disease, after extensive intestinal resection, or in vitamin D deficiency
Zinc	Decreased in extensive small intestinal mucosal disease or intestinal resection
Iron, ferritin	Decreased in celiac disease, in other extensive small intestinal mucosal diseases, and with chronic blood loss
Other Serum Tests	
Prothrombin time	Prolonged in vitamin K malabsorption
β-Carotene	Decreased in fat malabsorption from hepatobiliary or intestinal diseases
Immunoglobulins	Decreased in lymphangiectasia, diffuse lymphoma
Folic acid	Decreased in extensive small intestinal mucosal diseases, with anticonvulsant use, in pregnancy; may be increased in SIBO
Vitamin B_{12}	Decreased after gastrectomy, in pernicious anemia, terminal ileal disease, SIBO, and infection with *Diphyllobothrium latum*
Methylmalonic acid	Markedly elevated in vitamin B_{12} deficiency
Homocysteine	Markedly elevated in vitamin B_{12} or folate deficiency
Citrulline	May be decreased in destructive small intestinal mucosal disease or intestinal resection
Stool Tests	
Fat	Qualitative or quantitative increase in fat malabsorption
Elastase, chymotrypsin	Decreased concentrations and output in exocrine pancreatic insufficiency
pH	Less than 5.5 in carbohydrate malabsorption

SIBO, Small intestinal bacterial overgrowth; *TGs,* thyroglobulins.
From Feldman M et al: *Sleisenger and Fordtran's gastrointestinal and liver disease*, ed 10, Philadelphia, 2016, Elsevier.

ACUTE GENERAL Rx

- Control of the underlying disease should be primary goal.
- It is also essential to control any volume and electrolyte abnormalities that might exist.

CHRONIC Rx

- Control of chronic diarrhea with loperamide should be one of the goals in a chronic malabsorptive state.
- Correction of volume and electrolyte disturbance with oral rehydration therapy should be made a priority.
- Bile acid conjugates can decrease steatorrhea in some cases.
- Pancreatic insufficiency is typically treated with a low-fat diet and exogenous pancreatic enzymes.
- Teduglutide-homolog of GLP-2 has been shown to increase absorptive surface area in short bowel syndrome.
- Periodic DEXA scans are indicated in chronic malabsorption in the setting of vitamin D deficiency.
- Oral supplementation with vitamins and minerals is important, sometimes requiring parenteral therapy.

REFERRAL

- Gastroenterology consultation can help in diagnosis when initial laboratory testing is unclear.
- Nutrition consultation can help patients with diet modification to alleviate symptoms.

PEARLS & CONSIDERATIONS

COMMENTS

- Malabsorption should be considered a sign of an underlying disease.
- Treatment should focus on treating the underlying disorder.
- Nutrient and volume repletion should be priority in any treatment plan of malabsorption.

RELATED CONTENT

Celiac Disease (Related Key Topic)
Crohn Disease (Related Key Topic)
Cystic Fibrosis (Related Key Topic)
Irritable Bowel Syndrome (Related Key Topic)
Lactose Intolerance (Related Key Topic)
Chronic Pancreatitis (Related Key Topic)
Short Bowel Syndrome (Related Key Topic)
Small Bowel Intestinal Bacterial Overgrowth (Related Key Topic)
Ulcerative Colitis (Related Key Topic)

AUTHORS: **Rosann Cholankeril, MD, George Cholankeril, MD, Dimitri Gitelmaker, MD,** and **Alan Epstein, MD**

BASIC INFORMATION

DEFINITION

Malaria is a protozoan disease caused by intraerythrocytic protozoa of the genus *Plasmodium* and transmitted by female *Anopheles* spp. mosquitoes. It is endemic throughout most of the tropics and is characterized by hectic fever and often presents with classic malarial paroxysm. Five species of genus *Plasmodium* usually infect humans (Table 1):

- *P. falciparum*
- *P. vivax*
- *P. malariae*
- *P. ovale*
- *P. knowlesi*

SYNONYMS

Periodic fever
Tertian malaria
Quartan malaria
Tropical splenomegaly

ICD-10CM CODES

B50.9	*Plasmodium falciparum* malaria, unspecified
B51.9	*Plasmodium vivax* malaria without complications
B52.9	*Plasmodium malariae* malaria without complications
B53.0	*Plasmodium ovale* malaria
B53.8	Other parasitologically confirmed malaria, not elsewhere classified
B54	Unspecified malaria

EPIDEMIOLOGY & DEMOGRAPHICS

GLOBAL:

- ~219 million cases in 2018 in more than 100 countries (Fig. E1)
- Approximately 405,000 deaths in 2018, with more than 80% of the deaths occurring in children of sub-Saharan Africa
- Three billion people live in malaria-endemic areas

U.S.:

- ~2078 cases reported to the Centers for Disease Control and Prevention (CDC) in the U.S. in 2017 (Fig. E2). In the majority of reported cases, U.S. civilians who acquired infection abroad had not adhered to a chemoprophylaxis regimen that was appropriate for the country in which they acquired malaria
- More than 50% of the reported cases in the U.S. are *P. falciparum.* On average, there are six deaths per yr in the U.S.
- Most infections limited to:
  1. Immigrant population
  2. Returned travelers or troops from endemic area
- Occasionally, transmission through exposure to infected blood product or shared intravenous needles by users of injection drugs
- Congenital transmission possible
- Local mosquito-borne transmission reported
- Competent mosquito vectors present
  1. *A. albimanus* in Eastern U.S.
  2. *A. freeborni* in Western U.S.

GEOGRAPHIC DISTRIBUTION:

- *P. falciparum:* Sub-Saharan Africa, Papua New Guinea, Solomon Islands, Haiti, Indian subcontinent
- *P. vivax:* Central America, South America, North Africa, Middle East, Indian subcontinent
- *P. ovale:* West Africa
- *P. malariae:* Worldwide
- *P. knowlesi:* Southeast Asia

PARASITE LIFE CYCLE (FIG. E3):

- Human infection begins when a female anopheline mosquito bites (only female anopheline mosquito takes blood meal) and inoculates plasmodial sporozoites into bloodstream. The bite usually occurs between dusk and dawn.
- The sporozoites then travel to liver and invade to hepatocytes.
- In the hepatocytes, the sporozoites mature to tissue schizonts or become dormant hypnozoites.
- The tissue schizonts amplify the infection by producing a large number of merozoites (10,000-30,000).
- Each merozoite is capable of invading a RBC and can establish the asexual cycle of replication in RBCs.
- Asexual cycles produce and release 24 to 32 merozoites at the end of 48- or 72-hr *(P. malariae)* cycles.
- The hypnozoites are only found in relapsing malaria *P. vivax* or *P. ovale* and may remain dormant for up to 5 yr.
- Eventually some intraerythrocytic parasites develop into gametocytes. Male and female gametocytes are taken up by a female anopheline mosquito with a blood meal where they fertilize in the mosquito gut to produce a diploid zygote that matures to an ookinete; haploid sporozoites are generated that migrate to the salivary gland of the mosquito to infect another human.

PHYSICAL FINDINGS & CLINICAL PRESENTATION

- Fever is the hallmark of malaria, known as malarial paroxysm, initially daily until synchronization of infection after several wk, when fever may occur every other day (tertian) in *P. vivax, P. ovale,* or *P. falciparum* malaria or every third day (quartan) in *P. malariae* malaria. Table 2 describes the WHO criteria for severe malaria.
- Classic malarial paroxysm characterized by:
  1. Cold stage: Abrupt onset of cold feeling associated with rigors, shakes
  2. Hot stage: High fever (~40° C; 104° F) associated with restlessness
  3. Sweating stage: Patient defervesces
- Nonspecific symptoms are:
  1. Headache
  2. Cough
  3. Myalgia
  4. Vomiting
  5. Diarrhea
  6. Jaundice
- *P. falciparum:*
  1. Most pathogenic of the four species.
  2. Rapidly progresses to high-level parasitemia.
  3. Important cause of the fatal malaria.

TABLE 1 Characteristics of the *Plasmodium* Species Responsible for Human Malaria

	SPECIES				
Characteristic	***P. falciparum***	***P. vivax***	***P. ovale***	***P. malariae***	***P. knowlesi***
Incubation period in days (range)	12 (8-25)	14 (8-27)	17 (15 to ≥18)	28 (15 to ≥40)	11 (9 to >12)
Periodicity of febrile attacks (hours)	None	48	48	72	24
Earliest appearance of gametocytes (days)	10	3	?	?	?
Relapse	No	Yes	Yes	No	No
Duration of untreated infection (yrs)	1-2	1.5-4	1.5-4	3-50	?
RBC preference	Younger cells (but can invade cells of all ages)	Reticulocytes	Reticulocytes	Older cells	?
Characteristic morphology	Ring forms Multiply infected cells Banana-shaped gametocytes	Schüffner dots Enlarged RBCs	Schüffner dots Enlarged RBCs	Normal-sized cells Band or rectangular forms of trophozoites	Ring forms Occasional multiply infected cells Band forms

RBC, Red blood cell.
From Cherry JD et al: *Feigin and Cherry's textbook of pediatric infectious diseases,* ed 8, Philadelphia, 2019, Elsevier.

TABLE 2 World Health Organization Criteria for Severe Malaria, 2000

Impaired consciousness
Prostration
Respiratory distress
Multiple seizures
Jaundice
Hemoglobinuria
Abnormal bleeding
Severe anemia
Circulatory collapse
Pulmonary edema

From Kliegman RM et al: *Nelson textbook of pediatrics,* ed 19, Philadelphia, 2011, Saunders.

4. Classic malarial paroxysm is usually absent.
5. Incubation period after exposure is 12 days (range: 9-60 days).
6. Cytoadherence and resetting of RBCs play central role in pathogenesis.
7. The sequestration of RBCs in vital organs leads to fatal complications.
8. Cerebral malaria is a feared complication.
9. Invades erythrocytes of all ages.
10. Lacks hypnozoites (intrahepatic stage), does not relapse.
11. Blood smear usually shows ring form only.
12. Pigment color is black.
13. Banana-shaped gametocytes; if seen in blood, smear is diagnostic.
14. Chloroquine resistance is widely present.

- *P. vivax:*
  1. Known as tertian malaria: Fever occurs every other day.
  2. Duffy blood-group antigen FYA- or FYB-related receptor is needed for attachment to RBC.
  3. FyFy phenotype (most West African) individuals are resistant to P. vivax malaria.
  4. Incubation period after exposure is 14 days (range: 8 to 27 days).
  5. Hypnozoites may cause relapse of infection after yrs.
  6. Infects mainly reticulocytes.
  7. Irregularly shaped large rings and trophozoites, enlarged RBCs, and Schüffner dots are seen in peripheral blood smear.
  8. Pigment color is yellow-brown.
  9. P. vivax from Papua New Guinea has reduced sensitivity to chloroquine.
  10. Primaquine is needed to eradicate the hypnozoites.
- *P. ovale:*
  1. Also known as tertian malaria; fever occurs every other day.
  2. Occurs mainly in tropical Africa.
  3. Incubation period after exposure is 14 days (range: 8-27 days).
  4. Hypnozoites may cause relapse of infection.
  5. Infects mainly reticulocytes.
  6. Infected RBC is seen as enlarged, oval shape containing large ring or trophozoites with Schüffner dots.
  7. Pigment color is dark brown.
  8. Primaquine needed to eradicate the hypnozoites.
  9. No chloroquine resistance has been encountered.
- *P. malariae:*
  1. Known as quartan malaria; fever occurs every third day.
  2. Common cause of chronic malarial infection.
  3. May persist for 20 to 30 yr after leaving the endemic area.
  4. Worldwide distribution.
  5. Incubation period after exposure is 30 days (range: 16 to 60 days).
  6. Lacks hypnozoites (intrahepatic stage).
  7. May persist in blood for many yrs if treated inadequately.
  8. Chronic infection may cause soluble immune-complex, resulting in nephritic syndrome.
  9. Infects mainly mature RBCs.
  10. Band or rectangular forms of trophozoites are commonly seen in peripheral blood smear.
  11. Pigment color is brown-black.
- Cerebral malaria:
  1. Feared complication of *P. falciparum* infection.
  2. Mortality is ~20%.
  3. Pathogenesis is poorly understood.
  4. Ischemia as a result of sequestration of parasites or cytokines induced by parasite toxin(s) is the key debate.
  5. Seizure and altered mental status leading to coma are cardinal manifestation.
  6. Hypoglycemia, lactic acidosis, and elevated circulating tumor necrosis factor alpha (TNF-α) may be present.
  7. CSF studies: No increase of WBC count or protein, raised lactate concentrate, and increased opening pressure, especially in children, may be present.

Dx DIAGNOSIS

DIFFERENTIAL DIAGNOSIS

- Typhoid fever
- Dengue fever
- Yellow fever
- Viral hepatitis
- Influenza
- Brucellosis
- Urinary tract infection
- Leishmaniasis
- Trypanosomiasis
- Rickettsial diseases
- Leptospirosis
- Table 3 summarizes the differential diagnosis of uncomplicated malaria

WORKUP

- Clinical diagnosis is notoriously inaccurate.
- Demonstration of malarial parasites in blood smear is essential.
- Newer molecular diagnostic techniques (polymerase chain reaction, rapid diagnostic tests) are promising (Table 4).

LABORATORY TESTS

- The thick and thin blood film is required to identify malarial parasites (Fig. E4). A Giemsa-stained film of the patient's peripheral blood should be examined for parasites as soon as possible.
- The thick smears are more sensitive and primarily used to detect the presence of parasites.
- The thin smears are used for species differentiation and parasite density estimation.
- A patient who is suspected of having malaria but who has no parasite seen in blood smears should have blood smears repeated every 12 to 24 hr for 3 consecutive days.

PREPARATION OF BLOOD SMEAR:

- Must be prepared from fresh blood obtained by pricking the finger.
- The thin smear is fixed in methanol before staining.
- The thick smear is stained unfixed.
- The smear should be stained with a 3% Giemsa solution (pH of 7.2) for 30 to 45 min.
- The parasite density should be estimated by counting the percentage of RBCs infected, not the number of parasites, under an oil immersion lens on thin film.

COMMON ERRORS IN READING MALARIAL SMEARS:

- Platelets overlying an RBC
- Misreading artifacts as parasites
- Concern about missing a positive slide

MOLECULAR DIAGNOSIS OF MALARIA:

- Rapid diagnostic tests (RDT):
  1. Employ immunochromatographic lateral flow technology for antigen detection.
  2. Thus far only one RDT has been FDA approved: BinaxNOW Malaria test kit.
  3. This kit is based on antigens histidine-rich protein-2 (HRP-2) and aldolase.
  4. For *P. falciparum:* Sensitivity 95% and specificity 94%.
  5. For *P. vivax:* Sensitivity 69% and specificity 100%.
- Limitations of the BinaxNOW Malaria test:
  1. Not approved for mixed infections.
  2. Should not be used for *P. malariae* and *P. ovale* as data are limited.
  3. Positive test must be confirmed by microscopy.
  4. Negative results require confirmation by thick and thin smears.
  5. This test cannot be used to monitor therapy as antigen persists after the elimination of the parasite, causing false positives.
- Other diagnostic tests available include:
  1. Tagged monoclonal antibodies for malaria antigen detection.
  2. Nucleic acid amplification and detection: Polymerase chain reaction (PCR) can detect parasites down to a level of one to five parasites per microliter of blood. PCR can detect mixed species infection and is now considered the gold standard for diagnosis.
  3. Fluorescence microscopy with acridine orange or other staining.
  4. Dark field microscopy.

TABLE 3 Differential Diagnosis of Uncomplicated Malaria*

	Symptoms	Physical Examination	Laboratory Tests	Geography
Malaria	Fever Nonspecific myalgias, arthralgias, malaise, nausea, vomiting	Hepatomegaly Splenomegaly	Malaria smear positive Thrombocytopenia Hyperbilirubinemia	Primarily tropical areas
Viral syndromes (flu, pneumonia, early gastroenteritis)	Fever Nonspecific myalgias, arthralgias, malaise Nausea, vomiting	Lymphadenopathy	Low white cell count, lymphocyte predominant	Worldwide, frequently seen in local epidemics
Bacterial pneumonia	Fever Productive cough	Tachypnea Increased respiratory effort (intercostal and subcostal recession, use of accessory muscles) Crepitations (rales) Decreased oxygen saturation (<90%)	Leukocytosis	Worldwide
Meningitis (bacterial or viral)	Fever Altered mental status	Neck stiffness	Concomitant parasitemia uncommon in bacterial meningitis WBCs in CSF (>5-10/μl, or >10 times higher than the predicted CSF WBC count†)	Worldwide
Dengue	Retro-orbital pain Pain/tenderness of the extraocular eye muscles, particularly on extreme lateral gaze	Skin rash develops in at least 50% by day 2-3	Leukopenia Thrombocytopenia	Less common in sub-Saharan Africa
Leptospirosis	Fever, headache, dry cough, shaking, chills, nausea, vomiting, diarrhea, muscle pain, abdominal pain	Muscle tenderness (myositis), conjunctivitis, hepatosplenomegaly	Elevated creatinine kinase, abnormal urine sediment, proteinuria, normal to elevated WBC counts	Worldwide distribution Association with freshwater exposure
Typhus	High fever, dry cough, low back pain, headache, nausea, vomiting, abdominal pain, diarrhea, nausea, chills, delirium, photophobia, myalgia	Rash begins on the chest and spreads to the rest of the body (except the palms of the hands and soles of the feet) The early rash is a light rose color and fades when pressed Later, the rash becomes dull and red and does not fade People with severe typhus may also develop petechiae	Anemia Thrombocytopenia Twofold to fivefold elevation of liver enzymes	Worldwide distribution, murine typhus (*Rickettsia typhi)* seen in areas of poor hygiene and cold temperatures Epidemic typhus (*Rickettsia prowzekii*) associated with exposure to rat fleas or rat feces
Viral hemorrhagic fevers	Fever, bleeding diathesis, malaise, fatigue, myalgias, headache, vomiting, diarrhea, hypotension, shock	Flushing of the face and chest, frank bleeding, ecchymoses, renal failure, edema	Cytopenias seen early in illness with elevated WBC seen in late disease, coagulation abnormalities	Worldwide distribution and caused by several families of RNA viruses

CSF, Cerebrospinal fluid; *RBC,* red blood cell; *RNA,* ribonucleic acid; *WBC,* white blood cell.
*Individual patients may have more than one diagnosis.
†Predicted CSF WBC count/μl = CSF RBC count × (peripheral blood WBC count ÷ peripheral blood RBC count).
From Ryan ET: *Hunter's tropical medicine and emerging infectious diseases,* ed 10, Philadelphia, 2020, Elsevier.

Rx TREATMENT

NONPHARMACOLOGIC THERAPY

ANTIMOSQUITO MEASURES:

- Eradication of mosquito breeding places by chemical spray
- Use of mosquito nets properly in the endemic areas
- Use of protective clothing
- Use of insect spray (permethrin), mosquito coils, or repellents such as diethyltoluamide (DEET). For adults, DEET (30%-50%) is generally protective for at least 4 hr. For smaller children, use DEET at ≤20% concentration

ACUTE GENERAL Rx

A definitive diagnosis of malaria is essential for specific antimalarial chemotherapy.

UNCOMPLICATED CHLOROQUINE-SENSITIVE PLASMODIUM VIVAX, PLASMODIUM OVALE, OR PLASMODIUM MALARIAE (NON-FALCIPARUM MALARIA):

- Chloroquine:
  1. Adults: 600 mg base (= 1000 mg salt) orally immediately, followed by 300 mg base (= 500 mg salt) orally at 6, 24, and 48 hrs.
  2. Children: 10 mg base/kg orally immediately, followed by 5 mg base/kg orally at 6, 24, and 48 hrs.
  3. Maximum total dose: 1500 mg base (= 2500 mg salt).
  4. An alternative agent is hydroxychloroquine (Plaquenil): 620 mg base (= 800 mg salt) orally immediately, followed by 310 mg base (= 400 mg salt) orally at 6, 24, and 48 hrs.
- In the case of *P. vivax* and *P. ovale,* treatment with primaquine 15 mg daily for 14 days is needed to eradicate the exoerythrocytic forms, especially the hypnozoites responsible for relapses.
- G6PD should be measured before primaquine is given. Primaquine is not recommended for those who are glucose-6-phosphate dehydrogenase deficient, because primaquine can cause hemolysis and even death in G6PD-deficient persons. Normal G6PD levels must be documented before using primaquine for either chemoprophylaxis or treatment.
- Chloroquine-resistant *P. vivax* has been documented; in that case use quinine sulfate (10 mg/kg) plus either tetracycline or doxycycline or clindamycin for 7 days.

UNCOMPLICATED FALCIPARUM MALARIA OR SPECIES NOT IDENTIFIED:

- Chloroquine can be used cautiously for falciparum malaria acquired in chloroquine-sensitive areas (chloroquine is more rapidly effective than quinine).

TABLE 4 Malaria Rapid Diagnostic Tests Available in the U.S.[a]

RDT Name	Malaria Antigen Target	Malaria Species Detected	Sensitivity	Comment
BinaxNOW	HRP-2 and aldolase	*P. falciparum, P. vivax, P. malariae,* and *P. ovale*	94% for *P. falciparum* 84% for non-*P. falciparum* 87% for pure *P. vivax* infections 62% for pure *P. ovale* and *P. malariae* infections	Sensitivity increased to 96% for pure *P. falciparum* infection Overall specificity of 99% FDA-approved for use in the U.S.
ParaSight F	HRP-2	*P. falciparum*	96.5-100 in Kenya when >60 parasites/μL, lower with less parasitemia 40% in travelers when <50 parasites/μL, >93% when >100 parasites/μL	Antigen persists for 6-7 days 6 in 11.9%-20% of subjects whose blood smears had cleared Not FDA approved for use in the U.S.
ICT Malaria Pf/Pv	HRP-2 and aldolase	*P. falciparum* and *P. vivax*	97% for *P. falciparum* 44% for *P. vivax*	Specificity of 90% for *P. falciparum* Specificity of 100% for *P. vivax* Not FDA-approved for use in the U.S.
OptiMAL-IT	LDH	*P. falciparum, P. vivax, P. malariae,* and *P. ovale*	85-95%; decreased with lower parasite density	Specificity of 100% *P. falciparum*, 75%-85% for *P. vivax* Not FDA approved for use in the U.S.
Clearview	LDH	*P. falciparum, P. vivax, P. malariae,* and *P. ovale*	93% specificity of 100%, with sensitivities of 99%, 90.0%, 86%, and 60%, respectively, for *P. falciparum, P. vivax, P. malariae,* and *P. ovale*	Specificity of 100% for *P. falciparum*, 99% for *P. vivax*, 90% for *P. malariae*, and 60% for *P. ovale* Not FDA-approved for use in the U.S.

FDA, Food and Drug Administration; *HRP-2,* histidine-rich protein-2; *ICT,* immunochromatographic diagnostic test; *LDH,* lactate dehydrogenase; *RDT,* rapid diagnostic test.
[a]Direct microscopy should be performed where available with a negative RDT, given higher false-negative rates with low parasitemia, and when severe malaria is suspected.
From Cherry JD et al: *Feigin and Cherry's textbook of pediatric infectious diseases,* ed 8, Philadelphia, 2019, Elsevier.

- For uncomplicated *P. falciparum,* an oral artemisinin combination therapy (ACT), is recommended by the CDC as the first-line agent. While there are numerous ACT combinations, the only ACT approved in the U.S. is artemether-lumefantrine (Coartem), which is not widely available. Do not delay therapy in trying to obtain it; use another first-line agent. Dosage for adults: 4 tablets artemether-lumefantrine (20/120 mg) as a single dose, then 4 tablets again after 8 hr, then 4 tablets q12h for 2 days (take with food). Can cause prolongation of QT interval. Not recommended in infants <5 kg. Dose dependent on weight in children:
  1. 5 to 15 kg: 1 tablet (20/120 mg) as a single dose, then 1 tablet again after 8 hr, then 1 tablet q12h for 2 days
  2. 16 to 25 kg: 2 tablets (40/240 mg) as a single dose, then 2 tablets again after 8 hr, then 2 tablets q12h for 2 days
  3. 26 to 35 kg: 3 tablets (60/360 mg) as a single dose, then 3 tablets again after 8 hr, then 3 tablets q12h for 2 days
  4. >35 kg: Treat as adult
- Atovaquone-proguanil (Malarone): 250 mg atovaquone/100 mg proguanil: 4 adult tabs PO once a day for 3 days with food. Pediatric dosage: Pediatric tablets (62.5 mg atovaquone/25 mg proguanil) are used based on weight:
  1. 5 to 8 kg: 2 pediatric tabs PO once daily for 3 days
  2. 9 to 10 kg: 3 pediatric tabs PO once daily for 3 days
  3. 11 to 20 kg: 1 adult tab PO once daily for 3 days
  4. 21 to 30 kg: 2 adult tabs PO once daily for 3 days
  5. 31 to 40 kg: 3 adult tabs PO once daily for 3 days
  6. >40 kg: 4 adult tabs PO once daily for 3 days
- Another first-line option for treatment in adults is oral quinine sulfate 10 mg (salt)/kg (usually 650 mg) q8h for 3 to 7 days plus doxycycline 100 mg PO bid, both for 7 days. Pediatric dosage: Quinine sulfate 10 mg/kg PO tid plus clindamycin 20 mg/kg per day divided tid, both for 7 days.
- Table 5 summarizes some treatment guidelines for severe *Plasmodium falciparum* malaria.

ALTERNATIVES:

- Quinine sulfate plus clindamycin 900 mg tid for 7 days in adults
- Mefloquine 750 mg PO, then 500 mg PO 6 to 12 hr later in adults
- Atovaquone-proguanil (Malarone) or quinine sulfate plus doxycycline can be used when species is unknown. Artemether-lumefantrine is also recommended the World Health Organization (WHO) for treatment of unknown species, but in U.S. is only approved for *P.* falciparum
- Other ACT combinations not yet available in the U.S.: Artesunate-amodiaquine, artesunate-mefloquine, artesunate-sulfadoxine-pyrimethamine, dihydroartemisinin-piperaquine, artesunate-pyronaridine tetraphosphate

NOTE: Parasitemia may paradoxically rise in the first 24 to 36 hr and is not an indication of treatment failure.

SEVERE FALCIPARUM MALARIA:

- It is a medical emergency; intensive care is preferred. Features of complicated malaria are summarized in Table 6.
- Measurement of blood glucose, lactate, ABG is important.
- IV quinidine gluconate 10 mg salt/kg loading dose (maximum 600 mg) in normal saline (NS); infuse slowly over 1 to 2 hr, followed by continuous infusion of 0.02 mg/kg/min until patient can swallow.
- Need to monitor ECG for observation of QT interval as can prolong. Also need to monitor blood pressure and glucose to avoid hypoglycemia.
- Alternatively, IV artesunate: 2.4 mg/kg IV at hour 0, then at 12 and 24 hr followed by 2.4 mg/kg once daily. If <20 kg use 3.0 mg/kg per dose. This medication is now FDA approved for the initial treatment of severe malaria in children and adults regardless of the infecting species of malaria parasite. It has shown reduced mortality compared to parenteral quinine in clinical trials in patients with severe malaria in Asia and Africa.
- Plasmapheresis is an option for parasitemia >30% or in pregnant women and in elderly with severe malaria.

NOTE: WHO recommends IV artesunate as the treatment of choice for severe malaria in adults and children in area of low transmission. Data on children in high-transmission regions are limited, and WHO recommends treatment with artesunate, artemether, or quinine.

MULTIDRUG-RESISTANT MALARIA:

- Mefloquine 1250 mg as a single dose, *or*
- Halofantrine 500 mg every 6 hr for 3 doses, repeat same course after 1 wk
- Combination therapy usually preferred

DISPOSITION

RISK FACTORS FOR FATAL MALARIA:

- Failure to take chemoprophylaxis
- Delay in seeking medical care
- Misdiagnosis

COMPLICATIONS OF MALARIA:

- Anemia
- Acidosis
- Hypoglycemia
- Respiratory distress

TABLE 5 Treatment Guidelines for Severe *Plasmodium falciparum* Malaria

Drug	Dose	COMMENTS
Artemisinin compounds		
Artesunate Artemether	2.4 mg/kg IV bolus at 0, 12, 24 hours, then daily until patient is able to transition to the following oral regimen: 1. Artemether + lumefantrine: Tablets containing 20 + 120 mg, 40 + 240 mg of artemether and lumefantrine, respectively • Adults ≥35 kg: 80 + 480 mg twice daily for 3 days • Children: • 5 to <15 kg: 20 + 120 mg twice daily for 3 days • 15 to <25 kg: 40 + 240 mg twice daily for 3 days • 25 to <35 kg: 60 + 360 mg twice daily for 3 days 2. Artesunate + amodiaquine: A fixed-dose combination tablet containing 25 + 67.5 mg, 50 + 135 mg, 100 + 270 mg of artesunate and amodiaquine, respectively • Adults ≥36 kg, 200 + 540 mg daily for 3 days • Children: • 4.5 to <9 kg: 25 + 67.5 mg daily for 3 days • 9 to <18 kg: 50 + 135 mg daily for 3 days • 18 to <36 kg: 100 + 270 mg daily for 3 days 3. Dihydroartemisinin (DHA) + piperaquine (PPQ): Tablets containing 20 + 160 mg, 40 + 320 mg of DHA and PPQ, respectively • Adults: • 36 to <75 kg: 120 + 960 mg daily for 3 days • ≥75 kg: 160 + 1280 mg daily for 3 days (no data on dose recommendation >100 kg) • Children • 5 to <7 kg: 10 + 80 mg daily for 3 days • 7 to <13 kg: 20 + 160 mg daily for 3 days • 13 to <24 kg: 40 + 320 mg daily for 3 days • 24 to <36 kg: 80 + 640 mg daily for 3 days 4. Artesunate or quinine PO to complete 7 days plus doxycycline, 100 mg PO bid × 7 days 5. Artesunate or quinine PO to complete 7 days plus clindamycin, 20 mg base/kg/d PO, tid × 7 days Initial dose: 3.2 mg/kg IM (anterior tight); maintenance dose: 1.6 mg/kg IM daily until patient is able to transition to oral regimen as described earlier for artesunate	Artesunate has "investigational new drug" status in the U.S. and is available only on request to the CDC (770-488-7788). Eligibility requirements include inability to take oral medications, high levels of parasitemia, clinical evidence of severe malaria, intolerance of or contraindication to quinidine, failure of quinidine therapy, and lack of rapid access to quinidine. Where available, artesunate rectal suppositories (10 mg/kg) may be used in children <5 yr of age if IV or IM administration is not possible. Doxycycline is contraindicated in children <8 yr of age and in pregnancy. Atovaquone/proguanil is packaged in the U.S. in fixed-dose combination tablets of 250 mg atovaquone/100 mg proguanil for adults and 62.5 mg atovaquone/25 mg proguanil for children. Safety of atovaquone/proguanil in pregnancy has not been established.
Cinchona Alkaloid Regimens		
Quinine dihydrochloride	20 mg salt/kg IV or IM on admission, then 10 mg/kg q8h. Can be given IM if IV administration is not possible. One of the following drugs should also be given concurrently: 1. ACT as listed earlier. 2. Doxycycline as listed earlier. If patient unable to take PO, give 100 mg IV q12h and switch to PO when possible. Avoid rapid IV administration. 3. Clindamycin as listed earlier. If patient unable to take PO, give 10 mg base/kg loading dose IV followed by 5 mg base/kg IV q8h and switch to PO when possible. Avoid rapid IV administration.	The infusion rate of IV quinine should be rate controlled and not exceed 5 mg salt/kg per hour. The drug is usually diluted in 5% dextrose and infused over 4 hours. IV quinine is not available in the U.S. When administering IM, the dose should be split and diluted to a concentration of 60-100 mg/kg and delivered to each thigh. Reduce the quinine dose by one third (to 10 mg salt/kg q12h) after 48 hours in patients with severe renal and/or hepatic dysfunction. Doxycycline is contraindicated in children <8 yr old and in pregnancy.
Quinidine gluconate	6.25 mg base/kg (= 10 mg salt/kg) IV on admission over 1-2 hours, then 0.0125 mg base/kg minute (= 0.02 mg salt/kg per minute) continuous infusion. An alternative regimen is 15 mg base/kg (= 24 mg salt/kg) loading dose IV infused over 4 hours, followed by 7.5 mg base/kg (= 12 mg salt/kg) infused over 4 hours q8h, starting 8 hours after the loading dose. A second drug should be given concurrently as listed earlier for quinine.	The loading dose should be omitted if the patient received >40 mg/kg quinine in the preceding 48 hours or mefloquine in the previous 12 hours. Reduce the dose by one third after 48 hours in patients with severe renal and/or hepatic dysfunction.

ACT, Artemisinin combination therapy; *bid,* twice a day; *CDC,* Centers for Disease Control and Prevention; *IM,* intramuscular; *IV,* intravenous; *PO,* by mouth; *q,* every; *tid,* thrice a day.
From Vincent JL et al: *Textbook of critical care,* ed 7, Philadelphia, 2017, Elsevier.

- Disseminated intravascular coagulation
- Blackwater fever
- Renal failure
- Shock

REFERRAL

- To an infectious disease specialist or travel medicine expert for severe malaria complications
- To an intensive care specialist if severe cerebral malaria or other major organ failure develops
- All malaria cases are mandated to be reported to local and state health departments by health care providers or laboratory staff

PEARLS & CONSIDERATIONS

HOST RESPONSE

- The specific immune response to malaria confers protection from high-level parasitemia and disease, but not from infection.
- Asymptomatic parasitemia without illness (premunition) is common among adults in endemic areas.
- Immunity is specific for both the species and the strain of infecting malarial parasites.
- Immunity to all strains is never achieved.
- Normal spleen function is an important host factor because of immunologic as well as filtering functions of the spleen.
- Both humoral and cellular immunity is necessary for protection.

TABLE 6 Features of Complicated Malaria

Physical Findings	Laboratory Investigations
Impaired consciousness/unrousable coma (Blantyre Coma Score ≤2) (children > adults)	Hypoglycemia (<2.2 mmol/L or 40 mg/dl) (children > adults)
Prostration (unable to walk or sit up)	Metabolic acidosis (plasma bicarbonate <15 mmol/L) (children > adults)
Failure to feed	Severe anemia (hemoglobin <5 g/dl, PCV <15%) (children > adults)
Convulsions (more than 2 in 24 h) (children > adults)	Hemoglobinuria
Acidotic breathing (children > adults)	Hyperparasitemia (>2%, or 100,000/μl in low transmission setting, >5%, or 250,000/μl in high-transmission settings)
Shock (systolic blood pressure <70 mm Hg in adults, <50 mm Hg in children)	Hyperlactatemia (>5 mmol/L)
Clinical jaundice + evidence of another organ dysfunction (adults > children)	Renal impairment (creatinine >265 μmol/L) (adults > children)
Abnormal spontaneous bleeding	
Pulmonary edema (radiologic evidence) (adults > children)	

PCV, Packed cell volume.
From Ryan ET: *Hunter's tropical medicine and emerging infectious diseases,* ed 10, Philadelphia, 2020, Elsevier.

TABLE 7 Drug Regimens Used for Prevention of Malaria

Drug	Adult Dosage	Pediatric Dosage	Comments
Chloroquine-Sensitive Areas			
Chloroquine phosphate (drug of choice)	500 mg salt (300 mg base) orally once/wk	8.3 mg/kg salt (5 mg/kg base) once/wk, up to adult dose of 300 mg base	Begin 1-2 wk before exposure, continue during exposure, and continue for 4 wk after exposure May be used in pregnant women
Hydroxychloroquine sulfate	400 mg salt (310 mg base) orally once/wk	6.5 mg/kg salt (5 mg/kg base) orally once/wk	Begin 1-2 wk before exposure, continue during exposure, and continue for 4 wk after exposure An alternative to chloroquine for use only in areas with chloroquine-sensitive malaria
Chloroquine-Resistant Areas			
Atovaquone-proguanil	250 mg/100 mg (1 tablet) daily	5-8 kg: Pediatric tablet daily 9-10 kg: Pediatric tablet daily 11-20 kg: 1 Pediatric tablet daily 21-30 kg: 2 Pediatric tablets daily 31-40 kg: 3 Pediatric tablets daily >40 kg: 1 Adult tablet daily	Begin 1-2 days before exposure, continue during exposure, and continue for 7 days after exposure Pediatric tablets contain 62.5 mg atovaquone and 25 mg proguanil hydrochloride See text for contraindications
Mefloquine	250 mg salt (228 mg base) orally once/wk	≤9 kg: 5 mg/kg salt (4.6 mg/kg base) orally once/wk 10-19 kg: Tablet orally once/wk 20-30 kg: Tablet orally once/wk 31-45 kg: Tablet orally once/wk >45 kg: 1 Tablet orally once/wk	Begin 1-2 wk before exposure, continue during exposure, and continue for 4 wk after exposure
Or			
Doxycycline	100 mg daily	2.2 mg/kg/day up to 100 mg/day	Begin 1-2 days before exposure, continue during exposure, and for 4 wk after exposure; not to be used in children >8 yr or pregnant women
Or			
Alternative			
Primaquine	52.6 mg salt (30 mg base) orally daily	0.8 mg/kg salt (0.5 mg/kg base) up to adult dose orally daily	Begin 1-2 days before exposure, continue during exposure, and continue for 7 days after exposure Contraindicated in people with G6PD deficiency, in pregnancy, and during lactation Prophylaxis to areas principally with *P. vivax*
Tafenoquine (Krintafel)	300 mg tab once		Prevention of relapse of *P. vivax* 300 mg once

G6PD, Glucose-6-phosphate dehydrogenase.
From Cherry JD et al: *Feigin and Cherry's textbook of pediatric infectious diseases,* ed 8, Philadelphia, 2019, Elsevier.

- Polyclonal increase in serum level of immunoglobulin G (IgG), IgM, and IgA occurs in immune individuals.
- Antibody to antigenically variant protein PfEMP1 is important for protection in case of *P. falciparum* malaria.
- Passively transferred IgG from immune individuals has been shown to be protective.
- Maternal antibody confers relative protection of infants from severe disease.
- Genetic disorders (sickle cell disease, thalassemia, and G6PD deficiency) confer protection from death because parasites are unable to grow efficiently in low-oxygen tensions, thus preventing high-level parasitemias.
- Individuals deficient of Duffy factor in RBCs are resistant to infection by *P. vivax.*
- Nonspecific defense mechanisms, such as cytokines (TNF-α, IL-1, -6, -8), also play an important role in protection, causing fever (temperatures of 40° C (104° F) damage mature parasites) and other pathologic effects.

PREVENTION OF MALARIA: Medications are available for the prophylaxis of malaria and will vary depending on level of chloroquine resistance in a given area (Table 7).

Areas free of chloroquine-resistant Falciparum malaria:

Chloroquine 300 mg base (500 mg chloroquine phosphate) PO/wk. Start 1 wk prior to arrival in malaria area, then weekly while there and for 4 wk on leaving malaria area. Pediatric dose: 8.3 mg/kg (5 mg/kg base). Alternatives for adults include atovaquone-proguanil (Malarone): 1 adult tablet per day starting 1 to 2 days prior to arriving in malaria area, then daily while there and then for 7 days daily on leaving malaria area. For children, atovaquone-proguanil pediatric tablets based on weight:

- 11 to 20 kg: 1 pediatric tablet

TABLE 8 Sources for Malaria Prophylaxis, Diagnosis, and Treatment Recommendations

Type of Information	Source	Availability	Telephone Number, Internet Address, or Electronic Mail Address
Prophylaxis	CDC's Traveler's Health Internet site (includes online access to Health Information for International Travel)	24 hours/day	http://wwwnc.cdc.gov/travel
	(The Yellow Book)	Order from Oxford University Press, Inc. Order Fulfillment 198 Madison Avenue, New York, NY 10016-4314	800-451-7556 or http://www.oup.com/us/
	CDC's Malaria Branch Internet site with Malaria Information and Prophylaxis, By Country (Red Pages)	24 hours/day	http://www.cdc.gov/malaria/travelers/country_table/a.html
	CDC Malaria Map Application	24 hours/day	http://www.cdc.gov/malaria/map
Diagnosis	CDC's Division of Parasitic Diseases and Malaria diagnostic internet site (DPDx)	24 hours/day	http://www.cdc.gov/dpdx/index.html
	CDC's Division of Parasitic Diseases and Malaria diagnostic CD-ROM (DPDx)	Order by electronic mail from CDC Division of Parasitic Diseases and Malaria	dpdx@cdc.gov
Treatment	CDC Malaria Branch	9:00 A.M.-5:00 P.M. Eastern time, Monday-Friday	770-488-7788 or toll-free 855-856-4713*
	CDC Malaria Branch	5:00 P.M.-9:00 A.M. Eastern time on weekdays and all day weekends and holidays	770-488-7100* (This number is for the CDC's Emergency Operations Center. Ask a staff member to page the person on call for the Malaria Branch.) http://www.cdc.gov/malaria/diagnosis_treatment/treatment.html

CDC, Centers for Disease Control and Prevention.
*These numbers are intended for health care professionals only.
From Cullen KA et al: Malaria surveillance—United States, 2013, *MMWR Surveill Summ* 65:1-22, 2016.

- 21 to 30 kg: 2 pediatric tablets
- 31 to 40 kg: 3 pediatric tablets
- 40 kg: 1 adult tablet

Areas with chloroquine-resistant Falciparum malaria:
- Atovaquone-proguanil (Malarone): Dosing as previously
- Mefloquine 250 mg (228 mg base) PO/wk, starting 1 wk before arriving in malaria area, weekly while there and then weekly for 4 wk on return. In children, mefloquine dose is based on weight:
  1. <15 kg: 5 mg/kg
  2. 16 to 19 kg: ¼ adult dose
  3. 20 to 30 kg: ½ adult dose
  4. 31 to 45 kg: ¾ adult dose
  5. >45 kg: Adult dose
- Doxycycline 100 mg PO/day for adults and children aged >8. Start 1 to 2 days before travel, daily while in malaria area, and then daily for 4 wk on return.
- Tafenoquine (Arakoda, Krintafel) is a long-acting primaquine analog FDA approved in two different strengths: 300 mg single dose for antimalarial therapy (Krintafel) for *P. vivax* or *P. ovale* infection ; and 200 mg dose as chemoprophylaxis (Arakoda): Loading dose is 200 mg once/day for 3 days. Maintenance dose is 200 mg once/wk starting 7 days after last loading dose, terminal dose is 200 mg once (7 days after last maintenance dose). G6PD levels should be measured with tafenoquine.

SPECIAL CONSIDERATIONS:
- Long-term visitors or travelers
- Children aged <12 yr
- Immunocompromised host
- Pregnant women: Chloroquine and mefloquine are safe in pregnancy but not atovaquone-proguanil. A recent trial revealed that the burden of malaria in pregnancy was significantly lower among adolescent girls or women who received intermittent preventive treatment with dihydroartemisinin-piperaquine than among those who received sulfadoxine-pyrimethamine, and monthly treatment with dihydroartemisinin-piperaquine was superior to three-dose dihydroartemisinin-piperaquine with regards to several outcomes. Avoid doxycycline and primaquine.
- An increasing number of areas in southeast Asia have mefloquine-resistant malaria, including Cambodia, Thailand, and Vietnam. Therefore, in specific regions of these countries, mefloquine cannot be used for prophylaxis or treatment.

PREVENTION OF RELAPSE:
- Treatment of *P. vivax* requires the clearing of asexual parasites, but relapse can be prevented only if dormant hypnozoites are cleared from the liver (a treatment termed "radical cure").
- Tafenoquine, slowly eliminated, single dose 8-aminoquinoline is effective in significantly lowering the risk of *P. vivax* recurrence in patients with phenotypically normal GG PD activity.

VACCINATION:
- In 2015, Mosquirix (RTS,S), a recombinant protein-based vaccine, was approved in Europe to prevent malaria in babies in Africa. It showed an efficacy of about 30% in babies 6 to 12 wk old and about 46% in babies 5 to 17 mo old.
- New DNA-based vaccines are in development.

MALARIA INFORMATION:
- CDC Travelers' Health Hotline (877) 394-8747; CDC Travelers' Health Fax (888) 232-3299
- CDC Malaria Epidemiology (770) 488-7788; internet: http://www.cdc.gov
- Table 8 summarizes sources for malaria prophylaxis, diagnosis, and treatment recommendations.
- Box E1 describes useful malaria vocabulary

RELATED CONTENT

Malaria (Patient Information)

SUGGESTED READINGS

Available at ExpertConsult.com

AUTHOR: **Glenn G. Fort, MD, MPH**

BASIC INFORMATION

DEFINITION

Malignant hyperthermia (MH) is a rare life-threatening subclinical myopathy that can manifest clinical symptoms in MH-susceptible (MHS) individuals after exposure to triggering medications. These drugs include halogenated anesthetic gases, such as halothane, isoflurane, sevoflurane, and desflurane, as well as the depolarizing neuromuscular blocking agent succinylcholine. When given to genetically susceptible individuals, these agents may cause a hypermetabolic crisis. Initial signs include hypercarbia or rising end-tidal carbon dioxide ($ETCO_2$) levels in ventilated patients, tachypnea, and tachycardia, with subsequent hyperthermia, acidemia, arrhythmias, or skeletal muscle rigidity. Clinical presentation may be variable, especially during surgery and general anesthesia. Mortality has recently been reported to be 1.4% to 5%, down from 70% in the past, likely due to the prevalence of intraoperative temperature and $ETCO_2$ monitoring and the use of dantrolene for treatment.

SYNONYMS

Anesthesia-related hyperthermia
Hyperpyrexia, malignant
Hyperthermia, malignant
Malignant hyperpyrexia
MHS
MH

ICD-10CM CODES	
T88.3XXA	Malignant hyperthermia due to anesthesia
T88.3XXA	Initial encounter
T88.3XXD	Subsequent encounter
T88.3XXS	Sequelae
Z87.898	History of malignant hyperthermia
Z15.89	Malignant hyperthermia susceptibility
Z84.89	Family history of malignant hyperthermia

EPIDEMIOLOGY & DEMOGRAPHICS

Malignant hyperthermia results from a biochemical cascade within the skeletal muscle tissue of MHS individuals following exposure to one or more "triggering" medications, including halogenated volatile anesthetics and the skeletal muscle relaxant, succinylcholine. This is due to excessive release of sarcoplasmic calcium, which occurs because of a genetic anomaly. The result is a hypermetabolic and prolonged contractile state, with subsequent serious morbidity and possible mortality, especially without prompt diagnosis and treatment. A recent study comparing human muscle fiber mitochondria from non-MHS patients to those from MHS patients found that mitochondria from MHS patients displayed anatomic and physiologic differences when exposed to halothane, while the non-MHS fibers did not.

All ethnic groups are at risk. MH susceptibility is associated with, although distinct from, central core, multiminicore disease, and King-Denborough syndrome.

PREVALENCE: In the general population, the prevalence of MHS is estimated to be between 1:2000 to 1:3000. In family cohorts of patients who are susceptible, the prevalence of susceptibility ranges from 1:200 to 1:5000 due to incomplete penetrance and variable expressivity.

PREDOMINANT SEX AND AGE: MH male to female ratio is 2:1. Children account for up to half of cases.

PEAK INCIDENCE: Among patients undergoing general anesthesia, the incidence is approximately 1:100,000, considerably lower than its estimated prevalence.

RISK FACTORS:

- Preoperatively, the patient and family history is used to evaluate the risk of MH and other myopathies. It is important to note that previous exposure to triggering agents with no sequelae does not exclude the possibility of a future MH crisis since half of afflicted patients may have had a prior uneventful exposure to a triggering agent.
- Patients with other *RYR1* abnormalities, such as central core myopathy, multiminicore disease (*RYR1* or *SELENON*), or King-Denborough syndrome though not true MHS, should not receive succinylcholine or volatile anesthetics.
- Increased muscle mass, especially in bodybuilders, appears to be an independent predictor of increased susceptibility to, recurrence of, and death from MH episodes. This finding is independent of the increased incidence in males noted above.
- Patients with dystrophinopathies such as Duchenne and Becker muscular dystrophy, enzymopathies of skeletal muscle such as McArdle disease, or exercise- and heat-induced rhabdomyolysis, may develop rhabdomyolysis when exposed to these agents, especially succinylcholine.
  1. This pathophysiology, though different from that of MH, may result in similar signs and symptoms.
  2. However, it is important to understand that dantrolene is unlikely to be of value in treating these causes of rhabdomyolysis.

GENETICS:

- Three genes have been associated with MH susceptibility *(RYR1, CACNA1S,* and *STAC3),* all of which are inherited in an autosomal dominant pattern.
- Variants lead to at least six known susceptibility types.
  1. The most common is a mutation leading to MHS1 involving *RYR1* that encodes the ryanodine receptor-Ca^{2+} release channel of skeletal muscle sarcoplasmic reticulum.
  2. A *CACNA1S* mutation causes another form, *MHS5.*
  3. Other types are less common and in some cases (a *CACNA2D* mutation and *RYR1*) may interact (*MHS3*).
  4. However, the genetic basis of MH susceptibility may be unknown and unrelated to the three known genes.

PHYSICAL FINDINGS & CLINICAL PRESENTATION

- Within minutes to hours after a triggering agent is administered, the patient may develop tachycardia or hypercarbia.
- Hyperthermia or a rapidly increasing temperature is often a later finding as a result of hypermetabolism and is present in more than 50% of MH events. Higher core body temperature correlates with increased morbidity.
- Manifestations of increased skeletal muscle metabolism include increased CO_2 production, leading to elevated mixed venous and arterial pCO_2, and an elevated $ETCO_2$.
- Rhabdomyolysis, a condition of skeletal muscle injury and necrosis, is associated with an increased creatine kinase (CK), observed myoglobinuria (if a urinary catheter is present), and subsequent acute renal failure or DIC (disseminated intravascular coagulation) may develop.
- Masseter muscle rigidity in the context of succinylcholine use can be present. However, it may be unrelated to MHS, particularly if it is mild and not associated with generalized rigidity, and it is transient, terminating within minutes of succinylcholine dissipation.
- The skin may be erythematous initially, progressing to a mottled, cyanotic appearance.
- Box 1 summarizes the findings consistent with MH.

ETIOLOGY

Approximately 50% of cases of MH susceptibility (MHS) are inherited (primarily MH1 and MH5); the remainder are presumed to be the result of a new mutations. The majority of the mutations, either inherited or de novo, are on chromosome 19 (19q13.2, with at least 35 variants), but other mutations may be found at 1q32.1 (*CACNA1S* with at least five variants), 17q11.2-q24, 7q21.2, 3q13.1, or 5p. The result is the abnormality of skeletal muscle calcium homeostasis and susceptibility to MH, with significant clinical variability due to incomplete penetrance and variable expressivity.

Dx DIAGNOSIS

DIFFERENTIAL DIAGNOSIS

- Exertional heatstroke
- MH symptomology following excessive heat exposure to a MHS patient who did not receive a triggering agent
- Neuroleptic malignant syndrome
- Fever
- Thyrotoxicosis
- Pheochromocytoma
- Central nervous system infection or space-occupying lesion
- MDMA (Ecstasy), cocaine, alcohol withdrawal, or amphetamine use
- Serotonin syndrome
- Adverse reaction to monoamine oxidase inhibitors or anticholinergic drug

BOX 1 Positive Findings Consistent with Malignant Hyperthermia (MH)

History of recent exposure to trigger agent, including volatile anesthetic agents or succinylcholine
Family or personal history of MH susceptibility
Total body rigidity
Inappropriately elevated (38.8° C; 101.8° F) or rapidly increasing temperature (>1.5° C [34.7° F] over 5 min)
Inappropriate tachypnea
Profuse sweating
Mottled, cyanotic skin
Dark urine, urine dipstick testing shows a positive result from blood without red cells in the sediment and no hemolysis
Unexplained, excessive bleeding
Unexplained ventricular tachycardia or fibrillation
Inappropriate hypercarbia (venous $Paco_2$ >65 mm Hg, arterial $Paco_2$ >55 mm Hg) if the patient is receiving positive-pressure ventilation or is spontaneously breathing with greater than normal minute ventilation
Arterial base excess more negative than −8 mEq/L
Arterial pH <7.25
Potassium concentration >6 mEq/L
Creatine kinase >10,000 IU/L

$Paco_2$, Partial pressure of carbon dioxide.
From Fuhrman BP et al: *Pediatric critical care*, ed 4, Philadelphia, 2011, Saunders.

- Strychnine poisoning
- Sepsis
- Drug withdrawal
- Rhabdomyolysis
- Transfusion reactions

WORKUP

- MH can often be distinguished from other causes of hyperthermia based on a history of exposure to a triggering agent.
- A rapid rise in $ETCO_2$ with no change in minute ventilation under anesthesia, especially in the setting of tachycardia, should prompt consideration of MH until proven otherwise.

LABORATORY TESTS

Considerations for laboratory testing fall into three scenarios:

- In the acute setting, electrolytes, creatine kinase, arterial blood gas, and urine myoglobin.
- Once the diagnosis is presumptive, it is important to monitor serial lab data including:
  1. Blood gases
  2. Electrolytes, especially potassium and creatinine
  3. Creatine kinase
  4. Urine myoglobin
  5. Coagulation studies to evaluate for DIC
- If hyperthermia is less acute or the presentation atypical, thyroid function studies, CBC, toxicology screen, and plasma fractionated metanephrines or 24-hour urine fractionated metanephrines and catecholamines may be useful. Treatment should not be delayed while these labs are pending.

IMAGING STUDIES

A CT scan of the head may be obtained to evaluate for a space-occupying lesion if clinically indicated. Imaging should never delay prompt treatment of strongly suspected MH.

SUSCEPTIBILITY TESTING:

- Testing for MH susceptibility involves genetic evaluation or the *in vitro* muscle contracture test.
  1. The *in vitro* muscle contracture test is considered the gold standard and involves placing a muscle biopsy specimen in a bath of caffeine or halothane. Significant muscle contraction is 97% to 99% sensitive for MH susceptibility, with a specificity of 78% to 94%. Testing can be expensive since it is performed only in a few sites in the U.S. and must be performed on fresh tissue sample(s).
  2. Genetic testing, while noninvasive, has a sensitivity of <50%. Testing can be costly and prohibitive depending on insurance reimbursement and laboratory fees.
  3. Generally, a positive contracture test leads to genetic testing, unless there is a positive family history, in which case the patient may choose genetic testing directly.
- Testing for MHS can be performed preoperatively in patients deemed to be at risk or those with a personal or family history of anesthesia-induced complications suggestive of MH.
  1. Depending on the wishes of the patient and/or family following a thorough history and counseling, a decision to proceed with anesthesia and surgery without prior testing may be reasonable. If possible, the case should be scheduled as the first case in the room with the plan to avoid volatile agents or succinylcholine.
  2. In such a case, the patient should be counseled that forgoing testing may place them at risk if an intubation is required in an emergency setting, succinylcholine is used unknowingly, and the patient truly has MHS.
- After an acute event, the patient should be advised to undergo susceptibility testing to confirm the diagnosis and the need to test other immediate family members at risk. If positive, the patient should be given a letter and wear a medical alert bracelet.

Rx TREATMENT

NONPHARMACOLOGIC THERAPY

- The patient should be cooled to 38° C (100.4° F). This can be accomplished with ice packs to the axillae and groin, a cooling blanket, a fan with cool mist, or chilled IV fluids. In extreme situations, partial extracorporeal bypass or iced peritoneal lavage have proven helpful.
- Frequent evaluation of core temperature, hemodynamics, and gas exchange are imperative.

ACUTE GENERAL Rx (SEE BOX 2)

- Notify the surgeon to stop surgery immediately. Discontinue all triggering agents and switch to nontriggering agents if surgery must be continued.
- Call for help! Management of MH requires multiple personnel for various tasks.
- Request the facility's MH cart and have someone call MHAUS (Malignant Hyperthermia Association of the U.S.).
- Hyperventilate with 100% oxygen at flows of 10 L/min to flush volatile anesthetics and decrease $ETCO_2$. Insert charcoal filters, if available, into the inspiratory and expiratory limb of the breathing circuit to further absorb agent.
- Administer dantrolene as a rapid IV bolus at a dose of 2.5 mg/kg through a large bore catheter. Repeat every five minutes until an observable decrease is seen in muscle rigidity, tachycardia, or $ETCO_2$; a total dose greater than 10mg/kg may be required, especially in patients with greater muscle mass.
- Initiate cooling measures. Apply ice to the axilla, groin, or head.
- Up to 25% of patients will have recrudescence of their symptoms, on average 13 hours after the initiation of MH. Dantrolene, 1mg/kg IV every 4 to 6 hours or by continuous infusion at 0.1 to 0.3 mg/kg/hr IV, is recommended for at least 24 to 48 hours after an event. Additional boluses may be needed for breakthrough signs.
- Call ICU to arrange for continued observation. Place additional lines in the patient as necessary including an arterial line. Send and order serial labs for close monitoring.
- Recently, one study suggested that in at least one MH model involving the RyR receptor, dantrolene treatment may be ineffective in the setting of insufficient levels of cytoplasmic Mg^{++}. MgATP hydrolysis, a process that normally increases Mg^{++} during contraction, by itself may be insufficient to raise the Mg^{++} concentration in the setting of low resting Mg^{++} levels, thereby preventing dantrolene from being effective.
- Aggressive hydration with forced diuresis and alkalization of the urine should be instituted for rhabdomyolysis. Observe closely for the development of compartment syndrome, renal failure, and DIC. Use of calcium channel blockers should be avoided since the combination with dantrolene may produce

BOX 2 Management of an Acute Malignant Hyperthermia Episode in the Intensive Care Unit

1. Administer high-flow 100% oxygen via a nonrebreathing mask and consider endotracheal intubation.
2. For ventilated patients, administer an FiO_2 of 1.0 and increase minute ventilation to control $PaCO_2$.
3. Administer dantrolene (2.5 mg/kg intravenously) and repeat until acidosis and muscle rigidity have resolved. Repeat dantrolene (1 mg/kg) every 6 hr.
4. Initiate cooling with ice packs in the axillae and groin; decrease room temperature; use hypothermia blankets, iced intravenous saline solution, and lavage body cavities with cold saline solution if temperature is greater than 39° C (102.2° F). Stop cooling when core temperature falls to 38° C (100.4° F).
5. Correct metabolic acidosis with sodium bicarbonate (1 to 2 mEq/kg initially), and give subsequent doses based on base excess and body weight.
6. Administer calcium chloride (10 mg/kg) or calcium gluconate (100 to 200 mg/kg) for cardiotoxicity associated with hyperkalemia.
7. Give regular insulin (0.1 U/kg) and glucose (0.3 to 0.5 g/kg) to correct hyperkalemia if severe.
8. Administer lidocaine (1 mg/kg) to treat ventricular arrhythmias. Consider amiodarone (5 mg/kg IV) for refractory, stable ventricular tachycardia. Do not delay defibrillation or cardiopulmonary resuscitation if indicated for cardiovascular instability.
9. Maintain urine output of 2 ml/kg/hr with aggressive cold fluid administration, furosemide (0.5 to 1 mg/kg), and additional mannitol (0.25 to 0.3 g/kg) if needed.
10. Consider quantitative end-tidal CO_2 monitoring.
11. Monitor core temperature (pulmonary artery, esophageal temperature probe, rectal probe).
12. Place arterial catheter for invasive blood pressure monitoring and frequent blood sampling. Consider central venous catheter and/or pulmonary artery catheter if indicated by cardiovascular instability.
13. Repeat blood gases and electrolytes until these normalize. Repeat CK at least every 6 hours while the patient is in ICU and then daily until CK returns to normal. Assess glucose, clotting, hepatic, and renal functions. Repeat lactic acid measurement after each dantrolene administration.
14. Consider hemodialysis if indicated.
15. Consider intensive care monitoring for at least 24 hr after MH episode or after recrudescence of MH.
16. Refer the patient for muscle caffeine-halothane contracture testing and consider genetic testing. Pursue a pathologic diagnosis for other occult myopathies.

CK, Creatine kinase; *FiO_2,* fraction of inspired oxygen; *ICU,* intensive care unit; *IV,* intravenous; *MH,* malignant hyperthermia; *$Paco_2$,* partial pressure of carbon dioxide.

From Fuhrman BP et al: *Pediatric critical care,* ed 4, Philadelphia, 2011, Saunders.

profound hyperkalemia and significantly depress cardiac function.

CHRONIC Rx

- MH is an acute disease, resolving in 24 to 48 hours with appropriate treatment.
- The MHS patient should be aware that exercise in excessive heat and/or humidity could trigger an episode of MH without exposure to a pharmacologic triggering agent.
- The patient as well as immediate family members should be advised to undergo susceptibility testing.
- The patient should be given a letter by his/her anesthesiologist and wear a medical alert bracelet.

DISPOSITION

After MH crisis, patients should be admitted to the intensive care unit for at least 24 hours where close monitoring and supportive care can be maximized.

REFERRAL

Anesthesiology, cardiology, nephrology, and hematology consultation as appropriate. After the acute event, a genetics consult may be warranted to facilitate testing.

PEARLS & CONSIDERATIONS

COMMENTS

- MH is a life-threatening condition that requires prompt recognition to minimize illness, end-organ damage, and/or death.
- Family or personal history of problems with general anesthesia in the past are clues to susceptibility and should prompt careful preoperative evaluation.
- Prophylactic dantrolene is no longer recommended for known MHS patients undergoing general anesthesia with nontriggering agents.

PATIENT & FAMILY EDUCATION

- The patient and his/her family should be made aware of the diagnosis so that they can provide information to the anesthesiologist and other intraoperative caregivers when undergoing any type of surgery or procedure under sedation.
- The patient should be given a letter that can be shown to future care givers.
- A medical alert bracelet should be recommended.

SUGGESTED READINGS

Available at ExpertConsult.com

AUTHORS: **Eveline Mordehai, MD,** and **Edward Suh, MD, MPH**

BASIC INFORMATION

DEFINITION

A Mallory-Weiss tear (MWT) is a longitudinal mucosal laceration in the region of the gastroesophageal junction and gastric cardia typically occurring after repeated episodes of severe vomiting or retching.

SYNONYMS

Mallory-Weiss syndrome
MWT

ICD-10CM CODE

K22.6 Mallory-Weiss syndrome

EPIDEMIOLOGY & DEMOGRAPHICS

- Accounts for 5% to 15% of cases of upper gastrointestinal (GI) bleeding
- Reported from early childhood to old age; the majority of patients are age 40 to 60 yr
- More common in males
- Alcohol use is present in 30% to 60%

PHYSICAL FINDINGS & CLINICAL PRESENTATION

- Vomiting, retching, or vigorous coughing will often, but not always, precede hematemesis.
- Patients may be clinically stable or present with tachycardia, hypotension, melena, hematochezia, epigastric pain, back pain, syncope, or hemorrhagic shock.
- Bleeding may be self-limited or severe. Rebleeding is more common in patients with advanced alcoholic liver disease.
- Tears may be seen in association with other upper GI tract lesions, including hiatal hernia (present in as many as 90% of patients), ulcers, and esophageal varices, particularly in alcoholics.

ETIOLOGY

- An acute increase in intragastric and intraabdominal pressure is transmitted to the gastroesophageal junction and esophagus, resulting in mucosal laceration.
- Vomiting may be associated with alcohol use, cannabinoid use, ketoacidosis, ulcer disease, uremia, pancreatitis, chemotherapy, cholecystitis, pregnancy (in particular associated with hyperemesis gravidarum), bulimia, myocardial infarction, or the postoperative period.
- Infrequently reported causes include chest wall trauma (including CPR), hiccups, coughing, seizures, lifting/straining, blunt abdominal trauma, acute severe asthma, labor and delivery, and even primal scream therapy.
- Tears may be iatrogenic, related to routine endoscopy (especially in struggling, retching, or older patients, or in association with hiatal hernias or distal gastrectomy), enteroscopy with or without spiral or balloon overtubes, esophageal dilation, lower esophageal pneumatic disruption therapy for achalasia, endoscopic submucosal dissection, transesophageal echocardiography, or in association with polyethylene glycol electrolyte colonic lavage preparation.
- Tears are frequently found on the right lateral wall of the esophagus.

DIAGNOSIS

DIFFERENTIAL DIAGNOSIS

- Esophageal or gastric varices
- Esophagitis or esophageal ulcers (peptic or pill-induced)
- Gastric erosions
- Gastric or duodenal ulcer
- Dieulafoy lesion
- Arteriovenous malformations
- Neoplasms (usually gastric)
- Boerhaave syndrome

WORKUP

Endoscopy is the diagnostic method of choice.

LABORATORY TESTS

- Complete blood count, prothrombin time, partial thromboplastin time
- Electrolytes, blood urea nitrogen, creatinine, liver function tests, pregnancy test, tests to evaluate for predisposing conditions

IMAGING STUDIES

- Upper GI series is usually not sensitive.
- Patients with concurrent chest pain, dyspnea, shock, or physical examination findings of crepitus or pleural effusion should have a chest radiograph or CT to exclude Boerhaave syndrome.

TREATMENT

NONPHARMACOLOGIC THERAPY

- Supportive care
- Avoidance of aspirin, nonsteroidal antiinflammatory drugs, and anticoagulants

ACUTE GENERAL Rx

- Patients with active bleeding or hemodynamic instability require large-bore IVs, fluid resuscitation, transfusion of blood products (red blood cells, fresh frozen plasma, platelets), and holding or reversal of anticoagulation as appropriate.
- Nasogastric decompression and antiemetics may be considered.
- Endoscopic therapy for patients with active or ongoing hemorrhage (Fig. E1). Therapeutic modalities include electrocoagulation, argon plasma photocoagulation, heater probe coagulation, injection (e.g., 1:10,000 epinephrine, polidocanol), sclerotherapy (for bleeding associated with esophageal varices), band ligation, endoscopic hemoclips (Fig. E2), over-the-scope clips, and hemostatic sprays (therapies may be used alone or in combination) (Fig. E3). Hemoclips combined with a nylon snare ("tulip-bundle" technique) have been successfully used for refractory bleeding.
- Arterial embolization in patients with active bleeding who are poor surgical candidates.
- Laparotomy, with gastrotomy and oversewing of the tear, is required in a small percentage of patients with uncontrolled bleeding.

CHRONIC Rx

- Healing will usually occur without specific therapy.
- H_2 blockers or proton pump inhibitors may be given to help facilitate healing but should not be used long term unless appropriate indications are present.

DISPOSITION

- Prognosis is good, with spontaneous cessation of bleeding in upward of 90% of patients. Endoscopic features can guide treatment. Blatchford score <6 suggests no need for transfusion or endoscopic intervention.
  1. Blatchford score is calculated by certain indices (sex, blood urea nitrogen, hemoglobin, systolic blood pressure, pulse, and the presence of melena, syncope, hepatic disease, or cardiac failure) and is used to determine which patients need clinical intervention for acute upper gastrointestinal bleeding.
- Delayed rebleeding is described in patients with high-risk stigmata (shock at initial presentation, spurting, or oozing at initial endoscopy).
- Death has been reported in 3% to 12%, often in association with severe bleeding and underlying comorbid conditions such as advanced age, coagulopathy, elevated transaminases, thrombocytopenia, alcohol use, presentation with a very low hemoglobin level or melena, and multi-system organ failure. Over the past decade, associated mortality appears to be significantly declining.

REFERRAL

- Gastrointestinal referral for endoscopy
- Surgical referral for bleeding unresponsive to endoscopic treatment or in the setting of coexistent perforation

PEARLS & CONSIDERATIONS

Conditions predisposing to retching or vomiting should be identified and treated at presentation.

SUGGESTED READINGS

Available at ExpertConsult.com

RELATED CONTENT

Mallory-Weiss Tear (Patient Information)

AUTHOR: **Harlan G. Rich, MD, FACP, AGAF**

BASIC INFORMATION

DEFINITION

Mastitis is local painful inflammation of the breast that may or may not be accompanied by infection, flulike symptoms, and abscess formation.

ICD-10CM CODES

N61	Inflammatory disorders of breast
O91.12	Abscess of breast associated with the puerperium
O91.22	Nonpurulent mastitis associated with the puerperium

EPIDEMIOLOGY & DEMOGRAPHICS

- Mastitis is the most common cause of inflammatory breast disease, and most cases are related to lactation.
  1. Nonpuerperal cases of mastitis can affect either the periareolar (periductal) region or peripheral breast tissue.
  2. Periductal mastitis is most common in younger, reproductive-age women. The majority of those affected are active smokers.
- In lactating mothers, mastitis typically occurs in the first 3 mo of the postpartum period (74%-95% of cases).
- When severe, mastitis can lead to a breast abscess (5%-11%) or septicemia.
- Delayed diagnosis and treatment of lactational mastitis can lead to discontinuation of breastfeeding, breast tissue damage, or recurrence.
- In younger, nonlactating women, infection often presents as periductal mastitis (PM) and is caused by inflamed milk ducts near the nipple.
- Granulomatous mastitis (GM) is a rarer form of benign inflammation of the breast and also most commonly occurs in reproductive-age women. It generally affects the breast peripherally.
- Mastitis also can occur in infancy when there is breast hypertrophy from maternal hormone.

PREVALENCE: Lactational mastitis occurs in up to 33% of mothers.

PREDOMINANT SEX: Females

RISK FACTORS:

- Previous mastitis
- Milk stasis and missed feedings
- Cracked, fissured, or sore nipples
- Primiparity and infant attachment difficulties
- Cleft lip or palate or short frenulum in infant
- Use of manual breast pump
- Diabetes
- Breast implants
- Nipple piercings
- Rapid weaning
- Smoking (periductal mastitis)

PHYSICAL FINDINGS & CLINICAL PRESENTATION

- Warmth, redness, tenderness in breast
- Unilateral or bilateral
- Malaise, myalgias, fevers, chills
- Decreased milk output
- Breast is hard and swollen in a wedge-shaped area
- In PM, breast mass near nipple with retraction or discharge
- In GM, enlarged axillary lymph nodes or sinus tract formation

ETIOLOGY

- In lactational mastitis, infection occurs as a result of milk stasis and irritation of the milk ducts due to local immune response to milk proteins.
  1. Bacterial infection of subcutaneous tissue due to breaks in skin.
- Most commonly, *S. aureus;* less common, *S. epidermidis,* group A beta-hemolytic streptococci, *S. pneumoniae, E. coli, Candida albicans, M. tuberculosis.* GM results from inflammation with epithelioid histiocytes and multinucleated giant cells and can be caused by etiologies like tuberculosis, sarcoidosis, foreign body reaction, parasitic and mycotic infections, or idiopathic.
- Periductal mastitis occurs following inflammation around nondilated subareolar ducts and often can progress to abscess formation. Peripheral abscesses can result from trauma, usually in the setting of comorbid conditions impairing immunity such as diabetes or use of immunosuppressive medications.
- Neonatal mastitis caused by *S. aureus* or gram-negative enteric bacteria.

DIAGNOSIS

DIFFERENTIAL DIAGNOSIS

- Engorgement, plugged duct (see Table 1)
- Breast abscess
- Inflammatory or other breast cancer (3% of women diagnosed with breast cancer are lactating)
- Mastitis as a symptom of hyperprolactinemia or galactorrhea
- GM can be manifestation of systemic disease (sarcoidosis, Wegener granulomatosis, giant cell arteritis (GCA), polyarteritis nodosa, tuberculosis (TB), syphilis)

WORKUP

- History and clinical exam with thorough breast exam and assessment of axillary nodes and nipple discharge are sufficient for diagnosis.
- Recurrent mastitis should include workup for underlying breast disease.

LABORATORY TESTS

- Simple lactational mastitis requires no milk culture or laboratory studies.
- Obtain midstream sample of milk for culture and sensitivities in refractory mastitis or in methicillin-resistant *Staphylococcus aureus*-suspected cases.
- CBC and blood cultures in toxic patients.
- In abscess formation, culture of drainage or aspirate fluid.
- Inpatient intravenous antibiotics may be necessary in severe cases or recalcitrant to outpatient treatment.
- Gram stain and culture indicated in infant mastitis.

IMAGING STUDIES

- Not necessary unless refractory mastitis or abscess suspected
- Consider ultrasound (US) (Fig. E1) to evaluate for abscess or mammogram when appropriate to exclude carcinoma
- In GM, mammogram and US-guided fine needle aspiration (FNA) are standard

TREATMENT

NONPHARMACOLOGIC THERAPY

- Mainstay of therapy is effective milk removal through continued breastfeeding or pumping.
- Consider referral to a certified lactation consultant to improve breastfeeding technique.
- Warm compresses, increased fluid intake, good nutrition, and rest.
- In abscess formation (10% of women who are treated for bacterial mastitis), surgical drainage or needle aspiration is necessary, followed by antibiotic therapy based on sensitivities of culture.

ACUTE GENERAL Rx

NSAIDs and analgesics (e.g., acetaminophen, ibuprofen). There is insufficient evidence to support or refute the effectiveness of antibiotic therapy. Common regimens include:

- No history of MRSA (methicillin-resistant *Staphylococcus aureus*):
  1. Dicloxacillin 250 mg 4×/day for 7 days

TABLE 1 Comparison of Findings of Engorgement, Plugged Duct, and Mastitis

Characteristics	Engorgement	Plugged Duct	Mastitis
Onset	Gradual, immediately	Gradual, after feedings	Sudden, after 10 days postpartum
Site	Bilateral	Unilateral	Usually unilateral
Swelling and heat	Generalized	May shift/little or no heat	Localized red, hot, and swollen
Body temperature	<38.4° C; 101.1° F	<38.4° C; 101.1° F	>38.4° C; 101.1° F
Systemic symptoms	Feels well	Feels well	Flulike symptoms

From Lawrence RA, Lawrence RM: *Breastfeeding: a guide for the medical profession,* ed 5, St Louis, 1999, Mosby.

2. Cephalexin 500 mg 4×/day for 10 to 14 days
3. Inpatient: Nafcillin or oxacillin 2 g IV q4h
4. Erythromycin may be used in patients allergic to penicillin

- Suspected MRSA or high-risk penicillin allergy:
  1. Trimethoprim/sulfamethoxazole 160 mg/800 mg 2×/day for 10 to 14 days; should not be used when breastfeeding healthy infants <2 mo or compromised infants
  2. Clindamycin 300 mg 4×/day for 10 to 14 days
  3. Inpatient: Vancomycin 1 g IV q12h
- Oxytocin nasal spray if letdown reflex disturbed
- Consider treatment for candidal infection if bilateral symptoms and infant with thrush
  1. Topical clotrimazole for mother and oral nystatin for infant, with careful washing of all pacifiers and nipples
  2. If resistant to topical treatment, can consider oral fluconazole; however, data in breastfeeding are limited
- Infant mastitis typically is treated in an inpatient setting with parenteral antibiotics based on results of Gram stain.
- Most PM cases are treated adequately with a combination of antibiotics, needle aspiration/incision, and drainage. In recurrent cases, surgical removal of diseased ducts may be needed.
- If antibiotic and NSAID treatment for GM fails, immunosuppressive drugs (steroids, methotrexate) can be used. Surgical management is not recommended due to associated slow wound healing.

CHRONIC Rx

- No evidence proving benefit of prophylactic antibiotics to prevent lactational mastitis
- In GM, systemic corticosteroids or wide surgical resection

COMPLEMENTARY & ALTERNATIVE MEDICINE

- Complementary therapies not assessed in prospective studies: *Belladonna, Phytolacca, Chamomilla,* sulfur, *Bellis perennis.*
- Several strains of lactobacilli have shown promise as probiotic agents that might be useful in treating mastitis, including *L. fermentum* and *L. salivarius.* These results should be replicated before this approach is adopted widely.

REFERRAL

Refer to surgeon for severe PM or significant lactational abscess that does not resolve with conservative measures

PEARLS & CONSIDERATIONS

COMMENTS

- 25% of breastfeeding mothers with one episode of mastitis stop breastfeeding.
- Increasing incidence of MRSA mastitis.
- Lactational mastitis is a risk factor for vertical transmission of infections (i.e., HIV-1, cytomegalovirus, measles, hepatitis B and C).
- When reassessing refractory nonlactational mastitis, the most important consideration is the possibility of cancer.
- Nonlactational mastitis can be a manifestation of systemic disease.
- GM mimics breast cancer both clinically and radiologically (>50% of reported cases are initially mistaken for carcinoma). This includes fine needle aspiration, which is sometimes interpreted as malignant.

SUGGESTED READINGS

Available at ExpertConsult.com

RELATED CONTENT

Lactational Mastitis (Patient Information)
Mastitis (Patient Information)
Breast Abscess (Related Key Topic)
Fibrocystic Breast Disease (Related Key Topic)

AUTHOR: **Anthony Sciscione, DO**

BASIC INFORMATION

DEFINITION

Mediastinitis is an infection involving the connective mediastinal tissue that fills the interpleural spaces and surrounds the mediastinal organs. It can be acute or chronic.

SYNONYMS

Fibrosing mediastinitis
Sclerosing mediastinitis
Granulomatous mediastinitis

ICD-10CM CODE

J98.5 Mediastinitis

EPIDEMIOLOGY

Acute mediastinitis (Box 1) occurs most frequently as a postoperative infection after a median sternotomy and can be a life-threatening infection. Most infections are bacterial in nature.

Chronic mediastinitis is a chronic form of infection in the mediastinum characterized by an invasive and compressive inflammatory infiltrate. It is mostly caused by fungi and some bacteria.

INCIDENCE: Incidence of postoperative mediastinitis ranges from 0.4% to 5%.

RISK FACTORS: Mediastinal infections have four possible sources:

- Direct contamination as seen in trauma or surgery (e.g., open heart, esophageal)
- Hematogenous or lymphatic spread
- Extension of infection from the neck or retroperitoneum
- Extension from the lung, pleura, or chest wall

PHYSICAL FINDINGS & CLINICAL PRESENTATION

- Patients with acute mediastinitis present with acute onset of fever, tachycardia, chest pain, dysphagia, or respiratory distress. There may be signs of sternal wound infection or cellulitis and/or crepitus and edema of the chest wall.

BOX 1 Classification of Mediastinitis

Acute Mediastinitis
- A. Due to traumatic perforation of the esophagus
  1. Spontaneous or postemetic
  2. Foreign body–associated
  3. Instrumentation or surgery
- B. Due to extension of infection from adjacent structures
  1. Infection of the head and neck
  2. Infections of lungs, pleura, lymph nodes, or pericardium
  3. Subphrenic infection
  4. Vertebral osteomyelitis
  5. Hematogenous dissemination
- C. Postoperative

Chronic Mediastinitis

From Cherry JD et al: *Feigin and Cherry's textbook of pediatric infectious diseases*, ed 8, Philadelphia, 2019, Elsevier.

- Patients with chronic mediastinitis are mostly asymptomatic until symptoms develop related to invasion or obstructions of structures within the mediastinum or adjacent to the mediastinum, such as cough, dyspnea, wheezing, chest pain, dysphagia, or hemoptysis. Complications of chronic or sclerosing mediastinitis include:
- Superior vena cava syndrome. Histoplasma is the most common nonmalignant cause of this syndrome, marked by edema of face, neck, and torso; neck vein distention; and headache
- Pulmonary venous or arterial obstruction
- Esophageal obstruction, cor pulmonale, constructive pericarditis
- Thoracic duct obstruction

ETIOLOGY (TABLE 1)

Acute mediastinitis:

- Related to head and neck infections or esophageal perforation
  1. Anaerobic bacteria: *Peptostreptococci, Veillonella, Fusobacterium, Actinomyces, Prevotella, Eubacterium, Bacteroides*
  2. Aerobic bacteria: *Streptococcus, Staphylococcus, Corynebacterium, Moraxella,* enteric gram-negative rods
  3. Fungi: *Candida albicans*
- Related to cardiothoracic surgery
  1. Gram-positive bacteria: *Staphylococcus aureus, Staphylococcus epidermidis, Enterococcus, Streptococcus*
  2. Gram-negative bacteria: *Escherichia coli, Enterobacter, Klebsiella, Proteus, Pseudomonas,* other Enterobacteriaceae
  3. Fungi: *Candida albicans*

Chronic mediastinitis:

- *Histoplasma capsulatum,* a dimorphic fungus, is the most common and can cause mediastinal granuloma or fibrosing mediastinitis. A leakage of fungal antigens from lymph nodes into the mediastinal space is believed to cause a hypersensitivity reaction and subsequent exuberant fibrotic response.
- Other: *Mycobacterium tuberculosis, Nocardia,* actinomycosis, aspergillosis.

DIAGNOSIS

DIFFERENTIAL DIAGNOSIS

For chronic mediastinitis:

- Tumors that can also cause superior vena cava syndrome (e.g., Hodgkin and non-Hodgkin lymphomas, mesothelioma)
- Sarcoidosis
- Behçet syndrome
- Mediastinal fibrosis associated with radiation
- Silicosis

LABORATORY TESTS

- CBC with differential, C-reactive protein, and procalcitonin can point to bacterial infection.
- Obtain cultures: Aerobic and anaerobic bacteria and fungi, intraoperatively or of any purulent drainage.
- Pathologic examination: Distinguish between cancer and infection for chronic mediastinitis and allow for specific fungal stains on tissues.

IMAGING STUDIES

Chest x-ray: Can show diffuse mediastinal widening or evidence of mediastinal abscess, including gas bubbles or fluid level. Pneumomediastinum (Fig. E1) or pneumothorax can be seen with esophageal perforation (Table 2).

TABLE 1 Microbiology of Mediastinitis

Organisms Frequently Recovered in Mediastinitis Secondary to Infection of the Head and Neck or Esophageal Perforation

Anaerobic

Gram-positive cocci—*Peptostreptococcus* spp.
Gram-positive bacilli—*Actinomyces, Eubacterium, Lactobacillus*
Gram-negative cocci—*Veillonella*
Gram-negative bacilli—*Bacteroides* spp., *Fusobacterium* spp., *Prevotella* spp., *Porphyromonas* spp.

Aerobic or Facultative

Gram-positive cocci—*Streptococcus* spp., *Staphylococcus* spp.
Gram-positive bacilli—*Corynebacterium*
Gram-negative cocci—*Moraxella*
Gram-negative bacilli—Enterobacteriaceae, *Pseudomonas* spp., *Eikenella corrodens*
Fungi—*Candida albicans*

Representative Organisms Recovered in Mediastinitis Secondary to Cardiothoracic Surgery, with Representative Rate and Range

Gram-Positive Cocci
- *Staphylococcus aureus,* 25% (7.1%-66.7%)
- *Staphylococcus epidermidis,* 30% (6%-45.5%)
- *Enterococcus* spp., 10% (8%-18.8%)
- *Streptococcus* spp., 2% (0%-18.2%)

Gram-Negative Bacilli
- *Escherichia coli,* 5% (0%-12.5%)
- *Enterobacter* spp., 10% (4%-21.4%)
- *Klebsiella* spp., 3% (0%-21.1%)
- *Proteus* spp., 2% (0%-7.1%)
- Other Enterobacteriaceae, 2% (0%-20%)
- *Pseudomonas* spp., 2% (0%-54%)

Fungi
- *C. albicans,* <2 (0%-20.5%)
- Polymicrobial, 10% (0%-40%)

Others Occasionally Reported
- *Acinetobacter, Salmonella* spp., *Legionella* spp., *Bacteroides fragilis, Corynebacterium* spp., *Burkholderia cepacia, Mycoplasma hominis, Candida tropicalis, Aspergillus* spp., *Nocardia* spp., *Kluyvera, Gordonia sputi, Mycobacterium fortuitum, Mycobacterium chelonae, Rhodococcus bronchialis*

Other Unusual Causes of Mediastinitis

Anthrax, brucellosis, actinomycosis, paragonimiasis, *Streptococcus pneumonia*

From Bennett JE et al: *Mandell, Douglas, and Bennett's principles and practice of infectious diseases*, ed 8, Philadelphia, 2015, Saunders.

TABLE 2 Risk Factors for Surgical Site Infection/Mediastinitis Post–Cardiac Surgery

Preoperative Risk Factors	Operative Risk Factors	Postoperative Risk Factors
Increasing age	Emergent surgery	Need for reexploration
Diabetes	Heart transplant	Prolonged ICU stay
Staphylococcus aureus nasal colonization	Increasing complexity of surgery	Need for mechanical ventilation >48 hr
Previous sternotomy	Use of internal thoracic arteries in CABG	Lack of perioperative glucose control
COPD	Prolonged operative time	Placement of tracheostomy
Peripheral vascular disease	Hair removal by razor, not clippers	Postoperative myocardial infarction
Class 3-4 angina	Inappropriate timing of antibiotics	Receipt of multiple blood products
Renal failure requiring hemodialysis	Prolonged time on cardiopulmonary bypass	Postoperative low cardiac output state
History of endocarditis	High core temperature during bypass (>38° C; 100.4° F)	
Cigarette smoking		
Low cardiac output		
Concurrent infection		
Prolonged preoperative hospitalization		
Preoperative use of a ventricular assist device		

CABG, Coronary artery bypass grafting; *COPD,* chronic obstructive pulmonary disease; *ICU,* intensive care unit.
From Bennett JE et al: *Mandell, Douglas, and Bennett's principles and practice of infectious diseases,* ed 8, Philadelphia, 2015, Saunders.

- Chest CT (Fig. E2): Can show the same as x-ray but is more sensitive in determining degree of mediastinal involvement and may guide drainage procedures for treatment or diagnosis.
- MRI may be superior to CT for sclerosing mediastinitis.

Rx TREATMENT

NONPHARMACOLOGIC THERAPY

Surgery remains the gold standard treatment of mediastinitis for optimal drainage and debridement.

- Open techniques: Debridement of infected tissue and open packing of the wound with delayed closure or use of vacuum-assisted closure for acute mediastinitis
- Closed techniques: Debridement of infected tissues, closure of the sternum, and postoperative irrigation through drainage tubes for acute mediastinitis

ACUTE GENERAL Rx

- Intravenous antibiotics: Also a cornerstone of therapy but without surgery may fail. Broad-spectrum antibiotics should be used until cultures are finalized. Combination of piperacillin-tazobactam or meropenem plus vancomycin offers good initial coverage for acute mediastinitis. Other options include ciprofloxacin or cefepime for gram-negative rods, linezolid for gram-positive bacteria, metronidazole for anaerobic bacteria.
- Therapy is 2 to 3 wk, but some cases may require 4 to 6 wk.

CHRONIC Rx

There is no definitive cure for chronic fibrosing or sclerosing mediastinitis. Antifungal agents and steroids generally do not work. The goal of therapy is to palliate symptoms by relieving airway, vascular, or esophageal obstruction. Surgery in patients with extensive fibrosis has high morbidity and mortality.

DISPOSITION

Patients may need extensive wound care and possible vacuum-assisted closure and prolonged intravenous antibiotics.

REFERRAL

- Thoracic surgeon and/or head and neck surgeon for surgery and debridement
- Infectious diseases consultant for antibiotic selection and long-term management

PEARLS & CONSIDERATIONS

COMMENTS

Histoplasma capsulatum is a dimorphic fungus found commonly in bird and bat fecal material and is most prevalent in the Ohio and Mississippi river valleys of the United States.

PREVENTION

Antibiotic prophylaxis should be given within 60 min before incision for surgeries requiring sternotomy. Options include cefazolin 1 g IV if <80 kg and 2 g if >80 kg, or cefuroxime 1.5 g IV. If the patient is penicillin allergic or has a history of methicillin-resistant *S. aureus* (MRSA) infection or surgery is to be done in a hospital where MRSA infection is common, use vancomycin 1 g IV.

SUGGESTED READINGS

Available online at ExpertConsult.com

AUTHOR: **Glenn G. Fort, MD, MPH**

BASIC INFORMATION

DEFINITION

Medical marijuana or medical cannabis refers to the use of the unprocessed Cannabis sativa plant, part of the plant, or extracts from the plant as medical therapy to treat disease or alleviate symptoms.

SYNONYMS

Medical cannabis
Cannabinoids—are biologically active compounds that have affinity or activity to the cannabinoid receptors. They may be derived from the plant or be synthetic.
CBD—cannabinol
THC—Δ^9-tetrahydrocannabinol

ICD-10CM CODES

F12.9	Cannabis use, unspecified
Z02.79	Encounter for issue of other medical certificate
Z79.899	Other long term (current) drug therapy

BACKGROUND

- Medical use of marijuana has been restricted since classification as a Schedule I substance by the Controlled Substance Act in 1970.
- First medical marijuana law (MML) was enacted in California in 1996, allowing for use of medical cannabis despite lack of Food and Drug Administration (FDA) testing for safety and efficacy.
- In 2014, 0.8% of the U.S. population used medical marijuana exclusively, and 0.5% used medical and recreational marijuana.
- Of 2014 marijuana smokers, 6.2% used medical marijuana only and 3.6% used medical and recreational marijuana.
- In 2015, 1.57% U.S. population used medical marijuana; highest increase in prevalence noted to be in 2015.
- Residents of medical marijuana states were 1.3 times more likely to use medical marijuana in 2015 compared to 2013.
- As of July 2020, state-level referendum and legislation resulted in 42 U.S. states, DC, Guam, and Puerto Rico with policies that legalized marijuana use for medical purposes.

MECHANISM OF ACTION

- Cannabinoids elicit their effects by interacting with cannabinoid receptors in various central nervous system (CNS) locations, eliciting diverse CNS and peripheral nervous system (PNS) effects.
- Primarily bind to CB1 G-protein-coupled receptors in the basal ganglia, hippocampus, cortex, and cerebellum, eliciting antinociception, locomotor, and psychoactive effects.
- Marijuana contains >400 plant-derived compounds, >60 classified as cannabinoids, with the major phytocannabinoids being cannabidiol (CBD) and Δ^9-tetrahydrocannabinol (THC).

FORMULATIONS

Research has demonstrated a wide range of THC and CBD concentrations in various formulations, with frequent inaccurate labelling.

- Cigarettes
- Tinctures
- Capsules
- Vaporization cartridges
- Purified cannabinoids butane hash oil (BHO)
- Supercritical fluid extracts (SFEs or "dabs")
- Buccal sprays
- Edibles
- Lozenges
- Transdermal patches

INDICATIONS

- Variable evidence for treatment of:
  1. Chronic pain
  2. Chemotherapy-induced nausea/vomiting
  3. HIV-related anorexia
  4. Glaucoma
  5. Anxiety
  6. Multiple sclerosis (MS)
  7. Seizures
- Marijuana has not been FDA approved as safe and effective for any indication and remains a Schedule I drug.
- However, there are phytocannabinoids and synthetic phytocannabinoid analogs that are FDA approved.
  1. Dronabinol and Nabilone (synthetic THC analogs) are schedule II FDA approved medications for AIDS associated anorexia and chemotherapy induced nausea, respectively.
  2. Purified cannabidiol oral solution (Epidiolex) is FDA approved for seizures associated with Dravet or Lennox-Gastaut syndrome.
- Qualifying diagnoses for certification for prescription medical marijuana vary by state, but typically include:
  1. Cancer
  2. Glaucoma
  3. HIV/AIDS
  4. Hepatitis C
  5. Cachexia
  6. Severe, debilitating, chronic pain
  7. Severe nausea
  8. Seizures
  9. Severe muscle spasms
  10. Crohn disease
  11. Alzheimer disease
  12. PTSD
  13. Sickle cell disease

EFFICACY

- There is evidence in the medical literature demonstrating that marijuana improves non–cancer-related pain, chemotherapy-induced nausea and vomiting, and spasticity in multiple sclerosis.
  1. A 2011 systematic review of randomized controlled trials (RCTs) demonstrated statistically significant improvement in pain scores for non–cancer-related chronic pain in 15 of 18 trials with no serious adverse effects.
  2. A 2015 systematic review and meta-analysis showed improved response in nausea and vomiting compared to placebo (OR 3.82).
  3. A 2018 systematic review demonstrated a decrease in nausea and vomiting following chemotherapy (RR 3.60 compared to placebo), improved spasticity with MS (RR 1.45 compared to placebo), and a modest benefit with primarily neuropathic pain (RR 1.37 compared to placebo) with frequent adverse effects including psychosis, "feeling high," and somnolence (number needed to harm = 5 to 8).
     a. No statistically significant improvement was noted in acute pain.
  4. A Cochrane review in 2013 found no statistically significant weight gain with dronabinol in HIV/AIDS patients, and multiple RCTs have identified megestrol acetate as superior to dronabinol for weight gain in cancer patients.
  5. A 2020 systematic review and meta-analysis showed extremely limited evidence for benefits for Crohn disease and ulcerative colitis, with only three RCTs all showing no improvement of marijuana over placebo.
  6. In 2019, a systematic review determined that there was sufficient evidence from five reviews that cannabinoids may be effective for multiple sclerosis symptoms of pain and/or spasticity.

RISKS OF USE

- Marijuana use has been demonstrated to impair short-term memory consolidation, reaction time, and concept formation, and to increase incidence of road traffic accidents, ataxia, euphoria, disorientation, dry mouth, somnolence, and, at high doses, psychosis, panic, and paranoia.
- Marijuana has been shown to worsen preexisting anxiety, depression, and schizophrenia. It should be used with caution, particularly in combination with other drugs with similar effects.
- Meta-analyses demonstrate increased respiratory symptoms of cough, sputum production, and wheeze with smoking marijuana; however, there was no statistical difference in pulmonary function.
- Medical marijuana does have drug–drug interactions, and adverse effects can be potentiated by other medications. In particular, concomitant use of other medications such as opiates and benzodiazepines should be avoided as it could lead to somnolence and respiratory suppression.
- Acute marijuana intoxication is associated with reversible changes in P and T waves and ST segments (pseudo-Wellens syndrome).
- Medical marijuana should be stored away from children given the risk of toxic ingestion.

PRESCRIBING

- Marijuana remains classified as a schedule I drug under the Controlled Substance Act of 1970.

- However, the Justice Department declared it would not prosecute any physician who recommends medical marijuana for a legitimate medical indication in a state where it has been legalized.
- Medical marijuana card (MMC)
  1. MMC allows a patient to possess a certain amount of marijuana for medical use and not be prosecuted for possession of marijuana.
  2. In order to obtain an MMC, a patient must obtain physician certification confirming a clinical indication for medical marijuana.
  3. With an MMC, the patient can go to a licensed medical marijuana compassion center (dispensary), which will dispense a dose and formulation of medical marijuana appropriate for the patient's medical condition.
  4. Physicians do not prescribe the dose or formulation of medical marijuana.
- To certify a patient for a medical marijuana card, physicians must
  1. Complete a Department of Health certification form.
     a. Forms vary by state, but typically consist of a single-page form indicating a qualifying diagnosis that is to be signed by the physician.
  2. Complete and document a full medical history and physical exam.
  3. Explain the risks, benefits, and side effects of medical marijuana.
  4. Continue an ongoing role on the patient's health care team.
  5. Maintain accurate medical records and documentation of the patient's clinical indication for medical marijuana.
- Some states require additional physician training and registration with the state medical marijuana program prior to being able to certify patients.
- Physicians are under no obligation to issue medical marijuana certifications.

PEARLS & CONSIDERATIONS

- Medical marijuana has been shown to improve non–cancer-related pain, chemotherapy-induced nausea and vomiting, and spasticity in multiple sclerosis.
  1. Qualifying diagnoses for a medical marijuana card include cancer, glaucoma, HIV/AIDS, hepatitis C, cachexia, debilitating chronic pain, severe nausea, seizures, severe muscle spasms, Crohn disease, Alzheimer disease, PTSD, and sickle cell disease. Qualifying diagnoses may vary from state to state.
  2. Adverse effects include increased incidence of road traffic accidents and pulmonary and cognitive side effects. At high doses, psychosis, panic, and paranoia can occur.
  3. Hospitals may also have specific restrictions and policies regarding medical marijuana for inpatient stays.
- Medical marijuana laws and regulations permit patients to use medical marijuana if certified by a physician but vary by state.
  1. Physician certification involves documentation that a patient has a qualifying clinical condition.
  2. A medical marijuana card entitles a patient or designated caregiver to possess a given amount of marijuana and therefore will not be prosecuted for possession of marijuana.
  3. Medical marijuana can be obtained at state regulated medical marijuana compassion centers (dispensaries). Compassion centers obtain marijuana from licensed cultivators and offer a variety of formulations that are regulated by the state.
  4. There is no FDA oversight of the compassion centers.
- Physicians do not prescribe the dose or formulation of medical marijuana.
- Physicians are under no obligation to issue medical marijuana certifications.
- Emergency department (ED) visits attributable to inhaled cannabis are more frequent than those attributable to edible cannabis, although the latter is associated with more acute psychiatric visits and more ED visits than expected.

PATIENT & FAMILY EDUCATION

- Patients must possess a valid state-issued ID and apply for a state medical marijuana card.
- Patients can obtain medical marijuana from compassion centers without a medical marijuana card but could then be prosecuted for possession of marijuana.
- Patients should be aware that concomitant use of other medications such as opiates and benzodiazepines should be avoided as it could lead to somnolence and respiratory suppression.
- Patients should store medical marijuana away from children given the risk of toxic ingestions.

RELATED CONTENT

Pain Management in Chronic Pain (Related Key Topic)
Chemotherapy-Induced Nausea and Vomiting (Related Key Topic)

SUGGESTED READINGS

Available at ExpertConsult.com

AUTHORS: **Anjulika Chawla, MD,** and **Seth Clark, MD, MPH**

BASIC INFORMATION

DEFINITION

Melanoma is a skin neoplasm arising from the malignant degeneration of melanocytes. It is classically subdivided in four types (Table 1):
1. Superficial spreading melanoma
2. Nodular melanoma
3. Lentigo maligna melanoma
4. Acral lentiginous melanoma

SYNONYMS

Malignant melanoma
Cutaneous malignant melanoma

ICD-10CM CODES

C43.30	Malignant melanoma of unspecified part of face
C43.31	Malignant melanoma of nose
C43.4	Malignant melanoma of scalp and neck
C43.51	Malignant melanoma of anal skin
C43.52	Malignant melanoma of skin of breast
C43.59	Malignant melanoma of other part of trunk
C43.8	Malignant melanoma of overlapping sites of skin
C43.9	Malignant melanoma of skin, unspecified
D03.8	Melanoma in situ of other sites
D03.9	Melanoma in situ, unspecified

EPIDEMIOLOGY & DEMOGRAPHICS

- In 2020, an estimated 100,350 new cases were diagnosed in the United States. About 6850 people were expected to die of melanoma.
- Melanoma is more common in men.
- Melanoma is much more common in whites (17.2 per 100,000 white men) than in African Americans (1 per 100,000 African American men). Increased risk of developing melanomas is found in patients with fair skin, red hair, light eyes, abundance of freckles, atypical moles, or large amount of moles (>50). A personal history of any skin cancer or a family history of melanoma also increases the risk.
- Melanoma is the leading cause of death from skin cancer. Although it represents <10% of all skin-cancers, it accounts for at least 70% of deaths related to skin cancer.
- The median age at diagnosis is 53 yr.
- Individuals with high recreational/intermittent sun exposure, history of blistery sunburns in childhood or adolescence, and exposure to artificial UV radiation from use of tanning beds have a higher risk for developing melanoma. Risk factors for the development of cutaneous melanoma are summarized in Table 2.
- Superficial spreading melanoma occurs most often in young adults on sun-exposed areas.
- Acral lentiginous melanoma is most often found in Asian Americans and African Americans and is unrelated to sun exposure.
- Eight percent to 10% of melanomas arise in people with a family history of the disease.

PHYSICAL FINDINGS & CLINICAL PRESENTATION

Variable depending on the subtype of melanoma:
- Superficial spreading melanoma is most often found on the lower legs, arms, and upper back. It may have a combination of many colors or may be uniformly brown or black.
- Nodular melanoma can be found anywhere on the body, but it most frequently occurs on the trunk on sun-exposed areas. It has a dark-brown or red-brown appearance and can be dome shaped (or pedunculated). Lesions are frequently misdiagnosed because they may resemble a blood blister or hemangioma and may also be amelanotic.
- Lentigo maligna melanoma is generally found in older adults in areas continually exposed to the sun and frequently arising from lentigo maligna (Hutchinson freckle) or melanoma in situ. It might have a complex pattern and variable shape; color is more uniform than in superficial spreading melanoma.
- Acral lentiginous melanoma frequently occurs on soles, subungual mucous membranes, and palms (sole of the foot is the most prevalent site). Unlike other types of melanoma, it has a similar incidence in all ethnic groups.
- The warning signs that the lesion may be a melanoma can be summarized with the ABCDE mnemonic (Table E3):
  A: Asymmetry (e.g., lesion is bisected and halves are not identical)
  B: Border irregularity (uneven, ragged border) (Fig. E1)
  C: Color variegation (presence of various shades of pigmentation)
  D: Diameter enlargement (>6 mm)
  E: Evolving (mole changing in size, shape, or color, or mole that differs visibly from surrounding moles ["ugly duckling" sign])

TABLE 1 Histologic Subtypes of Cutaneous Melanoma

	Frequency	Location	Characteristics	Morphology
Superficial spreading melanoma 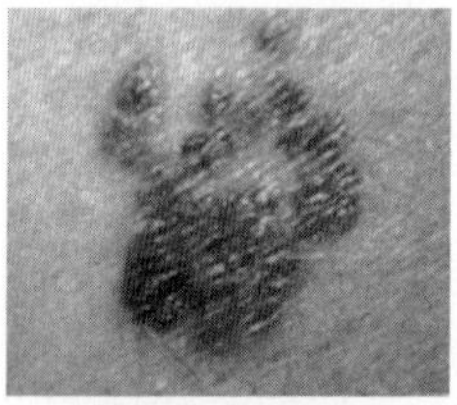	70% Women > men	Lower extremities	Slow radial growth phase	Flat during early phase, macule or papule
Nodular melanoma 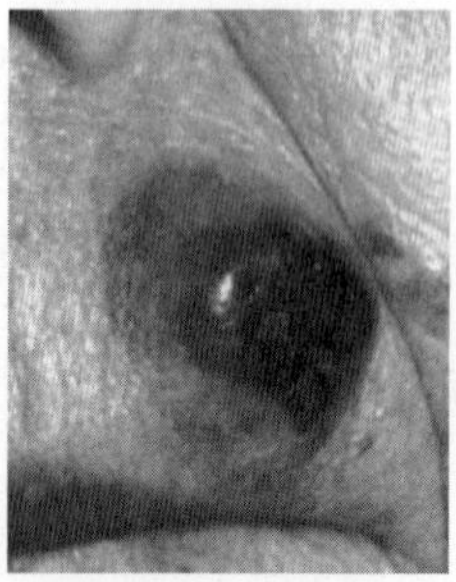	15%-30%	Trunk, head	Rapid vertical growth	Papule or nodule

Continued

TABLE 1 Histologic Subtypes of Cutaneous Melanoma—cont

	Frequency	Location	Characteristics	Morphology
Lentigo maligna 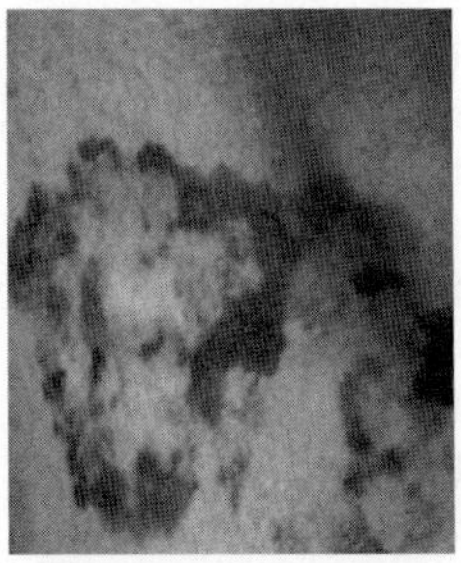	10%-15% More common in the elderly	Face, neck, arms Chronically sun-damaged skin	Slow radial growth, confirmed to the epidermis for many years	Large macule, arises in a preexisting nevus
Acral lentiginous 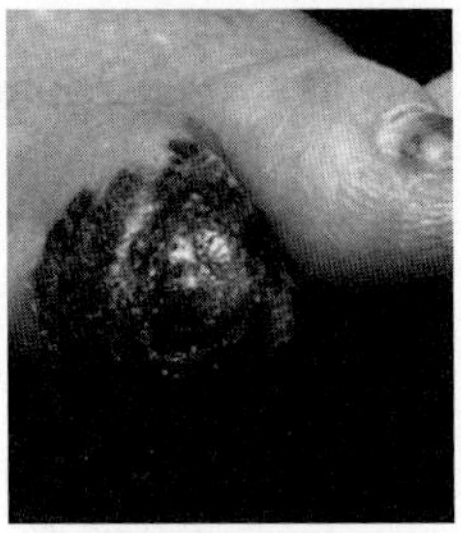	<5% More common in Asians and African Americans	Soles, palms Beneath nail beds (subungual)	Slow radial growth phase with vertical phase later on	Large dark patch, arising in a preexisting lesion

TABLE 2 Risk Factors for the Development of Cutaneous Melanoma

Genetic Factors
- Family history of cutaneous melanoma
- Lightly pigmented skin
- Tendency to burn, inability to tan
- Red hair color
- DNA repair defects (e.g., xeroderma pigmentosum)

Environmental Factors
- Intense intermittent sun exposure
- Chronic sun exposure
- Residence in equatorial latitudes
- PUVA (possible)
- Tanning bed use, especially under the age of 35 yr
- Iatrogenic or acquired immunosuppression

Phenotypic Expressions of Gene/Environment Interactions
- Melanocytic nevi and solar lentigines:
  - Increased total number of acquired melanocytic nevi (MN)
    >100 MN, relative risk ~ 8-10-fold increased
  - Atypical melanocytic nevi (AMN)
    > 5 AMN, relative risk ~ 4-6-fold increased
  - Multiple solar lentigines (SL)
    Multiple SL, relative risk ~3-4-fold increased

Relative risks (RR) are multiplicative: e.g., a person with >100 MN + >5 AMN + multiple SL has a relative risk ~ $10 \times 5 \times 3 = 150$-fold
- Personal history of cutaneous melanoma

From Bolognia J: *Dermatology,* ed 4, Philadelphia, 2018, Elsevier.

ETIOLOGY

- Ultraviolet light is the most important cause of malignant melanoma.
- There is a modest increase in melanoma risk in patients with small nondysplastic nevi and a much greater risk in those with dysplastic lesions.
- The *CDKN2A* gene, residing at the 9p21 locus, is often deleted in patients with familial melanoma.
- A mutated signal transduction molecule, v-raf murine sarcoma viral oncogene homolog B *(BRAF),* has been identified in 40% to 60% of patients with melanoma.

Dx DIAGNOSIS

DIFFERENTIAL DIAGNOSIS

- Dysplastic nevi
- Solar lentigo
- Vascular lesions
- Blue nevus
- Basal cell carcinoma
- Seborrheic keratosis

WORKUP

- Dermoscopy (use of an instrument that shines polarized light on skin surfaces and magnifies skin lesions) can increase the accuracy in diagnosing melanoma by 10% to 27%.
- Any suspicious lesion should be biopsied. Perform excisional biopsy with elliptical excision that includes 1 to 2 mm of normal skin surrounding the lesion and extends to the subcutaneous tissue; incisional punch biopsy is sometimes necessary in surgically sensitive areas (e.g., digits, nose). It is essential that the size of the specimen be adequate to determine the histologic depth of penetration, which is known as the Breslow depth.
- Sentinel lymph node excision (SLNE) is the most important staging and potentially prognostic procedure for patients with melanoma. It should be considered in patients with intermediate (1-4 mm) melanomas or high-risk skin tumors to obtain information regarding a patient's subclinical lymph node

status with minimal morbidity. The National Comprehensive Cancer Network (NCCN) recommends that SLNE be discussed with and offered to patients classified as stage IB or II, and should be considered for patients with stage IA melanoma and "adverse" features that might portend a higher risk of sentinel node tumor thickness of 0.8 mm or more with the presence of ulceration. SLNE involves the use of radiologic lymphoscintigraphy to map lymphatic drainage from the site of the primary melanoma to the first sentinel lymph node in the region. When properly performed, if the sentinel node is negative the remaining lymph nodes in the region will not have metastases in more than 98% of cases. If the sentinel nodes are negative, no additional regional surgery is recommended. The staging of intermediate thickness (1.2-3.5 mm) primary melanomas, according to the results of sentinel node biopsy, provides important prognostic information and identifies patients with nodal metastases whose survival can be prolonged by immediate lymphadenectomy.

- The staging system for melanoma adapted by the American Joint Committee on Cancer (AJCC) can be found in Table 4.

TABLE 4 The TNM Classification for Melanoma Adapted by the American Joint Committee on Cancer (AJCC, 8th edition)

T classification	Thickness	Ulceration status/mitoses
T_{is} (in situ)	n/a	n/a
T_1	<1.0 mm	Unknown or unspecified
T_{1a}	<0.8 mm	Without ulceration
T_{1b}	0.8 mm-1.0 mm	With/without ulceration
T_2	>1.0-2.0 mm	Unknown or unspecified
T_{2a}	>1.0-2.0 mm	Without ulceration
T_{2b}	>1.0-2.0 mm	With ulceration
T_3	>2.0-4.0 mm	Unknown or unspecified
T_{3a}	>2.0-4.0 mm	Without ulceration
T_{3b}	>2.0-4.0 mm	With ulceration
T_4	>4.0 mm	Unknown or unspecified
T_{4a}	>4.0 mm	Without ulceration
T_{4b}	>4.0 mm	With ulceration
Regional nodes (N)	**Number of nodes**	**Presence of in-transit, satellite, and/or microsatellite metastases**
N_0	0	None
N_1	One tumor-involved node or any number of in-transit, satellite, and/or microsatellite metastases with no tumor-involved nodes	
N_{1a}	One clinically occult (sentinel biopsy detected)	No
N_{1b}	One clinically detected	No
N_{1c}	No regional node	Yes
N_2	Two or three tumor-involved nodes or any number of in-transit, satellite, and/or microsatellite metastases with one tumor-involved node	
N_{2a}	Two or three clinically occult (sentinel biopsy detected)	No
N_{2b}	Two or three, at least one clinically detected	No
N_{2c}	One clinically occult or clinically detected	yes
N_3	Four or more tumor-involved nodes or any number of in-transit, satellite, and/or microsatellite metastases with two or more tumor-involved nodes, or any number of matted nodes without or with in-transit, satellite, and/or microsatellite metastases	
N_{3a}	Four or more clinically occult (sentinel biopsy detected)	No
N_{3b}	Four or more, at least one of which was clinically detected, or the presence of any number of matted nodes	No
N_{3c}	Two or more clinically occult or clinically detected and/or presence of any number of matted nodes	Yes
M category	**Anatomic site**	**LDH level**
M_0	No distant metastases	n/a
M_1	Evidence of distant metastases	
M_{1a}	Distant metastasis to skin, soft tissue including muscle, and/or nonregional lymph node	$M_{1a}(0)$: Normal $M_{1a}(1)$: Elevated
M_{1b}	Distant metastasis to lung with or without M_{1a} sites of disease	$M_{1b}(0)$: Normal $M_{1b}(1)$: Elevated
M_{1c}	Distant metastasis to non-CNS visceral sites with or without M_{1a} or M_{1b} sites of disease	$M_{1c}(0)$: Normal $M_{1c}(1)$: Elevated
M_{1d}	Distant metastasis to CNS with or without M_{1a}, M_{1b}, or M_{1c} sites of disease	$M_{1d}(0)$: Normal $M_{1d}(1)$: Elevated

CNS, Central nervous system; *LDH*, lactic dehydrogenase; *TNM*, tumor, nodes, metastases.

LABORATORY TESTS

The pathology report should indicate the following:

- Tumor thickness (Breslow microstage).
- Tumor depth: The depth of invasion is the most important histologic prognostic parameter in evaluating the primary tumor.
- Mitotic rate: Tabulated as mitoses per square millimeter in the dermal part of the tumor in which most mitoses are identified.
- Radial growth rates versus vertical growth rate: Radial growth phase describes the growth of melanoma within the epidermis and along the dermal-epidermal junction.
- Tumor infiltrating lymphocytes have a strong predictive value in vertical growth phase melanomas and are defined as brisk, nonbrisk, or absent.
- Histologic regression: Characterized by the absence of melanoma in the epidermis and dermis flanked on one or both sides by melanoma.
- Reverse-transcription polymerase chain reaction assay for tyrosine messenger RNA is a useful marker for the presence of melanoma cells. It is performed on sentinel lymph node biopsy and is useful for detection of submicroscopic metastases.

Rx TREATMENT (FIG. 2)

- Initial excision of the melanoma
- Re-excision of the involved area after histologic diagnosis: The margins of re-excision depend on the Breslow depth.
  1. For melanoma in situ, margin should be 5 mm.
  2. For melanomas with Breslow depth up to 1 mm, the recommended surgical margin is 1 cm.
  3. For melanomas of tumor thickness >1 mm and <4 mm, 2-cm excision margin is recommended.
  4. For melanomas >4 mm, a 2- to 4-cm margin is recommended.
- Lymph node dissection: Recommended in all patients with enlarged lymph nodes. Lymph node evaluation is important in patients with melanoma 1 mm in depth because it determines the overall prognosis and need for adjuvant treatment.
- Complete lymph node dissection is recommended for patients who present with palpable lymph nodes at the time of diagnosis.
- Sentinel node biopsy should be considered in those with a primary melanoma greater than 1 mm or any ulcerated melanomas.
- Adjuvant therapy:
  1. Interferon alfa-2b and Peginterferon alfa-2b have been previously used for the adjuvant treatment resected stage III melanoma despite modest benefits.

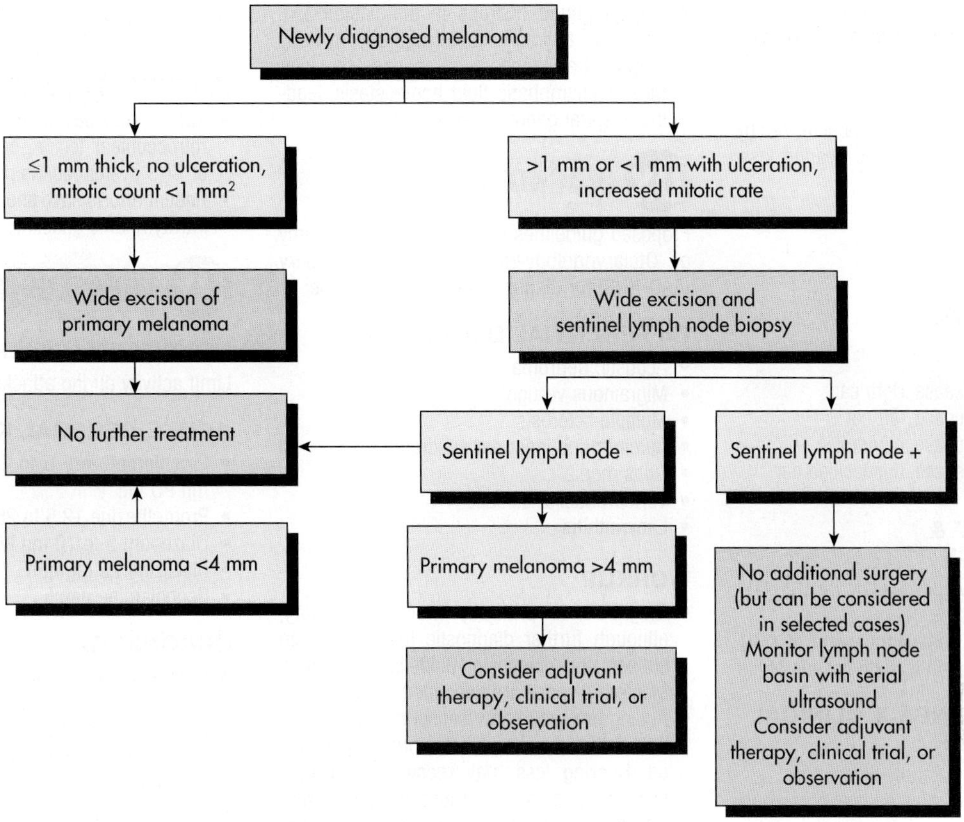

FIG. 2 Treatment algorithm for newly diagnosed melanoma. (From Goldman L, Schafer AI: *Goldman-Cecil medicine,* ed 26, Philadelphia, 2019, Elsevier.)

2. Ipilimumab, an antibody that blocks cytotoxic T-lymphocyte–associated antigen 4 (CTLA-4), improves survival in stage III high-risk resected melanoma but is associated with significant immune adverse events.
3. Immune checkpoint PD-1 (programmed death receptor-1) antibodies nivolumab and pembrolizumab have demonstrated superiority to ipilimumab in patients with resected high-risk stage III melanoma; currently only nivolumab is approved in this setting.
4. The combination regimen of BRAF inhibitor and MEK inhibitor (dabrafenib plus trametinib) has shown improved relapse-free survival in cases of resected BRAF V600-mutant stage III melanoma and is another option for these patients.

- Advanced or metastatic disease:
  1. The use of immune checkpoint inhibitors has improved overall survival in patients with previously treated or untreated metastatic melanoma irrespective of BRAF mutation status. Monotherapy with the PD-1 inhibitors nivolumab or pembrolizumab has been approved for the treatment of metastatic melanoma in treatment-naïve patients and also in cases of progression after initial therapy with ipilimumab.
  2. Combination immunotherapy with the use of nivolumab and ipilimumab in previously untreated patients with unresectable or metastatic melanoma has been shown to be more effective than ipilimumab alone as first-line treatment in high-risk patients though severe immune toxicity is seen in the majority of patients.
  3. In patients who carry the V600E *BRAF* mutation, the combination of oral BRAF inhibitors and oral MEK inhibitors improves overall survival in patients with previously untreated melanoma. Three such combination regimens (vemurafenib plus cobimetinib; dabrafenib plus trametinib; and encorafenib plus binimetinib) are approved by the FDA for use in this setting. Targeted therapy is useful in patients with rapidly growing melanoma with *BRAF* mutations, but resistance appears in almost all patients, and median progression-free survival is 15 to 18 mo. Interestingly, the majority of patients with melanoma central nervous system (CNS) metastases in this setting have similar response rates in the CNS as systemically.
  4. The combination of atezolizumab (PD-L1 checkpoint inhibitor), cobimetinib (MEK inhibitor), and vemurafenib (BRAF inhibitor) has been shown to improve progression-free survival compared with placebo in patients with *BRAF* mutated advanced melanoma and is likely to be another option in this setting.
- Patients with a history of melanoma should be followed up with skin examinations every 6 mo or sooner if patient detects any new lesions; the assessments usually consist of medical history, physical examination, laboratory values, and chest radiograph.

DISPOSITION

- Prognosis varies with the stage of the melanoma. The 5-yr survival related to thickness is as follows: <0.76 mm, 99% survival; 0.6 to 1.49 mm, 85%; 1.5 to 2.49 mm, 84%; 2.5 to 3.9 mm, 70%; >4 mm, 44%.
- The 5-yr survival in patients with distant metastasis was historically <10% but is improving with current therapeutic options and is now >20%.
- Treatment of advanced disease consists (in addition to surgical excision and lymph node dissection) of chemotherapy, immunotherapy, and radiation therapy. Nivolumab combined with ipilimumab has shown clinically meaningful activity in melanoma metastatic to the brain.

SUGGESTED READINGS

Available at ExpertConsult.com

RELATED CONTENT

Melanoma (Patient Information)

AUTHOR: **Maria Constantinou, MD**

Ménière Disease (PTG)

BASIC INFORMATION

DEFINITION

Ménière disease is a syndrome characterized by recurrent vertigo with fluctuating hearing loss, tinnitus, and fullness in the ear.

SYNONYMS

Endolymphatic hydrops
Lermoyez syndrome
Idiopathic endolymphatic hydrops

ICD-10CM CODES

H81.01	Ménière disease, right ear
H81.02	Ménière disease, left ear
H81.03	Ménière disease, bilateral
H81.09	Ménière disease, unspecified ear

EPIDEMIOLOGY & DEMOGRAPHICS

INCIDENCE (IN U.S.): Approximately 190/100,000 persons
PREDOMINANT SEX: Female:male ratio of 1.3:1
PEAK INCIDENCE: Fourth to sixth decade of life

PHYSICAL FINDINGS & CLINICAL PRESENTATION

- Hearing may be unilaterally decreased.
- Pallor, sweating, and nausea may occur during a severe attack.
- Usually the patient develops a sensation of fullness and pressure along with decreased hearing and tinnitus in a single ear.
- The patient typically experiences severe vertigo, which peaks within minutes, then slowly subsides over hours.
- May see spontaneous nystagmus on examination.
- Persistent sense of disequilibrium for days is typical after an acute episode.
- May have vestibulopathy demonstrable with a positive head thrust test.

ETIOLOGY

- Unknown; viral, autoimmune, and genetic causes have been suggested.
- Endolymphatic hydrops is the postmortem histologic hallmark. Endolymphatic hydrops may create cytochemical changes that disturb endolymphatic fluid homeostasis, leading to spiral ganglion cell death.

DIAGNOSIS

Proposed guidelines by the American Academy of Otolaryngology-Head and Neck Surgery (AAO-HNS) for diagnosis of Ménière disease:

DIFFERENTIAL DIAGNOSIS

- Acoustic neuroma
- Migrainous vertigo
- Multiple sclerosis
- Autoimmune inner ear syndrome
- Otitis media
- Vertebrobasilar disease
- Labyrinthitis

WORKUP

- Diagnosis is primarily made by history, although further diagnostic tests may help support the diagnosis. Guidelines to define Ménière disease are described in Table 1.
- Audiogram may show sensorineural hearing loss with lower frequencies primarily affected. Hearing loss may recover either partially or completely after an attack. Recurrent attacks may lead to a persistent and progressive sensorineural hearing loss.
- Electronystagmography may show peripheral vestibular deficit.
- Both vestibular-evoked myogenic potential (VEMP) studies and electrocochleography (ECoG) have low sensitivity and specificity for Ménière disease and are not clinically useful.

LABORATORY TESTS

No laboratory serologic test is specific for Ménière disease. A thyroid panel, glucose, hemoglobin A1C, antinuclear antibodies, urinalysis, chemistry panel, RPR, Lyme disease antibodies, and allergy testing can be ordered to screen for other disorders such as thyroid or autoimmune diseases, diabetes, otorenal syndrome, syphilis, Lyme disease, and allergy-mediated Ménière disease.

IMAGING STUDIES

- MRI to rule out acoustic neuroma or other retrocochlear lesion, especially if cerebellar or CNS dysfunction is present.
- Recent efforts have shown a role for MRI with intratympanic gadolinium.

TABLE 1 Guidelines to Define Ménière Disease

Definition	Symptoms
Certain Ménière disease	Histopathologic confirmation
Definite Ménière disease	≥2 definitive spontaneous episodes of vertigo 20 min to 12 hr Audiometrically documented low- to medium-frequency sensorineural hearing loss in one ear, defining the affected ear on at least one occasion before, during, or after one of the episodes of vertigo Fluctuating aural symptoms (hearing, tinnitus, or fullness) in the affected ear Not better accounted for by another vestibular diagnosis
Probable Ménière disease	One definite episode of vertigo Audiometrically documented hearing loss on at least one occasion Tinnitus or aural fullness in the treated ear Other causes excluded
Possible Ménière disease	Episodic vertigo without documented hearing loss, or sensorineural hearing loss (SNHL) fluctuating or fixed, with disequilibrium but nonepisodic Other causes excluded

TREATMENT

NONPHARMACOLOGIC THERAPY

Limit activity during attacks.

ACUTE GENERAL Rx

- Prochlorperazine 5 to 10 mg PO q6h or 25 mg PO bid
- Promethazine 12.5 to 25 mg PO q4 to 6h
- Diazepam 5 to 10 mg IV/PO for acute attack
- Meclizine 25 mg q6h
- Scopolamine patch

CHRONIC Rx

- Diuretics such as furosemide, hydrochlorothiazide, or acetazolamide.
- Lifestyle modification recommendations include salt restriction and avoidance of caffeine.
- For refractory cases, intratympanic gentamicin injections to the affected ear; endolymphatic sac surgery.

DISPOSITION

- Patients are usually followed by an otoneurologist or ENT specialist.
- Usual course of disease consists of alternating attacks and remissions.
- Majority of patients can be managed medically. Of all patients, 10% to 30% will undergo surgical intervention for persistent incapacitating vertigo.

REFERRAL

To an otolaryngologist for surgical intervention if attacks persist despite medical therapy

SUGGESTED READINGS

Available at ExpertConsult.com

RELATED CONTENT

Ménière Disease (Patient Information)

AUTHOR: **Joseph S. Kass, MD, JD, FAAN**

BASIC INFORMATION

DEFINITION

Meningiomas are generally slow-growing tumors arising from arachnoid cells of the arachnoid villi; 90% are benign.

ICD-10CM CODE

D32.0 Benign neoplasm of cerebral meninges

EPIDEMIOLOGY & DEMOGRAPHICS

INCIDENCE: 7.92/100,000 persons/yr, but increases with age. Most common primary type of central nervous system tumor, and most common nonmalignant primary central nervous system tumor.

PREDOMINANT SEX & AGE: Female:male ratio of almost 3:1 (in ages 35-54) in the brain and up to 6:1 in the spinal cord; 1:1 in childhood

PEAK INCIDENCE: Males: Sixth decade, females: Seventh decade, incidence increases with age, dramatic increase in incidence after age 65; rare in childhood

RISK FACTORS: Ionizing radiation results in increased incidence and a shorter latency period. Neurofibromatosis type 2 (NF2) is an autosomal dominant genetic disorder that predisposes to multiple intracranial tumors. Approximately half of all individuals with NF2 have meningiomas, most of which are intracranial. Studies have suggested a link between hormonal factors and development of meningioma, specifically estrogen exposure. Multiple prospective cohorts studies have also found an association between higher body mass index and meningioma, possibly relating to increased levels of circulating estrogen through increased adipose tissue. At present, there is no conclusive evidence to support a causal relationship with cell phone usage and subsequent development of meningioma.

GENETICS: Meningiomas may be isolated or found in association with other genetic diseases, such as NF2 and familial meningioma. Other genetic conditions associated with increased incidence of meningioma include BAP1 tumor predisposition syndrome, Rubinstein-Taybi syndrome, multiple endocrine neoplasia, type 1, Gorlin syndrome, Cowden syndrome 1, Werner syndrome, and familial meningiomatosis. Approximately half of meningiomas have allelic losses involving the *NF2* and *DAL-1* genes. Allelic losses of chromosomes 1p, 2p, 6q, 9q, 10q, 14q, 17p, and 18q may be associated with histologic progression. Genome-wide association studies (GWAS) have discovered two genomic variants associated with increased meningioma risk in genes for *MLLT10* and possibly *RIC8A*. Further, GWAS analysis also demonstrates an association between longer telomere length and increased risk of meningiomas.

PHYSICAL FINDINGS & CLINICAL PRESENTATION

- Neurologic symptoms vary with location and size (see Table 1); meningiomas can arise from the dura at any site, although they most commonly occur within the skull and at sites of dural reflection (i.e., the cerebral convexities and the falx). Other less common locations include the sphenoid wing, olfactory groove, and optic nerve sheath.
- The presence of focal symptoms such as vision loss, hearing loss, or mental status change depend on the site of origin and the time course of growth.
- Most common presentation is with a focal or generalized seizure or gradually worsening neurologic deficit. Seizures are present preoperatively in 30% to 40%.
- Typically are slow growing and asymptomatic; many meningiomas are asymptomatic and/or discovered incidentally on a neuroimaging study or at autopsy.

ETIOLOGY

- Meningiomas are thought to arise from a multistep progression of genetic changes.
- Mutations of the *NF2* gene on chromosome 22 are found in patients with neurofibromatosis type 2 and >50% of sporadic meningiomas. This gene is thought to act as a tumor suppressor gene; the protein product, merlin, is also involved in cytoskeletal organization.
- *DAL-1,* located on chromosome 18p, is another tumor suppressor gene that has been identified in a subset of the approximately 40% of sporadic meningiomas with neither the *NF2* gene mutations nor allelic loss of chromosome 22q.
- Cranial radiation may be responsible for some cases following an appropriate latency period from 10 to 20 yr. Meningiomas that result from radiation are generally more aggressive.
- The link with steroid hormones and their receptors is suggested by the increase in growth rate and/or development of meningiomas during pregnancy, increased incidence in women who use postmenopausal hormones, and in association with breast carcinomas.

TABLE 1 Locations and Presentations of Meningiomas

Location	Presenting Manifestation
Parasagittal	Urinary incontinence, dementia, gradual paraparesis, seizures
Lateral convexity	Variable depending on structures compressed, including slow hemiparesis, speech abnormalities
Olfactory groove	Anosmia, visual disturbance, dementia, Foster-Kennedy syndrome
Suprasellar	Hormonal failure, bitemporal hemianopsia, optic atrophy
Sphenoid ridge	Extraocular nerve paresis, exostoses, proptosis, seizures

From Goetz CG, Pappert EJ: *Textbook of clinical neurology,* Philadelphia, 1999, Saunders.

DIAGNOSIS

DIFFERENTIAL DIAGNOSIS

Other well-circumscribed intracranial tumors that involve the dura or subdural space:

- Acoustic schwannoma (typically at the pontocerebellar junction)
- Ependymoma, lipoma, and metastases within spinal cord
- Metastatic disease from lymphoma/adenocarcinoma
- Inflammatory disease such as sarcoidosis and Wegener granulomatosis
- Infections such as tuberculosis

WORKUP

Imaging studies with CT or MRI, followed by surgical removal with histologic confirmation

LABORATORY TESTS

According to the World Health Organization (WHO) classification, there are nine benign histologic variants (account for 90% of all meningiomas) and four variants associated with increased recurrence and rates of metastasis. 80% of meningiomas are classified as benign meningiomas or WHO grade I.

IMAGING STUDIES

- Cranial CT scanning or MRI can detect and determine the extent of meningiomas (Fig. 1). CT can show hyperostosis and/or intratumoral calcifications. MRI with contrast (Fig. 2) is the imaging modality of choice to demonstrate the dural origin of the tumor in most cases, with the characteristic "tail" sign that tracks along the dura outside brain parenchyma.
- On nonenhanced scans, meningiomas are typically isodense or slightly hyperdense to

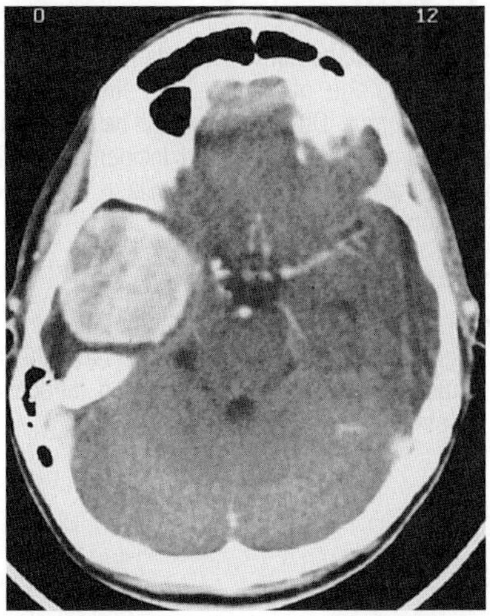

FIG. 1 Contrast-enhanced computed tomography scan demonstrates a large contrast-enhancing right sphenoid wing meningioma. (From Specht N [ed]: *Practical guide to diagnostic imaging,* St Louis, 1998, Mosby.)

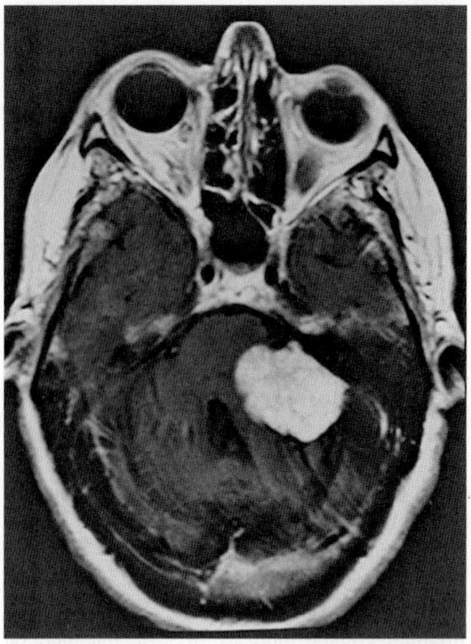

FIG. 2 Magnetic resonance imaging picture of a posterior fossa meningioma, demonstrated an extra-axial homogeneously contrast-enhanced mass arising from the tentorium and compressing the cerebellar hemisphere. (From Goetz CG, Pappert EJ: *Textbook of clinical neurology,* Philadelphia, 1999, Saunders.)

brain and are homogeneous in appearance. They show homogeneous contrast enhancement; gadolinium can facilitate imaging of smaller additional lesions that are missed on unenhanced images.
- Indistinct margins, marked edema, mushroom-like projections from tumor, brain parenchymal infiltration, and heterogeneous enhancement are suggestive of more aggressive behavior.
- Positron emission tomography (PET) scan may help in predicting the aggressiveness of the tumor and the potential for recurrence, but it is not used routinely.

Rx TREATMENT

Primary management depends on signs or symptoms, age of patient, and location and size of tumor. Observation may be appropriate if tumors are discovered incidentally and/or if growth is indolent and unlikely to cause symptoms.

PHARMACOLOGIC THERAPY

- Although a variety of chemotherapeutic agents, such as hydroxyurea, have been studied, there is no established effective systemic therapy.
- In 2020, the CEVOREM trial in France, a Phase 2 trial, demonstrated efficacy in treating recurrent meningioma with everolimus (an mTOR inhibitor) and octreotide (a somatostatin agonist).
- Inhibition of hormone receptors, such as progesterone, estrogen, and androgen, has failed to demonstrate clinical benefit.
- Treatment with molecularly targeted approaches, such as angiogenesis inhibition, is currently under way.

NONPHARMACOLOGIC THERAPY

- The mainstay of treatment for meningiomas remains surgical removal. Complete resection is usually attempted when feasible. After total excision, recurrence rates of 0% to 20% have been observed, while 20% to 50% of patients recur within 5 yr of a subtotal resection.
- Active surveillance to monitor for tumor recurrence is important.
- Radiation therapy is the only validated form of adjuvant therapy and may be beneficial in patients with incomplete resections or inoperable tumors. Stereotactic radiosurgery can provide local control with more limited toxicity.

ACUTE GENERAL Rx

- For lesions that cause significant mass effect, steroids are sometimes used to decrease brain edema.
- Anticonvulsants are used if the patient presents with seizures.

CHRONIC Rx

- Prophylactic use of anticonvulsants is not recommended in patients without a history of seizures.
- There is limited data on the efficacy of traditional chemotherapy, and the evidence is largely anecdotal. The most extensively evaluated agents are hydroxyurea, mifepristone (RU486), and interferon alfa-2b. Recently, somatostatin analogs and mTOR inhibitors have been evaluated in multicenter clinical trials, primarily in malignant recurrent meningiomas.

DISPOSITION

- Estimated surgical mortality is 7%. Significant morbidity and mortality can be observed in meningiomas with otherwise favorable pathology secondary to unfavorable location (e.g., skull base). 10-yr relative survival is 80.4% in the cerebral meninges vs. 93.2% in spinal meninges.
- Long-term outcome varies based on pathology, tumor grade, location, and completeness of resection. 10-yr relative survival for nonmalignant meningioma is 81.5%, with highest survivability in the youngest age group. 10-yr relative survival for malignant meningioma is 53.5%, with similar age-based effects.
- Most incidentally discovered meningiomas remain asymptomatic and have a slow rate of growth. Calcified tumors may be less likely to progress than noncalcified ones.
- Meningiomas may recur after surgical resection or progress to a higher grade. Risk factors for recurrence include multiple allelic chromosomal losses, local brain invasion, high rate of mitosis, and highly anaplastic features.

REFERRAL

- Neurosurgical consultation for all cases
- Neurology, radiation oncology, and oncology consults depending on presence of other sequelae or in the setting of recurrence

PEARLS & CONSIDERATIONS

COMMENTS

- Many meningiomas are discovered incidentally; most are benign and remain asymptomatic. A first follow-up MRI should be performed 3 to 6 mo after the tumor is identified to rule out an atypical meningioma with rapid growth.
- "Dural tail," which is the thickening of the dura adjacent to the mass, is a classic finding on neuroimaging studies.
- Individuals with neurofibromatosis type 2 are at high risk to develop meningiomas.

PATIENT & FAMILY EDUCATION

- Meningioma Mommas: meningiomamommas.com
- Meningioma Support and Patient Information Group
- National Brain Tumor Society
- Meningioma Online Support Group: braintrust.org/meningioma.html

SUGGESTED READINGS

Available at ExpertConsult.com

RELATED CONTENT

Meningioma (Patient Information)

AUTHORS: **Lily C. Pham, MD,** and **Jarey H. Wang, MD, PhD**

BASIC INFORMATION

DEFINITION

Bacterial meningitis is an inflammation of meninges with increased intracranial pressure, and pleocytosis or increased WBCs in cerebrospinal fluid (CSF) secondary to bacteria in the pia-subarachnoid space and ventricles, leading to neurologic sequelae and abnormalities.

SYNONYMS

Spinal meningitis
Bacterial meningitis

ICD-10CM CODES	
G00.9	Bacterial meningitis, unspecified
G00.8	Other bacterial meningitis
G01	Meningitis in bacterial diseases classified elsewhere

EPIDEMIOLOGY & DEMOGRAPHICS

INCIDENCE (IN U.S.): 1.3 to 2.0 cases/100,000 persons; 1.2 million cases per year in the world; 135,000 deaths annually worldwide. The rate of bacterial meningitis declined dramatically in the U.S. starting in the early 1990s with the introduction of the *Haemophilus influenzae* type b (Hib) vaccine and in 2000 with the introduction of the conjugate pneumococcal vaccine.
PREDOMINANT SEX: Male = female
PREDOMINANT AGE: All ages, neonate to geriatric

PHYSICAL FINDINGS & CLINICAL PRESENTATION

- Fever
- Headache
- Neck stiffness, nuchal rigidity, meningismus
- Altered mental state, lethargy
- Vomiting, nausea
- Photophobia
- Seizures
- Coma; lethargy, stupor
- Rash: Petechial and purpuric lesions (Fig. E1) associated with meningococcal infection, purpura fulminans
- Myalgia
- Cranial nerve abnormality (unilateral)
- Papilledema
- Dilated, nonreactive pupil(s)
- Posturing: Decorticate/decerebrate
- Physical examination findings of Kernig sign and Brudzinski sign (Fig. E2) in adults with meningitis are often seen later in the course of disease and may not be helpful in determining early meningeal inflammation

ETIOLOGY

The bacterial etiology of meningitis depends on the age of the patient. *Neisseria meningitidis* is now more common than *Haemophilus influenzae* as a cause of bacterial meningitis in children as well as adults, and streptococci *(Streptococcus pneumoniae)* are still common causes of community-acquired bacterial meningitis. *H. influenzae* is the cause of >30% of cases of meningitis (usually in infants and children <6 yr of age). It is associated with sinusitis, otitis media.

- Neonates: Group B streptococcus, gram-negative rods such as *E. coli, Listeria monocytogenes*
- Infants ≥1 mo and <3 mo: Group B streptococci (40%), gram-negative rods (30%), *Streptococcus pneumoniae* (14%), and *Neisseria meningitidis* (12%)
- Infants ≥3 mo and <3 yr:
  1. *S. pneumoniae* (45%)
  2. *N. meningitidis* (34%)
  3. *S. agalactiae* (group B streptococci) (11%)
  4. *H. influenzae*
  5. *E. coli*
- Ages ≥3 yr and <10 yr:
  1. *S. pneumoniae* (47%)
  2. *N. meningitidis* (32%)
- Ages ≥10 yr and <19 yr
  1. *N. meningitidis* (55%)
  2. *S. pneumoniae*
- Adults: *S. pneumoniae, N. meningitidis,* and *Streptococcus agalactiae* (third most common cause in adults).
- *Listeria monocytogenes* is uncommon in the general population but is often seen in older adults and in those with cell-mediated immune deficiencies.
- People with HIV/AIDS are at increased risk for invasive meningococcal disease (IMD).

DIAGNOSIS

An algorithm for early management of suspected bacterial meningitis is illustrated in Fig. 3. Lumbar puncture should be performed as soon as possible. Key elements to diagnosis are CSF evaluation and CT scan or MRI if the patient is in a coma or has focal neurologic deficits, pupillary abnormalities, or papilledema. Table 1 describes tests of CSF in patients with suspected CNS infection.

DIFFERENTIAL DIAGNOSIS (BOX E1)

- Endocarditis, bacteremia
- Intracranial tumor
- Lyme disease
- Brain abscess
- Partially treated bacterial meningitis
- Medications
- SLE
- Seizures
- Acute mononucleosis
- Other infectious meningitides
- Neuroleptic malignant syndrome
- Subdural empyema
- Subarachnoid hemorrhage (Table 2)
- Rocky Mountain spotted fever

WORKUP

CSF examination (Table 3):

- Opening pressure >100 to 200 mm Hg
- WBC usually $>1000/mm^3$
- Neutrophilic predominance: >80%
- Gram stain of CSF: Positive in 60% to 90% of patients
- CSF protein: >50 mg/dl
- CSF glucose: <40 mg/dl
- Culture: Positive in 65% to 90% of cases
- Multiplex PCR assay for detection of *S. pneumoniae, H. influenza, N. meningitidis,* and *L. monocytogenes* offer 100% sensitivity and 98% specificity

LABORATORY TESTS

Blood culturing, WBC with differential, and CSF examination (see "Workup")

IMAGING STUDIES

- Guidelines from the Infectious Society of America recommend CT of brain before lumbar puncture in patients presenting with:
  1. A high clinical suspicion for subarachnoid hemorrhage
  2. New focal neurologic deficit
  3. Papilledema
  4. Seizures within a week
  5. Altered mental status
  6. History of central nervous system disease (e.g., tumor, stroke)
  7. Immunodeficiency
  8. Age 60 or older

TREATMENT

Empiric therapy (Table 4) is necessary with IV antibiotic treatment if patient has purulent CSF fluid at time of lumbar puncture, is asplenic, or has signs of DIC/sepsis pending gram stain and culture results. Try to obtain blood and CSF cultures before starting antimicrobial therapy, but do not delay therapy if obtaining them is not possible. If CT scan is indicated (see "Imaging Studies" for indications) it should not delay empiric antibiotic therapy. Therapy after gram stain pending cultures is recommended for the following:

- Neonates: Ampicillin: 200 to 400 mg/kg per day divided q6 to 8 hr plus gentamicin: 7.5 mg/kg IV in three divided doses plus a third-generation cephalosporin: Cefotaxime or ceftriaxone
- 1 to 23 mo: Vancomycin: 60 mg/kg per day IV (maximum up to 4 g/day) divided in four doses plus third-generation cephalosporin: Ceftriaxone: 100 mg/kg (maximum dose 4 g/day) in one or two divided doses or cefotaxime: 300 mg/kg per day IV (maximum dose of 12 g/day) in three or four divided doses
- Children: Vancomycin: 60 mg/kg per day IV (maximum dose 4 g/day) in four divided doses plus third-generation cephalosporin: Ceftriaxone 100 mg/kg per day IV (maximum 4 g/day) or cefotaxime: 300 mg/kg IV (maximum dose of 12 g/day) in three or four divided doses
- Adults: Vancomycin: 15 to 20 mg/kg IV every 8 to 12 hr plus third-generation cephalosporin: Ceftriaxone: 2 g IV q12h or cefotaxime: 2 g IV q4 to 6 hr. For adults over 50 yr of age also add ampicillin 2 g IV every 4 hr to cover *Listeria*
- Immunocompromised patients: Vancomycin *plus* ampicillin *plus* either cefepime 2 g IV every 8 hr to cover *Pseudomonas* or meropenem 2 g IV q8h for adults, which also covers *Pseudomonas*

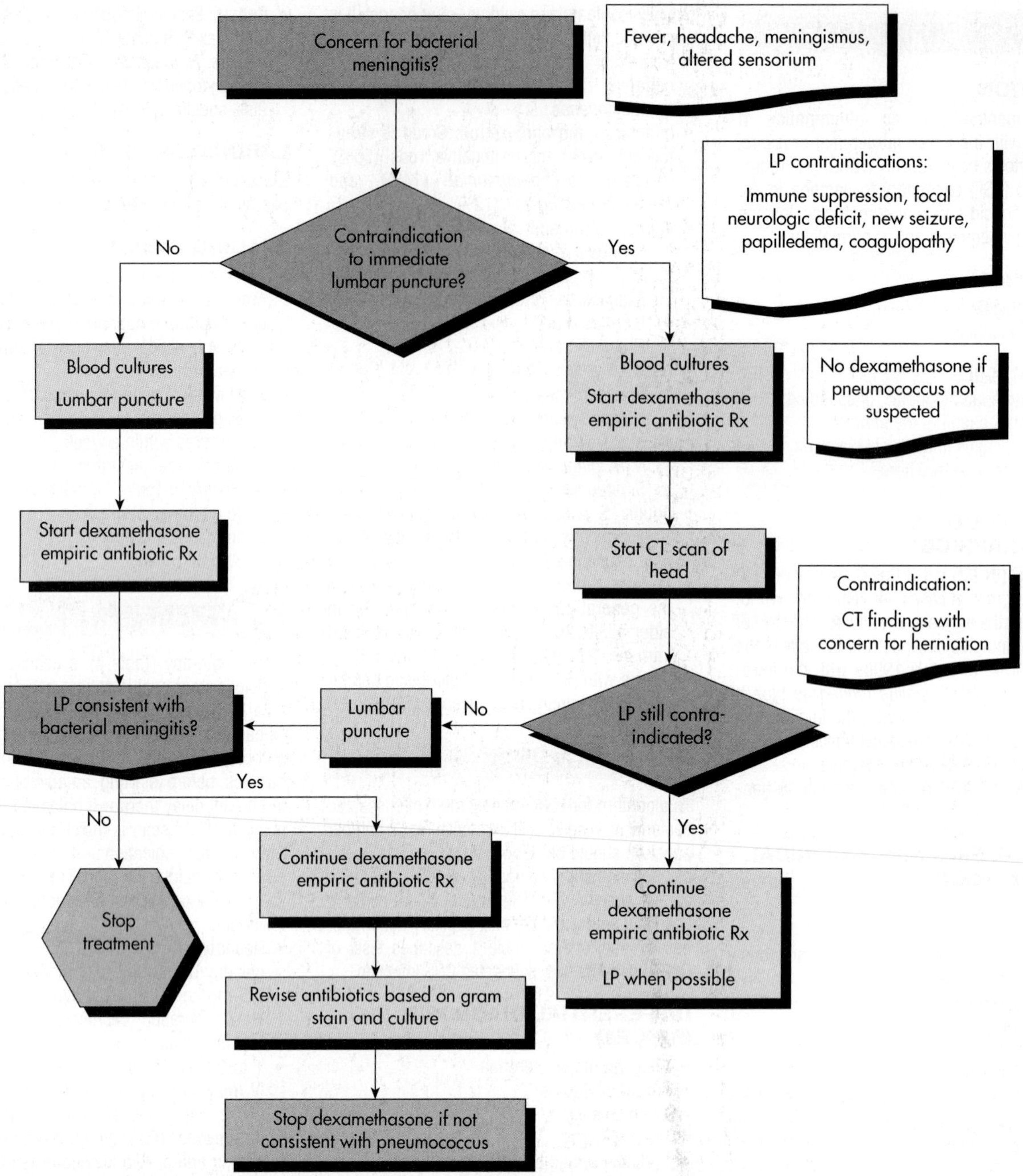

FIG. 3 Algorithm for early management of suspected bacterial meningitis including when to suspect the diagnosis, when imaging prior to lumbar puncture is appropriate, and when to initiate and discontinue empiric antibiotics and adjuvant dexamethasone. *CT,* Computed tomography; *LP,* lumbar puncture; *Rx,* treatment. (Based on Tunkel AR, Hartman BJ, Kaplan SL et al: Practice guidelines for the management of bacterial meningitis. *Clin Infect Dis* 39:1267-1284, 2004; and additional information from Hasbun R, Abrahams J, Jekel J et al: Computed tomography of the head before lumbar puncture in adults with suspected meningitis. *N Engl J Med* 345:1727-1733, 2001; Glimåker M, Johansson B, Grindborg Ö et al: Adult bacterial meningitis: earlier treatment and improved outcome following guideline revision promoting prompt lumbar puncture. *Clin Infect Dis* 60:1162-1169, 2015; and Brouwer MC, McIntyre P, Prasad K et al: Corticosteroids for acute bacterial meningitis. *Cochrane Database Syst Rev.* 12(9):CD004405, 2015.)

Use of corticosteroids in adults:

- Dexamethasone 0.15 mg/kg q6h for first 4 days of therapy should be used for adults in developed countries with known or suspected bacterial meningitis. Decreased mortality and neurologic sequelae (hearing loss, etc.) are seen with adjunct therapy in patients with pneumococcal meningitis but not other pathogens. The benefit of dexamethasone is less clear in developing countries with high HIV prevalence and malnutrition or with delayed clinical presentations.
- Dexamethasone also benefits children with Hib meningitis if given at the same time or before the first dose of the antibiotic: 0.15 mg/kg per dose q6h for 2 to 4 days. The use and benefit of corticosteroids in children with suspected or pneumococcal or meningococcal meningitis to prevent neurologic sequelae is not as clear and should be individualized after analysis of risk and benefits.

DISPOSITION

Bacterial meningitis is a reportable disease that needs to be reported to local health authorities. Droplet precautions should be used for first 24 hr of therapy for suspected or confirmed *N. meningitidis* infection.

REFERRAL

- To a neurologist if persistent neurologic sequelae develop after bacterial meningitis

M

Diseases and Disorders

TABLE 1 Tests of Cerebrospinal Fluid in Patients with Suspected Central Nervous System Infection

Routine Tests	
White blood cell count with differential	
Red blood cell count[a]	
Glucose concentration[b]	
Protein concentration	
Gram stain	
Bacterial culture	
Selected Specific Tests Based on Clinical Suspicion	
Viral culture[c]	
Smears and culture for acid-fast bacilli	
Venereal Disease Research Laboratory (VDRL)	
India ink preparation	
Cryptococcal polysaccharide antigen	
Fungal culture	
Antibody tests (IgM or IgG, or both)[d]	
Nucleic acid amplification tests (e.g., polymerase chain reaction)[e]	
Cytology[f]	
Flow cytometry	

[a]Should be checked in the first and last tubes; in patients with a traumatic tap, there should be a decrease in the number of red blood cells with continued flow of cerebrospinal fluid (CSF). See text for the formula for determining whether the numbers of CSF red blood cells and white blood cells are consistent with a traumatic tap.
[b]Compare with serum glucose drawn just before lumbar puncture.
[c]Yield of viral culture may be low.
[d]May be useful for specific causes of meningitis and encephalitis.
[e]Most useful for specific viral causes of encephalitis and causes of chronic meningitis.
[f]In patients with suspected malignancy.
From Bennett JE et al: *Mandell, Douglas, and Bennett's principles and practice of infectious diseases,* ed 8, Philadelphia, 2015, Saunders.

TABLE 2 Acute Bacterial Meningitis and Subarachnoid Hemorrhage

Finding	Frequency (%)
Acute Bacterial Meningitis	
Neck stiffness	84
Fever	66-97
Altered mental status	55-95
Kernig or Brudzinski sign	61
Focal neurologic signs	9-37
Seizures	5-28
Petechial rash	3-52
Subarachnoid Hemorrhage	
Neck stiffness	21-86
Seizures	7-32
Altered mental status	29-64
Focal neurologic findings	10-36
Fever	6
Preretinal hemorrhage	4

Diagnostic standard: For *meningitis,* cerebrospinal fluid pleocytosis and microbiologic or postmortem data supporting bacterial meningitis; for *subarachnoid hemorrhage,* computed tomography or lumbar puncture.
From McGee S: *Evidence-based physical diagnosis,* ed 4, Philadelphia, 2018, Elsevier.

TABLE 3 Typical Cerebrospinal Fluid Findings in Patients with Selected Infectious Causes of Meningitis

Cause of Meningitis	White Blood Cell Count (cells/mm³)	Primary Cell Type	Glucose (mg/dl)	Protein (mg/dl)
Viral	50-1000	Mononuclear[a]	>45	<200
Bacterial	1000-5000[b]	Neutrophilic[c]	<40[d]	100-500
Tuberculous	50-300	Mononuclear[e]	<45	50-300
Cryptococcal	20-500[f]	Mononuclear	<40	>45

[a]May be neutrophilic early in presentation.
[b]Range from <100 to >10,000 cells/mm³.
[c]About 10% of patients have cerebrospinal fluid lymphocyte predominance.
[d]Should always be compared with a simultaneous serum glucose; ratio of CSF to serum glucose is ≤0.4 in most cases.
[e]May see a "therapeutic paradox," in which a mononuclear predominance becomes neutrophilic during antituberculous therapy.
[f]More than 75% of patients with acquired immunodeficiency syndrome have <20 cells/mm³.
From Bennett JE et al: *Mandell, Douglas, and Bennett's principles and practice of infectious diseases,* ed 8, Philadelphia, 2015, Saunders.

- To an infectious disease consultant if a patient has recurrent bacterial meningitis; such patients deserve a workup for an anatomic (CSF dural leak) or immunologic defect (complement defect, hyposplenism, immunoglobulin deficiency)

PEARLS & CONSIDERATIONS

COMMENTS

- Patients with bacterial meningitis often require ICU care either to manage complications evident on presentation or for monitoring for any complications that may subsequently develop during their course. Criteria for admission to an ICU are summarized in Table 5.
- Nosocomial bacterial meningitis may result from invasive procedures (e.g., placement of ventricular catheters, lumbar puncture, craniotomy, spinal anesthesia). Treatment of this different spectrum of microorganisms requires empirical antimicrobial therapy with vancomycin plus either cefepime, ceftazidime, or meropenem. In cases of basilar skull fracture, effective empirical antimicrobial therapy consists of vancomycin plus a third-generation cephalosporin.
- False-positive elevations of CSF where blood cell counts can be found after traumatic lumbar puncture or in patients with intracerebral or subarachnoid hemorrhage in which RBCs and WBCs are introduced into the subarachnoid space. In those instances, the following formula should be used as a correction factor for the true WBC count in the presence of CSF RBCs:

$$\text{Adjusted WBC in CSF} = \text{Actual WBC in CSF} - \frac{\text{WBC in blood} \times \text{RBC in CSF blood}}{\text{RBC in blood}}$$

In the previous equation, the amount being subtracted is the predicted CSF WBC that would occur if all the CSF WBCs were the result of blood contamination.[1]

- Prevention of meningitis can be achieved through chemoprophylaxis of close contacts (household members and anyone exposed to oral secretions).
- Effective medications are rifampin 10 mg/kg PO bid for 2 days or ceftriaxone 250 mg IM single dose in patients older than age 12; 125 mg IM if age 12 or younger.
- Ciprofloxacin 500 mg for prevention of *Neisseria* meningitis can be given to patients older than 18 yr who cannot tolerate rifampin to eradicate pharyngeal colonization.
- Menactra: A protein-conjugate vaccine against serogroup A, C, Y, W-135 capsular polysaccharides is available for adults (up to 55 yr) and children older than 2 yr.
- Two new vaccines for *Neisseria* meningitis serogroup B (MenB) are now available: Bexsero and Trumenba.
- Children with cochlear implants are at increased risk of developing bacterial meningitis.
- Patients on eculizumab (Soliris) are at high risk for invasive meningococcal disease and should receive Menactra and a MenB vaccine and may need lifelong antibiotic prophylaxis as well.

SUGGESTED READINGS

Available at ExpertConsult.com

RELATED CONTENT

Meningitis (Patient Information)
Meningitis, viral (Related Key Topic)
Meningitis, fungal (Related Key Topic)

AUTHOR: **Glenn G. Fort, MD, MPH**

[1]Bennett JE et al: *Mandell, Douglas and Bennett's principles and practice of infectious diseases, ed 8,* Philadelphia, 2015, Saunders, p. 1093.

TABLE 4 Empiric Treatment of Suspected Bacterial Meningitis in Adults[a,1,2,3,4]

Host Factors to Consider	Age >50 yr? Risk for *Listeria monocytogenes* and aerobic gram-negative rods		
	Immune suppression? Includes host defects (e.g., HIV, alcoholism, lymphoma) and treatment-related (e.g., posttransplant, corticosteroids)		
	Health care–associated? Includes trauma, postneurosurgical, shunt- or ventriculostomy-related		
	Life-threatening penicillin/β-lactam allergy? Aztreonam or fluoroquinolone alternatives for gram-negative rods; trimethoprim-sulfamethoxazole an alternative for *L. monocytogenes*		
Host	**Likely Pathogens**	**Empiric Therapy**	**Additional Considerations**
Age 15-50 yr without Immune Suppression	*Streptococcus pneumoniae, Neisseria meningitidis*, group B β-hemolytic streptococci	Vancomycin + third-generation cephalosporin[b]	Adjuvant dexamethasone Consider rifampin if high rates of cephalosporin-resistant *S. pneumoniae*
Age ≥50 yr without Immune Suppression	*S. pneumoniae, N. meningitidis*, group B β-hemolytic streptococci, *L. monocytogenes*, aerobic gram-negative rods	Vancomycin + ampicillin + third-generation cephalosporin[b]	Adjuvant dexamethasone Consider rifampin if high rates of cephalosporin-resistant *S. pneumoniae*
Immune Suppression	*S. pneumoniae, N. meningitidis*, group B β-hemolytic streptococci, *L. monocytogenes*, *Staphylococcus aureus*, aerobic gram-negative rods including *Pseudomonas aeruginosa*	Vancomycin + ampicillin + cefepime or meropenum[c]	Adjuvant dexamethasone Consider rifampin if high rates of cephalosporin-resistant *S. pneumoniae*
Health Care–Associated: Trauma, Postneurosurgical, or Shunt-Associated[c]	*S. aureus*, coagulase-negative staphylococci, aerobic gram-negative rods including *P. aeruginosa*	Vancomycin + ceftazidime or cefepime or meropenem[c]	Dexamethasone not indicated Consider rifampin for staphylococci Consider intrathecal therapy for shunt-/ventriculostomy-associated infection
Health Care–Associated: Basilar Skull Fracture	*S. pneumoniae, Haemophilus influenzae*, group A β-hemolytic streptococci	Vancomycin + third-generation cephalosporin[b]	Adjuvant dexamethasone Consider rifampin if high rates of cephalosporin-resistant *S. pneumoniae*

[a]Age older than 15 yr.
[b]Third-generation cephalosporin: Ceftriaxone 2 g q12h or cefotaxime 2 g q4-6h.
[c]Dosing of other agents (modified for renal insufficiency): Vancomycin targeted to vancomycin trough levels of 15-20 μg/ml; ampicillin 2 g q4h; ceftazidime 2 g q8h; cefepime 2 g q8h; meropenem 2 g q8h.
HIV, Human immunodeficiency virus.

[1]van de Beek D et al: Community-acquired bacterial meningitis, *Nat Rev Dis Primers* 2, 16074, 1-20, 2016.
[2]Thigpen MC et al for the Emerging Infections Programs Network: Bacterial meningitis in the United States, 1998-2007, *N Engl J Med* 364(21):2016-2025, 2011.
[3]Tunkel AR et al: Practice guidelines for the management of bacterial meningitis, *Clin Infect Dis* 39(9):1267-1284, 2004.
[4]Tunkel AR et al: 2017 Infectious Diseases Society of America's Clinical Practice Guidelines for healthcare-associated ventriculitis and meningitis, *Clin Infect Dis* 64(6):e34-e65, 2017.
From Parrillo JE, Dellinger RP: *Critical care medicine, principles of diagnosis and management in the adult*, ed 5, Philadelphia, 2019, Elsevier.

TABLE 5 Major Complications of Bacterial Meningitis Requiring ICU Level of Care for Monitoring and Management[1,2,3,4,5]

Type of Complication	Etiologies, Prevalence	Management Strategies
Neurologic Complications		
Increasing intracranial pressure	Brain edema, 6%-10%	Strategies: Osmotic diuresis, intracranial pressure monitoring, head of bed elevation, prophylactic lumbar drain Glycerol and hypothermia not beneficial and may result in higher mortality
Hydrocephalus	Communicating hydrocephalus, 3%-8% Obstructive hydrocephalus uncommon	Repeated lumbar puncture, lumbar drain, ventriculostomy
Focal neurologic deficits	Arterial infarct or vasculitis, 10%-15% Venous infarction, 3%-5% Hearing loss, 14%-30% Cranial nerve deficits, especially eighth nerve, 15%-30% Hemorrhage, <1% Brain abscess, subdural empyema <1%	Radiographic studies to look for focal intracranial complications Administer dexamethasone for suspected pneumococcal meningitis to decreases risk of hearing loss
Seizures	Multiple etiologies, 14%-33%	Continuous EEG monitoring, antiepileptic agents Prophylactic antiepileptic agents not routinely recommended
Agitation	Common	Careful sedation
Other Complications		
Hyponatremia	Up to 25%-30%	? Hypertonic saline solution Presence of hyponatremia did not affect outcome
Sepsis and cardiorespiratory failure	38%	Hemodynamic support, mechanical ventilation
Pneumonia	17%, most often with *Streptococcus pneumoniae*	Ventilatory support

EEG, Electroencephalographic.

[1]van de Beek D et al: Community-acquired bacterial meningitis, *Nat Rev Dis Primers* 2(16074):1-20, 2016.
[2]Bijlsma MW et al: Community-acquired bacterial meningitis in adults in the Netherlands, 2006-2014: a prospective cohort study, *Lancet Infect Dis* 16(3):339-347, 2016.
[3]Durand ML et al: Acute bacterial meningitis in adults: review of 493 episodes, *N Engl J Med* 328(1):21-28, 1993.
[4]Tunkel AR et al: Practice guidelines for the management of bacterial meningitis, *Clin Infect Dis* 39(9):1267-1284, 2004.
[5]Brouwer MC et al: What's new in bacterial meningitis, *Intensive Care Med* 42(3):415-417, 2016.
From Parrillo JE, Dellinger RP: *Critical care medicine, principles of diagnosis and management in the adult*, ed 5, Philadelphia, 2019, Elsevier.

BASIC INFORMATION

DEFINITION

Viral meningitis is an acute febrile illness with signs and symptoms of meningeal irritation, usually with a lymphocytic pleocytosis of the cerebrospinal fluid (CSF) and negative CSF bacterial stains and cultures.

SYNONYMS

Aseptic meningitis
Viral meningitis

ICD-10CM CODES
A87.8 Other viral meningitis
A87.9 Viral meningitis, unspecified

EPIDEMIOLOGY & DEMOGRAPHICS (TABLE 1)

INCIDENCE (IN U.S.): 11 cases/100,000 persons; leads to 26,000 to 42,000 hospitalizations per yr
PREDOMINANT SEX: Male = female
GENETICS: Those with abnormal humoral immunity and agammaglobulinemia have associated difficulty with viral clearance

PHYSICAL FINDINGS & CLINICAL PRESENTATION

- Fever
- Headache
- Nuchal rigidity
- Photophobia
- Myalgias
- Vomiting
- Rash

ETIOLOGY

- Enterovirus: 85% to 95% of all cases. Most common are coxsackie viruses and echoviruses
- Parechoviruses
- Mumps virus
- Measles
- Arboviruses from mosquitoes: Eastern equine encephalitis (EEE), West Nile, St. Louis
- Herpes: HSV-1, HSV-2, VZV, HHV-6, and HHV-7
- Acute HIV
- Lymphocytic choriomeningitis virus
- Adenovirus
- Cytomegalovirus (CMV) and Epstein-Barr virus (EBV)
- Other arthropod-borne viruses: Powassan virus
- Influenza A and B virus
- Box E1 summarizes etiologic agents, factors, and diseases associated with aseptic meningitis

DIAGNOSIS

The diagnostic approach is similar to that for bacterial meningitis (see "Meningitis, Bacterial"); the foremost need is to rule out bacterial meningitis with CSF evaluation. Presentation may be similar to that of meningitis with bacterial involvement.

DIFFERENTIAL DIAGNOSIS

- Bacterial meningitis
- Meningitis secondary to Lyme disease, tuberculosis (TB), syphilis, amebiasis, leptospirosis
- Rickettsial illnesses: Rocky Mountain spotted fever
- Migraine headache
- Medications
- Systemic lupus erythematosus (SLE)
- Acute mononucleosis/EBV
- Seizures
- Carcinomatous meningitis

WORKUP

CSF examination:
- Usually shows pleocytosis
- Lymphocytic predominance (neutrophils in early stages)
- Opening pressure: 200 to 250 mm Hg H_2O (≤250 mm/H_2O)
- WBC: 100 to 1000 mm^3
- Increased CSF protein (<200 mg/dl)
- Slightly decreased or normal CSF glucose (>45 mg/dl)
- Negative Gram stain, cultures, CIE, latex agglutination
- Viral cultures or serologic testing may be diagnostic
- Polymerase chain reaction (PCR) for HSV or enterovirus (which could shorten duration of antibiotic treatment and hospitalization if bacterial meningitis was suspected); multiplex or panel-based PCR tests that test for multiple viruses and bacteria at the same time in a single CSF sample are available
- Antibody detection in CSF for diagnosis of West Nile virus meningitis

LABORATORY TESTS

CBC with differential, blood culturing, and CSF examination (see "Workup")

IMAGING STUDIES

CT scan or MRI: If cerebral edema, focal neurologic findings develop.

TREATMENT

- No specific antiviral therapy for most viruses. Treatment is supportive unless herpes simplex virus (HSV) is detected, which would be treated with IV acyclovir: 10 mg/kg q8h in adults for 14 to 21 days. Up to 20 mg/kg q8h in children >12 yr.
- Empiric antibiotics may be given until CSF cultures exclude bacterial meningitis.

DISPOSITION

Viral meningitis is almost always an uncomplicated illness that will resolve; however, relapsing headache, myalgia, and weakness may occur for 2 to 3 wk after onset of symptoms.

PEARLS & CONSIDERATIONS

- Enteroviruses are the most common cause of viral meningitis and are transmitted by fecal-oral route and less commonly by the respiratory route. They are more common in summer and fall mos. From 2000 to 2005, the most common serotypes were coxsackie viruses A9, B5, and B1 and echoviruses 6, 9, 13, 18, and 30.

TABLE 1 Epidemiology of Acute Viral Meningitis

EPIDEMIOLOGIC FACTORS*				
Season	Patient's Age (yr)	Patient's Sex	Risk Factor	Suggested Viral Agent
Summer-fall	Infant	—	Infected mother	Coxsackievirus B
	1-15	—	Swimming pools, closed communities	Enteroviruses
			Geographic area: California, southeastern U.S.	California serogroup virus
Winter	1-15	—	School exposure	Varicella virus, measles virus
		Male:female 3:1		Mumps virus
	16-21	—	College exposure	Measles virus
		Male:female 3:1		Mumps virus
				Epstein-Barr virus (mononucleosis)
	Any	—	Mice, rats, hamsters	Lymphocytic choriomeningitis virus
	Adults	—	Varicella-zoster	Varicella-zoster virus
Any	Any	—	Immunocompromise	Adenovirus
		—	Acquired immunodeficiency syndrome	Human immunodeficiency virus

*Epidemiologic factors are suggestive but should not be used to exclude diagnoses in individual cases.
From Gorbach SI: *Infectious diseases,* ed 2, Philadelphia, 1998, Saunders.

- Herpes simplex type 2 (HSV-2) can be a cause of a primary episode of meningitis and also be a cause of recurrent episodes of lymphocytic meningitis. HSV-2 meningitis presents most often without a history of genital herpes or genital symptoms. Recurrent aseptic meningitis, also known as Mollaret disease, is predominantly caused by HSV-2 infection.

SUGGESTED READINGS

Available at ExpertConsult.com

RELATED CONTENT

Meningitis (Patient Information)
Meningitis, Bacterial (Related Key Topic)

AUTHOR: **Glenn G. Fort, MD, MPH**

BASIC INFORMATION

DEFINITION

Menopause is the permanent cessation of menstrual periods for 1 yr after age 40 or permanent cessation of ovulation after lost ovarian activity without any other obvious pathologic or physiologic cause. It is the reproductive stage of life marked by waxing and waning estrogen levels followed by decreasing ovarian function. Primary ovarian insufficiency (previously also referred to as premature ovarian failure) and no menstrual periods may also occur because of depletion of ovarian follicles before the age of 40 yr.

SYNONYMS

Change of life
Climacteric ovarian failure

ICD-10CM CODES	
E28.310	Symptomatic premature menopause
E28.319	Asymptomatic premature menopause
N95.1	Menopausal and female climacteric states
N95.8	Other specified menopausal and perimenopausal disorders
Z78.0	Asymptomatic menopausal state

EPIDEMIOLOGY & DEMOGRAPHICS

- Average age of menopause in the U.S. is 51 yr.
- Age at which menopause occurs is primarily genetically determined.
- Smokers experience menopause an average of 1.5 yr earlier than nonsmokers.
- The menopausal transition, or perimenopause, begins on average 4 yr before the last menstrual period.
- Onset of perimenopause is usually in a woman's mid- to late-40s.
- Approximately 4000 women begin menopause each day.

PHYSICAL FINDINGS & CLINICAL PRESENTATION

- Menopausal vasomotor symptoms (VMS, hot flashes, flushes): Night sweats, cardiovascular disease, coronary artery disease, atherosclerosis, headaches, tiredness, and lethargy; the median duration of hot flashes is 7.4 yr, but that the length of hot flashes was largely dictated by how early they began in the perimenopause
- Either complete cessation of menses or a period of irregular cycles and diminished or heavier bleeding
- Atrophic vaginitis, which can cause burning, itching, bleeding, dyspareunia
- Osteoporosis
- Osteopenia
- Psychological dysfunction:
  1. Anxiety
  2. Depression
  3. Insomnia
  4. Nervousness
  5. Irritability
  6. Inability to concentrate
- Sexual changes, decreased libido, dyspareunia
- Urinary incontinence

ETIOLOGY

- The most common etiology: Physiologic, caused by depleted granulosa and theca cells that fail to react to endogenous gonadotropins, producing less estrogen; decreased negative feedback in the hypothalamic pituitary access, increased follicle-stimulating hormone (FSH), and increased luteinizing hormone (LH), which leads to stromal cells that continue to produce androgens as a result of the LH stimulation
- Surgical castration
- Other factors that contribute to menopause can be family history of early menopause, cigarette smoking, blindness, abnormal chromosomal karyotype (Turner syndrome, gonadal dysgenesis), precocious puberty, and left-handedness

DIAGNOSIS

DIFFERENTIAL DIAGNOSIS

- Primary ovarian insufficiency
- Asherman syndrome
- Hypothalamic dysfunction
- Hypothyroidism
- Pituitary tumors
- Adrenal abnormalities
- Ovarian abnormalities
- Polycystic ovarian syndrome
- Pregnancy
- Ovarian neoplasm
- Tuberculosis of the endometrium

WORKUP

- Physical examination, height, weight, blood pressure, breast examination, and pelvic examination are needed.
- If the clinical picture is highly suggestive of menopause, reassurance or hormone replacement therapy such as estrogen can be prescribed to help with menopausal symptoms (after appropriate counseling). If all symptoms resolve, then a diagnosis essentially has been made. Before estrogen is prescribed, however, a complete history and physical examination are needed. If a patient has an estrogen-dependent malignancy, unexplained abnormal uterine bleeding, a history of thrombophlebitis, or acute liver disease, estrogen therapy is contraindicated.
- Progesterone challenge test: Medroxy progesterone 10 to 20 mg PO or progesterone 100 mg IM to induce withdrawal bleeding. If no withdrawal bleeding is obtained, a hypoestrogenic state is assumed to be present.
- Assess risk for coronary artery disease, osteoporosis, cigarette smoking, personal history, history of breast cancer, liver disease, active coagulation disorder, or any unexplained vaginal bleeding.

LABORATORY TESTS

- No laboratory tests may be indicated if the patient fulfills clinical criteria of menopause at an anticipated average age.
- FSH, LH, and estrogen levels: Markedly elevated FSH and markedly depressed estrogen level constitute laboratory diagnosis of ovarian failure; LH only if polycystic ovarian disease is to be ruled out in a younger patient. It is not necessary to obtain an FSH if the patient fulfills the clinical criteria for menopause. Similarly, since estradiol levels vary during the menstrual cycle, estradiol levels are rarely necessary or informative.
- Anti-Müllerian hormone (produced by the granulosa cells) will demonstrate a decrease.
- TSH to rule out thyroid dysfunction and prolactin level if patient has symptoms of galactorrhea and if suspicion of pituitary adenoma exists.
- A general chemistry profile to check for any systemic diseases.
- Pap smear per standard guidelines, endometrial biopsy, or dilation and curettage in patients who have had irregular periods or intermenstrual or postmenopausal bleeding.
- Mammogram as recommended by American Congress of Obstetricians and Gynecologists for preventative care.

IMAGING STUDIES

- Per standard protocols, CT scan or MRI of sella if pituitary tumor is suspected
- Bone density studies if high-risk condition for osteoporosis exists
- Pelvic ultrasound to check endometrial stripe as determined by clinical history (i.e., in the setting of postmenopausal bleeding)

TREATMENT

NONPHARMACOLOGIC THERAPY

- A balanced diet: Low in fat, with total fat intake being <30% of calories; total calories sufficient to maintain body weight or produce weight loss if that is desired
- Avoidance of smoking and excessive alcohol or caffeine intake
- Exercise: Weight-bearing exercise for osteoporosis prevention
- Kegel exercises for strengthening the pelvic floor
- Adequate calcium intake: 1500 mg elemental calcium daily is necessary to maintain zero calcium balance in postmenopausal women
- Change in the ambient temperature (may ameliorate hot flashes and reduce night sweats)
- Vitamin E
- Avoidance of caffeine, alcohol, and spicy foods if they trigger hot flashes
- Vaginal lubricants to help with the dyspareunia attributable to vaginal dryness (e.g., Replens, K-Y Jelly, or Gyne-Moistrin cream)

ACUTE GENERAL Rx

Vasomotor symptoms are best managed with systemic hormone therapy given in the lowest dose and for the shortest period possible. Estrogen replacement in symptomatic patients can be administered in a variety of forms, including oral estrogen and transdermal estrogen patch. The lowest effective dose should be prescribed.

- Examples of oral estrogen include:
  1. Conjugated estrogens: Start with 0.3 mg daily and increase to 1.25 mg daily depending on symptoms.
  2. Estradiol: Start with 0.5 mg daily and increase up to 2 mg daily.
  3. Esterified estrogens: Start with 0.3 to 1.25 mg daily.
  4. Estropipate: Start with 0.75 to 3.0 mg daily.
  5. Esterified estrogen/testosterone combination: Give 1.25 mg and methyltestosterone 2.5 mg (Estratest) and esterified estrogen 0.625 mg and methyltestosterone 1.25 mg (Estratest HS [half-strength]). May improve sexual enjoyment and libido.
- If the patient has had a hysterectomy for benign disease, estrogen alone is sufficient. In patients who have an intact uterus, progestin is critical to prevent endometrial hyperplasia associated with unopposed estrogen, which is protective against endometrial cancer. Progestins can be prescribed as continual daily dose or cyclic fashion. Most commonly prescribed progestins include medroxyprogesterone acetate 2.5 mg, 5 mg, and 10 mg; Prometrium 100 mg, 200 mg, and 400 mg; and Aygestin 5 mg. Continuous hormone replacement therapy is preferred because after time the patient should be amenorrhoeic. Patients should be counseled that they may experience some irregular spotting for the first 6 to 9 mo after starting hormone replacement therapy. Cyclic therapy will cause withdrawal bleeding.
- Combination oral preparations Femhrt, Prefest, Prempro, Activella, Premphase are commonly used. However, the U.S. Preventive Services Task Force recommends against the use of combined estrogen and progestin for the prevention of chronic conditions such as cardiovascular disease in postmenopausal women.
- The combination of conjugated estrogen and bazedoxifene is approved for the treatment of moderate to severe vasomotor symptoms associated with menopause and also for prevention of postmenopausal osteoporosis in women with an intact uterus.
- Transdermal patches can be either estradiol (Estraderm, Vivelle, FemPatch) 0.025 to 0.1 mg applied twice weekly or Climara 0.025 to 0.1 mg used once a wk. With these preparations, progesterone should be used in a similar fashion. Apply CombiPatch twice weekly (combination estrogen and progesterone) or Climara Pro once per wk (one patch).
- Vaginal estrogen creams can be used; these should be reserved for local therapy of atrophic vaginitis. Minimal systemic absorption does occur; however, blood levels are unpredictable. Usual dose 0.5 to 2 g intravaginally daily, cyclically 3 wk on 1 wk off. When symptoms improve, once to twice weekly is adequate maintenance.
- Vagifem estradiol vaginal tablets. Initial dosage: One Vagifem tablet, inserted vaginally, daily for 2 wk. Maintenance dose: One Vagifem tablet, inserted vaginally, twice weekly.
- Femring vaginal ring delivering the equivalent of 0.5 mg/day inserted every 3 mo or Estring 0.0075 mg/day.
- EstroGel 0.06% (estradiol gel). One pump (1.25 g/day) applied to one arm from wrist to shoulder.
- The FDA contraindications to menopause hormone therapy include the following diseases and disorders: Active liver disease; current, past, or suspected breast cancer; active or recent anterior thromboembolic disease; cardiac disease (angina, myocardial infarction); known or suspected estrogen-sensitive malignant conditions; known hypersensitivity to the active substance of the therapy or to any of the excipients; porphyria cutanea tarda; previous idiopathic or current venous thromboembolism; undiagnosed genital bleeding; untreated hypertension; untreated endometrial hyperplasia.
- For women in whom estrogen is contraindicated or for those who do not wish to take estrogen, the following regimens can be used:
  1. Serotonin reuptake inhibitors, especially in women with menopausal mood disorders
  2. Depo-Provera 150 mg IM every mo (may be helpful in alleviating hot flashes)
  3. Clonidine 0.05 to 0.15 mg PO daily (questionable efficacy) or transdermal clonidine patch
  4. Bellergal-S (questionable efficacy)
- Tibolone significantly improves vasomotor symptoms, libido, and vaginal lubrication. Not available in the U.S.

CHRONIC Rx

Hormone replacement therapy should be used only for the short term unless benefits outweigh the risks of long-term use. As a result of the results of the Women's Health Initiative (WHI), the FDA has instituted a "black box" warning on postmenopausal hormone replacement products suggesting that the lowest dose should be used for the shortest period of time. This necessitates a considered counseling session with patients contemplating hormone replacement prior to the initiation of therapy and then on a periodic basis after that, usually at least on a yearly basis.

DISPOSITION

If treated, the patient should have resolution of her symptoms and reduced incidence of osteoporosis. Lifelong medical supervision is necessary to monitor adequacy of treatment and prevention of complications. This should include regular Pap smears in accordance with American Society for Colposcopy and Cervical Pathology (ASCCP) guidelines until the age of 65, pelvic examinations, breast examinations, mammography, and endometrial sampling of any type of abnormal bleeding. If untreated, the vasomotor symptoms will eventually dissipate; however, this may take several years in a small percentage of women. Some women who are in their 80s have experienced hot flashes. Urogenital atrophy will continue to worsen. Osteoporosis and coronary artery disease risks will increase with every passing yr.

REFERRAL

Most menopausal women are managed by their gynecologists. However, this condition can be managed adequately by the patient's primary care physician who has an interest in treating menopausal women.

PEARLS & CONSIDERATIONS

COMMENTS

- Short-term risks of hormone replacement therapy (HT) include an eighteenfold increased rise for cholecystitis, three-and-a-half-fold risk of a thrombo-cardiac event in the first yr, and possible increased risk of stroke and myocardial infarction.
- Results of the WHI study found that for every 10,000 women taking HT (combination of both estrogen and progesterone) for 1 yr (10,000 person-yr), seven more would have coronary events, eight would have more strokes, eight would have more pulmonary emboli, and eight would have earlier breast cancer than would 10,000 women taking placebo. Benefits of HT were six fewer cases of colorectal cancer and five fewer hip fractures per 10,000 women.
- HT should not be initiated or continued for the primary or secondary prevention of coronary heart disease.
- Estrogen-replacement therapy should only be prescribed for patients with sufficient menopausal symptoms that impact the patient's quality of life.
- Interestingly, women who start hormone therapy early in menopause may have cardiac and other benefits. A recent trial showed that oral estradiol therapy was associated with less progression of subclinical atherosclerosis (measured as change in carotid-artery intima media thickness [CIMT]) than with placebo when therapy was initiated within 6 yr after menopause but not when it was initiated 10 or more yr after menopause. Estradiol had no significant effect on cardiac CT measures of atherosclerosis in either postmenopause stratum.[1]

RELATED CONTENT

Menopause (Patient Information)
Hot Flashes (Related Key Topic)
Osteoporosis (Related Key Topic)

SUGGESTED READINGS

Available at ExpertConsult.com

AUTHORS: **Ghamar Bitar, MD,** and **Rachel Wright Heinle, MD, FACOG**

[1]Hodis HN et al: Vascular effects of early versus late postmenopausal treatment with estradiol, *N Engl J Med* 374:1221-1231, 2016.

BASIC INFORMATION

DEFINITION

Malignant mesothelioma is a neoplasm originating from the mesothelial surfaces of the pleural (80%) or peritoneal cavities (20%). The three major histologic subtypes are epithelial (most common), sarcomatous, and mixed (epithelial/sarcomatous).

SYNONYM

Malignant mesothelioma

ICD-10CM CODES

C45.0	Mesothelioma of pleura
C45.1	Mesothelioma of peritoneum
C45.2	Mesothelioma of pericardium
C45.7	Mesothelioma of other sites
C45.9	Mesothelioma, unspecified

EPIDEMIOLOGY & DEMOGRAPHICS

- Associated with asbestos exposure (all fiber types) and has a latency of 20 to 40 yr.
- About 3200 new cases are diagnosed in the U.S. annually with an incidence of 1.05 cases per 100,000 population.
- More common in men (5:1) as a result of workplace asbestos exposure; family members of exposed workers have a higher risk due to cleaning of contaminated clothes.
- Incidence in the U.S. has leveled off due to lack of asbestos use and mining.
- Incidence of mesothelioma increases with age; median age at presentation is >70 yr.
- More than 8 million persons in the U.S. are currently at risk for mesothelioma because of prior asbestos exposure.

PHYSICAL FINDINGS & CLINICAL PRESENTATION

- Dyspnea
- Nonpleuritic chest pain
- Fever, weight loss, sweats, fatigue, loss of appetite
- Dysphagia, superior vena cava syndrome, Horner syndrome in advanced stages
- Auscultation may reveal unilateral loss of breath sounds
- Dullness on percussion may be present

ETIOLOGY

- Asbestos exposure (>70% of patients).
- Other reported potentially causal factors include prior radiation therapy and extravasated thorotrast, zeolite, and erionite fibers.
- Mutations of BRCA1-associated protein 1 (BAP1) cyclin-dependent kinase inhibitor 2A gene *(CDKN2A)* have been causally linked to development of mesothelioma.

DIAGNOSIS

DIFFERENTIAL DIAGNOSIS

Metastatic adenocarcinomas (from lung, breast, ovary, kidney, stomach, prostate)

WORKUP

- Staging evaluation (Box 1) includes complete history (including occupational history), physical examination, and testing to determine potential operability (CT, bone scan, pulmonary function tests [PFTs]).
- Thoracoscopy, pleuroscopy, and open-lung biopsy are useful in obtaining adequate tissue samples for diagnosis.
- Pulmonary function tests.
- PET-CT scan (Figs. E1 and E2) is performed only in patients considered candidates for surgery to determine resectability.
- Staging: The TNM system categorizes mesothelioma in stages I to IV similar to that used for non–small cell lung cancer.

LABORATORY TESTS

- Diagnostic thoracentesis is generally insufficient for diagnosis because pleural effusions may only reveal atypical mesothelial cells.
- Immunohistochemistry is useful to distinguish adenocarcinoma from epithelial malignant mesothelioma (mesotheliomas are generally carcinoembryonic antigen negative and cytokeratin positive).
- Thrombocytosis and anemia may be found on initial laboratory evaluation.
- Serum osteopontin levels (when available) can also be used to distinguish persons with exposure to asbestos who do not have cancer from those with exposure to asbestos who have pleural mesothelioma.

BOX 1 International Mesothelioma Interest Group (IMIG) Staging System

T: Primary Tumor and Extent

T_1:
- a. Tumor limited to ipsilateral parietal pleura, including mediastinal and diaphragmatic pleura; no involvement of the visceral pleura
- b. Tumor involving the ipsilateral parietal pleura, including mediastinal and diaphragmatic pleura; scattered foci or tumor also involving the visceral pleura

T_2 Tumor involving each of the ipsilateral pleural surfaces (parietal, mediastinal, diaphragmatic pleura); scattered foci or tumor also involving the visceral pleura:
- a. Involvement of diaphragmatic muscle
- b. Confluent visceral pleura (including the fissures) or extension of tumor from visceral pleura into the underlying pulmonary parenchyma

T_3 Locally advanced but potentially resectable tumor; tumor involving all the ipsilateral pleural surfaces (parietal, mediastinal, diaphragmatic, and visceral pleura) with at least one of the following features:
- a. Involvement of the endothoracic fascia
- b. Extension into mediastinal fat
- c. Solitary, complete resectable focus or tumor extending into the soft tissues of the chest wall
- d. Nontransmural involvement of the pericardium

T_4 Locally advanced, technically nonresectable tumor; tumor involving all the ipsilateral pleural surfaces (parietal, mediastinal, diaphragmatic, and visceral pleura) with at least one of the following features:
- a. Diffuse extension or multifocal mass of tumor in the chest wall, with or without associated rib destruction
- b. Direct transdiaphragmatic extension of the tumor to the peritoneum
- c. Direct extension of tumor to the contralateral pleura
- d. Direct extension of tumor to one or more mediastinal organs
- e. Direct extension of tumor into the spine
- f. Tumor extending through the internal surface of the pericardium with or without a pericardial effusion or tumor involving the myocardium

N: Lymph Nodes

N_x Regional lymph nodes cannot be assessed
N_0 No regional lymph node metastases
N_1 Metastases in ipsilateral bronchopulmonary or hilar lymph nodes
N_2 Metastases in the subcarinal or the ipsilateral mediastinal lymph nodes, including the ipsilateral internal mammary nodes
N_3 Metastases in contralateral mediastinal, contralateral internal mammary, ipsilateral, or contralateral supraclavicular scalene lymph nodes

M: Metastases

M_x Presence of distant metastases cannot be assessed
M_0 No (known) metastasis
M_1 Distant metastasis present

Stage Grouping

I.
- a. $T_{1a}N_0M_0$
- b. $T_{1b}N_0M_0$

II. $T_2N_0M_0$
III. Any T_3M_0, any N_1M_0, any N_2M_0
IV. Any T_4, any N_3, any M_1

From Sellke FW et al: *Sabiston & Spencer surgery of the chest,* ed 9, Philadelphia, 2016, Elsevier.

BOX 2 Therapeutic Options for Malignant Pleural Mesothelioma

Single-Modality Therapy
- Debulking surgery (pleurectomy/decortication or extrapleural pneumonectomy)
- Radiation (external beam, brachytherapy)
- Chemotherapy (single- or double-agent approach: Doxorubicin, cyclophosphamide, cisplatinum; gemcitabine, pemetrexed, and cisplatin)

Multimodality Therapy
- Surgery and adjuvant radiation
- Surgery and adjuvant chemotherapy
- Surgery and adjuvant chemoradiotherapy

Innovative Therapies under Investigation
- Intracavitary lavage with hyperthermic chemotherapy
- Photodynamic therapy
- Gene therapy
- Angiogenesis
- Immunogenic therapy

From Sellke FW et al: *Sabiston & Spencer surgery of the chest,* ed 9, Philadelphia, 2016, Elsevier.

IMAGING STUDIES

- Chest radiographs may reveal pleural plaques (Fig. E3) or calcifications in the diaphragm.
- CT scans of the chest and abdomen, bone scan, and PET scan are used to assess the stage of disease.

Rx TREATMENT

GENERAL Rx

- Box 2 summarizes therapeutic options for malignant pleural mesothelioma.
- Operable patient (epithelial type, no positive nodes, confined to pleura, adequate PFTs): The two surgical techniques for therapeutic intervention are decortication (pleurectomy) and extrapleural pneumonectomy (EPP). Postoperative chemotherapy with cisplatin and pemetrexed and subsequent external-beam radiation are used with limited success. With EPP patients are eligible to be treated with either preoperative or postoperative radiation therapy radiation therapy to improve local control.
- Inoperable patient (elderly patient, extensive disease, sarcomatous or mixed histology type, poor PFTs): Chemotherapy is administered to improve survival; supportive care is a standard option. Combined modality therapies (radiation therapy, chemotherapy, and biologics) have also been used to reduce both local and distant recurrences.
- First-line chemotherapy options include the combination of cisplatin and pemetrexed with or without additional bevacizumab (antiangiogenic agent).
- Patients with progressive cancer after initial chemotherapy can often be treated with single-agent chemotherapy (gemcitabine or vinorelbine).
- The FDA has approved for first-line treatment for MPM patients a device called NovoTTF-100L, which is based on the delivery of specific electric frequencies (tumor treating fields [TTFs]) in combination with chemotherapy, to interfere with cancer cell proliferation. The reported median overall survival was 18.2 mo with no increase in systemic toxicity among patients treated with this approach.
- Recent data have shown improvement in survival with use of immune checkpoint inhibitors targeting the programmed death-1 (PD-1) pathway (pembrolizumab, durvalumab, nivolumab with or without ipilimumab).
- Intrapleural instillation of cisplatin or biologics (e.g., interferons, interleukin-2) is generally limited to very early disease because it can only penetrate a very limited depth of the tumor and there is a propensity of the pleural space to become progressively obliterated with advancing disease.
- In advanced stages, radiation therapy is often used for palliation of local chest pain.
- Obliteration of the pleural space (pleurodesis) with instillation of talc or tetracycline into the pleural cavity is done in the treatment of recurrent symptomatic pleural effusions.
- Several biomarkers have been evaluated extensively in mesothelioma management. Serum mesothelin is not sensitive or specific for diagnostic purposes, but serial measurements during chemotherapy can be useful as a monitoring tool. Recent data reveal that plasma fibulin-3 levels can distinguish healthy persons with exposure to asbestos from patients with mesothelioma. In conjunction with effusion fibulin-3 levels, plasma fibulin-3 levels can further differentiate mesothelioma effusions from other malignant and benign effusions.

DISPOSITION

- The overall prognosis of malignant mesothelioma is dismal, with a median survival of 8 mo. 5-yr survival is better for patients with lower stages: Localized (20%), regional (12%), and distant (8%).
- Patients who receive trimodality therapy (surgery, radiation therapy, systemic therapy) have improved survivals of ~18 mo; however, less than 10% of cases fit in this category.

PEARLS & CONSIDERATIONS

- Patients with early disease should be referred to treatment centers specializing in multidisciplinary therapy before attempts are made to obliterate the pleural space with pleurodesis.
- Patients with advanced or resected disease should be treated with appropriate combination chemotherapy as listed previously.

SUGGESTED READINGS

Available at ExpertConsult.com

RELATED CONTENT

Mesothelioma (Patient Information)
Asbestosis (Related Key Topic)

AUTHOR: **Bharti Rathore, MD**

BASIC INFORMATION

DEFINITION

An accidental or intentional ingestion of 1 gram per kg methanol or ethylene glycol is considered lethal, although smaller amounts can be toxic. Inhalational and dermal exposures rarely cause toxicity.

SYNONYMS

Toxic alcohols
Moonshine
Wood alcohol
Antifreeze

ICD-10CM CODES	
T51.8	Toxic effect of alcohols
T51.1X1	Toxic effect of methanol
T51.1X2	Toxic effect of methanol, intentional self-harm
T52.8X1	Ethylene glycol poisoning

EPIDEMIOLOGY & DEMOGRAPHICS

INCIDENCE:

- In 2016, the American Association of Poison Control Centers reported 6508 single-exposure cases of ethylene glycol poisoning and 1853 of methanol poisoning.
- Most cases are reported in adults and predominantly in men.
- Accidental exposure is common in children, while alcoholism, polysubstance abuse, depression, and suicide occur in adults.
- Suicide attempts involving toxic alcohols frequently involve the ingestion of multiple substances.
- Outbreaks or epidemic poisoning with methanol is frequently the result of bootleg distillation or counterfeit alcohol.

PHYSICAL FINDINGS & CLINICAL PRESENTATION

- Clinical manifestations depend on quantity of ingestion, duration of time since ingestion, and whether co-ingestion of other substances occurred.
- Early ingestion of either substance causes central nervous system (CNS) depression, nausea, and vomiting; inebriation can mimic ethanol ingestion. Late effects include progressive CNS dysfunction, including seizure and coma, as well as respiratory and cardiopulmonary failure.
- Visual symptoms ranging from blurry or snowy vision to complete visual loss and findings of papillary edema and, later, optic atrophy, fixed and dilated pupils, retinal hyperemia, and a Parkinson-like syndrome are indicative of methanol poisoning. Other CNS effects are hemorrhage and white matter lesions in the putamen, subcortical structures, brain stem, and cerebellum.
- Oliguria, hematuria, calcium oxalate crystalluria, tetany, cranial nerve palsy, and acute kidney injury suggest ethylene glycol toxicity.
- Abdominal pain may result from exposure to either substance, while methanol can cause acute pancreatitis.
- Kussmaul respirations (rapid, labored breathing) may be evident with severe acidosis.

PATHOPHYSIOLOGY

- Toxicity of these alcohols is related to their metabolites rather than the parent compound.
- Lethal dose for methanol is >15 to 30 ml and >1 to 1.5 ml/kg for ethylene glycol.
- Sequential metabolism by alcohol and aldehyde dehydrogenases converts methanol to formaldehyde and then formic acid, while ethylene glycol is converted to glycoaldehyde, glycolic acid, and then oxalate.
- Fig. E1 depicts the pathways involved in methanol metabolism.
- While methanol metabolites primarily cause retinal injury, ethylene glycol metabolites produce renal tubular injury and calcium oxalate stones.
  1. Formaldehyde binds to tissue proteins and is likely the major toxin in methanol poisoning involving necrosis of retinal and optic neurons and the basal ganglia (putamen). Formic acid, the acid produced in the largest quantity, inhibits cytochrome oxidase, preventing oxygen utilization by mitochondria and causing further organ dysfunction. Leukotriene has been implicated in the inflammation and neurotoxicity of acute methanol poisoning.
  2. Glycoaldehyde may be the major nephrotoxin, while glycolic acid is the acid produced in the largest quantity in ethylene glycol poisoning, with a small quantity converted to oxalic acid by lactate dehydrogenase. Oxalate subsequently forms calcium oxalate crystals that are deposited in the renal parenchyma, cerebral blood vessels, and meninges, causing hypocalcemic tetany.

DIAGNOSIS

DIFFERENTIAL DIAGNOSIS

- Other causes of a high anion gap metabolic acidosis include lactic acidosis, diabetic and alcoholic ketoacidosis, kidney failure (acute and chronic), early toluene toxicity, and salicylate intoxication. Importantly, L-lactate may be elevated in methanol toxicity due to cytochrome oxidase inhibition by formic acid and an increase of the NADH:NAD^+ ratio that is driven by methanol metabolism.
- Elevated plasma osmolal gap may be encountered in ethyl alcohol or isopropyl alcohol ingestion.

EVALUATION AND WORKUP

- Diagnosis depends on history, clinical presentation, and laboratory abnormalities.
- High anion gap metabolic acidosis (AG >12 mEq/L) with elevated plasma osmolal gap (>10 mOsm/kg H_2O; usually >25 mOsm/kg H_2O) in an appropriate clinical setting should raise the suspicion of methanol or ethylene glycol ingestion.
- In either intoxication, an osmolal gap will initially be positive, but as the parent compound is converted to its metabolites, the osmolal gap will normalize and the serum anion gap will increase.
- Serum methanol and ethylene glycol levels are elevated with their respective ingestions.
- Acute kidney injury, hypocalcemia with prolonged QTc interval, and calcium oxalate crystalluria are seen with ethylene glycol toxicity.
- Metabolic acidosis in the absence of acute kidney injury suggests methanol toxicity, i.e., ethylene glycol is more often associated with acute kidney injury.
- Wood's light uses ultraviolet light to detect fluorescein in urine because fluorescein is contained in some ethylene glycol preparations. However, fluorescence lacks sensitivity and specificity. Therefore, fluorescence is not considered a reliable clinical tool.

LABORATORY TESTS

- Calculation of anion and serum osmolal gaps
  1. Anion gap calculation
  2. Osmolal gap calculation: Measured minus calculated serum osmolalities. Measured plasma osmolality is performed by an osmometer using freezing point depression

     Calculated plasma osmolality = 2 × Serum sodium + BUN/2.8 + Glucose/18 + Ethanol/4.6 (units for BUN, glucose, ethanol in mg/dl)
- Arterial blood gas analysis, lactate, calcium, and creatine kinase
- Creatinine and urine microscopy for detection of tubular injury, typically acute tubular necrosis, and calcium oxalate crystals
- ECG to evaluate QTc interval
- Toxicology screen with quantification: Acetaminophen, salicylate, ethanol, methanol, ethylene glycol, and isopropyl alcohol

TREATMENT

High index of suspicion and immediate recognition with early treatment remain crucial to reduce mortality. Box 1 describes common commercial products that may contain ethylene glycol.

NONPHARMACOLOGIC THERAPY

- Cardiorespiratory support as required.

BOX 1 Common Commercial Products That May Contain Ethylene Glycol

Paints and lacquers
Polishes and detergents
Inks
Cosmetics
Hydraulic brake fluids
Solar collector fluids
Car wash fluids

Data from Kruse JA: Methanol, ethylene glycol, and related intoxications. In Carlson RW, Geheb MA (eds): *Principles and practice of medical intensive care,* Philadelphia, 1993, Saunders.

- Rapid (within 60 min) gastric decontamination (charcoal and/or gastric lavage). Later intervention is not beneficial due to rapid and complete invasion (methanol).
- Induction of vomiting is contraindicated even in conscious patients given the risks of development of central nervous system depression in these patients.

ACUTE GENERAL Rx

- Principles of therapy include prevention of formation of toxic metabolites, correction of acidosis, and toxin removal.
- Intravenous isotonic fluids can facilitate urinary excretion of volatile alcohol and its metabolites; when acidosis is present (pH <7.30), isotonic bicarbonate should be used because reversal of acidosis helps prevent end-organ damage from toxic metabolites (target pH: 7.35 to 7.45).
- Ethanol, a competitive substrate, and fomepizole (4-methylpyrazole or 4-MP), a competitive inhibitor of alcohol dehydrogenase, prevent formation of toxic metabolites of ethylene glycol and methanol.
- Fomepizole is preferred over ethanol given the increased incidence of GI and CNS adverse events with ethanol administration, greater inhibition of alcohol dehydrogenase, and ease of administration. Cost and availability of fomepizole may influence the decision to administer this agent versus ethanol.
- Ethanol: Dosing:
  1. Target ethanol concentration: 100 to 200 mg/dl with close monitoring
  2. Loading dose: 800 mg/kg in a 10% solution of 5% dextrose in water will raise serum ethanol by 100 mg/dl
  3. Maintenance dose: Infusion of 80 to 160 mg/kg per hr based on blood concentrations
  4. Dosing adjustment in patients receiving concomitant dialysis is required due to clearance of ethanol
- Fomepizole: Indications for use:
  1. Plasma concentration of methanol or ethylene glycol >20 mg/dl, or
  2. Documented ingestion with an osmolal gap >10 mOsm/kg H_2O, or
  3. Suspected ingestion with at least two of the following criteria:
     a. Arterial pH <7.30
     b. Serum bicarbonate <20 mEq/L
     c. Osmolal gap >10 mOsm/kg H_2O
     d. Urine microscopy for oxalate crystals in the case of ethylene glycol toxicity
- Fomepizole (4-methylpyrazole) dosing:
  1. Loading dose: 15 mg/kg body weight
  2. Maintenance dose: 10 mg/kg body weight every 12 hr for 4 doses, then 15 mg/kg every 12 hr (if blood levels do not reach goal by 48 hr)
  3. During hemodialysis: Add 1 to 1.5 mg/kg per hr, or repeat loading dose every 4 hr
- The half-lives of ethylene glycol and methanol increase with ethanol or fomepizole.
- The half-life of methanol metabolism during treatment with fomepizole is as long as 87 hr. Treatment with fomepizole alone is not recommended, and hemodialysis should be considered to prevent a prolonged requirement for intensive care.
- In contrast, the observed half-life of ethylene glycol during fomepizole use is approximately 34 hr. Ethylene glycol poisoning (even with levels greater than 50 mg/dl) in patients without kidney injury or acidosis can be managed with fomepizole alone, and without hemodialysis.
- Hemodialysis is indicated for likely or confirmed methanol poisoning in the setting of any of the following: New vision or neurologic deficit (particularly seizure or coma); metabolic acidosis or acidemia with pH ≤7.15; elevated anion gap >24 mmol/L; methanol concentration >70 mg/dl (or 21.8 mmol/L) in the context of fomepizole, or >50 mg/dl (or 15.6 mmol/L) in the absence of an ADH blocker.
- Hemodialysis is indicated for likely or confirmed ethylene glycol poisoning in the setting of any of the following: Acute kidney injury; anion gap metabolic acidosis; EG level >50 mg/dl (see earlier regarding use of fomepizole when elevated levels without acidosis or acute kidney injury are present).
- Hemodialysis should also be considered in patients with poisoning and electrolyte imbalances refractory to pharmacologic treatments, or hemodynamic instability.
- Average duration of dialysis in studies was 8.4±3.2 hr.
  1. Treatment with medications and/or hemodialysis is continued until the methanol or ethylene glycol concentration is <20 mg/dl.
  2. Intermittent hemodialysis is the preferred modality of dialysis, as continuous renal replacement therapy (CRRT) alone is ineffective in achieving rapid clearance of methanol and ethylene glycol. In the treatment of a mass outbreak of methanol poisoning, acidemia correction was faster with intermittent hemodialysis than CRRT.
  3. CRRT is an acceptable alternative when intermittent hemodialysis is not available.
  4. If blood concentration levels are not available, start by conducting an 8-hr intermittent hemodialysis session followed by 18 hr of continuous renal replacement therapy; adjust therapy afterward as clinically indicated.
  5. Do not use heparin with dialysis, as heparin may increase the risk for cerebral hemorrhage.

ADJUNCTIVE Rx

- In ethylene glycol poisoning, thiamine (100 mg IV q6h) and pyridoxine (100 mg IV daily) may decrease oxalic acid formation and direct metabolism to less toxic metabolites.
- In methanol poisoning, folinic acid doses (50 mg IV q6h) may increase formic acid metabolism to CO_2 and H_2O. Correct electrolyte abnormalities (hypocalcemia, etc.).
- Treat seizures.

DISPOSITION

Transfer to a hospital with an intensive care unit and hemodialysis capabilities that can mitigate early intoxication.

REFERRAL

- Regional poison center (toxicologist) and nephrology referrals are recommended to avoid treatment delays
- Ophthalmology referral for patients with visual symptoms
- Psychiatry referral if depression and suicidal ideation are present
- Detoxification centers for patients with substance abuse

PROGNOSIS

- Coma or seizures at presentation and prolonged severe acidosis correlate with increased mortality.
- High osmolal gap and high anion gap acidosis are associated with high mortality.
- Hyperglycemia may correlate with worse prognosis in methanol poisoning.

PEARLS & CONSIDERATIONS

- Profound plasma osmolal gap or anion gap metabolic acidosis should raise suspicion for ethylene glycol and/or methanol ingestion. A high index of suspicion and early treatment are crucial to reducing mortality. The metabolites of methanol and ethylene glycol produce the clinical toxidrome.
- Complaints of visual blurring, central scotomata, and blindness are consistent with methanol poisoning.
- Calcium oxalate crystalluria, oliguria, hematuria, and acute kidney injury are consistent with ethylene glycol poisoning.
- Fomepizole is preferred to ethanol due to complications associated with ethanol use.
- Emergent hemodialysis is indicated with end organ damage and/or severe metabolic acidosis.
- Elevated osmolal gap and anion gap metabolic acidosis may occur rarely with other toxic alcohols such as diethylene glycol and propylene glycol.

SUGGESTED READINGS

Available at ExpertConsult.com

RELATED CONTENT

Algorithm for the Management of Acute Poisoning (Algorithm, Section III)

AUTHOR: **Nikolas Harbord, MD**

BASIC INFORMATION

DEFINITION

Methicillin-resistant *Staphylococcus aureus* (MRSA) is a common bacterial pathogen with resistance to many antibiotics. It is defined as an *S. aureus* that shows a minimum inhibitory concentration (MIC) of greater than or equal to 4 mcg/ml to oxacillin. There are two types of MRSA (Table 1).

- HA-MRSA: Hospital-acquired MRSA, usually multidrug resistant
- CA-MRSA: Community-acquired MRSA; an emerging pathogen, usually acquired outside of the hospital setting; resistance may differ from HA-MRSA and is generally susceptible to more antibiotics than HA-MRSA

SYNONYMS

Multidrug-resistant *Staphylococcus aureus*
Oxacillin-resistant *Staphylococcus aureus*

ICD-10CM CODES

A41.02	Sepsis due to Methicillin resistant *Staphylococcus aureus*
A49.02	Methicillin resistant *Staphylococcus aureus* infection, unspecified site
B95.62	Methicillin resistant *Staphylococcus aureus* infection as the cause of diseases classified elsewhere
J15.212	Pneumonia due to Methicillin resistant *Staphylococcus aureus*
Z22.322	Carrier or suspected carrier of Methicillin resistant *Staphylococcus aureus*
Z86.14	Personal history of Methicillin resistant *Staphylococcus aureus* infection

EPIDEMIOLOGY & DEMOGRAPHICS

INCIDENCE: 1:3000

PREVALENCE: The national rate of MRSA colonization or infection is 46.3 per 10,000 inpatients. Hospital prevalence rate of MRSA is as high as 60% in hospitals, which means that 60% of *S. aureus* strains in that hospital will be MRSA

PREDOMINANT SEX & AGE: Both sexes and all ages

PEAK INCIDENCE: Occurs yr-round; may peak during summer and fall mos for CA-MRSA

RISK FACTORS:

- HA-MRSA: Hospitalization, invasive medical device, residing in long-term nursing facility
- CA-MRSA: Initially seen in young men engaged in athletic activities and in gyms, prisons, military barracks, etc., but has now spread to the entire age spectrum including neonates and the elderly

PHYSICAL FINDINGS & CLINICAL PRESENTATION

- CA-MRSA: Can present with skin infection, associated with opening in the skin; red bump, pustule, or boil; erythema, swelling; edema, often fluctuant and very painful
- HA-MRSA: Bacteremia; infection associated with intravenous device:
  1. Catheters: Pneumonia
  2. Skin: Cellulitis
  3. Bone: Osteomyelitis
  4. Endocarditis
  5. Abscesses: Skin or organ
  6. Pneumonia: Nosocomial

ETIOLOGY

- CA-MRSA: The most prevalent strain in the U.S. on pulse field electrophoresis (PFGE) is called USA 300.
  1. CA-MRSA: Common cause of skin and soft-tissue infections seen in the emergency room. It can, however, also cause necrotizing pneumonia, sepsis, osteomyelitis, etc.
  2. Virulence factors particular to CA-MRSA: Panton-Valentine leukocidin (PVL) toxin, alpha-hemolysin toxin, phenol-soluble modulins, etc., that enhance ability to cause infection.
- HA-MRSA: Most strains on PFGE are USA 100 or USA 200 and tend to have multidrug resistance. Patients with HA-MRSA infection have higher mortality and morbidity than patients with a methicillin-sensitive *S. aureus* (MSSA) infection.
- By definition, all MRSA strains carry the *mecA* gene, which confers resistance to all beta-lactam antibiotics, including cephalosporins and carbapenems.

DIAGNOSIS

LABORATORY TESTS

- Rapid detection methods for MRSA:
  1. Rapid culture methods: Chromogenic agar, which uses a culture media that changes color if *Staphylococcus aureus* is present and then has antibiotics incorporated into media that only allows MRSA strains to grow. This allows for early detection of MRSA in 24 to 48 hr.
  2. Molecular methods that target gene sequences of the bacteria: PCR and gene probe hybridization. Examples include IDI-MRSA, Genotype MRSA direct, and Gene Expert MRSA assay. The sensitivity and specificity of these assays compared to traditional cultures range from 90% to 98% and from 91% to 99%, respectively.
- PFGE is usually done only for epidemiologic or outbreak purposes.

IMAGING STUDIES

- Radiographs or computed tomography scan of suspected organ
- Echocardiogram: All adult patients with *S. aureus* bacteremia should undergo echocardiography

TREATMENT

- CA-MRSA: Oral antibiotics that may be effective include trimethoprim-sulfamethoxazole, doxycycline, minocycline, or clindamycin;

TABLE 1 Comparison of community-associated (CA) and healthcare-associated (HA) methicillin-resistant *Staphylococcal aureus* (MRSA)

	CA-MRSA	HA-MRSA
Epidemiology	• Favors children and young adults • More common in African Americans, Native Americans, and Pacific Islanders	• Favors adults age >65 years
Risk factors	• Close interpersonal contact, e.g., athletes, military personnel, prison inmates, children attending daycare • Men having sex with men • Injection drug use • Recent antibiotic use • Homelessness • HIV infection • Skin trauma, e.g., lacerations, abrasions, tattoos, body shaving/piercing • Dermatologic conditions (e.g., atopic dermatitis*)	• Underlying comorbidities (e.g., diabetes mellitus) • Recent surgery or hospitalization (especially if prolonged or in an ICU) • Residence in a long-term care facility • Dialysis • Indwelling percutaneous medical devices and catheters • Chronic wounds
Typical sites/ types of infection	• Skin and soft tissue, especially furuncles/ abscesses or purulent cellulitis	• Skin and soft tissue, especially in surgical sites • Urinary tract • Respiratory tract • Bloodstream
Molecular characteristics	• SCC*mec* types IV and V • Panton-Valentine leucocidin (PVL) genes • USA300 or USA400 PFGE	• SCC*mec* types I–III • USA100 or USA200 PFGE
Antibiotic susceptibility	• Usually multiple agents	• Limited

ICU, Intensive care unit; *PFGE*, pulsed-field electrophoresis pattern.
*Increased risk of staphylococcal infections, but not generally in the proportion due to MRSA.
From Bolognia JL: *Dermatology*, ed 4, 2018, Elsevier.

linezolid and tedizolid are other options but are very expensive
- HA-MRSA: Intravenous antibiotics, vancomycin, linezolid, tedizolid, daptomycin, tigecycline, and newer agent eravacycline

ACUTE GENERAL Rx

- Trimethoprim-sulfamethoxazole, one double-strength tablet PO bid, is useful in cases of CA-MRSA since 95% of community-acquired MRSA strains are susceptible to it in vitro. Other agents that can be used for CA-MRSA include:
  1. Clindamycin: 300 to 450 mg q6h to q8h also inhibits toxin production. If strain tests sensitive to clindamycin but resistant to erythromycin, then a D test must be done to ensure there will not be inducible resistance while on therapy with the clindamycin.
  2. Doxycycline: 100 mg PO q12h and minocycline also have some activity against MRSA.
  3. Rifampin: Never used alone but can be used with one of the other oral agents.
- Vancomycin 15 to 20 mg/kg IV q8 to 12h is the mainstay of parenteral therapy for MRSA infections. There is an increasing concern of MRSA strains developing tolerance to vancomycin, requiring higher doses to achieve eradication. True vancomycin-resistant strains (MIC ≥32 mg/L) remain rare. Vancomycin trough levels of at least 15 to 20 mcg/ml are recommended to treat MRSA infections.
- Linezolid 600 mg PO or IV bid is a synthetic oxazolidinone FDA-approved for MRSA skin and soft tissue infections and pneumonia. It has been shown to be more effective than vancomycin for MRSA pneumonia. A similar agent, tedizolid (200 mg IV or PO for 6 days), is approved for skin and soft-tissue infections. These agents are much more expensive than vancomycin.
- Daptomycin: 4 mg/kg/day to 6 mg/kg/day IV is approved for skin and soft tissue infections, bacteremia, and right-sided endocarditis but should not be used for pneumonia as it is inactivated by pulmonary surfactant.
- Tigecycline: 100 mg IV load, then 50 mg IV q12h, is approved for MRSA skin and soft tissue infections and intraabdominal abscess.
- Eravacycline, a derivative of tetracycline, does cover MRSA, VRE, and resistant GNRs but currently is approved only for complicated intraabdominal infections.
- Ceftaroline is a fifth-generation cephalosporin, also effective against MRSA but only skin and soft-tissue infections, not pneumonia: 600 mg IV q12h.
- Newer glycopeptide agents: Dalbavancin (1000 mg IV followed by 500 mg IV a wk later for complicated skin and soft-tissue infections) and telavancin (10 mg/kg IV daily for 7-14 days) to treat skin infections or pneumonia; these are expensive alternatives to vancomycin.

CHRONIC Rx

- Patients with MRSA colonization may have reexposure or may be unable to eradicate colonized state.
- Oral agents used to attempt eradication of nasal colonization of MRSA are rifampin, tetracycline, and minocycline.
- Topical agents used in an attempt to eradicate MRSA nares carriage include mupirocin nasal ointment 2% applied bid ×5 days. If mupirocin resistant, can use bacitracin or polymyxin.
- There are protocols for using an antiseptic on skin, such as chlorhexidine, along with mupirocin nasal ointment to eradicate MRSA carriage from the body. Postdischarge MRSA decolonization with chlorhexidine and mupirocin results in a 30% lower risk for MRSA infection than education alone.

PEARLS & CONSIDERATIONS

Adding a beta-lactam to vancomycin or daptomycin for MRSA bacteremia yeilds no clinical benefits and increases risk of acute kidney injury.[1]

SUGGESTED READINGS

Available at ExpertConsult.com

RELATED CONTENT

Methicillin-Resistant *Staphylococcus aureus* (Patient Information)

AUTHOR: **Glenn G. Fort, MD, MPH**

[1] Tong SYC et al: Effect of vancomycin or daptomycin with vs without an antistaphylococcal β-lactam on mortality, bacteremia, relapse, or treatment failure in patients with MRSA bacteremia: a randomized clinical trial. *JAMA* 323(6): 527-537, 2020.

BASIC INFORMATION

DEFINITION

Microangiopathic hemolytic anemia (MAHA) is used to describe any nonautoimmune hemolytic anemia that results in red blood cell fragmentation associated with small vessel disease. Several diseases, including thrombotic thrombocytopenic purpura (TTP), disseminated intravascular coagulation (DIC), hemolytic-uremic syndrome (HUS), atypical hemolytic-uremic syndrome (aHUS), hemolysis, elevated liver enzymes, and low platelets syndrome of pregnancy (HELLP), and malignant hypertension, are associated with MAHA.

SYNONYMS

MAHA
Thrombotic microangiopathy (TMA)
Mechanical hemolytic anemias
Nonautoimmune hemolytic anemias
Fragmentation hemolytic anemia

ICD-10CM CODE
D59.4 Other non-autoimmune hemolytic anemias

EPIDEMIOLOGY & DEMOGRAPHICS

- TTP: Increased incidence in women and African Americans
- Typical HUS:
  1. Associated with *E. coli* 0157:H7 in 80% of cases.
  2. Person-person transmission is implicated.
  3. Children are more commonly affected than adults.
- Atypical HUS:
  1. Diarrhea is not a presenting feature.
  2. Adults are more commonly affected.
- DIC:
  1. Always secondary to underlying causes, including sepsis, trauma, malignancy, surgery, or obstetrical complications.
  2. DIC can occur in about 20% of acute leukemias.
- HELLP syndrome:
  1. Occurs in 10% to 20% of pregnancies with preeclampsia.
  2. Develops between 28 and 36 wk of gestation.
  3. Can also present after delivery of fetus in 30% cases.
- Malignant hypertension: MAHA complicates about 25% of malignant hypertension cases.

PHYSICAL FINDINGS & CLINICAL PRESENTATION

- Mucosal pallor
- Fatigue
- Acute onset of generalized weakness
- Jaundiced skin
- Icteric sclera
- Dark-colored urine

ETIOLOGY

TTP	Idiopathic or familial deficiency of ADAMTS13 Acquired antibodies against ADAMTS13
Typical HUS	Shiga toxin–producing enterohemorrhagic *E. coli* 0157:H7
Atypical HUS	Inherited disorders of complement regulation
DIC	Secondary to multiple causes resulting in subendothelial tissue factor exposure and subsequent activation of coagulation cascade
HELLP syndrome	Mechanism not clearly identified, but endothelial injury from hypertension associated with preeclampsia has been implicated
Malignant hypertension	Endothelial damage

DIAGNOSIS

Pathognomonic findings in MAHA include anemia consistent with an intravascular hemolytic picture, including schistocytes (Fig. 1) on peripheral blood smear, elevated lactate dehydrogenase (LDH), increased indirect bilirubin, decreased serum haptoglobin, increased urinary urobilinogen, along with an elevated reticulocyte count and negative Coombs test.

DIFFERENTIAL DIAGNOSIS

- Immune-mediated hemolysis (positive Coombs test):
  1. Autoimmune hemolytic anemia
  2. Paroxysmal nocturnal hemoglobinuria
  3. Cold agglutinin disease
- Infections affecting red blood count (RBC):
  1. Malaria
  2. Babesiosis
  3. Bartonellosis
- Hemolysis due to mechanical stress or oxidative injury:
  1. G6PD deficiency
  2. Runner's anemia or march hemoglobinuria
- Extravascular hemolysis:
  1. Intrinsic RBC defects
  2. Liver disease
  3. Hypersplenism

WORKUP

- Peripheral blood smear showing schistocytes.
- Laboratory workup including CBC, liver function tests, LDH, haptoglobin, reticulocyte count, Coombs test, and urine analysis.
- MAHA and thrombocytopenia are sufficient to make a diagnosis of TTP or HUS; the classic "pentad" of fever, neurologic abnormalities, and renal failure is no longer necessary.
- In DIC, activated partial thromboplastin time and prothrombin time are prolonged, along with decreased fibrinogen levels and increased fibrin degradation products (including D-dimer).
- Blood pressure is greater than 180/120 mm Hg in malignant hypertension and usually associated with acute kidney injury (including hematuria and proteinuria).
- Additional specific tests:
  1. ADAMTS13 activity assay: Decreased activity is associated with idiopathic TTP, and ADAMTS13-directed antibodies are associated with secondary TTP.
  2. Stool culture for shiga toxin–producing *E. coli* in typical HUS.
  3. Although gold standard, renal biopsy is often not required for diagnosis of malignant hypertension.

TREATMENT

If specific etiology of MAHA is not readily identified, plasma exchange therapy should be instituted immediately, in presence of thrombocytopenia and appropriate clinical picture.

- TTP:
  1. Emergent plasma exchange (PEX) to remove unusually large von Willebrand factor (vWF) multimers and autoantibodies directed against ADAMTS13.
  2. Platelet transfusions reserved only for bleeding patients.
  3. If needed, PEX can be increased from once a day to twice daily, along with concomitant use of corticosteroids.
  4. Patients nonresponsive to PEX can be treated with second-line rituximab with or without cyclophosphamide.
- Typical HUS: Supportive care, including hemodialysis, for severe acute kidney injury and hypertension management.

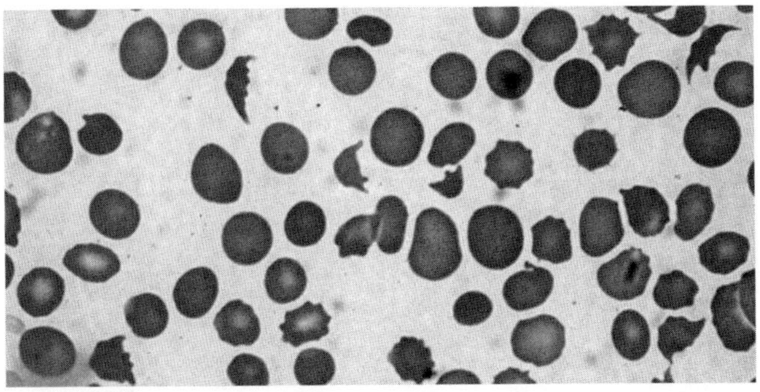

FIG. 1 Peripheral blood smear depicting schistocytes or fragmented red blood count.

- Atypical HUS: Eculizumab has been shown to be more effective than PEX. Eculizumab is an expensive drug, and current manufacturer recommendations include lifelong use, which can be cumbersome. Research is ongoing looking into shorter courses of treatments and outcomes.
- DIC:
  1. Treatment of underlying cause corrects the coagulopathy.
  2. Supportive care, including hemodynamic support and antimicrobial therapy, as indicated.
  3. Activated protein C (APC) is FDA approved for DIC complicated by sepsis.
- HELLP syndrome:
  1. Emergent delivery of fetus if more than 34 wk into gestation, preferably vaginal delivery.
  2. If less than 34 wk gestation, corticosteroids are recommended for expediting fetal lung maturation and delivery, but not beneficial to the mother.
- Malignant hypertension:
  1. Control blood pressure with medical therapy as indicated.
  2. Care should be taken to avoid rapid lowering of systolic blood pressure, which can lead to ischemia or hyperperfusion syndrome.

MONITORING & FOLLOW-UP

Serial laboratory monitoring of CBC, LDH, and presence of schistocytes on peripheral smear is required to asses MAHA disease activity.

- TTP:
  1. Idiopathic TTP has a relapse rate of 18%, which can happen up to 10 yr from initial presentation.
  2. Serial measurements of ADAMTS13 activity may have predictive value in assessing risk of relapse.
- Typical HUS: Full recovery of renal function, baseline neurologic status, and resolution of diarrhea.
- DIC: With adequate management of underlying cause, coagulopathy associated with DIC is reversible.
- HELLP syndrome:
  1. MAHA, thrombocytopenia, and liver injury are resolved within 48 hr after fetal delivery.
  2. Patients should be monitored for at least 2 days, with laboratory workup including CBC, LDH, and liver function.
- Malignant hypertension:
  1. Early adequate blood pressure control can reverse acute kidney injury.
  2. Patients can be discharged from the hospital after achieving adequate blood pressure control on an oral regimen.

PROGNOSIS

- TTP:
  1. If untreated, TTP has a high mortality rate of 90%.
  2. With PEX, mortality rate in idiopathic TTP is 15% and up to 59% in nonidiopathic TTP.
- Typical HUS:
  1. Typical HUS has a mortality rate of 5%, and younger children have better prognosis compared with adults.
  2. Central nervous system involvement or other extrarenal manifestations portend poor outcomes.
- Atypical HUS:
  1. Mortality ranges between 15% and 25%.
  2. Adults have poor prognosis compared with children.
  3. At 1-yr mark, about 25% of all patients have chronic renal failure.
- DIC:
  1. Prognosis of DIC depends on the severity of coagulopathy and underlying condition.
  2. DIC has been shown to be an independent predictor of mortality in sepsis and trauma, increasing the risk of death by a factor of 1.5 to 2.
- HELLP:
  1. Increased risk of preeclampsia in future pregnancies.
  2. Recurrence of HELLP with subsequent pregnancies is about 5%.
- Malignant hypertension:
  1. 10-yr overall survival is approximately 50%.
  2. MAHA in malignant hypertension predicts an increased likelihood of need for future hemodialysis.

REFERRAL

- Hematologist
- Nephrologist
- Neurologist
- Obstetrician

PEARLS & CONSIDERATIONS

- MAHA is not an individual clinical entity by itself, but rather includes many causes with different pathologic mechanisms, with a common phenomenon of small-vessel disease causing intravascular hemolysis.
- Presence of anemia with schistocytes and thrombocytopenia are key features in recognizing MAHA.
- If the etiology of MAHA is not readily apparent on initial evaluation, PEX must be immediately instituted for presumed TTP because it has a very high mortality rate of 90% if untreated.

SUGGESTED READING

Available at ExpertConsult.com

RELATED CONTENT

Disseminated Intravascular Coagulation (Related Key Topic)
HELLP Syndrome (Related Key Topic)
Hemolytic-Uremic Syndrome (Related Key Topic)
Thrombotic Thrombocytopenic Purpura (Related Key Topic)

AUTHOR: **Shiva Kumar R. Mukkamalla, MD, MPH**

BASIC INFORMATION

DEFINITION

Microscopic colitis (MC), also known as lymphocytic colitis, is an inflammatory condition of the colon that most often presents as chronic, watery, nonbloody diarrhea. Although clinically similar, lymphocytic colitis and collagenous colitis represent two histopathologic subtypes of microscopic colitis.

SYNONYMS

Lymphocytic colitis
Collagenous colitis
MC

ICD-10CM CODES	
K52.83	Microscopic colitis
K52.838	Other microscopic colitis
K52.832	Lymphocytic colitis
K52.831	Collagenous colitis
K52.9	Colitis, nonspecific

EPIDEMIOLOGY & DEMOGRAPHICS

INCIDENCE: Incidence of microscopic colitis is 24 to 103 in 100,000 person/yr.
PREVALENCE: Approximately 7.5% of patients who undergo workup for chronic watery diarrhea are diagnosed with MC.
PREDOMINANT SEX & AGE: Microscopic colitis, more specifically the collagenous variant, is often diagnosed later in life (>65 yr) and most commonly affects females.
PEAK INCIDENCE: Most cases of microscopic colitis are diagnosed in patients 60 to 70 yrs of age.
RISK FACTORS:
- Increased age
- Smoking: One study demonstrated that patients who smoke are diagnosed with MC an average of 10 yr earlier than their nonsmoker counterparts
- Autoimmune disorders such as rheumatoid arthritis, thyroid disease, type 1 diabetes
- Celiac disease
- Medications: NSAIDs, proton pump inhibitors (PPIs), selective serotonin reuptake inhibitors (SSRIs), HMG-COA reductase inhibitors (statins)

GENETICS: It is unclear how important specific genetic polymorphisms are in the pathophysiology of MC. However, a recent study described genetic similarities in human leukocyte antigen (HLA) genes for patients with microscopic colitis when compared with patients with Crohn disease.

PHYSICAL FINDINGS & CLINICAL PRESENTATION

- Most often presents with chronic watery diarrhea (>3 bowel movements daily). Classically, patients with microscopic colitis will experience nocturnal bowel movements.
- Other symptoms include abdominal pain, fecal incontinence, urgency, and less commonly, weight loss.
- Melena and hematochezia are not hallmarks of this disease.

ETIOLOGY

- The pathophysiology of MC remains unclear. Some studies suggest that colonic inflammation promotes a breakdown in electrolyte transport, leading to a combined osmotic and secretory diarrhea. Luminal agents including dietary items, bacterial flora, and medications may influence inflammation.
- Serotonin signaling also may play an important role in the development of MC as patients with a specific polymorphism in a serotonin receptor show a higher incidence of the disease.
- Microbiome studies show dysregulation and decreased bacterial diversity in patients with microscopic colitis.

DIAGNOSIS

DIFFERENTIAL DIAGNOSIS

- Irritable bowel syndrome (IBS)
- Inflammatory bowel disease (IBD)
- Ischemic colitis
- Infectious colitis (*C. difficile, E. coli, Giardia, Cryptosporidium, Entamoeba histolytica)*
- Pancreatic insufficiency
- Celiac sprue
- Intestinal lymphoma
- Carcinoid tumor
- Diverticulitis
- Small intestinal bacterial overgrowth

WORKUP

- Given the breadth of causes of watery diarrhea, the diagnostic workup is largely guided by clinical history.
- Infectious causes of symptoms should be ruled out first, particularly if the patient has specific risk factors including recent travel, recent sick contacts, consumption of untreated water, or recent antibiotic use or hospitalization.
- A careful history may elucidate specific dietary triggers such as lactose intolerance.
- Celiac disease is often comorbid with MC and should be ruled out in all patients with chronic watery diarrhea.

LABORATORY TESTS

- Complete blood count
- Hepatic function panel
- Electrolyte panel
- *C. difficile* stool PCR
- If the patient has been exposed to untreated drinking water, testing for Giardia, Cryptosporidium, and *E. histolytica* is indicated
- IgA tissue transglutaminase
- Consider fecal elastase if history is concerning for pancreatic insufficiency
- Fecal calprotectin: Unclear diagnostic benefit, but level significantly higher in active MC when compared to active IBD

IMAGING STUDIES

- MC is both a clinical and histopathologic diagnosis.
- Abdominal imaging is not helpful in diagnosing MC but may be warranted in patients with severe abdominal pain, evidence of obstruction, or a clinical history suggestive of infectious colitis or diverticulitis. Perforation is a rare complication of MC.
- Colonoscopy is a necessary part of MC diagnosis. On gross endoscopic examination, the colonic mucosa most often appears normal. Nonspecific findings such as erythema or mucosal cracking can be observed in a rare subset of patients.
- Obtaining multiple biopsies of each part of the large colon is foundational for endoscopic evaluation and maximizes diagnostic sensitivity. Lymphocytic colitis and collagenous colitis represent two histologic subtypes of MC. Lymphocytic colitis is marked by >20 intraepithelial lymphocytes to 100 surface epithelial cells in the presence of normal colonic mucosa (normal exhibits 5/100 ratio). Collagenous colitis is characterized by increased intraepithelial lymphocytes and a thickened (>1 mm, or 15-20 microns) subepithelial collagen band in the setting of normal colonic mucosa.

TREATMENT

There is no evidence to suggest that MC increases one's risk of colorectal cancer, nor is it believed to portend increased mortality. However, treatment is important to limit the significant burden on quality of life and healthcare costs. Both histopathologic subtypes of MC are clinically similar and managed using the same modalities. A treatment algorithm for collagenous and lymphocytic colitis is shown in Fig. E1.

NONPHARMACOLOGIC THERAPY

- The first step in management is to withdraw any medications that can provoke disease activity.
  1. NSAIDs are most notably associated with microscopic colitis and should be withheld.
  2. Other medications that may be associated with microscopic colitis include SSRIs, PPIs, statins, and bisphosphonates. Many of these medications are both common and effective, and a careful consideration of risk versus benefit should take place before halting medications.
- Smoking cessation.

ACUTE GENERAL Rx

- Antidiarrheal agents including loperamide or bismuth subsalicylate can be used in patients with mild symptoms. Nighttime dosing of these meds may curb nocturnal diarrhea.
- Budesonide (see Table 1): Shown to be the most effective first-line induction therapy and is often given for up to 8 wk.
  1. Induction therapy dose: 9 mg once daily for 6 to 8 wk.
  2. Remission therapy: After completing induction therapy for at least 8 wk, can be tapered over the course of approximately 1 mo and ultimately can be discontinued.
  3. Maintenance therapy dose: Administer in patients who relapse after completion of induction course. 6 mg daily tapered to lowest effective dose for duration of 6 to 12 mo OR alternating 3 mg and 6 mg daily dose for 12 mo.
- Mesalamine (see Table 1): Although several studies demonstrate that it is less effective than budesonide, mesalamine 3 g PO once daily also can be used for induction therapy in patients for whom budesonide therapy is

TABLE 1 Treatment Regimens for Lymphocytic Colitis

Medication	Induction	Maintenance
Budesonide	9 mg once daily for 6-8 wk	6 mg daily tapered to lowest effective dose for duration of 6-12 mo* OR Alternating 3 mg and 6 mg daily dose for 12 mo
Mesalamine	3 g PO once daily†	Not studied as a maintenance therapy
Bismuth subsalicylate	Nine 262-mg tablets daily, divided into three doses	Not studied as a maintenance therapy

*Administer in patients who relapse after completion of induction course.
†Shown to be inferior to budesonide in head-to-head randomized clinical trials.

not feasible. Limited, low-quality evidence demonstrates that combination therapy with cholestyramine can have favorable outcomes, and cholestyramine can have numerous potential interactions with other medications.

- Bismuth salicylate (see Table 1):
  For those with contraindications to budesonide and mesalamine, bismuth salicylate is another medication shown to be superior to watchful waiting in patients with mild symptomatic disease. The dose of bismuth salicylate is three 262-mg tablets taken three times daily.
- Bile acid sequestrants:
  There are limited data to suggest that bile acid sequestrants such as cholestyramine may be useful as single-agent or adjuvant induction therapy in patients with mild symptoms.
- Immune modulators:
  Although limited supporting evidence exists for their use, immune modulators such as azathioprine, vedolizumab, and anti-TNF-alpha inhibitors may also have a role for induction therapy in budesonide refractory disease.
- There is poor evidence supporting the role of systemic steroids such as prednisone in the treatment of microscopic colitis.
- Rarely, patients require surgical intervention with colonic diversion.

CHRONIC Rx

Approximately two thirds of patients with microscopic colitis experience relapsed disease and require maintenance therapy. Budesonide is the most studied maintenance agent that can be administered for up to 12 mo at doses lower than those used for induction. For less severe disease, patients also can continue using bismuth salicylate or cholestyramine.

COMPLEMENTARY & ALTERNATIVE MEDICINE

It is unclear whether probiotics provide benefit.

DISPOSITION

Symptoms associated with MC are often episodic. While induction therapy is highly effective, 66% of patients in remission will experience a subsequent disease flare.

REFERRAL

- Gastroenterology referral should be offered to patients with long standing chronic diarrhea whose workups have ruled out acute infectious causes.
- Nutrition referrals also may be helpful in patients with severe symptoms such as weight loss.

PEARLS & CONSIDERATIONS

COMMENTS

- MC poses a significant burden on patient quality of life and is often under-recognized.
- Chronic watery diarrhea in the older adult, particularly with nighttime symptoms, should prompt the provider to consider MC. Identification of MC through clinical history and endoscopic evaluation should not be delayed as induction therapy is highly effective at improving disease morbidity.
- Budesonide remains the most effective mainstay medication for both induction and maintenance therapy. Other medications such as bismuth salicylate and cholestyramine are well tolerated and suitable as adjunct or single-agent therapies. Refractory cases may require immunomodulator therapy such as azathioprine or anti-tumor necrosis factor biologic agents such as infliximab.

PREVENTION

As with many other chronic illnesses, smoking cessation is an important part of both management and prevention.

PATIENT & FAMILY EDUCATION

There is no known genetic abnormality, but presentation may trend in families.

SUGGESTED READINGS

Available at ExpertConsult.com

RELATED CONTENT

Irritable Bowel Syndrome (Related Key Topic)
Crohn Disease (Related Key Topic)
Ulcerative Colitis (Related Key Topic)
Traveler's Diarrhea (Related Key Topic)

AUTHORS: **Savan Kothadia, MD, Breton Roussel, MD,** and **Sarah Hyder, MD**

BASIC INFORMATION

DEFINITION

Microsporidiosis is an infection caused by single-celled intracellular spore-forming organisms previously classified as protozoan, but now classified as fungi. Infections occur more commonly in patients with HIV/AIDS, travelers, children, organ transplant recipients, contact lens wearers, and elderly adults.

SYNONYMS

Enterocytozoon bieneusi infection
Encephalitozoon species infection

ICD-10CM CODES	
A07.8	Microsporidiosis, intestinal
B60.8	Microsporidiosis
H16.8	Keratitis, microsporidia

EPIDEMIOLOGY & DEMOGRAPHICS

Microsporidia are a phylum of ubiquitous protists that exist worldwide in the environment and can infect vertebrate and invertebrate hosts, entering via ingestion or inhalation of spores and by direct contact through broken skin or lesions in the eyes.

PREVALENCE: Prevalence in immunocompetent persons is unclear, with rates varying from 5% to 45% in recent studies of stool from healthy human subjects.

In the postantiretroviral therapy era, prevalence rates have decreased; however, in a study of asymptomatic HIV patients, 15% had evidence of microsporidia on small bowel biopsy.

RISK FACTORS: Infections such as a nonbloody watery diarrhea and keratoconjunctivitis in contact lens wearers can occur in normal hosts, but immunocompromised hosts such as AIDS patients, organ transplant recipients, and bone marrow graft recipients are at greater risk for more severe disease, other organ involvement, and disseminated infection. Patients living with AIDS who have CD4 counts <200 should be advised to avoid untreated water and undercooked meat or seafood.

PHYSICAL FINDINGS & CLINICAL PRESENTATION

Each species of microsporidia has different reported infections:

- *Enterocytozoon bieneusi* can cause diarrhea, wasting syndrome, cholangitis, rhinitis, or bronchitis.
- *Encephalitozoon intestinalis* can cause diarrhea, intestinal perforation, cholangitis, nephritis, keratoconjunctivitis, and disseminated infection.
- *Encephalitozoon cuniculi* can cause hepatitis, peritonitis, encephalitis, urethritis, prostatitis, nephritis, sinusitis, keratoconjunctivitis, cystitis, cellulitis, and disseminated infection.
- *Encephalitozoon hellem* can cause keratoconjunctivitis, sinusitis, pneumonitis, nephritis, prostatitis, urethritis, cystitis, and disseminated infection.

ETIOLOGY

- There are 1200 species of Microsporidia, but only 14 infect humans from seven different genera. The four most common species to cause human disease are:
  1. *Enterocytozoon bieneusi*
  2. *Encephalitozoon intestinalis*
  3. *Encephalitozoon cuniculi*
  4. *Encephalitozoon hellem*
- These genotypes that infect humans have been identified in domestic, farm, and wild animals and thus may be a form of zoonotic disease.

DIAGNOSIS

DIFFERENTIAL DIAGNOSIS

- Other causes of watery nonbloody diarrhea: *Norovirus, Giardia, Cryptosporidia, Cyclospora, and Isospora belli*
- Other causes of keratoconjunctivitis: Herpetic keratoconjunctivitis and acanthamoeba keratitis

WORKUP

Consists of the microscopic detection of microsporidia spores (1-2 μm in diameter) in stool, body fluids, or tissue samples.

LABORATORY TESTS

- Modified trichrome stain with light microscopy can be used on stool, urine, mucus, or tissues. Spores stain pink against a blue-green background
- Fluorescent techniques: Calcofluor white stain, Uvitex 2B, and Fungi-Fluor kit
- Indirect immunofluorescence
- Serology: IgM and IgG antimicrosporidial antibodies
- For exact speciation: PCR

TREATMENT

ACUTE GENERAL Rx

Treatment will depend on organism and site involved.

- There is no available therapy currently for *E. bieneusi*; however, immune restoration through initiation of antiretroviral therapy (ART) has been shown to resolve symptoms in AIDS patients. ART should be offered as a part of initial management where applicable. Systemic fumagillin has shown some success.
- Intestinal or disseminated infection caused by microsporidia other than *E. bieneusi* and *V. corneae*: Albendazole 400 mg PO bid for 2 to 4 wk depending on level of immunosuppression. Children: 15 mg/kg/day PO in divided doses. For disseminated disease (especially *Trachipleistophora* or *Anncaliia* infections), consider the addition of itraconazole.
- Keratoconjunctivitis: Topical fumagillin 70 mcg/ml eye drops (2 drops every 2 hr for 4 days, then 2 drops 4 times a day). If associated with intestinal disease, add albendazole 400 mg PO bid for 2 to 4 wk depending on degree of immunosuppression.

CHRONIC Rx

- Antimotility agents are useful to control diarrhea.
- Recurrence or relapse may occur with ongoing immunosuppression; therefore, consider chronic maintenance therapy until CD4 counts remain >200 for 6 mo in those living with HIV.

REFERRAL

- Infectious diseases physician for antiretroviral therapy if positive for HIV/AIDS
- Ophthalmologist if keratoconjunctivitis is suspected

PEARLS & CONSIDERATIONS

COMMENTS

- Microsporidia infections occur particularly in HIV-positive patients with CD4+ cell counts <50/ml.
- Microsporidia spores can remain active in the environment for prolonged periods of time (e.g., months).

SUGGESTED READINGS

Available at ExpertConsult.com

AUTHORS: **Tara C. Bouton, MD, MPH, TM, Philip A. Chan, MD, MS,** and **Glenn G. Fort, MD, MPH**

BASIC INFORMATION

DEFINITION

Migraine headaches are recurrent severe headaches that either are preceded by a focal neurologic symptom (migraine with aura), occur independently without preceding focal neurologic symptoms (migraine without aura), or have atypical presentations (migraine variants). The migraine aura (Box 1) typically is characterized by visual or sensory symptoms that develop over 5 to 60 min. If the aura includes unilateral motor weakness, the migraine is referred to as hemiplegic. In migraine with and without aura, the headache is typically moderate to severe, unilateral, pulsatile, made worse with head movement, and associated with nausea and vomiting, photophobia, and phonophobia. Migraines that occur ≥15 days every mo for ≥3 mo are known as chronic; otherwise, they are referred to as episodic. Table 1 summarizes criteria for migraine.

ICD-10CM CODES

G43.909	Migraine, unspecified, not intractable, without status migrainosus
G43.1	Migraine with aura (classical migraine)
G43.0	Migraine without aura (common migraine)
G43.2	Status migrainosus
G43.3	Complicated migraine

EPIDEMIOLOGY & DEMOGRAPHICS

INCIDENCE: Increases from infancy, peaks during the third decade of life, then decreases.

PREVALENCE (IN U.S.): Migraine is the third-most prevalent disease in the world. It affects approximately 39 million people in the U.S.[1] Globally, it is estimated to affect 1 billion people and it has an estimated 1-yr prevalence of approximately 15% in the general population.[2]

BOX 1 Auras of Migraine

Sensory phenomena
- Special senses
  - Visual, olfactory, auditory, gustatory
- Paresthesias, especially lips and hand

Motor deficits
- Hemiparesis, hemiplegic

Neuropsychologic changes

Aphasia

Perceptual impairment, especially for size, shape, and time

Emotional and behavioral
- Anxiety, depression, irritability, (rarely) hyperactivity

From Kaufman DM et al: *Kaufman's clinical neurology for psychiatrists*, ed 8, Philadelphia, 2017, Elsevier.

[1] Spindler BL, Ryan M: Medications approved for preventing migraine headaches. *Am J Med* 133:664-667, 2020.

[2] Ashina M: Migraine. N Engl J Med 383:1866-1876, 2020.

PREDOMINANT SEX: Female:male ratio of 3:1.

PREDOMINANT AGE: Peak prevalence between ages of 18 and 49.

GENETICS: Familial predisposition: More than 50% of migraine sufferers have an affected family member.

- Autosomal-dominant transmission for some rare migraine variants (familial hemiplegic migraine, cerebral autosomal-dominant arteriopathy with subcortical infarcts and leukoencephalopathy [CADASIL]); familial hemiplegic migraines have been associated with calcium channelopathy, sodium channelopathy, and Na^+/K^+-ATPase dysfunction.

PHYSICAL FINDINGS & CLINICAL PRESENTATION

- Normal between episodes
- Normal for migraine without aura
- Focal motor or sensory abnormalities possible for migraine with aura or migraine variants
- Common aura types include scintillating scotoma, bright zigzags (fortifications), and other visual distortions such as macropsia or micropsia (enlargement or shrinkage of objects) that often cross visual fields. Homonymous visual disturbance, sensory phenomena such as hemibody paresthesia, speech disturbances, or hemiparesis (familial or sporadic hemiplegic migraine) also can occur independently or associated with visual symptoms

ETIOLOGY

The pathophysiology of migraines is not clearly understood, although the primary neuronal event results in a trigeminovascular reflex causing neurogenic inflammation. Calcitonin-gene related peptide (CGRP) is released by the trigeminal ganglion and binds receptors around meningeal vessels leading to inflammation. Serotonin, substance P, and nitric oxide also play a role, but the exact mechanism is unknown. Cortical spreading depressions also likely are responsible for the aura.

DIAGNOSIS

Migraine without aura:
- Five attacks fulfilling criteria
- Headache attacks lasting 4 to 72 hr
- Headache has at least two of the following characteristics:
  1. Unilateral location
  2. Pulsating quality
  3. Moderate or severe pain intensity
  4. Aggravation or causing avoidance of routine physical activity
- At least one of the following during headache:
  1. Nausea and/or vomiting
  2. Photophobia and phonophobia

Migraine with typical aura:
- At least two attacks
- Aura consisting of at least one of the following, but no motor weakness:
  1. Fully reversible visual symptoms, including positive and/or negative features
  2. Fully reversible sensory symptoms, including positive and/or negative features
  3. Fully reversible dysphasic speech disturbance
- At least two of the following:
  1. Homonymous visual symptoms and/or unilateral sensory symptoms
  2. At least one aura symptom develops gradually over >5 min and/or different aura symptoms occur in succession over >5 min
  3. Each symptom lasts between 5 and 60 min
- A migraine occurring during or within 60 min of the aura

DIFFERENTIAL DIAGNOSIS

- A diagnosis of migraine is possible only after five recurrent episodes.
- The first or the worst headache should always be investigated, and the differential includes headaches from all secondary causes.
- Headache red flags can be remembered by the mnemonic SSNOOP5:
  1. S: Systemic symptoms of fever, weight loss
  2. S: Secondary risk factors of immunosuppression from any cause, cancer
  3. N: Neurologic deficits, altered consciousness
  4. O: Onset is sudden, abrupt, split second thunderclap
  5. O: Older, age >50 for new-onset headache should be worked up for giant cell arteritis
  6. P: Pattern: Change in headache pattern
  7. P: Pregnancy
  8. P: Positional or postural
  9. P: Papilledema
  10. P: Precipitation with Valsalva maneuver or exertion

TABLE 1 Comparison of Tension-Type and Migraine Headaches

	Tension-Type	Migraine
Location	Bilateral	Hemicranial*
Nature	Dull ache	Throbbing*
Severity	Slight–moderate	Moderate–severe
Associated symptoms	None	Nausea, hyperacusis, photophobia
Behavior	Continues working	Seeks seclusion
Effect of alcohol	Reduces headache	Worsens headache

*In approximately half of patients, at least at onset.

From Kaufman DM et al: *Kaufman's clinical neurology for psychiatrists,* ed 8, Philadelphia, 2017, Elsevier.

- Section II describes the differential diagnosis of headaches. Table 1 compares tension-type and migraine headaches.
- Useful mnemonic for migraine is POUND: Pulsatile, One day in duration, Unilateral, Nausea/vomiting, Disabling.

WORKUP

- In general, no additional investigation is needed with recurrent, typical attacks with usual age of onset, family history, and a normal physical examination.
- Fundus examination is important to evaluate for the possibility of optic disk edema, which would suggest a secondary cause of headache such as idiopathic intracranial hypertension (IIH).
- If there is an unusual presentation, headache with red flags, and/or unexpected findings on examination, investigation for other causes is required.

LABORATORY TESTS

Lumbar puncture for history of abrupt-onset headaches and uncertain diagnosis of migraine

IMAGING STUDIES

- Imaging should be done in patients with any of the red flags for secondary headache such as described by the SSNOOP5 mnemonic (see "Differential Diagnosis" above).
- MRI brain with and without contrast is the imaging modality of choice for almost all headache types, although CT head without contrast may be used in the acute setting to evaluate for subarachnoid hemorrhage or other causes of acute intracranial hemorrhage.

Rx TREATMENT

Consider the use of a headache log/diary to identify triggers of headaches, record efficacy of treatments, and track history of headaches.

NONPHARMACOLOGIC THERAPY

- Avoid any identifiable provoking factors: Caffeine, tobacco, and alcohol may trigger attacks, as may dietary or other environmental precipitants (less common).
- Avoid emotional stressors and minimize variations in daily routine with regular sleep, meals, and exercise.
- Relaxation training, behavioral therapy, and biofeedback. Trials have shown that among young persons with chronic migraine, the use of cognitive-behavioral therapy (CBT) plus amitriptyline results in greater reductions in days with headaches and migraine-related disability compared with use of headache education plus amitriptyline.
- Trials in patients with migraine without aura have shown that acupuncture may be associated with long-term reduction in migraine recurrence.[1]

[1] Zhao L et al: The long-term effect of acupuncture for migraine prophylaxis: a randomized clinical trial. *JAMA Intern Med* 177(4):508-515, 2017.

ACUTE ANALGESIC Rx

- Many oral agents are ineffective because of poor absorption from migraine-induced gastric stasis. Nonoral route of administration should be selected in patients with severe nausea or vomiting.
- NSAIDs such as ketorolac, ibuprofen, and naproxen, or combination analgesics, may be used first line for mild migraine headaches.
- Barbiturate-containing compounds should be avoided because they are potentially addictive and promote medication overuse headaches.
- Opioids are not effective for treating patients with migraine headaches and should not be used.

ACUTE ABORTIVE Rx

- Triptans (SC, PO, and intranasal) are the drug class of choice for abortive therapy. Meta-analysis suggests that 10 mg rizatriptan, 40 mg eletriptan, and 12.5 mg almotriptan are most effective. Sumatriptan may also be given, especially in combination with naproxen. Early administration improves effectiveness. Triptans are relatively contraindicated in heart disease and hemiplegic migraine.
- Gepants (rimegepant, ubrogepant): Small-molecule CGRP antagonists newly approved for acute migraine abortive therapy, especially when triptans are ineffective or contraindicated. There have been no clear cardiac risks with this class.
- IV antiemetics (prochlorperazine, metoclopramide, chlorpromazine) may be used in addition to triptans. Acute dystonic reactions, QT prolongation, and akathisia are rare side effects. These are generally not used as monotherapy.
- Ergotamine, ergotamine combinations (PO/PR), and dihydroergotamine (DHE 45) (SC, IV, IM, intranasal) have well-documented efficacy against migraines. DHE is usually administered in combination with an antiemetic drug (Table 2) but cannot be given within 24 hr of a triptan.
- IV dexamethasone may be used to prevent recurrence but should not be used frequently due to risk for toxicity.
- Greater and lesser occipital nerve blocks may also be performed to alleviate pain in the acute setting. These injections may be combined with auriculotemporal, supraorbital, and supratrochlear nerve block to achieve anesthesia in the area of perceived pain.

PROPHYLAXIS Rx

- Prophylactic treatment is generally indicated when headaches are disabling more than 5 days of the mo or when symptomatic treatments are contraindicated or not effective. All prophylaxes should be maintained for at least 3 mo before deeming the medication a failure.
- Well-established options for prophylactic treatment include β-blockers (propranolol, timolol, atenolol, metoprolol), tricyclic antidepressants (amitriptyline, nortriptyline), and the antiepileptic drugs topiramate and sodium divalproate (valproic acid).
- CGRP monoclonal antibodies: A new class of injectable drugs that target the CGRP molecule or its receptor. There are currently four FDA-approved drugs in this class, erenumab (Aimovig, once-a-month injection), fremanezumab (Ajovy, once-a-month or quarterly injection), galcanezumab (Emgality, once-a-month injection), and eptinezumab (Vyepti, quarterly infusion), with more under study. These drugs can be used first line for episodic and chronic migraine but are usually used after failure of oral prophylactic treatment.
- Less-established options include calcium channel blockers, selective norepinephrine serotonin reuptake inhibitors, memantine, and other antiepileptic medications.
- Supraorbital transcutaneous electrical stimulation has been approved by the FDA for prophylaxis of episodic migraine and is widely available with a prescription in Europe and North America.
- For prevention of headaches in adult patients with chronic migraines only (≥15 headache days/mo for ≥3 mo), onabotulinum toxin A (Botox) injections are the only approved therapy.

DISPOSITION

With advancing age, many patients will have sustained reduction in frequency of migraine headaches.

REFERRAL

To neurologist if uncertain about diagnosis or treatment not effective

! PEARLS & CONSIDERATIONS

- Migraines that change in character or headaches that are different from the patient's typical ones need to be reevaluated.
- Long-term and frequent use of analgesic medications can result in medication overuse or rebound headaches. Early initiation of prophylactic medication is key.
- Avoid use of narcotics, barbiturates, and benzodiazepines because they are habit forming. Narcotics and barbiturates also promote medication overuse headaches.
- Migraine with aura is associated with excess stroke and thromboembolism risk, and is a relative contraindication to the use of combined oral contraceptives in women.

RELATED CONTENT

Migraine Headache (Patient Information)

SUGGESTED READINGS

Available at ExpertConsult.com

AUTHOR: **Corey Goldsmith, MD**

TABLE 2 Abortive and Analgesic Therapy for Migraine*

Drug	Route	Dose
Triptans (Serotonin Agonists)		
Sumatriptan	Subcutaneous	6 mg, repeat in 2 hr (max 2 doses/day)
Sumatriptan	Oral	25 mg, 50 mg, 100 mg, repeat in 2 hr (max 200 mg/day)
Sumatriptan	Nasal spray	5 mg, 20 mg, repeat in 2 hr (max 40 mg/day)
Zolmitriptan	Oral	1.25, 2.5 mg, 5 mg, repeat in 2 hr (max 10 mg/day)
Zolmitriptan	Nasal spray	5 mg, repeat in 2 hr (max 10 mg/day)
Zolmitriptan	Orally disintegrating tab	2.5, 5 mg, repeat in 2 hr (max 10 mg/day)
Naratriptan	Oral	1 mg, 2.5 mg, repeat in 4 hr (max 5 mg/day)
Rizatriptan	Oral	5 mg, 10 mg, repeat in 2 hr (max 30 mg/day)
Almotriptan	Oral	6.25 mg, 12.5 mg, may repeat in 2 hr (max 25 mg/day)
Eletriptan	Oral	20 mg, 40 mg, may repeat in 2 hr (max 80 mg/day)
Frovatriptan	Oral	2.5 mg, may repeat in 2 hr (max 7.5 mg/day); may also be used for mini prophylaxis
Ergotamine Preparations		
Ergotamine and caffeine	Oral	2 tablets, may repeat 1 tab q30 min (max 6/day)
Ergotamine and caffeine	Rectal	1 suppository, repeat in 1 hr (max 2/day)
Ergotamine	Sublingual	1 tablet, repeat in 1 hr (max 2/day)
Dihydroergotamine	Intramuscular	0.5-1.0 mg, repeat twice at 1-hr intervals (max 3 mg/attack)
	Subcutaneous	
	Intravenous	
	Nasal spray	
Isometheptene + dichloralphenazone + acetaminophen	Oral	1 to 2 capsules, repeat in 4 hr (max 8/day)
Nonsteroidal Antiinflammatory Drugs		
Acetaminophen + (should not be used alone)	Oral	2 tablets, repeat in 6 hr (max 8/day aspirin + caffeine)
Naproxen	Oral	550-750 mg, repeat in 1 hr (max 3 times/wk)
Meclofenamate	Oral	100-200 mg, repeat in 1 hr (max 3 times/wk)
Flurbiprofen	Oral	50-100 mg, repeat in 1 hr (max 3 times/wk)
Ibuprofen	Oral	200-300 mg, repeat in 1 hr (max 3 times/wk)
Antiemetics		
Promethazine	Oral	50-125 mg
	Intramuscular	No clear benefit in migraine, may be used
Prochlorperazine	Oral	1-25 mg
	Rectal	2.5-25 mg (suppository)
	Intramuscular/IV	5-10 mg, good evidence for strong benefit
Chlorpromazine	Oral	10-25 mg
	Rectal	50-100 mg (suppository)
	Intravenous	Up to 35 mg, use with monitoring, some evidence for good benefit
Trimethobenzamide	Oral	250 mg
	Rectal	200 mg
Metoclopramide	Oral	5-10 mg
	Intramuscular	10 mg
	Intravenous	5-10 mg
Dimenhydrinate	Oral	50 mg

*For side effects and contraindications, consult the manufacturer's drug insert before prescribing any of these drugs.
Modified from Wiederholt WC: *Neurology for non-neurologists*, ed 4, Philadelphia, 2000, Saunders.

BASIC INFORMATION

DEFINITION

Mitral regurgitation (MR) is retrograde blood flow into the left atrium resulting from any part of an incompetent mitral valve apparatus. This condition may cause left ventricular (LV) failure, as well as increased left atrial and pulmonary pressures leading to pulmonary hypertension and right-sided heart failure.

SYNONYMS

Mitral insufficiency
MR

ICD-10CM CODES

I34.0	Nonrheumatic mitral (valve) insufficiency
I05.1	Rheumatic mitral insufficiency
I05.9	Mitral valve disease, unspecified
I05.2	Rheumatic mitral stenosis with insufficiency
Q23.3	Congenital mitral insufficiency

EPIDEMIOLOGY & DEMOGRAPHICS

The incidence of MR has increased over the past 30 yr. However, this may be due to increasing availability of echocardiography leading to MR diagnosis rather than to an actual increase in the prevalence of this condition.

PHYSICAL FINDINGS & CLINICAL PRESENTATION

Heart sounds:
- Diminished S1 as valve leaflets fail to coapt properly
- Widely split S2 as A2 occurs earlier because of decreased LV ejection time
- Presence of an S3 as a result of increased flow into a dilated LV caused by severe MR with systolic impairment

Heart murmurs:
- Holosystolic, high-pitched, "blowing" murmur is most easily audible at apex with radiation to base, left axilla, or back. There is a poor correlation between the intensity of the systolic murmur and the degree of regurgitation. However, an early diastolic to middiastolic rumble (pseudomitral stenosis) suggests severe MR
- The murmur of acute MR (e.g., from papillary muscle rupture) can be very soft or inaudible because of a large regurgitant volume entering a noncompliant left atrium. This causes an acute rise in left atrial pressure and a decline in LV filling pressure, and thus a lack of significant gradient for an audible murmur
- Hyperdynamic apex, sometimes with palpable LV lift and apical thrill
- Symptomatic patients with MR generally present with the following:
  1. Symptoms suggestive of heart failure (fatigue, dyspnea, orthopnea, paroxysmal nocturnal dyspnea, edema)
  2. Hemoptysis (caused by pulmonary hypertension)
  3. Atrial fibrillation

ETIOLOGY

Primary MR:
- Idiopathic myxomatous degeneration of the mitral valve, mitral valve prolapse (most common cause of MR in industrialized countries)
- Papillary muscle dysfunction or rupture (typically as a result of an inferior wall myocardial infarction)
- Ruptured chordae tendineae
- Infective endocarditis
- Calcified mitral valve annulus
- Rheumatic valvulitis (may be combined with mitral stenosis; common in developing countries)
- Systemic lupus erythematosus (Libman-Sacks endocarditis)
- Drugs: Fenfluramine, dexfenfluramine, pergolide, cabergoline
- Congenital cleft valve
- Ischemic MR due to papillary muscle dysfunction from multivessel coronary artery disease (CAD)

Secondary MR:
- Hypertrophic cardiomyopathy
- LV dilation (e.g., secondary to dilated cardiomyopathy)

DIAGNOSIS

DIFFERENTIAL DIAGNOSIS

- Hypertrophic cardiomyopathy
- Tricuspid regurgitation
- Aortic stenosis
- Aortic sclerosis
- Ventricular septal defect
- Atrial septal defect

WORKUP

- Diagnostic workup consists of echocardiography, ECG, and chest radiograph; cardiac catheterization is sometimes needed to confirm severity of the disease.
- Tables 1 and 2 summarize stages of chronic primary and chronic secondary MR.
- Recent studies suggest that in patients with severe asymptomatic MR, normal LV function and elevations of brain natriuretic peptide (BNP) >105 pg/ml have an independent and additive prognostic value that may identify high-risk patients and aid in the selection of patients for early surgery.

IMAGING STUDIES

- Echocardiography (Fig. 1): Findings include dilated left atrium, hyperdynamic left ventricle, erratic motion of the leaflet in patients with ruptured chordae tendineae, and color flow Doppler with evidence of MR. The most important aspect of the echocardiographic examination is the quantification of the severity of MR (Table 3). A vena contracta width >0.7 cm, a regurgitant volume >60 ml, regurgitant orifice area >0.40 cm^2 by PISA (proximal isovelocity surface area), and systolic pulmonary vein flow reversal are all echocardiographic criteria of severe MR
- Chest x-ray:
  1. Left atrial enlargement, LV enlargement
  2. Possible pulmonary congestion, although most often normal
- ECG:
  1. Left atrial enlargement
  2. LV hypertrophy
  3. Atrial fibrillation
- Cardiac catheterization: To confirm severity of MR, or to rule out presence of coronary artery disease in patients being evaluated for surgical replacement
- Can consider cardiac MRI in cases where echocardiography is limited or LV function/dimensions are borderline, or when clinical condition and echocardiographic findings are discordant

TREATMENT

NONPHARMACOLOGIC THERAPY

- Salt restriction
- Surgical repair or replacement (see the following)

ACUTE GENERAL Rx

- Medical: Medical therapy is primarily directed toward treatment of the source or its complications (e.g., atrial fibrillation, ischemic heart disease, infective endocarditis, hypertension, and heart failure).
  1. The utility of afterload reduction to decrease the regurgitant fraction and increase cardiac output depends upon the etiology of MR. In acute MR, intravenous nitroprusside has shown some utility. Long-term use of oral afterload reducers (e.g., ACE inhibitors or angiotensin receptor blockers), while they do not slow the progression of MR, should be implemented when other indications such as hypertension and LV dysfunction are present.
  2. Control ventricular response in atrial fibrillation when rapid ventricular response is present. Use anticoagulants if atrial fibrillation occurs. Note that current guidelines do not consider atrial fibrillation in patients with MR "valvular," and non–vitamin K anticoagulation agents may be used for stroke prophylaxis.
  3. Diuresis and achieving a euvolemic state may significantly decrease the degree of functional MR caused by volume overload and heart failure.
- Surgery: Surgery is the only definitive treatment for MR. Although no randomized trial of mitral valve repair vs. replacement exists, repair is favored over replacement in degenerative mitral valve disease due to its lower perioperative risk, improved event-free survival, freedom from complications of prosthetic valves, and better postoperative LV function. It is a class I indication in patients with the following diagnoses (Fig. 2):
  1. Acute severe MR
  2. Symptomatic patients with severe primary MR despite optimal medical therapy and left ventricular ejection fraction (LVEF) >30%, LV dilation, severe MR by echo criteria

TABLE 1 Stages of Chronic Primary Mitral Regurgitation

Grade	Definition	Valve Anatomy	Valve Hemodynamics*	Hemodynamic Consequences	Symptoms
A	At risk for MR	Mild mitral valve prolapse with normal coaptation Mild valve thickening and leaflet restriction	No MR jet or small central jet area <20% LA on Doppler Small vena contracta <0.3 cm	None	None
B	Progressive MR	Severe mitral valve prolapse with normal coaptation Rheumatic valve changes with leaflet restriction and loss of central coaptation Previous IE	Central jet MR 20%-40% LA or late systolic eccentric jet MR Vena contracta <0.7 cm Regurgitant volume <60 ml Regurgitant fraction <50% ERO <0.40 cm^2 Angiographic grade 1-2+	Mild LA enlargement No LV enlargement Normal pulmonary pressure	None
C	Asymptomatic severe MR	Severe mitral valve prolapse with loss of coaptation or flail leaflet Rheumatic valve changes with leaflet restriction and loss of central coaptation Previous IE Thickening of leaflets with radiation heart disease	Central jet MR >40% LA or holosystolic eccentric jet MR Vena contracta ≥0.7 cm Regurgitant volume ≥60 ml Regurgitant fraction ≥50% ERO ≥0.40 cm^2 Angiographic grade 3-4+	Moderate or severe LA enlargement LV enlargement Pulmonary hypertension may be present at rest or with exercise C1: LVEF >60% and LVESD <40 mm C2: LVEF ≤60% and LVESD ≥40 mm	None
D	Symptomatic severe MR	Severe mitral valve prolapse with loss of coaptation or flail leaflet Rheumatic valve changes with leaflet restriction and loss of central coaptation Previous IE Thickening of leaflets with radiation heart disease	Central jet MR >40% LA or holosystolic eccentric jet MR Vena contracta ≥0.7 cm Regurgitant volume ≥60 ml Regurgitant fraction ≥50% ERO ≥0.40 cm^2 Angiographic grade 3-4+	Moderate or severe LA enlargement LV enlargement Pulmonary hypertension present	Decreased exercise tolerance Exertional dyspnea

ERO, Effective regurgitant orifice; *IE,* infective endocarditis; *LA,* left atrium; *LV,* left ventricle; *LVEF,* left ventricular ejection fraction; *LVESD,* left ventricular end-systolic dimension; *MR,* mitral regurgitation.

*Several valve hemodynamic criteria are provided for assessment of MR severity, but not all criteria for each category will be present in each patient. Classification of MR severity as mild, moderate, or severe depends on data quality and integration of these parameters in conjunction with other clinical evidence.

From Nishimura RA et al: 2014 AHA/ACCF guideline for the management of patients with valvular heart disease: a report of the American College of Cardiology Foundation/American Heart Association Task Force on Practice Guidelines, *J Am Coll Cardiol* 63:e57, 2014.

TABLE 2 Stages of Chronic Secondary Mitral Regurgitation

Grade	Definition	Valve Anatomy	Valve Hemodynamics*	Associated Cardiac Findings	Symptoms
A	At risk of MR	Normal valve leaflets, chords, and annulus in a patient with coronary disease or a cardiomyopathy	No MR jet or small central jet area <20% LA on Doppler Small vena contracta <0.30 cm	Normal or mildly dilated LV size with fixed (infarction) or inducible (ischemia) regional wall motion abnormalities Primary myocardial disease with LV dilation and systolic dysfunction	Symptoms due to coronary ischemia or HF may be present that respond to revascularization and appropriate medical therapy
B	Progressive MR	Regional wall motion abnormalities with mild tethering of mitral leaflet Annular dilation with mild loss of central coaptation of the mitral leaflets	ERO <0.20 cm^2† Regurgitant volume <30 ml Regurgitant fraction <50%	Regional wall motion abnormalities with reduced LV systolic function LV dilation and systolic dysfunction due to primary myocardial disease	Symptoms due to coronary ischemia or HF may be present that respond to revascularization and appropriate medical therapy
C	Asymptomatic severe MR	Regional wall motion abnormalities and/or LV dilation with severe tethering of mitral leaflet Annular dilation with severe loss of central coaptation of the mitral leaflets	ERO ≥0.20 cm^2† Regurgitant volume ≥30 ml Regurgitant fraction ≥50%	Regional wall motion abnormalities with reduced LV systolic function LV dilation and systolic dysfunction due to primary myocardial disease	Symptoms due to coronary ischemia or HF may be present that respond to revascularization and appropriate medical therapy
D	Symptomatic severe MR	Regional wall motion abnormalities and/or LV dilation with severe tethering of mitral leaflet Annular dilation with severe loss of central coaptation of the mitral leaflets	ERO ≥0.20 cm^2† Regurgitant volume ≥30 ml Regurgitant fraction ≥50%	Regional wall motion abnormalities with reduced LV systolic function LV dilation and systolic dysfunction due to primary myocardial disease	HF symptoms due to MR persist even after revascularization and optimization of medical therapy Decreased exercise tolerance Exertional dyspnea

ERO, Effective regurgitant orifice; *HF,* heart failure; *LA,* left atrium; *LV,* left ventricle; *MR,* mitral regurgitation.

*Several valve hemodynamic criteria are provided for assessment of MR severity, but not all criteria for each category will be present in each patient. Categorization of MR severity as mild, moderate, or severe depends on data quality and integration of these parameters in conjunction with other clinical evidence.

†The measurement of the proximal isovelocity surface area by two-dimensional transthoracic echocardiogram (TTE) in patients with secondary MR underestimates the true ERO because of the crescentic shape of the proximal convergence.

From Nishimura RA et al: 2014 AHA/ACCF guideline for the management of patients with valvular heart disease: a report of the American College of Cardiology Foundation/American Heart Association Task Force on Practice Guidelines, *J Am Coll Cardiol* 63:e57, 2014.

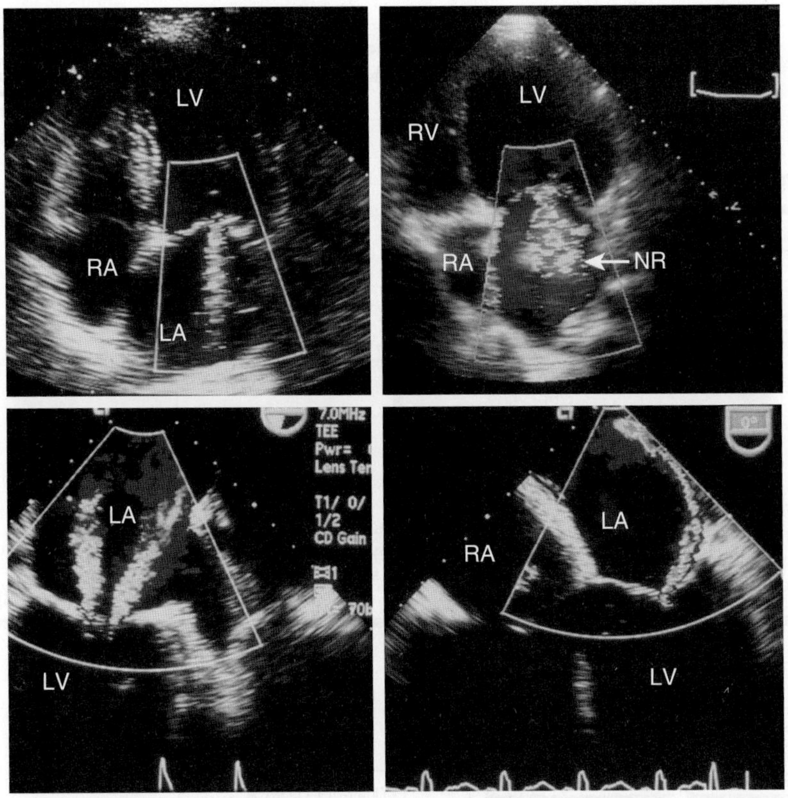

FIG. 1 Mitral regurgitation. Four panels depicting varying degrees of mitral regurgitation; the two top panels are apical four-chamber transthoracic views showing, on the left, mild mitral regurgitation and, on the right, moderate to severe mitral regurgitation. On the left, note the relatively narrow jet directed from the tips of the mitral valve toward the posterior left atrial wall. On the right, note the larger jet, filling approximately 40% of the left atrial cavity. The two bottom panels are transesophageal echocardiograms. On the left, note the mitral regurgitation occurring in two discrete jets and, on the right, the highly eccentric jet, which courses along the extreme lateral wall of the left atrium. *LA,* Left atrium; *LV,* left ventricle; *RA,* right atrium; *RV,* right ventricle. (From Zipes DP et al [eds]: *Braunwald's heart disease,* ed 7, Philadelphia, 2005, Saunders.)

TABLE 3 Mitral Regurgitation Severity*

	I (Mild)	II (Moderate)	III (Moderate)	IV (Severe)
MR = jet (%LA)	<15	15-30	35-50	>50
Spectral Doppler	Faint	—	—	Dense
Vena contracta	<3 mm	—	—	≥7 mm
Pulmonary vein flow	S > D	Normal to systolic blunting	Systolic blunting	Systolic reversal
RV (ml)	<30	30-44	45-59	≥60
ERO (cm2)	<0.2	0.2-0.29	0.3-0.39	≥0.40
PISA	Small	—	—	Large

D, Antegrade flow in diastole; *ERO,* effective regurgitant orifice; *%LA,* percentage of left atrial area encompassed by the MR jet with color flow Doppler; *MR,* mitral regurgitation; *PISA,* proximal isovelocity surface area; *RV,* regurgitant volume; *S,* antegrade flow in systole.

*For some parameters, the observation is valid at the extremes of MR severity and there may be marked overlap in intermediate (grades II, III) MR. In these instances, no value is presented.

From Zipes DP et al (eds): *Braunwald's heart disease,* ed 7, Philadelphia, 2005, Saunders; and the 2017

3. Asymptomatic patients with severe MR but with evidence of declining LV function (EF <60% but >30%) or progressive dilation (LV at end-systole >40 mm)
4. Concomitant mitral valve repair or MVR is indicated in patients with chronic severe primary MR undergoing cardiac surgery for other indications

- Surgery is a class IIa (reasonable) recommendation in:

1. Severe MR with new-onset atrial fibrillation, even if asymptomatic
2. Asymptomatic severe MR with pulmonary hypertension (≥50 mm Hg at rest or ≥60 mm Hg during exercise)
3. Asymptomatic severe MR secondary to flail leaflet
4. A recent study of early surgical intervention for severe MR secondary to a flail leaflet in patients with asymptomatic disease shows greater long-term survival and reduced rates of heart failure when compared with medical therapy alone
   a. Asymptomatic severe MR with preserved LVEF (>60%) and size (<40 mm in end-systole) in whom the likelihood of successful repair without residual MR is >95% and operative mortality is <1%

- Surgery is a class IIb recommendation in symptomatic patients (New York Heart Association [NYHA] class III to IV) with severe MR with severe LV dysfunction or dilatation (LVEF <30% or LV at end-systole >55 mm, respectively) in whom LV dysfunction is not the primary cause for the MR as well as functional MR where it is secondary to LV dysfunction.
- Quantitative grading of MR is a powerful predictor of the clinical outcome of asymptomatic MR. In general, patients with regurgitant orifice areas of ≥40 mm^2 should be considered for prompt surgery, whereas those with orifices between 20 and 39 mm^2 can be followed closely.
- Percutaneous mitral valve repair methods are continually being investigated. The MitraClip device is FDA approved for use in patients with significant symptomatic degenerative or primary MR (>3+) who are too high risk for surgery. In patients with secondary MR, repair should not be pursued until optimal medical therapy has been achieved. The device is a catheter-delivered clip that grasps and approximates the edges of the mitral leaflets at the origin of the regurgitant jet. Early data are limited and had not demonstrated a significant efficacy in MR reduction compared with surgical replacement. However, when comparing guideline-directed medical therapy (GDMT) alone vs. transcatheter mitral repair with MitraClip plus GDMT in patients with severe MR who were not surgical candidates, there was evidence of clinical efficacy. After 24 mo, heart failure hospitalizations were 36% in the MitraClip group versus 68% in the medical therapy group. Device therapy also improved symptoms and quality of life and decreased all-cause mortality (29% in device vs. 46% in the GDMT-only group).[1] Secondary analysis of the COAPT data showed presence of moderate to severe tricuspid regurgitation (TR) worsened clinical outcomes and should be considered when selected patients for this minimally invasive therapy vs. surgical repair.[2]
- Ischemic MR has been a source of controversy as to whether moderate or greater MR should be fixed at the time of revascularization with coronary artery bypass graft surgery (CABG). Mitral valve repair can be considered at the time of CABG in moderate MR, and mitral valve repair is reasonable for severe MR (class IIa) in the presence of a basal

[1] Stone GW et al: Transcatheter mitral-valve repair in patients with heart failure. *N Engl J Med* 379:2307-2318, 2018.

[2] Hahn RT et al: Impact of tricuspid regurgitation on clinical outcomes: The COAPT Trial. *JACC* 76(11):1305-1314, 2020.

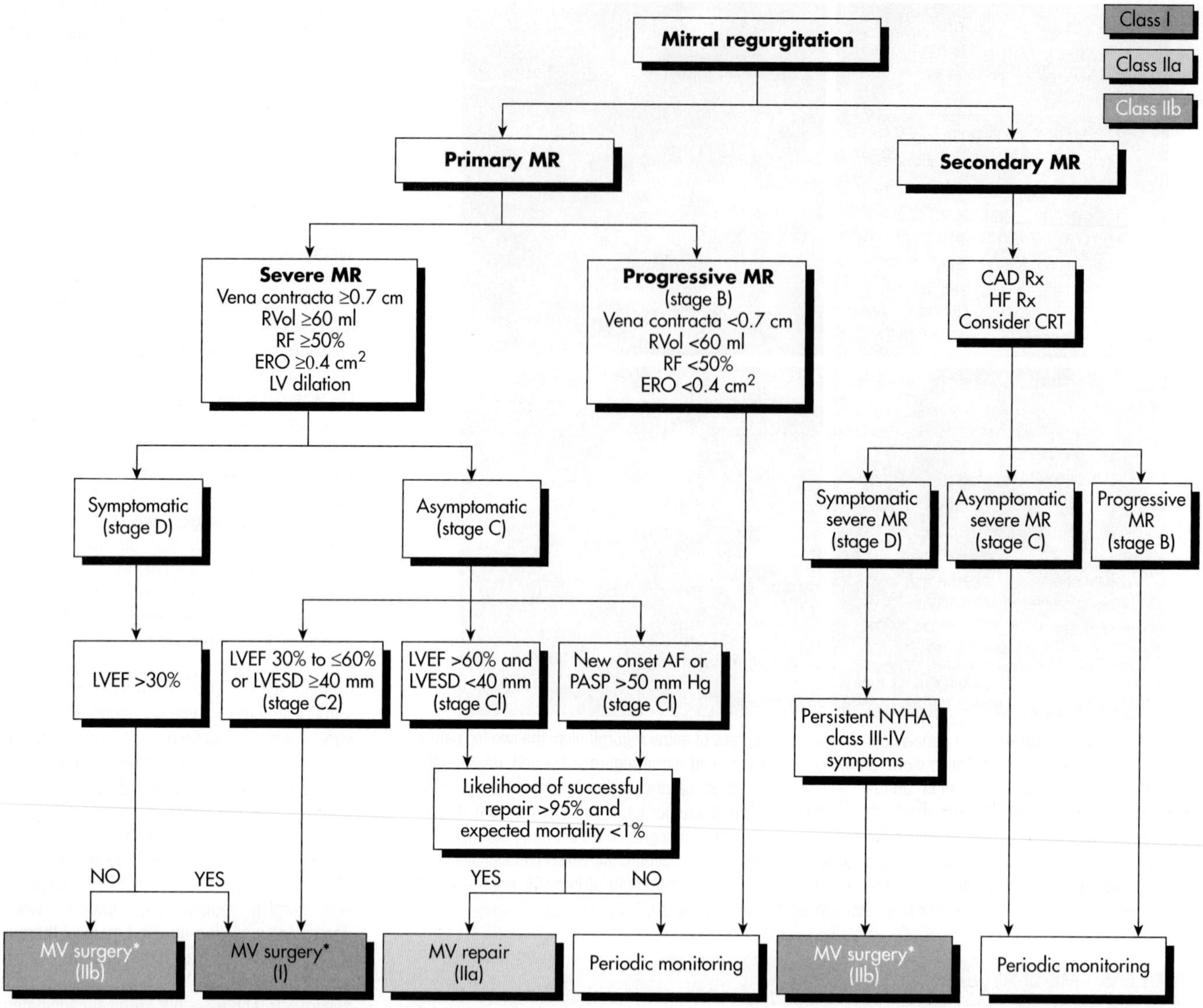

FIG. 2 Indications for surgery for MR. *Mitral valve repair is preferred over MVR when possible. *AF,* Atrial fibrillation; *CAD,* coronary artery disease; *CRT,* cardiac resynchronization therapy; *ERO,* effective regurgitant orifice; *HF,* heart failure; *LV,* left ventricle; *LVEF,* left ventricular ejection fraction; *LVESD,* left ventricle end-systolic dimension; *MR,* mitral regurgitation; *MV,* mitral valve; *MVR,* mitral valve replacement; *NYHA,* New York Heart Association; *PASP,* pulmonary artery systolic pressure; *RF,* regurgitant fraction; *RVol,* regurgitant volume; *Rx,* therapy. (From Nishimura RA et al: ACC/AHA focused update of valvular heart disease guideline, *J Am Coll Cardiol* 70:254-289, 2017.)

aneurysm or dyskinesis, significant leaflet tethering due to wall motion abnormalities, and moderate-to-severe LV remodeling (LV end-diastolic diameter >65 mm).

- American College of Cardiology/American Heart Association (ACC/AHA) guidelines for intervention for chronic primary MR are summarized in Table 4. Interventions for chronic secondary MR are described in Table 5.

DISPOSITION

Prognosis is generally good unless there is significant impairment of LV function or significantly elevated pulmonary artery pressures. Most patients remain asymptomatic for many yr (average interval from diagnosis to onset of symptoms is 16 yr). In patients with chronic severe MR, MR is commonly progressive, with onset of other symptoms or LV dysfunction within 6 to 10 yr. However, surgery should be advised well before the onset of symptoms in case of worsening LVEF and LV systolic dimensions and presence of pulmonary hypertension or atrial fibrillation, all of which are poor prognostic signs.

REFERRAL

- Surgical referral in selected patients (see "Acute General Rx"). Emergency surgery is usually necessary in patients with acute MR caused by ruptured papillary muscle or chordae tendineae after myocardial infarction.
- Mitral valve repair can also be accomplished with percutaneous implantation of a MitraClip device in patients who are too high risk for surgery.

PEARLS & CONSIDERATIONS

COMMENTS

- Although vasodilators and other agents should be used to treat hypertension in patients with severe MR, there is no evidence that they will delay the need for eventual valve surgery, which is the definitive treatment for severe MR.
- In 2007, the AHA guidelines for prevention of infectious endocarditis were revised and routine antibiotic prophylaxis to undergo dental or other invasive procedures is no longer recommended, unless the patient has had prior endocarditis.

SUGGESTED READINGS

Available at ExpertConsult.com

RELATED CONTENT

Mitral Regurgitation (Patient Information)

AUTHORS: **Maad M. Alhudairy, MD, MAS,** and **Uyen T. Lam, MD**

TABLE 4 American Society of Echocardiography Guidelines. Updated ACC/AHA Guidelines for Intervention for Chronic Primary Mitral Regurgitation (MR)[1]

Class	Indication	LOE
I	MV surgery for symptomatic patients with severe primary MR (stage D) and LVEF greater than 30%.	B
	MV surgery for asymptomatic patients with severe primary MR and LV dysfunction (LVEF 30%-60% and/or LVESD ≥40 mm, stage C2).	B
	MV repair in preference to MVR when surgical treatment for patients with severe primary MR limited to the posterior leaflet.	B
	MV repair in preference to MVR when surgical treatment for patients with severe primary MR involving the anterior leaflet or both leaflets when a successful and durable repair can be accomplished.	B
	Concomitant MV repair or replacement in patients with severe primary MR undergoing cardiac surgery for other indications.	B
IIa	MV repair is reasonable in asymptomatic patients with severe primary MR (stage C1) with preserved LV function (LVEF >60% and LVESD <40 mm) in whom the likelihood of a successful and durable repair without residual MR is greater than 95% with an expected mortality less than 1% when performed at a Heart Valve Center of Excellence.	B
	MV surgery is reasonable for asymptomatic patients with severe primary MR and preserved LV function (LVEF >60% and LVESD <40 mm) with a progressive increase in LV size or decrease in LVEF on serial imaging studies. (*New 2017*)	C
	MV repair is reasonable for asymptomatic patients with severe nonrheumatic primary MR (stage C1) and preserved LV function in whom there is a high likelihood of a successful and durable repair with (1) new onset of AF or (2) resting pulmonary hypertension (PA systolic pressure >50 mm Hg).	B
	Concomitant MV repair is reasonable in patients with moderate primary MR (stage B) undergoing cardiac surgery for other indications.	C
IIb	MV surgery may be considered in symptomatic patients with severe primary MR and LVEF of 30% or less (stage D).	C
	Transcatheter MV repair may be considered for severely symptomatic patients (NYHA class III/IV) with severe primary MR (stage D) who have a reasonable life expectancy, but a prohibitive surgical risk because of severe comorbidities.	B
III	MVR should not be performed for the treatment of isolated severe primary MR limited to less than one half of the posterior leaflet unless MV repair has been attempted and was unsuccessful.	B

ACC/AHA, American College of Cardiology/American Heart Association; *AF,* atrial fibrillation; *LOE,* level of evidence; *LV,* left ventricular; *LVEF,* LV ejection fraction; *LVESD,* LV end-systolic dimension; *MR,* mitral regurgitation; *MV,* mitral valve; *MVR,* mitral valve replacement; *NYHA,* New York Heart Association; *PA,* pulmonary artery.

[1]Kapadia S et al: Outcomes of inoperable symptomatic aortic stenosis patients not undergoing aortic valve replacement: insight into the impact of balloon aortic valvuloplasty from the PARTNER Trial (Placement of AoRtic TraNscathetER Valve Trial), *JACC Cardiovasc Interv* 8:324-333, 2015.

From Zipes DP: *Braunwald's heart disease, a textbook of cardiovascular medicine,* ed 11, Philadelphia, 2019,

TABLE 5 Elsevier. Updated ACC/AHA Guidelines for Intervention for Chronic Secondary Mitral Regurgitation (MR)[1]

Class	Indication	LOE
IIa	MV surgery is reasonable for patients with chronic severe secondary MR (stages C and D) who are undergoing CABG or AVR.	C
	It is reasonable to choose chordal-sparing MVR over downsized annuloplasty repair if operation is considered for severely symptomatic patients (NYHA class III/IV) with chronic severe ischemic MR (stage D) and persistent symptoms despite GDMT for heart failure. (*New 2017*)	B
IIb	MV surgery may be considered for severely symptomatic patients (NYHA class III-IV) with chronic severe secondary MR (stage D).	B
	In patients with chronic, moderate, or ischemic MR (stage B) undergoing CABG, the usefulness of mitral valve repair is uncertain. (*Modified 2017*)	B

ACC/AHA, American College of Cardiology/American Heart Association; *AVR,* aortic valve replacement; *CABG,* coronary artery bypass graft surgery; *GDMT,* guideline-directed medical therapy; *LOE,* level of evidence; *MV,* mitral valve; *NYHA,* New York Heart Association.

[1]Kapadia S, Stewart WJ, Anderson WN et al: Outcomes of inoperable symptomatic aortic stenosis patients not undergoing aortic valve replacement: insight into the impact of balloon aortic valvuloplasty from the PARTNER Trial (Placement of AoRtic TraNscathetER Valve Trial), *JACC Cardiovasc Interv* 8:324-333, 2015.

From Zipes DP: *Braunwald's heart disease, a textbook of cardiovascular medicine,* ed 11, Philadelphia, 2019, Elsevier

Mitral Stenosis

BASIC INFORMATION

DEFINITION

Mitral stenosis is a narrowing of the mitral valve orifice that prevents proper opening during diastole and obstruction of blood flow from the left atrium to the left ventricle. Due to thickening of the leaflets there is restricted movement. The obstruction leads to increased pressure in the left atrium, pulmonary vasculature, and the right side of the heart. The cross section of a normal orifice measures 4 to 6 cm^2. Symptoms usually develop with exercise when the orifice measures <2.5 cm^2, and symptoms may develop at rest when the orifice is <1.5 cm^2.

SYNONYM

MS

ICD-10CM CODES

I05.0	Rheumatic mitral stenosis
I05.2	Rheumatic mitral stenosis with insufficiency
I34.2	Nonrheumatic mitral (valve) stenosis
Q23.2	Congenital mitral stenosis

EPIDEMIOLOGY & DEMOGRAPHICS

- The predominant cause of mitral stenosis is rheumatic heart disease; however, the occurrence of mitral valve stenosis has decreased worldwide over the past 30 yr (particularly in developed countries) as a result of declining incidence of rheumatic fever due to appropriate antibiotic use.
- Rheumatic heart disease has a predilection for the mitral valve, aortic valve, and to some extent the tricuspid valve.
- The incidence of MS is higher in women (2:1 female-to-male ratio).
- There is high prevalence of rheumatic heart disease in developing countries.
- Outbreaks of rheumatic fever in the U.S. are due to increased virulence of a streptococcal strain or enhanced immigration from where rheumatic heart disease is prevalent.

PHYSICAL FINDINGS & CLINICAL PRESENTATION

- Dyspnea is the most common symptom, along with fatigue and decreased exercise capacity. These symptoms occur due to an inability to increase cardiac output, especially with exercise, and elevated pulmonary capillary wedge pressures, with resultant increase in pulmonary artery pressures. Stages of mitral stenosis are summarized in Table 1.
- "Mitral facies" that are pinkish-purple patches on the cheek due to low cardiac output and vasoconstriction, usually indicate severe MS.
- Paroxysmal nocturnal dyspnea (PND) and orthopnea secondary to elevated left atrial pressure may occur.
- Acute pulmonary edema may occur after an increase in flow across the mitral valve secondary to an increase in cardiac output or heart rate (exertion, tachyarrhythmias, fever, anemia, etc.).
- Pulmonary hypertension that results from chronically elevated pulmonary capillary wedge pressures can lead to right ventricular (RV) dysfunction and signs and symptoms of right heart failure (hepatomegaly, pulsatile liver, peripheral edema, ascites).
- The left ventricle is typically "protected" in mitral stenosis and exists in a low-pressure state; however, MS often coexists with mitral regurgitation and occasionally with aortic valve dysfunction, both of which can cause left ventricular dysfunction.
- Hemoptysis can be present secondary to rupture of thin-walled dilated bronchial veins due to an abrupt increase in left atrial pressure.
- Systemic embolic events are caused by left atrial thrombi. These are associated with atrial fibrillation 80% of the time, since mitral stenosis leads to left atrial enlargement, which is a predisposing factor for atrial arrhythmias.
- Atrial fibrillation is more prevalent in patients with more severe MS, increasing age, and other valvular abnormalities.
- Chest pain can be caused by RV pressure overload and/or concomitant coronary artery disease in up to 15% of patients.
- Loud first heart sound (S1) caused by delayed valve closure preceded by an opening snap and rapid rising left ventricular (LV) pressure.
- A low-pitched rumbling diastolic murmur is heard best at the apex. The intensity of the murmur is not related to the severity of the stenosis, but the duration is holodiastolic in severe MS.
- An opening snap (OS) caused by tensing of the valve leaflets after the cusps have opened completely. The OS follows S2 by 0.03 to 0.14 sec, and the shorter the S2 to OS interval, the more severe the MS, due to the increasing left atrial pressures.
- Prominent A wave on the pulmonary capillary wedge pressure tracing. This is analogous to the prominent A wave seen in systemic venous pressure tracings with tricuspid stenosis.
- A diastolic thrill may be palpable at the apex, especially with the patient in the left lateral recumbent position.
- A left parasternal heave secondary to RV hypertrophy and pulmonary hypertension.
- An accentuated P2 and/or a soft, early diastolic decrescendo murmur (Graham Steell murmur) caused by pulmonary regurgitation may be present in patients with pulmonary hypertension (not specific for mitral stenosis).
- Hoarseness due to the enlargement of the left atrium compressing the recurrent laryngeal nerve.
- Straightening of the left heart border seen on chest radiography indicative of left atrial enlargement.

TABLE 1 Stages of Mitral Stenosis

Stage	Definition	Valve Anatomy	Valve Hemodynamics	Hemodynamic Consequences	Symptoms
A	At risk for MS	Mild valve doming during diastole	Normal transmitral flow velocity	None	None
B	Progressive MS	Rheumatic valve changes with commissural fusion and diastolic doming of the mitral valve leaflets Planimetered MVA >1.5 cm^2	Increased transmitral flow velocities MVA >1.5 cm^2 Diastolic pressure half-time <150 msec	Mild to moderate LA enlargement Normal pulmonary pressure at rest	None
C	Asymptomatic severe MS	Rheumatic valve changes with commissural fusion and diastolic doming of the mitral valve leaflets Planimetered MVA ≤1.5 cm^2 (MVA ≤1 cm^2 with very severe MS)	MVA ≤1.5 cm^2 (MVA ≤1 cm^2 with very severe MS) Diastolic pressure half-time ≥150 msec (Diastolic pressure half-time ≥220 msec with very severe MS)	Severe LA enlargement Elevated PASP >30 mm Hg	None
D	Symptomatic severe MS	Rheumatic valve changes with commissural fusion and diastolic doming of the mitral valve leaflets Planimetered MVA ≤1.5 cm^2	MVA ≤1.5 cm^2 (MVA ≤1 cm^2 with very severe MS) Diastolic pressure half-time ≥150 msec (Diastolic pressure half-time ≥220 msec with very severe MS)	Severe LA enlargement Elevated PASP >30 mm Hg	Decreased exercise tolerance Exertional dyspnea

The transmitral mean pressure gradient should be obtained to determine the full hemodynamic effect of the MS and usually is >5 to 10 mm Hg in severe MS; however, because of the variability of the mean pressure gradient with heart rate and forward flow, it has not been included in the criteria for severity.

LA, Left atrium; *MS,* mitral stenosis; *MVA,* mitral valve area; *PASP,* pulmonary artery systolic pressure.

From Mann DL et al: *Braunwald's heart disease,* ed 10, Philadelphia, 2015, Elsevier.

- Fig. 1 shows schematic representations of LV, aortic, and left atrial (LA) pressures, showing normal relationships and alterations with mild and severe MS.

ETIOLOGY

- Rheumatic fever (RF) is the predominant cause of MS. RF causes thickening of the leaflet tips, commissure fusion, and chordal shortening and fusion. This leads to the classic doming of the leaflets in diastole due to fusion of the leaflet tips at the commissures. Rheumatic fever involves the leaflet tips first with progression toward the annulus. This is opposite of mitral annular calcification, which typically starts in the annulus and proceeds out to the leaflet tips, leading to mitral stenosis in severe cases.
- Congenital defect (parachute valve) has the usual two mitral leaflets, but the chordae, instead of diverging to insert into two papillary muscles, converge into one major papillary muscle, which allows little mobility of the leaflets, as in cor triatriatum (heart with three atria), in which there is a thin membrane that obstructs the pulmonary vein flow and simulates mitral stenosis.
- Rare causes are severe mitral annular calcification usually seen in end-stage renal disease patients, endomyocardial fibroelastosis, malignant carcinoid syndrome, systemic lupus erythematosus, Whipple disease, Fabry disease, rheumatoid arthritis, and 3,4-methylenedioxy-methamphetamine (MDMA) use.
- Atrial septal defect in association with rheumatic mitral stenosis is termed Lutembacher syndrome.
- Medications: Ergot alkaloids (methysergide and ergotamine).

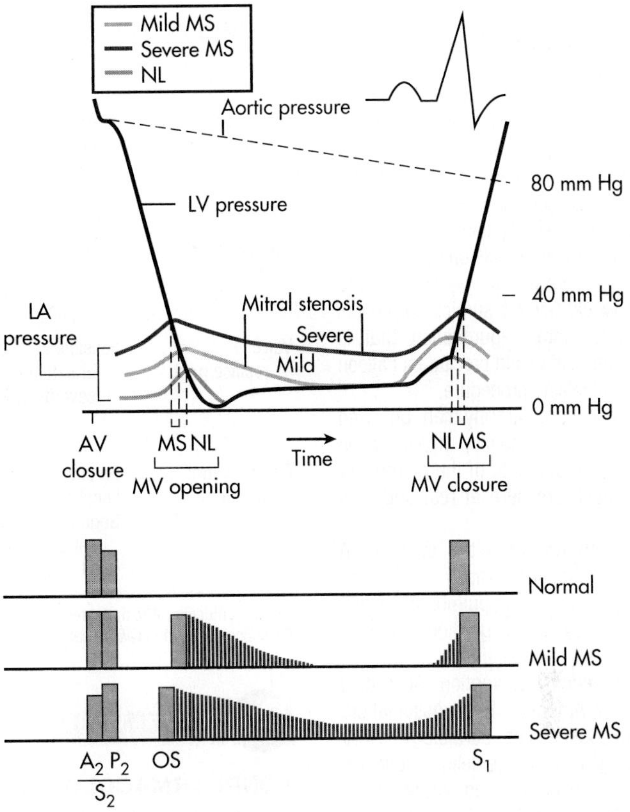

FIG. 1 Schematic representation of left ventricular *(LV)*, aortic, and left atrial *(LA)* pressures, showing normal relationships and alterations with mild and severe mitral stenosis *(MS)*. Corresponding classic auscultatory signs of MS are shown at the bottom. The higher left atrial V wave of severe MS causes earlier pressure crossover and earlier mitral valve *(MV)* opening, leading to a shorter time interval between aortic valve *(AV)* closure and the opening snap *(OS)*. The higher left atrial end-diastolic pressure with severe MS also results in later closure of the mitral valve. With severe MS, the diastolic rumble becomes longer and there is accentuation of the pulmonic component *(P_2)* of the second heart sound *(S_2)* in relation to the aortic component *(A_2)*. *NL,* Normal limits. (From Zipes DP: *Braunwald's heart disease, a textbook of cardiovascular medicine,* ed 11, Philadelphia, 2019, Elsevier.)

Dx DIAGNOSIS

DIFFERENTIAL DIAGNOSIS

- Left atrial myxoma
- Ball valve thrombus
- Other valvular abnormalities (e.g., tricuspid stenosis, mitral regurgitation)
- Atrial septal defect

IMAGING STUDIES

- Echocardiography (Fig. 2):
  1. Two-dimensional echocardiogram can measure valve area by direct planimetry or calculate it by the Doppler pressure half-time method (this may be inaccurate in patients with concomitant diastolic dysfunction, atrial septal defects, or aortic insufficiency, and those who recently have undergone mitral valvuloplasty), or the continuity equation can be used to calculate the valve area. It also can be measured using the proximal isovelocity surface area method. A valve area ≤ 1.5 cm^2 is consistent with severe MS (and ≤ 1.0 cm^2 with very severe MS). The transmitral gradient can also be calculated. A mean gradient of >10 mm Hg indicates severe MS, a gradient of 5 to 10 mm Hg is consistent with moderate MS, and 0 to 5 mm Hg is consistent with mild MS or no MS.
  2. M-Mode echocardiography will also show a markedly diminished E-to-F slope of the anterior mitral valve leaflet during diastole. There can be loss of the "A-wave" due to increased left atrial pressure or the presence of associated atrial fibrillation.

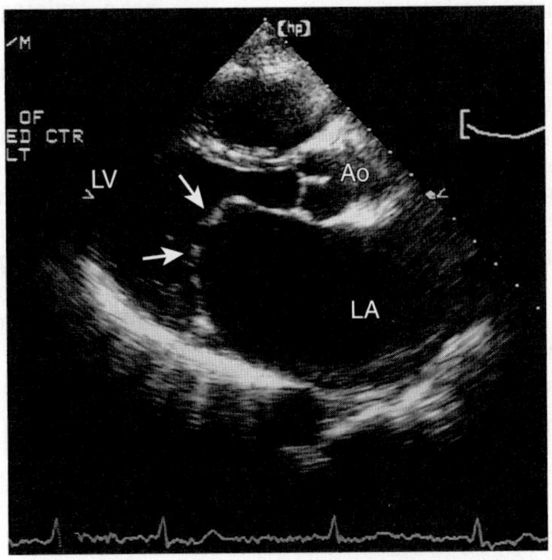

FIG. 2 Mitral stenosis. Parasternal long-axis view of a patient with mitral stenosis and a pliable noncalcified mitral valve leaflet. Note the "doming" motion of the mitral valve leaflets *(arrows)*. Valves with these morphologic features are excellent candidates for percutaneous balloon valvotomy. *Ao,* Aorta; *LA,* left atrium; *LV,* left ventricle. (From Zipes DP et al [eds]: *Braunwald's heart disease,* ed 7, Philadelphia, 2005, Saunders.)

There is also fusion of the commissures, resulting in "doming" of the leaflets during diastole.
3. Grading of leaflet thickness, mobility, calcification, and subvalvular thickening (Wilkins score) with a score of 0 to 4 for each characteristic can predict hemodynamic results and outcome of balloon mitral valvuloplasty (a low score of less than 8 is favorable for balloon valvuloplasty and a high score is unfavorable). A score above 8 would favor a surgical approach. In addition, mitral regurgitation that is greater than mild would preclude a balloon mitral valvuloplasty procedure.
4. Doppler echocardiography can be used to assess for pulmonary hypertension and to give an estimate of the pulmonary artery systolic pressure at rest and with exercise.
5. Patients with known mitral stenosis: A follow-up echocardiography is recommended to assess for pulmonary artery pressures and valve gradient, and to determine the optimal timing of surgical or percutaneous intervention. According to the 2017 American Heart Association/American College of Cardiology (AHA/ACC) Focused valve guideline, echocardiogram is recommended every yr for very severe MS with mitral valve area <1.0 cm^2, every 1 to 2 yr with severe MS with mitral valve area ≤1.5 cm^2, and every 3 to 5 yr with progressive MS with mitral valve area >1.5 cm^2.

- Chest radiograph:
  1. Straightening of the left cardiac border caused by enlarged left atrium
  2. Left atrial enlargement on lateral chest radiograph
  3. Prominence of pulmonary arteries that indicates pulmonary hypertension
  4. Possible pulmonary congestion and edema (Kerley B lines)
- ECG:
  1. RV hypertrophy; right axis deviation caused by pulmonary hypertension
  2. Left atrial enlargement (broad, biphasic P waves in lead V1 and duration of P-waves >0.11 sec in lead II); this is termed "P-mitrale"
  3. Atrial fibrillation
- Cardiac catheterization:
  1. Allows the measurement of pulmonary artery pressure and transmitral pressure gradients at rest or with exercise (supine biking or raising weights with arms while lying supine)
  2. Allows the measurement of transmitral flow and calculation of the valve area
  3. Is not routinely recommended for the evaluation of MS but is useful when the echocardiographic findings are nondiagnostic or discrepant with the clinical scenario
  4. Cardiac catheterization in addition to echocardiography can be used to monitor the hemodynamics during a balloon mitral valvuloplasty procedure

TABLE 2 Approaches to Mechanical Relief of Mitral Stenosis

Approach	Advantages	Disadvantages
Closed surgical valvotomy	Inexpensive Relatively simple Good hemodynamic results in selected patients Good long-term outcome	No direct visualization of valve Only feasible with flexible, noncalcified valves Contraindicated with MR grade higher than 2+ Surgical procedure with general anesthesia
Open surgical valvotomy	Visualization of valve allows directed valvotomy. Concurrent annuloplasty for MR is feasible.	Best results with flexible, noncalcified valves Surgical procedure with general anesthesia
Valve replacement	Feasible in all patients regardless of extent of valve calcification or severity of MR	Surgical procedure with general anesthesia Effect of loss of annular-papillary muscle continuity on LV function Prosthetic valve Chronic anticoagulation
Balloon mitral valvotomy	Percutaneous approach Local anesthesia Good hemodynamic results in selected patients Good long-term outcome	No direct visualization of valve Only feasible with flexible noncalcified valves Contraindicated with MR grade higher than 2+

LV, Left ventricular; *MR*, mitral regurgitation.
From Zipes DP: *Braunwald's heart disease, a textbook of cardiovascular medicine*, ed 11, Philadelphia, 2019, Elsevier.

Rx TREATMENT

NONPHARMACOLOGIC THERAPY

Decrease level of activity in symptomatic patients, and salt restriction if pulmonary congestion is present.

ACUTE GENERAL Rx

- Medical:
  1. Anticoagulation for the prevention of systemic embolic events in patients with MS and:
     a. Atrial fibrillation: In patients with atrial fibrillation and rheumatic mitral stenosis, anticoagulation with a vitamin K antagonist with a goal international normalized ratio (INR) of 2.5 is indicated. Further study is needed to establish the efficacy of direct oral anticoagulants (DOACs) in this setting
     b. Prior embolic event
     c. Documented left atrial thrombus or left atrial appendage thrombus
  2. Ventricular rate control (to increase diastolic filling period) with beta-blockers, nondihydropyridine calcium channel blockers, or digitalis and aggressive treatment of tachyarrhythmias.
  3. Treat congestive heart failure with loop diuretics and sodium restriction.
  4. Antibiotic prophylaxis to prevent recurrent rheumatic fever is usually not indicated unless presence of high-risk features such as prior endocarditis, prosthetic heart valves, valvulopathy of the transplanted heart, and certain cases of cyanotic congenital heart disease.
  5. Physical activity and exercise. Patients with mild MS in sinus rhythm with a peak pulmonary artery pressure <50 mm Hg can participate in all competitive sports. Patients with moderate MS and in sinus rhythm or atrial fibrillation with a peak pulmonary artery pressure of <50 mm Hg can participate in low to moderate static and dynamic sports. Patients in sinus rhythm with severe MS should not participate in any competitive sports. Patients in atrial fibrillation with any degree of MS and on anticoagulation should avoid all competitive sports.
  6. Pregnancy in females with advanced MS may be poorly tolerated due to the hemodynamic changes such as increased cardiac output occurring in pregnancy. Mild to moderate MS may be tolerated in pregnancy with medical therapy alone.
- Table 2 summarizes approaches to mechanical relief of mitral stenosis.
- Percutaneous mitral balloon commissurotomy (PMBC) is the therapy of choice for symptomatic patients with severe MS (valve area ≤1.5 cm^2) with a favorable valvuloplasty score, minimal or no mitral regurgitation, and no left atrial thrombus. PMBC is reasonable for asymptomatic patients with very severe MS (mitral valve area ≤1.0 cm^2) and favorable valve morphology in the absence of left atrial thrombus or moderate to severe MR (class IIa indication). PMBC is also considered the procedure of choice in pregnant women with rheumatic MS and in New York Heart Association (NYHA) class III to IV heart failure and/or unresponsive to adequate medical treatment. In addition, it may be considered for severely symptomatic (NYHA class III/IV) patients with very severe MS (mitral valve area ≤1.5 cm^2) who are not candidates for surgery or are at high risk for surgery, even if they have suboptimal valve anatomy (class IIb indication). Regular follow-up is needed after PMBC because restenosis may reoccur. Repeat intervention can be performed as long as valve anatomy remains favorable; however, there is usually more fibrosis and

TABLE 3 ACC/AHA Guidelines for Intervention for Mitral Stenosis (MS)[1]

Class	Indication	LOE
I	PMBC for symptomatic patients with severe MS (MVA ≤1.5 cm², stage D) and favorable valve morphology in the absence of contraindications.	A
	Mitral valve surgery in severely symptomatic patients (NYHA Class III/IV) with severe MS (MVA ≤1.5 cm², stage D) who are not high risk for surgery and who are not candidates for or failed previous PMBC.	B
	Concomitant mitral valve surgery for patients with severe MS (MVA ≤1.5 cm², stages C or D) undergoing other cardiac surgery.	C
IIa	PMBC is reasonable for asymptomatic patients with very severe MS (MVA ≤1 cm², stage C) and favorable valve morphology in the absence of contraindications.	C
	Mitral valve surgery is reasonable for severely symptomatic patients (NYHA class III/IV) with severe MS (MVA ≤1.5 cm², stage D) provided there are other operative indications.	C
IIb	PMBC may be considered for asymptomatic patients with severe MS (MVA ≤1.5 cm², stage C) and favorable valve morphology who have new onset of AF in the absence of contraindications.	C
	PMBC may be considered for symptomatic patients with MVA greater than 1.5 cm² if there is evidence of hemodynamically significant MS during exercise.	C
	PMBC may be considered for severely symptomatic patients (NYHA class III/IV) with severe MS (MVA ≤1.5 cm², stage D) who have suboptimal valve anatomy and are not candidates for surgery or at high risk for surgery.	C
	Concomitant mitral valve surgery may be considered for patients with moderate MS (MVA, 1.6-2.0 cm²) undergoing other cardiac surgery.	C
	Mitral valve surgery and excision of the left atrial appendage may be considered for patients with severe MS (MVA ≤1.5 cm², stages C and D) who have had recurrent embolic events while receiving adequate anticoagulation.	C

New York Heart Association (NYHA) *LOE,* level of evidence; *MVA,* mitral valve area; *NYHA,* New York Heart Association; *PMBC,* percutaneous mitral balloon commissurotomy.

[1]Nishimura R et al: 2013 AHA/ACCF guideline for valvular heart disease: a report of the American College of Cardiology Foundation/American Heart Association Task Force on Practice Guidelines, *J Am Coll Cardiol* 63:e57-e185, 2014.

From Zipes DP: *Braunwald's heart disease, a textbook of cardiovascular medicine,* ed 11, Philadelphia, 2019, Elsevier.

deformation of the valve with subsequent procedures. The approximate frequency of repeat intervention is 10% at 7 yr.

- Mitral valve surgery is indicated for patients with moderate to severe symptomatic MS when PMBC is not available or is contraindicated (valvuloplasty score greater than or equal to 8) or the valve is calcified, when MR is more than mild, when left atrial thrombus is present, and when the surgical risk is acceptable. The surgical approaches include closed mitral valvotomy, open valvotomy and repair (preferred), and mitral valve replacement when repair is not possible.
- Table 3 summarizes guidelines for intervention for mitral stenosis.

DISPOSITION

- Prognosis is generally good except in patients with chronic pulmonary hypertension.
- Operative mortality rates for mitral valve replacement are 1% to 5% at most institutions.

RELATED CONTENT

Mitral Stenosis (Patient Information)

SUGGESTED READING

Available at ExpertConsult.com

AUTHORS: **S. Hammad Jafri, MD, MMSCI,** and **Aravind Rao Kokkirala, MD, FACC**

Mitral Valve Prolapse

BASIC INFORMATION

DEFINITION

Mitral valve prolapse (MVP) is the bulging of one or both of the mitral valve leaflets ≥2 mm above the annular plane into the left atrium during systole. MVP syndrome refers to a constellation of MVP and associated symptoms (e.g., autonomic dysfunction, palpitations) or other physical abnormalities (e.g., pectus excavatum). Table 1 describes a classification of mitral valve prolapse.

SYNONYMS

MVP
Mitral click murmur syndrome
Barlow syndrome

ICD-10CM CODES

I34.1 Nonrheumatic mitral (valve) prolapse
I34.0 Nonrheumatic mitral (valve) insufficiency

EPIDEMIOLOGY & DEMOGRAPHICS

- MVP can be found by echocardiogram in 1% to 2.4% of the general population, with some studies suggesting that it is more common in women than in men.
- Increased incidence is seen with autoimmune thyroid disorders, Ehlers-Danlos syndrome, Marfan syndrome, osteogenesis imperfecta, pseudoxanthoma elasticum, pectus excavatum, anorexia nervosa, and bulimia.
- Compared to men, women with MVP have less posterior prolapse (22% vs. 31%), less flail (2% vs. 8%), more leaflet thickening (32% vs. 28%), and less frequent severe mitral regurgitation (MR) (10% vs. 23%).

TABLE 1 Classification of Mitral Valve Prolapse

Mitral Valve Prolapse Syndrome
Younger age (20-50 yr)
Predominantly female
Click or click-murmur on physical examination
Thin leaflets with systolic displacement on echocardiography
Associated with low blood pressure, orthostatic hypotension, palpitations
Benign long-term course
Myxomatous Mitral Valve Disease
Older age (40-70 yr)
Predominantly male
Thickened, redundant valve leaflets
Mitral regurgitation on physical exam and echocardiography
High likelihood of progressive disease requiring mitral valve surgery
Secondary Mitral Valve Prolapse
Marfan syndrome
Hypertrophic cardiomyopathy
Ehlers-Danlos syndrome
Other connective tissue diseases

Modified from Otto CM: *Valvular heart disease,* ed 2, Philadelphia, 2004, Saunders, p. 369.

- Although MVP is more common in women than men, men more often develop severe regurgitation requiring surgical intervention.

PHYSICAL FINDINGS & CLINICAL PRESENTATION

- The most common auscultatory finding in cardiac examination is a nonejection mid to late systolic click, heard best at the apex. It is caused by degeneration of the valve resulting in an abnormal ratio between the length of the mitral apparatus and left ventricle (LV) during contraction. When the valve prolapses, it gets caught by the subvalvular structures, causing an abrupt halt that creates the click.
- If regurgitation is present, a crescendo mid to late systolic murmur may be heard that worsens with standing and Valsalva maneuver.
- Timing of click within the cardiac cycle varies with loading conditions within the left ventricle (i.e., may occur earlier with standing or Valsalva and later with squatting or expiration).
- May be associated with small anteroposterior chest diameter, scoliosis, pectus excavatum, or low BMI.
- Most patients with MVP are asymptomatic; symptoms if present consist primarily of chest pain, palpitations, fatigue, dyspnea, and anxiety.
- Neurologic abnormalities (e.g., transient ischemic attack [TIA] or stroke) are rare.
- A spectrum of arrhythmias, mainly paroxysmal supraventricular tachycardia and atrial and ventricular premature beats, etc. is also observed with mitral valve prolapse. There is also an increased association with Wolff-Parkinson-White syndrome and QT prolongation.

ETIOLOGY

- Myxomatous degeneration of connective tissue within mitral valve, usually involving multiple leaflet segments (e.g., Barlow disease). In contrast, fibroelastic deficiency of single leaflet segment develops in elderly patients.
- Congenital deformity of mitral valve and supportive structures.
- Secondary to other disorders of connective tissue such as Ehlers-Danlos, Marfan, or pseudoxanthoma elasticum; association with other connective tissue disorders suggests MVP result of defective embryogenesis in cells of mesenchymal origin.

DIAGNOSIS

DIFFERENTIAL DIAGNOSIS

- Other valvular abnormalities (especially MR)
- Anxiety or panic disorders
- Pulmonary embolism
- Atypical chest pain

WORKUP

- Medical history and physical examination, with increased suspicion in patients with other findings of connective tissue disorder
- Two- or three-dimensional echocardiography in patients with a systolic click or murmur on careful auscultation
- Cardiac MRI is an emerging tool for the evaluation and diagnosis of MVP but has not yet been independently validated. However, MRI should be considered because it may be helpful in accurately quantifying the amount of mitral regurgitation when present. ECG is most often normal but may show nonspecific ST-T wave changes, prolonged QT interval, prominent Q waves, or early repolarization with J-point elevation in young patients

IMAGING STUDIES

Echocardiography (Fig. 1) shows one or more leaflets prolapsing >2 mm into the left atrium during systole in a long axis view. Mitral leaflets may be thickened (>5 mm) with myxomatous degeneration. MR is typically present but may only occur during late systole or with exertion. If moderate or severe MR is present findings of dilated left atrium, LV dilation and/or dysfunction, and elevated estimated RV systolic pressures may also be present. There is an increased incidence of secundum-type atrial septal defects (ASDs) in patients with MVP, which may also be identified with echocardiography.

TREATMENT

NONPHARMACOLOGIC THERAPY

Avoidance of stimulants (e.g., caffeine, nicotine) in patients with palpitations. Sometimes

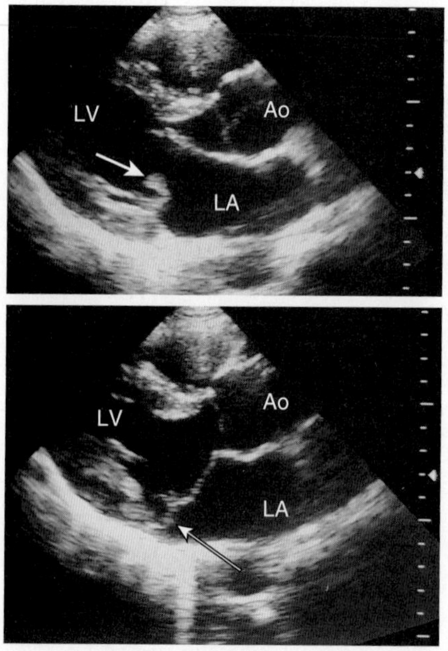

FIG. 1 Mitral valve prolapse. Parasternal long-axis view in diastole (*top*) and systole (*bottom*) in a patient with mitral valve prolapse and myxomatous changes. In the *upper panel,* note the open mitral valve and the diffuse thickening of the posterior mitral valve leaflet (*arrow*). The lower panel was recorded in systole. Note that both leaflets prolapse behind the plane of the mitral valve annulus. The prolapse of the posterior leaflet is somewhat more prominent (*arrow*). *Ao,* Aorta; *LA,* left atrium; *LV,* left ventricle. (From Zipes DP et al [eds]: *Braunwald's heart disease,* ed 7, Philadelphia, 2005, Saunders.)

TABLE 2 Predictors of Clinical Outcome in Mitral Valve Prolapse

Predictor	Survival	Valve Surgery	Arrhythmias or Sudden Death	Endocarditis
Age	+++	+++	–	–
Gender	++	++	–	–
Leaflet thickness or redundancy	+++	+++	++++	++++
Severity of mitral regurgitation	++++	++++	++++	++++
Systolic click	+	–	–	–
Left ventricular dilation	+	++++	++	–
Left atrial dilation	–	++	+	–

Symbols indicate the relative predictive value of each variable for the listed clinical outcomes on a scale of no predictive value (–) to strongly predictive (++++).

From Bonow RO et al: *Braunwald's heart disease: a textbook of cardiovascular medicine*, Philadelphia, 2012, Saunders.

reassurance is sufficient to reduce the severity of symptoms in many patients.

ACUTE GENERAL Rx

Beta-blockers may be used in symptomatic patients (e.g., palpitations, chest pain) to decrease the heart rate and contractility, thus potentially decreasing the stretch on the prolapsing valve leaflets.

CHRONIC Rx

Monitoring for complications:

- Mitral regurgitation (most common complication); on rare occasion may occur acutely due to rupture of chordae tendineae.
- Routine echocardiographic monitoring is indicated at the following intervals with patients with evidence of mitral regurgitation:
  1. Stage B with mild regurgitation: Every 3 to 5 yr
  2. Stage B with moderate regurgitation: Every 1 to 2 yr
  3. Stage C1 (asymptomatic severe MR without LV dysfunction): Every 6 to 12 mo
- Bacterial endocarditis (risk is three to eight times that of the general population); higher risk in patients with concomitant regurgitation. However, routine antibiotic prophylaxis is not recommended.
- TIA or stroke caused by embolic phenomena (from fibrin and platelet thrombi) in patients with thickened leaflets; risk in young patients is <0.05% per yr. If present, aspirin (75-325 mg) is indicated for secondary prevention.
- Cardiac arrhythmias with the vast majority being supraventricular and benign.
- Sudden death (rare); most often associated with acute flail leaflets or caused by ventricular arrhythmias associated with other structural heart disease.
- The incidence of complications of MVP is very low (<1% per yr). Mitral leaflet thickness is ≤0.5 mm, young patients <45 yr, and in the absence of mitral systolic murmur or MR on Doppler echocardiography. Table 2 lists variables that are predictors of favorable clinical outcome in mitral valve prolapse.
- Risk factors that predict higher risk of complications are presence of moderate to severe MR, LV ejection fraction <50%, LA dimension >40 mm, age >50 yr.

SURGICAL REFERRAL

Surgical referral may be necessary in patients who develop progressive MR with surgical indications as per guidelines for valvular heart disease (see topic on "Mitral Regurgitation").

PEARLS & CONSIDERATIONS

COMMENTS

- Recent studies suggest that the prevalence of MVP and its propensity to cause symptoms and serious complications have been overestimated in the past.
- The relationship between MVP syndrome and sudden cardiac death is unclear. The best evidence suggests that there is only a slight risk in subsets of patients with MVP who have severe MR, severe valvular deformity, complex ventricular arrhythmias, QT prolongation, and a history of syncope.
- Asymptomatic patients with MVP and mild or no MR can be evaluated clinically every 3 to 5 yr. High-risk patients (those with symptoms, arrhythmias, or significant regurgitation) should undergo a follow-up examination once a year.
- In 2007, the AHA guidelines for prevention of infectious endocarditis were revised, and prophylactic antibiotics are no longer recommended for patients with MVP without previous endocarditis.

PATIENT & FAMILY EDUCATION

http://www.themitralvalve.org

SUGGESTED READING

Available at ExpertConsult.com

RELATED CONTENT

Mitral Valve Prolapse (Patient Information)

AUTHORS: **Maad M. Alhudairy, MD, MAS,** and **Uyen T. Lam, MD**

BASIC INFORMATION

DEFINITION

Molluscum contagiosum is a poxvirus infection characterized by discrete skin lesions with central umbilication.

SYNONYM

MC

ICD-10CM CODE

B08.1 Molluscum contagiosum

EPIDEMIOLOGY & DEMOGRAPHICS

- Molluscum contagiosum spreads by autoinoculation, scratching, or touching a lesion.
- It usually occurs in young children. It is also common in sexually active adults and patients with HIV infection.
- Incubation period varies between 4 and 8 wk.
- Spontaneous resolution in immunocompetent patients can occur after several mo.

PHYSICAL FINDINGS & CLINICAL PRESENTATION

- The individual lesion appears initially as a small (2-3 mm), flesh-colored, firm, smooth-surfaced papule with subsequent central umbilication. Lesions are frequently grouped (Fig. 1). The size of each lesion generally varies from 2 to 6 mm in diameter.
- Typical distribution in children involves the face, extremities, and trunk. Mucous membranes are spared.
- Distribution in adults generally involves pubic and genital areas (Fig. E2).
- Erythema and scaling at the periphery of the lesions may be present as a result of scratching or hypersensitivity reaction.
- Lesions are not present on the palms and soles.

ETIOLOGY

Viral infection of epithelial cells caused by a poxvirus, molluscum contagiosum

DIAGNOSIS

Diagnosis is usually established by the clinical appearance of the lesions (distribution and central umbilication). A magnifying lens can be used to observe the central umbilication. If necessary, the diagnosis can be confirmed by removing a typical lesion with a curette and examining the content on a slide after adding potassium hydroxide and gentle heating. Staining with toluidine blue will identify viral inclusions.

DIFFERENTIAL DIAGNOSIS

- Verruca plana (flat warts): No central umbilication, not dome shaped, irregular surface, can involve palms and soles
- Herpes simplex: Lesions become rapidly umbilicated
- Varicella: Blisters and vesicles are present
- Folliculitis: No central umbilication, presence of hair piercing the pustule or papule
- Cutaneous cryptococcosis in AIDS patients: Budding yeasts will be present on cytologic examination of the lesions
- Basal cell carcinoma: Multiple lesions are absent
- Cellulitis

WORKUP

Careful examination of the papules

LABORATORY TESTS

Generally not indicated in children. Screening for other sexually transmitted diseases is recommended in all cases of genital molluscum contagiosum.

TREATMENT

GENERAL Rx

- Therapy is individualized depending on number of lesions, immune status, and patient's age and preference.
- Observation for spontaneous resolution is reasonable in patients with few, small, nonirritated, and nonspreading lesions. Genital lesions should be treated in all sexually active patients.
- Liquid nitrogen cryotherapy.
- Carbon dioxide laser.
- Curettage after pretreatment of the area with combination prilocaine 2.5% with lidocaine 2.5% cream (EMLA) for anesthesia is useful for treatment of a few lesions. Curettage should be avoided in cosmetically sensitive areas because scarring may develop.
- Treatments with liquid nitrogen therapy in combination with curettage are effective in older patients who do not object to some discomfort.
- Application of cantharidin 0.7% to individual lesions covered with clear tape will result in blistering over 24 hr and possible clearing without scarring. This medication should be avoided on facial lesions.
- Other treatment measures include use of imiquimod cream or tretinoin 0.025% gel or 0.1% cream at bedtime, daily use of salicylic acid (Occlusal) at bedtime, and use of laser therapy.
- Trichloroacetic acid peel generally repeated every 2 wk for several wk is useful in immunocompromised patients with extensive lesions.

DISPOSITION

Most patients respond well to the therapeutic modalities listed previously. Spontaneous resolution can occur after 6 to 9 mo in some immunocompetent patients.

REFERRAL

To dermatology when diagnosis is in doubt or in patients with extensive lesions

PEARLS & CONSIDERATIONS

COMMENTS

Genital molluscum contagiosum in children may be indicative of sexual abuse.

RELATED CONTENT

Molluscum Contagiosum (Patient Information)

AUTHOR: **Fred F. Ferri, MD**

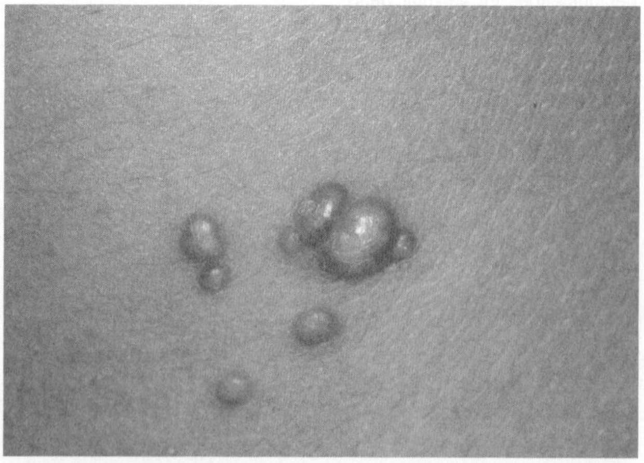

FIG. 1 Grouped molluscum. (From Kliegman RM et al: *Nelson textbook of pediatrics*, ed 19, Philadelphia, 2011, Saunders.)

BASIC INFORMATION

DEFINITION

MGUS is a premalignant disorder characterized by the clonal expansion of plasma cells or lymphoplasmacytic cells. It is typically detected incidentally when patients undergo testing with serum or urine protein electrophoresis. The term "monoclonal gammopathy of undetermined significance" (MGUS) is defined by the presence of a serum monoclonal (M) protein less than 3 g/dl and clonal plasma cells less than 10% in the bone marrow. In addition, there must be no evidence of end organ dysfunction such as renal insufficiency, anemia, hypercalcemia, or bony lesions on skeletal surveys (Table 1).

SYNONYMS

MGUS
Non-IgM MGUS
IgM MGUS
Light chain MGUS

ICD-10CM CODE
D47.2 Monoclonal gammopathy of undetermined significance (MGUS)

EPIDEMIOLOGY & DEMOGRAPHICS

INCIDENCE: In the U.S., the estimated age-adjusted incidence of MGUS is higher in men than in women. The annual incidence of MGUS in men is 120 per 100,000 at age 50 yr and increases to 530 per 100,000 at age 80 yr, whereas the incidence for women is 60 per 100,000 at age 50 yr and 370 per 100,000 at age 80 yr.

PREVALENCE: MGUS is associated with increasing age; approximately 1.5% of persons older than 50 yr and 3.0% of persons older than 70 yr have an elevated M protein level without end organ dysfunction. Studies have shown that at clinical diagnosis, MGUS is most likely to have been present undetected for a median duration of more than 10 yr. The prevalence of MGUS is also higher in African Americans. In one study, there was an almost threefold increase in prevalence among the African American population compared with the Caucasian population (8.6% vs. 3.6%).

PREDOMINANT SEX & AGE: The median age at diagnosis is about 70 yr. Prevalence is higher in men than in women at any given age.

RISK FACTORS: Race (African American), older age, male sex, or exposure to pesticides. Environmental and/or genetic defects play an important role, since the risk of MGUS in relatives of multiple myeloma or MGUS patients is increased twofold to threefold when compared to the general population. The cumulative risk of progression into multiple myeloma or related disorders is approximately 1% per yr. A variety of disorders (Table 2) are also associated with monoclonal gammopathy.

PHYSICAL FINDINGS & CLINICAL PRESENTATION

- MGUS typically is detected after a routine blood test reveals an elevated total protein concentration and is a common finding in medical practice.
- Patients are asymptomatic.
- Physical exam is normal.

ETIOLOGY

- The mechanism is unknown, and most cases are sporadic. The causes of malignant transformation of MGUS into multiple myeloma is still not well understood. Genetic predisposition, cytokine release, and bone marrow angiogenesis may play a role in the progression of MGUS into multiple myeloma.
- Characterized by a rearrangement of immunoglobulin genes resulting in the production of a monoclonal protein.

DIAGNOSIS

DIFFERENTIAL DIAGNOSIS

- Smoldering myeloma (Table E3)
- Multiple myeloma
- Waldenström agammaglobulinemia
- Secondary monoclonal gammopathies
  1. Chronic liver disease
  2. Rheumatologic diseases
  3. Chronic myelomonocytic leukemia
  4. Chronic neutrophilic leukemia
  5. Lichen myxedematosus
- Pyoderma gangrenosum
- AL amyloidosis
- Idiopathic Bence Jones proteinuria

LABORATORY TESTS

- Protein studies with serum free light chain assay
- Serum protein electrophoresis (Fig. E1): IgG most common, followed by IgM and IgA
- 24-hour urine protein excretion and urine electrophoresis
- Serum and urine immunofixation
- Determination of serum free light chain ratio (kappa and lambda free light chains)
- Hemoglobin
- Serum calcium and creatinine
- Examination of the bone marrow aspirate only when clinically indicated. It is not necessary in MGUS patients with low risk fractures (no end organ damage. Ig gammopathy less than 1.5 g/dl, normal serum free light chain ratio)

IMAGING STUDIES

- Skeletal survey
- Bone mineral density at baseline (MGUS is associated with increased risk of osteoporosis).

TREATMENT

- Risk stratification:
  1. Low risk: Serum M protein <1.5 g/dl, IgG subtype, normal genetics, free light chain ratio between 0.26 and 1.65. Absolute risk of progression (ARP) at 20 yr is 5%.
  2. Low-intermediate risk: Any 1 factor abnormal. ARP at 20 yr is 21%.
  3. High-intermediate risk: Any 2 factors abnormal. ARP at 20 yr is 37%.
  4. High risk: More than 3 factors abnormal. ARP at 20 yr is 58%.
- Follow-up by risk category: Patients with MGUS should be tested again within 4 to 6 mo from the time of first diagnosis to exclude evolving multiple myeloma. Those with low-risk MGUS can be followed up every 1 to 2 yr, whereas those with intermediate- or high-risk MGUS need to be followed up at least annually for life or until they develop a life-expectancy-threatening condition.
- Reevaluation consists of:
  1. Serum protein electrophoresis with immunofixation
  2. 24-hour urine protein excretion
  3. Serum free light chain assessment:
     a. Complete blood count
     b. Serum creatinine and calcium
     c. Careful history and physical examination to look for signs and symptoms known to evolve from MGUS

DISPOSITION

- Annual risk of progression to malignancy depends on type of M protein:
  1. Non-IgM MGUS: 1% per yr
  2. IgM MGUS: 1.5% per yr
  3. Light-chain MGUS: 0.3% per yr
- Non-IgM and light-chain MGUS tend to progress to myeloma or amyloidosis
- IgM MGUS tends to progress to Waldenstrom macroglobulinemia
- Risk of infection (bacterial and viral) is twofold compared with healthy controls
- Increased risk of mortality from bacterial infections

REFERRAL

To hematologist/oncologist for evaluation

PEARLS & CONSIDERATIONS

- Approximately 55% of 70-yr-old patients diagnosed as having MGUS have had the condition for more than 10 yr.
- Most patients with MGUS should be monitored every 6 to 12 mo for signs and symptoms of progression to a malignancy.
- There is no indicated treatment for asymptomatic MGUS, but some patients can develop monoclonal gammopathy of renal or neurological significance, and treatment sometimes is indicated in these cases.

SUGGESTED READINGS

Available at ExpertConsult.com

AUTHOR: **Jorge J. Castillo, MD**

TABLE 1 Disease Definitions for the Monoclonal Gammopathies: MGUS and Related Disorders

Type of Monoclonal Gammopathy	Premalignancy with a Low Risk of Progression (1%-2% per yr)	Premalignancy with a High Risk of Progression (10% per yr)	Malignancy
IgG and IgA (non-IgM) monoclonal gammopathies*	**Non-IgM MGUS** All 3 criteria must be met: Serum monoclonal protein <3 g/dl Clonal bone marrow plasma cells <10%, and Absence of end-organ damage such as hypercalcemia, renal insufficiency, anemia, and bone lesions (CRAB) that can be attributed to the plasma cell proliferative disorder	**Smoldering multiple myeloma** Both criteria must be met: Serum monoclonal protein (IgG or IgA) ≥3 g/dl and/or clonal bone marrow plasma cells ≥10%, and Absence of end-organ damage such as lytic bone lesions, anemia, hypercalcemia, or renal failure that can be attributed to a plasma cell proliferative disorder	**Multiple myeloma** All 3 criteria must be met except as noted: Clonal bone marrow plasma cells ≥10% Presence of serum and/or urinary monoclonal protein (except in patients with true nonsecretory multiple myeloma), and Evidence of end-organ damage that can be attributed to the underlying plasma cell proliferative disorder, specifically Hypercalcemia: Serum calcium >11.5 mg/dl or renal insufficiency: Serum creatinine >2 mg/dl or estimated creatinine clearance <40 ml/min Anemia: Normochromic, normocytic with a hemoglobin value of >2 g/dl below the lower limit of normal or a hemoglobin value <10 g/dl Bone lesions: Lytic lesions or severe osteopenia attributed to a plasma cell proliferative disorder or pathologic fractures
IgM monoclonal gammopathies	**IgM MGUS**[†] All 3 criteria must be met: Serum IgM monoclonal protein of any level Normal bone marrow and absence of end-organ damage such as anemia, constitutional symptoms, hyperviscosity, lymphadenopathy, or hepatosplenomegaly that can be attributed to the underlying lymphoproliferative disorder	**Smoldering Waldenström macroglobulinemia** Both criteria must be met: Serum IgM monoclonal protein of any level and/or bone marrow lymphoplasmacytic infiltration of any level, and No evidence of anemia, constitutional symptoms, hyperviscosity, lymphadenopathy, or hepatosplenomegaly that can be attributed to the underlying lymphoproliferative disorder	**Waldenström macroglobulinemia** All criteria must be met: IgM monoclonal gammopathy of any level, and any level of bone marrow lymphoplasmacytic infiltration (usually intratrabecular) by small lymphocytes that exhibit plasmacytoid or plasma cell differentiation and a typical immunophenotype (e.g., surface IgM+, CD5+/–, CD10–, CD19+, CD20+, CD23–) that satisfactorily excludes other lymphoproliferative disorders including chronic lymphocytic leukemia and mantle cell lymphoma Evidence of anemia, constitutional symptoms, hyperviscosity, lymphadenopathy, or hepatosplenomegaly that can be attributed to the underlying lymphoproliferative disorder. Presence of the *MYD88* L265P mutation **IgM myeloma** All criteria must be met: Symptomatic monoclonal plasma cell proliferative disorder characterized by a serum IgM monoclonal protein regardless of size Presence of 10% plasma cells on bone marrow biopsy Presence of lytic bone lesions related to the underlying plasma cell disorder and/or translocation t(11;14) on fluorescence in situ hybridization
Light-chain monoclonal gammopathies	**Light-chain MGUS** All criteria must be met: Abnormal FLC ratio (<0.26 or >1.65) Increased level of the appropriate involved light-chain (increased kappa FLC in patients with ratio >1.65 and increased lambda FLC in patients with ratio <0.26) No immunoglobulin heavy-chain expression on immunofixation Clonal bone marrow plasma cells <10%, and Absence of end-organ damage such as hypercalcemia, renal insufficiency, anemia, and bone lesions (CRAB) that can be attributed to the plasma cell proliferative disorder	**Idiopathic Bence Jones proteinuria** All criteria must be met: Urinary monoclonal protein on urine protein electrophoresis ≥500 mg/24 h and/or clonal bone marrow plasma cells ≥10% No immunoglobulin heavy-chain expression on immunofixation Absence of end-organ damage such as hypercalcemia, renal insufficiency, anemia, and bone lesions (CRAB) that can be attributed to the plasma cell proliferative disorder	**Light-chain multiple myeloma**[†] Same as multiple myeloma except no evidence of immunoglobulin heavy-chain expression

CRAB, Hypercalcemia, renal failure, anemia, and bone disease; *FLC,* free light chain; *Ig,* immunoglobulin; *MGUS,* monoclonal gammopathy of undetermined significance.
*Occasionally patients with IgD and IgE monoclonal gammopathies have been described and will be considered to be part of this category as well.
[†]Note that conventionally IgM MGUS is considered a subtype of MGUS, and similarly light-chain multiple myeloma is considered as a subtype of multiple myeloma. Unless specifically distinguished, when the terms MGUS and multiple myeloma are used in general, they include IgM MGUS and light-chain multiple myeloma, respectively.
Modified from Rajkumar SV et al: Advances in the diagnosis, classification, risk stratification, and management of monoclonal gammopathy of undetermined significance: implications for recategorizing disease entities in the presence of evolving scientific evidence, *Mayo Clin Proc* 85:945-948, 2010.

TABLE 2 Diseases Associated with Monoclonal Gammopathy

Plasma cell and related disorders	MGUS Solitary plasmacytoma: Bone Soft tissue Multiple myeloma Waldenström macroglobulinemia Primary amyloidosis	
Lymphoid disorders	Non-Hodgkin lymphoma	Monoclonal protein observed in CLL (>20% of cases with IgM, ≈50% with IgG, light chains also observed), extranodal marginal zone lymphomas (>30% of cases and correlated with BM involvement), follicular, mantle cell, and diffuse large B-cell lymphomas also reported with serum M proteins as has AITL
	Hodgkin lymphoma	Rare but reported
	Castleman disease	<2% with monoclonal gammopathy
Other hematologic disorders	Acquired von Willebrand disease	IVIG more effective than factor concentrate in increasing factor VIII coagulant and VWF levels
	Gaucher disease	Observed in 25% in one study; M protein declined after splenectomy
	Pernicious anemia, pure RBC aplasia, hereditary spherocytosis, MPD, MDS	
Connective tissue disorders	SLE	IgG, IgM, and IgA have been observed, no difference in disease activity or outcome
	Inclusion body myositis	80% with IgG M protein
	Polymyositis, RA, scleroderma	
Neurologic disorders	POEMS syndrome	Most have M-protein of λ light chain
	Peripheral neuropathy	Most common is IgM followed by IgG and IgA In half, IgM protein binds to myelin-associated glycoprotein Size of M protein not correlated with severity of neuropathy Some benefit from plasma exchange for those with IgG and IgA Fludarabine and rituximab with some benefit for IgM
	Myasthenia gravis, ALS, Alzheimer disease	
Dermatologic disorders	Schnitzler syndrome	Neutrophilic urticarial dermatitis, monoclonal IgM protein, and two of: Lymphadenopathy, fever, hepatosplenomegaly, joint pain, increased ESR, increased neutrophils, or abnormal bone imaging
	Scleredema	
	Pyoderma gangrenosum	Frequently an IgA protein
Infections	HIV	Both IgG and IgM M proteins observed
	HCV	M protein present in up to 10% of patients
Immunosuppression	Renal transplant	In children CMV infection associated with M protein
	Liver and heart transplant	Most patients with posttransplant lymphoproliferative disorders have M proteins
	BM transplant	Observed in both autologous and allogeneic transplants Appearance of M protein correlated with GVHD

AITL, Angioimmunoblastic T-cell lymphoma; *ALS,* amyotrophic lateral sclerosis; *BM,* bone marrow; *CLL,* chronic lymphocytic leukemia; *CMV,* cytomegalovirus; *ESR,* erythrocyte sedimentation rate; *GVHD,* graft-versus-host disease; *HCV,* hepatitis C virus; *HIV,* human immunodeficiency virus; *Ig,* immunoglobulin; *IVIG,* intravenous immunoglobulin; *MDS,* myelodysplastic syndrome; *MGUS,* monoclonal gammopathy of uncertain significance; *MPD,* myeloproliferative disorder; *POEMS,* polyneuropathy, organomegaly, endocrinopathy, monoclonal gammopathy, and skin changes; *RA,* rheumatoid arthritis; *RBC,* red blood cell; *SLE,* systemic lupus erythematosus; *VWF,* von Willebrand factor.

From Hoffman R et al: *Hematology: basic principles and practice,* ed 7, Philadelphia, 2018, Elsevier.

BASIC INFORMATION

DEFINITION

Infectious mononucleosis (IM) is a symptomatic infection most commonly caused by Epstein-Barr virus (EBV) and characterized by a classic triad of fever, tonsillar pharyngitis, and lymphadenopathy (predominantly cervical). Fatigue is also a very common finding. IM was first coined in 1920 to describe a syndrome characterized as an acute infectious process accompanied by atypical large peripheral blood lymphocytes.

SYNONYMS

Mononucleosis
EBV
Kissing disease

ICD-10CM CODES

B27	Infectious mononucleosis
B27.0	Gamma herpesviral mononucleosis
B27.1	Cytomegaloviral mononucleosis
B27.8	Other infectious mononucleosis
B27.9	Infectious mononucleosis

EPIDEMIOLOGY & DEMOGRAPHICS

INCIDENCE (IN U.S.): 500 cases/100,000 persons/yr; worldwide, approximately 90% lifetime prevalence by age 30 yr

PREDOMINANT SEX: Incidence is the same, but occurs earlier in females.

PREDOMINANT AGE: Symptomatic infection most common between the ages of 15 and 24 yr. The age at which primary EBV infection is acquired is potentially increasing in developed countries.

Young children rarely develop clinical signs of IM. Infection during childhood is more common in lower socioeconomic groups and may vary by geographic location or social factors, such as crowding, sharing a bedroom, maternal education, daycare attendance, and school catchment area.

PHYSICAL FINDINGS & CLINICAL PRESENTATION

- Following an incubation period of 4 to 7 wk, there are two common presentations. The first presentation represents the prodromal period with gradual onset of fever, chills, malaise, and anorexia for several days. This is followed by the second presentation of the classic triad of pharyngitis, fever, and lymphadenopathy. These patients often report the worst sore throat of their life. Pharyngitis (Fig. E1) is typically the most severe symptom and is characterized by white tonsillar exudates that may spread to the tongue. Up to half of patients may have palatal petechiae.
- Lymphadenopathy (nonnecrotic) can be diffuse, but most commonly occurs in both the anterior and posterior triangles of the neck.
- Splenomegaly may be palpable, most commonly during the second wk of illness. Most patients have some degree of splenomegaly on ultrasound assessment. Hepatomegaly with some degree of hepatitis is also common. In 75% of cases there is some increase in alanine aminotransferase (ALT).
- Rash (Fig. E2) is uncommon but will occur in nearly all patients who receive ampicillin or amoxicillin due to a transient penicillin hypersensitivity.
- IM is usually a self-limited illness (2 to 4 wk), but symptoms of malaise and fatigue may last mo before resolving.
- At times, IM can present as fever and adenopathy without pharyngitis.
- Although acute complications may be severe, they are uncommon and tend to resolve completely. Reported complications include cholestatic liver disease, chronic hepatitis, or even liver failure; hemolytic anemia; splenic rupture; or airway compromise.
- Splenic rupture is rare, with an incidence rate <1%, but it is the most feared. It should be suspected in anyone with confirmed or suspected IM who presents with acute abdominal or chest pain. Most cases occur in the first 3 wk of symptoms.
- Airway compromise, as evidenced by stridor, cyanosis, and/or tachypnea, is reported in 1% to 3% of cases and is an indication for hospitalization.
- Systemic corticosteroids are indicated for treating those at risk or with impending airway obstruction, and usually leads to improvement in 12 to 36 hr. Acute tonsillectomy may be pursued if steroids are not sufficient to mitigate the risk for obstruction.
- Late complications may include lymphoproliferative cancers (Burkitt lymphoma and Hodgkin lymphoma), multiple sclerosis, rheumatoid arthritis, and chronic active EBV infection (CAEBV).
- EBV may also cause hemophagocytic disease, alternatively referred to as EBV-associated hemophagocytic lymphohistiocytosis (EBV-HLH), characterized by fever, splenomegaly, and cytopenias with high ferritin and soluble CD25.
- Box 1 and Table 1 summarize the features of IM in immunocompetent patients.

ETIOLOGY

The most common cause of IM (90%) is primary infection with EBV. Cytomegalovirus (CMV) is the most common cause of the other 10% of IM, but CMV infection often occurs in infancy or early childhood and is minimally symptomatic. Other causes include human herpes virus-6, herpes simplex virus-1, and HIV. Primary EBV infection during childhood also often causes few or no symptoms; persistent fatigue and recurrent/persistent fevers are the most common reasons parents bring symptomatic children to medical care.

BOX 1 Summary of Features of Infectious Mononucleosis (IM) in Immunocompetent Patients

Epstein-Barr Virus (Human Herpesvirus-4)

Pathophysiology
- Virus enters through oropharyngeal epithelial and lymphoid cells.
- Virus attaches to CD21 on B cells.
- Viral antigens—viral capsid antigen (VCA), early antigen (EA), Epstein-Barr nuclear antigen (EBNA)—are produced and elicit antibody production.

Humoral Immune Response
- Immunoglobulin (Ig)M against VCA rises during incubation and prodrome, falls over few wk to mo.
- IgG against VCA rises during incubation, decreases during convalescence, remains detectable for life.
- Antibodies to EA rise 2-3 wk after onset of illness, then fall.
- Antibodies to EBNA rise during convalescence, detectable for life.

Cellular Immune Response
- T cells activated during second wk of illness.
- CD8-positive cytotoxic T cells kill infected B cells.
- Natural killer cells kill infected B cells.
- Some resting memory B cells remain latently infected.

Clinical Features
- 4- to 7-wk incubation period
- Vague onset of symptoms
- Fever, sore throat, lymphadenopathy
- Adolescents, young adults more often symptomatic than younger children

Laboratory Features
- Leukocytosis with absolute lymphocytosis and atypical lymphocytes
- Transient monocytosis
- Relative and absolute neutropenia early on
- Mild thrombocytopenia in half of cases
- Hemolytic anemia in 1%-3% of cases, often with anti-I specificity
- Elevated transaminases in 85%-100% of cases, but clinical jaundice rare
- Spot test is simple, rapid, specific, based on agglutination of horse red blood cells (RBCs)
- Heterophil antibody (HA) test is based on differential absorption of IM-specific HA by beef RBC stroma and guinea pig kidney

From McPherson RA, Pincus MR: *Henry's clinical diagnosis and management by laboratory methods,* ed 23, Philadelphia, 2017, Elsevier.

EBV infects epithelial cells and resting B cells of the oropharynx. It is then found in saliva, making it transmittable through coughing, sharing drink/food, and kissing; thus the pseudonym "kissing disease." IM is more prevalent during adolescence when these types of close contact increase. How it is transmitted in younger children is less clear.

EBV levels peak during the active phase of infection but can persist in the oropharynx for up to 18 mo. Transmission may also occur sexually because EBV can be isolated in cervical epithelial cells and male seminal fluid. It has also been shown to be transmitted by blood transfusion, solid organ transplantation, or hematopoietic cell transplantation.

Dx DIAGNOSIS

DIFFERENTIAL DIAGNOSIS

- Heterophile-negative IM caused by CMV
- Bacterial and viral causes of pharyngitis
- Toxoplasmosis
- Acute retroviral syndrome of HIV, lymphoma

WORKUP

Initial testing consists of heterophile antibody (monospot) and CBC with differential. Fig. 3 illustrates the serologic evaluation of patients with clinical symptoms of acute IM and atypical lymphocytosis.

LABORATORY TESTS

- About 85% of patients with EBV-related IM will have a positive heterophile antibody test, making it the best initial test for diagnosis of EBV infection (sensitivity of 71% to 90% for diagnosing IM). However, the test has a 25% false-negative rate in the first wk of illness because the amount of heterophile antibody may not be above the limit for detection early in the disease. A negative test should be repeated if clinical suspicion is high; negative results are common in patients symptomatic for <2 wk and children <4 yr. False-positive heterophile antibody tests have been reported in other acute infections, autoimmune diseases, and cancer.
- About 10% of patients will have a persistently negative heterophile antibody test. In this event, further testing may be pursued with EBV viral capsid antigen (VCA) IgG and IgM antibody testing, as well as EBV nuclear antigen (EBNA) antibodies for staging of infection. Early diagnosis in monospot-negative cases may be made by isolating IgM to the VCA, which is usually positive during the acute illness and disappears after 4 to 6 wk. If the monospot test remains negative (without evidence of acute infection with antibody testing) for 8 wk, alternative diagnoses should be considered. The monospot usually remains positive for 3 to 6 mo but can last >1 yr.
- Increased white blood count (WBC) is common, with a relative lymphocytosis and neutropenia. Atypical lymphocytes (Fig. E4) are the hallmark of IM but are not pathognomonic. Mild thrombocytopenia is common. A falling hematocrit may signal splenic rupture or severe immune-mediated hemolytic anemia. Elevated hepatocellular enzymes and cryoglobulins occur in many cases.

IMAGING STUDIES

Chest x-ray may rarely show infiltrates. An elevated left hemidiaphragm may occur in cases of splenic rupture.

Rx TREATMENT

NONPHARMACOLOGIC THERAPY

- No specific treatment exists; focus is on supportive care and symptomatic relief with analgesics, antipyretics, and hydration. Supportive rest is advocated by some, but the effect on outcome is not clear. Prolonged rest may result in deconditioning, which may contribute to further fatigue.
- Splenectomy if rupture occurs; transfusions for severe anemia or thrombocytopenia.

GENERAL Rx

- Pharmacologic therapy, including corticosteroids, is not indicated in mild illness or for symptomatic relief. Use of corticosteroids is controversial because they may impair clearance of the viral load.
- The use of steroids, however (Fig. E5), should be considered in patients who have severe acute complications, such as thrombocytopenia, hemolytic anemia, or impending airway obstruction.
- There is no role for antiviral agents such as acyclovir in the management of IM.

CHRONIC Rx

CAEBV is treated with hematopoietic cell transplantation.

DISPOSITION

Eventual resolution of all symptoms is the rule.

! PEARLS & CONSIDERATIONS

COMMENTS

- Contact sports should be avoided during the first mo of illness because splenic rupture can occur during this time, even in the absence of clinically detectable splenomegaly.
- Between 30% and 75% of college freshmen are seronegative for EBV. Each yr nearly 20% of susceptible persons become infected and up to 50% of these persons develop IM.

SUGGESTED READINGS

Available at ExpertConsult.com

RELATED CONTENT

Mononucleosis (Patient Information)
Epstein-Barr Virus Infection (Related Key Topic)

AUTHOR: **Russell J. McCulloh, MD**

TABLE 1 Clinical Manifestations of Infectious Mononucleosis in Children and Adults

Sign or Symptom	FREQUENCY (%) Age <4 yr	Age 4-16 yr	Adults (Range)
Lymphadenopathy	94	95	93-100
Fever	92	100	63-100
Sore throat or tonsillopharyngitis	67	75	70-91
Exudative tonsillopharyngitis	45	59	40-74
Splenomegaly	82	53	32-51
Hepatomegaly	63	30	6-24
Cough or rhinitis	51	15	5-31
Rash	34	17	0-15
Abdominal pain or discomfort	17	0	2-14
Eyelid edema	14	14	5-34

From Hoffman R et al: *Hematology, basic principles and practice*, ed 7, Philadelphia, 2018, Elsevier.

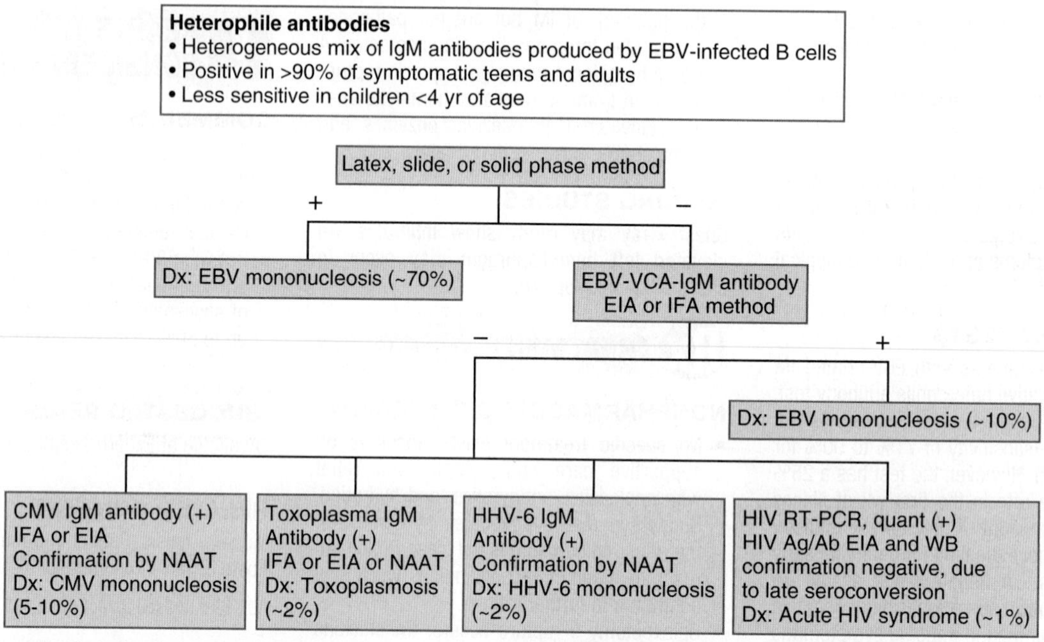

FIG. 3 Serologic evaluation of patients with clinical symptoms of acute infectious mononucleosis and atypical lymphocytosis. *Ab,* Antibody; *Ag,* antigen; *CMV,* cytomegalovirus; *Dx,* diagnosis; *EBV,* Epstein-Barr virus; *EIA,* enzyme immunoassay; *HHV-6,* human herpesvirus 6; *HIV,* human immunodeficiency virus; *IFA,* immunofluorescent assay; *IgM,* immunoglobulin M; *NAAT,* nucleic acid amplification testing; *quant,* quantitative; *RT-PCR,* reverse transcriptase polymerase chain reaction; *VCA,* viral capsid antigen; *WB,* Western blot. (From McPherson RA, Pincus MR: *Henry's clinical diagnosis and management by laboratory methods,* ed 23, Philadelphia, 2017, Elsevier.)

BASIC INFORMATION

DEFINITION

Multifocal atrial tachycardia (MAT) is a supraventricular tachyarrhythmia (rate greater than 100 beats per min) with organized atrial activity, showing P waves having at least three or more different morphologies and irregular P-P, P-R, and R-R intervals. MAT is differentiated from atrial fibrillation by discrete P wave depolarizations and an isoelectric baseline between P waves.

SYNONYMS

MAT
Chaotic atrial rhythm
Multiform atrial rhythm
Chronic atrial tachycardia
Repetitive multifocal paroxysmal atrial tachycardia
Multifocal ectopic atrial tachycardia
The term *wandering pacemaker* or multifocal atrial rhythm is used for a similar arrhythmia associated with heart rates less than 100 bpm.

ICD-10CM CODE
I47.1 Supraventricular tachycardia

EPIDEMIOLOGY & DEMOGRAPHICS

Estimated prevalence in hospitalized patients is 0.05% to 0.32%. The average age of onset is 70 yr of age. The entity is usually associated with underlying pulmonary disease with right atrial electromechanical delay. Chronic obstructive pulmonary disease (COPD) is present in approximately 55% of patients with MAT. Significant lung disease is associated in roughly 60% of cases. It may also be seen in patients with heart failure, valvular heart disease, pulmonary hypertension, and hypomagnesemia. These patients are in general quite ill and have an in-hospital mortality rate of 40% to 60% from pulmonary, cardiac, and/or other serious diseases.

PHYSICAL FINDINGS & CLINICAL PRESENTATION

Symptoms:
- Palpitations
- Lightheadedness
- Syncope
- Symptoms of the underlying pulmonary disease
- Physical findings associated with the underlying pulmonary disease

ETIOLOGY

- Exact mechanism unknown
- Potentially caused by right atrial distention such as in pulmonary hypertension due to underlying lung disease
- Also seen in other circumstances; therefore atrial distension may not be a universal mechanism
- Exacerbated by underlying pulmonary disease (COPD, hypoxia, pulmonary embolism, pneumonia), cardiac disease, hypercarbia, acidosis, electrolyte disturbances
- Hypomagnesemia can promote the development of atrial and ventricular arrhythmias

DIAGNOSIS

DIFFERENTIAL DIAGNOSIS

- Atrial fibrillation (up to 55% of patients with MAT will develop atrial fibrillation, MAT can degenerate into atrial fibrillation)
- Atrial flutter with variable AV conduction
- Sinus tachycardia
- Paroxysmal atrial tachycardia
- Sinus tachycardia with premature atrial or ventricular contractions

WORKUP

- ECG (Fig. 1)
- Chest x-ray
- Pulmonary function tests
- Electrolytes
- Arterial blood gases

TREATMENT

- Correction and/or improvement in the underlying pulmonary or metabolic dysfunction if possible.
- Correction of oxygenation and acid-base disorders.
- Avoid drugs such as theophylline, isoproterenol, etc.
- Electrolyte repletion, especially magnesium and potassium, to normal levels.
- Intravenous magnesium infusion may occasionally be helpful in patients with normal magnesium levels.
- Calcium channel blockers: Verapamil may be effective acutely and chronically and is often used as first line in patients with preserved LV function *if there are symptoms related to tachycardia.*
- β-blockers (metoprolol is relatively cardioselective) can be used if not contraindicated by obstructive lung disease, acute heart failure, hypotension, hypersensitivity, heart block, or sinus node dysfunction.
- If the arrhythmia is asymptomatic, it can be left untreated.
- Direct current cardioversion is ineffective.
- Antiarrhythmics are ineffective.
- Anticoagulation is not indicated, although some recent studies have linked frequent atrial ectopy on ambulatory monitoring with stroke risk
- No significant role for catheter ablation.
- In extreme cases of refractory MAT in symptomatic patients who cannot tolerate medical therapy or in MAT resistant to medical therapy, AV nodal ablation with pacemaker implantation has been performed.
- Table E1 summarizes the treatment of multifocal atrial tachycardia.

SUGGESTED READINGS
Available at ExpertConsult.com

AUTHOR: **Vybhav Jetty, MD, MHA**

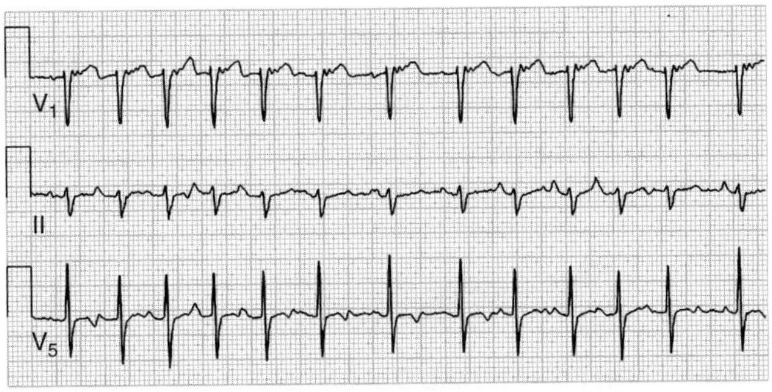

FIG. 1 Multifocal atrial tachycardia. This three-lead rhythm strip (leads II, V_1, and V_5) shows an irregularly irregular narrow QRS complex rhythm. However, unlike atrial fibrillation (AF), each QRS complex is preceded by discrete, conducted P waves. There are at least three different P wave morphologies and PR intervals, consistent with MAT. (From Olshansky B et al: *Arrhythmia essentials,* ed 2, Philadelphia, 2017, Elsevier.)

BASIC INFORMATION

DEFINITION

Multiple endocrine neoplasia (MEN) refers to a group of heritable genetic syndromes characterized by the development of specific groups of tumors of the endocrine glands.

SYNONYMS

MEN I: Wermer syndrome
MEN IIA: Sipple syndrome

ICD-10CM CODES

E31.2	Multiple endocrine neoplasia [MEN] syndromes
E31.20	Multiple endocrine neoplasia [MEN] syndrome, unspecified
E31.21	Multiple endocrine neoplasia [MEN] syndrome type I
E31.22	Multiple endocrine neoplasia [MEN] syndrome type IIA
E31.23	Multiple endocrine neoplasia [MEN] syndrome type IIB

EPIDEMIOLOGY & DEMOGRAPHICS

INCIDENCE:
- MEN I: 25 in 10,000
- MEN II: 1 in 30,000

PREVALENCE:
- MEN I: 1/30,000
- MEN II: 1/35,000 (predominantly MEN IIA)

RISK FACTORS: Family history of MEN syndrome, although it can also occur sporadically

GENETICS:
- MEN I: Autosomal-dominant mutation in MEN1 tumor-suppressor gene
- MEN IIA and MEN IIB: Autosomal-dominant mutations in RET proto-oncogene

PHYSICAL FINDINGS & CLINICAL PRESENTATION

- Patients may present due to screening or may present with a MEN-associated tumor. Tumors are found incidentally due to biochemical abnormalities or to symptoms.
- MEN I (PPP [pituitary, pancreas, parathyroid])
  1. Diagnostic criteria generally include two MEN-associated tumors, one tumor in a patient with a family history, or positive genetic testing.
  2. Primary hyperparathyroidism (parathyroid adenoma or hyperplasia) is the most common manifestation and can cause hypercalcemia (urolithiasis, GI disturbance, bone pain, neuropsychiatric disturbances) and also affect bone density.
  3. Pancreatic neuroendocrine tumors cause symptoms related to their secretory properties or metastases.
     a. Gastrinoma: Peptic ulcers, diarrhea, esophageal symptoms (see "Gastrinoma")
     b. Insulinoma: Hypoglycemic symptoms upon fasting and after exercise (see "Insulinoma")
     c. Glucagonoma: Necrolytic migratory erythema (a blistering skin lesion), diabetes/glucose intolerance, weight loss
     d. VIPoma: Diarrhea, hypokalemia, decreased gastric acid
     e. Somatostatinoma: Hyperglycemia, cholelithiasis, diarrhea, abdominal pain, weight loss
     f. Nonfunctioning tumors can metastasize (frequently to the liver), a frequent cause of death in MEN I
  4. Pituitary tumors may cause compressive symptoms, such as visual field defects or hypopituitarism (see "Pituitary Adenoma"). Hormonal secretion may also cause symptoms.
     a. Prolactinoma (most common pituitary tumor in MEN I): Menstrual irregularities, hypogonadism, gynecomastia, and/or galactorrhea (see "Prolactinoma").
     b. Somatotroph adenomas (producing growth hormone): Gigantism or acromegaly (frontal bossing, increased shoe/hat size, hyperglycemia, hyperhidrosis) depending on patient age (see "Acromegaly").
     c. Corticotroph adenomas (producing adrenocorticotropic hormone): Cushingoid features such as weight gain, moon facies, hyperglycemia, bone loss, proximal muscle weakness, hypertension, hypokalemia (see "Cushing Disease and Syndrome").
     d. Nonfunctioning (nonsecretory) tumors.
  5. Other manifestations: Carcinoid tumors, collagenomas, angiofibromas, meningiomas, lipomas
- MEN IIA:
  1. Medullary thyroid carcinoma (MTC) is a tumor of the thyroid's calcitonin-secreting C cells. It can present with a neck mass, as well as flushing and diarrhea due to elevated calcitonin levels.
  2. Primary hyperparathyroidism: See "MEN I." Less aggressive in "MEN IIA."
  3. Pheochromocytoma is an adrenal tumor producing catecholamines, which can lead to life-threatening hypertensive crises.
- MEN IIB:
  1. Medullary thyroid carcinoma (MTC)
  2. Pheochromocytoma
  3. Oral mucosal neuromas

ETIOLOGY

Tumor development facilitated by the previously described genetic mutations (Table E1).

DIAGNOSIS

DIFFERENTIAL DIAGNOSIS

Tumors associated with MEN may occur sporadically.

WORKUP

- MEN I: Note that opinions vary regarding the aggressiveness and frequency of screening for MEN-associated tumors.
  1. Genetic testing: Offered to patients meeting MEN I clinical criteria or to patients in whom there is high suspicion, as well as to first-degree relatives of MEN I patients.
  2. Hyperparathyroidism screening: Parathyroid hormone (PTH) and calcium annually.
  3. Pancreatic tumor screening: Annual pancreas imaging (endoscopic ultrasonography, CT, or MRI) and annual biochemical testing (glucose, gastrin, vasoactive intestinal peptide [VIP], glucagon, insulin, pancreatic polypeptide, chromogranin A). Notably, Gallium-68 DOTATATE PET-CT is an exciting new tool for neuroendocrine tumor localization, though it is not typically utilized in screening at this time.
  4. Pituitary tumor screening: Insulin-like growth factor 1 (IGF-1) and prolactin annually and pituitary MRI every 3 to 5 yr.
  5. Carcinoid tumor screening: Chest CT or MRI every 2 yr.
- MEN IIA:
  1. Genetic testing: At-risk members of families with known RET mutations should undergo screening for the specific mutation. Patients with MTC should have genetic testing of the tumor and genetic testing based on results. Cutaneous lichen amyloidosis (a skin finding) should prompt testing; Hirschsprung disease may also prompt testing.
  2. Hyperparathyroidism screening: PTH and calcium annually
  3. Pheochromocytoma: Plasma catecholamines and metanephrines annually for screening, age to begin depending on specific mutation; CT and MRI may localize; I-123 and PET (possibly including Gallium-68 DOTATATE PET-CT) also helpful for localization.
  4. MTC screening: Depends on risk category; physical exam, neck ultrasound, and calcitonin level yearly; carcinoembryonic antigen may also be indicated.
- MEN IIB:
  1. Genetic testing: See "MEN IIA"
  2. Pheochromocytoma: See "MEN IIA"
  3. MTC screening: Although there may be a role for monitoring, prophylactic thyroidectomy is typically performed early

LABORATORY TESTS

See "Workup."

IMAGING STUDIES

See "Workup."

TREATMENT

No therapy available at this time to reverse the underlying genetic cause. Treatment (both medical and surgical) focuses on tumor prevention and management.

NONPHARMACOLOGIC THERAPY

- MEN I:
  1. For hyperparathyroidism, surgical parathyroidectomy is indicated in patients

with significant hypercalcemia, osteoporosis, renal disease, or nephrolithiasis or found to be at high risk for nephrolithiasis. Hyperparathyroidism may be treated surgically with parathyroidectomy.
2. Pituitary tumors may be surgically excised via transsphenoidal approach; notably, medical therapy is first line for prolactinoma.
3. Pancreatic tumor treatment is extremely variable. Gastrinoma is frequently complicated by duodenal metastases, which are difficult to treat surgically, so treatment choice varies between centers. Ulcers caused by gastrinoma may require endoscopic or surgical management. Surgery is preferred for insulinoma, VIPoma, and glucagonoma. Nonfunctioning tumors may be treated surgically depending on tumor size and location. Conservative management for insulinoma may involve frequent carbohydrate intake. Cytotoxic chemotherapy and tyrosine kinase inhibitors are options for patients with metastatic disease. Peptide receptor radionucleotide therapy (PRRT) is an emerging and exciting therapeutic modality for metastatic disease.

- MEN IIA:
  1. MTC is generally treated surgically. Prophylactic thyroidectomy is considered based on genetic mutation. Almost all children with MEN IIA will require thyroidectomy (screening as previously described). Patients should undergo ultrasound and total thyroidectomy with cervical lymph node dissection. Extent of further neck dissection depends on metastases and may be guided by calcitonin levels. A more palliative surgical approach is considered in the setting of advanced disease.
  2. Hyperparathyroidism: Resection of only enlarged glands with intraoperative PTH monitoring is preferred.
  3. Pheochromocytoma is treated surgically. Unilateral adrenalectomy is preferred, although many patients will develop a contralateral pheochromocytoma. Preoperative blood pressure control with alpha blockade is key. If present, pheochromocytoma must be removed before thyroidectomy.
- MEN IIB:
  1. MTC: Prophylactic thyroidectomy offered in childhood.
  2. Pheochromocytoma: See "MEN IIA."

ACUTE GENERAL Rx

- MEN I:
  1. Hyperparathyroidism causes hypercalcemia that may be treated with IV hydration, diuretics, and bisphosphonates. Early vitamin D repletion prevents bone destruction postoperatively due to the "hungry bone syndrome."
  2. Gastrinoma may lead to peptic ulcers requiring IV proton-pump inhibitor (PPI).
  3. Supportive care (glucose for hypoglycemia caused by insulinoma; fluids and electrolytes for hypovolemia caused by diarrhea from VIPoma or gastrinoma) is required.
- MEN IIA:
  1. Hyperparathyroidism: See "MEN I."
  2. Pheochromocytoma: Preoperative blood pressure control is key; alpha blockers are first line. Phenoxybenzamine irreversibly blocks alpha adrenergic receptors; doxazosin may also be helpful. Calcium channel blockers can be utilized. There is concern that unopposed beta blockade may allow for alpha-medicated vasoconstriction.
- MEN IIB:
  1. Pheochromocytoma: See "MEN IIA."

CHRONIC Rx

- MEN I:
  1. Hyperparathyroidism may be amenable to agonists of the calcium-sensing receptor (cinacalcet), although surgery is preferred in patients who meet surgical criteria and are operative candidates.
  2. Pancreatic tumors may benefit from medical therapy.
     a. Gastrinoma: PPI or H2 antagonists, somatostatin agonists (such as octreotide)
     b. Insulinoma: Diazoxide or somatostatin agonists
     c. Glucagonoma and VIPoma: Somatostatin agonists
  3. Adjunctive medical therapy can be considered for pituitary tumors, although surgical treatment is first-line with the exception of prolactinoma (for which dopamine agonists are first line). Radiation therapy and/or medical therapy are considered in cases of incomplete resection or regrowth.
     a. Prolactinoma: Dopamine agonists (bromocriptine or cabergoline). Temozolomide is a chemotherapeutic agent for refractory cases.
     b. Somatotroph adenoma: Somatostatin or dopamine agonists, growth hormone receptor antagonist
     c. Corticotroph adenoma: Antiadrenal agents, adrenal enzyme blocker (such as ketoconazole), somatostatin or dopamine agonists, glucocorticoid receptor blockers
- MEN II A:
  1. Hyperparathyroidism: See "MEN I."
  2. MTC: Tyrosine kinase inhibitors and chemotherapy may help treat metastatic disease. After thyroidectomy, levothyroxine is indicated (TSH suppression not required).
- MEN IIB
  MTC: See "MEN II A."

COMPLEMENTARY & ALTERNATIVE MEDICINE

MEN is unlikely to be amenable to this.

DISPOSITION

Most workup can be done as an outpatient (multidisciplinary team); inpatient stays may be required due to acute complications or for surgical procedures.

REFERRAL

Patients with MEN should be followed by a multispecialty team, including endocrinologists, endocrine surgeons, and genetic counselors.

PEARLS & CONSIDERATIONS

COMMENTS

MEN is a group of genetic syndromes that requires close monitoring and intervention to prevent and treat tumor development, as well as genetic counseling of patients and family members.

PREVENTION

Prevention focuses on screening for MEN in persons at risk and early identification of MEN-associated tumors.

PATIENT & FAMILY EDUCATION

- American Multiple Endocrine Neoplasia Support: www.amensupport.org/
- Association for Multiple Endocrine Neoplasia Disorders: www.amend.org.uk/

RELATED CONTENT

Acromegaly (Related Key Topic)
Cushing Disease and Syndrome (Related Key Topic)
Gastrinoma (Related Key Topic)
Hyperparathyroidism (Related Key Topic)
Insulinoma (Related Key Topic)
Pheochromocytoma (Related Key Topic)
Pituitary Adenoma (Related Key Topic)
Prolactinoma (Related Key Topic)
Thyroid Carcinoma (Related Key Topic)

SUGGESTED READINGS

Available at ExpertConsult.com

AUTHORS: **Harikrashna B. Bhatt, MD,** and **Russell E. Bratman, MD**

BASIC INFORMATION

DEFINITION

Multiple myeloma (MM) is a plasma cell neoplasm characterized by clonal proliferation of malignant plasma cells in the bone marrow, production of a monoclonal protein in the blood or urine leading to end-organ dysfunction. The transition from normal cells to genomic instability is not well understood, but current evidence suggests that antigenic stimulation may be a key factor (Fig. E1). Diagnostic criteria for the diagnosis of MM was updated by the International Myeloma Working Group (IMWG) in 2014 and requires the following:

- Presence of ≥10% plasma cells on examination of the bone marrow (or biopsy of a tissue with monoclonal plasma cells) and any one or more of the following myeloma-defining events:
  1. Evidence of end-organ damage (calcium elevation, renal insufficiency, anemia, or bone lesions [CRAB criteria])
  2. Clonal bone marrow plasma cell percentage ≥60%
  3. Involved: Uninvolved serum free light ratio ≥100
  4. >1 focal lesion on MRI studies

SYNONYM

MM

ICD-10CM CODES

C90.00	Multiple myeloma not having achieved remission
C90.01	Multiple myeloma in remission
C90.02	Multiple myeloma in relapse

EPIDEMIOLOGY & DEMOGRAPHICS

INCIDENCE:

- Five cases/100,000 persons (African Americans affected twice as frequently as whites, males more than females).
- MM accounts for 10% of all hematologic cancers and is the second most common hematologic malignancy
- More than 30,770 new cases and 12,770 deaths occurred in 2018 in the U.S.

PREDOMINANT AGE: The peak incidence is in the seventh decade at a median age of 70 yr.

PHYSICAL FINDINGS & CLINICAL PRESENTATION

The patient usually comes to medical attention because of one or more of the following:

- Bone pain (58%) commonly in the back and thorax or pathologic fractures (30%) caused by osteolytic lesions
- Anemia from bone marrow infiltration by plasma cells
- Recurrent infections as a result of impaired neutrophil function and deficiency of normal immunoglobulins (humoral deficiency)
- Nausea and vomiting caused by constipation and uremia
- Delirium resulting from hypercalcemia
- Neurologic complications, such as spinal cord or nerve root compression
- Purpura, epistaxis from thrombocytopenia
- Paresthesias, weight loss, generalized weakness

DIAGNOSIS

DIFFERENTIAL DIAGNOSIS

- Metastatic carcinoma to bone marrow
- Lymphoma, non-Hodgkin
- Bone neoplasms (e.g., sarcoma)
- Monoclonal gammopathy of undetermined significance
- Primary amyloidosis
- Waldenström macroglobulinemia
- Table 1 compares diagnostic criteria for multiple myeloma, myeloma variants, and monoclonal gammopathy of unknown significance (MGUS)

LABORATORY TESTS

- The evaluation of patients with multiple myeloma is summarized in Table 2.
- Normochromic, normocytic anemia; rouleaux formation on peripheral smear (Fig. 2).
- Hypercalcemia is present in 15% of patients at diagnosis.
- Elevated blood urea nitrogen, creatinine, uric acid, and total protein.
- Urine protein immunoelectrophoresis: Proteinuria from overproduction and secretion

TABLE 1 Diagnostic Criteria for Multiple Myeloma, Myeloma Variants, and Monoclonal Gammopathy of Unknown Significance

Monoclonal Gammopathy of Undetermined Significance (MGUS) or Monoclonal Gammopathy, Unattributed/Unassociated (MG[u])
M protein in serum <30 g/L
Bone marrow clonal plasma cells <10%
No evidence of other B-cell proliferative disorders
No myeloma-related organ or tissue impairment (no end-organ damage, including bone lesions)
Asymptomatic Myeloma (Smoldering Myeloma)
M protein in serum >30 g/L and/or
Bone marrow clonal plasma cell ≥10%-60%
No related organ or tissue impairment (no end-organ damage, including bone lesions) or symptoms
Symptomatic Multiple Myeloma (MM)
M protein in serum and/or urine[a]
Bone marrow (clonal) plasma cells[a] or plasmacytoma
Related organ or tissue impairment (end-organ damage, including bone lesions)
Clonal bone marrow plasma cell percentage ≥60%
Involved: Uninvolved serum free light ratio ≥100
>1 focal lesion on MRI studies
Solitary Plasmacytoma of Bone
No M protein in serum and/or urine[b]
Single area of bone destruction caused by clonal plasma cells
Bone marrow not consistent with MM
Normal skeletal survey (and MRI of spine and pelvis if done)
No related organ or tissue impairment (no end-organ damage other than solitary bone lesion)[b]
Nonsecretory Myeloma
No M protein in serum and/or urine with immunofixation
Bone marrow clonal plasmacytosis ≥10% or plasmacytoma
Related organ or tissue impairment (end-organ damage, including bone lesions)
Extramedullary Plasmacytoma
No M protein in serum and/or urine[c]
Extramedullary tumor of clonal plasma cells
Normal bone marrow
Normal skeletal survey
No related organ or tissue impairment (end-organ damage including bone lesions)
Multiple Solitary Plasmacytomas (Recurrent or Not)
No M protein in serum and/or urine[d]
More than one localized area of bone destruction or extramedullary tumor of clonal plasma cells that may be recurrent
Normal bone marrow
Normal skeletal survey and MRI of spine and pelvis if done
No related organ or tissue impairment (no end-organ damage other than the localized bone lesions)
Myeloma-Related Organ or Tissue Impairment (End-Organ Damage)
Calcium levels increased: Serum calcium >0-25 mmol/L above the upper limit of normal or >2-75 mmol/L
Renal insufficiency: Creatinine >173 mmol/L
Anemia: Hemoglobin 2 g/dl below the lower limit of normal or hemoglobin <10 g/dl
Bone lesions: Lytic lesions or osteoporosis with compression fractures (MRI or CT may clarify)
Other: Symptomatic hyperviscosity, amyloidosis, recurrent bacterial infections (more than two episodes in 12 mo)

CT, Computed tomography; *MRI,* magnetic resonance image.
[a]If flow cytometry is performed, most plasma cells (>90%) will show a neoplastic phenotype.
[b]A small M component may sometimes be present.
[c]A small M component may sometimes be present.
[d]A small M component may sometimes be present.
From Hoffman R et al: *Hematology, basic principles and practice,* ed 7, Philadelphia, 2018, Elsevier.

TABLE 2 Evaluation of Patients with Multiple Myeloma

Evaluation for Diagnosis
Evaluation for Monoclonal Protein
Serum protein electrophoresis, immunofixation
Quantitative immunoglobulin by nephelometric method
24-hr urine collection for electrophoresis and Bence Jones protein assessment and immunofixation
Serum free light chain and ratio
Evaluation for Clonal Plasma Cells
Bone marrow aspirate and biopsy for
Histology
Clonality by immunostaining or flow cytometry by κ/λ staining
Fine-needle aspiration of plasmacytoma if indicated
Evaluation for End-Organ Damage
Hemogram to detect anemia
Chemistry panel for renal function and calcium
Radiologic evaluation: Skeletal survey
PET-CT or MRI as indicated for bone lesions or extramedullary disease
Evaluation for Risk Stratification
β_2-Microglobulin and serum albumin for ISS stage
Cytogenetics and fluorescence in situ hybridization on bone marrow sample
LDH
C-reactive protein
Other Investigations for Selected Patients
Abdominal fat pad or rectal biopsy for amyloid
Solitary lytic lesion biopsy
Serum viscosity if IgM component or high IgA levels or serum M component >7 g/dl
Immunofixation for IgD or IgE in select cases

CT, Computed tomography; *Ig,* immunoglobulin; *ISS,* International Staging System; *LDH,* lactate dehydrogenase; *MRI,* magnetic resonance imaging; *PET,* positron emission tomography.

From Hoffman R et al: *Hematology, basic principles and practice,* ed 7, Philadelphia, 2018, Elsevier.

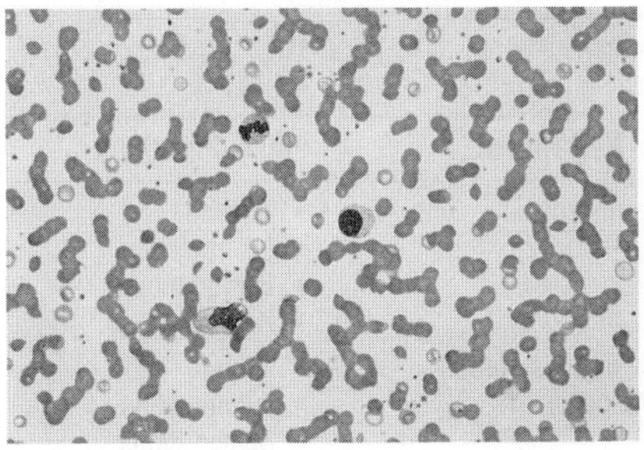

FIG. 2 Increased rouleaux formation is seen in this blood smear from a patient with a large M protein. Marked rouleaux formation is often a clue to the diagnosis of a plasma cell neoplasm but may also be observed in other conditions (Wright-Giemsa stain). (From Jaffe ES et al: *Hematopathology,* Philadelphia, 2011, Saunders.)

of free monoclonal kappa or lambda chains (Bence Jones protein).

- Serum protein immunoelectrophoresis: Monoclonal spike (M spike) on protein immunoelectrophoresis in approximately 75% of patients (Fig. 3); decreased levels of normal immunoglobulins (Ig).
  1. The increased immunoglobulins are generally IgG (70%) and IgA (20%).

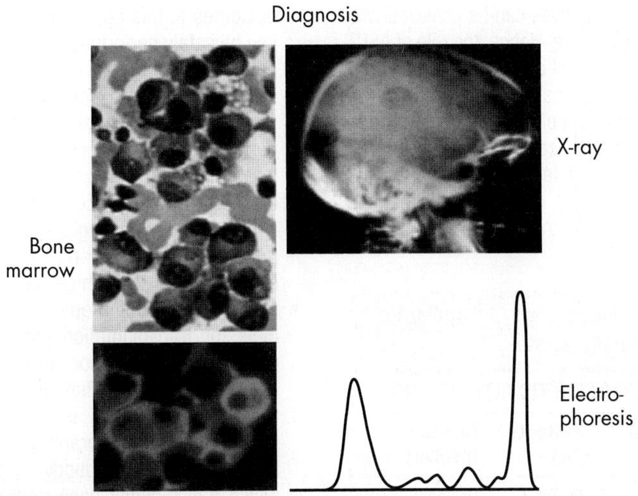

FIG. 3 Common diagnostic features in multiple myeloma. Light chain–restricted plasma cells in a bone marrow aspirate; multiple lytic lesions in a skull radiograph; large monoclonal spike in the g-globulin area in serum electrophoresis. (From Hoffman R et al: *Hematology, basic principles and practice,* ed 5, Philadelphia, 2009, Churchill Livingstone.)

  2. Approximately 5% to 10% of patients have only increased light chains in the urine by electrophoresis (light chain MM).
  3. A small percentage (<2%) of patients have nonsecretory MM (no increase in immunoglobulins and no light chains in the urine) but have other evidence of the disease (e.g., positive bone marrow examination).
- Elevated serum free light chains (kappa or lambda types) with abnormally elevated or decreased kappa:lambda ratios suggestive of the presence of monoclonal light chain proteins.
- Hyponatremia, increased serum viscosity (more common with production of IgM).
- Bone marrow examination demonstrates nests or sheets of plasma cells, which comprise >10% of the bone marrow.
- Serum beta 2-microglobulin is useful for prognosis, and elevated levels indicate high tumor mass and advanced stage disease.
- Elevated serum lactate dehydrogenase at diagnosis defines a subgroup of myeloma patients with very poor prognosis.
- Nearly all patients with MM present with abnormal chromosomes (Table 3) identified by fluorescence in situ hybridization (FISH). High-risk patients (<25% of patients at diagnosis) are those with any of the following: Deletion 17p, translocation 4:14, translocation 14:16, translocation 14;20, and gain of chromosome 1q21.

IMAGING STUDIES

Imaging modalities for disease assessment in myeloma are summarized in Table 4. Radiograph films of painful areas often demonstrate punched-out lytic lesions or osteoporosis (Figs. 3, E4, E5, and E6). CT can identify rib involvement not evident on plain films and differentiate it from osteoporotic and traumatic fractures (Fig. E7). MRI is the preferred technique for suspected spinal compression or soft tissue plasmacytomas. Bone scans may not be useful because MM lesions are not blastic. Positron emission tomography (PET) scans are increasingly used for detection of osseous and extraosseous disease.

STAGING

Table 5 describes the Revised International Staging System (R-ISS) for multiple myeloma that incorporates traditional laboratory parameters alongside high-risk chromosomal abnormalities detected by FISH techniques on bone marrow samples. This system provides important prognostic assessment and classifies patients into three risk groups (high, intermediate, and standard). Risk stratification in multiple myeloma is summarized in Tables 6 and 7.

Rx TREATMENT

NONPHARMACOLOGIC THERAPY

Prevention of renal failure with adequate hydration and avoidance of nephrotoxic agents and dye contrast studies.

ACUTE GENERAL Rx

- Treatment strategy is initially related to the determination of transplant-eligibility.
- Transplant-eligible patients generally receive approximately 4 to 6 mo of induction chemotherapy with triplet regimens such as the RVD regimen (bortezomib, lenalidomide, and dexamethasone) or the CyBorD regimen (cyclophosphamide, bortezomib, and dexamethasone). Upon demonstration of at least a partial response, these patients can undergo stem cell mobilization and collection followed by high-dose melphalan chemotherapy and autologous stem cell transplantation.
- ASCT has been associated historically with improvement in overall survival, and most recent studies have demonstrated a continued improvement in progression-free survival in favor of early transplantation. With the discovery of numerous novel agents, including monoclonal antibodies, next-generation proteasome inhibitors, and immunomodulatory

agents, deep responses can be achieved with these therapies alone. Hence, the role of ASCT in the current era will continue to evolve.

- Patients with high-risk features (high R-ISS stage, poor cytogenetics) should be offered autologous stem cell transplant (ASCT) subsequently, provided they have adequate cardiac, pulmonary, and hepatic function based on demonstrated improvement in outcomes in this population. Currently, ASCT can be safely performed in most centers in fit patients up to age 75 yr.
- Patients should be offered maintenance chemotherapy with either lenalidomide and/or bortezomib after recovery from ASCT for at least 2 yr or until disease progression. The choice of maintenance therapy depends on risk category, with single-agent maintenance preferred for standard-risk patients and doublet maintenance for high-risk patients.
- Induction chemotherapy in patients ineligible for transplantation (age >75 yr, high comorbidity index, poor performance status) can be identical to that offered transplant-eligible patients but is dose modified to allow for better tolerability. Daratumumab is a monoclonal antibody targeting CD38, which has recently been approved in combination with lenalidomide and dexamethasone in transplant-ineligible myeloma and is increasingly used, as it carries a lower risk of peripheral neuropathy compared to bortezomib-based therapy. Alternatively, less aggressive regimens (doublet regimens or single agents) can be recommended, including the following:
  1. Lenalidomide and dexamethasone (RD)
  2. Bortezomib and dexamethasone (VD)
- Therapy for relapsed and refractory myeloma can include second- or third-generation proteasome inhibitors (carfilzomib and ixazomib), immunomodulatory drugs (thalidomide, pomalidomide), and monoclonal antibodies elotuzumab (targeting signaling lymphocytic activation molecule F7 [SLAMF7]), daratumumab, and isatuximab. All of these agents have shown improved progression-free survival in relapsed or refractory multiple myeloma in various combinations and are useful options in this setting. The histone deacetylase inhibitor panobinostat is also approved in this setting, along with recent drug approval of nuclear protein transport inhibitor selinexor. In 2020, the first B-cell maturation antigen (BCMA)–targeted agent belantamab-mafodotin was approved for relapsed and refractory myeloma, and additional approvals of anti-BCMA chimeric antigen receptor therapy (CAR T-cell therapy) is anticipated.
- If the relapse occurs more than 6 mo after conventional therapy is stopped, the initial chemotherapy regimen can be reinstituted.
- ASCT can be considered as salvage therapy in patients who had stem cells cryopreserved early in the course of the disease, as this approach has been studied leading to similar survival compared to up-front transplantation.
- Approximately 15% of patients with newly diagnosed MM are recognized incidentally and present without significant symptoms (asymptomatic MM, formerly known as smoldering myeloma). The rate of progression of smoldering MM to symptomatic disease is 10% per yr for the initial 5 yr, decreasing to 5% for the next 5 yr, and decreasing further to 1.5% per yr thereafter. A subset of smoldering myeloma patients are considered high risk if they have 2 of the following criteria:
  1. Bone marrow plasmacytosis ≥20%
  2. Involved: Uninvolved serum free light chain ratio ≥20
  3. Monoclonal protein ≥2 g/dl
- Recent phase 3 studies of lenalidomide and lenalidomide and dexamethasone in treatment of high-risk smoldering myeloma have

TABLE 3 Recurrent Cytogenetic Changes in Myeloma

COMMON CYTOGENETIC ALTERATIONS

Chromosomal Abnormality	Patients (%)	Genes Involved
Hyperdiploidy	50-60	Unclear
Hypodiploid	20	Unclear
Pseudodiploid	15	Unclear
del(17p)	8	p53
t(4:14)	15	*FGFR3, MMSET*
t(11;14)	20	Cyclin D1
t(14;16)	3	*c-MAF*
t(14;20)	1	*MAFB*
t(6p25 or 6p21;14)	1	*IRF4* or *CCND3*
t(8;14)	5	*c-Myc*
t(9;14)	<1%	*PAX5*
del(13 or 13q)	50%	Unclear
Recently Identified Alterations		
1q+	35%	
1p–	30%	
5q+	50%	
12p–	10%	

From Hoffman R et al: *Hematology, basic principles and practice*, ed 7, Philadelphia, 2018, Elsevier.

TABLE 4 Imaging Modalities for Disease Assessment in Myeloma

	Use	Sensitivity/Specificity	False-Negatives	False-Positives
Bone scan	• For diagnostic screening, except for multiple myeloma	Varies	• Pure osteolytic lesions	• Trauma • Inflammation • Benign tumor • Healing
X-ray	• Can clarify nonspecific findings on bone scan • Assesses risk of fracture • Possible follow-up of tumor response, but evidence of response takes considerable time to appear	Low sensitivity	• Low disease burden • Osteopenia	• Trauma • Inflammation • Benign tumor • Healing
CT	• For anatomic detail in axial skeleton • Possible follow-up of tumor response, but role is still undefined	High sensitivity	• Low disease burden	• Trauma • Inflammation • Benign tumor • Healing
MRI	• Detection of spinal cord compression • Can help distinguish benign from malignant vertebral compression fracture • Possible follow-up of tumor response, but role is still undefined	High sensitivity and specificity	• Lesion only in cortex	• Edema
PET scan	• May eventually become first-line screening test for bone metastases • Possible follow-up of tumor response, but role is still undefined	High specificity	• Lesion only in cortex	• After chemotherapy
Bone density	• Measure osteoporosis • Response to bisphosphonates	High specificity and sensitivity		• Age-related osteoporosis

CT, Computed tomography; *MRI,* magnetic resonance imaging; *PET,* positron emission tomography.
From Hoffman R et al: *Hematology, basic principles and practice,* ed 7, Philadelphia, 2018, Elsevier.

TABLE 5 Revised International Staging System (R-ISS) for Multiple Myeloma Staging System

Stage	Criteria
I	ALL of the following: • Serum β-2 microglobulin <3.5 mg/L • Serum albumin >3.5 mg/dl • No high-risk chromosomal abnormalities by FISH • Normal LDH level
II	• Fitting neither stage I nor III
III	• Serum β-2 microglobulin >5.5 mg/L *AND* either elevated LDH *OR* high-risk chromosomal abnormalities by FISH [(del 17(p) and/or translocation t(14;16) and/or translocation t(4;14)]

FISH, Fluorescence in situ hybridization; *LDH,* lactate dehydrogenase.

TABLE 6 Risk Stratification in Multiple Myeloma

Investigations Recommended for Risk Stratification

Serum albumin and β_2-microglobulin to determine ISS stage
Bone marrow examination for t(4;14), t(14;16), and del(17p) on identified PCs by FISH
LDH
Immunoglobulin type: IgA
Histology: Plasmablastic disease or plasma cell leukemia

Additional Investigations for Risk Stratification

Cytogenetics
Gene expression profiling
Labeling index
MRI/PET scan
DNA copy number alteration by CGH/SNP array

CGH/SNP, Comparative genomic hybridization/single-nucleotide polymorphism; *DNA,* deoxyribonucleic acid; *FISH,* fluorescence in situ hybridization; *IgA,* immunoglobulin A; *ISS,* International Staging System; *LDH,* lactate dehydrogenase; *MRI,* magnetic resonance imaging; *PC,* plasma cell; *PET,* positron emission tomography.
From Hoffman R et al: *Hematology, basic principles and practice,* ed 7, Philadelphia, 2018, Elsevier.

TABLE 7 Standard Risk Factors for Multiple Myeloma and the Revised International Staging System

Prognostic Factor	Criteria
ISS stage	
I	Serum β_2-microglobulin <3.5 mg/L, serum albumin ≥3.5 g/dl
II	Not ISS stage I or III
III	Serum β_2-microglobulin ≥5.5 mg/L
CA by iFISH	
High risk	Presence of del(17p) and/or translocation t(4;14) and/or translocation t(14;16)
Standard risk	No high-risk CA
LDH	
Normal	Serum LDH below the upper limit of normal
High	Serum LDH above the upper limit of normal
A New Model for Risk Stratification for MM R-ISS stage	
I	ISS stage I and standard-risk CA by iFISH and normal LDH
II	Not R-ISS stage I or III
III	ISS stage III and either high-risk CA by iFISH or high LDH

CA, Chromosomal abnormalities; *iFISH,* interphase fluorescence in situ hybridization; *ISS,* International Staging System; *LDH,* lactate dehydrogenase; *MM,* multiple myeloma; *R-ISS,* Revised International Staging System.
From Greipp PR et al: International staging system for multiple myeloma, *J Clin Oncol* 23:3412, 2005. In Hoffman R et al: *Hematology, basic principles and practice,* ed 7, Philadelphia, 2018, Elsevier.

demonstrated an improvement in progression-free survival, prompting its use in this population.

CHRONIC Rx

- Promptly diagnose and treat infections. Common bacterial agents are *Streptococcus pneumoniae* and *Haemophilus influenzae.* Prophylactic therapy against *Pneumocystis jiroveci* with trimethoprim-sulfamethoxazole must be considered in patients receiving chemotherapy and high-dose corticosteroid regimens. Vaccinate against *S. pneumoniae,* influenza, and *H. influenzae.*
- Hypercalcemia is aggressively treated with IV fluids, bisphosphonates, and corticosteroids. Monthly infusions of the bisphosphonate pamidronate or zoledronate provide significant protection against skeletal complications and improve the quality of life of patients with advanced MM. The receptor activator of nuclear factor kappa B (RANK)-ligand inhibitor denosumab is effective in the treatment of hypercalcemia in this setting and in cases in which bisphosphonates are contraindicated (e.g., renal failure). Denosumab has also been studied in a large phase III study and has been shown to be noninferior to zoledronic acid.
- Control pain with analgesics; radiation therapy to treat painful bone lesions or cord compression. Perform surgical stabilization of pathologic fractures. Consider vertebroplasty or kyphoplasty for selected vertebral lesions.
- Anemia is treated with erythropoietin.

DISPOSITION

- In patients presenting at an age <60 yr, the 10-yr survival is approximately 30%. The median length of survival after diagnosis is now 7 to 8 yr and is rapidly increasing due to novel agents. Prognosis is better in asymptomatic patients with indolent or smoldering myeloma. Median survival time is approximately 10 yr in persons with no lytic bone lesions and a serum myeloma protein concentration <3 g/dl. Adverse outcome is associated with increased levels of beta-2 microglobulin, low levels of serum albumin, circulating plasma cells, plasmablastic features in bone marrow, increased plasma cell labeling index, poor cytogenetics (t (4;14) or t (14;16) translocation, deletion 17p).
- Tandem transplantation (two successive ASCT) improves survival among patients with MM who do not have a very good partial response after undergoing a single transplantation.
- Recent trials reveal that among patients with newly diagnosed myeloma, survival in recipients of a hematopoietic stem cell autograft followed by a stem cell allograft from an human leukocyte antigen (HLA)-identical sibling is superior to that in recipients of tandem stem cell autografts.

REFERRAL

To hematologist for management of disease, and bone marrow transplant specialist for transplantation options and management

SUGGESTED READINGS

Available at ExpertConsult.com

RELATED CONTENT

Multiple Myeloma (Patient Information)

AUTHORS: **Omar Nadeem, MD,** and **Bharti Rathore, MD**

BASIC INFORMATION

DEFINITION

Multiple sclerosis (MS) is a chronic predominantly autoimmune demyelinating disease of the central nervous system (CNS) characterized by subacute neurologic deficits correlating with CNS lesions separated in time and space, excluding other possible disease.

Subtypes include:

- **Relapsing-remitting MS (RRMS)** (82%): Relapses followed by complete or near-complete recovery, 50% to 85% of which later transition to SPMS
- **Secondary progressive MS (SPMS):** Progression of disability with few or no relapses
- **Primary progressive MS (PPMS)** (18%): Progression from the onset, rare relapses
- Progressive relapsing or relapsing progressive courses can be incorporated into PPMS or SPMS, respectively
- Relapses are defined as a subacute onset of neurologic dysfunction that lasts for at least 24 hr due to inflammatory demyelination

Classic rare MS variants include:

- **Marburg variant:** MRI reveals a tumor-like lesion with notable edema in one cerebral hemisphere. Pathology shows severe inflammation with necrosis: Typically acute onset with a fulminant, often malignant, course. May also involve peripheral nerves.
- **Balo concentric sclerosis:** Neuroimaging and pathology show alternating rings of myelination and demyelination resembling an onion bulb macroscopically and microscopically.
- **Schilder diffuse sclerosis:** Childhood onset with one to two large confluent lesions. Some cases were later found to be due to metabolic defects, and many have thus abandoned this disorder.

Neuromyelitis optica spectrum disorder (NMOSD): NMOSD is a distinct demyelinating disease with unique pathophysiology, treatment, and prognosis. Unlike MS, NMOSD usually involves extensive portions of the optic nerves and spinal cord (typically three or more spinal segments). Other areas of the CNS may also be involved, including the area postrema (presenting with intractable hiccups or nausea/vomiting), the brain stem, or the cerebral cortex. Additionally, patients may present with symptomatic narcolepsy. The lesions look very different on MRI than typical MS demyelinating lesions. The majority of patients are aquaporin-4 receptor Ab positive (NMO immunoglobulin G [IgG] positive) while some are antibody negative or are myelin oligodendrocyte glycoprotein Ab positive (MOG-IgG positive), which has a better prognosis. The actual diagnostic criteria for NMOSD vary depending on the patient's aquaporin-4 receptor antibody status. Prognosis is typically worse than MS, and this condition does not respond to MS-specific therapies. Steroids, plasma exchange, rituximab, mycophenolate mofetil, and azathioprine are among the treatments that may be used.

SYNONYMS

MS

Disseminated sclerosis

ICD-10CM CODE

G35 Multiple sclerosis

EPIDEMIOLOGY & DEMOGRAPHICS

PREVALENCE: More common in people raised in northern latitudes and in certain genetic clusters. Prevalence per 10,000 varies from 20 in southern Europe to 150 to 180 in Canada, northern United States, and northern Europe; and <10 in Asia, Central America, and most of Africa.

PREDOMINANT SEX & AGE: Female/male ratio is 2 to 3:1.

PEAK INCIDENCE: 20 to 40 yr in two thirds of patients; it is the most common permanently disabling disorder of the central nervous system in young adults; mean age of onset is 30 yr, range is infancy to 70 yr.

GENETICS: Frequency of MS in dizygotic twins and siblings is 3% to 5%, and 20% to 40% in monozygotic twins. Most common associations include human leukocyte antigen classes I and II (DRB1*1501, DQA1*0102, DQB1*0602), (DRB1*0405-DQA1*0301-DQB1*0302 in Mediterranean population). A notable epigenetic interaction between vitamin D and the main MS-linked HLA-DRB1*1501 allele has been elucidated.

PHYSICAL FINDINGS & CLINICAL PRESENTATION

Findings depend on the location of the CNS lesion(s) and may include the following:

- Common: Nonspecific complaints such as fatigue, blurred vision, diplopia, vertigo, falls, hemiparesis, paraparesis, monoparesis, numbness, paresthesias, ataxia, cognitive deficits, depression, sexual dysfunction, and urinary dysfunction
- Visual abnormalities: Horizontal nystagmus, visual field defects, ***Marcus Gunn pupil*** (i.e., relative afferent papillary defect—normal direct and consensual light reflexes; however, when swinging flashlight from one eye to the other, direct light causes dilatation of pupil of affected eye), ***internuclear ophthalmoplegia*** (paresis of the adducting eye on conjugate lateral gaze with horizontal nystagmus of the abducting eye) (Fig. 1)
- Corticospinal tract(s) involvement: Leads to upper motor neuron signs such as spasticity, hyperreflexia, clonus, extensor plantar responses, and upper motor neuron pattern of weakness
- Sensory loss: May include partial or full dermatomal loss of pain and temperature, loss of vibration (common) and position sense, or a thoracic band of sensory loss
- Ataxia: Intention tremor, dysmetria, dysdiadochokinesis, titubation, inability to tandem gait
- Bladder dysfunction: Detrusor hyperreflexia (urge incontinence), flaccidity (neurogenic bladder), and dyssynergia (bladder contracts against a closed sphincter)
- ***Lhermitte* sign:** Flexion of the neck elicits an electrical sensation extending down the spine and occasionally into the extremities
- ***Uhthoff* phenomenon:** Transient worsening of preexisting symptoms with small elevations in body temperature (e.g., during exercise or warm bathing)

ETIOLOGY

Remains unknown but multifactorial with evidence for autoimmunity (autoreactive T and B cells), environmental factors, and genetics (Mendelian and epigenetic). Environmental risk factors during childhood include certain viruses (e.g., Epstein-Barr virus and human herpes virus 6), low UV exposure, and month of birth (higher in spring). Other risk factors include low vitamin D level and smoking.

DIAGNOSIS

- MS: Based on revised 2017 McDonald criteria (Table 1)
- RRMS: See Table 1
- PPMS: Insidious progression of disability for at least 1 yr with a positive CSF and MRI evidence of >1 brain or >2 spinal cord MS-like lesions

DIFFERENTIAL DIAGNOSIS (TABLE 2)

- Autoimmune: Acute disseminated encephalomyelitis (ADEM), postvaccination encephalomyelitis, neuromyelitis optica spectrum disorder
- Degenerative: Subacute combined degeneration of the cord (vitamin B_{12} deficiency), amyotrophic lateral sclerosis, primary lateral sclerosis
- Infections: Lyme disease, neurosyphilis, HIV, tropical spastic paraparesis, progressive multifocal leukoencephalopathy, Whipple disease, acute flaccid myelitis, CNS tuberculosis, or fungal disease

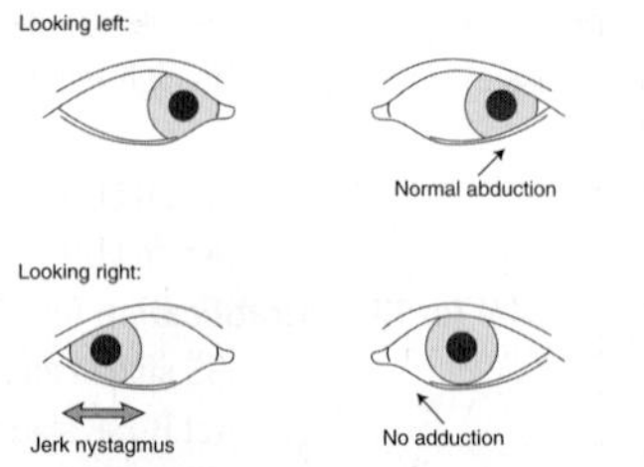

FIG. 1 Internuclear ophthalmoplegia. When the patient in the figure looks to the left (*top* row), both eyes move normally, but when the patient looks to the right (*bottom* row), the left eye fails to adduct ("weak" medial rectus) and the contralateral eye develops a jerk nystagmus. The finding is named for the side with weak adduction (i.e., in this example, a *left* internuclear ophthalmoplegia), and the lesion is in the *ipsilateral* medial longitudinal fasciculus (i.e., *left* medial longitudinal fasciculus in this example). See the text. (From McGee S: *Evidence-based physical diagnosis*, ed 4, Philadelphia, 2018, Elsevier.)

TABLE 1 Summary of Revised 2017 McDonald Criteria for Diagnosis of Multiple Sclerosis

RRMS/Clinical Attacks	Clinical Lesions	Paraclinical Testing Needed
2	2	None
2	1	MRI dissemination in space *or* a second clinical attack at a different CNS site
1	2	MRI dissemination in time *or* CSF-specific oligoclonal bands
1	1	1. Additional clinical attack at a different CNS site or MRI dissemination in space 2. MRI dissemination in time or CSF-specific oligoclonal bands

Evidence of clinical lesions by physical examination or evoked potentials.
CNS, Central nervous system; *CSF,* cerebrospinal fluid; *MRI dissemination in space,* ≥1 T2 lesions in 2 of the 4 typical areas for MS lesions—periventricular, juxtacortical, infratentorial, or spinal cord; *MRI dissemination in time,* a new lesion at follow-up MRI at any time, or presence of both an enhancing and nonenhancing lesion at any time; *RRMS,* relapsing-remitting multiple sclerosis.

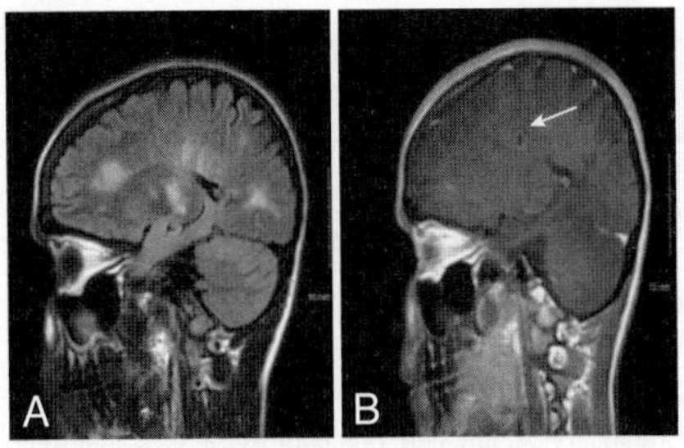

FIG. 2 Multiple sclerosis. A, Sagittal fluid-attenuated inversion recovery (FLAIR) image magnetic resonance scan shows multiple lesions in corpus callosum, "Dawson fingers" (periventricular finger-like lesions oriented toward the ventricles), along with ovoid and punctuate lesions in the deep white matter. **B,** Gadolinium-enhanced scan shows an enhancing lesion *(arrow).*

- Inflammatory: Systemic lupus erythematosus, vasculitis, sarcoidosis, Sjögren disease, Behçet disease, celiac disease
- Inherited metabolic disorders: Leukodystrophies
- Mitochondrial: Leber hereditary optic neuropathy, mitochondrial encephalopathy, lactic acidosis, and strokelike episodes (MELAS)
- Neoplasms: CNS lymphoma, metastases
- Vascular: Subcortical infarcts, Binswanger disease

WORKUP

- Lumbar puncture for cases that are atypical and to evaluate for mimics of MS. Typical CSF abnormalities may include increased protein (less than 100 mg/dl), mild elevation of mononuclear white blood cells, and increased IgG synthesis rate. 70% of clinically definite MS (CDMS) have elevated CSF IgG index, and 90% have CSF oligoclonal bands. (Serum for a serum protein electrophoresis needs to be sent to lab simultaneously with CSF for both tests.) False-positive results with IgG index and rarely with positive OCBs can be seen in CNS infections, parainfections, vasculitis, and CNS lymphoma.
- Serum: Complete blood count (CBC), chemistry panel, liver function tests, vitamin B_{12}, 25-OH vitamin D_3.
- Consider in the proper clinical setting: Aquaporin-4 IgG, MOG-IgG, antinuclear antibody (ANA), ACE (a test with low specificity and sensitivity for sarcoidosis) thyroid stimulating hormone (TSH), free T_4, very-long-chain fatty acids, arylsulfatase A.
- Consider optical coherence tomography or evoked potentials (visual, somatosensory, and brain stem auditory evoked response).

IMAGING STUDIES

Brain MRI with and without gadolinium is recommended in all cases. Fig. 2 illustrates imaging features of MS. MRI with and without contrast of the cervical (Fig. E3) and thoracic spine can be helpful. MRI assesses acute and chronic lesions as well as atrophy. A normal MRI of the brain does not conclusively exclude early MS but makes it extremely unlikely.

Rx TREATMENT

NONPHARMACOLOGIC THERAPY

Patient education regarding disease characteristics, treatment options, risks and benefits of treatment, and prognosis. Often patients need intermittent rest periods on a daily basis and when physically active, and avoid exposure to heat, which typically worsens symptoms (not the disease).

Recommend physical therapy for new or worsening weakness, incoordination, or spasticity.

ACUTE GENERAL Rx

Relapses: High-dose IV methylprednisolone (3 to 5 days of 1 g/day), often followed by a 7- to 10-day prednisone or methylprednisolone taper. High-dose corticosteroids do not alter the long-term course of disease. May consider plasmapheresis for refractory cases.

CHRONIC Rx

- The vast majority of FDA-approved therapies are only for relapsing MS; the FDA-approved ocrelizumab is the first medication for primary progressive MS.
- Disease-modifying injection therapy includes interferon beta-1a (intramuscular injection [IM Avonex, IM] Plegridy, subcutaneous [SC] Rebif), interferon beta-1b (SC Betaseron, SC Extavia), and glatiramer acetate (SC Copaxone, SC Glatopa). These medications are the first generation of multiple sclerosis drugs and have a low risk of side effects but are not as efficacious in preventing future relapses. Common side effects for interferons include flulike symptoms, depression, liver toxicity, and leukopenia; CBC and liver function tests (LFTs) (initially q1mo, then q3mo). Common side effects for glatiramer acetate include injection site reactions and benign chest tightness; no serum studies are needed.
- Disease-modifying oral therapy: These medications are newer and more efficacious in preventing multiple sclerosis relapses; however, they have a higher risk of serious side effects and infections. Consider baseline pregnancy test and infectious tests for all oral therapies, although not required by the FDA, such as VZV Ab, Lyme Ab, tuberculosis (TB) test, JC virus Ab, hepatitis Ab panel. Also review general risk of infections (hx UTIs, kidney stones, smoking, diabetes, bronchitis, disability, pulmonary function, and age). Typically monthly CBC and liver function tests for 6 mo then q3mo; pregnancy test.
  1. Fingolimod (Gilenya), siponimod (Mayzent), or ozanimod (Zeposia): Sphingosine-1-phosphate receptor modulators and lymphocyte sequesters. Possible side effects: Liver toxicity, bradycardia with first dose (requiring cardiac monitoring and ECG for at least 8 hr after administration of first dose), arrhythmia, pancytopenia, macular edema (ophthalmologic exam at baseline, at 3 mo, and thereafter for those with hx DM or uveitis), increased infections, and reduced pulmonary function. Obtain varicella-zoster virus (VZV) serology.
  2. Teriflunomide (Aubagio) - reversible inhibitor of pyrimidine synthesis (enzyme dihydroorotate dehydrogenase). Possible side effects: Diarrhea, abnormal liver function tests, nausea, and hair loss; pregnancy category X. Men should not impregnate their partners while on teriflunomide. Serum levels can be measured, and drug can be eliminated by charcoal or cholestyramine. Obtain TB test.
  3. Dimethyl fumarate (Tecfidera), diroximel fumarate (Vumerity), or monomethyl fumarate (Bafiertam): Mechanism includes inhibition of transcription of Nuclear factor-κB NF-κB. Frequent side effects include nausea, abdominal discomfort, and flushing—especially during the first month—and rarely leukopenia.
  4. Siponimod (Mayzent): A selective sphingosine-1-phosphate receptor modulator and lymphocyte sequester. Possible side effects: Liver toxicity but does not cause first-dose bradycardia and requires observation. Obtain VZV serology.

TABLE 2 Conditions that Can Be Mistaken for Multiple Sclerosis and Other Diseases of Myelin

Vascular Disease
Small-vessel cerebrovascular disease
Vasculitis
CADASIL
Antiphospholipid antibody syndrome
Structural Lesions
Craniocervical junction, posterior fossa, or spinal tumors
Cervical spondylosis or disc herniation
Chiari malformation or syrinx
Degenerative Diseases
Hereditary myelopathy
Spinocerebellar degeneration
Infections
HTLV-1 infection
HIV myelopathy or HIV-related cerebritis
Neuroborreliosis (e.g., Lyme disease)
John Cunningham (JC) JC virus/progressive multifocal leukoencephalopathy
Neurosyphilis
Other Inflammatory Conditions
Systemic lupus erythematosus
Sjögren syndrome
Sarcoidosis
Monofocal or Monophasic Demyelinating Syndromes
Neuromyelitis optica spectrum disorder
Acute disseminated encephalomyelitis
Other Conditions
Hashimoto thyroiditis with or without encephalopathy
Nonspecific MRI abnormalities related to migraine, aging, or trauma

CADASIL, Cerebral autosomal dominant arteriopathy with subcortical infarcts and leukoencephalopathy; *HIV,* human immunodeficiency virus; *HTLV,* human T-cell lymphotropic virus; *MRI,* magnetic resonance imaging.
From Goldman L, Schafer AI: *Goldman's Cecil Medicine,* ed 24, Philadelphia, 2012, Saunders.

5. Cladribine (mavenclad) is a purine antimetabolite. Possible side effects: Neutropenia, increased infections, thrombocytopenia, weight loss, increased risk of malignancy.

- Disease-modifying IV therapy: These medications are newer and more efficacious in preventing multiple sclerosis relapses; however, they have a higher risk of serious side effects and infections.
  1. Natalizumab (Tysabri) is a monoclonal humanized Ab that binds integrin-$\alpha 4$ interfering with binding to VCAM-1. It has been associated with a *higher* risk of progressive multifocal leukoencephalopathy (JC virus) than other immunomodulatory therapies. Test for JC virus Ab at least annually because conversion to a positive antibody occurs at increased frequency while on this drug. If positive, progressive multifocal leukoencephalopathy (PML) is still rare, but risk increases with increased length of therapy (>2 yr), history of chemotherapy, and concomitant immunosuppressants.
  2. Alemtuzumab (Lemtrada): An anti-CD52 humanized monoclonal antibody and second-line therapy for patients who have failed at least two FDA-approved MS therapies. The medication is delivered in two treatment courses. After an initial series of five daily infusions, the medication is administered 1 yr later for 3 days. Serious side effects include the development of autoimmune conditions (34% developed autoimmune thyroid disorders), infusion reactions, and certain cancers. The medication is only available through a restricted access program.
  3. Ocrelizumab (Ocrevus): A first-line therapy that is a humanized monoclonal antibody to CD20+ B cells. This is the only drug approved not only for relapsing forms of MS but also for primary progressive MS. Infections are the most common side effects.
  4. Ofatumumab (Kesimpta): CD20 monoclonal antibody delivered as a monthly SC injection.
- Symptomatic therapy:
  1. Dalfampridine (Ampyra) is a potassium channel blocker recently approved to improve walking speed in patients with MS. This medication is contraindicated in patients with epilepsy.
  2. Treat spasticity with baclofen or tizanidine. Onabotulinum toxin type A injection for focal intractable spasticity. Intrathecal baclofen pump for generalized intractable spasticity. Acute worsening may be due to infections such as urinary tract infection (UTI), injury, recent surgery, or colder temperatures.
  3. Treat urge incontinence with anticholinergic/muscarinic therapy such as oxybutynin, tolterodine, or solifenacin. Treat urinary retention with tamsulosin. In both cases, rule out a bladder infection.
  4. Treat dysesthesias with gabapentin or pregabalin.
  5. Fatigue: Consider amantadine 100 mg bid, modafinil, or a stimulant.
  6. Tremor: Clonazepam, propranolol, or gabapentin.
  7. Depression and anxiety are common. Consider referring to both a counselor and psychiatrist.

DISPOSITION

Most patients have complete or near-complete recovery weeks to months after a relapse. Typically, two relapses occur in RRMS patient per yr (75% will have >1 relapse). Although the rate of disease progression is highly variable, there is higher risk of greater long-term disability with higher relapse rate during the first 2 to 5 yr, poor recovery from initial relapses, older age of onset, involvement of multiple systems, male sex, African American, and primary progressive disease.

Disease-modifying treatment has improved, and the current treatment goal is no relapses and no disease progression on imaging.

REFERRAL

- Referral to neurologist is highly recommended. Referral to MS specialist should be considered in cases of poor response to therapy and/or if there is concern about complications of therapies.
- Consider referrals for physical, speech, and occupational therapy.
- Consider referral to urology if bladder-sphincter dyssynergia is possible or if not responsive to treatment.

PEARLS & CONSIDERATIONS

- Clinically isolated syndrome (CIS): Isolated demyelinating event and assessing risk of CDMS 1) in optic neuritis, if brain MRI is completely normal, there is 20% to 25% chance of CDMS over 15 yr. 2) In CIS, if there are >1 T2 hyperintensity on brain MRI, there is 84% risk, and if there are >2 Gd + lesions there is a 96% risk of CDMS over 18 mo.
- Pseudorelapses may occur with heat, fever, or infections (urinary tract infections common in patients with MS).
- Headache, fever, altered mental status, elevated CSF WBCs, or recurrent relapses over days to weeks raises concern for CNS infection or ADEM.

SUGGESTED READINGS

Available at ExpertConsult.com

RELATED CONTENT

Multiple Sclerosis (Patient Information)

AUTHOR: **Corey Goldsmith, MD**

BASIC INFORMATION

DEFINITION

Mushroom poisoning is intoxication resulting from ingestion of poisonous mushrooms.

ICD-10CM CODE

T62.0X1A Toxic effect of ingested mushrooms, accidental (unintentional), initial encounter

EPIDEMIOLOGY & DEMOGRAPHICS

- 5% of all mushrooms are poisonous. Distinction between poisonous and edible mushrooms may be difficult even by experienced persons.
- Common poisonous species include *Amanita, Russula, Gyromitra,* and *Omphalotus* (see Table 1). *Amanita phalloides* (Fig. E1), colloquially known as the "death cap," belongs to the *Phalloideae* section of the *Amanita* family of mushrooms and is responsible for most deaths following ingestion of foraged mushrooms worldwide.
- Identification of syndromes is more important than knowing the associated species (Table 2).

PHYSICAL FINDINGS & CLINICAL PRESENTATION

- *Russula* causes confusion, delirium, visual disturbance, tachycardia, and diarrhea within a few hours of ingestion. Prognosis: Spontaneous recovery (mortality rate >1%).
- *Amanita* and *Gyromitra* intoxication begins with symptoms of gastroenteritis (nausea, vomiting, diarrhea, and abdominal cramps) approximately 10 hr after ingestion. *Amanita* then causes cardiomyopathy and hepatic and renal failure. *Gyromitra* produces jaundice and seizures. Both mushrooms are associated with a 50% mortality rate.
- *Omphalotus* causes symptoms of gastroenteritis that subside spontaneously within 24 hr.

ETIOLOGY

- *Amanita* contains cytotoxic substances and isoxazoles that are gamma-aminobutyric acid neurotransmitter analogs. Amatoxins, consisting of alpha-, beta-, and gamma-amanitin, account for >90% of deaths related to mushroom poisoning. The amanitas are heat stable and not inactivated by cooking.
- *Gyromitra* contains a pyridoxine antagonist that disrupts the gastrointestinal mucosa and causes hemolysis.
- *Russula* contains a cholinergic substance.
- Table 3 provides an overview of fungal toxins and main symptoms

DIAGNOSIS

DIFFERENTIAL DIAGNOSIS

- Food poisoning
- Overdose of prescription or illegal drug
- Other intoxications
- See topic on specific organ failure (e.g., renal or hepatic failure) for differential diagnosis of those conditions

WORKUP

- History
- Inspection and identification of suspected mushrooms
- Mushroom or gastric content analysis (by thin-layer chromatography or radioimmunoassay)

TREATMENT

- Gastric lavage.
- Repeated administration of activated charcoal.
- Penicillin G or silibinin can be used for *Amanita* mushroom intoxication. Silibinin interferes with hepatic uptake of alpha-amanitin. IV silibinin is not currently available in the U.S. Where available, it is given at a rate of 5 mg/kg IV over 1 hr, followed by 20 mg/kg/day. An oral form of silibinin is available in health food stores as an extract from milk thistle called silymarin. Dose is 1 g PO qid. IV benzyl penicillin reduces hepatocyte uptake of amatoxin.
- Supportive care as needed (may require respiratory assistance, hemodialysis, or emergency liver transplantation) in the event of irreversible fulminant liver failure.
- In patients with severe *Amanita* poisoning, early contact with the nearest liver transplant center is recommended.
- Box 1 summarizes the general management of mushroom poisoning.

RELATED CONTENT

Mushroom Poisoning (Patient Information)

SUGGESTED READING

Available at ExpertConsult.com

AUTHOR: **Fred F. Ferri, MD**

TABLE 1 Mushroom Groups

Group/Toxin	Representative Example	Clinical Effects
Early Onset of Symptoms		
Coprine	*Coprinus atramentarius*	Disulfiram reaction with alcohol
GI toxin	Many species	Nausea, vomiting, diarrhea, abdominal pain
Ibotenic acid and muscimol	*Amanita muscaria*	Diverse CNS effects, including hallucinations, seizures, delirium, coma, agitation
Muscarine	*Clitocybe dealbata*	Peripheral cholinergic toxidrome
Psilocybin	*Psilocybe cubensis*	CNS effects, including hallucinations and euphoria
Late Onset of Symptoms		
Cyclopeptides	*Amanita phalloides*	GI effects followed by hepatotoxicity
Gyromitrin	*Gyromitra esculenta*	GI effects followed by seizures
Orellanine	*Cortinarius orellanus*	GI effects followed by renal toxicity

CNS, Central nervous system; *GI,* gastrointestinal.
From Marx J: *Rosen's emergency medicine: concepts and clinical practice*, ed 7, Philadelphia, 2010, Elsevier.

TABLE 2 Summary Common Mushroom-Associated Syndromes

Syndrome	Clinical Course	Toxin(s)	Typical Causative Mushroom(s)
Delayed gastroenteritis followed by hepatorenal syndrome	Stage 1: 24 hr after ingestion: Onset of nausea, vomiting, profuse cholera-like diarrhea, abdominal pain, hematuria Stage 2: 12-48 hr after ingestion: Apparent recovery; levels of hepatic enzymes are rising during this stage Stage 3: 24-72 hr after ingestion: Progressive hepatic and renal failure, coagulopathy, cardiomyopathy, encephalopathy, convulsions, coma, death	Cyclopeptides, principally amatoxins	"Deadly *Amanitas*," *Galerina* species
Hyperactivity, delirium, coma	30 min to 2 hr after ingestion: Delirium, hallucinations, and coma	Muscimol, ibotenic acid	*Amanita muscaria, Amanita pantherina*

continued

TABLE 2 Summary Common Mushroom-Associated Syndromes—cont'd

Syndrome	Clinical Course	Toxin(s)	Typical Causative Mushroom(s)
Delayed gastroenteritis with central nervous system abnormalities	6-24 hr after ingestion: Nausea, vomiting, diarrhea, abdominal pain, muscle cramps, delirium, convulsions, coma; hemolysis and methemoglobinemia may occur	Gyromitrin	*Gyromitra esculenta* ("false morel")
Cholinergic syndrome	30 min to 2 hr after ingestion: Bradycardia, bronchorrhea, bronchospasm, salivation, perspiration, lacrimation, convulsions, coma	Muscarine	*Boletus* species, *Clitocybe* species, *Inocybe* species, *Amanita* species
Disulfiram-like reaction with ethanol	30 min after drinking ethanol (may occur up to 1 wk after eating coprine-containing mushrooms): Flushing of skin of face and trunk, hypotension, tachycardia, chest pain, dyspnea, nausea, vomiting, extreme apprehension	Coprine	*Coprinus atramentarius*
Hallucinations	30 min to 3 hr after ingestion: Hallucinations, euphoria, drowsiness, compulsive behavior, agitation	Psilocybin and psilocin	*Psilocybe* species
Delayed gastritis and renal failure	Abdominal pain, anorexia, vomiting starting over 30 hr after ingestion, followed by progressive renal failure 3-14 days later	Orelline, orellanine	*Cortinarius* species
Immune-mediated hemolytic anemia	Syncope, gastroenteritis, oliguria, hemoglobinuria, back pain, hemolysis	Immunoglobulin mediated	*Paxillus involutus*
General gastrointestinal irritants	30 min to 2 hr after ingestion: Nausea, vomiting, abdominal cramping, diarrhea; may recover without treatment	Unidentified, probably multiple	*Chlorophyllum molybdites*, backyard mushrooms ("little brown mushrooms"), many others

From Brent J et al (eds): *Haddad and Winchester's clinical management of poisoning and drug overdose*, ed 4, Philadelphia, 2007, Saunders, Table 23-1.

TABLE 3 Overview of Fungal Toxins, Examples of Poisonous Mushrooms and Main Symptoms

Toxins	Fungi	Symptoms
Cytotoxic Agents		
Amatoxins	*Amanita phalloides, A. virosa, A. verna, Galerina marginata, Lepiota* spp.	Intense gastroenteritis after 8-24 hr, liver and kidney damage
Nephrotoxins		
Aminohexadienoic acid	*Amanita smithiana, A. proxima*	Early renal damage
Orellanine	*Cortinarius orellanus, C. speciocissimus*	Late renal damage
Neurotoxins		
Psilocybins	*Psilocybe* and *Panaeolus* spp., etc.	Euphoria, anxiety, agitation, hallucinations, depersonalization, tachycardia, flushing etc.
Muscarine	*Inocybe* and *Clitocybe* spp., etc.	Nausea, diarrhea, diaphoresis, salivation, miosis, bradycardia, hypotension, lacrimation, chills, tremor, bronchospasm, etc.
Isoxazoles	*Amanita muscaria, A. pantherina, A. regalis, A. strobiliformis*	Inebriation, euphoria, confusion, agitation, anxiety, delusions, hallucinations, violent behavior, seizures, tachycardia, mydriasis, urinary retention, etc.
Myotoxins		
Cycloprop-2-ene carboxylic acid	*Russula subnigricans*	Early myotoxicity
Saponaceolide B and M	*Tricholoma equestre*	Late myotoxicity
Metabolic Toxins		
Gyromitrin	*Gyromitra esculenta*	Neurological, gastrointestinal and hepatic symptoms, hemolysis
Coprine	*Coprinus, Clitocybe, Boletus*	Antabuse syndrome
γ-guanidinobutyric acid, etc.	*Trogia venenata*	Hypoglycemia
Gastrointestinal Irritants		
Not identified	*Agaricus, Entoloma, Boletus, Hebeloma, Tricholoma, Russula, Lactarius, Ramaria* spp., etc.	Gastrointestinal symptoms

From Ryan ET et al: *Hunter's tropical medicine and emerging infectious diseases*, ed 10, Philadelphia, 2019, Elsevier.

BOX 1 General Management of Mushroom Ingestion

1. Determine history of ingestion: How many types of mushrooms ingested, what time, if anyone else ate them, and what symptoms are present.
2. Attempt to determine which of the possible syndromes (see Table 2) the patient may have. For example, gastrointestinal symptoms occurring more than 6 hr after ingestion strongly suggest cyclopeptide, gyromitrin, or *Cortinarius* poisoning.
3. Administer activated charcoal. If the patient has diarrhea, do not give a cathartic. If a cathartic is used, give it only with the first dose of activated charcoal. Use repeated doses of activated charcoal for suspected amatoxin poisonings.
4. If feasible and when indicated, send gastric aspirate or emesis, along with any remaining mushrooms, to a mycologist for identification.
5. Try to perform a preliminary identification of mushroom and spores. Start to develop a spore print as soon as possible.
6. Maintain supportive measures, including airway support, intravenous fluids, and vasopressors (if needed). Monitor volume status.
7. Avoid antispasmodics for gastrointestinal symptoms.
8. Anticipate the clinical course.

From Brent J et al (eds): *Haddad and Winchester's clinical management of poisoning and drug overdose*, ed 4, Philadelphia, 2007, Saunders.

BASIC INFORMATION

DEFINITION

Myasthenia gravis (MG) is an autoimmune disorder affecting postsynaptic neuromuscular transmission, most commonly mediated by antibodies directed against the nicotinic acetylcholine receptor (AChR) of the neuromuscular junction. Anti-AChR antibodies cause a decrease in functional postsynaptic ACh receptors, resulting in fatigable weakness. A small percentage of MG patients lack AChR antibodies, and a subset of these patients possess antibodies against muscle-specific tyrosine kinase (MuSK), impacting both pre- and postsynaptic function of the neuromuscular junction. A classification of MG is described in Table 1.

SYNONYM

MG

ICD-10CM CODES

G70.00	Myasthenia gravis without (acute) exacerbation
G70.01	Myasthenia gravis with (acute) exacerbation
P94.0	Transient neonatal myasthenia gravis

EPIDEMIOLOGY & DEMOGRAPHICS

INCIDENCE (IN U.S.): 8 to 10 cases annually per 1 million persons. It is the most common disorder of neuromuscular junction transmission.

PREVALENCE (IN U.S.): 150 to 250 cases per 1 million

PREDOMINANT SEX: Females are affected more often than males (3:2) in adults; they are equally affected in the elderly.

PEAK INCIDENCE: Female, second to third decades; male, sixth to eighth decades

GENETICS: Increased frequency of HLA-B8, DR3

PHYSICAL FINDINGS & CLINICAL PRESENTATION

- The hallmark of MG is weakness worsened with exercise and improved with rest.
- Generalized weakness involving proximal muscles, diaphragm, and neck extensors is common.
- Weakness is confined to eyelids and extraocular muscles in approximately 15% of patients (Fig. 1).
- Bulbar symptoms of ptosis, diplopia, dysarthria, and dysphagia are common.
- Reflexes, sensation, and coordination are normal.

ETIOLOGY

Antibody-mediated decrease in nicotinic AChR in the postsynaptic neuromuscular junction resulting in defective neuromuscular transmission and subsequent muscle weakness and fatigue. Early-onset MG is associated with *HLA-DR3, HLA-B8,* and non-*HLA* genes. Late-onset MG is associated with *HLA-DR2, HLA-B27,* and *HLA-DRB1*. MuSK antibodies have been recognized since 2001 and present with a similar syndrome to AChR MG although they may have more bulbar weakness, proximal muscle atrophy, and either lack of or paradoxical response to pyridostigmine. Serologic and clinical presentation of myasthenia gravis subgroups are summarized in Table 2.

DIAGNOSIS

DIFFERENTIAL DIAGNOSIS

Lambert-Eaton myasthenic syndrome, botulism, medication-induced myasthenia, chronic progressive external ophthalmoplegia, congenital myasthenic syndromes, thyroid disease, basilar meningitis, intracranial mass lesion with cranial neuropathy, Miller-Fisher variant of Guillain-Barré syndrome

WORKUP

- Edrophonium (Tensilon) test (Fig. 2): Useful in MG patients with ocular symptoms, although uncommonly used now. Cardiac monitoring and atropine ready at the bedside are essential. Patients with MG may also have a positive ice pack test (Fig. E3).
- Repetitive nerve stimulation: Successive stimulation shows decrement of muscle action potential in clinically weak muscle; may be negative in up to 50%.
- Single-fiber electromyography: Highly sensitive; abnormal in up to 95% of patients.
- Serum AChR antibodies found in up to 90% of patients.
- A subset of patients with seronegative MG may have MuSK antibodies.

LABORATORY TESTS

- Forced vital capacity (FVC) is the most useful test for assessing neuromuscular respiratory status. Patients with an FVC of <20 ml/kg are at high risk of respiratory failure and should be monitored in an ICU setting. Although the decision of when to intubate is a clinical one, FVC falling below 10 to 15 ml/kg generally requires intubation.
- CT scan with contrast of anterior chest to look for thymoma or residual thymic tissue. 10% of patients with MG have a thymoma and the prevalence increases with age.
- Thyroid-stimulating hormone, free T_4 to rule out thyroid disease.

TREATMENT

NONPHARMACOLOGIC THERAPY

- Patient education to facilitate recognition of worsening symptoms and impress need for medical evaluation at onset of clinical deterioration
- Avoidance of selected drugs (Table 3) known to provoke exacerbations of MG (beta-blockers, aminoglycoside and quinolone antibiotics, penicillamine, interferons,

TABLE 1 Osserman Classification Used by the Myasthenia Gravis Foundation of America to Standardize Clinical Symptoms[1]

Class I	Any ocular muscle weakness
Class II	Ocular muscle weakness of any severity, MILD limb weakness
Class IIa	Predominantly limb and/or axial muscle weakness
Class IIb	Predominantly bulbar and/or respiratory muscle weakness
Class III	Ocular muscle weakness of any severity, MODERATE weakness of other muscles
Class IIIa	Predominantly limb and/or axial muscle weakness
Class IIIb	Predominantly bulbar and/or respiratory muscle weakness
Class IV	Ocular muscle weakness of any severity, SEVERE weakness of other muscles
Class IVa	Predominantly limb and/or axial muscle weakness
Class IVb	Predominantly bulbar and/or respiratory muscle weakness
Class V	Intubation with or without mechanical ventilation

[1]Jaretzki A et al: Myasthenia gravis: recommendations for clinical research standards. Task Force of the Medical Scientific Advisory Board of the Myasthenia Gravis Foundation of America, *Neurology* 55:16-23, 2000.

From Parrillo JE, Dellinger RP: *Critical care medicine: principles of diagnosis and management in the adult,* ed 5, Philadelphia, 2019, Elsevier.

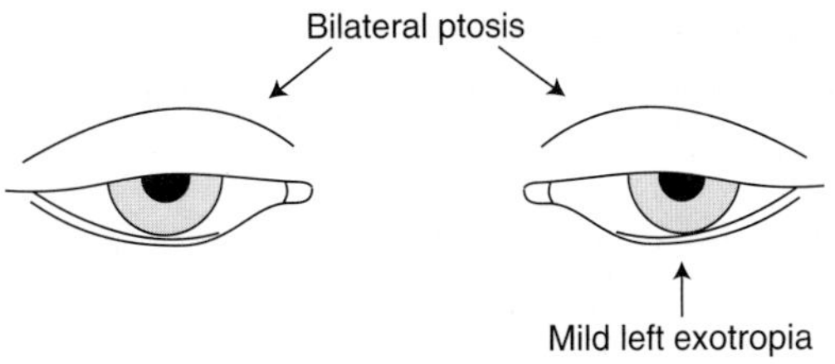

FIG. 1 Myasthenia gravis. Myasthenia gravis may mimic any ocular disorder causing diplopia, although most often it mimics weakness of the superior rectus muscle or medial rectus muscle (i.e., difficulty with sustained elevation or adduction of the eye, respectively). Clues to the diagnosis of myasthenia gravis are associated ptosis, fluctuating course, and normal pupils. (From McGee S: *Evidence-based physical diagnosis,* ed 4, Philadelphia, 2018, Elsevier.)

TABLE 2 Serologic and Clinical Presentation of Myasthenia Gravis Subgroups[1-7]

	AChR Antibody	MuSK Antibody	Striated Muscle Antigens Titin Antibody RyR Antibody	Age at Onset Sex	Clinical Findings	Response to Therapy	Response to Thymectomy	Prognosis
Ocular MG	50%-75%	None	None	Older Male	Ocular	Good	Good	Good (but 50% can develop generalized MG in 2 yr)
Early-onset generalized MG	80%-85% (high titer)	None	None-rare	<50 yr	General	Rarely needs immuno-suppression	Good	Less severe Low mortality
Late-onset generalized MG	None-rare	None	50% 54% titin 33% RyR	≥50 yr	General	Often requires immuno-suppression	Poor	Severe
Thymomatous-associated MG	Positive, nearly 100% (low titer)	None	95% 50% titin 47% RyR	Ranges: Older but <40 yr if RyR	General If RyR: Ocular, bulbar, respiratory weakness	Often requires immuno-suppression	Fair	RyR: Invasive, malignant thymoma Severe Higher mortality
Generalized MG MuSK positive	None	100%	None	Younger Female	Facial, bulbar, neck, respiratory weakness paraspinal, esophageal muscles	Poor response to AChE inhibitors	Poor (no thymic changes)	Severe, progressive course
MG with thymic hyperplasia	89%	None	None	Younger Female	General	Good	Good	Good
ACh antibody negative	Negative	Negative	Present	Younger Female	General	Poor		Fair

ACh, Acetylcholine; *AChE*, acetylcholinesterase; *AChR*, acetylcholine receptor; *MG*, myasthenia gravis; *MuSK*, muscle-specific tyrosine kinase; *RyR*, ryanodine receptor.
[1]Romi F et al: Myasthenia gravis patients with ryanodine receptor antibodies have distinctive clinical features, *Eur J Neurol* 14:617-620, 2007.
[2]Romi F et al: Myasthenia gravis: clinical, immunological, and therapeutic advances, *Acta Neurol Scand* 111:134-141, 2005.
[3]Akaishi T et al: Response to treatment of myasthenia gravis according to clinical subtype, *BMC Neurol* 16:225, 2016.
[4]Gilhus NE, Verschuuren JJ: Myasthenia gravis: subgroup classification and therapeutic strategies, *Lancet Neurol* 14:1023-1036, 2015.
[5]Hong Y et al: Autoantibody profile and clinical characteristics in a cohort of Chinese adult myasthenia gravis patients, *J Neuroimmunol* 298:51-57, 2016.
[6]Gilhus NE et al: Myasthenia gravis-autoantibody characteristics and their implications for therapy, *Nat Rev Neurol* 12:259-268, 2016.
[7]Roberts PF et al: Thymectomy in the treatment of ocular myasthenia gravis, *J Thorac Cardiovasc Surg* 122:562-568, 2001.
From Parrillo JE, Dellinger RP: *Critical care medicine: principles of diagnosis and management in the adult*, ed 5, Philadelphia, 2019, Elsevier.

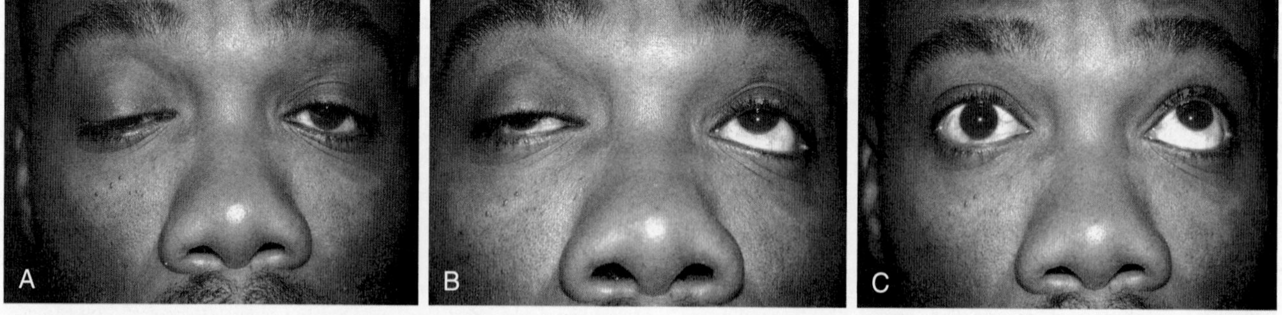

FIG. 2 Positive edrophonium test in myasthenia gravis. A, Asymmetric ptosis in the primary position. **B,** Defective upgaze. **C,** Following injection of edrophonium, there is marked bilateral improvement of ptosis and modest improvement of left upgaze. (From Kanski JJ et al: *Clinical ophthalmology: a systematic approach*, ed 7, Philadelphia, 2010, Saunders.)

TABLE 3 Medications to Avoid in Myasthenia Gravis[1]

Medications to Avoid	Examples	Recommendation for Avoidance	Mechanism of Weakness
Antibiotics			
Aminoglycosides	Gentamycin Streptomycin	Contraindicated	Blocks ACh receptor, prevents release of ACh
	Tobramycin Amikacin	Less likely problematic	
Antimalarials	Quinine Chloroquine	Contraindicated	Presynaptic blockage of voltage-dependent sodium channels and postsynaptic potentiation of depolarization
Macrolides	Erythromycin, Tetracycline Azithromycin	Relative	Affects presynaptic transmission
Fluoroquinolones	Moxifloxacin Ciprofloxacin Levofloxacin Ofloxacin	FDA black box warning	Unknown
Ketolide	Telithromycin	FDA black box warning	Unknown
	Polymyxins	Contraindicated	Presynaptic and postsynaptic effects
Cardiovascular			
Antiarrhythmics	Procainamide Propafenone	Contraindicated	Decreases the release of ACh Sodium influx blocker
β-Blockers	Propranolol Atenolol Ophthalmic timolol	Relative	Unclear—may be at the neuromuscular junction or muscle membrane
Calcium channel blocker	Verapamil Amlodipine	Relative	Presynaptic and postsynaptic blockade of L-type calcium channels
Anticonvulsants			
	Phenytoin	Relative	Depressed postsynaptic response to ACh; inhibition of calcium channel; increase in muscle membrane threshold
	Carbamazepine	Relative	Triggers immune response
	Gabapentin	Relative	Binds voltage-gated calcium channel
Chemotherapeutic Agents			
	Doxorubicin Etoposide Cisplatin	Relative	Unknown
Others			
	Interferon	Relative	Autoantibody production
Neuromuscular blocking agents	Atracurium Cisatracurium Vecuronium	Relative	Blocks ACh receptors
Statins		Relative	Unknown
Corticosteroids		Relative	Direct blocking of ACh receptor through ionic channels
Botulinum toxin		Contraindicated	Impairs synaptic transmission
Magnesium		Relative	Impairs synaptic transmission
Penicillamine		Contraindicated	Binds the ACh receptor; induces antibodies to receptor

[1]Ahmed A, Simmons Z: Drugs which may exacerbate or induce myasthenia gravis: a clinician's guide. *Internet J Neurol* 10:1-8, 2008.
ACh, Acetylcholine; *FDA,* Food and Drug Administration.
From Parrillo JE, Dellinger RP: *Critical care medicine: principles of diagnosis and management in the adult,* ed 5, Philadelphia, 2019, Elsevier.

class I antiarrhythmics [procainamide, quinidine, etc.])
- Prompt treatment of infections, diet modification, and speech evaluation with dysphagia

ACUTE GENERAL Rx

- Symptomatic treatment with acetylcholinesterase inhibitors:
  1. Pyridostigmine 30 to 60 mg PO q4 to 6h initially; onset of effects is 30 min, duration 4 hr. May be titrated up to 120 mg every 4 hr. GI upset is not uncommon with higher doses and may respond to hyoscyamine.
- Immunosuppressive treatment with corticosteroids and azathioprine is first-line treatment:
  1. Prednisone initiated at 10 to 20 mg daily titrated by 5-mg increments to effect or dose of 1 mg/kg/day with improvement in 2 to 4 wk and maximal response by 3 to 6 mo.
  2. Azathioprine initiated at 50 mg daily titrated to 2 to 3 mg/kg/day with clinical effect in 6 to 12 mo. Azathioprine is not recommended in patients with no thiopurine methyltransferase activity.
- Alternative secondary agents:
  1. Eculizumab, a first-in-class compliment inhibitor, is FDA-approved for adult patients who are acetylcholine-antibody positive and continue to suffer from severe symptoms despite current immunotherapy use.
  2. Cyclosporine initiated at 5 mg/kg/day with clinical effect within 1 to 2 mo.
  3. Mycophenolate mofetil 500 mg twice a day titrated to 2 g/day with clinical effect in 3 to 6 mo, but can be up to 12 mo.
  4. Rituximab.
- Plasmapheresis and IV immunoglobulin are short-term options for immunotherapy during an exacerbation. There is no significant difference in efficacy between intravenous immunoglobulin (IVIG) and plasmapheresis.
- Mechanical ventilation is lifesaving in setting of a myasthenic crisis. Consider elective intubation if forced vital capacity <10 to 15 ml/kg.

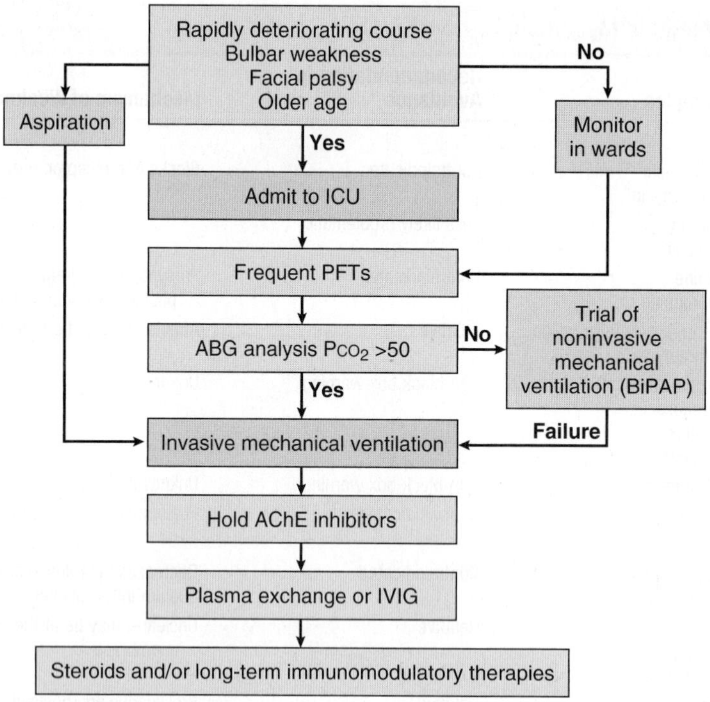

FIG. 4 Clinical flowchart for the management of myasthenic crisis. *ABG,* Arterial blood gas; *AChE,* acetyl cholinesterase; *BiPAP,* bilevel positive airway pressure; *ICU,* intensive care unit; *IVIG,* intravenous immunoglobulin; *PFT,* pulmonary function test. (From Parrillo JE, Dellinger RP: *Critical care medicine, principles of diagnosis and management in the adult,* ed 4, Philadelphia, 2014, Elsevier.)

- Fig. 4 illustrates a flowchart for the management of myasthenic crisis.

SURGICAL Rx

- In thymomatous MG, thymectomy is indicated in all patients. If the tumor cannot be surgically resected, chemotherapy can be considered for prevention of local invasion and symptom relief.
- For nonthymomatous autoimmune MG, thymectomy improves clinical outcomes and reduces the need for steroids sustained over at least a 5-yr period. Surgical referral should be considered in patients <60 yr old without significant medical comorbidities even if no frank thymic tissue seen on imaging, especially if they are refractory to therapy.
- MuSK myasthenia is not associated with thymic pathology.

DISPOSITION

Course of disease is highly variable. Mortality rate has decreased from 75% to 4.5% over the past four decades.

REFERRAL

- Referral to a general neurologist or neuromuscular specialist is appropriate.
- Surgical referral for thymectomy in selected cases (see "Surgical Rx").

PEARLS & CONSIDERATIONS

- Sustained upward or lateral gaze and arm abduction for 120 sec may be necessary to elicit subtle signs on examination.
- Myasthenic patients can worsen rapidly and warrant careful observation during an exacerbation or when ill.

SUGGESTED READINGS

Available at ExpertConsult.com

RELATED CONTENT

Myasthenia Gravis (Patient Information)

AUTHOR: **Corey Goldsmith, MD**

BASIC INFORMATION

DEFINITION

Myelodysplastic syndromes (MDS) are a group of acquired clonal disorders affecting hematopoietic stem cells and are characterized by altered differentiation and proliferation. Patients present with peripheral blood cytopenias and the bone marrow reveals hypercellularity with morphologic abnormalities. The increased bone marrow cellularity reflects ineffective hematopoiesis with inadequate maturation resulting in cytopenias.

CLASSIFICATION

- In 1982, the French-American-British (FAB) classification included refractory anemia (RA), refractory anemia with ringed sideroblasts (RARS), refractory anemia with excess blasts (RAEB), chronic myelomonocytic leukemia (CMML), and refractory anemia with excess blasts in transformation (RAEB-T).
- In 1999, the World Health Organization (WHO) modified the FAB by incorporating newer morphologic insights and cytogenetic findings. It reduced the blast percentage for the diagnosis of acute myeloid leukemia (AML) to 20%, added refractory cytopenia with multilineage dysplasia (RCMD), refined refractory anemia with excessive blasts into types 1 and 2 (RAEB-1, RAEB-2), and added unclassified MDS, and MDS associated with isolated del(5q).
- In 2008, the WHO further modified the classification by subcategorizing MDS into six different categories (Table 1).

SYNONYMS

MDS
Preleukemia

ICD-10CM CODES

D46.9	Myelodysplastic syndrome, unspecified
D46.C	Myelodysplastic syndrome with isolated del(5q) chromosomal abnormality
D46.Z	Other myelodysplastic syndromes

EPIDEMIOLOGY & DEMOGRAPHICS

INCIDENCE (IN U.S.): Approximately 4 new cases/100,000 persons per yr. An estimated 30,000 new cases are diagnosed annually in the U.S.

PREDOMINANT AGE: More common in elderly patients; median age >65 yr

PHYSICAL FINDINGS & CLINICAL PRESENTATION

- Patients often present with fatigue due to anemia
- Patients can present with thrombocytopenia and leukopenia.
- Skin pallor, mucosal bleeding, and ecchymosis may be present.
- Fever, infection, and dyspnea are common.

ETIOLOGY

Exposure to radiation, chemotherapeutic agents, benzene, or other organic compounds is associated with myelodysplasia. Table 2 describes predisposing factors and epidemiologic associations of patients with MDS. Up to 40 genes that affect specific functional pathways are mutated in MDS, with 90% of patients having at least one mutation and a median of two to three mutations detected per patient. The most common mutations occur in genes involved in RNA splicing *(SF3B1, SRSF2, U2AF1,* and *ZRSR2),* epigenetic modification *(TET2, ASXL1,* and *DNMT3A),* regulators of signal transduction *(NRAS* and *JAK2),* and transcription factors *(RUNX1* and *TP53).*

DIAGNOSIS

DIFFERENTIAL DIAGNOSIS

- Hereditary dysplasias (e.g., Fanconi anemia, Diamond-Blackfan syndrome)

TABLE 1 2008 World Health Organization Classification of the Adult Myelodysplastic Syndromes

Refractory Cytopenia with Unilineage Dysplasia	
Dysplasia	≥10% of cells from a single lineage
Blasts	<5% in marrow; <1% in peripheral blood; no Auer rods
Notes	Includes refractory anemia (RA), refractory neutropenia, refractory thrombocytopenia; RA is by far the most common subtype
Refractory Anemia with Ring Sideroblasts	
Dysplasia	Isolated erythroid dysplasia
Blasts	<5% in marrow; <1% in peripheral blood; no Auer rods
Notes	≥15% of erythroid precursors are ring sideroblasts
	Frequently associated with SF3B1 mutations
MDS with Isolated del(5q)	
Dysplasia	Normal or increased megakaryocytes with hypolobated nuclei
Blasts	<20% (though usually much less)
Notes	del(5q31) must be sole chromosomal abnormality
Refractory Cytopenia with Multilineage Dysplasia	
Dysplasia	≥10% of cells from two or more myeloid lineages
Blasts	<5% in marrow; <1% in peripheral blood; no Auer rods
Notes	Peripheral monocyte count must be $<1 \times 10^9$/L; ring sideroblasts may be present
Refractory Anemia with Excess Blasts	
Dysplasia	No specific requirement
Blasts	RAEB-1: 5%-9% in marrow, <5% in peripheral blood, AND no Auer rods
	RAEB-2: 10%-19% in marrow, 5%-19% in peripheral blood, OR Auer rods
Notes	Old designation of RAEB-t (20%-30% blasts) now considered AML
Unclassifiable MDS	
Dysplasia	Minimal, or not meeting criteria for another subtype
Blasts	<5% in marrow; <1% in peripheral blood; no Auer rods
Notes	In presence of *clonal cytogenetic finding* considered diagnostic of MDS

Excludes refractory cytopenias of childhood. MDS/myeloproliferative neoplasms such as chronic myelomonocytic leukemia and RARS with thrombocytosis are classified separately. *AML,* Acute myeloid leukemia; *MDS,* myelodysplastic syndrome; *RAEB,* refractory anemia with excess blast.
From Hoffman R et al: *Hematology, basic principles and practice,* ed 7, Philadelphia, 2018, Elsevier.

TABLE 2 Predisposing Factors and Epidemiologic Associations of Patients with Myelodysplastic Syndrome

Heritable

Constitutional Genetic Disorders

Trisomy 8 mosaicism
Familial monosomy 7
Down syndrome (trisomy 21)
Neurofibromatosis 1
Germ cell tumors [embryonal dysgenesis del(12p)]

Congenital Neutropenia

Kostmann syndrome
Shwachman-Diamond syndrome

DNA Repair Deficiencies

Fanconi anemia
Ataxia-telangiectasia
Bloom syndrome
Xeroderma pigmentosum
Pharmacogenomic polymorphisms (GSTq1-null)

Acquired

Senescence

Mutagen Exposure

Alkylator therapy (chlorambucil, cyclophosphamide, melphalan, N-mustards)
Topoisomerase II inhibitors (anthracyclines)
β Emitters (32p)
Autologous stem cell transplantation
Environmental/occupational (benzene)
Tobacco
Aplastic anemia
Paroxysmal nocturnal hemoglobinuria

DNA, Deoxyribonucleic acid.
From Hoffman R et al: *Hematology, basic principles and practice,* ed 7, Philadelphia, 2018, Churchill Livingstone.

- Vitamin B_{12}/folate deficiency
- Exposure to toxins (drugs, alcohol, chemotherapy)
- Renal failure
- Irradiation
- Autoimmune disease
- Paroxysmal nocturnal hemoglobinuria

WORKUP

Diagnostic workup includes laboratory evaluation and bone marrow examination (Fig. E1). Cytogenetic analysis (Box E1) by conventional metaphase karyotyping or by MDS FISH assessment should be performed in patients with MDS. Next-generation sequencing (NGS) can be performed on bone marrow to provide additional information on mutations. Genes recurrently mutated in myelodysplastic syndrome are summarized in Table 3. Physical examination, medical history, and laboratory tests aiding in diagnosis of MDS are described in Table 4. Key features of the major myelodysplastic syndromes are summarized in Table 5.

Rx TREATMENT

NONPHARMACOLOGIC THERAPY

- Packed red blood cell transfusions in patients with severe symptomatic anemia
- Platelet transfusions in patients with severe thrombocytopenia or those with bleeding episodes

ACUTE GENERAL Rx

- The initial focus of MDS therapy involves stratification of patients into low-, intermediate-, and high-risk states using well-defined and validated risk stratification systems. The original International Prognostic Scoring System (IPSS), which incorporated cytopenias, cytogenetics, and blast percentage, is still clinically used. The revised IPSS (IPSS-R) has been created from an evaluation of more than 7000 patients and utilizes a five-tier risk grouping that accounts for the degree of cytopenias and bone marrow blast percentage and has 15 cytogenetic subtypes.
- Fig. 2 and Table 6 summarize a treatment approach for MDS.
- Low-risk patients are treated with supportive care or growth factors.
- Intermediate- and high-risk patients are offered treatment with hypomethylating agents along with supportive care.
- Appropriate patients are offered allogeneic donor stem cell transplantation as a potentially curative option, with high-volume centers treating patients <80 yr old.
- Erythropoietin (10,000-40,000 units/week) or pegylated erythropoietin (200-500 mg every 1-3 wk) is used in patients with symptomatic anemia. Responses with increase in hemoglobin and decreased transfusion

TABLE 3 Genes Recurrently Mutated in Myelodysplastic Syndrome

Gene	Frequency (%)	Notes
Splicing Factors		
SF3B1	20-30	Strong association with RARS
SRSF2	10-15 (MDS) 40 (CMML)	Enriched in CMML
U2AF1	5-12	Association with del(20q)
Epigenetic Modifiers		
TET2	20-30 (MDS) 40-50 (CMML)	Enriched in CMML Mutually exclusive with IDH
DNMT3A	8-13	
ASXL1	10-20 (MDS) 30-40 (CMML)	Enriched in CMML
EZH2	5-10 (MDS) 20-30 (CMML)	Enriched in CMML May be functionally involved in 7q−
IDH1/2	<5	More frequent in AML
ATRX	Rare	Associated with acquired thalassemia
Transcription Factors		
RUNX1	10-15	Can be somatic or germline
GATA2	Rare	Mostly germline
ETV6	<5	Can be somatic or germline
TP53	10-12	Association with complex karyotype, therapy-related disease
Kinases and Receptors		
JAK2	<5	Enriched in RARS-T
NRAS	5-10	Seen in progression to AML
CBL	<5	Enriched in JMML
PTPN11	<5	More common in JMML
BRAF	Rare	Also seen in hairy cell leukemia
Cohesin Complex		
STAG2	5-10	Cohesin class mutations enriched in high-risk MDS and secondary AML
RAD21	<5	
SMC3	<2	
SMC1A	<2	
GCPR Complex		
GNAS	Rare	Mutations recently described in wide range of hematologic malignancies, including MDS
GNB1	Rare	

AML, Acute myeloid leukemia; *CMML*, chronic myelomonocytic leukemia; *GCPR*, G-coupled protein receptor; *IDH*, isocitrate dehydrogenase; *JMML*, juvenile myelomonocytic leukemia; *MDS*, myelodysplastic syndrome; *RARS*, refractory anemia with ring sideroblasts; *RARS-T*, RARS with thrombocytosis.
From Hoffman R et al: *Hematology, basic principles and practice*, ed 7, Philadelphia, 2018, Elsevier.

TABLE 4 Physical Examination, Medical History, and Laboratory Tests Aiding in Diagnosis of Myelodysplastic Syndrome

Medical History
- Duration of symptoms
- History of blood disease
- History of exposure to occupational toxins or cytotoxic agents
- Medication history
- Alcohol intake
- Comorbid conditions

Physical Examination
- Pallor
- Petechiae
- Purpura
- Bruising
- Tachypnea
- Signs of infection
- Splenomegaly

Laboratory Testing
- Complete blood count with a manual differential
- Reticulocyte count
- Vitamin B_{12} and folate levels
- Consider methylmalonic acid and red blood cell folate levels
- Iron, total iron-binding capacity, and ferritin level
- Thyroid-stimulating hormone level
- Lactate dehydrogenase
- Antinuclear antibody
- Coombs test and haptoglobin
- Serum erythropoietin level
- Human leukocyte antigen (histocompatibility antigens) typing in appropriate patients
- Paroxysmal nocturnal hemoglobinuria screen

Bone Marrow Testing
- Hematopathology
- Percentage of blasts on 200 cell aspirate differential
- Presence or absence of Auer rods
- Percentage of cellularity of bone marrow biopsy
- Iron stain on aspirate (ringed sideroblasts)
- Iron stain on biopsy (storage)
- Dysplastic features (% and number of dysplastic lineages)
- Cytogenetics (karyotype of 20 metaphase cells)
- Fluorescent in situ hybridization
- Flow cytometry (not useful for quantitation)

From Hoffman R et al: *Hematology, basic principles and practice*, ed 7, Philadelphia, 2018, Churchill Livingstone.

TABLE 5 Diagnostic Criteria for Myelodysplastic Syndrome

A. Presence of at Least One Unexplained Cytopenia for at Least 6 Mo[a]

Hemoglobin <11 g/dl, *or*

Absolute neutrophil count <1.5 × 10^9/L, *or*

Platelet count <100 × 10^9/L

plus B. Presence of One or More MDS-Qualifying Criteria:

>10% dysplasia in one or more hematopoietic lineage, *or*

5%-19% blasts in bone marrow, *or*

MDS-defining cytogenetic abnormality, such as:

t(1;3)(p36.3;q21.1)	t(2;11)(p21;q23)	inv(3)(q21;q26.2)
t(3;21)(q26.2;q22.1)	−5 or del(5q)	t(6;9)(p23;q34)
−7 or del(7q)		del(9q)
del(11q)	t(11;16)(q23;p13.3)	del(12p) or t(12p)
−13 or del(13q)	i(17q) or del(17p)	idic(X)(q13)

***plus* C. Exclusion of Alternative Diagnoses**

AML (i.e., <20% blasts, and no t(8;21), inv(16), t(16;16), t(15;17), or erythroleukemia) or *ALL*

Other hematologic diseases (aplastic anemia, PNH, LGL, lymphoma, myelofibrosis and other MPN)

Viral infections (HIV, EBV, parvovirus)

Nutritional deficiencies (iron, copper, B_{12}, folate)

Medications (methotrexate, azathioprine, isoniazid, cytotoxic chemotherapy)

Alcohol or other toxins

Autoimmune diseases (SLE, Felty syndrome, ITP, autoimmune hemolytic anemia)

Congenital disorders (Diamond-Blackfan anemia, Shwachman-Diamond syndrome, Fanconi anemia, and others)

[a]Diagnosis can be made earlier than 6 mo if no other cause is apparent for cytopenias, or there are excess blasts or an MDS-defining cytogenetic abnormality.

ALL, Acute lymphoblastic leukemia; *AML*, acute myeloid leukemia; *EBV*, Epstein-Barr virus; *HIV*, human immunodeficiency virus; *ITP*, immune thrombocytopenic purpura; *LGL*, large granular lymphocyte leukemia; *MDS*, myelodysplastic syndrome; *MPN*, myeloproliferative neoplasm; *PNH*, paroxysmal nocturnal hemoglobinuria; *SLE*, systemic lupus erythematosus.

From Hoffman R et al: *Hematology, basic principles and practice*, ed 7, Philadelphia, 2018, Elsevier.

requirements are achieved typically in patients who have serum erythropoietin levels <500 U/L and adequate iron stores.

- DNA methyltransferase inhibitors: Azacitidine, a pyrimidine nucleoside analogue of cytidine, has been shown to improve the quality of life for patients and to prolong overall survival. Decitabine, another nucleoside analogue, has also been FDA approved for patients with MDS. These agents may also be useful in preventing the transition of MDS to AML.
- Recently, the FDA approved a fixed-dose oral combination of decitabine and cedazuridine for adults with myelodysplastic syndromes (MDS), including those with previously treated and untreated, *de novo*, and secondary MDS with the following FAB subtypes: Refractory anemia, refractory anemia with ringed sideroblasts, refractory anemia with excess blasts, and chronic myelomonocytic leukemia (CMML). Also included in the approval were patients with intermediate-1, intermediate-2, and high-risk International Prognostic Scoring System (IPSS) disease.
- Immunomodulators: Lenalidomide, a novel analogue of thalidomide, has demonstrated hematologic activity in patients with low-risk MDS who have no response to erythropoietin or who are unlikely to benefit from conventional therapy. Lenalidomide can also reduce transfusion requirements and reverse cytologic and cytogenetic abnormalities in patients who have MDS with the 5q31 deletion.
- Results of chemotherapy are generally disappointing. Combination chemotherapy regimens that are used to treat AML generally induce a complete response in only a minority of patients, and the average duration of response is <1 yr.
- The use of myeloid growth factors (granulocyte colony-stimulating factor [G-CSF], granulocyte-macrophage colony-stimulating factor [GM-CSF]) is reserved for patients with severe neutropenias and high infection risk. Additionally, these provide a synergistic effect when used in combination with erythropoietin in terms of improvement in the hemoglobin levels.

CHRONIC Rx

- Monitor for infections, bleeding, and complications of anemia.
- Supportive measures include packed red blood cell (PRBC) transfusions and erythropoietin for anemia and antimicrobials to treat opportunistic infections.
- Iron overload from frequent transfusions (>100 PRBC units) requires iron chelation therapy.

DISPOSITION

- The 5-yr overall survival is approximately 30%. Median overall survival rates are best for patients with refractory anemia (56 mo), refractory anemia with ring sideroblasts (48 mo), and deletion 5q subtype (32 mo). The International Prognostic Scoring System (IPSS) for MDS is summarized in Tables 7 and 8. Table 9 describes survival based on IPSS.
- Long-term remission rates in young patients with allogeneic stem cell transplantation approach 40% to 50%.
- The risk of transformation to AML varies with cytogenetics and bone marrow blast percentage.

REFERRAL

- Hematology referral for all patients
- Bone marrow transplant evaluation for stem cell transplant eligibility as a potentially curative modality

PEARLS & CONSIDERATIONS

COMMENTS

- Somatic point mutations in *TP53, EZH2, ETV6, RUNX1,* and *ASXL1* are predictors of poor overall survival in patients with MDS independent of established risk factors. Patients with cytogenetic abnormalities associated with poor prognosis should be considered for upfront allogeneic stem cell transplantation.
- Many younger patients who respond to immunosuppressive therapy with drugs

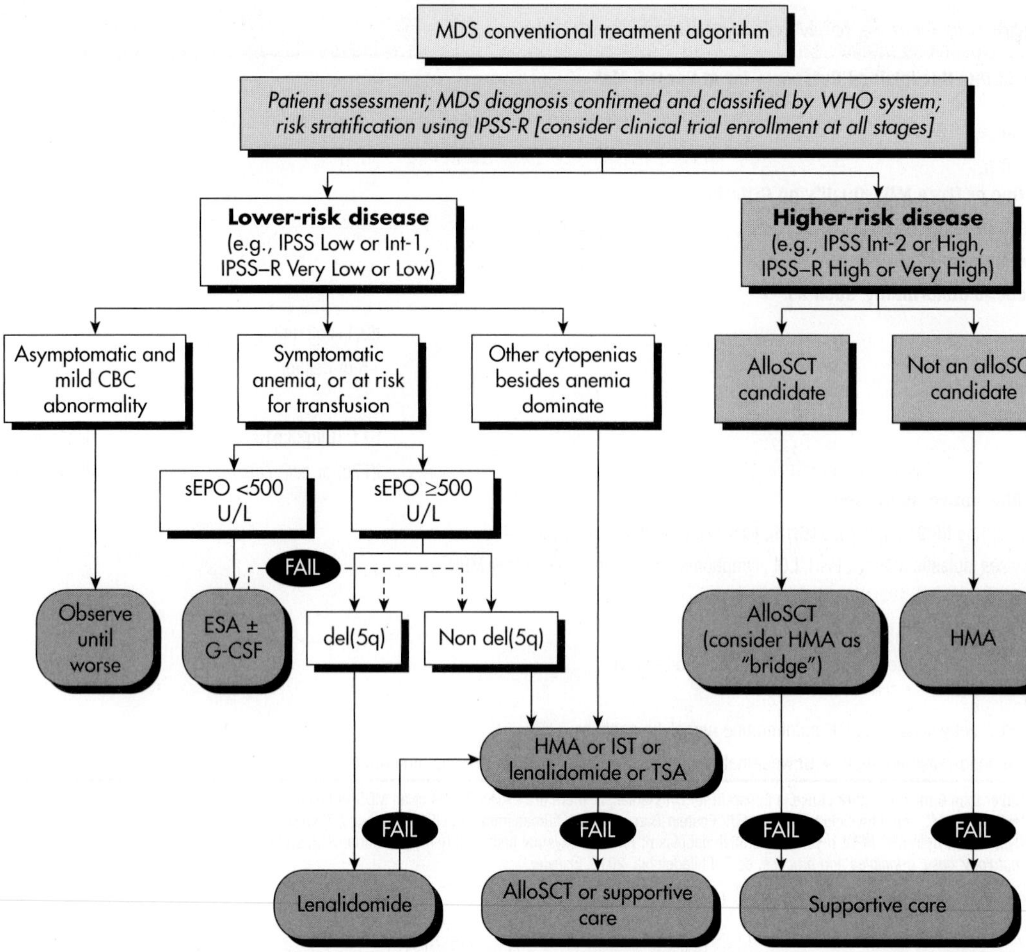

FIG. 2 A suggested treatment algorithm for myelodysplastic syndrome *(MDS)*, described further in the text and in Table 6. Risk assessment has traditionally been based on the International Prognostic Scoring System *(IPSS)* (and more recently the IPSS-R), but that is likely to change with the advent of new prognostic scoring systems and molecular markers. IPSS-R intermediate-risk disease may follow the track for lower- or higher-risk disease. Disease classification should use the 2016 World Health Organization *(WHO)* system. Clinical trial enrollment should be considered at each step. Some clinicians would proceed to lenalidomide without a trial of an ESA if del(5q) is present, even if the serum erythropoietin level is less than 500 U/L. *alloSCT,* Allogeneic stem cell transplantation; *CBC,* complete blood count; ESA, erythropoiesis-stimulating agent (epoetin or darbepoetin—off-label uses); *G-CSF,* granulocyte colony-stimulating factor (e.g., filgrastim or tbo-filgrastim); *HMA,* hypomethylating agent (azacitidine or decitabine); *IPSS-R,* revised International Prognostic Scoring System; *IST,* immunosuppressive therapy (antithymocyte globulin with cyclosporine A or tacrolimus—off-label uses); *SCT,* stem cell transplantation; *sEPO,* serum erythropoietin level; *TSA,* thrombopoiesis-stimulating agent (e.g., eltrombopag, romiplostim—off-label uses). (From Niederhuber JE: *Abeloff's clinical oncology,* ed 6, Philadelphia, 2020, Elsevier.)

TABLE 6 Available Therapies for Myelodysplastic Syndromes in the U.S. and Preferred Dosage Regimen[a]

1. Erythropoiesis-stimulating agents (should hold if hemoglobin ≫10 g/dl)
   a. Epoetin alfa 20-60,000 mIU/wk subcutaneously; dose can be adjusted every 1-2 mo depending on response; or
   b. Darbepoetin alfa 200-300 μg subcutaneously every 1-2 wk or 500 μg subcutaneously every 3 wk; or
   c. Epoetin alfa as per (a) plus G-CSF (filgrastim) 0.5 μg /kg subcutaneously 1-3 times per wk (pegfilgrastim is commonly substituted in the U.S., but data are absent, and splenic rupture and leukemoid reactions are risks).
2. Iron chelation therapy
   a. Deferoxamine (starting dose ~20 mg/kg/day; a typical effective dose for an adult is 6 g/day subcutaneously or intravenously, administered by infusion pump over 8-16 h daily); or
   b. Deferasirox, tablet for oral suspension 20-30 mg/kg/day orally once daily oral tablet, 14-28 mg/kg/day, adjust as tolerated and according to efficacy.
   c. Deferiprone (L1) is available outside the U.S., but is only approved for thalassemia in the U.S. and is a weaker chelator than the other two and cytopenias can be problematic.
3. Lenalidomide: 10 mg orally once daily for 21-28 days per 28-day cycle (dose reduction due to cytopenias is commonly required)
4. Azacitidine: 75 mg/m^2/day subcutaneously or intravenously for 7 days, repeat every 28 days; "weekend-sparing" schedules may also be effective
5. Decitabine: 15 mg/m^2/dose over 3-4 h intravenously every 8 h × 9 doses (=3 days); or 20 mg/m^2/day intravenously over 1-2 h daily × 5 consecutive days; repeat every 4-6 wk
6. Immunosuppression: Equine ATG per aplastic anemia regimens (e.g., 40 mg/kg/day × 4 days intravenously, after test dose), with corticosteroids to prevent serum sickness, with or without cyclosporine A or tacrolimus
7. Miscellaneous therapies such as antifibrinolytics (aminocaproic acid, tranexamic acid) and androgens (danazol) can be useful in some cases.

[a]Consult the package insert in each case. Only azacitidine, lenalidomide, and decitabine are approved by the U.S. Food and Drug Administration for myelodysplastic syndrome–related indications in the U.S.

ATG, Antithymocyte globulin; *G-CSF,* granulocyte colony-stimulating factor.

From Niederhuber JE: *Abeloff's clinical oncology,* ed 6, Philadelphia, 2020, Elsevier.

such as antithymocyte globulin and cyclosporine have clonal expansions of cytotoxic CD8+ T cells that suppress normal hematopoiesis, as well as expansion of CD4+ helper T cell subsets that promote and sustain autoimmunity.

- Nearly 50% of the deaths that result from MDS are the result of cytopenias associated with bone marrow failure.

RELATED CONTENT

Myelodysplastic Syndrome (Patient Information)

SUGGESTED READINGS

Available at ExpertConsult.com

AUTHOR: **Ritesh Rathore, MD**

TABLE 7 1997 International Prognostic Scoring System for Myelodysplastic Syndromes (IPSS)

	SCORE			
Variable	**0**	**0.5**	**1**	**1.5**
Marrow blasts (%)	<5	5-10	–	11-20
Karyotype	Good	Intermediate	Poor	–
Cytopenias	0-1	2-3	–	–

From Hoffman R et al: *Hematology, basic principles and practice*, ed 7, Philadelphia, 2018, Elsevier.

TABLE 8 2012 Revised International Prognostic Scoring System for Myelodysplastic Syndrome (IPSS-R)

CYTOGENETIC RISK	INCLUDED KARYOTYPIC ABNORMALITIES
Very good	del(11q), −Y
Good	Normal, del(20q), del(5q) alone or +1 other abnormality, del(12p)
Intermediate	+8, del(7q), i(17q), +19, +21 Any other single or double abnormality Two or more independent clones
Poor	der(3q), −7, double with del(7q), complex with exactly 3 abnormalities
Very poor	Complex with >3 abnormalities

Scoring Table

Parameter	Category/Score				
Cytogenetic risk	Very good 0	Good 1	Intermediate 2	Poor 3	Very poor 4
Marrow blasts (%)	≤2 0	3-4 1	5-10 2	>10 3	
Hemoglobin (g/dl)	≥10 0	8-9.9 1	<8 1.5		
Platelet count (×10^9/L)	≥100 0	50-99 0.5	<50 1		
Neutrophil count (×10^9/L)	≥0.8 0	<0.8 0.5			

IPSS-R Risk Group	Total Score	% of Patients	Median Survival (Years)	25% With AML (Years)
Very low	≤1.5	19	8.8	NR
Low	2-3	38	5.3	10.8
Intermediate	3.5-4.5	20	3	3.2
High	5-6	13	1.6	1.4
Very high	>6	10	0.8	0.73

AML, Acute myeloid leukemia; *NR,* not reached.
From Hoffman R et al: *Hematology, basic principles and practice*, ed 7, Philadelphia, 2018, Elsevier.

TABLE 9 Survival Based on International Prognostic Scoring System for Myelodysplastic Syndromes (Percent)

IPSS Risk Group	# Patients	2 Yr	5 Yr	10 Yr	15 Yr
Low	267 (33%)	85	55	28	20
Intermediate-1	314 (38%	70	35	17	12
Intermediate-2	179 (22%)	30	8	0	–
High	56 (7%)	5	0	–	–

IPSS, International Prognostic Scoring System.
From Hoffman R et al: *Hematology, basic principles and practice*, ed 7, Philadelphia, 2018, Elsevier.

BASIC INFORMATION

DEFINITION

Myocardial infarction (MI) is a clinical syndrome characterized by symptoms of myocardial ischemia, persistent electrocardiographic (ECG) changes, and release of biomarkers of myocardial necrosis resulting from an insufficient supply of oxygenated blood to an area of the heart. MI may be classified as ST-segment elevation MI (STEMI) and non–ST-segment elevation MI (NSTEMI) depending on the ECG findings on MI presentation. Acute coronary syndrome (ACS) refers to acute myocardial ischemia without myocardial necrosis (unstable angina) or myocardial infarction (NSTEMI or STEMI). According to the European Society of Cardiology/American College of Cardiology guidelines, the following criteria for acute evolving or recent MI (NSTEMI and STEMI) satisfies the diagnosis:

- Detection of the rise and/or fall of cardiac biomarker values (preferably cardiac troponin [cTn]) with at least one value above the 99th percentile upper reference limit and with at least one of the following:
  1. Symptoms of ischemia
  2. Development of pathologic Q waves in the ECG
  3. Imaging evidence of new loss of viable myocardium or a new regional wall motion abnormality
  4. Identification of an intracoronary thrombus by angiography or autopsy pathologic findings of acute MI
  5. Electrocardiogram criteria:
     a. STEMI:
        (1) New, or presumed new, significant ST-T changes or new left bundle branch block (LBBB)
        (2) New ST elevation at the J-point in at least 2 contiguous leads of ≥2 mm (0.2 mV) in men or ≥1.5 mm (0.15 mV) in women in leads V2 to V3 and/or of ≥1 mm (0.1 mV) in another contiguous chest leads or the upper limb leads
     b. NSTEMI:
        (1) New ST-segment depression ≥0.5 mV (0.5 mm) and T-wave abnormalities

New generation troponin assays are extremely sensitive to small changes in serum troponin levels at the cost of diagnostic specificity for MI related to plaque rupture or erosion.

Universal classification of acute MI:

- Type 1: Spontaneous MI related to ischemia due to a primary coronary event such as plaque erosion and/or rupture, fissuring, or dissection.
- Type 2: MI secondary to ischemia, other than coronary artery disease, due to either increased oxygen demand or decreased supply (e.g., coronary endothelial dysfunction, coronary artery spasm, coronary embolism, anemia, arrhythmias, respiratory failure, hypertension with/without left ventricular hypertrophy (LVH), or hypotension). Also in critically ill patients or in patients undergoing major noncardiac surgery, elevated values of cardiac biomarkers may appear due to the direct toxic effects of endogenous or exogenous high circulating catecholamine levels.
- Type 3: Sudden unexpected cardiac death, including cardiac arrest, often with symptoms suggestive of myocardial ischemia, accompanied by presumed new ST elevation, new left bundle branch block, or evidence of fresh thrombus in a coronary artery by angiography and/or at autopsy, or death occurring before blood samples could be obtained or at a time before the appearance of cardiac biomarkers in the blood.
- Type 4a: MI associated with percutaneous coronary intervention. Elevation of cTn >5× percentile of upper reference limit (URL) in patients with normal baseline value, or a rise of cTn >20% if the baseline values are stable and are stable or falling. In addition to either symptoms of ischemia, new ischemic ECG changes or new LBBB, or angiographic loss of a patent coronary artery, persistent slow or no-flow, or embolization, or imaging of new wall motion abnormality.
- Type 4b: MI associated with stent thrombosis as documented by angiography or at autopsy in the setting of myocardial ischemia and with a rise/fall of cardiac biomarker values.
- Type 5: MI associated with coronary artery bypass grafting. Elevation of cardiac biomarker values >10× 99% URL in patients with normal baseline cTn values, in addition to either new pathological Q waves or new LBBB, or new native coronary artery occlusion or imaging of new abnormal wall motion abnormality.
- Myocardial Infarction with Nonobstructive Coronary Arteries (MINOCA): It is defined as acute myocardial infarction in the absence of obstructive coronary artery disease. Conditions like takotsubo cardiomyopathy, spontaneous coronary artery dissection, coronary artery spasm, microvascular dysfunction, and pulmonary embolism come under this novel category.

SYNONYMS

MI
Myocardial infarction
ST-elevation MI
Heart attack
Acute myocardial infarction
AMI
Coronary thrombosis
Coronary occlusion

ICD-10CM CODES

I21.01	ST elevation (STEMI) myocardial infarction involving left main coronary artery
I21.02	ST elevation (STEMI) myocardial infarction involving left anterior descending coronary artery
I21.09	ST elevation (STEMI) myocardial infarction involving other coronary artery of anterior wall
I21.11	ST elevation (STEMI) myocardial infarction involving right coronary artery
I21.19	ST elevation (STEMI) myocardial infarction involving another coronary artery of inferior wall
I21.21	ST elevation (STEMI) myocardial infarction involving left circumflex coronary artery
I21.29	ST elevation (STEMI) myocardial infarction involving other sites
I21.3	ST elevation (STEMI) myocardial infarction of unspecified site
I21.4	Non-ST elevation (NSTEMI) myocardial infarction
I22.0	Subsequent ST elevation (STEMI) myocardial infarction of anterior wall
I22.1	Subsequent ST elevation (STEMI) myocardial infarction of inferior wall
I22.2	Subsequent non-ST elevation (NSTEMI) myocardial infarction
I22.8	Subsequent ST elevation (STEMI) myocardial infarction of other sites
I22.9	Subsequent ST elevation (STEMI) myocardial infarction of unspecified site

EPIDEMIOLOGY & DEMOGRAPHICS

INCIDENCE & PREVALENCE (IN U.S.):

- According to data from National Health and Nutrition Examination Survey (NHANES) 2009 to 2012 (National Heart, Lung, and Blood Institute [NHLBI] tabulation), the overall prevalence for MI is 2.8% in U.S. adults ≥20 yr of age. MI prevalence is 4.0% for men and 1.8% for women.
- In 2013 in the U.S., coronary heart disease alone caused ≈1 of every 7 deaths. In 2013, 370,213 Americans died of coronary heart disease. Each yr, an estimated 660,000 Americans have a new coronary attack (defined as first hospitalized myocardial infarction or coronary heart disease death), and 305,000 have a recurrent attack. It is estimated that an additional 160,000 silent myocardial infarctions occur each yr. Approximately every 34 seconds, one American has a coronary event, and approximately every 1 minute 24 seconds, an American will die of one.
- Community incidence rates as well as mortality rates from STEMI have declined over the past decade, whereas those for NSTEMI have increased. At present, STEMI comprises approximately 30% to 40% of MI presentations. In-hospital mortality (approximately 5% to 6%) and 1-yr mortality (approximately 7% to 18%). The most common cause of death in adults over the age of 40 is myocardial infarction. A heart attack takes the life of >1,500,000 people each yr in the U.S.
- Modifiable risk factors such as hypertension, diabetes, and cigarette smoking have recently declined, although hyperlipidemia has shown no significant change, and obesity has steadily increased.
- Tobacco use remains the second-leading cause of total deaths and disability. The percentage of adults who reported current cigarette use declined from 24.1% in 1998 to 15.5% in 2016. Still, almost one third of coronary heart disease deaths are attributable to smoking and exposure to secondhand smoke. Patients with first acute MI were

found to have an almost threefold increase in cigarette smoking from 2002 to 2009. Cigarette smoking is associated with endothelial dysfunction, prothrombotic defects, and increased oxidative stress.
- It is more prevalent in males between the ages of 45 and 65 yr old; there is no predominant sex differential after the age of 65.
- Women comprised 30% of STEMI patients. They experience more lethal and severe first acute MIs than men regardless of comorbidity, previous angina, or age. Studies have suggested that women are less likely to receive reperfusion therapy, have longer reperfusion times, are often given the standard of care treatment within 24 hr of presentation, and have higher risk of bleeding with antithrombotic therapy.
- At least one fourth of all MIs are clinically unrecognized. Approximately 23% of patients with STEMI in the U.S. have diabetes mellitus, and three quarters of all deaths among patients with diabetes mellitus are related to coronary artery disease. Diabetes mellitus is associated with higher short- and long-term mortality after STEMI. In the CRUSADE (Can Rapid risk stratification of Unstable angina patients Suppress ADverse outcomes with Early implementation of the ACC/AHA guidelines) trial, 7% of eligible patients did not receive reperfusion therapy. The most important factor for not providing reperfusion therapy in eligible patients was increasing age.

PHYSICAL FINDINGS & CLINICAL PRESENTATION

The clinical presentation of myocardial infarction is usually based on a history of substernal pressure type chest pain radiated to the neck, lower jaw, left arm, or mid-back lasting 20 min or more that is not completely relieved by sublingual nitroglycerin. The pain may not be severe. Some patients may present with atypical symptoms such as nausea/vomiting, shortness of breath, fatigue, palpitations, and diaphoresis. The elderly in particular may present with dizziness, or syncope. The patients who tend to present with atypical symptoms are more likely to be women, diabetic patients, or elderly patients and less frequently receive reperfusion therapy and other evidence-based therapies than patients with a typical chest pain presentation. Records show that up to 30% of patients with STEMI present with atypical symptoms.

Physical findings:
- Skin may be diaphoretic and exhibit pallor (because of decreased oxygen).
- Rales may be present at the bases of lungs (indicative of heart failure [HF]).
- Cardiac auscultation may reveal an apical systolic murmur caused by mitral regurgitation from papillary muscle dysfunction; S_3 or S_4 may also be present.
- Up to 10% of patients may present with acute pulmonary edema and/or cardiogenic shock.
- Physical examination may be completely normal.

ETIOLOGY

- Coronary atherosclerosis and plaque rupture
- Coronary artery spasm
- Coronary embolism (caused by infective endocarditis, rheumatic heart disease, intracavitary thrombus, atrial fibrillation)
- Periarteritis and other coronary artery inflammatory diseases
- Dissection into coronary arteries (aneurysmal or iatrogenic or spontaneous)
- Anomalous origin of coronary artery, especially interarterial (aorta and pulmonary artery) course of coronary artery
- MI with normal coronaries: More frequent in younger patients and cocaine addicts. The risk of acute MI is increased by a factor of 24 during the 60 min after the use of cocaine in persons who are otherwise at relatively low risk. Most patients with cocaine-related MI are young, nonwhite, male cigarette smokers without other risk factors for coronary heart disease and who have a history of repeated cocaine use. Blood and urine toxicology screen for cocaine is recommended in all young patients who present with acute MI
- Hypercoagulable states, increased blood viscosity (polycythemia vera and autoimmune diseases such as systemic lupus, antiphospholipid syndrome)

Dx DIAGNOSIS

DIFFERENTIAL DIAGNOSIS

The various causes of myocardial ischemia are described along with the differential diagnosis of chest pain.

LABORATORY TESTS

- Electrocardiogram (Fig. 1): A 12-lead ECG should be performed and shown to an experienced emergency physician within 10 min of emergency department (ED) arrival for all patients with chest discomfort (or anginal equivalent) or other symptoms suggestive of MI. Table 1 and Table 2 describe ECG

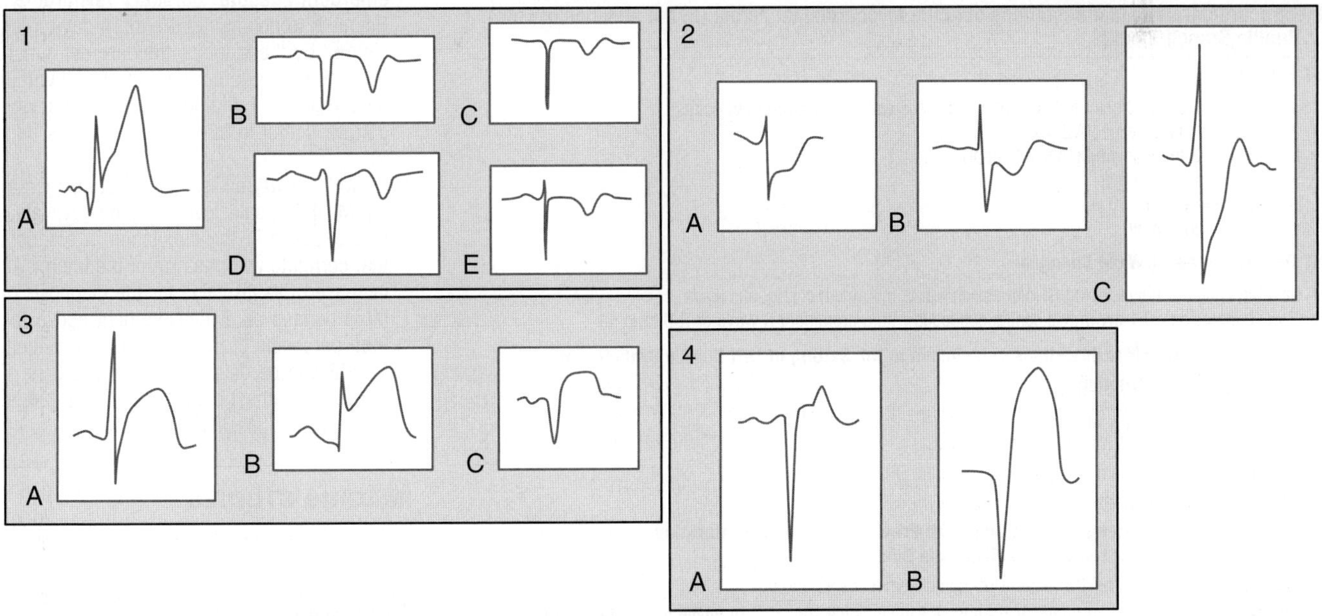

FIG. 1 Electrocardiographic findings of acute myocardial infarction (AMI). 1, T-wave abnormalities of AMI. *A,* Prominent "hyperacute" T wave. *B* through *E,* T-wave inversions of non–ST-segment elevation MI (NSTEMI). **2,** ST-segment depression. *A,* Flat. *B,* Downsloping. *C,* Upsloping. **3,** ST-segment elevation. *A,* Convex ST-segment elevation. *B,* Obliquely straight ST-segment elevation. *C,* Convex ST-segment elevation. **4,** Pathologic Q waves. *A,* Pathologic Q wave of completed myocardial infarction. *B,* Simultaneous ST-segment elevation with pathologic Q wave 2 hr into the course of ST-segment elevation MI (STEMI). (From Vincent JL et al: *Textbook of critical care,* ed 6, Philadelphia, 2011, Saunders.)

findings in myocardial infarction. If the initial ECG is not diagnostic for MI but the patient remains symptomatic and there is a high clinical suspicion for MI, serial ECGs at 5- to 10-min intervals or continuous 12-lead ST-segment monitoring should be performed to detect the potential development of ST deviation. In patients with inferior STEMI, right-sided ECG leads should be obtained to look for ST elevation suggestive of right ventricular (RV) infarction. The joint ESC/ACCF/AHA committee for the definition of MI

TABLE 1 Leads Showing Abnormal Electrocardiographic Findings in Myocardial Infarction

	Limb Leads	Precordial Leads
Lateral	I, aVL	V5, V6
Anterior		V1, V2, V3
Anterolateral	I, aVL	V2-V6
Diaphragmatic	II, III, aVF	
Posterior		V1-V3*

aVF, Augmented vector foot; *aVL,* augmented vector left.
*None of the leads is oriented toward the posterior surface of the heart. Therefore, in posterior infarction, changes that would have been present in the posterior surface leads will be seen in the anterior leads as a mirror image (e.g., tall and slightly wide R waves in V1 and V2, comparable to abnormal Q waves, and tall and wide, symmetric T waves in V1 and V2).
From Park MK: *Park's pediatric cardiology for practitioners,* ed 6, Philadelphia, 2014, Elsevier.

established the definition for the diagnosis of ST-elevation MI, which is considered to be present when there is an ST-segment elevation in two contiguous leads, ≥2 mm for men and ≥1.5 mm for women in precordial leads and/or ≥1 mm in limb leads. ST-segment elevation is measured at 0.08 sec after the J point (the junction between the end of the QRS and the beginning of the ST segment). In addition, ST depression in >2 precordial leads (V1 to V4) may indicate transmural posterior injury; multilead ST depression with coexistent ST elevation in lead aVR has been described in patients with left main or proximal left anterior descending artery involvement.

- New or presumably new LBBB at presentation occurs infrequently, may interfere with ST-elevation analysis, and should not be considered diagnostic of acute myocardial infarction (MI) in isolation.
- Diagnosing new STEMI in patients with old left bundle branch block could be challenging. Sgarbossa and colleagues emphasized that concordant 1 mm ST-segment elevation in any lead with a positive QRS deflection or discordant ST-segment elevation >5 mm in any lead with negative QRS deflection suggest STEMI.
- New ST-segment depression ≥0.5 mV (0.5 mm) and T-wave abnormalities suggest NSTEMI. ECG findings alone, without laboratory results, are sufficient to diagnose STEMI; therefore, treatment should not be delayed until biomarkers are available.

TABLE 2 Electrocardiographic Manifestations of Myocardial Infarction

Electrocardiographic Manifestations of Acute Myocardial Ischemia (In the Absence of Left Bundle Branch Block)

ST Elevation

New ST elevation at the J point in two contiguous leads with the following cut points:
- ≥0.1 mV in all leads (except V2-V3)
- In leads V2-V3 the following cut points apply:
  - ≥0.2 mV in men ≥40 yr
  - ≥0.25 mV in men <40 yr
  - ≥0.15 mV in women

ST Depression and T Wave Changes

- New horizontal or downsloping ST depression ≥0.05 mV in two contiguous leads
- T-wave inversion ≥0.1 mV in two contiguous leads with a prominent R wave or R/S ratio >1

Electrocardiographic Manifestations of Ischemia In the Setting of Left Bundle Branch Block

Electrocardiographic Criterion	Points
ST-segment elevation ≥1 mm and concordant with the QRS complex	5
ST-segment depression ≥1 mm in lead V1, V2, or V3	3
ST-segment elevation ≥5 mm and discordant with the QRS complex	2

A score of ≥3 had a specificity of 98% for acute MI

Electrocardiographic Changes Associated with Previous Myocardial Infarction (In the Absence of Left Ventricular Hypertrophy and Left Bundle Block)

Any Q wave in leads V2-V3 ≥0.02 sec or a QS complex in leads V2 and V3

Q wave ≥0.03 sec and ≥0.1-mV deep or QS complex in leads I, II, aVL, aVF, or V4-V6 in any 2 leads of a contiguous lead grouping (I, aVL; V1-V6; II, III, aVF)

R wave ≥0.04 sec in V1-V2 and R/S ≥1 with a concordant positive T wave in absence of a conductions defect.

aVF, Augmented vector foot; *aVL,* augmented vector left; *MI,* myocardial infarction.
Based on criteria from O'Gara PT et al: 2013 ACCF/AHA guideline for the management of ST-elevation myocardial infarction: a report of the American College of Cardiology Foundation/American Heart Association Task Force on Practice Guidelines, *J Am Coll Cardiol* 61:e78, 2013. In Zipes DP: *Braunwald's heart disease, a textbook of cardiovascular medicine,* ed 11, Philadelphia, 2019, Elsevier.

- Cardiac troponin levels: Cardiac-specific troponin T (cTnT) and cardiac-specific troponin I (cTnI) are generally indicative of myocardial injury with increases in serum levels of >99th percentile of a normal reference population. Detection of a rise and fall pattern of the measurements is essential to the diagnosis of AMI. The rise may occur relatively early after muscle damage (3-6 hr), peak at 12 to 16 hr, and may be present for several days after MI (up to 7 days for cTnI and more than 14 days for cTnT). Earlier peaking and rapid decline of cardiac enzymes may present in light of successful revascularization (Fig. 2). cTnT or cTnI tests can be falsely positive for myocardial infarction in patients with renal failure, heart failure, myocarditis, aortic dissection, and pulmonary embolism. Recently, highly sensitive troponin assays (hs-cTnI, hs-cTnT) have also been developed to facilitate an early diagnosis of AMI. Most patients can be diagnosed with AMI within the first 2 to 3 hr of presentation. However, an initial negative high-sensitivity troponin at the time of presentation is not sensitive enough to completely rule out AMI. MI can be excluded in most patients by 6 hr of presentation, and guidelines suggest serial samples be obtained every 3 to 6 hr after an initial sample if there is a high degree of suspicion for AMI.
- Troponin is the preferred marker for the diagnosis of myocardial necrosis. A single high-sensitivity assay for cardiac troponin (hs-cTnT) concentration below the limit of detection in combination with a nonischemic ECG may successfully rule out an MI in patients presenting to EDs with possible emergency acute coronary syndrome.[1] Because troponins need 7 to 14 days to be cleared by the kidneys, they are not sensitive enough to detect a recurrent MI within days from the initial MI. CK-MB isoenzyme can be useful in such circumstances (Fig. 2).
- CK-MB isoenzyme is also a useful marker for MI if troponin levels are not available. It is released in the circulation in amounts that correlate with the size of the infarct. An increased CK-MB value for the diagnosis of MI is defined as a measurement above the 99th percentile of the upper reference limit. CK-MB can be detected within 3 to 8 hr of the onset of chest pain, peak at 12 to 24 hr, and return to baseline levels within 24 to 48 hr.

IMAGING STUDIES

Imaging studies such as a high-quality portable chest x-ray, transthoracic echocardiography, and a contrast chest CT scan should be used to differentiate MI from aortic dissection, pulmonary embolism, and other intrathoracic causes

[1] Pickering JW et al: Rapid rule-out of acute myocardial infarction with a single high-sensitivity cardiac troponin T measurement below the limit of detection: a collaborative meta-analysis. *Ann Intern Med* 166:715-724, 2017.

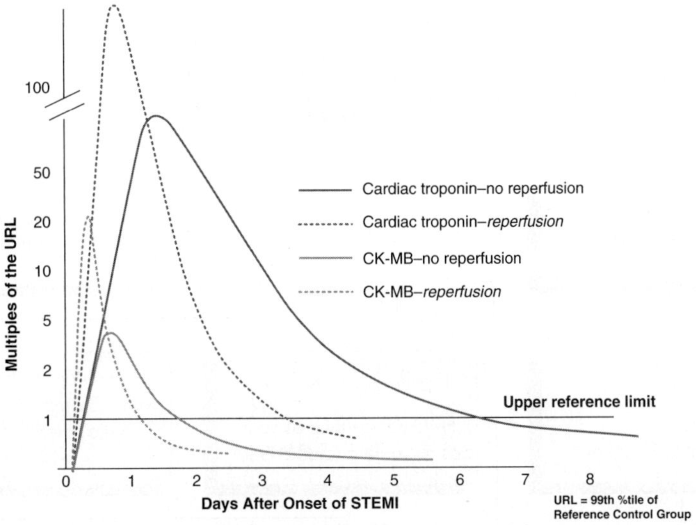

FIG. 2 Trends of Troponin and CK-MB following revascularization in MI. *CK-MB,* Creatine kinase-MB; *STEMI,* ST-segment elevation myocardial infarction; *URL,* upper reference limit. (Modified from Shapiro BP, Jaffe AS: Cardio biomarkers. In: Murphy JG, Lloyd MA [eds]: *Mayo Clinic cardiology: concise textbook,* ed 3, Rochester, MN, 2007, Mayo Clinic Scientific Press, and New York, 2007, Informa Healthcare USA. Used with permission of Mayo Foundation for Medical Education and Research.)

of chest pain (i.e., pneumonia and pneumothorax) in patients for whom this distinction is initially unclear, or to assess for complications of AMI such as pulmonary edema. Transthoracic echocardiography may provide evidence of focal wall motion abnormalities and facilitate triage in patients with ECG findings that are difficult to interpret.

RISK ASSESSMENT

For STEMI patients, TIMI (Thrombolysis in Myocardial Infarction) risk index, TIMI risk score (30-day outcomes), and GRACE (Global Registry of Acute Coronary Events) risk score (6-mo outcomes) are commonly available risk assessment models. In the TIMI risk score for STEMI, the mean 30-day mortality was 6.7%. It is composed of eight baseline variables. The risk score showed a >40-fold graded increase in mortality, with scores ranging from 0 to >8 (P <0.0001); 30-day mortality was 0.1% among patients with a score of 0, 2.25 with a score of 5, and >8.8% among patients with a score of 8 or greater. The higher the score, the higher the 30-day mortality rate. The variables are divided between historic, exam, and presentation:

Historic:

- Age 65 to 74 (2 points), >75 (3 points)
- Diabetes/HTN or angina (1 point)

Exam:

- SBP <100 mm Hg (3 points)
- Heart rate >100 bpm (2 points)
- Killip 2 to 4 (2 points)
- Weight <67 kg (1 point)

Presentation:

- Anterior ST elevation or LBBB (1 point)
- Time to reperfusion >4 hr (1 point)

For NSTEMI patients, TIMI risk score (14-day outcomes) and GRACE (Global Registry of Acute Coronary Events) risk score (in hospital outcomes) are available.

- Age ≥65 yr
- Presence of ≥3 risk factors for CAD
- Known CAD (coronary artery stenosis ≥50%)
- Aspirin use in the past 7 days
- ≥2 episodes of angina within 24 hr
- ST changes ≥0.05 mV
- Positive cardiac enzymes

In TIMI score for the NSTEMI patients, each variable scores one point. The risk score of 6 to 7 carries estimated major acute coronary event (MACE) rate of 41% during 14 days of post-MI. Risk assessment is a continuous process that should be repeated throughout hospitalization and at time of discharge.

Rx TREATMENT

NONPHARMACOLOGIC THERAPY

- Limit patient's activity: Bed rest with bedside commode for the initial 12 to 24 hr. If the patient remains stable, gradually increase.
- Diet: Nothing by mouth until stable, then clear liquids as tolerated to advance gradually to a diet tailored to the patient's comorbidities (i.e., diabetes, hypertension, heart failure, hyperlipidemia, renal failure, chronic obstructive pulmonary disease [COPD], etc.).
- Patient education to decrease the risk of subsequent cardiac events, counseling on smoking cessation, dietary restrictions, regular exercise, and medication compliance should be initiated when the patient is medically stable.

ACUTE GENERAL Rx

- Fig. 3 shows a treatment algorithm for STEMI. Assessment and treatment algorithm for non–ST-segment MI is described in Fig. 4. Rationale of the treatment of a patient with STEMI is based on "time is muscle." Therefore, all communities should create and maintain a regional system of STEMI care that includes assessment and continuous quality improvement of EMS and hospital-based activities. A 12-lead ECG must be done by EMS personnel at the site of first medical contact (FMC).
- Reperfusion therapy should be administered to all eligible patients with STEMI with symptom onset within 12 hr. Indications for primary angioplasty and comparison with fibrinolytic therapy are described in Table 3. Primary PCI (Fig. E5) is the recommended method of reperfusion when it can be performed in a timely fashion by experienced operators with an ideal FMC-to-device time system goal of 90 min or less.
- In the absence of contraindications, fibrinolytic therapy (Table 4) should be administered to patients with STEMI at non–PCI-capable hospitals when the anticipated FMC-to-device time at a PCI-capable hospital exceeds 120 min because of unavoidable delays. Door-in door-out time (DIDO) for fibrinolytic therapy should be less than 30 min. If more than 30 min delay, transfer the patient to a PCI-capable hospital.
- Among STEMI patients who were treated with fibrinolytics, patients with >50% ST-segment resolution on EKG were at much lower risk for cardiac-related mortality compared with those with <50% resolution at 30 days.

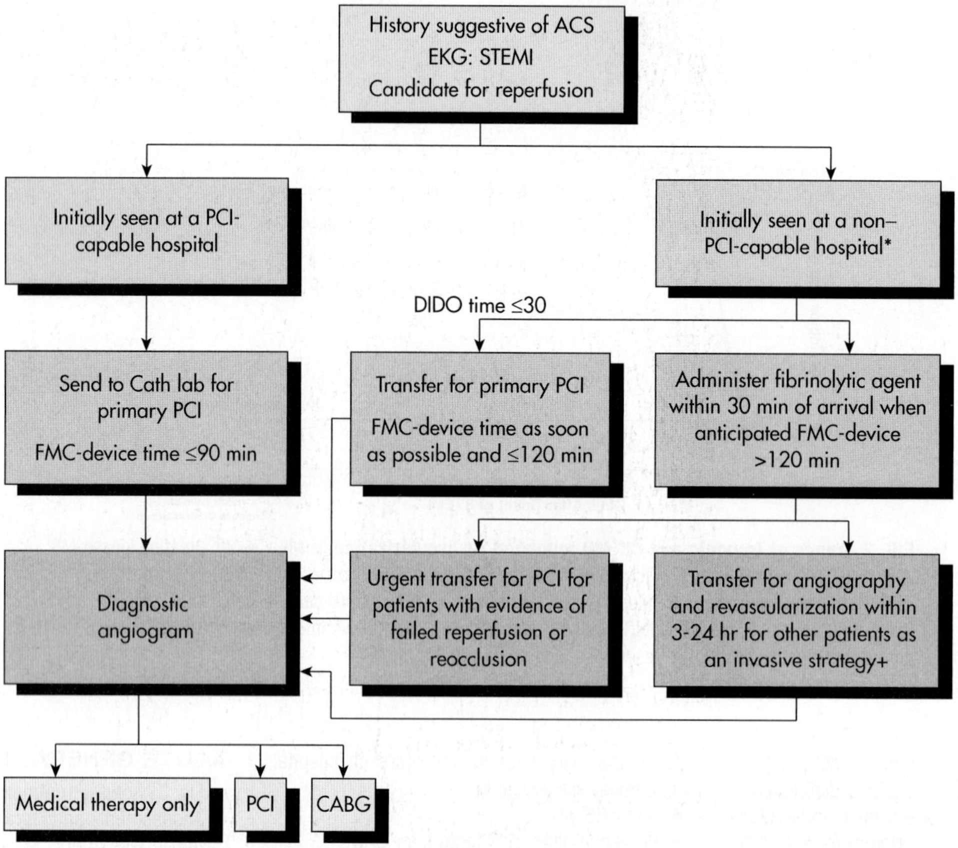

FIG. 3 Reperfusion therapy for patients with STEMI. *Patients with cardiogenic shock or severe heart failure initially seen at a non–PCI-capable hospital should be transferred for cardiac catheterization and revascularization as soon as possible, irrespective of time delay from MI onset. +Angiography and revascularization should not be performed within the first 2 to 3 hr after administration of fibrinolytic therapy. *ACS,* Acute coronary syndrome; *CABG,* coronary artery bypass graft; *Cath,* catheterization; *DIDO,* door-in to door-out; *EKG,* electrocardiogram; *FMC,* first medical contact; *MI,* myocardial infarction; *PCI,* percutaneous coronary intervention; *STEMI,* ST-elevation myocardial infarction. (Modified from O'Gara PT et al: 2013 ACCF/AHA guideline for the management of ST-elevation myocardial infarction, *JACC* 61(4):e78-e140, 2013.)

- PCI is superior to thrombolytic therapy and is the standard of care. It is effective and generally results in more favorable outcomes than thrombolytic therapy.
- Primary PCI should be performed in patients with STEMI and persistent ischemic symptoms and who have contraindications to fibrinolytic therapy, irrespective of the time delay from FMC, or in patients with cardiogenic shock or acute severe HF irrespective of time delay from myocardial infarction (MI) onset, first medical contact to balloon time is <90 minutes or door to balloon/door to needle time is <1 hr, symptoms onset was >3 hr ago and when diagnosis of STEMI in doubt. Coronary stents (drug-eluting or bare-metal) are useful in patients with STEMI.
- The question of culprit vessel vs. complete revascularization during PCI has been brought up since the stent technology was applied to the management of STEMI. The most recent clinical trials (CuLPRIT, PRAMI and DANAMI3-PRIMULTI [FFR-driven revascularization]) appear to favor complete revascularization in the setting of STEMI. However, CULPRIT-SHOCK trial showed culprit vessel only PCI associated with 9.5% absolute reduction in the rate of death or renal replacement therapy at 30 days compared to multivessel PCI in acute MI patients with cardiogenic shock. One-yr outcomes did not show significant difference in mortality between two groups. Korea Acute Myocardial Infarction-National Institutes of Health (KAMIR-NIH) Registry data showed better outcomes with multivessel PCI in cardiogenic shock patients compared to culprit vessel-only PCI. Thus, multivessel PCI should be reserved for few selective patients.
- For patients presenting to a non–PCI-capable hospital, rapid assessment should be done of (1) the time from onset of symptoms, (2) the risk of complications related to STEMI, (3) the risk of bleeding with fibrinolysis, (4) the presence of shock or severe HF, and (5) the time required for transfer to a PCI-capable hospital and a decision about administration of fibrinolytic therapy reached. Because the effectiveness of thrombolytics is time dependent, these agents should ideally be administered either in the field or within 30 min of the patient's arrival to the emergency department (door-to-needle time).
- Fibrinolytic therapy: If tissue plasminogen activator (t PA) or reteplase is used, anticoagulants, such as heparin, are given to increase the likelihood of patency in the infarct-related artery for 48 hr and preferably for the duration of the index hospitalization, up to 8 days. In patients receiving fibrinolysis for STEMI, treatment with enoxaparin is superior to treatment with unfractionated heparin for 48 hr but is associated with an increase in major bleeding episodes. In patients receiving streptokinase or APSAC, heparin after thrombolysis is not indicated because it does not offer any additional benefit and can result in increased bleeding complications. Tenecteplase and reteplase are comparable with accelerated infusion recombinant t-PA in terms of efficacy and safety but are more convenient because they are administered by bolus injection. Lanoplase and heparin bolus plus infusion are as effective as tPA with

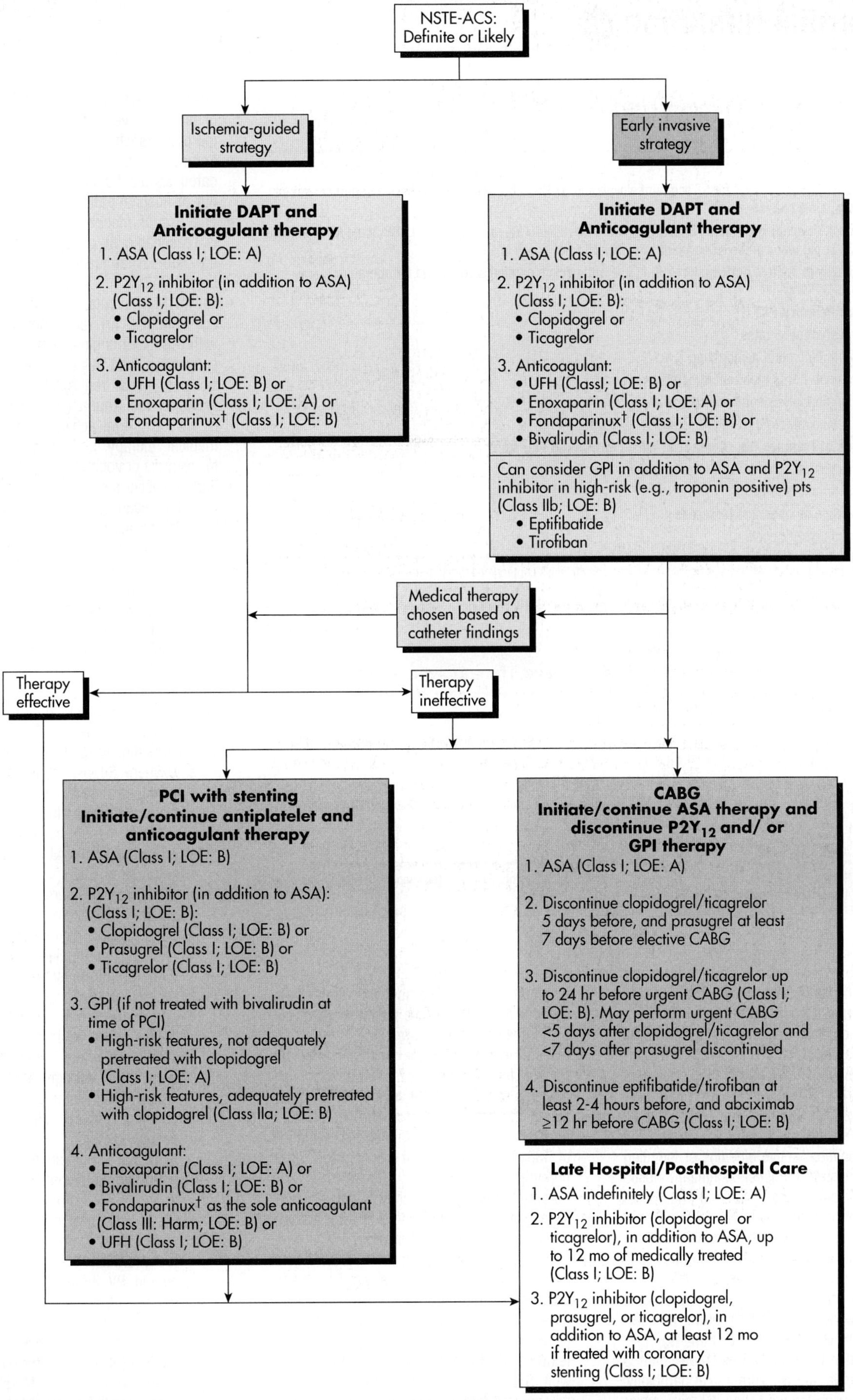

FIG. 4 Algorithm for management of patients with definite of likely non–ST-elevation acute coronary syndromes *(NSTE-ACS)*. †In patients who have been treated with fondaparinux (as upfront therapy) who undergo percutaneous coronary intervention (PCI), an additional anticoagulant with anti-IIa activity should be administered at the time of PCI because of the risk of catheter thrombosis. *ASA,* Acetylsalicylic acid (aspirin); *CABG,* coronary artery bypass grafting; *DAPT,* dual-antiplatelet therapy; *GPI,* glycoprotein inhibitor; *LOE,* level of evidence; *pts,* patients; *UFH,* unfractionated heparin. (From Amsterdam EA et al: 2014 AHA/ACC guideline for the management of patients with non–ST-elevation acute coronary syndromes: a report of the American College of Cardiology/American Heart Association Task Force on Practice Guidelines, *J Am Coll Cardiol* 64:e139-228, 2014. In Zipes DP: *Braunwald's heart disease, a textbook of cardiovascular medicine*, ed 11, Philadelphia, 2019, Elsevier.)

TABLE 3 Indications for Primary Angioplasty and Comparison with Fibrinolytic Therapy

Indications

Alternative recanalization strategy for ST segment elevation or LBBB acute MI within 12 hr of symptom onset (or >12 hr if symptoms persist)

Cardiogenic shock developing within 36 hr of ST segment elevation/Q wave acute MI or LBBB acute MI in patients >75 yr old who can be revascularized within 18 hr of shock onset

Recommended only at centers performing >200 PCI/yr with backup cardiac surgery and for operators performing <75 PCI/yr

Advantages of Primary PCI

Higher initial recanalization rates

Reduced risk of intracerebral hemorrhage

Less residual stenosis; less recurrent ischemia or infarction

Usefulness when fibrinolysis contraindicated

Improvement in outcomes with cardiogenic shock

Disadvantages of Primary PCI (Compared with Fibrinolytic Therapy)

Access, advantages restricted to high-volume centers, operators

Longer average time to treatment

Greater dependence on operators for results

Higher system complexity, costs

LBBB, Left bundle branch block; *MI,* myocardial infarction; *PCI,* percutaneous coronary intervention (includes balloon angioplasty, stenting).

From Goldman L, Schafer AI: *Goldman's Cecil medicine,* ed 24, Philadelphia, 2012, Saunders.

TABLE 4 Dosing Regimens of Commonly Used Thrombolytic Agents

Thrombolytic Agents	Dosing Regimen
t-PA (alteplase)	15 mg bolus IV, followed by 0.75 mg/kg body weight (not to exceed 50 mg) over 30 min, followed by 0.5 mg/kg (not to exceed 35 mg) over 60 min
r-PA (reteplase)	Two 10-U IV boluses, given 30 min apart
TNK–t-PA (tenecteplase)	Single bolus IV 0.5 mg/kg (dose rounded to the nearest 5 mg, ranging from 30 to 50 mg)
Streptokinase	1.5 million U IV over 60 min

IV, Intravenous; *PA,* plasminogen activator; *r-PA,* recombinant plasminogen activator; *TNK–t-PA,* tenecteplase tissue plasminogen activator; *t-PA,* tissue plasminogen activator; *U,* units.

From Andreoli TE et al: *Andreoli and Carpenter's Cecil essentials of medicine,* ed 8, Philadelphia, 2010, Saunders.

regard to mortality rate, but the rate of intracranial hemorrhage is significantly higher.

- Absolute contraindications to thrombolytic therapy (Table 5) include history of intracranial hemorrhage, known intracranial malignant neoplasm or arteriovenous malformation, ischemic stroke within 3 mo (except acute ischemic stroke within 4.5 hr), suspected aortic dissection, active bleeding or bleeding diathesis (except menses), significant closed head or facial trauma within 3 mo, intracranial or intraspinal surgery within 2 mo, or severe uncontrolled hypertension (unresponsive to therapy). For streptokinase, this applies to prior treatment within 6 mo.
- Relative contraindications: History of chronic severe, poorly controlled hypertension, SBP >180 mm Hg, DBP >110 mm Hg, history of prior ischemic stroke more than 3 mo, dementia, known intracranial pathology, traumatic or prolonged CPR (>10 min), major surgery <3 wk, recent internal bleeding within 2 to 4 wk, noncompressible vascular punctures, pregnancy, active peptic ulcer, oral anticoagulant therapy. After the administration of thrombolytics, immediate transfer to a PCI-capable facility is advisable without waiting for lytic results.
- Transfer to a PCI-capable hospital: Immediate transfer for STEMI patients who develop cardiogenic shock or acute severe HF, irrespective of the time delay from MI onset. Urgent transfer if the patient demonstrates evidence of failed reperfusion or reocclusion after fibrinolytic therapy.
- Coronary angiography should not be performed within the first 2 to 3 hr after administration of fibrinolytic therapy.
- Coronary artery bypass graft (CABG): Urgent CABG is indicated in patients with STEMI and coronary anatomy not amenable to PCI who have ongoing or recurrent ischemia, cardiogenic shock, severe HF, or other high-risk features. CABG is recommended in patients with STEMI at time of operative repair of mechanical defects. Box 1 summarizes CABG in patients with MI.
- Therapeutic hypothermia should be started as soon as possible in comatose patients with STEMI and out-of-hospital cardiac arrest caused by ventricular fibrillation (VF) or pulseless ventricular tachycardia, including patients who undergo primary PCI.
- Immediate angiography and PCI when indicated should be performed in resuscitated out-of-hospital patients.
- The use of mechanical circulatory support is reasonable in patients with STEMI who are hemodynamically unstable and require urgent CABG.
- For NSTEMI patients, immediate invasive strategy (within 2 hr) recommended in patients with refractory angina, signs or symptoms of congestive heart failure or new or worsening ischemic mitral regurgitation, hemodynamic instability, recurrent angina or ischemia at rest or with low level activities despite intensive medical therapy and sustained ventricular tachycardia or ventricular fibrillation.
- Early invasive strategy (<24 hr) for NSTEMI patients recommended if GRACE risk for more than 140, dynamic ST changes on EKG and temporal change in troponin levels.
- NSTEMI patient with low-risk TIMI score (0 or 1) and/or low GRACE score (<109) and/or troponin-negative female patients can benefit from ischemia-guided strategy. Fibrinolytic therapy is contraindicated in NSTEMI patients.
- Medical therapy should be initiated immediately in the emergency department for all MI patients. This includes:
  1. Routine measures
     a. Oxygen: Supplemental oxygen should be administered to patients with arterial oxygen desaturation (SaO_2 less than 90%). No benefit has been demonstrated to supplemental oxygen in patients with normal SaO_2.
     b. Nitroglycerin: Increase oxygen supply by reducing coronary vasospasm and decrease oxygen consumption by reducing ventricular preload. Patients with ongoing ischemic discomfort should receive sublingual nitroglycerin every 5 min for a total of three doses, after which an assessment should be made about the need for intravenous nitroglycerin. Intravenous nitroglycerin is indicated for relief of ongoing ischemic discomfort, control of hypertension, or management of pulmonary congestion. Nitrates should not be administered to patients whose systolic blood pressure is <90 mm Hg or ≥30 mm Hg below baseline or severe bradycardia (<50 beats/min), tachycardia (>100 beats/min), or suspected RV infarction. Nitrates should not be administered to patients who have received a phosphodiesterase inhibitor for erectile dysfunction within the last 24 hr (48 hr for tadalafil).
     c. Adequate analgesia: Morphine sulfate 2 to 4 mg IV initially with increments of 2 to 8 mg IV at 5- to 10-min intervals can be given for severe pain unrelieved by nitroglycerin. Morphine can reduce the catecholamine surge caused

TABLE 5 Contraindications to and Cautions in the Use of Fibrinolytics for Treating ST-Elevation Myocardial Infarction*

Absolute Contraindications

Any previous intracranial hemorrhage
Known structural cerebral vascular lesion (e.g., arteriovenous malformation)
Known malignant intracranial neoplasm (primary or metastatic)
Ischemic stroke within 3 mo *except* acute ischemic stroke within 4.5 hr
Suspected aortic dissection
Active bleeding or bleeding diathesis (excluding menses)
Significant closed-head or facial trauma within 3 mo
Intracranial or intraspinal surgery within 2 mo
Severe uncontrolled hypertension (unresponsive to emergency therapy)
For streptokinase, previous treatment within the previous 6 mo

Relative Contraindications

History of chronic, severe, poorly controlled hypertension
Significant hypertension at initial evaluation (SBP >180 mm Hg or DBP >110 mm Hg)†
History of previous ischemic stroke >3 mo
Dementia
Known intracranial pathology not covered in Absolute Contraindications
Traumatic or prolonged (>10 min) cardiopulmonary resuscitation
Major surgery (<3 wk)
Recent (within 2 to 4 wk) internal bleeding
Noncompressible vascular punctures
Pregnancy
Active peptic ulcer
Oral anticoagulant therapy

DBP, Diastolic blood pressure; *MI,* myocardial infarction; *SBP,* systolic blood pressure.
*Viewed as advisory for clinical decision making and may not be all-inclusive or definitive.
†Could be an absolute contraindication in low-risk patients with MI.
From O'Gara PT et al: 2013 ACCF/AHA guideline for the management of ST-elevation myocardial infarction: a report of the American College of Cardiology Foundation/American Heart Association Task Force on Practice Guidelines, *J Am Coll Cardiol* 61:e78, 2013. In Zipes DP: *Braunwald's heart disease, a textbook of cardiovascular medicine,* ed 11, Philadelphia, 2019, Elsevier.

BOX 1 CABG in Patients with Acute MI

Class I

1. Emergency CABG is recommended in patients with acute MI in whom (1) primary PCI has failed or cannot be performed, (2) coronary anatomy is suitable for CABG, and (3) persistent ischemia of a significant area of myocardium at rest or hemodynamic instability refractory to nonsurgical therapy is present.
2. Emergency CABG is recommended in patients undergoing surgical repair of a postinfarction mechanical complication of MI, such as ventricular septal rupture, mitral valve insufficiency because of papillary muscle infarction or rupture, or free wall rupture.
3. Emergency CABG is recommended in patients with cardiogenic shock and who are suitable for CABG irrespective of the time interval from MI to onset of shock and time from MI to CABG.
4. Emergency CABG is recommended in patients with life-threatening ventricular arrhythmias (believed ischemic in origin) in the presence of left main stenosis greater than or equal to 50% or three-vessel CAD.

Class IIa

1. The use of CABG is reasonable as a revascularization strategy in patients with multivessel CAD with recurrent angina or MI within the first 48 hr of STEMI presentation as an alternative to a more delayed strategy.
2. Early revascularization with PCI or CABG is reasonable for selected patients older than 75 yr of age with ST-segment elevation or left bundle branch block who are suitable for revascularization irrespective of the time interval from MI to onset of shock.

Class III

1. Emergency CABG should not be performed in patients with persistent angina and a small area of viable myocardium who are stable hemodynamically.
2. Emergency CABG should not be performed in patients with no reflow (successful epicardial reperfusion with unsuccessful microvascular reperfusion).

CABG, Coronary artery bypass graft; *CAD,* coronary artery disease; *MI,* myocardial infarction; *PCI,* percutaneous coronary intervention; *STEMI,* ST-segment elevation myocardial infarction.

From Hillis LD et al: 2011 ACCF/AHA guideline for coronary artery bypass graft surgery: a report of the American College of Cardiology Foundation/American Heart Association Task Force on Practice Guidelines, *J Am Coll Cardiol* 58:e123-e210, 2011. In Parrillo JE et al: *Critical care medicine, principles of diagnosis and management in the adult,* ed 5, Philadelphia, 2019, Elsevier.

by anxiety and pain, particularly in patients with anterior myocardial infarctions, which in turn can reduce heart rate and pulmonary capillary wedge pressure (PCWP), the increased cardiac workload and oxygen demand, leading to decreased ischemia and pulmonary congestion. Hypotension from morphine can be treated with careful IV hydration with saline solution. If sinus bradycardia accompanies hypotension, use atropine (0.5 to 1.0 mg IV q5min prn to a total dose of 2.5 mg). Respiratory depression caused by morphine can be reversed with naloxone 0.8 mg. Morphine sulfate and nitroglycerine should be avoided in patients with RV involvement who usually present with bradycardia and hypotension. Pain management in these cases should be provided preferentially with meperidine 25 to 50 mg intravenously q4h, in combination with Phenergan 12.5 mg to prevent nausea and/or vomiting. Blood pressure support with normal saline solution is of critical importance to maintain adequate hemodynamics until optimal revascularization is accomplished.

d. Aspirin 162 to 325 mg PO should be crushed and chewed to enhance drug absorption and delivery. It should be given as soon as possible and continued indefinitely, at 81 mg daily. Depending on the clinical and ECG findings, if the patient is suspected to have a coronary anatomy that needs CABG rather than PCI, aspirin should be continued. P2Y12 receptor antagonists should be avoided (except cangrelor) because they increase the perioperative bleeding risk; on-pump surgery should be deferred for at least 24 hr after clopidogrel and ticagrelor. Off-pump surgery might be considered within 24 hr of clopidogrel or ticagrelor if the benefits of revascularization outweigh the risk of bleeding. However, if the coronary artery disease is likely to benefit from PCI alone, then a loading dose of clopidogrel 600 or 300 mg or ticagrelor 180 mg PO or prasugrel 60 mg should be given as early as possible and no later than 1 hr after PCI. P2Y12 receptor antagonist should be continued for at least 1 yr after acute coronary syndrome or after primary PCI. Prasugrel showed significant net clinical benefit (MACE vs. bleeding complications) only in patients with MI who underwent revascularization. It shouldn't be given for nonrevascularized patients. Ticagrelor or clopidogrel can be given in patients with MI with or without catheter-based revascularization. Cangrelor is the newest direct-acting P2Y12 platelet receptor inhibitor. It has a similar chemical structure to ATP, with a half-life of 3 to 6 min. It is given IV as a bolus plus 120 min of infusion at the time of

TABLE 6 Recommendations for Beta-Blocker Therapy for ST-Elevation Myocardial Infarction (STEMI)

Recommendation	COR	LOE
Oral beta-blockers should be initiated in the first 24 hr in patients with STEMI who do not have any of the following: Signs of heart failure or evidence of a low-output state Increased risk for cardiogenic shock*: • Age >70 yr • Systolic blood pressure <120 mm Hg • Sinus tachycardia >110 beats/min or heart rate <60 beats/min • Increased time since the onset of symptoms of STEMI Other relative contraindications to use of oral beta-blockers: • PR interval longer than 0.24 second • Second- or third-degree heart block • Active asthma or reactive airways disease	I	B
Beta-blockers should be continued during and after hospitalization for all patients with STEMI and no contraindications to their use.	I	B
Patients with initial contraindications to the use of beta-blockers in the first 24 hr after STEMI should be reevaluated to determine their subsequent eligibility.	I	C
It is reasonable to administer IV beta-blockers at initial encounter to patients with STEMI and no contraindications to their use who are hypertensive or have ongoing ischemia.	IIa	B

COR, Class of recommendation; *IV*, intravenous; *LOE*, level of evidence.
*The greater the number of risk factors present, the higher the risk for development of cardiogenic shock.
Modified from O'Gara PT et al: 2013 ACCF/AHA guideline for the management of ST-elevation myocardial infarction: a report of the American College of Cardiology Foundation/American Heart Association Task Force on Practice Guidelines, *J Am Coll Cardiol* 61:e78, 2013. In Zipes DP: *Braunwald's heart disease, a textbook of cardiovascular medicine*, ed 11, Philadelphia, 2019, Elsevier.

primary PCI in patients who are naïve to P2Y12 receptor antagonists. It was approved by the FDA in 2015 after the CHAMPION PHOENIX trial. Clopidogrel and prasugrel should be started after its infusion is finished. The ticagrelor loading dose can be given during the infusion. Considering rapid onset action and clearance, cangrelor can be started in the emergency room at the time of high-risk acute myocardial infarction diagnosis irrespective surgical or catheter-based revascularization.

2. In patients receiving fibrinolytics only or balloon angioplasty without stent, P2Y12 antagonists can be given for as little as 14 days. Clopidogrel is recommended for postfibrinolytic patients.
3. Unfractionated heparin (UFH) is recommended in all patients with NSTEMI and STEMI (fibrinolysis or invasive revascularization). UFH infusion should not exceed more than 48 hr after PCI or fibrinolysis in the absence of an ongoing indication due to risk of heparin-induced thrombocytopenia. NSTEMI patients who underwent ischemia-guided therapy, low molecular weight heparin (LMWH) showed better MACE outcomes compared with UFH. The benefit was not significant in revascularized patients. Bivalirudin was associated with lower MACE and bleeding events in STEMI patients compared with UFH. However, it increased the risk of stent thrombosis. In NSTEMI patients who are undergoing PCI, LMWH, bivalirudin, and UFH are acceptable.
4. Beta-adrenergic blocking agents should generally be given to all patients who do not exhibit evidence of shock. Table 6 summarizes recommendations for beta-blocker therapy for STEMI. Beta-blockers are useful to reduce myocardial oxygen consumption and prevent tachyarrhythmias. Early IV beta blockage (in the initial 24 hr) followed by institution of an oral maintenance regimen is also effective in reducing recurrent infarction and ischemia. Oral beta-blockers should be initiated in the first 24 hr in patients with MI who do not have any of the following: Signs of HF, evidence of a low-output state, sinus tachycardia, increased risk for cardiogenic shock, or other contraindications for its use (bradycardia, PR interval more than 0.24 seconds, second- or third-degree heart block, active asthma, or reactive airways disease).
5. They should be continued during and after hospitalization for all patients with MI and with no contraindications to their use for at least 2 yr. Patients with initial contraindications to the use of beta-blockers in the first 24 hr after MI should be reevaluated to determine their subsequent eligibility. It is reasonable to administer intravenous beta-blockers at the time of presentation to patients with MI and no contraindications to their use who are hypertensive or have ongoing ischemia.
6. In patients with acute MI, treatment with drug-eluting stents is associated with decreased mortality rates and a reduction in the need for repeated revascularization procedures compared with treatment including bare-metal stents.
7. Gp IIb/IIIa inhibitors in the era of DAPT therapy and primary PCI have failed to show benefit with "upstream" treatment. Abciximab might be useful in the presence of large thrombus burden during primary PCI. For patients receiving bivalirudin as the primary anticoagulant, routine adjunctive use of GP IIb/IIIa inhibitors is not recommended but may be considered as adjunctive or "bail-out" therapy in selected cases. In patients with acute coronary syndrome with high-risk features and not adequately pretreated with P2Y12 inhibitors, it is useful to administer GP IIb/IIIa inhibitors at the time of PCI.

CHRONIC Rx

- Discharge medications in all patients with MI (unless contraindicated) should include antiischemic medications (e.g., nitroglycerin, beta-blocker), lipid-lowering agents, and antiplatelet therapy (aspirin and/or P2Y12 antagonists).
- Aspirin, 81 mg PO daily, but should be continued indefinitely unless not tolerated (e.g., GI bleed). In MI patients, clopidogrel 75 mg PO daily; ticagrelor, 90 mg bid, or prasugrel, 10 mg PO daily, can be combined with aspirin and should be continued without interruption for a minimum of 12 mo after drug-eluting stent placement; however, aspirin should be continued indefinitely. In cases of high bleeding risk or significant overt bleeding, consider discontinuation of P2Y12 inhibitor after 6 mo (Fig. 6). Combining P2Y12 antagonists with aspirin reduces risk for repeat myocardial infarction and stent thrombosis. If there is an elective surgical intervention pending, it is recommended to defer the surgery until completion of the full course of the P2Y12 antagonist treatment.
- Angiotensin-converting enzyme inhibitors (ACEIs) should be started within the first 24 hr of MI to all patients having MI with anterior infarction, pulmonary congestion, or LV EF <40%, in the absence of hypotension. They reduce LV dysfunction and dilation and slow the progression to HF during and after acute MI. Angiotensin receptor blockers (ARBs) should be given to patients who have indication but are intolerant of ACEIs. IV formulations of ACEIs should not be given within the first 24 hr of STEMI due to risk of hypotension. ARBs offer no advantage over ACEIs and should be considered only in patients who are intolerant to ACEIs.
  1. Commonly used ACEIs are ramipril 2.5 mg PO bid, captopril 12.5 mg PO bid, enalapril 2.5 mg PO bid, and lisinopril 2.5 to 5 mg PO qd initially, with subsequent titration as needed. Ramipril is associated with a lower mortality rate than most ACEIs.
  2. ACEIs may be stopped in patients without complications and no evidence of LV dysfunction after 6 to 8 wk.
  3. ACEIs should be continued indefinitely in patients with impaired LV function (EF <40%) or clinical HF.
- Long-term aldosterone antagonist therapy should be prescribed for post-MI patients without significant renal dysfunction

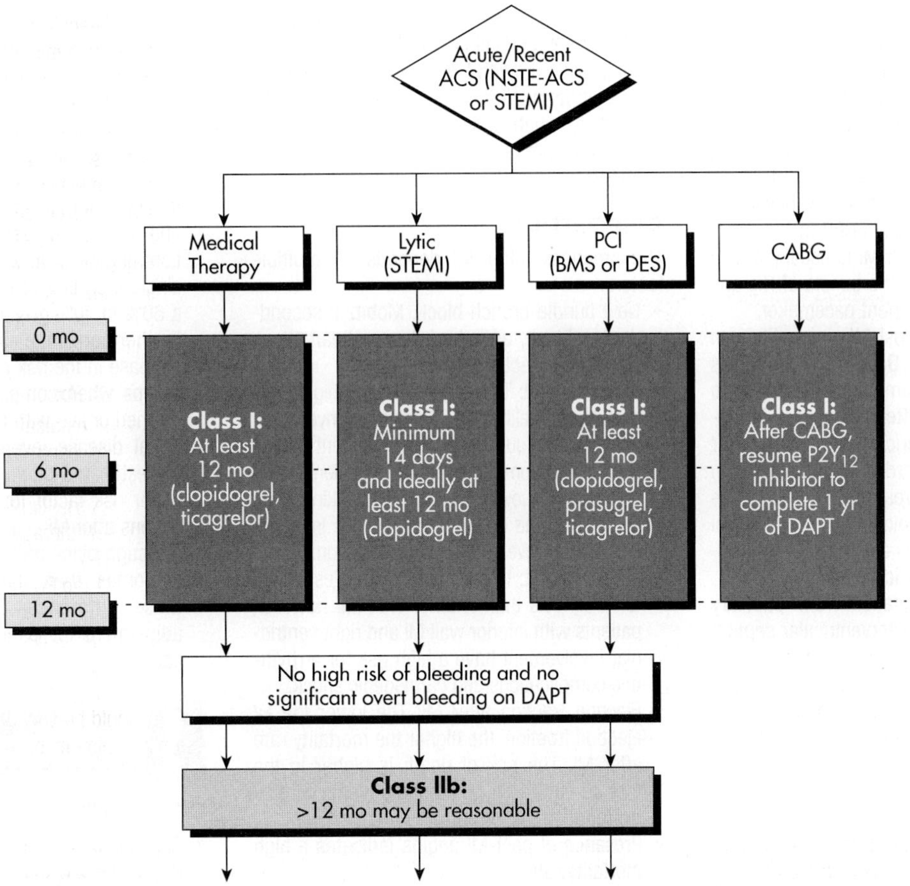

FIG. 6 ACC/AHA guideline recommendation for duration and choice of antiplatelet agent in patients with recent acute coronary syndrome (ACS), including STEMI aspirin therapy is generally continued indefinitely post-ACS. In patients treated with dual-antiplatelet therapy (DAPT) after DES implantation who have a high risk of bleeding (e.g., use of oral anticoagulant therapy, major intracranial surgery) or develop significant overt bleeding, discontinuation of P2Y12 inhibitor therapy after 6 mo for ACS may be reasonable. The optimal duration of prolonged DAPT is not established. *BMS,* Bare-metal stent; *CABG,* coronary artery bypass grafting; *DES,* drug-eluting stent; *lytic,* fibrinolytic therapy; *NSTE-ACS,* non–ST-elevation acute coronary syndrome; *PCI,* percutaneous coronary intervention; *STEMI,* ST-elevation myocardial infarction. (Modified from Levine GN et al: 2016 ACC/AHA guideline focused update on duration of dual antiplatelet therapy in patients with coronary artery disease, *J Am Coll Cardiol* 68(10):1082-115, 2016. In Zipes DP: *Braunwald's heart disease, a textbook of cardiovascular medicine,* ed 11, Philadelphia, 2019, Elsevier.)

(creatinine ≤2.5 mg/dl in men and ≤2.0 mg/dl in women) or hyperkalemia who are already taking an ACEI, a beta-blocker, and have LV EF <40% with symptomatic HF or diabetes.

- In late 2018, American College of Cardiology (ACC) recommended LDL goal of <70 mg/dl for secondary prevention of atherosclerotic cardiovascular disease. High-intensity statins (atorvastatin 40 to 80 mg or rosuvastatin 20 to 40 mg) should be started as early as possible in all patients with MI regardless of lipid panel, not only for their lipid-lowering effects, but also their antiinflammatory properties (JUPITER trial), which can stabilize the ruptured plaque. Atorvastatin 80 mg can be used (PROVE IT-TIMI 22 and MIRACL trials). IMPROVE-IT trial showed adding ezetimibe to statin treatment could decrease recurrent MI and ischemic stroke in MI patients. FDA also approved two PCSK9 (proprotein convertase subtilisin/kexin type 9) inhibitors (alirocumab and evolocumab) for heterozygous familial hypercholesterolemia patients who are receiving maximally tolerated statins or patients with clinical atherosclerotic cardiovascular disease who require lowering LDL levels. Newer 2018 lipid guidelines suggested starting PCSK9 inhibitor in very high-risk atherosclerotic cardiovascular disease patients who did not meet the LDL goal on high intensity statin and ezetimibe. One should always consider adding ezetimibe to high intensity statin prior to initiation of PCSK9 inhibitor due to cost issues. A fasting lipid panel should be checked during the first 24 hr of hospital course, and the intensive therapy can be stepped down if appropriate.
- In diabetic patients, HbA1c goal should be aimed at below or around 7.0% to reduce micro- and macrovascular complications. Oral hypoglycemic agents GLP1 (glucagon-like peptide) agonist (liraglutide) and SGLT2 (sodium-glucose cotransporter) inhibitor (empagliflozin) showed significant mortality benefit in type 2 diabetic patients with history of CAD.
- ACC/AHA 2017 hypertension guidelines recommend initiation of blood pressure (BP)-lowering medications in patients with clinical CVD and an average SBP ≥130 mm Hg or a DBP ≥80 mm Hg for goal BP of <130/80.

COMPLICATIONS OF MI

- Cardiogenic shock: Emergent revascularization with either PCI or CABG is the recommended treatment.
- Sustained ventricular tachycardia: Implantable cardioverter-defibrillator therapy (ICD) is indicated before discharge in patients who develop sustained ventricular tachycardia/ventricular fibrillation more than 48 hr after STEMI, provided the arrhythmia is not due to transient or reversible ischemia, reinfarction, or metabolic abnormalities.

- Pacing in MI: Temporary pacing is indicated for symptomatic bradyarrhythmias unresponsive to medical treatment and after revascularization. AV block and bradyarrhythmias in the setting of inferior wall MI are usually transient, will not require long-term pacing, and usually resolve within 2 to 4 wk of the event. On the contrary, AV block and bradyarrhythmias or new LBBB in the presence of an anterior wall MI is usually a sign of severe disruption of the bundle of His and often requires a permanent pacemaker.
- Pericarditis after MI: Post-MI pericarditis can occur early after MI. Dressler syndrome is an autoimmune inflammatory reaction to myocardial antigen after myocardial infarction. Symptoms of pericarditis usually occur 2 to 3 wk after myocardial infarction. Aspirin is recommended for treatment of pericarditis after MI. Glucocorticoids and nonsteroidal antiinflammatory drugs are potentially harmful for treatment of pericarditis after STEMI.
- Severe mitral regurgitation from papillary muscle rupture (1%), interventricular septum rupture (0.2%), and free wall rupture (1% to 3%) are the three major mechanical complications that can occur after acute myocardial infarction. Echocardiogram is helpful in diagnosing papillary muscle rupture, ventricular septal rupture, and free wall rupture. Right heart catheterization is needed to show "step-up" in oxygen saturation at the level of right ventricle. Emergent surgical repair is the treatment of choice for ventricular free wall rupture, intraventricular septum rupture, and papillary muscle rupture.

EVALUATION OF POST-MI PATIENTS

- Noninvasive testing for ischemia should be performed before discharge to assess the presence and extent of inducible ischemia in patients with STEMI who have not had coronary angiography and do not have high-risk clinical features for which coronary angiography would be warranted. It might be considered before discharge to evaluate the functional significance of a noninfarct artery stenosis previously identified at angiography and/or before discharge to guide the postdischarge exercise prescription.
- Assessment of LV function: LV ejection fraction should be measured in all patients with STEMI. Echocardiography to rule out presence of mural thrombi in patients suspected of having an extensive infarction (more common with anterior wall MI); contrast echocardiography is added if mural thrombus is suspected.
  1. Assessment of risk for sudden cardiac death: Patients with an initially reduced LV ejection fraction, <40%, who are possible candidates for implantable cardiovert-er-defibrillator therapy should undergo reevaluation of LV ejection fraction at 90 days (or 42 days if no revascularization was performed). ICD is recommended when LVEF remains <35% in the presence of NYHA class II or III heart failure, or in patients with LVEF <30% regardless of symptoms, if the life expectancy is >1 yr.
- Cardiac rehabilitation/secondary prevention programs are recommended for patients with STEMI.

DISPOSITION

The prognosis after MI depends on multiple factors:

- New bundle branch block, Mobitz II second-degree block, and third-degree heart block adversely affect outcome.
- Size of infarct: The larger it is, the higher the post-MI mortality rate. Significant myocardial stunning with subsequent improvement of ventricular function occurs in most patients after anterior MI. A lower level of creatine kinase, an estimate of the extent of necrosis, is independently predictive of recovery of function.
- Site of infarct: Inferior wall MI carries a better prognosis than anterior wall MI; however, patients with inferior wall MI and right ventricular involvement have a high risk for arrhythmic complications and cardiogenic shock.
- Ejection fraction after MI: The lower the LV ejection fraction, the higher the mortality rate after MI. The risk of death is higher in the first 30 days after MI among patients with LV dysfunction, HF, or both.
- Presence of post-MI angina indicates a high mortality rate.
- Performance on low-level exercise test: The presence of ST-segment changes during the test is a predictor of high mortality rate during the first yr.
- Presence of pericarditis during the acute phase of MI increases mortality rate at 1 yr.
- Type A behavior (competitive drive, ambitiousness, hostility) is associated with a lower mortality rate after symptomatic MI.
- The Killip classification is an independent predictor of all-cause 30-day mortality:
  1. Killip class I includes individuals with no clinical signs of HF. Mortality rate is 6%.
  2. Killip class II includes individuals with rales or crackles in the lungs, S_3 gallop, and elevated jugular venous pressure. Mortality rate is 17%.
  3. Killip class III describes individuals with frank acute pulmonary edema. Mortality rate is 38%.
  4. Killip class IV describes individuals in cardiogenic shock or hypotension (measured as systolic blood pressure <90 mm Hg) and evidence of peripheral vasoconstriction (oliguria, cyanosis, or sweating). Mortality rate is 67%.
- Self-reported moderate alcohol consumption in the yr before acute MI is associated with reduced 1-yr mortality rate.
- Discharge medication in patients with MI should include lipid-lowering agents. Statins may also lower vascular inflammation and damage by mechanisms other than reduction of low-density lipoprotein cholesterol. Early initiation of statin treatment in patients with acute MI is associated with reduced 1-yr mortality rate.
- Additional poor prognostic factors include cigarette smoking, history of hypertension or prior MI, presence of ST-segment depression in acute MI, older age, diabetes mellitus, and female sex (especially women >50 yr). Lammintausta and Fonarow reported that single men and women who live alone have a 60% to 70% greater risk of a heart attack. Furthermore, the study showed >160% increase in the risk of sudden death in these groups when compared to people who are married or live with family.
- Renal disease, even mild, as assessed by the estimated glomerular filtration rate, is a major risk factor for cardiovascular complications after MI.
- Although black patients with MI have worse outcomes than their white counterparts, these differences did not persist after adjustment for patient factors and site of care.

PEARLS & CONSIDERATIONS

COMMENTS

- Approximately 1.5 million patients undergo PCI in the U.S. each yr. Depending on local practices and the diagnostic criteria used, 5% to 30% of these patients have evidence of a periprocedural MI.
- The 12-lead ECG has low sensitivity for the detection of MI if the culprit lesion is in the left circumflex artery (LCX). If the initial 12-lead ECG is not diagnostic and high clinical suspicion for acute coronary syndrome exists, it is reasonable to obtain additional posterior chest leads (V_7 to V_9) to detect LCX occlusion.
- Triad of hypotension, elevated jugular venous pressure, and clear lungs are suggestive of RV infarction in patients with inferior AMI. Administration of nitroglycerin is contraindicated due to hypotension. IV fluids, inotropic support, and early reperfusion are the mainstays of treatment.

SUGGESTED READINGS

Available at ExpertConsult.com

RELATED CONTENT

Heart Attack (Patient Information)
Acute Coronary Syndrome (Related Key Topic)
Angina Pectoris (Related Key Topic)
Coronary Artery Disease (Related Key Topic)

AUTHOR: **Maheswara Satya Gangadhara Rao Golla, MD**

BASIC INFORMATION

DEFINITION

Myocarditis broadly refers to inflammatory disease of the heart muscle (myocardium). Disease severity may range from benign and self-limiting illness to severe, acute decompensation requiring intensive care. Myocarditis may result from exposure to a variety of infectious and noninfectious triggers.

ICD-10CM CODES	
I40.0	Infective myocarditis
I40.1	Isolated myocarditis
I40.8	Other acute myocarditis
I40.9	Acute myocarditis, unspecified
A39.52	Meningococcal myocarditis
B26.82	Mumps myocarditis
B33.22	Viral myocarditis
B58.81	Toxoplasma myocarditis
D86.85	Sarcoid myocarditis
I01.2	Acute rheumatic myocarditis
I09.0	Rheumatic myocarditis
I41	Myocarditis in diseases classified elsewhere
I51.4	Myocarditis, unspecified

EPIDEMIOLOGY & DEMOGRAPHICS

- Myocarditis is often underdiagnosed.
- The incidence of focal myocarditis reported at autopsy is 1% to 9% in asymptomatic patients and 50% in patients infected with HIV.
- Myocarditis is the third leading cause of sudden unexpected death (as high as 8% to 9%), especially in competitive athletes, Approximately 1% to 5% of patients that test positive for viral infections may develop myocarditis.

PHYSICAL FINDINGS & CLINICAL PRESENTATION

- Clinical symptoms are heterogeneous, ranging from asymptomatic to severe forms resulting in cardiogenic shock and arrhythmias.
- The most common presentations in patients are new onset heart failure (<6 mo), chest pain, and arrhythmias, which include sinus tachycardia as well as atrial and ventricular premature contractions.
- Chest pain, especially pleuritic and positional, presents when the pericardium is involved.
- Persistent tachycardia may be present, out of proportion to fever.
- Bradyarrhythmia and new-onset unexplained heart block may also occur both in infectious (e.g., Lyme disease) and in immune-mediated forms of myocarditis.
- Faint S_1, S_3, and S_4 gallops on auscultation are important signs of impaired ventricular function.
- Murmur of functional mitral regurgitation and functional tricuspid regurgitation caused by severe left ventricular and right ventricular dilation.
- Pericardial friction rub if associated with pericarditis as in the clinical syndrome of myopericarditis.
- Patients may present with a history of a recent flulike syndrome or nonspecific viral prodrome (fever, arthralgias, malaise, fatigue); children often have a more fulminant presentation than adults. Difficulty breathing is the most common presentation of pediatric myocarditis.
- Congestive heart failure (CHF) symptoms that usually manifest with fatigue and decreased exercise capacity and appetite.
- Signs of biventricular failure (hypotension, hepatomegaly, peripheral edema, distention of neck veins, S_3 sounds, and pulmonary edema).
- Presyncope or syncope can occur secondary to ventricular arrhythmias.
- Sudden cardiac death from ventricular tachycardia/ventricular fibrillation mediated by inflammation and/or a scar, which sets up a reentry-mediated pathway for ventricular arrhythmias.
- Acute coronary syndrome, which can occur due to local coronary spasm and inflammation and can present on ECG as acute injury pattern or ischemic changes.

ETIOLOGY

- Infection:
  1. Viral (adenovirus, parvovirus B19, hepatitis C virus [HCV], Coxsackie B virus, cytomegalovirus, enterovirus, poliovirus, mumps, HIV, and Epstein-Barr virus, etc.). Viruses are the most common cause of myocarditis in developed countries. In the 1980s and 1990s, enteroviruses and adenoviruses were frequently associated with myocarditis and dilated cardiomyopathy. In the past 20 yr, however, other viruses such as HCV, parvovirus B19, herpesvirus 6 (HH6), and HIV have emerged as the significant pathogens (Box E1)
  2. Bacterial (*Staphylococcus aureus, Clostridium perfringens,* diphtheria, mycoplasma, and any severe bacterial infection)
  3. Mycotic (*Candida, Mucor, Aspergillus, Blastomyces, Histoplasma*)
  4. Parasitic (*Trypanosoma cruzi*—most common worldwide, *Trichinella, Echinococcus, Amoeba, Toxoplasma*)
  5. *Rickettsia rickettsii*
  6. Spirochetal (*Borrelia burgdorferi*–Lyme carditis)
- Rheumatic fever
- Systemic lupus erythematosus
- Granulomatosis with polyangiitis (Wegener granulomatosis)
- Giant cell arteritis and Takayasu arteritis
- Drugs (e.g., cocaine, emetine, doxorubicin, sulfonamides, isoniazid, methyldopa, amphotericin B, tetracycline, phenylbutazone, lithium, 5-fluorouracil, phenothiazines, interferon-alfa, nivolumab, ipilimumab, tricyclic antidepressants, cyclophosphamides, smallpox vaccination)
- Toxins (carbon monoxide, ethanol, diphtheria toxin, lead, arsenicals)
- Systemic and collagen-vascular disease (scleroderma, sarcoidosis, celiac disease, Sjögren syndrome, Kawasaki syndrome, etc.)
- Celiac disease: Two reports from Italy suggest that celiac disease, which is often clinically unsuspected, accounts for as many as 5% of patients with autoimmune myocarditis or idiopathic DCM
- Radiation
- Postpartum status
- Post–stem cell transplantation
- Hypersensitivity reactions from insect bites, such as bee and wasp bites; from snake bites; and from tetanus toxoid

DIAGNOSIS (TABLE 1)

DIFFERENTIAL DIAGNOSIS

- Ischemic cardiomyopathy and nonischemic cardiomyopathies, including dilated idiopathic cardiomyopathy
- Acute coronary syndromes
- Valvular heart disease
- Infiltrative diseases of the myocardium, such as sarcoidosis, amyloidosis, hemochromatosis, and Chagas disease

The differential diagnosis of chest pain is described in Section II.

WORKUP

- Medical history: The clinical presentation of myocarditis is nonspecific and can consist of fatigue, palpitations, dyspnea, precordial discomfort, and myalgias.
- Diagnostic workup includes chest x-ray examination, ECG, laboratory evaluation, echocardiogram, cardiac catheterization, cardiac MRI with late gadolinium enhancement, and endomyocardial biopsy (in selected patients on the basis of the likelihood of finding specific treatable disorders such as giant cell myocarditis). Of note, endomyocardial biopsy has a sensitivity of only 10% to 35% using standard histologic criteria. This is due to variability in interpretation and sampling error.

LABORATORY TESTS

- Elevated cardiac troponin is suggestive of myocarditis in patients with clinically suspected myocarditis. Troponin I specificity is 89%; sensitivity is 34% to 53%. Elevated troponin aids in diagnosis but does not confer a prognostic value. A normal level does not rule out the diagnosis.
- Increased creatine kinase (CK) (with elevated MB fraction, lactate dehydrogenase), and aspartate aminotransferase from myocardial necrosis
- Elevation of cardiac troponin I or T is more common than CK-MB elevation in patients with biopsy-proven myocarditis
- The elevations of cardiac troponin I were correlated with a short duration (typically less than 1 mo) of CHF symptoms, indicating that

TABLE 1 Expanded Criteria for Diagnosis of Myocarditis

Suggestive of myocarditis:	2 positive categories
Compatible with myocarditis:	3 positive categories
High probability of being myocarditis:	all 4 categories positive

(Any matching feature in category = positive for category)

Category I: Clinical Symptoms

- Clinical heart failure
- Fever
- Viral prodrome
- Fatigue
- Dyspnea on exertion
- Chest pain
- Palpitations
- Presyncope or syncope

Category II: Evidence of Cardiac Structural or Functional Perturbation *in the Absence* of Regional Coronary Ischemia

- Echocardiography evidence
- Regional wall motion abnormalities
- Cardiac dilation
- Regional cardiac hypertrophy
- Troponin release
- High sensitivity (>0.1 ng/ml)
- Positive indium In 111 antimyosin scintigraphy
- Normal coronary angiography *or*
- Absence of reversible ischemia by coronary distribution on perfusion scan

Category III: Cardiac Magnetic Resonance Imaging

- Increased myocardial T2 signal on inversion recovery sequence
- Delayed contrast enhancement after gadolinium-DTPA infusion

Category IV: Myocardial Biopsy—Pathologic or Molecular Analysis

- Pathology findings compatible with Dallas criteria
- Presence of viral genome by polymerase chain reaction or in situ hybridization

DTPA, Diethylenetriamine penta-acetic acid.
From Bonow RO et al: *Heart disease,* 9th ed, Philadelphia, 2012, Saunders.

the majority of myocardial necrosis occurs early in the disease course

- Persistent elevations of cardiac biomarkers are indicative of ongoing myocardial necrosis
- BNP or NT-proBNP is recommended if patient has heart failure symptoms
- Increased erythrocyte sedimentation rate (nonspecific but may be of value in following the progress of the disease and the response to therapy)
- Increased white blood cell count, again, nonspecific (increased eosinophils if parasitic infection)
- Viral titers (acute and convalescent)
- Cold agglutinin titer, antistreptolysin O titer, blood cultures
- Lyme disease antibody titer
- RPR, VDRL
- Histology on endomyocardial biopsy may reveal histiocytic and mononuclear cellular infiltrates, fulfilling the Dallas criteria, which were developed by a panel of cardiac pathologists as a working standard to define the disease; active myocarditis is defined as "an inflammatory infiltrate of the myocardium with necrosis and/or degeneration of adjacent myocytes not typical of the ischemic damage associated with coronary artery disease"
- Based on the European Society of Cardiology Working Group on Myocardial and Pericardial Diseases, immunohistochemical criteria of myocarditis are abnormal inflammatory infiltrates defined as >14 leukocytes/mm^2 including up to 4 monocytes/mm^2 with the presence of >7 CD^3 positive T lymphocytes/mm^2

IMAGING STUDIES

- Chest x-ray: Enlargement of cardiac silhouette with or without pulmonary congestion may be present.
- ECG: May be normal or show nonspecific findings. Sinus tachycardia with nonspecific ST-T wave changes unless there is concomitant pericarditis in which the ECG changes are more specific; intraventricular conduction defects and bundle branch blocks are uncommon in typical viral myocarditis but are common manifestations in cardiac sarcoid and idiopathic giant cell myocarditis. The presence of Q waves or left bundle branch block was associated with higher rates of death or transplantation in some patients.
  1. Lyme disease and diphtheria can cause varying degrees of heart block.
  2. Changes mimicking acute myocardial infarction (regional ST elevations and Q waves) can occur with focal necrosis from myocarditis.
- Echocardiogram:
  1. The most useful test in detecting decreased ventricular function in suspected myocarditis even when subclinical.
  2. Acute severe myocarditis is associated with systolic dysfunction with decreased ejection fraction.
  3. Dilated and hypokinetic chambers.
  4. The systolic dysfunction is generally global but may be regional or segmental as in the case of focal myocarditis.
  5. Exercise-induced wall motion abnormalities may also be seen. This is usually due to microvascular dysfunction.
  6. Abnormal tissue Doppler signal can provide additional evidence for the presence of myocarditis.
  7. The echocardiogram can also be helpful with diagnosing coexisting pericardial involvement.
  8. The spheroid dysfunctional ventricle in acute myocarditis tends to remodel to the more normal elliptical shape over several months.
- Cardiac catheterization and angiography:
  1. To rule out coronary artery disease and valvular disease. Coronary angiography is most commonly normal with evidence of minimal or no coronary artery disease.
  2. A right ventricular endomyocardial biopsy can confirm the diagnosis, although a negative biopsy result does not exclude myocarditis owing to the low sensitivity of this test. Recent studies have shown that myocardial biopsy may be unnecessary because immunosuppression therapy based on biopsy results is generally ineffective. However, if idiopathic giant cell myocarditis is suspected, biopsy can confirm this diagnosis, and immunosuppression therapy is often helpful in this patient cohort.
- Cardiac MRI (Fig. E1):
  1. Can be used to detect myocardial edema and myocyte injury in myocarditis.
  2. Increased focal or global signal intensity can be used to calculate an edema ratio. Edema in the absence of necrosis or scar represents reversible injury and thus can predict functional recovery.
  3. Late gadolinium enhancement (LGE) and the presence of increased focal and global myocardial contrast enhancement relative to skeletal muscle.
  4. Any combination of two of the above has a sensitivity and specificity of 76% and 96%, with 85% diagnostic accuracy, and is probably the gold standard for diagnosis of myocarditis, as opposed to routine biopsy.
  5. Cardiac MRI has demonstrated that myocarditis tends to start as a focal process and becomes a more global process over time, with the extent of myocardial enhancement correlating with clinical status and left ventricular function.
  6. The pattern of LGE is different from that in ischemic cardiomyopathy. LGE in myocarditis tends to involve the epicardium with variable extension into the midmyocardium and sparing of the endocardium. This is in contrast to ischemic injury, which involves endocardium first with extension outward.

- Indium-111-labeled antimyosin antibody scintigraphy is positive in myocarditis with a sensitivity of up to 65%.

Rx TREATMENT

NONPHARMACOLOGIC THERAPY

- Supportive care is the first line of therapy for patients with myocarditis.
- Restrict physical activity (to decrease cardiac work). Bed rest is advisable during viremia.
- Avoid heavy use of alcohol.
- Nonsteroidal antiinflammatory drugs (NSAIDs) should be avoided in patients with HF generally, given the risk of HF exacerbation and possible risk of increased mortality. NSAIDs in the lowest required dose are reserved for patients with perimyocarditis in whom LV function is clearly normal and who have prominent chest pain from pericarditis.

ACUTE GENERAL Rx

- Treat underlying cause (e.g., use specific antibiotics for bacterial infection).
- Treat congestive heart failure (CHF) with diuretics, angiotensin-converting enzyme inhibitors (ACE inhibitors), and salt restriction. A beta-blocker may be added once clinical stability has been achieved. Digoxin should be used with caution and only at low doses.
- In patients with myocarditis associated with severe left ventricular dysfunction, major treatment decisions such as referral for heart transplant, left ventricular assist device, and with implantable cardioverter-defibrillator (ICD) implantation should be deferred for 3 to 6 mo when feasible to allow for improvement with optimal medical therapy.
- Patients who are left with an LVEF ≤35% despite optimal medical therapy for 3 to 6 mo, and who have good functional status with prognosis >1 yr, will benefit from primary prevention therapy with ICD implantation as in patients with ischemic cardiomyopathy and other nonischemic cardiomyopathies.
- Antiarrhythmics if needed for ventricular arrhythmias. When antiarrhythmic therapy is necessary, options include amiodarone, dofetilide, and, in patients without class IV HF, cautious use of beta-blockers or calcium channel blockers. ICD implantation for secondary prevention in patients who have life-threatening ventricular arrhythmias and have good functional status with prognosis >1 yr.
- Complete heart block and/or symptomatic bradycardia are indications for pacing during the acute phase of myocarditis but are usually transient, so temporary pacing is sufficient.
- In patients with chronic CHF from myocarditis, only ACE inhibitors, beta-blockers, and possibly aldosterone receptor antagonists will decrease their mortality in the long term (as with all CHF etiologies).
- Anticoagulation is indicated in patients with evidence of systemic embolism or presence of acute left ventricular thrombus. Standard criteria for anticoagulation for atrial fibrillation should also be applied. Heart failure and/or low EF with normal sinus rhythm are generally not indications for anticoagulation.
- Inotropes or mechanical assist devices such as intraaortic balloon pumps, Impella device, and left ventricular assist device (LVAD) if acute heart failure or if cardiogenic shock persists despite medical therapy.
- Cardiac transplantation in patients with chronic or acute fulminant myocarditis with intractable cardiomyopathy and persistent CHF.
- Corticosteroid use is contraindicated in early infectious myocarditis; it may be justified in only selected patients with intractable CHF, severe systemic toxicity, and severe life-threatening arrhythmias.
- Immunosuppressive drugs (prednisone with cyclosporine/Cytoxan or azathioprine) do not have any significant effect on the prognosis of myocarditis and should not be used in the routine treatment of patients with myocarditis. Immunosuppression may have a role in the treatment of myocarditis from systemic autoimmune disease (e.g., lupus, scleroderma); in idiopathic giant cell myocarditis, sarcoidosis, or myocarditis caused by hypersensitivity reactions; or in severe hemodynamic compromise.
- Observational data suggest that patients with giant cell myocarditis treated with certain immunosuppressive regimes have improved survival compared with patients who do not receive immunosuppressive treatment.
- In patients with ongoing viral genomic expression, preliminary data suggest that treatment with interferons may improve both symptoms and left ventricular function when compared with standard heart failure therapy.
- IV immunoglobulins have been studied, but because of lack of efficacy data, at present there is no indication for their use except in some pediatric cases or those refractory to immunosuppressive therapy.
- Improved cardiac function and arrhythmias have been reported in patients with celiac disease and myocarditis or DCM following a gluten-free diet with or without immunosuppressive therapy, but controlled data are lacking.
- A treatment algorithm for patients with myocarditis is described in Fig. E2.

DISPOSITION

- The natural history of myocarditis is illustrated in Fig. E3. Most patients with acute myocarditis and mild cardiac involvement have a partial or a full clinical recovery. In some cases, however, the process may continue subclinically with eventual progression to a cardiomyopathy. Therefore all patients with myocarditis should be followed up at least initially at intervals of 1 to 3 mo, depending on their initial severity of illness. Of those with advanced cardiac dysfunction, one third will have residual cardiac dysfunction, and 25% may progress to cardiac transplantation or death.
- Prognosis is best for patients with fulminant lymphocytic myocarditis (severe hemodynamic compromise, rapid onset of symptoms, or high fever). These patients tend to have complete recovery with total resolution of myocarditis on repeat biopsy.
- In contrast, patients with giant cell myocarditis have an extremely poor prognosis with a median survival of <6 mo, and most require cardiac transplantation.
- The American Heart Association recommends 3 to 6 mo abstinence from competitive sports after myocarditis.

REFERRAL

Consider heart transplant if intractable CHF develops.

RELATED CONTENT

Myocarditis (Patient Information)

SUGGESTED READINGS

Available at ExpertConsult.com

AUTHORS: **Vrinda Trivedi, MBBS,** and **Aravind Rao Kokkirala, MD, FACC**

BASIC INFORMATION

DEFINITION

Narcolepsy is a chronic neurologic sleep disorder characterized by excessive daytime sleepiness and dysregulation of rapid eye movement (REM) sleep. It is the second most common cause of disabling daytime sleepiness after obstructive sleep apnea. Symptoms of REM sleep dysregulation include cataplexy, sleep paralysis, and hallucinations during transition between wake and sleep. Difficulty sleeping with either frequent awakenings or disrupted sleep may also occur. An international classification of sleep disorders is summarized in Table 1.

SYNONYMS

Hypersomnia of central origin
Narcolepsy with cataplexy
Narcolepsy-cataplexy syndrome
Narcolepsy with hypocretin deficiency
Gélineau syndrome

ICD-10CM CODES
G47.411 Narcolepsy with cataplexy
G47.419 Narcolepsy without cataplexy

EPIDEMIOLOGY & DEMOGRAPHICS

INCIDENCE: 0.74/100,000 persons/yr
PREVALENCE: 1 in 2000 people
PREDOMINANT SEX: Males and females equally affected
AGE OF ONSET: Peak 15 to 30 yr (range, 10 to 55 yr)
RISK FACTORS: Anesthesia, head injury, history of meningitis or encephalitis, family history of narcolepsy, tumor, vascular malformations, stroke, and obesity
GENETICS:
- Associated with human leukocyte antigen (HLA) subtypes, specifically, *DQB1*0602,* which is present in 95% of patients with cataplexy and 96% of patients with hypocretin deficiency.
- Risk of narcolepsy increases 20 to 40 times if a family member is affected.
- Monozygotic twin concordance rate is 17% to 36%, thus indicating an incomplete penetrance and suggesting an environmental factor in the disease process.

PHYSICAL FINDINGS & CLINICAL PRESENTATION

- Overwhelming urge to sleep with chronic hypersomnia may occur during the day.
- Cataplexy occurs in 60% to 100% of patients with narcolepsy and is reported as a partial or complete loss of voluntary muscle control with preserved consciousness that is precipitated by a strong emotion, more commonly with laughter. This is the most specific symptom and is considered pathognomonic for narcolepsy.
- Hypnagogic (wake to sleep) or hypnopompic (sleep to wake) hallucinations have been reported in 60% to 80% of patients with narcolepsy.
- Sleep paralysis, defined as loss of muscle tone during the transition between sleep and wakefulness, occurs in 60% to 80% of patients with narcolepsy. It may occur with hallucinations and can be interrupted by sensory stimuli.
- Only about one third of patients will have all four symptoms of narcolepsy: Chronic daytime sleepiness, cataplexy, hypnagogic hallucinations, and sleep paralysis.
- Fragmented sleep is seen in 60% to 80% of narcolepsy patients and can often be mistaken for insomnia or other intrinsic sleep disorder.
- Other symptoms that have been reported in narcolepsy include automatic behavior or semipurposeful movements in 40% of patients and memory disturbance in 50% of patients.

ETIOLOGY

The loss of hypocretin/orexin signaling, genetic factors, and brain lesions are presently identified factors in the development of narcolepsy. May be a manifestation of neuromyelitis optica spectrum disorder.
HYPOCRETIN/OREXIN:
- Loss of hypocretin-1 and hypocretin-2 (also known as orexin-A and orexin-B) producing neurons in the lateral hypothalamus.
- Human cerebrospinal fluid (CSF) levels of hypocretin-1 are low to undetectable in narcoleptics with cataplexy.
- Narcolepsy without cataplexy may have a different cause because CSF hypocretin levels are usually normal in these patients, so there may be a completely separate mechanism in these patients, or it may result from less extensive loss of hypocretin neurons or impaired signaling.

SECONDARY ETIOLOGIES:
- Central nervous system lesions including tumors, vascular malformations, and strokes have all been reported to cause secondary narcolepsy.
- Direct injury to the hypocretin neurons or their projections is the most likely cause of secondary narcolepsy due to central nervous system lesions.
- Narcolepsy has been reported in genetic syndromes, including Prader-Willi syndrome and Niemann-Pick disease type C, as well as neuromyelitis optica spectrum disorder and paraneoplastic syndromes.

TABLE 1 International Classification of Sleep Disorders: Definitions and Pathophysiology

Condition	Diagnostic Criteria*	Pathophysiology
Type 1 narcolepsy	Presence of two or more of the following: Cataplexy, positive MSLT, and low CSF hypocretin-1	Hypocretin deficiency 98% HLA-DQB1*06:02
Type 2 narcolepsy	Positive MSLT; most often with no or unclear cataplexy	Unknown, heterogenous ~16% Hypocretin deficiency ~40% HLA-DQB1*0602
Secondary narcolepsy	As above, but due to neurologic conditions	With or without hypocretin deficiency, various disorders
Idiopathic hypersomnia	No cataplexy, no SOREMPs during the MSLT	Unknown, likely heterogeneous

CSF, Cerebrospinal fluid; *HLA,* human leukocyte antigen; *REM,* rapid eye movement.
*Abnormal Multiple Sleep Latency Test (MSLT): Sleep latency ≤8 min, ≥2 sleep-onset REM periods (SOREMPs), including a nocturnal SOREMP. For details, see *International Classification of Sleep Disorders,* third edition. (American Academy of Sleep Medicine: *International classification of sleep disorders,* ed 3, Darien, IL, 2014, American Academy of Sleep Medicine.)
From Kryger M et al: *Principles and practice of sleep medicine,* ed 6, Philadelphia, 2017, Elsevier.

DIAGNOSIS

DIFFERENTIAL DIAGNOSIS

Excessive daytime somnolence:
- Autism
- Autosomal dominant cerebellar ataxia, deafness, and narcolepsy
- Behaviorally induced insufficient sleep syndrome
- Central or obstructive sleep apnea (sleep-disordered breathing)
- Circadian rhythm disorder
- Depression
- Diencephalic lesions
- Drug or alcohol abuse
- Hypothyroidism
- Idiopathic hypersomnia with long or short sleep time
- Inadequate sleep hygiene
- Insufficient sleep
- Increased intracranial pressure

Insomnia:
- Kleine-Levin syndrome
- Medication effect
- Menstrual-related hypersomnia
- Posttraumatic narcolepsy
- Seizures
- Sleep fragmentation (multiple causes)

Cataplexy:
- Seizures
- Periodic paralysis
- Cardiovascular insufficiency
- Psychogenic (multiple causes)
- Lesions of the hypothalamus or brain stem

WORKUP

- Because persistent sleepiness can occur with many conditions, it is important to rule out other sleep disorders.
- Narcolepsy is often diagnosed by clinical history. The Epworth Sleepiness Scale is very useful in determining the degree of excessive daytime sleepiness (Table 2).

- The diagnosis of narcolepsy can be made without the need for further testing if there is a clear history of cataplexy in the setting of excessive daytime somnolence. Sleep laboratory testing is otherwise necessary if cataplexy does not exist, if a diagnosis needs to be confirmed, or if concerns exist for another sleep disorder.
- The medical history should include questions regarding severity of daytime hypersomnia while also evaluating for sleep-disordered breathing, transient muscle weakness triggered by emotion, hallucinations while falling asleep or upon awakening, and inability to move after awakening. The clinical evaluation should also address symptoms of seizures and paraneoplastic disorders while also asking about previous stroke or genetic disorders. A detailed family history is imperative. Hypothalamic dysfunction such as unexplained weight gain, endocrine abnormalities, circadian dysrhythmias, and autonomic nervous system problems may provide useful insight.
- A thorough examination including a detailed neurologic examination should be performed.
- Nocturnal polysomnography followed by a multiple sleep latency test (MSLT) remains the gold standard for the diagnosis of narcolepsy. A drug screen should also be performed to rule out pharmacologic modulations of sleep.

LABORATORY TESTS

None

Rx TREATMENT

Narcolepsy can be treated with a combination of behavioral and pharmacologic approaches. Examples of initial treatment packages for adults are summarized in Table 3.

NONPHARMACOLOGIC THERAPY

Avoidance of over-the-counter drugs and illicit drugs, optimal sleep hygiene and scheduled daily naps, and psychosocial support can be used for symptoms of excessive daytime somnolence. However, nonpharmacologic therapy is typically not sufficient for treatment of narcolepsy alone but is often used as adjunct therapy with medications.

PHARMACOLOGIC THERAPY (TABLE 4)

For excessive daytime somnolence:

- Sodium oxybate: A central nervous system depressant that can be used for the treatment of cataplexy and REM-related symptoms
- Modafinil 200 to 600 mg PO every morning or divided bid
- Armodafinil 150 or 250 mg PO as a single dose in the morning
- Methylphenidate 5 to 15 mg PO bid to tid
- Methylphenidate SR 18 to 54 mg PO every morning or divided bid
- Dextroamphetamine 10 to 60 mg PO qd
- Eldepryl 5 mg PO bid

TABLE 2 Epworth Sleepiness Scale

How likely are you to doze off or fall asleep in the following situations, in contrast to just feeling tired? This refers to your usual way of life in recent time. Even if you have not done some of these things recently, try to work out how they would have affected you. Use the following scale to choose the most appropriate number for each situation.

0 = Would never doze
1 = Slight chance of dozing
2 = Moderate chance of dozing
3 = High chance of dozing

Situation	Chance of Dozing
Sitting and reading	
Watching TV	
Sitting and inactive in a public place (theater or meeting)	
As a passenger in a car for an hour without a break	
Lying down to rest in the afternoon when circumstances permit	
Sitting and talking to someone	
Sitting quietly after lunch (without alcohol)	
In a car, while stopped for a few minutes in traffic	
Total	

From Johns MW: A new method for measuring daytime sleepiness: the Epworth Sleepiness Scale, *Sleep* 14:540-545, 1991.

TABLE 3 Examples of Initial Treatment Packages for Adults

General Measures

Avoid shifts in sleep schedule
Avoid heavy meals and alcohol intake
Regular timing of nocturnal sleep: 10:30 P.M. to 7 A.M.
Naps: Strategically timed naps if possible (e.g., 15 min at lunchtime, 15 min at 5:30 P.M.)

Medications for Sleepiness

The effects of stimulant medications vary widely among patients. The dosing and timing of medications should be individualized to optimize performance. Additional doses, as needed, may be suggested for periods of anticipated sleepiness.

Modafinil* 100-200 mg (taken when waking up in the morning) and 100-200 mg at lunchtime *or* sodium oxybate† at bedtime: Dosage must start low at 2.25 g taken twice while in bed (at bedtime and 2.5-4 hr after bedtime); increase to total dosage of 5-6 g within 2-4 wk. This initial dose is usually ineffective, so increase to 3 g at bedtime and 3 g approximately 2.5-4 hr after bedtime if tolerated. Depending on response, dosage can be increased to as high as 9 g total nightly dose. Do not increase above 9 g because of risk of serious side effects during sleep. It may take more than 2 mo for daytime symptoms to improve, and cataplexy ma improve faster than excessive daytime sleepiness. If the patient is already taking a daytime stimulant, it may be possible to reduce the stimulant dose or to discontinue it once a therapeutic dosage of sodium oxybate has been reached.

Methylphenidate 5 mg (three or four tablets; 10 mg when waking up; 5 mg 30 min before lunch; 5 mg near 3 P.M.; better action is always obtained if the drug is taken on an empty stomach) or 20 mg SR in the morning (on an empty stomach)

If Persistent Difficulties

Modafinil 200 mg in the morning and 200 mg at lunch (total daily dosage, 400 mg) *or* add sodium oxybate (GHB) at bedtime: Dosage must start low as indicated above.

Methylphenidate (SR): 20 mg in the morning; 5 mg after noon nap; 5 mg at 4 P.M. *or* Possibly (more in teenagers) atomoxetine: Start at 0.5 mg/kg within 1 wk to appropriate dosage of 1-1.2 mg/kg taken in the morning

If No Response

Dextroamphetamine sulfate: 15 mg on awakening; 5 mg after noon nap; 5 mg at 3:30 or 4 P.M. (or 15 mg at awakening and 15 mg after noon nap)

Medications for Cataplexy‡

Sodium oxybate (see above)
Venlafaxine 150-300 mg
Fluoxetine 20-60 mg
Duloxetine 60 mg

If No Response

Clomipramine 75-125 mg, *or* Viloxazine 150-200 mg, *or* Imipramine 75-125 mg

SR, Sustained-release tablet.
*Modafinil works best in naive subjects. It should be the drug of first choice in children and adults.
†Response to sodium oxybate is slow.
‡Medications may be taken in the evening near bedtime (sodium oxybate, clomipramine, imipramine), only in the morning (fluoxetine), or in the morning and at lunchtime (viloxazine, venlafaxine). The only medications specifically approved for use in narcolepsy by the Food and Drug Administration are modafinil and sodium oxybate.
From Kryger M et al: *Principles and practice of sleep medicine,* ed 6, Philadelphia, 2017, Elsevier.

TABLE 4 Narcolepsy Drugs Currently Available

Drug	Usual Dosage* (All Drugs Administered Orally)
Treatment of EDS	
Stimulants†	
Modafinil	100-400 mg/day
Sodium oxybate	6-9 g/day (divided in two doses)
Methylphenidate	10-60 mg/day
Atomoxetine	10-25 mg/day
Dextroamphetamine	5-60 mg/day
Methamphetamine	20-25 mg/day
Treatment of Auxiliary Effects (e.g., Cataplexy)	
Sodium oxybate (gamma-hydroxybutyrate)	6-9 g/day (divided in two doses)
Antidepressants	
Without Atropinic Side Effects	
Venlafaxine XR	75-300 mg/day
Fluoxetine	20-60 mg/day
Viloxazine	50-200 mg/day
Duloxetine	60 mg/day
With Atropinic Side Effects	
Protriptyline	2.5-20 mg/day
Imipramine	25-200 mg/day
Clomipramine	25-200 mg/day
Desipramine	25-200 mg/day

EDS, Excessive daytime somnolence.
*On occasion, depending on clinical response, the dose may be outside the usual dosage range.
†Most stimulants should be administered in divided doses, commonly in the morning and at lunchtime. This is recommended for amphetamines and modafinil. Methylphenidate has a fast elimination rate, so the slow-release (SR) formula may be helpful in the morning (e.g., 20 mg SR). If it is administered by 5-mg increments, the usual timing of methylphenidate administration is every 3 to 4 hr until 3 P.M.
From Kryger M et al: *Principles and practice of sleep medicine,* ed 6, Philadelphia, 2017, Elsevier.

- Pitolisant: Initial does is 8.9 mg (two 4.45 mg tablets) taken once daily upon waking. It is the first FDA approved histamine-3 (H3) receptor antagonist/inverse agonist for narcolepsy. It is a noncontrolled substance for narcolepsy

For cataplexy:

- Sodium oxybate: A central nervous system depressant that can be used for the treatment of cataplexy and rapid eye movement (REM) related symptoms
- Fluoxetine 20 mg PO qd initially
- Sertraline 25 mg PO qd initially
- Venlafaxine 25 mg PO qd initially
- Clomipramine 25 mg/day initially
- Protriptyline 5 mg tid initially
- Imipramine 25 to 50 mg/day initially
- Desipramine 10 mg bid initially

DISPOSITION

This is a chronic sleep disorder that may worsen for the first few years and then persist for life.

REFERRAL

Because of the complexity of this disorder and its ever-changing management and treatment, patients should be referred to centers or programs with highly trained sleep specialists with expertise caring for these patients, especially if sodium oxybate (Xyrem) therapy is needed.

PEARLS & CONSIDERATIONS

Many narcoleptics report the onset of symptoms beginning in childhood to early adulthood, with a long delay of actual diagnosis on the order of 10 to 15 yr. Typically, excessive daytime sleepiness is the initial symptom, followed by REM dysregulation (e.g., cataplexy, sleep paralysis, hypnagogic hallucinations). Patients with narcolepsy also have higher than expected incidence of other sleep disorders, including obstructive sleep apnea, periodic limb movements of sleep, and REM sleep behavior disorder.

COMMENTS

Narcolepsy is a rare disorder that is underdiagnosed. The average time from onset of symptoms to diagnosis is 5 to 15 yr. Cataplexy is specific for narcolepsy, but other symptoms of REM dysregulation, including sleep paralysis and hypnagogic or hypnopompic hallucinations, can occur even in normal patients. Sleep-onset REM or REM periods on an MSLT may occur as a result of sleep deprivation or withdrawal from REM-suppressing drugs.

SUGGESTED READINGS

Available at ExpertConsult.com

RELATED CONTENT

Narcolepsy (Patient Information)

AUTHOR: **Don Hayes Jr, MD, MS, MEd**

BASIC INFORMATION

DEFINITION

Nasopharyngeal carcinoma (NPC) is an epithelial carcinoma originating in the nasopharynx that is clinically distinct from other head and neck carcinomas.

SYNONYM

Nasopharynx cancer

ICD-10CM CODE

C11.9 Malignant neoplasm of nasopharynx, unspecified

EPIDEMIOLOGY & DEMOGRAPHICS

- NPC is an uncommon cancer that is endemic to east and southeast Asia (70% of cases). The worldwide incidence and deaths were estimated at 129,079 and 72,987, respectively, in 2018. Incidence is decreasing steadily in the endemic regions in Asia.
- Incidence rate of 3 per 100,000 population in China and 0.4 per 100,000 in Caucasian population.
- Incidence is higher in males (2.5 times than females).

RISK FACTORS:

- Epstein-Barr virus (EBV) infection
- Tobacco smoking
- Alcohol consumption
- Family history
- Consumption of preserved foods
- Poor oral hygiene

GENETICS:

- HLA genes residing at the MHC region on chromosome 6p21 have been widely recognized as major risk loci conferring nasopharyngeal carcinoma risk.
- Genomic changes involved in the development of NPC include: Multiple loss-of-function mutations in the NFkB–negative regulators, recurrent genetic lesions such as loss of the *CDKN2A/CDKN2B* locus, *CCND1* amplification, *TP53* mutation, and mutations in the PI3K/MAPK signaling pathways.

ETIOLOGY

- Pathological subtypes of squamous NPC are: Keratinizing, nonkeratinizing, and basaloid type. The keratinizing subtype accounts for less than 20% of cases worldwide and is seen in nonendemic areas. The nonkeratinizing subtype constitutes most cases in endemic areas (>95%) and is predominantly associated with Epstein-Barr virus (EBV) infection.
- Persistent EBV infection in genetically mutated epithelial cells and the proliferation of infected cells lead to tumorigenic transformation. Chronic exposure of the nasopharyngeal mucosa to environmental carcinogens increases DNA damage and leads to somatic genetic changes in the nasopharyngeal epithelial cells. EBV infection in turn facilitates inactivation of a variety of cancer-related genes. During tumor development, acquired mutations of regulatory factors in the NF-κB signaling pathway alter the activity of additional cancer-related genes. Mutations in the MHC class I genes, PI3K/MAPK pathways as well as somatic mutations of *TP53* and *RAS* genes may be at play in the development of tumor recurrence and metastasis.

CLINICAL PRESENTATION

- Chronically blocked or stuffy nose
- Recurrent epistaxis and bloody rhinorrhea
- Hearing impairment and tinnitus
- Headache
- Ear pain
- Palpable neck adenopathy
- Cranial nerve palsies

Dx DIAGNOSIS

DIFFERENTIAL DIAGNOSIS

- Nasal polyps
- Nasopharyngeal lymphoma
- Nasopharyngeal sarcoma

WORKUP

- Direct nasopharyngoscopy by ENT physician followed by biopsy (Fig. E1) and imaging studies (Figs. E2 and E3)

LABORATORY TESTS

- Complete blood count
- Comprehensive chemistry panel
- Circulating cell-free EBV DNA is a biomarker for nasopharyngeal carcinoma. Pretreatment plasma EBV-DNA levels may add to the prognostic value of conventional TNM staging systems (Table 1)

IMAGING STUDIES

- CT or MRI of the head and neck; MRI is better than CT for soft-tissue extent assessment and retropharyngeal nodal detection
- PET/CT is used to assess for detection of distant metastasis and for detection of residual cancer after completion of therapy

Rx TREATMENT

The mainstay of therapy is concurrent chemotherapy and radiation therapy. Both adjuvant chemotherapy and to a lesser extent neoadjuvant chemotherapy are routinely utilized after and before chemoradiotherapy in the clinical setting.

NONPHARMACOLOGIC THERAPY

- Surgery is utilized for diagnostic biopsies and for neck dissection in the setting of residual neck lymphadenopathy after completion of definitive chemoradiotherapy.
- Supportive care with gastrostomy tube nutrition is often required to maintain nutritional and hydration status during treatment.

ACUTE GENERAL Rx

- Intensity modulated radiotherapy (IMRT) with concurrent every 3-wk cycles of cisplatin and 5-fluorouracil chemotherapy over a period of 6 to 7 wk is a standard approach in patients with locoregionally advanced NPC. Adjuvant chemotherapy with cisplatin and gemcitabine is routinely administered with benefits seen in reduction of distant metastases and improvement in overall survival.
- Neoadjuvant (induction) chemotherapy with the a multiagent chemotherapy regimen prior to definitive chemoradiotherapy has been shown to improve survival but with increased hematologic and gastrointestinal toxicity in a recent meta-analysis of seven randomized controlled trials involving 2311 patients.
- Besides systemic chemotherapy and anti–epidermal growth factor receptor inhibitor (EGFR) approaches, the use of immune checkpoint inhibitors (pembrolizumab, nivolumab, camrelizumab) has demonstrated significant antitumor efficacy in patients with recurrent or metastatic disease.
- Significant supportive care with nutrition, hydration, and mucositis management (especially pain control) is required.
- Post-therapy rehabilitation with swallowing therapy, dental care, endocrinology care, and lymphedema care are often required.

DISPOSITION

Patients with early stage disease typically have a good outcome (5-yr survival is 60% to 75%), whereas patients with stage IV disease have a poor outcome (5-yr survival is <40%).

REFERRAL

Diagnosis is usually confirmed by biopsy performed by otorhinolaryngology physician. Referrals include to medical oncology, radiation oncology, dietitian, and gastroenterology.

PEARLS & CONSIDERATIONS

- Analysis of EBV DNA in plasma samples has been found to be useful in screening for early asymptomatic cases. NPC was detected significantly earlier and outcomes were better in participants who were identified by screening compared to those in a historical cohort.
- Higher pre-treatment, mid-treatment, and post-treatment EBV DNA levels have been significantly correlated with poor outcomes for patients afflicted with NPC.

SUGGESTED READINGS

Available at ExpertConsult.com

RELATED CONTENT

Head and Neck Squamous Cell Carcinoma (Related Key Topic)

AUTHOR: **Ritesh Rathore, MD**

TABLE 1 Current TNM Staging Systems for Nasopharyngeal Carcinoma

Carcinoma: Comparison of the Seventh and Eighth Editions of the UICC/AJCC Staging System for Nasopharyngeal Carcinoma		
	Seventh Edition	**Eighth Edition**
Primary tumor (T)		
T_X	Primary tumor cannot be assessed	Primary tumor cannot be assessed
T_0		No tumor identified, but there is EBV-positive cervical node(s) involvement
T_1	Nasopharynx, oropharynx, or nasal cavity without parapharyngeal extension	Nasopharynx, oropharynx, or nasal cavity without parapharyngeal extension
T_2	Parapharyngeal extension	Parapharyngeal extension, adjacent soft tissue involvement (medial pterygoid, lateral pterygoid, prevertebral muscles)
T_3	Bony structures of skull base and/or paranasal sinuses	Bony structures (skull base, cervical vertebra) and/or paranasal sinuses
T_4	Intracranial, cranial nerves, hypopharynx, orbit, infratemporal fossa or masticator space	Intracranial extension, cranial nerve, hypopharynx, orbit, extensive soft tissue involvement (beyond the lateral surface of the lateral pterygoid muscle, parotid gland)
Regional lymph nodes (N)		
N_X	Regional lymph nodes cannot be assessed	Regional lymph nodes cannot be assessed
N_0	No regional lymph node metastasis	No regional lymph node metastasis
N_1	Unilateral cervical, unilateral, or bilateral retropharyngeal lymph nodes, above the supraclavicular fossa; ≤6 cm	Unilateral cervical, unilateral, or bilateral retropharyngeal lymph nodes, above the caudal border of cricoid cartilage; ≤6 cm
N_2	Bilateral metastasis in lymph node(s), ≤6 cm in greatest dimension, above the supraclavicular fossa	Bilateral metastasis in lymph node(s), ≤6 cm in greatest dimension, above the caudal border of cricoid cartilage
N_{3a}	>6 cm in dimension	>6 cm and/or below caudal border of cricoid cartilage (regardless of laterality)
N_{3b}	Supraclavicular fossa	
Distant metastasis (M)		
M_0	No distant metastasis	No distant metastasis
M_1	Distant metastasis	Distant metastasis
Stage group		
I	T_1 N_0 M_0	T_1 N_0 M_0
II	T_2 N_{0-1} M_0, T_1 N_1 M_0,	T_2 N_{0-1} M_0, T_{0-1} N_1 M_0
III	T_{1-3} N_2 M_0, T3 N_{0-1} M_0	T_3 N_{0-2} M_0, T_{0-2} N_2 M_0
IVA	T_4 N_{0-2} M0	T_4 or N_3 M_0
IVB	Any T, N_3 M_0	Any T, any N, M_1
IVC	Any T, any N, M_1	

EBV, Epstein-Barr virus; *UICC/AJCC,* International Union Against Cancer/American Joint Committee on Cancer. T category: T_0 is added for EBV-positive cervical node(s) involvement despite unidentified primary tumor. Involvement of medial pterygoid, lateral pterygoid, and prevertebral muscles is now staged as T_2. In T_4, the original "infratemporal fossa or masticator space" has been replaced by specific description of soft tissue involvement to avoid potential ambiguity. N category: The previous N_{3b} criterion of "supraclavicular fossa" has been changed to "below caudal border of cricoid cartilage." N_{3a} and N_{3b} have been merged into a single N_3. Stage group: The previous stages IVA and IVB have been merged into IVA. The previous IVC has been upstaged to IVB.
From Chen YP et al: Nasopharyngeal carcinoma, *Lancet* 394(10192):64-80, 2019.

BASIC INFORMATION

DEFINITION

Necrotizing fasciitis (NF) is a rapidly spreading bacterial infection of the deep fascia, with associated inflammation, leading to necrosis of subcutaneous tissue planes. This infection can occur in wounds from trauma or surgical wounds or can be spontaneous or idiopathic. There are two clinical types, both of which carry a high rate of morbidity and mortality.

SYNONYMS

NF
Soft tissue gangrene
Flesh-eating bacteria
Fournier gangrene
Hemolytic streptococcal gangrene

ICD-10CM CODE
M72.6 Necrotizing fasciitis

EPIDEMIOLOGY & DEMOGRAPHICS

INCIDENCE: Invasive group A *Streptococcus* infection occurs at a rate of 3.5 cases per 100,000 persons, with a case fatality rate of around 24%.

PREDOMINANT SEX: Male > female

PREDOMINANT AGE: 6 to 50 yr; less common in children

PHYSICAL FINDINGS & CLINICAL PRESENTATION

CLINICAL TYPES OF NECROTIZING FASCIITIS:

- Type I: Necrotizing fasciitis: At least one anaerobic species is isolated in conjunction with one or more facultative anaerobic species, such as streptococci (not group A), *and* members of the *Enterobacteriaceae* (gram-negative rods)
- Anaerobic bacteria, most commonly *Bacteroides* or *Peptostreptococcus* spp.
- *Enterobacteriaceae: Escherichia coli, Klebsiella* spp., *Proteus* spp., *Enterobacter* spp.
- Usually associated with diabetes or peripheral vascular disease
- Example of type I: Fournier gangrene of the perineum
- Type II: Necrotizing fasciitis: Group A *Streptococcus* is isolated alone or in combination with other bacteria, most likely *Staphylococcus aureus.* Also known as hemolytic streptococcal gangrene
  1. Example of type II: Invasive group A *Streptococcus*, associated with virulence factors type 1 and type 3 M protein

EXAMPLES OF NECROTIZING FASCIITIS:

- Fournier gangrene: Aggressive type I infection of the perineum usually caused by penetration of the gastrointestinal or urethral mucosa by enteric organisms. It can rapidly spread to involve the scrotum, penis, and abdominal wall or gluteal muscles, causing gangrene. Use of sodium-glucose cotransporter-2 (SGLT2) inhibitors in diabetics has been associated with Fournier gangrene.
- Clostridial cellulitis: Caused by *Clostridium perfringens* associated with local trauma or surgery and crepitus caused by gas production; generally noted in the skin, with deeper tissues generally spared.

PHYSICAL FINDINGS

Minor skin trauma, toxic-appearing patient:

- Open skin wound
- Severe pain at injury or surgical site
- Fever, confusion, weakness, diarrhea
- Early skin erythema, quickly spreading in hours to days
- Skin redness changes to purple discoloration
- Gangrenous skin changes may develop
- Loosening of skin and subcutaneous skin in association with deep fascial necrosis (Fig. E1). "Woody" induration and crepitus of involved area are characteristics
- Muscle involvement, thrombosis of blood vessels, and myonecrosis may develop
- Bullae and gas formation at site

ETIOLOGY

- NF usually arises from skin damage or trauma. Risk is increased with presence of comorbidities (diabetes mellitus, cancer, liver disease, immunosuppression, use of SGLT2 inhibitors)
- Polymicrobial: Mixture of anaerobes and aerobic enteric gram-negative rods
- Group A streptococci *(S. pyogenes)*
- *S. aureus*
- *C. perfringens*
- *Bacteroides fragilis*
- *Vibrio vulnificus*
- Methicillin-resistant *S. aureus* (MRSA), especially community-acquired MRSA

DIAGNOSIS

DIFFERENTIAL DIAGNOSIS

- Cellulitis
- Pyomyositis
- Gas gangrene
- A classification of necrotizing skin, soft-tissue, and muscle infections is described in Table 1

WORKUP

- Diagnosis of necrotizing fasciitis generally requires incision and probing. In patients with necrotizing fasciitis, there is no resistance to probing subcutaneously, and there is fascial plane involvement. Fig. 2 is an algorithm for assessment and treatment of suspected necrotizing fasciitis.
- Laboratory tests:
  1. The laboratory risk indicator for necrotizing fasciitis (LRINEC) consists of the following six variables (Table 2). When present, the reported positive predictive value is 92%: Complete blood cell count (CBC) with differential (leukocytosis [white blood count >15,000], anemia [Hb <13.5]), elevated C-reactive protein (≥15 mg/dl), hyponatremia (sodium <135 mEq/L), elevated creatinine (>1.6 mg/dl), hyperglycemia (glucose >180 mg/dl).
  2. Cultures of skin, soft tissue, or debrided tissue, aerobically and anaerobically. Blood cultures are positive in 60% of patients with type II infections and 20% with type I infections.
- Imaging:
  1. Radiographs may show subcutaneous gas in fascial planes (Fig. 3).
  2. Computed tomography (CT) or magnetic resonance imaging (MRI) may be helpful because they can detect gas in the tissues. MRI with contrast is more sensitive than CT.

TREATMENT

- Aggressive surgical debridement of involved necrotic tissues is essential *as soon as possible* to reduce mortality.
- Fasciotomies of extremities may be necessary.
- Immediate start of empiric antibiotics:
  1. Type I: Vancomycin, daptomycin, or linezolid plus piperacillin/tazobactam; a carbapenem (such as imipenem, meropenem, or doripenem); and third-generation cephalosporin + metronidazole or a fluoroquinolone plus metronidazole (ceftriaxone) are reasonable choices pending cultures. Empiric clindamycin may also be added to suppress toxin production by staphylococci and streptococci. It is important to always have anaerobic coverage. Use the highest dosages possible for age and CrCl.
  2. Type II: For group A *Streptococcus*, give intravenous (IV) penicillin G, 4 million U q4h in patients who weigh >60 kg with clindamycin, 600 to 900 mg IV q8h.
     a. Clindamycin has the added effect of suppressing toxin production. If MRSA is suspected, add vancomycin, daptomycin, or linezolid.
- Intravenous gammaglobulin (IVIG): 1 g/kg on day 1 and 0.5 g/kg on days 2 and 3 neutralizes circulating streptococcal toxins and has been shown beneficial in severe forms of invasive group A streptococcal infections, although data are not definitive.
- For *Vibrio vulnificus* use doxycycline plus ceftazidime; for *Aeromonas hydrophila* use doxycycline plus ciprofloxacin.
- Hyperbaric oxygen evaluation as an adjunct to surgery and IV antibiotics.

SUGGESTED READINGS

Available at ExpertConsult.com

AUTHOR: **Glenn G. Fort, MD, MPH**

TABLE 1 Classification of Necrotizing Skin, Soft-Tissue, and Muscle Infections

Disease	Bacteriology	Comments
Necrotizing Cellulitis		
Clostridial cellulitis	*Clostridium perfringens*	Local trauma, recent surgery; fascial/deep muscle spared
Nonclostridial cellulitis	Mixed: *Escherichia coli, Enterobacter, Peptostreptococcus* spp., *Bacteroides fragilis*	Diabetes mellitus predisposes; produces foul odor
Meleney synergistic gangrene	*Staphylococcus aureus,* microaerophilic streptococci	Rare infection; postoperative; slowly expanding, indolent, ulceration in superficial fascia
Synergistic necrotizing cellulitis	Mixed aerobic and anaerobic, including *B. fragilis, Peptostreptococcus* spp.	Diabetes mellitus predisposes; variant of necrotizing fasciitis type I; involves skin, muscle, fat, and fascia
Necrotizing Fasciitis		
Type I	Mixed aerobic and anaerobic; staphylococci, *B. fragilis, E. coli,* group A streptococci, *Peptostreptococcus* spp., *Prevotella, Porphyromonas* spp., *Clostridium* spp.	Usually requires a breach in the mucous membrane layer either through surgery or penetrating injuries or from chronic medical conditions such as diabetes, peripheral vascular disease, malignancy, and anal fissures
Type II	Group A streptococci	Increasing in frequency and severity since 1985; very high mortality; often begins at site of nonpenetrating minor trauma such as a bruise or muscle strain but often no identified precursor Predisposing factors: Blunt/penetrating trauma, varicella (chickenpox), intravenous drug abuse, surgical procedures, childbirth, nonsteroidal antiinflammatory drug use
Myonecrosis		
Clostridial myonecrosis	*Clostridium* spp.	Predisposing factors: Deep/penetrating injury, bowel and biliary tract surgery, improperly performed abortion and retained placenta, prolonged rupture of the membranes, and intrauterine fetal demise or missed abortion in postpartum patients. Recurrent gas gangrene occurs at sites of previous gas gangrene
Streptococcal myonecrosis	Streptococci	
Special Type of Necrotizing Soft-Tissue Infection		
Fournier gangrene	Polymicrobial, with *E. coli* the predominant aerobe and *Bacteroides* the predominant anaerobe. Other microflora: *Proteus, Staphylococcus, Enterococcus,* aerobic and anaerobic *Streptococcus, Pseudomonas, Klebsiella,* and *Clostridium*	Necrosis of the scrotum or perineum that starts with scrotal pain and erythema and rapidly spreads onto anterior abdominal wall and gluteal muscle. It is more often seen in diabetics and can be associated with trauma

From Vincent JL et al: *Textbook of critical care,* ed 6, Philadelphia, 2011, Saunders.

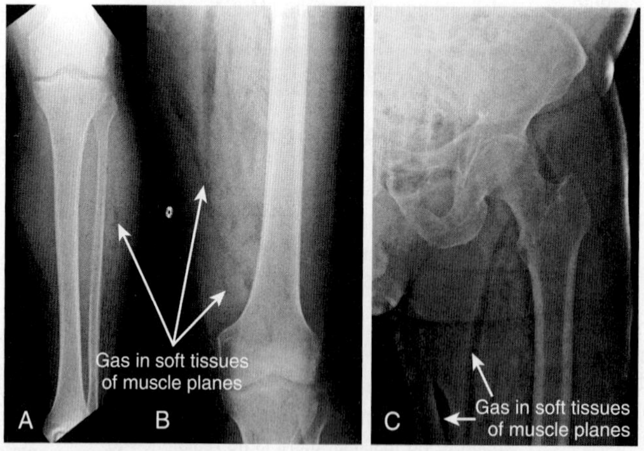

FIG. 2 Necrotizing fasciitis. This 71-yr-old man with aplastic anemia presented with fevers to 38.9° C (102.02° F), leg weakness, and extreme leg pain. Initially, the patient was thought to have neuropathic pain and weakness, possibly indicating spinal disease such as epidural abscess. He rapidly developed crepitus of his legs. Radiographs of the patient's legs were obtained, followed by noncontrast computed tomography. **A,** Anterior-posterior (AP) tibia and fibula. **B,** AP femur. **C,** AP hip. Air is seen dissecting in muscle planes of the legs. On radiograph, air appears black. Given the wide distribution of air, a focal abscess is unlikely, and necrotizing fasciitis with gas-producing organisms should be suspected. (From Broder JS: *Diagnostic imaging for the emergency physician,* Philadelphia, 2011, Saunders.)

TABLE 2 Laboratory Risk Indicator for Necrotizing Fasciitis (LRINEC)[a]

Variable	Points
CRP >150 mg/L	4
Leukocytosis	1
WBC count between 15,000 and 25,000/mm^3	2
WBC count >25,000/mm^3	
Anemia	1
Hgb between 11 and 13.5 g/dl	2
Hgb <11 g/dl	
Hyponatremia	2
Na <135 mmol/L	
Renal insufficiency	2
Cr >1.6 mg/dl	
Serum glucose >180 mg/dl	1

Cr, Creatinine; *CRP,* C-reactive protein; *Hgb,* hemoglobin; *WBC,* white blood cell.

[a]LRINEC score <6 points is considered low risk for necrotizing soft tissue infection but does not rule out the diagnosis. High clinical suspicion for necrotizing soft tissue infection warrants surgical debridement, irrespective of LRINEC score.

From Spec, A et al. *Comprehensive review of infectious diseases,* Philadelphia, 2019, Elsevier.

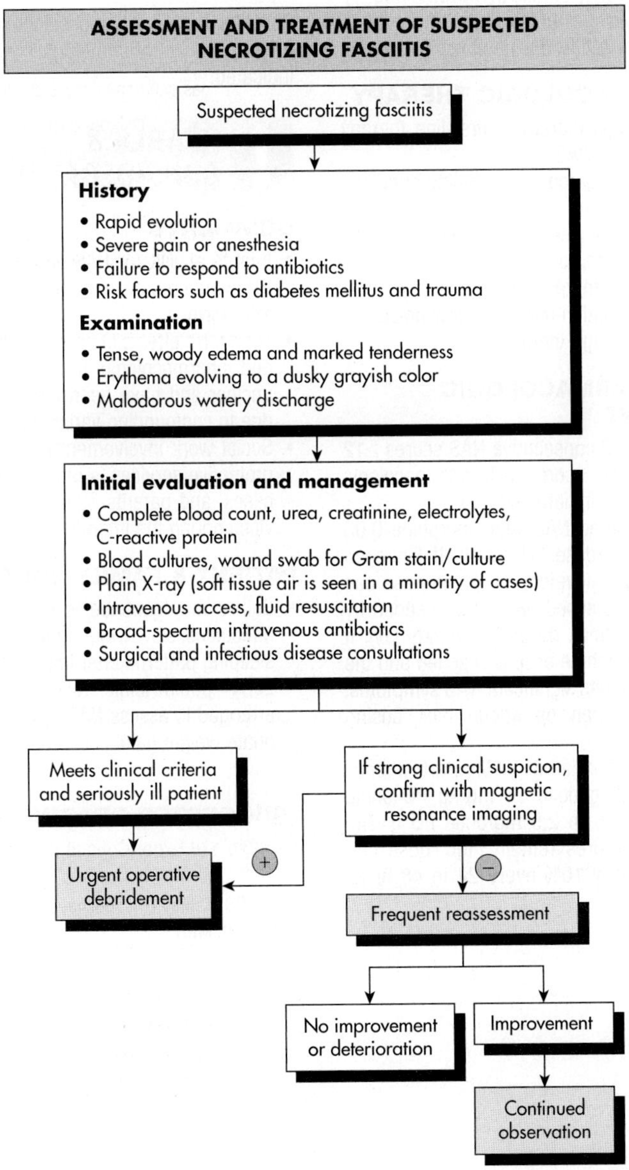

FIG. 3 Algorithm for assessment and treatment of suspected necrotizing fasciitis. (From Bolognia J: *Dermatology*, ed 4, Philadelphia, 2018, Elsevier.)

Neonatal Abstinence Syndrome (ALG)

BASIC INFORMATION

DEFINITION

Neonatal abstinence syndrome (NAS) is a postnatal withdrawal syndrome. NAS is most commonly attributed to in-utero opioid exposure, although other substances have also been associated with NAS.

SYNONYMS

NAS
Neonatal opioid withdrawal syndrome (NOWS)
NOWS

ICD-10CM CODE
P96.1 Neonatal withdrawal symptoms from maternal use of drugs of addiction

EPIDEMIOLOGY & DEMOGRAPHICS

More than 50% of newborns born to mothers with perinatal substance use will develop NAS.
INCIDENCE: The rate of NAS is 7 per 1,000 newborn hospitalizations in the U.S.
PEAK INCIDENCE: In the U.S., the incidence of NAS continues to increase.
RISK FACTORS: Most cases of NAS are associated with antenatal exposure to opioids. Antenatal cumulative drug exposure, type of opioid, tobacco use, and SSRI use may increase the risk of NAS.

PHYSICAL FINDINGS & CLINICAL PRESENTATION

- History of prenatal substance exposure
- The severity and presentation of NAS is highly variable. The main signs and symptoms of NAS are sleep and wake cycle disturbances, hyperarousal, irritability, hypertonicity, tremors, jitteriness, sweating, sneezing, yawning, feeding difficulties and loose stools.
- The timing of onset of NAS depends upon the drug's half-life and timing of most recent exposure. Symptoms usually begin within 24 to 72 hr after birth; however, symptom onset may be delayed until 5 days of age.

ETIOLOGY

- Transmission of drug(s) across placenta in utero
- Majority of cases are due to maternal opioid use
- Barbiturates, benzodiazepines, selective serotonin reuptake inhibitors (SSRIs), selective norepinephrine reuptake inhibitors (SNRIs), tricyclic antidepressants, ethanol, and less commonly, stimulants, have also been implicated in NAS.

Dx DIAGNOSIS

DIFFERENTIAL DIAGNOSIS

- Seizures
- Hypoglycemia
- Infection
- Hyperthyroidism

WORKUP

Diagnosis is clinical

LABORATORY TESTS

Neonatal urine or meconium drug testing

Rx TREATMENT

The modified Finnegan scoring system is the most common scoring tool used to monitor and assess severity of NAS symptoms (Fig. 1). Scoring should be performed after feeds every 3 to 4 hr while the newborn is awake.

NONPHARMACOLOGIC THERAPY

Nonpharmacologic therapy is first-line therapy for all infants with NAS:
- Swaddling, kangaroo care, holding/cuddling, rocking, pacifiers
- Frequent, small feedings (support breastfeeding when appropriate)
- Modify environment: Room-in with mother, minimal stimulation (dim light, low noise)
- Neonatal massage therapy

ACUTE PHARMACOLOGIC TREATMENT

If the infant has 2 consecutive NAS scores ≥12 or 3 consecutive scores ≥8, pharmacologic therapy should be initiated (Fig. 2).
- For opioid-related NAS, start morphine 0.05 to 0.08 mg/kg/dose PO q3-4h. If Finnegan scores remain elevated, morphine dose can need to be increased q8-12h as needed by 10% to 20% (max dose: 1.3 mg/kg/day). If maximum morphine dose is reached and the infant still exhibits significant NAS symptoms, phenobarbital can be added (see dosing below).
- For nonopioid related NAS, start phenobarbital (loading dose 16 mg/kg PO once, followed by 1.5 to 2.5 mg/dose PO q12h). If Finnegan scores remain high, dose can be increased by 10% every 24 to 48 hr as needed.

WEANING PHARMACOLOGIC THERAPY

Once NAS scores are <8 for 24 hr, begin to wean pharmacotherapy.
- Wean morphine dose by 10% every 12 to 24 hr. Discontinue morphine when infant tolerates morphine 0.02 mg/kg/dose for 24 to 48 hr.
- If infant is receiving morphine and phenobarbital, begin by weaning morphine as above. Once morphine dose reaches 0.3 mg/kg/day, maintain the dose and discontinue phenobarbital. If scores remain stable for 48 hr, resume morphine wean.
- If receiving phenobarbital monotherapy, wean phenobarbital dose by 20% q24h.

DISPOSITION

Neonates may be discharged to a safe home environment when scores are stable off pharmacotherapy for 24 to 48 hr.

REFERRAL

Consider future neurodevelopmental assessment and ophthalmologic evaluation as indicated.

PEARLS & CONSIDERATIONS

COMMENTS

- Infants at risk for NAS should be monitored for symptoms of withdrawal for 3 to 5 days after birth.
- Long term effects of prenatal opioid exposure and pharmacologic treatment of NAS are unclear and have been difficult to elucidate due to confounding variables.
- Social work involvement is needed, as child protective services is often involved in these cases, and parents often require social services during the infant's hospitalization.

PATIENT & FAMILY EDUCATION

- Babies may continue to have some feeding difficulties, slow weight gain, and/or irregular sleeping patterns after leaving the hospital.
- Early pediatrician follow-up should be arranged to assess NAS symptoms and adequate weight gain.

SUGGESTED READINGS

Available at ExpertConsult.com

AUTHORS: **Ashley D. Osborne, MD,** and **Melissa D. Patel, MD, MPH**

NEONATAL ABSTINENCE SCORE

Date: ____________________ **Weight:** ______

System	Signs & Symptoms	Score	Time (AM / PM)	Comments
Central Nervous System Disturbances	Excessive High Pitched Cry	2		
	Continuous High Pitched Cry	3		
	Sleeps < 1 Hour After Feeding	3		
	Sleeps < 2 Hours After Feeding	2		
	Sleeps < 3 Hours After Feeding	1		
	Hyperactive Moro Reflex	2		
	Markedly Hyperactive Moro Reflex	3		
	Mild Tremors Disturbed	1		
	Moderate - Severe Tremors Disturbed	2		
	Mild Tremors Undisturbed	3		
	Moderate - Severe Tremors Undisturbed	4		
	Increased Muscle Tone	2		
	Excoriation (Specific Area)	1		
	Myoclonic Jerks	3		
	Generalized Convulsions	5		
Metabolic / Vasomotor / Respiratory Disturbances	Sweating	1		
	Fever < 101° F (37.2° - 38.2° C)	1		
	Fever ≥ 101.1° F (≥38.4° C)	2		
	Frequent Yawning (> 3 - 4 Times/Interval)	1		
	Mottling	1		
	Nasal Stuffiness	1		
	Sneezing (> 3 - 4 Times/Interval)	1		
	Nasal Flaring	2		
	Respiratory Rate - 60/min	1		
	Respiratory Rate - 60/min with Retractions	2		
Gastrointestinal Disturbances	Excessive Sucking	1		
	Poor Feeding	2		
	Regurgitation	2		
	Projectile Vomiting	3		
	Loose Stools	2		
	Watery Stools	3		
	TOTAL SCORE			
	Initials of Scorer			

FIG. 1 Modified Finnegan Scoring System. Score used to assess severity of infant's NAS symptoms. Add scores for total at each evaluation. (Adapted from Finnegan LP, Kaltenbach K: The assessment and management of neonatal abstinence syndrome. In Hoekelman RA et al [eds.]: *Primary pediatric care*, ed 3, St Louis, 1992, Mosby, p. 1367.)

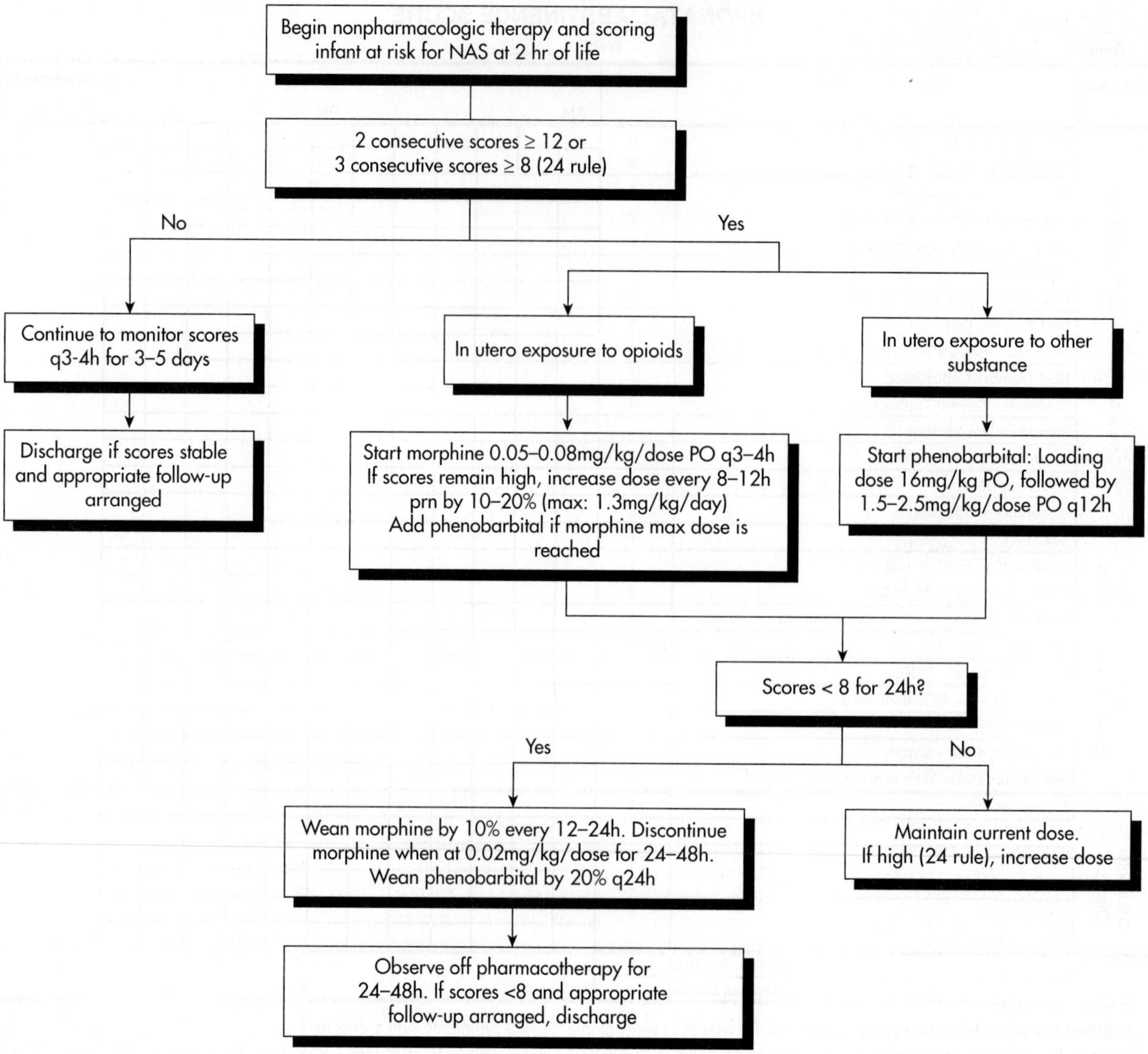

FIG. 2 A management plan for neonates with NAS. Medications should be increased or decreased based on the infant's Finnegan score. *PO,* By mouth.

BASIC INFORMATION

DEFINITION

Nephrotic syndrome is characterized by heavy proteinuria (usually defined as >3.5 g/24 hr), hypoalbuminemia, hyperlipidemia, lipiduria, and edema. Nephrotic-range proteinuria involves urine protein excretion of >3.5 g/24 hr without other features of the nephrotic syndrome. Proteinuria, primarily in the form of albuminuria, can have many causes that share a common mechanism of glomerular injury , the most common being diabetes, focal segmental glomerulosclerosis, membranous nephropathy, minimal change disease, and amyloidosis. Though less common, disorders that are classically categorized under the nephritic syndrome also may lead to nephrotic-range proteinuria.

ICD-10CM CODES

N04.9	Nephrotic syndrome with unspecified morphologic changes
N04.0	Nephrotic syndrome with minor glomerular abnormality
N04.1	Nephrotic syndrome with focal and segmental glomerular lesions
N04.2	Nephrotic syndrome with diffuse membranous glomerulonephritis
N04.3	Nephrotic syndrome with diffuse mesangial proliferative glomerulonephritis
N04.4	Nephrotic syndrome with diffuse endocapillary proliferative glomerulonephritis
N04.5	Nephrotic syndrome with diffuse mesangiocapillary glomerulonephritis
N04.6	Nephrotic syndrome with dense deposit disease
N04.7	Nephrotic syndrome with diffuse crescentic glomerulonephritis
N04.8	Nephrotic syndrome with other morphologic changes

EPIDEMIOLOGY & DEMOGRAPHICS

- Among children (especially <6 yr of age), the most common causes of nephrotic syndrome are:
  1. Minimal change disease (MCD) (75% of pediatric cases)
  2. Focal and segmental glomerulosclerosis (FSGS) (7% to 20% of cases)
- Among adults, diabetes is the most common cause of nephrotic syndrome. FSGS is the most common *primary* (nonsystemic) cause of nephrotic-range proteinuria. Membranous nephropathy is the second most common primary cause of nephrotic syndrome. FSGS is more common in persons of African ancestry, and membranous nephropathy is seen more commonly in Caucasians.

PHYSICAL FINDINGS & CLINICAL PRESENTATION

- Patients usually present with severe lower extremity, periorbital edema, and weight gain.
- Ascites and anasarca may occur.
- Hypercoagulability is a potential clinical manifestation.
- Patients are at higher risk for infections due to urinary immunoglobulin loss.

ETIOLOGY

Glomerular diseases can be thought of as diseases affecting one of five elements that comprise the renal corpuscle: Endothelium, basement membrane, podocyte, mesangium, or parietal epithelium. In general, disorders that involve the endothelium and/or mesangial compartment activate inflammatory mediators. Disorders that exclusively affect the basement membrane or podocyte generally have a noninflammatory pathology. Compromised structural integrity of the glomerulus produces an impairment of the normal mechanisms that prevent abnormal filtration, leading to proteinuria as primarily albuminuria, the hallmark of glomerular disease.

Traditionally, the clinical correlate to this pathological schema has been a subdivision of patients into those with a nephrotic versus nephritic presentation. "Nephritic" disorders have subnephrotic proteinuria, low glomerular filtration rates, and hematuria. "Nephrotic" disorders have greater proteinuria, often normal glomerular filtration rates, and lack hematuria. While generally true, this schema may cause diagnostic confusion because nephritic disease may present with nephrotic-range proteinuria, *especially earlier in the disease course before glomerular filtration is substantially reduced.* It is better to categorize these disorders as "nephrotic" with a noninflammatory urine sediment (i.e., proteinuria without casts or cellular elements) versus "nephritic" with an inflammatory sediment (i.e., proteinuria plus RBC casts and/or dysmorphic RBCs).

Fig. 1 details this breakdown. In this chapter, we focus on primary diseases that present with a noninflammatory sediment (namely, minimal change disease, focal segmental glomerulosclerosis, membranous nephropathy, and amyloidosis) and on primary disorders with inflammatory sediment often with nephrotic-range proteinuria, membranoproliferative glomerulonephritis (MPGN). The evaluation of "nephritic syndrome" is noted by worsening glomerular filtration in the setting of proteinuria and hematuria. Important points regarding the most common etiologies of nephrotic syndrome are detailed in the following text (Table 1).

- MCD has a bland urine sediment with abrupt onset of disease and abrupt remission. Proteinuria may exceed 20 g daily. Nonsteroidal antiinflammatory drug (NSAID) use, chronic lithium ingestion, viral infections, and lymphomas are associated with secondary forms of MCD.

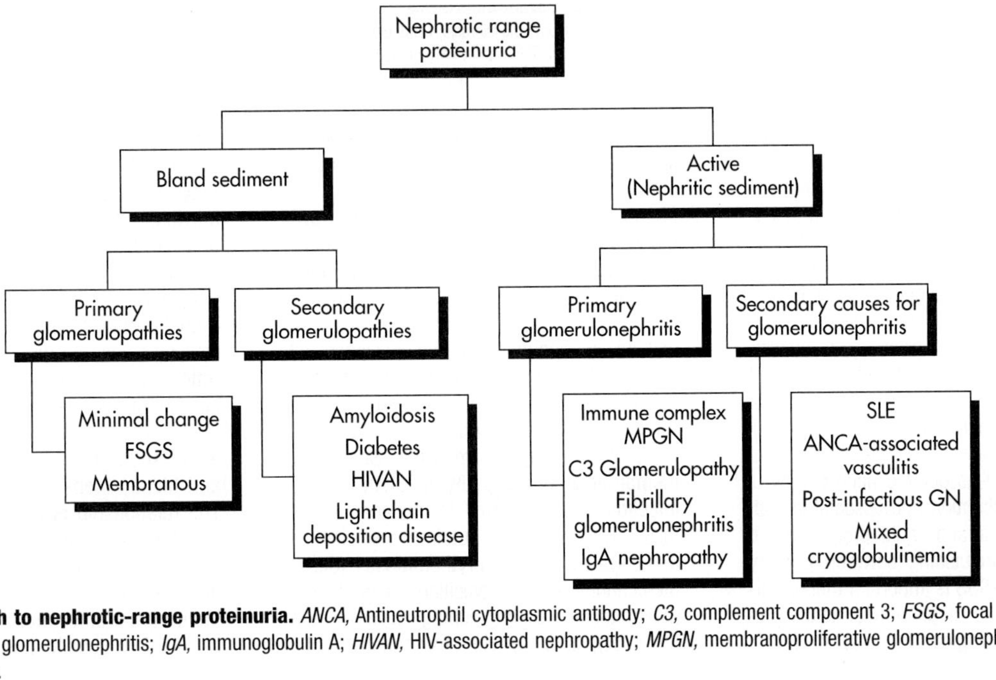

FIG. 1 An approach to nephrotic-range proteinuria. *ANCA,* Antineutrophil cytoplasmic antibody; *C3,* complement component 3; *FSGS,* focal and segmental glomerulosclerosis; *GN,* glomerulonephritis; *IgA,* immunoglobulin A; *HIVAN,* HIV-associated nephropathy; *MPGN,* membranoproliferative glomerulonephritis; *SLE,* systemic lupus erythematosus.

TABLE 1 Important Clinical, Serological, and Pathological Features of Selected Diseases Causing Nephrotic Syndrome

Disease	Important Clinical Features	Serological Features	Pathological Features
Minimal change disease	Rapid onset with heavy proteinuria and rapid remission with therapy. True steroid resistance is rare and should prompt repeat biopsy to rule out FSGS.	Complements are normal.	Light microscopy (LM) shows completely normal kidney architecture. Immunofluorescence microscopy: Normal. Electron microscopy (EM): Diffuse podocyte effacement.
Primary FSGS	Often heavier proteinuria and low serum albumin and edema. Tip lesion subtype and collapsing FSGS often have more explosive onset. Sediment usually bland, but RBCs can be seen. Usually no cellular casts.	Complements are normal.	LM: Only one glomerulus need show features of FSGS to make diagnosis. Immunofluorescence microscopy: Often devoid of immunoglobulin, although IgM can be seen. EM: Often has diffuse podocyte effacement.
Secondary FSGS	Proteinuria is often subnephrotic, or if nephrotic, serum albumin levels are maintained. Minimal edema.	HIV and parvovirus infection can cause phenotype identical to idiopathic collapsing FSGS.	LM: Often shows evidence of glomerulomegaly. EM: Foot process effacement is less diffuse.
Primary membranous nephropathy	Often seen in older Caucasian patients. More likely than other forms of nephrotic syndrome to be associated with thrombotic complications Sediment: Bland. RBCs can be found, although RBC casts are usually found.	Serum antiphospholipase A2 receptor antibodies are found in 70% of patients with idiopathic primary membranous nephropathy. Antineutral endopeptidase antibodies are found in a minority of others.	LM: Characterized by thickening of the GBM; "spikes" can be seen on silver stain. Immunofluorescence microscopy: C3 and IgG noted in granular pattern. Newer techniques stain for antiphospholipase A2 receptor antibody in situ. EM: Associated with subepithelial deposits.
Secondary membranous nephropathy	Associated with malignancy, lupus, syphilis, hepatitis B and C, medications (gold, captopril, penicillamine, etc.).	Notable for the absence of antiphospholipase A2 antibodies. ANA, hepatitis B, HCV serologies are helpful. RPR can be sent in context of appropriate history.	Morphology is exactly the same except when examined by EM. On high power, one sees both subendothelial and mesangial deposits in addition to classic subepithelial deposits.
Amyloidosis	Often found with massive proteinuria. Kidney size is enlarged. Bland sediment.	UPEP, SPEP, serum free light chains may be positive. The UPEP will show glomerular proteinuria, which can help differentiate from myeloma kidney.	LM: Often notable for nodular pattern. Diagnosis can be made by staining using Congo red or thioflavin T. Immunofluorescence microscopy: Antibody use can differentiate AA from AL amyloid. EM: Shows characteristic random 10-nm fibrils.
Diabetes	Often associated with nephrotic-range proteinuria in the setting of retinopathy. Kidney sizes are preserved.	No specific serologic tests are positive.	LM: Nodular pattern often seen, thickened GBM.
MPGN	Often associated with nephrotic-range proteinuria with a "nephritic" sediment. RBC casts often seen along with dysmorphic RBC.	C3 and C4 are often low in immune complex MPGN. Immune complex GN warrants checking SPEP and UPEP, as gammopathy is associated with MPGN. Hepatitis B, HCV, ANA, and cryoglobulins are also warranted. C3 alone is low in dense deposit disease and C3 glomerulonephritis, which may prompt specific tests for complement dysregulation.	The key point here is to look at the IF. If immunofluorescence shows both immunoglobulin and complement deposition, the diagnosis is immune complex MGPN. If only complement, the diagnosis is most likely C3 glomerulopathy (either dense deposit disease or C3 glomerulonephritis).

ANA, Anti-nuclear antibody; *C3,* complement component 3; *FSGS,* focal and segmental glomerulosclerosis; *GBM,* glomerular basement membrane; *GN,* glomerulonephritis; *HCV,* hepatitis C virus; *Ig,* immunoglobulin; *MPGN,* membranoproliferative glomerulonephritis; *RBC,* red blood cell; *RPR,* rapid plasma reagin; *SPEP,* serum protein electrophoresis; *UPEP,* urine protein electrophoresis.

- FSGS, primary or secondary: Primary FSGS denotes an idiopathic cause that typically manifests with heavy proteinuria and nephrotic syndrome and requires immunosuppressive therapy. FSGS is more prevalent in persons of African ancestry. Secondary FSGS is caused by a known etiology, including heroin use, sickle cell disease, scarring of any kind from prior injury, obesity, low nephron mass, HIV, etc. Most cases of secondary FSGS are associated with lower levels of proteinuria (often subnephrotic), higher albumin levels, and less significant edema (e.g., HIV-associated nephropathy is an important exception and associated with heavy proteinuria and rapid progression if untreated). Distinguishing between primary and secondary FSGS is important therapeutically. Many forms of glomerular injury can produce morphological features of FSGS, and worsening proteinuria attributable to secondary FSGS generally portends worse outcomes.
- Membranous nephropathy may be primary or secondary. Primary membranous nephropathy is due to in situ deposition of antibodies directed against a glomerular antigen. In 70% or more cases, the epitope is identified as phospholipase A2 receptor. A second, less-common epitope is thrombospondin type-1 domain-containing 7A (THSD7A). Proteinuria in membranous nephropathy may be massive. Secondary membranous nephropathy is often due to infection (e.g., hepatitis B, malaria, schistosomiasis, syphilis), autoimmune disease (e.g., systemic lupus erythematosus [SLE]), medications (e.g., D-penicillamine, gold), and malignancies. Distinguishing between the two subtypes is important for management.
- Amyloidosis is frequently due to overproduction of immunoglobulin light chains (AL amyloid) or chronic inflammatory state (AA amyloid). Kidney size is often enlarged, and proteinuria may be massive. Congo red staining of amyloid can establish the diagnosis.
- Diabetic nephropathy is often characterized by slowly progressive proteinuria with retinopathy and preserved kidney size. The correlation between retinopathy, proteinuria, and diabetic nephropathy is well-established in type 1 diabetic patients, and kidney biopsies are usually not done. The relationship is less well-established in type 2 diabetes, and absence of retinopathy does not preclude a diagnosis of diabetic nephropathy.
- Membranoproliferative glomerulonephritis (MPGN) usually has immune complex

deposition with complement, or alternate complement system activation without immune complex formation (e.g., C3 glomerulopathy). The prior classification of types 1, 2, and 3 MPGN is obsolete, and a pathophysiological scheme is used now. Common immune complex causes are from infections (e.g., hepatitis C), autoimmune disorders (e.g., SLE), disorders of the alternative complement pathway (C3 glomerulopathy), or dysproteinemias (e.g., monoclonal gammopathies). Distinguishing between these possibilities guides therapy. The urine is associated with heavy proteinuria. Urinary sediment often contains dysmorphic erythrocytes and erythrocyte casts, and is also associated with heavy proteinuria.

Dx DIAGNOSIS

DIFFERENTIAL DIAGNOSIS

- Other states that present with edema (CHF, cirrhosis, protein-losing enteropathy, severe malnutrition)
- Glomerulonephritis from disorders commonly associated with inflammatory urinary sediment and glomerular inflammation
- Mimickers of glomerulonephritis (thrombotic microangiopathy due to malignant HTN, preeclampsia, or antiphospholipid syndrome)

WORKUP

- Evaluation includes determining the rate of change of serum creatinine, quantification of proteinuria by 24-hr collection, and urinary sediment examination.
- Abnormalities in any of the above tests should prompt nephrology consultation.
- Serologic testing may include urine and serum electrophoresis, HIV, hepatitis B surface antigen, hepatitis C virus (HCV) antibody, and antinuclear antibody (ANA). As urinary sediment examination is not 100% sensitive in ruling out an inflammatory process, C3 and C4 can be checked, as complement levels are often low in many inflammatory glomerulonephritides and often low in MPGN. Low complement levels may change the nature of the differential diagnosis before kidney biopsy. Depending on practice patterns, these tests are used selectively before or (in some cases) after biopsy to better define an etiology.
- Antiphospholipase A2 receptor antibody (anti-PLA2R) titer. Elevated titers are found in primary membranous nephropathy and less commonly in secondary membranous nephropathy. With treatment, patients may go into an immunologic remission (decreasing titers) prior to a clinical remission based on urine proteinuria. Thus, monitoring titers during the course of treatment may help guide treatment duration and limit toxic side effects of therapy.
- Patients should undergo a kidney ultrasound to document organ presence and sizes before biopsy.

TABLE 2 Important Definitions in Dealing with Treatment of Primary Nephrotic Syndrome

	Adults	Children
Definition		
Complete Remission	Reduction in proteinuria to <0.3 g/24 hr	<4 mg/m^2 per hr on at least 3 occasions within 7 days and serum albumin >3.5 g/dl
Partial Remission	Reduction in proteinuria between 0.3 g/24 hr and 3.5 g daily with ≥50% decrease in proteinuria from baseline	Disappearance of edema, increase in serum albumin >3.5 g/dl, and persistent proteinuria >4 mg mg/m^2 per hr or >100 mg/m^2 per hr
Relapse*	Increase in proteinuria to >3.5 g daily after one mo of complete or partial remission	Urine dipstick 3+ or proteinuria >40 mg/m^2 per hr occurring on 3 days within 1 wk
Steroid Dependent*	Two consecutive relapses occurring during therapy or within 14 days of completing therapy	Two relapses of proteinuria within 14 days after stopping or during alternate-day steroid therapy
Steroid Resistant*	Persistence of proteinuria without significant reduction despite prednisone therapy at 1 mg/kg for 16 wk	Persistence of proteinuria despite prednisone therapy at 60 mg/m^2 for 4 wk

*These definitions only truly apply to diseases such as minimal change disease and focal and segmental glomerulosclerosis (FSGS).
Adapted from Cattran DC et al: Cyclosporine in idiopathic glomerular disease associated with the nephrotic syndrome: workshop recommendations, *Kidney Int* 72(12):1429-1447, 2007, and *KDIGO clinical practice guidelines for glomerulonephritis.*

Rx TREATMENT

NONIMMUNOSUPPRESSIVE THERAPY

- Control of proteinuria is key to progressive kidney disease. Nearly all trials of nondiabetic chronic kidney disease demonstrate that reducing proteinuria improves renal survival. Angiotensin-converting enzyme inhibitors (ACEIs) or angiotensin II type 1 receptor blockers (ARBs) should be used at maximally tolerated doses. The exception is MCD where proteinuria reduction may rapidly occur during therapy. Generally, a strategy of dual ACEI and ARB therapy is not recommended due to increased risks of hyperkalemia and elevating the serum creatinine. Nondihydropyridine calcium channel blockers (verapamil, diltiazem) can be used in lieu of ACEIs or ARBs when these agents are contraindicated.
- For proteinuria >1 g per day, target blood pressure is <125/75 mm Hg.
- With the exception of MCD, patients with nephrotic-range proteinuria and hyperlipidemia should be treated with HMG CoA synthetase inhibitors (statins).
- Although some patients with nephrotic syndrome are hypercoagulable (particularly, membranous nephropathy), the role of prophylactic anticoagulation is not well-defined and controversial. For patients with membranous nephropathy and serum albumin levels <2.0 g/dl, anticoagulation should be considered if bleeding risk is low.
- Low sodium diet (<2 g daily) with diuretics.
- Diuretic resistance is common due to gut wall edema and hypoalbuminemia. More bioavailable diuretics (bumetanide, torsemide) may increase urine output better than furosemide. Thiazide diuretics can be added to loop agents to augment diuresis.
- Loop diuretics should be dosed at least on a twice-daily basis.

IMMUNOSUPPRESSIVE THERAPY

Important terms in dealing with the management of nephrotic-range proteinuria due to primary glomerular diseases are listed in Table 2. First-line therapies for each disease are highlighted in the following.

- MCD: First-line therapy in adults is prednisone (1 mg/kg per day to a maximum of 80 mg per day) for a minimum of 4 wk and maximum of 16 wk. Steroids are tapered over 6 mo for favorable responses. Second-line options include cyclophosphamide and/or calcineurin inhibitors. Newer, randomized controlled trial data from children reveal efficacy of rituximab in steroid-dependent patients with recurrent relapsing MCD. Consequently, rituximab may become a reasonable option for patients who do not respond to conventional therapy.
- FSGS: Primary FSGS is often treated with high-dose prednisone (maximum, 80 mg daily in adults) tapered over 6 mo. Alternative regimens include low-dose prednisone with cyclosporine. Mycophenolate mofetil (MMF) has also been used in primary FSGS. Treatment of secondary FSGS is based on arresting the underlying cause and nonspecific therapy with an ACEI or ARB, BP control, weight loss, and dietary protein restriction. Immunosuppression is avoided. A recent clinical trial, DUET, demonstrated superior antiproteinuric therapy of sparsentan, endothelin type A inhibitor and angiotensin II type 1 receptor antagonist, versus irbesartan, an ARB.
- Membranous nephropathy: Acceptable treatments include alternating months of cyclophosphamide and steroids, calcineurin inhibitors with low-dose steroids or without steroids, and rituximab. Currently, exogenous

ACTH is a last-line resort and not standard of care. Therapy for secondary membranous nephropathy is directed at treating the underlying cause (malignancy, SLE, etc.).

- Amyloidosis, diabetes, and immune complex MPGN: Treatment is specific for the underlying disorder. In rapidly progressive HCV-related MPGN, immunosuppressive therapy with rituximab or glucocorticoids and cyclophosphamide can be administered during direct-acting antiviral therapy.
- MPGN: A reclassification of MPGN highlights alternative complement cascade activation (C3 glomerulonephritis) as etiologic. MPGN is considered immune complex mediated or complement mediated by immunofluorescent microscopy. Treatment may now involve agents (e.g., eculizumab) that inhibit the complement cascade. Prior nontargeted approaches (e.g., steroids) for MPGN have been largely unsuccessful except in selected pediatric cases.

REFERRAL

Nephrology consultation is recommended for all cases of nephrotic syndrome.

PEARLS & CONSIDERATIONS

- Albuminuria generally implies glomerular disease is present. The urine protein electrophoresis defines the type(s) of proteins excreted: Albumin, immunoglobulins, and tubular.
- Massive proteinuria (>20 g daily) is rarely encountered with inflammatory glomerulonephritis and generally indicates MCD, FSGS, membranous nephropathy, or amyloidosis.
- Partial remissions and steroid resistance are rarely seen in primary minimal change disease. These circumstances require repeat kidney biopsy because FSGS is often revealed.
- Proteinuria is quantitated by a 24-hr urine collection with evaluation of urinary creatinine excretion to document adequacy of collection. Spot collections have not been validated for heavy proteinuria or patients with rapidly changing creatinine values. A "spot" urine protein-to-creatinine ratio directly obtained from the 24-hr collection defines the relationship between spot and "true" ratios for therapeutic monitoring.
- Most noninflammatory processes progress slowly. If a sediment without red blood cell casts is detected with a rapidly increasing serum creatinine and heavy proteinuria, the differential is relatively narrow:
  1. MCD with acute tubular necrosis or acute interstitial nephritis, as occurs with nonsteroidal antiinflammatory drug administration
  2. Any form of nephrotic syndrome associated with acute tubular necrosis from hypovolemia
  3. Bilateral renal vein thrombosis superimposed on nephrotic syndrome
  4. Myeloma cast nephropathy
  5. Collapsing FSGS

SUGGESTED READINGS

Available at ExpertConsult.com

RELATED CONTENT

Nephrotic Syndrome (Patient Information)

AUTHOR: **Rupali Avasare, MD**

BASIC INFORMATION

DEFINITION

The American Psychiatric Association's *Diagnostic and Statistical Manual of Mental Disorders,* 5th edition (DSM-5), includes delirium and major and mild neurocognitive disorders, as well as their subtypes, under the grouping *neurocognitive disorders.*

The core features of neurocognitive disorders (NCDs) are deficits in cognitive function. The cognitive dysfunction is acquired rather than developmental and thus represents a decline from a previously attained level of functioning. The NCDs are subtyped according to known or presumed etiologic/pathologic entities underlying the decline. The subtypes may be distinguished by clinical characteristics such as time course, physical examination, and cognitive domains affected. It is possible for more than one NCD to be identified in a given patient at a given time.

In major and mild NCDs, the cognitive deficits are present in one or more cognitive domains. The initial evidence is based on concern brought forth by the patient, a knowledgeable informant, or the clinician and is often supported by performance on objective standardized assessments such as neuropsychological testing. In major NCDs, the deficits interfere with independence in everyday activity, whereas in minor NCDs, the impairment is more modest and does not interfere with capacity for independence in everyday activity.

In the DSM-5, *delirium* (acute encephalopathy) is subsumed under the category *neurocognitive disorders.* Although it shares the core feature of acquired deficit in cognitive function, it is discussed as a distinct entity from major and minor neurocognitive disorders and is discussed separately in this text. The DSM-IV term *dementia* (chronic encephalopathy) is subsumed under the entity *major neurocognitive disorder* in the DSM-5, and the DSM-IV term *amnestic disorder* and its subtypes are subsumed under the category *major neurocognitive disorder due to another medical condition* in the DSM-5.

Some of the more commonly seen NCDs include major or mild NCD due to Alzheimer disease, major or mild vascular NCD, and major or mild NCD due to Lewy body disease. ICD-10CM coding classified NCDs under F02 (dementia in other diseases classified elsewhere), and they are coded alongside underlying physiologic conditions, such as Alzheimer disease (G30), frontotemporal dementia (G31.09), or Parkinson disease (G20).

ICD-10CM CODES

F02.80	Major or mild neurocognitive disorder, without behavior disturbance
F02.81	Major or mild neurocognitive disorder, with behavior disturbance

DSM-5 CODES

294.10	Major or mild neurocognitive disorder, without behavior disturbance
294.11	Major or mild neurocognitive disorder, with behavior disturbance

EPIDEMIOLOGY & DEMOGRAPHICS

The prevalence varies depending on the etiology of the neurocognitive disorder and age of the patient. Among patients >60 yr, the prevalence tends to increase sharply for the most common neurocognitive disorders. Overall prevalence estimates for major NCDs are approximately 1% to 2% at 65 yr old and as high as 30% at 85 yr. Mild NCD prevalence is variable, ranging from 2% to 10% at age 65 and 5% to 25% at age 85. The strongest risk factor for major and mild NCD is age. Female gender is associated with a higher prevalence in major and mild NCD due to Alzheimer disease, though this association is confounded by increased female longevity. African-American and Latinx populations may be at increased risk for particular neurodegenerative diseases, such as Alzheimer disease, but these populations remain underrepresented in epidemiologic research at this time.

PHYSICAL FINDINGS & CLINICAL PRESENTATION

Neurocognitive domains that are affected in NCDs include:

- Complex attention, including sustained attention, divided attention, selective attention, and processing speed
- Executive functioning, such as planning, decision making, working memory, and mental flexibility
- Learning and memory, including immediate memory, recent memory
- Language expression and reception, including word recall, grammar, and syntax
- Perceptual motor skills, including visual construction, praxis, and gnosis
- Social cognition, including recognition of emotions

Associated physical findings, time course of illness, and response to treatment depend on etiology of the NCD. Mood disturbance, psychosis, and behavior disturbances are recognized as common neuropsychiatric symptoms associated with NCDs. Mood symptoms are common early in the course of NCDs due to Alzheimer disease, NCD with Lewy bodies, and vascular NCD. Psychoses, including delusions and paranoia, may present across the spectrum of illness but are more common in mild to moderate stages of NCD with Lewy bodies and in moderate to severe stages of NCD due to Alzheimer disease. Psychosis, agitation, and other behavioral disturbances lead to increased rate of hospitalization, early admission to assisted living environments or nursing homes, and increased level of caregiver depression and distress. Apathy manifests early in the course of NCDs and is the most common neuropsychiatric symptom of NCD due to Alzheimer disease across the spectrum of the disease.

ASSOCIATED SIGNS AND SYMPTOMS BY ETIOLOGY

(For each etiology, the criteria are met for major or mild neurocognitive disorder.)

- **Major or mild neurocognitive disorder due to Alzheimer disease:** Insidious onset and gradual progression, occasionally with brief plateaus. Impairment in memory, learning, and executive function are prominent early in the disease. In moderate to severe disease, language deficits manifest and problematic behaviors, including agitation, combativeness, and psychosis, may arise. Apathy, agitation, and psychosis are often more distressing to caregivers than the cognitive deficits.
- **Major or mild frontotemporal neurocognitive disorder:** Behavior and language variants are characterized by progressive development of personality changes, behavior changes including disinhibition, and/or language impairment. Patients with behavior variant may present with impaired insight, socially inappropriate behaviors, apathy, hyperorality, or compulsive behaviors. Learning and memory dysfunction may be spared in the early stages. Symptoms of FTD usually come before motor symptoms. Behavioral variant frontotemporal lobar degeneration (bv-FTLD), corticobasal degeneration, primary progressive aphasia, progressive supranuclear palsy, and Pick disease are often considered variants of frontotemporal neurocognitive disorders.
- **Major or mild neurocognitive disorder with Lewy bodies:** Cognitive decline occurs prior to or within 1 yr of the onset of parkinsonism motor symptoms. Recurrent, well-formed, and detailed visual hallucinations and fluctuating cognition that can resemble delirium are core features. Mood disturbances, autonomic dysfunction, and REM sleep disorder are suggestive of this diagnosis. Individuals with major or mild neurocognitive disorder with Lewy bodies are typically functionally more impaired than would be expected for their cognitive deficits because of the motor and autonomic impairments. They can present with multifocal myoclonus and visual hallucinations.
- **Major or mild neurocognitive disorder due to Parkinson disease:** Parkinson disease onset precedes the onset of major neurocognitive decline by at least 1 yr. Apathy, depression, hallucinations, and REM sleep disorder are suggestive of this diagnosis. The atypical parkinsonian syndrome progressive supranuclear palsy presents with early postural instability and retropulsion, supranuclear gaze palsy, and early cognitive impairment with depression, apathy, and anxiety.
- **Major or mild vascular neurocognitive disorder:** The onset of cognitive decline is temporally related to one or more cerebrovascular events. The diagnosis is supported by neuroimaging evidence of parenchymal injury, including large vessel infarcts or hemorrhages, two or more lacunar infarcts outside the brainstem, or confluent white matter lesions attributed to cerebrovascular disease. Patients typically present with decline in processing speed, complex attention, and executive dysfunction. Stepwise and/or

fluctuating decline is described. Prominent depression, apathy, and personality changes are common.

- **Major or mild neurocognitive disorder due to traumatic brain injury (TBI):** This NCD presents immediately after the occurrence of or can be attributed to a traumatic brain injury that causes loss of consciousness, posttraumatic amnesia, disorientation, or neurologic signs such as seizure or hemiparesis. Cognitive presentation may be variable but may include difficulty with complex attention, executive dysfunction, or deficits in learning and memory. Associated findings include disturbances in emotional function and personality change. The features of major or mild NCD due to TBI vary by age of patient and specifics of the injury as well as other factors, such as premorbid functioning of the patient. Chronic traumatic encephalopathy results from multiple concussive episodes (e.g., sports-related injuries).
- **Substance/medication-induced major or mild neurocognitive disorder:** A NCD that persists beyond the duration of intoxication and acute withdrawal from a substance. NCD due to alcohol frequently manifests with memory, learning, and executive impairments. Wernicke syndrome is an acute neurologic disorder caused by thiamine deficiency manifesting with a clinic triad of encephalopathy, oculomotor dysfunction, and gait ataxia. Korsakoff syndrome is a late manifestation of Wernicke syndrome manifesting with dense anterograde amnesia and confabulation. MRI may show mammillary body or medial dorsal thalamic nucleus atrophy. Major or mild NCD may be induced by medication or combinations of medications, including those with sedating and pain-ameliorating properties and those with anticholinergic properties. Particular attention should be paid to review of medications in any patient with major or mild NCD, especially those in the geriatric population.
- **Major or mild neurocognitive disorder due to Prion disease:** Neurocognitive deficits occur rapidly, typically over 6 mo as occurs in Creutzfeldt-Jakob disease. In some variants, prominent psychiatric symptoms such as depression and anxiety may occur prior to neurocognitive deficits. Ataxia, myoclonus, chorea, and a prominent startle reflex are typically present.
- **Major or mild neurocognitive disorder due to Huntington disease:** Early prominent changes in processing speed, organization, and planning rather than learning and memory are common. Behavior changes, changes in mood, anxiety, obsessive-compulsive symptoms, irritability, and apathy often precede motor symptoms.
- **Major or mild neurocognitive disorder due to another medical condition:** Many medical conditions can cause NCDs. Examples include structural brain lesions such as primary or secondary brain tumors, subdural hematomas or those seen in normal pressure hydrocephalus, hypoxia, infectious causes (e.g., HIV), endocrine conditions, immune disorders, and metabolic conditions. The temporal association between the onset or exacerbation of the medical condition and the development of the cognitive deficit supports the diagnosis.

Dx DIAGNOSIS

DIFFERENTIAL DIAGNOSIS

Etiology is assessed by a detailed history from the patient, family members, or other informants, physical examination, and neuropsychological testing and imaging studies. Rule out other causes of dementia-like presentations, including depression and untreated sleep apnea.

LABORATORY TESTS & IMAGING STUDIES

- A focal neurologic examination and often neuropsychological testing and neuroimaging are indicated. In some cases, serology and lab testing, including B12, complete blood count, and thyroid-stimulating hormone (TSH) levels, reveal abnormalities which upon treatment can improve cognition. Biomarkers and genetic screening tests are diagnostic in some cases. Particular attention should be paid to rule out underlying medical causes of the major or mild NCD.
- Alzheimer disease: Detailed history and physical examination including neuropsychological tests often points to the diagnosis. MRI findings include general as well as focal (hippocampal and temporoparietal cortical) atrophy, and can reveal alternative or additional diagnoses (e.g., cerebrovascular disease). FDG-PET may show hypometabolism in temporoparietal regions. Amyloid PET scanning may have diagnostic value, and tau PET imaging is under development. Cerebrospinal fluid biomarkers include elevated total and phosphorylated tau levels with reduced amyloid beta-42 (Aβ-42) or a low Aβ-42:40 ratio. *APOE* testing may detect APOE4, a risk factor for development of Alzheimer disease. For early onset, autosomal dominant inheritance mutation in *APP, PSEN1,* or *PSEN2* may be detected.
- Frontotemporal dementia: In cases with early-onset behavior or language disorders, an MRI or CT scan may show atrophy in frontal lobes and/or corresponding parts of anterior or inferior temporal lobes either bilaterally or asymmetrically. Functional imaging may show hypoperfusion in the corresponding regions. In familial cases, genetic mutations in genes encoding the microtubule-associated protein tau and the granulin gene may confirm the diagnosis.
- Dementia with Lewy bodies: A sleep study may help to confirm a diagnosis of REM sleep behavior disorder. Nuclear medicine testing (SPECT/DaTscan or PET) may reveal reduced perfusion or metabolism in the occipital lobe, or low dopamine transporter or dopaminergic activity levels in the striatum.
- Parkinson disease: Physical examination and abnormal dopamine transporter scans are supportive of the diagnosis.
- Vascular disorder: Neurologic assessment often reveals a history of stroke or transient ischemic attack (TIA). MRI or CT scan may show significant parenchymal injury attributed to cerebrovascular disease.
- TBI: May be associated with abnormal CT or MRI scan showing petechial hemorrhages, diffuse axonal injury, subdural or subarachnoid hemorrhage, or evidence of contusion.
- Prion disease: May be suspected in patients with appropriate clinical presentation, including rapidly progressive course. MRI may show gray matter hyperintensities in the subcortical region, particularly in the putamen and head of caudate nuclei. Electroencephalogram (EEG) reveals periodic synchronous biphasic or triphasic sharp waves complexes. Cerebrospinal fluid (CSF) biomarkers including 14-3-3, tau, S100 protein, or neuron-specific enolase are suggestive, though not diagnostic.
- Huntington disease: Genetic testing for trinucleotide cytosine-adenine-guanine (CAG) repeat expansion in the gene that encodes Huntington protein on chromosome 4 is diagnostic.

Rx TREATMENT

- Modifiable risk factors to reduce cognitive decline in dementia include social engagement, exercise, improved diet, reduced alcohol intake, quitting smoking, managing hypertension and diabetes, and treating hearing loss. Cognitive training and stimulation (e.g., cognitive-behavioral therapy, music-based therapies) can improve mood and memory early in the course of neurocognitive disease.
- Acetylcholinesterase inhibitors and memantine can be prescribed for cognitive enhancement. Disease-modifying drugs such as passive antibody infusions (e.g., anti-Aβ and anti-tau) are in clinical trials for Alzheimer disease.
- Agitation is notoriously difficult to treat. Pharmacologic treatments for behavior disturbance have a limited role in improving overall quality of life for most causes of major or minor NCD, and nonpharmacologic approaches (e.g., behavioral strategies) are first line for most behavioral manifestations. Identify and treat underlying causes first, including infection (e.g., UTI), medication toxicity, sleep disorders, and pain. Antidepressants such as SSRIs have shown mixed benefits to risk (QTc prolongation, orthostasis, and falls). Atypical antipsychotics such as olanzapine, risperidone, and quetiapine can effectively reduce agitation symptoms. A risk/benefit conversation is necessary when initiating neuroleptic treatment, given the possible side effects of increased all-cause mortality, risk for arrhythmias, extrapyramidal symptoms, and

stroke. Attempts to taper or discontinue these medications should be done when feasible. Patients with dementia with Lewy bodies are highly sensitive to antidopaminergic effects of antipsychotics, and agitation in these patients should be managed cautiously. Recently, dextromethorphan/quinidine (Nuedexta), a nonneuroleptic, has been trialed with evidence of benefit in dementia-related agitation and aggression.

- Care coordination and family education and support may help reduce the need for a skilled nursing facility and reduce caregiver stress and burnout. Patient safety, including risks associated with driving, wandering, and cooking, should be addressed throughout the course of the illness. Supervised living may ensure appropriate long-term care in late stages of progressive illness.

SUGGESTED READINGS

Available at ExpertConsult.com

RELATED CONTENT

Alzheimer Disease (Related Key Topic)
Delirium (Related Key Topic)
Human Immunodeficiency Virus (Related Key Topic)
Huntington Disease (Related Key Topic)
Parkinson Disease (Related Key Topic)
Progressive Supranuclear Palsy (Related Key Topic)
Traumatic Brain Injury (Related Key Topic)
Wernicke Syndrome (Related Key Topic)

AUTHORS: **Jennifer J. Holiman, MSN, APRN, PMHNP-BC, Michael Friedman, MD,** and **Marc S. Weinberg, MD, PhD**

BASIC INFORMATION

DEFINITION

Neurofibromatosis (NF) is an autosomal-dominant disorder affecting bone, the nervous system, soft tissue, and skin. There are three major subtypes of NF disorders: NF type 1 (NF1), NF type 2 (NF2), and schwannomatosis (SWN). SWN has only recently been recognized as a distinct disorder; currently very little is known about it.

SYNONYMS

NF1: von Recklinghausen disease, peripheral NF
NF2: Bilateral acoustic neurofibromatosis, central NF

ICD-10CM CODES	
Q85.00	Neurofibromatosis, unspecified
Q85.01	Neurofibromatosis, type 1
Q85.02	Neurofibromatosis, type 2

EPIDEMIOLOGY & DEMOGRAPHICS

- Incidence of NF1 (one case/3000 live births), NF2 (one case/25,000 live births).
- Prevalence of NF1 (one case/5000 persons), NF2 (one case/210,000 persons).
- NF1 and NF2 are autosomal dominant; approximately 50% of cases have no family history.
- The two disorders affect approximately 100,000 people in the U.S.
- Affects males and females equally.
- NF1 may be associated with optic gliomas, astrocytomas, spinal neurofibromas, pheochromocytomas, and chronic myeloid leukemia.
- NF2 may be associated with meningiomas, spinal schwannomas, and cataracts.
- For SWN, the incidence is one per 30,000 persons, and the disease is mostly sporadic in nature.

PHYSICAL FINDINGS & CLINICAL PRESENTATION

- Common features of NF1 include:
  1. Café-au-lait macules (100% of children by age 2 yr)
     a. Hyperpigmented skin lesions (Fig. E1) occurring anywhere on the body except the face, palms, and soles
     b. Appear early in life and increase in size and number during puberty
     c. Are focal or diffuse
  2. Axillary and inguinal freckling (70%)
  3. Multiple neurofibromas (Fig. 2) can be soft or firm; three subtypes:
     a. Cutaneous: Circumscribed, not specific for NF1
     b. Subcutaneous: Circumscribed, not specific for NF1
     c. Plexiform: Noncircumscribed, thick and irregular; can cause disfigurement of supportive structures and specific for NF1

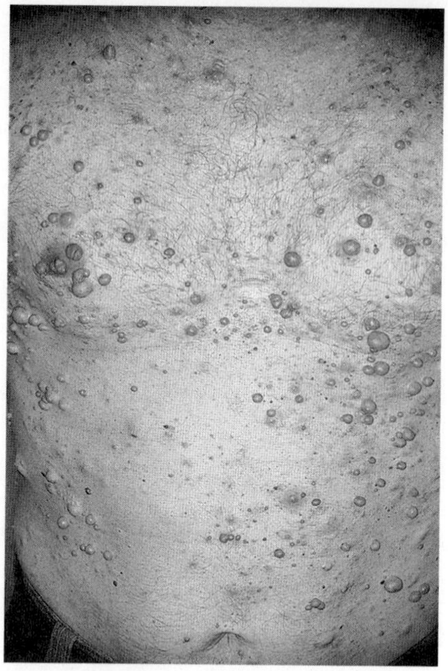

FIG. 2 Multiple neurofibromas are present in this individual. (From Callen JP et al: *Dermatological signs of systemic disease,* ed 5, Philadelphia, 2017, Elsevier.)

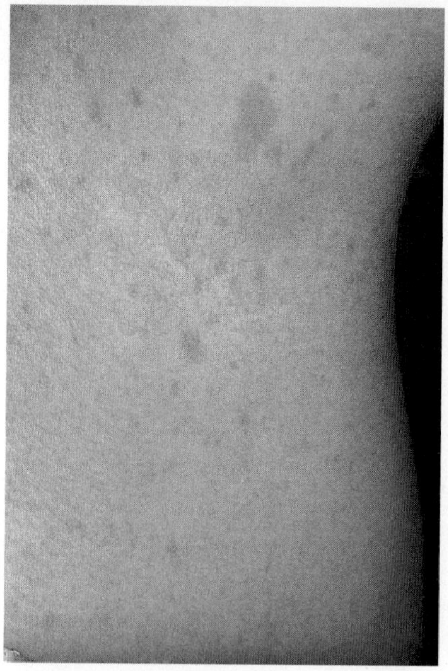

FIG. 3 A café-au-lait spot and multiple freckles (Crowe sign) in the axillary vault is seen in this patient with neurofibromatosis. (From Callen JP et al: *Dermatological signs of systemic disease,* ed 5, Philadelphia, 2017, Elsevier.)

  4. Lisch nodule (small hamartoma of the iris) found in >90% of adult cases
  5. Visual defects possibly related to optic gliomas (2% to 5%)
  6. Neurodevelopment problems such as learning disability and mental retardation (30% to 40%)
  7. Skeletal disorders, including long bone dysplasia, pseudoarthrosis, scoliosis, short stature, and decreased bone mineral density
- Common features of NF2 include:
  1. Hearing loss and tinnitus related to bilateral acoustic neuromas (>90% of adults)
  2. Cataracts (81%)
  3. Headache (may be due to intracranial meningiomas, which are present in 80% of patients)
  4. Unsteady gait
  5. Cutaneous and subcutaneous neurofibromas but fewer than in NF1
  6. Café-au-lait macules (1%) (Fig. 3)
- Common features of SWN include painful multiple schwannomas of the spinal (74%), peripheral (89%), or cranial nerves *except* the vestibular nerve (9%)

ETIOLOGY

- NF1 is caused by DNA mutations located on the long arm of chromosome 17 responsible for encoding the protein neurofibromin.
- NF2 is caused by DNA mutations located in the middle of the long arm of chromosome 22 responsible for encoding the protein merlin, which is a potent inhibitor of glioma growth.
- Both proteins are speculated to act as tumor suppressors.
- The etiology of SWN remains unclear; however, most cases are attributed to mutations on chromosome 22, which inactivate two distinct tumor-suppressor genes.

DIAGNOSIS

- The major clinical features of NF1 are summarized in Table 1. NIH diagnostic criteria for NF1 are described in Table 2. NF1 is diagnosed if the person has two or more of the following features:
  1. Six or more café-au-lait macules >5 mm in prepubertal patients and >15 mm in postpubertal patients
  2. Two or more neurofibromas of any type or one plexiform neurofibroma
  3. Axillary or inguinal freckling
  4. Optic glioma
  5. Two or more Lisch nodules (iris hamartomas)
  6. Sphenoid wing dysplasia or cortical thinning of long bones, with or without pseudoarthrosis
  7. A first-degree relative (parent, sibling, or child) with NF1 based on the previous criteria
- NF2 is diagnosed if the person has either of the following two criteria:
  1. Bilateral eighth nerve masses seen by appropriate imaging studies (e.g., CT, MRI)
  2. A first-degree relative with NF2 and either a unilateral eighth nerve mass or two of the following: Neurofibroma, meningioma, glioma, schwannoma, or juvenile posterior subcapsular lenticular opacity

TABLE 1 Major Clinical Features of Neurofibromatosis Type 1

Cutaneous
- Neurofibromas (60%-90%)
- Café-au-lait macules (>90%)
- Axillary and/or inguinal freckling (~80%)
- Plexiform neurofibroma (25%)
- Nevus anemicus (30%-50%)
- Juvenile xanthogranuloma (15%-35% in first 3 yr of life)

Ocular
- Lisch nodules (~90% by 20 yr of age)
- Choroidal nodules (>80% of adults)
- Neovascular glaucoma, retinal vasoproliferative tumors

Skeletal

Cranial
- Macrocephaly (20%-50%)
- Hypertelorism (25%)
- Sphenoid wing dysplasia (<5%)

Spinal
- Scoliosis (5%-10%)
- Spina bifida

Limbs
- Dysplasia of long bone cortex (5%), pseudarthrosis (2%)

Other
- Generalized osteopenia (~50%), osteoporosis (~20%)
- Short stature (~30% <3rd percentile)
- Pectus deformity (30%-50%)

Tumors
- Optic glioma (10%-15%) (with or without precocious puberty)
- Malignant peripheral nerve sheath tumors (3%-15%)
- Pheochromocytoma (~1%)
- Juvenile myelomonocytic leukemia
- CNS tumors other than optic gliomas (~5%)
- Rhabdomyosarcoma, especially of the genitourinary tract
- Duodenal carcinoid
- Somatostatinoma
- Parathyroid adenoma
- Gastrointestinal stromal tumors (GIST)
- Breast cancer (~5-fold increased risk in women <50 yr of age)

Neurologic
- Unidentified bright objects (UBO) on MRI (50%-75%)
- Learning difficulties (30%-50%)
- Seizures (~5%)
- Intellectual impairment (severe in <5%)
- Aqueductal stenosis and hydrocephalus (~2%)

Cardiovascular
- Hypertension (~30%): Essential > renal artery stenosis or pheochromocytoma
- Pulmonic stenosis (~1%)
- Renal artery stenosis (~2%)
- Cerebrovascular anomalies (2%-5%), including vascular stenoses and aneurysms

JXGs, Juvenile xanthogranulomas; *MRI,* magnetic resonance imaging.
From Bolognia JL: *Dermatology,* ed 4, Philadelphia, 2018, Elsevier.

TABLE 2 NIH Diagnostic Criteria for Neurofibromatosis Type 1

Two or more of the following must be present:
- Six or more café-au-lait macules >5 mm in prepubertal individuals and >15 mm in postpubertal individuals
- Two or more neurofibromas of any type or one plexiform neurofibroma
- "Freckling" in the axillary or inguinal regions
- Optic gliomas
- Two or more Lisch nodules (iris hamartomas)
- Osseous lesion, such as sphenoid wing dysplasia or thinning of long bone cortex, with or without pseudarthrosis
- First-degree relative (parent, sibling, or offspring) with NF1 by the above criteria

Updated diagnostic criteria including recently recognized manifestations (e.g. nevus anemicus, choroidal nodules) and *NF1* gene testing are under development. When a multistep, comprehensive analysis of the *NF1* gene is performed, an underlying mutation can be detected in ≥95% of nonfounder patients who fulfill these diagnostic criteria.
From Bologna JL: *Dermatology,* ed 4, Philadelphia, 2018, Elsevier.

TABLE 3 Evaluation and Management of Neurofibromatosis 1 (NF1) Patients

At time of diagnosis and annually during childhood and adolescence (unless otherwise indicated)

Dermatologic examination (especially if a plexiform neurofibroma [PNF] is present)
- Surgical consultation if painful or disfiguring neurofibromas
- PET-CT if rapid growth, increased firmness, or persistent pain within an established PNF or the development of a new neurologic deficit*
- Ophthalmologic examination with visual assessment (prior to age 8 yr)
- Orbital/brain MRI if signs/symptoms of optic glioma
- Evaluation for scoliosis and tibial bowing
- Referral to orthopedics if scoliosis develops
- Neurologic examination, developmental/behavioral evaluation, and (in young children) measurement of head circumference
- Orbital/brain and/or spinal MRI if neurologic signs/symptoms develop†
- Comprehensive developmental assessment prior to starting school and if problems arise
- Cardiac assessment and measurement of blood pressure
- Referral to cardiology if murmur is detected
- Renal arteriography and 24-hour urine collection for catecholamines and metanephrines if hypertension develops
- Assessment for pubertal development
- Orbital/brain MRI and referral to endocrinology if precocious puberty develops

Minimum annual evaluation for adults with uncomplicated disease

Dermatologic evaluation if PNF is present
  PET-CT for indications described above
Neurologic examination (especially if a PNF is present)
  MRI and/or other studies as indicated if neurologic signs/symptoms develop
Measurement of blood pressure
  Evaluation as described above if hypertension develops
In women, screening for breast cancer with clinical examination + mammography ± MRI (beginning by age 40 yr)

Potentially affected family members

Dermatologic examination for cutaneous manifestations of NF1
Ophthalmologic examination for Lisch nodules
Consider genetic testing if a mutation has been identified in the proband

CT, Computed tomography; *MRI,* magnetic resonance imaging; *PET-CT,* positron emission tomography–computed tomography.
*Immediate assessment is required for any of these findings.
†The role of neuroimaging in asymptomatic patients is controversial.
From Bolognia JL: *Dermatology,* ed 4, Philadelphia, 2018, Elsevier.

- SWN is diagnosed in an individual >30 yr having either of the following two criteria:
  1. Two nonintradermal schwannomas, no vestibular tumor found on MRI scan, no NF2 mutation
  2. One nonvestibular schwannoma and a first-degree relative fitting the above criteria

DIFFERENTIAL DIAGNOSIS

- Abdominal NF
- Myxoid lipoma
- Nodular fasciitis
- Fibrous histiocytoma
- Segmental NF

WORKUP

The evaluation and management of NF1 patients are summarized in Table 3. The diagnosis of NF is usually self-evident. Workup is dictated by clinical symptoms in NF1 and usually includes MRI evaluation of the head and spine in NF2 and SWN. In fact, if NF2 is suspected but no vestibular nerve schwannomas are found, the diagnosis points to SWN.

LABORATORY TESTS

- Genetic testing is possible in individuals who desire prenatal diagnosis for NF1. There is no single standard test and multiple tests are required. Results can only tell if an individual is affected but cannot predict the severity of the disease due to variable expression.
- In NF2, linkage analysis testing provides a >99% certainty the individual has NF2.

IMAGING STUDIES

- MRI with gadolinium is the imaging study of choice in both NF1 and NF2 patients. MRI increases detection of optic gliomas, tumors of the spine, acoustic neuromas, and "bright spots" believed to represent hamartomas.
- MRI of the spine is recommended in all patients diagnosed with NF2 to exclude intramedullary tumors.

OTHER TESTS

- Wood's lamp examination may be useful in patients with very pale skin for visualizing café-au-lait spots.
- Slit-lamp examination is recommended for children >6 yr to confirm the presence of Lisch nodules and subcapsular opacity.

Rx TREATMENT

Treatment is directed primarily at symptoms and complications of NF1 and NF2. As for SWN, resection should be reserved for tumors that are symptomatic or threaten to cause spinal cord compression.

NONPHARMACOLOGIC THERAPY

- Counseling addressing prognosis and genetic, psychological, and social issues.
- Hearing testing and speech pathology evaluation.

ACUTE GENERAL Rx

- Surgery is usually not done on skin tumors unless cosmetically requested or if suspicion of malignant transformation exists.
- Surgery may be indicated for spinal or cranial neurofibromas, gliomas, or meningiomas.
- Acoustic neuromas can be treated by surgical excision.

CHRONIC Rx

- Radiation may be indicated in optic nerve gliomas and patients whose central nervous system tumors show radiographic progression.
- Stereotactic radiosurgery with a gamma knife may be an alternative approach to surgery for acoustic neuromas.
- Bevacizumab continues to be studied as a treatment option for NF2 meningiomas (which express vascular endothelial growth factor [VEGF]).

DISPOSITION

- Prognosis varies according to the severity of involvement.
- There is no cure for NF.

REFERRAL

A multidisciplinary team of consultants is needed in patients with NF, including neurosurgeon, otolaryngologist, dermatologist, neurologist, audiologist, speech pathologist, geneticist, and neuropsychologist.

PEARLS & CONSIDERATIONS

- Friedrich Daniel von Recklinghausen first reported his cases in 1882, although there had been similar accounts dating back to the 1600s.
- A high SPRED1 mutation detection rate has been identified in NF1 mutation-negative families with an autosomal dominant phenotype of café-au-lait macules with or without freckling and no other NF1 features.

COMMENTS

For additional information and patient resources, refer to the Neurofibromatosis Network or Neurofibromatosis Inc. (www.nfnetwork.org).

SUGGESTED READINGS

Available at ExpertConsult.com

RELATED CONTENT

Neurofibromatosis Type 1 (Patient Information)
Neurofibromatosis Type 2 (Patient Information)

AUTHOR: **Craig Blakeney, MD**

BASIC INFORMATION

DEFINITION

Neuroleptic malignant syndrome (NMS) is a disorder characterized by hyperthermia, muscular rigidity, autonomic dysfunction, and depressed/fluctuating levels of arousal that evolve over 24 to 72 hr. This occurs as an idiosyncratic adverse reaction to medications that affect the central dopaminergic system, usually D2 receptors blockade.

SYNONYM

NMS

ICD-10CM CODE

G21.0 Malignant neuroleptic syndrome

EPIDEMIOLOGY & DEMOGRAPHICS

INCIDENCE (IN U.S.): 0.02% to 0.2% annual incidence in psychiatric population

PREDOMINANT SEX: More than two thirds of patients are male.

PREDOMINANT AGE: Young and middle-aged adults

PREDISPOSING FACTORS: History of intake of dopamine antagonists, e.g., antipsychotics

PHYSICAL FINDINGS & CLINICAL PRESENTATION

- Syndrome typically begins abruptly while the patient is taking therapeutic (not toxic) dosages of neuroleptics and reaches maximum severity within 72 hr
- Severe muscle rigidity (hypertonia, cogwheeling, or "lead pipe" rigidity)
- Hyperthermia (38.6° to 42.3° C [101.48° to 108.14° F], usually <40° C [104° F])
- Autonomic symptoms: Diaphoresis, dysphagia, sialorrhea, skin pallor, urinary incontinence
- Tachycardia, tachypnea
- Labile blood pressure (hypertension or postural hypotension)
- Agitation, catatonia, fluctuating consciousness, obtundation

ETIOLOGY

- Exact etiology is unknown, but it has been suggested that sudden and marked dopamine receptor blockade in nigrostriatal, hypothalamic, mesolimbic, and mesocortical pathways leads to clinical manifestations seen in NMS.
- Neuroleptic drugs have different potencies for inducing NMS:
  1. Typical neuroleptics:
     a. High potency: Haloperidol
     b. Medium potency: Chlorpromazine, fluphenazine
     c. Low potency: Levomepromazine, loxapine
  2. Atypical neuroleptics:
     a. Low potency: Risperidone, olanzapine, clozapine, quetiapine

DIAGNOSIS

DIFFERENTIAL DIAGNOSIS

- Infectious: Encephalitis, meningitis, brain abscess, rabies, tetanus, sepsis
- Endocrine: Pheochromocytoma, thyrotoxicosis
- Toxic: Substances of abuse (ecstasy, phencyclidine), heavy metals (lead, arsenic), lithium, salicylates
- Pharmacologic (Table 1): Serotonin syndrome, malignant hyperthermia, drug withdrawal, or overdose
- Environmental: Heatstroke, spider envenomation
- Neuropsychiatric: Catatonia, acute psychosis with agitation, status epilepticus
- Table E2 summarizes the differential diagnosis of neuroleptic malignant syndrome

WORKUP

A careful and thorough drug history should be obtained. There is a significant overlap in the features of NMS and serotonin syndrome. The major difference is the presence of hyperreflexia and myoclonus with serotonin syndrome.

LABORATORY TESTS

- Elevated creatine phosphokinase (CPK) (sensitivity 0.71)
- Urinary myoglobin
- Leukocytosis, usually 10,000 to 40,000/mm^3
- Electrolytes and renal function
- Blood gases
- Drug levels

TREATMENT

NONPHARMACOLOGIC THERAPY

- Stop all neuroleptic drugs and reinstitute any recently discontinued dopaminergic agonists.

TABLE 1 Clinical Features of Serotonin Toxicity, Neuroleptic Malignant Syndrome, and Anticholinergic Syndrome

	Anticholinergic Toxicity	Neuroleptic Malignant Syndrome	Serotonin Syndrome	Adrenergic Toxicity
Tempo	**Rapid onset**	**Slow onset (1-3 days)**	**Rapid onset (min-hr)**	
Mental state:	+++	+++	+ (late stage)	+
1. Confusion	+++	Akathisia	+++	+++
2. Agitation/restlessness	+	++ (severe)		
3. Coma				
Motor system:	+	++	---	---
1. Bradykinesia	+	+	+++	+++
2. Tremor		++ (lead pipe)	+	---
3. Rigidity		0	++	---
4. Hypertonia		--	+++	+++
5. Hyperreflexia		--	+++ (LL > UL)	++
6. Clonus (ankle/eye)		--	+	---
7. Myoclonus			+ (rare)	++
8. Seizures				
Autonomic system[a,b]**:**	---	+++		---
1. Instability	++	Labile (systolic blood pressure >30 mm Hg	+	++
2. Hypertension	++	above baseline)	+	+++
3. Tachycardia	---	Labile (>30 beats/min above baseline)	+++	++
4. Diaphoresis	+++ [c]	+++	++	++
5. Hyperthermia		+++	++	
Others:	---	+++	++	++
1. Rhabdomyolysis	++	---	+++	++
2. Mydriasis				

[a]These features are nonspecific and do not assist in differentiating between syndromes.
[b]Mechanism is excess serotonin.
[c]Mechanism is inability to sweat and unopposed dopamine centrally, leading to dysregulation. +: mild, ++: moderate, +++: severe, ---: not affected.
LL, Lower limbs; UL, upper limbs.
From Cameron P et al: *Textbook of adult emergency medicine*, ed 5, Philadelphia, 2020, Elsevier.

- Remember that metoclopramide is also an antidopaminergic drug that must be discontinued and avoided.
- Respiratory and nutritional support as required.
- Careful fluid balance monitoring with adequate hydration (intravenous in severe cases).
- Active cooling (cooling blanket and antipyretics).
- Skilled nursing care is necessary to prevent decubitus ulcers in bed-confined patients.

ACUTE GENERAL Rx

- Bromocriptine, a dopamine receptor agonist, is the mainstay of therapy for patients with NMS. Initial doses of 2.5 to 10 mg are given IV q8h and are increased by 5 mg/day until clinical improvement is seen. The drug should be continued for at least 10 days after the syndrome has been controlled and then tapered slowly.
- Dantrolene, which blocks calcium efflux from the sarcoplasmic reticulum of skeletal muscles, inhibits the excessive muscle contractions that generate myoglobinemia. Initially, patients can be given 0.25 mg/kg IV q6 to 12h, followed by a maintenance dose up to 3 mg/kg/day. After 2 to 3 days, patients may be given the drug orally (25 to 600 mg/day in divided doses). Oral dantrolene therapy (50 to 600 mg/day) may be continued for several days afterward.
- Amantadine, an N-Methyl-D-aspartate (NMDA) receptor antagonist with possible dopaminergic properties, can be administered orally at doses of 100 to 200 mg PO bid for moderate to severe cases. As an adjunctive treatment, it has been shown to reduce mortality in comparison to supportive therapy alone.
- IV benzodiazepines (e.g., diazepam 2 to 10 mg, with total daily dose of 10 to 60 mg) to relax muscles and control agitation.
- Electroconvulsive therapy with neuromuscular blockage may be beneficial in pharmacologically refractory cases. Succinylcholine should not be used because it may cause hyperkalemia and cardiac arrhythmias in patients with rhabdomyolysis or dysautonomia.

CHRONIC Rx

- Respiratory care, nutritional support, and physical therapy may be required in more severe cases.
- Appropriate therapy would be required in patients with persistent neuropsychiatric sequelae of NMS (e.g., antidepressants for depression, cognitive behavioral therapy for cognitive deficits, rehabilitation for contractures).

DISPOSITION

- Mortality rate is currently 5% to 10% despite therapeutic measures. Serious sequelae may occur in a further 20%. Complete recovery occurs in >70% of patients.
- Rhabdomyolysis is the most common complication. Other complications include acute kidney injury, respiratory failure, pneumonia, and sepsis.
- Causes of death include cardiac arrhythmias, myocardial infarction, renal failure secondary to rhabdomyolysis, seizures, pulmonary edema, and bronchopneumonia.
- Factors adversely affecting mortality are increased age, acute respiratory failure, renal failure, and core temperature >104° F (40° C).
- Patients should be monitored closely for future complications of pharmacologic therapy.

REFERRAL

If the patient's condition is critical, it is preferable to treat the patient in a medical/neurologic ICU.

PEARLS & CONSIDERATIONS

COMMENTS

- Early detection and diagnosis lead to a more favorable outcome. Refer to recent consensus diagnostic criteria as a guide. Treatment is a medical emergency.
- Sudden withdrawal from dopaminergic agents (such as those used in Parkinson disease) may lead to "levodopa withdrawal syndrome" that presents with similar clinical manifestations.
- Patients with dementia with Lewy bodies have increased susceptibility to neuroleptic malignant syndrome.

SUGGESTED READING

Available at ExpertConsult.com

AUTHORS: **Joseph S. Kass, MD, JD, FAAN,** and **Fariha Jamal, MD**

BASIC INFORMATION

DEFINITION

Neuropathic pain is not itself a disease but rather a symptom that is associated with multiple different diseases and localizations within the nervous system. Thus, it is not enough to define its presence without searching for a cause. It is defined as the sensation derived from the abnormal discharges of impaired or injured neural structures in either the peripheral or central nervous system. Descriptors include:

- Hyperesthesia: Heightened sensitivity to nonpainful stimuli (e.g., light touch)
- Hyperalgesia: Heightened sensitivity to painful stimuli (e.g., pinprick), or reduced threshold to feel pain
- Allodynia: Pain provoked by a stimulus that is not normally painful
- Paresthesias: Abnormal sensations, typically "tingling" or "prickling," present with or without any tactile stimulation

SYNONYM

Neuralgia

ICD-10CM CODES

B02.29	Postherpetic neuralgia
G50.0	Trigeminal neuralgia
G58.0	Intercostal neuropathy
G58.7	Mononeuritis multiplex
G58.8	Other specified mononeuropathies
G58.9	Mononeuropathy, unspecified
G61.9	Inflammatory polyneuropathy, unspecified
G62.0	Drug-induced polyneuropathy
G62.1	Alcoholic polyneuropathy
G62.9	Polyneuropathy, unspecified
G63.2	Diabetic polyneuropathy
G63.5	Polyneuropathy in systemic connective tissue disease
G63.8	Polyneuropathy in other diseases classified elsewhere
M79.2	Neuralgia and neuritis, unspecified

EPIDEMIOLOGY & DEMOGRAPHICS

- Estimates of the prevalence of neuropathic pain in the general population range from 1.6% to 8.2%
- Demographics vary widely depending on etiology, for example:
  1. Postherpetic neuralgia: Affects elderly, pain seen in almost 100% of cases
  2. AIDS: 30% of patients affected
  3. Diabetes mellitus: 20% to 24% affected (prevalence rates vary, increasing with longer disease duration); most diabetic neuropathy is painless (although, given the prevalence of diabetes and diabetic neuropathy, it is a common cause of neuropathic pain)
  4. Fabry disease: Affects mostly children, pain in 81% to 90% of patients

PHYSICAL FINDINGS & CLINICAL PRESENTATION

- History: Localize the disease with questions
  1. Quality (description) of neuropathic pain: Burning, hot or cold, "icy hot," "pins and needles," stinging, lancinating, sharp, shooting
  2. Distribution of symptoms may aid in localization (i.e., "stocking-glove" symptoms in generalized neuropathy, numbness in a peripheral nerve territory in focal neuropathy)
  3. Generalized small fiber neuropathy: Dysesthesias without numbness common, but many etiologies (e.g., diabetes) cause both small and large fiber dysfunction
  4. Large fiber neuropathy (LFPN): Coexisting numbness, hyporeflexia, or weakness may be seen, usually worse distally
  5. Nerve root: Coexisting neck or low back pain that radiates along a specific dermatome; most common cause is structural compression
  6. Spinal cord symptoms: Coexisting spasticity, bowel or bladder involvement, sensory level
  7. Prior history of thalamic stroke in central thalamic pain syndrome (Dejerine-Roussy syndrome)
  8. Family history may suggest a genetic cause
- Examination: See Table 1. Table 2 describes joint involvement in neuropathic arthropathy.

Fig. 1 illustrates a diagnostic approach to neuropathic pain. Fig. E2 shows a neuropathic ankle

ETIOLOGY & LABORATORY EVALUATION (TABLE 3)

- Metabolic: Diabetes mellitus; malnutrition and alcoholism; vitamin B_{12} deficiency; thiamine deficiency; porphyria; Fabry disease
- Vascular: Prior stroke usually in the thalamus.
- Inflammatory: Autoimmune diseases (systemic vasculitides, systemic lupus erythematosus, Sjögren syndrome, etc.), acute inflammatory demyelinating polyneuropathy (classically presents with ascending weakness and numbness, although pain is also a common feature), chronic inflammatory demyelinating polyneuropathy, sarcoidosis, multiple sclerosis
- Infiltrative: Amyloidosis, paraproteinemias (e.g., monoclonal gammopathy of uncertain significance [MGUS] associated neuropathy)
- Infectious: Postviral (brachial neuritis), HIV/AIDS, HSV, varicella-zoster virus (VZV; postherpetic neuralgia), Lyme disease, leprosy (thickened nerves and skin lesions), syphilis
- Neoplastic and paraneoplastic-carcinomatous infiltration of nerve/nerve root, anti-Hu
- Drugs/toxins: History of exposure to alcohol, chemotherapeutic agents (paclitaxel,

TABLE 1 Examination

Exam Finding	Localization
Pinprick/temperature loss alone	Small fibers only
Pinprick/temperature loss + vibratory/proprioceptive loss	Small and large fibers
Sensory loss and motor dysfunction worse distally than proximal	Large fiber neuropathy
Sensory loss and motor dysfunction along single nerve distribution	Single nerve
Sensory loss and motor dysfunction along multiple single nerves	Multiple mononeuropathies (i.e., mononeuropathy multiplex)
Motor and sensory loss involving multiple nerves belonging to specific region of brachial or lumbar plexus	Plexopathy
Sensory loss along dermatome with multiple myotomal muscles affected	Nerve root lesion
Asymmetric sensory loss without weakness and pseudoathetosis	Dorsal root ganglion
Vibratory/proprioceptive loss without pinprick/temperature loss	Dorsal column dysfunction (from compressive lesion, B_{12} deficiency, or tabes dorsalis from neurosyphilis)
Sensory level with weakness below the level of lesion and long tract signs (spasticity/Babinski sign)	Spinal cord lesion
Hemisensory hyperalgesia	Contralateral thalamus

TABLE 2 Joint Involvement in Neuropathic Arthropathy

Disease	Site of Involvement
Diabetes mellitus	Midtarsal, metatarsophalangeal, tarsometatarsal
Syringomyelia	Shoulder, elbow, wrist
Amyloidosis	Knee, ankle
Congenital sensory neuropathy	Knee, ankle, intertarsal, metatarsophalangeal
Tabes dorsalis	Knee, hip, ankle
Leprosy	Tarsal, tarsometatarsal

From Hochberg MC et al: *Rheumatology,* ed 5, St Louis, 2011, Mosby.

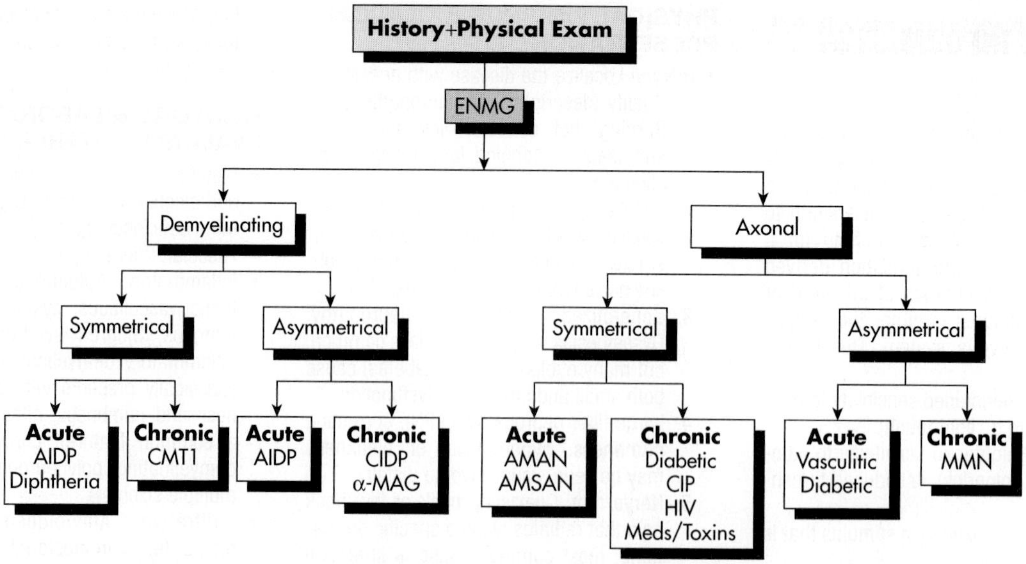

FIG. 1 A systematic approach to evaluate neuropathy. The diseases listed are examples of neuropathies associated with specific neurophysiologic and clinical findings. Diabetic distal, predominantly sensory neuropathies are manifested as chronic axonal neuropathies; acute asymmetric neuropathies can also occur with diabetes. Most neuropathies caused by toxins or by side effects of medication are chronic, symmetric axonal neuropathies. AIDP, AMAN, and AMSAN are subtypes of Guillain-Barré syndrome. These and other examples are discussed in more detail in the text. *AIDP,* Acute inflammatory demyelinating polyradiculoneuropathy; *AMAN,* acute motor axonal neuropathy; *AMSAN,* acute motor and sensory axonal neuropathy; *CIDP,* chronic inflammatory polyradiculoneuropathy; *CIP,* chronic illness polyneuropathy; *CMT1,* Charcot-Marie-Tooth disease type 1, a genetic disorder; *ENMG,* electroneuromyography; *HIV,* human immunodeficiency virus–related neuropathy; *α-MAG,* alpha-myelin-associated glycoprotein; *MMN,* multifocal motor neuropathy. (From Goldman L, Schafer AI: *Goldman's Cecil medicine,* ed 24, Philadelphia, 2012, Saunders.)

vincristine), isoniazid, metronidazole, or heavy metals (thallium, arsenic)

Dx DIAGNOSIS

LABORATORY TESTS

- Fasting blood glucose (FBG)
- 2-hour oral glucose tolerance test (OGTT)
- Vitamin B_{12} level
- If B_{12} level normal: Serum methylmalonic acid and homocysteine levels
- Serum erythrocyte sedimentation rate (ESR), ANA, SS-A and SS-B, c-ANCA, p-ANCA
- RPR or FTA-ABS
- Serum ACE level (sarcoid)
- HIV antibody
- SPEP, UPEP, immunofixation
- Urine and stool protoporphyrins, if porphyria is suspected clinically
- Hu antibody: Can be seen in both small cell and non–small cell lung cancers, may be positive without evidence of lung cancer
- Lumbar puncture: Protein elevation, oligoclonal bands, CSF/serum IgG index

ELECTROPHYSIOLOGY STUDIES

- Electrophysiologic testing (electromyography with nerve conduction studies): May be normal in small fiber neuropathies or CNS lesion, but is often abnormal in large fiber neuropathies
- Quantitative sensory testing: Abnormal in small and large fiber neuropathy
- Evoked potentials (only if suspicion for spinal cord lesion)

PATHOLOGY STUDIES

- Nerve biopsy is occasionally useful in selected cases, particularly when vasculitis, sarcoidosis, or amyloid neuropathy are in the differential.
- Skin biopsy for intraepidermal nerve fiber (IENF) density may be useful for small fiber neuropathy when other studies are normal.
- Rectal or abdominal fat pad biopsy may show amyloid deposition in systemic amyloidosis.

IMAGING STUDIES

Based on localization:
- MRI (with and without contrast):
  1. Of the brain to exclude thalamic pathology if symptoms and signs are consistent with thalamic lesion (hemibody pain)
  2. Of the spinal cord and nerve roots to exclude structural, inflammatory, neoplastic, or infectious causes
  3. Of the lumbar spine to evaluate for arachnoiditis
- If MRI cannot be performed, consider:
  1. CT of the brain for thalamic pathology
  2. CT myelography of the spinal cord to evaluate for structural/neoplastic disease, but only if clinical signs of spinal or nerve root compromise are present

Rx TREATMENT

NONPHARMACOLOGIC THERAPY

- Counseling should be initiated at the beginning of therapy to address psychological issues exacerbating physiologic pain
- Physical therapy: Especially in cases of chronic neck and low back pain
- Cognitive behavioral therapy

ACUTE GENERAL Rx

- Treatment of the underlying cause if possible will help slow or prevent worsening.
- Medications may reduce or alleviate pain but do not affect numbness.
- Antidepressants:
  1. Tricyclic antidepressants (TCAs): Nortriptyline preferred over amitriptyline (fewer anticholinergic side effects with nortriptyline). Begin 25 mg PO qd in adults, or 10 mg qd in elderly. Increase dose by 25 mg every wk as tolerated until usual maximal effective dose of 150 mg/day.
  2. Duloxetine: Begin 30 mg daily, increase to 60 to 120 mg daily. Duloxetine is effective in diabetic neuropathy, post-herpetic neuropathy, and chemotherapy-induced painful peripheral neuropathy.
  3. Venlafaxine.
- Antiepileptics:
  1. Gabapentin: Begin 300 mg PO qd, advance to 300 mg PO tid by the end of the first wk. Effective dose: Higher than 1600 mg/day. Max dose: 1200 mg PO tid.
  2. Carbamazepine: For trigeminal neuralgia. Begin 400 mg PO bid, increase to tid if necessary. Side effects and drug levels help to determine optimal dosing. Risk of aplastic anemia and hyponatremia (monitor CBC and chemistries). Risk of Stevens-Johnson syndrome, especially in Asian population (check HLA before starting).

TABLE 3 Clinical Presentation and Laboratory Findings

Neuropathy Type	Predisposition	Examination Findings	EMG/NCS	Laboratory Analysis
Idiopathic small fiber PN	Age >50	Strength: Normal Reflexes: Normal Pos/vib: Normal Pain/temp: Decreased distally	Normal	Serum studies: Normal skin biopsy: Abnormal sudomotor studies: Abnormal
Diabetic PN	Long-standing disease, family history	Strength normal to reduced, sensation reduced distally	Abnormal	Abnormal glucose tolerance: High fasting glucose
Inherited PN	Family history	Pes cavus, hammer toes, reduced reflexes, sensation reduced distally	Abnormal	Genetic studies may be abnormal, other studies normal
Familial amyloid PN	Family history	Pain/temp loss, reduced reflexes, orthostasis	Abnormal if large fibers affected; also carpal tunnel syndrome	Transthyretin genetic study
Acquired amyloid PN	Monoclonal gammopathy	Pain/temp loss, reduced reflexes, orthostasis	Abnormal if large fibers affected; also carpal tunnel syndrome	SPEP, UPEP, immunofixation abnormal
Fabry disease	Age, renal failure, strokes	Normal; possible reduced pain/temp sensation	Normal	α-Galactosidase levels in cultured fibroblasts
PN + mixed connective tissue disease	History of lupus, rheumatoid arthritis, Sjögren syndrome	Reduced reflexes and distal sensation	Abnormal	ANA, RF, SS-A/SS-B may be abnormal
Peripheral nerve vasculitis	Asymmetric disease	Multiple peripheral nerves involved	Abnormal	ANA, RF, SS-A/SS-B, ANCA, cryoglobulins may be abnormal
Paraneoplastic neuropathy	Lung cancer risk factors, chemical exposures	Asymmetric sensory loss, pseudoathetosis, relatively preserved strength	Abnormal	Anti-Hu
Sarcoidosis	Pulmonary sarcoid	Multiple mononeuropathies	Abnormal	Abnormal biopsy, elevated serum ACE, CXR abnormal
Arsenic	Pesticides, copper smelting	Reduced reflexes and distal sensation	Abnormal	Elevated arsenic in plasma, urine, and hair
HIV	Promiscuity, unprotected sex, IV drug abuse, blood transfusion	Variable, but most often reduced reflexes and distal sensation	Abnormal if large fibers involved	HIV antibody

ACE, Angiotensin-converting enzyme; *ANA*, antibody to nuclear antigens; *ANCA*, antineutrophil cytoplasmic antibodies; *CXR*, chest x-ray; *EMG*, electromyography; *HIV*, human immunodeficiency virus; *IV*, intravenous; *NCS*, nerve conduction studies; *PN*, polyneuropathy; *Pos*, position sensation; *RF*, rheumatoid factor; *SPEP*, serum protein electrophoresis; *SS-A*, Sjögren syndrome A; *SS-B*, Sjögren syndrome B; *Temp*, temperature sensation; *UPEP*, urine protein electrophoresis; *Vib*, vibration sensation.
Adapted from Mendell JR, Sahenk Z: Painful sensory neuropathy, *N Engl J Med* 348(13):1243, 2003.

3. Oxcarbazepine: Better tolerated than carbamazepine. Start 150 mg PO bid and gradually increase to a dose of 600 mg bid. Maximum dose is 1200 mg bid.
4. Pregabalin: Begin 50 mg PO tid, increase slowly to 100 to 200 mg PO tid.

- Analgesics: When first-line agents are ineffective. While effective, the use of opioids is associated with substantial adverse effects as well as novel pain syndromes. Chronic use of opioids leads to tolerance and escalation of dose:
  1. Tramadol: 150 mg/day (50 mg tid), increase by 50 mg/wk, max 200 to 400 mg/day
  2. Morphine (oral): 15 to 30 mg q8h, max 90 to 360 mg/day
  3. Oxycodone: 20 mg q12h, increase by 10 mg/wk, max 40 to 160 mg/day
  4. Fentanyl patch: 25 to 100 mcg transdermally q3 days
- Topical anesthetics:
  1. 5% lidocaine patch, apply to area of pain, max three patches every 12 hr.
  2. Capsaicin cream and patches are inconsistent in their ability to relieve pain and may exacerbate it. A capsaicin 8% patch is approved specifically for post-herpetic neuralgia and is applied for 60 min under medical supervision.
- Procedural/surgical: This option is considered mostly when the patient suffers from pain secondary to spinal cord or cauda equina injury. Procedures should be considered only when all other therapeutic modalities have failed. In addition, the patient should be cautioned that surgical procedures may not result in pain relief and may be associated with significant morbidity and even mortality.
  1. Dorsal root rhizotomy
  2. Nerve blocks
  3. Spinal cord stimulator

DISPOSITION

Prognosis depends on multiple factors, including:

- Etiology of pain
- Treatment of any underlying condition
- Initiation of appropriate (often multiple) therapeutic modalities
- Patient compliance with prescribed regimen

Most care is accomplished in the outpatient setting, except when surgery is required.

REFERRAL

- Pain clinic
- Neurology
- Psychiatry
- Psychology
- Physiatry
- Anesthesiology (nerve blocks)
- Neurosurgery if considering surgical management

PEARLS & CONSIDERATIONS

- Factitious disorder and malingering frequently manifest with pain complaints. These are diagnoses of exclusion and require negative evaluation for organic etiologies before diagnosis is made.
- Peripheral neuropathy in diabetics increases the risk of foot ulceration by sevenfold. Abnormal results in monofilament testing and vibratory perception (alone or in combination with the appearance of the feet, ulceration, and ankle reflexes) are the most helpful sign for the detection of LFPN.

SUGGESTED READINGS

Available at ExpertConsult.com

AUTHOR: **Corey Goldsmith, MD**

BASIC INFORMATION

DEFINITION

An unprovoked seizure is a seizure that occurs without triggers or precipitating factors. In contrast, an acute symptomatic seizure occurs in the setting of an insult to the brain (infectious, toxic, etc.). The presentation of a new seizure can vary greatly depending on the type (focal or generalized), progression, and severity.

SYNONYM

Convulsions

ICD-10CM CODES

G40.001	Localization-related (focal) (partial) idiopathic epilepsy and epileptic syndromes with seizures of localized onset, not intractable, with status epilepticus
G40.009	Localization-related (focal) (partial) idiopathic epilepsy and epileptic syndromes with seizures of localized onset, not intractable, without status epilepticus
G40.10	Localization-related (focal) (partial) symptomatic epilepsy and epileptic syndromes with simple partial seizures, not intractable
G40.101	Localization-related (focal) (partial) symptomatic epilepsy and epileptic syndromes with simple partial seizures, not intractable, with status epilepticus
G40.109	Localization-related (focal) (partial) symptomatic epilepsy and epileptic syndromes with simple partial seizures, not intractable, without status epilepticus
G40.201	Localization-related (focal) (partial) symptomatic epilepsy and epileptic syndromes with complex partial seizures, not intractable, with status epilepticus
G40.209	Localization-related (focal) (partial) symptomatic epilepsy and epileptic syndromes with complex partial seizures, not intractable, without status epilepticus
G40.301	Generalized idiopathic epilepsy and epileptic syndromes, not intractable, with status epilepticus
G40.309	Generalized idiopathic epilepsy and epileptic syndromes, not intractable, without status epilepticus
G40.A01	Absence epileptic syndrome, not intractable, with status epilepticus
G40.A09	Absence epileptic syndrome, not intractable, without status epilepticus
G40.4	Other generalized epilepsy and epileptic syndromes
G40.401	Other generalized epilepsy and epileptic syndromes, not intractable, with status epilepticus
G40.409	Other generalized epilepsy and epileptic syndromes, not intractable, without status epilepticus
G40.501	Epileptic seizures related to external causes, not intractable, with status epilepticus
G40.509	Epileptic seizures related to external causes, not intractable, without status epilepticus
G40.909	Epilepsy, unspecified, not intractable, without status epilepticus

EPIDEMIOLOGY & DEMOGRAPHICS

INCIDENCE: 29 to 39 per 100,000 per yr for acute symptomatic seizures. 23 to 61 per 100,000 person-yr for unprovoked seizures. Approximately 8% to 10% of the population will experience a seizure during their lifetime; however, less than 3% go on to develop epilepsy.

PREVALENCE: 5 to 8.4 cases per 1000 persons

PREDOMINANT SEX & AGE: Males younger than 12 mo and older than 65 yr

RISK FACTORS:

- Age of onset
- Family history of epilepsy
- Excessive sleep deprivation, use of alcohol, or illicit drugs
- History of head trauma, diseases of the brain, brain surgeries, and strokes
- History of congenital cerebral anomalies or developmental delay

GENETICS: Although some new onset seizures are related to specific genes, most are not.

PHYSICAL FINDINGS & CLINICAL PRESENTATION

- Patients with generalized seizures will typically have normal physical exams. Patients with focal seizures due to persistent structural CNS damage may have exam findings consistent with the location of the lesion.
- A generalized seizure may start without warning and can typically last from 30 to 120 seconds, during which the patient will be unconscious and may have increased rigidity and/or jerking of the whole body, or staring spells. Cyanosis (especially of the lips and face) can result from temporary airway compromise due to muscle spasms. Tonic-clonic seizures can cause injuries, tongue biting, and bladder incontinence. Patients are usually unaware of the seizure afterwards. A postictal state characterized by confusion, lethargy, headaches, or drowsiness may result and can last from min to hours depending on the severity of the seizure.
- During a focal seizure, a patient may be aware (focal aware seizure) or have impaired consciousness (focal impaired awareness seizures). A focal impaired awareness seizure may be associated with an aura (itself a focal aware seizure) and lasts between 30 and 120 seconds. Motor or nonmotor symptoms may predominate in focal seizures, including jerking of one limb, automatisms, head turning, auditory hallucinations, or feelings of derealization. A focal seizure may progress to a generalized seizure, which usually involves the head and eye turning to one side. Postictal weakness may result after focal seizures and can last for hours but usually resolves within 1 day. Persistent neurological deficits beyond this time may indicate other causes and should be investigated.

ETIOLOGY

- New, unprovoked seizures are often idiopathic.
- Acute symptomatic seizures can be due to cerebral abnormalities (e.g., infections/abscesses, subarachnoid hemorrhages, ischemic strokes, tumors, arteriovenous malformations, venous malformations) or systemic causes (e.g., systemic infections, electrolyte abnormalities, hypoglycemia, hyperthyroidism, malignant hypertension, drug intoxication or withdrawal).

Dx DIAGNOSIS

DIFFERENTIAL DIAGNOSIS

- Syncope
- Transient ischemic attacks
- Migraines
- Sleep disorders
- Paroxysmal movement disorders
- Panic attacks, hallucinations, and other psychiatric disorders

WORKUP

- Ambulatory 30-min EEG if patient fully recovers after seizure within 30 to 60 min. May be delayed if treatment does not depend on EEG result.
- Consider inpatient continuous EEG if patient does not fully recover within 60 min or for recurrent seizures.
- ECG.
- Fig. 1 illustrates an algorithm for the approach to the child with a suspected convulsive disorder.

LABORATORY TESTS

Comprehensive metabolic panel and urine drug screen

IMAGING STUDIES

- Acutely, CT of the head with and without contrast to evaluate for hemorrhage and space-occupying lesions
- Brain MRI with and without contrast with epilepsy protocol in patients with no clear provoking cause of a seizure, in consultation with a neurologist

Rx TREATMENT

ACUTE Rx

- The immediate management of a seizure focuses on stabilization of the patient with focus on the airway and vital signs and rapid identification and correction of reversible causes.

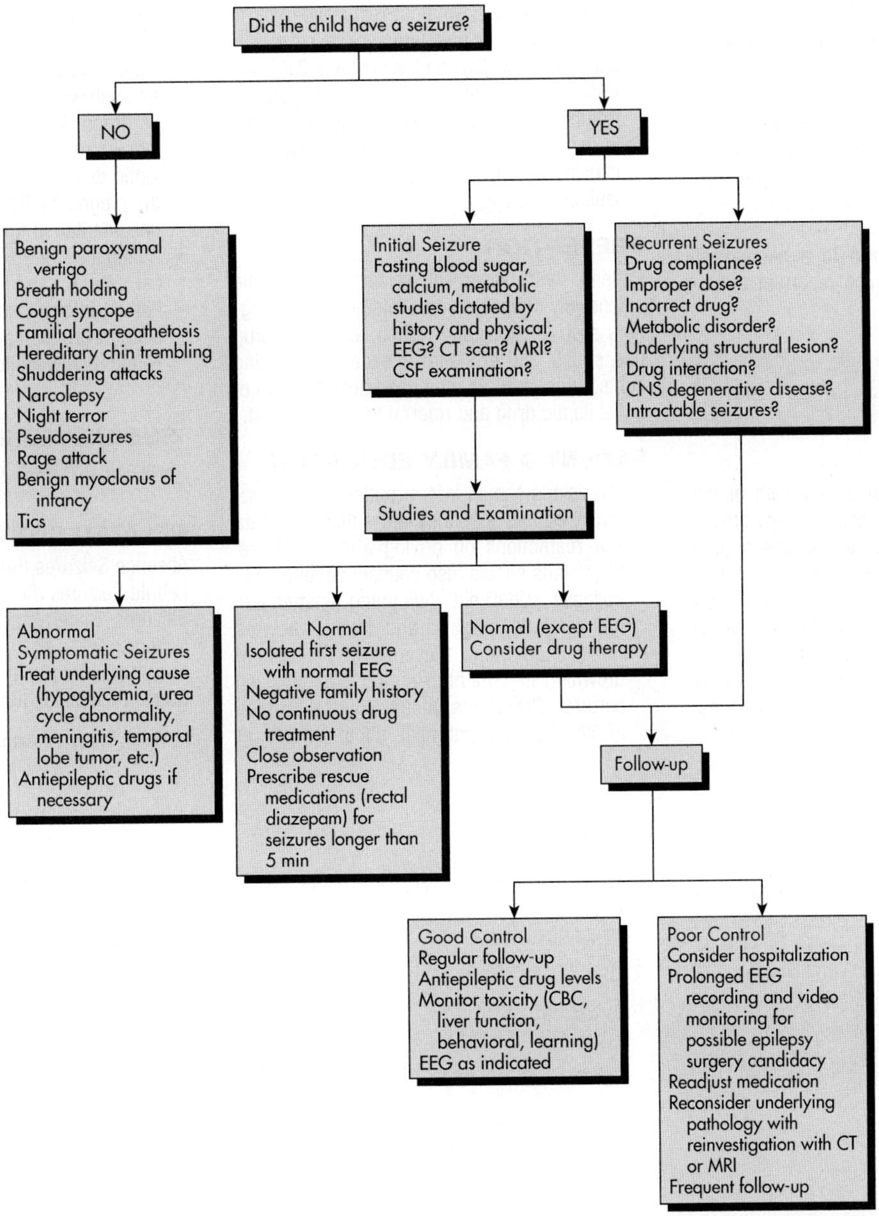

FIG. 1 Algorithm for the approach to the child with a suspected convulsive disorder. *CBC,* Complete blood count; *CT,* computed tomography; *CNS,* central nervous system; *CSF,* cerebrospinal fluid; *EEG,* electroencephalogram; *MRI,* magnetic resonance imaging. (From Kliegman RM: *Nelson textbook of pediatrics,* ed 21, Philadelphia, 2020, Elsevier.)

- Seizures lasting >5 min or multiple seizures without return to baseline in between should be treated as status epilepticus.
- Treatment is based on the type and etiology of seizures (i.e., metabolic disturbance, infectious, unprovoked, etc.).

CHRONIC Rx

- Provoked seizures do not need long-term treatment.
- Patients with a first unprovoked seizure who have a normal EEG, imaging, lab values, and physical exam do not require treatment with antiepileptic drugs but may be offered therapy because the use of an antiepileptic drug after a first unprovoked seizure in an adult reduces the absolute risk of seizure recurrence at 2 yr by 35%. However, there is no difference at 3 yr. This decision should be made in conjunction with the patient and should take into consideration the patient's job, risks of medications, and individual preferences.
- Patients with two or more unprovoked seizures, or those with one seizure and an abnormal workup consistent with epilepsy findings, should be started or continued on antiepileptic drugs. Patients on antiepileptic therapy with negative workup may be considered for weaning off antiepileptic drug if seizure-free after 2 yr.
- The choice of treatment depends largely on seizure type and etiology. Antiepileptics may be thought of as narrow- or wide-spectrum drugs. Treatment with wide-spectrum antiepileptics is advisable in generalized seizures or those of unknown type, whereas partial seizures are better controlled with narrow-spectrum antiepileptics.
- Narrow-spectrum drugs include carbamazepine, oxcarbazepine, gabapentin, pregabalin, lacosamide, and phenytoin. Wide-spectrum drugs include valproate, topiramate, zonisamide, lamotrigine, and levetiracetam.
- In patients with significant comorbidities, the use of antiepileptics with limited drug interactions is advised (lamotrigine, levetiracetam, lacosamide).
- Older patients may benefit from lamotrigine, levetiracetam, or gabapentin due to a lower risk of adverse events.

DISPOSITION

- Patients should avoid swimming unobserved, bathing alone, working at heights, using heavy machinery, or other activities that may be high-risk in the event of a seizure.
- Discontinue driving until seizures are well controlled and in accordance with state laws.

REFERRAL

Patients should be referred to a neurologist, especially if they experience recurrent unprovoked seizures.

PEARLS & CONSIDERATIONS

COMMENTS

- Driving: Physicians should be aware of the law in their jurisdiction about driving after a seizure. Although a few U.S. states require physicians to notify the state government authority that issues driver's licenses, most do not impose such an obligation on physicians. However, states do require patients to self-report and abstain from driving until seizure-free for a specified period of time, depending on the state.
- Recurrence risk: Greatest recurrence risk in an adult with a first unprovoked seizure is within the first 2 yr and is between 21% and 45%. The recurrence risk is lower in patients treated with an antiepileptic drug and higher in patients with a brain MRI abnormality causing the seizure or an EEG showing epileptiform activity.

PREVENTION

Patients with recurrent seizures should be extensively counseled on avoiding seizure triggers such as sleep deprivation, alcohol or drug use, stress, and exposure to excessive flashing lights. Such patients may need dose titration of antiepileptic drug and referral to a neurologist.

PATIENT & FAMILY EDUCATION

- Physicians should inform patients with first-time seizures that they are subject to state law restrictions on driving after a seizure. Physicians should also counsel patients with epilepsy about not swimming unattended, not climbing heights, and taking showers rather than baths (because of the risk of drowning in a bathtub during a generalized seizure). Physicians should counsel women of childbearing potential about effects of antiepileptic drugs on both oral contraceptive efficacy and on a developing fetus. They should recommend supplemental folic acid for such women if they are taking antiepileptic drugs. They should also recommend that women plan pregnancy if they are on antiepileptic drugs to minimize adverse effects on the pregnancy. All such counseling should be documented in the medical record.
- A diagnosis of epilepsy has significant medical, social, and emotional consequences. Patient information on seizures and locating support groups can be found at the Epilepsy Foundation website: www.epilepsy.com.

SUGGESTED READINGS

Available at ExpertConsult.com

RELATED CONTENT

Absence Seizures (Related Key Topic)
Febrile Seizures (Related Key Topic)
Seizures, Generalized Tonic-Clinic (Related Key Topic)
Focal Seizures (Related Key Topic)
Status Epilepticus (Related Key Topic)

AUTHOR: **Corey Goldsmith, MD**

BASIC INFORMATION

DEFINITION

- *Nonalcoholic fatty liver disease* (NAFLD) is a spectrum of diseases based on histopathologic findings and representing a morphologic rather than a clinical diagnosis. It is liver disease occurring in patients who do not abuse alcohol and manifesting histologically by mononuclear cells and/or polymorphonuclear cells, hepatocyte ballooning, and spotty necrosis. Nonalcoholic steatohepatitis (NASH) is a subset of NAFLD. Patients with NASH have progressive disease that can result in fibrosis and cirrhosis. A diagnosis of NAFLD is contingent on the following factors:
  1. Alcohol consumption in amounts less than those considered hepatotoxic.
  2. Absence of serologic evidence of other hepatic diseases or disorders.
  3. Liver biopsy showing predominant macrovesicular steatosis or steatohepatitis.
- NAFL is defined as ≥5% hepatic steatosis without evidence of hepatocellular injury or fibrosis.
- NASH is ≥5% hepatic fibrosis with inflammation and hepatocellular injury with or without fibrosis.
- *NASH cirrhosis* is the presence of cirrhosis with current or past evidence of steatosis.

SYNONYMS

Nonalcoholic steatohepatitis (NASH)
NAFLD
Fatty liver hepatitis
Diabetes hepatitis
Alcohol-like liver disease
Laënnec disease

ICD-10CM CODE
K76.0 Fatty (change of) liver, not elsewhere classified

EPIDEMIOLOGY & DEMOGRAPHICS

- NAFLD affects 30% of the adult general population in the U.S.
- Increased prevalence in obese persons (57% to 74%), type 2 diabetes mellitus, and hyperlipidemia (primarily hypertriglyceridemia).
- Most common cause of abnormal liver test results in adults in the United States (accounts for up to 90% of cases of asymptomatic ALT elevations).
- NAFLD is more prevalent in men than women.
- NAFLD is more prevalent in the Hispanic population.
- Approximately 20% of patients with NAFLD have NASH, and 10% to 30% of patients with NASH have NASH cirrhosis.

PHYSICAL FINDINGS & CLINICAL PRESENTATION

- Most patients are asymptomatic.
- Patients may report a sensation of fullness or discomfort on the right side of the upper abdomen.
- Nonspecific complaints of fatigue or malaise may be reported.
- Hepatomegaly (Table 1) is generally the only positive finding on physical examination.
- Acanthosis nigricans may be found in children.

ETIOLOGY

- Metabolic syndrome and insulin resistance are the most reproducible factors in the development of NAFLD and accumulation of triglycerides within the liver. High baseline and continuously increasing fasting insulin levels are independent determinants for

TABLE 1 Symptoms, Signs, and Laboratory Features of Nonalcoholic Fatty Liver Disease

Symptoms	Signs	Laboratory Features
Common		
None (48%-100% of patients)	Hepatomegaly	2- to 4-fold elevation of serum ALT and AST levels AST/ALT ratio <1 in most patients Serum alkaline phosphatase level slightly elevated in one third of patients Normal serum bilirubin, serum albumin, and prothrombin time Elevated serum ferritin level
Uncommon		
Vague right upper quadrant pain Fatigue Malaise	Splenomegaly Spider telangiectasias Palmar erythema Ascites	Low-titer (<1:320) antinuclear antibodies

ALT, Alanine aminotransferase; *AST,* aspartate aminotransferase.
From Feldman M et al: *Sleisenger and Fordtran's gastrointestinal and liver disease,* ed 10, Philadelphia, 2016, Elsevier.

BOX 1 Causes of Fatty Liver Disease

Acquired Metabolic Disorders
Diabetes mellitus
Dyslipidemia
Kwashiorkor and marasmus
Obesity
Rapid weight loss
Starvation

Cytotoxic and Cytostatic Drugs
L-Asparaginase
Azacitidine
Bleomycin
Cisplatin
5-Fluorouracil
Methotrexate
Tetracyclines (inhibit mitochondrial beta oxidation)

Other Drugs and Toxins
Amiodarone
Camphor
Chloroform
Cocaine
Ethanol
Ethyl bromide
Estrogens
Glucocorticoids
Griseofulvin
HAART (zidovudine, stavudine, didanosine)
Lycopodium serratum (Jin Bu Huan, an herbal supplement)
Nifedipine
Nitrofurantoin
NSAIDs (piroxicam, ibuprofen, indomethacin, sulindac)
Tamoxifen
Valproic acid

Metals
Antimony
Barium salts
Chromates
Mercury
Phosphorus
Rare earth metals of low atomic number
Thallium compounds
Uranium compounds

Inborn Errors of Metabolism
Abetalipoproteinemia
Familial hepatosteatosis
Galactosemia
Glycogen storage disease
Hereditary fructose intolerance
Homocystinuria
Systemic carnitine deficiency
Tyrosinemia
Weber-Christian syndrome
Wilson disease

Surgical Procedures
Biliopancreatic diversion
Extensive small bowel resection
Jejunoileal bypass

Miscellaneous Conditions
Industrial exposure to petrochemicals
IBD
Jejunal diverticulosis with bacterial overgrowth
Partial lipodystrophy
TPN

HAART, Highly active antiretroviral therapy; *IBD,* inflammatory bowel disease; *NSAIDs,* nonsteroidal antiinflammatory drugs; *TPN,* total parenteral nutrition.
From Feldman M et al: *Sleisenger and Fordtran's gastrointestinal and liver disease,* ed 10, Philadelphia, 2016, Elsevier.

TABLE 2 NAFLD Activity Score on a Liver Biopsy Specimen

Steatosis	
5%	1
5%-33%	2
33%-66%	3
Ballooning	
None	0
Few	1
Many	2
Lobular Inflammation	
Mild	1
Moderate	2
Severe	3
Total Score	
0-2	Likely not NASH
3-4	Intermediate
5-8	Likely NASH

NAFLD, Nonalcoholic fatty liver disease; *NASH,* nonalcoholic steatohepatitis.

From Feldman M et al: *Sleisenger and Fordtran's gastrointestinal and liver disease,* ed 10, Philadelphia, 2016, Elsevier.

future development of NAFLD. The transition from NAFLD to NASH is poorly understood; there may be a genetic component. The presence of the I48M variant of PNPLA3 increases risk for and severity of NAFLD. Genetic polymorphism (TM6SF2) also increases NAFLD risk.

- Risk factors are obesity (especially truncal obesity), diabetes mellitus, hyperlipidemia.

Dx DIAGNOSIS

DIFFERENTIAL DIAGNOSIS

- Alcohol-induced liver disease (a daily alcohol intake of 20 g in females and 30 g in males [three 12-oz beers or 12 oz of wine] may be enough to cause alcohol-induced liver disease)
- Viral hepatitis
- Autoimmune hepatitis
- Toxin- or drug-induced liver disease
- Box 1 summarizes the various causes of fatty liver disease

WORKUP

Diagnosis is usually suspected on the basis of hepatomegaly, asymptomatic elevations of transaminases, or "fatty liver" on sonogram of abdomen in obese patients with little or no alcohol use. Fig. E1 describes an algorithm for the diagnostic approach to NAFLD. Transient elastography is a noninvasive imaging modality that can be used to screen for the development of hepatic fibrosis. In obese patients newer "XL" FibroScan machines are more accurate. Liver biopsy can confirm diagnosis and provide prognostic information. It should be considered in patients with suspected advanced liver fibrosis (presence of obesity or type 2 diabetes, AST/ALT ratio 1, age 45 yr). NAFLD activity score on liver biopsy is described in Table 2.

LABORATORY TESTS

- Elevated ALT, AST: AST/ALT ratio is usually <1, but can increase as fibrosis advances. In advanced fibrosis AST to ALT ratio is >1 and platelet count is low.
- Negative serology for infectious hepatitis; generally normal GGTP and serum alkaline phosphatase.
- Hyperlipidemia (primarily hypertriglyceridemia) may be present.
- Elevated glucose levels may be present.
- Prolonged prothrombin time, hypoalbuminemia, and elevated bilirubin may be present in advanced stages.
- Elevated serum ferritin and increased transferrin saturation may be found in up to 10% of patients; however, hepatic iron index and hepatic iron level are normal.
- Antismooth muscle antibodies and antinuclear antibodies at low titer are not uncommon.

IMAGING STUDIES

- Ultrasound generally reveals diffuse increase in echogenicity as compared with that of the kidneys; CT scan reveals diffuse low-density hepatic parenchyma. The sensitivity of ultrasound and CT scan for detection of fat in liver is over 90% if hepatic steatosis exceeds 33%.
- Occasionally patients may have focal rather than diffuse steatosis, which may be misinterpreted as a liver mass on ultrasound or CT (Fig. E2); use of MRI in these cases will identify focal fatty infiltration.
- Vibration-controlled elastography (FibroScan) can also be used to evaluate hepatic fibrosis and to further stratify patients.

Rx TREATMENT

NONPHARMACOLOGIC THERAPY

- Weight reduction in all obese patients. The American Gastroenterological Association recommends that the initial target weight loss be 10% of baseline weight at a rate of 1 to 2 lb (0.45 to 0.90 kg) per week.
- Increase physical activity. Vigorous and moderate exercise are equally effective in reducing intrahepatic triglyceride content, the effect being largely mediated by weight loss.
- Alcohol has a deleterious effect on NAFLD and should be avoided.

ACUTE GENERAL Rx

- There are no drugs currently approved by FDA for NAFLD. Medications to control hyperlipidemia (e.g., fenofibrates for elevated triglycerides) and hyperglycemia (e.g., pioglitazone, insulin, metformin) can lead to improvement in abnormal liver test results.
- A 3-yr trial with pioglitazone (30 mg/day), an insulin-sensitizing thiazolidinedione, revealed that pioglitazone treatment was associated with long-term metabolic and histologic improvement in patients with prediabetes or type 2 diabetes mellitus and NASH. These results suggest that NASH progression may be halted and the natural history of the disease may be modified with the use of pioglitazone in patients with prediabetes or type 2 diabetes mellitus.[1] Glucagon-like peptide-1 receptor agonists (GLP-1RA) like liraglutide have shown modest improvement in reduction of plasma aminotransferase and steatosis.[3]

DISPOSITION

- Patients with pure steatosis on liver biopsy generally have a relatively benign course.
- The presence of steatohepatitis or advanced fibrosis on liver biopsy is associated with a worse prognosis.

REFERRAL

Liver transplantation should be considered in patients with decompensated, end-stage disease; however, in these patients there may be a recurrence of NAFLD posttransplantation.

PEARLS & CONSIDERATIONS

COMMENTS

- NAFLD is closely associated with metabolic disorders, even in nonobese, nondiabetic subjects. It can be considered an early predictor of metabolic disorders, particularly in the normal-weight population. The presence of metabolic syndrome is a strong predictor of NAFLD.
- NAFLD is associated with an increased risk of incident cardiovascular disease that is independent of the risk conferred by traditional risk factors and components of the metabolic syndrome.
- 10% of patients with NASH have progression to advanced fibrosis. Most common in patients older than 50, ALT > twice normal, BMI >28, triglycerides >150 mg/dl.
- Statins are not contraindicated in patients with NASH and should be considered in hypercholesterolemic patients.
- A recent trial has shown that daily aspirin use is associated with reduced risk for fibrosis progression in patients with NAFLD.[2]

SUGGESTED READINGS

Available at ExpertConsult.com

RELATED CONTENT

Fatty Liver (Patient Information)

AUTHOR: **Fred F. Ferri, MD**

[1]Cusi K et al: Long-term pioglitazone treatment for patients with nonalcoholic steatohepatitis and prediabetes or type 2 diabetes mellitus: a randomized trial, *Ann Intern Med* 165:305-315, 2016.

[2]Simon TG et al: Daily aspirin use associated with reduced risk for fibrosis progression in patients With nonalcoholic fatty liver disease, *Clin Gastroenterol Hepatol* 17(13):2776-2784.e4, 2019.

[3]Cusi K: Incretin-based therapies for the management of nonalcoholic fatty liver disease in patients with type 2 diabetes, *Hepatology* 69(6):2318-2322, 2019.

BASIC INFORMATION

DEFINITION

Non-allergic rhinitis (NAR) involves dysfunction and inflammation of nasal mucosa defined as a pathogenically distinct process from allergic rhinitis (AR) in that it is not driven by IgE-mediated events. However, symptoms may be similar to those with AR, with patients presenting with acute or chronic rhinorrhea, severe congestion, and postnasal drainage. Triggers of NAR symptoms vary and can include infections, medications, foods, hormones, airborne irritants, temperature changes, and chronic health conditions.

SYNONYMS

Vasomotor rhinitis
Non-allergic, non-infectious rhinitis
Atrophic rhinitis
Eosinophilic nonallergic rhinitis
Gustatory rhinitis
Hypertrophic rhinitis
Irritant rhinitis
Mixed rhinitis
Rhinitis medicamentosa

ICD-10CM CODES

J30.0	Vasomotor rhinitis
J31.0	Chronic rhinitis (atrophic rhinitis, granulomatous rhinitis, hypertrophic rhinitis, obstructive rhinitis, ozena, purulent rhinitis, rhinitis NOS, ulcerative rhinitis)

EPIDEMIOLOGY & DEMOGRAPHICS

- NAR affects approximately 7% of the U.S. population (approximately 23 million people).
- Approximately 50% of patients presenting with rhinitis symptoms may have NAR alone or a mixed form of rhinitis that includes both allergic and nonallergic components.
- Unlike AR that typically presents in childhood, NAR usually presents in adulthood with 70% of patients presenting after the age of 20.
- Risk factors include female sex (hormonal changes), chronic health conditions (hypothyroid, diabetes mellitus), genetic predisposition in individuals whose parents have AR, prolonged use of nasal decongestants, exposure to irritants (smoke, smog, fumes), and occupational exposures.

PHYSICAL FINDINGS & CLINICAL PRESENTATION

- NAR is a clinical diagnosis that is distinguished from AR in that it has a later age of onset, absence of nasal and ocular itching, and absence of prominent sneezing.
- Physical exam may be completely unremarkable but typically presents with:
  1. Nasal and pharyngeal discharge that may be clear or mucopurulent (as in infectious rhinitis)
  2. Nasal congestion, sometimes with pain and pressure
  3. Cough
- Nasal mucosa is typically boggy and edematous with hypertrophic, congested turbinates.

ETIOLOGY

- NAR involves a heterogeneous group of diseases without a clear unifying theory of pathogenesis, but most subtypes involve variable autonomic dysregulation with nasal hyperresponsiveness to environmental triggers (e.g., smog, perfume, tobacco smoke, chemical fumes, mining dust, temperature or humidity changes) or chronic health conditions (hypothyroidism, diabetes mellitus) with subsequent inflammatory or nociceptive responses that culminate in increased vasodilation, glandular hypersecretion, and acute or chronic nasal congestion.
- NAR includes both non-infectious rhinitis (vasomotor rhinitis, food-induced rhinitis, hormonal rhinitis, atrophic rhinitis, drug-induced rhinitis, non-allergic occupational rhinitis, non-allergic rhinitis with eosinophilia, and senile rhinitis) and infectious rhinitis. Specific subtypes likely have unique pathophysiologies:
  1. Vasomotor rhinitis: Diagnosis of exclusion after AR has been ruled out, sometimes referred to as idiopathic rhinitis. Likely involves hypersensitivity to triggers (temperature changes, airborne irritants like tobacco smoke, and exercise).
  2. Food-induced (gustatory) rhinitis: Abnormal vagally-mediated rhinitis typically after ingestion of hot or spicy foods (but can occur with any foods) or alcohol (alcohol-induced rhinitis) that produces primarily rhinorrhea and congestion sometimes with lacrimation, sweating, and flushing.
  3. Hormone-induced rhinitis: Vascular engorgement and airway obstruction due to hormonal changes during pregnancy, menstruation, oral contraceptive (OCP) use, or severe hypothyroidism. Typically resolves after delivery or discontinuation of estrogen-containing OCPs.
  4. Atrophic rhinitis: Unknown etiology of progressive atrophy of the nasal mucosa with foul-smelling nasal crusts likely related to bacterial colonization with Klebsiella ozaenae. In developed countries, more commonly seen in patients with repeated nasal surgery.
  5. Drug-induced rhinitis: Sensitivity to specific drugs or disruption of certain drug classes (e.g., sympatholytics). Rhinitis medicamentosa refers to rebound nasal congestion and rhinorrhea from prolonged use (typically more than 7 to 10 days) of decongestants. Medications that can cause chronic nasal symptoms are summarized in Table E1.
  6. Non-allergic occupational rhinitis: Occupations with increased prevalence of work-related rhinitis are summarized in Table E2.
  7. Non-allergic rhinitis with eosinophilia syndrome (NARES): Unknown etiology with AR symptoms (in the absence of facial pain or nasal obstruction) and elevated nasal eosinophils but without positive skin prick testing or specific IgE blood tests.
  8. Senile rhinitis (rhinitis of the elderly): Frequently drug-induced, but also secondary to poorly understood physiologic changes likely due to imbalances in parasympathetic and sympathetic tone.
  9. Infectious rhinitis/rhinosinusitis: Due to viral infections in 98% of cases, less commonly bacterial or fungal infections. Very common in pediatric populations.

DIAGNOSIS

DIFFERENTIAL DIAGNOSIS

- Allergic rhinitis (sensitivity to pollens, indoor allergens, occupational allergens)
- Mixed rhinitis (components of both AR and NAR)
- Mechanical obstruction (e.g., deviated septum, nasal polyps, nasal neoplasms, adenoid or turbinate hypertrophy, foreign bodies)
- Ciliary dyskinesia
- Local allergic rhinitis (localized nasal allergic response with nasal specific immunoglobulin E in the absence of systemic atopy)
- Systemic diseases with nasal manifestations (e.g., systemic lupus erythematosus, granulomatous disease, pharyngonasal reflux, GERD)
- Cerebral spinal fluid (CSF) leak (typically unilateral clear fluid after sustaining head trauma or as a postoperative complication)

WORKUP

- Because many patients with NAR may also have AR or present with a "mixed form" of rhinitis including both allergic and non-allergic types, NAR can be challenging to diagnose. Questionnaires, including the Cincinnati Irritant Index Scale, have proven useful in differentiating NAR from AR.
- A diagnosis of NAR is typically made after an allergic cause is ruled out via skin prick testing or specific IgE blood testing. Given the common overlap between NAR and AR, it may be reasonable to revisit diagnostic testing if patients do not respond to therapy as expected.
- In severe or refractory cases, nasal endoscopy can be considered to rule out nasal polyps, anatomic deformities, and rare life-threatening diagnoses (e.g. intranasal tumors) that could be contributing to the chronic rhinitis.
- Plain x-ray films are not helpful in diagnosing chronic rhinosinusitis and should not be ordered. Sinus CT changes are similar in viral and bacterial rhinosinusitis and should not be routinely ordered.
- Utility of other testing approaches (nasal provocation tests, nasal lavage cytology, mucosal histopathological alterations) are not regularly performed in the clinical setting.

Rx TREATMENT

NONPHARMACOLOGIC THERAPY

- Identification and avoidance of specific triggers may provide relief.
- Discontinuing any medication/drugs that could be contributing (Table E1).
- Daily nasal lavage (distilled water mixed with saline packets) and over-the-counter nasal saline sprays improve symptoms in most types of NAR.
- Cryosurgical ablation of the posterior nasal nerve is an increasingly utilized office-based procedure that decreases NAR symptoms in 67 to 97% of patients without significant complications.
- Surgical intervention (turbinoplasty, deviated nasal septum, polyp removal, parasympathetic nerve resection [vidian or posterior nasal neurectomy]) may be considered if medical measures fail, but data illustrating symptom reduction is limited and such surgeries are not commonly performed in the U.S.

PHARMACOLOGIC THERAPY

- If patients still have symptoms despite avoidance of inciting factors, a trial intranasal application of corticosteroids, antimuscarinics, or antihistamines can be considered. Clinicians should offer an intranasal corticosteroid or intranasal antihistamine as first-line therapy in NAR. Combined therapy with intranasal antihistamine and intranasal corticosteroid is now available and may be both more efficacious and convenient, though the cost is often prohibitive.
  1. Intranasal corticosteroids sprays (fluticasone, triamcinolone, mometasone, beclomethasone) prevent and treat inflammation.
  2. Intranasal antihistamines (azelastine, olopatadine) are faster-acting than intranasal corticosteroids in controlling nasal congestion. While first-generation oral antihistamines may improve rhinorrhea in select cases, topical therapies have been shown to be most efficacious as first-line therapy. Second-generation oral antihistamines have not been shown to be beneficial in NAR.
  3. Intranasal antimuscarinics (ipratropium bromide) reduce rhinorrhea by decreasing cholinergic secretion in most types of NAR and can be added to an intranasal corticosteroid/antihistamine regimen if symptoms are not well controlled.
- Some subtypes may require individualized therapies to address underlying pathophysiology:
  1. Gustatory: Many patients have persistent symptoms regardless of dietary modification and may require utilization of a pre-prandial intranasal antimuscarinic administered 30 min prior to each meal.
  2. Rhinitis medicamentosa: It may take up to 2 wk for receptor densities to return to their pre-drug state after discontinuation of a topical decongestant. During this withdrawal period, patients may benefit from a short course of intranasal and oral (e.g., prednisone 0.5 mg per kg for 5 days) corticosteroids to relieve severe congestion.
  3. Senile rhinitis: Intranasal antimuscarinics are first line.
  4. Infectious: Avoid antibiotics treatment for 7 to 10 days after symptom onset as bacterial infections are uncommon and antibiotics are consistently overprescribed with resultant increasing antibiotic resistance. It may take up to 6 to 8 wk of supportive care for symptoms to subside after resolution of acute infection.
- Decongestants reduce congestion via vasoconstriction and may be helpful temporarily for refractory congestion, though increase the risk for rhinitis medicamentosa as discussed above. Similarly, alpha agonist may improve nasal flow for several hours due to nasal vasoconstriction and decreased nasal edema, but are not recommended for continuous use due to the risk of developing rhinitis medicamentosa.
- Several studies have shown administration of topical capsaicin decreases nasal congestion, rhinorrhea, and postnasal drainage in NAR (but not AR) patients. Comparative studies on NAR with capsaicin versus steroids demonstrate the superiority of capsaicin; however, the exact dose and frequency have not been determined.
- There is no evidence to support the use of leukotriene receptor antagonists or intranasal cromolyn in NAR.

DISPOSITION

Most patients experience mild to moderate symptomatic relief with avoidance of triggers and appropriate use of medications. Up to 52% of patients with NAR report worsening symptoms at 3- to 7-yr follow-ups. Periodic reevaluations should be performed, as there is evidence supporting increased development of asthma, AR, nasal polyps, middle ear infections, turbinate hypertrophy, and sinusitis in patients with chronic NAR.

REFERRAL

Referral to allergist and/or ENT may be appropriate when severe symptoms are unresponsive to standard therapy and/or diagnosis is uncertain.

PEARLS & CONSIDERATIONS

- NAR symptoms are nonspecific, and a specific trigger is often never identified. Compared to AR, patients typically lack symptoms of sneezing, nasal pruritus, and conjunctival symptoms.
- Second-generation oral antihistamines are typically not efficacious and while the treatment of NAR usually includes intranasal corticosteroids and/or intranasal antihistamines, it should be individualized based on underlying pathophysiology whenever possible.

SUGGESTED READINGS

Available at ExpertConsult.com

RELATED CONTENT

Allergic Rhinitis (Patient Information)
Allergic Rhinitis (Related Key Topic)

AUTHORS: **Alexa Papaila, MD, MPH,** and **Shyam Joshi, MD**

BASIC INFORMATION

DEFINITION

Non-celiac gluten sensitivity (NCGS) is an intestinal and/or extraintestinal reaction to ingested gluten or wheat that improves once gluten-containing foods have been eliminated from the diet. Gluten is a group of proteins found in grains (wheat, rye, barley, and oats). The two main protein components of gluten are gliadin and glutenin. Celiac disease and wheat allergy must be excluded before the diagnosis of NCGS can be made.

SYNONYMS

Non-celiac wheat sensitivity (NCWS)
NCGS

ICD-10CM CODE

K90.41 Non-celiac gluten sensitivity

EPIDEMIOLOGY & DEMOGRAPHICS

- Global prevalence of NCGS is about 10%, although this number is not well established due to the absence of diagnostic markers. Prevalence is based primarily on self-reported questionnaires for gluten sensitivity.
- The reported prevalence has increased significantly over the past decade.
- NCGS is reported more often in women than in men.
- It is more commonly reported in urban areas.
- The median age of diagnosis is in the fourth decade of life.

PHYSICAL FINDINGS & CLINICAL PRESENTATION

- Intestinal symptoms include abdominal pain, bloating, diarrhea (with or without alternating constipation), and flatulence.
- Extraintestinal findings may include constitutional symptoms such as fatigue and weight loss as well as neurological changes (headache, brain fog, numbness) and psychological changes (anxiety). Less commonly, anemia and dermatological findings such as eczema may be seen.
- Symptoms of NCGS greatly overlap with IBS and therefore may be difficult to distinguish.

ETIOLOGY

- There is no known biomarker or diagnostic test for NCGS, making the pathogenesis unclear.
- It has been suggested that in patients with NCGS, ingestion of gluten may lead to increased intestinal permeability by increasing serum concentration of zonulin, a protein that increases permeability through changes in epithelial tight junctions. The rise in zonulin leads to breaks and leakage through the intestinal epithelial wall in predisposed people.
- Several studies have found changes in the intestinal microbiome of patients with NCGS compared with those in healthy controls. Compared with asymptomatic controls, patients with gluten sensitivity have a higher number of gut bacteria with more harmful than beneficial bacteria. These changes revert back to normal following initiation of a gluten-free diet (GFD).

Dx DIAGNOSIS

DIFFERENTIAL DIAGNOSIS

- Celiac disease
- Wheat allergy
- Irritable bowel syndrome (IBS)

WORKUP

- There are no strict diagnostic criteria; therefore, there is a great deal of dependence on the patient's perception of symptoms and nocebo effect.
- Salerno Experts' Criteria is the most widely used method for diagnosing NCGS.
  1. Patient must be on a normal gluten-containing diet for at least 6 wk. During this time, the patient is assessed by a diagnostic questionnaire (Table E1) at wk −2, −1, and 0 to establish baseline symptoms.
  2. At time 0, patient begins a strict GFD as instructed by a dietician. Patient will remain on GFD for 6 wk with weekly data recording via the questionnaire.
  3. Response is assessed, with a positive result defined as a decrease of ≥30% in the baseline score in 1 to 3 categories for ≥50% of the observation time.
  4. The diagnosis of NCGS is excluded in subjects failing to show symptomatic improvement after 6 wk. These patients should be worked up for other causes of IBS-like symptoms, including intolerance to fermentable oligo-, di- and monosaccharides and polyols (FODMAPS) or small bowel bacterial overgrowth.
  5. This 6-wk test study is followed by a double-blind placebo-controlled challenge of ≥8 g/day of gluten (or placebo) for a week of each. Gluten is given in a "vehicle" such as a bar, bread, or muffin. Gluten and placebo must be indistinguishable in look, texture, and taste.
  6. Again, a positive result is defined as a variation of ≥30% between gluten and placebo.
  7. While the Salerno Expert Criteria is the proposed method for diagnosis of NCGS, it is often impractical to perform in the primary care setting. Therefore, simply asking the patient to adopt a GFD will achieve the same desired clinical outcome.

LABORATORY TESTS

- Mainly a clinical diagnosis as there are no diagnostic tests or biomarkers for NCGS.
- Celiac disease and wheat allergy must be excluded through their respective laboratory tests prior to the diagnosis of NCGS.

Dx TREATMENT

NONPHARMACOLOGIC THERAPY

Treatment of NCGS is strict elimination of gluten from the diet. A low-FODMAPS diet may be indicated if symptoms are not responding to a GFD.

ACUTE GENERAL Rx

- Correct nutritional deficiencies
- Lifelong elimination of gluten or wheat

DISPOSITION

Unlike celiac disease, which requires a strict, lifelong gluten-free diet, it is unclear whether NCGS is a permanent condition. Some authors have suggested reintroduction of gluten after 1 to 2 yr.

REFERRAL

A multidisciplinary team approach is recommended for patients with NCGS, with involvement of the primary doctor, gastroenterologist, and nutritionist.

PEARLS AND CONSIDERATIONS

COMMENTS

- The gluten-free market is rising, likely due to the perceived health benefits of a GFD. This, however, is debatable, as grains should be the main energy source in the human diet. A GFD is poor in trace elements and vitamins such as zinc, iron, magnesium, calcium, vitamin D, vitamin B_{12}, folate, and fiber. It is also high in calories, fat, sugar, and salt.
- Studies show that intake of gluten through whole grains is associated with a lower risk of elevated triglycerides and lower risk of cardiovascular disease.

SUGGESTED READINGS

Available at ExpertConsult.com

RELATED CONTENT

Celiac Disease (Related Key Topic)
Irritable Bowel Syndrome (Related Key Topic)

AUTHOR: **Christina M. Bortz, MD**

Non-Hodgkin Lymphoma PTG ALG

BASIC INFORMATION

DEFINITION

Non-Hodgkin lymphoma (NHL) is a heterogeneous group of malignancies of the lymphoreticular system. There are approximately 60 different NHL subtypes. The WHO classification of lymphomas is summarized in Table 1 and Fig. 1.

SYNONYM

NHL

ICD-10CM CODES

C85.90	Non-Hodgkin lymphoma, unspecified, unspecified site
C85.91	Non-Hodgkin lymphoma, unspecified, lymph nodes of head, face, and neck
C85.92	Non-Hodgkin lymphoma, unspecified, intrathoracic lymph nodes
C85.93	Non-Hodgkin lymphoma, unspecified, intra-abdominal lymph nodes
C85.94	Non-Hodgkin lymphoma, unspecified, lymph nodes of axilla and upper limb
C85.95	Non-Hodgkin lymphoma, unspecified, lymph nodes of inguinal region and lower limb
C85.96	Non-Hodgkin lymphoma, unspecified, intrapelvic lymph nodes
C85.97	Non-Hodgkin lymphoma, unspecified, spleen
C85.98	Non-Hodgkin lymphoma, unspecified, lymph nodes of multiple sites
C85.99	Non-Hodgkin lymphoma, unspecified, extranodal and solid organ sites

EPIDEMIOLOGY

- Sixth most common neoplasm in the U.S. (>70,000 new cases annually). Incidence increases with age; majority of patients are above 60 yr of age.
- In the U.S. and Europe, diffuse large B-cell lymphoma (DLBCL) is the most common subtype (30% of the cases), and follicular lymphoma (FL) is the second most common subtype (25% of the cases).
- In patients with HIV, NHL is the most common tumor (followed by Kaposi sarcoma). DLBCL accounts for 80% to 90% of the cases of HIV-associated NHL.
- Factors associated with an increased risk of non-Hodgkin lymphoma are summarized in Box 1.

PHYSICAL FINDINGS & CLINICAL PRESENTATION

- Patients often present with lymphadenopathy.
- Approximately one third of the NHL involve extranodal sites, which can result in unusual presentations (e.g., gastrointestinal tract involvement can simulate peptic ulcer disease).

TABLE 1 World Health Organization Classification of Lymphomas[a]

Mature B-Cell Neoplasms

Chronic Lymphocytic Leukemia/Small Lymphocytic Lymphoma
- B-cell prolymphocytic leukemia
- Splenic B-cell marginal zone lymphoma
- Hairy cell leukemia
- *Splenic B-cell lymphoma/leukemia, unclassifiable*
- *Splenic diffuse red pulp small B-cell lymphoma*
- *Hairy cell leukemia-variant*
- Lymphoplasmacytic lymphoma
- Waldenström macroglobulinemia
- Heavy chain diseases
- Alpha heavy chain disease
- Gamma heavy chain disease
- Mu heavy chain disease

Plasma Cell Myeloma
- Solitary plasmacytoma of bone
- Extraosseous plasmacytoma

Extranodal Marginal Zone Lymphoma of Mucosa-Associated Lymphoid Tissue (MALT Lymphoma)
- Nodal marginal zone lymphoma
- *Pediatric nodal marginal zone lymphoma*

Follicular Lymphoma
- *Pediatric-type follicular lymphoma*
- Primary cutaneous follicle center lymphoma

Mantle Cell Lymphoma

Diffuse Large B-Cell Lymphoma (DLBCL), NOS
- T-cell/histiocyte–rich large B-cell lymphoma
- Primary DLBCL of the CNS
- Primary cutaneous DLBCL, leg type
- EBV-positive DLBCL
- DLBCL associated with chronic inflammation
- Lymphomatoid granulomatosis
- Primary mediastinal (thymic) large B-cell lymphoma
- Intravascular large B-cell lymphoma
- ALK-positive large B-cell lymphoma
- Plasmablastic lymphoma
- HHV8-positive diffuse large B-cell lymphoma and primary effusion lymphoma
- Burkitt lymphoma
- High grade B-cell lymphomas, with *MYC* and *BCL2* and/or *BCL6* rearrangements
- B-cell lymphoma unclassifiable, with features intermediate between diffuse large B-cell lymphoma and classic Hodgkin lymphoma

Mature T-Cell and NK-Cell Neoplasms
- T-cell prolymphocytic leukemia
- T-cell large granular lymphocytic leukemia
- *Chronic lymphoproliferative disorder of NK-cells*
- Aggressive NK leukemia
- Systemic EBV-positive T-cell lymphoma of childhood
- Hydroa vacciniforme-like lymphoma
- Adult T-cell leukemia/lymphoma
- Extranodal NK/T-cell lymphoma, nasal type
- Enteropathy-associated T-cell lymphoma
- Monomorphic epitheliotropic intestinal T-cell lymphoma
- Hepatosplenic T-cell lymphoma
- Subcutaneous panniculitis-like T-cell lymphoma

Mycosis Fungoides
- Sézary syndrome
- Primary cutaneous CD30-positive T-cell lymphoproliferative disorders
- Lymphoid papulosis
- Primary cutaneous anaplastic large cell lymphoma
- Primary cutaneous gamma-delta T-cell lymphoma
- Primary cutaneous CD8-positive aggressive epidermotropic cytotoxic T-cell lymphoma
- Primary cutaneous CD4-positive small/medium T-cell lymphoproliferative disease

Peripheral T-Cell Lymphoma, NOS

Angioimmunoblastic T-Cell Lymphoma

Anaplastic Large Cell Lymphoma, ALK-Positive
- Anaplastic large cell lymphoma, ALK-negative

Hodgkin Lymphoma

Nodular Lymphocyte Predominant Hodgkin Lymphoma

Classic Hodgkin Lymphoma

Nodular Sclerosis Hodgkin Lymphoma
- Lymphocyte-rich classic Hodgkin lymphoma
- Mixed cellularity classic Hodgkin lymphoma
- Lymphocyte-depleted classic Hodgkin lymphoma

ALK, Anaplastic lymphoma kinase; *CNS,* central nervous system; *EBV,* Epstein-Barr virus; *HHV-8,* human herpesvirus-8; *NK,* natural killer; *NOS,* not otherwise specified.
[a]Most common entities are underlined. Provisional entities are in italics. Some rare entities or variants are omitted.
From Hoffman R et al: *Hematology: basic principles and practice,* ed 7, Philadelphia, 2018, Elsevier.

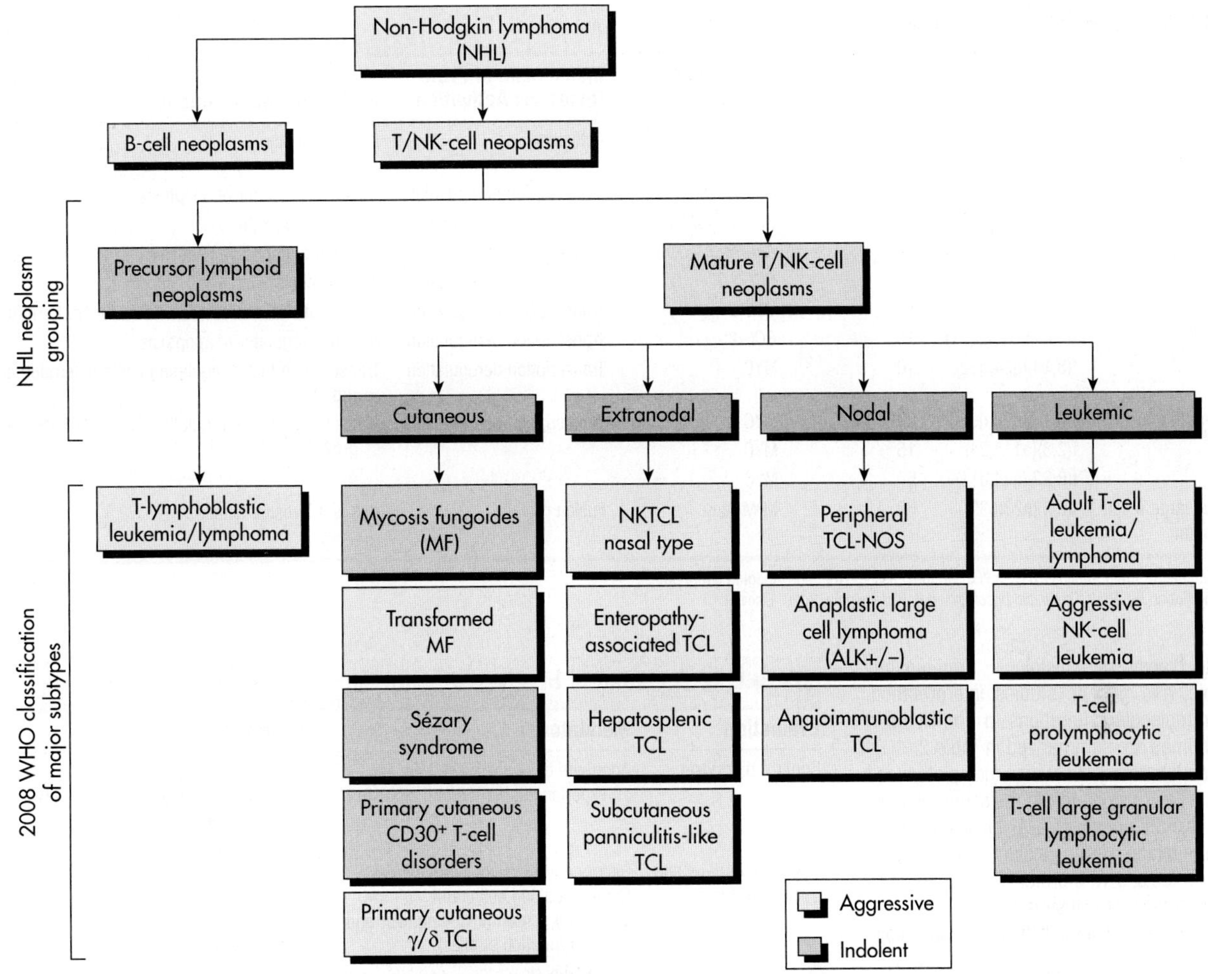

FIG. 1 World Health Organization *(WHO)* classification of the mature T-cell neoplasms. *NK,* Natural killer; *NKTCL,* nasal NK/T-cell lymphoma; *NOS,* not otherwise specified; *TCL,* T-cell lymphoma; *WHO,* World Health Organization. (From Hoffman R et al: *Hematology: basic principles and practice,* ed 7, Philadelphia, 2018, Elsevier.)

BOX 1 Factors Associated with an Increased Risk of Non-Hodgkin Lymphoma

Immunosuppression, acquired
- After solid-organ or hematopoietic stem cell transplantation
- HIV/AIDS

Congenital immunodeficiency syndromes
Increasing age (waning immunity)
Previous history of HL or NHL
Family history of NHL
Drugs
- Methotrexate
- TNF-α inhibitors

Occupational exposures
- Herbicides, pesticides, wood dust, epoxy glue, organic solvents
- Farming, forestry, painting, carpentry, tanning

AIDS, Acquired immunodeficiency syndrome; *HIV,* human immunodeficiency virus; *HL,* Hodgkin lymphoma; *NHL,* non-Hodgkin lymphoma; *TNF,* tumor necrosis factor.

From Niederhuber JE: *Abeloff's clinical oncology,* ed 6, Philadelphia, 2020, Elsevier.

- Presence of B symptoms like unexplained weight loss, fever, fatigue, and night sweats are seen typically in aggressive or highly aggressive lymphomas.
- Aggressive lymphomas have acute or subacute presentation with increasing size of the mass and B symptoms.
- Indolent lymphomas have a more chronic course, with asymptomatic lymphadenopathy and/or slowly progressive cytopenias.
- Hepatomegaly and splenomegaly may be present.
- Cough, dyspnea with bulky mediastinal involvement

Dx DIAGNOSIS

DIFFERENTIAL DIAGNOSIS

- Hodgkin lymphoma
- Viral infections
- Metastatic carcinoma
- Autoimmune conditions
- Sarcoidosis

WORKUP

Initial laboratory evaluation may be entirely normal. Elevated LDH may be seen in aggressive lymphoma or in indolent lymphoma with high disease bulk. In cases of highly aggressive NHL (e.g., Burkitt lymphoma), spontaneous tumor lysis syndrome (TLS) may be seen, characterized by hyperkalemia, hyperuricemia, hypocalcemia, hyperphosphatemia, and acidosis. TLS can be life threatening and is considered a medical emergency. Acute management includes aggressive IV fluid repletion and/or rasburicase. Proper staging of NHL includes the following:

- A thorough history and physical examination
- Excisional or incisional surgical biopsy is preferred. Image-guided core needle biopsies may be acceptable in patients without peripheral adenopathy. Fine needle aspirates are not adequate for precise lymphoma subclassification. Laparoscopic lymph node biopsy or mediastinoscopy can be used on an outpatient basis for most patients with intraabdominal or mediastinal lymphoma, respectively.

TABLE 2 Major Molecular Alterations in Non-Hodgkin Lymphomas

NHL Histologic Type	Alteration	Cases Affected (%)	Proto-Oncogene Involved	Mechanism of Proto-Oncogene Activation	Proto-Oncogene Function
Lymphoplasmacytic lymphoma	*MYD88* L265P mutation	95	*MYD88*	Activation	B-cell signaling
Follicular lymphoma	t(14;18)(q32;q21)	90	*BCL-2*	Transcription deregulation	Negative regulator of apoptosis
Mantle cell lymphoma	t(11;14)(q13;q32)	70	*BCL-1/cyclin D1*	Transcription deregulation	Cell cycle regulator
MALT lymphoma	t(11;18)(q21;q21)	50	*API_2/MLT*	Fusion protein	*API_2* has antiapoptotic activity
	t(1;14)(p22;q32)		*BCL-10*	Transcription deregulation	Antiapoptosis
Diffuse large B-cell lymphoma	der(3)(q27)	35	*BCL-6*	Transcription deregulation	Transcriptional repressor required for GC formation
	t(14;18)(q32;q21)	15	*BCL-2*	Transcription deregulation	Negative regulator of apoptosis
	t(8;14)(q24;q32)	10	MYC	Transcription deregulation	Transcription factor regulating cell proliferation and growth
Burkitt lymphoma	t(8;14)(q24;q32)	80	MYC	Transcription deregulation	Transcription factor regulating cell proliferation and growth
	t(2;8)(p11;q24)	15	MYC		
	t(8;22)(q24;q11)	5	MYC		
Anaplastic large T-cell lymphoma	t(2;5)(p23;q35)	60	NPM/ALK	Fusion protein	*ALK* is a tyrosine kinase

GC, Gastric cancer; *MALT,* mucosa-associated lymphoid tissue; *NHL,* non-Hodgkin lymphoma.
From Niederhuber JE: *Abeloff's clinical oncology,* ed 6, Philadelphia, 2020, Elsevier.

- Tissue biopsy with histologic, immunophenotypic, and genetic studies interpretation. Major molecular alterations in non-Hodgkin lymphomas are summarized in Table 2.
- Routine laboratory evaluation (complete blood count, flow cytometry in selected circumstances, ESR, urinalysis, LDH, blood urea nitrogen, creatinine, serum calcium, uric acid, liver function tests, serum protein electrophoresis).
- HIV and hepatitis B testing.
- Bone marrow evaluation (aspirate and biopsy) (Fig. E2)
- CT scan of chest, abdomen, and pelvis with IV contrast, if possible
- Fluorine-18 fluorodeoxyglucose (FDG) positron emission tomography (PET) integrated with CT (Fig. E3) has emerged as a tool for staging, response evaluation, and posttreatment surveillance in patients with aggressive subtypes of NHL.
- Depending on the histopathology, the results of the previous studies, and the planned therapy, some other tests may be performed.
- Lumbar puncture is needed in some patients with aggressive NHL, and most patients with HIV-associated NHL, to evaluate for CNS involvement by lymphoma.
- The evaluation of a new patient with non-Hodgkin lymphoma is summarized in Table 3.

CLASSIFICATION: For clinical approach, NHL is subdivided lymphomas into indolent, aggressive, and highly aggressive disease.

STAGING: The Ann Arbor staging system that was initially developed for Hodgkin lymphoma (HL) was revised as the Lugano criteria and remains the current standard; but unlike HL, NHL does not spread predictably via lymphatic channels to contiguous nodal regions, so stage is only one of multiple contributors to prognosis (Table 4). Histopathology has greater therapeutic implications in NHL than in Hodgkin lymphoma. Fig. 4 illustrates a diagnostic algorithm outlining the steps in classification of B-cell lymphomas composed of cells of small to intermediate size.

TABLE 3 Evaluation of a New Patient with Non-Hodgkin Lymphoma

Evaluation	Mandatory	As Indicated
Confirm diagnosis	Adequate biopsy reviewed by experienced hematopathologists	Immunophenotyping with immunohistochemistry +/− flow cytometry Cytogenetics/molecular studies
General overview and risks of therapy	History and physical examination Complete blood cell count Chemistry screen (including liver and renal function studies) HIV serology Hepatitis B serologies	Blood coagulation studies EBV serology and PCR assay Hepatitis C serology Serum electrolytes, uric acid Assessment of cardiac ejection fraction Pregnancy testing in women Discussion of fertility issues
Prognostic categorization	Serum lactate dehydrogenase Serum albumin	Erythrocyte sedimentation rate Serum β_2-microglobulin
Anatomic disease	Chest, abdominal, and pelvic CT with contrast enhancement	Ultrasonography FDG-PET/CTMRI
Occult sites of involvement		Unilateral bone marrow biopsy with aspirate Lumbar puncture with flow cytometry of CSF Biopsy of suspicious sites Blood flow cytometry

CSF, Cerebrospinal fluid; *CT,* computed tomography; *EBV,* Epstein-Barr virus; *FDG-PET,* fluorodeoxyglucose-18–labeled positron emission tomography; *HIV,* human immunodeficiency virus; *MRI,* magnetic resonance imaging; *PCR,* polymerase chain reaction.
From Niederhuber JE: *Abeloff's clinical oncology,* ed 6, Philadelphia, 2020, Elsevier.

TABLE 4 Non-Hodgkin Lymphoma: Lugano Staging Classification

Stage	Features
I	Involvement of a single lymph node region or lymphoid structure (e.g., spleen, thymus, Waldeyer ring), or a single extranodal location without nodal involvement (IE)
II	Involvement of two or more lymph node regions on the same side of the diaphragm or limited nodal disease with limited contiguous extranodal involvement (IIE)
III	Involvement of lymph node regions or structures on both sides of the diaphragm
IV	Involvement of diffuse or noncontiguous extranodal site(s)

From Niederhuber JE: *Abeloff's clinical oncology,* ed 6, Philadelphia, 2020, Elsevier.

Rx TREATMENT

ACUTE GENERAL Rx

The therapeutic regimen varies with specific lymphoma subtype and pathologic stage.

Following are the commonly used therapeutic modalities:

INDOLENT NHL:

- Deferment of therapy and careful observation in asymptomatic patients with low volume disease.

- Local radiotherapy for stage I disease
- Rituximab, an anti-CD20 monoclonal antibody, with or without chemotherapy is used in patients with symptomatic or progressive disease.
- The addition of rituximab to chemotherapy is generally well tolerated and has increased response and survival rates in NHL patients. Patients who received rituximab, cyclophosphamide, doxorubicin, vincristine, and prednisone (R-CHOP) had higher response rates (96% vs. 90%) with a better 2-yr overall survival rate (95% vs. 90%) than patients who received CHOP without rituximab. Similarly, patients who received rituximab, cyclophosphamide, vincristine, and prednisone (R-CVP) had higher response rates (81% vs. 57%) and better overall survival at 4 yr (83% vs. 77%) than patients who were treated with CVP without rituximab.
- In a recent phase III noninferiority study, the combination of bendamustine and rituximab was associated with better progression-free survival rates than R-CHOP (70 vs. 31 mo) with fewer toxic effects. Subset analyses showed better progression-free survival in patients with follicular lymphoma, mantle cell lymphoma, and lymphoplasmacytic lymphoma.
- The combination of obinutuzumab and chemotherapy followed by obinutuzumab maintenance was approved by the FDA in previously untreated patients with follicular lymphoma based on a randomized study, in which obinutuzumab and chemotherapy were associated with longer median progression-free survival than rituximab and chemotherapy.
- Combination regimens containing cytarabine such as R-CHOP alternating with R-DHAP or the NORDIC regimen are used for the frontline treatment of aggressive mantle cell lymphoma. Bendamustine and rituximab, R-CHOP, and lenalidomide and rituximab are less aggressive regimens for mantle cell lymphoma.
- Maintenance rituximab after rituximab-containing regimens has been associated with better progression-free survival rates than observation in follicular and mantle cell lymphoma.
- The combination of obinutuzumab and bendamustine followed by obinutuzumab maintenance was approved by the FDA for the treatment of patients with rituximab-refractory follicular lymphoma.
- The oral BTK inhibitor ibrutinib is FDA-approved for the treatment of patients with relapsed mantle cell lymphoma, lymphoplasmacytic lymphoma, and marginal zone

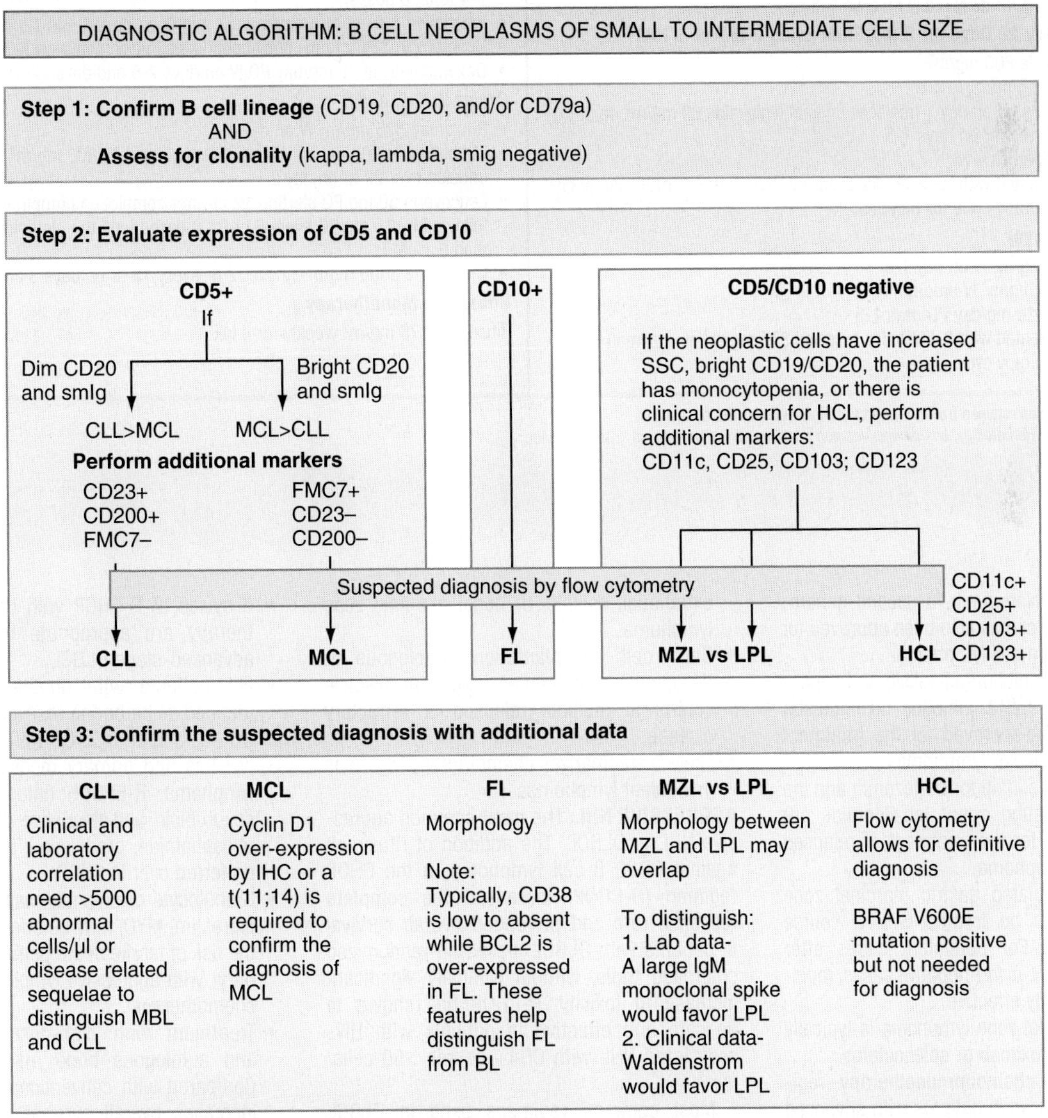

FIG. 4 This diagnostic algorithm outlines the steps in classification of B-cell lymphomas composed of cells of small to intermediate size. *BL,* Burkitt lymphoma; *CLL,* chronic lymphocytic leukemia; *FL,* follicular lymphoma; *HCL,* hairy cell leukemia; *IgM,* immunoglobulin M; *IHC,* immunohistochemistry; *LPL,* lymphoplasmacytic lymphoma; *MBL,* monoclonal B-cell lymphocytosis; *MCL,* mantle cell lymphoma; *MZL,* marginal zone lymphoma; *SmIg,* surface immunoglobulin; *SSC,* scleroderma and systemic sclerosis. (From McPherson RA, Pincus MR: *Henry's clinical diagnosis and management by laboratory methods,* ed 23, Philadelphia, 2017, Elsevier.)

TABLE 5 Chemotherapy Regimens in Indolent Lymphomas

BR (Every 28 Days)
- Bendamustine 120 mg/m² days 1 and 2
- Rituximab 375 mg/m² IV day 1

CVP-R (Every 21 Days)
- Cyclophosphamide 750 mg/m² IV on day 1
- Vincristine 1.4 mg/m², up to a maximal dose of 2 mg IV, on day 1
- Prednisone 40 mg/m² daily PO days 1-5
- Rituximab 375 mg/m² IV day 1[32]

R-CHOP (Every 21 Days)
- Cyclophosphamide 750 mg/m² IV on day 1
- Doxorubicin 50 mg/m² IV on day 1
- Vincristine 1.4 mg/m², up to a maximal dose of 2 mg IV, on day 1
- Prednisone 100 mg daily orally on days 1-5
- Rituximab 375 mg/m² IV on day 1 of each therapy cycle[33] or by alternate schedule[34]

CNOP (Every 21 Days)
- Cyclophosphamide 750 mg/m² IV on day 1
- Mitoxantrone 10 mg/m² IV on day 1
- Vincristine 1.4 mg/m², up to a maximal dose of 2 mg IV, on day 1
- Prednisone 50 mg/m² daily orally on days 1-5

R-CHVP-IFN (Every 28 Days for 6 Mo, Then Every 2 Mo for 6 Mo)[35]
- Cyclophosphamide 600 mg/m²
- Doxorubicin 25 mg/m²
- Etoposide 100 mg/m² on day 1 (replaces original teniposide 60 mg/m² on day 1)
- Prednisolone 40 mg/m² on days 1-5
- Interferon-α 5-3 times a wk
- Patients being treated with R-CHVP also received 375 mg/m² of rituximab IV on day 1 of each therapy cycle for 6 cycles

FMD (Every 28 Days)
- Fludarabine 25 mg/m² IV on day 1-3
- Mitoxantrone 10 mg/m² IV on day 1
- Dexamethasone 20 mg/day PO days 1-5
- Patients being treated with R-FMD also received 375 mg/m² of rituximab IV on day 1 of each therapy cycle

ProMACE-MOPP
- Cycles repeated every 28 days

Day 1
- Cyclophosphamide 650 mg/m² IV
- Doxorubicin 25 mg/m² IV
- Etoposide 120 mg/m² IV
- Prednisone 60 mg/m² orally daily days 1-14

Day 8
- Mechlorethamine 6 mg/m² IV
- Vincristine 1.4 mg/m² (maximum 2 mg) IV on day 8
- Procarbazine 100 mg/m² orally daily days 8-14

Day 15
- Methotrexate 500 mg/m² IV on day 15 with leucovorin 50 mg/m² orally every 6 hr for four doses beginning 24 hr after methotrexate

R-Hyper-CVAD (Every 21 Days)[36]

Cycles 1, 3, 5, and 7
- Rituximab 375 mg/m² IV on day 1
- Cyclophosphamide (with mesna) 300 mg/m² IV over 3 hr every 12 hr on days 2-4 (total 6 doses)
- Vincristine 1.4 mg/m² (maximum 2 mg) IV on days 5 and 12
- Doxorubicin 16.6 mg/m² IV by continuous infusion on days 5-7
- Dexamethasone 40 mg/day PO/IV on days 2-5 and days 12-15

Cycles 2, 4, 6, and 8
- Rituximab 375 mg/m² IV on day 1
- Methotrexate 200 mg/m² IV over 2 hr, followed by 800 mg/m² IV continuous infusion over 22 hr on day 2
- Leucovorin 50 mg PO starting 12 hr after completion of methotrexate infusion, followed by 15 mg PO every 6 hr for 8 dosed until the methotrexate level is less than 0.1 μM/L
- Cytarabine 3000 mg/m² IV over 2 hr every 12 hr on days 3 and 4 (4 doses total)

Rituximab Monotherapy

Rituximab 375 mg/m² weekly for 4 wk

NOTE: Reference endnotes retained from the source. *IV,* Intravenous; *PO,* by mouth.
From Hoffman R et al: *Hematology, basic principles and practice,* ed 7, Philadelphia, 2018, Elsevier.

lymphoma. Acalabrutinib, a second-generation BTK inhibitor, has also been approved for relapsed mantle cell lymphoma.
- The oral PI3K inhibitors idelalisib and copanlisib and the EZH2 inhibitor tazemetostat have been FDA-approved for the treatment of relapsed follicular lymphoma.
- The proteasome inhibitor bortezomib and the immunomodulating agent lenalidomide are FDA-approved for the treatment of relapsed mantle cell lymphoma.
- *H. pylori*-associated gastric marginal zone lymphoma can be treated with a course of antibiotics. For persistent cases after eradication or *H. pylori*-negative cases, radiotherapy is highly effective.
- Splenic marginal zone lymphoma is typically treated with rituximab or splenectomy.
- Rituximab or chemoimmunotherapy regimens can be used in patients with advanced stage extranodal, splenic, or nodal marginal zone lymphoma.
- Ibrutinib has been FDA approved for the treatment of relapsed and/or refractory extranodal, splenic, or nodal marginal zone lymphoma.
- Stem cell transplantation (autologous or allogeneic) may confer long-term disease control in multiple relapsed or refractory disease.
- Table 5 summarizes chemotherapy regimens in indolent lymphomas.

AGGRESSIVE NHL: The most common aggressive NHL is DLBCL. The addition of rituximab against CD20 B-cell lymphoma to the CHOP regimen (R-CHOP) increased the complete response rate and prolonged overall survival in patients with DLBCL, based on randomized controlled trials, without clinically significant increase in toxicity. R-CHOP has shown to be safe and effective in patients with HIV-associated NHL with CD4+ counts >50 cells/mm³.

Most common regimens used in DLBCL include:
- Three to four cycles of R-CHOP followed by involved-field radiotherapy or 6 cycles of R-CHOP alone are appropriate approaches in patients with localized DLBCL.
- 6 cycles of R-CHOP with or without radiotherapy are appropriate in patients with advanced-stage DLBCL.
- For patients with double-hit lymphomas (defined as harboring rearrangement of MYC, BCL-2, and/or BCL-6), HIV-associated lymphomas and primary mediastinal large cell lymphoma, R-EPOCH (infusional etoposide, doxorubicin, and vincristine, along with cyclophosphamide, prednisone, and rituximab) is preferred over R-CHOP.
- Granulocyte-colony stimulating factor (e.g., filgrastim, MYC) may be effective in reducing the risk of febrile neutropenia in patients over 65 yr with aggressive lymphoma undergoing chemotherapy.
- Treatment with high-dose chemotherapy and autologous bone marrow transplant: Compared with conventional chemotherapy, increases overall survival in patients with chemotherapy-sensitive relapsed DLBCL.
- Chimeric antigen receptor T-cell therapy agents (axicabtagene ciloleucel and tisagenlecleucel) have been FDA approved for patients with relapsed or refractory diffuse

TABLE 6 Combination Chemotherapy Regimens for Non-Hodgkin Lymphoma

Regimen	Dose	Days of Administration	Frequency
R-Bendamustine			**Every 28 days**
Bendamustine	90 mg/m_2 IV	1-2	
Rituximab	375 mg/m_2 IV	1	
R-CHOP			**Every 21 days**
Cyclophosphamide	750 mg/m_2 IV	1	
Doxorubicin	50 mg/m_2 IV	1	
Vincristine	1.4 mg/m_2 IV	1	
Prednisone, fixed dose	100 mg PO	1-5	
Rituximab	375 mg/m_2 IV	1	
R-CVP			**Every 21 days**
Cyclophosphamide	1000 mg/m_2 IV	1	
Vincristine	1.4 mg/m_2 IV	1	
Prednisone, fixed dose	100 mg PO	1-5	
Rituximab	375 mg/m_2 IV	1	

IV, Intravenous; *PO,* by mouth.
Adapted from Goldman L, Schafer AI: *Goldman's Cecil medicine,* ed 24, Philadelphia, 2012, Saunders.

TABLE 7 Clinical Prognostic Indexes

International Prognostic Index (IPI) for Aggressive Lymphomas[1]

Risk Group	IPI Score[a]	CR Rate (%)	5-Yr OS Rate (%)
Low	0, 1	87	73
Low intermediate	2	67	51
High intermediate	3	55	43
High	4,5	44	26

Follicular International Prognostic Index (FLIPI)[2]

Risk Group	FLIPI Score[b]	Distribution (%)	5-Yr OS Rate (%)
Low	0-1	36	90.6
Intermediate	1-2	37	77.6
Poor	≥3	27	52.5

Mantle Cell International Prognostic Index (MIPI)[3]

Risk Group	MIPI Score[c]	Distribution (%)	Median Survival Rate
Low	0-3	44	Not reached
Intermediate	4-5	35	51 mo
High	6-11	21	29 mo

CR, Complete response; *OS,* overall survival.
[a]One point is given for the presence of each of the following characteristics: Age older than 60 yr, elevated serum lactate dehydrogenase (LDH) level, Eastern Cooperative Oncology Group performance status ≥2, Ann Arbor stage III or IV, and more than two extranodal sites.
[b]One point is given for the presence of each of the following characteristics: Age older than 60 yr, elevated serum LDH level, hemoglobin level <12 g/dl, Ann Arbor stage III or IV, and number of nodal sites ≥5.
[c]Points are based on age, ECOG performance status, white blood cell count, and serum LDH level.
(1)The International Non-Hodgkin's Lymphoma Prognostic Factors Project: A predictive model for aggressive non-Hodgkin's lymphoma, *N Engl J Med* 329:987-994, 1993.
(2)Solal-Celigny P et al: Follicular lymphoma international prognostic index, *Blood* 104:1258-1265, 2004.
(3)Hoster E et al: A new prognostic index (MIPI) for patients with advanced-stage mantle cell lymphoma, *Blood* 111:558-565, 2008.
From Niederhuber JE: *Abeloff's clinical oncology,* ed 6, Philadelphia, 2020, Elsevier.

large B-cell lymphoma after two prior lines of chemotherapy.
- The anti-CD79 antibody drug conjugate polatuzumab vedotin, in combination with bendamustine and rituximab; the selective inhibitor of nuclear export selinexor; and the anti-CD19 monoclonal antibody tafasitamab, in combination with lenalidomide, have been FDA approved for the treatment of relapsed and/or refractory diffuse large B-cell lymphoma.
- Combination chemotherapy regimens for NHL are described in Table 6.

HIGHLY AGGRESSIVE NHL: The most common high-grade NHL subtype is Burkitt lymphoma (BL). BL affects younger patients than DLBCL and is common in HIV-infected individuals. Regimens more intensive than R-CHOP are needed to cure patients with high-grade NHL. The most commonly used multi-agent regimens include hyper-CVAD, CODOX-M/IVAC, and dose-adjusted EPOCH, usually in combination with rituximab. The 5-yr survival approximates 75%.

DISPOSITION

- Patients with indolent NHL in the rituximab era experience long survival despite the lack of curative potential of chemoimmunotherapy. Patients with aggressive NHL may achieve a cure with chemoimmunotherapy.
- Complete remission occurs in 50% to 60% of patients with aggressive NHL. Prognostic factors include the lymphoma subtype, age of patient, and extent of disease. Table 7 describes the International Prognostic Index (IPI) for aggressive lymphomas. More recently, studies of the IPI in the modern era incorporating the anti-CD20 monoclonal antibody rituximab show an overall improved prognosis with 33% of the highest-risk patients alive 5 yr from diagnosis and 96% in the lowest risk.
- Patients who present with HIV-related NHL and low CD4+ cell count have a poor prognosis (median duration of survival is 15 to 34 mo). Despite therapeutic advances, the management of HIV-associated lymphomas is challenging due to potential pharmacologic interactions and increased risk of infectious complications. It is important to optimize the CD4 cell count during treatment. Referral to an HIV oncologist is recommended.

SUGGESTED READINGS

Available at ExpertConsult.com

RELATED CONTENT

Non-Hodgkin Lymphoma (Patient Information)

AUTHORS: **Jorge J. Castillo, MD,** and **Ann S. LaCasce, MD, MMSc**

Nummular Dermatitis

BASIC INFORMATION

DEFINITION

Well-marginated, coin-shaped lesions of eczema

ETYMOLOGY

From the Latin *nummus* ("piece of money")

SYNONYM(S)

Nummular eczema
Discoid eczema
Microbial eczema

ICD-10CM CODE
L30.0 Nummular Dermatitis

EPIDEMIOLOGY & DEMOGRAPHICS

INCIDENCE: 0.1% to 9.1%
PREVALENCE: About 1 in 500
PREDOMINANT SEX & AGE: There are two peaks. Men >50 yr old predominate in the older peak, women <30 yr old predominate in the younger peak.
PEAK INCIDENCE: Men, slightly more often affected later >50 yr old, women usually <30 yr old
RISK FACTORS: Coexisting allergic contact dermatitis or atopic dermatitis
GENETICS: Multifactorial

PHYSICAL FINDINGS & CLINICAL PRESENTATION

Eruption of 1- to 3-cm, well-demarcated, round/annular eczematous patches (Fig. 1), which are almost exclusively on the extremities. Lesions commonly occur on the lower legs of men and the forearms and dorsal aspects of the hands in women. Lesions can be single or multiple. They are typically acutely or subacutely inflamed with vesicles and weeping but later become lichenified and hyperkeratotic (Figs. 2 & E3-E7). In patients with darker skin types often can present with scaly annular areas of hyperpigmentation and lichenification.

ETIOLOGY

Exact etiology is unknown. External irritants, cold, dry weather and source of infection may aggravate nummular dermatitis. Stasis and autoeczematization are other possible etiologic factors. Several medications have been cited as provoking nummular eczema (methyldopa, latanoprost eye drops, gold, interferon with ribavirin, mercury dental fillings). There is an association between allergic contact dermatitis and leading allergens such as nickel sulfate, potassium dichromate, and cobalt chloride. Coexisting infection with *Staphylococcus aureus* may occur but its role in pathogenesis is unclear.

DIAGNOSIS

DIFFERENTIAL DIAGNOSIS

- Atopic dermatitis
- Contact dermatitis
- Psoriasis
- Tinea corporis
- Mycosis fungoides
- Pityriasis rosea
- Stasis dermatitis.

WORKUP

None needed with a typical presentation. Most frequently, these lesions are mistaken for tinea corporis, but plaques of nummular eczema are distinguished by the lack of a raised, sharply circumscribed border. Skin biopsy can be helpful in clinically atypical or refractory cases to exclude entities in the differential diagnosis.

LABORATORY TESTS

None needed in typical cases. Patch testing is useful if an underlying contact allergy is suspected.

TREATMENT

Medium to high-potency topical corticosteroid ointments used judiciously and intermittently so as to avoid side effects. A tapering course of oral corticosteroid therapy can be considered in severe cases. In refractory and extensive cases, a steroid sparing immunosuppressant such as methotrexate or cyclosporine may be considered. Most recently, a case series using dupilumab (an IL-4Rα monoclonal antibody) for refractory nummular eczema showed a durable response in five out of six patients.

NONPHARMACOLOGIC THERAPY

Phototherapy or natural sunlight can help.

ACUTE GENERAL Rx

High potency topical corticosteroid ointment 2× a day for 2 wk, if severe 3-wk oral corticosteroid taper

CHRONIC Rx

High-dose topical corticosteroid taper 4 days a wk, alternating with a steroid-sparing agent

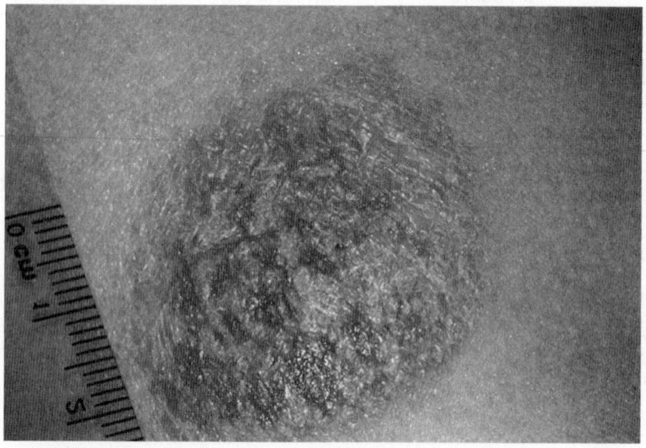

FIG. 1 Typical well-demarcated, 1-3 cm eczematous patch. (From Kliegman RM et al: *Nelson textbook of pediatrics*, ed 19, Philadelphia, 2018, Elsevier.)

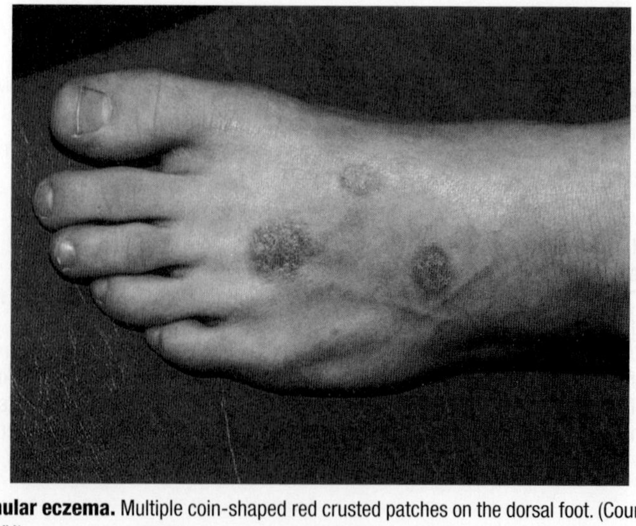

FIG. 2 Nummular eczema. Multiple coin-shaped red crusted patches on the dorsal foot. (Courtesy Dr. Robert Kalb, Buffalo, NY.)

such as a topical calcineurin inhibitor (tacrolimus or pimecrolimus), as well as topical emollient creams

COMPLEMENTARY & ALTERNATIVE MEDICINE

Tar preparations have been used with some success

DISPOSITION

Affected individuals will usually respond well to judicious use of topical steroids, but often will have a chronic course with intermittent relapses and exacerbations. Maintenance with intermittent use of topical steroids or topical calcineurin inhibitors may be required.

REFERRAL

Dermatology referral may be useful if lesions are refractory to topical corticosteroids, if contact allergy is suspected, or the presentation is atypical and other entities such as psoriasis or mycosis fungoides need to be excluded.

PEARLS & CONSIDERATIONS

COMMENTS

Lesions of nummular eczema are extremely pruritic and often take a chronic course. Nummular eczema can be frustrating for patients and physicians alike and often comes back when therapy is discontinued. Clarifying expectations and indicating that the goal is often control rather than cure is important for framing risk versus benefit management decisions.

PREVENTION

Application of emollients, such as Vaseline or Aquaphor after a bath or a shower can help prevent transepidermal water loss and lessen the severity of the eczema. Patients should be counseled to avoid exposure to irritants and common allergens and avoid the unnecessary use of topical antibiotics.

PATIENT & FAMILY EDUCATION

Nummular eczema often presents later in life than atopic dermatitis. Patients should be reassured and counseled that nummular eczema is not caused by anything that the patient "did." It is helpful to understand that improvement with topical medication can be expected, nummular eczema will often follow a chronic course. It is not the manifestation of systemic disease or anything "wrong" internally. The goal should be to gain control and maintain control with maintenance therapy coupled with sensitive skin care that improves quality of life.

SUGGESTED READINGS

Available at ExpertConsult.com

RELATED CONTENT

Atopic Dermatitis (Related Key Topic)

AUTHORS: **Leesha A. Helm, MD, MPH,** and **Matthew F. Helm, MD**

BASIC INFORMATION

DEFINITION

Obesity refers to having an excess amount of body fat in relation to lean body mass, or a body mass index (BMI) of ≥30 kg/m^2. Overweight is defined as BMI of 25 to 29.9 kg/m^2, and morbid obesity refers to adults with a BMI ≥40 kg/m^2. BMI is used as a surrogate measure of obesity. Weight classification by BMI is summarized in Table E1 Abdominal obesity is defined as waist circumference >102 cm (40 in) in men and >88 cm (35 in) in women.

ICD-10CM CODES	
E66.01	Morbid (severe) obesity due to excess calories
E66.09	Other obesity due to excess calories
E66.1	Drug-induced obesity
E66.2	Morbid (severe) obesity with alveolar hypoventilation
E66.8	Other obesity
E66.9	Obesity, unspecified
099.210	Obesity complicating pregnancy, unspecified trimester
099.211	Obesity complicating pregnancy, first trimester
099.212	Obesity complicating pregnancy, second trimester
099.213	Obesity complicating pregnancy, third trimester
099.214	Obesity complicating childbirth
099.215	Obesity complicating the puerperium

EPIDEMIOLOGY & DEMOGRAPHICS

- The World Health Organization first recognized obesity as a worldwide epidemic in 1997. As of 2005, 1.6 billion adults worldwide were classified as overweight, 400 million of whom were obese. It is predicted that the combination of overweight and obesity will soon eclipse public health issues such as malnutrition and infectious diseases as the most significant cause of poor health.
- Worldwide, data from the Global Burden of Disease Study from 1980 to 2013 indicate the prevalence of adult obesity has increased from 28.8% to 36.9% in men and 29.8% to 38% in women. The prevalence of childhood and adolescent obesity has also substantially increased.
- Based on U.S. NHANES data from 2011 to 2012, the prevalence of abdominal obesity was 54%. It is estimated that by 2020, 2 in every 5 adults and 1 in every 4 children in the U.S. will be categorized as obese.
- The present cost of obesity in the U.S. population is estimated at $100 billion annually. Approximately two thirds of people living in the U.S. are overweight, which is the highest percentage in the world (Marie Ng, 2014).
- For persons with a BMI ≥30 kg/m^2, all-cause mortality is increased by 50% to 100% above that of persons with BMI in the range of 20 to 25 kg/m^2.
- Obesity is an independent risk factor for cardiovascular disease (CVD), type 2 diabetes, hypertension, cancer (particularly colon, prostate, breast, and gynecologic malignancies), sleep apnea, degenerative joint disease, thromboembolic disorders, digestive tract diseases (gallstones), and dermatologic disorders.
- Significant morbidity and risk of death are projected to begin in young adulthood, resulting in >100,000 excess cases of CHD by 2035, even with the most modest projection of future obesity.
- When children enter kindergarten, 12.4% are obese, and another 14.9% are overweight. Data show that incident obesity between the ages of 5 and 14 yr is more likely to have occurred at younger ages.[1]
- Obesity in adolescence is significantly associated with increased risk of incident severe obesity in adulthood, with variations by sex and race/ethnicity. Overweight or obese adults who were obese as children have increased risk of type 2 DM, dyslipidemia, hypertension, and carotid artery atherosclerosis.
- Obesity is a major preventable cause of death and disability in the U.S. (the other is tobacco).
- Extensive data indicate that weight loss can reverse or arrest the harmful effects of obesity.
- In 2013 nearly 180,000 bariatric surgery procedures were performed in the U.S. Of these procedures 42% were laparoscopic sleeve gastrectomy, 34% were Roux-en-Y gastric bypass, and 15% were laparoscopic adjustable gastric banding.

PHYSICAL FINDINGS & CLINICAL PRESENTATION

- Physical examination should assess the degree and distribution of body fat, signs of secondary causes of obesity, and obesity-related comorbidities.
- Increased waist circumference is apparent. Excess abdominal fat is clinically defined as a waist circumference >40 in (>102 cm) in men and >35 in (>88 cm) in women (in Asian men and women, >36 in and >33 in, respectively). Central obesity is a risk factor for mortality even among individuals with normal BMIs.
- Symptoms associated with hypertension, coronary artery disease (CAD), and diabetes (e.g., polyuria, polydipsia, acanthosis nigricans, retinopathy, and neuropathy) may be present.
- Obesity is associated with cardiac hypertrophy, diastolic dysfunction, and decreased aortic compliance, which are independent predictors of cardiovascular risk.
- Joint pain and swelling are associated with degenerative joint disease secondary to obesity.
- The physical exam and ECG often underestimate the presence and extent of cardiac dysfunction in obese patients. Jugular venous distention and hepatojugular reflux may not be seen and heart sounds are frequently distant.
- A large quantity of fluid is present in the interstitial space of adipose tissue, as the interstitial space is ~10% of the tissue wet weight. This excess fluid in this compartment, if redistributed into the circulation, can have negative repercussions in obese individuals with heart failure. Obese individuals have higher cardiac output and a lower total peripheral resistance than do lean individuals, and obesity is associated with persistence of elevated cardiac filling pressure during exercise.
- Obesity predisposes to heart failure through several different mechanisms: Increased total blood volume, increased cardiac output, LVH, left ventricular diastolic dysfunction, and adipositas cordis (excessive epicardial fat and fatty infiltration of the myocardium).

ETIOLOGY

- The pathophysiology of obesity is complex and poorly understood, but includes social, nutritional, physiologic, psychological, and genetic factors.
- Environmental factors such as a sedentary lifestyle and chronic ingestion of excess calories can cause obesity.
- Obesity may be related to genetic factors, which are thought to be polygenic. Genetic studies with adopted children have demonstrated that they have similar BMIs to their biologic parents but not their adoptive parents. Twin studies also demonstrate a genetic influence on BMI.
- Secondary causes of obesity can result from medications (antipsychotics, steroids, and protease inhibitors being common ones) and neuroendocrine disorders (like Cushing syndrome and hypothyroidism).

Dx DIAGNOSIS

- BMI will establish the diagnosis of obesity. BMI is defined as the adult's weight in kilograms divided by the square of his or her height—and is closely correlated with total body fat content.
- BMI values can categorize patients into three classes of obesity:
    1. Class I (mild): BMI of 30.0 to 34.9 kg/m^2
    2. Class II (moderate): BMI of 35.0 to 39.9 kg/m^2
    3. Class III (severe): BMI of ≥40 kg/m^2
- Although BMI is commonly used to define obesity, it is not a highly accurate indicator of body fat composition in children, who are undergoing rapid changes in height, or in bodybuilders or athletes who have large amounts of muscle tissue.

[1]Cunningham SA et al: Incidence of childhood obesity in the United States, *N Engl J Med,* 370:403-411, 2014.

- Waist circumference or waist-hip ratio is indicative of visceral adipose tissue/intraabdominal fat, which may be more deleterious than overall overweight or obesity.

DIFFERENTIAL DIAGNOSIS

It is important to evaluate obese patients for secondary medical causes of obesity. Hypothalamic disorders, hypothyroidism, Cushing syndrome, insulinoma, depression, and drugs (corticosteroids, antidepressants, second-generation antipsychotics, sulfonylureas, and HIV protease inhibitors) can cause obesity. In children, certain genetic conditions, such as Prader-Willi syndrome, are associated with obesity.

WORKUP

History should be obtained regarding weight change, family history of obesity, and eating and exercise behavior. Assessment for eating disorders and depression should be made. Attention should be directed to the use of nutritional supplements, over-the-counter medications, hormones, diuretics, and laxatives. The workup of an obese patient typically requires laboratory work to assess for risks and complications as well as to rule out underlying causative medical conditions.

LABORATORY TESTS

- Obese patients should be assessed for medical consequences of their obesity by screening for metabolic syndrome. This includes measurement of fasting lipid profile, blood pressure, and waist circumference and screening for diabetes or prediabetes (oral glucose tolerance test, fasting glucose, or hemoglobin A1C).
- Polycythemia might warrant screening for sleep apnea. Liver function tests should be obtained to screen for hepatic steatosis.
- In the proper clinical setting, thyroid function studies and dexamethasone suppression testing will exclude hypothyroidism and Cushing syndrome as underlying causes of obesity. If insulinoma is suspected, the patient will need to undergo a 72-hr fast to confirm hypoglycemia with inappropriate insulin secretion.
- Obesity is associated with changes in the ECG, including a reduction in voltage and nonspecific ST-T changes that may interfere with diagnosis of left ventricular hypertrophy (LVH) or CAD.

IMAGING STUDIES

- Several methods are available for determining or calculating total body fat but offer no significant advantage over the BMI. These include measurement of total body water, total body potassium, bioelectrical impedance, and dual-energy x-ray absorptiometry.
- Buoyancy testing is an accurate method for determining total body fat composition.

OTHER STUDIES

Obesity increases the risk of obstructive sleep apnea, which, in turn, increases the risks of hypertension, cardiac arrhythmias, CVD, stroke, and heart failure. Therefore, one should have a low threshold to screen obese patients for obstructive sleep apnea via sleep study/polysomnography.

Rx TREATMENT

The National Heart, Lung, and Blood Institute (NHLBI) developed guidelines for selecting treatment strategies for overweight and obese patients based on BMI and comorbidities. They recommend a combination of dietary management, physical activity management, and behavior therapy for anyone with a BMI ≥25 or with a high-risk waist circumference and two or more obesity-associated comorbidities. Pharmacotherapy should be considered for patients with a BMI ≥30 or ≥27 with comorbidities.

Bariatric surgery is indicated for patients with a BMI ≥35 with comorbidities and for any patient with a BMI ≥40 (Table 2).

NONPHARMACOLOGIC THERAPY

- The cornerstones for weight management and reduction are calorie restriction, exercise, and behavioral modification. Assessment of patient's willingness to make changes must be evaluated, as treatment is more likely to succeed in motivated patients.
- The NHLBI guidelines recommend an initial diet to produce a calorie deficit of 500 to 1000 kcal/day. This has been shown to reduce total body weight by an average of 8% over 3 to 12 mo.
- These guidelines recommend the use of a food diary to focus on dietary substitutes.
- Thirty min of moderate-intensity activity on 5 or more days of the wk results in health benefits for obese individuals. Moreover, several studies indicate that 60 to 80 min of moderate to vigorous physical activity may provide additional benefit.
- Increased physical activity without caloric restriction (minimal or no weight loss) can reduce abdominal (visceral) adipose tissue and improve insulin resistance.
- The key features of the standard behavioral modification program include goal setting, self-monitoring, stimulus control (modification of one's environment to enhance behaviors that will support weight management), cognitive restructuring (increased awareness of perceptions of oneself and one's weight), and prevention of relapse (weight regain).
- Mammalian sleep is closely integrated with the regulation of energy balance. Trials have shown that the amount of human sleep contributes to the maintenance of fat-free body mass at times of decreased energy intake. Lack of sufficient sleep may compromise the efficacy of typical dietary interventions for weight loss and related metabolic risk reduction.

ACUTE GENERAL Rx

- According to the NHLBI *Guidelines on the Identification, Evaluation, and Treatment of Overweight and Obesity in Adults* and the U.S. Food and Drug Administration (FDA), pharmacotherapy is indicated for:
  1. Obese patients with a BMI ≥30
  2. Overweight patients with a BMI of ≥27 and concomitant obesity-related risk factors or diseases, such as hypertension, diabetes, or dyslipidemia
- Pharmacologic treatment options include:
  1. Gastrointestinal lipase inhibitors: Orlistat is the only drug available for long-term treatment of obesity. It blocks the digestion and absorption of ingested dietary fat. It is a reversible inhibitor of pancreatic, gastric, and carboxyl ester lipases and phospholipase A2, which are required for the hydrolysis of dietary fat in the gastrointestinal tract. Side effects include flatulence, fecal incontinence, cramps, and oily spotting. There can also be impairment of absorption of fat-soluble vitamins (A, D, E, K) and

TABLE 2 Weight-Loss Treatment Guidelines from the National Heart, Lung, and Blood Institute*

	BMI				
Treatment	**25.0-26.9**	**27.0-29.9**	**30.0-34.9**	**35.0-39.9**	**>40.0**
Diet, physical activity, behavioral therapy, or all three	Yes	Yes	Yes	Yes	Yes
Pharmacotherapy†		In patients with obesity-related diseases	Yes	Yes	Yes
Surgery‡				In patients with obesity-related diseases	Yes

*Data are from www.nhlbi.nih.gov/science/obesity-nutrition-and-physical-activity. These guidelines are generally consistent with those from the American Heart Association, the American Medical Association, the American Diabetic Association, the Obesity Society (Practical Guide), the American Diabetes Association, the American Academy of Family Physicians, the American College of Sports Medicine, and the American Cancer Society. *BMI* denotes body mass index, calculated as the weight in kilograms divided by the square of the height in meters.

†Pharmacotherapy should be considered only in patients who are not able to achieve adequate weight loss with available conventional lifestyle modifications and who have no absolute contraindications for drug therapy.

‡Bariatric surgery should be considered only in patients who are unable to lose weight with available conventional therapy and who have no absolute contraindications for surgery.

beta-carotene. Oxalate-associated acute kidney injury and rare severe liver injury have also been reported.

2. C serotonin agonists: Lorcaserin is a selective serotonin agonist that acts centrally to reduce appetite, aiding weight loss. Adverse effects include headache, upper respiratory infections, dizziness, and nausea. While there is little evidence of serotonin-associated cardiac valvular disease or pulmonary hypertension (as seen with nonselective serotonergic agonists fenfluramine and dexfenfluramine), long-term data is currently limited.
3. Sympathomimetic medications: Phentermine and diethylpropion are currently approved for short-term treatment of obesity. They reduce food intake by causing early satiety. Side effects include increased blood pressure and increased pulse. They are Schedule IV drugs with a potential for abuse. Other sympathomimetic drugs that have been removed from the market due to concerns about cardiovascular safety are sibutramine, phenylpropanolamine, and ephedrine.
4. Antidepressants: While not FDA-approved for treatment of obesity alone, bupropion and fluoxetine are antidepressants that have been associated with modest weight loss. The FDA has recently approved a fixed-dose combination of bupropion with the opioid receptor antagonist naltrexone. It is called Contrave and approved for use as an adjunct to diet and exercise in patients with BMI ≥30 kg/m² or a BMI ≥27 kg/m² and one or more weight-related comorbidities (e.g., diabetes, hypertension, dyslipidemia).
5. Antiepileptic drugs: Zonisamide and topiramate (also used in migraine therapy) have been associated with weight loss in clinical trials but are not currently FDA-approved for treatment of obesity alone.
6. Diabetes drugs: While not FDA-approved for treatment of obesity alone, metformin, pramlintide (synthetic human amylin), and glucagon-like polypeptide-1 agonists (GLP-1) (exenatide) have been associated with weight loss in the treatment of individuals with diabetes. The GLP-1 receptor agonist liraglutide (Victoza) is now FDA approved at a higher dose as Saxenda for chronic weight management in adults with BMI ≥30 or a BMI ≥27 with a weight-related comorbidity such as hypertension, dyslipidemia, or diabetes.

CHRONIC Rx

- According to the NHLBI guidelines, surgical intervention is an option for selected patients with clinically severe obesity (a BMI ≥40 or a BMI ≥35 with comorbid conditions), when patients are at high risk for obesity-associated morbidity or death, and when less invasive methods of weight loss have failed. Box 1 summarizes patient requirements for bariatric surgery.
- Eligible patients should also be at an acceptable risk for surgery, well informed, and motivated.
- Restrictive surgeries limit the amount of food the stomach can hold and slow the rate of gastric emptying. These include vertical banded gastroplasty and laparoscopic adjustable silicone gastric banding (LAGB). Band slippage is the most common LAGB complication. Other potential complications include port or tubing malfunction, stomal obstruction, band erosion, pouch dilatation, and port infection. Gastric necrosis of the stomach wall is a rarer late complication that results from ischemia caused by a combination of gastric prolapse—the part of the stomach below the band herniates up through the device —and pressure from the band. Complications of bariatric surgery are summarized in Box E2.
- Gastric bypass has better outcomes than gastric band procedures for long-term weight loss, type 2 diabetes control and remission, hypertension, and hyperlipidemia. These procedures have benefits that include lower perioperative mortality rate, a quicker recovery period, and no malabsorption issues. However, they are not as effective as gastric bypass for weight reduction and comorbidity improvement.
  1. Malabsorptive surgeries reduce nutrient absorption by shortening the length of small intestine. These include jejunoileal bypass and the duodenal switch operation (DS).
  2. Restrictive malabsorptive bypass procedures combine the elements of gastric restriction and selective malabsorption. These include Roux-en-Y gastric bypass (considered the gold standard because of its high level of effectiveness and durability) and biliopancreatic diversion. These procedures have higher rates of comorbidity improvement than restrictive surgeries, but can be complicated by malabsorption and nutritional deficiencies.
- Compared with usual care, bariatric surgery is associated with reduced number of cardiovascular deaths and lower incidence of cardiovascular events and cancer mortality[2] in obese adults. A study on bariatric surgery patients demonstrated a significant reduction in long-term cardiovascular events. Ten-yr follow-up estimated relative risk reductions ranging from 18% to 79% according to the Framingham risk score, and 8% to 62% with the PROCAM risk score.
- A long-term observational study of obese patients with type 2 diabetes showed that bariatric surgery was associated with higher diabetes remission rates and fewer complications than usual care (Sjöström et al., 2014). Remission of type 2 DM occurs in 60% to 80% of patients 2 yr after surgery and persists in about 30% of patients 15 yr after Roux-en-Y gastric bypass.
- Liposuction is removal of fat by aspiration after injection of physiologic saline. This technique reduces the subcutaneous fat but has failed to improve insulin sensitivity or risk factors for CHD.
- The Maestro Rechargeable System is a subcutaneously implanted device FDA approved for weight loss in adults with a BMI of 40 to 45 or with a BMI of ≥35 and at least one obesity-related comorbidity. It utilizes high-frequency electrical pulses to block vagus nerve signals between the brain and stomach. It is less effective than bariatric surgery for weight loss. The list price for the Maestro system exceeds $15,000.
- The AspireAssist device is FDA approved for weight loss in adults ≥22 yr old with a BMI of 35 to 55. It requires the insertion of a PEG tube endoscopically and pulled through a percutaneous incision. Thirty min after a meal, the patient attaches a connector to it and drains a portion of their stomach content into a toilet. The tube is then flushed with potable water. The connector stops working after 115 cycles (6 wk) and is replaced at a follow-up appointment. Estimated cost for procedure and follow-ups are $13,000 for the first yr.

DISPOSITION

- The incidence of venous thromboembolism in the upper tertile of BMI was 2.42 times that of the lowest BMI tertile. Obese patients have a higher incidence of postoperative thromboembolic events when undergoing noncardiac surgery.
- Obesity may be associated with higher rates of postoperative pulmonary complications and poor wound healing.

BOX 1 Patient Requirements for Bariatric Surgery

1. Patients with a BMI of 40 kg/m² or greater are potential candidates for bariatric surgery.
2. Patients with a BMI of 35 to 40 kg/m² with significant obesity-related comorbidity are also potential candidates for bariatric surgery.
3. Patients with a history of dieting.
4. Patients with no recent substance abuse.
5. Patients should be evaluated by a multidisciplinary team that includes a dietician and psychologic evaluation before surgery.

BMI, Body mass index.

From Cameron JL, Cameron AM: *Current surgical therapy,* ed 12, Philadelphia, 2017, Elsevier.

[2]Doumouras AG et al: Association Between Bariatric Surgery and All-Cause Mortality: A Population-Based Matched Cohort Study in a Universal Health Care System. *Ann Intern Med* 173(9):694-703, 2020.

- Weight-stable obese subjects have an increased risk of arrhythmias and sudden death even in the absence of cardiac dysfunction.
- Obesity and the cardiac autonomic nervous system are intrinsically related. A 10% increase in body weight is associated with a decline in parasympathetic tone accompanied by a rise in mean heart rate. Conversely, a 10% weight loss in severely obese patients is associated with significant improvement in autonomic nervous system cardiac modulation, including decreased heart rate and increased heart rate variability.
- Postmortem Determinants of Atherosclerosis in Youth (PDAY) study data provided convincing evidence that obesity in adolescents and young adults accelerates the progression of atherosclerosis decades before the appearance of clinical manifestations.
- Obesity accelerates the progression of native coronary atherosclerosis and after coronary artery bypass grafting.
- In older adults, obesity is associated with protection against hip fracture, but this protective effect on bone status does not offset the extensive array of potential adverse effects on conditions common in the older population.
- A 3-yr trial comparing midterm effects of bariatric surgery on patients with obesity and hypertension revealed roux-en-Y gastric bypass (RYGB) is an effective strategy for midterm blood pressure control and hypertension remission, with fewer medications required in patients with hypertension and obesity.[4]
- A study on the effects of diet vs. gastric bypass on metabolic function in type 2 diabetes revealed that the metabolic benefits of gastric bypass surgery and diet are similar and related to weight loss itself, with no evident clinically important effects independent of weight loss.[5] A 10-yr trial in obese diabetic patients comparing bariatric surgery versus medical treatment for promoting remission and preventing diabetes-related complications revealed that surgery patients had fewer diabetes-related complications but more digestive and metabolic complications.[6]

[4] Schiavon CA et al: Three-year outcomes of bariatric surgery in patients with obesity and hypertension: a randomized clinical trial. *Ann Intern Med* 173(9):685-693, 2020.

[5] Yoshino M et al: Effects of diet versus gastric bypass on metabolic function in diabetes. *N Engl J Med* 3838:721-732, 2020.

[6] Mingrone G et al: Metabolic surgery versus conventional medical therapy in patients with type 2 diabetes: 10-year follow-up of an open-label, single-centre, randomised controlled trial. *Lancet* 397(10271):293-304, 2021.

REFERRAL

Obesity is commonly seen in the primary care setting. If pharmacologic therapy is considered, consultation with physicians specializing in obesity and experienced with the use of the drug is recommended. In addition, consultation with nutritionists and behavioral therapists is helpful. A consultation with general surgery is indicated in patients being considered for surgical intervention.

PEARLS & CONSIDERATIONS

COMMENTS

- Enhanced weight-loss counseling helps about one third of obese patients achieve long-term, clinically meaningful weight loss. Adults can lose 1 to 2 lb (0.45 to 0.9 kg per wk) by consuming 500 to 1000 fewer calories per day.
- The NHLBI launched the Obesity Education Initiative in January 1991. The overall purpose of the initiative is to help reduce the prevalence of overweight along with the prevalence of physical inactivity to reduce the risk of CHD and overall morbidity and mortality rates from CHD.
- A recent study on BMI and all-cause mortality in a large prospective study suggests that optimal BMI range is between 20 and 24.9 (Patel AV, 2014).
- Recent research indicates that brown adipose tissue represents a natural target for the modulation of energy expenditure. The presence of brown adipose tissue in humans may be quantified with the use of ^{18}F-FDG PET-CT. The amount of brown adipose tissue is inversely correlated with BMI, suggesting a potential role of brown adipose tissue in adult human metabolism.
- Obesity, glucose intolerance, and hypertension in childhood are strongly associated with increased rates of premature death from endogenous causes in this population.
- Recent trials have shown that among persons living in a controlled setting, calories alone account for the increase in fat. Protein affected energy expenditure and storage of lean body mass, but not body fat storage.
- There have been no evidence-based studies supporting combination medical therapy for weight loss.
- Data are lacking for the role of pharmacotherapy and bariatric surgery in the elderly population.

PREVENTION

- Prevention of overweight and obesity involves both increasing physical activity and dietary modification to reduce caloric intake.
- There is compelling evidence that prevention of weight regain in formerly obese individuals requires 60 to 90 min of moderate-intensity activity or lesser amounts of vigorous intensity activity.
- Moderate-intensity activity of approximately 45 to 60 min per day, or 1.7 physical activity level (PAL), is required to prevent the transition to overweight or obesity. For children, even more activity time is recommended.
- Clinicians can help guide patients to develop personalized eating plans and help them recognize the contributions of fat, concentrated carbohydrates, and large portion sizes.
- Clinicians must work with patients to modify other risk factors such as tobacco use, high glycemic intake, and elevated blood pressure to prevent the long-term chronic disease sequelae of obesity. Generally lower carbohydrate, moderate fat intake, with stable protein and energy intake results in higher energy expenditure during weight-loss maintenance.[3]
- Regular screening of body weight and BMI measurements at routine office visits can help identify early weight gain.
- Among obese adolescents, the most rapid weight gain occurs between 2 and 6 yr of age. Most children who are obese at that age are obese in adolescence.[3]

PATIENT & FAMILY EDUCATION

Information can be obtained on the American Obesity Association website (www.obesity.org) and the American Medical Association website (www.ama-assn.org).

SUGGESTED READINGS

Available at ExpertConsult.com

RELATED CONTENT

Obesity, Female (Patient Information)
Obesity, Male (Patient Information)
Obesity, Child (Patient Information)

AUTHOR: **Fred F. Ferri, MD**

[3] Ebbeling CB et al: Effects of a low carbohydrate diet on energy expenditure during weight loss maintenance: randomized trial, *BMJ* 363:k4583, 2018.

BASIC INFORMATION

DEFINITION

Excessive use of an opioid, either derived from the opium poppy or semi- or fully synthetic, resulting in respiratory depression, central nervous system depression, and/or death

SYNONYMS

Opiate overdose
Heroin overdose
Narcotic overdose
Opioid poisoning

ICD-10CM CODES	
T40.0X1	Poisoning by opium, accidental (unintentional)
T40.0X2	Poisoning by opium, intentional self-harm
T40.0X3	Poisoning by opium, assault
T40.0X4	Poisoning by opium, undetermined
T40.0X5	Adverse effect of opium
T40.1X	Poisoning by heroin
T40.4	Poisoning by other synthetic narcotics

EPIDEMIOLOGY & DEMOGRAPHICS

INCIDENCE: Drug overdose deaths and opioid-involved deaths continue to increase in the U.S. The majority of drug overdose deaths (more than six out of ten) involve an opioid. 91 Americans die every day from an opioid overdose.

PREVALENCE: From 1999 to 2017 more than 700,000 U.S. residents died from drug overdoses. From 2013 to 2017, the number of opioid-involved overdose deaths (opioid deaths) in the U.S. increased 90% from 25,052 to 47,600. This increase was primarily driven by substantial increases in deaths involving illicitly manufactured fentanyl (IMF) or fentanyl analogs mixed with heroin, sold as heroin, or pressed into counterfeit prescription pills.

PREDOMINANT SEX & AGE: The "typical" heroin death involves experienced users in their 20s to 30s using coingestants, with a male predilection.

RISK FACTORS: The majority of drug-overdose deaths are unintentional or accidental (74%). The following increase risk for opioid overdose:

- Opioid dependence, in particular following reduced tolerance (following detoxification, release from incarceration, cessation of treatment)
- Injecting opioids
- Using prescription opioids, in particular taking higher doses
- Using opioids in combination with other sedating substances
- Using opioids and having comorbidities such as HIV, liver or lung disease, or suffering from depression
- Household members of people in possession of opioids (including prescription opioids)

The highest drug-induced mortality is associated with the following factors: 40 to 49 yr of age, male gender, non-Hispanic whites, and living in the South, all of which account for approximately 38.2% of drug-induced deaths in the U.S.

PHYSICAL FINDINGS & CLINICAL PRESENTATION

Patients with opioid overdose classically present with the triad of altered mental status, pinpoint pupils, and respiratory depression. Patients may be apneic or with low respiratory rate and tidal volumes. Respiratory depression becomes profound enough to cause anoxia, leading to death. Little to no response will be elicited from painful stimuli. Look for clinical clues, such as "track marks" or darkening along the length of veins from injection drug use that may suggest opioid overdose. The use of coingestants, which is exceedingly common in opioid overdose, can alter the classic exam findings one may expect. For example, use of sympathomimetics like cocaine can cause pupillary dilation. Respiratory rate <12 breaths/min is most sensitive for predicting response to naloxone. Once the patient is hemodynamically stable, examine for other sequelae of drug use, including pulmonary rales suggestive of aspiration pneumonia or murmurs and skin lesions associated with endocarditis in IV drug abusers.

DIAGNOSIS

DIFFERENTIAL DIAGNOSIS

- Hypoglycemia
- Alcohol or sedative overdose
- Postictal state
- Infectious or metabolic encephalopathy
- Clonidine overdose
- Phenothiazine overdose
- Organophosphate exposure

WORKUP

Opioid overdose requires little workup if the patient's altered mental status can be completely attributed to the overdose (i.e., by full recovery with naloxone). However, if the patient remains altered or with significant respiratory compromise after adequate treatment, continue appropriate workup. Obtain an ECG in the following scenarios: Use of methadone, oxycodone, loperamide or a coingestant tricyclic antidepressant to screen for QTc prolongation; coingestion of a sympathomimetic to rule out arrhythmias.

LABORATORY TESTS

- Serum glucose should be quickly obtained as with any resuscitation.
- Urine drug screen is not routinely required unless the history or physical exam raises suspicion for coingestants that would alter management.
- Tylenol and aspirin levels in intentional overdoses or when used in a combination formulation with an opioid.

IMAGING STUDIES

Not required unless guided by your physical exam and/or response to therapy:

- Computed tomography of the head and cervical spine for suspected trauma
- Chest x-ray if signs of aspiration
- Echocardiogram if concerned for endocarditis

TREATMENT

The principal goals of treatment for opioid overdose are support of ventilation and reversal of the drug.

NONPHARMACOLOGIC THERAPY

Support the airway and breathing. For apneic or bradypneic patients, use bag-valve-mask ventilation.

ACUTE GENERAL Rx

Administer naloxone, a short-acting opioid antagonist, as soon as possible. Intravenous is the preferred route; however, in November 2015, Narcan Nasal Spray became the first FDA-approved non-injectable naloxone product for the treatment of opioid overdose. Higher concentration intranasal naloxone 2 mg/ml seems to have efficacy similar to IM naloxone for reversal of opioid overdose. Via the IV route, onset of action is within 1 to 2 min. Dosing is as follows:

- For most adult patients, 0.4 to 1.2 mg should yield recovery of consciousness.
- For patients in cardiac arrest, 2 mg is the starting dose.
- Younger than 5 yr or body weight 20 kg or less: 0.1 mg/kg administered by IV push, intraosseous (IO) push, or by endotracheal tube (ETT).
- 5 yr and older or body weight more than 20 kg: 2 mg administered by IV push, IO, or ETT.

Prepare for adverse effects of acute withdrawal, including agitation, nausea, vomiting, piloerection, diarrhea, lacrimation, yawning, and rhinorrhea after naloxone administration to chronic opioid users, especially with higher doses. Naloxone continues to block binding of additional opioids to the receptor for 20 to 90 min.

CHRONIC Rx

- Naloxone autoinjectors and nasal sprays are available in some states and intended for buddy administration. Patients can buy these formulations over-the-counter in some states, whereas others require a prescription. Check your state's legislature for continual updates on this matter.
- A 2016 nonrandomized study demonstrated that patients prescribed opioids plus naloxone had 47% fewer opioid-related emergency department visits within 6 mo than those not prescribed naloxone.

REFERRAL

Patients can be offered referral to drug rehabilitation services. Otherwise, follow up with the primary care physician is appropriate.

SUGGESTED READINGS

Available at ExpertConsult.com

RELATED CONTENT

Drug Use Disorder (Related Key Topic)
Opioid Use Disorder (Related Key Topic)

AUTHORS: **Amanda Box, MD, MS,** and **Mark F. Brady, MD, MPH, MMSc**

BASIC INFORMATION

DEFINITION

- Opioid use disorder is defined as a cluster of cognitive, behavioral, and physiologic symptoms in which the individual continues use of opiates despite significant opiate-induced problems. Opiate use disorder is a chronic, relapsing disorder characterized by repeated self-administration that usually results in opiate tolerance, withdrawal, and compulsive drug use. Tolerance is the need to increase dose to achieve the same effect. Dependence may occur with or without the physiologic symptoms of tolerance and withdrawal.
- There are four stages of addiction:
  1. Stage I, acute drug effects: Rewarding effects of drug result from neurobiologic changes in response to the acute drug use. Duration varies from hours to days.
  2. Stage II, transformation to addiction: Associated with changes in neuronal function that accumulate with repeated administration and diminish over days or weeks after discontinuation of drug use.
  3. Stage III, relapse after extended periods of abstinence: Precipitated by an incubation of cue-induced craving (people, places, and things as triggers) and priming (relapse precipitated by drug exposure).
  4. Stage IV, end-stage addiction: Vulnerability to relapse endures for yr and results from prolonged changes at the cellular level.
- Pseudoaddiction: Undertreatment of pain resulting in "opiate-seeking" behaviors such as "doctor shopping" and multiple emergency department visits. These behaviors disappear with adequate treatment of pain.

SYNONYMS

Opioid dependence
OUD (opioid use disorder)
Opiate addiction
Opiate abuse
Narcotic addiction
Narcotic abuse
Substance use disorder

ICD-10CM CODES

F11.10	Opioid abuse, uncomplicated
F11.120	Opioid abuse with intoxication, uncomplicated
F11.121	Opioid abuse with intoxication delirium
F11.122	Opioid abuse with intoxication with perceptual disturbance
F11.129	Opioid abuse with intoxication, unspecified
F11.14	Opioid abuse with opioid-induced mood disorder
F11.150	Opioid abuse with opioid-induced psychotic disorder with delusions
F11.151	Opioid abuse with opioid-induced psychotic disorder with hallucinations
F11.159	Opioid abuse with opioid-induced psychotic disorder, unspecified
F11.181	Opioid abuse with opioid-induced sexual dysfunction
F11.182	Opioid abuse with opioid-induced sleep disorder
F11.188	Opioid abuse with other opioid-induced disorder
F11.19	Opioid abuse with unspecified opioid-induced disorder

EPIDEMIOLOGY & DEMOGRAPHICS

INCIDENCE: It is estimated that more than 2.5 million Americans have an opioid use disorder.

PREVALENCE:

- In 2018, U.S. retail pharmacies dispensed 170 million prescriptions for opioid pain relievers.
- In 2014, 10.3 million persons reported using prescription opioids nonmedically.
- Admissions to substance-abuse treatment programs linked to prescription opioids more than quadrupled between 2002 and 2012.
- In 2016, 948,000 Americans used heroin.
- The percentage of eighth-, tenth-, and twelfth-graders who have used heroin has more than doubled since the late 1990s. This increase has largely been attributed to decreased price and increased purity in the last decade.
- In 2017, >40% of suicide and overdose deaths involved opioids.
- In 2018, approximately 47,000 Americans died of opioid-related overdose.
- In March and October 2015, the Drug Enforcement Administration and Centers for Disease Control and Prevention issued nationwide alerts identifying fentanyl, particularly illicitly manufactured fentanyl, as a threat to public health and safety. Illicitly manufactured fentanyl is pharmacologically similar to pharmaceutical fentanyl but is unlawfully produced in clandestine laboratories and obtained via illicit drug markets; it also includes fentanyl analogs. Fentanyl is a synthetic opioid 50 to 100 times more potent than morphine and approved for the management of surgical/postoperative pain, severe chronic pain, and breakthrough cancer pain.
- In the U.S., approximately 10 million adults are prescribed long-term opioid therapy (LTOT) for chronic pain despite inadequate evidence of long-term benefit and growing evidence of harm.

PREDOMINANT SEX: Males abuse opioids more commonly than females, with a male:female ratio of 3:1 for heroin and 1.5:1 for prescription opiates.

PEAK INCIDENCE: The majority of new abusers of opiates are <26 yr.

RISK FACTORS:

- Family history
- Prior history of addiction
- Psychiatric disorders

GENETICS:

- Genetic epidemiologic studies suggest a high degree of heritable vulnerability for opioid dependence.
- Gene polymorphism for dopamine receptor/transporters, opioid receptors, serotonin receptors/transporters, proenkephalin, and catechol-*O*-methyltransferase all appear to be associated with vulnerability to opioid dependence. Future interventions for opiate dependence may include medications identified through genetic research.

PHYSICAL FINDINGS & CLINICAL PRESENTATION

- Physical examination is often noncontributory.
- Small-sized pupils may be the only observable sign of use because only mild tolerance develops for miosis.
- Scars or tracks from chronic IV use may be visible over the veins of the arms, hands, ankles, neck, and breasts.
- Inflamed nasal mucosa or respiratory wheezing may be apparent in patients who are snorting heroin or OxyContin.
- Patients in withdrawal may have more dramatic findings such as tachycardia, hypertension, fever, piloerection (goose flesh), mydriasis, lacrimation, central nervous system (CNS) arousal, irritability, and repeated yawning. In patients with sympathetic overactivity and panic attacks, use of CNS stimulants, such as amphetamines or cocaine, should also be ruled out.
- Although gastrointestinal symptoms of nausea, vomiting, and abdominal pain are common in opioid withdrawal, other causes such as gastroenteritis, pancreatitis, peptic ulcer disease, and intestinal obstruction need to be ruled out.
- The history may provide relevant information in making the diagnosis. Significant findings may include:
  1. A long history of opioid self-administration, typically by the IV or intranasal route but sometimes through smoking as well.
  2. Polysubstance use. Intoxication by drugs other than narcotics (e.g., benzodiazepines, barbiturates) should be ruled out in unconscious patients.
  3. A high incidence of nonopioid-related psychiatric disorders (>80%).
  4. History of problems at work, school, or relationships associated with drug use.
  5. History of legal problems associated with drug use, such as arrest for possession, robbery, or prostitution.
  6. History of interpersonal violence (as perpetrator or victim).
  7. History of physical problems such as skin infections, phlebitis, endocarditis, or liver diseases attributable to acetaminophen toxicity (Vicodin/Percocet) or viral hepatitis. Hepatitis C is the most prevalent bloodborne pathogen. It is present in approximately 90% of opiate-dependent people and is often spread by sharing IV drug paraphernalia or snorting devices. There is also a higher incidence of HIV infection.

ETIOLOGY

Opioid use disorder is a biopsychosocial disorder. Pharmacologic, social, genetic, and psychodynamic factors interact to influence abusive

TABLE 1 CAGE-AID

1. Have you ever tried to **C**ut down on your alcohol or drug use?
2. Do you get **A**nnoyed when people comment about your drinking or drug use?
3. Do you feel **G**uilty about things you have done while drinking or using drugs?
4. Do you need an **E**ye-opener to get started in the morning?

Two or more questions answered in the affirmative require further assessment. *AID,* adapted to include drugs.
From Bowman S et al: Reducing the health consequences of opioid addiction in primary care, *Am J Med* 126:565-571, 2013.

TABLE 2 Drug Abuse Screening Test (DAST-10)

1. Have you used drugs other than those required for medical reasons?
2. Do you abuse more than one drug at a time?
3. Are you unable to stop using drugs when you want to?
4. Have you ever had blackouts or flashbacks as a result of drug use?
5. Do you ever feel bad or guilty about your drug use?
6. Does your spouse (or parents) ever complain about your involvement with drugs?
7. Have you neglected your family because of your use of drugs?
8. Have you engaged in illegal activities in order to obtain drugs?
9. Have you ever experienced withdrawal symptoms (felt sick) when you stopped taking drugs?
10. Have you had medical problems as a result of your drug use (e.g., memory loss, hepatitis, convulsions, bleeding)?

Two or more questions answered in the affirmative require further assessment.
From Bowman S et al: Reducing the health consequences of opioid addiction in primary care, *Am J Med* 126:565-571, 2013.

behaviors. Pharmacologic factors are especially prominent in opiate addiction because these drugs are strong reinforcing agents due to their euphoric effects and their ability to reduce anxiety and increase self-esteem and the patient's subjective feelings of improved ability to cope with daily challenges.

Dx DIAGNOSIS

DIFFERENTIAL DIAGNOSIS

- Psychiatric disorders (e.g., anxiety, depression, bipolar disorder).
- Acute medical illness (e.g., hypoglycemia, seizure disorder, sepsis, renal or hepatic insufficiency) may mimic opiate withdrawal symptoms.

WORKUP

The history is the most important part of the workup. Useful screening tools are the CAGE-AID (Table 1), the DAST-10 (Table 2), and the CRAFFT (Table 3). The CAGE-AID has a sensitivity of 70% and a specificity of 85% when two questions are answered in the affirmative. The DAST-10 can

TABLE 3 CRAFFT Screening Tool for Adolescents

1. Have you ever ridden in a **C**ar driven by someone (including yourself) who was high or had been using alcohol or drugs?
2. Do you ever use alcohol or drugs to **R**elax, feel better about yourself, or fit in?
3. Do you ever use alcohol or drugs while you are by yourself **A**lone?
4. Do you ever **F**orget things you did while using alcohol or drugs?
5. Do your **F**amily or Friends ever tell you that you should cut down on your drinking or drug use?
6. Have you ever gotten into **T**rouble while you were using alcohol or drugs?

Two or more questions answered in the affirmative require further assessment.
From Bowman S et al: Reducing the health consequences of opioid addiction in primary care, *Am J Med* 126:565-571, 2013.

discriminate between current users versus former users. The CRAFFT is a useful screening tool for adolescents. A CRAFFT score of 2 or higher is optimal for identifying any problem (sensitivity 76%, specificity 94%), any disorder (sensitivity 80%, specificity 86%), and drug dependence (sensitivity 92%, specificity 80%).

- Observation of opioid withdrawal is indicative of opioid addiction.
- Observation of purposeful behaviors such as complaints and manipulations directed at getting more drugs and anxiety during withdrawal is suggestive of opioid addiction.
- Screen blood and urine for opioid metabolites.
- Screen for communicable diseases: HIV, hepatitis B and hepatitis C, tuberculosis.
- Screen for endocarditis in patients with newly diagnosed murmurs.

LABORATORY TESTS

- Urine and serum toxicology screen
- Complete blood count
- Chemistries (alanine aminotransferase, aspartate aminotransferase, serum creatinine): Elevated liver function test (LFT) results may be from viral hepatitis or acetaminophen toxicity
- Hepatitis screen: If hepatitis C antibody positive, follow up with hepatitis C polymerase chain reaction (viral load) even in patients with normal LFTs
- HIV
- PPD

IMAGING STUDIES

Generally not helpful in routine diagnosis and treatment. Consider echocardiography in patients with heart murmurs and liver sonography or CT scan in patients with elevated LFTs or who are positive for hepatitis C or B (increased risk of hepatocellular carcinoma).

Rx TREATMENT

NONPHARMACOLOGIC THERAPY

- Brief counseling interventions during a visit with their primary care physician or OB/GYN have proved efficacious in motivating patients for treatment
- Therapeutic communities (residential)
- 12-step or other self-help groups (e.g., Alcoholics Anonymous, Narcotics Anonymous)
- Relapse prevention (counseling)
- Opioid prevention education (Table 4)

TABLE 4 Basic Components of Opioid Overdose Prevention Education Curriculum

1. Know the signs of an opioid overdose (e.g., unresponsive, limp, slow, shallow breathing, pale or clammy, finger nails or lips turning blue, gurgling).
2. Call 911.
3. Administer rescue breathing.
4. Administer naloxone if no response and Emergency Medical Services has not yet arrived.
5. Stay with the person until help arrives.

From Bowman S et al: Reducing the health consequences of opioid addiction in primary care, *Am J Med* 126:565-571, 2013.

ACUTE GENERAL Rx

- Medical withdrawal (not overdosed). Opioid withdrawal alone is not recommended for treatment of opioid use disorder in most patients because of increased risk of overdose death and infectious disease (e.g., HIV through IV drug use) following detoxification.
- Short- (30 days) or long-term (30 to 180 days) protocols.
- Buprenorphine (opioid partial agonist) or methadone (opioid agonist) is initiated in tapering doses.
- Clonidine 0.1 mg bid to tid can be used to minimize autonomic symptoms (sweating) and craving.
- Nonsteroidal antiinflammatory drugs for body and muscle aches.
- The anticholinergic dicyclomine can be used to minimize gastrointestinal hyperactivity.
- Nonbenzodiazepine hypnotics, low-dose atypical antipsychotics (e.g., quetiapine), or low-dose tricyclic antidepressants are effective for promoting adequate sleep.
- Psychosocial supports tailored to patient needs should be offered as an adjunct to medical treatment.

CHRONIC Rx

Opioid antagonist treatment:

- Buprenorphine/naloxone is the preferred first-line treatment. Methadone is an alternative in certain populations.
- Naltrexone: Does not stabilize neuronal circuitry like partial or full opioid agonists and generally results in poor outcomes, much like Antabuse for alcohol.
- Opioid partial agonist therapy: Buprenorphine (Suboxone, Bunavail).
- Opioid agonist therapy: Methadone.
- NOTE: Buprenorphine and methadone are both metabolized by the cytochrome P-450 3a4 and 2d6 I isoenzyme pathways. Prescribers should be aware of multiple possible drug

interactions. Methadone and buprenorphine produce similar improvements during opioid withdrawal, although buprenorphine is associated with less sedation and respiratory depression. To avoid precipitating more intense withdrawal, buprenorphine should be initiated 12 to 18 hr after the last administration of opioids in patients who misuse shorter-acting opioids (48 hr in patients who are receiving long-acting drugs such as methadone), with initial doses of 4 to 8 mg.[1]

PATIENT SELECTION FOR BUPRENORPHINE OR METHADONE

- Appropriate patients for buprenorphine office-based treatment:
  1. Patients interested (highly motivated) in treatment
  2. Have no major contraindications (see following)
  3. Can be expected to be reasonably compliant with treatment
  4. Understand the benefits and risks of buprenorphine treatment
  5. Willing to follow safety precautions
- Less likely to be appropriate for office-based treatment:
  1. Have comorbid dependence on benzodiazepines or other CNS depressants (including ethylene alcohol)
  2. Have significant untreated psychiatric comorbidities
  3. Have active or chronic suicidal or homicidal ideation or attempts
  4. Have multiple previous treatments with frequent relapses
  5. Have poor response to previous treatment with buprenorphine
  6. Have significant medical complications (e.g., hepatic insufficiency, bacterial endocarditis, active tuberculosis)
- Methadone maintenance: Narcotic treatment program (clinic setting) indications:
  1. Evidence of opiate addiction >1 yr
  2. Two failed previous treatment attempts
  3. Patients not appropriate for office-based treatment
  4. Eligible without active "use" if prior methadone maintenance patient within previous 2 mo
  5. Pregnancy

DISPOSITION

- Opioid addiction is a chronic, relapsing disease
- High rate of relapse after "detox"
- Relapse potential after medically supervised withdrawal from methadone:
  1. 90% after 1 yr stable in treatment
  2. 80% after 3 yr stable in treatment
  3. 70% after 5 yr stable in treatment
- Postmarketing surveillance indicates that the diversion and abuse of prescription opioid medications increased between 2002 and 2010 and plateaued or decreased between 2011 and 2013. These findings suggest that the U.S. may be making some progress in controlling the abuse of opioid analgesics[2]

[1] Schuckit MA: Treatment of opioid-use disorders, *N Engl J Med* 375:357-368, 2016.

TABLE 5 Organizations Providing Referral Information for Patients

Organization	Resources/Website
Substance Abuse and Mental Health Services Administration (SAMHSA)	Opioid treatment program directory: dpt2.samhsa.gov/treatment/
Physicians who provide buprenorphine	Buprenorphine physician and treatment program locator: www.samhsa.gov/medication-assisted-treatment/treatment/buprenorphine
Pain Action	Chronic pain management materials for patients: www.painaction.com/
Substance abuse treatment facilities	Substance Abuse treatment facility locator: http://dasis3.samhsa.gov/
Harm Reduction Coalition	Local risk reduction resources and programs, overdose prevention education, and naloxone prescribing information: www.harmreduction.org/
Narcotics Anonymous (NA)	General information and meeting information for NA, a 12-step program modeled after Alcoholics Anonymous: www.na.org

From Bowman S et al: Reducing the health consequences of opioid addiction in primary care, *Am J Med* 126:565-571, 2013.

REFERRAL

Refer to addiction medicine specialist or narcotic treatment program when the neurobiologic disease of opioid addiction is identified.

PEARLS & CONSIDERATIONS

COMMENTS

- Methadone maintenance is the gold standard for the pregnant opioid-addicted patient regardless of the duration of the addiction or prior treatment attempts. Detoxification is contraindicated during pregnancy.
- Breastfeeding is encouraged in mothers on methadone maintenance. The American Academy of Pediatrics statement regarding "Transfer of Drugs and Other Chemicals into Human Milk" has placed methadone into the "usually compatible with breastfeeding" group based on the assumption that maternal urine is monitored to detect use of illicit drugs. The U.S. Department of Health and Human Services also recommends that mothers on methadone be encouraged to breastfeed.
- When a physician identifies a patient as a "drug seeker," it is imperative that the physician avoid abruptly stopping the opioid prescription because this will often result in the patient's buying the drugs illegally. These patients should be counseled and referred for treatment.
- Patients on methadone or buprenorphine who have pain resulting from an acute injury will need pain medication in addition to their daily dose of methadone or buprenorphine. They will require higher than usual doses of pain medications because of opioid receptor blockade attributable to their methadone or buprenorphine use.
- Opioid-dependent patients have a lower pain threshold resulting from hyperalgesia caused by the long-term use of opioids.

[2] Dart RC et al: Trends in opioid analgesic abuse and mortality in the United States, *N Engl J Med* 372:241-248, 2015.

PREVENTION

Education is the hallmark of prevention:
- School drug prevention education programs.
- Educate children about their family medical history, including diseases of addiction.
- Address childhood psychiatric disorders to prevent self-medicating.
- Educate patients on nonopioid analgesics for pain management.

Opioid overdose:
- Naloxone (Narcan) is a competitive mu-opioid receptor antagonist in the brain and is effective for opioid overdose. It is available for IM/IV and intranasal administration. It begins to reverse respiratory depression, sedation, and hypotension 2 to 5 min after IM administration and 1 to 2 min after IV administration.

PATIENT & FAMILY EDUCATION

- Stigma of addictions and treatment often interferes with good treatment.
- Family needs to be educated so they can support the patient's efforts.
- Encourage family meeting with addiction specialist, counselor.
- Recommend support groups for family members. Table 5 identifies organizations providing referral information for patients. Recommendations for integrating risk reduction strategies for addressing opioid misuse in the primary care setting are summarized in Table E6.

RELATED CONTENT

Drug Use Disorder (Patient Information)
Opioid Overdose (Related Key Topic)

SUGGESTED READINGS

Available at ExpertConsult.com

AUTHORS: **Tracy Cherian, BA,** and **Joshua Justice, MD**

BASIC INFORMATION

DEFINITION

Optic neuritis is an inflammation of the optic nerve resulting in impaired visual function.

SYNONYMS

Optic papillitis
Retrobulbar neuritis

ICD-10CM CODES
H46.8 Other optic neuritis
H46.9 Unspecified optic neuritis

EPIDEMIOLOGY & DEMOGRAPHICS

INCIDENCE (IN U.S.): 1 to 5/100,000 person(s) per yr; rates vary according to incidence of multiple sclerosis (MS). Optic neuritis affects 1% to 5% of patients with neurosarcoid.
PREVALENCE (IN U.S.): Common in patients with MS
PREDOMINANT SEX: Female:male ratio: 1.8:1
PEAK INCIDENCE: 20 to 49 yr, mean 30
GENETICS: Unknown. If due to MS, it is more common in patients with certain human lymphocyte antigen (HLA) blood types and in monozygotic twins of affected siblings.

PHYSICAL FINDINGS & CLINICAL PRESENTATION

- Presentation with acute or subacute (days) visual loss, often accompanied by periocular tenderness that worsens with eye movements.
- **Marcus Gunn pupil** (relative afferent pupillary defect [RAPD]): Direct and consensual response is normal; however, when flashlight is swung from eye to eye, the affected eye's pupil dilates to direct light.
- Decreased visual acuity.
- Unilateral visual field abnormalities—often a central scotoma (Fig. E1).
- Color desaturation; red is most often affected.
- Normal fundus examination in 66% cases; disc edema is noted in 33%. Other abnormalities include uveitis or periphlebitis. In neurosarcoid, the optic nerve head may exhibit a lumpy appearance suggestive of granulomatous infiltration, and there may be associated vitritis (Fig. E2).
- May have movement or light-induced phosphenes (flashes of light lasting 1-2 sec).
- Uhthoff phenomenon (benign exercise- or heat-induced deterioration of vision) is seen in some. Vision may also worsen in bright sunlight.
- Over time the optic disc may atrophy and become pale.

ETIOLOGY

An inflammatory response associated with an infection or autoimmune disease (such as collagen vascular disease, granulomatous disease, MS, or neuromyelitis optica).

DIAGNOSIS

Diagnosis is clinically established in a young patient with acute onset of monocular vision loss associated with retroorbital pain associated with eye movements and presence of RAPD lasting more than 24 hr. Absence of other orbital or ocular pathology is based on clinical examination.

DIFFERENTIAL DIAGNOSIS

For optic neuritis:
- Inflammatory: MS, neuromyelitis optica spectrum disorder (NMOSD), sarcoidosis, lupus: MS, neuromyelitis optica, acute disseminated encephalomyelitis, paraneoplastic, autoimmune optic neuropathy
- Infectious: Syphilis, TB, Lyme disease, *Bartonella,* HIV, cytomegalovirus (CMV), herpes, helminths, chickenpox, Q fever, periorbital infections, *Toxocara* sp.
- Ischemic: Anterior and posterior ischemic optic neuropathies, diabetic papillopathy, branch or central retinal artery or vein occlusion
- Drugs and toxins: Arsenic, methanol, ethambutol, cyclosporine, etc.
- Mitochondrial: Leber hereditary optic neuropathy, other mitochondrial

WORKUP

A thorough neurologic examination; dilated ophthalmoscopy

LABORATORY TESTS

Acute optic neuritis is a clinical diagnosis based on presentation with classical features: Acute, painful unilateral loss of vision associated with RAPD in a young person with no other apparent causes such as trauma. In atypical cases additional studies may be considered.
- CBC, antinuclear antibody (ANA), ACE, erythrocyte sedimentation rate (ESR)
- Consider HIV Ab, Lyme titer, rapid plasma reagin (RPR), other autoimmune or infectious causes
- Bilateral or recurrent optic neuritis (ON): Neuromyelitis optica (NMO) immunoglobulin (IgG), myelin oligodendrocyte glycoprotein (MOG IgG), paraneoplastic CRMP-5-IgG

IMAGING STUDIES

- Contrast-enhanced MRI of the brain is performed to assess the risk of developing MS. Often enhancement of the optic nerve is seen. MRI orbits with thin sections of fat suppressed sequences may be needed if the patient demonstrates atypical features (Fig. E3).
- Consider using optical coherence tomography to follow optic nerve atrophy objectively longitudinally.

TREATMENT

NONPHARMACOLOGIC THERAPY

Assure patient that in most cases of typical optic neuritis, there is near complete recovery of vision.

ACUTE GENERAL Rx

Treat if the visual loss is significant, atypical features, or if there is an abnormal MRI (higher risk of MS). Treatment is with methylprednisolone (MP) 250 mg IV every 6 hr (or 1 g IV daily) for 3 days followed by an oral prednisone taper of 11 days. Optic neuritis from NMOSD is often more severe and has a worse prognosis; therefore plasma exchange can be considered.

CHRONIC Rx

Depends on underlying cause. Disease-modifying treatment when increased risk of developing MS or neuromyelitis optica spectrum disorder. See topic "Multiple Sclerosis."

DISPOSITION

Most often vision is worst at the end of wk 1, followed by recovery over months. In the Optic Neuritis Treatment Trial (ONTT), 90% had 20/40 or better vision at 1 yr and 3% had 20/200 or worse. Of initial 20/200 or worse cases, only 5% remained in that group at 6 mo.

REFERRAL

- To neurologist for other neurologic signs and to assess risk of developing MS. In ONTT (Optic Neuritis Treatment Trial), risk of MS >15 yr was 72% with ≥1 lesion(s) on MRI, and 25% with a normal MRI.
- To ophthalmologist when atypical features or slowly progressive; urgently when other ocular pathology is present or if vision worsens or does not improve after several wk, or pain is severe.

PEARLS & CONSIDERATIONS

- Bilateral optic neuritis suggests a systemic inflammatory disorder, infection, NMOSD, or paraneoplastic, but can also occur in MS.
- Acute bilateral loss of vision with a severe headache or diplopia should raise concern for pituitary apoplexy and/or giant cell arteritis.

RELATED CONTENT

Idiopathic Intracranial Hypertension (Related Key Topic)
Multiple Sclerosis (Related Key Topic)

AUTHORS: **Sachin Kedar, MBBS, MD,** and **Corey Goldsmith, MD**

BASIC INFORMATION

DEFINITION

Oral cancers refer to malignant transformation of the oral tissues usually preceded by a process of sequential dysplastic changes leading to the development of squamous carcinoma. Oral squamous cell cancers (OSCC) include oral cavity cancers (lip, floor of mouth, buccal mucosa, anterior tongue, gingivae, hard palate, retromolar trigone), oropharynx cancers (base of tongue, tonsils, soft palate, pharyngeal walls), and hypopharynx cancers (pyriform sinus, postcricoid area, posterior pharyngeal wall).

SYNONYMS

Head and neck cancer
Oral malignant neoplasm
OSCC

ICD-10CM CODES	
C01	Malignant neoplasm of base of tongue
C03	Malignant neoplasm of gum
C04	Malignant neoplasm of floor of mouth
C05	Malignant neoplasm of palate
C06	Malignant neoplasm of other and unspecified parts of mouth
C09	Malignant neoplasm of tonsil
C10	Malignant neoplasm of oropharynx
C11	Malignant neoplasm of nasopharynx
C12	Malignant neoplasm of piriform sinus
C13	Malignant neoplasm of hypopharynx
C14	Malignant neoplasm of other and ill-defined sites of lip, oral cavity and larynx
C14.0	Malignant neoplasm of pharynx, unspecified
C14.2	Malignant neoplasm of Waldeyer ring
C14.8	Malignant neoplasm of overlapping sites of lip, oral cavity and pharynx

EPIDEMIOLOGY & DEMOGRAPHICS

INCIDENCE & PREVALENCE: It was estimated that in 2020, approximately 53,260 new cases and 10,750 deaths would occur in the U.S. The incidence of oral cancers linked to alcohol and tobacco use has been declining in the U.S., whereas those linked to human papillomavirus (HPV), primarily HPV type 16, are on the rise, especially for cancers located in the tonsils and base of tongue. In developed countries across the world, HPV is increasingly implicated in the growing incidence of oral cancer. In Asian countries where chewing betel nut is customary, oral cancer accounts for up to 40% of cancers in some regions. Squamous cell carcinoma is the most common malignancy that occurs in the oral cavity.

PREDOMINANT SEX & AGE: The ratio of oral cancer in males:females is 2.5:1 in the U.S. Black males have a higher early incidence in the 50- to 60-yr age group, but with increasing age, white men predominate.

RISK FACTORS (Fig. 1)**:** The following factors are implicated in the development of oral cancer:

- Tobacco use
- HPV infection (primarily types 16 and 18)
- Alcohol
- Immune deficiency
- Radiation
- Betel nut consumption
- Solar radiation

GENETICS: The genes that are critically altered in OSCC include *TP53,* the retinoblastoma family, *p16* and cyclin *D1*. The *TP53, CCND1,* and *CDKN2A* genes are established cancer genes in HPV-negative cancers. *TP53* and the genes encoding the Rb family are established cancer genes in HPV-positive cancers. Signaling pathways that are involved in the pathogenesis of oral cancers include that of the human epidermal receptor (HER) family, vascular endothelial growth factor (VEGF) receptor, and signal transducer and activator of transcription 3 (STAT 3). The tumor suppressor gene *TP53* is frequently mutated in HPV-negative tumors.

PHYSICAL FINDINGS & CLINICAL PRESENTATION

- Specific patient complaints may include the following: Oral ulcers or mass, choking, difficulty breathing, dysphagia, odynophagia, voice hoarseness, globus sensation, otalgia, ear or nose stuffiness, hemoptysis, trismus, neck mass, and pain in the head/neck region.
- Generalized symptoms and signs may include weight loss, fatigue, anorexia, altered mood, and sleep.
- Clinically, oral cancers can present as:
  1. Erythroplakia (flat red patch); can mimic inflammatory or traumatic lesions
  2. Leukoplakia (white patch; Fig. E2)
  3. Raised lesion
  4. Ulcerated lesion
  5. Warty lesion or growth

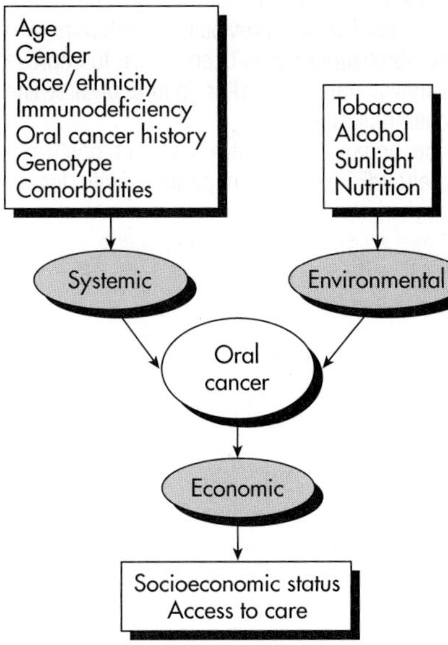

FIG. 1 Risk model for oral cancer. Oral cancer is a multifactorial disease process that includes systemic, environmental, and economic effects. The interplay of these variables ultimately leads to the incidence of this disease. The multifactorial nature of oral cancer should be addressed in the assessment of a patient's risk. (From Jones DL, Rankin KV: Oral cancer and associated risk factors. In Cappelli D, Mobley C [eds]: *Prevention in clinical oral health care,* St Louis, 2008, Elsevier, pp. 68-77.)

Dx DIAGNOSIS

DIFFERENTIAL DIAGNOSIS

- Oral leukoplakia
- Invasive fungal infections
- Chancre of early syphilis and gumma of tertiary syphilis
- Chronic ulcer
- Metastatic or locally invading cancers from sinuses or other sites of the body

WORKUP

- Primary workup includes either biopsy or fine-needle aspiration (FNA) of the presenting lesion or suspected neck lymph node for histopathologic analysis. HPV assessment with p16 immunohistochemical staining and confirmatory in situ hybridization (ISH) testing is performed when indicated for oropharynx primary tumors.
- Detailed examination of the oral cavity, pharynx, larynx, neck, ears, nose, and cranial nerves should be performed.
- Laryngoscopy and examination under anesthesia are commonly performed.
- Pretreatment evaluation of tumor size, the extent of invasion, and the presence or absence of regional lymph node metastases is critical for planning treatment.
- Laboratory workup can include complete blood count, complete chemistry panel, and thyroid function.
- Staging workup includes CT or MRI imaging of the head and neck and a chest x-ray. If locoregional or advanced disease is a consideration, a PET scan is typically completed.
- The TNM system is used for staging of OSCC and is subdivided according to primary tumor sites: (1) lip and oral cavity, (2) pharynx.

Rx TREATMENT

- Surgery, radiation therapy, and chemotherapy are treatment modalities involved in the treatment plan for OSCC.
- The use of supportive and special therapeutic modalities such as nutritional therapy including feeding gastrostomy, speech and swallowing therapy, reconstructive surgery, and speech prosthesis is required often.
- For treatment purposes OSCC are classified as early (T1 or T2 lesions), locoregional (T3-4 or any N), or metastatic (M1) stages. Site-specific TNM staging is done as per the primary tumor site (e.g., oral cavity, oropharynx, hypopharynx, etc.).
- After staging completion, the initial treatment considerations include:
  1. Determination of primary tumor resectability (resectable vs. unresectable)
  2. Management of neck nodes

3. Intent of radiation therapy (curative vs. palliative)
4. Need for organ preservation
5. Need for reconstructive surgery
6. Need for chemotherapy
7. HPV status of tumor

- Localized tumors (stage I or II) can be approached by initial surgical resection or definitive radiotherapy. Locoregionally advanced tumors (stage III and localized IV) that are resectable are typically approached by upfront surgery followed by adjuvant radiation and/or chemotherapy. Unresectable patients are typically treated with definitive chemotherapy and radiotherapy. Patients with distant metastatic disease are treated with systemic chemotherapy, while locally recurrent tumors can be approached with either surgery or chemotherapy or both.
- Surgery is typically associated with less long-term morbidity than radiation therapy. Surgical therapy traditionally involved wide-exposure approaches (mandibulotomy, transpharyngeal access). Newer surgical techniques allow tumor resection through the mouth. Recently, transoral robotic surgery (TORS) has been developed to improve access to oropharyngeal squamous cell carcinomas with excellent oncologic outcomes.
  1. Acute surgical complications can include infection, bleeding, aspiration, wound breakdown, fistula, and flap loss.
  2. Surgical procedures can cause functional deficits in speech and swallowing, but these adverse effects can be minimized by appropriate reconstruction and prostheses.
- Definitive radiation therapy is reserved for patients who cannot tolerate surgery or for whom surgical resection would result in particularly severe functional impairment.
  1. Radiation therapy can include external beam radiation and brachytherapy.
  2. Radiation therapy side effects include mucositis, radiation dermatitis, loss of taste, dysphagia, dental caries and decay, and xerostomia.
  3. Late complications can include skin/soft tissue atrophy and fibrosis, osteoradionecrosis, and trismus.
- Systemic chemotherapy can be administered alone or in combination with radiotherapy, depending on the disease stage. Agents typically used include cisplatin, carboplatin, 5-fluorouracil, taxanes, and the epidermal growth factor receptor (EGFR) antibody cetuximab.
- For locally advanced OSCC, the combination of cisplatin and radiotherapy is the regimen of choice. Recent reports have demonstrated similar outcomes with standard every-3-wk administered cisplatin and lower doses of once-weekly administered cisplatin, but with lower toxicity rates. In selected patients with large primary tumors or bulky nodal disease, neoadjuvant chemotherapy may be utilized prior to chemoradiotherapy administration.
- Patients who have metastatic cancers or unresectable locoregional recurrences usually are treated with systemic chemotherapy.
- Front-line chemoimmunotherapy with a regimen consisting of platinum plus 5-fluorouracil chemotherapy in combination with the checkpoint inhibitor, pembrolizumab has been demonstrated to be a superior regimen in patients with recurrent or metastatic head and neck cancer. Alternatively, doublet chemotherapy regimens (platinum plus either 5-fluorouracil or a taxane) can be combined with the epidermal growth factor receptor (EGFR)–targeting antibody cetuximab in this setting.
- In patients who have not received checkpoint inhibitor therapy previously, nivolumab and pembrolizumab have been shown to improve survival outcomes after failure of first-line chemotherapy.
- The negative predictive value of posttreatment PET imaging in patients with locally advanced cancer who have been treated with chemoradiotherapy is 98% to 99%.

DISPOSITION

- Prognosis depends on the staging and resectability of the primary tumor as well as on patient performance status.
- Tumor HPV status is a strong and independent prognostic factor for survival among patients with base of tongue and oropharyngeal cancer.

REFERRAL

Referral to multidisciplinary head and neck cancer team consisting of ENT or head/neck surgeon, radiation oncologist, and medical oncologist

PEARLS & CONSIDERATIONS

COMMENTS

- Oral and pharyngeal cancer is the sixth most common cancer globally.
- Biopsy with HPV-status assessment is the key for accurate diagnosis.
- Posttreatment rehabilitation and surveillance is important.

PREVENTION

- Encourage patients to stop using any type of tobacco and drinking alcohol.
- Examine oral cavities at annual checkups and work up suspicious lesions.

SUGGESTED READINGS

Available at ExpertConsult.com

RELATED CONTENT

Mouth Cancer (Patient Information)

AUTHOR: **Ritesh Rathore, MD**

BASIC INFORMATION

DEFINITION

Oral hairy leukoplakia (OHL) is a painless, white, nonremovable, plaquelike lesion typically located on the lateral aspect of the tongue.

SYNONYMS

Oral hairy leukoplakia
OHL

ICD-10CM CODE

K13.3 Hairy leukoplakia

EPIDEMIOLOGY & DEMOGRAPHICS

INCIDENCE AND PREVALENCE: Epstein-Barr virus (EBV) is implicated in the etiology of OHL, and the incidence of EBV seroprevalence is high in individuals who are HIV seropositive. However, OHL occurs in only 25% of these cases but may also occur in other immunosuppressed individuals, for example, organ transplant recipients, as well as individuals who may be receiving systemic or inhaled steroids.

RISK FACTORS: OHL is usually found in HIV-seropositive individuals (median CD4 count is 468/ml) but may also be identified in smokers and other immunocompromised patients such as transplant recipients (particularly renal) and patients taking steroids. Diagnosing OHL is an indication to institute a workup to evaluate and manage HIV disease.

PHYSICAL FINDINGS & CLINICAL PRESENTATION

- Varying morphology and appearance, which may change daily.
- May be unilateral or bilateral.
- White plaques can be small with fine, vertical corrugations on the lateral margin of the tongue (Fig. 1). The plaques from OHL are adherent to the tongue surface (in contrast to candidal plaques, which may be easily scraped off).
- Irregular surface; may have prominent folds or projection, occasionally markedly resembling hairs.
- May spread to cover the entire dorsal surface or spread onto the ventral surface of the tongue where the lesions usually appear flat.
- Rarely, lesions can manifest on the soft palate, buccal mucosa, or posterior oropharynx.
- Usually asymptomatic, but some patients have mouth pain, soreness, or a burning sensation; impaired taste, or difficulty eating; others complain of its unsightly appearance.

ETIOLOGY

EBV is implicated in its etiology, and OHL is a result of unchecked lytic replication of EBV in the epithelium of keratinized cells. OHL differs from most EBV-related diseases in that infection is predominantly lytic rather than latent, with abundant virus production resulting in cell lysis.

OHL should be differentiated from oral leukoplakia, which is a potentially premalignant condition.

DIAGNOSIS

DIFFERENTIAL DIAGNOSIS

- Oral homogenous/nonhomogenous leukoplakia
- *Candida albicans*
- Lichen planus
- Idiopathic leukoplakia
- White sponge nevus
- Dysplasia
- Squamous cell carcinoma

WORKUP

Requires physical examination and evaluation of HIV disease

LABORATORY TESTS

The *provisional* diagnosis is clinical and based on:

- Visual inspection
- Inability to scrape the lesion off the tongue with a blade
- Failure to respond to antifungal therapy

The *presumptive* diagnosis requires biopsy and histologic demonstration of:

- Epithelial hyperplasia with hairs
- Absence of inflammatory cell infiltrate

The *definitive* diagnosis requires:

- In situ hybridization of histologic or cytologic specimens revealing EBV DNA *or*
- Electron microscopy of specimens revealing herpeslike particles
- Measurement of the DNA content in cells of oral leukoplakia may be used to predict the risk of oral carcinoma

NOTE: Specimens obtained from lesions may demonstrate hyphae of *Candida albicans,* which may coexist and potentiate EBV-induced OHL

TREATMENT

NONPHARMACOLOGIC THERAPY

OHL is usually asymptomatic and requires no specific therapy. It may resolve spontaneously and is generally benign in HIV-seropositive patients.

ACUTE GENERAL Rx

- Antiretroviral therapy (ART) has considerably changed the frequency of oral lesions caused by opportunistic infections in HIV-seropositive individuals.
- Topical retinoids (0.1% vitamin A) may improve the appearance of OHL-affected oral surfaces through their dekeratinizing and immunomodulation effects; however, they are expensive, and prolonged use may result in a burning sensation over the treated area.
- Topical podophyllin resin 25% solution has been reported to induce resolution.
- Surgical excision and cryotherapy may help, but the lesions may recur.
- High-dose acyclovir 800 mg five times per day, valacyclovir 1000 mg tid, famciclovir 500 mg tid, ganciclovir 1000 mg tid, or foscarnet 40 mg/kg IV tid will cause lesions to resolve but only temporarily.

REFERRAL

Referral to ENT or oral surgeon for biopsy of tongue to confirm diagnosis

PEARLS & CONSIDERATIONS

- OHL may be the presenting sign of patients infected with HIV who are unaware of their status.
- The incidence has decreased significantly in the era of antiretroviral therapy.

RELATED CONTENT

Acquired Immunodeficiency Syndrome (Related Key Topic)
Oral Hairy Leukoplakia (Patient Information)
Epstein-Barr Virus Infection (Related Key Topic)
Human Immunodeficiency Virus (Related Key Topic)

AUTHOR: **Sajeev Handa, MD, SFHM**

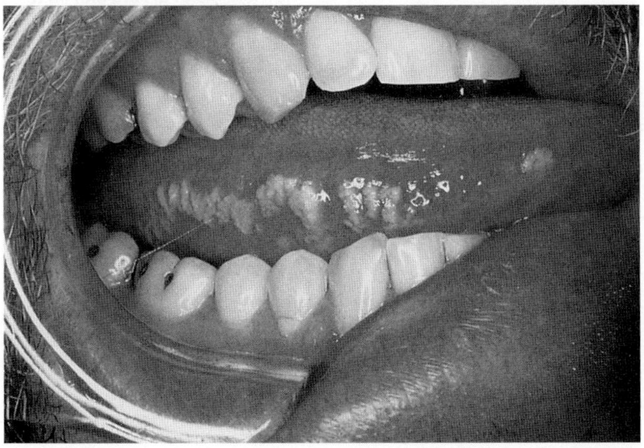

FIG. 1 Oral hairy leukoplakia. (From Callen JP et al: *Dermatological signs of systemic disease,* ed 5, Philadelphia, 2017, Elsevier.)

Orchitis

BASIC INFORMATION

DEFINITION

Orchitis is an inflammatory process (usually infectious) involving the testicles. Infection may be viral or bacterial and can be associated with infection of other male sex organs (prostate, epididymis, or bladder) or lower urogenital tract or sexually transmitted diseases often via hematogenous spread. Common causes are:

- Viral: Mumps—20% postpubertal; Coxsackie B virus
- Bacterial: Pyogenic via spread from involving epididymis; bacteria include *Escherichia coli, Klebsiella pneumoniae, P. aeruginosa, Staphylococcus, Streptococcus* or *Rickettsia, Brucella* spp.; in sexually active men: *Neisseria gonorrhoeae* and *Chlamydia trachomatis*
- Other:
  1. Viral—HIV-associated, CMV, Zika
  2. Fungi
     a. Cryptococcosis
     b. Histoplasmosis
     c. *Candida*
     d. Blastomycosis
     e. Syphilis
  3. *Mycobacterium tuberculosis* and *M. leprae*
  4. Parasitic causes: Toxoplasmosis, filariasis, schistosomiasis
- Table 1 describes a classification of epididymitis and orchitis based on etiology.

SYNONYMS

Epididymo-orchitis
Testicular infection
Testicular inflammation

ICD-10CM CODES

N45.9	Orchitis, epididymitis, and epididymo-orchitis without abscess
A54.1	Gonococcal orchitis
A56.1	Chlamydial orchitis
N51.1	Mumps orchitis

EPIDEMIOLOGY & DEMOGRAPHICS

PREDOMINANT SEX: Male
PREDOMINANT ORGANISM: The leading cause of viral orchitis is mumps. The mumps virus rarely causes orchitis in prepubertal males but involves one or both testicles in nearly 30% of postpubertal males.

PHYSICAL FINDINGS & CLINICAL PRESENTATION

- Testicular pain, unilateral or bilateral swelling
- May have associated epididymitis, prostatitis, fever, scrotal edema, erythema, cellulitis
- Inguinal lymphadenopathy
- Acute hydrocele (bacterial)
- Rare development: Abscess formation, pyocele of scrotum, testicular infarction
- Spermatic cord tenderness may be present
- Granulomatous

Dx DIAGNOSIS

Clinical presentation as described previously with possible history of acute viral illness or concomitant epididymitis

DIFFERENTIAL DIAGNOSIS

- Epididymo-orchitis-gonococcal
- Autoimmune disease
- Vasculitis
- Epididymitis
- Mumps, with or without parotitis
- Neoplasm
- Hematoma
- Spermatic cord torsion
- Behçet disease

LABORATORY TESTS

- CBC with differential
- Urinalysis
- Viral titer—mumps. Mumps IgM will be detectable after 5 days of onset of clinical mumps and remain positive for up to 4 wk. A reverse-transcriptase PCR (RT-PCR) on serum or buccal or oral swab is another option
- Urine culture for mumps virus
- Ultrasound of testicle to rule out abscess
- Urine NAAT for *Neisseria gonorrhoeae* and *Chlamydia trachomatis*

IMAGING STUDIES

Ultrasound if abscess suspected

Rx TREATMENT

- Dependent on cause
- Viral (mumps): Observation; bed rest, ice packs, analgesics, and a scrotal sling for support may provide some relief of discomfort that accompanies mumps orchitis
- Bacterial: Empiric antibiotic treatment with parenteral antibiotic treatment until pathogen identified:
  1. Ceftriaxone 500 mg IM as a single dose for persons weighing <150 kg (300 lb), 1 g of IM ceftriaxone for persons weighing ≥150 kg (300 lb) plus doxycycline (100 mg PO bid for 10 days), in men <35 yr old to cover *Neisseria gonorrhoeae* and *Chlamydia trachomatis.* In men who have sex with men or men >35 yr old: Levofloxacin 500 to 750 mg IV/PO qd for 10 to 14 days *or* ampicillin-sulbactam *or* third-generation cephalosporin or piperacillin/tazobactam
- Surgery for abscess, pyogenic process

DISPOSITION

Follow-up for evidence of recurrence, hypogonadism, and infertility may be needed with bilateral orchitis.

REFERRAL

- To a urologist if surgical drainage is needed
- To an endocrinologist if hypogonadism develops
- To a fertility specialist if infertility develops

PEARLS & CONSIDERATIONS

Consider tuberculous orchitis if symptoms fail to respond to standard antibacterial therapy, even in the absence of chest radiographic evidence of pulmonary tuberculosis.

SUGGESTED READINGS

Available at ExpertConsult.com

RELATED CONTENT

Orchitis (Patient Information)
Epididymitis (Related Key Topic)
Mumps (Related Key Topic)

AUTHOR: **Glenn G. Fort, MD, MPH**

TABLE 1 Classification of Epididymitis and Orchitis

Acute Epididymitis or Epididymo-orchitis	Granulomatous Epididymitis or Orchitis	Viral Orchitis
Neisseria gonorrhoeae	*Mycobacterium tuberculosis*	Mumps
Chlamydia trachomatis	*Treponema pallidum*	Enteroviruses
Escherichia coli		
Streptococcus pneumoniae	*Brucella* spp.	
Klebsiella spp.	Sarcoid	
Salmonella spp.	Fungal	
Other urinary tract pathogens	Parasitic	
Idiopathic	Idiopathic	

From Cohen J, Powderly WG: *Infectious diseases,* ed 2, St Louis, 2004, Mosby.

BASIC INFORMATION

DEFINITION

Orthostatic hypotension (OH) is defined as the presence of at least one of the following:

- Decrease in systolic blood pressure by ≥20 mm Hg *or*
- Decrease in diastolic blood pressure by ≥10 mm Hg, within 3 min of standing

It is a physical sign that requires further investigation to discern its underlying etiology.

Recent studies have shown that blood pressure measurements within 1 min might be more useful in predicting fractures, falls, and other adverse events and for most patients, assessment within 1 min of standing rather than waiting for 3 min may be sufficient.[1]

SYNONYMS

Postural hypotension
OH

ICD-10CM CODE

I95.1 Orthostatic hypotension

EPIDEMIOLOGY & DEMOGRAPHICS

- The incidence of OH is increased in older people. Surveys have shown OH to be present in approximately 20% of adults over 65 yr of age.
- Also, higher incidence noted in those with diseases associated with autonomic dysfunction (e.g., Parkinson disease, diabetes mellitus).
- OH may cause up to 30% of all syncopal events in the elderly, and OH is associated with an increased risk of heart failure among those aged 45 to 55 yr and an increased risk of cardiovascular disease and all-cause mortality among those aged 55 yr and older.
- OH can be a common cause and/or a contributor to hospitalization in older adult patients.
- There is an association between orthostatic hypotension and cognitive dysfunction among older adults.

PHYSICAL FINDINGS & CLINICAL PRESENTATION

- Symptoms may include dizziness, lightheadedness, syncope, visual and auditory disturbances, weakness, diaphoresis, pallor, and nausea.
- OH may be asymptomatic, especially in older hypertensive patients with autonomic dysfunction. These patients tend to have systolic hypertension when seated or supine.
- Associated with increased autonomic activity during meals (from increased splanchnic blood flow), exercise, prolonged standing, and hot weather.
- Supine and nocturnal hypertension in patients with OH may indicate an underlying autonomic dysfunction.

ETIOLOGY

- There are two main mechanisms for OH: Autonomic dysfunction and volume depletion.
- Normal response: Assumption of an upright posture results in the pooling of approximately 500 ml of blood in the lower extremities due to gravity and decreased venous return, decreased cardiac output, and decreased arterial pressure. The consequent increase in sympathetic tone due to increased carotid baroreceptor activity causes arterial and venous constriction as well as positive inotropic and chronotropic effects, thereby limiting the fall in upright blood pressure. Peripheral vasoconstriction is also mediated by increased activity of the renin-angiotensin system and decreased activity of atrial natriuretic factor.
- Autonomic Dysfunction: Impairment of the baroreceptor reflex, as in central (such as Parkinson disease) or peripheral autonomic dysfunction (such as diabetes) and aging, may cause OH because decreased blood pressure cannot be counteracted by the aforementioned regulatory mechanisms.
- Volume depletion: May be caused by diuretics, vomiting, hemorrhage, and hyperglycemia. Mechanism of OH in these patients is similar to what is described earlier, with failure of the regulatory mechanisms kicking in.

DIAGNOSIS

DIFFERENTIAL DIAGNOSIS

Common:

- Medications: Antihypertensives, antidepressants (tricyclics), antipsychotics (phenothiazines), alcohol, narcotics, barbiturates, insulin, nitrates, PDE-5 inhibitors, alpha-adrenergic antagonists
- Reduced intravascular volume (hemorrhage, dehydration, hyperglycemia, hypoalbuminemia)
- Postprandial effect (especially in the elderly)
- Vasovagal syncope
- Deconditioning
- Central autonomic dysfunction (Parkinson disease)
- Peripheral autonomic dysfunction (diabetes mellitus, Guillain-Barré syndrome)

Uncommon:

- Central autonomic dysfunction (Shy-Drager syndrome)
- Postganglionic autonomic dysfunction: Impaired norepinephrine release
- Autoimmune autonomic dysfunction: Nicotinic acetylcholine receptor autoantibodies
- Paraneoplastic autonomic dysfunction: Anti-Hu antibodies (in small-cell lung cancer)
- Postural tachycardia syndrome (POTS): Usually occurs in young women; an abnormally large increase in heart rate is observed in the upright position, caused by increased venous pooling from autonomic dysfunction of the lower extremities, but blood pressure is not affected because of an excess of plasma norepinephrine
- Impaired cardiac output (myocardial infarction, aortic stenosis, arrhythmias)
- Cerebrovascular accident
- Adrenal insufficiency
- Deconditioning
- Carotid sinus hypersensitivity
- Anxiety, panic attacks
- Seizures
- Sepsis
- Idiopathic

WORKUP

- Obtain a detailed history including medication list, recent history of potential volume loss, medical history of congestive heart failure, malignancy, diabetes and alcoholism, evidence on history and physical examination of parkinsonism, ataxia, peripheral neuropathy, or dysautonomia.
- Measure supine blood pressure after the patient has been resting comfortably. The duration of time that the patient should spend supine and standing when measuring orthostatic hypotension is controversial. Limited evidence supports having the patient remain supine for 5 to 10 min before obtaining the supine blood pressure, followed by blood pressure measurement within 1 min of standing and again after 3 min of standing. The blood pressure cuff must be held at the level of the right atrium; holding the cuff below this level will result in a 5 to 10 mm Hg underestimation of blood pressure.
- Thorough neurologic examination should be performed.

LABORATORY TESTS

- Hemoglobin and hematocrit
- Consider BUN/creatinine if suspecting dehydration as the cause
- ECG if suspecting underlying cardiac cause
- Consider when treatable causes of OH have been ruled out:
  1. Blood pressure and heart rate monitoring with a tilt table test
  2. Plasma norepinephrine measurements (to distinguish postganglionic from preganglionic autonomic dysfunction)
  3. Other methods, which use the Valsalva maneuver or measure sweating as indirect means of evaluating the autonomic nervous system

IMAGING STUDIES

None

TREATMENT

NONPHARMACOLOGIC THERAPY

- Patient education (leg crossing, prolonged sitting before first standing in the morning, avoid excessive straining and hot baths)
- High-salt diet (e.g., bouillon cubes); caution if history of heart failure
- Liberal fluid intake

[1] Juraschek SP et al: Associated of history of dizziness and long-term adverse outcomes with early vs. later orthostatic hypotension assessment times in middle-aged adults, *JAMA Intern Med* 2017.

TABLE 1 Management of Orthostatic Hypotension in Older Adults

Identify and treat correctable causes.

Reduce or eliminate drugs causing orthostatic hypotension.

Avoid situations that may exacerbate orthostatic hypotension.

- Standing motionless
- Prolonged recumbency
- Large meals
- Hot weather
- Hot showers
- Straining at stool or with voiding
- Isometric exercise
- Ingesting alcohol
- Hyperventilation
- Dehydration

Raise the head of the bed to a 5- to 20-degree angle.

Wear waist-high, custom-fitted, elastic stockings and an abdominal binder.

Participate in physical conditioning exercises.

Participate in controlled postural exercises using the tilt table.

Avoid diuretics and eat salt-containing fluids (unless congestive heart failure is present).

Drug therapy:

- Caffeine
- Fludrocortisone
- Midodrine
- Desmopressin
- Erythropoietin

From Fillit HM: *Brocklehurst's textbook of geriatric medicine and gerontology*, ed 8, *Philadelphia*, 2017, Elsevier.

- Take needed antihypertensive medications at different times of the day
- Raise the head of the bed at night
- Compression stockings (to include splanchnic circulation)
- Multiple low-carbohydrate meals to avoid postprandial OH
- Avoid large carbohydrate loads and excess alcohol consumption

ACUTE GENERAL Rx

- Correction of volume status and impairment of cerebral perfusion.
- Review medication list and attempt to eliminate those potentially contributing to OH.

CHRONIC Rx

- Fludrocortisone: 0.1 mg/day (may combine with an alpha-1 agonist to lower the dose of each); monitor for electrolyte disturbances and supine hypertension
- Midodrine (alpha-1 agonist): 10 mg three times a day; monitor for supine hypertension
- Erythropoietin (consider if anemic)
- Caffeine (for postprandial hypotension)
- Table 1 summarizes management of orthostatic hypotension in older adults.

OTHER TREATMENTS

- Pyridostigmine (enhances renal sodium reabsorption): 0.2 to 0.6 mg/day (not FDA-approved for this indication)
- Octreotide: 300 to 600 mg/day (not FDA-approved for this indication)
- Indomethacin (prostaglandin inhibitor)
- DDAVP (experimental)
- Droxidopa (used for patients with autonomic dysfunction to increase the availability of norepinephrine) has been FDA approved for treatment of adults with symptomatic neurogenic orthostatic hypotension caused by primary autonomic failure or nondiabetic autonomic neuropathy

PEARLS & CONSIDERATIONS

COMMENTS

- The presence of OH should always trigger a search for an underlying etiology.
- OH is diagnosed by observing changes in blood pressure, not heart rate.
- Volume depletion should cause an increased heart rate on standing; a lack of heart rate response in this setting suggests autonomic dysfunction.
- Pharmacotherapy with mineralocorticoids may require concomitant potassium replenishment and monitoring for hypertension.
- Evidence to support the efficacy of pharmacologic interventions to treat OH, including midodrine, is limited.
- The etiology of OH is often multifactorial in older patients, but increased susceptibility to volume depletion due to decreased baroreceptor reflexes frequently contributes. Chronic vitamin D deficiency is associated with the development of OH.
- Intensive blood pressure control did not increase injurious falls compared with controls among community-dwelling older adults participating in the Systolic Blood Pressure Intervention Trial (SPRINT).
- The physical examination of patients with dizziness, gait disturbance, and/or falls should include an assessment for OH. OH is an independent predictor of unexplained falls in older adults.
- Because OH may be asymptomatic, physical examination of those at risk must include assessment of blood pressure in both the supine and upright positions.

SUGGESTED READINGS

Available at ExpertConsult.com

AUTHOR: **Hussain R. Khawaja, MD, FACP**

BASIC INFORMATION

DEFINITION

Osteoarthritis (OA) is a progressive disease of the joint representing failed repair of joint damage. It is a complex disorder involving the articular cartilage, the subchondral bone, ligaments, menisci, periarticular muscles, peripheral nerves, and synovium. The process often starts with "micro-cracks" in the articular cartilage with resultant inflammatory cascade perpetuated by the cartilage, synovium, and other joint structures. It results in pain, stiffness, and functional disability often leading to reduced health-related quality of life. It also has a significant economic burden (up to 2.5% of the GDP in the U.S.) and is the leading cause of analgesic consumption and joint replacement surgeries. The American College of Rheumatology Classification criteria for osteoarthritis is described in Table 1.

SYNONYMS

Degenerative joint disease (DJD)
DJD
Arthrosis
OA

ICD-10CM CODES

M15.1	Heberden nodes (with arthropathy)
M15.2	Bouchard nodes (with arthropathy)
M15.3	Secondary multiple arthritis
M15.4	Erosive OA
M15.8	Other polyosteoarthritis
M15.9	Polyarthrosis, unspecified
M17	Gonarthrosis (arthrosis of knee)
M18	Arthrosis of first metacarpal joint
M19	Other arthrosis
M19.8	Other specified arthrosis
M19.9	Arthrosis, unspecified

EPIDEMIOLOGY & DEMOGRAPHICS

PREVALENCE: Affects more than 30 million individuals in the U.S. Approximately 10% of men and 18% of women over the age of 60 yr are affected.

PREDOMINANT SEX: Prior to age 50, there is almost no gender discrepancy. After age 50, there is increased incidence of OA in females compared to males.

PREDOMINANT AGE: Occurs more frequently after 50 yr of age, but it is increasingly being recognized that OA may occur as early as 30 yr of age.

RISK FACTORS: Osteoarthritis is considered predominantly a mechanical noninflammatory form of arthritis (Fig. 1). OA is thought to be the result of hostile biomechanics on an already susceptible joint (Fig. E2). Risk factors may be classified as either local or systemic. Local or biomechanical factors include obesity leading to increased load on the articular cartilage, mechanical environment of the joint (includes deformities like pes planus, genu varus and valgus, proprioception at the joint), local joint activity/occupation (textile worker leading to hand OA, high-impact runners leading to knee OA), and muscle weakness (quadriceps weakness leading to knee OA). Other deformities, such as femoro-acetabular impingement and limb length inequality, can confer significant risk of developing end-stage OA. Systemic risk factors include nutritional factors such as antioxidant and vitamin D deficiency, hormonal status, high bone mineral density, and genetics (candidate genes being evaluated include IGF-1 gene, cartilage oligomeric protein gene, vitamin D receptor gene). That said, there is no concrete evidence showing that preventing the disease or reducing disease progression can be achieved by supplemental vitamin D, antioxidants, or estrogen. Obesity also increases the susceptibility of developing osteoarthritis via systemic adipokines.

GENETICS: 39% to 65% heritability rate in twin studies of women who have generalized OA, concordance rate of 0.64 in monozygotic twins. In genome-wide association studies, 11 candidate loci have been identified, but all with a very small effect size.

PHYSICAL FINDINGS & CLINICAL PRESENTATION

- Similar symptoms in most forms: Pain generally with activity, stiffness, or gelling (generally short-lived and morning stiffness lasting less than 30 min), crepitus

TABLE 1 American College of Rheumatology Classification Criteria for Osteoarthritis

Hip	Knee (Clinical Criteria)	Hand
Pain in the hip and two of the following: ESR <20 mm/hr Radiographic joint space narrowing Radiographic osteophytes	Pain in the knee and five of the following: Age >50 <30 min morning stiffness Crepitus Bony enlargement Bony tenderness No synovial warmth	Pain, aching, and stiffness in the hand and three of the following: Fewer than three MCP joints swollen Hard tissue enlargement of two or more DIP joints Hard tissue enlargement of two or more of the following joints: Second and third DIP, second and third PIP, both CMC joints Deformity of at least one of the following joints: Second and third DIP, second and third PIP, both CMC joints

CMC, Carpometacarpal; *DIP,* distal interphalangeal; *ESR,* erythrocyte sedimentation rate; *MCP,* metacarpophalangeal joint; *PIP,* proximal interphalangeal.

Modified from (1) Altman R et al: The American College of Rheumatology criteria for the classification and reporting of osteoarthritis of the hand, *Arthritis Rheum* 33:1601-1610, 1990; (2) Altman R et al: The American College of Rheumatology criteria for the classification and reporting of osteoarthritis of the hip, *Arthritis Rheum* 34:505-514, 1991; (3) Altman R et al: Development of criteria for the classification and reporting of osteoarthritis. Classification of osteoarthritis of the knee, *Arthritis Rheum* 29:1039-1049, 1986. In Fillit HM: *Brocklehurst's textbook of geriatric medicine and gerontology,* ed 8, Philadelphia, 2017, Elsevier.

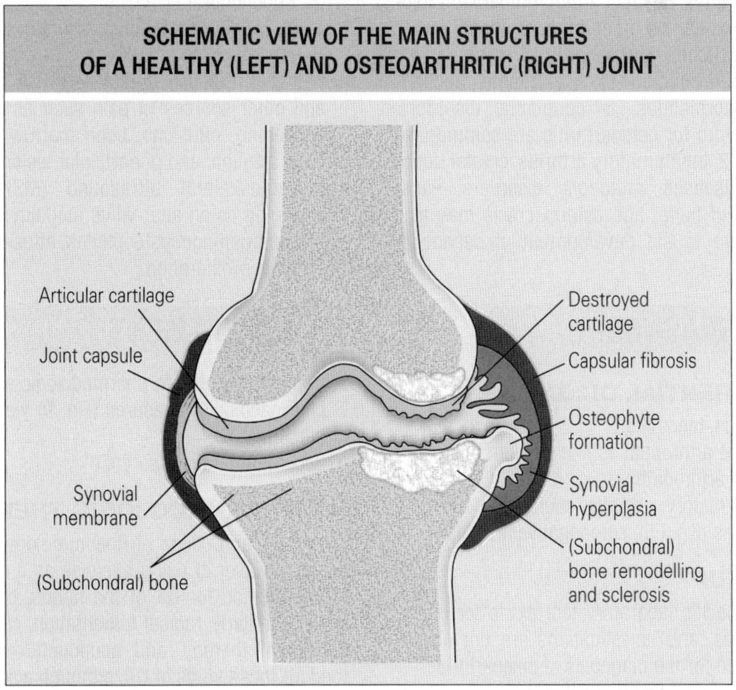

FIG. 1 In osteoarthritis (OA), the articular cartilage is lost or severely thinned, the subchondral bone is sclerotic, the joint capsule is thickened, and the synovial membrane is activated. (Courtesy of E. Bartnik, Frankfurt, Germany. In Hochberg MC: *Rheumatology,* ed 7, Philadelphia, 2019, Elsevier.)

TABLE 2 Risk Factors for Osteoarthritis

HOST FACTORS		ENVIRONMENTAL FACTORS	
Genetic factors	Familial clustering has also been found at the hip and knee	Biomechanics	Repetitive ergonomic and biomechanical demands may create joint stresses leading to OA Hemiparesis associated with reduction of expression of OA in the affected limb and overexpression in the remaining functional limb Chopstick use associated with OA of the IP joint of the thumb, second and third MCP, and PIP joints
Age	The strongest identifiable risk factor	Trauma	Injuries to the joint, such as dislocations, fractures, ligament ruptures, and meniscal tears
Gender	The age association is strongest in women: Possibly a hormonal influence Hand OA has a peak incidence in menopausal women		
Hormones	Controversial Hand OA has a peak in menopausal women; however, the Chingford and Framingham studies suggested estrogen has protective effect		
Bone mineral density	Negative relationship between bone mineral density and OA at some sites		
BMI	Obesity is strongly associated with the incidence of knee OA Hand OA likely to be related to biomechanical factors		
Joint alignment	Varus deformity of the knee is associated with progressive OA, as is varus/valgus ligamentous instability at the knee joint Developmental problems leading to altered joint biomechanics such as congenital dysplasias		

BMI, Body mass index; *IP,* interphalangeal; *MCP,* metacarpophalangeal joint; *OA,* osteoarthritis; *PIP,* proximal interphalangeal.
Modified from Fillit HM: *Brocklehurst's textbook of geriatric medicine and gerontology,* ed 8, Philadelphia, 2017, Elsevier.

- Loss of function in joints (e.g., loss of dexterity in patients with hand osteoarthritis, with or without significant pain)
- Joint tenderness (Fig. E3), swelling
- Crepitus with motion, pain with range of motion
- Bouchard and Heberden nodes (bony enlargement of the proximal interphalangeal [PIP] and distal interphalangeal [DIP] joints of the hand, respectively) (Fig. E4)

ETIOLOGY

Osteoarthritis is most often primary or idiopathic and can be monoarticular, oligoarticular, or polyarticular. Secondary OA is due to an identifiable condition such as trauma, mechanical abnormalities, or congenital disorders. Risk factors for osteoarthritis are summarized in Table 2. Inflammatory arthritis, crystal deposition diseases, metabolic disorders, Paget disease of bone, and osteonecrosis may also contribute to the development of secondary OA.

Dx DIAGNOSIS

DIFFERENTIAL DIAGNOSIS

- Bursitis, tendinitis
- Crystal arthropathies like calcium pyrophosphate arthropathy
- Inflammatory arthritis such as rheumatoid arthritis (Fig. E5), seronegative arthritis

WORKUP

- No specific laboratory test exists for osteoarthritis, and investigations are not always needed for the diagnosis of osteoarthritis.
- Rheumatoid factor, ESR, CBC, and antinuclear antibody tests may be required if inflammatory component is suggested by history and are normal in patients with OA.
- Arthrocentesis of swollen joints: Synovial fluid examination is noninflammatory (clear, viscous fluid with normal white cell count).

IMAGING STUDIES

- Plain x-ray of the involved joints is the first step and usually of high diagnostic value.
- Radiographic evaluation (Fig. E6) reveals:
  1. Joint space narrowing (Fig. E7)
  2. Subchondral sclerosis
  3. New bone formation in the form of osteophytes
- MRI (Fig. E8) can detect early OA changes and other sources of pain such as synovial thickening, effusions, bone marrow edema, bony attrition, and periarticular lesions.
- Musculoskeletal ultrasound (MSKUS) is emerging as an alternative modality to identify joint damage, osteophytes, effusions, and synovial proliferation.

Rx TREATMENT

- Optimal use of both pharmacologic and nonpharmacologic measures (Fig. 9) yields best outcome
- Education and reassurance

NONPHARMACOLOGIC THERAPY

The American College of Rheumatology recommends in favor of using exercise as a modality of intervention for OA of the hands, hips, and knees. Similarly, topical fomentation, cognitive-behavioral therapy, and acupuncture can be tried for these kinds of OA, although evidence is limited. Additional recommendations are summarized in the following.

HAND OA:
- First CMC orthosis and other orthotic devices
- Paraffin baths/soaks
- Kinesiotaping

HIP AND KNEE OA:
- Weight loss for overweight patients is probably the most crucial recommendation
- Pedometer step-count of more than 10,000 steps per day has been shown to prevent osteoarthritis; a dose-response curve has been noted for this modality with benefits seen at step counts as low as 6000 per day
- Physical therapy includes closed-chain quadriceps strengthening, aerobics, aquatics, and resistance exercises. A recent trial revealed that patients with osteoarthritis of the knee who undergo physical therapy have less pain and functional disability at 1 yr than patients who receive an intra-articular glucocorticoid injection[1]
- Kinesiotaping
- Tibiofemoral and patellofemoral knee brace
- Tai-chi, yoga, and balance training

It should be noted that the American College of Rheumatology recommends *against* using a TENS unit, iontophoresis, massage therapy, modified shoes, wedged insoles, and pulsed vibration therapy for management of hip, knee, or hand OA.

GENERAL Rx/ PHARMACOLOGIC Rx

The following pharmacologic interventions should be used after failure of or adjunct to the conservative measures; Topical applications of capsaicin or topical application of NSAIDs (diclofenac gel).

[1]Deyle GD et al: Physical therapy versus glucocorticoid injection for osteoarthritis of the knee, *N Engl J Med* 382:1420-1429, 2020.

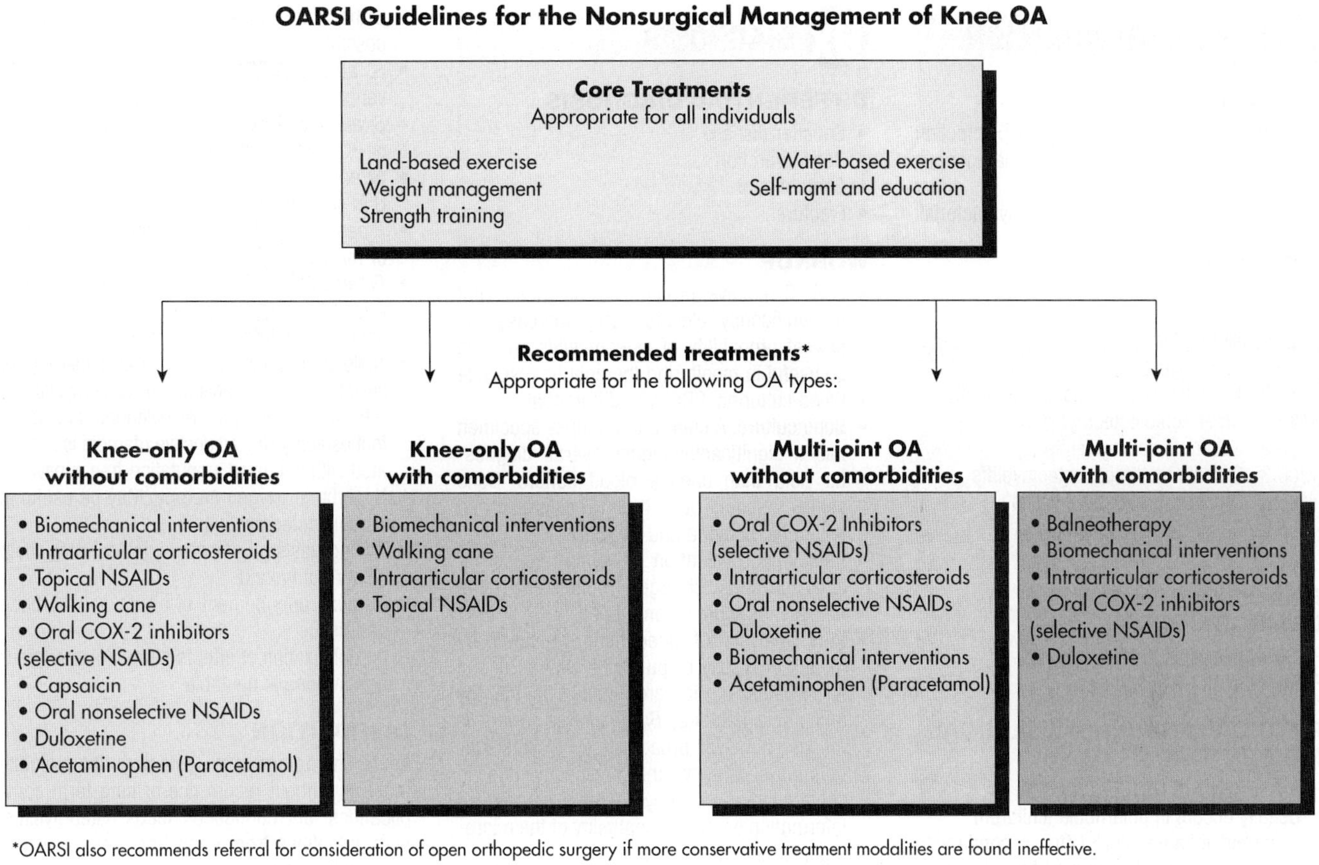

FIG. 9 Appropriate treatments summary. *COX-2,* Cyclooxygenase-2; *NSAID,* nonsteroidal antiinflammatory drug; *OA,* osteoarthritis; *OARSI,* Osteoarthritis Research Society International. (From McAlindon TE et al: OARSI guidelines for the non-surgical management of knee osteoarthritis, *Osteoarthritis Cartilage* 22:363-388, 2014.)

- Oral acetaminophen can be used given the safety of medication, but the analgesic effect is significantly lower than NSAIDs.
- Oral NSAIDs can be tried. One must consider side effects of NSAIDs, including GI bleeding, cardiovascular toxicity, and renal toxicity.
- Duloxetine can be used for treatment of osteoarthritis.
- Tramadol is recommended only for severe pain that is unresponsive to other treatment modalities. Other opioid analgesics are not typically recommended for treatment of osteoarthritis. Similarly, pregabalin has not been recommended for treatment of OA.
- Arthrocentesis of the involved joint, followed by intraarticular steroid injection, has been shown to provide short-term relief of symptoms.
- Nutritional supplements such as glucosamine and chondroitin are not recommended. Most trials indicate that neither glucosamine sulfate nor glucosamine hydrochloride reduces pain compared with placebo in knee or hip osteoarthritis. Similarly, there is no role of fish oils or vitamin D supplementation in the treatment of OA.
- Use of intraarticular hyaluronan injection for knee OA is also not generally recommended given lack of consistent benefit.

It should be noted that injections of stem cells, platelet-rich plasma, and biologic and nonbiologic disease-modifying agents are not helpful for management of osteoarthritis. Anti–nerve growth factor (anti-NGF) molecule is being investigated for treatment of osteoarthritis.

SURGICAL TREATMENT

Orthopedic interventions can be considered if there is failure of conservative and pharmacologic therapy. Joint arthroplasties are a potential option. It should be noted that surgeries such as meniscectomy, arthroscopic debridement, and lavage in the setting of osteoarthritis have not been shown to be associated with improved outcomes.

DISPOSITION

Progression of OA is not always inevitable, and the prognosis is variable depending on the site and extent of disease. Research is currently very active to find other targets to treat OA pain.

PEARLS & CONSIDERATIONS

COMMENTS

Surgical intervention is generally helpful in degenerative joint disease. Arthroplasty, arthrodesis, and realignment osteotomy are the most common procedures performed. Arthroscopic debridement of the knee appears to be of questionable value.

SUGGESTED READINGS

Available at ExpertConsult.com

RELATED CONTENT

Osteoarthritis (Patient Information)
Osteoarthritis of the Knee (Patient Information)

AUTHOR: **Deepan S. Dalal, MD, MPH**

BASIC INFORMATION

DEFINITION

Osteomyelitis is an acute or chronic infection of the bone secondary to the hematogenous or contiguous source of infection or direct traumatic inoculation, which is usually bacterial.

SYNONYM

Bone infection

ICD-10CM CODES

M86	Osteomyelitis
M86.0	Acute hematogenous osteomyelitis
M86.1	Other acute osteomyelitis
M86.2	Subacute osteomyelitis
M86.3	Chronic multifocal osteomyelitis
M86.6	Other chronic osteomyelitis
M86.9	Osteomyelitis, unspecified

EPIDEMIOLOGY & DEMOGRAPHICS

PREDOMINANT SEX: Male > female
PREDOMINANT AGE: All ages

PHYSICAL FINDINGS & CLINICAL PRESENTATION

HEMATOGENOUS OSTEOMYELITIS:
- Usually occurs in tibia/fibula (children)
- Localized inflammation: Often secondary to trauma with accompanying hematoma or cellulitis
- Abrupt fever
- Lethargy
- Irritability
- Pain in involved bone

VERTEBRAL OSTEOMYELITIS:
- Usually hematogenous
- Fever: 50%
- Localized pain/tenderness. Back pain is the most common initial symptom (86% of cases)
- Neurologic defects: Motor/sensory (sensory loss, weakness, radiculopathy)

CONTIGUOUS OSTEOMYELITIS:
- Direct inoculation
- Associated with trauma, fractures, surgical fixation
- Chronic infection of skin/soft tissue
- Fever, drainage from surgical site

CHRONIC OSTEOMYELITIS:
- Bone pain
- Sinus tract drainage, nonhealing ulcer
- Chronic low-grade fever
- Chronic localized pain

ETIOLOGY

- MSSA: Methicillin-sensitive *Staphylococcus aureus*
- MRSA: Methicillin-resistant *S. aureus*
- *Pseudomonas aeruginosa*
- *Enterobacteriaceae*
- *Streptococcus pyogenes*
- Enterococcus
- Mycobacteria
- Fungi
- Coagulase-negative staphylococci
- *Salmonella* (in sickle cell disease)

DIAGNOSIS

DIFFERENTIAL DIAGNOSIS

- Gaucher disease
- Bone infarction
- Charcot joint
- Fracture

WORKUP

- ESR, C-reactive protein: Nondiagnostic but if significantly elevated they increase the pretest probability of osteomyelitis and can be useful in monitoring therapeutic response
- Blood culturing, CRC with differential
- Bone culture. A culture of a biopsy specimen has a significantly higher overall diagnostic yield than does a blood culture. Bone samples should be cultured for aerobic and anaerobic bacteria and for fungi
- Pathologic evaluation of bone biopsy for acute/chronic changes consistent with necrosis or acute inflammation
- PCR analysis of specimens obtained by means of biopsy or puncture may be useful for organisms that are difficult to identify (anaerobic bacteria, *Bartonella* sp., *Kingella kingae*); however, broad-range PCR has suboptimal sensitivity and specificity due to contamination and may not provide sufficient information on the susceptibility of the microorganisms to antibiotics

IMAGING STUDIES

- Bone radiograph examination (Fig. E1): Initial study but not sensitive in early osteomyelitis as may not show changes for as much as 2 wks
- MRI with and without contrast (Fig. E2): Most accurate imaging study. CT only if patient has contraindication to MRI
- Triple-phase technetium-99m bone scan (Fig. E3) when MRI is unavailable or contraindicated. Typically positive within a few days after onset of symptoms but accuracy is lower than that of MRI
- Gallium scan (Ga-67) scintigraphy with single-photon emission CT (SPECT) has higher accuracy than bone scan but is less sensitive for detection of epidural abscess in vertebral osteomyelitis
- Indium-111–labeled leukocyte scintigraphy scan; low sensitivity (<20%) for vertebral osteomyelitis
- Positron emission tomography (PET) scanning with ^{18}F-fluorodeoxyglucose has high accuracy (similar to MRI) and is useful in patients with metallic implants
- Table 1 summarizes imaging findings in osteomyelitis

TREATMENT

- Surgical debridement in biopsy-positive cases will guide direction for antibiotic therapy. This will vary with type of osteomyelitis. Duration of therapy is usually 4 to 6 wk for acute osteomyelitis; chronic osteomyelitis may need a longer course of medication
- Orthopedic hardware should be removed if possible
- *S. aureus* (MSSA): Cefazolin IV, nafcillin IV, vancomycin IV (in patient allergic to penicillin)
- *S. aureus* (MRSA): Vancomycin IV, linezolid IV or PO, daptomycin IV
- *Streptococcus* spp: Ceftriaxone, IV penicillin G in sensitive species
- *P. aeruginosa:* Cefepime, imipenem/cilastatin, or meropenem
- *Enterobacteriaceae:* Ceftriaxone or ertapenem
- Anaerobes: Clindamycin, piperacillin-tazobactam, cefotetan, or metronidazole
- Table 2 summarizes antimicrobial therapy for selected microorganisms in osteomyelitis. A retrospective analysis[1] revealed that in diabetic foot osteomyelitis adjunctive rifampin is associated with improved amputation-free survival
- Hyperbaric oxygen therapy: May be useful in chronic osteomyelitis
- Wound-assisted vacuum device may help closure of wound
- Surgical debridement of all devitalized bone and tissue
- Immobilization of affected bone (plaster, traction) if bone is unstable

DISPOSITION

Acute hematogenous osteomyelitis usually resolves without recurrence or long-term complications, but contiguous focus osteomyelitis, bone infections from open fractures, or osteomyelitis frequently recurs.

REFERRAL

- To an orthopedic surgeon if chronic osteomyelitis with need for bone debridement, bone grafting, or stabilization of infected tissue adjacent to a bone fracture
- To an infectious disease specialist for appropriate treatment for difficult-to-treat or recalcitrant infections
- To a hyperbaric oxygen chamber service for nonhealing, chronic osteomyelitis

PEARLS & CONSIDERATIONS

- Chronic osteomyelitis is one of the most challenging infections to treat; the high failure rate is a consequence of poor vascular supply, nondistensible bone tissue, and limited penetration of bone tissue.
- Parenteral antibiotics are usually chosen initially, but oral fluoroquinolones have good bone penetration and may be used in stable patients. A recent trial comparing oral versus IV antibiotics for bone and joint infections found that oral antibiotic therapy is not inferior to IV antibiotic therapy when used during the first 6 wk for complex orthopedic infections.[2]

---

[1] Wilson BM et al: Adjunctive rifampin therapy for diabetic foot osteomyelitis in the veterans health administration, *JAMA Netw Open* 2(11)e1916003, 2019.
[2] Li HK, et al: Oral versus intravenous antibiotics for bone and joint infection, *N Engl J Med* 380(5):425–436, 2019.

TABLE 1 Imaging Findings in Osteomyelitis

	Plain Radiograph	CT	MRI	NM
Acute	Minimal findings Soft-tissue swelling may be seen	Not useful	Bone marrow edema can occur as early as 24-48 h, seen as low T1, and high T2 signal	May show increased uptake, but takes a few days
Subacute	Lucent or sclerotic lesion, periosteal reaction, soft-tissue swelling	Cortical and marrow abnormalities including abscess, periosteal reaction, soft-tissue edema, and abscess	Bone marrow changes, cortical abnormalities seen as thickening, bone abscess, periosteal reaction, increased T2 signal in soft tissues, abscess formation. Postgadolinium T1W sequences outline abscess cavities clearly	Three-phase bone scintigram, indium-111 WBC scan and combined studies are useful, especially to assess multifocal involvement. PET-CT generally not used in this context, but may be useful in exceptional circumstances
Chronic	Bone sclerosis, cortical thickening, sequestrum and cloaca, bone destruction, resorption, and deformities	Much better than plain radiographs to demonstrate cloaca and sequestrum, periosteal new bone formation, and abscess	Better soft-tissue and bone marrow resolution to demonstrate medullary and cortical changes, sequestra and cloaca well demonstrated, useful to outline soft-tissue abscess, and sinus tracts	Generally useful if there is a problem with diagnosis. Combined WBC and bone marrow scintigram is useful. May highlight multiple sites of involvement

CT, Computed tomography; *MRI,* magnetic resonance imaging; *NM,* nuclear medicine; *PET,* positron emission tomography; *WBC,* white blood cell.
From Grant LA: *Grainger & Allison's diagnostic radiology essentials,* ed 2, Philadelphia, 2019, Elsevier.

TABLE 2 Antimicrobial Therapy for Selected Microorganisms in Chronic Osteomyelitis in Adults

Microorganism	First Choice*	Alternative Choice
Methicillin/oxacillin/nafcillin-sensitive staphylococci	Nafcillin sodium or oxacillin sodium 1.5-2 g IV q4h for 4-6 wk *or* cefazolin 1-2 g IV q8h for 4-6 wk	Vancomycin 15 mg/kg IV q12h for 4-6 wk
Methicillin/oxacillin/nafcillin-resistant staphylococci (MRSA)	Vancomycin† 15 mg/kg IV q12h for 4-6 wk *or* daptomycin 6 mg/kg IV q24h	Linezolid 600 mg PO/IV q12h *or* levofloxacin† 500-750 mg PO/IV daily, plus rifampin 600-900 mg PO for 6 wk if susceptible to both drugs
Penicillin-sensitive streptococci	Aqueous penicillin G 20 epto^6 U/24 hr IV either continuously or in six equally divided daily doses *or* ceftriaxone 1-2 g IV q24h *or* cefazolin 1-2 g IV q8h for 4-6 wk	Vancomycin 15 mg/kg IV q12h for 4-6 wk
Enterococci	Aqueous crystalline penicillin G 20×10^6 U/24 hr IV either continuously or in six equally divided daily doses *or* ampicillin sodium 12 g/24 hr IV either continuously or in six equally divided daily doses; the addition of gentamicin sulfate 1 mg/kg IV or IM q8h for 1-2 wk is *optional*	Vancomycin† 15 mg/kg IV q12h; the addition of gentamicin sulfate 1 mg/kg IV or IM q8h for 1-2 wk is *optional*
Enterobacteriaceae	Ceftriaxone 1-2 g IV q24h for 4-6 wk or ertapenem 1 g IV q24h	Ciprofloxacin 500-750 mg PO q12h for 4-6 wk or levofloxacin 500-750 mg PO q24h
Pseudomonas aeruginosa	Cefepime 2 g IV q12h, meropenem 1 g IV q8h, or imipenem 500 mg IV q6h for 4-6 wk	Ciprofloxacin 750 mg PO q12h for 4-6 wk or ceftazidime 2 g IV q8h

IM, Intramuscular; *IV,* intravenous; *MRSA,* methicillin-resistant *Staphylococcus aureus; PO,* by mouth.
*Antimicrobial selection should be based on in vitro sensitivity data, as well as allergies, intolerances, and drug interactions in individual patients.
†Doses shown are based on normal renal and hepatic function and may need to be adjusted or serum levels monitored (vancomycin).

- The optimal duration of therapy for vertebral osteomyelitis is unclear. Trials comparing 6 wk to 12 wk of antibiotic treatment in pyogenic vertebral osteomyelitis showed similar cure rates (91%) in both groups.

SUGGESTED READINGS

Available at ExpertConsult.com

RELATED CONTENT

Osteomyelitis (Patient Information)

AUTHOR: **Glenn G. Fort, MD, MPH**

BASIC INFORMATION

DEFINITION

Osteonecrosis, also known as avascular necrosis (AVN), is ischemic death of bone due to insufficient blood supply. It is not a specific disease entity but a final common pathway to several disorders that impair blood supply to the femoral head and other locations.

SYNONYMS

AVN
Avascular necrosis
Aseptic necrosis

ICD-10CM CODES

M87	Idiopathic aseptic necrosis of bone
M87.1	Osteonecrosis due to drugs
M87.2	Osteonecrosis due to previous trauma
M87.3	Other secondary osteonecrosis
M87.9	Osteonecrosis, unspecified

EPIDEMIOLOGY & DEMOGRAPHICS

- 15,000 new cases per yr in the U.S. It is most commonly associated with the hip and accounts for 10% of total hip replacements in the U.S.
- Usually occurs in middle age and is more frequent in males than females
- Associated conditions:
  1. Corticosteroid treatment: 35%
  2. Alcohol abuse: 22%
  3. Idiopathic and other: 43%
  4. Hemoglobinopathies, pancreatitis, chronic renal failure, SLE, chemotherapy, decompression sickness
- Common sites involved
  1. Femoral head
  2. Femoral condyle
  3. Humeral head
  4. Navicular and lunate wrist bones
  5. Talus

PHYSICAL FINDINGS & CLINICAL PRESENTATION

- May be asymptomatic in early stages
- Pain in the involved area exacerbated by movement or weight bearing in later stages
- Decreased range of motion as the disease progresses
- Functional limitation

ETIOLOGY

Final common pathway of conditions that lead to impairment of the blood supply to the involved bone. Trauma disrupting the blood supply is the most common cause of osteonecrosis. Arterial factors are considered the most common cause of osteonecrosis. Table 1 describes proposed mechanism of disease of common conditions associated with osteonecrosis.

STAGING

Tables 2 and 3 and Box 1 illustrate various staging systems for osteonecrosis.

DIAGNOSIS

DIFFERENTIAL DIAGNOSIS

- None in late stages
- Early: Any condition causing focal musculoskeletal pain, including arthritis, bursitis, tendinitis, myopathy, neoplastic bone and joint diseases, traumatic injuries, pathologic fractures

WORKUP

Fig. 1 describes a diagnostic algorithm for osteonecrosis.

IMAGING STUDIES (FIG. 2)

- MRI: The most sensitive technology to diagnose early aseptic necrosis. The first sign is a margin of low signal. An inner border of high signal associated with a low-signal line is specific for aseptic necrosis ("double line sign"). Sensitivity is 75% to 100%.
- Radiography: Insensitive early in the course. The earliest changes include diffuse osteopenia, areas of radiolucency with sclerotic border, and linear sclerosis. Later, a subchondral lucency (crescent sign) indicates subchondral fracture. More advanced cases reveal flattening, collapsed bone, and abnormal bone contour. In late disease, osteoarthritic changes are seen.
- Bone scan:
  1. Early: "Cold" area
  2. Later: Increased radionuclide uptake as a result of remodeling
  3. Sensitivity in early disease is only 70% and specificity is poor
- CT scan: May reveal central necrosis and area of collapse before those are visible on radiographs.

TREATMENT

PREVENTION

- Manage etiologic conditions
- Minimize corticosteroid use

NONPHARMACOLOGIC THERAPY

- Core decompression: Effectiveness 35% to 95% in early phases
- Bone grafting
- Osteotomies
- Joint replacement

ACUTE GENERAL Rx

- Decrease weight bearing of affected area.
- Pulsing electromagnetic fields applied externally (still experimental).
- Peripheral vasodilators (e.g., dihydroergotamine) (unproven).
- Late-stage AVN is most often treated by total joint arthroplasty.

PROGNOSIS

- When diagnosed at an early stage treatment is appropriate in all cases because 85% to 90% can be expected to progress to a more advanced stage.
- Contralateral joint involvement is common (30% to 70%).

RELATED CONTENT

Avascular Necrosis (Patient Information)

AUTHOR: **Fred F. Ferri, MD**

TABLE 1 Proposed Mechanism of Disease of Common Conditions Associated with Osteonecrosis

	MECHANISM OF OSTEONECROSIS							
Associated Condition	**Apoptosis**	**Osteoblast/ Osteoclast Homeostasis**	**Lipid Abnormalities**	**Coagulation Abnormalities**	**Oxidative Stress**	**Parathyroid/ Calcium Imbalance**	**Vascular Plugging**	**Vasoactive Substances**
Corticosteroids	X	X	X	X	X			X
Bisphosphonates	X	X	X					
Alcohol abuse	X	X	X	X	X			
Trauma	X	X						X
Renal transplantation	X	X		X		X		
Dialysis						X		
Sickle cell disease							X	

From Firestein GS et al: *Kelley's textbook of rheumatology,* ed 9, Philadelphia, 2013, Saunders.

TABLE 2 Ficat Staging System

Stage	Description
I	Normal radiographic findings
II	Sclerotic or cystic lesions
III	Subchondral collapse
IV	Osteoarthritis with articular collapse

From Hochberg MC: *Rheumatology,* ed 7, Philadelphia, 2019, Elsevier.

TABLE 3 Steinberg Staging System

Stage	Description
I	Normal radiographic findings; abnormal bone scan and/or magnetic resonance imaging findings • Mild (<15% of head affected) • Moderate (15%-30% of head affected) • Severe (>30% of head affected)
II	Lucent and sclerotic changes in the femoral head • Mild (<15% of head affected) • Moderate (15%-30% of head affected) • Severe (>30% of head affected)
III	Subchondral collapse without flattening • Mild (<15% of head affected) • Moderate (15%-30% of head affected) • Severe (>30% of head affected)
IV	Flattening of the femoral head • Mild (<15% of head affected) • Moderate (15%-30% of head affected) • Severe (>30% of head affected)
V	Joint narrowing and/or acetabular changes • Mild • Moderate • Severe
VI	Advanced degenerative changes

From Hochberg MC: *Rheumatology,* ed 7, Philadelphia, 2019, Elsevier.

BOX 1 International Classification of Osteonecrosis of the Femoral Head (Association Research Circulation Osseous)

- Stage 0: Bone biopsy results consistent with osteonecrosis; other test results normal
- Stage I: Positive findings on bone scan, magnetic resonance imaging (MRI), or both
  - A: <15% involvement of the femoral head (MRI)
  - B: 15%-30% involvement
  - C: >30% involvement
- Stage II: Mottled appearance of femoral head, osteosclerosis, cyst formation, and osteopenia on radiographs; no signs of collapse of femoral head on radiographic or computed tomographic study; positive findings on bone scan and MRI; no changes in acetabulum
  - A: <15% involvement of the femoral head (MRI)
  - B: 15%-30% involvement
  - C: >30% involvement
- Stage III: Presence of crescent sign lesions classified on basis of appearance on anteroposterior and lateral radiographs
  - A: <15% crescent sign or <2-mm depression of femoral head
  - B: 15%-30% crescent sign or 2- to 4-mm depression
  - C: >30% crescent sign or >4-mm depression
- Stage IV: Articular surface flattened; joint space shows narrowing; changes in acetabulum with evidence of osteosclerosis, cyst formation, and marginal osteophytes

From Hochberg MC: *Rheumatology,* ed 7, Philadelphia, 2019, Elsevier.

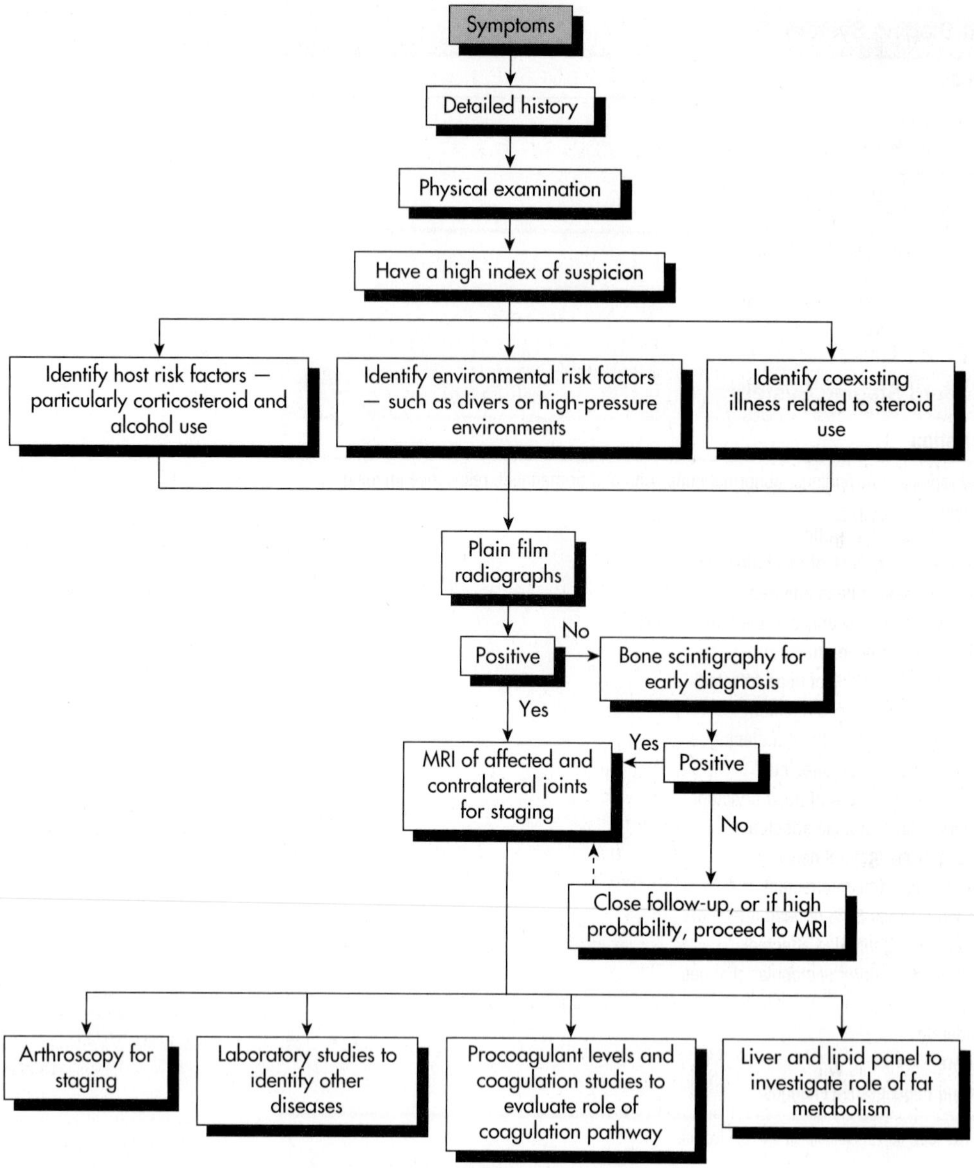

FIG. 1 Diagnostic algorithm for osteonecrosis. *MRI*, Magnetic resonance image. (From Firestein GS et al: *Kelley's textbook of rheumatology*, ed 9, Philadelphia, 2013, Saunders.)

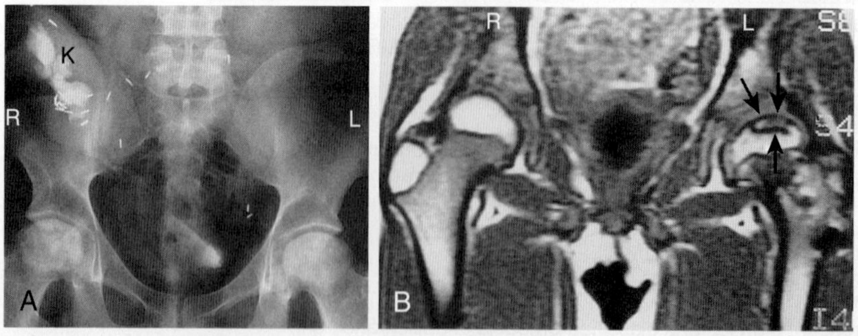

FIG. 2 Aseptic necrosis of the hips. A, Aseptic necrosis can occur from a number of causes, including trauma and steroid use. In this patient, an anteroposterior view of the pelvis shows a transplanted kidney *(K)* in the right iliac fossa. Use of steroids has caused this patient to have bilateral aseptic necrosis. The femoral heads are somewhat flattened, irregular, and increased in density. **B,** Aseptic necrosis in a different patient is demonstrated on an MRI scan as an area of decreased signal *(arrows)* in the left femoral head. This is the most sensitive method for detection of early aseptic necrosis. (From Mettler FA [ed]: *Primary care radiology,* Philadelphia, 2000, Saunders.)

BASIC INFORMATION

DEFINITION

Osteoporosis is a skeletal disorder characterized by a progressive loss of bone mass and a decline in bone quality that results in increased bone fragility and a higher fracture risk. Poor bone mass acquisition during adolescence and bone loss during the sixth decade of life are the main processes responsible for osteoporosis. The various types are as follows:

PRIMARY OSTEOPOROSIS: Primary osteoporosis is the loss of bone mass due to aging and decreased gonadal function, not to any other chronic illness.

- Idiopathic osteoporosis: Unknown pathogenesis; may occur in children and young adults.
- Type I osteoporosis (postmenopausal women): Occurs after menopause due to an abrupt decline in estrogen production. It is characterized by accelerated and disproportionate trabecular bone loss and is associated with fractures of the spine, hip, and wrist.
- Type II osteoporosis (involutional): Occurs in both men and women aged >70 yr due to the progressively negative balance between bone formation and resorption. It is characterized by both trabecular and cortical bone loss and associated with fractures of the spine, long bones, and hip.

SECONDARY OSTEOPOROSIS: Secondary osteoporosis is bone loss due to another chronic condition such as thyroxine excess, hyperparathyroidism, malignancies, gastrointestinal disease, medications, renal failure, and connective tissue diseases (see "Differential Diagnosis").

ICD-10CM CODES

M81.0	Age-related osteoporosis without current pathological fracture
M81.4	Drug-induced osteoporosis
M81.5	Idiopathic osteoporosis
M81.6	Localized osteoporosis

EPIDEMIOLOGY & DEMOGRAPHICS

PREVALENCE (IN U.S.):

- Affects more than 10 million people in the U.S.
- Annual incidence of osteoporotic fractures exceeds 1.5 million in the U.S. (70% women)
- Twice as common in women than in men
- Results: Institutionalization, death, and health care costs in excess of $17 billion annually

RISK FACTORS:

- Female sex
- Postmenopausal state
- Advanced age
- Petite body frame, low body weight (<58 kg)
- White or Asian ancestry
- Sedentary lifestyle
- Nulliparity
- Calcium deficiency
- Previous low-trauma fracture
- Parental history of hip fracture
- Tobacco use
- Excess alcohol or caffeine use
- Long-term glucocorticoid use
- Chronic disease states; e.g., primary ovarian insufficiency, diabetes mellitus, androgen deficiency, inflammatory bowel disease, hyperthyroidism, hypercortisolism

PHYSICAL FINDINGS & CLINICAL PRESENTATION

- Most commonly silent with no signs or symptoms.
- Insidious and progressive development of dorsal kyphosis *(dowager's hump),* loss of height, and skeletal pain typically associated with fracture; reduced gait speed or grip strength; other physical findings related to other conditions with associated increased risk for osteoporosis such as nodular thyroid, hepatic enlargement, jaundice, cushingoid features (see "Risk Factors" and Boxes 1 and 2).

ETIOLOGY

Normal bone turnover involves balance between process of bone resorption and bone formation. Osteoclasts resorb bone, and osteoblasts secrete bone matrix for building bone. In postmenopausal women, rate of bone turnover increases after loss of ovarian function, leading to progressive bone loss.

Several fracture risk calculation tools have been developed. FRAX is the leading tool among them. Clinical risk factors used in the World Health Organization Fracture Risk Assessment Tool (WHO FRAX) 10-yr fracture risk calculator are summarized in Box 3.

DIAGNOSIS

DIFFERENTIAL DIAGNOSIS

- Malignancy (multiple myeloma, lymphoma, leukemia, metastatic carcinoma)
- Primary hyperparathyroidism
- Osteomalacia
- Paget's disease
- Osteogenesis imperfecta: Types I, III, and IV

WORKUP

- History and physical examination, with appropriate evaluation for identified risk factors and secondary causes. Medications associated with osteoporosis are summarized in Table 1. Investigations for secondary osteoporosis are summarized in Box 4.

BOX 1 Major Clinical Risk Factors for Osteoporotic Fracture

- Age
- Gender
- Previous fragility fracture
- Glucocorticoid therapy
- History of falls
- Family history of hip fracture
- Other causes of secondary osteoporosis
- Low body mass index
- Smoking
- High alcohol intake

From Hochberg MC: *Rheumatology,* ed 7, Philadelphia, 2019, Elsevier.

BOX 2 Causes of Secondary Osteoporosis

- Endocrine
  1. Hypogonadism in either sex, including untreated, premature menopause and treatment with aromatase inhibitors or androgen deprivation therapy
  2. Hyperthyroidism
  3. Hyperprolactinemia
  4. Cushing disease
  5. Diabetes
- Gastrointestinal
  1. Celiac disease
  2. Inflammatory bowel disease
  3. Chronic liver disease
  4. Chronic pancreatitis
  5. Other causes of malabsorption
- Rheumatologic
  1. Rheumatoid arthritis
  2. Other inflammatory arthropathies
- Hematologic
  1. Multiple myeloma
  2. Hemoglobinopathies
  3. Systemic mastocytosis
  4. Chronic heparin treatment
- Respiratory
  1. Cystic fibrosis
  2. Chronic obstructive pulmonary disease
- Metabolic
  1. Homocystinuria
- Chronic renal disease
- Immobility

From Hochberg MC: *Rheumatology,* ed 7, Philadelphia, 2019, Elsevier.

BOX 3 Clinical Risk Factors Included in the FRAX Case-Finding Algorithm

- Age (50 to 90 yr)
- Sex
- Weight (in kilograms) and height (in centimeters). Body mass index is automatically computed from height and weight
- Previous fragility fracture (yes/no)
- Parental history of hip fracture (yes/no)
- Current tobacco smoking (yes/no)
- Long-term use of oral glucocorticoids (over 3 mo) (yes/no)
- Rheumatoid arthritis (yes/no)
- Alcohol consumption of 3 or more units daily (yes/no)
- Other causes of secondary osteoporosis (yes/no): Includes type I diabetes, osteogenesis imperfecta, longstanding untreated hyperthyroidism, hypogonadism or premature menopause (<45 yr), chronic malnutrition, malabsorption, chronic liver disease

From World Health Organization. WHO risk fracture assessment tool. www.sheffield.ac.uk/FRAX/. From Hochberg MC: *Rheumatology,* ed 7, Philadelphia, 2019, Elsevier.

TABLE 1 Medications Associated with Osteoporosis

System	Medication
Endocrine	Aromatase inhibitors (e.g., anastrozole) Excess thyroxine replacement Glucocorticoids Gonadotropin-releasing hormone agonists Ovarian-suppressing drugs (e.g., medroxyprogesterone acetate) Thiazolidinediones SGLT2 inhibitors
Gastrointestinal	Proton pump inhibitors
Hematologic	Heparin Warfarin
Infectious disease	Antiretroviral therapy
Immunosuppressant	Cyclosporine Cytotoxic drugs Tacrolimus
Neurologic	Anticonvulsants—phenytoin, phenobarbital, carbamazepine
Psychiatric	Selective serotonin reuptake inhibitors
Renal	Loop diuretics (e.g., furosemide)

From Hochberg MC: *Rheumatology,* ed 7, Philadelphia, 2019, Elsevier.

BOX 4 Investigations for Secondary Osteoporosis in Older People with Low Trauma Fractures or Low Bone Mineral Density

CBC
ESR or CRP
Biochemical profile: Including renal function, adjusted serum calcium, and alkaline phosphatase
Thyroid function tests
Serum testosterone, sex hormone–binding globulin, LH, FSH (men)
Serum and urine electrophoresis (vertebral fractures)
Serum 25OHD and PTH

CRP, C-reactive protein; *ESR,* erythrocyte sedimentation rate; *FSH,* follicle-stimulating hormone; *LH,* luteinizing hormone; *PTH,* parathyroid hormone; *25OHD,* 25 hydroxyvitamin.

From Fillit HM: *Brocklehurst's textbook of geriatric medicine and gerontology,* ed 8, Philadelphia, 2017, Elsevier.

- WHO guidelines for the diagnosis of osteoporosis are based on bone mineral density (BMD) measurements of the hip or spine in g/cm^2 and are reported as a T score.
  1. Dual-energy x-ray absorptiometry (DEXA) is the gold standard for screening and monitoring changes in BMD due to excellent precision, widespread availability, low cost, and minimal radiation exposure.
  2. DEXA (Fig. 1) is indicated in all women 65 yr and older and in postmenopausal women younger than 65 yr of age who are at risk for fracture (e.g., weight <127 lbs, parental history of hip fracture, use of medications that cause bone loss, current smoking, excessive alcohol use (>2 drinks per day), rheumatoid arthritis, or presence of diseases that cause bone loss). Causes of erroneous bone mineral density measures by DEXA in the lumbar spine are summarized in Table 2.
  3. FRAX questionnaire (Fig. 2): Use of FRAX calculator (www.sheffield.ac.uk/FRAX/) is proposed by the U.S. Preventive Services Task Force (USPSTF) to determine the need for screening in women between the ages of 50 and 64. If the FRAX 10-yr major osteoporotic risk is greater than or equal to 9.3%, the USPSTF recommends screening with DEXA scan.
  4. Currently, routine testing in men for osteoporosis is not recommended unless there are clinical manifestations of low bone mass.
  5. Quantitative ultrasound can be used as an adjunctive tool to predict risk of fracture in both men and women. It is cheaper than DEXA and has no radiation. However,

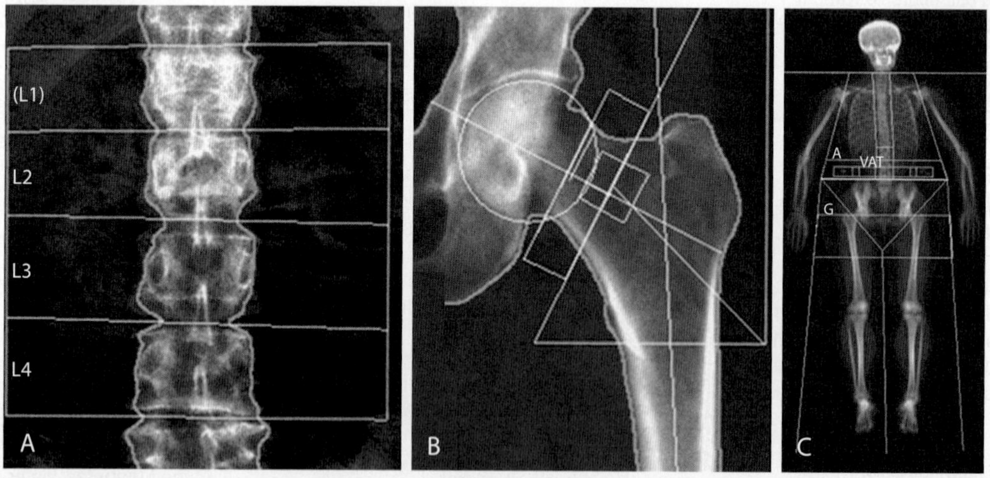

FIG. 1 Dual-energy x-ray absorptiometry (DEXA) provides "areal" bone mineral density (BMD) (g/cm^2) and is currently the gold standard for diagnosis of osteoporosis by bone densitometry (World Health Organization definition T score −2.5 or below) in (**A**) posteroanterior lumbar spine *(L1 through L4)* or (**B**) hip (femoral neck or total). **C,** DEXA of the whole body can provide information on total and regional BMD and body composition (fat and muscle mass). Recent additional parameters measured are android *A*/gynoid *G* ratio and visceral adipose tissue *(VAT).* (From Pope TL et al: *Musculoskeletal imaging,* ed 2, Philadelphia, 2014, Saunders.)

TABLE 2 Causes of Erroneous Bone Mineral Density Measures by DEXA in the Lumbar Spine

Overestimation of Bone Mineral Density
Extraneous calcification (lymph nodes, aorta)
Degenerative disk and spine disease (osteophytes)
Ankylosing spondylitis
Vertebral fracture
Sclerotic metastases
Vertebral hemangioma
Overlying metal artifacts (navel rings)
Surgical interventions (metallic rods, spinal fusion)
Vertebroplasty
Paget disease
Treatment with strontium ranelate
Underestimation of Bone Mineral Density
Laminectomy

DEXA, Dual-energy x-ray absorptiometry.
From Pope TL et al: *Musculoskeletal imaging*, ed 2, Philadelphia, 2014, Saunders.

at this point, additional research and trials are needed to establish its utility in diagnosis and management of osteoporosis.

- Recommendations as to when to repeat bone density testing should be based on initial T scores (Fig. 3). Data from the Study of Osteoporotic Fractures indicates that in women with normal bone density or mild osteopenia, repeat testing might not be necessary for another 10 to 15 yr. For women with moderate osteopenia, a screening interval of 3 to 5 yr may be appropriate. For women with advanced bone loss/osteoporosis, testing every 1 to 2 yr is recommended.

LABORATORY TESTS (BOX 5)

- Biochemical profile to evaluate renal and hepatic function, primary hyperparathyroidism, and malnutrition.
- CBC for nutritional status and myeloma.
- TSH to rule out the presence of hyperthyroidism.
- 24-hr urinary calcium levels and 26-hydroxyvitamin D level may be helpful in evaluating for secondary causes of osteoporosis.
- Consider celiac panel and serum protein electrophoresis.
- Biochemical markers of bone remodeling may be useful to predict rate of bone loss and/or follow therapy response. Specific biochemical markers (listed below) are followed (e.g., 3-mo interval) to document normalization as a response to therapy.
  1. High-turnover osteoporosis: High levels of resorption markers (lysyl pyridinoline, deoxy lysyl pyridinoline, n-telopeptide of collagen cross-links, C-telopeptide of collagen cross-links) and formation markers (osteocalcin and bone-specific alkaline phosphatase); accelerated bone loss responding best to antiresorptive therapy
  2. Low-normal-turnover osteoporosis: Normal or low levels of the markers of resorption and formation (see "high-turnover osteoporosis" listed previously); no accelerated bone loss; responds best to drugs that enhance bone formation

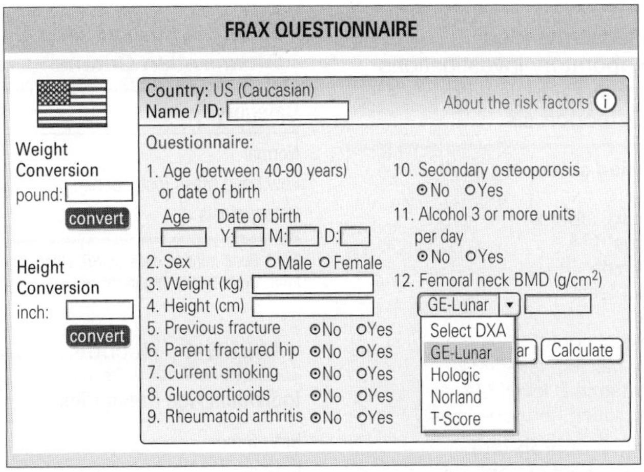

FIG. 2 FRAX questionnaire. (From Hochberg MC: *Rheumatology*, ed 7, Philadelphia, 2019, Elsevier.)

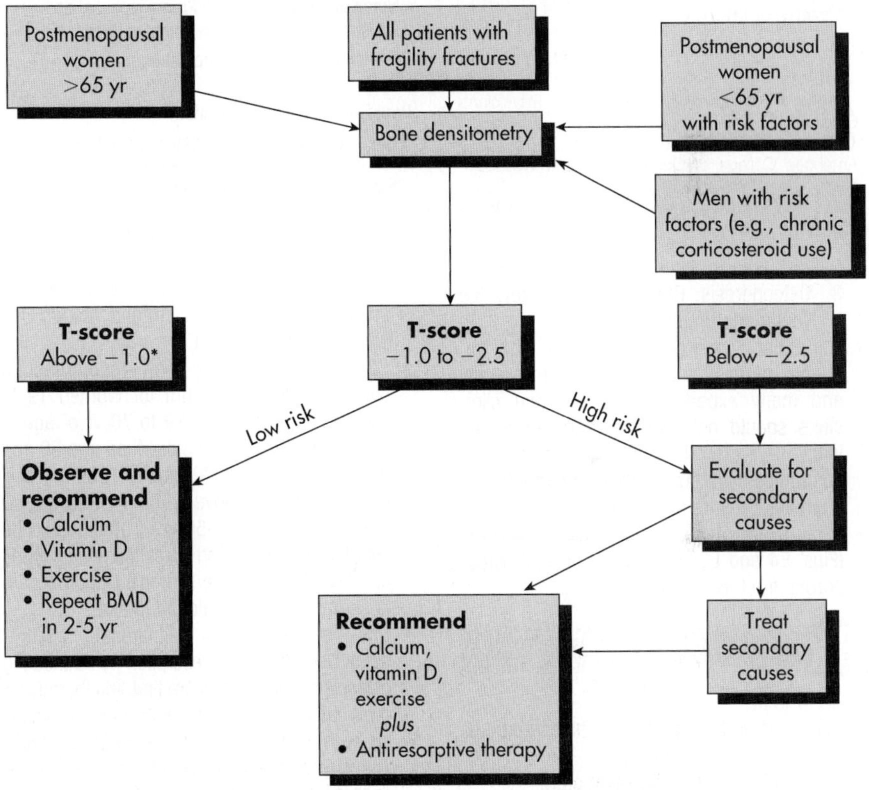

*Patients with fragility fractures and a T-score above −1.0 should be evaluated for other causes of pathologic fracture.

FIG. 3 Diagnosis and management of osteoporosis.

IMAGING STUDIES

- Bone mineral density (BMD) determination (see "Workup") should be performed on all women with determined risk factors and/or associated secondary causes. Criteria for the diagnosis of osteoporosis based on measurement of bone density and T score are summarized in Table 3.
  1. Normal: BMD <1 SD below the young adult reference mean
  2. Osteopenia: BMD 1 to 2.5 SD below the young adult reference mean

BOX 5 Recommended Laboratory Investigations for Individuals with Osteoporosis

Recommended screening in all patients
Serum calcium, albumin, phosphorus*,†,‡,§
Serum creatinine*,†,‡,§
Liver function tests*
Bicarbonate*
Complete blood count*
24-hr urinary calcium level*,†,‡,§
25-hydroxyvitamin D level*,†,‡,§
Thyroid-stimulating hormone level*,†,‡,§

Other testing, if appropriate
Biochemical markers of bone turnover*,†,‡,§
Cortisol levels*,‡
Protein electrophoresis*,†,§
Parathyroid hormone level*,§

*American Association of Clinical Endocrinologists guidelines.
†National Osteoporosis Foundation Physician's Guide.
‡U.S. Surgeon General's report.
§American College of Obstetricians and Gynecologists.
From Hochberg MC: *Rheumatology,* ed 7, Philadelphia, 2019, Elsevier.

TABLE 3 Diagnostic Categories for Osteoporosis Based on World Health Organization Criteria

Category	Definition
Normal	BMD not more than 1 SD below the young adult mean value
Low bone mass (osteopenia)	BMD lying between 1 and 2.5 SD below the young adult mean value
Osteoporosis	BMD more than 2.5 SD below the young adult mean value

BMD, Bone mineral density; *SD,* standard deviation.
From World Health Organization data, 1994. In Hochberg MC: *Rheumatology,* ed 7, Philadelphia, 2019, Elsevier.

TABLE 4 Recommended Supplementation of Calcium and Vitamin D

Individual Age Categories	Elemental Calcium	Vitamin D*
Birth-6 mo	400 mg	200 IU
6-12 mo	600 mg	200 IU
1-10 yr	800 mg	200 IU
11-24 yr	1200-1500 mg/day	400 IU
Women and men 25-65 yr: Premenopausal or postmenopausal women taking estrogen	1000 mg/day	400-600 IU
Postmenopausal women, no estrogen	1500 mg/day	400-600 IU for men and women >65 yr
Pregnant and lactating women	1200-1500 mg/day	400 IU
National Osteoporosis Foundation guidelines	1200 mg	800-1000 IU

*These recommendations are guidelines and may be sufficient for healthy individuals with normal 25-hydroxyvitamin D levels. In many circumstances, however, they are insufficient.
From Hochberg MC: *Rheumatology,* ed 7, Philadelphia, 2019, Elsevier.

3. Osteoporosis: BMD >2.5 SD below the young adult reference mean

- For patient undergoing treatment: The frequency of BMD monitoring is controversial and many experts recommend that clinicians should not monitor BMD during the initial 5-yr drug treatment period because no studies have proven that such monitoring improves fracture outcomes.
- X-ray exam of appropriate part of skeleton (Figs. E4 and E5) to evaluate clinical osteoporotic fracture only.

Rx TREATMENT

When to treat:
- Osteoporosis based on DEXA measurements of BMD
- History of hip and vertebral fracture
- Osteopenia on DEXA + 10-yr FRAX score of greater than or equal to 3% at hip or greater than or equal to 20% of major osteoporotic fracture

NONPHARMACOLOGIC THERAPY

Prevention:
- Identification and minimization of risk factors
- Appropriate diagnosis and treatment of secondary causes
- Behavioral modification: Proper nutrition, physical activity (specifically weight-bearing activity), fracture prevention strategies, fall risk reduction

ACUTE GENERAL Rx

- Vitamin D supplement: 600 IU/day for persons 19 to 70 yr of age and 800 IU/day for persons 71 yr and older. Recommended supplementation of calcium and vitamin D is summarized in Table 4.
- Calcium supplement: The recommended dietary intake of calcium for women 19 to 50 yr of age and men 19 to 70 yr of age is 1000 mg/day; women older than age 50 and men older than age 70 require 1200 mg/day. Calcium intake above 2500 mg/day (2000 mg/day in persons >50 yr of age) should be avoided. Consumption of calcium-rich foods and beverages is the preferred approach to ensuring adequate calcium intake.[1]
- Oral bisphosphonates (alendronate, risedronate): Decrease bone resorption by attenuating osteoclast activity. They are first-line therapy for the treatment of most patients with osteoporosis, with proven efficacy to reduce fracture risk. The bisphosphonates differ in binding affinity, dose frequency, and route of administration. To facilitate absorption, most oral bisphosphonates are taken on an empty stomach with a full glass of water. Patients are instructed to remain in a sitting or standing position for 30 to 60 min. Contraindications include esophageal disorders, inability to remain standing for 30 to 60 min after taking the medication, chronic kidney disease, and Roux-en-Y gastric bypass procedures. Adverse side effects include gastroesophageal reflux disease, esophagitis, transient hypocalcemia, musculoskeletal pain, renal impairment, ocular side effects, jaw necrosis, and atypical femur fracture. Zoledronic acid: A bisphosphonate given by IV infusion over at least 15 min, 5 mg once per year may be used in patients who are unable to tolerate oral bisphosphonates. It is contraindicated in patients with acute renal failure. IV ibandronate has only been shown to reduce the risk of vertebral fractures and is not indicated for reduction of risk of hip and nonvertebral fractures.
- Biologic agents: Denosumab is a human monoclonal antibody that inhibits osteoclast formation and prevents resorption for treatment of postmenopausal osteoporosis. Dosage is 60 mg subcutaneously every 6 mo. Romosozumab is a monoclonal antibody that increases bone formation and decreases bone resorption by binding to sclerostin. It may be considered for patients who are at high risk for fracture and cannot tolerate any other osteoporotic therapies. Dosage is two consecutive subcutaneous injections (105 mg each) for a total dose of 210 mg once monthly. It should not be used in patients who have had a myocardial infarction or stroke in the past yr.
- Teriparatide is a recombinant human parathyroid hormone used for postmenopausal women with osteoporosis who are at high risk for fracture, especially vertebral fractures. It is also used in men with primary or hypogonadal osteoporosis who are at high risk of fracture. It is administered by injection 20 mcg daily, subcutaneously into the thigh or abdominal wall. Use for more than 2 yr is not recommended. It stimulates bone formation and reduces the risk of fracture but may increase the risk of stroke in older women with osteoporosis. Common side effects include headaches, myalgia, hypercalcemia, and hypercalciuria. Trials involving abaloparatide, a selective activator of the parathyroid hormone type 1 receptor have also shown reduced risk

[1]Bauer DC: Calcium supplements and fracture prevention, *N Engl J Med* 369:1537-1543, 2013.

of new vertebral and nonvertebral fractures in postmenopausal women with osteoporosis.

- Estrogen prescription drugs or raloxifene (selective estrogen receptor modulator [SERM]) should not be prescribed as first line to treat women with osteoporosis. Raloxifene can reduce the risk of vertebral fractures, but not nonvertebral fractures. It's useful in women at high risk for invasive breast cancer.
- Romosuzab is an anabolic sclerostin inhibitor that stimulates bone formation and decreases bone resorption. It may be useful in women at very high risk of fracture.

CHRONIC Rx

- Lifelong attention to behavior modification issues (nutrition, physical activity, fracture prevention strategies) and compliance with pharmacologic intervention. Recommendations include weight-bearing and muscle-strengthening exercises, smoking cessation, reduced alcohol intake, and adoption of fall prevention strategies.
- There is little evidence to guide physicians about long-term bisphosphonate therapy. The decision to continue drug therapy beyond 5 yr should reflect reassessment of risk and benefit. The risk of atypical fracture of the femur increases after 5 yr of bisphosphonate use. It is reasonable to consider a drug holiday in postmenopausal women who are not at high fracture risk after 3 yr (IV) to 5 yr (oral) of bisphosphonate therapy. Continued treatment may be advisable in those at highest risk.
- Continuing need to eliminate high-risk factors when possible and to optimally manage secondary causes of osteoporosis.

DISPOSITION

Goals for diagnosis and treatment include identification of women at risk; initiation of preventive measures for all women lifelong; institution of treatment modalities that will result in a decrease in fracture risk; and reduction of morbidity, mortality, and unnecessary institutionalization, thereby improving quality of independent life and productivity. Table 5 summarizes the effect of major treatment options on the risk of vertebral, nonvertebral, and hip fractures.

TABLE 5 Effect of Major Treatment Options on the Risk of Vertebral, Nonvertebral, and Hip Fractures

	Vertebral Fractures	Nonvertebral Fractures	Hip Fractures
Alendronate	A	A	A
Etidronate	A	ND	ND
Risedronate	A	A	A
Raloxifene	A	ND	ND
Strontium ranelate	A	A	(A)
Teriparatide	A	A	ND
Denosumab	A	A	A
Zoledronate*	A	A	A
Ibandronate*	A	(A)	ND
Calcium and vitamin D*	ND	A	A

A indicates evidence from randomized, controlled trials and/or meta-analysis; *(A)* reflects that a beneficial effect on fracture risk was found only in post hoc subgroup analysis; *ND* indicates that fracture reduction has not been demonstrated.
*Not included in current National Institute for Health and Clinical Excellence (NICE) guidance.
From Fillit HM: *Brocklehurst's textbook of geriatric medicine and gerontology,* ed 8, Philadelphia, 2017, Elsevier.

REFERRAL

- To reproductive endocrinologist, medical endocrinologist, gynecologist, or rheumatologist if unfamiliar with diagnosis and management of osteoporosis
- If multidisciplinary management is required, to other specialties depending on presence of acute fracture and/or secondary associated disorders

PEARLS & CONSIDERATIONS

COMMENTS

- Osteonecrosis of the jaw is a known complication of high-dose IV bisphosphonate therapy for cancer; however, there is considerable debate on whether low-dose bisphosphonates used for osteoporosis also cause this disorder. Evidence for this is inconclusive.
- Long-term use (>10 yr) of bisphosphonates has been reported to increase risk of atypical subtrochanteric or femoral shaft fractures in several uncontrolled case series. Prodromal symptoms of thigh pain, lack of trauma, and specific radiologic characteristics (cortical thickening) have been reported. The evidence remains inconclusive. Patients can be reassured that short or intermediate use of bisphosphonates does not increase the risk of atypical femoral fractures. Current strategies should include considering a 12-mo interruption in therapy after 5 yr in patients who are clinically stable and considering teriparatide treatment in individuals who experience an atypical fracture while receiving bisphosphonate therapy.
- Increased risk of esophageal cancer and atrial fibrillation have been reported as possible adverse effects of bisphosphonate therapy.

SUGGESTED READINGS

Available at ExpertConsult.com

RELATED CONTENT

Osteoporosis (Patient Information)
Medication-Related Osteonecrosis of the Jaw (Related Key Topic)
Vertebral Compression Fractures (Related Key Topic)

AUTHORS: **Sydney Ford, MD, MPH,** and **Rachel Wright Heinle, MD, FACOG**

BASIC INFORMATION

DEFINITION

Otitis externa refers to a variety of conditions causing inflammation and/or infection of the external auditory canal (and/or auricle and tympanic membrane). There are six subgroups of otitis externa:

1. Acute localized otitis externa (furunculosis)
2. Acute diffuse bacterial otitis externa (i.e., "swimmer ear")
3. Chronic otitis externa
4. Eczematous otitis externa
5. Fungal otitis externa (otomycosis)
6. Invasive or necrotizing (malignant) otitis lexterna

SYNONYMS

See "Definition."

ICD-10CM CODES

H60.90	Unspecified otitis externa, unspecified ear
H60.2	Malignant otitis externa
H60.3	Other infective otitis externa
H60.5	Acute otitis externa, non-infective
H60.8	Other otitis externa

EPIDEMIOLOGY & DEMOGRAPHICS

INCIDENCE (IN U.S.):

- Among the most common disorders
- An estimated 10% of people develop external otitis during their lifetime
- Affects 3% to 10% of patients seeking otologic care

PREVALENCE (IN U.S.):

- Diffuse otitis externa is most often seen in swimmers and in hot, humid climates, conditions that lead to water retention in the ear canal. In the U.S., 44% of AOE-related healthcare visits occur June to August.
- Necrotizing otitis externa is more common in elderly, diabetics, and immunocompromised patients.

PREDOMINANT SEX: None

PREDOMINANT AGE:

- Occurs at all ages, however incidence is highest during childhood and decreases with age
- Necrotizing otitis externa: Typically occurs in elderly: Mean age >65 yr

PHYSICAL FINDINGS & CLINICAL PRESENTATION

The two most common symptoms are otalgia, ranging from pruritus to severe pain exacerbated by motion (e.g., chewing), and otorrhea. Patients may also experience aural fullness and hearing loss as a result of swelling with occlusion of the canal. More intense symptoms may occur with bacterial otitis externa, with or without fever, and lymphadenopathy (anterior to tragus). Findings unique to specific forms of the infection include:

- Acute localized otitis externa (furunculosis):
  1. Occurs from infected hair follicles, usually in the outer third of the ear canal, forming pustules and furuncles
  2. Furuncles are superficial and pointing or deep and diffuse
- Impetigo:
  1. In contrast to furunculosis, this is a superficial spreading infection of the ear canal that may also involve the concha and the auricle
  2. Begins as a small blister that ruptures, releasing straw-colored fluid that dries as a golden crust
- Erysipelas:
  1. Caused by group A streptococcus (*Streptococcus pyogenes*, GAS)
  2. May involve the concha and canal
  3. May involve the dermis and deeper tissues
  4. Area of cellulitis, often with severe pain
  5. Fever, chills, malaise
  6. Regional adenopathy
- Eczematous or seborrheic otitis externa:
  1. Stems from a variety of dermatologic problems that can involve the external auditory canal
  2. Severe itching, erythema, scaling, crusting (Fig.E1), and fissuring possible
- Acute diffuse otitis externa (swimmer ear):
  1. Begins with itching and a feeling of pressure and fullness in the ear that becomes increasingly tender and painful
  2. Mild erythema and edema of the external auditory canal, which may cause narrowing and occlusion of the canal (Fig.E2), leading to hearing loss
  3. Minimal serous secretions, which may become profuse and purulent
  4. Tympanic membrane may appear dull and infected
  5. Usually absence of systemic symptoms such as fever, chills
- Otomycosis:
  1. Chronic superficial infection of the ear canal and tympanic membrane
  2. In primary fungal infection, major symptom is intense itching
  3. In secondary infection (fungal infection superimposed on bacterial infection), major symptom is pain
  4. Fungal growth of variety of colors
- Chronic otitis externa:
  1. Dry and atrophic canal
  2. Typically lack of cerumen
  3. Itching, often severe, and mild discomfort rather than pain
  4. Occasionally mucopurulent discharge
  5. With time, thickening of the walls of the canal, causing narrowing of the lumen
- Necrotizing otitis externa (also known as malignant otitis externa). Typically seen in older patients with diabetes or in patients who are immunocompromised
  1. Redness, swelling, and tenderness of the ear canal
  2. Classic finding of granulation tissue on the floor of the canal and the bone–cartilage junction
  3. Small ulceration of necrotic soft tissue at bone–cartilage junction
  4. Most common symptoms: Pain (often severe) and otorrhea
  5. Lessening of purulent drainage as infection advances
  6. As the infection advances, osteomyelitis of the base of the skull and temporomandibular joint osteomyelitis can develop
  7. Facial nerve palsy often the first and only cranial nerve defect
  8. Possible involvement of other cranial nerves

ETIOLOGY

- Box 1 summarizes common pathogens in otitis externa
- Acute localized otitis externa: *Staphylococcus aureus*
- Impetigo:
  1. *S. aureus* including MRSA
  2. *Streptococcus pyogenes* (GAS)
- Erysipelas: GAS
- Eczematous otitis externa:
  1. Seborrheic dermatitis
  2. Atopic dermatitis
  3. Psoriasis
  4. Neurodermatitis
  5. Lupus erythematosus
- Acute diffuse otitis externa:
  1. Swimming
  2. Hot, humid climates
  3. Tightly fitting hearing aids
  4. Use of ear plugs
  5. *Pseudomonas aeruginosa*
  6. *S. aureus* including MRSA
- Otomycosis:
  1. Prolonged use of topical antibiotics and steroid preparations
  2. Uncontrolled diabetes mellitus can contribute to risk
  3. *Aspergillus* (80% to 90%)
  4. *Candida*
- Chronic otitis externa: Persistent low-grade infection and inflammation
- Necrotizing otitis externa (NOE):
  1. Complication of persistent otitis externa

BOX 1 Common Pathogens in Otitis Externa

Gram-negative Organisms
Pseudomonas aeruginosa
Pseudomonas spp. Nov. "otitidis"
Proteus mirabilis
Serratia marcescens

Gram-positive Organisms
Staphylococcus aureus
Staphylococcus epidermidis
Corynebacterium auris
Enterococcus faecalis

Fungi and Yeasts
Aspergillus fumigatus
Candida albicans
Candida parapsilosis

From Cherry JD et al: *Feigin and Cherry's pediatric infectious diseases*, ed 8, Philadelphia, 2019, Elsevier.

2. Extends through Santorini fissures, small apertures at the bone-cartilage junction of the canal, into the mastoid and along the base of the skull
3. *P. aeruginosa*

Dx DIAGNOSIS

DIFFERENTIAL DIAGNOSIS

- Acute otitis media
- Bullous myringitis
- Mastoiditis
- Foreign bodies
- Neoplasms
- Contact dermatitis
- Eczema
- Ramsey-Hunt syndrome
- Seborrhea
- Otomycosis
- Referred pain
- Table 1 describes the differential diagnosis of painful external ear and auditory canal disorders.

WORKUP

Thorough history and physical examination

LABORATORY TESTS

- Cultures from the canal are usually not necessary unless the condition does not respond to treatment.
- Leukocyte count normal or mildly elevated.
- Erythrocyte sedimentation rate is often quite elevated in malignant otitis externa.

IMAGING STUDIES

- CT scan is the best technique for defining bone involvement and extent of disease in malignant otitis externa.
- MRI is slightly more sensitive in evaluation of soft tissue changes and intracranial extension of infection.
- Gallium scans are more specific than bone scans in diagnosing NOE.
- Follow-up scans are helpful in determining efficacy of treatment. NOTE: Expert opinion supports history and physical examination as the best means of diagnosis. Persistent pain that is constant and severe should raise the question of NOE (particularly in the elderly, diabetics, and immunocompromised patients).

Rx TREATMENT

NONPHARMACOLOGIC THERAPY

- Cleansing and debridement of the ear canal with cotton swabs and hydrogen peroxide or other antiseptic solution allows a more thorough examination of the ear.
- If the canal lumen is edematous and too narrow to allow adequate cleansing, a cotton wick or gauze strip inserted into the canal serves as a conduit for topical medications to be drawn into the canal. Usually remove wick after 2 days.
- Local heat is useful in treating deep furunculosis.
- Incision and drainage is indicated in treatment of superficial pointing furunculosis.

TABLE 1 Differential Diagnosis of Painful External Ear and Auditory Canal Disorders

Disorder	Clinical Features
Acute otitis externa	Diffuse redness, swelling, and pain of the canal with greenish to whitish exudate; often very tender pinna
Malignant otitis externa	Rapidly progressive, severe swelling and redness of pinna, which may be laterally displaced
Dermatitis	
Eczema	History of atopy, presence of lesions elsewhere; lesions are scaly, red, pruritic, and weeping
Contact	History of cosmetic use or irritant exposure; lesions are scaly, red, pruritic, and weeping
Seborrhea	Scaly, red, papular dermatitis; scalp may have thick, yellow scales
Psoriasis	History or presence of psoriasis elsewhere; erythematous papules that coalesce into thick, white plaques
Cellulitis	Diffuse redness, tenderness, and swelling of the pinna
Furuncles	Red, tender papules in areas with hair follicles (distal third of the ear canal)
Infected periauricular cyst	Discrete, palpable lesions; history of previous swelling at same site; cellulitis may develop, obscuring cystic structure
Insect bites	History of exposure; lesions are red, tender papules
Herpes zoster	Painful, vesicular lesions in the ear canal and tympanic membrane in the distribution of cranial nerves V and VII
Perichondritis	Inflammation of the cartilage, usually secondary to cellulitis
Tumors	Palpable mass, destruction of surrounding structures
Foreign body	Foreign body may cause secondary trauma to the ear canal or become a nidus for an infection of the ear canal
Trauma	Bruising and swelling of external ear; there may be signs of basilar skull fracture (cerebrospinal fluid otorrhea, hemotympanum)

From Kliegman RM et al (eds): *Nelson pediatric symptom-based diagnosis,* Philadelphia, 2018, Elsevier, Table 4.1, p. 62, in Kliegman RM: *Nelson textbook of pediatrics,* ed 21, Philadelphia, 2020, Elsevier.

ACUTE GENERAL Rx

Topical medications:

- An acidifying agent such as 2% acetic acid (Vosol) inhibits growth of bacteria and fungi.
- Topical antibiotics (in the form of otic or ophthalmic solutions) or antifungals, often in combination with an acidifying agent and a steroid preparation. Direct application of topical agents to the infected site is a key element in the treatment of external otitis regardless of severity. Proper installation of eardrops entails tilting the head toward the opposite shoulder, pulling the superior aspect of the auricle upward, and filling the ear canal with drops. In young children, the earlobe should be pulled downward to fill the canal.
- The ideal antibiotic regimen should have coverage against the most common pathogens, *S. aureus* and *P. aeruginosa.*
- Side effect profile can also influence choice of treatment. Ototoxicity is the most important concern with aminoglycoside drugs, including neomycin, tobramycin, and gentamicin. Aminoglycosides are a significant potential source for iatrogenic hearing loss and balance dysfunction, particularly in the presence of tympanic membrane perforation. Allergic contact dermatitis is commonly associated with neomycin when used for prolonged courses. Topical fluoroquinolones can cause local irritation.
- The following are some of the available preparations:
  1. Neomycin otic solutions and suspensions:
     a. With polymyxin-B-hydrocortisone (Cortisporin)
     b. With hydrocortisone-thonzonium (Coly-Mycin S)
  2. Polymyxin-B-hydrocortisone (Otobiotic)
  3. Quinolone otic solutions:
     a. Ofloxacin 0.3% solution (Floxin Otic)
     b. Ciprofloxacin 0.3% with hydrocortisone (Cipro HC)
  4. Quinolone ophthalmic solutions:
     a. Ofloxacin 0.3% (Ocuflox)
     b. Ciprofloxacin 0.3% (Ciloxan)
  5. Aminoglycoside ophthalmic solutions:
     a. Gentamicin sulfate 0.3% (Garamycin)
     b. Tobramycin sulfate 0.3% (Tobrex)
     c. Tobramycin 0.3% and dexamethasone 0.1% (TobraDex)
  6. Chloramphenicol 0.5% otic solution or 0.25% ophthalmic solution (Chloromycetin)
  7. Gentian violet (methylrosaniline chloride 1%, 2%)
  8. Antifungals:
     a. Amphotericin B 3% (Fungizone lotion)
     b. Clotrimazole 1% solution (Lotrimin)
     c. Tolnaftate 1% (Tinactin)
- Topical preparations should be applied qid (bid for quinolones, antifungals), generally for 3 days after cessation of symptoms (average 10-14 days total).

Systemic antibiotics:

- Reserved for when the infection has spread beyond the ear canal.

- Treatment usually for 10 days with ciprofloxacin 750 mg q12h or ofloxacin 400 mg q12h, or with antistaphylococcal agent (e.g., dicloxacillin or cephalexin 500 mg q6h). Use Bactrim or clindamycin when MRSA suspected or cultured at one DS twice a day instead of cephalexin or dicloxacillin. For malignant otitis externa (due to *Pseudomonas aeruginosa* in >90% of cases), effective agents are meropenem 1 g IV q8h or ciprofloxacin 400 mg IV q12h or 750 mg PO q12h or cefepime 2 g q12h.

Treatment for NOE:
- Requires prolonged therapy up to 3 mo; whether to use oral parenteral therapy is based on clinical judgment.
- Oral quinolones, ciprofloxacin 750 mg q12h or ofloxacin 400 mg q12h may be appropriate initial therapy or used to shorten the course of IV therapy.
- Intravenous antipseudomonals with or without aminoglycosides are also appropriate.
- Local debridement.

Pain control:
- May require NSAIDs or opioids
- Topical corticosteroids to reduce swelling and inflammation

CHRONIC Rx

- Patients prone to recurrent infections should try to identify and avoid precipitants to infection.
- Swimmers should try tight-fitting ear plugs or tight-fitting bathing caps and remove all excess water from the ears after swimming.
- Treat underlying systemic diseases and dermatologic conditions that predispose to infection.
- Hearing aids should be removed nightly and regularly cleaned.

DISPOSITION

Inadequate treatment of otitis externa may lead to NOE and mastoiditis.

REFERRAL

To an otolaryngologist:
- NOE
- Treatment failure
- Severe pain

PEARLS & CONSIDERATIONS

Otitis externa varies in severity from a mild irritation of the external acoustic canal (swimmer ear) that resolves spontaneously by simply removing the offending agent (stay out of freshwater or wear ear plugs when swimming) to a life-threatening infection with the risk of intracranial extension, gram-negative bacterial meningitis, and severe neurologic impairment with multiple cranial neuropathy. Do not miss severe malignant otitis externa in patients who are diabetic or immunocompromised.

SUGGESTED READINGS

Available at ExpertConsult.com

RELATED CONTENT

Otitis Externa (Patient Information)

AUTHOR: **Russell J. McCulloh, MD**

BASIC INFORMATION

DEFINITION

Acute otitis media (AOM) is defined by infected middle ear fluid resulting in moderate to severe bulging of the tympanic membrane (TM) or new onset of otorrhea not due to acute otitis externa. Care should be taken to differentiate AOM from serous otitis media, which involves noninfected middle ear fluid that does not result in bulging of the TM. Serous otitis media does not require antibiotic treatment.

SYNONYMS

Acute suppurative otitis media
Purulent otitis media
Acute otitis media
AOM

ICD-10CM CODES

H65.3	Chronic mucoid otitis media
H66.0	Acute suppurative otitis media
H66.4	Suppurative otitis media, unspecified
H66.9	Otitis media, unspecified
H66.1	Chronic tubotympanic suppurative otitis media
H66.2	Chronic atticoantral suppurative otitis media

EPIDEMIOLOGY & DEMOGRAPHICS

INCIDENCE (IN U.S.):

- Affects patients of all ages but is largely a disease of infants and young children
- Affects approximately 80% of all children by age 5 yr
- Occurs three or more times in one third of all children by age 3 yr
- Costs associated with otitis media exceed $5 billion, with 40% of the costs occurring from patients ages 1 to 3
- One of the most common indications for antibiotic prescription among children

PEAK INCIDENCE:

- AOM occurs at all ages but is most prevalent between 6 and 24 mo of age.
- A second peak in incidence occurs between 4 and 6 yr of age.
- AOM is most frequent in the fall, winter, and early spring (coincident with peak respiratory virus prevalence in the community).
- Incidence of infection declines with age; AOM is seen infrequently in adults.

RISK FACTORS:

- Daycare attendance
- Limited or no breastfeeding
- Tobacco smoke exposure
- Pacifier use
- Craniofacial anomalies
- Immune globulin G (IgG) or subclass deficiencies

PHYSICAL FINDINGS & CLINICAL PRESENTATION

- Moderate to severe bulging of the TM.
- Fluid in the middle ear along with signs and symptoms of local inflammation.
  1. Erythema with diminished light reflex (Fig. E1)
- As infection progresses, middle ear exudation occurs (exudative phase); the exudate rapidly changes from serous to purulent (suppurative phase).
- Retraction and poor mobility of the TM ensues, and the TM begins to bulge.
- At any time during the suppurative phase, the TM may rupture, releasing the middle ear contents (otorrhea).
- Erythema of the TM without other abnormalities is not a diagnostic criterion for acute otitis media (AOM) because it may occur with any inflammation of the upper respiratory tract, crying, or nose blowing.
- Symptoms:
  1. Rapid- or recent-onset otalgia, ranging from slight discomfort to severe, is the most common presenting symptom.
  2. Hearing loss while middle ear fluid is present.
  3. Otorrhea (if TM has ruptured).
  4. Systemic symptoms such as fever, listlessness, irritability, decreased appetite, vomiting, and diarrhea are common. Although vertigo, facial swelling, nystagmus, tinnitus, lethargy, and facial nerve palsies can occur as rare complications of AOM; these symptoms should prompt consideration of an alternate diagnosis.
  5. Table 1 summarizes symptom scoring systems designed to aid in diagnosis.
- After an episode of AOM:
  1. Persistence of effusion for weeks or months (called secretory, serous, or nonsuppurative otitis media)
  2. Fever and otalgia usually absent
  3. Hearing loss possible (10 to 50 dB, with predominant involvement of the low frequencies)
  4. Manifestations of the sequelae and complications of otitis media are summarized in Table E2

ETIOLOGY

- Most common etiology is a viral upper respiratory tract infection, which causes inflammation and dysfunction of the eustachian tube and transient aspiration of nasopharyngeal secretions into the middle ear (Fig. 2). Bacterial colonization from the nasopharynx in conjunction with eustachian tube dysfunction leads to infection.
- May occasionally develop as a result of hematogenous spread or by direct invasion from the nasopharynx.
- Conjugated pneumococcal vaccination of children has resulted in decreases in *Streptococcus pneumoniae* causing AOM.
- Most common bacterial pathogens:
  1. *S. pneumoniae* causes up to half of cases and is the least likely of the major pathogens to resolve without treatment.
  2. *Haemophilus influenzae.*
  3. *Moraxella catarrhalis.*
  4. Of increasing importance, infection caused by penicillin-nonsusceptible *S. pneumoniae* (MIC >0.1 mg/ml), ranging from 8% to 34%. About 50% of PNSSP isolates are penicillin-intermediate (MIC 0.1 to 2.0 mg/ml).
  5. Group A streptococci is associated with higher rates of TM perforation than AOM caused by other pathogens.
- Viral pathogens:
  1. Respiratory syncytial virus (RSV)
  2. Rhinovirus
  3. Adenovirus
  4. Influenza
- Others:
  1. *Mycoplasma pneumoniae*
  2. *Chlamydia trachomatis*
  3. *Streptococcus pyogenes* (Latin America)

Dx DIAGNOSIS

DIFFERENTIAL DIAGNOSIS

- Otitis externa
- Otitis media with effusion (OME): An algorithm for distinguishing between acute otitis media and otitis media with effusion is illustrated in Fig. 3
- Referred pain from mouth, nasopharynx, or throat
- Section II describes the differential diagnosis of earache

WORKUP

Thorough otoscopic examination. AOM is a visual diagnosis based on viewing the tympanic membrane. Adequate visualization of the tympanic membrane may require removal of cerumen and debris.

- Tympanometry
  1. Measures compliance of the tympanic membrane and middle ear pressure
  2. Detects the presence of fluid, but cannot determine whether the fluid is infected
- Acoustic reflectometry
  1. Measures sound waves reflected from the middle ear
  2. Is useful in infants >3 mo
  3. Increased reflected sound correlated with the presence of effusion, but cannot determine whether the fluid is infected

LABORATORY TESTS

- Tympanocentesis.
  1. Not necessary in most cases because the microbiology of middle ear effusions has been shown to be extremely consistent
  2. May be indicated in:
     a. Patients who do not respond to treatment in 72 hr or those who experience multiple treatment failures
     b. Immunocompromised patients
- Cultures of the nasopharynx are not helpful.
- Blood counts (generally unnecessary) usually reveal leukocytosis with polymorphonuclear elevation.
- Plain mastoid radiographs (generally unnecessary) reveal haziness in the periantral cells that may extend to entire mastoid.
- CT or MRI may be indicated if serious complications are suspected (meningitis, brain abscess, severe mastoiditis).

Rx TREATMENT

ACUTE GENERAL Rx

Hydration, avoidance of irritants (e.g., tobacco smoke), nasal decongestants, cool mist

TABLE 1 Acute Otitis Media Symptom Scoring Systems Designed to Aid in Diagnosis

3-Item Otitis Media Score (OM-3)	Ear Treatment Group Symptom Questionnaire (ETG-5)	Acute Otitis Media Faces Scale (AOM-FS)	Otoscopic Severity Scale (OS-8)	Acute Otitis Media Severity of Symptom Scale (AOM-SOS)	Otitis Media Clinical Severity Index (OM-CSI) 30-Point Scale[a]	Otitis Media Clinical Severity Index (OM-CSI) 10-Point Scale[a]
Physical suffering	Ear pain	Seven facial expressions ranging from no problem to extreme problem	Eight categories of TM inflammation[b]	Ear pain	Ear pain	Ear pain
Emotional distress	Fever			Ear tugging	Fever	Fever
Limitation of activities	Irritability			Irritability	Irritability	Irritability
	Appetite			Decreased play	Fever at examination	Fever at examination
	Sleep quality			Decreased appetite	TM erythema	TM erythema
				Difficulty sleeping	TM mobility	TM mobility
				Fever	TM position	TM position
					Effusion color	Effusion color
					Otorrhea	Otorrhea

TM, Tympanic membrane.
[a]The 30-point scale used a 2- to 5-point Likert scale and the 10-point scale used a 2- to 3-point Likert scale.
[b]0 = normal; 1 = erythema only; 2 = erythema, air-fluid level, clear fluid; 3 = erythema, complete effusion, no opacification; 4 = erythema, opacification with air-fluid level or air bubbles, no bulging; 5 = erythema, complete effusion, opacification, no bulging; 6 = erythema, bulging rounded doughnut appearance of the tympanic membrane; 7 = erythema, bulging, complete effusion and opacification with bulla formation.
From Cherry JD et al: *Feigin and Cherry's pediatric infectious diseases,* ed 8, Philadelphia, 2019, Elsevier.

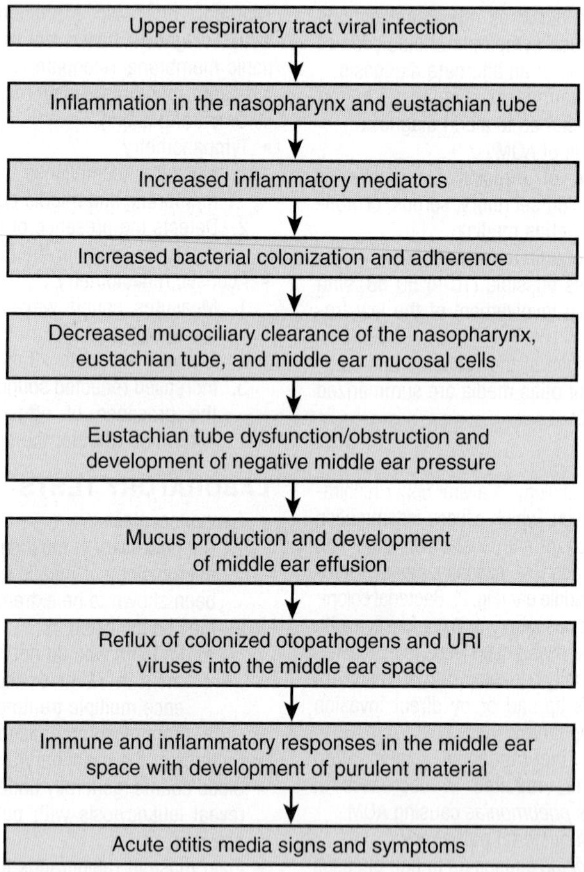

FIG. 2 Pathogenesis of virus-induced acute otitis media. *URI,* Upper respiratory infection. (From Cherry JD et al: *Feigin and Cherry's pediatric infectious diseases*, ed 8, Philadelphia, 2019, Elsevier.)

humidifier, and oral ibuprofen or acetaminophen. Topical procaine or lidocaine preparations (if available) are an alternative to oral analgesics for children ≥2 yr but should not be used in children with tympanic membrane perforation.

Antimicrobials:

NOTE: Most uncomplicated cases of AOM resolve spontaneously, without complications. Studies have demonstrated limited therapeutic benefit from antibiotic therapy. Watchful waiting is appropriate for children who look well, can be comforted with supportive care, and are old enough to easily evaluate. Children <24 mo with bilateral AOM should receive antibiotic therapy. Children with severe signs or symptoms (moderate or severe otalgia or otalgia for ≥48 hr or temperature ≥39° C) should also receive antibiotic therapy. Fig. E4 illustrates an algorithm for management of acute otitis media in pediatric populations.

When opting to use antibiotic therapy:

- Amoxicillin remains the drug of choice for first-line treatment of uncomplicated AOM despite the increasing prevalence of drug-resistant *S. pneumoniae.*
- Treatment failure is defined by lack of clinical improvement of signs or symptoms after 3 days of therapy.
- With treatment failure, in the absence of an identified etiologic pathogen, therapy should be redirected to cover:
  1. Drug-resistant *S. pneumoniae*
  2. β-lactamase–producing strains of *H. influenzae* and *M. catarrhalis*
- Agents fulfilling these criteria include amoxicillin/clavulanate, second-generation (e.g., cefuroxime axetil, cefaclor) or third-generation (e.g., oral cefdinir or cefpodoxime or IM ceftriaxone) cephalosporins. Cefaclor, cefixime, loracarbef, and ceftibuten should be avoided given their limited activity against pneumococci.
- Cross-resistance between TMP/SX and macrolides and the β-lactams exists; therefore patients who do not respond to amoxicillin are more likely to have infections resistant to TMP/SMX and macrolides.
- Fluoroquinolones are not indicated as first- or second-line therapy for AOM and should be avoided in young children due to risks of musculoskeletal effects and limited dosing guidance.
- Treatment should be modified according to cultures and sensitivities when available.
- Treatment course is 10 days for children <2 yr and those with severe symptoms, 7 days for children age 2 to 5 yr, and 5 to 7 days for children ≥6 yr.
- Follow-up should be tailored to clinical improvement and concern for neurocognitive developmental delays in at-risk children.

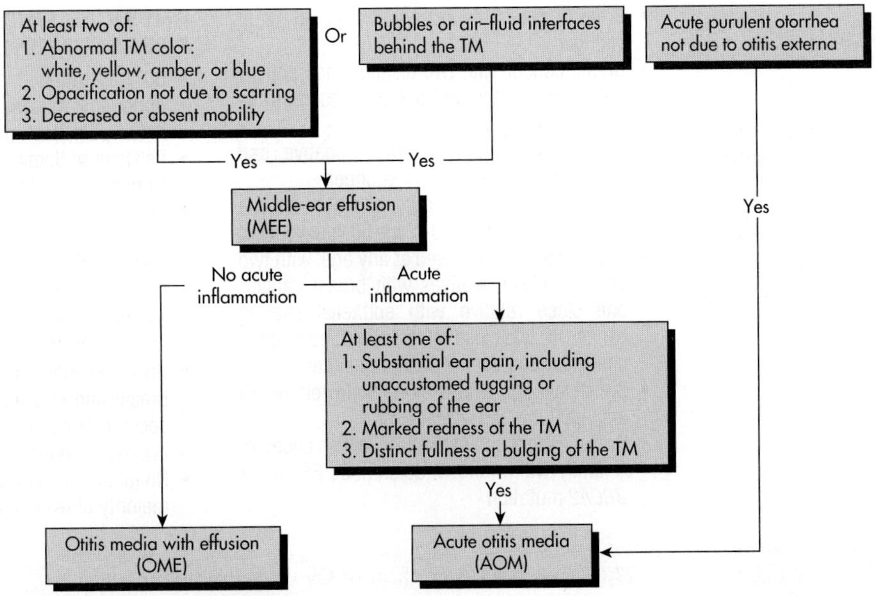

FIG. 3 Algorithm for distinguishing between acute otitis media and otitis media with effusion. *TM,* tympanic membrane. (From Kliegman RM: *Nelson textbook of pediatrics*, ed 21, Philadelphia, 2020, Elsevier.)

Standard follow-up of all cases is no longer recommended.

- Antibiotic prophylaxis to reduce the frequency of AOM episodes in children with recurrent AOM is not recommended.
- Table E3 summarizes suggested antibiotics for treatment of otitis media and for patients who have failed first-line antibiotic treatment.

NOTE: Effusions may persist for 8 wk or longer in many cases of adequately treated otitis media.

SURGICAL Rx

- There is no evidence to support the routine use of myringotomy, but in severe cases it provides prompt pain relief and accelerates resolution of infection.
- Purulent secretions retained in the middle ear can lead to increased pressure that may lead to spread of infection to contiguous areas. Myringotomy to decompress the middle ear is sometimes necessary to avoid complications such as mastoiditis, facial nerve paralysis, labyrinthitis, meningitis, and brain abscess.

CHRONIC Rx

- Myringotomy and tympanostomy tube placement for persistent or recurrent middle ear effusion unresponsive to medical therapy can be considered if fluid has persisted for ≥3 mo if bilateral or ≥6 mo if unilateral.
- Adenoidectomy, with or without tonsillectomy, often is advocated for treatment of recurrent otitis media, although evidence for this procedure is controversial.
- Long-term complications include tympanic membrane perforations, cholesteatoma, tympanosclerosis, ossicular necrosis, toxic or suppurative labyrinthitis, hearing loss, and intracranial suppuration.

DISPOSITION

Patients can be treated at home as outpatients with the rare exception of patients with evidence of local suppurative complications (e.g., meningitis, acute mastoiditis, brain abscess, cavernous sinus, or lateral sinus thrombosis).

REFERRAL

- To otorhinolaryngologist in cases of:
  1. Medical treatment failure
  2. An uncertain diagnosis; adults with one or more episodes of AOM should be referred for evaluation to rule out an underlying process (e.g., malignancy)
  3. Any of the above-mentioned acute and chronic complications

PEARLS & CONSIDERATIONS

COMMENTS

- Otoscopic findings are critical for accurate AOM diagnosis.
- AOM microbiology has changed with use of pneumococcal conjugate vaccine (PCV13).
- Antibiotics are modestly more effective than no treatment but cause adverse effects in 4 to 10% of children.
- Most antibiotics have comparable clinical success.

Prevention:

- Vaccinate against common pathogens.
- Breastfeed and bottle-feed infants in an upright position.
- Avoid irritants (e.g., tobacco smoke).

SUGGESTED READINGS

Available at ExpertConsult.com

AUTHOR: **Stephen Dolter, MD**

Ovarian Cancer (PTG) (ALG)

BASIC INFORMATION

DEFINITION

Ovarian cancer is not one disease but a constellation of distinct cancer subtypes classified according to their tissue of origin. About 90% of tumors are epithelial ovarian cancers, 5% are germ cell tumors, and 5% are sex cord-stromal tumors. A classification of ovarian epithelial tumors is summarized in Table 1.

SYNONYMS

Epithelial ovarian cancer
Germ cell tumor
Sex cord stromal tumor
Ovarian tumor of low malignant potential

ICD-10CM CODES

C56.9	Malignant neoplasm of unspecified ovary
C56.1	Malignant neoplasm of right ovary
C56.2	Malignant neoplasm of left ovary

EPIDEMIOLOGY & DEMOGRAPHICS

INCIDENCE: 12.9 to 15.1 cases/100,000 persons; ~25,000 new cases annually. Lifetime risk for developing ovarian cancer is 1.3%. It is the leading cause of gynecologic cancer-related deaths.

PREVALENCE: Median age at time of diagnosis: 63 yr

RISK FACTORS:
- Low parity
- Delayed childbearing
- Smoking
- Polycystic ovary syndrome
- Endometriosis
- High-fat diet
- Lynch II syndrome (nonpolyposis colon cancer, endometrial cancer, breast cancer, and ovarian cancer clusters in first- and second-degree relatives)
- Breast-ovarian familial cancer syndrome
- Site-specific familial ovarian cancer
- The **strongest** risk factors are advancing age and family history of ovarian and breast cancer
- Factors that **decrease** the risk of ovarian cancer include previous pregnancy, oral contraceptive pill use, hysterectomy, tubal ligation, or salpingectomy
- Table 2 summarizes risk and protective factors for ovarian cancer

GENETICS: The greatest risk factors of ovarian cancer are a family history and associated genetic syndromes. More than 90% of inherited ovarian malignancies are associated with *BRCA1* and *BRCA2* mutations. *BRCA* mutations interact with and affect DNA repair proteins. The estimated lifetime risk of ovarian cancer for patients with either of these mutations is 65% to 74%.

Genetic counseling is recommended for certain patients, including those with:
- Epithelial ovarian cancer at any age
- Breast cancer diagnosed at age 45 yr or younger
- Breast cancer with two distinct and sequential primaries, the first one diagnosed at age 50 yr or younger
- Breast cancer that is triple-negative and diagnosed at age 60 yr or younger
- Breast cancer at any age, with at least one close relative diagnosed at age 50 yr or younger
- Breast cancer diagnosed at any age, with two or more close relatives with breast cancer; one close relative with epithelial ovarian cancer; or two close relatives with pancreatic cancer or aggressive prostate cancer
- Breast cancer, with a close male relative at any age who has breast cancer
- Breast cancer and Ashkenazi Jewish ancestry
- A family with a known deleterious *BRCA1* or *BRCA2* mutation

PHYSICAL FINDINGS & CLINICAL PRESENTATION

- 60% present with advanced disease
- Abdominal fullness, early satiety, dyspepsia
- Pelvic pain, back pain, constipation
- Pelvic or abdominal mass
- Lymphadenopathy (inguinal)
- Sister Mary Joseph nodule (umbilical mass)

ETIOLOGY

- Can be inherited as site-specific familial ovarian cancer (two or more first-degree relatives have ovarian cancer)
- Breast-ovarian cancer syndrome (clusters of breast and ovarian cancer among first- and second-degree relatives)
- Lynch syndrome
- No family history and unknown etiology in the majority of ovarian cancer cases

TABLE 1 Classification of Ovarian Epithelial Tumors

Terminology	Notes
Serous Tumors	Most common epithelial tumor group
Adenocarcinoma	More than 85% involve the ovarian surface or adjacent structures Includes low (~10%) and high (~90%) grade carcinomas
Noninvasive low-grade serous carcinoma (LGSC)	Grade 1, synonymous with micropapillary/cribriform borderline
Borderline	Can be intracystic or involve the ovarian surface
Benign	Includes adenofibroma
Mucinous Tumors	Include intestinal (common) and müllerian (less common) types
Adenocarcinoma	Includes borderline tumors with "intraepithelial carcinoma"
Borderline	
Benign	
With mural nodules	
Endometrioid Tumors	
Adenocarcinoma	High-grade carcinomas overlap with high-grade serous carcinomas (HGSCs)
Carcinosarcoma	
Adenosarcoma	
Borderline	Also known as *proliferative cystadenoma/adenofibroma;* including squamous morules
Benign	
Clear Cell Tumors	
Adenocarcinoma	Papillary and adenofibromatous types
Borderline	Occur in adenofibromas
Benign	Very rare
Transitional Cell Tumors	
Malignant	Includes malignant Brenner tumors and the rare transitional cell carcinoma
Borderline	Typically proliferating Brenner tumors
Benign	Usually Brenner tumors
Squamous Cell Tumors	
Malignant	Rare squamous carcinomas with or without a coexisting teratoma
Benign	Epidermoid cysts
Mixed Epithelial Tumors	
Malignant	Commonly a mixture of high-grade serous and endometrioid (high-grade commonly)
Borderline and benign	Overlap with serous and overlap w mucinous tumors, also called "seromucinous borderline tumors"
Benign	
Undifferentiated or Unclassified	

Modified from the World Health Organization in Crum CP et al: *Diagnostic gynecologic and obstetric pathology,* ed 3, Philadelphia, 2018, Elsevier.

Dx DIAGNOSIS

DIFFERENTIAL DIAGNOSIS

- Primary peritoneal cancer mesothelioma
- Benign ovarian tumor
- Functional ovarian cyst
- Endometriosis
- Ovarian torsion
- Pelvic kidney
- Pedunculated uterine fibroid
- Primary cancer from breast, gastrointestinal tract, or other pelvic organ metastasized to the ovary

TABLE 2 Risk and Protective Factors for Ovarian Cancer

Increased Risk	Protective
Lifestyle and diet factors	Lifestyle and diet factors
Aging	Soy intake
Obesity	Flavonoids
Tall stature	High calcium
Animal fat intake	Sun exposure
α-linolenic acid	Long sleep
Dairy foods	Metformin
Lactose product	
Cigarette use	
Diabetes mellitus	
Reproductive factors	Reproductive factors
Menopausal hormone therapy	Oral contraceptive
Menopausal age	Breastfeeding
Infertility	Tubal sterilization
Polycystic ovarian syndrome	Salpingectomy
Endometriosis	Hysterectomy
Pelvic inflammatory disease	Parity
Genetic factors	

From Niederhuber JE: *Abeloff's clinical oncology,* ed 6, Philadelphia, 2020, Elsevier.

WORKUP

- Definitive diagnosis made at laparotomy; epithelial ovarian cancer most common type of ovarian cancer (90% of ovarian cancer)
- Careful physical and history, including family history
- Exclusion of nongynecologic etiologies
- Observation of small cystic masses in premenopausal women for regression for 2 mo
- FIGO classification of ovarian carcinoma is described in Table 3
- Referral to specialists who have extensive training and experience in treating ovarian cancer significantly increases survival after an ovarian cancer diagnosis

LABORATORY TESTS

- Complete blood count.
- Chemistry profile including liver tests and calcium (to evaluate for paraneoplastic syndrome).
- CA-125 or lysophosphatidic acid level. Use of these tests for annual screening is controversial, and most experts warn against universal screening with this marker. Only about 50% of early-stage ovarian cancers will be associated with elevated CA-125. Additionally, false elevations may occur with uterine leiomyoma, endometriosis, pregnancy, and intraabdominal infections. The PLCO cancer screening trial revealed that annual screening based on CA-125 and vaginal ultrasound is ineffective, and diagnostic follow-up of false positives resulted in 15% serious complication rate.
- Consider: Human chorionic gonadotropin, inhibin, alpha-fetoprotein, neuron-specific enolase, and lactate dehydrogenase in patients at risk for germ cell tumors.
- A panel of three serum biomarkers (apolipoprotein A-1 [ApoA-1], transthyretin [TTR], and transferrin [TF]) has been reported useful in distinguishing normal samples from early-stage ovarian cancer with a sensitivity of 84% and normal samples from late-stage ovarian cancer with a sensitivity of 97%.
- *BRCA1/2* testing is recommended for all women with ovarian cancer.

IMAGING STUDIES

- Ultrasound
- Chest x-ray
- CT or MRI of abdomen and pelvis help evaluate extent of disease (Fig. E1)
- Mammogram

Rx TREATMENT

NONPHARMACOLOGIC THERAPY

Virtually all cases of ovarian cancer involve surgical exploration. This includes:

- Abdominal cytology
- Total abdominal hysterectomy and bilateral salpingo-oophorectomy (except in early stages in which fertility preservation is an issue)
- Omentectomy
- Diaphragm sampling
- Selective lymphadenectomy (pelvic and paraaortic nodes)
- Primary cytoreduction with a goal of residual tumor diameter <2 cm
- Bowel surgery, splenectomy if needed to obtain optimal (<2 cm) cytoreduction
- Conventional treatment includes surgical debulking (cytoreduction) followed by chemotherapy. However, patients with low-grade, well-differentiated stage I ovarian cancer do not benefit from adjuvant chemotherapy

ACUTE GENERAL Rx

- Optimal cytoreduction (debulking) is generally followed by chemotherapy (except in some early-stage disease [stage I without high-risk features is treated with surgery alone]).
- Cisplatin-based combination chemotherapy is used for stage II or greater, 6-mo treatment. Compared with IV paclitaxel plus cisplatin, IV paclitaxel plus intraperitoneal cisplatin and paclitaxel improves survival rates in patients with optimally debulked stage III ovarian cancer.
- Chemotherapy regimens continue to change as research continues. Bevacizumab, a humanized antivascular endothelial growth factor monoclonal antibody, has been shown to be effective in improving progression-free survival in women

TABLE 3 International Federation of Gynecology and Obstetrics (FIGO) Classification of Ovarian Carcinomas

Stage I	Growth limited to the ovaries:
	Stage I_A: Growth limited to one ovary, no ascites and no tumor present on the external surface; capsule intact
	Stage I_B: Growth limited to both ovaries, no ascites and no tumor present on the external surface; capsule intact
	Stage I_C: Stage 1_A or 1_B where there is tumor on the surface of either ovary; or with ruptured capsules or with ascites containing malignant cells or positive peritoneal washings. Surgical spillage of a malignant cyst upgrades the patient to I_C, although it is unlikely that this event affects prognosis
Stage II	Growth involving one or both ovaries with pelvic extension:
	Stage II_A: Extension and/or metastases to the uterus and tubes
	Stage II_B: Extension to other pelvic tissues
	Stage II_C: Stage II_A or II_B with tumor on the surface of either ovary or positive peritoneal washings or malignant ascites
Stage III	Growth involving one or both ovaries with peritoneal implants outside the pelvis or positive retroperitoneal or inguinal lymph nodes:
	Stage III_A: Microscopic seeding of abdominal peritoneal surfaces
	Stage III_B: Macroscopic disease outside the pelvis less than 2 cm in diameter
	Stage III_C: Abdominal implants greater than 2 cm and/or positive nodes
Stage IV	Growth involving one or both ovaries with distant metastases including parenchymal (but not superficial) liver metastases and pleural effusions containing malignant cells

From Symonds EM, Symonds IM: *Essential obstetrics and gynaecology,* ed 4, London, 2004, Churchill Livingstone.

with ovarian cancer. Trials using bevacizumab during and up to 10 mo after carboplatin and paclitaxel chemotherapy have shown prolongation of the median progression-free survival by about 4 mo in patients with advanced epithelial ovarian cancer.

- PARP inhibitors are up-and-coming chemotherapeutic agents that have been used for maintenance therapy and have been shown to improve progression-free survival among patients with platinum-sensitive high-grade serous cancers. PARP inhibitors work by pharmacologically inhibiting the enzyme poly (ADP-ribose) polymerase. Three PARP inhibitors are currently FDA approved for different indications. Olaparib, an oral polymerase inhibitor, was approved in 2014 and has shown antitumor activity in patients with high-grade serous ovarian cancer with or without *BRCA1* and *BRCA2* germline mutations. Rucaparib was approved in 2016 to treat high-grade serous cancers with *BRCA1* and *BRCA2* germline or somatic mutations. Lastly, niraparib was approved in 2017 for use in high-grade serous cancers with or without *BRCA1* and *BRCA2* mutations.
- Second-look surgery when chemotherapy is complete generally is no longer recommended because this has not been shown to improve survival.
- In most cases, neoadjuvant (presurgical) chemotherapy has no advantage over postsurgical initiation of chemotherapy. However, some trials have shown that neoadjuvant chemotherapy followed by interval debulking surgery is not inferior to debulking surgery followed by chemotherapy as a treatment option for patients with bulky stage IIIC or IV ovarian carcinoma. Complete resection of all macroscopic disease, whether performed as primary treatment or after neoadjuvant chemotherapy, remains the objective whenever cytoreductive surgery is performed.

CHRONIC Rx

- If CA-125 elevated, may have recurrent disease
- Physical and pelvic examinations every 2 to 4 mo for 2 yr, every 3 to 6 mo during third yr, then annually after 5 yr
- Routine monitoring of CA-125 at every visit does not improve survival and should be reserved for addressing specific clinical concerns
- Yearly Pap smear
- A treatment approach algorithm for recurrent ovarian cancer is illustrated in Fig. 2

DISPOSITION

- Overall 5-yr survival rates remain low because of the preponderance of late-stage disease:
  1. Stage I and II: 80% to 100%
  2. Stage III: 15% to 20%
  3. Stage IV: 5%
- Younger patients (<50 yr) in all stages have a considerably better 5-yr survival than older patients (40% vs. 15%).
- Among women with high-grade serous ovarian cancer, *BRCA2* mutation, but not *BRCA1* deficiency, is associated with improved survival, improved chemotherapy response, and genome instability compared with *BRCA* wild-type.
- Among patients with invasive epithelial ovarian cancer (EOC), having a germline mutation in *BRCA1* or *BRCA2* is associated with improved 5-yr overall survival. *BRCA2* carriers have the best prognosis.

COMMENTS

- The U.S. Preventive Services Task Force has concluded that current evidence does not show any mortality benefit to routine screening for ovarian cancer with transvaginal ultrasonography or single-threshold serum CA-125 testing and that the harms of such screening are at least moderate. This recommendation applies to asymptomatic women who are not known to have a high-risk hereditary cancer syndrome.
- Oral contraceptives reduce the risk of ovarian cancer by 40% to 50%. The greatest risk reduction is present after ≥15 yr of oral contraceptive use.
- Patients at high risk for developing ovarian cancer (*BRCA1/BRCA2* gene mutation, hereditary nonpolyposis colorectal cancer syndrome) should consider prophylactic salpingo-oophorectomy after childbearing is complete. Prophylactic bilateral salpingo-oophorectomy reduces ovarian cancer by 80%. It is recommended by age 35 to 40 yr for *BRCA1* carriers and by age 45 for *BRCA2* carriers. If surgery is declined, the National Comprehensive Cancer Network guidelines recommend intensive surveillance with pelvic and abdominal sonogram and serum CA-125 every 6 mo starting at age 35 or 10 yr earlier than cancer diagnosis in family member.

SUGGESTED READINGS

Available at ExpertConsult.com

RELATED CONTENT

Ovarian Cancer (Patient Information)
Ovarian Neoplasm, Benign (Related Key Topic)

AUTHORS: **Helen Toma, MD, MSPH,** and **Anthony Sciscione, DO**

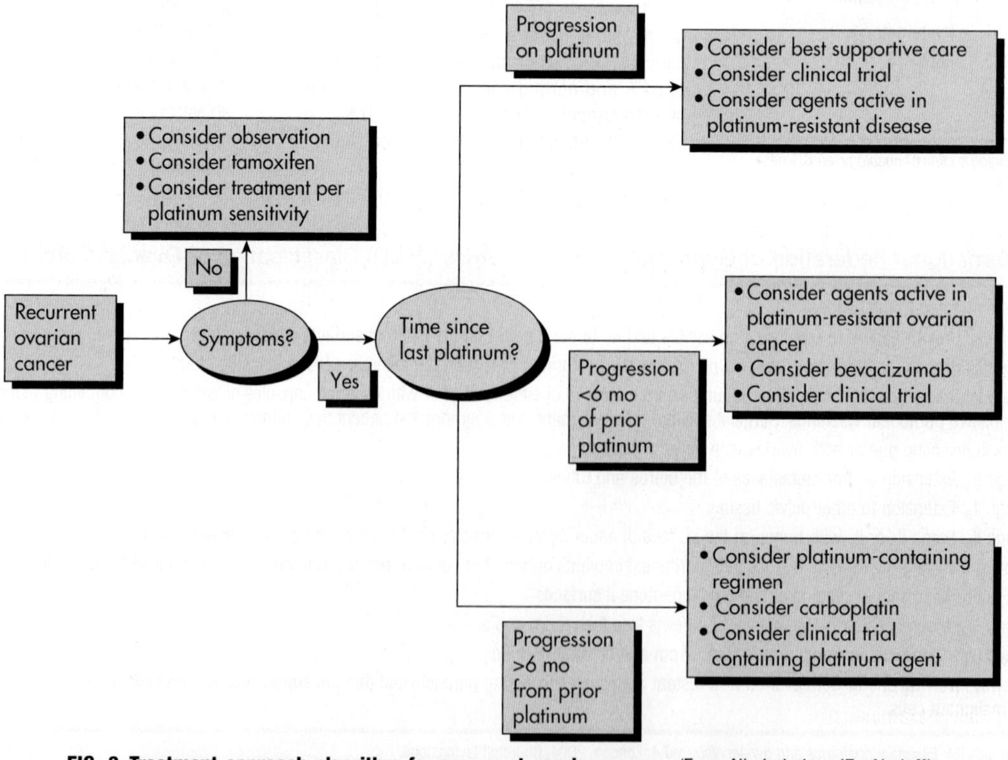

FIG. 2 Treatment approach algorithm for recurrent ovarian cancer. (From Niederhuber JE: *Abeloff's clinical oncology,* ed 6, Philadelphia, 2020, Elsevier.)

BASIC INFORMATION

DEFINITION

Benign ovarian neoplasms are often clinically indistinguishable from their malignant counterparts. Therefore, all persistent adnexal masses must be considered malignant until proven otherwise. Nonneoplastic tumors include:

- Germinal inclusion cyst
- Follicle cyst
- Corpus luteum cyst
- Pregnancy luteoma
- Theca lutein cysts
- Sclerocystic ovaries
- Endometrioma

Neoplastic tumors derived from coelomic epithelium include:

- Cystic tumors: Serous cystadenoma, mucinous cystadenoma, mixed forms
- Tumors with stromal overgrowth: Fibroma, adenofibroma, Brenner tumor

Tumors derived from germ cells are dermoids (benign cystic teratomas)

ICD-10CM CODES	
D27.0	Benign neoplasm of right ovary
D27.1	Benign neoplasm of left ovary
D27.9	Benign neoplasm of unspecified ovary

EPIDEMIOLOGY & DEMOGRAPHICS

REPRODUCTIVE YEARS:

- Most common benign ovarian neoplasms: Serous cystadenoma and benign cystic teratoma
- Most common adnexal mass: Functional cyst
- Risk of malignancy increases after age 40 yr

INFANTS:

Adnexal masses are usually follicular cysts attributable to maternal hormone stimulation that regress during first few months of life.

CHILDHOOD:

- Adnexal masses are rare.
- 9% to 11% malignant.
- Almost always dysgerminomas or teratomas (germ cell origin).
- Frequency of malignancy is inversely correlated with age.

ADOLESCENCE:

- Most common adnexal mass is a functional cyst.
- Most common neoplastic ovarian tumor is a benign cystic teratoma.
- Solid/cystic adnexal tumors are rare and almost always dysgerminomas or malignant teratomas.

PHYSICAL FINDINGS & CLINICAL PRESENTATION

- Usually asymptomatic
- Pelvic pain or pressure
- Dyspareunia
- Abdominal pain ranging from mild to severe peritoneal irritation
- Increasing abdominal girth or distention
- Adnexal mass of pelvic examination
- Children: Abdominal or rectal mass, early-onset puberty

ETIOLOGY

- Physiologic
- Endometriosis
- Unknown

DIAGNOSIS

DIFFERENTIAL DIAGNOSIS

- Ovarian torsion
- Endometrioma
- Uterine fibroid
- Ectopic pregnancy
- Tubo-ovarian abscess
- Paratubal or paraovarian cyst
- Hydrosalpinx
- Malignancy: Ovary, fallopian tube, colon
- Diverticular abscess, diverticulitis
- Appendiceal abscess, appendicitis (especially in children)
- Urethral diverticulum
- Nerve sheath tumors
- Distended bladder
- Pelvic kidney
- Retroperitoneal cyst or neoplasm

WORKUP

- Complete history and physical examination
- Pelvic or rectovaginal examination to reveal firm, irregular, mobile mass
- Pelvic ultrasound
- Laparoscopy or laparotomy to establish diagnosis

LABORATORY TESTS

- Pregnancy test
- Serum tumor markers if there is high suspicion for malignancy:
  1. Cancer antigen 125 (CA-125)
  2. Alpha-fetoprotein (endodermal sinus tumor, immature teratoma)
  3. Beta-human chorionic gonadotropin
  4. Lactate dehydrogenase (dysgerminoma)

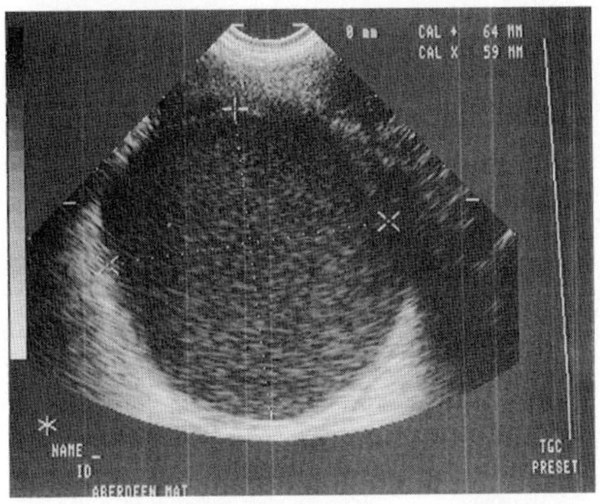

FIG. 1 Ultrasonogram reveals a cyst 6.5 cm across, which was found at laparotomy to be an endometrioma full of altered blood, the so-called chocolate cyst. This may cause cyclical or chronic pelvic pain. (From Greer IA et al: *Mosby's color atlas and text of obstetrics and gynecology,* London, 2000, Harcourt.)

IMAGING STUDIES

Ultrasound (Fig. 1):

- May differentiate adnexal mass from other pelvic masses
- Features that increase risk of malignancy include solid component, papillae, multiple septations or solitary thick septa, ascites, matted bowel, bilaterality, irregular borders
- CT scan with contrast
- Colonoscopy or barium enema, if symptomatic

TREATMENT

NONPHARMACOLOGIC THERAPY

Repeat pelvic examination, typically with transvaginal pelvic ultrasound, for premenopausal women in 4 to 6 wk to rule out persistent cyst.

ACUTE GENERAL Rx

Indications for surgery:

- Postmenopausal or premenarchal palpable adnexal mass
- Adnexal mass with suspicious ultrasound features
- Adnexal mass greater than 10 cm
- Suspected torsion or rupture

CHRONIC Rx

- Depends on diagnosis
- Possible suppression of formation of new cysts by oral contraceptives

DISPOSITION

- Depends on diagnosis.
- One study showed that all malignant masses demonstrated growth within 7 mo. Expert opinion recommends limiting observation of stable masses without solid components to 1 yr and with solid components to 2 yr.

REFERRAL

- If malignancy suspected
- If surgery required

SUGGESTED READING

Available at ExpertConsult.com

RELATED CONTENT

Ovarian Cysts (Patient Information)
Ovarian Cancer (Related Key Topic)

AUTHORS: **Helen Toma, MD, MSPH,** and **Anthony Sciscione, DO**

Paget Disease of Bone (ALG) (PTG)

BASIC INFORMATION

DEFINITION

Paget disease of bone is a focal disorder of chaotic bone remodeling with increased osteoblastic and osteoclastic activity that results in disorganized woven and lamellar bone (Fig. E1) in one or more skeletal sites. The end result is bone of poor quality that is enlarged, hypervascular, and susceptible to deformation and fracture.

SYNONYM

Osteitis deformans

ICD-10CM CODES

M88.9	Osteitis deformans of unspecified bone
M88.0	Osteitis deformans of skull
M88.1	Osteitis deformans of vertebrae
M88.869	Osteitis deformans of unspecified lower leg
M88.89	Osteitis deformans of multiple sites
M90.60	Osteitis deformans in neoplastic diseases, unspecified site
M90.679	Osteitis deformans in neoplastic diseases, unspecified ankle and foot
M90.68	Osteitis deformans in neoplastic diseases, other site
M90.69	Osteitis deformans in neoplastic diseases, multiple sites

EPIDEMIOLOGY & DEMOGRAPHICS

Epidemiologic data suggest an origin of Paget disease in Great Britain spreading to other areas by English colonists beginning in the seventeenth century. Highest prevalence occurs in Eastern and Western Europe and in those who have emigrated to New Zealand, Australia, South Africa, and North America. Paget is rarely seen in Japanese, Chinese, Asian Indians, sub-Saharan Africans, and Middle Eastern Arabs.

- Most commonly diagnosed in those aged >50 yr and rare before 40 yr.
- Prevalence estimates of up to 3% of population aged >50 yr and up to 10% in those aged >90 yr.

PREDOMINANT SEX: Variable preponderance of males

PREDOMINANT AGE: Middle or advanced years

FAMILIAL INCIDENCE: Common, family history positive in up to 40% of cases

PHYSICAL FINDINGS & CLINICAL PRESENTATION

- Most common sites of involvement: Pelvis (70%), lumbar spine (53%), sacrum, femur (55%), skull (42%), tibia (30%) (Fig. E2), humerus, scapula
- Uncommon: Hand, foot, fibula
- Lesions in one (monostotic) or more bones (polyostotic)
- Gradual progression of disease in affected bone(s) with rare appearance at new site(s)
- Many patients are asymptomatic, but up to 40% of patients who come to medical attention present with bone pain
- Symptoms and signs include bone and articular pain often related to secondary arthritis, bone deformities and enlargement, increased warmth over pagetic bone, skull enlargement, nerve entrapment or compression syndromes, cranial nerve deficits especially deafness (Fig. E3), spinal cord compression and vascular steal syndromes, fissure fractures, fractures, and neoplastic degeneration

ETIOLOGY

Fig. E4 illustrates the pathophysiology of Paget disease. Extensive epidemiologic and laboratory data are in keeping with potential role of paramyxoviral infection of osteoclasts in a genetically susceptible individual with or without documented genetic mutations.

DIAGNOSIS

Diagnosis is often suspected in asymptomatic patients with isolated elevation of alkaline phosphatase without evidence of liver disease.

DIFFERENTIAL DIAGNOSIS

- Osteosclerosis
- Hyperphosphatasia
- Familial expansile osteolysis
- Fibrous dysplasia
- Skeletal neoplasm (primary or metastatic)
- Osteomalacia with secondary hyperparathyroidism

LABORATORY TESTS

- Increase in serum alkaline phosphatase or bone-specific alkaline phosphatase
- Increase in urine NTx/creatinine ratio or plasma CTx
- Bone biopsy is rarely needed but may be necessary in selected cases to rule out sarcomatous degeneration or metastatic disease

IMAGING STUDIES

Bone scintigraphy (Fig. E5) is the most sensitive test for delineating the extent and site of pagetic lesions but nonspecific in that areas of uptake may be related to arthritis or metastatic lesions. Radiographs (Fig. E6) will further delineate characteristic pagetic changes (thickening of cortical bone, coarsened trabecular markings, distortion and expansion of involved bone).

TREATMENT

Indications for therapy include extensive or symptomatic disease; neurologic complications; involvement of weight-bearing bones, skull, vertebrae, and other areas of critical involvement (e.g., in proximity to joints); prevention of excess bleeding from an orthopedic procedure on pagetic bone; and if serum alkaline phosphatase is more than 4 times the upper limit of normal.

NONPHARMACOLOGIC THERAPY

- Optimization of calcium and vitamin D intake and appropriate guidance regarding ambulatory needs.
- Orthopedic stabilization may be required for patients with pseudofractures.

SPECIFIC THERAPY

Bisphosphonates are the mainstay of therapy and include oral alendronate or risedronate and intravenous pamidronate or zoledronic acid. A one-time dose of zoledronic acid (5 mg IV) may be effective in controlling symptoms for over 3 yr.

- SC salmon calcitonin when bisphosphonates are not tolerated or are contraindicated as in those with GFR of <35 ml/min
- Acetaminophen, aspirin, and nonsteroidal drugs for relief of pain

DISPOSITION

- Without treatment, progression of disease is common.
- With treatment, remissions of varying duration in most patients. For most patients with PD, a single infusion of zoledronic acid will provide a prolonged suppression of pagetic activity and for many elderly patients a possible lifelong remission. Careful and regular clinical and biochemical follow-up at 3- to 6-mo intervals with necessity of retreatment in patients with continued pagetic activity or reactivation.
- With first-ever intravenous dose of pamidronate or zoledronic acid, patients may experience a flulike syndrome that may be prevented with acetaminophen.

SUGGESTED READINGS

Available at ExpertConsult.com

RELATED CONTENT

Paget Disease of Bone (Patient Information)

AUTHOR: **Joseph R. Tucci, MD, FACP, FACE**

BASIC INFORMATION

DEFINITION

Paget disease of the breast is a malignant disease that presents itself as a scaly, sore, eroding, bleeding ulcer of the nipple. It represents an extension of a ductal adenocarcinoma of the breast. Microscopically, typical large clear cells (Paget cells) with pale and abundant cytoplasm and hyperchromatic nuclei with prominent nucleoli are found in the epidermal layer. Paget disease is more often associated with primary invasive or in situ carcinoma of the breast.

ICD-10CM CODES

C50.0	Malignant neoplasm of nipple and areola
C50.011	Malignant neoplasm of nipple and areola, right female breast
C50.012	Malignant neoplasm of nipple and areola, left female breast
C50.019	Malignant neoplasm of nipple and areola, unspecified female breast
C50.021	Malignant neoplasm of nipple and areola, right male breast
C50.022	Malignant neoplasm of nipple and areola, left male breast
C50.029	Malignant neoplasm of nipple and areola, unspecified male breast

EPIDEMIOLOGY & DEMOGRAPHICS

- 1% to 3% of new female breast cancer cases in the United States
- Peak incidence ages 50s through 60s, although it has been diagnosed in ages 26 to 88
- Subclinical Paget's found on histology may be more frequent

PHYSICAL FINDINGS & CLINICAL PRESENTATION

- Variable; most often an erythematous, irregularly bordered plaque that can be vesicular or ulcerated that starts on the nipple and spreads to the areola.
- Itching or burning nipple and/or reported lump. Itching/burning may occur before lesion.
- Very minimal scaly lesion that may bleed when scales are lifted.
- Typical ulcer located on nipple with serous fluid weeping or small amount of bleeding coming from it (Fig. E1). Bloody discharge may also occasionally occur.
- Palpable carcinoma in the breast in 50% of patients.
- 20% with no palpable mass will have suspicious finding on mammogram.

ETIOLOGY

- Exact origin unknown
- Possibly migration of either in situ or invasive carcinoma cells in breast to nipple skin to produce Paget disease

Dx DIAGNOSIS

DIFFERENTIAL DIAGNOSIS

- Chronic dermatitis
- Florid papillomatosis of the nipple or nipple adenoma
- Eczema
- Skin cancer

WORKUP

- Clinically apparent
- Careful breast examination
- Palpable mass or mammographic lesions in 50% of patients

LABORATORY TESTS

Biopsy of nipple lesion: Scraping, punch biopsy, or wedge biopsy

IMAGING STUDIES

Mammograms to search for possible primary carcinoma

Rx TREATMENT

NONPHARMACOLOGIC THERAPY

- Paget disease without palpable mass and negative mammogram:
  1. Consideration of wide excision of nipple with radiation
  2. Mastectomy is also an option
- Paget disease with palpable mass or abnormal mammogram findings:
  1. Mastectomy
  2. Breast conservation surgery and whole breast radiation
- Presence of underlying in situ or invasive carcinoma in mastectomy specimen of majority of patients.
- Evaluation of axilla is the same for other breast cancers and depends on underlying type.

ACUTE GENERAL Rx

Systemic adjuvant therapy depending on extent of invasive carcinoma found

DISPOSITION

- Parallel prognosis to that of breast cancer patient without Paget disease
- Prognosis is better in those without palpable mass
- Regular follow-up as in other invasive or in situ carcinoma patients

REFERRAL

At outset, all suspicious nipple lesions should be referred for evaluation and treatment.

SUGGESTED READINGS

Available at ExpertConsult.com

RELATED CONTENT

Paget Disease of the Breast (Patient Information)
Breast Cancer (Related Key Topic)

AUTHORS: **Gina Ranieri, DO,** and **Anthony Sciscione, DO**

BASIC INFORMATION

DEFINITION

Chronic pain is pain that persists for longer than the expected time frame (typically >3 mo) or that is associated with progressive, nonmalignant disease. Pain is an unpleasant sensory and emotional experience associated with actual or potential tissue damage or described in terms of such damage. The perception of pain is influenced by physiologic, psychological, and social factors. Chronic pain may be the direct result of an underlying disease process, or it may be a separate condition in its own right.

SYNONYMS

Chronic pain management
Nonmalignant chronic pain
Pain management

ICD-10CM CODES

G89.21	Chronic pain due to trauma
G89.22	Chronic post-thoracotomy pain
G89.3	Neoplasm-related pain (acute) (chronic)
G89.4	Chronic pain syndrome
G89.28	Other chronic post-procedural pain
G89.29	Other chronic pain

EPIDEMIOLOGY & DEMOGRAPHICS

Estimates of the prevalence of chronic pain in the U.S. vary widely. A 2011 report from the Institute of Medicine, *Relieving Pain in America*, estimates that 116 million adults live with chronic pain at a cost of almost $635 billion per yr. Chronic pain is the third-leading cause of physical impairment in the U.S. and the leading cause of disease burden and disability globally. Patients with chronic pain may also experience mood changes, depression, sleep disturbances, fatigue, and decreased overall physical functioning.

CLINICAL PRESENTATION

- History: Comprehensive patient assessment, including history of present illness (cause of pain, location, timing, characteristics, exacerbating/relieving factors, triggers), past therapies (pharmacologic and nonpharmacologic and outcomes of these therapies), medical history, family and social history, psychiatric history (including history of depression, anxiety, abuse, and/or other psychological disorders), substance use history, allergies, sleep patterns and disturbances, and current medications. Social supports, coping mechanisms, and spirituality can also help guide development of a treatment plan.
- Pain assessment should be performed at each visit; includes pain intensity (1-10), response to medication, and attributes of pain. Standardized templates for both initial and follow-up pain assessment have been developed by various organizations. The Brief Pain Inventory is an example of a widely used assessment tool. In addition, a functional assessment should be performed. Tools such as the Functional Ability Questionnaire (FAQ5) can guide the clinician in determining a patient's functional status. Lastly, consider assessment of a patient's risk for substance abuse.
- Physical examination: Directed at systems affected by pain (often musculoskeletal) and neurologic examination.
- Look for contributing factors (e.g., comorbidities, lifestyle factors) and barriers to effective care (e.g., behavioral, social, insurance). Increasing evidence points to a relation between obesity and chronic pain.
- Components of a comprehensive assessment of cancer pain are summarized in Box 1.

ETIOLOGY

Mechanisms of chronic pain can be divided into three broad categories:

- Nociceptive: Pain arising from damage to peripheral tissue from injury or inflammatory, mechanical, or metabolic causes
- Neuropathic: Peripheral nerve impairment
- Central: Central disturbance in pain processing

DIAGNOSIS

DIFFERENTIAL DIAGNOSIS

- Depends on etiology:
  1. Nociceptive: Osteoarthritis, rheumatoid arthritis, postsurgical pain, posttraumatic, cancer pain
  2. Neuropathic: Postherpetic neuralgia, diabetic neuropathy, nerve root compression
  3. Central: Fibromyalgia, irritable bowel syndrome, chronic headache, phantom limb
- Many chronic pain syndromes may involve one or more of the previously named mechanisms. The etiology of pain in cancer patients is summarized in Box 2.
- Depression and anxiety disorders can be both a cause and a result of chronic pain, so temporal association of these disorders is important.
- Coping mechanisms also can contribute to the risk of developing chronic pain. For example, anxiety and fear about pain is associated with an increased likelihood of developing chronic pain. Patients with a passive attitude toward treating pain (e.g., rest,

BOX 1 Components of a Comprehensive Assessment of Cancer Pain

I. Detailed history of current pain problem
   A. Catalog of pain (number and locations)
   B. Information for each type of pain
      1. Intensity (0-10)
      2. Locations and radiation
      3. Onset and changes over time
      4. Temporal pattern (e.g., constant or intermittent) and quality (e.g., burning)
      5. Exacerbating and relieving factors
      6. Associated neurologic or vasomotor abnormalities
      7. Other associated factors
      8. Interference with the patient's life
      9. Current therapeutic modalities (e.g., schedule, efficacy, and adverse effects)
      10. Prior therapeutic modalities (e.g., schedule, efficacy, and adverse effects)
II. Oncologic history
   A. Histologic type
   B. Presentation: Date, stage, and sites of involvement
   C. Antineoplastic therapies: Dates, types, doses, toxicities, and response to each therapy
   D. Current sites of disease: Stable, responding, or progressive
   E. Patient expectations and goals
III. Medical history—may be affected by pain therapies
   A. Coexisting diseases
   B. Medications and allergies
   C. Substance abuse history
   D. Other constitutional symptoms such as anorexia, fatigue, sedation and other changes in mental status, nausea, vomiting, dysphagia, dyspnea, constipation, urinary and sexual dysfunction, depression, dry mouth; also, the ability to take medications by mouth and the presence of a central venous catheter
IV. Personal and social history
   A. Background: Age, education, employment, marital status, place of residence, religious affiliation, and cultural and ethnic background
   B. Current status: Functional status, caregivers and their health and availability, support system
V. Physical examination
VI. Review of additional information
   A. Medical records, radiologic and laboratory studies
   B. Family members, physicians and/or nurses who know the patient and his or her illness
VII. Differential diagnosis
VIII. Recommendations regarding workup and therapy
XI. Reassessment

From Niederhuber JE: *Abeloff's clinical oncology,* ed 6, Philadelphia, 2020, Elsevier.

medication use) also are associated with higher rates of chronic pain than those with active attitudes.

- Genetic factors play a role. There are at least 150 genes that contribute to chronic pain. It has been shown to be a heritable phenotype, although no one set of genes has been identified as the culprit.
- Factors such as socioeconomic background, employment status, physical activity, sleep disorders, and weight can have a bidirectional effect on chronic pain.

WORKUP

- Workup should be directed at identifying the source of pain. Identification of the mechanism of pain will guide the development of an appropriate treatment plan.
- Laboratory testing, imaging studies, and/or electromyographic (EMG) studies should be used when etiology of chronic pain is unknown or unclear, when comorbidities are suspected, and as the history and physical examination direct.
- Consider use of random urine drug screens or other tests to screen for presence of illegal drugs, unreported prescribed medications, or alcohol use.

Rx TREATMENT

- Studies increasingly support the application of a multidisciplinary, biopsychosocial approach that addresses the multiple facets of pain and includes the patient's perspective and goals.
- Therapeutic goal is the reduction of pain (elimination of chronic pain is generally unlikely, and providers establish expectations and treatment goals from the outset).
- A written care plan that includes methods to address the patient's personal goals, improve sleep, increase physical activity, manage stress, and reduce pain. Increasing evidence re-enforces the role of patient education, self-management, and active coping skills in reducing pain perception and self-efficacy.

NONPHARMACOLOGIC THERAPY

- Exercise (recommended for all patients and tailored to individual abilities and needs). Recent studies demonstrate the benefit of tai chi for patients with osteoarthritis and therapeutic exercise for those with all forms of chronic pain
- Modalities: Heat therapy, cold therapy, transcutaneous electrical nerve stimulation (TENS) units, manipulative therapy, cognitive behavioral therapy, psychological counseling, and physical therapy
- Electrostimulation therapy: TENS units (mixed evidence)
- Behavioral therapies: Cognitive behavioral therapy, hypnosis, biofeedback, relaxation therapy, mindfulness
- Music therapy (in conjunction with other types of therapy)
- Virtual reality programs (through distraction and dissociation techniques therapy[ies]), biofeed
- Surgery (rarely considered a first-line therapy for chronic pain)

GENERAL PHARMACOLOGIC Rx

- Short-acting antiinflammatory and analgesic medications (e.g., acetaminophen/NSAIDs/opioids). Avoid use of NSAIDs in patients with hypertension, congestive heart failure (CHF), or any type of chronic kidney disease (CKD). These medications should be considered first-line therapy for all patients without contraindications
- Topical analgesics (lidocaine, NSAIDs, capsaicin)
- Trigger-point or joint injections (immediate anesthetic plus long-acting corticosteroids)
- Epidural steroid injections
- Nerve blocks (Table 1)
- Antidepressants (tricyclic and selective serotonin reuptake inhibitors)
- Anticonvulsant medications (e.g., carbamazepine, valproic acid, gabapentin, pregabalin); particularly helpful for neuropathic conditions
- Ketamine (N-methyl-d-aspartate [NMDA] receptor antagonist). Recent studies have been done on its use in patients with opioid tolerance and hyperalgesia. The efficacy of ketamine is moderate to weak, and it only should be considered as third-line treatment. Ketamine also requires regular infusion, and its efficacy is limited by side effects (mainly psychological)

BOX 2 Etiology of Pain in Patients with Cancer

A. Direct tumor involvement (70%)
1. Invasion of bone
2. Invasion or compression of neural structures
3. Obstruction of hollow viscus or ductal system of solid viscus
4. Vascular obstruction or invasion
5. Mucous membrane ulceration or involvement

B. Cancer-induced syndromes (<10%)
1. Paraneoplastic syndromes
2. Pain associated with debility (e.g., bedsores, constipation, rectal or bladder spasms)
3. Other (e.g., postherpetic neuralgia)

C. Diagnostic or therapeutic procedures (20%)
1. Procedure-related pain (e.g., bone marrow aspiration or biopsy and lumbar puncture)
2. Acute postoperative pain or postsurgical syndromes (e.g., postmastectomy, postthoracotomy, and postamputation syndromes)
3. After radiation (e.g., injury to plexus or spinal cord, mucositis, and enteritis)
4. After chemotherapy (e.g., mucositis, peripheral neuropathy, and aseptic necrosis)

D. Pain unrelated to the malignancy or its treatment (<10%)

From Niederhuber JE: *Abeloff's clinical oncology,* ed 6, Philadelphia, 2020, Elsevier.

TABLE 1 Regional Anesthetic Techniques

	Types of Blocks	Examples	Indications	Comments
Local anesthetic blocks	Diagnostic	Intercostal nerve block	Determine etiology of pain and the response and adverse effects following local therapies	Analgesic effect will last only hours
	Treatment of sympathetically maintained pain	Stellate ganglion block	Sympathetically maintained pain	Repeated blocks might be needed
	Trigger point injections	Trigger point injection	Myofascial pain syndrome	Repeated blocks might be needed
Neurolytic (alcohol or phenol) blocks	Peripheral	Intercostal nerve blocks	Chest wall tumor	Pain relief usually lasts several mo
	Visceral	Celiac plexus block Superior hypogastric block Ganglionic impar block	Pancreatic cancer Gastrointestinal or genitourinary cancers	Pain relief usually lasts several mo
	Neuraxial	Epidural Intrathecal neurolysisSpinal cord stimulator	Pain localized to two or three dermatomes	Pain relief usually lasts several mo

From Niederhuber JE: *Abeloff's clinical oncology,* ed 6, Philadelphia, 2020, Elsevier.

TABLE 2 Commonly Used Adjuvant Analgesics for Cancer Pain

Drug Category	Indications	Drugs	Common Toxicities	Comments
Antidepressants	Neuropathic pain	AmitriptylineNortriptyline Desipramine Duloxetine Venlafaxine	Sedation, dry mouth, constipation, postural hypotension, urinary retention	Begin with low doses and increase the dose every few days
Anticonvulsants	Neuropathic pain	CarbamazepinePregabalin Clonazepam Gabapentin	Drowsiness, dizziness, nausea, rash, bone marrow depression	Monitor platelets with carbamazepine
Corticosteroids	Spinal cord compression, increased intracranial pressure, visceral distention	Dexamethasone Methylprednisolone Prednisone	Gastritis, insomnia, fluid retention, hyperglycemia, myopathy, increased appetite	
Muscle relaxants	Muscle spasm	Diazepam Baclofen Methocarbamol Cyclobenzaprine	Sedation, dizziness, nausea, weakness, confusion	
Benzodiazepines	Muscle spasm, myoclonus, anxiety, insomnia	Diazepam Lorazepam Alprazolam Midazolam Temazepam	Sedation, delirium, hypotension, headache, respiratory depression	Not analgesics; synergistic effect with opioids can cause respiratory depression
Antispasmodics	Gastrointestinal or bladder spasm	Diphenoxylate and atropine Loperamide Scopolamine patch Dicyclomine	Sedation, dry mouth, constipation	
Neuroleptics	Delirium, agitation, nausea and vomiting, hiccups	Olanzapine Risperidone Quetiapine Haloperidol Prochlorperazine	Sedation, orthostatic hypotension, confusion, extrapyramidal reactions	Useful for symptoms other than pain
Bisphosphonates	Bone pain	Pamidronate Zoledronic acid Alendronate Risedronate Ibandronate Etidronate Denosumab	Hypocalcemia, fever, gastrointestinal disturbances, anemia	Delays time to painful skeletal events; also used with analgesics for bone pain

From Niederhuber JE: *Abeloff's clinical oncology,* ed 6, Philadelphia, 2020, Elsevier.

- Implantable methods, epidural and intrathecal drug delivery systems, dorsal column stimulators
- Treatment of insomnia and sleep disorders to reduce pain with standard sleep-inducing agents (trazodone, antihistamines)
- Many patients may require combination drug therapy (CDT) for adequate control of pain, with appropriate attention given to interactions and side effects. Commonly used adjuvant analgesics for cancer pain are summarized in Table 2

OPIOID THERAPY

- Although a mainstay of treatment over the past two decades, limited evidence is available demonstrating the efficacy of both immediate- and long-acting opioid preparations. Some patients with severe chronic pain syndromes may still benefit from this form of treatment. Full opioid agonists are generally the drug of choice for severe chronic cancer pain. Tenets of opioid prescribing are summarized in Box 3.
- Opioids are rarely beneficial in the treatment of inflammatory or mechanical pain and are not indicated for treatment of headaches. Recent studies also have demonstrated the development of hyperalgesia with long-term opioid use.
- The Centers for Disease Control and Prevention has published detailed guidelines for prescribing opioids for chronic pain in light of rising rates of opioid addiction and overdose. The guidelines include when and with whom to use opioid therapy, opioid selection, dosing, duration, and follow-up, along with assessment of the risks, benefits, and discontinuation of therapy.
- Current recommendations include aiming for daily opioid doses of <50 morphine milligram equivalents (MMEs)/day to limit the risk of overdose and side effects, prescribing naloxone to patients receiving daily doses >50 MMEs/day due to risk of overdose, avoiding concomitant use with benzodiazepines, and avoiding doses >90 MMEs/day, or referral to a pain management specialist for close monitoring.
- Sustained-release opioids (used for moderate to severe pain that has failed other therapeutic interventions): Oxycodone, morphine sustained release(SR), methadone (use with caution), or fentanyl patch; short-acting opioids can be used in conjunction with these agents for management of breakthrough pain. Conversion to a long-acting opioid should be based on an equianalgesic conversion. Table E3 compares MME doses for commonly prescribed opioids.

Table E4 describes common opioids used for cancer pain management. Titration of these medications should not exceed the equivalent of 100 mg morphine/day to avoid risk of overdose. Box E4 summarizes CDC recommendations for prescribing opioids for chronic pain outside of active cancer and palliative and end-of-life care. Box E5 summarizes the interpretation of recommendation categories and evidence types.

MEDICAL MARIJUANA

- Preclinical studies demonstrate potential benefits of cannabinoids, with a good safety profile; however, the evidence for use in the clinical setting is limited because of nonclinical factors.
- Some small, randomized controlled trials (RCTs) show benefit of low-dose cannabinoids for chronic neuropathic pain.
- Newer RCTs note a positive impact of cannabidiol (CBD) on reduction of opiate medication use and improvement of quality-of-life indicators.

COMPLEMENTARY & ALTERNATIVE MEDICINE

Acupuncture and massage (evidence-based for some indications). Acupuncture is most likely to benefit patients with low back pain, neck pain, chronic idiopathic or tension headache, migraine, and knee osteoarthritis. Recent evidence has demonstrated the benefit of modalities such as yoga, tai chi, and music therapies. Supplements, although popular, do not have substantial evidence to recommend for or against their use.

BOX 3 Management Approach: Tenets of Opioid Prescribing

- Order opioids on a scheduled "around-the-clock" basis to optimize relief.
- Order an as-needed opioid to treat breakthrough or incidental pain.
- Initiate a prophylactic bowel regimen at the same time opioids are prescribed. Patients usually require a combination of stool softeners and stimulant laxatives to treat opioid-induced constipation.
- Treat opioid-induced nausea and vomiting with aggressive antiemetic management, which includes giving patients antiemetics on an around-the-clock basis. Patients often become tolerant to this adverse effect several days after beginning opioids.
- Once baseline opioid requirements are determined, sustained-release opioid preparations can be used to reduce the number of pills taken each day.
- Teach the patient and family about the purpose and benefits of opioids to allay their fears about adverse effects and addiction. This instruction will improve patient compliance.
- Frequent assessment of pain relief is paramount during the opioid titration period. Titrate doses based on the patient's report of pain relief and/or the amount of as-needed opioid that has been required for patient comfort.
- Maximize the doses of one opioid before changing to another agent or route. Changes should be made primarily because of toxicities. For example, a patient taking 200 mg of controlled-release morphine every 12 hr and 200 mg of immediate-release morphine daily for breakthrough pain should have the dose of controlled-release morphine increased to 300 mg every 12 hr if he or she is not experiencing significant opioid adverse effects. This approach is more likely to be beneficial than beginning titration with subcutaneous or intravenous morphine or oral hydromorphone.
- Refer to equianalgesic tables when initiating or changing a patient's analgesic regimen.
- Avoid chronic administration of intramuscular or rectal opioids.
- Avoid chronic administration of meperidine, which can be associated with the accumulation of normeperidine, a neurotoxic metabolite.

From Niederhuber JE: *Abeloff's clinical oncology,* ed 6, Philadelphia, 2020, Elsevier.

REFERRAL

- Pain medicine specialist or multidisciplinary pain clinic: Useful when primary therapies fail, in patients with complex pain conditions, in patients requiring a high daily MME, or for invasive therapies
- Consider referral to an addiction specialist if patient has a history of substance abuse or addiction
- Psychiatry/psychological services for counseling, if needed

PEARLS & CONSIDERATIONS

- Patient consent should be obtained in the form of a written treatment agreement before initiating treatment. This agreement should outline the goals of therapy, use of a single provider or treatment team and a single pharmacy, limitations on dose and number of prescribed medications, prohibition on use with alcohol or sedating medications, keeping medication safe and secure, prohibition on selling or sharing medication, limitations on refills, compliance with all components of the treatment plan, the role of drug screening, and consequences of nonadherence.
- Follow-up assessment should occur every 1 to 6 mo and include a complete pain assessment (see earlier), review of the type of long-acting analgesic used and dosage, use of breakthrough analgesics, side effects and their management, use of nonpharmacologic therapies, and adjunct medication use.

COMMENTS

- Medication dependence and addiction should not be confused. Most patients receiving chronic opioid therapy can become dependent on these medications for pain relief without developing opioid addiction. Patients exhibiting signs of addiction often will seek escalating doses of medication, request refills of prescriptions earlier than planned, and engage in drug-seeking activities (e.g., emergency department visits between prescriptions, seeking multiple prescriptions).
- Side effects need not preclude use of opioid medications and should be anticipated. Antiemetics can aid in controlling nausea. Constipation can be managed with stool softeners and laxatives.
- The emphasis of comprehensive pain management for non–cancer-related chronic pain has led to a fourfold increase in prescribing of opioid medications in the U.S. This increase in opiate use has also led to a rise in the misuse and abuse of these medications. Providers should proceed with caution before initiating pain management with opiate medications and should familiarize themselves with processes and tools for pain assessment and medication management. Forty-two states have developed prescription drug monitoring programs (PDMPs) to assist providers in identifying issues of abuse, polypharmacy, and misuse of controlled substances.

PATIENT & FAMILY EDUCATION

- National Pain Foundation (http://www.painconnection.org)
- National Institutes of Health (http://www.nih.gov)

SUGGESTED READINGS

Available at ExpertConsult.com

RELATED CONTENT

Pain Medications (Patient Information)

AUTHOR: **AnnGene Anthony, MD, MPH, FAAFP**

Pancreatic Cancer (Exocrine) ALG PTG

BASIC INFORMATION

DEFINITION

Pancreatic cancer is an adenocarcinoma derived from pancreatic duct epithelium. Microscopic premalignant pancreatic lesions in the pancreatic ducts are referred to as pancreatic intraepithelial neoplasia (PIN) in which there is a stepwise progression from low grade to high grade associated with accumulating genetic alterations. Intraductal papillary mucinous neoplasms (IPMN) are a second type of precursor to pancreatic cancer that are associated with an overall risk of invasive cancer of approximately 25%, especially in those arising from the main pancreatic duct.

ICD-10CM CODES

C25.9	Malignant neoplasm of pancreas, unspecified
C25.0	Malignant neoplasm of head of pancreas
C25.1	Malignant neoplasm of body of pancreas
C25.2	Malignant neoplasm of tail of pancreas
C25.3	Malignant neoplasm of pancreatic duct

EPIDEMIOLOGY & DEMOGRAPHICS

INCIDENCE: In the U.S. it is estimated that there were 57,600 new cases and 47,050 deaths in 2020. It is the third-leading cause of cancer-related death in the U.S. The majority of patients present with advanced disease, and less than 20% of patients present with potentially resectable tumors.

PREDOMINANT SEX: Male:female ratio of 2:1.

PREDOMINANT AGE: Median age at diagnosis is 71 yr.

PHYSICAL FINDINGS & CLINICAL PRESENTATION

Presenting symptoms are generally related to location:

- Jaundice (60% to 70% of pancreatic cancers are located in the head of the pancreas)
- Abdominal pain: Generally dull upper abdominal pain or vague abdominal discomfort
- Weight loss
- Anorexia/change in taste, asthenia
- Nausea
- Uncommonly: Depression, gastrointestinal bleeding, acute pancreatitis (from obstruction of the pancreatic duct), back pain
- Trousseau syndrome (hypercoagulability in the setting of malignancy) may be initial presentation in some patients
- Table 1 summarizes demographic features and presenting symptoms in pancreatic cancer patients

Physical Findings

- Icterus
- Cachexia, temporal wasting
- Ascites, peripheral lymphadenopathy, hepatomegaly
- Excoriations from scratching pruritic skin

ETIOLOGY

Unknown, but several conditions have been associated with pancreatic cancer:

- Smoking
- Alcoholism
- Genetics: Up to 20% of patients have a family history of the disease
- Genetic syndromes and associated genes: Hereditary pancreatitis (*PRSS1, SPINK1*), Peutz-Jeghers syndrome (*STK11[LKB1]*), familial atypical multiple mole and melanoma syndrome (*p16*), hereditary breast and ovarian cancer syndromes (*BRCA1, BRCA2, PALB2*), ataxia telangiectasia (*ATM*), and Li-Fraumeni syndrome (*P53*)
- Gallstones
- Diabetes mellitus (present in at least 50% of patients with pancreatic cancer)
- Chronic pancreatitis
- Diet rich in animal fat
- Occupational exposure: Oil refining, paper manufacturing, chemical industry
- Overweight or obesity during early adulthood is associated with a greater risk of pancreatic cancer and a younger age of disease onset. Obesity at an older age is associated with a lower overall survival in patients with pancreatic cancer
- There are four major driver genes for pancreatic cancer: *KRAS*, *CDKN2A*, *TP53*, and *SMAD4*. *KRAS* mutation and alterations in *CDKN2A* are early events in pancreatic cancer tumorigenesis
- Table 2 summarizes nongenetic and genetic risk factors for pancreatic cancer

Dx DIAGNOSIS

DIFFERENTIAL DIAGNOSIS

- Common duct cholelithiasis
- Cholangiocarcinoma
- Common duct stricture
- Sclerosing cholangitis
- Primary biliary cirrhosis
- Autoimmune pancreatitis
- Drug-induced cholestasis (e.g., phenothiazines)
- Other pancreatic tumors (islet cell tumor, cystadenocarcinoma, epidermoid carcinoma, sarcomas, lymphomas)

WORKUP

- Initial laboratory testing includes complete blood count, serum chemistries. The bile duct antigen CA 19-9 is not used as a screening test but can be utilized as a modality for detecting recurrence and for therapeutic monitoring in patients undergoing therapy.
- As per updated consensus guidelines, all patients diagnosed with pancreatic cancer should undergo assessment of risk for hereditary syndromes known to be associated with an increased risk of cancer. Germline genetic testing for cancer susceptibility should be considered even if family history is unremarkable.

Routine Laboratory Tests	% Abnormal
Alkaline phosphatase	80
Bilirubin	55
Total protein	15
Amylase	15
Hemoglobin	60

IMAGING STUDIES

- Multidetector helical CT (Fig. E1) with IV administration of contrast is the imaging procedure of choice for initial evaluation.
- Endoscopic ultrasonography (Fig. E2) is useful when the diagnosis is strongly suspected and tissue is required for diagnostic purposes. Fine-needle aspiration biopsy combined with endoscopic ultrasonography is the preferred modality for evaluation of cystic or mass lesions to determine malignancy.
- Endoscopic retrograde cholangiopancreatography (ERCP, Fig. E3) is useful in patients with jaundice needing an endoscopic stent to relieve obstruction.
- PET scans are of limited value in pancreatic cancer and are not part of standard management.

TABLE 1 Demographic Features and Presenting Symptoms and Signs in Patients with Unresectable (Palliated) and Resectable (Resected) Pancreatic Cancer

	Palliated (*N* = 256)	Resected (*N* = 512)
Demographic Features		
Age, average (yr)	64.0	65.8
Men/women	57%/43%	55%/45%
Race	91% white	91% white
Symptoms and Signs (%)		
Abdominal pain	64	36*
Jaundice	57	72*
Weight loss	48	43
Nausea/vomiting	30	18*
Back pain	26	2*

*P = 0.001 vs. palliated group.

From Feldman M et al: *Sleisenger and Fordtran's gastrointestinal and liver disease*, ed 10, Philadelphia, 2016, Elsevier.

TABLE 2 Nongenetic and Genetic Risk Factors for Pancreatic Cancer

Variable	Risk Increase
Nongenetic Risk Factors	
Chronic pancreatitis	13.3
New onset type 2 diabetes	7.9
Long-standing diabetes mellitus	2.0
Obesity	2.0
Smoking	1.8
Alcohol abuse	1.2
Non–O blood group	1.3
Genetic Syndrome and Associated Genes	
Familial pancreatic cancer (unknown gene)	
One first-degree relative	9
Three first-degree relatives	32
Familial adenomatous polyposis *(APC)*	4.5-6
Breast and ovarian cancer syndrome *(BRCA1, BRCA2, PALB2)*	2-3.5
Peutz-Jeghers syndrome *(STK11/LKB1)*	132
Hereditary pancreatitis *(PRSS1, SPINK1)*	69
Familial atypical multiple mole melanoma pancreatic carcinoma syndrome *(P16INK4A/CDKN2A)*	47
Lynch syndrome *(MLH1, MSH2, MSH6, PMS2, EPCAM)*	8.6
Cystic fibrosis *(CFTR)*	3.5
Ataxia-telangiectasia *(ATM)*	Unknown
Genetic Polymorphisms	
ABO	1.3
NR5A2	1.3
TERT	1.2
PDX1	1.2
BCAR1, CTRB1, CTRB2	1.5
ZNRF3	1.2
LINC00673	1.3
ETAA1	1.1
TP63	1.1
SUGCT	1.1

From Niederhuber JE: *Abeloff's clinical oncology*, ed 6, Philadelphia, 2020, Elsevier.

Noninvasive Imaging	% Abnormal
Abdominal ultrasonography	60
Abdominal CT scan (with contrast) (Fig. E4)	90
Abdominal MRI scan	90

Invasive Imaging	% Abnormal
ERCP	90
CT scan or ultrasonography-guided needle aspiration cytology	90-95

STAGING

2018 AJCC eighth edition of staging system for pancreatic cancer

PRIMARY TUMOR (T):

T_X	Primary Tumor Cannot Be Assessed
T_0	No evidence of primary tumor
T_1	Tumor <2 cm
T_2	Tumor >2 cm and <4 cm
T_3	Tumor >4 cm
T_4	Tumor involves celiac axis or superior mesenteric artery (unresectable primary)

LYMPH NODES (N):

N_0	No regional lymph nodes
N_1	Metastasis in 1-3 regional lymph nodes
N_2	Metastasis in >4 regional lymph nodes

DISTANT METASTASES (M):

M_X	Presence of distant metastasis cannot be assessed
M_0	No distant metastasis
M_1	Distant metastasis

STAGING GROUPS:

I_A	T_1, N_0, M_0
I_B	T_2, N_0, M_0
II_A	T_3, N_0, M_0
II_B	T_{1-3}, N_1, M_0
III	T_{1-3}, N_2, M_0 T_4, any N, M_0
IV	Any T, any N, M_1

Rx TREATMENT

Treatment sequencing strategies are summarized in Fig. 5 and Table 3.

SURGERY FOR RESECTABLE DISEASE

- Classification of resectability of pancreatic cancer per the National Comprehensive Cancer Network and Surgical Oncology Expert Consensus Statement is summarized in Table 4.
- Curative cephalic pancreaticoduodenectomy (Whipple procedure) for tumors in the head and neck of the pancreas is appropriate for only 10% to 20% of patients whose lesion is <5 cm, solitary, and without locoregional invasion. Surgical mortality rate can be up to 5%. Tumors in the body or tail of the pancreas are removed by means of a distal pancreatectomy, which often includes a splenectomy. Due to the complexity of surgery and risk for significant morbidity and mortality, current guidelines recommend that pancreatic resections be carried out in centers that perform at least 15 to 20 cases annually. In addition, a recent review concluded that high-volume institutions are associated with higher negative-margin status and higher 5-yr survival rates, and that patients are more likely to receive multimodality therapy at these centers.

ADJUVANT THERAPY

Adjuvant chemotherapy has been demonstrated to improve postoperative survival in multiple randomized trials and is considered the standard of care in patients with resected cancers.

- The use of single agent 5-fluorouracil (5-FU) or gemcitabine is reserved for patients with older age or borderline performance status. The combination of gemcitabine and capecitabine is superior to gemcitabine alone, with median overall survival in the 28-mo range.
- Currently, the use of the modified FOLFIRNOX (5-FU, oxaliplatin, and irinotecan) regimen in this setting strikingly improves outcomes with median overall survival reported at 54 mo and is the standard of care for patients with adequate performance status.

The use of adjuvant radiotherapy in this setting is controversial and is best limited to patients with poor risk features, margin-positive surgery, or with multiple nodal or extra-nodal tumor involvement. Palliative therapeutic ERCP with metal or plastic stents is performed for biliary decompression.

NEOADJUVANT THERAPY

The current treatment paradigm in patients with resectable and borderline-resectable pancreatic cancer involves the use of upfront combination chemotherapy, and possibly chemoradiotherapy, to achieve improved resectability and survival outcomes. Both FOLFIRINOX and gemcitabine-based regimens are routinely used in this setting for 2 to 4 mo.

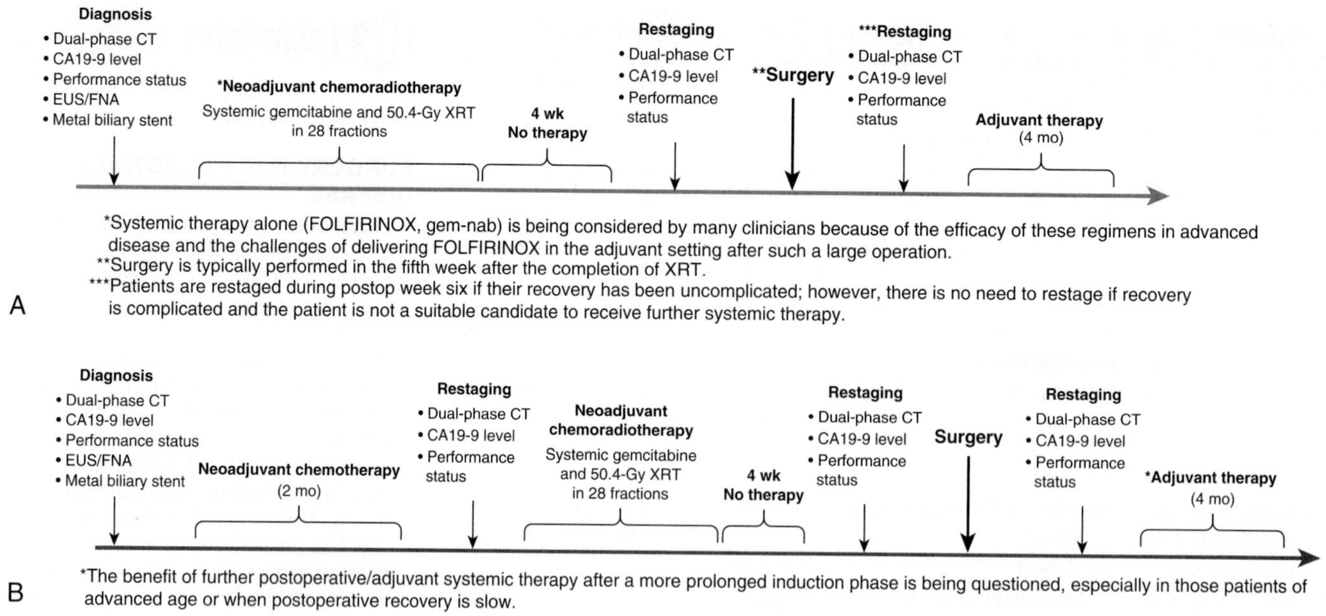

FIG. 5 Schematic representation of treatment sequencing in **(A)** resectable and **(B)** borderline resectable pancreatic cancer (PC). *CA 19-9*, Cancer antigen 19-9; *CT*, computed tomography; *EUS*, endoscopic ultrasound scan; *FNA*, fine-needle aspiration; *FOLFIRINOX*, 5-fluorouracil, leucovorin, irinotecan, and oxaliplatin; *gem-nab*, gemcitabine/nab-paclitaxel; *XRT*, external radiotherapy. (From Cameron JL, Cameron AM: *Current surgical therapy*, ed 12, Philadelphia, 2017, Elsevier.)

TABLE 3 Comparison of Treatment Sequencing Strategies for Patients with Pancreatic Cancer (outside of a clinical trial)

Stage	NCCN	MCW
Resectable	• Surgery • Restaging • Adjuvant therapy (+/− chemoradiotherapy; 6 mo)	• Neoadjuvant chemoradiotherapy (5.5 wk)* • Restaging • Surgery • Restaging • Adjuvant therapy (4 mo)
Borderline resectable	• Neoadjuvant therapy (regimen not specified) • Restaging • Surgery • Restaging • Consider adjuvant therapy	• Neoadjuvant chemotherapy (2 mo) • Restaging • Neoadjuvant chemoradiotherapy (5.5 wk) • Restaging • Surgery • Restaging • Adjuvant therapy (4 mo)
Locally advanced	• Chemotherapy • Restaging • Chemoradiotherapy in selected patients	• Chemotherapy (minimum 4 mo) • Restaging • Chemoradiotherapy • Restaging • Surgery in highly selected patients
Metastatic	• Systemic therapy • Clinical trial	• Systemic therapy • Clinical trial

NOTE: Clinical trials are preferred in all patients with pancreatic cancer (regardless of stage of disease) who have a performance status acceptable for treatment.

FOLFIRINOX, 5-fluorouracil, leucovorin, irinotecan, and oxaliplatin; *gem-nab*, gemcitabine/nab-paclitaxel; *MCW*, Medical College of Wisconsin; *NCCN*, National Comprehensive Cancer Network.

*Systemic therapy alone (FOLFIRINOX, gem-nab) is being considered by many clinicians because of the efficacy of these regimens in advanced disease and the challenges of delivering FOLFIRINOX in the adjuvant setting after such a large operation.

From Cameron JL, Cameron AM: *Current surgical therapy*, ed 12, Philadelphia, 2017, Elsevier.

RECURRENT/METASTATIC DISEASE

In patients with metastatic disease, accepted upfront chemotherapy treatment approaches have demonstrated improvement in survival outcomes. Acceptable chemotherapy regimens for locally advanced and metastatic disease are summarized in Table 5.

- Treatment options can include the administration of gemcitabine alone, combination regimen consisting of 5-fluorouracil, leucovorin, irinotecan, and oxaliplatin (FOLFIRINOX), or the combination of nab-paclitaxel plus gemcitabine. Multiagent regimens have an improved survival outcome compared with single-agent therapy. Liposomal irinotecan in combination with infusional 5-fluorouracil is now also approved in the setting of progressive cases.
- The use of maintenance olaparib (after systemic chemotherapy) among patients with a germline *BRCA* mutation in metastatic pancreatic cancer has demonstrated improvement in progression-free survival compared with placebo.
- Poor survival outcomes are seen in patients with poor performance status, significant weight loss, and with liver metastases.
- Combined chemotherapy and radiotherapy can be utilized in the case of patients with locally advanced but unresectable cases and confers a modest improvement in median overall survival.

DISPOSITION

- Adjuvant postoperative chemotherapy has a significant survival benefit in patients with resected pancreatic cancer.
- Adjuvant chemotherapy with FOLFIRINOX regimen significantly delays the development of recurrence and results in median survival of approximately 54 mo.
- The role of radiotherapy in the adjuvant setting is best restricted to patients who have a high risk for locoregional recurrence.

PEARLS & CONSIDERATIONS

COMMENTS

- Risk factors for pancreatic cancer and recommendations for screening of individuals at risk are summarized in Tables 6 and 7. New onset diabetes (NOD) after age 50 yr confers a 6- to 8-fold increased risk for sporadic (nonfamilial) pancreatic ductal

P

TABLE 4 Classification of Resectability of Pancreatic Cancer per the National Comprehensive Cancer Network and Surgical Oncology Expert Consensus Statement

Resectability Status	Criteria
Resectable	• No distant metastases • No radiographic evidence of SMV and portal vein abutment, distortion, tumor thrombus, or venous encasement • Clear fat planes around the celiac axis, hepatic artery, and SMA
Borderline resectable	• For tumors of the head or uncinate process: 1. Solid tumor contact with the SMV or portal vein of >180 degrees with contour irregularity of the vein or thrombosis of the vein but with suitable vessel proximal and distal to the site of involvement, allowing for safe and complete resection and vein reconstruction 2. Solid tumor contact with the IVC 3. Solid tumor contact with the common hepatic artery without extension to the celiac axis or hepatic artery bifurcation, allowing for safe and complete resection and reconstruction 4. Solid tumor contact with the SMA ≤180 degrees 5. Solid tumor contact with variable anatomy (e.g., accessory right hepatic artery, replaced right hepatic artery, replaced common hepatic artery, and the origin of replaced or accessory artery), and the presence and degree of tumor contact should be noted if present, as it may affect surgical planning • For tumors of the body or tail: 1. Solid tumor contact with the celiac axis of ≤180 degrees 2. Solid tumor contact with the celiac axis >180 degrees without involvement of the aorta and with an intact and uninvolved gastroduodenal artery, thereby permitting a modified Appleby procedure (although some members of the consensus committee preferred this criterion to be in the unresectable category)
Unresectable/locally advanced	• Head of pancreas or uncinate lesions: 1. Solid tumor contact with the SMA >180 degrees 2. Solid tumor contact with the celiac axis >180 degrees 3. Solid tumor contact with the first jejunal SMA branch 4. Unreconstructable SMV or portal vein because of tumor involvement or occlusion (can be because of tumor or bland thrombus) 5. Contact with the most proximal draining jejunal branch into the SMV • Body and tail lesions: 1. Solid tumor contact of >180 degrees with the SMA or celiac axis 2. Solid tumor contact with the celiac axis and aortic involvement 3. Unreconstructable SMV or portal vein because of tumor involvement or occlusion (can be because of tumor or bland thrombus) • For all sites: 1. Distant metastases 2. Metastases to lymph nodes beyond the field of resection
Metastatic	• Any presence of distant metastases

IVC, Inferior vena cava; *SMA,* spinal muscular atrophy; *SMV,* superior mesenteric vein.
From Niederhuber JE: *Abeloff's clinical oncology*, ed 6, Philadelphia, 2020, Elsevier.

Diseases and Disorders

adenocarcinoma (PDAC) in the 3 yr after diagnosis. About 20% of patients with PDAC have NOD, and about 1% of patients with NOD will be diagnosed with PDAC in the 3 yr after NOD.[1]

- The U.S. Preventive Services Task Force (USPSTF) recommends against routine screening for pancreatic cancer in asymptomatic adults by abdominal palpation, ultrasonography, or serologic markers. The USPSTF found no evidence that screening for pancreatic cancer is effective in reducing mortality rates. There is potential for significant harm because of the low prevalence of pancreatic cancer, limited accuracy of available screening tests, invasive nature of diagnostic tests, and poor outcome of treatment. Alcohol consumption, specifically liquor consumption of three or more drinks per day, increases pancreatic cancer mortality independent of smoking.
- Patients should be referred for pancreatic cancer surgery to high-volume medical centers that perform at least 15 to 20 cases a yr.

[1]Chari ST et al: Early detection of sporadic pancreatic ductal adenocarcina: problems, promise, and prospects, *Ann Intern Med* 172(8):558-559, 2020.

SUGGESTED READINGS

Available at ExpertConsult.com

RELATED CONTENT

Pancreatic Cancer (Patient Information)

AUTHOR: **Ritesh Rathore, MD**

TABLE 5 Acceptable Chemotherapy Regimens for Locally Advanced and Metastatic Disease[a]

Locally Advanced or Unresectable	Metastatic Disease
Options for patients with good performance status: • FOLFIRINOX • Gemcitabine + albumin bound-paclitaxel • Gemcitabine + erlotinib • Gemcitabine + capecitabine • Gemcitabine + cisplatin (especially in patients with *BRCA1/2* mutation and/or family history) • Capecitabine single agent • CI 5-FU • Fixed-dose gemcitabine/docetaxel/capecitabine (GTX regimen) • Fluoropyrimidine + oxaliplatin • Chemotherapy (any of above) followed by chemoradiation or SBRT • Chemoradiation or SBRT	Options for patients with good performance status: • FOLFIRINOX (category 1) • Gemcitabine + albumin bound-paclitaxel (category 1) • Gemcitabine + erlotinib (category 1) • Gemcitabine (category 1) • Gemcitabine + capecitabine • Gemcitabine + cisplatin (especially in patients with *BRCA1/2* mutation and/or family history) • Fixed-dose gemcitabine/docetaxel/capecitabine (GTX regimen) (category 2B) • Fluoropyrimidine + oxaliplatin (category 2B)
Options for patients with poor performance status: • Gemcitabine • Capecitabine • CI 5-FU	Options for patients with poor performance status: • Gemcitabine (category 1) • Capecitabine (category 2B) • CI 5-FU (category 2B)

[a]Level of Recommendation is based on National Comprehensive Cancer Network (NCCN) Guidelines. Category 1 is based on high-level evidence with uniform NCCN consensus that the intervention is appropriate. Category 2B is based on lower level evidence with NCCN consensus that the intervention is appropriate.
CI, Continuous infusion; *5-FU,* 5-fluoroacil; *FOLFIRINOX,* 5-FU, irinotecan, oxaliplatin; *GTX,* gemcitabine, docetaxel, capecitabine; *SBRT,* stereotactic body radiation therapy.
From Niederhuber JE: *Abeloff's clinical oncology*, ed 6, Philadelphia, 2020, Elsevier.

TABLE 6 Risk Factors for Pancreatic Cancer

Risk Factor	Relative Increase in Risk
High Risk (>10-fold)	
FAMMM	13- to 47-fold
Hereditary pancreatitis	50- to 83-fold
Peutz-Jeghers syndrome	132-fold
Three or more first-degree relatives with PC	14- to 32-fold
Moderate Risk (5- To 10-fold)	
Two first-degree relatives with PC	4- to 6.4-fold
Cystic fibrosis	5.3-fold
Chronic pancreatitis	2- to 19-fold
BRCA2 mutation carrier	3.5- to 10-fold
PALB2 mutation carrier	6-fold
Low Risk (<5-fold)	
Cigarette smoking	1.5- to 3-fold
Alcohol consumption	None to 1.2-fold
Obesity	None to 1.7-fold
Diabetes mellitus	1.3- to 2.6-fold
One first-degree relative with PC	3-fold
BRCA1 mutation carrier	None to 2-fold
Familial adenomatous polyposis	4-fold
Li-Fraumeni syndrome	2-fold
Lynch syndrome	2- to 8-fold

FAMMM, Familial atypical multiple-mole melanoma; *PC,* pancreatic cancer.
From Niederhuber JE: *Abeloff's clinical oncology*, ed 6, Philadelphia, 2020, Elsevier.

TABLE 7 Recommendations for Screening

HRIs To Consider for Screening
FAMMM patients with *CDKN2A*
Patients with hereditary pancreatitis
Patients with hereditary PJS
Three or more first-, second-, or third-degree relatives with PC with at least one being a first-degree relative
Two or more first-degree relatives with PC
BRCA1, BRCA2, or *PALB2* mutation carriers with at least one first- or second-degree relative with PC

Age to Start Screening
Age 45-50 yr *or* 15 yr before age of earliest occurrence of PC in the family (whichever is earliest)
Consider age 30 yr for patients with PJS

FAMMM, Familial atypical multiple-mole melanoma; *HRI,* high-risk individual; *PC,* pancreatic cancer; *PJS,* Peutz-Jeghers syndrome.
From Niederhuber JE: *Abeloff's clinical oncology*, ed 6, Philadelphia, 2020, Elsevier.

BASIC INFORMATION

DEFINITION

- Acute pancreatitis is an inflammatory process of the pancreas with intrapancreatic activation of enzymes that may also involve peripancreatic tissue and/or remote organ systems. The diagnosis of acute pancreatitis requires at least two of the following criteria: Serum amylase or lipase ≥3 times normal, abdominal pain consistent with pancreatitis, and radiographic findings (CT or MRI) of acute pancreatitis.
- Commonly used scoring systems for acute pancreatitis are described in Table 1.
- The **Revised Atlanta Criteria**[1] use early prognostic signs, organ failure, and local complications to define disease severity:
  1. **Mild pancreatitis:** No organ failure, no local or systemic complications, pancreatitis typically resolves in first wk
  2. **Moderate pancreatitis:** Transient organ failure (≤48 hr) *or* local complications (e.g., pancreatic necrosis, peripancreatic fluid collections, peripancreatic necrosis) *or* exacerbation of comorbid disease
  3. **Severe pancreatitis:** Persistent organ failure (>48 hr)
- The **BALI Score**[2] evaluates only four variables:
  1. BUN ≥25 mg/dl
  2. Age ≥65 yr
  3. LDH ≥300 U/L
  4. Interleukin-6 level ≥300 pg/ml
- These measurements are taken at admission and at 48 hr. Mortality is >25% for a score of 3 and exceeds 50% with a score of 4.
- **Severe acute pancreatitis (SAP)** is diagnosed by the presence of any of the following four criteria:
  1. Organ failure with one or more of the following: Shock (systolic blood pressure <90 mm Hg), pulmonary insufficiency (Pao_2 ≤60 mm Hg), renal failure (serum creatinine >2 mg/dl after rehydration), and gastrointestinal bleeding (>500 ml/24 hr)
  2. Local complications such as necrosis, pseudocyst, or abscess
  3. At least three of Ranson criteria (see tables) *or*
  4. At least eight of the Acute Physiology and Chronic Health Evaluation II (APACHE II) criteria

ICD-10CM CODES

K85.0 Idiopathic acute pancreatitis
K85.1 Biliary acute pancreatitis
K85.2 Alcohol-induced acute pancreatitis
K 85.3 Drug-induced pancreatitis
K85.6 Other acute pancreatitis
K85.9 Acute pancreatitis, unspecified

EPIDEMIOLOGY & DEMOGRAPHICS

- The incidence of pancreatitis is increasing in the U.S. Admissions for acute pancreatitis have increased dramatically, and acute pancreatitis was the number-one GI-related cause for admission across U.S. hospitals in 2012. There are >270,000 cases of acute pancreatitis reported annually in the U.S., with 40%+ resulting from gallstone disease (most common cause) and 30% caused by alcohol consumption.
- Incidence in urban areas is twice that of rural areas (20/100,000 persons in urban areas).
- 20% of patients have necrotizing pancreatitis; the remainder have interstitial, or edematous, pancreatitis.
- Drugs are responsible for less than 5% of all cases of acute pancreatitis.

PHYSICAL FINIDINGS & CLINICAL PRESENTATION

- Epigastric tenderness and guarding, often radiating to the back; pain usually developing suddenly, reaching peak intensity within 10 to 30 min, severe and lasting several hours without relief. Rarely, some patients can have painless severe pancreatitis
- Nausea and vomiting (up to 90% of cases)
- Hypoactive bowel sounds (from ileus)
- Tachycardia, shock (from decreased intravascular volume)
- Confusion (from metabolic disturbances)
- Fever (SIRS response or infection when pancreatic necrosis is present)
- Decreased breath sounds (pleural effusions) or rales (atelectasis, acute respiratory distress syndrome [ARDS])
- Jaundice (from obstruction or compression of biliary tract)
- Ascites (from tear in pancreatic duct, leaking pseudocyst)
- Palpable abdominal mass (pseudocyst, phlegmon, abscess, carcinoma)
- Evidence of hypocalcemia (Chvostek sign, Trousseau sign)
- Evidence of retroperitoneal bleeding (hemorrhagic pancreatitis):
  1. Ecchymosis around the umbilicus **(Cullen sign)**
  2. Ecchymosis involving the flanks **(Grey Turner sign)**
- Tender subcutaneous nodules (caused by subcutaneous fat necrosis)

TABLE 1 Commonly Used Scoring Systems: Advantages and Disadvantages

System	Scoring	Advantages	Disadvantages
Ranson criteria on admission: 1. Age >55 yr 2. WBC >16 × 10^9/L 3. LDH >350 U/L 4. AST >250 U/L 5. Glucose >200 mg/dl During initial 48 hr: 1. Hgb falls below 10 mg/dl 2. BUN rises by >5 mg/dl 3. Ca <8 mg/dl 4. Pao_2 <60 mm Hg 5. Base deficit >4 mEq/L 6. Fluid sequestration >6 L	One point for each factor listed; score >3 indicates SAP	Well known, relatively easy to calculate	Requires 48 hr to complete evaluation
APACHE II*	Score >8 predicts SAP	Can be calculated within 24 hr of admission	Requires large dataset for processing
BISAP 1. BUN >25 mg/dl 2. Altered mental status 3. Presence of SIRS 4. Age >60 yr 5. Pleural effusions	One point for each factor listed; score >3 indicates SAP	Ease of use, available within 24 hr of admission	Significantly lower sensitivity than either Ranson or APACHE II; results in greater likelihood of missing severe AP
CTSI	Based on radiographic data	Excellent predictor of local complications; can show infected pancreatic necrosis	Requires 72 to 96 hr, making it a poor test for guiding decisions at admission

*Based on diverse variables, including age, physiology, and long-term health; equation available at https://sfar.org/scores2/apache22.php. Adding body mass index (BMI) to APACHE II (the APACHE 0 score) increases discrimination (1 point added for BMI 26-30; 2 points for BMI >30).

AP, Acute pancreatitis; *APACHE,* Acute Physiology and Chronic Health Evaluation; *AST,* aspartate aminotransferase; *BISAP,* Bedside Index for Severity in Acute Pancreatitis; *BUN,* blood urea nitrogen; *Ca,* serum calcium; *CTSI,* Computed Tomography Severity Index; *Hgb,* hemoglobin; *LDH,* lactate dehydrogenase; *SAP,* severe acute pancreatitis; *SIRS,* systemic inflammatory response syndrome; *WBC,* white blood cell count.

From Cameron JL, Cameron AM: *Current surgical therapy,* ed 10, Philadelphia, 2011, Saunders.

[1] Banks PA et al: Acute Pancreatitis Classification Working Group: classification of acute pancreatitis-2012: revision of the Atlanta classification and definitions by international consensus, *Gut* 62(1):102-111, 2013.

[2] Spitzer AL et al: Applying Ockham's razor to pancreatitis prognostication: a four-variable predictive model, *Ann Surg* 243(3):380-388, 2006.

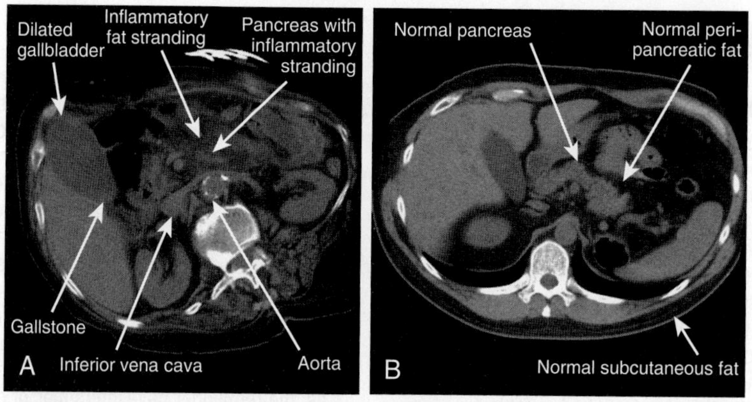

FIG. 1 Gallstone pancreatitis and normal pancreas for comparison, axial computed tomography without contrast. A, Gallstone pancreatitis CT. A dilated gallbladder is visible with a hyperdense dependent lesion consistent with a gallstone. The region of the pancreas shows significant inflammatory stranding. In this patient the pancreas lies just anterior to the left renal vein, which can be seen crossing anterior to the aorta and entering the inferior vena cava. **B,** A normal pancreas is visible. This pancreas is surrounded by uninflamed fat, which is dark (nearly black). Compare this normal fat with normal subcutaneous fat. (From Broder JS: *Diagnostic imaging for the emergency physician,* Philadelphia, 2011, Saunders.)

ETIOLOGY

- The most common causes of acute pancreatitis are gallstones (40% of cases) and excessive alcohol consumption (30% of cases). Alcohol-related pancreatitis is most common after long term (>10 yr of heavy drinking)
- Hypertriglyceridemia (usually >1000 mg/dl) from any cause
- Drugs (e.g., thiazides, furosemide, corticosteroids, tetracycline, estrogens, valproic acid, metronidazole, azathioprine, methyldopa, pentamidine, ethacrynic acid, procainamide, amiodarone, sulindac, nitrofurantoin, angiotensin-converting enzyme inhibitors, danazol, cimetidine, piroxicam, gold, ranitidine, sulfasalazine, isoniazid, acetaminophen, cisplatin, didanosine, opiates, erythromycin, metformin, GLP-1 receptor agonists, incretin mimetics)
- Abdominal trauma
- Surgery
- Endoscopic retrograde cholangiopancreatography (ERCP), especially with manipulation of the pancreatic duct
- Infections (predominantly viral)
- Peptic ulcer (penetrating duodenal ulcer)
- Pancreas divisum (congenital failure to fuse of dorsal or ventral pancreas)
- Idiopathic
- Pregnancy
- Vascular (vasculitis, ischemic)
- Hypercalcemia
- Pancreatic carcinoma (primary or metastatic)
- Renal failure
- Hereditary pancreatitis, such as in patients with cystic fibrosis
- IgG4 disease
- Occupational exposure to chemicals: Methanol, cobalt, zinc, mercuric chloride, creosol, lead, organophosphates, chlorinated naphthalenes
- Others: Scorpion venom, obstruction at ampulla region (neoplasm, duodenal diverticula, Crohn disease, rarely celiac disease), hypotensive shock, autoimmune pancreatitis

DIAGNOSIS

DIFFERENTIAL DIAGNOSIS

- PUD
- Acute cholangitis, biliary colic
- High intestinal obstruction
- Early acute appendicitis
- DKA
- Pneumonia (basilar)
- Myocardial infarction (inferior wall)
- Renal colic
- Ruptured or dissecting aortic aneurysm
- Mesenteric ischemia

LABORATORY TESTS

Pancreatic enzymes:

- Amylase is increased, usually elevated in the initial 3 to 5 days of acute pancreatitis. Isoamylase determinations (separation of pancreatic cell isoenzyme components of amylase) are useful in excluding occasional cases of salivary hyperamylasemia. The use of isoamylase rather than total serum amylase reduces the risk of erroneously diagnosing pancreatitis and is preferred by some as initial biochemical test in patients suspected of having acute pancreatitis.
- Urinary amylase determinations are useful to diagnose acute pancreatitis in patients with lipemic serum, to rule out elevated serum amylase caused by macroamylasemia, and to diagnose acute pancreatitis in patients whose serum amylase is normal.
- Serum lipase levels are elevated in acute pancreatitis; the elevation is less transient than serum amylase and more sensitive in patients with alcoholic pancreatitis. Concomitant evaluation of serum amylase and lipase does not improve diagnostic accuracy of acute pancreatitis. Serial measurements have limited usefulness because levels are not predictors of severity. Elevated serum trypsin levels are diagnostic of pancreatitis (in absence of renal failure).
- Serum C-reactive protein is an excellent laboratory marker of severity; a level >150 mg/dl at 48 hr is associated with severe pancreatitis.
- Rapid measurement of urinary trypsinogen-2 (if available) is useful in the emergency department as a screening test for acute pancreatitis in patients with abdominal pain; a negative dipstick test for urinary trypsinogen-2 rules out acute pancreatitis with a high degree of probability, whereas a positive test indicates need for further evaluation.
- Interleukin-6 level: Worse prognosis with level ≥300 pg/ml.

ADDITIONAL TESTS

- Complete blood count: Reveals leukocytosis; hematocrit (Hct) may be initially increased as a result of hemoconcentration; decreased Hct may indicate hemorrhage or hemolysis.
- Blood urea nitrogen (BUN) is increased because of dehydration. Serial BUN measurements are the most valuable lab test for predicting mortality during the initial 48 hr.
- Elevation of serum glucose in a previously normal patient correlates with the degree of pancreatic malfunction and may be related to increased release of glycogen, catecholamines, and glucocorticoid release and decreased insulin release.
- Liver profile: Aspartate aminotransferase (AST) and lactate dehydrogenase (LDH) are increased as a result of tissue necrosis; bilirubin and alkaline phosphatase may be increased from common bile duct obstruction. A threefold or greater rise in serum alanine aminotransferase concentrations is an excellent indicator (95% probability) of biliary pancreatitis.
- Serum calcium is decreased because of saponification, precipitation, and decreased parathyroid hormone response.
- Arterial blood gases: Pa_{O_2} may be decreased as a result of ARDS, pleural effusion(s); pH may be decreased as a result of lactic acidosis, respiratory acidosis, and renal insufficiency.
- Serum electrolytes: Potassium may be increased from acidosis or renal insufficiency; sodium may be increased from dehydration.

IMAGING STUDIES

- Abdominal plain films are useful initially to distinguish other conditions that may mimic pancreatitis (perforated viscus). They may reveal localized ileus (sentinel loop), pancreatic calcifications (chronic pancreatitis), blurring of left psoas shadow, dilation of transverse colon, calcified gallstones.
- Chest x-ray may reveal elevation of one or both diaphragms, pleural effusions, basilar infiltrates, or platelike atelectasis.
- Abdominal ultrasonography is useful in detecting gallstones (sensitivity of 60% to 70% for detecting stones associated with pancreatitis). Its availability and noninvasive nature make it the initial imaging study of choice; its major limitation is the presence

TABLE 2 Computed Tomography (CT) Severity Index Score for Pancreatitis*

Grade†	CT Findings	Score
A	Normal pancreas	0
B	Focal or diffuse enlargement of the pancreas, contour irregularities, heterogeneous attenuation, no peripancreatic inflammation	1
C	Grade B plus peripancreatic inflammation	2
D	Grade C plus a single fluid collection	3
E	Grade C plus multiple fluid collections or gas	4
Percent Necrosis Present on CT		
0		
<33		
33-50		
>50		

*Severity Index Score = Grade score + Percent necrosis score. Maximum score = 10; severe disease = 6 or higher.
†Severity of the acute inflammatory process.
From Adams JG et al: *Emergency medicine, clinical essentials,* ed 2, Philadelphia, 2013, Elsevier.

of distended bowel loops overlying the pancreas.

- CT scan (Fig. 1) is less sensitive than ultrasound in identifying gallstones and exposes the patient to risk of contrast-induced nephropathy. It is, however, superior to ultrasonography in identifying pancreatitis and defining its extent, and it also plays a role in diagnosing pseudocysts (they appear as a well-defined area surrounded by a high-density capsule); gastrointestinal fistulization or infection of a pseudocyst can also be identified by the presence of gas within the pseudocyst. Sequential contrast-enhanced CT is useful for detection of pancreatic necrosis. The severity of pancreatitis can also be graded by CT scan (Table 2). (A = normal pancreas, B = enlarged pancreas [1 point], C = pancreatic and/or peripancreatic inflammation [2 points], D = single peripancreatic collection [3 points], E = at least two peripancreatic collections and/or retroperitoneal air [4 points]. Percentage of pancreatic necrosis <30% [2 points], 30% to 50% [4 points], >50% [6 points]. The CT severity index is calculated by adding grade points to points assigned for percentage of necrosis.)
- Magnetic resonance cholangiopancreatography (MRCP) has >90% sensitivity for choledocholithiasis and can identify other anatomic abnormalities.
- Endoscopic ultrasonography (EUS) is a minimally invasive test that provides high-resolution imaging of the pancreas. It is useful to identify anatomic abnormalities of the pancreas and has good sensitivity and specificity for small gallstones (≤5 mm).
- ERCP indications: Useful to perform biliary sphincterotomy and stone removal in the presence of a retained bile duct stone seen on imaging. The role and timing of ERCP in patients with acute biliary pancreatitis has been controversial. Guidelines from the American College of Gastroenterology suggest that urgent ERCP (within 24 hr of admission) is indicated in patients with biliary pancreatitis who have concurrent acute cholangitis, but it is not needed in most patients who do not have evidence of ongoing biliary obstruction.[3,4,5]

Rx TREATMENT

NONPHARMACOLOGIC THERAPY

- Bowel rest with avoidance of liquids or solids during the acute illness. Limited data suggest that early feeding in patients with acute pancreatitis does not seem to increase adverse events and, for patients with mild to moderate pancreatitis, may reduce length of hospital stay.[6]
- Avoidance of alcohol and any drugs associated with pancreatitis.

ACUTE GENERAL Rx

GENERAL MEASURES:

- Assess severity of pancreatitis (see Table 1).
- An algorithm for the management of acute pancreatitis is described in Fig. 2.
- Maintain adequate intravascular volume with vigorous IV hydration. Aggressive fluid resuscitation (250 to 500 ml/hr) with isotonic crystalloids is critical in managing acute pancreatitis, unless cardiac or renal disease precludes it.
- Patient should remain NPO until clinically improved, stable, and hungry. Enteral feedings are preferred over total parenteral nutrition if supplemental nutrition is necessary. Enteral nutrition reduces mortality, multiple organ failure, systemic infections, and operative interventions more than total parenteral nutrition does in patients with acute pancreatitis. Parenteral nutrition may be necessary in patients who do not tolerate enteral feeding or in whom an adequate infusion rate cannot be reached within 2 to 4 days. Early (within 24 to 48 hr of admission) enteral feeding through a nasogastric (NG) feeding tube has limited evidence to support this strategy. A recent trial did not show superiority of early NG tube feeding, as compared with oral diet after 72 hr, in reducing the rate of infection or death in patients with acute pancreatitis at high risk for complications.
- Nasogastric suction is useful only in severe pancreatitis to decompress the abdomen in patients with ileus.
- Control pain: IV hydromorphone or fentanyl. Meperidine and morphine are also commonly used narcotics for pain control, although morphine has been shown to increase sphincter of Oddi pressure and has delayed metabolite clearance in patients with concomitant renal failure.
- Correct metabolic abnormalities (e.g., replace calcium and magnesium as necessary).
- Prophylactic antibiotics are not recommended, regardless of the severity or presence of pancreatic necrosis.
- An algorithm for the management of acute pancreatitis at various stages is described in Fig. 2.

SPECIFIC MEASURES:

- Pancreatic or peripancreatic infection develops in 30% of patients with pancreatic necrosis. The use of antibiotics is justified if the patient has evidence of septicemia, pancreatic abscess, or pancreatitis caused by biliary calculi with concomitant cholangitis. Their use should generally be limited to 5 to 7 days to prevent development of fungal superinfection. Appropriate empiric antibiotic therapy should penetrate pancreatic necrosis. Options include a carbapenem alone (due to anaerobic coverage) or a quinolone, ceftazidime, or cefepime, combined with an enteric anaerobic agent such as metronidazole. CT-guided fine-needle aspiration (FNA) can be performed to culture the infected necrosis and tailor antibiotic therapy. If sampling of infected necrosis occurs and is sterile, antibiotics should be discontinued
- Surgical therapy has a limited role in acute pancreatitis; it is indicated in the following:
  1. Gallstone-induced pancreatitis: Cholecystectomy when acute pancreatitis subsides. However, randomized trials have shown that patients with mild gallstone pancreatitis can undergo cholecystectomy safely during the first 48 hr of hospitalization
  2. Perforated peptic ulcer
  3. Necrotizing pancreatitis with infected necrotic tissue is associated with an elevated rate of complications and increased risk of death. Traditional treatment has been open necrosectomy; surgical necrosectomy induces a proinflammatory response and is associated with a high complication rate. Recent trials have shown that a step-up approach consisting of percutaneous drainage followed, if necessary, by minimally invasive retroperitoneal necrosectomy may have a lower rate of complications and

[3] Fogel EL, Sherman S: ERCP for gallstone pancreatitis, *N Engl J Med* 370:150-157, 2014.
[4] Tenner S et al: American College of Gastroenterology guidelines: management of acute pancreatitis, *Am J Gastroenterol* 108:1400-1415, 2013.
[5] Bakker OJ et al: Early versus on-demand nasogastric tube feeding in acute pancreatitis, *N Engl J Med* 371:1983-1993, 2014.
[6] Vaughn VM et al: Early versus delayed feeding in patients with acute pancreatitis, a systematic review, *Ann Intern Med* 66:883-892, 2017.

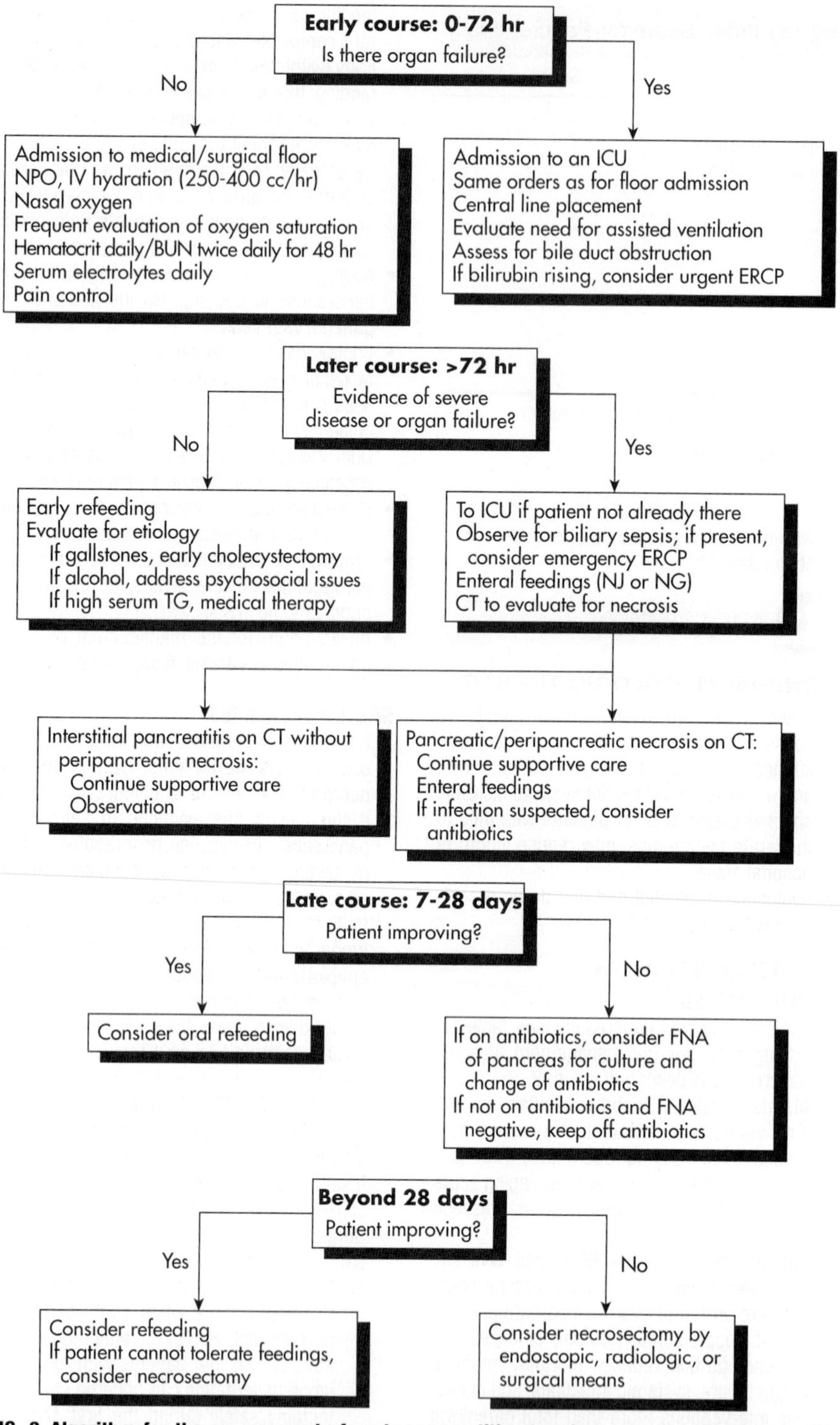

FIG. 2 Algorithm for the management of acute pancreatitis at various stages in its course. *NJ,* Nasojejunal. (From Feldman M et al: *Sleisenger and Fordtran's gastrointestinal and liver disease*, ed 10, Philadelphia, 2016, Elsevier.)

death. Endoscopic transgastric necrosectomy, a form of natural orifice transluminal endoscopic surgery, has been shown in recent trials to be effective in reducing the proinflammatory response as well as reducing complications

- Identification and treatment of complications:
  1. **Pseudocyst:** Round or spheroid collection of fluid, tissue, pancreatic enzymes, and blood
     a. Diagnosed by CT scan or sonography.
     b. Treatment: Pancreatic pseudocysts can be drained surgically or endoscopically. The endoscopic approach is preferable when the patient's anatomy is suitable and an experienced endoscopist is available. CT scan or ultrasound-guided percutaneous drainage (with a pigtail catheter left in place for continuous drainage) can be used, but the recurrence rate is high; the conservative approach is to reevaluate the pseudocyst (with CT scan or sonography) after 6 to 7 wk and surgically drain it if the pseudocyst has not decreased in size.
     c. Generally, pseudocysts <5 cm in diameter are reabsorbed without intervention, whereas those >5 cm require surgical intervention after the wall has matured.
  2. **Phlegmon:** Represents pancreatic edema. It can be diagnosed by CT scan or sonography. Treatment is supportive as it usually resolves spontaneously
  3. **Pancreatic abscess:** Diagnosed by CT scan (presence of air in the retroperitoneum); Gram staining and cultures of fluid obtained from guided percutaneous aspiration usually identify bacterial organism. Therapy is surgical (or catheter) drainage and IV antibiotics (carbapenem is the drug of choice)
  4. **Pancreatic ascites:** Usually caused by leaking of pseudocyst or tear in pancreatic duct. Paracentesis reveals very high amylase and lipase levels in the pancreatic fluid; ERCP may demonstrate the lesion. Treatment is surgical correction if exudative ascites from severe pancreatitis does not resolve spontaneously
  5. **Abdominal compartment syndrome:** Caused by intraabdominal leakage of fluids from volume resuscitation or ascites. Diagnosed with sustained intraabdominal pressure >20 mm Hg with new-onset organ failure
  6. **Gastrointestinal bleeding:** Caused by alcoholic gastritis, bleeding varices, stress ulceration, or disseminated intravascular coagulation (DIC)
  7. **Renal failure:** Caused by hypovolemia, resulting in oliguria or anuria, cortical or tubular necrosis (shock, DIC), or thrombosis of renal artery or vein
  8. **Hypoxia:** Caused by ARDS, pleural effusion, or atelectasis
  9. **Vascular:** Splenic, portal, or superior mesenteric vein thrombosis; pseudoaneurysm

THERAPY OF UNCOMMON FORMS OF PANCREATITIS

- **Autoimmune pancreatitis (AIP):** Fibroinflammatory disease characterized by an IgG4 lymphoplasmacytic infiltrate. It is a variant of chronic pancreatitis and has been associated with other autoimmune disorders (e.g., primary sclerosing cholangitis, Sjögren syndrome). The inflammatory process is generally responsive to corticosteroid therapy. Older men aged 60 to 70 yr are primarily affected. Patients present with abdominal pain, weight loss, anorexia, and obstructive jaundice. Immunoglobulin G_4 levels are elevated. Radiographically on CT, the pancreas is diffusely enlarged, with a characteristic smooth, capsulelike rim ("sausage pancreas"). Features of type 1 and type 2

TABLE 3 Features of Type 1 and Type 2 Autoimmune Pancreatitis

Feature	Type 1	Type 2
Histology	Lymphoplasmacytic infiltration Dense periductal infiltrate without damage to ductal epithelium Storiform fibrosis Obliterative phlebitis Abundant (>10 cells/HPF) IgG4-positive cells Fibroinflammatory process may extend to peripancreatic region	Periductal lymphoplasmacytic and neutrophilic infiltration Destruction of the duct epithelium by neutrophils (granulocytic epithelial lesion, or GEL) Obliterative phlebitis is rare No IgG4-positive cells
Average age at presentation	60-70 yr	40-50, but may present in young adults and even children
Gender predominance	Male	Equal
Usual clinical presentations	Obstructive jaundice (75%) Acute pancreatitis (15%)	Obstructive jaundice (50%) Acute pancreatitis (33%)
Pancreatic imaging	Diffuse pancreatic enlargement (40%) Focal pancreatic enlargement (60%)	Diffuse pancreatic enlargement (15%) Focal pancreatic enlargement (85%)
IgG4	Level elevated in serum (~2/3 of patients) Positive in staining of involved tissues	Not associated
Other organ involvement	Biliary strictures Pseudotumors Kidney Lung Others Retroperitoneal fibrosis Sialoadenitis	Not associated
Associated diseases	See above (other organ involvement)	IBD
Long-term outcome	Frequent relapses	Rare or no relapse

HPF, High power field; *IBD,* inflammatory bowel disease; *IgG4,* Immunoglobulin G, subclass 4.
From Feldman M et al: *Sleisenger and Fordtran's gastrointestinal and liver disease,* ed 10, Philadelphia, 2016, Elsevier.

TABLE 4 Prognostic Criteria for Acute Pancreatitis

Ranson Criteria*	Simplified Glasgow Criteria†	Computed Tomography Criteria‡
On admission: Age >55 yr	*Within 48 hr of admission:* Age >55 yr	Normal
WBC >16,000/μL	WBC >15,000/μL	Enlargement
AST >250 U/L LDH >350 U/L	LDH >600 U/L	Pancreatic inflammation
Glucose >200 mg/dl	Glucose >180 mg/dl	Single fluid collection
48 hr after admission:	Albumin <3.2 g/dl	Multiple fluid collection
Hematocrit decrease by >10	Ca^{2+} <8 mg/dl	
BUN increase by >5 mg/dl	Arterial Po_2 <60 mm Hg	
Ca^{2+} <8 mg/dl	BUN >45 mg/dl	
Arterial Po_2 <60 mm Hg		
Base deficit >4 mEq/L		
Fluid sequestration >6 L		

*Three or more Ranson criteria predict a complicated clinical course. Data from Ranson JH et al: Prognostic signs and nonoperative peritoneal lavage in acute pancreatitis, *Surg Gynecol Obstet* 143:209-219, 1976.
†Data from Blamey SL et al: Prognostic factors in acute pancreatitis, *Gut* 25:1340, 1984.
‡Grades A and B represent mild disease with no risk of infection or death. Grade C represents moderately severe disease with a minimal likelihood of infection and essentially no risk of mortality. Grades D and E represent severe pancreatitis with an infection rate of 30% to 50% and mortality rate of 15%. Data from Balthazar EJ et al: Acute pancreatitis value of CT in establishing prognosis, *Radiology,* 174:331, 1990.
AST, Aspartate aminotransferase; *BUN,* blood urea nitrogen; *LDH,* lactate dehydrogenase; *WBC,* white blood cells.
From Goldman L, Ausiello D (eds): *Cecil textbook of medicine,* ed 24, Philadelphia, 2012, Saunders.

autoimmune pancreatitis are summarized in Table 3. Type II autoimmune hepatitis (idiopathic duct-centric chronic pancreatitis) is associated with inflammatory bowel disease and not related to IgG4 cell deposition.

- **Hypertriglyceridemic pancreatitis (HTGP):** IV insulin therapy is the cornerstone of immediate treatment, with supplemental IV glucose infusion if the serum glucose levels are not elevated. IV heparin was previously used as well, but its effectiveness has come into question. Antihyperlipidemic agents (fibrates) should be initiated as adjuvant therapy as soon as possible for long-term control. Beneficial results have been reported with early (within 48 hr) initiation of apheresis with therapeutic plasma exchange when there is concomitant hypocalcemia, lactic acidosis, or other signs of organ dysfunction.

DISPOSITION

Prognosis varies with the severity of pancreatitis; overall mortality rate in acute pancreatitis is 5% to 10%. Prognostic criteria for acute pancreatitis are described in Table 4.

REFERRAL

- Hospitalization is indicated in moderate to severe cases of pancreatitis.
- Surgical consultation is needed in suspected gallstone pancreatitis, perforated peptic ulcer, or presence of necrotic or infected foci. Acute pancreatitis can generally be attributed to gallstones when patients have both abnormal liver enzymes and gallstones (or sludge) on imaging. Such patients should consider cholecystectomy prior to discharge to prevent recurrent pancreatitis.
- Gastroenterology consultation in severe or recurrent pancreatitis, when ERCP is needed for gallstone pancreatitis, or when the cause of pancreatitis is unclear.
- Consider intensive care unit transfer for patients who require aggressive fluid resuscitation and are at risk of volume overload from cardiac or renal causes. Similarly, consider transfer for patients with developing ARDS, patients with abdominal compartment syndrome (with surgical consultation), and those who require apheresis.

PEARLS & CONSIDERATIONS

- Acute pancreatitis is the most common major complication of ERCP. NSAIDs are potent inhibitors of phospholipase A_2, cyclooxygenase, and neutrophil-endothelial interactions, which play an important role in the pathogenesis of acute pancreatitis. Preliminary trials show that among patients at high risk for post-ERCP pancreatitis, rectal indomethacin (given as two 50-mg indomethacin suppositories administered immediately after ERCP) significantly reduced the incidence of post-ERCP pancreatitis.
- Pancreatic stent placement decreases the risk of post-ERCP pancreatitis.
- Statins reduce risk for pancreatitis in adults. Fibrates do not affect risk for pancreatitis other than in patients with hypertriglyceridemia-induced pancreatitis.
- Diabetes mellitus may develop from extensive pancreatic necrosis.

SUGGESTED READINGS

Available at ExpertConsult.com

RELATED CONTENT

Acute Pancreatitis (Patient Information)

AUTHOR: **David J. Lucier Jr, MD, MBA, MPH**

BASIC INFORMATION

DEFINITION

- A **panic attack** is a relatively brief, sudden episode of intense fear or apprehension, often associated with a sense of impending doom and various uncomfortable and disquieting physical symptoms. Panic attacks may be unexpected ("out of the blue") or expected (i.e., triggered by a particular object or situation). Panic attacks may be present in a variety of different anxiety-related disorders (e.g., phobias, social anxiety, obsessive-compulsive disorder). Table E1 describes criteria for diagnosis of panic attack.
- **Panic disorder** is diagnosed after at least two uncued panic attacks have occurred followed by at least 1 mo (or more) of significant concern about future attacks, worry about their implications, or a major change in behavior related to these attacks. The criteria for diagnosis of panic disorder are summarized in Table E2.
- **Agoraphobia** is anxiety about, and avoidance of, places or situations in which the ability to escape is perceived to be limited or embarrassing or in which help might not be available in the event of having a panic attack. Starting with DSM-5, agoraphobia is considered a disorder separate from panic disorder (Table E3).

SYNONYMS

Anxiety attacks
Fear attacks
Ataque de nervios

ICD-10CM CODES
F41.0 Panic disorder
F40.0 Agoraphobia
DSM-5 CODES
300.01 Panic disorder
300.22 Agoraphobia

EPIDEMIOLOGY & DEMOGRAPHICS

INCIDENCE (IN U.S.): 1% 1-mo incidence of panic attacks

PREVALENCE (IN U.S.):
- 15% to 20% lifetime prevalence of one or more panic attacks.
- Panic disorder is much less common, with a lifetime prevalence of 3.8%; the chronicity of panic disorder is reflected in a similar 1-yr prevalence rate of 2.4%.
- Agoraphobia with or without panic disorder is relatively rare; 2.5% lifetime prevalence.
- Lower rates of panic disorder are reported among Latinos, African Americans, Caribbean blacks, and Asian Americans (DSM-5).
- Estimates of panic disorder prevalence for Asian, African, and Latin American countries are lower (0.2% to 1.7%; WHO).

PREDOMINANT SEX:
- Panic disorder twice as common in women.
- Panic disorder with comorbid agoraphobia three times as common in women.

PREDOMINANT AGE:
- Age of onset is typically late adolescence to mid-30s. Onset earlier in males (24 yr) than females (28 yr). Some may experience onset later in life.
- Onset after age 45 yr is rare and should raise suspicion of different etiology.

PEAK INCIDENCE:
- Chronic condition with a waxing and waning course.
- Bimodal incidence peaks noted, with the first peak between ages 15 and 24 yr and second peak between ages 35 and 44 yr.

GENETICS:
- Risk of developing panic disorder in first-degree relatives of individuals with panic disorder is four to seven times that of general population.
- Findings in twin studies: Heritability estimates for panic disorder range from 28% to 50%.

PHYSICAL FINDINGS & CLINICAL PRESENTATION

Panic disorder:
- Presents either with a panic attack or with fear and anxiety related to anticipation of a future panic attack or its implications.
- Typical presentation: Unexpected, untriggered periods of intense anxiety and fear with associated physiologic changes (e.g., palpitations, sweating, tremulousness, shortness of breath, chest pain, gastrointestinal distress, faintness, derealization, paresthesia). This is accompanied by associated fear of dying, heart attack, stroke, passing out, losing control, or losing one's mind. Panic attacks are often described as "the most terrifying" episode an individual has experienced.
- Emergency or physician visits often occasioned by physical symptoms such as chest pain, palpitations, dizziness, or difficulty breathing. Thirty percent of patients presenting with chest pain have panic disorder.
- In a recent study of 1327 patients reporting noncardiac chest pain, 77.1% had visited the emergency department following a panic attack.
- Patients reporting a fear of dying from a panic attack tend to have more symptomatic panic attacks and agoraphobia.

Agoraphobia:
- Rare complaints to physician. May manifest in missed office visits or tardiness. Patients may request home visits or telephone care.
- Fear or anxiety about situations or activities such as the following:
  1. Crowded public areas (stores, public transportation, flying, church)
  2. Individual interactions (hairdresser, dentist, meetings)
  3. Driving (especially if alone, far from home, over bridges, through tunnels, on highways, or on isolated roads)
- This fear is a result of the belief that he or she might experience a panic attack and would be unable to exit readily. Patients may also experience fear of other symptoms, beyond the paniclike symptoms, such as falling or incontinence.
- On exposure to or anticipation of exposure to feared situations, significant anxiety occurs. Anxiety may generate somatic symptoms that trigger a full- or limited-symptom panic attack. Patients believe that escape from these situations reduces the alarming symptoms, thus reinforcing future avoidance. In actuality, symptom relief stems from adrenaline breaking down in the body after approximately 20 minutes.

ETIOLOGY

Hypotheses (NOTE: There are sufficient data to support each model. Models are not mutually exclusive.):
- Central dyscontrol of autonomic arousal (typically localized to the locus ceruleus); similar symptoms may be chemically induced with yohimbine, caffeine, or cholecystokinin.
- Cognitive overreaction (i.e., "catastrophic misinterpretation") to relatively mild or benign physiologic cues that then triggers a genuine autonomic cascade and further misinterpretations.
- Dysfunction of a central suffocation alarm mechanism; some signs of compensated respiratory alkalosis. Can be experimentally induced with sodium lactate or carbon dioxide.

RISK FACTORS

- Temperamental: Negative affect and anxiety sensitivity are risk factors for the onset of panic attacks. Severe separation anxiety in childhood may precede the panic disorder.
- Environmental: Early life stress such as sexual and physical abuse in childhood is common in panic disorder. Most panic sufferers are able to identify a coalescence of stressors preceding their first panic attack.
- Genetic and physiological: Although the exact genes are unknown, it is believed that multiple genes contribute to the vulnerability to panic attacks.

Dx DIAGNOSIS

DIFFERENTIAL DIAGNOSIS

Medical conditions:
- Endocrinopathies:
  1. Hyperthyroidism
  2. Hyperparathyroidism
  3. Pheochromocytoma
  4. Carcinoid tumor
- Cardiac and respiratory diseases:
  1. Arrhythmias
  2. Myocardial infarction
  3. Chronic obstructive pulmonary disease
  4. Asthma
  5. Mitral valve prolapse
  6. Pulmonary embolism
- Metabolic:
  1. Hypoglycemia
  2. Electrolyte imbalances
  3. Porphyria
- Seizure disorders: Ictal fear happens with simple partial seizures of meso-temporal lobe origin and lasts for seconds to minutes. May evolve to a focal seizure with impaired awareness.

- Psychiatric disorders (NOTE: Panic attacks are common in a variety of psychiatric disorders. Panic disorder could be conceptualized as a phobia of the somatic sensations or situations that have become paired with panic attacks.):
  1. Phobias (e.g., specific phobia or social phobia). Note that fear of going on a plane because of crashing would be a specific phobia, whereas fear of going on a plane because one is then trapped and worries about panic is more suggestive of panic disorder with comorbid agoraphobia
  2. Obsessive-compulsive disorder (cued by exposure to the object of the obsession)
  3. Posttraumatic stress disorder (cued by recall of a trauma)
  4. Generalized anxiety disorder (cued by excessive worry)
- Therapeutic (theophylline, steroids) and recreational (cocaine, amphetamine, caffeine, diet pills) drugs and drug withdrawal (alcohol, cannabis, barbiturates, benzodiazepines)

WORKUP

- Emergency presentation: Cardiac, respiratory, or neurologic symptoms
- History and physical examination to rule out a concomitant medical or substance-related condition

NOTE: Panic disorder and agoraphobia are not diagnoses of exclusion, but exclusion of other conditions is usually required.

LABORATORY TESTS

- Thyroid profile
- Electrolyte measures, including calcium
- Toxicology screen
- ECG
- Acute cases: Possible monitoring and cardiac enzymes to rule out arrhythmia or ischemia

IMAGING STUDIES

- For temporal lobe dysfunction (e.g., temporal lesions or as ictal or interictal manifestation of temporal lobe focal seizures): Brain CT scan or MRI or an electroencephalogram in some patients
- Holter monitor to rule out occult or episodic arrhythmias
- Chest x-ray, arterial blood gases, or pulmonary function tests if respiratory compromise suspected

Rx TREATMENT

NONPHARMACOLOGIC THERAPY

- Cognitive-behavioral therapy (CBT), in particular panic control treatment (PCT), is generally very effective, with strongest results for cognitive restructuring (i.e., challenging catastrophic misinterpretations of somatic symptoms), in vivo or imaginal exposures (i.e., exposure to panic triggers in a controlled graded hierarchical fashion from least to most difficult with the goal of habituation and extinction of the fear response), and interoceptive exposures (i.e., repeated recreation and management of feared somatic sensations via activities such as chair spinning, straw breathing, and hyperventilation).
- CBT effect sizes are equal to or larger than for pharmacotherapy, attrition rates are lower, and relapse rates are lower. Treatment may take several sessions spread over weeks and may require referral to a behavioral specialist. CBT has been shown to be the most effective intervention for panic disorder with or without agoraphobia across treatment sites. CBT may also be effectively delivered online (e.g., iCBT).
- A recent dismantling study of cognitive-behavioral therapy components for panic disorder suggests that interoceptive exposure and a face-to-face setting were associated with better treatment efficacy whereas muscle relaxation and virtual reality exposure were associated with significantly lower efficacy.

ACUTE GENERAL Rx

- Benzodiazepines, particularly clonazepam and alprazolam: Highly effective in the acute setting, although long-term use is contraindicated for effective outcome and due to addictive potential.
- Low-dose clonazepam for patients with rare panic attacks and asymptomatic periods (0.25 to 0.5 mg PO or sublingually PRN).
- Start patient on selective serotonin reuptake inhibitor (SSRI) or similar agent and taper patient off benzodiazepine by wk 2 to 3.

CHRONIC Rx

- Preferred pharmacologic agents: Antidepressants with a significant serotonin reuptake inhibitory action. Generally, start at low dose and titrate upward. Minimum treatment duration is 6 to 8 mo, but many patients need to take medications indefinitely. These medications should not be discontinued abruptly; they should be tapered due to withdrawal effects including rebound anxiety.
  1. SSRIs: Sertraline (50 to 200 mg/day), citalopram (20 to 60 mg/day), escitalopram (5 to 30 mg/day), fluoxetine (5 to 60 mg/day), fluvoxamine (50 to 300 mg/day) and paroxetine (10 to 60 mg/day)
  2. Imipramine (100 to 300 mg/day)
  3. SNRIs: Venlafaxine (37.5 to 225 mg/day)
- Combination CBT plus SSRI has shown good long-term effects and is somewhat better than antidepressants or CBT alone. Combination CBT plus benzodiazepine does not provide any added benefit and may undermine CBT (interoceptive and in vivo exposures may be less effective if the benzodiazepine is completely controlling the anxiety).

DISPOSITION

- Typical course is chronic but with significant waxing and waning (common to have long periods of remission).
- Presence of agoraphobia associated with a more chronic course.
- Findings with long-term follow-up studies: 6 to 10 yr after treatment some 30% are in remission, 40% to 50% have improved with residual symptoms, and the remainder are either unchanged or worse.

REFERRAL

- If patients do not respond to an SSRI.
- Cognitive-behavioral therapy is the preferred treatment.

PEARLS & CONSIDERATIONS

- Patient and family education is an important first step in the management of panic disorder. Psychoeducation provides more adaptive explanations for the benign somatic sensations paired with panic. Presentation of genetic information and explanation of the nonthreatening nature of the physiology of each of the symptoms the patient experiences serve as a good start to allay fears and reduce stigma. It may also ensure compliance with treatment.
- Resumption of avoided activities or situations is a positive prognostic sign and may promote further therapeutic gains. Patients should be encouraged to resume such activities after treatment is stabilized.
- Additional types of interventions such as mindfulness meditation through programs like Mindfulness Based Stress Reduction (MBSR) may be helpful in treating panic disorder and agoraphobia.
- The therapist's adherence to the treatment protocol and the therapeutic alliance established during the first session predict a better outcome for the long-term success of CBT for panic disorder with or without comorbid agoraphobia.

RELATED CONTENT

Panic Disorder (Patient Information)

SUGGESTED READINGS

Available at ExpertConsult.com

AUTHORS: **Perla M. Romero Gómez, MD, Ilana Ander, BA, and John Denninger, MD, PhD**

BASIC INFORMATION

DEFINITION

Panniculitis refers to inflammation of subcutaneous fat. Most cases are found in association with a systemic disease. Panniculitis can be separated into groups based on histopathologic characteristics. Panniculitis is classified into lobular or septal panniculitis based on whether the inflammation is seen in the fat lobules or septae, respectively. It can be further classified based on whether the inflammation is found with or without vasculitis (Table 1) and by predominant cell type. A classification of the panniculitides is summarized in Box 1.

ICD-10CM CODES

M79.3	Unspecified panniculitis
M5400	Panniculitis affecting regions of neck and back, site unspecified
M5401	Panniculitis affecting regions of neck and back, occipito-atlanto-axial region
M5402	Panniculitis affecting regions of neck and back, cervical region
M54.03	Panniculitis affecting regions of neck and back, cervicothoracic region
M54.04	Panniculitis affecting regions of neck and back, thoracic region
M54.05	Panniculitis affecting regions of neck and back, thoracolumbar region
M54.06	Panniculitis affecting regions of neck and back, lumbar region
M54.07	Panniculitis affecting regions of neck and back, lumbosacral region
M54.08	Panniculitis affecting regions of neck and back, sacral and sacrococcygeal region
M54.09	Panniculitis affecting regions, neck and back, multiple sites in spine

EPIDEMIOLOGY & DEMOGRAPHICS

The epidemiology of the various panniculitides varies with each disease process. The most common panniculitis is erythema nodosum (refer to topic "Erythema Nodosum"). Another common panniculitis seen in the clinical setting is lipodermatosclerosis (LDS), which is usually seen in young, overweight females with associated venous insufficiency.

PHYSICAL FINDINGS & CLINICAL PRESENTATION

- Skin lesions can appear as nonspecific areas of erythema or erythematous nodules and/or plaques. The nodules can be palpated beneath the dermis. Ulceration, atrophy, and sclerosis can be associated clinical features of these lesions.
- The lesions are frequently painful and tender to palpation.
- Associated constitutional symptoms such as low-grade fevers, malaise, fatigue, myalgias, and arthralgias may be present.
- These skin findings usually are found on the lower limbs; however, the location of these lesions can vary with each specific panniculitis, that is, erythema nodosum is found on the pretibial areas of the lower extremities (Fig. E1), erythema induratum occurs on the calf, and lupus panniculitis occurs on the upper arms, shoulders, and face.
- Skin findings tend to evolve as the types of inflammatory cells change over the course of a few days.

ETIOLOGY

Panniculitis can be either primary/idiopathic or secondary. Common secondary etiologies can be classified into the following broad categories:

- Infections: Bacterial (streptococci), mycobacterial, fungal, parasitic, and viral
- Inflammatory/connective tissue disease: Erythema nodosum, erythema induratum, lipodermatosclerosis, lupus panniculitis, cutaneous polyarteritis nodosa, dermatomyositis-associated panniculitis
- Malignancy: Subcutaneous panniculitis-like type T cell lymphoma
- Pancreatic disease: Pancreatic panniculitis, which is associated with pancreatitis or pancreatic carcinoma
- Immunodeficiency states: Alpha-1 antitrypsin deficiency panniculitis, which is associated with pulmonary and hepatic disease
- Trauma: Cold panniculitis (due to exposure to the cold), traumatic panniculitis, and factitial panniculitis (due to injection of medication or foreign substances into the subcutaneous fat)
- Deposition: Calciphylaxis, gout

Panniculitis can be a sign of an underlying systemic disease. Lupus panniculitis can occur alone or may present before or after the onset of either discoid lupus erythematosus or systemic lupus erythematosus.

Dx DIAGNOSIS

DIFFERENTIAL DIAGNOSIS

- The skin lesions of panniculitis need to be distinguished from other skin lesions that may manifest similarly, such as insect bites, thrombophlebitis, and cellulitis.
- Disorders affecting the deep dermis or fascia (i.e., plaque morphea, eosinophilic fasciitis), benign or malignant tumors manifesting as subcutaneous nodules, and nodules with deep bruising may have similar clinical findings and be difficult to distinguish from panniculitis.

WORKUP

- Diagnosis of panniculitis depends on a thorough history and physical examination, evaluation of patient's risk factors, skin lesion appearance and distribution, as well as any associated clinical findings.
- If the diagnosis is unclear or needs to be confirmed, a deep skin biopsy should be performed. The preferred biopsy is an excisional biopsy, but a large 6- to 8-mm punch biopsy may be sufficient.

Although the above often establishes a diagnosis, there are times when it is difficult to accurately diagnose a specific panniculitis. Different forms of panniculitides have similar clinical findings while others are rare, complicating the presentation. Biopsy specimens may be too superficial to assess for the involvement of the subcutaneous fat or to assess for the presence of vasculitis. Inflammation of the subcutaneous fat is a changing process, with varying histologic findings as well as physical characteristics of skin lesions based on the stage of evolution. Cellular infiltrates may not be confined to one location in the subcutaneous fat, and may overlap between septa and lobules (Fig. E2).

TABLE 1 Classification of Panniculitis

I. Without prominent vasculitis
  A. Septal inflammation
    1. Lymphocytic and mixed: Erythema nodosum and variants
    2. Granulomatous: Palisaded granulomatous diseases, sarcoidosis, subcutaneous infection: Tuberculosis, syphilis
    3. Sclerotic: Scleroderma, eosinophilic fasciitis, lipodermatosclerosis, toxins
  B. Lobular inflammation
    1. Neutrophilic: Infection, ruptured folliculitis and cysts, pancreatic fat necrosis
    2. Lymphocytic: Lupus panniculitis, poststeroid panniculitis, lymphoma/leukemia
    3. Macrophagic: Histiocytic cytophagic panniculitis
    4. Granulomatous: Erythema induratum/nodular vasculitis, palisaded granulomatous diseases, sarcoidosis, Crohn disease
    5. Mixed inflammation with many foam cells: α1-antitrypsin deficiency, traumatic fat necrosis
    6. Eosinophilic: Eosinophilic panniculitis, arthropod bites, parasites
    7. Enzymatic fat necrosis: Pancreatic enzyme panniculitis
    8. Crystal deposits: Scleredema neonatorum, subcutaneous fat necrosis of the newborn, gout, oxalosis
    9. Embryonic fat pattern: Lipoatrophy, lipodystrophy
II. With prominent vasculitis (septal or lobular)
  A. Neutrophilic: Leukocytoclastic vasculitis, subcutaneous polyarteritis nodosa, thrombophlebitis, ENL
  B. Lymphocytic: Nodular vasculitis, perniosis, angiocentric lymphomas
  C. Granulomatous: Nodular vasculitis/erythema induratum, ENL, granulomatosis with polyangiitis, Churg-Strauss allergic granulomatosis
III. Mixed patterns

ENL, Erythema nodosum leprosum.
From Lee L, Werth V: The skin and rheumatic diseases: panniculitis, In Firestein G et al (eds): *Kelley's textbook of rheumatology,* ed 9, Philadelphia, 2013, Elsevier Saunders, p. 611.

BOX 1 Classification of the Panniculitides

Mostly septal panniculitis without vasculitis
- Erythema nodosum
- Vilanova disease: Subacute nodular migratory panniculitis

Mostly lobular panniculitis without vasculitis
- Idiopathic neutrophilic panniculitis
- Subcutaneous fat necrosis of the newborn
- Postcorticosteroid panniculitis
- Calcifying panniculitis
- Pancreatic panniculitis
- α_1-Antitrypsin deficiency
- Physical or factitial panniculitis
- Histiocytic cytophagic panniculitis
- Lipodystrophy syndromes
- Connective tissue panniculitis
- Subcutaneous panniculitis–like T-cell lymphoma
- Sclerosing panniculitis: Lipodermatosclerosis

Mixed panniculitis
- Lupus profundus: Lupus erythematosus panniculitis
- Erythema nodosum–like lesions of Behçet syndrome

Panniculitis with vasculitis
- Small-vessel vasculitis (postcapillary venule), also known as *leukocytoclastic vasculitis*
- Medium-sized-vessel vasculitis (arterioles or small arteries): Polyarteritis nodosa
- Erythema induratum, also known as *nodular vasculitis*

From Hochberg MC: *Rheumatology*, ed 7, Philadelphia, 2019, Elsevier.

LABORATORY TESTS

Depending on the suspected underlying disorder, the following workup may be considered:
- Throat swab for rapid streptococcal screen, ASO titer, CBC, PPD, chest radiograph, tissue cultures, and histologic stains for organisms
- Amylase, lipase
- Serum alpha-1 antitrypsin level
- ESR, CRP
- Laboratory evaluation for possible connective tissue disease
- Further special studies of biopsy sample if malignancy is suspected

IMAGING STUDIES

- Chest radiography
- Ankle-brachial index for assessment of peripheral vascular disease
- Further imaging based on clinical suspicion (i.e., CT scan of abdomen for pancreatitis)

Rx TREATMENT

Treatment of panniculitis is toward treatment of the underlying etiology. Any suspected medications should be discontinued. Appropriate antibiotics to treat underlying infections should be prescribed.

NONPHARMACOLOGIC THERAPY

- Leg elevation, bed rest
- Support stockings

ACUTE GENERAL Rx

- Nonsteroidal antiinflammatory medications (NSAIDs)
- Oral corticosteroids

CHRONIC Rx

- Oral potassium iodide (300 to 900 mg per day)
- Oral corticosteroids
- Colchicine
- Hydroxychloroquine
- Immunosuppressive medications

REFERRAL

- Dermatology for biopsy of skin lesions
- Specific specialists based on underlying etiology

SUGGESTED READINGS

Available at ExpertConsult.com

RELATED CONTENT

Erythema Nodosum (Related Key Topic)

AUTHOR: **Joanne Szczygiel Cunha, MD**

BASIC INFORMATION

DEFINITION

Paraneoplastic syndromes are a large group of disorders caused by either an abnormal immune response to a malignancy or as a result of hormonal or other soluble factors produced by these malignancies. They often affect areas of the body distant from the site of the original tumor or metastases, which is in contrast to syndromes that are direct complications of tumor invasion, compression, or metastasis (e.g., superior vena cava syndrome). Findings and symptoms are specific to each syndrome. Paraneoplastic syndromes affect multiple organ systems and remain a challenging diagnostic entity.

ICD-10CM CODES

E22.2	Syndrome of inappropriate secretion of antidiuretic hormone
E83.5	Disorders of calcium metabolism
G13.0	Paraneoplastic neuromyopathy and neuropathy
G13.1	Other systemic atrophy primarily affecting central nervous system in neoplastic disease
G73.1	Lambert-Eaton syndrome in neoplastic disease
G73.3	Myasthenic syndromes in other diseases classified elsewhere

EPIDEMIOLOGY & DEMOGRAPHICS

- Paraneoplastic syndromes may affect as many as 8% of cancer patients.
- See Table 1 for epidemiology of each syndrome.

PHYSICAL FINDINGS & CLINICAL PRESENTATION

Hypercalcemia of malignancy:
- Nausea/vomiting
- Constipation
- Abdominal pain
- Anorexia
- Hypertension
- Fatigue
- Altered mental status (from confusion to coma)
- Depression/anxiety
- Polyuria
- Acute kidney injury
- Bone pain

Syndrome of inappropriate antidiuretic hormone (SIADH):
- Headache
- Weakness
- Anorexia
- Nausea, vomiting
- Memory impairment, irritability, restlessness, seizures
- Obtundation or coma may be seen with hyponatremia <125 mEq/L

Cushing syndrome:
- Muscle weakness
- Rapid weight gain
- Centripetal fat distribution, progressing to obesity; limbs are often spared or wasted
- Characteristic "moon facies" resulting from accumulation of fat deposition in the cheeks
- Skin atrophy, easy bruising, and purple abdominal striae due to skin fragility
- Hyperpigmentation, notably in sun-exposed areas
- Menstrual irregularity, mild hirsutism in women
- Hypertension
- Depression, anxiety, irritability

Paraneoplastic thrombocytosis:
- Thrombosis
- Nausea, vomiting
- Paresthesias, visual disturbances, headache

Paraneoplastic erythrocytosis:
- Erythroderma
- Postshower (aquagenic) pruritus
- Plethora

Paraneoplastic glomerulonephritis:
- Renal failure: Oliguric or anuric
- Malaise
- Nausea, vomiting

Paraneoplastic Neurological Syndromes: (Table 2 and Table 3)

Paraneoplastic cerebellar degeneration (PCD):
- May develop prodrome of dizziness, nausea, vomiting
- Ataxia
- Diplopia
- Dysphagia, dysarthria

Lambert-Eaton myasthenic syndrome (LEMS):
- Gradual onset of symmetric proximal muscle weakness and fatigability; lower extremity involvement is more common. Uniquely, strength improved after exercise.
- Hyporeflexia also can be improved after exercise.
- Mild bulbar dysfunction, although respiratory failure can occur late in the disease process.
- Dysautonomia, especially erectile dysfunction.

Myasthenia gravis (MG):
- Ocular symptoms: Ptosis and diplopia
- Weakness of facial muscles, notably with fatigable chewing
- Weakness of neck extensor and flexor muscles; proximal and distal extremities may also be involved
- May progress to involve muscles of respiration and respiratory crisis

Opsoclonus myoclonus syndrome (OMS):
- Truncal ataxia and unsteady gait
- Involuntary and conjugate gaze rapid eye movements (opsoclonus)
- Muscle twitching (myoclonus)
- Other symptoms: Irritability, sleep disturbance, dysarthria or mutism

Limbic encephalitis (LE):
- Insidious mood or psychiatric changes; hallucinations
- Short-term memory loss
- Hyperthermia or somnolence if hypothalamic involvement
- Seizures occur in up to half of patients

Paraneoplastic dermatologic and rheumatologic syndromes:
- Acanthosis nigricans
- Dermatomyositis (DM)
- Necrolytic migratory erythema
- Hypertrophic osteoarthropathy
- Leukocytoclastic vasculitis
- Paraneoplastic pemphigus (PNP)
- Polymyalgia rheumatica (PMR)
- Sweet syndrome (acute febrile neutrophilic dermatosis)
- Sign of Leser-Trélat (explosive onset of multiple seborrheic keratoses)

TABLE 1 Epidemiology of Each Paraneoplastic Syndrome

Condition	Prevalence	Risk Factors
Hypercalcemia of malignancy	Up to 20% of all cancer patients	Squamous cell cancers (lung, head, and neck), breast, kidney, bladder, and ovarian cancers, lymphoma
Syndrome of inappropriate antidiuretic hormone (SIADH)	Up to 2% of all cancer patients Found in 10%-45% of SCLC patients	SCLC
Cushing syndrome	Approximately 2% of all cancer patients (50% of these are SCLC)	SCLC Pituitary adenoma, benign and malignant adrenal tumors, carcinoid tumors
Limbic encephalitis (LE)	Less than 1%	SCLC Testicular germ cell tumor Breast cancer Ovarian teratoma
Paraneoplastic cerebellar degeneration	Less than 1%	SCLC Hodgkin lymphoma Breast cancer
Lambert-Eaton myasthenic syndrome (LEMS)	3% of SCLC patients	SCLC, prostate cancer, lymphoma
Paraneoplastic thrombocytosis	5%-20% of patients with solid tumors	Lung, colorectal, mesothelioma
Paraneoplastic erythrocytosis	4% of patients	Renal cell carcinoma, hepatocellular carcinoma
Paraneoplastic glomerulonephritis	2%-4% of patients	Hodgkin lymphoma, thymoma, prostate cancer
Myasthenia gravis (MG)	15% of thymoma patients	Thymoma
Opsoclonus myoclonus syndrome (OMS)	Less than 1%	SCLC, breast cancer, ovarian teratoma in adults; neuroblastoma in children

SCLC, Small cell lung cancer.

TABLE 2 Paraneoplastic Syndromes

Syndrome	Tumor	Associated Antibodies
Cerebellar degeneration	SCLC Gynecologic Breast Lymphoma Thymoma	Anti-Hu Anti-Yo Anti-Ri Anti-CV2 Anti-TR
Limbic encephalitis	SCLC Testes Breast Ovarian teratoma Thymoma	Anti-Hu Anti-Ma Anti-Amphiphysin Anti-NMDA receptor Anti-VGKC Anti-GAD
Lambert–Eaton myasthenic syndrome	SCLC	Anti-VGCC
Sensory neuronopathy	SCLC	Anti-Hu
Stiff-person syndrome	SCLC Breast Thymoma	Anti-GAD Anti-Amphiphysin
Opsoclonus-myoclonus	Neuroblastoma SCLC Gynecologic Breast	Most cases do not have an established antibody, small subset with Anti-Ri
Dermatomyositis/ polymyositis	Ovary Pancreas Stomach Colorectal Non-Hodgkin lymphoma	Variety of antibodies have been associated, including anti-TIF1

GAD, Glutamic acid decarboxylase; *NMDA,* N-methyl-D-aspartate; *SCLC,* small cell lung cancer; *VGCC,* voltage-gated calcium channel; *VGKC,* voltage-gated potassium channel.
Adapted from Kaufman DM et al: *Kaufman's clinical neurology for psychiatrists,* ed 8, Philadelphia, 2017, Elsevier.

TABLE 3 Paraneoplastic Syndromes of the Nervous System

Classical
Limbic encephalitis
Encephalomyelitis
Cerebellar degeneration
Opsoclonus-myoclonus
Sensory neuronopathy
Gastrointestinal pseudoobstruction/autonomic neuropathy
Lambert–Eaton myasthenic syndrome
Inflammatory myopathy
Nonclassical
Brain stem encephalitis
Stiff-person syndrome
Motor neuron disease
Necrotizing myelopathy
Optic neuropathy/retinopathy
Acute sensorimotor neuropathy
Chronic sensorimotor neuropathy
Myasthenia gravis
Autoimmune Encephalitides
NMDAR encephalitis
AMPAR encephalitis

AMPAR, Alpha-amino-3-hydroxy-5-methyl-4-isoxazolepropionic acid receptor; *NMDAR,* anti-*N*-methyl-D-aspartate receptor.
From Swaiman KF: *Swaiman's pediatric neurology, principles and practice,* ed 6, 2017, Elsevier.

ETIOLOGY

Paraneoplastic endocrine syndromes (PES) are caused by ectopic production of bioactive substances (e.g., hormones or peptides) that lead to metabolic derangements:

- **Hypercalcemia of malignancy:**
  1. *Humoral hypercalcemia of malignancy (HHM):* Due to production of parathyroid hormone-related peptide (PTHrP). Accounts for 80% of hypercalcemia of malignancy cases. Most common in lung (Table 4) and breast cancer (also seen in renal, bladder, and ovarian cancer).
  2. *Other etiologies of hypercalcemia of malignancy:* 1,25-dihydroxyvitamin D production from increased 1α-hydroxylase activity causes hypercalcemia in most Hodgkin and some non-Hodgkin lymphomas.
  3. *Osteolytic activity:* 20% of hypercalcemia of malignancy cases. Tumor cells produce local factors that stimulate osteoclast activation, resulting in increased bone resorption.
  4. *True ectopic parathyroid hormone (PTH):* Rare. Thyroid and nonthyroid tumors can also produce PTH, leading to hypercalcemia.
- **SIADH:** Ectopic production of antidiuretic hormone (ADH) (arginine vasopressin, atrial natriuretic peptide) by tumor cells leads to inappropriately concentrated urine and natriuresis.
- **Cushing syndrome:** Ectopic ACTH promotes excess production of cortisol and other glucocorticoids from the adrenal glands, which do not respond to normal HPA feedback.
- **Paraneoplastic erythrocytosis**: Mediated by inappropriate production of erythropoietin (EPO) and is associated most commonly with renal cell carcinoma and hepatocellular carcinoma.

TABLE 4 Hypercalcemia of Malignancy

Cancer	Frequency (%)	Mechanism
Lung	35	PTHrP Local osteolysis
Breast	25	PTHrP Local osteolysis
Head and neck	6	PTHrP
Renal	3	PTHrP Local osteolysis
Multiple myeloma	15	PTHrP (rare) Local osteolysis 1,25-Dihydroxyvitamin D
Prostate	7	Local osteolysis
Lymphoma	15	1,25-Dihydroxyvitamin D PTHrP

PTHrP, Parathyroid hormone-related protein.
From Skorecki K et al: *Brenner and Rector's the kidney,* ed 10, Philadelphia, 2016, Elsevier.

- **Paraneoplastic thrombocytosis**: Overproduction of inflammatory cytokines, especially IL-6, which induces thrombopoietin (TPO) mRNA expression and protein synthesis in the liver. Unlike secondary (reactive) thrombocytosis, TPO levels are not elevated.
- **Paraneoplastic glomerulonephritis**: Acute renal failure in the setting of newly diagnosed malignancy that is not explained by direct tumor involvement of the kidneys or genitourinary system. Diseases include minimal change disease, rapidly progressive glomerulonephritis, focal segmental glomerulonephritis, IgA nephropathy, and membranous nephropathy.
- **Paraneoplastic neurologic syndromes (PNS):** Due to immune cross-reactivity between tumor cells and components of the nervous system. Tumor-directed antibodies (onconeural antibodies) are produced by the patient in response to a developing cancer. These onconeural antibodies and associated onconeural antigen-specific T lymphocytes attack components of the nervous system because of antigenic similarity (molecular mimicry). Diagnostic criteria for paraneoplastic neurologic syndromes is summarized in Table 5.
- **LE, PCD, LEMS, MG, OMS:** Cross-reactive autoantibodies against various components of the central and peripheral nervous system.

Dx DIAGNOSIS

DIFFERENTIAL DIAGNOSIS

- **Hypercalcemia of malignancy:** Primary hyperparathyroidism, familial hypocalciuric hypercalcemia, excess calcium intake, vitamin D toxicity, chronic granulomatous disorders, thiazide diuretics. It is important to differentiate between HHM and osteolytic causes of malignancy-associated hypercalcemia because prognosis and response to treatment differ

TABLE 5 Diagnostic Criteria for Paraneoplastic Neurologic Syndromes

Definite Paraneoplastic Neurologic Syndromes
- A classical syndrome and cancer that develops within 5 yr of the diagnosis of the neurologic disorder
- A nonclassical syndrome that resolves significantly after cancer treatment without concomitant immunotherapy provided that the syndrome is not susceptible to spontaneous remission
- A nonclassical syndrome with onconeural antibodies (well characterized or not) and cancer that develops within 5 yr of the diagnosis of the neurologic disorder
- A neurologic syndrome (classical or not) with well-characterized onconeural antibodies (anti-Hu, Yo, CV2, Ri, Ma2, or amphiphysin) and no cancer

Possible Paraneoplastic Neurologic Syndromes
- A classical syndrome, no onconeural antibodies, no cancer, but at high risk to have an underlying tumor
- A neurologic syndrome (classical or not) with partially characterized onconeural antibodies and no cancer
- A nonclassical syndrome, no onconeural antibodies, and cancer present within 2 yr of diagnosis

From Swaiman KF et al: *Swaiman's pediatric neurology: principles and practice*, ed 6, Philadelphia, 2017, Elsevier.

BOX 1 Evaluation and Diagnosis of Paraneoplastic Syndromes

- Characterize abnormality; obtain laboratory studies, imaging, and biopsy, as necessary.
- Carefully elicit any additional symptoms and signs.
- Eliminate common causes.
- If there is no obvious etiology, consider a paraneoplastic syndrome.
- If signs and symptoms are consistent with a paraneoplastic syndrome, undertake a search for an unknown primary cancer or recurrence or progression of a known primary tumor.
- Screening should include a careful physical examination with breast, gynecologic, and prostate evaluations; basic hematology, chemistry, and urine studies; chest radiograph; and mammography.
- Computed tomography (CT) of the chest, abdomen and pelvis, or positron emission tomography/CT is indicated if there are any suspicious symptoms, signs, or laboratory abnormalities. Antibody testing for paraneoplastic neurologic syndromes and/or skin biopsy should be performed as indicated.
- Consider treatment of cancer and/or appropriate palliative treatment, including immunosuppressive therapy for paraneoplastic symptoms when possible.

- **SIADH:** Hypovolemic hyponatremia, volume overload, reset osmostat, adrenal insufficiency, hypothyroidism, psychogenic polydipsia
- **Cushing syndrome:** Excess glucocorticoid administration, pituitary adenoma, benign or malignant adrenal tumors
- **Paraneoplastic thrombocytosis**: Reactive thrombocytosis from iron deficiency anemia, infection, inflammation, essential thrombocythemia
- **Paraneoplastic erythrocytosis**: Polycythemia vera, secondary polycythemia from smoking, high-affinity hemoglobinopathies, or chronic hypoxia (e.g., obstructive sleep apnea)
- **Paraneoplastic glomerulonephritis**: Renal failure from intrinsic injury from nephrotoxic agents (e.g., chemotherapy), postrenal failure from bladder obstruction, or rarely direct metastatic invasion from a primary tumor
- **LE, PCD, LEMS, MG, OMS:** Multiple sclerosis, stroke, meningitis, encephalitis, neurodegenerative diseases, myelitis, mixed connective tissue disease

WORKUP

- History and physical examination. Box 1 summarizes the evaluation and diagnosis of paraneoplastic syndromes.
- Age-appropriate cancer screening
- Chest-abdomen-pelvis CT
- Paraneoplastic neurologic syndromes: Lumbar puncture, PET, EEG, EMG

LABORATORY TESTS

Hypercalcemia of malignancy:
- Serum calcium and albumin levels to measure corrected calcium (HHM more common when serum Ca^{2+} >13 mg/dl)
- Ionized serum calcium
- PTH (low to normal)
- PTHrP (elevated)
- 1,25$(OH)_2$D levels (if the above values are inconclusive)

SIADH:
- Serum (corrected for glucose) and urine sodium (serum sodium <135 mEq/L or urine sodium >40 mEq/L)
- Serum and urine osmolality (serum osm <280 mOsm/kg of water and/or urine osm >100 mOsm/kg of water)

Cushing syndrome:
- Initial testing: Low-dose dexamethasone suppression test, late-night salivary cortisol, 24-hr urinary free cortisol excretion.
- Once diagnosis is confirmed: High-dose dexamethasone suppression tests can help to distinguish Cushing syndrome (pituitary hypersecretion of ACTH) from patients with ectopic ACTH production.
- Potassium and glucose should be monitored closely due to increased risk of hypokalemia and hyperglycemia.

LE: Anti-Hu, Anti-Ma2, Anti-CRMP5, Anti-LGI1, Anti-AMPAR, Anti-mGluR5, CSF analysis, Anti-NMDAR, Anti-GABA-AR, Anti-GABA-BR

PCD: Anti-Yo, Anti-Tr Anti-Hu, Anti-Ma, Anti-Ri, Anti-CV2, Anti-VGCC, Anti-mGluR1, CSF analysis

LEMS: Anti-VGCC (P/Q), CSF analysis

MG: Anti-AChR, Anti-MuSK, CSF analysis

Paraneoplastic thrombocytosis: CBC, liver panel, iron panel, *JAK2* mutation, *CALR* mutation, *MPL* mutation

Paraneoplastic erythrocytosis: CBC, EPO level, *JAK2* mutation, peripheral blood smear

Paraneoplastic glomerulonephritis: BMP, urinalysis, urine protein to creatinine ratio, 24-hr urine protein collection, urine sediment analysis

IMAGING STUDIES

- **Hypercalcemia of malignancy:** CT imaging to evaluate for breast lesion, lung mass, or lymphadenopathy
- **SIADH:** CT imaging to evaluate for brain or lung mass
- **Cushing syndrome:** CT scan, MRI, or octreotide scan
- **LE, PCD, LEMS, MG:** CT chest, FDG-PET scan, MRI
- **Paraneoplastic erythrocytosis**: CT renal mass protocol or renal ultrasound to evaluate for renal cell carcinoma

Rx TREATMENT

NONPHARMACOLOGIC THERAPY

Hypercalcemia of malignancy:
- Treatment of underlying malignancy, either surgical resection or chemotherapy/radiation of identified tumors
- Fluid resuscitation, typically with initial 1 L bolus of isotonic saline followed by 200 to 300 ml/hr to achieve euvolemia, followed by maintenance hydration

SIADH:
- Surgical resection of identified tumors
- Fluid restriction
- Maintain adequate dietary protein and salt intake

Cushing syndrome: Surgical resection of identified tumors

LE, PCD, LEMS, MG
- IVIG
- Plasma exchange

ACUTE GENERAL Rx

Hypercalcemia of malignancy:
- Aggressive fluid hydration with normal saline to promote renal calcium excretion
- Bisphosphonates, either pamidronate or zoledronic acid intravenous infusions (treatment side effects are renal dysfunction and osteonecrosis of the jaw)
- Calcitonin weight-based dosing, although tachyphylaxis occurs after 48 hr of administration
- Loop diuretics if concurrent heart failure or renal failure

- Corticosteroids in cases of myeloma and lymphoma
- Hemodialysis in severe cases

SIADH:
- If patient develops seizure or obtundation in cases of severe hyponatremia, then sodium replacement with hypertonic saline (3%) is indicated
- Sodium should be corrected at a rate less than 8 mEq/L in any 24-hr period to decrease chances of osmotic demyelination syndrome (ODS). Desmopressin, free water, and/or nephrology consultation may be required for an overly rapid correction

Cushing syndrome:
- Diuretics and antihypertensive agents for blood pressure and volume status management

CHRONIC Rx

- Chronic treatment is centered on treatment of the underlying malignancy
- **Hypercalcemia of malignancy:**
  1. Bisphosphonate therapy every 4 wk in cases of bone metastasis
  2. Chronic calcitonin use can be considered
  3. Denosumab, a monoclonal antibody that inhibits osteoclastic bone resorption by blocking RANKL from binding to osteoclastic RANK receptors, can be used in patients refractory to bisphosphonate therapy
- **SIADH:**
  1. Demeclocycline and vasopressin receptor antagonists (vaptans: Conivaptan and tolvaptan, although tolvaptan should not be used for longer than 30 days and should be avoided in patients with liver disease)
  2. Cessation of any possible causative medications
  3. Oral salt tablets if dietary salt intake insufficient
- **Cushing syndrome:** If surgery contraindicated, consider inhibition of adrenal enzymes with ketoconazole, mitotane, metyrapone
- **LE/PCD:** Glucocorticoids, cyclophosphamide, rituximab
- **LEMS:** Pyridostigmine, azathioprine, glucocorticoids
- **MG:** Pyridostigmine, azathioprine, cyclosporine, mycophenolate, rituximab
- **Paraneoplastic thrombocytosis**: Consider prophylactic low-molecular-weight heparin or aspirin if no contraindications exist, siltuximab (antibody against IL-6)

DISPOSITION

Specific to each condition; however, humoral hypercalcemia of malignancy carries a poor overall prognosis with 30-day mortality of 50%.

REFERRAL

Oncology, endocrinology, neurology, nephrology

PEARLS & CONSIDERATIONS

COMMENTS

- Signs or symptoms of a paraneoplastic syndrome may manifest prior to the identification of a malignancy.
- If paraneoplastic syndrome is suspected, a thorough workup for a tumor is indicated.
- With treatment of the primary tumor, the clinical effects of hypercalcemia of malignancy, SIADH, and Cushing syndrome may improve or resolve.
- Neurologic paraneoplastic syndromes can have long-term effects due to permanent CNS or PNS damage. Tumor detection can also be difficult as these immune-mediated syndromes may also be keeping the tumor in check.
- New neurologic deficits after starting a checkpoint inhibitor (e.g., PD-1 inhibitor) may indicate drug-induced autoimmunity rather than a paraneoplastic syndrome.

PREVENTION

- Smoking cessation
- Age-appropriate cancer screening

PATIENT & FAMILY EDUCATION

In conditions with autoimmune etiology (LE, PCD, LEMS, MG, OMS), symptoms may not improve even if the tumor is identified and treated, as damage to the nervous system may be sustained or permanent.

SUGGESTED READINGS

Available at ExpertConsult.com

AUTHORS: **Mark Godding, MD,** and **John L. Reagan, MD**

BASIC INFORMATION

DEFINITION

Idiopathic Parkinson disease (PD) is a progressive neurodegenerative disorder characterized clinically by rigidity, tremor, postural instability, and slowness of movement (bradykinesia).

SYNONYMS

PD
Paralysis agitans

ICD-10CM CODES	
G20	Parkinson disease
G21.1	Other drug-induced secondary parkinsonism
G21.11	Neuroleptic induced parkinsonism
G21.2	Secondary parkinsonism due to other external agents
G21.3	Postencephalitic parkinsonism
G21.4	Vascular parkinsonism
G21.8	Other secondary parkinsonism
G21.9	Secondary parkinsonism, unspecified

EPIDEMIOLOGY & DEMOGRAPHICS

PREVALENCE:

- It is the second most common neurodegenerative disease worldwide and is found in every country.
- Affects more than 1 million people in North America at 0.3% of the population and 1% of people over the age of 60. Prevalence increases with age.
- In those aged >70 yr, 700/100,000 are affected.
- Lifetime risk of Parkinson disease is 2% in men and 1.3% in women.

PHYSICAL FINDINGS & CLINICAL PRESENTATION

- Tremor (Fig. 1)—typically a resting tremor with a frequency of 4 to 6 Hz that is often first noted in the hand as a pill-rolling tremor (thumb and forefinger). Can also involve the leg and lip. Tremor improves with purposeful movement. Usually starts asymmetrically.
- Rigidity—increased muscle tone that persists throughout the range of passive movement of a joint. Rigidity, like resting tremor, is usually asymmetric at onset.
- Akinesia/bradykinesia—slowness in initiating movement and decrement with repeated movements.
- Postural instability—tested by "pull test." Ask patient to stand in place with back to examiner. Examiner pulls patient back by the shoulders, and proper response would be to take no steps back or very few steps back without falling. Retropulsion is a positive test, as is falling straight back. Postural instability is not usually severe early on. If falls and postural reflexes are greatly impaired early on, then consider other disorders, such as progressive supranuclear palsy.
- Masked facies (hypomimia)—face seems expressionless, giving the appearance of depression. Decreased blink; often there is excess drooling.
- Gait disturbance.
- Stooped posture, decreased arm swing.
- Difficulty initiating the first step; small shuffling steps that increase in speed (festinating gait). Steps become progressively faster and shorter while the trunk inclines further forward.
- Other complaints and findings early on include handwriting becoming smaller (micrographia), and voice becoming softer and often "gruffer" (hypophonia).
- Nonmotor symptoms in Parkinson disease include neuropsychiatric (depression, apathy, impulse control disorders, hallucinations), cognitive, dysautonomia (especially orthostatic hypotension, sexual dysfunction, and anosmia), and sensory abnormalities. These symptoms also may be subject to fluctuations during "on" vs. "off" states.
- Common premotor symptoms of Parkinson disease include constipation, anosmia, depression, and REM sleep behavior disorder.

ETIOLOGY

- Most cases are sporadic. Age is the most common risk factor, although a combination of both environmental and genetic factors likely contributes to disease expression.
- Approximately 5% to 10% have a genetic etiology. Several different genes have been identified; these include the parkin gene, a significant cause of early-onset autosomal recessive PD, and *LRRK2,* the most common cause of familial and sporadic parkinsonism.

Dx DIAGNOSIS

- A clinical diagnosis can be made based on a comprehensive history and physical examination. The four cardinal signs used to diagnose PD are (mnemonic = TRAP):
  1. **T**remor (resting, typically 4-6 Hz)
  2. **R**igidity, of the cogwheel type
  3. **A**kinesia/bradykinesia—slowing and decrement of movement
  4. **P**ostural instability—failure of postural "righting" reflexes leading to poor balance and falls
- Bradykinesia plus at least one other sign are necessary, but all four cardinal signs do not need to be present to make a presumptive diagnosis of PD and begin treatment

DIFFERENTIAL DIAGNOSIS

- Multiple system atrophy—distinguishing features include early autonomic dysfunction (including urinary incontinence, orthostatic hypotension, and erectile dysfunction), parkinsonism, cerebellar signs, and normal cognition
- Dementia with Lewy bodies—parkinsonism with concomitant dementia: Patients often have early hallucinations and fluctuations in level of alertness and mental status
- Corticobasal syndrome—often begins asymmetrically with apraxia, cortical sensory loss in one limb, and sometimes, alien limb phenomenon
- Progressive supranuclear palsy—tends to have axial rigidity greater than appendicular (limb) rigidity. These patients have early and severe postural instability. Hallmark is supranuclear gaze palsy that usually involves vertical gaze (especially downward) before horizontal
- Essential tremor—bilateral postural and action tremor
- Secondary (acquired) parkinsonism (Box 1):
  1. Iatrogenic—many, including any of the neuroleptics and antipsychotics. The high-potency D_2-blocker neuroleptics are most likely to cause parkinsonism. Quetiapine is an atypical antipsychotic with lower risk of parkinsonism. Metoclopramide can also cause parkinsonism. Abuse of methamphetamine has been linked to risk of PD
  2. Postinfectious parkinsonism—von Economo encephalitis

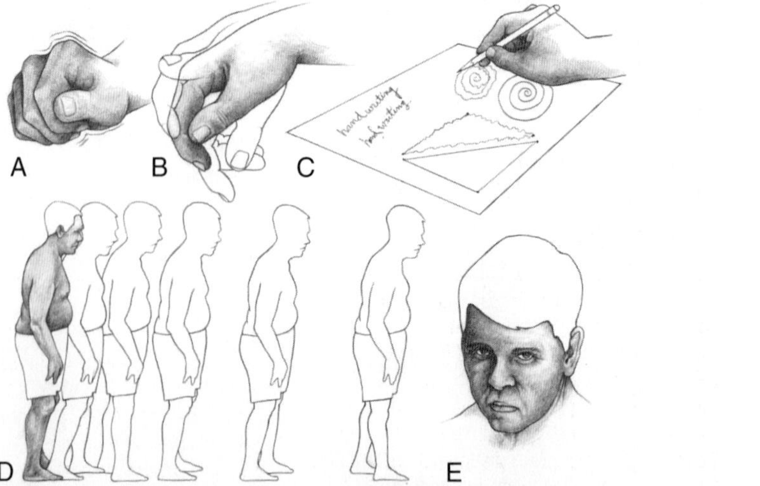

FIG. 1 The parkinsonian syndrome. A, The "pill-rolling" tremor. **B,** Tremor that can worsen with emotional stress. **C,** Handwriting abnormalities, including micrographia. **D,** Typical posture and gait, which becomes faster (festination). **E,** Lack of facial expression as well as "stare" from decreased blinking.

BOX 1 Causes of Parkinsonism

Primary Parkinsonism
- Parkinson disease (idiopathic/sporadic parkinsonism)

Secondary Parkinsonism
- Drug-induced parkinsonism
  1. Neuroleptic drugs
  2. Calcium blocker cinnarizine
- Vascular parkinsonism (pseudoparkinsonism)
  1. Multi-infarct states
  2. Single basal ganglia/thalamic infarct
  3. Binswanger disease
- Multisystem degenerative diseases
  1. Progressive supranuclear palsy
  2. Multiple system atrophy (striatonigral type)
  3. Corticobasal degeneration
  4. Alzheimer disease
  5. Wilson disease (young-onset parkinsonism)
  6. Dementia with Lewy bodies
  7. Neurofibrillary tangle parkinsonism
- Toxins
  1. MPTP
  2. Manganese
- Familial parkinsonism
- Postinfectious parkinsonism
  1. Creutzfeldt-Jakob disease
  2. AIDS
  3. Postencephalitis (encephalitis lethargica)
- Miscellaneous causes
  1. Hydrocephalus
  2. Posttraumatic
  3. Tumors
- Metabolic causes (postanoxic)

AIDS, Acquired immunodeficiency syndrome; *MPTP,* 1-methyl-4-phenyl-1,2,2,6-tetrahydropyridine.
From Fillit HM: *Brocklehurst's textbook of geriatric medicine and gerontology,* ed 8, Philadelphia, 2017, Elsevier.

3. Chronic traumatic encephalopathy (dementia pugilistica)—parkinsonism and dementia after repeated head trauma
4. Toxins (e.g., MPTP, manganese, carbon monoxide)
5. Cerebrovascular disease "vascular parkinsonism" (basal ganglia infarcts); often lower limbs (especially gait) affected more than upper extremities

WORKUP

- Identification of clinical signs and symptoms associated with PD (see "Physical Findings"), and elimination of conditions that may mimic it with a comprehensive history and physical examination.
- Routine genetic testing is not recommended.

IMAGING STUDIES

- Computed tomographic (CT) scan has almost no role in investigations. Magnetic resonance imaging (MRI) of the head may sometimes distinguish between idiopathic PD and other conditions that present with signs of parkinsonism (see "Differential Diagnosis").
- Dopamine transporter imaging (DaTscan with [^{123}I]β-CIT SPECT) evaluates the level of dopamine in the striatum and can be used to confirm parkinsonism in atypical cases. DaTscan is approved to distinguish essential tremor from parkinsonism but cannot distinguish between different causes of parkinsonism. Interpretation can be tricky, and routine use is not recommended at this time.

Rx TREATMENT

NONPHARMACOLOGIC THERAPY

- Physical therapy, patient education and reassurance, treatment of associated conditions (e.g., depression) are important. A safe, practical, and reasonable exercise regimen must be encouraged.
- Avoidance of drugs that can induce or worsen parkinsonism: Neuroleptics (especially high potency), certain antiemetics (prochlorperazine, trimethobenzamide), metoclopramide, nonselective MAO inhibitors (may induce hypertensive crisis), reserpine, methyldopa.

ACUTE GENERAL Rx

- There continues to be controversy whether levodopa or dopamine agonists should be the initial treatment. In younger patients, agonists may be favored; in patients >65 yr, levodopa is typically the preferred initial therapy.
- It is appropriate to initiate pharmacotherapy when required by symptoms; prior practice of waiting for limitation of ADLs is now outdated. Fig. 2 describes an approach to patients with parkinsonism.
- Motor complications do develop during the course of the disease and likely reflect the combination of disease progression together with the side effects of dopaminergic medications.

CHRONIC Rx

- Levodopa therapy:
  1. The most efficacious treatment and cornerstone of symptomatic therapy—should be used with a peripheral dopa decarboxylase inhibitor (carbidopa) to minimize side effects (nausea, light-headedness, postural hypotension). The combination of the two drugs is marketed under the trade name Sinemet. Levodopa therapy has been found to reduce morbidity and mortality in PD patients.
  2. Usual starting dose is 25/100 mg (carbidopa/levodopa) tid 1 hr before (or after) meals.
  3. Controlled-release (Sinemet CR) and extended-release (Rytary) preparations are also available, but their use should be supervised by a neurologist.
  4. Stalevo (combination Sinemet and entacapone, a COMT inhibitor). Useful for patients with motor fluctuations (wearing off); has no role in treating early patients with PD.
  5. Duopa (carbidopa/levodopa), administered via a 16-hr infusion to the jejunum through either a nasojejunal tube (short-term) or PEG-J tube (long-term), is used for treating motor fluctuations in patients with advanced PD.
- Dopamine receptor agonists (ropinirole, pramipexole, rotigotine) are not as potent as levodopa, but they are often used as initial treatment in younger patients in an attempt to delay the onset of complications (dyskinesias, motor fluctuations) associated with levodopa therapy. In general, they cause more side effects than levodopa, including nausea, vomiting, light-headedness, peripheral edema, confusion, and somnolence. They can also cause impulse control behaviors such as hypersexuality, binge eating, and compulsive shopping and gambling. Presence of these must be assessed at each visit as the appearance of these side effects is often under-reported and their consequences can be severe. Dopamine agonists also can be associated with a prolonged withdrawal syndrome.
  1. Ropinirole: Initial dose is 0.25 mg tid but must be titrated over the course of 4 wk to 1 mg tid and then may be increased by 1.5 mg/wk to a maximum of 24 mg/day. An extended-release formulation is also available.
  2. Pramipexole: Initial dose is 0.125 mg tid but must be titrated over the course of weeks to 1.5 to 4.5 mg/day in three doses. An extended-release formulation is also available.
  3. Rotigotine: 2 mg to 6 mg/24 hr transdermal patch.
  4. Apomorphine: A dopamine agonist used for acute, intermittent treatment of unpredictable "off" episodes with advanced Parkinson disease.
- COMT inhibitors (entacapone, opicapone, and tolcapone) are used as adjunct to levodopa therapy to treat end-of-dose wearing off.

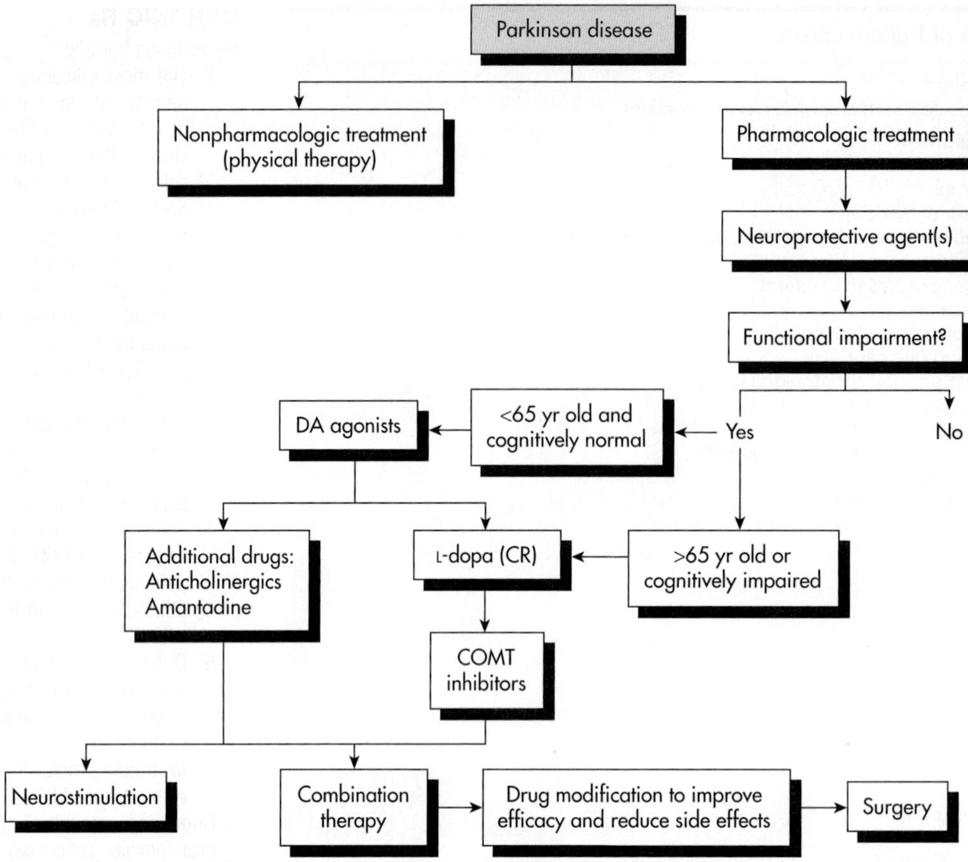

FIG. 2 Diagrammatic representation of a therapeutic approach to patients with parkinsonism. *COMT,* Catechol-O-methyl transferase; *CR,* controlled release; *DA,* dopamine. (Modified from Goldman L, Ausiello D [eds]: *Cecil textbook of medicine,* ed 24, Philadelphia, 2012, WB Saunders.)

- MAO-B inhibitors can be used as monotherapy early in the disease or as adjunctive therapy in later stages; they have been shown to have milder symptomatic benefit than dopamine agonists or levodopa. They are well tolerated and easy to titrate. Concurrent use of stimulants and sympathomimetics should be avoided. Certain food restrictions may apply.
  1. Rasagiline: Initial dose is 0.5 mg qd, then 1 mg daily. The ADAGIO study suggests that 1-mg rasagiline may have disease-modifying benefits, but results must be interpreted with caution.
  2. Selegiline: Usual dose, 5 mg bid with breakfast and lunch. Has amphetamine byproduct so has mild stimulant-like effects, which can be beneficial in some patients.
  3. Safinamide: FDA approved as add-on therapy for carbidopa-levodopa that reduces "off time" and increases "on time" with fewer dyskinesias. Starting dose is 50 mg daily for 2 wk, which can be increased if needed to 100 mg daily.
- Istradefylline is the first FDA-approved adenosine A 2A receptor agonist for use as an adjunct to carbidopa/levodopa in adults with Parkinson disease experiencing "off" episodes.
- Amantadine (unclear mechanism of action, but reported to modulate the dopamine and glutamate systems in the CNS) can be used alone early in the disease. Later in the disease, it is especially useful in the treatment of dyskinesias. Dosage is 100 mg tid (titrate q wk from 100 mg qd). Must adjust for elderly and renal impairment. The most notable side effect, especially in the elderly, is confusion. An extended-release version is now FDA approved for the treatment of dyskinesia.
- Anticholinergic agents are only helpful in treating tremor but may be more effective than levodopa for tremor in some circumstances. They can also be used to treat drooling in patients with PD. Potential side effects include constipation, urinary retention, memory impairment, and hallucinations. They should be avoided in the elderly.
  1. Trihexyphenidyl: Initial dose, 1 mg PO tid.
  2. Benztropine: Usual dose, 0.5 to 1 mg qd or bid.
- Treatment of nonmotor symptoms: Nonmotor symptoms such as depression, anxiety, irritability, dementia, psychosis, urinary and sexual dysfunction, sleep disturbances such as REM behavior disorder, decreased sense of smell, and impulsive behavior among others often cause a great deal of distress for patients and caretakers alike. Treatable symptoms should be addressed pharmacologically using medications appropriate for elderly patients sensitive to antidopaminergic medications.
- Psychosis: Dopamine agonists and anticholinergics can cause hallucinations, so adjustment of these medication should be the first step. Pimavanserin (Nuplazid) is FDA approved for the treatment of Parkinson disease psychosis and has been shown effective for the treatment of hallucinations and delusions associated with Parkinson disease psychosis. The medication is an inverse agonist of 5-HT2A and 5-HT2C receptors without any evidence of dopamine blockade.
- Parkinson disease dementia: Rivastigmine (Exelon), a cholinesterase inhibitor available both orally and transdermally as a patch (with few GI side effects), is approved to treat not only Alzheimer disease but also Parkinson disease dementia.

SURGICAL OPTIONS

- Pallidal (globus pallidus interna) and subthalamic deep-brain stimulation (subthalamic nucleus) are currently the surgical options of choice for patients with advanced PD; similar improvement in motor function and adverse effects have been reported after either procedure. Compared with ablative procedures, DBS has the advantage of being reversible and adjustable. Thalamic DBS may be useful for refractory tremor. It improves the cardinal motor symptoms, extends medication "on" time, and reduces motor fluctuations during the day. In general, patients are likely to benefit from this therapy if they show a clear response to levodopa. Therefore, when considering DBS, patients should be evaluated for motor response to levodopa by stopping levodopa overnight and evaluating motor response before and after a dose of levodopa.

- Focused ultrasound (FUS) is an imaging-guided method for creating therapeutic lesions in dead-brain structures including the subthalamic nucleus. A recent trial of focused ultrasound subthalamotomy in one hemisphere improved motor features of Parkinson Disease in selected patients with asymmetric signs.[1]
- Surgery is often limited to patients with disabling, medically refractory problems, and patients must still have a good response to L-dopa to undergo surgery. Yet for many patients, earlier stimulation might provide an improved motor benefit before disability from other symptoms has occurred and should be considered at an earlier stage of PD. DBS results in decreased dyskinesias, fluctuations, rigidity, and tremor.

[1]Martinez-Fernandez R et al: Randomized trial of focused ultrasound subthalamotomy for Parkinson's Disease. *N Engl J Med* 383(26): 2501-2513, 2020.

DISPOSITION

PD usually follows a slowly progressive course leading to disability over the course of several years. However, every patient will progress individually, and patients should be reassured that this diagnosis does not, by definition, result in being either wheelchair or bed bound.

REFERRAL

- Neurology consultation is recommended at initial diagnosis of PD.
- Exercise is important for all patients with PD.
- Participation in outpatient physical therapy program is recommended for patients with moderate to advanced disease.

PEARLS & CONSIDERATIONS

- Asymmetry of symptoms at onset is typical of PD and therefore very useful in distinguishing PD from other causes of parkinsonism.
- Although resting tremor is a common presenting symptom, up to 25% of patients with idiopathic PD do not have classic resting tremor.

SUGGESTED READINGS

Available at ExpertConsult.com

RELATED CONTENT

Parkinson Disease (Patient Information)

AUTHOR: **Corey Goldsmith, MD**

BASIC INFORMATION

DEFINITION

Coronavirus Disease 2019 (COVID-19) is an infectious disease caused by a recently discovered coronavirus named severe acute respiratory syndrome coronavirus 2 (SARS-CoV-2).

SYNONYMS

Multisystem inflammatory syndrome in children (MIS-C)
MIS-C
Pediatric inflammatory multisystem syndrome temporally associated with SARS-CoV-2 (PIMS-TS).

ICD10-CM CODE
U07.1 COVID-19

EPIDEMIOLOGY & DEMOGRAPHICS

- The emergence of COVID-19 is the third coronavirus outbreak in humans since 2000; included are the 2002 severe acute respiratory syndrome coronavirus (SARS-CoV) and 2012 Middle East respiratory syndrome coronavirus (MERS-CoV).
- Severe pneumonia caused by SARS-CoV-2 was first identified in December 2019. The primary cluster was connected with a seafood and live animal market in Wuhan, the capital city of Hubei province, in China.
- COVID-19 disease in children tends to be milder than in adults. The reasons for this milder course are not yet understood.
- The incubation period ranges from 2 to 14 days with a median of 5 days.
- On March 11, 2020, COVID-19 was declared a pandemic by the World Health Organization (WHO).
- On April 27, 2020, the United Kingdom National Health Service issued an alert highlighting a multisystem inflammatory syndrome in children and citing a possible link to SARS-CoV-2. This became known as the pediatric inflammatory multisystem syndrome temporally associated with SARS-CoV-2 (PIMS-TS).
- On May 14, 2020, the Centers for Disease Control and Prevention (CDC) issued a public health advisory and case definition for a hyperinflammatory syndrome associated with COVID-19, termed multisystem inflammatory syndrome in children (MIS-C).
- Most patients with MIS-C develop symptoms 2 to 4 wk after suspected infection. MIS-C tends to affect older children (>5 yr) and adolescents, with a median age 8 yr and has a higher prevalence in the Black and Hispanic/Latino communities.

ROUTE OF TRANSMISSION

- SARS-CoV-2 is highly contagious and transmitted from person-to-person via respiratory droplets. The droplets containing virus can reach the mouth, nose or eyes of a susceptible person which can lead to infection.
- Airborne transmission can occur during medical procedures ("aerosol-generating procedures").
- Transmission may occur through fomites.
- Transplacental transmission from pregnant woman to their fetus has not been excluded. Limited data suggest that breastfeeding is not likely to be a source of transmission. Neonatal disease due to postnatal exposure is documented.

RISK FACTORS

- Infants and children with underlying medical conditions are among the most commonly hospitalized. Childhood obesity may be linked to a higher risk of hospitalization.
- Medical conditions that increase the risk of severe disease at any age include: Serious heart conditions, chronic kidney disease, diabetes, sickle cell disease, cancer, and immunosuppression.

PHYSICAL FINDINGS & CLINICAL PRESENTATION

ACUTE COVID-19 INFECTION:

- The disease severity can be classified as asymptomatic, mild, moderate, severe (e.g., pneumonia with hypoxemia or respiratory distress) and critical (acute respiratory distress syndrome [ARDS], septic shock, and/or multiple organ dysfunction).
- In children less than 1 yr, the most common clinical presentation is fever without a source.
- Most children are asymptomatic or have symptoms of a common viral upper respiratory infection.
- Signs and symptoms of laboratory-confirmed COVID-19 in U.S. children:
    1. More frequent: Fever, cough, shortness of breath
    2. Less frequent: Headache, myalgia, diarrhea, nausea, vomiting, rhinorrhea, abdominal pain, sore throat, conjunctivitis, fatigue, ageusia, and anosmia
- Coinfection with viral or bacterial respiratory pathogens is documented.
- In the critically ill population, myocarditis or myocardial dysfunction was noted in patients with no medical history of cardiovascular disease; in some cases, myocarditis was noted in patients who presented with gastrointestinal symptoms.

MULTISYSTEM INFLAMMATORY SYNDROME IN CHILDREN (MIS-C):

- Myocardial dysfunction and gastrointestinal symptoms are more prevalent than respiratory disease.
- CDC Case definition
    1. An individual aged <21 yr presenting with:
        a. Fever (24 hr or more);
        b. Laboratory evidence of inflammation (1 or more of the following: elevations of C-reactive protein [CRP], erythrocyte sedimentation rate [ESR], fibrinogen, procalcitonin, D-dimer, ferritin, lactate dehydrogenase [LDH] or interleukin-6 [IL-6], elevated neutrophils; lymphopenia, low albumin);
        c. Evidence of clinically severe illness requiring hospitalization;
        d. Multisystem (≥2) organ involvement (cardiac, renal, respiratory, hematologic, gastrointestinal, dermatologic or neurological); AND
    2. No alternative plausible diagnoses; AND
    3. Positive for current or recent SARS-CoV-2 infection by polymerase chain reaction (PCR), serology, or antigen test; or COVID-19 exposure within the 4 wk prior to the onset of symptoms.

ETIOLOGY

The WHO has classified SARS-CoV-2 as a new betacoronavirus that infects humans. Bats are the suspected natural reservoir of SARS-CoV-2.

DIAGNOSIS

DIFFERENTIAL DIAGNOSIS

ACUTE COVID-19 INFECTION:

- Influenza virus, parainfluenza virus, adenovirus, respiratory syncytial virus, rhinovirus, human metapneumovirus, non-COVID-19cc coronavirus, and other known viral respiratory infections
- Atypical organisms: *Mycoplasma pneumoniae*, chlamydia pneumonia, and legionellosis
- Bacterial pneumonia
- Streptococcal pharyngitis
- Viral and bacterial gastrointestinal infections

MIS-C:

- Kawasaki disease or Kawasaki disease shock syndrome
- Toxic shock syndrome
- Myocarditis or heart failure
- Macrophage activation syndrome
- Hemophagocytic lymphohistiocytosis

WORKUP

ACUTE COVID-19 INFECTION:

- SARS-CoV-2 polymerase chain reaction (PCR) on upper and/or lower respiratory secretions.
- Rapid antigen test using nasal swab can detect viral proteins but with less sensitivity than PCR.

HISTORY OF COVID-19 INFECTION:

- Antibody testing should not be used as the sole basis for diagnosing an acute infection. Children with MIS-C tend to have positive serologic tests more often than PCR; serology testing must be sent prior to intravenous immunoglobulin (IVIG) administration.

LABORATORY TESTS

- Laboratory tests are frequently nonspecific.
- SARS-CoV-2 PCR on stool samples can be positive but is not used for routine diagnosis.
- Common findings include lymphopenia, thrombocytopenia, and elevations in C-reactive protein, procalcitonin, D-dimer, ferritin, troponin, and B-type natriuretic peptide.
- Additional MIS-C laboratory testing is listed with the diagnostic criteria above.

IMAGING STUDIES

- Chest radiograph may be normal in early or mild disease. The most common abnormalities are bilateral, peripheral patchy airspace consolidation, peribronchial thickening, or ground glass opacities.
- Chest computed tomography (CT) images show bilateral, peripheral and subpleural ground glass opacities. A consolidation with surrounding halo sign is considered typical in children.
- If MIS-C is suspected, cardiac evaluation with echocardiogram to evaluate myocardial function and coronary arteries is warranted.

Rx TREATMENT

- Treatment is supportive and symptomatic.
- Vaccines are now available for adults but are not yet FDA approved for children.

NONPHARMACOLOGIC THERAPY

- Patients with mild disease usually recover at home with supportive care and appropriate isolation guidelines.
- Patients with moderate or severe COVID-19 often require hospitalization.
- Respiratory support can include: Supplemental oxygen, high flow nasal cannula (HFNC), noninvasive ventilation, mechanical ventilation, extracorporeal membrane oxygenation (ECMO).
- Prone positioning should be considered in patients with severe hypoxemia.

ACUTE GENERAL Rx

- Empiric antibacterial therapy is reasonable if there is concern for a bacterial pneumonia.
- Empiric treatment for influenza during the influenza season is reasonable until influenza test results are known.
- No current data connect the use of NSAIDs to worsening COVID-19 symptoms.
- On May 1, 2020, the U.S. Food and Drug Administration issued an emergency use authorization for remdesivir—an investigational antiviral drug for the treatment of suspected or laboratory confirmed COVID-19. Remdesivir for 5 or 10 days should be considered for children hospitalized with severe or critical disease.
- Corticosteroids should be considered in mechanically ventilated patients.
- Other therapies to consider for severe or critical disease: Convalescent plasma, interleukin-6 inhibitor (e.g., tocilizumab), or interleukin-1Ra inhibitor (e.g., anakinra).
- Pharmacologic anticoagulation prophylaxis should be considered in critically ill children because of the prothrombotic state described in adults.
- MIS-C patients have been treated most commonly with IVIG, corticosteroids, and antiplatelet and/or anticoagulant therapy.
- Children with severe myocardial dysfunction (EF<30%) have been treated with enoxaparin and/or aspirin.
- Treatment of MIS-C is evolving, and recommendations are likely to change pending further research.

DISPOSITION

- Most children infected with COVID-19 experience mild, self-limiting illness.
- The duration of hospitalization is usually less than 7 days. Of the patients requiring intensive care, the majority recover well.
- Except for rare situations, a test-based strategy is no longer recommended to determine when an individual with a COVID-19 infection is no longer infectious.
- Patients recovering from MIS-C who had significant myocardial involvement require pediatric cardiology follow-up.

PEARLS & CONSIDERATIONS

- The optimal clinical management for COVID-19 is evolving.
- Cytopenias distinguish MIS-C from Kawasaki and the degree of hyperferritinemia and pattern of cytokine production differ between MIS-C and macrophage activation syndrome.
- SARS-CoV-2 enters human cells through the angiotensin-converting–enzyme 2 (ACE2) receptor which is highly expressed on type II alveolar epithelial cells, myocardial cells, proximal tubule cells of the kidney, enterocytes of the small intestine, neurons in the brain, and vascular endothelial cells. This may explain the multiple organ involvement.
- During times of high community spread of COVID-19, universal face mask wearing (excluded are children under age 2 yr), frequent handwashing, routine cleaning/disinfecting of frequently touched surfaces, and maintaining social distancing lower the risk of transmission.
- Health care providers should wear personal protective equipment (PPE) and eye protective equipment during patient encounters.
- During aerosol-generating procedures in patients with COVID-19, current guidelines recommend that clinicians wear gowns, gloves, N95 masks, and eye protection and place patients in negative-pressure rooms whenever possible.

SUGGESTED READINGS

Available at ExpertConsult.com

AUTHORS: **Sheyla Richards, MD,** and **Margaret Priestley, MD**

BASIC INFORMATION

DEFINITION

Pediculosis is lice infestation. Human beings can be infested with three kinds of lice: *Pediculus capitis* (head louse, Fig. 1), *Pediculus corporis* (body louse), and *Phthirus pubis* (pubic, or crab, louse). Lice inject saliva into the skin and feed on human blood, causing local inflammation. They deposit eggs (nits) on hair shafts (head lice and pubic lice) and along the seams of clothing (body lice). Nits remain firmly attached, and generally hatch within 7 to 10 days. Lice are obligate human parasites and cannot survive away from their hosts for longer than 7 to 10 days. Fig. 2 illustrates the life cycle of the head louse.

SYNONYM

Lice

ICD-10CM CODES

B85.0	Pediculosis due to *Pediculus humanus capitis*
B85.1	Pediculosis due to *Pediculus humanus corporis*
B85.2	Pediculosis, unspecified
B85.3	Phthiriasis
B85.4	Mixed pediculosis and phthiriasis
Z11.8	Screening for head lice
Z20.7	Exposure to head lice
Z83.1	Family history of lice
Z86.19	History of lice

EPIDEMIOLOGY & DEMOGRAPHICS

- There are 6 to 12 million cases of head lice in the United States annually in children between ages 3 and 11 yr, with infection more common in females.
- Head lice affect children of all socioeconomic levels. Risk factors include sharing hair care items and attending daycare. Frequency of hair washing, brushing, and hair length do not modify risk of infestation.
- Risk factors for body lice include poor hygiene, homelessness, and crowded living conditions. Unlike head and pubic lice, body lice can transmit disease.
- Pubic lice in a child, including infestation of the eyelashes, may indicate sexual abuse.
- The chance of acquiring pubic lice from one sexual exposure with an infested partner is >90% (the most contagious sexually transmitted infection [STI] known) and diagnosis should prompt additional STI evaluation.
- Pets are not implicated in the transmission of lice.

PHYSICAL FINDINGS & CLINICAL PRESENTATION

- Infections may be asymptomatic. However, pruritis is the most common symptom, caused by hypersensitivity to lice saliva and fecal material. Secondary bacterial infections may develop from excoriation sores.
- Nits can be identified by examining hair shafts (Fig. E3) in cases of head and pubic lice or on clothing in instances of body lice.
- Head lice are most frequently found on the nape of the neck and behind the ears.
- Lymphadenopathy may be present (cervical adenopathy with head lice, inguinal lymphadenopathy with pubic lice).
- Pubic lice may affect the hair around the anus.

ETIOLOGY

Lice are most commonly transmitted by close personal contact and less commonly by use of contaminated objects (e.g., combs, clothing, bed linen, hats). Lice cannot jump or fly.

DIAGNOSIS

DIFFERENTIAL DIAGNOSIS

- Seborrheic dermatitis
- Scabies
- Eczema
- Other: Pilar casts, trichonodosis (knotted hair), monilethrix (beaded hair)
- Table 1 describes the differential diagnosis of nits

WORKUP

Diagnosis is made by seeing live, adult lice (Fig. 4), which are typically 1 to 3 mm in length, as nits alone may be hatched or nonviable. Combing hair with a fine-toothed comb is recommended because visual inspection of the hair and scalp may miss more than 50% of infestations.

LABORATORY TESTS

Wood's light examination is useful to screen a large number of children: Live nits fluoresce, empty nits have a gray fluorescence, and nits with unborn lice reveal white fluorescence.

TREATMENT

ACUTE GENERAL Rx

The following products are available for treatment of head and pubic lice. Generally, body lice can be treated with nonpharmacologic therapies. Because head and pubic lice present minimal health risk, therapy should prioritize safety and cost. Side effects of topical therapy include pruritis, erythema, and mild burning. These side effects do not indicate treatment failure and do not necessitate retreatment. Additionally, clinicians should heed local resistance patterns, and if patients fail standard therapy, consultation with an infectious disease specialist may be beneficial.

- Permethrin is available over the counter (1% permethrin [Nix]) or by prescription (5% permethrin [Elimite]). It should be applied to damp hair and rinsed out after 10 min. Repeat application is generally not necessary in patients with head lice, but if required, it is most efficacious when performed 9 days after first treatment. Permethrin is nontoxic and FDA approved for use in children >2 mo old. Resistance to permethrin is now widespread.
- Malathion, an organophosphate, is effective in head lice, but is available by prescription only. It is applied to dry hair but is not commonly used due to its objectionable odor, risk of flammability, and prolonged application time (8 to 12 hr). It is contraindicated in children <2 yr old.
- Spinosad (Natroba) is a newer, FDA-approved product for head lice. It is a topical suspension applied to dry hair for 10 min, then rinsed out. Its application may be repeated 7 days later if necessary. It is more effective than permethrin, but more expensive. It is

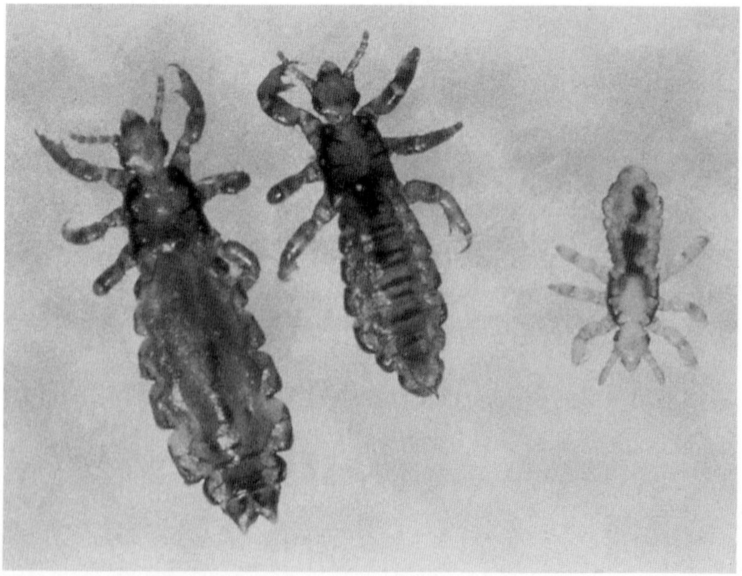

FIG. 1 Head louse family. From left to right: Female, male, and nymph. (With permission from Taplin D, Meinking TL: Infestations. In Schachner LA, Hansen RC [eds]: *Pediatric dermatology*, ed 4, Edinburgh, 2011, Mosby, pp. 1141-80; Bolognia JL et al: *Dermatology*, ed 4, Philadelphia, 2018, Elsevier.)

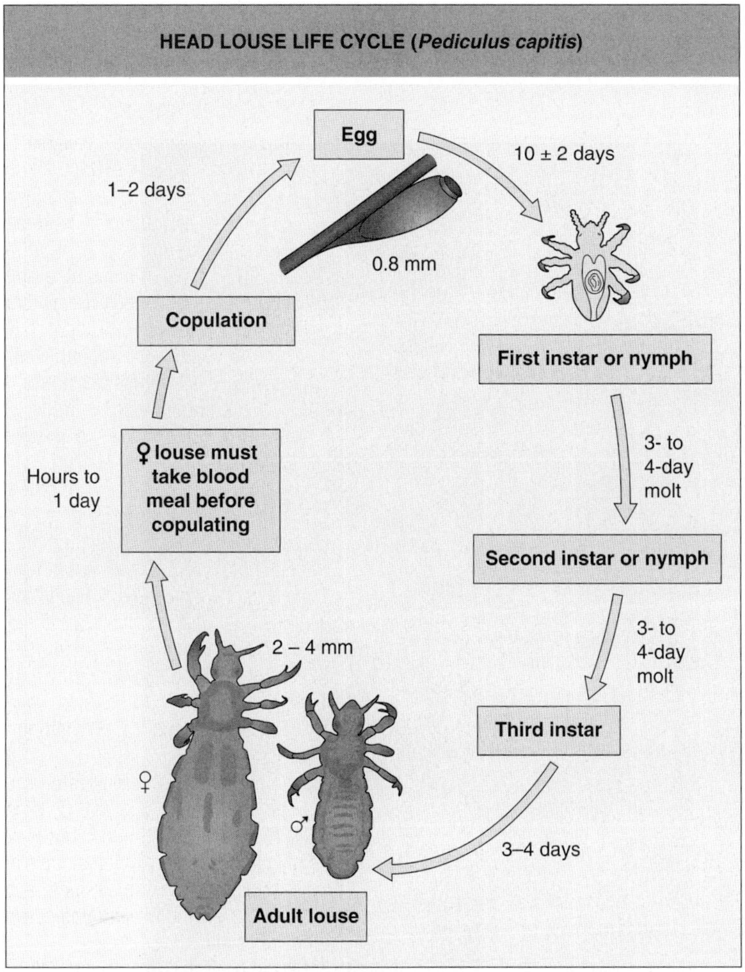

FIG. 2 Head louse life cycle *(Pediculus capitis).* (From Bolognia JL et al: *Dermatology,* ed 4, Philadelphia, 2018, Elsevier.)

TABLE 1 Differential Diagnosis of Nits

Diagnosis	Comment
Nits	Firmly adherent to hair shaft; not easily removed with fingers
Seborrheic dermatitis (dandruff)	Diffuse scalp scaling; scales occasionally adhere to hair but easy to remove; scalp erythema may be present
Hair casts	Keratin protein that encircles hair shaft; easily removed
Piedra	Fungal infection of hair; firm nodules attached to hair shafts, white or black in color
Psoriasis	Thick silvery scales, often present overlying red plaques on the scalp
Hair products	Hairspray, mousse, gel

From Paller AS, Mancini AJ: *Hurwitz clinical pediatric dermatology, a textbook of skin disorders of childhood and adolescence,* ed 5, Philadelphia, 2016, Elsevier.

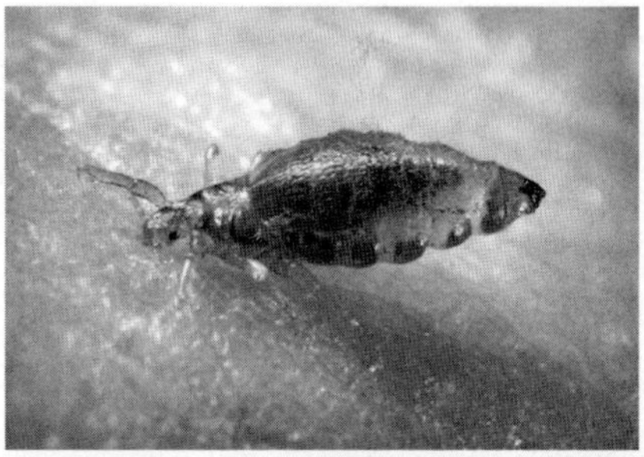

FIG. 4 Body louse, *Pediculus humanus* var. *corporis,* as it was obtaining a blood meal from human host. (Courtesy Public Health Image Library, Centers for Disease Control and Prevention. From Vincent JL et al: *Textbook of critical care,* ed 6, Philadelphia, 2011, Saunders.)

safe for use in pregnant persons (category B—no evidence of risk in humans) and in children >6 mo old.
- Benzyl alcohol lotion, 5% (Ulesfia) can be used for treatment of head lice in patients >6 mo old. The lotion is applied to dry hair and left on for 10 min. Treatment must be repeated after 7 days because the drug is not ovicidal. It is FDA approved for children >6 mo old.
- Eyelash infestation can be treated with the application of ophthalmic-grade, prescription petroleum jelly rubbed into the eyelashes 2 to 4 times a day for 10 days.
- In patients with resistance to 1% permethrin cream rinse, a 10-day course of trimethoprim-sulfamethoxazole (TMP-SMX) 8 mg/kg/day in divided doses is an effective treatment for head lice infestation, especially for eyelash infestations with *Phthirus pubis.* However, the risk of Stevens-Johnson syndrome should be weighed against the minimal health risk posed by lice, especially in the setting of other efficacious regimens.
- Ivermectin, an antiparasitic drug, given as an oral dose of 400 mcg/kg of body weight on days 1 and 9, is effective for head lice resistant to other treatments. It is currently not FDA approved for pediculosis and should not be used in children <15 kg given risk of neurotoxicity. Ivermectin 0.5% lotion is FDA approved as a single-use topical treatment for head lice in patients >6 mo, but may be cost prohibitive.
- Fig. 5 summarizes treatments for head lice.

COMPLEMENTARY & ALTERNATIVE MEDICINE

- Wet combing is a widely recommended but unproven adjunctive therapy.
- Personal items such as combs and brushes should be soaked in hot water for 15 to 30 min. Clothing, towels, and bed linens used in the 48 hr prior to treatment should be washed in hot water (>130 °F [>54.4 °C]), and then dried for 10 min at the hottest setting. Items that cannot be washed should be sealed in a plastic bag for 2 wk.
- Vacuuming floors and furniture is recommended, but excessive, costly household cleaning is not needed.
- Gaseous pesticides are toxic and should not be used.

PEARLS & CONSIDERATIONS

COMMENTS

- Given the low risk of classroom transmission, the American Academy of Pediatrics does not support exclusion from school because of head lice.
- Close contacts and household members should also be examined for the presence of lice.
- Patients with pubic lice should notify their sexual contacts. Sexual partners within the last month should be treated.

TREATMENTS FOR HEAD LICE				
Treatment	Group	Administration on days 1 and 8	Concerns	Efficacy & resistance
Pyrethrins (0.33%) synergized with piperonyl butoxide (4%), various formulations*	Natural botanicals	Topical application for 10 minutes to dry hair	Allergic reactions in individuals with sensitivity to chrysanthemums, ragweed, and related plants	Poor–fair; resistance common
Permethrin cream rinse or lotion (1%)*	Synthetic pyrethroid	Topical application for 10 minutes to clean, dry hair	None	Poor–fair; resistance common
Permethrin cream (5%)†	Synthetic pyrethroid	Topical overnight application to clean, dry hair	Allergic contact dermatitis in individuals with sensitivity to formaldehyde	Poor–fair; resistance common
Lindane shampoo (1%)	Organochlorine	Topical application for 4 minutes to clean, dry hair, then add water to lather and rinse	Potential CNS toxicity; not recommended for infants, children, breastfeeding mothers or pregnant women (category C)	Poor; resistance common
Carbaryl shampoo (0.5%)	Carbamate cholinesterase inhibitor	Topical application for 8–12 hours	Possible carcinogen	Poor–fair; resistance common (not approved in the U.S.)
Benzyl alcohol lotion (5%)§	Alcohol	Topical application for 10 minutes to dry hair	Potential skin irritation	Good; no resistance noted to date
Dimethicone (4%)	Silicone oil	Topical application for 15 minutes or overnight	None	Good
Spinosad cream rinse (0.9%)§	Bacterial fermentation product	Topical application for 10 minutes to dry hair	None	Good; no resistance noted to date
Malathion lotion or gel (0.5%)‡	Organophosphate cholinesterase inhibitor	Topical application for 8–12 hours to dry hair (Ovide® and gel products with isopropyl alcohol base are effective at 20 minutes)	Flammable isopropyl alcohol base; burning or stinging at sites of eroded skin	Excellent (in U.S.); resistance noted in Europe and Australia, but to date not in U.S.
Ivermectin solution (0.5%)§	Avermectin	Topical application for 10 minutes to dry hair	Potential skin and eye irritation	Excellent; no resistance noted to date
Oral ivermectin (available as 3 mg tablets)		Oral dose of 200–400 mcg/kg	Potential CNS toxicity; not recommended for children weighing <33 pounds (15 kg), breastfeeding mothers or pregnant women (category C)	

*Over-the-counter products.
†Approved for individuals ≥2 mo of age; pregnancy category B.
‡Approved for individuals ≥6 yr of age; pregnancy category B.
§Approved for individuals ≥6 mo of age; pregnancy category B.

FIG. 5 Treatments for head lice. In general, treatments should be given on two separate occasions, with optimal timing of the second dose on day 9. However, the FDA-approved regimen for treatment of head lice with 0.5% ivermectin solution is a single application. AirAllé® is an FDA-cleared medical device that uses hot air to treat head lice via dehydration of their eggs and, to a lesser degree, hatched lice. Abametapir 0.74% lotion, an ovicidal metalloprotease inhibitor, has been shown in phase 3 clinical trials to have efficacy in the treatment of head lice. *CNS,* Central nervous system; *FDA,* U.S. Food and Drug Administration. (From Bolognia JL et al: *Dermatology*, ed 4, Philadelphia, 2018, Elsevier.)

- Finding nits without live, adult lice, especially >0.25 inches from the scalp, suggests past infection.
- Lice-removal companies may be helpful for some families, but no studies exist comparing efficacy of professional vs. home removal.

RELATED CONTENT

Lice (Patient Information)

SUGGESTED READINGS

Available at ExpertConsult.com

AUTHORS: **Eileen Everly, MD,** and **Leora Lieberman, MD**

Pelvic Abscess (PTG)

BASIC INFORMATION

DEFINITION

Pelvic abscess is an acute or chronic infection, most commonly involving the pelvic viscera. Treatment requires directed therapy including broad-spectrum antimicrobials and, if medical therapy fails, surgical intervention. There are four categories based on etiologic factors:

- Ascending infection, spreading from cervix through endometrial cavity to adnexa, forming a tuboovarian complex
- Infection occurring in the puerperium, which spreads to the adnexa from the endometrium or myometrium by a hematogenous or lymphatic route
- Abscess complicating pelvic surgery
- Involvement of the pelvic viscera as a result of spread from contiguous organs, such as appendicitis or diverticulitis

SYNONYMS

Tuboovarian abscess (TOA)
Vaginal cuff abscess

ICD-10CM CODES	
K63.0	Abscess of intestine
K65.1	Peritoneal abscess
K68.11	Postprocedural retroperitoneal abscess
K68.12	Psoas muscle abscess
K68.19	Other retroperitoneal abscess
N70.93	Salpingitis and oophoritis, unspecified
N70.0	Acute salpingitis and oophoritis
N70.1	Chronic salpingitis and oophoritis

EPIDEMIOLOGY & DEMOGRAPHICS

INCIDENCE:

- 34% of hospitalized patients with pelvic inflammatory disease
- 1% to 2% of patients undergoing hysterectomy, most frequently with vaginal approach
- Peak incidence in third to fourth decade

RISK FACTORS: Same risk factors as for pelvic inflammatory disease, although in 30% to 50% of patients there is no prior history of salpingitis before abscess forms.

PHYSICAL FINDINGS & CLINICAL PRESENTATION

- Abdominal or pelvic pain (90%)
- Fever or chills (50%)
- Abnormal bleeding (21%)
- Vaginal discharge (28%)
- Nausea (26%)
- Up to 60% to 80% present without fever or leukocytosis; absence of these findings should not exclude diagnosis

ETIOLOGY

- Mixed flora of anaerobes, aerobes, and facultative anaerobes, such as *Escherichia coli, Bacteroides fragilis, Prevotella* spp., aerobic streptococci, and *Peptococcus* and *Peptostreptococcus* spp.
- *Neisseria gonorrhoeae* and *Chlamydia* are the major etiologic bacteria in cervicitis and salpingitis but are rarely found in abscess cavity cultures.
- In elderly patients consider diverticular disease.

DIAGNOSIS

DIFFERENTIAL DIAGNOSIS

- Pelvic neoplasms, such as ovarian tumors and leiomyomas.
- Ovarian torsion.
- Inflammatory masses involving adjacent bowel or omentum, such as ruptured appendicitis or diverticulitis.
- Pelvic hematomas, as may occur after cesarean section or hysterectomy.
- Ectopic pregnancy.

LABORATORY TESTS

- CBC with differential
- Aerobic as well as anaerobic cultures of cervix, blood, urine, sputum, peritoneal cavity (if entered), and abscess cavity before starting antibiotics
- Pregnancy test in patients of reproductive age

IMAGING STUDIES

- Sonogram: Noninvasive, inexpensive study to confirm diagnosis, estimate size of abscess, and monitor response to therapy; sensitivity >90%
- CT scan: Used for both diagnosis and therapy (CT-guided drainage) (Fig. E1)
  1. Useful where sonogram provides insufficient information, as with intraabdominal abscesses
  2. Success rate with CT-guided abscess drainage: Unilocular, 90%; multilocular, 40%

TREATMENT

Major concerns:

- Desire for future fertility
- Likelihood of rupture of abscess, with resulting peritonitis, septic shock, and morbid sequelae

ACUTE GENERAL Rx

- Clinical quandary is whether patient requires immediate laparoscopic surgery (uncertain diagnosis or suspicion of rupture) or management with IV antibiotics, reserving surgery for those with inadequate clinical response (e.g., 48 to 72 hr of therapy, with persistent fever or leukocytosis, increasing size of mass, or suspicion of rupture).
- Surgery indicated in poor response to medical therapy. Early surgery may be needed in those with large adnexal masses (>8 cm), or in immunocompromised patients.
- Antibiotic combinations:
  1. Ampicillin-sulbactam 3 g IV q6h or cefoxitin 2 g IV q6h or cefotetan 2 g IV q12h plus doxycycline 100 mg IV q12h
  2. For penicillin allergic patients: Clindamycin 900 mg IV q8h or metronidazole 500 mg IV q6 to 8h plus gentamicin either 5 to 7 mg/kg q24h or 1.5 mg/kg q8h
- During medical management, high index of suspicion for acute rupture, such as acute worsening of abdominal pain or new-onset tachycardia and hypotension, mandating immediate surgical intervention after patient stabilization.
- Surgical options:
  1. Laparoscopy with drainage and irrigation
  2. CT-guided drainage (interventional radiology)
  3. Transvaginal colpotomy (abscess must be midline, dissect rectovaginal septum, and be adherent to vaginal fornix)
  4. Laparotomy, including total abdominal hysterectomy with bilateral salpingo-oophorectomy or unilateral salpingo-oophorectomy
  5. Evidence of ruptured tuboovarian abscess is a surgical emergency

DISPOSITION

- Of patients treated with medical therapy, response in 75%, with a 50% pregnancy rate. Pregnancy rate decreases with recurrent episodes.
- No response in 30% to 40%; can be treated with either CT-guided drainage or surgical intervention, keeping in mind that unilateral adnexectomy may give equal chance of cure versus hysterectomy, yet preserve reproductive potential.

REFERRAL

If patient has a tuboovarian abscess, refer to gynecologist.

PEARLS & CONSIDERATIONS

COMMENTS

- If *Actinomyces* species is isolated from culture, treatment with penicillin is required for an extended period (6 wk to 3 mo).
- Most common cause of preventable death: Physician delay in diagnosis.

SUGGESTED READING

Available at ExpertConsult.com

RELATED CONTENT

Pelvic Abscess (Patient Information)
Pelvic Inflammatory Disease (Related Key Topic)

AUTHORS: **Ella Stern, MD,** and **Simone Sweeney, MD**

BASIC INFORMATION

DEFINITION

Pelvic inflammatory disease (PID) is infection and inflammation of the upper female genital tract (including uterus, fallopian tubes, ovaries, and/or pelvic peritoneum) unrelated to pregnancy or surgical intervention. PID can be classified as acute (≤30 days duration), subclinical, or chronic (>30 days' duration).

SYNONYMS

PID
Salpingitis
Oophoritis
Adnexitis
Pyosalpinx
Tuboovarian abscess
TOA

ICD-10CM CODES

A18.17	Tuberculous female pelvic inflammatory disease
A52.76	Syphilitic pelvic inflammatory disease
A54.2*	Gonococcal pelviperitonitis and other gonococcal genitourinary infections
A54.24	Gonococcal female pelvic inflammatory disease
A56.1*	Chlamydial infection of pelviperitoneum and other genitourinary organs
A56.11	Chlamydial female pelvic inflammatory disease
A56.19	Other chlamydial genitourinary infection
N70*	Salpingitis and oophoritis
N70.0*	Acute salpingitis and oophoritis
N70.01	Acute salpingitis
N70.02	Acute oophoritis
N70.03	Acute salpingitis and oophoritis
N70.1*	Chronic salpingitis and oophoritis
N70.11	Chronic salpingitis
N70.12	Chronic oophoritis
N70.13	Chronic salpingitis and oophoritis
N70.9*	Salpingitis and oophoritis, unspecified
N70.91	Salpingitis, unspecified
N70.92	Oophoritis, unspecified
N70.93	Salpingitis and oophoritis, unspecified
N71*	Inflammatory disease of uterus, except cervix
N71.0	Acute inflammatory disease of uterus
N71.1	Chronic inflammatory disease of uterus
N71.9	Inflammatory disease of uterus, unspecified
N72	Inflammatory disease of cervix uteri
N73*	Other female pelvic inflammatory diseases
N73.0	Acute parametritis and pelvic cellulitis
N73.1	Chronic parametritis and pelvic cellulitis
N73.2	Unspecified parametritis and pelvic cellulitis
N73.3	Female acute pelvic peritonitis
N73.4	Female chronic pelvic peritonitis
N73.5	Female pelvic peritonitis, unspecified
N73.6	Female pelvic peritoneal adhesions (postinfective)
N73.8	Other specified female pelvic inflammatory diseases
N73.9	Female pelvic inflammatory disease, unspecified
N74	Female pelvic inflammatory disorders in diseases classified elsewhere

*Indicates nonbillable codes

EPIDEMIOLOGY & DEMOGRAPHICS

INCIDENCE & PREVALENCE: Pelvic inflammatory disease is most often diagnosed in young, sexually active women. The incidence of PID is difficult to ascertain given its broad diagnostic criteria, its propensity to be missed as a diagnosis, and the challenges with follow-up due to patients seeking urgent or emergent care for this condition. The Centers for Disease Control and Prevention estimates 1 million new cases of PID are diagnosed yearly. The incidence may be rising given recent sharp increases in STDs associated with PID in the United States. PID has long-term health risks for women, including recurrent infection, chronic pelvic pain, pelvic adhesive disease, and tubal disease resulting in ectopic pregnancy and infertility.

RISK FACTORS:
- Sexually active adolescent and young women
- Previous episode of PID
- Prior chlamydial infection
- Multiple or new sexual partners within past 12 mo
- Sexual partner diagnosed with sexually transmitted infection (STI)
- Nonuse of barrier contraception

PHYSICAL FINDINGS & CLINICAL PRESENTATION

- Lower abdominal pain
- Abnormal vaginal discharge
- Abnormal uterine bleeding
- Postcoital bleeding
- Dysuria
- Dyspareunia
- Fever
- Nausea and vomiting (suggestive of peritonitis)

PHYSICAL FINDINGS

- Fever
- Abdominal tenderness
- Abnormal vaginal discharge
- Cervical friability
- Cervical motion tenderness
- Adnexal tenderness
- Adnexal mass
- Right upper quadrant tenderness (perihepatitis): 5% of PID cases

NOTE: Women with PID may be asymptomatic and/or have a benign physical examination.

ETIOLOGY

Pelvic inflammatory disease occurs as a result of ascending infection from the lower genital tract. Infections are often polymicrobial, and although gonorrheal and chlamydial infections are commonly implicated in the development of PID, fewer than 50% of women test positive for these organisms. This is likely due in part to increased STI screening efforts. PID may also arise in the setting of organisms associated with normal vaginal flora such as:
- *Bacteroides fragilis*
- *Escherichia coli* and other enteric gram-negative rods
- *Gardnerella vaginalis*
- *Haemophilus influenzae*

Rarer infectious causes include the following: *Mycoplasma hominis, Ureaplasma urealyticum, Mycoplasma genitalium* (a concern because of antibiotic resistance), *Mycobacterium tuberculosis* (an important cause in developing countries), and cytomegalovirus (CMV).

Dx DIAGNOSIS

Diagnosis of PID is made when a patient has clinical or pathologic evidence of upper genital tract infection and inflammation. Although no single test or measure reliably diagnoses the spectrum of disorders that comprise PID:
- Providers should maintain a low threshold for diagnosis and treatment of PID given significant long-term health risks associated with the disease, especially if untreated
- Definitive criteria for diagnosis of PID include:
  1. Laparoscopic abnormalities consistent with PID
  2. Histopathologic evidence of endometritis in women with clinical suspicion for PID
  3. Transvaginal sonography or other imaging techniques showing thickened, fluid-filled tubes, with or without free pelvic fluid or tuboovarian complex
- The CDC suggests that women with risk factors, abdominal or pelvic pain, and any pelvic tenderness (cervical, uterine, and/or adnexal) be treated for PID

DIFFERENTIAL DIAGNOSIS

- Appendicitis
- Ectopic pregnancy
- Intrauterine/other pregnancy
- Ovarian cyst
- Adnexal torsion
- Endometriosis
- Urinary tract infection (cystitis or pyelonephritis)

WORKUP

- History—as in risk factors and clinical presentation, previously
- Physical examination—as in physical findings, previously

LABORATORY TESTS

- Wet mount: Clue cells, increased white cells
- Gram stain of endocervical exudate: >30 polymorphonuclear cells per high-power field correlates with chlamydial or gonococcal infection
- Endocervical cultures for *N. gonorrhoeae* and *C. trachomatis*
- Fallopian tube aspirate or peritoneal exudate culture if laparoscopy performed
- WBC: Leukocytosis
- Elevated acute phase reactants: ESR >15 mm/hr, C-reactive protein
- HCG to rule out intrauterine or ectopic pregnancy
- HIV, with consideration for other STI screening such as RPR, HBsAg, Hep C Ab (HIV increases incidence of TOA)

IMAGING STUDIES

Ultrasonography is commonly used to assess for PID and can be used to determine inpatient vs. outpatient treatment by presence or absence of TOA. Findings include:

- Thick-walled adnexal mass with heterogenous or cystic contents suggestive of abscess
- Dilated fallopian tubes (note that normal fallopian tubes are rarely identified on ultrasonography)
- "Cogwheel sign" indicating thickened fallopian tube walls
- Heterogenous fluid within the endometrium

CT or MRI scan may be useful to better characterize adnexal masses and/or rule out other pathology, such as appendicitis or renal calculus. Choice of imaging modality will depend on clinical suspicion, logistical access, and associated cost.

PROCEDURES

Endometrial biopsy that reveals endometritis may support a diagnosis of PID. Laparoscopy has been utilized as a gold standard for diagnosing PID, but due to the invasive nature of this procedure and the risks and costs associated, it is rarely indicated as a diagnostic tool.

Rx TREATMENT

Primary management of PID is medical, with broad-spectrum antibiotics administered in an outpatient setting. Inpatient treatment should be initiated when:

- Surgical emergency is not excluded
- Tuboovarian abscess is present
- Patient is unable or unwilling to complete outpatient treatment (including medication regimen and clinical follow-up)
- Outpatient treatment fails to improve symptoms in 48 to 72 hr
- Pregnancy, immunodeficiency, or other complicating medical condition exists

Evidence-based guidelines recommended by the CDC for acute PID are as follows:

INPATIENT REGIMENS

RECOMMENDED PARENTERAL REGIMENS:

- Cefotetan 2 g IV q12h *PLUS* doxycycline 100 mg PO or IV q12h OR
- Cefoxitin 2 g IV q6h *PLUS* doxycycline 100 mg PO or IV q12h OR
- Clindamycin 900 mg IV q8h *PLUS* gentamicin loading dose IV or IM (2 mg/kg of body weight), followed by a maintenance dose (1.5 mg/kg) q8h. Single daily dosing (3 to 5 mg/kg) can be substituted.

ALTERNATIVE PARENTERAL REGIMEN:

- Ampicillin/sulbactam 3 g IV q6h *PLUS* doxycycline 100 mg PO or IV q12h
- When clinical improvement is apparent based on symptoms, physical exam, and laboratory criteria, antibiotics may be transitioned from IV to PO with doxycycline PO or clindamycin PO (depending on the regimen selected) administered to complete 14 days of total antibiotic therapy. If a patient does not improve despite use of a recommended antibiotic regimen, further workup and potential procedural intervention are warranted.

OUTPATIENT REGIMENS

RECOMMENDED INTRAMUSCULAR/ORAL REGIMENS:

- Ceftriaxone 250 mg IM in a single dose *PLUS doxycycline* 100 mg PO bid for 14 days
  WITH or WITHOUT metronidazole 500 mg PO bid for 14 days
  OR
- Cefoxitin 2 g IM in a single dose and probenecid, 1 g PO administered concurrently in a single dose *PLUS* doxycycline 100 mg PO bid for 14 days
  WITH or WITHOUT metronidazole 500 mg PO bid for 14 days
  OR
- Other third-generation cephalosporin (ceftizoxime or cefotaxime) *PLUS* doxycycline 100 mg orally bid for 14 days
  WITH or WITHOUT metronidazole 500 mg orally twice a day for 14 days

ALTERNATIVE INTRAMUSCULAR/ORAL REGIMEN:

- Azithromycin 1 g PO once weekly for 2 wk *PLUS* ceftriaxone 250 mg IM in a single dose

TREATMENT CONSIDERATIONS

- Antimicrobials should include coverage against *N. gonorrhoeae* and *C. trachomatis* even if these organisms are not identified on culture.
- Due to increasing antibiotic resistance of *N. gonorrhoeae*, fluoroquinolones should be avoided in the treatment of PID. If gonorrhea is isolated in a woman with PID, addition of azithromycin 1 g orally one time should be considered in treatment.
- Women should avoid sexual activity until they and their sexual partners have been adequately treated and symptoms have resolved.
- TOA may require drainage, which may be accomplished by interventional radiology via aspiration or placement of a drain, or by a gynecologist via vaginal or laparoscopic means. Recurrent/persistent TOAs may be managed by total abdominal hysterectomy with bilateral salpingo-oophorectomy after acute treatment of infection.
- Treatment of PID in women with intrauterine devices (IUDs) does not include/require removal of the device unless there is no clinical improvement after 48 to 72 hr of treatment with an approved regimen. IUDs rarely serve as a source for PID, especially >3 wk after insertion.
- Sexual partners of patients diagnosed with PID or other STIs should be evaluated and treated appropriately. In the setting of PID, treat all sexual partners within 60 days of onset of symptoms. Some states allow for expedited partner therapy (EPT), such that a woman's provider is able to supply her with enough medication to treat herself and her partner(s).
- Treatment of chronic PID may be aimed at a different spectrum of microbes and should be tailored appropriately.

DISPOSITION

- Given the risk of reinfection, all women should be retested for gonorrhea and chlamydia 3 to 6 mo after treatment.
- Follow-up includes confirmation of partner treatment, education on use of barrier contraception, and risks of PID and long-term sequelae, including:
  1. Recurrent PID
  2. Chronic pelvic pain
  3. Fallopian tube damage that leads to infertility and/or ectopic pregnancy
  4. Fitz-Hugh-Curtis syndrome
  5. Potential risk for cancer: Limited studies have suggested a small association between PID and ovarian, endometrial, and colon cancer

PEARLS & CONSIDERATIONS

COMMENTS

- Maintain a low threshold for the diagnosis and treatment of PID given the risks for progression to severe infection and to significant and chronic medical and reproductive complications.
- Most patients are candidates for outpatient therapy, but inpatient hospitalization is recommended in select cases.
- Use only CDC-recommended treatment regimens unless contraindicated due to severe patient allergy; in such cases, check local susceptibilities of suspected pathogen.
- Offer HIV and other STI screening to all women with suspected or diagnosed PID.
- IUDs may be retained unless women have failed to improve with 48 to 72 hr of treatment.
- Treat sexual partners of women with PID, with EPT if possible.
- Counsel patients on abstinence until they and their partners have completed treatment.
- Test for reinfection with gonorrhea and chlamydia 3 to 6 mo after treatment.

PREVENTION

Women aged <25 yr and/or participating in high-risk sexual behavior should be screened annually for chlamydia; studies have shown such screening to reduce cases of PID by >50%. The importance of minimizing partner exposures and using barrier contraception (either alone or in conjunction with another method) should also be emphasized.

SUGGESTED READINGS

Available at ExpertConsult.com

RELATED CONTENT

Pelvic Inflammatory Disease (Patient Information)
Chlamydia Genital Infections (Related Key Topic)
Gonorrhea (Related Key Topic)
Pelvic Abscess (Related Key Topic)

AUTHOR: **Gretchen Makai, MD**

BASIC INFORMATION

DEFINITION

Pelvic organ prolapse (POP) refers to descent of vaginal tissue and/or the uterus into the vaginal canal. It results from injury to or weakness in the connective tissue and muscles of the pelvic floor. Modern definitions of POP describe anterior and posterior vaginal wall defects, as well as apical defects in pelvic floor connective tissue. Synonyms for POP include cystocele (Fig. E1), rectocele (Fig. E2), uterine prolapse (Fig. E3), enterocele (Fig. E4), and vaginal vault prolapse. Descriptions of this condition as a "dropped bladder," "dropped uterus," or defects in other pelvic organs should be avoided. These types of descriptions do not accurately reflect the pathophysiology of POP and often create confusion and unnecessary stress for patients. Table 1 describes the various types of POP affecting each vaginal compartment with corresponding ICD-10 codes.

SYNONYMS

Vaginal prolapse
Uterine prolapse
Genital prolapse
Uterine descensus
POP
Pelvic floor disorder
PFD

ICD-10CM CODES	
N81.11	Cystocele, midline
N81.12	Cystocele, lateral
N81.2	Incomplete uterovaginal prolapse
N81.3	Complete uterovaginal prolapse
N81.4	Uterovaginal prolapse, unspecified
N81.5	Vaginal enterocele
N81.6	Rectocele
N81.89	Other female genital prolapse

EPIDEMIOLOGY & DEMOGRAPHICS

INCIDENCE AND PREVALENCE: Prevalence estimates are difficult to determine due to varying definitions of POP and various diagnostic criteria. Based on self-reported symptoms in the National Health and Nutrition Examination Survey, the prevalence of POP is 3% to 4%. However, based on physical examination, the prevalence of POP is much higher. The incidence of POP surgery is 1.5 to 1.8 surgeries per 1000 women years. Annual direct health care costs are high, and repeat operations are common.

RISK FACTORS: POP has a long latency and is multifactorial. Multiple risk factors have been identified. Some are modifiable, suggesting POP may be preventable; however, many risk factors are not. Some of the most common risk factors include:

- Parity, labor, and vaginal childbirth
- Age
- Chronic increased intraabdominal pressure (chronic coughing due to COPD, chronic constipation, chronic heavy lifting)
- Smoking
- Chronic steroid use
- Connective tissue diseases (Marfan syndrome, Ehlers-Danlos syndrome)
- Pelvic surgery
- Menopause
- Family history
- Caucasian and Hispanic race

GENETICS: Data suggest a heritable component to POP; however, no specific genes or genetic factors outside of specific connective tissue diseases have been identified. Connective tissue disorders associated with an increased risk include Marfan syndrome and Ehlers-Danlos syndrome. In general, a genetic susceptibility exists in certain families, which is then affected by external factors to increase an individual woman's risk of POP.

ETIOLOGY

- The cause of pelvic organ prolapse is usually multifactorial, but pregnancy is the most commonly associated risk factor.
- Muscle injury (levator ani) and connective tissue damage (pubocervical fascia) cause failure of pelvic floor support.
- Increased intraabdominal pressure results in strain on pelvic floor support structures.
- Injury to pelvic floor muscles or connective tissue supports results in uncompensated forces on pelvic floor, resulting in further injury to pelvic floor support structures.
  1. Acute (traumatic) injury to pelvic floor support can result from vaginal delivery, labor, or surgery.
  2. Chronic injury or strain on pelvic floor connective tissue and muscle can result from conditions such as COPD with chronic coughing or chronic constipation.
  3. Neurologic injury from acute or chronic strain on pelvic floor can result in denervation and subsequent muscular atrophy.
  4. Diseases or medications that weaken connective tissue (Marfan syndrome, corticosteroids) can predispose to injury.
  5. Hypoestrogenism may weaken pelvic floor tissue and impair ability to heal from injury.
- With injury to pelvic floor support structures, vaginal tissue becomes subject to the forces of intraabdominal pressure and will be displaced downward into the vaginal canal, resulting in clinical symptoms. In certain cases, the bladder, uterus, rectum, or peritoneal contents may be inferiorly displaced further, exacerbating symptoms and functional abnormalities.

PHYSICAL FINDINGS & CLINICAL PRESENTATION

- Bulge symptoms
  1. Vaginal pressure
  2. Protrusion from vagina (Fig. E5)
- Urinary symptoms
  1. Urinary hesitancy, frequency, or urgency
  2. Manual reduction of prolapse to complete urination (splinting)
  3. Incomplete emptying
  4. Weak urinary stream
- Bowel symptoms
  1. Incomplete defecation
  2. Altered rectal sensation (urgency, lack of sensation)
  3. Splinting of vagina/perineum to defecate
- Sexual symptoms
  1. Dyspareunia
  2. Difficulty with vaginal penetration
- Other
  1. Vaginal bleeding from exteriorized vaginal epithelium
  2. Incarcerated prolapse with inability to be manually reduced

Dx DIAGNOSIS

WORKUP

- Elicit specific symptoms. Determine the degree of bother with symptoms.
- Perform detailed pelvic exam. Examine anterior, posterior, and apical segments of vagina independently using a split speculum. Assess pelvic floor muscle tone.
  1. Exam is done in standard lithotomy position, and POP is assessed with Valsalva during exam.
  2. If symptoms are out of proportion to findings, repeat exam in standing position.
- Describe exam findings objectively (Boxes 1, 2, and 3).
  1. Quantitatively with POP-Q (more precise and reproducible than Baden-Walker system)
  2. Descriptively with Baden-Walker halfway systems

TABLE 1 Types of Genital Prolapse

Original Position of Organs	Prolapse	Symptoms (in addition to the general symptoms of discomfort, dragging, the feeling of a "lump," and, rarely, coital problems)
Anterior	Urethrocele Cystocele	Urinary symptoms (stress incontinence, urinary frequency)
Central	Cervix/uterus: 1st, 2nd, and 3rd degree Procidentia	Bleeding and/or discharge from ulceration in association with procidentia
Posterior	Rectocele Enterocele	Bowel symptoms, particularly the feeling of incomplete evacuation and sometimes having to press the posterior wall backward to pass stool

BOX 1 Points of Reference for POP-Q

Point	Description	Range of Values
Aa	3 cm above the hymen on anterior vaginal wall roughly corresponds with the urethrovesical junction.	−3 cm to +3 cm
Ba	The lowest extent of the segment of vagina between point Aa and the apex of the vagina. Unlike point Aa, it is not fixed but will be the same as Aa if point Aa is the most protruding point. In maximal prolapse, it will be the same as point C.	−3 cm to + TVL
C	Most distal edge of cervix (vaginal cuff if uterus/cervix absent).	
D	Posterior fornix (n/a if hysterectomy).	
Ap	3 cm above the hymen on posterior vaginal wall.	−3 cm to +3 cm
Bp	The lowest extent of the segment of vagina between point Ap and the apex of the vagina. Unlike point Ap, it is not fixed but will be the same as Ap if point Ap is the most protruding point. In maximal prolapse it will be the same as point D.	−3 cm to + TVL
GH (Genital Hiatus)	From urethral meatus to inferior hymenal ring.	
PB (Perineal Body)	From inferior hymenal ring to middle of anal orifice.	
TVL (Total Vaginal Length)	Without stretch or Valsalva.	

Key Points: Measure position of six points with respect to the position of the hymen. Points above the hymen (inside) are negative, points below the hymen are positive, and points at the hymen are 0.
Modified from Pemberton J (ed): *The pelvic floor,* Philadelphia, 2002, Saunders; and Bump RC et al: The standardization of terminology of female pelvic organ prolapse and pelvic floor dysfunction. *Am J Obstet Gynecol* 175(1):13, 1996.

BOX 2 POP-Q Examination and Staging

Stage 0	No prolapse
Stage I	Leading edge ≥1 cm above hymenal ring
Stage II	Leading edge ≤1 cm above hymenal ring but ≤1 cm below hymenal ring
Stage III	Most distal point is >1 cm but < (TVL-2) cm below the hymenal ring
Stage IV	Leading edge ≥ (TVL-2) cm below hymenal ring

BOX 3 Baden Walker Halfway System

Grade 0	Normal position for each respective site
Grade 1	Descent halfway to the hymen
Grade 2	Descent to the hymen
Grade 3	Descent halfway past the hymen
Grade 4	Maximum possible descent for each site

- Urinary symptoms should be evaluated separately.
  1. POP is associated with urinary incontinence but *does not cause* urinary incontinence.
  2. If lower urinary tract symptoms are present, perform urinalysis with culture
  3. Urodynamic testing may help with surgical planning in patients who have incontinence and >stage II prolapse or voiding dysfunction
- Evaluate postvoid residual urine volume in advanced POP (stage 3 and stage 4).
  1. Bladder ultrasound or catheterization at time of exam

LABORATORY TESTS

Not indicated for routine evaluation of POP

IMAGING STUDIES

- Not indicated for routine evaluation of POP. Imaging studies for other gynecologic or urologic conditions may be indicated.
- Pelvic ultrasound may be considered in the *absence of POP* in patients with specific symptoms (i.e., pelvic pressure) (Fig. E6).

Rx TREATMENT

PRIMARY PREVENTION:

- Diagnosis and treatment of chronic cough
- Correction of constipation
- Weight control, nutrition, and smoking cessation counseling
- Pelvic muscle exercises
- Proper management of vaginal apex at time of hysterectomy in patients without POP such as McCall culdoplasty to prevent vaginal vault prolapse
- Cesarean delivery NOT indicated for prevention of POP

POP TREATMENT OPTIONS:

- Only indicated if prolapse is bothersome to the patient
- Expectant management: Can be appropriate, except in cases of incomplete bladder emptying.
- Pessaries (Fig. E7):
  1. Silicone support device
  2. Exists in various shapes and sizes
     a. Use the simplest and smallest pessary that works
  3. Up to 92% of women can be fitted successfully with a pessary (Fig. E8)
     a. Includes sexually active women
  4. Self-care can be learned by the majority of women
     a. Usually remove and clean once per month; otherwise, office visit every 3 mo for cleaning and exam
  5. Side effects/complications:
     a. Increased risk of UTI
     b. Small vaginal erosions and very mild bleeding or spotting are common
        1) First episode of vaginal bleeding needs evaluation in postmenopausal patients
     c. Neglected pessaries can cause vaginitis, odor, severe vaginal erosion/bleeding, and fistula
     d. Vaginal estrogen may prevent or treat erosions and minimize risk of vaginitis and UTI
- Surgery:
  1. Indicated for bothersome POP and when patients fail or decline nonsurgical treatments.
  2. Goals of surgery are to eliminate vaginal bulge and improve associated symptoms.
     a. Resolution of bladder and bowel symptoms is not routinely associated with surgical correction of POP.
     b. Choice of operation should be tailored to patient's presenting problems, lifestyle, and goals for the surgery.
  3. Evaluate and treat all defects present on exam.
     a. Multiple defects are the most common presentation of POP. Seen in 60% of patients.
     b. Anterior and apical combination is most common.
  4. There are multiple ways to classify operations for POP
     a. Obliterative:
        1) Narrow, shorten, or completely close off the vagina.
        2) High success rates with low morbidity.
        3) First-line treatment for women with significant medical comorbidities who do not desire future vaginal intercourse.

TABLE 2 Procedures for POP

Classification		Procedure	Compartment(s)
Obliterative		Le Fort colpocleisis	All
		Total colpocleisis	All
Reconstructive	Restorative	Uterosacral ligament suspension	Apex
		Hysteropexy	Apex
		Paravaginal defect repair	Anterior
		Anterior colporrhaphy	Anterior
		Posterior colporrhaphy	Posterior
		Defect-directed posterior repair	Posterior
		Perineorrhaphy	Posterior
	Compensatory		
	Mesh	Sacral colpopexy	All
		Sacral hysteropexy	Apex
		Transvaginal mesh	All
	Nonmesh	Sacrospinous ligament suspension	Apex
		Iliococcygeus suspension	Apex
		Enterocele repair	Posterior

4) Associated with high rates of postoperative incontinence; most surgeons offer antiincontinence procedure at the same setting.

b. Reconstructive:
   1) Restorative procedures use normal anatomic relationships and structures.
   2) Compensatory procedures utilize nonanatomic relationships.
   3) Reconstructive procedures may or may not use synthetic meshes or biologic grafts.

5. Table 2 categorizes various common procedures for POP.
6. Hysterectomy alone does not treat POP.
   a. Often performed concomitantly with POP repair as necessary step to expose critical anatomy.
   b. During hysterectomy, vaginal apex suspension should be performed to reduce risk of recurrent POP.
7. Hysteropexy is option for women who wish to preserve uterus.
   a. Patient preference or desire for future childbearing.
   b. Short term comparative studies with hysterectomy procedures show equal efficacy.
8. Women without stress incontinence undergoing vaginal surgery for POP are at risk for postoperative urinary incontinence.
   a. Use of a prophylactic midurethral sling inserted during vaginal prolapse surgery has been shown to result in a lower rate of urinary incontinence at 3 and 12 mo, but also in a higher rate of adverse events (UTIs, major bleeding complications, incomplete bladder emptying).
9. Abdominal or laparoscopic mesh-based repairs (sacral colpopexy) have superior durability but higher risk and potential for unique complications.
10. In April 2019, the U.S. FDA ordered that the sale of all transvaginal mesh products for pelvic organ prolapse be halted in the U.S. due a lack of data showing clinical superiority (https://www.fda.gov/medical-devices/implants-and-prosthetics/urogynecologic-surgical-mesh-implants, last accessed September 2020).

DISPOSITION

- Surgical success rates range between 70% and 95%.
- Up to 30% of patients may require a second operation for POP.
- Untreated POP does not necessarily worsen.

REFERRAL

To a urogynecologist/gynecologist if surgical intervention is needed or for complex cases involving bladder dysfunction or recurrent symptoms.

PEARLS & CONSIDERATIONS

- POP rarely, if ever, causes pain.
- Stage of POP does not dictate treatment or prognosis or predict symptoms.
- Treatment for POP is based on symptoms, patient bother, and patient goals
- Options for most patients are no treatment, pessary, or surgery.

SUGGESTED READINGS

Available at ExpertConsult.com

RELATED CONTENT

Pelvic Organ Prolapse (Patient Information)
Uterine Prolapse (Patient Information)
Incontinence, Urinary (Related Key Topic)

AUTHORS: **Ashley Hodges, MD,** and **Matthew J. Fagan, MD, FACOG**

BASIC INFORMATION

DEFINITION

Peptic ulcer disease (PUD) is an ulceration in the stomach or duodenum resulting from an imbalance between mucosal protective factors and various mucosal damaging mechanisms (see "Etiology").

SYNONYMS

PUD
Duodenal ulcer (DU)
Gastric ulcer (GU)

ICD-10CM CODES

K25.3	Acute gastric ulcer without hemorrhage or perforation
K25.7	Chronic gastric ulcer without hemorrhage or perforation
K26.3	Acute duodenal ulcer without hemorrhage or perforation
K26.7	Chronic duodenal ulcer without hemorrhage or perforation
K27.0	Acute peptic ulcer, site unspecified, with hemorrhage
K27.1	Acute peptic ulcer, site unspecified, with perforation
K27.2	Acute peptic ulcer, site unspecified, with both hemorrhage and perforation
K27.3	Acute peptic ulcer, site unspecified, without hemorrhage or perforation
K27.4	Chronic or unspecified peptic ulcer, site unspecified, with hemorrhage
K27.5	Chronic or unspecified peptic ulcer, site unspecified, with perforation
K27.6	Chronic or unspecified peptic ulcer, site unspecified, with both hemorrhage and perforation
K27.7	Chronic peptic ulcer, site unspecified, without hemorrhage or perforation
K27.9	Peptic ulcer, site unspecified, unspecified as acute or chronic, without hemorrhage or perforation
P78.82	Peptic ulcer of newborn
Z87.11	Personal history of peptic ulcer disease

EPIDEMIOLOGY & DEMOGRAPHICS

- Incidence: 250,000 to 500,000 (200,000 to 400,000 duodenal; 50,000 to 100,000 gastric) annually; duodenal ulcer/gastric ulcer ratio is 4:1.
- Anatomic location: <90% of duodenal ulcers occur in the first portion of the duodenum; gastric ulcers occur most frequently in the lesser curvature near the incisura angularis.

PHYSICAL FINDINGS & CLINICAL PRESENTATION

- Epigastric pain is the most frequently reported symptom of PUD. The pain is typically improved with food or antacids and worsened by fasting.
- Physical examination is often unremarkable.
- Patient may have epigastric tenderness, tachycardia, pallor, hypotension (from acute or chronic blood loss), nausea and vomiting (if pyloric channel is obstructed), boardlike abdomen and rebound tenderness (if perforated), and hematemesis or melena (with a bleeding ulcer). Box 1 describes key symptoms and signs of peptic ulcer.

ETIOLOGY

Often multifactorial. The following are common mucosal damaging factors:

- *Helicobacter pylori* infection. *H. pylori* is the major cause of PUD. It is found in more than 70% of patients with duodenal ulcers and gastric ulcers in the U.S. Rates are much higher (>90%) in other parts of the world. Eradication of *H. pylori* markedly reduces peptic ulcer recurrence
- Medications (NSAIDs, glucocorticoids). Risk factors for development of NSAID-related ulcers are described in Box 2
- Incompetent pylorus or lower esophageal sphincter
- Bile acids
- Impaired proximal duodenal bicarbonate secretion
- Decreased blood flow to gastric mucosa
- Acid secreted by parietal cells and pepsin secreted as pepsinogen by chief cells
- Cigarette smoking
- Alcohol

BOX 1 Key Symptoms and Signs of Peptic Ulcer

Uncomplicated Ulcer
- No symptoms ("silent ulcer" in up to 40% of cases)
- Epigastric pain
- Pain may radiate to the back, thorax, other parts of abdomen (cephalad most likely, caudad least likely)
- Pain may be nocturnal (most specific), "painful hunger" relieved by food, or continuous (least specific)
- Nausea
- Vomiting
- Heartburn (mimics or associated with gastroesophageal reflux)

Complicated Ulcer
- Acute perforation
  - Severe abdominal pain
  - Shock
  - Abdominal boardlike rigidity (and rebound and other signs of peritoneal irritation)
  - Free intraperitoneal air
- Hemorrhage
  - Hematemesis and/or melena
  - Hemodynamic changes, anemia
  - Previous history of ulcer symptoms (80%)
- Gastric outlet obstruction
  - Satiation, inability to ingest food, eructation
  - Nausea, vomiting (and related disturbances)
  - Weight loss

From Goldman L, Schafer AI: *Goldman's Cecil medicine,* ed 24, Philadelphia, 2012, Saunders.

Dx DIAGNOSIS

DIFFERENTIAL DIAGNOSIS

- Gastroesophageal reflux disease
- Cholelithiasis syndrome
- Pancreatitis
- Gastritis
- Nonulcer dyspepsia
- Neoplasm (gastric carcinoma, lymphoma, pancreatic carcinoma)
- Angina pectoris, myocardial infarction, pericarditis
- Dissecting aneurysm
- Other: High small-bowel obstruction, pneumonia, subphrenic abscess, early appendicitis

WORKUP

Comprehensive history and physical exam to exclude other diagnoses. Diagnostic modalities include endoscopy or upper GI series. Endoscopy is preferred and remains the gold standard for diagnosis of PUD. The presence of a mucosal break ≥5 mm in the stomach or duodenum confirms the diagnosis.

BOX 2 Risk Factors for Development of NSAID-Related Ulcers

Definite
- Advanced age
- History of ulcer
- Concomitant corticosteroid therapy
- Concomitant anticoagulation therapy
- High doses of NSAIDs
- Serious systemic disorders

Possible
- Concomitant infection with *Helicobacter pylori*
- Cigarette smoking
- Consumption of alcohol

NSAIDs, Nonsteroidal antiinflammatory drugs.
From Andreoli TE et al: *Andreoli and Carpenter's Cecil essentials of medicine,* ed 8, Philadelphia, 2010, Saunders.

LABORATORY TESTS

- Routine laboratory evaluation is usually unremarkable.
- Anemia may be present in patients with significant GI bleeding.
- *H. pylori* testing by endoscopic biopsy, urea breath test, or stool antigen test (*H. pylori* stool antigen) is recommended:
  1. The urea breath test documents active infection (sensitivity and specificity >90%). The patient ingests a small amount of urea labeled with carbon 13 or carbon 14. If urease is present (produced by the organism), the urea is hydrolyzed and the patient exhales labeled carbon dioxide that is then collected and measured. Use of proton pump inhibitors (PPI) within 2 wk of the urea breath test may interfere with test results.
  2. Stool antigen test is an ELISA that identifies *H. pylori* antigen in a stool specimen through a polyclonal anti–*H. pylori* antibody. It is as accurate as the urea breath test for diagnosis of active infection and follow-up evaluation of patients treated for *H. pylori.* A negative result on the stool antigen test 6 wk after completion of therapy identifies patients in whom eradication of *H. pylori* was successful.
  3. Serologic testing for antibodies to *H. pylori* is easy and inexpensive; however, the presence of antibodies demonstrates previous but not necessarily current infection. Antibodies to *H. pylori* can remain elevated for mos to yrs after infection has cleared; therefore antibody levels must be interpreted in light of the patient's symptoms and other test results (e.g., PUD seen on upper GI series).
  4. Histologic evaluation of endoscopic biopsy samples is considered by many the gold standard for accurate diagnosis of *H. pylori* infection. However, detection of *H. pylori* depends on the site and number of biopsy samples, the method of staining, and experience of the pathologist.
- Additional laboratory evaluation is indicated only in specific cases (e.g., amylase level in suspected pancreatitis, serum gastrin level in suspected Zollinger-Ellison [ZE] syndrome).

IMAGING STUDIES

- Conventional upper GI barium studies identify approximately 70% to 80% of PUD; accuracy can be increased to approximately 90% by using double contrast.
- Abdominal CT is helpful when suspecting perforating peptic ulcer disease (sensitivity >95%).

Rx TREATMENT

NONPHARMACOLOGIC THERAPY

- Stop smoking; smoking increases the risk of PUD, decreases the healing rate, and increases the frequency of recurrence.
- Avoid NSAIDs and alcohol.
- Special diets have been proved unrelated to ulcer development and healing; however, avoid foods that cause symptoms.

ACUTE GENERAL Rx

Eradication of *H. pylori,* when present, can be accomplished with various regimens (see "*Helicobacter pylori* Infection").

PUD patients testing negative for *H. pylori* should be treated with antisecretory agents:

- H_2-receptor antagonists (H_2RAs): Famotidine and nizatidine are effective; they are usually given in split dose or at nighttime.
- PPIs: Can also induce rapid healing; they are usually given 30 min before meals.

Antacids and sucralfate are also effective agents for the treatment and prevention of PUD.

CHRONIC Rx

Maintenance therapy in peptic ulcer patients is indicated in the following situations:

- Persistent smokers
- Recurrent ulcerations
- Long-term treatment with NSAIDs, glucocorticoids
- Elderly or debilitated patients
- Aggressive or complicated ulcer disease (e.g., perforation, hemorrhage)
- Asymptomatic bleeders

DISPOSITION

- The recurrence rate for untreated PUD is ~60% (>70% in smokers). Treatment decreases the recurrence rate by nearly 30%.
- Patients with recurrent ulcers should be re-treated for an additional 8 wk and then placed on maintenance therapy with H_2RAs, PPIs, sucralfate, or antacids.
- An ulcer is considered refractory to treatment if healing is not evident after 8 wk for duodenal ulcers and 12 wk for gastric ulcers. In these patients, maximum acid inhibition (e.g., esomeprazole 40 mg bid) is preferred over continued therapy with standard antiulcer therapy.
- Eradication of *H. pylori* (when present) is indicated in all patients. A negative stool antigen test for *H. pylori* 6 wk after treatment accurately confirms cure of *H. pylori* infection with reasonable sensitivity in initially seropositive healthy subjects.
- Screening for ZE syndrome should also be considered in patients with multiple recurrent ulcers; in patients with ZE, the serum gastrin level is >1000 pg/ml and the basal acid output is usually >15 mEq/hr.
- Surgery for refractory ulcers is now only rarely performed; it consists of highly selective vagotomy for duodenal ulcers or ulcer removal with antrectomy or hemigastrectomy without vagotomy for gastric ulcers.

REFERRAL

- GI referral for patients requiring endoscopy
- Surgical referral for patients with nonhealing ulcers despite appropriate medical therapy

PEARLS & CONSIDERATIONS

COMMMENTS

- Patients with gastric ulcers should generally have repeat endoscopy after 8 to 12 wk of antisecretory therapy to document healing and test exfoliative cytology for gastric carcinoma. Patients with duodenal ulcers and those with low-risk gastric ulcers, such as young patients on NSAIDs, generally do not require endoscopic surveillance.
- After endoscopic treatment of bleeding peptic ulcers, bleeding recurs in up to 20% of patients. PPI administration intravenously by continuous infusion substantially reduces the risk of recurrent bleeding. High-dose IV esomeprazole (80 mg IV bolus followed by 8 mg/hr infusion over 72 hr) given after successful endoscopic therapy to patients with high-risk peptic ulcer bleeding has been reported to reduce recurrent bleeding at 72 hr and to maintain sustained clinical benefits for up to 30 days.
- Among low-dose aspirin recipients who had peptic ulcer bleeding, continuous aspirin therapy may increase the risk for recurrent bleeding.

RELATED CONTENT

Peptic Ulcer (Patient Information)
Helicobacter pylori Infection (Related Key Topic)

AUTHOR: **Fred F. Ferri, MD**

BASIC INFORMATION

DEFINITION

Acute pericarditis is the inflammation (or infiltration) of the pericardium. The pericardium is a rigid, avascular fibrous sac with both visceral and richly innervated parietal layers where fluid resides for lubrication. It is characterized by at least two of the following four criteria: (1) chest pain, (2) specific electrocardiographic changes, (3) pericardial friction rub, and (4) new or worsening pericardial effusion.

ICD-10CM CODES

I30.0	Acute nonspecific idiopathic pericarditis
I30.1	Infectious pericarditis
I30.8	Other forms of acute pericarditis
I30.9	Acute pericarditis, unspecified
I301.0	Chronic adhesive pericarditis
I31.1	Chronic constrictive pericarditis
I31.3	Pericardial effusion (non-inflammatory)
I31.9	Diseases of pericardium, unspecified (tamponade)
I31.2	Hemopericardium

EPIDEMIOLOGY & DEMOGRAPHICS

- Most common form of pericardial disease worldwide
- It is diagnosed in 0.1% to 0.2% of hospitalized patients and is responsible for 5% of emergency room admissions for chest pain.
- Acute pericarditis can have recurrences in as high as 20% to 30% of cases, and nearly 50% of recurrent pericarditis cases persist. Four definitions: Acute (<4 to 6 wk), incessant (>4 to 6 wk), recurrent (after symptom-free interval), and chronic (>3 mos).

PHYSICAL FINDINGS & CLINICAL PRESENTATION

- Chest pain: Characteristically sharp, pleuritic, positional (improved by sitting up and leaning forward).
- Pericardial rub: A triphasic (ventricular systole, early diastole, atrial contraction), scratchy sound best heard at the lower left sternal border is pathognomonic. Unlike pleural friction rub, the rub of pericarditis is not affected by respiration.
- Pericardial effusion: Beck's triad (hypotension, elevated jugular venous pressure, and muffled heart sounds) suggests pericardial tamponade.

ETIOLOGY

- In developed countries, viral and idiopathic etiologies are the most common.
- Viral causes can include common gastrointestinal or respiratory flulike illnesses, whereas Parvovirus B19, Epstein-Barr, and HIV are also quite common precipitants. Recently, the novel coronavirus (COVID-19) has emerged as a cause of pericarditis.
- Tuberculosis accounts for 80% to 90% of pericarditis in developing countries, with a high prevalence in HIV-positive patients.
- Neoplastic etiologies (7% to 13%) are typically of lung, breast, esophageal, hematologic, and melanoma origin.
- Autoimmune syndromes (3% to 4%) include systemic lupus erythematosus and rheumatoid arthritis, Sjögren syndrome, sarcoidosis, scleroderma
- Drug-induced: Procainamide, hydralazine, phenytoin, isoniazid, rifampin, doxorubicin, mesalamine, adalimumab, immune checkpoint inhibitors.
- Radiation-induced pericarditis prevalence is improving, with better radioprotective techniques. Morbidity is closely related to the radiation dose due to damage of capillary endothelial cells, lymphatic stenosis or occlusion.
- Metabolic: Uremia, myxedema, anorexia nervosa.
- Postcardiac injury syndrome: Post-pericardiotomy, post-pacemaker lead placement, postcatheter ablation, post-CPR, post-PCI, perimyocardial infarction, or Dressler syndrome.

Dx DIAGNOSIS

DIFFERENTIAL DIAGNOSIS

- Angina pectoris and acute coronary syndrome
- Myopericarditis, perimyocarditis, Takotsubo stress cardiomyopathy syndrome
- Dissecting aortic aneurysm
- Pulmonary and thoracic causes: Thromboembolism, infarction, pneumothorax, pneumonia with pleurisy, costochondritis
- Gastrointestinal causes: Hepatitis, cholecystitis, GERD, esophageal spasm or rupture
- Box 1 summarizes the differential diagnosis of pericardial effusion by etiology

WORKUP (TABLE 1)

Table 2 summarizes an initial approach to acute pericarditis. Diagnosis of pericarditis requires at least two of the four following clinical criteria:

- Typical pleuritic chest pain
- Pericardial friction rub
- Suggestive ECG changes (diffuse concave ST segment elevation, PR depression in all leads except for AVR where there is elevation)
- New or worsening pericardial effusion

LABORATORY TESTS

Initial laboratory tests may determine severity of inflammation and acuity of patient's condition, while also guiding workup and treatment timeline:

- Inflammatory markers: Erythrocyte sedimentation rate, (high-sensitivity) C-reactive protein (CRP), and complete blood count with differential
- Cardiac biomarkers (Troponin T and I) will help determine myocardial involvement
- Basic metabolic profile

Additional lab studies:

- HIV
- PPD
- Antinuclear antibody, rheumatoid factor
- TSH
- Routine viral studies are not indicated since they are low yield

PERICARDIAL FLUID AND TISSUE SAMPLING

Indications for pericardiocentesis are:

- Tamponade physiology
- Moderate to large pericardial effusion with symptoms, or refractory to medical therapy
- Suspicion of a neoplastic, bacterial, or tuberculous process
- Evidence of constrictive or effusive-constrictive pericarditis
- Pericardiocentesis is for diagnostic and therapeutic purposes. The pericardial fluid

BOX 1 Major Differential Diagnosis of Pericardial Effusion by Etiology

Noninfectious
- Malignancy (usually metastatic)
- Myocardial infarction associated (Dressler syndrome)
- Uremia
- Myxedema (rare cause of tamponade physiology)
- Trauma (penetrating or nonpenetrating)
- Chylopericardium
- Acute idiopathic
- Rheumatic fever
- Collagen vascular disease (systemic lupus erythematosus, rheumatoid arthritis, scleroderma, Wegener granulomatosis)
- Postsurgical (cardiac and intrathoracic)
- Drug induced (procainamide, hydralazine, phenytoin, doxorubicin, isoniazid)

Infectious
- Viral (coxsackievirus, echovirus, mumps, adenovirus, hepatitis, human immunodeficiency virus)
- Bacterial (pneumococcus, streptococcus, staphylococcus)
- Tuberculous
- Fungal (histoplasmosis, coccidiomycosis, *Candida*, particularly in immunosuppressed patients)

From Niederhuber JE: *Abeloff's clinical oncology*, ed 6, Philadelphia, 2020, Elsevier.

TABLE 1 Diagnostic Pathway and Sequence of Performance in Acute Pericarditis

Diagnostic Measure	Characteristic Findings
Obligatory	
Auscultation	Pericardial rub (monophasic, biphasic, or triphasic)
ECG*	*Stage I:* Anterior and inferior concave ST segment elevation. PR segment deviations opposite to P wave polarity
	Early stage II: All ST junctions return to the baseline. PR segments deviated
	Late stage II: T waves progressively flatten and invert
	Stage III: Generalized T-wave inversions in most or all leads
	Stage IV: ECG returns to prepericarditis state
Echocardiography	Effusion types B to D (Horowitz)
	Signs of tamponade
Blood analyses	Erythrocyte sedimentation rate, C-reactive protein, lactate dehydrogenase, leukocytes (inflammation markers)
	Troponin I,† CK-MB (markers of myocardial involvement)
Chest radiograph	Ranging from normal to "water bottle" shape of the heart shadow
	Performed primarily to reveal pulmonary or mediastinal pathology
Mandatory in Tamponade, Optional in Large/Recurrent Effusions or if Previous Tests Inconclusive in Small Effusions	
Pericardiocentesis/drainage	Polymerase chain reaction and histochemistry for etiopathogenetic classification of infection or neoplasia
Optional or if Previous Tests Inconclusive	
CT	Effusions, pericardium, and epicardium
MRI	Effusions, pericardium, and epicardium
Pericardioscopy, pericardial/epicardial biopsy	Establishing the specific etiology

*Typical lead involvement: I, II, aVL, aVF, and V3-V6. The ST segment is always depressed in aVR, frequently in V1, and occasionally in V2. Stage IV may not occur, and there are permanent T-wave inversions and flattenings. If an ECG is first recorded in stage III, pericarditis cannot be differentiated by ECG from diffuse myocardial injury, "biventricular strain," or myocarditis. ECG in early repolarization is very similar to stage I. Unlike stage I, this ECG does not acutely evolve, and J-point elevations are usually accompanied by a slur, oscillation, or notch at the end of the QRS just before and including the J point (best seen with tall R and T waves—large in an early repolarization pattern). Pericarditis is likely if, in lead V6, the J point is greater than 25% of the height of the T-wave apex (using the PR segment as a baseline).

†A rise in cardiac muscle troponin I (cTnI) is detected in 32.2% of patients, more frequently in younger, male patients, with ST segment elevation and pericardial effusion at presentation. An increase beyond 1.5 ng/ml is uncommon (7.6%) and associated with CK-MB elevation. cTnI increase and is not a negative prognostic marker for the incidence of recurrences, constrictive pericarditis, cardiac tamponade, or residual left ventricular dysfunction.

CK-MB, Creatine kinase-MB; *CT,* computed tomography; *ECG,* electrocardiogram; *MRI,* magnetic resonance imaging.

From Vincent JL et al: *Textbook of critical care,* ed 7, Philadelphia, 2017, Elsevier.

TABLE 2 Initial Approach to the Patient with Definite or Suspected Acute Pericarditis

1. If the diagnosis is suspected but not certain, listen often for pericardial rub and obtain ECGs frequently to check for diagnostic findings.
2. If the diagnosis is suspected or certain, obtain the following tests to help confirm the diagnosis (if necessary) and determine whether a specific causative diagnosis and/or significant associated conditions and/or complications are present:
   Hemogram
   hsCRP
   Troponin I
   Chest radiograph
   Echocardiogram
   Consider additional testing on the basis of clinical suspicion of a specific etiology.
3. If the diagnosis is likely or certain, initiate therapy with an NSAID plus colchicine.

From Zipes DP: *Braunwald's heart disease, a textbook of cardiovascular medicine,* ed 11, Philadelphia, 2019, Elsevier.

should be analyzed for RBC, WBC, Gram stain, culture, cytology, glucose, pH, LDH, and protein. In select cases, consider checking triglyceride for chylopericardium, adenosine deaminase (ADA), or PCR for tuberculosis

- Pericardial biopsy can be performed for cases of recurrent pericardial effusion when pericardial fluid analysis does not reveal etiology, and especially if malignancy or tuberculosis is suspected.

IMAGING STUDIES

- ECG (Fig. 1): Changes in the ECG reflect inflammation of the epicardium, because the parietal pericardium is electrically inert. The ECG changes are staged as follows:
  1. Stage I (Acute phase): Hours to few days. PR-segment depression in all leads except aVR (where PR elevation is seen) and diffuse concave ST-segment elevations
  2. Stage II (Intermediate phase): Seen in first wk with return of PR and ST segments to baseline
  3. Stage III (Intermediate): T-wave inversion in leads previously showing ST-segment elevation
  4. Stage IV (Late phase): Normalization of the ECG or indefinite persistence of T-wave inversions
- Echocardiogram is used to evaluate for pericardial effusion (present in 50% to 60% of patients) (Fig. 2). Echocardiogram can help exclude STEMI (through absent wall motion abnormality) and support the diagnosis of constrictive pericarditis or tamponade. Echocardiogram is also recommended for guidance for pericardiocentesis.
- Chest x-ray: Performed to rule out abnormalities of the mediastinum or lung fields. Cardiac silhouette may appear enlarged when pericardial effusion accumulates over ≥200 ml of fluid (Fig. 3). Calcifications around the heart may be seen with chronic constrictive pericarditis.
- Computed tomography: Evaluation of associated pleuropulmonary and extra thoracic diseases and pericardial calcifications.
- Cardiac MRI (Fig. 4) is recommended in patients with elevated troponin I or T and can also be helpful in cases of chronic constrictive pericarditis and malignancy.

TREATMENT

NONPHARMACOLOGIC THERAPY

- Physical activity should be restricted until pain resolves and inflammatory markers, ECG, and echocardiogram normalize.
- Athletes should avoid competitive activity for 3 mo at a minimum. Exercise intensity, HR >100 bpm, and shear stress on pericardium are thought to worsen inflammation. With myocardial involvement (positive troponin), athletic activity must be avoided for at least 6 mo.

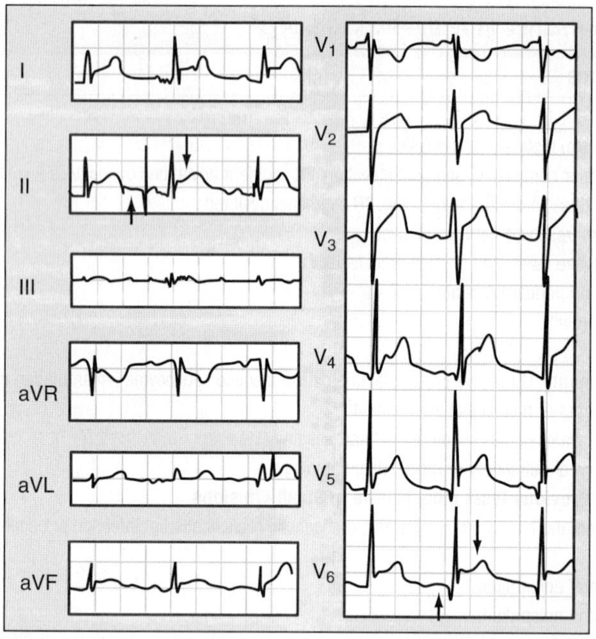

FIG. 1 Typical electrocardiographic changes in acute pericarditis: PR depression *(small arrow)* and concave ST-segment elevation *(large arrow)*. *aVF,* Augmented vector foot; *aVL,* augmented vector left; *aVR,* augmented vector right. (From Vincent JL et al: *Textbook of critical care,* ed 7, Philadelphia, 2017, Elsevier.)

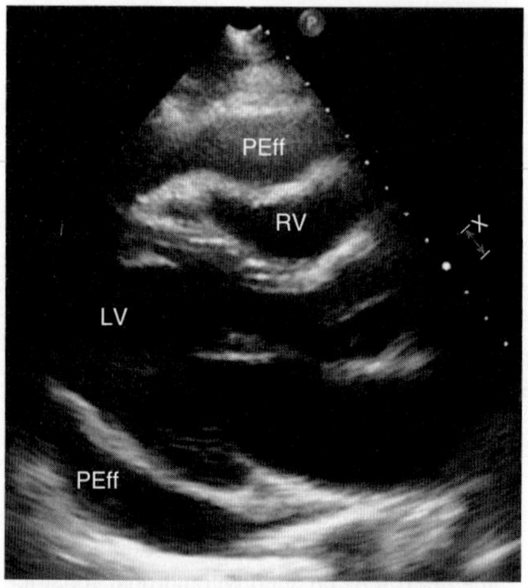

FIG. 2 Bedside echocardiogram showing pericardial effusion compressing the right ventricle during diastole, consistent with cardiac tamponade. *LV,* Left ventricle; *PEff,* pericardial effusion; *RV,* right ventricle.

- Patient education should be provided of potential warning signs of complications such as cardiac tamponade, recurrent pericarditis (which can occur in up to one third of patients), and chronic constrictive pericarditis.

ACUTE GENERAL Rx

- High-dose aspirin (750 to 1000 mg tid) or NSAIDs (e.g., ibuprofen 600 to 800 mg tid, indomethacin 50 mg tid) for 1 to 2 wk. Proton pump inhibitor should be provided for gastric protection. NSAIDs should be avoided in patients with recent MI, CHF, acute renal failure, and upper GI bleed.
- Colchicine 0.5 to 0.6 mg once daily (<70 kg) or bid (>70 kg) for 3 mo. Current evidence (COPE, CORE, CORP, ICAP, CORP-2 trials) supports the effectiveness of colchicine in symptomatic relief and prevention of recurrent pericarditis.
- Corticosteroids should be used only as second-line treatment and typically prescribed for refractory recurrent pericarditis. Other circumstances include cases of established rheumatologic disease, renal failure, or other contraindications to NSAID or colchicine therapies. They can be associated with severe adverse effects, more hospitalizations, and high rate of recurrence.

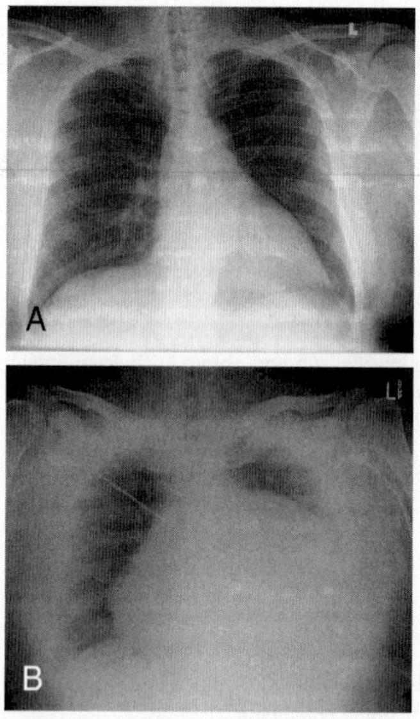

FIG. 3 Chest x-ray. A, patient's chest radiograph 1 yr before presentation with cardiac tamponade. **B,** same patient's chest radiograph on presentation to the emergency department with cardiac tamponade. (From Adams JG et al: *Emergency medicine, clinical essentials,* ed 2, Philadelphia, 2013, Elsevier.)

- In tuberculous pericarditis, adjunctive corticosteroids can prevent development of constriction with tapering dose of 120 mg prednisolone over 6 wk in patients without HIV. Because of increased risk of malignancy, corticosteroids should be avoided in persons with combined TB and HIV infection.
- When corticosteroids are indicated, recommended dosing is as follows: Low- to moderate-dose (0.25 to 0.5 mg/kg/day) systemic steroid therapy for 1 mo, followed by a long taper (6 to 12 wk).
- Azathioprine, intravenous immunoglobulins, and anti-IL-1 therapies (e.g., anakinra) can be considered for patients with refractory recurrent pericarditis.
- Pericardiectomy and pericardiotomy at specialized centers are a last-resort procedure reserved for recurrent cardiac tamponade, refractory pericarditis, and hemodynamically significant constrictive pericarditis.
- Avoidance of anticoagulants (increased risk of hemopericardium).

TREATMENT OF UNDERLYING CAUSE:

- Purulent bacterial pericarditis: Systemic antibiotics and drainage of pericardium
- Collagen vascular disease: Corticosteroid therapy (prednisone)
- Tuberculous pericarditis: Rifampicin, isoniazid, pyrazinamide, and ethambutol for 2 mo, then isoniazid and rifampicin for 6 mo. Isoniazid is the most effective agent in penetrating the pericardial space.
- Thyroid-related pericardial effusion: Thyroid replacement therapy
- Uremic: Dialysis
- Malignant pericardial effusion: Fig. 5

POTENTIAL COMPLICATIONS FROM PERICARDITIS:

- **Chronic constrictive pericarditis:** Occurs in <1% of patients with acute idiopathic pericarditis. New awareness of subset of patients with "transient constrictive pericarditis" who have an initial hyperacute stage of inflammation that must be identified before progression to fibrosis and calcification of the pericardium.
  1. Physical examination: Signs of right heart failure—hepatomegaly, splenomegaly, ascites, pedal edema, scrotal edema, possible anasarca, jugular venous pressure, Kussmaul sign (paradoxical increase in jugular venous pressure during inspiration), pericardial knock (early diastolic filling sound heard 0.06 to 0.1 sec after S2), and clear lungs.
  2. ECG: Low QRS voltage, nonspecific ST-segment changes, biatrial enlargement.
  3. Chest radiograph: Mild alveolar edema, pleural effusions, biatrial enlargement, pericardial calcification (seen in tuberculous pericarditis).
  4. Echocardiography: May show thickened pericardium (>4 mm), >25% mitral and >50% tricuspid valve inflow variation with respiration, interventricular septal bounce; and mitral annulus reversus

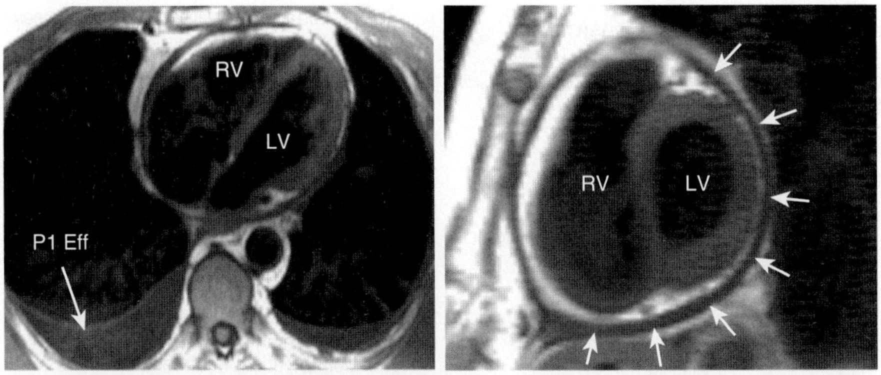

FIG. 4 Cardiovascular magnetic resonance imaging in a patient with constrictive pericarditis. On the *right* is a basal short-axis view of the ventricles showing a thickened pericardium encasing the heart *(arrows)*. On the *left* is a transaxial view, again showing the thickened pericardium, particularly over the right heart, but also a pleural effusion *(Pl Eff)*. *LV,* Left ventricle; *RV,* right ventricle. (From Zipes DP et al [eds]: *Braunwald's heart disease,* ed 7, Philadelphia, 2005, Saunders.)

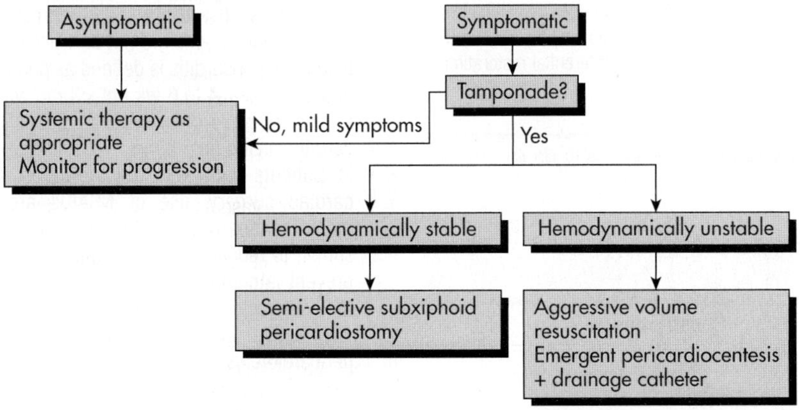

FIG. 5 Treatment approach algorithm to malignant pericardial effusions. (From Niederhuber JE: *Abeloff's clinical oncology*, ed 6, Philadelphia, 2020, Elsevier.)

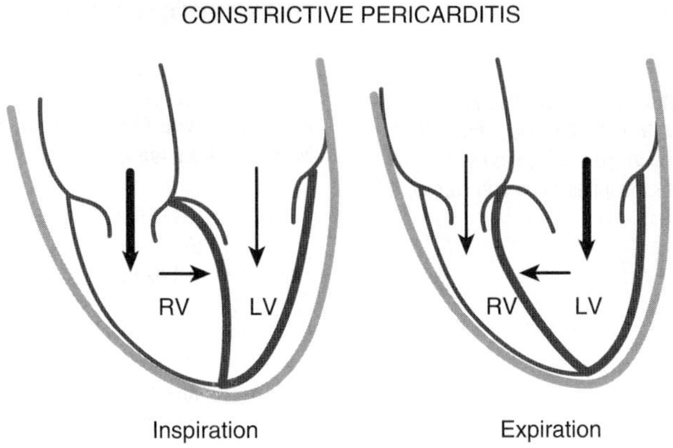

FIG. 6 Ventricular interdependence in constrictive pericarditis. *LV,* left ventricle; *RV,* right ventricle. (Courtesy Miguel Quinones, MD, Houston Methodist DeBakey Heart and Vascular Center. In Parrillo JE, Dellinger RP: *Critical care medicine, principles of diagnosis and management in the adult,* ed 5, Philadelphia, 2019, Elsevier.)

(medial e' velocity > lateral e' velocity) suggests constrictive pericarditis.

5. Hemodynamics (Fig. 6): Elevation of right-sided filling pressures, equalization of diastolic pressures, as well as prominent "x" and rapid "y" descent in the atrial tracing are seen in constrictive pericarditis. Right ventricular pressure tracing typically shows a "dip and plateau" (square root sign) that is a result of the unimpeded early filling of the RV with an abrupt halt to the late diastolic filling by the stiff pericardium. Discordance of right ventricular and left ventricular systolic pressures during respiration is also suggestive of constrictive pericarditis.

6. Therapy: Complex surgical stripping or removal of both layers of the constricting pericardium improves the functional class in majority of late survivors, but has high operative mortality.

- **Cardiac tamponade:** Occurs in 5% to 15% of patients with idiopathic pericarditis, but in up to 60% of those with neoplastic, tuberculous, or purulent pericarditis.
  1. Signs and symptoms: Dyspnea, orthopnea, chest pain, fatigue
  2. Physical examination: Beck's triad (distended neck veins, distant heart sounds, hypotension), reduced apical impulse, diaphoresis, tachypnea, tachycardia, narrowed pulse pressure, or pulsus paradoxus (decrease in systolic blood pressure ≥10 mm Hg during inspiration; most specific sign)
  3. ECG: Decreased amplitude of the QRS complex, electrical alternans (occurs more frequently with large neoplastic effusions)
  4. Chest x-ray: Cardiomegaly ("water-bottle" configuration of the cardiac silhouette may be seen) with clear lungs
  5. Echocardiography (Table 3): Pericardial effusion, >25% mitral and >50% tricuspid valve inflow variation with respiration, paradoxical motion of interventricular septum, diastolic right or left atrium collapse, diastolic right ventricular collapse (pathognomonic).
  6. Hemodynamics: Equalization of diastolic pressures within chambers of the heart, elevation of right atrial pressure with a prominent "x" but blunted "y" descent. Table 4 summarizes hemodynamics in cardiac tamponade and constrictive pericarditis
  7. Therapy: Cardiac tamponade is a life-threatening condition usually requiring emergent pericardiocentesis. Avoid drugs (diuretics, nitrates) or therapies (high PEEP) that reduce the preload. Fluid resuscitation can temporize hemodynamics while awaiting pericardiocentesis. In patients with recurrent effusions (e.g., neoplasms), placement of a percutaneous drainage catheter or pericardial window may be necessary.
- **Effusive-constrictive pericarditis:** Uncommon syndrome characterized by concomitant tamponade caused by tense pericardial effusion and constriction caused by the visceral pericardium.
  1. Signs and symptoms of both tamponade and/or constriction. Pulsus paradoxus is present, but Kussmaul sign and pericardial knock are typically absent.
  2. Echocardiography: Low sensitivity to distinguish effusive-constrictive pericarditis from other types.
  3. Cardiac catheterization: Before drainage, "y" descent is usually less prominent than expected, and right atrial "v" wave persists. After drainage, may continue to have elevated right atrial and pulmonary wedge pressures.

TABLE 3 Hemodynamic and Echocardiographic Features of Constrictive Pericarditis Compared with Restrictive Cardiomyopathy

	Constriction	Restriction
Prominent y descent in venous pressure	Present	Variable
Paradoxical pulse	~1/3 cases	Absent
Pericardial knock	Present	Absent
Equal right- and left-sided filling pressures	Present	Left at least 3-5 mm Hg higher than right
Filling pressures >25 mm Hg	Rare	Common
Pulmonary artery systolic pressure >60 mm Hg	No	Common
"Square root" sign	Present	Variable
Respiratory variation in left-sided and-right-sided pressures/flows	Exaggerated	Normal
Ventricular wall thickness	Normal	Usually increased
Pericardial thickness	Increased	Normal
Atrial size	Possible LA enlargement	Biatrial enlargement
Septal bounce	Present	Absent
Tissue Doppler E′velocity	Increased	Reduced
Speckle tracking	Normal longitudinal, decreased circumferential restoration	Decreased longitudinal, normal circumferential restoration

From Zipes DP: *Braunwald's heart disease, a textbook of cardiovascular medicine,* ed 11, Philadelphia, 2019, Elsevier.

TABLE 4 Hemodynamics in Cardiac Tamponade and Constrictive Pericarditis

	Tamponade	Constriction
Paradoxical pulse	Usually present	Present in ~1/3
Equal left/right-sided filling pressure	Present	Present
Systemic venous wave morphology	Absent y descent	Prominent y descent (M or W shape)
Inspiratory change in systemic venous pressure	Decrease (normal)	Increase or no change (Kussmaul sign)
"Square root" sign in ventricular pressure	Absent	Present

From Mann DL et al: *Braunwald's heart disease,* ed 10, Philadelphia, 2015, Elsevier.

4. Therapy: Extensive epicardiectomy (with disruption of the visceral layer of pericardium) is the procedure of choice in symptomatic patients.

- **Myopericarditis**: Defined by an elevated cardiac biomarker. Myocarditis and pericarditis may coexist in 20% to 30% of patients presenting with pericarditis. Hospitalization and cardiac MRI are favored in these patients. Overall, myopericarditis has a good prognosis with appropriate guideline medical therapies and has very low rates of morbidity, mortality, and heart failure.

DISPOSITION

- Complete resolution of pain and other signs and symptoms during the initial 3 wk of therapy occurs in 70% to 90% of cases.
- Admission is highly recommended if any of the following high risk and poor prognostic features exist: Fever >38° C (>100.4° F) during thion/tamponade, failure to respond to 1 wk of outpatient treatment.
- The following are considered moderate risk factors but should also prompt admission: Myopericarditis, trauma, immunosuppression, oral anticoagulant therapy.
- Recurrent pericarditis occurs after a symptom-free interval (4 to 6 wk) following the initial episode of pericarditis. Incidence is reported as 10% to 15% and increases to 50% in patients who are not on colchicine.
- Incessant pericarditis is defined as pericarditis lasting for >4 to 6 wk but <3 mo without remission, while chronic pericarditis is pericarditis lasting for >3 mo.
- In patients with pericardial effusion after cardiac surgery, use of NSAIDs are not recommended because they have not been shown to reduce the size of the effusions or prevent late cardiac tamponade. The COPPS trial suggested that prophylactic colchicine may reduce the risk of developing a post-pericardiotomy pericarditis.

SUGGESTED READINGS

Available at ExpertConsult.com

RELATED CONTENT

Pericarditis (Patient Information)
Cardiac Tamponade (Related Key Topic)

AUTHORS: **Amy E. Riviere, DO, MA,** and **Maxwell Eyram Afari, MD**

Periodic Limb Movement Disorder (PLMD)

BASIC INFORMATION

DEFINITION

A disorder characterized by periodic episodes of involuntary repetitive limb movements during sleep, causing sleep disturbances that are not due to a primary sleep disorder. They consist of triple flexion movements of the legs that repeat in 5- to 90-second cycles during sleep.

SYNONYMS

PLMD
Periodic leg movements of sleep (PLMS)
Nocturnal myoclonus

ICD-10CM CODE

G47.61 Periodic limb movement disorder

EPIDEMIOLOGY & DEMOGRAPHICS

INCIDENCE: Unknown
PREVALENCE: 5% to 8%
PREDOMINANT SEX AND AGE: Prevalence is higher in females and increases with age
PEAK INCIDENCE: None
RISK FACTORS:

- Musculoskeletal disease, heart disease, obstructive sleep apnea, narcolepsy, psychiatric disorders, diabetes mellitus
- Shift work
- Snoring
- Stress
- Restless legs syndrome
- Parkinson disease, idiopathic REM sleep behavior disorder

GENETICS: Unknown, but may share autosomal dominant inheritance pattern if concurrent with restless legs syndrome

PHYSICAL FINDINGS & CLINICAL PRESENTATION

- Patients may complain of excessive daytime sleepiness, fatigue, and unrestful sleep.
- During an episode of periodic limb movements, the patient may experience repetitive dorsiflexion of the ankle and extension of the big toe, but other movements may occur, such as kicking. These movements last up to 5 sec and may recur every 5 to 90 sec, with the total episode lasting min to an hr. The movements are typically involuntary, and the patient is unaware of their occurrence, in contrast to those of restless legs syndrome (RLS).
- Neurologic examination is usually normal but may reveal an associated neuropathy or myelopathy.
- Periodic leg movements of sleep are present in most patients with RLS but are not specific nor sensitive for RLS.

ETIOLOGY

The exact etiology is unknown. It is hypothesized that PLMD may share a common pathophysiology with RLS, which involves iron metabolism and dopaminergic pathways in the brain.

DIAGNOSIS

DIFFERENTIAL DIAGNOSIS

- Restless legs syndrome
- Neuroleptic-induced akathisia
- Positional discomfort
- Nocturnal leg cramps

WORKUP

In addition to a history of excessive daytime sleepiness or sleep disturbance, the diagnosis of PLMD requires a polysomnographic study to exclude other sleep disorders and to document the periodic limb movements resulting in sleep disturbances. During the study the movements must occur in a series of at least four, recurring every 5 to 90 sec, each with a duration of 0.5 to 5 sec.

LABORATORY TESTS

- No laboratory tests are required to diagnose PLMD.
- A CBC, iron panel, and BMP may be ordered if RLS is suspected.

IMAGING STUDIES

Imaging studies are not required for diagnosis of PLMD.

TREATMENT

- Patients with periodic limb movements only, without sleep disturbances of insomnia or excessive daytime sleepiness, do not require treatment.
- The treatment of PLMD is the same as that for RLS.
- Calcium channel ligands such as gabapentin or pregabalin are effective and do not worsen symptoms with long-term use.
- Dopaminergic agonists such as pramipexole or ropinirole have been shown to decrease PLMS, but long-term use may be associated with worsening of symptoms (augmentation).
- Iron replacement should be started in case of iron deficiency, and the cause of iron-deficiency investigated.

NONPHARMACOLOGIC THERAPY

- Follow good sleep hygiene.
- Minimize shift work.
- Avoid caffeine, alcohol, nicotine.

ACUTE GENERAL Rx

- Treatment is indicated when PLMD is suspected and causing significant sleep fragmentation
- For calcium channel ligands: Gabapentin initial dose of 100 to 300 mg/day before bedtime, with therapeutic range of 300 to 2400 mg/day. Pregabalin initial dose of 50 to 75 mg/day, with therapeutic range of 75 to 450 mg/day
- For dopamine agonists: Pramipexole initial dose of 0.125 mg before bedtime, with a therapeutic range of 0.125 to 0.75 mg/day. Ropinirole initial dose of 0.25 mg/day, with a therapeutic range of 0.25 to 4 mg/day

CHRONIC Rx

For patients treated with dopamine agonists, close monitoring is recommended to screen for augmentation of symptoms.

COMPLEMENTARY & ALTERNATIVE MEDICINE

None

REFERRAL

Refer to neurologist if diagnosis is uncertain or an underlying disorder is suspected.

PEARLS & CONSIDERATIONS

COMMENTS

- Periodic limb movements disorder is a diagnosis of exclusion. PLMS occur during many sleep disorders and do not support a diagnosis of PLMD until all possible underlying causes are excluded.
- Certain medications such as antihistamines, dopamine receptor blockers, selective serotonin reuptake inhibitors, and stimulants may worsen PLMS and should be avoided if possible.

PREVENTION: As mentioned in "Nonpharmacologic Therapy."

PATIENT & FAMILY EDUCATION

Patient information on PLMD and other sleep disorders can be found at the National Sleep Foundation website: www.sleepfoundation.org.

SUGGESTED READINGS

Available at ExpertConsult.com

RELATED CONTENT

Restless Legs Syndrome (Related Key Topic)

AUTHOR: **Corey Goldsmith, MD**

BASIC INFORMATION

DEFINITION

Peripheral artery disease (PAD) refers to atherosclerotic, inflammatory, occlusive, and aneurysmal diseases involving the noncerebral and noncoronary arteries. (This topic focuses on lower-extremity PAD.)

SYNONYMS

PAD
Peripheral vascular disease (PVD)
Arteriosclerosis obliterans
Atherosclerotic occlusive disease
Atherosclerosis of the extremities
Peripheral arterial stenosis
Vasoocclusive disease of the legs
Chronic critical limb ischemia

ICD-10CM CODES

I70	Atherosclerosis
I70.2	Atherosclerosis of native arteries of the extremities
I70.21	Atherosclerosis of native arteries of extremities with intermittent claudication
I70.22	Atherosclerosis of native arteries of extremities with rest pain
I70.3	Atherosclerosis of unspecified type of bypass graft(s) of the extremities
I73	Other specified peripheral vascular diseases
I73.8	Other specified peripheral vascular diseases
I73.9	Peripheral vascular disease, unspecified
I79	Disorders of arteries, arterioles, and capillaries in diseases classified elsewhere

EPIDEMIOLOGY & DEMOGRAPHICS

- There are more than 200 million patients afflicted with PAD globally (ABI ≤0.9); it affects approximately 8 to 12 million Americans.
- The prevalence is nearly equal in men and women. It increases with age, from 5.28% in those aged 40 to 49 yr to 18.83% in those aged 70 to 79 yr. However, symptoms of claudication are more likely to be present in males with PAD (50%) vs. women with PAD (25%).
- As per the PARTNERS study, the prevalence of PAD in patients >70 yr or 50 to 69 yr with history of smoking or diabetes was 29%.
- Risk factors that increase risk of PAD according to a 2013 meta-analysis of 112,027 studied patients include:
  1. Smoking (odds ratio 2.72)
  2. Diabetes (odds ratio 1.88)
  3. Hypertension (odds ratio 1.55)
  4. Hypercholesterolemia (odds ratio 1.19)
  5. Older age
- Smoking is three times more likely to lead to PAD than CAD. Conversely, the association of HTN and hyperlipidemia with PAD is lower than that with CAD and cerebrovascular disease.
- Patients at increased risk of PAD include those aged greater than 65 yr, those aged 50 to 64 yr with risk factors of atherosclerosis, those aged less than 50 yr with diabetes and an additional risk factor, as well as those individuals with known atherosclerotic disease in another vascular bed.
- Black race/ethnicity has greater prevalence according to NHANES data (odds ratio 2.83).
- Patients with newly diagnosed PAD are six times more likely to die within the next 10 yr when compared with patients without PAD.
- Patients with heart failure and PAD have increased risk of mortality (HR 1.36), increased risk of MI, and less improvement in a structural physical exercise program.
- Concomitant renal failure (Cr >2) is associated with worse overall cardiovascular prognosis in addition to lower rates of amputation-free survival to the point that the *European Journal of Vascular Medicine* guidelines recommend a special attention to be paid to atherosclerosis in lower extremities in these patients.
- The total annual costs associated with the hospitalization of patients with PAD in the U.S. exceed $21 billion, and account for ~13% of all Medicare Part A and B expenditures.

PHYSICAL FINDINGS & CLINICAL PRESENTATION

- Peripheral artery disease may present in a variety of ways:
  1. 20% to 50%: Asymptomatic (estimated 3 times more than symptomatic patients)
  2. 10% to 35%: Intermittent claudication (IC), defined as aching pain, cramping, weakness, numbness, or heaviness of the leg induced by exercise, relieved by rest
  3. 1% to 2%: Critical limb ischemia (CLI), defined as chronic (>2 wk) rest pain, or tissue loss with nonhealing ulceration, necrosis, or gangrene (Fig. E1)
  4. 40% to 50%: Atypical symptoms involving the calf, thigh, or buttock
  5. Acute limb ischemia (ALI) will be present in 14 per 100,000 individuals in the general population. It is defined as acute (<2 wk) onset of symptoms due to severe poor perfusion of the extremities, and further categorized into the following:
     a. Viable: No sensory or muscle weakness with audible Doppler pulses
     b. Threatened: Mild to moderate sensory or motor loss; inaudible arterial Doppler
     c. Irreversible: Severe sensory loss and muscle weakness; inaudible arterial Doppler
        (1) Claudication can be categorized using the Rutherford and Fontaine classification symptoms.
- Physical findings include:
  1. Diminished pulses and/or cool skin temperature of lower extremities
  2. Bruits heard over the distal aorta, iliac, or femoral arteries (femoral bruit is an independent marker for ischemic cardiac events)
  3. Change in skin color:
     a. Dependent rubor in critical limb ischemia
     b. Livedo reticularis, or a mottled reticulated vascular pattern that appears lacelike
  4. Trophic changes of hair loss, brittle nails, and muscle atrophy

ETIOLOGY

- PAD is primarily the result of atherosclerotic narrowing of the arterial lumen that results in impaired blood flow to the lower-extremity tissues. Fig. 2 illustrates the pathophysiology of intermittent claudication.
- Symptoms initially manifest with exercise as metabolic demands increase. Critical limb ischemia (CLI) may develop gradually from progressive atherosclerosis or in a subacute fashion from multisegmental atherothrombosis or atheroembolization. In contrast, acute limb ischemia (ALI) is marked by a sudden onset of symptoms (<2 wk) due to poor perfusion of the extremities.

Dx DIAGNOSIS

DIFFERENTIAL DIAGNOSIS

- Vasculitis
- Musculoskeletal disorder
- Spinal stenosis or nerve root compression (neurogenic or pseudoclaudication)
- Peripheral neuropathy
- Reflex sympathetic dystrophy
- Raynaud phenomenon
- Compartment syndrome
- Deep venous thrombosis
- Popliteal entrapment syndrome
- Direct vascular injury

WORKUP

- Thorough history, including symptoms regarding walking impairment, claudication, ischemic rest pain, or nonhealing wounds in patients ≥70 yr or those ≥50 yr with a history of smoking and/or diabetes
- Careful physical examinations include:
  1. Measurement of blood pressure in both arms; pressure difference of >15 to 20 mm Hg is abnormal and suggestive of subclavian artery stenosis (marker of vascular disease risk and death)
  2. Palpation and recording of carotid pulses, upstroke, amplitude, and presence of bruits
  3. Auscultation and palpation of abdomen for bruits, aortic pulsation, and diameter
  4. Palpation of brachial, radial, ulnar, femoral, popliteal, dorsalis pedis, and posterior tibial pulses. Pulse intensity should be recorded as follows: 0, absent; 1+, diminished; 2+, normal; 3+, bounding
  5. Auscultation of femoral arteries for the presence of bruits

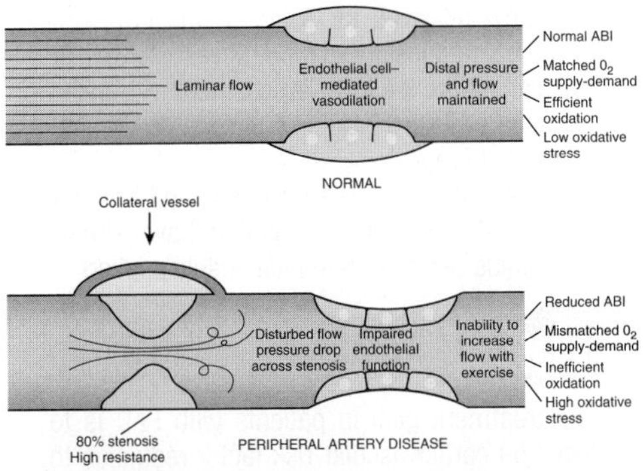

FIG. 2 Pathophysiology of intermittent claudication. In healthy arteries *(top),* flow is laminar and endothelial function is normal; therefore blood flow and oxygen delivery match muscle metabolic demand at rest and during exercise. Muscle metabolism is efficient and results in low oxidative stress. In contrast, in peripheral artery disease *(PAD) (bottom),* arterial stenosis results in disturbed flow, and the loss of kinetic energy results in a drop in pressure across the stenosis. Collateral vessels have high resistance and only partially compensate for the arterial stenosis. In addition, endothelial function is impaired, thereby resulting in further loss of vascular function. These changes limit the blood flow response to exercise and result in a mismatch of oxygen delivery to muscle metabolic demand. Changes in skeletal muscle metabolism further compromise the efficient generation of high-energy phosphates. Oxidant stress, the result of inefficient oxidation, further impairs endothelial function and muscle metabolism. *ABI,* Ankle-brachial index. (From the text *Anatomie, physiologie, pathologie des vaisseaux lymphatiques* by PC Sappey [1874], courtesy Harvard Medical Library, Francis A. Countway Library of Medicine. In Hiatt WR, Brass EP: Pathophysiology of intermittent claudication. In Creager MA et al [eds]: *Vascular medicine, a companion to Braunwald's heart disease,* ed 2, Philadelphia, 2013, Elsevier.)

TABLE 1 Fontaine Classification of Peripheral Artery Disease

Stage	Symptoms
I	Asymptomatic
II	Intermittent claudication
IIa	Pain free, claudication walking >200 m
IIb	Pain free, claudication walking <200 m
III	Rest and nocturnal pain
IV	Necrosis, gangrene

From Bonow RO et al: *Braunwald's heart disease: a textbook of cardiovascular medicine,* ed 9, Philadelphia, 2012, Saunders.

6. Extremities should be inspected for color, temperature, integrity of the skin, hair loss, and hypertrophic nails

- Classification/staging system for PAD
  1. Fontaine staging system (Table 1):
     a. I: Asymptomatic
     b. IIa: Mild claudication
     c. IIb: Moderate-severe claudication
     d. III: Ischemic rest pain
     e. IV: Ulceration or gangrene
- Resting ankle-brachial index (ABI) is the first-line noninvasive test to establish a diagnosis of PAD in individuals with symptoms or signs suggestive of disease (individuals with one or more of the following exertional leg symptoms: Nonhealing wounds, age >65 yr, or age >50 yr with smoking or diabetes history)
- ABI of each leg is calculated by dividing the highest dorsalis pedis or posterior tibial systolic blood pressure by the highest systolic brachial pressure obtained from either the right or left arm
  1. Noncompressible/calcified: >1.40
  2. Normal: 1.00 to 1.40 at rest

How to Perform and Calculate the ABI

Partners Program ABI Interpretation
Above 0.90—Normal
0.71-0.90—Mild Obstruction
0.41-0.70—Moderate Obstruction
0.00-0.40—Severe Obstruction

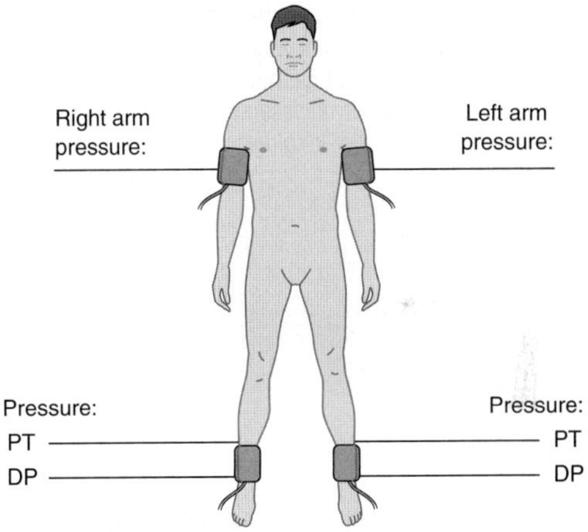

RIGHT ABI | **LEFT ABI**

Higher right ankle pressure / Higher arm pressure = mm Hg / mm Hg = ______ Higher left ankle pressure / Higher arm pressure = mm Hg / mm Hg = ______

EXAMPLE

Higher ankle pressure / Higher arm pressure = 92 mm Hg / 164 mm Hg = 0.56 See ABI Chart

FIG. 3 Performing pressure measurements and calculating the ankle-brachial index *(ABI).* To calculate the ABI, systolic pressures are determined in both arms and both ankles with the use of a handheld Doppler instrument. The highest readings for the dorsalis pedis (DP) and posterior tibial (PT) arteries are used to calculate the index. (From Goldman L, Schafer AI: *Goldman's Cecil medicine,* ed 24, Philadelphia, 2012, Saunders.)

  3. Borderline: 0.91 to 0.99 at rest
  4. Abnormal: ≤0.90
     a. ABI <0.5 severe PAD
     b. 0.5 <ABI <0.75 moderate PAD
     c. 0.75 <ABI <0.9 mild PAD
- ABI should be measured in both legs in all new patients (Fig. 3)
- Exercise ABI is recommended if resting ABI is borderline or normal (>0.9) and symptoms of claudication are suggestive
- Toe-brachial index should be used in patients suspected of PAD with ABI of >1.4. A TBI of <0.70 is abnormal and diagnostic of PAD. TBI may be used to assess perfusion in patients with suspected CLI
- Routine screening for lower-extremity PAD in the absence of risk factors, history, signs, or symptoms is not recommended
- PAD is recognized as a risk factor for abdominal aortic aneurysm (AAA), and in

observational studies the prevalence of AAA was higher in patients with symptomatic PAD

LABORATORY TESTS

Laboratory tests can help identify risk factors or other potential causative etiologies. These include lipid profile, hemoglobin A_{1C}, D-dimer, and CRP/ESR.

PHYSIOLOGIC TESTING & IMAGING STUDIES

- Rest or exercise pulse volume recordings (PVRs) and segmental limb pressures are also useful. PVRs measure volume of limb flow per pulse in different segments of the limb (e.g., thigh, calf, ankle, metatarsal, and toes). They help to assess the location and severity of the lesion with alterations in the pulse volume contour and amplitude indicating proximal arterial obstruction.
- Duplex ultrasound (DUS) incorporates anatomic and physiologic evaluation by combining 2D ultrasound to visualize arterial segments and pulse wave Doppler to sample blood flow velocities at specific locations in the arterial lumen.
- Conventional contrast angiography remains the gold standard, but duplex ultrasonography, computed tomography angiography (CTA), and magnetic resonance angiography (MRA) have largely replaced catheter-based angiography in anatomic assessment for revascularization. Contrast angiography (Fig. E4) is now reserved for patients with PAD who are being considered for endovascular revascularization. It allows assessment of translesional pressure gradients prior to percutaneous intervention.
- Carotid intima-media thickness and brachial artery flow–mediated dilation have shown promise but have not been widely applied.

Rx TREATMENT

The treatment goal in patients with PAD is to focus on cardiovascular risk factor reduction to decrease morbidity and mortality as well as to improve limb-related symptoms. There are also medical and surgical approaches to management of limb-related symptoms. Fig. 5 illustrates an approach to a patient with PAD. 2016 ACCF/AHA guidelines for medical management of patients with peripheral artery disease are summarized in Table 2.

MEDICAL THERAPY (TABLE 3)

LOWERING CARDIOVASCULAR RISK FACTORS, MORBIDITY, AND MORTALITY:

- Smoking cessation or avoidance of secondhand smoke should be emphasized in patients with PAD at each visit with assistance of behavioral and pharmacologic treatment (Class I).
- E-cigarettes may be considered an interim activity to reduce habituation and making smoking cessation possible.
- Proper foot care, including use of appropriate footwear, chiropody/podiatric medicine, daily foot inspection, skin cleansing, and use of topical moisturizing creams, should be encouraged, and skin lesions and ulcerations should be addressed urgently in all patients with diabetes and lower-extremity PAD (Class I).
- A foot infection should be suspected in patients presenting with local pain, periwound erythema, edema, or discharge; these patients should undergo prompt diagnosis and treatment with an interdisciplinary care team to avoid amputation.
- Antiplatelet therapy is indicated to reduce risk of myocardial infarction, stroke, and vascular death in individuals with symptomatic PAD with either aspirin (75 to 325 mg) or clopidogrel (75 mg) (Class I) and in asymptomatic patients (Class IIa). Uncertain benefit has been observed with combination aspirin and clopidogrel therapy (Class IIb). Limited data on use of newer P2Y12 receptor antagonists in PAD. In the EUCLID trial, ticagrelor was not shown to be superior to clopidogrel for the reduction of cardiovascular events, with major bleeding being similar in the two groups. Uncertain benefit with vorapaxar (Class IIb).
- Anticoagulation with low-dose (2.5 mg twice daily) rivaroxaban (Xarelto) plus aspirin 100 mg daily showed significant reductions in both major cardiovascular and limb events,

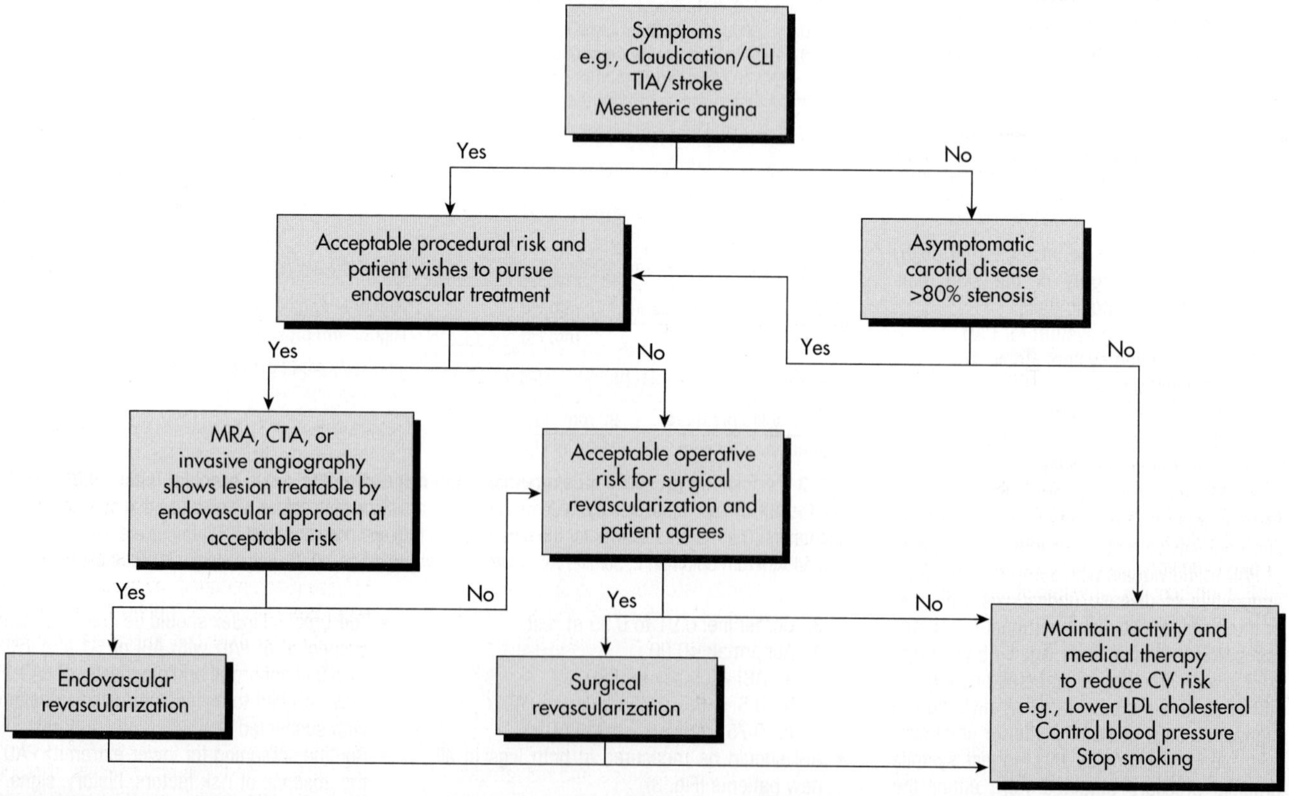

FIG. 5 Approach to a patient with peripheral artery disease. This strategy is based on assessment of the risk for adverse events with and without treatment by taking into consideration procedural or operative risks and the patient's informed decision to proceed with revascularization. *CLI*, Critical limb ischemia; *CTA*, computed tomographic angiography; *CV*, cardiovascular; *LDL*, low-density lipoprotein; *MRA*, magnetic resonance angiography; *TIA*, transient ischemic attack. (From Zipes DP: *Braunwald's heart disease, a textbook of cardiovascular medicine*, ed 11, Philadelphia, 2019, Elsevier.)

TABLE 2 ACCF/AHA Guidelines for Medical Therapy for Patients with Peripheral Artery Disease

COR	Indication	LOE
I	1. Antiplatelet therapy with aspirin alone (range, 75 to 325 mg/day) or clopidogrel alone (75 mg/day) is recommended to reduce MI, stroke, and vascular death in patients with symptomatic PAD.	A
	2. Treatment with a statin medication is indicated for all patients with PAD.	A
	3. Antihypertensive therapy should be administered to patients with hypertension and PAD to reduce the risk of MI, stroke, heart failure, and cardiovascular death.	A
	4. Patients with PAD who smoke cigarettes or use other forms of tobacco should be advised at every visit to quit.	A
	5. Patients with PAD who smoke cigarettes should be assisted in developing a plan for quitting that includes pharmacotherapy (varenicline, bupropion, and/or nicotine replacement therapy) and/or referral to a smoking cessation program.	A
	6. Patients with PAD should avoid exposure to environmental tobacco smoke at work, at home, and in public places.	B-NR
	7. Management of diabetes mellitus in the patient with PAD should be coordinated between members of the health care team.	C-EO
	8. Cilostazol is an effective therapy to improve symptoms and increase walking distance in patients with claudication.	A
	9. Patients with PAD should have an annual influenza vaccination.	C-EO
IIa	1. In asymptomatic patients with PAD (ABI ≤0.90), antiplatelet therapy is reasonable to reduce the risk of MI, stroke, or vascular death.	C-EO
	2. The use of angiotensin-converting enzyme inhibitors or angiotensin receptor blockers can be effective to reduce the risk of cardiovascular ischemic events in patients with PAD.	A
	3. Glycemic control can be beneficial for patients with CLI to reduce limb-related outcomes.	B-NR
IIb	1. In asymptomatic patients with borderline ABI (0.91-0.99), the usefulness of antiplatelet therapy to reduce the risk of MI, stroke, or vascular death is uncertain.	B-R
	2. The effectiveness of dual-antiplatelet therapy (aspirin and clopidogrel) to reduce the risk of cardiovascular ischemic events in patients with symptomatic PAD is not well established.	B-R
	3. Dual-antiplatelet therapy (aspirin and clopidogrel) may be reasonable to reduce the risk of limb-related events in patients with symptomatic PAD after lower extremity revascularization.	C-LD
	4. The overall clinical benefit of vorapaxar added to existing antiplatelet therapy in patients with symptomatic PAD is uncertain.	B-R
	5. The usefulness of anticoagulation to improve patency after lower extremity autogenous vein or prosthetic bypass is uncertain.	B-R
III	1. Anticoagulation should not be used to reduce the risk of cardiovascular ischemic events in patients with PAD.	A
	2. Pentoxifylline is not effective for treatment of claudication.	B-R
	3. Chelation therapy (e.g., ethylenediaminetetraacetic acid) is not beneficial for treatment of claudication.	B-R
	4. B-complex vitamin supplementation to lower homocysteine levels for prevention of cardiovascular events in patients with PAD is not recommended.	B-R

ABI, Ankle-brachial index; *ACCF*, American College of Cardiology Foundation; *AHA*, American Heart Association; *CLI*, critical limb ischemia; COR, class of recommendation; *LOE*, level of evidence; *MI*, myocardial infarction.
From Zipes DP: *Braunwald's heart disease, a textbook of cardiovascular medicine*, ed 11, Philadelphia, 2019, Elsevier.

including amputations, in patients with peripheral arterial disease in the COMPASS trial. (Class IIa – Level B per 2019 *European Journal of Vascular Medicine* PAD guidelines.)

- Anticoagulation is not indicated except in select postsurgical bypass conditions.
- Lipid-lowering therapy in patients with lower limb PAD has been shown to help slow disease progression, alleviate symptoms, and improve walking distance. The 2018 ACC/AHA Guideline on the Treatment of Blood Cholesterol recommends that patients with atherosclerotic PAD receive high-intensity statin therapy in order to lower risk of cardiovascular events regardless of baseline cholesterol values (Class I). In patients who are judged to be very high risk and considered for PCSK9 inhibitor therapy, maximally tolerated LDL-C lowering therapy should include maximally tolerated statin therapy and ezetimibe (Class I). 2019 *European Journal of Vascular Medicine* PAD guidelines also recommends addition of ezetimibe to get better tolerance of the statin medication (with reduced dose) or to achieve target level of LDL <70 mg/dl or >50% decrease.
- Management of hypertension should be in accordance with current HTN guidelines. Control of blood sugar in diabetic patients with PAD is recommended (hemoglobin A_{1C} goal <6.5), although studies have failed to demonstrate a beneficial effect on intensive insulin therapy in lowering risk of PAD. Annual influenza vaccination reduces CV event rates in patients with PAD (Class I).

TREATMENT OF CLAUDICATION:

- Exercise therapy: Supervised exercise-training may be as beneficial as stent revascularization in symptomatic improvement. Patients should be prescribed exercise for a minimum of 30 to 45 min, in sessions performed at least three times per week for a minimum of 12 wk (Class I). ACCF/AHA guidelines for exercise therapy in patients with peripheral artery disease are summarized in Table 4.
  1. Pharmacologic therapy:
     a. Cilostazol (100 mg bid) is indicated as effective therapy for enabling pain-free and maximal walking distance (Class 1). It is a phosphodiesterase (PDE-3) inhibitor that reduces platelet aggregation and causes vasodilatation. It may have an added benefit of reducing restenosis and repeat revascularization following endovascular therapy. Cilostazol is contraindicated in patients with systolic heart failure.
     b. Pentoxifylline, prostanoids, L-arginine, buflomedil, ginkgo biloba, and chelation therapy are no longer considered effective in treatment of claudication
     c. No clear evidence exists for effectiveness of hyperbaric oxygen therapy as an adjunctive therapy for wound treatment in severe PAD

REVASCULARIZATION

In general, there is no difference in clinical outcomes in percutaneous vs. surgical revascularization in iliac and femoropopliteal disease except for the higher morbidity with surgery and greater re-interventions in the percutaneous approach.

- The 2016 ACC/AHA guidelines on PAD (Table 5) have recommended revascularization as a reasonable treatment option for the patient with lifestyle-limiting claudication with inadequate response to guideline-directed medical therapy. A multidisciplinary approach by vascular specialists in all chronic limb ischemia patients for management of pain, risk factors, and comorbidities is appropriate. ACCF/AHA guidelines for wound healing therapies for patients with critical limb ischemia are summarized in Table 6.
- The following approach is discussed:

TABLE 3 Approved Medical Therapies for Patients with Peripheral Artery Disease (PAD)

			Indications			
Therapy	**Mechanism of Action**	**Key Clinical Trials**	**European Medicines Agency**	**European Society of Cardiology**	**FDA**	**ACC/AHA**
Statin (Class effect)	Cholesterol lowering HMG-CoA reductase inhibitor	Heart Protection Study 13% RRR with simvastatin 40 mg daily vs. placebo in all-cause mortality, 18% RRR in coronary heart death Approval for PAD based on subgroup of 6748 patients, 2700 had PAD and no CHD	Reduction in MACE and mortality	Class I for lipid lowering with LDL <2.5 mmol/L, optimally <1.8 mmol/L	Reduction in MACE and mortality	Class I, LOE A
ACEI or ARB (Class effect)	Blood pressure lowering and other vascular effects Renin-angiotensin system inhibition	HOPE 22% RRR with ramipril 10 mg daily vs. placebo for composite of MI, stroke, or CV death Approval for PAD based on subgroup of 4051 patients, 1725 with "clinical PAD"	Reduction in MACE	Class I for blood pressure lowering to ≤140/90 mm Hg	Reduction in MACE	Class I, LOE A for antihypertensive therapy Class IIa, LOE A for ACEI/ARB specifically
Clopidogrel	Antiplatelet $P2Y_{12}$ inhibitor	CAPRIE 8.7% RRR vs. aspirin for composite of ischemic stroke, MI, or vascular death Approval for PAD based on subgroup of 6452 patients	As monotherapy Reduction in MACE	Class I monotherapy for risk reduction Class I added to ASA after lower extremity stenting	As monotherapy Reduction in MACE	Class I, LOE A for monotherapy Class IIb, LOE B-R, C-LD, when added to aspirin as DAPT
Vorapaxar	Antiplatelet PAR-1 antagonist	TRA2P-TIMI 50 20% RRR vs. placebo for composite of MI, stroke, or CV death Approval for PAD based on subgroup of 3787 patients	Added to aspirin or clopidogrel Reduction in MACE, limb benefits mentioned	Approved after most recent guidelines	Added to aspirin and/or clopidogrel Reduction in MACE	Class IIb, LOE B-R added to aspirin and/or clopidogrel
Pentoxifylline	Decreases blood viscosity Mechanism not fully understood	Meta-analysis of six studies including 788 patients who showed minimal increase in maximal walking distance with (+59 m)	Improve function and symptoms in patients with intermittent claudication	Described but no clear recommendation	Improve function and symptoms in patients with intermittent claudication	Class III, LOE B-R
Cilostazol	Antiplatelet and vasodilator Mechanism not fully understood	50 mg bid (n = 303), 100 mg bid (n = 998), and placebo (n = 973) Improvement in maximal walking distance with 100 mg bid, expressed as the percent mean change from baseline, 28%-100% vs. placebo, which were −10%-41%	Reduction of symptoms of intermittent claudication, as indicated by an increased walking distance	Class I for symptoms	Reduction of symptoms of intermittent claudication, as indicated by an increased walking distance	Class I, LOE A

ACC/AHA, American College of Cardiology/American Heart Association; *ACEI,* angiotensin-converting enzyme inhibitor; *ARB,* angiotensin receptor blocker; *bid,* twice daily; *ASA,* acetylsalicylic acid; *CAPRIE,* Clopidogrel versus Aspirin in Patients at Risk of Ischaemic Events; *CHD,* coronary heart disease; *CV,* cardiovascular; *DAPT,* dual-antiplatelet therapy; *FDA,* U.S. Food and Drug Administration; *HOPE,* Heart Outcomes Prevention Evaluation; *LDL,* low-density lipoprotein; *LOE,* level of evidence *(B-R,* moderate-quality evidence from one or more randomized clinical trials; *C-LD,* randomized or nonrandomized observational/registry studies or a meta-analysis); *MACE,* major adverse cardiovascular events; *MI,* myocardial infarction; *PAR-1,* protease-activated receptor 1; *RRR,* relative risk reduction; *TRA2P-TIMI 50,* Thrombin Receptor Antagonist in Secondary Prevention of Atherothrombotic Ischemic Events–Thrombolysis in Myocardial Infarction.
From Zipes DP: *Braunwald's heart disease, a textbook of cardiovascular medicine,* ed 11, Philadelphia, 2019, Elsevier.

1. Considerations in percutaneous/endovascular treatment:
   a. In patients with a vocational- or lifestyle-limiting disability due to claudication or limb ischemia from either significant aortoiliac or femoropopliteal disease despite optimal medical therapy when clinical features suggest a reasonable likelihood of symptomatic improvement with endovascular intervention.
   b. Endovascular intervention is not indicated as prophylactic therapy in an asymptomatic patient with lower-extremity PAD.
   c. Durability of endovascular intervention is greater in iliac and proximal (including proximal popliteal) artery than in the femoropopliteal segment.
2. Considerations in surgical revascularization:
   a. Individuals with claudication symptoms who have a significant functional disability that is vocational or lifestyle limiting. These patients need to also be unresponsive to exercise or pharmacotherapy and should have a reasonable likelihood of symptomatic improvement with an acceptable surgical risk and technical factors favoring surgical vs. endovascular approach.
   b. Autogenous vein graft is superior to prosthetic graft if surgical revascularization is performed (Class I).
   c. Iliac or femoropopliteal disease with long segments; multifocal segments; long segment occlusions; and

TABLE 4 ACCF/AHA Guidelines for Exercise Therapy in Patients with Peripheral Artery Disease

COR	Indication	LOE
I	1. In patients with claudication, a supervised exercise program is recommended to improve functional status and quality of life and to reduce leg symptoms.	A
	2. A supervised exercise program should be discussed as a treatment option for claudication before possible revascularization.	B-R
IIa	1. In patients with PAD, a structured community- or home-based exercise program with behavioral change techniques can be beneficial to improve walking ability and functional status.	A
	2. In patients with claudication, alternative strategies of exercise therapy, including upper-body ergometry, cycling, and pain-free or low-intensity walking that avoids moderate to maximum claudication while walking, can be beneficial to improve walking ability and functional status.	A

COR, Class of recommendation; *LOE,* level of evidence.
From Zipes DP: *Braunwald's heart disease, a textbook of cardiovascular medicine,* ed 11, Philadelphia, 2019, Elsevier.

TABLE 5 ACCF/AHA Guidelines for Revascularization of Patients with Peripheral Artery Disease

COR	Indication	LOE
I	1. In patients with CLI, revascularization should be performed when possible to minimize tissue loss.	B-NR
	2. An evaluation for revascularization options should be performed by an interdisciplinary care team before amputation in the patient with CLI.	C-EO
	3. Endovascular procedures are recommended to establish in-line blood flow to the foot in patients with nonhealing wounds or gangrene.	B-R
	4. Surgical procedures are recommended to establish in-line blood flow to the foot in patients with nonhealing wounds or gangrene.	C-LD
	5. When surgery is performed for CLI, bypass to the popliteal or infrapopliteal arteries (i.e., tibial, pedal) should be constructed with suitable autogenous vein.	A
	6. Endovascular procedures are effective as a revascularization option for patients with lifestyle-limiting claudication and hemodynamically significant aortoiliac occlusive disease.	A
	7. When surgical revascularization is performed, bypass to the popliteal artery with autogenous vein is recommended in preference to prosthetic graft material.	A
IIa	1. Revascularization is a reasonable treatment option for the patient with lifestyle-limiting claudication with an inadequate response to GDMT.	A
	2. Endovascular procedures are reasonable as a revascularization option for patients with lifestyle-limiting claudication and hemodynamically significant femoropopliteal disease.	B-R
	3. Surgical procedures are reasonable as a revascularization option for patients with lifestyle-limiting claudication with inadequate response to GDMT, acceptable perioperative risk, and technical factors suggesting advantages over endovascular procedures.	B-NR
	4. A staged approach to endovascular procedures is reasonable in patients with ischemic rest pain.	C-LD
	5. Evaluation of lesion characteristics can be useful in selecting the endovascular approach for CLI.	B-R
	6. In patients with CLI for whom endovascular revascularization has failed and a suitable autogenous vein is not available, prosthetic material can be effective for bypass to the below-knee popliteal and tibial arteries.	B-NR
	7. A staged approach to surgical procedures is reasonable in patients with ischemic rest pain.	C-LD
IIb	1. The usefulness of endovascular procedures as a revascularization option for patients with claudication due to isolated infrapopliteal artery disease is unknown.	C-LD
	2. Use of angiosome-directed endovascular therapy may be reasonable for patients with CLI and nonhealing wounds or gangrene.	B-NR
III	1. Endovascular procedures should *not* be performed in patients with PAD solely to prevent progression to CLI.	B-NR
	2. Surgical procedures should *not* be performed in patients with PAD solely to prevent progression to CLI.	B-NR
	3. Femoral-tibial artery bypasses with prosthetic graft material should not be used for the treatment of claudication.	B-R

COR, Class of recommendation; *LOE,* level of evidence; *CLI,* critical limb ischemia; *GDMT,* guideline-directed medical therapy.
From Zipes DP: *Braunwald's heart disease, a textbook of cardiovascular medicine,* ed 11, Philadelphia, 2019, Elsevier.

eccentric, calcified stenosis, which are less amenable to percutaneous interventions.
   d. Surgical intervention is not indicated to prevent progression to limb-threatening ischemia in patients with intermittent claudication as generally claudication does not progress to severe ischemia.
3. Revascularization for acute limb ischemia (Table 7):
   a. Management approach is dependent on whether affected limb is viable, threatened, or irreversible. Initial management will depend on the absence of sensation and movement. If absent, then urgent surgery should be considered.
   b. Heparin should be given to all patients with ALI; direct thrombin inhibitor is used if patient has history of HIT.
   c. Catheter-based thrombolysis is effective in ALI with salvageable limb.
   d. Amputation should be performed in patients with irreversible damage.

DISPOSITION

Risk factors for atherosclerosis should be assessed, and appropriate modification instituted. Focus should be placed on smoking cessation, dietary adjustment, and pharmacotherapy for dyslipidemia, hyperglycemia, and hypertension. All patients with PAD should receive aspirin therapy unless contraindicated. Revascularization should be considered for refractory lifestyle-limiting symptoms.

- More than 1 in 6 patients with peripheral arterial disease who undergo peripheral arterial revascularization have unplanned readmission within 30 days with high associated mortality risks and costs. Procedure- and patient-related factors were the primary reasons for readmission.[1]

[1] Secemsky EA et al: Readmissions after revascularization procedures for peripheral arterial disease, *Ann Int Med* 168:93-99, 2018.

TABLE 6 ACCF/AHA Guidelines for Wound Healing Therapies for Patients with Critical Limb Ischemia (CLI)

COR	Indication	LOE
I	1. An interdisciplinary care team should evaluate and provide comprehensive care for patients with CLI and tissue loss to achieve complete wound healing and a functional foot.	B-NR
	2. In patients with CLI, wound care after revascularization should be performed with the goal of complete wound healing.	C-LD
IIb	1. In patients with CLI, intermittent pneumatic compression (arterial pump) devices may be considered to augment wound healing and/or ameliorate severe ischemic rest pain.	B-NR
	2. In patients with CLI, the effectiveness of hyperbaric oxygen therapy for wound healing is unknown.	C-LD
III	Prostanoids are not indicated in patients with CLI.	B-R

COR, Class of recommendation; *LOE,* level of evidence.
From Zipes DP: *Braunwald's heart disease, a textbook of cardiovascular medicine,* ed 11, Philadelphia, 2019, Elsevier.

TABLE 7 ACCF/AHA Guidelines for Management of Patients with Acute Limb Ischemia (ALI)

COR	Indication	LOE
I	1. Patients with ALI should be emergently evaluated by a clinician with sufficient experience to assess limb viability and implement appropriate therapy.	C-EO
	2. In patients with suspected ALI, initial clinical evaluation should rapidly assess limb viability and potential for salvage and does not require imaging.	C-LD
	3. In patients with ALI, systemic anticoagulation with heparin should be administered unless contraindicated.	C-EO
	4. In patients with ALI, the revascularization strategy should be determined by local resources and patient factors (e.g., etiology, degree of ischemia).	C-LD
	5. Catheter-based thrombolysis is effective for patients with ALI and a salvageable limb.	A
	6. Amputation should be performed as the first procedure in patients with a nonsalvageable limb.	C-LD
	7. Patients with ALI should be monitored and treated (e.g., fasciotomy) for compartment syndrome after revascularization.	C-LD
	8. In the patient with ALI, a comprehensive history should be obtained to determine the cause of thrombosis and/or embolization.	C-EO
IIa	1. In patients with ALI with a salvageable limb, percutaneous mechanical thrombectomy can be useful as adjunctive therapy to thrombolysis.	B-NR
	2. In patients with ALI due to embolism and with a salvageable limb, surgical thromboembolectomy can be effective.	C-LD
	3. In the patient with a history of ALI, testing for a cardiovascular cause of thromboembolism can be useful.	C-EO
IIb	The usefulness of ultrasound-accelerated catheter-based thrombolysis for patients with ALI with a salvageable limb is unknown.	C-LD

ACCF, American College of Cardiology Foundation; *AHA,* American Heart Association; *COR,* class of recommendation; *LOE,* level of evidence.
From Zipes DP: *Braunwald's heart disease, a textbook of cardiovascular medicine,* ed 11, Philadelphia, 2019, Elsevier.

REFERRAL

Consultation with vascular medicine, vascular surgery, interventional cardiology, or other physicians with expertise in PAD is recommended in patients with rest pain, functional disability from pain, ABI <0.90 at rest, or any physical signs of limb ischemia or gangrene.

PEARLS & CONSIDERATIONS

COMMENTS

- PAD is a highly prevalent disease process that remains underdiagnosed and undertreated.
- Patients with PAD are at markedly higher risk of future coronary, cerebrovascular, and other vascular events.
- Medical treatment is aimed mainly at cardiovascular risk factor modification, except for cilostazol.
- Studies of the natural history of claudication show the relative safety of initial conservative treatment of PAD in the absence of critical limb ischemia.
- When PAD limits a patient's ability to walk and exercise, revascularization should be considered.
- Exercise training is an important and often neglected treatment strategy that has proven beneficial in improving functional status, reducing symptoms, and improving quality of life. Exercise capacity alone is the strongest predictor of mortality in patients with PAD.
- Surgical intervention should be considered in patients who meet the criteria for intervention but have lesions that are not amenable to PTA/stenting or in older patients with a low surgical risk. Advances in endovascular therapy have broadened the range of revascularization options for refractory claudication and critical and acute limb ischemia in patients with multiple comorbidities.

PREVENTION

Cardiovascular disease is the major cause of death in patients with intermittent claudication. Therefore, the treatment of claudication is directed not only at improving walking distance but also at reducing cardiovascular risk.

PATIENT & FAMILY EDUCATION

The following organizations offer more information about PAD:
- American College of Cardiology (www.acc.org)
- Vascular Disease Foundation (www.vdf.org)

SUGGESTED READINGS

Available at ExpertConsult.com

RELATED CONTENT

Peripheral Arterial Disease (Patient Information)

AUTHORS: **Ali Ashtiani, MD,** and **Pranav M. Patel, MD, FACC, FAHA, FSCAI**

BASIC INFORMATION

DEFINITION

A perirectal abscess is a localized inflammatory process that can be associated with infections of soft tissue and anal glands based on anatomic location. Perianal and perirectal abscesses may be simple or complex, causing suppuration. Infections in these spaces may be classified as superficial perianal or perirectal with involvement in the following anatomic spaces: Ischiorectal, intersphincteric, perianal, and supralevator. The Parks classification of anorectal abscess is subdivided into intersphincteric, transsphincteric, suprasphincteric, and extrasphincteric abscess (Fig. 1).

SYNONYMS

Rectal abscess
Perianal abscess
Anorectal abscess

ICD-10CM CODES
K61.0 Anal abscess
K61.1 Rectal abscess

EPIDEMIOLOGY & DEMOGRAPHICS

INCIDENCE (IN U.S.): Commonly encountered
PREDOMINANT SEX: Male > female
PREDOMINANT AGE: All ages
PEAK INCIDENCE: Not seasonal; common
GENETICS: None known

PHYSICAL FINDINGS & CLINICAL PRESENTATION

- Localized perirectal or anal pain—often worsened with movement or straining
- Perirectal erythema or cellulitis
- Perirectal mass by inspection or palpation
- Fever and signs of sepsis with deep abscess
- Urinary retention

ETIOLOGY

- Polymicrobial aerobic and anaerobic bacteria involving one of the anatomic spaces (see "Definition"), often associated with localized trauma
- Microbiology: Most infections are polymicrobial, mixed enteric, and skin flora
- Predominant anaerobic bacteria:
  1. *Bacteroides fragilis*
  2. *Peptostreptococcus* spp.
  3. *Prevotella* spp.
  4. *Porphyromonas* spp.
  5. *Clostridium* spp.
  6. *Fusobacterium* spp.
- Predominant aerobic bacteria:
  1. *Staphylococcus aureus*
  2. *Streptococcus* spp.
  3. *Escherichia coli*
  4. *Enterococcus* spp.

Dx DIAGNOSIS

Many patients will have predisposing underlying conditions including:
- Malignancy or leukemia
- Immune deficiency
- Diabetes mellitus
- Recent surgery
- Steroid therapy

DIFFERENTIAL DIAGNOSIS

- Neutropenic enterocolitis
- Crohn disease (inflammatory bowel disease)
- Pilonidal disease
- Hidradenitis suppurativa
- Tuberculosis or actinomycosis; Chagas disease
- Cancerous lesions
- Chronic anal fistula
- Rectovaginal fistula
- Proctitis—often STD-associated, including syphilis, gonococcal, chlamydia, chancroid, condylomata acuminata
- AIDS-associated: Kaposi sarcoma, lymphoma, CMV

WORKUP

- Examination of rectal, perirectal/perineal areas
- Rule out necrotic process and crepitance suggesting deep tissue involvement
- Local aerobic and anaerobic culture
- Blood cultures if toxic, febrile, or compromised
- Possible sigmoidoscopy

IMAGING STUDIES

Usually not indicated unless extensive disease is suspected. CT has a sensitivity of 77% and is relatively poor in detecting a perirectal abscess in immunocompromised patients.

Rx TREATMENT

ACUTE GENERAL RX

- Incision and drainage of abscess
- Debridement of necrotic tissue
- Rule out need for fistulectomy
- Local wound care—packing
- Sitz baths
- Antibiotic treatment: Directed toward coverage for mixed skin and enteric flora

OUTPATIENT—ORAL:
- Trimethoprim/sulfamethoxazole DS bid or ciprofloxacin 500 mg bid or levofloxacin 500 mg q24h plus metronidazole 500 mg q8h x 7 to 10 days
- Amoxicillin/clavulanic acid 875 to 1000 mg 1 tabs bid
- Clindamycin 150 to 300 mg PO q6 to 8h 0 mg 1 tabs bid

INPATIENT—INTRAVENOUS:
- Piperacillin/tazobactam 3.375 g IV q6 to 8h
- Ampicillin/sulbactam 1.5 to 3 g IV q6h
- Cefotetan 1 to 2 g IV q8h
- Imipenem or meropenem 500 to 1000 mg IV q8h

DISPOSITION

Follow-up with a general surgeon or infectious disease physician is often warranted.

REFERRAL

- General surgeon or colorectal surgeon for drainage.
- AIDS specialist may be needed for perirectal complications of HIV infection.
- Gastroenterologist follow-up may be warranted in Crohn disease with perirectal fistula and other complications.
- Endoscopic ultrasound–guided perirectal abscess drainage is a recently described promising alternative treatment.

PEARLS & CONSIDERATIONS

Perirectal abscess may be a presenting manifestation of type 2 diabetes mellitus in older adults. Check the blood sugar in patients to exclude the possibility of undiagnosed diabetes mellitus.

SUGGESTED READINGS

Available at ExpertConsult.com

RELATED CONTENT

Perirectal Abscess (Patient Information)

AUTHOR: **Glenn G. Fort, MD, MPH**

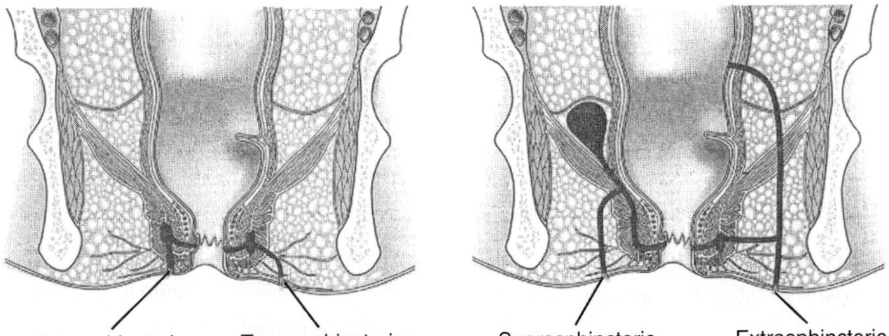

FIG. 1 Parks classification of anorectal abscess. (From Cameron JL, Cameron AM: *Current surgical therapy*, ed 10, Philadelphia, 2011, Saunders.)

BASIC INFORMATION

DEFINITION

Peritonitis refers to the acute onset of severe abdominal pain caused by peritoneal inflammation.

Secondary peritonitis is peritonitis stemming from another condition; commonly a defect in an abdominal viscus.

SYNONYMS

Acute abdomen
Surgical abdomen

ICD-10CM CODES	
K65.0	Generalized (acute) peritonitis
K65.8	Other peritonitis
K65.9	Peritonitis, unspecified
A18.31	Tuberculous peritonitis
A54.85	Gonococcal peritonitis
A74.81	Chlamydial peritonitis
K35.2	Acute appendicitis with generalized peritonitis
K35.3	Acute appendicitis with localized peritonitis
K65.2	Spontaneous bacterial peritonitis
N73.3	Female acute pelvic peritonitis
N73.4	Female chronic pelvic peritonitis
N73.5	Female pelvic peritonitis, unspecified
P78.1	Other neonatal peritonitis

EPIDEMIOLOGY & DEMOGRAPHICS

Common presentation as a result of diverse etiologies; for example, 5% to 10% of the population has acute appendicitis at some point in their lives.

PHYSICAL FINDINGS & CLINICAL PRESENTATION

- Acute abdominal pain
- Abdominal distention and ascites
- Abdominal rigidity, rebound, and guarding
- Altered mental status
- Fever, chills
- Exacerbation with movement
- Anorexia, nausea, and vomiting
- Constipation or diarrhea
- Decreased bowel sounds
- Hypotension and tachycardia
- Tachypnea, dyspnea

ETIOLOGY

- One of the early steps is disturbance in gut flora with overgrowth and extraintestinal organismal overtake. Most common are gram-negative bacteria (*Escherichia coli, Enterobacter, Klebsiella, Proteus*), gram-positive bacteria (enterococci, streptococci, staphylococci), anaerobic bacteria (*Bacteroides, Clostridium*), and fungi
- It can be acute perforation peritonitis: Gastrointestinal perforation, intestinal ischemia, pelvic peritonitis, and other forms
- Postoperative peritonitis: Anastomotic leak, accidental perforation, and devascularization
- Posttraumatic peritonitis: After blunt or penetrating abdominal trauma

Dx DIAGNOSIS

DIFFERENTIAL DIAGNOSIS

- Postoperative: Abscess, sepsis, bowel obstruction, injury to internal organs
- Gastrointestinal: Perforated viscus, appendicitis, inflammatory bowel disease, infectious colitis, diverticulitis, acute cholecystitis, peptic ulcer perforation, pancreatitis, bowel obstruction
- Gynecologic: Ruptured ectopic pregnancy, pelvic inflammatory disease, ruptured hemorrhagic ovarian cyst, ovarian torsion, degenerating leiomyoma
- Urologic: Nephrolithiasis, interstitial cystitis
- Miscellaneous: Abdominal trauma, penetrating wounds, infections caused by intraperitoneal dialysis

WORKUP

- Acute peritonitis is mainly a clinical diagnosis based on patient history and physical examination.
- Laboratory and imaging studies assist in determining the need for and type of intervention. Typical pretreatment peritoneal fluid and blood culture results in peritonitis are summarized in Table E1.
- If patient is hemodynamically unstable, immediate diagnostic laparotomy should be performed in lieu of adjuvant diagnostic studies.

LABORATORY TESTS

- Ascitic fluid testing
  1. Anaerobic and aerobic cultures
  2. Cell count and differential
  3. Albumin, protein, amylase, bilirubin
  4. Glucose
  5. LDH
- Complete blood count: Leukocytosis, left shift, anemia
- SMA7: Electrolyte imbalances, kidney dysfunction
- Liver function tests: Indicative of cirrhosis as ascites from liver disease, cholelithiasis
- Amylase: Pancreatitis
- Blood cultures: Bacteremia, sepsis
- Blood gas: Respiratory versus metabolic acidosis
- Urinalysis and culture: Urinary tract infection
- Cervical cultures for gonorrhea and *Chlamydia*
- Urine/serum human chorionic gonadotropin

IMAGING STUDIES

- Abdominal series: Free air from perforation, small or large bowel dilation from obstruction, identification of fecalith
- Chest x-ray examination: Elevated diaphragm, pneumonia
- Pelvic/abdominal ultrasound: Abscess formation, abdominal mass, intrauterine versus ectopic pregnancy, identify free fluid suggestive of hemorrhage or ascites
- CT: Mass, ascites

Rx TREATMENT

NONPHARMACOLOGIC THERAPY

- IV hydration to correct dehydration, hypovolemia
- Blood transfusion to correct anemia from hemorrhage
- Nasogastric decompression, especially if obstruction is present
- Oxygen: Intubation if necessary
- Bed rest

ACUTE GENERAL Rx

- Surgery to correct underlying pathology, such as controlling hemorrhage, correcting perforation, and draining abscess
- Broad-spectrum antibiotics to cover both gram-negative aerobic and gram-negative anaerobic bacteria:
  1. Mild-moderate disease: Piperacillin-tazobactam 3.375 g IV q6h or 4.5 g IV q8h *or* ticarcillin-clavulanate 3.1 g IV q6h. Alternative agents are ciprofloxacin 400 mg IV q12h or levofloxacin 750 mg IV q24h *plus* metronidazole 1 g IV q12h.
  2. Severe life-threatening disease: Imipenem 500 mg IV q6h or meropenem 1 g IV q8h. Alternative agents are ampicillin *plus* metronidazole *plus* ciprofloxacin.
  3. Antibiotic therapy should be tailored to culture results and sensitivities.
- Pain control: Morphine or meperidine as needed (hold until diagnosis confirmed)

DISPOSITION

Depends on etiology of peritonitis, age of patient, coexisting medical disease, and duration of process before presentation.

REFERRAL

Surgical consultation is required in all cases of acute peritonitis.

PEARLS & CONSIDERATIONS

Computed tomographic scan guides therapeutic approach and should be considered as the primary imaging study if available. As with forms of sepsis, early administration of broad-spectrum antibiotics, fluid resuscitation, and rapidly obtaining anatomic source control (when appropriate) will lead to improved outcomes.

AUTHORS: **Ghamar Bitar, MD,** and
Anthony Sciscione, DO

BASIC INFORMATION

DEFINITION

Peritonsillar abscess is an acute infection located between the capsule of the palatine tonsil and the superior constrictor muscle of the pharynx.

SYNONYMS

Quinsy
PTA

ICD-10CM CODE
J36 Peritonsillar abscess

EPIDEMIOLOGY & DEMOGRAPHICS

INCIDENCE (IN U.S.): 30:100,000/yr for ages 5 to 59. For adolescents, the incidence is 40:100,000/yr. It is the most common deep infection of the head and neck in children and adolescents, accounting for at least 50% of cases.
PREVALENCE: 45,000 cases/yr in the U.S.
PREDOMINANT SEX: Male > female
PREDOMINANT AGE: Highest incidence is adults ages 20 to 40 yr
PEAK INCIDENCE: Bimodal frequency during the year, with highest occurrence from November to December and April to May
RISK FACTORS: Smoking, periodontal disease, oropharyngeal or dental infection, male gender

PHYSICAL FINDINGS & CLINICAL PRESENTATION

- There is often a delay of 2 to 5 days between abscess formation and local and systemic symptoms
- Sore throat, which may be severe and unilateral (Table 1)
- Dysphagia and odynophagia
- Otalgia on the side of abscess
- Foul-smelling breath
- Facial swelling
- Drooling
- Headache
- Fever
- Trismus: The examination of the pharynx can be limited by trismus
- Hoarseness, muffled voice (also called "hot potato voice")
- Tender submandibular and anterior cervical lymph nodes
- Tonsillar hypertrophy with likely peritonsillar edema
- Contralateral deflection of the uvula: The distinguishing feature of peritonsillar abscess is inferior medial displacement of the infected tonsil with contralateral deviation of the uvula (Fig. E1)
- Stridor

ETIOLOGY

- Peritonsillar abscess is usually a complication of tonsillitis or acute bacterial pharyngitis caused by blockage of salivary ducts. Tonsillitis → peritonsillar cellulitis → peritonsillar abscess.
- Group A β-hemolytic *Streptococcus* is the most common bacterial cause, accounting for 15% to 30% of cases in children and 5% to 10% of cases in adults.
- Less common aerobic causes are *Staphylococcus aureus, Haemophilus influenzae, are Neisseria* spp.
- The most common anaerobic organism is *Fusobacterium.*

DIAGNOSIS

DIFFERENTIAL DIAGNOSIS

- Hypertrophic tonsillitis
- Infectious mononucleosis
- Peritonsillar cellulitis
- Retropharyngeal abscess
- Epiglottitis
- Dental abscess (retromolar)
- Lymphoma
- Ludwig angina
- Tubercular granuloma
- Cervical adenitis
- Diphtheria
- Foreign body
- Neoplasm

WORKUP

- Based on history and physical exam. Aspiration of pus established diagnosis of peritonsillar abscess.
- Consider additional testing if presentation is less clear.

LABORATORY TESTS

- Consider rapid strep antigen testing and/or pharyngeal culture and sensitivity.
- Aspiration of the abscess for culture and sensitivity (see "Treatment" for role of aspiration in Tx).
- Consider lab testing for mononucleosis (patients with peritonsillar abscess have a 20% incidence of mononucleosis).

IMAGING STUDIES

- Consider ultrasound, CT scan (Fig. 2), or MRI (Fig. 3) to help differentiate abscess from cellulitis or mass when diagnosis is unclear.
- Intraoral ultrasound may improve diagnosis and aspiration of PTA compared with visual inspection in adult patients.
- MRI provides better soft-tissue differentiation than CT.

TABLE 1 Clinical Differentiation of Common Conditions Arising as Sore Throat

Feature	Viral Pharyngitis	Bacterial Tonsillitis	Peritonsillar Abscess	Epiglottitis
Tonsillar enlargement	Usual	Rare	None	None
Tonsillar exudates	Occasional (mononucleosis)	Usual	Often	None
Tonsillar asymmetry	None	None	Usual	None
Trismus (inability to open jaw)	None	None	Usual	None
Cervical adenopathy	Occasional	Usual (tender)	Usual (tender)	None
Tender larynx	Rare	None	None	Usual

From Goldman L, Schafer AI: *Goldman's Cecil medicine*, ed 24, Philadelphia, 2012, Saunders.

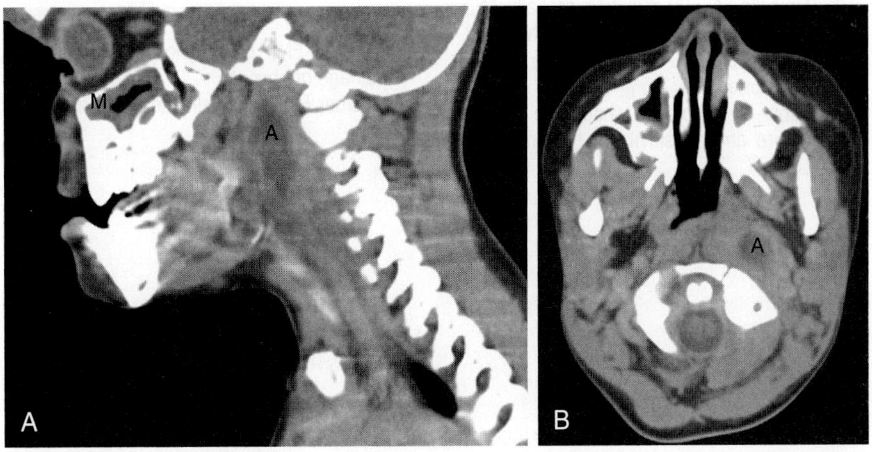

FIG. 2 Computed tomography of parapharyngeal abscess in a 3-yr-old child. A, Sagittal section demonstrating parapharyngeal abscess *(A)* and mucosal swelling *(M)* in the maxillary sinus. **B,** Coronal section of parapharyngeal abscess *(A)*. (From Kliegman RM et al: *Nelson textbook of pediatrics,* ed 19, Philadelphia, 2011, Saunders.)

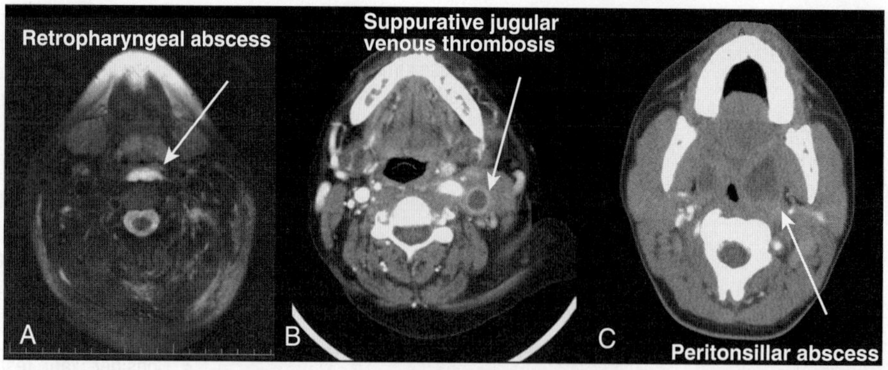

FIG. 3 Magnetic resonance imaging and computed tomography images showing a variety of life-threatening head and neck infections, including retropharyngeal abscess (A), suppurative jugular venous thrombosis (B), and peritonsillar abscess (C). (Images provided by Dr. Joshua Brody, Department of Radiology, the Cooper Health System, Camden, NJ. In Parrillo JE, Dellinger RP: *Critical care medicine, principles of diagnosis and management in the adult,* ed 5, Philadelphia, 2019, Elsevier.)

Rx TREATMENT

NONPHARMACOLOGIC THERAPY

Drainage of the abscess by needle aspiration or by surgical incision and drainage. Intraoral ultrasound-guided needle aspiration is a useful adjunct in the presence of trismus.

ACUTE GENERAL Rx

- Aspiration or surgical drainage AND antibiotics for 10 to 14 days
- Initial antibiotics should cover group A *Streptococcus* and anaerobes
- Intravenous
  1. Piperacillin/tazobactam or ticarcillin/clavulanate. If penicillin allergic, use IV clindamycin (600-900 mg IV q8h)
  2. Ampicillin-sulbactam 3 g q6h
  3. Penicillin G 10 million units q6h AND metronidazole 500 mg q6h (may use clindamycin 900 mg q8h if penicillin allergic)
- OR oral
  1. Amoxicillin-clavulanic acid 875 mg twice daily
  2. Penicillin VK 500 mg 4 times daily AND metronidazole 500 mg 4 times daily
  3. Clindamycin 600 mg twice daily or 300 mg 4 times daily
- Selection of antibiotics should be guided by culture and sensitivity of the organism. Consulting local antimicrobial guidelines for resistance profiles is also advisable for empiric coverage before culture results are available

CHRONIC Rx

- Tonsillectomy can be considered 3 to 6 mo after diagnosis of peritonsillar abscess with or without the diagnosis of recurrent tonsillitis.
- Though rare, in adults and children with an acute case of peritonsillar abscess and a history of recurrent pharyngitis or previous peritonsillar abscess, a specialist may recommend a *quinsy or hot tonsillectomy,* an immediate removal of the tonsils after starting IV antibiotics.

DISPOSITION

- Successful treatment is defined by symptomatic improvement in sore throat, fever, and/or tonsillar swelling within 24 hr of intervention.
- Treatment failure is defined by lack of symptomatic improvement or worsening despite 24 hr of antimicrobial therapy (with or without surgical drainage).

REFERRAL

- Consider ENT or diagnostic radiology for drainage of abscess.
- Consider ENT for tonsillectomy if criteria are met.

PEARLS & CONSIDERATIONS

COMMENTS

- Risk for a recurrence is immediate (within 4 days) and long term (2-3 yr).
- Most recurrences occur shortly after the initial presentation, suggesting continued infection rather than recurrence.
- Overall recurrence rate is 10% to 15%.
- Supportive treatment for pain control and hydration. Newer reports suggest a single dose of dexamethasone (10 mg) administered after needle aspiration will reduce pain at 24 hr as compared with placebo (see "Suggested Readings").

PREVENTION

- Adequate treatment of peritonsillar abscess.
- Up to 30% of patients with peritonsillar abscess meet criteria for tonsillectomy.

PATIENT & FAMILY EDUCATION

Advise family members to call with any trouble breathing, swallowing, or talking.

SUGGESTED READINGS

Available at ExpertConsult.com

AUTHORS: **Peter J. Sell, DO, Amity Rubeor, DO, CAQSM,** and **Glenn G. Fort, MD, MPH**

BASIC INFORMATION

DEFINITION

Pertussis is a prolonged bacterial infection of the upper respiratory tract characterized by paroxysms of an intense cough.

SYNONYM

Whooping cough

ICD-10CM CODES	
A37.00	Whooping cough due to Bordetella pertussis without pneumonia
A37.01	Whooping cough due to Bordetella pertussis with pneumonia
A37.10	Whooping cough due to Bordetella parapertussis without pneumonia
A37.11	Whooping cough due to Bordetella parapertussis with pneumonia
A37.80	Whooping cough due to other Bordetella species without pneumonia
A37.81	Whooping cough due to other Bordetella species with pneumonia
A37.90	Whooping cough, unspecified species without pneumonia
A37.91	Whooping cough, unspecified species with pneumonia

EPIDEMIOLOGY & DEMOGRAPHICS

INCIDENCE (IN U.S.): Case reports from 2018 totaled 15,609, including five deaths. This represents a decrease in the number of case reports compared with 2017. The reported rates were 18,975 and 17,972 in 2017 and 2016, respectively. In 2012 there were 48,277 cases reported, which is the highest rate reported since 1955. The highest incidence in 2018 was among infants <6 mo (72.8/100,000), with a second peak in adolescents ages 11 to 19 yr (13.0/100,000).

PREDOMINANT AGE:
- 20% in children aged <1 yr
- 50% in children aged >10 yr
- Classically an infection of infants and young children, pertussis is often overlooked as a cause of chronic cough in adults. However, nearly 50% of all cases are identified in adolescents and adults, likely resulting from waning immunity and decreased effectiveness of acellular vaccines in early childhood compared to older, whole-cell-derived vaccines.

PEAK INCIDENCE:
- Childhood
- Usually affects children aged <1 yr
- Increasing infections seen in adolescence

PHYSICAL FINDINGS & CLINICAL PRESENTATION

- Infection is characterized by three phases: Catarrhal, paroxysmal, and convalescent.
- Catarrhal phase: Usually begins with a 1- to 2-wk prodrome that resembles a common cold. This phase may be mild or absent in adolescents and adults given partial immunity from prior immunization.
- After this initial phase, increased production of mucus occurs. Excessive lacrimation and conjunctival infection should heighten the suspicion for pertussis.
- Paroxysmal phase: Increased mucus production is followed by an intense, paroxysmal cough, ending with gasps and an inspiratory whoop. Note that infants with pertussis may not whoop.
- In some children, apnea, cyanosis, and anoxia are noted; posttussive gagging and vomiting are characteristic of pertussis.
- Cases can be severe and life-threatening in young infants, particularly children <6 mo old.
- When prolonged, frank exhaustion and even apnea occur. The paroxysmal phase lasts from 2 wk to 2 mo.
- Convalescent phase: Lasts over 2 mo and is characterized by cough of decreasing severity.
- See Box 1 for complications of pertussis.

ETIOLOGY

Bordetella pertussis, a gram-negative rod that adheres to human cilia and respiratory epithelia

DIAGNOSIS

DIFFERENTIAL DIAGNOSIS

- Croup
- Epiglottitis
- Foreign body aspiration
- Bacterial pneumonia
- Viral pneumonia

WORKUP

Pertussis is often overlooked as a cause of chronic cough, especially in adolescents and adults. The presence of posttussive emesis and/or inspiratory whoop increases the likelihood of pertussis, but only modestly. Therefore clinicians must use their overall impression in pursuing the diagnosis.

- Polymerase chain reaction (PCR) is the most sensitive method for rapid detection of pertussis. PCR testing should be used only to confirm a diagnosis in persons with signs and symptoms consistent with pertussis. PCR testing sensitivity declines and is unlikely to be positive after 1 mo of infection. PCR testing after 5 days of treatment with antibiotics can cause false-negative results and is generally not recommended
- Blood cultures in hospitalized patients
- Chest x-ray
- Culture of bacteria, usually from nasopharynx by aspiration or by swabbing the posterior nasopharynx with a polyester-tipped, rayon-tipped, or nylon-flocked swab
- Serologic tests for immunoglobulin G (IgG) or A (IgA) are available. A twofold increase between acute and convalescent sera is considered proof of seroconversion. A single elevated IgG or IgA titer is considered diagnostic when no acute serum is available. Can be useful for diagnosis later in illness

BOX 1 Pertussis Complications

- Periorbital edema
- Subconjunctival hemorrhage
- Petechiae
- Epistaxis
- Hemoptysis
- Subcutaneous emphysema
- Pneumothorax
- Pneumomediastinum
- Diaphragmatic rupture
- Umbilical and inguinal hernias
- Rectal prolapse

From Marx J et al: *Rosen's emergency medicine: concepts and clinical practice,* ed 7, Philadelphia, 2010, Mosby.

LABORATORY TESTS

Complete blood count, which usually demonstrates marked lymphocytosis:
- 15,000 white blood cells or greater
- 70% to 80% lymphocytes

IMAGING STUDIES

Chest x-ray examination is of value if secondary bacterial pneumonia is suspected. The classic finding of a "right shaggy heart border" is neither sensitive nor specific for pertussis.

TREATMENT

ACUTE GENERAL Rx

- Intensive supportive care:
  1. Adequate hydration
  2. Control of secretions
  3. Maintenance of airway
- Antibiotics (Table 1) are indicated, even though their ability to alter the course of the disease is controversial
  1. Azithromycin 500 mg on day 1, followed by 250 mg for days 2 to 5. Erythromycin 50 mg/kg/day for 14 days. Recent literature reports indicate that a 7-day treatment regimen may be as effective as a 14-day course of erythromycin. TMP/SMX 320/1600 mg per day in divided doses can be used in patients with allergy or intolerance to macrolides
  2. Although unproved, dexamethasone 1 mg/kg/day in four doses for severe, life-threatening paroxysms
  3. Ceftriaxone 75 mg/kg/day in two doses for broad coverage of secondary bacterial pneumonias
  4. Close observation of infants <6 mo old, as risk for apnea is high in this age group
- Vaccination is successful in preventing the disease: Universal vaccination is advised for all children and adults. Children are recommended to receive the five-dose DTaP series at months 2, 4, 6, and 15 to 18, and at ages 4 to 6 yr
- The Advisory Committee on Immunization Practices (ACIP) updated Tdap recommendations to include a single dose of Tdap vaccine in place of routine Td for adults ages 19 to 64 yr and a single-dose Tdap for adults ages 65 yr and older who have or will have close

TABLE 1 Recommended Antimicrobial Treatment and Postexposure Prophylaxis for Pertussis, by Age Group

	PRIMARY AGENTS		ALTERNATE AGENT*	
Age Group	**Azithromycin**	**Erythromycin**	**Clarithromycin**	**TMP-SMZ**
<1 mo	Recommended agent. 10 mg/kg/day in a single dose for 5 days (only limited safety data available)	Not preferred. Erythromycin is substantially associated with infantile hypertrophic pyloric stenosis. Use if azithromycin is unavailable; 40-50 mg/kg/day in 4 divided doses for 14 days	Not recommended (safety data unavailable)	Contraindicated for infants aged <2 mo (risk for kernicterus)
1-5 mo	10 mg/kg/day in a single dose for 5 days	40-50 mg/kg/day in 4 divided doses for 14 days	15 mg/kg/day in 2 divided doses for 7 days	Contraindicated at age <2 mo. For infants aged ≥2 mo: TMP 8 mg/kg/day plus SMZ 40 mg/kg/day in 2 divided doses for 14 days
Infants aged ≥6 mo and children	10 mg/kg in a single dose on day 1 (maximum 500 mg), then 5 mg/kg/day (maximum 250 mg) on days 2-5	40 mg/kg/day (maximum 1-2 g/day) in 4 divided doses for 14 days	15 mg/kg/day in 2 divided doses (maximum 1 g/day) for 7 days	TMP 8 mg/kg/day plus SMZ 40 mg/kg/day in 2 divided doses for 14 days
Adolescents and adults	500 mg in a single dose on day 1, then 250 mg/day on days 2-5	2 g/day in 4 divided doses for 14 days	1 g/day in 2 divided doses for 7 days	TMP 320 mg/day, SMZ 1600 mg/day in 2 divided doses for 14 days

*Trimethoprim-sulfamethoxazole (TMP-SMZ) can be used as an alternative agent to macrolides in patients aged ≥2 mo who are allergic to macrolides, who cannot tolerate macrolides, or who are infected with a rare, macrolide-resistant strain of *Bordetella pertussis.*

SMZ, Sulfamethoxazole; *TMP,* trimethoprim.

From Centers for Disease Control and Prevention: Recommended antimicrobial agents for treatment and postexposure prophylaxis of pertussis: 2005 CDC guidelines, *MMWR Morbid Mortal Wkly Rep* 54:1-16, 2005.

contact with an infant (<12 mo). The ACIP also recommends that all pregnant women receive a dose of Tdap with every pregnancy, preferably during weeks 27 to 36 of gestation

- Azithromycin, clarithromycin, or erythromycin is recommended for all household contacts and should be given to all persons at high risk of severe disease from pertussis and were in contact with a pertussis case within 21 days of cough onset: TMP/SMX in two oral doses per day for those intolerant to macrolides

DISPOSITION

Close attention to accepted vaccination schedules is the best prevention.

REFERRAL

To intensive care setting for life-threatening infections:

- Pulmonologist
- Infectious disease specialist

PEARLS & CONSIDERATIONS

- The diagnosis of pertussis in a young child is easily recognized, but in adults pertussis can be a subtle diagnosis and is often missed. The tip-off is often a persistent, hacking, and productive cough with minor or no fever in a previously healthy person that lasts <2 wk.
- Approximately 11% of pertussis cases in the pediatric population are attributable to vaccine refusal, dispelling the myth that herd immunity protects children whose parents refuse pertussis vaccine.

SUGGESTED READINGS

Available at ExpertConsult.com

RELATED CONTENT

Pertussis (Patient Information)

AUTHOR: **Russell J. McCulloh, MD**

BASIC INFORMATION

DEFINITION

- A hamartomatous polyp is a benign intestinal growth that may contain all components of the intestinal mucosa. In Peutz-Jeghers syndrome (PJS), hamartomas are found primarily in the small bowel but can also be present in the colon and stomach. In gastrointestinal polyposis, multiple such polyps coexist within the intestinal tract, and associated manifestations are usually also present.
- Juvenile polyps are benign polyps composed of cystic dilations of glandular structures within the fibroblastic stroma of the lamina propria. They may cause bleeding or intussusception.
- Commonly recognized syndromes are Peutz-Jeghers syndrome, juvenile polyposis syndrome, Cowden disease, Bannayan-Ruvalcaba-Riley syndrome, and Cronkhite-Canada syndrome. Other, lesser-known inherited hamartomatous polyposis syndromes are hereditary mixed polyposis syndrome, intestinal ganglioneuromatosis and neurofibromatosis (variant of von Recklinghausen syndrome), Devon family syndrome, basal cell nevus syndrome, and tuberous sclerosis (may involve gastrointestinal tract). Table 1 describes general features of some inherited colorectal cancer syndromes.

ICD-10CM CODE
D12.6 Colon, unspecified (adenomatosis of colon, hereditary polyposis)

EPIDEMIOLOGY & DEMOGRAPHICS

- The incidence of PJS is 1 in 200,000.
- Colonic adenomas, the precursors of nearly all colorectal cancers, are found in nearly 40% of patients by age 60 yr.
- 25% of men and 15% of women who undergo colonoscopy are found to have one or more adenomas.
- Detection of any adenoma in patients <60 yr confers an increased risk of colorectal cancer (by a factor of 2.6) in their first-degree relatives.

PHYSICAL FINDINGS & CLINICAL PRESENTATION

PEUTZ-JEGHERS SYNDROME:

- Transmission: Autosomal dominant with incomplete penetrance. The syndrome is caused in the majority of patients by a germline mutation of the *STK11/LKB1* tumor suppression gene on chromosome 19P13.
- Disease expression:
  1. Stomach, small and large intestinal hamartomas with bands of smooth muscle in the lamina propria
  2. Pigmented lesions around mouth (lips and buccal mucosa [Fig. E2]), nose, hands, feet, genitals, and perineal areas
  3. Ovarian tumors
  4. Sertoli cell testicular tumors
  5. Airway polyps
  6. Pancreatic cancer
  7. Breast cancer
  8. Urinary tract polyps
- Cumulative lifetime cancer risk:
  1. Colon cancer: 39%
  2. Stomach cancer: 29%
  3. Small intestine cancer: 13%
  4. Pancreatic cancer: 36%
  5. Breast cancer: 54%
  6. Ovarian cancer: 10%
  7. Sertoli cell tumor: 9%
  8. Overall cancer risk: 93%
- Clinical manifestation:
  1. Gastrointestinal, small-bowel obstruction, intussusception, gastrointestinal bleeding
  2. See chapters on relevant malignancies for their signs and symptoms

DIAGNOSIS: The diagnosis of PJS is made with any of four major criteria:

1. Two or more histologically confirmed PJS polyps
2. Any number of PJS polyps and a family history of PJS
3. Characteristic mucocutaneous pigmentation and a family history of PJS, or
4. Any number of PJS polyps and characteristic mucocutaneous pigmentation

JUVENILE POLYPOSIS SYNDROME:

- Transmission: Autosomal dominant
- Disease expression:
  1. Solitary juvenile polyps numbering 10 or more in the rectum or throughout the gastrointestinal tract; the polyps are smooth and covered with normal epithelium
  2. Various congenital abnormalities coexist in 20%
- Cumulative cancer risk is increased (may be as high as 50%)
- Clinical manifestation:
  1. Intestinal obstruction
  2. Intussusception
  3. Gastrointestinal bleeding

COWDEN DISEASE:

- Transmission: Autosomal dominant, rare
- Disease expression:
  1. Juvenile intestinal polyposis
  2. Orocutaneous hamartomas
  3. Fibrocystic breast disease and breast cancer
  4. Goiter and thyroid cancer
  5. Facial tricholemmomas (papules) in 83%
- Cumulative cancer risk:
  1. Gastrointestinal: Same as general population
  2. Thyroid: 3% to 10%
  3. Breast: 25% to 50%

BANNAYAN-RUVALCABA-RILEY SYNDROME:

- Transmission: Autosomal dominant, rare
- Disease expression:
  1. Juvenile intestinal polyposis
  2. Macrocephaly
  3. Developmental delay
  4. Penile pigmented spots
  5. Cumulative cancer risk unknown

CRONKHITE-CANADA SYNDROME:

- Transmission: Acquired
- Age of onset: Midlife
- Disease expression:
  1. Diffuse gastrointestinal juvenile polyposis (50% to 95% of cases)
  2. Chronic diarrhea and protein-losing enteropathy (the entire intestinal mucosa may

TABLE 1 General Features of Some Inherited Colorectal Cancer Syndromes

Syndrome	Polyp Histology	Polyp Distribution	Age of Onset	Risk of Colon Cancer	Genetic Lesion	Clinical Manifestations	Associated Lesions
Familial adenomatous polyposis (Fig. E1)	Adenoma	Large intestine, duodenum	16 yr (range, 8-34 yr)	100%	5q (*APC* gene)	Rectal bleeding, abdominal pain, bowel obstruction	Desmoids, CHRPE
Peutz-Jeghers syndrome	Hamartoma	Large and small intestine	First decade	Slightly above average	19p (*STK11* gene)	Possible rectal bleeding, abdominal pain, intussusception	Orocutaneous melanin pigment spots, other tumors
MUTYH-associated polyposis	Adenoma	Large intestine, duodenum	45-50 yr (range, 13-60 yr)	75% (range, 50%-100%)	1p (*MYH* gene)	Rectal bleeding, abdominal pain, bowel obstruction	CHRPE, osteomas
Juvenile polyposis	Hamartoma (rarely adenoma)	Large and small intestine	First decade	~9%	*PTEN, SMAD4, BMPR1*	Possible rectal bleeding, abdominal pain, intussusception	Pulmonary AVMs
Hereditary nonpolyposis colon cancer	Adenoma	Large intestine	40 yr (range, 18-65 yr)	30%	Mismatch repair genes+*	Rectal bleeding, abdominal pain, bowel obstruction	Other tumors (e.g., ovary, uterus, pancreas, stomach)

*Including *hMSH2, hMSH3, hMSH6, hMLH1, hPMS1*, and *hPMS2*.
AVM, Arteriovenous malformation; *CHRPE*, congenital hypertrophy of the retinal pigment epithelium; *MUTYH*, mutY homolog (*Escherichia coli*).
From Goldman L, Schafer AI: *Goldman's Cecil medicine*, ed 24, Philadelphia, 2012, Saunders.

be inflamed), which leads to abdominal pain, weight loss, and various complications of malnutrition
3. Dystrophic nails
4. Alopecia
5. Hyperpigmentation
- Cumulative cancer risk: Same as the average population

Dx DIAGNOSIS

Diagnosis is suggested in many cases by family history and confirmed by colonoscopy and physical findings described previously.

Rx TREATMENT

GENERAL Rx/SURVEILLANCE

Peutz-Jeghers syndrome:
- Colonoscopies with polypectomies and upper endoscopy every 2 to 3 yr beginning in teen yr
- MRI or endoscopic ultrasound of the pancreas every 1 to 2 yr beginning at age 30
- Screening for breast cancer, testicular cancer, possibly ovarian cancer
- Surveillance of small bowel with capsule endoscopy or CT or magnetic resonance enterography every 2 to 3 yr starting at age 8 to 10 yr

Juvenile polyposis syndrome:
- Colonoscopies with polypectomies and upper endoscopy every 2 to 3 yr beginning at age 15
- Total colectomy if numerous polyps
- Esophagogastroscopies and polypectomies

Cowden disease:
- Rigorous breast cancer screening or prophylactic simple bilateral mastectomy with reconstruction

Cronkhite-Canada syndrome:
- Progressive malabsorption syndrome is the hallmark of this syndrome, and no specific treatment exists. Enteral or parenteral feeding is the cornerstone of management and can result in remission
- Other syndromes:
  1. Serrated polyposis syndrome: Colonoscopy yearly
  2. PTEN hamartoma tumor syndrome: Colonoscopy every 5 yr beginning at age 35

DISPOSITION

- The screening of first-degree relatives of patients with colonic adenomas detected before 60 yr of age is controversial. Some recommend beginning colonoscopic screening at age 40 yr, or 10 yr younger than the age at diagnosis of the youngest person in the family with an adenoma.
- Recommended intervals between colonoscopies from the U.S. Consensus Guidelines for Colonoscopic Surveillance after Polypectomy are as follows:
  1. 10 yr for small, rectal hyperplastic polyps
  2. 5 to 10 yr for one to two low-risk adenomas (tubular adenomas <1 cm)
  3. 3 yr for low-risk adenomas or any high-risk adenoma (large [≥1 cm] or histologically advanced adenomas [tubulovillous or villous adenomas or villous adenomas and those with high-grade dysplasia])
  4. <3 yr for presence of >10 adenomas
  5. 2 to 6 mo for inadequately removed adenomas

RELATED CONTENT

Peutz-Jeghers Syndrome (Patient Information)
Colorectal Cancer (Related Key Topic)
Familial Adenomatous Polyposis and Gardner Syndrome (Related Key Topic)
Lynch Syndrome (Related Key Topic)

AUTHOR: **Fred F. Ferri, MD**

BASIC INFORMATION

DEFINITION

Sore throat may represent pain or soreness in the pharynx or surrounding anatomy. Pharyngitis specifically refers to inflammation of the pharynx. Tonsillitis refers to inflammation of the tonsils, which are situated in the rear of the pharynx. Either pharyngitis or tonsillitis may present with pain, erythema, edema, exudates or enanthems (e.g., ulcers, vesicles).

SYNONYMS

Sore throat
Acute Pharyngitis
Pharyngitis
Tonsillitis
Group A streptococcus (GAS)
Group A beta-hemolytic streptococcus (GABHS)

ICD-10CM CODES

J02.9	Acute pharyngitis, unspecified
J03.0	Acute tonsillitis
J03.9	Acute tonsillitis, unspecified

EPIDEMIOLOGY & DEMOGRAPHICS

Acute pharyngitis accounts for 1% to 2% of all ambulatory care visits and 12 million outpatient visits each year in the United States.

PREDOMINANT SEX: Females = males

PREDOMINANT AGE:

- All ages are affected (children younger than age 3 have atypical symptoms and rarely complain of sore throat).
- Incidence peaks in childhood and adolescence, with 50% of cases before age 18 yr.
- Streptococcal pharyngitis is the most common among school-age children (ages 5 to 15 yr). GAS infections are responsible for 5% to 15% of cases of pharyngitis in adults and 35% to 40% of cases in children (ages 5 to 15 yr).

PEAK INCIDENCE:

- Late winter/early spring (GAS infections)

PHYSICAL FINDINGS & CLINICAL PRESENTATION

- Pharynx:
  1. May appear normal to severely erythematous (Fig. E1).
  2. Tonsillar hypertrophy and exudates are commonly seen but do not confirm etiology.
- Common associated viral symptoms:
  1. Coryza
  2. Conjunctivitis
  3. Cough
  4. Cervical lymphadenopathy
     a. Findings associated with specific viral etiology
        (1) Herpes simplex or *Enterovirus* infection: Exudates and vesicles
        (2) Severe acute respiratory syndrome coronavirus 2 (SARS-CoV-2): Fever, cough, diarrhea and vomiting
        (3) Epstein-Barr virus (EBV): Malaise, cervical node enlargement
  5. Rhinorrhea
- Common candidal symptoms:
  1. Pseudomembranous white plaques on buccal mucosa, palate, tongue
- Common bacterial symptoms, especially for GAS:
  1. High fever >38° C (100.4° F)
  2. Tonsillar exudate
  3. Scarlatiniform rash
  4. Strawberry tongue
  5. Systemic signs of infection
  6. Rare complications associated with GAS infection:
     a. Scarlet fever
     b. Rheumatic fever
     c. Acute glomerulonephritis
     d. Streptococcal toxic shock syndrome
     e. Pediatric autoimmune neuropsychiatric disorders associated with streptococcal infections (PANDAS) syndrome
  7. Extension of infection (Fig. E2): Tonsillar, parapharyngeal, or retropharyngeal abscess presenting with severe pain, high fever, trismus, respiratory distress, difficulty swallowing, and drooling.
- Streptococcal tonsillitis is manifested as acute onset of fever, headache, neck pain, dysphagia, odynophagia, sore throat, otalgia, red tongue with enlargement of papillae, sore throat, red swollen uvula, palatal petechiae, and tender anterior cervical adenitis.
- Peritonsillar abscess (accumulation of pus between the tonsil and its capsule) is the most common complication of acute tonsillitis. Clinical signs include dysphagia, odynophagia, drooling, neck stiffness, deformed posterior pharynx, medial displacement of the uvula, trismus, muffled voice (hot-potato voice), and respiratory distress.
- Lingual tonsillitis is a rarely diagnosed cause of pharyngitis that predominantly occurs in patients who have had their palatine tonsils removed. The lingual tonsils are located below the inferior pole of the palatine tonsils and anterior to the vallecula at the base of the tongue. The lymphoid tissue may enlarge after tonsillectomy and repeated infections. Patients have a sore throat that worsens with movement of the tongue. Physical findings often include a normal-appearing pharynx and hyperemia. Lateral soft tissue neck films reveal a normal-appearing epiglottis and a scalloped appearance of the lingual tonsil (Fig. E3).
- Box 1 describes seven danger signs in patients with sore throat.

ETIOLOGY

- Viruses:
  1. Adenovirus
  2. Coronavirus, including SARS-CoV-2
  3. Cytomegalovirus
  4. Enterovirus
  5. Epstein-Barr virus
  6. Herpes simplex virus
  7. Human metapneumovirus
  8. Influenza
  9. Parainfluenza
  10. Respiratory syncytial virus
  11. Rhinovirus
- Bacteria:
  1. GAS: The most common cause of acute tonsillitis
  2. *Fusobacterium necrophorum* (10% of pharyngitis): Highest incidence in patients ages 15 to 30 yr
  3. *Haemophilus influenzae B*
  4. *Neisseria gonorrhoeae*
  5. *Peptostreptococcus*
  6. *Prevotella*
- Other organisms:
  1. *Arcanobacterium haemolyticum*
  2. *Candida albicans*
  3. *Chlamydophila pneumoniae*
  4. *Chlamydia trachomatis*
  5. *Mycoplasma pneumoniae*

DIAGNOSIS

DIFFERENTIAL DIAGNOSIS

- Infectious: Viral, bacterial, fungal, peritonsillar abscess, Lemierre syndrome, epiglottitis, tracheitis, croup, lateral or retropharyngeal abscess, uvulitis
- Allergic/inflammatory: Allergic rhinitis/sinusitis, gastroesophageal reflux disease, Kawasaki disease, periodic fever with aphthous stomatitis, Stevens-Johnson syndrome, Behçet syndrome, angioedema, anaphylaxis, sore throat associated with granulocytopenia, thyroiditis
- Environmental exposure: Foreign body ingestion, chemical exposure (e.g., smoke), irritative pharyngitis, trauma
- Referred pain: Psychogenic pharyngitis, referred pain from dental abscess, otitis media, cervical adenitis
- Oncologic: Tonsillar hypertrophy associated with lymphoma, lymphangioma, or hemangioma of airway
- Section II describes the differential diagnosis of sore throat

BOX 1 Seven Danger Signs in Patients with Sore Throat

1. Persistence of symptoms longer than 1 wk without improvement
2. Respiratory difficulty, particularly stridor
3. Difficulty in handling secretions
4. Difficulty in swallowing
5. Severe pain in the absence of erythema
6. A palpable mass
7. Blood, even in small amounts, in the pharynx or ear

From Andreoli TE et al: *Andreoli and Carpenter's Cecil essentials of medicine,* ed 8, Philadelphia, 2010, Saunders.

BOX 2 Centor Criteria for Determining Group A Beta-Hemolytic Streptococcal Pharyngitis

- Tonsillar exudates
- Tender anterior lymphadenopathy or lymphadenitis
- Absence of cough
- History of fever

From Marx JA et al: *Rosen's emergency medicine*, ed 8, Philadelphia, 2014, Elsevier.

WORKUP

The Centor criteria (Box 2 and Table 1) identifies patients at risk for GAS and consists of (1) fever subjective or measured >38° C [100.5° F], (2) absence of cough, (3) tonsillar exudates, and (4) tender anterior cervical lymphadenopathy. Patients with ≤1 criteria are at low risk and do not need additional testing. Patients with 3 or more criteria warrant testing. The McIsaac criteria adds one point for ages 3 to 14 and subtracts one point for ages ≥45 yr.

- Rapid antigen detection test (RADT) (culture should be performed if RADT negative)
- Gold Standard: Throat swab for culture

LABORATORY TESTS

- Testing for bacteria other than GAS is performed infrequently.
- Reserved for patients with persistent signs or symptoms suggestive of a specific non–GAS bacteria.
- For example, gonococcal testing in a sexually active patient. In a patient with suspected EBV, a complete blood count may show atypical lymphocytes or a mononucleosis slide agglutination test (monospot) may confirm clinical diagnosis of EBV. When indicated based on population prevalence and supply availability, a nasal swab for a general respiratory viral panel or specifically SARS-CoV-2 will help indicate a viral etiology.

IMAGING STUDIES

- Seldom indicated.
- Imaging is not necessary to make the diagnosis of a peritonsillar abscess.
- If there is concern for parapharyngeal or retropharyngeal space infection, CT or MRI are preferred over plain radiographs.

Rx TREATMENT

NONPHARMACOLOGIC THERAPY

- Rest
- Soft diet

TABLE 1 Centor Criteria Scoring for Determining Testing and Treatment for Group A Beta-Hemolytic Streptococcal Pharyngitis

Centor Score	Testing and Treatment
0-1	None
2-3	Treatment based on results of rapid streptococcal test results
4	Treat without testing

- Hydration
- Warm saltwater gargles
- Warm beverages with honey or lemon (avoid honey in children <12 mo of age due to risk of infantile botulism)
- Cold beverages/ice chips
- Anesthetic spray/lozenges

ACUTE GENERAL Rx

- Analgesics: Acetaminophen (adults and children) or ibuprofen (adults and children >6 mo of age). Systemic glucocorticoids are not recommended in uncomplicated pharyngitis/tonsillitis because of increased risk of adverse events; analgesics are effective for pain.
- The primary benefit and intent of antibiotic treatment in GAS pharyngitis is the prevention of acute rheumatic fever.
- If streptococcal infection is proven or suspected:
  1. Amoxicillin 500 mg BID or penicillin V 500 mg PO BID for 10 days or benzathine penicillin 1.2 million U IM once (adults and children >27 kg). Children ages 3 to 18 yr: Amoxicillin 50 mg/kg daily or 25 mg/kg BID for 10 days (maximum dose 1000 mg daily). Benzathine penicillin 600,000 U IM in children <27 kg
  2. If avoiding penicillin, cephalexin 500 mg orally twice daily for 10 days in adults
- If uncomplicated gonococcal pharyngitis infection:
  1. Children >45 kg, adolescents, and adults: IM ceftriaxone 250 mg once in addition to azithromycin
  2. Infants and children ≤45 kg: IM/IV 25 to 50 mg/kg/dose, maximum dose 125 mg/dose
- Treatment of peritonsillar abscess is drainage through needle or incision.

CHRONIC Rx

- Recurrent streptococcal infections are common and may represent chronic carrier status, reinfection prior to antibody development, new infection to a different GAS M subtype, poor compliance to antibiotic, or rarely, an immune disorder.
- Recurrence in children is defined as 7 or more infections in 1 yr, 5 or more infections in 2 yr, or 3 or more infections in 3 yr.
- Chronic carrier: Oral treatment options include clindamycin, amoxicillin-clavulanate, and penicillin plus rifampin.
- In adults, tonsillectomy is rarely indicated for patients with recurrent GAS.
- In children, tonsillectomy may lower the incidence for recurrent pharyngitis.
- In both children and adults, each individual case is reviewed based on patient age, frequency or severity of infections, history of antibiotic use, and patient preferences.

DISPOSITION

- Tonsillopharyngitis is generally managed in an outpatient setting with follow-up arranged in 1 to 2 wk.
- Admission to the hospital is indicated for local suppurative complications (peritonsillar abscess; lateral pharyngeal, posterior or retropharyngeal abscess; concern for impending airway closure or respiratory distress; or inability to swallow food, medications, or water).

REFERRAL

- To otolaryngologist:
  1. If peritonsillar or other abscess is suspected
  2. If tonsillar hypertrophy persists

PREVENTION

- Hand hygiene.
- Antimicrobial prophylaxis is only recommended in patients with a history of acute rheumatic fever and is based on the risk of recurrence and severity of disease.

SUGGESTED READINGS

Available at ExpertConsult.com

RELATED CONTENT

Sore Throat (Patient Information)
Strep Throat (Patient Information)
Tonsillitis (Patient Information)

AUTHORS: **Shivali Choxi, MD,** and **Carol Duh-Leong, MD**

BASIC INFORMATION

DEFINITION

Pheochromocytomas are catecholamine-producing tumors that originate from the chromaffin cells of the adrenergic system. While they generally secrete both norepinephrine and epinephrine, norepinephrine is usually the predominant amine.

SYNONYM

Paraganglioma

ICD-10CM CODES

C74.9 Malignant neoplasm of adrenal gland, unspecified
C75.9 Malignant neoplasm of endocrine gland, unspecified
E27.5 Adrenomedullary hyperfunction

EPIDEMIOLOGY & DEMOGRAPHICS

- Incidence: 0.05% of population; peak incidence in 30s and 40s.
- Approximately 25% of patients with apparently sporadic pheochromocytoma may be carriers of mutations.
- Approximately 25% of pheochromocytomas are familial and associated with genetic disorders (Table 1). Pheochromocytoma is a feature of two disorders with an autosomal-dominant pattern of inheritance:
  1. Multiple endocrine neoplasia (MEN) type 2
  2. von Hippel-Lindau disease: Angioma of the retina, hemangioblastoma of the central nervous system, renal cell carcinoma, pancreatic cysts, and epididymal cystoadenoma
- Pheochromocytomas occur in 5% of patients with neurofibromatosis type 1.

PHYSICAL FINDINGS & CLINICAL PRESENTATION

- Hypertension: Can be sustained (55%) or paroxysmal (45%).
- Headache (80%): Usually paroxysmal in nature and described as "pounding" and severe.
- Palpitations (70%): Can be present with or without tachycardia.
- Hyperhidrosis (60%): Most evident during paroxysmal attacks of hypertension.
- Physical examination may be entirely normal if done in a symptom-free interval; during a paroxysm the patient may demonstrate marked increase in both systolic and diastolic pressure, profuse sweating, visual disturbances (caused by hypertensive retinopathy), dilated pupils (from catecholamine excess), paresthesias in the lower extremities (caused by severe vasoconstriction), tremor, and tachycardia.
- Orthostatic hypotension is common among patients with pheochromocytoma due to reduction of blood volume and desensitization of adrenergic receptors by the chronic excess of catecholamines.
- Box E1 summarizes features suggestive of pheochromocytoma.

ETIOLOGY

- Catecholamine-producing tumors that are usually located in the adrenal medulla.
- Specific mutations of the RET protooncogene cause familial predisposition to pheochromocytoma in MEN-2.
- Mutations in the von Hippel-Lindau tumor suppressor gene (VHL gene) cause familial disposition to pheochromocytoma in von Hippel-Lindau disease.
- Recently identified genes for succinate dehydrogenase subunit D (SDHD) and succinate dehydrogenase subunit B (SDHB) predispose carriers to pheochromocytoma and globus tumors.

DIAGNOSIS

DIFFERENTIAL DIAGNOSIS

- Anxiety disorder
- Thyrotoxicosis
- Amphetamine or cocaine abuse
- Carcinoid
- Essential hypertension
- The differential diagnosis of pheochromocytoma-type spells is summarized in Box 2

WORKUP

Laboratory evaluation and imaging studies to locate the neoplasm (Fig. 1). Anatomic and functional imaging studies that can be used to localize pheochromocytomas are summarized in Table E2. Misdiagnosis of pheochromocytoma is common. Correct interpretation of biochemical tests and imaging is crucial to a correct diagnosis.

LABORATORY TESTS

- Although there is no consensus on the best test, plasma-free metanephrines have been suggested as the test of first choice for excluding the tumor. Elevated plasma concentrations of normetanephrine or metanephrine have a sensitivity of up to 100%, but the specificity is markedly lower (85%).
- 24-hr urine collection will also show increased metanephrines (90% sensitivity, 95% specificity); the accuracy of the 24-hr urinary levels for metanephrines can be improved by indexing urinary metanephrine levels by urine creatinine levels.
- Medications that may increase measured levels of fractionated catecholamines and metanephrines are summarized in Box 3.

TABLE 1 Autosomal Dominant Syndromes Associated with Pheochromocytoma and Paraganglioma

Syndrome	Gene	Gene Locus	Protein Product	Protein Function	Gene Mechanism	Typical Tumor Location
SDHD (familial paraganglioma type 1)*	SDHD	11q23	SDH D subunit	ATP production	Tumor suppressor	Skull base and neck; occasionally adrenal medulla, mediastinum, abdomen, pelvis
Familial paraganglioma type 2*	SDHAF2	11q13.1	Flavination cofactor	ATP production	Tumor suppressor	Skull base and neck; occasionally abdomen and pelvis
SDHC (familial paraganglioma type 3)	SDHC	1q21	SDH C subunit	ATP production	Tumor suppressor	Skull base and neck
SDHB (familial paraganglioma type 4)	SDHB	1p36.1-35	SDH B subunit	ATP production	Tumor suppressor	Abdomen, pelvis and mediastinum; rarely adrenal medulla, skull base, and neck
MEN-1	MEN-1	11q13	Menin	Transcription regulation	Tumor suppressor	Adrenal medulla
MEN-2A and MEN-2B	RET	10q11.2	RET	Tyrosine kinase receptor	Protooncogene	Adrenal medulla, bilaterally
Neurofibromatosis type 1	NF1	17q11.2	Neurofibromin	GTP hydrolysis	Tumor suppressor	Adrenal-periadrenal
von Hippel-Lindau disease	VHL	3p25-26	VHL	Transcription elongation suppression	Tumor suppressor	Adrenal medulla, bilaterally; occasionally paraganglioma
Familial pheochromocytoma	FP/TMEM127	2q11	Transmembrane protein	Regulation of the mTORC1 signaling complex	Tumor suppressor	Adrenal medulla

*Associated with maternal imprinting.
ATP, Adenosine triphosphate; *GTP,* guanosine triphosphate; *MEN,* multiple endocrine neoplasia; *mTORC1,* mammalian target of rapamycin complex 1; *RET,* "rearranged during transfection" proto-oncogene; *SDH,* succinate dehydrogenase; *VHL,* von Hippel-Lindau disease.
From Melmed S: *Williams textbook of endocrinology,* ed 12, Philadelphia, 2011, Saunders, Elsevier.

BOX 2 Differential Diagnosis of Pheochromocytoma-Type Spells

Endocrine Causes
- Carbohydrate intolerance
- Hyperadrenergic spells
- Hypoglycemia
- Pancreatic tumors (e.g., insulinoma)
- Pheochromocytoma
- Primary hypogonadism (menopausal syndrome)
- Thyrotoxicosis

Cardiovascular Causes
- Angina
- Cardiovascular deconditioning
- Labile essential hypertension
- Orthostatic hypotension
- Paroxysmal cardiac arrhythmia
- Pulmonary edema
- Renovascular disease
- Syncope (e.g., vasovagal reaction)

Psychologic Causes
- Factitious (e.g., drugs, Valsalva maneuver)
- Hyperventilation
- Severe anxiety and panic disorders
- Somatization disorder

Pharmacologic Causes
- Chlorpropamide-alcohol flush
- Combination of a monoamine oxidase inhibitor and a decongestant
- Illegal drug ingestion (cocaine, phencyclidine, lysergic acid diethylamide)
- Sympathomimetic drug ingestion
- Vancomycin (red man syndrome)
- Withdrawal of adrenergic-inhibitor

Neurologic Causes
- Autonomic neuropathy
- Cerebrovascular insufficiency
- Diencephalic epilepsy (autonomic seizures)
- Migraine headache
- Postural orthostatic tachycardia syndrome
- Stroke

Other Causes
- Carcinoid syndrome
- Mast cell disease
- Recurrent idiopathic anaphylaxis
- Unexplained flushing spells

From Melmed S et al: *Williams textbook of endocrinology*, ed 14, 2020, Elsevier.

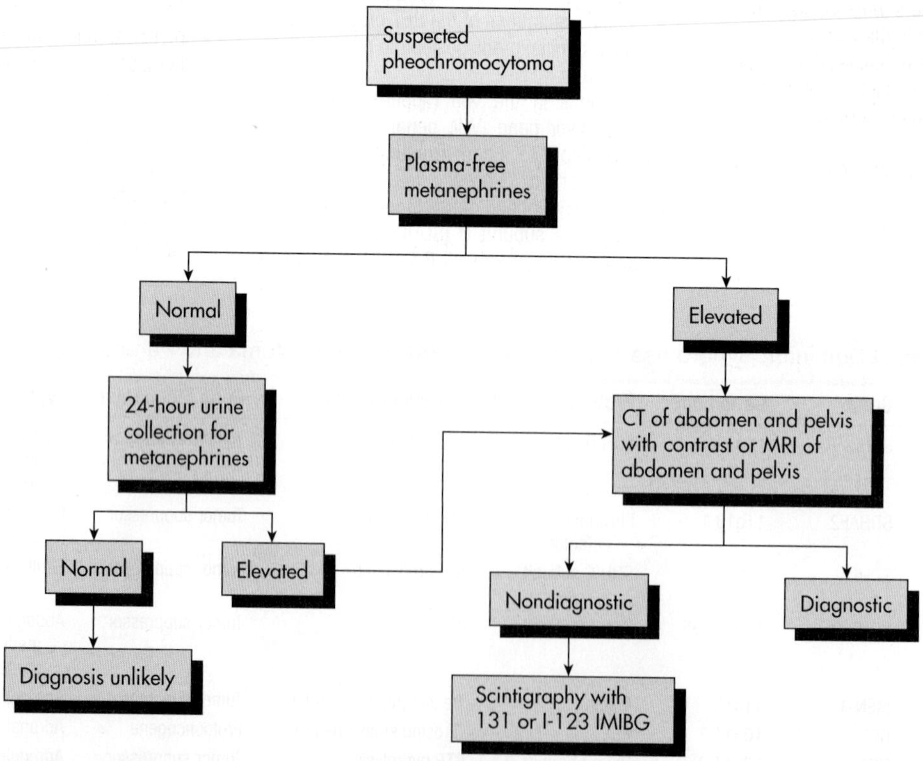

FIG. 1 Pheochromocytoma. *CT,* Computed tomography; *IMIBG,* iodine metaiodobenzylguanidine; *MRI,* magnetic resonance imaging.

BOX 3 Medications That May Increase Measured Levels of Fractionated Catecholamines and Metanephrines

Tricyclic antidepressants (including cyclobenzaprine)
Levodopa
Drugs containing adrenergic receptor agonists (e.g., decongestants)
Amphetamines
Buspirone and antipsychotic agents
Prochlorperazine
Reserpine
Withdrawal from clonidine and other drugs (e.g., illicit drugs)
Illicit drugs (e.g., cocaine, heroin)
Ethanol

From Melmed S et al: *Williams textbook of endocrinology,* ed 14, 2020, Elsevier.

IMAGING STUDIES

- Abdominal CT scan (Fig. E2) with and without contrast (88% sensitivity) is useful in locating pheochromocytomas >0.5 inch in diameter (90% to 95% accurate).
- MRI with contrast: Pheochromocytomas demonstrate a distinctive MRI appearance (up to 100% sensitivity); MRI may become the diagnostic imaging modality of choice.
- Scintigraphy with 131 or 1-123 I-MIBG (up to 100% sensitivity) (see Fig. E2): This norepinephrine analog localizes in adrenergic tissue; it is particularly useful in locating extraadrenal pheochromocytomas.
- 6-[18F]Fluorodopamine positron emission tomography is reserved for cases in which clinical symptoms and signs suggest pheochromocytoma, and results of biochemical tests are positive but conventional imaging studies cannot locate the tumor. It is also used for identification of metastatic disease.

TREATMENT

GENERAL Rx

Laparoscopic adrenalectomy (surgical resection for both benign and malignant disease):

- Preoperative stabilization with combination of alpha-adrenergic blocking agents (phenoxybenzamine, prazosin, doxazosin, or terazosin), beta-blocker, and liberal fluid and salt intake starting 10 to 14 days before surgery. Beta-blockers should be avoided until patients receive adequate alpha-adrenergic blockade for several days to avoid hypertensive crisis due to unopposed alpha stimulation. Amlodipine or verapamil can be added to beta-blockers if blood pressure control is still inadequate. Table E3 describes orally administered drugs to treat pheochromocytoma.
- Hypertensive crisis preoperatively and intraoperatively can be controlled with nitroprusside. Table E4 summarizes intravenously administered drugs used to treat pheochromocytoma.

PEARLS & CONSIDERATIONS

COMMENTS

- Obtaining a detailed family history is important because 25% of pheochromocytomas are familial.
- Screening for pheochromocytoma should be considered in patients with any of the following:
  1. Malignant hypertension
  2. Poor response to antihypertensive therapy
  3. Paradoxical hypertensive response
  4. Hypertension during induction of anesthesia, parturition, surgery, or thyrotropin-releasing hormone testing
  5. Hypertension associated with imipramine or desipramine
  6. Neurofibromatosis (increased incidence of pheochromocytoma)
- All patients with pheochromocytoma should be screened for MEN-2 and von Hippel-Lindau disease with the pentagastrin test, serum parathyroid hormone, ophthalmoscopy, MRI of the brain, CT scan of the kidneys and pancreas, and ultrasonography of the testes.
- In patients with pheochromocytoma, routine analysis for mutations of RET, VHL, SDHD, and SDHB is indicated to identify pheochromocytoma-associated syndromes.

SUGGESTED READINGS

Available at ExpertConsult.com

RELATED CONTENT

Pheochromocytoma (Patient Information)
Hypertension (Related Key Topic)

AUTHORS: **Brett Patrick, MD, Mark F. Brady, MD, MPH, MMSc,** and **Fred F. Ferri, MD**

BASIC INFORMATION

DEFINITION

Enterobius vermicularis is a small (6 to 13 mm) helminth of the nematode (roundworm) family that can cause noninvasive infestation of the large intestine. Females have a notably long and pointed tail that is similar in appearance to a pin; therefore, *E. vermicularis* is also referred to as pinworms. Other species such as *Enterobius gregorii* and *Syphacia obvelata* have been described to cause pinworms, although *E. vermicularis* is the most frequent culprit.

SYNONYMS

Enterobiasis
Oxyuriasis
Threadworms

ICD-10CM CODE
B80 Enterobiasis

EPIDEMIOLOGY & DEMOGRAPHICS

- *E. vermicularis* is the most prevalent helminth infection in the United States, with an estimated prevalence of 20 to 40 million infected individuals.
- There are approximately 30,000 cases diagnosed annually in the United States alone.
- *E. vermicularis* is found worldwide, although most common in temperate climates.
- Preschool and early grade school age children are at the highest risk of infection given close proximity to one another and poor hand hygiene.
- Pinworms are easily spread in day cares, institutions, within homes, and in the community of men who have sex with men.

PHYSICAL FINDINGS & CLINCIAL PRESENTATION

- Many individuals (30% to 50%) with pinworms are asymptomatic.
- The most common symptom is perianal pruritus, which can lead to excoriation and secondary infection.
- Symptomatic individuals may endure insomnia, enuresis, teeth-grinding, and irritability. Anorexia secondary to pinworms has been described.
- In addition to the gastrointestinal tract, pinworms can also cause vaginal infestations.
- Immunocompromised individuals are at risk for pinworm-associated appendicitis and eosinophilic enteritis.

ETIOLOGY & PATHOGENESIS

- Humans are the definitive host for *E. vermicularis,* which has a fecal-oral transmission pattern. The pinworm species that infect human and animals are different from each other and do not spread between species.
- Upon ingestion of embryonated eggs, larvae hatch in the small intestine and then migrate to the large intestine after they have matured (this occurs over 1 to 2 mo). Gravid females tend to occupy the more distal aspects of the large intestine; each gravid female migrates to the perianal region at night to release approximately 10,000 eggs.
- The larvae within the eggs mature and become infectious within 4 to 6 h of deposition and remain infectious for 2 to 3 wk. Embryonated eggs are pruritic, and when the host scratches the perianal region, the eggs are deposited under the fingernails and lead to infection via contamination of food. Autoinfection is common.
- Retroinfection, when newly hatched larvae migrate from the perianal region into the rectum, can occur but is not believed to be common.
- Because of their small size, pinworm eggs can become airborne and subsequently ingested.
- *E. vermicularis* may be transmitted between sexual partners, especially those engaging in oral-anal sex.

DIAGNOSIS

DIFFERENTIAL DIAGNOSIS

- Perianal itching related to poor hygiene. Section II describes the causes of pruritus ani, which includes infectious and inflammatory pathologies
- Hemorrhoidal disease and anal fissures
- Perineal yeast/fungal infections

WORKUP

E. vermicularis ova are elongated with one flattened side and surrounded by a thick, smooth, and colorless shell (Fig. 1). The eggs can be identified when transparent tape (Fig. 2) is placed on the perianal skin. The test is most effective upon awakening. This is known as the cellophane (Scotch) tape test. (NOTE: Five consecutive negative tests rule out the diagnosis.) A single examination detects 50% of infections, three examinations detect 90%, and five examinations detect 99%. Pinworm paddles are clear plastic paddles that have been developed and can used in place of transparent tape. It is important to keep in mind that the ova will not be present in the stool because the eggs are not passed in stool. On rare occasions, adult *E. vermicularis* can be identified in the stool and confirm the diagnosis. No serologic testing for *E. vermicularis* is available.

TREATMENT

- Treatment for *E. vermicularis* should be repeated 2 wk after first treatment. It can be difficult to eradicate the infestation due to reinfection and autoinfection. Additionally, retreatment at 2 wk targets newly hatched pinworms before they can lay eggs.
- Treatment options include mebendazole (100 mg), albendazole (400 mg), or pyrantel pamoate (11 mg/kg up to 1 gram). Mebendazole and albendazole require a prescription and pyrantel pamoate is available over the counter.
- Other infected family members and close contacts should be treated at the same time as the initial case.

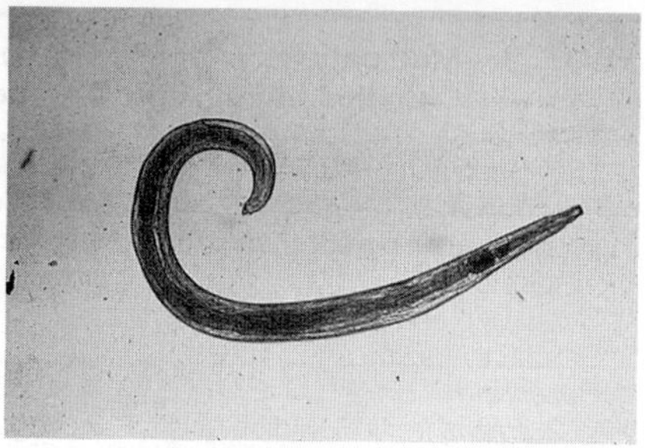

FIG. 1 Adult male pinworm, *Enterobius vermicularis,* with curved posterior end; note prominent esophageal bulb (4x). (From McPherson RA, Pincus MR: *Henry's clinical diagnosis and management by laboratory methods,* ed 23, Philadelphia, 2017, Elsevier.)

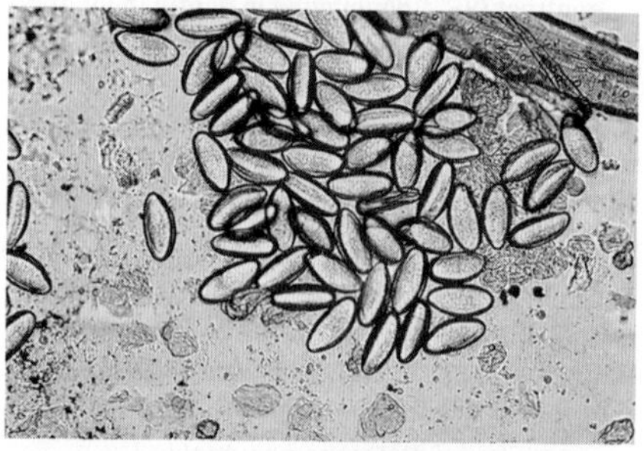

FIG. 2 Numerous eggs of *Enterobius vermicularis* as seen on a cellophane tape preparation (400x). (From McPherson RA, Pincus MR: *Henry's clinical diagnosis and management by laboratory methods,* ed 23, Philadelphia, 2017, Elsevier.)

PEARLS & CONSIDERATIONS

- Eosinophilia is not observed in most cases because *E. vermicularis* is noninvasive.
- Good hand hygiene is the most effective method of prevention.
- Control of *E. vermicularis* infection requires treatment of contacts and family members and decontamination of the environment by frequent changing of underclothes, bed clothes, and bedsheets to reduce risk of autoinfection.
- Personal hygiene and cleanliness are crucial. Fingernails should be cut short and scrubbed frequently as pinworm eggs can reside beneath the nails.

RELATED CONTENT

Pinworms (Patient Information)

AUTHORS: **Ajibike Lapite, MD, MPTM,** and **Jeremy Michel, MD, MHS**

BASIC INFORMATION

DEFINITION

Pituitary adenoma is a benign neoplasm of the anterior lobe of the pituitary that causes symptoms, either by excess secretion of hormones or by a local mass effect as the tumor impinges on other, nearby structures (e.g., optic chiasm, hypothalamus, pituitary stalk). Pituitary adenomas are classified by their size, function, and features that characterize their appearance. Microadenomas are <10 mm in size, macroadenomas are ≥10 mm in size, and giant adenomas are ≥40 mm in size.

- *Nonsecretory pituitary adenomas* are those in which the neoplasm is a space-occupying lesion whose secretory products do not cause a specific disease state.
- *Secretory pituitary adenomas* can cause endocrine manifestations related to what they are secreting.

Endocrine manifestations of secretory adenomas include:

- *Acromegaly,* a disease state characterized by a pituitary adenoma that secretes growth hormone (GH)
- Galactorrhea, which is the result of a *prolactinoma* that secretes prolactin (PRL)
- *Cushing disease,* a disease state of hypersecretion of adrenocorticotropic hormone (ACTH)
- *Hyperthyroidism* due to a thyrotropin-secreting pituitary adenomas, which secrete primarily thyroid-stimulating hormone (TSH)

ICD-10CM CODE
D35.2 Benign neoplasm of pituitary gland

EPIDEMIOLOGY & DEMOGRAPHICS

CLASSIFICATION (BY HORMONE SECRETED):

- PRL only: 35%
- No hormone: 30%
- GH only: 20%
- PRL and GH: 7%
- ACTH: 7%
- Luteinizing hormone (LH), follicle-stimulating hormone (FSH), TSH: 1%

INCIDENCE & PREVALENCE:

- Pituitary adenomas: Up to 15% of all intracranial neoplasms; 3% to 27% at autopsy series. The prevalence of pituitary adenomas has increased to 100 cases per 100,000 over the past decades, probably as a result of enhanced awareness and improved diagnostic imaging and hormone assays.[1] True prevalence is likely underestimated due to nonfunctioning pituitary adenomas going undiagnosed until they are large
- Prolactinomas: Up to 20% in women with unexplained primary or secondary amenorrhea
- GH-secreting pituitary adenoma: 50 to 60 cases per 1 million persons. They account for 8% to 16% of pituitary tumors and are most common in men over age 50
- Thyrotropin-secreting pituitary adenoma: 1% of pituitary adenomas with a slight female/male predominance of 1.7:1
- Corticotropin-secreting pituitary adenomas: Female/male predominance of 8:1 but overall uncommon diagnosis, accounting for 2% to 6% of adenomas

PHYSICAL FINDINGS & CLINICAL PRESENTATION

All sellar masses can cause visual defects by compression of the optic chiasm (bitemporal hemianopsia) or headaches.

PROLACTINOMAS:

- Females:
  1. Galactorrhea
  2. Amenorrhea
  3. Oligomenorrhea with anovulation
  4. Infertility
  5. Estrogen deficiency and associated osteopenia
  6. Decreased vaginal lubrication
- Males:
  1. Large tumors more common as a result of delayed diagnosis
  2. Possible impotence, decreased libido, or hypogonadism
  3. Galactorrhea rare because males lack the estrogen-dependent breast growth and differentiation

GH-SECRETING PITUITARY ADENOMA—ACROMEGALY:

- Coarse facial features
- Oily skin
- Prognathism
- Carpal tunnel syndrome
- Osteoarthritis
- History of increased hat, glove, or shoe size
- Decreased exercise capacity
- Visual field deficits
- Diabetes mellitus

CORTICOTROPIN-SECRETING PITUITARY ADENOMA—CUSHING DISEASE:

- Usually present when the tumor is small (1 to 2 mm)
- 50% of the tumors are <5 mm
- Other symptoms:
  1. Truncal obesity
  2. Round facies (moon face)
  3. Dorsocervical fat accumulation (buffalo hump)
  4. Hirsutism
  5. Acne
  6. Menstrual disorders
  7. Hypertension
  8. Striae
  9. Bruising
  10. Thin skin
  11. Hyperglycemia

THYROTROPIN-SECRETING PITUITARY ADENOMA:

- In males, larger, more invasive, and more rapidly growing tumors that present later in life
- Other symptoms: Thyrotoxicosis, goiter, visual impairment

NONSECRETORY PITUITARY ADENOMAS (ENDOCRINE INACTIVE PITUITARY ADENOMA):

- Usually large at the time of diagnosis
- Symptoms:
  1. Bitemporal hemianopsia as a result of compression of the optic chiasm
  2. Hypopituitarism from compression of the pituitary gland
  3. Hypogonadism in men and in premenopausal women
  4. Cranial nerve deficits caused by extension into the cavernous sinus
  5. Hydrocephalus from extension into the third ventricle, compressing the foramen of Monro
  6. Diabetes insipidus resulting from compression of the hypothalamus or pituitary stalk (a rare complication)

ETIOLOGY

Benign neoplasms of epithelial origin linked to genetic mutations of *MEN1, Gs-Alpha,* and *AIP*

Dx DIAGNOSIS

DIFFERENTIAL DIAGNOSIS

PROLACTINOMA:

- Pregnancy
- Postpartum puerperium
- Primary hypothyroidism
- Breast disease
- Breast stimulation
- Drug ingestion (especially phenothiazines, antidepressants, haloperidol, methyldopa, reserpine, opiates, amphetamines, and cimetidine)
- Chronic renal failure
- Liver disease
- Polycystic ovarian disease
- Chest wall disorders
- Spinal cord lesions
- Previous cranial irradiation

ACROMEGALY: Ectopic production of GH-releasing hormone from a carcinoid or other neuroendocrine tumor

CUSHING DISEASE:

- Diseases that cause ectopic sources of ACTH overproduction (including small-cell carcinoma of the lung, bronchial carcinoid, intestinal carcinoid, pancreatic islet cell tumor, medullary thyroid carcinoma, or pheochromocytoma)
- Adrenal adenomas, adrenal carcinoma
- Nelson syndrome

THYROTROPIN-SECRETING PITUITARY ADENOMAS: Primary hypothyroidism

NONSECRETORY PITUITARY ADENOMA: Nonneoplastic mass lesions of various etiologies (e.g., infectious, granulomatous)

WORKUP

- Pituitary adenomas should be identified at an early stage so that effective treatment can be implemented.
- Screening tests for functional pituitary adenomas are described in Table 1.

PROLACTINOMA: First step: Measurement of basal PRL levels (practitioners should be aware of discriminatory values in their own institutions).

[1]Melmed S: Pituitary-tumor endocrinopathies, *N Engl J Med* 382:937-950, 2020.

TABLE 1 Screening Tests for Functional Pituitary Adenomas

Disorder	Test	Comments
Acromegaly	IGF-1 OGTT with GH obtained at 0, 30, and 60 min	Interpret IGF-1 relative to age- and gender-matched controls. Normal subjects should suppress GH to <1 μg/L.
Prolactinoma	Serum PRL level	A level >500 μg/L is pathognomonic for macroprolactinoma. If >200 μg/L, prolactinoma is likely.*
Cushing disease	24-hr UFC nighttime salivary cortisol dexamethasone (1 mg) at 11 P.M. and fasting plasma cortisol measured at 8 A.M. ACTH assay	Ensure that urine collection is total and accurate by measuring urinary creatinine. Free salivary cortisol reflects circadian rhythm, and elevated levels may indicate Cushing disease. Normal subjects suppress to <1.8 μg/dl. Distinguishes adrenal adenoma from ectopic ACTH or Cushing disease.
TSH-secreting tumor	TSH measurement free T_4 by dialysis total T_3	If T_4 or T_3 is elevated and TSH is measurable or elevated, a TSH-secreting tumor may be present.

ACTH, Adrenocorticotropic hormone; *GH*, growth hormone; *IGF-1*, insulin-like growth factor type 1; *OGTT*, oral glucose tolerance test; *PRL*, prolactin; *T_3*, triiodothyronine; *T_4*, thyroxine; *TSH*, thyroid-stimulating hormone; *UFC*, urinary free cortisol.
*Risperidone may result in prolactin levels >200 μg/L.
From Melmed S et al: *Williams textbook of endocrinology*, ed 12, Philadelphia, 2011, Saunders.

- Elevated PRL levels are correlated with tumor size.
- Level >200 ng/ml indicates likely prolactinoma, with levels of 100 to 200 ng/ml being equivocal and possibly associated with medications or other sources.
- Basal PRL levels between 20 and 100 suggest a microadenoma but can be due to common medications (estrogen, antidepressants, metoclopramide, Aldomet, and others) or recent breast stimulation.
- Basal level <20 ng/ml is usually considered normal. Each laboratory should develop its own normative values, however, and practitioners should refer to these values.
- Threshold level for obtaining imaging such as MRI should be developed by individual providers depending on the level of specificity and sensitivity desired.

ACROMEGALY:

- First screening tests are the measurement of the serum insulin-like growth factor I level, postprandial serum GH, and thyrotropin-releasing hormone (TRH) stimulation test.
- Follow with an oral glucose tolerance test.
- Failure to suppress serum GH to <2 ng/ml with an oral load of 100 g glucose is considered conclusive.
- A GH-releasing hormone level >300 ng/ml is indicative of an ectopic source of GH.

CUSHING DISEASE:

- Measurement of late-night salivary cortisol level is the best screening test.
- Normal or slightly elevated corticotropin levels ranging from 20 to 200 pg/ml; normal is 10 to 50 pg/ml (normative data should be developed by each institution for its population).
- Level <10 pg/ml usually indicates an autonomously secreting adrenal tumor.
- Level >200 pg/ml suggests an ectopic corticotropin-secreting neoplasm.
- Cushing disease can be assessed by absence of cortisol suppression with the low-dose dexamethasone test but with the presence of cortisol suppression after the high-dose test. As a method to distinguish Cushing disease from an ectopic source of ACTH, this test is robust.
- 24-hr urine collection should demonstrate an increased level of cortisol excretion.

THYROTROPIN-SECRETING PITUITARY ADENOMA:

- Highly sensitive thyrotropin assays, which evaluate the presence of thyrotoxicosis, are one way to detect a thyrotropin-secreting tumor.
- Free alpha subunit is secreted by >80% of tumors, with the ratio of the alpha subunit to thyrotropin <1.
- With central resistance to thyroid hormone, ratio is <1, and the sella is normal.
- Laboratory tests show elevated serum levels of both T^3 and T^4.

NONSECRETORY PITUITARY ADENOMA:

- Visual field testing
- Assessment of the pituitary and organ function to determine if there is hypopituitarism or hypersecretion of hormones (even if the effects of hypersecretion are subclinical)
- TRH to provoke secretion of FSH, LH, and LH-beta-subunit; will not elicit response in normal persons
- Exclusion of Klinefelter syndrome in patient with longstanding primary hypogonadism, elevated gonadotropin levels, and enlargement of the sella

IMAGING STUDIES

Study of choice: MRI of the pituitary (Fig. E1) and hypothalamus. If an MRI shows the tumor impinging on the optic chiasm, then formal visual field testing is indicated.

- When evaluating Cushing disease, small size at the onset of symptoms noted.
- MRI, in this case, only 60% sensitive at best and may yield false-positive results.
- CT scan only when MRI is unavailable or is otherwise contraindicated.

TABLE 2 Transsphenoidal Pituitary Surgery

Primary Indications
General
Visual tract or central nervous system compression arising from within sella
Relief of compressive hypopituitarism by presenting, residual, or recurrent tumor tissue
Tumor recurrence after surgery or irradiation
Pituitary hemorrhage
Cerebrospinal fluid leak
Resistance to medical therapy
Intolerance of medical therapy
Personal choice
Desire for immediate pregnancy with macroadenoma
Requirement for diagnostic tissue histology
Specific
Acromegaly
Cushing disease
Clinically nonfunctioning macroadenoma
Prolactinoma
Nelson syndrome
TSH-secreting adenoma
Side Effects
Transient
Diabetes insipidus
Cerebrospinal fluid leak and rhinorrhea
Inappropriate ADH secretion
Arachnoiditis
Meningitis
Postoperative psychosis
Local hematoma
Arterial wall damage
Epistaxis
Local abscess
Pulmonary embolism
Narcolepsy
Permanent (up to 10%)
Diabetes insipidus
Total or partial hypopituitarism
Visual loss
Inappropriate ADH secretion
Vascular occlusion
CNS damage: Oculomotor palsy, hemiparesis, encephalopathy
Nasal septum perforation
Surgery-Related Mortality (up to 1%)
Brain, hypothalamic
Vascular damage
Postoperative meningitis
Cerebrospinal fluid leak
Pneumocephalus
Acute cardiopulmonary disease
Anesthesia-related
Seizure

ADH, Antidiuretic hormone; *CNS*, central nervous system; *TSH*, thyroid-stimulating hormone.
From Melmed S et al: *Williams textbook of endocrinology*, ed 12, Philadelphia, 2011, Saunders.

Rx TREATMENT

NONPHARMACOLOGIC THERAPY

SURGERY:

- Selective transsphenoidal resection of the adenoma (Table 2) is the treatment of choice for acromegaly, Cushing disease, and thyrotropin-secreting pituitary adenomas, all of

which tend to be microadenomas at the time of onset of symptoms.
- Macroadenomas, such as the nonsecretory pituitary adenoma, may also be surgically removed, but risk of recurrence is greater with these tumors and adjunctive therapy such as irradiation may also be necessary.
- Bilateral adrenalectomy has been performed in patients with Cushing disease after failure of other therapies; complications requiring lifelong hormone replacement or Nelson syndrome (rapid enlargement of pituitary tumor due to adrenal resection) may occur.

RADIOTHERAPY:
- Radiotherapy is used primarily as adjuvant treatment. It is reserved for patients who have not responded to surgical treatment and who still have symptoms of the adenoma.
- Used with varying degrees of success in all the different pituitary adenomas.
- Radiotherapy complications include long-term hypopituitarism (40% of patients) and secondary neoplasms (1.5% of patients).

ACUTE GENERAL Rx

PROLACTINOMA:
- For prolactinomas, initial therapy is generally dopamine agonists. Bromocriptine, a dopamine analogue, is generally given orally in divided doses of 1.5 to 10 mg. Cabergoline is given once or twice weekly. It is better tolerated and more effective than bromocriptine for tumor shrinkage but more expensive.
- Side effects include orthostatic hypotension, nausea, and dizziness; avoided by beginning with low-dose therapy.
- Other compounds include pergolide mesylate, a long-acting ergot derivative with dopaminergic properties, as well as other nonergot derivatives.

ACROMEGALY:
- Somatostatin analogues: Octreotide, lanreotide administered as monthly injections.
- Cabergoline or bromocriptine can also be used. They have modest activity but can be administered orally and are less expensive than somatostatin analogues.
- Pegvisomant can also be used to normalize IGF-1 levels.

CUSHING DISEASE:
- Ketoconazole, which inhibits the cytochrome P-450 enzymes involved in steroid biosynthesis, is effective in managing mild to moderate disease in daily oral doses of 600 to 1200 mg.
- Metyrapone and aminoglutethimide can be used to control hypersecretion of cortisol but are generally used when preparing a patient for surgery or while waiting for a response to radiotherapy.

THYROTROPIN-SECRETING PITUITARY ADENOMA:
- Ablative therapy with either radioactive iodide or surgery is indicated.
- Treatment directed to the thyroid alone may accelerate growth of the pituitary adenoma.
- Octreotide has been shown to be effective in doses similar to those used for acromegaly.
- Fig. E2 illustrates the management of thyrotrophic hormone–secreting pituitary tumors.

NONSECRETORY PITUITARY ADENOMA:
- There is no role for medical therapy at this time.
- Surgery and radiotherapy may be indicated. An algorithm for the management of nonfunctioning pituitary adenomas is described in Fig. 3.

CHRONIC Rx

For all pituitary adenomas:
- Careful follow-up is important. Patients undergoing transsphenoidal microsurgical resection should be seen in 4 to 6 wk to ensure that the adenoma has been completely removed and that the endocrine hypersecretion is resolved.
- If there is good clinical response, patient should be monitored yearly for recurrence and to follow the level of the hypersecreted hormone.
- Patients who have undergone irradiation should have close follow-up with backup medical therapy because response to radiotherapy may be delayed; incidence of hypopituitarism also increases with time.
- Surgical resection is not indicated in pituitary incidentalomas that are microadenomas since only 10% will experience tumor growth.
- Approximately 30% of surgically resected adenomas have persistent or progressive postoperative growth for several decades. Tumors particularly prone to invasive growth and recurrence include those arising from sparsely granulated somatotrophs, silent corticotrophs, corticotroph Crooke cells, and lactotrophs in middle-aged or older men.

SUGGESTED READINGS

Available at ExpertConsult.com

RELATED CONTENT

Pituitary Adenoma (Patient Information)
Acromegaly (Related Key Topic)
Amenorrhea (Related Key Topic)
Cushing Disease and Syndrome (Related Key Topic)
Galactorrhea (Related Key Topic)
Prolactinoma (Related Key Topic)

AUTHORS: **Ghamar Bitar, MD,** and **Anthony Sciscione, DO**

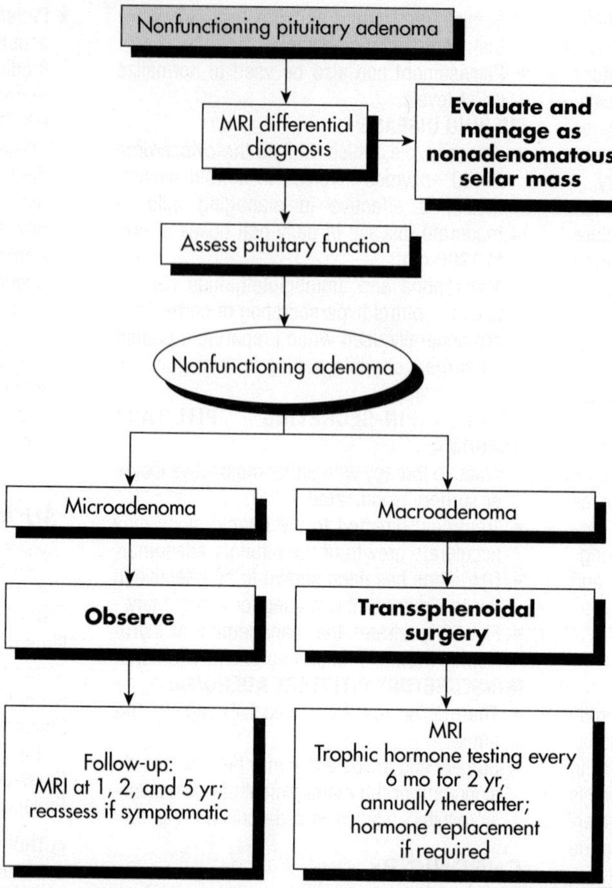

FIG. 3 Management of nonfunctioning pituitary adenomas. Skilled interpretation of magnetic resonance images is crucial to diagnosing a nonadenomatous mass such as a meningioma, aneurysm, or other sellar lesion. *MRI,* Magnetic resonance imaging. (From Melmed S et al: *Williams textbook of endocrinology*, ed 12, Philadelphia, 2011, Saunders.)

BASIC INFORMATION

DEFINITION

The diagnosis of placenta previa is based on sonography and requires the identification of echogenic homogeneous placental tissue over the internal cervical os. When the placental edge is <2 cm from the internal os, the placenta is called "low-lying." The historic terms "marginal" and "partial" for characterizing a placenta previa are no longer used. A classification of placenta previa in "major" or "minor" is described in Table 1 and illustrated in Fig. 1.

One hypothesis is that the lower uterine cavity contains more vascularized decidua, which promotes implantation of trophoblast toward the cervical os. Another hypothesis is that a particularly large placental surface area increases the probability that the placenta will implant over the cervical os.

ICD-10CM CODES

O44	Placenta previa
O44.0	Complete placenta previa NOS or without hemorrhage
O44.1	Complete placenta previa with hemorrhage
O44.2	Partial placenta previa without hemorrhage
O44.3	Partial placenta previa with hemorrhage
O44.4	Low-lying placenta NOS or without hemorrhage
O44.5	Low-lying placenta with hemorrhage

TABLE 1 Classification of Placenta Previa

Minor	I	Encroaches the lower uterine segment
	II	Reaches internal os of the cervix (marginal)
Major	III	Covers part of internal os (partial)
	IV	Completely covers the internal os (complete)

From Magowan BA. *Clinical obstetrics and gynecology*, ed 4, London, 2019, Elsevier.

EPIDEMIOLOGY & DEMOGRAPHICS

INCIDENCE: The pooled prevalence of major placenta previa was 4.3 cases per 1000 pregnancies. Prevalence was highest among Asian studies (12.2 per 1000) and lower among studies from Europe (3.6 per 1000), North America (2.9 per 1000), and sub-Saharan Africa (2.7 per 1000).

RISK FACTORS:

- Previous placenta previa (recurs in 4% to 8% of subsequent pregnancies)
- Previous cesarean delivery (increases incidence by 47% to 60%)
- Multiparity
- Multiple gestation (increases prevalence by 40%)
- Smoking and cocaine use
- Previous intrauterine surgical procedure or Asherman syndrome
- Abnormal or large placenta

PHYSICAL FINDINGS & CLINICAL PRESENTATION

The classic presentation of placenta previa is painless vaginal bleeding, usually in the second or third trimester. 10% to 20% of women present with uterine contractions, pain, and bleeding. On physical examination, the uterus is soft and pain free. The fetus is often in breech, transverse lie, or high. Fetal distress is usually not present.

Dx DIAGNOSIS

DIFFERENTIAL DIAGNOSIS

- Morbidly adherent placenta (accreta, increta, percreta)
- Vasa previa
- Abruptio placentae
- Vaginal or cervical trauma
- Labor
- Local malignancy

WORKUP

- Do *not* perform a digital vaginal examination.
- Perform a speculum examination in a hospital setting to exclude any local bleeding.
- Perform a transvaginal ultrasonography to assess for placental location.
- Exclude the presence of placenta previa-accreta in patients with a history of cesarean sections. In a prospective study, the frequency of placenta accreta increased with an increasing number of cesarean deliveries: 3% for first cesarean, 11% for second cesarean, 40% for third cesarean, 61% for fourth cesarean, and up to 67% for fifth or more cesarean sections.

LABORATORY TESTS

- A complete blood count can be used to monitor hemoglobin and hematocrit.
- A Kleihauer-Betke preparation of maternal blood in all Rh-negative women and Rh-immune globulin when indicated

IMAGING STUDIES

- The simplest and safest method of placental localization is transabdominal sonography with confirmatory imaging by transvaginal ultrasonography (TVUS). Transabdominal ultrasonography alone is inaccurate in the diagnosis of placenta previa and should be used only as a screening tool. TVUS (Fig. 2) has become the gold standard for the diagnosis of placenta previa. It is safe even in the presence of active bleeding.
- MRI has also been effective in detecting placenta previa, although sonography remains the preferred method due to lower cost, widespread availability, and well-established accuracy.

Rx TREATMENT

MANAGEMENT OF ASYMPTOMATIC PLACENTA PREVIA

- Avoid sexual activity, digital exams, and extraneous exercise.
- Review bleeding precautions and anticipatory guidance, including the need for cesarean section and the risk for hysterectomy early in pregnancy.

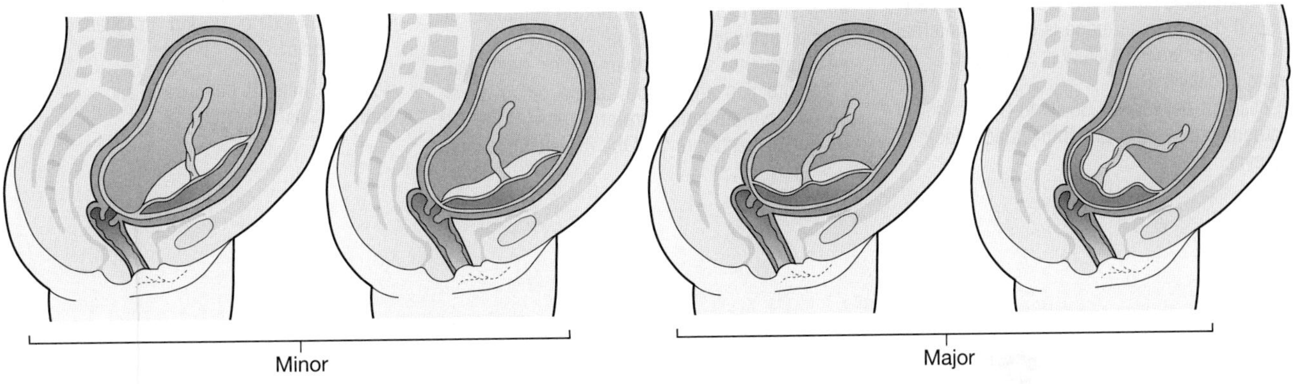

FIG. 1 Classification into "major" and "minor" placenta previa depends on the distance of the placenta from the internal os of the cervix. In the presence of a caesarean section scar, an anterior placenta previa may result in abnormal invasion (morbidly adherent placenta, placenta accreta). (From Magowan BA: *Clinical obstetrics and gynecology*, ed 4, London, 2019, Elsevier.)

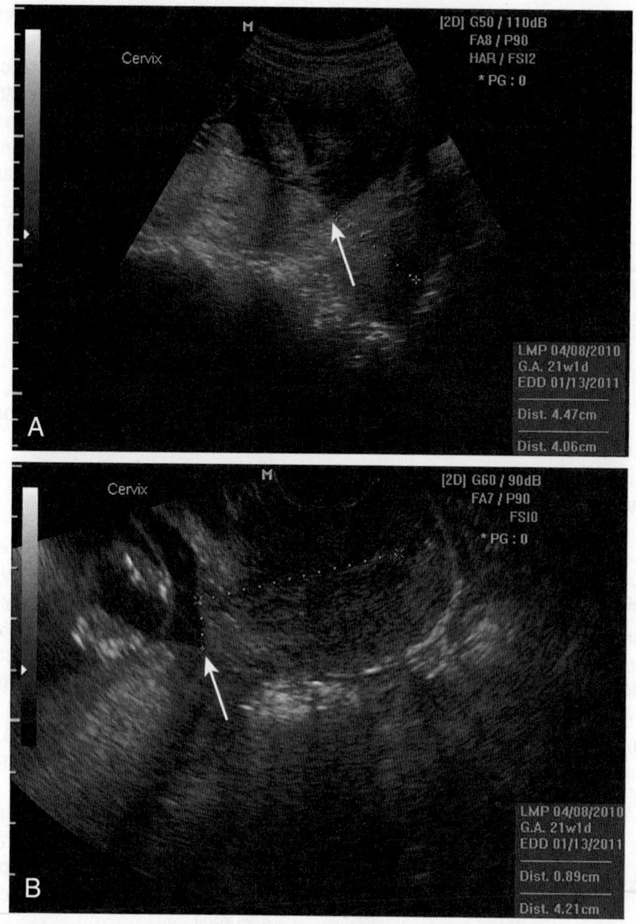

FIG. 2 Transabdominal ultrasonography and transvaginal ultrasonography of marginal placenta previa. *Arrows* identify placental edge. (Courtesy K. Francois. From Gabbe SG: *Obstetrics*, ed 6, Philadelphia, 2012, Saunders.)

Sequential assessment of placental location:

- At 32 wks, follow-up is indicated:
  1. If the placental edge is ≥2 cm from the internal os, placenta previa has resolved and no further assessment is required.
  2. If the placental edge is over or <2 cm from the internal os, placenta previa persists and repeat at 36 wks is indicated.
- At 36 wks:
  1. If the placental edge is ≥2 cm, the patient is consented for vaginal delivery.
  2. If the placental edge is over the internal os, cesarean delivery is scheduled.

Timing of delivery:

- Cesarean delivery at 36+0 to 37+6 wks in pregnancies with uncomplicated placenta previa

MANAGEMENT OF SYMPTOMATIC PLACENTA PREVIA

- Initial assessment for signs of maternal hemodynamic compromise or hemorrhagic shock; large-bore IV access with crystalloid fluid resuscitation.
- Assess fetal status and gestational age by sonogram and continuous fetal heart rate monitoring.
- Cross-matched blood should be made available during bleeding episodes.
- Tocolytic therapy should not be administered in an actively bleeding patients.
- Magnesium sulfate therapy for fetal neuroprotection should be considered in those with symptomatic preterm (less than 32 wks) placenta previa if the decision has been made to likely deliver the patient within 24 hr. Emergent delivery should not be delayed to administer magnesium.
- Cesarean delivery is indicated for active labor, nonreassuring fetal heart rate tracing, active bleeding with hemodynamic instability, and significant bleeding after 34 wks' gestation.

Expectant management after a resolved bleed:

- Antenatal corticosteroid should be administered to symptomatic women between 23+0 and 36+6 wks of gestation to enhance fetal pulmonary maturity.
- Correct anemia.
- Administer anti-D immune globulin to D-negative women.

DISPOSITION

Inpatient versus outpatient: Consider discharge for women whose bleeding has stopped for 24 hr and live in close proximity to the hospital, demonstrate compliance with medical management, can maintain bed rest, understand bleeding precautions, and have an adult companion available for transport 24 hr a day.

PEARLS & CONSIDERATIONS

COMMENTS

- Placenta previa is diagnosed by TVUS, with repeat assessment at 32 and 36 wks when indicated.
- Asymptomatic placenta previa can be managed expectantly with a planned cesarean delivery at 36+0 to 37+6 wks.
- Symptomatic placenta previa is managed by assessing hemodynamic stability, considering steroids for fetal lung maturity, magnesium sulfate for fetal neuroprotection when indicated, and cesarean delivery.

SUGGESTED READINGS

Available at ExpertConsult.com

RELATED CONTENT

Placenta Previa (Patient Information)
Vaginal Bleeding During Pregnancy (Related Key Topic)

AUTHORS: **Helen B. Gomez, MD,** and **Anthony Sciscione, DO**

BASIC INFORMATION

DEFINITION

A pleural effusion is the pathologic accumulation of fluid in the pleural space, stemming from a wide range of etiologies.

SYNONYMS

Exudates
Transudates
Hydrothorax
Hemothorax
Chylothorax
Empyema

ICD-10CM CODES

J90	Pleural effusion, not elsewhere classified
J91.8	Pleural effusion in other conditions classified elsewhere

PHYSICAL FINDINGS & CLINICAL PRESENTATION

- Subjective symptoms largely depend on the underlying etiology and may include dyspnea, cough, fatigue, fever, chest pain.
- Box 1 summarizes signs and symptoms of pleural effusion.
- Physical examination findings include dullness to percussion, decreased tactile fremitus, and decreased breath sounds.

ETIOLOGY

A pleural effusion may be caused by a number of factors, including increased capillary permeability, increased vascular hydrostatic pressure, decreased vascular oncotic pressure, inflammation of the pleurae, traumatic/iatrogenic causes, and/or obstruction of normal pleural fluid efflux. Box 2 summarizes causes of pleural effusion.

DIAGNOSIS

DIFFERENTIAL DIAGNOSIS

Differential diagnosis for causes of pleural effusion includes the following:

- ***Transudate***—effusions that stem from hydrostatic and oncotic imbalances (pleural to serum LDH (lactate dehydrogenase) ratio <0.6 or total protein ratio <0.5 or pleural to upper limit of normal for serum LDH ratio <2/3)
  1. Heart failure
  2. Cirrhosis (hepatic hydrothorax)
  3. Chronic renal insufficiency
  4. Hypoalbuminemia
  5. Pericardial disease
  6. Urinothorax
- ***Exudate***—effusions that stem from an infiltrative or inflammatory process (typically characterized by pleural to serum LDH ratio ≥0.6 or total protein ratio ≥0.5 or pleural to upper limit of normal for serum LDH ratio ≥$^2/_3$). Box 3 describes cellular differential of pleural effusions.
- Malignancy (secondary to metastatic cancer or primary; e.g., mesothelioma)
- Infection
  1. Parapneumonic effusion (simple = pH >7.2, complicated = ≤7.2)
  2. Empyema (pus in the pleural space, positive pleural fluid cultures or Gram stain from pleural fluid) [*see section on "Empyema"*]
  3. Tuberculous effusion
  4. Viral pleurisy
- Pulmonary embolism (rarely can present as transudate)
- Hemothorax
- Chylothorax
- Esophageal perforation
- Pleuropancreatic fistula
- Connective tissue disease

WORKUP

Thoracentesis can help to establish the etiology of a pleural effusion. Light criteria should be used for classification of the pleural effusion (summarized in Box 4.) Fig. 1 illustrates a diagnostic algorithm for pleural effusions. A thorough history and physical examination can avoid unnecessary instrumentation, as it is important to remember that not all pleural effusions need to be immediately sampled (e.g., clear history of heart failure). Fig. E2 illustrates an approach to malignant pleural effusions.

LABORATORY TESTS

See Table 1.

BOX 1 Signs and Symptoms of Effusion

Dyspnea
Cough (dry, nonproductive)
Chest pain (pleuritic or nonpleuritic)
Chest wall discomfort
Decreased breath sounds
Dullness to percussion
Egophony, decreased tactile fremitus
Pleural friction rub
Disease-specific signs and symptoms may include:
  Orthopnea
  Paroxysmal nocturnal dyspnea
  Fever
  Night sweats

From Adams JG et al: *Emergency medicine, clinical essentials*, ed 2, Philadelphia, 2013, Elsevier.

BOX 2 Causes of Pleural Effusions

Transudates
Atelectasis (early)
Congestive heart failure
Central venous occlusion
Glomerulonephritis
Hepatic hydrothorax
Hypoalbuminemia
Myxedema
Nephrotic syndrome
Peritoneal dialysis
Pulmonary embolism
Veno-occlusive disease

Exudates
Infectious
Bacterial infection
Fungal infection
Lung abscess
Parasitic infection
Traumatic hemothorax
Tuberculosis
Viral illness

Malignancies
Lymphoma
Mesothelioma
Primary lung cancer
Pulmonary metastasis

Connective Tissue Disease
Rheumatoid arthritis
Systemic lupus erythematosus

Abdominal/Gastrointestinal
Esophageal rupture
Pancreatic disorders
Subphrenic abscess

Other
Asbestos
Atelectasis (chronic)
Chylothorax
Drug reactions (amiodarone, nitrofurantoin)
Hemothorax
Meigs syndrome
Postpartum state
Postsurgical (abdominal, cardiac bypass)
Pulmonary infarction or embolism
Thoracic endometriosis
Uremia
Superior vena cava syndrome
Yellow nail syndrome

From Adams JG et al: *Emergency medicine, clinical essentials*, ed 2, Philadelphia, 2013, Elsevier.

BOX 3 Cellular Differential of Pleural Effusions

Neutrophilia (>50%)
- Bacterial pneumonia (parapneumonic effusion)
- Pulmonary infarction
- Pancreatitis
- Subphrenic abscess
- Early tuberculosis
- Transudates (>10%)

Lymphocytosis (>50%)
- Tuberculosis
- Viral infection
- Malignancy (lymphoma, other neoplasms)
- True chylothorax
- Rheumatoid pleuritis
- Systemic lupus erythematosus
- Uremic effusions
- Transudates (≈30%)

Eosinophilia (>10%)
- Pneumothorax (air in pleural space)
- Trauma
- Pulmonary infarction
- Congestive heart failure
- Infection (especially parasitic, fungal)
- Hypersensitivity syndromes
- Drug reaction
- Rheumatologic diseases
- Hodgkin disease
- Idiopathic

From McPherson RA, Pincus MR: *Henry's clinical diagnosis and management by laboratory methods*, ed 23, St. Louis, 2017, Elsevier.

IMAGING STUDIES

- ***Chest x-ray*** (Fig. 3): Blunting of the costophrenic angle, ipsilateral atelectasis, contralateral shift of the mediastinum with large effusions, elevated hemidiaphragm with subpulmonic effusions, "spine sign" on lateral chest x-ray, may be free-flowing or fixed on lateral decubitus film depending on etiology.
- ***Ultrasonography*** (Fig. E4): Bedside transthoracic ultrasound can be helpful to identify characteristics of pleural effusions, including:
  1. Size, location, and laterality
  2. Presence of loculations, pleural adhesions, or implants
  3. Procedure planning (e.g., thoracentesis, chest tube)
  4. Underlying lung parenchymal pathology (e.g., pulmonary edema, consolidation, pneumothorax)
- ***Computed tomography*** (Fig. E5): Useful to identify loculated effusions and to assess underlying lung parenchyma to aid in establishing a diagnosis. In empyema, can demonstrate heterogeneity and gas bubbles. (See chapter on "Empyema.")

BOX 4 Light Criteria for Classification of Pleural Effusions

In 1972, Light et al developed the currently accepted benchmark for classifying pleural fluid, as follows:
Pleural fluid protein to serum protein ratio >0.5:1
Pleural fluid lactate dehydrogenase (LDH) to serum LDH ratio >0.6:1
Pleural fluid LDH greater than two thirds the upper limit of normal for serum LDH (a cutoff value of 200 IU/L was used previously)

Pleural fluid is classified as an exudate if it meets any of the aforementioned criteria. Conversely, if all three characteristics are absent, the fluid is classified as a transudate. These researchers achieved a diagnostic sensitivity of 99% and a specificity of 98% for classification of an exudate.

From Adams JG et al: *Emergency medicine, clinical essentials*, ed 2, Philadelphia, 2013, Elsevier.

Rx TREATMENT

- Table 2 summarizes treatment options for pleural effusions.
- Fig. 6 describes a treatment approach to malignant pleural effusions.

REFERRAL

Negative diagnostic workup after initial pleural fluid sampling should be followed by referral to a pulmonologist for further evaluation (including consideration for thoracoscopy for pleural biopsy).

PEARLS & CONSIDERATIONS

- One-time drainage of a pleural effusion is seldom a definitive therapy. Early identification of the underlying etiology of new effusions should be pursued.
- Managing patients with malignant pleural effusion can be challenging. A recent trial showed that, among patients with malignant pleural effusion, outpatient administration of talc via an indwelling tunneled pleural

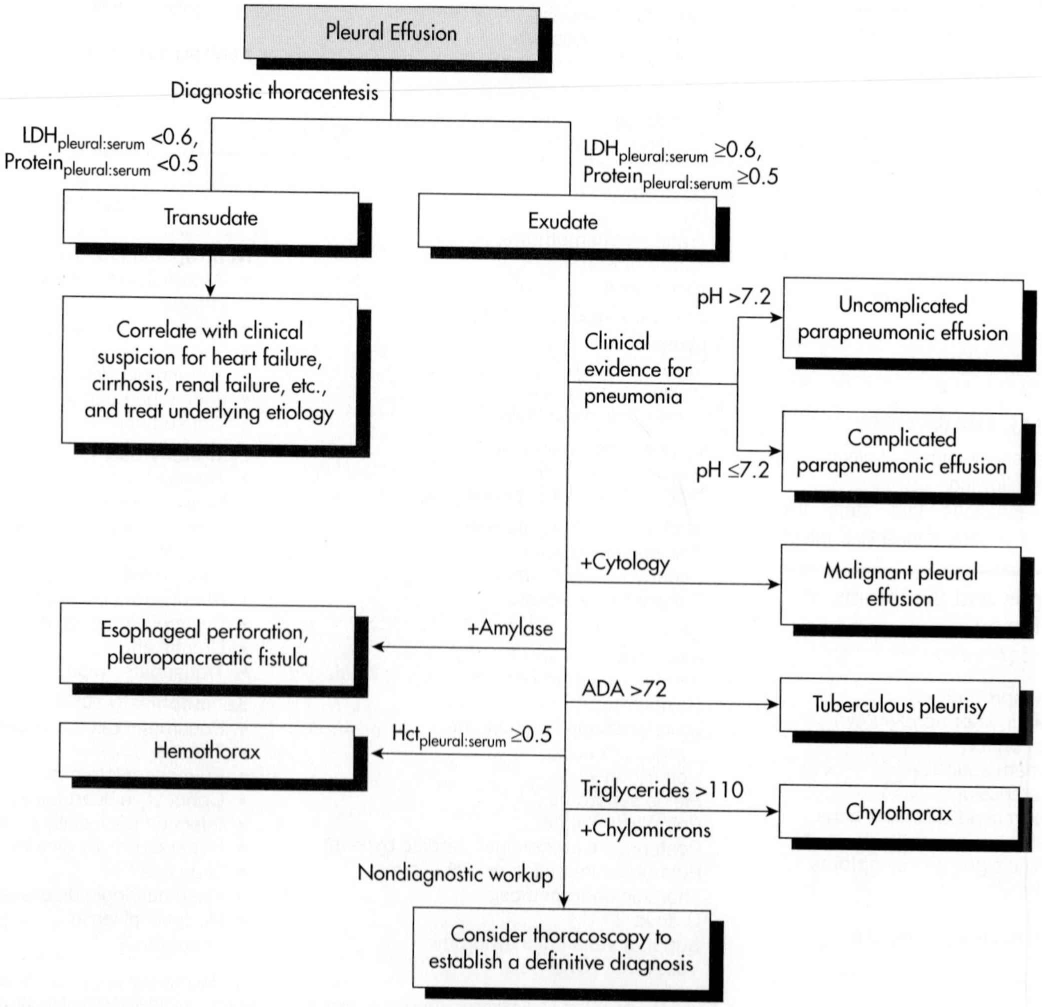

FIG. 1 Diagnostic algorithm. *ADA,* Adenosine deaminase; *Hct,* hematocrit; *LDH,* lactate dehydrogenase.

TABLE 1 Selected Laboratory Tests Used to Diagnose Pleural Effusion

Test	Diagnostic Utility	Comments
Adenosine deaminase (ADA)	<40 IU/L excludes tuberculous pleurisy	Values >72 IU/L highly specific for tuberculosis, with improved yield with pleural biopsy and PCR, can also be elevated in lymphoma and parapneumonic effusions
Albumin	Pleural: Serum albumin ratio <0.83 more consistent with transudate	Can be used to corroborate mixed findings from LDH and protein ratios
Amylase	Esophageal perforation, pancreatitis, malignancy	
Cell count	**Lymphocyte** predominance suggestive of tuberculosis, lymphoma, malignancy, pulmonary embolism **Neutrophil** predominant effusions seen with bacterial infection, occasionally with malignancy (20%) **Eosinophil** (>10%) predominance is suggestive of air or blood	Helpful in distinguishing causes of exudative effusions
Chylomicrons	Positive finding adds to specificity of triglycerides for establishing chylothorax	Consider thoracic duct defect (due to malignancy, trauma or iatrogenic)
Creatinine	Pleural: Serum creatinine >1 suggests urinothorax	
Culture	Positive findings used to narrow therapy	Should be sent from every suspected parapneumonic effusion to guide antimicrobial selection
Cytology	Sensitivity for malignancy of ~65%	Increment in diagnostic yield with up to three serial samples (~90%)
Glucose	<60 mg/dl suggests complicated parapneumonic effusion, malignancy, tuberculous pleurisy or rheumatoid effusion	
Hematocrit	Pleural fluid hematocrit >50% peripheral blood hematocrit consistent with hemothorax	Pleural fluid with relatively low hematocrit can appear bloody on gross exam, does not necessarily represent hemothorax
Lactate dehydrogenase (LDH)	Pleural to serum LDH ratio >0.6 or pleural LDH >2/3 the upper limit of normal serum LDH suggests exudate	
pH	≤7.2 with clinical suspicion highly suggestive of complicated parapneumonic effusion	Can also have low pH with malignant pleural effusions and esophageal perforation
Protein	Pleural to serum protein ratio ≥0.5 suggests exudate	Very low pleural protein (<0.5g/dl) suggests urinothorax or periteonal dialysis associated effusion
NT-proBNP	>1500 pg/ml suggests heart failure even if effusion meets criteria for exudate	Chronic pleural effusions related to heart failure in patients on diuretic therapy may appear exudative
Triglycerides	Triglycerides >110 mg/dl seen with chylothorax <50 mg/dl argues against the presence of a chylothorax	Absent triglycerides w/high suspicion for chylothorax can be confirmed with pleural chylomicrons

NT-proBNP, N-terminal pro b-type natriuretic peptide; *PCR,* polymerase chain reaction.

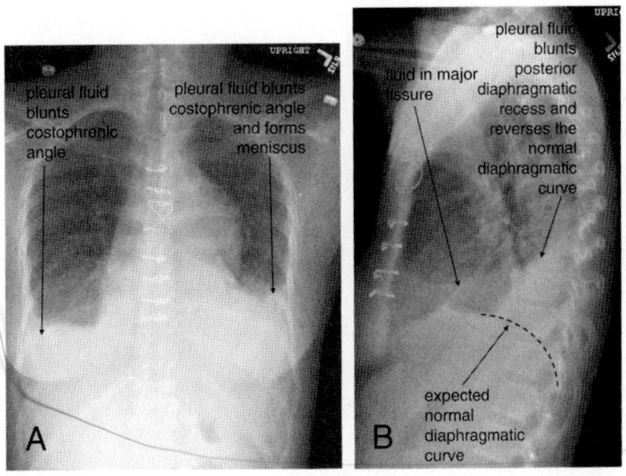

FIG. 3 Pleural effusions. A, Posterior-anterior upright view in which a pleural effusion is most evident on this patient's left side. Both costophrenic angles are blunted. The pleural effusion forms a meniscus against the left lateral chest wall. **B,** Lateral upright view shows two meniscus densities, suggesting bilateral pleural effusions. The posterior diaphragmatic recess is filled with pleural fluid, which forms a meniscus with the posterior chest wall. (From Broder JS: *Diagnostic imaging for the emergency physician*, Philadelphia, 2011, Saunders.)

TABLE 2 Treatment Options for Pleural Effusion

Thoracentesis	Site selection should be guided by ultrasonography whenever possible; evacuation of pleural fluid can be limited when the lung cannot fully re-expand, including central airway obstruction, chronic atelectasis, and the presence of extensive pleural adhesions; aspiration in these circumstances can lead to pneumothorax ex vacuo
Tube thoracostomy	Consider when ongoing drainage will be needed, especially for empyema or hemothorax
Indwelling tunneled pleural catheter	A cuffed pleural drainage catheter tunneled through subcutaneous tissue, drained regularly on an outpatient basis, most commonly used to manage malignant pleural effusions
Pleurodesis	Instillation of a chemical irritant under direct thoracoscopic visualization (e.g., talc poudrage) or via tube thoracostomy to adhere the visceral and parietal pleurae, can also be done with mechanical pleurodesis via video-assisted thoracic surgery (VATS)
Pharmacotherapy	Based on underlying etiology (e.g., diuretics, antimicrobials, chemotherapy)

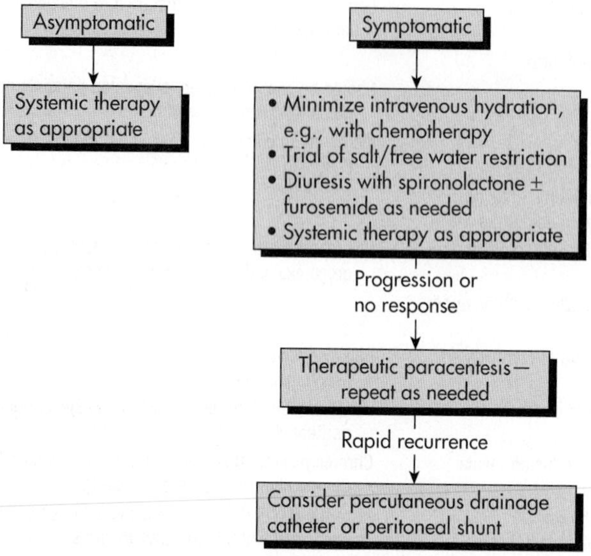

FIG. 6 Treatment approach algorithm to malignant pleural effusions. (From Niederhuber JE: *Abeloff's clinical oncology*, ed 6, Philadelphia, 2020, Elsevier.)

catheter resulted in a higher rate of pleurodesis and catheter removal than placement of a tunneled catheter alone.[1]

- In the few patients with malignant pleural effusion and slow accumulation of fluid near the end of life, repeated thoracentesis, as needed, is a reasonable strategy.
- Pleural biopsy should be considered when the underlying etiology is uncertain.

SUGGESTED READINGS

Available at ExpertConsult.com

RELATED CONTENT

Empyema (Related Key Topic)
Heart Failure (Related Key Topic)
Lung Neoplasms, Primary (Related Key Topic)

AUTHORS: **Yaron B. Gesthalter, MD,** and **Katherine Malcolm, MD, MPH**

[1] Bhatnagar R et al: Outpatient talc administration by indwelling pleural catheter for malignant effusion, *N Engl J Med* 378:1313-1322, 2018.

BASIC INFORMATION

DEFINITION

Pleurisy refers to a condition that leads to stimulation of pain receptors in the parietal pleura, resulting in pleuritic chest pain (pain that is worsened by respiration or movement). This pleuritic pain is usually caused by inflammation that may be caused by a number of different disorders. Thus, the key to management depends on determining the underlying etiology.

SYNONYMS

Pleuritis
Pleuritic chest pain

ICD-10CM CODE
R09.1 Pleurisy

EPIDEMIOLOGY & DEMOGRAPHICS

INCIDENCE: Incidence of pleurisy in undetermined as there are a variety of disorders that may result in pleurisy.

PHYSICAL FINDINGS & CLINICAL PRESENTATION

- Pleurisy is characterized by chest pain that worsens with respiration, coughing, or sneezing. This pleuritic chest pain is typically described as sharp or stabbing; however, it also may be described as dull pain, burning pain, or a "catch" while breathing. Movement of the trunk or chest wall may exacerbate pain, thus many patients with pleurisy will identify and remain in the position that minimizes discomfort.
- Depending on the underlying etiology, dyspnea may be present.
- Physical exam may disclose a pleural friction rub.
- Decreased breath sounds, rhonchi, or egophony may be appreciated if pneumonia is the underlying etiology of the patient's pleurisy.

ETIOLOGY

- Pathophysiology: Only the parietal pleura, not the visceral pleura, has nociceptors. Thus pleurisy results from inflammation of the parietal pleura. However, injury or inflammation at the periphery of the lung parenchyma may result in inflammation of the overlying parietal pleura. The parietal pleura, which lines the rib cage and the lateral portion of each hemidiaphragm, is innervated by intercostal nerves; therefore, pain is localized to the cutaneous distribution of those nerves (over the chest wall). The parietal pleura of the central diaphragm is innervated by fibers that travel with the phrenic nerve; therefore pain associated with inflammation in this area is referred to the ipsilateral shoulder or neck.
- Various underlying etiologies may result in pleurisy, including the following:
  1. Pulmonary embolism
  2. Viral pneumonia (adenovirus, coxsackieviruses, influenza, respiratory syncytial virus [RSV], parainfluenza, human metapneumovirus, cytomegalovirus , Epstein-Barr virus [EBV])
  3. Bacterial infection (pneumonia or tuberculous pleuritis)
  4. Fungal infection (coccidioidomycosis, histoplasmosis)
  5. Rheumatologic disease (rheumatoid arthritis, systemic lupus erythematosus [SLE])
  6. Medications
  7. Malignancy of the lung or pleura
  8. Trauma (rib fracture)
  9. Hereditary (familial Mediterranean fever, sickle cell disease)
  10. Other etiologies that result in an inflammatory or exudative pleural effusion

Dx DIAGNOSIS

DIFFERENTIAL DIAGNOSIS

- Cardiac: Myocardial infarction, ischemia, pericarditis
- Intraabdominal process: Pancreatitis, cholecystitis
- Traumatic/mechanical: Rib fracture or pneumothorax
- Epidemic pleurodynia (pain resulting from infection and inflammation of the intercostal muscles). Most common virus implicated is coxsackieviruses

WORKUP

- A thorough history and physical exam of all patients presenting with pleuritic chest pain should be taken. The time course of the patient's symptoms can provide valuable diagnostic clues. Acute onset of symptoms is suggestive of traumatic injuries, spontaneous pneumothorax, pulmonary embolism, or myocardial infarction. Subacute onset of symptoms suggests a potential infectious, rheumatologic, or medication-induced cause. Viral pleurisy is often associated with prodromal symptoms of upper respiratory infection. Chronic or recurrent symptoms suggest a potential malignant, tuberculous, or hereditary cause.
- Chest x-ray to evaluate for pneumonia, pneumothorax, or pleural effusion.
- ECG to evaluate for infarction, ischemia, or pericarditis.
- Evaluation for pulmonary embolism should be undertaken if clinical suspicion exists.
- If tuberculous pleurisy is suspected, pleural biopsy by pleuroscopy or video-assisted thoracoscopic surgery may help to establish a diagnosis.

LABORATORY TESTS

- Laboratory testing varies based on suspected underlying etiology. Consider CBC, Chem 7, and D-Dimer testing depending on clinical presentation.
- If a pleural effusion is present, diagnostic thoracentesis may provide valuable diagnostic clues to the underlying etiology.

IMAGING STUDIES

- Chest x-ray results may be normal or may show consolidation in cases of associated pneumonia, hazy opacities if viral pneumonia, wedge-shaped defect in cases of pulmonary embolism/infarction, or small pleural effusion.
- Chest CT chest in select patients can evaluate lung parenchyma and pleura, particularly in cases where underlying malignancy might be suspected.
- CT pulmonary angiogram should be obtained in cases where pulmonary embolism is considered.
- Transthoracic ultrasound can be helpful to evaluate the pleural space to identify and characterize a pleural effusion, to assess for pleural or underlying lung parenchymal pathology (e.g., pulmonary edema, consolidation, pneumothorax), and to plan for a procedure such as a diagnostic thoracentesis.

Rx TREATMENT

- Treatment of pleurisy consists of (1) pain control and (2) treating the underlying condition.
- NSAIDs are the preferred first-line agent to control pain associated with pleurisy. Human studies have been limited to trials using indomethacin for pain control, although an NSAID class effect is presumed.
- Indomethacin 50 mg orally up to three times a day has been found to be effective in relieving pain and is associated with an improvement in mechanical lung function.

REFERRAL

Pulmonary consultation is indicated if prolonged pleurisy without an established etiology.

PEARLS & CONSIDERATIONS

Pleurisy is not a diagnosis. It is a symptom caused by a number of disorders leading to inflammation of the parietal pleura. Attempt should be made to discern the etiology for the pleurisy.

SUGGESTED READINGS

Available at ExpertConsult.com

RELATED CONTENT

Pleural Effusion (Related Key Topic)

AUTHOR: **Lorriana E. Leard, MD**

BASIC INFORMATION

DEFINITION

Pneumonia is defined as inflammation of the pulmonary parenchyma caused by an infectious agent (in this case, bacteria). It can be further categorized as community-acquired or health care-associated. The definition of community-acquired pneumonia (CAP), traditionally referred to alveolar infection that develops in the outpatient setting or within 48 hr of admission, now includes patients previously categorized as having health care-associated pneumonia (HCAP) since the microbiology and treatment is similar. Hospital-acquired pneumonia (HAP) is pneumonia occurring ≥48 hr after hospital admission and not incubating at the time of admission.

SYNONYMS

Community-acquired pneumonia
CAP

ICD-10CM CODES	
J15.9	Unspecified bacterial pneumonia
J13	Pneumonia due to *Streptococcus pneumoniae*
J15.1	Pneumonia due to *Pseudomonas*
J15.20	Pneumonia due to staphylococcus, unspecified
J15.0	Pneumonia due to *Klebsiella pneumoniae*
J14	Pneumonia due to *Haemophilus influenzae*
J15.211	Pneumonia due to methicillin-susceptible *Staphylococcus aureus*
J15.212	Pneumonia due to methicillin-resistant *Staphylococcus aureus*
J15.6	Pneumonia due to other aerobic gram-negative bacteria
J15.7	Pneumonia due to *Mycoplasma pneumoniae*

EPIDEMIOLOGY & DEMOGRAPHICS

- The annual incidence of pneumonia in the U.S. is 24.8 cases per 10,000 adults, with the highest rates among adults between 65 and 79 yr of age (63 cases per 10,000 adults) and those 80 yr or older (164.3 cases per 10,000 adults). Health care expenditures for CAP exceed $10 billion annually.
- Hospitalization rate for pneumonia is 15% to 20%. Incidence is highest among the oldest adults.
- In 2017, the tenth leading cause of mortality in the U.S. reported by the National Center for Health Statistics was influenza and pneumonia together. Deaths per 100,000 population: 15.1.
- Globally, *Streptococcus pneumoniae* (pneumococcus) is the most common pathogen causing community-acquired pneumonia.

PHYSICAL FINDINGS & CLINICAL PRESENTATION

- Fever, tachypnea, chills, tachycardia, cough; pleurisy in the case of pleural effusion.
- Presentation varies with the cause of pneumonia, the patient's age, and the clinical situation:
  1. Patients with streptococcal pneumonia usually present with high fever, chills, atypical chest pain, cough, and copious production of rusty-appearing purulent sputum. Pleurisy in the setting of parapneumonic effusions can also occur. Potential complications include bacteremia, empyema, and distant infections (e.g., meningitis).
  2. *Mycoplasma pneumoniae:* Insidious onset; headache; dry, paroxysmal cough that is worse at night; myalgias; malaise; sore throat; extrapulmonary manifestations (e.g., erythema multiforme, aseptic meningitis, urticaria, erythema nodosum) may be present. (See chapter on "Mycoplasma pneumonia.")
  3. *Chlamydia pneumoniae:* Persistent, nonproductive cough, low-grade fever, headache, sore throat.
  4. *Legionella pneumophila:* High fever, mild cough, mental status change, myalgias, diarrhea, respiratory failure. (See chapter on "Legionnaires disease.")
  5. MRSA pneumonia: Often preceded by influenza, may present with shock and respiratory failure.
  6. Elderly or immunocompromised hosts with pneumonia may initially present with only minimal symptoms (e.g., low-grade fever, confusion); respiratory and nonrespiratory symptoms are less commonly reported by older patients with pneumonia.
  7. In general, auscultation of patients with pneumonia reveals crackles and diminished breath sounds.
  8. Dullness on percussion may be an indication that pleural effusion is present.
  9. The clinical impression of pneumonia has an overall sensitivity of 70% to 90%; specificity ranges from 40% to 70%.

ETIOLOGY

- Table 1 summarizes common pathogens causing CAP
- *Streptococcus pneumoniae* (5% to 15% of hospitalized CAP cases): Incidence has been declining due to widespread use of pneumococcal vaccination and reduced rate of cigarette smoking
- *Haemophilus influenzae* (3% to 10% of CAP cases)
- *L. pneumophila* (1% to 5% of adult pneumonias) (2% to 8% of CAP cases)
- *Klebsiella pneumoniae, Pseudomonas aeruginosa, Escherichia coli*
- *Staphylococcus aureus* (3% to 5% of CAP cases)
- Atypical organisms such as *Mycoplasma pneumoniae, Chlamydia pneumoniae,* and *Legionella pneumophila* implicated in up to 40% of cases of CAP
- Influenza infection is one of the important predisposing factors to *S. pneumoniae* and *S. aureus* pneumonia; gram-negative organisms cause >80% of nosocomial pneumonias
- Predisposing factors (Table 2 and Table 3):
  1. Chronic obstructive pulmonary disease: *H. influenzae, S. pneumoniae, Legionella, Moraxella catarrhalis*
  2. Seizures: Aspiration pneumonia
  3. Compromised hosts: *Legionella*, gram-negative organisms
  4. Alcoholism: *K. pneumoniae, S. pneumoniae, H. influenzae*
  5. HIV: *S. pneumoniae*
  6. IV drug addicts with right-sided bacterial endocarditis: *S. aureus*
  7. Older patient with comorbid diseases: *C. pneumoniae*

Dx DIAGNOSIS

DIFFERENTIAL DIAGNOSIS

- Viral pneumonias (see chapter on "viral pneumonia")
- Aspiration pneumonia (see chapter on "aspiration pneumonia")
- Exacerbation of chronic bronchitis
- Pulmonary embolism or infarction (see chapter on "pulmonary embolism")
- Lung neoplasm
- Bronchiolitis
- Sarcoidosis (see chapter on "sarcoidosis")
- Hypersensitivity pneumonitis (see chapter on "hypersensitivity pneumonitis")
- Pulmonary edema
- Drug-induced lung injury
- Fungal pneumonias
- Parasitic pneumonias
- Atypical pneumonia
- Tuberculosis
- Cryptogenic organizing pneumonia

WORKUP

Diagnostic testing for CAP is summarized in Table 4. Useful tools for assessing severity of illness are the *CURB-65* (see "Disposition") and *Pneumonia Severity Index* (Fig. 1 and Box 1). Poor prognostic indicators are hypotension (SBP <90 or DBP <60), respiratory rate >30/min, fever (>40° C; 104° F), or hypothermia (<35° C; 95° F). None of these indices is as valuable as clinical judgment.

LABORATORY TESTS

- Complete blood count with differential; white blood cell count is elevated, usually with left shift or the presence of bandemia
- Blood cultures (hospitalized patients only): Positive in approximately 20% of cases of pneumococcal pneumonia
- Pneumococcal urinary antigen test can be used to detect the C-polysaccharide antigen of *S. pneumoniae* (70% sensitivity). It is a useful tool in the treatment of hospitalized adult patients with CAP
- When suspecting *Legionella,* a respiratory specimen culture on special media and/or a urinary antigen should be requested
- Serologic testing for HIV in selected patients

TABLE 1 Common Pathogens Causing Community-Acquired Pneumonia

Inpatient, with No Cardiopulmonary Disease or Modifying Factors

Streptococcus pneumoniae, Haemophilus influenzae, Mycoplasma pneumoniae, Chlamydophila pneumoniae, mixed infection (bacteria plus atypical pathogen), viruses (including influenza), *Legionella* spp., and others *(Mycobacterium tuberculosis,* endemic fungi, *Pneumocystis jirovecii)*

Inpatient, with Cardiopulmonary Disease and/or Modifying Factors

All of the above, but drug-resistant *S. pneumoniae* (DRSP) and enteric gram-negative organisms are more of a concern

Severe Community-Acquired Pneumonia, with No Risks for *Pseudomonas Aeruginosa*

S. pneumoniae (including DRSP), *Legionella* spp., *H. influenzae*, enteric gram-negative bacilli, *Staphylococcus aureus* (including methicillin-resistant *S. aureus*), *M. pneumoniae*, respiratory viruses (including influenza), others (*C. pneumoniae, M. tuberculosis*, endemic fungi)

Severe CAP, with Risks for *P. Aeruginosa*

All of the pathogens above plus *P. aeruginosa*

From Vincent JL et al: *Textbook of critical care,* ed 7, Philadelphia, 2017, Elsevier.

TABLE 2 Risk Factors for Developing Severe Community-Acquired Pneumonia

Advanced age
Comorbid illness (e.g., chronic respiratory illness, cardiovascular disease, diabetes mellitus, neurologic illness, renal insufficiency, malignancy)
Cigarette smoking
Alcohol abuse
Absence of antibiotic therapy before hospitalization
Failure to contain infection to its initial site of entry
Immune suppression
Genetic polymorphisms in the immune response

From Vincent JL et al: *Textbook of critical care,* ed 7, Philadelphia, 2017, Elsevier.

TABLE 3 Clinical Associations with Specific Pathogens

Condition	Commonly Encountered Pathogens
Alcoholism	*Streptococcus pneumoniae* (including penicillin-resistant), anaerobes, gram-negative bacilli (possibly *Klebsiella pneumoniae*), tuberculosis
Chronic obstructive pulmonary disease/ current or former smoker	*S. pneumoniae, Haemophilus influenzae, Moraxella catarrhalis*
Residence in nursing home	*S. pneumoniae*, gram-negative bacilli, *H. influenzae, Staphylococcus aureus, Chlamydophila pneumoniae;* consider *M. tuberculosis.* Consider anaerobes, but these are less common
Poor dental hygiene	Anaerobes
Bat exposure	*Histoplasma capsulatum*
Bird exposure	*Chlamydophila psittaci, Cryptococcus neoformans, H. capsulatum*
Rabbit exposure	*Francisella tularensis*
Travel to southwestern United States	*Coccidioidomycosis;* hantavirus in selected areas
Exposure to farm animals or parturient cats	*Coxiella burnetii* (Q fever)
Postinfluenza pneumonia	*S. pneumoniae, S. aureus* (including the community-acquired strain of methicillin-resistant *S. aureus*), *H. influenzae*
Structural disease of the lung (e.g., bronchiectasis, cystic fibrosis)	*Pseudomonas aeruginosa, Pseudomonas cepacia,* or *S. aureus*
Sickle cell disease, asplenia	Pneumococcus, *H. influenzae*
Suspected bioterrorism	Anthrax, tularemia, plague
Travel to Asia	Severe acute respiratory syndrome, tuberculosis, melioidosis

From Vincent JL et al: *Textbook of critical care,* ed 7, Philadelphia, 2017, Elsevier.

- Serum electrolytes (hyponatremia in suspected *Legionella* pneumonia), BUN, creatinine
- Test for and treat influenza during flu season1
- Serum procalcitonin level: Often used to distinguish pneumonia from heart failure in patients presenting to the emergency department with acute dyspnea. The procalcitonin level is significantly higher in patients with pneumonia than in those without.[1] However, serum procalcitonin should not be used to determine initiation or duration of antibiotic therapy in patients with radiographically confirmed CAP unless antibiotic therapy is being extended beyond 5 to 7 days. Recent trials regarding procalcitonin-guided use of antibiotics for lower respiratory tract infections did not result in less use of antibiotics than did usual care among patients with suspected lower respiratory tract infection[2]
- Pulse oximetry or arterial blood gases: Hypoxemia with partial pressure of oxygen <60 mm Hg while the patient is breathing room air, a standard criterion for hospital admission
- Fig. 2 illustrates an algorithm for the diagnosis and treatment of nosocomial pneumonia

[1]Alba GA et al: Diagnostic and prognostic utility of procalcitonin in patients presenting to the emergency department with dyspnea, *Am J Med* 129:96, 2016.

IMAGING STUDIES

Chest x-ray (PA and lateral) (Fig. 3): Findings vary with the stage and type of pneumonia and the hydration of the patient:

- Classically, pneumococcal pneumonia presents with a segmental lobe infiltrate (Fig. E4).
- Diffuse infiltrates on chest x-ray can be seen with *L. pneumophila* (Fig. 5), *M. pneumoniae*, viral pneumonias, *P. jirovecii (carinii)*, miliary tuberculosis, aspiration, aspergillosis.
- An initial chest x-ray is also useful to rule out the presence of any complications (pneumothorax, empyema, abscesses).

Rx TREATMENT

NONPHARMACOLOGIC THERAPY

- Avoidance of tobacco use
- Oxygen to maintain partial oxygen pressure in arterial blood >60 mm Hg or oxygen saturation >88% in COPD patients and >92% in non-COPD patients
- IV hydration, correction of dehydration
- Assisted ventilation in patients with significant respiratory failure

ACUTE GENERAL Rx

- Antibiotic therapy should be based on clinical, radiographic, and laboratory evaluation. Empiric therapy regimens for severe community-acquired pneumonia are summarized in Table 5.
- Macrolides (azithromycin or clarithromycin) or doxycycline can be used for empiric outpatient treatment of CAP as long as the patient has not received antibiotics within the past 3 mo and does not reside in a community in which the prevalence of macrolide resistance is high. Updated guidelines from the American Thoracic Society and Infectious Diseases Society of America[3] have added amoxicillin as a first-line agent for healthy adult outpatients with CAP. Fig. 6 summarizes

[2]Huang DT et al: Procalcitonin-guided use of antibiotics for lower respiratory tract infection, *N Engl J Med* 379:236-249, 2018.

[3]Metlay JP et al: Diagnosis and treatment of adults with community-acquired pneumonia. An official clinical practice guideline of the American Thoracic Society and Infectious Diseases Society of America, *Am J Respir Crit Care Med* 200:e45-e67, 2019.

TABLE 4 Diagnostic Testing for Community-Acquired Pneumonia

Test	Sensitivity	Specificity	Comment
Chest radiograph	65%-85%	85%-95%	Computed tomography is more sensitive to infiltrates. Recommended for all patients.
Computed tomography	Gold standard	Not infection specific	Should not be performed routinely but helpful to identify cavitation and loculated pleural fluid. Recommended in the evaluation of nonresponding patients.
Blood cultures	10%-20%	High when positive	Usually shows pneumococcus (in 50%-80% of positive samples) and defines antibiotic susceptibility. Recommended in patients with severe CAP, particularly if not on antibiotic therapy at the time of testing.
Sputum Gram stain	40%-100% depending on criteria	0%-100% depending on criteria	Can correlate with sputum culture to define predominant organism and can be used to identify unsuspected pathogens. Recommended if sputum culture is obtained. May not be able to narrow empiric therapy choices.
Sputum culture			Use if suspect drug-resistant or unusual pathogen, but a positive result cannot differentiate colonization from infection. Obtain via tracheal aspirate in all intubated patients.
Oximetry or arterial blood gas			Define both severity of infection and need for oxygen; if hypercarbia is suspected, a blood gas sample is needed. Recommended in severe community-acquired pneumonia.
Serologic testing for *Legionella, Chlamydophila pneumoniae, Mycobacterium pneumoniae,* viruses			Accurate, but usually requires acute and convalescent titers collected 4 to 6 wk apart. Not routinely recommended.
Legionella urinary antigen	50%-80%		Specific to serogroup 1, but the best acute diagnostic test for *Legionella.*
Pneumococcal urinary antigen	70%-100%	80%	False positives if recent pneumococcal infection. Can increase sensitivity with concentrated urine.
Serum procalcitonin			Not a routine test, but if performed, should be measured with the highly sensitive Kryptor assay. May help guide duration of therapy and need for ICU admission.

From Vincent JL et al: *Textbook of critical care,* ed 7, Philadelphia, 2017, Elsevier.

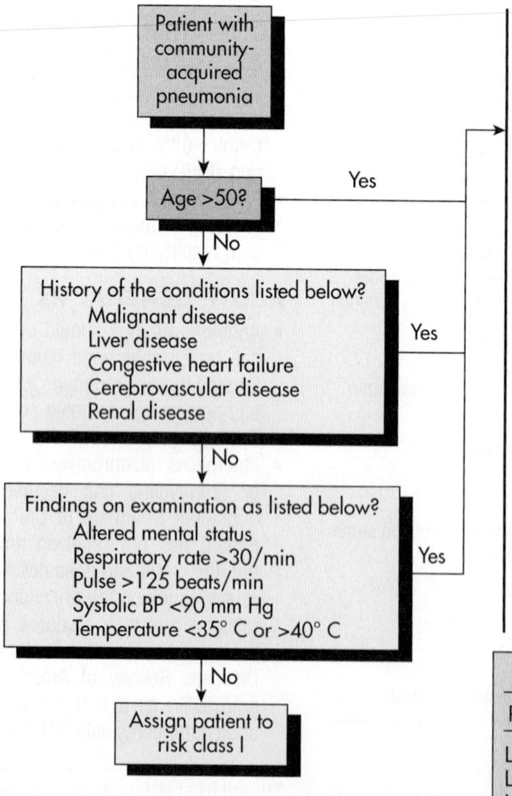

Characteristic	Assigned points
Age	
Male	Age (in years)
Female	Age (in years) – 10
Nursing home resident	+10
Comorbidities	
Malignant disease	+30
Liver disease	+20
Congestive heart failure	+10
Cerebrovascular disease	+10
Renal disease	+10
Altered mental status	+20
Respiratory rate >30/min	+20
Pulse >125	+10
Systolic blood pressure <90 mm Hg	+20
Temperature <35° C or >40° C	+15
Arterial pH <7.35	+30
Blood urea nitrogen >30 mg/dL	+20
Sodium <130 mmol/liter	+20
Glucose >250 mg/dL	+10
Hematocrit <30%	+10
Po_2 <60 mm Hg or O_2 saturation <90%	+10
Pleural effusion	+10

Stratification of risk score

Risk	Risk class	Score	Mortality
Low	I	Based on algorithm	0.1%
Low	II	≤70	0.6%
Low	III	71–90	0.9%
Moderate	IV	91–130	9.3%
High	V	>130	27.0%

FIG. 1 The pneumonia severity index. *BP,* Blood pressure; *O_2,* oxygen; *Po_2,* partial pressure of oxygen. (From Sellke FW et al: *Sabiston & Spencer surgery of the chest,* ed 9, Philadelphia, 2016, Elsevier.)

BOX 1 Severe Pneumonia: Diagnostic Criteria[1]

Major Criteria
Invasive mechanical ventilation
Use of vasopressors to maintain blood pressure

Minor Criteria
Respiratory rate ≥30 breaths/min
Multilobar infiltrates
New-onset confusion/disorientation
Uremia (BUN >20 mg/dl)
Leukopenia (WBC count <4000 cells/μL)
Pa_{O_2}/F_{IO_2} ratio ≥250
Thrombocytopenia (platelet count <100,000 cells/μL)
Hypothermia (core temperature <36°C; 96.8º F)
Hypotension requiring aggressive fluid resuscitation

ATS/IDSA, American Thoracic Society/Infectious Diseases Society of America; *BUN*, blood urea nitrogen; *WBC*, white blood cell.
[1]According to ATS/IDSA 2007 guidelines.
From Parrillo JE, Dellinger RP: *Critical care medicine: principles of diagnosis and management in the adult*, ed 4, Philadelphia, 2014, Saunders.

empiric therapy for CAP. The treatment of choice in suspected *Legionella* pneumonia is either a quinolone (e.g., moxifloxacin) or a macrolide (e.g., azithromycin) antibiotic. A beta-lactam antibiotic is usually added to macrolides.

- In the hospital setting, patients admitted to the general ward can be treated empirically with a second- or third-generation cephalosporin (ceftriaxone, cefotaxime, or cefuroxime) plus a macrolide (azithromycin or clarithromycin) or doxycycline. An antipseudomonal quinolone (levofloxacin or moxifloxacin) can be substituted in place of the macrolide or doxycycline.
- Empiric therapy in ICU patients: IV beta-lactam (ceftriaxone, cefotaxime, ampicillin-sulbactam) plus an IV quinolone (levofloxacin, moxifloxacin) or IV azithromycin.
- In hospitalized patients at risk for *P. aeruginosa* infection, empiric treatment should consist of an antipseudomonal beta-lactam (meropenem, doripenem, imipenem, or piperacillin-tazobactam) with or without a second antipseudomonal agent such as an aminoglycoside or an antipseudomonal quinolone.
- In patients with suspected methicillin-resistant *S. aureus,* vancomycin or linezolid is effective.
- Corticosteroids: Clinical trials evaluating adjunctive use of corticosteroids in severe CAP have produced mixed results. There is no evidence that adjunctive use of corticosteroids improves outcomes in mild to moderate CAP. Guidelines advise against adjunctive treatment of CAP with corticosteroids except in patients with other indications for their use such as asthma, COPD, an autoimmune disease or CAP with septic shock that is refractory to fluid resuscitation and vasopressor support.[4]
- Duration of antibiotic treatment ranges from 5 to 14 days. Trials have shown that in adults hospitalized with CAP, stopping antibiotic treatment after 5 days in clinically stable patients is reasonable and noninferior to usual care. Hematogenous *Staphylococcus* infection, abscesses, and cavitary lesions might require prolonged antibiotic therapy, sometimes until radiological resolution is documented.

CHRONIC Rx

Parapneumonic effusion and empyema can be managed with chest tube placement for drainage. (See chapters on "pleural effusion" and "empyema".)

DISPOSITION

Risk factors for a poor outcome from CAP are summarized in Table E6. Indications for hospital admission are:

- Hypoxemia (oxygen saturation <90% while patient is breathing room air)
- Hemodynamic instability
- Inability to tolerate medications
- Active coexisting condition requiring hospitalization. A criterion often used to determine hospital admission is known as the "CURB-65": **C**onfusion, B**U**N >19.6 mg/dl, **R**espiratory rate >30 breaths/min, systolic **B**P <90 mg Hg, and diastolic BP ≤60 mm Hg, age ≥**65.** Patients are generally admitted to the hospital if they fulfill 2 or more criteria and to the ICU if they have 3 or more criteria

PEARLS & CONSIDERATIONS

COMMENTS

- Causes of slowly resolving or nonresolving pneumonia:
  1. Difficult to treat infections: Viral pneumonia, *Legionella,* pneumococci or staphylococci with impaired host response, tuberculosis, atypical mycobacteria, nocardia, or fungi
  2. Neoplasm: Lung, lymphoma, metastasis
  3. Congestive heart failure
  4. Pulmonary embolism
  5. Immunologic or idiopathic: Cryptogenic organizing pneumonia, eosinophilic pneumonia, granulomatosis with polyangiitis,
  6. Drug toxicity (e.g., amiodarone, methotrexate)
- Repeat imaging: If patients with pneumonia are not improving, repeat thoracic imaging should be done promptly. In those with complete clinical recovery, it is reasonable to wait 6 to 8 wk before repeating the imaging study to document clearing of the infiltrate. The benefit of routine imaging after pneumonia has been questioned due to the low 1-yr incidence of lung cancer. Opponents propose a selective approach limiting follow-up imaging to middle-aged and older adults.
- Prevention: Two pneumococcal vaccines are currently available: The 23-valent pneumococcal polysaccharides vaccine (PPSV23) and the pneumococcal conjugated vaccine (PCV13. The Centers for Disease Control and Prevention (CDC) recommends giving the PCV13 to all children. PPSV23 is recommended for all adults over the age of 65 yr and any other individual with risk factors (including smoking, alcoholism, diabetes mellitus, or chronic heart, lung, or liver disease.) In addition, it is recommended that adults with certain medical conditions (including end-stage renal disease, sickle cell disease, congenital or acquired asplenia, HIV infection, congenital or acquired immunodeficiency, nephrotic syndrome, leukemia, lymphoma, Hodgkin disease, generalized malignancy, iatrogenic immunosuppression, solid organ transplant, multiple myeloma, CSF leak, cochlear implant) receive the PCV13 vaccine, followed by PPSVS3. During the influenza season, patients should also receive influenza vaccination.

[4]Rhodes A et al: Surviving Sepsis Campaign: International Guidelines for Management of Sepsis and Septic Shock: 2016, *Intensive Care Med* 43:304-377, 2017.

SUGGESTED READINGS

Available at ExpertConsult.com

RELATED CONTENT

Bacterial Pneumonia (Patient Information)
Aspiration Pneumonia (Related Key Topic)
Pneumonia, Mycoplasma (Related Key Topic)

AUTHOR: **Jorge Mercado, MD**

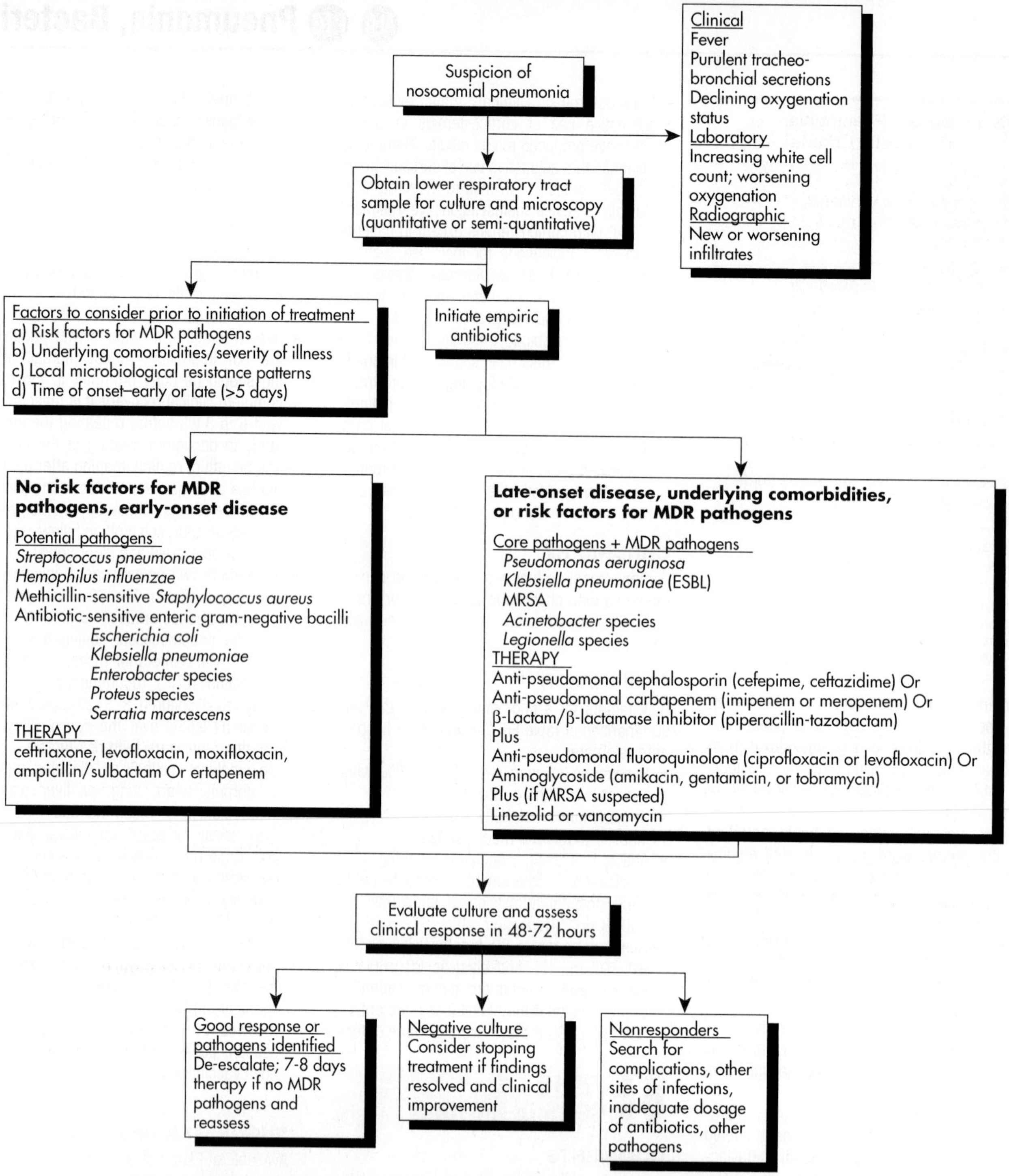

FIG. 2 A suggested algorithm for the diagnosis and treatment of nosocomial pneumonia. (From Parrillo JE, Dellinger RP: *Critical care medicine, principles of diagnosis and management in the adult*, ed 4, Philadelphia, 2014, Elsevier.)

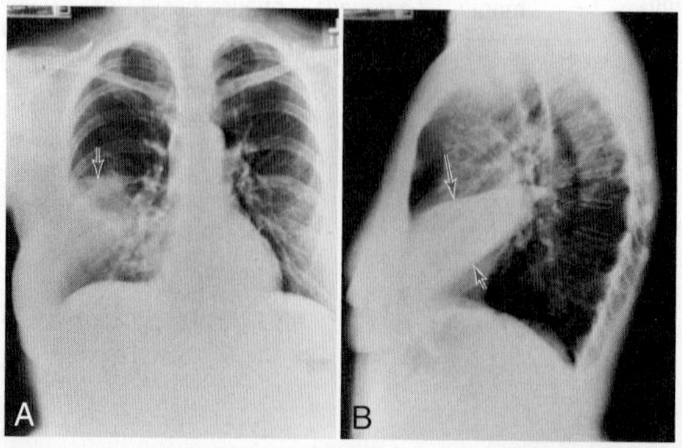

FIG. 3 Posteroanterior (A) and lateral (B) chest radiographs show lobar pneumonia (probably caused by *Streptococcus pneumoniae*) affecting the right middle lobe. In **A,** the arrow points to a minor fissure, which defines the upper border of the middle lobe. In **B,** the long arrow points to a minor fissure, and the short arrow points to a major fissure. (From Weinberger SE: *Principles of pulmonary medicine*, ed 7, Philadelphia, 2019, Elsevier.)

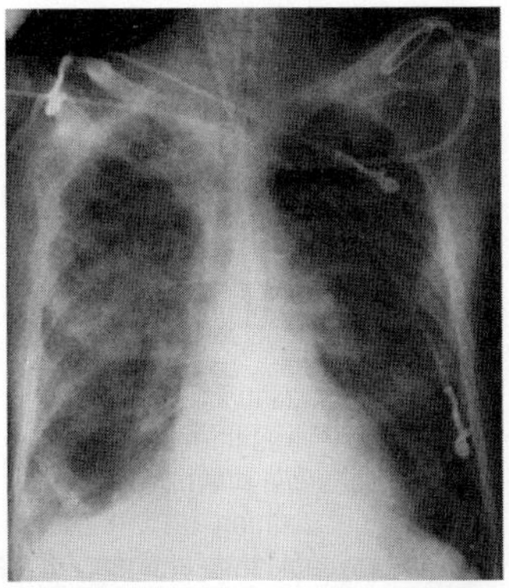

FIG. 5 Chest radiograph of a patient with extensive gram-negative pneumonia. Note the patchy infiltrates throughout both lungs, which are more prominent on the right. (From Weinberger SE: *Principles of pulmonary medicine,* ed 7, Philadelphia, 2019, Elsevier.)

TABLE 5 Empiric Therapy Regimens for Severe Community-Acquired Pneumonia

No Pseudomonal Risk Factors
Selected IV beta-lactam (cefotaxime, ceftriaxone, ampicillin/sulbactam)
Plus
Intravenously administered macrolide (azithromycin) *or* quinolone (moxifloxacin or levofloxacin*)
Pseudomonal Risk Factors Present
Selected IV antipseudomonal beta-lactam (cefepime, piperacillin/tazobactam, imipenem, meropenem)
Plus
IV levofloxacin or moxifloxacin
Or
Selected antipseudomonal beta-lactam
Plus
Aminoglycoside
Plus
Intravenously administered macrolide or antipneumococcal quinolone (moxifloxacin or levofloxacin*)

NOTE: Although routine methicillin-resistant *Staphylococcus aureus* (MRSA) coverage is NOT recommended for all severe community-acquired pneumonia, consider community-acquired MRSA, especially after influenza and with bilateral necrotizing pneumonia, and if suspected, treat by adding either linezolid or the combination of vancomycin and clindamycin.
*For patients with normal renal function, the recommended dose of levofloxacin is 750 mg daily.
Modified from Vincent JL et al: *Textbook of critical care,* ed 7, Philadelphia, 2017, Elsevier.

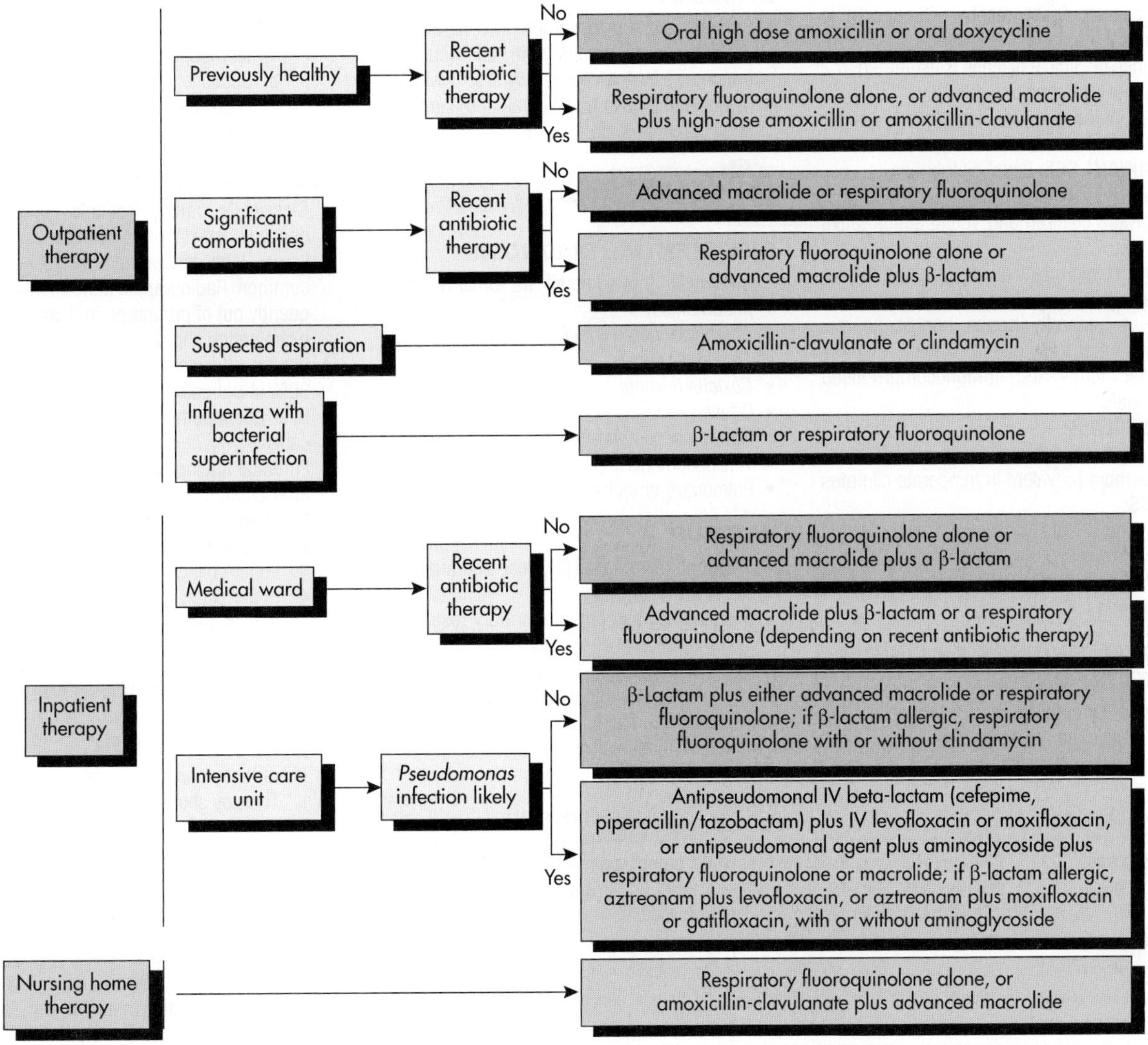

FIG. 6 Empiric therapy for community-acquired pneumonia. (Modified from Sellke FW et al: *Sabiston & Spencer surgery of the chest,* ed 9, Philadelphia, 2016, Elsevier.)

BASIC INFORMATION

DEFINITION

Mycoplasma pneumonia is an infection of the lung parenchyma caused by a small rod-shaped bacterium, *Mycoplasma pneumoniae.*

SYNONYMS

Primary atypical pneumonia
Walking pneumonia

ICD-10CM CODE

J15.7 Pneumonia due to *Mycoplasma pneumoniae*

EPIDEMIOLOGY & DEMOGRAPHICS

INCIDENCE (IN U.S.):
- Frequent cause of community-acquired pneumonia (CAP); particularly in persons ages 5 to 20 yr.
- Endemic worldwide, also causes periodic outbreaks with high secondary attack rate among household contacts because it is easily transmitted.
- Many cases probably resolve without coming to medical attention.
- Incidence of clinical disease is estimated at 2 cases per 1000 persons annually.
- Asymptomatic carriage, increasingly recognized, contributes to disease spread.

PREDOMINANT SEX: Equal distribution
PREDOMINANT AGE:
- School-age children and young adults (ages 5-20 yr)
- Occurs in older adults as well, especially after household exposure to a young child
- While it generally has a benign course, mycoplasma can cause severe disease in older adults and immunocompromised individuals

PEAK INCIDENCE:
- More common in late summer and fall
- Seems more prevalent in temperate climates

GENETICS:
Familial disposition:
- None known
- May be more severe in patients with sickle cell anemia

PHYSICAL FINDINGS & CLINICAL PRESENTATION

- Common symptoms include cough, headache, otalgia, and fever
- Exam findings include rhonchi or rales, especially in the lower lung fields, conjunctivitis, lymphadenopathy, splenomegaly, and muscle tenderness
- Less common presenting symptoms and physical findings include bullous myringitis and rashes, which occur in 10% to 25% of infected individuals. Rashes can be:
  1. Morbilliform
  2. Urticarial
  3. Erythema nodosum (unusual)
  4. Erythema multiforme (unusual)
  5. Stevens-Johnson syndrome (rare)
- Neurologic and autoimmune sequelae of infection occur occasionally, including:
  1. Mononeuritis or polyneuritis
  2. Transverse myelitis
  3. Cranial nerve palsies
  4. Meningoencephalitis
  5. Pancreatitis
  6. Glomerulonephritis
  7. Myocarditis/Pericarditis
  8. Hemolytic anemia
- Table 1 summarizes the clinical manifestations of *Mycoplasma pneumoniae*

TABLE 1 Clinical Manifestations of *Mycoplasma pneumoniae* Infection

Respiratory tract	**Pharyngitis, laryngitis, acute bronchitis, bronchopneumonia**
Skin and mucosa	Maculopapular and vesicular exanthema, urticaria, purpura, erythema nodosum, erythema multiforme, Stevens-Johnson syndrome
Central nervous system	Meningitis, meningoencephalitis, acute psychosis, cerebellitis, Guillain-Barré syndrome*
Other organ involvement	Pancreatitis, diabetes mellitus, nonspecific reactive hepatitis, subacute thyroiditis*
Autoimmune and other phenomena	Hemorrhagic bullous myringitis, hemolytic anemia, pericarditis, thromboembolism*

*Some association remains uncertain.
From Cohen J, Powderly WG: *Infectious diseases,* ed 2, St Louis, 2004, Mosby.

ETIOLOGY

- Spreads person-to-person via respiratory droplets or secretions with an incubation period of 1 to 4 wk (generally 2 to 3 wk.)
- Mycoplasma have no cell wall and cannot be seen on Gram stain

DIAGNOSIS

DIFFERENTIAL DIAGNOSIS

- *Chlamydia* (now known as *Chlamydophila pneumoniae*)
- *Chlamydophila psittaci*
- *Legionella* spp.
- *Coxiella burnetii*
- Q fever
- *Streptococcus pneumoniae*
- Viral pneumonia (e.g., influenza, RSV, COVID-19)
- Pulmonary embolism or infarction

WORKUP

- Thorough history and physical examination
- Chest x-ray (Fig. 1)
- Microbiology and other laboratory tests
  1. White blood cells (WBCs):
     a. WBC count >10,000/mm^3 in approximately one fourth of patients
     b. Differential count nonspecific
     c. Leukopenia rare
  2. Cold agglutinins:
     a. Detected in approximately 50% to 70% of all patients within 1 to 2 wk of infection
     b. Neither sensitive nor specific, so are of limited diagnostic utility
     c. Cold agglutinins are also found in:
        (1) Lymphoproliferative diseases
        (2) Influenza
        (3) Mononucleosis
        (4) Adenovirus infections
        (5) *Legionella pneumonia*
  3. Complement fixation testing assay specific for mycoplasma antigens of paired sera (fourfold rise) or a single titer ≥1:32 in patients with a compatible syndrome:
     a. Considered diagnostic in the appropriate clinical setting
     b. Other assays include enzyme-linked immunosorbent assay (ELISA), antigen capture-enzyme immunoassay, and polymerase chain reaction (PCR).
  4. Culture of the organism from specimens
     a. Most specific test, but technically difficult and not widely performed
     b. May require weeks to get results
  5. Sputum is of limited use:
     a. Often no sputum produced for laboratory testing
     b. Because there is no cell wall, Gram stain can show inflammatory cells (PMN) but not mycoplasma itself.

IMAGING STUDIES

- Classically patchy, reticular opacities but dense consolidation is possible
- Lower lobe involvement of lungs is most common. Radiographic abnormalities are frequently out of proportion to those on physical examination (Fig. 2)
- Pleural effusions are seen in approximately 30% of patients, typically small
- Hilar adenopathy present in 20% to 25% of cases
- Potential findings in late-stage of infection or after acute infection resolves:
  1. Lung abscess
  2. Pneumatoceles
  3. Lobar collapse
  4. Hyperlucent lung syndrome (aka Swyer-James or postinfectious bronchiolitis)

TREATMENT

ACUTE GENERAL Rx

- Therapeutic considerations:
  1. Therapy shortens illness duration, but the disease is self-limiting in most children and nonimmunocompromised adults.
  2. Macrolide resistance is becoming a concern. One study showed resistance of 5% to 13% in France and U.S.
- Antimicrobial options:
  1. Azithromycin: 500 mg daily × 3 days or 500 mg initially, then 250 mg daily for 4 days for adults. For children: 10 mg/kg in one dose on first day, then 5 mg/kg in daily for 4 days.

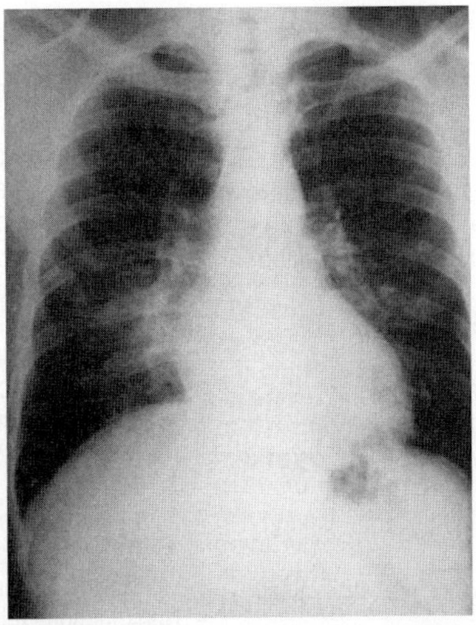

FIG. 1 Radiographic findings in *Mycoplasma pneumoniae* pneumonia are nonspecific. Bilateral bronchopneumonia occurred in this patient. (From Mason RJ et al: *Murray and Nadel's textbook of respiratory medicine*, ed 5, Philadelphia, 2010, Saunders.)

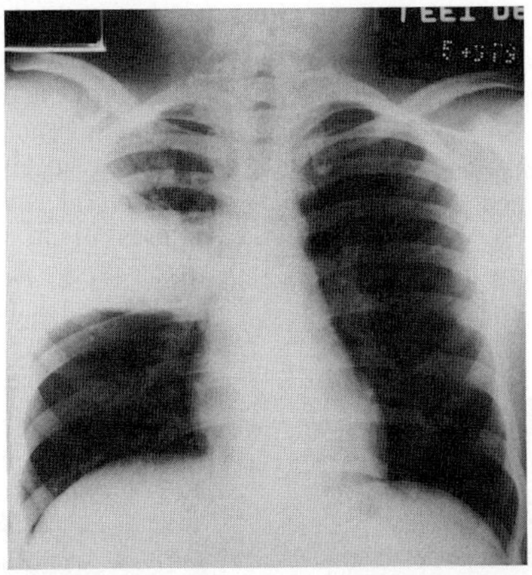

FIG. 2 Localized airspace opacification resulting from *Mycoplasma pneumoniae*. (From Specht N [ed]: *Practical guide to diagnostic imaging,* St Louis, 1998, Mosby.)

2. Clarithromycin: 500 mg bid for 10 days in adults, 15 mg/kg per day in two divided doses for 10 days in children.
3. Erythromycin (500 mg 4x per day) for adults or 30 to 40 mg/kg per day in four divided doses in children.
4. Doxycycline: 2 to 4 mg/kg per day in one or two divided doses for 10 days, maximum daily dose: 100 to 200 mg, but this agent cannot be used in young children or women of childbearing age.
5. Respiratory fluoroquinolones such as levofloxacin or moxifloxacin are alternatives for treatment in adults, but should not be used in young children.

CHRONIC Rx

- Effective antimicrobial therapy does not eliminate the organism from the respiratory secretions, which may remain positive for weeks.
- Serum antibody response does not necessarily provide lifelong immunity.
- Chronic symptoms do not occur, although clinical relapses may occur 7 to 10 days after the initial response and may be associated with new areas of infiltration.

DISPOSITION

- Clinical improvement is almost universal within 10 days.
- Chest imaging generally improves within 5 to 8 wk.
- Rare deaths are likely attributable to underlying medical diseases.
- Person-to-person spread can be minimized by avoiding open coughing, especially in enclosed areas. Azithromycin prophylaxis has efficacy in close contacts of patients.

REFERRAL

- To infectious disease specialist for patients not responding to treatment, for severe infection (including multilobar involvement), or for severe extrapulmonary manifestations.
- To pulmonologist, if diagnosis is unclear or alternate diagnosis being considered.

PEARLS & CONSIDERATIONS

COMMENTS

- Outbreaks occur in military recruits, group homes, nursing homes, and in the community.
- Infection control: In the hospital these patients should be on droplet precautions.
- Chest x-ray resolution is complete by 8 wk in approximately 90% of patients.

SUGGESTED READINGS

Available at ExpertConsult.com

RELATED CONTENT

Mycoplasma Pneumonia (Patient Information)
Pneumonia, Bacterial (Related Key Topic)

AUTHOR: **Brian Block, MD**

BASIC INFORMATION

DEFINITION

Pneumocystis jirovecii pneumonia (PJP) or *Pneumocystis* pneumonia (PCP) is a respiratory infection caused by the fungal pathogen *P. jirovecii* (formerly known as *P. carinii*).

SYNONYMS

Pneumocystis jirovecii pneumonia
PJP
Pneumocystis pneumonia
PCP

ICD-10CM CODE
B59 Pneumocystosis

EPIDEMIOLOGY & DEMOGRAPHICS

INCIDENCE (IN U.S.):

- Approximately 90% to 95% of cases occur in HIV-infected individuals with CD4 cell counts <200/mm^3.
- Risk factors for infection include CD4 cell count <200/mm^3 or CD4% <14%, elevated HIV RNA levels, and history of PCP. Early in the epidemic, risk factors included oral thrush and unintentional weight loss.
- Since the advent of antiretroviral therapy (ART), PCP incidence has plummeted in the U.S. Incidence remains high in those who are unaware of their HIV-infected status and those not on ART or PCP prophylaxis.
- Infection can also occur in other immunocompromised patients, including those with severe cell-mediated immune deficiency (congenital T-cell deficiency, acute leukemia, lymphoma, bone marrow or organ transplant deficiency), as well as patients treated with antilymphocyte monoclonal antibodies, TNF alpha inhibitors, and idelalisib for hematologic cancers or rheumatologic disease.
- Associated with defects in cellular and/or humoral immunity, either acquired or due to immunosuppressive drugs such as glucocorticoids (with incidence related to dose and duration of immunosuppression, seen with doses of prednisone greater than 30 mg/day for 12 or more wk) or other immunomodulating medications (see above).
- *Pneumocystis* is ubiquitous in the environment and is also frequently found as a colonizer in the airways of infants, children, and adults.

PREDOMINANT SEX: Equal incidence when adjusted for HIV status

PREDOMINANT AGE: 20 to 50 yr (parallel to AIDS epidemic)

PEAK INCIDENCE: Age 20 to 50 yr (parallel to AIDS epidemic)

GENETICS:

- Most frequent opportunistic infection among HIV-infected children.
- Up to two-thirds of healthy children from ages 2 to 4 have antibodies to *P. jirovecii.*

PHYSICAL FINDINGS & CLINICAL PRESENTATION

- PCP can be acute (3 to 5 days) or subacute (2 to 4 wk) pneumonia with fever, nonproductive cough, and dyspnea that is progressive. Progresses to respiratory failure if not treated. Fulminant pneumonia is observed more commonly in immunosuppressed patients without HIV.
- Purulent sputum argues against PCP.
- Hemoptysis is unusual.
- Extrapulmonary manifestations are rare and can involve nearly any organ.
- Vital signs: Febrile, tachypneic, low oxygen saturation.
  1. Oxygen desaturation with ambulation/exertion.
- Pulmonary exam is often normal. Dry rales can be auscultated.
- Spontaneous pneumothorax is possible, so beware unilateral decreased or absent breath sounds.

ETIOLOGY

- *P. jirovecii* (formerly *P. carinii*) reclassified as a fungal organism (previously classified as a protozoan) (Fig. E1).
- Infection can occur either as a result of activation of latent infection or by new acquisition.
- Infection occurs via airborne transmission.
- No transmission from vertebrate animals (mammals) to humans.

DIAGNOSIS

DIFFERENTIAL DIAGNOSIS

- Other opportunistic respiratory infections:
  1. Tuberculosis (especially in low- and middle-income countries)
  2. Bacterial pneumonia
  3. Cryptococcal pneumonia
  4. Histoplasma pneumonia (in endemic areas and advanced AIDS with CD4 cell count <50 cells/mm^3)
  5. Coccidioides pneumonia (in endemic areas and advanced AIDS with CD4 cell count <50 cells/mm^3)
  6. CMV pneumonitis (in CD4 cell count <50 cells/mm^3)
  7. Mycobacterium avium complex (MAC) (in CD4 cell count <50 cells/mm^3)
  8. Toxoplasmosis
- Nonopportunistic infections:
  1. Viral pneumonia, including COVID-19 (SARS CoV-2)
  2. Mycoplasma pneumonia
  3. *Legionella* pneumonia
  4. Other fungal pneumonias, such as *Aspergillus* and *Blastomycosis*
- Noninfectious etiologies:
  1. Kaposi sarcoma
  2. Non-Hodgkin lymphoma

WORKUP

- Chest x-ray (Fig. 2) or chest CT (Fig. E3).
- Arterial blood gas for evaluation of severity of hypoxemia and risk stratification.
- Because *Pneumocystis* cannot be cultured, diagnosis must be made through histopathologic or cytopathologic visualization of the organism from induced sputum, bronchoalveolar lavage (BAL) fluid, or tissue. Induced sputum is a common first diagnostic procedure. If negative, bronchoscopy with BAL is performed, which has sensitivity >90% to 97%, and rarely a transbronchial biopsy can be done to augment BAL results and exclude other pathogens.
- Several stains can be performed (Fig. E4), such as Giemsa, Diff-Quik, and Wright (all stain both the cystic and the trophic forms of the organism but not the cyst wall); Grocott-Gomori methenamine silver, Gram-Weigert, toluidine blue, and cresyl violet stain (stain

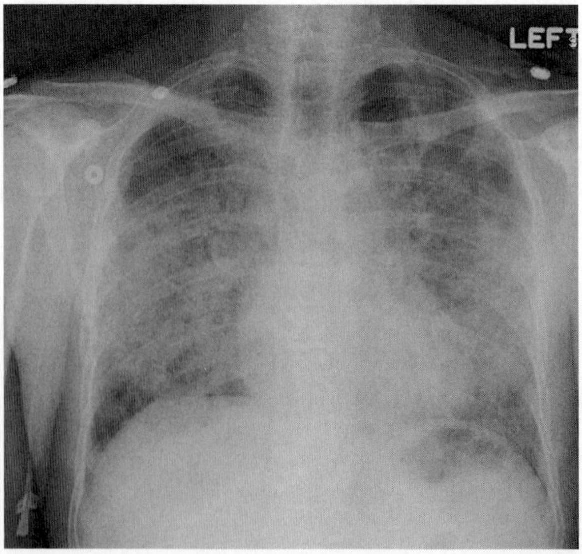

FIG. 2 Chest radiograph showing diffuse interstitial infiltrate in a patient with *Pneumocystis jirovecii* pneumonia. (From Firestein GS et al [eds]: *Kelly's textbook of rheumatology,* ed 9, Philadelphia, 2013, Saunders.)

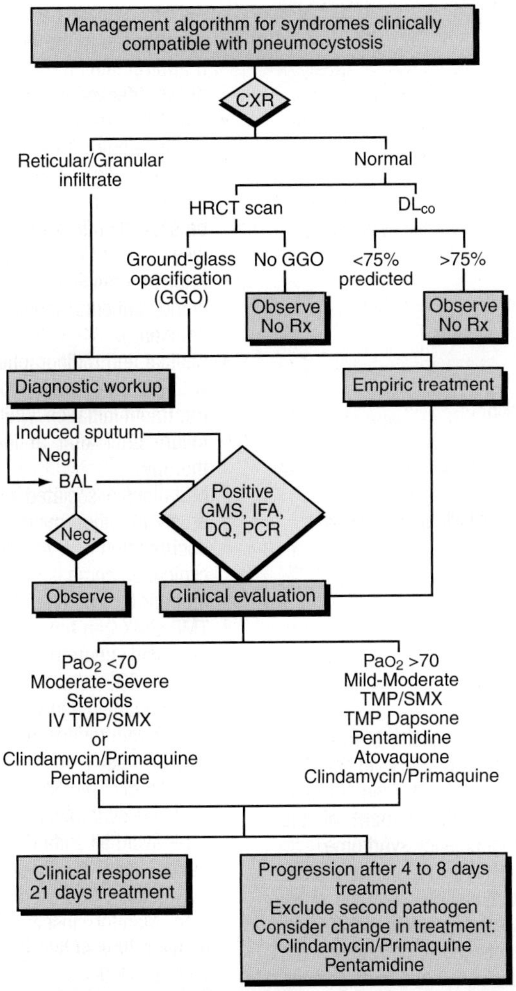

FIG. 5 Algorithm for the diagnostic evaluation and management of patients with suspected *Pneumocystis* pneumonia. *BAL*, Bronchoalveolar lavage; *CXR*, chest x-ray; DL_{CO}, single-breath diffusing capacity for carbon monoxide; *DQ*, Diff-Quik (stain); *GGO*, ground-glass opacities; *GMS*, Gomori methenamine silver (stain); *HRCT*, high-resolution computed tomography; *IFA*, immunofluorescent antibody (stain); *IV*, intravenous; *Neg.*, negative; PaO_2, partial pressure of oxygen in arterial blood; *PCR*, polymerase chain reaction; *Rx*, treatment; *TMP/SMX*, trimethoprim-sulfamethoxazole. (Bennett JE et al: *Mandell, Douglas, and Bennett's principles and practice of infectious diseases*, ed 8, Philadelphia, 2015, Saunders.)

the cyst wall), as well as immunofluorescent stains, with results depending on the lab experience and the quality of the specimen.
- Polymerase chain reaction (PCR) can be used; however, this cannot distinguish between colonization and active disease.
- Serum 1,3 beta-D glucan has good negative predictive value (very sensitive, less specific).
- Lactate dehydrogenase (LDH) is nonspecific; it is often elevated, but a normal LDH does not rule out PCP. Persistently elevated LDH may be predictive of mortality or lack of response to treatment.
- Fig. 5 describes an algorithm for the diagnostic evaluation and management of patients with suspected *Pneumocystis* pneumonia.

LABORATORY TESTS

- HIV antibody test and CD4 cell count (and CD4%) if cause of underlying immune deficiency state is unclear.
- Arterial blood gas and calculation of the alveolar-arterial (A-a) oxygen gradient for determination of disease severity and need for adjunctive corticosteroids:
  1. Mild disease: A-a gradient <35 mm Hg and/or PaO_2 >70 mm Hg
  2. Moderate disease: A-a gradient 35 to 45 mm Hg and PaO_2 >60 mm Hg and <70 mm Hg
  3. Severe disease: A-a gradient >45 mm Hg and PaO_2 <60 mm Hg
- Elevated 1,3 beta-D-glucan (>80 pg/ml).
- Elevated lactate dehydrogenase.

IMAGING STUDIES

- Early in the disease course, the chest x-ray can be normal. In these cases, a high-resolution chest CT is recommended.
- Classically, PCP presents as bilateral, symmetric interstitial, reticular, or granular infiltrates in the perihilar region ("butterfly pattern") on chest x-ray, and CT chest typically shows ground-glass opacities; however, variable radiographic presentations are possible (unilateral, asymmetric, nodular, miliary, etc.). Pneumatoceles, or cysts, which may cause pneumothorax, are common.
- A high-resolution chest CT without ground-glass opacities strongly argues against PCP.

OTHER STUDIES

If diagnostic uncertainty, PFTs can be used as adjunctive test. Low DLCO is highly sensitive but not specific for PCP infection. A normal DLCO argues against PCP.

Rx TREATMENT

NONPHARMACOLOGIC THERAPY

- Supplemental oxygen
- Noninvasive or invasive ventilatory support if needed
- Prompt chest tube placement if pneumothorax develops

ACUTE GENERAL Rx

For confirmed or suspected PCP:
- Preferred therapy: Trimethoprim-sulfamethoxazole (TMP-SMX; 15 to 20 mg/kg trimethoprim and 75 to 100 mg/kg sulfamethoxazole) divided and given q6 to q8h.
  1. Mild PCP can be treated with PO formulation of TMP-SMX, usually two double-strength (DS) tablets PO tid.
  2. Moderate and severe disease should be treated with intravenous (IV) formulation of TMP-SMX at first, but can be switched to PO after clinical improvement.
- Alternative therapies: Use only if severe contraindication to TMP-SMX (e.g., Stevens-Johnson syndrome or toxic epidermal necrolysis [TEN]) and after development of treatment-limiting adverse reaction.
  1. Mild-moderate disease:
     a. TMP 15 mg/kg/day split into tid dosing plus dapsone 100 mg PO daily, OR
     b. Clindamycin 600 mg PO q8hr plus primaquine 30 mg (base) PO daily, OR
     c. Atovaquone 750 mg PO bid (with food).
  2. Moderate-severe disease:
     a. Clindamycin (600 mg q6h or 900 q8h) IV and primaquine 30 mg (base) PO daily, OR
     b. Pentamidine (4 mg/kg) IV daily. May reduce dose to 3 mg/kg IV daily if toxicity develops. Careful monitoring is required, as IV pentamidine can cause nephrotoxicity, numerous electrolyte disturbances, and cardiac arrhythmias.
- Adjunctive corticosteroids are indicated in moderate to severe PCP (PaO_2 <70 mm Hg and A-a gradient >35 mm Hg):
  1. Prednisone 40 mg bid × 5 days, followed by 40 mg daily × 5 days, followed by 20 mg daily × 11 days (for total of 21 days).
  2. Alternative: IV methylprednisolone at 75% of prednisone dose.
- Therapy continued for 21 days.
- Antiretroviral therapy should be initiated as soon as possible. Monitor for IRIS.
- Table 1 summarizes causes of deterioration in an HIV-infected patient receiving treatment for PCP.

TABLE 1 Causes of Deterioration in an HIV-Infected Person Receiving Treatment for PCP

Etiology	Explanation
Severe Progressive PCP	
Iatrogenic	Pulmonary edema due to IV fluid overload when giving TMP-SMX IRIS following early initiation of ART
Side effects of therapy	Anemia (e.g., caused by TMP-SMX), methemoglobinemia (e.g., caused by dapsone, primaquine)
Inadequate therapy	Incorrect dosage or route of administration Adjuvant glucocorticoids not given for treatment of moderate or severe PCP
Post bronchoscopy	Sedation Pneumothorax
Pneumothorax	Spontaneous Associated with intubation and positive pressure ventilation
Co-pathology in lung	Bacterial infection Pulmonary Kaposi sarcoma Intercurrent pulmonary embolism
Wrong diagnosis	Empiric diagnosis of PCP, and correct diagnosis is another pathology (e.g., bacterial pneumonia)

ART, Antiretroviral therapy; *HIV*, human immunodeficiency virus; *IRIS*, immune reconstitution inflammatory syndrome; *IV*, intravenous; *PCP*, *Pneumocystis jirovecii* pneumonia; *TMP-SMX*, trimethoprim-sulfamethoxazole.

Bennett JE et al: *Mandell, Douglas, and Bennett's principles and practice of infectious diseases*, ed 8, Philadelphia, 2015, Saunders.

CHRONIC Rx (SECONDARY PROPHYLAXIS)

- After completion of therapy, secondary prophylaxis should be maintained with TMP-SMX (one single-strength tablet PO daily OR one double-strength tablet PO daily OR [alternative] one double-strength tablet PO three times weekly) until the CD4 cell count is >200 cells/mm^3 for at least 3 mo as a result of ART.
  1. Can consider discontinuation of prophylaxis if CD4 cell count between 100 and 200/mm^3 with undetectable HIV viral load for 3 to 6 mo as a result of ART.
  2. If PCP occurs at a CD4 cell count >200 cells/mm^3 while on ART, continue PCP prophylaxis for life, regardless of how high the CD4 cell count rises as a result of ART.
- Patients intolerant of this therapy should be treated with dapsone (100 mg PO daily) or atovaquone (1500 mg PO daily) with food.
- Inhaled pentamidine (300 mg monthly by standardized nebulizer) is less effective and is reserved for patients intolerant to other forms of prophylaxis. Inhaled pentamidine or dapsone without pyrimethamine should not be used for PCP prophylaxis in patients who are also seropositive for *Toxoplasma gondii*.

DISPOSITION

- After completion of therapy, long-term ambulatory follow-up is mandatory to provide secondary prophylaxis of PCP (see "Chronic Rx" previously) and management of the underlying immunodeficiency syndrome.
- Many patients have chronic respiratory complaints such as exertional dyspnea and many develop chronic obstructive pulmonary disease (COPD). These patients should be referred to a pulmonologist for evaluation and management.

REFERRAL

- To pulmonologist for bronchoscopy if diagnosis cannot be confirmed by sputum examination.
- To an infectious disease specialist if case is severe or difficult to manage and to evaluate for underlying immune deficiency.
- To pulmonologist for evaluation if persistent respiratory complaints such as exertional dyspnea after PCP treatment.

PEARLS & CONSIDERATIONS

COMMENTS

- All patients, especially those with severe infection or intolerant of conventional therapy, should be followed by a physician experienced in the management of PCP and, if appropriate, in the long-term management of HIV infection or other underlying disease.
- Patients with suspected PCP should be started on empiric PCP therapy (and adjunctive corticosteroids if indicated) without waiting for diagnostic procedures. *Pneumocystis* can be seen on microscopic examination days to weeks into PCP therapy.
- Prior to administration of dapsone or primaquine, patients should be tested for G6PD deficiency.
- Clinical and radiographic findings in patients with PCP may worsen in the first 5 days after treatment initiation. Wait to declare treatment failure until after at least 7 to 10 days of therapy.
- Mutations associated with resistance to sulfa drugs in other microorganisms have been documented in *P. jirovecii*, but their effect on clinical outcome is uncertain.
- Monitor for IRIS after ART initiation.
- TMP-SMX can have a range of side effects, including neutropenia (absolute neutrophil count <500 cells/mm^3), fever, hyperkalemia, acute kidney injury, rash. May be able to slowly reintroduce medication after resolution of most mild side effects. Most severe and deadly TMP-SMX side effect is Stevens-Johnson syndrome/toxic epidermal necrolysis—avoid all sulfa drugs thereafter.
- Severe and life-threatening hypoglycemia may occur 1 or 2 wk after start of IV pentamidine. Monitor closely and advise the patient of symptoms of hypoglycemia.

SUGGESTED READING

Available at ExpertConsult.com

RELATED CONTENT

Pneumocystis Pneumonia (Patient Information)
Acquired Immunodeficiency Syndrome (Related Key Topic)

AUTHORS: **Rebecca A. Abelman, MD, Katerina L. Byanova, MD, MS,** and **Lawrence Huang, MD, FCCP, ATSF**

BASIC INFORMATION

DEFINITION

Viral pneumonia is a lung infection caused by any of a large number of viral pathogens. Some of the most important viruses are discussed in this chapter.

SYNONYMS

Viral pneumonia
Nonbacterial pneumonia

ICD-10CM CODES

J12.9	Viral pneumonia, unspecified
J12.89	Other viral pneumonia

EPIDEMIOLOGY & DEMOGRAPHICS

INCIDENCE (IN U.S.):
- SARS-CoV-2 virus:
  1. The novel coronavirus disease (COVID-19) was first detected in December 2019, and became a worldwide pandemic in 2020. (See "COVID-19" chapter for further information.)
- Influenza virus:
  1. The CDC estimated ~35.5 million illnesses, ~16.5 million medical visits, ~490,600 hospitalizations, and 34,200 deaths caused by influenza in the 2018-2019 influenza season.
  2. Secondary bacterial pneumonia develops in a small percentage of infected persons.
- Incidence of other important viral pathogens can vary widely depending on setting, geography, and testing modalities. With the more widespread use of rapid molecular testing of respiratory secretions, an increase in the detection of viral pathogens has been observed. However, determining causality of the identified virus to the suspected pneumonia remains challenging because respiratory viruses remain detectable for several weeks after initial infection, and the pneumonia may be due to secondary bacterial infection.

PREVALENCE (IN U.S.):
- Often related to immune status of the population or presence of an epidemic/pandemic
- Normal hosts (estimates):
  1. Viral pneumonia requiring children's hospitalization accounts for ~66% cases.
  2. Viruses have been detected in ~23% of adults with clinical pneumonia.

PREDOMINANT SEX:
- Equal predominance.
- Male sex may predispose to more severe respiratory disease in RSV infection.
- Case fatality ratio of COVID-19 is greater among men than among women.

PREDOMINANT AGE:
- COVID-19:
  1. Hospitalization and death increase with age
  2. More prevalent in adults >30 yr
- Influenza:
  1. Overall incidence greatest in children <5 yr
  2. In general, lower incidence with increasing age
  3. Hospitalizations are greatest in infants and children aged <5 yr and adults aged >64 yr
  4. Mortality is greater in adults >64 yr
- RSV and parainfluenza virus:
  1. Young children (as the major cause of pneumonia)
  2. Occurs throughout life
- Human metapneumovirus:
  1. Children: Peak incidence 11 mo
  2. Increasingly detected in adults (bronchitis, chronic obstructive pulmonary disease [COPD] exacerbation, pneumonia)
  3. Frequent cause of lower respiratory tract infection (LRTI) in lung transplant recipients
- Adenoviruses:
  1. Young children
  2. Adults, primarily military recruits
- Varicella:
  1. Approximately 16% of adults (not infected in childhood) who contract varicella develop pneumonia
  2. Acute varicella during pregnancy is more likely to be complicated by severe pneumonia
  3. 90% of reported varicella pneumonia cases are in adults (highest incidence ages 20 to 60 yr)
- Measles:
  1. Young adults and older children who only received a single vaccination (5% failure rate)
  2. Currently most cases are seen in unvaccinated individuals
  3. Measles during pregnancy more likely to be complicated by pneumonia
  4. Underlying cardiopulmonary diseases and immunosuppression predispose to serious pneumonia
  5. Before availability of measles vaccine, 90% of pneumonias in those <10 yr
  6. ~6% of measles cases are complicated by pneumonia
- Cytomegalovirus (CMV):
  1. Neonatal through adult
  2. Immunosuppression is key predisposing factor
  3. Hematopoietic stem cell transplant recipients are at highest risk

PEAK INCIDENCE:
- COVID-19:
  1. Onset in December 2019 without clear seasonal variation
- Influenza:
  1. Winter months for influenza A
  2. Year-round for influenza B
  3. Peak of pneumonia seen weeks into the outbreak of infection
- Respiratory syncytial virus (RSV) and parainfluenza virus: Winter and spring
- Human metapneumovirus: Winter months
- Adenovirus: Endemic (military)
- Varicella: Spring in temperate zones
- Measles: Year-round
- Cytomegalovirus (CMV): Year-round

GENETICS: Familial disposition:
- Close contact, not genetics, is important in acquisition
- Congenital anomalies and immunosuppression worsen course of RSV pneumonia

Congenital infection:
- CMV is the most common intrauterine infection in the U.S.
- Pneumonia occurs occasionally in infants with symptomatic congenital infection

Neonatal infection:
- Severe RSV pneumonia
- Adenovirus pneumonia
  1. 5% to 20% mortality rate
  2. Can lead to residual restrictive or obstructive functional abnormalities
- "Varicella neonatorum"
  1. Disseminated visceral disease including pneumonia
  2. May develop in neonates whose mothers develop peripartum chickenpox
- CMV pneumonia:
  1. Generally fatal
  2. Associated with severe cerebral damage in this population

PHYSICAL FINDINGS & CLINICAL PRESENTATION

- COVID-19:
  1. Fever, chills, fatigue, myalgias, headache
  2. Cough, shortness of breath, sore throat, congestion, rhinorrhea
  3. Loss of taste or smell
  4. Nausea, vomiting, diarrhea
- Influenza:
  1. Fever, cough, or sore throat (referred to as influenza-like illness [ILI])
  2. Uncomfortable or lethargic appearance
  3. Prominent dry cough (rarely hemoptysis)
  4. Flushed integument and erythematous mucous membranes
  5. Rales or rhonchi
- RSV, parainfluenza, and human metapneumovirus:
  1. Fever
  2. Tachypnea
  3. Prolonged expiration
  4. Wheezes and rales
- Adenoviruses:
  1. Hoarseness
  2. Pharyngitis
  3. Tachypnea
  4. Cervical adenitis
- Measles:
  1. Conjunctivitis
  2. Rhinorrhea
  3. Koplik spots (white lesions on the buccal mucosa)
  4. Exanthem (maculopapular rash that starts on the head, then moves down to rest of body)
  5. Pneumonitis (coincident with rash, may also develop after apparent recovery from measles)
  6. Fever
  7. Dry cough
- Varicella:
  1. Fever

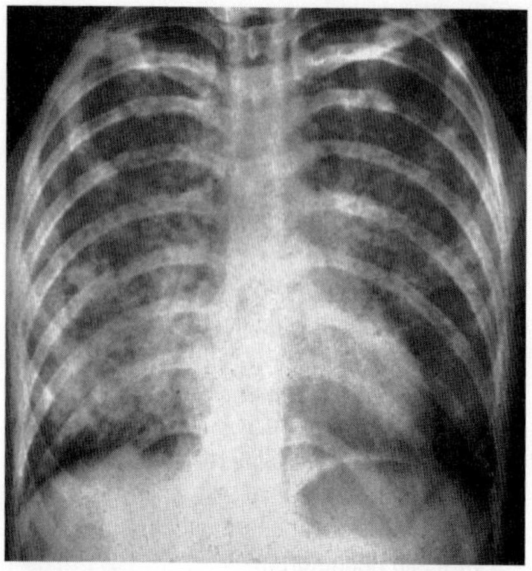

FIG. 1 This chest radiograph demonstrates bilateral nodular and interstitial pneumonia characteristic of varicella pneumonia. The patient, a 27-yr-old gravida 6, para 2, abortus 3, was exposed to varicella infection in her two children. Characteristic skin vesicles of varicella occurred several days before the development of pulmonary symptoms. She required endotracheal intubation and mechanical ventilation for 6 days. She was treated with intravenous acyclovir and ceftazidime for possible superimposed infection. The patient recovered fully and delivered a healthy infant at term. (From Gabbe SG: *Obstetrics,* ed 6, Philadelphia, 2012, Saunders.)

2. Maculopapular or vesicular rash (all lesions at the same stage) becomes encrusted
3. Pneumonia typical 1 to 6 days after rash appears. Pneumonia (Fig. 1) may be accompanied by cough and occasionally hemoptysis
4. Few auscultatory abnormalities noted on examination of the lungs

- CMV:
  1. Fever
  2. Paroxysmal cough
  3. Occasional hemoptysis
  4. Diffuse adenopathy when pneumonia occurs after transfusion

ETIOLOGY

Viral infection can lead to pneumonia in both immunocompetent and immunocompromised hosts.

Dx DIAGNOSIS

DIFFERENTIAL DIAGNOSIS

- Bacterial pneumonia; primary bacterial, secondary bacterial infection, or bacterial coinfection.
- Other causes of atypical pneumonia:
  1. *Mycoplasma* spp.
  2. *Chlamydia* spp.
  3. *Coxiella* spp.
  4. Legionnaires' disease
  5. In certain patient populations (e.g., immunocompromised) consider fungal infections, pneumocystis, tuberculosis, or atypical mycobacterium.
  6. Acute respiratory distress syndrome (ARDS)
- Pulmonary emboli

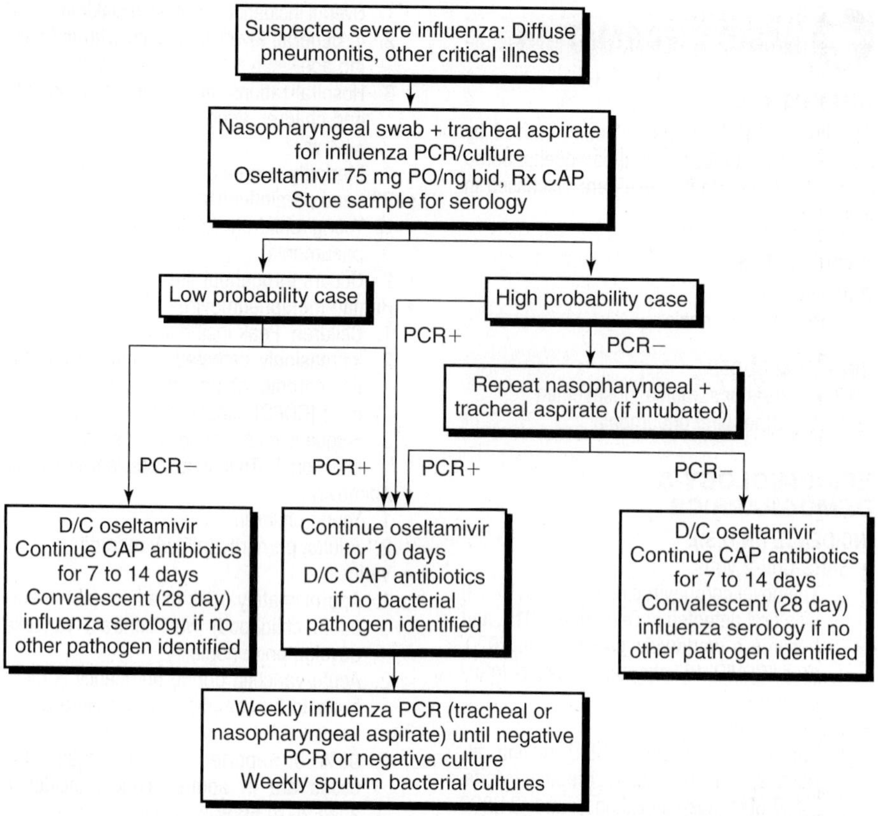

FIG. 2 Suggested algorithm in the workup and management of suspected severe influenza pneumonia in the critical care unit. *CAP,* Community-acquired pneumonia; *D/C,* discontinue; *PCR,* polymerase chain reaction; *PO,* by mouth; *Rx,* prescription. (From Vincent JL et al: *Textbook of critical care,* ed 6, Philadelphia, 2011, Saunders.)

WORKUP

- Information about the current prevalent strain of influenza virus or local prevalence of COVID-19 can be obtained from local health departments or from the Centers for Disease Control and Prevention.
- Influenza and other viruses may be cultured from respiratory secretions during the initial few days of the illness (special media and techniques necessary).
- Respiratory viral panels that use PCR-based assays to test for a variety of viruses are extremely sensitive and are becoming the test of choice.
- Rapid flu tests have a 50% to 70% sensitivity in diagnosing influenza (a negative test does not mean the patient does not have influenza).
- Measles and adenovirus pneumonia are usually diagnosed clinically and can be confirmed with serology.
- CMV may be grown in culture or PCR amplified from bronchoalveolar lavage samples.
- An algorithm for the workup and management of suspected severe influenza pneumonia in the critical care unit is described in Fig. 2.
- COVID-19 can be assessed by nasopharyngeal or tracheal aspirate PCR tests for diagnostic work-up. Antibody serology testing is not generally useful for acute diagnosis.

LABORATORY TESTS

- COVID-19, influenza, RSV, and several other respiratory viruses can be assessed by nasopharyngeal or tracheal aspirate PCR tests for diagnostic work-up.
- Sputum Gram stain (usually produced in scanty amounts) typically shows few polymorphonuclear leukocytes and few bacteria.
- White blood cell count may vary from leukopenic to modest elevation, usually without a leftward shift. COVID-19 is particularly characterized by leukopenia.
- Disseminated intravascular coagulation occasionally complicates adenovirus type 7 pneumonia.
- Multinucleated giant cells on Tzanck preparation of an unroofed vesicular lesion are useful in diagnosing varicella (also found in herpes simplex).
- Severe immunosuppression is associated with symptomatic CMV pneumonia (may be reactivation of latent infection or in previously seronegative recipients from the donor).
- Hypoxemia may be profound.
- Cultures may be helpful in identifying superinfecting bacterial pathogens.
- When they occur, parapneumonic pleural effusions are exudative.

IMAGING STUDIES

- Chest x-rays may demonstrate a spectrum of findings from ill-defined, patchy, or generalized interstitial opacities, which can be associated with ARDS.
- Chest CT most commonly demonstrates ground glass opacities, which are usually patchy and peripheral in COVID-19.
- A localized dense alveolar opacification suggests a superimposed bacterial pneumonia.
- Small calcified nodules may develop as a radiographic residual of varicella pneumonia.

Rx TREATMENT

NONPHARMACOLOGIC THERAPY

General:
- Measures to diminish person-to-person transmission
- Modified bed rest
- Maintenance of adequate hydration
- Possible ventilation support for severe pneumonia or ARDS

COVID-19:
- Facial coverings, social distancing, and quarantine are important in limiting spread of disease

Influenza:
- Yearly prophylactic strain-specific influenza vaccination can be given to prevent infection

RSV:
- Isolation techniques are important in limiting spread of RSV infections
- Immunoglobulins with a high RSV-neutralizing antibody titer are beneficial in treatment

Adenoviruses:
- Intestinal inoculation of respiratory adenoviruses has been used to successfully immunize military recruits
- Although they produce no disease in recipients, the viruses may be shed chronically and may infect others at a later date
- These vaccines are not available for civilian populations

Varicella:
- Live, attenuated varicella vaccine has been successfully used in clinical trials
- Varicella-zoster immune globulin should be administered within 4 days of exposure to prevent or modify the disease in susceptible persons
- Nonimmunized persons exposed to varicella are potentially infectious between 10 and 21 days after exposure

Measles:
- Effective measles vaccine (MMR) is available
  1. The vaccine should be administered at age 15 mo
  2. A second dose should be administered at the time of school entry
- Live, attenuated vaccine or gamma-globulin can prevent measles in unvaccinated persons if administered early after exposure
- Vitamin A given PO for 2 days reduces morbidity and mortality rates from measles in exposed children

ACUTE GENERAL Rx

- General: Administer antibiotics for bacterial superinfections when appropriate.
- COVID-19:
  1. Supportive care is the mainstay of treatment in outpatient and inpatient cases.
  2. Remdesivir obtained emergency use authorization from FDA to be used in patients with severe infection.
  3. Dexamethasone decreases mortality in patients requiring respiratory support.
- Influenza:
  1. Oseltamivir is recommended in patients of any age suspected or confirmed to have Influenza.
  2. Oseltamivir is recommended in outpatients with complicated disease or exacerbation of pre-existing conditions with suspected or confirmed influenza.
  3. Baloxavir, oseltamivir, peramivir, or zanamivir may be used in uncomplicated outpatients suspected or confirmed to have influenza.
  4. Amantadine and rimantadine are not recommended for treatment in the United States due to high resistance.
- RSV and parainfluenza:
  1. Ribavirin aerosol may be effective for severe RSV pneumonia.
  2. No approved antiviral therapy for parainfluenza virus pneumonia.
- Human metapneumovirus: No specific antiviral treatment is available.
- Adenoviruses: No approved antiviral therapy for adenovirus; cidofovir has been used in severe cases.
- Varicella:
  1. Patients over age 12 yr who develop chickenpox should be treated with acyclovir or valacyclovir, which may prevent the development of pneumonia.
  2. Varicella pneumonia can be treated with IV acyclovir.
- Measles:
  1. No effective antiviral agent.
  2. Vitamin A should be given to children with measles.
- CMV:
  1. Acyclovir, ganciclovir, and valganciclovir are used to prevent CMV infection in transplant recipients.
  2. Ganciclovir and foscarnet, with or without CMV hyperimmune globulin, are used to treat CMV infection, including pneumonia.

DISPOSITION

- Supportive therapy is useful.
- Death is possible during acute illness.
- Residual functional abnormalities may be persistent or develop into or predispose to chronic respiratory diseases in later life.
- Morbidity and mortality rates after most viral pneumonias are increased by bacterial superinfection.

REFERRAL

- To infectious disease specialist and/or pulmonologist if uncertainty about the diagnosis.
- If symptoms or findings are progressive, with severe respiratory compromise, diffuse infiltrates, or the development of ARDS, referral for supportive care on extracorporeal life support could be considered in select patients.

PEARLS & CONSIDERATIONS

COMMENTS

- Facial coverings, social distancing, and quarantine are important in reduction of COVID-19 transmission, which is spread by droplets and aerosols.
- Influenza spreads through close contact and by small droplets transmitted by cough.
- RSV is effectively transmitted by fomites and by direct contact (little by aerosol).
- Varicella is transmitted by direct contact or by aerosol.
- Of the three major forms of parainfluenza viruses (types 1 to 3), type 3 is the most common cause of viral pneumonia; types 1 and 2 primarily cause laryngotracheitis.
- Human metapneumovirus is a recently identified common cause of upper respiratory infections and pneumonia.

SUGGESTED READINGS

Available at ExpertConsult.com

RELATED CONTENT

Viral Pneumonia (Patient Information)
Cytomegalovirus Infection (Related Key Topic)
Influenza (Related Key Topic)
Varicella (Related Key Topic)
COVID-19 (Related Key Topic)

AUTHOR: **Arturo Gasga, MD,** and **Lekshmi Santhosh, MD, MAEd**

BASIC INFORMATION

DEFINITION

A spontaneous pneumothorax (SP) is defined as air in the pleural space, collapsing the lung without a precipitating event. This can be primary SP (otherwise healthy people without any obvious underlying lung disease) or secondary SP (with underlying lung disease).

SYNONYMS

Primary spontaneous pneumothorax (PSP)
Secondary spontaneous pneumothorax (SSP)
SP
PSP
SSP

ICD-10CM CODES	
J93.0	Spontaneous tension pneumothorax
J93.11	Primary spontaneous pneumothorax
J93.12	Secondary spontaneous pneumothorax
J93.81	Chronic pneumothorax
J93.83	Other pneumothorax
J93.9	Pneumothorax, unspecified
J95.811	Postprocedural pneumothorax
P25.1	Pneumothorax originating in the perinatal period
S27.0XXA	Traumatic pneumothorax, initial encounter
S27.0XXD	Traumatic pneumothorax, subsequent encounter
S27.0XXS	Traumatic pneumothorax, sequela

EPIDEMIOLOGY & DEMOGRAPHICS

- Approximately 20,000 new cases of SP occur each yr in the U.S.
- SP is more common in men than women (6:1).
- Incidence of primary SP is 7.4 per 100,000 in men and 1.2 per 100,000 in women.
- Incidence of secondary SP is 6.3 per 100,000 in men and 2.0 per 100,000 in women.
- SP is commonly seen in tall, thin young men aged 20 to 40 yr.
- Risk factors include smoking, family history, Marfan syndrome, homocystinuria, and thoracic endometriosis.
- Anorexia nervosa is thought to be a risk factor due to pulmonary parenchymal consequences of malnutrition.

PHYSICAL FINDINGS & CLINICAL PRESENTATION

- Sudden onset of pleuritic chest pain (90%), usually at rest and no relationship between the onset of pneumothorax and physical activity, which often becomes dull after a few hours
- Pain is usually unilateral and can be sharp and agonizing and associated with considerable apprehension
- Dyspnea (80%), which often resolves within 24 hr, despite persistence of pneumothorax
- Cough (10%)
- Asymptomatic (5%); may take up to 7 days to come to medical attention
- Tachycardia
- Hypoxemia
- Hypercapnia is rare because the alveolar ventilation is maintained by the contralateral lung
- Decreased chest excursion on the affected side (Fig. 1)
- Diminished breath sounds
- Subcutaneous emphysema may be present
- Hyperresonance on percussion

Tension pneumothorax (Fig. 2) is a medical emergency and should be suspected when the patient is hemodynamically unstable. Other signs of tension pneumothorax include jugular venous distention and contralateral tracheal deviation.

ETIOLOGY

- In primary SP, rupture of small blebs and bullae, usually located near the apex of the upper lobes, is a common cause.
- In secondary SP, chronic obstructive pulmonary disease is the most common cause, but it can also be associated with pneumonia, bronchogenic carcinoma, mesothelioma, sarcoidosis, tuberculosis, cystic fibrosis, and many other lung diseases. Causes of secondary spontaneous pneumothorax are summarized in Box 1.

DIAGNOSIS

Established by the chest x-ray (CXR) (Fig. 3) or bedside ultrasound.

DIFFERENTIAL DIAGNOSIS

- Pleurisy
- Pulmonary embolism
- Myocardial infarction
- Pericarditis
- Asthma
- Pneumonia

WORKUP

CXR

LABORATORY TESTS

Arterial blood gases may show hypoxemia and hypocapnia as a result of hyperventilation.

IMAGING STUDIES

- SP is usually confirmed by upright CXR:
  1. A white visceral pleural line. The absence of vessel markings peripheral to this line helps differentiate from mimicking conditions such as an overlying skin fold. A lateral width of 1 cm corresponds to 27% pneumothorax, and 2 cm occupies 49% of the hemithorax.
  2. The left lateral decubitus position is the most sensitive and the supine position the least sensitive. Inspiratory and expiratory films have equal sensitivities.

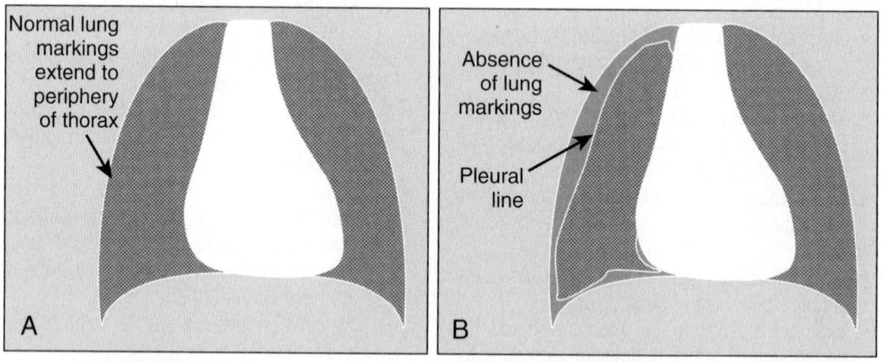

FIG. 1 Pneumothorax. A, Schematic of normal lung. **B,** Schematic of pneumothorax. Pneumothoraces can range in size from tiny to massive. Because of the variability in their size and location, pneumothoraces can be difficult to detect on chest x-ray. For example, a pneumothorax that is anterior or posterior rather than lateral may be hidden on frontal chest x-ray, particularly one taken in the supine position. An upright chest x-ray should be obtained if possible. An expiratory film is thought to be more sensitive, because the lung and thorax decrease in size during expiration, but air trapped in the pleural space remains the same size and thus appears relatively larger. Subtle pneumothoraces may not be visible on chest x-ray. In some cases, subcutaneous air may be the only visible clue to underlying lung injury. CT is extremely sensitive for pneumothorax, although controversy remains over the proper management of pneumothoraces seen only on CT. Ultrasound is also thought to be more sensitive than chest x-ray for detection of pneumothorax, although, again, the management of pneumothorax seen only on ultrasound is uncertain because this is a relatively newly described method of detection. The chest x-ray findings of pneumothorax include a lack of the normal lung markings, which should be visible to the periphery of the chest wall. Sometimes a line marking the boundary of the lung and visceral pleura is visible, although this can be confused with ribs and with the medial margin of the scapula. Depending on the degree of pneumothorax and lung collapse, the lung parenchyma may appear denser than the opposite side. In extreme cases of tension pneumothorax, the pressure exerted by the air in the pleural space may begin to displace other structures, including the diaphragm and mediastinum. In tension pneumothorax, the hyperinflated hemithorax may also have abnormally positioned ribs, with a position more horizontal than usual. (From Broder JS: *Diagnostic imaging for the emergency physician,* Philadelphia, 2011, Saunders.)

3. As little as 50 ml of air can be detected on upright film.

- Tension pneumothorax should be suspected with contralateral tracheal and mediastinal deviation and ipsilateral flattening or inversion of the diaphragm on the CXR (Fig. 4).
- Chest CT scan should be considered for a patient with recurrent pneumothorax or persistent air leak, and for planning surgery.
- Lung ultrasound has emerged as a rapid and accurate screening tool for pneumothorax.

The absence of lung sliding and a positive "stratosphere sign" on M-mode are suggestive of pneumothorax. The lung point sign, a sonographic representation of the point of the chest wall where the pleural layers re-adhere, is 100% specific to confirm the diagnosis.[1]

Rx TREATMENT

INITIAL MANAGEMENT

- When tension pneumothorax is suspected or the patient has severe respiratory distress, emergent needle decompression or tube thoracostomy should be performed. Needle decompression can be done at the bedside using a large-bore angiocatheter needle. The needle is introduced in the second intercostal space midclavicular line. The needle is retracted and the catheter is left in place and attached to a three-way stopcock and a three-chamber system connected to suction. Alternative sites for needle decompression include the fourth or fifth intercostal space in the anterior axillary line.
- 100% oxygen administration reduces the partial pressure of nitrogen in pleural capillaries, consequently quadrupling the rate of pneumothorax absorption, and should be administered to all patients with pneumothorax.
- When the patient is hemodynamically stable and tension pneumothorax is not suspected, further treatment is based on the size of the pneumothorax and the presence or absence of associated symptoms.
- If the pneumothorax is small (<2 cm between lung and chest wall on CXR) and the patient is asymptomatic, the patient can be treated with observation alone. Repeat imaging should be performed to ensure stability/resorption of the pneumothorax. Some studies have shown that using a cutoff of 35 mm for deciding which patients can be managed with observation is reasonable in selected patients with nonoccult traumatic pneumothoraces after consultation with trauma consultants.
- If the pneumothorax is large (>2 cm), or if the patient is symptomatic with chest pain and dyspnea, initial management should focus on removing air from the pleural space.
- Needle aspiration is the treatment of choice in the clinically stable patient with a large primary spontaneous pneumothorax. Needle aspiration can be done at the bedside using a large-bore angiocatheter needle or a commercially available catheter aspiration kit. The needle is introduced in the second intercostal space midclavicular line. The needle is retracted and the catheter is left in place and attached to a three-way stopcock and a large syringe. Air is aspirated until resistance is met or the patient experiences significant coughing. Repeat CXR is done immediately after aspiration and again in 4 to 24 hours to document reexpansion of the lung.
- If there is improvement but not complete resolution of pneumothorax after the aspiration, the catheter can be attached to a Heimlich (one-way) valve or to waterseal to allow further lung expansion. Some stable patients can be discharged home with a Heimlich valve in place if close follow-up monitoring can be obtained.
- Tube thoracostomy is the treatment of choice for patients with a large secondary spontaneous pneumothorax or in patients with large primary spontaneous pneumothorax that did not resolve with needle aspiration. Tube thoracostomy can be performed at the bedside preferably using the Seldinger technique with a small to medium bore chest tube (<14 Fr). The chest tube should be inserted in the second intercostal space in the midclavicular line. Alternate sites for tube thoracostomy include the fourth or fifth intercostal space in the anterior axillary line.
- An algorithmic approach to the treatment of primary spontaneous pneumothorax is outlined in Fig. 5.

PREVENTION

- Approximately 25% to 50% of patients with primary SP with have a recurrence within 5 yr. The recurrence rate is higher in patients with secondary spontaneous pneumothorax.
- Surgical bullectomy and pleurodesis can decrease rate of recurrence. These interventions should be considered in all patients after their first instance of secondary spontaneous pneumothorax, as well as in patients with recurrent primary spontaneous pneumothorax.
- Additional indications for intervention include simultaneous bilateral SP, persistent air leak (>5 to 7 days), failure of lung reexpansion by the chest tube, and professions at risk (e.g., pilots, divers).
- The current recommended surgical approach is the use of video-assisted thoracoscopy (VATS) with bullectomy and/or pleurodesis. Surgical chemical pleurodesis is best achieved with sterile talc. The overall recurrence rate is estimated at <5% after VATS.
- Chemical pleurodesis can also occur via instillation of a sclerosing agent through a chest tube. Talc slurry is the preferred agent; doxycycline and minocycline are considered to be acceptable alternatives. The recurrence rates for the instillation of sclerosing agents are higher than for VATS-guided therapy (<25%). Therefore, this mode of therapy should be reserved for patients who are poor surgical candidates.

DISPOSITION

- Smoking cessation should be advised.

BOX 1 Causes of Secondary Spontaneous Pneumothorax

Airway Disease
Chronic obstructive pulmonary disease
Asthma
Cystic fibrosis

Infections
Necrotizing bacterial pneumonia, lung abscess
Pneumocystis jirovecii pneumonia
Tuberculosis

Interstitial Lung Disease
Sarcoidosis
Idiopathic pulmonary fibrosis
Lymphangiomyomatosis
Tuberous sclerosis
Pneumoconioses

Neoplasms
Primary lung cancers
Pulmonary or pleural metastases

Miscellaneous
Connective tissue diseases
Pulmonary infarction
Endometriosis, catamenial pneumothorax

From Marx JA et al: *Rosen's emergency medicine,* ed 8, Philadelphia, 2014, Elsevier.

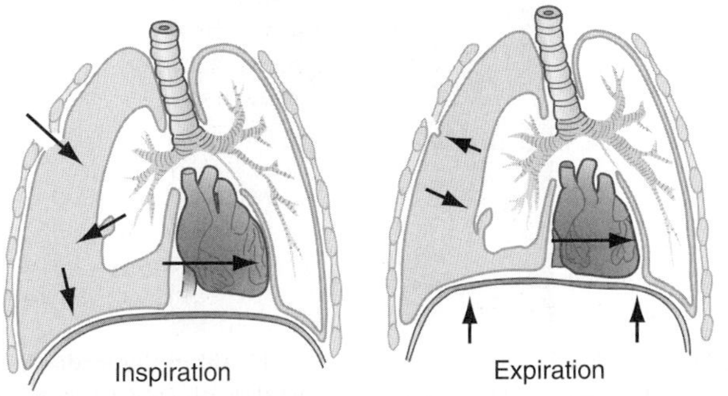

FIG. 2 Tension pneumothorax with total collapse of the right lung and shift of mediastinal structures to the left. Air is forced into the pleural space during inspiration and cannot escape during expiration. (From Marx JA et al: *Rosen's emergency medicine,* ed 8, Philadelphia, 2014, Elsevier.)

[1]Aspler A et al: Double-lung point sign in traumatic pneumothorax, *Am J Emerg Med* 32:819, 2014.

- Death from primary SP is uncommon.
- In patients with secondary SP and chronic obstructive pulmonary disease, mortality rates range from 1% to 16%.

REFERRAL

Pulmonary and surgical consultations are recommended.

PEARLS & CONSIDERATIONS

- The rate of pleural air absorption is approximately 1.25% of the volume of the hemithorax per day. This rate can be used to estimate the time interval for complete resolution of pneumothorax with observation.
- Catamenial pneumothorax is a rare condition characterized by recurrent SP coinciding with the onset of menses. It usually affects the right lung and is believed to be caused by endometriosis with involvement of the diaphragm and/or pleura. It is believed to be hormonally related, and treatment is aimed at endometrial suppression.
- Air travel should be avoided until complete resolution of pneumothorax.
- Scuba diving is contraindicated following spontaneous pneumothorax. It may be considered on a case by case basis in patients who have had surgical pleurectomy.

COMMENTS

- A recent trial revealed that conservative management of spontaneous pneumothorax is safe and effective and noninferior to interventional management, and it also has a lower risk of serious adverse events.[2]
- Patients with AIDS and *Pneumocystis jirovecii* infection have a high incidence of SP. Treatment typically requires chest tube placement and either thoracoscopy or open thoracotomy.

SUGGESTED READINGS

Available at ExpertConsult.com

RELATED CONTENT

Pneumothorax (Patient Information)

AUTHOR: **Mihir Parikh, MD**

[2]Brown SGA et al: Conservative versus interventional treatment for spontaneous pneumothorax, *N Engl J Med* 382(5):405-415, 2020.

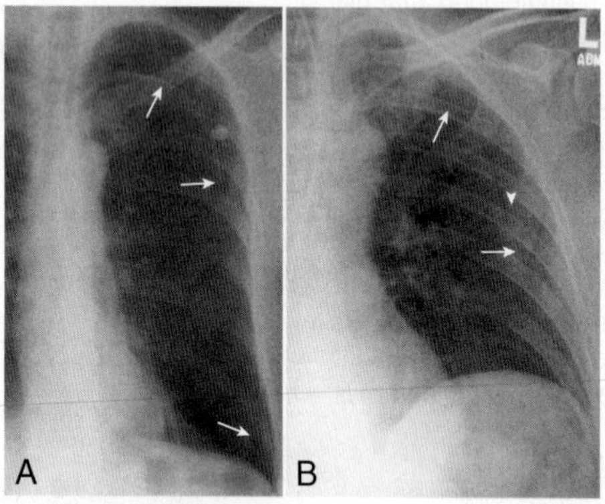

FIG. 3 A, Chest radiograph of a pneumothorax. The pleural line has lucency on either side, representing air in the pleural space on one side of the line and air in the lung on the other. The line is sharply demarcated and can be traced along its course *(lower arrow)*. No blood vessels can be seen beyond the superior *(upper arrow)* and lateral *(middle arrow)* extent of the line. **B,** Chest radiograph of a skinfold *(arrows)* that could be mistaken for a pneumothorax. The border is more of an edge, with lucency on only one side. The edge is poorly defined and cannot be followed continuously *(lower arrow)*. Blood vessels can be traced beyond the border of the fold *(arrowhead)*. (Courtesy Michael B. Gotway, MD, Scottsdale Medical Imaging, and the Department of Radiology, University of California, San Francisco. From Mason RJ et al: *Murray & Nadel's textbook of respiratory medicine*, ed 5, Philadelphia, 2010, Saunders.)

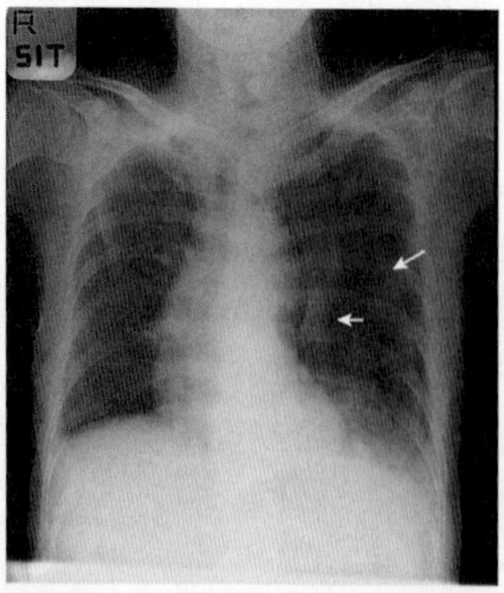

FIG. 4 Chest radiograph showing left pneumothorax with shift of the mediastinum and trachea to the right side *(white arrows)*. The left lung is not completely collapsed, suggesting the presence of a loculated tension pneumothorax. (From Chan SSW: Tension pneumothorax managed without immediate needle decompression, *Am J Emerg Med* 36[3]:242-245, 2009.)

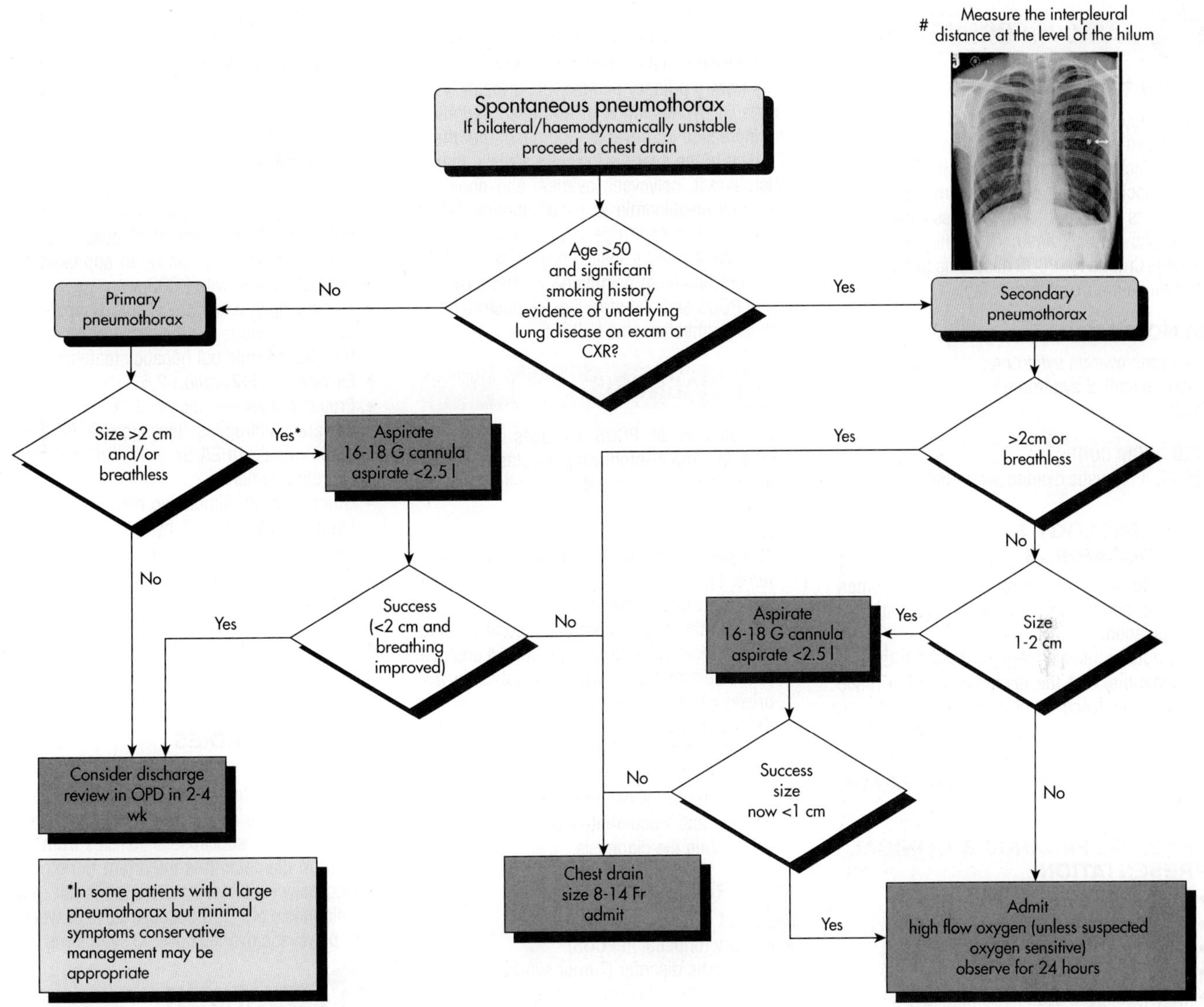

FIG. 5 Management of spontaneous pneumothorax. *CXR,* Chest radiograph; *PTX,* pneumothorax. (From Macduff A et al. Management of spontaneous pneumothorax: British Thoracic Society pleural disease guideline 2010, *Thorax* 65:ii18-ii31, 2010.)

BASIC INFORMATION

DEFINITION

Polycystic ovary syndrome (PCOS) is characterized by an accumulation of incompletely developed follicles in the ovaries due to anovulation and associated with ovarian androgen production. In its complete form, it is associated with polycystic ovaries, amenorrhea, hirsutism, and obesity. Criteria for PCOS according to published definitions are described in Table 1.

SYNONYMS

Polycystic ovarian syndrome
Stein-Leventhal syndrome
PCOS

ICD-10CM CODE
E28.2 Polycystic ovarian syndrome

EPIDEMIOLOGY & DEMOGRAPHICS

- 6% to 25% of reproductive-age women (most common endocrine disorder in this population).
- Symptoms usually begin around the time of menarche, and the diagnosis is often made during adolescence or young adulthood.
- Increased risk of endometrial and ovarian cancers.
- PCOS is the most common cause of anovulatory infertility.

PHYSICAL FINDINGS & CLINICAL PRESENTATION

- Oligomenorrhea or amenorrhea
- Dysfunctional uterine bleeding
- Infertility
- Hirsutism
- Acne, alopecia, acanthosis nigricans (Fig. E1)
- Obesity (40% only), predominantly abdominal obesity
- Insulin resistance (type 2 diabetes mellitus)
- Hypertension

ETIOLOGY & PATHOGENESIS

Elevated serum luteinizing hormone (LH) concentrations and an increased serum LH/follicle-stimulating hormone (FSH) ratio result either from an increased gonadotropin-releasing hormone hypothalamic secretion or less likely from a primary pituitary abnormality. This results in dysregulation of androgen secretion and increased intraovarian androgen, the effect of which in the ovary is follicular atresia, maturation arrest, polycystic ovaries, and anovulation. Hyperinsulinemia is a contributing factor to ovarian hyperandrogenism, independent of LH excess. A role for insulin growth factor (IGF) receptors has been postulated for the association of PCOS and diabetes. Fig. E2 illustrates the pathologic mechanisms in PCOS.

DIAGNOSIS

The diagnosis of PCOS excludes secondary causes (androgen-producing neoplasm, hyperprolactinemia, adult-onset congenital adrenal hyperplasia).
Clinical:

- The symptoms, signs, and biochemical features of PCOS vary greatly among women and may change over time.
- PCOS is the most common cause of chronic anovulation with estrogen present. A positive progesterone withdrawal test establishes the presence of estrogen. Medroxyprogesterone (Provera) 10 mg qd is administered for 5 days and bleeding occurs if estrogen is present.
- The presence of oligomenorrhea, hirsutism, obesity, and documented polycystic ovaries establishes the diagnosis.

DIFFERENTIAL DIAGNOSIS

Causes of amenorrhea:

- Primary (unusual in PCOS):
  1. Genetic disorder (Turner syndrome)
  2. Anatomic abnormality (e.g., imperforate hymen)
- Secondary:
  1. Pregnancy
  2. Functional (cause unknown, anorexia nervosa, stress, excessive exercise, hyperthyroidism, less commonly hypothyroidism, adrenal dysfunction, pituitary dysfunction, severe systemic illness, drugs such as oral contraceptives, estrogens, or dopamine agonists)
  3. Abnormalities of the genital tract (uterine tumor, endometrial scarring, ovarian tumor)

LABORATORY TESTS

- Glucose tolerance test at the initial presentation and every 2 yr thereafter (rule out diabetes mellitus). Impaired glucose tolerance is very common, occurring in approximately 30% of women with PCOS
- Fasting lipid panel (rule out dyslipidemia), alanine aminotransferase, aspartate aminotransferase (rule out hepatic steatosis)
- Elevated LH/FSH ratio >2.5
- Prolactin level elevation in 25%
- Elevated androgens (testosterone [free and total levels], DHEA-S) (rule out androgen-secreting tumor)
- Other: Thyroid-stimulating hormone (rule out hypothyroidism), 17-hydroxyprogesterone (rule out congenital adrenal hyperplasia), 24-hr urine for cortisol and creatinine (rule out Cushing syndrome)
- TSH
- Table 2 summarizes laboratory testing to exclude other causes of ovulatory dysfunction and hyperandrogenism

IMAGING STUDIES

Pelvic ultrasound (Fig. E3) reveals the presence of twofold to fivefold ovarian enlargement with a thickened tunica albuginea, thecal hyperplasia, and 20 or more subcapsular follicles from 1 to 15 mm in diameter. It is important to note that having polycystic ovaries alone does not make the diagnosis of PCOS because 20% of women with polycystic ovaries have no symptoms.

TREATMENT

The goal is to interrupt the self-perpetuating abnormal hormone cycle:

- Reduction of ovarian androgen secretion by laparoscopic ovarian wedge resection. Laparoscopic ovarian surgery (laparoscopic ovarian drilling [LOD]) is a useful alternative that does not trigger ovarian hyperstimulation.

TABLE 1 Criteria for Polycystic Ovary Syndrome According to Published Definitions

	NICHD/NIH/1990	Rotterdam 2003	AE-PCOS/2009
Diagnostic criteria	Requires simultaneous presence of: • Clinical and/or biochemical hyperandrogenism • Menstrual dysfunction	Requires the presence of at least two criteria: • Clinical and/or biochemical hyperandrogenism • Ovulatory dysfunction • PCOM	Requires the presence of: • Hyperandrogenism and/or hyperandrogenemia • Ovarian dysfunction: Oligoovulation or anovulation and/or polycystic ovaries
Exclusion criteria	Congenital adrenal hyperplasia, androgen-secreting tumors, Cushing syndrome, and hyperprolactinemia	Congenital adrenal hyperplasia, androgen-secreting tumors, and Cushing syndrome	21-hydroxylase-deficient nonclassic adrenal hyperplasia, androgen-secreting neoplasms, androgenic–anabolic drug use or abuse, the hyperandrogenic-insulin resistance-acanthosis nigricans syndrome, thyroid dysfunction, and hyperprolactinemia
Clinical traits	Hirsutism, acne, and alopecia	Hirsutism, acne, and androgenic alopecia	Hirsutism
PCOM	Not included	At least one ovary showing either: • Twelve or more follicles of 2-9 mm in diameter • Ovarian volume, 10 ml	At least one ovary showing either: • Twelve or more follicles of 2-9 mm in diameter • Ovarian volume, 10 ml

AE-PCOS, Androgen Excess and PCOS Society; *NICHD/NIH*, National Institute for Child Health and Human Development/National Institutes of Health; *PCOM*, polycystic ovarian morphology.
From Fielding JR et al: *Gynecologic imaging*, Philadelphia, 2011, Saunders.

TABLE 2 Laboratory Testing to Exclude Other Causes of Ovulatory Dysfunction and Hyperandrogenism

Lab	Evaluation for:	Comment
Total and/or bioavailable testosterone	Androgen-secreting tumor	Measure if there are symptoms concerning for an androgen-secreting tumor or if biochemical evidence of hyperandrogenism is needed to make the diagnosis of polycystic ovary syndrome. Rapid progression or a total testosterone >200 ng/dl should prompt a workup for an androgen-secreting tumor.
Dehydroepiandrosterone sulfate	Androgen-secreting tumor	Measure if there are symptoms concerning for an androgen-secreting tumor. Although modest elevations in dehydroepiandrosterone sulfate can be seen in polycystic ovary syndrome, rapid progression or greater elevations should prompt a workup for an adrenal androgen-secreting tumor.
Morning 17-hydroxyprogesterone	Late-onset congenital adrenal hyperplasia	This disorder is caused by a partial adrenal enzyme defect that leads to impaired cortisol production, compensatory elevation in adrenocorticotropic hormone, and subsequent excess androgen production. Symptoms may mimic polycystic ovary syndrome. Normal values <200 ng/dl. If higher than this, adrenocorticotropic hormone stimulation test recommended.
24-hour urine for cortisol and creatinine; dexamethasone suppression test; salivary cortisol	Cushing syndrome	Consider ruling out Cushing syndrome in women with an abrupt change in menstrual pattern, later-onset hirsutism, or other evidence of cortisol excess such as hypertension, facial plethora, supraclavicular fullness, hyperpigmented striae, and fragile skin.
Prolactin	Hyperprolactinemia	May be accompanied by galactorrhea. Consider ruling this out in all women with irregular menstrual cycles.
Thyroid function studies	Hyperthyroidism or hypothyroidism	Consider ruling out thyroid dysfunction in all women with irregular menstrual cycles.

From Setji TL, Brown AJ: Polycystic ovary syndrome: update on diagnosis and treatment, *Am J Med* 127:912-919, 2014.

- Reduction of ovarian androgen secretion by using oral contraceptives or LH-releasing hormone (LHRH) analogs.
- Weight reduction for all obese women with PCOS. Loss of abdominal fat seems to be crucial to restore ovulation.
- FSH stimulation with clomiphene HMG or pulsatile LHRH.
- Urofollitropin (pure FSH) administration.
- Metformin improves ovulation, insulin sensitivity, and possibly hyperandrogenemia.

Choice of treatment:

- The management of hirsutism without risking pregnancy includes oral contraceptives, glucocorticoids, LHRH analogs, or spironolactone (an antiandrogen). Finasteride and flutamide may be similarly effective in reducing hirsutism as spironolactone.
- Pregnancy can be achieved with clomiphene (alone or with glucocorticoids, human chorionic gonadotropin, or bromocriptine), HMG, urofollitropin, pulsatile LHRH, or ovarian wedge resection. Metformin may also induce ovulation. Recent trials comparing the aromatase inhibitor letrozole to clomiphene for infertility have shown higher live-birth and ovulation among infertile women with PCOS treated with letrozole. When considering in vitro fertilization (IVF), the transfer of fresh embryos is generally preferred over the transfer of frozen embryos; however, a recent trial among infertile women with PCOS undergoing IVF revealed that frozen-embryo transfer is associated with a higher rate of live birth, a lower risk of the ovarian hyperstimulation syndrome, and a higher risk of preeclampsia after the first transfer than with fresh-embryo transfer.[1]

[1]Chen ZJ et al: Fresh versus frozen embryos for infertility in the polycystic ovary syndrome, *N Engl J Med* 375:523-533, 2016.

- Psychological screening for depression is recommended. Women with PCOS are fourfold more likely to have abnormal depression scores.
- Table 3 describes a mnemonic for assessment and management of PCOS.

DISPOSITION

Table 4 summarizes metabolic complications in PCOS.

SUGGESTED READINGS

Available at ExpertConsult.com

RELATED CONTENT

Polycystic Ovarian Syndrome (Patient Information)
Amenorrhea (Related Key Topic)
Abnormal Uterine Bleeding (Related Key Topic)

AUTHOR: **Fred F. Ferri, MD**

TABLE 3 MY PCOS: Mnemonic for Assessment and Management of Polycystic Ovary Syndrome (PCOS)

	Assessment	Management
Metabolic	2-hour glucose tolerance test with 75 g oral glucose, measuring serum glucose at time 0 and 120 min. Lipid profile Liver function tests (if other risk factors for nonalcoholic fatty liver disease)	Lifestyle intervention: Diet, exercise, and weight loss (if overweight or obese) Metformin for abnormal glucose tolerance not controlled with lifestyle Statin therapy if patient meets criteria (Adult Treatment Panel-III or American College of Cardiology/American Heart Association guidelines)
Cycle control	Ask about menstrual pattern; normal cycle length is 28 days (range 21-35)	If amenorrhea for 3 mo or more, induce withdrawal bleed with progesterone (after negative pregnancy test) Hormonal therapy Examples: • Estrogen-containing oral contraceptives (monthly cycling, seasonal cycling, continuous use) • Vaginal ring • Patch • Progestin-only pill (smokers, hypertension) • Progestin-eluting intrauterine device (Mirena) • Progesterone prn to induce withdrawal bleeding (medroxyprogesterone acetate 10 mg daily for 10-14 days, micronized progesterone 400 mg daily for 10-14 days) • Metformin (second-line therapy)
Psychosocial	Screen for depression, disordered eating Affirm that polycystic ovary syndrome is an important medical issue; provide nonjudgmental support Discuss stress management Reinforce self-care behaviors	Mental health referral and/or antidepressant therapy may be warranted if depression or disordered eating is identified
Cosmetic	Ferriman-Gallwey score as guide to assess hirsutism Evaluate for acne and male pattern hair loss Serum androgen levels if uncertain about degree of hirsutism or atypical symptoms	Estrogen-containing hormonal contraception Antiandrogens such as spironolactone or finasteride. Teratogenic; only use with contraception Cyproterone acetate (not available in the U.S.) Eflornithine hydrochloride 13.9% cream Laser or electrolysis Topical treatment for acne Minoxidil 2.5% or 5% for male pattern hair loss
Ovulation and fertility	Counsel that fertility is reduced in polycystic ovary syndrome, but patients typically not infertile Assess fertility goals	If subfertility is an issue, consider referral to Reproductive Endocrine for possible clomiphene citrate therapy Metformin has limited role
Sleep apnea	Screen for sleep apnea: Daytime somnolence, morning headache, reflux symptoms, snoring, observed interrupted breathing	Refer for sleep study Continuous positive airway pressure therapy recommended if sleep apnea diagnosed

PCOS, Polycystic ovary syndrome.
From Setji TL, Brown AJ: Polycystic ovary syndrome: update on diagnosis and treatment, *Am J Med* 127:912-919, 2014.

TABLE 4 Metabolic Complications in Polycystic Ovary Syndrome

Abnormal glucose tolerance (impaired glucose tolerance or type 2 diabetes)	30% of obese polycystic ovary syndrome women have impaired glucose tolerance, and 10% have type 2 diabetes by age 40. In thin women with polycystic ovary syndrome, 10% have impaired glucose tolerance, and 1.5% have type 2 diabetes.
Obesity	Prevalence of obesity varies considerably in women with polycystic ovary syndrome. Previously, prevalence rates of obesity were estimated based on populations of women with polycystic ovary syndrome seeking care. A recent study comparing patients presenting for care in a polycystic ovary syndrome clinic with an unselected population evaluated during a preemployment physical suggests that obesity and overweight may not be more common in polycystic ovary syndrome. In that study, 63.7% of polycystic ovary syndrome clinic patients were obese, compared with 28% of unselected women with polycystic ovary syndrome identified during screening, and 28% of nonpolycystic ovary syndrome controls. Polycystic ovary syndrome symptoms, including hyperandrogenism and oligo-ovulation, are exacerbated by obesity.
Metabolic syndrome	33%-50% of U.S. women with polycystic ovary syndrome have metabolic syndrome compared to only 12% in a similarly aged National Health and Nutrition Examination Survey population. In contrast, only 8.2% of women with polycystic ovary syndrome in Italy met criteria for metabolic syndrome. Thus, metabolic syndrome varies by geographic location, a finding likely related to different body mass index, though other causes including genetics and diet could also be playing a part.
High blood pressure	Data have been conflicting, but a large Kaiser Permanente study demonstrated that hypertension or elevated blood pressure was more than twice as common in women with polycystic ovary syndrome (27% vs. 12%).
Dyslipidemia	Dyslipidemia is more prevalent in women with polycystic ovary syndrome compared to controls (15% vs. 6%). In a meta-analysis, triglyceride values were 26 mg/dl higher (95% CI 17-35), low-density lipoprotein cholesterol was 12 mg/dl higher (95% CI 10-16), and high-density lipoprotein-cholesterol was 6 mg/dl lower (95% CI 4-9) in women with polycystic ovary syndrome compared with controls. Women with polycystic ovary syndrome also have higher concentrations and proportions of small, dense low-density lipoprotein cholesterol.
Nonalcoholic fatty liver disease and nonalcoholic steatohepatitis	Nonalcoholic fatty liver disease and nonalcoholic steatohepatitis have recently been recognized as a potential complication in women with polycystic ovary syndrome. Prevalence of fatty liver disease in polycystic ovary syndrome women has been estimated to be 15%-55%, depending on the diagnostic parameter used (level of serum alanine aminotransferase or ultrasound). Individuals that may be at higher risk of nonalcoholic fatty liver disease including nonalcoholic steatohepatitis include those with metabolic syndrome, insulin resistance, and possibly hyperandrogenemia.
Cardiovascular disease	Many studies demonstrate abnormal surrogate markers of cardiovascular disease in women with polycystic ovary syndrome. However, data regarding cardiovascular disease risk are conflicting with some studies suggesting an increased risk in women with polycystic ovary syndrome, whereas other studies have not found this difference in cardiovascular risk. While it is important to recognize and treat cardiovascular risk factors in this population, further research of cardiovascular risk and complications is still needed to clarify the long-term risk.

CI, Confidence interval.
From Setji TL, Brown AJ: Polycystic ovary syndrome: update on diagnosis and treatment, *Am J Med* 127:912-919, 2014.

BASIC INFORMATION

DEFINITION

Polycythemia vera is a clonal disorder of aberrant myeloid/erythroid stem cells resulting in erythropoietin-independent proliferation of erythrocytes.

SYNONYMS

PV
Primary polycythemia

ICD-10CM CODE
D45 Polycythemia vera

EPIDEMIOLOGY & DEMOGRAPHICS

INCIDENCE:

- 1 to 2 cases per 100,000 persons
- Occurs most commonly in patients ages 50 to 75 yr
- Mean age at onset is 60 yr; men are affected more often than are women

PHYSICAL FINDINGS & CLINICAL PRESENTATION

Polycythemia vera has a latent, proliferative, and spent phase. The patient generally comes to medical attention because of symptoms associated with increased blood volume and viscosity or impaired platelet function:

- Impaired cerebral circulation resulting in headache, vertigo, blurred vision, dizziness, transient ischemic attack, cerebrovascular accident
- Fatigue, poor exercise tolerance
- Pruritus, particularly after bathing (caused by overproduction of histamine)
- Bleeding: Epistaxis, upper gastrointestinal bleeding (increased incidence of peptic ulcer disease)
- Abdominal discomfort from splenomegaly; hepatomegaly may be present
- Hyperuricemia may result in nephrolithiasis and gouty arthritis
- Up to 40% of patients experience arterial or venous thrombosis during the course of their disease. Cerebral and splanchnic thrombotic events occur commonly and can be presenting events

The physical examination may reveal:

- Facial plethora, congestion of oral mucosa, ruddy complexion
- Enlargement and tortuosity of retinal veins
- Erythromelalgia—painful redness, swelling, and warmth of the skin of the hands and feet
- Splenomegaly (found in >75% of patients)

DIAGNOSIS

DIFFERENTIAL DIAGNOSIS

Smoking:

- Polycythemia is caused by increased carboxyhemoglobin, resulting in left shift in the hemoglobin (Hgb) dissociation curve.
- Laboratory evaluation shows increased hematocrit (Hct), RBC mass, erythropoietin level, and carboxyhemoglobin.
- Splenomegaly is not present on physical examination.

Hypoxemia (secondary polycythemia):

- Living for prolonged periods at high altitudes, pulmonary fibrosis, congenital cardiac lesions with right-to-left shunts.
- Laboratory evaluation shows decreased arterial oxygen saturation and elevated erythropoietin level.
- Splenomegaly is not present on physical examination.

Erythropoietin-producing states:

- Renal cell carcinoma, hepatoma, cerebral hemangioma, uterine fibroids, polycystic kidneys.
- The erythropoietin level is elevated in these patients, and the arterial oxygen saturation is normal.
- Splenomegaly may be present with metastatic neoplasms.

Stress polycythemia (Gaisböck syndrome, relative polycythemia):

- Laboratory evaluation demonstrates normal RBC mass, arterial oxygen saturation, and erythropoietin level; plasma volume is decreased.
- Splenomegaly is not present on physical examination.

Hemoglobinopathies associated with high oxygen affinity:

- An abnormal oxyhemoglobin-dissociation curve (P50) is present.

WORKUP

- The revised 2016 WHO diagnostic criteria for PV use a hemoglobin/hematocrit level exceeding 16.5 g/dl/49% in men or 16 g/dl/48% in women after secondary causes have been excluded. Initial myelofibrosis (present in up to 20% of patients) can only be detected by performing a biopsy, and this finding may predict a more rapid progression to overt post-polycythemia myelofibrosis.
- Janus kinase 2 *(JAK2)* gene mutations are detected with the polymerase chain reaction (PCR) assay in approximately 99% of patients with polycythemia vera and can be used for diagnostic purposes. The exon 14 JAK2V617F mutation is seen in 97% cases and the remainder 3% of JAK2 mutations are spread across exons 12, 13, and 14. In patients with high hematocrit (>52% in men or >48% in women) and in the absence of coexisting secondary erythrocytosis, the presence of a *JAK2* mutation is sufficient for the diagnosis of polycythemia vera.
- The World Health Organization diagnostic criteria for polycythemia vera are described in Table 1.

LABORATORY TESTS

- Elevated Hgb (>16.5 g/dl in men, >16 g/dl in women), elevated Hct (>49% in men, >48% in women), or elevated red cell mass (RCM)
- Increased white blood cell count (often with basophilia; basophilia is a strong predictor of PV instead of a reactive state)
- Thrombocytosis is found in the majority of patients
- Elevated leukocyte alkaline phosphatase, serum vitamin B_{12}, and uric acid levels testing have been supplanted by molecular testing
- Low serum erythropoietin level
- Peripheral blood smear: May reveal basophils or immature myeloid forms
- Bone marrow aspiration: May reveal hypercellularity, panmyelosis (growth of all three cell lines), pleomorphic megakaryocytes, reticulin fibrosis, and absent iron stores

TREATMENT

NONPHARMACOLOGIC THERAPY

Phlebotomy to keep Hct <45% in men and <42% in women is the mainstay of therapy. Phlebotomy, however, has no effect on the development of myelofibrosis.

TABLE 1 World Health Organization 2016 Diagnostic Criteria for Polycythemia Vera

Major Criteria

- Hemoglobin (Hgb) >16.5 g/dl (men), >16.0 (women); *or* Hematocrit (Hct) >49% (men), >48% (women); *or* elevated red cell mass (>25% above mean normal predicted value)
- BM biopsy showing hypercellularity for age with trilineage growth (panmyelosis) including prominent erythroid, granulocytic, and megakaryocytic proliferation with pleomorphic, mature megakaryocytes (differences in size)
- Presence of *JAK2 V617F* or similar mutation

Minor Criterion

- Subnormal serum erythropoietin level

1. Diagnosis of PV requires meeting either all three major criteria, or the first two major criteria and the minor criterion
2. BM biopsy may not be required in cases with sustained absolute erythrocytosis: hemoglobin levels >18.5 g/dl in men (hematocrit, 55.5%) or >16.5 g/dl in women (hematocrit, 49.5%) if major criterion 3 and the minor criterion are present.

From Arber DA et al: *Blood,* 127(20):2391-2405, 2016.

BOX 1 Algorithm for Management of Patients with Polycythemia Vera

Low-Risk Young Patients (Age <60 Yr) and No History of Thrombosis, Platelet Count <1.5 × 10^6 mm^{-3}

Phlebotomy + low-dose aspirin (81 mg/day) to maintain hematocrit lower than 45%. Aspirin should not be used in patients with histories of a hemorrhagic episode or with extreme thrombocytosis (>1.5 × 10^6 mm^{-3}) or acquired von Willebrand syndrome.

↓

Thrombosis or hemorrhage
Systemic symptoms
Severe pruritus refractory to histamine antagonists
Painful splenomegaly

↓

Hydroxyurea 15-20 mg/kg (unless age <40 yr, pregnant, intolerant to hydroxyurea; consider pegylated interferon [IFN])

↓

Pegylated IFN 45-180 μg/wk or IFN-α (3 × 10^6 units three times a week; alter dose depending on response and toxicity) or ruxolitinib 10 mg twice daily and titrate dose depending on the response. →

In a patient with a prior thrombosis or a history of bleeding due to acquired von Willebrand syndrome, normalization of platelet numbers is necessary. If platelet control is inadequate or the patient cannot tolerate interferon, one option is the use of anagrelide. In this case, supplemental phlebotomy is required to maintain hematocrit lower than 45%, and the use of hydroxyurea should be considered, especially if the patient continues to have thrombotic episodes.

↓

If the patient has increasing splenomegaly, systemic symptoms, or repeated thromboses despite adequate dose of hydroxyurea (2 to 3 g/day) or if unable to tolerate hydroxyurea, start ruxolitinib 10 mg twice daily and titrate up or down based on hematologic parameters.

For patients unable to tolerate ruxolitinib or resistant to it, start low doses of busulphan or melphalan, which should be administered until the blood counts are normalized. Therapy should be then discontinued because patients frequently enjoy drug-free prolonged remissions lasting months. Therapy should be reinstituted only at the time the blood counts begin to be elevated again. Such therapy with alkylating agents should be rarely used in young patients. It should be mentioned that the sequential use of hydroxyurea and alkylating agents may be associated with an increased risk of leukemia. Supplemental phlebotomy may be required.

Painful splenomegaly

↓

Patients should be treated with ruxolitinib
If unable to tolerate or insufficient response
Splenectomy + continued systemic therapy

↓

High-risk patients (age >60 yr), previous thrombosis, platelet count >1.5 × 10^6 mm^{-3}
Phlebotomy to hematocrit of 45%
Aspirin (81 mg/day) to be given only in patients with platelet counts <1.5 × 10^6 mm^{-2}
Myelosuppressive therapy with hydroxyurea 30 mg/kg orally for 1 wk
Then 15-20 mg/kg

↓

If patient continues to have thrombotic episodes and has extreme thrombocytosis or cannot tolerate hydroxyurea

Consider pegylated IFN 45-180 μg/wk, anagrelide, or ruxolitinib 10 mg twice daily, or add intermittent busulphan or melphalan (in older patients).

If on busulphan or melphalan, stop when blood counts are normalized or platelet count is lower than 300,000 mm^{-3}.

Occasional supplemental phlebotomy if hematocrit is >45%; when patient relapses (patient is symptomatic), initiate busulphan therapy again at same dose.

Patient Age >70 yr

Phlebotomy + low-dose aspirin + hydroxyurea

↓

No response or poor compliance
Ruxolitinib, melphalan, or busulfan.

From Hoffman R et al: *Hematology: basic principles and practice,* ed 7, Philadelphia, 2018, Elsevier.

ACUTE GENERAL Rx

- Patients are stratified into low risk (<60 yr and no prior thrombosis) or high risk (>60 yr and/or prior thrombosis).
- Low-dose aspirin can safely prevent thrombotic complications in patients with polycythemia vera and reduces rates of cardiovascular events and death by 60%. Twice-daily dosing may be superior to once-daily dosing, especially in patients at high risk for arterial thrombosis.
- Hydroxyurea can be used in conjunction with phlebotomy in patients older than 60 yr to decrease the incidence of thrombotic events.
- Pegylated interferon-alpha-2b is effective in achieving noninferior rates of complete hematologic remission compared to hydroxyurea without major side effects and is approved in Europe for initial therapy. Response rates with peg-interferon continue to increase over time and surpassed those with hydroxyurea at the 36-mo mark in a recent randomized trial.
- Box 1 describes an algorithm for management of patients with polycythemia vera.
- Ruxolitinib, a Janus kinase (JAK) 1 and 2 inhibitor, is superior to standard therapy in controlling the hematocrit, reducing the spleen volume and improving symptoms associated with polycythemia vera.
- Newer agents with promising early results include murine double minute 2 (MDM2) antagonists (idasanutlin) and histone deacetylase (HDAC) inhibitors (givinostat).

CHRONIC Rx

- Patient education regarding need for lifelong monitoring and treatment
- Adjunctive therapy:
  1. Treatment of pruritus with antihistamines
  2. Control of significant hyperuricemia with allopurinol
  3. Reduction of gastric hyperacidity with antacids of H_2 blockers
  4. Low-dose aspirin to treat vasomotor symptoms in patients without bleeding diathesis

DISPOSITION

- The median survival time with standard antiplatelet and cytoreductive therapy extends the median survival time to 14 yr (range 11 to 28 yr).
- Prognosis is worse in patients >60 yr and those with a history of thrombosis.

SUGGESTED READINGS

Available at ExpertConsult.com

RELATED CONTENT

Polycythemia Vera (Patient Information)

AUTHOR: **Bharti Rathore, MD**

BASIC INFORMATION

DEFINITION

Polymyalgia rheumatica (PMR) is an inflammatory condition characterized by muscle pain and stiffness of the neck, shoulder, and pelvic girdle. PMR primarily affects the elderly and can occur alone or in conjunction with giant cell arteritis (GCA).

SYNONYMS

Anarthritic rheumatoid syndrome
PMR

ICD-10CM CODES

M31.5 Polymyalgia rheumatica with giant cell arteritis
M35.3 Polymyalgia rheumatica

EPIDEMIOLOGY & DEMOGRAPHICS

- PMR almost exclusively occurs above age 50 with peak incidence between ages 70 and 79 yr. Female:male ratio 2:1.
- In the U.S., incidence is 52.5 cases per 100,000; increases with advancing age. Prevalence is 0.5% to 0.7%. Scandinavian and Northern European populations have higher incidence.

PHYSICAL FINDINGS & CLINICAL PRESENTATION

- Patients with PMR often have symptoms for 1 to 3 mo before a diagnosis is made.
- Onset of symmetric muscle pain and stiffness, which is worst in the morning and recurs with periods of inactivity.
- Neck, shoulders, lower back, hips, thighs, and occasionally trunk and arms are involved. Shoulders are usually affected first. Pain distribution in PMR is illustrated in Fig. 1.
- Constitutional symptoms of fatigue, malaise, weight loss, loss of appetite, and low-grade fever may accompany pain and stiffness.
- Physical exam may reveal limited range of motion of shoulder (most common), cervical spine, and hips. May have subdeltoid and subacromial bursitis and peripheral joint synovitis. Motor exam is normal, although can be limited by pain.
- High-spiking fevers, night sweats, visual disturbances, headaches, or jaw claudication should raise suspicion of giant cell arteritis and be further evaluated promptly.

ETIOLOGY

The cause is unknown, but both PMR and GCA are associated with HLA-DRB1 haplotype. With both conditions, also see elevated Th17 cells and decreased Treg cells.

Dx DIAGNOSIS

DIFFERENTIAL DIAGNOSIS

See Box 1.

WORKUP

- Initial laboratory evaluation: ESR, CRP, CBC, CPK.
- ESR >30 mm/hr in majority of patients. CRP elevation may be more common than high ESR.
- CBC may show a normocytic anemia and thrombocytosis.
- CPK is normal. Antibodies (ANA, RF, CCP) are typically negative.
- An algorithm for diagnosing polymyalgia rheumatica without giant cell arteritis (GCA) is described in Fig. E2, and Tables 1 and 2 describe various classification criteria for PMR.
- Ultrasonography, MRI and PET may identify bursitis or tenosynovitis, (features of the 2012 PMR classification of criteria), which increase sensitivity and specificity.

Rx TREATMENT

- Start prednisone 12.5 to 25 mg/day, with dramatic improvement usually within 3 days.
- Dosage should be tailored to patient's weight, symptom severity, and comorbidities (e.g., diabetes, hypertension, or heart failure). If nighttime side effects are experienced, can divide prednisone dose. If symptoms persist after 1 wk, increase dose by 5 mg. Ongoing symptoms require consideration of alternative diagnosis.
- Initial prednisone dose should be maintained for 4 to 8 wk. Steroid dose is then tapered every 2 to 4 wk as tolerated to minimum amount required to remain symptom free. When dose reaches 10 mg/day, taper slowly, usually by 1 mg/month.
- Flares are typical during tapering, can manage by increasing prednisone 10% to 20%. Most require treatment for 1 to 2 yr with steroids; others are unable to taper off fully.
- Monitor both clinical response and ESR and CRP intermittently.
- Gastroprotection should be considered. Start calcium and vitamin D supplementation for bone health. Start prophylactic bisphosphonates if indicated.
- Although routine use of adjunctive therapy is not recommended, up to one-third of patients have incomplete response to oral prednisone. Consider methotrexate for refractory disease or those at risk of steroid-related side effects. TNFi has not been shown to have benefit. Tocilizumab (IL6i) is potentially beneficial in patients with contraindications to methotrexate, and it is FDA approved to treat GCA. Additional studies on the role of biologics are ongoing.

PEARLS & CONSIDERATIONS

Patients with PMR should be monitored closely for the development of GCA. Patients who have incomplete response to prednisone or have an evolving pattern of pain and swelling should be re-evaluated for the possibility of a different diagnosis such as rheumatoid arthritis.

SUGGESTED READINGS

Available at ExpertConsult.com

RELATED CONTENT

Polymyalgia Rheumatica (PMR) (Patient Information)
Giant Cell Arteritis (Related Key Topic)
Vasculitis, Systemic (Related Key Topic)

AUTHOR: **Yvonne Lee, MD**

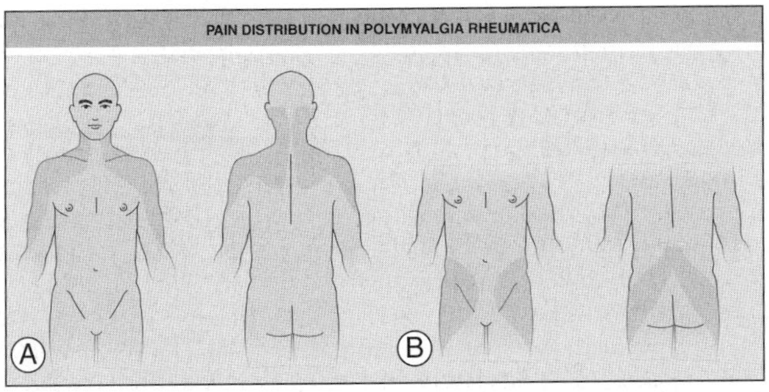

FIG. 1 Typical distribution of pain in patients with polymyalgia rheumatica (PMR). Shaded areas demonstrate typical sites of pain in individuals with PMR, including **(A)** shoulder girdle and neck pain distribution and **(B)** pelvic girdle pain distribution. (From Hochberg MC: *Rheumatology,* ed 7, Philadelphia, 2019, Elsevier.)

BOX 1 Differential Diagnosis of Polymyalgia Rheumatica

- Rheumatoid arthritis
- Rotator cuff syndrome
- Osteoarthritis of shoulder and hip joints
- Fibromyalgia
- Polymyositis/dermatomyositis
- Spondyloarthritis
- Systemic lupus erythematosus
- Vasculitides
- Paraneoplastic myalgias
- Infection-associated myalgias
- RS3PE (remitting seronegative symmetric synovitis and pitting edema)
- Parkinson disease
- Hypothyroidism

TABLE 1 2012 European League Against Rheumatism/American College of Rheumatology Classification Criteria for Polymyalgia Rheumatica*

Criteria	Points with Ultrasonography	Points without Ultrasonography
1. Morning stiffness duration >45 min	2	2
2. Hip pain or limited range of movement	1	1
3. Absence of rheumatoid factor or anticitrullinated protein antibody	2	2
4. Absence of other joint involvement	1	1
5. ≥1 shoulder with subdeltoid bursitis and/or biceps tenosynovitis and/or glenohumeral synovitis (either posterior or axillary) and ≥1 hip with synovitis and/or trochanteric bursitis	1	Not applicable
6. Both shoulders with subdeltoid bursitis, biceps tenosynovitis, or glenohumeral synovitis	1	Not applicable

*Score ≥4 without ultrasonography or ≥5 with ultrasonography is categorized as polymyalgia rheumatica.

TABLE 2 Classification Criteria for Polymyalgia Rheumatica

Chuang Criteria

1. Patients aged 50 yr or older
2. Bilateral aching and stiffness persisting for 1 month or more involving two of the following areas: Neck or torso, shoulders or proximal regions of the arms, and hips or proximal aspects of the thighs
3. ESR >40 mm/hr
4. Exclusion of other diagnoses except GCA

The presence of all these criteria defines diagnosis of PMR.

Healey Criteria (22)

1. Persistent pain (for at least 1 month) involving two of the following areas: Neck, shoulders, and pelvic girdle
2. Morning stiffness lasting >1 hr
3. Rapid response to prednisone (≤20 mg/day)
4. Absence of other diseases capable of causing the musculoskeletal symptoms
5. Age >50 yr
6. ESR >40 mm/hr

The diagnosis of PMR is made if all the above criteria are satisfied.

Bird Criteria (23)*

1. Bilateral shoulder pain and/or stiffness
2. Onset of illness within 2 wk
3. Initial ESR >40 mm/hr
4. Morning stiffness >1 hr
5. Age >65 yr
6. Depression or loss of weight
7. Bilateral upper arm tenderness

ESR, Erythrocyte sedimentation rate; *GCA,* giant cell arteritis.

*A diagnosis of probable polymyalgia rheumatica (PMR) is made if any three or more of these criteria are fulfilled. The presence of any three or more criteria yields a sensitivity of 92% and a specificity of 80%.

From Hochberg MC: *Rheumatology,* ed 7, Philadelphia, 2019, Elsevier.

BASIC INFORMATION

DEFINITION

Clinically significant portal hypertension is defined as a portal vein pressure >10 mm Hg, most commonly attributable to liver disease.

ICD-10CM CODE
K76.6 Portal hypertension

EPIDEMIOLOGY & DEMOGRAPHICS

- Incidence of portal hypertension is not known.
- Cirrhosis is the most common cause of portal hypertension in the U.S.
- Portal hypertension is developed by >90% of patients with cirrhosis.
- Alcoholic and viral liver diseases are the most common causes of cirrhosis and portal hypertension in the U.S.
- Schistosomiasis is the main cause of portal hypertension outside the U.S.
- Esophageal varices may appear when portal vein pressure rises to >10 mm Hg.
- Variceal hemorrhage is the most serious complication of portal hypertension and may occur when portal pressures rise >12 mm Hg.

PHYSICAL FINDINGS & CLINICAL PRESENTATION

- Jaundice
- Ascites (Fig. 1)
- Spider angiomata
- Testicular atrophy
- Gynecomastia
- Palmar erythema
- Dupuytren contracture
- Asterixis (with advanced liver failure)
- Irritability, encephalopathy
- Splenomegaly
- Dilated veins in the anterior abdominal wall
- Venous pattern on the flanks
- Caput medusae (tortuous collateral veins around the umbilicus)
- Hemorrhoids
- Hematemesis
- Melena
- Pruritus

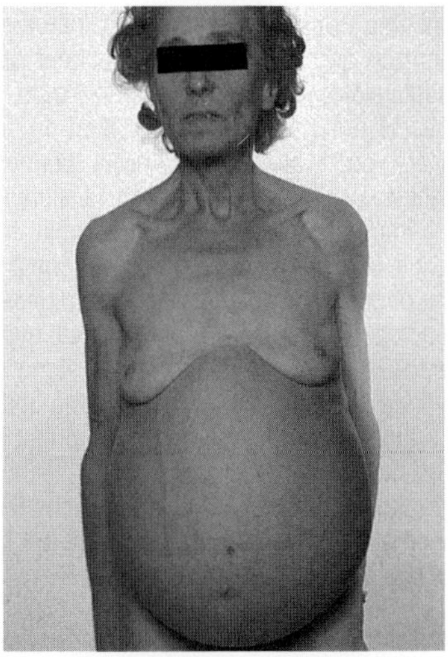

FIG. 1 Ascites secondary to portal hypertension. Note the dilated collateral vein running up the right side of the abdomen. (From Forbes A et al [eds]: *Atlas of clinical gastroenterology,* ed 3, Oxford, 2005, Mosby.)

ETIOLOGY

Pathophysiologically caused by:
- Conditions resulting in an increased resistance to flow:
  1. **Prehepatic** (e.g., portal vein thrombosis, splenic vein thrombosis, congenital stenosis)
  2. **Hepatic** (e.g., cirrhosis, alcoholic liver disease, primary biliary cirrhosis, schistosomiasis)
  3. **Posthepatic** (e.g., Budd-Chiari syndrome, constrictive pericarditis, inferior vena cava obstruction, cor pulmonale, tricuspid regurgitation)
- Conditions leading to increase in portal blood flow:
  1. Splanchnic arterial vasodilation accompanying portal hypertension, mediated by local release of nitric oxide
  2. Arterial-portal venous fistulae

Table 1 describes the pathophysiologic changes in portal hypertension and Table 2 summarizes the etiologies of portal hypertension.

DIAGNOSIS

- The diagnosis of portal hypertension is made on clinical grounds after a comprehensive history and physical examination.
- Noninvasive and invasive procedures confirm diagnosis and determine the severity of portal hypertension.

DIFFERENTIAL DIAGNOSIS

- Ascites from infection, neoplasm, or other inflammatory processes
- Obesity
- Abdominal organomegaly

WORKUP

The workup of portal hypertension includes blood tests and noninvasive imaging studies to determine if the cause of portal hypertension is prehepatic, hepatic, or posthepatic. Ascitic fluid analysis is a key part of the diagnosis.

LABORATORY TESTS

- Complete blood count with platelets
- Liver function tests with serum albumin
- Prothrombin and partial thromboplastin times
- Hepatitis B surface antigen and antibody
- Hepatitis C antibody
- In selected cases: Iron, total iron-binding capacity, and ferritin; antinuclear antibody, anti–smooth muscle antibodies, antimitochondrial antibody, ceruloplasmin, alpha-1 antitrypsin
- Ascitic fluid analysis: A serum-ascites albumin gradient ≥1.1 mg/dl suggests portal hypertension. Polymorphonuclear cells ≥250 cells/ml or positive Gram stain or culture suggest complicating spontaneous bacterial peritonitis (SBP)

IMAGING STUDIES

- Duplex-Doppler ultrasound is effective in screening for portal hypertension.
- Less commonly, CT/MRI/MRA scanning (Figs. E2 and E3) or liver-spleen nuclear medicine scanning can be used if the results from ultrasound are equivocal.
- Upper endoscopy is the most reliable test documenting the presence of esophageal varices.

TREATMENT

The treatment of portal hypertension is complex and involves measures to reduce the hypertension directly, minimize volume overload, correct underlying disorders, and prevent complications (most notably SBP and variceal bleeding).

TABLE 1 Pathophysiologic Changes in Portal Hypertension

Pathophysiologic Change	Specifics
Hepatic resistance	
	Passive, mechanical component: 60%-70%
	Active, dynamic component: 30%-40%
Portal hypertension	
Shunts	
Splanchnic vasodilation	
Increased portal inflow	
Decrease in effective circulating volume; redistribution total blood volume	
Increase in endogenous vasopressors (RAA, SNS, VP)	
	Increase in endothelin-1
	Angiotensin II
	Norepinephrine
	Vasopressin
	PGF-2 alpha
Decrease in NO, CO	

CO, Carbon monoxide; *NO,* nitrogen monoxide; *PGF,* prostaglandin; *RAA,* renin-angiotensin-aldosterone; *SNS,* sympathetic nervous system; *VP,* vasopressin.
From Vincent JL et al: *Textbook of critical care,* ed 7, Philadelphia, 2017, Elsevier.

TABLE 2 Etiology of Portal Hypertension Grouped by Location of Insult

Site of Increased Resistance	Condition	FHVP	WHVP	HVGP	SPP
Presinusoidal (extrahepatic)	Extrahepatic portal, splenic, or mesenteric vein thrombosis	Normal	Normal	Normal	Increased
Presinusoidal (intrahepatic)	Early primary biliary cirrhosis	Normal	Normal/raised (?)	Normal/raised (?)	Increased
Presinusoidal (intrahepatic)	PSC	Normal	Normal/raised (?)	Normal/raised (?)	Increased
Presinusoidal (intrahepatic)	Sarcoid	Normal	Normal/raised (?)	Normal/raised (?)	Increased
Presinusoidal (intrahepatic)	Schistosomiasis	Normal	Normal/raised (?)	Normal/raised (?)	Increased
Presinusoidal (intrahepatic)	Congestive heart failure	Normal	Normal/raised (?)	Normal/raised (?)	Increased
Presinusoidal (intrahepatic)	Noncirrhotic portal fibrosis	Normal	Normal/raised (?)	Normal/raised (?)	Increased
Intrahepatic sinusoidal	Cirrhosis (any etiology)	Normal	Increased	Increased	Increased
Intrahepatic sinusoidal	Alcoholic hepatitis	Normal	Increased	Increased	Increased
Intrahepatic sinusoidal	Fulminant liver failure (any etiology)	Normal	Increased	Increased	Increased
Extrahepatic postsinusoidal hypertension	Budd-Chiari syndrome	Increased	Increased	Normal	Increased
Extrahepatic postsinusoidal hypertension	Constrictive pericarditis	Increased	Increased	Normal	Increased
Extrahepatic postsinusoidal hypertension	Inferior vena cava obstruction	Increased	Increased	Normal	Increased
Extrahepatic postsinusoidal hypertension	Congenital inferior vena cava web	Increased	Increased	Normal	Increased
Extrahepatic postsinusoidal hypertension	Right heart failure	Increased	Increased	Normal	Increased

FHVP, Free hepatic venous pressure; *HVPG,* hepatic venous pressure gradient; *PSC,* primary sclerosing cholangitis; *SPP,* systolic pulse pressure; *WHVP,* wedged hepatic venous pressure.
From Vincent JL et al: *Textbook of critical care,* ed 7, Philadelphia, 2017, Elsevier.

NONPHARMACOLOGIC THERAPY

Dietary sodium restriction to generally 2000 mg/day forms the basis of therapy to limit fluid overload.

ACUTE GENERAL Rx

- For tense ascites, serial large-volume paracentesis (LVP) is generally recommended. The use of albumin infusion (8 to 10 g/L of ascites fluid removed) during LVP >5 L has been shown to reduce the incidence of postparacentesis circulatory dysfunction, although its use remains somewhat controversial.
- IV diuretics, typically furosemide and spironolactone, are used to achieve natriuresis and net negative salt and water balance. Renal function and serum electrolytes are monitored frequently, with transition to an oral regimen for long-term therapy.
- SBP is treated with IV antibiotics directed against enteric bacteria.
- Acute variceal hemorrhage is treated with crystalloid and blood product resuscitation, IV octreotide, terlipressin/vasopressin or somatostatin, and urgent upper endoscopy, often with sclerotherapy or band ligation. Patients with acute variceal hemorrhage should receive empiric antibiotic therapy for SBP.
- Traditionally, a transjugular intrahepatic portosystemic shunt (TIPS) or surgical shunt placement may be considered in patients not responding to above measures. However, recent data show *early* TIPS placement improved outcomes in acute variceal hemorrhage. Table 3 summarizes indications, contraindications, and complications of the TIPS procedure.
- Table 4 compares treatment modalities for portal hypertension.

CHRONIC Rx

- Dietary sodium restriction in combination with diuretics: The typical ratio of furosemide 40 mg to spironolactone 100 mg retains normal serum potassium levels in most patients.
- Nonselective beta-blockers (propranolol and nadolol) in dosages sufficient to reduce the resting heart rate by 25% have been shown to be effective in primary prophylaxis for first-time variceal bleeding and for preventing recurrent variceal bleeding. Dosages are usually given bid and decreased if heart rate falls to <55 beats/min or systolic blood pressure drops to <90 mm Hg. The addition of a long-acting nitrate (e.g., isosorbide-5-mononitrate) has been shown to improve portal hemodynamics. Findings of a prospective trial of beta-blockers to prevent the formation of varices were negative. The combination of beta-blockade plus endoscopic esophageal variceal banding is superior to either intervention alone.
- Intermittent LVP may be needed in "diuretic-resistant" patients.
- Patients with prior SBP merit lifelong antibiotics for secondary prevention.
- Abstinence from alcohol or treatment for hepatitis B or hepatitis C. Vaccination for hepatitis A and B as appropriate.
- Hepatic transplantation is an option in selected patients.

DISPOSITION

- The most common complication associated with portal hypertension is variceal bleeding. The risk of bleeding from varices is approximately 15% at 1 yr.
- Development of the hepatorenal syndrome (HRS) is associated with high near-term mortality. In particular, HRS may complicate SBP, which emphasizes the importance of making the diagnosis of SBP and instituting appropriate prophylaxis.

REFERRAL

Consultation with a gastroenterologist is recommended in all patients with portal hypertension to screen for esophageal varices.

PEARLS & CONSIDERATIONS

Splanchnic arterial vasodilation is increasingly recognized as an important component of the pathophysiology of portal hypertension and ascites. There may be vasodilation in other capillary beds as well; of note, pulmonary arteriolar vasodilation can create a significant shunt fraction and resultant hypoxemia in the absence of chest radiograph or CT chest evidence of parenchymal disease. The diagnosis is suspected when otherwise unexplained hypoxia arises in a patient with cirrhosis, along with platypnea (dyspnea worse when sitting upright) and orthodeoxia (desaturation with upright posture). The diagnosis is confirmed by echocardiography with agitated saline, in which there is delayed appearance of bubbles in the left heart after injection into a peripheral vein.

COMMENTS

Portal hypertension and its complications carry significant morbidity and mortality rates. Emphasize ethanol abstinence, provide

TABLE 3 Indications, Contraindications, and Complications of the TIPS Procedure

Indications	Relative Contraindications	Contraindications	Acute Complications	Chronic Complications
Upper GI bleeding	Pulmonary hypertension	Right-sided heart failure	Neck hematoma	Congestive heart failure
Ascites	Severe liver failure	Biliary tract obstruction	Arrhythmia	Portal vein thrombosis
Hepatic hydrothorax	Portal vein thrombosis	Uncontrolled infection	Stent displacement	Progressive liver failure
	Multiple hepatic cysts	Chronic recurrent disabling hepatic encephalopathy	Hemolysis	Chronic recurrent encephalopathy
		Hepatocellular carcinoma involving hepatic veins	Bilhemia	Stent dysfunction
			Hepatic vein obstruction	TIPSitis
			Shunt thrombosis	
			Hemoperitoneum	
			Hemobilia	
			Liver ischemia	
			Cardiac failure	
			Sepsis	

GI, Gastrointestinal; *TIPS,* transjugular intrahepatic portosystemic shunt.
From Vincent JL et al: *Textbook of critical care,* ed 7, Philadelphia, 2017, Elsevier.

TABLE 4 Comparison of Treatment Modalities

Treatment Modality	No (%), N = 77	Age, Yr (Mean)	Female %	Initial Meld (Mean, Range)	Child-Pugh Score (N = 74)	Ascites Size	Death (No, %) (N = 44)	Days from Presentation Until Death or End of Study
Medical management	64/77 (83%)	52	23/64 (36%)	16 (4-46)	A = 1 B = 31	None: 6 Small: 34 Moderate: 16 Large: 8	40/64 (63%)	321 ± 463
TIPS	8/77 (10%)	56	5/8 (63%)	12 (7-28)	A = 0 B = 5 C = 2	None: 1 Small: 3 Moderate: 3 Large: 1	4/8 (50%)	845 ± 407
Transplant	5/77 (7%)	54	0	21 (10-40)	A = 1 B = 1 C = 1	Large: 1	0	1896 ± 1752

TIPS, Transjugular intrahepatic portosystemic shunt.
From Vincent JL et al: *Textbook of critical care,* ed 7, Philadelphia, 2017, Elsevier.

vaccinations and prophylactic therapy where indicated, and consider early referral to a specialist for assistance with management and consideration for hepatic transplantation.

SUGGESTED READING

Available at ExpertConsult.com

AUTHOR: **Fred F. Ferri, MD**

BASIC INFORMATION

DEFINITION

Portal vein thrombosis (PVT) is thrombotic occlusion of the portal vein. The thrombus can also involve segments of the mesenteric veins and/or the splenic vein.

SYNONYMS

Pylethrombosis
PVT

ICD-10CM CODE
I81 Portal vein thrombosis

EPIDEMIOLOGY & DEMOGRAPHICS

- Occurs with equal frequency in children (peak age: 6 yr) and adults (peak age: 40 yr)
- Occurs in 8% to 25% of patients with decompensated cirrhosis

PHYSICAL FINDINGS & CLINICAL PRESENTATION

- Acute PVT may present with sudden onset of fever and abdominal pain (when there is mesenteric extension).
- Upper gastrointestinal hemorrhage (hematemesis and/or melena) caused by esophageal varices.

ETIOLOGY & PATHOPHYSIOLOGY

In children: Umbilical sepsis (pathophysiology unknown). In adults:

- Hypercoagulable states:
  1. Antiphospholipid syndrome
  2. Neoplasm (common cause)
  3. Paroxysmal nocturnal hemoglobinuria
  4. Myeloproliferative diseases
  5. Oral contraceptives
  6. Polycythemia vera
  7. Pregnancy
  8. Protein S or C deficiency
  9. Sickle cell disease
  10. Thrombocytosis
- Inflammatory diseases:
  1. Crohn disease
  2. Pancreatitis
  3. Ulcerative colitis
- Complications of medical intervention:
  1. Ambulatory dialysis
  2. Chemoembolization
  3. Liver transplantation
  4. Partial hepatectomy
  5. Sclerotherapy
  6. Splenectomy
  7. Transjugular intrahepatic portosystemic shunt
- Infections:
  1. Appendicitis
  2. Diverticulitis
  3. Cholecystitis
- Miscellaneous:
  1. Cirrhosis (common cause)
  2. Bladder cancer

Pathophysiology: PVT results in portal hypertension, leading to esophageal and gastrointestinal varices. The liver sustained by the hepatic artery maintains normal function.

Dx DIAGNOSIS

DIFFERENTIAL DIAGNOSIS

Causes of upper gastrointestinal hemorrhage and abdominal pain are described in Section II.

WORKUP

- Abdominal ultrasound with Doppler (Fig. 1) or MRI may show the PVT. Abdominal ultrasound color Doppler imaging has a 98% negative predictive value and is considered the imaging modality of choice in diagnosing PVT.
- Determination of underlying cirrhosis of the liver should be the foremost step. It is crucial to differentiate acute from chronic PVT because chronic PVT does not require treatment.
- Esophagogastroscopy typically shows esophageal varices.
- Laboratory evaluation for hypercoagulable state is not cost-effective in patients with cirrhosis.

Rx TREATMENT

- Anticoagulation data on thrombolytic therapy are inconclusive and there is no formal recommendation for or against anticoagulation in acute PVT. However, anticoagulation is generally recommended for patients with extension of PVT into the superior mesenteric vein to prevent intestinal infarction. In patients with chronic PVT and concomitant cirrhosis, long-term anticoagulation is generally not recommended.
- Variceal sclerotherapy or banding.
- Surgical mesocaval or splenorenal shunt.
- The roles of thrombolysis and transjugular intrahepatic portosystemic shunt continue to evolve.

REFERRAL

- To surgeon to rule out intestinal infarction
- To gastroenterologist

SUGGESTED READING
Available at ExpertConsult.com

AUTHOR: **Fred F. Ferri, MD**

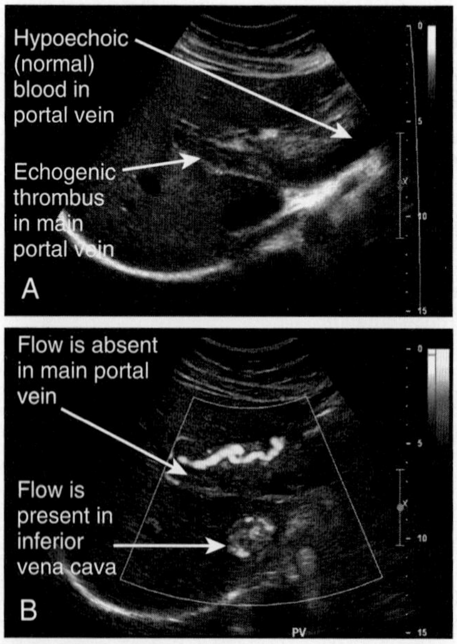

FIG. 1 Portal vein thrombosis: Ultrasound. This 22-yr-old female, 2 mo postpartum, presented with 1 wk of right upper quadrant pain. Ultrasound was performed to evaluate for suspected cholecystitis or symptomatic cholelithiasis. Instead, portal vein thrombosis was discovered. The postpartum state is a risk factor for this condition. Hypercoagulable states and inflammatory or neoplastic abdominal conditions, including pancreatitis and abdominal malignancies, also can result in portal vein thrombosis. **A,** Ultrasound gray scale image showing thrombus in the main portal vein. **B,** Doppler ultrasound showing no flow within the portal vein. (From Broder JS: *Diagnostic imaging for the emergency physician,* Philadelphia, 2011, Saunders.)

BASIC INFORMATION

DEFINITION

Postconcussion syndrome (PCS) refers to nonspecific neurologic, cognitive, and psychological symptoms that result from traumatic brain injury (TBI) and persist beyond the expected recovery period. Concussion is an acute trauma-induced alteration of mental function lasting <24 hours, with or without preceding loss of consciousness. Approximately 90% of concussion symptoms resolve within 10 to 14 days, but some may linger. The extent and severity of lingering symptoms are highly dependent on the testing and reporting used. PCS can also follow moderate and severe brain injury, although it is more commonly associated with mild brain injury or concussion.

SYNONYMS

PCS
Postconcussive syndrome
Posttraumatic nervous instability or brain injury
Postcontusion syndrome or encephalopathy
Status post commotio cerebri

ICD-10CM CODE
F07.81 Postconcussional syndrome

EPIDEMIOLOGY & DEMOGRAPHICS

- Incidence is approximately 27 cases per 100,000 persons/yr.
- From 30% to 80% of patients with mild to moderate brain injury will experience some symptoms of PCS.
- Usually reported in the young, ages 20 to 30 yr old.
- Risk factors include female sex, low socioeconomic status, anxiety sensitivity, previous TBI, severe bodily injury from TBI, headaches, and unsettled court cases.
- Recurrent TBI, especially when symptoms of previous injuries still exist, significantly increases the risk and severity of future postconcussive syndrome.
- Acute post-injury symptoms such as headache, dizziness, photophobia, diplopia, or tinnitus are associated with development of persistent symptoms.

PHYSICAL FINDINGS & CLINICAL PRESENTATION

- Symptoms start within a few days to weeks after the head injury and usually persist after 3 mo; 15% of patients or more will have persistent symptoms 1 yr later.
- At least three of the following symptoms after TBI are required to meet ICD-10 criteria:
  1. Headache (usually of frontooccipital location and showing characteristics of tension or migraine headache). The International Headache Society suggests that coding and attribution of headaches with characteristics of primary headaches but in the setting of an inciting event should be attributed to the event, unless there was a known history of the headache and the inciting event was seen as aggravating/initiating the preexisting migraine/tension headache.
  2. Fatigue
  3. Dizziness and/or vertigo
  4. Impaired memory
  5. Difficulty in concentrating
  6. Insomnia
  7. Irritability/frustration
  8. Lowered tolerance of stress, emotion, or alcohol
- Other associated symptoms: Noise sensitivity, neck pain, nondermatomal paresthesias, interference with social role functioning.
- Focal neurologic deficits are typically absent on examination.

ETIOLOGY

- The inciting TBI may occur as a result of events such as falls, motor vehicle accidents, military injuries, and contact sports.
- The primary injury triggers a slew of pathophysiological changes at the cellular level secondary to the axonal stretching and injury, leading to alterations in membrane and intracellular physiology, thereby affecting neurotransmission. These changes are believed to be a factor in determining whether the outcome will be an apparent normal recovery or persistent postconcussion symptoms.
- Postmortem findings reveal diffuse axonal injury as the primary pathologic finding, along with small petechial hemorrhages and local edema.
- Prior history of anxiety is a strong risk factor for occurrence of PCS.

Dx DIAGNOSIS

A careful history, a nonfocal neurologic examination, and normal neurologic testing will usually establish the diagnosis.

DIFFERENTIAL DIAGNOSIS

- Headache (dissection of the vertebral artery, occipital neuralgia)
- Epidural hematoma
- Subdural hematoma
- Skull fracture
- Cervical spine disk disease
- Whiplash
- Cerebrovascular accident
- Benign paroxysmal positional vertigo—common after head injury
- Depression
- Anxiety
- Posttraumatic stress disorder

WORKUP

- Neuropsychological testing, which often reveals difficulties in concentration, memory, language, and executive function
- To exclude other causes of neurologic symptoms after TBI:
  1. Normal results of electroencephalography
  2. Normal evoked potentials

LABORATORY TESTS

Various biomarkers in blood and cerebrospinal fluid and genetic testing have been proposed and studied in patients with TBI, but these tests are not specific and are not routinely used in clinical practice.

IMAGING STUDIES

- There is no imaging modality to diagnose PCS. PCS is primarily a clinical diagnosis. The American College of Emergency Physicians' clinical policy regarding neuroimaging in adults with mild traumatic brain injury is summarized in Box 1.
- 10% of CT scans of the head following mild TBI are abnormal, showing mild subarachnoid hemorrhage, subdural hemorrhage, or contusions.

BOX 1 American College of Emergency Physicians' Clinical Policy Regarding Neuroimaging in Adults with Mild Traumatic Brain Injury

A noncontrast head CT is indicated (level one recommendation) in adults with LOC or posttraumatic amnesia only if at least one of the following is present:
- Headache
- Vomiting
- Age older than 60 yr
- Drug or alcohol intoxication
- Deficits in short-term memory
- Physical evidence of trauma above the clavicle
- Posttraumatic seizure
- GCS score below 15
- Focal neurologic deficit
- Coagulopathy

A noncontrast head CT should be considered (level two recommendation) in head trauma patients with no LOC or posttraumatic amnesia if any of the following is present:
- Focal neurologic deficit
- Vomiting
- Severe headache
- Age 65 yr or older
- Physical signs of a basilar skull fracture
- GCS score below 15
- Coagulopathy
- A dangerous mechanism (e.g., ejection from motor vehicle, pedestrian struck, fall of more than 3 feet or 5 stairs)

CT, Computed tomography; *GCS,* Glasgow Coma Scale; *LOC,* loss of consciousness.
From Marx J et al: *Rosen's emergency medicine: concepts and clinical practice,* ed 7, Philadelphia, 2010, Mosby.

- MRI of the head after a mild traumatic brain injury (mTBI) is abnormal in 30% of patients with normal CT scans and may show irregular brain contours or old cerebral contusions.
- More advanced imaging modalities, including diffuse tensor imaging (DTI) and susceptibility weighted imaging (SWI) in MRI, functional MRI (fMRI), and metabolic imaging such as magnetic resonance spectroscopy (MRS), positron emission tomography (PET), and single-photon emission computed tomography (SPECT) imaging, can show acute and chronic changes even after one mTBI, although they have not found a major role in clinical practice yet.
- None of the imaging modalities have been able to predict the occurrence of PCS in patients with mild TBI.

Rx TREATMENT

PCS must be recognized as a physiologic and psychological problem and treated accordingly. Treatment should be individualized to target the patient's particular symptoms and is typically completed on an outpatient basis. Some symptoms may be refractory to treatment.

NONPHARMACOLOGIC THERAPY

- Early reassurance and patient education are major components of treatment. Explanation of symptoms and expectations, combined with early follow-up with reassurance, may hasten resolution of symptoms.
- Early and graduated physical activity is preferred over prolonged cognitive and physical rest. Light aerobic activity that avoids risk for reinjury has been shown beneficial in mitigating refractory concussion symptoms. Physical and occupational therapy may be beneficial.
- Cognitive behavioral therapy may be effective in treating symptoms.
- Avoidance of alcohol, narcotics, and sleep deprivation.

PHARMACOLOGIC THERAPY

- Supportive symptomatic care may include the use of nonnarcotic analgesics and antiemetics.
- Amitriptyline has been widely used for posttraumatic tension-type headaches as well as for nonspecific symptoms such as irritability, dizziness, insomnia, and depression. Amantadine is also a consideration.
- Posttraumatic migraine-type headaches can be treated with a trial of propranolol or amitriptyline alone or in combination.
- Depression can be treated with selective serotonin reuptake inhibitors but may not respond as well when compared with patients without PCS who have depression.

DISPOSITION

- Most patients improve after mild TBI without any residual deficits within 3 mo, though the cognitive and emotional symptoms resolve more slowly.
- Although good improvement is typically seen within the first 6 mo, patients can continue to show improvement for up to 12 to 18 mo.
- Patients with very severe brain injuries (low Glasgow Coma Scale [GCS] score) and prolonged anterograde amnesia are at increased risk of development of some degree of permanent cognitive and personality disturbance.
- Predictors for the development of persistent PCS include:
  1. Female sex
  2. Ongoing litigation (conflicting studies)
  3. Low socioeconomic status
  4. Prior headaches
  5. Prior TBI
  6. Prior psychiatric illnesses, particularly anxiety

REFERRAL

Early consultations with psychologists, psychiatrists, neurologists, and rehabilitation specialists in an outpatient setting may be beneficial.

PEARLS & CONSIDERATIONS

- PCS starts within a few days after the injury.
- Recognizing depression and treating pain symptoms early in the course may help prevent the development of persistent PCS (>1 yr).
- The severity of the trauma does not clearly predict the risk of PCS and symptoms do not cluster in a predictable manner.
- The severity of brain injury is usually documented by initial GCS score, duration of loss of consciousness, and duration of amnesia; however, there is a move toward tests of function, such as neuropsychological testing or fMRI.

COMMENTS

- Attempts to determine how much of a role psychological and/or neurologic factors play in PCS are important but very difficult.
- No medication at hospital discharge has been proved to change the natural course of the disease.
- Engaging in physical activity within 2 days after concussion is associated with a lower rate of persistent postconcussive symptoms.

RELATED CONTENT

Post-concussion Syndrome (Patient Information)
Concussion (Related Key Topic)
Traumatic Brain Injury (Related Key Topic)

AUTHORS: **Chloe Mander Nunneley, MD,** and **Corey Goldsmith, MD**

BASIC INFORMATION

DEFINITION

Postherpetic neuralgia (PHN) is a pain syndrome that results as a complication of herpes zoster (HZ). HZ, also known as shingles, is a painful vesicular eruption in a dermatomal distribution. HZ is caused by the reactivation of varicella zoster virus (VZV) in someone with a known history of varicella. PHN is pain and/or dysesthesia that persist for 3 or more mo at the site of resolved HZ.

ICD-10CM CODE

B02.29 Other postherpetic nervous system involvement

EPIDEMIOLOGY & DEMOGRAPHICS

INCIDENCE: PHN occurs in approximately 9% to 34% of HZ patients. It is the most frequent chronic complication of herpes zoster and the most common neuropathic pain disorder resulting from infection. In one study, approximately 60% of patients with HZ developed PHN at age 60 yr, and 75% developed PHN at age 70 yr. In another study, the incidence of PHN at 9 yr post-HZ eruption was 21%.

PEAK INCIDENCE: Unknown

PREDOMINANT SEX & AGE:

- PHN occurs equally in males and females.
- The likelihood of developing PHN significantly increases with advancing age.

GENETICS: Family history of HZ is considered a risk factor for HZ, with higher risk if multiple family members have had HZ.

RISK FACTORS:

- Advanced age
- Greater severity of HZ prodromal pain
- Greater severity of pain during acute HZ eruption
- Location—specifically ophthalmic (V1) location and brachial plexus
- Severe immunosuppression

PHYSICAL FINDINGS & CLINICAL PRESENTATION

- HZ typically presents as a painful vesicular eruption in a dermatomal distribution. Rarely, HZ can occur subclinically with dermatomal pain in the absence of a rash.
- PHN is pain that continues for 3 mo at the dermatomal site of the resolved HZ. The pain may be described as burning, stabbing, shooting, or shock-like.
- Patients may note an amplified response to stimuli at the site of PHN, with increased pain response (hyperalgesia), pain to typically nonnoxious stimuli (allodynia), or focal changes in autonomic function (e.g., increased sweating).
- Physical examination should include a comparison of sensory function in the affected dermatome with that on the contralateral side.

ETIOLOGY

PHN is associated with damage and scarring to the dorsal root ganglion secondary to inflammation related to active herpes zoster infection.

DIAGNOSIS

DIFFERENTIAL DIAGNOSIS

Zoster sine herpete (subclinical HZ without skin eruption)

TREATMENT

ACUTE GENERAL Rx

- Administration of acyclovir or valacyclovir within 72 hours of HZ onset is thought to help reduce the likelihood of developing PNH. However, one Cochrane review paper found no difference with acyclovir administration.
- A single published study supports the use of amitriptyline (25 mg daily) as an adjunct to an antiviral agent in acute HZ to decrease the incidence of PHN and the pain associated with subsequent PHN.
- A suggestive noncontrolled study with co-administration of valacyclovir and gabapentin during acute HZ reduced the incidence of PHN as well.
- Corticosteroids do NOT prevent PHN.

CHRONIC Rx

TOPICAL TREATMENTS:

- Lidocaine 5% patches may be used for mild pain.
- Capsaicin 0.075% cream (although little reported efficacy) 5 times per day.
- Capsaicin 8% patch has greater efficacy, but overall analgesia may be minimal at best, with one third of patients unable to tolerate the agent due to burning, stinging, and erythema. However, a single 60-minute treatment with high concentration capsaicin patch was found in one study to reduce PHN for up to 12 wk regardless of concomitant systemic neuropathic pain medication use.

ORAL TREATMENTS: First line:

- Gabapentinoids (gabapentin, pregabalin) are the only FDA-approved oral therapy for PHN and are some of the most commonly used first-line therapies for chronic PHN pain. Gabapentin may be administered in the immediate-release or extended-release formulation. Dosing includes gabapentin 300 mg 3 times a day (titrating up to max 3600 mg/day) and pregabalin 75 mg nightly (titrating up to 300 mg twice daily).
- Tricyclic antidepressants such as amitriptyline (25 mg/day, increased by 25 mg every night to a maximum of 75 mg/night), desipramine (10-25 mg/day, increased by 25 mg/day every 3 days as needed to a maximum of 150 mg/day), and nortriptyline (10-25 mg/day, increased by 25 mg/day weekly as needed to maximum of 75 mg day) are other first-line treatments. These medications have a delayed onset of action and may not work as well in patients with certain types of pain, such as burning pain or allodynia. They have a considerable side effect profile. Their use in elderly patients should be carefully considered. A recent study showed the combination of gabapentin and nortriptyline was more efficacious than either drug as monotherapy for neuropathic pain.

Second line:

- Opiates (e.g., controlled-release oxycodone): Side effects, the possibility of misuse, and the potential for abuse must be weighed.

Other modalities:

- Dorsal root entry zone (DREZ) lesions have been used with an improvement rate of 20% in long-term studies.
- For recalcitrant cases, epidural corticosteroids and nerve blocks, botulinum toxin, and cryotherapy.
- Fig. 1 describes a treatment algorithm for HZ and PHN.

COMPLEMENTARY & ALTERNATIVE MEDICINE

Acupuncture: Studies on acupuncture and PHN pain have had varying results; however, the only randomized, controlled study showed no significant difference in pain reduction between control and treatment groups.

REFERRAL

For complicated cases, dermatology, neurology, and/or pain management input can be helpful.

PEARLS & CONSIDERATIONS

COMMENTS

- Careful consideration of treatment side effects and drug interactions is needed.
- The natural history of PHN is slow resolution, and most individuals respond to medical therapy. However, a subtype of patients may develop severe, long-lasting pain that is recalcitrant to medical therapy.
- In a questionnaire study of 385 adults age >65 yr with persistent acute pain, the mean duration of PHN was 3.3 yr.

PREVENTION

- Vaccination:
  1. A nonlive VZV vaccine (Shingrix®) is approved by the FDA for individuals age 50 and older. It is administered as two shots spaced 2 mo apart and is 97% effective against shingles in people ages 50 to 69, and 91% effective against PHN in people 50 and older. It is more effective than the live attenuated VZV vaccine (zostvax).
  2. The CDC recommends that those who received Zostavax be revaccinated with Shingrix.

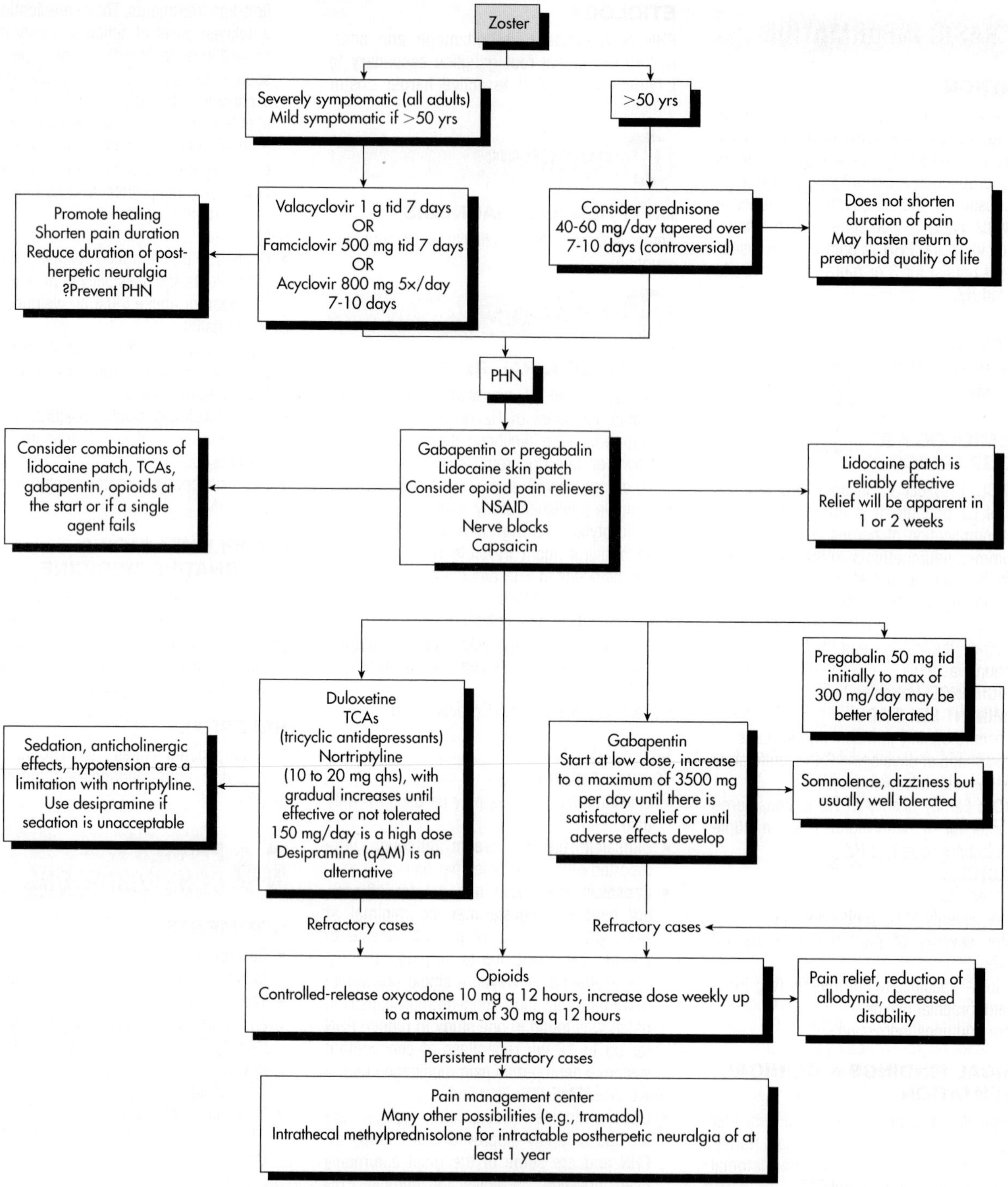

FIG. 1 Treatment of herpes zoster and postherpetic neuralgia. *NSAID,* Nonsteroidal antiinflammatory drug; *PHN,* postherpetic neuralgia. (Modified from Habif TA: *Clinical dermatology,* ed 6, St Louis, 2016, Elsevier.)

3. Those who have had HZ should still receive the vaccine.

PATIENT & FAMILY EDUCATION

- The only well-documented means of preventing PHN is the prevention of herpes zoster through vaccination.
- Patients should understand both the benefits and the potential adverse effects of treatment.
  1. They should be informed that pain relief will likely not be immediate.
  2. Frequent reassessment may be needed, and drug doses should be increased as necessary.

SUGGESTED READINGS

Available at ExpertConsult.com

RELATED CONTENT

Herpes Zoster (Related Key Topic)

AUTHOR: **Lisa Pappas-Taffer, MD**

BASIC INFORMATION

DEFINITION

Major or minor depressive episodes that are severe enough to affect activities of daily living and occur most commonly within 1 to 3 wk after delivery but can also present up to 12 mo postpartum.

SYNONYMS

Spectrum of disease presentation
Postpartum blues
Postpartum depression
Postpartum psychosis

ICD-10CM CODES	
F53	Includes postpartum depression and postpartum psychosis
090.6	Includes postpartum blues, postpartum dysphoria and sadness

EPIDEMIOLOGY & DEMOGRAPHICS

INCIDENCE: Approximately 800,000 women who deliver in the U.S. or 20% of all live births are affected by postpartum depression annually.
PREVALENCE: Perinatal depression affects approximately 10% to 15% of women.
RISK FACTORS: Risk factors include depression or anxiety during pregnancy, traumatic birth experiences, stressful life events during pregnancy or the postpartum period, infant NICU admission or preterm delivery, poor social support, history of depression, and problems with breastfeeding.
GENETICS: A family history of mood disorders is a risk factor for postpartum depression.

PHYSICAL FINDINGS & CLINICAL PRESENTATION

Patients present with depressed or irritable mood, decreased interest in activities, appetite and sleep changes, weight changes, decreased energy, excessive guilt or feelings of worthlessness, psychomotor agitation or retardation, and possibly suicidal/homicidal ideation. The diagnosis of major depressive episode requires that symptoms be present nearly every day for 2 wk and that the woman experiences a decline from a previous level of functioning.

ETIOLOGY

The decline in reproductive hormones following delivery is believed to contribute to the development of postpartum depression in some women. In addition, women with a history of depression, premenstrual syndrome or dysphoric disorder, stressful life events, and a family history of mood disorders have an increased risk of both depression and postpartum depression.

DIAGNOSIS

DIFFERENTIAL DIAGNOSIS

- Hyperthyroid
- Hypothyroid
- Postpartum blues: Syndrome involving symptoms of depression, anxiety, or anger that usually occurs 2 to 3 days after delivery and resolves within a few days to 1 to 2 wk postpartum without treatment
- Postpartum psychosis: Usually occurs between 1 to 2 wk postdelivery and is characterized by extreme disorganization of thought, hallucinations, and bizarre behavior. It requires rapid intervention, as there is a real risk of suicide or infanticide
- Bipolar disorder

WORKUP

- History and physical examination
- Screening all postpartum women with a screening instrument such as the Edinburgh Postnatal Depression Scale (specific to the postpartum period and takes less than 5 min to complete) or the Patient Health Questionnaire-9
- In any patient with postpartum depression, screening for bipolar disorder

LABORATORY TESTS

Thyroid screening tests (if high suspicion for thyroid disorder)

TREATMENT

NONPHARMACOLOGIC THERAPY

Psychotherapy: Studies have shown psychotherapy to be equally effective to fluoxetine.

ACUTE GENERAL Rx

- Therapy with a selective serotonin reuptake inhibitor should be considered as first-line treatment because of low risk of toxic effects with overdose and ease of dosing. However, if the patient has had good success with another medication in the past, then it is appropriate to restart that medication. Start at half the recommended dose and increase after 4 days, with gradual up-titration until therapeutic effects are seen.
- A single medication is favored over multiple medications in order to decrease exposure to the fetus/neonate.
- Sertraline is the first-line selective serotonin reuptake inhibitor recommended for breastfeeding mothers secondary to existing evidence suggesting little risk for infants. There is, however, no evidence of adverse infant effects from mothers taking sertraline, paroxetine, or fluvoxamine. Fluoxetine may be present in higher levels in breast milk and breastfed infants.
- Tricyclic antidepressants do not appear to pass in significant amounts into breastfeeding infants and their use appears to be safe. Data regarding atypical antidepressants and breastfeeding are limited.
- The FDA recently approved an IV infusion of the drug brexanolone (Zulresso). It is administered as a single 60-hr IV drip and is currently only available to patients through a restricted distribution program at certified health care facilities.

CHRONIC Rx

- Medical therapy should be continued until at least 6 mo after remission.
- Long-term therapy should be considered for women with a history of three or more episodes of depression.

DISPOSITION

- Without treatment, the duration of postpartum depression averages 7 mo.
- 15% to 85% of women will experience at least one relapse after completing medical therapy.

REFERRAL

- Consider referral to psychiatrist if a patient demonstrates no improvement after 6 wk of drug therapy or experiences a relapse.
- Prompt or urgent referral to psychiatrist is indicated if a patient has signs/symptoms of postpartum psychosis, bipolar disorder, or expresses suicidal/homicidal ideation.

PEARLS & CONSIDERATIONS

COMMENTS

- Depression and anxiety both during and after pregnancy can have negative effects not only on the mother but also on her fetus, new baby, and family. Low birth weight, decreased fetal growth, increased NICU admission rates, increased neonate crying, and decreased developmental scores have been seen with these disorders when untreated. In addition, depression is associated with increased smoking, alcohol, and drug use, which can have negative effects on the infant and family. These factors should be taken into account when counseling women about medical therapy.
- Selective serotonin reuptake inhibitors do pass through breast milk but are present in very small quantities compared with the transplacental exposure infants receive in utero. Adverse infant effects are extremely rare; however, long-term data are lacking.

PREVENTION

In a patient with a history of postpartum depression, recurrence risk is approximately 25%. These patients should be screened for depression both during and after pregnancy. It is reasonable to initiate prophylactic therapy in patients with a history of depression, and they should have close postpartum follow-up for early identification of depressive episodes.

PATIENT & FAMILY EDUCATION

- National Women's Health Information Center: www.womenshealth.gov
- Postpartum Support International: www.postpartum.net
- Centers for Disease Control and Prevention: www.cdc.gov/reproductivehealth/depression/

SUGGESTED READINGS

Available at ExpertConsult.com

RELATED CONTENT

Depression, Major (Related Key Topic)

AUTHOR: **Anthony Sciscione, DO**

BASIC INFORMATION

DEFINITION

Postpartum hemorrhage (PPH) is defined, for both vaginal and cesarean deliveries, as an estimated blood loss ≧1000 ml OR blood loss resulting in signs/symptoms of hypovolemia within 24 hr following delivery. PPH is further categorized into primary or secondary. Primary PPH occurs within the first 24 hr after delivery. Secondary PPH occurs >24 hr after delivery but within 12 wk following delivery.

SYNONYMS

Obstetric hemorrhage
Maternal hemorrhage
PPH

ICD-10CM CODES

072.0	Third stage hemorrhage
072.1	Other immediate postpartum hemorrhage
072.2	Delayed and secondary postpartum hemorrhage
072.3	Postpartum coagulation defects

EPIDEMIOLOGY & DEMOGRAPHICS

INCIDENCE: Depending on definitions used and scope considered, anywhere from 1% to 6% of obstetric patients will experience postpartum hemorrhage. Postpartum hemorrhage is the leading cause of maternal mortality worldwide and is implicated in >10% of maternal deaths in the U.S.

PREDOMINANT SEX & AGE: Female of reproductive age

RISK FACTORS:

- Antepartum factors: History of PPH, primiparity or high parity, macrosomic infant, multiple gestation, polyhydramnios, uterine fibroids, prior uterine surgery, abnormal placentation, bleeding disorder
- Intrapartum factors: Prolonged labor, augmented labor, rapid labor, preeclampsia, chorioamnionitis, operative delivery, episiotomy, lacerations, retained products, placental abruption, fetal demise

PHYSICAL FINDINGS & CLINICAL PRESENTATION (TABLE 1)

- Bleeding is generally brisk at time of delivery.
- Examination findings can include a boggy uterus with continued passage of clot or blood with fundal pressure.
- Objective findings can also include hypotension, tachycardia, and oliguria with substantial blood loss.

ETIOLOGY

- Primary: Uterine atony (70%-80%), retained placenta, lacerations, and coagulopathies
- Secondary: Subinvolution of placental site, retained products (includes abnormal placentation), infection, and coagulopathies

DIAGNOSIS

WORKUP

- Bimanual examination to evaluate for atony; remove clots; massage if it is present
- Bladder should be emptied
- Examination to verify that placenta is intact
- Ensure adequate IV access
- Consider ultrasonography at bedside to evaluate for retained tissue or clot
- Examination to verify that no lacerations are present, including cervical examination with necessary lighting and retractors (may require examination in OR for adequate exposure)

LABORATORY TESTS

Significant hemorrhage can lead to disseminated intravascular coagulation (DIC). If DIC is suspected, complete blood count and coagulation panels should be ordered. Similarly, if coagulopathy is suspected, evaluation of clotting factors should be ordered. Thromboelastography (TEG) is a useful test to guide product replacement in association with coagulation cascade dysfunction.

IMAGING STUDIES

Ultrasonography can be used to scan for retained products, including clot or placenta. It can be performed to assess the need for more invasive measures, such as instrumentation or a manual sweep.

TREATMENT

The most effective strategy for the prevention of postpartum hemorrhage is active management of the third stage of labor (AMTSL). Medical management with uterotonics is generally the first line of treatment. None of the following medications has been demonstrated to be superior in treating PPH compared with the others.

- Oxytocin (IV, 10-40 units diluted into IV solution, or 10 units IM); often given prophylactically immediately after delivery to minimize EBL with delivery of placenta
- Methergine (IM, 0.2 mg)—contraindicated in hypertensive patient
- Hemabate (IM, 0.25 mcg)—contraindicated in patient with history of asthma
- Misoprostol (400-800 mcg sublingually, buccally, or rectally)

Other medical management:

- Tranexamic acid (IV, 1 g)

NONPHARMACOLOGIC THERAPY

- Active management of third stage of labor: Controlled cord traction (Brandt-Andrews maneuver) and uterine massage after delivery of placenta (in addition to Pitocin)
- Uterine tamponade (Fig. E1): Packing with gauze, Foley catheter, or tamponade balloon (Bakri)
- Uterine curettage for suspected retained products
- Uterine artery embolization
- Surgical management with laparotomy:
  1. Hypogastric artery ligation
  2. Bilateral uterine artery ligation (O'Leary sutures)
  3. B-lynch sutures
  4. Hysterectomy

ACUTE GENERAL Rx

- Uterotonics, surgical management, embolization, blood transfusion. Fig. E2 outlines the management of postpartum hemorrhage.
- Table 2 describes therapeutic response to initial fluid resuscitation. Dosing regimen for oxytocic drugs is summarized in Table 3. Blood product replacement is described in Box 1.

TABLE 1 Presentation of Symptoms in Postpartum Hemorrhage

% Blood loss (ml)	Systolic blood pressure (mm Hg)	Signs and symptoms
10-15 (500-1000)	Normal	Tachycardia, palpitations, dizziness
15-25 (1000-1500)	Low-normal	Tachycardia, weakness, diaphoresis
25-35 (1500-2000)	70-80	Restlessness, pallor, oliguria
35-45 (2000-3000)	50-70	Collapse, air hunger, anuria

From Vincent JL et al: *Textbook of critical care,* ed 6, Philadelphia, 2011, Saunders.

TABLE 2 Therapeutic Response to Initial Fluid Resuscitation

Response	Description	Follow-up treatment
Rapid response	<20% of blood volume lost	No additional fluids or blood are needed.
Transient response	20%-40% of blood volume lost; responds to initial fluid bolus but later has worsening vital signs	Continue fluids and consider blood transfusions.
Minimal or no response	Ongoing severe hemorrhage with >40% blood volume lost	Continue aggressive fluid and blood product replacements.

From Vincent JL et al: *Textbook of critical care,* ed 6, Philadelphia, 2011, Saunders.

TABLE 3 Dosing Regimens for Oxytocic Drugs

Drugs	Regimens
Oxytocin (Pitocin)	5-unit IV bolus
	Add 20-40 units oxytocin to 1 L of fluids for continuous infusion
	10 units intramyometrially
Methylergonovine (Methergine)	0.2 mg IM every 2-4 h
Ergonovine maleate (Ergotrate)	100-125 μg IM or intramyometrially every 2-4 h
	200-250 μg IM
	Total dose 1.25 mg
Carboprost (Hemabate)	250 μg IM or intramyometrially every 15-90 min
	Total dose 2 mg (8 doses maximum)
Misoprostol	800-1000 μg PR, oral, or sublingual

IM, Intramuscular; *IV,* intravenous; *PR,* per rectum.
From Vincent JL et al: *Textbook of critical care,* ed 7, Philadelphia, 2017, Elsevier.

CHRONIC Rx

For anemia (Hb <10 g/dl) – Ferrous sulfate and ascorbic acid supplementation to support new red blood cell production. Can also consider IV iron replacement.

DISPOSITION

- The patient should be closely watched for at least 24 hr after a postpartum hemorrhage. Vital signs should be monitored for evidence of hemodynamic stability and appropriate response to anemia. Serial laboratory tests can be performed in the setting of concern for ongoing bleeding.
- Morbidity can include: Shock, acute respiratory distress syndrome, Sheehan syndrome, thromboembolic disease, and loss of fertility.
- For cases with large blood loss (e.g., >2 L) and hemodynamic instability, intensive care unit admission may be warranted.

REFERRAL

During the course of a postpartum hemorrhage, the anesthesiology department, blood bank, and OR staff should be notified, and adequate nursing should be available. Early considerations should be made to notify obstetricians. If bleeding is brisk or estimated blood loss is considerable, preparation should be made for transfusion of blood products, including drawing blood for typing and notifying the blood bank.

PEARLS & CONSIDERATIONS

PREVENTION

- Active management of third stage of labor
- Implementation of institution-specific PPH risk assessment tools effective for identifying patients at increased risk, though clinical suspicion should be maintained in all patients

BOX 1 Blood Product Replacement

Crossmatched blood.
Type-specific or "saline crossmatched" blood.
Compatible ABO and Rh blood types.
Rh-negative blood is preferable.
- Warm the blood, if possible, especially if the rate of infusion is >100 ml/min or if the total volume transfused is high; cold blood is associated with an increased incidence of arrhythmias and paradoxic hypotension.
- Administer calcium if blood is transfused rapidly at >100 ml/min because of binding of calcium by anticoagulants in banked blood.
- Give 6-10 units fresh frozen plasma (FFP) for every 10 units of packed red blood cell (PRBC) transfusions.

Give 10-12 units of platelets if the platelet count decreases to <50 × 10^9/L.
Cryoprecipitate can be given to replace fibrinogen in addition to the FFP.
Consider 60-120 μg/kg intravenous bolus injection of recombinant activated factor VII (rFVIIa).

From Vincent JL et al: *Textbook of critical care,* ed 7, Philadelphia, 2017, Elsevier.

SUGGESTED READINGS

Available at ExpertConsult.com

AUTHORS: **Anthony Sciscione, DO,** and **Scott J. Merrill, MD**

BASIC INFORMATION

DEFINITION

Postthrombotic syndrome (PTS) is a delayed complication of deep vein thrombosis (DVT) that leads to signs and symptoms of venous insufficiency.

SYNONYMS

Postphlebitic syndrome
Chronic venous insufficiency
PTS

ICD-10CM CODES

I87.001	Postthrombotic syndrome without complications of right lower extremity
I87.002	Postthrombotic syndrome without complications of left lower extremity
I87.003	Postthrombotic syndrome without complications of bilateral lower extremities

EPIDEMIOLOGY & DEMOGRAPHICS

INCIDENCE: 23% to 60% of people with DVT will experience postthrombotic syndrome, often within 2 yr of onset of DVT.
PREVALENCE: Unknown
PREDOMINANT SEX: Slightly female predominance
RISK FACTORS: Symptomatic DVT, postoperative DVT, recurrent DVT, underlying primary venous insufficiency, older age, obesity, presence of varicose veins, proximal DVT, residual thrombus after 6 mo of treatment, and inadequate antithrombotic treatment

PHYSICAL FINDINGS & CLINICAL PRESENTATION

Symptoms can be intermittent or constant and often appear weeks to months following DVT, but can occur up to years later. Symptoms are generally progressive over time and include pain in the extremity, heaviness of effected limb, itching, cramps, and paresthesia. Physical signs include edema of extremity, changes in skin pigmentation, venous dilation, telangiectasia, and ulceration (Fig. E1).

ETIOLOGY

Venous insufficiency results from chronic venous hypertension due to obstruction from thrombus and to reflux related to valvular incompetence. Inflammatory cytokines such as interleukin-6 are thought to play a role.

DIAGNOSIS

DIFFERENTIAL DIAGNOSIS

DVT, primary venous insufficiency, Baker cyst, tumor, lymphedema, lipedema, and injury to extremity.

WORKUP

Clinical diagnosis based on history of DVT and signs and symptoms of chronic venous insufficiency. The Villalta scale can be used in cases when the diagnosis is uncertain. It is the most widely used scoring system for both diagnosing PTS and assessing its severity.

- Entails five patient symptoms (pain, leg cramps, heaviness in extremity, paresthesia, and pruritus) and six physical signs (pretibial edema, skin induration, hyperpigmentation, pain with calf compression, venous ectasia, and redness).
- Scored on a scale of 0 to 3 (0 = none, 1 = mild, 2 = moderate, 3 = severe).
- Total score ranges from 0 to 33; a score ≥5 is consistent with a diagnosis of PTS.
  1. PTS can also be diagnosed if a venous ulcer is present independent of total score.
- Severity is assessed based on score:
  1. Mild = score of 5 to 9
  2. Moderate = score of 10 to 14
  3. Severe = score of 15 to 33

LABORATORY TESTS

None presently used

IMAGING TESTS

Venous duplex ultrasonography or compression ultrasonography can be done to look for prior evidence of DVT but is not necessary to make the diagnosis.

Rx TREATMENT

- First-line treatment includes compression stockings, regular exercise, and elevation of extremity.
- Lymphedema therapy and intermittent pneumatic compression devices can be used as well.
- Skin care is important, particularly in cases with eczematous changes. Moisturizing lotions can be used in conjunction with mild potency corticosteroids.
- Diuretics have a limited role but can decrease edema in some patients.
- No evidence that new oral anticoagulation medications work better than warfarin or low-molecular-weight heparin at preventing PTS.
- Endovascular recanalization can be considered for cases that are refractory to treatment and where pain control is difficult. Two randomized controlled trials have been done to study the benefits.
  1. A 2007 randomized controlled trial, Catheter Directed Venous Thrombolysis in Acute Iliofemoral Vein Thrombosis, sought to answer the question of whether early endovascular recanalization would reduce long-term venous disease or improve quality of life. After 2 yr of follow up, there was no significant difference between groups with respect to either primary end point.
  2. A second trial, Acute Venous Thrombosis: Thrombus Removal with Adjunctive Catheter-Directed Thrombolysis (ATTRACT), was a randomized multicenter trial conducted to assess whether catheter-directed thrombolysis (CDT) along with a device that aspirates and breaks down thrombus was superior to standard therapy at preventing postthrombotic syndrome. However, no significant difference was found between groups (47% in the treatment group vs 48% in the control group developed PTS; risk ratio, 0.96; 95% confidence interval, 0.82 to 1.1; P=0.56).
- The American College of Cardiology does not recommend routine use of CDT as first-line treatment but states it may be useful for patients at low risk of bleeding or for those with limb-threatening complications.
- Surgical repair is generally reserved for severe cases causing acute limb-threatening circulatory compromise and for those with nonhealing ulcers. Surgical options include angioplasty, venous bypass, or endophlebectomy.

DISPOSITION

- Chronic venous insufficiency can impair quality of life and is often a chronic condition.
- Early treatment with anticoagulation may decrease the risk of postthrombotic syndrome.
- Early use of compression stockings can reduce symptoms of venous insufficiency and halt progression.

REFERRAL

Lymphedema clinic, interventional radiology, and vascular surgery

PEARLS & CONSIDERATIONS

COMMENTS

Compression stockings have the most evidence both for preventing postthrombotic syndrome and for treatment once the syndrome has developed.

PREVENTION

There is evidence both for and against early treatment with thrombolytic drugs to prevent postthrombotic syndrome. Reducing the recurrence of DVT is the best way to prevent PTS. With each subsequent DVT the risk of PTS increases. Periodic leg elevation, weight loss, smoking cessation, and regular exercise are all thought to prevent PTS; however, no randomized controlled trial has been done to evaluate.

SUGGESTED READINGS

Available at ExpertConsult.com

RELATED CONTENT

Deep Vein Thrombosis (Related Key Topic)
Venous Insufficiency, Chronic (Related Key Topic)

AUTHOR: **Lynn Dado, MD**

BASIC INFORMATION

DEFINITION

Posttraumatic stress disorder (PTSD) is a syndrome that develops in a significant minority of people after witnessing or experiencing a traumatic event that involves actual or threatened harm to the self or others. Symptoms continue longer than 1 mo after the event, or may have delayed onset, and include intrusive, distressing memories; nightmares; dissociation (such as flashbacks); avoidance of reminders; hyperarousal; and negatively altered mood and cognition. These symptoms cause distress and a decline in interpersonal, social, and occupational functioning. People with PTSD may feel numb or irritable, may be easily startled or frightened, and often isolate themselves from others. They are at high risk for comorbid psychiatric illness, substance abuse, and suicide.

SYNONYMS

PTSD
Soldier's heart (Civil War–era term)
Shell shock (World War I–era term)
Battle fatigue or combat neurosis
Concentration camp syndrome

ICD-10CM CODES	
F43.10	Post-traumatic stress disorder, unspecified
F43.11	Post-traumatic stress disorder, acute
F43.12	Post-traumatic stress disorder, chronic
DSM-5 CODES	
309.81/F43.10	Posttraumatic stress disorder
308.3/F43.0	Acute stress disorder
309.89/F43.8	Other specified trauma and related disorder
309.9/F43.9	Unspecified trauma and stressor-related disorder

EPIDEMIOLOGY & DEMOGRAPHICS

INCIDENCE: About 10% of individuals who have experienced a significant traumatic event will develop syndromal PTSD; however, there is considerable variability in prevalence rates associated with specific trauma types. The most frequently reported traumas in the U.S. are physical and sexual assaults (52% lifetime prevalence).

PREVALENCE (IN U.S.):
- 12-mo prevalence in the U.S. is 3.5% to 4.7%. Estimated lifetime prevalence 6.1% to 9.2%.
- Prevalence among high-risk populations (e.g., combat veterans or victims of violent crimes) is up to 58%.
- Delayed expression, most frequently among military veterans, accounts for 25% of chronic PTSD cases.
- Comorbidity is the rule, not the exception: Depression, anxiety/panic, substance use, agoraphobia, anger/rage, violence/suicide, development of personality disorders (e.g., avoidant PD, paranoid PD).
- Factors most associated with development of PTSD are previous traumatic experience(s), subsequent life stress, social vulnerability, perceived lack of social support/communalization, lack of intrinsic resiliency.
- Prevalence varies widely across the globe and may be lowest in lower-middle-income countries (which may be due to access to care, stigma in reporting, and cultural validity issues in the DSM-5 criteria of PTSD itself).

PREDOMINANT AGE & SEX:
- Younger age at trauma exposure—and repetitive trauma—predisposes to PTSD.
- Twice as many women as men are affected (prevalence 10%-14% for women and 5%-6% for men). More than 50% of cases in women are related to sexual violence.
- Intellectual disability appears to predispose to higher risk for developing PTSD after traumatic exposure.
- Human-engineered and repeated, violent traumas (especially sexual violence) are the most potent in inducing PTSD.

GENETICS: Heritability for PTSD is predicted at 30% to 40%. The biologic correlates studied include genes, epigenetic regulation, neuroendocrine factors, inflammatory markers, and autonomic regulation. Genes related to heart-rate variability and adrenergic response to perceived threat, for example, have been studied.

PHYSICAL FINDINGS & CLINICAL PRESENTATION

Core symptom clusters include intrusion, avoidance, negatively altered mood and cognition, hyperarousal, and dissociative symptoms. Individuals present with different variations of these symptoms. Individuals who display these core symptom clusters within the first post-trauma month are diagnosed with acute stress disorder. In PTSD, these symptoms must be present >1 mo after the trauma and result in significant distress and functional impairment.

Key PTSD symptoms:
- Distressing memories or dreams of the trauma(s)
- Dissociation (e.g., depersonalization, derealization, flashbacks)
- Intense distress with reminders
- Efforts at avoidance of reminders (both environmental and cognitive)
- Persistent negative affect and cognition (hopelessness, helplessness, nihilism, anger, despair, numbing, etc.)
- Aggressive or reckless behavior (e.g., short fuse in interpersonal situations, road rage)
- Hyperarousal (e.g., low startle threshold, vigilance, difficulty being in crowds or confined spaces)
- Problems with concentration, executive functioning, and sleep

ETIOLOGY

- Common types of trauma: Interpersonal violence (physical, sexual, psychologic, gaslighting), natural disasters, military combat, motor vehicle accident, childhood abuse and neglect, critical illness or hospitalization in ICU, physical injury, diagnosis of life-threatening illness—and direct knowledge or witnessing of any of these phenomena in a close contact.
- Risk factors: Previous trauma, initial severity of reaction to event, psychiatric history, traumatic brain injury, childhood abuse or neglect, poor social support, limited resiliency factors.
- Human-engineered (especially repeated), interpersonal violence is more likely to cause PTSD than events such as motor vehicle accidents or natural disasters, where there can be more ability to communalize the experience with other survivors (and understand the experience as random rather than perpetrated).
- Severity of physical injury is a weaker predictor of PTSD than the associated psychological distress.
- Proposed mechanisms include activation of the amygdala; disruption of prefrontal, insular, and anterior cingulate regulation of the amygdala; abnormal sympathetic and HPA axis regulation; and associated derangements in dopaminergic, GABAergic, serotonergic, and adrenergic neurotransmission.
- Classical fear conditioning is involved in pairing hyperarousal symptoms to a painful stimulus (trauma); operant conditioning is involved in the negative reinforcement, or avoidance, of a painful stimulus.

DIAGNOSIS

Diagnosis is made when the stressor is consistent with the DSM-5 criteria. The symptoms must be present for >1 mo, must cause impairment in functioning, and must not be attributable to substance use or other medical conditions. Subtypes include dissociative PTSD (criteria + depersonalization or derealization) and delayed onset PTSD (criteria starting at least 6 mo after the event). There is also a non–DSM-5 term called "complex PTSD," which involves severe and persistent symptoms across developmental phases as the result of severe and prolonged trauma (e.g., profound emotional and cognitive dysfunction after prolonged captivity or torture).

Definition of stressor:
- Exposure to actual or threatened death, injury, or violence; directly experiencing the event, witnessing the event occur to others, or learning that a close contact was exposed to such trauma. If the event involved actual or threatened death, it must have been violent or accidental (not dying from old age, for example).
- Repeated or extreme indirect exposure to aversive details of the event(s), usually in the course of professional duties (e.g., first responders' exposure to dead bodies or horrific narrative details of violence).

DIFFERENTIAL DIAGNOSIS

- Adjustment disorders: Precipitating stress is less catastrophic and psychological reaction is less specific and in constellation
- Mood disorder: Depression or the bipolar spectrum, which would involve specific constellations of mood symptoms in isolation

- Anxiety disorders: Generalized or specific anxiety symptoms that lack the specific trauma precursor and specific set of psychologic reactions
- Somatic symptom or functional neurological symptom disorder (formerly "conversion disorder")
- Psychotic disorder
- Traumatic brain injury: Can co-occur with PTSD and each can make the other worse (for example, being concussed while also witnessing the deaths of comrades in warfare may make the symptoms of each phenomenon worse in combination)

WORKUP

- Validated self-report questionnaires and structured diagnostic instruments include the Posttraumatic Diagnostic Scale and Clinician Administered PTSD Scale (CAPS).
- Although numerous potential biomarkers have been identified and are under investigation, at this time evidence is not conclusive. To date, laboratory and imaging are not clinically useful.
- Primary care PTSD (PC-PTSD) screen recommended by the Veterans' Administration.
- "Yes" answer to three of four of the following questions is a positive screen. In your life, have you ever had any experience that was so frightening, horrible, or upsetting that, in the past month, you:
    1. Have had nightmares about it or thought about it when you did not want to?
    2. Tried hard not to think about it or went out of your way to avoid situations that reminded you of it?
    3. Were constantly on guard, watchful, or easily startled?
    4. Felt numb or detached from others, activities, or your surroundings?

Rx TREATMENT

- Cognitive-behavioral therapy approaches, including prolonged exposure (PE) and cognitive processing therapy (CPT), have the greatest empirical support to date among psychotherapy approaches.
- Prolonged exposure (PE) includes psychoeducation on the stress response, imaginal exposure focused on recounting trauma memories, and in vivo exposure focusing on reducing avoidance of fear-provoking situations associated with the trauma.
- CPT adds further skills development to the exposure methods.
- A recent clinical trial found that brief written exposure therapy intervention was noninferior to standard CPT and had fewer dropouts.
- Group therapy: Current standards recommend individual therapy as first-line treatment, with more mixed data on group over individual interventions.
- Eye movement desensitization and reprocessing (EMDR) demonstrates comparable efficacy to traditional CBT approaches in clinical trials. However, to date it is unclear whether it offers advantages over, or operates through distinct mechanisms from, traditional CBT approaches.
- A growing number of studies have demonstrated efficacy of CBT approaches for PTSD delivered through novel formats, including exposure therapy integrating virtual reality technology and Internet- and telephone-delivered CBT.
- Couples therapy, occupational therapy, or vocational rehabilitation when appropriate.
- There are specialized, multidisciplinary treatment programs provided by the Veterans Administration and the philanthropic organization Home Base for veterans, and similar programs are provided at the community level for first responders.

MEDICATIONS

There is no definitive cure for PTSD, and individuals have varying responses to different medications. Sertraline and paroxetine, both SSRIs, are the only FDA-approved medications for PTSD. Other medication use is off-label with differing levels of evidence to support use. Medications are used to target symptoms and the physiologic changes associated with PTSD and with psychiatric disorders that are frequently comorbid with PTSD. SSRIs and SNRIs are currently considered the first-line medication treatments for PTSD, and it is recommended that they be prescribed for duration of at least 8 to 12 wk, with some studies demonstrating maximum benefit reached as late as 36 wk.

- SSRIs: Sertraline, paroxetine, fluoxetine, citalopram, escitalopram, fluvoxamine
- SNRIs: Venlafaxine, duloxetine, milnacipran/levomilnacipran
- Other antidepressants: Mirtazapine has shown efficacy in small randomized trials.
- Alpha-adrenergic receptor blockers: Prazosin has demonstrated some efficacy in reducing nightmares, but the most recent RCT in military veterans with PTSD did not show efficacy. Clonidine is also frequently used for this purpose.
- Atypical antipsychotics (e.g., risperidone, quetiapine, olanzapine) have demonstrated efficacy as augmenting agents for individuals with partial response to SSRIs and may be particularly beneficial for individuals with paranoia, extreme anxiety, or angry outbursts. They should not be used for insomnia in isolation.
- Mood stabilizers (e.g., valproic acid, lamotrigine, carbamazepine) can be used if there are significant mood symptoms such as extreme irritability, explosiveness, or anger. They are fairly commonly used when there is comorbid brain injury.
- Transcranial magnetic stimulation (TMS) is being evaluated as a possible effective treatment modality.
- Ketamine: Recent clinical trials of intravenous ketamine infusion showed quick-onset but time-limited PTSD and depression symptom reduction, although more research is needed.
- *N*-methyl-D-aspartate (NMDA) agonists and partial agonists have shown some efficacy in early clinical trials, although more research is needed. These agents may help with plasticity and learning, which could synergize with psychotherapy.
- Recent efforts are underway to examine the efficacy of pharmacologic interventions in preventing development of PTSD early after exposure to trauma, with GABAergic sedatives, beta-blockers, or opioids, for example. These are not currently recommended as standard of care.

ACUTE Rx

- Immediate post-incident debriefing may worsen outcomes.
- Benzodiazepines are not currently recommended as monotherapy for the treatment of PTSD, as there is no evidence that they reduce reexperiencing and avoidance/numbing symptoms. There is also concern for misuse and addiction, with substance use being commonly comorbid with PTSD.
- Beta-adrenergic blockers may be helpful if given within hours after the trauma to disrupt the physiologic stress response, although more research is needed.
- Sedating antidepressants or sleep aids may be helpful for initial insomnia.

DISPOSITION

- Recovery rates are highest in the first 12 mo after onset.
- Average duration of symptoms is 36 mo for those who undergo treatment and 64 mo for those never treated.
- 50% chance of remission at 2 yr; 50% have chronic symptoms.
- Predictors of chronic course include previous trauma, premorbid psychiatric function, panic reaction at time of event, prolonged terror, or dissociation at time of event.

REFERRAL

Because early intervention improves outcomes, refer to a specialist as soon as the diagnosis is made.

PEARLS & CONSIDERATIONS

- PTSD is associated with increased occurrence of suicidal ideation and attempts.
- PTSD can be associated with aggressive and violent behavior.
- Traumatic medical experiences such as being in the ICU, myocardial infarction, or an emergent cesarean section can cause PTSD.
- Individuals with PTSD present with comorbid psychiatric disorders in >50% of cases, including substance abuse, major depression, anxiety disorders, and personality disorders.
- Among combat veterans of recent wars, there is a 41% cooccurrence with mild TBI. TBI and PTSD can make the symptoms of each other worse.

- PTSD may vary culturally and present with specific idioms of distress.
- Treatment can be effective even if it begins years after the traumatic event occurred. In fact, 25% of chronic cases have a significantly delayed onset of symptoms. Cognitive changes with age and psychosocial changes in circumstance may account for this.

SUGGESTED READINGS

Available at ExpertConsult.com

RELATED CONTENT

Posttraumatic Stress Disorder (PTSD) (Patient Information)

AUTHOR: **Bryce Wininger, MD**

BASIC INFORMATION

DEFINITION

Preeclampsia involves the presence of new-onset hypertension (after 20 wk of gestation) with other associated comorbidities in a pregnant woman. In 2013, the American College of Obstetrics and Gynecology (ACOG) Task Force on Hypertension in Pregnancy revised the criteria, making preeclampsia a hypertensive disorder and one where the presence of proteinuria was no longer needed to make the diagnosis. The task force reinforced the importance of hypertension as a necessary condition and deemphasized proteinuria. In the absence of proteinuria, other criteria, including thrombocytopenia, new development of renal insufficiency, impaired liver function, pulmonary edema, and new-onset cerebral or visual symptoms, could substitute.

Additionally, the task force emphasized the categories employed in prior ACOG bulletins:

- Preeclampsia: Hypertension with or without proteinuria, but with the presence of one of the previously mentioned comorbidities
- Preeclampsia with severe features (Table 1)
- Chronic hypertension: Hypertension predating pregnancy or present at <20 wk gestation
- Gestational hypertension: Hypertension in pregnancy after 20 wk without proteinuria or any of the previously mentioned comorbidities
- Chronic hypertension with superimposed preeclampsia: The presence of chronic hypertension with sudden increase in blood pressure or escalation of medication when previously well controlled or with development of new onset of signs or symptoms meeting criteria for severe preeclampsia. Table 1 summarizes the criteria for the diagnosis of severe preeclampsia
- Hemolysis, elevated liver enzymes, and low platelet count (HELLP) syndrome: A severe form of preeclampsia defined by LDH greater than 600 IU/L, liver enzymes (AST, ALT) greater than twice the upper limit of normal, and a platelet count less than 100×10^9/L.

SYNONYMS

Pregnancy-induced hypertension (PIH)
Hypertensive disorders of pregnancy (HDP)
Severe gestational hypertension

ICD-10CM CODES

O11.1	Pre-existing hypertension with pre-eclampsia, first trimester
O11.2	Pre-existing hypertension with pre-eclampsia, second trimester
O11.3	Pre-existing hypertension with pre-eclampsia, third trimester
O11.9	Pre-existing hypertension with pre-eclampsia, unspecified trimester
O14.00	Mild to moderate pre-eclampsia, unspecified trimester
O14.02	Mild to moderate pre-eclampsia, second trimester
O14.03	Mild to moderate pre-eclampsia, third trimester
O14.10	Severe pre-eclampsia, unspecified trimester
O14.12	Severe pre-eclampsia, second trimester
O14.13	Severe pre-eclampsia, third trimester
O14.90	Unspecified pre-eclampsia, unspecified trimester
O14.92	Unspecified pre-eclampsia, second trimester
O14.93	Unspecified pre-eclampsia, third trimester

EPIDEMIOLOGY & DEMOGRAPHICS

INCIDENCE: The global incidence of preeclampsia is 2% to 8%.
RISK FACTORS: See Table 2.
GENETICS: Positive correlation with maternal and paternal family history

PHYSICAL FINDINGS & CLINICAL PRESENTATION

- Preeclampsia typically presents with hypertension and proteinuria, most commonly in the third trimester of pregnancy.
- May be asymptomatic.
- Generalized swelling or nondependent edema, possibly manifested by rapid weight gain (>4 lb/wk), even in the absence of edema, is common but is nonspecific and is seen in many normal pregnancies.
- Auscultation of pulmonary rales.
- Cerebral symptoms: Headache, vision changes
- Right upper quadrant pain (HELLP syndrome or subcapsular liver hematoma).
- Hyperreflexia or clonus.
- Vaginal bleeding (placental abruption).
- Chronic fetal compromise manifested by fetal growth restriction or acute fetal compromise manifested by nonreassuring fetal testing.
- Wide range of symptoms attributable to multiorgan system dysfunction, involving hepatic, hematologic, renal, pulmonary, and central nervous systems.
- Possibility of severe disease despite "normal" blood pressure readings, so a high index of suspicion must be maintained in high-risk situations.

ETIOLOGY

- Exact etiology is unknown.
- Theories:
  1. Imbalance between thromboxane A_2 (vasoconstrictor and platelet aggregator) and prostacyclin (vasodilator)
  2. Abnormal trophoblastic invasion of spiral arteries and exaggerated maternal inflammatory response to deported trophoblasts
  3. Increased sensitivity to angiotensin II by the muscular walls of the arteries
  4. Excess circulating soluble FMS-like tyrosine kinase 1 (*sFlt1*), which binds placental growth factor (PIGF) and vascular endothelial growth factor (VEGF), may have a pathogenic role
- Potential secondary effects of the metabolic, inflammatory endothelial alternatives in preeclampsia are described in Table 3.

DIAGNOSIS

DIFFERENTIAL DIAGNOSIS

- Acute fatty liver of pregnancy
- Appendicitis
- Diabetic ketoacidosis
- Gallbladder disease
- Gastroenteritis
- Glomerulonephritis
- Hemolytic-uremic syndrome
- Hepatic encephalopathy
- Hyperemesis gravidarum
- Idiopathic thrombocytopenia
- Thrombotic thrombocytopenic purpura
- Nephrolithiasis
- Pyelonephritis
- Peptic ulcer disease

TABLE 2 Risk Factors for Preeclampsia

- Nulliparity
- Multifetal gestations
- Preeclampsia in a previous pregnancy
- Chronic hypertension
- Pregestational diabetes
- Gestational diabetes
- Thrombophilia
- Systemic lupus erythematosus
- Prepregnancy body mass index greater than 30
- Antiphospholipid antibody syndrome
- Maternal age 35 yr or older
- Kidney disease
- Assisted reproductive technology
- Obstructive sleep apnea

From Gestational hypertension and preeclampsia. ACOG Practice Bulletin No. 222. American College of Obstetricians and Gynecologists, *Obstet Gynecol* 135:e237–e260, 2020.

TABLE 1 Criteria for the Diagnosis of Preeclampsia with Severe Features

In patients with preeclampsia, **preeclampsia with severe features** can be diagnosed if any one of the following criteria is present:
Blood pressure ≥160 mm Hg systolic or ≥110 mm Hg diastolic on two separate occasions at least 4 hr apart (unless antihypertensive therapy is initiated before this time)
Serum creatinine >1.1 mg/dl or a doubling of the serum creatinine
New onset of visual disturbances
New-onset headache unresponsive to medication and not accounted for by alternative diagnoses
Pulmonary edema
Hepatocellular injury (serum transaminases at least twice the upper limit of normal) or severe persistent right upper quadrant or epigastric pain unresponsive to medications
Thrombocytopenia (platelet count $<100 \times 10^9$/L)

- Systemic lupus erythematosus
- Viral hepatitis
- Medications or medication withdrawal

WORKUP

Hypertension: After at least 20 wk of gestation, with the patient sitting or semireclined with back support

- Two blood pressure measurements at least 4 hr apart, with a systolic BP of 140 mm Hg or more or a diastolic blood pressure of 90 mm Hg or more.
- Systolic BP of 160 mm Hg or more or a diastolic blood pressure of 110 mm Hg or more.
- Severe hypertension can be confirmed in a brief period to allow for immediate treatment of severe range blood pressure.

Proteinuria:

- ≥300 mg per 24-hr urine collection
- Protein/creatinine ratio ≥0.3
- 2+ on dipstick ONLY IF OTHER METHODS NOT AVAILABLE
- In the absence of proteinuria, preeclampsia (with severe features) may be diagnosed with new onset of hypertension and one of the following:
  1. Platelet count less than 100×10^9/L
  2. Serum creatinine concentrations greater than 1.1 mg/dl, or doubling of serum Cr levels in the absence of other renal disease
  3. Elevated serum liver transaminases to twice the normal concentration
  4. Pulmonary edema
  5. New-onset headache unresponsive to medication and not accounted for by alternative diagnoses or visual symptoms
- Because of the insidious nature of the disease with potential for multiple organ involvement, as well as its prevalence, complete evaluation for preeclampsia in any pregnant patient presenting with central nervous system derangement or gastrointestinal symptoms after 20 wk of gestation
- Evaluation for associated conditions such as disseminated intravascular coagulation, hepatic dysfunction, or subcapsular hematoma
- Fig. 1 outlines a management plan for patients with severe preeclampsia

TABLE 3 Potential Secondary Effects of the Metabolic, Inflammatory Endothelial Alternatives in Preeclampsia

CVS	Increased peripheral resistance leading to hypertension; increased vascular permeability and reduced maternal plasma volume.
Lungs	Laryngeal and pulmonary edema.
Renal	Glomerular damage leading to proteinuria, hypoproteinemia, and reduced oncotic pressure, which further exacerbates the hypovolemia. May develop acute renal failure ± cortical necrosis.
Clotting	Hypercoagulability, with increased fibrin formation and increased fibrinolysis (i.e., disseminated intravascular coagulation).
Liver	HELLP syndrome hepatic rupture.
CNS	Thrombosis and fibrinoid necrosis of the cerebral arterioles. Eclampsia (convulsions), cerebral hemorrhage, and cerebral edema.
Fetus	Impaired uteroplacental circulation, potentially leading to FGR, hypoxemia, and intrauterine death.

CVS, Cardiovascular system; *CNS*, central nervous system; *FGR*, fetal growth restriction; *HELLP*, hemolysis, elevated liver enzymes, low platelets.
From Drife J, Magowan B: *Clinical obstetrics and gynecology*, Philadelphia, 2004, Saunders.

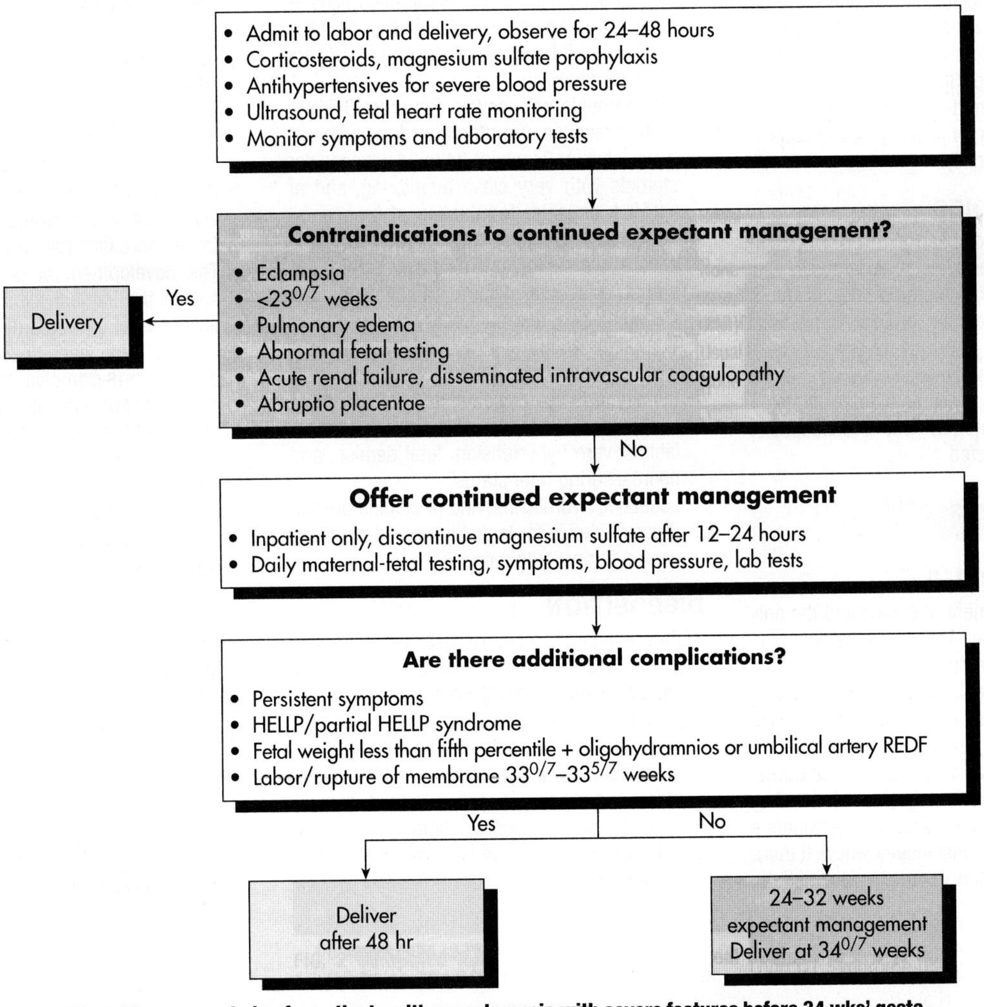

FIG. 1 Management plan for patients with preeclampsia with severe features before 34 wks' gestation. *HELLP*, Hemolysis, elevated liver enzymes, and low platelets; *REDF*, reversed end-diastolic flow. (From Gabbe SG et al: *Obstetrics: normal and problem pregnancies*, ed 7, Philadelphia, 2017, Elsevier.)

LABORATORY TESTS

- High-risk patients: Baseline assessment of renal function (24-hr urine collection for total protein and creatinine clearance or protein:creatinine ratio), complete blood count, serum creatinine, liver function tests (LFTs), and uric acid should be obtained at the first prenatal visit.
- Complete blood count (hemoglobin, hematocrit, platelets) may show signs of hemoconcentration or HELLP syndrome.
- LFTs (aspartate aminotransferase, alanine aminotransferase, lactate dehydrogenase) are useful in evaluation for HELLP syndrome or to exclude important differentials.
- Hyperuricemia or increased creatinine may indicate decreasing renal function.
- Prothrombin time, partial thromboplastin time, and fibrinogen can be checked to rule out disseminated intravascular coagulation, if clinically appropriate.
- Peripheral smear may demonstrate microangiopathic hemolytic anemia.
- Complement levels can be used to differentiate from an acute exacerbation of a collagen-vascular disease.
- The ratio of soluble FMS-like tyrosine kinase 1 (sFlt-1) to placental growth factor (PIGF) is elevated in pregnant women before the clinical onset of preeclampsia. Increased levels of sFlt1 and reduced levels of PIGF predict subsequent development of preeclampsia. An sFlt-1:PIGR ratio of 38 or lower can be used to predict the short-term absence of preeclampsia in women in whom the syndrome is suspected clinically.

IMAGING STUDIES

- CT or MRI scan of head if atypical presentation of eclampsia or preeclampsia with atypical cerebral symptoms, possibility of intracerebral bleed, or prolonged postictal state
- Sonogram of fetus to evaluate for intrauterine growth restriction amniotic fluid, placenta
- Sonogram of maternal liver if subcapsular hematoma suspected

Rx TREATMENT

ACUTE GENERAL Rx

Delivery is the treatment of choice and the only cure for the disease. This must be taken in the context of the gestational age of the fetus, severity of the preeclampsia, and the likelihood of a successful induction and reliability of patient, if pursuing expectant management.

- For preeclampsia with severe features, administer magnesium sulfate 4 to 6 g IV loading dose, with 2 g/hr maintenance (adjust dosage for renal insufficiency). If there is a contraindication to magnesium sulfate, such as myasthenia gravis, then use phenytoin at 10 to 15 mg/kg loading dose, then 200 mg IV q8h starting 12 hr after loading dose.
- Treat blood pressure (BP) >160 mm Hg systolic or >110 mm Hg diastolic either with hydralazine 5 to 10 mg IV, then 10 mg, every 20 min to a max dose of 20 mg; or with labetalol hydrochloride 20, 40, 80, 80 mg IV, escalating dosage every 10 min to a max dose of 300 mg IV; or with nifedipine 10 to 20 mg orally every 20 min to a max dose of 180 mg/day for acute blood pressure control. If maximum dose of one medication is reached, add an additional medication to reach goal of BP 140 to 150/90 to 100 mm Hg.
- Continuous fetal monitoring.
- Epidural is anesthesia of choice for pain management in labor or cesarean section.
- All patients undergoing induction of labor or cesarean section should receive antiseizure medications (magnesium sulfate) if disease with severe features, for delivery and 12 to 24 hr postpartum.

CHRONIC Rx

- Preeclampsia without severe features <37 wk: Close observation for worsening maternal or fetal condition, with delivery at 37 wk. If 24 to 36 wk, consider antenatal corticosteroids. If severe features develop or there is evidence of fetal compromise, earlier delivery is appropriate.
- Preeclampsia with severe features: Delivery in the presence of maternal or fetal compromise, labor, or 34 wk; at 24 to 34 wk consider steroids with very close monitoring, and at <24 wk consider termination of pregnancy. Risks of expectant management include severe worsening of disease, eclampsia, abruptio placenta, stillbirth, HELLP syndrome, ICU admission, and pulmonary edema.
- Contraindications to expectant management include eclampsia, HELLP syndrome, pulmonary edema, disseminated intravascular coagulation, abruptio placenta, uncontrollable severe hypertension, fetal demise, and nonreassuring fetal status.
- Labetalol, hydralazine, and nifedipine are the drugs of choice for long-term blood-pressure control during pregnancy.

DISPOSITION

- Preeclampsia is a progressive and unpredictable disease process; a course of expectancy should be managed with caution. Up to 20% of patients who have seizures are normotensive.
- The reoccurrence rate for preeclampsia in a subsequent pregnancy is approximately 20%, and higher in cases with a second trimester presentation or complications. This risk may be decreased with the use of low-dose aspirin.

REFERRAL

Obstetric management is indicated because of the insidious nature of the disease, with transfer of all cases <34 wk to a facility with appropriate maternal and neonatal care facilities.

! PEARLS & CONSIDERATIONS

COMMENTS

- Low-dose aspirin, beginning as early as the second trimester, decreases the risk of preeclampsia, preterm birth, and intrauterine growth retardation in women who are at high risk of preeclampsia. The American College of Obstetricians and Gynecologists (ACOG) and the U.S. Preventive Services Task Force (USPSTF) recommend the use of low-dose aspirin as preventive medication starting after 12 wk of gestation (ideally before 16 wk) in women who are at high risk for preeclampsia (previous preeclampsia, multifetal gestation, chronic hypertension, type 1 or 2 diabetes, renal disease, or autoimmune disease).
- The use of low-dose aspirin, 150 mg/day started at 11 to 14 wk gestation, has been demonstrated to decrease the incidence of preterm preeclampsia in a selected high-risk population. In the U.S., low-dose aspirin is available as an 81 mg tablet. U.S. clinicians who recommend aspirin for preeclampsia prevention could consider prescribing two 81 mg tablets daily.
- Although the absolute risk of end-stage renal disease (ESRD) in women who have had preeclampsia is low, preeclampsia is a marker for an increased risk of subsequent ESRD.
- The development of preeclampsia may be one of the earliest identifiable risk markers for potential future cardiovascular disease in women. It has been shown that women who develop preeclampsia have a higher incidence of cardiovascular risk factors including components of the metabolic syndrome within 1 yr of delivery. Women with a history of preeclampsia, particularly preterm or recurrent, are at increased risk for cardiovascular disease and appropriate follow-up should be encouraged.

SUGGESTED READINGS

Available at ExpertConsult.com

RELATED CONTENT

Preeclampsia (Patient Information)
Eclampsia (Related Key Topic)
Hypertension (Related Key Topic)

AUTHORS: **Emily E. Nuss, MD,** and **Philip A. Shlossman, MD**

BASIC INFORMATION

DEFINITION

Premenstrual syndrome (PMS) consists of various somatic and physical complaints that develop during the luteal phase of the menstrual cycle and that are of sufficient severity to interfere with daily functioning and/or interpersonal relationships. The symptoms resolve shortly after the onset of menses.

SYNONYM

PMS

ICD-10CM CODE

N94.3 Premenstrual tension syndrome

EPIDEMIOLOGY & DEMOGRAPHICS

- Premenstrual disorders affect about 12% of reproductive-age women, although as many as 80% of women will report at least one somatic or affective symptom during their luteal phase (Table 1).
- Severe cases of premenstrual dysphoric disorder (PMDD), which is more of a psychiatric diagnosis, occur in approximately 1.3% to 5.3% of women.
- The prevalence of PMS is not associated with age, race, or socioeconomic status.
- Those seeking treatment for PMS are usually in their 30s or 40s.
- Based on some identical twinning studies, a genetic component is thought to exist, but no genes have been identified.
- The natural history of PMS has not been clearly elucidated.

PHYSICAL FINDINGS & CLINICAL PRESENTATION

- Diverse and potentially disabling symptoms. Table 1 summarizes common symptoms of PMS
- Associated with multiple psychologic, physical, and behavioral symptoms
- Most frequent reason for seeking treatment: Emotional symptoms
- Most common emotional symptoms: Depression, irritability, anxiety, labile moods, anger, crying easily, sadness, extreme sensitivity, nervous tension
- Most common physical symptoms: Headache, bloating, cramps, breast tenderness, migraines, fatigue, weight gain, aches and pains, palpitations
- Most common behavior symptom: Food cravings
- Other behavioral symptoms: Increased appetite, increased alcohol intake, decreased motivation, decreased efficiency, avoidance of activities, staying home, sleep changes, libido changes, forgetfulness, decreased concentration

ETIOLOGY

- Etiology is poorly understood. The syndrome is thought to result from steroid hormone effects on serotonin, ϒ-aminobutyric acid, dopamine systems, and the renin-aldosterone system, thus causing some of the bloating symptoms.
- Because of the multifactorial, multiorgan nature of PMS, a single etiologic cause is unlikely.

DIAGNOSIS

DIFFERENTIAL DIAGNOSIS

- A diagnosis of exclusion, so other medical or psychologic disorders should be ruled out
- Common disorders to rule out: Depression or anxiety, anemia, migraines, endometriosis, thyroid disease

WORKUP

- History.
- Physical examination.
- Laboratory studies to rule out alternative diagnosis.
- If no alternative diagnosis, confirm by either history of regular menses, basal body temperature charting, or elevated luteal progesterone that patient is ovulatory.
  1. If she is not ovulating, it is not PMS.
  2. A prospective questionnaire given over two menstrual cycles has been found to be the most accurate way to assess the presence of PMS or PMDD. If symptoms are not occurring only in the luteal phase, it is not PMS, and further investigation is needed.
     a. If symptoms occur in the follicular phase, patient has premenstrual exacerbation of another condition.
     b. If symptoms do not occur in the follicular phase, diagnosis of PMS is confirmed.

LABORATORY TESTS

- None available to specifically confirm the diagnosis of PMS
- Thyroid function tests to rule out thyroid disease

TREATMENT

NONPHARMACOLOGIC THERAPY

- Individualization of the treatment plan to maximize therapeutic response.
- Psychosocial intervention:
  1. Education
  2. Stress management
  3. Environmental changes
  4. Adequate rest and sleep
  5. Regular exercise
- Nutritional recommendations:
  1. Regularly eaten, well-balanced meals
  2. Adequate amounts of protein, fiber, and complex carbohydrates; low fat
  3. Avoidance of foods that are high in salt and simple sugars; may promote water retention, weight gain, and physical discomfort
  4. Avoidance of alcohol and illicit drugs; may worsen emotional lability
  5. Calcium supplementation (1000 mg/day for women 19-50 yr, 1300 mg/day for girls 14-18 yr) to reduce the physical and emotional symptoms
  6. The data are mixed regarding the benefits of vitamin D supplementation in reducing PMS symptoms, so more studies are needed
  7. Pyridoxine (vitamin B_6) 80 mg qd to improve depression, fatigue, and irritability has been suggested in small studies

ACUTE GENERAL Rx

Suppression of ovulation:

- Oral contraceptives: One pill per day; continuous use associated with better treatment effect
- Progestin-only oral contraceptive: One pill per day
- Oral micronized progesterone: 100 mg every morning and 200 mg every evening on days 17 through 28 of menstrual cycle
- Progestin suppository: 200 to 400 mg bid on days 17 through 28 of menstrual cycle
- Medroxyprogesterone: 150 mg IM q3mo
- Levonorgestrel implants: Surgical insertion every 5 yr

TABLE 1 Common Symptoms of Cyclic Premenstrual Syndrome

Somatic Symptoms	
Abdominal bloating	Constipation or diarrhea
Acne	Headache
Alcohol intolerance	Peripheral edema
Breast engorgement and tenderness	Weight gain
Clumsiness	
Emotional and Mental Symptoms	
Anxiety	Insomnia
Change in libido	Irritability
Depression	Lethargy
Fatigue	Mood swings
Food cravings (especially salt and sugar)	Panic attacks
Hostility	Paranoia
Inability to concentrate	Violence toward self and others
Increased appetite	Withdrawal from others

From Goldman L, Schafer AI: *Goldman's Cecil medicine*, ed 24, Philadelphia, 2012, Saunders.

- Transdermal estradiol: One or two 100-μg patches every 3 days
- Danazol: 100 to 200 mg/day (ovulation not suppressed at this dose); has significant side-effect profile
- Gonadotropin-releasing hormone (GnRH) agonists: Daily by intranasal spray or monthly by depot injection; profound hypoestrogenism, concerns for osteoporosis and vasomotor symptoms

Suppression of physical symptoms:

- Spironolactone: 25 to 50 mg bid on days 14 through 28 of menstrual cycle—need a reliable form of birth control
- Mefenamic acid
  1. For fluid retention: 250 mg tid on days 24 through 28 of cycle
  2. For pain: 500 mg tid on days 19 through 28 of cycle
- Bromocriptine: 5 mg/day on days 10 through 26 of cycle
- Naproxen: 550 mg bid on days 17 through 28 of cycle, Naprosyn-500 mg bid on days 17 through 28 of cycle

Suppression of psychologic symptoms:

- SSRI, or serotonergic antidepressants, are first-line treatment for PMS/PMDD, treating mostly the psychologic aspects but also some physical aspects
- Sertraline, paroxetine, fluoxetine, citalopram, escitalopram
- In 2013 the *Cochrane Reviews* reported a statistically significant benefit over placebo when taken either continuously or in the luteal phase
- Serotonin-norepinephrine reuptake inhibitors (SNRI) such as venlafaxine; use is off-label, but onset of action is quick and has been found to be helpful
- Seroquel: Smaller studies
- Wellbutrin: Not as effective as the other options

CHRONIC Rx

- Therapy is largely trial and error, with the goal of providing effective treatment with the safest therapy. Provider should initially attempt to ameliorate the most pronounced symptom(s).
- Limited evidence exists that acupuncture and/or acupressure may ameliorate some symptoms associated with PMS and improve quality of life. More studies are needed to determine if this option is as good as or better than conventional therapies such as treatment with an SSRI.
- For severe intractable PMS: Bilateral oophorectomy; give trial of GnRH therapy or danazol before surgery (bilateral oophorectomy should be exceedingly rare).
- Estrogen replacement therapy recommended postoperatively to reduce the risk of osteoporosis, heart disease, and genitourinary atrophy.

DISPOSITION

Improved symptoms in 90% of women over time

REFERRAL

- For counseling with a psychologist or psychiatrist if underlying psychiatric disorder is discovered (cognitive-behavioral therapy)
- To a gynecologist if surgical therapy is contemplated

SUGGESTED READINGS

Available at ExpertConsult.com

RELATED CONTENT

Premenstrual Syndrome (Patient Information)
Dysmenorrhea (Related Key Topic)
Premenstrual Dysphoric Disorder (Related Key Topic)

AUTHOR: **Adrienne B. Neithardt, MD**

BASIC INFORMATION

DEFINITION

The 2019 International Guideline for Prevention and Treatment of Pressure Ulcers/Injuries defines a pressure injury as localized damage to the skin and/or underlying tissue as a result of pressure or pressure in combination with shear. A pressure injury is caused by prolonged mechanical deformation of soft tissues between internal stiff anatomical structures such as bones, cartilages, and tendon and the external stiff support surfaces (e.g., mattresses or seats or contact with medical and other devices). The tolerance of soft tissue for pressure and shear may also be affected by other factors such as microclimate, nutrition, perfusion, comorbidities, moisture, and condition of the soft tissue. Common sites (Fig. 1) include the sacrum (Fig. E2), heels, elbows, lateral malleoli, occiput, scapula, ischium, and calcaneus among others. It can present as an intact skin or an open ulcer that could be painful. This revised nomenclature allows for the recognition of lesser degrees of skin damage that are not necessarily associated with pressure injuries.

SYNONYMS

Decubitus ulcers
Pressure sores
Bed sores
Pressure ulcers
Pressure-induced skin injury
Pressure-induced soft tissue injury

ICD-10CM CODES
L89 Pressure ulcers
Subcategories of codes determined by stage and location of ulcer
L89.153 Example: Stage 3 ulcer of sacral area

New codes for Deep Tissue Injury [DTI]: introduced 10/1/19 for all patient encounters and discharges. Determined by location:
L89.016 Example: Pressure-induced deep tissue damage of the right elbow

EPIDEMIOLOGY & DEMOGRAPHICS

- An estimated 2.5 million cases of pressure injuries are treated each year in acute care facilities across the U.S.
- Worldwide, the prevalence of pressure injury in the acute care setting ranges from 6% to 18%. According to the 2019 National Pressure Ulcer Advisory Panel, the prevalence of pressure injuries in acute care settings has shown a gradual and progressive decline over the past 20 yr.
- Pressure injuries resulted in 28,500 documented deaths globally in 2013, more than double from 13,700 deaths in 1990.
- Development of pressure injury results in increased hospital length of stay by 7 to 10 days. These patients are three times more likely to be discharged to long-term care facilities.
- In the U.S., the Centers for Medicare and Medicaid (CMS) do not provide any reimbursement to hospitals for treatment of stage 3 and 4 pressure injuries acquired during hospitalization.
- In 2016, the national cost for pressure injury management was $22 billion. Hospital-acquired pressure injuries added $8200 to the cost of the surgical stay, which conferred an additional 44% increase in surgical stay costs.
- Patients who develop pressure injuries tend to be older patients (mean age of 71 yr), debilitated, immobile, and have multiple medical problems such as dementia, lung disease, diabetes mellitus, urinary or fecal incontinence, spinal cord injuries, and nutritional deficiencies to include a few. A cohort study observed that pressure injuries occurred in 36% of older patients with hip fracture.
- Occur in all health care settings including hospitals, nursing homes, and residential homes. The reported rates upon admission to a nursing home range from 10% to 35%. The incidence rate is highest in institutions with lower staffing levels of registered nurses and certified nursing assistants, reflecting the importance of health care resources rather than medical decision-making.
- Associated with impaired quality of life and significant morbidity and mortality. 1-yr mortality rate approaches 40%, and if complicated by bacteremia may exceed 55%. Emotional and psychological trauma often accompany pressure injury, leading to more significant reduction in overall well-being and quality of life.
- Significant pain occurs in two thirds of patients with stage 2 or greater pressure injury.

CLINICAL PRESENTATION

There are a number of pressure injury classification systems that have been developed and utilized to describe the stages of pressure injury. The most commonly used system is from the National Pressure Ulcer Advisory Panel (NPUAP). The European Pressure Ulcer Advisory Panel (EPUAP) recommends similar staging except for the presence of suspected deep tissue injury and unstageable ulcers. The staging of the wound should be based according to the extent or depth of injury. Common locations of pressure injury have been demonstrated in the following settings: Supine position, prone position, lying in bed with head elevated, and sitting position. In order of prevalence, sites most commonly involved are those over the sacrum, calcaneus, ischium, and greater trochanter. In

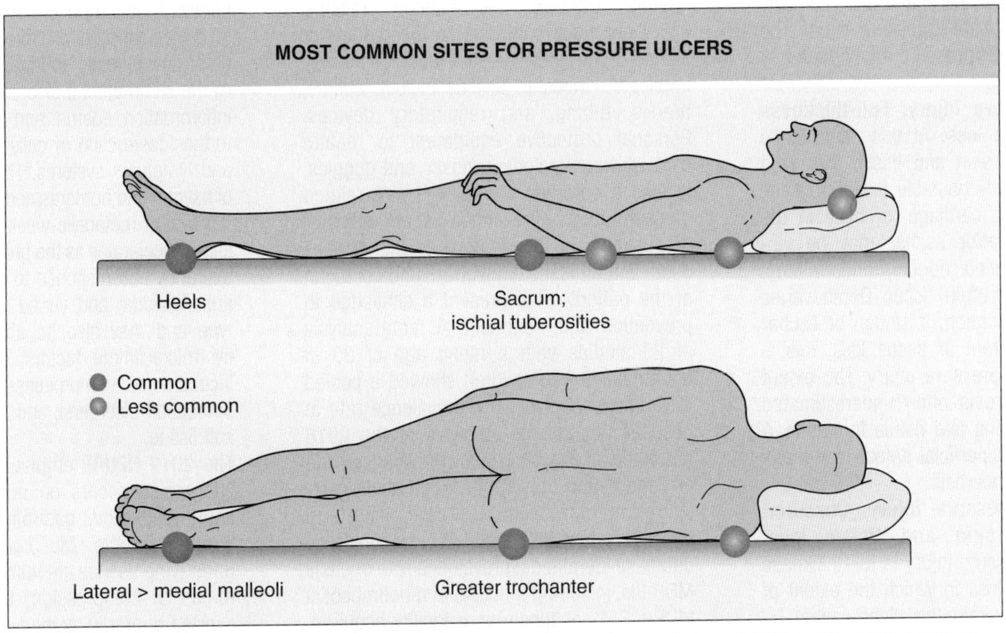

FIG. 1 Most common sites for pressure ulcers. (From Bolognia J. *Dermatology*, ed 4, Philadelphia, 2018, Elsevier.)

general, up to 75% of all pressure injuries are located around the pelvic girdle. Heel is the second most common site after the sacrum and the most common site in the case of suspected deep tissue injuries.

The NPUAP 2016 guidelines (Fig. E3) described the staging system as follows:

- **Stage 1 pressure injury: Nonblanchable erythema of intact skin.** Skin is intact with a localized area of nonblanchable erythema, which may appear differently in patients with darkly pigmented skin color. The presence of blanchable erythema or changes in sensation, temperature, or firmness may precede visual changes. Color changes do not include purple or maroon discoloration; these may indicate deep tissue pressure injury.
- **Stage 2 pressure injury: Partial-thickness skin loss with exposed dermis.** The wound bed is viable, pink or red, moist, and may also present as an intact or ruptured serum-filled blister. Adipose tissue is not visible, and deeper tissues are not visible. Granulation tissue, slough, and eschar are not present. These injuries commonly result from adverse microclimates and shear in the skin over the pelvis and shear in the heel. This stage should not be used to describe moisture-associated skin damage, including incontinence-associated dermatitis, intertriginous dermatitis, medical adhesive–related skin injury, or traumatic wounds (skin tears, burns, abrasions).
- **Stage 3 pressure injury: Full-thickness skin loss.** At this stage there is full-thickness loss of skin with adipose tissue visible in the ulcer; granulation tissue and epibole (rolled wound edges) are often present. Slough and/or eschar may be visible. The depth of tissue damage varies by anatomical location; areas of significant adiposity can develop deep wounds. Undermining and tunneling may occur. Fascia, muscle, tendon, ligament, cartilage, and/or bone are not exposed. If slough or eschar obscures the extent of tissue loss, this is an unstageable pressure injury. The depth of a stage 3 pressure injury varies by anatomic location.
- **Stage 4 pressure injury: Full-thickness skin and tissue loss.** At this stage there is full-thickness skin and tissue loss with exposed or directly palpable fascia, muscle, tendon, ligament, cartilage, or bone in the ulcer. Slough and/or eschar may be visible. Epibole (rolled edges), undermining, and/or tunneling often occur. Depth varies by anatomical location. If slough or eschar obscures the extent of tissue loss, this is an unstageable pressure injury. The extent of stage 4 ulcers is often underestimated due to undermining and fistula formation. A relatively small superficial defect may mask extensive tissue necrosis.
- **Unstageable pressure injury: Obscured full-thickness skin and tissue loss.** Unstageable pressure injury is full-thickness skin and tissue loss in which the extent of tissue damage within the ulcer cannot be confirmed because it is obscured by slough or eschar. If slough or eschar is removed, a stage 3 or stage 4 pressure injury will be revealed. Stable eschar (i.e., dry, adherent, intact without erythema or fluctuance) on the heel or ischemic limb should not be softened or removed.
- **Deep tissue pressure injury: Persistent nonblanchable deep red, maroon, or purple discoloration:** New ICD-10 subcategory for DTPI: Separates this category of pressure injury from unstageable wounds.
  1. Deep tissue pressure injury consists of intact or nonintact skin with a localized area of persistent nonblanchable deep red, maroon, or purple discoloration, or with epidermal separation revealing a dark wound bed or blood-filled blister. Pain and temperature changes often precede skin color changes. Discoloration may appear differently in darkly pigmented skin. This injury results from intense and/or prolonged pressure and shear forces at the bone-muscle interface. Early stage deep tissue pressure injuries do not have an outer layer of slough or eschar and are not debrided. The wound may evolve rapidly to reveal the actual extent of tissue injury, or it may resolve without tissue loss. If necrotic tissue, subcutaneous tissue, granulation tissue, fascia, muscle, or other underlying structures are visible, a full-thickness pressure injury is present (unstageable, stage 3 or stage 4). Deep tissue pressure injury should not be used to describe vascular, traumatic, neuropathic, or dermatologic conditions.
  2. Deep tissue injury (DTI) prevalence is highest in the ICU. It accounts for about 14% of all ulcers. Common areas affected include coccyx, sacrum, buttocks, and heels.
- **Medical device–related pressure injury:** Medical device–related pressure injuries (MDR PIs) result from the use of devices designed and applied for diagnostic or therapeutic purposes. The resultant pressure injury generally conforms to the pattern or shape of the device. The most commonly implicated medical devices include splints, braces, tubing, and respiratory devices. Personal protective equipment for health care workers, including masks and goggles, is also a common cause of device-related pressure injury. Prevention is an indicator of quality care. The nature of the devices used, anatomical site involved, and condition of the patient often present a challenge to prevention and treatment. A meta-analysis of 29 studies with a mean age of 39 in adults and 5.9 in children showed a pooled 12% incidence and 10% prevalence rate in hospitalized patients. Analysis of the 2016 International Pressure Ulcer Prevalence Data in Canada and the U.S. included acute care, long-term care, subacute care, long-term acute care hospitals, and hospice. This large database identified a prevalence rate of 0.6% MDR PIs, including mucosal and nonmucosal MDRs. 75% of these were facility-acquired. Over half (>50%) were stage 1 to 2, 22% stage 3 to 4, and 15% deep tissue PI. These injuries tend to form up to 3 days faster than non-MDR pressure injuries. The most common site is the ears, associated with respiratory cannulas, tubings and masks. Meatal pressure injury is associated with prolonged use of urinary catheters, but may occur as early as day 1 of insertion. Another common site is the feet, associated with casts and splints. The resultant pressure injury generally conforms to the pattern or shape of the device. The injury should be classified using the staging system.
- **Mucosal membrane pressure injury:** Mucosal membrane pressure injury is found on mucous membranes with a history of a medical device use at the location of the injury. Due to the anatomy of the tissue, these ulcers cannot be staged. Unique characteristics of mucosa include difficulty to detect nonblanchable erythema and absence of scar formation that in turn lead to an underappreciation of the severity of the injuries.
- **Incontinence-associated dermatitis (IAD):** There is intense and diffuse erythema of specific sites such as perineum, buttocks, and inner thighs. Associated symptoms include itching, burning sensation, pain, and concomitant fungal infections. The presentation can be varied. This includes ulcers with diffuse and irregular edges, papules, scaling, and weeping lesions. These are not classified as pressure injuries; however, they serve as a significant risk factor for the evolution to pressure injury.

PATHOGENESIS

- The development of a pressure injury is a complex interaction of external forces and host-specific (intrinsic) factors. The 2019 NPUAP Clinical Practice Guideline describes the mechanism for tissue damage as a direct and indirect result of compression (applied perpendicular to the tissue surface) and/or tension or shear (applied parallel to the surface). When these forces are sustained beyond a critical load, the tissue deformation leads to direct cellular damage. At the same time, it also initiates a cascade of inflammation, edema, and ischemia leading to further destruction of cells in the endothelium and lymphatic systems. This reduces delivery of oxygen and nutrients and inhibits or prevents removal of metabolic waste. The rate of tissue injury accelerates as the process continues. The tolerance and response to pressure and shear are individual and varied. It differs by tissue type and may also be affected by immobility, microclimate factors, nutrition, perfusion, incontinence, comorbidities (including sensory perception disorders), and the condition of the soft tissue.
- The 2019 NPUAP emphasizes that pressure injury also occurs on mucous membranes lining respiratory, gastrointestinal, and genitourinary tracts. Mucous membranes and underlying tissues are vulnerable to the same forces of compression, friction, and shear exerted primarily by medical devices such as tubes and stabilization devices.

- The 2016 NPUAP consensus statement identified risk factors in specific situations that may lead to the development of unavoidable pressure injuries. These include the following: Impaired tissue oxygenation, cardiovascular instability, hypovolemia, sepsis, anasarca, peripheral vascular disease, sensory impairment, immobility, end-of-life skin failure, and multiorgan failure. Body mass index (BMI) has an important role in the risk for pressure injury. Underweight (BMI <19 kg/m^2) and morbidly obese (BMI >40 kg/m^2) patients are at high risk for pressure injury formation. Other contributing mechanisms for the development of pressure injury include reperfusion injury, increased capillary permeability, soft tissue edema, lymphatic impairment, direct mechanical cellular injury, up-regulated autophagy, and accelerated cell senescence. Diseases that affect tissue perfusion such as peripheral vascular disease, diabetes mellitus, and heart failure pose a heightened risk for pressure injury development. However, it is important to note that patients with poor hemodynamics in addition to liver failure, sepsis, and acute respiratory distress syndrome may present with acute skin failure (ASF) rather than pressure injury. This is most commonly observed in the ICU setting.
- Unlike other wounds, pressure injuries do not often follow the normal phases of healing (i.e. initial inflammatory phase, proliferative phase, and final remodeling and maturation phase). Instead, they become arrested in the inflammatory phase.
- Complications of untreated pressure injuries include cellulitis, osteomyelitis, abscess formation, sinus tract formation/fistulas, heterotopic ossification, systemic amyloidosis from chronic inflammation, rhabdomyolysis, renal dysfunction, chronic nonhealing wounds, and malignant transformation such as squamous cell cancer, particularly in a nonhealing pressure injury.
- Recurrence rates described in the literature are limited to pressure injuries occurring after surgical wound closure. Injuries involving closure after secondary intention have not been widely studied but postulated to be significant. Overall, there is a wide variation in recurrence rates from 3% to 100%.

Dx DIAGNOSIS

DIFFERENTIAL DIAGNOSIS

- Venous insufficiency ulcers
- Arterioocclusive ulcers
- Diabetic foot ulcers
- Neuropathic ulcers
- Skin cancer
- Cellulitis and erysipelas
- Skin abscess
- Kennedy terminal ulcers (KTU)
- Acute skin failure (ASF)
- Incontinence-associated dermatitis (IAD)
- Perineal dermatitis
- Device-related pressure injury

WORKUP

- Begin with a comprehensive assessment, including evaluation of medical, social, and psychological history, medications, functional status (including mobility and continence), cognition, nutrition, vascular status, pressure injury risk, physical exam, and other elements affecting wound healing should be implemented.
- A proper documentation of wound history is a must. This includes etiology, onset, duration, prior treatments, and procedures.
- A thorough physical examination of the identified areas of skin damage and of a minimum of 4 cm of periwound tissue should be performed.
- These areas should be evaluated for their length, width, and depth and for the presence of sinus tracts, undermining, tunneling, fistulas, exudate, and necrotic tissue as well as any evidence for healing such as the formation of granulation tissue.
- Adequate documentation such as the use of photographs for comparison can be extremely helpful to track changes over time.
- It is essential to rule out infection, as this would impair wound healing. The presence of cellulitis, abscess, and osteomyelitis should be explored.
- Clinical signs of osteomyelitis include exposed bone, persistent sinus tracts, tissue necrosis, and signs of local and systemic infection.

LABORATORY TESTS

- Directed at identifying causes, risk factors, and/or any complications arising from the pressure injury (e.g., abscess or osteomyelitis). May include complete blood count, blood cultures, erythrocyte sedimentation rate, and C-reactive protein.
- Cultures of wound bed are not believed to be helpful and should be avoided. Deep tissue biopsy is the gold standard to rule out osteomyelitis.
- Potentially useful markers for nutritional status include prealbumin, albumin, transferrin, lymphocyte count, and total cholesterol level.
- Complete blood count may be obtained if systemic infection is suspected.

IMAGING STUDIES

- Ultrasound is not proven to be effective.
- Plain radiographs, MRI, and triple-phase bone scan may help identify osteomyelitis when clinically suspected. A comparison study of 44 patients scheduled for open biopsy showed that MRI has superior diagnostic benefit over plain radiography.

Rx TREATMENT

- The most effective strategies for prevention and resolution of pressure injuries are designed to provide a systematic approach involving risk assessment, continuous monitoring, education, and multiple interventions.
- Conduct a structured and individualized risk assessment on a regular basis, especially when the clinical condition changes.
- Identify high-risk patients using standardized risk assessment scales and risk prediction tools (e.g., Braden and Norton in the U.S.; Waterlow scale in the UK; Cubbin and Jackson scale for ICU patients).
- Use standardized assessment tools to monitor wound healing on a weekly basis. Examples include the Pressure Sore Status Tool (PSST), Pressure Ulcer Scale for Healing (PUSH), Wound Healing Scale, and the Sessing Scale. The PUSH tool in conjunction with the NPUAP staging system is the most readily applied tool.
  1. Use of prophylactic dressings in high-risk patients resulted in an 88% reduction in pressure injury when included in a skin care bundle.
  2. A high-quality U.S. and Australian study suggests that foam and silicone dressings may be effective in reducing the incidence of pressure injury in high-risk patients when used for prevention.
  3. Focus on controlling the microclimate (moisture and temperature).
  4. Minimize prolonged skin exposure to moisture, urine, or stool.
  5. Treat dry, cracked skin.
- Use of repositioning and pressure-reducing devices (e.g., foam mattresses, air-fluidized beds, low–air-loss beds, pillows, gel pads, or foam wedges when in bed or in a chair).
  1. Patient repositioning (based on individual tissue tolerance): Current studies assume repositioning is effective for prevention and healing. Expert opinion has traditionally advised repositioning every 2 hr, but recent guidelines from NPUAP have rescinded this recommendation because of a lack of evidence. Two important risk factors that are relevant to this intervention include the angle of incline and the specific position of the body. Focus is on education, positioning devices, most effective position, and turning frequency. Studies range from basic techniques and devices such as pillows to pressure mapping imaging and ultrasound to detect changes indicating deep tissue injury. Pilot studies continue in acute care hospitals, critical care, rehabilitation facilities, nursing homes, and in home-bound populations.
  2. Bed surface:
     a. There is consensus that pressure-reducing mattresses are effective in prevention and healing of pressure injuries compared with standard bed surfaces. Data comparing reactive vs. nonreactive support surfaces are inconsistent and inconclusive.
     b. Two randomized controlled trials (RCTs) found that use of air-fluidized beds contributed to the healing of a greater number of pressure injuries after 15 days compared with standard care.
     c. A systematic review revealed no differences in the rate of pressure injury healing with the use of either

alternating-pressure mattresses or low–air-loss beds compared with standard care. A small Belgian prospective RCT compared a static air mattress vs alternating pressure mattress in high risk, bed or chair-dependent nursing home residents over age 65. Results noted pressure injuries presented 50% sooner in the alternating pressure mattress group compared with the static air mattress.

3. Support surface:
   a. The first meta-analysis of support surfaces and pressure injury prevention concluded with moderate certainty that powered active air surfaces and powered hybrid air surfaces probably reduced the incidence of pressure injuries by 58% and 78% when compared with standard hospital surfaces.
   b. There is low certainty that nonpowered reactive surfaces reduce pressure injuries.
   c. Based on the results of 19 RCTs, a Cochrane Review concluded based on current evidence: No support surface is more effective at healing pressure injuries than standard support surfaces.
   d. Pressure-relieving overlays: One RCT demonstrated that a viscoelastic pad on the operating table significantly reduced incidence of postoperative pressure injuries compared with a standard operating table.
   e. Use adequate support surfaces while in bed or in a chair to prevent "bottoming out" (defined as less than 1 inch between patient and support surface; measured by putting hand under support surface and feeling thickness to patient).
4. Foam alternatives:
   a. Forty-one RCTs demonstrated that patients lying on standard hospital mattresses are more likely to develop pressure injuries than those patients lying on higher-specification foam mattresses.

- A small, open-label, multicenter hospital study in China compared the effectiveness of two pressure injury prevention protocols. They found no increased risk or incidence of pressure injury with use of a viscoelastic mattress and every 4-hr repositioning schedule versus the control, powered air pressure redistribution mattress at a standard every 2-hr positioning schedule. Total incidence of pressure injury was 13 (1.1%) of 1204 participants.
- Recent extensive systematic reviews including a meta-synthesis of 25 Cochrane reviews of pressure injury prevention and treatment trials show poor methodology in most studies. The low certainty of evidence results in few recommendations for clinical practice. Use of support surfaces, repositioning, optimized nutrition, and sacral skin moisturizing was most appropriate.

NONPHARMACOLOGIC THERAPY

- Pressure injuries and the surrounding skin should be cleaned at each dressing change.
- Avoid agents that are cytotoxic to epithelial cells (e.g., iodine, iodophor, sodium hypochlorite, hydrogen peroxide, acetic acid, alcohol).
- Wound irrigation should not exceed 15 psi and is best done with an 18-gauge angiocatheter.
- Necrotic tissue debridement is essential to wound bed preparation. Methods include sharp debridement, autolytic, biological, and mechanical. There is strong consensus for early debridement to prevent wound infection and delayed wound healing.
- Do not debride hard, dry, stable eschar on heels or ischemic limbs unless infection is suspected.
- No single dressing or product is superior; keep the wound bed moist and protect it from urine/stool. Silver dressings, topical phenytoin, and growth factors should be limited to difficult-to-heal wounds, chronic ulcers, and extensive burns given their extra cost and limited scientific validation. Reduce pressure by using foam mattress, dynamic support surface (e.g., low–air-loss bed), and frequent repositioning (e.g., every 2 hr or, in case of poor perfusion, more frequently).
- Hyperbaric oxygen therapy when used for some wounds provided temporary benefit. There have been no studies specifically looking at treatment of pressure injuries. Moreover, serious adverse events such as pneumothorax and seizures can occur.
- The data on the efficacy of ultrasound as wound therapy is limited. Results were not statistically significant when compared to standard therapy. Similarly RCTs on electromagnetic therapy found no evidence of benefit on wound healing.
- Use of topical agents such as phenytoin, becaplermin gel, sucralfate, and medicinal manuka honey showed limited evidence for the healing of stage 2 ulcers.
- Negative-pressure wound therapy (NPWT) may be useful for wounds that have significant drainage and third-space edema. They help improve healing by promoting angiogenesis, improving tissue perfusion, and decreasing bacterial count. Calcium alginate and foam dressings may also be beneficial for such wounds. Randomized studies have not identified any significant differences to quantitative wound healing; however, it provided some level of patient and provider comfort and shortened the rate of healing.
- Although controlling poor nutrition has been shown to be beneficial, a recent large investigation demonstrated that feeding tubes did not prevent or heal pressure injuries, but increased the risk for their development.
- Minimize or promptly remove urinary and/or fecal contamination.
- No RCTs have compared debridement versus no debridement in the treatment of pressure injuries.
  1. Thirty-two RCTs have compared different debridement agents, but there is insufficient evidence to promote the use of one particular agent.
  2. One RCT demonstrated pressure injuries treated with collagenase healed significantly more quickly than those treated with hydrocolloid.
  3. One RCT comparing honey-treated dressings with saline-soaked dressings showed faster healing times with the honey-treated group.
  4. A meta-analysis and one RCT found significant benefit in rates of healing with use of hydrocolloid dressings versus traditional saline gauze dressings but not over other forms such as hydrogels, foam dressings, or collagenase.
- Malnutrition is an independent risk factor for pressure injury. However no benefit was found with nutritional and vitamin supplementation for those without known nutritional deficiencies. There is inconclusive evidence that vitamin C and zinc are effective in wound healing. Data is limited to support enteral or parenteral nutrition for patients whose oral intake is inadequate.
- There is insufficient data to recommend the use of anabolic steroids such as oxandrolone therapy to promote weight gain and repletion of protein stores.

ACUTE GENERAL Rx

- The cornerstone of therapy involves the use of appropriate wound dressings, pressure-reducing devices, treatment of infection, debridement, and surgical consultation when appropriate.
- Traditional bedside debridement provides excellent results in reducing the surface area for a majority of the wounds. Sharp debridement can effectively remove devitalized tissue and is a proven significant component to advancing wound closure.
- All pressure injuries are colonized with bacteria. Clinically evident infections should be assessed with culture and treated appropriately with topical and systemic antibiotics.
- A randomized controlled trial in 2017 showed significant reduction in stage 2 to 4 pressure injuries using anode and cathode high-voltage electrical stimulation.
- Pain medications are necessary if pressure injuries are present. One study found that excruciating pain was more prevalent in nursing home residents with pressure injuries. Local factors that may be contributing to pain such as ischemia, infection, or breakdown of surrounding skin should be properly addressed.

CHRONIC Rx

- Continue vigilance with pressure reduction because pressure injuries can recur with minimal trauma.

- There are no randomized trials available to identify whether repositioning makes a difference in the healing rates of pressure injuries or what the optimal repositioning regimen should be.
- Consider radiologic evaluation for infected ulcer bed, occult osteomyelitis, or abscess.

DISPOSITION

- When systematic risk assessments are done and preventive measures are followed, most pressure injuries can be prevented. Most injuries heal when appropriate management strategies are followed.
- Stage 4 pressure injuries in high-risk patients (e.g., paraplegics) can take mo to yr to heal.

REFERRAL

- Physical and occupational therapists to help improve bed and chair mobility, as well as basic activities of daily living
- Wounds with necrotic tissue may need referral to providers trained in sharp debridement
- Role of plastic surgeons for operative repair for large stage 3 or 4 pressure injuries that do not respond to optimal care
- To a specialty wound care center for nonhealing complex pressure injuries

PATIENT & FAMILY EDUCATION

- Educate patient and family members on the risk factors for pressure injury formation.
- Encourage mobility and adequate nutritional intake as well as avoidance of bed rest.
- There is a need for patient involvement and education during periods of care transition and service changes by health care providers.

Considerations for palliative wound care for pressure injuries that exist and occur in serious illness to include the end-of-life stage

- Palliative patient populations have the highest incidence of all types of wounds. Pressure injuries comprise about 60% of them.
- Pressure injuries are unavoidable at the end of life. The term SCALE (skin changes at life's end) was introduced in 2008 to describe the group of wound phenomena that result from the complex failure of homeostatic mechanisms at the end of life.
- Kennedy Terminal Ulcer (KTU) has been described in the literature as an unavoidable and rapid onset skin breakdown or skin failure that occurs as part of the dying process. Poor circulation is the main trigger. It occurs in the sacrococcygeal area, heel, calf, and elbows. Its classic configuration could be shaped like a pear, butterfly, or horseshoe. In contrast, the 3:30 syndrome of KTU was coined due to the rapidity of change, i.e., the patient's skin was normal when examined in the morning and by 3:30 pm shift change, the ulcer had emerged.
- The basic steps in pressure injury management at the end of life mirror that of conventional pressure injury except that the primary intent is not necessarily for wound healing. Rather, emphasis on quality of life and symptom control is the overarching goal. These steps include cleansing/debridement; management of exudate, slough, or infection; protection of the periwound skin; and dead space management.
- Common wound cleansing solutions used in this population include Dakin solution, cadexomer iodine, acetic acid, and topical phenytoin. All promote some improvement in inflammation, bacterial burden, healing, odor, pain, and granulation tissue development.
- The factors associated with increased likelihood of healing include age less than 70 yr, palliative performance score >30, and in exceptional circumstances, the use of artificial nutrition for those with good performance status.

PEARLS & CONSIDERATIONS

COMMENTS

SARS-COV2/COVID 19-related considerations:

- Personal protective equipment used by health care professionals and patients across all settings has dramatically increased with the COVID-19 pandemic. Prolonged wear time is associated with dermatitis and rising incidence of pressure injuries.
  1. The nasal bridge, ears, and cheekbones are most affected.
  2. A case series of five health care workers using N95 masks revealed the presence of pressure ulcers over the dorsum of the nose following prolonged usage.
  3. On average, N95 respirators were used over 5 hr after each donning procedure.
  4. Principles of prevention and treatment focus on adequate training on proper donning and doffing of protective equipment, offloading pressure (proper fit, and scheduled breaks), protective silicone and other barrier dressings to reduce pressure and friction, and moisturizers.
- Prone positioning is used to enhance oxygenation levels in patients with severe acute respiratory distress. Proning minimizes ventral alveolar distention and reduces dorsal alveolar collapse by decreasing the difference between dorsal and ventral transpulmonary pressure. Moreover, it prevents lung compression thereby improving gas exchange and blood perfusion.
  1. Up to 28% of patients admitted to intensive care units with confirmed COVID-19 are cared for in the prone position.
  2. According to international data, up to 57% of patients treated with this postural therapy developed pressure injuries grade 2 to 4 on the face and other weight-bearing areas. This is an additional risk in critically vulnerable patients already challenged with stressors of reduced tissue tolerance in periods of hypoxia and hypoperfusion, combined with immobility and use of medical devices, including masks, tubings, and catheters.
     a. A multidisciplinary approach to prevent and treat pressure injuries in prone COVID-19 patients in Brazil is a promising strategy to take care of at-risk patients.
- Up to 10% of older persons will have a pressure injury.
- Because 70% of pressure injuries occur in older persons, the approach should be similar to other multifactorial geriatric syndromes with an interprofessional team approach.
- Identify and reduce all modifiable risk factors for pressure injuries.
- Treat the pain associated with pressure injuries.
- Proper skin care, use of support surfaces, mobilization, and nutritional support are integral for prevention and treatment. Of these, pressure redistribution is the most important factor for prevention.
- Effective prevention practices consist of timely wound reassessments, regular communication with team members, patient and caregiver empowerment, and utilization of clinical decision support tools for health care providers.
- Clinical studies have not revealed that any one dressing product is superior to another.
- Nonhealing pressure injuries require assessment for debridement, infection, abscess, and/or referral to a wound center.

SUGGESTED READINGS

Available at ExpertConsult.com

RELATED CONTENT

Bed Sores (Patient Information)

AUTHORS: **Mary-Beth Walesko, MS, APRN-BC, WCC,** and **Noelle Marie Javier, MD**

BASIC INFORMATION

DEFINITION

Preterm labor is defined as regular contractions that result in cervical dilation or effacement prior to 37 wk gestation. Preterm birth is one that occurs after 20 wk gestation and before the completion of 37 wk gestational age.

SYNONYM

Premature labor

ICD-10CM CODES

O60.0	Preterm labor without delivery
O60.1	Preterm spontaneous labor with preterm delivery
O60.2	Preterm spontaneous labor with term delivery

EPIDEMIOLOGY & DEMOGRAPHICS

INCIDENCE: The incidence of preterm births in the U.S. increased from 9.5% in 1981 to 12.7% in 2006 before falling gradually to 11.4% by 2013. The increase since 1981 is attributed to improvements in pregnancy dating by ultrasound, increased use of assisted reproductive technology, and increased preterm induction or preterm operative delivery for maternal or fetal indications. Between 40% and 45% of these births follow spontaneous preterm labor; either the remaining preterm births result from preterm premature rupture of membranes (PPROM), or they occur secondary to intentional delivery for maternal or fetal indications.

PREDOMINANT AGE & RACIAL DIFFERENCES: Pregnant women at the extremes of reproductive age (<17 yr and >35 yr) are at greatest risk. Black race is one of the most significant risk factors with the rate of preterm birth averaging 13.9% between 2016 and 2018 compared to 8.7% among Asian Americans and 9.6% in white women. The disparity between African-American and other ethnic American races persists after adjusting for income, education, and other medical risk factors.

GENETICS: A genetic component has been suggested. Women with sisters who have had preterm births and women with grandparents who were born preterm may be at increased risk for having preterm deliveries themselves. Single-nucleotide polymorphisms have also been associated with preterm labor.

RISK FACTORS: Risk factors for premature labor include a prior preterm delivery, intrauterine infection, systemic or genital tract infections, periodontal disease, short interpregnancy interval (<6 mo), short cervical length (<25 to 30 mm), low pre-pregnancy body mass index (BMI) (<19.8 kg/m^2), age (<17 yr or >35 yr), a history of elective pregnancy termination, history of prior stillbirth, African-American ethnicity, vaginal bleeding, polyhydramnios or oligohydramnios, multiple gestation, structural abnormalities of the uterus, history of cervical cone biopsy or loop electrocautery excision, in vitro fertilization or ovulation induction, tobacco use, heavy alcohol consumption, cocaine use, heroin use, and psychological or social stress. The strongest historic risk factor for preterm birth is a previous birth between 16 and 36 wk gestation.

PHYSICAL FINDINGS & CLINICAL PRESENTATION

Presenting symptoms include increased pelvic pressure, abdominal cramping or contractions, increased vaginal discharge, vaginal bleeding or spotting, or leakage of fluid.

ETIOLOGY

Causes of premature labor are varied and often difficult to determine. Premature labor may be secondary to infection, systemic illness, trauma, anatomic abnormalities (i.e., uterine anomaly), or a combination of factors. It is thought that cervical ripening is the most common first step to premature labor or delivery. Subsequently, decidual-membrane activation occurs followed by contractions (Box 1).

DIAGNOSIS

DIFFERENTIAL DIAGNOSIS

The differential diagnosis for preterm labor should include preterm rupture of membranes, preterm contractions (contractions before 37 wk gestation that do not result in cervical change), and abdominal pain or cramping secondary to other medical conditions. There are many medical conditions that may cause preterm contractions or premature labor. Treating some of these underlying conditions may improve the prognosis for stopping the preterm labor.

Possible medical conditions include:

- Infection
  1. Chorioamnionitis
  2. Genital tract infections, including bacterial vaginosis, gonorrhea, chlamydia
  3. Urinary tract infections, including pyelonephritis, cystitis, or asymptomatic bacteriuria
  4. Gastroenteritis
- Trauma
- Placental abruption
- Illicit drug use
- Preterm premature rupture of membranes
- Appendicitis
- Nephrolithiasis
- Pancreatitis
- Cholelithiasis
- Uterine fibroids

WORKUP

- History and physical exam to rule out trauma, abuse, other causes of abdominal pain, and infection
- Fetal heart rate monitoring and tocometry to determine fetal status and contraction frequency
- Speculum exam to visually assess the cervix and assess for rupture of membranes, bleeding, infection, or advanced cervical dilation
  1. If the patient is <35 wk gestation, a Fetal Fibronectin (FFN) test should be collected prior to performing a digital exam or transvaginal ultrasound. A FFN test can help predict preterm delivery.
- Digital exam in the unruptured patient with normal placentation to determine cervical dilation and effacement, and fetal station

LABORATORY TESTS

- CBC
- Urine analysis and culture

BOX 1 Factors Linked to Preterm Labor

Demographic and Psychosocial
- Extremes of age (>40 yr, teenagers)
- Lower socioeconomic status
- Tobacco use
- Cocaine abuse
- Prolonged standing (occupation)
- Psychosocial stressors

Reproductive and Gynecologic
- Prior preterm delivery
- Diethylstilbestrol exposure
- Multiple gestations
- Anatomic endometrial cavity anomalies
- Cervical incompetence
- Low pregnancy weight gain
- First-trimester vaginal bleeding
- Placental abruption or previa

Surgical
- Prior reproductive organ surgery
- Prior paraendometrial surgery other than genitourinary (appendectomy)

Infectious
- Urinary tract infections
- Nonuterine infections
- Genital tract infections (bacterial vaginosis)

From Marx JA et al: *Rosen's emergency medicine: concepts and clinical practice,* ed 7, Philadelphia, 2010, Elsevier.

- Urine toxicology screen
- Collect tests for GBS, gonorrhea, and *Chlamydia*
- Perform a wet prep for yeast, bacterial vaginosis, and *Trichomonas*
- Fetal fibronectin swab as described earlier
- Consider PT, PTT, INR, CMP, amylase, and lipase
- Amniocentesis may be performed if an intraamniotic infection is suspected

IMAGING STUDIES

- A formal ultrasound is indicated to determine estimated fetal weight, fetal presentation, amniotic fluid volume, placental location and appearance, and cervical length.
- The diagnosis of preterm labor is confirmed in the presence of regular contractions with subsequent cervical change. Suspicion for preterm labor may be heightened if FFN is positive.

Rx TREATMENT

Patients with premature labor should be delivered promptly when an intraamniotic infection is suspected or when they have advanced cervical dilation >5 cm, a persistently nonreassuring fetal heart rate tracing, or significant vaginal bleeding concerning for placental abruption having maternal or neonatal implications.

NONPHARMACOLOGIC THERAPY

- Smoking cessation.
- Bedrest, activity restriction, and pelvic rest are often recommended by clinicians, but there are insufficient data to support this practice.

ACUTE GENERAL Rx

- Antenatal administration of corticosteroids between 24 wk and 33 6/7 wk gestation is recommended for women at risk of preterm delivery to prevent neonatal respiratory distress syndrome and decrease the incidence of intraventricular hemorrhage and necrotizing enterocolitis. It is also recommended between 34.0 and 36.6 wk gestation if there is no prior steroid exposure.
- Numerous tocolytic agents have been used in an attempt to inhibit contractions (Box 2). Although efficacy is unclear, they can be utilized during an observation period in an effort to prolong gestation for administration and exposure of steroids or to transfer the mother to a facility capable of caring for preterm infants. This, of course, assumes there are no maternal or fetal medical contraindications to use of tocolytic drugs and no indications for rapid delivery. The most commonly used tocolytics are beta-mimetics (terbutaline), magnesium sulfate, calcium channel blockers (nifedipine), or prostaglandin synthetase inhibitors (indomethacin, ketorolac, sulindac). Table E1 summarizes side effect profiles of tocolytic agents.
- Routine antibiotic use has failed to show benefit in the absence of a known infection. But all mothers in preterm labor (without a documented negative group B strep culture) should be given antibiotics to prevent neonatal GBS infection.
- Intravenous magnesium sulfate has been shown to decrease cerebral palsy in children exposed antenatally with premature labor or premature rupture of the membranes at less than 32 wks' gestation.

BOX 2 Commonly Used Tocolytic Agents

Magnesium sulfate
- 4-6 g IV bolus over 30 min
- 2-4 g/hr IV infusion

Terbutaline
- 5-10 mg PO q4-6h
- 0.25-0.5 mg SC q30 min-6 h
- 10-80 μg/min IV

Ritodrine*
- 10 mg PO q2-4 h
- 5-10 mg IM q2-4 h
- 50-350 μg/min IV

Isoxsuprine
- 20 mg PO q4-6 h
- 0.05-0.5 mg/min IV

IV, Intravenously; *PO,* orally; *SC,* subcutaneously.
*Ritodrine is currently discontinued in the U.S.
From Marx JA et al: *Rosen's emergency medicine: concepts and clinical practice,* ed 7, Philadelphia, 2010, Elsevier.

PROPHYLACTIC OR CHRONIC Rx

- Patients with a history of prior spontaneous preterm birth may be candidates for prophylactic use of 17 alpha-hydroxyprogesterone caproate between 16 wk and 36 wk gestation. These patients may also benefit from transvaginal cervical length screening in pregnancy to monitor for short cervix.
- Patients with a history of preterm birth and short cervix may also be candidates for prophylactic or rescue cerclage.
- Patients with a short cervix may be candidates for vaginal progesterone for prevention and, in some clinical studies, vaginal pessary.
- There is no evidence supporting the use of maintenance tocolytic therapy.

REFERRAL

- Women who present in preterm labor should be referred to an obstetrician and transferred to a facility with a neonatal intensive care unit.
- For women who present for prenatal care with a history of preterm delivery, early referral to an obstetrician is also recommended.

SUGGESTED READINGS

Available at ExpertConsult.com

RELATED CONTENT

Abruptio Placentae (Related Key Topic)
Breech Birth (Related Key Topic)

AUTHORS: **Ghamar Bitar, MD,** and **Anthony Sciscione, DO**

BASIC INFORMATION

DEFINITION

Primary biliary cholangitis (PBC), previously known as primary biliary cirrhosis is a chronic, variably progressive cholestatic liver disease most often affecting middle-aged women and characterized by autoimmune destruction of intralobular bile ducts leading to portal inflammation, hepatic cell necrosis, fibrosis, cirrhosis and, ultimately, liver failure.

SYNONYMS

PBC
Primary biliary cirrhosis
Biliary cirrhosis
Nonsuppurative destructive cholangitis
Autoimmune cholangiopathy (AIC)

ICD-10CM CODE
K74.3 Primary biliary cholangitis

EPIDEMIOLOGY & DEMOGRAPHICS

INCIDENCE:

- Annual incidence rates range from 3.3 to 58 cases per million.
- PBC accounts for up to 2% of deaths from cirrhosis worldwide.

PREVALENCE: Prevalence is greatest in North America and Northern Europe and varies tremendously by time and geographic areas, ranging globally from 2.7 to 492 cases per million. Disease burden seems to be increasing, which may be a result of better detection rather than true rise in disease incidence.

PREDOMINANT SEX: Female:male ratio of 9:1

PREDOMINANT AGE: Onset typically occurs between the ages of 30 and 65 yr and is uncommon before age 25 yr.

PREDOMINANT RACE: Most often described in Caucasians but PBC affects all races.

GENETICS:

- Pathogenesis is unknown, but it is thought to be in the setting of environmental influences and genetic predisposition.
- There are no clearly identified genetic factors associated with PBC; however, there is a clear familial occurrence. Prevalence among familial clustering of PBC is approximately 3% to 9% in the U.S., Brazil, Japan, and Europe. The concordance rate among monozygotic twins is 63%.
- Up to 73% of patients with PBC have at least one other extrahepatic autoimmune disorder such as thyroiditis, Sjögren syndrome, rheumatoid arthritis, cutaneous scleroderma (which can include CREST syndrome), systemic lupus erythematosus, pernicious anemia, celiac disease, autoimmune thrombocytopenia purpura, autoimmune diabetes mellitus, and/or other autoimmune diseases.
- A variant form of PBC exists as an overlap syndrome with autoimmune hepatitis (AIH).
- PBC is closely associated with a greater risk of hepatocellular carcinoma as well as an overall greater risk of cancer.

ETIOLOGY

- Although the cause of PBC remains unknown, it is believed to require both a genetic susceptibility as well as an environmental trigger ultimately leading to the modification of mitochondrial proteins triggering a persistent T lymphocyte–mediated attack on intralobular bile ducts.
- PBC is associated most strongly with HLA alleles DRA, DRB1, DPB1, DQB1, BTNL2 and c6orf10. PBC is also associated with ORMDL3, CD80, STAT1/STAT4, IL12A, NF-κB, and RPL3/SYNGR1. However, there is variation across ethnic groups.
- Possible environmental triggers include infectious agents, cigarette smoking, environmental pollutants, radiation, urinary tract infections, reproductive hormone replacement, prior pregnancy, toxic waste sites (particularly exposure to halogenated hydrocarbons), electrophilic drugs, and xenobiotics found in food additives and cosmetics.
- The enzyme complex subunit PDC-E2 is an autoantigen that plays a major role in the early pathogenesis of PBC. Patients with PBC have a tenfold increased concentration of PDC-E2-specific cytotoxic $CD8^+$ lymphocytes in their livers compared to their blood, and antimitochondrial antibodies (AMAs), which are the serologic hallmark of this disease, react to the PDC-E2 subunit leading to a strong inflammatory response. In addition, biliary epithelial cells handle PDC-E2 in a unique way that exposes them to immune-mediated attack. Future therapies may be specific immunomodulation directed at these peptides.
- In addition, secondary damage to hepatocytes results from the chronic accumulation of bile acids.

PHYSICAL FINDINGS & CLINICAL PRESENTATION

Clinical stages:

- Asymptomatic
- Symptomatic
- Cirrhotic
- Hepatic failure

Symptoms:

- 50% to 65% of patients may be asymptomatic; 50% of patients develop symptoms in 5 yr, 80% in 10 yr, and 95% in 20 yr.
- Fatigue (20%-85% of patients) and pruritus (40%-80% of patients) are the usual presenting symptoms and are independent of disease severity.
- Fatigue can be chronic and correlate with daytime somnolence and autonomic dysfunction.
- Pruritus is worse at night, with constricting, coarse garments, and in association with dry skin and hot, humid weather. The cause is unknown but elevated histamine, bile salt concentration, endogenous opioids, lysophosphatidic acid, and female steroid hormones and their metabolites have been discussed as potential causes. Pruritus may first occur during pregnancy but is distinguished from pruritus of pregnancy because it persists into the postpartum period and beyond.
- Symptoms include jaundice (10%-60%), unexplained right upper quadrant pain (10%), manifestations of portal hypertension, dyslipidemia (76%-96%), xanthomas (15%-50%), osteoporosis (20%-44%), Sjögren syndrome (4%-73%), rheumatoid arthritis (2%-6%), systemic lupus erythematosus (up to 4%), celiac disease (up to 6%), and thyroid disorders (6%-24%) with the most common being Hashimoto thyroiditis.
- Other symptoms can include steatorrhea, fat-soluble vitamin deficiencies, and anemia.

Physical examination:

- Variable: Findings depend on stage of disease at time of presentation; patients at the early stage may be completely unaffected.
- Excoriations may be present due to extensive scratching from pruritus and can be severe enough to cause bleeding.
- Hepatomegaly and splenomegaly can worsen with disease progression.
- Xanthomas and jaundice generally appear in advanced disease. Kayser-Fleischer rings are rare and result from copper retention. Hyperpigmentation of the skin due to melanin deposition may also occur.
- Late physical findings mirror those of cirrhosis: Spider nevi, caput medusae, temporal and proximal limb wasting, ascites, palmar erythema, digital clubbing, gynecomastia, and edema.

Dx DIAGNOSIS

The diagnosis of PBC can be established when two of the following three criteria are met.

- Positive serum AMA, titer >1:40 or PBC-specific anti-nuclear antibody reactivity
- Biochemical evidence of cholestasis (mainly alkaline phosphatase elevation [ALP] ≥1.5 times the upper limit of normal [ULN])
- Characteristic liver histology demonstrating nonsuppurative destruction of small to medium-sized interlobular biliary ducts

DIFFERENTIAL DIAGNOSIS

- Drug-induced cholestasis (common medications: Phenothiazines, anabolic steroids, some antibiotics as TMP-SMX, oxacillin, and ampicillin)
- PBC-AIH overlap syndrome; reported in 2% to 20% of patients initially diagnosed with PBC. Transition from stable PBC to AIH and vice versa also seen
- Other etiologies of chronic liver disease and cirrhosis, such as alcoholic cirrhosis, chronic viral hepatitis, primary sclerosing cholangitis, AIH, sarcoidosis, hepatic amyloidosis, chemical/toxin-induced cirrhosis, other hereditary or familial disorders (e.g., cystic fibrosis, α-1-antitrypsin deficiency)
- Biliary obstruction
- Secondary biliary cirrhosis or secondary sclerosing cholangitis

WORKUP

History, physical examination, laboratory evaluation, liver biopsy

LABORATORY TESTS

- AMAs found in 90% to 95% of patients with PBC and are 98% specific.
- Antinuclear antibodies (ANAs) and AMAs found in 53% of patients. In approximately 5% to 10% of patients, AMAs are absent (AMA-negative PBC). Nearly all patients have ANA or AMAs, or both.
- Cholestatic pattern of liver biochemical markers; markedly increased ALP (of hepatic origin). ALP levels along with bilirubin levels correlate with the risk of liver transplantation or death.
- γ-Glutamyl transpeptidase is increased (indicates biliary origin of ALP).
- Serum IgM levels are increased (lower in AMA-negative PBC).
- Bilirubin level is normal early on and increases with disease progression (direct and indirect). Increased serum bilirubin level is a poor prognostic indicator.
- Rising serum hyaluronate levels correlate with the serum bilirubin and histologic worsening of the disease.
- Aminotransferase level may be normal and, if increased, is rarely more than 5x ULN.
- Bile acids are strikingly elevated, whose accumulation is thought to cause foamy degeneration of hepatocytes due to its toxic effect.
- Serum ceruloplasmin may also be elevated.
- Markedly increased serum lipids in more than 50% of patients is largely due to increased lipoprotein X (LpX). Total cholesterol may surpass 1000 mg/dl (with increased xanthomas rather than xanthelasmas). In the early stages of PBC, patients can have relatively higher HDL in comparison to LDL and VLDL. This rise in HDL might explain the lack of increased risk for cardiovascular disease. However, cardiovascular risk may still exist due to other risk factors (e.g., family history and metabolic syndrome).
- Percutaneous liver biopsy confirms or rules out the diagnosis, allows staging, but is not essential to make the diagnosis or to initiate medical therapy in patients with typical liver chemistry and positive AMA test.
- Histology is not uniform, so histologic stage is based on the most advanced lesion present.
  1. Stage I: Nonsuppurative cholangitis indicated by lymphocytic infiltration of small bile ducts with or without epithelioid granulomas or plasma cells, limited to portal areas
  2. Stage II: Extension of inflammatory cells to periportal parenchyma, ductular proliferation
  3. Stage III: Bridging necrosis or fibrous septa linking portal triads
  4. Stage IV: Frank cirrhosis with regenerative nodules

IMAGING STUDIES

If history, physical examination, blood tests, and liver biopsy are all consistent with PBC neither imaging nor cholangiography is necessary (Fig. E1).

PROGNOSIS

- Median survival is 7.5 to 16 yr in untreated patients but is getting longer with earlier diagnosis and initiation of treatment. Table 1 summarizes time course of histologic progression to a higher stage in patients with PBC.
- 80% of patients progress one stage within 3 yr, and 31% of patients progress from stage I to stage IV within 4 yr.
- Neither presence nor total titer level of AMAs predicts survival, disease progression, or response to therapy.
- Prognostic laboratory measures: Serum bilirubin is the best predictor of survival and the most heavily weighted factor in prognostic models. Box 1 summarizes independent predictors of survival in patients with PBC.
- Response to ursodeoxycholic acid (UDCA) therapy can be prognostic, with approximately 40% of patients failing to respond. There are multiple biochemical response criteria that, if met after 1 yr of treatment with UDCA, are associated with improved clinical outcomes. Three of these criteria are Barcelona (decrease in ALP level of at least 40% or to the reference range), Paris I (ALP <3 × ULN, AST <2 × ULN and bilirubin within normal limits), and Paris II (ALP <1.5 × ULN, ALT <1.5 × ULN and bilirubin within normal limits). Similarly, the Mayo Risk score, a predictor of short-term survival probability in nontransplanted patients (www.mayoclinic.org/medical-professionals/transplant-medicine/calculators/the-updated-natural-history-model-for-primary-biliary-cirrhosis/itt-20434724), can also reliably predict life expectancy when calculated after 6 mo of UDCA therapy.
- Several predictive models based upon laboratory and clinical data have been proposed, and two such models (GLOBE score and UK-PBC score) are based on multicenter studies including large cohorts of patients with PBC.
  1. GLOBE score: Includes the following five variables: Serum bilirubin, albumin, serum ALP, platelet count after 1 yr of UDCA treatment, and age at start of therapy. It estimates the duration of transplant-free survival.
  2. UK-PBC score: Includes serum ALP, aminotransferases, and bilirubin after 12 mo of UDCA therapy, in addition to baseline albumin and platelet count. This model estimates the risk of liver transplantation or liver-related death.
- Poorer prognosis is associated with jaundice, advanced histologic stage, elevated bilirubin or ALP, low albumin, hepatocellular carcinoma, nonresponse to UDCA, and esophageal varices.

TABLE 1 Time Course of Histologic Progression to a Higher Stage in Patients with PBC

Histologic Progression*	Initial Histologic Stage 1	2	3
1 yr	41	43	35
2 yr	62	62	50

*Percent of patients in whom the histologic stage increases at 1 yr and 2 yr.

From Feldman M et al: *Sleisenger and Fortran's gastrointestinal and liver disease,* ed 10, Philadelphia, 2016, Elsevier.

BOX 1 Independent Predictors of Survival in Patients with PBC in Various Clinical Studies

Clinical
Age
Ascites
Edema
Hepatomegaly
Variceal bleeding

Laboratory
Serum albumin level
Serum alkaline phosphatase level
Serum bilirubin level
Prothrombin time

Liver Histology
Cholestasis
Cirrhosis
Fibrosis
Mallory hyaline

PBC, Primary biliary cholangitis.

From Feldman M et al: *Sleisenger and Fortran's gastrointestinal and liver disease,* ed 10, Philadelphia, 2016, Elsevier.

Rx TREATMENT

- Treatment is according to the clinical stage of the disease.
- Asymptomatic stage:
  1. Follow liver function tests every 3 mo.
  2. Once ALP is elevated up to 1.5 × ULN, begin UDCA at 13 to 15 mg/kg/day in two to four divided doses regardless of histologic stage.
     a. Side effects may include headaches, dizziness, diarrhea or constipation, dyspepsia, nausea, weight gain, back pain, and upper respiratory infections.
     b. Watch for interactions with fibric acid derivatives, bile acid sequestrants, estrogen derivatives, as well as aluminum hydroxide, which may interfere with the therapeutic effect or serum concentration of UDCA.
     c. Efficacy is best if started during stage I or II disease but should be started at any stage of disease. Lifelong therapy is currently recommended.
- Treatment also includes treatment of associated conditions such as fatigue, pruritus, osteoporosis, hypercholesterolemia, malabsorption, fat-soluble vitamin deficiencies, anemia, hypothyroidism, and any complications of cirrhosis.

ACUTE GENERAL Rx

- Symptomatic stage: Goals of treatment are resolution of symptoms such as pruritus, treatment of chronic cholestatic complications, and delay of liver failure.
- Obeticholic acid has recently been approved as a second line treatment for PBC.
  1. It is a farnesoid X receptor agonist and is used in combination with UDCA for patients who have an inadequate response to UDCA or as monotherapy for patients who are UDCA nonresponders.
  2. It is initially dosed at 5 mg once daily and can be increased to 10 mg once daily after 3 mo if there has been an inadequate decrease in bilirubin and/or ALP.
  3. The most common adverse event noted is pruritus and therefore this drug may not be ideal for patients with that symptom.
- Prednisone, azathioprine, colchicine, methotrexate, fibrates, penicillamine, cyclosporine, silymarin, and mycophenolate mofetil are no longer used because of limited efficacy and/or significant toxicity.
- For the pruritus of PBC, cholestyramine resin (4 to 16 g/day) reduces pruritus in most patients but must be given at least 4 hr before UDCA to avoid reducing the efficacy of that drug. Antihistamines at bedtime help nighttime symptoms. Rifampin (150-300 mg bid), oral opiate antagonists such as naltrexone (12.5-50 mg daily) and sertraline (75-100 mg daily) can be used for pruritus refractory to bile acid sequestrants. Table 2 summarizes treatment recommendations for pruritus in PBC. Intractable pruritus can be an indication for liver transplantation.
- Newer agents that are being investigated for pruritus include ileal bile acid transporter inhibitors and fibrates. In a study of 48 patients with PBC treated with UDCA, adjuvant therapy with bezafibrate (400 mg daily) resulted in partial or complete relief from itching in 23 of 24 patients (96%) in whom itching was assessed.

CHRONIC Rx

- Liver function tests should be checked every 3 to 6 mo.
- Management of sicca syndrome: Artificial tears can be used initially for dry eyes. Saliva substitutes can be used for xerostomia and dysphagia; pilocarpine or cevimeline can be used for refractory cases. Moisturizers can be given for vaginal dryness.
- Treatment/Prevention of osteopenia/osteoporosis: Patients with PBC should be given 1000 to 1200 mg calcium daily in divided doses and 1000 IU of vitamin D daily in the diet and as supplements if needed. Weight-bearing exercises are also recommended. Bone densitometry should be done at time of diagnosis, after a fragility fracture, in patients with cirrhosis, prior to transplant, or in patients receiving steroids more than 3 mo. It should then be performed every 2 to 4 yr. Alendronate (70 mg weekly) or other bisphosphonates should be considered if patients have osteopenia in the absence of acid reflux or known varices.
- Hyperlipidemia is common in patients with PBC. However, there is no elevated risk of cardiovascular disease. Statins are safe and effective in patients who may need treatment even if liver chemistry is abnormal.
- Vitamin A, K, and E deficiencies can be clinically important in advanced cases and respond to oral replacement.
- Upper endoscopy to assess for varices is indicated every 1 to 3 yr in patients with cirrhosis or Mayo risk score >4.1. Nonselective beta-blockers or endoscopic banding can be considered for prevention of variceal hemorrhage.
- Regular screening for hepatocellular carcinoma with ultrasound and α-fetoprotein every 6 mo is recommended for patients with cirrhosis.
- Liver transplantation is the only effective treatment for patients with liver failure, and approximately 25% of PBC patients ultimately need a liver transplant. Indications for transplantation include hepatic decompensation (encephalopathy, recurrent variceal bleeding, intractable ascites and spontaneous bacterial peritonitis), hepatocellular carcinoma fulfilling Milan criteria (see "Hepatocellular Carcinoma"), and intractable pruritus. Liver transplant should also be considered with a Mayo risk score >7.8, MELD score >12, and bilirubin ≥6 mg/dl.
- The outcome of liver transplantation for patients with PBC is more favorable than that of nearly all other liver disease categories. The survival rates at 1 yr are now up to 90% to 95%. Although recurrent disease may develop in 11% to 42% of patients after liver transplantation within a median of 47 mo, patient and graft survival is usually not affected.

DISPOSITION

Definitive treatment requires liver transplantation. Among untreated patients transplant-free survival is 79%, 59%, and 32% at 5, 10, and 15 yr, respectively.

REFERRAL

Gastroenterology and/or hepatology for treatment, evaluation for liver transplantation, and management of portal hypertension.

SUGGESTED READINGS

Available at ExpertConsult.com

RELATED CONTENT

Primary Biliary Cirrhosis (PBC) (Patient Information)

AUTHORS: **Jeanette G. Smith, MD,** and **Dina A. Ibrahim, MD**

TABLE 2 Current Recommendations for Treatment of Pruritus in Primary Biliary Cholangitis

Approach	Drug	Mechanism of Action	Dose	Adverse Effects	Comments
First line	Cholestyramine	Bile acid resin	4-16 g/day	Unpleasant taste, bloating, constipation, and diarrhea	Morning dose preferred; separate at least 3 hr from other drugs
	Colesevelam	Bile acid resin	3.75 g/day in two or three divided doses	As above (but less frequent), headache, myalgia	Separate at least 3 hr from other drugs
Second line	Rifampicin (rifampin)	Pregnane X receptor (PXR) agonist and enzyme inducer	150-600 mg/day	Hepatitis, liver failure, hemolysis	150 mg/day when serum bilirubin level <3 mg/dl; 300 mg/day when serum bilirubin level >3 mg/dl; regular monitoring of blood count and liver biochemistry
Third line	Naltrexone	Opiate mu receptor antagonist	50 mg/day	Opioid withdrawal–like reaction—abdominal pain, high blood pressure, tachycardia, goose bumps, nightmares	Start at 12.5 mg/day; increase gradually; regular monitoring of liver biochemistry
Fourth line	Sertraline	Serotonin reuptake inhibitor (SSRI)	100 mg/day	Nausea, dizziness, diarrhea, visual hallucinations, increased fatigue	Start at 25 mg/day; increase gradually

From Fillit HM: *Brocklehurst's textbook of geriatric medicine and gerontology,* ed 8, 2017, Elsevier.

BASIC INFORMATION

DEFINITION

Primary central nervous system lymphoma (PCNSL) is a rare form of non-Hodgkin lymphoma which originates in the brain parenchyma, spinal cord, eyes, and cerebrospinal fluid. PCNSL is a disease limited to a single extranodal organ with morphology consistent with diffuse large B-cell lymphoma in most cases.

SYNONYMS

PCNSL
CNS lymphoma
Primary diffuse large B-cell lymphoma of the CNS
Cerebral lymphoma
Brain lymphoma
Reticulum cell sarcoma

ICD-10CM CODE

C72.9 Malignant neoplasm of central nervous system, unspecified

EPIDEMIOLOGY & DEMOGRAPHICS

INCIDENCE:
- PCNSL represents 4% to 6% of extra-nodal lymphomas.
- There are approximately 1500 new cases in the U.S. annually.

PREDOMINANT SEX & AGE:
- It generally occurs in the fifth or sixth decade of life.
- The male:female ratio is 1.2:1.7.

PEAK INCIDENCE:
- PCNSL incidence increased in the 1970s to 1980s due to an initially growing elderly population
- A spike in incidence the 1990s was due to the HIV epidemic.
- Recently, the incidence in the elderly (>65 yr) has been gradually increasing.

RISK FACTORS: Immunodeficiency states:
- Can be acquired or inherited
- In patients with HIV infection, PCNSL is seen with CD4 <50 cells/ml and EBV infection
- Solid organ transplant patients (renal, cardiac, liver, and lung)
- Congenital disorders such as Wiskott-Aldrich syndrome (WIS), Combined Variable Immunodeficiency state (CVID), and Ataxia telangiectasia carry an increased risk

PHYSICAL FINDINGS & CLINICAL PRESENTATION

- Classic B-symptoms such as fever, sweats, and weight loss as observed in systemic lymphoma patients are uncommon.
- PCNSL causes focal neurologic deficits in 70% of patients.
- Nonspecific behavioral or neurocognitive changes are the presenting deficits in 40% to 45% cases.
- Signs of increased intracranial pressure including headache, confusion, nausea, and vomiting are common (33%).
- Seizures are uncommon (14%) because the cortex is less frequently involved by PCNSL lesions.
- Leptomeningeal dissemination is generally asymptomatic.
- Lymphomatous spinal cord lesions can cause sensory changes, limb weakness, and bladder or bowel dysfunction.
- Patients with ocular involvement can have decreased acuity, blurry vision, and floaters.

ETIOLOGY

- Most PCNSLs are diffuse large B-cell lymphomas (90%) and on rare occasions Burkitt, T-cell, or low-grade lymphomas. T-cell PCNSL cases are found in eastern Asia.
- Pathologic review reveals highly proliferating lymphoma cells that diffusely infiltrate the brain parenchyma in a perivascular growth pattern. This phenomenon is called angiotropism and likely results in disruption of the blood-brain barrier.
- Most cases (>80%) are of the activated B-cell–like (ABC)/nongerminal center (NGC) subtype.
- Next-generation sequencing has revealed that recurrent mutations, particularly *MYD88* and *CD79B,* are detected in PCNSL and affect the B cell receptor (BCR) signaling pathway with resultant activation of nuclear factor kappa B. These mutations are enriched in ABC/NGC subtypes of non-Hodgkin lymphomas as in other immune-privileged sites like the testes. A recently described gain at chromosome 9p24.1, which includes the PDL-1 and PDL-2 loci, suggests that immune evasion and response modulation likely play a role in pathogenesis. Inactivation of *p14ARF* and *p16INK4a* genes may represent an important step in the molecular pathogenesis of PCNSL.

DIAGNOSIS

DIFFERENTIAL DIAGNOSIS

- Primary high-grade glioma
- Cerebral abscess
- CNS involvement by systemic lymphoma
- Solid tumor metastases
- Infectious disease (e.g. toxoplasmosis, cysticercosis)
- Granulomatous disease (e.g. neurosarcoidosis)

WORKUP

Pathologic confirmation of diagnosis requires either a stereotactic biopsy of the brain lesion, or, if ocular involvement is present, vitrectomy. CSF sampling demonstrating lymphoma cells on cytology or flow cytometry may also be sufficient. Fig. 1 is an algorithm for diagnosis and management of PCNSL.

LABORATORY TESTS

- Complete blood count
- Complete chemistry panel including tumor lysis labs (LDH, uric acid, urinalysis)
- Coagulation panel including DIC labs (PT, PTT, D-dimer, fibrinogen, FDP)
- HIV testing

IMAGING STUDIES

- Magnetic resonance imaging (MRI) with gadolinium (Fig. E2) is the imaging modality of choice. PCNSL can appear as either solitary or multifocal disease. Lesions frequently are surrounded by moderate edema and are restricted on diffusion weighted images.
- Ophthalmologic examination including a slit lamp evaluation to detect vitreal or subretinal lymphoma infiltrates.
- Systemic lymphoma needs to be excluded with either a PET scan or whole-body CT examination
- Bone marrow examination is performed

TREATMENT

The treatment of PCNSL involves a multi-modal approach and has evolved from a historical reliance on radiotherapy to relying on intensive, high dose methotrexate-containing regimens.

NONPHARMACOLOGIC THERAPY

- Surgery:
  1. Stereotactic biopsy conducted by experienced neurosurgical teams is essential for early and accurate diagnosis
  2. In many cases, maximum safe resection of lesions may provide immediate relief of mass effect, facilitate glucocorticoid taper, and theoretically eliminate drug-resistant tumor clones.
- Radiotherapy: Historically, whole brain radiation therapy (WBRT) has been utilized to achieve major tumor responses in PCNSL. However, when used as definitive therapy, this approach results in short-lived responses and overall survival of 11 to 12 mo. In addition to local failure, WBRT results in delayed neuro-cognitive toxicity including incontinence as well as gait and memory disturbances, especially in elderly patients.

ACUTE GENERAL Rx

- The International Extranodal Lymphoma Study Group (IELSG) identified five clinical variables that correlate with prognosis in PCNSL: Elevated LDH, age > 60 yr, ECOG performance status > 1, elevated CSF protein, tumor location within the deep regions of the brain (periventricular, basal ganglia, brainstem and/or cerebellum). The presence of 0 to 1, 2 to 3, or 4 to 5 adverse risk factors respectively correlates with 2-yr survival rates of 80%, 48%, or 15%.
- The Memorial Sloan Kettering Cancer Center (MSKCC) score utilizes two clinical variables: Karnofsky performance status and age. The low, intermediate, and high-risk prognostic groups as defined by this MSKCC score correlated with a median overall survival of 5.2 yr, 2.1 yr, and 0.9 yr in a validation cohort.
- Newly diagnosed PCNSL: Treatment generally involves induction and consolidation phases.
  1. Induction therapy typically consists of a chemoimmunotherapy regimen. The IELSG-32 study utilized a novel regimen (MATrix) containing high-dose methotrexate, cytarabine, thiotepa, and rituximab with resultant

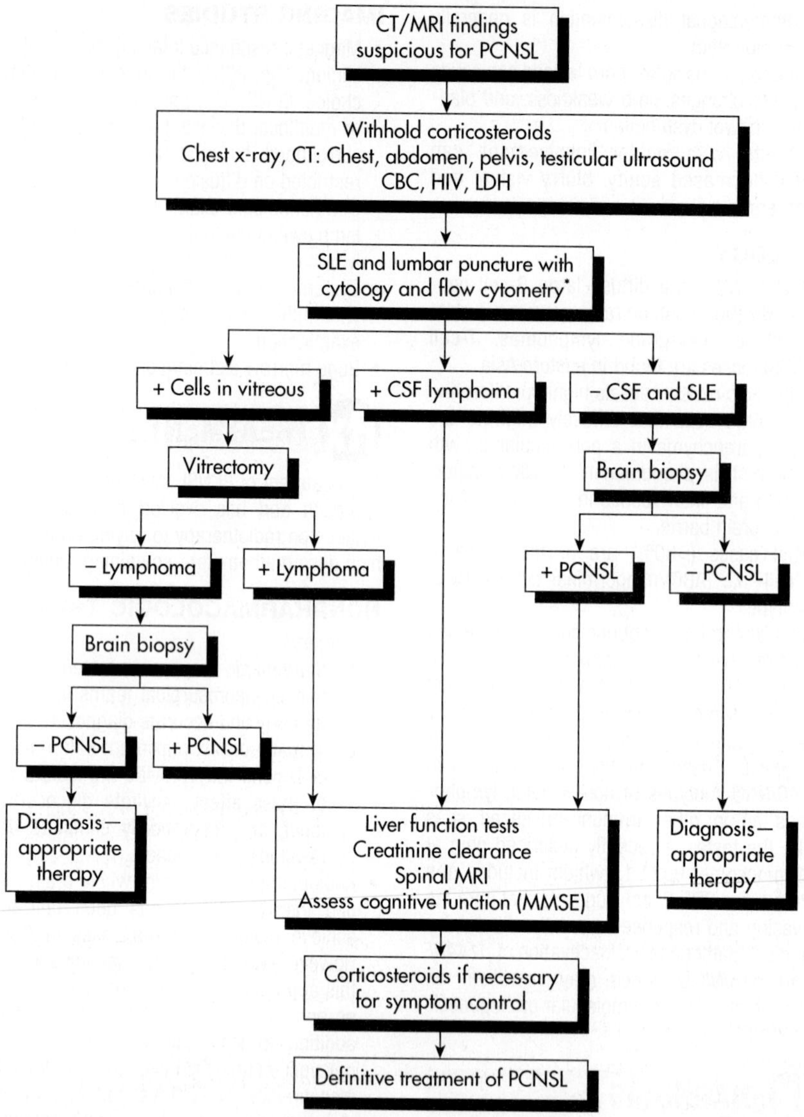

FIG. 1 Algorithm for diagnosis and management of primary central nervous system lymphoma (PCNSL) at the University of Pennsylvania. *CBC,* Complete blood cell count; *CSF,* cerebrospinal fluid; *CT,* computed tomography; *HIV,* human immunodeficiency virus; *LDH,* lactate dehydrogenase; *MMSE,* Mini Mental State Examination; *MRI,* magnetic resonance imaging; *SLE,* slit-lamp examination. *See text for other CSF investigations. (From Niederhuber JE: *Abeloff's clinical oncology*, ed 6, Philadelphia, 2020, Elsevier.)

complete remission rates of 49% and this represents a current standard of care approach in clinical practice.

2. Consolidation therapy with WBRT or autologous stem cell transplant (ASCT) have been evaluated in prospective studies and found to have equivalent survival outcomes. ASCT is associated with higher hematological toxicity while WBRT results in neurocognitive toxicity. Both approaches are only well tolerated in patients < 70 yr only. Less intensive consolidative chemotherapy infusional regimens instead of ASCT have also shown promising progression-free survival outcomes.
3. Maintenance therapy approaches for long term use (1 yr or until progression) have shown promise utilizing oral chemotherapy temozolomide and oral immunomodulatory agent lenalidomide. This approach is useful in elderly or unfit patients who cannot receive WBRT or ASCT as consolidation therapy.

- Recurrent PCNSL:
  1. Therapy is dependent on whether patients are candidates for rechallenge with high-dose methotrexate regimens and/or are candidates for ASCT. Patients with relapse 1 yr after completion of prior chemotherapy are candidates for methotrexate rechallenge and can demonstrate high response rates.
  2. Otherwise, patients are approached with salvage regimens incorporating alternative chemotherapy (temozolomide, pemetrexed, high dose cytarabine) and targeted therapy (ibrutinib, lenalidomide, temsirolimus) approaches.
  3. Novel immunotherapy approaches are being investigated in this setting including checkpoint inhibitors (nivolumab, pembrolizumab) as well as CAR-T cell therapy.

DISPOSITION

- The median OS of patients with PCNSL in the U.S. (from the SEER database) significantly increased from 12.5 mo in the 1970s to 26 mo in the 2010s.
- Five-yr survival in PCNSL was improved from 19% to 30% between 1990 and 2000. This survival benefit was limited to patients <70 yr of age only. The median survival of the elderly population is approximately 6 mo and has not changed in the last 40 yr.

REFERRAL

To Neurosurgery, Radiation Oncology, Hematology/Oncology

RELATED CONTENT

Non-Hodgkin Lymphoma (Related Key Topic)

SUGGESTED READINGS

Available at ExpertConsult.com

AUTHOR: **Bharti Rathore, MD**

BASIC INFORMATION

DEFINITION

- Women younger than 40 yr of age with amenorrhea, oligomenorrhea, or dysfunctional uterine bleeding for 4 mo or more along with follicle stimulating hormone (FSH) levels in the menopausal range meet diagnostic criteria for primary ovarian insufficiency.
- Menopause younger than the age of 40 yr.

SYNONYMS

POI
Hypergonadotropic hypogonadism
Premature ovarian failure
Premature menopause
Gonadal dysgenesis

ICD-10CM CODES

E28.3	Primary ovarian failure
E28.310	Symptomatic premature menopause
E28.39	Other primary ovarian failure
E28.9	Ovarian dysfunction, unspecified

EPIDEMIOLOGY & DEMOGRAPHICS

INCIDENCE: Affects 1% to 4% of the female population in the U.S.

PREDOMINANT AGE: 1:250 incident cases by age 35 and 1:100 by age 40

PHYSICAL FINDINGS & CLINICAL PRESENTATION

- The most common presentation is disturbance in menstrual pattern due to intermittent ovarian function.
- Between 5% and 30% of affected women have another affected female relative.
- Between 10% and 30% of affected women already have a concurrent autoimmune condition, the most common of which is hypothyroidism.
- Symptoms of estrogen deficiency include hot flashes, night sweats, poor concentration, drying of the vagina, and infertility.
- Physical exam may reveal stigmata of an autoimmune condition such as vitiligo, thyroid enlargement, or Turner syndrome (webbed neck, short stature, and high-arched palate).

ETIOLOGY (See Table 1)

Idiopathic in 95% of cases

DIAGNOSIS

DIFFERENTIAL DIAGNOSIS

- Pregnancy.
- Causes of secondary amenorrhea include eating disorder, exercise, drugs, sarcoidosis, polycystic ovarian disease, hypothalamic amenorrhea, hyperprolactinemia/prolactinoma, and Cushing disease.

WORKUP

- After pregnancy is ruled out, the initial evaluation should include the measurement of serum prolactin, FSH, and thyrotropin (TSH) levels.
- If the FSH level is in the menopausal range (>40 μIU/ml by radioimmunoassay), the test should be repeated in 1 mo along with a serum estradiol measurement to confirm the diagnosis of primary ovarian insufficiency.

LABORATORY TESTS

Once a diagnosis of premature ovarian failure is made, other evaluations include:

- Autoimmune disorders, adrenal insufficiency (seen in 3% of cases): Serum anti-adrenal and anti-21 hydroxylase antibodies should be measured.
- Hypothyroidism: Serum TSH, T_4, and anti-TPO antibodies.
- All cases should be screened for osteoporosis by DXA for bone mineral density.
- A karyotype analysis should be performed for all patients to look for chromosomal defects including Turner variant or deletions of the X chromosome.
- Permutations for the fragile X syndrome (*FMR1* gene) should be checked for as well.

IMAGING STUDIES

Pelvic ultrasound has no proven benefit in the management of these patients.

TREATMENT

NONPHARMACOLOGIC THERAPY

Counseling or patient support group should be offered to all women with low self-esteem and depression due to the psychological scar left by the diagnosis.

ACUTE GENERAL Rx

- Physiologic estrogen and progestin replacement is reasonable in the cases of young women until they reach the age of natural menopause.
- A dose of 100 mcg of estradiol per day, administered by transdermal patch, achieves average estradiol level observed in normal menstruating women and effectively treats symptoms.

TABLE 1 Mechanisms and Causes of Primary Ovarian Insufficiency

Accelerated Follicular Depletion	
Genetic: Turner syndrome, fragile X premutations, galactosemia	
Toxic: Chemotherapy, radiation, infections such as mumps or cytomegalovirus	
Autoimmune: Polyglandular failure, hypothyroidism, Addison disease, vitiligo, myasthenia gravis	
Abnormal Follicular Stimulation	
Gonadotropin receptor function: Follicle stimulating hormone/luteinizing hormone receptor mutation	
Enzyme defects: Aromatase deficiency, luteinized follicles	

- Cyclic medroxyprogesterone at a dose of 10 mg per day for 12 days each month is the preferred progestin to provide protection against endometrial cancer.
- Pregnancy may occur while a woman is taking estrogen and progesterone therapy and the therapy should be stopped immediately if the pregnancy test is found to be positive.

CHRONIC Rx

- Intake of 1200 mg of elemental calcium and 800 units of vitamin D_3 per day should be encouraged to prevent bone loss. A serum 25-hydroxyvitamin D level of 30 ng per ml or higher should be maintained.
- Patients with positive tests for adrenal antibodies should be evaluated annually for adrenal insufficiency by corticotropin stimulation test.
- Patients who wish to avoid pregnancy should use a barrier method or an IUD.
- Options for parenthood include adoption, foster parenthood, egg donation, and embryo donation.

DISPOSITION

Women with the known diagnosis should be encouraged to maintain a lifestyle that optimizes bone and cardiovascular health, including regular weight-bearing exercises, adequate intake of calcium (1200 mg daily) and vitamin D (800 IU daily), healthy diet to prevent obesity, and screening for cardiovascular risk factors.

REFERRAL

Referral to gynecologist and reproductive endocrinologist may be helpful in patients who decide to pursue parenthood.

PEARLS & CONSIDERATIONS

COMMENTS

- Common etiologies should be ruled out, including chromosomal abnormalities, fragile X premutations, and autoimmune causes.
- Management directed at symptom resolution and bone protection primarily, but should include psychosocial support for women facing this devastating diagnosis.

PREVENTION

Early diagnosis of primary ovarian insufficiency important for osteoporosis prevention and possibly prevention of coronary artery disease.

PATIENT & FAMILY EDUCATION

- https://medlineplus.gov/primaryovarianinsufficiency.html
- www.earlymenopause.com
- www.nichd.nih.gov/health/topics/poi/resources/patients

RELATED CONTENT

Amenorrhea (Related Key Topic)

AUTHOR: **Fred F. Ferri, MD**

BASIC INFORMATION

DEFINITION

Primary sclerosing cholangitis (PSC) is a chronic cholestatic liver disease characterized by segmental inflammation and fibrosis of the intrahepatic and extrahepatic bile ducts. PSC has a strong association with inflammatory bowel disease (IBD) and may be complicated by recurrent cholangitis, cholangiocarcinoma (CCA), and cirrhosis.

SYNONYMS

Chronic obliterative cholangitis
Fibrosing cholangitis
Stenosing cholangitis
PSC

ICD-10CM CODES

K83.0 Cholangitis
K83.9 Disease of biliary tract, unspecified

EPIDEMIOLOGY & DEMOGRAPHICS

- The incidence and prevalence of PSC are 0.9 to 1.3 cases per 100,000 persons per yr and 8.5 to 16.2 cases per 100,000 persons, respectively.
- About 65% of patients with PSC are men.
- Mean age of presentation is 30 to 40.
- Over 80% of patients with PSC also have IBD. 4% to 5% of patients with ulcerative colitis (UC) will develop PSC. A PSC-IBD phenotype may be present which carries a higher risk of colon cancer and is characterized by mild pancolitis, rectal sparing, and backwash ileitis. PSC is an independent risk factor for developing colon cancer in patients with IBD.
- PSC can coexist with other autoimmune liver diseases. Autoimmune hepatitis (AIH) and PSC overlap syndrome can be seen and is more common in young adults and children.
- CCA is present in 1% to 2% of PSC patients at diagnosis. PSC should be considered a premalignant disease with a lifetime risk of developing CCA between 5% and 10%.
- Box 1 summarizes a classification of diseases associated with sclerosing cholangitis.
- The median survival from time of diagnosis is 10 to 15 yr without liver transplantation.

PHYSICAL FINDINGS & CLINICAL PRESENTATION

- Many patients are asymptomatic (up to 50%) at the time of diagnosis with normal physical examination findings. However, many patients will have abnormal liver tests and a known diagnosis of IBD.
- The most common symptoms on presentation include pruritus and fatigue. Additional symptoms may include abdominal pain, abdominal distension, confusion, jaundice, or other symptoms related to decompensated liver disease or cholangitis. On physical exam patients may have jaundice, skin excoriation and hyperpigmentation from scratching, hepatosplenomegaly, and xanthelasma.

ETIOLOGY

- The cause of PSC is unknown, but the most likely mechanism is immunologic priming in a genetically susceptible patient causing phenotypic expression of PSC.
- Genetic and immunologic factors are supported by reports of familial occurrence of this disorder and increased frequency of HLA B8 and DR3. Genome-wide association studies have discovered novel loci associated with PSC, but the functional aspects of these genes are still unknown.
- Portosystemic inflammation caused by translocation of the gut microbiota is an increasing area of research. The close association with UC and PSC may be secondary to gut-activated T lymphocytes in IBD causing portal inflammation because of overlapping adhesion molecules in the gut and liver. Furthermore, intestinal dysbiosis in PSC has also been seen and remains an area of ongoing research.
- Dysregulated inflammatory cytokine production by cholangiocytes is also more recently suggested to be playing a role in the pathogenesis of PSC.

DIAGNOSIS

DIFFERENTIAL DIAGNOSIS

- IgG4-associated cholangitis (IAC)
- Surgical biliary trauma
- Ischemic cholangitis, recurrent pyogenic cholangitis, recurrent pancreatitis
- Choledocholithiasis, cholangiocarcinoma
- Intraarterial chemotherapy (5-FU/floxuridine)
- Diffuse intrahepatic metastasis, sarcoidosis, or amyloidosis
- AIDS-related, eosinophilic, or mast cell cholangiopathy
- Histiocytosis X, graft-versus-host disease
- Hepatic inflammatory pseudotumor, portal hypertensive biliopathy

WORKUP

Diagnosis is based on characteristic cholangiographic findings in combination with clinical and biochemical features. Though liver biopsy is now rarely used to diagnose PSC, histologic confirmation may be indicated in patients with normal cholangiograms and high suspicion of PSC. Table 1 describes the staging of PSC.

LABORATORY TESTS

- Liver function tests are abnormal in approximately 75% of patients with PSC, with a predominantly cholestatic pattern and an elevation in the serum alkaline phosphatase (3 to 10 times the upper limit of normal for more than 6 mo). However, this value can vary and be normal during the disease course. Serum aminotransferase levels are elevated in the majority of patients (2 to 3 times the upper limits of normal). Serum bilirubin is usually normal at the time of diagnosis unless the patient has advanced stricturing disease or advanced liver disease. Initial elevation of bilirubin at diagnosis may be related to a worse prognosis.
- A wide range of autoantibodies can be detected in patients with PSC including perinuclear antineutrophil cytoplasmic antibody (pANCA), antinuclear antibody (ANA), and anti-smooth muscle antibody (ASMA). These antibodies are nonspecific for PSC.
  1. Perinuclear antineutrophil cytoplasmic antibody (pANCA) is positive in 33% to 88% of those with PSC but is not specific.
  2. Anti-mitochondrial antibody (AMA), which is characteristic of primary biliary cholangitis (PBC), is *NOT* found in PSC and can be helpful in excluding PSC.
  3. Serum IgG levels are useful in the diagnosis of PSC-AIH overlap syndrome (more common in pediatric patients) and IAC with autoimmune pancreatitis.
  4. In particular, elevated levels of IgG4 are found in 10% to 20% of PSC patients, with a subset of these patients displaying features of autoimmune pancreatitis. PSC patients with elevated IgG4 tend to have worse outcomes and seem to respond to corticosteroid therapy; hence, IgG4 levels should be checked at least once in all patients with PSC.

IMAGING STUDIES

- Cholangiography with magnetic resonance cholangiopancreatography (MRCP), endoscopic retrograde cholangiopancreatography (ERCP), or percutaneous transhepatic cholangiography (PTC) is considered to be the gold standard for the diagnosis of PSC. Characteristic findings reveal segmental fibrosis of bile ducts with saccular dilatation of normal intervening areas resulting in a "beads-on-a-string" appearance (Fig. E1).
- MRCP has largely supplanted ERCP and PTC as the diagnostic study of choice because it is noninvasive, less expensive, and has a high diagnostic accuracy of 90%.
- Noninvasive measurements of liver elastography including MR elastography are promising methods for evaluating for cirrhosis but have not yet been validated in this patient cohort.

TREATMENT

- No medical therapy has been established to be effective in treating PSC. Management of PSC patients is aimed at symptom relief and management of complications from PSC (i.e., obstruction/strictures, cirrhosis, portal hypertension).

BOX 1 Classification of and Diseases Associated with Sclerosing Cholangitis

Primary Sclerosing Cholangitis
Principal Disease Associations
Inflammatory bowel disease:
- Crohn colitis or ileocolitis
- Ulcerative colitis

Other Disease Associations
Systemic diseases with fibrosis:
- Inflammatory pseudotumor
- Mediastinal fibrosis
- Peyronie disease
- Pseudotumor of the orbit
- Retroperitoneal fibrosis
- Riedel thyroiditis

Autoimmune or collagen vascular disorders:
- Autoimmune hemolytic anemia
- Celiac disease
- Chronic sclerosing sialadenitis
- Membranous nephropathy
- PSS
- Rapidly progressive glomerulonephritis
- RA
- Sjögren syndrome
- SLE
- Type 1 diabetes mellitus

Alloimmune diseases:
- Hepatic allograft rejection
- Hepatic graft-versus-host disease after bone marrow transplantation

Infiltrative diseases:
- Hypereosinophilic syndrome
- Histiocytosis X
- Sarcoidosis
- Systemic mastocytosis

Immunodeficiency:
- Congenital immunodeficiency
  - Combined immunodeficiency
  - Dysgammaglobulinemia
  - X-lined agammaglobulinemia
- Acquired immunodeficiency:
  - AIDS
  - Angioimmunoblastic lymphadenopathy
  - Opportunistic infections (e.g., cryptosporidiosis, cytomegalovirus, microsporidiosis)
  - Selective IgA deficiency

Secondary Sclerosing Cholangitis
Obstructive
Autoimmune pancreatitis
Biliary parasites
Caroli disease
Choledocholithiasis
Chronic pancreatitis
Congenital abnormalities:
- CF
- Choledochal cyst

Fungal infection
Recurrent pyogenic cholangitis
Surgical stricture

Toxic
Intraarterial floxuridine (FUDR)
Intraductal formaldehyde or hypertonic saline (echinococcal cyst treatment)

Ischemic
Hepatic allograft arterial occlusion
Paroxysmal nocturnal hemoglobinuria
Toxic vasculitis (FUDR)
Vascular trauma

Neoplastic
Cholangiocarcinoma
Hepatocellular carcinoma
Lymphoma
Metastatic cancer

AIDS, Acquired immunodeficiency syndrome; *CF*, cystic fibrosis; *FUDR*, 5-fluorouracil deoxyribonucleoside; *Ig*, immunoglobulin; *PSS*, progressive systemic sclerosis; *RA*, rheumatoid arthritis; *SLE*, systemic lupus erythematosus.
From Feldman M et al: *Sleisenger and Fordtran's gastrointestinal and liver disease,* ed 10, Philadelphia, 2016, Elsevier.

- Ursodeoxycholic acid (UDCA) has shown variable benefit in randomized controlled trials. Although biochemical improvement has been seen with UDCA, there has been no proven benefit on survival. The American Association for Liver Diseases (AASLD) currently recommends against the use of UDCA in PSC.
- The use of corticosteroids and other immunosuppressive agents is not recommended in patients with PSC alone; however, it is recommended in patients with PSC-AIH overlap syndrome or elevated IgG4.
- Oral vancomycin may show clinical and biochemical response in pediatric patients, but no randomized clinical trial has been performed. The benefit seen from the use of oral vancomycin may be related to the antibiotic effect on the microbiome of the gut. Investigations are ongoing.
- Manipulation of the microbiome is an exciting area being explored as a future treatment for PSC. Recent studies have shown that fecal microbiota transplantation (FMT) in PSC is safe, improves liver biochemistries, and improves microbiome diversity. This is a rapidly expanding area of gastroenterology that shows promise. However, larger studies are needed to determine if such treatments can affect mortality or reduce liver transplantation.

ACUTE GENERAL Rx

- For mild pruritus, skin emollients and antihistamines are recommended as the first-line treatment.
- For moderate or severe pruritus, bile acid sequestrants such as cholestyramine are preferred for initial management. Alternative agents for pruritus refractory to bile acid sequestrants include rifampicin, naltrexone, sertraline, and phenobarbital.
- Patients who present with increasing serum bilirubin, worsening pruritus, progressive bile duct dilation on imaging studies, or cholangitis should be evaluated for dominant strictures with imaging. A dominant stricture is a stenosis <1.5 mm in the common bile duct or <1 mm in the hepatic duct.
- ERCP with brushings, cytology, and fluorescent in situ hybridization (FISH) is recommended to evaluate dominant strictures for CCA, which is found in 15% to 20% of cases. Once malignancy is excluded, balloon dilation with or without stenting is recommended to treat symptomatic patients. Routine stenting is not required, but short-term stenting may be helpful in patients with severe stricture. If ERCP is unsuccessful, percutaneous cholangiopancreatography with stenting should be considered.
- In noncirrhotic patients with dominant strictures refractory to endoscopic or percutaneous management, surgery should be considered, although this may complicate future liver transplantation surgery.
- Antibiotic usage is recommended in patients with dominant strictures/obstructions both acutely and for long-term prophylaxis in patients with recurrent cholangitis.

TABLE 1 Staging of Primary Sclerosing Cholangitis

Stage	Description
I—Portal	Portal edema, inflammation, ductal proliferation; abnormalities do not extend beyond the limiting plate
II—Periportal	Periportal fibrosis with or without inflammation extending beyond the limiting plate
III—Septal	Septal fibrosis, bridging necrosis, or both
IV—Cirrhotic	Biliary cirrhosis

From Cameron JL, Cameron AM: *Current surgical therapy,* ed 10, Philadelphia, 2011, Saunders.

CHRONIC Rx

- Avoidance of alcohol and vaccination against hepatitis A and B is advised.
- Patients with PSC are at risk for osteoporosis and osteopenia; therefore DEXA scan should be performed at diagnosis and repeated every 2 to 4 yr. The pathophysiology of osteopathy in PSC is not well understood, but has been hypothesized to be related to decreased absorption of fat-soluble vitamins and impairment of osteoblasts by bilirubin.
- With advanced disease, fat-soluble vitamin deficiencies such as A, E, and D should be assessed.
- Patients with newly diagnosed PSC should undergo colonoscopy with biopsies to exclude concurrent IBD and for surveillance of colorectal cancer. In patients with IBD, continued surveillance colonoscopy with biopsies, or chromoendoscopy, at 1- to 2-yr intervals is recommended. In patients without IBD, a 3- to 5-yr surveillance interval has been recommended due to an increased risk of colorectal cancer.
- CCA development is common in PSC with a 10-yr cumulative incidence of approximately 7% to 9%. Screening for CCA should be performed every 6 to 12 mo with ultrasound, CT, or MRI, with or without serum CA 19-9. CCA screening is not indicated in PSC patients <20 yr of age or those who have small duct PSC. ERCP with brush cytology or cholangioscopy should be performed in patients who have biochemical or symptomatic deterioration or dominant stricture to rule out CCA.
- Annual transabdominal ultrasound is recommended due to the increased risk of gallbladder malignancy, even in patients who are not cirrhotic. The AASLD recommends cholecystectomy for all gallbladder masses/polyps in PSC patients, while the American College of Gastroenterology (ACG) recommends cholecystectomy only for lesions >8 mm.
- Patients with PSC and cirrhosis are recommended to have hepatocellular carcinoma (HCC) surveillance with ultrasound, with or without α-fetoprotein, every 6 mo and gastroesophageal variceal surveillance at regular intervals.
- In patients with HCC and CCA, resection versus liver transplantation may be indicated depending on the extent of disease.

DISPOSITION

Liver transplantation is the only effective treatment for patients with end-stage liver disease, portal hypertension, liver failure, and recurrent or intractable bacterial cholangitis. Survival is excellent, with 90% and 80% survival rates at 1 and 5 yr, respectively. The recurrence of PSC after transplant is reportedly 5% to 20%. Transplant referral is warranted in patients with MELD score ≥14, refractory cholangitis, and early stage HCC/CCA.

REFERRAL

All patients with suspected PSC should be referred to a gastroenterologist or hepatologist for formal diagnosis, management of complications, surveillance of associated malignancies, and evaluation for liver transplantation.

PEARLS & CONSIDERATIONS

- Diagnosis of PSC is made by a combination of clinical presentation, cholestatic liver function tests, and cholangiographic evidence of multifocal biliary strictures.
- There is currently no effective medical treatment of PSC. Management of PSC targets symptom relief, complications of PSC, cirrhosis, early carcinoma detection, and timely referral for liver transplantation.
- Patients are at increased risk for the development of colorectal cancer, gallbladder cancer, and cholangiocarcinoma and need surveillance.
- In patients with cirrhosis, surveillance for gastroesophageal varices and HCC is recommended.
- Liver transplant remains the only definitive therapy for complications of PSC.

SUGGESTED READINGS

Available at ExpertConsult.com

RELATED CONTENT

Ulcerative Colitis (Related Key Topic)

AUTHORS: **May Min, MD,** and **Amanda Pressman, MD**

BASIC INFORMATION

DEFINITION

Prolactinomas are monoclonal tumors that secrete prolactin.

ICD-10CM CODES
D35.2 Benign neoplasm of pituitary gland
E22.8 Other hyperfunction of pituitary gland

EPIDEMIOLOGY & DEMOGRAPHICS

INCIDENCE: Most common pituitary tumor; nearly 30% of all pituitary adenomas secrete enough prolactin to cause hyperprolactinemia

PREDOMINANT SEX: Microadenomas are more common in women; macroadenomas are found more frequently in men.

PHYSICAL FINDINGS & CLINICAL PRESENTATION

- Men: Decreased facial and body hair, infertility, small testicles; may also have decreased libido, erectile dysfunction, and delayed puberty (caused by decreased testosterone as a result of inhibition of gonadotropin secretion).
- Women: Physical examination may be normal; history may reveal amenorrhea, galactorrhea (Fig. E1), oligomenorrhea, and anovulation.
- Both sexes: Visual field defects and headache may occur depending on size of tumor and its expansion.

ETIOLOGY

Prolactin-secreting pituitary adenomas: Microadenomas (<10 mm diameter) or macroadenomas (>10 mm diameter). No risk factors have been identified for sporadic prolactinomas. Rarely prolactinomas can be part of multiple endocrine neoplasia (MEN) type 1 syndrome.

DIAGNOSIS

DIFFERENTIAL DIAGNOSIS

Secretion of prolactin is under tonic inhibitory control by hypothalamic dopamine. Hyperprolactinemia may be caused by the following:

- Drugs: Risperidone, phenothiazines, methyldopa, reserpine, monoamine oxidase inhibitors, androgens, progesterone, cimetidine, tricyclic antidepressants, haloperidol, meprobamate, chlordiazepoxide, estrogens, narcotics, metoclopramide, verapamil, amoxapine, cocaine, oral contraceptives
- Hepatic cirrhosis, renal failure, primary hypothyroidism
- Ectopic prolactin-secreting tumors (hypernephroma, bronchogenic carcinoma)
- Infiltrating diseases of the pituitary (sarcoidosis, histiocytosis)
- Head trauma, chest wall injury, spinal cord injury
- Polycystic ovary disease, pregnancy, nipple stimulation
- Idiopathic hyperprolactinemia, stress, exercise

WORKUP

- The diagnosis of prolactinoma is established by demonstration of an elevated serum prolactin level (after exclusion of other causes of hyperprolactinemia) and radiographic evidence of a pituitary adenoma.
  1. Normal mean prolactin levels are 8 ng/ml in women and 5 ng/ml in men.
  2. Prolactin levels >100 ng/ml are suspicious for prolactinomas. Most macroprolactinomas raise prolactin levels >250 ng/ml and levels >500 ng/ml are virtually diagnostic of macroprolactinomas.
  3. Prolactin levels can vary with time of day, stress, sleep cycle, and meals. More accurate measurements can be obtained 2 to 3 hr after awakening, preprandially, and when patient is not distressed.
  4. Serial measurements are recommended in patients with mild prolactin elevations.
- TSH, free T_4, BUN, Creat, ALT, AST are useful tests. Pregnancy test in all women of childbearing age.
- All patients with prolactinomas should undergo visual field testing. Serial evaluation is recommended, particularly during pregnancy in patients with macroadenomas.

IMAGING STUDIES

- MRI with gadolinium enhancement is the procedure of choice in the radiographic evaluation of pituitary disease.
- In absence of MRI, a radiographic diagnosis is best accomplished with a high-resolution CT scanner and special coronal cuts through the pituitary region.

Rx TREATMENT

NONPHARMACOLOGIC THERAPY

Pregnancy and breastfeeding should be avoided because they can encourage tumor growth. The management of patients with prolactinoma planning pregnancy is summarized in Table E1.

ACUTE GENERAL Rx

- Management of prolactinomas depends on their size and encroachment on the optic chiasm and other vital structures, the presence or absence of gonadal dysfunction, and the patient's desires regarding fertility. Patients with microprolactinomas without symptoms of hypogonadism do not require treatment. Fig. 2 describes a management algorithm for prolactinomas. Women with hypogonadism related to a microadenoma who do not desire fertility can be treated with a combined oral contraceptive.
- Medical therapy is preferred when fertility is an important consideration. Prolactinomas are treated with the dopamine agonists (DA) bromocriptine and cabergoline.
  1. Bromocriptine: Initial dose is 0.625 mg at bedtime for the first week. After 1 wk, add morning dose of 1.25 mg. Gradually increase dose by 1.25 mg/wk until dose of 5 to 10 mg/day is achieved. Bromocriptine decreases size of the tumor and generally lowers the prolactin level into the normal range when the initial serum prolactin is <500 ng/ml. Side effects of bromocriptine are nausea, constipation, dizziness, and nasal stuffiness. Bromocriptine appears to be safe during pregnancy.
  2. Cabergoline is a longer-acting dopamine agonist that is more expensive but may be more effective and better tolerated than bromocriptine; initial dose is 0.25 mg twice weekly.
  3. After therapy is initiated, MRI should be repeated in 1 yr for microprolactinomas if the prolactin level normalizes. For macroprolactinomas, MRI is repeated after 2 mo and every 6 to 12 mo until stable on serial studies.
- Transsphenoidal resection: Option in an infertile patient who cannot tolerate bromocriptine or cabergoline or when medical therapy is ineffective. The success rate depends on the location of the tumor (entirely intrasellar), experience of the neurosurgeon, and size of the tumor (<10 mm in diameter); the recurrence rate may reach 80% within 5 yr. Possible complications of transsphenoidal surgery vary with experience and skill of the neurosurgeon and tumor anatomy and include transient diabetes insipidus, hypopituitarism, cerebrospinal fluid rhinorrhea, and infections (meningitis, wound infection).
- Pituitary irradiation is useful as adjunctive therapy of macroadenomas (>10 mm in diameter) and in patients with persistent hypersecretion after surgery. Potential complications include cranial nerve damage, radionecrosis, and cognitive abnormalities.
- Stereotactic radiosurgery (gamma knife) has become popular as a modality in the treatment of prolactinomas. A high dose of ionizing radiation is delivered to the tumor through multiple ports. Its advantage is minimal irradiation to surrounding tissues. Proximity of the tumor to the optic chiasm limits this therapeutic modality.

CHRONIC Rx

- Patients on medical therapy require periodic measurement of prolactin levels. An attempt to reduce the dose of bromocriptine or cabergoline can be made after the prolactin level has been normal for 2 yr. An MRI scan of the pituitary should be obtained to rule out tumor enlargement within 6 mo of initiation of tapering regimen.
- Evaluation and monitoring of pituitary function are recommended after transsphenoidal surgery.

DISPOSITION

- Transsphenoidal surgery will result in a cure in nearly 50% to 75% of patients with microadenomas and 10% to 20% of patients with macroadenomas.
- Nearly 20% of microprolactinomas resolve during long-term dopamine agonist treatment.

PEARLS & CONSIDERATIONS

COMMENTS

- Patients must be monitored for several years after surgery because up to 50% of

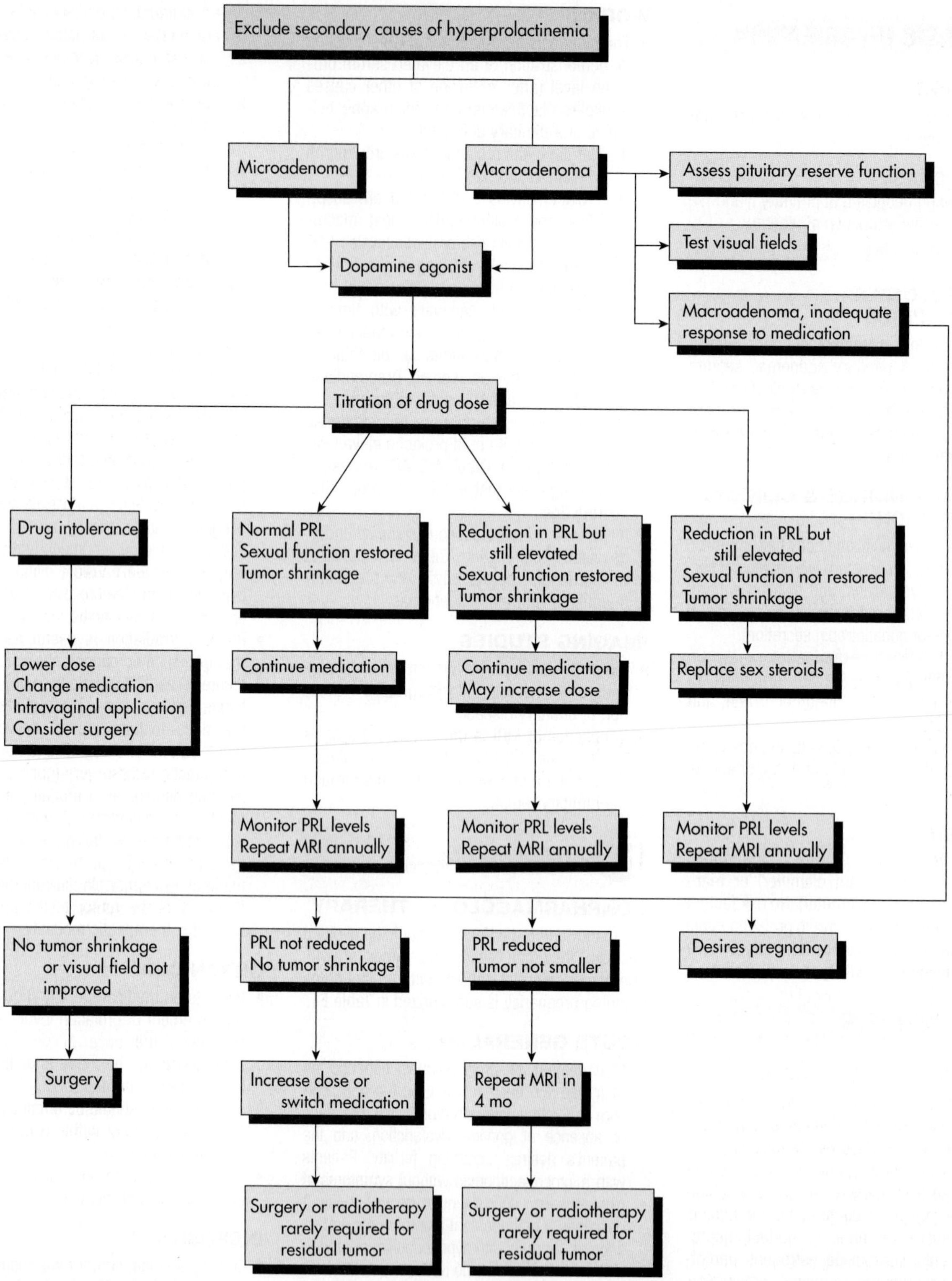

FIG. 2 Prolactinoma management. After secondary causes of hyperprolactinemia have been excluded, subsequent management decisions are based on clinical imaging and biochemical criteria. *MRI,* Magnetic resonance imaging; *PRL,* prolactin. (From Melmed S et al: *Williams textbook of endocrinology,* ed 14, Philadelphia, 2020, Saunders.)

microadenomas and nearly 90% of macroadenomas can recur.
- Pituitary microadenomas are found in 10.9% of autopsies, and 44% of these microadenomas are prolactinomas.

SUGGESTED READING

Available at ExpertConsult.com

RELATED CONTENT

Prolactinoma (Patient Information)
Pituitary Adenoma (Related Key Topic)

AUTHOR: **Fred F. Ferri, MD**

BASIC INFORMATION

DEFINITION & CLASSIFICATION

Prostate cancer is a neoplasm involving the prostate. Various classifications have been developed to evaluate malignancy potential and prognosis.

- The degree of malignancy varies with the stage:
  1. Stage A: Confined to the prostate, no nodule palpable.
  2. Stage B: Palpable nodule confined to the gland.
  3. Stage C: Local extension.
  4. Stage D: Regional lymph nodes or distant metastases.
- In the Gleason classification (Box 1 and Fig. E1), two histologic patterns are independently assigned numbers 1 to 5 (best to least differentiated). These numbers are added to give a total tumor score between 2 and 10. Prognosis is best for highly differentiated tumors (e.g., Gleason score 2 to 4) compared with most poorly differentiated tumors (Gleason score 7 to 10).
- Another commonly used classification is the Tumor-Node-Metastasis (TNM) classification of prostate cancer (Table 1).
- Table 2 summarizes the definition of risk groups and biopsy criteria.

ICD-10CM CODES

C61	Malignant neoplasm of prostate
D07.5	Carcinoma in situ of prostate

EPIDEMIOLOGY & DEMOGRAPHICS

- Prostate cancer has surpassed lung cancer as the most common nonskin cancer in men.
- In the United States, more than 220,000 new cases are diagnosed yearly, and nearly 30,000 males die from prostate cancer each year (second leading cause of death from cancer in U.S. men).
- Incidence of prostate cancer increases with age: Uncommon <50 yr; 80% of new cases are diagnosed in patients aged ≥65 yr. Widespread prostate-specific antigen (PSA) testing has doubled the incidence of prostate cancer and the lifetime risk for prostate cancer to approximately 16%. Prostate cancer is also diagnosed earlier, and the incidence of clinically "silent" T_1 tumors has increased from 17% in 1989 to 48% in 2001 since the advent of PSA screening. Currently, approximately 80% of prostate cancer cases are diagnosed as localized disease and only 4% as metastatic disease.
- Prostate cancer is found at autopsy in more than half of U.S. men older than 50 yr but is the cause of death in only 3%.
- Average age at time of diagnosis is 72 yr.
- Blacks in the United States have the highest incidence of prostate cancer in the world (one in every nine males).
- Incidence is low in Asians.
- Approximately 9% of all prostate cancers may be familial. Obesity is a risk factor for prostate cancer. High-fat, low-fiber diet increases risk. High insulin levels may also increase the risk of prostate cancer. Dietary supplementation with vitamin E has been reported to significantly increase the risk of prostate cancer among healthy men. Linkage studies have implicated chromosome 17p21-22 as a possible location of a prostate-cancer susceptibility gene. Germline mutations in *HOXB13* are associated with a significantly increased risk of hereditary prostate cancer.
- Mortality rates of prostate cancer have declined substantially in the past 15 yr from 34% in 1990 to <20% currently.

PHYSICAL FINDINGS & CLINICAL PRESENTATION

- Generally silent disease until it reaches advanced stages.
- Bone pain and pathologic fractures may be initial symptoms of prostate cancer.
- Local growth can cause symptoms of outflow obstruction.
- Digital rectal examination (DRE) may reveal an area of increased firmness; 10% of patients will have a negative DRE.
- Prostate may be hard, fixed, with extension of tumor to the seminal vesicles in advanced stages.

Dx DIAGNOSIS

DIFFERENTIAL DIAGNOSIS

- Benign prostatic hypertrophy
- Prostatitis
- Prostate stones

LABORATORY TESTS

- Measurement of PSA is controversial in early diagnosis of prostate cancer. PSA screening is associated with psychological harm, and its potential benefits remain uncertain. In asymptomatic men with no history of prostate cancer, screening using PSA does not reduce all-cause mortality or death from prostate cancer. Normal PSA is found in >20% of patients with prostate cancer, whereas only 20% of men with PSA levels between 4 ng/ml and 10 ng/ml have prostate cancer. Most guidelines encourage a shared decision-making approach between patient and physician regarding PSA testing. Available evidence favors clinician discussion of the pros and cons of PSA screening with average-risk men aged 65 to 69 yr. Only men who express a definite preference for screening should have PSA testing. Rather than widespread annual PSA screening, a reasonable approach may be to focus on high-risk men (those with PSA levels ≥2 ng/ml at age 60). The American Cancer Society recommends offering the PSA test and DRE yearly to men aged ≥50 yr who have a life expectancy of at least 10 yr. Earlier testing, starting at age 40 to 45 yr, is recommended for men at high risk (e.g., blacks, men with family history of prostate cancer). An isolated elevation in PSA level should be confirmed several weeks later before proceeding with further testing, including prostate biopsy. Screening for prostate cancer in men aged ≥75 yr is controversial and generally not recommended. The American College of Physicians (ACP) recommends that clinicians should not screen for prostate cancer using the PSA in average-risk men under age 50, men over age 69, or men with a life expectancy of <10 to 15 yr. The U.S. Preventive Services Task Force (USPSTF) recommends against PSA-based screening for prostate cancer in all age groups. According to the USPSTF:

BOX 1 2005 International Society of Urological Pathology Modified Gleason System

Pattern 1
Circumscribed nodule of closely packed but separate, uniform, rounded to oval, medium-sized acini (larger glands than pattern 3)

Pattern 2
Like pattern 1, fairly circumscribed, yet at the edge of the tumor nodule there may be minimal infiltration
Glands are more loosely arranged and not quite as uniform as Gleason pattern 1

Pattern 3
Discrete glandular units
Typically smaller glands than seen in Gleason pattern 1 or 2
Infiltrates in and among nonneoplastic prostate acini
Marked variation in size and shape

Pattern 4
Fused microacinar glands
Ill-defined glands with poorly formed glandular lumens
Large cribriform glands
Cribriform glands
Hypernephromatoid

Pattern 5
Essentially no glandular differentiation, composed of solid sheets, cords, or single cells
Comedocarcinoma with central necrosis surrounded by papillary, cribriform, or solid masses

From Wein AJ et al: *Campbell-Walsh urology,* ed 11, Philadelphia, 2016, Elsevier.

1. The magnitude of harms from screening (e.g., falsely high PSA levels, psychological effects, unnecessary biopsies, overdiagnosis of indolent tumors) is "at least small."
2. The magnitude of treatment-associated harms (i.e., adverse effects of surgery, radiation, and hormonal therapy) is "at least moderate."
3. The 10-yr mortality benefit of PSA-based prostate cancer screening is "small to none."
4. The overall balance of benefits and harms results in "moderate certainty that PSA-based screening has no net benefit."

- Free PSA: The use of serum free PSA for prostate screening has been proposed by some urologists as a means to decrease unwarranted biopsies without missing a significant number of prostate cancers. This approach is based on the higher free PSA in men with benign prostatic hyperplasia and the higher protein-bound PSA levels in men with prostate cancer. For example, in men with total PSA levels of 4 to 10 ng/ml, the cancer probability is 0.25, but if the percentage of free PSA is ≤17%, the probability of cancer increases to 0.45.
- PSA velocity: The rate of increase of serum PSA over time (PSA velocity) can aid in the diagnosis of prostate cancer. A yearly PSA velocity >0.75 ng/ml increases the likelihood of later malignancy when total PSA is still within normal range. Proper interpretation of PSA velocity requires at least three PSA measurements over an 18-mo period because most PSA variations are physiologic. Recent trials have cast a doubt on the value of PSA velocity by showing that adding PSA velocity as a trigger for biopsy did not improve predictive accuracy beyond that of using PSA threshold values alone.
- Age-adjusted PSA: There is evidence that the current threshold of 4.0 ng/ml is inadequate for younger men, because in a recent study 22% of men with PSA levels between 2.6 and 4.0 were found to have prostate cancer. The concept of age-related cutoffs remains controversial. Lowering the upper limit of normal for PSA would improve sensitivity but decrease specificity.
- Prostatic acid phosphatase can be used for evaluation of nonlocalized disease.
- Prostate cancer gene 3 (*PCA3*) is overexpressed in prostate cancer cell, and high levels are suggestive of prostate cancer. Measurement of *PCA3* in urine specimens collected after digital exams is helpful to make decisions about prostate biopsy in men with elevated PSA.
- Ultrasound-guided transrectal biopsy and fine-needle aspiration of prostate can confirm the diagnosis. Indications for biopsy include an abnormal PSA level, an abnormal DRE, or a previous biopsy specimen that showed prostatic intraepithelial neoplasia or prostatic atypia. The number of cores taken is patient specific, typically including a minimum of 10 cores. Prostate volume negatively affects cancer detection rate (23% in glands >50 cm^3, 38% in glands <50 cm^3). MRI-targeted biopsy identifies clinically significant prostate cancers more accurately than conventional systematic biopsy in men with suspected localized prostate cancer.[1]

TABLE 1 Prostate Cancer

T Stage		
T_x	Primary tumor is not assessable	
T_0	There is no evidence of primary tumor	
T_1	Tumor is not clinically palpable or detected with imaging	
	T_{1a}	*An incidental histological finding in ≤5% of resected tissue (e.g., TURP)*
	T_{1b}	*An incidental histological finding in >5% of resected tissue (e.g., TURP)*
	T_{1c}	*Tumor is identified by needle biopsy*
T_2	Prostate-confined tumor that is clinically palpable or detected with imaging	
	T_{2a}	*Tumor involves ≤1/2 of one prostate lobe*
	T_{2b}	*Tumor involves >1/2 of one prostate lobe (but not both lobes)*
	T_{2c}	*Tumor involves both lobes*
T_3	There is tumor extension through the prostate capsule	
	T_{3a}	*Unilateral or bilateral tumor extension through the prostate capsule*
	T_{3b}	*Seminal vesical involvement*
T_4	Tumor invades structures other than the seminal vesicles (e.g., the bladder neck, rectum, or pelvic wall)	
N Stage		
N_x	The lymph nodes are not assessable	
N_0	There is no tumor spread	
N_1	There is tumor spread to one or more regional pelvic nodes	
M Stage		
M_0	There is no tumor spread beyond the regional pelvic nodes	
M_1	There is tumor spread beyond the regional pelvic nodes	
	M_{1a}	*Tumor spread to nodes outside of the pelvis*
	M_{1b}	*Tumor spread to bones*
	M_{1c}	*Tumor spread to other organs (e.g., lung, liver and brain) ± bone involvement*

From Grant LA: *Grainger & Allison's diagnostic radiology essentials*, ed 2, Philadelphia, 2019, Elsevier.

IMAGING STUDIES (FIGS. E2 TO E5)

- Bone scan is useful to evaluate bone metastasis (present or eventually develops in almost 80% of patients). However, according to the American Urological Association (AUA), the routine use of bone scanning is not required for staging of prostate cancer in asymptomatic men with clinically localized cancer if the PSA level is ≤20 ng/ml.
- CT scan, MRI, and transrectal ultrasonography may be useful in selected patients to assess extent of prostate cancer. High-resolution MRI with magnetic nanoparticles

[1]Ahdoot M et al: MRI-targeted, systematic, and combined biopsy for prostate cancer diagnosis, *N Engl J Med* 382:917, 2020.

TABLE 2 Definition of Risk Groups

Risk Group	Clinical Stage	PSA (ng/ml)	Gleason Score	Biopsy Criteria
Low	T_{1a} or T_{1c}	<10	2-6	Unilateral or <50% of core involved
Intermediate	T_{1b}, T_{1c}, or T_{2a}	<10	3 + 4 = 7	Bilateral
High	T_{1b}, T_{1c}, T_{2b}, or T_3	10-20	4 + 3 = 7	>50% of core involved or perineural invasion or ductal differentiation
Very high	T_4	>20	8-10	Lymphovascular invasion or neuroendocrine differentiation

From Wein AJ et al: *Campbell-Walsh urology*, ed 11, Philadelphia, 2016, Elsevier.

has been used for the detection of small and otherwise undetectable lymph node metastases in patients with prostate cancer. However, according to the AUA, transrectal ultrasonography adds little to the combination of PSA and DRE. Similarly, CT and MRI imaging are generally not indicated for cancer staging in men with clinically localized cancer and PSA <25 ng/ml. With regard to pelvic lymph node dissection in staging, the AUA states that it may not be required in patients with PSA levels <10 ng/ml and when PSA level is <20 ng/ml and the Gleason score is <6.

Rx TREATMENT

NONPHARMACOLOGIC THERAPY

Watchful waiting is reasonable in selected patients with early-stage (T_{1a}) and projected life expectancy <10 yr or in patients with focal and moderately differentiated carcinoma.

ACUTE GENERAL Rx

- Therapeutic approach varies with the following:
  1. Stage of the tumor
  2. Patient's life expectancy
  3. General medical condition
  4. Patient's treatment preference (e.g., patient may be opposed to orchiectomy)
- The optimal treatment of clinically localized prostate cancer is unclear. It is important to remember that all forms of treatment have potential adverse effects. Management requires careful consideration of the potential benefits and harms of intervention, the patient's age, health status, and individual preferences. A treatment algorithm for prostate cancer is described in Fig. 6. Table 3 summarizes recommended treatment based on risk group and life expectancy.
  1. Radical prostatectomy is generally performed in patients with localized prostate cancer and life expectancy >10 yr. Radical prostatectomy reduces disease-specific mortality, overall mortality, and the risks of metastasis and local progression. The absolute reduction in the risk of death after 10 yr is small, but the reductions in the risks of metastasis and local tumor progression are substantial. A 29 yr follow-up comparing radical prostatectomy with watchful waiting showed that men with clinically detected, localized prostate cancer and a long life expectancy benefited from radical prostatectomy with a mean 2.9 yr of life gained. Postoperative complications of radical prostatectomy include urinary incontinence (10% to 20% depending on degree of neurovascular bundle and urethral preservation, patient age, and correct mucosal apposition) and erectile dysfunction (percentage >50% and varies with patient age, preoperative erectile dysfunction, stage of tumor at time of surgery, and preservation of neurovascular bundle). Lower complication rates occur in hospitals that perform a large number of prostatectomies. Fewer men will have postsurgical erectile dysfunction after unilateral or bilateral nerve-sparing surgery. In men undergoing prostatectomy, robotic-assisted laparoscopic surgery represents an alternative to open retropubic radical prostatectomy. Despite advertisements that suggest that there are fewer complications after robotic surgery, data show that sexual dysfunction occurs postoperatively in about 88% of patients who have undergone robotic-assisted or conventional prostatectomy and that incontinence problems are more prevalent (33%) with robotic surgery than with open retropubic radical prostatectomy (RPP) (27%). Trials have shown that prostatectomy is preferred over "watchful waiting" in patients with localized prostate cancer detected by PSA if the PSA level is >10 ng/ml. In this subgroup, the 10-yr mortality is 48.4% with prostatectomy versus 61.6% with watchful waiting. In men who have low-risk disease (PSA level <10 mcg/L, stage <T_{2a}, Gleason score ≤3 + 3), and <6% risk for prostate cancer–specific death at 15 yr, watchful waiting (WW) and active surveillance (AS) are reasonable and underutilized options.
  2. Radiation therapy (external-beam irradiation or brachytherapy with implantation of radioactive pellets [iodine-125 or palladium-103 seeds] into the prostate gland) represents an alternative in patients with localized prostate cancer, especially poor surgical candidates or patients with a high-grade malignancy. The efficacy of brachytherapy is comparable to external radiation and radical prostatectomy.[2] In patients receiving external-beam radiation, a total dose of 79.2 Gy (high dose) compared with a total dose of 70.2 Gy (conventional dose) has been reported to lower the risk of recurrence without increased risk of morbidity and mortality. Newer radiation treatments such as intensity-modulated radiation therapy (IMRT) and proton therapy are becoming increasingly popular and replacing the older technique of conformal radiation therapy over the past 10 yr. Trials have shown that among patients with nonmetastatic prostate cancer, the use of IMRT compared with conformal therapy is associated with less gastrointestinal morbidity and fewer hip fractures but more erectile dysfunction; IMRT compared with proton therapy is associated with less GI morbidity. Patients with localized prostate cancer and high risk for extraprostatic disease and disease recurrence (e.g., Gleason score ≤7 with multiple positive biopsy cores and clinical stage T_{1b}-T_{2b}) may benefit (increased overall survival) with the addition of 6 mo of androgen suppression therapy to radiation therapy. High-intensity focused ultrasound (HIFU) is a newer treatment option for patients with prostate cancer. It ablates localized areas of the prostate with the goal of sparing patients the morbidity of whole-gland therapy.[3] Longer-term studies comparing HIFU with standard therapy are needed. Hemigland cryoablation is another newer treatment modality for intermediate-risk prostate cancer.[4] Longer studies are needed before drawing conclusions.
  3. Watchful waiting is reasonable in patients who are too old or too ill to survive longer than 10 yr. If the cancer progresses to the point where it becomes symptomatic, palliation can be attempted with several methods. Conservative management is also reasonable for patients with Gleason score of 2 to 4 because these patients do not have a shortened life expectancy and treatment is associated with long-term side effects. Watchful waiting also appears to be safe in older men with less-aggressive disease. Individual preferences play a central role in the decision whether to treat or to pursue active surveillance.
- Patients with advanced disease and projected life expectancy <10 yr are candidates for radiation therapy and hormonal therapy (diethylstilbestrol, luteinizing hormone–releasing hormone analogues, antiandrogens, bilateral orchiectomy).
- Recommended treatment of patients with regional metastatic prostate cancer with projected life expectancy ≥10 yr includes radiation therapy and hormonal therapy.
- Prostate cancer is an androgen-receptor-dependent disease, and the blocking of androgen-receptor signaling is an effective treatment modality. Table 4 summarizes major circulating androgens. Androgen deprivation therapy (ADT) is the mainstay of treatment for metastatic prostate cancer. Adverse effects of ADT include decreased libido, impotence, hot flashes, osteopenia with increased fracture risk, metabolic alterations, and changes in mood and cognition. Adjuvant treatment with luteinizing hormone-releasing hormone (LHRH) agonists (goserelin, leuprolide, or triptorelin) plus antiandrogens (flutamide, bicalutamide, or nilutamide), when started simultaneously with external-beam radiation, improves local control and survival in patients with locally advanced prostate cancer. Pamidronate inhibits osteoclast-mediated bone resorption and prevents bone loss in the hip and lumbar spine in men receiving treatment for prostate cancer. Gonadotropin-releasing hormone (GnRH)

[2]Goy BW et al: Ten-year outcomes of radical prostatectomy vs external beam radiation therapy vs brachytherapy for 1503 patients with intermediate-risk prostate cancer, *Urology* 136:180, 2020.

[3]Nahar B et al: Prospective evaluation of focal high intensity focused ultrasound for localized prostate cancer, *J Urol* 204:483, 2020.

[4]Chuang R et al: Hemigland cryoablation of clinically significant prostate cancer: intermediate-term followup via magnetic resonance imaging guided biopsy, *J Urol* 209:941, 2020.

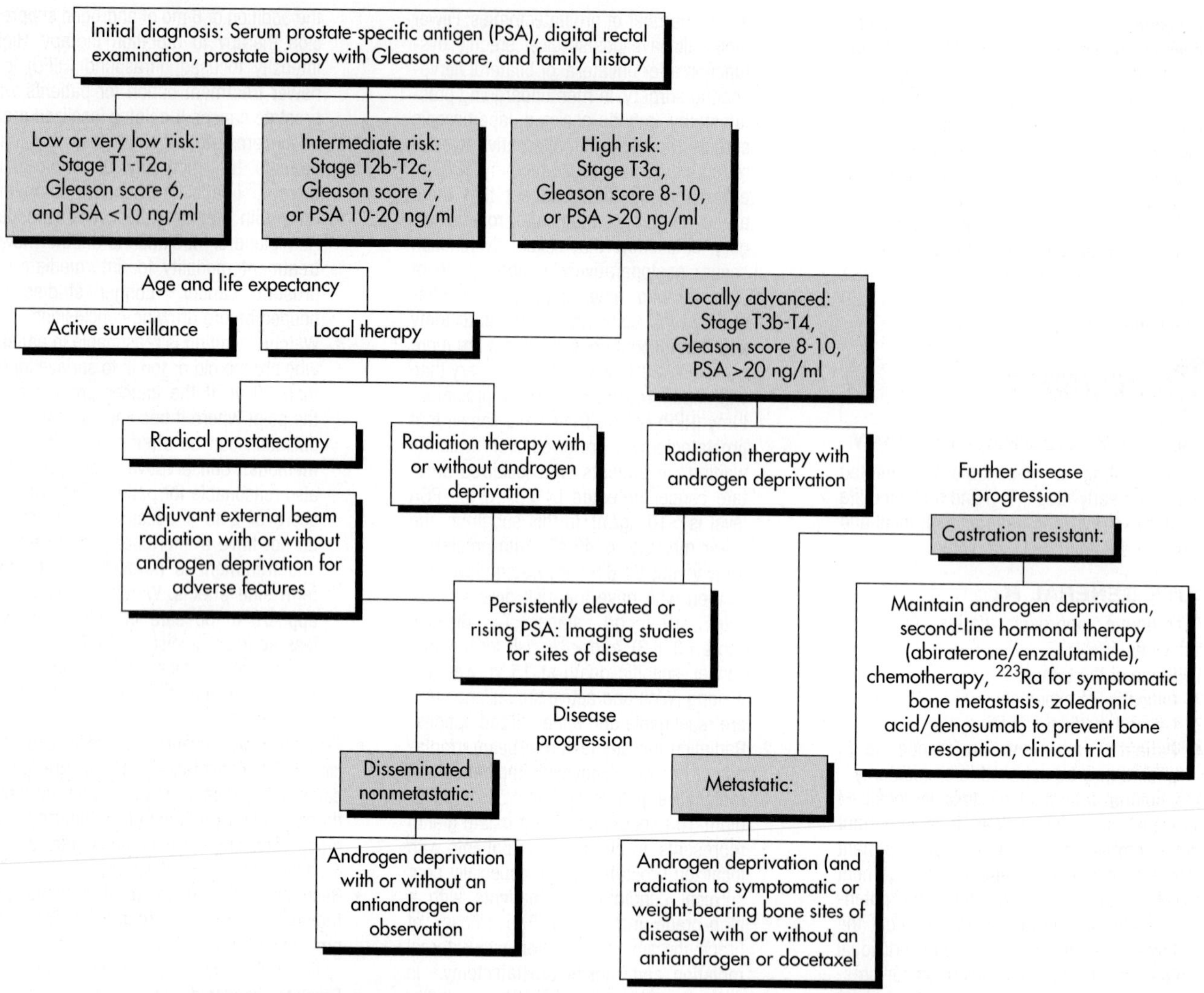

FIG. 6 Treatment algorithm. ^{223}*Ra,* Radium-223. (From Niederhuber JE: *Abeloff's clinical oncology,* ed 6, Philadelphia, 2020, Elsevier.)

TABLE 3 Recommended Treatment

Risk Group	Life Expectancy (Yr)	Recommended Treatment
Low	0-5	AS, HT
	5-10	AS, RT, HT, O
	>10	RP, RT, AS, O
Intermediate*	0-5	AS, HT, RT, O
	5-10	RT, HT, RP, O
	>10	RP, RT, O, HT
High*	0-5	AS, RT + HT, O
	5-10	RT + HT, HT, RP, O
	>10	RT + HT, RP + RT + HT, HT
Very high*	0-5	AS, RT + HT, O
	5-10	H, RT + HT, ST
	>10	RT + HT, RP + RT + HT, HT, ST, IT

AS, Active surveillance; *HT,* hormone therapy; *IT,* investigational multimodal therapy; *O,* others; *RP,* radical prostatectomy; *RT,* radiation therapy; *ST,* systemic therapy.
*If there is more than a 20% probability of positive lymph nodes, AS, HT, ST + HT.
From Wein AJ et al: *Campbell-Walsh urology,* ed 11, Philadelphia, 2016, Elsevier.

receptor antagonists can be used for rapid medical castration of men with advanced prostate cancer. Degarelix is an injectable GnRH agonist useful to suppress testosterone in patients with prostate cancer who are not good candidates for LHRH agonists and refuse surgical castration. Assessment of bone density and treatment with once-weekly oral alendronate can prevent and improve the bone loss that occurs in men receiving ADT for prostate cancer.

- Docetaxel plus prednisone or docetaxel plus estramustine can be used in metastatic hormone–refractory prostate cancer. Newer treatments for hormone–refractory prostate cancer (castration-resistant cancer) include immunotherapy with sipuleucel and cabazitaxel, a microtubule inhibitor that interferes with cell mitosis and replication. Both agents can prolong survival but adverse effects can be severe and both agents are very expensive. Abiraterone is an oral agent that

TABLE 4 Major Circulating Androgens

Source	Androgen	Amount Produced/Day (mg)	Relative Potency	Relative Potency/Amount Produced
Testes	Testosterone	6.6	100	15.2
Testes and peripheral tissues	Dihydrotestosterone	0.3	160-190	533-633
Adrenal glands	Androstenedione	1.4	39	27.9
Adrenal glands	Dehydroepiandrosterone	29	15	0.5

From Wein AJ et al: *Campbell-Walsh urology,* ed 11, Philadelphia, 2016, Elsevier.

blocks biosynthesis of androgens by inhibiting CYP17, an enzyme required for androgen biosynthesis. It has been FDA approved for oral treatment, in combination with prednisone, of metastatic castration-resistant prostate cancer in patients previously treated with docetaxel. Darolutamide is an androgen-receptor inhibitor approved for the treatment of nonmetastatic castration-resistant prostate cancer.[5]

- Enzalutamide is a newer nonsteroidal antiandrogen. Trials have shown it to be highly effective in extending survival in patients with metastatic castration-resistant prostate cancer. It can be used sequentially with other agents such as docetaxel, abiraterone, cabazitaxel, and immunotherapy.
- Radium-223, an alpha emitter, selectively targets bone metastases and has been found effective in improving survival in men with castration-resistant prostate cancer and bone metastases.
- The polyadenosine diphosphate [ADP]-ribose) polymerase (PARP) inhibitor olaparib has shown a high response rate in trials[6] in patients whose prostate cancers were no longer responding to standard treatments with enzaculamide or abiraterone and who had defects in DNA-repair genes.

CHRONIC Rx

- Patients should be monitored at 3- to 6-mo intervals with clinical examination and PSA for the first yr, then every 6 mo for the second yr, then yearly if stable. For patients who have undergone radical prostatectomy, a rising PSA level suggests evidence of residual or recurrent prostate cancer. A recent study revealed that if the PSA level remains undetectable 3 to 5 yr after radical prostatectomy, the probability of biochemical recurrence is extremely low, and it is reasonable to stop PSA monitoring.[7] Salvage radiotherapy may potentially cure patients with disease recurrence after radical prostatectomy. Recent trials have shown that addition of 24 mo of antiandrogen therapy with daily bicalutamide to salvage radiation therapy results in significantly higher rates of long-term overall survival and lower incidences of metastatic prostate cancer and death from prostate cancer than radiation therapy plus placebo.[8]
- Chest radiography and bone scan should be performed yearly or sooner if patient develops symptoms.

DISPOSITION

- Prognosis varies with the stage of the disease and the Gleason classification (see "Definition"). For patients between ages 65 and 69 yr at diagnosis and a Gleason score of 2 to 4, the probability of dying from prostate cancer 15 yr after diagnosis is 0.06 and that of dying from other causes is 0.56. If the Gleason score is 7 to 10, the probability of dying from prostate cancer increases to 0.72 and from other causes varies from 0.25 to 0.36.
- The ploidy of the tumor also has prognostic value; prognosis is better with diploid tumor cells and worse with aneuploid tumor cells.
- For grade 1 tumors, the extended 10-yr, disease-specific survival is similar for patients with prostatectomy (94%), radiotherapy (90%), and conservative management (93%); survival rate is better with surgery than with radiotherapy or conservative management in patients with grade 2 or 3 localized prostate cancer.
- Expression of the gene *EZH2* has been identified as an important factor in the determination of the aggressiveness of prostate cancer. A recent study revealed that expression of the *EZH2* gene may be a better predictor of clinical failure than Gleason score, tumor stage, or surgical margin status. Testing for EZH2 protein in prostate cancer tissue may be useful to determine prognosis and direct treatment.
- Preoperative PSA level and PSA velocity have prognostic significance. Men whose PSA level increases by >2.0 mcg/ml during the year before the diagnosis of cancer may have a relatively high risk of death from prostate cancer despite undergoing radical prostatectomy.
- Extraprostatic disease is detected at radical prostatectomy in 38% to 52% of patients and is associated with a risk of disease recurrence, progression, and death. In these patients, adjuvant radiotherapy results in significantly reduced risk of PSA relapse and disease recurrence; however, the improvements in metastases-free survival and overall survival are not statistically significant. Table 5 summarizes common pain syndromes in metastatic castration-resistant prostate cancer.
- The Prostate Cancer Prevention trial revealed that the use of 5-alpha-reductase inhibitors lowers the incidence of prostate cancer but also increases the incidence of high-grade tumors (Gleason score >7). It is possible that these agents delay diagnosis of prostate cancer by lowering PSA levels and decreasing prostate size. The trade-off inherent in using 5-alpha-reductase inhibitors for prostate cancer prevention is risk of one additional high-grade cancer in order to avert three or four lower-grade cancers. Based on these results, the FDA's Oncologic Drugs Advisory Committee concluded that finasteride and dutasteride do not have a favorable risk-benefit profile for chemoprevention of prostate cancer in healthy men.
- Patients undergoing prostatectomy are more likely to have urinary incontinence than those undergoing radiotherapy at 2 yr and 5 yr. However, at 15 yr there are no significant relative differences in disease-specific functional outcomes among men undergoing prostatectomy or radiotherapy.
- Bone health is a significant concern in men with prostate cancer. Trials involving bisphosphonates and denosumab reveal that both improve bone mineral density (BMD) in men with nonmetastatic prostate cancer receiving androgen deprivation therapy. Denosumab has also been shown to reduce the risk of vertebral fractures.

SUGGESTED READINGS

Available at ExpertConsult.com

RELATED CONTENT

Prostate Cancer (Patient Information)

AUTHOR: **Fred F. Ferri, MD**

[5]Fizazi K et al: Nonmetastatic, castration-resistant prostate cancer and survival with darolutamide, *N Engl J Med* 383:1040-9, 2020.
[6]de Bono J et al: Olaparib for metastatic castration-resistant prostate cancer, *N Engl J Med* 382:2091-102, 2020.
[7]Matsumoto K et al: Determining when to stop prostate specific antigen monitoring after radical prostatectomy: the role of ultrasensitive prostate specific antigen, *J Urol* 197:655, 2017.
[8]Shirley WV et al: Radiation with or without antiandrogen therapy in recurrent prostate cancer, *N Engl J Med* 376:417-428, 2017.

TABLE 5 Common Pain Syndromes in Metastatic Castration-Resistant Prostate Cancer

Pain Syndrome	Initial Management	Other Therapeutic Alternatives
Localized bone pain	Pharmacologic pain management Localized radiotherapy (special attention to weight-bearing areas, lytic metastasis, and extremities)	Surgical stabilization of pathologic fractures or extensive bone erosions Epidural metastasis and cord compression should be evaluated in all patients with focal back pain Radiopharmaceuticals should be considered if local radiation therapy fails
Diffuse bone pain	Pharmacologic pain management "Multispot" or wide-field radiotherapy Radiopharmaceuticals	Corticosteroids Bisphosphonates or RANK ligand inhibitors Calcitonin Chemotherapy
Epidural metastasis and cord compression	High-dose corticosteroids Radiation therapy Surgical decompression and stabilization are indicated in high-grade epidural compressions, extensive bone involvement, or recurrence after irradiation.	Pharmacologic pain management Physical therapy for recovery of neurologic function
Nerve plexopathies caused by direct tumor extension or previous therapy (rare)	Pharmacologic pain management Radiation therapy (if not previously used) Neurolytic procedures (nerve blocks)	Tricyclic antidepressants (amitriptyline) Anticonvulsants (gabapentin, pregabalin)
Miscellaneous neurogenic causes: Postherpetic neuralgia, peripheral neuropathies	Complete neurologic evaluation Pharmacologic pain management Discontinuation of neurotoxic drugs: Docetaxel, platinum compounds	Tricyclic antidepressants (amitriptyline) Anticonvulsants (gabapentin, pregabalin)
Other uncommon pain syndromes: Extensive skull metastasis with cranial nerve/skull base involvement, extensive painful liver metastasis, or pelvic masses	Radiation therapy Pharmacologic pain management Corticosteroids (cranial nerve involvement)	Chemotherapy Intrathecal chemotherapy may ameliorate symptoms of meningeal involvement

RANK, Receptor activator of nuclear factor-κB.
From Wein AJ et al: *Campbell-Walsh urology,* ed 11, Philadelphia, 2016, Elsevier.

BASIC INFORMATION

DEFINITION

Prostatitis refers to inflammation of the prostate gland. There are four major categories (Table 1):

1. Acute bacterial prostatitis (type I)
2. Chronic bacterial prostatitis (type II)
3. Chronic prostatitis/pelvic pain syndrome (CP/CPPS) (type III): Subdivided into type IIIA (inflammatory) and IIIB (noninflammatory)
4. Asymptomatic inflammatory prostatitis (type IV)

ICD-10CM CODES

N41.0 Acute prostatitis
N41.1 Chronic prostatitis

EPIDEMIOLOGY & DEMOGRAPHICS

- 50% of men will have symptoms of prostatitis in their lifetime.
- Prostatitis accounts for >8% of visits to urologists and 1% of visits to primary care physicians.
- The prevalence of chronic bacterial prostatitis is 5% to 10%.
- CP/CPPS is the most common of the clinically defined prostatitis syndromes, with prevalence ranging from 9% to 12% of men.
- Acute bacterial prostatitis accounts for 10% of all cases of prostatitis.

PHYSICAL FINDINGS & CLINICAL PRESENTATION

- Acute bacterial prostatitis:
  1. Sudden or rapidly progressive onset of:
     a. Dysuria
     b. Frequency
     c. Urgency
     d. Nocturia
     e. Perineal pain that may radiate to the back, rectum, or penis
  2. Hematuria or a purulent urethral discharge may occur.
  3. Occasionally urinary retention complicates the course.
  4. Fever, chills, and signs of sepsis can also be part of the clinical picture.
  5. On rectal examination the prostate is typically tender.
- Chronic bacterial prostatitis:
  1. Characterized by positive culture of expressed prostatic secretions. May cause symptoms such as suprapubic, low back, or perineal pain; mild urgency, frequency, and dysuria with urination; and possibly recurrent urinary tract infections.
  2. May be asymptomatic when the infection is confined to the prostate.
  3. May present as an increase in severity of baseline symptoms of benign prostatic hypertrophy (BPH).
  4. When cystitis is also present, urinary frequency, urgency, and burning may be reported.
  5. Hematuria may be a presenting complaint.
  6. In elderly men, new onset of urinary incontinence may be noted.
- CP/CPPS:
  1. Presents similarly with pain in the pelvic region lasting >3 mo. Symptoms also can include pain in the suprapubic region, low back, penis, testes, or scrotum.
  2. The symptoms can be of variable severity and may include lower urinary tract symptoms, sexual dysfunction, and reduced quality of life.

ETIOLOGY

- Acute bacterial prostatitis:
  1. Acute, usually gram-negative infection of the prostate gland. *E. coli* is the most commonly isolated organism.
     a. Generally associated with cystitis.
     b. Results from the ascent of bacteria into the urethra.
  2. Occasionally the route of infection is hematogenous or a lymphatogenous spread of rectal bacteria.
  3. Consider *Neisseria gonorrhoeae* or *Chlamydia trachomatis* in young patients (age <35 yr) with risk of sexually transmitted disease (STD).
- Chronic bacterial prostatitis:
  1. Often asymptomatic. *E. coli* is the most commonly isolated organism.
  2. Exacerbation of symptoms of BPH caused by the same mechanism as in acute bacterial prostatitis.
- CP/CPPS:
  1. Type IIIA: Refers to symptoms of prostatic inflammation associated with the presence of white blood cells in prostatic secretions with no identifiable bacterial organism.
  2. *Chlamydia* infection may be etiologically implicated in some cases.
  3. Type IIIB: Refers to symptoms of prostatic inflammation with no or few white blood cells in the prostatic secretion. Its cause is multifactorial (Fig. 1).

DIAGNOSIS

DIFFERENTIAL DIAGNOSIS

- BPH with lower urinary tract symptoms
- Prostate cancer
- Interstitial cystitis/bladder pain syndrome
- Pelvic floor dysfunction
- Bladder cancer
- Urolithiasis
- UTI
- Proctitis

WORKUP

- Rectal examination:
  1. Tender prostate most suggestive of acute bacterial prostatitis
  2. Enlarged prostate common in chronic bacterial prostatitis
  3. Normal prostate is consistent with chronic bacterial prostatitis and CP/CPPS
- Expression of prostatic secretions by prostate massage is contraindicated in acute bacterial prostatitis but is appropriate in the other three situations.

LABORATORY TESTS

- Urinalysis
- Urine culture and sensitivity
- Bacterial localization studies can be performed but are cumbersome and impractical in most clinical settings
- Cell count and culture of expressed prostatic secretions
- Prostate-specific antigen (PSA) is not used to diagnose prostatitis and is not recommended unless a nodule is present on digital examination. A rapid rise over baseline should raise the possibility of prostatitis even in the absence of symptoms. In such cases, a follow-up PSA after treatment of prostatitis is appropriate
- Complete blood count and blood cultures if fever, chills, or signs of sepsis exist

TABLE 1 Classification System for the Prostatitis Syndromes

Traditional	National Institutes of Health	Description
Acute bacterial prostatitis	Category I	Acute infection of the prostate gland
Chronic bacterial prostatitis	Category II	Chronic infection of the prostate gland
N/A	Category III Chronic pelvic pain syndrome (CPPS)	Chronic genitourinary pain in the absence of uropathogenic bacteria localized to the prostate gland employing standard methodology
Nonbacterial prostatitis	Category IIIA Inflammatory CPPS	Significant number of white blood cells in expressed prostatic secretions, postprostatic massage urine sediment (VB3), or semen
Prostatodynia	Category IIIB Noninflammatory CPPS	Insignificant number of white blood cells in expressed prostatic secretions, postprostatic massage urine sediment (VB3), or semen
N/A	Category IV Asymptomatic inflammatory prostatitis (AIP)	White blood cells (and/or bacteria) in expressed prostatic secretions, postprostatic massage urine sediment (VB3), semen, or histologic specimens of prostate gland

From Wein AJ et al: *Campbell-Walsh urology*, ed 11, Philadelphia, 2016, Elsevier.

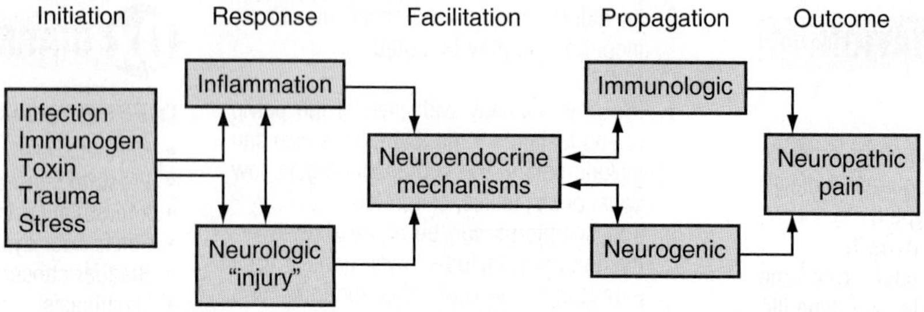

FIG. 1 The cause and pathogenesis of chronic prostatitis/chronic pelvic pain syndrome (category III chronic pelvic pain syndrome) appears to involve a pluricausal, multifactorial mechanism. An initiating stimulus, such as infection, reflux of some toxic or immunogenic urine substance, or perineal or pelvic trauma, starts a cascade of events in an anatomically or genetically susceptible man, resulting in a local response of inflammation or neurogenic injury or both. Further interrelated immunologic, neuropathic, endocrinologic, and psychologic mechanisms propagate or sustain the chronicity of the initial (or ongoing) event. The final outcome is the clinical manifestation of chronic perineal or pelvic pain and associated symptoms with local and central neuropathic mechanisms involving areas outside the prostate or pelvic area. (From Wein AJ et al: *Campbell-Walsh urology,* ed 11, Philadelphia, 2016, Elsevier.)

BOX 1 Suggested Therapies for Chronic Prostatitis and Chronic Pelvic Pain Syndrome (National Institutes of Health Category III)

Recommended
1. α-Blocker therapy as part of a multimodal treatment strategy for newly diagnosed, α-blocker–naive patients who have voiding symptoms
2. Antimicrobial therapy trial for selected newly diagnosed, antimicrobial-naive patients
3. Selected phytotherapies: Cernilton and quercetin
4. Multimodal therapy directed by clinical phenotype
5. Directed physiotherapy. Although level 1 evidence is not available, evidence from multiple weak trials and vast clinical experience strongly suggests benefit for selected patients

Not Recommended
1. α-Blocker monotherapy, particularly in patients previously treated with α-blockers
2. Antiinflammatory monotherapy
3. Antimicrobial therapy as primary therapy, particularly for patients in whom treatment with antibiotics has previously failed
4. 5α-Reductase inhibitor monotherapy; can be considered in older patients with coexisting benign prostatic hyperplasia
5. Most minimally invasive therapies such as transurethral needle ablation (TUNA), laser therapies
6. Invasive surgical therapies such as transurethral resection of the prostate (TURP) and radical prostatectomy

Requiring Further Evaluation
1. Low-intensity shock wave treatment
2. Acupuncture
3. Biofeedback
4. Invasive neuromodulation (e.g., pudendal nerve modulation)
5. Electromagnetic stimulation
6. Botulinum toxin A injection
7. Medical therapies including mepartricin, muscle relaxants, neuromodulators, and immunomodulators

Modified from Nickel JC et al: Male chronic pelvic pain syndrome (CPPS). In Chapple C, Abrams P (eds): *Male lower urinary tract symptoms (LUTS). An international consultation on male LUTS, Fukuoka, Japan, Sept 30–Oct 4, 2012,* Montreal, 2013, Société Internationale d'Urologie. From Wein AJ et al: *Campbell-Walsh urology,* ed 11, Philadelphia, 2016, Elsevier.

Rx TREATMENT

- Acute bacterial prostatitis:
  1. Uncomplicated (with risk of STD, age <35 yr): Ceftriaxone 250 mg IM × 1 dose *or* cefixime 400 mg PO × 1 *then* doxycycline 100 mg bid × 10 days.
  2. Uncomplicated with low risk of STD: Levofloxacin 500 mg qid or ciprofloxacin 500 mg bid × 10 to 14 days.
- Chronic bacterial prostatitis:
  1. First-line choice is a quinolone (ciprofloxacin or levofloxacin) for 4 wk.
  2. Trimethoprim-sulfamethoxazole (TMP-SMX) is second-line choice for 1 to 3 mo if the organism is sensitive. Tissue penetration for TMP-SMX is not as good as quinolones, and there is evidence of increasing uropathogenic resistance.
- CP/CPPS:
  1. Suggested therapies for CP/CPPS are summarized in Box 1.

SUGGESTED READINGS

Available at ExpertConsult.com

RELATED CONTENT

Prostatitis (Patient Information)

AUTHOR: **Fred F. Ferri, MD**

BASIC INFORMATION

DEFINITION

Psoriasis is a chronic skin disorder characterized by excessive proliferation of keratinocytes, resulting in the formation of thickened scaly plaques, itching, and inflammatory changes of the epidermis and dermis. Psoriasis is also associated with cardiovascular, metabolic, and neuropsychiatric effects. The various forms of psoriasis include plaque (most common), guttate, erythrodermic, pustular, inverse, and arthritis variants.

ICD-10CM CODES

L40	Psoriasis
L40.0	Psoriasis vulgaris
L40.1	Generalized pustular psoriasis
L40.4	Guttate psoriasis
L40.8	Other psoriasis
L40.9	Psoriasis unspecified
L40.54	Psoriatic juvenile arthropathy

EPIDEMIOLOGY & DEMOGRAPHICS

- Psoriasis affects 2% to 4% of the world's population. Most patients have limited psoriasis involving <5% of their body surface.
- There is a strong association between psoriasis and human leukocyte antigens (HLAs) B13, B17, and B27 (pustular psoriasis).
- Peak age of onset is bimodal (age 30-39 yr and at age 60 yr). Mean age at diagnosis is 34 yr.
- Men and women are affected equally. Approximately 20% of patients with psoriasis also have psoriatic arthritis. Median time from development of joint symptoms to diagnosis of psoriatic arthritis is 5 yr. Nail psoriasis affects over 50% of patients with psoriasis and can occur with any of the subtypes.

PHYSICAL FINDINGS & CLINICAL PRESENTATION

- Approximately 67% of patients with psoriasis have mild-to-moderate disease.
- The primary psoriatic lesion is an erythematous papule topped by a loosely adherent scale. Scraping the scale results in several bleeding points *(Auspitz sign).*
- Chronic plaque psoriasis generally manifests with symmetric, sharply demarcated, erythematous, silver-scaled patches affecting primarily the intergluteal folds, elbows, scalp, fingernails, toenails, and knees (Figs. 1 and 2). This form accounts for 80% of psoriasis cases. Psoriasis may also involve the forehead, particularly contiguous to the scalp (Fig. E3).
- Psoriasis can also develop at the site of any physical trauma (sunburn, scratching). This is known as *Koebner phenomenon.*
- Nail involvement is common (pitting of the nail plate), resulting in hyperkeratosis, onychodystrophy with onycholysis (Fig. E4).
- Pruritus is variable; soreness and bleeding may occur.
- Joint involvement can result in sacroiliitis and spondylitis.
- Guttate psoriasis is generally preceded by streptococcal pharyngitis and manifests with multiple droplike lesions on the extremities and the trunk.
- Erythrodermic psoriasis is characterized by widespread cutaneous erythema and scaling.
- Pustular psoriasis manifests with widespread pustules. Localized forms may affect palms and soles.
- Inverse psoriasis is characterized by red and sharply demarcated thinner patches involving intertriginous areas (axillae, inguinal areas).
- Adverse effect on psychologic and social functioning, with affected persons often feeling stigmatized.

ETIOLOGY

- Unknown, but there is a strong genetic component and high heritability. There are at least nine chromosomal loci with linkage to psoriasis. These loci are called psoriasis susceptibility 1 through 9 (PSORS1-PSORS9). PSORS1 locus in the major histocompatibility complex (MHC) region on chromosome 6 is considered the most important susceptibility locus and is believed to account for 35% to 50% of the heritability of the disease.
- Familial clustering (genetic transmission with a dominant mode with variable penetrants).
- One third of persons affected have a positive family history.
- A high prevalence of celiac disease has been noted in patients with psoriasis.

Dx DIAGNOSIS

DIFFERENTIAL DIAGNOSIS

- Contact dermatitis
- Atopic dermatitis
- Stasis dermatitis
- Tinea
- Nummular dermatitis
- Candidiasis
- Mycosis fungoides, Sezary syndrome
- Cutaneous systemic lupus erythematosus
- Secondary and tertiary syphilis

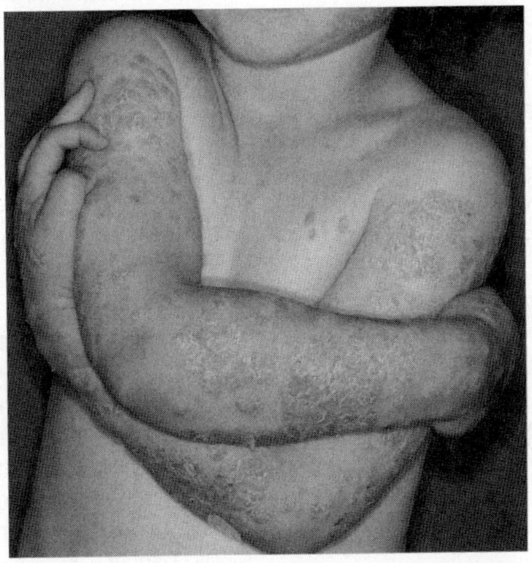

FIG. 1 Psoriasis. Variably sized erythematous plaques with moderately thick overlying scale. (From Paller AS, Mancini AJ: *Hurwitz clinical pediatric dermatology: a textbook of skin disorders of childhood and adolescence,* ed 5, Philadelphia, 2016, Elsevier.)

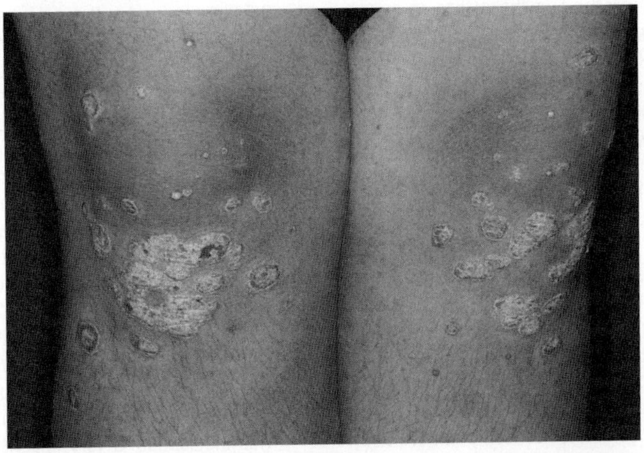

FIG. 2 Typical plaques of psoriasis with thick, micaceous scale overlying erythema. (From Paller AS, Mancini AJ: *Hurwitz clinical pediatric dermatology: a textbook of skin disorders of childhood and adolescence,* ed 5, Philadelphia, 2016, Elsevier.)

- Drug eruption
- Dermatomyositis (DM)
- Lupus erythematosus (LE)
- Seborrheic dermatitis
- Pityriasis rosea
- Lichen planus
- Pityriasis rubra pilaris

WORKUP

- Diagnosis is clinical. Blood work is rarely needed. A rapid plasma regain test is useful when ruling out syphilis. Antinuclear antibody (ANA) and anti-Ro and anti-La antibodies are helpful in ruling out subacute cutaneous lupus.
- Skin biopsy is rarely necessary.

LABORATORY TESTS

Generally not necessary for diagnosis

Rx TREATMENT

NONPHARMACOLOGIC THERAPY

- Sunbathing generally leads to improvement.
- Eliminate triggering factors (e.g., stress, certain medications [e.g., lithium, beta-blockers, antimalarials]). Severe emotional stress tends to aggravate psoriasis.
- Patients with psoriasis benefit from a daily bath in warm water followed by application of a cream or ointment moisturizer. Regular use of an emollient moisturizer limits evaporation of water from the skin and allows the stratum corneum to rehydrate itself.
- Psoralen and ultraviolet A (PUVA) therapy (see "General Rx").
- Local hyperthermia has been used successfully to clear psoriatic plaques, but relapse is common.
- Occlusive treatment with surgical tape or dressings is effective as monotherapy or in combination with topical medications.
- Avoidance of tobacco. Smoking tobacco may worsen psoriasis.

GENERAL Rx

Therapeutic options vary according to the extent of disease and comorbidities. Topical therapies remain the cornerstone for treating mild psoriasis. Treatment of psoriasis in the setting of comorbidities is described in Table E1. Treatment of psoriasis at specific sites is summarized in Table E2. Approximately 70% to 80% of all patients can be treated adequately with topical therapy.

- Patients with limited disease (<20% of the body) can be treated with the following:
  1. Topical steroids: Disadvantages are brief remissions, expense, and decreased effect with continued use. Salicylic acid can be compounded by pharmacist in concentrations of 2% to 10% and used in combination with a corticosteroid to decrease the amount of scale.
  2. Calcipotriene: A vitamin D analogue effective for moderate plaque psoriasis. Adults should comb the hair, apply solution to the lesions, and rub it in, avoiding uninvolved skin. Disadvantages include its cost and potential burning and skin irritation. It should not be used concurrently with salicylic acid because calcipotriene is inactivated by the acidic nature of salicylic acid. Taclonex ointment and Enstilar aerosol foam formulation are a combination of calcipotriene and the high-potency corticosteroid betamethasone dipropionate. They are well tolerated and more effective than either agent used alone but also much more expensive.
  3. Tar products (Estar, liquor carbonis detergens [LCD], Psorigel) can be used overnight and are most effective when combined with ultraviolet B (UVB) light (Goeckerman regimen).
  4. Anthralin: Useful for chronic plaques; can result in purple-brown staining; best used with UVB light.
  5. Retinoids such as tazarotene 0.05%, 0.1% cream or gel, are effective in thinning plaques but are expensive and can cause irritation.
  6. Other useful measures include tape or occlusive dressing, UVB and lubricating agents, and interlesional steroids.
- Therapeutic options for persons with generalized disease (affecting >20% of the body) and for those with inadequate response to topical agents:
  1. UVB light exposure three times a wk: This therapy does not require administration of a systemic drug (unlike psoralen plus ultraviolet A [PUVA]), but to be effective, it requires removal of scale with keratolytic agents and emollients.
  2. Oral PUVA administered two to three times weekly is effective for generalized disease. It is often considered in patients for whom narrow-band UVB therapy is ineffective. However, many PUVA treatments are required, necessitating frequent office visits, and it may be associated with phototoxicity, such as erythema and blistering, and increased risk of skin cancer.
- Systemic treatments include methotrexate 25 mg/wk for severe psoriasis. Etretinate (a synthetic retinoid) is most effective for palmar-plantar pustular psoriasis. Dose is 0.5 to 1 mg/kg/day. It can cause liver enzyme and lipid abnormalities and is teratogenic.
- Apremilast is a phosphodiesterase type-4 inhibitor used in moderate to severe plaque psoriasis. Side effects include diarrhea, nausea, headache, and worsening depression.
- Cyclosporine is also effective in severe psoriasis; however, relapses are common.
- Chronic plaque psoriasis may be treated with alefacept, a recombinant protein that selectively targets T lymphocytes. Treatment with alefacept for 12 wk (0.025, 0.075, or 0.150 mg/kg of body weight IV weekly) may result in significant improvement. Some patients also demonstrate a sustained clinical response after the cessation of treatment. This medication is very expensive (a 12-wk course can cost >$8000).
- Biologic therapies are now routinely used when traditional systemic agents are ineffective or poorly tolerated. Screening for tuberculosis is necessary before initiating treatment with these agents. Active, serious infection is a contraindication to the use of biologics.
- Tumor necrosis factor (TNF) inhibitors (adalimumab [Humira], etanercept [Enbrel], infliximab [Remicade]): Trials revealed a reduction in severity of plaque psoriasis. Efalizumab, a humanized monoclonal antibody that inhibits the activation of T cells, has also been reported to produce significant improvement in plaque psoriasis treatment period. Adalimumab has been reported to be effective for joint and skin manifestations of psoriasis.
- Newer biologic agents in patients with moderate to severe plaque psoriasis are ustekinumab (Stelara; an interleukin-12 and interleukin-23 blocker), brodalumab (SILIQ), ixekizumab (Taltz), secukinumab (Cosentyx) anti–interleukin-17 receptor antagonists, and guselkumab (Tremfya), risankizumab (Skyrizi), and tildrakizumab (ILUMYA) interleukin-23 blockers. Cost is a limiting factor with all these agents.
- A phase 2 trial of the topical PDE4 inhibitor Roflumilast in chronic plaque psoriasis revealed modest efficacy rate of Roflumilast with an Investigator's Global Assessment (IGA) score of 23% to 28% when compared to potent corticosteroids (up to 77%).[1]

DISPOSITION

The course of psoriasis is chronic, and the disease may be refractory to treatment.

REFERRAL

- Dermatology referral is recommended in all patients with generalized disease.
- Hospital admission may be necessary for severe diffuse or poorly responsive psoriasis. The Goeckerman regimen combines daily application of tar with UVB exposure and can result in prolonged remissions.

PEARLS & CONSIDERATIONS

COMMENTS

Psoriasis is more emotionally than physically disabling for most patients. Counseling may be indicated, particularly when it affects younger patients.

SUGGESTED READINGS

Available at ExpertConsult.com

RELATED CONTENT

Psoriasis (Patient Information)
Psoriatic Arthritis (Related Key Topic)

AUTHOR: **Fred F. Ferri, MD**

[1]Lebwohl MG et al: Trial of Roflumilast Cream for Chronic Plaque Psoriasis, New England Journal of Medicine 383:229-239, 2020.

BASIC INFORMATION

DEFINITION

Psoriatic arthritis (PsA) is an inflammatory arthropathy, often included in a class of disorders called the *seronegative spondyloarthropathies (SpA),* a family of diseases characterized by inflammation of the spine, peripheral joints, and entheses (sites of insertion of tendon into bone). Both the Moll and Wright and CASPAR classification criteria are described in Table 1.

ICD-10CM CODES

L40.5+	Arthropathic psoriasis
L40.54	Psoriatic juvenile arthropathy
L40.52	Psoriatic arthritis mutilans

EPIDEMIOLOGY & DEMOGRAPHICS

INCIDENCE: 6 per 100,000 per yr

PREVALENCE: One to two per 1000 in the general population. Variable estimates of 4% to 30% of patients with underlying psoriasis

PREDOMINANT SEX: Equal male-to-female distribution

PREDOMINANT AGE: Symptom onset generally between age 30 to 55

PHYSICAL FINDINGS & CLINICAL PRESENTATION

- Psoriasis precedes arthritis in 67% of cases by an average of 8 to 10 yr.
- Arthritis precedes psoriasis or occurs concomitantly in 33% of patients.
- Arthritis, dactylitis, spondylitis, and enthesitis are main features.
- On examination, about 15% of patients will have psoriasis without prior diagnosis of skin disease.
- Arthritis is inflammatory, commonly characterized by prolonged morning stiffness, improvement with activity, joint erythema, warmth, or swelling.
- There are five classically described patterns of joint involvement (Box 1, Table 2).
- Some patients may present with more than one pattern, and patterns can evolve over time. The distal interphalangeal (DIP) joints (Fig. E1) and spine are each affected in 40% to 50% of cases. It is rare to have spondyloarthritis alone, and it usually occurs with peripheral involvement.
- Dactylitis, also known as "sausage digit," refers to diffuse swelling of a finger or toe (Fig. E2); it is fairly common and occurs in approximately 30% to 40% of patients during the disease course. It is associated with increased risk of radiographic joint damage.
- Enthesitis commonly occurs at the Achilles and plantar fascia (Fig. E3), and swelling and tenderness may be seen on exam. Subclinical disease may be evident by ultrasonography.
- Dystrophic changes of the nails (pitting, onycholysis, leukonychia) may occur in association with joint inflammation in involved digits.
- Spondyloarthritis may include sacroiliitis but is generally less likely to cause fusion to the extent seen in ankylosing spondylitis. More common to have asymmetric sacroiliac joint involvement (usually bilateral in ankylosing spondylitis).
- Ocular inflammation including conjunctivitis and uveitis can be seen.

ETIOLOGY

Remains unknown, but felt to be interplay of genetic, immunologic, and environmental factors. Fig. E4 illustrates the pathogenetic pathways in PsA. There is a higher frequency of HLA-B12, HLA-B17, HLA_B57, HLA-Cw*0602 in PsA. Those with PsA versus psoriasis alone have higher frequency of HLA-B7, HLA-B27.

DIAGNOSIS

DIFFERENTIAL DIAGNOSIS

- Rheumatoid arthritis (RA)
- Erosive osteoarthritis
- Crystalline arthritis, including gout and pseudogout
- Other seronegative spondyloarthropathies, which include reactive arthritis, enteropathic arthritis, and ankylosing spondylitis (also see differential diagnosis of SpA in Section III)

WORKUP

- Diagnosis is generally made on clinical grounds based on history, exam, and radiographic findings given lack of specific lab findings. An algorithm for the diagnosis of psoriatic arthritis is described in Fig. 5.
- Early diagnosis can be difficult to establish when the joint symptoms develop before skin and nail findings.

LABORATORY TESTS

- No specific diagnostic lab tests.
- Acute phase reactants such as ESR and CRP may be elevated, although less commonly than in patients with rheumatoid arthritis.
- Anemia of chronic disease may be seen.
- Rheumatoid factor (RF) and anti-CCP are generally negative but can be present in up to 15% of patients.
- *HLA-B27* is significantly more common in patients with axial inflammation.
- Arthrocentesis generally demonstrates inflammatory synovial fluid without crystals.

IMAGING STUDIES

Radiographic findings of involved joints may include soft tissue swelling, joint space

BOX 1 Subtypes of Psoriatic Arthritis

- Distal interphalangeal joint–predominant arthritis (10%)
- Symmetric polyarthritis–predominant arthritis (5%-20%)
- Asymmetric oligoarthritis or monoarthritis (70%-80%)
- Axial disease predominant (spondylitis, sacroiliitis, or both) (5%-20%)
- Arthritis mutilans (rare)

From Hochberg MC: *Rheumatology,* ed 7, Philadelphia, 2019, Elsevier.

TABLE 1 Classifications of Psoriatic Arthritis

	CASPAR*		
Moll and Wright	Points	Category	Description
Presence of PsO and an inflammatory arthritis (peripheral arthritis and/or sacroiliitis or spondylitis)	2	Current PsO	Psoriatic skin or scalp disease confirmed by a dermatologist or rheumatologist; history of PsO from the patient, family physician, dermatologist, rheumatologist, or other qualified practitioner; patient-reported history of PsO in a first- or second-degree relative
	1	Personal or family history of PsO	
The (usual) absence of serologic tests for RF	1	Psoriatic nail dystrophy on current physical examination	Includes onycholysis, pitting, and hyperkeratosis
	1	Negative test for RF	ELISA or nephelometry preferred (no latex) using the local laboratory reference range
	1	Current dactylitis or history of dactylitis documented by a rheumatologist	Swelling of the entire digit
	1	Radiographic evidence of juxtaarticular new bone formation	Ill-defined ossification near joint margins in the hand or foot, excluding osteophyte formation on plain radiographs

*Psoriatic arthritis is diagnosed when three or more points are assigned in the presence of inflammatory articular disease (joint, spine, or entheseal).
CASPAR, Classification Criteria for the Study of Psoriatic Arthritis; *ELISA,* enzyme-linked immunosorbent assay; *PsO,* psoriasis; *RF,* rheumatoid factor.
From Hochberg MC: *Rheumatology,* ed 7, Philadelphia, 2019, Elsevier.

TABLE 2 Five Major Types of Psoriatic Arthritis*

Type	Clinical Findings
Mono- and asymmetric oligoarthritis (most common type)	• Inflammation of the DIP and PIP joints of the hands and feet • Involvement of the PIP or both the DIP and PIP joints of a single digit can result in the classic "sausage" digit • MCP joint involvement unusual (unlike RA) • May be accompanied by inflammation of larger joints
Arthritis of the distal interphalangeal joints	• Exclusive involvement of the DIP joints • Classic but uncommon presentation • The joints may become fixed in a flexed position
Rheumatoid arthritis–like presentation (difficult to distinguish from RA clinically**)	• *Symmetric* polyarthritis that involves small and medium-sized joints, in particular the PIP, MCP, wrist, ankle, and elbow • Most patients are seronegative for RF
Arthritis mutilans*** (least common type)	• Severe, rapidly progressive joint inflammation that results in destruction of the joints and permanent deformity • Digits become shorter, wider, and softer to palpation because of osteolysis and a telescoping phenomenon
Spondylitis and sacroiliitis (also have peripheral joint involvement)	• Spondylitis resembles that seen in ankylosing spondylitis, with axial arthritis as well as involvement of the knees and sacroiliac joints • Patients are often HLA-B27-positive and may have associated inflammatory bowel disease and/or uveitis

*Patients with psoriatic arthritis can have tendonitis, enthesitis, and dactylitis.
**Whether some seropositive patients have an overlap of the two disorders is possible.
***Also occurs in multicentric reticulohistiocytosis.
DIP, Distal interphalangeal; *MCP,* metacarpophalangeal; *PIP,* proximal interphalangeal; *RA,* rheumatoid arthritis; *RF,* rheumatoid factor.
(From Bolognia JL: *Dermatology,* ed 4, Philadelphia, 2018, Elsevier.)

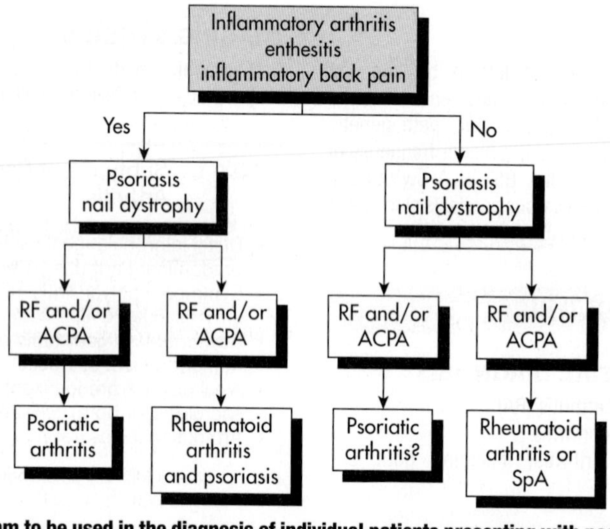

FIG. 5 Algorithm to be used in the diagnosis of individual patients presenting with possible psoriatic arthritis. Some patients may present with typical articular manifestations of psoriatic arthritis but in the absence of skin or nail disease. They can be diagnosed as having definite psoriatic arthritis only when psoriasis subsequently develops. *ACPA,* Anticitrullinated protein antibody; *RF,* rheumatoid factor; *SpA,* spondyloarthropathy. (From Firestein GS et al: *Kelly's textbook of rheumatology,* ed 9, Philadelphia, 2013, Saunders.)

narrowing, subluxation, erosive changes, and new bone formation (periostitis, fusion). As opposed to RA, see more asymmetric joint involvement and DIP joint changes.

Severe digital erosive change with adjacent heterotopic bone formation may give rise to "pencil in cup" deformity. Can see whittling of the phalanges.

With axial involvement can see sacroiliac joint changes (sclerosis, erosions, pseudo-widening, ankylosis) and bridging vertebral syndesmophytes.

Musculoskeletal ultrasonography can be used in the evaluation of enthesitis or arthritis.

MRI may be helpful in further evaluation of sacroiliac and spinal involvement.

Rx TREATMENT

PHARMACOLOGIC THERAPY

The choice of therapeutic agent depends on the type of clinical manifestations, as not all agents are effective for all manifestations. For example, enthesis and spinal involvement are not responsive to traditional oral disease-modifying agents such as methotrexate or leflunomide but are responsive to tumor necrosis factor blocking agents (TNFi).

- NSAIDs may be used for mild or limited disease.
- Intraarticular corticosteroid injections can be used as adjunctive Rx for involved joints.
- Oral glucocorticoids should generally be avoided, given increased risk for development of erythrodermic or pustular psoriasis.
- In patients with active peripheral joint disease, elevated acute phase reactants, or evidence of changes on imaging, traditional DMARDs such as methotrexate, sulfasalazine, and leflunomide should be considered early on, though data supporting their use is limited.
- Apremilast is an oral phosphodiesterase 4 (PDE 4) inhibitor and is safe to use, especially in those with multiple comorbidities. Can also be beneficial for enthesitis and dactylitis.
- In patients with peripheral arthritis who fail to respond to nonbiologic DMARDs, escalation of therapy should be considered. All five TNFi are FDA-approved to treat psoriatic arthritis (etanercept, infliximab, adalimumab, golimumab, certolizumab pegol). In those resistant to a TNFi, a second TNFi can be tried. If adequate response is still not achieved, a different mechanism of action (IL-17i, IL-12/23 blockade) can be tried.
- Secukinumab, an IL-17 inhibitor, is approved to treat psoriasis, PsA, and AS. Ixekizumab, an anti-IL-17 monoclonal antibody, can also be used to treat psoriasis, PsA, and now AS. Brodalumab, an anti-IL17RA monoclonal antibody, treats psoriasis alone currently. Guselkumab, an anti-IL23 antibody, has recently been approved to treat psoriatic arthritis.
- Ustekinumab is a human IgG monoclonal antibody that binds to the p40 subunit of interleukin (IL)-12 and -23 and is approved to treat psoriasis, psoriatic arthritis, and Crohns.
- Abatacept (selective T-cell costimulation modulator) was approved to treat PsA, but has shown limited efficacy in treatment of psoriasis. It can help with peripheral arthritis. Tofacitinib (oral Janus kinase inhibitor) has also been approved.
- In patients with predominantly axial disease not responsive to NSAIDs, TNFi or IL17i can be tried. For enthesitis/dactylitis TNFi, IL17i, IL12/23, and apremilast can be considered.

REFERRAL

Rheumatology, dermatology

PEARLS & CONSIDERATIONS

COMMENTS

- Patients frequently have a positive family history of psoriasis or psoriatic arthritis.
- Severity of skin psoriasis and activity of inflammatory arthritis can be discordant.

SUGGESTED READINGS

Available at ExpertConsult.com

RELATED CONTENT

Psoriatic Arthritis (Patient Information)

AUTHOR: **Daphne Scaramangas-Plumley, MD**

BASIC INFORMATION

DEFINITION

Psychosis is a state in which a patient's experience of reality is distorted by delusions and/or hallucinations (a delusion is a fixed false idiosyncratic belief; a hallucination is a false auditory, visual, olfactory, tactile, or taste perception). Delusions take a variety of forms, and include persecutory, referential, somatic, religious, grandiose, erotomanic, bizarre, and others. In addition to delusions and hallucinations, disorganized speech and behavior are often seen in psychosis regardless of etiology.

Psychosis is a key finding in many mental illnesses, such as brief psychotic disorder, delusional disorder, schizoaffective disorder, schizophrenia, schizophreniform disorder, or shared psychotic disorder. Psychosis can also present as part of the evolution of a mood disorder (depression and bipolar disorder), a decompensated personality or trauma disorder, a sign of an underlying general medical or neurologic condition, or as the result of substance intoxication or withdrawal. It is important to note that primary psychiatric illnesses (i.e., idiopathic diseases) are largely diagnoses of exclusion, and that general medical etiologies should be considered and ruled out in an early presentation of psychosis.

ICD-10CM CODES

F05	Delirium not induced by alcohol and other psychoactive substances
F06.0	Organic hallucinosis
F09	Unspecified organic or symptomatic mental disorder
F10.5	Psychotic disorder due to psychoactive substance use
F30.2 and F31.2	Manic episode with psychosis and bipolar affective disorder with psychosis
F32.3	Major depressive disorder, single episode, severe with psychotic features

DSM-5 CODES

Depends on specific diagnosis

ICD-11CM CODES

6D70	Delirium
6E61	Secondary psychotic syndrome
6C4G.5	Delirium induced by unknown or unspecified psychoactive substance
6C4G.6	Psychosis induced by unknown or unspecified psychoactive substance
6A60.1	Bipolar type 1 disorder, current episode manic, with psychotic symptoms
6A70.4	Single episode depressive disorder, severe, with psychotic features
6A71.4	Recurrent depressive disorder, current episode severe, with psychotic symptoms
6D86.0	Psychotic symptoms in dementia
6E21	Mental or behavioral disorders associated with pregnancy, childbirth, or the puerperium, with psychotic symptoms

For primary psychotic disorders, see "Schizophrenia" chapter

EPIDEMIOLOGY & DEMOGRAPHICS

1-yr prevalence is roughly 4 per 1000 people. Approximately 3% of the worldwide population will be diagnosed with a psychotic disorder. The (demographics of) psychosis depends on the underlying disorder.

PHYSICAL FINDINGS & CLINICAL PRESENTATION

GENERAL:
- Collateral sources of information will likely be essential for understanding a full history of presentation.
- The patient may be unpredictable or easily agitated. Focus on mutual safety and rapport building. Do not challenge delusional material early on or in an uncontrolled setting.

HISTORY:
- Past and current medical history important to identify potential general medical etiologies
- Medication use
- Use of illicit substances or alcohol
- Identification of functional and social impairment, including time course
- Behavior that is odd or unpredictable; patient may be acting based on misinterpretation of their reality or false perceptions (delusions or hallucinations)

EXAMINATION:
- Examine for symptoms of:
  1. Mood disorder: Delusions or hallucinations are often congruent with the mood (e.g., auditory hallucinations in a depressed patient may tell the patient what a terrible person he is, or a delusion that they are dead or part of them is rotten [the Cotard delusion]; or grandiose delusions found in mania)
  2. Altered or disorganized thought pattern: Usually reflected in disorganized speech (including word salad, thought blocking, rhyming, clang associations), or disorganized behavior
  3. Poor insight and judgment, odd behavior
  4. Motor examination, including signs of Parkinsonism and catatonia
  5. Full cognitive examination, in particular memory and attention

PATHOPHYSIOLOGY

- Involves an interaction among:
  1. Dopaminergic overactivity (particularly in the mesocortical, mesolimbic, and nigrostriatal systems)
  2. Environmental, social, or childhood factors
  3. Genetic predisposition
  4. Disease-specific factors

Dx DIAGNOSIS

Differential diagnosis (including for delirium and psychotic symptoms without delirium)
- General medical conditions: Infections ranging from urinary tract infections (UTIs) to HIV/AIDS and COVID-19, hypo- and hyperthyroidism, shock (all causes), leprosy, malaria, sarcoidosis, systemic lupus erythematosus, hypoglycemia, hypercarbia and hypoxemia, DKA and HHS, porphyria, pheochromocytoma, paraneoplastic syndrome and brain metastasis, vitamin deficiency (including Wernicke encephalopathy), pain
- Medications: Systemic steroids, anticonvulsants, anticholinergic medications (including diphenhydramine, scopolamine), antibiotics, some chemotherapy
- Neurodegenerative diseases: Alzheimer disease, dementia with Lewy bodies and Parkinson disease (and associated dementia), vascular dementia
- Other neurologic diseases: Huntington disease, cerebrovascular accident (stroke), epilepsy (ictal, postictal, interictal psychoses), multiple sclerosis, prion disease, brain tumors, autoimmune encephalitis, infectious encephalitis (e.g., HSV), traumatic brain injury, posterior reversible encephalopathy syndrome (PRES)
- Illicit drugs (usually with chronic use; can be caused by intoxication or withdrawal): Lysergic acid diethylamide (LSD), phencyclidine (PCP), cocaine, gamma-hydroxybutyrate (GHB; withdrawal), alcohol (delirium tremens and alcoholic hallucinosis), amphetamines, and marijuana. New substances of abuse (e.g., "bath salts," synthetic cannabinoids) may not be detected by current toxicology panels
- Psychiatric:
  1. Primary psychotic disorders: Schizophrenia, major depression, brief psychotic disorder, delusional disorder, schizoaffective disorder, schizophreniform disorder
  2. Mood disorders: Major depression with psychotic features; bipolar disorder, manic/depressed, with psychotic features
  3. Trauma disorders: Complex PTSD
  4. Personality disorders: Borderline, paranoid, schizoid, schizotypal
  5. Other: Peripartum psychosis (80% of patients go on to be diagnosed with bipolar disorder), autism spectrum disorders (acute decompensation can appear psychotic in some cases)

WORKUP

- On the initial workup, for psychotic symptoms (with or without delirium), consider a comprehensive metabolic panel and expanded electrolytes, complete blood count with urine toxicology, urinalysis, urine/serum toxicology, TSH, CXR, and blood cultures/procalcitonin if clinically appropriate.
- If the initial workup is unrevealing, follow-up testing of vitamin B_{12}/methylmalonic acid, folate, thiamine (vs. empiric treatment), AM cortisol, HIV, RPR, SARS-CoV-2 PCR, ESR/CRP, serum ANA is appropriate.
- For rapidly progressing psychotic symptoms and encephalopathy, and EEG and LP for CSF cell counts, glucose, immunoglobulins, and Mayo autoimmune encephalopathy panel is appropriate.
- A head CT is appropriate in the workup for delirium but is rarely useful for isolated psychotic symptoms. If laboratory workup is

unrevealing, brain MRI +/- contrast may be useful.

- In the appropriate clinical context, consider also 24-hour urine collection for metanephrines and porphobilinogens, serum angiotensin-converting enzyme.

Rx TREATMENT

NONPHARMACOLOGIC THERAPY

- Cognitive-behavioral therapy
- Social and behavioral skills training
- Training for self-management of disease
- Aforementioned strategies favored over psychoanalytic techniques given the relative inability for abstract thought and lack of insight in psychotic patients
- Family intervention, including education and strategies to reduce emotional expression
- Counseling for substance abuse

ACUTE PHARMACOLOGIC TREATMENT

- The treatment of psychosis will depend greatly on the etiology.
- Antipsychotics in schizophrenia, schizoaffective disorders, and bipolar or major depressive disorder with psychosis have been well studied. See dedicated chapters in this text for more details, but briefly:
  1. Schizophrenia-spectrum illness: Risperidone is a commonly prescribed first-line medication, although according to several meta-analyses olanzapine and clozapine may be more effective. First-generation antipsychotics are useful if SGAs are poorly tolerated and generally all have similar efficacy, but the risk of motor side effects (both acutely and chronically) is higher.
  2. Delusional disorder has roughly equivalent responsiveness to antipsychotics as schizophrenia, although treatment uptake is often more limited.
  3. Bipolar disorder, mania with psychotic features: Olanzapine, risperidone, and haloperidol all demonstrate excellent efficacy, with tolerability profiles in that order. Consider initiating a mood stabilizer (especially lithium or valproic acid), as well as ECT.
  4. Major depressive disorder with psychotic features: ECT is both efficacious and cost-effective and should be considered early. Treatment involves both antidepressants and antipsychotics; sertraline or escitalopram and olanzapine or quetiapine are reasonable first choices. Aripiprazole is also commonly used in the treatment of depression.
- The treatment of delirium primarily involves the general medical management of the underlying condition. For example, the treatment of sepsis associated with a UTI with antibiotics can be reasonably expected to improve the mental status in time. Otherwise, the mitigation of delirious symptoms is best approached nonpharmacologically with frequent reorientation, engagement with family members to ensure comfort, minimization of discomfort and maximization of senses (e.g., glasses, hearing aids), and maintaining appropriate cues for an appropriate sleep-wake cycle. Melatonin-receptor agonists are commonly used in prevention and may have modest benefits. The role of antipsychotics in delirium is limited to the management of behavioral disturbances (including aggression and interfering with general medical care) or terror associated with psychotic experiences. Antipsychotics, though useful for the aforementioned indications, do not promote the resolution of delirium nor do they shorten hospital stays. Benzodiazepines and anticholinergic agents, though often useful in schizophrenia and other primary psychiatric illnesses, will worsen delirium.
- Psychotic symptoms related to other medical conditions (in the absence of delirium) may also be managed with antipsychotics. There are few randomized trials available to guide treatment and they depend on the etiology.
- Substance-induced psychosis is typically self-limited, although persistent symptoms may occur, particularly in methamphetamine-induced psychosis. In these cases, antipsychotics and cognitive-behavioral therapy can be helpful.
- For all agents, use the minimum effective dose to limit side effects.
- Multiple formulations are available, including oral, dissolvable, intravenous, short- and long-acting intramuscular injections, and recently transcutaneous.
- Obtain baseline labs and studies, including BMP and magnesium and ECG (especially when treating behavioral disturbance in delirium), lipid profile, fasting glucose/A_{1c}, and CBC.
- Use antipsychotics with caution in elderly patients because of the higher risk of adverse events, including death.
- For medications with stronger D2 blockade (i.e., first-generation antipsychotics, risperidone/paliperidone), combination with anticholinergic agents (e.g., benztropine) reduce motor side effects if such arise but should not be used in the long term.
- Benzodiazepines can be useful for concurrent agitation if severe (if no contraindications).

CHRONIC PHARMACOLOGIC TREATMENT

- There are few studies of antipsychotics for all causes of psychosis, although for conditions such as schizophrenia, long-term treatment with antipsychotics can decrease all-cause mortality in spite of the side-effect burden.
- Consider economic factors, including insurance formulary, when selecting a maintenance regimen.
- Second-generation antipsychotics have a lower incidence of tardive dyskinesia but increase the likelihood metabolic disorders compared with first-generation antipsychotics.

OTHER:

- ECT is commonly used in the treatment of mood and psychotic disorders.

DISPOSITION

Prognosis varies according to etiology of psychosis. In general, the more severe and longer the psychotic episode, the worse the prognosis.

REFERRAL

Once delirium and general medical causes of isolated psychosis have been ruled out, patients should be admitted psychiatrically for acute stabilization if actively psychotic to prevent harm to self and others as well as ensure administration of medications. Legal barriers to compelling admission and treatment will vary geographically. Consider looking up local laws regarding compulsory mental health treatment.

PEARLS & CONSIDERATIONS

- Delusions and/or hallucinations are hallmarks of psychosis.
- Rule out medical or drug causes of psychosis, including delirium, which is characterized by altered sensorium, inattention, and commonly visual hallucinations or paranoia.
- Antipsychotics are the mainstay of acute and chronic treatment.
- Brief psychotic disorder DSM-5 298.8 (F23) (brief reactive psychosis), which is a psychotic response to a severe stressor, usually responds well to low-dose neuroleptic treatment.
- Consider alternatives to antipsychotics in elderly or intellectually disabled patients (see "Nonpharmacologic Therapy").

SUGGESTED READINGS

Available at ExpertConsult.com

RELATED CONTENT

Psychosis (Patient Information)
Delirium (Related Key Topic)

AUTHORS: **Nathan Praschan, MD, MPH,** and **Arnaldo A. Berges, MD**

BASIC INFORMATION

DEFINITION

Acute cardiogenic pulmonary edema (ACPE) is a clinically observed consequence of increased capillary leakage of fluid into the interstitial space in the pulmonary vasculature, resulting in the constellation of clinical signs and symptoms of decreased gaseous exchange in the alveoli.

SYNONYMS

Cardiogenic pulmonary edema (CPE)
Acute cardiogenic pulmonary edema (ACPE)
Acute decompensated heart failure (ADHF) with pulmonary edema
Acute diastolic heart failure with pulmonary edema
Acute systolic heart failure with pulmonary edema
Acute combined heart failure with pulmonary edema

ICD-10CM CODES

J81.0	Acute pulmonary edema
J81.1	Chronic pulmonary edema
I50.1	Left ventricular failure
J68.1	Pulmonary edema due to chemicals, gases, fumes and vapors

EPIDEMIOLOGY & DEMOGRAPHICS

- The prevalence of heart failure (HF) is estimated around 6.5 million people in the United States and about 23 million people globally. In the United States this number is expected to increase to 8 million by the year 2030.
- In 2012, 1.7 million HF-related visits to U.S. physician offices, and half a million emergency department visits were reported.
- Approximately 20% of all-cause admissions in the age group older than 65 was related to HF.
- Within 30 days, 25% to 30% of these patients are readmitted with recurrent ADHF.
- In-hospital mortality rate is 10% to 20%, particularly when associated with acute MI.

CLINICAL PRESENTATION

- Altered mental status
- Dyspnea (exertional or at rest, paroxysmal nocturnal dyspnea, orthopnea)
- Cough and wheezing (cardiac asthma)
- Diaphoresis
- Perioral and peripheral cyanosis
- Pink, frothy sputum

PHYSICAL EXAMINATION FINDINGS

- Hypertension (in cardiogenic shock could be hypotensive)
- Tachycardia
- Elevated jugular venous pressure with hepatojugular reflex
- Bilateral pulmonary rales/decreased or pleural effusions
- S3 gallop/S4 and/or laterally displaced apex
- Abdominal distension/ascites
- Peripheral edema
- Cold and clammy skin
- Weight gain

ETIOLOGY

Common causes of acute pulmonary edema include the following:

- Acute myocardial infarction
- Poor dietary compliance or medication nonadherence
- Atrial and ventricular arrhythmias
- Valvular heart disease (mitral, aortic, tricuspid, and pulmonary valve disease)
- Renal and liver disease
- Endocrine (thyrotoxicosis, obesity, metabolic syndrome, diabetes)
- Toxin mediated (cocaine, alcohol, chemotherapy agents, ephedra)
- Peripartum cardiomyopathy/heart failure of pregnancy
- Infections (myopericarditis, endocarditis, HIV, Chagas)
- Uncontrolled hypertension
- Structural heart disease (ventricular septal defect, infiltrative heart disease, hypertrophic cardiomyopathy)
- Pulmonary embolism
- Postcardioversion syndrome
- Box 1 summarizes common causes of cardiogenic and noncardiogenic pulmonary edema

DIAGNOSIS

DIFFERENTIAL DIAGNOSIS

- Noncardiogenic pulmonary edema (see Fig. E1 and Table 1)

BOX 1 Common Causes of Cardiogenic and Noncardiogenic Pulmonary Edema

Cardiogenic Pulmonary Edema
- Acute exacerbation of heart failure
- Acute valve dysfunction (e.g., mitral valve chordae tendineae rupture)
- Arrhythmia/myocardial infarction
- Hypertensive crisis
- Fluid overload following aggressive volume resuscitation (e.g., postoperative)
- Ventricular septal rupture
- Pericardial tamponade

Noncardiogenic Pulmonary Edema
- Direct lung injury
  - Pneumonia
  - Gastric aspiration
  - Toxic inhalation
  - Negative pressure related (e.g., strangulation)
- Indirect causes of lung injury
  - Sepsis
  - Trauma
  - Pancreatitis
  - Multiple blood transfusions
  - Burn injury

From Vincent JL et al: *Textbook of critical care,* ed 7, Philadelphia, 2017, Elsevier.

- Viral pneumonitis and other pulmonary infections
- Pulmonary embolism
- Exacerbation of asthma/chronic obstructive pulmonary disease
- High altitude pulmonary edema (HAPE)
- Sarcoidosis
- Pulmonary fibrosis
- Lymphangitic carcinomatosis

LABORATORY TESTS

- Arterial blood gases (ABGs): Respiratory and metabolic acidosis, decreased Pa_{O_2}, increased Pa_{CO_2}, low pH. (NOTE: The patient may initially show respiratory alkalosis as a result of hyperventilation in attempts to maintain Pa_{O_2}.)
- BNP and NT-pro BNP add diagnostic value to the history and physical examination as evidenced in the Breathing Not Properly (BNP) study.
- Cardiac biomarkers: Troponin T or I if suspicion for acute coronary syndrome.
- Basic metabolic profile: Assess for electrolyte abnormalities and kidney function.
- Elevated LFTs are indicative of congestive hepatopathy or shock liver.
- Serology for suspected inciting agents, including HIV, Chagas, adenovirus, enterovirus, parvovirus, herpes virus, and more recently the novel Coronavirus disease (COVID-19).
- Complete blood count: Anemia can trigger acute pulmonary edema.
- Glucose, Hb A1C, fasting lipid profile, TSH for risk stratification.
- Urinalysis and urine toxicology if indicated.

IMAGING STUDIES

NONINVASIVE IMAGING:

- ECG: May elucidate the etiology of pulmonary edema. Causes may include ischemia/infarct, arrhythmias, LV hypertrophy, and atrial enlargement.
- Chest x-ray (Fig. 2):
  1. Bilateral interstitial and alveolar infiltrates
  2. Cephalization of the pulmonary vessels
  3. Kerley B lines; fluffy perihilar infiltrates
  4. Pleural effusions
  5. Enlarged cardiac silhouette
- Echocardiogram:
  1. Assess left and right ventricular systolic/diastolic function.
  2. Structural abnormalities (VSD, LV rupture).
  3. Evaluate valvular abnormalities including endocarditis.
  4. Engorged inferior vena cava (IVC) and IVC plethora, based on bedside ultrasound, suggests elevated filling pressures.
- Computed tomography of the chest; may differentiate between cardiogenic and noncardiogenic pulmonary edema.
- Lung ultrasound has emerged as a tool to diagnose pulmonary edema. It is easy to use, accessible, and noninvasive, and has a high accuracy. Kerley B lines and pleural effusions are suggestive of pulmonary edema.

TABLE 1 Distinguishing Cardiogenic and Noncardiogenic Pulmonary Edema

	History	Exam	Labs	Imaging	Pulmonary Artery Catheter
Cardiogenic	Heart disease Renal disease Uncontrolled HTN Edema Orthopnea Recent administration of IV fluids or blood products	Heart failure exam findings: Distended neck veins S3 heart sound Dependent edema Elevated blood pressure Cool extremities	↑BNP >1200 pg/ml ↑Creatinine (in setting of volume overload) ↑Troponin	CXR: CMG Pleural effusions Kerley B lines TEE: ↓LVEF Diastolic filling defect Severe mitral or aortic valvular disease Pericardial effusion with tamponade VSD	PCWP >18 mm Hg Prominent V-waves (mitral regurgitation) Elevation and equilibration of right atrial pressure, pulmonary artery diastolic and PCWP (tamponade physiology) CVP >12 mm Hg
Noncardiogenic	Sepsis Aspiration event Trauma (long bone fractures) Burn injury Pancreatitis Multiple transfusions	Signs of active infection Extensive burn injury Evidence of trauma (absence of heart failure exam findings)	↑WBC BNP <200 pg/ml	CXR: Diffuse central and peripheral infiltrates Normal heart size No or minimal pleural effusions TEE: Normal LV and valvular function No evidence of volume overload	PCWP <18 mm Hg CVP <12 mm Hg

BNP, Brain natriuretic peptide; *CVP,* central venous pressure; *CXR,* chest x-ray; *HTN,* hypertension; *IV,* intravenous; *LVEF,* left ventricle ejection fraction; *PCWP,* pulmonary capillary wedge pressure; *S3,* third heart sound; *TEE,* transesophageal echocardiogram; *VSD,* ventricular septal defect; *WBC,* white blood count.
From Vincent JL et al: *Textbook of critical care,* ed 7, Philadelphia, 2017, Elsevier.

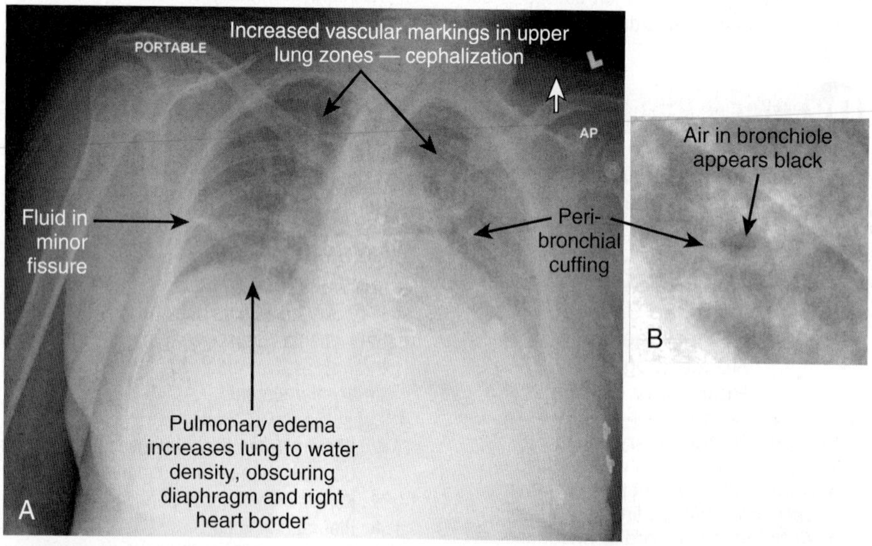

FIG. 2 Pulmonary edema. A, Anterior-posterior chest x-ray. **B,** Close-up from **A.** This 53-yr-old female with end-stage renal disease missed dialysis and presented to the emergency department. Her examination demonstrated bilateral rales. Her x-ray shows mild cardiomegaly, bilateral interstitial opacities, and cephalization of the pulmonary vascular markings. The minor fissure appears thickened. These findings are consistent with pulmonary edema. In addition, peribronchial cuffing is present. As discussed elsewhere, this is a nonspecific thickening of the bronchial wall that can occur from edema in the setting of heart failure, asthma, viral illness, or even infections such as pertussis. The thickened wall appears white, whereas the air-filled bronchiole appears black and has a circular short-axis cross section. (From Broder JS: *Diagnostic imaging for the emergency physician,* Philadelphia, 2011, Saunders.)

INVASIVE IMAGING:

- Right heart catheterization (RHC): Obtain estimated filling pressures, assess cardiac output, differentiate between different shocks, and used to guide tailored inotropic and pressor therapy. Despite the widespread availability of Swan-Ganz catheters the ESCAPE trial failed to demonstrate the utility of pulmonary artery catheters in acute decompensated heart failure.
- Coronary angiogram: Rule out acute MI/progressive coronary artery disease.
- Left heart catheterization (LHC): Measure left ventricular end-diastolic pressure (LVEDP) to estimate left-sided filling pressure.
- CardioMEMS (St. Jude Medical) is an invasive pulmonary artery pressure monitoring device that can provide remote monitoring capability and aid in reduction of frequency of heart failure hospitalizations.

Rx TREATMENT

ACUTE GENERAL Rx (FIG. 3)

Nonpharmacologic treatment:

- Heart failure teaching.
- Sodium restriction in ACC/AHA class C and D heart failure patients has conflicting data.
- Restrict 1.5 to 2 L of free water in the setting of hyponatremia.
- Risk factor modification (BP and glucose control, dietary modifications).
- Oxygen supplementation if signs of hypoxia are present.
- Noninvasive ventilation (continuous positive airway pressure [CPAP]) or bilevel noninvasive positive-pressure ventilation [NPPV]) reduces dyspnea and may reduce the need for endotracheal intubation. Positive pressure ventilation (invasive or noninvasive) decreases preload and afterload and reduces the work of breathing, while positive end expiratory pressure improves oxygenation.

Pharmacologic treatment

- Loop diuretics such as furosemide, torsemide, bumetanide, and ethacrynic acid are the cornerstones of the treatment of volume overload. Intravenous treatment might be required in acute pulmonary edema due to coexistent gut edema that is a barrier to effective gastrointestinal absorption. There is no difference in symptoms or kidney function whether the diuretic is given as a bolus versus continuous infusion (DOSE trial; *New England Journal of Medicine,* March 3, 2011).
- Nitrates: Particularly useful if the patient has concomitant chest pain or is hypertensive.

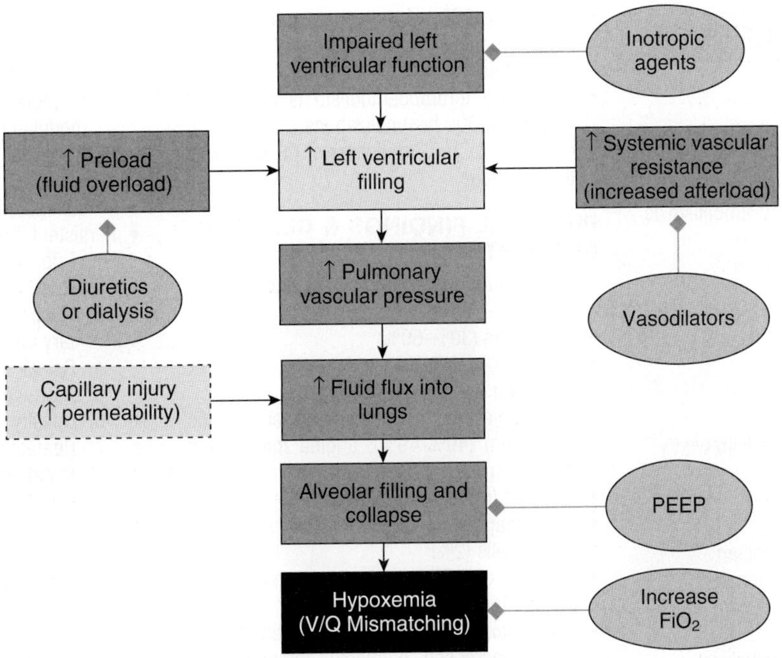

FIG. 3 Acute management of pulmonary edema. This schematic represents basic mechanisms distinguishing cardiogenic and noncardiogenic pulmonary edema and the contributing factors *(blue boxes)* that ultimately lead to impaired gas exchange *(black box)*. The *green circles* represent treatments that are available in the intensive care unit setting to reduce pulmonary edema or to mitigate its adverse consequences. *FiO2*, Fraction of inspired oxygen; *PEEP*, post end-expiratory pressure; *V/Q*, ventilation/perfusion. (From Vincent JL et al: *Textbook of critical care*, ed 7, Philadelphia, 2017, Elsevier.)

1. Nitroglycerin: 0.4 to 0.8 mg SL or nitroglycerin spray may be given immediately on arrival and repeated every 5 min up to three times if the patient remains symptomatic and blood pressure remains stable.
2. 2% nitroglycerin ointment: 1 to 3 inches out of the tube applied continuously; absorption may be erratic.
3. IV nitroglycerin for refractory chest pain or and hypertension: Start at 0.2 to 0.4 mcg/kg/min.

- Nitroprusside is useful for afterload reduction in severe hypertension, acute mitral regurgitation, or acute aortic regurgitation.
  1. Start at low-dose 0.5 μg/kg/min with an arterial line in place.
  2. Monitor for cyanide toxicity.
- ACE inhibitors, angiotensin II receptor blockers, aldosterone antagonist, and angiotensin receptor–neprilysin inhibitors are vasodilators with long-term mortality benefit in patients with heart failure with reduced ejection fraction.
- In patients with heart failure with reduced ejection fraction, with and without type 2 diabetes, SGLT2 inhibitors decrease frequency of hospitalization for HF, an urgent visit resulting in intravenous therapy for HF, or death from cardiovascular causes (EMPA-REG OUTCOME, DAPA HF trial). They can be initiated before discharge during acute hospitalizations for ADHF.
- Ultrafiltration/aquapheresis if diuretic resistant.

Pharmacologic-vasopressors:
- Patients with profound hypotension benefit from vasopressors.
  1. Norepinephrine: Powerful vasoconstrictor with small inotropic effect.
  2. Dopamine: Low doses (0.5-3 μg/kg/min) increase blood flow to coronary, renal, and cerebral beds. Intermediate doses (3-10 μg/kg/min) increase cardiac contractility while high doses (10-20 μg/kg/min) have a pressor effect.

Pharmacologic-inotropes:
- Dobutamine: Potent inotrope, mild chronotropic effects. Dose ranges from 2.5 to 20 mcg/kg/min.
- Phosphodiesterase inhibitors (amrinone, milrinone, and enoximone [not available in U.S.]) may be useful in refractory cases.

Mechanical support:
- Intra-aortic balloon pump (IABP): Decreases afterload, increases coronary blood flow.
- Impella: Axial-flow pump on a pigtail catheter that crosses the aortic valve and unloads the left ventricle.
- Tandem heart device: Oxygenated blood is pumped from the left atrium into the femoral artery. It can provide 3.5 to 4.5 L/min of cardiac output.
- Extracorporeal membrane oxygenation (ECMO) as a bridge to heart transplant or recovery.
- Durable mechanical circulatory support such as left ventricular assist device can be considered for those in cardiogenic shock refractory to medical therapy.

DISPOSITION

Admit to ICU/CCU if:
- Need for intubation
- Signs and symptoms of hypoperfusion
- SpO_2 <90% despite supplemental oxygen
- Use of accessory muscles/RR >25/min
- Heart rate <40 or >130, SBP <90

PEARLS & CONSIDERATIONS

COMMENTS

Accumulated evidence still favors the use of noninvasive ventilation, especially CPAP, in patients with ACPE, especially as this therapy reduces dyspnea and helps correct metabolic abnormalities more rapidly than standard oxygen therapy. The role of morphine in the treatment of ACPE has come into question.

SUGGESTED READINGS

Available at ExpertConsult.com

RELATED CONTENT

Heart Failure (Related Key Topic)

AUTHORS: **Gemini Yesodharan, MD,** and **Maxwell Eyram Afari, MD**

BASIC INFORMATION

DEFINITION

Pulmonary embolism (PE) refers to the lodging of a thrombus or other embolic material from a distant site in the pulmonary circulation. A classification of acute pulmonary embolism is described in Table 1.

SYNONYMS

Pulmonary thromboembolism
PE

ICD-10CM CODES

I26	Pulmonary embolism
I26.01	Septic pulmonary embolism with acute cor pulmonale
I26.09	Other pulmonary embolism with acute cor pulmonale
I26.90	Septic pulmonary embolism without acute cor pulmonale
I26.99	Other pulmonary embolism without acute cor pulmonale
I27.82	Chronic pulmonary embolism
Z86.711	Personal history of pulmonary embolism

EPIDEMIOLOGY & DEMOGRAPHICS

- Approximately 650,000 cases of PE occur in the U.S. each year (increased incidence in women and with advanced age); annually, as many as 100,000 people in the U.S. die from acute PE, and the diagnosis is often not made until after autopsy. The incidence of PE is increasing with the increasing use of spiral CT scans, with a lower severity of illness and lower mortality, suggesting that the increase is the result of earlier diagnosis.
- More than 90% of pulmonary emboli originate in the deep venous system of the lower extremities.
- Pulmonary thromboembolism is associated with >200,000 hospitalizations.
- Up to 8% to 10% of victims of PE die within the first hour.

PHYSICAL FINDINGS & CLINICAL PRESENTATION

- Most common symptom: Dyspnea (82%-85%)
- Tachypnea (30%-60%)
- Cough (30%-40%)
- Wheezing (20%)
- Chest pain: May be nonpleuritic or pleuritic (infarction) (40%-49%); angina may reflect right ventricle (RV) ischemia
- Syncope (massive PE) (10%-14%)
- Fever, diaphoresis, apprehension
- Hemoptysis (2%)
- Evidence of DVT may be present (e.g., swelling and tenderness of extremities)
- Cardiac examination may reveal: Tachycardia (23%), increased pulmonic component of S2, murmur of tricuspid insufficiency, right ventricular heave, right-sided S3
- Pulmonary examination: May demonstrate rales, localized wheezing, friction rub

ETIOLOGY

- Thrombus, fat, air, tumor, or other foreign material
- Major transient risk factors for PE:
  1. Postoperative state, major surgery including hip or knee replacement
  2. Trauma to lower extremities, immobilizer, or cast
  3. Prolonged immobilization, reduced mobility
  4. Central venous catheter
  5. Pregnancy and early puerperium
- Minor transient risk factors for PE:
  1. Estrogen-containing birth control pills, hormone replacement therapy, estrogen-modulators (e.g., raloxifene, tamoxifen)
  2. Prolonged air travel
  3. Acute medical illness (e.g., infection, disseminated intravascular coagulation)
- Persistent risk factors for PE:
  1. Prior history of DVT or PE
  2. Heart failure
  3. Visceral cancer (lung, pancreas, alimentary and genitourinary tracts)
  4. Spinal cord injury
  5. Advanced age
  6. Obesity
  7. Hematologic disease (e.g., factor V Leiden mutation, antithrombin III deficiency, protein C deficiency, protein S deficiency, lupus anticoagulant, polycythemia vera, dysfibrinogenemia, paroxysmal nocturnal hemoglobinuria, acquired protein C resistance without factor V Leiden, G20210A prothrombin mutation)
  8. Chronic obstructive pulmonary disease (COPD)
  9. Diabetes mellitus
  10. Autoimmune diseases (Systemic lupus erythematosus, inflammatory bowel disease, rheumatoid arthritis)

DIAGNOSIS

DIFFERENTIAL DIAGNOSIS

- Myocardial infarction
- Pericarditis
- Pneumonia
- Pneumothorax
- Chest wall pain
- GI abnormalities (e.g., peptic ulcer, esophageal rupture, gastritis)
- Heart failure
- Pleuritis
- Anxiety disorder with hyperventilation
- Pericardial tamponade
- Dissection of aorta
- Asthma or COPD exacerbation
- Chronic thromboembolic pulmonary hypertension (CTEPH)

WORKUP

- Guidelines from the Clinical Guidelines Committee of the American College of Physicians for the Evaluation of Patients with Suspected Acute Pulmonary Embolism recommend the following:[1]
  1. Use of validated clinical prediction rules to estimate pretest probability in patients in whom acute PE is being considered.
  2. Not obtaining a D-dimer measurement or imaging studies in patients with

TABLE 1 Classification of Acute Pulmonary Embolism

Category (Frequency)	Presentation	Therapy
Massive PE (5%-10%)	Systolic blood pressure <90 mm Hg or drop ≥40 mm Hg or poor tissue perfusion or multisystem organ failure plus extensive thrombosis, such as "saddle" PE or right or left main pulmonary artery thrombus	Anticoagulation (usually with high-dose intravenous UFH), plus advanced therapy: Systemic thrombolysis, pharmacomechanical catheter–directed therapy, surgical embolectomy, and/or inferior vena cava (IVC) filter.
Submassive PE, high risk (15%)	Hemodynamically stable but moderate or severe RV dysfunction or enlargement, coupled with biomarker elevation indicative of RV microinfarction and/or RV pressure overload	Anticoagulation until decision made regarding implementation of advanced therapy; controversy centers on this group. For systemic thrombolysis, reducing the rate of cardiovascular collapse and death must be balanced against the increased rate of hemorrhagic stroke.
Submassive PE, low risk (5%-10%)	Hemodynamically stable with RV dysfunction or biomarker elevation, but not both	Anticoagulation followed by "watch and wait." Implement advanced therapy if there is clinical deterioration.
Small to moderate PE (70%)	Normal hemodynamics and normal RV size and function	Anticoagulation and consider brief hospital stay or entirely outpatient therapy.

PE, Pulmonary embolism; *RV*, right ventricular; *UFH*, unfractionated heparin.
From Zipes DP: *Braunwald's heart disease, a textbook of cardiovascular medicine*, ed 11, Philadelphia, 2019, Elsevier.

[1] Raja AS et al: Evaluation of patients with suspected acute pulmonary embolism: best practice advice from the Clinical Guidelines Committee of the American College of Physicians, *Ann Intern Med* 163:701-711, 2015.

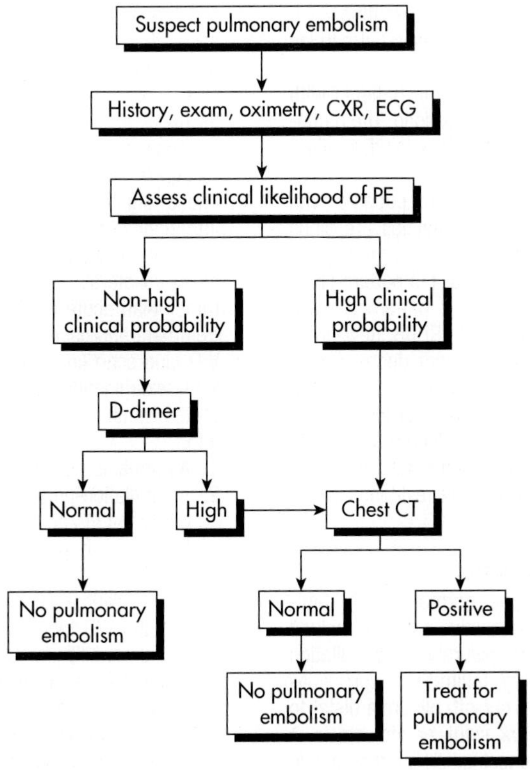

FIG. 1 Integrated diagnostic approach. *CT,* Computed tomography; *CXR,* chest x-ray [examination]; *ECG,* electrocardiogram; *PE,* pulmonary embolism. (From Zipes DP: *Braunwald's heart disease, a textbook of cardiovascular medicine,* ed 11, Philadelphia, 2019, Elsevier.)

TABLE 2 Wells Score for Pulmonary Embolism*

Characteristic	Points
Risk Factors	
Previous pulmonary embolism or deep venous thrombosis	1.5
Immobilization or surgery in the previous 4 wk	1.5
Cancer	1
Clinical Findings	
Hemoptysis	1
Heart rate >100/min	1.5
Clinical signs of deep venous thrombosis	3
Other	
Alternative diagnosis is less likely than pulmonary embolism	3

Interpretation of total score: 0-1 point, low probability; 2-6 points, moderate probability; 7 or more points, high probability.

*Wells PS et al: Derivation of a simple clinical model to categorize patients probability of pulmonary embolism: increasing the models utility with the SimpliRED d-dimer, *Thromb Haemost* 83:416-420, 2000.

From McGee S: *Evidence-based physical diagnosis,* ed 4, Philadelphia, 2018, Elsevier.

TABLE 3 Revised Geneva Score for Pulmonary Embolism*

Characteristic	Points
Risk Factors	
Age >65 yr	1
Previous pulmonary embolism or deep venous thrombosis	3
Surgery (under general anesthesia) or fracture (of lower limbs) within 1 mo	2
Cancer (active or considered cured <1 yr)	2
Clinical Findings	
Unilateral leg pain	3
Hemoptysis	2
Heart Rate	
75-94 beats/min	3
≥95 beats/min	5
Pain on palpation of lower-limb deep veins and unilateral edema	4

Interpretation of total score: 0-3 points, low probability; 4-10 points, moderate probability; ≥11 points, high probability.

*Le Gal G et al: Prediction of pulmonary embolism in the emergency department: the revised Geneva score, *Ann Intern Med* 144:165-171, 2006.

From McGee S: *Evidence-based physical diagnosis,* ed 4, Philadelphia, 2018, Elsevier.

low pretest probability of PE and who meet all pulmonary embolism rule-out criteria.

3. Obtaining a high-sensitivity D-dimer measurement as the initial diagnostic test in patients who have an intermediate pretest probability of PE or in patients with low pretest probability of PE who do not meet all pulmonary embolism rule-out criteria. Clinicians should not use imaging studies as the initial test in patients who have a low or intermediate pretest probability of PE.
4. Use of age-adjusted D-dimer thresholds (age × 10 ng/ml rather than a generic 500 ng/ml) in patients older than 50 yr to determine whether imaging is warranted.
5. Clinicians should not obtain any imaging studies in patients with a D-dimer level below the age-adjusted cutoff.
6. CT pulmonary angiography (CTPA) should be obtained in patients with high pretest probability of PE. Ventilation-perfusion scans should be reserved for patients who have a contraindication to CTPA or if CTPA is not available.
7. A D-dimer measurement should not be obtained in patients with a high pretest probability of PE.

- Clinical assessment alone is insufficient to diagnose or rule out PE. It is also important to remember that no single noninvasive test has both high sensitivity and high specificity for PE. Consequently, in addition to clinical assessment, most patients require an imaging test to diagnose PE. An integrated diagnostic approach to PE is illustrated in Fig. 1. The Wells prediction rules (Table 2) and the revised Geneva score (Table 3) can be used to estimate the probability of PE. In the Wells prediction rules, each of the following findings is assigned a score:
  1. Clinical signs/symptoms of deep vein thrombosis (score = 3.0).
  2. No alternate diagnosis as likely or more likely than PE (score = 3.0).
  3. Heart rate >100/min (score = 1.5).
  4. Immobilization or surgery in last 4 wk (score = 1.5).
  5. Previous history of DVT or PE (score = 1.5).
  6. Hemoptysis (score = 1.0).
  7. Cancer actively treated within last 6 mo (score = 1.0).
- The probability of PE is high if total score is >6, moderate if 2 to 6, and low if <2.
- The modified Wells score divides PE as likely (>4 points) or unlikely (<4 points).
- A low clinical probability of PE in association with a normal plasma D-dimer measurement essentially rules out PE, and further imaging is not needed. If clinical probability is intermediate or high, and/or the D-dimer measurement is abnormal, further workup with imaging is needed.
- The YEARS algorithm is a risk-adjusted D-dimer tool to rule out DVT that allows a threshold of 1000 ng/ml in patients without signs of DVT, no hemoptysis, and in whom PE is considered not to be the most likely diagnosis.
- CT pulmonary angiography (CTPA) (Fig. E2) is an excellent diagnostic modality (83% sensitivity and 96% specificity).
- V/Q scan is reserved for patients with clinically significant contrast allergies or renal insufficiency, or when CTPA is not available.
- Pulmonary angiogram (gold standard) can confirm the diagnosis in equivocal cases, but is rarely used.

- Serial compressive duplex ultrasonography of lower extremities can be used in patients with "low-probability" V/Q scans and high clinical suspicion (see "Imaging Studies"). It is useful if positive; negative results do not exclude PE.

LABORATORY TESTS

- ABGs may reveal hypoxemia and respiratory alkalosis (decreased Pa_{O_2} and Pa_{CO_2} and increased pH); normal results do not rule out PE.
- Alveolar-arteriolar (A-a) oxygen gradient, a measure of the difference in oxygen concentration between alveoli and arterial blood, may be elevated. However, a normal A-a gradient does not rule out PE.
- High-sensitivity plasma D-dimer measurement: D-dimer assays by ELISA detect the presence of plasmin-mediated degradation products of fibrin that contain cross-linked D fragments in the whole blood or plasma. A normal plasma D-dimer level is useful to exclude PE in patients with a low pretest probability of PE. However, it cannot be used to "rule in" the diagnosis because it increases with many other disorders (e.g., metastatic cancer, trauma, sepsis, postoperative state). Plasma D-dimer can also be used in conjunction with lower-extremity compression ultrasonography in patients with indeterminate V/Q and spiral CT scans. Absence of DVT and presence of a normal D-dimer level in these settings generally rule out clinically significant PE.
- Elevated cardiac troponin levels also occur in patients with PE because of right ventricular dilation and myocardial injury; therefore, PE should be considered in the differential diagnosis of all patients presenting with chest pain or dyspnea and elevated cardiac troponin levels.
- Elevated serum BNP levels in patients with acute PE may reflect RV overload. The pathophysiology of RV dysfunction in PE is illustrated in Fig. 3.
- ECG is abnormal in 85% of patients with acute PE. Frequent abnormalities are sinus tachycardia; nonspecific ST-segment or T-wave changes; S-1, Q-3, T-3 pattern (10% of patients); S-1, S-2, S-3 pattern; T-wave inversion in V_1 to V_6; acute RBBB; new-onset atrial fibrillation; ST segment depression in lead II; RV strain. A RV strain pattern on ECG in patients with PE and normal blood pressure is associated with adverse short-term outcome and adds incremental prognostic value to echocardiographic evidence of RV function.

IMAGING STUDIES

- Chest x-ray can be normal but is typically abnormal; suggestive findings include elevated diaphragm, pleural effusion, dilation of pulmonary artery, infiltrate or consolidation, abrupt vessel cut-off, oligemia distal to the PE *(Westermark sign),* or atelectasis. A wedge-shaped consolidation in the middle and lower lobes is suggestive of a pulmonary infarction and is known as *Hampton hump.*
- CT pulmonary angiography (CTPA) is an accurate, noninvasive tool in the diagnosis of PE at the main, lobar, and segmental pulmonary artery levels. A major advantage of CTPA over standard pulmonary angiography is its ability to diagnose intrathoracic disease other than PE that may account for the patient's clinical picture. It is also less invasive, less costly, and more widely available. Its major shortcoming is its poor sensitivity for subsegmental emboli. It is important to recognize signs of chronic clot on CT scan. These signs include eccentric thrombus, intraluminal webs/bands, mosaic attenuation of lung fields, and presence of bronchial artery collaterals, which may suggest chronic rather than acute PE, warranting a different treatment approach.
- V/Q lung scan (in patient with normal chest x-ray examination): This test must be interpreted within the pretest probability of having a PE.
  1. A normal lung scan rules out PE.
  2. A ventilation-perfusion mismatch is suggestive of PE, and a lung scan interpretation of high probability is confirmatory (Fig. E4).
  3. If the clinical suspicion of PE is high and the V/Q lung scan is interpreted as low probability, moderate probability, or indeterminate, a pulmonary angiogram is diagnostic. A positive angiogram confirms diagnosis. A positive compressive duplex ultrasonography for DVT obviates the need for an angiogram, because treatment with anticoagulants is indicated in these patients. The overall sensitivity of compressive ultrasonography for DVT in patients with PE is 29% with a specificity of 97%. Adding ultrasonography in patients with a nondiagnostic lung scan

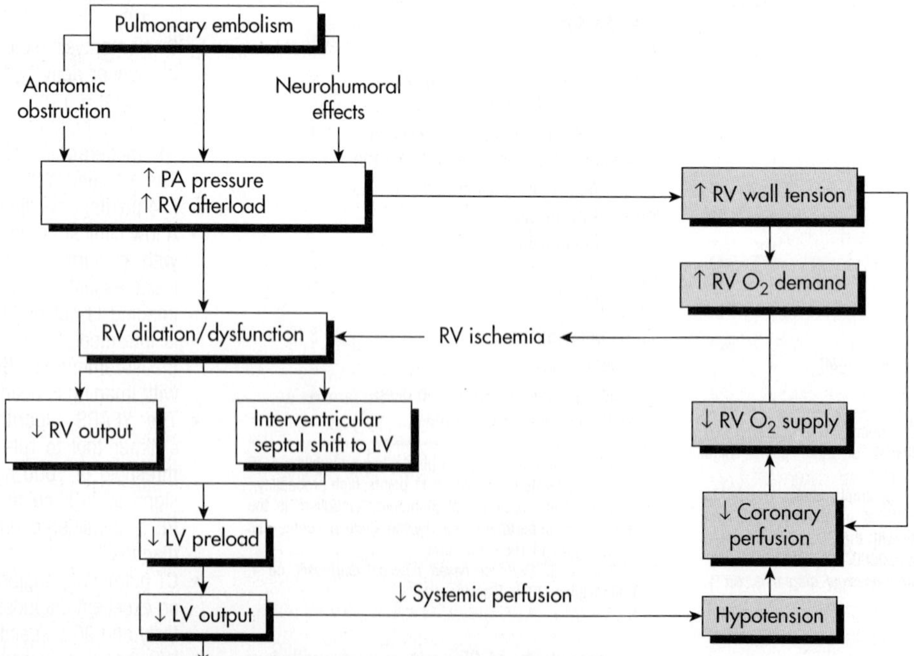

FIG. 3 Pathophysiology of right ventricular dysfunction and its deleterious effects of causing decreased systemic arterial pressure, decreased coronary perfusion, and deteriorating ventricular function. *LV,* Left ventricle/ventricular; *PA,* pulmonary artery; *RV,* right ventricle/ventricular. (From Zipes DP: *Braunwald's heart disease, a textbook of cardiovascular medicine,* ed 11, Philadelphia, 2019, Elsevier.)

prevents 9% of angiographies; however, this improvement in efficacy is achieved at the cost of unnecessary anticoagulant therapy in 26% of patients who have false-positive ultrasonography results.

- Pulmonary angiography is the historic gold standard; however, it is invasive, expensive, and not readily available in some clinical settings. False-positive pulmonary angiograms may result from mediastinal disorders such as radiation fibrosis and tumors.
- Echocardiography is useful for identifying patients with PE who are high risk for poor outcomes. Moderate or severe RV hypokinesis, persistent pulmonary hypertension, patent foramen ovale, and free-floating right heart thrombus are markers of increased risk of death or recurrent thrombosis. RV pressure overload may be inferred from a RV:LV ratio ≥1.0 and predicts higher rates of in-hospital death or clinical deterioration. McConnell's sign, akinesia of mid-free wall with normal motion at apex, is 77% sensitive and 94% specific for acute PE.
- Gadolinium-enhanced magnetic resonance angiography (MRA/MRV) of the pulmonary arteries has a moderate sensitivity and high specificity for the diagnosis of PE at experienced centers, but obtaining acceptable images is technically challenging and should only be performed if other imaging tests are contraindicated.

Rx TREATMENT

NONPHARMACOLOGIC THERAPY

Correction of risk factors (see "Etiology") to prevent future PE.

ACUTE GENERAL Rx

Patients with acute PE should be initially stratified according to risk (see Table 1) so that higher-risk therapies (e.g., thrombolysis, embolectomy) are offered to patients with the greatest chance of benefit. Many tertiary and quaternary care centers deploy a multidisciplinary Pulmonary Embolism Response Team (PERT) to determine the optimal course of treatment for patients with intermediate and high risk PE, given the highly variable mortality risk in the intermediate risk group.

Anticoagulation is recommended as initial therapy in all patients with small to moderate PE without a contraindication.

- For patients with low risk or intermediate-low risk PE, anticoagulation can be initiated right away with the direct oral anticoagulant (DOAC) rivaroxaban or apixaban; subcutaneous low–molecular-weight heparin (LMWH) or fondaparinux; or IV Unfractionated heparin (UFH). When oral anticoagulation is initiated, a DOAC is recommended over a vitamin K antagonist.
  1. Oral rivaroxaban, a factor Xa inhibitor (15 mg bid for 3 wk, then 20 mg/d), has been studied as a treatment for DVT and PE, without prior parenteral therapy. For both DVT and PE, treatment with rivaroxaban alone was noninferior to treatment with LMWH followed by a vitamin K antagonist with regard to the endpoint of recurrent venous thromboembolism. Use of rivaroxaban should be avoided in patients with severe renal failure.
  2. Apixaban, a factor Xa inhibitor (10 mg bid for a week, followed by 5 mg bid), is approved for the treatment of acute PE based on the data in the AMPLIFY and AMPLIFY-EXT trials, in which apixaban met its noninferiority mark in terms of efficacy and improved safety compared to warfarin.
  3. Dabigatran, a direct thrombin inhibitor (150 mg bid following 5-10 days of parenteral anticoagulation), is approved for treatment of DVT and PE in patients with CrCl >30 mL/min based on data in the RE-COVER and RE-COVER II trials where it was non-inferior to warfarin.
  4. Edoxaban, a factor Xa inhibitor (60 mg daily, or 30 mg daily if CrCl 15-50 ml/min or body weight ≤60 kg or if on certain P-glycoprotein inhibitors, following 5-10 days of parenteral anticoagulation) is approved for treatment of DVT and PE based on the Hokusai VTE trial where it was noninferior to warfarin.
  5. UFH, subcutaneous LMWH, or subcutaneous fondaparinux can be used for initial treatment for at least 5 days when used with warfarin, dabigatran, or edoxaban. If IV unfractionated heparin is used, a bolus dose (80 U/kg) followed by a weight-based (18 U/kg/hr) continuous infusion to achieve therapeutic anti-factor Xa (or aPTT) levels should be used. LMWH and fondaparinux should be avoided in patients with severe renal failure.
- For patients with intermediate-high risk or high risk PE, anticoagulation with LMWH or IV UFH (if LMWH is contraindicated due to renal failure or bleeding concerns) is recommended and can be transitioned to an oral agent prior to hospital discharge.
- For patients with contraindications to anticoagulation, consider placement of a *temporary* inferior vena cava (IVC) filter and frequent reassessment of safety for initiation of anticoagulation as soon as possible.
- For patients with intermediate-high risk PE (demonstrating RV strain by imaging and myocardial injury with positive biomarkers), attempts should be made to risk stratify individual patients as this cohort may have multiple therapeutic options including anticoagulation alone, catheter-directed therapies, or systemic thrombolysis at a reduced dose. In high volume centers, the distinction between treatment strategies in this group may occur via a multidisciplinary PERT team, often consisting of pulmonary and critical care, cardiology, hematology, and interventional radiology specialists.
- For patients with massive or high risk PE without contraindications to thrombolytics (Box 1), thrombolytic agents (urokinase, tPA, streptokinase) provide rapid resolution of clots with some increased risk of major bleeding (up to 3% incidence of intracranial hemorrhage with systemic thrombolytic administration). The standard dosing for systemic thrombolytic is 100 mg of alteplase (synthetic tPA), administered over 2 hr.

BOX 1 Contraindications to systemic thrombolysis

Absolute contraindication to systemic thrombolytics tPA:
(Prior intracranial hemorrhage, known structural intracranial cerebrovascular disease, known malignant intracranial neoplasm, ischemic CVA within 3 mo, suspected aortic dissection, active bleeding, recent surgery encroaching on spinal canal or brain, recent significant closed head or facial trauma)
Relative contraindication to systemic thrombolytics
(Age >75, current use of anticoagulation, pregnancy, noncompressible vascular punctures, CPR >10 min, recent internal bleeding, dementia, remote history of CVA [<3 mo], major surgery within 3 wk)

Modified from Parrillo JE, Dellinger RP: *Critical care medicine, principles of diagnosis and management in the adult,* ed 5, Philadelphia, 2019, Elsevier.

- In high risk patients with absolute contraindications to thrombolytics, catheter-directed thrombectomy or surgical embolectomy should be considered at centers with the appropriate level of expertise. Finally, in high risk PE patients in refractory shock or with cardiac arrest, additional mechanical support, such as extracorporeal membrane oxygenation (ECMO), may serve as a bridge to advanced therapies or recovery. Fig. 5 describes treatment of submassive pulmonary embolism. Fig. 6 illustrates the approach to high risk or massive pulmonary embolus.
- Long-term treatment for PE not associated with malignancy can be carried out with a DOAC, LMWH, or warfarin.
- For PE associated with malignancy, DOACs or LMWH are recommended for long-term therapy.
- If thrombolytics and anticoagulants are contraindicated (e.g., GI bleeding, recent CNS surgery, recent trauma) or if the patient continues to have recurrent PE despite anticoagulation therapy, an IVC filter is recommended.
- In older adults, IVC filters are associated with higher 30-day and 1-yr mortality (11.6% and 20.5%, respectively, versus 9.3% and 13.4% in those who do not); however, these patients tended to be sicker. An IVC filter is not advised for patients with recurrent venous thromboembolism, unless risk for cardiopulmonary deterioration outweighs risk for IVC filter replacement.[2]
- For PE occurring in the setting of pregnancy, LMWH is the treatment of choice. Dosing is based on early pregnancy weight. Planned

[2] Kaufman JA et al: Society of International Radiology Clinical Practice Guidelines for Inferior Vena Cava Filters in the Treatment of Patients with Venous Thromboembolic Disease, *J Vasc Interv Radiol* 31:1529, 2020.

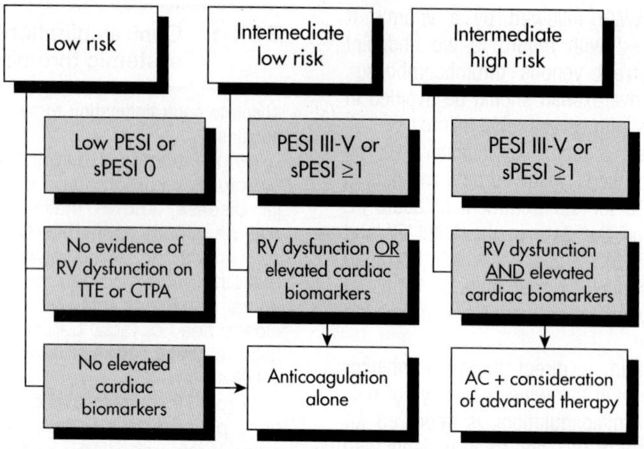

FIG. 5 Acute PE management in non-high-risk patients (SBP >90 mm Hg and no cardiac arrest). Submassive pulmonary embolism algorithm. *SBP,* Systolic blood pressure; *CTPA,* computed tomography pulmonary angiography; *PESI,* Pulmonary Embolism Severity Index; *sPESI,* simplified Pulmonary Embolism Severity Index; *RV,* right ventricular; *TTE,* transthoracic echocardiogram; *AC,* anticoagulation.

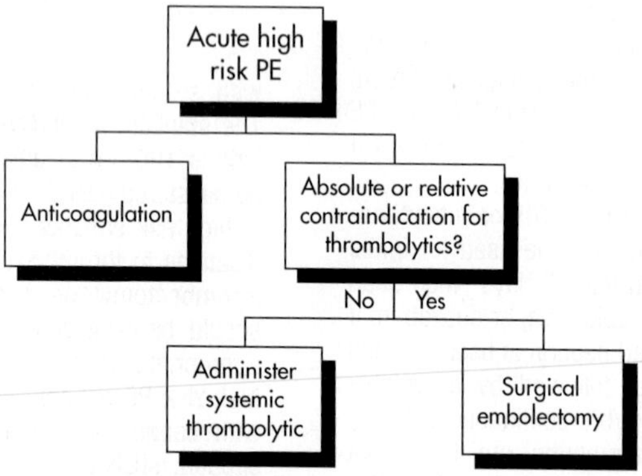

FIG. 6 Acute PE management in massive or high-risk patients (SBP <90 mm Hg or cardiac arrest). *PE,* Pulmonary embolism.

delivery should be strongly considered to avoid complications with anticoagulation and spinal anesthesia. For a patient with a recent PE, LMWH should be switched to UFH approximately 36 hr prior to planned delivery and the drip should be stopped 4 to 6 hr prior to delivery, with a normal partial thromboplastin time (PTT) at the time of spinal anesthesia initiation. LMWH should be restarted as soon as it is deemed safe by the obstetrician. Duration of anticoagulation should be at least 3 mo total with at least 6 wk of anticoagulation after delivery. Breastfeeding mothers can be prescribed either LMWH or warfarin. Thrombolytic therapy should only be used for life-threatening PE during pregnancy due to the high risk of peri-partum and post-partum bleeding.

CHRONIC Rx

- Elimination of risk factors (see "Etiology").
- Duration of anticoagulation:
  1. Patients with PE occurring in the setting of a minor transient risk factor should complete at least 6 mo of therapeutic anticoagulation. If bleeding risk is low and patient is tolerating therapy well, consider low dose extended DOAC (apixaban 2.5 mg PO bid or rivaroxaban 10 mg daily) indefinitely.
  2. Patients with PE occurring in the setting of persistent risk factors such as hematologic thrombotic disorders, antiphospholipid syndrome, and ongoing active malignancy, therapeutic anticoagulation should continue during the presence of the persistent risk factor.
  3. For unprovoked PE, lifelong anticoagulation should be considered, as long as bleeding risk is low. If bleeding risk is moderate or high after a single unprovoked PE, stopping anticoagulation can be considered. Indefinite long-term anticoagulation should be used in patients with recurrent unprovoked PE.
  4. Recurrence risk calculators help inform the risk/benefit discussion with patients interested in avoiding indefinite anticoagulation. Such calculators include the modified Vienna prediction model, the HERDOO-2 score, the DASH model, and the Louzada score.
- Patients with unprovoked DVT/PE have a high rate of recurrent VTE. Longer durations of chronic anticoagulation after unprovoked DVT/PE result in lower rates of recurrent DVT/PE while on anticoagulation, but benefits are lost once anticoagulation is halted. The use of indefinite anticoagulation in select individuals with apparently unprovoked DVT/PE must be weighed against ongoing bleeding risk and other factors.
- Aspirin (100 mg daily) is superior to placebo in preventing recurrence of venous thromboembolism (VTE) in patients with a first-ever unprovoked VTE who had completed 6 to 18 mo of oral anticoagulation. This suggests that aspirin could be offered as an alternative to oral anticoagulants for prevention of recurrent VTE in patients who refuse to or cannot continue oral anticoagulant therapy but who have a high risk of recurrent VTE.

DISPOSITION

- Mortality can be reduced to <10% by rapid and effective treatment. Stratification of risk of death associated with PE and severity-adjusted treatment is described in Table 4. Indicators of poor prognosis include hemodynamic instability/hypotension, signs of RV dysfunction, elevated BNP, elevated troponin, thrombus burden, coexisting DVT, and RV thrombus. The Pulmonary Embolism Severity Index (PESI) is summarized in Table 5.
- Mortality from recurrent pulmonary emboli is 8% with effective treatment and >30% in patients with untreated pulmonary emboli.

OUTPATIENT FOLLOW-UP

- Monitor for recurrent, persistent, or progressive symptoms after PE.
- Determine appropriate plan for type, dosing, duration, and monitoring of anticoagulation.
- Ensure appropriate evaluation of underlying factors contributing to the development of the PE, including hypercoagulable workup and age-appropriate cancer screening.
- Facilitate appropriate and expeditious removal of temporary IVC filters.
- Monitor for sequelae of PE, such as post-PE syndrome, chronic thromboembolic disease (CTED), and chronic thromboembolic pulmonary hypertension (CTEPH).
  1. Between 0.1% and 9% of patients who experience PE develop CTEPH, which can be a life-threatening disease if not identified and treated in a timely fashion.

PEARLS & CONSIDERATIONS

COMMENTS

- A recent study detected PE in about 6% of patients hospitalized with acute exacerbations of COPD.[3]
- Use of clinical prediction rules in association with D-dimer testing may reduce the use of unnecessary imaging in patients in whom PE is unlikely. A combination of a low clinical pretest probability and a D-dimer level less

[3] Couturand F et al: Prevalence of pulmonary embolism among patients with COPD hospitalized with acutely worsening respiratory symptoms, *JAMA* 325:59, 2021.

TABLE 4 Stratification of Risk of Death Associated with Pulmonary Embolism and Severity-Adjusted Treatment*

	Risk Factor			
Early Risk of Death	**Shock or Hypotension (on Clinical Examination)**	**Right Ventricular Dysfunction (on Echocardiography or Multidetector CT)**	**Myocardial Injury (on Cardiac Troponin Testing)**	**Recommended Treatment**
High	Present	Present†	NA‡	LMWH or unfractionated heparin plus thrombolysis or embolectomy
Intermediate-high	Absent	Both present		LMWH, fondaparinux, or UFH; consideration of reperfusion therapy
Intermediate-low	Absent	Only one present		LMWH, fondaparinux, or UFH; avoid early thrombolysis; monitor clinical status and right ventricular function
Low	Absent	Absent	Absent	DOAC, LMWH, fondaparinux, or UFH; consider outpatient treatment

CT, Computed tomography; *RV,* right ventricle; *LMWH,* low-molecular-weight-heparin; *UFH,* unfractionated heparin; *DOAC,* direct oral anticoagulant.
*Adapted with modifications from the 2019 Guidelines on the Diagnosis and Management of Acute Pulmonary Embolism of the European Society of Cardiology. NA denotes not applicable.
†If RV function is normal on echocardiography, or if a CT scan shows no RV dilation in a patient with hemodynamic compromise and clinically suspected pulmonary embolism, an alternative diagnosis should be sought.
‡Troponin test results do not influence risk assessment or treatment in hemodynamically compromised patients with acute pulmonary embolism.
From Konstantinides S: Acute pulmonary embolism, *N Engl J Med* 359:2804-2813, 2008.

TABLE 5 Original and Simplified Pulmonary Embolism Severity Index (PESI)

Variable	Original PESI	Simplified PESI
Age	Age, in yr	1 (if age >80 yr)
Male sex	+10	—
History of cancer	+30	1
History of heart failure	+10	1 for either or both of these items
History of chronic lung disease	+10	
Pulse >110 beats/min	+20	1
Systolic blood pressure <100 mm Hg	+30	1
Respiratory rate >30 breaths/min	+20	—
Temperature <36 °C	+20	—
Altered mental status	+60	—
Arterial oxyhemoglobin saturation (SaO_2) <90%	+20	1
30-DAY MORTALITY RISK STRATA (BASED ON THE SUM OF POINTS)		
LOW-RISK PESI	**LOW-RISK sPESI**	
Class I: <65 Points	**0 Points**	
(event rate 95% CI, 0-1.6)	(event rate 95% CI, 0-2.1)	
Class II: 66-85 Points		
(event rate 95% CI, 1.7-3.5)		
HIGH-RISK PESI	**HIGH-RISK sPESI**	
Class III: 86-105 Points	**≥1 Point**	
(event rate 95% CI, 3.2-7.1)	(event rate 95% CI, 8.5-13.2)	
Class IV: 106-125 Points		
(event rate 95% CI, 4.0-11.4)		
Class V: >125 Points		
(event rate 95% CI, 10.0-24.5)		

CI, Confidence interval; *PESI,* Pulmonary Embolism Severity Index; *sPESI,* simplified Pulmonary Embolism Severity Index.
From Vincent JL et al: *Textbook of critical care,* ed 7, Philadelphia, 2017, Elsevier.

than 1000 mg per milliliter can identify patients at low risk for pulmonary embolism.

- Massive PE (PE associated with hypotension, shock, or circulatory arrest) remains the clearest situation in which thrombolytics should be employed. Submassive PE (PE associated with RV dysfunction or injury but without hypotension) remains an area of controversy with regard to thrombolytic use.
- The outpatient follow-up of PE is crucial for comprehensive care. Between 0.1% and 9% of patients who experience PE will go on to develop CTEPH.

SUGGESTED READINGS

Available at ExpertConsult.com

RELATED CONTENT

Pulmonary Embolism (PE) (Patient Information)
Deep Vein Thrombosis (Related Key Topic)
Hypercoagulable State (Related Key Topic)

AUTHORS: **Alexander Sherman, MD, Sonia Jasuja, MD,** and **Tisha Wang, MD**

BASIC INFORMATION

DEFINITION

Pulmonary hypertension (PH) is defined as the presence of an elevated mean pulmonary arterial pressure (PAP) ≥20 mm Hg at rest (previously ≥25 mm Hg). Pulmonary hypertension is classified into five major groups: Pulmonary arterial hypertension (Group 1), pulmonary hypertension due to left heart disease (Group 2), pulmonary hypertension due to lung disease (Group 3), pulmonary hypertension due to chronic thromboembolic disease (Group 4), and miscellaneous (Group 5).

Pulmonary arterial hypertension (PAH) is a syndrome defined as mean pulmonary pressure ≥20 mm Hg with pulmonary capillary wedge pressure <15 mm Hg and a pulmonary vascular resistance ≥3 Wood units on right heart catheterization. Idiopathic pulmonary arterial hypertension (IPAH) is diagnosed when PAH is present without any apparent cause. It is a highly morbid disease characterized by progressive obliteration of precapillary arterioles. This topic will mostly focus on pulmonary arterial hypertension.

SYNONYMS

PH
Pulmonary arterial hypertension
Idiopathic pulmonary arterial hypertension
IPAH
Associated pulmonary arterial hypertension
PAHA, also known as secondary pulmonary hypertension
Heritable pulmonary arterial hypertension
HPAH
Group I pulmonary hypertension

ICD-10CM CODES

I27.0	Primary pulmonary hypertension
I27.2	Other secondary pulmonary hypertension

EPIDEMIOLOGY & DEMOGRAPHICS

- IPAH is rare, occurring in one to two cases per 1 million people per year, with an overall prevalence estimated at 15 to 50 per 1 million.
- IPAH is more common in women than men (3:1), usually presenting in the third to fourth decades of life.
- In adults the most common cause of pulmonary hypertension is due to left-sided heart disease (Group 2).
- Prevalence of secondary PAH could range from 8% to 12% in cases of scleroderma, 0.5% of HIV, 23% to 53% of mixed connective tissue disorders, and 1% to 4% cases of systemic lupus erythematosus.

PHYSICAL FINDINGS & CLINICAL PRESENTATION

- Insidious, may go undetected for years
- Exertional dyspnea most common presenting symptom (60%)
- Fatigue and weakness
- Anorexia/abdominal pain
- Syncope, classically exertion-related or after a warm shower with peripheral vasodilation
- Chest pain
- Hoarse voice from compression of recurrent laryngeal nerve by an enlarged pulmonary artery (Ortner syndrome)
- Hemoptysis
- Rarely, palpitations due to atrial fibrillation or atrial flutter
- Loud P2 component of the second heart sound and paradoxical splitting of second heart sound
- Right-sided S4
- Jugular venous distension
- Abdominal distension and ascites
- Prominent parasternal (right ventricular [RV]) impulse
- Holosystolic tricuspid regurgitation murmur heard best along the left fourth parasternal line that increases in intensity with inspiration
- Peripheral edema
- Features of the physical exam pertinent to the evaluation of pulmonary hypertension are summarized in Table 1

ETIOLOGY

- The etiology of IPAH is unknown.
- Associated PAH (APAH) has several known risk factors: Connective tissue disorders such as systemic sclerosis, portal hypertension and liver cirrhosis, appetite-suppressant drugs (e.g., fenfluramine), and infections, including schistosomiasis and HIV disease. High altitude, schistosomiasis, and HIV disease are common causes of PH worldwide; however, pulmonary venous hypertension from left ventricular failure and PH related to COPD are more common causes of PH in developed nations.
- Several genetic abnormalities have been associated with HPAH (heritable PAH), many of which are mutations in the genes that code for members of the tumor growth factor-beta family of receptors (BMPR-II, ALK-1, endoglin) on chromosome 2q33.
- Up to 25% of patients with IPAH have abnormal BMPR-II structure or function, while up to 80% of hereditary PAH is due to mutations in BMPR-II.
- Mutations in *KCNK3*, *SMAD9*, and *CAV1* have also been associated with both familial and idiopathic pulmonary arterial hypertension.
- Heritable PAH is an autosomal-dominant disease with variable penetrance, affecting only about 10% to 20% of carriers.
- Several factors play a role in the pathogenesis of PAH, including a genetic predisposition, endothelial cell dysfunction, abnormalities in vasomotor control, thrombotic obliteration of the vascular lumen, and vascular remodeling through cell proliferation and matrix production.
- SSRI use in late pregnancy is associated with increased persistent PAH in newborns.
- The updated clinical classification of pulmonary hypertension is described in Table 2.

DIAGNOSIS

- PAH is a hemodynamic diagnosis involving the detection of elevated pressure in the pulmonary arteries and elevated pulmonary vascular resistance in the pulmonary vascular bed, occurring in the absence of significant pulmonary venous hypertension.
- Right-sided heart catheterization must be performed in all patients suspected of having PAH to establish the diagnosis and to assess pulmonary hemodynamics including reactivity response to vasodilators.
- One of the most challenging differential diagnoses of IPAH is heart failure with preserved EF (HFpEF). In such patients, the PCWP may be at the higher limit of normal at rest. Exercise or fluid challenge at the time of right heart catheterization can result in disproportionate rise in PCWP, which favors group 2 pulmonary hypertension.
- IPAH is a diagnosis of exclusion; causes that lead to groups 2 to 5 pulmonary hypertension must be ruled out. Transthoracic echocardiogram (TTE), high-resolution computed tomography (HR-CT), pulmonary function tests (PFTs), and ventilation-perfusion (V/Q) scan must be performed before the diagnosis of IPAH is established and treatment started.

DIFFERENTIAL DIAGNOSIS

The differential diagnosis is as listed under "Etiology." Table 3 summarizes distinguishing pulmonary arterial hypertension from heart failure with preserved ejection fraction.

EVALUATION

- Consists of establishing the diagnosis and etiology.
- Echocardiography with Doppler technique can provide a noninvasive but limited estimation of systolic PAP. Common findings include tricuspid regurgitation, right heart enlargement, abnormal movement of septum and, rarely, pericardial effusion. However, the diagnosis of PH cannot be established by echocardiography alone, as echocardiography can overestimate or underestimate PAP.
- ECG shows RV enlargement, strain pattern, and right axis deviation.
- Chest radiograph (Fig. 1) shows enlarged central pulmonary arteries and right heart enlargement. Chest radiography is abnormal in 90% of patients at diagnosis.
- A normal chest radiograph does not rule out the diagnosis. HR-CT (Fig. E2) can assist in the evaluation for emphysema or interstitial lung disease. V/Q lung scan has high sensitivity for chronic thromboembolic disease. CT angiography is less sensitive for diagnosing chronic thromboembolic disease. The diagnosis can be confirmed by pulmonary angiography, which has high specificity.
- Cardiac magnetic resonance imaging (CMR) can provide accurate noninvasive evaluation of the right ventricular size, morphology, and function.

TABLE 1 Features of the Physical Examination Pertinent to the Evaluation of Pulmonary Hypertension

Sign	Implication
PHYSICAL SIGNS THAT REFLECT THE SEVERITY OF PULMONARY HYPERTENSION	
Accentuated pulmonary component of S_2 (audible at the apex in >90%)	High pulmonary pressure that increases force of pulmonic valve closure
Early systolic click	Sudden interruption of opening of the pulmonary valve into a high-pressure artery
Midsystolic ejection murmur	Turbulent transvalvular pulmonary outflow
Left parasternal lift	High right ventricular pressure and hypertrophy present
Right ventricular S4 (in 38%)	High right ventricular pressure and hypertrophy present
Increased jugular A wave	Poor right ventricular compliance
PHYSICAL SIGNS THAT SUGGEST MODERATE TO SEVERE PULMONARY HYPERTENSION	
Moderate to severe pulmonary hypertension	
Holosystolic murmur that increases with inspiration	Tricuspid regurgitation
Increased jugular V waves	
Pulsatile liver	
Diastolic murmur	Pulmonary regurgitation
Hepatojugular reflux	High central venous pressure
Advanced pulmonary hypertension with right ventricular failure	
Right ventricular S_3 (in 23%)	Right ventricular dysfunction
Distension of jugular veins	Right ventricular dysfunction or tricuspid regurgitation, or both
Hepatomegaly	Right ventricular dysfunction or tricuspid regurgitation, or both
Peripheral edema (in 32%)	
Ascites	
Low blood pressure, diminished pulse pressure, cool extremities	Reduced cardiac output, peripheral vasoconstriction
PHYSICAL SIGNS THAT SUGGEST A POSSIBLE UNDERLYING CAUSE FOR OR ASSOCIATIONS WITH PULMONARY HYPERTENSION	
Central cyanosis	Abnormal ventilation-perfusion ratio, intrapulmonary shunt, hypoxemia, pulmonary-to-systemic shunt
Clubbing	Congenital heart disease, pulmonary venopathy
Cardiac auscultatory findings, including systolic murmurs, diastolic murmurs, opening snap, and gallop	Congenital or acquired heart or valvular disease
Rales, dullness, or decreased breath sounds	Pulmonary congestion or effusion, or both
Fine rales, accessory muscle use, wheezing, protracted expiration, productive cough	Pulmonary parenchymal disease
Obesity, kyphoscoliosis, enlarged tonsils	Possible substrate for disordered ventilation
Sclerodactyly, arthritis, telangiectasia, Raynaud phenomenon, rash	Connective tissue disorder
Peripheral venous insufficiency or obstruction	Possible venous thrombosis
Venous stasis ulcers	Possible sickle cell disease
Pulmonary vascular bruits	Chronic thromboembolic pulmonary hypertension
Splenomegaly, spider angiomas, palmar erythema, icterus, caput medusae, ascites	Portal hypertension

From McLaughlin VV et al: ACCF/AHA 2009 expert consensus document on pulmonary hypertension: a report of the American College of Cardiology Foundation Task Force on Expert Consensus Documents and the American Heart Association developed in collaboration with the American College of Chest Physicians; American Thoracic Society, Inc., and the Pulmonary Hypertension Association, *J Am Coll Cardiol* 53:1573, 2009; In Mann DL et al: *Braunwald's heart disease,* ed 11, Philadelphia, 2019, Elsevier.

TABLE 2 Updated Clinical Classification of Pulmonary Hypertension

1 PAH
- 1.1 Idiopathic PAH
- 1.2 Heritable PAH
- 1.3 Drug- and toxin-induced PAH
- 1.4 PAH associated with:
  - 1.4.1 Connective tissue disease
  - 1.4.2 HIV infection
  - 1.4.3 Portal hypertension
  - 1.4.4 Congenital heart disease
  - 1.4.5 Schistosomiasis
- 1.5 PAH long-term responders to calcium channel blockers
- 1.6 PAH with overt features of venous/capillaries (PVOD/PCH) involvement
- 1.7 Persistent PH of the newborn syndrome

2 PH due to left heart disease
- 2.1 PH due to heart failure with preserved LVEF
- 2.2 PH due to heart failure with reduced LVEF
- 2.3 Valvular heart disease
- 2.4 Congenital/acquired cardiovascular conditions leading to postcapillary PH

3 PH due to lung disease and/or hypoxia
- 3.1 Obstructive lung disease
- 3.2 Restrictive lung disease
- 3.3 Other lung disease with mixed restrictive/obstructive pattern
- 3.4 Hypoxia without lung disease
- 3.5 Developmental lung disorders

4 PH due to pulmonary artery obstructions
- 4.1 Chronic thromboembolic PH
- 4.2 Other pulmonary artery obstructions

5 PH with unclear and/or multifactorial mechanisms
- 5.1 Hematologic disorders
- 5.2 Systemic and metabolic disorders
- 5.3 Others
- 5.4 Complex congenital heart disease

HIV, Human immunodeficiency virus; *LVEF,* left ventricular ejection fraction; *PAH,* pulmonary arterial hypertension; *PCH,* pulmonary capillary hemangiomatosis; *PH,* pulmonary hypertension; *PVOD,* pulmonary veno-occlusive disease.

From Simonneau G et al: Haemodynamic definitions and updated clinical classification of pulmonary hypertension, *Eur Respir J* 53(1):1801913, 2019, http://doi.org/10.1183/13993003.01913-2018.

TABLE 3 Distinguishing Pulmonary Arterial Hypertension (PAH) from Heart Failure with Preserved Ejection Fraction (HFpEF)

Characteristic	PAH More Likely	HFpEF More Likely
Age	Younger	Older
Comorbid conditions—DM, HTN, CAD, obesity (metabolic syndrome)	Often absent	Often multiple present
Symptoms—PND, orthopnea	Often absent	Often present
Cardiac examination	RV heave, loud P_2, TR murmur	Sustained LV impulse, LS4
CXR	Clear lung fields	Pulmonary vascular congestion, pleural effusions, pulmonary edema
Chest CT	Often clear lungs	Mosaic perfusion pattern, ground-glass opacities consistent with chronic interstitial edema
ECG	RAD, RVE	LAE, LVE, atrial fibrillation, no RAD
Natriuretic peptides	Often elevated	Often elevated
Echo—LAE, LVH	Absent	Often present
Echo—diastolic dysfunction	Grade 1 common	Grade 2, 3 common
Echo—right ventricle	Often enlarged, may share the apex	Often normal, mildly enlarged
Echo—pericardial effusion	Sometimes	Rare

CAD, Coronary artery disease; *CT,* computed tomography; *CXR,* chest x-ray; *DM,* diabetes mellitus; *ECG,* electrocardiogram; *Echo,* echocardiography; *HTN,* hypertension; *LAE,* left atrial enlargement; *LS4,* left-sided fourth heart sound; *LV,* left ventricular; *LVE,* left ventricular enlargement; *LVH,* left ventricular hypertrophy; *PND,* paroxysmal nocturnal dyspnea; *RAD,* right-axis deviation; *RV,* right ventricular; *RVE,* right ventricular enlargement; *TR,* tricuspid regurgitation.
From Mann DL et al: *Braunwald's heart disease,* ed 10, Philadelphia, 2015, Elsevier.

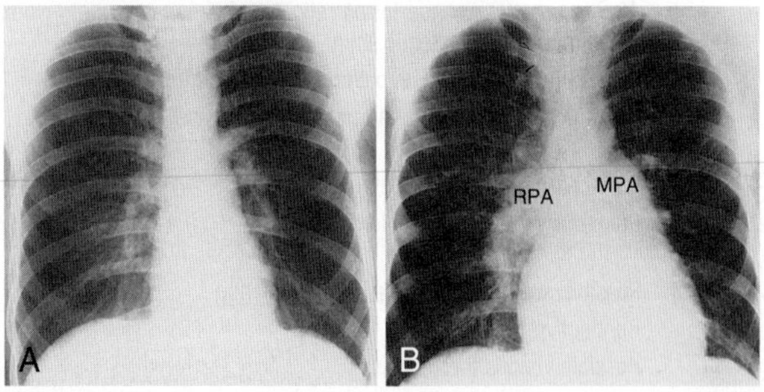

FIG. 1 Progressive pulmonary arterial hypertension. This patient initially presented with a relatively normal chest radiograph **(A).** However, several years later **(B)** there is increasing heart size and marked dilation of the main pulmonary artery *(MPA)* and right pulmonary artery *(RPA).* Rapid tapering of the arteries as they proceed peripherally is suggestive of pulmonary hypertension and is sometimes referred to as pruning. (From Mettler FA [ed]: *Primary care radiology,* Philadelphia, 2000, Saunders.)

- PFTs may show obstructive (airway disease) and/or restrictive disease (parenchymal disease) depending on etiology. Diffusion capacity of carbon monoxide in the lung is reduced due to pulmonary vascular destruction in PAH.
- In asymptomatic patients the severity of pulmonary arterial hypertension (PAH) disease should be evaluated in a systematic and consistent manner, using a combination of World Health Organization (WHO) functional class (FC), exercise capacity, and echocardiographic, laboratory, and hemodynamic variables to inform therapeutic decisions.
- Right heart catheterization is required to assess pulmonary hemodynamics, exclude shunts and left heart disease, and perform acute vasoreactivity response testing.
- Symptomatic patients with PAH, in the absence of contraindications, should undergo acute vasoreactivity testing using a short-acting agent at a center with experience in the performance and interpretation of vasoreactivity testing.
- Screening for the presence of PAH with Doppler echocardiography is warranted in individuals with a known predisposing genetic mutation or first-degree relative with IPAH, connective tissue diseases (especially scleroderma), congenital heart disease with left-to-right shunt, HIV, sickle cell disease, or portal hypertension undergoing evaluation for orthotopic liver transplantation.
- Determining the degree of functional impairment, as assessed by the WHO functional classification system (Classes I-IV) and the 6-min walk test (6MWT), is a useful way to monitor disease progression and assess response to treatment.
- The longitudinal evaluation of patients with pulmonary arterial hypertension is summarized in Table 4.

LABORATORY AND DIAGNOSTIC TESTS

- Complete blood count is usually normal in PAH but may show secondary polycythemia.
- Other blood tests: Antinuclear antibody (ANA), antineutrophil cytoplasmic antibodies (ANCA), anti-Scl-70, anticentromere, antitopoisomerase, anti-Ro, anti-La, anti-RNA polymerase III, ribonucleoprotein antibody levels, and rheumatoid factor (RF) to screen for underlying connective tissue disease, HIV serology, liver function tests, and antiphospholipid antibodies.
- Schistosoma stool serologies.
- Brain natriuretic peptide (BNP) level can provide prognostic information, with elevation in BNP level being associated with increased mortality.

Rx TREATMENT (FIG. 3)

- Most of the evidence in management of PAH is limited to IPAH/HPAH. There is some evidence in treatment of APAH associated with connective tissue disease, especially scleroderma, and congenital heart disease. The recommendations for treating PAH associated with other causes are limited to case studies and expert opinions.
- There is some evidence for the use of advanced therapies for sarcoidosis-associated PH. The heterogeneity of sarcoid-associated PH complicates the interpretation.

GENERAL MEASURES AND TREATMENT:

- Patients should be encouraged to remain active within symptom limits and avoid excessive physical activity.
- Exercise training appears to be beneficial for patients with PH. It is associated with improved exercise capacity, muscular function, quality of life, and possibly right ventricular function and pulmonary hemodynamics.
- PAH is a contraindication to pregnancy as it carries a 30% to 50% mortality risk.
- PAH patients have a higher risk of death from infections and should receive age-appropriate vaccines as well as be vaccinated against influenza and pneumococcal pneumonia.
- Although patients with pulmonary hypertension were found to have a similar incidence of SAR-COV-2 as the general population, a higher mortality rate (12%) was noted in this patient population.
- Although there are no randomized data to suggest that long-term O_2 therapy is beneficial, oxygen administration has shown to reduce PVR. Ambulatory O_2 may be considered for exercise-induced desaturations to maintain oxygen saturations of >90%.
- Diuretics (e.g., furosemide 40-80 mg qd) improve dyspnea by reducing preload and peripheral edema. Avoid excessive diuresis in patients who are preload dependent.
- Digoxin has been used in patients with IPAH with inconclusive benefits. It can be considered in patients who develop atrial tachyarrhythmia. There is no conclusive data regarding the use of beta-blockers, ACE

TABLE 4 Longitudinal Evaluation of Patients with Pulmonary Arterial Hypertension*

	Low Risk	High Risk
Clinical course	Stable; no increase in symptoms and/or decompensation	Unstable; increase in symptoms and/or decompensation
Physical examination	No evidence of right-sided heart failure	Signs of right-sided heart failure
Functional class†	I/II	IV
6MW distance†	>400 m	<300 m
Echocardiogram	RV size/function normal	RV enlargement/dysfunction
Hemodynamics	RAP normal CI normal	RAP high CI low
BNP	Nearly normal/remaining stable or decreasing	Elevated/increasing
Treatment	Oral therapy	Intravenous prostacyclin and/or combination treatment
Frequency of evaluation	Every 3-6 mo‡	Every 1-3 mo
FC assessment	Every clinic visit	Every clinic visit
6MW distance	Every clinic visit	Every clinic visit
Echocardiogram§	Yearly or center dependent	Every 6-12 mo or center dependent
BNP¶	Center dependent	Center dependent
RHC	Clinical deterioration and center dependent	Every 6-12 mo or clinical deterioration

BNP, Brain natriuretic peptide; *CI,* cardiac index; *FC,* functional class; *IV,* intravenous; *RAP,* right atrial pressure; *RV,* right ventricle; *6MW,* 6-min walk.
*For patients in the high-risk category, consider referral to a PAH specialty center for consideration of advanced therapies, clinical trials, and/or lung transplantation.
†The frequency of follow-up evaluation for patients in functional class III and/or 6MW distance between 300 and 400 m would depend on a composite of detailed assessments of the other clinical and objective characteristics listed.
‡For patients who remain stable with established therapy, follow-up assessments can be performed by referring physicians or PH specialty centers.
§Echocardiographic measurement of pulmonary artery systolic pressure is an estimation only, and it is strongly advised that its evaluation not be relied on as the sole parameter to make therapeutic decisions.
¶The usefulness of serial BNP levels to guide management in individual patients has not been established.
From McLaughlin VV et al: ACCF/AHA 2009 expert consensus document on pulmonary hypertension. A report of the American College of Cardiology Foundation Task Force on Expert Consensus Documents and the American Heart Association developed in collaboration with the American College of Chest Physicians; American Thoracic Society, Inc.; and the Pulmonary Hypertension Association, *J Am Coll Cardiol* 53:1573, 2009.
From Mann DL et al: *Braunwald's heart disease,* ed 10, Philadelphia, 2015, Elsevier.

inhibitors, or ARB in IPAH unless required by comorbidities such as concurrent hypertension or cardiomyopathy.
- Evidence for the use of oral anticoagulation with warfarin for IPAH is derived mostly from retrospective single-center experience. Data from RCT and registries remain heterogenous and inconclusive. A large multicenter observational longitudinal registry of patients with IPAH (REVEAL Registry) assessed the effect of warfarin treatment on survival and found no benefit; it also found poorer survival in patients with PAH associated with systemic sclerosis. Generally, patients with IPAH who are undergoing IV prostaglandin therapy are anticoagulated if there are no contraindications to anticoagulation, as they are at high risk for catheter-related thrombosis. There are no data regarding the role of direct oral anticoagulants in IPAH.
- Iron deficiency with or without anemia is common and is associated with reduced exercise capacity; it should be closely monitored and replenished as needed.

CHRONIC Rx

Calcium channel blocker (CCB):
- Acute vasoreactivity response testing should be done in all patients at the time of right heart catheterization. Epoprostenol, adenosine, or nitric oxide is generally used to assess the response. A positive response is a fall in mean PAP of ≥10 mm Hg to a value of <40 mm Hg, with increased or unchanged cardiac output. Fewer than 10% of patients are responders in IPAH, and they are the only patients who can be safely treated with this type of therapy. Acute vasoreactivity study is not recommended for patients in groups 2 to 5.
- The positive responders may benefit from treatment with calcium channel blockers (diltiazem, amlodipine, or nifedipine). All patients should be reassessed in 6 to 8 wk to demonstrate sustained benefit from the calcium channel blocker.
- CCBs should not be used empirically to treat PAH in the absence of demonstrated acute vasoreactivity because of potential severe side effects.
- If patients do not show an adequate response, additional PAH therapy should be started.

PROSTANOIDS

- These synthetic prostacyclin analogues act as potent vasodilators of pulmonary arteries and inhibitors of platelet aggregation. They all have shown improvement in symptoms, exercise capacity including 6MWD, and hemodynamics. They are ideal for WHO functional class III and IV patients.
  1. Epoprostenol: IV formulation with very short half-life (3-5 min). It is the most studied drug, and it is the only one that has shown to improve mortality. It requires long-term IV access with associated risks of infection and thrombosis. Rapid tachyphylaxis with dose escalation is seen. Common side effects include flushing, headache, jaw pain, abdominal cramping, and diarrhea. Limited evidence exists for use in secondary PAH patients.
  2. Treprostinil: IV and SQ formulation with longer half-life. Main disadvantage is pain at SQ pump site (no long-term evidence for IV formulation). Treprostinil is also available as an oral or nebulized inhaled solution.
  3. Iloprost: Aerosolized formulation with short half-life requiring 6 to 8 treatments/day. Oral and IV forms are also available. Well tolerated, with flushing and jaw pain being the most frequent side effects.
  4. Beraprost: PO formulation. Not approved in the U.S.

RIOCIGUAT: GUANYLATE CYCLASE STIMULATORS

Guanylate cyclase stimulators enhance cGMP production and in preclinical studies show antiproliferative and antiremodeling properties in animal models. These oral agents are useful for class II and III patients and have shown favorable results on exercise capacity, hemodynamics (decrease in PVR), WHO functional class, and time to clinical worsening without any mortality benefit. There has also been reported benefit in patients with inoperable and persistent chronic group IV pulmonary hypertension with improvement in 6MWD and reduction in PVR. The most serious side effect is syncope.

Endothelin receptor antagonists (ERAs): Activation of the endothelin system results in vasoconstriction of the pulmonary vascular smooth muscles. Most of these oral pulmonary vasodilators require monthly liver function tests, and often the response is delayed by weeks. Thus it is not an ideal starting therapy for WHO class IV patients. It is effective in class II and III patients and improves symptoms, exercise capacity, and hemodynamics without any improvement in mortality.
- Bosentan is an oral nonselective endothelin A and B receptor blocker, whereas sitaxsentan and ambrisentan are oral selective endothelin A receptor blockers. Ambrisentan does not require monitoring of liver function tests.
- ERAs have been shown to cause improvement in exercise capacity, WHO functional class, hemodynamic and echocardiographic variables without affecting mortality.
- Macitentan is a nonselective endothelin receptor antagonist that showed significant reduction in composite end point of death in patients with IPAH. It was thought not to

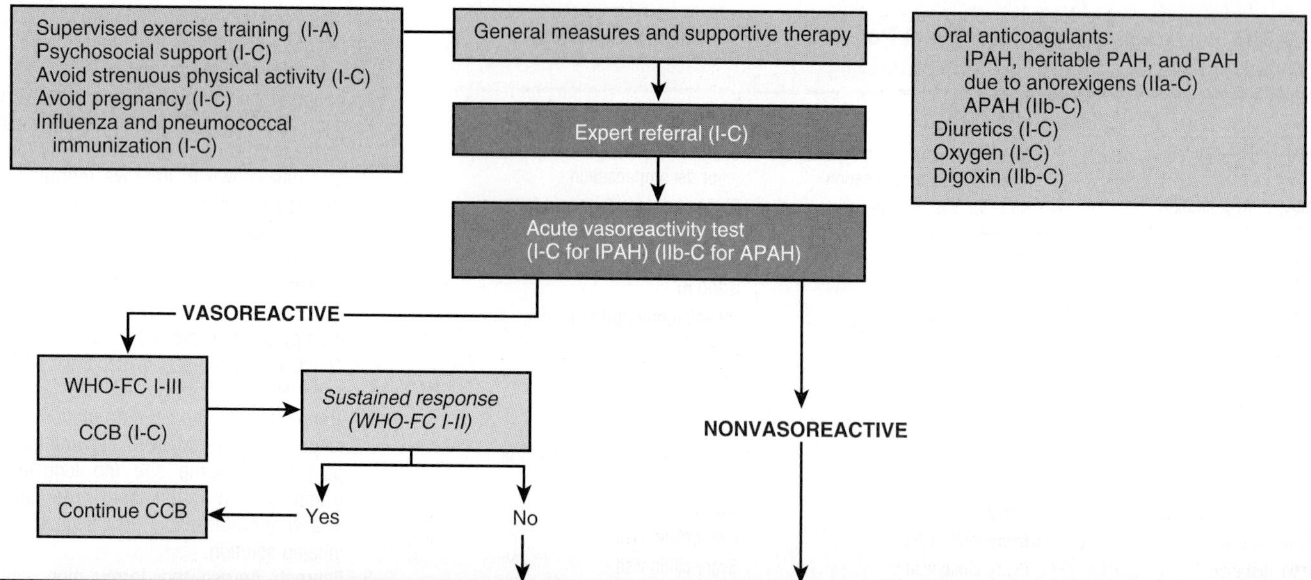

INITIAL THERAPY WITH PAH-APPROVED DRUGS

RED: Morbidity and mortality as primary endpoint in randomized controlled study or reduction in all-cause mortality (prospectively defined)
* Level of evidence is based on the WHO-FC of most of the patients in the studies
† Approved only, in the United States (treprostinil inhaled), in New Zealand (iloprost IV), in Japan and S. Korea (beraprost)
‡ Drugs under regulatory approval

Recommendation	Evidence*	WHO-FC II	WHO-FC III	WHO-FC IV
I	A or B	Ambrisentan Bosentan Macitentan‡ Riociguat‡ Sildenafil Tadalafil	Ambrisentan Bosentan Epoprostenol IV Iloprost inhaled Macitentan‡ Riociguat‡ Sildenafil Tadalafil Treprostinil SC, inhaled†	Epoprostenol IV
IIa	C		Iloprost IV† Treprostinil IN	Ambrisentan, bosentan Iloprost inhaled, and IV† Macitentan‡ Riociguat‡ Sildenafil, tadalafil Treprostinil SC, IV, inhaled†
IIb	B		Beraprost†	
	C		Initial combination therapy	Initial combination therapy

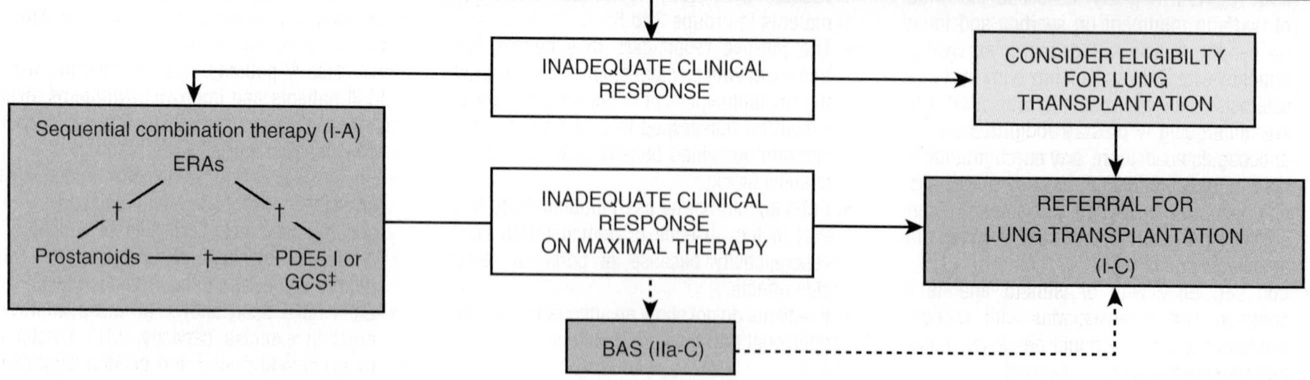

FIG. 3 Treatment algorithm for pulmonary arterial hypertension *(PAH)*. Background therapies include warfarin anticoagulation, which is recommended in all patients with IPAH and no contraindication. Diuretics are used for the management of right-sided heart failure. Oxygen is recommended to maintain oxygen saturation higher than 90%. Acute vasodilator testing should be performed in all patients with IPAH who may be potential candidates for long-term therapy with calcium channel–blocking agents (CCBs). Patients with PAH caused by conditions other than IPAH have a very low rate of long-term responsiveness to oral CCBs, and the value of acute vasodilator testing in such patients needs to be individualized. Patients with IPAH in whom CCB therapy would not be considered, such as those with right-sided heart failure or hemodynamic instability, should not undergo acute vasodilator testing. CCBs are indicated only for patients who have a positive acute vasodilator response, and such patients need to be monitored closely for both safety and efficacy. For patients who did not have positive acute vasodilatory testing and are considered to be at lower risk based on clinical assessment (see Table 5), oral therapy with an endothelin receptor antagonist (ERA) or phosphodiesterase-5 inhibitor (PDE5 I) would be the first line of therapy recommended. If an oral regimen is not appropriate, consideration of the other treatments would need to be based on the patient's profile, side effects, and risk associated with each therapy. For patients who are considered high risk based on clinical assessment (Table 5), continuous treatment with an intravenous prostacyclin (epoprostenol or treprostinil) would be the first line of therapy recommended. If a patient is not a candidate for continuous intravenous treatment, consideration of the other therapies would have to be based on the patient's profile and the side effects and risk associated with each treatment. Epoprostenol improves exercise capacity, hemodynamics, and survival in patients with IPAH and is the preferred treatment option for the most critically ill patients. Combination therapy should be considered when patients are not responding adequately to initial monotherapy. *APAH,* Associated PAH; *BAS,* balloon atrial septostomy; *GCS,* guanylate cyclase stimulators; *IPAH,* idiopathic pulmonary arterial hypertension; *IV,* intravenous; *SC,* subcutaneous; *WHO-FC,* World Health Organization functional class. (From Galiè N et al: Updated treatment algorithm of pulmonary arterial hypertension, *J Am Coll Cardiol* 62[25 Suppl]:D60, 2013. (From Mann DL et al: *Braunwald's heart disease*, ed 10, Philadelphia, 2015, Elsevier.)

TABLE 5 Pulmonary Arterial Hypertension: Determinants of Prognosis*

Determinants of Risk (estimated 1-yr mortality)	Lower Risk (<5%)	Intermediate Risk (5%-10%)	Higher Risk (>10%)
Clinical evidence of RV failure	No	No	Yes
Progression of symptoms	No	Gradual	Rapid
WHO class†	I, II	III	IV
6MW distance‡	>440 m	164-440 m	<165 m
CPET	Peak V_{O_2} >15 ml/kg/min	Peak V_{O_2} 11-15 ml/kg/min	Peak V_{O_2} <11 ml/kg/min
Echocardiography	No pericardial effusion, no RA enlargement, Minimal RV dysfunction	No or minimal pericardial effusion, minimal RA enlargement	Pericardial effusion, significant RV enlargement/ dysfunction, right atrial enlargement
Hemodynamics	RAP <8 mm Hg, CI >2.5 L/min/m^2	RAP 8-14 mm Hg CI 2-2.4 L/min/m^2	RAP >14 mm Hg, CI <2.0 L/min/m^2
BNP§	Not elevated	Mildly elevated	Significantly elevated

BNP, Brain natriuretic peptide; *CI,* cardiac index; *CPET,* cardiopulmonary exercise testing; *peak V_{O_2},* average peak oxygen uptake during exercise; *RA,* right artrial; *RAP,* right atrial pressure; *RV,* right ventricular; *WHO,* World Health Organization.
*Most data available pertain to IPAH, with little data available for other forms of PAH. One should not rely on any single factor to make risk predictions.
†The WHO class is the functional classification for PAH and is a modification of the NHYA functional class.
‡6MW distance is also influenced by age, sex, and height.
§Because data regarding the influence of BNP on prognosis are currently limited and many factors, including renal function, weight, age, and sex, may influence BNP, absolute numbers are not given for this variable.
From McLaughlin VV et al: ACCF/AHA 2009 expert consensus document on pulmonary hypertension. A report of the American College of Cardiology Foundation Task Force on Expert Consensus Documents and the American Heart Association developed in collaboration with the American College of Chest Physicians; American Thoracic Society, Inc.; and the Pulmonary Hypertension Association, *J Am Coll Cardiol* 53:1573, 2009. In Mann DL et al: *Braunwald's heart disease,* ed 10, Philadelphia, 2015, Elsevier.

cause liver toxicity, but postmarketing analysis suggested it can cause liver toxicity. It however more frequently can cause anemia and pharyngitis.

Phosphodiesterase (PDE-5) inhibitors:

- These are oral agents that act by inhibiting phosphodiesterase type 5 enzyme (PDE-5), resulting in increased concentration of nitric oxide causing vasodilation through the cGMP/NO pathway. In addition, they exert antiproliferative effects. Highly effective in WHO class II patients, both in IPAH and scleroderma-associated PAH. Improve symptoms, exercise capacity including 6MWD, hemodynamics, and time to clinical worsening. Mortality benefit was not studied. Most side effects are related to vasodilion including headache, flushing, and epistaxis.
- Sildenafil is administered as 20 mg PO tid. Tadalafil dose is 40 mg once daily. They are also used as combination therapy with epoprostenol and endothelin receptor antagonists.

Prostacyclin agonists:

Selexipag is an oral selective nonprostanoid prostacyclin IP receptor agonist approved for PAH. The IP receptor promotes vasodilation and antiproliferation. Selexipag has been shown to decrease disease progression and hospitalizations without any effect on mortality. Side effects are mild and consist of headache, jaw pain, flushing, and diarrhea.

Treatment considerations depending on WHO functional class:

- According to consensus definition, patients with PAH who demonstrate acute vasoreactivity should be considered candidates for therapy with an oral CCB, except in the case of right heart failure or other contraindications.
- CCBs should not be used empirically to treat PAH in the absence of demonstrated acute vasoreactivity, as described previously.
- For treatment-naïve PAH patients with WHO functional class (FC) II or III symptoms who are not candidates for, or who have failed, CCB therapy, monotherapy should be initiated with an approved ERA, phosphodiesterase-5 (PDE5) inhibitor, or the soluble guanylate cyclase stimulator riociguat.
- For treatment-naïve PAH patients with WHO FC IV, prostanoids are first line.
- For treatment-naïve PAH patients with WHO FC III symptoms who have evidence of rapid progression of their disease or other markers of a poor clinical prognosis, consideration of initial treatment with a parenteral prostanoid is recommended.
- For treatment-naïve PAH patients in WHO FC IV who are unable, or do not desire, to manage parenteral prostanoid therapy, treatment with an inhaled prostanoid in combination with an ERA is recommended.
- For WHO FC III or IV PAH patients with unacceptable clinical status despite established PAH-specific monotherapy, addition of a second class of PAH therapy to improve exercise capacity is recommended. Such patients should be evaluated at centers with expertise

in the evaluation and treatment of complex patients with PAH.

- Combination therapies: Considered when there is no improvement or deterioration on monotherapy. The FDA has approved the use of ambrisentan and tadalafil together as the first two-drug regimen for PAH because it is associated with a significant reduction in the rate of clinical failure compared with monotherapy with either drug alone (AMBITION trial). Starting dose is 5 mg for ambrisentan and 20 mg for tadalafil once daily.
- Bosentan + inhaled iloprost (STEP trial) showed some benefit over monotherapy.
- IV epoprostenol + oral bosentan (BREATH-2 trial) did not show a statistically significant difference when compared with monotherapy.
- IV epoprostenol + oral sildenafil (PACES trial) showed benefit over monotherapy.
- Inhalation of Treprostinil, a stable analogue of Prostacyclin, impaired exercise capacity in patients with pulmonary hypertension due to interstitial lung disease in a recent trial.[1]

INVASIVE Rx

- Lung transplantation and heart-lung transplantation are other options in patients with end-stage class IV disease.
- Atrial septostomy may be performed as a bridge to transplant. It involves creation of an interatrial communication, resulting in right-to-left shunt, which decreases right-sided pressure and increases LV preload and cardiac output. Atrial septostomy is recommended for individuals with a room air SaO_2 >90% who have severe right-sided heart failure (with refractory ascites) despite maximal diuretic therapy, or who have signs of impaired systemic blood flow (such as syncope) from reduced left heart filling.
- Extracorporeal membrane oxygenation (ECMO) is also commonly used as a bridge to transplant.
- Patients should be referred for lung transplant if:
  1. They have WHO FC III or IV during escalating treatment
  2. They have rapidly progressive disease
  3. Parenteral therapy is utilized
  4. Pulmonary venoocclusive disease (PVOD) or pulmonary capillary hemangiomatosis is known or suspected

Lung transplant recipients with IPAH have survival rates of 52% to 75% at 5 yr and 45% to 66% at 10 yr.

TREATMENT OF SECONDARY PAH, APAH:

- Directed toward cause. Some situations merit mention:
  1. PAH with uncorrected congenital heart disease: Eisenmenger syndrome. Medical treatment generally ineffective. Heart-lung transplantation required in most patients. PH may persist after surgical correction of congenital heart disease, and pulmonary vasodilators can be effective therapies in this patient population.
  2. PAH with scleroderma: Selective pulmonary vasodilators are effective.
  3. PAH with lung disease or hypoxia: Oxygen therapy for hypoxemia, CPAP for OSA, control of primary disease process.
  4. PAH with chronic thromboembolic disease: Pulmonary endarterectomy is curative; may consider pulmonary vasodilators, notably riociguat, after anticoagulation (for at least 3 mo and if endarterectomy is not an option) if continued symptoms and elevation in PVR and transpulmonary gradient.
  5. PAH with HIV: Control of viral load by antiretroviral therapy.

[1]Wakman A et al: Inhaled Treprostinil in pulmonary hypertension due to interstitial lung disease, *N Engl Med* 384:325-334, 2021.

DISPOSITION

- The 6MWT is predictive of survival in patients with idiopathic PAH. A baseline 6MWT <250 m is associated with a 50% risk of death at 2 yr. Drop in O_2 saturation >10% during the test increases mortality risk 2.9 times over a median follow-up of 26 mo.
- Cardiopulmonary exercise testing (CPET) is also performed, during which gaseous exchange and ventilation are continuously measured during incremental exercise. A peak oxygen uptake (pVO_2) of <10 ml/kg/min independently predicts a worse prognosis.
- WHO class II and III patients with PAH have a mean survival of 3.5 yr.
- WHO class IV patients have a mean survival of 6 mo.
- As per the REVEAL 2.0 (Registry to Evaluate Early and Long-term Pulmonary Arterial Hypertension Disease Management) risk score, poor prognostic signs include:
  1. PAH associated with portopulmonary hypertension
  2. WHO functional class IV
  3. Walk a distance of <165 meters in 6-min walk test
  4. Elevated BNP levels >800 pg/ml or NT-proBNP >1100 pg/ml
  5. Presence of pericardial effusion
  6. Right atrial pressure >20 mm Hg within 1 yr on right heart catheterization
  7. Increased heart rate >96 or BP <110 mm Hg
  8. Male gender >60 yr of age
  9. Concomitant renal dysfunction with estimated glomerular filtration rate <60 ml/min/m
  10. Diffusion capacity of lung for carbon monoxide (DLCO) <40%
  11. All-cause hospitalization within the last 6 mo

REFERRAL

If the diagnosis of IPAH/HPAH is suspected, a consultation with a pulmonary specialist is recommended. PHA may require disease-specific consultations. Advanced cases need to be transferred to transplant centers.

PEARLS & CONSIDERATIONS

- The exertional dyspnea of PAH is typically described by patients as being relentlessly progressive over several months to a year, often out of proportion to, or in the absence of, underlying heart or lung disease.
- Over 20% of patients in the Registry to Evaluate Early and Long-term PAH Disease Management had symptoms for more than 2 yr before PAH was recognized. Consideration of the diagnosis of PAH in the differential diagnosis of unexplained dyspnea, especially in younger individuals, is essential.
- Chest x-ray may reveal evidence of interstitial fluid or fibrosis within the lungs in cases of secondary PH. IPAH is not associated with infiltrates on chest radiograph.

COMMENTS

- RV systolic pressure (RVSP) as estimated by echocardiography is not a good indicator of the presence of PAH because RVSP increases with age and body mass index. Athletically conditioned men also have a higher resting RVSP. Thus these measurements can be misleading.
- Abrupt development of pulmonary edema during acute vasodilator testing suggests pulmonary venoocclusive disease or pulmonary capillary hemangiomatosis and is a contraindication to long-term vasodilator treatment.
- In advanced PAH, heart rate increase is the main compensatory mechanism and reflects increased sympathetic tone. A higher heart rate at rest is an important marker of prognosis and should be assessed at frequent intervals after initiation of treatment for PAH.
- Current therapies significantly improve exercise capacity, quality of life, and pulmonary hemodynamics, but none of these therapies is curative and long-term prognosis remains poor. Many therapies are still under clinical development and there are some promising results. These therapies include tyrosine kinase inhibitors, rho kinase inhibitors, and pulmonary artery denervation, among others.

SUGGESTED READINGS

Available at ExpertConsult.com

RELATED CONTENT

Pulmonary Hypertension (Patient Information)

AUTHOR: **Caroline Zahm, MD**

BASIC INFORMATION

DEFINITION

Ascending infection of a bacterial pathogen that infects the renal pelvis and kidney. It primarily presents as a urinary tract infection (UTI) characterized by painful urination (dysuria) with associated flank pain/tenderness, nausea, vomiting, and/or fever. The elderly may also present with failure-to-thrive, unexplained anorexia, other organ system decompensation, or generalized deterioration.

CONSISTS OF TWO GROUPS:

- ***Uncomplicated:*** Can be treated as an outpatient with oral antibiotics.
- ***Complicated:*** Inpatient treatment with intravenous antibiotics is required. Hospitalization is indicated for persistent vomiting, progression of uncomplicated UTI, suspected sepsis, immunosuppression, or urinary tract obstruction. This is a potentially life-threatening infection that can lead to renal parenchymal damage. Timely diagnosis and management can significantly impact patient outcomes.

SYNONYMS

Acute pyelonephritis
Pyonephrosis
Renal carbuncle
Lobar nephronia
Acute bacterial nephritis

ICD-10CM CODES

N10	Acute pyelonephritis
N11	Chronic tubulo-interstitial nephritis
N11.0	Nonobstructive reflux-associated chronic pyelonephritis
N11.1	Chronic obstructive pyelonephritis
N11.8	Other chronic tubulo-interstitial nephritis
N11.9	Chronic tubulo-interstitial nephritis, unspecified
N12	Tubulo-interstitial nephritis, not specified as acute or chronic
N20.9	Calculus pyelonephritis

Use additional code (B95-B97) to identify infectious agent.

EPIDEMIOLOGY & DEMOGRAPHICS

INCIDENCE: Pyelonephritis is common in the U.S. at approximately 450,000 cases per yr with the highest incidence in the summer. Pyelonephritis accounts for 9.1% to 31% of severe sepsis cases annually depending on geographic area. Mortality averages 16.1% annually, ranging from 5% for ages <25 yr to 43% for ages >64 yr.

PREDOMINANT SEX: Women are 5 times more likely to be hospitalized than men until the age of 65 yr. In males beyond age 65 yr, the difference in prevalence narrows. Risk factors associated with pyelonephritis in healthy women are sexual intercourse (3 or more times weekly over the previous 30 days), a new sex partner in the past year, use of spermicide, urinary tract infection (UTI) during the past 12 mo, mother with a history of UTI, diabetes mellitus, and urinary incontinence. Urinary tract obstruction is the most important risk factor for a complicated UTI.

PREDOMINANT AGE: Trimodal distribution described in females

- Girls, ages 0 to 4 yr
- Women, ages 15 to 35 yr, especially if sexually active
- Gradual increase in frequency after age 50 yr, with peak incidence at 80 yr

Bimodal distribution in males:

- Boys, ages 0 to 4 yr
- Gradual increase in prevalence after age 35 yr, with peak incidence at 85 yr

GENETICS: Congenital urologic structural disorders associated with vesicoureteral reflux predispose to infections at an early age (<5 yr) and produce renal scarring in most males and some females. Pyelonephritis may produce an Ask-Upmark kidney (segmental renal hypoplasia) that is found more often in young females with severe hypertension.

PHYSICAL FINDINGS & CLINICAL PRESENTATION

Diagnosis established by clinical presentation, history, and physical examination.

Pyelonephritis is suspected in cases of lower urinary tract symptoms (e.g., urinary frequency, urgency, and dysuria) and frequently accompanied by any of the following:

- Fever, rigors, chills (fever may not be present in the elderly or immunosuppressed)
- Flank pain
- Hematuria: Gross hematuria occurs rarely in acute pyelonephritis and raises suspicion for acute cystitis, papillary necrosis, or lower genitourinary malignancy
- Toxic appearance
- Nausea and vomiting
- Headache
- Diarrhea

Physical examination may elicit costovertebral angle tenderness with flank pain, a nearly universal finding. Its absence suggests an alternative diagnosis. Patients presenting with nephrolithiasis/ureterolithiasis usually do not present with costovertebral angle tenderness. Usually, abdominal or suprapubic tenderness is present.

ETIOLOGY

Ascending infections from intestinal bacteria that colonize the perineum and vulvae in women account for most infections. Less commonly, bacteria, viruses, or fungal pathogens may produce hematogenously induced pyelonephritis.

- Gram-negative bacilli cause 95% of cases (e.g., *E. coli* and *Klebsiella* species).
- Less common gram-negative bacteria may produce infection, particularly after urinary tract instrumentation (e.g., *Enterobacter, Serratia,* and *Proteus mirabilis, Pseudomonas,* among others).
- Resistant gram-negative organisms or fungi such as *Candida* may colonize indwelling catheters.
- Gram-positive organisms such as enterococci and rarely, *Staphylococcus saprophyticus.*
- *Staphylococcus aureus* indicates hematogenous spread to the kidneys.
- Viruses generally are limited to the lower urinary tract.
- Urea-splitting organisms generate alkaline urine that fosters production of staghorn calculi. These stones may grow to large size and cause infection, obstruction, or both.

In the elderly, *E. coli* is less common (60%). Diabetics develop infections from *Klebsiella* species, *Enterobacteriaceae*, *Clostridia* species, or *Candida* species.

During the past decade, community-acquired bacteria (particularly *E. coli*) that produce extended-spectrum beta-lactamases have emerged as a cause of acute pyelonephritis worldwide. The most common risk factors for these uropathogens include frequent visits to health care centers, recent use of antimicrobials (e.g., cephalosporins and fluoroquinolones), older age, immunosuppression, recurrent pyelonephritis, nephrolithiasis, and comorbid conditions such as diabetes mellitus and recurrent UTIs.

DIAGNOSIS

DIFFERENTIAL DIAGNOSIS

Differential diagnosis includes the following:

- Abdominal abscess
- Acute abdomen
- Appendicitis
- Basilar pleural process
- Diverticulitis
- Endometriosis
- Herpes zoster
- Lower rib fracture
- Metastatic disease
- Musculoskeletal disorders
- Nephrolithiasis
- Pancreatitis
- Papillary necrosis
- Pelvic inflammatory disease
- Prostatitis
- Pulmonary infarctions
- Renal corticomedullary necrosis
- Renal vein thrombosis
- Retroperitoneal hemorrhage or abscess
- Splenic abscess or infarct
- Urinary tract obstruction
- Vascular pathology

WORKUP

Evaluation includes prostate health assessment in older males.

URINALYSIS

Obtained from and conducted on a clean-catch voided or catheterized specimen, if unable to void or cooperate. Dipstick and microscopic examination must be performed on a fresh specimen for preservation of formed elements (e.g., cells, casts, and microorganisms). Most cases demonstrate pyuria and positive leukocyte esterase in association with a positive blood reaction and microhematuria. Leukocyte casts are generally of kidney origin but may be absent.

URINE CULTURE

Historically, clean, midstream cultures are obtained from all patients suspected of having acute pyelonephritis to guide antibiotic therapy. However, a clean-catch specimen may not be necessary. Recent evidence demonstrates no significant difference in the number of contaminated or unreliable culture results when collected with or without preparatory cleansing. Obtain a catheterized urine sample if the patient is unable to void, uncooperative, or has an altered mental status. There is no difference in colony counts or organisms between catheterized and midstream voiding samples.

More than 95% of acute pyelonephritis cases exhibit more than 10^5 colony-forming units of a single bacterium per ml of urine. However, it is important to obtain an accurate history regarding the timing of culture acquisition and prior antibiotic administration. A negative culture with classic clinical and radiologic findings does not rule out acute pyelonephritis as proven by a prospective study where only 23.5% of 196 patients with clinical and radiologic evidence of acute pyelonephritis demonstrated positive urine cultures. A urine Gram stain may aid in the choice of empiric antimicrobial therapy pending urine culture. If Gram-positive cocci are seen, consider *Enterococcus* species or *Staphylococcus saprophyticus* as causative.

Post-treatment urinalysis and culture are unnecessary if symptomatic improvement occurs, but these studies should be obtained when symptomatic improvement does not occur after 2 or 3 days of antibiotic treatment, or symptoms recur within 2 wk of treatment. Urinary tract imaging is recommended in such cases.

BLOOD CULTURES

Cultures are obtained from hospitalized patients but may not be routinely required in uncomplicated cases. Approximately 15% to 30% of patients with acute pyelonephritis are bacteremic. The elderly and individuals with complicated acute pyelonephritis are more likely to develop bacteremia and sepsis.

Urine cultures yield a causative organism in nearly all cases of acute pyelonephritis. Therefore, a positive blood culture may be diagnostically redundant. However, in unclear cases, or when an alternative diagnosis to acute pyelonephritis is considered, blood cultures should be obtained.

RADIOLOGY

Most uncomplicated cases of acute pyelonephritis do not require imaging studies unless symptoms do not improve, recurrence occurs, or the patient has prolonged fever (>72 hr) or persistent bacteremia. Abdominal radiographs (i.e., kidney, ureter, and bladder x-ray [KUB]) are of limited utility in acute pyelonephritis, unless staghorn calculi are present. Retrograde or antegrade pyelography may be helpful in severe obstruction that is not evident after noninvasive evaluations. Voiding cystourethrography demonstrates vesicoureteral reflux and generally conducted routinely only in children.

Recommendations for radiologic tests:

- Healthy patients with uncomplicated pyelonephritis typically do not require radiologic evaluation when therapeutic responses occur within 72 hr of antibiotic therapy.
- If no response to therapy occurs within 72 hr, abdominal CT is the study of choice.
- Diabetics and immunocompromised patients should undergo precontrast and postcontrast abdominal and pelvic CT scans (Fig. 1) within 24 hr of diagnosis when response to therapy is not prompt.
- Ultrasound (Fig. E2) is reserved for patients in whom exposure to contrast or radiation is considered hazardous. There is a high false-negative rate for renal abscess with ultrasound. In a prospective study of acute pyelonephritis of 213 patients submitted for CT/NMR study, 50 patients (23.5%) had a renal abscess, yet only two were detected by ultrasound.
- All other adults with complicated cases (i.e., history of stones or other urologic conditions, prior urologic surgery, repeated episodes of pyelonephritis) should be evaluated early by CT.
- Helical CT detects calculi with high sensitivity.
- Urologic imaging studies should be conducted in all young men and boys.

Although the risk of contrast nephropathy has declined substantially, exert caution during contrast administration to patients with chronic kidney disease or for those taking metformin. When evaluating kidney function, diagnostic decision-making must include estimated glomerular filtration rate trends, not serum creatinine levels, especially in the elderly with reduced muscle mass. Patients with acute pyelonephritis and acutely elevated baseline serum creatinine concentrations may warrant CT imaging to rule out obstruction. If the risk of radiocontrast media administration outweighs its benefits, consider retrograde or antegrade pyelography.

The purpose of imaging is to identify underlying structural abnormalities such as occult obstruction from a stone or abscess and serious complications such as emphysematous pyelonephritis. In a prospective study of 213 patients with acute pyelonephritis, there were no differences in frequency of fever, leukocytosis, C-reactive protein, pyuria, urine cultures, and duration of symptoms before hospitalization for positive or negative CT. Accordingly, systematic CT or magnetic resonance imaging is not required to exclude an anatomic abnormality. Such abnormalities cannot be predicted based on clinical, biochemical, or culture parameters.

Emphysematous pyelonephritis is a necrotizing infection that produces intraparenchymal kidney gas visualized by renal imaging. This disorder is associated with high mortality. Risk factors include diabetes mellitus and/or urinary tract obstruction. Gas-forming bacteria, most commonly *E. coli,* produce gas typically restricted within the Gerota fascia. If gas is localized to the kidney, mortality is 60%. If gas spreads to the perinephric space, mortality is 80%. In emphysematous pyelitis, mortality is 20%. This must be differentiated from a renal abscess that can also be associated with a gas collection. With drainage and antibiotic treatment, a renal abscess has a favorable prognosis.

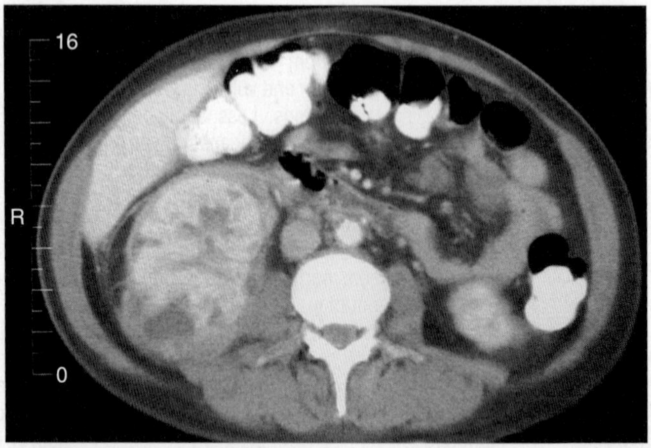

FIG. 1 Acute pyelonephritis: Contrast material–enhanced computed tomographic (CT) scan. The heterogeneous CT nephrogram shows the diffuse involvement of the right kidney. Stranding and some fluid are visible in the perinephric space with thickening of Gerota fascia. (From Skorecki K et al: *Brenner & Rector's the kidney,* ed 10, Philadelphia, 2016, Elsevier.)

P

LABORATORY TESTS

A basic metabolic profile and CBC with differential count are required for patients with suspected acute pyelonephritis to estimate kidney function. If the diagnosis is in doubt, other laboratory tests may be appropriate to clarify the differential diagnosis (e.g., lipase, transaminase, and β-HCG levels).

Rx TREATMENT

ACUTE GENERAL Rx

UNCOMPLICATED ACUTE PYELONEPHRITIS: Close outpatient follow-up is possible with minimal gastrointestinal symptoms and the ability to maintain fluid intake and oral medications. Prompt antibiotic therapy prevents progression of infection and must be initiated following acquisition of appropriate cultures. Begin empiric therapy based on risk of adverse effects, local community bacterial profiles, and resistance rates. Antibiotics are revised after urine culture results are available.

The concept of requiring long-term treatment of acute pyelonephritis has been questioned. Women with acute pyelonephritis were randomized to oral treatment with ciprofloxacin 500 mg twice daily for 7 days or 14 days, and 27% of these patients experienced bacteremia from *E. coli.* No differences in the cure rates were found (87% and 96%, respectively).

Outpatient regimens:

- Fluoroquinolones are preferred in communities where the local prevalence of resistant *E. coli* is ≤10%.
- Ciprofloxacin 500 mg by mouth twice daily or a single, 1000-mg dose in the extended-release form by mouth daily for 7 days.
- Levofloxacin 750 mg by mouth daily for 5 days.
- The initial dose may be administered intravenously (ciprofloxacin 400 mg or levofloxacin 500 mg).
- When a fluoroquinolone is contraindicated, alternative treatment with trimethoprim/sulfamethoxazole 160/800 mg by mouth twice daily for 10 to 14 days may be administered if the pathogen is susceptible. Recent data suggest that stopping treatment at 7 days may be equally effective.

Because of the high prevalence of resistance to oral beta-lactam antibiotics and trimethoprim/sulfamethoxazole, these agents usually are reserved for cases where susceptibility results are known. Additional factors (e.g., allergy history, potential drug–drug interactions, drug availability) may require empiric treatment with these agents before susceptibility testing results are known. In this circumstance, a long-acting, broad-spectrum parenteral drug (e.g., ceftriaxone 1 g or gentamicin 5 mg/kg) may be administered as a one-time dose or longer, until sensitivities of the organism are known. If the local prevalence of fluoroquinolone resistance to *E. coli* exceeds 10%, an initial intravenous dose of ceftriaxone or gentamicin is recommended, followed by an oral fluoroquinolone regimen.

Significant clinical improvement during appropriate empiric antibiotic therapy should occur within 48 to 72 hr. If improvement does not occur, a complication of acute pyelonephritis or an alternative diagnosis such as an abscess, emphysematous pyelonephritis, or an obstructing calculus should be considered. Any unexpected change in the clinical picture warrants immediate investigation with a CT scan.

COMPLICATED ACUTE PYELONEPHRITIS: Hospitalization is indicated for the following reasons:

- Toxic patients
- Complicated infections
- Diabetes or otherwise immunosuppressed
- Suspected bacteremia

Inpatient care includes supportive care, monitoring of culture results, adjustment of antibiotic regimen, and intravenous volume repletion as required. Intravenous antibiotics are continued until defervescence occurs and clinical improvement occurs. Next, there is conversion to an oral antibiotic regimen for a total duration of 10 to 14 days.

- Intravenous antibiotic options for more toxic patients pending cultures include ceftriaxone (1-2 g once daily), IV ciprofloxacin (400 mg every 12 hr) or IV levofloxacin (500-750 mg IV once daily), piperacillin/tazobactam (3.375 g IV every 6 hr), or carbapenems such as meropenem or imipenem (500 mg IV every 6-8 hr).
- Ceftazidime 1 to 2 g IV every 8 hr, piperacillin/tazobactam, or carbapenems are optimal choices for *Pseudomonas* because of increasing ciprofloxacin resistance.
- Aminoglycosides (2 mg/kg IV loading dose followed by 1 mg/kg IV every 8-12 hr, adjusted for kidney function) are potentially nephrotoxic. These agents should be used only if no better alternative exists. Vancomycin 1 g IV every 12 hr, linezolid 600 mg IV or PO every 12 hr, or daptomycin 4 to 6 mg/kg IV daily for gram-positive cocci (e.g., enterococci, staphylococci).
- Ampicillin 1 to 2 g IV every 4 to 6 hr for ampicillin-sensitive enterococci with aminoglycoside for synergy. Urinary obstruction is promptly drained by nephrostomy tube. Surgical drainage of abscess formation(s).
- Pregnant females with acute pyelonephritis are hospitalized and treated initially with a second- or third-generation cephalosporin.

RENAL ABSCESSES (RENAL CARBUNCLES)

Cortical abscesses historically required surgical drainage; however, using current antibiotics is commonly sufficient for cure.

- Semisynthetic penicillin, cephalosporin, fluoroquinolone, or vancomycin, with guidance from culture and sensitivity results.
  1. Parenteral therapy for 10 to 14 days followed by oral therapy for 2 to 4 wk.
  2. Fever should resolve in 5 to 6 days and pain within 24 hr.
  3. If no clinical response occurs within 48 hr, percutaneous or open drainage should be considered. More extreme measures are occasionally required, including enucleation or nephrectomy.

CORTICOMEDULLARY ABSCESSES

- Parenteral therapy for at least 48 hr is generally successful.
- May require incision and drainage and possibly, nephrectomy.
- If defervescence occurs, IV antibiotic treatment may be switched to complete a 2-wk course of oral antibiotic therapy.

PERINEPHRIC ABSCESSES

- Serious complication with mortality in the 25% to 50% range.
- Lesions require early recognition, surgical drainage, and parenteral antibiotics (not adequate alone) to reduce mortality.
- Initial antibiotic therapy should include an aminoglycoside and an antistaphylococcal agent.
  1. If *Pseudomonas* species grow in culture or are suspected, an antipseudomonal beta-lactam antibiotic should be administered with the aminoglycoside.
  2. For enterococcui, an aminoglycoside and ampicillin are recommended.
- Reported with tuberculosis or fungi as rare causes.
- Nephrectomy may be considered with clinical deterioration despite aggressive therapy.

CALCULI-RELATED INFECTIONS

Chronic pyelonephritis may lead to formation of struvite stone, magnesium ammonium phosphate (struvite) stones. Formation requires infection with a urease-producing organism such as *Proteus* or *Klebsiella.* Symptoms directly attributable to struvite stones are uncommon. Typically, patients will present with symptoms of a urinary tract infection, mild flank pain, or hematuria. The stone may grow rapidly over a period of weeks to months if treatment is inadequate. Medical treatment for struvite stones is often ineffective and only indicated when surgery is not an option. Mortality is 28% with observation alone versus 7.2% with surgical therapy. The most common surgical intervention is percutaneous nephrolithotomy. Open surgery, once the gold standard, is rarely used now.

Surgical intervention is generally recommended in patients with newly discovered stones or in patients with a solitary kidney or two equally functioning kidneys. Nephrectomy is a reasonable option in patients with a nonfunctional kidney, particularly when chronic infection is present.

RENAL PAPILLARY NECROSIS

- Admission for parenteral antibiotics:
  1. Initial therapy should cover *E. coli, Enterobacter, Proteus,* and *Klebsiella* species, pending culture results.
  2. For more serious infections, *Pseudomonas* and *Enterococcus* should also be covered.
  3. Empiric therapy agent options include the following:

a. Aminoglycosides
b. Cefotaxime
c. Ceftriaxone
d. Ceftazidime
e. Cefepime
f. Piperacillin-tazobactam
g. Imipenem-cilastatin
h. Meropenem
i. Ciprofloxacin
4. Continue parenteral therapy until fever and clinical symptoms improve.

Xanthogranulomatous pyelonephritis is a rare variant of chronic pyelonephritis with destruction of renal parenchyma.

- Generally, unilateral
- Usually in individuals with obstructing stones
- CT is the diagnostic modality of choice and provides staging information
- Can be confused with malignancy
- Treatment is surgical nephrectomy

CHRONIC Rx

- Repair underlying structural problems especially when kidney function is compromised.
  1. Reflux
  2. Obstruction
  3. Suspect nephrolithiasis
- Avoid urinary catheters.

DISPOSITION

- If pyelonephritis is uncomplicated with no significant GI symptoms, treatment may be initiated on an outpatient basis with close monitoring of therapeutic response(s) in 48 to 72 hr.
- If pyelonephritis is complicated and symptoms persist for >48 to 72 hr, admission is recommended for any of the following: Significant GI symptoms that preclude oral therapy, pregnancy, urinary tract obstruction, suspected renal or perinephric abscess, bacterial sepsis, diabetes or other immunocompromised states, recurrent or refractory pyelonephritis, or infection with unusual or antibiotic-resistant microorganisms.
- If sepsis is present, consider intensive care unit hospitalization.
- Acute pyelonephritis may be fatal when complications develop such as emphysematous pyelonephritis (mortality rate, 20%-80%), perinephric abscess (mortality rate, 20%-50%), or sepsis syndrome (>25% overall mortality rate).
- Acute deterioration or nonresponse to conventional therapy may be due to a complication, resistant organism, or unrecognized comorbidity.
- Diabetic patients with acute pyelonephritis are prone to bacteremia, longer hospital stays, and greater mortality. Diabetics should be considered complicated patients.
- Patients older than 65 yr experience greater mortality, septic shock, bedridden status, and immunosuppression. In males, mortality is also increased with the use of antibiotics in the previous month.

REFERRAL

- General surgery or urology for suspected abscess
- Infectious disease for resistant organisms and poor response to routine antibiotic therapy as outlined
- Urology to correct underlying urologic problems (e.g., reflux and hydronephrosis)
- Nephrology consult for renal dysfunction or nephrolithiasis evaluation
- Critical care monitoring, if ICU admission is required

PEARLS & CONSIDERATIONS

- Consider acute pyelonephritis in patients with urinary symptoms, flank pain, and fever.
- Obtain a urinalysis and culture before starting empiric antibiotic therapy. Adjust treatment, pending antibiotic sensitivity testing.
- Evaluate clinical response in 48 to 72 hr during outpatient therapy. If there is no or delayed improvement, continue evaluation to rule out urinary tract obstruction.
- Urology consultation in all cases of urinary tract obstruction or detection of urinary tract gas (e.g., emphysematous pyelonephritis).
- Treat all diabetics as complicated acute pyelonephritis.

SUGGESTED READINGS

Available at ExpertConsult.com

RELATED CONTENT

Pyelonephritis (Patient Information)

AUTHORS: **James P. Reichart MD,** and **Nelson Kopyt, DO**

BASIC INFORMATION

DEFINITION

- Radiation induced lung injury (RILI) results from exposure to ionizing radiation. Following radiation therapy (RT), there is a *latent phase* of 1 to 2 mo in which usually there are no microscopic, clinical, or radiographic findings. (Electron microscopy will show degeneration of pneumocytes.) This is followed by an *acute phase* 1 to 6 mo after RT and may progress to a *chronic phase* > 9 mo after RT. RILI that develops in the acute phase is usually acute radiation pneumonitis (RP). RILI that more commonly develops in the chronic phase is radiation fibrosis.
- *Radiation recall pneumonitis*, a rare reaction, may occur > 2 yr after RT. It occurs when radiation therapy is followed at a later date by chemotherapy, immunotherapy, or by a variety of other drugs including antituberculous agents, antibiotics, tamoxifen, and simvastatin. The infiltrate conforms to the treatment portals.
- Very high doses (> 70 Gy) are associated with bronchostenosis, bronchomalacia, mediastinal fibrosis and laryngeal nerve injury.

SYNONYMS

Acute radiation pneumonitis (RP)
Radiation pneumonia
Radiation pulmonary fibrosis (RPF)

ICD-10CM CODES

J70.0	Acute pulmonary manifestations due to radiation
J70.1	Chronic and other pulmonary manifestations due to radiation

EPIDEMIOLOGY & DEMOGRAPHICS

Incidence & Prevalence: RILI occurs in about 15% of patients receiving RT to the lung area. It is dose intensity and lung volume dependent. Certain risk factors increase individual risk.

RISK FACTORS

- See Table 1.
- In addition to the above, electron beam radiation to the chest wall or breast tissue may sensitize the lung to radiation.
- Radiation recall pneumonitis may be seen when RT is followed by consolidative chemotherapy and with postradiation immunotherapy

PREVENTION

Conformal radiation techniques that limit lung exposure to radiation may reduce the incidence of RILI:

- Intensity-modulated radiation therapy (IMRT) uses multiple small photon or proton beams to conform to the shape of the tumor.
- Volumetric arc radiation therapy (VMAT) delivers radiation via a continuously molded cone-shaped beam which rotates around the patient.
- Stereotactic body radiosurgery (SBRT) utilizes multiple static beams delivered from different points using 3-D imaging of the target. X-ray, gamma ray and proton beam therapy are delivered in this manner.
- Proton (particle) beam energy is deposited mainly at the target and has no exit path. This method itself has not been shown to reduce acute radiation pneumonitis.

CLINICAL FINDINGS AND PRESENTATION

- Acute radiation pneumonitis: Dyspnea (sometimes out of proportion to radiographical findings), cough, mild fever represent the classic triad. Pleuritic pain may also occur. Physical findings include dullness to percussion, rales, and a pleural friction rub.
- Radiation fibrosis: Symptoms include dyspnea, and a nonproductive cough. Dullness and rales may be heard over the affected area.
- Radiation recall pneumonitis. Similar to RP.

Radiation pneumonitis grading system: See Table 2.

TABLE 1 Risk Factors for Radiation-Induced Lung Injury

Radiation risk factors	
% Total lung volume receiving ≥20 Gy (V20), ≥30%	
% Total lung volume receiving ≥5 Gy (V5), ≥65%	
Mean lung dose, >20 Gy	
Absolute volume lung spared >5 Gy (AVS5), <500 cc	
Target location, lower lobe	
Disease risk factors	
Refractory or relapsed disease (lymphoma)	
Supraclavicular field (breast cancer)	
Bulky disease	
Chemotherapy	
Re-irradiation	
Host risk factors	
Age ≥50 yr	
Autoimmune disease	
Interstitial lung disease	
Former or current smoker	
COPD	

From Hanania A et al: Radiation-induced lung injury assessment and management, *Chest* 156:150, 2019, Elsevier. Table 1.

DIAGNOSIS

DIFFERENTIAL DIAGNOSIS

Infection, recurrent tumor, and medication-induced lung injury.

WORKUP

- The clinical and temporal presentation along with a typical radiographical image is often sufficient to make the diagnosis of acute, chronic, or recall radiation pneumonitis
- There are no specific laboratory findings, although serum inflammatory markers are often elevated. Procalcitonin is low.
- Chest CT is the best imaging technique. In acute RP, an opacity is seen in the target region. Cavitation may also occur. A small pleural ipsilateral effusion may develop. Rarely, acute RP presents as bilateral disease resembling hypersensitivity pneumonitis. With radiation fibrosis, retraction with volume loss is seen on chest x-ray or CT scan. The retraction usually conforms to the irradiated area.
- PET/CT shows low uptake in radiation fibrosis (> 9 mo after treatment completion).
- Pulmonary function studies show a restrictive pattern with a proportionate reduction in flow rates, reduced total lung capacity and residual volume, and a reduction in the diffusing capacity.
- Additional studies including bronchoscopy with BAL, thoracentesis, and open biopsy are only occasionally required.

TABLE 2 Radiation Pneumonitis Grading Systems

Grading System	RTOG	CTCAE
Grade 1	Asymptomatic or mild symptoms (dry cough). Slight radiographic appearances	Mild; asymptomatic. Clinical and diagnostic observations only. Intervention not indicated
Grade 2	Moderate symptomatic fibrosis or pneumonitis (severe cough). Low-grade fever. Patchy radiographic appearances	Moderate. Minimal, local, or noninvasive intervention indicated. Limiting age-appropriate instrumental ADL
Grade 3	Severe symptomatic fibrosis or pneumonitis. Dense radiographic changes	Severe or medically significant but not immediately life-threatening. Hospitalization or prolongation of hospitalization indicated. Disabling. Limiting self-care ADL
Grade 4	Severe respiratory insufficiency/ continuous oxygen/assisted ventilation	Life-threatening consequences. Urgent intervention indicated
Grade 5	Death related to adverse events	Death related to adverse events

ADL, Activities of daily living; *CTCAE*, Common Terminology Criteria for Adverse Events; *RTOG*, Radiation Therapy Oncology Group.
From Hanania A et al: Radiation-induced lung injury assessment and management, *Chest* 156:150, 2019, Elsevier. Table 2.

Rx TREATMENT

- Acute radiation pneumonitis: There are no controlled studies on treatment. Most experts recommend prednisone 1 mg/kg for 2 to 4 wk with slow taper over 6 to 12 wk. Relapse may occur after discontinuation of steroids. Steroid-sparing agents azathioprine and cyclosporine have also been used.
- Radiation fibrosis: No available treatment.
- Radiation recall pneumonitis: Steroids with slow taper as in acute RP.
- Supportive care includes oxygen, antipyretics, and cough suppressants.

PREVENTION

- Amifostine, a prodrug, is the only FDA-approved radioprotective agent. Hydrolyzed by alkaline phosphatase, its thiol metabolite scavenges free radicals and reduces lung radiation injury of grade 2 or higher. Its side effect profile limits its use. (Hypotension 62%.)
- Pentoxifylline, not FDA-approved, inhibits proinflammatory molecules (TNF-α, leukotrienes). It has been demonstrated to reduce radiation pneumonitis.

SUGGESTED READINGS

Available at ExpertConsult.com

AUTHOR: **Jerome L. Slate, MD, FCCP**

BASIC INFORMATION

DEFINITION

Raynaud phenomenon (RP) is a vasospastic disorder that causes an exaggerated response to cold temperatures and/or emotional stress, resulting in episodic digital ischemia. It presents as a cold-induced, symmetric, sharply demarcated white or blue discoloration of the distal fingers or toes, followed by erythema at a variable time after rewarming.

SYNONYMS

Primary Raynaud phenomenon or Raynaud disease
Secondary Raynaud phenomenon
RP

ICD-10CM CODES

I73.0	Raynaud syndrome
I73.00	Raynaud syndrome without gangrene
I73.01	Raynaud syndrome with gangrene

EPIDEMIOLOGY & DEMOGRAPHICS

- RP is classified clinically into primary or secondary forms and affects approximately 3% to 5% of the general population, 15% of children younger than 12 yr, and less than 1% of adults older than 60 yr.
- Occurs more commonly in colder climates.
- Primary RP usually occurs between the ages of 12 and 25 yr.
- It is more likely to affect more women than men (4:1).
- 5% to 15% of patients with primary Raynaud phenomenon develop a secondary cause later in the course of the disease (mostly a connective tissue disorder).
- Secondary RP tends to begin after age 35 to 40 yr.
- Secondary RP occurs in more than 90% of patients with scleroderma and in approximately 30% of patients with systemic lupus erythematosus or Sjögren syndrome.

PHYSICAL FINDINGS & CLINICAL PRESENTATION

- The typical manifestation of RP is the biphasic color response of the digits to cold exposure and rewarming, which may or may not be accompanied by pain. RP most often affects the hand (Fig. E1).
  1. White (pallor) or blue (cyanotic) discoloration of the digit(s) resulting from vasospasm on cold or vibration exposure.
  2. Red (rubor) with or without pain and paresthesia when vasospasm resolves and blood returns to the digit.
- Color changes can sometimes be induced by placing the hand in an ice bath, although this is not recommended as a diagnostic maneuver because responses may be inconsistent even in patients with definite RP.
- Color changes are well delineated, symmetric, and usually bilateral, involving the fingers and toes. The index, middle, and ring fingers are commonly involved and the thumb infrequently; however, if the thumb is involved, that suggests secondary causes of RP.
- Fingertips are most often involved, but feet, ears, nose, tongue, and nipples can also be affected.
- Patients with RP may exhibit a violaceous or reticular pattern of skin of arms and legs, sometimes with regular, unbroken circles (livedo reticularis).
- Duration of attacks can range from seconds to hours and averages 15 to 20 min.
- Chronic skin changes resulting from repeated attacks may include skin thickening and brittle nails. Ulcerations and, rarely, gangrene may occur.
- Physical examination should also include examination for symptoms associated with autoimmune disease, such as fever, rash, arthritis, dry eyes, dry mouth, myalgias, or cardiopulmonary abnormalities.

ETIOLOGY

- Primary RP can also be called idiopathic Raynaud phenomenon, primary Raynaud syndrome, or Raynaud disease. It occurs in the absence of any associated disease.
- With primary RP, the possibility that another first-degree family member is affected is reported as approximately 25%.
- Secondary RP is associated with an underlying pathologic condition or disorder, use of certain drugs, or related occupation. Secondary causes of Raynaud phenomenon are summarized in Box 1.

Dx DIAGNOSIS

Clinical criteria:
- Definite RP: Repeated episodes of biphasic color change on cold exposure
- Possible RP: Uniphasic color changes plus numbness or paresthesia on cold exposure
- No RP: No color change on cold exposure

The suggested criteria for primary RP are:
- Symmetric attacks
- Absence of tissue necrosis, ulceration, gangrene, or peripheral vascular disease
- Absence of a secondary cause on the basis of a patient's history and general physical examination
- Negative nail-fold capillary examination
- Negative test for antinuclear antibody (ANA)
- Normal erythrocyte sedimentation rate (ESR)

Secondary RP is suggested by the following findings:
- Onset of symptoms after age 30 yr
- Male gender
- Episodes that are painful, asymmetric, or associated with ischemic skin lesions
- Clinical features suggestive of a connective-tissue disease
- Elevated specific autoantibody tests and ESR

BOX 1 Secondary Causes of Raynaud Phenomenon

Rheumatologic
Systemic sclerosis (CREST syndrome)
Sjogren syndrome
Systemic lupus erythematosus
Ehlers-Danlos syndrome
Rheumatoid arthritis
Dermatomyositis
Polymyositis
Mixed connective tissue disease

Autoimmune
Reiter syndrome
Vasculitis (polyarteritis nodosa, Henoch-Schönlein purpura)
Antiphospholipid syndrome
Primary pulmonary hypertension

Endocrine
Hypothyroidism
Pheochromocytoma
Carcinoid

Infectious
Hepatitis B and C infection
Mycoplasma pneumonia

Medications
Cyclosporine
Ergotamine
Beta-blockers
Cytotoxic (bleomycin, cisplatin, vinblastine)
Bromocriptine
Nicotine
Cocaine
Sulfasalazine
Interferon-alpha and interferon-beta
Clonidine
Sympathomimetics
Estrogen in oral contraceptives
Caffeine

Occlusive Vascular
Arteriosclerosis
Vascular trauma (hypothenar hammer syndrome)
Buerger disease
Thoracic outlet syndrome
Thromboembolism

Hematologic Proliferative
Leukemia
Lymphoma
Polycythemia vera
Multiple myeloma
Disseminated intravascular coagulation
Cryoglobulinemia
Cold agglutinin disease

Neurologic
Migraines
Carpal tunnel syndrome
Polyneuropathy

Environmental
Emotional stress
Frostbite
Repetitive trauma or injuries to hand

Malignancy
Lung, stomach, small bowel
Paraneoplastic syndrome
Neurofibromatosis

From Cameron JL, Cameron AM: *Current surgical therapy,* ed 12, Philadelphia, 2017, Elsevier.

TABLE 1 Characteristics of Primary and Secondary Raynaud Phenomenon

Characteristic	Primary	Secondary
Age	Younger (<30 yr)	Older (>30 yr)
Gender preference	Female	Male (depending on secondary cause)
Incidence	Most common	Less common
Familial predisposition	Yes	Yes
Combination with other disease	No, idiopathic	Associated with systemic disease
Vascular defect	Functional dysregulation of autonomic nervous system	Structural changes in connective tissue or vessels
Associated signs	None	Arthritis, sclerodactyly, cardiopulmonary abnormality, rash
Frequency	Precipitated by stimuli	Periodic and stimuli trigger
Severity of symptoms	Long history of mild attacks	Severe and disabling pain
Distribution	Symmetric	Asymmetric
Duration	Self-limited	Need for additional treatment (pharmacologic, surgery)
Critical complications	None	Ischemia and ulcers
Capillaroscopy	Normal (symmetric, thin, and uniform)	Abnormal (dilated, irregular, elongated, and tortuous vessel)
Vascular examination	Normal pulses	Abnormal pulses
Erythrocyte sedimentation rate	Normal	Elevated
Serologic studies	Negative	Antinuclear antibody, autoantibodies
C-reactive protein	Normal	Elevated

From Cameron JL, Cameron AM: *Current surgical therapy*, ed 12, Philadelphia, 2017, Elsevier.

- Evidence of microvascular disease on microscopy of nail-fold capillaries
- It is critical to differentiate primary and secondary RP since management is significantly different for the two conditions. Table 1 summarizes characteristics of primary and secondary Raynaud phenomenon

DIFFERENTIAL DIAGNOSIS

- Neurogenic thoracic outlet syndrome or carpal tunnel syndrome
- Frostbite or cold weather injury
- Medication reaction (ergotamine, chemotherapeutic agents)
- Atherosclerosis, thromboembolic disease
- Buerger disease, embolic disease
- Acrocyanosis
- Livedo reticularis
- Injury from repetitive motion

WORKUP

- An algorithm for the evaluation of Raynaud phenomenon is illustrated in Fig. 2.
- Once the diagnosis of RP is established, differentiating primary from secondary is helpful in treatment and prognosis.
- Patients who are younger when their symptoms occur, have a normal history and physical examination and normal nail-fold capillaries, and have no history of digital ischemic lesions can be considered as having primary RP. These patients can be monitored clinically without any further testing.
- If a secondary cause of RP is suspected, appropriate laboratory testing is recommended (see "Laboratory Tests"). Secondary RP has associated abnormal nail-fold microscopy.

LABORATORY TESTS

- CBC, serum electrolytes, blood urea nitrogen, creatinine, ESR, ANAs, VDRL antibody test, rheumatoid factor, and urinalysis should be included in the initial evaluation.
- If the history, physical examination, and initial laboratory tests suggest a possible secondary cause, specific serologic testing (e.g., anticentromere antibodies, anti-Scl 70, cryoglobulins, complement testing, and serum protein electrophoresis) may be indicated.
- Noninvasive vascular testing includes finger systolic blood pressures, segmental blood pressure measurements, cold recovery time (measure vasoconstrictor and vasodilator responses of finger to cold), fingertip thermography, and laser Doppler with thermal challenge (measures relative change in skin blood flow with ambient warming).

IMAGING STUDIES

- The diagnosis of RP should not be made on the basis of laboratory tests, and imaging studies should not replace a good history and physical examination.
- Duplex ultrasound can image the palmar arch and digital arteries for patency.
- Magnetic resonance angiography is useful for imaging larger arteries.
- Contrast angiography is the gold standard for arterial imaging.
- Nail-fold capillary microscopy can differentiate primary from secondary RP.
- Videomicroscopy and thermography are also useful for diagnosis of RP.

Rx TREATMENT

NONPHARMACOLOGIC THERAPY

- Avoid drugs that may precipitate RP (see "Etiology").
- Avoid cold exposure and sudden temperature shifts. Use warm gloves, hats, and garments during the winter months or before going into cold environments (e.g., air-conditioned rooms).
- Avoid stressful situations, and use relaxation techniques in preventing RP attacks.

ACUTE GENERAL Rx

- Acute measures to terminate an attack include rotating the arms in a windmill pattern, placing the hands under warm water or in a warm body fold such as the axilla, and the swing-arm maneuver.
- Medications are indicated in the treatment of RP if there are signs of critical ischemia or if the quality of life of the patient is affected to the degree that activities of normal living are no longer possible and preventive techniques do not work. Table 2 summarizes drugs commonly used in Raynaud phenomenon.

CHRONIC Rx

- Dihydropyridine calcium channel blockers (e.g., nifedipine, amlodipine, felodipine, nisoldipine, isradipine) are the most effective pharmacologic treatment for RP and are the drugs of choice. Amlodipine or nifedipine are commonly used.
- Amlodipine dosage ranges from 2.5 to 10 mg/day. Nifedipine is most often prescribed at a dose of 10 to 20 mg 30 min before cold exposure. If symptoms occur with long duration, nifedipine XL 30 to 180 mg PO qd is often effective.
- When calcium channel blockers do not appropriately control symptoms, phosphodiesterase inhibitors (cilostazol, pentoxifylline, and sildenafil) can be added or substituted. Sildenafil can be started at a dosage of 20 mg/day. Angiotensin 2 receptor antagonists (losartan), and selective serotonin reuptake inhibitors (fluoxetine) have also been used with some limited success.
- Some potential therapeutic options include direct vasodilators such as nitroprusside, hydralazine, papaverine, minoxidil, niacin, and griseofulvin. Topical 1% nitroglycerin or topical l-arginine, ethyl nicotinate, hexyl nicotinate, thurfyl salicylate may also be useful, particularly if low blood pressure is a concern.
- Alpha receptor antagonists such as prazosin and phenoxybenzamine have also shown some effectiveness in treating RP.
- The prostaglandins, including inhaled iloprost, IV epoprostenol, alprostadil, and tadalafil, may be promising in severe RP. However, additional experience and controlled studies are needed.

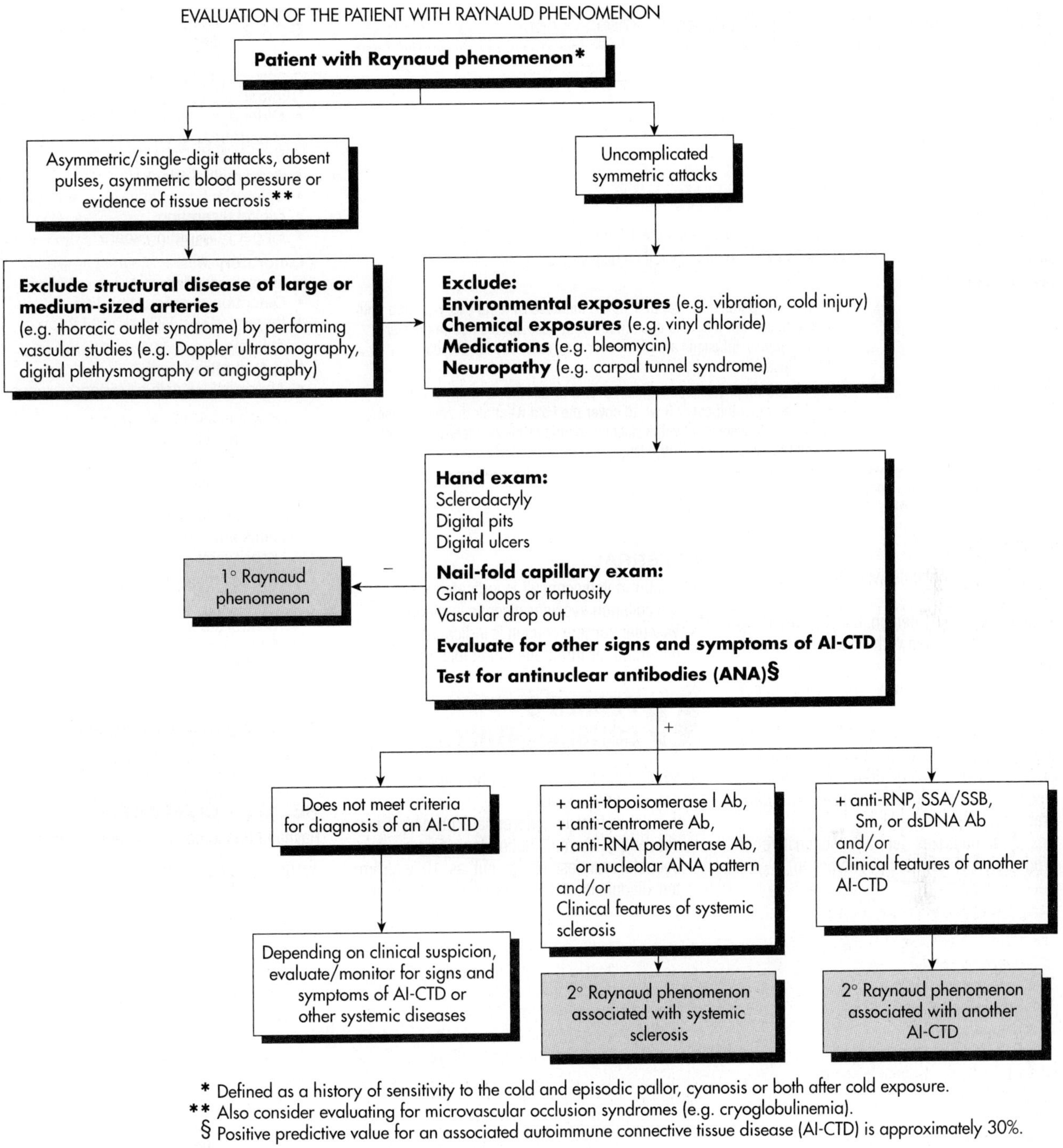

FIG. 2 Evaluation of the patient with Raynaud phenomenon. *ds*, Double-stranded; *RNP*, ribonucleoprotein; *Sm*, Smith. (From Bolognia J. *Dermatology*, ed 4, Philadelphia, 2018, Elsevier.)

- Antioxidants like zinc gluconate have been used to decrease tissue damage.
- *N*-Acetylcysteine and probucol have been shown to lead to improvement in RP.
- Anticoagulation with IV unfractionated heparin or subcutaneous low–molecular-weight heparin and addition of aspirin can be considered during the acute phase of a severe ischemic event. Aspirin (81 mg/day) therapy can be considered in all patients with secondary RP with a history of ischemic ulcers or thrombotic events; however, caution should be exercised because aspirin can theoretically worsen vasospasm by the inhibition of prostacyclin. Long-term anticoagulation with heparin or warfarin is not recommended unless there is evidence of a hypercoagulable state.
- Bypass surgery can be performed for severe RP associated with reconstructible arterial occlusive disease.
- Sympathectomy is available for unreconstructible occlusive disease or pure vasospastic disease refractory to medical treatment.
- Microsurgical revascularization of the hand and digital reconstruction may improve digital vascular perfusion and heal digital ulcers when proximal arterial occlusion is associated with digital vasospasm.
- Ischemic digital lesions should be treated with topical antibiotics and daily cleansing with soap and water. Digits that progress to dry gangrene should be permitted to undergo autoamputation. Surgical amputation is limited for intractable pain or deep tissue infection.

TABLE 2 Drugs Commonly Used in Raynaud Phenomenon

Drug	Dosage
Oral	
Nifedipine (or other long-acting calcium channel blocker)	10-20 mg bid or tid
Sildenafil	25-50 mg tid
Naftidrofuryl oxalate	100-200 mg tid
Inositol nicotinate	1 g tid or inositol nicotinate forte 1.5 g bid
Thymoxamine	40-80 mg qid (stop after 2 wk if no response)
Intravenous Infusion	
Iloprost	Start infusion (peripheral line) at 1 μg/hr; increase by 1 μg every 30 min until reach maximum tolerable dose (maximum dose should not be greater than 3 μg/hr). Infusions are given over 6 hr each day for 3-7 days on each occasion.
Prostaglandin E_1	60 μg in 250-ml physiologic infusion over 3 hr daily for 5-6 days. This could be repeated every 6 wk to cover the cold weather in severe cases, especially if associated with critical ischemia or digital ulceration, and should be given via a central line.

bid, Twice a day; *qid,* four times a day; *tid,* three times a day.
From Hochberg MC: *Rheumatology,* ed 7, Philadelphia, 2019, Elsevier.

BOX 2 Features Suggestive of Progression of RP

Clinical
- Older age at onset (>35 yr)
- Recurrence of chilblains as adult
- Vasospasm all year round
- Asymmetric attacks
- Sclerodactyly or any other sign of CTD
- Digital ulceration
- Finger pulp pitting scars

Laboratory
- Increased inflammatory markers
- Detection of autoantibodies
- Increased von Willebrand factor antigen

Nail-fold Microscopy
- Abnormal vessels on videomicroscopy

CTD, Connective tissue disorder.
From Hochberg MC: *Rheumatology,* ed 7, Philadelphia, 2019, Elsevier.

DISPOSITION

The prognosis of patients with RP depends on the etiology.

- Primary RP is fairly benign, usually remaining stable and controlled with nonpharmacologic medical treatment.
- Remission of primary RP can occur spontaneously.
- Patients with secondary RP, specifically those with scleroderma, CREST syndrome, or thromboangiitis obliterans, may develop severe ischemic digits with ulceration, gangrene, and autoamputation.
- Box 2 summarizes features suggestive of progression of Raynaud phenomenon.

REFERRAL

- Rheumatology consult is indicated if secondary collagen vascular disease is diagnosed.
- Vascular surgery consult is indicated if ulcers, gangrene, or threatened digit loss is noted.

PEARLS & CONSIDERATIONS

- Most patients with RP can be managed by a primary care provider.
- It is important to differentiate primary from secondary forms. Secondary forms may become manifest as far out as 10 yr from the diagnosis of RP. It is important to take immediate action during an attack, and patients are encouraged to:
  1. Keep warm
  2. Not use tobacco products
  3. Avoid aggravating medications
  4. Control stress
  5. Exercise
  6. Follow up with a physician

SUGGESTED READINGS

Available at ExpertConsult.com

RELATED CONTENT

Raynaud Phenomenon (Patient Information)

AUTHOR: **Fred F. Ferri, MD**

BASIC INFORMATION

DEFINITION

Renal abscess and perinephric abscess are purulent complications of an underlying urinary infection of the ascending tract with an obstructed pyelonephritis. Predisposing factors include diabetes and renal stones. There is lobar necrosis with renal abscess and perirenal fat necrosis in perinephric abscess.

SYNONYMS

Intrarenal abscess
Perinephric abscess
Kidney abscess

ICD-10CM CODE

N15.1 Renal and perinephric abscess

EPIDEMIOLOGY & DEMOGRAPHICS

INCIDENCE: Ranges from 1 to 10 per 10,000 hospital admissions

PREDOMINANT SEX & AGE: In one study, median age was 59.8 yr

RISK FACTORS: Diabetes and renal stones

PHYSICAL FINDINGS & CLINICAL PRESENTATION

- Symptoms include fever, flank pain, abdominal pain, and urinary frequency or dysuria.
- At times, renal abscess can present insidiously in the elderly or persons with diabetes.

ETIOLOGY

These infections may be a complication of a urinary tract infection that ascends to the upper tract, usually due to gram-negative bacteria, or a complication of a bacteremia with hematogenous seeding to the kidney, usually secondary to a *Staphylococcus aureus* infection.

DIAGNOSIS

DIFFERENTIAL DIAGNOSIS

- Acute pyelonephritis with papillary necrosis
- Acute lobar nephronia: Acute nonsuppurative renal infection
- Renal cell carcinoma
- Malakoplakia: Rare granulomatous inflammatory disease seen with *Escherichia coli* infection
- Emphysematous pyelonephritis: Gas formation within the renal parenchyma caused by infection by facultative anaerobes or *Candida* spp.

WORKUP

Combination of laboratory tests and imaging

LABORATORY TESTS

- Blood cultures, urine cultures, urinalysis, and CBC are basic tests.
- Elevated ESR or C-reactive protein may be marker for a deep-seated infection.

IMAGING STUDIES

- Ultrasound may show thick-walled fluid-filled cavity in renal parenchyma. A perinephric abscess is confined to the perinephric space by Gerota fascia.
- CT with contrast (Fig. E1) is preferred over ultrasound for the diagnosis.
- MRI and nuclear scans are of limited value.

TREATMENT

Antibiotic therapy and, when necessary, interventional radiology or surgical drainage procedure

NONPHARMACOLOGIC THERAPY

- Therapy for a renal abscess greater than 5 cm in diameter should be percutaneous drainage by CT- or US-guided therapy along with intravenous antibiotics.
- A perinephric abscess should be drained percutaneously with CT or US guidance.
- At times a nephrectomy may be required for severe cases, usually in diabetic patients.

ACUTE GENERAL Rx

A renal abscess less than 5 cm in diameter can be treated successfully with targeted intravenous therapy (92% success rate for abscess 3-5 cm in diameter). Antibiotic choices are based on culture results but initially should target gram-negative bacteria unless infection is secondary to staphylococcal bacteremia. Empiric antibiotic therapy in geographic areas where fluoroquinolone resistance rates are <10% consists of ciprofloxacin 400 mg IV loading dose. In areas with high fluoroquinolone resistance rates, ceftriaxone 1 g IV is appropriate. If perinephric abscess is associated with staphylococcal bacteremia, give IV nafcillin if methicillin-susceptible *Staphylococcus aureus* (MSSA) or vancomycin 1 g IV q12h if methicillin-resistant *S. aureus*.

CHRONIC Rx

Antibiotic therapy generally continues for 2 to 3 wk, some of which can be completed with oral therapy.

DISPOSITION

Antibiotics such as trimethoprim-sulfamethoxazole and quinolone antibiotics penetrate well in the kidney and are ideal oral agents for therapy.

REFERRAL

Interventional radiology, urologic surgeon, and infectious diseases consult

PEARLS & CONSIDERATIONS

COMMENTS

This diagnosis should be considered in patients who are being treated for pyelonephritis with appropriate antibiotics and fail to respond clinically after 5 days.

PREVENTION

Early and targeted therapy for urinary tract infections, especially in diabetic patients

SUGGESTED READINGS

Available at ExpertConsult.com

RELATED CONTENT

Pyelonephritis (Related Key Topic)
Urinary Tract Infection (Related Key Topic)

AUTHOR: **Glenn G. Fort, MD, MPH**

Renal Artery Stenosis

BASIC INFORMATION

DEFINITION

Renal artery stenosis (RAS) is the progressive narrowing of the renal artery, which is most commonly due to atherosclerosis or fibromuscular dysplasia (FMD). RAS is an important, potentially reversible cause of hypertension, ischemic nephropathy, and destabilizing cardiac syndromes. RAS increases the risk of renal artery occlusion via progressive stenosis.

SYNONYMS

Fibromuscular disease
FMD
RAS
Renovascular disease

ICD-10CM CODES

Q27.1	Congenital renal artery stenosis
I70.1	Atherosclerosis of renal artery
I15.0	Renovascular hypertension
I77.9	Disorder of arteries and arterioles, unspecified

EPIDEMIOLOGY & DEMOGRAPHICS

- ARAS:
  1. Atherosclerotic RAS (ARAS) accounts for about 90% of cases. Its true prevalence is unknown.
     a. General population autopsy studies: 10%, 27% over 50 yr; hypertensive patients, 0.2% to 5%.
     b. In a general population older than 65 yr, the prevalence is 6.8% by Doppler ultrasound (5.5% of women, 9.1% of men; 6.7% of African Americans and 6.9% of Caucasians). Bilateral disease was present in 12% of afflicted individuals.
     c. In patients with malignant hypertension, the prevalence is 43% in Caucasians and 7% in African Americans. In patients with mild hypertension, the prevalence is <1%.
     d. In patients with peripheral artery disease, the prevalence is 22% to 59%.
- FMD:
  2. FMD accounts for approximately 10% of chronic RAS and typically encountered in women (90%). FMD was previously thought to be a disease of the young and healthy with few risk factors. Recent data suggest the average age of onset of hypertension is 43 yr. Bilateral renal artery involvement is seen in 25% to 35% of cases.

ETIOLOGY

- Atherosclerosis: ARAS has similar risk factors to atherosclerosis in other vascular beds, including family history, smoking, diabetes, hypertension, and hyperlipidemia. ARAS most often involves the ostium and proximal third of the main renal artery.
- Fibromuscular dysplasia (FMD) (Figs 1 and 2): Etiology unknown. Classified into three categories based on the affected layer of arterial wall: Medial (>90%), intimal (<10%), adventitial (<1%). FMD typically involves the distal main renal artery and intrarenal branches.

PATHOGENESIS

- Pathogenesis of fibromuscular dysplasia is unknown. Fibromuscular dysplasia involves abnormal constrictions and dilations of the renal artery, leading to a typical "string of beads" appearance on angiography.
- The pathogenesis of atherosclerotic RAS is similar to that of atherosclerosis in other vascular beds.
- The pathogenesis of renovascular hypertension is related to the neurohormonal cascade resulting from renal ischemia. Renal hypoperfusion or ischemia secondary to arterial stenosis produces an increase in plasma renin and secondary elevations of angiotensin II, with consequent vasoconstriction, aldosterone elevation, sodium retention, and potassium wasting. Hypertension results and can be self-sustaining, even in the case of unilateral RAS due to hypertensive damage of the contralateral kidney.
- The pathogenesis of ischemic nephropathy is due to the activation of numerous mechanisms of tissue injury resulting in progressive tubular cell loss and fibrosis. On histology, glomeruli are usually preserved but often collapsed.
- "Flash" or sudden-onset pulmonary edema, a manifestation usually seen in bilateral ARAS, results from sodium and water retention as well as upregulation of the sympathetic nervous system.

NATURAL HISTORY

- RAS caused by fibromuscular dysplasia rarely causes renal artery occlusion or ischemic nephropathy.
- ARAS rarely progresses to total occlusion. One study of serial ultrasounds of patients with RAS demonstrated that those with >60% stenosis progressed to total occlusion in 1 yr in just 5% of cases; an additional 11% progressed to total occlusion by 2 yr.

PHYSICAL FINDINGS & CLINICAL PRESENTATION

Progressive RAS:
- RAS should be considered in any white female of age <30 yr with hypertension not attributed to any other cause, any patient of age >50 yr with new-onset refractory hypertension, or a patient with stable hypertension that has abruptly and/or significantly worsened.
- RAS most often presents as a clinically asymptomatic finding. Manifestations can include renovascular hypertension, ischemic nephropathy, or flash pulmonary edema.
- Flash pulmonary edema in the absence of cardiac disease most often indicates severe bilateral renal artery stenosis.
- Renovascular hypertension should be considered if blood pressure control remains suboptimal on a medication regimen that includes 3 maximally dosed medications, one of which is a diuretic.
- Ischemic nephropathy should be considered if kidney function is rapidly deteriorating or kidney sizes are decreasing on serial imaging, particularly with bilateral disease.
- Acute elevations of serum creatinine (>30%) after starting angiotensin–converting-enzyme inhibitors (ACEIs) or angiotensin receptor blockers (ARBs) may be seen in bilateral disease.
- A bruit heard in either upper quadrant on abdominal auscultation may suggest RAS. Patients with atherosclerotic RAS will often have bruits heard in other vascular beds.

Dx DIAGNOSIS

SCREENING

American College of Cardiology and American Heart Association (ACC/AHA) guidelines

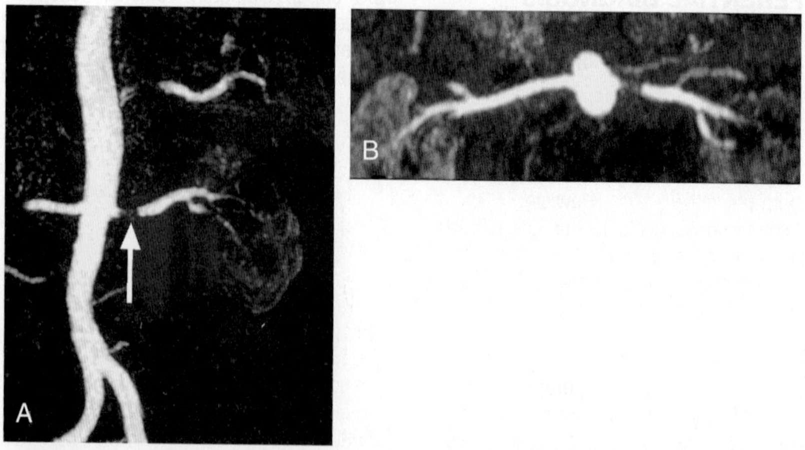

FIG. 1 Magnetic resonance angiogram. A, Coronal maximum intensity projection (MIP) of a patient with significant left renal artery stenosis *(white arrow).* **B,** Axial MIP of the same patient. (From Adam A et al: *Grainger & Allison's diagnostic radiology,* ed 5, 2007, Churchill Livingstone. In Grant LA: *Grainger & Allison's diagnostic radiology essentials,* ed 2, 2019, Elsevier.)

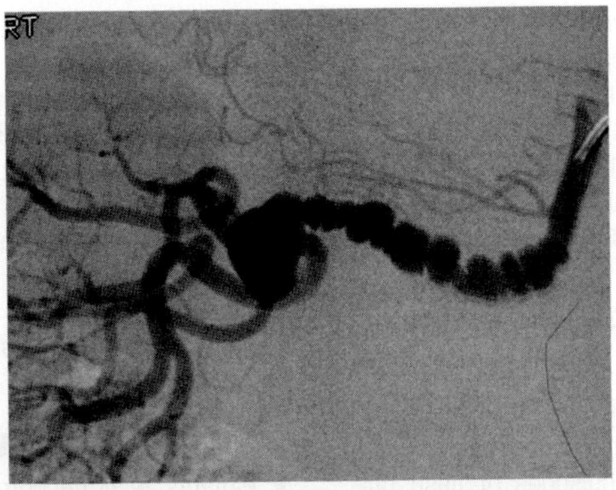

FIG. 2 Fibromuscular dysplasia. On a selective right anterior oblique (RAO) digital subtraction angiogram, the characteristic saccular dilatations and web-like stenoses are clearly evident. (From Adam A et al: *Grainger & Allison's diagnostic radiology,* ed 5, 2007, Churchill Livingstone. In Grant LA: *Grainger & Allison's diagnostic radiology essentials,* ed 2, 2019, Elsevier.)

for identification of patients who should be screened for RAS:

- Onset of hypertension at age <30 yr or severe hypertension at age >55 yr
- Clinical findings that suggest secondary hypertension as opposed to essential hypertension in the absence of a more likely cause of secondary hypertension such as pheochromocytoma
- Malignant hypertension: Hypertension with coexistent evidence of acute end-organ damage (acute renal failure, acute decompensated heart failure, new visual or neurologic disturbance, and/or advanced retinopathy)
- Accelerated hypertension: Sudden and persistent worsening of previously controlled hypertension
- Resistant hypertension: Full doses of a 3-drug regimen that includes a diuretic
- Sudden unexplained pulmonary edema
- New acute kidney injury following initiation of an ACEI or ARB
- Unexplained atrophic kidney or variation in size of both kidneys by >1.5 cm, smaller kidney likely affected by RAS

LABORATORY TESTS

- Basic chemistry panel including sodium, potassium, blood urea nitrogen, and serum creatinine
- Urinalysis
- Renal vein renin sampling helps determine whether one or both kidneys are overproducing renin in cases of suspected renovascular hypertension (RVH). A positive result has strong predictive value. However, 50% of patients with no evidence for lateralization can still respond to unilateral intervention. This procedure is rarely performed except in specialized hypertension centers

IMAGING STUDIES

Renal Duplex Doppler ultrasonography, CT angiography, and magnetic resonance angiography (MRA) are effective diagnostic screening methods. The choice of imaging modality will depend on the availability of the diagnostic tool, the experience and local accuracy of each modality, patient characteristics including body size, renal function, and contrast allergy, and the presence of prior stents.

RENAL DOPPLER ULTRASOUND:

- Renal Doppler is a noninvasive, inexpensive screening study, and it can determine whether a stenosis of >60% is present.
- Abnormal results in RAS:
  1. Peak systolic velocity (PSV) >250 cm/sec
  2. Peak diastolic velocity >150 cm/sec
  3. Renal-to-aortic ratio (RAR) >3.5
  4. Acceleration time >100 msec
  5. Exact definitions of a positive renal Doppler for RAS varies by institution
- Compared to renal angiography, Doppler studies have shown varied performance, with a sensitivity of 84% to 98% and a specificity of 62% to 99%.
- Limitations include high user variability. Valid test performance requires technicians who perform a high volume of these tests to reduce user error. If significant user variability exists at certain institutions, renal Doppler may be excluded from the diagnostic algorithm. Patients with a large body habitus may have limited imaging results. It is not as sensitive or specific as MR or CT methods. Detection of RAS is limited to identifying whether stenosis of 60% to 99% is present.
- Duplex Doppler is a good modality for monitoring patency following therapeutic, vascular stent insertion.

MAGNETIC RESONANCE ANGIOGRAPHY (MRA):

- MRA provides good visualization of main and accessory renal arteries. The test has high sensitivity (90%-100%) and a specificity (76%-94%). MRA is superior to renal Doppler ultrasonography and equivalent to CT angiography.
- Benefits include the lack of exposure to iodine contrast or radiation.
- Limitations include claustrophobia, high cost, and inability to image within a previously placed metallic stent.

COMPUTED TOMOGRAPHY ANGIOGRAPHY (CTA):

- CTA is rapid and effective. When compared with angiography, this modality has a sensitivity of 59% to 96% and a specificity of 82% to 99%. It is superior to renal Doppler ultrasonography and equivalent to MRA. Contrast uptake in kidneys can also be used to estimate the viability of affected kidneys.
- CTA has good spatial resolution and can detect restenosis through metal stents.
- CTA can be used more easily than MRA in obese or claustrophobic patients.
- Limitations include radiation exposure and potentially nephrotoxic, iodinated radiocontrast exposure to CKD patients. Heavily calcified arteries may appear narrower than in actuality.

DIRECT ANGIOGRAPHY:

- IV digital subtraction angiography (DSA) has an 88% sensitivity and 90% specificity. It is the gold standard for anatomic diagnosis of RAS. It is not a first-line screening tool and recommended after a positive noninvasive test. DSA is used when there is a high clinical suspicion for RAS with inconclusive noninvasive tests and when the decision has already been made that correction of stenosis will produce clinical benefit. DSA allows for angioplasty with stenting during the same procedure. Renal fractional flow reserve at the time of DSA can evaluate the severity of RAS during maximal vasodilatation.
- This modality is reserved for patients with a high likelihood of intervention.
- Limitations include its invasive nature, i.e., requirement for intraaortic catheterization that may lead to aortic and renal artery trauma and/or dissection, rupture, thrombosis, or embolization.
- Procedure requires a certified interventionalist (radiologist, cardiologist, nephrologist, or vascular surgeon).
- Procedure requires iodinated contrast that must be used cautiously with CKD. Carbon dioxide contrast imaging and limiting image acquisition number reduce kidney injury risk.

NUCLEAR RENOGRAPHY (WITHOUT CAPTOPRIL): A noninvasive test conducted when renal atrophy is present to document differential kidney function. This test is useful when determining whether to revascularize an atrophic kidney or to remove it. Atrophic kidneys with <20% differential renal function are unlikely contributing to overall renal functional decline, but may still contribute to renovascular hypertension.

Rx TREATMENT

ACUTE GENERAL Rx

The treatment of RAS is targeted to the clinical presentation:

- Asymptomatic disease requires no treatment.
- Patients with chronic hypertension in the setting of incidentally discovered RAS require only antihypertensive medical therapy.
- When RVH is suspected, initial therapy is by antihypertensive therapy, specifically medications that block the renin-angiotensin-aldosterone system (RAAS). As discussed later, failure to control blood pressure on an aggressive regimen is a reason to consider renal revascularization.

- Patients with ischemic nephropathy should be considered for intervention only if the renal function is declining rapidly or flash pulmonary edema occurs in the setting of bilateral RAS.

PHARMACOLOGIC THERAPY

- Because of RAAS activation, ACEIs or ARBs are recommended and well-tolerated (92%) as treatment of RVH. Kidney function should be monitored carefully when initiating or titrating these medications, particularly when bilateral RAS (78% tolerability) or unilateral stenosis with a solitary kidney is present to avoid precipitating AKI.
- Diuretics should be considered in patients with congestive heart failure or flash pulmonary edema.
- Antiplatelet therapy and statin therapy.

NONPHARMACOLOGIC THERAPY

- If blood pressure is not controlled by medications alone, flash pulmonary edema occurs, or kidney function rapidly declines, referral for renal angiography, angioplasty, or stenting may be indicated.
- Angioplasty without stenting is insufficient for atherosclerotic lesions due to a high failure rate of adequate dilation of the artery or a high rate of restenosis.
- Occasionally, a kidney that has lost function from RAS may cause refractory hypertension. This situation would be discovered only by renal vein renin sampling in a patient with unilateral renal atrophy. In such cases, nephrectomy of the atrophied kidney may be the best method to control blood pressure.
- Renal artery bypass is rarely required.
- If RAS is suspected as the cause of flash pulmonary edema or rapidly declining kidney function, bilateral disease is likely. If confirmed by angiography, both renal arteries should be stented.
- Hypertension is rarely cured with revascularization of RAS due to longstanding hypertension. The goal of intervention is blood pressure control and its reduction.
- The ACC/AHA guidelines for clinical indications of renal artery revascularization in the presence of significant stenosis include:
  1. Accelerated, resistant, or malignant hypertension (class IIa)
  2. Hypertension with unilateral small kidney (class IIa)
  3. Hypertension with intolerance to medication (class IIa)
  4. Treatment of cardiac destabilization syndromes such as unexplained heart failure exacerbations or episodes of flash pulmonary edema (class I) and refractory or unstable angina (class IIa)
  5. Progressive chronic kidney disease with bilateral RAS or RAS associated with a solitary functioning kidney (class IIa)
- Many patients who meet these criteria will not demonstrate a beneficial response to renal revascularization. Careful patient selection for angiography and intervention is obvious.
- Multiple randomized controlled trials (e.g., ASTRAL, CORAL, DRASTIC, and STAR) have shown no benefit of revascularization versus medical therapy, with end points of blood pressure control, renal function, and cardiovascular events. Therefore, it is recommended that the decision to refer a patient for revascularization be made by specialists who are practiced and skilled in handling hypertension and RAS.

FIBROMUSCULAR DYSPLASIA

- Medical therapy should include an ACEI or ARB to control blood pressure unless severe bilateral disease is present (rare).
- RVH from fibromuscular dysplasia (FMD) is often cured by renal artery revascularization because many younger patients do not have background essential hypertension.
- In most cases, patients should be referred for renal artery angioplasty regardless of whether blood pressure can be controlled medically.
- Stenting is not appropriate in patients with FMD because angioplasty alone usually yields a durable result. In addition, recurrence of FMD is common, and the presence of stents may hinder additional interventions.
- Renal artery bypass may be necessary in patients whose FMD recurs multiple times or in whom angioplasty failed to yield an improvement in blood pressure.

DISPOSITION & REFERRAL

- Patients with uncontrolled hypertension on multiple agents should be referred for management by a hypertension specialist.
- Percutaneous intervention for atherosclerotic RAS must be reserved for selected patients until further data are available.

PEARLS & CONSIDERATIONS

- Renal artery stenosis is most commonly an incidental finding and clinically silent.
- Renal artery stenosis may present as hypertension, renal dysfunction, or both, or flash pulmonary edema.
- Stenting is inappropriate for most patients with RAS. Consideration should be made only in high-risk patients and after consultation with a specialist in the field.
- The modality for the type of imaging should depend on the expertise of the institution.

SUGGESTED READINGS

Available at ExpertConsult.com

RELATED CONTENT

Renal Artery Stenosis (Patient Information)
Hypertension (Related Key Topic)

AUTHOR: **Kausik Umanth, MD, MS, FASN**

BASIC INFORMATION

DEFINITION

Renal cell carcinoma (RCC) is a primary carcinoma originating in the renal parenchyma from the malignant transformation of proximal renal tubular epithelial cells. The majority of renal cell cancers are of clear cell type; papillary tumors comprise 15%, and chromophobe cancers comprise 10%.

SYNONYMS

Hypernephroma
RCC
Renal cell adenocarcinoma

ICD-10CM CODES

C64.9	Malignant neoplasm of kidney, except renal pelvis
C64.1	Malignant neoplasm of right kidney, except renal pelvis
C64.2	Malignant neoplasm of left kidney, except renal pelvis
C64.9	Malignant neoplasm of unspecified kidney, except renal pelvis
C65.9	Malignant neoplasm of renal pelvis

EPIDEMIOLOGY & DEMOGRAPHICS

INCIDENCE: In 2020, there were an estimated 73,750 new cases and 14,830 deaths in the U.S. Two percent of cases of renal cancer are associated with inherited syndromes.

PREDOMINANT SEX: Male:female ratio is approximately 2:1.

PREDOMINANT AGE: Peak incidence is at age 50 to 70 yr.

PHYSICAL FINDINGS & CLINICAL PRESENTATION

Patients are often asymptomatic until they have advanced disease. Paraneoplastic syndromes such as hypercalcemia, erythrocytosis, anemia, and hepatic dysfunction may occur with renal cell carcinoma. The classic triad of flank pain, hematuria, and a palpable abdominal mass currently represents an unusual presentation. Current presenting findings in RCC include:

Hematuria	50%-60%
Elevated erythrocyte sedimentation rate	50%-60%
Abdominal mass	25%-45%
Anemia	20%-40%
Flank pain	35%-40%
Hypertension	20%-40%
Weight loss	30%-35%
Fever	5%-15%
Hepatic dysfunction	10%-15%
Classic triad (hematuria, abdominal mass, flank pain)	5%-10%
Hypercalcemia	3%-6%
Erythrocytosis	3%-4%
Varicocele	2%-3%

ETIOLOGY

Hereditary forms:
- Familial renal carcinoma
- Renal carcinoma associated with Von Hippel-Lindau disease
- Hereditary papillary renal cell carcinoma

Risk factors:
- Cigarette smoking
- Obesity
- Phenacetin-containing analgesics
- Asbestos, lead, Thorotrast, and chromium exposure
- Gasoline and other petroleum products
- Role of the *VHL* gene on chromosome 3

DIAGNOSIS

DIFFERENTIAL DIAGNOSIS

- Transitional cell carcinomas of the renal pelvis (8% of all renal cancers)
- Wilms tumor
- Other primary renal carcinomas and sarcomas
- Renal cysts
- Retroperitoneal tumors

WORKUP

LABORATORY TESTS:
- Urinalysis: Hematuria
- Complete blood count: Anemia or erythrocytosis
- Chemistry panel: Renal failure and electrolyte issues, including hypercalcemia
- Liver function tests: Hepatic dysfunction with elevated alkaline phosphatase, prolonged prothrombin time, and hypoalbuminemia

IMAGING STUDIES

Nearly 50% of renal cancers are now detected because a renal mass is incidentally detected on radiographic evaluation.
- Renal ultrasound
- Abdominal CT scan with contrast (Fig. E1 and Fig. E2); CT-guided biopsy is generally not necessary for diagnosis of solid masses >4 cm (high likelihood of cancer)
- MRI
- Renal arteriogram
- Intravenous pyelography

STAGING

See Table 1.

COMMON SITES OF METASTASES

Lung	50%-60%
Bone	30%-40%
Regional nodes	15%-30%
Main renal vein	15%-20%
Perirenal fat	10%-20%
Adrenal (ipsilateral)	10%-15%
Vena cava	10%-15%
Brain	10%-15%
Adjacent organs (colon, pancreas)	10%
Kidney (contralateral)	2%

TREATMENT

- Surgery:
  1. Surgical nephrectomy (open procedure or laparoscopic approach) is the only effective management for stages I, II, and some stage III tumors. Although radical nephrectomy had long been the standard treatment, retrospective studies have shown that partial rather than radical nephrectomy is associated with improved survival and is appropriate for patients with renal cell neoplasms <4 cm that are not adjacent to the renal pelvis or invading the vena cava.
  2. Laparoscopic robotic-assisted nephrectomy has been adopted in multiple centers, primarily for nephron-sparing surgery in the case of tumors <4 cm. Advantages include less blood loss, minimal effects on renal function, and similar oncologic outcomes. Disadvantages include increased costs and limitations in tumor size and locations eligible for robotic surgery.
  3. Various forms of partial nephrectomy may be available for patients with bilateral cancers or with a solitary kidney.
  4. Cytoreductive nephrectomy in patients with metastatic RCC before immunotherapy improved survival in patients compared with immunotherapy alone on the basis of randomized trials data. However, recent results from the randomized Clinical Trial to Assess the Importance of Nephrectomy (CARMENA) demonstrated no benefit for intermediate- and poor-risk patients in the setting of modern tyrosine kinase inhibitor (sunitinib) therapy. Additional trials data are awaited to assess the role of nephrectomy in favorable risk patients and with the use of neoadjuvant tyrosine kinase inhibitor therapy.
- Angioinfarction, cryoablation, or radiotherapy (for palliation).
- Systemic therapy:
  1. Risk stratification using prognostic scoring systems such as the International mRCC Database Consortium Prognostic Model (IMDC score) is the initial step in planning systemic therapy. Absence of any of the following risk factors confers the most favorable risk status (IMDC-Fav), one to two risk factors increase this to intermediate risk (IMDC-Int), and a patient with three or more risk factors has poor-risk disease (IMDC-Poor):
     a. Karnofsky performance status less than 80%
     b. Time from diagnosis to treatment <1 yr
     c. Hemoglobin concentration < lower limit of normal
     d. Serum calcium > upper limit of normal
     e. Neutrophil count > upper limit of normal
     f. Platelet count > upper limit of normal

TABLE 1 TNM Staging of Renal Cell Carcinomas as per the AJCC Eighth Edition

T Stage	Description
T_x	Tumor cannot be assessed
T_1: Tumor ≤7 cm, limited to kidney	T_{1a}: Tumor <4 cm T_{1b}: Tumor ≥4 cm to ≤7 cm
T_2: Tumor >7 cm, limited to kidney	T_{2a}: Tumor >7 cm but ≤10 cm T_{2b}: Tumor >10 cm
T_3: Tumor extending into major veins or perinephric tissue but not into ipsilateral adrenal gland or beyond Gerota fascia	T_{3a}: Tumor extends to renal vein/branches or invades perirenal and/or renal sinus fat T_{3b}: Tumor extends into IVC below diaphragm T_{3c}: Tumor extends into IVC above diaphragm or wall of IVC
T_4	Tumor invades beyond Gerota fascia (including contiguous extension into ipsilateral adrenal gland)
N stage	**Description**
N_x	Regional nodes cannot be assessed
N_1	No regional nodes involved
N_2	Metastasis in regional node(s)
M stage	**Description**
M_0	No distant metastases
M_1	Distant metastasis present
Stage	**TNM grouping**
I	$T_1N_0M_0$
II	$T_2N_0M_0$
III	$T_3N_0M_0$ or $T_{1-3}N_1M_0$
IV	$T_4N_{any}M_{any}$ or $T_{any}N_{any}M_1$

AJCC, American Joint Committee on Cancer; *IVC*, intravenous cholangiography; *TNM*, tumor, node, metastases.

2. Until recently, monotherapy with multi-targeted kinase inhibitors was the initial option for treatment of metastatic cancers followed by the use of mTOR inhibitors as second-line therapy. However, the evolving data with the use of immunotherapy has now moved combinations of dual immunotherapy combinations or immunotherapy/targeted therapy combinations to the frontline as initial therapy in this setting:
   a. Checkpoint inhibitors: The checkpoint inhibitors have demonstrated efficacy in both treatment-naïve and previously treated patients. Combination checkpoint inhibition with ipilimumab plus nivolumab has demonstrated superior efficacy for patients with IMDC intermediate and poor risk treatment-naïve patients. Furthermore, therapeutic regimens combining tyrosine kinase inhibition plus immune checkpoint inhibition (axitinib plus pembrolizumab, axitinib plus avelumab) also have demonstrated superiority in all risk groups for compared to sunitinib monotherapy.
   b. Tyrosine kinase inhibitors: In patients with unresectable disease, therapy with the multi-targeted inhibitors axitinib, sunitinib, pazopanib, cabozantinib, lenvatinib, and sorafenib and also mTOR kinase inhibitors such as everolimus and temsirolimus can be used as therapy. The combination of lenvatinib plus everolimus has also been approved in second-line therapy after demonstrating improved outcomes compared to single-agent everolimus use. The majority of responses with these agents are typically either partial or stable disease, and relapse is the norm.
   c. Immunotherapy: High-dose interleukin-2 therapy may achieve a 15% response rate, which is often durable and associated with long-term survival in highly selected patients with excellent performance status. Severe toxicities associated with this therapy have limited the use of this approach.

PROGNOSIS

The 5-yr survival rate among patients with kidney cancer has increased from 57% in 1987 to 1989 to 74% in 2006 to 2012. The prognosis of surgically treated patients is shown in the following:

TNM Stage	5-yr Survival (%)
I	95
II	88
III (renal vein or vena cava)	50-60
III (nodal involvement)	15-25
IV	5-20

REFERRAL

- To urologist for staging and surgery
- To medical oncologist if metastatic disease is present

PEARLS & CONSIDERATIONS

- Patients should be considered for nephron-sparing surgery in case of smaller tumors (<4 cm).
- Laparoscopic robotic-assisted surgery is utilized for standard nephron-sparing surgery routinely; it is utilized for central tumors and tumors >4 cm in some experienced centers.
- Adjuvant therapy utilizing tyrosine kinase inhibitors has showed mixed results when used in the postresection setting and is not approved for use in this setting. An intergroup study showed no survival benefit, whereas a smaller study limited to high-risk patients showed a progression-free survival benefit.
- High-dose interleukin-2 can lead to long-term remissions in 10% to 15% of carefully selected patients.

SUGGESTED READINGS

Available at ExpertConsult.com

RELATED CONTENT

Kidney Cancer (Patient Information)

AUTHOR: **Bharti Rathore, MD**

BASIC INFORMATION

DEFINITION

Systemic lupus erythematosus (SLE) is a chronic autoimmune inflammatory disease that commonly results in a renal complication termed lupus nephritis (LN). There are several patterns of kidney injury, but the hallmark finding on a kidney biopsy is immune complex deposition containing IgG, IgA, IgM, C3, and C1q, a "full-house" immunofluorescence pattern.

SYNONYMS

Renal-limited lupus
LN
Lupus nephritis

ICD-10CM CODES

M32.14 Glomerular disease in systemic lupus erythematosus
M32.15 Tubulo-interstitial nephropathy in systemic lupus erythematosus
M32.10 Systemic lupus erythematosus, organ or system involved unspecified
M32.8 Other forms of systemic lupus erythematosus
M32.9 Systemic lupus erythematosus, unspecified

EPIDEMIOLOGY & DEMOGRAPHICS

INCIDENCE & PREVALENCE: The prevalence of SLE is highly variable worldwide. The incidence in U.S. is estimated at 144 per 100,000 persons with a female-to-male ratio as high as 15:1 during reproductive years and as low as 4:3 during prepubertal years. The frequency with which SLE patients develop LN is highly variable among different races and ethnicities (range, 29%-69%). Within the U.S., the LN frequency is higher in African Americans (up to 69%) after adjusting for socioeconomic factors. African-American and Hispanic SLE patients compared to Caucasian counterparts also have earlier onset of LN and overall poorer outcomes, including death and end-stage kidney disease (ESKD). The poorer outcomes and more aggressive LN may be explained by the higher incidence of diffuse proliferative LN. These differences are thought to arise from genetic predispositions that exist in the African American population, including APOL1, Fcγ RIIA-R131, and HLA-DRB181503. Developing LN conveys significant risk of morbidity and mortality for SLE patients. Although, 10% of LN patients progress to ESKD overall, 44% of class IV proliferative LN can progress to ESKD over 15 yr. Patients with LN survive less than other SLE patients without LN, resulting in a higher standardized mortality ratio of 6 as opposed to 2.4. Survival can be significantly improved (46%-95%) if disease remission is achieved. Other important factors contributing to increased risk of progression include delay in diagnosis and/or therapy, disease relapse, and medication non-compliance.

PHYSICAL FINDINGS & CLINICAL PRESENTATION

LN can present in isolation or with other manifestations of SLE. Clinical presentation is often discovered on urine examination rather than physical findings. Depending on the degree of proteinuria, patients may also have clinical manifestations of nephrotic syndrome including significant peripheral edema, foamy urine, and thrombotic events. If SLE is also present, patients can have a wide range of symptoms, including but not limited to fatigue, fever, arthralgia, rashes, oral ulcer, myalgias, photosensitivity, alopecia, and pleuritic chest pain.

ETIOLOGY

SLE is thought to arise from a genetic predisposition to autoimmunity combined with environmental triggers. This combination leads to neutrophil activation, increased interferon levels, upregulation of proinflammatory factors, and autoantibody production. Autoantibodies commonly target DNA and bind with self-antigens to form circulating immune complexes that deposit in glomeruli, especially in the mesangium, subendothelial, and/or subepithelial space. The location of deposition and type of immune complex differentiates the findings on kidney biopsy. Immune complexes promote inflammation and cellular injury via proinflammatory cytokines, recruitment of proinflammatory leukocytes, and mesangial cellular proliferation. Additional contributory mechanisms that enhance inflammation include direct anti–double-stranded DNA binding to glomerular structures, anti-C1q and C3b antibodies, neutrophil extracellular traps (NETs), and complement system activation. After the autoimmune inflammatory process is initiated, it self-perpetuates and amplifies with more pronounced symptoms and organ damage.

DIAGNOSIS

DIFFERENTIAL DIAGNOSIS

- ANCA vasculitis
- Anti-glomerular basement membrane disease
- Membranoproliferative glomerulonephritis
- Cryoglobulinemic vasculitis
- Infection-related glomerulonephritis
- IgA nephropathy

As SLE patients have multiple other complaints and comorbidities, other non-lupus causes of kidney dysfunction should be explored, especially if urinalysis and microscopy are unrevealing.

WORKUP

- Given the high frequency of kidney involvement, all SLE patients with should undergo annual evaluation of the kidney function and urinalysis with repetition if there is an SLE flare.
- If LN is considered, a kidney biopsy should be done to guide treatment and determine whether other injury types are present that require a different treatment approach. Some of these patterns of injury include thrombotic microangiopathy, lupus podocytopathy, and acute tubular necrosis.
- Histological classification of LN (Table 1) characterizes extent and degree of activity. For example, class II disease limited to the mesangium may not require kidney specific therapy but may benefit from treatment for extrarenal manifestations. Similarly, LN without evidence of ongoing inflammation and activity may not require immunosuppressive therapy.
- Repeat kidney biopsy is when the therapeutic response is suboptimal, a disease flare has occurred, or there is an unexplained reduction in renal function.

LABORATORY TESTS

In addition to a careful history and exam, the initial evaluation includes laboratory testing to narrow the differential diagnosis, characterize the extent of lupus involvement, and define baseline serologies. Laboratory evaluations include the following:

- Complete blood count with differential count
- Renal function panel

TABLE 1 International Society of Nephrology/Renal Pathology Society (2003) Classification of Lupus Nephritis (LN)

Class	Description
I	Minimal mesangial LN
II	Mesangial proliferative LN
III	Focal LN* (<50% of glomeruli)
III (A)	Active lesions
III (A/C)	Active and chronic lesions
III (C)	Chronic lesions
IV	Diffuse LN† (≥50% of glomeruli) Diffuse segmental (IV-S) or global (IV-G) LN
IV (A)	Active lesions
IV (A/C)	Active and chronic lesions
IV (C)	Chronic lesions
V‡	Membranous LN
VI	Advanced sclerosing LN (≥ globally sclerosed glomeruli without residual activity)

*Indicate the proportion of glomeruli with active and with sclerotic lesions.
†Indicate the proportion of glomeruli with fibrinoid necrosis and with cellular crescents.
‡Class V may occur in combination with III or IV, in which case both may be diagnosed.
From Skorecki K, Chertow GM, Marsden PA, et al: *Brenner & Rector's the Kidney*, ed 10, Elsevier, Philadelphia, 2016.

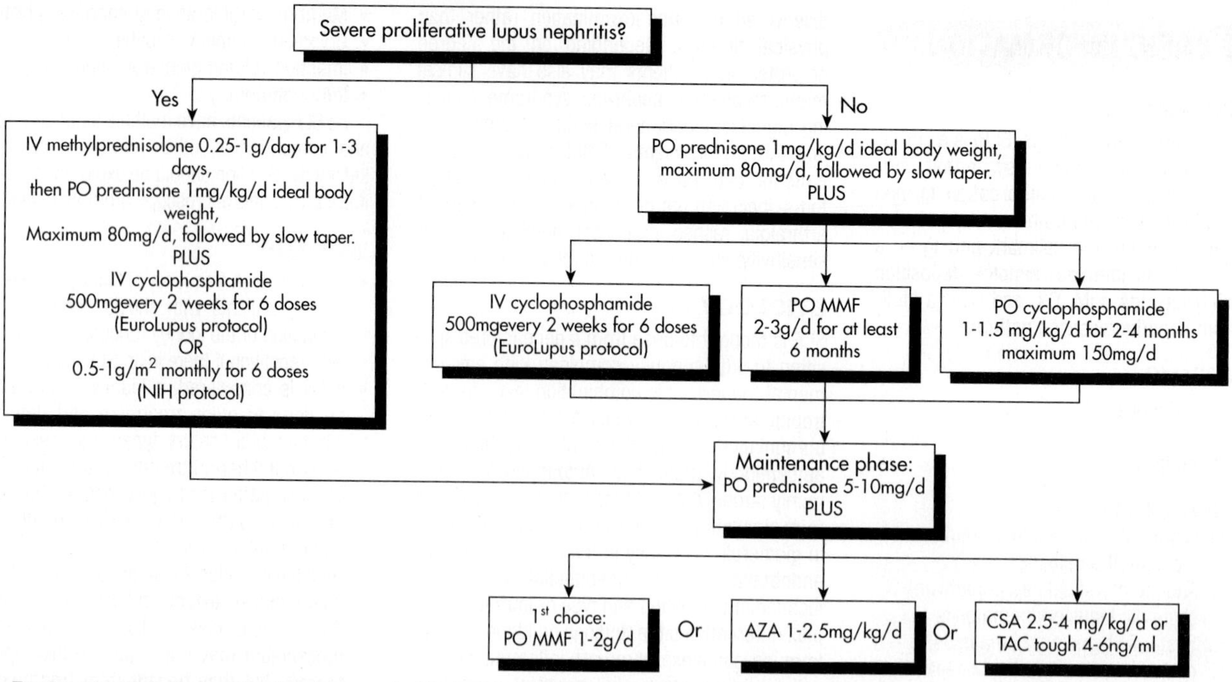

FIG. 1 Treatment options for proliferative lupus nephritis. (Data from Almaani S et al: Update on lupus nephritis, *Clin J Am Soc Nephrol* 12(5):825-835, 2017 and Hahn BH et al: American College of Rheumatology guidelines for screening, treatment, and management of lupus nephritis, *Arthritis Care Res (Hoboken)* 64(6):797-808, 2012.)

- Liver function tests
- Urinalysis with microscopy
- Urine protein-to-creatinine ratio
- Antinuclear antibody
- C3 and C4 complement levels
- Anti-double-stranded DNA
- Extractable nuclear antigen panel (antibodies: Anti-RNP, anti-SSA/Ro, anti-SSB/La, anti-SCL70, anti-Jo1, and anti-Smith)

Rx TREATMENT

Treatment depends on the histologic class of LN.

- Strategy: Achieve and maintain renal remission
- Class I and II lupus nephritis: Therapy is directed toward extrarenal manifestations of the disease.
- Proliferative immune complex LN (Class III and IV LN): The treatment is divided into two phases (Fig. 1).
  1. Induction phase: Initial immunosuppressive therapy aimed at stopping the inflammatory process (usually 3 to 6 mo duration).
  2. Maintenance phase: Less intensive immunosuppression that facilitates healing process (usually years in duration).
- Severe proliferative LN is considered if glomerular crescents and/or fibrinoid necrosis affecting several glomeruli are present on kidney biopsy
  1. Induction phase: Multiple approaches can be considered but usually consists of high-dose corticosteroids with mycophenolate mofetil (MMF) or cyclophosphamide. Cyclophosphamide can be administered in a standard-dose (NIH) or lower dose (Euro-lupus) protocol.
  2. Maintenance phase: Glucocorticoid steroids are weaned gradually to lowest possible dose with the assistance of a steroid sparing agent, preferably, MMF; alternative agents are used.
- LN flares: Repeat renal biopsy should be considered to help guide therapy decisions.
- Hydroxychloroquine: Minimizes flares and improves overall SLE outcomes.
- Other therapeutic agents: Cyclosporin, tacrolimus, azathioprine, belimumab (human monoclonal antibody), and abatacept (modified anti-CTLA-4 antibody).
- Membranous LN (Class V LN): Additive treatments should include anti-proteinuric drugs, including calcineurin inhibitors and angiotensin–converting-enzyme inhibitors or angiotensin II type 1 receptor blockers.

REFERRAL

Optimal LN management should be done with a nephrologist to assist with the initial work-up and subsequent management. When persistent renal dysfunction exists, a nephrologist can facilitate chronic kidney disease management.

When extrarenal manifestations are present, comanagement with a Rheumatology subspecialist is recommended.

PEARLS & CONSIDERATIONS

- LN patients must maintain up-to-date vaccination status because of ongoing immunosuppression.
- Female LN patients of reproductive age should receive counseling regarding the risks for pregnancy complications and of medications used to treat SLE. Individuals who do not desire pregnancy or taking medications incompatible with pregnancy should receive contraception counseling.
- The selection of contraception modality may require modification when antiphospholipid antibodies are and hypercoagulability are present. Patients desiring pregnancy should be referred to a maternal-fetal medicine subspecialist for preconception counseling.
- SLE patients are encouraged to wear sunscreen regularly.

SUGGESTED READINGS

Available at ExpertConsult.com

AUTHORS: **Jia Yi, MD,** and **Koyal Jain, MD, MPH**

BASIC INFORMATION

DEFINITION

Renal tubular acidosis (RTA) is a group of chronic diseases characterized by hyperchloremic metabolic acidosis (HCMA) produced by the inability of the renal tubules to either excrete hydrogen ion (H^+) or retain bicarbonate ion (HCO_3^-). Factors differentiating the four major types of RTA are described in Table 1:

- Type 1 (classic, distal RTA): Abnormality in distal tubule hydrogen secretion, resulting in hypokalemic HCMA
- Type 2 (proximal RTA): Decreased proximal tubule bicarbonate reabsorption, resulting in hypokalemic HCMA
- Type 3 (mixed RTA): Rare autosomal recessive disorder with features of distal and proximal RTA
- Type 4 (hyporeninemic, hypoaldosteronism RTA): Aldosterone deficiency or a disease of the cortical collecting duct characterized by decreased distal sodium reabsorption and decreased distal tubule acidification hyperkalemic HCMA

SYNONYM

RTA

ICD-10CM CODE

N25.89 Other disorders resulting from impaired renal tubular function

EPIDEMIOLOGY & DEMOGRAPHICS

RTA type 4 affects primarily adults, whereas RTA types 1 and 2 are more frequent in children.

PHYSICAL FINDINGS & CLINICAL PRESENTATION

- Physical examination may be normal.
- Reduced skin turgor may be present from polyuria and dehydration.
- Muscle weakness and aches, paralysis, and cardiac arrhythmias from hypokalemia may occur.
- Low back pain and bone pain may be present in patients with abnormalities of calcium and phosphorus metabolism (RTA type 2).
- Failure to thrive or delayed growth in children.
- Some patients may present with sensorineural deafness in RTA type 1 (H^+–ATPase mutations).

ETIOLOGY

- Type 1 RTA: Inherited as a primary disorder with mutation of the basolateral chloride-bicarbonate exchanger (*SLC4A1* gene) or apical proton-ATPase (H^+-ATPase). Acquired causes: Autoimmune disorders (SLE, Sjögren syndrome); primary biliary cirrhosis and other liver diseases; medications (amphotericin, NSAIDs, lithium carbonate, ifosfamide); genetic disorders (Ehlers–Danlos syndrome, Marfan syndrome, hereditary elliptocytosis); toxins (toluene); disorders with nephrocalcinosis (primary hyperparathyroidism, vitamin D intoxication, idiopathic hypercalciuria); and tubulointerstitial disease (renal transplantation, renal medullary cystic disease, obstructive uropathy, chronic urinary tract infections, and analgesic nephropathy)
- Type 2 RTA: Inherited defects of the proximal tubule cell sodium bicarbonate co-transporter (NBCe1) defect, carbonic anhydrase type 2, and Fanconi syndrome (caused by cystinosis, Wilson disease, hereditary fructose intolerance, Lowe syndrome, Fanconi–Bickel syndrome, Dent disease, tyrosinemia, and galactosemia). Acquired causes include primary hyperparathyroidism, multiple myeloma, amyloidosis, light chain deposition diseases, heavy metals (copper, lead, mercury, and cadmium), chronic rejection of a transplanted kidney, and medications (acetazolamide, topiramate, outdated tetracycline, ifosfamide, zidovudine, didanosine, aminoglycosides)
- Type 3 RTA: Rare inherited recessive disorder with carbonic anhydrase 2 deficiency, drugs (topiramate).
- Type 4 RTA: Inherited disorders such as pseudohypoaldosteronism types 1 or 2 (Gordon syndrome). Acquired causes include diabetes mellitus, HIV/AIDS, sickle cell disease, obstructive uropathy, lupus, amyloidosis, adrenal insufficiency, kidney transplant rejection, drugs (spironolactone, eplerenone, amiloride, angiotensin–converting-enzyme [ACE] inhibitors, angiotensin II type 1 receptor blockers [ARBs], trimethoprim, pentamidine, heparin, NSAIDs, and calcineurin inhibitors [cyclosporine, tacrolimus])

Dx DIAGNOSIS

DIFFERENTIAL DIAGNOSIS: EXTRARENAL ETIOLOGY

- Diarrhea with significant bicarbonate loss
- External loss of biliary and pancreatic secretions
- Bowel-urinary diversion procedures (e.g., ureterosigmoidostomy, ileal conduit)
- Respiratory acidosis
- Drugs: Calcium chloride, magnesium sulfate, cholestyramine

WORKUP

Detection of HCMA by serum electrolyte and arterial blood gas (ABG) analysis followed by evaluation of potential causes (see "Etiology"). Fig 1 describes an approach to the patient with RTA.

LABORATORY TESTS

- ABG reveals metabolic acidosis.
- Anion gap is normal, i.e., Anion Gap = $[Na^+] - ([Cl^-] + [HCO_3^-]) = 6$ to 10 mEq/L
- Serum potassium is low in RTA types 1 and 2, normal in type 3, and high in type 4.
- First-morning urine pH is >5.5 in RTA type I, <5.5 in types 2 and 3, and <5.5 (low mineralocorticoid secretion) or >5.5 (collecting duct abnormality) in RTA type 4.
- Urine Anion Gap (UAG = Urine $[Na^+ + K^+]$ – Urine $[Cl^-]$ is an indirect evaluation of urinary ammonium excretion, and can differentiate renal from extrarenal causes of normal anion gap metabolic acidosis (e.g., diarrhea). UAG is 0 or positive in all types of RTA.
- UAG should be calculated only if U_{Na} >20 mEq/L and urine pH <6.5.
- Urine osmolar gap (UOG) is an independent surrogate of urinary ammonium concentration and not affected by the presence of other non-reabsorbable anions (e.g., keto-acids, 5-oxoproline/pyroglutamic acid, bicarbonate, or hippurate).
- Calculated $U_{NH4}{}^+$ (mmol/L) = 0.5 (Measured Uosm – Calculated Uosm [2 (Na + K) + Urine Urea Nitrogen (mg/dl; divided by 2.8) + glucose (mg/dl/18]).
- Calculated urine ammonium ≥75 mEq/L denotes intact renal tubular function and supports an extrarenal origin of HCMA.

TABLE 1 Contrasting Features and Diagnostic Studies in Renal Tubular Acidosis

	TYPES OF RENAL TUBULAR ACIDOSIS		
Finding	Proximal (Type 2)	Classical Distal (Type 1)	Generalized Distal Dysfunction (Type 4)
Plasma potassium	Low	Low	High
Urine pH during metabolic acidosis (ABG pH <7.3)	<5.5	>5.5	<5.5 or >5.5
Urine net charge	Positive	Positive	Positive
Fanconi lesion	Present	Absent	Absent
Fractional bicarbonate excretion	10%-15%	2%-5%	5%-10%
Urine–Blood PCO_2	Normal	Low	Low
H^+–ATPase defect		Low	
HCO_3^-/Cl^- transporter defect		High	
Amphotericin B		Normal	
Response to therapy	Least responsive	Responsive	Less responsive
Associated features	Fanconi syndrome	Nephrocalcinosis/ hypergammaglobulinemia	Chronic kidney disease

ATPase, Adenosine triphosphatase; (U – B) PCO_2, urine–blood CO_2 tension difference, <30 is low.
Modified from DuBose TD: Disorders of acid-base balance. In *Brenner and Rector's the kidney,* ed 9, Philadelphia, 2011, Saunders.

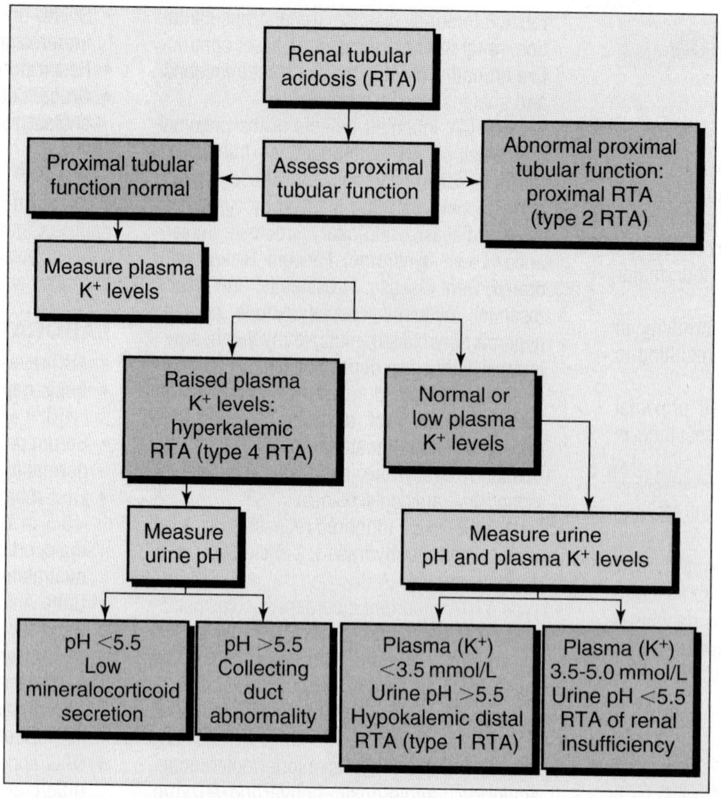

FIG. 1 Approach to the patient with renal tubular acidosis. (From Floege J et al: *Comprehensive clinical nephrology*, ed 4, Philadelphia, 2010, Saunders.)

- Calculated urine ammonium ≤25 mEq/L denotes inappropriately low concentration.
- UOG cannot be used if there are other neutral substances in the urine (e.g., mannitol, alcohols) or during a urinary tract infection urease-producing bacteria.
- Additional studies include urine and serum calcium concentrations.
- Intact parathyroid hormone measurement when primary hyperparathyroidism is suspected (type 2 RTA).

IMAGING STUDIES

- Plain abdominal radiographs for evaluation of nephrocalcinosis
- Kidney ultrasound to determine kidney sizes and/or presence of stones
- Non-contrast-enhanced CT scan in patients with nephrocalcinosis or nephrolithiasis

Rx TREATMENT

ACUTE GENERAL Rx

- RTA types 1 and 2 are treated with oral sodium bicarbonate (1 to 2 mEq/kg per day in RTA types 1, and 2 to 4 mEq/kg per day in RTA type 2) titrated to correct metabolic acidosis (serum total carbon dioxide >22 mEq/L).
- Potassium supplementation is required for hypokalemic patients.
- Type 4 RTA can be treated with diuretics to lower elevated potassium levels and sodium bicarbonate to correct significant acidosis. Fludrocortisone 0.1 to 0.3 mg/day can be used to correct mineralocorticoid deficiency.

CHRONIC Rx

- Monitor potassium levels in RTA type 4.
- Monitor for bone disease (osteomalacia) in RTA type 2.
- Monitor for nephrolithiasis and nephrocalcinosis in RTA type 1.

DISPOSITION

- Prognosis varies with the associated conditions (see "Etiology").
- Untreated distal RTA may result in hypocalcemia, hypophosphatemia, nephrolithiasis, and nephrocalcinosis.

PEARLS & CONSIDERATIONS

- Non-anion gap metabolic acidosis: Evaluate urine ammonium (urine anion and osmolar gaps) to differentiate nonrenal vs. renal causes of HCMA.
- Examine serum potassium to differentiate between RTA types 1 or 2 vs. type 4.
- In type 4 hyperkalemic RTA, review medication list and rule out urinary obstruction, especially in elderly males.

COMMENTS

Patient education material can be obtained from the National Kidney and Urologic Diseases Information Clearinghouse, Box NKUDIC, Bethesda, MD 20893.

SUGGESTED READINGS

Available at ExpertConsult.com

AUTHOR: **Jian Li, MD, PhD**

BASIC INFORMATION

DEFINITION

Renal vein thrombosis (RVT) is the thrombotic occlusion of one or both renal veins.

ICD-10CM CODE
I82.3 Embolism and thrombosis of renal vein

EPIDEMIOLOGY & DEMOGRAPHICS

- Incidence unknown; probably an underdiagnosed condition
- May occur at any age with no gender preference
- Epidemiology tied to the underlying cause

PHYSICAL FINDINGS & CLINICAL PRESENTATION

Acute bilateral renal vein thrombosis:
- Back and bilateral flank pain
- Acute renal failure

Acute unilateral renal vein thrombosis:
- Flank pain
- Decline in renal function
- Hematuria
- Increase in the amount of proteinuria if associated with nephrotic syndrome

Chronic unilateral renal vein thrombosis:
- May be silent
- Pulmonary emboli and hemolysis
- Back pain
- Deep vein thrombosis in lower extremities
- Edema
- Glycosuria
- Hyperchloremic acidosis
- Left varicocele (if the left renal vein is thrombosed)
- Dilated abdominal veins

ETIOLOGY & PATHOGENESIS

- Nephrotic syndrome, especially when the serum albumin is <2 g/dl
- Extrinsic compression by a tumor or retroperitoneal mass
- Invasion of the renal vein or inferior vena cava by tumor (almost always renal cell cancer)
- Trauma
- Other hypercoagulable states
- Severe dehydration

NOTE: For unknown reasons, diabetic nephropathy is not commonly associated with renal vein thrombosis, even if the nephrotic syndrome is present.

Controversy has existed regarding whether the renal vein thrombosis association with nephrotic syndrome is a complication of nephrotic syndrome or whether renal vein thrombosis occurring in the setting of increased renal vein pressure (e.g., with congestive heart failure, constrictive pericarditis, or extrinsic compression) can independently cause proteinuria. Current evidence is that renal vein thrombosis does not cause nephrotic syndrome.

Dx DIAGNOSIS

DIFFERENTIAL DIAGNOSIS

The diagnosis of renal vein thrombosis does not include any differential consideration. The differential diagnosis is that of proteinuria. Renal vein thrombosis should be considered if proteinuria worsens or if renal function worsens in a patient with glomerulonephritis. Renal vein thrombosis should also be considered in patients with pulmonary emboli and no lower-extremity deep vein thrombosis.

WORKUP

Clinical suspicion (see "Differential Diagnosis") and imaging studies

IMAGING STUDIES

- Abdominal ultrasound with Doppler (Fig. E1)
- Abdominal MRI or CT with contrast (Fig. 2) in the absence of significant renal failure
- Renal arteriography (delayed films during venous phase)
- Selective renal vein venography
- Renal biopsy may be indicated if evidence of nephritis is present (e.g., active urinary sediment)

Rx TREATMENT

- Anticoagulation with heparin or low-molecular-weight heparin as a bridge to coumadin in acute renal vein thrombosis to prevent pulmonary emboli and in attempt to improve renal function and decrease proteinuria.
- Note that patients with nephrotic syndrome can be resistant to heparin because of antithrombin III deficiency.
- Direct thrombin and factor Xa inhibitors have not been studied in patients with nephrotic syndrome. However, there are case reports of their effectiveness in patients who have contraindications or refuse warfarin or low-molecular-weight heparin.
- Local thrombolytic therapy with or without endovascular thrombectomy has also been reported to be effective, particularly for patients with acute renal vein thrombosis with evidence of acute renal failure.
- The value of anticoagulation in chronic renal vein thrombosis is dubious. The exception is in nephrotic patients with membranous glomerulonephritis with profound hypoalbuminemia, where prolonged prophylactic anticoagulation may be of benefit even if renal vein thrombosis has not been documented.

PROGNOSIS

Probable worsening of the underlying nephropathy by acute renal vein thrombosis; the effect of chronic renal vein thrombosis is unclear.

AUTHOR: **David J. Lucier Jr, MD, MBA, MPH**

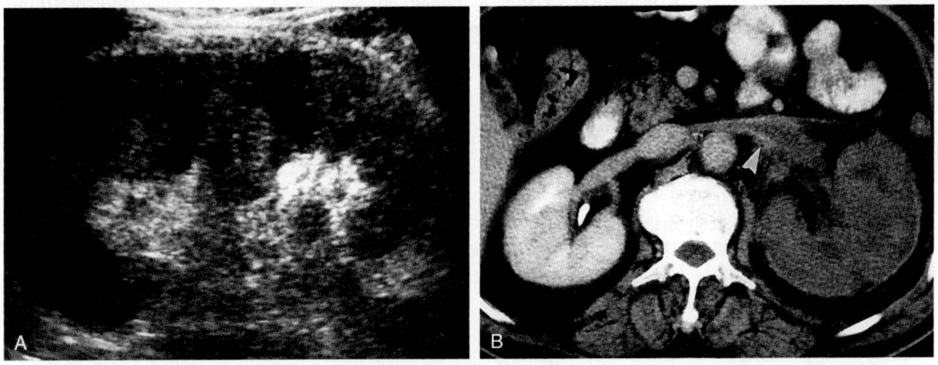

FIG. 2 Renal vein thrombosis. A, Sagittal sonogram demonstrates a diffusely enlarged, edematous left kidney with loss of corticomedullary differentiation. **B,** Confirmatory contrast-enhanced computed tomography shows a large, poorly perfused left kidney and thrombus in the left renal vein *(arrowhead)*. (From Rumack CM et al: *Diagnostic ultrasound,* ed 4, Philadelphia, 2011, Elsevier.)

BASIC INFORMATION

DEFINITION

Restless legs syndrome (RLS) is an awake phenomenon consisting of an urge to move legs, usually associated with feeling of discomfort in legs. Symptoms typically are present only at rest and at least partially improve with movement. Additionally, symptoms are usually worse at night. RLS can result in sleep disturbance with associated executive dysfunction and depression.

SYNONYMS

RLS
Wittmaack-Ekbom syndrome

ICD-10CM CODE

G25.81 Restless legs syndrome

EPIDEMIOLOGY & DEMOGRAPHICS

PREVALENCE: Average prevalence rate is 1% to 29%. Prevalence estimates in Europe are around 10%, and 0.1% to 12% in East Asian population.
PREDOMINANT SEX: Early-onset RLS is more common in females, with 2:1 female/male ratio.
PREDOMINANT AGE: Prevalence of RLS increases with age, and it is more commonly seen in the elderly population but can occur in children.
PEAK PREVALENCE: 10% in persons aged 30 to 79 and 19% in persons aged 80 or above
RISK FACTORS:
- Iron deficiency anemia (IDA)—25% to 35%
- Pregnancy: Increases in severity and prevalence with each passing trimester
- End-stage renal disease (ESRD) requiring hemodialysis: Improves with transplant but not dialysis
- Many neurologic diseases such as Parkinson disease, multiple sclerosis, neuropathy, and myelopathy increase risk as do mood disorders, other inflammatory disease, and cardiovascular disease

GENETICS: Genetic basis of RLS has been reported, particularly in early-onset RLS.
- Autosomal dominant disorder
- Common among first-degree relatives
- RLS associated with certain sequences in chromosomes 6p, 12q, 14q, 9p, 20p, 2p, 16p
- These include polymorphisms in the genes *BTBD9*, *MEIS1*, *PTPRD*, *MAP2K5*, *SKOR1*, and *TOX3*

CLASSIFICATION

- Primary RLS is without any obvious cause, with no associated disorder.
- Secondary RLS results from other medical conditions.

PHYSICAL FINDINGS & CLINICAL PRESENTATION

- Wide spectrum of severity of clinical manifestations has been reported in RLS.
- Most common symptom is unpleasant sensations in legs ("dysesthesias"), reported as discomfort or "creepy-crawling" sensations, mostly bilateral. Arms are occasionally involved.
- There is an extreme urge to move legs, and relief is sustained as long as the movement continues.
- Symptoms are worse at night or evening. Best sleep is usually early in the morning.

ETIOLOGY

The exact etiology remains unknown. Pharmacologic, pathologic, physiologic, and imaging studies have implicated dopaminergic pathways, brain iron metabolism, and endogenous opioid pathways.

DIAGNOSIS

DIFFERENTIAL DIAGNOSIS

- Periodic limb movement disorder (PLMD)
- Nocturnal leg cramps
- Painful peripheral neuropathy
- Akathisia
- Positional discomfort
- Volitional movements, foot tapping, leg rocking

WORKUP

- Diagnosis of RLS is based on established clinical criteria (Table 1) and normal neurologic examination.
- Testing is done to determine possible cause of secondary RLS. All patients with RLS should be screened for iron deficiency because iron supplementation in patients with iron deficiency may resolve the symptoms.
- Polysomnography with leg activity monitors to determine limb movements during sleep, but they are unable to distinguish periodic limb movements from periodic movements associated with sleep apnea.
- Nerve conduction studies and electromyography for associated peripheral neuropathy.

LABORATORY TESTS

- Iron status: Serum ferritin, total iron binding capacity, percent saturation
- CBC for anemia in case of iron deficiency
- Metabolic panel: Blood urea nitrogen and serum creatinine for renal insufficiency

IMAGING STUDIES

No imaging studies are required for diagnosis of RLS.

TREATMENT

NONPHARMACOLOGIC THERAPY

- Avoidance of caffeine, alcohol, and nicotine, which can exacerbate RLS
- Review and adjustment of medications that may exacerbate or cause RLS (selective serotonin reuptake inhibitors, dopamine blocking agents, stimulants)
- Physical and mental activity
- Good sleep hygiene
- Monitoring for depression as RLS has an elevated suicide risk. Bupropion may be the best agent for depression in RLS due to lack of dopamine effects

CHRONIC Rx

Once the diagnosis of RLS is considered based on clinical criteria as mentioned in Table 1 and causes impairment of quality of life, an anticonvulsant (gabapentin enacarbil or pregabalin) or dopamine agonist (bromocriptine, pramipexole, or ropinirole) should be started at low dose and then gradually tapered depending on tolerance.

Treatment options (Table 2) for RLS include:
- Anticonvulsants, such as gabapentin, have been shown to be effective in multiple studies. Gabapentin enacarbil and pregabalin would now be considered first-line agents in the treatment of RLS. These agents do not cause iatrogenic worsening (augmentation) of RLS with long-term treatment. Limited case reports support use of lamotrigine and topiramate in patients who are intolerant of other agents.
- Dopaminergic agents such as levodopa and dopamine agonists help to ameliorate RLS symptoms, decrease periodic limb movements, and improve sleep. Dopamine agonists, pramipexole and ropinirole, can be first-line agents in the treatment of RLS but often cause augmentation of RLS with long-term treatment.

TABLE 1 Diagnostic Criteria for Restless Legs Syndrome

Minimal Criteria
- Desire to move the legs usually associated with paresthesias
- Motor restlessness, as characterized by floor pacing, leg rubbing, stretching, and flexing
- Worse at rest, with relief by activity
- Worse at night

Additional Criteria
- Sleep disturbances, as difficulty in sleep onset and maintaining sleep, daytime fatigue, or somnolence
- Involuntary movements, as periodic limb or leg movements in sleep and periodic or aperiodic limb movements while awake
- Neurologic examination is normal in idiopathic restless legs syndrome
- Clinical course may begin at any age but most severe in middle and older age
- Family history suggests autosomal dominant mode of inheritance in one third of the cases

From Stiansy K et al: Clinical symptomatology and treatment of restless leg syndrome and periodic limb movement disorder, *Sleep Med Rev* 6(4):253-265, 2002.

TABLE 2 Management of Restless Legs Syndrome LS/WED

Agent and Daily Dosage	Side Effects	Countermeasures
Step 1: α2δ Agents		
First-line treatment, particularly if sleep disturbance, pain, or anxiety is present		
Gabapentin enacarbil, 300-600 mg Pregabalin, 50-450 mg* Gabapentin, 100-1800 mg*	Dizziness	Reduce dose and add alternate medication class as needed. If fall risk, then discontinue and change to alternate medication class.
	Somnolence, daytime fatigue	Reduce dose and add alternate medication class as needed. If significant, discontinue and change to alternate medication class.
	Tolerance	Discontinue, take drug holiday with return to medication. Switch to alternate medication class.
	Weight gain	Reduce dose and add alternate medication class as needed. If significant, discontinue and change to alternate medication class.
Step 2: Dopamine Agonists		
Alternative first-line treatment if depression is present and dose kept low.		
Pramipexole, 0.125-0.5 mg* (0.75 mg in Europe), Ropinirole, 0.5-4.0 mg* Rotigotine, 1-3 mg/24 h	Nausea and orthostatic hypotension	Slowly increase dosage or use domperidone if available (10-30 mg).
	Insomnia	Add or switch to α2δ agent. Use a small dose of benzodiazepines in association with dopamine agonists.
	Daytime fatigue and somnolence	Reduce dosage or discontinue dopamine agonists.
	Compulsive or impulsive behavior	Reduce dose and add alternate medication class as needed. If significant, discontinue and change to alternate medication class.
	Tolerance	Discontinue and switch to longer-acting dopamine agonist or alternate medication class.
	Augmentation	Discontinue and switch to alternate medication class or longer-acting dopamine agonist.
Step 3: Dopamine Precursors		
Useful for intermittent treatment, such as twice a wk		
Levodopa-benserazide or levodopa-carbidopa (regular or slow release), 100/25 or 200/50 mg†	Same as for dopamine agonists	See "Countermeasures" for dopamine agonists.
	Morning rebound or augmentation of restless legs syndrome in early evening	Use small extra dose of levodopa during daytime or reduce dosage or combine levodopa with dopamine agonists or benzodiazepines or discontinue levodopa (if severe and persistent).
	Augmentation	Do not use daily. Discontinue and switch to dopamine agonists or a nondopamine medication.
Benzodiazepines		
Useful for sleep promotion		
Clonazepam, 0.5-2.0 mg‡ Temazepam, 15-30 mg‡ Nitrazepam, 5-10 mg*	Daytime somnolence Tolerance	Reduce dosage. Take drug holiday for 2 wk then return to lower dosage.
Opiates		
Second-line treatment		
Oxycodone-naloxone, 10/5 to 40/20 mg/day Methadone, 2.5-20 mg Oxycodone, 5-40 mg	Constipation Dependency	Use for symptom treatment. Take a drug holiday. Discontinue and switch to alternate medication.
Oral Iron		
Always consider if serum iron ≤75 mcg/L or transferrin saturation ≤17%		
Ferrous sulfate, 650 mg (325 mg with vitamin C, 100 mg twice a day)	Constipation, stomach upset and pain Diarrhea, nausea, vomiting	Reduce dose, discontinue, take with food. Reduce dose, discontinue, take with food.

*One hour before onset of symptoms in the evening or 1-2 hours before bedtime if symptoms are not present in the evening.
†Considered most appropriate for PRN dosing not more than 3 times a wk rather than daily use.
‡Before bedtime usually to promote sleep with restless legs syndrome.
From Kryger M et al: *Principles and practice of sleep medicine*, ed 6, Philadelphia, 2017, Elsevier.

- Rotigotine patch (Neupro) is also effective and FDA approved for moderate to severe RLS.
- Opiates, mostly methadone, are generally reserved as last line of treatment.
- Iron replacement should be started concurrently in case of iron deficiency. Iron supplements are indicated even with low-normal ferritin levels (<45 ng/ml). Sometimes IV iron replacement is used.

REFERRAL

Refer to neurologist if diagnosis is uncertain or an underlying disorder is suspected.

SUGGESTED READINGS

Available at ExpertConsult.com

RELATED CONTENT

Restless Legs Syndrome (Patient Information)

AUTHORS: **Fariha Jamal, MD,** and **Corey Goldsmith, MD**

BASIC INFORMATION

DEFINITION

Retropharyngeal abscess is a soft tissue infection of the throat that involves retropharyngeal space and that primarily affects children. The anatomic boundaries of the retropharyngeal space are the buccopharyngeal fascia (middle layer of the deep cervical fascia) anteriorly and the alar fascia (deep layer of the deep cervical fascia) posteriorly. The space begins at the skull base superiorly and ends inferiorly where the two fasciae fuse at the level between the first and second thoracic vertebrae.

ICD-10CM CODE
J39.0 Retropharyngeal and parapharyngeal abscess

EPIDEMIOLOGY & DEMOGRAPHICS

Retropharyngeal abscess occurs most commonly in children between the ages of 2 and 4 yr, analogous to suppurative cervical adenitis. 70% of cases are in patients under the age of 6, and 50% are in patients under the age of 3. This represents the peak age group for numerous viral upper respiratory tract infections and their attendant complications, acute otitis media and sinusitis. Retropharyngeal space infection is less common in older children and adults because the lymph nodes generally atrophy by puberty.

PHYSICAL FINDINGS & CLINICAL PRESENTATION

- The onset of a retropharyngeal infection may be insidious, with little more than fever, irritability, drooling, a muffled voice (dysphonia), or possibly nuchal rigidity.
- The acute symptoms relate to pressure and inflammation produced by the abscess on either the airway or the upper digestive tract and pharynx. The patient may have intense dysphagia, drooling, and odynophagia, or there may be some element of respiratory distress from edema and inflammation of the airway (stridor, tachypnea, or both).
- Unwillingness to move the neck because of discomfort is often a prominent presenting feature and should lead to consideration of retropharyngeal abscess if the child is febrile and irritable.
- Extension of the neck is usually affected more than flexion. This causes the patient to hold his or her neck stiffly or to present with torticollis.
- Trismus is unusual.
- On physical examination it may be possible to appreciate midline or unilateral swelling of the posterior pharyngeal wall. The mass may be fluctuant to the examining finger, and care must be taken to avoid rupture of the abscess into the upper airway.
- Complications are numerous and could be fatal; these include airway obstruction, septicemia, thrombosis of the internal jugular vein, carotid artery rupture, and acute necrotizing mediastinitis. Aspiration with resultant pneumonia may complicate retropharyngeal abscess if rupture of the abscess occurs and empties into the airway. Infection can spread from one space in the neck to another.
- The most dreaded complication is jugular vein suppurative thrombophlebitis (Lemierre syndrome), in which the vessels of the carotid sheath become infected, leading to bacteremia and spread of infection to the lungs, brain, and mediastinum.

ETIOLOGY

- The retropharyngeal space comprises two chains of lymph nodes that drain the nasopharynx, adenoids, posterior paranasal sinuses, middle ear, and Eustachian tube. Accordingly, suppurative infections in these areas may provide the seeds for infection for retropharyngeal abscess.
- The predominant bacterial species are *Streptococcus pyogenes* (group A *Streptococcus*), *Staphylococcus aureus,* and respiratory anaerobes (including *Fusobacteria, Prevotella,* and *Veillonella* species). *Haemophilus* species are also occasionally found.
- In young children, infection usually reaches this space by lymphatic spread from a septic focus in the pharynx or sinuses.
- In adults, infection may reach the retropharyngeal space from either local or distant sites. Penetrating trauma (e.g., from chicken bones or iatrogenic) is the usual source of local spread. More distant sources of infection include odontogenic sepsis and peritonsillar abscess (now a rare cause).

DIAGNOSIS

DIFFERENTIAL DIAGNOSIS

- Cervical osteomyelitis
- Pott disease
- Meningitis
- Calcific tendonitis of the long muscle of the neck
- Differentiating features of deep neck infections are summarized in Table 1

LABORATORY TESTS

- CBC with differential.
- Blood cultures may be considered in refractory cases or for severe symptoms.

IMAGING STUDIES

- A lateral neck film should be obtained and can be helpful in delineating the presence of a retropharyngeal abscess and may demonstrate cervical lordosis; the retropharyngeal space is considered widened and pathologic if it is greater than 7 mm at C2 or 14 mm at C6 (Fig. E1).
  1. There must be attention to technical issues when performing the study, especially in children. The film should be a perfect lateral, and the child must keep the neck in extension during inspiration to avoid a false thickening of the retropharyngeal space. Crying, particularly in infants, may also cause false thickening of the retropharyngeal space.
- CXR should be considered to evaluate for mediastinitis or aspiration pneumonia.
- A CT scan of the neck is useful for patients with moderate or high suspicion of having a deep neck space abscess. It is the most useful imaging modality to identify abscesses in the retropharyngeal space, but it is not perfect. Both the sensitivity and specificity of the CT scan in predicting the presence of drainable purulent material are quite variable from study to study, ranging between 68% and 100%.
  1. The CT scan provides more information than the plain radiograph because it can generally differentiate between retropharyngeal cellulitis and retropharyngeal abscess and can demonstrate extension of the retropharyngeal abscess to contiguous spaces in the neck. Findings on CT common to both cellulitis and abscess are a low-density core, soft tissue swelling, obliterated fat planes, and mass effect. Findings on CT scan that

TABLE 1 Differentiating Features of Deep Neck Infections

Space	Clinical Features*
Submandibular space (Ludwig angina)	Woody submental induration, protruding swollen/necrotic tongue, no trismus, rotted lower molars commonly present
Lateral pharyngeal space (anterior)	Fever, toxicity, trismus, neck swelling
Lateral pharyngeal space (posterior)	No trismus, no swelling (unless ipsilateral parotid is involved), cranial nerve IX-XII palsies, Horner syndrome, carotid artery erosion
Retropharyngeal space (retropharynx)	Neck stiffness, decreased neck range of motion, soft-tissue bulging of posterior pharyngeal wall, sore throat, dysphagia, dyspnea
Retropharyngeal space ("danger space")	Mediastinal or pleural involvement
Retropharyngeal space (prevertebral)	Neck stiffness, decreased neck range of motion, cervical instability, possible spread along length of vertebral column
Jugular vein septic thrombophlebitis (Lemierre syndrome)	Sore throat, swollen tender neck, dyspnea, chest pain, septic arthritis

*Fever and signs of systemic toxicity are common to all.
From Vincent JL et al: *Textbook of critical care*, ed 7, Philadelphia, 2017, Elsevier.

TABLE 2 Therapeutic Options for Deep Neck Infections

Syndrome	Likely Flora	Therapeutic Options*
Submandibular space infection (community acquired)	Anaerobes, streptococci, *Staphylococcus aureus*	Ampicillin-sulbactam (3 g IV q6h) Ceftriaxone (1-2 g IV q24h) *plus* clindamycin (300-900 mg IV q8h) *or* metronidazole (500 mg IV q6h) Ertapenem (1 g IV q day)
Submandibular space infection (hospital/ICU acquired)	*Pseudomonas aeruginosa,* methicillin-resistant *S. aureus* (MRSA), anaerobes	Imipenem (500 mg IV q6h) *or* piperacillin-tazobactam (3.375 g IV q8h by continuous infusion) *plus* vancomycin (1 g IV q12h)
Retropharyngeal space infection	Anaerobes, streptococci, *S. aureus*	Ampicillin-sulbactam (3 g IV q6h) Ceftriaxone (1-2 g IV q24h) *plus* clindamycin (300-900 mg IV q8h) *or* metronidazole (500 mg IV q6h) Ertapenem (1 g IV q day)
Lateral pharyngeal space infection	Anaerobes, streptococci, *S. aureus*	Ampicillin-sulbactam (3 g IV q6h) Ceftriaxone (1-2 g IV q24h) *plus* clindamycin (300-900 mg IV q8h) *or* metronidazole (500 mg IV q6h) Ertapenem (1 g IV q day)
Internal jugular vein septic thrombophlebitis	*Fusobacterium necrophorum*	Metronidazole (500 mg IV q6h) Clindamycin (300-900 mg IV q8h) Ampicillin-sulbactam (3 g IV q6h)

ICU, Intensive care unit; *IV,* intravenous.
*Antibiotic choices listed are examples, because for most infections, multiple different antibiotics are effective; individual choice will be influenced by patient factors (e.g., allergies, concurrent medications), local hospital bacterial resistance rates, and microbiologic culture results.
From Vincent JL et al: *Textbook of critical care*, ed 7, Philadelphia, 2017, Elsevier.

are indicative of abscess are "complete rim enhancement" and scalloping of the abscess borders (Fig. E2). The abscess may be seen as a mass impinging on the posterior pharyngeal wall.

- MRI of the neck is rarely used for diagnosis, especially in the pediatric population because of the longer time to acquire the study and the need for sedation in the younger population. T2-weighted images may identify and localize areas of pus for drainage or aspiration. Gadolinium enhancement is important to accurately define the soft tissue component. It also can be useful for distinguishing inflammatory from congenital or neoplastic lesions. Magnetic resonance angiography can be helpful for imaging vascular lesions, such as jugular thrombophlebitis.

Rx TREATMENT

ACUTE GENERAL & CHRONIC Rx

- When the CT findings suggest cellulitis or phlegmon, a trial of IV antibiotic therapy without drainage is initiated, and the child is monitored as an inpatient for 48 hr. If the child is clinically improved, consider discharge home with a course of oral antibiotics. If the clinical course is not improved or is worse, a repeat CT scan should be obtained, and surgical drainage or prolonged IV antibiotic therapy may be warranted. Some investigators also support a trial of IV antibiotic therapy alone when small abscesses are identified by CT scans, as long as the airway is not compromised.
  1. Ampicillin-sulbactam (300 mg/kg/day IV divided q6h) or clindamycin (25 to 40 mg/kg/day IV divided q8h) are effective antimicrobial selections. In adults, ampicillin-sulbactam 3 g IV q6h or clindamycin 600 mg IV q8h. Antibiotics should be adjusted as culture data become available, and oral therapy is continued to complete at least a 14-day course. Therapeutic options for deep neck infections are summarized in Table 2.
- Surgical intervention has historically played a prominent role in the management of retropharyngeal abscess in conjunction with antibiotic therapy. Prompt surgical drainage is indicated when there is a large hypodense area suggestive of an abscess or when a patient has not responded to parenteral therapy alone.

PEARLS & CONSIDERATIONS

PREVENTION

The complications of deep neck infection in any space are numerous and potentially fatal. Early diagnosis, with prompt and appropriate management, is key to avoiding these complications.

SUGGESTED READING

Available at ExpertConsult.com

AUTHOR: **Louis F. Insalaco, MD**

BASIC INFORMATION

DEFINITION

Rhabdomyolysis is a syndrome characterized by striated muscle lysis with resulting muscle damage and leakage of intracellular contents into the circulation. The presentation may range from asymptomatic elevation of creatine kinase (CK) to severe muscle injury with irreversible kidney failure. In general, 5- to 10-fold elevations of CK levels, muscle pain, and myoglobinuria in an appropriate clinical setting (see below) are sufficient criteria for the diagnosis of rhabdomyolysis. Acute kidney injury, which is not a diagnostic criterion of rhabdomyolysis, typically results from multiple factors, including volume depletion, tubular obstruction, direct heme pigment-induced proximal tubular cell injury, and renal vasoconstriction.

ICD-10CM CODES

M62.82	Rhabdomyolysis (idiopathic)
T79.6	Traumatic ischemia of muscle
M62.89	Other specified disorders of muscle

EPIDEMIOLOGY & DEMOGRAPHICS

PREDOMINANT AGE: Incidence is approximately 1 per 10,000 persons in the U.S.
- Rare in children, with increased risk with age, i.e., >80 yr
- Reported incidence of acute kidney injury (AKI) with rhabdomyolysis is 10% to 55%
- 7% to 10% of cases of AKI are due to rhabdomyolysis

MORTALITY RATE: 5% to 8%, with better prognosis when AKI is absent

ONSET:
- Evidence is limited regarding the onset of physical exertion-induced rhabdomyolysis. Exercise levels exceeding usual exercise tolerance levels for individuals are commonly causative. Extracellular volume depletion and vasoconstriction are common predisposing features. Patients with risk factors (e.g., metabolic myopathies, advanced age) develop symptoms associated with rhabdomyolysis within 2 to 6 hr after activity. Patients without such risk factors generally become symptomatic 12 to 36 hr after muscle injury. The presence of concurrent electrolyte abnormalities such as hypokalemia, hyponatremia, hypernatremia, hypomagnesemia, hypophosphatemia, and hypocalcemia increase the risk for rhabdomyolysis.
- CK levels rise within 2 to 12 hr of onset of muscle injury, generally peak after 24 to 72 hr, and decline within 3 to 5 days after cessation of muscle injury. Peak CK concentrations may predict development of renal injury.
- Rhabdomyolysis from cholesterol-lowering therapy by HMG-CoA synthetase inhibitors (statins) requires hospitalization in less than 0.1% of cases. The mechanism of damage is multifactorial: Uptake efficacy of transport proteins in hepatocytes, level of systemic circulation of statins, level of extrahepatic inhibition of mitochondrial respiration, bioavailability, and lipophilicity. Among the statins, pravastatin has a lower risk for induction of rhabdomyolysis than other statins, presumably due to lower lipid solubility. The average duration of statin therapy before onset of myopathy is 6 mo. Symptom resolution with normalization of serum CK concentrations occurs in days to weeks following drug discontinuation. The average time for onset of rhabdomyolysis after addition of fibrate to statin therapy is 32 days. Rare genetic variants are associated with statin-induced myopathy.

PHYSICAL FINDINGS & CLINICAL PRESENTATION

- Classic triad of muscle pain, weakness, and dark urine from myoglobinuria
- Muscle tenderness is present in only half of cases
- Muscle swelling that occurs after intravenous fluid repletion
- Muscular rigidity
- Fever
- In statin-induced rhabdomyolysis, fatigue (74%) is nearly as common as muscle pain (88%)
- Oliguria or anuria with acute kidney injury

ETIOLOGY

Causes can be divided into three categories:
- Traumatic or muscle compression
  1. High-current electrical injury
  2. Crush injury and compartment syndrome
  3. Tourniquet and limb ischemia
  4. Reperfusion after revascularization procedures for ischemia
  5. Extensive surgical (spinal) dissection, bariatric surgery
- Nontraumatic exertional
  1. Exercise: More than 10 genetically predisposing mutations are associated with exertional rhabdomyolysis
  2. Sickle cell trait, rarely; usually additional predisposing factors are involved (e.g., BMI >30 kg/m^2, tobacco use, statin use, antipsychotic use, high altitude)
  3. Heat stroke
  4. Metabolic myopathies
  5. Malignant hyperthermia and neuroleptic malignant syndrome
  6. Seizure activity
- Nontraumatic, nonexertional
  1. Drug-induced (statins alone, combination of statins with fibrates, or erythromycin, simvastatin and amiodarone, amphetamines, haloperidol, levofloxacin, macrolide antibiotics)
  2. Alcoholism
  3. Hypothyroidism
  4. Infectious and inflammatory myositis

Table 1 summarizes various causes of rhabdomyolysis.

DIAGNOSIS

DIFFERENTIAL DIAGNOSIS

"Creatine Kinase Elevation" in Section IV describes a clinical algorithm for the evaluation of CK elevation.

LABORATORY TESTS

- Creatine kinase: Usually CK is 5 to 10 times the upper limit of normal and typically peaks 24 to 72 hr after the initial insult (Fig. 1). Levels >15,000 IU/L are more likely associated with renal injury. However, in patients with concomitant risk factors such as hypokalemia or volume depletion, CK levels as low as 5000 U/L have been associated with AKI.
- Myoglobin: Excreted in urine with visible changes in urine ("port wine" color) at levels >100 to 300 mg/dl. Myoglobinuria can be suspected by a positive urine dipstick test for blood and minimal or no microhematuria. Due to rapid hepatic metabolism, myoglobin lacks sensitivity in detecting rhabdomyolysis. Therefore, serum and/or urine myoglobin measurement is not recommended to establish diagnosis. Blood urea nitrogen and creatinine help monitor the severity of AKI.
- Potassium, calcium, phosphorus, and uric levels are released from damaged muscle, and levels should be monitored. Hyperkalemia is less common in nontraumatic rhabdomyolysis.
- Calcium: Hypocalcemia from deposition of calcium phosphate complexes in damaged muscle tissue. Hypercalcemia may follow resolution of rhabdomyolysis from liberation of calcium from damaged muscle into the circulation and increased gut calcium absorption from enhanced vitamin D production.
- Anion gap metabolic acidosis may occur from release of organic acids and phosphates from damaged muscle. Metabolic acidosis is less common in nontraumatic rhabdomyolysis.
- Urinalysis: Myoglobin is detected as blood on dipstick, but erythrocytes are absent on

TABLE 1 Causes of Rhabdomyolysis

Muscle injury/ ischemia	Trauma, pressure necrosis, electric shock, burns, acute vascular disease
Myofiber exhaustion	Seizures, excessive exercise, heat exhaustion
Toxins	Alcohol, cocaine, heroin, amphetamines, ecstasy, phencyclidine, snakebite
Drugs	Statins, fibrates, zidovudine, neuroleptic malignant syndrome, azathioprine, theophylline, lithium, diuretics, colchicine
Electrolyte disorders	Hypophosphatemia, hypokalemia, excess water shifts (hyperosmolality)
Infections	Viral (influenza, HIV, coxsackievirus, Epstein-Barr virus), bacterial (*Legionella, Francisella, Streptococcus pneumoniae, Salmonella, Staphylococcus aureus*)
Familial	McArdle disease, carnitine palmitoyl transferase deficiency, malignant hyperthermia
Other	Hypothyroidism, polymyositis, dermatomyositis

From Floege J et al: *Comprehensive clinical nephrology*, ed 4, Philadelphia, 2010, Saunders.

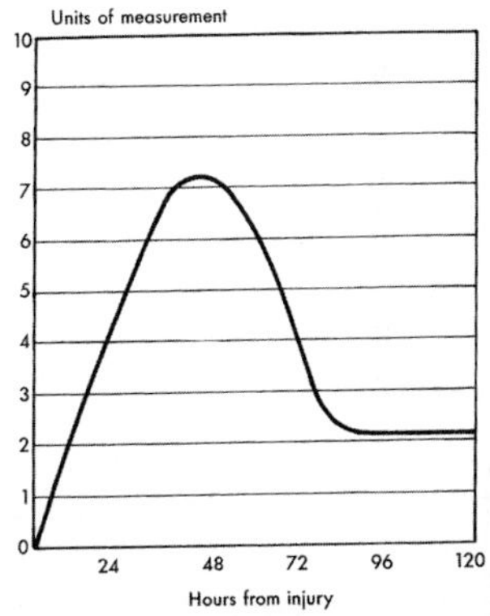

FIG. 1 Typical creatine kinase elimination curve.

microscopy. Presence of pigmented tubular casts establishes acute tubular necrosis.
- Rhabdomyolysis-induced acute tubular necrosis may occur with a low fractional excretion of sodium (FENa <1%)
- Box 1 summarizes laboratory abnormalities observed with rhabdomyolysis.

BOX 1 Laboratory Abnormalities Observed with Rhabdomyolysis

Potassium
Elevated
Risk for acute kidney injury

Bicarbonate
Decreased (20 mEq/L)
Metabolic acidosis

Uric Acid
Elevated (>7 mg/dl)
Marker of acute renal failure

Sodium
Usually normal
Can decrease with mannitol therapy
Use serum osmolality values as a guide

Phosphate
Elevated
Risk for precipitation of calcium phosphate
May need phosphate binders if phosphate >7 mg/dl

Creatine Kinase
Elevated
Associated with creatine kinase level of 15 to 75,000

Blood Urea Nitrogen
Elevated (>20 mg/dl)

Creatinine
Elevated

Calcium
Initially low
Rebound phase may demonstrate hypercalcemia

Liver Function Tests
Occasionally elevated
Serum aspartate transaminase, lactate dehydrogenase, aldolase, muscle enzyme levels elevated

Troponin
Normal
Suspect myocardial damage as a cause (or effect) if elevated
7% false-positive rate for troponin I

Anion Gap
Sometimes elevated
May predict acute kidney injury

Prothrombin Time, Partial Thromboplastin Time, D-Dimer
Disseminated intravascular coagulation in up to 30% of severe cases
Associated with greater mortality

From Adams JG et al: *Emergency medicine, clinical essentials,* ed 2, Philadelphia, 2013, Elsevier.

Rx TREATMENT

ACUTE GENERAL Rx

- Identify precipitating factor(s) and discontinue potentially contributory drugs or toxins
- Early, aggressive, high-volume IV fluid replacement with normal saline. Extracellular fluid volume loading and diuresis reduce the risk for renal damage by elimination of urate and phosphate that can precipitate in the kidneys. Fig. 2 describes a treatment algorithm for rhabdomyolysis.
- Fasciotomy is indicated in compartment syndrome for preservation of muscle and nerve function.
- Initiate volume repletion with normal saline at a rate of 200 to 1000 ml per hr depending on clinical circumstances and severity of muscle damage. Titrate to maintain a urine output of at least 200 ml per hr. Consider treatment with mannitol (up to 200 g per day with cumulative dose up to 800 g) to glomerular filtration rate, diuresis, and scavenge free radicals. Typically, a 20% mannitol infusion at a dose of 0.5 g/kg is given over a 15-min period followed by an infusion at 0.1 gram/kg per hr. Discontinue mannitol and volume resuscitation if diuresis (>20 ml/hr) is not established. Maintain volume repletion until myoglobinuria stops (negative urine dipstick blood test) or plasma CK levels decrease to <5000 U/L.
- Correct hypocalcemia if symptomatic or hyperkalemia that produces electrocardiographic changes.
- Treatment of all electrolyte imbalances.
- Urine alkalinization: Maintain urine pH at 6 to 7 pH units and serum pH at ~7.50. This recommendation is controversial. Early volume resuscitation and expansion are the most important treatments.
- Initiation of renal replacement therapy is determined by severity of kidney injury and/or electrolyte imbalances. The use of continuous renal replacement therapy or specialized hemodialysis membranes to enhance myoglobin clearance have not been proven superior to intermittent hemodialysis or systematically studied.

DISPOSITION

Early diagnosis and management are required to prevent AKI.

REFERRAL

Renal consultation and surgical consultation if compartment syndrome develops

PEARLS & CONSIDERATIONS

COMMENTS

- Statin-induced rhabdomyolysis occurs 12 times more frequently when statins are combined with fibrates than when used alone.
- Short-term, high-dose glucocorticoid steroid administration (500 to 1000 mg methylprednisolone) has been used for treatment of alcohol-induced rhabdomyolysis, refractory to volume repletion. This treatment may be efficacious in cases of severe rhabdomyolysis by retarding secondary leukocyte inflammatory muscle injury.

SUGGESTED READINGS

Available at ExpertConsult.com

RELATED CONTENT

Rhabdomyolysis (Patient Information)
Statin-Induced Muscle Syndrome (Related Key Topic)

AUTHORS: **Hesham Shaban, MD,** and **Junior Uduman, MD**

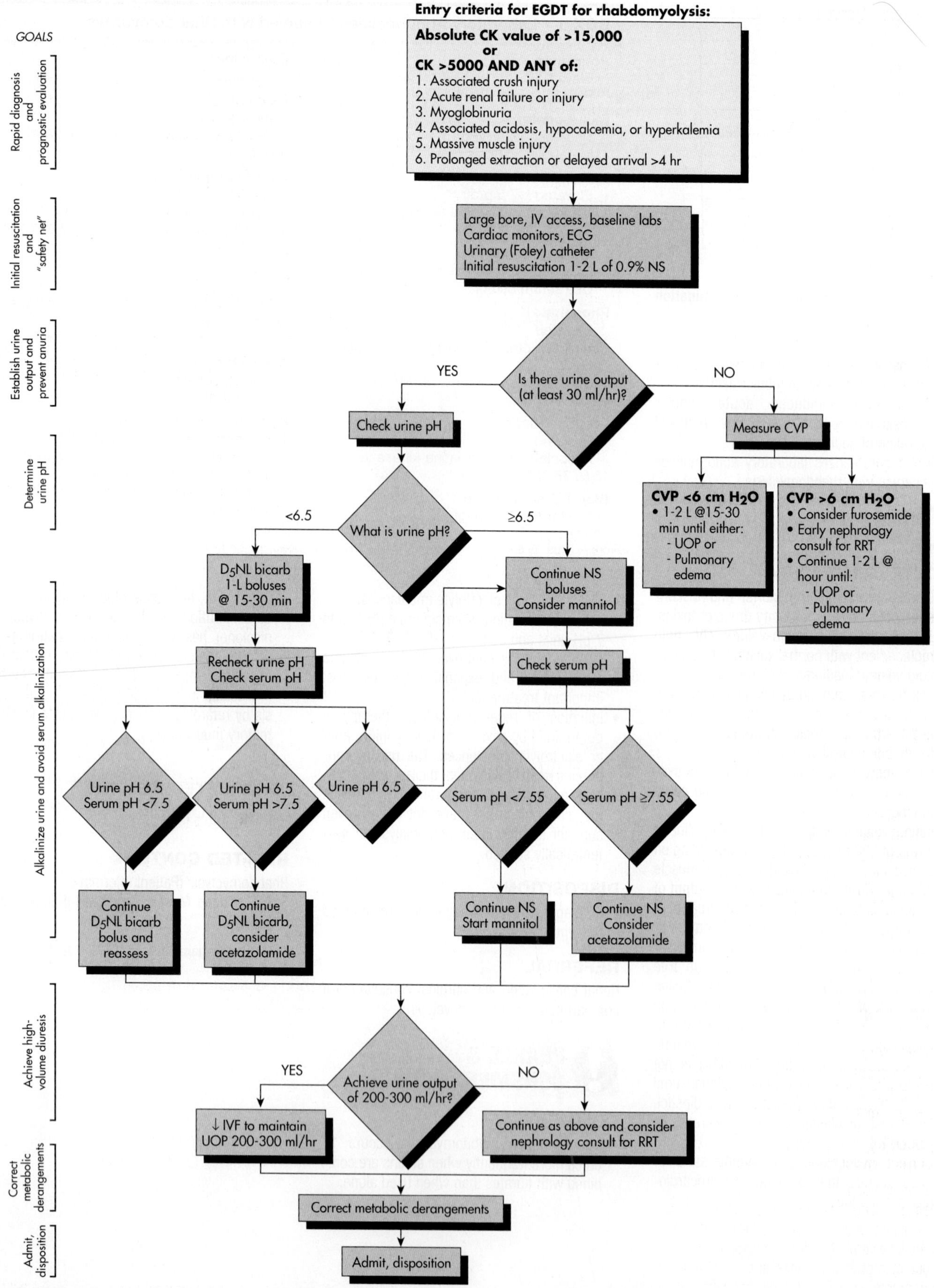

FIG. 2 Early goal-directed therapy for rhabdomyolysis. *CK,* Creatine kinase; *CVP,* central venous pressure; *D5NL bicarb,* 5% dextrose in normal sodium bicarbonate solution; *EGDT,* early goal-directed therapy; *IV,* intravenous; *IVF,* intravenous fluid; *NS,* normal saline; *RRT,* renal replacement therapy; *UOP,* urinary output. (From Adams JG et al: *Emergency medicine, clinical essentials*, ed 2, Philadelphia, 2013, Elsevier.)

BASIC INFORMATION

DEFINITION

Rheumatoid arthritis (RA) is a systemic autoimmune disease characterized by inflammatory polyarthritis that affects peripheral joints, especially the small joints of the hands and feet. It is a chronic, progressive disease in which untreated inflammation may lead to cartilage and bone erosions and joint destruction resulting in functional impairment.

SYNONYM

RA

ICD-10CM CODES

M06.9	Rheumatoid arthritis, unspecified
M05.10	Rheumatoid lung disease with rheumatoid arthritis of unspecified site
M05.20	Rheumatoid vasculitis with rheumatoid arthritis of unspecified site
M05.39	Rheumatoid heart disease with rheumatoid arthritis of multiple sites
M05.49	Rheumatoid myopathy with rheumatoid arthritis of multiple sites
M05.59	Rheumatoid polyneuropathy with rheumatoid arthritis of multiple sites
M05.69	Rheumatoid arthritis of multiple sites with involvement of other organs and systems
M05.79	Rheumatoid arthritis with rheumatoid factor of multiple sites without organ or systems involvement
M05.80	Other rheumatoid arthritis with rheumatoid factor of unspecified site

EPIDEMIOLOGY & DEMOGRAPHICS

INCIDENCE: Annual incidence in northern Europe and the U.S. 0.15 to 0.60 per 1000

TYPICAL AGE AT DIAGNOSIS: Usually between age 30 and 60. Steadily increases with age until the mid-70s

PREVALENCE: 0.5% to 1.0% of the worldwide population, with different rates in different ethnic groups

PREDOMINANT SEX: Females > males (2 to 3:1)

RISK FACTORS: Female gender, age, tobacco use, silica exposure, and obesity, family history. Smoking has an additive detrimental effect in RA patients (two-fold excess mortality risk).

PHYSICAL FINDINGS & CLINICAL PRESENTATION

Initial presentation:

- Pain, swelling, warmth in one or more peripheral joints, frequently with symmetric small joint involvement, often associated with >1 hour of morning stiffness and constitutional symptoms such as fatigue, malaise, low-grade fevers, and weight loss occurring over a period of weeks to months. A subset of patients can also present with acute-onset polyarthritis instead of insidious symptoms.
- Most common joints involved include metacarpophalangeal (MCP) joints, proximal interphalangeal (PIP) joints (Fig. E1), and metatarsophalangeal (MTP) joints (Fig. E2), as well as wrists.
- Other affected joints involved include elbows, shoulders, hips, knees, and ankles.
- Distal interphalangeal (DIP) joints are spared.
- Sacroiliac and vertebral joints are spared, except for the C1 and C2 articulations.

Chronic longstanding disease:

- "Swan-neck" (DIP flexion and PIP hyperextension) (Fig. E3), "boutonniere" (DIP hyperextension and PIP flexion), and "Z-thumb" (MCP flexion and IP hyperextension) deformities (Fig. 4), ulnar deviation, and subluxation of the MCP joints as well as radial deviation of the wrists.
- C1-C2 (atlantoaxial) inflammation can lead to odontoid erosion and transverse ligament laxity/rupture, resulting in atlantoaxial subluxation and cord compression.
- Joint damage of wrists, elbows, shoulders, hips, and knees can lead to severe secondary osteoarthritis, necessitating joint surgery and/or replacement.

Extraarticular manifestations:

- Secondary Sjögren syndrome (~35%): Immune-mediated inflammation of lacrimal and salivary glands, resulting in dry mouth (xerostomia) and eyes (keratoconjunctivitis sicca).
- Rheumatoid nodules (25%): Nontender, firm nodules on extensor surfaces and pressure points, usually in rheumatoid factor positive (RF+) disease. Histopathology demonstrates palisading histiocytes surrounding a central area of fibrinoid necrosis.
- Felty syndrome: RA with splenomegaly and leukopenia. Most patients are positive for HLA-DR4 and RF.

Pulmonary disease:

- Pleural disease (exudative effusions, pleuritis)
- Interstitial lung disease (up to 10% clinically significant)
- Bronchiolitis obliterans
- Cryptogenic organizing pneumonia
- Pulmonary nodules: A combination of RA and pneumoconiosis is called Caplan syndrome

Neuromuscular:

- Entrapment neuropathy (carpal tunnel, tarsal tunnel, cubital tunnel most commonly involved)
- Mononeuritis multiplex
- Peripheral neuropathy
- Cervical myelopathy and cord compression in atlantoaxial subluxation
- Pachymeningitis (rare)

Vasculitis

Cardiac disease:

- Pericarditis (most common)
- Myocarditis
- Valvular nodules
- There is an increased risk of cardiovascular disease compared to the general population, probably due to accelerated atherosclerosis from systemic inflammation

Ocular disease:

- Keratoconjunctivitis sicca (dry eye, without dry mouth) (10%)
- Episcleritis, scleritis, scleral thinning, scleromalacia perforans, ulcerative keratitis

Amyloidosis: Occurs in longstanding, poorly controlled RA. Usually presents as nephrotic syndrome. Can affect heart, kidney, liver, spleen, intestines, and skin

Osteoporosis

ETIOLOGY

The exact cause of RA remains unknown despite extensive research. It is likely that a combination of genetic, hormonal, and environmental factors lead to aberrant immune activation and inflammatory response in the joint. A common genetic background plays a role in susceptibility to disease, as twins and first-degree relatives of RA patients are at increased risk of developing the disease compared to the general population. Patients with HLA-DR4, DR1, and DR14 alleles have increased susceptibility to RA; in particular, one amino acid sequence in the DR β chain, known as the shared epitope, is overrepresented in these patients. Other identified genetic associations include polymorphisms

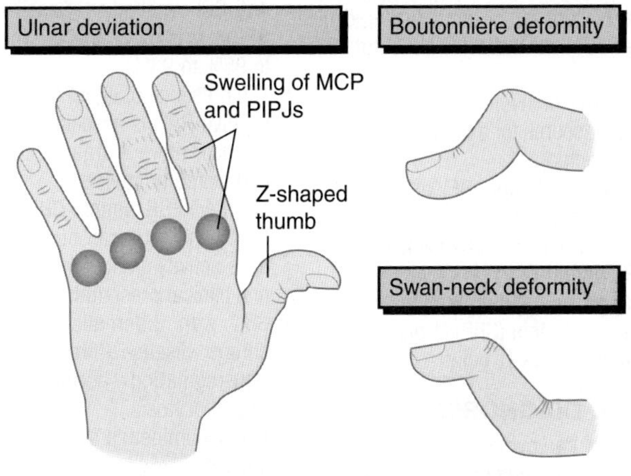

FIG. 4 Characteristic hand deformities in rheumatoid arthritis. *MCP,* Metacarpophalanges; *PIPJs,* proximal interphalangeal joints. (From Ballinger A: *Kumar & Clark's essentials of clinical medicine,* ed 6, Edinburgh, 2012, Saunders.)

in *PTPN22, PADI4, CTLA4, TRAF1-C5, STAT4, TNFAIP3*. Epigenetic factors are also likely to be involved. Multiple environmental factors have also been implicated as possible etiologic factors, including cigarette smoking, silica exposure, and low socioeconomic class. Infectious agents such as *P. gingivalis*, Epstein-Barr virus, and parvovirus B19 have also been reported as possible triggers.

Stages of disease development presumably include:

- Initiation of the innate immune response through toll-like receptor (TLR) activation by a stimulating signal.
- Perpetuation of inflammatory response through activation of the adaptive immune system. There is migration of inflammatory cells (autoreactive B and T cells, monocytes) into the joint space, activation of macrophage-like and fibroblast-like synoviocytes, and development of a "synovial pannus," a thickened synovial membrane.
- The pannus releases pro-inflammatory cytokines (tumor necrosis factor alpha [TNF-α], interleukin [IL]-1, IL-6, IL-15, IL-17, IL-18) as well as proteases, which erode cartilage and bone. Bone erosions are caused mainly by osteoclasts, which express the receptor activator of NF-κB (RANK). TNF-α, IL-1, IL-6, and IL-17 promote the expression of RANK ligand (RANKL) on T cells and fibroblast-like synoviocytes, thus creating a positive feedback loop. IL-6 and TNF-α act synergistically to increase vascular endothelial growth factor levels, which in turn stimulate angiogenesis, thereby maintaining pannus formation. B-cell differentiation is also promoted by IL-6, leading to the production of autoantibodies.
- Many of the new "biologic" disease-modifying antirheumatic drugs (DMARDs) are engineered to target these cytokines (see "Treatment" section).

TABLE 1 Factors Useful for Differentiating Early Rheumatoid Arthritis from Osteoarthritis

	Rheumatoid Arthritis	Osteoarthritis
Age at onset	Childhood and adults, peak incidence in 50s	Increases with age
Predisposing factors	Susceptibility epitopes (HLA-DR4, HLA-DR1, HLA-DR14)	Trauma
	Polymorphisms, epigenetic factors, infectious agents	Congenital abnormalities (e.g., shallow acetabulum)
	Smoking, silica exposure	
Early symptoms	Morning stiffness, pain, swelling	Pain increases through the day and with use
Joints involved	Wrists, MCP, PIP, and MTP joints; DIP joints are almost never involved.	DIP joints (Heberden nodes), PIP joints (Bouchard nodes), carpometacarpal joints, weight-bearing joints (hips, knees)
Physical findings	Soft tissue swelling, warmth	Bony osteophytes, minimal soft tissue swelling early on, crepitus
Radiologic findings	Periarticular osteopenia, marginal erosions	Subchondral sclerosis, osteophytes
Laboratory findings	Increased CRP, RF, and anti-CCP antibody, anemia, thrombocytosis	Normal

anti-CCP, Anticitrullinated protein; *CRP-RF,* C-reactive protein-rheumatoid factor; *DIP,* distal interphalangeal joint; *MCP,* metacarpophalangeal joint; *MTP,* metatarsophalangeal joint; *PIP,* proximal interphalangeal joint.

Dx DIAGNOSIS

The American College of Rheumatology (ACR) and the European League against Rheumatism (EULAR) developed new classification criteria for RA in 2010. These are based on a point system where patients with score ≥6/10 are considered to have "definite RA." Four variables constitute the new criteria:

- The number and size of involved joints (0 to 5 points, with higher scores for a larger number of small joints affected)
- Levels of rheumatoid factor (RF) and anti-cyclic citrullinated peptide (CCP) antibody (0 to 3 points, with a higher score for a high-titer positive RF or anti-CCP)
- Elevated erythrocyte sedimentation rate (ESR) or C-reactive protein (CRP) (1 point)
- Symptom duration ≥6 wk (1 point)

DIFFERENTIAL DIAGNOSIS

- Infectious causes: Parvovirus B19, hepatitis B, hepatitis C, poststreptococcal reactive arthritis, acute rheumatic fever
- Connective tissue diseases: Systemic lupus erythematosus, scleroderma, mixed connective tissue disease, Sjögren syndrome
- Seronegative spondyloarthropathies
- Calcium pyrophosphate deposition (CPPD or "pseudo-RA")
- Polyarticular gout
- Polymyalgia rheumatica
- Remitting seronegative symmetric synovitis with pitting edema (RS3PE) can resemble seronegative RA in elderly patients
- Hemochromatosis
- Paraneoplastic syndromes
- Osteoarthritis, a degenerative arthritis that lacks prolonged morning stiffness and that usually lacks synovitis, should not be confused with RA (see Table 1)

LABORATORY TESTS

- RF (sensitivity ~60%; specificity ~80%). False positives are seen with hepatitis C, subacute bacterial endocarditis, primary biliary cirrhosis, sarcoidosis, malignancy, Sjögren syndrome, SLE, and increasing age.
- Anti-CCP antibodies. Sensitivity is similar to RF, but it is more specific for RA than RF (up to 95% to 98%).
- The presence of either RF or anti-CCP ("seropositive RA") is associated with more severe disease, more extraarticular manifestations, and worse prognosis.
- Elevated ESR and/or CRP. Will decline with treatment; thus can be used to monitor disease activity along with physical examination and clinical presentation.
- CBC with differential. Possible anemia of chronic disease (through production of the iron-regulating hormone, hepcidin) and thrombocytosis.
- Hypoalbuminemia and hypergammaglobulinemia.
- ANA is present is 20% to 30% of patients. However, complement will usually be normal or increased, in contrast to patients with systemic lupus erythematosus. Many patients will have secondary Sjögren syndrome (positive ANA with negative SSA and SSB).
- Inflammatory synovial fluid with >2000 PMNs. Of note, patients with RA have an increased risk of developing septic arthritis. Hence, synovial fluid with white blood cells >50,000 cells/mm^3 is concerning for an infectious process and must always be ruled out.

IMAGING STUDIES

Plain radiography (Table E2):

- Early changes include soft tissue swelling, symmetric joint space narrowing, and periarticular osteopenia.
- Later changes include periarticular erosions and deformities. This reflects cartilage and bone destruction secondary to pannus formation (Fig. E5).
- Radiographs of hands and feet should be obtained at disease onset and repeated to monitor disease progression and to ensure that adequate treatment is achieved.

MRI and musculoskeletal US:

- More sensitive for detecting erosive disease and joint effusions/synovitis

Rx TREATMENT

- Early identification and treatment of RA with DMARDs is crucial. More than half of patients have radiographic joint damage within 2 yr of disease onset, but early aggressive treatment with DMARDs and/or biologic agents is associated with decreased progression of synovitis and bone erosions, and with decreased disability. Fig. 6 describes the American College of Rheumatology recommendations for treatment of rheumatoid arthritis. Goal of therapy is to "treat to a target" of low disease activity or remission.

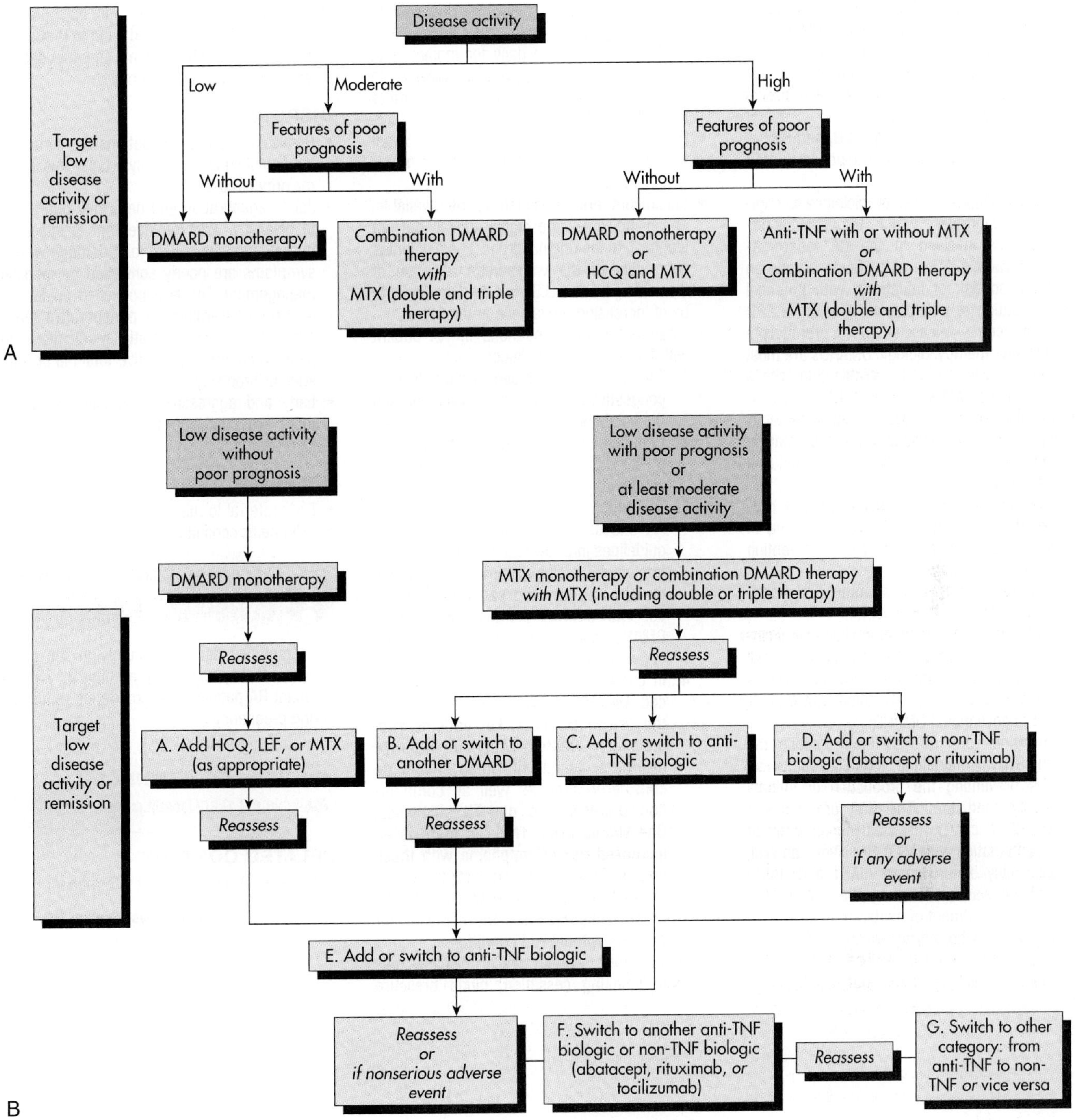

FIG. 6 American College of Rheumatology recommendations for treatment of rheumatoid arthritis. A, Early disease. **B,** Established disease. *DMARD,* Disease-modifying antirheumatic drug; *HCQ,* hydroxychloroquine; *LEF,* leflunomide; *MTX,* methotrexate; *TNF,* tumor necrosis factor. (From Firestein GS et al [eds]: *Kelly's textbook of rheumatology,* ed 9, Philadelphia, 2013, Saunders.)

- There are several tools to measure disease activity and define remission in rheumatoid arthritis, including (but not limited to) the following: Clinical Disease Activity Index (CDAI), Simplified Disease Activity Index (SDAI), Disease Activity Score (DAS) 28, Routine Assessment of Patient Index Data 3 (RAPID3), Stanford Health Assessment Questionnaire (HAQ), and Patient Activity Scale (PAS).

ACUTE GENERAL Rx

- NSAIDs: Can be used initially to relieve pain and mild inflammation or used later in the disease course for additional control of mild pain. NSAIDs are not disease modifying.
- Corticosteroids: Oral or intraarticular, frequently used initially to reduce inflammation rapidly until oral DMARD treatments take effect. They may also be used during acute flares or in low doses for additional control of inflammation. The use of corticosteroids at the lowest dose possible and shortest duration is recommended. Corticosteroids have many side effects, including but not limited to weight gain, increased risk of diabetes, osteoporosis, cataract formation, peptic ulcer disease (especially when used in combination with NSAIDs), and avascular necrosis.

CHRONIC Rx

- DMARDs: Can be classified into "nonbiologic" and "biologic" treatments.
  1. Nonbiologic DMARDs: Most commonly used agents are methotrexate (MTX), hydroxychloroquine (HCQ), sulfasalazine (SSZ), and leflunomide (LEF). Most of these are associated with potential toxicity and require close monitoring. They

are also slow-acting drugs that generally require >8 wk to start taking effect.
2. MTX is the most commonly used DMARD worldwide for the treatment of RA. It is effective as monotherapy in about 30% of patients with RA.
3. "Triple therapy"—MTX, HCQ, and SSZ—has been shown to be superior to MTX alone.

- Biologic DMARDs: Newer biologically engineered therapies, which target cytokines and cells involved in the RA inflammatory response. Major side effects include an increased risk of infections, with potential reactivation of tuberculosis. A negative PPD or interferon γ-release assay is a prerequisite to initiate therapy. Biologic DMARDs are most effective when used in combination with a nonbiologic DMARD, usually MTX.
- The five approved tumor necrosis factor α inhibitors (TNFI) include infliximab, etanercept, adalimumab, certolizumab pegol, and golimumab.
- Abatacept (CTLA-4Ig) is a recombinant protein that prevents costimulatory binding of antigen presenting cell to T cell, preventing T-cell activation.
- Tocilizumab (anti–IL-6) is a monoclonal antibody against the IL-6 receptor.
- Sarilumab is another IL-6 inhibitor monoclonal antibody, approved by the FDA in 2017 for treatment of RA, and can be used as monotherapy or in combination with MTX or other conventional DMARDs.
- Tofacitinib (JAK1/2/3 inhibitor) inhibits the JAK-STAT intracellular signaling pathway, thus preventing the production of inflammatory mediators. The first oral biologic DMARD, it can be used as monotherapy or in combination with MTX. Baricitinib, an oral, once-daily Janus kinase (JAK1 and JAK2) inhibitor, was approved by the FDA in May 2018 for treatment of moderate to severe RA in patients who did not respond adequately to one or more TNFIs. A dose of 2 mg was approved, with concerns that higher doses had increased adverse events. Upadacitinib (JAK1 > JAK2/3 inhibitor) was approved in 2019 at 15 mg once daily for moderate to severely active RA resistant or intolerant to MTX, or in combination with MTX with other nonbiologic DMARDs.
- Rituximab (anti-CD20) is a monoclonal antibody against the CD20 antigen on B lymphocytes.
- Biosimilars are beginning to be available. These molecules are highly similar, but not identical, to the original drugs. Legal disputes have delayed the widespread adoption of these drugs in the U.S., but they are likely to be of increasing prevalence in the future.
- Treatment recommendations in RA patient with high-risk comorbidities:
  1. TNFI should be avoided in patients with congestive heart failure, as it can worsen the condition.
  2. In patients with hepatitis B, immunosuppressive therapy can be safely prescribed along with concomitant antiviral therapy.
  3. Treatment of hepatitis C patients with RA should be done following standard guidelines in collaboration with gastroenterology/hepatology. Immunosuppressive therapy can be used safely in conjunction with antiviral therapy; avoidance of DMARDs such as MTX and LEF should be taken into consideration.
  4. In patients with a history of skin cancer, DMARDs are recommended over the use of biologics. For patients with previously treated lymphoproliferative disorders, use of rituximab should be considered first, as well as combination DMARDs and non-TNF biologics. One should avoid TNFI, as there is an increased risk of lymphoma with these agents. Recommendations for treatment of patients with previously treated solid organ malignancy are the same as for patients without the condition.

Immunization, cardiovascular disease prevention (smoking cessation, blood pressure control, cholesterol control), and osteoporosis prevention (with calcium and vitamin D supplementation and bisphosphonate therapy) should be addressed in all RA patients.

DISPOSITION

- Remissions and exacerbations are common, but condition is chronically progressive in the majority of cases.
- Joint degeneration and deformity often lead to disability. Joint replacement is indicated for patients with severe joint damage whose symptoms are poorly controlled by medical management. The ACR published guidelines in 2017 concerning the perioperative management of antirheumatic medications in patients undergoing elective total hip or total knee arthroplasty.
- Early and aggressive diagnosis and treatment are crucial in preventing or slowing joint destruction.

REFERRAL

- Early referral to rheumatologist
- Orthopedic consultation for corrective surgery

PEARLS & CONSIDERATIONS

RA sometimes develops acutely in the postpartum patient; conversely, as high as 75% of pregnant RA patients will experience remission during pregnancy.

SUGGESTED READINGS

Available at ExpertConsult.com

RELATED CONTENT

Rheumatoid Arthritis (Patient Information)

AUTHOR: **Daphne Scaramangas-Plumley, MD**

BASIC INFORMATION

DEFINITION

Rosacea is a chronic skin disorder characterized by papules and pustules affecting the face and often associated with flushing and erythema.

SYNONYM

Acne rosacea

ICD-10CM CODES	
L71	Rosacea
L71.9	Rosacea unspecified
L71.1	Rhinophyma
L71.8	Other rosacea
L71.0	Perioral dermatitis

EPIDEMIOLOGY & DEMOGRAPHICS

- Rosacea occurs in 1 in 20 Americans
- Onset often between ages 30 and 50 yr
- More common in people of Celtic origin; however, this disease may be overlooked in nonwhites because skin pigmentation results in atypical presentation
- Female:male ratio of 3:1

PHYSICAL FINDINGS & CLINICAL PRESENTATION

- Facial erythema, presence of papules, pustules, and telangiectasia (Fig. E1).
- Excessive facial warmth and redness are the predominant presenting symptoms.
- Itching is generally absent.
- Comedones are absent (unlike acne).
- Women are more likely to show symptoms on the chin and cheeks, whereas in men the nose is commonly involved.
- Ocular findings (mild dryness and irritation with blepharitis, conjunctival injection, burning, stinging, tearing, eyelid inflammation, swelling, and redness) are present in 50% of patients.

Rosacea can be classified into four major subtypes (Table E1):

1. Erythematotelangiectatic (vascular): Erythema in central part of face, telangiectasia, flushing
2. Papulopustular (inflammatory): Presence of dome-shaped erythematous papules and small pustules, in addition to facial erythema, flushing, and telangiectasia
3. Phymatosis/glandular rosacea (Fig. E2): Presence of thickened skin with prominent pores that may affect the nose (rhinophyma) (Fig. E3), chin (gnathophyma), forehead (metophyma), eyelids (blepharophyma), and ears (otophyma)
4. Ocular: Conjunctival injection, sensation of foreign body in the eye, telangiectasia and erythema of lid margins, scaling

ETIOLOGY

- The pathophysiology of rosacea is incompletely understood but believed to involve the vasculature.
- Hot drinks, alcohol, and sun exposure may accentuate the erythema by causing vasodilation of the skin.
- Flare-ups may also result from reactions to medications (e.g., simvastatin, angiotensin-converting enzyme inhibitors, vasodilators, fluorinated corticosteroids), stress, extreme heat or cold, wind, humidity, strenuous exercise, spicy drinks, menstruation.

Dx DIAGNOSIS

The presence of at least one of the following primary features in a central distribution of the face is generally sufficient to diagnose rosacea: Papules and pustules, telangiectasia, flushing (transient erythema), nontransient erythema.

DIFFERENTIAL DIAGNOSIS

- Drug eruption
- Acne vulgaris
- Contact dermatitis
- Systemic lupus erythematosus
- Carcinoid flush
- Idiopathic facial flushing
- Seborrheic dermatitis
- Facial sarcoidosis
- Photodermatitis
- Mastocytosis
- Perioral dermatitis
- Granulomas of the skin

WORKUP

Diagnosis is based on clinical findings. Distinguishing features between acne and rosacea are the presence of telangiectasia and deep diffuse erythema and absence of comedones in rosacea.

Rx TREATMENT

NONPHARMACOLOGIC THERAPY

- Instruct patients to keep a diary to identify stimuli and triggers that exacerbate rosacea (e.g., spicy foods, drugs, cosmetics) and avoid identified triggers.
- Avoid alcohol, excessive sun exposure, and hot drinks of any type.
- Use of mild, nondrying soap or soap-free cleansers and nonoily moisturizers is recommended; local skin irritants should be avoided. General recommendations for skin care in patients with rosacea are summarized in Table 2.
- Sunscreens are an important component of therapy and should be applied each morning.
- Daily circular massage for several minutes of the central portion of the face is helpful in decreasing lymphedema and inflammation in this area.
- Reassure patient that rosacea is completely unrelated to poor hygiene.
- Vascular laser surgery is effective for telangiectasia.
- Surgical options are available for telangiectasia and rhinophyma and include dermabrasion, laser ablation, heated scalpel, electrocautery, and radiofrequency electrosurgery.

GENERAL Rx

- Several classes of drugs are used in treatment of rosacea, including the metronidazole family, the tetracycline family, ivermectin cream, and azelaic acid.
- Vascular rosacea: Topical therapy with metronidazole aqueous gel is effective as initial therapy for mild cases. Clindamycin lotion (Cleocin), sulfacetamide, or erythromycin 2% solution may also be effective. A 1.5% topical foam formulation of minocycline is also available for treatment of inflammatory lesions of rosacea in adults. Cost is a limiting factor. Brimonidine is a selective alpha$_2$-adrenergic receptor agonist FDA-approved as a gel preparation for topical treatment of adults with persistent facial erythema of rosacea. Oxymetazoline 1% cream is also an FDA-approved selecting alpha1a-adrenergic receptor agonist for topical treatment of persistent facial erythema in adults. Neither brimonidine or oxymetazoline are indicated for the treatment of inflammatory lesions of rosacea.
- Pustular and ocular rosacea: Systemic antibiotics (doxycycline 100 mg qd or tetracycline 250 mg qid until symptoms diminish, then taper off). Minocycline 50 to 100 mg is useful qd in resistant cases. Oral metronidazole (200 mg qd to bid) for 4 to 6 wk is also effective. A 1% cream formulation of the antiparasitic drug ivermectin is effective for papulopustular rosacea with minimal adverse effects. After 3 mo of therapy, it will produce clearing of rosacea lesions in up to 80% of patients with moderate to severe symptoms. Its mechanism of action is unknown, but it may be due to the combination of its antiinflammatory effects and its antiparasitic effects on the Demodex mite, which may contribute to the symptoms of rosacea.
- Isotretinoin 0.5 to 1 mg/kg/day in two divided doses for 15 to 20 wk can be used for refractory papular and pustular rosacea; use of retinoids may, however, worsen erythema and telangiectasis.
- Erythema and flushing may respond to low-dose clonidine (0.05 mg bid).
- Treatment of phymatous rosacea: Oral tetracyclines, oral isotretinoin, ablative/pulsed dye laser therapy, electrosurgery.
- Treatment of ocular rosacea: Topical or oral tetracyclines, artificial tears, and/or lid cleansing for eyelid hygiene. Medical and surgical therapies for rosacea are summarized in Table E3.

DISPOSITION

- Rosacea is often resistant to initial treatment and recurrent. Periods of remission and relapse are common.
- The progression of rosacea is variable. Typical stages include:
  1. Facial flushing
  2. Erythema and/or edema and ocular symptoms
  3. Papules and pustules
  4. Rhinophyma

TABLE 2 General Recommendations for Facial Skin Care and Education in Patients with Rosacea

Facial Skin Care

- Wash with lukewarm water and use soap-free cleansers that are pH balanced.
- Cleansers are applied gently with fingertips.
- Use sunscreens with both UVA and UVB protection and an SPF ≥30.
- Sunscreens containing the inorganic filters titanium dioxide and/or zinc oxide are usually well tolerated.
- Use cosmetics and sunscreens that contain protective silicones.
- Water-soluble facial powder containing inert green pigment helps to neutralize the perception of erythema.
- Moisturizers containing humectants (e.g., glycerin) and occlusives (e.g., petrolatum) help to repair the epidermal barrier.
- Avoid astringents, toners, and abrasive exfoliators.
- Avoid cosmetics that contain alcohol, menthols, camphor, witch hazel, fragrance, peppermint, and eucalyptus oil.
- Avoid waterproof cosmetics and heavy foundations that are difficult to remove without irritating solvents or physical scrubbing.
- Avoid procedures such as glycolic peels or dermabrasion.

Patient Education

- Reassure the patient about the benign nature of the disorder and the rarity of rhinophyma, particularly in women.
- Emphasize the chronicity of the disease and the likelihood of exacerbations.
- Direct patients to information websites such as those of the National Rosacea Society (http://www.rosacea.org) or the American Academy of Dermatology (http://www.aad.org).
- Advise to avoid recognized triggers.
- Explain the importance of compliance with topical regimens.
- Educate on the importance of sun avoidance.

SPF, Sun protective factor; *UVA,* ultraviolet A; *UVB,* ultraviolet B.

Adapted from Del Rosso JQ, Baum EW: Comprehensive medical management of rosacea: an interim study report and literature review, *J Clin Aesthet Dermatol* 1:20-25, 2008; Powell FC: Rosacea, *N Engl J Med* 352:793-803, 2005; and Pelle MT et al: Rosacea: II. Therapy, *J Am Acad Dermatol* 51:499-512, 2004; In Bolognia J: *Dermatology,* ed 4, Philadelphia, 2018, Elsevier.

PEARLS & CONSIDERATIONS

COMMENTS

- The course of the disease is typically chronic, with remissions and relapses.
- Patients with resistant cases may have *Demodex folliculorum* mite infestation or tinea infection (diagnosis can be confirmed with potassium hydroxide examination); the role of *D. folliculorum* in rosacea is unclear. These mites can sometimes be found in large numbers in the lesions; however, their numbers do not generally decline with treatment.
- Rosacea can result in emotional and social stigmas, especially because many people associate rosacea and rhinophyma with alcohol abuse.
- Early consultation with an ophthalmologist is recommended in patients with suspected ocular involvement.

SUGGESTED READINGS

Available at ExpertConsult.com

RELATED CONTENT

Rosacea (Patient Information)

AUTHOR: **Fred F. Ferri, MD**

BASIC INFORMATION

DEFINITION

Salmonellosis is an infection caused by one of several serotypes of a gram-negative bacillus of the genus *Salmonella.* Salmonella infection can be typhoidal (serotype Typhi or Paratyphi) or nontyphoidal. Current *Salmonella* nomenclature is described in Box 1.

SYNONYMS

Typhoid fever
Paratyphoid fever
Enteric fever

ICD-10CM CODES

A02.0 *Salmonella* enteritis
A02.1 *Salmonella* sepsis
A02.2 Localized *Salmonella* infections
A02.8 Other specified *Salmonella* infections
A0.9 *Salmonella* infection, unspecified

EPIDEMIOLOGY & DEMOGRAPHICS

INCIDENCE (IN U.S.):

- Epidemiologically, the clinical syndromes are divided into those that cause a typhoidal type of infection (systemic illness with fever and abdominal pain) such as *Salmonella typhi* and those that do not: Nontyphoidal *Salmonella* infections (gastroenteritis) such as *S. enteritidis, S. newport,* and *S. typhimurium.*
- Estimated 1 million cases/yr of nontyphoidal salmonellosis in the United States (leading cause of foodborne illness in the U.S.). In 2017 an outbreak occurred linked to live poultry in backyard flocks with over 960 cases in 48 states caused by several different *Salmonella* bacteria. In 2020 an outbreak associated with onions occurred in the U.S.
- Largest outbreak of gastroenteritis syndrome (nontyphoidal): 200,000 who ingested contaminated milk.
- Approximately 500 cases of *Salmonella typhi* infection are reported each yr, of which nearly 80% is associated with foreign travel.

PREDOMINANT AGE:

- <20 yr old
- >70 yr old
- Highest rates of infection in infants, especially neonates

PEAK INCIDENCE: Summer and fall

GENETICS:

Neonatal Infection:

- Highly susceptible to infection with nontyphoidal *Salmonella*

PHYSICAL FINDINGS & CLINICAL PRESENTATION (TABLE 1)

- Infections:
  1. Localized to GI tract (gastroenteritis)
  2. Systemic (typhoid fever)
  3. Localized outside of GI tract
- Gastroenteritis:
  1. Incubation period: 12 to 48 hr
  2. Nausea, vomiting
  3. Diarrhea, abdominal cramps
  4. Fever
  5. Bacteremia: Occurs mostly in the immunocompromised host or those with underlying conditions, including HIV infection
  6. Self-limited illness lasting 3 or 4 days
  7. Colonization of GI tract persistent for months, especially in those treated with antibiotics
- Typhoid fever:
  1. Incubation period of few days to several wk
  2. Prolonged fever, often with a stepwise-increasing temperature pattern
  3. Myalgias
  4. Headache, cough, sore throat
  5. Malaise, anorexia
  6. Abdominal pain
  7. Hepatosplenomegaly
  8. Diarrhea or constipation early in the course of illness
  9. Rose spots (faint, maculopapular, blanching lesions) sometimes seen on chest or abdomen
- Untreated disease:
  1. Fever lasting 1 to 2 mo
  2. Main complication: GI bleeding caused by perforation from ulceration of Peyer patches in the ileum
  3. Rare complications:
     a. Mental status changes
     b. Shock
  4. Relapse rate of approximately 10%
- Infections outside GI tract:
  1. Can occur in virtually any location
  2. Usually occur in patients with underlying diseases
  3. Endocarditis, endovascular infections are caused by seeding of atherosclerotic plaques or aneurysms
  4. Hepatic or splenic abscesses in patients with underlying disease in these organs
  5. Urinary tract infections in patients with renal tuberculosis (TB) or schistosomiasis
  6. *Salmonellae* are a frequent cause of gram-negative meningitis in neonates

BOX 1 Nomenclature of *Salmonella* Infections

The multiple microbiologic, serologic, and clinical designations applied to *Salmonella* infections are confusing.[1] Most pathogenic *Salmonella* belong to a single subspecies designated *Salmonella enterica* subspecies enterica. In addition to this species designation, *Salmonella* are classified serologically. The serogroup is assigned based on the O antigen alone, whereas the serotype designation, from which the name is derived, is based on both the O and H antigens.

Salmonella enterica subsp. enterica includes over 1400 serotypes. Although the full name of the cause of typhoid fever is *Salmonella enterica* subsp. enterica serotype Typhi, it is normally shortened to *S.* Typhi. Although serogroup designation is performed routinely in many laboratories, the test lacks clinical utility. Complete serotype identification is often performed in a reference laboratory; however, *S.* Typhi and Paratyphi A can also be identified by biochemical tests in a routine microbiology laboratory. Identification of *S.* Typhi and Paratyphi A are reviewed in detail in the World Health Organization's, "The Diagnosis, Treatment and Prevention of Typhoid Fever."[2]

Clinically *Salmonella* are classified as typhoidal or nontyphoidal. The typhoidal serotypes are *S.* Typhi and Paratyphi A, B, and C. All others are classified as nontyphoidal. However, this is also misleading, as many nontyphoidal strains also cause invasive infection, which may mimic typhoid fever.

Examples of Clinical and Serologic Classification of Pathogenic *Salmonella*

Clinical Classification	Serotype	Formal Designation	Serogroup
Typhoidal	Typhi	*S. enterica* subsp. enterica ser. Typhi	D
	Paratyphi A	*S. enterica* subsp. enterica ser. Paratyphi A	A
	Paratyphi B (schottmuelleri)	*S. enterica* subsp. enterica ser. Paratyphi B	B
	Paratyphi C (hirschfeldii)	*S. enterica* subsp. enterica ser. Paratyphi C	C
Nontyphoidal	Typhimurium	*S. enterica* subsp. enterica ser. Typhimurium	B
	Enteritidis	*S. enterica* subsp. enterica ser. Enteritidis	D
	Newport	*S. enterica* subsp. enterica ser. Newport	C

[1]Brenner FW et al: Salmonella nomenclature, *J Clin Microbiol* 38:2465-2467, 2000.
[2]World Health Organization: Background document: the diagnosis, treatment and prevention of typhoid fever, 2003.
From Ryan ET et al: *Hunter's tropical medicine and emerging infectious diseases,* ed 10, Philadelphia, 2019, Elsevier.

TABLE 1 Clinical Features of Typhoid and Paratyphoid Fever

	Clinical Feature	Approx. Frequency*
	Fever	>95%
Flulike symptoms	Headache	80%
	Chills	40%
	Cough	30%
	Myalgia	20%
	Arthralgia	<5%
Abdominal symptoms	Anorexia	50%
	Abdominal pain	30%
	Diarrhea	20%
	Constipation	20%
Physical findings	Coated tongue	50%
	Hepatomegaly	10%
	Splenomegaly	10%
	Abdominal tenderness	5%
	Rash	<5%
	Generalized adenopathy	<5%

*The proportion of patients demonstrating these clinical features of enteric fever varies depending on the time, region, and type of clinical population (hospitalized or ambulatory) assessed. Estimates are drawn from case series in an endemic area presenting for ambulatory or inpatient care.
From Ryan ET et al: *Hunter's tropical medicine and emerging infectious diseases*, ed 10, Philadelphia, 2019, Elsevier.

TABLE 2 Complications of Typhoid and Paratyphoid Fever

System	Complication	Notes
Gastrointestinal	Hemorrhage	10%-15% hospitalized patients
	Perforation	3% hospitalized patients
Hepatobiliary	Jaundice	1%-3% hospitalized patients
	Hepatitis	Usually subclinical (↑ ALT/AST)
	Acute cholecystitis	Rare, gallbladder may perforate
Neurologic	Mild encephalopathy	Confusion or apathy common
	Severe encephalopathy	Delirium, stupor, or coma
	Seizures	Common in children ≤5 yr
	Meningitis	Rare, primarily infants
	Guillain–Barré syndrome	Reported
Respiratory	Bronchitis	Cough is common
	Pneumonia	May be other concomitant bacterial infection (e.g., *S. pneumoniae*)
Cardiovascular	Myocarditis	Usually subclinical (ECG changes)
	Shock	Uncommon
Hematologic	Anemia	Usually subclinical
	DIC	Usually subclinical (↑ PT/PTT)
Other	Pyogenic infections	Uncommon
	Hemolytic uremic syndrome	Reported
	Miscarriage	Reported

ALT, Alanine aminotransferase; *AST,* aspartate aminotransferase; *DIC,* disseminated intravascular coagulation; *ECG,* echocardiogram; *PT,* prothrombin time; *PTT,* partial thromboplastin time.
From Ryan ET et al: *Hunter's tropical medicine and emerging infectious diseases*, ed 10, Philadelphia, 2019, Elsevier.

7. Osteomyelitis in children with hemoglobinopathies (particularly sickle cell disease)
8. Complications of typhoid and paratyphoid fever are summarized in Table 2

ETIOLOGY

- More than 2000 serotypes of *Salmonella* exist, but only a few cause disease in humans. Host factors and conditions predisposing to the development of systemic disease with nontyphoidal *Salmonella* strains are described in Table 3 and Table 4.
- Raw produce is an increasingly recognized vehicle for salmonellosis. In 2008 there was a large outbreak due to contaminated jalapeno and Serrano peppers with *Salmonella Saintpaul* involving 1500 persons, of whom 21% were hospitalized and two died. In 2009 there was an outbreak associated with contaminated peanut butter and peanuts. In 2017 there was an outbreak associated with papaya.

TABLE 3 Host Factors and Conditions Predisposing to the Development of Systemic Disease with Nontyphoidal *Salmonella* Strains

Neonates and young infants (≤3 mo of age)
HIV/AIDS
Other immunodeficiencies and chronic granulomatous disease
Immunosuppressive and corticosteroid therapies
Malignancies, especially leukemia and lymphoma
Hemolytic anemia, including sickle cell disease, malaria, and bartonellosis
Collagen vascular disease
Inflammatory bowel disease
Achlorhydria or use of antacid medications
Impaired intestinal motility
Schistosomiasis, malaria
Malnutrition

AIDS, Acquired immunodeficiency syndrome; *HIV,* human immunodeficiency virus.
From Kliegman RM et al: *Nelson textbook of pediatrics*, ed 19, Philadelphia, 2011, Saunders.

- Some found only in humans are the cause of enteric fever:
  1. *S. typhi*
  2. *S. paratyphi*
- Some responsible for gastroenteritis and frequently isolated from raw meat and poultry and uncooked or undercooked eggs:
  1. *S. typhimurium*
  2. *S. enteritidis*
- *S. choleraesuis* is a prototype organism that causes extraintestinal nontyphoidal disease.
- Transmission generally via ingestion of contaminated food or drink.
- Outbreaks of gastroenteritis related to contaminated poultry, meat, and dairy products are common.
- Typhoid fever is a systemic illness caused by serotypes exclusive to humans:
  1. Acquisition by ingestion of food or water contaminated by other humans.
  2. Most cases in the United States are:
     a. Acquired during foreign travel: 80% of cases.
     b. Acquired by ingestion of food prepared by chronic carriers, many of whom have acquired the organism outside of the United States.

Dx DIAGNOSIS

DIFFERENTIAL DIAGNOSIS

- Other causes of prolonged fever:
  1. Malaria
  2. TB
  3. Brucellosis
  4. Amebic liver abscess
- Other causes of gastroenteritis:
  1. Bacterial: *Shigella, Yersinia, Campylobacter* spp.
  2. Viral: Norwalk virus, rotavirus
  3. Parasitic: *Entamoeba histolytica, Giardia lamblia*
  4. Toxic: *Enterotoxigenic E. coli, Clostridium difficile*

TABLE 4 Susceptibility to *Salmonella* spp. Infection

Patient Group at Risk	Mechanism
Newborn	Achlorhydria, rapid gastric emptying Poorly developed cell-mediated immunity Complement deficiency Immunoglobulin deficiency in premature infants
Sickle-cell anemia	Reticuloendothelial system overload owing to hemolysis Functional asplenia Tissue infarcts Defective opsonization
Neutropenia (congenital or acquired)	Polymorphonuclear neutrophils needed for killing
Chronic granulomatous disease	Defective killing by polymorphonuclear neutrophils
Defects of immune system IL-12/ interferon-γ axis	Defective signaling resulting in failure to activate macrophages and recurrent/persistent infection by nontyphoid *Salmonella*
Acquired immunodeficiency syndrome	Low CD4 Effects of malnutrition on cell-mediated immunity Survival of organisms in macrophages (owing to *Salmonella* genes *PhoP/PhoQ, spvA-D, R*)
Organ transplantation, immunosuppression	Defective cell-mediated immunity
Gastrectomy	Loss of stomach acid barrier
Malaria	Reticuloendothelial overload during hemolysis Abnormal complement levels Abnormal macrophage function
Bartonellosis (verruga peruana)	Reticuloendothelial overload during hemolysis
Schistosomiasis	*Salmonella* sequestered in schistosomes protected from host defenses and antibiotics

From Cherry JD et al: *Feigin and Cherry's textbook of pediatric infectious diseases,* ed 8, Philadelphia, 2019, Elsevier.

TABLE 5 Treatment of Salmonella Gastroenteritis in Children

Organism and Indication	Dose and Duration of Treatment
Salmonella infections in infants <3 mo of age or immunocompromised persons (in addition to appropriate treatment for underlying disorder)	Cefotaxime 100-200 mg/kg/day every 6 hr for 5-14 days *or* Ceftriaxone 75 mg/kg/day once daily for 7 days *or* Ampicillin 100 mg/kg/day every 6 hr for 7 days *or* Cefixime 15 mg/kg/day for 7-10 days

From Kliegman RM et al: *Nelson textbook of pediatrics,* ed 19, Philadelphia, 2011, Saunders.

WORKUP

- Typhoid fever:
  1. Cultures of blood, stool, urine; repeat if initially negative.
  2. Blood cultures are more likely to be positive early in the course of illness.
  3. Stool and urine cultures are more commonly positive in the second and third wk of illness.
  4. Highest yield with bone marrow biopsy cultures: 90% positive.
  5. Serology using Widal test is helpful in retrospect, showing a fourfold increase in convalescent titers.
- Gastroenteritis: Stool cultures
- Extraintestinal localized infection:
  1. Blood cultures.
  2. Cultures from the site of infection.

LABORATORY TESTS

- Neutropenia is common.
- Transaminitis is possible.
- Culture to grow organism: Blood, body fluids, biopsy specimens.

IMAGING STUDIES

- Not routinely indicated.
- Radiographs of bone may be suggestive of osteomyelitis (particularly in patients with sickle cell disease and bone infarctions).
- Computed tomography (CT) scan or sonogram of abdomen:
  1. May reveal hepatic or splenic abscesses or pleural involvement
  2. May reveal aortic aneurysm

Rx TREATMENT

NONPHARMACOLOGIC THERAPY

Adequate hydration and electrolyte replacement in people with diarrhea.

ACUTE GENERAL Rx

Treatment decisions must consider the severity of infection and the risk for extraintestinal disease.

- Typhoid fever:
  1. Levofloxacin 750 mg PO/intravenous (IV) q24h or ciprofloxacin 500 mg PO bid or 400 mg IV bid for 7 to 10 days. Should not be used as first line in patients from South Asia due to resistance unless known to be susceptible
  2. Ceftriaxone 2 g IV qd for 7 to 14 days or cefixime (20-30 mg/kg/day orally divided into q12h dosing for 7 to 14 days)
  3. Another alternative agent: Azithromycin (1 g orally then 500 mg daily for 5 to 7 days)
  4. Children: See Table 5. In general, quinolones are avoided in children unless a multidrug-resistant strain is involved due to concerns of possible cartilage damage. Another alternative for children: Azithromycin (10-20 mg/kg to 1 g maximum once daily for 5-7 days)
  5. If tests show susceptibility, can also use amoxicillin or trimethoprim/sulfamethoxazole in adults and children (Table 6)
  6. Dexamethasone 3 mg IV initially, followed by 1 mg IV q6h for eight doses for patients with shock or mental status changes
- Gastroenteritis:
  1. Usually not indicated for gastroenteritis alone because this illness usually self-limited
  2. Treatment may prolong the carrier state and is discouraged for healthy patients <50 yr of age who have relatively mild disease
  3. Prophylactic treatment for patients who are at high risk of developing complications from bacteremia (see Table 5):
     a. Neonates
     b. Patients with hemoglobinopathies
     c. Patients with atherosclerosis
     d. Patients with aneurysms
     e. Patients with prosthetic devices
     f. Immunocompromised patients

CHRONIC Rx

- Carrier states are possible in those with typhoid fever.
- More common in people >60 yr of age and in people with gallstones.
- Usual site of colonization is the gallbladder.
- Treatment should be considered for those with persistently positive stool cultures and for food handlers.
- Suggested regimens for eradication of carrier state:
  1. Ciprofloxacin 500 mg PO bid for 4 wk.
  2. SMX/TMP 1 to 2 DS tabs PO bid for 6 wk (if susceptible).
  3. Amoxicillin 2 g PO q8h for 6 wk (if susceptible).
- Cholecystectomy may be required in carriers with gallstones who fail medical therapy, but this is rarely indicated for nontyphoidal salmonellosis currently.
- Prolonged course of oral therapy or lifetime suppression for patients with AIDS who have chronic infection.

TABLE 6 Antibiotics Commonly Used in the Treatment of *Salmonella* Infections

Drug	Dose	Comments
Ciprofloxacin	20-30 mg/kg per day in 2 doses PO or IV	First-line therapy[a]
Ceftriaxone	75-100 mg/kg per day in 1 or 2 doses IM or IV	First-line therapy
Cefotaxime	100-300 mg/kg per day in 3-4 doses IM or IV	First-line therapy
Cefixime	20-30 mg/kg per day in 1 or 2 doses PO	Alternative therapy
Azithromycin	10 mg/kg per day in 1 dose PO	Alternative therapy
Chloramphenicol	50-100 mg/kg per day in 4 doses PO	High frequency of resistance; use only for susceptible strains
Ampicillin	200-400 mg/kg per day in 4 doses PO, IM, or IV	High frequency of resistance; use only for susceptible strains
TMP-SMX	10 mg/kg per day TMP, 50 mg/kg per day SMX in 2 doses PO or IV	High frequency of resistance; use only for susceptible strains

IM, Intramuscular; *IV,* intravenous; *PO,* by mouth; *TMP-SMX,* trimethoprim-sulfamethoxazole.
[a]Not approved by the US Food and Drug Administration in children <18 yr; current expert opinion agrees in recommending this agent as an effective therapy for regions with susceptible *Salmonella* strains and especially for severe infections.
From Cherry JD et al: *Feigin and Cherry's textbook of pediatric infectious diseases,* ed 8, Philadelphia, 2019, Elsevier.

DISPOSITION

- Typhoid fever:
  1. Treated patients usually respond to therapy; small percentage of chronic carriers.
  2. Untreated patients may have serious complications.
- Gastroenteritis:
  1. Usually self-limited
  2. May be recurrent or persistent in AIDS patients

PEARLS & CONSIDERATIONS

COMMENTS

- Fluoroquinolones remain the most reliably effective class of antibiotics for empiric therapy despite increasing resistance. They should not be used in children or pregnant women.
- Infections should be reported to local health departments.
- Other recent outbreaks in the U.S. have been traced back to raw tomatoes, peanut butter, pet turtles, frozen pot pies, and onions.
- Vaccine is available for *Salmonella typhi*: Oral live weakened vaccine (four doses, one every other day) for age >6 yr and lasts for 5 yr or one dose of inactivated injectable vaccine for persons >2 yr old that lasts for 2 yr, but neither vaccine is greater than 75% effective.
- Outbreaks of extensively drug resistant (XDR) typhoid fever have occurred in Pakistan (resistant to ampicillin, sulfa, chloramphenicol, quinolones, and ceftriaxone). Drug of choice for these cases has been azithromycin for milder cases and carbapenems for more severe cases. Some of these cases have been detected in travelers returning from Pakistan.

SUGGESTED READINGS

Available at ExpertConsult.com

RELATED CONTENT

Salmonellosis (Patient Information)
Typhoid Fever (Related Key Topic)

AUTHOR: **Glenn G. Fort, MD, MPH**

BASIC INFORMATION

DEFINITION

Sarcoidosis is a chronic multisystem granulomatous disease characterized histologically by the presence of noncaseating granulomas.

SYNONYM

Boeck sarcoid

ICD-10CM CODES

D86	Sarcoidosis
D86.0	Sarcoidosis of lung
D86.1	Sarcoidosis of lymph nodes
D86.2	Sarcoidosis of lung with sarcoidosis of lymph nodes
D86.3	Sarcoidosis of skin
D86.8	Sarcoidosis of other and combined sites
D86.9	Sarcoidosis, unspecified

EPIDEMIOLOGY & DEMOGRAPHICS

INCIDENCE (IN U.S.): Incidence is 11 in 100,000 in whites and 35 in 100,000 in blacks; presents most commonly in the winter and early spring. (The adjusted annual incidence among black Americans is roughly three times higher than among white Americans [35.5 cases/100,000, as compared with 10.9/100,000] and is likely more chronic and fatal in black Americans.)

PREDOMINANT SEX: Increased incidence in females.

PREDOMINANT AGE: 20 to 40 yr.

GENETICS: Familial clustering has been described. Having a first-degree relative with sarcoidosis increases the risk for disease fivefold (ACCESS study). There have been reports of association between sarcoidosis and gene products, specifically human leukocyte antigen (HLA) class II antigens, encoded by HLA-DRB1 and DQB1 alleles.

PHYSICAL FINDINGS & CLINICAL PRESENTATION

- Clinical manifestations often vary with the stage of the disease and degree of organ involvement. Patients may be asymptomatic, but a chest radiograph may demonstrate findings consistent with sarcoidosis (see "Imaging Studies"). Nearly 50% of patients with sarcoidosis are diagnosed by incidental findings on chest radiograph. Lung involvement occurs in >90% of patients with sarcoidosis.
- Frequent manifestations:
  1. Pulmonary manifestations: Dry, nonproductive cough; dyspnea; chest discomfort.
  2. Constitutional symptoms: Fatigue, weight loss, anorexia, malaise, night sweats.
  3. Visual disturbances: Blurred vision, ocular discomfort, conjunctivitis, iritis, uveitis (65% of patients).
  4. Dermatologic manifestations (30% of patients): Erythema nodosum (10% of patients), macules, papules, subcutaneous nodules, hyperpigmentation, lupus pernio (indurated violaceous lesions on the nose, lips, ears, and cheeks that can erode into underlying cartilage and bone) (Fig. E1).
  5. Myocardial disturbances, arrhythmias, cardiomyopathy, various conduction abnormalities, and pericardial effusion. Cardiac sarcoidosis is much more common than clinically appreciated and is found in up to 25% of patients in the U.S.
  6. Splenomegaly, hepatomegaly.
  7. Rheumatologic manifestations: Arthralgias have been reported in up to 40% of patients. It typically affects the ankles but can also involve the knees, wrists, and small joints of the hands and feet.
  8. **Löfgren syndrome,** consisting of the triad of arthritis, erythema nodosum, and bilateral hilar adenopathy, occurs in 9% to 34% of patients. Fever is frequently present.
  9. Neurologic and other manifestations: Cranial nerve palsies, diabetes insipidus, meningeal involvement, parotid enlargement, hypothalamic and pituitary lesions, peripheral adenopathy. Neurosarcoidosis is detected in up to 25% of patients and can occur in the absence of apparent disease elsewhere.
  10. The presence of anterior uveitis, parotiditis, fevers, and facial nerve palsy is known as **Heerfordt syndrome.**

ETIOLOGY & PATHOGENESIS

A cardinal feature of sarcoidosis is the presence of CD4+ T cells that interact with antigen-presenting cells to initiate the formation and maintenance of granulomas (Fig. 2). Multiple lines of evidence suggest that sarcoidosis may result from the interaction of multiple genes with environmental exposures or infection.

GENETIC PREDISPOSITION TO SARCOIDOSIS

Various HLA antigens have been implicated in diverse patient populations. Familial predisposition has been reported dating back to 1923, with a wide percentage of variability of affected relatives (0.4% to 21%) and heterogeneity based on genetic background. A more recent study was published by the ACCESS (A Case Controlled Etiologic Survey of Sarcoidosis) study group, which confirmed increased risk for family members with an odds ratio of 4.6 for all relatives. Absolute risk, however, for a family member to be affected was less than 1%. This study also showed a higher risk in white versus black American siblings and parents.

IMMUNOPATHOGENESIS OF SARCOIDOSIS: Numerous chemokines and cytokines have been implicated in the development and/or resolution of the disease. In sarcoidosis, the alveolitis seen at disease presentation represents an increase in primarily lymphocytic cellularity, predominated by CD4 cells. Presence of increased neutrophils in the bronchoalveolar lavage of patients with sarcoidosis has been associated with persistence of disease, with spontaneous remission noted in 36% of patients with elevated neutrophil counts.

DIAGNOSIS

DIFFERENTIAL DIAGNOSIS

- Berylliosis
- Tuberculosis
- Lymphoma
- Metastases
- Pneumoconioses
- Enlarged pulmonary arteries
- Infectious mononucleosis
- Lymphangitic carcinomatosis
- Idiopathic hemosiderosis
- Alveolar cell carcinoma
- Pulmonary eosinophilia
- Hypersensitivity pneumonitis
- Fibrosing alveolitis
- Collagen disorders
- Parasitic infection

Section II describes the differential diagnosis of granulomatous lung disease and a classification of granulomatous disorders.

WORKUP

- No pathognomonic diagnostic test exists for sarcoidosis, so the diagnosis remains one of exclusion. The presence of noncaseating granulomas does not establish the diagnosis, because conditions such as tuberculosis and malignancies, among others, can cause granulomas. Workup is aimed at excluding critical organ involvement, determining extent and severity of disease, and excluding other disease. A complete neurologic and ophthalmologic examination is mandatory. A complete occupational and environmental exposure history is recommended.
- Initial laboratory evaluation should include complete blood count, serum chemistries (alanine aminotransferase, aspartate aminotransferase, alkaline phosphatase, electrolytes, blood urea nitrogen, creatinine, serum calcium), urinalysis, 24-hour urinary excretion of calcium, C-reactive protein (CRP), erythrocyte sedimentation rate (ESR), and tuberculin skin test or QuantiFERON gold test for tuberculosis. Routine vitamin D screening is generally not recommended; if done it should measure both 25-hydroxyvitamin D and 1,25-dihydroxyvitamin D because sarcoidosis increases conversion of the former to the latter.[1]
- Chest radiograph and ECG should also be obtained in all patients with sarcoidosis.
- Pulmonary function testing: Spirometry, diffusion capacity of carbon monoxide–single breath.
- Biopsy in symptomatic patients should be done on accessible tissues suspected of sarcoid involvement (conjunctiva, skin, lymph nodes); bronchoscopy with transbronchial biopsy (85% diagnostic yield) is often performed in patients without any readily

[1]Crouser ED et al: Diagnosis and detection of sarcoidosis. An official American Thoracic Society Clinical Practice Guideline, *Am J Respir Crit Care Med* 201(8):e26-e51, 2020.

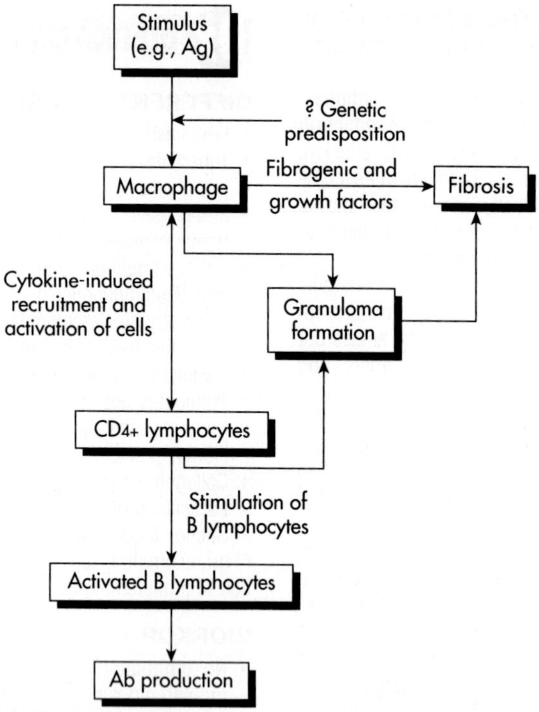

FIG. 2 Simplified proposed pathogenetic sequence in sarcoidosis. *Ab*, Antibody; *Ag*, antigen. (From Weinberger SE: *Principles of pulmonary medicine*, ed 7, Philadelphia, 2019, Elsevier.)

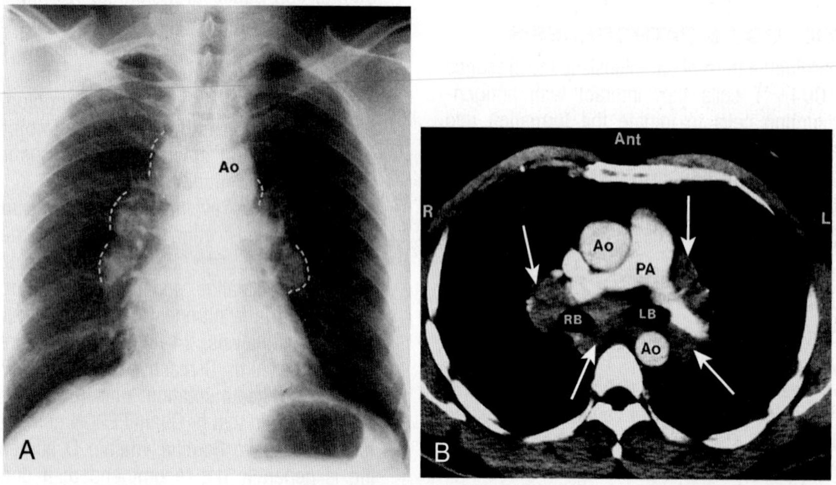

FIG. 3 Sarcoid. Marked lymphadenopathy *(dotted lines)* is seen in the region of both hila in the right paratracheal region **(A).** The transverse contrast-enhanced computed tomography (CT) scan of the upper chest **(B)** clearly shows the ascending and descending aorta *(Ao)* as well as the pulmonary artery *(PA)* and superior vena cava. The right and left mainstem bronchus area is also seen. The *arrows* indicate the extensive lymphadenopathy. *LB*, Left bronchus; *RB*, right bronchus. (From Mettler FA [ed]: *Primary care radiology*, Philadelphia, 2000, Saunders.)

accessible site. Endobronchial ultrasound-guided fine-needle aspiration of intrathoracic lymph nodes also has high diagnostic yield. Among patients with suspected Stage I/II pulmonary sarcoidosis undergoing tissue confirmation, the use of endosonographic nodal aspiration compared with bronchoscopic biopsy resulted in greater diagnostic yield.

LABORATORY TESTS

Laboratory abnormalities:

- Hypergammaglobulinemia, anemia, leukopenia may be present.
- Liver function test abnormalities are common, e.g., elevated alkaline phosphatase.
- Hypercalcemia (11% of patients), hypercalciuria (40% of patients; attributable to increased gastrointestinal absorption, abnormal vitamin D metabolism, and increased calcitriol production by sarcoid granuloma).
- Angiotensin-converting enzyme: Elevated in approximately 75% of patients with untreated sarcoidosis; nonspecific and poor sensitivity; generally not useful as a diagnostic tool or in following the course of the disease.
- Serum adenosine deaminase (ADA); serum amyloid A (SAA) elevated but nonspecific.
- In patients with a history of beryllium exposure, beryllium lymphocyte proliferation testing should be obtained to assess for berylliosis.

IMAGING STUDIES

- Chest radiograph (Fig. 3): Pulmonary sarcoidosis is classified based on radiographic pattern. Adenopathy of the hilar and paratracheal nodes is a frequent finding. Parenchymal changes may also be present, depending on the stage of the disease (stage 0, normal radiograph; stage I, bilateral hilar adenopathy; stage II, stage I plus pulmonary infiltrate; stage III, pulmonary infiltrate without adenopathy; stage IV, advanced fibrosis with evidence of "honeycombing," hilar retraction, bullae, cysts, and emphysema).
- Computed tomography (CT) imaging: High-resolution CT may help detect early parenchymal abnormalities. A chest CT scan with contrast can better define mediastinal adenopathy.
- For patients without apparent lung involvement, ^{18}F-fluorodeoxyglucose positron emission tomography (FDG-PET) is useful in identifying sites for diagnostic biopsy.
- FDG-PET and MRI with gadolinium are useful in patients with suspected cardiac and neurologic involvement.
- Gallium-67 scan: Represents an older testing modality. It will localize in areas of granulomatous infiltrates; however, it is not specific and not necessary. The "panda" sign (localization in the lacrimal and salivary glands, giving a "panda" appearance to the face) is suggestive of sarcoidosis.

Additional diagnostic tests:

- Pulmonary function tests (spirometry, lung volumes, and diffusing capacity of the lung for carbon dioxide): May be normal or may reveal a restrictive ventilatory defect with reduced forced vital capacity, reduced DLCO, or both. Endobronchial sarcoidosis may exhibit obstructive physiology, depending on severity.
- Bronchoscopy: Flexible bronchoscopy and bronchoalveolar lavage (BAL) with transbronchial biopsy (showing noncaseating granulomas) are traditional methods for the minimally invasive diagnosis of sarcoidosis. With hilar adenopathy, endobronchial ultrasound (EBUS) is the preferred method for lymph node sampling. BAL may show predominantly lymphocytosis, elevated ADA levels, and elevated CD4:CD8 ratio (4:1).
- Mediastinoscopy: Rarely used nowadays for lymph node sampling and diagnosis.
- Routine eye examination is recommended, even for patients without ocular symptoms.
- Echocardiogram is indicated only in patients with suspected pulmonary hypertension. If confirmed, right heart catheterization can be performed.

TABLE 1 Indications for Use of Corticosteroids in Sarcoidosis

Disorder	Treatment
Iridocyclitis	Corticosteroid eye drops; local subconjunctival deposit of cortisone
Posterior uveitis	Oral prednisone
Pulmonary involvement	Steroids rarely recommended for stage I; typically used if infiltrate remains static or worsens over 3-mo period or the patient is symptomatic
Upper airway obstruction	Rare indication for intravenous steroids
Lupus pernio	Oral prednisone shrinks the disfiguring lesions
Hypercalcemia	Responds well to corticosteroids
Cardiac involvement	Corticosteroids usually recommended if patient has arrhythmias or conduction disturbances
Central nervous system involvement	Response is best in patients with acute symptoms
Lacrimal/salivary gland involvement	Corticosteroids recommended for disordered function, not gland swelling
Bone cysts	Corticosteroids recommended if symptomatic

From Andreoli TE (ed): *Cecil essentials of medicine,* ed 8, Philadelphia, 2010, Saunders.

Rx TREATMENT

ACUTE GENERAL Rx

- Many patients with sarcoidosis will not require any treatment. In general, treatment should be instituted when organ function is threatened. Corticosteroids (Table 1) are the mainstay of therapy when treatment is required (e.g., prednisone 40 mg qd for 8-12 wk with gradual tapering of the dose to 10 mg qod over 8-12 mo). Corticosteroids should be considered in patients with severe symptoms (e.g., dyspnea, chest pain); hypercalcemia; ocular, central nervous system, or cardiac involvement; or progressive pulmonary disease. Patients with interstitial lung disease benefit from oral steroid therapy for 6 to 24 mo.
- A lack of benefit from steroid therapy may be due to the presence of irreversible fibrotic disease. Patients with progressive disease refractory to corticosteroids may be treated with methotrexate 7.5 to 15 mg once per week or another immunosuppressant such as azathioprine or mycophenolate mofetil.
- Methotrexate, at a dose of 7.5 to 10 mg per week, has been demonstrated to be relatively safe and can also be used as a steroid-sparing agent. Additional agents that have been used with limited clinical experience include mycophenolate, pentoxifylline, infliximab, cyclosporine, minocycline, and leflunomide.
- Immunomodulators: Etanercept has not been found to be useful in sarcoidosis. Infliximab has been used with some benefits in cutaneous, pulmonary, and neurologic disease.
- NSAIDs are useful for musculoskeletal symptoms and erythema nodosum.
- Pulmonary rehabilitation in patients with significant respiratory insufficiency. Consider liver and lung transplantation in patients unresponsive to conventional treatment.
- Pulmonary hypertension is a dreaded complication of advanced pulmonary sarcoidosis. The prognosis for patients with sarcoidosis-associated pulmonary hypertension is not known.

DISPOSITION

- The majority of patients with sarcoidosis have spontaneous remission within 2 yr and do not require treatment. Their course can be followed by periodic clinical evaluation, chest radiographs, and pulmonary function tests.
- Blacks have increased rates of pulmonary involvement, a worse long-term prognosis, and more frequent relapses.
- Up to one third of patients have unrelenting disease, leading to clinically significant organ impairment. Adverse prognostic factors in sarcoidosis include age of onset >40 yr, cardiac involvement, neurosarcoidosis, progressive pulmonary fibrosis, chronic hypercalcemia, chronic uveitis, involvement of nasal mucosa, nephrocalcinosis, and presence of cystic bone lesions and lupus pernio.
- Prognosis for Loeffler syndrome is good with remittance within 16 wk in most patients. Symptoms can generally be controlled with NSAIDs. Low-dose glucocorticoids, hydroxychloroquine, and colchicine are also effective.

REFERRAL

- Patients with progressive pulmonary disease despite therapy should be referred for consideration of lung transplant candidacy.
- Ophthalmologic examination is indicated in all patients with suspected sarcoidosis because ocular findings (iridocyclitis, uveitis, conjunctivitis, and keratopathy) are found in ≥25% of documented cases.

PEARLS & CONSIDERATIONS

COMMENTS

- Serial spirometry and measurement of DLCO can be useful in following response to therapy and disease progression.
- Approximately 15% to 20% of patients with lung involvement advance to irreversible lung impairment (bronchiectasis, cavitation, progressive fibrosis, pneumothorax, and respiratory failure). Death from pulmonary failure occurs in 5% to 7% of patients with sarcoidosis.
- Newer treatment approaches are aimed at targeting mechanisms involving CD4 type 1 helper T cells.
- The diagnosis of sarcoidosis should be reconsidered in the presence of atypical manifestations or persistent/progressive disease despite appropriate therapy.
- Diagnostic biopsy may not be necessary in most patients presenting with asymptomatic bilateral lymphadenopathy (with no other evidence of malignancy), in those with Lofgren syndrome, or in those with Heerfordt syndrome.

SUGGESTED READINGS

Available at ExpertConsult.com

RELATED CONTENT

Sarcoidosis (Patient Information)

AUTHOR: **Imrana Qawi, MD**

BASIC INFORMATION

DEFINITION

Scabies is a skin infestation caused by the mite *Sarcoptes scabiei.*

ICD-10CM CODE

B86 Scabies

EPIDEMIOLOGY & DEMOGRAPHICS

- Scabies is generally acquired by prolonged direct skin-to-skin contact with an infected individual.
- Scabies is endemic in many developing countries; however, it can affect individuals of any age and socioeconomic status.
- Prevalence is 100 to 200 million people worldwide.
- Risk factors include living in crowded conditions (homes, shelters, nursing homes, child care facilities, and prisons). More common in resource-limited areas and in tropical climates.

PHYSICAL FINDINGS & CLINICAL PRESENTATION

- Primary lesions are caused when the female mite burrows within the stratum corneum, laying eggs within the tract she leaves behind; burrows (linear or serpiginous tracts, see Fig. E1) end with a minute papule or vesicle.
- The distribution of primary lesions (Fig. E2) is usually widespread, and lesions are most commonly found in the web spaces of the hands, flexor aspects of wrists, buttocks, genitalia, breasts, axillae, and knees. In children, they can also involve the head, neck, face, palms of the hands, and soles of the feet. They are often confused with eczema (Fig. E3).
- Secondary lesions result from repeatedly scratching or secondary staphylococcal or streptococcal infections.
- Intense pruritus, especially nocturnal, is the hallmark of this condition; it is caused by a delayed hypersensitivity to the mite or fecal pellets and is usually noted 2 to 6 wk after the primary infestation.
- Examination of the skin may reveal burrows, tiny vesicles, excoriations, or inflammatory papules.
- Widespread and crusted lesions (Norwegian or crusted scabies) may be seen in the elderly, in immunocompromised patients, or in patients who do not have the ability to scratch (Fig. E4). Pruritus may be mild or absent due to impaired host immune response.
- Table 1 summarizes the different presenting forms of scabies.

ETIOLOGY

- Human scabies is caused by the mite *Sarcoptes scabiei,* var. *hominis* (Fig. 5). After impregnation on the skin surface, the gravid female burrows in the stratum corneum and gradually extends the tract along the boundary with the stratum granulosum laying 2 to 3 eggs per day for 4 to 6 wk. The eggs hatch in 3 to 4 days, and larvae move to the skin surface and mature in 2 to 3 wk, resuming the cycle (Fig. 6).
- Transmission is usually due to prolonged skin-to-skin contact. Transmission can occasionally be due to fomites (especially in crusted scabies) as they can survive off a host for 24 to 36 hr.
- Clinical manifestations result from a delayed type IV hypersensitivity reaction to the mite, eggs, saliva, or scybala (fecal pellets).

Dx DIAGNOSIS

DIFFERENTIAL DIAGNOSIS

- Pediculosis
- Atopic dermatitis
- Flea bites
- Seborrheic dermatitis
- Dermatitis herpetiformis
- Contact dermatitis
- Nummular eczema
- Infantile acropustulosis
- Langerhans cell histiocytosis
- Arthropod bites

WORKUP

Diagnosis is made based on the clinical appearance of the rash and burrows and should be suspected if the patient presents with intense itching out of proportion to skin findings or there is a history of other family members with similar symptoms. Diagnosis can be confirmed by microscopic detection of mites, eggs, or mite feces.

LABORATORY TESTS

- Microscopic demonstration of the mites, feces, or eggs: A drop of mineral oil may

TABLE 1 Different Presenting Forms of Scabies

Presenting Forms of Scabies	Specific High-Risk Populations	Clinical Manifestations	Limited Differential Diagnoses
Classic scabies (scabies vulgaris)	Infants and children; sexually active adults; men who have sex with men	Intense generalized pruritus, worse at night; inflammatory pruritic papules localized to finger webs, flexor aspects of wrists, elbows, axillae, buttocks, genitalia, female breasts; lesions and pruritus spare the face, head, and neck; secondary lesions include eczematization, excoriation, impetigo	Dermatitis herpetiformis, drug reactions, eczema, pediculosis corporis, lichen planus, pityriasis rosea
Scalp scabies	Infants and children; institutionalized older adults; AIDS patients; patients with preexisting crusted scabies	Atypical crusted papular lesions of the scalp, face, palms, and soles	Dermatomyositis, ringworm, seborrheic dermatitis
Crusted scabies (Norwegian scabies, scabies norvegica, scabies crustosa)	Institutionalized older adults; institutionalized developmentally disabled (Down syndrome); homeless, especially HIV-positive; all immunocompromised patients, particularly those with AIDS or positive for HIV or HTLV-1; transplant recipients; patients on prolonged systemic corticosteroids and chemotherapy	Psoriasiform hyperkeratotic papular lesions of the scalp, face, neck, hands, feet, with extensive nail involvement; eczematization and impetigo common	Contact dermatitis, drug reactions, eczema, erythroderma, ichthyosis, psoriasis
Nodular scabies	Sexually active adults; men who have sex with men; HIV-positive men > HIV-positive women	Violaceous pruritic nodules localized to male genitalia, groin, axillae, representing hypersensitivity reaction to mite antigens	Acropustulosis, atopic dermatitis, Darier disease, lupus erythematosus, lymphomatoid papulosis, papular urticaria, necrotizing vasculitis, secondary syphilis

AIDS, Acquired immunodeficiency syndrome; *HIV,* human immunodeficiency virus; *HTLV-1,* human T-cell lymphotropic virus type 1.
From Bennett JE et al: *Mandell, Douglas, and Bennett's principles and practice of infectious diseases,* ed 8, Philadelphia, 2015, Saunders.

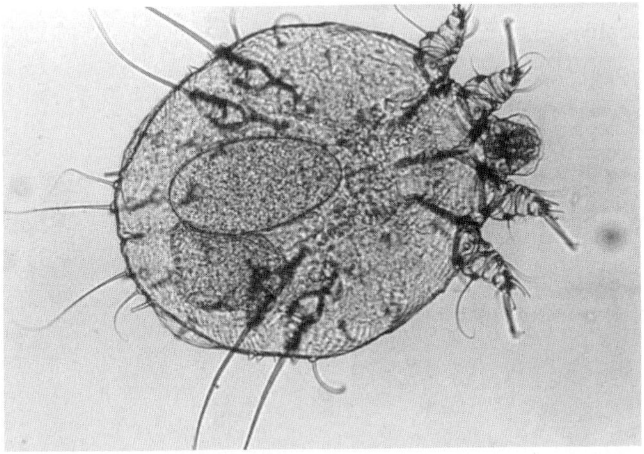

FIG. 5 Scabies mite. Note the eggs within the body of the mite. (Live scabies mite, ×40 magnification.) (From Paller AS, Mancini AJ: *Hurwitz clinical pediatric dermatology: a textbook of skin disorders of childhood and adolescence,* ed 5, Philadelphia, 2016, Elsevier.)

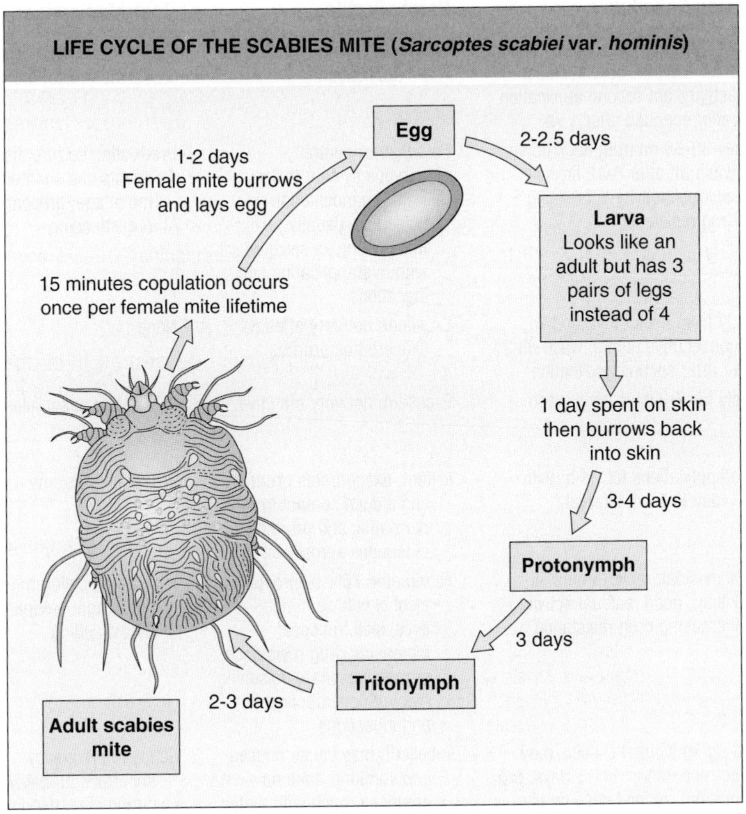

FIG. 6 Life cycle of the scabies mite (*Sarcoptes scabiei* var. *hominis*). (From Bolognia J: *Dermatology,* ed 4, Philadelphia, 2018, Elsevier.)

be placed over the suspected lesion before removal (Box 1); the scrapings are transferred directly to a glass slide; a drop of potassium hydroxide is added and a cover slip is applied.
- Skin biopsy is rarely necessary to make the diagnosis.

Rx TREATMENT

NONPHARMACOLOGIC THERAPY

Clothing, underwear, bedding, and towels used 72 hr before treatment must be washed in hot water and dryer or sealed in a plastic bag for at least 72 hr.

ACUTE GENERAL Rx

- Permethrin 5% cream is usually effective with one treatment; it should be massaged into the skin from head to soles of feet and applied under fingernails and toenails. Cream should be applied overnight and then washed off after 8 to 14 hr. In children, cream should also be applied to the scalp and face. May need a second application in 1 to 2 wk. Permethrin is safe for children >2 mo old.
- A single dose of ivermectin (200 μg/kg), an antiparasitic agent, can be used for those who have failed topical treatment. Repeat doses, along with topical therapy, are recommended for Norwegian (crusted) scabies.
- Pruritus generally abates 24 to 48 hr after treatment but can last up to 2 wk; oral antihistamines can be effective. Retreatment may be necessary if pruritis is persistent for 2 to 4 wk or if new burrows or rash appears.
- It is essential that all close contacts and household members are treated at the same time whether symptomatic or not. If the patient is a resident of an extended care facility, it is important to educate the patients, staff, family, and frequent visitors about scabies and the need to have full cooperation in treatment.
- Table 2 summarizes currently recommended treatment for scabies.

DISPOSITION

Treatment failure is often result of poor adherence to treatment regimen or reinfestation. Refractory cases are usually only seen with immunocompromised hosts or patients with underlying skin diseases. ***Norwegian scabies (crusted scabies)*** refers to a highly contagious, severe variant often found in institutions caring for the elderly or physically and mentally disabled individuals.

PEARLS & CONSIDERATIONS

COMMENTS

- Symptoms can take 4 to 6 wk to develop; however, individuals can still spread scabies before symptoms arise.
- Sexual partners and household members should be notified and treated.
- Lindane is potentially neurotoxic and should not be used on infants or pregnant women (permethrin is safe in pregnancy and infants over 2 mo old).

SUGGESTED READINGS

Available at ExpertConsult.com

RELATED CONTENT

Scabies (Patient Information)

AUTHORS: **Julianna Lau, MD,** and **Mary E. Bove, MD**

BOX 1 Performing a Mineral-Oil Examination for Scabies

1. Apply a drop of mineral oil to the lesion(s) to be scraped.
2. Scrape through the lesion with a number 15 scalpel blade (a small amount of bleeding is expected with appropriately deep scrapings).
3. Smear contents of scraping on a clean glass slide.
4. Add a few more drops of mineral oil.
5. Place cover slip over oil and examine under microscope at low power.
   Criteria for a positive mineral oil examination:
   Scabies mite.
   or
   Ova (eggs).
   or
   Scybala (feces).

From Paller AS, Mancini AJ: *Hurwitz clinical pediatric dermatology: a textbook of skin disorders of childhood and adolescence*, ed 5, Philadelphia, 2016, Elsevier.

TABLE 2 Currently Recommended Treatment for Scabies

Scabicides	FDA Approved?	Pregnancy Category*	Dosing Schedule	Safety Profile	Contraindications
5% Permethrin cream (Actin, Nix, Elimite)	Yes	B	Apply from neck down; wash off after 8-14 hr; good residual activity, but second application recommended after 1 wk	Excellent; itching and stinging on application	Prior allergic reactions; infants <2 mo of age; breastfeeding
1% Lindane lotion or cream	Yes	B	Apply 30-60 ml from neck down; wash off after 8-12 hr; no residual activity; increasing drug resistance	Potential for central nervous system toxicity from organochloride poisoning, usually manifesting as seizures, with overapplication and ingestions	Preexisting seizure disorder; infants and children <6 mo of age; pregnancy; breastfeeding
10% Crotamiton cream or lotion (Eurax)	Yes	C	Apply from neck down on two consecutive nights; wash off 24 hr after second application	Excellent; not very effective; exacerbates pruritus	None
2%-10% Sulfur in petrolatum ointments	No	C	Apply for 2-3 days, then wash	Excellent; not very effective	Preexisting sulfur allergy
10%-25% Benzoyl benzoate lotion	No	None	Two applications for 24 hr with 1-day to 1-wk interval	Irritant; exacerbates pruritus; can induce contact irritant dermatitis and pruritic cutaneous xerosis	Preexisting eczema
0.5% Malathion lotion (Ovide), 1% malathion shampoo (unavailable in the U.S.)	No	B	95% ovicidal; rapid (5 min) killing; good residual activity; increasing drug resistance	Flammable 78% isopropyl alcohol vehicle stings eyes, skin, mucosa; increasing drug resistance; organophosphate poisoning risk with overapplication and ingestions	Infants and children <6 mo of age; pregnancy; breastfeeding
Ivermectin (Stromectol)	Yes	C	200 μg/kg single PO dose, may be repeated in 14-15 days; not ovicidal, second dose on day 14 or 15 highly recommended; recommended for endemic or epidemic scabies in institutions and refugee camps	Excellent; may cause nausea and vomiting; take on empty stomach with water	Safety in pregnancy uncertain; probably safe during breastfeeding; not recommended for children younger than 5 yr of age or weighing <15 kg

FDA, U.S. Food and Drug Administration; *PO*, by mouth.
*U.S. Food and Drug Administration (FDA) safety in pregnancy categories: A, safety established; B, presumed safe; C, uncertain safety; D, unsafe; X, highly unsafe.
From Bennett JE et al: *Mandell, Douglas, and Bennett's principles and practice of infectious diseases*, ed 8, Philadelphia, 2015, Saunders.

BASIC INFORMATION

DEFINITION

Sciatica is a clinical diagnosis of neuralgia along the sciatic nerve distribution. Sciatica usually occurs unilaterally. Pain is described as sharp or aching and typically radiates from the buttock down the leg posteriorly, laterally, or anteriorly depending on the level of nerve root compression.

SYNONYMS

Radicular pain
Lumbosacral radicular syndrome
Deep gluteal syndrome
Ischialgia
Low back pain—sciatica
Lumbago with sciatica
Lumbar nerve root pain
Neuropathy—sciatic nerve
Sciatic nerve dysfunction
Sciatic neuritis

ICD-10CM CODES	
G57.00	Lesion of sciatic nerve, unspecified lower limb
G57.01	Lesion of sciatic nerve, right lower limb lesion
G57.02	Lesion of sciatic nerve, left lower limb
M54.30	Sciatica, unspecified side
M54.31	Sciatica, right side
M54.32	Sciatica, left side
M54.40	Lumbago with sciatica, unspecified side
M54.41	Lumbago with sciatica, right side
M54.42	Lumbago with sciatica, left side

EPIDEMIOLOGY & DEMOGRAPHICS

INCIDENCE: Very few studies have determined the incidence of sciatica. However, 2% to 11% of patients with low back pain have sciatica.

PREVALENCE: Annual prevalence of disc-related sciatica in the general population is estimated at 2.2%.

PEAK INCIDENCE: Fourth decade

RISK FACTORS:

- Increasing risk with height in the 50 to 60 age group.
- Physical activity in those with prior sciatic symptoms
- Smoking
- Diabetes
- Obesity
- Prolonged sitting and sedentary lifestyle
- Occupational factors:
  1. Strenuous physical activity (e.g., frequent lifting while bending and twisting)
  2. Driving

PHYSICAL FINDINGS & CLINICAL PRESENTATION

- Unilateral leg pain worse than low back pain
- Pain radiating to foot or toes
- Numbness and paresthesia in the same distribution
- Straight leg raise test induces more leg pain
- Localized neuropathy limited to one nerve root

ETIOLOGY

- Sciatica is caused by inflammation or compression of the sciatic nerve roots (L4 to S2). L4 root involvement causes pain localized to the frontal and lateral sides of the thigh.
- The most common cause is from disc herniation resulting from age-related degenerative changes.
- Other causes include lumbar spinal stenosis, facet joint osteoarthritis or other arthropathies, sacroiliac joint dysfunction, isthmic spondylolisthesis, soft tissue stenosis, neoplasm, trauma, spinal cord infection, gynecological conditions, and muscle entrapment (e.g., piriformis syndrome).

Dx DIAGNOSIS

DIFFERENTIAL DIAGNOSIS

- Nonspecific low back pain
- Piriformis syndrome
- Muscular problems (e.g., sprain, spasm)
- Vascular problems (e.g., claudication, compartment syndrome)
- Pott's disease Chronic edema
- Box 1 summarizes the differential diagnosis for low back pain

WORKUP

Sciatica is a clinical diagnosis. Historical clues to the cause of low back pain are summarized in Table 1. Red flags indicating cauda equina or spinal infection mandate emergent workup. Fig. 1 summarizes an algorithm for the management of low back pain.

HISTORY TAKING:

- Onset and duration
- Leg pain more severe than back pain
- Severity of pain
- Complaints of radiating pain in the leg following a dermatomal pattern, generally below the knee, into the foot
- Sensory symptoms (e.g., tingling, numbness)
- Muscle weakness in the legs
- Influence of coughing, movement, or rest on severity of pain

PHYSICAL EXAMINATION: Neurological testing

- Myotomes
- Reflexes (patellar - L4, medial hamstring - L5, Achilles - S1)
- Sensations (dermatomes; see Fig. E2)

LUMBAR MOBILITY ASSESSMENT: Neural tension tests

- Straight leg raise test (L5 to S1)
- Reversed straight leg raise test (L2 to L4)
- Bragard test
- Crossed straight leg raise test
- Slump test
- Femoral nerve tension test

BOX 1 Differential Diagnosis for Low Back Pain

Localized and Common
Uncomplicated musculoskeletal back pain
Intervertebral disk herniation
Spinal stenosis
Spondylolisthesis
Osteoarthritis
Fracture

Localized and Uncommon
Infection
Spondylitis
Epidural abscess
Discitis
Herpes zoster

Malignancy
Metastatic
Breast
Lung
Prostate
Kidney, thyroid, colon (less common)
Primary
Multiple myeloma
Lymphoma
Leukemia
Primary cord or extradural tumors
Osteoid osteoma
Other primary bone tumors

Pediatric
Spondylolisthesis, spondylolysis
Severe scoliosis
Scheuermann disease
Rheumatologic
Ankylosing spondylitis
Psoriatic arthritis
Polymyalgia rheumatica
Reiter syndrome

Vascular
Arteriovenous malformation of spinal cord
Epidural hematoma
Life-threatening referred pain
Abdominal aortic aneurysm

Gastrointestinal System
Biliary pathology
Pancreatitis
Peptic ulcer disease
Diverticulitis

Genitourinary System
Renal colic
Pyelonephritis
Prostatitis
Cystitis

Gynecologic System
Menstrual cramps
Spontaneous abortion
Labor
Ectopic pregnancy
Pelvic inflammatory disease
Endometriosis
Ovarian cyst
Ovarian torsion

Hematologic System
Sickle cell vaso-occlusive crisis

Functional
Somatization disorder
Depression
Fibrositis
Malingering

From Marx JA et al: *Rosen's emergency medicine*, ed 8, Philadelphia, 2014, Elsevier.

TABLE 1 Historical Clues to the Cause of Low Back Pain

Questions for Patient	Potential Diagnosis
Does the back pain radiate down past the knees?	Radiculopathy and likely a herniated disk
Is the pain worse with walking and better with bending forward and sitting?	Spinal stenosis
Do you have morning back stiffness that improves with exercise?	Ankylosing spondylitis
Are you older than 50 yr?	Osteoporotic fracture, spinal malignancy
Has there been any recent history of blunt trauma?	Fracture
Do you take long-term corticosteroids?	Fracture, spinal infection
Do you have a history of cancer?	Spinal metastatic malignancy
Does your pain persist at rest?	Spinal malignancy, spinal infection
Has there been persistent pain for longer than 6 wk?	Spinal malignancy
Has there been unexplained weight loss?	Spinal malignancy
Is the pain worse at night?	Spinal malignancy, spinal infection
Are you immunocompromised (e.g., HIV infection, alcoholism, diabetes)?	Spinal infection
Have you had fevers or chills?	Spinal infection
Do you have pain, weakness, or numbness in both legs?	Cauda equina syndrome
Do you have bladder or bowel control problems?	Cauda equina syndrome

HIV, Human immunodeficiency virus.
From Walls RM et al: *Rosen's emergency medicine: concepts and clinical practice*, ed 9, Philadelphia, 2018, Elsevier.

Major maneuvers:
- Knee extension (L4)
- Lumbar lateral bending
- Hip flexion
- Lasègue test
- Bechterew test
- Fajersztajn test

Minor maneuvers:
- Ankle dorsal flexion (L5)
- Ankle plantar flexion (S1)
- Cervical flexion
- Spinal flexion
- Hip internal rotation
- Hip adduction
- Great toe dorsiflexion
- Increased intrathecal/intradiscal pressure

LABORATORY TESTS

No laboratory tests specifically identify sciatica.
- Occasionally, laboratory tests such as complete blood count (CBC) and erythrocyte sedimentation rate may suggest infection or inflammation, anemia due to certain cancers, or other unusual causes of sciatica.
- Urinalysis may suggest a kidney stone if hematuria is present or infection if bacteria and white blood cells are present.

IMAGING STUDIES

- Routine imaging is not advised in nonspecific low back pain.
- If pain lasts for longer than 12 wk or if neurological deficits or pain progress, magnetic resonance imaging (MRI) scans of the spine can evaluate for other causes. A repeat MRI is not helpful.
- Computed tomography (CT) is not preferred. Plain radiography is not useful.
- If the patient has a history of cancer, HIV infection, or IV drug use, or has been taking steroids chronically, imaging is recommended.
- Electromyography (EMG).

Rx TREATMENT

Initial treatment for sciatica includes managing pain and maintaining activity and function. Surgery can be considered if there are anatomical abnormalities or pain progresses. If pain is severe and not relieved by previous measures, then narcotic medications may be prescribed for a short period.

NONPHARMACOLOGIC THERAPY

- Exercise minimally reduces intensity of pain. Individual pain and ability to exercise must be considered.
- Bed rest is not recommended.
- Physical and exercise therapy
- Manual therapy (e.g., spinal mobilization)
- Ice or heat on affected area for 20 min every 2 hours
- Reducing pressure on the nerve root

ACUTE GENERAL Rx

- Pain medications should be used sparingly, in minimal doses, and for a short time period due to their uncertain benefit for sciatica and possible adverse effects.
- Acetaminophen for mild pain
- Corticosteroids may improve symptoms for a short term. However, adverse effects limit usage.
- Benzodiazepines, opioids, and antidepressants are not recommended for sciatica.
- Anticonvulsants or biological agents have uncertain benefits.
- Gabapentin or pregabalin are frequently prescribed, but trials have failed to show reduced intensity of leg pain or improved outcomes.

Procedures
- Epidural injection of local anesthetic and steroids in the lumbar nerve root area may be considered in acute, severe sciatica. However, evidence is limited and beneficial effect is low.
- Surgery may be recommended if the pain continues for more than 6 to 8 wk despite conservative treatment and if imaging shows an anatomic problem with disc or bone. Surgery is also indicated in serious or progressive neurologic deficits (e.g., motor weakness, bladder dysfunction).
- In a recent trial involving patients with sciatica lasting more than 4 mo and caused by lumbar disk herniation, micro discectomy was superior to nonsurgical care with respect to pain intensity at 6 mo of follow-up.[1]

COMPLEMENTARY & ALTERNATIVE MEDICINE

- Acupuncture is not recommended in sciatica.
- Traction and electrotherapy are not recommended in back pain.

CHRONIC Rx

If pain is severe and unrelieved by previous measures, then consider a short course of narcotics; however, the medical community is increasingly turning away from long-term opioids due to the associated morbidity and mortality.

DISPOSITION

Outpatient workup and assessment, including:
- Screening for red flags that may indicate malignancies, osteoporotic fractures, trauma, infection, or cauda equina syndrome
- Taking a history to determine localization, severity, loss of strength, sensation, duration, course, influence of coughing, rest or movement
- Physical examination, including straight leg raising test
- Imaging or laboratory diagnostic testing if red flags are present
- Prescribing medication as needed

REFERRAL

- Physical therapist
- Pain management
- Orthopedic surgeon
- Refer to neurosurgeon immediately in cases of cauda equina syndrome or acute severe paresis or progressive paresis (within a few days)
- Refer to neurosurgeon or orthopedic surgeon for consideration of surgery in cases of intractable radicular pain or if pain does not diminish after 12 wk of conservative care.

PEARLS & CONSIDERATIONS

COMMENTS

- Most patients will recover fully from sciatica and often without treatment, but permanent nerve damage can occur. The following

[1] Bailey CS et al: Surgery versus conservative care for persistent sciatica lasting 4 to 12 months, *N Engl J Med* 382(12):1093-1102, 2020.

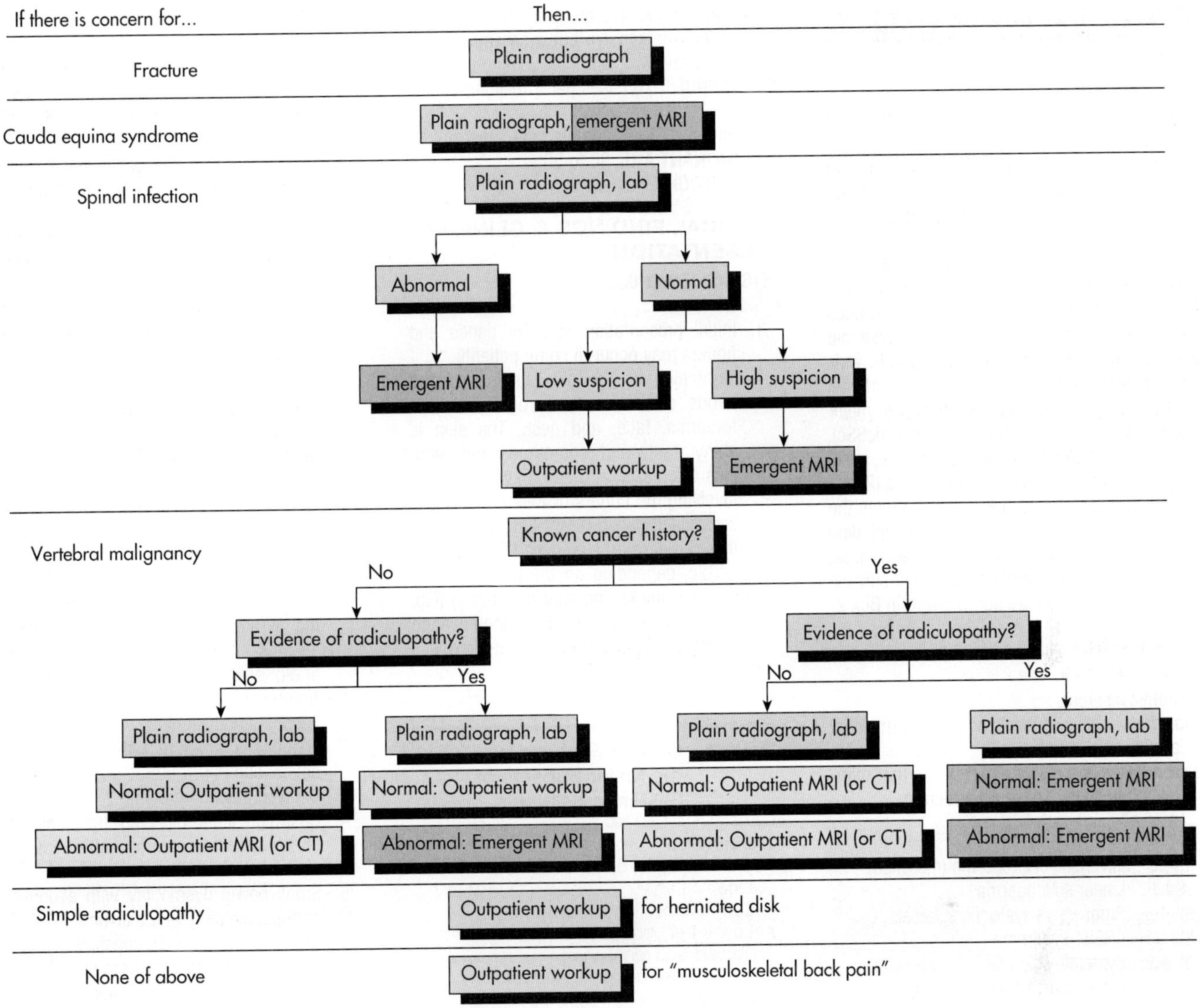

FIG. 1 Algorithm for management of low back pain. The patient's history may be concerning for more than one red flag diagnosis. *CT*, Computed tomography; *MRI*, magnetic resonance imaging. (From Marx JA et al: *Rosen's emergency medicine*, ed 8, Philadelphia, 2014, Elsevier.)

should prompt emergent workup as these symptoms could indicate spinal cord compression: Loss of feeling in affected leg; weakness in affected leg; or loss of bowel or bladder function.

- Sciatica does tend to recur.
- Bed rest is not recommended.

PREVENTION

- Exercise regularly.
- Maintain proper posture when you sit.
- Use good body mechanics.

SUGGESTED READINGS

Available at ExpertConsult.com

RELATED CONTENT

Lumbar Disk Syndrome (Related Key Topic)
Piriformis Syndrome (Related Key Topic)

AUTHORS: **Diana Zhou, MD,** and **Amanda Box, MD, MS**

BASIC INFORMATION

DEFINITION

Scleroderma or systemic sclerosis (SSc) is a term used to describe a connective tissue disorder that is characterized by thickening and fibrosis of the skin. Scleroderma is divided into two forms: Localized scleroderma and systemic sclerosis. Systemic sclerosis is a multiorgan disease characterized by fibrosis and vasculopathy. Skin thickening without any organ involvement is known as localized scleroderma and includes three subset conditions (see Box 1). Systemic sclerosis includes skin fibrosis along with variable severe involvement of diverse internal organs. It is further divided into two major subgroups: (1) Limited cutaneous SSc (lcSSc), which involves skin thickening of the face, neck, and distal to the elbows and knees; and (2) diffuse cutaneous SSc (dcSSc), which affects the skin in a more generalized distribution including the proximal and distal extremities, face, neck, and trunk. Clinical features of the major subsets of systemic sclerosis are summarized in Box 2.

SYNONYMS

SSc

Systemic sclerosis

Morphea applies to localized scleroderma that affects only the skin.

Scleredema is a disease of the skin that mimics but is distinct from scleroderma.

ICD-10CM CODES

L94.0	Localized scleroderma (morphea)
L94.1	Linear scleroderma
M34.0	Progressive systemic sclerosis
M34.1	CREST syndrome
M34.2	Systemic sclerosis induced by drug and chemical
M34.81	Systemic sclerosis with lung involvement
M34.82	Systemic sclerosis with myopathy
M34.83	Systemic sclerosis with polyneuropathy
M34.89	Other systemic sclerosis
M34.9	Systemic sclerosis, unspecified

EPIDEMIOLOGY & DEMOGRAPHICS

Incidence and prevalence of SSc differs between studies due to variations between geographic regions and time periods.

BOX 1 Classification of Scleroderma

I. Localized scleroderma
  A. Morphea
  B. Linear scleroderma
  C. Scleroderma en coup de sabre
II. Systemic sclerosis
  A. Limited cutaneous systemic sclerosis
  B. Diffuse cutaneous systemic sclerosis

From Hochberg MC et al: *Rheumatology,* ed 5, St Louis, 2011, Mosby.

INCIDENCE: There are an estimated 19 cases per 1 million persons/yr, but many mild cases go unrecognized.

PREVALENCE: 276 cases per 1 million persons per yr

PREDOMINANT SEX: Female/male ratio of 4:1

PREDOMINANT AGE: 30 to 50 yr

DISTRIBUTION: Worldwide

PHYSICAL FINDINGS & CLINICAL PRESENTATION

PHYSICAL FINDINGS:

- Skin:
  1. Initial presentation of puffy hands and fingers may occur in some patients.
  2. Tightening of the skin begins on the hands and then can progress to the forearms, face, and neck. The skin is shiny, taut, and sometimes red, with loss of creases and hair. Skin thickening involving the fingers or toes is known as sclerodactyly (Fig. E1). Skin involvement in scleroderma is classified as lcSSc or dcSSc, depending on the distribution of the skin thickening (see previously) (Fig. E2). Fig. E3 illustrates the method used to quantify skin thickness in scleroderma.
  3. Skin tightening may limit movement by causing flexion contractures of the fingers, wrists, and elbows. Perioral skin tightening (Fig. E4) results in decreased oral aperture, furrowing around the lips, and dry membranes.
  4. Pigmentary skin changes (hypo or hyperpigmentation) may occur (e.g., "salt and pepper").
  5. Telangiectasias (dilated capillaries) may be seen on face, hands, mucous membranes (Fig. E4), and trunk.
  6. Subcutaneous calcinosis, calcinosis cutis
  7. In dcSSc patients, the skin fibrosis can soften over time (generally occurring at least 2 yr after onset of skin manifestation), with improved joint mobility.
  8. Skin atrophy and thinning can also occur in the late stages of SSc.
- Musculoskeletal:
  1. Arthralgias and swelling
  2. Inflammatory arthritis, tendinitis
  3. Myalgias, myopathy
  4. Joint contractures
  5. Tendon friction rubs (physical exam finding of a palpable rub felt over tendon sheaths—fingers, wrists, elbows, knees, and/or ankles)
- Gastrointestinal involvement:
  1. Esophageal dysmotility with heartburn
  2. Esophageal stricture with dysphagia and odynophagia
  3. Delayed gastric emptying
  4. Gastrointestinal bleeding from mucosal telangiectasias, gastric antral vascular ectasias, or gastritis
  5. Small bowel dysmotility with abdominal cramps, bloating, and diarrhea
  6. Colon dysmotility with constipation
  7. Intestinal bacterial overgrowth resulting in irregular bowel movements (diarrhea alternating with constipation)
  8. Pseudo-obstruction (functional ileus)
  9. Primary biliary cholangitis
- Pulmonary:
  1. Interstitial lung disease (ILD): Pulmonary fibrosis with symptoms of dyspnea and nonproductive cough as well as fine inspiratory crackles on examination. Seen in both lcSSc and dcSSc, but it is more common and severe in dcSSc
  2. Pulmonary arterial hypertension (PAH): Presenting with dyspnea and/or fatigue. Can be identified in both lcSSc and dcSSc, but it is more commonly seen in lcSSc
- Cardiac:
  1. Pericarditis or pericardial effusion
  2. Myocardial fibrosis or ischemia that can lead to CHF or arrhythmias
  3. Left or right systolic or diastolic dysfunction
- Renal:
  1. Rapidly progressive renal failure also known as scleroderma renal crisis (SRC): New-onset hypertension, anemia with schistocytes on peripheral blood smear, thrombocytopenia and renal insufficiency with active urinary sediment and proteinuria

BOX 2 Clinical Features of the Major Subsets of Systemic Sclerosis

Limited SSc
- Skin sclerosis, distal limbs and face
- Long preexisting RP symptoms
- Lower frequency of severe lung fibrosis and renal crisis
- High burden of nonlethal morbidity

Diffuse SSc
- Proximal skin sclerosis
- Shorter preexisting RP history
- High frequency of severe lung fibrosis
- Increased risk of scleroderma renal crisis
- Inflammatory skin changes and pruritus common for first 1-3 yr

Sine SSc
- Features of RP with scleroderma-associated ANA reactivity and at least one internal organ manifestation of SSc
- Frequency uncertain because of likely underdiagnosis

Overlap SSc
- Cases that fulfill classification criteria for SSc and that are diagnosed as SSc but also show features of another autoimmune rheumatic disease
- Most often myositis
- Other cases of lupus, arthritis, or vasculitis
- Comprise up to 20% of SSc cohorts

ANA, Antinuclear antibody; *RP*, Raynaud phenomenon; *SSc*, systemic sclerosis.

From Hochberg MC: *Rheumatology*, ed 7, Philadelphia, 2019, Elsevier.

- Vascular:
  1. Raynaud phenomenon (RP): Vasospasm of the fingers with exposure to cold, resulting in color changes of the digits along with numbness/tingling and discomfort
  2. Complications of vascular involvement can include digital pitted scars or ulcers, nonreversible ischemic changes with impending tissue loss, dry gangrene, and auto-amputation
  3. Nailfold capillary abnormalities: Seen with nailfold capillaroscopy, including capillary dilatation, avascularity, or "drop out" of capillaries
- Other organ involvement:
  1. Hypothyroidism
  2. Erectile dysfunction
  3. Sjögren syndrome
  4. Entrapment neuropathies
  5. Depression

CLINICAL PRESENTATION

- Raynaud phenomenon: Initial complaint in 70% of patients (NOTE: The prevalence of Raynaud phenomenon is 5%-10% in the general population; most cases do not progress to scleroderma)
- Finger or hand swelling that is sometimes associated with carpal tunnel syndrome
- Arthralgias/arthritis
- Internal organ involvement (Table 1, Table E2, Fig. E5, Fig. E6)
- LcSSc (previously known as CREST syndrome): Calcinosis, Raynaud phenomenon, Esophageal dysmotility, Sclerodactyly telangiectasias—skin fibrosis is limited to the distal extremities. This acronym is now considered obsolete by many because it does not accurately reflect the burden of internal organ involvement

ETIOLOGY

The etiology of this condition is unknown, but genetic and environmental factors (infectious agents, occupational exposures, drugs) contribute to the manifestation of the disease. Genetic profiles show clustering of different alleles according to the subtype of SSc.

Pathologically, small- and medium-sized arteries become injured, leading to fibrin deposition and ultimately luminal occlusion, causing chronic tissue hypoxia. There is also an abnormal selection of fibroblasts and aberrant control of connective tissue synthesis by fibroblasts and other cells. This fibrosis occurs in different organs, causing dysfunction and eventual failure. Although there are characteristic autoantibodies detected, it is not clear that they directly participate in the pathogenesis of the disease.

Dx DIAGNOSIS

The American College of Rheumatology (ACR) and European League Against Rheumatism (EULAR) have created criteria as a guide in diagnosing and classifying SSc (Table 3). These include a scoring system for both clinical and laboratory findings (sclerodactyly, fingertip lesions, telangiectasias, abnormal nailfold capillaries, Raynaud phenomenon, PAH/ILD, and SSc-related autoantibodies).

DIFFERENTIAL DIAGNOSIS

DERMATOLOGIC:

- Scleredema
- Amyloidosis

TABLE 3 ACR/EULAR 2013 Classification Criteria for Systemic Sclerosis*

Item	Subitem	Weight or Score
Skin thickening of fingers on both hands extending proximal to the MCP joints (sufficient criterion)	—	9
Skin thickening on the fingers (only count the higher score)	Puffy fingers Sclerodactyly of fingers (distal to MCP joints but proximal to proximal interphalangeal joints)	2 4
Fingertip lesions (only count higher score)	Digital tip ulcers Fingertip pitting scars	2 3
Telangiectasia	—	2
Abnormal nailfold capillaries	—	2
Pulmonary arterial hypertension or ILD (maximum score, 2)	PAH ILD	2 2
Raynaud phenomenon	—	3
SSc-related antibodies (anticentromere, antitopoisomerase 1 [anti–SCL-70], anti-RNA polymerase III (max score 3)	Anticentromere Antitopoisomerase I Antipolymerase III	3

ACR, American College of Rheumatology; *EULAR*, European League Against Rheumatism; *ILD*, interstitial lung disease; *MCP*, metacarpophalangeal; *PAH*, pulmonary arterial hypertension; *SSc*, systemic sclerosis.
*The score is determined by adding the maximum weight or score in each category. Patients with scores ≥9 have definite systemic sclerosis (SSc).
From Hochberg MC: *Rheumatology*, ed 7, Philadelphia, 2019, Elsevier.

TABLE 1 Overview of Musculoskeletal Complications of Systemic Sclerosis

Manifestation	Clinical Features	Serologic Associations
Contractures	Typical feature of dcSSc Associated with ARA positivity Palmar fibrosis	ARA, ATA, RF, ACPA
Tendonitis or tendon friction rubs	Overlap arthritis	ARA
Arthritis	May resemble RA in overlap Associated with RF positivity and ACPA positivity More with U1RNP reactivity Contributes to deformity and contractures May have Jaccoud pattern but with fixed deformity	U1RNP, ACPA, RF
Myositis	Minor elevation in CK common, especially in dcSSc Weakness and loss of muscle bulk Severe myositis less frequent Overlap syndromes with myositis most common Serologic associations include anti–PM-Scl, antiU1RNP, antifibrillarin	U1RNP, PM-Scl, U3RNP
Acro-osteolysis	More common in environmentally triggered SSc Association with vasculopathy and Raynaud phenomenon Possible association with calcinosis	ACA, ATA

ACA, Anticentromere; *ACPA*, anticyclic citrullinated protein antibody; *ARA*, anti-RNA polymerase III antibody; *ATA*, antitopoisomerase; *CK*, creatine kinase; *dcSSc*, diffuse cutaneous systemic sclerosis; *PM-Scl*, antipolymyositis scleroderma antibody; *RA*, rheumatoid arthritis; *RF*, rheumatoid factor; SSc, systemic sclerosis; *U1RNP*, anti-U1-ribonucleoprotein antibody; *U3RNP*, anti–U3-ribonucleoprotein antibody.
From Hochberg MC: *Rheumatology*, ed 7, Philadelphia, 2019, Elsevier.

TABLE 4 Distinguishing Features of Scleroderma and Scleroderma-like Conditions

Condition	Skin Changes and Distribution	Extradermal Involvement	Dermatopathology	Other
Localized scleroderma	Amorphous plaques (morphea) or lines involving the face (linear) and extremities and sparing the fingers	None	Dermal sclerosis, mononuclear inflammation	Linear especially common in children, autoantibodies common
Scleredema	Trunk, back, neck	Rare	Swollen collagen bundles, mucin accumulation	
Scleromyxedema	Induration, sclerodactyly Limited mouth opening	Rare	Excessive dermal mucin deposition	Serum paraprotein (especially IgG λ)
Nephrogenic systemic fibrosis	Extremities, fingers; symmetric	Frequent, mild (muscle, fascia, lungs)	Fibroblast proliferation, mucin deposition, dermal spindle cell proliferation	After gadolinium exposure in end-stage renal disease
Eosinophilic fasciitis	Extremities, trunk; spares fingers	Rare; low-grade myositis	Dermal and hypodermal sclerosis, normal epidermis, muscle inflammation occasionally	Peripheral blood eosinophilia frequent

From Hochberg MC: *Rheumatology*, ed 7, Philadelphia, 2019, Elsevier.

TABLE 5 Autoantigens and Autoantibodies in Scleroderma

Autoantigen	Molecular Structure	Autoantibody Frequency
Scl-70	100-kD native and 70-kD degradation product; DNA topoisomerase I	75% in diffuse scleroderma; 20%-59% in all patients; 13% in CREST
Centromere	Proteins 17, 80, and 140 kD; localized at inner and outer kinetochore plates	57%-82% in CREST; 8% in diffuse form
RNA Pol I	RNA Pol I complex of subunit proteins, 210-211 kD	4%-30% in scleroderma; 13% in diffuse form
RNA Pol II	Transcripts mRNA	4%
RNA Pol III	Transcripts 5S rRNA, tRNA	23% in scleroderma; 45% in diffuse form; 6% in CREST
Fibrillarin	Protein 34 kD, component of U3 RNP particle	6%-8%; 5% in diffuse form; 10% in CREST
U1nRNP	Spliceosome complex	2%-5% in all patients; 24% in PM/scleroderma overlap
PM-Scl	Complex of 11 proteins, 110-120 kD	4%-11%; 24% in PM/scleroderma overlap
Ku	DNA-binding protein	1%-14% in scleroderma; 26%-55% in PM/scleroderma overlap
Th/To	Protein 40 kD, complexes with 7S and 8S RNAs	1%-13% in scleroderma; 1%-11% in diffuse form; 8%-19% in CREST; up to 3% in PM/scleroderma overlap
NOR-90	Protein 90 kD, human upstream binding factor, localized in nucleolus organizer region	Rare

CREST, Calcinosis, Raynaud phenomenon, esophageal dysfunction, sclerodactyly, and telangiectasia; *DNA,* deoxyribonucleic acid; *mRNA,* messenger RNA; *PM,* polymyositis; *RNA,* ribonucleic acid; *RNP,* ribonucleoprotein; *rRNA,* ribosomal RNA; *tRNA,* transfer RNA.
From McPherson RA, Pincus MR: *Henry's clinical diagnosis and management by laboratory methods,* ed 23, Philadelphia, 2017, Elsevier.

- Porphyria cutanea tarda
- Eosinophilic fasciitis
- Reflex sympathetic dystrophy
- Nephrogenic systemic fibrosis
- Table 4 summarizes distinguishing features of scleroderma and scleroderma-like conditions

SYSTEMIC:
- Idiopathic pulmonary fibrosis
- Primary pulmonary hypertension
- Primary biliary cirrhosis
- Cardiomyopathies
- Gastrointestinal dysmotility problems
- Systemic lupus erythematosus and overlap syndromes

WORKUP

Laboratory tests and imaging studies

LABORATORY TESTS

- Antinuclear antibodies (ANA): Nucleolar (more common), homogeneous, or speckled patterns
- Rheumatoid factor positive in 20% of patients
- Routine biochemistry tests may indicate specific organ involvement (e.g., liver, kidney, muscle); should check CBCD, CK, CMP, UA

The following extractable nuclear antigens are either present or absent in SSc:
- Anticentromere antibodies: Generally positive in one third of patients with lcSSc
- Anti–Scl-70 antibody (antitopoisomerase I): Positive in 40% of patients with dcSSc and has an increased risk of developing ILD
- AntiRNA polymerase III antibody: Portends a worse prognosis, with rapidly progressive skin fibrosis and increased risk of developing SRC. May also indicate increased cancer risk
- Antiribonucleoprotein (anti-RNP): Positive in 20%, can see with overlap conditions
- Other possible antibodies include U3 RNP, U1 RNP, PM-Scl, Th/To, Anti-Ku
- Table 5 summarizes autoantigens and autoantibodies in scleroderma

IMAGING & OTHER STUDIES

- Arthritis: Joint radiographs
- Gastrointestinal:
  1. Upper endoscopy (diagnostic procedure of choice; may be therapeutic)
  2. Cine-esophagography (in rare circumstances)
  3. Barium swallow (occasionally indicated)
  4. Esophageal manometry
- Pulmonary:
  1. Chest x-ray
  2. Pulmonary function tests (especially single-breath diffusion capacity for carbon monoxide—DLCO)
  3. Thoracic high-resolution computed tomography (HRCT) scan
  4. Bronchoscopy with biopsy, bronchoalveolar lavage
- Cardiac:
  1. ECG
  2. Ambulatory (Holter) ECG monitoring
  3. Echocardiography (screen for pulmonary arterial hypertension)
  4. Cardiac catheterization
- Kidney: Renal biopsy
- Skin: Skin biopsy
- Vascular: Nailfold capillaroscopy

Rx TREATMENT

Currently, there is no disease-modifying therapy available for SSc. Generally, the internal organ involvement of the disease is treatable. Fig. 7 illustrates management strategies in SSc. Immunosuppressive agents are used in individual patients. Prednisone should be used with extreme caution, especially in doses >20 mg/day (can precipitate SRC).
- Raynaud phenomenon:
  1. Keep hands and body warm

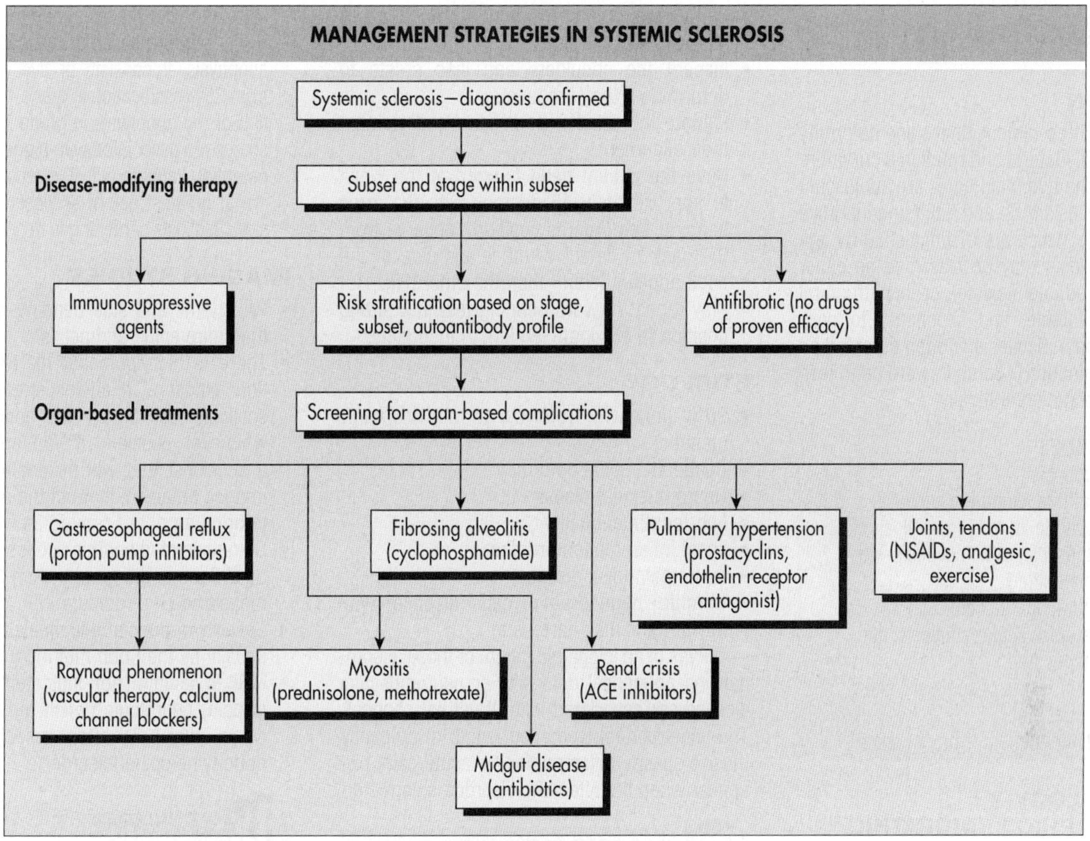

FIG. 7 Management of scleroderma requires multiple strategies depending on the specific problems that are present in individual patients. *ACE,* Angiotensin-converting enzyme; *NSAID,* nonsteroidal antiinflammatory drug. (From Hochberg MC: *Rheumatology*, ed 7, Philadelphia, 2019, Elsevier.)

2. Avoid smoking and using vasoconstricting drugs
3. Calcium channel blockers (i.e., long-acting dihydropyridines)
4. Peripheral α1-adrenergic blockers
5. Angiotensin II receptor blockers
6. Topical nitrate
7. Phosphodiesterase inhibitors
8. Stellate ganglion blockades
9. Digital sympathectomy
10. Table E6 summarizes vascular therapies for Raynaud phenomenon

- Arthralgias: NSAIDs or low-dose corticosteroids (5-10 mg of prednisone per day)
- Myositis: Methotrexate or azathioprine with low-dose corticosteroids
- Skin: For skin fibrosis, immunomodulatory drugs have been used, generally started within 3 yr of onset (methotrexate, mycophenolate mofetil). Cyclophosphamide can be used for refractory or rapidly progressive involvement. Table E7 summarizes immunomodulatory and antifibrotic strategies for disease-modifying treatment of systemic sclerosis skin disease
- GI tract: Table E8 summarizes treatment of GI tract complications in systemic sclerosis
- Esophageal reflux:
  1. H_2-receptor blockers
  2. Proton pump inhibitors
- Interstitial lung disease:
  1. Mycophenolate mofetil or cyclophosphamide for symptomatic ILD
  2. Nintedanib, a small molecule that inhibits several kinases linked to the pathogenesis of interstitial lung diseases (receptor tyrosine kinases and nonreceptor tyrosine kinases), recently received FDA approval for the treatment of ILD associated with systemic sclerosis
  3. Lung transplantation for patients with advanced pulmonary involvement
- Pulmonary hypertension:
  1. Oxygen
  2. Diuretics (with caution)
  3. Prostacyclins (epoprostenol, iloprost, treprostinil)
  4. Endothelin-1 receptor inhibitors (bosentan, ambrisentan)
  5. Phosphodiesterase 5 inhibitors (sildenafil, tadalafil)
  6. Table E9 summarizes approved therapies for treatment of pulmonary arterial hypertension
- Renal involvement:
  1. Angiotensin-converting enzyme inhibitors
  2. Dialysis
  3. Renal transplantation

REFERRAL

Rheumatology consultation is indicated. Consider pulmonary, cardiology, or gastrointestinal consultations depending on organ involvement.

PEARLS & CONSIDERATIONS

COMMENTS

Autologous hematopoietic stem cell therapy (HSCT) has shown some benefit in patients with severe diffuse cutaneous systemic sclerosis, but there was greater treatment-related mortality and morbidity associated with HSCT.

SUGGESTED READINGS

Available at ExpertConsult.com

RELATED CONTENT

Scleroderma (Patient Information)

AUTHOR: **Joanne Szczygiel Cunha, MD**

BASIC INFORMATION

DEFINITION

Scoliosis is a three-dimensional spine deformity characterized by lateral and rotational curvature of the spine. The two main types are adolescent idiopathic scoliosis (AIS) and adult degenerative scoliosis (ADS), which are distinguished by age of onset. Scoliosis may be classified as either structural (fixed, nonflexible) or nonstructural (flexible, correctable, and secondary to nonspinal pathology). Scoliosis is often detected on physical examination (Adams forward bend test) and confirmed radiographically.

ICD-10CM CODES	
M41	Scoliosis
M41.0	Infantile idiopathic scoliosis
M41.1	Juvenile idiopathic scoliosis
M41.20	Other idiopathic scoliosis, site unspecified
M41.3	Thoracogenic scoliosis
M41.40	Neuromuscular scoliosis, site unspecified
M41.80	Other forms of scoliosis, site unspecified
Q67.5	Congenital deformity of spine

EPIDEMIOLOGY & DEMOGRAPHICS (IDIOPATHIC FORM)

PREVALENCE: 1.5% to 3% of adolescents

PREDOMINANT SEX: The incidence of AIS is similar in males and females; however, females have up to a tenfold greater risk of curve progression. Females are roughly seven times as likely to require orthopedic surgical intervention for idiopathic scoliosis. ADS has an equal gender distribution.

PREDOMINANT AGE:
- Onset variable
- Most curves found in adolescents (age ≥11 yr)

PHYSICAL FINDINGS & CLINICAL PRESENTATION

- Typical presentation involves postural complaints rather than pain or neurologic symptoms.
- Record patient age (in years plus months) and height.
- Perform neurologic examination to rule out neuromuscular disease.
- Inspect the shoulders and iliac crests to determine if they are level.
- Palpate the spinous processes to determine their alignment.
- Have the patient bend forward at the waist to approximately 45 degrees with the arms hanging free (Adams position); observe from the back to detect whether one side of the back appears higher than the other (Fig. 1).
- May repeat forward bending test in a sitting position to eliminate leg length inequality.

ETIOLOGY

- 90% unknown, referred to as *idiopathic* (genetic)
- Congenital spine deformity
- Neuromuscular disease
- Leg-length inequality
- Local inflammation or infection
- Acute pain (disk disease)
- Chronic degenerative disk disease with asymmetric disk narrowing

Curves of an idiopathic nature or those accompanying congenital deformity or neuromuscular disease are associated with structural changes. The nonstructural types (leg-length discrepancy, muscle spasm, inflammation, or acute pain) disappear when the offending disorder is corrected.

DIAGNOSIS

WORKUP

- Curvatures associated with congenital spine abnormalities, neuromuscular disease, and other less common forms of scoliosis can usually be identified by history or associated radiographic or physical findings.
- The diagnosis of scoliosis is suspected on the basis of physical examination and confirmed by radiography performed while the patient is in a standing position. Physical examination with the Adams forward bend test and scoliometer measurement can identify scoliosis, and the radiologic testing for Cobb angle measurement can confirm the diagnosis. The Cobb angle is measured on a thoraco-lumbar radiograph and is defined as the intersecting angle between lines drawn parallel to the endplates of the two vertebrae with the greatest amount of tilt. The Risser grade measures ossification of the iliac apophysis. It consists of five grades ranging from 25% ossification in grade 1 to full ossification of the apophysis in grade 5. Lower Risser scores are associated with higher spinal growth potential. Patients with Risser scores of 0 or 1 are at greatest risk of scoliosis curve progression. Scoliosis screening is described in Fig. 2.

IMAGING STUDIES

- PA, lateral, and side-bending radiographs of the entire spine and pelvis.
- There is high potential for repeated radiation exposure in adolescents evaluated for scoliosis. Use breast and gonadal shielding whenever possible. If you are referring to a specialist that will be unable to view the images obtained, instruct the patient's family to bring a printed copy to their visit.
- Diagnosis of idiopathic scoliosis is confirmed by a Cobb angle greater than 10 degrees as measured on a radiograph.
- Severity of the curve is measured in degrees, usually by the Cobb method (Fig. 3).
- MRI is usually not indicated unless there is pain, neurologic deficit, or a left thoracic curve (which is often associated with an underlying spinal disorder).

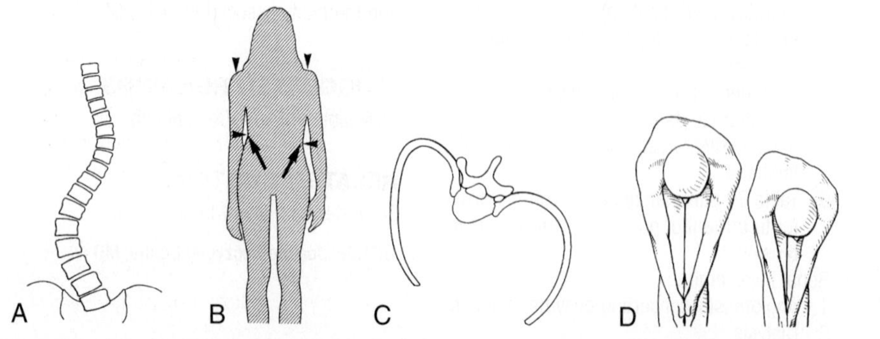

FIG. 1 Structural changes in idiopathic scoliosis. A, As curvature increases, alterations in body configuration develop in both the primary and compensatory curve regions. **B,** Asymmetries of shoulder height, waistline, and the elbow-to-flank distance are common findings. **C,** Vertebral rotation and associated posterior displacement of the ribs on the convex side of the curve are responsible for the characteristic deformity of the chest wall in scoliosis patients. **D,** In the school screening examination for scoliosis, the patient bends forward at the waist. Rib asymmetry of even a small degree is obvious.

Rx TREATMENT

ACUTE GENERAL Rx

- Treatment or correction of cause if curve is nonstructural
- Early detection is key in treating genetic (idiopathic) curve
- Regular observation for curves <20 degrees
- If no curve progression, repeat imaging may be limited to once per yr
- Bracing for idiopathic curves of 25 to 45 degrees in patients with an immature skeleton (Risser score 0-2) to prevent progression
- Surgery (Fig. E4) for idiopathic curves >45 degrees in patients with an immature skeleton

DISPOSITION

- The larger the curve at detection, the greater the chance of progression.
- Progression is more common in young children who are beginning their growth spurt.
- Curves in females are more likely to progress.
- Curves <20 degrees will improve spontaneously >50% of the time.
- Failure to diagnose and treat these curves may allow progressive deformity, pain, and cardiopulmonary compromise to develop.
- Spinal deformities >50 degrees in adults may progress and eventually become painful or compromise pulmonary function.
- There is no difference in the rate of back pain in the general population and patients with adolescent idiopathic scoliosis.

REFERRAL

Refer for orthopedic consultation if structural curve >20 degrees is present or if structural curve <20 degrees progresses 5 degrees or more upon follow-up evaluation.

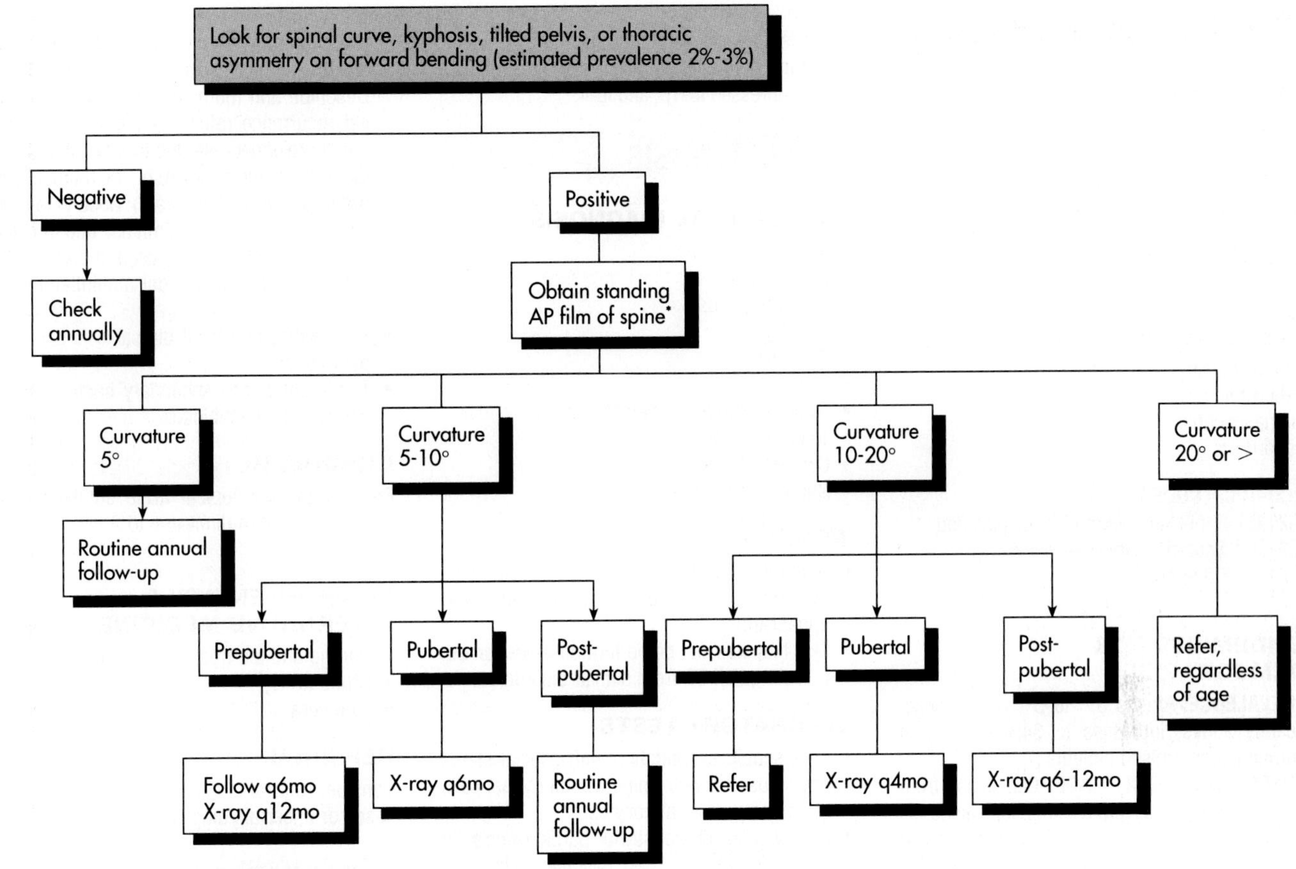

*Cobb method of angle measurement.

1. Find the lowest vertebra whose bottom tilts toward concavity of curve.
2. Erect a perpendicular line from extension of bottom surface.
3. Find highest vertebra as in #1 and erect perpendicular from extension of top surface.
4. Measure intersecting angle = angle of scoliosis.

FIG. 2 Scoliosis screening and follow-up. *AP,* Anteroposterior.

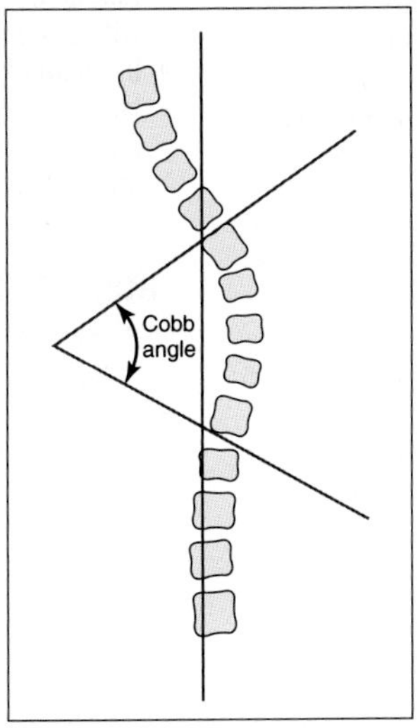

FIG. 3 Cobb angle. This is measured using the superior and inferior end plates of the most tilted vertebrae at the end of each curve. (From Tschudy MM, Arcara KM: *The Harriet Lane handbook,* ed 19, Philadelphia, 2012, Mosby.)

PEARLS & CONSIDERATIONS

COMMENTS

- Congenital scoliosis has a high incidence of cardiac and urinary tract abnormalities.
- Bracing is not intended to completely straighten the idiopathic curve. It may improve the curvature but is mainly used to stabilize and prevent progression.
- The initial Cobb angle magnitude (≥25 degrees) is the most important predictor of long-term curve progression.

SUGGESTED READINGS

Available at ExpertConsult.com

RELATED CONTENT

Scoliosis (Patient Information)

AUTHORS: **Michael Bergen, MD, Shyam A. Patel, MD,** and **Eren O. Kuris, MD**

Seborrheic Dermatitis (SD) PTG

BASIC INFORMATION

DEFINITION

Seborrheic dermatitis (SD) is a common, inflammatory skin condition characterized by a mild to severe rash with scaling and erythema that occurs in areas of the skin rich in sebaceous glands.

SYNONYMS

SD
Dandruff
Cradle cap (Fig. E1)
Sebopsoriasis
Seborrheic eczema
Pityriasis capitis
Seborrhea

ICD-10CM CODES

L21.9	Seborrheic dermatitis, unspecified
L21.1	Seborrheic infantile dermatitis
L21.8	Other seborrheic dermatitis

EPIDEMIOLOGY & DEMOGRAPHICS

PREVALENCE: Affects 3% to 5% of otherwise healthy adults; increases to 34% to 83% in immunocompromised patients

PREDOMINANT SEX & AGE: Can occur from infancy through old age, with peak incidence in adolescents and young adults and increasing again after age 50 yr. More common in men than women.

RISK FACTORS: More common in patients with HIV/AIDS, Parkinson disease, other neurologic disorders, mood disorders, chronic alcoholic pancreatitis, hepatitis, cancer, and genetic disorders (e.g., Down syndrome). Recent evidence linking obesity and metabolic syndrome with an increased occurrence of SD. Occurs more often during winter season and during periods of increased stress.

PHYSICAL FINDINGS & CLINICAL PRESENTATION

- Mild, greasy scaling of the scalp and nasolabial folds (Fig. E2); postauricular skin, beard area, eyebrows, trunk, and sometimes the central face. Blepharitis, otitis externa, and coexisting acne vulgaris or pityriasis may also be present. Itching and stinging of lesions can occur. Increased occurrence during times of stress or sleep deprivation.
- The scale often has a yellow, greasy appearance.

ETIOLOGY

Newer studies indicate that defects in the immune system may trigger proliferation of the *Malassezia yeast* and the associated skin changes. Patients with SD may show upregulation of interferon (IFN)-α, expressed interleukin-6 (IL-6), expressed IL-1β, and IL-4.

Dx DIAGNOSIS

DIFFERENTIAL DIAGNOSIS

- Atopic dermatitis
- Candidiasis
- Dermatophytosis
- Impetigo
- Psoriasis
- Rosacea
- Systemic lupus erythematosus
- Tinea infection
- Contact dermatitis
- Nummular dermatitis

WORKUP

- Diagnosis usually based on clinical identification of lesions (distribution and appearance).
- Skin biopsies can be performed, if warranted, to distinguish SD from similar disorders.

LABORATORY TESTS

- Microscopic examination with special stains can be used to determine whether yeast cells are present in keratinocytes.
- Biopsy can demonstrate parakeratosis in the epidermis, plugged follicular ostia, and spongiosis.
- HIV testing.

Rx TREATMENT

NONPHARMACOLOGIC THERAPY

- Patient education that SD is a chronic condition and treatment is aimed at resolving lesions but does not prevent recurrence.
- General recommendations: Wash skin regularly, soften and remove scales, and apply moisturizing emollients after washing.
- Scale removal can be accomplished through the application of mineral or olive oil and removed with a comb or brush after 1 hr.

ACUTE GENERAL Rx

- Antifungals (e.g., Nizoral, selenium sulfide, ketoconazole [the most evidence for effectiveness among antifungals], ciclopirox, fluconazole). Considered first-line therapy. Shampoos should be kept on the skin for 5 min before washing off.
- Reserve oral antifungal therapy for patients with widespread SD, or SD that is refractory to topical therapy.
- Topical steroids: Can be in the form of shampoos, creams, or ointments. Can be used alone or in more severe SD with antifungals. Desonide and mometasone display the lowest recurrence rates and highest clearance. Avoid prolonged use due to side effects.
- Calcineurin inhibitors (e.g., tacrolimus ointment, pimecrolimus cream): Good when face and ears are affected. Limit use due to potential side effects. Can be used in combination with topical nonsteroidal antiinflammatory agents
- Keratolytics (e.g. coal tar, salicylic acid, zinc pyrithione).
- Treatment of any secondary bacterial infection with oral antibiotics.

CHRONIC Rx

Recalcitrant SD: Topical azole combined with desonide regimen (limit use to 2 wk), pimecrolimus cream

COMPLEMENTARY & ALTERNATIVE MEDICINE

- Borage and tea tree oil (melaleuca oil)
- Crude honey
- Aloe vera

REFERRAL

Consider referral to dermatology for recalcitrant cases or uncertain diagnosis.

PEARLS & CONSIDERATIONS

- Use a combination of topical steroids and antifungal cream for severe SD.
- Limit use of steroids to 2-wk course of treatment due to risk of cutaneous atrophy and telangiectasias.
- SD of the scalp can be treated with an antifungal (e.g., 2% ketoconazole) or keratolytic shampoo. Limit use of antifungal shampoos to twice a wk to prevent drying of the scalp. Alternate the use of antifungal shampoos with a moisturizing shampoo.
- In patients with widespread SD, consider testing for HIV infection. In patients with HIV/AIDS, the severity of seborrheic dermatitis is inversely correlated with the CDs counts.

SUGGESTED READINGS

Available at ExpertConsult.com

RELATED CONTENT

Seborrheic Dermatitis (Patient Information)

AUTHOR: **AnnGene Anthony, MD, MPH, FAAFP**

BASIC INFORMATION

DEFINITION

Tonic clonic seizures are characterized by sudden loss of consciousness, muscle contraction (tonic phase), followed by rhythmic jerking activity (clonic phase).

SYNONYMS

Bilateral tonic-clonic seizures
Convulsive seizures
Grand mal seizures
Generalized tonic clonic seizures

ICD-10CM CODES

G40.6 Grand mal seizures, unspecified
G41.0 Grand mal status epilepticus

EPIDEMIOLOGY & DEMOGRAPHICS

INCIDENCE: 30 to 50 cases per 100,000 person-yr (epilepsy incidence)
PREVALENCE: 5 to 8 cases/1,000 persons (epilepsy incidence)
PREDOMINANT SEX & AGE: No gender preference
PEAK INCIDENCE: Not applicable

PHYSICAL FINDINGS & CLINICAL PRESENTATION

- Patients with unprovoked tonic clonic seizures usually have normal physical and neurologic examinations.
- A generalized seizure may start without warning and can typically last from 30 to 120 seconds, during which the patient will be unconscious and may have increased rigidity and/or jerking of the whole body, or staring spells. Cyanosis (especially of the lips and face) can result from temporary airway compromise due to muscle spasms. Tonic-clonic seizures can cause injuries, tongue biting, and bladder incontinence. Patients are usually unaware of the seizure afterwards. A postictal state characterized by confusion, lethargy, headaches, or drowsiness may result and can last from minutes to hours depending on the severity of the seizure (Fig. 1).
- Tonic clonic seizures are associated with injuries, bladder incontinence, and tongue biting.
- Any warning or aura before onset of the seizure or focal postictal weakness (Todd paralysis) may point toward a focal neurologic lesion.

ETIOLOGY

- Seizures are a cardinal sign of cortical neurologic injury. Generalized seizures include both hemispheres of the brain at onset. However, seizures can start focally and then quickly generalize across both hemispheres of the brain and be almost identical to primary generalized seizures. Any warning or aura symptoms before the generalized seizure starts would point to a focal onset.
- Acute symptomatic generalized seizures can be due to systemic causes (e.g., systemic infections, meningitis, encephalitis, electrolyte abnormalities, hypoglycemia, hyperthyroidism, malignant hypertension, eclampsia, drug intoxication or withdrawal).
- Generalized seizures are seen in many epilepsy syndromes with genetic causes.

DIAGNOSIS

DIFFERENTIAL DIAGNOSIS

- Convulsive syncope
- Psychogenic nonepileptic spells, conversion disorder, somatic symptom disorder, dissociative disorder
- Focal seizure with secondary generalization
- TIA
- Vertigo
- Factitious disorder
- Malingering
- Myoclonus (from metabolic disturbance)

WORKUP

- EEG (Fig. 2). An EEG can help confirm the presence of epilepsy but cannot be used to exclude the diagnosis.
- Ambulatory EEG and/or video EEG recommended for patients with diagnostic uncertainty.

LABORATORY TESTS

- Routine blood workup (CBC, CMP, glucose, electrolytes)
- Urine drug screen
- Lumbar puncture is recommended in patients with suspicion of meningitis

IMAGING STUDIES

- Neurodiagnostic imaging studies such as CT of the head or, preferably, MRI of the brain should be performed in all patients with first unprovoked seizure.
- CT scans of the head should be avoided in children due to unnecessary exposure to radiation and the low yield of the test. CT scans of the head are reserved for neurologic emergencies and are adjusted for weight in children.

TREATMENT

ACUTE Rx

- The immediate management of a seizure focuses on stabilization of the patient with focus on the airway and vital signs and rapid identification and correction of reversible causes.
- Seizures lasting >5 minutes or multiple seizures without return to baseline in between should be treated as status epilepticus.
- Treatment is based on the type and etiology of seizures (i.e., metabolic disturbance, infectious, etc.).
- Provoked seizures due to metabolic derangements, infections, fever, alcohol, or drug-withdrawal are typically generalized and likely do not need long-term treatment.
- Multiple antiepileptic medication choices are available. Choice depends on side effect profile as well as whether the seizure started focally or is secondary to an idiopathic generalized epilepsy syndrome.

NONPHARMACOLOGIC THERAPY

Not applicable

GENERAL Rx

- Patients with a first unprovoked seizure who have a normal EEG, imaging, lab values, and physical exam do not require treatment with antiepileptic drugs but may be offered therapy because the use of an antiepileptic drug after a first unprovoked seizure in an adult reduces the absolute risk of seizure recurrence at 2 yr by 35%. However, there is no difference at 3 yr. This decision should be made in conjunction with the patient and should take into consideration the patient's job, risks of medications, and individual preferences.
- Patients with two or more unprovoked seizures, or those with one seizure and an abnormal workup consistent with epilepsy findings, should be started or continued on antiepileptic drugs. Patients on antiepileptic therapy with negative workup may be considered for weaning off antiepileptic drug if seizure-free after 2 yr.
- Primary generalized epilepsies:
  1. Levetiracetam (Keppra): Initial dose 250 to 500 bid, maximum dose 1500 mg bid.
  2. Lamotrigine (Lamictal): Initial dose 25 mg daily and increase slowly to goal dose 150 to 250 mg daily (depends on combination of other medications).
  3. Topiramate (Topamax): Initial dose 25 mg bid and increase to usual dose of 100 to 200 mg bid.
  4. Perampanel (Fycompa): Initial dose of 2 mg once daily at bedtime, increments of 2 mg once daily at weekly intervals to a recommended maintenance dose of 8 to 12 mg (adjunctive treatment in patients with epilepsy 12 yr of age and older).
  5. Valproic acid (Depakote): Initial dose: 10 to 15 mg/kg/day (divided bid), maximum dose 60 mg/kg/day. Valproic acid should be avoided in girls and women with childbearing potential due to the risk of teratogenicity.
- Focal epilepsies with secondary generalization: Almost all antiepileptic drugs are approved for focal seizures, either in monotherapy or in adjunct. Carbamazepine, oxcarbazepine, eslicarbazepine, lamotrigine, levetiracetam, or lacosamide are all possibilities, among others.
- Patients who continue to have seizures despite adequate trials on at least two antiepileptic medications should be referred to a tertiary care epilepsy center for evaluation of surgical treatment of epilepsy.

DISPOSITION

- Patients should avoid situations that may cause injuries or accidents in the event of a

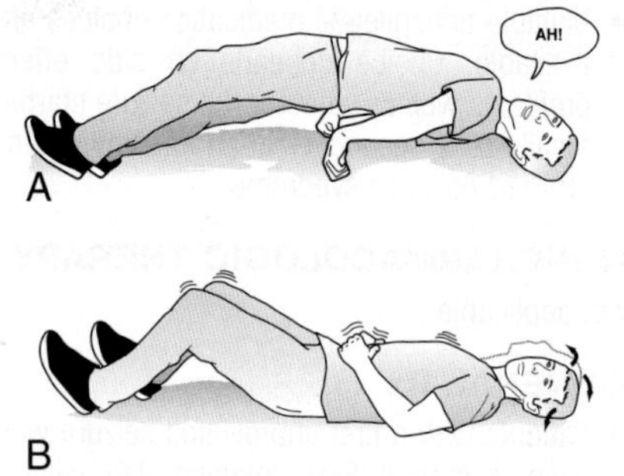

FIG. 1 A, This man in the tonic phase of a tonic-clonic seizure arches his torso and extends his arms and legs. He assumes this position because of the relatively greater strength of the extensor muscles compared to the flexor muscles. Simultaneous diaphragm, chest wall, and laryngeal muscle contractions force air through his tightened larynx to produce the shrill "epileptic cry." During this phase, he may also bite his tongue and lose control of his urine. **B,** In the clonic phase, his head, neck, and legs contract symmetrically and forcefully for about 10 to 20 seconds. Saliva, aerated and often blood-tinged from tongue lacerations, froths from his mouth. His pupils dilate, and he sweats profusely. Finally, his muscular contractions lose strength. The seizure usually ends with stertorous breathing. In the immediate postictal period, he remains unresponsive. Before regaining consciousness, he may pass through a state of confusion and agitation. (From Kaufman DM et al: *Kaufman's clinical neurology for psychiatrists*, ed 8, Philadelphia, 2017, Elsevier.)

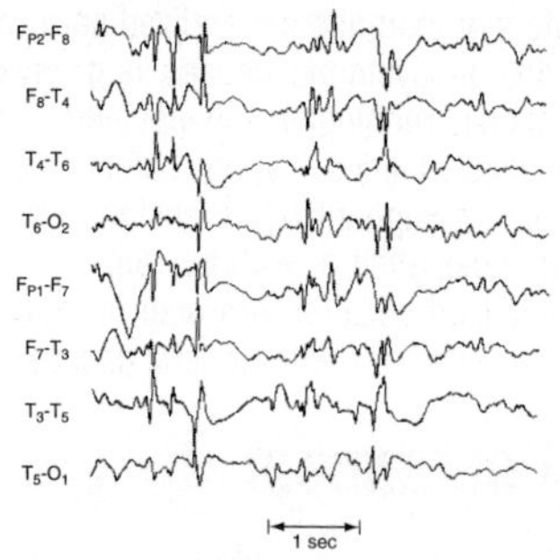

FIG. 2 During a tonic-clonic seizure, the EEG ideally shows paroxysms of spikes, polyspikes, and occasional slow waves in all channels; however, muscle artifact can obscure this pattern. Even during interictal periods, the EEG contains multiple bursts of generalized spikes in the background. In contrast to occasional temporal lobe spikes, this pattern confirms a diagnosis of epilepsy in patients with seizures. (From Kaufman DM et al: *Kaufman's clinical neurology for psychiatrists*, ed 8, Philadelphia, 2017, Elsevier.)

seizure, such as climbing ladders, swimming unsupervised, or taking baths (rather than showers).

- No driving until seizure-free in accordance with local laws and regulations.

REFERRAL

Patients with epilepsy and seizures should be referred for a consultation by a neurologist.

PEARLS & CONSIDERATIONS

COMMENTS

- It is crucial to understand that tonic clonic seizures can occur in variety of acute neurologic diseases.
- Successful treatment depends on the correct choice of antiepileptic drugs based on the type (focal onset versus generalized onset) and etiology of the seizures.
- All women of childbearing age taking antiepileptic drugs should take folic acid supplementation (1 to 4 mg/day) for the prevention of neural tube defects.
- Many antiepileptic drugs also affect vitamin D absorption or metabolism, prompting attention to patients' bone health.

PREVENTION

Sleep deprivation and alcohol consumption should be avoided.

PATIENT & FAMILY EDUCATION

Patients with ongoing seizures are forbidden to drive; check your state regulations and laws regarding driving and epilepsy.

SUGGESTED READING

Available at ExpertConsult.com

RELATED CONTENT

Generalized Tonic-Clonic Seizures (Patient Information)
Status Epilepticus (Related Key Topic)

AUTHOR: **Corey Goldsmith, MD**

BASIC INFORMATION

DEFINITION

Sepsis is an exaggerated inflammatory response to an infectious stimulus. It is usually caused by generalized bacterial or fungal infection and characterized by evidence of infection, fever or hypothermia, hypotension, and evidence of end-organ compromise. The Sepsis Definitions Task Force in 2016 updated definitions for sepsis and septic shock (Table 1). A major change in the definitions is the elimination of mention of SIRS*. According to the new definitions, sepsis is now defined as evidence of infection plus life-threatening organ dysfunction, clinically codified by an acute change in 2 points or greater in the SOFA score (Table 2). The new clinical criteria for septic shock include sepsis with fluid, unresponsive hypotension, serum lactate level greater than 2 mmol/L, and the need for vasopressors to maintain mean arterial pressure of 65 mm Hg or greater.[1,2]

SYNONYMS

Septicemia
Sepsis syndrome
Severe sepsis
Systemic inflammatory response syndrome
Septic shock

*SIRS (Systemic Inflammatory Response Syndrome): Variables in SIRS criteria include respiratory rate (breaths/min), white blood cell count (109/L), hands (%), heart rate (beats/min), temperature (°C), and arterial carbon dioxide tension (mm Hg). Score range is 0 to 4.

[1]Abraham E: New definitions for sepsis and septic shock: continuing evolution but with much still to be done, *JAMA* 315(8):757-759, 2016.

[2]Shankar-Hari M et al: Developing a new definition and assessing new clinical criteria for septic shock: for the Third International Consensus Definitions for Sepsis and Septic Shock (Sepsis-3), *JAMA* 315(8):775-787, 2016.

ICD-10CM CODES

A41.9	Sepsis, unspecified organism
A41.50	Gram-negative sepsis, unspecified
A41.2	Sepsis due to unspecified *Staphylococcus*
A41.4	Sepsis due to anaerobes
A41.51	Sepsis due to *Escherichia coli* [E. coli]
A41.52	Sepsis due to Pseudomonas
A54.86	Gonococcal sepsis
B37.7	Candidal sepsis
A32.7	Listerial sepsis
A40.0	Sepsis due to streptococcus, group A
A40.1	Sepsis due to streptococcus, group B
A40.3	Sepsis due to Streptococcus pneumoniae
A40.8	Other streptococcal sepsis
A40.9	Streptococcal sepsis, unspecified
A41.01	Sepsis due to Methicillin susceptible *Staphylococcus aureus*
A41.02	Sepsis due to Methicillin resistant *Staphylococcus aureus*

EPIDEMIOLOGY & DEMOGRAPHICS

INCIDENCE (IN U.S.):
- Sepsis occurs in 6% of hospitalized patients; approximately half require ICU admission.
- More than 1 million cases of sepsis occur each year in the U.S. 15% of sepsis patients die in the hospital; 6% are discharged to hospice.

PREDOMINANT SEX: Males are slightly more commonly affected than females.

PREDOMINANT AGE:
- Neonatal period.
- Patients >65 yr of age account for 60% of all cases of sepsis.

GENETICS:
- Familial disposition: A great variety of congenital immunodeficiency states and other inherited disorders may predispose to septicemia.
- Neonatal infection: Incidence is high in neonatal period.

PHYSICAL FINDINGS & CLINICAL PRESENTATION

- Fever or hypothermia
- Hypotension
- Tachycardia
- Tachypnea
- Altered mental status
- Bleeding diathesis
- Skin rashes
- Symptoms that reflect primary site of infection: Urinary tract, GI tract, CNS, respiratory tract
- Table 3 describes some clinical signs and symptoms of sepsis

ETIOLOGY

- Disseminated infection with a great variety of bacteria:
  1. Gram-negative bacteria:
     a. *Escherichia coli*
     b. *Klebsiella spp.*
     c. *Pseudomonas aeruginosa*
     d. *Proteus spp.*
     e. *Neisseria meningitides*
  2. Gram-positive bacteria:
     a. *Staphylococcus aureus (including MRSA)*
     b. *Streptococcus spp.*
     c. *Enterococcus spp.*
- Less common infections:
  1. Fungal
  2. Viral
  3. Rickettsial
  4. Parasitic
- Sepsis is a complex dysregulation of both inflammation and coagulation (Fig. E1). There is activation of coagulation, inflammatory cytokines, complement, and kinin cascades with release of a variety of vasoactive endogenous mediators. The innate immune system recognizes pathogens by means of pattern-recognition receptors (toll-like receptors [TLRs], Table 4). TLRs bind to structures on microorganisms and,

TABLE 1 Proposed New Definitions of Sepsis

Term	Definition	Criteria	Notes
Sepsis[a] (previously severe sepsis)	Life-threatening organ dysfunction caused by a dysregulated host response to infection	Organ dysfunction is identified as an acute change in the SOFA score, ≥2 points from the baseline consequent to the infection.	qSOFA (quick Sequential Organ Failure Assessment) Prolonged ICU stay or in-hospital mortality can be identified at the bedside with qSOFA. 1. Respiratory rate ≥22 breaths/min 2. Acute mental status change 3. Systolic blood pressure ≤100 mm Hg An increase in SOFA of ≥2 predicts a 10% mortality in the general hospital population. Presume a baseline SOFA of 0 unless the patient has known (acute or chronic) organ dysfunction before the onset of infection.
Septic shock	It is a subset of sepsis in which the underlying circulatory and cellular/metabolic abnormalities are profound enough to substantially increase mortality.	A clinical construct of sepsis with persisting hypotension requiring vasopressors to maintain MAP ≥65 mm Hg and having a serum lactate level ≥2 mmol/L despite adequate volume resuscitation	Septic shock portends hospital mortality in excess of 40%.

MAP, Mean arterial pressure.
[a]Note that the proposed new definitions abandon the previous term "severe sepsis" to describe infection-induced organ dysfunction and now use "sepsis" in its place. The previous condition called "sepsis" is now just called "infection," and when infection is not associated with organ dysfunction, there is no differentiation between infection with or without systemic manifestations.
From Parrillo JE, Dellinger RP: *Critical care medicine, principles of diagnosis and management in the adult,* ed 5, Philadelphia, 2019, Elsevier.

TABLE 2 The Sequential Organ Failure Assessment (SOFA) Score

Score	0	1	2	3	4
Respiration					
PaO_2/FiO_2, mm Hg	>400	≤400	≤300	≤200 With respiratory support	≤100
Coagulation					
Platelets × $10^3/mm^3$	>150	≤150	≤100	≤50	≤20
Liver					
Bilirubin, mg/dl (μmol/L)	<1.2 (<20)	1.2-1.9 (20-32)	2.0-5.9 (33-101)	6.0-11.9 (102-204)	>12.0 (>204)
Cardiovascular					
Hypotension	No hypotension	MAP <70 mm Hg	Dopamine ≤5 or dobutamine (any dose)*	Dopamine >5 or epinephrine ≤0.1 or norepinephrine ≤0.1*	Dopamine >15 or epinephrine >0.1 or norepinephrine >0.1*
Central Nervous System					
Glasgow coma score	15	13-14	10-12	6-9	<6
Renal					
Creatinine, mg/dl (μmol/L) OR urine output	<1.2 (<110)	1.2-1.9 (110- 170)	2.0-3.4 (171-299)	3.5-4.9 (300-440) <500 ml/d	>5.0 (>440) <200 ml/d

*Adrenergic agents administered for at least 1 hour (doses given are in mcg/kg per min).
From Ronco C et al: *Critical care nephrology,* ed 3, Philadelphia, 2019, Elsevier.

TABLE 3 Clinical Signs and Symptoms of Sepsis

Infection	General	Inflammatory	Hemodynamic	Tissue Perfusion
Documented or suspected	Temperature >38° C (100.4° F) or <36° C (96.8° F) Heart rate >90 beats/min Respiratory rate ≥20 breaths/min Altered mental status Hyperglycemia Third spacing of fluid	WBC count <4000 or >12,000 cells/μL or ≥10% bands	Hypotension: Systolic blood pressure <90 mm Hg MAP <70 mm Hg SVo_2 >70 CI >3.5 L/min/m²	Hypoxemia: (Pao_2/Fio_2 <300) Acute oliguria (urine output <0.5 ml/kg/hr) Coagulopathy Abnormal liver function tests Platelet count <100,000 cells/μL Lactic acidosis Skin mottling

CI, Cardiac index; *MAP,* mean arterial pressure; *SVo_2,* mixed venous oxygen saturation; *WBC,* white blood cell.
From Cameron JL, Cameron AM: *Current surgical therapy,* ed 10, Philadelphia, 2011, Saunders.

based on the composite information gained, generate a tailored response to the invading pathogen.
- Predisposing host factors:
  1. General medical condition
  2. Extremes of age
  3. Immunosuppressive therapy
  4. Recent surgery
  5. Granulocytopenia
  6. Hyposplenism
  7. Diabetes
  8. Instrumentation

Dx DIAGNOSIS

DIFFERENTIAL DIAGNOSIS

- Cardiogenic shock
- Acute pancreatitis
- Pulmonary embolism
- Systemic vasculitis
- Toxic ingestion
- Exposure-induced hypothermia
- Fulminant hepatic failure
- Collagen-vascular diseases

WORKUP

- Evaluation should focus on identifying a specific pathogen and localizing the site of primary infection. Box 1 summarizes a general approach to shock.
- Hemodynamic, metabolic, coagulation disorders should be carefully characterized.
- Intensive monitoring.

LABORATORY TESTS

- Cultures of blood and examination and culture of sputum, urine, wound drainage, stool, and CSF, depending on the presenting signs and symptoms for each patient
- CBC with differential, coagulation profile
- Routine chemistries, LFTs
- ABGs, lactic acid level
- Procalcitonin can be useful as a serum marker of bacterial infection as a cause of the sepsis, and has been shown to improve survival and facilitate earlier discontinuation of antibiotics
- Urinalysis

IMAGING STUDIES

- Chest x-ray
- Other radiographic and radioisotope procedures according to suspected site of primary infection

Rx TREATMENT

NONPHARMACOLOGIC THERAPY

- Tissue oxygenation: Mixed venous oxygen saturation maintained >70% if possible; early mechanical ventilation with low tidal volume (6 ml/kg predicted body weight) to protect lung parenchyma from overstretching and "volutrauma." Recommended plateau pressure for sepsis-related ARDS is ≤30 cm H_2O.
- Focal infection should be drained if possible, and potentially infected catheters should be removed.

ACUTE GENERAL Rx

- Blood pressure support, rapid IV fluid resuscitation and vasopressors (Table 5), if needed, with the goal of reestablishing a mean arterial blood pressure >65 mm Hg; reduction in blood lactate and improved mixed venous oxygen saturation >70% within 6 hr of recognition of septic shock is associated with improved survival. If possible, measure vena cava oxygen saturation ($ScvO_2$) to assess adequacy of resuscitation. If the $ScvO_2$ is <70%, consider packed red blood cell transfusion to achieve Hct >30%. Start inotropic agents if $ScvO_2$ is <70% despite transfusion and adequate fluid resuscitation.
  1. IV hydration; patients receiving balanced crystalloids as resuscitation fluids. appear to have a lower 30-day mortality compared with patients who received saline (26% versus 31%) in a recent trial. Use the fluid challenge technique to evaluate the effect (and safety) of fluid

TABLE 4 Toll-Like Receptors

Toll-Like Receptor	Pathogen or Disease State
TLR1	Lyme disease
	Neisseria meningitidis
TLR2	*Mycobacterium tuberculosis*
	Chagas disease
	Leptospirosis
	Fungal sepsis
	CMV viremia
TLR3	Many
TLR4	Gram-negative bacteria
	Septic shock
	Chlamydia trachomatis
	Chlamydia pneumoniae
	Certain viruses
	Mycobacterium tuberculosis
TLR5	Flagellated bacteria (e.g., *Salmonella*)
TLR7	Viral infections
TLR8	Viral infections
TLR9	Bacterial and viral infections
TLR10	Unknown

CMV, Cytomegalovirus; *TLR*, toll-like receptor.
From Parrillo JE, Dellinger RP: *Critical care medicine, principles of diagnosis and management in the adult,* ed 5, Philadelphia, 2019, Elsevier.

BOX 1 General Approach to Shock: Initial Diagnosis and Evaluation

Clinical (primary diagnosis)
- Tachycardia, hypotension (systolic blood pressure <90 mm Hg) tachypnea, oliguria, encephalopathy (confusion), peripheral hypoperfusion (mottled extremities), cyanosis

Laboratory (confirmatory)
- Hemoglobin, WBC, platelets

Prothrombin time/partial thromboplastin time
- Electrolytes, arterial blood gases, Ca, Mg, BUN, creatinine, serum lactate
- ECG

Monitoring (continuous ECG and respiratory monitors)
- Pulse oximetry
- Urinary catheter (urine output)
- Point-of-care ultrasonography (heart, lung, abdominal, and major vessels)
- Arterial pressure catheter
- Central venous pressure monitor (uncomplicated shock)
- Pulmonary artery flotation catheter
  - Cardiac output
  - Pulmonary artery occlusion pressure
  - Central and/or mixed venous oxygen saturation (intermittent or continuous)
- Oximetry[a]

Imaging (chest x-ray)
- X-ray views of abdomena
- Computed tomographic scan: Abdomen or chest[a]
- Formal transthoracic and/or transesophageal echocardiogram[a]

BUN, Blood urea nitrogen; *Ca*, calcium; *ECG*, electrocardiogram; *Mg*, magnesium; *WBC*, white blood cell.
[a]Optional.
From Parrillo JE, Dellinger RP: *Critical care medicine, principles of diagnosis and management in the adult,* ed 5, Philadelphia, 2019, Elsevier.

TABLE 5 Relative Potency of Intravenously Administered Vasopressors/Inotropes Used in Shock[a]

		Cardiac		Peripheral Vasculature			
Drug	**Dose**	**Heart Rate**	**Contractility**	**Vasoconstriction**	**Vasodilation**	**Dopaminergic**	**Typical Clinical Use**
Dopamine	1-4 μg/kg/min	1+	1-2+	0	1+	4+	All shock
	5-10 μg/kg/min	2+	2+	1-2+	1+	4+	
	11-20 μg/kg/min	2+	2+	2-3+	1+	4+	
Norepinephrine	0.01-0.3 μg/kg/min	2+	2+	4+	0	0	Refractory shock
Dobutamine	1-20 μg/kg/min	1-2+	3+	1+	2+	0	CHF; cardiogenic, obstructive and septic shock
Dopexamine[b]	0.5-6 μg/kg/min	2+	1+	0	3-4+	4+	CHF; cardiogenic shock
Epinephrine	0.05-0.2 μg/kg/min	4+	4+	4+	3+	0	Refractory or anaphylactic shock
Phenylephrine	0.1-1 μg/kg/min	0	1+	4+	0	0	Neurogenic or septic shock
Isoproterenol	1-8 μg/min	4+	4+	0	4+	0	Cardiogenic shock (bradyarrhythmia), torsades de pointes, ventricular tachycardia
Vasopressin	0.02-0.04 U/min	0	0	4+	0	0	Vasodilatory (e.g., septic) shock
Milrinone	37.5-75 μg/kg bolus over 10 min; 0.375-0.75 μg/kg/min infusion	1+	3+	0	2+	0	CHF; cardiogenic shock

CHF, Congestive heart failure.
[a]The 1 to 4+ scoring system represents an arbitrary quantitation of the comparative potency of different vasopressors/inotropes.
[b]Not clinically released in the U.S.
From Parrillo JE, Dellinger RP: *Critical care medicine, principles of diagnosis and management in the adult,* ed 5, Philadelphia, 2019, Elsevier.

administration. For sepsis-induced hypoperfusion, give 30 ml/kg of IV crystalloids within 3 hr, with additional fluid based on frequent reassessment using dynamic variables (e.g., passive leg raise test or pulse or stroke volume variations induced by mechanical ventilation) rather than previous guidelines using target-specific values of central venous pressure. Fluid administration should be discontinued when the response to fluids is no longer beneficial. Most patients need 4 to 6 L of fluid in the first 6 hr. Trials have shown that resuscitation with balanced crystalloids or albumin compared with other fluids seems to be associated with reduced mortality, and that albumin replacement in addition to crystalloids alone does not improve the rate of survival at 28 and 90 days.

2. Therapy with vasopressors if mean arterial blood pressure of >65 mm Hg cannot be maintained by hydration alone. Use norepinephrine as a first-choice vasopressor and target a mean arterial pressure (MAP) of 65 mm Hg.

- Correction of acidosis by improving the tissue perfusion, not by giving bicarbonate. Mechanical ventilation as needed.

TABLE 6 Empirical Antibiotic Options for Patients with Severe Sepsis or Septic Shock

	Suspected Source				
	Lung	**Abdomen**	**Skin/Soft Tissue**	**Urinary Tract**	**Source Uncertain**
Major Community-Acquired Pathogens	*Streptococcus pneumoniae* *Haemophilus influenzae* *Legionella* *Chlamydia pneumoniae*	*Escherichia coli* *Bacteroides fragilis*	*Streptococcus pyogenes* *Staphylococcus aureus* Polymicrobial	*E. coli* *Klebsiella* species *Enterobacter* species *Proteus* spp. *Enterococci*	
Empirical Antibiotic Therapy	Moxifloxacin *or* levofloxacin *or* azithromycin *plus* cefotaxime *or* ceftazidime *or* cefepime *or* piperacillin-tazobactam	Imipenem *or* meropenem *or* doripenem *or* Piperacillin-tazobactam ± aminoglycoside If biliary source: Piperacillin-tazobactam, ampicillin-sulbactam, *or* ceftriaxone with metronidazole	Vancomycin *or* daptomycin *plus either* imipenem *or* meropenem *or* piperacillin-tazobactam; ± clindamycin (see text)	Ciprofloxacin *or* levofloxacin (if gram-positive cocci, use ampicillin *or* vancomycin ± gentamicin)	Vancomycin *plus either* doripenem *or* ertapenem *or* imipenem *or* meropenem
Major Commensal or Nosocomial Microorganisms	Aerobic gram-negative bacilli	Aerobic gram-negative rods Anaerobes *Candida* spp.	*Staphylococcus aureus* (? MRSA) Aerobic gram-negative rods	Aerobic gram-negative rods *Enterococci*	Consider MDRO if in area of high prevalence. Consider echinocandin if neutropenic or indwelling intravascular catheter
Empirical Antibiotic Therapy	Imipenem *or* meropenem *or* doripenem *or* cefepime (if *Acinetobacter baumannii* or carbapenem-resistant *Klebsiella* in ICU, add colistin)	Imipenem *or* meropenem ± aminoglycoside (consider echinocandin)	Vancomycin *or* daptomycin *plus* imipenem-cilastatin *or* meropenem *or* cefepime, ± clindamycin	Vancomycin *plus* imipenem *or* meropenem *or* cefepime	Cefepime *plus* vancomycin ± caspofungin

Dosages for intravenous administration (normal renal function):
- Imipenem-cilastatin, 0.5-1.0 g q6-8h
- Meropenem, 1-2 g q8h
- Doripenem, 0.5 g q8h
- Piperacillin-tazobactam, 3.375 g q4h or 4.5 g q6h
- Vancomycin, load 25-30 mg/kg, then 15-20 mg/kg q8-12h
- Cefepime, 1-2 g q8h
- Levofloxacin, 750 mg q24h
- Ciprofloxacin, 400 mg q8-12hr
- Moxifloxacin, 400 mg qd
- Ceftriaxone, 2 g q24h
- Caspofungin, 70 mg, followed by 50 mg q24h
- Colistin: loading dose = 5 mg/kg body weight

ICU, Intensive care unit; *MDRO*, multidrug-resistant organisms; *MRSA*, methicillin-resistant *Staphylococcus aureus*.
For MDRO, resistance usually includes carbapenems. Carbapenems are less susceptible to extended-spectrum β-lactamases; base choice on local resistance pattern.
From Bennett JE et al: *Mandell, Douglas, and Bennett's principles and practice of infectious diseases,* ed 8, Philadelphia, 2015, Saunders.

- Antibiotics:
  1. Directed at the most likely sources of infection. Table 6 describes initial antibiotic recommendations for septic patients.
  2. Should generally provide broad coverage of gram-positive and gram-negative bacteria (or fungi if clinically indicated).
  3. Antibiotics should be administered within 1 hr of the diagnosis of septic shock—this is a medical emergency.
- The role of corticosteroids in the acute management of septicemia has long been debated. Previous trials had shown that corticosteroid therapy improved hemodynamic outcomes in patients with severe septic shock. Patients with relative adrenal insufficiency may benefit from low-dose therapy with hydrocortisone (200 mg IV by continuous infusion for 7 days). Recent trials, however, revealed that hydrocortisone did not improve survival or reversal of shock, either overall or in patients who did not have a response to corticotropin, although hydrocortisone hastened reversal of shock in patients in whom shock was reversed. Until definitive data are available, the decision to administer corticosteroids for septic shock should be based on the individual patient's severity of illness versus risk of corticosteroid administration. Current evidence and guidelines support limiting the use of IV hydrocortisone for patients with septic shock to these instances with fluid resuscitation and vasopressor therapy are inadequate to restore hemodynamic stability.[3] A recent meta-analysis revealed that although 28-day mortality is lower with corticosteroids in adult patients with sepsis, that effect does not persist at 90 days.[4] The corticotropin (ACTH) stimulation test is not helpful and should not be used to determine the need for corticosteroid in these patients. During the COVID 19 pandemic, the RECOVERY trial provided evidence that treatment with dexamethasone in hospitalized patients at a dose of 6 mg once

[3]Yende S, Thompson T: Evaluating glucocorticoids for sepsis. Time to change course, *JAMA* 316(17):1769-1770, 2016.
[4]Fang F et al: Association of corticosteroid treatment with outcomes in adult patients with sepsis: a systematic review and meta-analysis, *JAMA Intern Med* 179(2):213-223, 2019.

a day (IV or oral) for up to 10 days reduced 28-day mortality in patients with COVID 19.

- Blood transfusion: A lower hemoglobin threshold is preferred. Trials have shown that among patients with septic shock, mortality at 90 days and rates of ischemic events and use of life support is similar among those assigned to blood transfusion at a higher hemoglobin threshold (hemoglobin level of 9 g/dl or less) and those assigned to blood transfusion at a lower threshold (hemoglobin level of 7 g/dl or less).

CHRONIC Rx

- Adjust antibiotic therapy on the basis of culture results.
- In general, continue antibiotic therapy for a minimum of 7 to 10 days.
- Infection source control (e.g., removal of catheter/device suspected to be infected).
- If hyperglycemia develops during treatment, start continuous insulin IV infusion, maintain blood glucose in the 110 to 180 mg/dl level, and avoid insulin-induced hypoglycemia.

DISPOSITION

- All patients with sepsis should be hospitalized and given access to intensive monitoring and nursing care.
- Among adults with suspected infection admitted to an ICU, an increase in SOFA score of 2 or more has greater prognostic accuracy for in-hospital mortality than SIRS criteria or the qSOFA score (quick SOFA).[5] The qSOFA can be done at bedside and consists of increased respiratory rate ≥22/min, altered mentation and systolic BP ≤100 mm Hg with each allocated 1 point.

REFERRAL

- To infectious diseases expert
- To physician experienced in critical care

PEARLS & CONSIDERATIONS

COMMENTS

- Mortality rises quickly if antibiotic therapy is not instituted promptly (preferably within 1 hr of onset of shock) and metabolic derangements are not treated aggressively.
- The Surviving Sepsis Campaign hour-1 bundle 2018 update recommends: Measure lactate level. Re-measure if initial lactate is >2 mmol/L. [weak recommendation, low quality of evidence] Obtain blood cultures prior to administration of antibiotics. [best practice statement] Administer broad spectrum antibiotics. [strong recommendation, moderate quality of evidence] Rapidly administer 30 ml/kg crystalloid for hypotension or lactate ≥4 mmol/L [strong recommendation, low quality of evidence] and apply vasopressors if patient is hypotensive during or after fluid resuscitation to maintain MAP ≥65 mm Hg. [strong recommendation, moderate quality of evidence]
- Recent trials have shown that early, goal-directed therapy (EGDT) does not result in better outcomes than usual care and is associated with higher hospitalization costs across a broad range of patient and hospital characteristics.[6]
- A recent trial (ACTS Randomized Clinical Trial) in which patients with septic shock were given the combination of ascorbic acid, corticosteroids, and thiamine did not show significant reduction in SOFA score in first 72 hr and thus this combination should not be used in septic shock.

SUGGESTED READINGS

Available at ExpertConsult.com

AUTHORS: **Glenn G. Fort, MD, MPH,** and **Fred F. Ferri, MD**

[5]Raith EP et al: Prognostic accuracy of the SOFA score, SIRS criteria, and qSOFA score for in-hospital mortality among adults with suspected infection admitted to the intensive care unit, *JAMA* 310(3):290 -300, 2016.

[6]The PRISM Investigators: Early, goal-directed therapy for septic shock–a patient-level meta-analysis, *N Engl J Med* 376:2223-2234, 2017.

BASIC INFORMATION

DEFINITION

Septic arthritis is a highly destructive form of joint disease most often caused by hematogenous spread of organisms from a distant site of infection. Direct penetration of the joint as a result of trauma or surgery and spread from adjacent osteomyelitis may also cause bacterial arthritis. Any joint in the body may be affected.

SYNONYMS

Infectious arthritis
Bacterial arthritis
Pyogenic arthritis

ICD-10CM CODE
M00.9 Pyogenic arthritis, unspecified

EPIDEMIOLOGY & DEMOGRAPHICS

INCIDENCE (IN U.S.): Between 2 and 6 cases per 100,000 people per yr
PREVALENCE (IN U.S.): Unknown
PREDOMINANT SEX: Gonococcal arthritis in females
PREDOMINANT AGE: Gonococcal arthritis in sexually active adults
PEAK INCIDENCE:
- Gonococcal arthritis: Young adults
- Other bacterial causes: All ages

PHYSICAL FINDINGS & CLINICAL PRESENTATION

- Hallmark: Acute onset of monoarticular joint pain, erythema, heat, and immobility
- Limited range of motion of the joint
- Effusion, with varying degrees of erythema and increased warmth around the joint
- Single joint affected in 80% to 90% of cases of nongonococcal arthritis
- Gonococcal dermatitis-arthritis syndrome:
  1. Typical pattern is a migratory polyarthritis or tenosynovitis
  2. Small pustules on the trunk or extremities
- Febrile patient at presentation
- Most commonly affected joints in adult: Knee and hip, but any joint may be involved; in children—hip

ETIOLOGY

- Bacteria spread from another locus of infection.
  1. Highly vascular synovium is invaded by hematogenously spread bacteria.
  2. WBC enzymes cause necrosis of synovium, cartilage, and bone.
  3. Extensive joint destruction is rapid if infection is not treated with appropriate IV antibiotics and drainage of necrotic material.
- Predisposing factors: Rheumatoid arthritis, prosthetic joints, advanced age, immunodeficiency (HIV, DM, immunosuppressive drugs), gout, sexual activity (gonococcal arthritis), skin infections, cutaneous ulcers (contiguous spread), recent joint surgery, recent intraarticular infection. Fig. E1 illustrates routes by which bacteria can reach the joint.
- The most common nongonococcal organisms are staphylococci (40%), streptococci (28%), and gram-negative bacilli (19%). Less common are mycobacteria (8%), gram-negative cocci (3%), anaerobes (1%), and gram-positive bacilli (1%).
- Staphylococci (*S. aureus* and coagulase-negative staphylococcal species) account for >50% of prosthetic-hip and prosthetic-knee infections. *S. aureus* is very common in patients with rheumatoid arthritis.

DIAGNOSIS

DIFFERENTIAL DIAGNOSIS

- Gout
- Pseudogout
- Trauma
- Hemarthrosis
- Rheumatic fever
- Adult or juvenile rheumatoid arthritis
- Spondyloarthropathies such as reactive arthritis (Reiter syndrome)
- Osteomyelitis
- Viral arthritides
- Septic bursitis
- Lyme disease caused by *Borrelia burgdorferi*

WORKUP

- Joint aspiration, Gram stain, and culture of the synovial fluid. Fig. 2 describes an algorithm for synovial fluid analysis in septic arthritis.
- Immediate arthrocentesis before other studies are undertaken or antibiotics instituted. Synovial fluid should be evaluated at bedside and then sent for lab evaluation.

LABORATORY TESTS

- Joint fluid analysis:
  1. Synovial fluid leukocyte count is usually elevated >50,000 cells/mm^3 with >80% polymorphonuclear cells.
  2. Counts are highly variable, with similar findings in gout, pseudogout, or rheumatoid arthritis. Lower WBC counts can occur in joint replacement, disseminated gonococcal disease, and peripheral leukopenia.
  3. Synovial fluid glucose or protein is not helpful because results are not specific for septic arthritis. The differential diagnosis of synovial fluid abnormalities is described in Section IV.
  4. PCR testing: Useful for detection of uncommon organisms (e.g., Lyme disease).
  5. Crystal analysis: Septic arthritis can coexist with crystal arthropathy; therefore, the presence of crystals does not preclude a diagnosis of septic arthritis.
- Blood cultures: Positive in 25% to 50% of patients with septic arthritis.
- Culture of possible extraarticular sources of infection.
- Elevated peripheral WBC count, ESR (nonspecific), C-reactive protein (CRP) (nonspecific). When elevated, ESR and CRP may be useful to monitor therapeutic response.
- If gonococcus is suspected, perform nucleic acid amplification tests (NAATs) on synovial fluid.

IMAGING STUDIES

- Radiograph of the affected joint (Fig. E3): Useful to rule out osteomyelitis, fractures, chondrocalcinosis, or inflammatory arthritis
- MRI: Findings that suggest an acute intraarticular infection include the combination of bony erosions with marrow edema
- CT scan: Useful for early diagnosis of infections of the spine, hips, and sternoclavicular and sacroiliac joints
- Ultrasound: Can be useful for detecting effusions in joints that are more difficult to examine (e.g., hip)

TREATMENT

NONPHARMACOLOGIC THERAPY

- Affected joints aspirated daily to remove necrotic material and to follow serial WBC counts and cultures
- If no resolution with IV antibiotics and closed drainage: Open debridement and lavage, particularly in nongonococcal infections
- Prevention of contractures:
  1. After acute stage of inflammation, range-of-motion exercises of the affected joint
  2. Physical therapy helpful

ACUTE GENERAL Rx

- IV antibiotics immediately after joint aspiration and Gram stain of the synovial fluid. Empiric antibiotic therapy (Table E1) is based on organism found on Gram stain of synovial fluid:
  1. Gram-positive cocci: Vancomycin: 15 to 20 mg/kg IV q8 to 12h. Keep trough levels at 15 to 20 mcg/ml. Alternatives include daptomycin and linezolid
  2. Gram-negative cocci: Ceftriaxone: 1 to 2 g IV q day in adults (children: 50-100 mg/kg IV q day). Alternative includes cefotaxime
  3. Gram-negative rods: Ceftriaxone, cefepime: 1 to 2 g IV q8 to 12h in adults (children: 100-150 mg/kg/day divided in q8h dosing), piperacillin-tazobactam: 3.375 g IV to 4.5 g IV q6h. Aztreonam or fluoroquinolones can be used in patients with allergy to penicillin or cephalosporins
  4. Negative Gram stain: Vancomycin plus either cefepime or a carbapenem such as meropenem: 1 g IV q8h in adults (children: 60 mg/kg/day divided in q8h dosing) or ertapenem
- The optimal duration of antibiotic use in septic arthritis has traditionally been 3 to 6 wk usually following surgical drainage. Recent trials (Gjika et al, *Ann Rheum Dis* Aug 2019, 78: 1114) support a 2-wk course in conjunction with surgery.

SUGGESTED READINGS
Available at ExpertConsult.com

RELATED CONTENT

Septic Arthritis (Patient Information)

AUTHOR: **Glenn G. Fort, MD, MPH**

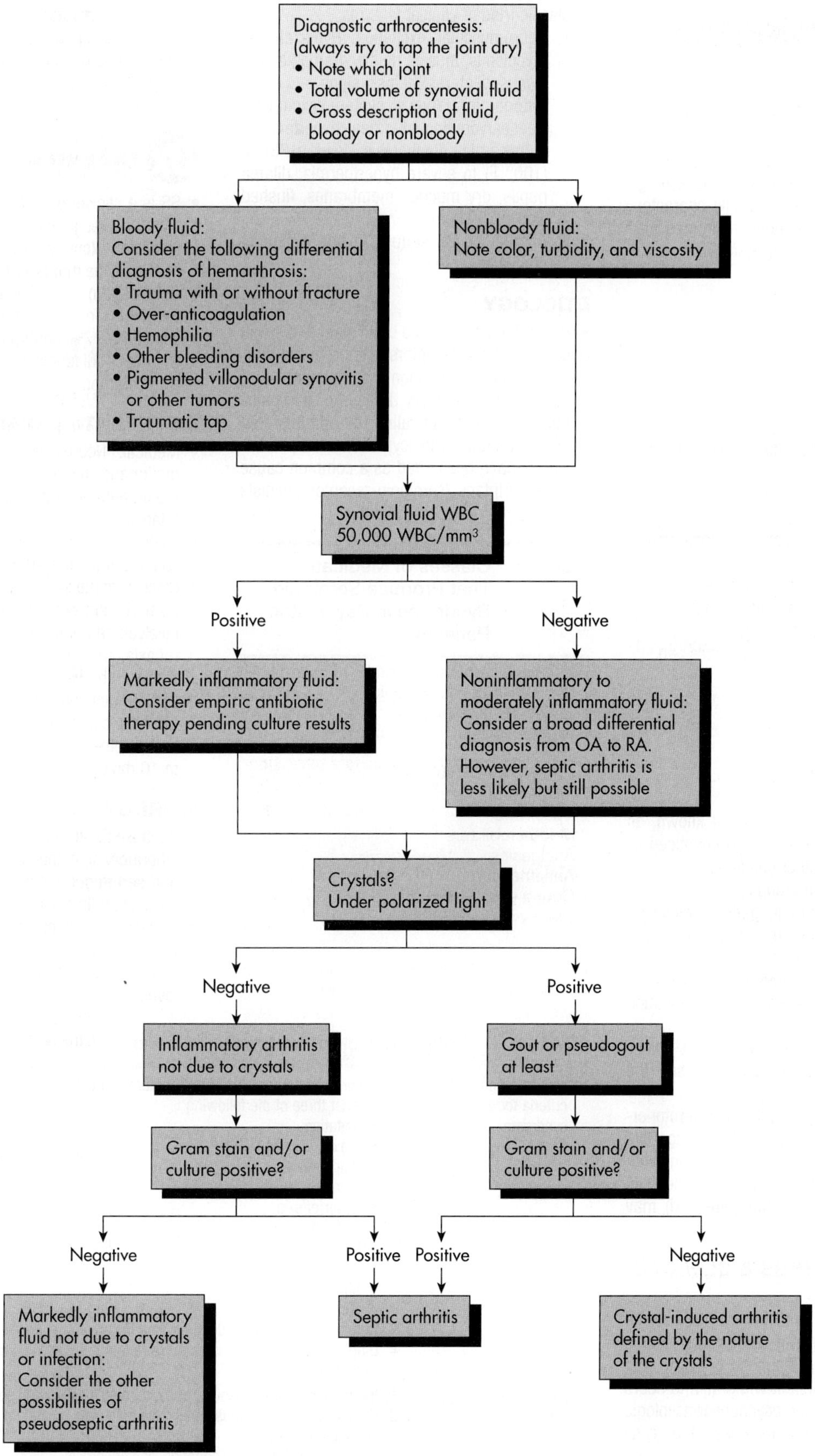

FIG. 2 Algorithm for synovial fluid analysis in septic arthritis. *OA,* Osteoarthritis; *RA,* rheumatoid arthritis; *WBC,* white blood cell count. (From Harris ED et al: *Kelley's textbook of rheumatology,* ed 7, Philadelphia, 2005, Saunders.)

Serotonin Syndrome

BASIC INFORMATION

DEFINITION

Serotonin syndrome (SS) is a potentially life-threatening condition resulting from excessive serotonergic stimulation of 5-HT_{1A} and 5-HT_{2A} receptors in the CNS and PNS. SS is a drug-induced disorder that is classically characterized by mental status changes, neuromuscular hyperactivity, and autonomic dysfunction.

SYNONYMS

SS
Hyperserotonemia
Serotonergic syndrome
Serotonin toxicity

ICD-10CM CODES

Y49	Adverse effects due to psychotropic drugs
Y49.0	Adverse effects due to tricyclic and tetracyclic antidepressants
Y49.1	Adverse effects due to monoamino-oxidase-inhibitor antidepressants
Y49.2	Adverse effects due to other and unspecified antidepressants
Y49.3	Adverse effects due to phenothiazine antipsychotics and neuroleptics
G25.89	Other specified extrapyramidal and movement disorders

EPIDEMIOLOGY & DEMOGRAPHICS

- The true incidence of SS is not known, as clinical manifestations may go unnoticed or be attributed to another condition.
- SS is seen in all age groups.
- SS classically occurs in patients receiving two or more serotonergic drugs, but it can also occur with monotherapy
- Selective serotonin reuptake inhibitor (SSRI) is the most commonly implicated medication associated with SS.
- Concomitant use of an SSRI with a monoamine oxidase inhibitor (MAOI) poses the greatest risk of developing SS.
- Combination of SSRIs with other serotonergic drugs (e.g., tryptophan, illicit drugs like cocaine and MDMA, "Ecstasy") or drugs with serotonergic properties (e.g., methylene blue, lithium, meperidine, triptans, linezolid) may also lead to SS.

PHYSICAL FINDINGS & CLINICAL PRESENTATION

- Findings of clonus with hyperreflexia in the setting of recent use of serotonergic agents strongly suggest the diagnosis of SS.
- Symptoms can manifest within min to hours after starting a new psychopharmacologic treatment, increasing the dose of a serotonergic drug, or administering a second serotonergic drug. Nearly all patients develop symptoms within 24 hours of exposure.
- Clonus (inducible, spontaneous, and ocular) is the key finding in establishing a diagnosis of SS.
- Classic triad of clinical features:
  1. Neuromuscular excitation: Hyperreflexia, myoclonus, muscle rigidity, tremor, ocular clonus, bilateral Babinski signs
  2. Autonomic nervous system excitation: Nausea/vomiting, diarrhea, hypertension, tachycardia, diaphoresis, fever >38° C (100° F) to severe hyperthermia, dilated pupils, dry mucous membranes, flushed skin
  3. Altered mental status: Anxiety, agitation, confusion, coma

ETIOLOGY

- Hyperstimulation of the brain stem and spinal cord serotonin receptors leading to the neuromuscular and autonomic symptoms.
- Psychopharmacologic drugs—in particular, fluoxetine and sertraline co-administered with MAOI (e.g., tranylcypromine and phenelzine)—have been cited as a common cause of SS. Triptans (serotonin-receptor agonists used in the treatment of migraines) may also precipitate the SS when used in combination with SSRIs and serotonin-norepinephrine reuptake inhibitors (SNRIs). Box 1 describes classes of medications that produce SS.

BOX 1 Classes of Medications That Produce Serotonin Syndrome in Psychiatric Patients

Selective serotonin reuptake inhibitors
Monoamine oxidase inhibitors
Atypical antipsychotics
Heterocyclic antidepressants
Trazodone
Dual-uptake inhibitors
Psychostimulants
Buspirone
Mood stabilizers
Analgesics
Antiemetics
Cough suppressants
Dietary supplements
Linezolid

From Goldman L, Schafer AI: *Goldman-Cecil medicine*, ed 24, Philadelphia, 2012, Saunders.

DIAGNOSIS

- SS is a clinical diagnosis. There are no specific laboratory tests for SS. A high index of suspicion along with a detailed medication history is the mainstay of diagnosis.
- Diagnostic criteria: Most accurate is Hunter Serotonin Toxicity Criteria (sensitivity 84%, specificity 97%, confirmation by toxicologist). Sternbach diagnostic criteria (Table 1) are also commonly used.

DIFFERENTIAL DIAGNOSIS

- Medical: Neuroleptic malignant syndrome, malignant hyperthermia, infection (e.g., meningitis, encephalitis), hyperthyroidism, tetanus
- Toxins: Anticholinergic, amphetamines, cocaine, lithium, LSD, PCP, salicylates
- Classic features in differentiation of NMS from SS are that SS develops over 24 hr, involves neuromuscular hyperactivity (hyperreflexia, myoclonus), and begins to resolve within 24 hr with appropriate therapy, whereas NMS develops gradually over days to wks, involves sluggish neuromuscular response, and resolves over an average period of 1 wk to 10 days.

WORKUP

- Because SS is a clinical diagnosis, there is no laboratory test that confirms the diagnosis, and serum serotonin concentration does not correlate with the clinical picture.
- However, patients with SS may develop leukocytosis, elevated creatinine phosphokinase, and decreased sodium bicarbonate levels.

TABLE 1 Criteria to Determine Serotonin Syndrome and Toxicity

Sternbach diagnostic criteria for serotonin syndrome	1. Recent addition or increase of proserotonergic medication 2. At least three of the following: • Agitation • Ataxia • Diaphoresis • Diarrhea • Hyperreflexia • Hyperthermia • Mental status changes • Myoclonus • Shivering • Tremor 3. Neuroleptic agent not added or dose increased before the onset of symptoms 4. Diagnosis of infections, withdrawal, and other poisoning or metabolic disruptions excluded
Hunter criteria for serotonin toxicity (context of serotonergic medications)	1. If patient has spontaneous clonus, serotonin toxicity present 2. If no spontaneous clonus, one of the following needed for a diagnosis of serotonin toxicity: 1. Inducible clonus *and* agitation *or* diaphoresis 2. Ocular clonus *and* agitation *or* diaphoresis 3. Tremor *and* hyperreflexia 4. Temperature >38° C *and* ocular clonus *or* inducible clonus

From Adams JG et al: *Emergency medicine, clinical essentials*, ed 2, Philadelphia, 2013, Elsevier.

- Patients with severe SS may develop complications including disseminated intravascular coagulation, rhabdomyolysis, metabolic acidosis, renal failure, myoglobinuria, and acute respiratory distress syndrome.
- All patients should receive more extensive workup to rule out other life-threatening illnesses.

LABORATORY TESTS (USED TO NARROW DIFFERENTIAL DIAGNOSIS)

- CBC with differential when considering sepsis
- Urine and blood cultures
- Electrolytes, BUN, and creatinine to rule out acidosis and renal failure
- Coagulation studies to rule out disseminated intravascular coagulation
- Blood and urine toxicology screen, including acetaminophen and salicylate levels if overdose was intentional
- Thyroid function tests
- Creatine-phosphokinase (CPK) with isoenzymes
- ECG because ventricular rhythm disturbance is a potentially fatal complication
- CSF studies to rule out meningitis

IMAGING STUDIES (USED TO NARROW DIFFERENTIAL DIAGNOSIS)

- Plain chest radiograph
- Head computed tomography

Rx TREATMENT

- Once a diagnosis of SS is established, consultation with a medical toxicologist, clinical pharmacologist, and/or poison control center should be considered.
- Management includes:
  1. Discontinue use of all potential precipitating drugs.
  2. Provide supportive management.
  3. Control agitation.
  4. Administer serotonin antagonists.
  5. Control autonomic instability.
  6. Control hyperthermia.
  7. Reassess the need to resume the use of the serotonergic agent once the symptoms have resolved.

NONPHARMACOLOGIC THERAPY

- Discontinuation of the drug is the mainstay of therapy.
- Supportive treatment aimed at normalizing vital signs.
- Patients who are severely hyperthermic with temperatures >41°C (106°F) should be given IV sedation, paralyzed, and intubated. Cooling blankets can be used for patients with mild to moderate hyperthermia. There is no role for acetaminophen.
- Intubation is recommended for patients unable to protect their airways as a result of mental status changes or seizures.

ACUTE GENERAL Rx

- Benzodiazepines for control of agitation are preferred to physical restraints.
  1. Lorazepam 1 to 2 mg IV every 30 min has been used effectively in treating agitation, muscle rigidity, myoclonus, and seizure complications.
  2. Diazepam is an alternative choice.
- Patients may have rapid changes in blood pressure and heart rate. Hypertensive patients should be treated with short-acting agents (e.g., esmolol or nitroprusside). Hypotensive patients may require both IV fluids and vasopressor therapy.
- Serotonin antagonists should be titrated to clinical effectiveness in patients for whom nonpharmacologic therapy and benzodiazepines are not achieving adequate response. Although, limited evidence is available for these treatments.
  1. Cyproheptadine (4 mg tablet or 2 mg/5 ml syrup available) – widely accepted as standard of care
     a. Adults: 12 mg initially followed by 2 mg every 2 hr until therapeutic response (up to 32 mg/day)
     b. Children (ages 7-14): 4 mg every 6 hr (up to 16 mg/day)
     c. Children (ages 2-6): 2 mg every 6 hr (up to 12 mg/day)
     d. Children (younger than 2 yr): 0.06 mg/kg every 6 hours (up to 0.25 mg/kg/day)
  2. Atypical antipsychotic agents with serotonin antagonist properties (e.g., olanzapine 10 mg SL) have been tried with some success, but efficacy is unproven.
  3. Chlorpromazine 50 to 100 mg IM may be considered in severe cases, but intravenous fluid loading is essential to prevent hypotension. This may also worsen hyperthermia.

CHRONIC Rx

For patients not requiring hospital admission, lorazepam can be given in an oral dose on a prn basis with close follow-up.

DISPOSITION

- SS is a potentially life-threatening condition if not recognized early, although it does exist on a spectrum.
- Prompt diagnosis and withdrawal of the medication results in improvement of symptoms within 24 hr.
- Seizures, rhabdomyolysis, hyperthermia, ventricular arrhythmia, respiratory arrest, and coma are all complicating features of SS.

REFERRAL

All cases of SS secondary to psychotropic medications should be referred to a psychiatrist.

PREVENTION

Modify prescription practices by avoiding multidrug regimens.

Detailed pharmacy review before starting high risk drugs (Box 1).

PEARLS & CONSIDERATIONS

The combined use of SSRIs and MAOIs is contraindicated.

COMMENTS

- The use of SSRIs and other serotonergic agents is not an absolute contraindication; however, prompt withdrawal of the medication is recommended if any symptoms suggesting SS occur.
- SS is usually found in patients being treated for depression, bipolar disorders, obsessive-compulsive disorder, attention deficit disorder, and Parkinson disease.

SUGGESTED READINGS

Available at ExpertConsult.com

AUTHORS: **James Earl Corley III, MD,** and **Alan Taylor, MD**

Short Bowel Syndrome (ALG) (PTG)

BASIC INFORMATION

DEFINITION

Short bowel syndrome (SBS) is a malabsorption syndrome that results from extensive small intestinal resection or congenital causes (Table 1).

SYNONYMS

Short bowel
SBS

ICD-10CM CODE
K91.2 Postsurgical malabsorption, not elsewhere classified

EPIDEMIOLOGY & DEMOGRAPHICS

- Parallels Crohn disease (see "Crohn Disease" in Section I), which is the most common cause of the syndrome in adults.
- In children, two thirds of short bowels are related to congenital abnormalities (intestinal atresia, gastroschisis, volvulus, aganglionosis) and one third are related to necrotizing enterocolitis.
- Prevalence: 10,000 to 20,000 cases are estimated to exist in the U.S.

PHYSICAL FINDINGS & CLINICAL PRESENTATION

- Diarrhea and steatorrhea
- Weight loss
- Anemia related to iron or vitamin B_{12} absorption
- Bleeding diathesis related to vitamin K malabsorption
- Osteoporosis/osteomalacia related to vitamin D and calcium malabsorption
- Hyponatremia, hypokalemia
- Hypovolemia
- Other macronutrient or micronutrient deficiency states

TABLE 1 Daily Stomal or Fecal Losses of Electrolytes, Minerals, and Trace Elements in Severe Short Bowel Syndrome*

Component	Amount Lost
Sodium	90-100 mEq/L
Potassium	10-20 mEq/L
Calcium	772 (591-950) mg/day
Magnesium	328 (263-419) mg/day
Iron	11 (7-15) mg/day
Zinc	12 (10-14) mg/day
Copper	1.5 (0.5-2.3) mg/day

*For sodium and potassium, the average concentration per liter of stomal effluent is given. Values for minerals and trace elements are mean 24-hr losses, with the range in parentheses.
From Feldman M et al: *Sleisenger and Fordtran's gastrointestinal and liver disease*, ed 10, Philadelphia, 2016, Elsevier.

ETIOLOGY

- Extensive bowel resection for treatment of the conditions mentioned previously (see "Epidemiology"). SBS typically does not occur until less than 200 cm of healthy small intestine remains. Risk for SBS is decreased if colon is intact.
- Congenital.
- Box 1 summarizes causes of short bowel syndrome.

The human intestine is 3 to 8 m in length. Removal of up to half of the small intestine produces no disruption in nutrient absorption, and most patients can maintain nutritional balance on oral feeding if they have more than 100 cm (3 ft) of jejunum. Similarly, 100 cm of intact jejunum can maintain a normal water, sodium, and potassium balance under normal circumstances. The presence of an intact colon can compensate for some small intestine loss.

Site-specific functions (Fig. 1):

- Calcium, magnesium, phosphorus, iron, and vitamins are absorbed in the duodenum and proximal jejunum.
- Vitamin B_{12} and bile acids are absorbed in the ileum. The resection of more than 60 cm of ileum results in vitamin B_{12} malabsorption. The loss of more than 100 cm results in fat malabsorption (from the loss of bile acids).
- The loss of gastrointestinal endocrine hormones can affect intestinal motility.
- Intestinal bacterial overgrowth may also occur, especially if the ileocecal valve is lost.

BOX 1 Causes of Short Bowel Syndrome (SBS) and Intestinal Failure in Adults and Children

Adults
Catastrophic vascular accidents:
  Superior mesenteric arterial embolism
  Superior mesenteric arterial thrombosis
  Superior mesenteric venous thrombosis
Chronic intestinal pseudoobstruction
Intestinal resection for tumor or trauma
Midgut volvulus
Multiple intestinal resections for Crohn disease
Radiation enteritis
Refractory sprue
Scleroderma and mixed connective tissue disease

Children
Congenital villus atrophy
Extensive aganglionosis
Gastroschisis
Jejunal or ileal atresia
*Necrotizing enterocolitis

*Functional SBS can also occur in conditions associated with severe malabsorption and intact bowel length.
From Feldman M et al: *Sleisenger and Fordtran's gastrointestinal and liver disease,* ed 10, Philadelphia, 2016, Elsevier.

- Macronutrient requirements in patients with short bowel syndrome are summarized in Table 2.

DIAGNOSIS

Presence of macronutrient and/or micronutrient loss in a patient with a known history of bowel resection. Daily stromal or fecal losses of electrolytes, minerals, and trace elements in SBS are summarized in Table 1.

DIFFERENTIAL DIAGNOSIS

Because the history of significant bowel resection is typically known, there is no differential diagnosis. If that history is not known, all causes of weight loss, malabsorption, and diarrhea must be considered.

TREATMENT

Extensive small bowel resection with colectomy (<100 cm of jejunum):

- Rx: Long-term total parenteral nutrition (TPN). Some patients can switch to oral intake after 1 to 2 yr of TPN. In jejunostomy patients, excessive fluid loss can be reduced with H_2 blockers, proton pump inhibitors, or octreotide. Micronutrients are supplemented.

Extensive small bowel resection with partial colectomy (usually patients with Crohn disease):

- Rx: Oral intake alone is possible in all patients with >100 cm of jejunum. In addition to vitamin B_{12} deficiency, these patients often have diarrhea. Consider lactose malabsorption and bacterial overgrowth treated, respectively, with lactose restriction and antibiotics (tetracycline 250 mg tid or metronidazole 500 mg tid for 2 wk). Nonspecific antidiarrheal agents may also be indicated (e.g., Imodium

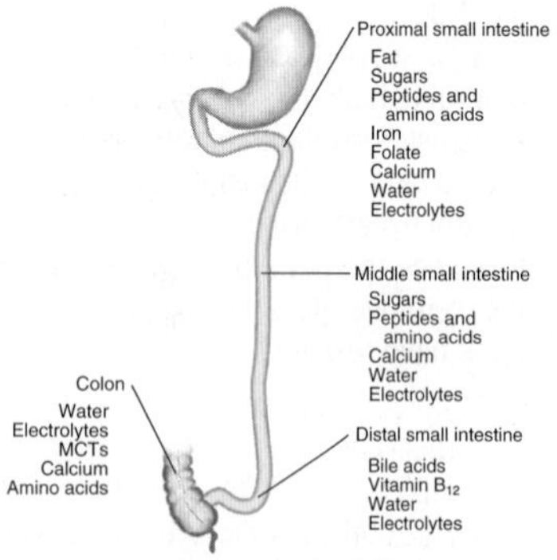

FIG. 1 Specific areas of absorption of dietary constituents and secretions in the small intestine and colon. Macronutrients and micronutrients are absorbed predominantly in the proximal jejunum. Bile acids and vitamin B_{12} (cobalamin) are absorbed only in the ileum. Electrolytes and water are absorbed in both the small and large intestine. Medium-chain triglycerides *(MCTs),* calcium, and some amino acids can be absorbed in the colon. (From Feldman M et al: *Sleisenger and Fordtran's gastrointestinal and liver disease,* ed 10, Philadelphia, 2016, Elsevier.)

TABLE 2 Macronutrient Requirements in Patients with Short Bowel Syndrome

Colon Present	Colon Absent
Carbohydrate	
Complex carbohydrates/starches	Variable types
30-35 kcal/kg per day	30-35 kcal/kg per day
Soluble fiber	
Fat	
MCT/LCT	LCT
20%-30% of caloric intake	20%-30% of caloric intake
Protein	
Intact protein	Intact protein
1.0-1.5 g/kg per day	1.0-1.5 g/kg per day

LCT, Long-chain triglycerides; *MCT,* medium-chain triglycerides.
From Feldman M et al: *Sleisenger and Fordtran's gastrointestinal and liver disease,* ed 10, Philadelphia, 2016, Elsevier.

TABLE 3 Management Strategies for Short Bowel Syndrome

1. Acute phase
   a. Treat postoperative complications
   b. Maintain full support via the parenteral route
   c. Initiate low-rate trophic enteral feeds
   d. Document amount and site of remaining bowel and underlying disease
2. Early adaptation (up to 1 yr postsurgery)
   a. Increase enteral nutrition to tolerance; supplement with glutamine
   b. Achieve permanent parenteral access, if indicated
   c. Maximize antiperistaltic agents
   d. Octreotide for high-output ostomy or fistula
   e. Dietary counseling
   f. Clinical trials of trophic growth factors
3. Long-term adaptation (>1 yr postsurgery)
   a. Recruit bypassed bowel
   b. Bowel-lengthening procedure (Bianchi or STEP)
   c. Monitor for development of TPN-associated complications, and refer for transplant before recurrent sepsis, thrombosis, or end-stage liver disease

STEP, Serial transverse enteroplasty; *TPN,* total parenteral nutrition.
From Cameron JL, Cameron AM: *Current surgical therapy,* ed 10, Philadelphia, 2011, Saunders.

or codeine). The patient must be monitored for micronutrient losses.

- Table 3 and Fig. 2 summarize management strategies for SBS. Intestinal transplantation is performed mostly in children at selective centers.
- Therapeutic agents used to decrease intestinal transit and diarrheal volume are summarized in Table E4.
- FDA-approved medications for SBS in patients receiving nutritional support are:
  1. Recombinant growth hormone somatropin (Zorbtive): Effective in increasing weight and reducing parenteral nutrition volume. These effects do not persist when the drug is stopped.
  2. Teduglutide (Gattex), a recombinant DNA analog of glucagon-like peptide-2. It promotes mucosal growth in the small bowel through stimulation of crypt cell proliferation and inhibition of enterocyte apoptosis. This drug may have to be continued indefinitely for effects to persist.

COMPLICATIONS

- Oxalate kidney stones
- Cholesterol gallstones
- D-Lactic acidosis

PROGNOSIS

- Directly dependent on the extent of the bowel resection and in the case of Crohn disease by the underlying illness.
- Whether the colon remains in continuity with the small bowel is an important factor in the patient's ability to adapt after significant small bowel resection.

RELATED CONTENT

Short Bowel Syndrome (Patient Information)
Malabsorption (Related Key Topic)

AUTHOR: **Fred F. Ferri, MD**

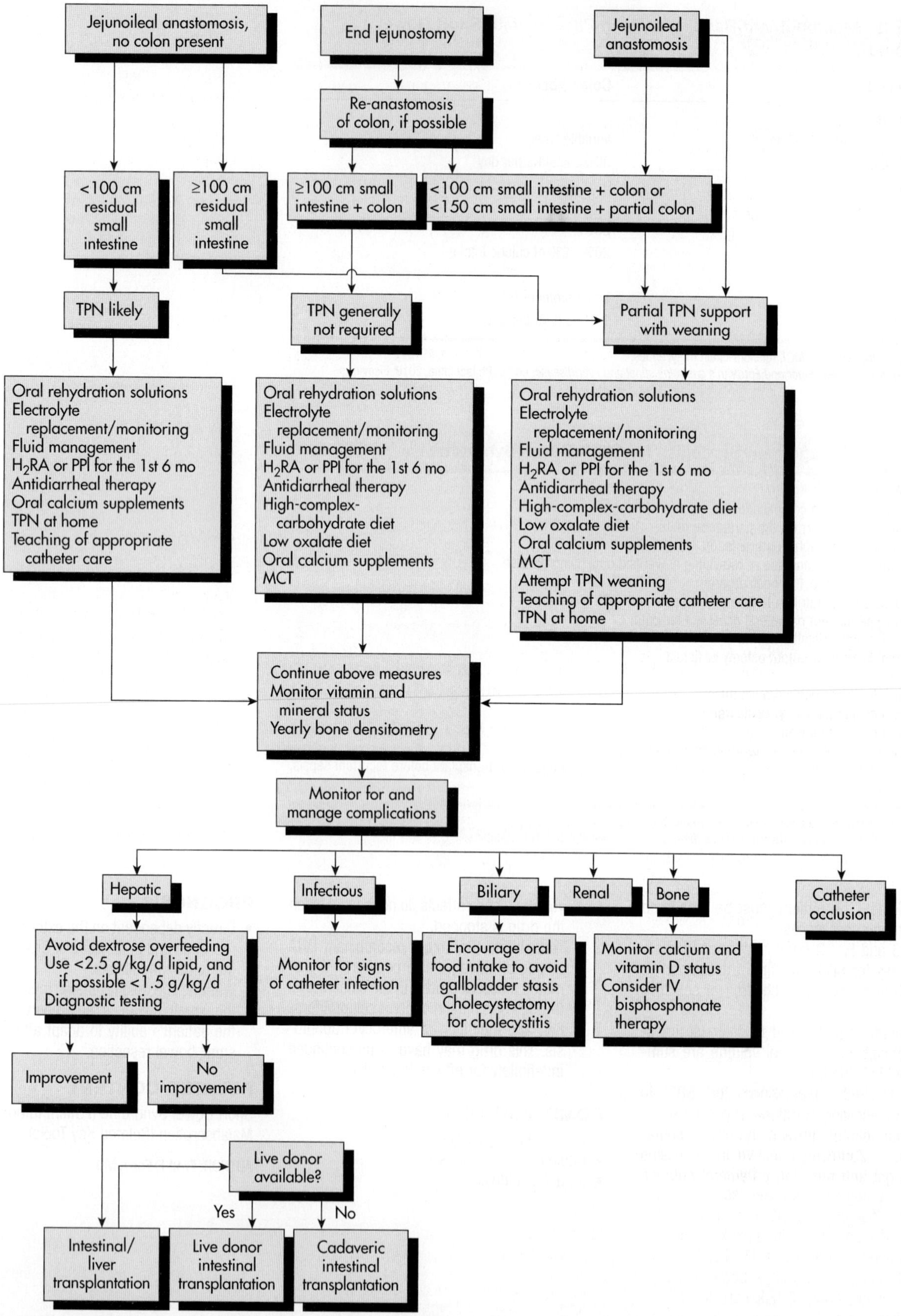

FIG. 2 Algorithm for management of the patient with short bowel syndrome. *H2RA,* Histamine 2 receptor antagonist; *IV,* intravenous; *MCT,* medium-chain triglycerides; *PPI,* proton pump inhibitor; *TPN,* total parenteral nutrition. (From Feldman M et al: Sleisenger and Fordtran's gastrointestinal and liver disease, ed 10, Philadelphia, 2016, Elsevier.)

BASIC INFORMATION

DEFINITION

Short QT syndrome (SQTS) is a genetically inherited disorder of cardiac repolarization characterized by a severely shortened QT interval on the ECG, leading to atrial and ventricular arrhythmias and sudden cardiac death in affected individuals. This is a primary electrical disorder and patients have structurally normal hearts.

SYNONYM

SQTS

ICD-10CM CODE

I45.89 Other specified conduction disorders

EPIDEMIOLOGY & DEMOGRAPHICS

- The disease is a relative new entity, first documented in 2000. In most (but not all) cases of SQTS, the QT or QTc (correct QT interval) has been <360 ms; however, there are many individuals with that QT interval who are clinically unaffected. Although poorly defined, the estimated prevalence of short QTc ≤340 ms is estimated to be 5 in 10,000 in persons less than 21 yr of age. Males are more commonly affected. Approximately 250 cases have been described across 150 affected families. The low number of cases presents challenges mainly in risk stratifying asymptomatic individuals with SQTS.
- Genetics: The disease is genetically heterogeneous and transmitted in an autosomal dominant fashion. Different genes encoding various cardiac ion channels have been attributed to SQTS, including a carnitine transporter and a chloride-bicarbonate anion exchanger. Based on this, eight SQTS have been described, from SQTS 1 to SQTS 8. SQT 1 is the most common variant described, due to a mutation in the cardiac ion channel KCNH2(HERG). SQTS 2 has been described to be sporadic, while the others are familial in nature.

PHYSICAL FINDINGS & CLINICAL PRESENTATION

- Seen across all age groups, though most patients are children or young adults.
- Syncope and cardiac arrest are the most common presenting features. Syncope is likely due to ventricular arrhythmias. Sudden death can happen with exercise as well as at rest. Cardiac arrest is often the first manifestation of the disease with a peak incidence in the first year of life, with a 4% risk for cardiac arrest, and a second peak between 20 and 40 yr of age; overall risk cardiac arrest is 40% before age 41.
- Atrial fibrillation and flutter are well described as being part of the syndrome.
- A significant percentage of patients are asymptomatic.

ETIOLOGY

- Cardiac repolarization abnormality
- A total of 22 different mutations have been found in 9 different genes, 15 in single families. At present, the chance of finding a causative mutation in a family with SQTS is approximately 20%. Mutations cause an increase in net outward current from either a reduction in inward depolarizing currents INa or ICa or augmentation of outward repolarizing currents I to I K1, I K-ATP, I ACh, I Kr or I Ks as well as defects in Cl/HCO_3 exchanger. The resultant shortening of the action potential causes a shortening of myocyte repolarization and the effective refractory period, with subsequent increased susceptibility of both atrial and ventricular muscle to premature depolarizations that lead to AF and VF
- Acquired causes—see "Differential Diagnosis"

DIAGNOSIS

- Current diagnostic criteria for SQTS are from 2013 HRS guidelines
  1. SQTS is diagnosed in the presence of a QTc ≤330 ms.
  2. SQTS can be diagnosed in the presence of a QTc ≤360 ms and one or more of the following: a pathogenic mutation, family history of SQTS, family history of sudden death at age ≤40, survival of a ventricular tachycardia/ventricular fibrillation episode in the absence of heart disease.
  3. Notably, more recent studies suggest the use of somewhat more liberal cutoffs of 340 ms as standalone and 370 ms in combination with additional risk factors.
- A proposed scoring system (Table 1) for the diagnosis of SQTS incorporates the above criteria but has not yet been fully endorsed by the current guidelines.
- The differential diagnosis of a short QT includes various conditions such as hyperkalemia, hypercalcemia, acidosis, digitalis toxicity, effect of acetylcholine or epinephrine, sinus tachycardia, or hyperthermia. All these are possible causes of an acquired short QT interval that must be ruled out before a diagnosis of SQTS can be entertained.

WORKUP

- Evaluation of any survivor of sudden death starts with a detailed history and physical examination, with particular emphasis on family history. Many patients with SQTS have unexplained syncope or palpitations prior to resuscitated sudden death. Atrial fibrillation is common in SQTS patients and a family history of lone AF should also be sought, in addition to resuscitated VF arrest.
- Physical examination is mostly normal in patients with SQTS.
- ECG findings in SQTS include not only an abnormally short QT interval (usually <360 msec), but usually also a short or even absent ST interval, with the T-wave appearing to emanate directly from the S-wave. T-waves are usually any combination of tall, narrow, and symmetric, with a prolonged Tpeak-Tend ratio (Fig. E1). Additionally, PQ-segment depression (PQD), defined as 0.05-mV PQ depression from the isoelectric TP segment, is more typically present in patients with

TABLE 1 SQTS Diagnostic Criteria

	Points
QTc, msec	
<370	1
<350	2
<330	3
Jpoint-Tpeak interval <120 msec	1
Clinical history	
History of sudden cardiac arrest	2
Documented polymorphic VT or VF	2
Unexplained syncope	1
Atrial fibrillation	1
Family history	
First- or second-degree relative with high-probability SQTS	2
First- or second-degree relative with autopsy-negative sudden cardiac death	1
Sudden infant death syndrome	1
Genotype	
Genotype positive	2
Mutation of undetermined significance in a culprit gene	1

SQTS, Short QTS syndrome; *VF,* ventricular fibrillation; *VT,* ventricular tachycardia.
A minimum of 1 point must be obtained in the electrocardiographic section in order to obtain additional points.
High-probability SQTS: ≥4 points; intermediate-probability SQTS: 3 points; low-probability SQTS: ≤2 points. Electrocardiogram: Must be recorded in the absence of modifiers known to shorten the QT. Jpoint-Tpeak interval must be measured in the precordial lead with the greatest amplitude T-wave. Clinical history: Events must occur in the absence of an identifiable etiology, including structural heart disease. Points can only be received for 1 of cardiac arrest, documented polymorphic VT, or unexplained syncope. Family history: Points can only be received once in this section.
Adapted from Gollob MH, Redpath CJ, Roberts JD: The short QT syndrome: proposed diagnostic criteria, *J Am Coll Cardiol* 57(7):802-812, 2011.

SQTS. Another feature to look for is the lack of adaptation of the QT interval to the heart rate (diminished rate dependence) as a result of which the corrected QT interval can be misleading; therefore, QT measurement on resting ECG in SQTS is more accurate with heart rate as close to 60 as possible.

- Echocardiogram and cardiac MRI should be performed to confirm a lack of structural heart disease.
- Holter recordings and stress tests can document a lack of variation of the QT interval in relation to the RR cycle; this is an important aspect of establishing the diagnosis. The QT interval shortens only slightly with increasing heart rates, so the QT and QTc values approach normal levels during faster heart rates. The QT fails to lengthen at slower heart rates.
- At electrophysiology study (EPS), the atrial and ventricular refractory periods are usually very short (140 to 200 msec at a CL of 400 to 600 msec). Sustained atrial fibrillation or flutter with rapid ventricular rates is often induced with programmed stimulation in the atrium. The inducibility of VF in SQTS patients at EPS is about 60%. EPS has a role in adding to the diagnosis by demonstrating short A and V refractory periods (also seen in other channelopathies such as Brugada syndrome), but given its low sensitivity, it cannot be used for risk stratification.

LABORATORY TESTS

- Genetic testing is recommended for all patients in whom a diagnosis of SQTS is suspected. This is especially true if they have a clinical or family history of syncope or sudden death.
- Screening family members: Mutation-specific genetic testing is recommended for all first-degree relatives of a patient diagnosed with a genotype-positive short QT syndrome.

Rx TREATMENT

- There is no significant clinical data on how to approach patients with an isolated short QT interval ≤330 but no family or clinical history or genotype criterion (low and intermediate probability of SQTS). Risk stratification of these patients is not possible at this time; however, they should be referred to an electrophysiologist with expertise on this topic for comprehensive testing, including genetic testing.
- Asymptomatic patients with incidentally found SQTS should be followed without any prophylactic medication.
- Patients with QT <330 msec and one criterion from clinical/family history or genetic testing fall in the high probability category of SQTS and hence a higher-risk subgroup for sudden cardiac death. An ICD implant is recommended in this group for secondary and possibly also primary prevention against sudden cardiac death.
- ICD implantation is a class I indication in patients with the diagnosis of SQTS and who are survivors of cardiac arrest or have sustained ventricular arrhythmia if meaningful survival greater than 1 yr is expected.
- A peculiar issue in patients with SQTS implanted with an ICD is double counting of peaked T-waves that are closely coupled to the QRS complex. This may lead to inappropriate ICD shocks. Most ICDs have programming modifications that can be made to avoid this problem.
- Pharmacologic therapy is usually only advised in patients with multiple and frequent appropriate ICD shocks. Quinidine is the preferred agent in these cases.
- However, medications may be the mainstay of therapy in patients in whom an ICD cannot be implanted for various reasons, including in children in whom technical challenges are significant.
- Isoproterenol infusion is effective in the setting of refractory VF storm and SQTS.
- While many drugs, such as flecainide, sotalol, ibutilide, hydroquinone, and amiodarone, have been used in an attempt to increase the QT interval, most of the available data favor hydroquinidine as the drug of choice across all forms of the SQTS.
- On a special note, primary carnitine deficiency, which presents with SQTS and is associated with VF, is a rare autosomal recessive disorder caused by a defective transport of carnitine into the cell. Administration of oral DL-carnitine or L-carnitine 5g/day over time abolishes the changes on ECG.

REFERRAL

Consultation with an electrophysiologist is strongly recommended if SQTS is suspected.

PEARLS AND CONSIDERATIONS

- SQTS is a rare genetic syndrome causing arrhythmias and sudden death.
- Should be suspected in patients with QT interval <370 msec presenting with syncope, sudden cardiac death, or atrial fibrillation and a family history of the same.

SUGGESTED READINGS

Available at ExpertConsult.com

AUTHOR: **Hrak Chemchirian, MD**

BASIC INFORMATION

DEFINITION

Sialadenitis is an inflammation of one or multiple salivary glands. It may present as acute or chronic disease with multiple potential etiologies. This section focuses mainly on the workup and management of acute sialadenitis.

ICD-10CM CODE
K11.20 Sialadenitis, unspecified

EPIDEMIOLOGY & DEMOGRAPHICS

INCIDENCE:
- Accounts for approximately 0.01% to 0.02% of hospital admissions.
- 30% to 40% of affected patients are postoperative patients.
- Parotid gland is most frequently affected, followed by the submandibular glands (Fig. E1).

PREDOMINANT SEX & AGE:
- Affects men and women equally.
- Patients are usually in the sixth and seventh decades of life.

PHYSICAL FINDINGS & CLINICAL PRESENTATION

- Pain and swelling of the affected salivary gland
- Increased pain with meals
- Erythema and localized tenderness at the duct opening
- Massage may express purulent discharge from duct orifice
- Induration and pitting of the skin, with involvement of the masseteric and submandibular spatial planes in severe cases

ETIOLOGY

- Ductal obstruction is generally from salivary stasis and increased salivary viscosity as a result of dehydration, medication-induced xerostomia, or poor dental hygiene. This predisposes patients to retrograde migration of bacteria, which can then lead to suppurative sialadenitis.
- Acute suppurative sialadenitis is a bacterial infection of the salivary gland. Most frequent infecting organisms are *Staphylococcus aureus* (50% to 90% of cases), streptococcal species, *Haemophilus influenzae,* and *E. coli;* more recently, anaerobic infections have been increasing in prevalence.
- Recent surgery, Sjögren syndrome, diabetes mellitus, hypothyroidism, renal failure, trauma, radiation therapy, chemotherapy, dehydration, and chronic illness are predisposing factors.
- Mumps is the most common cause of nonsuppurative acute sialadenitis. Majority of cases (>80%) occur in children younger than 15 yr.

DIAGNOSIS

DIFFERENTIAL DIAGNOSIS

- Salivary gland neoplasm
- Ductal stricture
- Sialolithiasis
- Decreased salivary secretion as a result of medications (e.g., amitriptyline, diphenhydramine, anticholinergics)
- Dental infections
- Lymphoma
- Cervical adenitis
- Infected branchial cleft or sebaceous cysts

WORKUP

- Generally not necessary. Fig. E2 describes a diagnostic algorithm.
- Ultrasound or CT scan in patients not responding to medical treatment.

LABORATORY TESTS

- Generally not indicated
- Complete blood count with differential to possibly reveal leukocytosis with left shift
- Mumps antibodies if there is clinical suspicion
- Culture of purulent drainage from salivary duct opening or percutaneously should be obtained to provide useful information in tailoring antibiotic therapy if the patient is not responding to empiric therapy

IMAGING STUDIES

- Ultrasound or CT scan (Fig. E3) may be needed in patients with no improvement or clinical worsening after 48 to 72 hr of medical therapy. This can provide information on the presence of a drainable collection.
- Sialography should not be performed during the acute phase, as it can worsen symptoms.
- MRI is also of little utility in acute sialadenitis.

TREATMENT

Nonpharmacologic therapy—these interventions are crucial in expediting resolution of symptoms.
- Massage of the gland: May express pus and relieve some of the pressure
- Hydration with intravenous fluid or aggressive oral hydration along with electrolyte repletion
- Warm compresses
- Oral cavity irrigations
- Administration of sialagogues such as lemon drops or vitamin C lozenges

ACUTE GENERAL Rx

- Amoxicillin-clavulanate 500 to 875 mg bid or cefuroxime 250 to 500 mg bid should be given for 10 days. Clindamycin is an alternative choice in patients allergic to penicillin.
- In patients coming from nursing homes or in cases of nosocomial infections, consider empiric treatment with vancomycin given the prevalence of methicillin-resistant *S. aureus.*
- IV antibiotics (e.g., cefoxitin, nafcillin) can be given in severe cases.
- Patients generally improve with 48 to 72 hr of medical treatment. If there is no improvement, consider imaging with CT or ultrasound.
- Surgical drainage is indicated for the rare cases that are refractory to medical management and that are found to have an abscess on CT or ultrasound.

DISPOSITION

Complete recovery unless the patient has underlying obstruction (e.g., ductal stricture, tumor, or stone)

REFERRAL

- To ear-nose-throat specialist for cases refractory to appropriate medical therapy
- For salivary gland incision and drainage, which may be necessary in resistant cases

PEARLS & CONSIDERATIONS

COMMENTS

Prevention of dehydration will decrease the risk of sialadenitis.

SUGGESTED READINGS
Available at ExpertConsult.com

RELATED CONTENT

Salivary Gland Inflammation (Patient Information)
Sialolithiasis (Related Key Topic)
Salivary Gland Neoplasms (Related Key Topic)

AUTHOR: **Louis F. Insalaco, MD**

BASIC INFORMATION

DEFINITION

Sialolithiasis is the existence of hardened intraluminal deposits in the ductal system of a salivary gland.

SYNONYMS

Salivary gland stone
Salivary calculus

ICD-10CM CODE

K11.5 Sialolithiasis

EPIDEMIOLOGY & DEMOGRAPHICS

Affects patients mostly in the fifth to eighth decades and occurs most commonly in the submandibular gland (85%); 15% of occurrences are located in a parotid gland (Table E1).

PHYSICAL FINDINGS & CLINICAL PRESENTATION

- Symptoms: Colicky postprandial pain and swelling of a salivary gland. Tends to have a remitting/relapsing course.
- Signs: Swelling and tenderness of a salivary gland. The stone may be felt with bimanual palpation of the floor of the mouth or inner cheek.

ETIOLOGY

- The cause is unknown. Contributing factors include saliva stagnation, sialadenitis (inflammation of a salivary gland), ductal inflammation, or injury (Fig. 1).
- Gout is a known cause of salivary gland calculi.
- Salivary calculus composition is mainly calcium phosphate and carbonate, often combined with small proportions of magnesium, zinc, ammonium salts, and organic materials or debris.

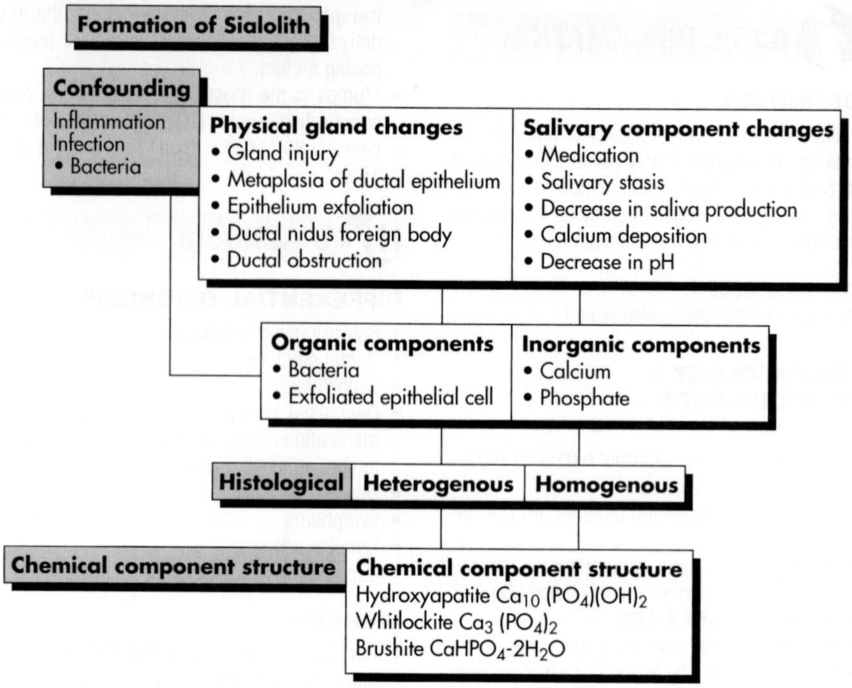

FIG. 1 Algorithm of clinical findings and pathogenesis of sialolithiasis. (From Lee LT, Wong YK: Sialolithiasis in minor salivary glands, *J Oral Maxillofac Surg*, 2010.)

Dx DIAGNOSIS

DIFFERENTIAL DIAGNOSIS

- Lymphadenitis
- Salivary gland tumor
- Salivary gland bacterial (*Staphylococcus* or *Streptococcus*), viral (mumps), or fungal infection (sialadenitis)
- Noninfectious salivary gland inflammation (e.g., Sjögren syndrome, sarcoidosis, lymphoma)
- Salivary duct stricture
- Dental abscess

IMAGING STUDIES

- X-ray: 90% of submandibular stones are radiopaque and will show up on x-ray. 90% of parotid stones are radiolucent and will not show up on x-ray.
- Non–contrast-enhanced computed tomography is very useful in detecting nearly all salivary stones.
- Ultrasound can detect 90% of salivary stones >2 mm.
- Sialography has a 95% to 100% sensitivity in detecting stones (Figs. E2 and E3), although it is more invasive than the above options and requires contrast injection into the affected duct.

Rx TREATMENT

- Nonsurgical management is usually the first-line treatment.
  1. Warm compresses, gland massages, sialogogues (lemon wedges, sour candies), IV or oral hydration.
  2. Antibiotics if associated bacterial sialadenitis is present.
- Surgical treatment:
  1. The surgical approach depends on the location of the stone. Submandibular stones in the distal aspect of the duct that are palpable may be excised transorally under local anesthesia. More proximal stones may require removal of the submandibular gland. Sialoendoscopy is a newer technique where a rigid endoscope and specialized instruments and/or lasers are used to visualize and remove the stones. Stones in the parotid duct also may be accessible via the transoral approach or may require parotidectomy. Sialoendoscopy is also an option for parotid stones.
  2. Extracorporeal shock wave lithotripsy is an alternative technique that breaks up the stones into smaller fragments that can be secreted naturally through the duct.

REFERRAL

To otorhinolaryngologist

SUGGESTED READINGS

Available at ExpertConsult.com

RELATED CONTENT

Salivary Gland Stones (Patient Information)
Sialadenitis (Related Key Topic)

AUTHOR: **Louis F. Insalaco, MD**

BASIC INFORMATION

DEFINITION

Sinus node dysfunction is a group of cardiac rhythm disturbances characterized by abnormalities of the sinus node leading to the inability of the SA node to react to heart rate changes to meet physiological demands. This entity includes (1) chronic, inappropriate bradycardia; (2) sinus pauses or arrest; (3) sinoatrial exit block; and (4) alternating sinus bradycardia with paroxysmal supraventricular tachyarrhythmias (frequently atrial fibrillation) known as tachycardia-bradycardia syndrome. When sinus node dysfunction is associated with symptoms, it is called sick sinus syndrome (SSS).

SYNONYMS

Sinus pause
Sinus arrest
Inappropriate persistent sinus bradycardia
Tachycardia-bradycardia syndrome
Sinoatrial exit block
SSS
Bradycardia-tachycardia syndrome

ICD-10CM CODE

I49.5 Sick sinus syndrome

EPIDEMIOLOGY & DEMOGRAPHICS

- In children: Associated with congenital and acquired heart disease, particularly after cardiac surgery.
- In adults: It is primarily a disease of the elderly secondary to progressive idiopathic degenerative disease. A modern population study has suggested that white race, increased BMI, prolonged baseline QRS or right bundle branch block, elevated N-terminal pro-B-type natriuretic peptide, HTN, or other cardiovascular diseases are associated with increased incidence of sick sinus syndrome. With an aging population, the annual incidence of SSS is projected to increase significantly.

PHYSICAL FINDINGS & CLINICAL PRESENTATION

- Fatigue, light-headedness, syncope, presyncope, palpitations. Other manifestations include dyspnea on exertion and worsening angina.
  1. Usually symptoms are progressive; however, abrupt symptoms are not uncommon (i.e., syncope).
- Physical examination may be normal or reveal abnormalities (e.g., irregular heart rhythm, signs of congestive heart failure, heart murmurs or gallop sounds) associated with the underlying heart disease.

ETIOLOGY

- Sinus node fibrosis is the primary etiology, which may also affect the atrioventricular node, the His bundle, or its branches. Polypharmacy should be considered and obtaining an accurate medicine list is essential.
  1. Common medications include beta blockers, nondihydropyridine calcium channel blockers, digoxin, and antiarrhythmic medications.
- Additional etiologies include acute coronary syndromes, diseases of the SA nodal artery, inflammatory and infiltrative diseases such as hemochromatosis, amyloidosis, sarcoidosis, collagen vascular diseases (SLE and scleroderma), epicardial and pericardial diseases, trauma following cardiac surgery, hypothyroidism, hypothermia, hypoxia, sepsis, muscular dystrophies (e.g., myotonic dystrophy, Friedreich ataxia), infectious etiologies such as Lyme disease, increased intracranial pressure.
  1. The sinus node artery arises from right coronary artery in 60% of people and the left circumflex artery in 40%.

TABLE 1 Indications for Permanent Pacing in Chronic Sinus Node Dysfunction

Class	Indications
I	• In patients who are symptomatic due to sinus node dysfunction, permanent pacing is indicated to increase heart rate and improve symptoms. • In patients with symptomatic sinus bradycardia as a consequence of necessary therapy for which there is no alternative treatment, permanent pacing is recommended to increase heart rate and improve symptoms.
IIa	• For patients with tachy-brady syndrome and symptomatic bradycardia, permanent pacing is reasonable to increase heart rate and reduce symptoms attributable to hypoperfusion. • In patients with symptomatic chronotropic incompetence, permanent pacing with rate-responsiveness is reasonable to improve symptoms and increase exertional heart rates.
IIb	• In patients with symptoms that are likely attributable to SND, a trial of oral theophylline may be considered to increase heart rate, improve symptoms, and help determine the potential benefits of permanent pacing.
III	• In asymptomatic patients with sinus bradycardia or sinus pauses that are secondary to physiologically elevated parasympathetic tone, permanent pacing should not be performed. • In patients with sleep-related sinus bradycardia or transient sinus pauses occurring during sleep, permanent pacing should not be performed in the absence of other indications for pacing. • In patients with asymptomatic SND, or in those in whom the symptoms have been documented to occur in the absence of bradycardia or chronotropic incompetence, permanent pacing is not indicated.

ACC, American College of Cardiology; *AHA*, American Heart Association; *HRS*, Heart Rhythm Society.
Adapted from 2018 ACC/AHA/HRS guideline on the evaluation and management of patients with bradycardia and cardiac conduction delay.

Dx DIAGNOSIS

DIFFERENTIAL DIAGNOSIS

- Bradycardia: Atrioventricular block
- Tachycardia: Atrial fibrillation or atrial flutter, sinus tachycardia
- Medication toxicity
- Carotid sinus hypersensitivity
- Metabolic abnormality (e.g., hyperkalemia in acute kidney injury)

WORKUP

- ECG (Fig. E1)
- Ambulatory cardiac rhythm monitoring with diary to correlate symptoms to findings:
  1. Event recorder or an implantable loop recorder if symptoms are less frequent.
  2. Establishment of diagnosis is more effective with longer-term recording (at least 2 to 4 wk) compared with 24-hr ambulatory ECG.
  3. Exercise stress testing to evaluate the severity of chronotropic incompetence.

The term *chronotropic incompetence* is thought to represent the inability to augment heart rates appropriately in response to exercise or activities of daily living.

- Electrophysiologic testing, including sinus node recovery time and sinoatrial conduction time

Rx TREATMENT

- Permanent pacemaker placement is primarily indicated if bradycardia is symptomatic and a reversible etiology is not identified. Indications for permanent pacemaker in sinus node dysfunction are described in Table 1.
- In tachycardia-bradycardia syndrome, drug treatment is indicated for tachycardia, primarily with AV node blocking agents, after placement of the permanent pacemaker.

SUGGESTED READINGS

Available at ExpertConsult.com

AUTHORS: **Daniel R. Frisch, MD, Max Weiss, MD,** and **Ryan Watson, MD**

BASIC INFORMATION

DEFINITION

- Sickle cell disease (SCD) is a hemoglobin synthesis disorder in which the substitution of valine for glutamic acid at position six of the beta-globin chain yields a variant molecule, hemoglobin S. In its deoxygenated form, hemoglobin S (deoxy HgbS) polymerizes into long strands, deforming red blood cells (RBCs) into a characteristic sickle shape. Chronic RBC membrane damage from this process locks cells into an abnormal sickle shape; along with abnormal adherence to vascular endothelium, this leads to obstruction in the microcirculation and causes painful crises—the hallmark of sickle cell disease.
- SCD patients include those who are homozygous for sickle cell hemoglobin (HbS), and those with one sickle hemoglobin gene inherited with other hemoglobin abnormalities, notably beta thalassemia (Hgb S/β^0 or Hgb S/β^+ thalassemia) and hemoglobin C (HbSC).

SYNONYMS

Sickle cell anemia
SCD
Hemoglobin S disease

ICD-10CM CODES

D57.1	Sickle-cell disease without crisis
D57.20	Sickle-cell/Hb-C disease without crisis
D57.211	Sickle-cell/Hb-C disease with acute chest syndrome
D57.212	Sickle-cell/Hb-C disease with splenic sequestration
D57.219	Sickle-cell/Hb-C disease with crisis, unspecified
D57.3	Sickle-cell trait
D57.40	Sickle-cell thalassemia without crisis
D57.411	Sickle-cell thalassemia with acute chest syndrome
D57.412	Sickle-cell thalassemia with splenic sequestration
D57.419	Sickle-cell thalassemia with crisis, unspecified
D57.80	Other sickle-cell disorders without crisis
D57.811	Other sickle-cell disorders with acute chest syndrome
D57.812	Other sickle-cell disorders with splenic sequestration
D57.819	Other sickle-cell disorders with crisis, unspecified

EPIDEMIOLOGY & DEMOGRAPHICS

- SCD is an autosomal-recessive disorder. In African Americans the incidence at birth is 1 in 400 and the incidence of all genotypes is 1 in 300. Approximately 100,000 people in the U.S. have SCD.
- Sickle cell trait occurs in approximately 300 million people worldwide, with the highest prevalence of approximately 30% to 40% in sub-Saharan Africa, but also in the southern Mediterranean region (usually as Hgb S/β^0 or Hgb S/β^+), parts of the Middle East, and India. In the U.S., it is found in nearly 10% of African Americans.
- An estimated 2000 babies are born with sickle cell disease in the U.S. each yr, and worldwide 275,000 infants are born with the disease annually.
- There is no predominant sex.

PHYSICAL FINDINGS & CLINICAL PRESENTATION

- Physical examination is variable depending on the degree of anemia and presence of acute vasoocclusive syndromes, as well as acute pulmonary, neurologic, cardiovascular, genitourinary, and musculoskeletal complications. Table 1 summarizes organ damage seen in sickle cell disease. Table 2 summarizes acute problems in sickle cell disease.
- A study of the prevalence of pain in sickle cell patients found that they complained of pain on 55% of days surveyed; another study showed 40% to 80% complained. Chronic pain may be due to avascular necrosis of joints and is sometimes poorly explained.
- There is no clinical laboratory finding that is pathognomonic of an episode of painful SCD crisis. The diagnosis is made solely on the basis of the medical history and physical examination. Elevated total bilirubin and lactate dehydrogenase (LDH) are sometimes seen with crisis due to increased hemolysis. However, hemolytic anemia is typical for sickle cell disease at baseline. "Aplastic crisis" refers to crisis presenting with severe anemia and low reticulocyte count, usually caused by B19 parvovirus infection.
- Bones are the most common site of pain. Dactylitis, or hand-foot syndrome (acute, painful swelling of the hands and feet), is the first manifestation of sickle cell disease in many infants. Irritability and refusal to walk are other common symptoms. After infancy, musculoskeletal pain can be symmetric, asymmetric, or migratory, and it may or may not be associated with swelling, low-grade fever, redness, or warmth.
- In both children and adults, sickle vasoocclusive episodes are difficult to distinguish from osteomyelitis, septic arthritis, synovitis, rheumatic fever, or gout.
- Cholecystitis presents with abdominal pain commonly in patients with chronic hemolysis. In general, localizing symptoms for infections should be evaluated because these can trigger sickle crisis. Adult patients with severe SCD have splenic atrophy, whereas patients with milder disease (e.g., Hgb S/C) may have splenic infarct-related pain.
- Acute chest syndrome is a potentially life-threatening complication that manifests with chest pain, fever, wheezing, tachypnea, and cough and pulmonary infiltrates on imaging. Causes include infection (*Mycoplasma, Chlamydia,* viruses), infarction, and fat embolism; often no cause is identified.
- Musculoskeletal and skin abnormalities include leg ulcers (particularly on the malleoli) and limb-girdle deformities caused by avascular necrosis of the femoral and humeral heads. Osteonecrosis of the heads of the femur and humerus is found in nearly 50% of adults with Hgb S/S disease.
- Endocrine abnormalities include delayed sexual maturation and late physical maturation, especially evident in boys.
- Neurologic abnormalities on examination may include seizures and altered mental status. Strokes occur in about 10% of children and adults with sickle cell anemia and approximately 35% of children with sickle cell anemia have cerebrovascular disease.
- Infections, particularly involving *Salmonella, Staphylococcus aureus, Mycoplasma,* and *Streptococcus,* are relatively common. Catheter-associated bacteremia should be considered if a vascular access device is present; these may present without fever.
- Severe splenomegaly as a result of sequestration often occurs in children before splenic atrophy.

TABLE 1 Organ Damage Seen in Sickle Cell Disease

Organ or System	Injury
Skin	Stasis ulcer
Central nervous system	Cerebrovascular accident
Eye	Retinal hemorrhage, retinopathy
Cardiac	Congestive heart failure
Pulmonary	Intrapulmonary shunting, embolism, infarct, infection
Vascular	Occlusive phenomenon at any site
Liver	Hepatic infarct, hepatitis resulting from transfusion, hepatic sequestration, intrahepatic cholestasis
Gallbladder	Increased incidence of bilirubin gallstones caused by hemolysis
Spleen	Acute sequestration
Urinary	Hyposthenuria, hematuria
Genital	Decreased fertility, impotence, priapism
Skeletal	Bone infarcts, osteomyelitis, aseptic necrosis
Placenta	Insufficiency with fetal wastage
Leukocytes	Relative immunodeficiency
Erythrocytes	Chronic hemolysis

From Marx J et al: *Rosen's emergency medicine: concepts and clinical practice,* ed 7, Philadelphia, 2010, Mosby.

DIAGNOSIS

DIFFERENTIAL DIAGNOSIS

- Thalassemia
- Other hemolytic anemias
- The differential diagnosis of patients presenting with a painful crisis is discussed in "Physical Findings"

TABLE 2 Acute Problems in Sickle Cell Disease

Dactylitis. Typically the bones of the hands and feet are affected, with fever and leukocytosis. It is often the first event in young children and can occur multiple times until the age 3 yr.
Painful crises. Typically occurs after the first few years in bones or occasionally abdominal viscera. Pain is caused by ischemia and can be very severe. Crises are associated with low-grade fever and mild leukocytosis compared with osteomyelitis, in which fever and leukocytosis are more pronounced. Pain relief with paracetamol, nonsteroidal antiinflammatory drugs, or opioids, as appropriate, should be instigated immediately. Supportive measures such as hydration, intravenously if necessary, and oxygen also help to reduce the duration of the pain crisis. Any precipitating cause such as infection should be treated.
Central nervous system events. Strokes occur in up to 17% of children and young adults. The pathogenesis is unclear, but angiography often shows occlusions or stenosis. Recurrence is likely unless a long-term transfusion program is initiated.
Acute chest syndrome. This is a common cause of death presenting with fever, tachypnea, chest pain, and leukocytosis, often with a sudden drop in hemoglobin. It can be difficult to differentiate among infection, infarction, and embolism. Common precipitating causes are pulmonary fat embolism and infections. Treatment is with transfusion (simple or exchange), antibiotics, and aggressive treatment of hypoxia.
Splenic sequestration. This occurs in children between ages 6 mo and 2 yr. It is caused by sudden trapping of red cells within the spleen, producing a sudden drop in hemoglobin and rapidly enlarging spleen, eventually leading to hypovolemic shock and death. Management includes early detection of the rapidly enlarging spleen and blood transfusion.
Priapism. Engorgement of the penis can be short-lived and self-terminating, or it can last in excess of 24 hr and may lead to impotence. Initial management is with fluids and analgesia, but persistent priapism (>12 hr) may need partial exchange transfusion and corporal aspiration.
Infections. Overwhelming infection with *Streptococcus pneumoniae* is the most common cause of death in children. Other common causes of infections in sickle cell disease include *Haemophilus influenzae* and *Salmonella*. A significant reduction in the number of deaths from sepsis has resulted from the routine use of vaccinations against these organisms and antibiotic prophylaxis. Malaria prophylaxis should be considered in endemic areas.

From Ryan ET et al: *Hunter's tropical medicine and emerging infectious diseases*, ed 10, Philadelphia, 2019, Elsevier.

WORKUP (TABLE 3)

- Screening of all newborns regardless of racial background is performed in the U.S. Screening can be performed with sodium metabisulfite reduction test (Sickledex test).
- Hemoglobin electrophoresis will also confirm the diagnosis and is useful to identify hemoglobin variants such as fetal hemoglobin and hemoglobin C.
- Patients will have evidence of hemolysis (elevated reticulocyte count, low haptoglobin, variable elevation of LDH and total bilirubin).
- Chest x-ray often reveals typical vertebral body changes ("fish mouth" vertebrae) caused by chronic vasoocclusive injury to vertebral bodies.
- For prenatal diagnosis, initial step is identification of parenteral globin gene mutation by DNA-based testing. If positive, then DNA-based testing of chorionic villus sampling or amniotic fluid cells is performed.

LABORATORY TESTS

- Anemia (from chronic hemolysis), reticulocytosis, leukocytosis, and thrombocytosis are common. Hgb S/β^0 and Hgb S/β^+ thalassemia will have microcytosis; Hgb S/C is also typically microcytic. Hgb S/C may have normal or near-normal hematocrit but will have characteristic changes on peripheral smear (target cells).
- Elevations of bilirubin, lactate dehydrogenase, and low haptoglobin are consistent with chronic hemolysis.
- Peripheral blood smear may reveal sickle cells, target cells, poikilocytosis, and hypochromia (Fig. 1).
- Elevated blood urea nitrogen and creatinine may be present in patients presenting acutely with dehydration or chronically with progressive renal insufficiency.
- Urinalysis may reveal hematuria and proteinuria. Patients with SCD should be screened for microalbuminuria and proteinuria with spot urine testing by 10 yr of age.

IMAGING STUDIES (FIGS. E2 AND E3)

- Chest x-ray or noncontrast chest CT scan to evaluate acute and chronic lung changes is helpful.
- Routine skeletal imaging is rarely helpful in acute crisis and should usually be reserved for pain that is not consistent with transient acute crisis.
- MRI or bone scan is useful to address chronic avascular necrosis or, in the acute setting, osteomyelitis.
- CT or MRI scan of brain is not indicated in asymptomatic adults and children with SCD but is often needed in patients with neurologic complications, such as transient ischemic attack, cerebrovascular accident, seizures, or altered mental status.
- Transcranial Doppler ultrasonography (TCD) is used to identify children with sickle cell anemia who are at risk for stroke. There should be an annual screening starting at age 2 until age 16. Patients determined to be at risk (transcranial Doppler velocity ≥200 cm/s) should be enrolled in long-term transfusion programs. These transfusions are effective in reducing risk of stroke by >90%. In adults, magnetic resonance angiography (MRA) can be used instead of TCD to identify those at risk for stroke.
- Doppler echocardiography should be performed in patients with unexplained respiratory symptoms to evaluate for pulmonary hypertension, with right heart catheterization performed if abnormal. Screening for vasculopathy is done by estimating the tricuspid regurgitant jet velocity (TRV). Elevated values are predictive of early mortality. The prevalence of pulmonary hypertension when right heart catheterization is performed is approximately 6% in adults with sickle cell disease.

Rx TREATMENT

NONPHARMACOLOGIC THERAPY

- Patients should be instructed to avoid conditions that may precipitate sickling crisis, such as extremes of cold and heat and dehydration.
- Maintain adequate hydration (PO or IV).
- Correct hypoxia when present.

ACUTE GENERAL Rx

- Initiate aggressive IV or oral hydration; most patients in crisis have evidence of dehydration.
- Aggressively diagnose and treat suspected infections such as urinary infection, respiratory infections, or catheter-associated line infections. Table 4 summarizes bacteria and viruses that most frequently cause serious infection in patients with sickle cell disease.
- Provide pain relief during the vasoocclusive crisis (Table 5). Most patients will have a treatment history that can guide dosing. Opiate management is complicated by high levels of tolerance in patients often treated over many years. Patient-controlled analgesic pumps are often helpful; caution should be used when employing continuous infusions, which are usually not necessary or helpful. Morphine and hydromorphone are most commonly used. Meperidine is rarely used now and generally discouraged because of neurologic side effects, although some patients state a preference for it.
- Oral diphenhydramine is used to control pruritus, which is commonly associated with opiate analgesics; preferred to IV therapy in guidelines.
- Table 6 summarizes overall strategies for the management of acute chest syndrome.
- Follow oxygenation in patients presenting with chest pain or respiratory symptoms; assess for evolving acute chest syndrome if oxygenation deteriorates.
- Urology evaluation for priapism.

CHRONIC Rx

- Hydroxyurea increases hemoglobin F levels, reduces the incidence of vasoocclusive complications, and improves survival. It is helpful in patients with Hgb S/S and S/β^0 thalassemia; its value in other variants is less certain. There is strong evidence to support use of hydroxyurea therapy in children ages 9 mo and older to decrease the frequency of vasoocclusive crises and acute chest syndrome. Hydroxyurea is also strongly

TABLE 3 Baseline Evaluations to Consider

	Tests
Blood tests	CBC with differential
	Reticulocyte count
	Hemoglobin HPLC or electrophoresis
	LDH
	Renal function tests
	Liver function tests
	Mineral panel
	Serum iron, ferritin, TIBC
	Vitamin D level
	Hepatitis B sAg
	Hepatitis C antibody
	RBC alloantibody screen
	RBC typing
	D-dimer[a]
	C-reactive protein[a]
	Brain natriuretic peptide
Urine and kidney tests	Urinalysis
	Renal ultrasonography[b]
Radiology	MRI or MRA brain (adults)[c] or transcranial Doppler ultrasonography starting at age 2 yr (children)
	Chest radiography[d]
	Hip or shoulder radiograph or MRI (or both)[c]
	Bone density in teenagers and adults
Cardiology and pulmonary	Echocardiogram
Neurocognitive	Neurocognitive testing[d]

CBC, Complete blood count; *HPLC*, high-performance liquid chromatography; *LDH*, lactate dehydrogenase; *MRA*, magnetic resonance angiography; *MRI*, magnetic resonance imaging; *RBC*, red blood cell; *sAg*, surface antigen; *TIBC*, total iron-binding capacity.
[a]Consider following as surrogate markers after initiation of disease-modifying intervention.
[b]If hematuria with red blood cells in urine.
[c]As clinically indicated.
[d]If the patient has poor school performance, an abnormal memory, or abnormal MRI findings.
From Hoffman R et al: *Hematology: basic principles and practice*, ed 7, Philadelphia, 2018, Elsevier.

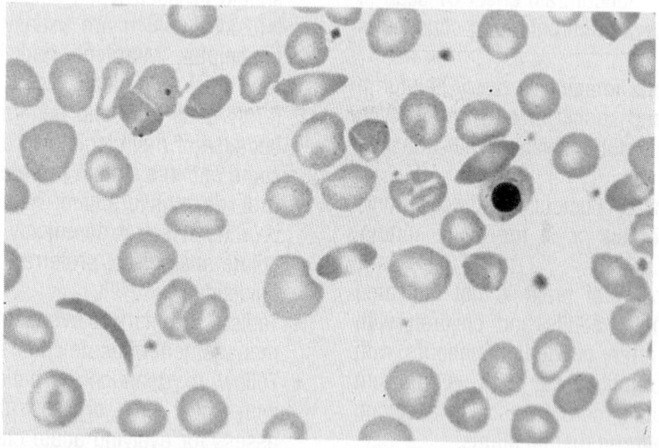

FIG. 1 Photomicrograph of a blood film. Sickle cell anemia (homozygosity for hemoglobin S). Shown are a sickle cell, boat-shaped cells, a nucleated red cell, and target cells. (From Bain BJ et al: *Dacie and Lewis practical haematology*, ed 12, Philadelphia, 2017, Elsevier.)

recommended for adults with three or more crises during any 12-mo period, with SCD pain or chronic anemia interfering with daily activities, or with severe or recurrent episodes of acute chest syndrome. It should be stopped in pregnancy, and contraception counseling should be given to all patients.

- Recommended starting doses for hydroxyurea are 15 mg/kg/day in adults and 5 to 10 mg/kg/day in patients with renal disease. A recent randomized study has shown markedly superior efficacy with a dose escalation strategy of up to 30 mg/kg/day compared with traditional dosing of 20 mg/kg/day.
- Pharmaceutical grade L-glutamine is approved for use to decrease crisis symptoms in patients with Hgb S/S and Hgb S/β° thalassemia; benefits include decrease in acute crisis episodes, reduced hospitalization, and decrease in episodes of acute chest syndrome. Dosing is 5 to 15 g tid, taken with food or 8 oz of cold or room-temperature fluid. Constipation, nausea, headache, and abdominal discomfort were common side effects, occurring in approximately 15% to 20% of patients. It may work with or without concomitant use of hydroxyurea. Caution may be warranted in prescribing L-glutamine to patients with clinically significant renal or hepatic dysfunction.
- Replace folic acid (1 mg PO daily) to replace increased utilization of folic acid stores from chronic hemolysis. Patients also have mineral and vitamin deficiencies (calcium, zinc, and vitamins A, C, D, and E) and may need oral supplementation.
- Chronic pain management represents an enduring challenge, made more difficult by the current opiate addiction and overdose epidemic. In one study, patients reported pain in 55% of days. Review of guidelines for safe opiate prescribing is strongly recommended and management with pain management specialists is also strongly recommended.
- Indications for PRBC transfusion in SCD are described in Table 7. Urgent exchange transfusion for acute chest syndrome with progressive hypoxia (arterial oxygen saturation <90%) or multiorgan failure may be lifesaving. Simple transfusion may be adequate in milder cases with a target Hgb of 10 g/dl. Transfusion therapy is appropriate for patients with stroke or at high risk by transcranial Doppler study (see earlier) if possible. Transfusion has shown to be beneficial in children with silent infarcts by MRI in preventing progression. Transfusion to Hgb 10 g/dl is recommended in anemic patients undergoing general anesthesia to reduce crisis and respiratory complications after surgery. Patients on chronic transfusion therapy should receive RBC matched at C, E, and K antigens to avoid alloimmunization. Transfusion is not recommended for asymptomatic anemia. Serum ferritin level should be monitored quarterly. Iron overload due to blood transfusions (transfusional hemosiderosis) can be treated with chelating agents (deferoxamine [SC infusion], deferasirox [PO], and deferiprone [PO]).
- Annual screening for proteinuria is recommended. ACE inhibitor therapy should be started for microalbuminuria in adults with SCD to prevent progression of renal injury. Progressive renal injury may cause worsening anemia and responds to erythropoietin.
- Annual retinopathy screening should be performed beginning at age 10, especially for patients with Hgb S/C variant, in whom proliferative retinopathy occurs in about 30% to 50%. It is less common in Hgb S/S and other variants.
- Gene therapy for SCD patients represents a novel approach. Clinical trials with lentiviral vector-mediated addition of an antisickling β-globin gene into autologous hematopoietic stem cells are ongoing with encouraging early results in terms of reduction of sickle cell crises and correction of the biologic hallmarks of the disease. A level of erythrocyte

TABLE 4 Bacteria and Viruses That Most Frequently Cause Serious Infection in Patients with Sickle Cell Disease

Microorganism	Type of Infection	Comments
Streptococcus pneumoniae	Septicemia	Common despite prophylactic penicillin and pneumococcal vaccine
	Meningitis	Less frequent than in yrs past
	Pneumonia	Rarely documented except in infants and young children
	Septic arthritis	Uncommon
Haemophilus influenzae type b	Septicemia	
Meningitis		
Pneumonia	Much less common in recent yr because of immunization with conjugate vaccine	
Salmonella species	Osteomyelitis	
Septicemia	Most common cause of bone and joint infection	
Escherichia coli and other gram-negative enteric pathogens	Septicemia	
Urinary tract infection		
Osteomyelitis	Focus sometimes not apparent	
Staphylococcus aureus	Osteomyelitis	Uncommon
Mycoplasma pneumoniae	Pneumonia	Pleural effusions; multilobe involvement
Chlamydia pneumoniae	Pneumonia	
Parvovirus B19	Bone marrow suppression (aplastic crisis)	High fever common; rash and other organ involvement infrequent
Hepatitis viruses (A, B, and C)	Hepatitis	Marked hyperbilirubinemia

Data from Buchanan GR, Glader BE: Benign course of extreme hyperbilirubinemia in sickle cell anemia: analysis of six cases, *J Pediatr* 91:21, 1977. From Hoffman R et al: *Hematology: basic principles and practice*, ed 7, Philadelphia, 2018, Elsevier.

fetal hemoglobin (HbF) comprising alpha and gamma globins may ameliorate the hemolytic anemia of sickle cell disease by mitigating sickle hemoglobin polymerization and erythrocyte sickling. BCL11A is a repressor of gamma-globin expression and HbF production in adult erythrocytes. Its downregulation is a promising therapeutic strategy for induction of HbF.[1]

- Allogeneic stem cell transplantation can be curative in young patients with symptomatic SCD.
- Crizanlizumab, an antibody against the adhesion molecule p-selectin, revealed a significantly lower rate of sickle cell–related pain crisis than placebo and was associated with a low incidence of adverse events in a recent study. It has been approved for the prevention of vasoocclusive crises in adults and pediatric patients ages 16 yr and older.
- Voxelotor, an inhibitor of sickle hemoglobin (HbS) polymerization, significantly increases hemoglobin levels and reduces markers of hemolysis and is approved for the therapy of adults and children over age 12 yr.[2]

[1]Esrick EB et al: Post-transcriptional genetic silencing of BCL11A to treat sickle cell disease, N Engl J Med 384(3)205-215, 2021.
[2]Vichinsky E et al: A phase 3 randomized trial of Voxelotor in sickle cell disease, *N Engl J Med* 381:509-519, 2019.

TABLE 5 Recommended Dose and Interval of Analgesics Necessary to Obtain Adequate Pain Control in Patients with Sickle Cell Disease

	Dose/Rate	Comments
Severe to Moderate Pain		
Morphine	Parenteral: 0.1-0.15 mg/kg every 3-4 hr Recommended maximum single dose, 10 mg PO: 0.3-0.6 mg/kg every 4 hr	Drug of choice for pain; lower doses in elderly adults and infants and in patients with liver failure or impaired ventilation
Meperidine	Parenteral: 0.75-1.5 mg/kg every 2-4 hr Recommended maximum dose, 100 mg PO: 1.5 mg/kg every 4 hr	Increased incidence of seizures; avoid in patients with renal or neurologic disease and those who receive MAOIs
Hydromorphone	Parenteral: 0.01-0.02 mg/kg every 3-4 hr PO: 0.04-0.06 mg/kg every 4 hr	
Oxycodone	PO: 0.15 mg/kg/dose every 4 hr	
Ketorolac	IM: Adults: 30 or 60 mg initial dose followed by 15-30 mg; children: 1 mg/kg load followed by 0.5 mg/kg every 6 hr	Equal efficacy to 6 mg MS; helps narcotic-sparing effect; not to exceed 5 days; maximum, 150 mg first day, 120 mg maximum on subsequent days; may cause gastric irritation
Butorphanol	Parenteral: Adults: 2 mg every 3-4 hr	Agonist–antagonist; can precipitate withdrawal if given to patients who are being treated with agonists
Mild Pain		
Codeine	PO: 0.5-1 mg/kg every 4 hr Maximum dose, 60 mg	Mild to moderate pain not relieved by aspirin or acetaminophen; can cause nausea and vomiting
Aspirin	PO: Adults: 0.3-6 mg every 4-6 hr; children: 10 mg/kg every 4 hr	Often given with a narcotic to enhance analgesia; can cause gastric irritation; avoid in febrile children
Acetaminophen	PO: Adults: 0.3-0.6 g every 4 hr; children: 10 mg/kg	Often given with a narcotic to enhance analgesia
Ibuprofen	PO: Adults: 300-400 mg every 4 hr; children: 5-10 mg/kg every 6-8 hr	Can cause gastric irritation
Naproxen	PO: Adults: 500 mg/dose initially and then 250 every 8-12 hr; children: 10 mg/kg/day (5 mg/kg every 12 hr)	Long duration of action; can cause gastric irritation
Indomethacin	PO: Adults: 25 mg every 8 hr; children: 1-3 mg/kg/day given 3 or 4 times	Contraindicated in psychiatric, neurologic, renal diseases; high incidence of gastric irritation; useful in gout

IM, Intramuscular; *MAOI*, monoamine oxidase inhibitor; *MS*, morphine sulphate; *PO*, oral.
Adapted from Charache S et al: Effect of hydroxyurea on the frequency of painful crises in sickle cell anemia: investigators of the multicenter study of hydroxyurea in sickle cell anemia, *N Engl J Med* 332:1317, 1995. In Hoffman R et al: *Hematology: basic principles and practice*, ed 7, Philadelphia, 2018, Elsevier.

TABLE 6 Overall Strategies for the Management of Acute Chest Syndrome

Prevention
Incentive spirometry and periodic ambulation in patients admitted for sickle cell pain, surgery, or febrile episodes
Watchful waiting in any hospitalized child or adult with sickle cell disease (pulse oximetry monitoring and frequent respiratory assessments)
Cautious use of intravenous fluids
Intense education and optimum care of patients who have sickle cell anemia and asthma
Diagnostic Testing and Laboratory Monitoring
Blood cultures, if febrile
Nasopharyngeal samples for viral culture (respiratory syncytial virus, influenza), depending on clinical setting
Complete blood counts every day and appropriate chemistries
Continuous pulse oximetry
Chest radiographs for persistent or progressive illness
Treatment
Blood transfusion (simple or exchange) depending on clinical features; consider maintaining an active type and crossmatch
Supplemental O_2 for drop in pulse oximetry by 4% over baseline, or values <90%
Empirical antibiotics (third-generation cephalosporin and macrolide)
Continued respiratory therapy (incentive spirometry and chest physiotherapy as necessary)
Bronchodilators and corticosteroids for patients with asthma
Optimum pain control and fluid management

From Kliegman RM: *Nelson textbook of pediatrics,* ed 21, Philadelphia, 2020, Elsevier.

TABLE 7 Indications for Transfusion in Sickle Cell Disease

	Duration	Consensus	Method	Goal*
Stroke, acute	Single	+	Ex	HbS <30%
Stroke, ongoing care	Chronic	+	Either	HbS <30%
High-velocity transcranial Doppler	Chronic	+	Either	HbS <30%
ACS, initial episode	Single	+	Dir > Ex	Hgb 10
ACS, recurrent	6-12 mo	+	Either	
Pulmonary hypertension	Chronic	+	Either	
Multiorgan failure	Single	+	Ex	
Major surgery	Single	+	Dir	Hgb 10
Acute anemia	Single	+	Dir	
Recurrent spleen sequestration	Chronic	+		
Sepsis/meningitis	Single	+	Dir	
Severe chronic pain	6-12 mo	+		
Congestive heart failure	Chronic	+		
Silent infarct with abnormal neuropsychology	Chronic	–		
Pregnancy		–		
Anemia/renal failure	Chronic	–		
Leg ulcers	6-12 mo	–		
Severe growth delay		–		
Severe eye disease		–		
Priapism		–		

ACS, Acute chest syndrome; *Dir,* direct; *Ex,* exchange; *Hb,* hemoglobin type; *Hgb,* hemoglobin concentration; +, consensus reached; –, consensus not reached.
*Goal of transfusion if a consensus has been reached.
From Fuhrman BP et al: *Pediatric critical care,* ed 4, Philadelphia, 2011, Saunders.

- Penicillin V 125 mg PO bid should be administered by age 2 mo and increased to 250 mg bid by age 3 yr. Penicillin prophylaxis can be discontinued after age 5 yr, except in children who have had splenectomy.
- Table 8 summarizes disease-modifying treatments to consider.

REFERRAL

- Hospitalization for pain crisis unresponsive to oral analgesics, or involving fever, respiratory symptoms, or vomiting and diarrhea.
- Optimal management requires coordination with hematology, blood banking, pain management, and psychosocial counseling and support.
- Referral for patients with organ-specific complications, notably pulmonary hypertension, acute/chronic kidney disease, and ophthalmologic complications.
- Referral to an ophthalmologist for an annual dilated retinal examination beginning at 10 yr of age.

PEARLS & CONSIDERATIONS

COMMENTS

- The average life span of individuals with sickle cell trait is similar to that of the general population. It may be associated with hematuria, often painless, and rhabdomyolysis under extreme conditions. Chronic pain and acute pain are not typical of sickle cell trait. It is also associated with a higher incidence of renal medullary cancer. Chronic problems in sickle cell disease are summarized in Table 9.
- Regular immunizations, especially pneumococcal vaccination, are recommended. The prophylactic administration of penicillin soon after birth and the timely administration of pneumococcal and *Haemophilus influenzae* type b vaccines have resulted in a significant decline in the incidence of these infections. The heptavalent conjugated pneumococcal vaccine (Prevnar) should be administered from 2 mo of age. The 23-valent unconjugated pneumococcal vaccine (Pneumovax) is given from age 2 yr and can be boosted once 3 yr later. Influenza vaccination can be given after 6 mo of age.
- Pulmonary hypertension is a complication of chronic hemolysis and is associated with a high risk of death. It can be detected by Doppler echocardiography in more than 30% of adult patients with sickle cell disease. Cardiac catheterization will confirm the diagnosis. It is resistant to hydroxyurea therapy.
- Metformin increases fetal hemoglobin (HbF) levels in patients with SCD. A recent study revealed that metformin use in SCD patients with diabetes is associated with fewer episodes of consequential SCD complications and with lower health care utilization.[3]

SUGGESTED READINGS

Available at ExpertConsult.com

RELATED CONTENT

Sickle Cell Anemia (Patient Information)

AUTHOR: **Bharti Rathore, MD**

[3] Badawy SM, Payne AB: Association between clinical outcomes and metformin use in adults with sickle cell disease and diabetes mellitus, *Blood Adv* 3:3297-3306, 2019.

TABLE 8 Disease-Modifying Treatments to Consider[a]

Robust clinical data	Penicillin prophylaxis
	Streptococcus pneumoniae vaccination
	Hydroxyurea
	Chronic exchange transfusion
	Iron chelation for chronic iron overload[b]
Limited clinical data	Daily multivitamin without iron or folate supplementation *and* vitamin D replacement[c]
	Haemophilus influenzae vaccination
	Influenza vaccination
	Erythropoietin
	Phlebotomy
Experimental	Hb F reactivation with decitabine, histone deacetylase inhibitors, or imids
	Erythropoietin for chronic relative reticulocytopenia
	Nutritional supplements and antioxidants (e.g., glutamine, zinc, multivitamins)
	N-acetylcysteine

[a]See text for specific indications and limitations.
[b]Best data from thalassemia patient experience.
[c]Risks minimal; therefore it is generally done.
Hb F, Fetal hemoglobin.
From Hoffman R et al: *Hematology: basic principles and practice,* ed 7, Philadelphia, 2018, Elsevier.

TABLE 9 Chronic Problems in Sickle Cell Disease

Growth and development	Reduced height and weight
	Pubertal delay
	Cognitive impairment (recurrent small strokes)
Locomotor	Osteonecrosis of humeral and femoral heads
	Chronic leg ulcers
Cardiovascular	Myocardial infarction
	Left and right ventricular dilatation
Pulmonary	Pulmonary fibrosis
	Pulmonary hypertension
	Cor pulmonale
Genitourinary	Renal papillary necrosis—hematuria and tubular defects
	Chronic renal failure
	Frequent urinary tract infections in women
	Impotence (secondary to priapism)
Ocular	Proliferative retinopathy (30% of patients)
	Blindness (especially in SC disease)
	Retinal detachment

SC, Sickle cell.
From Ryan ET et al. *Hunter's tropical medicine and emerging infectious diseases,* ed 10, Philadelphia, 2019, Elsevier.

BASIC INFORMATION

DEFINITION

Silicosis is a spectrum of lung disease attributable to the inhalation of silica (silicon dioxide) in crystalline form.

SYNONYM

Pneumoconiosis caused by silica

ICD-10CM CODE

J62.8 Pneumoconiosis due to other dust containing silica

EPIDEMIOLOGY & DEMOGRAPHICS

- Occupational disease affecting men and women involved in gathering, milling, processing, or using silica-containing rock or sand. Jobs that can lead to silicosis are described in Box 1.
- According to the Occupational Safety and Health Administration (OSHA), an estimated 200,000 miners and 1.7 million others have experienced an occupational exposure to silica.
- African Americans have a seven times greater rate of developing silicosis compared to whites at the same level of exposure. The annual number of silicosis deaths declined 40% from 185 in 1999 to 111 in 2013, but the decline appears to have leveled off during 2010 to 2013, according to the Centers for Disease Control and Prevention.

PHYSICAL FINDINGS & CLINICAL PRESENTATION

- There are three patterns of silicosis: acute, chronic, and accelerated. The chronic form can be further subdivided in chronic simple silicosis and chronic complicated silicosis (progressive massive fibrosis).
- Acute silicosis is also known as silicoproteinosis. Develops several weeks to 5 yr after silica exposure. Presents with rapid onset of cough, weight loss, fatigue, and pleuritic chest pain.
- Chronic silicosis is the most common clinical presentation, and onset occurs after decades of repeated exposure. It has two types:
  1. Simple silicosis, which may be asymptomatic, with the only manifestation being an abnormal chest radiograph. Latency period is 10 to 20 yr and progression to massive fibrosis is rare.
  2. Progressive massive fibrosis characterized by radiographic progression and resulting fibrosis.
- Accelerated silicosis may have an initial asymptomatic phase followed by rapidly increasing frequency of symptoms parallel with worsening radiographic abnormalities. Develops <10 yr after initial high-level exposure.

BOX 1 Jobs That Can Lead to Silicosis

Mining: Surface or underground mining (tunneling)
Milling: Ground silica for abrasives and filler
Quarrying
Sandblasting (e.g., of buildings, preparing steel for painting)
Pottery; ceramic or clay work
Grinding, polishing using silica wheels
Stone work: Strong fabrication, especially with engineered stone.
Foundry work: Grinding, molding, chipping
Refractory brick work
Glass making: To polish and as an abrasive
Boiler work: Cleaning boilers
Manufacture of abrasives

From Goldman L, Schafer AI: *Goldman's Cecil medicine*, ed 24, Philadelphia, 2012, Saunders.

ETIOLOGY

- Silica particles are ingested by alveolar macrophages, which in turn release oxidants causing cell injury and cell death, attract fibroblasts, and activate lymphocytes, increasing immunoglobulins in the alveolar space.
- Hyperplasia of alveolar epithelial cells occurs.
- Collagen accumulates in the interstitium.
- Neutrophils also accumulate and secrete proteolytic enzymes, which leads to tissue destruction and emphysema.
- Silica dust may be carcinogenic (not proven).
- Exposure to silicosis predisposes to tuberculosis.
- Some patients develop rheumatoid silicotic pulmonary nodules and may have arthritic symptoms of rheumatoid arthritis (Caplan syndrome). Scleroderma has also been associated with silicosis.

DIAGNOSIS

DIFFERENTIAL DIAGNOSIS

- Other pneumoconiosis, berylliosis, hard metal disease, asbestosis
- Sarcoidosis
- Tuberculosis
- Interstitial lung disease
- Hypersensitivity pneumonitis
- Lung cancer
- Langerhans cell granulomatosis (histiocytosis X)
- Granulomatous pulmonary vasculitis

WORKUP

- History that identifies occupational exposure
- Chest radiograph (Fig. E1)
- Pulmonary function testing

Acute silicosis:

- Chest x-ray demonstrates typical pattern of perihilar or basilar opacities.
- Chest CT demonstrates diffuse nodular and patchy consolidative opacities with enlargement of hilar lymph nodes.
- Bronchoscopy: Milky and lipoproteinaceous effluent is seen on bronchoalveolar lavage (BAL).
- Lung biopsy is not necessary in the setting of a definite exposure history.
- Exclusion of other causes like pulmonary edema, alveolar hemorrhage, and pulmonary alveolar proteinosis is necessary.

Chronic silicosis:

- Chest x-ray demonstrates multiple small, rounded opacities (<10 cm in diameter) distributed in the upper lung zones. Often progresses from lower lobe opacities to more dense consolidation in the mid and lower zones.
- Progressive massive fibrosis (PMF) refers to coalescence of the nodules of chronic silicosis with calcified hilar adenopathy.
- Pulmonary function tests (PFT) show mixed obstructive and restrictive defect.
- High resolution CT scan (HRCT), bronchoscopy, and lung biopsies have limited diagnostic role unless atypical radiographic features are noted.

Accelerated silicosis:

- Radiographic pattern is that of simple silicosis, although development of radiographic abnormalities is more rapid. This has greater risk for PMF.

TREATMENT

- Treatment is symptomatic (supplemental O_2 for hypoxemia, bronchodilators, antibiotics for infections).
- Prevention (industrial hygiene).
- Smoking cessation.
- Vaccination against influenza and pneumococcus.
- Whole-lung lavage may have a role in acute silicoproteinosis.
- Treatment of associated tuberculosis if present.
- Consider lung transplant for patients who develop chronic respiratory failure.
- Once patients progress to fibrosis, no therapies can alter the course of the disease.

ASSOCIATED COMPLICATIONS

Silicosis is associated with increased risk of mycobacterial infections, including tuberculosis, chronic necrotizing aspergillosis, lung cancer, rheumatic disorders, and chronic airflow obstruction.

RELATED CONTENT

Interstitial Lung Disease (Key Topic)
Silicosis (Patient Information)

AUTHORS: **Javeryah Safi, MD,** and **Samaan Rafeq, MD**

BASIC INFORMATION

DEFINITION

Sinus arrhythmia is a common variation of normal sinus rhythm when, despite the presence of sinus rhythm, the variation in the R-R interval is >0.12 sec. P waves should be uniform, and their morphology consistent with sinus node origin (Fig. 1). There are three types of sinus arrhythmia: Respiratory-phasic (also known as respiratory); nonrespiratory-nonphasic, and nonrespiratory-ventriculophasic (for more, see below, on etiology).

ICD-10CM CODE
I49.9 Cardiac arrhythmia, unspecified

EPIDEMIOLOGY & DEMOGRAPHICS

PREVALENCE: Any type of sinus arrhythmia is present in 16% ± 10% of young, healthy individuals. Respiratory sinus arrhythmia is 20% less common in the elderly as compared to younger individuals. Ventriculophasic sinus arrhythmia is present in more than 40% of patients with third-degree AV block.

PREDOMINANT SEX & AGE: No significant difference between genders. Respiratory sinus arrhythmia is less common in the elderly.

PEAK INCIDENCE: Peak incidence is highest among younger individuals. This holds true especially for respiratory sinus arrhythmia.

RISK FACTORS:
- Respiratory-phasic: Younger age
- Nonrespiratory-nonphasic: Underlying heart disease, digitalis overdose, intracranial hypertension
- Nonrespiratory-ventriculophasic: Typically in patients with third-degree AV block

GENETICS: There is evidence of some genetic contribution to variation in heart rate, mainly deriving from twin design cohorts. Sinus arrhythmia is unlikely to be attributed to a single gene, but some genes have been shown to affect resting heart rate. Ser49Gly polymorphism in the β-1 adrenoreceptor gene is one such example; Ser49 homozygotes have average heart rates that are 5 bpm lower than the Gly49 homozygotes.

PHYSICAL FINDINGS & CLINICAL PRESENTATION

No physical exam findings directly correlate directly to the diagnosis of sinus arrhythmia other than the finding of a slightly irregular pulse.

- Respiratory sinus arrhythmia is a common incidental finding on electrocardiograms. Lack of sinus arrhythmia in young individuals may be a sign of underlying chronic disease requiring further investigation. Symptoms and physical findings are rare, if any.
- Nonrespiratory-nonphasic sinus arrhythmia can be considered a normal finding, or underlying structural heart disease might be present, causing dyspnea and edema. Additionally, history of trauma to the head or neck, especially in the setting of anticoagulation, increases suspicion for intracranial hemorrhage.
- Nonrespiratory-ventriculophasic: Rule out 3rd-degree heart block.

ETIOLOGY

- There are three types of sinus arrhythmia: Respiratory-phasic; nonrespiratory-nonphasic, and nonrespiratory-ventriculophasic.
- Respiratory-phasic sinus arrhythmia: Intermittent vagus nerve activation during respiration results in beat-to-beat variations of the RR interval.
- Nonrespiratory-nonphasic sinus arrhythmia can occur in healthy individuals but more often is a result of underlying heart disease or digitalis overdose. Traumatic intracerebral hemorrhage has been reported as a cause as well. The actual mechanism is not fully understood.
- Nonrespiratory-ventriculophasic sinus arrhythmia occurs in third-degree AV heart block or after a compensatory pause following a premature ventricular beat. The two P waves surrounding a QRS complex occur at a faster rate compared to consecutive P waves that occur without an intervening QRS complex. The prolongation of the PP interval is probably attributed to enhanced cardiac filling, resulting in increased stroke volume, which in turn triggers a carotid baroreceptor response. The elevated arterial blood pressure caused by ventricular ejection activates the arterial baroreceptors, resulting in a vagal reflex, which lengthens the following PP interval without a QRS complex.

DIAGNOSIS

DIFFERENTIAL DIAGNOSIS

- Premature atrial contractions
- Sinoatrial exit block
- Sick sinus syndrome

WORKUP

- Evaluation (Figs. 2 and 3) is limited because respiratory sinus arrhythmia is often an asymptomatic and normal finding.
- When reading an electrocardiogram, care should be taken to rule out other causes of group beating, such as atrial fibrillation, flutter, or multifocal atrial tachycardia.
- The presence of nonrespiratory-nonphasic sinus arrhythmia or nonrespiratory-ventriculophasic sinus arrhythmia (Fig. 4) should prompt further investigation for underlying heart disease, such as with an echocardiogram.
- Especially in nonrespiratory-ventriculophasic sinus arrhythmia, which usually occurs in third-degree heart block, causes of the block should be investigated. (See topic "Complete Heart Block".)

LABORATORY TESTS

In isolated respiratory sinus arrhythmia without other findings or symptoms, no laboratory workup is needed.

IMAGING STUDIES

In isolated sinus arrhythmia without other findings or symptoms, imaging is redundant.

TREATMENT

In isolated sinus arrhythmia without other findings or symptoms, no treatment is necessary.

NONPHARMACOLOGIC THERAPY

In asymptomatic patients with isolated respiratory sinus arrhythmia, no therapy is required. In cases of nonrespiratory-ventriculophasic sinus arrhythmia, which happens in the setting of third-degree AV block, permanent pacemaker might be needed in the absence of a reversible cause.

ACUTE GENERAL Rx

In asymptomatic patients with isolated respiratory sinus arrhythmia, no acute therapy is required. In respiratory-phasic sinus arrhythmia and nonrespiratory-ventriculophasic sinus arrhythmia, treat the underlying cause.

CHRONIC Rx

In asymptomatic patients with isolated respiratory sinus arrhythmia, no chronic therapy is required. In respiratory-phasic sinus arrhythmia and nonrespiratory-ventriculophasic sinus arrhythmia, treat the underlying cause.

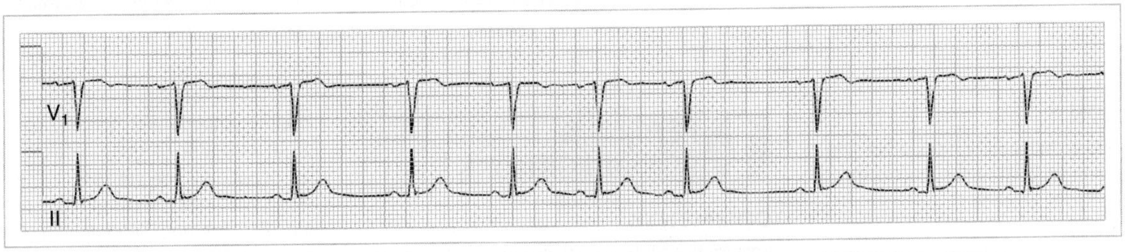

FIG. 1 Normal sinus rhythm with sinus arrhythmia. This lead V 1 and II rhythm strip shows normal sinus rhythm with sinus arrhythmia, in which the P-P intervals vary by >0.16 sec. Sinus arrhythmia is often related to respiratory cycles. (From Olshansky B et al: *Arrhythmia essentials,* ed 2, Philadelphia, 2017, Elsevier.)

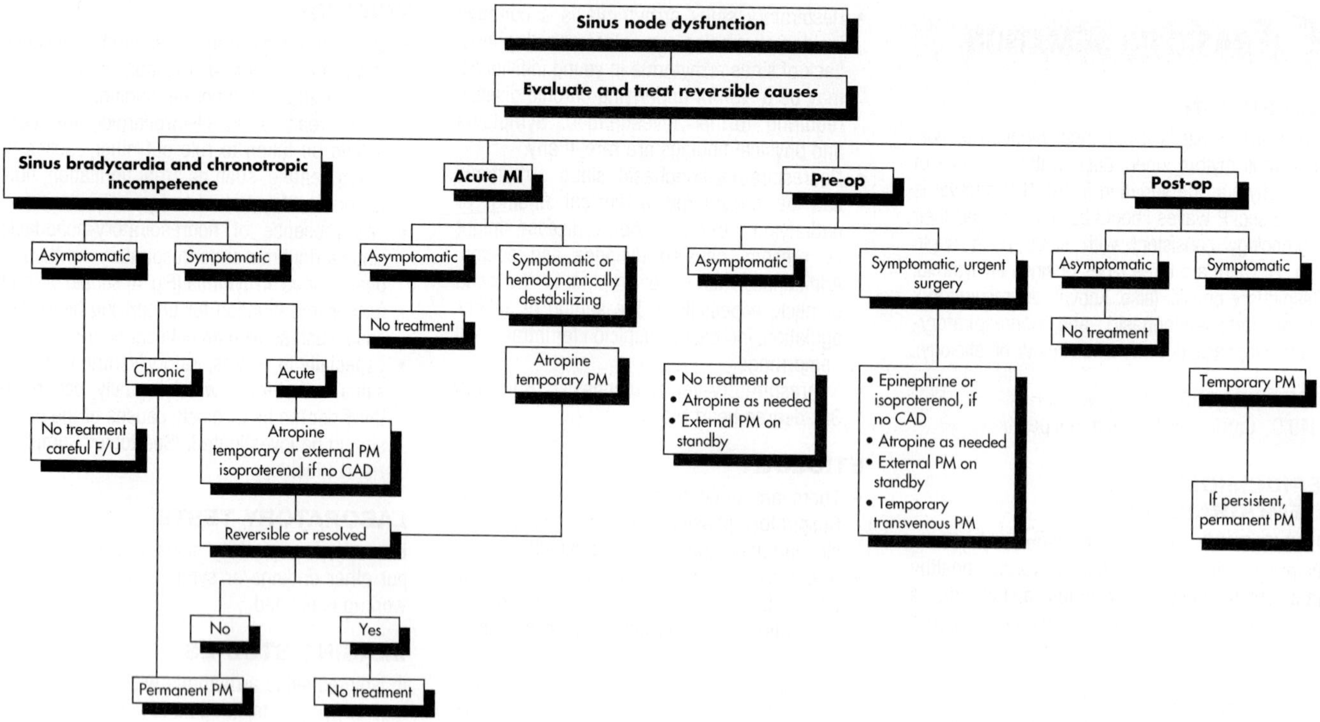

FIG. 2 Sinus node dysfunction. *CAD*, Coronary artery disease; *PM*, pacemaker. (From Olshansky B et al: *Arrhythmia essentials*, ed 2, Philadelphia, 2017, Elsevier.)

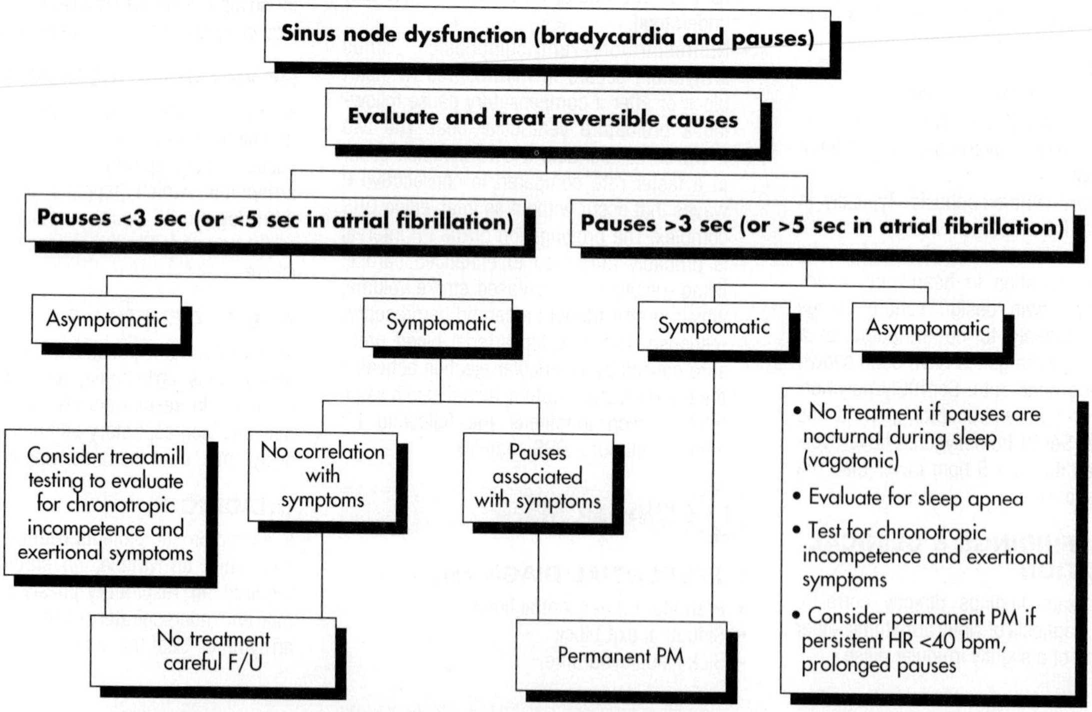

FIG. 3 Sinus node dysfunction (bradycardia and pauses). *HR*, Heart rate; *PM*, pacemaker. (From Olshansky B et al: *Arrhythmia essentials*, ed 2, Philadelphia, 2017, Elsevier.)

DISPOSITION

In isolated sinus arrhythmia without other findings or symptoms, no treatment is necessary.

REFERRAL

Upon confirming sinus arrhythmia as an isolated finding on EKG, no further recommendations are needed. Cardiology consultation is not a requirement.

PEARLS & CONSIDERATIONS

COMMENTS

Respiratory sinus arrhythmia is a common incidental finding on EKG, most prevalent in young, healthy patients and typically asymptomatic. It is an indicator of good cardiovascular health. Its prevalence decreases in the elderly, and those with multiple comorbid conditions including diabetes and heart failure. Patients rarely require evaluation by a cardiologist or additional treatment.

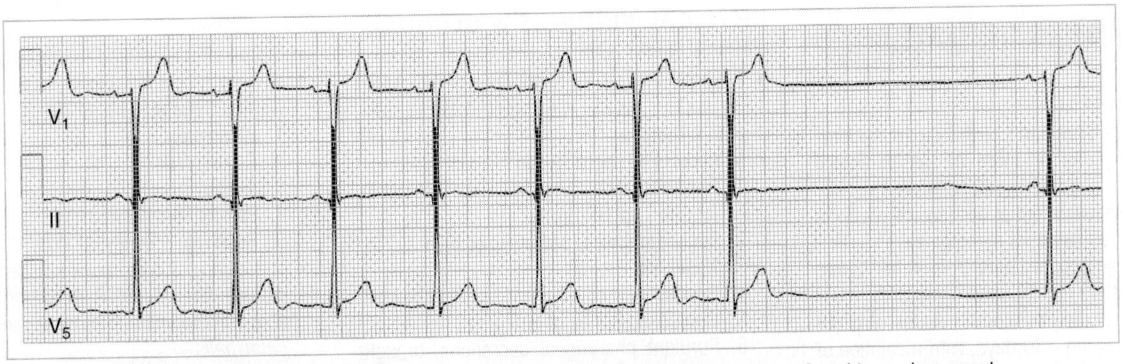

FIG. 4 Sinus pause. Sinus pauses can be prolonged, in which case they can be referred to as sinus arrest. In this lead V1, VII, and V5 rhythm strip, following 7 beats of sinus rhythm (rate ~68 bpm), there is a 3-second sinus pause, followed by a sinus beat. (From Olshansky B et al: *Arrhythmia essentials,* ed 2, Philadelphia, 2017, Elsevier.)

PATIENT & FAMILY EDUCATION

Patients with sinus arrhythmia should be informed that this is a common finding seen in young, healthy persons. It rarely requires further evaluation.

SUGGESTED READING

Available at ExpertConsult.com

RELATED CONTENT

Sick sinus syndrome (Related Key Topic)
Complete heart block (Related Key Topic)

AUTHOR: **Ioannis Koulouridis, MD, MS**

BASIC INFORMATION

DEFINITION

Sinusitis is inflammation of the mucous membranes lining one or more of the paranasal sinuses. The various presentations are:
- Acute sinusitis: Infection lasting <4 wk, with complete resolution of symptoms.
- Subacute infection: Lasts from 4 to 12 wk, with complete resolution of symptoms.
- Recurrent acute infection: Episodes of acute infection lasting <30 days, with resolution of symptoms, which recur at intervals at least 10 days apart.
- Chronic sinusitis: Inflammation of the paranasal sinuses and nasal cavities lasting >12 wk, with persistent upper respiratory symptoms. It accounts for 1% to 2% of total physician encounters.
- Acute bacterial sinusitis superimposed on chronic sinusitis: New symptoms that occur in patients with residual symptoms from prior infection(s). With treatment, the new symptoms resolve but the residual ones do not.

SYNONYM

Rhinosinusitis: Sinusitis is almost always accompanied by inflammation of the nasal mucosa; thus it is now the preferred term.

ICD-10CM CODES

J32.9	Chronic sinusitis, unspecified
J01.90	Acute sinusitis, unspecified
J01.00	Acute maxillary sinusitis, unspecified
J01.01	Acute recurrent maxillary sinusitis
J01.10	Acute frontal sinusitis, unspecified
J01.11	Acute recurrent frontal sinusitis
J01.20	Acute ethmoidal sinusitis, unspecified
J01.21	Acute recurrent ethmoidal sinusitis
J01.30	Acute sphenoidal sinusitis, unspecified
J01.31	Acute recurrent sphenoidal sinusitis
J01.80	Other acute sinusitis
J01.81	Other acute recurrent sinusitis
J01.91	Acute recurrent sinusitis, unspecified
J32.0	Chronic maxillary sinusitis
J32.1	Chronic frontal sinusitis
J32.2	Chronic ethmoidal sinusitis
J32.3	Chronic sphenoidal sinusitis
J32.8	Other chronic sinusitis

EPIDEMIOLOGY & DEMOGRAPHICS

INCIDENCE (IN U.S.): Seems to correlate with the incidence of upper respiratory tract infections and higher in women than men; 30 million cases per year in the U.S.

PEAK INCIDENCE:
- Fall, winter, spring: September through March
- In adults: Greatest incidence between 45 and 74 yr of age
- Approximately 6% to 7% of children presenting with respiratory symptoms have acute sinusitis

PHYSICAL FINDINGS & CLINICAL PRESENTATION

- Patients often give a history of a recent upper respiratory illness with some improvement, then a relapse
- Mucopurulent secretions in the nasal passage:
  1. Purulent nasal and postnasal discharge lasting 7 to 10 days
  2. Facial tightness, pressure, or pain
  3. Nasal obstruction
  4. Headache
  5. Decreased sense of smell
  6. Purulent pharyngeal secretions, brought up with cough, often worse at night
- Erythema, swelling, and tenderness over the infected sinus in a small proportion of patients:
  1. Diagnosis cannot be excluded by the absence of such findings.
  2. These findings are not common, and do not correlate with number of positive sinus aspirates.
- Intermittent low-grade fever in about half of adults with acute bacterial sinusitis
- Toothache is a common complaint when the maxillary sinus is involved
- Periorbital cellulitis and excessive tearing with ethmoid sinusitis:
  1. Orbital extension of infection: Chemosis, proptosis, impaired extraocular movements
- Characteristics of acute sinusitis in children with upper respiratory tract infections:
  1. Persistence of symptoms
  2. Cough
  3. Bad breath
- Symptoms of chronic sinusitis (may or may not be present):
  1. Nasal or postnasal discharge
  2. Fever
  3. Facial pain or pressure
  4. Headache
- Nosocomial sinusitis is typically seen in patients with nasogastric tubes or nasotracheal intubation

ETIOLOGY

- Each of the four paranasal sinuses is connected to the nasal cavity by narrow tubes (ostia), 1 to 3 mm in diameter; these drain directly into the nose through the turbinates. The sinuses are lined with a ciliated mucous membrane (mucoperiosteum).
- Acute viral infection:
  1. Infection with the common cold or influenza
  2. Mucosal edema and sinus inflammation
  3. Decreased drainage of thick secretions/obstruction of the sinus ostia
  4. Subsequent entrapment of bacteria
     a. Multiplication of bacteria
     b. Secondary bacterial infection
- Other predisposing factors:
  1. Tumors
  2. Polyps
  3. Foreign bodies
  4. Congenital choanal atresia
  5. Other entities that cause obstruction of sinus drainage
  6. Allergies
  7. Asthma
- Dental infections lead to maxillary sinusitis.
- Viruses recovered alone or in combination with bacteria (in 16% of cases):
  1. Rhinovirus
  2. Coronavirus
  3. Adenovirus
  4. Parainfluenza virus
  5. Respiratory syncytial virus
- The principal bacterial pathogens in sinusitis are *Streptococcus pneumoniae,* nontypable *Haemophilus influenzae,* and *Moraxella catarrhalis.*
- In the remainder of cases *Streptococcus pyogenes, Staphylococcus aureus,* beta-hemolytic streptococci, and mixed anaerobic infections (*Peptostreptococcus, Fusobacterium, Bacteroides, Prevotella* spp.) are found.
- Infection is polymicrobial in about one third of cases.
- Anaerobic infections are seen more often in cases of chronic sinusitis and in cases associated with dental infection; anaerobes are unlikely pathogens in sinusitis in children.
- Fungal pathogens are isolated with increasing frequency in immunocompromised patients but remain uncommon pathogens in the paranasal sinuses. Fungal pathogens include *Phaeohyphomycosis, Aspergillus, Pseudallescheria, Sporothrix, and Zygomycetes spp.*
- Nosocomial infections: Occur in patients with nasogastric tubes, nasotracheal intubation, cystic fibrosis, and immunocompromised state.
  1. *S. aureus* (including MRSA)
  2. *Pseudomonas aeruginosa*
  3. *Klebsiella pneumoniae*
  4. *Enterobacter* spp.
  5. *Proteus mirabilis*
- Organisms typically isolated in chronic sinusitis:
  1. *S. aureus*
  2. *S. pneumoniae*
  3. *H. influenzae*
  4. *P. aeruginosa*
  5. Anaerobes

DIAGNOSIS

DIFFERENTIAL DIAGNOSIS

- Temporomandibular joint disease
- Migraine headache
- Cluster headache
- Dental infection
- Trigeminal neuralgia
- Allergic rhinitis
- Drugs (cocaine, decongestant overuse)
- Gastroesophageal reflux disease
- Wegener granulomatosis
- Cystic fibrosis

WORKUP

- The diagnosis is generally based on clinical signs and symptoms (purulent rhinorrhea and facial pain). Radiologic tests and cultures are not recommended initially and should be considered only when treatment is ineffective and sinusitis persists.

- In the normal healthy host, the paranasal sinuses should be sterile. Although the contiguous structures are colonized with bacteria and likely contaminate the sinuses, the mucociliary lining functions to remove these bacteria.
- Gold standard for diagnosis: Recovery of bacteria in high-density ≥10^4 colony-forming units/ml from a paranasal sinus, in the setting of a patient with history of upper respiratory infection and symptoms persisting for 7 to 10 days. Sinus aspiration is the best method for obtaining cultures; however, it must be performed by an otorhinolaryngologist and is not practical for the primary care practitioner. Therefore, most diagnoses are based on the clinical history and presentation, possibly supported by radiologic evaluations.
  1. Overall, standard radiographs are of limited use in diagnosis, although negative films are strong evidence against the diagnosis
  2. CT scans:
     a. Much more sensitive than plain radiographs in detecting acute changes and disease in the sinuses
     b. Recommended for patients requiring surgical intervention, including sinus aspiration; it is a useful adjunct to guide therapy
  3. Transillumination:
     a. Used for diagnosis of frontal and maxillary sinusitis
     b. Absence of light transmission indicates that sinus is filled with fluid
     c. Dullness (decreased light transmission) is less helpful in diagnosing infection
  4. Endoscopy:
     a. Used to visualize secretions coming from the ostia of infected sinuses
     b. Culture collection via endoscopy often contaminated by nasal flora; not nearly as good as sinus puncture
  5. Sinus puncture:
     a. Gold standard for collecting sinus cultures
     b. Generally reserved for treatment failures, suspected intracranial extension, and nosocomial sinusitis

Rx TREATMENT

NONPHARMACOLOGIC THERAPY

To help promote sinus drainage:
- Air humidification with vaporizers (for steam) or humidifiers (for a cool mist)
- Application of hot, wet towel over the face
- Sipping hot beverages
- Hydration

ACUTE GENERAL Rx

- Sinus drainage:
  1. Nasal vasoconstrictors, such as phenylephrine nose drops, 0.25% or 0.5%.
  2. Topical decongestants should not be used for more than a few days because of the risk of rebound congestion.
  3. Systemic decongestants.
  4. Corticosteroids: Nasal or systemic corticosteroids, such as nasal beclomethasone. Oral corticosteroids combined with antibiotics may be associated with modest benefit for short-term relief of symptoms in adults with severe symptoms of acute sinusitis compared with antibiotics alone. Oral corticosteroids as monotherapy are not associated with improved clinical outcomes in adults with clinically diagnosed acute sinusitis.[1]
  5. Nasal irrigation, with hypertonic or normal saline (saline may act as a mild vasoconstrictor of nasal blood flow).
  6. Use of antihistamines has no proven benefit, and the drying effect on the mucous membranes may cause crusting, which blocks the ostia, thus interfering with sinus drainage.
- Analgesics, antipyretics

Antimicrobial therapy:
- Most cases of acute sinusitis have a viral cause and will resolve within 2 wk without antibiotics.
- Current treatment recommendations favor symptomatic treatment for those with mild symptoms. 85% of persons have a reduction or resolution of symptoms within 7 to 15 days without antibiotic therapy. Physicians grossly overprescribe antibiotics for presumed bacterial sinusitis despite a much higher prevalence of viral infections.
- Antibiotics should not be prescribed for mild to moderate sinusitis within the first wk of illness. They should be reserved for those with persistent symptoms for more than 10 days, high fever and purulent nasal discharge or facial pain lasting for at least 3 consecutive days, or worsening symptoms after a typical viral illness lasting >5 days that had initially improved ("double sickening").
- Antibiotic therapy is usually empiric, targeting the common pathogens:
  1. First-line antibiotics in children include amoxicillin or amoxicillin/clavulanate. For adults amoxicillin/clavulanate or doxycycline is first-line agent, with quinolones (levofloxacin or moxifloxacin) reserved as second-line agents unless patient is penicillin allergic.
  2. Second-line antibiotics include the newer macrolides: clarithromycin, and oral cephalosporins: cefuroxime axetil, cefprozil, cefaclor, loracarbef, but high rate of resistance of *S. pneumoniae* is a concern with these agents as is *H. influenzae* resistance with TMP-SMX and azithromycin such that they should no longer be used as first-line agents.
  3. For patients with uncomplicated acute sinusitis, the less expensive first-line agents appear to be as effective as the costlier second-line agents.
- Hospitalization and IV antibiotics may be required for more severe infection and those with suspected intracranial complications. Broader-spectrum antibiotic coverage may be indicated in severe cases, to cover for MRSA, *Pseudomonas*, and fungal pathogens.
- Duration of therapy generally 5 to 7 days in adults rather than 10 to 14 days as recommended in the past.
  1. Optimal duration of treatment in children varies from 10 to 28 days.

Surgery:
- Surgical drainage indicated
  1. If intracranial or orbital complications suspected
  2. Many cases of frontal and sphenoid sinusitis
  3. Chronic sinusitis recalcitrant to medical therapy
- Surgical debridement imperative in the treatment of fungal sinusitis

Complications:
- Untreated, sinusitis may lead to a number of serious, life-threatening complications.
- Intracranial complications include meningitis, brain abscess, and epidural and subdural empyema.
- Intracranial sequelae are more common with frontal and ethmoid infections.
- Extracranial complications include orbital cellulitis, blindness, orbital abscess, osteomyelitis.
- Extracranial sequelae are more commonly seen with ethmoid sinusitis.

CHRONIC Rx

- Chronic sinusitis: Evidence supports daily high-volume saline irrigation with topical corticosteroid therapy as a first-line therapy for chronic sinusitis. A short course of systemic corticosteroids (1 to 3 wk), short course of doxycycline (3 wk), or a leukotriene antagonist may be considered in patients with nasal polyps. A prolonged course (3 mo) of macrolide antibiotic may be considered for patients without polyps.
- Dupilumab (Dupixent), a monoclonal antibody that targets interleukin (IL)-4 and -13 was recently FDA approved for chronic rhinosinusitis with nasal polyps (CRSwNP). Cost is a limiting factor.
- Surgical intervention may be necessary in nonresponders.

REFERRAL

- To infectious disease specialist if failure to respond to initial therapy
- To otorhinolaryngologist for:
  1. Failure to respond to therapy
  2. Suspected fungal infection
  3. Suspected intracranial or orbital complications

SUGGESTED READINGS

Available at ExpertConsult.com

RELATED CONTENT

Sinusitis (Patient Information)

AUTHOR: **Glenn G. Fort, MD, MPH**

[1] Venekamp RP et al: Systemic corticosteroid therapy for acute sinusitis, *JAMA* 313(12):1258-1259, 2015.

BASIC INFORMATION

DEFINITION

Sinusoidal Obstruction Syndrome (SOS) is the constellation of hepatomegaly, ascites, right upper quadrant pain, and jaundice that results from toxic injury to the endothelium of terminal hepatic venules and sinusoids and can lead to multiorgan dysfunction (MOD) (Table 1).

SYNONYMS

Hepatic venoocclusive disease (VOD)
SOS

ICD-10CM CODE

K76.5 Hepatic venoocclusive disease

EPIDEMIOLOGY & DEMOGRAPHICS

Most commonly following:
- Hematopoietic stem cell transplantation (HSCT)

Less commonly following:
- Nontransplant chemotherapy
- Ingestion of alkaloid toxins
- High-dose radiation therapy
- Liver transplantation

INCIDENCE:
- 13.7% incidence on average in the post-HSCT population

PREDOMINANT SEX & AGE:
- The incidence of SOS in children and infants (estimated at 22% and 30%, respectively) after HSCT is twofold to threefold higher than in adults.

RISK FACTORS (TABLE 2):
- The Center for Blood and Marrow Transplant Research (CIBMTR) maintains an online risk calculator.
- No factor alone or in combination can explain the variability in risk for developing SOS.

GENETICS: The following factors have been implicated in some cases of SOS:
- GSTM1-null genotype
- Hemochromatosis *C282Y* allele
- MTHFR 677CC/1298CC haplotype in patients receiving high-dose oral busulfan

PHYSICAL FINDINGS & CLINICAL PRESENTATION

- Hepatomegaly
- Right upper quadrant tenderness/pain
- Ascites
- Weight gain >5% of baseline
- Jaundice
- Peripheral edema

ETIOLOGY

Impaired metabolism of chemotherapy and metabolites leads to accumulation in zone 3 of the hepatic acinus, causing toxic sinusoidal endothelial cell injury. Direct injury of the endothelial cells leads to compromise of the fenestrated endothelium, which allows erythrocytes into the space of Disse. This causes extraluminal compression of the sinusoidal tract, sinusoidal thrombosis, and sloughing of endothelial cells, which then leads to central venous and sinusoidal obstruction. Collagen deposition and fibrotic obstruction occurs later in small and central hepatic veins. This ultimately leads to portal hypertension, reversal of hepatic venous flow, hepatorenal dysfunction, and multiorgan dysfunction.

DIAGNOSIS

DIFFERENTIAL DIAGNOSIS

- Budd-Chiari syndrome
- Graft-versus-host disease (GVHD)
- Acute drug toxicity
- Viral hepatitis
- Heart failure

WORKUP

- SOS should be considered in all patients who develop hepatic dysfunction after HSCT, especially within the first mo.
- SOS is a clinical diagnosis, with use of imaging and labs helpful for earlier diagnosis and to narrow the differential diagnosis. The European Group for Blood and Marrow Transplantation (EBMT) criteria for severity grading of a suspected SOS in adults is summarized in Table 1.
- Liver biopsy can be diagnostic but not required, and it is often impractical given elevated risks of bleeding in most HSCT patients. If liver biopsy is performed, the

TABLE 2 Risk Factors for Development of SOS

Pretransplant-Related Risk Factors	Odds Ratio
Bilirubin >1.5mg/dl	23.5
Inotuzumab treatment	22
Gemtuzumab treatment	19.8
Norethisterone treatment	10.1
Young age	5.2-9.5
Acyclovir	4.8
GSTM1-null genotype	4.1
Thalassemia	4.0
Preexisting liver disease	3.4
Immunodeficiency	3.3
Ferritin levels >1000	3.1
CMV (+)	3.0
Prior abdominal radiation	2.9
Karnofsky score <90%	2.7
Transaminases >2.5 ULN	2.4-4.6
Vancomycin during cytopreduction	2.4
Impaired pulmonary function	2.4
Hepatitis C (+)	2.2
Underlying leukemia	2.2
Previous HSCT	1.9
Inborn errors of metabolism	1.8
Myelodysplasia	1.5
Transplant-Related Risk Factors	**Odds Ratio**
Allogenic vs autologous	2.8
Parental	4.6
Sibling	2.8
Unrelated donor/HLA mismatch	1.4
Haploidentical	1.9
High-dose/myeloablative therapy	2.3-7.9
Busulfan + thiotepa	8.8
Fludarabine	4.0
Busulfan + cyclophosphamide (CY)	3.9-5.1
BCNU + CY + etoposide	2.8
Busulfan vs. others	2.6-4.5
Busulfan based	2.43
Total body irradiation based	1.73
GVHD prophylaxis	4.2
Cyclosporine	3.3
Methotrexate + CY	~3
Sirolimus + methotrexate + tacrolimus	2.8
High-dose total body irradiation	
>12 Gy + CY	

TABLE 1 European Group for Blood and Marrow Transplantation (EBMT) Criteria for Severity Grading of a Suspected SOS in Adults

	Mild	Moderate	Severe	Very Severe
Time since initial symptoms	>7 days	5-7 days	≤4 days	Anytime
Bilirubin (mg/dl)	≥2 and <3	≥3 and <5	≥5 and <8	≥8
Bilirubin kinetics			Doubling with 48 hr	
Transaminases	≤2x normal	>2 and ≤5x normal	>5 and ≤8x normal	>8x normal
Weight increase	<5%	≥5% and <10%	≥5% and <10%	≥10%
Renal function	<1.2x baseline at transplant	≥1.2 and <1.5x baseline at transplant	≥1.5 and <2x baseline at transplant	≥2x baseline at transplant or other signs of MOD
Treatment	Supportive care; Pharmacologic therapy if progression of symptoms	Pharmacologic therapy if signs/symptoms persist or progress after 2 days or portal-hepatic venous gradient ≥10 mm Hg	Pharmacologic therapy	Pharmacologic therapy; hemodialysis if required

From Mohty et al: Prophylactic, preemptive, and curative treatment for sinusoidal obstruction syndrome/veno-occlusive disease in adult patients: a position statement from an international expert group, *Bone Marrow Transplantation* 55:485-495, 2020.

TABLE 3 Criteria Established for Diagnosis of SOS Patients

Modified Seattle	Baltimore	EBMT - Classical	EBMT – Late Onset	EBMT - Pediatric
At least 2 of the following before day 20 post-HSCT	Bilirubin ≥2 mg/dl before day 21 post-HSCT AND at least 2 of the following:	Bilirubin ≥2 mg/dl before day 21 post-HSCT AND at least 2 of the following:	Classical SOS beyond day 21 OR Histologically proven SOS OR At least 2 of the following:	Presence of at least 2 of the following with no limitation for time of onset:
Bilirubin ≥2 mg/dl			Bilirubin ≥2 mg/dl	Rising bilirubin on at least 3 consecutive days OR Bilirubin ≥2 mg/dl within 72 hr
Hepatomegaly, RUQ pain	Hepatomegaly	Painful hepatomegaly	Painful hepatomegaly	Hepatomegaly
Ascites with or w/o unexplained weight gain >2% from baseline	Ascites	Ascites	Ascites AND Hemodynamical and/or ultrasound evidence of SOS	Ascites Unexplained consumptive and transfusion-refractory thrombocytopenia
	Weight gain >5% from baseline	Weight gain >5% from baseline	Weight gain >5% from baseline	Unexplained weight gain on 3 consecutive days (despite diuretics) OR Weight gain >5% from baseline

EBMT, European Society for Blood and Marrow Transplantation.
From Richardson PG et al: Defibrotide sodium for the treatment of hepatic veno-occlusive disease/sinusoidal obstruction syndrome, *Expert Rev Clin Pharmacol*, 11(2):113-124, 2018.

TABLE 4 Different Imaging Modalities for SOS and Their Findings

Modality		Role	Findings
Ultrasound	B-mode	Screening and early differential diagnosis, especially in asymptomatic or late-onset cases	Hepatosplenomegaly Gallbladder wall thickening >6 mm Portal diameter >12 mm Hepatic vein diameter <3 mm Ascites
	Doppler	Surveillance and diagnostic, revealing morphologic changes, and flow velocity fluctuations	Hepatic vein diameter <3 mm Collateral circulatory visualization Demodulation of portal vein flow Spectral density decline Congestion index <0.1 Portal vein flow <10 cm/s Hepatic artery resistive index >0.75 Monophasic flow in hepatic veins
	Contrast enhanced	Rapid diagnosis and differential diagnosis	Diffuse/geographic enhancement of parenchyma Scattered hypoechoic areas Hypoechoic lesion with hypervascularity in the arterial phase and rapid wash-out in portal phase
CT		Diagnostic	Cloverleaf or clawlike shapes Lesion with peritumoral enhancement and central low attenuation
MRI	Gadolinium enhanced	Diagnostic	Cloverleaf or clawlike shapes; peritumoral enhancement lesion with central low-signal intensity
	Gadoxetate enhanced	Diagnostic and provides information about liver function	Diffuse or geographic hypointensity
	Susceptibility-weighted imaging	Differential diagnosis	Geographic or nodular hypointensity

From Zhang Y et al: Noninvasive imaging diagnosis of sinusoidal obstruction syndrome: a pictorial review, *Insights Imaging* 10:110, 2019.

transjugular approach is preferred for safety reasons and because it allows for measurement of the portal-hepatic venous pressure gradient. A portal-hepatic venous pressure gradient >10 mm Hg is consistent with SOS, with a high specificity and high positive-predictive value.

- Three diagnostic criteria have been proposed. The Baltimore criteria has a higher specificity and is included as part of the EBMT criteria (Table 3) for classical SOS. However, multiple analyses have demonstrated improved outcomes using the modified Seattle criteria because it does not require waiting for hyperbilirubinemia to develop when disease may be more severe.

LABORATORY TESTS

- Liver function panel, including GGT
- Complete blood count
- Prothrombin time (PTT)/International Normalized Ratio (INR)
- Comprehensive metabolic panel including magnesium, phosphate, and lactate dehydrogenase
- Lipase, amylase
- Ammonia
- Viral serologies (HBV, HCV, HSV, CMV)

IMAGING STUDIES

Hepatosplenomegaly, ascites, a thickened gallbladder wall, and periportal edema are the hallmark imaging features of SOS. However, SOS is a clinical diagnosis and does not require imaging except in late onset. Imaging (Table 4) is most helpful in narrowing down the differential diagnosis early on and provide timely treatment.

Rx TREATMENT

NONPHARMACOLOGIC THERAPY

- Fluid and sodium balance
- Avoidance of hepatotoxic and nephrotoxic medications
- Symptomatic treatment (analgesia, oxygen, thoracentesis, paracentesis)
- Hemodialysis (~25% of patients)
- Transjugular intrahepatic portosystemic shunt (TIPS) or liver transplant can be considered in severe cases of refractory ascites or portal hypertension

ACUTE GENERAL Rx

- Defibrotide is the only approved therapy for SOS. It augments plasmin enzymatic activity to hydrolyze fibrin clots and generally acts to protect endothelial cells and restore the thrombolytic-fibrinolytic balance.
  - In the U.S., it is indicated for adult and pediatric patients with renal or pulmonary dysfunction and has been shown to improve survival at day +100.
  - Earlier initiation has been linked to improved survival.
  - It has a safety profile similar to that of best supportive care.
  - It is dosed at 25 mg/kg/day divided into 4 doses daily for 21 days.
  - Evidence is lacking for alternative pharmacological therapies to defibrotide.

DISPOSITION

- Mortality for patients who develop severe SOS with multiorgan dysfunction, characterized by renal and pulmonary dysfunction, is estimated at >80%.
- Late-onset SOS will occur in ~20% of children, but is unusual in adults.

REFERRAL

- Gastroenterology and hematology/oncology consultation to confirm diagnosis
- Nephrology consultation for patients who may require dialysis
- Critical care consultation for patients with multiorgan failure

PEARLS & CONSIDERATIONS

COMMENTS

- Early recognition and treatment are essential for patient survival; SOS should be considered in any patient after HSCT who develops liver dysfunction.
- Hepatomegaly, right upper quadrant pain, ascites, weight gain, and jaundice are the hallmarks of SOS.
- Defibrotide is the only approved treatment for SOS.

PREVENTION

- Defibrotide is not currently approved for use as prophylaxis for SOS, but previous studies have shown promising results and phase 3 trials are ongoing (ClinicalTrials.gov identifier NCT02851407).

SUGGESTED READINGS

Available at ExpertConsult.com

AUTHOR: **Brian D. Mikolasko, MD**

BASIC INFORMATION

DEFINITION

Sjögren syndrome (SS) is a chronic autoimmune disorder that targets exocrine glands. It is characterized by lymphocytic and plasma cell infiltration and destruction of salivary, lacrimal, and parotid glands, resulting predominantly in dry eyes and dry mouth, but it can affect other organ systems as well.

Primary and secondary forms have been described:

- Primary: Dry mouth (xerostomia) and dry eyes (xerophthalmia) develop as isolated entities. Is immunogenetically associated with HLA-DRB1*0301 and DRB1*1501 and serologically associated with antibodies to Ro/SS-A and La/SS-B.
- Secondary: Associated with other autoimmune connective tissue diseases. The immunogenetic and serologic findings are usually those of the accompanying disease (e.g., HLA-DR4 if associated with RA).

SYNONYMS

SS
Sicca syndrome
Keratoconjunctivitis sicca
Sicca complex
Dry eye syndrome/dysfunctional tear syndrome

ICD-10CM CODES

M35.00	Sicca syndrome, unspecified
M35.01	Sicca syndrome with keratoconjunctivitis
M35.02	Sicca syndrome with lung involvement
M35.03	Sicca syndrome with myopathy
M35.04	Sicca syndrome with tubulo-interstitial nephropathy
M35.09	Sicca syndrome with other organ involvement

EPIDEMIOLOGY & DEMOGRAPHICS

INCIDENCE: 4 per 100,000; of these cases, 70% had primary SS.

PREVALENCE: Prevalence is 0.2% to 2.7% of population; secondary SS is also common and can affect up to 19% of patients with systemic lupus erythematosus (SLE) and 26% to 31% of rheumatoid arthritis (RA) and scleroderma patients.

PREDOMINANT SEX: Female:male ratio is approximately 10:1.

PREDOMINANT AGE: Peak incidence is the fourth and fifth decade, but can occur in all ages. Rarely reported in children.

RISK FACTOR: Seen in all races/ethnicities, but more common in Caucasians.

PHYSICAL FINDINGS & CLINICAL PRESENTATION

SS is one of the most common autoimmune diseases and should be considered in any patient with unexplained symptoms and a positive antinuclear antibody.

2016 American College of Rheumatology/European League Against Rheumatism classification criteria for primary SS: A score of >4 when the weights from the criteria are summed:

- Labial salivary gland with focal lymphocytic sialadenitis and focus of >1 foci/4 mm^2—score 3
- Anti-SSA/Ro positive—score 3
- Ocular staining score >5 in at least one eye—score 1
- Schirmer test <5 mm/5 min in at least one eye—score 1
- Unstimulated whole saliva flow rate <0.1 ml/min—score 1
- Diagnosis of SS based on the prior diagnostic criteria was presence of at least two of three objective diagnostic tests below:
  1. Positive serum levels of anti-SS-A/Ro and/or anti-SS-B/La or a positive rheumatoid factor and antinuclear antibody (ANA) titer of at least 1:320
  2. Salivary gland biopsy exhibiting focal sites of inflammation. One or more sites of inflammation per 4 mm^2 are considered to be positive
  3. Keratoconjunctivitis sicca with ocular staining score of three or more (the dissipation rate of a specialized dye that is applied to the tear film that bathes the surface of the eye; a score of three or more is considered to be positive)

Manifestations:

- Dry mouth, dry lips (cheilosis), erythema, and hyperlobulation of tongue (Fig. E1) and other mucosal surfaces, carious teeth
- Dry eyes (conjunctival injection, corneal ulceration, blurred vision, decreased luster, enlargement of lacrimal glands, and irregularity of the corneal light reflex)
- Salivary gland enlargement (Fig. E2) and dysfunction, with subsequent difficulty in chewing and swallowing food and in speaking without frequent water intake, thickened saliva, and burning sensation in mouth
- Extraglandular involvement occurs in 50% of patients. There are multiple systemic manifestations associated with SS, which include the following:
  1. Fever/fatigue.
  2. Cutaneous vasculitis may be present, usually of lower extremities.
  3. Skin ulceration, photosensitivity, Raynaud phenomenon.
  4. Dyspareunia and pruritus can occur secondary to vaginal dryness.
  5. Pulmonary involvement includes interstitial lung disease (NSIP, UIP); lymphocytic interstitial pneumonitis (LIP) and cryptogenic organizing pneumonia (COP); chronic obstructive pulmonary disease; fibrosis; and xerotrachea.
  6. Gastrointestinal: Celiac disease, esophageal dysmotility, type I autoimmune hepatitis, primary biliary cirrhosis, and pancreatitis can occur.
  7. Renal manifestations: Type 1 renal tubular acidosis, Fanconi syndrome, glomerulonephritis, and interstitial nephritis.
  8. Neurologic involvement: Peripheral, cranial, or autonomic neuropathy; CNS involvement also possible, cognitive dysfunction ("brain fog").
  9. Musculoskeletal: Arthralgias and myopathy.
  10. Hematologic: Cytopenias, hypergammaglobulinemia, cryoglobulins. Increased lymphoma risk, with 5% to 10% developing non-Hodgkin lymphoma.
  11. RA and other connective tissue diseases are seen commonly with secondary SS.
  12. Autoimmune thyroiditis may be observed in patients with SS.
  13. Pregnancy: Patients with anti-SSA antibodies have an increased risk of delivering a baby with neonatal lupus, with cutaneous manifestations or congenital heart block.

ETIOLOGY

Sjögren syndrome is an autoimmune disorder of unclear etiology. It is associated with certain HLA-DQ and HLA-DR alleles. It has been postulated that viral agents (e.g., hepatitis C and Epstein-Barr virus) may trigger the clinical manifestations. The pathogenesis involves a complex interplay of several factors, including genetic and epigenetic controls of immune homeostasis and gene expression, age, gender, and environmental insults.

Over 90% of the infiltrating cells are CD4+ T lymphocytes with memory phenotype (70%) and B lymphocytes (20%). The remaining 10% are an admixture of plasma cells, CD8+ T lymphocytes, T regulatory cells, natural killer cells, and dendritic cells. Predominantly Th1- and Th17-driven response.

Dx DIAGNOSIS

DIFFERENTIAL DIAGNOSIS

- Medication-related dryness (e.g., anticholinergics, antihistamines, diuretics, benzodiazepines, antidepressants)
- Age-related exocrine gland dysfunction
- Mouth breathing, anxiety
- Infections such as viruses, HIV, hepatitis C
- Diabetes mellitus, acromegaly, type V hyperlipidemia
- Chronic sialadenitis
- Graft-versus-host disease
- IgG4-related disease
- Ocular herpetic lesions, blepharitis, corneal abrasions, contact lens irritation
- Vitamin A deficiency
- Other: Sarcoidosis, primary salivary hypofunction, radiation injury, amyloidosis
- An algorithm for the diagnosis of SS is provided in Fig. 3

WORKUP

Workup involves ocular and oral examination and laboratory and radiographic testing to demonstrate the following criteria for diagnosis of primary and secondary SS.

- Symptoms and objective signs of ocular dryness:

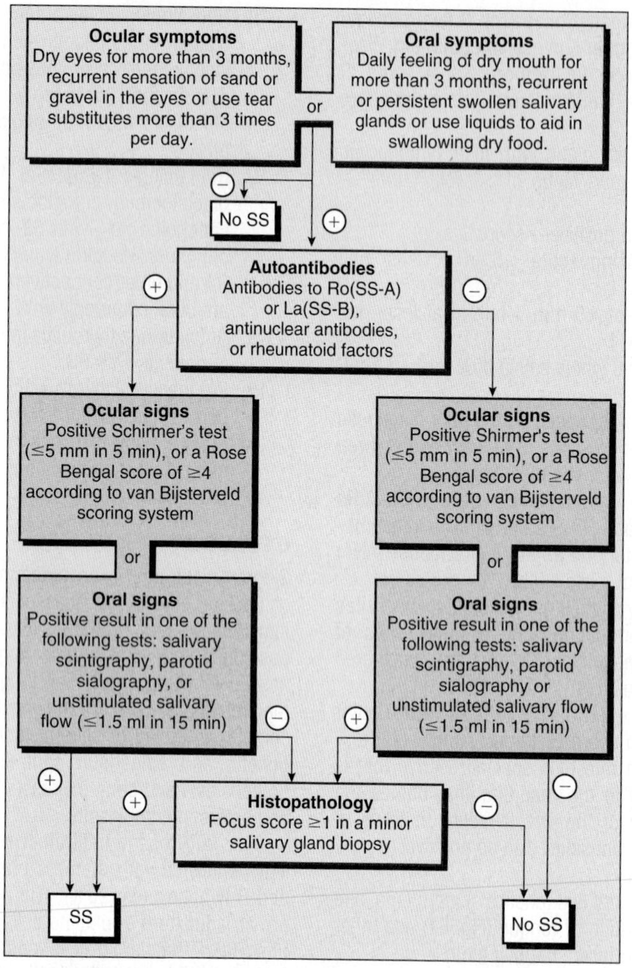

FIG. 3 Suggested algorithm for the diagnosis of Sjögren syndrome. Exclusion criteria include hepatitis C or human immunodeficiency virus infection, sarcoidosis, graft-versus-host disease, preexisting lymphoma, previous head or neck irradiation, and use of anticholinergic drugs. (From Hochberg MC et al: *Rheumatology*, ed 5, St Louis, 2011, Mosby.)

1. Schirmer test (Fig. E4): <5 mm wetting per 5 min. (Normal wetting is >15 mm in 5 min). There is a 15% false-positive and false-negative rate.
2. Zone-quick diagnostic threads: A sterile cotton thread with pH indicator, phenol red. Yellow turns to red in contact with tears.
3. Positive Rose Bengal stains dead/dying cells.
4. Tear breakup time and tear osmolality measured after instillation of fluorescein.

- Symptoms and objective signs of dry mouth:
  1. Decreased parotid flow using Lashley cups or other methods
  2. Abnormal biopsy result of minor salivary gland (focus score >1 based on average of four assessable lobules)
  3. Sialometry (sensitivity 56%, specificity 81%): Assessment of rate of saliva production in which collection of ≤1.5 ml after two expectorations 15 min apart is considered positive
- Evidence of systemic autoimmune disorder:
  1. Elevated rheumatoid factor (70% to 90% of patients)
  2. Elevated titer of ANA >1:320 (80% of patients)
  3. Presence of anti-SS-A (Ro) (>60% of patients) or anti-SS-B (La) antibodies (40% of patients)

SECONDARY:
- Characteristic signs and symptoms of SS
- Clinical features sufficient to allow a diagnosis of RA, SLE, polymyositis, or scleroderma

LABORATORY TESTS
- Positive ANA (80% of patients) with autoantibodies anti-SS-A and anti-SS-B may be present.
- Additional laboratory abnormalities may include elevated erythrocyte sedimentation rate, anemia, leukopenia, thrombocytopenia, abnormal liver function studies, elevated serum beta$_2$ microglobulin levels, rheumatoid factor (50% to 60%), hypergammaglobulinemia, antibodies to double-stranded DNA (in cases with proteinuria), depressed C3 and C4, and the presence of cryoglobulins (30% of patients).
- A definite diagnosis of SS can be made with a salivary gland biopsy (gold standard) showing focal lymphocytic sialadenitis with focus score of 1 per 4 mm^2 of glandular tissue.
- Salivary gland ultrasound can be done to characterize changes in salivary gland parenchyma (sensitivity 75%, specificity 78%). Diseased gland shows hypoechoic areas with convex borders.
- MRI of the gland shows inhomogeneous parenchyma. Finding generally correlates with biopsy of the gland.

Rx TREATMENT

NONPHARMACOLOGIC THERAPY
- Adequate fluid replacement: Ameliorate skin dryness by gently blotting dry after bathing, leaving a small amount of moisture, and then applying a moisturizer
- Increased environmental moisture by using humidifiers
- Proper oral hygiene (daily topical fluoride use, antimicrobial mouth rinses, and stabilization of oral cavity pH) to reduce the incidence of caries
- Sugar-free chewing gum and sour lemon lozenges to stimulate salivary secretion
- Periodic dental and ophthalmologic evaluations to screen for complications
- Exercise: Education about self-care measures to reduce fatigue
- Reduce caffeine intake and smoking

GENERAL Rx
- Use artificial tears frequently.
- Muscarinic agonists: Pilocarpine (5 mg PO qid) or cevimeline (30 mg PO tid) can be useful to improve oral dryness.
- Ophthalmic cyclosporine and lifitegrast drops may be useful for dry eyes.
- Hydroxychloroquine alone or in conjunction with methotrexate may be useful for arthralgias and cutaneous manifestations.
- Oral cyclosporine only improves the symptoms of subjective dryness.
- Tumor necrosis factor (TNF) antagonists have not shown benefit in short-duration placebo-controlled trials.
- Dehydroepiandrosterone (DHEA) is not recommended for treatment of fatigue.
- Rituximab (RTX) has been shown to affect some improvement in oral dry mouth symptoms, relieving marked salivary and lacrimal gland swelling in a retrospective review.
- Propionic acid gel can be used for vaginal dryness.
- Systemic manifestations are treated according to symptoms and complications.
- Cyclophosphamide, azathioprine, and mycophenolate mofetil are generally reserved for life-threatening extraglandular manifestations.
- Fig. 5 describes a treatment algorithm for Sjögren syndrome.

REFERRAL
- Rheumatology referral is generally indicated.

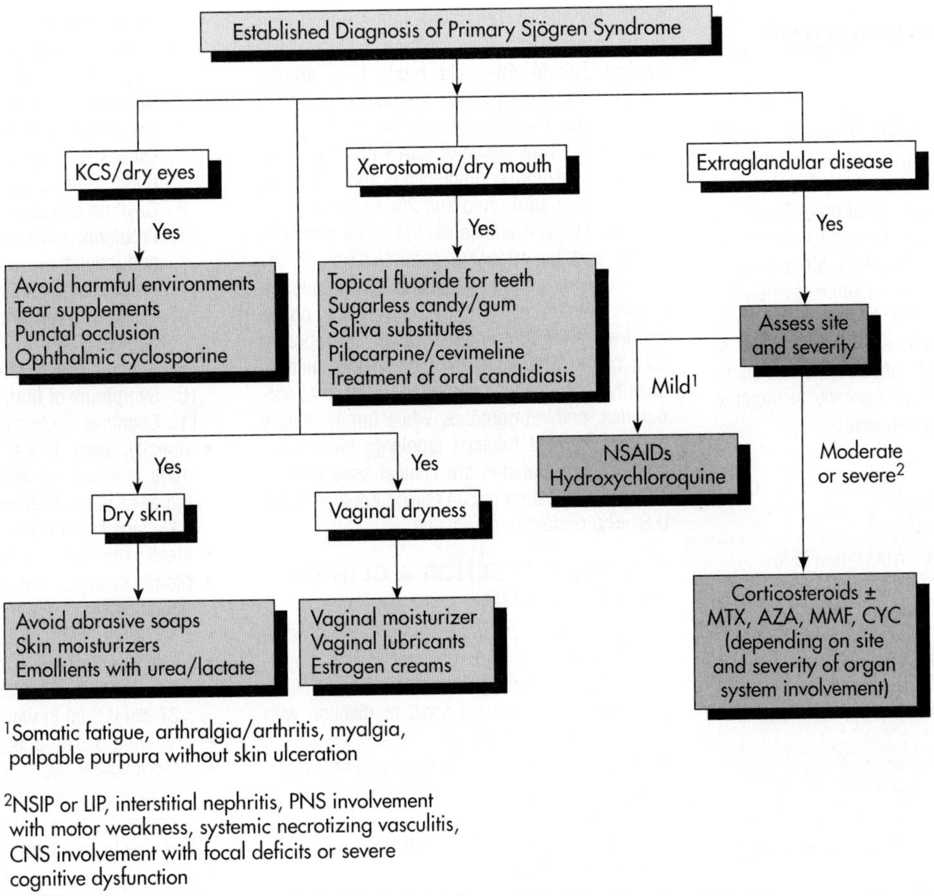

FIG. 5 Treatment algorithm for Sjögren syndrome. The treatment of Sjögren syndrome usually requires a multidisciplinary approach involving rheumatologists, ophthalmologists, dentists/oral surgeons, otolaryngologists, and other subspecialists, depending on the extent of extraglandular disease. In all cases, it is prudent to minimize the use of medications that can exacerbate the symptoms of dryness, such as antihistamines, antidepressants, muscle relaxers, and other drugs with anticholinergic properties. The treatment of extra-glandular disease is individualized according to the site and severity of organ system involvement. The approaches indicated in the algorithm for the treatment of extra-glandular disease are not supported by evidence from randomized, controlled trials, but rather from expert opinion based on retrospective case series and clinical experience. *AZA,* Azathioprine; *CNS,* central nervous system; *CYC,* cyclophosphamide; *KCS,* keratoconjunctivitis sicca; *LIP,* lymphocytic interstitial pneumonitis; *MMF,* mycophenolate mofetil; *MTX,* methotrexate; *NSAIDs,* nonsteroidal antiinflammatory drugs; *NSIP,* nonspecific interstitial pneumonitis; *PNS,* peripheral nervous system. (From Firestein GS et al: *Kelly's textbook of rheumatology,* ed 9, Philadelphia, 2013, Saunders.)

- Referral should be made to an oncologist when lymphoma is suspected.
- During pregnancy, if patient tests positive for SSA/SSB antibody, should seek consultation with a perinatologist.

PEARLS & COSIDERATIONS

COMMENTS

- Unusual presentations of SS may occur in association with polymyalgia rheumatica, chronic fatigue syndrome, fever of unknown origin, and inflammatory myositis.
- The most serious complication of primary SS is the development of non-Hodgkin lymphoma and other lymphoproliferative disorders, which occur at a tenfold to forty-fourfold increased rate as compared to age-matched controls.
- The presence of parotid gland enlargement, rheumatoid factor, low C4, cryoglobulinemia, lymphopenia, and higher levels of disease activity as measured by EULAR Sjögren Syndrome Disease Activity Index (ESSDAI) predicts a higher lymphoma risk.

SUGGESTED READINGS

Available at ExpertConsult.com

RELATED CONTENT

Sjögren Syndrome (Patient Information)

AUTHOR: **Pieusha Malhotra, MD, MPH**

BASIC INFORMATION

DEFINITION

The *International Classification of Sleep Disorders, Third Edition,* classifies sleep-disordered breathing disorders into five categories: central sleep apnea syndrome (Table 1), obstructive sleep apnea disorders (OSA), sleep-related hypoventilation disorders, sleep-related hypoxemia disorder, and isolated symptoms and normal variants. The American Academy of *Sleep Medicine* defines OSA as repetitive episodes of upper airway obstruction that occur during sleep and that are typically associated with oxyhemoglobin desaturations.

SYNONYMS

Sleep apnea syndrome
Sleep-disordered breathing
Obstructive sleep apnea syndrome (OSA)
Obstructive sleep apnea–hypopnea syndrome

ICD-10CM CODES

G47.30	Sleep apnea, unspecified
G47.31	Primary central sleep apnea
G47.33	Obstructive sleep apnea (adult) (pediatric)
G47.37	Central sleep apnea in conditions classified elsewhere
G47.39	Other sleep apnea
P28.3	Primary sleep apnea of newborn

EPIDEMIOLOGY & DEMOGRAPHICS

OSA is a common disease in the U.S. Data from the Wisconsin Cohort Study indicated that the current prevalence of moderate to severe sleep-disordered breathing (apnea-hypopnea index, measured as events/hour, ≥15) is 10% among 30- to 49-yr-old men; 17% among 50- to 70-yr-old men; 3% among 30- to 49-yr-old women; and 9% among 50- to 70-yr-old women. The prevalence of OSA with associated excessive daytime somnolence is approximately 3% to 7% in adult men and 2% to 5% in adult women. The prevalence seems to be higher in obese and hypertensive patients. The prevalence of OSA in the general pediatric population is estimated to be 1% to 6%. However, in obese children and adolescents, OSAH is reported to occur in 19% to 61%. Risk factors include obesity, craniofacial and upper airway abnormalities, and retrognathia, while family history of OSA, current tobacco smoking, nasal congestion, and diabetes are clinical associations. There are an estimated 24 million persons in the U.S. who remain undiagnosed.

PHYSICAL FINDINGS & CLINICAL PRESENTATION

- Many patients are unaware that their breathing is affected and may not visit a physician for evaluation. Others may not consider sleepiness a relevant topic to discuss with their health care provider.
- Nocturnal symptoms, including gastroesophageal reflux symptoms, nocturia, and angina pectoris
- Snoring (potentially loud, habitual, and bothersome to others)
- Witnessed apneas that often interrupt snoring and end with a snort
- Gasping, choking, or smothering sensations that arouse the patient from sleep
- Restless sleep associated with frequent arousals
- Daytime symptoms:
  1. Nonrestorative sleep
  2. Not feeling refreshed upon awakening
  3. Morning headache
  4. Dry mouth or throat upon awakening
  5. Excessive daytime sleepiness, typically during quiet activities
  6. Daytime fatigue or tiredness
  7. Problems with memory, concentration, and cognitive function, especially with executive functioning
  8. Easily angered, short tempered, and inattentive
  9. Hyperactivity in children
  10. Symptoms of fibromyalgia
  11. Cognitive decline (older population)
- Obesity (body mass index >30 kg/m2). A 10% increase in weight predicts a sixfold increase in the likelihood of developing clinically significant OSA
- Insulin resistance or type 2 diabetes mellitus
- Mood swings, irritability, anxiety, and/or depression
- Decreased libido and/or impotence
- Neck circumference (surrogate marker for central obesity) of >43 cm (17 in) in men and >37 cm (15 in) in women
- Erythematous oropharynx because of snoring
- Adenotonsillar hypertrophy, excessive soft tissue, high-arched hard palate, pendulous uvula, prominent tongue, large degree of overjet, and retrognathia or micrognathia can be present
- Narrowing of lateral airway walls is independent predictor of OSA in men but not women
- Craniofacial skeletal abnormalities can lead to OSA, particularly among children and nonobese adults
- Systemic hypertension (HTN)
- Pulmonary HTN
- Family history of OSA increases risk with each additional close family member further increasing odds
- Table 2 summarizes clinical characteristics of patients with sleep apnea

TABLE 1 Pathophysiologic Classification of Central Sleep Apneas

Physiologic	Pathologic
• Sleep transition • Phasic REM	Nonhypercapnic • Medical condition related 1. Congestive heart failure 2. Poststroke 3. ESRD 4. PAH 5. Atrial fibrillation • High altitude • Idiopathic Hypercapnic • Congenital central hypoventilation syndrome • Primary chronic alveolar hypoventilation syndromes • Other CNS disorders associated with CSA 1. Encephalitis, tumors, strokes 2. Anatomic abnormalities 3. Neurodegenerative disorders • Muscular and PNS disorders associated with CSA (selected examples) 1. Muscular dystrophies 2. Acid maltase deficiency 3. Charcot-Marie-Tooth disease and other neuropathies 4. Postpolio syndrome 5. Myasthenia gravis Disintegrative (e.g., brainstem injury, opioid induced) CSA with OSA or upper airway disorders (including treatment emergent CSA)

CNS, Central nervous system; *CSA,* central sleep apnea; *ESRD,* end-stage renal disease; *OSA,* obstructive sleep apnea; *PAH,* pulmonary arterial hypertension, *PNS,* peripheral nervous system; *REM,* rapid eye movements.
From Kryger M et al: *Principles and practice of sleep medicine,* ed 6, Philadelphia, 2017, Elsevier.

ETIOLOGY

- Narrowing of upper airway as a result of obesity or increased peripharyngeal fat deposition, retrognathia and/or micrognathia, adenotonsillar hypertrophy, macroglossia, or neuromuscular weakness (Fig. E1)
- Upper airway muscular weakness as a result of neuromuscular disorders, primary CNS disorders (e.g., stroke), or metabolic disorders
- Other diseases associated with the development of OSAH (e.g., hypothyroidism, acromegaly)
- Fig. E2 illustrates the pathophysiologic consequences of OSA

Dx DIAGNOSIS

DIFFERENTIAL DIAGNOSIS

- Anemia
- Anxiety or panic disorder
- Behaviorally induced insufficient sleep syndrome
- Cardiac or heart disease
- Central sleep apnea
- Circadian rhythm disorder

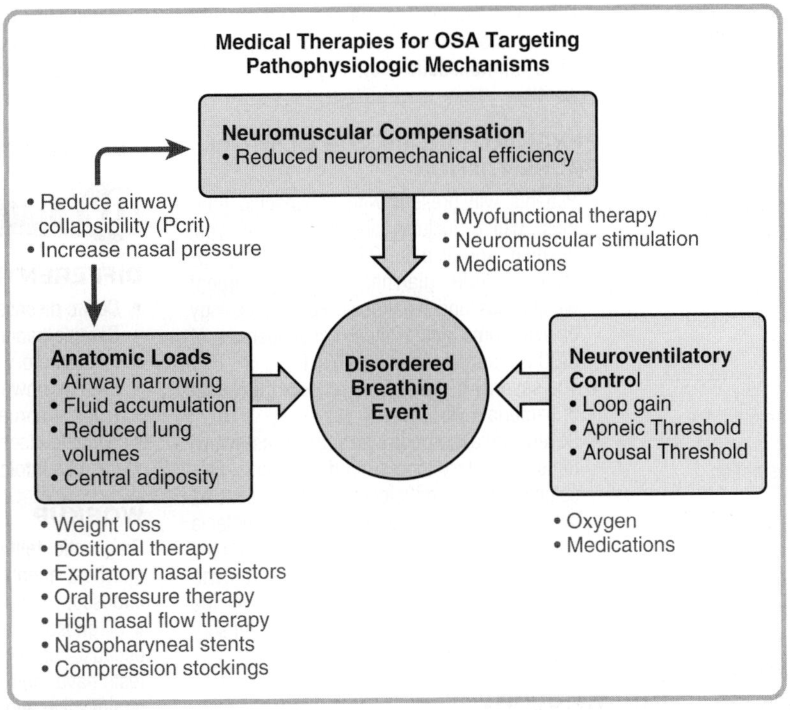

FIG. 5 Medical therapies for obstructive sleep apnea *(OSA)*, stratified by mechanisms targeted. Certain therapies can be considered on the basis of the pathophysiologic mechanisms targeted. OSA is thought to occur as a consequence of increases in anatomic loads on the upper airway, impairments in neuromuscular compensation, or alterations in neuroventilatory control. Traditional therapies such as continuous positive airway pressure (CPAP) use nasal pressure to overcome anatomic loads. By contrast, upper airway surgery or weight loss results in reduced airway collapsibility (Pcrit). Other therapies that may relieve anatomic loads on the upper airway include positional therapy, use of expiratory nasal resistors, oral pressure therapy, nasopharyngeal stenting, and application of compression stockings. Therapies that address impairments in neuromuscular function include myofunctional therapies, use of certain medications, and neuromuscular stimulation. Therapies that may affect neuroventilatory control include use of medications to increase the arousal threshold and supplemental oxygen, which can affect loop gain. (From Kryger M et al: *Principles and practice of sleep medicine,* ed 6, Philadelphia, 2017, Elsevier.)

- Surgical treatment:
  1. Surgery is done to correct specific anatomic areas of narrowing: nasal, pharyngeal, and tongue base/hypopharynx.
  2. Adenotonsillectomy is often curative for children with OSA.
  3. Nasal septoplasty/turbinectomy should be considered for patients with nasoseptal deformities.
  4. Uvulopalatopharyngoplasty, which involves resection of the uvula and soft palate, is effective for a small number of patients. Predicting which patients will benefit from this surgical treatment is difficult.
  5. Palatal implant surgery and distraction osteogenesis maxillary expansion (DOME) for high-arched palates are other surgical options.
  6. Hypoglossal nerve stimulation (by surgical placement of an implant in the upper chest) helps recruit lingual muscles, reduce pharyngeal collapsibility, and decrease upper airway resistance.
  7. Tracheostomy is typically reserved for patients with very severe OSA who failed medical therapy or who have cor pulmonale.

DISPOSITION

- The short-term prognosis for excessive daytime sleepiness and snoring is good to excellent with the regular use of CPAP, but no studies have been performed to address the long-term effects in a large population of patients.
- Residual symptoms of excessive daytime sleepiness can occur in some patients with OSA despite regular CPAP use. This has led the FDA to approve modafinil for the management of residual sleepiness.

REFERRAL

- Highly trained sleep specialists with expertise in caring for patients with OSA are recommended, especially for complex cases.
- Surgical referral to otolaryngology should be considered for children with adenotonsillar hypertrophy and for adults who are unresponsive to weight loss and CPAP therapy.
- Referral to a qualified dentist for treatment with an oral appliance may be useful for certain patients with mild OSA.

PEARLS & CONSIDERATIONS

- OSAH is a common disorder that is underrecognized and underdiagnosed, so the identification of risk factors is crucial for making the correct diagnosis.
- The prevalence of OSA increases among women after menopause.
- The single most effective therapy for OSA is CPAP administered by nasal or facial masks or other interfaces if required.
- Patients with OSA are more vulnerable than healthy persons to the effects of alcohol consumption and sleep restriction with regard to various driving performance variables.
- OSA is a risk factor for systemic and pulmonary HTN, stroke, atrial fibrillation, and coronary artery disease. In patients with untreated HTN and OSA, the use of CPAP results in small but statistically significant reductions in blood pressure. Therapy with CPAP has not been shown to prevent cardiovascular events in patients with moderate-to-severe obstructive sleep apnea and established cardiovascular disease.
- OSA may also be an independent risk factor for peptic ulcer bleeding.
- Ethnic differences may exist for some populations, with South Asians having a higher prevalence and risk for cardiovascular side effects.

SUGGESTED READINGS

Available at ExpertConsult.com

RELATED CONTENT

Sleep Apnea (Patient Information)

AUTHORS: **Grace Rebecca Paul, MBBS, MD,** and **Don Hayes Jr, MD, MS, Med**

Small Bowel Bacterial Overgrowth (SIBO) PTG

BASIC INFORMATION

DEFINITION

Small bowel bacterial overgrowth (SIBO) is the presence of excessive native and/or nonnative bacteria in the small intestine (bacterial count >10^5/ml per jejunal aspirate) causing chronic diarrhea and malabsorption.

SYNONYMS

Bacterial overgrowth syndrome
SIBO

ICD-10CM CODES	
K90.4	Malabsorption due to intolerance, NEC
K90.89	Other intestinal malabsorption

EPIDEMIOLOGY & DEMOGRAPHICS

PREVALENCE: The prevalence of SIBO is varied based on the population studied and the diagnostic tests used. It has shown to be prevalent in up to 12.5% to 20% of the healthy population using glucose and lactulose breath test.

PREDOMINANT SEX & AGE: SIBO affects predominantly the elderly population or those with recent UGI surgery, including bariatric surgery. The elderly population has decreased gastric secretion and hypomotility due to age-associated decline as well as increased use of motility-altering medications.

RISK FACTORS:

- Advanced age is a known risk factor as there is thought to be an age-associated decline in GI motility.
- Patients with irritable bowel syndrome have a higher prevalence of SIBO compared to the general population. Initial studies have shown up to 65% to 80% of IBS patients with confirmed SIBO with an abnormal lactulose breath test.
- Other risk factors include UGI tract surgery, inflammatory bowel disease, chronic pancreatitis, immunodeficiency, liver disease, and obesity.

PHYSICAL FINDINGS & CLINICAL PRESENTATION

- Patients will present with nonspecific findings, which include abdominal distention, bloating, and/or pain. Other common symptoms include diarrhea and subsequent weight loss and weakness. Pathophysiology of symptoms and clinical consequences of SIBO are summarized in Table 1.
- The severity of symptoms reflects the extent of bacterial overgrowth.
- Severe malabsorption can present as symptoms secondary to vitamin deficiencies. Fat-soluble vitamin deficiencies can present as night blindness (vitamin A), osteomalacia and hypocalcemia (vitamin D), or prolonged bleeding (vitamin K). Bacterial overgrowth can affect vitamin B_{12} absorption in the ileum, leading to neuropathies with sensory ataxia.

ETIOLOGY

Disorders that disrupt protective mechanisms against bacterial burden predispose patients to SIBO. Box 1 summarizes diseases and disorders linked to SIBO based on pathophysiology.

- Patients with structural or anatomical abnormalities are at greater risk. These include patients with small bowel diverticula, small intestinal strictures, surgical blind loops, ileocecal resections, or gastric resections (increasing common cause of SIBO).
- Motility disorders predispose to SIBO because of the ineffective clearance of bacteria from the proximal bowel into the colon. Examples of this include gastroparesis and small bowel dysmotility, both suggestive of poorly controlled diabetes. Long-standing celiac disease can also interfere with small bowel motility.
- It is thought that recent antibiotic use as well as antacid medication can alter the normal bacterial flora in the small intestine, contributing to SIBO.

Dx DIAGNOSIS

DIFFERENTIAL DIAGNOSIS

- Celiac disease
- Chronic pancreatitis
- Inflammatory bowel disease
- Irritable bowel syndrome
- Tropical sprue
- Whipple disease
- Lactose intolerance

WORKUP

Diagnostic testing should include workup for diarrhea, anemia, and malabsorption. Although endoscopy with jejunal aspirate and culture was a diagnostic tool of choice, its role is limited because of low specificity. Hydrogen breath tests have their limitations as well, but they are noninvasive and easy to perform.

LABORATORY TESTS

- Breath tests have become more commonplace in diagnosing SIBO. Typically fermenting bacteria reside in the colon. In SIBO, fermenting bacteria is present in the small intestine as well. A carbohydrate test dose (typically lactulose or glucose) is given and its byproduct (hydrogen) is measured as it is excreted in the breath. In SIBO, exhaled hydrogen concentrations rise early.
- Standard anemia workup is essential. CBC may suggest macrocytic anemia secondary to B_{12} deficiency.
- Nutritional status should be evaluated with albumin levels.

TABLE 1 Pathophysiology of Symptoms and Clinical Consequences in Small Bowel Bacterial Overgrowth

Process	Mechanisms of Action	Clinical Consequences
Mucosal injury induced by bacteria and/or their toxins or products	Loss of brush-border enzymes	Carbohydrate maldigestion
	Injury to epithelial barrier leading to enhanced intestinal permeability	Protein-losing enteropathy; bacterial translocation and portal and systemic endotoxemia
	Inflammatory response generating inflammatory cytokines	Liver injury and inflammation, systemic inflammatory responses
Luminal competition with the host for nutrients	Consumption of dietary protein	Hypoproteinemia, edema
	Consumption of vitamin B_{12}	B_{12} deficiency, megaloblastic anemia, neurologic symptoms
	Consumption of thiamine	Thiamine deficiency
	Consumption of nicotinamide	Nicotinamide deficiency
Bacterial metabolism	Fermentation of unabsorbed carbohydrates	Bloating, distension, flatulence
	Deconjugation of primary bile acids	Diarrhea due to the effects of deconjugated bile acids in the colon; depletion of the bile acid pool leading to fat and fat-soluble vitamin malabsorption
	Synthesis of vitamin K	Interference with dosing of vitamin K antagonists (e.g., warfarin)
	Synthesis of folate	High serum folate levels
	Synthesis of D-lactic acid	D-lactic acidosis
	Synthesis of alcohol	Liver injury
	Synthesis of acetaldehyde	Liver injury

From Feldman M et al: *Sleisenger and Fordtran's gastrointestinal and liver disease*, ed 10, Philadelphia, 2016, Elsevier.

BOX 1 Diseases and Disorders Linked to Small Bowel Bacterial Overgrowth (SIBO) Based on Pathophysiology

Dysmotility
Acromegaly:
- Amyloidosis
- Chronic opiate use
- Diabetic autonomic neuropathy
- Gastroparesis
- Hypothyroidism
- Idiopathic intestinal pseudo-obstruction
- Long-standing use of motility-suppressing drugs
- Myotonic muscular dystrophy
- Systemic sclerosis/scleroderma

Altered Anatomy
Blind loops:
- Gastrocolic or jejunocolic fistula
- Ileocecal valve resection
- Small intestinal diverticulosis
- Strictures (Crohn disease, radiation, surgery)
- Surgically induced alterations in anatomy (Billroth II gastrectomy, end-to-side anastomosis)

Hypochlorhydria
Long-term acid suppression (?)
- Postsurgical

Immune Deficiency
Acquired immune deficiency syndrome (e.g., AIDS, severe malnutrition)
- Inherited immune deficiencies

Multifactorial Causes
Advanced age:
- Celiac disease
- Chronic pancreatitis
- Crohn disease
- Cystic fibrosis
- End-stage kidney disease
- Intestinal failure
- Liver disease
- Radiation enteropathy
- Tropical sprue

Unclear or Undefined Relationship to SIBO
Erosive esophagitis:
- Interstitial cystitis
- IBS
- Parkinson disease
- Restless legs syndrome
- Rosacea
- Severe obesity

From Feldman M et al: *Sleisenger and Fordtran's gastrointestinal and liver disease,* ed 10, Philadelphia, 2016, Elsevier.

- Stool evaluation can aid in the diagnosis as well. An increase in fecal fat may be suggestive of SIBO. Stool WBC, culture, ova, and parasites should be ordered as well to rule out other infectious etiology.

IMAGING STUDIES

- Endoscopic evaluation of the small intestine can be useful in finding structural and motility causes of bacterial overgrowth such as diverticula and strictures. Small bowel biopsy may aid in the diagnosis of celiac disease as well.
- Jejunal aspirate cultures via endoscopy are considered a standard of diagnosis. Aspirate cultures that exceed 10^5 organisms/ml suggest the presence of SIBO.
- There are several limitations to jejunal aspirate cultures. Bacterial overgrowth is not uniform and may be in inaccessible areas to endoscopist and can easily be missed. Contamination from oropharyngeal flora can lead to false-positive tests. Also, endoscopy is an invasive test and other methods of testing such as a breath test may be a more practical initial approach.

Rx TREATMENT

The goal is to treat the underlying cause and treat the bacterial overgrowth with antibiotic therapy.

NONPHARMACOLOGIC THERAPY

Structural disorders such as strictures, fistula, and diverticula may require surgical intervention.

ACUTE GENERAL Rx

- 7- to 10-day course of antibiotic therapy with rifaximin, amoxicillin-clavulanate, or metronidazole and ciprofloxacin has been shown to be beneficial.
- Nutritional support with vitamin replacement and dietary modification (lactose-free diet).

CHRONIC Rx

- Recurrence is common after antibiotic therapy. These patients may require subsequent courses of antibiotic therapy.
- Avoid using antacid medication.
- Avoid drugs that reduce GI motility (opioids).
- Consider lactose-free diet if the response to antimicrobial agents is incomplete.

DISPOSITION

Prognosis is dependent on underlying cause of SIBO. Although recurrence rate is high, antibiotic therapy remains the mainstay of therapy often requiring repeated courses if the underlying condition cannot be resolved.

REFERRAL

- Gastroenterology consultation for small bowel evaluation
- Surgical consultation with an underlying structural disorder

PEARLS & CONSIDERATIONS

COMMENTS

- SIBO is due to a disruption of protective mechanisms against bacterial burden.
- Look for risk factors including UGI tract surgery, structural disorders, IBD, IBS, and disorders decreasing GI motility.
- Diagnosis can be made with hydrogen breath test or endoscopic jejunal aspirate culture.
- Treatment is with antibiotics.
- The combination of vitamin B_{12} deficiency (due to bacterial consumption) and an elevated serum folate level (due to bacterial production) is suggestive of SIBO.
- SIBO can contribute to symptoms of IBS or IBD.

SUGGESTED READINGS

Available at ExpertConsult.com

RELATED CONTENT

Small Intestinal Bacterial Overgrowth (Patient Information)
Irritable Bowel Syndrome (Related Key Topic)
Malabsorption (Related Key Topic)

AUTHOR: **George Cholankeril, MD**

BASIC INFORMATION

DEFINITION

- Small bowel obstruction can be **functional** (as a result of intrinsic abnormal intestinal pathology; dysfunction peristalsis, also called "ileus") or **mechanical** (which may occur acutely or may be chronic).
- Small bowel obstruction is due to intraluminal or extraluminal mechanical compression.
- Mechanical obstruction means the blockage of the intestinal lumen, preventing the passage of luminal contents through the gut tube. Adhesion disease is the most common cause of mechanical small bowel obstruction in developed countries.
- Mechanical obstruction may be either:
  1. **Simple obstruction:** In which the lumen may be *partially* or *completely blocked* but with intact intestinal blood flow *OR*
  2. **Strangulated obstruction:**
     a. This is a surgical emergency.
     b. Usually the obstruction is complete; blood flow to the obstructed segment is cut off; and tissue necrosis, gangrene, and perforation may occur.

ICD-10CM CODES

K56	Paralytic ileus and intestinal obstruction
K56.1	Intussusception
K56.2	Volvulus
K56.3	Gallstone ileus
K56.4	Other impaction of intestine
K56.5	Intestinal adhesions (bands) with obstruction
K56.6	Other and unspecified intestinal obstruction
K56.9	Ileus, unspecified

EPIDEMIOLOGY & DEMOGRAPHICS

- The most frequently encountered surgical disorder of the small intestines is mechanical small bowel obstruction (SBO). This is a common surgical emergency accounting for 2% to 4% of emergency room visits and 15% of hospital admissions.
- 75% of all cases of small bowel obstruction result from intraabdominal adhesion related to prior abdominal surgery, such as appendectomy, colorectal surgery, and gynecologic procedures.

PREDOMINANT SEX & AGE: None—incidence is similar for males and females.

RISK FACTORS:

- Previous abdominal or pelvic surgery—most important risk factor for mechanical SBO in the U.S.
- Hernia (abdominal wall or groin)
- Prior abdominal irradiation
- Bowel neoplasm
- Foreign-body ingestion
- Parasitic infestation
- Gallstones
- Inflammatory/ischemic stricture

PHYSICAL FINDINGS & CLINICAL PRESENTATION

PHYSICAL FINDINGS: These may include:

- Dehydration (manifested by tachycardia, decreased urine output, orthostatic hypotension, dry mucous membrane)
- Abdominal distention may suggest an abnormal accumulation of air or fluid
- Hyperactive bowel sounds (an early occurrence)
- Tympany to abdominal percussion over a distended abdomen may indicate the presence of air
- Percussion dullness over a distended abdomen may indicate fluid
- High-pitched "tinkling" sound on auscultation of the abdomen
- Hypoactive bowel sounds (late finding)
- Hernia
- Rectal examination may reveal:
  1. Blood (suggestive of neoplasm or strangulation or mucosal ischemia)
  2. Masses (may suggest obturator hernia)
  3. Fecal impaction

CLINICAL PRESENTATION: There are four key symptoms: Abdominal pain, vomiting, distention, and constipation

- Abdominal pain (abrupt onset):
  1. Intermittent, crampy, or colicky
  2. Constant pain (that is, change in pain's character) signifies serious complication
- Abdominal distension: Indicates abnormal accumulation of air or fluid
- Nausea
- Vomiting (bilious vomiting seen in proximal obstructions)
- Diarrhea (early finding)
- Constipation (a late finding)
- Obstipation (inability to pass gas or stool)
- Hypotension, fever, tachycardia, leukocytosis, and peritoneal signs (these late findings may be seen with strangulation or intestinal ischemia) should compel urgency toward operative management
- It is important to perform serial abdominal examinations to detect changes early

ETIOLOGY

- Postoperative adhesions, especially prior abdominopelvic operations (may cause acute obstruction usually within 1 mo of surgery; or chronic obstructions can occur yrs later)
- Incarcerated inguinal hernia
- Malignant tumor
- IBD
- Gallstone ileus
- Stricture
- Cystic fibrosis
- Volvulus
- In children consider pyloric stenosis, intussusception, congenital atresia

DIAGNOSIS

DIFFERENTIAL DIAGNOSIS

- Paralytic ileus
- Pseudoobstruction
- Acute cholangitis
- Cholecystitis
- Gastroenteritis
- Inflammatory bowel disease
- Diverticulitis
- Endometriosis
- Mesenteric ischemia
- Pancreatitis
- Dysmenorrhea
- Ovarian torsion

WORKUP

During the initial evaluation of patients with suspected SBO, the primary objectives are to gauge the degree of metabolic derangement and volume depletion and to assess the need for and expediency of surgery. It is also important to exclude sepsis, perforation, and bowel ischemia. As with many surgical conditions, determining the correct diagnosis and management strategy hinges on a focused, yet thorough history and physical examination.

LABORATORY TESTS

- Laboratory abnormalities are not diagnostic of bowel obstruction but instead may indicate complications of obstruction. Essential laboratory tests include:
  1. Basic metabolic panel (hyponatremia, hypokalemia)
  2. CBC: Hemoconcentration, leukocytosis
  3. Urinalysis
  4. Serum amylase: May be elevated
  5. LDH
  6. Hepatic panel
  7. Check serum lactate, blood cultures, ABG in patients with signs such as fever, hypotension, or change in mental status
  8. Type and cross-match (in anticipation of possible surgical intervention)

IMAGING STUDIES

- Image to confirm diagnosis, identify the location of the obstruction, and access the type of obstruction.
- Imaging also helps identify complications (perforation, necrosis, etc.) and possible cause of the obstruction.
- Initial radiographic evaluation begins with plain x-ray films of the abdomen (supine and upright) and an upright chest radiograph. An upright chest radiograph is of paramount importance to inspect for pneumoperitoneum and also for evidence of aspiration in a patient with a history of vomiting. A supine and upright plain abdominal x-ray in patients with suspected small bowel obstruction may show:
  1. Ladderlike pattern of dilated small bowel loops with air-fluid levels (Fig. 1) indicating small bowel obstruction
  2. Accumulation of air and fluid proximal and clearance of fluid and air distal to the point of obstruction
  3. Proximal small bowel dilation with distal loop collapse
- Enteroclysis (a fluoroscopic x-ray of the small intestine) is useful in detecting obstruction and can distinguish partial from complete blockage and adhesions from metastases.
- CT scan is the study of choice if the patient has fever, tachycardia, abdominal pain, and

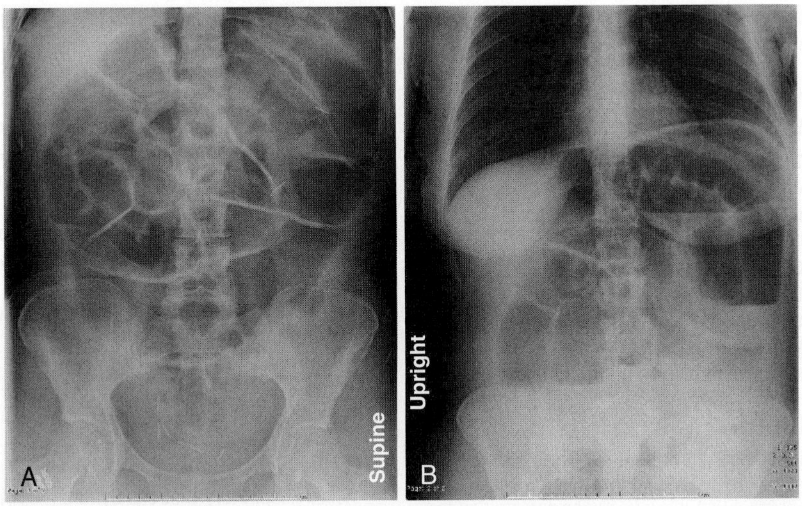

FIG. 1 A, Supine film showing dilated loops of small bowel in a patient with small bowel obstruction. **B,** Upright abdominal film revealing multiple air-fluid levels and small bowel dilation, consistent with a diagnosis of small bowel obstruction. (From Marx J: *Rosen's emergency medicine: concepts and clinical practice*, ed 6, Philadelphia, 2006, Saunders.)

leukocytosis. It can reveal the etiology of the obstruction: Abscess, inflammatory process, extra-luminal pathology, and/or metastases.
- CT can elucidate the cause, such as the presence of a mass (Fig. E2) or a hernia with subsequent obstruction (Fig. E3). In addition, CT has high sensitivity for detecting strangulation and pneumoperitoneum indicative of a perforation and is particularly useful in the early postoperative setting to rule out ischemia, intraabdominal abscess, or morbidity as the underlying cause. It is also useful in patients with a history of malignancy to differentiate potentially recurrent disease from adhesions (Fig. 4).
- CT enterography, in which intraluminal distention is achieved with administration of large volumes of oral contrast such as water-methylcellulose solution, can be useful. This modality is most often used to diagnose patients with Crohn disease–related strictures, and its benefit is high-resolution imaging of the bowel wall; however, it is impractical in the patient with gastrointestinal (GI) distress who is nauseated and vomiting.

Rx TREATMENT

- Immediate admission to the hospital if acute small bowel obstruction is suspected.
- Prompt surgical consultation to determine if surgical intervention is needed.

EMERGENCY ROOM CARE

- Vigorous fluid resuscitation and correction of electrolyte disorders underpin the initial therapeutic goals of both nonoperative and preoperative management strategies. Placing a Foley catheter to measure urinary output, establishing adequate intravenous access, and reassessing hemodynamic and electrolyte status are all essential in the initial management.
- Initial treatment:
  1. Designate the patient nothing by mouth; *nil per os* ("NPO")
  2. Fluid resuscitation (with isotonic Ringer or normal saline solution)
  3. Bowel decompression (via nasogastric [NG] tube placement): A standard NG tube provides symptomatic relief, prevents added gas and fluid accumulation proximally, and enables the serial assessment of antegrade fluid movement
  4. Correction of metabolic and electrolyte abnormalities
  5. Pain management
  6. Antiemetic administration
  7. Surgical consultation: Must be done early
  8. Antibiotic administration

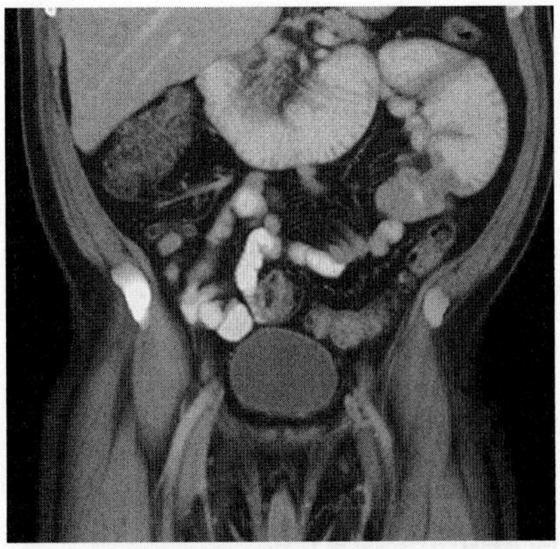

FIG. 4 Coronal image of computed tomographic scan showing mass in proximal small bowel with decompressed loops of small bowel distal to obstruction. (From Cameron JL, Cameron AM: *Current surgical therapy,* ed 10, Philadelphia, 2011, Saunders.)

NONSURGICAL INPATIENT CARE

General principles:
- Bowel rest
- Continue NG suction for decompression
- Serial abdominal examination (q4 to 6h)
- Check labs, for example, CBC, BMP, lactic acid q6h
- Provide adequate fluid

Patients with low-grade partial SBOs are prone to spontaneous resolution with conservative interventions such as bowel rest, NG decompression, and appropriate fluid resuscitation. For partial or simple obstructions resolution usually occurs within 72 hr.

SURGICAL CARE

More than 25% of inpatients admitted because of SBO will require an operation. Patients with complete or high-grade partial SBO are most likely to need surgery, with less than 20% successfully managed nonoperatively. Surgery is indicated in:
- Strangulated obstruction (which is a surgical emergency)
- Patients with signs of necrosis or perforation (require prompt surgery)
- Simple complete obstruction: After failed nonoperative care

AUTHOR: **Daniel K. Asiedu, MD, PhD, FACP**

BASIC INFORMATION

DEFINITION

Respiratory damage caused by breathing in harmful gases, vapors, and particle pollution contained in smoke

SYNONYM

Inhalation Injury

ICD-10CM CODE

J70.5 Smoke Inhalation Injury

EPIDEMIOLOGY & DEMOGRAPHICS

- 5% to 10% of burn patients suffer from smoke inhalation injury (SII), with a higher number seen in patients with facial burns.
- SII is the most common cause of fire-related deaths.
- The most vulnerable age groups are children and the elderly.
- Individuals with a physical or cognitive disability have a higher mortality rate.
- Other risk factors for SII correlate to risk of fires in general, such as substandard housing conditions, cold winter months, and homes lacking smoke detectors.

PHYSICAL FINDINGS & CLINICAL PRESENTATION

- Voice change, hoarseness, stridor
- Cough
- Burns to the face, oral or nasal mucosa, pharynx
- Soot in the sputum, nose, or mouth
- Respiratory distress
- Decreased consciousness or confusion
- Hypoxemia
- Increased carboxyhemoglobin levels

ETIOLOGY

- SII is the result of heat exposure and inhalation of the combustion products of smoke, such as carbon monoxide (CO) and cyanide (CN).
- Mechanism of injury can be organized by anatomic location:
  1. Damage to the upper airway is caused by thermal injury. Exposure to heat initiates an inflammatory cascade and leads to edema of mucosal tissue, causing airway obstruction.
  2. Injury to the lower airway and lung parenchyma occurs from toxic chemicals in the inhaled smoke. Damaged tissues slough off and create casts. Impaired mucociliary transport contributes to physical obstruction in the lower airways. Surfactant is also inactivated, leading to alveolar collapse and atelectasis.
  3. Systemic effects occur from metabolic and cellular dysfunction from agents such as CO and CN.
  4. Fig. 1 illustrates the pathophysiology of smoke inhalation injury.

Dx DIAGNOSIS

DIFFERENTIAL DIAGNOSIS

- Acute Respiratory Distress Syndrome (ARDS)

WORKUP

- Diagnosis is mainly clinical, which stresses the importance of a careful history and physical exam.
- Physical exam should include a detailed pulmonary evaluation as well as examination of the oral airway to look for tissue edema and soot in the oropharynx.

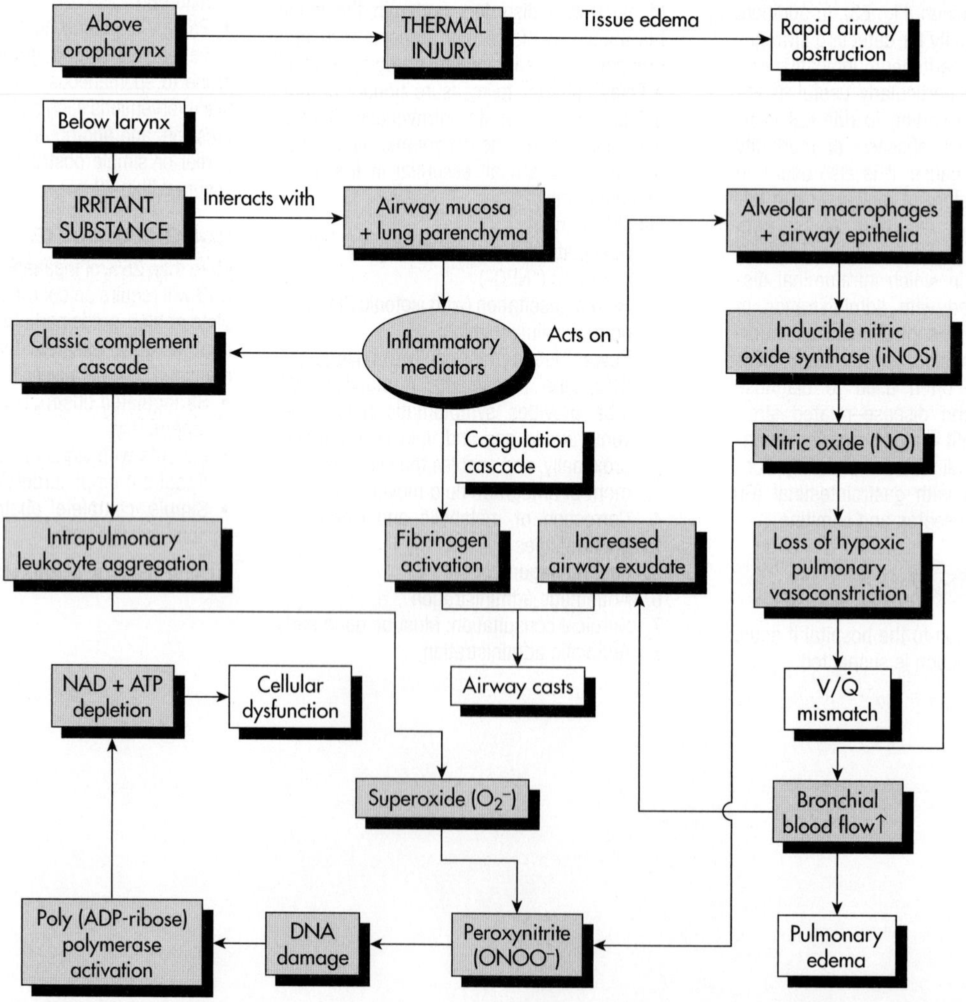

FIG. 1 Pathophysiology of acute smoke inhalation injury. *ADP,* Adenosine diphosphate; *ATP,* adenosine triphosphate; *NAD,* nicotinamide adenine dinucleotide; *V̇/Q̇,* ventilation-perfusion. (From Parrillo JE, Dellinger RP; *Critical care medicine, principles of diagnosis and management in the adult,* ed 5, Philadelphia, 2019, Elsevier.)

LABORATORY TESTS

- Arterial blood gas (ABG) to evaluate for retention of carbon dioxide and metabolic acidosis.
- In victims of fire, lactate of 10 mmol/L is an indicator of CN toxicity.
- COHb levels are tested by blood CO oximetry. Pulse oximetry may be falsely normal despite significant CO poisoning.
- BMP to evaluate anion gap.
- CBC to trend Hgb/Hct.
- Creatinine phosphokinase (CPK) is elevated in rhabdomyolysis.
- Troponin levels should be monitored because CO exposure increases the risk of dysrhythmias and myocardial ischemia.

IMAGING STUDIES

- Chest x-ray may show perivascular haziness, atelectasis, pulmonary edema, bronchial wall thickening.
- CT of chest may reveal consolidation, bronchial wall thickening, or ground-glass opacities similar to ARDS.
- The gold standard for diagnosing SII is fiberoptic bronchoscopy. Positive findings include mucosal erythema, edema, ulcerations or blistering, fibrin casts, charred tissue, or soot.

TABLE 1 Treatment Strategies for Acute Smoke Inhalation

Current	Under Investigation
Rescue victim from source	Activated protein C
High-flow 100% oxygen	Antiinflammatory drugs Methylprednisolone Phenytoin
Body check	Nitric oxide synthase inhibitors
Intravenous access	Antioxidants γ-Tocopherol 21-Aminosteroid
± Intubation	Endothelin-1–receptor antagonist tezosentan
If upper airway edema: Nebulized adrenaline Nebulized corticosteroids	P-selectin blockade
If bronchospasm: Nebulized α_2-agonists	Nebulized deferoxamine-pentastarch complex
If elevated COHb: High-flow 100% oxygen Hyperbaric oxygen	Mechanical ventilation: High-frequency percussive ventilation Airway pressure release ventilation Volumetric diffuse ventilator
If cyanide intoxication: Amyl nitrate Sodium thiosulfate Hydroxocobalamin Cyanokit	Extracorporeal membrane oxygenation
Mechanical ventilation Low tidal volume	Arteriovenous carbon dioxide removal
Nebulized heparin	Pulmonary decontamination with nebulized amphoteric chelating agents
Nebulized N-acetylcysteine	

COHb, Carboxyhemoglobin
From Parrillo JE, Dellinger RP: *Critical care medicine, principles of diagnosis and management in the adult,* ed 5, Philadelphia, 2019, Elsevier.

Rx TREATMENT

NONPHARMACOLOGIC THERAPY

Treatment includes airway and respiratory support, lung protective ventilation, 100% oxygen or hyperbaric oxygen therapy for CO poisoning, and hydroxycobalamin for CN toxicity.

ACUTE GENERAL Rx

- Respiratory support and endotracheal intubation are indicated if there is a threat of acute airway obstruction, respiratory failure not responding to noninvasive interventions, or altered mental status in which the patient is unable to protect his/her airway.
- Noninvasive positive-pressure ventilation (NIPPV) can be used in patients with mild to moderate respiratory distress.
- Bronchoscopy can be used therapeutically to suction particulate matter, secretions, and fibrin casts.
- Treatment strategies for acute smoke inhalation are summarized in Table 1.

DISPOSITION

- Complications are the result of direct mucosal injury and the subsequent inflammatory response. These include vocal cord dysfunction, pneumonia, pulmonary edema, and ARDS.
- Endobronchial polyps can form acutely or in a delayed manner.
- Tracheal stenosis is a delayed complication that can develop mo after injury.

REFERRAL

- Intensive care unit (ICU) admission will likely be required.

PEARLS & CONSIDERATIONS

COMMENTS

- Inhalation injury is one of the criteria for transfer to a burn center.

SUGGESTED READING

Available at ExpertConsult.com

RELATED CONTENT

Acute Respiratory Distress Syndrome (ARDS) (Related Key Topic)
Acute Respiratory Failure (ARF) (Related Key Topic)
Carbon Monoxide Poisoning (Related Key Topic)

AUTHOR: **Christine M. Bortz, MD**

BASIC INFORMATION

DEFINITION

- Spinal cord compression is characterized by direct compression of the spinal cord within the spinal canal. This may result in loss of neurologic function from compression of the spinal cord in the cervical, thoracic, and upper lumbar spinal canal. Compression may also occur at the cauda equina in the lower lumbar spinal canal, which is anatomically below the level of the spinal cord. Fig. 1 illustrates a schematic demarcation of principal dermatomes shown as distinct segments. Depending on the underlying etiology, symptoms may develop gradually or acutely and may result in complete or incomplete deficits. Neurologic deficits related to compression of the cord itself are referred to as myelopathy, whereas deficits caused by compression on nerve roots are described as radiculopathy.
- Signs and symptoms of myelopathy:
  1. Upper motor neuron signs (Hoffman sign, inverted radial reflex, Babinski sign, spasticity, hyperreflexia, clonus) in chronic cases
  2. Weakness
  3. Sensory deficits
  4. Clumsiness, difficult ambulation, ataxic gait (secondary to loss of proprioception in legs)
  5. Signs and symptoms of radiculopathy:
     a. Lower motor neuron signs (hyporeflexia, hypotonicity, fasciculations, muscle atrophy)
     b. Weakness
     c. Sensory deficits

Incomplete spinal cord lesions may classically present in distinct syndromic patterns (Table 1), for example, as follows:

- Anterior cord syndrome
- Central cord syndrome (most common)
- Cauda equina syndrome (not a true example of spinal cord compression but rather of cauda equina compression, affecting lower motor neurons in lumbosacral nerve roots)
- Conus medullaris syndrome
- Brown-Séquard syndrome

SYNONYMS OR RELATED TERMS

- Central cord syndrome
- Anterior cord syndrome
- Brown-Séquard syndrome
- Acute spinal cord compression
- Cauda equina syndrome
- Conus medullary syndrome

ICD-10CM CODES	
S14.13XX	Anterior cord syndrome
G83.81	Brown-Séquard syndrome
G83.4	Cauda equina syndrome
S14.12XX	Central cord syndrome
G95.81	Conus medullaris syndrome

EPIDEMIOLOGY & DEMOGRAPHICS

Dependent on etiology of cord compression

DEGENERATIVE SPINE DISORDERS

May affect the cervical, thoracic, and/or lumbar spine. Underlying pathology involves changes in keratin sulfate-to-chondroitin sulfate ratio in intervertebral disks with aging. This leads to a cascade of secondary events, including loss of disk height, disk herniation, spondylosis, increased intersegmental motion, formation of osteophytes, ligamentum flavum hypertrophy, and arthrosis of the facet joints. Compression of the nerve roots and/or spinal cord may result.

Spinal cord and nerve root compression from degenerative conditions are more common with increasing age, although any age group may be affected. Specific epidemiology and demographics are dependent on the type of degenerative changes.

TUMOR

Epidemiology dependent entirely on tumor type. Malignant tumors in the spine are most commonly metastatic disease, although primary musculoskeletal tumors are possible. The spine is the third-most common site for tumor metastases, after the lung and liver. Common metastatic lesions to the spine include lung cancer, breast cancer, prostate cancer, cancer of the GI tract, multiple myeloma, and lymphoma.

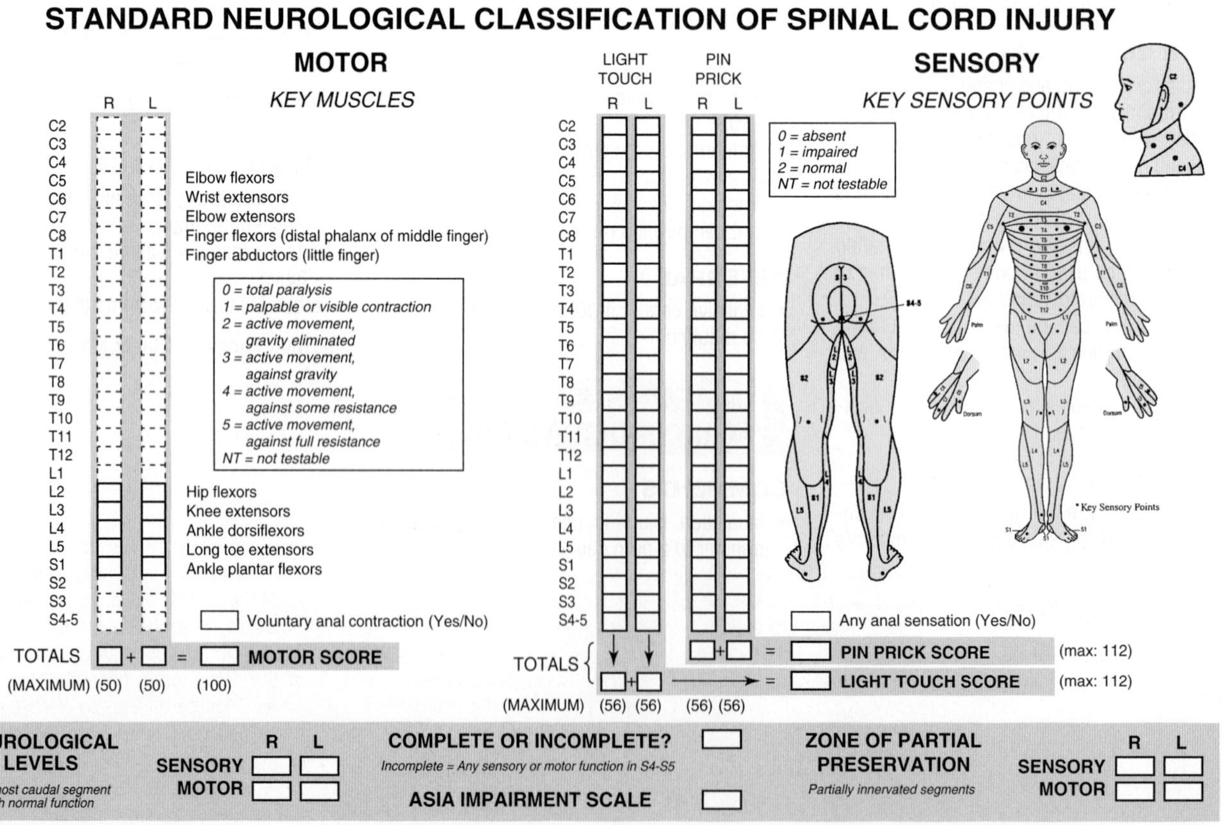

FIG. 1 The American Spinal Injury Association (ASIA) neurological classification of spinal cord injury and the ASIA impairment scale are useful tools for precisely mapping motor and sensory deficits to a specific spinal cord level. (From Browner B et al: *Skeletal trauma: basic science, management, and reconstruction,* ed 6, Philadelphia, 2019, Elsevier.)

TABLE 1 Spinal Cord Syndromes

Syndrome	Sensory	Motor	Sphincter Involvement
Central cord syndrome	Variable	Upper extremity weakness, distal > proximal	Variable
Brown-Séquard syndrome	Ipsilateral position and vibration sense loss Contralateral pain and temperature sensation loss	Motor loss ipsilateral to cord lesion	Variable
Anterior cord syndrome	Loss of pin and touch sensation Vibration, position sense preserved	Motor loss or weakness below cord level	Variable
Transverse cord syndrome—complete	Loss of sensation below level of cord injury	Loss of voluntary motor function below cord level	Sphincter control lost
Cauda equina syndrome	Saddle anesthesia may be present, or sensory loss may range from patchy to complete transverse pattern	Weakness may be of lower motor neuron type	Sphincter control impaired

From Marx JA et al: *Rosen's emergency medicine*, ed 8, Philadelphia, 2014, Saunders.

TABLE 2 Physical Examination Findings Associated with Vertebral Fractures and Spinal Cord Injuries

Injury	Physical Examination Area	Associated Findings
Vertebral fracture	Spine	Tenderness of the neck and/or back. Examine the entire spine because vertebral fractures may occur in multiples.
	Neurologic	See "Spinal cord injury" later.
	Chest	*Thoracic spine fractures:* Check for chest tenderness, unequal breath sounds, and arrhythmia, which are suggestive of an associated intrathoracic injury or myocardial contusion.
	Abdomen/pelvis	*Thoracolumbar and lumbar spine fractures:* Check for abdominal or pelvic tenderness. A transverse area of ecchymosis on the lower abdominal wall (seat belt sign) increases the chance of an abdominopelvic injury.
	Extremity	*Thoracolumbar and lumbar spine fractures*: Check for calcaneal tenderness because 10% of calcaneal fractures are associated with a low thoracic or lumbar fracture. Mechanistically, these areas are fractured as a result of axial loading.
Spinal cord injury	Neurologic, motor (anterior column)	Assess motor function on a scale of 0-5. The *motor level* is defined as the most caudal segment with at least 3/5 strength. Injuries to the first eight cervical segments result in tetraplegia (previously known as quadriplegia); lesions below the T1 level result in paraplegia.
	Neurologic, sensory (spinothalamic tract)	Assess sensory function via pinprick and light touch on the following scale: 0 = absent; 1 = impaired; 2 = normal. The *sensory level* is defined as the most caudal segment of the spinal cord with normal sensory function. The highest intact sensory level should be marked on the patient's spine to monitor for progression.
	Neurologic, sensory (dorsal column)	Assess vibratory sensory function on a scale of 0-2 by using a tuning fork over bony prominences. Assess position sense (proprioception) by flexing and extending the great toe.
	Neurology, deep tendon reflex	On a scale of 0-4, assess the deep tendon reflexes in the upper (biceps, triceps) and lower (patellar, Achilles) extremities.
	Anogenital	Assess rectal tone, sacral sensation, signs of urinary or fecal retention or incontinence, and priapism. Also check the anogenital reflexes. An *anal wink* (S2-S4) is present if the anal sphincter contracts in response to stroking the perianal skin area. The *bulbocavernosus reflex* (S3-S4) is elicited by squeezing the glans penis or clitoris (or pulling on an inserted Foley catheter), which results in reflexive contraction of the anal sphincter.
	Head-to-toe examination	A spinal cord injury may mask a patient's ability to perceive and localize pain. Imaging of high-risk areas, such as the abdomen, and areas of bruising or swelling may be required to exclude occult injuries.

From Adams JG et al: *Emergency medicine, clinical essentials*, ed 2, Philadelphia, 2013, Elsevier.

INFECTION

Diskitis/osteomyelitis may progress to epidural abscess, causing spinal cord or cauda equina compression. If not adequately addressed in a timely manner, this may result in permanent neurologic deficit. Epidural abscess incidence is approximately 0.2 to 3.0 per 10,000 hospital admissions. *Staphylococcus aureus* is the most common offending organism. Risk factors include increasing age, diabetes mellitus, end-stage renal disease, chronic hepatitis/cirrhosis, known endocarditis, immunocompromise, and IV drug abuse.

SPINAL CORD INJURY

Occurred most commonly in males with a mean age of 37 yr in 2010. Alcohol plays a major role in at least 25% of spinal cord injury (SCI).

INCIDENCE: 12,400 new cases/yr in 2010 in the U.S.

PREVALENCE: 250,000 persons in 2005 in the U.S.

COST (IN U.S.): >$5 billion/yr

RISK FACTORS: Underlying spinal disease can predispose to SCI:
- Inflammatory spondyloarthropathies, especially ankylosing spondylitis
- Diffuse idiopathic skeletal hyperostosis (DISH)
- Congenital spinal disorders
- Preexisting spinal canal stenosis or compromise
- Atlantoaxial instability
- Osteoporosis
- Rheumatoid arthritis (cervical spine)

PHYSICAL FINDINGS & CLINICAL PRESENTATION

Clinical features reflect the amount of spinal cord involvement:
- Weakness, sensory changes (dependent on level of compression/lesion/injury). Motor strength is tested bilaterally in each of five upper extremity muscle groups (Fig. E2) and five lower extremity muscle groups (Fig. E3).
- Myelopathy if cord involvement, radiculopathy if nerve root involvement (may involve both).
- ***Central cord syndrome (most common incomplete spinal cord injury):*** Motor impairment greater in upper than in lower extremities, variable degree of sensory loss below the injury level. Weakness and poor hand dexterity are especially common. Classically occurs after mild trauma including cervical hyperextension in the setting of preexisting cervical spondylosis.
- ***Anterior cord syndrome (worst prognosis of incomplete spinal cord injury):*** Affects the anterior or ventral two thirds of the spinal cord, sparing the dorsal columns. May be caused by a vascular injury to the anterior spinal artery or by a flexion/compression injury. Impairment usually is worse in the lower extremities than upper extremities. Physical manifestations include motor, pain, and temperature loss below the lesion. Proprioception and vibratory sense may be preserved as dorsal columns are preserved.

TABLE 3 Cervical Spine Clearance in Blunt Trauma Patients

Category	Characteristics	Diagnostic Recommendations
Alert and asymptomatic	Awake and alert No cervical pain or tenderness Normal neurologic examination findings No distracting injuries No intoxication	Remove cervical collar and perform functional range-of-motion test If functional test is pain free, discontinue cervical restrictions Otherwise, evaluate as a symptomatic patient
Short-term cognitive impairment	No neck pain or tenderness Normal neurologic examination findings Intoxicated or has distracting injuries Expect resolution in 24-48 hr	If urgent clearance is not needed, clinically reassess after return of normal cognition and treating distracting injuries If urgent clearance needed, evaluate as an obtunded patient
Symptomatic	Cervical pain or tenderness Neurologic deficits	Cervical spine imaging (plain films or CT) Also MRI if there are neurologic deficits or suspected ligamentous injury
Long-term cognitive impairment	Abnormal cognition that precludes reliable clinical examination	Cervical spine CT read by two qualified reviewers independently

CT, Computed tomography; *MRI,* magnetic resonance imaging.
From Browner B et al: *Skeletal trauma: basic science, management, and reconstruction,* ed 6, Philadelphia, 2019, Elsevier.

TABLE 4 Thoracolumbar Spine Clearance in Blunt Trauma Patients

Category	Characteristics	Diagnostic Recommendations
Asymptomatic and low risk	Awake and alert (GCS score = 15) Normal neurologic examination findings No thoracolumbar pain, tenderness, deformity, or ecchymosis No cervical spine fracture No intoxication or distracting injuries No high-energy mechanism (see following description)	No thoracolumbar imaging needed
Symptomatic or high risk	Thoracolumbar pain or tenderness Neurologic deficits High-energy mechanism (fall ≥10 ft, vehicular accident with ejection or ≥50 mph) Cervical spine fracture	Thoracolumbar CT (+ MRI if any neurologic deficits)
Not examinable	Any alteration in cognition (GCS score <15) or distracting injury that precludes reliable clinical examination	Thoracolumbar CT (+ MRI if any neurologic deficits)

CT, Computed tomography; *GCS,* Glasgow Coma Scale; *MRI,* magnetic resonance imaging.
From Browner B et al: *Skeletal trauma: basic science, management, and reconstruction,* ed 6, Philadelphia, 2019, Elsevier.

- ***Brown-Séquard syndrome:*** Rare in isolation. Caused by injury to half of the spinal cord and resulting in the loss of motor function, position, vibration, and light touch on the side of injury, as well as loss of pain and temperature sense on the contralateral side. Typically, secondary to a knife wound.
- ***Conus medullaris syndrome:*** Results in variable motor loss in the lower extremities with loss of bowel and bladder function. In general, more bowel and bladder is affected earlier than motor.
- ***Cauda equina syndrome:*** Low back pain, weakness in bilateral lower extremities, saddle anesthesia, and loss of voluntary bladder and/or bowel control, often presenting as bladder retention and/or bowel incontinence.

ETIOLOGY

- Trauma (most SCIs result from high-speed motor vehicle accidents, falls, sports injuries, or violence)
- Tumor
- Infection (e.g., epidural abscess)
- Inflammatory processes
- Degenerative disk disease with associated spinal stenosis
- Acute disk herniation
- Cystic abnormalities
- Ankylosing spondylitis, DISH. Patients with underlying DISH or ankylosing spondylitis are at high risk of SCI with otherwise relatively minor fractures of the spine
- Table 2 summarizes physical examination findings associated with vertebral fractures and spinal cord injuries

Dx DIAGNOSIS

DIFFERENTIAL DIAGNOSIS

See "Synonyms or Related Terms."

WORKUP

- Signs and symptoms of spinal cord or cauda equina compression often indicate urgent surgical conditions and thus require urgent imaging and early referral for assessment by a spine specialist.
- In cases of acute trauma in which spinal cord injury is suspected, patient should undergo full trauma evaluation following advanced trauma life support protocol in emergency room setting. With suspected injury to the cervical spine, the patient should be immobilized in a hard cervical collar or in-line traction at all times during evaluation. Log-roll precautions may be indicated as well to immobilize the spine during acute injury evaluation. The goal of "clearing the cervical spine" (Table 3) is to establish the absence of an injury that would put the spinal cord at risk after the collar is removed and the patient is mobilized. Table 4 summarizes thoracolumbar spine clearance in blunt trauma patients.
- Inflammatory labs will usually be elevated both in cases of trauma and infectious processes. Laboratory tests ordered should be specific to the suspected etiology or differential diagnosis for spinal cord compression.

IMAGING STUDIES

- Signs and symptoms of spinal cord compression in most cases will mandate advanced imaging, often including CT and CT myelogram and/or MRI.
- Plain x-rays may be helpful; however, normal plain films do not negate the need for further advanced imaging in the setting of signs and symptoms of spinal cord compression or spinal cord injury. This is especially true in the setting of ankylosing spondylitis or DISH.
- In the trauma setting, after primary and secondary surveys, fine-cut helical CT scans with axial, coronal, and sagittal reconstructions have replaced plain cervical radiographs in most trauma centers as the initial evaluation of choice in detecting fractures of the cervical spine.
- Detection of injury to any part of the spine during trauma evaluation mandates full imaging evaluation of the entire spine, as noncontiguous injuries are common.
- Although CT scan is excellent at imaging bony structures and detecting fractures, MRI provides more detailed imaging of the soft-tissue structures, including neural structures, discoligamentous structures, the posterior ligamentous complex, and paraspinal soft tissues. MRI is very sensitive for detecting ligamentous injury, spinal cord edema, spinal cord compression from soft-tissue structures, epidural hematoma, diskitis, osteomyelitis, and epidural abscess. Of note,

gadolinium contrast may increase the sensitivity of the MRI study for the detection of tumors or infections.

Rx TREATMENT

- Depending on the etiology of spinal cord compression as well as the specific signs and symptoms during physical examination and history-taking, urgent surgical decompression and/or stabilization may be indicated. Referral to a spine specialist is indicated in most cases of spinal cord compression.
- Corticosteroids: Controversial in cases of acute spinal cord injury. Methylprednisolone was thought to reduce the amount of secondary injury that occurs after SCI and was previously used in many trauma centers. However, current evidence is insufficient to support corticosteroids for this use, and most spine trauma centers no longer utilize steroids in cases of acute spinal cord injury.
- Vasopressors: Current evidence supports the use of vasopressors in cases of spinal cord injury to maintain spinal cord perfusion and to prevent ischemic damage to the cord. The ideal mean arterial pressure and duration of treatment are yet to be defined. Both the treatment modality and the injury itself mandate admission to ICU level of care in most cases for close monitoring.

DISPOSITION

Indicators regarding prognosis:

- Patients with acute traumatic SCI need monitoring in the ICU and evaluation for potential life-threatening complications, including cardiovascular instability and respiratory failure.
- In general the greater the distal motor and sensory sparing, the greater the expected recovery.
- In most cases of spinal cord compression and/or spinal cord injury, the primary goal of surgical decompression and/or stabilization should be to spare the remaining functional levels and to prevent worsening of the injury. Return of function should not be guaranteed.
- Prophylaxis against deep vein thrombosis and pulmonary embolism should always be provided. In acute injuries to the spine or postoperatively, this may consist of mechanical prophylaxis including TEDs and SCDs. Pharmacologic deep vein thrombosis/pulmonary embolism prophylaxis is often held initially to prevent development of epidural hematoma. The optimal timing for initiation of pharmacologic prophylaxis is controversial, and no strict guidelines are currently in place.

REFERRAL

Signs and symptoms of spinal cord or cauda equina compression often indicate urgent surgical conditions and thus require urgent imaging and early referral for assessment by a spine specialist.

SUGGESTED READINGS

Available at ExpertConsult.com

RELATED CONTENT

Spinal Stenosis (Patient Information)
Lumbar Disk Syndrome (Related Key Topic)
Spinal Epidural Abscess (Related Key Topic)
Spinal Stenosis, Lumbar (Related Key Topic)

AUTHORS: **Shyam A. Patel, MD,** and **Eren O. Kuris, MD**

Spinal Epidural Abscess

BASIC INFORMATION

DEFINITION

A spinal epidural abscess (SEA) is a focal suppurative infection occurring in the spinal epidural space.

SYNONYM

SEA

ICD-10CM CODE

G06.1 Intraspinal abscess and granuloma

EPIDEMIOLOGY & DEMOGRAPHICS

INCIDENCE (IN U.S.):

- 2 to 25 cases/100,000 hospitalized patients/yr
- May be increasing over the past 3 decades

PREDOMINANT AGE:

- Median age of onset approximately 50 yr (35 yr in intravenous drug users)
- Peak incidence in seventh and eighth decades of life

PHYSICAL FINDINGS & CLINICAL PRESENTATION

- The presentation of SEA can be nonspecific.
- Fever, malaise, and back pain are the most consistent early symptoms.
- Pain is often focal. It may initially be mild but can progress to become severe.
- As the disease progresses, root pain can occur, followed by motor weakness, sensory changes, bladder and bowel dysfunction, and paralysis.
- Physical findings may be limited to fever or spinal tenderness.
- The evolution to neurologic deficits can occur as quickly as a few hours, or over wk to mo.
- Once paralysis occurs, it may quickly become irreversible without the appropriate intervention.

ETIOLOGY

- SEA most commonly results from hematogenous dissemination.
- Pyogenic bacteria account for the majority of cases in the U.S. Immigrants from TB-endemic areas may present with tuberculous SEAs. Fungi and parasites can also cause this condition. The most common causative organism is *Staphylococcus aureus.* Gram-negative bacilli and anaerobes may be seen if the infection has a urinary or GI source.
- Most posterior SEAs are thought to originate from distant focus (e.g., skin and soft tissue infections), whereas anterior SEAs are commonly associated with diskitis or vertebral osteomyelitis. No source was found in approximately one third of cases.
- Associated predisposing conditions include diabetes mellitus, alcoholism, cancer, AIDS, and chronic renal failure, or following epidural anesthesia, spinal surgery or trauma, prolonged epidural catheter placement, paraspinal glucocorticoid or analgesic injections, acupuncture, or IV drug use. No predisposing condition is found in approximately 20% of patients.
- Damage to the spinal cord can be caused by direct compression of the spinal cord, vascular compromise, bacterial toxins, and inflammation.

DIAGNOSIS

DIFFERENTIAL DIAGSNOSIS

- Herniated disk
- Vertebral osteomyelitis and diskitis
- Metastatic tumors
- Meningitis

LABORATORY TESTS

- WBC may be normal or elevated.
- ESR and C-reactive proteins are usually elevated.
- Blood cultures are positive in approximately 60% of patients with SEA and should be obtained before starting antibiotics.
- CSF cultures are positive in 19%, but lumbar puncture is unnecessary, and may be contraindicated.
- Once imaging is done, CT-guided aspiration or open biopsy should be done to determine

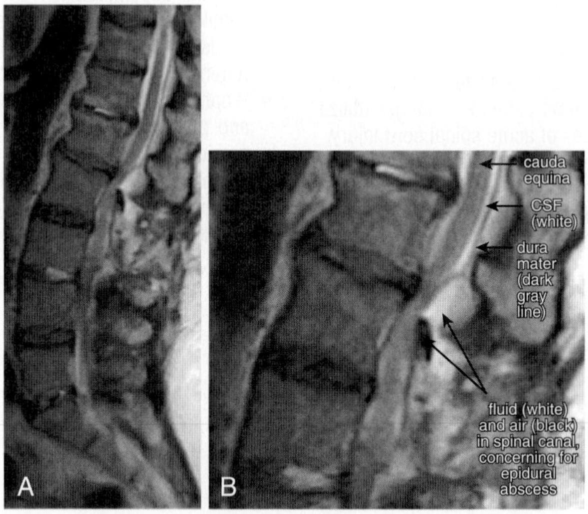

FIG. 1 Same patient as in Fig. 2, in whom noncontrast computed tomography showed air in the spinal canal, concerning for epidural abscess. Magnetic resonance imaging (MRI) of the lumbar spine without contrast was performed, as the patient was in acute renal failure. **A,** This T2-weighted sagittal MRI provides useful information even without gadolinium contrast. **B,** Close-up. On T_2-weighted MRI sequences, fluid including cerebrospinal fluid *(CSF)* appears white. Fat-containing tissues such as bone marrow and the spinal cord or cauda equina appear dark gray. Calcified bone appears nearly black due to an absence of resonating protons. Air appears completely black for the same reason. The midline sagittal image shows the cauda equina to be impinged upon by an epidural fluid collection containing air—an epidural abscess. The dura mater is visible as a thin, dark-gray line parallel to the spinal cord. It is indented in the region of the epidural abscess. (From Broder JS: *Diagnostic imaging for the emergency physician*, Philadelphia, 2011, Saunders.)

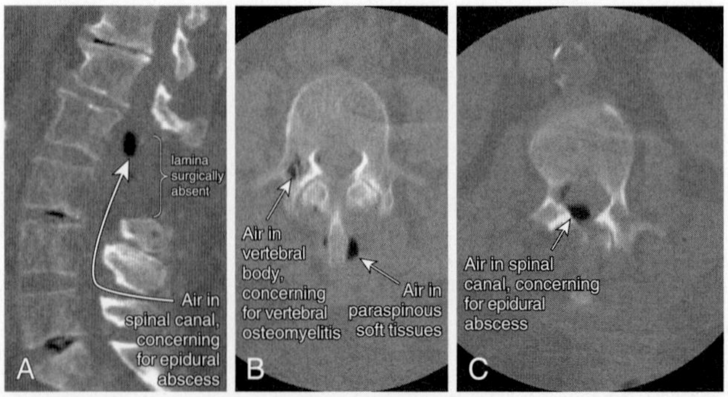

FIG. 2 This 67-yr-old female presented with delirium and fever. She had undergone lumbar laminectomy 3 mo prior, and her wound had been treated with a wound VAC dressing. Magnetic resonance imaging was not initially available, so noncontrast computed tomography (CT) was performed. Noncontrast CT is excellent at delineating air, which appears black on bone windows. **A,** The midsagittal view demonstrates air *(black)* in the spinal canal at the L2 and L3 levels. On the axial views **(B, C)**, air is visible in the spinal canal, in paraspinal soft tissues, and within the vertebral body. These findings are concerning for a paraspinal infection that has developed into an epidural abscess with vertebral osteomyelitis. (From Broder JS: *Diagnostic imaging for the emergency physician*, Philadelphia, 2011, Saunders.)

causative organism. Abscess content culture is positive in 90% of patients.

IMAGING STUDIES

- MRI with gadolinium is the imaging modality of choice (Fig. 1); CT scan with contrast may show the abscess (Fig. 2) but is less sensitive than MRI.
- CT with myelography is more sensitive for cord compression.

Rx TREATMENT

NONPHARMACOLOGIC THERAPY

- Surgical decompression is the mainstay of treatment. Decompression within the first 24 hr has been related to an improved prognosis.
- Nonsurgical treatment is effective in some patients, but failure rate may be excessive. This approach should not be considered and should only be attempted in the absence of signs of compressive myelopathy and with very careful follow-up.

ACUTE GENERAL Rx

- In addition to surgery, antibiotics directed at the most likely organism should be initiated. Fig. 3 describes an algorithm for the management of patients with SEA.
- If the organism is unknown, broad coverage against staphylococci, streptococci, and gram-negative bacilli should be initiated. Empiric antimicrobial intravenous therapy typically includes vancomycin (loading dose: 25 to 30 mg/kg, then 15 to 20 mg/kg q8-12h, aiming for trough levels of 15 to 20) plus an antipseudomonal cephalosporin such as piperacillin/tazobactam at high dose (4.5 g IV q6h) or carbapenem such as meropenem (1 to 2 g IV q8h) or imipenem. The regimen can be adjusted according to culture results. Therapy should continue for at least 4 to 6 wk.

CHRONIC Rx

Neurologic deficits may remain despite aggressive treatment.

DISPOSITION

Irreversible paralysis and death can occur in up to 25% of patients.

REFERRAL

All cases should be referred to a neurosurgeon and an infectious disease specialist.

PEARLS & CONSIDERATIONS

- Follow-up imaging with MRI is not necessary unless patient develops new neurologic signs or symptoms, has poor clinical response, or has persistent elevation of inflammatory markers.
- It is critically important to recognize this process early; the prognosis is generally excellent if treatment is initiated while symptoms are localized and before evidence of myelopathy develops.
- The likelihood of success postsurgery is low in patients who have developed complete paralysis for longer than 36 hr.

SUGGESTED READINGS

Available at ExpertConsult.com

AUTHOR: **Glenn G. Fort, MD, MPH**

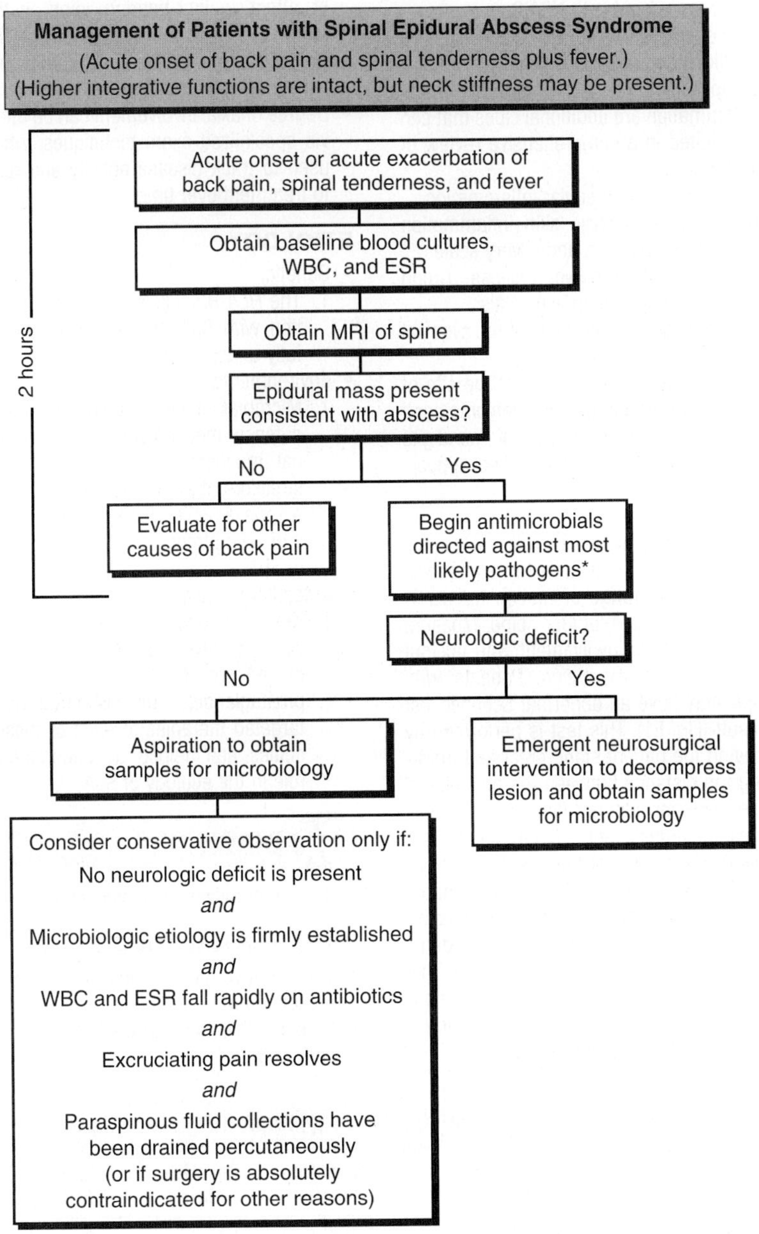

FIG. 3 Algorithm for the management of patients with spinal epidural abscess syndrome. If MRI cannot be performed, myelography, high-contrast computed tomography (CT), or CT-myelography may be an acceptable alternative to localize an epidural abscess. If abscess drainage can be performed promptly, antimicrobial drugs may be withheld until specimens for microbial analysis are obtained. *ESR,* Erythrocyte sedimentation rate; *MRI,* magnetic resonance imaging; *WBC,* white blood cell. (From Vincent JL et al: *Textbook of critical care,* ed 6, Philadelphia, 2011, Saunders.)

BASIC INFORMATION

DEFINITION

Spondyloarthropathies (SpAs) are a group of interrelated systemic autoinflammatory conditions that are serologically negative for rheumatoid factor, connected by an underlying genetic risk with similar patterns of inflammation. This group encompasses ankylosing spondylitis, psoriatic arthritis, reactive arthritis, enteropathic arthritis, and undifferentiated spondyloarthritis (Table 1). SpAs are broadly classified by axial versus peripheral joint involvement, and with or without radiographic progression.

SYNONYMS

Spondyloarthritis
Spondylopathy
Spondylitis
SPAs

ICD-10CM CODES

M46.80 Other specified inflammatory spondylopathies, unspecified site
M46.82 Other specified inflammatory spondylopathies, cervical region
M46.83 Other specified inflammatory spondylopathies, cervicothoracic region
M46.86 Other specified inflammatory spondylopathies, lumbar region
M46.87 Other specified inflammatory spondylopathies, lumbosacral region
M46.89 Other specified inflammatory spondylopathies, multiple sites
M46.81 Other specified inflammatory spondylopathies, occipito-atlanto-axial region
M46.88 Other specified inflammatory spondylopathies, sacrococcygeal region
M46.84 Other specified inflammatory spondylopathies, thoracic region
M46.85 Other specified inflammatory spondylopathies, thoracolumbar region

EPIDEMIOLOGY & DEMOGRAPHICS

PREVALENCE: Worldwide prevalence of SpA is 0.2% to 1.6%, with approximately 1% of the U.S. population affected. Varies regionally with prevalence of HLA-B27.

PREDOMINANT SEX & AGE: Males younger than age 45 yr are predominantly affected. Previously, male:female ratio was thought to be 10:1; more recently, approximately 3:1.

Patients >45 yr may present with chronic, severe disease due to diagnostic delays.

RISK FACTORS: *HLA-B27* allele,* male sex,* smoking,* ethnic background, family history of SpA, and certain infections. (*Associated with more severe disease.)

GENETICS: Association with the *HLA-B27* allele is the strongest known genetic risk factor.

PHYSICAL FINDINGS & CLINICAL PRESENTATION

- History:
  1. Inflammatory low back pain may be the primary presenting symptom:
     a. Pain and stiffness in low back or buttocks that is worst in the morning, may awaken the patient from sleep, and improves with exercise
     b. Morning stiffness generally lasting longer than 1 hr
     c. Improvement with NSAIDs
     d. Sensitivity up to 90% and positive likelihood ratio up to 2.2 for axial SpA
  2. Symptoms of systemic and peripheral inflammation are additional clues that can be elicited in a comprehensive review of systems:
     a. Uveitis: Painful ocular inflammation
     b. Psoriasis: Chronic skin inflammation with red patches and silvery scales
     c. Inflammatory bowel disease: Crohn disease and ulcerative colitis
     d. Synovitis: Inflammation of the synovial membrane of joints
     e. Enthesitis: Inflammation at the site of tendon or ligament insertion onto bone
     f. Dactylitis: Tenosynovitis of the digits causing classic sausage-like appearance
- Physical exam:
  1. Axial joints: Spine and sacroiliac (SI) joints
  2. Inspect curvature, palpate for tenderness, and evaluate range of motion for cervical, thoracic, and lumbar spine. Measure degree of axial involvement with occiput wall, thoracic expansion. Patients with SpA may have an abnormal Schober test result (Fig. E1). This test is performed by having the patient stand erect and marking the distance between the midpoint of the posterior superior iliac spines ("dimples of Venus") and 10 cm above that point. The patient is then asked to maximally flex forward while the more caudal spot is kept stationary. The more cephalad point on the tape measure should demonstrate at least 5 cm of excursion. This abnormality also can be seen with lumbar degenerative disk disease. Test for sacroiliitis with Patrick and Gaenslen tests
  3. Peripheral joints: Lower extremity predominance
  4. Inspect for signs of inflammation, including dactylitis, synovitis, and enthesitis
  5. Evaluate for systemic involvement manifesting as anterior uveitis and psoriasis:
     a. Slit lamp is necessary to diagnose anterior uveitis
     b. Full skin exam is critical to detect occult psoriasis; look for nail changes
- Musculoskeletal manifestations commonly affect weight-bearing joints with high mechanical stress; thus it is particularly important to examine the lumbar spine, SI joints, and lower extremities
- Degree of axial involvement can be measured via specialized exam techniques, which are used to track disease activity and response to treatment over time

ETIOLOGY

- Genetic:
  1. The *HLA-B27* allele has a strong association with SpA, through mechanisms not fully understood.
- Environmental:
  1. Microbial infections, disruptions in barrier defense mechanisms (skin and intestinal mucosa), and mechanical articular stressors may trigger an inflammatory response, which then develops into signs and symptoms specific to each type of SpA.
- Autoinflammatory:
  1. Key components of the inflammatory cascade involved in the pathogenesis of SpA are TNF, IL-12, IL-17, IL-23, and prostaglandins. Success in treatment with targeted therapies to each of these molecules has helped us understand their role in the etiology of SpA.

DIAGNOSIS

Table 2 summarizes diagnostic criteria for SpA.

DIFFERENTIAL DIAGNOSIS

- Seronegative rheumatoid arthritis (peripheral presentation)
- Degenerative disc disease (axial presentation) or DISH

TABLE 1 Comparison of Ankylosing Spondylitis and Related Disorders

Feature	Ankylosing Spondylitis	Psoriatic Arthritis	Reactive Arthritis	Enteropathic Arthropathy
Sex (male:female)	2-3:1	1:1	1:1	1:1
Age of onset	<40 yr	35-55 yr	20-40 yr	Any age
Sacroiliitis or spondylitis (%)	100	~20	~40	<20
Symmetry of sacroiliitis	Symmetrical	Asymmetrical	Asymmetrical	Symmetrical
Peripheral arthritis (%)	~25	95	90	5-20
Distribution	Axial and lower limbs	Variable	Lower limbs	Variable
HLA-B27 positivity (%)	85-95	25-60*	30-70	7-70†
Uveitis	0-40	~20	~50	<15

*60% when spondylitis is present.
†70% when spondylitis is present.
From Hochberg MC: *Rheumatology*, ed 7, Philadelphia, 2019, Elsevier.

TABLE 2 Criteria for Spondyloarthritis (SpA)*

Amor Criteria	ESSG Criteria
Past or current clinical manifestations:	Inflammatory back pain *or* synovitis:
1. Back pain at night and/or back stiffness in the morning (1 point)	• Asymmetric synovitis or • Predominantly lower limb synovitis
2. Asymmetric oligoarthritis (2 points)	AND
3. Gluteal pain without other details (1 point) or alternating gluteal pain (2 points)	One or more of the following: • Positive family history • Psoriasis
4. Sausage-like digit or toe (2 points)	• Inflammatory bowel disease
5. Heel pain or other enthesopathy (2 points)	• Urethritis, cervicitis, or acute diarrhea within 1 mo before arthritis
6. Iritis (2 points) 7. Nongonococcal urethritis within 1 mo before the onset of arthritis (1 point)	• Buttock pain alternating between right and left gluteal areas • Enthesopathy • Sacroiliitis (radiography)
8. Acute diarrhea within 1 mo before the onset of arthritis (1 point)	
9. Past or current psoriasis and/or balanitis and/or inflammatory bowel disease (2 points)	
Radiographic changes:	
1. Sacroiliitis grade 2 or more if bilateral, grade 3 or more if unilateral (3 points)	
Predisposing genetic factors:	
2. Presence of HLA-B27 antigen and/or family history of ankylosing spondylitis, Reiter syndrome, psoriasis, uveitis, or chronic bowel disease (2 points)	
Responsiveness to treatment:	
3. Improvement within 48 hours after initiation of an NSAID and/or recurrence within 48 hours after discontinuation of an NSAID (2 points)	

ESSG, European Spondyloarthropathy Study Group; *NSAID,* nonsteroidal antiinflammatory drug.
*Definite SpA if ≥6 points; probable SpA if 5 points.
From Hochberg MC: *Rheumatology*, ed 7, Philadelphia, 2019, Elsevier.

- Inflammatory osteoarthritis (axial or peripheral presentation)
- Hypertrophic osteoarthropathy (peripheral presentation)

WORKUP

- Young patients, particularly men <45 yr, with chronic inflammatory low back pain responsive to NSAIDs should be screened.
- Patients with psoriasis, inflammatory bowel disease, or recent gastrointestinal or genitourinary infections presenting with new-onset low back or peripheral joint pain should also be screened.
- Screening begins with a comprehensive history and physical exam.
- HLA-B27 testing and imaging of SI joints and/or lumbar spine are indicated based on clinical suspicion.

LABORATORY TESTS

- HLA-B27:
  1. Negative test does not rule out SpA.
  2. Sensitivity: 95% for ankylosing spondylitis, 80% for reactive arthritis, 70% for psoriatic arthritis, and 50% for enteropathic arthritis
- Elevated ESR and CRP, anemia of chronic disease, leukocytosis, and thrombocytosis may reflect active inflammation. A normal CRP or ESR does not rule out spondyloarthropathies
- Testing for rheumatoid arthritis antibodies is generally negative (RF, CCP)
- Synovial fluid is inflammatory and nonspecific, with WBC >2,000/mm^2

IMAGING STUDIES

- **X-Ray:** SI joints and lumbar spine:
  1. May not detect early inflammation
  2. 20% to 80% have nonradiographic disease at time of presentation
  3. May show signs of structural damage such as erosions, syndesmophytes, sclerosis, and ankylosis in chronic axial disease
- **MRI:** SI joints and lumbar spine:
  1. Subchondral bone marrow edema in early disease
  2. Useful when x-ray and clinical findings are nondiagnostic but clinician's suspicion for axial SpA remains high

Rx TREATMENT

Improvement in symptoms, preservation of function, and prevention of structural damage can be achieved through a multidisciplinary approach.

NONPHARMACOLOGIC THERAPY

- Physical and occupational therapies improve functional outcomes
- Surgery:
  1. Joint replacements (high-impact joints such as hips)
  2. Spinal wedge osteotomy (advanced axial disease)
  3. Colectomy (advanced enteropathic arthritis)

ACUTE GENERAL Rx

- NSAIDs are first line.
- Avoid steroids in psoriatic arthritis due to risk of life-threatening pustular psoriasis and erythroderma.

CHRONIC Rx

- **NSAIDs:**
  1. Up to 35% of patients may achieve remission
  2. Best response in early disease
  3. Continuous dosing may prevent radiographic progression of axial disease
- **DMARDs:** Effective for peripheral involvement only, not effective in axial disease
  1. Methotrexate, leflunomide, sulfasalazine
- **TNF inhibitors:** NSAID or DMARD failure
  1. Infliximab, adalimumab, golimumab, etanercept, certolizumab pegol
- **IL-17 and IL-12/23 inhibitors:** 2nd TNF inhibitor failure
  1. Recent studies show similar efficacy compared to TNF inhibitors
  2. Ixekizumab (IL-17 inhibitor) recently approved for ankylosing spondylitis
  3. Ustekinumab (IL-12/23 inhibitor) and secukinumab (IL-17 inhibitor) are effective in psoriatic arthritis. Secukinumab also is approved for ankylosing spondylitis
  4. Ustekinumab is also effective in Crohn-enteropathic arthritis
- **JAK inhibitors:** Phase II clinical trial Tofacitinib (JAK 1, 2, 3 inhibitor) was shown to improve clinical and imaging outcomes in axial SpA, with phase III trial data pending Tofacitinib is approved to treat both UC and psoriatic arthritis

COMPLEMENTARY & ALTERNATIVE MEDICINE

- Strong clinical trials are lacking.
- Small studies have shown Pilates, t'ai chi, deep tissue massage, and hydroelectric therapy can be beneficial in axial SpA.

DISPOSITION

- Function and mobility may be limited in advanced axial disease.
- Psoriatic arthritis is an independent risk factor for cardiovascular disease.

REFERRAL

Rheumatology, dermatology, ophthalmology, gastroenterology, infectious disease

PEARLS & CONSIDERATIONS

COMMENTS

Young patients with chronic inflammatory low back pain deserve referral to a rheumatologist. HLA-B27 positivity is not required for diagnosis if strong clinical features are present. MRI may be needed to detect early axial disease. Repeated spinal x-rays at scheduled intervals (e.g., every 2 yr) are not recommended in patients with active or stable nonradiographic axial SpA. Track axial disease activity with clinical scoring systems and physical exam measurements. Traditional DMARDs are not effective in axial disease.

PREVENTION

High index of suspicion and prompt referral allows for early diagnosis. Early treatment with treat-to-target approach may prevent symptomatic and radiographic progression.

PATIENT & FAMILY EDUCATION

Smoking cessation is key. Discuss with family the implications of strong genetic component. Educate patients with psoriasis and inflammatory bowel disease about symptoms of inflammatory low back or peripheral joint pain to monitor for development of SpA in these high-risk individuals.

SUGGESTED READINGS

Available at ExpertConsult.com

RELATED CONTENT

Ankylosing Spondylitis (Related Key Topic)
Psoriatic Arthritis (Related Key Topic)
Reactive Arthritis (Reiter Syndrome) (Related Key Topic)
Enteropathic Arthritis (Related Key Topic)

AUTHOR: **Matthew J. White, DO**

BASIC INFORMATION

DEFINITION

Spontaneous abortion is fetal loss before wk 20 of pregnancy, calculated from the patient's last menstrual period, or the delivery of a fetus weighing <500 g. Early loss is before menstrual wk 12, whereas late loss refers to losses from wk 12 to 20.

Spontaneous abortion can also be classified as incomplete (partial passage of fetal tissue through partially dilated cervix), complete (spontaneous passage of all fetal tissue), threatened (uterine bleeding without cervical dilation or passage of tissue), inevitable (bleeding with cervical dilation without passage of fetal tissue), or missed abortion (intrauterine fetal demise without passage of tissue).

Recurrent spontaneous abortion involves three or more spontaneous pregnancy losses before wk 20. It affects approximately 1% of couples attempting to conceive. However, in actual practice, most reproductive experts consider two spontaneous pregnancy losses sufficient to initiate an evaluation for habitual or recurrent spontaneous abortion, since the risk of another loss is similar at this point, and the emotional stress is high. As many as 5% of couples and probably even a higher proportion of couples in which the woman is over age 35 are affected by two or more consecutive spontaneous abortions.

SYNONYMS

Spontaneous miscarriage
Miscarriage
Spontaneous pregnancy loss

ICD-10CM CODES

003.89	Complete or unspecified spontaneous abortion with other complications
003.9	Complete or unspecified spontaneous abortion without complication

EPIDEMIOLOGY & DEMOGRAPHICS

INCIDENCE: 10% to 20% of clinically recognized pregnancies; 80% of miscarriages occur in the first trimester. Recurrent miscarriage occurs in <1% of couples attempting to have children.

MATERNAL CAUSES:

- Uterine anomalies: Müllerian abnormalities such as unicornuate, bicornuate, or septated uterus are associated with increased miscarriage risk, although rates vary in different studies. A septated uterus is most highly associated with recurrent loss and can be surgically corrected and thus is important to diagnose. Other intrauterine pathologies such as synechiae, leiomyomas, or prior DES exposure are important to rule out also.
- Incompetent cervix (iatrogenic or congenital, associated with 20% of midtrimester losses).
- Antiphospholipid antibody syndrome.
- Uncontrolled diabetes mellitus.
- Rare or controversial causes include HLA associations between mother and father; infections such as tuberculosis, *Chlamydia*, and *Ureaplasma;* smoking and alcohol use; irradiation; progesterone deficiency; and environmental toxins. Most of the literature is observational in nature, which may skew risk factor data.
- With two or more spontaneous miscarriages, a karyotype can be performed on the products of conception to evaluate for aneuploidy, which may be associated with a balanced translocation in one of the parents, and which has a substantially increased risk for abortion (depending on the actual type of translocation); if the pregnancy is carried to term, it has a 3% to 5% risk for an unbalanced karyotype. In patients with habitual abortion, evaluation for anatomic defects such as uterine septum and for antiphospholipid syndrome (lupus anticoagulant, beta 2 glycoprotein IgG/IgM, and anticardiolipin antibody IgG/IgM) should also be obtained.

RISK FACTORS:

- Vaginal bleeding, especially >3 days, carries with it a 15% to 20% chance of miscarriage
- Advancing maternal age
- Two or more prior miscarriages
- Significant underlying maternal health issues such as uncontrolled diabetes, thyroid disease, or other endocrine disturbances
- Illicit substance use
- Obesity
- Alcohol, smoking, and excessive caffeine intake
- Use of fluconazole in pregnancy is associated with a statistically significant increased risk of spontaneous miscarriage

GENETICS:

- Fetal chromosomal aneuploidy and polyploidy account for the overwhelming majority of first-trimester losses.
- Autosomal trisomy accounts for the majority of abnormalities, followed by monosomy X, tetraploidy, and, lastly, structural chromosomal abnormalities.
- The incidence of trisomy increases as maternal age increases.

PHYSICAL FINDINGS & CLINICAL PRESENTATION

- Profuse bleeding and cramping have a higher association with miscarriage than bleeding without cramping, which is more consistent with a threatened miscarriage.
- Cervical dilation with history or finding of fetal tissue at cervical os may be present.
- In cases of missed abortion, uterine size may be smaller than menstrual dating, in contrast to molar gestation, where size may be greater than dates.
- The presence of nausea and vomiting in early pregnancy is associated with a reduced risk for pregnancy loss.

ETIOLOGY

In a general overview the etiology can be classified in terms of maternal (environmental) and fetal (genetic) factors, with the majority of miscarriages being related to genetic or chromosomal causes.

Dx DIAGNOSIS

DIFFERENTIAL DIAGNOSIS

- Normal pregnancy
- Hydatidiform molar gestation
- Ectopic pregnancy
- Dysfunctional uterine bleeding
- Pathologic endometrial or cervical lesions

WORKUP

- All patients with bleeding in the first trimester should have an evaluation for possible ectopic pregnancy.
- If there are three early, prior pregnancy losses, a workup and treatment for recurrent miscarriage should begin before next conception. If there is a strong history for second-trimester loss, consideration for cerclage should be given if the history is consistent with incompetent cervix (e.g., painless cervical dilation).
- Most providers will initiate an evaluation for couples who have had two previous losses.
- One unexplained fetal loss beyond 10 wk or 1 birth before 34 wk because of preeclampsia should prompt an evaluation for antiphospholipid antibody syndrome.

LABORATORY TESTS

- Type and antibody screen are used to evaluate the need for Rh immune globulin.
- Recurrent pregnancy loss: During the preconception period in patients with recurrent pregnancy loss, hemoglobin A_{1c}, TSH, prolactin, anticardiolipin antibody, lupus anticoagulant, 20210A beta 2 glycoprotein antibodies, karyotyping, and anatomic evaluation with hysterosalpingography, or saline ultrasonography to assess for uterine septum. With increasing age, oocyte quality is a factor, and some practitioners will perform day 3 of the menstrual cycle FSH and antimüllerian hormone to assess for diminished ovarian reserve. Progesterone level <5 mg/dl suggests nonviable gestation vs. >25 mg/dl, which suggests a good prognosis.

IMAGING STUDIES

Transvaginal sonogram (preferred) (Figs. 1 through 3) can be used with menstrual dating and serum quantitative human chorionic gonadotropin to document pregnancy location, fetal heart presence, gestational sac size, and adnexal pathology.

Rx TREATMENT

NONPHARMACOLOGIC THERAPY

Depending on the patient's clinical status, desire to continue the pregnancy, and certainty of the diagnosis, expectant management can be considered. In pregnancies <6 wk or >14 wk, complete expulsion of fetal tissue usually occurs, and surgical intervention such as D&C can be avoided.

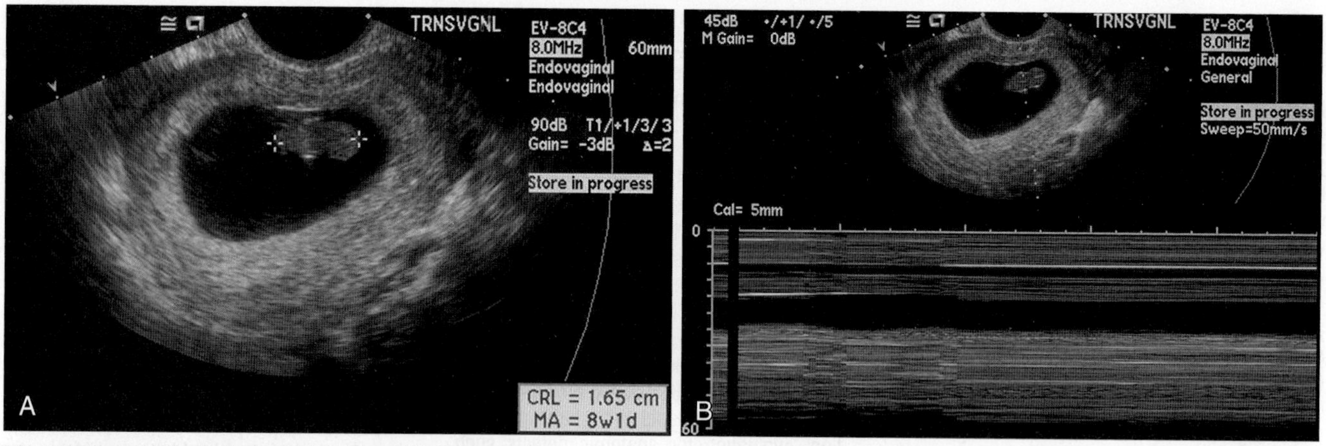

FIG. 1 Embryonic demise. Transvaginal **(A)** and M-mode **(B)** ultrasound. There was no cardiac activity in an embryo measuring more than the threshold of 5 mm. (From Fielding JR et al: *Gynecologic imaging*, Philadelphia, 2011, Saunders.)

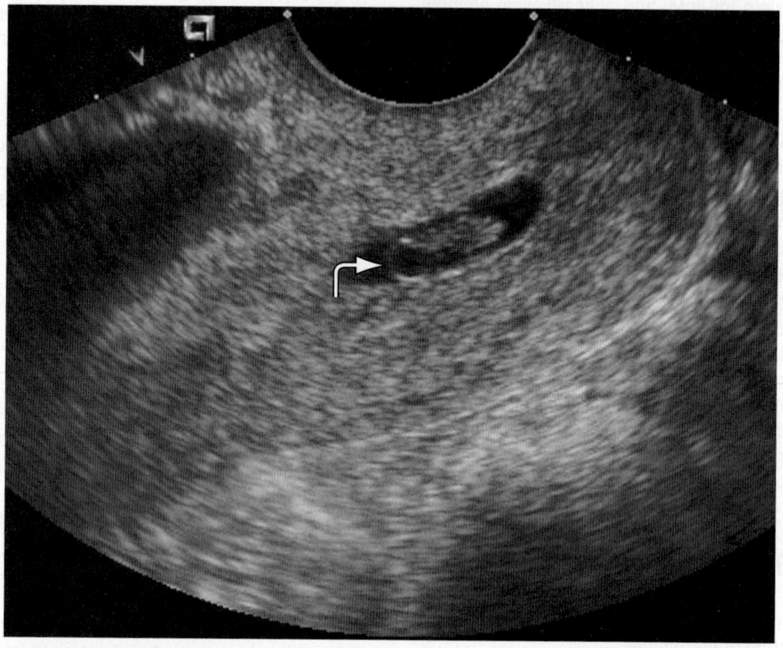

FIG. 2 Inevitable abortion. Transvaginal ultrasonography shows a sac in the cervical canal, past the internal os. The embryo *(curved arrow)* was nonviable. (From Fielding JR et al: *Gynecologic imaging*, Philadelphia, 2011, Saunders.)

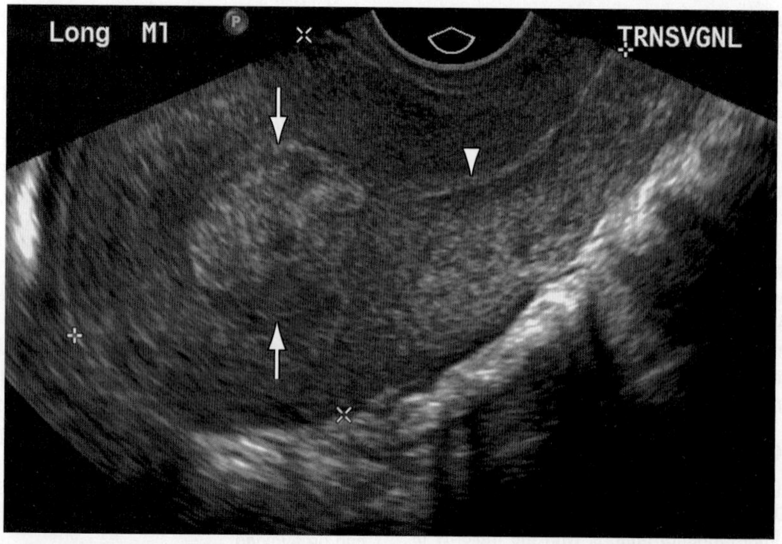

FIG. 3 Incomplete abortion. Transvaginal ultrasonography shows an echogenic mass *(arrows)* in the fundal endometrial cavity. The lower-segment endometrium *(arrowhead)* is normal. (From Fielding JR et al: *Gynecologic imaging*, Philadelphia, 2011, Saunders.)

ACUTE GENERAL Rx

- Incomplete miscarriage between 6 and 14 wk can be associated with great blood loss; these patients should undergo D&C.
- In cases of missed abortion, if fetal demise has occurred >6 wk before or gestational age is >14 wk, there is an increased risk of hypofibrinogenemia with disseminated intravascular coagulation. Thus D&C or manual vacuum aspiration should be performed early in the disease course. Consider use of misoprostol (Cytotec) in appropriate cases where the patient wishes to avoid surgery.
- There is evidence that a surgical approach leads to quicker resolution of the pregnancy event with fewer visits being required.
- Rh-negative patients should be given RhoGAM 50 mcg IM to prevent Rh isoimmunization.

PEARLS & CONSIDERATIONS

Spontaneous pregnancy loss is recommended as a replacement for the term *abortion* and to acknowledge the emotional aspects of losing a pregnancy.

RELATED CONTENT

Miscarriage (Patient Information)

SUGGESTED READINGS

Available at ExpertConsult.com

AUTHOR: **Adrienne B. Neithardt, MD**

BASIC INFORMATION

DEFINITION

Spontaneous bacterial peritonitis (SBP) is an inflammatory reaction of the peritoneum secondary to the presence of bacteria or other microorganisms. More specifically, SBP is defined as an ascitic fluid infection without an evident intraabdominal surgically treatable source occurring primarily in patients with advanced cirrhosis of the liver.

SYNONYMS

Primary peritonitis
SBP
Peritonitis, spontaneous bacterial

ICD-10CM CODE

K65.2 Spontaneous bacterial peritonitis

EPIDEMIOLOGY & DEMOGRAPHICS

PREVALENCE: The prevalence of SBP in cirrhotic patients admitted to the hospital has been estimated at 10% to 30%.
PREDOMINANT SEX: Males are affected more often than females.

PHYSICAL FINDINGS & CLINICAL PRESENTATION

- Acute fever with accompanying abdominal pain/ascites, nausea, vomiting, diarrhea.
- In cirrhotic patients, presentation may be subtle with a low-grade temperature (100° F [37.8° C]) with or without abdominal abnormalities.
- In patients with ascites, a heightened degree of awareness is necessary for detection.
- Jaundice and encephalopathy.
- Deterioration of mental status and/or renal function.
- Table E1 summarizes symptoms and signs of ascetic fluid infection.

ETIOLOGY

- *Escherichia coli*
- *Klebsiella pneumoniae*
- *Streptococcus pneumoniae*
- *Streptococcus* and *Enterococcus* spp.
- *Staphylococcus aureus*
- Anaerobic pathogens: *Bacteroides, Clostridium* organisms
- Other: Fungal, mycobacterial, viral

Dx DIAGNOSIS

The diagnosis of SBP is established by a positive ascitic fluid bacterial culture and an elevated ascitic fluid absolute polymorphonuclear leukocyte count (≥250 cells/mm^3).

DIFFERENTIAL DIAGNOSIS

- Appendicitis (in children)
- Perforated peptic ulcer
- Secondary bacterial peritonitis
- Peritoneal abscess
- Splenic, hepatic, or pancreatic abscess
- Cholecystitis
- Cholangitis

WORKUP

Paracentesis and ascitic fluid analysis will confirm diagnosis (see "Laboratory Tests").

LABORATORY TESTS

Ascitic fluid analysis reveals the following:

- Cell count with an absolute polymorphonuclear cell count >250/mm^3
- Presence of bacteria on Gram stain
- pH <7.31
- Lactic acid >32 mg/dl
- Protein <1 g/dl
- Glucose >50 mg/dl
- Lactate dehydrogenase <225 μU/ml
- Positive culture of peritoneal fluid
- Measurement of the serum/ascites/albumin gradient: The serum/ascites/albumin gradient indirectly measures portal pressure. The albumin concentration of ascitic fluid and serum must be obtained on the same day. The ascitic fluid value is subtracted from the serum value to obtain the gradient. If the difference (not a ratio) is >1.1 g/dl, the patient has portal hypertension, with 97% accuracy. If the difference is <1.1 g/dl, portal hypertension is not present. The majority of patients with SBP have portal hypertension as a result of cirrhosis

IMAGING STUDIES

- Abdominal ultrasound: If there is clinical difficulty in performing paracentesis
- CT scan: To rule out secondary peritonitis (if indicated) and to exclude abscess, mass

Rx TREATMENT

ACUTE GENERAL Rx

- Cefotaxime (2 g IV q8h) or ceftriaxone (2 g IV q24h). Alternative agents include ticarcillin-clavulanate, piperacillin-tazobactam, cefoxitin, and meropenem. Continue therapy for 5 to 7 days. Repeat diagnostic paracentesis can be done at day 2. Repeat paracentesis at 48 hr will demonstrate a significant decrease in polymorphonuclear count in patients with SBP. If ascites PMN count decreases by at least 25% at day 2, IV therapy can be switched to PO (levofloxacin 500 to 750 mg qd) to complete 7 days of therapy if organisms are susceptible.
- IV albumin (1.5 g/kg of body weight upon initial diagnosis and 1 g/kg of albumin on day 3) if BUN >30 mg/dl, serum creatinine >1 mg/dl, bilirubin >4 mg/dl.

PROPHYLAXIS

- Ciprofloxacin 500 mg PO qd or levofloxacin 250 mg PO qd.
- Alternative therapy: TMP-SMX one double-strength tablet PO qd.
- Rifaximin 1200 mg a day was shown in a recent study to be superior to norfloxacin.
- Prophylaxis should be continued until disappearance of ascites or until liver transplantation.

DISPOSITION

The overall mortality rate from an episode of SBP is 20%, and following an episode, the 1-yr mortality rate approaches 70%. Patients that develop SBP should be considered for liver transplantation.

PEARLS & CONSIDERATIONS

COMMENTS

- Renal failure is a major cause of morbidity in cirrhotic patients with SBP. The use of IV albumin (1.5 g/kg at the time of diagnosis and 1 g/kg on day 3) may lower the rate of renal failure and mortality in patients with SBP.
- The criteria for the diagnosis of SBP require that abdominal paracentesis be performed and ascitic fluid be analyzed before a diagnosis of SBP can be made.
- Culturing ascitic fluid as if it were blood (with bedside inoculation of at least 10 ml of ascitic fluid directly into blood culture bottles at the bedside) has been shown to significantly increase the culture positivity of the ascitic fluid in the 80% to 100% range.
- Avoid therapeutic paracenteses during active infection.
- Positive blood cultures in an individual with ascites require exclusion of a peritoneal source by paracentesis.
- Follow-up paracentesis is indicated only in selected cases (worsening clinical status, nosocomial SBP, infection with atypical organism, recent β-lactam exposure).

SUGGESTED READINGS

Available at ExpertConsult.com

AUTHOR: **Glenn G. Fort, MD, MPH**

BASIC INFORMATION

DEFINITION

Squamous cell carcinoma (SCC) is a malignant neoplasm of keratinocytes.

SYNONYMS

SCC
Skin cancer

ICD-10CM CODES

C44.5	Malignant neoplasm of skin of trunk
C44.4	Malignant neoplasm of skin of scalp and neck
D04	Carcinoma in situ of skin
C44.9	Malignant neoplasm of skin, unspecified
C44.0	Malignant neoplasm of skin of lip
C44.2	Malignant neoplasm of skin of ear and external auricular canal
C44.3	Malignant neoplasm of skin of other and unspecified parts of skin
C44.02	Squamous cell carcinoma of skin of lip
C44.121	Squamous cell carcinoma of skin of unspecified eyelid, including canthus
C44.122	Squamous cell carcinoma of skin of right eyelid, including canthus
C44.129	Squamous cell carcinoma of skin of left eyelid, including canthus
C44.221	Squamous cell carcinoma of skin of unspecified ear and external auricular canal
C44.222	Squamous cell carcinoma of skin of right ear and external auricular canal
C44.229	Squamous cell carcinoma of skin of left ear and external auricular canal
C44.320	Squamous cell carcinoma of skin of unspecified parts of face
C44.321	Squamous cell carcinoma of skin of nose
C44.329	Squamous cell carcinoma of skin of other parts of face
C44.42	Squamous cell carcinoma of skin of scalp and neck
C44.520	Squamous cell carcinoma of anal skin
C44.521	Squamous cell carcinoma of skin of breast
C44.529	Squamous cell carcinoma of skin of other part of trunk
C44.621	Squamous cell carcinoma of skin of unspecified upper limb, including shoulder
C44.622	Squamous cell carcinoma of skin of right upper limb, including shoulder
C44.629	Squamous cell carcinoma of skin of left upper limb, including shoulder
C44.721	Squamous cell carcinoma of skin of unspecified lower limb, including hip
C44.722	Squamous cell carcinoma of skin of right lower limb, including hip
C44.729	Squamous cell carcinoma of skin of left lower limb, including hip
C44.82	Squamous cell carcinoma of overlapping sites of skin

EPIDEMIOLOGY & DEMOGRAPHICS

- SCC is the second most common cutaneous malignancy, comprising 20% of all cases of nonmelanoma skin cancer.
- Incidence is highest in lower latitudes (e.g., southern U.S., Australia).
- Male:female ratio is 2:1.
- Incidence increases with age and sun exposure.
- In black patients, SCC are 20% more common than basal cell carcinomas (BCC).
- Average age at diagnosis is 66 yr.

PHYSICAL FINDINGS & CLINICAL PRESENTATION

- SCC frequently begins at the site of actinic keratosis and commonly affects the scalp, neck region, back of hands (Fig. E1), superior surface of the pinna, and the lip (Fig. E2). On the lower lip, SCC often develops on actinic cheilitis. A history of smoking is a significant predisposing factor.
- Bowen disease refers to SCC in situ (Fig. E3).
- SCC lesions may have a scaly, erythematous macule or plaque (Fig. E4).
- Telangiectasia, central ulceration may also be present. The ulcer may be superficial and hidden by a crust. Removal of the crust may reveal a well-defined papillary base.
- Most SCCs present as exophytic lesions that grow over a period of mo.
- Although most SCCs are relatively slow growing and nonaggressive, some (2% to 5%) can exhibit rapid growth and metastases. Aggressive tumors are more common in immunocompromised patients and when arising from scars, burns, or prior injury (Marjolin ulcer). Presence of SCC on ears, lips, or size >2 cm are high-risk features of SCC.

ETIOLOGY

Risk factors include ultraviolet B radiation, immunosuppression (kidney transplant recipients have a significantly increased risk), arsenic exposure, HPV infection, medications (azathioprine, sorafenib, tumor necrosis factor [TNF] inhibitors), discoid LE, erosive lichen planus, chronic ulcers, prior radiation exposure, and tobacco abuse.

Dx DIAGNOSIS

DIFFERENTIAL DIAGNOSIS

- Keratoacanthomas
- Actinic keratosis
- Amelanotic melanoma
- Basal cell carcinoma
- Benign tumors
- Healing traumatic wounds
- Spindle cell tumors
- Warts

WORKUP

Diagnosis is made by full-thickness skin biopsy (incisional or excisional).

Rx TREATMENT

ACUTE GENERAL Rx

- Electrodesiccation and curettage for small SCCs (<2 mm in diameter), superficial tumors, and lesions located in extremity and trunk.
- Tumors thinner than 4 mm can be managed by simple local removal.
- Lesions 4 to 8 mm thick or those with deep dermal invasion should be excised.
- Tumors penetrating the dermis can be treated with several modalities, including excision and Mohs surgery, radiation therapy, and chemotherapy. Mohs surgery is commonly used for lesions on the face.
- Metastatic SCC can be treated with cryotherapy and combination of chemotherapy using 13-*cis*-retinoic acid and interferon-alpha 2A.
- A treatment algorithm for squamous cell carcinoma is illustrated in Fig. 5.
- In a recent phase 1 study of PD-1 blockade with cemiplimab among patients with advanced cutaneous squamous cell carcinoma, cemiplimab induced a response in approximately half the patients.[1]

DISPOSITION

- Survival is related to size, location, degree of differentiation, immunologic status of the patient, depth of invasion, and presence of metastases. Risk factors for metastasis include lesions on the lip or ear, increasing lesion depth, and poor cell differentiation. Table 1 summarizes risk factors for metastasis of invasive squamous cell carcinoma.
- Patients whose tumors penetrate through the dermis or exceed 8 mm in thickness are at risk of tumor recurrence.
- The most common metastatic locations are regional lymph nodes, liver, and lung.
- Tumors on the scalp, forehead, ears, nose, and lips also carry a higher risk.
- The rate of SCC metastasis from all skin sites ranges from 0.5% to 5.2%.
- SCCs originating in the lip and pinna metastasize in 10% to 20% of cases.
- 5-yr survival for metastatic SCC is 34%.

REFERRAL

Oncology referral for metastatic SCC

PEARLS & CONSIDERATIONS

COMMENTS

- SCC arising in areas of prior radiation, thermal injury, and areas of chronic ulcers or chronic draining sinuses are more aggressive and have a higher frequency of metastasis than those originating in actinic damaged skin.

[1]Migden MR et al: PD-1 blockade with cemiplimab in advanced cutaneous squamous-cell carcinoma, *N Engl J Med* 379:341-51, 2018.

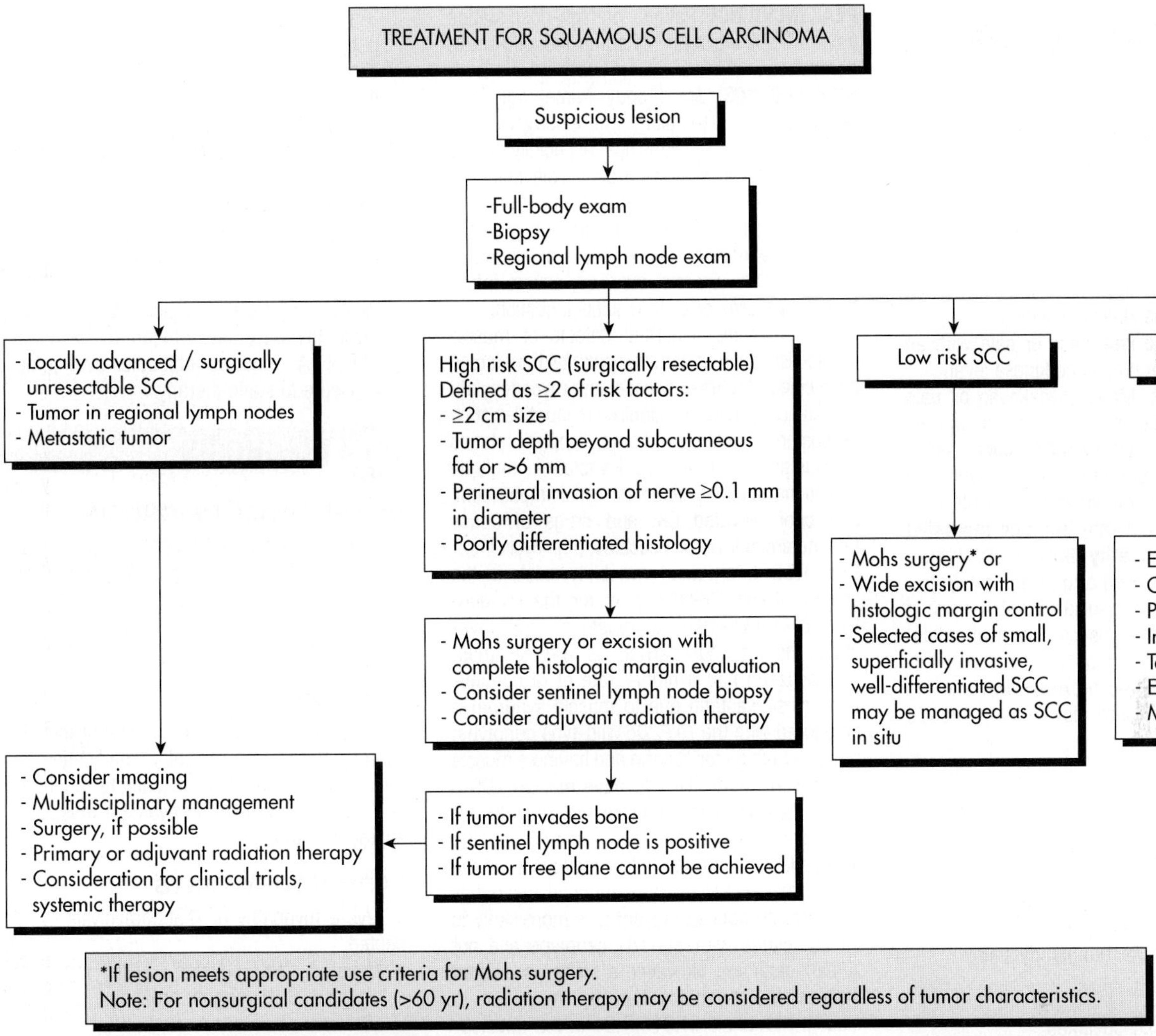

FIG. 5 Treatment algorithm for squamous cell carcinoma *(SCC)*. *EDC,* Electrodesiccation and curettage; *5-FU,* 5-fluorouracil; *PDT,* photodynamic therapy. (From Niederhuber JE: *Abeloff's clinical oncology,* ed 6, Philadelphia, 2020, Elsevier.)

TABLE 1 Risk Factors for Metastasis of Invasive Squamous Cell Carcinoma

Tumor thickness: >2 mm (high risk: Tumor thickness >6 mm)
Diameter: >2 cm
Location: Ear, lips, and mucosae, including tongue, vulva, and penis (perineural growth may be an additional risk factor in these locations)
Arising within a scar (e.g., burn, radiation)
Histopathologic features: Poorly differentiated or undifferentiated, acantholytic,* developing within Bowen disease
Immunosuppression

*Recently questioned Ogawa T et al: Acantholytic squamous cell carcinoma is usually associated with hair follicles, not acantholytic actinic keratosis, and is not "high risk": Diagnosis, management, and clinical outcomes in a series of 115 cases, *J Am Acad Dermatol* 76:327-333, 2017.

Based in part on Brantsch KD et al: Analysis of risk factors determining prognosis of cutaneous squamous-cell carcinoma: a prospective study, *Lancet Oncol* 9:713-720, 2008.

- Oral retinoids may be useful as a preventive strategy in patients with immunosuppression.
- Nicotinamide (500 mg bid, available over the counter) mitigates some of the deleterious effects of UV radiation and has been reported to lower the incidence of nonmelanoma skin cancer (NMSCO) by 23%.[2]

RELATED CONTENT

Squamous Cell Carcinoma (Patient Information)

AUTHOR: **Fred F. Ferri, MD**

[2]Chen AC et al: A phase 3 randomized trial of nicotinamide for skin cancer chemoprevention, *N Engl J Med* 373:1618, 2015.

BASIC INFORMATION

DEFINITION

Statin-induced muscle syndromes (SIMS) include myopathy, myalgia, myositis, and rhabdomyolysis. Definitions for these syndromes are inconsistent in the medical literature.

- Myopathy: A general term defined as any disease of muscles.
- Myalgia: Muscle weakness or pain without serum creatinine kinase elevation.
- Myositis: Muscle weakness or pain with an increased serum creatinine kinase level.
- Rhabdomyolysis: Muscle weakness or pain and a marked serum creatinine kinase level usually greater than 10× the upper limit of normal and serum creatinine elevation as well as signs of brown urine and elevated urine myoglobin. A rare **immune-mediated necrotizing myopathy (IMNM)**, also known as **statin-associated autoimmune myopathy**, has also been associated with the use of statins with symptoms persisting after discontinuation of the drug. This condition presents with symmetric proximal arm and leg weakness and severe elevations of muscle enzymes.

SYNONYMS

SIMS
Statin-induced myopathies
Statin-induced myositis
Statin-induced myalgias
Statin-induced rhabdomyolysis
Statin-associated autoimmune myopathy

ICD-10CM CODES	
M60.9	Myositis, unspecified
M62.82	Rhabdomyolysis
G72.2	Myopathy due to other toxic agents
G72.9	Myopathy, unspecified
G72.81	Critical illness myopathy
G72.89	Other specified myopathies
M60.89	Other myositis, multiple sites

EPIDEMIOLOGY & DEMOGRAPHICS

INCIDENCE: Risk of statin-induced rhabdomyolysis is 1.2 per 10,000 persons/yr. Rhabdomyolysis risk of death is 0.15 deaths per 1 million prescriptions. SIMS most commonly occur in people aged 51 to 75, which may reflect the pattern of statin use. Statin-associated autoimmune myopathy occurs in an estimated 2 or 3 of every 100,000 patients treated with statins.

PREVALENCE: The prevalence of statin-induced myalgias is about 1% to 5%, similar to placebo in clinical trials, although observational studies have suggested a prevalence of 10% or higher. Statins may cause elevated transaminases (ALT, AST) at a prevalence of 0.5% to 2.0% and rhabdomyolysis ~0.08%.

PREDOMINANT SEX & AGE: The mean age of hospitalized patients with statin-induced myopathy or rhabdomyolysis was 64 yr old and was slightly more common in women (56%).

PEAK INCIDENCE: Patients on high-dose statins have a 0.9% incidence of statin-induced rhabdomyolysis.

RISK FACTORS: Small body frame; age over 80 yr; women, particularly frail elderly women; patients taking multiple drugs, especially gemfibrozil, niacin, cyclosporine, itraconazole, ketoconazole, erythromycin, clarithromycin, verapamil, amiodarone; renal or liver impairment; pharmacogenetic variability; hypothyroidism; excessive alcohol intake; vigorous exercise; severe infections; excessive grapefruit juice ingestion; low vitamin D levels; inherited defects of muscle metabolism such as carnitine palmityl transferase II deficiency, McArdle disease, and myoadenylate deaminase deficiency; acquired myopathies such as postpoliomyelitis syndrome; lipophilic statins (simvastatin, atorvastatin, lovastatin); multiple conditions such as diabetes; renal impairment, and prior elevated CK; and drugs of abuse (amphetamines, heroin, cocaine, phencyclidine).

GENETICS: Interpatient variability exists in the activity of the *CYP3A4* gene for the metabolism of simvastatin, atorvastatin, and lovastatin. Homozygous carriers of *CYP2D6* (poor metabolizers) had a higher rate of discontinuation of simvastatin due to muscle syndromes compared with the *CYP2D6* wild-type genotype; patients taking atorvastatin and having a muscle event were more likely to have the CYP2D6*4 allele. *SLCO1B1* polymorphisms encode for the organic anion transport of statins into the liver cells. The variant C allele may increase the risk of the *SLCO1B1* statin–induced myopathy. Simvastatin-induced myopathy is more likely to be associated with *SLO1B1* genotype and not *ABCB1* genotype. However, a statin-associated autoimmune myopathy has shown a link to class II HLA allele DRB1*11:01 in the development of anti-HMG CoA reductase antibodies, leading to an increase in expression of the antibodies in the muscles of patients exposed to statins. Deficiencies in ubiquinone (coenzyme Q10) may exist in patients with a mutation in the *COQ2* gene. The *EYS* gene can affect neuromuscular tissue and may have a role. In addition, *RYR1* and *CACNA1S* genetic variants may be associated with statin-induced muscle syndromes and elevated CK levels.

PHYSICAL FINDINGS & CLINICAL PRESENTATION

- Myopathy can occur at any time, although it is more common within the first 4 wk of therapy; statin-associated necrotizing myopathy may occur after months of using statins
- Proximal generalized muscle aches, body aches, and pains, and may be mild or severe
- Dark-colored urine
- Muscle cramps, spasms, tenderness, or stiffness
- Unusually tired or weak
- Nocturnal cramping
- Tendon pain

ETIOLOGY

- History of current statin use.
- May be explained by one of three deficiencies of end products of the 3-hydroxy-3-methyl-glutaryl-coA reductase pathway: Cell signaling and apoptosis, mitochondrial function and ubiquinone concentrations, and cholesterol concentrations and cell membrane integrity.
- The risk may be enhanced by drug interactions that interfere with hepatic metabolism and gut wall transport of interacting medications and by pharmacodynamic effects.
- Underlying metabolic muscle disorder may predispose a patient to develop myopathy.
- Patients with statin-associated autoimmune myopathy have been found to have anti–HMG-CoA reductase antibodies even prior to exposure to statin therapy.

Dx DIAGNOSIS

DIFFERENTIAL DIAGNOSIS

Bursitis, tendinitis, radiculopathy, osteoarthritis, muscle strain, myofascial pain, hypothyroidism, proton pump inhibitor–induced polymyositis, viral illness, polymyositis, idiopathic inflammatory myositis, and polymyalgia rheumatica

WORKUP

Workup consists of a thorough history, including exercise history, urine color, medication history, and physical exam to palpate tenderness and obtain blood tests to evaluate muscle and kidney damage.

LABORATORY TESTS

If severe myopathy or rhabdomyolysis is suspected:

- Elevated CPK, positive serum myoglobin, elevated BUN, serum creatinine, AST, ALT, LDH, and potassium
- Urine creatinine, positive casts, and hemoglobin in urine with absence of red blood cells
- Anti-3-hydroxy-3-methylglutaryl-conenzyme A (anti–HMG-CoA) antibody
- Consider electrocardiogram and assessment of calcium, phosphate, and uric acid

If mild to moderate myopathy is suspected:

- Monitor TSH and CPK levels; CPK may only be elevated when sudden severe myopathy occurs.
- If the patient has brown or dark urine or elevated CPK, monitor BUN and serum creatinine.
- In statin-associated autoimmune myopathy, the creatine kinase level is usually ≥10 times the upper limit of normal. In these patients, muscle biopsy specimens will be positive for autoantibodies against HMG-CoA reductase and may have necrosis.

IMAGING STUDIES

- Not recommended.
- In statin-associated autoimmune myopathy, electromyography shows small-amplitude motor-unit potentials with increased spontaneous activity characteristic of an active myopathic process. Muscle edema is evident on MRI.[1]

[1]Mammen AL: Statin-associated autoimmune myopathy, *N Engl J Med* 374:664-669, 2016.

- Statin Intolerance Tool:
  1. The American College of Cardiology has created a tool to assess statin muscle symptoms and to guide clinicians that can be of value: http://tools.acc.org/statintolerance/#!/

Rx TREATMENT

NONPHARMACOLOGIC THERAPY

Treatment of rhabdomyolysis is generally supportive in nature (see "Rhabdomyolysis" topic).

ACUTE GENERAL Rx

- Stop statin therapy immediately if muscle symptoms occur. Check history, potential drug-drug interactions, CPK, TSH, renal function, hepatic function, and urinalysis.
- If patients have suspected rhabdomyolysis, they should be hospitalized and treated with supportive therapy and monitoring of complications.
- If CPK <10× the upper limit of normal without symptoms, continue statin therapy at the same or lower dosage.
- If CPK <10× the upper limit of normal with intolerable symptoms, discontinue statin.
- If CPK >10× the upper limit of normal, discontinue statin.

Box E1 describes recommendations of the National Lipid Association Statin Safety Assessment Task Force regarding statin and muscle safety.

CHRONIC Rx

- After stopping the statin and symptom or CPK resolution, which may take up to 4 mo, consider the same statin at a lower dosage or a different statin at an equivalent or lower dosage.
- When restarting therapy, consider statins such as low-dose rosuvastatin; pravastatin; and alternate-day dosing of rosuvastatin or atorvastatin.
- If patient had rhabdomyolysis secondary to statin therapy, consider nonstatin treatments.
- If the patient develops myopathy after a second trial of therapy, statin treatment should be permanently discontinued and nonstatin cholesterol-lowering therapy initiated.
- Bempedoic acid may offer a safe and effective lipid-lowering therapeutic option for patients unable to tolerate statins.
- For IMNM (statin-associated autoimmune myopathy and idiopathic inflammatory myositis), immunosuppressive therapy with prednisone (1 mg per kg of body weight per day) and at least one agent (methotrexate, azathioprine, or mycophenolate mofetil) have been used. In resistant cases, IV immune globulin or another agent such as rituximab may be added.

INTEGRATIVE MEDICINE

- The effect of coenzyme Q10 on reducing or preventing SIMS remains controversial; although it may be effective in reducing muscle pain, weakness, cramps, and tiredness, it has no effect on lowering CK levels. Given its safety, coenzyme Q10 can be recommended if the actions listed under "Chronic Rx" are insufficient to continue the use of the statin and if the muscle symptoms have been limited to myalgias. Use coenzyme Q10 with caution in patients taking warfarin, as its anticoagulant effect may be decreased.
- A 2015 meta-analysis of observational studies reported that vitamin D levels were lower in patients with statin-induced myalgias than in individuals who did not have these symptoms.
- In a study of 282 patients with vitamin D levels less than 32 ng/ml and with myalgia-myositis from statins, vitamin D supplementation (median 50,000 IU D_3/wk) for 6 mo improved symptoms and statin tolerance in 74% to 85% of patients; another study showed that replacement of vitamin D in patients with low-serum vitamin D may be able to maintain or restart previously failed statin therapy.

DISPOSITION

- Usually resolves within 1 wk up to 4 mo after discontinuing statin therapy.
- Once the patient has a full recovery, an alternative statin can be tried.
- Statins should not be restarted in IMNM or idiopathic inflammatory myositis.

REFERRAL

If rhabdomyolysis is suspected, immediate referral for hospitalization is suggested.

PEARLS & CONSIDERATIONS

COMMENTS

SIMS are usually mild and will resolve within a few wk after discontinuing statin therapy. However, such syndromes may progress to rhabdomyolysis.

PREVENTION

- Follow the 2013 AHA/ACC treatment guidelines and the 2017 ACC focused update on nonstatin therapies for LDL cholesterol and limit the concomitant use of fibrates with statins.
- Discontinue statin therapy prior to and during surgical procedures.
- If patient requires a short-term therapy with an interacting medication such as an azole antifungal, temporarily discontinue statin therapy until interacting therapy is completed.
- If statin–fibric acid therapy is warranted, fenofibrate is preferred over gemfibrozil to decrease risk of myopathy.
- Baseline liver function testing before initiation of statin therapy and only if clinically indicated thereafter.

PATIENT & FAMILY EDUCATION

- Inform patients to promptly report muscle weakness, unexpected muscle pain, or brownish urine.
  1. Providers should be cautious of the impact of media coverage of statin-induced side effects, which may include the nocebo effect.
- Ensure that the pharmacist and/or primary care physician checks for drug-drug interactions with every new prescription, including those from dentists and physicians from other specialties.
- Coenzyme Q10 may lessen milder muscle symptoms from statins, but patients should inform their physician and pharmacist if they decide to use this supplement.
- A recent clinical trial comparing lipid-lowering efficacy for two nonstatin therapies, ezetimibe and evolocumab, among patients with statin intolerance revealed that evolocumab resulted in a significantly greater reduction in LDL-C levels after 24 wk. Further studies are needed to assess long-term efficacy and safety.

SUGGESTED READINGS

Available at ExpertConsult.com

RELATED CONTENT

Rhabdomyolysis (Related Key Topic)

AUTHORS: **Lisa Cohen, PharmD,** and **Anne L. Hume, PharmD**

BASIC INFORMATION

DEFINITION

Status epilepticus is a medical neurologic emergency. It is historically defined as 30 min of continuous seizure activity or two or more seizures without full recovery of consciousness between seizures. However, in practice a continuous seizure that lasts >5 min is treated as status epilepticus.

SYNONYMS

Convulsive status epilepticus
Nonconvulsive status epilepticus

ICD-10CM CODES

G41	Status epilepticus
G40.301	Generalized idiopathic epilepsy and epileptic syndromes, not intractable, with status epilepticus

EPIDEMIOLOGY & DEMOGRAPHICS

INCIDENCE: 40 to 100 cases per 100,000 persons
PREDOMINANT SEX & AGE: No gender preference
PEAK INCIDENCE: It is most common among children younger than 1 yr and adults older than 60 yr.

PHYSICAL FINDINGS & CLINICAL PRESENTATION

- Patients can present with repetitive tonic-clonic movements of the body (convulsive status epilepticus); other patients are comatose and nonresponsive (nonconvulsive status epilepticus).
- Patients may also present with lethargy, intermittent confusion, and involuntary movements.

ETIOLOGY

- Status epilepticus can be the result of an acute neurologic injury, such as stroke, meningitis, brain tumor, etc. Table 1 summarizes causes of status epilepticus in adults presenting in the community.
- In patients with epilepsy, abrupt discontinuation of antiepileptic drugs can result in status epilepticus.

DIAGNOSIS

DIFFERENTIAL DIAGNOSIS

- Convulsive syncope
- Encephalopathies: Metabolic, infectious, toxic, etc.
- Nonepileptic spells

WORKUP

- ABCs
- ICU admission
- Emergent electroencephalogram (EEG), especially if the patient does not start returning to baseline
- Continuous EEG in refractory cases
- Table 2 describes a suggested timetable for emergency diagnosis and treatment of status epilepticus. A treatment approach is summarized in Table 3 and Fig. 1.

LABORATORY TESTS

- Routine blood workup (CBC, CMP, glucose, electrolytes)
- Urine drug screen
- Lumbar puncture and CSF analysis in patients with suspected infectious meningitis or encephalitis or suspected autoimmune or paraneoplastic encephalitis

TABLE 1 Causes of Status Epilepticus in Adults Presenting from the Community

Previous Seizures	No Previous Seizures
Common	
Subtherapeutic anticonvulsant	Ethanol-related
Ethanol-related	Drug toxicity
Intractable epilepsy	CNS infection
	Head trauma
	CNS tumor
Less Common	
CNS infection	Metabolic aberration
Metabolic aberration	Stroke
Drug toxicity	
Stroke	
CNS tumor	
Head trauma	

CNS, Central nervous system.
From Vincent JL et al: *Textbook of critical care,* ed 7, Philadelphia, 2017, Elsevier.

IMAGING STUDIES

- Immediate CT scan of the head.
- MRI of the brain with and without contrast should be performed once the patient is in a stable condition.

TREATMENT

- The longer a patient is in status epilepticus, the harder it is to treat and the more likely permanent damage is done.
- Patients with continuous seizure activity over 5 min should be given intravenous lorazepam 0.1 mg/kg at 2 mg/min (or diazepam 0.2 mg/kg at 5 mg/min only when lorazepam is not available).
- In the absence of intravenous access, intramuscular administration of midazolam 10 mg in an adult is a superior alternative.
- It is not uncommon for patients in convulsive status epilepticus to transition to nonconvulsive status epilepticus with time or with benzodiazepine treatment. If a patient does not start improving or has any subtle signs of ongoing seizures, consider nonconvulsive status epilepticus.
- Failure of response to lorazepam or midazolam is referred to as established status

TABLE 2 Suggested Timetable for Emergency Diagnosis and Treatment of Status Epilepticus

Time	Exam/Intervention	Testing
Initial presentation: 0 min	Airway, breathing, circulation, IV access, monitoring	Glucose, oxygenation via pulse oximetry ± blood gas analysis
Primary survey: 5 min	Neurologic exam Administer antiepileptic drugs Lorazepam, 0.1 mg/kg IV Phenobarbital, 20 mg/kg IV Normal saline maintenance IV Reduce fever	Electrolytes, renal and liver function, ammonia, anticonvulsant levels, toxicology, complete blood cell count, urinalysis
Secondary survey: 15-30 min	Evaluate treatment results Second-line antiepileptic drug if seizure persists Fosphenytoin, 20 mg/kg IV, or phenytoin, 20 mg/kg IV	Patient-specific: Cranial imaging (CT vs. MRI), lumbar puncture, EEG, ECG
Status epilepticus: >30 min	Intubation and mechanical ventilation	
Refractory status epilepticus: >60 min	Titrate antiepileptic drug to burst suppression Pentobarbital, 10 mg/kg IV given over 30 min, then 5 mg/kg every hour for 3 doses, then 1 mg/kg/h; titrate to effect Midazolam, 0.15 mg/kg IV, then 1-2 μg/kg/min, titrate to effect Phenobarbital, 5-10 mg/kg IV every 20 minutes to achieve burst suppression, then every 12 hours Evaluate need for vasopressors	Continuous EEG Neurologic consultation Consider anesthesia consultation for treatment with inhaled anesthetic

CT, Computed tomography; *ECG,* electrocardiogram; *EEG,* electroencephalogram; *IV,* intravenous; *MRI,* magnetic resonance imaging.
From Vincent JL et al: *Textbook of critical care,* ed 7, Philadelphia, 2017, Elsevier.

TABLE 3 Treatment Approach to Status Epilepticus

1. Appropriate critical care treatment should be provided as soon as possible and simultaneously with emergent initial therapy for seizures. Treatment should be escalated quickly until seizures are controlled.
2. Critical care treatment (dictated by clinical circumstances):
   a. Intubation for airway protection and mechanical ventilation
   b. Vital sign monitoring
   c. Peripheral IV access
   d. Treatment of hypotension with vasopressors
   e. Finger stick blood glucose
   f. Nutrient resuscitation (thiamine before dextrose)
   g. Hypertension may be related to ongoing seizure activity, and termination of status epilepticus often substantially corrects it. Additionally, many agents used to terminate status epilepticus can produce hypotension.
3. Emergent initial therapy with benzodiazepines:
   a. Lorazepam 0.1 mg/kg up to 4 mg per dose, may repeat after 5-10 min
   b. Midazolam 0.2 mg/kg IM/IV up to 10 mg
   c. Diazepam 0.15 mg/kg up to 10 mg per dose, may repeat after 5 min
4. Urgent control therapy—antiseizure drugs available in IV formulations:
   a. Fosphenytoin/phenytoin 20 mg PE/kg IV, may repeat bolus of 5 mg/kg IV:
   b. Valproic acid 20-40 mg/kg IV, may repeat bolus of 20 mg/kg IV
   c. Levetiracetam 1000-3000 mg IV
   d. Phenobarbital 20 mg/kg IV, may repeat bolus of 5-10 mg/kg
   e. Lacosamide 200-400 mg IV
   f. Midazolam bolus 0.2 mg/kg IV, followed by 0.05-2 mg/kg/h continuous infusion
5. Refractory therapy–continuous infusion of antiseizure drugs, titrated to either seizure cessation, suppression-burst, or complete suppression on EEG:
   a. Midazolam bolus 0.2 mg/kg IV, followed by 0.05-2 mg/kg/h continuous infusion
   b. Propofol bolus 1-2 mg/kg, followed by 20 mcg/kg/min continuous infusion, titrate up to 30-200 mcg/kg/min
   c. Pentobarbital 5-15 mg/kg, may repeat bolus of 5-10 mg/kg, followed by 0.5-5 mg/kg/h continuous infusion
6. Treat complications.
7. Complications of status epilepticus are numerous and can involve multiple organ systems. In particular, convulsive status epilepticus is associated with cardiac complications such as hypertension and tachycardia, as well as rhabdomyolysis and hyperthermia. Respiratory complications, including respiratory failure, hypoxia, and neurogenic pulmonary edema, may be seen. Status epilepticus is associated with neuronal damage and cerebral edema with increased intracranial pressure, which may require intracranial pressure monitoring and aggressive treatment with hypertonic agents.

From Vincent JL et al: *Textbook of critical care,* ed 7, Philadelphia, 2017, Elsevier.

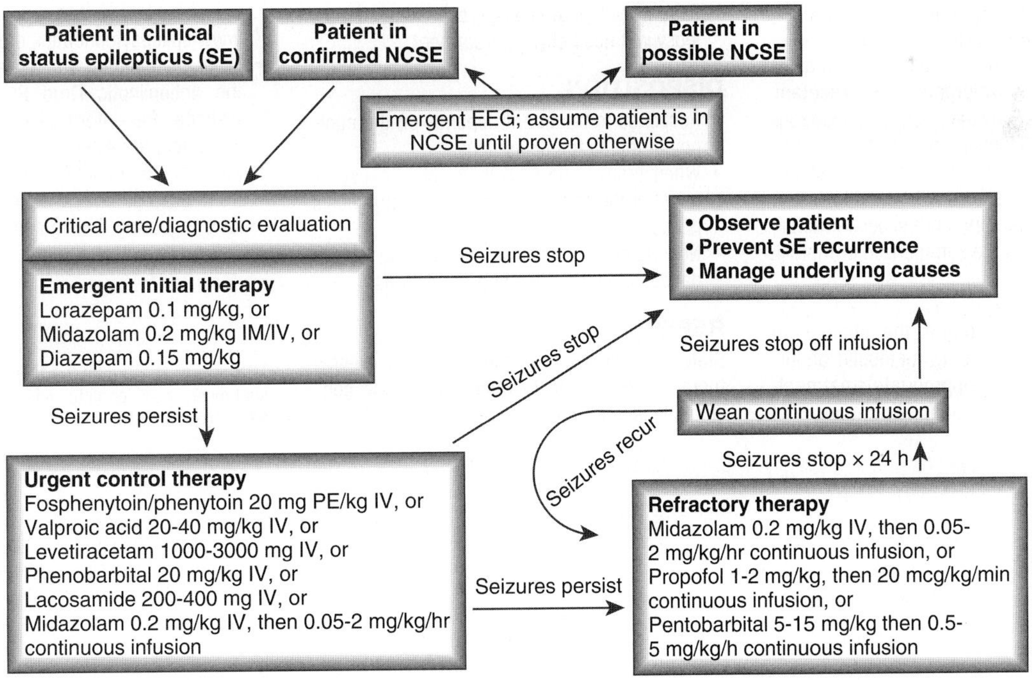

FIG. 1 Management algorithm for status epilepticus. *EEG,* Electroencephalogram; *IM,* intramuscular; *IV,* intravenous; *NCSE,* nonconvulsive status epilepticus; *SE,* status epilepticus. (From Vincent JL et al: *Textbook of critical care,* ed 7, Philadelphia, 2017, Elsevier.)

TABLE 4 Treatment Alternatives for Refractory and Super-Refractory Status Epilepticus

	Comments	Adverse Events
Thiopental	Metabolized to pentobarbital	Hypotension Respiratory depression Cardiac depression
Ketamine	Mechanism of action particularly well-suited to treat refractory and super-refractory SE (NMDA receptor antagonist)	High intracranial pressure Hypotension Hallucinations
Inhaled anesthetics	High rate of complications Needs closed system (gas recovery)	Hypotension Infection Paralytic ileus
Ketogenic diet	Relatively safe (no respiratory and cardiocirculatory instability) Slow onset of action Requires skilled dietician	Gastroesophageal reflux Constipation Acidosis Hypertriglyceridemia
Lidocaine	Minor respiratory depression compared with other drugs	Cardiocirculatory instability Possible induction of seizures
Hypothermia	Only transitory control (cannot be a prolonged therapy)	Hypotension Cardiovascular instability Impaired coagulation (bleeding risks)
Resective surgery	Long-term treatment of seizures Not all patients are eligible	Surgical risks

NMDA, N-methyl-D-aspartate; *SE,* status epilepticus.
From Swaiman KF et al: *Swaiman's pediatric neurology, principles and practice,* ed 6, Philadelphia, 2017, Elsevier. See original table for references.

epilepticus and should be followed by second-line therapy of intravenous fosphenytoin 20 mg/kg (PE) at a rate not greater than 150 mg/min, phenytoin 20 mg/kg IV at up to 50 mg/min as tolerated, intravenous valproic acid 40 mg/kg IV, or intravenous levetiracetam 60 mg/kg IV. Vital signs should be monitored during the infusion.

- If seizures continue, an additional infusion of intravenous valproate, levetiracetam, lacosamide, or brivaracetam or continuous infusions of phenobarbital, midazolam, and propofol are alternatives. Superiority of any one agent is not established. Treatment alternatives for refractory and super-refractory status epilepticus are summarized in Table 4.

GENERAL Rx

It is important to find out the etiology of the status epilepticus (e.g., metabolic disturbance, infection). The appropriate treatment/understanding of the underlying cause of the status epilepticus will impact successful treatment.

CHRONIC Rx

- Chronic treatment of status epilepticus depends on underlying etiology.
- Patient with status epilepticus due to epilepsy will need chronic treatment.

DISPOSITION

- Response to treatment depends on the etiology of the status epilepticus.
- When there is no CNS injury as a cause or result of the status epilepticus, the prognosis is good.
- No driving until seizure freedom in accordance with local laws and regulations.

REFERRAL

Status epilepticus is a neurologic emergency; therefore immediate inpatient neurologic consultation is warranted.

PEARLS & CONSIDERATIONS

COMMENTS

- Status epilepticus is a medical emergency that carries a high risk of mortality. Mortality among patients who present in status epilepticus is 15% to 22%. Among those who survive, functional ability will decline in 25% of cases.
- Continuous video EEG is crucial in the treatment of these patients because some of them may not be clinically seizing (convulsing) but electrographically they may still have subclinical repetitive seizures or subclinical status epilepticus.
- In the context of benzodiazepine-refractory convulsive status epilepticus, the anticonvulsant drugs levetiracetam, fosphenytoin, and valproate each led to seizure cessation and improved alertness by 60 min in approximately half the patients, and the three drugs were associated with similar incidences of adverse events.[1]

PREVENTION

Medication compliance is crucial in patients with epilepsy.

PATIENT & FAMILY EDUCATION

- Patients with epilepsy have normal lives.
- The goal of treatment is no seizures and no side effects to medications.
- Patient education and information can be obtained at the Epilepsy Foundation: www.epilepsyfoundation.org
- Pregnant women with epilepsy should visit the Antiepileptic Drug Pregnancy Registry website for information and assistance: www.aedpregnancyregistry.org
- Patients with ongoing seizures are forbidden from driving; check state regulations and laws regarding driving and epilepsy.

AUTHOR: **Corey Goldsmith, MD**

[1] Kapur J et al: Randomized trial of three anticonvulsant medications for status epilepticus, *N Engl J Med,* 381:2103-13, 2019.

BASIC INFORMATION

DEFINITION

Stickler syndrome is a group of hereditary connective tissue diseases, which are characterized by various ocular signs, bone and joint disorders, distinct facial features, and sensorineural deafness (seen in 10% of cases).

SYNONYMS

Stickler syndrome type 1: STL1, vitreous type 1, membranous vitreous type, arthroopthalmopathy, hereditary progressive, AOM

Stickler syndrome type 2: STL2, vitreous type 2, beaded vitreous type

Stickler syndrome type 3: STL3, Stickler syndrome nonocular type

ICD 10-CM CODES

Q87	Congenital malformation syndromes predominantly affecting facial appearance
Q89.8	Other specified congenital malformations

EPIDEMIOLOGY & DEMOGRAPHICS

INCIDENCE: At birth estimated around 1/7500

PREVALENCE: 1 to 9 per 100,000

PREDOMINANT SEX & AGE: Pediatric population

RISK FACTORS: Family history given inheritance patterns

GENETICS: Inheritance is primarily autosomal dominant, though it can also be autosomal recessive and is genetically heterogeneous. Prenatal diagnosis is possible in families in which the mutation has been identified.

PHYSICAL FINDINGS & CLINICAL PRESENTATION

- Clinical features include facial changes, eye abnormalities, hearing loss, and arthritis.
- Facies: Flat midface, depressed nasal bridge, short nose, anteverted nares, micrognathia. Soft palate cleft is possible, associated with Pierre Robin sequence.
  1. Pierre Robin sequence can be an isolated abnormality or be a part of another syndrome; it results from hypoplasia of the mandible, leading to posterior displacement of the tongue (glossoptosis).
- Eyes: Abnormal architecture of the vitreous gel is pathognomonic, associated with high myopia; retinal detachment (ablatio retinae) is common (occurs in nearly 50%, bilateral in 40%); cataracts.
- Joint/bone: Joint hypermobility, early age of onset of arthritis.
- Hearing: Hearing loss can be sensorineural and/or conductive. Deafness can occur.
- Other: Mitral valve prolapse.

ETIOLOGY

The following mutations are autosomal dominant:

- Stickler syndrome type 1: Mutations in *COL2A1* gene (12q13.11-q13.2)
- Stickler syndrome type 2: Mutations in *COL11A1* gene (1p21)
- Stickler syndrome type 3: Mutations in *COL11A2* gene (6p21.3)
- Mutations in *COL9A1, COL9A2, and COL9A3* are inherited in autosomal recessive manner

DIAGNOSIS

DIFFERENTIAL DIAGNOSIS

- Marshall syndrome
- Wagner syndrome
- Weissenbacher-Zweymuller syndrome
- Marfan syndrome

WORKUP

- Diagnosis is based on clinical features
- Ophthalmology evaluation; slit-lamp evaluation is difficult in infants and young children
- Maxillofacial assessment if evidence of midline cleft
- Hearing testing

LABORATORY TESTS

Genetic testing can be done to confirm the diagnosis when there is clinical suspicion. Given inheritance patterns other family members may also be tested for further information.

IMAGING STUDIES

Joint x-rays (Figs. 1, 2, and 3) can be considered depending on symptoms.

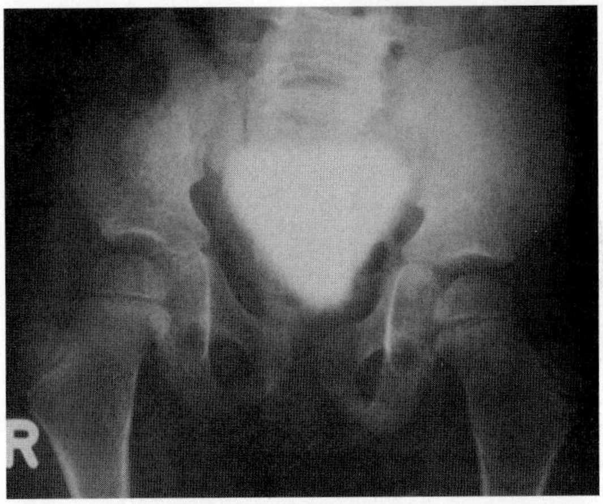

FIG. 1 Stickler syndrome. Anteroposterior pelvis. Tilted acetabular roofs render easy visualization of the posterior walls. (From Pope TL et al: *Musculoskeletal imaging,* ed 2, Philadelphia, 2015, Elsevier.)

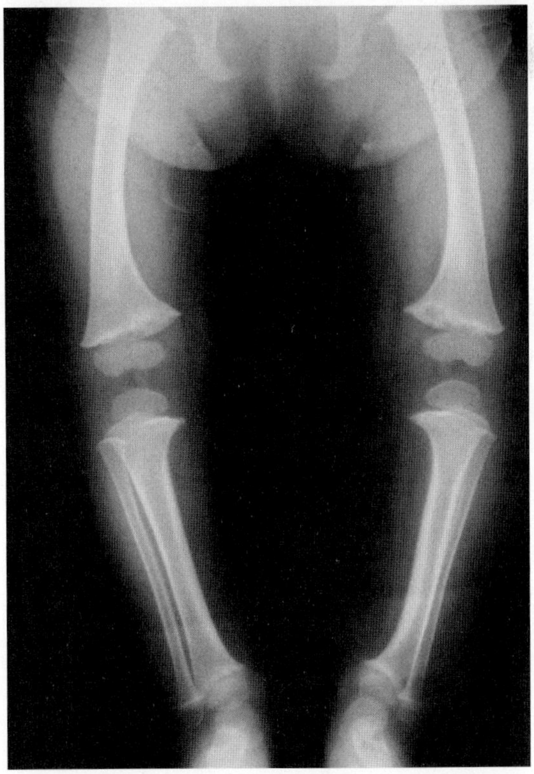

FIG. 2 Schmid metaphyseal chondrodysplasia. Anteroposterior radiograph of the lower limbs shows flared irregular metaphyses with widened growth plates. This patient has coxa vara and normal bone density. (From Pope TL et al: *Musculoskeletal imaging,* ed 2, Philadelphia, 2015, Elsevier.)

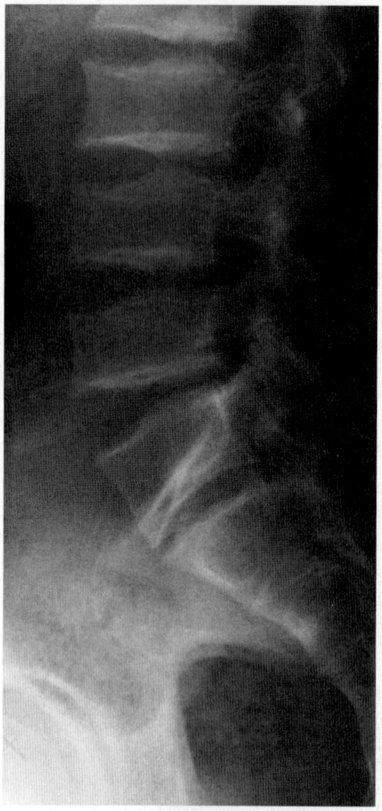

FIG. 3 X-linked spondyloepiphyseal dysplasia tarda. Lateral radiograph of lumbosacral spine shows characteristic vertebral humps, which become less apparent with increasing age and are best seen between ages 4 and 12 yr. (From Pope TL et al: *Musculoskeletal imaging,* ed 2, Philadelphia, 2015, Elsevier.)

Rx TREATMENT

Treatment is primarily supportive and depends on involvement.

- Ophthalmology evaluation with routine long-term follow-up given the high risk of retinal detachment.
- Corrective lenses to be prescribed as early as possible. May need laser photocoagulation, surgical interventions of retinal detachment or tears.
- Surgical evaluations and treatment if cleft palate is present.
- Rheumatology or orthopedic evaluation if joint complaints. Physical therapy can be helpful. Joint replacements may ultimately be required.
- Potential hearing aids. Speech therapy if cleft is present.
- Educational assessments, though intelligence is normal. Hearing or visual impairments can lead to difficulties.

DISPOSITION

Prognosis is generally good, but varies based on organ involvement and symptoms.

REFERRAL

Ophthalmology, craniofacial, ENT, rheumatology

PEARLS & CONSIDERATIONS

COMMENTS

Stickler syndrome is fairly common, but because many people have mild symptoms and may only have a few features (phenotypic variability), they are not always diagnosed or aware of the condition.

PREVENTION

Consider genetic counseling if known family history

PATIENT & FAMILY EDUCATION

Stickler Involved People (U.S. support group; https://stickler.org)

SUGGESTED READINGS

Available at ExpertConsult.com

AUTHOR: **Daphne Scaramangas-Plumley, MD**

BASIC INFORMATION

DEFINITION

Ischemic stroke is the sudden onset of a focal neurologic deficit as a result of cerebral ischemia resulting in cell death. The purpose of this chapter is to help the provider make decisions about the management of the acute stroke patient within the first several hours of symptoms; this is the crucial time for definitive treatment interventions.

SYNONYMS

Stroke
Brain attack
Cerebrovascular accident (this is a nonspecific term and should not be used)

ICD-10CM CODES	
I63	Cerebral infarction
I63.3	Cerebral infarction due to thrombosis of cerebral arteries
I63.4	Cerebral infarction due to embolism of cerebral arteries
I63.5	Cerebral infarction due to unspecified occlusion or stenosis of cerebral arteries
I63.6	Cerebral infarction due to cerebral venous thrombosis, nonpyogenic
I63.8	Other cerebral infarction
I63.9	Cerebral infarction, unspecified
I67.89	Other cerebrovascular disease

EPIDEMIOLOGY & DEMOGRAPHICS

INCIDENCE:

- ~795,000 new or recurrent strokes occur each yr in the U.S.
- Stroke is the number five cause of death (165,000 deaths every yr) and the leading cause of long-term disability in the U.S.

PREVALENCE: There are ~4.5 million stroke survivors in the U.S.

RISK FACTORS: Hypertension, dyslipidemia, diabetes mellitus, and smoking are the four major modifiable risk factors. Other risk factors include age, gender, atrial fibrillation (most common cause of cardioembolic stroke), mechanical heart valve, patent foramen ovale, recent myocardial infarction, metabolic syndrome, carotid artery stenosis, vertebral artery stenosis, intracranial artery stenosis, hypercoagulable states, subclinical atrial tachyarrhythmias without clinical atrial fibrillation, sickle cell disease, and obesity.

GENETICS: Multifactorial

PHYSICAL FINDINGS & CLINICAL PRESENTATION

When a patient presents with an acute ischemic stroke acutely, the most important considerations are determination of the time the patient was last known normal, the etiology (ischemic or hemorrhagic), and the severity, because these aspects will determine acute treatment. The time last known normal was when the patient was last seen normal (by themselves or by someone else). If they awoke with the deficits, the time last seen normal was when they went to bed.

Clinical presentation varies with the artery and region of CNS affected. Clinical presentation cannot reliably distinguish between hemorrhagic and ischemic causes, and so imaging must be done. Below is a noncomprehensive list of common stroke syndrome presentations based on the cerebral vascular territory affected. Please note that this list is not comprehensive and that all findings for a particular syndrome may not be listed here.

- Large- to medium-sized arteries:
  1. Dominant middle cerebral artery (MCA): Dominant face and arm > leg weakness and sensory loss with aphasia (expressive, receptive, or both); possible hemianopia
  2. Nondominant MCA: Nondominant face and arm > leg weakness and sensory loss with hemineglect; possible hemianopia
  3. Anterior cerebral artery (ACA): Contralateral leg weakness and sensory loss
  4. Internal carotid artery: Combination of contralateral MCA and ACA
  5. Basilar artery: Typically an acute loss of consciousness preceded by vertigo, nausea, vomiting, and diplopia; quadriparesis or quadriplegia may be seen, including "locked-in" syndrome
  6. Posterior cerebral artery: Unilateral hemianopia; blindness with anosognosia (Anton syndrome) if bilateral
  7. Posterior inferior cerebellar artery: Lateral medullary (Wallenberg) syndrome—ipsilesional loss of pinprick and temperature on the face and contralateral loss of pinprick and temperature on the body; ipsilesional Horner syndrome and ipsilesional palatal weakness with resulting dysphagia, dysarthria. Also with vertigo, nystagmus, ataxia.
- **Small arteries: Lacunar syndromes;** no cortical signs are present in lacunar syndromes.
  1. Pure motor hemiparesis: Typically due to an ischemic lesion in either the internal capsule or pons.
  2. Pure hemisensory loss: Typically due to an ischemic lesion of the thalamus.
  3. Ataxic hemiparesis: Ataxia out of proportion to the hemiparesis; typically due to an ischemic lesion of either the internal capsule or pons.
  4. Sensorimotor stroke: Typically due to ischemic lesion involving both the thalamus and internal capsule.
  5. Dysarthria–clumsy hand syndrome: Multiple localizations possible but typically the pons; facial weakness, dysarthria, and mild clumsiness and weakness of the hand.

ETIOLOGY

Etiologies include atherosclerosis, cardioembolism, artery-to-artery embolism, small-vessel lipohyalinosis, arteritis, arterial dissection, and vasospasm.

Dx DIAGNOSIS

DIFFERENTIAL DIAGNOSIS

The differential diagnosis of acute ischemic stroke includes hemorrhagic stroke (intracerebral hemorrhage), subarachnoid or subdural hemorrhage, seizure with postictal paralysis, migraine with hemiparesis or other aura, syncope, hypoglycemia, hypertensive encephalopathy, and conversion disorder.

LABORATORY TESTS

- Immediate (Box 1): Complete blood count, metabolic panel that includes blood glucose

BOX 1 Immediate Diagnostic Studies: Evaluation of a Patient with Suspected Acute Ischemic Stroke

All Patients
Noncontrast brain computed tomographic scan (magnetic resonance imaging, if available)
Blood glucose level
Serum electrolyte and renal function tests
Electrocardiography
Markers of cardiac ischemia
Complete blood count, including platelet count
Prothrombin time/international normalized ratio
Activated partial thromboplastin time
Oxygen saturation

Selected Patients
CT angiogram head and neck or MR angiogram head and neck
CT or MR perfusion
Hepatic function tests
Toxicology screen
Blood alcohol level
Pregnancy test
Arterial blood gas tests (if hypoxia is suspected)
Chest radiography (if lung disease is suspected)
Lumbar puncture (if subarachnoid hemorrhage is suspected and computed tomography scan is negative for blood)
Electroencephalogram (if seizures are suspected)

CT, Computed tomography; *MR,* magnetic resonance.

From Christensen H et al: Abnormalities on ECG and telemetry predict stroke outcome at 3 months, *J Neurol Sci* 234:99–103, 2005.

TABLE 1 National Institutes of Health Stroke Scale

1A. Level of Consciousness (LOC) 0 = Alert 1 = Not alert, but arousable 2 = Not alert, obtunded 3 = Coma	**1B. LOC Questions** Ask the month and his/her age. 0 = Answers both correctly 1 = Answers one correctly 2 = Answers neither correctly	**1C. LOC Commands** Open and close the eyes. Open and close the nonparetic hand. 0 = Performs both tasks correctly 1 = Performs one task correctly 2 = Performs neither task correctly
2. Best Gaze (Horizontal) 0 = Normal 1 = Partial gaze palsy 2 = Forced deviation or total gaze paresis	**3. Visual Fields** 0 = No visual loss 1 = Partial hemianopia 2 = Complete hemianopia 3 = Bilateral hemianopia	**4. Facial Palsy** 0 = Normal 1 = Minor paralysis 2 = Partial paralysis (total or near total paralysis of lower face) 3 = Complete paralysis of upper and lower face
5. Motor Arm **Right** Arm extended with palms down 90 degrees (if sitting) or 45 degrees (if supine) for 10 s 0 = No drift 1 = Drift; limb drifts down from position and does not hit bed or support in 10 s 2 = Some effort against gravity 3 = No effort against gravity 4 = No movement **Left**	**6. Motor Leg** **Right** Leg extended at 30 degrees, always tested supine for 5 s 0 = No drift 1 = Drift; limb drifts down from position and does not hit bed or support in 5 s 2 = Some effort against gravity 3 = No effort against gravity 4 = No movement **Left**	**7. Limb Ataxia** The finger-nose-finger and heel-shin tests 0 = Absent 1 = Present in one limb 2 = Present in two limbs
8. Sensory **To Pinprick or Noxious Stimuli** 0 = Normal 1 = Mild to moderate sensory loss 2 = Severe to total sensory loss	**9. Best Language** 0 = No aphasia, normal 1 = Mild-to-moderate aphasia 2 = Severe aphasia 3 = Mute, global aphasia, coma	**10. Dysarthria** 0 = Normal 1 = Mild-to-moderate 2 = Severe (including mute/anarthric due to aphasia) Do not score if intubated.
11. Extinction and Inattention 0 = No abnormality 1 = Present 2 = Profound (two modalities)		**Total Score:**

From Vincent JL et al: *Textbook of critical care*, ed 7, Philadelphia, 2017, Elsevier.

and renal function, PT/INR, aPTT, troponin I, and urinalysis. Blood glucose is the only test required before initiation of IV t-PA
- National Institutes of Health Stroke Scale (Table 1): A brief, focused neurologic examination aimed at providing a numeric estimate of the severity of stroke; can be performed by any health care provider trained in its use
- ECG and telemetry monitoring
- Echocardiogram to look for potential cardiogenic source of embolism, infective endocarditis, and intracardiac shunts

IMAGING STUDIES

- Immediate (Fig. 1): Computed tomography (CT) of the head without contrast to rule out hemorrhage.
- CT angiogram of the head and neck is necessary acutely in selected patients if deficits are severe to assess whether there is a thrombus that is amenable to intervention as well as CT head perfusion to assess for the degree of salvageable tissue (Table 2).
- MRI of the brain with stroke protocol to assess the extent of stroke (because CT typically will not show an ischemic stroke for several hours), but it is rarely needed in the hyperacute setting to determine appropriateness of reperfusion strategy.

Cross reference: See "Transient Ischemic Attack" for general workup, which is identical to that for ischemic stroke.

Rx TREATMENT

NONPHARMACOLOGIC THERAPY

GENERAL CONSIDERATIONS:
- Airway and breathing should be maintained.
- Supplemental oxygen should be provided to keep the oxygen saturation at ≥92%.
- Pneumatic compression devices or pharmacologic means should be applied to help prevent deep venous thrombosis.
- Avoid any and all oral intake until swallowing is evaluated and found to be unimpaired; this helps to avoid aspiration pneumonia.
- Early mobilization for rehabilitation is desirable.
- Consider neurosurgical intervention for craniectomy in select cases. Typical cases in which craniectomy may be performed include cerebellar ischemia with compression of the brain stem and/or the fourth ventricle as well as large middle cerebral artery ischemia. Available evidence suggests that it may be better to perform early hemicraniectomy (<48 hr) to achieve better outcomes in malignant hemispheric strokes. Decompressive hemicraniectomy has shown good benefit in terms of mortality and morbidity.

ACUTE GENERAL Rx

INTRAVENOUS THROMBOLYSIS:
- IV t-PA, or alteplase, is the only medical therapy approved by the U.S. FDA for the treatment of acute ischemic stroke.
- The time window for administration is generally accepted to be within 4.5 hours of symptom onset, although the FDA indication is still within 3 hours. The American Heart Association/American Stroke Association recommends a t-PA administration window of up to 4.5 hours with certain additional exclusion criteria when compared to the 3-hour administration. Time goals for evaluation and treatment of patients with acute ischemic stroke are summarized in Table 3.
- There are strict criteria for the administration of IV t-PA (see Tables 4 and 5).
- The protocol is weight based, with 90 mg being the maximum allowable dose.
- The risk of brain hemorrhage with IV t-PA is about 6% in stroke patients. The management of suspected intracranial hemorrhage after use of t-PA is summarized in Box 2.
- Endovascular intervention is useful only for large, accessible thrombi. Therefore if a stroke patient is a candidate for IV t-PA, treatment with IV t-PA should be started and then the patient should be assessed for possible endovascular therapy. Table 6 summarizes AHA recommendations for endovascular therapy in patients with acute ischemic stroke.

IMMEDIATE CATHETER CEREBRAL ANGIOGRAPHY FOR ENDOVASCULAR INTERVENTION

(Figs. E2 and E3): Methods available:
- The American Heart Association/American Stroke Association 2018 guidelines now recommend mechanical thrombectomy with a stent-retriever device for highly selected patients who present with large vessel occlusion (LVO) up to 16 hours after last known normal and suggest that it is reasonable up to 24 hours.
  1. IV t-PA should be administered in this group if eligible.
  2. All patients should be assessed with CT angiogram head and neck or MRA head and neck for possible LVO if they have an NIHSS of ≥6 or suspicion of a large vessel stroke.
  3. In selected patients with acute ischemic stroke within 6 to 24 hours of last known normal who have LVO on noninvasive angiogram, obtaining a CT perfusion, DW-MRI, or perfusion is recommended to aid in patient selection for mechanical thrombectomy.
- Adult patients should receive mechanical thrombectomy with a stent retriever if they

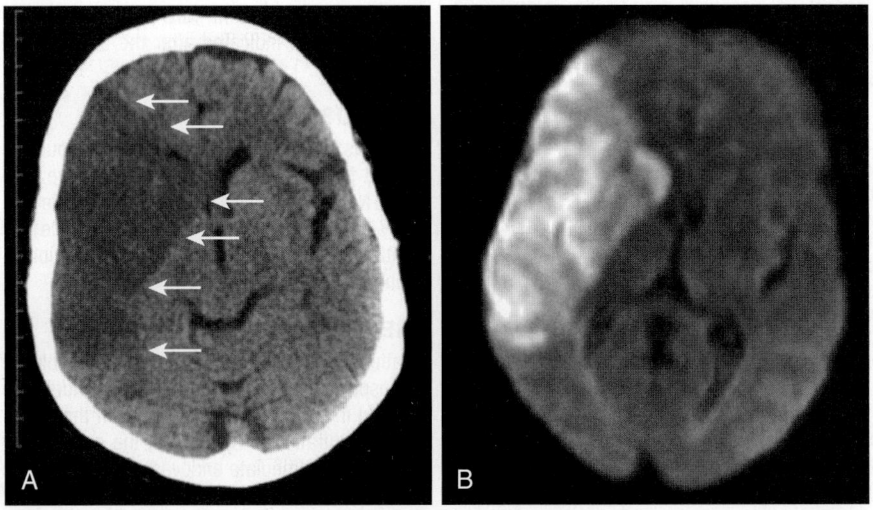

FIG. 1 Large right middle cerebral artery infarct on an unenhanced computed tomographic scan **(A)** and a diffusion-weighted magnetic resonance image **(B).** There is a mass effect, and this patient is at risk for cerebral herniation syndromes.

TABLE 2 Imaging Modalities for Stroke

Imaging Modality	Advantage	Disadvantage
Cerebral catheter angiography	• Allows for the definitive assessment of cerebral circulation (gold standard) • Allows for the deployment of intra-arterial thrombolysis and thrombectomy devices if a thrombus is found • Allows for the assessment of collateral circulation	• Invasive (significant risks) • High cost • Not available at all facilities
Doppler studies	• Noninvasive • May be performed at the patient's bedside	• Can be limited by the patient's body habitus • Operator dependent
Magnetic resonance angiography	• Excellent view of the large arteries of the neck and brain • No contrast material needed	• Cannot be performed in patients who are critically ill, who are unable to tolerate supine positioning, who have a pacemaker or other ferromagnetic hardware, or who are claustrophobic
Magnetic resonance perfusion	• Assesses cerebral hemodynamics • May show ischemic penumbra (i.e., the area of the brain that may be saved by timely intervention)	• Not commonly available • Not well standardized
CT angiography	• Excellent view of the large arteries of the neck and brain • Similar to magnetic resonance angiography with regard to resolution	• Requires intravenous contrast
CT perfusion	• Assesses cerebral hemodynamics • May show ischemic penumbra (i.e., the area of the brain that may be saved by timely intervention)	• Challenging to interpret in some cases • Not routinely available at many facilities • Requires intravenous contrast

CT, Computed tomography.

present within 6 hours of last known normal with a causative LVO (especially of the internal carotid artery or MCA segment 1 [M1] but reasonable in the setting of a causative MCA segment 2 or 3 [M2/3] or other large vessel cerebral artery) if they were relatively independent before the stroke and have an NIHSS score of ≥6 and an ASPECTS score of ≥6. Treatment needs to be able to be initiated (groin puncture) within 6 hours of symptom onset.

- Patients should receive mechanical thrombectomy with a stent retriever if treatment can be initiated within 16 hours (and possibly up to 24 hours) of last known normal with a large anterior circulation LVO and they meet the DAWN or DEFUSE-3 criteria (a defined mismatch between clinical severity and/or infarct volume compared to the penumbra [tissue at risk]). The number needed to treat to improve functional outcomes is only 2.8, and so patients should be aggressively evaluated for possible treatment.
- Complications can ensue from the endovascular procedure itself, including an intracerebral hemorrhage rate that is similar to that associated with IV t-PA. A recent meta-analysis revealed that among patients with acute ischemic stroke, endovascular therapy with mechanical thrombectomy versus standard medical care with t-PA was associated with improved functional outcomes and higher rates of angiographic revascularization, but no significant difference in symptomatic intracranial hemorrhage or all-cause mortality at 90 days.[1,2]
- Endovascular intervention is typically available only at comprehensive stroke centers.

HYPERTENSION: Elevated blood pressure is common during acute stroke, and it often subsides without specific therapy. In general, hypertension is not treated acutely unless it is extremely high (e.g., >220 mm Hg systolic blood pressure); there is evidence of hypertension-induced organ damage; or thrombolysis is being considered, in which case the blood pressure needs to be reduced (if it can be safely accomplished) to <185/110 mm Hg. It is risky to decrease blood pressure dramatically and quickly in the presence of acute ischemic stroke as it can cause an extension of the infarcted tissue into the ischemic penumbra. A 15% to 25% decrease over the first 24 hours is recommended when more acute lowering is not required.

HYPOTENSION: The presence of systemic hypotension in acute ischemic stroke portends a poor outcome. The cause should be sought, and volume depletion should be corrected with normal saline. Cardiac arrhythmias should be treated. Induced hypertension with vasopressor agents may be useful for select cases with an ischemic penumbra that is at risk, but caution is strongly advised.

HYPOGLYCEMIA: Hypoglycemia can mimic stroke. Prompt assessment of serum glucose level and replacement as necessary are important.

HYPERGLYCEMIA: Hyperglycemia should be treated with sliding scale insulin, taking into consideration the patient's oral intake. The presence of hyperglycemia worsens ischemic stroke outcomes, but recent evidence has not shown that aggressive treatment with an insulin pump improves outcomes.

FEVER: Fever is harmful during acute stroke. Ascertaining and addressing the cause while lowering an elevated temperature is strongly advised.

ANTIPLATELET THERAPY: Oral, rectal, or feeding tube administration of aspirin (325 mg/day) within 48 hours of stroke onset is advised to decrease the likelihood of a repeat ischemic stroke. Other oral antiplatelet regimens approved for secondary stroke prophylaxis (e.g., clopidogrel, aspirin plus extended-release

[1] Only test recommended before initiation of IV rtPA.

[2] Although it is desirable to know the results of these tests before giving a patient tissue plasminogen activator, thrombolytic therapy should not be delayed while awaiting the results unless (1) there is clinical suspicion of a bleeding abnormality or thrombocytopenia; (2) the patient has received heparin or warfarin; or (3) the patient's use of anticoagulants is not known.

TABLE 3 Time Goals for Evaluation and Treatment of Patients with Acute Ischemic Stroke

Time after Emergency Department Arrival	Goals
10 minutes	Assess ABCs, vital signs Provide oxygen if hypoxemic Obtain intravenous access Obtain laboratory studies CBC, coagulation, electrolytes Check glucose level, treat if indicated Perform screening neurologic assessment Activate stroke team Order "stroke code" brain CT or MRI Obtain 12-lead ECG
25 minutes	Review history Establish time at onset or last known normal Perform neurologic examination NIH Stroke Scale
45 minutes	Review laboratory studies Review brain CT or MRI results Evaluate inclusion and exclusion criteria (see Table 4)
60 minutes	Review risks and benefits Obtain consent Begin infusion

ABCs, Airway, breathing, circulation; *CBC*, complete blood count; *CT*, computed tomography; *ECG*, electrocardiogram; *MRI*, magnetic resonance imaging; *NIH*, National Institutes of Health.
From Goldman L, Schafer AI: *Goldman-Cecil medicine*, ed 26, Philadelphia, 2019, Elsevier.

TABLE 4 Eligibility Criteria for Acute Thrombolysis in Acute Ischemic Stroke

Eligibility Criteria

- Diagnosis of ischemic stroke causing measurable neurological deficit
- The neurological signs should not be minor and isolated. Caution should be exercised in treating a patient with major deficits
- Onset of symptoms <4.5 hours before beginning treatment
- The neurologic signs should not be clearing spontaneously
- The symptoms of stroke should not be suggestive of subarachnoid hemorrhage
- The patient or family members should understand the potential risks and benefits from treatment

Contraindications for Thrombolysis

- Evidence of intracranial hemorrhage on CT
- Head trauma or prior stroke in previous 3 months
- Myocardial infarction in the previous 3 months
- Gastrointestinal or urinary tract hemorrhage in previous 21 days
- Arterial puncture at a noncompressible site in the previous 7 days
- Major surgery in the previous 14 days
- History of previous intracranial hemorrhage
- Elevated blood pressure (systolic >185 mm Hg and diastolic >110 mm Hg)
- Evidence of active bleeding or acute trauma (fracture) on examination
- Taking an oral anticoagulant or, if taking anticoagulant, INR ≥1.7 is a contraindication
- If receiving heparin in previous 48 hours, aPTT must be in normal range
- Platelet count ≤100,000 mm^3
- Blood glucose concentration ≥50 mg/dl (2.7 mmol/L)
- Seizure with postictal residual neurologic impairments
- CT shows a multilobar infarction (hypodensity >1/3 cerebral hemisphere)

aPTT, Activated partial thromboplastin time; *CT*, computed tomography; *INR*, international normalized ratio.
From Hoffman R et al: *Hematology: basic principles and practice*, ed 7, Philadelphia, 2018, Elsevier.

dipyridamole) may also be used. Patients who have received t-PA cannot be given antithrombotic or anticoagulant agents within the first 24 hr after administration. In patients with acute ischemic stroke and atrial fibrillation, full dose anticoagulation with heparin infusion or low molecular weight heparin should be avoided in the acute setting, as this could potentially harm the patient by causing symptomatic intracranial hemorrhage, and there is very little evidence to suggest any benefit. However, chronic anticoagulation is indicated after the acute period has passed.

DISPOSITION

Patients with acute ischemic stroke should be cared for in a stroke unit or an intensive care unit. Nurses with skills in stroke care and telemetry monitoring should be routine. Once the patient is stable and the workup is complete, rehabilitation should be arranged.

REFERRAL

Patients with acute ischemic stroke should be transported to a hospital in which providers are skilled in stroke care. Depending on the severity and duration of symptoms, the patient may qualify for immediate endovascular intervention at a comprehensive stroke center, even if he or she is not a candidate for IV t-PA. If complications from brain edema develop, further evaluation by a neurosurgeon may be helpful during the acute phase.

PEARLS & CONSIDERATIONS

PREVENTION

- The prevention of acute ischemic stroke depends on the aggressive management of risk factors in individual patients.
- Cross reference: Stroke, secondary prevention.
- Paroxysmal atrial fibrillation is common in patients with cryptogenic stroke. A recent study found that noninvasive ambulatory ECG monitoring for 30 days significantly improved the detection of atrial fibrillation by a factor of >5 and nearly doubled the rate of anticoagulant treatment compared to the standard practice of short-duration ECG monitoring.

PATIENT & FAMILY EDUCATION

Patients and families need to be taught about ways to reduce the risk for recurrent stroke, including lifestyle modifications. Education about rehabilitation goals, when appropriate, should also be accomplished.

RELATED CONTENT

Stroke (Patient Information)
Stroke, Secondary Prevention (Related Key Topic)
Transient Ischemic Attack (Related Key Topic)
Atrial Fibrillation (Related Key Topic)

SUGGESTED READINGS

Available at ExpertConsult.com

AUTHORS: **Corey Goldsmith, MD,** and **Prashanth Krishnamohan, MBBS, MD**

TABLE 5 Administration of rtPA for Acute Ischemic Stroke

Infuse 0.9 mg/kg (maximum dose 90 mg) over 60 min, with 10% of the dose given as a bolus over 1 min.

Admit the patient to an intensive care or stroke unit for monitoring.

If the patient develops severe headache, acute hypertension, nausea, or vomiting or has a worsening neurologic examination, discontinue the infusion (if IV rtPA is being administered) and obtain emergent CT scan.

Measure blood pressure and perform neurologic assessments every 15 min during and after IV rtPA infusion for 2 h, then every 30 min for 6 h, then hourly until 24 h after IV rtPA treatment.

Increase the frequency of blood pressure measurements if systolic blood pressure is >180 mm Hg or if diastolic blood pressure is >105 mm Hg; administer antihypertensive medications to maintain blood pressure at or below these levels.

Delay placement of nasogastric tubes, indwelling bladder catheters, or intraarterial pressure catheters if the patient can be safely managed without them.

Obtain a follow-up CT or MRI scan at 24 h after IV rtPA before starting anticoagulants or antiplatelet agents.

CT, Computed tomography; *IV*, intravenous; *MRI*, magnetic resonance imaging; *rtPA*, recombinant tissue plasminogen activator.

From Jauch EC et al: Guidelines for the early management of patients with acute ischemic stroke: a guideline for healthcare professionals from the American Heart Association/American Stroke Association, *Stroke* 44:870–947, 2013. In Goldman L, Schafer AI: *Goldman-Cecil medicine*, ed 26, Philadelphia, 2019, Elsevier.

BOX 2 Management of Suspected Intracerebral Hemorrhage after Use of Tissue Plasminogen Activator

Discontinue the t-PA infusion if it remains in progress.
Obtain noncontrast CT scan of the head stat.
Order PT, PTT, platelet count, fibrinogen level, type and cross-match stat.
In event of hemorrhage, consult hematology and neurosurgery.
Give 6 to 8 units of cryoprecipitate, then 6 to 8 units of platelets.
Administer aminocaproic acid 4 to 5 gm IV over 1 hour, followed by 1 gm PO or IV per hour.
Check fibrinogen every 4 hours and give cryoprecipitate to keep fibrinogen >150 mg/dl.
Monitor blood pressure every 15 min.
Periodically repeat CBC, PT, PTT.
Consider repeat head CT.

CBC, Complete blood cell count; *CT*, computed tomography; *IV*, intravenous; *PO*, oral; *PT*, prothrombin time; *PTT*, partial thromboplastin time; *stat*, immediately; *t-PA*, tissue plasminogen activator.

From Parrillo JE, Dellinger RP: *Critical care medicine: principles of diagnosis and management in the adult*, ed 5, Philadelphia, 2019, Elsevier.

TABLE 6 AHA Recommendations for Endovascular Therapy in Patients with Acute Ischemic Stroke

Patients should receive endovascular therapy with a stent retriever if they meet all of the following criteria (class I; level of evidence, A):

1. Prestroke modified Rankin score 0 to 1 (functionally independent)
2. Acute ischemic stroke receiving intravenous recombinant tissue plasminogen activator within 4.5 hours of onset according to guidelines from professional medical societies
3. Causative occlusion of the internal carotid artery or proximal middle cerebral artery
4. Age 18 years or older
5. National Institutes of Health Stroke Scale (NIHSS) score of 6 or greater
6. Alberta Stroke Program Early CT Score (ASPECTS) of 6 or greater
7. Treatment can be initiated (groin puncture) within 6 hours of symptom onset

CT, Computed tomography.

From Zipes DP: *Braunwald's heart disease: a textbook of cardiovascular medicine*, ed 11, Philadelphia, 2019, Elsevier.

BASIC INFORMATION

DEFINITION

Hemorrhagic stroke is the sudden onset of a focal neurologic deficit caused by hemorrhage into or around the brain.

SYNONYMS

Intracerebral hemorrhage (ICH)
Intracranial hemorrhage
Cerebrovascular attack (this is a nonspecific term and should not be used)
The term *subarachnoid hemorrhage* refers to a specific location for hemorrhage, which commonly occurs as a result of a ruptured aneurysm. Please see "Subarachnoid Hemorrhage" for additional information.

ICD-10CM CODES

I61	Intracerebral hemorrhage
I61.0	Intracerebral hemorrhage in hemisphere, subcortical
I61.1	Intracerebral hemorrhage in hemisphere, cortical
I61.2	Intracerebral hemorrhage in hemisphere, unspecified
I61.3	Intracerebral hemorrhage in brainstem
I61.4	Intracerebral hemorrhage in cerebellum
I61.5	Intracerebral hemorrhage, intraventricular
I61.6	Intracerebral hemorrhage, multiple localized
I61.9	Nontraumatic intracerebral hemorrhage, unspecified

EPIDEMIOLOGY & DEMOGRAPHICS

INCIDENCE: There are approximately 795,000 new or recurrent strokes per yr in the U.S., of which approximately 10% are hemorrhagic.[1]

RISK FACTORS:
- Hypertension
- Anticoagulant use
- Thrombolysis
- Alcoholism
- Illicit drug use (e.g., cocaine)
- Cerebral amyloid angiopathy
- Increased age
- African American race
- Low cholesterol, low-density lipoprotein, and triglycerides
- Minuscule increase in absolute risk from antiplatelet therapy
- Questionable effect of chronic kidney disease and selective use of serotonin reuptake inhibitors

GENETICS: Multifactorial

PHYSICAL FINDINGS & CLINICAL PRESENTATION

The presentation varies with the region of the brain that is affected. Table 1 summarizes correlation between levels of brain function and clinical signs. There is no clinical way to distinguish between a primary cerebral hemorrhage and an ischemic stroke; therefore imaging is required. Imaging can also help determine if the diagnosis is ischemic stroke with hemorrhagic conversion versus primary hemorrhage.

The following are common locations for hypertensive hemorrhage:
- Basal ganglia
- Cerebellum
- Pons

Lobar hemorrhage in an older adult is likely due to amyloid angiopathy.

A systematic, detailed examination is necessary when approaching a comatose patient (Box 1). The ICH score is a widely used grading scale to estimate mortality based on CT scan results. Parameters used to calculate the ICH score include Glasgow Coma Scale (GCS) (0-2 points) at presentation, patient age ≥80 (1 point), ICH volume ≥30 ml (1 point), presence of intraventricular blood (1 point), and infratentorial origin of blood (1 point). Scores range from 0 to 6, with a score of 0 conferring 0% mortality and a score of 6 with estimated 100% mortality.

ETIOLOGY

- Rupture of vessels
- Aneurysm
- Arteriovenous malformation
- Brain tumor
- Amyloid angiopathy

DIAGNOSIS

DIFFERENTIAL DIAGNOSIS

- Ischemic stroke
- Seizure with postictal paralysis
- Syncope
- Migraine with hemiparesis
- Conversion disorder

LABORATORY TESTS

- Complete blood count, metabolic panel including blood glucose and renal function, prothrombin time/international normalized ratio, activated partial thromboplastin time, urinalysis, and toxicology screens
- ECG and telemetry monitoring

IMAGING STUDIES

- Immediate: CT scan of the head without contrast is highly sensitive for hemorrhage (Fig. E1).
- CT or MR angiogram to rule out an underlying vascular malformation. CT spot sign on the CTA has been shown to be a reliable early predictor of hematoma expansion.

TABLE 1 Correlation between Levels of Brain Function and Clinical Signs

Structure	Function	Clinical Sign
Cerebral cortex	Conscious behavior	Speech (including any sounds) Purposeful movement Spontaneous To command To pain
Brainstem activating and sensory pathways (reticular activating system)	Sleep-wake cycle	Eye opening Spontaneous To command To path
Brainstem motor pathways	Reflex limb movements	Flexor posturing (decorticate) Extensor posturing (decerebrate)
Midbrain CN III	Innervation of ciliary muscle and certain extraocular muscles	Pupillary reactivity
Pontomesencephalic MLF	Connects pontine gaze center with CN III nucleus	Internuclear ophthalmoplegia
Upper pons		
CN V	Facial and corneal	Corneal reflex-sensory
CN VIII	Facial muscle innervation	Corneal reflex-motor response Blink Grimace
Lower pons		
CN VIII (vestibular portion) connects by brainstem pathways with CN III, IV, VI	Reflex eye movements	Doll's eyes Caloric responses
Pontomedullary junction pressure	Spontaneous breathing Maintained blood pressure	Breathing and blood pressure do not require mechanical or chemical support
Spinal cord	Primitive protective responses	Deep tendon reflexes Babinski response

CN, Cranial nerve; *MLF,* medial longitudinal fasciculus.
Parrillo JE, Dellinger RP: *Critical care medicine: principles of diagnosis and management in the adult,* ed 4, Philadelphia, 2014, Elsevier.

[1]Chatterjee S et al: New oral anticoagulants and the risk of intracranial hemorrhage: traditional and Bayesian meta-analysis and mixed treatment comparison of randomized trials of new oral anticoagulants in atrial fibrillation, *JAMA Neurol* 70(12):1486-1490, 2013.

BOX 1 Neurologic Profile: A Modified Glasgow Coma Scale

Verbal Response	**Spontaneous Eye Movement**
Oriented speech	Orienting
Confused conversation	Roving conjugate
Inappropriate speech	Roving disconjugate
Incomprehensible speech	Miscellaneous abnormal movements
No speech	None
Eye Opening	**Oculocephalic Response**
Spontaneous	Normal (unpredictable)
Response to verbal stimuli	Full
Response to noxious stimuli	Minimal
None	None
Motor Response	**Oculovestibular Response**
Obeys	Normal (nystagmus)
Localizes	Tonic conjugate
Withdraws (flexion)	Minimal or disconjugate
Abnormal flexion	None
None	**Deep Tendon Reflexes**
Pupillary Reaction	Normal
Present	Increased
Absent	Absent

From Parrillo JE, Dellinger RP: *Critical care medicine: principles of diagnosis and management in the adult,* ed 4, Philadelphia, 2014, Elsevier.

TABLE 2 Medical Management Protocol for Acute Intracranial Hemorrhage

Blood pressure	• Maintain mean arterial pressure <140 mm Hg with continuous infusion labetolol (2-10 mg/min), nicardipine (5-15 mg/hr), or clevidipine (2-6 mg/hr) • If stuporous or comatose, measure ICP and maintain CPP >70 mm Hg.
Reversal of anticoagulation	• For elevated INR: Vitamin K 10 mg IV push and 4F-PCC 1. INR 2 to <4: 25 units/kg; not to exceed 2500 units 2. INR 4-6: 35 units/kg; not to exceed 3500 units 3. INR >6: 50 units/kg; not to exceed 5000 units • For heparin: protamine sulfate 10 to 50 mg slow IV push (1 mg reverses approximately 100 units of heparin) • For dabigatran: Idarucizumab 5g IV (Praxbind®) • For the factor Xa inhibitors (rivaroxaban, apixaban and edoxaban): Andexanet-alpha IV. Low dose (≤10 mg rivaroxaban or ≤5 mg apixaban per dose): 400 mg IV bolus, followed by 4 mg/kg for 2 hrs. High dose (higher doses given within 8 hr): 800 mg bolus, followed by 8 mg/kg for 2 hrs. • For thrombocytopenia or platelet dysfunction: Desmopressin 0.3 μg/kg intravenous push. Platelet transfusion is reasonable in the setting of thrombocytopenia but is not effective and may be harmful when given to patients on NSAIDs or other antiplatelet agents. • Expedited INR reversal for life-saving neurosurgical intervention: recombinant activated factor VII 40-80 μg/kg (approximately 3.0-6.0 mg) intravenous push
Intracranial hypertension	• Elevate head of bed to 30° • Mannitol 1.0-1.5 g IV • Hyperventilate to pCO_2 of 30 mm Hg
Fluids and nutrition	• Normal (0.9%) saline at 1.0 ml/kg/hr • Begin enteral feeding via nasoduodenal tube within 24 hr
Seizure prophylaxis	• For coma with intracranial hypertension or acute seizures: fosphenytoin or phenytoin IV load (15-20 mg/kg); 300 mg IV daily for 7 days
Physiologic homeostasis	• Cooling blankets to maintain temperature ≤37.5° C • Insulin drip as needed to maintain glucose 120-180 mg/dl

CPP, Cerebral perfusion pressure; *FEIBA,* factor VIII inhibitor bypass activity; *4F-PCC,* four factor prothrombin complex concentrate, containing factors II, VII, IX, and X; *NSAIDs,* nonsteroidal antiinflammatory drugs.
From Goldman L, Schafer AI: *Goldman-Cecil medicine,* ed 26, Philadelphia, 2019, Elsevier.

- MRI of the brain with a gradient echo sequence is also highly sensitive for hemorrhage, including intracerebral microhemorrhages that may not be visible with computed tomography scanning. MRI may also help to identify underlying brain tumors or vascular malformations, especially if the bleeding occurs at atypical sites. In the acute setting the MRI may show only the hematoma, but repeat MRI approximately 6 wk after initial hemorrhage may help exclude these other etiologies.

Rx TREATMENT

NONPHARMACOLOGIC THERAPY

- Urgent neurosurgical evaluation is needed in many cases either for evacuation of the hematoma or for relieving raised intracranial pressure by procedures such as EVD placement or decompressive surgeries.
- Surgery should be performed promptly for cases of cerebellar hemorrhage of >3 cm when the patient is deteriorating clinically, showing brain stem edema or hydrocephalus.
- Surgery for lobar or deep brain clots may be considered for select cases, although the level of evidence for efficacy is not high. Surgery is often considered in lobar hemorrhages close to the surface and/or when the patient is neurologically deteriorating.
- Recent innovative surgical techniques, such as instillation of thrombolytic agents for intraventricular hemorrhage and minimally invasive surgery for hematoma evacuation, appear to be promising. Clinical trials are currently in progress to assess whether these approaches improve mortality and neurologic outcomes.

ACUTE GENERAL Rx

The cornerstones of medical management of acute intracerebral hemorrhage (Table 2) include:

- Control of hypertension
- Correction of coagulopathy
- Management of elevated intracranial pressure
- Treatment of seizures

HYPERTENSION (BOX 2): Blood pressure should be quickly lowered by 15% and then gradually and safely brought to the individual patient's target range. In theory, this may diminish the expansion of the hematoma. More aggressive control of systolic blood pressure (SBP) to 140 or less in the acute setting has been shown to be safe in clinical trials (INTERACT2 trial) with nonsignificant improvement in outcomes compared to less aggressive BP control (target SBP <180 mm Hg). ATACH 2 studied aggressive blood pressure lowering in patients randomized within 4.5 hr of symptom onset. Patients were randomized to aggressive blood pressure lowering to a target SBP of 110 to 139 mm Hg compared to standard blood pressure lowering to target SBP of 179 to 140 mm Hg. The trial was stopped early because there was no difference in neurological outcome or death, but patients in the aggressive blood pressure lowering arm suffered more kidney injury.

The most recent guidelines, published in 2015, state that for ICH patients presenting with SBP between 150 and 220 mm Hg and without contraindication to acute BP treatment, acute lowering of SBP to 140 mm Hg is safe and can be effective for improving functional outcome. For ICH patients presenting with SBP >220 mm Hg, it may be reasonable to consider aggressive reduction of BP with a continuous intravenous infusion and frequent BP monitoring.

CORRECTION OF COAGULOPATHY:

- Early hematoma expansion has been associated with poor outcome. Hemostatic therapy has not been shown convincingly to improve outcomes, despite reducing hematoma expansion, but is clinically reasonable.
- Protamine sulfate is used to treat cases of heparin-induced intracerebral hemorrhage.

BOX 2 Suggested Recommended Guidelines for the Treatment of Elevated Blood Pressure in Patients with Spontaneous Intracerebral Hemorrhage

1. SBP of >200 mm Hg or MAP of >150 mm Hg: Consider the aggressive reduction of BP with continuous intravenous infusion, with BP monitoring every 5 min.
2. SBP of >180 mm Hg or MAP of >130 mm Hg with evidence or suspicion of elevated ICP: Consider ICP monitor and reducing BP with intermittent or continuous intravenous medications to keep cerebral perfusion pressure >60 to 80 mm Hg.
3. SBP of >180 mm Hg or MAP of >130 mm Hg without evidence or suspicion of elevated ICP: Consider a modest reduction of BP (e.g., MAP of 110 mm Hg or target blood pressure of 160/90 mm Hg) with intermittent or continuous intravenous medications, and clinically reexamine the patient every 15 min.

BP, Blood pressure; *ICP,* intracranial pressure; *MAP,* mean arterial pressure; *SBP,* systolic blood pressure.

Modified from Broderick J et al: Guidelines for the management of spontaneous intracerebral hemorrhage in adults: 2007 update, *Stroke* 38:2001–2023, 2007.

Protamine dosage is 1 mg IV for every 100 units of heparin administered in the previous 2 to 3 hr (maximum dose is 50 mg).

- Prothrombin concentrate complex (PCC) is now recommended for reversal of warfarin-associated ICH. FFP may also be used for this purpose, although it carries the disadvantage of administering more volume, potentially leading to complications such as pulmonary edema and slightly longer times to reversal of coagulopathy compared to PCC. Vitamin K should be administered IV along with flash-frozen plasma (FFP)/PCC for sustained effects. Routine use of recombinant factor VII concentrates is not recommended due to insufficient evidence and concern for increased risk of thromboembolic events.
- Idarucizumab (Praxbind) is a humanized monoclonal antibody fragment that can be used for urgent reversal of the anticoagulant effect of the direct thrombin inhibitor dabigatran (Pradaxa). PCC infusion is also recommended.
- Andexanet alfa, a recombinant modified human factor X2 decoy protein, has been effective for reversion of the anticoagulant effect of apixaban (Eliquis), rivaroxaban (Xarelto), and edoxaban (Savaysa), though it requires continuous infusion. PCC infusion is also recommended.
- Recommendations for thrombolytic-associated intracerebral hemorrhage treatment include the consideration of the infusion of platelets and cryoprecipitate.
- Platelet transfusion for patients experiencing ICH while on aspirin appears to result in worse outcomes than no platelet transfusion according to the PATCH trial.

ELEVATED INTRACRANIAL PRESSURE: This condition should be treated with a graded approach, which may include the elevation of the head of the bed, analgesia/sedation, hyperventilation, and osmotic therapy. In patients clinically suspected to have elevated ICP or with GCS <8, invasive monitoring of the ICP may be required. If conservative treatment fails to control ICP, external ventricular drain (EVD) placement or other decompressive procedures like craniotomy should be pursued.

SEIZURES: If seizures occur, they should be treated aggressively, including with intravenous medications, if needed. Although widely practiced, routine use of prophylactic antiepileptic medications is not recommended. Continuous EEG monitoring should be employed in patients with suspected seizures or unexplained low levels of consciousness.

SUPPORTIVE TREATMENT:

- Hyperglycemia: A high blood glucose level predicts a worse outcome. Markedly elevated glucose levels should be lowered to <200 mg/dl.
- Antipyretics should be administered for fever in addition to searching for a cause of the fever.
- Care should be taken to avoid hypoxia. Airway and ventilatory management should happen early and concurrently with the primary management of ICH.
- Pneumatic compression devices should be applied to help prevent deep venous thrombosis. Chemical deep venous thrombosis prophylaxis can be started after 48 to 72 hr in most situations once the bleed has been determined to be stable.
- Early mobilization for rehabilitation is desirable.

DISPOSITION

For large hemorrhages or unstable patients, immediate referral to a stroke center

REFERRAL

Patients with hemorrhagic stroke should be transported to a hospital where providers are skilled in the treatment of stroke and cerebrovascular diseases including the availability of neurosurgery services and neurocritical care. Depending on the severity and duration of symptoms, the patient may require neurosurgical intervention.

PEARLS & CONSIDERATIONS

- Outcomes are inversely correlated with hemorrhage size.
- Specific reversal agents may be useful for warfarin-, heparin-, direct oral anticoagulant- (DOAC), or thrombolysis-associated hemorrhage.
- No procoagulant medications have yet been shown to be safe and effective for the mitigation of spontaneous intracerebral hemorrhage in placebo-controlled trials.

PREVENTION

- Prevention depends on the aggressive management of risk factors in individual patients, including hypertension, smoking, alcohol use, and cocaine use.
- DOACs dabigatran, apixaban, rivaroxaban, and edoxaban are uniformly associated with an overall reduced risk of iatrogenic ICH when used for stroke prevention in atrial fibrillation when compared to warfarin. Any of the currently available DOACs can be considered first line for patients at high risk for ICH.

PATIENT & FAMILY EDUCATION

Patients and families need to understand that most patients will not soon achieve functional independence and that rehabilitation will be a long process. Education about avoiding antithrombotic agents should be stressed as appropriate for individual circumstances.

SUGGESTED READINGS

Available at ExpertConsult.com

RELATED CONTENT

Stroke (Patient Information)

AUTHORS: **Corey Goldsmith, MD,** and **Prashanth Krishnamohan, MBBS, MD**

BASIC INFORMATION

DEFINITION

Secondary prevention of stroke involves preventing the recurrence of a cerebral vascular ischemic or hemorrhagic stroke after a primary event (including transient ischemic attack) and early rehabilitation.

SYNONYMS

Brain attack
Stroke
Cerebral thrombosis
Cerebral hemorrhage
Brain infarct

ICD-10CM CODES

I65.2	Occlusion and stenosis of carotid artery
I65.0	Occlusion and stenosis of vertebral artery
I65.9	Occlusion and stenosis of unspecified precerebral artery
I66	Occlusion and stenosis of cerebral artery, not resulting in cerebral infarction
I65.1	Occlusion and stenosis of basilar artery

EPIDEMIOLOGY & DEMOGRAPHICS

Stroke is the fifth leading cause of death in the U.S. and the leading cause of disability. Each yr, there are a total of 795,000 strokes, of which 185,000 are recurrent strokes. Thus, secondary prevention of ischemic stroke remains good treatment strategy. Secondary prevention is specifically targeted toward modifiable risk factors.

RISK FACTORS: Age is the most important nonmodifiable risk factor. Modifiable risk factors include hypertension, hyperlipidemia, cigarette smoking, excessive alcohol consumption, physical inactivity, obesity (i.e., a body mass index of >25 kg/m^2), obstructive sleep apnea, illegal drug use (amphetamines, cocaine), and diabetes mellitus.

GENETICS: Multifactorial and strong family correlation if idiopathic strokes occur in parents <65 yr old.

PHYSICAL FINDINGS & CLINICAL PRESENTATION

- Stroke can have a varied presentation. Typically, the individual has a sudden definable loss of motor, sensory, visual, or cognitive functions that have a clear time of onset and that are noticed by others or by the individuals themselves.
- Physical findings such as weakness and/or numbness in one limb or on one side of the body, facial droop, visual field loss, or the inability to understand or communicate with others raises one's suspicion of a stroke event.

ETIOLOGY

- Strokes are broadly divided into ischemic or hemorrhagic (i.e., intraparenchymal or subarachnoid hemorrhage). It is impossible to distinguish ischemic from hemorrhagic intracerebral hemorrhage by history alone; therefore imaging is required to confirm stroke subtype.
- Ischemic strokes can be caused by large-vessel atherosclerosis, cardioembolism due to atrial fibrillation or cardiomyopathy, or small vessel disease such as lacunar stroke. Rare causes such as recreational drug use (e.g., cocaine abuse), arterial dissection, and hypercoagulable states need to be considered when ischemic stroke occurs in younger individuals.
- The most common cause of intracerebral hemorrhage is uncontrolled hypertension. Older patients with lobar hemorrhages likely have amyloid angiopathy as the cause of their hemorrhagic stroke. Spontaneous rupture of a brain aneurysm causes subarachnoid hemorrhage.

DIAGNOSIS

DIFFERENTIAL DIAGNOSIS

- Seizure and postictal states
- Brain tumor
- Complicated migraine
- Hypoglycemia
- Psychogenic disorder

WORKUP

- Blood glucose level, HBA_{1c}
- Activated partial thromboplastin time, prothrombin time/international normalized ratio complete blood count, and comprehensive metabolic panel
- Fasting lipid panel
- Hypercoagulability tests for young stroke patients with no obvious risk factors

IMAGING STUDIES

- Computed tomography scanning of the head without contrast can differentiate between ischemic and hemorrhagic stroke. MRI of the brain is a more specific and prognostic study.
- Carotid ultrasound and transcranial Doppler are used to detect large-vessel extracranial carotid atherosclerosis but are not useful for visualizing the intracranial vasculature or the posterior circulation. Magnetic resonance angiography (MRA) and computed tomography angiography (CTA) of the head and neck provide imaging of the entire extracranial and intracranial vascular supplying both the anterior and posterior circulations. MRA can be performed without contrast, whereas CTA requires iodinated contrast and may be inappropriate for patients with renal dysfunction.
- Echocardiogram to look for structural abnormalities that could be the source of cardioembolism.
- Heart rhythm monitoring to detect atrial fibrillation. It is rare for an isolated ECG to detect paroxysmal atrial fibrillation that may be the source of the ischemic stroke or transient ischemic attack (TIA). It can even be missed under 24 hr of telemetry in many patients. If a high index of suspicion for a cardioembolic source exists, working with a cardiologist to place a monitoring device should be considered because many cases of paroxysmal atrial fibrillation require more prolonged monitoring for detection.

TREATMENT

The secondary prevention of stroke is targeted toward modifiable risk factors. These include lifestyle modifications such as appropriate diet, exercise, weight loss, and smoking cessation, avoidance of heavy alcohol use, and risk factor modification as listed in the following.

Antiplatelet or Anticoagulant Choice:

All patients with noncardioembolic ischemic stroke or TIA should be on aspirin (50 to 325 mg/day), a combination of aspirin and extended-release dipyridamole, or clopidogrel. Long-term treatment with a combination of clopidogrel and aspirin in secondary stroke prevention when no other pressing medical conditions require their use is no longer recommended due to increased mortality from intracerebral hemorrhage. In some circumstances, short-term treatment with the combination of clopidogrel and aspirin is reasonable in the first 30 to 90 days. Ticagrelor failed to show benefit for secondary stroke prevention compared with aspirin in general, though it may have an improved efficacy in intracranial stenosis. Prasugrel is contraindicated in patients with a history of stroke or TIA. If a patient is already on an antiplatelet drug at the time of stroke or TIA, then consideration of switching to another agent is reasonable, although a holistic approach that includes assessment of compliance with the antiplatelet agent and the extent other risk factors have been controlled is recommended.

PREVENTING STROKE IN SPECIFIC CONDITIONS

- Cardioembolic strokes as a result of nonvalvular atrial fibrillation (AF): All patients with an ischemic stroke secondary to nonvalvular atrial fibrillation would have a CHA2DS2-VASc score of >2, and therefore anticoagulation is recommended. Two first-line drug therapies can be recommended: Direct oral anticoagulants (DOACs) such as apixaban, dabigatran, edoxaban, and rivaroxaban; and warfarin with an international normalized ratio (INR) between 2.0 and 3.0. DOACs have been shown to result in a lower rate of intracerebral hemorrhage. Although more expensive than warfarin, DOACs do not require monitoring, do not have the dietary issues associated with warfarin, and have fewer drug-drug interactions. However, patients on enzyme-inducing medications such as phenytoin or HIV patients on protease inhibitors cannot use DOACs. Warfarin is still preferred in patients with marked renal impairment (see specific information available from the FDA about renal impairment and dosing for each DOAC) and in patients with mechanical heart valves or valvular causes of atrial fibrillation. Reversible therapies for some of the DOACs have recently been made available. There is no evidence that aspirin monotherapy is helpful in reducing cardioembolic events. The Active-A trial suggested that a combination of aspirin and clopidogrel is slightly better than aspirin alone for those unable to tolerate warfarin, but patients on dual therapy experienced an increased risk of hemorrhagic complications. Because dual-antiplatelet therapy and DOACs have similar rates of bleeding complications but different levels of efficacy for prevention of cardioembolic stroke, the use of aspirin/clopidogrel dual therapy instead of a DOAC is almost never indicated. Furthermore, apixaban and aspirin monotherapies have been shown to have similar rates of bleeding. Thus, patients at risk of bleeding who previously were put on aspirin rather than warfarin could now be prescribed apixaban and experience the same bleeding risk but with actual benefit in terms of stroke risk reduction.

- Cardioembolic strokes as a result of a prosthetic metallic valve: Anticoagulant therapy with warfarin is recommended with a goal INR between 2.5 and 3.5.
- Strokes as a result of large-vessel extracranial atherosclerosis (i.e., symptomatic carotid stenosis): For patients with recent TIA or ischemic stroke and ipsilateral severe (70% to 99%) carotid artery stenosis, carotid endarterectomy (CEA) or carotid stenting is recommended, preferably within 14 days of the event if no contraindication. For patients with recent TIA or ischemic stroke and ipsilateral moderate (50% to 69%) carotid stenosis, intervention is recommended on a case-by-case basis only if the surgeon's perioperative morbidity and mortality rate is <6%.When the degree of stenosis is <50%, there is no indication for CEA. Carotid stenting can be an alternative to CEA in patients with low or average risk of periprocedural complications. In older patients (>70), CEA is associated with better outcomes.
- Symptomatic intracranial atherosclerosis (i.e., cavernous carotid stenosis, basilar stenosis): The symptomatic intracranial artery stenosis stenting trial (SAMMPRIS) demonstrated superiority of aggressive medical management of intracranial atherosclerosis compared with angioplasty and stenting for secondary stroke prevention. Therefore the use of aspirin plus clopidogrel 75 mg daily for 90 days is reasonable in addition to modifiable risk factor management, including high-intensity statin and SBP <140. There is no advantage to using warfarin over aspirin.
- Small vessel or lacunar: The CHANCE and POINT trials support short-term use of dual antiplatelet with aspirin plus clopidogrel 75 mg for 21 to 30 days after a TIA or small vessel (NIHSS ≤3) followed by long-term single antiplatelet.
- Patent foramen ovale (PFO): The American Academy of Neurology's 2016 guidelines recommend medical therapy with antiplatelets for stroke patients with PFO though recent trials (CLOSE and REDUCE trials) suggest a benefit for PFO closure devices especially in the setting of an atrial septal aneurysm or large interatrial shunt.
- Intracerebral hemorrhage: For immediate management, please refer to the chapter on intracerebral hemorrhage. Anticoagulation or antiplatelet agents should be held for 3 to 4 wk and can be restarted if there is a compelling indication such as nonvalvular atrial fibrillation. The American Stroke Association/American Heart Association 2014 guideline recommends avoiding long-term anticoagulation (e.g., warfarin, heparin) after spontaneous lobar intracerebral hemorrhage, but antiplatelet therapy (e.g., aspirin, clopidogrel, Aggrenox) may be considered in all cases of intracerebral hemorrhage where there is a definite indication, a recommendation that is supported by recent clinical trials.
- Antiplatelet therapy is recommended in cases of cryptogenic strokes. A consultation with a neurologist should be considered for young stroke patients and for patients with no obvious cause or with stroke from unusual causes (e.g., hypercoagulable states, dissections).

PREVENTING LONG-TERM COMPLICATIONS AFTER A STROKE

- Evaluation by a physical, occupational, and speech therapist will reduce the long-term disability that can follow a stroke event. The American Stroke Association 2014 guideline recommends a multidisciplinary approach to rehabilitation. Studies have shown an improved survival and recovery. Home-based rehabilitation can be considered after discussion with the rehabilitation specialist.
- Depression rates are high after an ischemic stroke, and patients should be screened.

RISK FACTOR MODIFICATION

- Hypertension: Antihypertensive treatment is recommended for both the prevention of recurrent stroke and the prevention of other vascular events in persons who have had an ischemic stroke or a TIA. Absolute target blood pressure level and reduction should be individualized, but a target of <140/90 is reasonable. Blood pressure should be lowered gradually over the first several days after an ischemic stroke to prevent cerebral hypoperfusion and extension of stroke. After a hemorrhagic stroke, blood pressure should be lowered quickly. Lifestyle modifications as listed previously should be included as part of a comprehensive antihypertension treatment plan.
- Diabetes: Uncontrolled hyperglycemia can lead to acceleration of both intracranial and extracranial arteriosclerosis. The goal for the hemoglobin A_{1c} level should be <7%.
    1. In a recent trial involving patients with a history of ischemic stroke or TIA, the risk of stroke or MI was lower among patients who received pioglitazone than among those who received placebo. Pioglitazone was also associated with a lower risk of diabetes but with a higher risk of weight gain, edema, and fracture.
- Hyperlipidemia: For patients with ischemic stroke or TIA with elevated cholesterol levels, statin agents are recommended with a goal low-density lipoprotein <70 mg/dl. The SPARCL study demonstrated that, compared with patients taking placebo, patients taking atorvastatin 80 mg daily experienced a statistically significant reduction in the risk of experiencing a recurrent ischemic stroke.
- Cigarette smoking: Absolute cessation is required. Try to offer pharmacologic therapy or counseling services to the patient. Secondhand tobacco exposure is just as dangerous, so inquire about secondhand exposure.
- Obesity: Weight reduction may be considered for all overweight ischemic stroke and TIA patients to maintain the goal of a body mass index of between 18.5 and 24.9 kg/m^2 and a waist circumference of <35 in for women and <40 in for men.
- Excessive alcohol consumption: Patients with ischemic stroke or TIA who are heavy drinkers should eliminate or reduce their consumption of alcohol. Light to moderate levels of no more than two drinks per day for men and one drink per day for nonpregnant women may be considered.
- Obstructive sleep apnea: A sleep study should be considered due to high prevalence of obstructive sleep apnea in this population and improvement in outcomes.

DISPOSITION

Secondary stroke prevention is a multifaceted approach of lifestyle modification and pharmacologic intervention that is aimed at preventing or limiting disability.

REFERRAL

For complicated recurrent strokes, a referral to a neurologist who specializes in stroke is recommended.

PEARLS & CONSIDERATIONS

The modification of risk factors is the best preventive measure for stroke. Lifestyle modification is a very important aspect of secondary stroke prevention. Always consider the patient's ability to afford the therapy and prescribed follow-up tests. Experience teaches us that patients sometimes will not let us know about their ability to afford therapies unless we inquire.

PREVENTION

Prevention is the goal of treatment, and compliance is the most important factor. Review risk factor reduction and pharmacologic therapy as previously discussed.

PATIENT & FAMILY EDUCATION

More information can be obtained from the following sources:

- American Heart Association, National Center, 7272 Greenville Avenue, Dallas, TX 75231
- American Stroke Association, 1-888-4-STROKE or 1-888-478-7653
- H.O.P.E. for Stroke, 250 Duck Pond Drive, Wantagh, NY 11793, 516-804-8495

SUGGESTED READINGS

Available at ExpertConsult.com

RELATED CONTENT

Stroke (Patient Information)
Transient Ischemic Attack (Related Key Topic)

AUTHORS: **Joseph S. Kass, MD, JD, FAAN,** and **Corey Goldsmith, MD**

BASIC INFORMATION

DEFINITION

Subarachnoid hemorrhage (SAH) is defined as hemorrhage into the subarachnoid space surrounding the brain. This can be either nontraumatic (typically due to cerebral aneurysm rupture) or traumatic in nature. Here we will focus upon nontraumatic subarachnoid hemorrhage. Box 1 describes the Hunt and Hess clinical classification of patients presenting with aneurysmal SAH.

SYNONYMS

Subarachnoid bleed
SAH

ICD-10CM CODES

I60	Subarachnoid hemorrhage
I60.1	Subarachnoid hemorrhage from middle cerebral artery
I60.2	Subarachnoid hemorrhage from anterior communicating artery
I60.3	Subarachnoid hemorrhage from posterior communicating artery
I60.4	Subarachnoid hemorrhage from basilar artery
I60.5	Subarachnoid hemorrhage from vertebral artery
I60.7	Subarachnoid hemorrhage from intracranial artery, unspecified

EPIDEMIOLOGY & DEMOGRAPHICS

INCIDENCE: Nontraumatic: 6 to 8 cases/100,000 persons per yr.

PREDOMINANT SEX: Women aged >55 yr were found to have a 25% greater risk of developing SAH compared with men of the same age.

PREDOMINANT AGE: The mean age at onset is 55 yr.

PEAK INCIDENCE: Most aneurysmal SAH occurs in people who are between the ages of 55 and 60 yr.

RISK FACTORS: Although genetics seem to play a factor in SAH, lifestyle factors are more important for determining overall risk. These risk factors include smoking, hypertension, oral contraception, pregnancy, and amphetamine/cocaine use.

BOX 1 Hunt and Hess Clinical Classification of Subarachnoid Hemorrhage

I	Asymptomatic or mild headache and neck stiffness
II	Moderate to severe headache and neck stiffness ± cranial nerve palsy
III	Mild focal deficit, lethargy, or confusion
IV	Stupor, moderate to severe hemiparesis
V	Deep coma, extensor posturing

From Vincent JL et al: *Textbook of critical care*, ed 6, Philadelphia, 2011, Saunders.

GENETICS:

- First-degree relatives have a 5 to 12 times greater risk of developing SAH compared with the general population.
- Autosomal dominant polycystic kidney disease is known to be associated with cerebral aneurysms in 8% of cases; screening is recommended in families with this condition. in which one family member has experienced a ruptured aneurysm.
- Collagen vascular diseases such as Marfan syndrome, Ehler Danlos syndrome have also been implicated in the formation of aneurysms.

PHYSICAL FINDINGS & CLINICAL PRESENTATION

- The primary symptom is a sudden, severe headache in >90% of cases. About 50% have a headache that is classically described as the "worst headache of my life" and reaches maximal intensity within 1 min—the so-called thunderclap headache. This headache may be associated with nausea/vomiting, neck pain, seizure, or complete loss of consciousness.
- 30% to 60% of patients report a history of headaches during the weeks preceding the actual hemorrhage event. These are most likely sentinel bleeds that represent microhemorrhages.
- Altered mental status and coma may result from the direct effect (hemorrhagic mass effect), but more likely is the result of acutely increased intracranial pressure.
- A posterior communicating artery aneurysm may present as oculomotor (cranial nerve III) palsy, typically involving the pupillary fibers, even in a nonruptured setting.
- Table 1 describes the World Federation of Neurologic Surgeons clinical classification of SAH.

ETIOLOGY

- A ruptured saccular (berry) aneurysm is the most common cause of spontaneous SAH (75%-80% of spontaneous SAH).
- Idiopathic SAH, also known as angiogram-negative SAH, accounts for 5% to 20% of spontaneous SAH. In these cases, no angiographic cause of the hemorrhage is found. This entity is also known as benign perimesencephalic SAH and is thought to occur due to rupture of venous plexus in the cisterns surrounding the brain stem.
- Other causes of spontaneous SAH include arteriovenous malformations, bleeding into preexisting tumors, vasculitis, and rarely reversible cerebral vasoconstriction syndrome, cerebral venous sinus thrombosis, or intracranial cerebral artery dissection.
- Cocaine abuse, sickle cell anemia, coagulopathies, and pituitary apoplexy can also result in SAH.
- Trauma.
- Table 2 summarizes non-aneurysmal causes of subarachnoid hemorrhage.

DIAGNOSIS

DIFFERENTIAL DIAGNOSIS

- Intracerebral hemorrhage as a result of spontaneous rupture of intracerebral arteries or arterioles (rather than arteries passing through the subarachnoid space) due to hypertension or amyloid angiopathy, as well as trauma, intratumoral bleed, ischemic stroke with hemorrhagic conversion, cerebral venous sinus hemorrhage associated with venous sinus thrombosis, mycotic aneurysm rupture.
- Other headache syndromes: Thunderclap headaches due to reversible cerebral vasoconstriction syndrome (often with recurrent thunderclap headaches), migraine headache, sexual headache, cough headache, exertional headache, secondary causes including, but not limited to, pituitary apoplexy or acute hydrocephalus.

WORKUP

IMAGING STUDIES:

- If a patient who presents with acute headache peaking within one hour of onset has none of the features on the Ottawa Subarachnoid Hemorrhage Rule (Fig. 1), subarachnoid hemorrhage is effectively excluded and imaging is not needed.
- Computed tomography (CT) of the head (Fig. E2) shows hemorrhage in more than 95% of cases, especially during the acute phase (i.e., 24-48 hr) after the onset of bleeding. Box 2 describes the Fisher grade of SAH on initial CT (Fisher III being associated with highest risk of vasospasm). About 3% to 5% of SAH may be missed on initial CT of the head. MRI brain, specifically FLAIR sequence, is helpful in detecting subarachnoid blood if clinically suspected.

TABLE 1 World Federation of Neurologic Surgeons Clinical Classification of Subarachnoid Hemorrhage

Grade	Glasgow Coma Scale	Motor Deficits
I	15	Absent
II	13-14	Absent
III	13-14	Present
IV	7-12	Present or absent
V	3-6	Present or absent

From Vincent JL et al: *Textbook of critical care*, ed 6, Philadelphia, 2011, Saunders.

TABLE 2 Non-aneurysmal Causes of Subarachnoid Hemorrhage

Trauma
Idiopathic perimesencephalic subarachnoid hemorrhage
Arteriovenous malformation
Intracranial arterial dissection
Cocaine and amphetamine use
Mycotic aneurysm
Pituitary apoplexy
Moyamoya disease
Central nervous system vasculitis
Sickle cell disease
Coagulation disorders
Primary or metastatic neoplasm

Causes are listed in approximate order of frequency.
From Goldman L. Shafer AI. *Goldman-Cecil Medicine*, ed 26, 2019, Elsevier.

- Lumbar puncture should be performed in all cases of suspected SAH with "normal CT of the head" between 6 and 12 hours after the onset of the headache for highest yield. The following suggest SAH:
  1. An RBC count of more than 100,000/m^3 in tubes 1 AND 4. This is to differentiate from a traumatic tap in which there will be a drop in RBC count from tube 1 to 4.
  2. Presence of xanthochromia or bilirubin in the cerebrospinal fluid.
  3. SAH can also be excluded by the following two criteria: CSF RBC count $<2000 \times 10^6$/L and no xanthochromia.
- CT angiogram of the brain (Fig. E3).
- Digital subtraction angiography with 3D processing when indicated is the gold standard for diagnosis of etiology in subarachnoid hemorrhage.

LABORATORY TESTS

- Basic laboratory values, including CBC, chemistry panel, prothrombin time, partial thromboplastin time, and platelet count.
- Serum troponin to evaluate for severe cardiac stress; elevated troponins indicate cardiac ischemia secondary to catecholamine surge and is associated with poor outcome.
- Patients with SAH are prone to developing cerebral salt wasting, resulting in hyponatremia. Sodium levels should be monitored frequently.

Rx TREATMENT

NONPHARMACOLOGIC THERAPY

- Airway, breathing, and circulation
- Once stabilized, good neurologic exam
- Cerebrospinal fluid (CSF) drainage may be required for patients who develop hydrocephalus and increased intracranial pressure. It is also recommended for patients with Hunt and Hess grade 3 or higher.

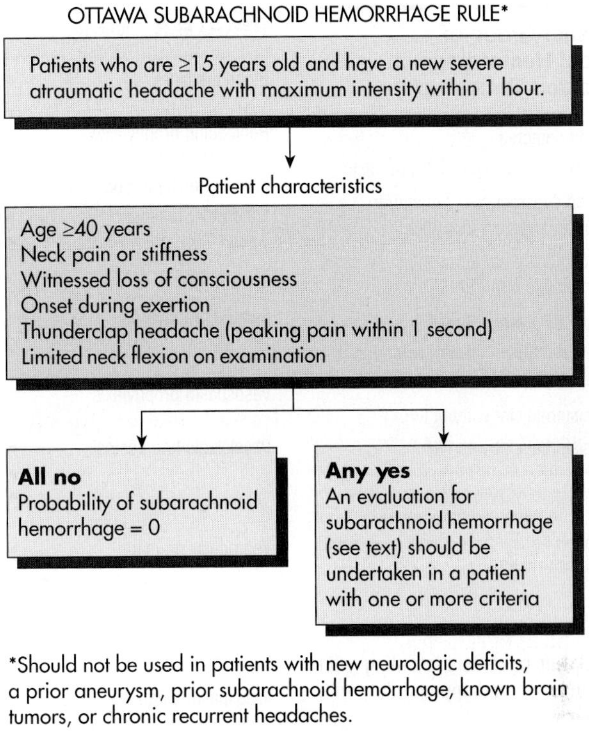

FIG. 1 The Ottawa Subarachnoid Hemorrhage Rule. (From Goldman L. Shafer AI. *Goldman-Cecil Medicine*, ed 26, 2019, Elsevier.)

ACUTE GENERAL Rx

- Critical care management: Initial management strategies are geared toward stabilizing the patient and preventing re-hemorrhage and hydrocephalus. Re-hemorrhage occurs within 72 hours in up to 23% and is associated with very high mortality rates.
- Blood pressure control: Tight blood pressure control is paramount before securing the aneurysm to protect against re-rupture. Blood pressure control can be achieved with the use of antihypertensive infusions such as intravenous nicardipine. A systolic blood pressure of less than 140 mm Hg is recommended. Placement of arterial line is recommended. After securing of the aneurysm, liberalization of blood pressure parameters is the standard.
- Intracranial pressure control: Raised intracranial pressure occurs in more than 50% of patients with subarachnoid hemorrhage secondary to hydrocephalus, cerebral edema, cerebral infarction or other causes. Insertion of a ventricular catheter to treat acute hydrocephalus and maintain intracranial pressure <20 mm Hg can be lifesaving. Patients who are unable to be weaned may require permanent CSF diversion.
- In cases of aneurysmal SAH, treatment focuses on occlusion/exclusion of the aneurysm to prevent rebleeding. The most common treatment methods are:
  1. Microsurgical clipping: Performed through a craniotomy by placing a clip around the neck of the aneurysm
  2. Endovascular coiling (Fig. E4): Performed via digital subtraction angiography; it consists of deploying platinum coils inside the aneurysm or stents in the parent artery to cause thrombosis of the aneurysmal sac. Most aneurysms currently are treated endovascularly.
- Vasospasm: Cerebral vasospasm is a morbid complication leading to cerebral ischemia, disability, and death after SAH. It typically develops between day 4 and 14 (but may occur up to day 21) after the hemorrhage, and it reaches a peak on day 6 to 8. Treatment strategies include:
  1. Current medical therapy for vasospasm focuses upon hypertension, with typical mean arterial pressure goals of 90 to 100 (after aneurysm is secured) and with euvolemia instead of hypervolemia, as the latter was found to lead to significant cardiopulmonary and hemodynamic complications. "Triple H" therapy—*H*ypertension, *H*ypervolemia, and *H*emodilution—was originally employed to maintain cerebral perfusion, but it has fallen out of favor due to its many complications.
  2. Nimodipine (60 mg q4h or 30 mg q2h if blood pressure is low) has been shown to improve outcomes if it is administered between days 4 and 21 after the hemorrhage, even if it does not significantly reduce the amount of vasospasm detected on angiography.
  3. Intraarterial therapies such as intraarterial calcium channel blockers and balloon angioplasty may be employed as needed.
- Seizures occur in about 3% of patients during the acute phase; use of prophylactic antiepileptics is controversial and not

BOX 2 Fisher Grade of Subarachnoid Hemorrhage on Initial Computed Tomography

1	No blood detected
2	Diffuse or vertical layers <1 mm thick
3	Localized subarachnoid clot and/or vertical layers ≥1 mm thick
4	Intraparenchymal or intraventricular clot with diffuse or no SAH
Modified Fisher CT Rating Scale	
1	Minimal or diffuse thin SAH without IVH
2	Minimal or thin SAH with IVH
3	Thick cisternal clot without IVH
4	Thick cisternal clot with IVH

CT, Computed tomography; *IVH,* intraventricular hemorrhage; *SAH,* subarachnoid hemorrhage.

From Vincent JL et al: *Textbook of critical care,* ed 6, Philadelphia, 2011, Saunders.

TABLE 3 Management Protocol for Acute Subarachnoid Hemorrhage

Blood pressure	• Control elevated blood pressure during the preoperative phase (systolic BP <160 mm Hg) with IV labetalol or nicardipine to prevent rebleeding
Rebleeding prophylaxis	• ε-aminocaproic acid 4 g IV upon diagnosis followed by 1 g/hr until aneurysm repair, for a maximum of up to 72 hours after ictus
Intravenous hydration	• Normal (0.9%) saline at 1.0-1.5 ml/kg/hr
Laboratory testing	• Periodically check complete blood count and electrolytes • Obtain serial ECGs and check admission cardiac troponin level to evaluate for cardiac injury; perform echocardiography in poor-grade patients (i.e., Hunt-Hess IV-V), ECG findings, or elevated cardiac troponin level.
Seizure prophylaxis	• Fosphenytoin or phenytoin IV load (15-20 mg/kg); discontinue on post-op day 1 unless patient has seized, is poor grade, or has focal cortical pathology or is otherwise unstable.
Vasospasm prophylaxis	• Nimodipine 60 mg PO every 4 hours until day subarachnoid hemorrhage 21 or discharge
Physiologic homeostasis	• Cooling blankets to maintain temperature ≤37.5° C • Insulin drip if needed to maintain glucose 100-120 mg/dl • Transfuse to maintain hemoglobin >7.0 g/dl (in the absence of active cerebral or cardiac ischemia)
Ventricular drainage	• Emergent external ventricular drain placement in all stuporous/comatose patients (Hunt-Hess IV/V), as well as lethargic patients with hydrocephalus • Begin trials of clamping external ventricular drain and monitoring intracranial pressure on day 3 after placement. • Perform ventriculoperitoneal shunting during subacute phase of illness in patients with persistent cognitive dysfunction and ventriculomegaly
Vasospasm diagnosis	• Transcranial Doppler sonography every one to two days until the tenth day after subarachnoid hemorrhage • Computed tomographic angiography and perfusion on day 4-8 after subarachnoid hemorrhage or for neuroworsening
Therapy for symptomatic vasospasm	• Place patient in Trendelenberg (head down) position. • Infuse 1 liter normal saline over 30 minutes. • If the deficit persists, raise the systolic blood pressure with phenylephrine or norepinephrine until the deficit resolves (target 180-220 mm Hg). • If refractory, monitor cardiac output and add dobutamine or milrinone to maintain cardiac index ≥4.0 L/min/m^2. • Transfuse to maintain hemoglobin >10.0 g/dl • Emergency angiogram for intra-arterial verapamil or cerebral angioplasty unless the patient responds well to the above measures.

From Goldman L. Shafer Al. *Goldman-Cecil Medicine,* ed 26, 2019, Elsevier.

recommended, but patients presenting with seizures should be treated appropriately with anticonvulsants.
- Pain control: Use short-acting and less-sedating medications (e.g., codeine, low-dose morphine).
- Monitor and treat for cerebral salt wasting and any other electrolyte abnormalities or anemia.
- Maintain normothermia.
- Table 3 summarizes a management protocol for acute subarachnoid hemorrhage.

CHRONIC Rx

- Management of reversible risk factors mentioned above (smoking, hypertension, drug use)
- Management of neurologic disability through physical therapy and rehabilitation

DISPOSITION

- SAH is often associated with a poor outcome with a death rate between 30% and 40%; 10% to 15% of patients die before they reach the hospital though outcomes have been improving over the past two decades.
- Almost half of those who survive hospitalization have cognitive impairments or disability that affect their lifestyles.

REFERRAL

Patients should be managed in a cerebrovascular center that maintains capacity to perform open surgical and endovascular procedures, with a critical care unit experienced in caring for neurosurgical patients.

PEARLS & CONSIDERATIONS

COMMENTS

- "Thunderclap" headaches should be considered SAH until proven otherwise and evaluated by CT of the head with/without LP. MRI FLAIR sequence is also a helpful modality.
- All SAH should be managed in a critical care setting (preferably neurocritical care unit) with neurosurgical care available.
- Measures to prevent rebleeding include adequate control of blood pressure and aneurysm treatment with the use of coiling or clipping.

PREVENTION

Controlling some of the modifiable risk factors, especially smoking and blood pressure, may help to decrease the risk of aneurysmal rupture.

PATIENT & FAMILY EDUCATION

- SAH is a devastating condition, with most survivors developing significant neurologic or cognitive deficits. A good support system and an adequate physical and cognitive rehabilitation program may prove useful to survivors.
- Screening may be useful for patients with two or three first-degree relatives with SAH.

SUGGESTED READINGS

Available at ExpertConsult.com

RELATED CONTENT

Subarachnoid Hemorrhage (Patient Information)

AUTHORS: **Farhan A. Mirza, MD,** and **Justin F. Fraser, MD**

BASIC INFORMATION

DEFINITION

Subclavian steal syndrome is an occlusion or severe stenosis of the proximal subclavian artery leading to decreased antegrade flow or retrograde flow in the ipsilateral vertebral artery and neurologic symptoms referable to the posterior circulation.

SYNONYM

Proximal subclavian (or innominate) artery stenosis or occlusion

ICD-10CM CODE

G45.8 Other transient cerebral ischemic attacks and related syndromes

EPIDEMIOLOGY & DEMOGRAPHICS

- Similar to that of other manifestations of atherosclerosis (coronary artery disease, cerebrovascular disease, or peripheral vascular disease)
- Affects middle-aged persons (men somewhat younger than women on average) with arteriosclerotic risk factors, including family history, smoking, diabetes mellitus, hyperlipidemia, hypertension, and sedentary lifestyle

PHYSICAL FINDINGS & CLINICAL PRESENTATION

Symptoms:

- Many patients are asymptomatic.
- Upper-extremity ischemic symptoms: Fatigue, exercise-related aching, coolness, numbness of the involved upper extremity.
- Neurologic symptoms are reported by 25% of patients with known unilateral subclavian steal. These include brief spells of:
  1. Vertigo
  2. Diplopia
  3. Decreased vision
  4. Oscillopsia
  5. Gait unsteadiness

  These spells are only occasionally provoked by exercising the ischemic upper extremity (classic subclavian steal). Left subclavian steal is more common than right, but the latter is more serious.
- Posterior circulation stroke related to subclavian steal is rare.
- Innominate artery stenosis can cause decreased right carotid artery flow and cerebrovascular symptoms of the anterior cerebral circulation, but this is uncommon.

Physical findings:

- Delayed and smaller volume pulse (wrist or antecubital) in the affected upper extremity
- Lower blood pressure in the affected upper extremity
- Supraclavicular bruit

NOTE: Inflating a blood pressure cuff will increase the bruit if it originates from a vertebral artery stenosis and decrease the bruit if it originates from a subclavian artery stenosis.

ETIOLOGY & PATHOGENESIS

Etiology:

- Atherosclerosis
- Arteritis (Takayasu disease and temporal arteritis)
- Embolism to the subclavian or innominate artery
- Cervical rib
- Long-term use of a crutch
- Occupational (baseball pitchers and cricket bowlers)

Pathogenesis: The vertebral artery originates from the subclavian artery. For subclavian steal to occur, the occlusion must be proximal to the takeoff of the vertebral artery. On the right side, only a small distance separates the bifurcation of the innominate artery and the takeoff of the vertebral artery, explaining why the condition occurs less commonly on the right side. Occlusion of the innominate artery must affect right carotid artery flow.

DIAGNOSIS

The carotid arteries should be evaluated at least noninvasively in all cases.

DIFFERENTIAL DIAGNOSIS

- Posterior circulation transient ischemic attack or stroke
- Upper-extremity ischemia:
  1. Distal subclavian artery stenosis or occlusion
  2. Raynaud phenomenon
  3. Thoracic outlet syndrome

WORKUP

- Noninvasive upper-extremity arterial flow studies
- Doppler sonography of the vertebral, subclavian, and innominate arteries
- Arteriography, magnetic resonance arteriogram (Fig. 1)

TREATMENT

- In most patients the disease is benign and requires no treatment other than atherosclerosis risk factor modification and aspirin. Symptoms tend to improve over time as collateral circulation develops.
- Vascular surgical reconstruction requires a thoracotomy; it may be indicated in innominate artery stenosis or when upper-extremity ischemia is incapacitating.

AUTHOR: **Fred F. Ferri, MD**

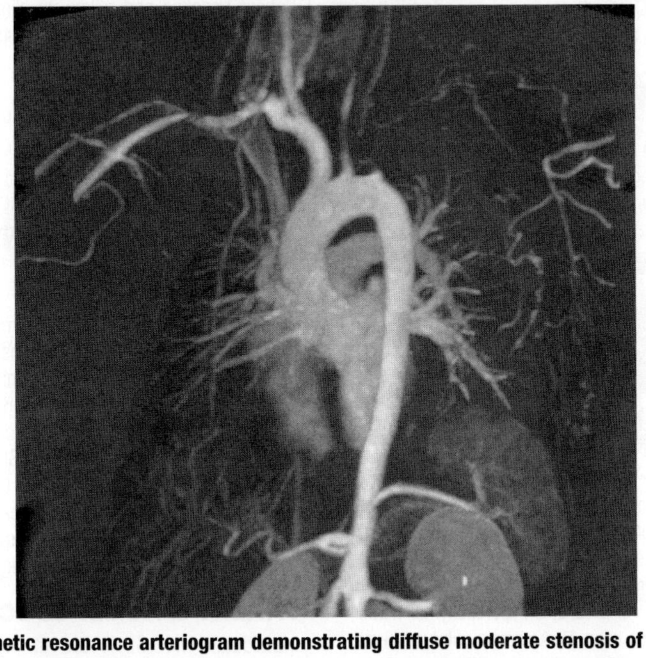

FIG. 1 Magnetic resonance arteriogram demonstrating diffuse moderate stenosis of the proximal left common carotid and proximal occlusion of the left subclavian artery coming off the aortic arch with development of an extensive collateral network. (From Hochberg MC et al: *Rheumatology,* ed 5, St Louis, 2011, Mosby.)

BASIC INFORMATION

DEFINITION

A subdural hematoma (SDH) is a collection of blood or blood products between the brain and dura mater. Subdural hematomas can be acute (ASDH) or chronic (CSDH) and vary significantly in presentation and treatment.

SYNONYM

Acute subdural hematoma
ASDH
Chronic subdural hematoma
CSDH
Subdural hemorrhage

ICD-10CM CODES

I62.01	Acute subdural hematoma
I62.03	Chronic subdural hematoma
S06.5	Traumatic subdural hemorrhage

EPIDEMIOLOGY & DEMOGRAPHICS

INCIDENCE:

- The exact incidence of ASDH is unknown, but it is commonly seen in patients with head injury.
- CSDH is most common in the elderly with an estimated incidence of 1.72 to 13.1 per 100,000.

PREVALENCE: Unknown

PREDOMINANT AGE & SEX:

- Peak incidence of CSDH is in the eighth decade and is notably higher in males.
- ASDHs usually present in the trauma setting and can happen in all age groups. In particular, shaken baby syndrome can be associated with SDH in the infant population.

RISK FACTORS:

- Trauma and antithrombotic therapy are the most common risk factors for ASDH and CSDH.
- Brain atrophy secondary to advanced age and alcoholism are common risk factors, especially with the coagulopathy/thrombocytopenia seen in chronic alcoholics.
- Intracranial hypotension associated with CSF shunts or leaks is uncommon but can result in acute or chronic SDH.

PHYSICAL FINDINGS & CLINICAL PRESENTATION

- Symptoms vary on the basis of acuity, size, and location. Acute traumatic SDHs are often seen in traumatic brain injury patients, and their Glasgow Coma Scale may vary according to the extent of brain injury, size of hematoma, and associated compression. When associated with a midline shift (i.e., >5 mm), they can cause signs of cerebral herniation (e.g., ipsilateral pupil dilation, contralateral weakness) requiring prompt surgical evacuation.
- Patients with CSDH may present with diverse nonspecific symptoms such as headaches, confusion, gait disturbance, incontinence, aphasia, hemiparesis, transient ischemic attack-like symptoms, and seizures.

ETIOLOGY

SDH is usually the result of shearing and tearing of a bridging vein between the brain parenchyma and the dura mater. Other causes of bleeding into the subdural space include contusion, extension of parenchymal hemorrhage. In the setting of spontaneous SDH, other vascular abnormalities, such as arteriovenous (AV) malformation, aneurysm, and dural AV fistula, should be kept in mind.

DIAGNOSIS

DIFFERENTIAL DIAGNOSIS

Cerebrospinal fluid (CSF) hygromas, abscesses, and tumor infiltrations

WORKUP

- Clinical assessment: Patient history, including medications, specifically anticoagulants/antiplatelets; alcohol abuse; recent trauma; cancer; and recent bacterial infections
- Neurologic examination: Glasgow Coma Scale, cranial nerves, motor/sensory exam CT head

LABORATORY TESTS

Assessment of the patient's coagulation status including CBC with platelet count, prothrombin time, partial thromboplastin time, and liver function test (especially with a history of alcoholism or liver failure)

IMAGING STUDIES

CT head (Fig. 1): Demonstrates the classic crescentic collection between the brain and inner table. For comatose and trauma patients, include a cervical spine CT scan. ASDH is usually hyperdense, whereas a CSDH is usually hypodense on noncontrast CT. Contrast is only needed if there are concerns about tumor or infection.

TREATMENT

- Correction of underlying coagulopathy, if present (e.g., warfarin/DOAC/ASA/clopidogrel reversal).

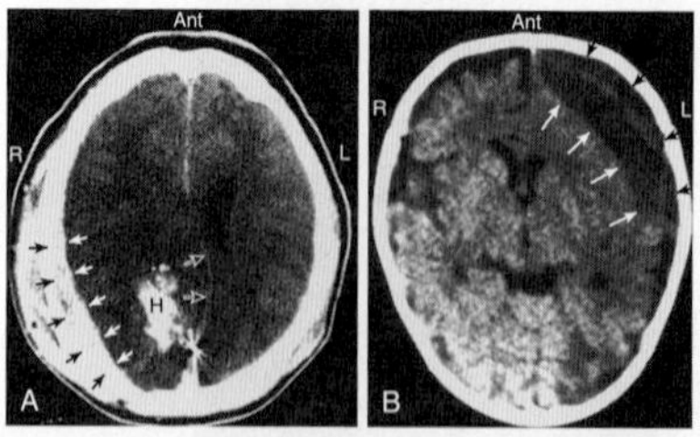

FIG. 1 A, Noncontrast computed tomography scan of an acute subdural hematoma shows a crescentic area of increased density in the right posterior parietal region between the brain and the skull *(black and white arrows).* An area of intraparenchymal hemorrhage *(H)* is also seen. **B,** A chronic subdural hematoma for a different patient is shown. There is an area of decreased density in the left frontoparietal region *(arrows)* that effaces the sulci, compresses the anterior horn of the left lateral ventricle, and shifts the midline somewhat to the right. (From Mettler FA [ed]: *Primary care radiology,* Philadelphia, 2000, WB Saunders.)

- Admission for monitoring in the setting of acute SDH.
- The majority of SDH can be managed without surgery in awake patients with normal neurologic examinations.
- Medical management of CSDH using antifibrinolytic therapy with tranexamic acid 650 mg per day has shown promising results, although a small, randomized, placebo-controlled trial showed no statistically significant difference.
- Seizure prophylaxis with phenytoin or levetiracetam for seven days should be considered in almost all cases, as there is underlying injury to the brain tissue associated with acute subdural hematoma. The irritative effects of blood products on the brain can also contribute to seizures, in both acute and chronic subdural hematomas. If seizures do occur, video EEG monitoring should be instituted and aggressive treatment undertaken.

NONPHARMACOLOGIC THERAPY

Surgical treatment is indicated in:

- ASDHs measuring >10 mm in thickness with a midline shift >5 mm on CT scan and a compromised neurologic status (Glasgow Coma Scale <9, pupillary asymmetry or fixation) should be immediately evacuated.
- In CSDH with a mass effect, a clear change in the neurologic examination from baseline, and/or enlargement of the hematoma size, evacuation via craniotomy or burr hole should be considered.

DISPOSITION

Depending on the size and location of the SDH and the examination of the patient, observation can range from the ICU to outpatient management. When observation of the patient is considered, clinical examinations should be serially performed. Patient baseline and follow-up clinical examinations are more important than CT scan findings.

REFERRAL

Neurosurgical and operative consultation should be made available.

PEARLS & CONSIDERATIONS

COMMENTS

- Many elderly patients have small CSDHs or hygromas. Unless these are associated with seizures or clinical or radiographic progression, they are usually not emergent and usually do not require neurosurgical intervention. Recurrence after surgical management for CSDH is common.
- SDHs in elderly patients can have a mixed hyperdense and hypodense appearance on noncontrast CT scan; this finding is suggestive of subdural membranes and chronic components.

PATIENT & FAMILY EDUCATION

Individuals with SDHs are at higher risk for seizure, so surveillance is important.

RELATED CONTENT

Subdural Hematoma (Patient Information)

AUTHORS: **Farhan A. Mirza, MD,** and **Justin F. Fraser, MD**

BASIC INFORMATION

DEFINITION

A localized accumulation of infected fluid, often encapsulated, located under the diaphragm and may also involve the liver and spleen

SYNONYMS

Subdiaphragmatic abscess
Infradiaphragmatic abscess

ICD-10CM CODES

K65.1	Peritoneal abscess
K68.11	Postprocedural retroperitoneal abscess

EPIDEMIOLOGY & DEMOGRAPHICS

INCIDENCE: Not well known but intraabdominal abscess occurs in 1% to 2% of all cases of abdominal surgery. It increases to 10% to 30% in cases with preoperative perforation of a hollow viscus, spillage of fecal material into peritoneum, or intestinal ischemia.

RISK FACTORS:
- Abdominal surgery, especially with accidental viscus perforation
- Peptic ulcer perforation
- Appendiceal perforation
- Diverticulitis with perforation
- Mesenteric ischemia with bowel infarction
- Abdominal trauma especially penetrating trauma
- Foreign body ingestion with subsequent viscus perforation

PHYSICAL FINDINGS & CLINICAL PRESENTATION

- Constitutional symptoms include:
  1. Fever, malaise, or chills
  2. Cough, increased respiratory rate with shallow or grunting respiration
  3. Shoulder-tip pain on affected side (referred pain)
- Physical findings can include:
  1. Dullness to percussion on affected side
  2. Diminished or absent breath sounds on affected side
  3. Tenderness over the eighth to eleventh ribs

ETIOLOGY

Infection is usually polymicrobial: Aerobic gram-negative rods, most commonly *Escherichia coli, Klebsiella* species, *Enterobacter* species, and *Pseudomonas aeruginosa,* and gram-positive cocci: *Streptococcus viridians,* enterococci and *Staphylococcus aureus,* and anaerobes (found in 60% to 70% of cases) such as *Bacteroides fragilis* and *Clostridia* species.

DIAGNOSIS

DIFFERENTIAL DIAGNOSIS

- Liver abscess
- Subhepatic abscess
- Lesser sac abscess
- Empyema of the lung
- Diaphragmatic hernia

WORKUP

Should be started in patients with recent abdominal surgery (weeks to months) with the constitutional symptoms and physical findings mentioned above

LABORATORY TESTS

- Complete blood count with differential may show an elevated white blood count with left shift.
- Blood cultures may be positive in up to 50% of the cases.
- Gram stain and culture, aerobically and anaerobically, of any aspiration procedure.

IMAGING STUDIES

- Plain x-ray films can suggest the location of the abscess in about 50% of the cases and can demonstrate elevation of the hemidiaphragm and/or subphrenic air-fluid level.
- Ultrasonography and CT (Fig. 1) are more sensitive.
- Other options include leukocyte tagged with gallium 67 and indium 111 scans and MRI.

TREATMENT

Includes source control with either percutaneous drainage or surgery and intravenous antibiotics:

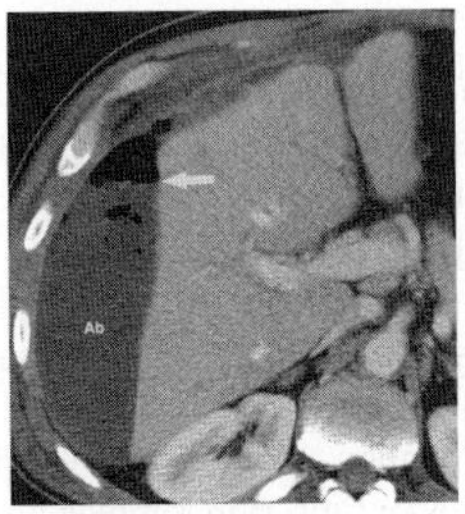

FIG. 1 SUBPHRENIC ABSCESS. A postoperative abscess *(Ab)* is seen as a fluid collection between the diaphragm and the liver. Mass impression on the liver is evidence of fluid loculation. An air–fluid level *(arrow)* is evident, caused by gas-producing *Escherichia coli.* This abscess was successfully treated using percutaneous catheter drainage guided by computed tomography. (From Webb WR et al: *Fundamentals of body CT,* ed 4, Philadelphia, 2015, Saunders.)

- Percutaneous drainage via interventional radiology:
  1. Percutaneous drainage with catheter placement remains the preferred treatment despite the fact that the subphrenic location can be problematic for imaging-guided percutaneous drainage.
  2. Approaches include subcostal approach or intercostal approach. The intercostal approach is associated with a higher risk for pleural complications, but these tend to be minor.
  3. Radiographic modalities used include ultrasonography, CT, and fluoroscopy.
  4. Complications of drainage procedures can include pleural effusion, pneumothorax, or empyema.
- Surgery: May be required in recurrence of abscess or due to multiple abscesses not amenable to percutaneous drainage procedure
- Antibiotics: Broad-spectrum antibiotics should be used to cover gram-negative rods, gram-positive bacteria, and anaerobes until cultures are resulted and should be continued at least 4 to 7 days after adequate drainage procedure. Examples include:
  1. Piperacillin/tazobactam 3.375 g IV q6h or 4.5 g IV q8h
  2. Meropenem 1 g IV q8h or imipenem 0.5 to 1 g IV q6h
  3. Ciprofloxacin IV 400 mg IV q12h plus IV metronidazole 500 mg IV q8h for penicillin allergic patients

REFERRAL

- Interventional radiology
- General surgery
- Infectious diseases

PEARLS & CONSIDERATIONS

COMMENTS

Success of percutaneous drainage procedures is greater than 85%, and recurrence rates are about 1% to 10%.

SUGGESTED READINGS

Available at ExpertConsult.com

RELATED CONTENT

Peritonitis, Secondary (Related Key Content)

AUTHOR: **Glenn G. Fort, MD, MPH**

BASIC INFORMATION

DEFINITION

The *Diagnostic and Statistical Manual of Mental Disorders, Fifth Edition (DSM-5)* renamed "Dementia, Delirium, Amnestic, and Other Cognitive Disorders" as "Neurocognitive Disorders (NCDs)," which includes three conditions: Delirium, major neurocognitive disorder, and mild neurocognitive disorder. **Substance/medication-induced major or mild neurocognitive disorder (NCD),** a subtype of NCDs, is associated with several neurocognitive impairments caused by excessive substance consumption or medication abuse and not explained by delirium, episodes of intoxication or withdrawal, or another co-occurring medical or mental health condition.

Major NCD assumes two standard deviations below normal scores on cognitive testing.

- Significant cognitive decline
- Interferes with independence
- Not due to delirium
- Not due to other mental disorder

Mild NCD assumes one standard deviation below normal scores on cognitive testing.

- Moderate cognitive decline
- Does *not* interfere with independence
- Not due to delirium
- Not due to other mental disorder

SYNONYMS

DSM-IV diagnoses of substance-induced persisting dementia and amnestic disorder.
DSM-IV category for "alcohol-induced persisting dementia" characterized by neurocognitive decline associated with alcohol use, in the absence of other causes of dementia; alcohol-related dementia (ARD)
DSM-IV category of "alcohol-induced persisting amnestic disorder" or Wernicke-Korsakoff syndrome (WKS)
Medication induced neurocognitive disorder
Substance induced neurocognitive disorder

ICD 10-CM CODES

F10.97	Alcohol use, unspecified with alcohol-induced persisting dementia
F10.27	Alcohol dependence with alcohol-induced persisting dementia
F10.6	Amnesic syndrome
F10.73	"Residual and late-onset psychotic disorder"
F19.97	Other psychoactive substance use, unspecified with psychoactive substance-induced persisting dementia
F19.17	Other psychoactive substance abuse with psychoactive substance-induced persisting dementia
F19.27	Other psychoactive substance dependence with persisting dementia
	Other (or unknown) substance use disorder, moderate, with other (or unknown) substance-induced major neurocognitive disorder
	Other (or unknown) substance use disorder, severe, with other (or unknown) substance-induced major neurocognitive disorder

EPIDEMIOLOGY & DEMOGRAPHICS

INCIDENCE & PREVALENCE:

- Most cases of NCD are attributed to Alzheimer disease (AD), vascular dementia, and Lewy body dementia.
- **Alcohol use disorder with alcohol-induced major NCD (ARD)** and other substance/medication use NCDs are largely overlooked or seen as a comorbid factor. The incidence and prevalence of ARD vary across studies.
- Heavy use of alcohol appears to contribute in approximately 24% of cases of dementia.
- The prevalence rate estimates for WKS based on postmortem studies are 1% to 2% of the general population and 10% of alcohol consumers. WKS cases are estimated to be approximately 0.05% (Korsakoff) and 0.03% (Wernicke) of all hospital admissions.
- Information about prevalence of NCDs related to other psychoactive substances is very limited.

PREDOMINANT SEX & AGE:

- Elderly are at increased risk for substance/medication-induced NCDs.
- Individuals with ARD are often male, have comorbid mental and physical conditions, and are often identified during hospital admissions.
- Patients are often single or are socially isolated leading to poor case tracking and limited treatment.
- There is little study of the prevalence of comorbid polysubstance abuse, head injuries, or psychiatric comorbidities in the ARD population.

RISK FACTORS:

- Risks for neurodegenerative and cerebrovascular diseases are elevated with increasing age, thus making age a strong risk factor for both major and mild NCD.
- Older drinkers show greater cognitive dysfunction and less recovery once they become abstinent.
- Poor education is associated with poorer recovery over time, and females appear to be more vulnerable despite less alcohol intake than men.
- Occupation and education are potentially important risk factors, with more demanding occupational or recreational activity more likely to cause allostatic loading, oxidative stress, and ultimately increased risk of cognitive decline, especially at a mild level.
- Higher education as well as environmental and lifestyle factors such as physical exercise and mentally stimulating activities have been associated with decreased risk of major or mild NCD of various subtypes.
- Poor nutritional intake leading to thiamine deficiency related to alcohol abuse, gastrointestinal disorders, and systemic diseases contributes to WKS risk.

GENETICS:

- Apolipoprotein E (APOE) ε4 is a well-known risk factor for major or mild NCD due to AD.
- Genetic mutations, polygenic risk factors, vascular risk factors (e.g., stroke, atrial fibrillation, and hypertension), and family history are other risk factors for several NCD subtypes.
- Genetic vulnerabilities for alcoholism and substance abuse must be considered and may contribute to a polygenic risk factor effect in NCD.

PHYSICAL FINDINGS & CLINICAL PRESENTATION

Persons with major NCD experience a substantial decline in function (loss of independence) as a result of profound cognitive impairment, whereas subjects with mild NCD experience only a modest cognitive decline and, as a result, function relatively independently. There are four categories of criteria (criteria A, B, C, and D) and three specifiers (etiologies, presence or absence of behavioral problems, and severity of functional decline).

DSM-5 DIAGNOSTIC CRITERIA

- Cognitive impairment in one or more domains (e.g., complex attention, executive function, learning and memory, language, perceptual-motor, and social cognition). First, there is subjective concern reported by the patient, an informant, or a clinician for a cognitive change from a previous level of cognitive function. Second, cognitive impairment is confirmed by neuropsychological testing or quantitative clinical assessment at the bedside.
- Neurocognitive impairments do not occur exclusively during the course of delirium and persist beyond the usual duration of intoxication and acute withdrawal.
- The involved substance or medication and duration and extent of use are capable of producing the neurocognitive impairment.
- The temporal course of the neurocognitive deficits is consistent with the timing of substance or medication use and deficits remain stable or improve after a period of abstinence.
- The NCD is not attributable to another medical condition or better explained by another mental disorder. For example, syndromes such as major depressive disorder need to be ruled out before making a diagnosis of NCD.
- If a mild substance use disorder is comorbid with the substance-induced NCD, the clinician records "mild [substance] use disorder" before the substance-induced NCD (e.g., "mild inhalant use disorder with inhalant-induced major neurocognitive disorder").
- If a moderate or severe substance use disorder is comorbid with the substance-induced NCD, the clinician should record "moderate [substance] use disorder" or "severe [substance] use disorder."
- If there is no comorbid substance use disorder, the clinician should record only the substance-induced NCD.
- For some classes of substances (i.e., alcohol; sedatives, hypnotics, anxiolytics), it is

not permissible to record a comorbid mild substance use disorder with a substance-induced NCD; only a comorbid moderate or severe substance use disorder, or no substance use disorder, can be diagnosed.

- *DSM-5* describes three specifiers:
  1. *Etiologies*, such as AD, frontotemporal lobar degeneration, Lewy body disease, vascular disease, traumatic brain injury, **substance/medication use**, HIV infection, prion disease, Parkinson disease, Huntington disease, "another medical condition," multiple etiologies, and unspecified.
  2. Presence or absence of *behavioral abnormalities* in both major and mild NCD, such as psychotic or mood symptoms, sleep disturbances, agitation, apathy, and other symptoms. In such cases, the clinician or researcher needs to document the behavioral abnormality (e.g., mild NCD with apathy).
  3. *Severity* of symptoms and severity of functional decline. The severity specifier clearly distinguishes between major NCD and mild NCD. *DSM-5* classifies the severity of symptoms in major NCD into three categories: Mild (impairment only in instrumental activities of daily living), moderate (impairment in basic day-to-day functions such as clothing and feeding), and severe (completely dependent on others).
- Patients with NCDs often experience neuropsychiatric symptoms (NPSs) at some point in their illness.
- NCD etiology plays a role in frequency of different clinical manifestations of NPSs. Apathy and agitation become more prevalent with progression of NCDs, especially when the frontal network is affected. Affective symptoms tend to decrease in severity as NCDs progress whereas delusions, hallucinations, agitation, anxiety, apathy, disinhibition, irritability, and aberrant motor behavior tend to be more severe with disease progression.
- Intoxication with alcohol impairs most cognitive skills and in excess may lead to stupor and respiratory depression.
- Alcohol withdrawal can result in tremor, fluctuating alertness, hallucinations, seizures, and agitation. Patients with ARD are unlikely to demonstrate as much language impairment as in other dementia syndromes.
- ARD patients show poorer performance on visuospatial measures, including clock drawing and copying tasks. Deficits in working memory, motor speed, and executive function (verbal abstract reasoning and letter fluency) have also been observed in ARD patients.
- Clinical profile of ARD reflects both cortical and subcortical pathology.
- Patients with WKS suffer with anterograde and retrograde amnesia, have poor working memory, and show impaired executive functions and visuoperceptual changes. These deficits may reflect damaged frontocortico-cerebellar circuit functions.

ETIOLOGY

- *DSM-5* lists 10 causes of major or mild NCD: (1) AD, (2) frontotemporal lobar degeneration, (3) Lewy body disease, (4) vascular disease, (5) traumatic brain injury, (6) **substance/medication-induced**, (7) HIV infection, (8) prion disease, (9) Parkinson disease, and (10) Huntington disease.
- *DSM-5* presents three other etiologic categories: (1) major or mild NCD due to multiple etiologies, (2) major or mild NCD due to "another medical condition," and (3) major or mild NCD with unclear etiology.
- *DSM-5* looks at associated features supporting a diagnosis; prevalence estimates; development and course; risk and prognostic factors; culture-related diagnostic issues; diagnostic markers; functional consequences; differential diagnosis; and comorbidity. This is crucial in teasing apart **substance/medication-induced NCD** from NCD due to probable AD.
- There is controversy whether dementia can be the direct result of alcohol neurotoxicity—a primary alcoholic dementia—or whether another underlying pathology (thiamine deficiency) or several factors (alcohol neurotoxicity along with nutritional deficiencies) lead to the NCD. Confounding factors include hypertension and other vascular dementia risk factors, other maladaptive behaviors, head trauma, psychiatric factors, and other substance abuse comorbidities.
- Medications with anticholinergic activity can cause **substance/medication-induced NCD** (Table 1). Narcotics (meperidine, codeine), first-generation antihistamines (diphenhydramine, hydroxyzine), antispasmodics, antinausea medications, histamine (H2)–receptor blockers (ranitidine), psychoactive medicines (tricyclic antidepressants, lithium), sedative-hypnotics such as benzodiazepines and barbiturates, fluoroquinolone antibiotics, chemotherapeutic agents, cardiovascular drugs including digoxin and beta blockers, and corticosteroids all have been associated with NCDs.
- In a recent systematic review that assessed drug effect on cognition in individuals over 50 yr old, it was found that there were significant increases in dementia risk for anticholinergic antidepressants, antiparkinsonian drugs, antipsychotics, bladder antimuscarinic drugs, and antiepileptic drugs.
- Evidence also suggests that benzodiazepine use may be a modifiable risk factor for dementia, particularly in patients 65 yr of age or older. This suggests that benzodiazepine use in the elderly population is associated with cognitive decline and dementia. There is also conflicting evidence in this regard perhaps related to causation bias.

PATHOGENESIS:

- Varied NCD symptom complexes makes correlation between the cognitive symptoms and NPSs of NCDs difficult.
- NPSs may be common pathway effects of NCDs and not etiologically specific to one NCD or another. On the other hand, certain symptoms may associate with subtypes of NCDs. For example, patients with vascular NCD show more depression with anxiety than AD patients.
- Studies have shown generalized reductions in cortical and subcortical gray and white matter in patients with chronic alcohol abuse, suggesting pathogenic vulnerabilities for NCD as well as NPSs.
- Symptoms common to the NPSs of NCDs and psychiatric disorders share certain neuroanatomic similarities.
- NPSs may therefore be helpful in understanding the underpinnings of primary psychiatric disorders. Examples: Delusions in schizophrenia and NCDs share frontal corticostriato-thalamocortical (CSTC) and temporal network dysfunction; apathy and abulic syndrome, seen in both NCDs and primary psychotic and mood disorders, have been shown to involve dysfunction in the anterior cingulate cortex (ACC)/medial prefrontal cortical (mPFC) CSTC loop regardless of the etiology; perceptual changes correlate with neuroimaging changes in sensory and association regions regardless of NCD versus schizophrenia diagnosis; catatonic symptoms in NCDs and primary psychiatric disorders share GABA and dopamine hypofunction and glutamate hyperfunction in certain CTSC circuits and respond to the same treatments; anxiety and depressive symptoms in NCDs and primary psychiatric disorders also share a similar syndrome of the aminergic neuron establishing the relationship between the dementia of depression and NCDs.
- The WKS has a classic pathogenesis related to nutritional deficiency of thiamine with

TABLE 1 Medications with Anticholinergicity

Antiarrhythmic	Disopyramide
Antidepressants	Amitriptyline, clomipramine, despiramine, doxepin, imipramine, nortriptyline, paroxetine, protriptyline, trimipramine
Antiemetics	Prochlorperazine, promethazine
Antihistamines	Brompheniramine, carbinoxamine, chlorpheniramine, clemastine, cyproheptadine, dexbrompheniramine, dexchlorpheniramine, dimenhydrinate, homatropine (excludes ophthalmic), hyoscyamine, methscopolamine, propantheline, promethazine, pyrilamine, triprolidine; newer antihistamines, including cetirizine (Zyrtec), may have less anticholinergic and therefore less cognitive effects, but sedation may still be problematic
Antimuscarinic	Darifenacin, festerodine, flavoxate, oxybutynin, solifenacin, tolterodine, trospium
Antiparkinsonian Agents	Benztropine, trihexyphenidy

From Updated 2019 American Geriatric Society Beers Criteria.

damage specifically in the mammillary bodies and the medial dorsal nucleus of the thalamus that will disturb functioning in CSTC tracks.

Dx DIAGNOSIS

DIFFERENTIAL DIAGNOSIS

- Patients with substance use disorders, intoxication, and withdrawal have increased relative risk for other conditions. This situation may worsen neurocognitive function. For example, traumatic brain injury and infections are prevalent conditions in substance use disorder and may independently or in combination cause cognitive dysfunction. Therefore, NCDs secondary to conditions outside the context of substance use, intoxication, and withdrawal, including these accompanying conditions, must be differentiated from substance/medication-induced major or mild NCD.
- Early-onset dementia must be differentiated from ARD. Alcohol use may play a large role in the development of early-onset dementia.
- A broad differential diagnosis is required when assessing NPSs that are possibly secondary to NCDs. Medications and drugs, infections, inflammatory responses, space-occupying lesions, and toxic-metabolic causes of delirium need to be considered as causes of cognitive and behavioral NPSs.
- Patients with NCDs are at increased risk for delirium with resulting acute cognitive dysfunction and NPSs.
- Pain, bowel retention, and urinary retention can worsen mental status in patients with NCDs.
- Sensory changes with reductions in eyesight and hearing, along with environmental alterations in living circumstances, interpersonal conflict, and change in caregivers, can all result in dysfunction in NCD patients.
- Painstaking history and physical examination accompanied by laboratory testing, electroencephalography, and neuroimaging studies as guided by the clinical findings should be pursued to rule out reversible causes of cognitive and behavioral symptoms. Assessment of risk of harm to self and others is required in this patient population.

WORKUP

- Changes in cognition and behavior require a delirium workup, including routine blood work, investigations for "treatable dementias" (including thyroid-stimulating hormone screen and vitamin B12 and folate levels), and a blood test for syphilis. A vitamin D level is often added. A PHQ-2 screen for depression, with PHQ-9 to follow with positive screen in, is done to check for depression as a treatable dementia. Coinciding with clinical examination findings and baseline blood work, other studies, including electroencephalography, structural and functional neuroimaging, and cerebrospinal fluid studies, may be indicated.
- Neuropsychological studies are important given criteria for NCDs. Psychometric tests for memory measure learning and recall; tests for language, executive function, and visuospatial function can be employed to objectively measure cognitive function.
- ARD patients exhibit similar frontal executive dysfunction to vascular dementia patients but perform more poorly than subcortical patients on delayed word recall and recognition. The ARD patients do not display as much memory impairment as the AD patients.

IMAGING STUDIES

- Substances responsible for NCDs can cause neuroimaging changes. For example, inhalant abuse is shown to cause abnormalities in the thalamus, basal ganglia, pons, and cerebellum. Solvent abusers also had more extensive and more severe abnormalities in brain white matter (WM). The diffuse WM abnormalities found among solvent abusers have been associated with greater cognitive impairment.
- Although no common neuroimaging findings exist for the multiple substance/medication causes of NCD, imaging biomarkers can distinguish several etiologic subtypes of major and mild NCD. For example, chemical and neuroimaging biomarkers are present from the asymptomatic phase through the major NCD phase of AD. These include amyloid-β (Aβ), tau-mediated neuronal injury, and loss of neurons. Aβ and tau and neuronal injury can be measured by employing various types of ligands developed for positron emission tomography (FDG-PET) studies. Structural magnetic resonance imaging is used to document cortical atrophy in brain regions characteristic of NCDs. Functional neuroimaging techniques are essential when structural neuroimaging is normal. For example, glucose hypometabolism can be detected in AD signature areas by using FDG-PET (parietotemporal, posterior cingulate cortex, frontal cortex, and medial temporal lobe hypometabolism).
- Neuroimaging in ARD may suggest atrophy in the mammillary bodies, anterior thalamus, and cerebellum, and ventricular enlargement. Single-photon emission computed tomography (SPECT) results suggest reduced regional cerebral blood flow in the frontal cortices, basal ganglia, and thalami of patients with ARD.

Rx TREATMENT

DSM-5 codes for the presence of NPSs, among patients with NCDs, by using the descriptor "with behavioral disturbances." Psychiatrists try to map these NPSs onto specific disorders—such as anxiety, depression, or psychosis—and plan treatment accordingly, though there is no consensus on the appropriate treatment for NPSs among patients with NCDs. Usefulness in neurodegenerative NCDs is sometimes used to suggest treatments for substance use/medication-induced NCDs.

ACUTE AND CHRONIC PHARMACOLOGIC TREATMENT APPROACHES

Cognitive Enhancers: Acetylcholinesterase inhibitors have shown some very modest efficacy for NPSs in NCDs such as AD, vascular dementia, and Lewy body disease in addition to cognitive enhancing effects. Rivastigmine has shown some effectiveness in preventing psychotic and nonpsychotic symptoms (such as apathy and agitation) associated with AD and in helping to manage agitation in Lewy body disease, but effects are modest at best. Memantine may also be mildly effective for agitation and psychosis, and it is generally well tolerated. Patients with ARD and WKS have preliminarily shown cognitive improvement following treatment with memantine. Cognitive enhancers may be considered in cases of substance use/medication-induced NCD or in multimorbid NCD if the side-effect profile permits. Monitoring closely for side effects such as gastrointestinal (GI) distress, bradycardia, and syncope is important.

Antidepressants: Several studies show that antidepressants, citalopram in particular, are effective in treating agitation in patients with AD. Sertraline has a significant benefit for treating depression in AD but not other symptoms. There is evidence of significant benefit in reduction and remission of depressive symptoms in NCD patients. SSRIs and trazodone may also have benefit for NPSs in NCDs.

Evidence exists to suggest that SSRIs can be of benefit in managing depression and agitation in NCDs. The Citalopram for Agitation in Alzheimer Disease study reported significant improvement in agitation, but prolonged QT interval changes and some confusion were seen, requiring caution. More research is needed to better understand the effects of antidepressants for NPSs of patients with NCDs.

Antiepileptic Drugs: Anticonvulsants, such as valproate and carbamazepine, have been used to manage NPSs, especially agitation, in NCDs. In systematic reviews, valproate preparations have been shown to be ineffective in treating agitation and are associated with a high rate of adverse effects. Small trials of carbamazepine show modest effect in management of agitation, but there is a black box warning for hematologic toxicity and the potential drug-drug interactions. There is limited evidence supporting use of gabapentin.

Antipsychotics: First-generation antipsychotics have limited efficacy and have increased risk of extrapyramidal side effects (EPSs), tardive dyskinesia, dystonia, and corrected QT interval prolongation. Atypical antipsychotics (AAs) are more widely used due to side-effect profile and tolerability. Nevertheless, there is known risk of mortality, stroke, and other cerebrovascular risks, which has resulted in a black box warning.

American Psychiatric Association guidelines recommend against haloperidol as a first-line nonemergent treatment for patients with dementia without delirium. Haloperidol was associated with highest mortality followed by olanzapine, risperidone, valproic acid, and quetiapine. Aripiprazole, at a 10 mg/day dose, has been found to be effective for psychosis and for agitation of patients with AD with fewer side effects. Clozapine, the antipsychotic medication with the lowest risk of causing EPSs, can be effective for treatment-resistant agitation of patients with NCDs of multiple etiologies, though cardiac and GI side effects are significant.

In summary, personalizing the medication regimen for selected target symptoms of NCDs, after getting informed consent from the patient or health care proxy, and starting medications at low doses and titrating doses gradually, appears to be the best approach. In addition, vigorous monitoring for side effects and response is required.

OTHER POTENTIAL INTERVENTIONS: Benzodiazepines continue to be used for patients with NCDs despite limited evidence of efficacy and potential adverse cognitive and other side effects. The use of lithium has limited published evidence. A retrospective study reported on the benefits of dronabinol for agitation in patients with NCDs who were acutely hospitalized. Electroconvulsive therapy has also been reported from some centers for selected patients with NCDs.

The management of individuals with ARD and WKS should involve consideration of parenteral thiamine. WKS patients have potential for recovery with abstinence and thiamine supplementation. Improvements in general knowledge, visual long-term memory, and verbal fluency have been found in abstinent individuals with KS over 2 yr, and cognitive improvement is associated with higher premorbid education and fewer detoxifications in the past. Early observations suggest that a large proportion (21%) of individuals with KS can make a full recovery. Treatment with oral thiamine does not achieve an adequate plasma level. Although there is no consensus on dose of thiamine treatment, it is usually given in doses of 200 mg three times daily, preferably intravenously. This treatment should be continued until improvement in signs and symptoms plateaus.

Pimavanserin (Nuplazid) and dextromethorphan-hydrobromide/quinidine (Nuedexta) have recently been tried for NPSs secondary to dementia, but results are preliminary.

NONPHARMACOLOGIC THERAPY

- Psychoeducation: Social interaction, initiating enjoyable activities, complementary therapies, and minimizing conflict.
- Environmental interventions: Optimizing noise level and light, maintaining sleep/wake cycle, providing orientation cues and maintaining routines in a familiar environment, encouraging physical exercise, and accessing adult day services.
- Cognitive-behavioral therapy may be used in an effort to manage NPSs.
- Although meta-analyses are not encouraging with little evidence to recommend routine use for NPSs in NCDs, given low risk coupled with side effects of pharmacotherapy, nonpharmacologic therapies as initial management approaches for NPSs in nonemergent situations are reasonable considerations.
- It is important to emphasize that caregiver support, education, and training can be beneficial in reducing caregiver burnout but also secondarily for patient NPSs.

COMPLEMENTARY & ALTERNATIVE MEDICINE

Music and art therapies, aromatherapy, pet therapy, bright light therapy, and reminiscence therapy have all been used, though the evidence base is meager.

DISPOSITION

Depending on outcomes of management of the offending agents and condition and abstinence, patients may require rehabilitation stays or, if the NCD is major and chronic, longitudinal care facility placement.

REFERRAL

Referral for behavioral neurologic and neuropsychiatric care, as well as physical or occupational therapy and social work, may be necessary.

PEARLS & CONSIDERATIONS

Personalized treatment and management with special attention to medication side effects is essential.

PREVENTION

Public health approaches should include education about NCDs and NPSs associated with substance abuse.

PATIENT & FAMILY EDUCATION

Education focuses on substance use disorder approaches and on caregiver advice and stress management.

SUGGESTED READINGS

Available at ExpertConsult.com

RELATED CONTENT

Neurocognitive Disorders (Related Key Topic)
Substance Use Disorder (Related Key Topic)

AUTHOR: **Gregory L. Fricchione, MD**

Superior Vena Cava Syndrome (ALG)

BASIC INFORMATION

DEFINITION

Superior vena cava (SVC) syndrome is a set of symptoms that results when a mediastinal mass compresses the SVC or the veins that drain into it, resulting in obstruction of blood flow from the head, neck, upper torso, or extremities to the right atrium.

SYNONYM

SVC

ICD-10CM CODES

I87.1	Compression of vein
S25.20XA	Unspecified injury of superior vena cava, initial encounter
S25.29XA	Other specified injury of superior vena cava, initial encounter

EPIDEMIOLOGY & DEMOGRAPHICS

- SVC syndrome occurs in 15,000 persons in the U.S. every yr.
- More than 50% of patients present with SVC on presentation of malignancy.
- Mirrors lung cancer (especially small cell carcinoma) and lymphoma.

PHYSICAL FINDINGS & CLINICAL PRESENTATION

The pathophysiology of the syndrome involves increased pressure in the venous system draining into the SVC producing edema of the head, neck, and upper extremities. Symptoms develop over a period of 2 wk in one third of patients and include:

- Shortness of breath
- Chest pain
- Cough
- Dysphagia, hoarseness, stridor
- Headache
- Syncope
- Visual trouble

Signs:

- Chest wall vein distention (Fig. E1)
- Neck vein distention
- Facial edema, facial plethora
- Upper-extremity swelling
- Cyanosis

ETIOLOGY

- Lung cancer (65% of all cases, of which half are small cell lung cancer)
- Lymphoma (15%)
- Thymoma
- Tuberculosis
- Goiter
- Aortic aneurysm (arteriosclerotic or syphilitic)
- SVC thrombosis:
  1. Primary: Associated with a central venous catheter
  2. Secondary: Complication of SVC syndrome associated with one of the abovementioned causes
- Inflammatory process, fibrosing mediastinitis
- Fig. E2 illustrates the anatomy of superior vena cava syndrome. Table 1 summarizes common malignancies associated with SVC syndrome in adults.

Dx DIAGNOSIS

Diagnostic imaging (Fig. E3 and E4): CT scan of the chest with contrast is the most useful diagnostic study. MRI is usually adequate to establish the diagnosis of SVC obstruction and to assist in the differential diagnosis of probable cause.

DIFFERENTIAL DIAGNOSIS

The syndrome is characteristic enough to exclude other diagnoses. The differential diagnosis concerns the underlying etiologies listed previously.

WORKUP

- Chest x-ray usually shows mediastinal widening and pleural effusion.
- Chest CT with contrast or MRI (in patient who cannot tolerate contrast medium) usually confirms the diagnosis.
- Venography is rarely needed and is warranted only when an intervention (e.g., stent or surgery) is planned.
- Percutaneous needle biopsy, endobronchial ultrasound-guided needle biopsy, and mediastinoscopy are usually the initial diagnostic modalities used to establish a histologic diagnosis.
- Box 1 summarizes an approach to patients with superior vena cava obstruction.

TABLE 1 Malignancies Associated with Superior Vena Cava (SVC) Syndrome in Adults*

Neoplastic Diagnosis	Percentage of SVC	Percentage of Disease-Associated SVC
Lung cancer, stage 3B or 4:	48-81	
Small cell lung cancer		15-45
Squamous cell cancer		20-25
Adenocarcinoma		5-25
Large cell carcinoma		4-30
Lymphoma:	2-21	
Diffuse large cell lymphoma		64
Lymphoblastic lymphoma		33
Breast cancer	11	

*Includes lung cancer, lymphomas, and metastases from other solid tumors. 75% to 85% of patients with SVC have neoplastic disease.

From Zipes DP et al (eds): *Braunwald's heart disease,* ed 7, Philadelphia, 2005, Saunders.

BOX 1 Approach to Patients with Superior Vena Cava Obstruction

The diagnosis is established by physical examination and clinical presentation (see text).

- Respiratory status should be assessed promptly. Only patients in extremis should be treated urgently with radiation therapy or stent placement without a histologic diagnosis. Emergency therapy is necessary in fewer than 5% of all superior vena cava (SVC) obstruction cases.
- Diagnostic evaluation should proceed with the least invasive procedures performed initially followed by more invasive procedures as needed to obtain histologic diagnosis:
  1. Chest radiography
  2. Sputum cytology
  3. Thoracentesis with cytologic evaluation of fluid
  4. Node biopsy if a palpable node is present; avoid fine-needle aspiration if lymphoma is suspected
  5. Fiber-optic bronchoscopy with endobronchial ultrasound
  6. Mediastinoscopy with video-assisted imaging
  7. Thoracostomy with video-assisted imaging
- Evaluation may vary depending on the age and sex of the patient:
  1. In older adults (i.e., ≥50 years), the most common cause of SVC obstruction is lung cancer; lymphoma and metastatic cancer are less common, and benign processes are uncommon.
  2. In young adults (<50 years old), the most common cause of SVC obstruction is lymphoma (usually large cell lymphoma or lymphoblastic lymphoma; rarely Hodgkin disease). Lung cancer and thoracic malignancy are less common. Germ cell cancer (almost never in female patients) and benign causes are uncommon. The preceding evaluation should be modified to include the following studies before more invasive procedures are performed:
     a. Serum tumor markers (i.e., β-human chorionic gonadotropin, α-fetoprotein, and lactate dehydrogenase)
     b. Bone marrow aspiration and biopsy

From Niederhuber JE: *Abeloff's clinical oncology,* ed 6, Philadelphia, 2020, Elsevier.

TABLE 2 Comparison of Treatment Modalities for Malignancy-Related Superior Vena Cava Obstruction

Modality	Time to Symptom Relief	Percentage with Symptom Response	Potential for Combined Modality Therapy
Radiation therapy	3-30 days	56-96	Yes
Chemotherapy	1-2 weeks	59-77	Yes
Stent placement	0-72 hours	78-95	Yes

From Niederhuber JE: *Abeloff's clinical oncology*, ed 6, Philadelphia, 2020, Elsevier.

Rx TREATMENT

- Tissue diagnosis is usually needed before commencing therapy. EBUS is now considered the first step in evaluation. Mediastinoscopy would be considered if EBUS is nondiagnostic or there is high clinical suspicion for lymphoma.
- Management is guided by the severity of the symptoms and the underlying etiology. Table 2 compares treatment modalities for malignancy-related superior vena cava obstruction.
- Most patients with SVC do not require emergency intervention. Emergency empiric radiation is indicated in critical situations such as respiratory failure or central nervous system signs associated with increased intracranial pressure.
- Treatment of the underlying malignancy:
  1. Radiotherapy: The majority of tumors causing SVC syndrome are sensitive to radiotherapy
  2. Systemic chemotherapy
- Anticoagulant or fibrinolytic therapy in patients who do not respond to cancer treatment within a week or if an obstructing thrombus has been documented.
- Loop diuretics are often used, but their effect is limited.
- Upright positioning and fluid restriction until collateral channels develop and allow for clinical regression are useful modalities for SVC syndrome secondary to benign disease.
- Steroids (dexamethasone 4 mg q6h) may be useful in reducing the tumor burden in lymphoma and thymoma after definitive diagnosis is made.
- Percutaneous self-expandable stents that can be placed under local anesthesia with radiologic manipulation are useful in the treatment of SVC syndrome to bypass the obstruction, especially in cases associated with malignant tumors.
- Surgical bypass grafting is infrequently used to treat SVC syndrome.
- Fig. 5 illustrates a management algorithm for superior vena cava obstruction.

REFERRAL

To a thoracic surgeon, pulmonary specialist, and/or oncologist

AUTHOR: **Gaetane Michaud, MD**

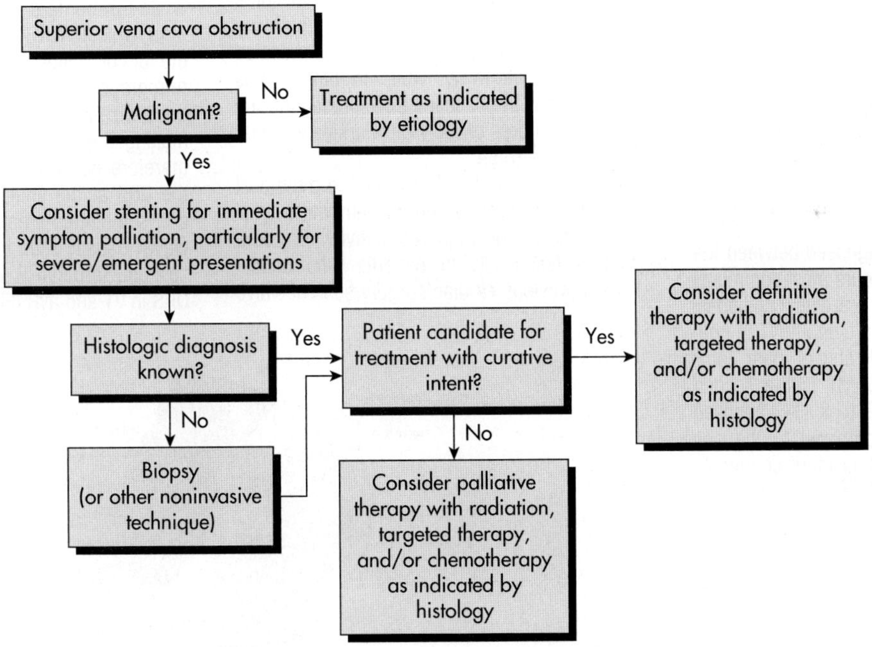

FIG. 5 A management algorithm for superior vena cava obstruction. (From Niederhuber JE: *Abeloff's clinical oncology*, ed 6, Philadelphia, 2020, Elsevier.)

BASIC INFORMATION

DEFINITION

Supraventricular tachycardia (SVT) is a group of rapid regular tachyarrhythmia. There are three major categories of SVT:

1. Atrial tachycardia (AT): An arrhythmia that originates from the atrium and does not involve the AV node. This is usually a focal arrhythmia. In some cases, the underlying mechanism may be a reentry circuit, either a small circuit (microreentry) or a large circuit (macroreentry)
2. AV nodal reentrant tachycardia (AVNRT)
3. AV reentrant tachycardia (AVRT) (Fig. 1)

The latter two are reentrant arrhythmia that always involve the AV node as part of the circuit (Fig. 1).

Other forms of arrhythmia that involve the atria, such as atrial fibrillation and atrial flutter, have distinct electrocardiographic features and are covered in separate chapters. Rare forms of SVT such as inappropriate sinus tachycardia, sinus mode reentry tachycardia, and junctional tachycardia are beyond the scope of this chapter.

SYNONYMS

SVT
Paroxysmal supraventricular tachycardia
PSVT

ICD-10CM CODE	
I47.1	Supraventricular tachycardia

EPIDEMIOLOGY & DEMOGRAPHICS

SVT is most commonly diagnosed between the ages of 12 and 30. SVT occurs most commonly in patients with no prior cardiac conditions. AVNRT is the most common type of SVT in both genders and in all ages. It occurs most commonly in young women. AVRT is the second most common SVT, and it is typically diagnosed in younger patients as compared to the age of patients with AVNRT. AT is more commonly associated with structural heart disease.

PHYSICAL FINDINGS & CLINICAL PRESENTATION

- Patients may be either symptomatic or asymptomatic.
- Patient may be aware of "fast" regular heartbeat (but sometimes complain of irregular heartbeat, palpitations); may complain of weakness, dyspnea, dizziness, chest pain, presyncope or, rarely, syncope.
- Patients with AVNRT may complain of neck pounding during the episode due to simultaneous contraction of the atria and ventricles with closed AV valves causing a sharp increase in atrial and jugular venous pressure.
- In some cases the episodes can be triggered by physical activity or psychological stress, but in others there may not be an obvious trigger. In patients with AVNRT, sometimes the arrhythmia is reproducibly initiated when bending forward to pick up an item from the floor.
- Hemodynamic status during the arrhythmia may vary and depend on the patient's comorbidities and presence of underlying structural heart disease. Usually, patients are hemodynamically stable.
- Physical examination is most commonly normal and unrevealing, except rapid regular heart rate and occasionally hypotension. In patients with AVNRT sharp tall jugular vein A waves may be seen when the right atrium contracts against a closed tricuspid valve.

ETIOLOGY (SEE FIG. 1)

- AVNRT: Dual electrical pathways within the AV node. In typical AVNRT the anterograde limb conducts slowly (slow pathway) and the retrograde limb has fast conduction properties (fast pathway), and vice versa in atypical AVNRT.
- AVRT is accessory pathway mediated, either orthodromic (antegrade through the AV node and retrograde through the accessory pathway) or, much less commonly, antidromic (antegrade through the accessory pathway and retrograde through the AV node). In the case of antidromic tachycardia, the QRS will be wide and fully preexcited. In some patients, the presence of accessory pathway is not evident on the baseline ECG (concealed accessory pathway), while in others it is manifest in the baseline ECG, presenting the typical features of the Wolff-Parkinson-White (WPW) syndrome.
- Paroxysmal atrial tachycardia and multifocal atrial tachycardia: Abnormal automaticity of atrial tissue or triggered activity. In some cases (especially in patients who underwent previous cardiac surgery such as valve replacement or ASD closure), the underlying mechanism is macroreentrant AT.

DIAGNOSIS

The diagnosis of SVT relies principally on the 12-lead ECG. Every patient suspected of having an episode of SVT should have a 12-lead ECG done immediately. Typically, patients with SVT will present with a narrow complex QRS tachycardia with a ventricular rate faster than 100 beats per minute (bpm) and typically faster than 130 to 150 bpm.

P wave morphology can be useful in discriminating rhythms. P waves with a similar axis to the sinus node can be atrial tachycardias and sinus tachycardias. P waves with retrograde depolarization of the atria (seen as inverted in the inferior leads) can be seen in AVNRT, AVRT, and atrial tachycardia. Sawtooth P waves are indicative of classical counterclockwise typical type I flutter, and an absence of P waves with irregular R-R intervals points to atrial fibrillation. Variable (>3) morphologies of P wave are suggestive of multifocal atrial tachycardia. Wide QRS complex (>0.12 sec) with initial slurring (delta wave) during sinus rhythm and short PR (<0.12 sec) is characteristic of Wolff-Parkinson-White syndrome.

In typical AVNRT, due to the small size of the circuit within the AV node and the fast retrograde conduction, there is simultaneous depolarization of the ventricles and atria, thus making the P wave "buried" in the QRS and therefore not visible or inscribed very close to the QRS at the final part of the QRS complex, and sometimes creating a "pseudo terminal S wave" usually seen in leads II, III, and aVF and "pseudo terminal R waves" at the end of the QRS in V1 and avR (Fig. 1).

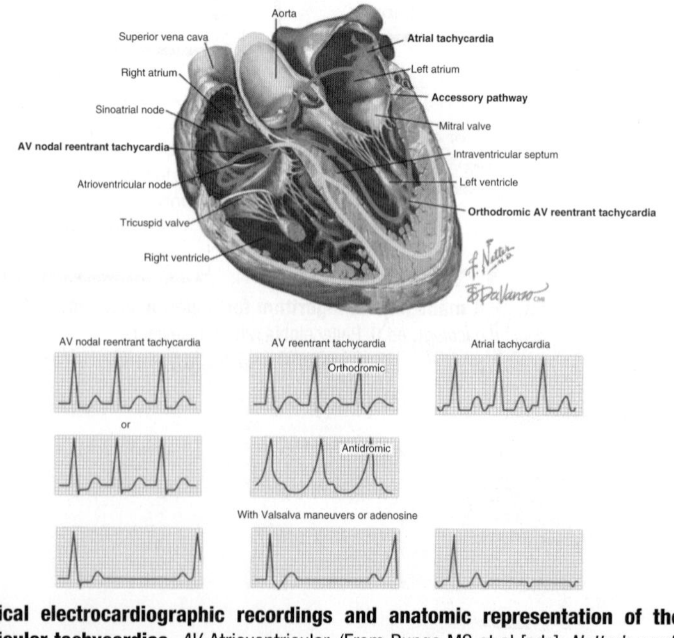

FIG. 1 Typical electrocardiographic recordings and anatomic representation of the common supraventricular tachycardias. *AV,* Atrioventricular. (From Runge MS et al [eds]: *Netter's cardiology,* ed 2, Philadelphia, 2010, Saunders. Adapted from Delacretaz E: Clinical practice: supraventricular tachycardia, *N Engl J Med* 354:1039-1051, 2006.)

In orthodromic AVRT, the P wave is usually visible close after the QRS due to the rapid conduction properties of the accessory pathway (short RP tachycardia). In AT, the P wave is usually noticed farther away after the QRS (long RP tachycardia) (Fig. 1). A unique form of orthodromic AVRT termed *paroxysmal junctional reentrant tachycardia* (PJRT) involves a concealed accessory pathway, usually located in the posteroseptal region, and typically presents with deeply inverted retrograde P waves in leads II, III, and aVF, with a long RP interval.

Other diagnostic maneuvers that may assist in the differential diagnosis are vagal maneuvers (such as carotid sinus massage) or giving intravenous AV nodal blocking agents (such as adenosine or verapamil) to produce AV nodal conduction block. This will terminate reentrant arrhythmia dependent on the AV node—AVNRT and AVRT—but not AT, which will continue, albeit with nonconducted P waves.

Other arrhythmias that present with narrow complex tachycardia like PSVT are:

- Fascicular VT
- Junctional tachycardias
- Artifact such as with Parkinson disease

SVT can conduct with bundle branch block (BBB) and wide QRS either due to preexisting BBB on the baseline ECG or due to aberrant conduction (rapid rate–dependent BBB). When a patient presents with wide QRS tachycardia, VT must be excluded first. Features to distinguish SVT from ventricular tachycardia are outlined in Table 1.

WORKUP

- Electrocardiography
- Echocardiography to exclude structural heart disease
- Thyroid function tests
- Complete blood count to exclude anemia or infection as an underlying trigger for the event
- In most cases the workup will be negative, with no underlying cardiac or systemic pathology and no clear triggers for an acute episode
- Holter or event monitor to document the arrhythmias if they are paroxysmal and not documented yet

TABLE 1 Features That May Differentiate Ventricular Tachycardia from Supraventricular Tachycardia with Aberrancy

Helpful Features	Implications
Positive QRS concordance	Diagnostic of VT
Presence of AV dissociation, capture beats, or fusion beats	Diagnostic of VT
R to S interval >100 ms in any one precordial lead	Suggests VT
Atypical RBBB (monophasic R, QR, RS, or triphasic QRS in V_1; R:S ratio <1, QS or QR, monophasic R in V_6)	Suggests VT
Atypical LBBB (R >30 min or R to S [nadir or notch] >60 min in V_1 or V_2; R:S ratio <1, QS or QR in V_6)	Suggests VT
Shift of axis from baseline	Suggests VT
History of CAD	Suggests VT
QRS during tachycardia identical to QRS during sinus rhythm	Suggests SVT
Termination with adenosine	Suggests SVT

AV, Atrioventricular; *CAD,* coronary artery disease; *LBBB,* left bundle branch block; *RBBB,* right bundle branch block; *SVT,* supraventricular tachycardia; *VT,* ventricular tachycardia.

From Stambler BS et al: Etripamil nasal spray for rapid conversion of supraventricular tachycardia to sinus rhythm, *J Am Coll Cardiol* 72:489-497, 2018.

Rx TREATMENT (FIG. 2)

NONPHARMACOLOGIC THERAPY

Acute termination: If the patient is hemodynamically unstable, prompt synchronized cardioversion with an external defibrillator using 50 to 100 J should be performed.

If the patient is stable, Valsalva maneuver in the supine position is the most effective way to terminate most types of SVT; carotid sinus massage (after excluding occlusive carotid disease and murmurs over the carotid arteries) is also commonly used to elicit vagal efferent impulses. These are effective in terminating AVRT, AVNRT, and may occasionally terminate some types of atrial tachycardia, but in the case of sinus tachycardia, atrial flutter, and atrial fibrillation, they only transiently slow down AV conduction without terminating the actual tachycardia.

PHARMACOLOGIC THERAPY

- Adenosine is useful to terminate acutely orthodromic AVRT and AVNRT and can uncover the underlying rhythm in paroxysmal atrial tachycardia (Fig. 3); it is the first choice of therapy for treatment of almost all episodes of SVT unresponsive to vagal maneuvers. The dose is 6 mg given as a rapid IV bolus; tachycardia is usually terminated within a few seconds. If this fails, one may repeat with 12 mg IV bolus for up to two times. Contraindications

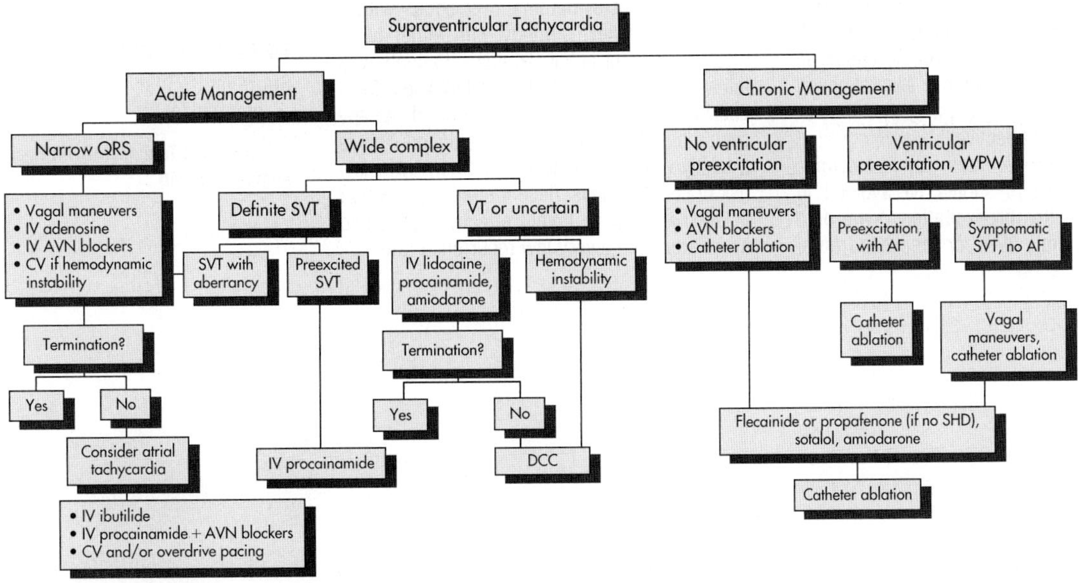

FIG. 2 Supraventricular tachycardia. *AF,* Atrial fibrillation; *AVN,* atrioventricular node; *CV,* cardioversion; *IV,* intravenous; *DCC,* direct current cardioversion; *SHD,* structural heart disease (no overt evidence of myocardial, valvular, congenital, or coronary heart disease); *SVT,* supraventricular tachycardia; *VT,* ventricular tachycardia; *WPW,* Wolff-Parkinson-White. (From Olshansky B et al: *Arrhythmia essentials,* ed 2, Philadelphia, 2017, Elsevier.)

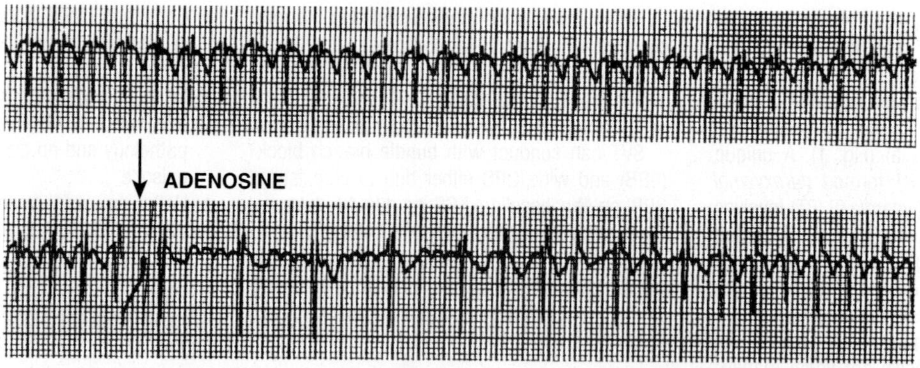

FIG. 3 Adenosine can uncover the mechanism of supraventricular tachycardia. A 3-month-old infant developed an extremely fast, narrow QRS complex tachycardia and a heart rate of 220 beats/min after insertion of a central line through a jugular vein. Adenosine produced a transient atrioventricular block and unmasked very rapid atrial fibrillation waves (570 beats/min). (From Park MK: *Park's pediatric cardiology for practitioners*, ed 6, Philadelphia, Elsevier, 2014.)

are second- or third-degree atrioventricular block; WPW with atrial fibrillation; sick sinus syndrome; and chronic use of drugs such as dipyridamole, theophylline, or aminophylline; and heart transplant. Adenosine may cause bronchospasm in asthmatics as well as chest discomfort, flushing, and shortness of breath, but these usually last for a very short time and serious adverse effects are extremely rare due to the drug's very short half-life.

- Verapamil 5 to 10 mg IV is given over 5 min; if no effect, may repeat in 30 min.
  1. Verapamil should be used cautiously in patients with SVT associated with hypotension and should not be used in patients with heart failure with reduced ejection fraction or those who are under regular beta-blocker treatment.
  2. Slow injection of calcium chloride (10 ml of a 10% solution given over 5-8 min before verapamil administration) decreases the hypotensive effect without compromising its antiarrhythmic effect.
- Metoprolol (IV 5 mg/2 min up to 15 mg) or esmolol (500 μg/kg IV bolus, then 50 μg/kg/min) may be effective in the treatment of SVT.
  1. IV digoxin (0.75-1 mg slow IV loading in increments of 0.25 mg over several hours) is rarely used in SVT but may tried if other agents are not effective.
  2. Digoxin, beta-blockers, and calcium-channel blockers should be avoided in patients with preexcitation syndrome and antidromic AVRT or preexcited atrial fibrillation to avoid increased conduction through the accessory pathway.
- Recently a new rapidly acting intranasal calcium-channel blocker—etripamil—was reported to be effective in rapid conversion of SVT to sinus rhythm. This may prove in the future to be an important treatment modality but is not yet available for routine clinical use.

CHRONIC TREATMENT

The goal is prevention of recurrent episodes. In patients with infrequent and minimally symptomatic episodes without preexcitation, it is optional to provide treatment only during acute episodes. In patients with recurrent symptomatic episodes, regular treatment with beta-blockers or nondihydropyridines calcium channel blockers can be tried; if these fail, class Ic antiarrhythmics are an option. Rarely, in cases in which all other treatments fail or are contraindicated, class III antiarrhythmics such as amiodarone or sotalol may be tried. It is also possible to treat patients who have infrequent symptomatic episodes with a "pill-in-the-pocket" strategy with either beta-blockers or other antiarrhythmics. Patients who fail antiarrhythmic therapy, develop side effects due to medications, or refuse medical therapy should be referred for catheter ablation. This is a highly effective mode of treatment with low risk of complications. Recent studies show that ablation therapy is highly effective, safe, and associated with a very low recurrence rate.

DISPOSITION

Most patients respond well with resolution of the SVT upon treatment (see "Acute General Rx"). Some patients may need chronic AV blocking agents for recurrence.

REFERRAL

Radiofrequency ablation (RFA) is the procedure of choice in symptomatic patients who are refractory to medical therapy especially in AVRT, AVNRT, and atrial flutter. RFA has high efficacy rates (single procedure success is 93.2%), low all-cause mortality (0.1%), and low adverse events (2.9%). Recent technologic developments provided the ability to perform RFA with no to minimal radiation using advanced electroanatomic mapping systems and intracardiac echocardiography. Despite high reported success rates and high safety profile, RFA appears to be underused in clinical practice.

SUGGESTED READINGS

Available at ExpertConsult.com

RELATED CONTENT

Supraventricular Tachycardia (Patient Information)

AUTHORS: **Gal Tsaban, MD, MPH,** and **Yuval Konstantino, MD**

BASIC INFORMATION

DEFINITION

Syncope is the transient loss of consciousness with spontaneous recovery that results from an acute global reduction in cerebral blood flow. There are three major types: Neurocardiogenic, orthostatic, and cardiac. Syncope is a symptom, and the goal is to distinguish lethal causes from benign causes of transient loss of consciousness.

ICD-10CM CODE
R55 Syncope and collapse

EPIDEMIOLOGY & DEMOGRAPHICS

- Syncope accounts for 3% to 5% of emergency department visits.
- 30% of the adult population will experience at least one syncopal episode during their lifetimes.
- Incidence of syncope is highest in elderly men and young women.
- 15% of children and adolescents experience syncope; fewer than 5% have cardiac causes.

PHYSICAL FINDINGS & CLINICAL PRESENTATION

- Blood pressure: If low, consider orthostatic hypotension; if unequal in both arms (difference >20 mm Hg), consider subclavian steal or dissecting aneurysm. (NOTE: Blood pressure [BP] and heart rate should be recorded in the supine and standing positions, waiting at least 5 minutes between each position.) If there is a drop in BP but no change in heart rate (HR), the patient may be taking a beta-blocker or may have an autonomic neuropathy.
- Pulse: If patient has tachycardia, bradycardia, or irregular rhythm, consider arrhythmia.
- Heart: If there are murmurs present, consider syncope attributable to left ventricular outflow obstruction (aortic stenosis or idiopathic hypertrophic subaortic stenosis); if there are jugular venous distention and distal heart sounds, consider cardiac tamponade.
- Carotid sinus pressure: Can be diagnostic if it reproduces symptoms and other causes are excluded; a pause >3 sec or a systolic BP drop >50 mm Hg without symptoms or <30 mm Hg with symptoms when sinus pressure is applied separately on each side for <5 sec is considered abnormal. This test should be avoided in patients with carotid bruits or cerebrovascular disease. ECG monitoring, IV access, and bedside atropine should be available when carotid sinus pressure is applied.

ETIOLOGY

- Neurocardiogenic or neurally mediated syncope: Most common type, accounting for two thirds of cases. It includes vasovagal, situational, carotid hypersensitivity, and postexertional syncope (Box 1).
  1. Psychophysiologic (emotional upset, panic disorders, hysteria, hyperventilation)
  2. Visceral reflex (micturition, defecation, food ingestion, coughing, ventricular contraction, glossopharyngeal neuralgia)
  3. Carotid sinus pressure
  4. Reduction of venous return caused by Valsalva maneuver
  5. Postural tachycardia syndrome (POTS)
- Orthostatic hypotension (10% of cases):
  1. Hypovolemia
  2. Vasodilator medications
  3. Autonomic neuropathy (diabetes, amyloid, Parkinson disease, multisystem atrophy)
  4. Pheochromocytoma
  5. Carcinoid syndrome
- Cardiac (10%-20%):
  1. Reduced cardiac output:
     a. Left ventricular outflow obstruction (aortic stenosis, hypertrophic cardiomyopathy)
     b. Obstruction to pulmonary flow (pulmonary embolism, pulmonic stenosis, primary pulmonary hypertension)
     c. Myocardial infarct with pump failure
     d. Cardiac tamponade
     e. Mitral stenosis
     f. Reduction of venous return (atrial myxoma, valve thrombus)
     g. Beta-blocker therapy
  2. Arrhythmias or asystole:
     a. Extreme tachycardia (>160-180 beats/min)
     b. Severe bradycardia (<30-40 beats/min)
     c. Sick sinus syndrome
     d. Atrioventricular block (second or third degree)
     e. Ventricular tachycardia or fibrillation
     f. Long QT syndrome
     g. Pacemaker malfunction
     h. Psychotropic medications and beta-blockers (Table 1)

Dx DIAGNOSIS

DIFFERENTIAL DIAGNOSIS

- Seizure (Table 2).
- Vertebrobasilar transient ischemic attack (TIA) usually manifests as diplopia, vertigo, or ataxia but not loss of consciousness. Isolated episodes of transient loss of consciousness

BOX 1 Causes of Syncope

Reflex Syncopal Syndromes
- Vasovagal faint (common faint)
- Carotid sinus syncope
- Situational faint:
  1. Acute hemorrhage
  2. Cough, sneeze
  3. Gastrointestinal stimulation (swallow, defecation, visceral pain)
  4. Micturition (postmicturition)
  5. Postexercise
  6. Pain, anxiety
- Glossopharyngeal and trigeminal neuralgia

Orthostatic
- Aging
- Antihypertensives
- Autonomic failure:
  1. Primary autonomic failure syndromes (e.g., pure autonomic failure, multiple system atrophy, Parkinson disease with autonomic failure)
  2. Secondary autonomic failure syndromes (e.g., diabetic neuropathy, amyloid neuropathy)
- Medications
- Volume depletion:
  1. Hemorrhage, diarrhea, Addison disease, diuretics, febrile illness, hot weather

Cardiac Arrhythmias
- Sinus node dysfunction (including bradycardia-tachycardia syndrome)
- Atrioventricular conduction system disease
- Paroxysmal supraventricular and ventricular tachycardias
- Implanted device (pacemaker, implantable cardioverter defibrillator) malfunction
- Drug-induced proarrhythmias

Structural Cardiac or Cardiopulmonary Disease
- Cardiac valvular disease:
  1. Acute myocardial infarction, ischemia
  2. Obstructive cardiomyopathy
  3. Atrial myxoma
  4. Acute aortic dissection
  5. Pericardial disease, tamponade
  6. Pulmonary embolus, pulmonary hypertension

Cerebrovascular
- Vascular steal syndromes

Multifactorial

Fillit HM: *Brocklehurst's textbook of geriatric medicine and gerontology*, ed 8, Philadelphia, 2017, Elsevier.

TABLE 1 Drugs That Can Cause or Contribute to Syncope

Drug	Mechanism
Diuretics	Volume depletion
Vasodilators: • Angiotensin-converting enzyme inhibitors • Calcium channel blockers • Hydralazine • Nitrates • α-Adrenergic blockers • Prazosin	Reduction in systemic vascular resistance and venodilation
Other antihypertensive drugs: • α-Methyldopa • Clonidine • Guanethidine • Hexamethonium • Labetalol • Mecamylamine • Phenoxybenzamine	Centrally acting antihypertensives
Drugs associated with torsades de pointes: • Amiodarone • Disopyramide • Encainide • Flecainide • Quinidine • Procainamide • Sotalol	Ventricular tachycardia associated with a prolonged QT interval
Digoxin	Cardiac arrhythmias
Psychoactive drugs: • Tricyclic antidepressants • Phenothiazines • Monamine oxidase inhibitors • Barbiturates	Central nervous system effects causing hypotension; cardiac arrhythmias
Alcohol	Central nervous system effects causing hypotension; cardiac arrhythmias

Fillit HM: *Brocklehurst's textbook of geriatric medicine and gerontology*, ed 8, Philadelphia, 2017, Elsevier.

(TLOC, Fig. E1) without accompanying neurologic symptoms are unlikely to be TIAs.
- Recreational drugs or alcohol.
- Functional causes such as somatoform disorders.
- Sleep disorders, such as sleep attacks and narcolepsy, are also in the differential for TLOC.
- Head trauma.

WORKUP

The history is crucial to diagnosing the cause of syncope and may suggest a diagnosis that can be evaluated with directed testing. History is also important to determine other etiologies for TLOC, such as seizure.
- Sudden loss of consciousness (LOC): Consider cardiac arrhythmias.
- Gradual LOC: Consider orthostatic hypotension, vasodepressor syncope, hypoglycemia.
- History of aura before LOC or prolonged confusion (>1 min), amnesia, or lethargy after LOC suggests seizure rather than syncope.
- Patient's activity at the time of syncope:
  1. Micturition, coughing, defecation: Consider syncope caused by decreased venous return.
  2. Turning head or while shaving: Consider carotid sinus syndrome.
  3. Physical exertion in a patient with murmur: Consider aortic stenosis.
  4. Arm exercise: Consider subclavian steal syndrome.
  5. Assuming an upright position: Consider orthostatic hypotension.
- Associated events:
  1. Chest pain: Consider myocardial infarction, pulmonary embolism.
  2. Palpitations: Consider arrhythmias or POTS.
  3. Incontinence (urine or fecal) and tongue biting are associated with seizure or syncope.
  4. Brief, transient shaking after LOC may represent myoclonus from global cerebral hypoperfusion and not seizures. However, sustained tonic/clonic muscle action is more suggestive of seizure.
  5. Focal neurologic symptoms or signs point to a neurologic event such as a seizure with residual deficits (e.g., Todd paralysis) or cerebral ischemic injury.
  6. Psychologic stress: Syncope may be vasovagal.
  7. Multiple nonspecific symptoms (fatigue, diffuse weakness, headache, "brain fog," exercise intolerance, "coat hanger sign") can be seen in POTS and neurogenic orthostatic hypotension and may have psychophysiologic or functional causes.
- Review current medications, particularly antihypertensive and psychotropic drugs.
- Carotid sinus massage (CSM) may be reasonable in patients older than 40 with syncope of unknown origin and possibly due to vasovagal mechanism. It is contraindicated in patients with carotid disease.
- Table 3 differentiates syncope caused by neutrally mediated hypotension, arrhythmias, seizures, and psychogenic causes.
- Fig. 2 illustrates an approach to the evaluation of syncope.

LABORATORY TESTS

Routine blood tests rarely yield diagnostically useful information and should be done only if they are specifically suggested by the results of the history and physical examination. The following are commonly ordered tests:
- Pregnancy test in women of childbearing age
- Complete blood count to look for anemia and signs of infection
- Electrolytes, blood urea nitrogen, creatinine, magnesium, and calcium to look for electrolyte abnormalities and evaluate fluid status
- Serum glucose level
- Cardiac troponins, especially if the patient gives a history of chest pain before the syncopal episode
- Drug and alcohol levels with suspected toxicity

IMAGING STUDIES

- ECG to rule out arrhythmias; may be diagnostic in 5% to 10% of patients.
- Echocardiography. Indicated in patients where initial evaluation suggests structural heart disease (based on physical exam and/or ECG) or have known heart disease.
- If seizure is suspected, MRI of the brain and electroencephalogram may be useful.
- If head trauma or neurologic signs on examination, CT or MRI may be helpful.
- If arrhythmias are suspected, a 24-hr Holter monitor or admission to a telemetry unit in high risk patients is appropriate. In general, Holter monitoring is rarely useful, revealing a cause for syncope in <3% of cases. Loop recorders that can be activated after syncopal episode to retrieve information about the cardiac rhythm during the preceding 4 min add considerable diagnostic yield in patients with unexplained syncope.
- Implantable cardiac monitors that function as permanent loop recorders or implantable cardioverter-defibrillators, which are placed subcutaneously in the pectoral region with the patient under local anesthesia, are useful in patients with cardiac syncope.
- Electrophysiologic studies may be indicated in patients with structural heart disease and/or recurrent syncope.

TILT-TABLE TESTING

- Useful to support a diagnosis of neurocardiogenic syncope. Patients age >50 yr should have stress testing before tilt-table testing. Positive results would preclude tilt-table testing.
- Indicated in patients with recurrent episodes of unexplained syncope as well as patients in high-risk occupations (e.g., pilots, bus

TABLE 2 Clinical Features That Help Distinguish a Generalized Tonic-Clonic Seizure from Syncope

	Seizure	Syncope
Clinical context and circumstances	Neurologic or systemic conditions that predispose to seizures, family history of seizures. Mental fatigue, sleep deprivation, alcohol use or withdrawal, systemic illness	Cardiovascular disorders, dehydration, anemia. Family history of syncope
Triggers	Usually none (unless reflex epilepsy)	Orthostatic hypotension, venipuncture, painful and noxious stimuli, emotional stress, micturition, Valsalva maneuver
Clinical features		
• Onset	No warning unless there is a warning symptom. Abrupt loss of consciousness, generalized stiffening, and fall. Occurs in any position	Tiredness, nausea, diaphoresis, tunneling of vision. Loss of consciousness over few seconds and fall. Occurs usually standing
• Course	Prominent tonic phase then clonic movements lasting about 1 minute, cyanosis, labored breathing, may bite tongue or cheeks, sometimes urinary incontinence	Usually loss of tone, pallor, multifocal myoclonic jerks lasting <15 seconds, sometimes urinary incontinence, usually no tongue or cheek biting
• Offset	Postictal sleepiness and confusion lasting up to hours, headache, myalgia	Rapid recovery over seconds to less than few minutes, no confusion, headache, or myalgia. May have fatigue

From Goldman L, Schafer AI: *Goldman-Cecil medicine,* ed 26, Philadelphia, 2019, Elsevier.

TABLE 3 Differentiation of Syncope Caused by Neurally Mediated Hypotension, Arrhythmias, Seizures, and Psychogenic Factors

	Neurally Mediated Hypotension	Arrhythmias	Seizures	Psychogenic
Demographics and clinical setting	Female > male sex Younger age (<55 yr) More episodes (>2) Standing, warm room, emotional upset	Male > female sex Older age (>54 yr) Fewer episodes (<3) During exertion or when supine Family history of sudden death	Younger age (<45 yr) Any setting	Female > male sex Occurs in presence of others Younger age (<40 yr) Many episodes (often many episodes in a day) No identifiable trigger
Premonitory symptoms	Longer duration (>5 sec) Palpitations Blurred vision Nausea Warmth Diaphoresis Lightheadedness	Shorter duration (<6 sec) Palpitations less common	Sudden onset or brief aura (déjà vu, olfactory, gustatory, visual)	Usually absent
Observations during the event	Pallor Diaphoresis Dilated pupils Slow pulse, low BP Incontinence may occur Brief clonic movements may occur	Blue, not pale Incontinence may occur Brief clonic movements may occur	Blue face, no pallor Frothing at the mouth Prolonged syncope (duration >5 min) Tongue biting Horizontal eye deviation Elevated pulse and BP Incontinence more likely* Tonic-clonic movements if grand mal	Normal color Not diaphoretic Eyes closed Normal pulse and BP No incontinence Prolonged duration (minutes) common
Residual symptoms	Residual symptoms common Prolonged fatigue common (>90%) Oriented	Residual symptoms uncommon (unless prolonged unconsciousness) Oriented	Residual symptoms common Aching muscles Disorientation Fatigue Headache Slow recovery	Residual symptoms uncommon Oriented

BP, Blood pressure.
*May be observed with any of these causes of syncope but more common with seizures.
From Zipes DP: *Braunwald's heart disease: a textbook of cardiovascular medicine,* ed 11, Philadelphia, 2019, Elsevier.

drivers). The test is also useful for identifying patients with prominent bradycardic response who may benefit from implantation of a permanent pacemaker. The test is contraindicated in patients with recent stroke, MI, and severe coronary or carotid disease.
- It is performed by keeping the patient strapped in an upright posture on a tilt table with footboard support. The angle of the tilt table varies from 60 to 80 degrees. The duration of upright posture during tilt-table testing varies from 25 to 45 min.
- The hallmark of neurocardiogenic syncope is severe hypotension associated with a paradoxic bradycardia triggered by a specific stimulus. The diagnosis of neurocardiogenic syncope is likely if upright tilt testing reproduces these hemodynamic changes in <15 min and causes presyncope or syncope.
- Postural orthostatic tachycardia syndrome is diagnosed if there is a sustained heart rate increase of not less than 30 beats/minute or above 120 beats/min within 10 min of active standing or head-up tilt without associated orthostatic hypotension and with reproduction of symptoms.

PSYCHIATRIC EVALUATION

- May be indicated in young patients without heart disease who have frequently recurring transient loss of consciousness and other somatic symptoms.
- Generalized anxiety disorder, pain disorder, and major depression predispose patients to neurally mediated reactions and may result in syncope.

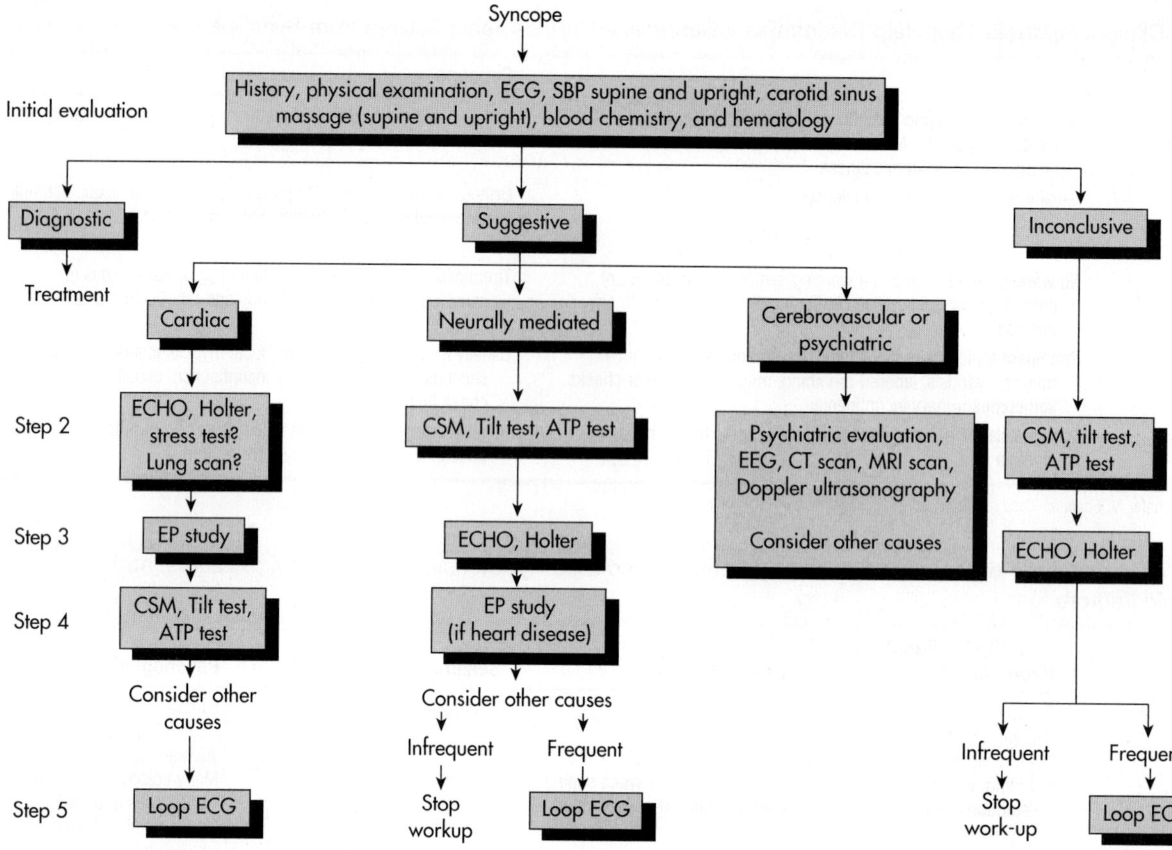

FIG. 2 An approach to the evaluation of syncope for all age groups. *ATP test,* Adenosine provocation test; *CSM,* carotid sinus massage; *ECG,* electrocardiogram; *ECHO,* echocardiogram; *EEG,* electroencephalography; *EP study,* electrophysiologic study; *SBP,* systolic blood pressure. (Fillit HM: *Brocklehurst's textbook of geriatric medicine and gerontology,* ed 8, Philadelphia, 2017, Elsevier.)

Rx TREATMENT

NONPHARMACOLOGIC THERAPY

- Ensure proper hydration; consider compression stockings and salt tablets in appropriate patients.
- Eliminate medications that may induce hypotension.
- Elevate the head of the bed by 10 to 30 degrees while sleeping.

ACUTE GENERAL Rx

- Varies with the underlying etiology of syncope (e.g., pacemaker in patients with syncope resulting from complete heart block). Clinical variables for identification of high-risk syncope patients who may benefit from hospitalization or an accelerated outpatient evaluation are summarized in Table E4.
- Syncope caused by orthostatic hypotension is treated with volume replacement in patients with intravascular volume depletion. Also consider midodrine to promote venous return by adrenergic-mediated vasoconstriction and fludrocortisone for its mineralocorticoid effects to increase intravascular volume, although these medications can cause supine hypertension. Droxidopa is approved for neurogenic orthostatic hypotension in pure autonomic failure or multiple system atrophy.

DISPOSITION

Prognosis varies with the age of the patient and the etiology of the syncope. In general:

- Benign prognosis (very low 1-yr morbidity rate) in patients:
  1. Age <30 yr and having noncardiac syncope
  2. Age <70 yr and having vasovagal or psychogenic syncope or syncope of unknown cause
- Poor prognosis (high mortality and morbidity rates) in patients with cardiac syncope, with presenting systolic BP <90 mm Hg.
- Patients with the following risk factors have a higher 1-yr mortality rate: Abnormal ECG, history of ventricular arrhythmia, history of congestive heart failure.

REFERRAL

Hospital admission in elderly patients without prior history of syncope or unknown etiology of their syncope and in any patients suspected of having cardiac syncope, with presenting systolic BP <90 mm Hg.

PEARLS & CONSIDERATIONS

COMMENTS

- The etiology of syncope is identified in <50% of cases during the initial evaluation.
- A thorough history and physical examination are the most productive means of establishing a diagnosis in patients with syncope.
- Driving restrictions vary based on state but consider restricting driving if syncope is frequent or unpredictable.

SUGGESTED READINGS

Available at ExpertConsult.com

RELATED CONTENT

Syncope (Patient Information)
Orthostatic Hypotension (Related Key Topic)

AUTHORS: **Corey Goldsmith, MD,** and **Tzu-Ching (Teddy) Wu, MD, MPH**

BASIC INFORMATION

DEFINITION

In healthy individuals, the expected physiologic response to serum hypotonicity is inhibition of antidiuretic hormone/arginine vasopressin (ADH/AVP) hypothalamic synthesis and posterior pituitary gland release. Decreased binding to renal medullary collecting duct vasopressin (V2) receptors results in the increased excretion of urine that is dilute (low osmolality) and hypotonic (low sodium and potassium concentrations). The syndrome of inappropriate antidiuresis (SIAD) is defined by "inappropriately" concentrated urine in patients with hypotonic hyponatremia and normal extracellular fluid (ECF) volume. In the absence of an elevated serum glucose or exogenous osmole such as mannitol, the serum sodium concentration (S_{Na}) is essentially determined by the ratio of total body exchangeable sodium and potassium ($Na_e + K_e$) (mmol) to total body water (TBW) (L):

$$S_{Na} = \frac{(Na + K)e}{TBW}$$

Hyponatremia results from a reduction of the numerator, increase of the denominator, or both. To correct hyponatremia, the normal, appropriate renal response is excretion of urine with Na and K concentrations significantly less than S_{Na}. In SIAD, TBW is increased primarily by expansion of the volume of electrolyte-free water (EFW), which is water essentially devoid of Na and K. The severity of hyponatremia in SIAD reflects a urinary dilution defect and the magnitude of electrolyte-free fluid intake. The definition of SIAD excludes hemodynamic stimuli that stimulate ADH, including ECF volume (decreased total body sodium content), hypotension, and disorders characterized by decreased effective arterial blood volume. The latter group is characterized by increased ECF volume (edema or ascites) from increased total body sodium content. This group includes cardiac disease (e.g., congestive heart failure or chronic pericardial disease), nephrotic syndrome, and cirrhosis.

The term *syndrome of inappropriate antidiuretic hormone* (SIADH) has fallen into disfavor because 10% to 15% of so-called SIADH patients manifest suppressed or undetectable serum ADH concentrations. The group with suppressed ADH may have increased sensitivity of renal collecting duct cells to ADH, secretion of other ADH-like peptides, or altered renal hemodynamics that reduce sodium and water delivery to distal diluting sites, thereby preventing maximal urinary dilution. Establishing a diagnosis of SIAD does not require the measurement of ADH levels. Patients with adrenal insufficiency are excluded from the definition of SIAD. Hypothyroidism has been considered a cause of SIADH previously but is no longer because bioscientific proof of thyroid hormone influencing water metabolism is lacking. Instead, hyponatremia may result from impaired cardiac output (heart failure) in severe cases of hypothyroidism (i.e., myxedema). SIAD should not be diagnosed in acute or chronic kidney disease.

SYNONYMS

SIADH
SIAD
Syndrome of inappropriate antidiuretic hormone secretion
Syndrome of inappropriate ADH release
Inappropriate secretion of antidiuretic hormone

ICD-10CM CODE
E22.2 Syndrome of inappropriate secretion of antidiuretic hormone

EPIDEMIOLOGY & DEMOGRAPHICS

INCIDENCE: Hyponatremia occurs in nearly 14% of hospitalized patients and represents an acquired disorder in the majority of cases. Nearly half of these patients have SIAD. The adjusted odds ratio for in-hospital mortality in patients with hyponatremia at hospital admission is 1.47 (95% Confidence Interval, 1.33-1.62).

PHYSICAL FINDINGS & CLINICAL PRESENTATION

- Chronic hyponatremia is defined as an S_{Na} <130 mmol/L persisting for more than 48 hours with normal ECF volume. Patients are hemodynamically stable with no evidence of edema, ascites, pleural, or pericardial effusion.
- Manifestations: Marathon running or other extreme endurance exercise, fever and delirium after 3,4-methylenedioxy-methamphetamine (MDMA, ecstasy) administration, stigmata of alcoholism or malnutrition, fever and/or localizing symptoms related to pneumonia or other pulmonary disease, or headaches and visual field defects from an intracranial mass.
- If hyponatremia occurs rapidly, namely, in less than 24 hr, delirium, lethargy, or seizures may occur. Diminished reflexes and extensor plantar responses may occur with severe hyponatremia or an S_{Na} <120 mmol/L.
- Neurologic abnormalities, including ataxia, mood changes, and proximal muscle weakness, are frequent in chronic hyponatremia. Abnormalities may be subtle despite severe hyponatremia.
- Drugs: Thiazide diuretics and selective serotonin reuptake inhibitor (SSRI) antidepressants are the two most common causes of drug-related hyponatremia. Narcotic analgesics, carbamazepine, phenothiazines, tricyclic antidepressants, MDMA (ecstasy), nicotine, clofibrate, haloperidol, nonsteroidal antiinflammatory drugs (NSAIDs), monoamine oxidase inhibitors, chlorpropamide, vasopressin, desmopressin, oxytocin, and chemotherapeutic agents (vincristine, cyclophosphamide) represent additional etiologies.
- Neoplasms: Lung, oropharynx, stomach, duodenum, pancreas, brain, thymus, bladder, prostate, endometrium, mesothelioma, lymphoma, and Ewing sarcoma.
- Pulmonary disorders: Pneumonia, aspergillosis, pulmonary abscess, tuberculosis, bronchiectasis, emphysema, cystic fibrosis, status asthmaticus, and respiratory failure associated with positive-pressure breathing.
- Intracranial pathology: Trauma, neoplasms, infections (meningitis, encephalitis, brain abscess), hemorrhage, hydrocephalus, multiple sclerosis, and Guillain-Barré syndrome.
- Postoperative period: Surgical stress, positive pressure ventilation, anesthetic agents, and pain.
- Other: Acute intermittent porphyria, psychosis, delirium tremens, general anesthesia, and endurance exercise.
- Table 1 summarizes common etiologies of SIAD.

DIFFERENTIAL DIAGNOSIS

- Hyponatremia associated with subclinical hypovolemia
- Solute-limited water excretion (e.g., "tea-and-toast" diet, beer-drinker's potomania); an acquired disorder in which the renal capacity to excrete sufficient electrolyte-free water is impaired from an insufficient osmolar intake (sodium and potassium) and/or metabolism (generation of urea from protein metabolism).
- Primary polydipsia or water intake that exceeds renal dilutional capability and is frequently accompanied by solute-limited water excretion
- Endocrine disorders, including hypothyroidism and adrenal insufficiency
- Severe hypokalemia produces hyponatremia because the exchangeable potassium pool is twice the size of the exchangeable sodium pool. When intracellular potassium is in severe deficit, sodium ions exit the plasma, enter cells, and cause hyponatremia.
- Hypertonic hyponatremia (hyperglycemia, iatrogenic administration of mannitol, sorbitol, glycine)
- Hyponatremia from subclinical heart or liver disease
- Pseudohyponatremia caused by extreme hyperglobulinemia or hyperlipidemia
- Reset osmostat: ADH regulation occurs at a lower-than-normal osmotic threshold, with intact urinary dilution and concentration

WORKUP

- Normal ECF volume by history and physical examination. No history of large-volume fluid losses. No generalized edema, ascites, or large pleural effusions.
- Laboratory evaluation (see "Laboratory Tests") is consistent with excessive ADH secretion or sensitivity in the absence of osmotic or hemodynamic stimuli for ADH secretion.
- Normal thyroid, adrenal, and cardiac function.
- No recent or concurrent use of loop diuretics.
- Failure to correct hyponatremia after ECF volume repletion by isotonic 0.9% saline solution.
- Correction of hyponatremia by solely fluid restriction is generally unsuccessful.
- Diagnostic criteria for SIADH are described in Table 2.

TABLE 1 Common Etiologies of the Syndrome of Inappropriate Antidiuretic Hormone Secretion (SIADH)

Tumors
Pulmonary/mediastinal (bronchogenic carcinoma, mesothelioma, thymoma)
Extrapulmonary (duodenal carcinoma, pancreatic carcinoma, ureteral/prostate carcinoma, uterine carcinoma, nasopharyngeal carcinoma, leukemia)
Central Nervous System Disorders
Mass lesions (tumors, brain abscesses, subdural hematoma)
Inflammatory diseases (encephalitis, meningitis, systemic lupus erythematosus, acute intermittent porphyria, multiple sclerosis)
Degenerative/demyelinating diseases (Guillain-Barré syndrome, spinal cord lesions)
Miscellaneous (subarachnoid hemorrhage, head trauma, acute psychosis, delirium tremens, pituitary stalk section, transsphenoidal adenomectomy, hydrocephalus)
Drug-Related
Stimulated release of AVP (nicotine, phenothiazines, tricyclics)
Direct renal effects and/or potentiation of AVP antidiuretic effects (desmopressin, oxytocin, prostaglandin synthesis inhibitors)
Mixed or uncertain actions (ACE inhibitors, carbamazepine and oxcarbazepine, chlorpropamide, clofibrate, clozapine, cyclophosphamide, 3,4-methylenedioxy-methamphetamine (ecstasy), omeprazole; serotonin reuptake inhibitors (SSRIs), vincristine
Pulmonary
Infections (tuberculosis, acute bacterial and viral pneumonia, aspergillosis, empyema)
Mechanical/ventilatory causes (acute respiratory failure, COPD, positive-pressure ventilation)
Other Causes
Acquired immunodeficiency syndrome (AIDS) and AIDS-related complex
Prolonged strenuous exercise (marathon, triathlon, ultramarathon, hot-weather hiking)
Senile atrophy
Idiopathic

ACE, Angiotensin-converting enzyme; *AVP,* arginine vasopressin; *COPD,* chronic obstructive pulmonary disease.
From Melmed S: *Williams textbook of endocrinology,* ed 12, Philadelphia, 2011, Saunders.

TABLE 2 Diagnostic Criteria for the Syndrome of Inappropriate Antidiuretic Hormone Release

Essential Diagnostic Criteria
Decreased extracellular fluid effective osmolality (<270 mOsm/kg H_2O)
Inappropriate urinary concentration (>100 mOsm/kg H_2O)
Clinical normovolemia
Elevated urinary sodium concentration under conditions of normal salt and water intake
Absence of adrenal, thyroid, or pituitary insufficiency
Absence of chronic kidney disease
Absence of diuretic use
Supplemental Criteria
Abnormal water loading test (inability to excrete at least 90% of a 20 ml/kg H_2O load in 4 hours and/or failure to dilute urine osmolality to <100 mOsm/kg H_2O)
Plasma vasopressin level inappropriately elevated relative to the plasma osmolality
No significant correction of S_{Na} with volume expansion, but improvement after fluid restriction

S_{Na}, Serum sodium.
From Floege J et al: *Comprehensive clinical nephrology,* ed 4, Philadelphia, 2010, Saunders.

LABORATORY TESTS

- Normal or low BUN and/or serum creatinine
- S_{Na} lower than the limit of the normal range
- Decreased serum osmolality (<275 mOsm/kg H_2O) corrected for serum glucose and exogenous osmoles
- Decreased serum uric acid concentration
- Urine osmolality >100 mOsm/kg H_2O with simultaneous plasma hypo-osmolality, that is, plasma osmolality <270 mOsm/kg H_2O
- Urine Na concentration is generally >40 mmol/L with normal dietary salt intake

IMAGING STUDIES

Imaging is not routinely required for diagnosis. Imaging may facilitate the diagnosis of an associated underlying pulmonary or CNS disease or rule out intracranial pathology.

Rx TREATMENT

NONPHARMACOLOGIC THERAPY

With mild SIAD, fluid restriction (10-15 ml/kg per day) combined with increased solute loads (diets high in protein, urea powder, sodium chloride, and potassium chloride) may normalize S_{Na}. The enhanced solute load produces an osmotic diuresis that increases electrolyte-free water loss. Urea administration should be undertaken with a consulting nephrologist; it has been proven safe for decades.

ACUTE GENERAL Rx

PHARMACOLOGIC THERAPY:

Rate of Correction: In chronic hyponatremia, rapid S_{Na} correction rates are avoided to prevent brain injury from osmotic demyelination syndrome. Patients with moderate-to-severe hyponatremia should undergo serial monitoring of S_{Na} and serum potassium concentration (S_K), urine volumes, and urine chemistries (osmolality, K, and Na). Most SIAD patients have chronic hyponatremia (developing over more than 24 hours) and mild symptoms. Target S_{Na} correction rates are 6 to 8 mmol/L per day in chronic hyponatremia. The S_{Na} should be actively lowered in patients who experience increases of >10 mmol/L during a 24-hour period. The rate of S_{Na} change during conservative therapy or 0.9% infusion is often slow or flat because sodium is excreted while water is mostly retained. In cases of hyponatremia from undiagnosed ECF volume depletion or a limitation of EFW excretion due to inadequate urinary solute (tea and toast diet or beer potomania), administration of saline may produce rapid excretion of large volumes of hypotonic urine with overly rapid S_{Na} correction. Therefore, close monitoring of serum and urine electrolytes, osmolality, and volume is always recommended.

Acute Hyponatremia: In patients with acute hyponatremia (duration <24 hours), the goal of therapy is to increase S_{Na} sufficiently to prevent or reduce the severity of cerebral edema. S_{Na} should be increased by up to 6 mmol/L within the first 3 hours if symptoms are mild-to-moderate and within the initial hour with severe symptoms (seizures, coma, obtundation).

Rapid correction of S_{Na} in acute hyponatremia may involve hypertonic saline therapy (3% saline, 513 mmol/L). As a rule of thumb, 1 ml/kg body weight of 3% saline is expected to increase S_{Na} by 1 mmol/L. S_{Na} correction rates may be greater than anticipated when unrecognized ECF volume depletion is concurrently corrected. The simultaneous delivery of the synthetic ADH analog desmopressin can mitigate S_{Na} overcorrection. Intravenous furosemide therapy may augment urinary EFW loss and prevent unintended ECF volume expansion during hypertonic saline therapy, which is contraindicated in individuals with heart failure.

Chronic Hyponatremia: The therapeutic goals of chronic hyponatremia from SIAD are normalization of TBW and restoration of Na and K stores to their respective normal levels. These goals may be achieved as follows.

- Choose a 24-hour target S_{Na}, based on current S_{Na} and safe rates of correction (see "Rate of Correction").
- Estimate TBW and total body cation content. Estimation of current TBW should consider the patient's baseline TBW, volume of additional retained water, and changes in total body content of sodium and potassium (see example below).
- Account for all sources of EFW intake and loss (including insensible losses). Add/subtract this total volume to/from net target EFW to determine total EFW volume loss required to attain the target S_{Na}.
- Select strategy that achieves target EFW volume loss: Collecting duct arginine vasopressin receptor-2 antagonist (e.g., tolvaptan), urea therapy, or loop diuretic combined with electrolyte replacement such as sodium chloride ("salt") tablets with 17 mmol Na per 1 gram of NaCl.

The following example demonstrates the method to determine the target TBW and EFW loss required to reach an appropriate S_{Na} target after 24 hours of therapy in a patient with chronic hyponatremia.

- S_{Na} is 115 mmol/L in 75 kg, minimally symptomatic elderly woman who chronically takes an SSRI and hydrochlorothiazide.
  1. *Step 1: Establish target S_{Na}:*
     a. Target S_{Na} after 24 hours = Current S_{Na} + 6 = 121 mmol/L
  2. *Step 2: Estimate current TBW and total body cations:*
     a. Current weight = 75 kg
     b. Estimated TBW fraction = 0.55 (55%)
     c. Current TBW = 0.55 × 75 = 41.2 L
     d. Current total body cation quantity = Current TBW × S_{Na} = 41.2 × 115 = 4743 mmol
  3. *Step 3: Calculate target TBW:*
     a. Target TBW (L) = Current Na and K cation/Target S_{Na} = 4743 mmol/121 mmol/L = 39.2 L
  4. *Step 4: Calculation of net EFW loss:*
     a. Target *net EFW loss* after 24 hours = Current TBW − Target TBW = 41.2 L − 39.2 L = 2 L
  5. *Step 5: Calculate total urine EFW volume:*
     a. Target *total urine EFW excretion* (estimate: 1 L oral fluid intake and 0.5 L net insensible loss) Urine EFW volume = 2 + (1 − 0.5) = 2.5 L
  6. *Step 6: Choose therapeutic strategy*
  7. *Step 7: Implement strategy and monitor results frequently*

A 24-hour net EFW loss of 2.5 L is required. With loop diuretic administration, roughly a 5 L urine output is required to reduce total body water appropriately. The urine can be functionally considered half-normal saline (0.45% saline). The urine may be considered as two proportions: An electrolyte-free fraction, representing 2.5 L of pure water, and 2.5 L of isotonic saline, with the urine cation concentrations of Na and K equaling a concentration of sodium in 0.9% saline. Cation losses can be repaired with 0.9% saline or 3% saline. Administration of the latter requires 70% less volume than 0.9% saline and elevates S_{Na} more rapidly. Alternatively, cation replacement may be carried out by oral administration of NaCl and KCl tablets. Periodic monitoring of S_{Na}, S_K, urine volume, and urine chemistries (osmolality, sodium, and potassium) is recommended to prevent overly rapid correction of S_{Na}.

Loop Diuretic Plus Saline Strategy: Before the advent of specific arginine vasopressin receptor-2 antagonists, SIAD was typically treated by increasing urine volume and EFW loss with a loop diuretic. Half of the urine volume can be assumed to consist of electrolyte-free water because the sum of urine sodium and potassium cation concentrations will approximate 75 mmol/L, i.e, half-normal saline concentration. Isotonic or hypertonic IV fluids can be administered to correct urine sodium loss. A 1 L volume 0.9% saline is equivalent to 0.3 L of 3% saline. The use of hypertonic saline solutions should be guided by an expert. Urine potassium loss cannot be ignored, and these losses are corrected separately.

Arginine Vasopressin Receptor (V2R) Antagonists: Selective V2 receptor antagonist therapy is straightforward and convenient for patients and medical personnel. Currently, two agents are available in the U.S.: IV conivaptan (20 mg IV × 1 followed by continuous IV infusion of 20-40 mg/day for 2-4 days) and oral tolvaptan (15-90 mg/day, as needed). Tolvaptan must be initiated in-hospital. Urinary electrolyte losses are minimal, meaning that administration produces virtually electrolyte-free urines.

CHRONIC Rx

- When SIAD is chronic, fluid restriction (<15 ml/kg per day) may be required indefinitely and combined with high dietary electrolyte and protein.
- NaCl tablets, electrolyte supplements, protein powders to generate urea production, and pharmaceutical-grade urea may be used to correct hyponatremia. Periodic monitoring of electrolytes is recommended in patients with chronic SIAD.
- Tolvaptan has been administered successfully in clinical trials. FDA labeling states that initial therapy must take place in-hospital. Tolvaptan use is restricted to 30 days due to concerns regarding hepatotoxicity, which was detected during clinical trials for polycystic kidney disease. Additional contraindications include volume contraction and concomitant use of strong cytochrome P3A inhibitors. Patients undergoing tolvaptan therapy are not fluid-restricted.
- Demeclocycline variably increases urine electrolyte-free water losses. This agent is contraindicated in hepatic disease and rarely used today.

DISPOSITION

- Mortality exceeding 40% has been reported in patients with S_{Na} <110 mmol/L.
- Hospital readmission rates are common in chronic SIAD when an underlying cause cannot be eliminated, especially if patients are unwilling or unable to restrict their fluid intake and follow dietary recommendations.
- Chronic, mild-to-moderate hyponatremia is associated with bone loss, falls, and increased fracture risk, particularly in elderly patients.

REFERRAL

Emergency department evaluation and hospital admission are appropriate for moderate-to-severe hyponatremia due to SIAD, especially when acute or symptomatic. Due to a high complication risk from overly aggressive or ineffective treatment, consultation by a nephrologist, endocrinologist, or critical care physician is recommended.

SUGGESTED READINGS

Available at ExpertConsult.com

RELATED CONTENT

Syndrome of Inappropriate Secretion of Antidiuretic Hormone (Patient Information)

AUTHORS: **Mark D. Faber, MD,** and **Jerry Yee, MD**

BASIC INFORMATION

DEFINITION

Syphilis is a systemic sexually transmitted disease caused by the bacteria *Treponema pallidum*, with acute and chronic manifestations, characterized by primary skin lesions; secondary eruption involving skin and mucous membranes; long periods of latency; and late lesions of the skin, bone, viscera, central nervous system, and cardiovascular system.

SYNONYM

Lues

ICD-10CM CODES

A50	Congenital syphilis
A51.0	Primary genital syphilis
A51.1	Primary anal syphilis
A51.2	Primary syphilis of other sites
A51.3	Secondary syphilis of skin and mucous membranes
A51.4	Other secondary syphilis
A51.5	Early syphilis, latent
A51.9	Early syphilis, unspecified
A52	Late syphilis
A52.0	Cardiovascular and cerebrovascular syphilis
A52.1	Symptomatic neurosyphilis
A52.2	Asymptomatic neurosyphilis
A52.3	Neurosyphilis, unspecified
A52.8	Late syphilis, latent
A52.9	Late syphilis, unspecified
A53.9	Syphilis, unspecified

EPIDEMIOLOGY & DEMOGRAPHICS

- Most commonly diagnosed in people 20 to 30 yr old.
- Slightly more prevalent in men than women.
- Rates reached historic lows in the U.S. in 2000 but began increasing among males in 2001, and increase has continued. The number of cases reported to the CDC increased by 71% from 2014 to 2018. In 2018 men accounted for 86% of all patients with syphilis. Rates are disproportionately higher among black and Hispanic men who have sex with men (MSM), compared with white MSM and among young MSM. Rates are also increasing in women, with highest rates in black women compared with Hispanic and white women. The rates of primary and secondary syphilis among women more than doubled between 2014 and 2018. Congenital syphilis rates also have been increasing, with 1306 cases reported in 2018.
- Usually more prevalent in urban areas and among people of lower socioeconomic status.
- Communicability is indefinite and variable. Communicable during primary, secondary, and latent mucocutaneous lesions in up to first 4 yr of latency. Most probable congenital transmission occurs in early maternal syphilis. Adequate penicillin treatment ends infectivity within 24 to 48 hr.

PHYSICAL FINDINGS & CLINICAL PRESENTATION

PRIMARY SYPHILIS:

- Characteristic lesion is a painless chancre on genitalia (Figs. E1 and E2), mouth, or anus; atypical primary lesions may occur.
- May appear 3 days to 12 wk (usually 3 wk) after exposure and may resolve without treatment within 6 wk.

SECONDARY SYPHILIS:

- Bacteremia associated with generalized lymphadenopathy and a characteristic maculopapular rash including palms, soles, trunk, and mucous membranes. Lesions may also be pustular, involve the mucosal surfaces. Constitutional, flulike symptoms may also occur, as well as mild disturbances of multiple organ systems.
- 60% to 80% have maculopapular lesions on palms and soles (Fig. E3).
- 21% to 58% have mucocutaneous or mucosal lesions (pharyngitis, tonsillitis, "mucous patch" lesion on oral and genital mucosa).
- Condylomata lata intertriginous papules (raised, gray-white lesions) form at areas of friction and moisture, such as the vulva (Fig. E4).
- Occurs 4 to 6 wk after appearance of chancre. Resolves within 1 wk to 12 mo. Can have relapsing episodes up to 5 yr after initial episode.
- Clinical features of secondary syphilis are summarized in Table 1.

LATENT SYPHILIS—EARLY VS. LATE LATENT:

- Generally asymptomatic, can occur between 1 and 30 yr after a primary infection
- Seroreactivity without other evidence of primary or secondary disease
- Not sexually transmitted but may be transmitted from a pregnant woman to her fetus for up to 4 yr after acquiring the disease
- In early latent syphilis, disease can be transmitted even without the current presence of an active lesion. This is not the case in late latent syphilis
- Early latent: <12 mo from acquisition
- Late latent: >12 mo from acquisition, or time since infection is unknown

TERTIARY SYPHILIS:

- A form of late syphilis characterized by gummas (nodular, ulcerative lesions) that can involve the skin, mucous membranes, skeletal system, and viscera.
- Manifestations of cardiovascular syphilis include aortitis, aneurysm, or aortic regurgitation.
- Neurosyphilis may be asymptomatic or symptomatic. Tabes dorsalis, meningovascular syphilis, general paralysis, or insanity may occur.
- Ocular syphilis can affect any part of the eye. Posterior uveitis is the most common. Iritis, choroidoretinitis, and leukoplakia may also occur.
- A classification of neurosyphilis is described in Table 2.

CONGENITAL SYPHILIS:

- Mother-to-child transmission of untreated syphilis and its consequences are described in Table 3.
- Table 4 summarizes the stigmata of congenital syphilis.

ETIOLOGY

- *Treponema pallidum,* a spirochete
- Spread by sexual intercourse or by intrauterine transfer

TABLE 1 Clinical Features of Secondary Syphilis

- **Prodromal symptoms and signs:**
  Weight loss
  Low-grade fever
  Malaise
  Headache (meningeal irritation)
  Sore throat
  Conjunctivitis (iridocyclitis)
  Arthralgia (periostitis)
  Myalgias
  Hepatosplenomegaly (mild hepatitis)
- **Generalized lymphadenopathy with indolent enlargement of lymph nodes** (50%-85%)
- **Skin manifestations:**
  Early (10%): Generalized eruption; nonpruritic, roseola-like, discrete macules, initially distributed on the flanks and shoulders
  Late (70%): Generalized maculopapular and papulosquamous eruptions; more infiltrated lesions, often copper-colored; annular plaques on the face; corymbose arrangement (satellite papules around a larger central lesion); occurs in successive waves and is polymorphic
  Localized syphilids (specific infiltrations of treponemes; positive darkfield examination):
    - Palms and soles: symmetric papules and plaques with a collarette of scale (collarette of Biett)
    - Anogenital area: condylomata lata
    - Seborrheic area: "corona veneris" along the hairline
  Hypopigmented macules, mainly on the neck (postinflammatory; "necklace of Venus")
- **Manifestations involving mucous membranes** (30%):
  Syphilitic perlèche, split papules
  Mucous patches: "plaques muqueuses" in the oropharynx (equivalent to condylomata lata in the genital area)
  Syphilitic sore throat: Inflammation of the whole pharynx
- **Patchy alopecia** (7%): "Moth-eaten" localized areas of hair loss; toxic telogen effluvium

From Bolognia J: *Dermatology,* ed 4, Philadelphia, 2018, Elsevier.

TABLE 2 Classification of Neurosyphilis

- **Asymptomatic**
  - Early
  - Late
- **Meningeal**
  - Acute syphilitic meningitis
  - Meningovascular
  - Cerebrovascular
  - Spinal form
- **Parenchymatous**
  - General paresis (dementia paralytica)
  - Tabes dorsalis
  - Taboparesis (mixed)
  - Optic atrophy
- **Gummatous**
  - Cerebral form
  - Spinal form
  - Both spinal and cerebral

From Bolognia J: *Dermatology,* ed 4, Philadelphia, 2018, Elsevier.

TABLE 3 Mother-to-Child Transmission of Untreated Syphilis and Its Consequences

Risk
- Infection of the mother from conception to 7th month of pregnancy: Risk of transmission is nearly 100% (often fetal demise or severe congenital syphilis)
- Infection at least 2 yr before pregnancy: Reduced risk of transmission to 50%
- Infection during 7th, 8th, or early 9th month: Reduced risk of transmission
- Infection 3-6 wk before labor: No placental transmission; risk of perinatal transmission

Consequences of Infection
- Spontaneous abortion (second or third trimester) (10%)
- Stillbirth (10%)
- Infant death (20%)
- Congenital syphilis (20%)
- Healthy child (40%)

From Bolognia J: *Dermatology,* ed 4, Philadelphia, 2018, Elsevier.

TABLE 4 Stigmata of Congenital Syphilis

Cutaneous
- Rhagades—radial periorificial (mouth, nose, eyes, anus) scars at sites of previous fissures

Dental
- Hutchinson teeth—peg-shaped, notched permanent incisors*
- Mulberry molars—multiple rounded rudimentary cusps on the permanent first molars
- Caries due to defective enamel

Skeletal
- Saddle nose—depression of the nasal root due to destruction of cartilage/bone
- Frontal bossing of Parrot ("Olympian brow")
- Hypoplastic maxilla, relatively prominent mandible
- High palatal arch ± perforation
- Higouménakis' sign—thickening of the medial clavicle
- Scaphoid scapulae
- Saber shins—anterior tibial bowing
- Clutton's joints—painless synovitis and effusions of the knees

Other
- Eighth nerve deafness*
- Interstitial keratitis leading to corneal ulcers and opacities*

*Components of Hutchinson triad.
From Bolognia J: *Dermatology,* ed 4, Philadelphia, 2018, Elsevier.

TABLE 5 Genital Ulcer Disease

Disease	Lesions	Lymphadenopathy	Systemic Symptoms
Primary syphilis	**Painless,** indurated, with a clean base, usually singular	Nontender, rubbery, nonsuppurative bilateral lymphadenopathy	None
Genital herpes	**Painful** vesicles, shallow, usually multiple	Tender, bilateral inguinal adenopathy	Present during primary infection
Chancroid	Tender papule, then **painful,** undermined purulent ulcer, single or multiple	Tender, regional, painful, suppurative nodes	None
Lymphogranuloma	Small, **painless** vesicle or papule progresses to an ulcer	Painful, matted, large nodes with fistulous tracts	Present after genital lesion heals

From Wein AJ et al: *Campbell-Walsh urology,* ed 11, Philadelphia, 2016, Elsevier.

TABLE 6 Differential Diagnoses for Syphilis

Primary Syphilis
Other causes of genital ulcers should be considered:
- Genital herpes
- Genital trauma
- Fixed drug eruption
- Ulcerative genital carcinoma (e.g., squamous cell carcinoma)
- Chancroid: Jagged border, yellow exudate, painful
- Lymphogranuloma venereum: Transient, indurated, painless
- Primary EBV infection
- Behçet disease

Secondary syphilis
- Cutaneous: Pityriasis rosea, guttate psoriasis, viral exanthems, lichen planus, pityriasis lichenoides chronica, primary HIV infection, drug eruption, nummular eczema, folliculitis
- Mucous membranes: Lichen planus; chronic aphthae; hand, foot and mouth disease; herpangina; perlèche
- Condylomata lata: Warts due to HPV, bowenoid papulosis, squamous cell carcinoma

Tertiary syphilis
- Cutaneous: Lupus vulgaris, chromoblastomycosis, dimorphic fungal infections, leishmaniasis, lupus erythematosus, mycosis fungoides, sarcoidosis, tumors, venous ulcer

From Bolognia J: *Dermatology,* ed 4, Philadelphia, 2018, Elsevier.

Dx DIAGNOSIS

DIFFERENTIAL DIAGNOSIS

- Other genitoulcerative diseases such as herpes, chancroid (see Tables 5 and 6)
- See Section III for a clinical algorithm for the evaluation of genital ulcer disease

WORKUP

Confirmation is primarily through laboratory diagnosis.
- Culture of lesions
- Serologic testing (see the following lab tests)
- Cerebrospinal fluid (CSF) testing

LABORATORY TESTS

- Dark-field microscopy of fluid from lesion to look for treponeme is the definitive method for diagnosis of early syphilis.
- Serologic testing:
  1. Nontreponemal tests: Venereal disease research laboratory (VDRL) or rapid plasma reagin (RPR).
  2. Treponemal tests: Fluorescent treponemal antibody absorbed (FTA-ABS) tests, the *T. pallidum* passive particle agglutination (TP-PA) assay, various enzyme immunoassays (EIAs), chemiluminescence immunoassays, immunoblots, or rapid treponemal assays.
  3. Limitations of nontreponemal and treponemal tests are summarized in Table E7.

4. Antibody titers can assess for response to treatment and for reinfection in previously treated patients.

- Screening methods:
  1. Traditional: Screen with nontreponemal tests; confirmation with treponemal testing.
  2. Alternative: Screen with treponemal testing, confirm with nontreponemal testing. More false positives, less likely to miss early or latent syphilis.
- When the nontreponemal test is negative despite a positive screen, an additional treponemal screen may be helpful. Trials have shown that two positive treponemal screens help identify a population with likely prior or current syphilis, and treatment of these patients may be justifiable.
- In patients with neurosyphilis, serologic criteria for response to therapy is a fourfold or greater decrease in VDRL titer over 6 to 12 mo.
- Lumbar puncture (LP) for cerebrospinal fluid VDRL (CSF-VDRL) in patients with evidence of latent syphilis (good specificity, poor sensitivity). If negative with high suspicion, can also perform a CSF FTA-ABS (good sensitivity, less specificity). When reactive in the absence of substantial contamination of CSF with blood, it is considered diagnostic of neurosyphilis. The Centers for Disease Control and Prevention indications for LP are neurologic symptoms, treatment failure, any eye or ear involvement, or evidence of active syphilis (aortitis, gumma, iritis).
- HIV testing in all patients.

Rx TREATMENT

ACUTE GENERAL Rx

- Primary, secondary, early latent:
  1. Penicillin G benzathine 2.4 million U IM once.
  2. Infants and children: Benzathine penicillin G 50,000 units/kg IM, up to the adult dose of 2.4 million units in a single dose.
  3. Nonpregnant penicillin-allergic patients: Doxycycline 100 mg bid × 14 days.
  4. Alternative regimens (contraindicated in MSM, persons with HIV, or pregnant women):
     a. Azithromycin 2 g PO × 1 dose
     b. Ceftriaxone 1 to 2 g IM or IV for 10 to 14 days
     c. Tetracycline 500 mg PO QID for 14 days
     d. Amoxicillin 3 g PO BID + probenecid 500 mg PO BID for 14 days
  5. Careful clinical and serologic follow-up of persons receiving any alternative therapy is essential.
  6. Persons with a penicillin allergy whose compliance with therapy or follow-up cannot be ensured should be desensitized and treated with benzathine penicillin.
- Late latent syphilis, tertiary syphilis (not neurosyphilis):
  1. Penicillin G benzathine 2.4 million U IM qwk × 3 wk.
  2. Infants and children: Benzathine penicillin G 50,000 units/kg IM, up to the adult dose of 2.4 million units in a single dose.
  3. Nonpregnant penicillin-allergic patients: Doxycycline 100 mg PO BID × 4 wk.
- Neurosyphilis:
  1. Aqueous crystalline penicillin G 18 to 24 million U/day, administered as 3 to 4 million U IV q4h or continuous infusion for 10 to 14 days.
  2. Alternative regimen: Procaine penicillin 2.4 million U IM/day plus probenecid 500 mg PO qid, both for 10 to 14 days.
- Congenital syphilis:
  1. Aqueous crystalline penicillin G 50,000 U/kg/dose IV q12h × first 7 days of life and q8h after that for a total of 10 days OR procaine penicillin G 50,000 U/kg/dose IM/day × 10 days.
  2. An algorithm for evaluation and treatment of infants born to mothers with reactive serologic tests for syphilis is illustrated in Fig. E5.

DISPOSITION

- Repeat quantitative nontreponemal tests at 6 and 12 mo to ensure adequate treatment. For HIV-infected patients, repeat testing at 3, 6, 9, 12, and 24 mo. Pregnancy requires monthly tests until delivery.
- Findings indicating need for retreatment of syphilis and additional testing for HIV:
  1. If a fourfold increase in titer occurs and is sustained over testing performed >2 wk apart
  2. If initial high titer fails to drop by fourfold within a yr for early syphilis or 24 mo for late syphilis
  3. If signs persist, or patient develops new signs of infection
- Because treatment failure may be the result of unrecognized CNS infection, CSF examination can be considered in such situations. For retreatment, weekly infusions of benzathine penicillin G 2.4 million units IM for 3 wk is recommended, unless CSF examination indicates that neurosyphilis is present.
- Pregnant women without a fourfold drop in titer by 6 mo compared to pretreatment titer need to be retreated. Inadequate treatment is likely if patient delivers fewer than 30 days after treatment, or if titers are fourfold higher than pre-treatment at delivery. Titers should be repeated monthly during pregnancy for those infected.
- Cases should be reported to local or state health department for referral, follow-up, and partner notification.

REFERRAL

- Pregnant and possible congenital syphilis
- Pregnant and allergic to penicillin, who need to be desensitized for treatment
- Late latent syphilis with serious central nervous system, cardiovascular, or other organ system compromise

PEARLS & CONSIDERATIONS

- Jarisch-Herxheimer reaction (fever, myalgia, tachycardia, hypotension) may occur within 24 hr of treatment.
- Fig. E6 illustrates the course of untreated syphilis. One third of untreated patients develop CNS and/or cardiovascular sequelae.
- Up to 80% of those treated during late stages remain seropositive indefinitely.
- Treponemal tests remain positive even after adequate therapy.
- Male circumcision does not decrease the incidence of syphilis (unlike HIV, HSV-2, and HPV infection).
- Partner notification and treatment:
  1. Persons who are exposed within 90 days preceding the diagnosis of primary, secondary, or early latent syphilis in a sex partner might be infected even if seronegative; therefore, such persons should be treated presumptively.
  2. Persons who were exposed ≥90 days before the diagnosis of syphilis in a sex partner should be treated presumptively if serologic test results are not available immediately and the opportunity for follow-up is uncertain.

SUGGESTED READINGS

Available at ExpertConsult.com

RELATED CONTENT

Syphilis (Patient Information)
Tabes Dorsalis (Related Key Topic)

AUTHORS: **Anthony Sciscione, DO,** and **Ashwini U. Dhokte, MD**

BASIC INFORMATION

DEFINITION

Systemic lupus erythematosus (SLE) is a chronic inflammatory disorder characterized by autoantibody production responsible for antibody-mediated and immune complex deposition tissue damage. SLE involves multiple organs and systems and has heterogeneous disease patterns. Relapses and remissions are a common feature.

SYNONYMS

SLE
Lupus

ICD-10CM CODES	
M32	Systemic lupus erythematosus
M32.0	Drug-induced systemic lupus erythematosus
M32.8	Other forms of systemic lupus erythematosus
M32.9	Systemic lupus erythematosus, unspecified
M32.10	Systemic lupus erythematosus, organ or system involvement unspecified
M32.11	Endocarditis in systemic lupus erythematosus
M32.12	Pericarditis in systemic lupus erythematosus
M32.13	Lung involvement in systemic lupus erythematosus
M32.14	Glomerular disease in systemic lupus erythematosus
M32.15	Tubulo-interstitial nephropathy in systemic lupus erythematosus
M32.19	Other organ or system involvement in systemic lupus erythematosus

EPIDEMIOLOGY & DEMOGRAPHICS

INCIDENCE: Varies across gender, race/ethnic groups, and geography from 20 to 70 cases per 100,000 persons. Prevalence higher among African Americans, Asian Americans, and Hispanics. There are an estimated 350,000 people with SLE in the U.S.

PREDOMINANT SEX: Female:male ratio is 9:1. The ratio is highest in reproductive age group, and about half of that in patients younger than 16 and older than 55.

PREDOMINANT AGE: Mean age at diagnosis is 31.

PHYSICAL FINDINGS & CLINICAL PRESENTATION

- Constitutional: Unexplained fever, fatigue (80%-100% patients), malaise (Table 1)
- Mucocutaneous lesions (more than 80% of patients): Acute (associated with + Ro antibody): Malar rash (Fig. E1) sparing nasolabial folds (acute cutaneous lupus); annular or papulosquamous rash (subacute cutaneous lupus); Chronic: Raised erythematous patches with subsequent edematous plaques and adherent scales (discoid cutaneous lupus), lupus profundus, lupus tumidus; alopecia, photosensitivity, nasal, or oropharyngeal ulcerations (classically painless, but discoid lesions [Fig. E2] may be painful); Raynaud phenomenon; leukocytoclastic vasculitis, chilblains; livedo reticularis or livedo racemosa (secondary to antiphospholipid antibody syndrome); skin biopsy hallmark: Interface dermatitis
- Musculoskeletal (about 90% of lupus patients): Arthralgias are more common than true arthritis, but nonerosive deforming arthritis is not rare; myositis
- Cardiac: Pericardial rub (pericarditis) is most common; valvular heart disease: Valve nodules and thickening (Libman-Sacks endocarditis); congestive heart failure, myocarditis, premature atherosclerotic heart disease
- Pulmonary: Pleuritis (most common), acute or chronic pneumonitis, diffuse alveolar hemorrhage, pulmonary hypertension
- Gastrointestinal: Dysphagia, mesenteric vasculitis, peritonitis, pancreatitis, hepatitis
- Neuropsychiatric: Headache, psychosis, seizure, acute confusional states, peripheral or cranial neuropathy, transverse myelitis, stroke (may be associated with antiphospholipid syndrome), cognitive dysfunction
- Hematologic (about 50% of lupus patients): Anemia (hemolytic, anemia of chronic disease, aplastic anemia), thrombocytopenia, leukopenia, lymphadenopathy, secondary antiphospholipid antibody syndrome
- Renal: Acute renal failure, proteinuria, nephritic syndrome, nephrotic syndrome

ETIOLOGY

Lupus may develop in genetically susceptible individuals, triggered by endogenous and exogenous factors. SLE susceptibility involves MHC class II polymorphism with commonly observed association with *HLA-DR-2, DR3, DR4,* and *DR8.* SLE is also associated with inherited deficiencies of C1q, C2, C4a, others. There is predilection for familial clustering of SLE with risk in monozygotic twins—about 25% to 50%—and 5% in dizygotic twins. Environmental factors such as UV light, Epstein-Barr virus infection, and tobacco smoking may have a triggering role. Autoantibody production is the hallmark of disease development and diagnosis of SLE. Evidence supports the improper processing of nuclear proteins and nucleic acid from cell death. Impairments in neutrophil cell death via a process termed NET-osis (nuclear extracellular trap) contribute to the accumulation of nuclear debris. This, in turn, can lead to the presentation of self-nuclear material to plasmacytoid dendritic cells. Plasmacytoid dendritic cells propagate antibody and immune complex production via a type I interferon-dependent mechanism.

DIAGNOSIS

DIFFERENTIAL DIAGNOSIS

- Rheumatoid arthritis, mixed connective tissue disease, systemic vasculitis
- Neoplastic disorder
- Hematologic malignancy, paraneoplastic syndrome
- Systemic infection
- Other: Thrombotic thrombocytopenic purpura/hemolytic uremic syndrome, primary antiphospholipid antibody syndrome

EVALUATION

The diagnosis of SLE is clinical. The 2019 European League Against Rheumatism/American College of Rheumatology (ACR) classification criteria for SLE include positive antinuclear antibody (ANA) at least once as obligatory entry criterion, followed by additive weighted criteria grouped in 7 clinical (constitutional, hematologic, neuropsychiatric, mucocutaneous, serosal, musculoskeletal, renal) and 3 immunologic (antiphospholipid antibodies, complement proteins, SLE-specific antibodies) domains, and weighted from 2 to 10. Patients accumulating ≥10 points are classified as having

TABLE 1 Potential Clinical Manifestations of Systemic Lupus Erythematosus

Target Organ	Potential Clinical Manifestations
Constitutional	Fatigue, anorexia, weight loss, fever, lymphadenopathy
Musculoskeletal	Arthritis, myositis, arthralgias, myalgias, avascular necrosis, osteoporosis
Skin	Malar rash, discoid rash, photosensitive rash, cutaneous vasculitis, livedo reticularis, periungual capillary abnormalities, Raynaud phenomenon, alopecia, oral and nasal ulcers
Renal	Hypertension, proteinuria, hematuria, edema, nephrotic syndrome, renal failure
Cardiovascular	Pericarditis, myocarditis, conduction system abnormalities, Libman-Sacks endocarditis
Neurologic	Seizures, psychosis, cerebritis, stroke, transverse myelitis, depression, cognitive impairment, headaches, pseudotumor, peripheral neuropathy, chorea, optic neuritis, cranial nerve palsies
Pulmonary	Pleuritis, interstitial lung disease, pulmonary hemorrhage, pulmonary hypertension, pulmonary embolism
Hematologic	Immune-mediated cytopenias (hemolytic anemia, thrombocytopenia or leukopenia), anemia of chronic inflammation, hypercoagulability, thrombocytopenic thrombotic microangiopathy
Gastroenterology	Hepatosplenomegaly, pancreatitis, vasculitis affecting bowel, protein-losing enteropathy
Ocular	Retinal vasculitis, scleritis, episcleritis, papilledema

systemic lupus. The new criteria had a sensitivity of 96.1% and specificity of 93.4%, compared with 82.8% sensitivity and 93.4% specificity of the ACR 1997 (see below) and 96.7% sensitivity and 83.7% specificity of the Systemic Lupus International Collaborating Clinics 2012 criteria.

1997 ACR Criteria:
- Malar rash
- Discoid rash
- Photosensitivity (recurrence of unusual skin rash in sun-exposed areas)
- Oral or nasopharyngeal painless ulceration, observed by physician
- Arthritis (nonerosive)
- Serositis (pleuritis, pericarditis)
- Renal disorder (persistent proteinuria >0.5 g/day, or ≥3+ on dipstick if quantification not performed; cellular casts)
- Neurologic disorder (seizures, psychosis [in absence of offending drugs or metabolic derangement])
- Hematologic disorder:
  1. Hemolytic anemia with reticulocytosis
  2. Leukopenia (<4000/mm^3 total on two or more occasions)
  3. Lymphopenia (<1500/mm^3 on two or more occasions)
  4. Thrombocytopenia (<100,000/mm^3 in the absence of offending drugs)
- Immunologic disorder:
  1. Anti–double-stranded DNA antibody (anti-dsDNA)
  2. Anti-Smith antibody (anti-Sm)
  3. Antiphospholipid antibodies (anticardiolipin IgM or IgG, lupus anticoagulant, anti-beta-2 glycoprotein IgM or IgG, or false-positive fluorescent treponemal antibody absorption test or *Treponema pallidum* immobilization for 6 mo)
- ANA: An abnormal titer of ANA by immunofluorescence or equivalent assay at any time in the absence of drugs known to be associated with drug-induced lupus syndrome

2012 SLICC Criteria: SLE can be diagnosed if:
- Biopsy-proven nephritis with either ANA or anti-dsDNA antibodies *or*
- Patient satisfies four clinical criteria, requiring at least one clinical and at least one immunologic criterion
- Clinical criteria:
  1. Acute cutaneous lupus (malar rash, bullous lupus, toxic epidermal necrolysis, photosensitive lupus rash, maculopapular lupus, subacute cutaneous lupus)
  2. Chronic cutaneous lupus (discoid, hypertrophic verrucous, panniculitis, mucosal lupus, lupus tumidus, chilblains lupus, lichen planus)
  3. Oral ulcers or nasal ulcers
  4. Nonscarring alopecia
  5. Synovitis (more than two joints or inflammatory arthralgias of more than two joints)
  6. Serositis (pleurisy for more than 1 day, pericardial pain for more than 1 day)
  7. Renal (>500 mg proteinuria/24 hr) or RBC casts)
  8. Neurologic (seizures, psychosis, mononeuritis multiplex, myelitis, peripheral or cranial neuropathy, acute confusional state)
  9. Hemolytic anemia
  10. Lymphopenia (<1000/mm^3 at least once)
  11. Thrombocytopenia (<100,000/mm^3 at least once)
- Immunologic criteria:
  1. ANA
  2. Anti-dsDNA (>2× laboratory reference range)
  3. Anti-Smith
  4. Antiphospholipid antibodies (lupus anticoagulant, RPR, anti-cardiolipin IgA, IgG, IgM, anti-β2 glycoprotein IgA, IgG, IgM)
  5. Low complement
  6. Direct Coombs test in the absence of hemolytic anemia

Definitions of SLE classification criteria are included in Table 2.

LABORATORY TESTS

Suggested initial laboratory evaluation of suspected SLE:
- ANA by immunofluorescence or similar high-quality method
  1. Complete blood count with differential, blood urea nitrogen and serum creatinine, urinalysis, ESR, PTT, complements (C3, C4)

TABLE 2 Definitions of SLE Classification Criteria 2019

Criteria	Definition
Antinuclear antibodies (ANA)	ANA at a titer of ≥1:80 on HEp-2 cells or an equivalent positive test at least once. Testing by immunofluorescence on HEp-2 cells or a solid-phase ANA screening immunoassay with at least equivalent performance is highly recommended.
Fever	Temperature >38.3° C (100.9° F)
Leukopenia	White blood cell count <4000/mm^3
Thrombocytopenia	Platelet count <100,000/mm^3
Autoimmune hemolysis	Evidence of hemolysis, such as reticulocytosis, low haptoglobin, elevated indirect bilirubin, elevated LDH, *AND* positive Coombs (direct antiglobulin) test
Delirium	Characterized by 1) change in consciousness or level of arousal with reduced ability to focus, 2) symptom development over hours to <2 days, 3) symptom fluctuation throughout the day, 4) either 4a) acute/subacute change in cognition (e.g., memory deficit or disorientation), or 4b) change in behavior, mood, or affect (e.g., restlessness, reversal of sleep/wake cycle)
Psychosis	Characterized by 1) delusions and/or hallucinations without insight and 2) absence of delirium
Seizure	Primary generalized seizure or partial/focal seizure
Non-scarring alopecia	Non-scarring alopecia observed by a clinician†
Oral ulcers	Oral ulcers observed by a clinician†
Subacute cutaneous OR discoid lupus	Subacute cutaneous lupus erythematosus observed by a clinician:† Annular or papulosquamous (psoriasiform) cutaneous eruption, usually photodistributed If skin biopsy is performed, typical changes must be present (interface vacuolar dermatitis consisting of a perivascular lymphohistiocytic infiltrate, often with dermal mucin noted). OR Discoid lupus erythematosus observed by a clinician:† Erythematous-violaceous cutaneous lesions with secondary changes of atrophic scarring, dyspigmentation, often follicular hyperkeratosis/plugging (scalp), leading to scarring alopecia on the scalp If skin biopsy is performed, typical changes must be present (interface vacuolar dermatitis consisting of a perivascular and/or periappendageal lymphohistiocytic infiltrate. In the scalp, follicular keratin plugs may be seen. In longstanding lesions, mucin deposition may be noted.)
Acute cutaneous lupus	Malar rash or generalized maculopapular rash observed by a clinician† If skin biopsy is performed, typical changes must be present (interface vacuolar dermatitis consisting of a perivascular lymphohistiocytic infiltrate, often with dermal mucin noted. Perivascular neutrophilic infiltrate may be present early in the course).
Pleural or pericardial effusion	Imaging evidence (such as ultrasound, x-ray, CT scan, MRI) of pleural or pericardial effusion, or both
Acute pericarditis	≥2 of 1) pericardial chest pain (typically sharp, worse with inspiration, improved by leaning forward), 2) pericardial rub, 3) EKG with new widespread ST elevation or PR depression, 4) new or worsened pericardial effusion on imaging (such as ultrasound, x-ray, CT scan, MRI)

TABLE 2 Definitions of SLE Classification Criteria 2019—cont'd

Criteria	Definition
Joint involvement	Either 1) synovitis involving two or more joints characterized by swelling or effusion, or 2) tenderness in two or more joints and at least 30 min of morning stiffness
Proteinuria >0.5 g/24 hr	Proteinuria >0.5 g/24 hr by 24-hr urine or equivalent spot urine protein-to-creatinine ratio
Class II or V lupus nephritis on renal biopsy according to ISN/RPS 2003 classification	Class II: Mesangial proliferative lupus nephritis: Purely mesangial hypercellularity of any degree or mesangial matrix expansion by light microscopy, with mesangial immune deposit. A few isolated subepithelial or subendothelial deposits may be visible by immunofluorescence or electron microscopy, but not by light microscopy. Class V: Membranous lupus nephritis: Global or segmental subepithelial immune deposits or their morphologic sequelae by light microscopy and by immunofluorescence or electron microscopy, with or without mesangial alterations
Class III or IV lupus nephritis on renal biopsy according to ISN/RPS 2003 classification	Class III: Focal lupus nephritis: Active or inactive focal, segmental, or global endocapillary or extracapillary glomerulonephritis involving <50% of all glomeruli, typically with focal subendothelial immune deposits, with or without mesangial alterations Class IV: Diffuse lupus nephritis: Active or inactive diffuse, segmental, or global endocapillary or extracapillary glomerulonephritis involving ≥50% of all glomeruli, typically with diffuse subendothelial immune deposits, with or without mesangial alterations. This class includes cases with diffuse wire loop deposits but with little or no glomerular proliferation.
Positive antiphospholipid antibodies	Anticardiolipin antibodies (IgA, IgG, or IgM) at medium or high titer (>40 APL, GPL, or MPL, or >the 99th percentile) or positive anti-β_2GPI antibodies (IgA, IgG, or IgM) or positive lupus anticoagulant
Low C3 OR low C4	C3 OR C4 below the lower limit of normal
Low C3 AND low C4	Both C3 AND C4 below their lower limits of normal
Anti-dsDNA antibodies OR anti-Sm antibodies	Anti-dsDNA antibodies in an immunoassay with demonstrated ≥90% specificity for SLE against relevant disease controls OR anti-Sm antibodies

anti-β_2GPI, Anti–β_2-glycoprotein I; *anti-dsDNA*, anti-double-stranded DNA; *CT*, computed tomography; *EKG*, electrocardiography; *ISN*, International Society of Nephrology; *LDH*, lactate dehydrogenase; *MRI*, magnetic resonance imaging; *RPS*, Renal Pathology Society; *SLE*, systemic lupus erythematosus.
†This may include physical examination or review of a photograph.

TABLE 3 Autoantibodies and Clinical Significance in Systemic Lupus Erythematosus (SLE)

Autoantibody	Prevalence in SLE	Clinical Significance
Antinuclear Antibody		
Anti-dsDNA	60%	95% specificity for SLE; fluctuates with disease activity; associated with glomerulonephritis
Anti-Smith	20%-30%	99% specificity for SLE; associated with anti-U1RNP antibodies
Anti-U1RNP	30%	Antibody associated with mixed connective tissue disease and lower frequency of glomerulonephritis
Anti-Ro/SSA	30%	Associated with Sjögren syndrome, photosensitivity, SCLE, neonatal lupus, congenital heart block
Anti-La/SSB	20%	Associated with Sjögren syndrome, SCLE, neonatal lupus, congenital heart block, anti-Ro/SSA
Antihistone	70%	Also associated with drug-induced lupus
Antiphospholipid	30%	Associated with arterial and venous thrombosis, pregnancy morbidity

Anti-dsDNA, Anti-double-stranded deoxyribonucleic acid; *SSA*, anti-Sjögren-syndrome-related antigen A; *SSB*, anti-Sjögren-syndrome-related antigen B; *SCLE*, subacute cutaneous lupus erythematosus.
From Firestein GS et al: *Kelley's textbook of rheumatology*, ed 9, Philadelphia, 2013, Saunders.

Consider additional laboratory testing in a patient with strong suspicion for systemic lupus:

- Anti-dsDNA, anti-Smith, anti-SSA, anti-SSB, anti-RNP antibodies. Table 3 summarizes autoantibodies and clinical significance in SLE
- Lupus anticoagulant, RPR, anticardiolipin antibodies, anti-beta-2 glycoprotein antibodies especially in patients with thrombotic events or recurrent miscarriages
- Urinalysis for RBC, cellular casts
- Random spot urine protein: Urine creatinine ratio, 24-hr urine protein collection if proteinuria; >0.5 or >500 mg/24 hr is abnormal, respectively. Evaluation of renal biopsy specimens in lupus nephritis is summarized in Table E4.
- Direct Coombs test

IMAGING STUDIES

- Chest x-ray for evaluation of pulmonary involvement (pleural effusion, infiltrates)
- Electrocardiogram for chest pain
- Echocardiogram if murmur, evidence of new or unexplained congestive heart failure, or suspected pericarditis

Rx TREATMENT

NONPHARMACOLOGIC THERAPY

- Avoidance of sunlight and use of high-SPF sunscreen (>35).
- Screening and counseling for modifiable cardiovascular risk factors such as cigarette smoking, diet, exercise, cholesterol, and uncontrolled HTN.
- Counseling for pregnancy planning for patients of childbearing age.
- Calcium and vitamin D supplementation for prevention of early osteoporosis (see "Clinical Pearls").

GENERAL Rx

- There are only four FDA-approved SLE medications: Aspirin, steroids, hydroxychloroquine (1955), and belimumab (2011).
- Treatment should be targeted toward the involved organ(s).
- Limited and defined courses of corticosteroids are useful for a variety of SLE symptoms. Steroid therapy should be restricted to acute or subacute control of symptoms, due to the increased cardiovascular risk and increased organ damage associated with chronic steroid use.
- Consider checking G6PD in certain ethnic groups more predisposed to antimalarial-induced hemolytic anemia.
- Hydroxychloroquine has best evidence for reducing flares, organ damage, lipids, thrombosis; improving survival; augmenting action of mycophenolate mofetil (MMF) in lupus nephritis; and preventing seizures. Currently recommend not to exceed dose of 5 mg/kg/day to decrease risk of retinal toxicity.
- Methotrexate and azathioprine are used as steroid-sparing agents. Indications include cutaneous and joint involvement.
- Joint pain and mild serositis are generally well controlled with NSAIDs or low-dose corticosteroids. Hydroxychloroquine and methotrexate are also effective for arthritis. Belimumab does well for joint and cutaneous manifestations. Leflunomide and rituximab

TABLE 5 Treatment Approach for Musculoskeletal Features of Systemic Lupus Erythematosus

	First-Line Therapy	Second-Line Therapy	Third-Line Therapy	Experimental Therapy
Arthritis	HCQ or CQ Low doses of glucocorticoids	MTX Leflunomide	Belimumab RTX Anti-TNF	Abatacept Sifalimumab
AVN	Avoid high doses of corticosteroid	Antiaggregation in aPL positivity	Core decompression Percutaneous drilling Arthroplasty	
Myositis	High-dose corticosteroid	MTX Azathioprine	IVIG RTX	

aPL, Antiphospholipid; *AVN,* avascular necrosis; *CQ,* chloroquine; *HCQ,* hydroxychloroquine; *IVIG,* intravenous immunoglobulin; *MTX,* methotrexate; *RTX,* rituximab; *TNF,* tumor necrosis factor.
From Hochberg MC: *Rheumatology,* ed 7, Philadelphia, 2019, Elsevier.

may be considered for refractory arthritis. Treatment approach for musculoskeletal features of SLE is summarized in Table 5.

- Cutaneous manifestations:
  1. Topical or intradermal corticosteroids are helpful for individual discoid lesions, especially in the scalp.
  2. Hydroxychloroquine alone or in combination with quinacrine and/or chloroquine can be considered for refractory skin disease.
  3. Refractory cases may be treated with belimumab, MMF, dapsone, or combination treatment.
  4. Table 6 summarizes general management of cutaneous lesions in SLE.
- Hematologic manifestations:
  1. Corticosteroids are first-line therapy. Table E7 summarizes the treatment and main hematologic features of SLE.
  2. Azathioprine can be used for thrombocytopenia or hemolytic anemia. Check for TPMT genetic mutation before the first use.
  3. Intravenous immunoglobulin (IVIG) or rituximab may be considered for severe leukopenia, autoimmune hemolytic anemia, or autoimmune thrombocytopenia.
- Central nervous system manifestations:
  1. Headaches are treated symptomatically. Most headaches will not be SLE-related and should be treated according to underlying cause.
  2. Anticonvulsants and antipsychotics may be indicated.
  3. Standard therapy for other neuropsychiatric SLE symptoms is not established.
- Renal disease: The histologic classification of lupus nephritis according to the International Society of Nephrology/Renal Pathology Society is summarized in Table E8. Severity of lupus nephritis is described in Table E9. Treatment recommendations for lupus nephritis are summarized in Table E10. (Class III, IV or IV/V with cellular crescents lupus nephritis; see Table E11). INDUCTION: 6-mo treatment
- The typical treatment induction period is 6 mo. The use of intravenous cyclophosphamide (CYC) with corticosteroids given at monthly intervals is more effective in preserving renal function than is treatment with glucocorticoids alone. Low-dose "Euro-Lupus" protocol may be equally efficacious and less toxic for certain populations (e.g., Caucasians, Blacks) than high-dose regimen. MMF is considered equivalent to CYC based on high-quality studies, with better tolerability and fertility profile. MMF may be preferred in African Americans and Hispanics. MMF and azathioprine are good options for maintenance treatment.
- There is interest in and positive data for use of calcineurin inhibitors, such as tacrolimus, for treatment of LN. Newer and possibly less toxic voclosporin has entered phase III trial and when added to MMF showed better results in renal responses compared with MMF alone.
- Severe nonrenal organ disease:
  1. Evidence from systematic randomized controlled trials for nonrenal lupus treatment is comparatively limited.
  2. High-dose intravenous CYC is used as induction treatment. Azathioprine or MMF may be used as maintenance.
  3. IVIG may be considered in severe disease especially when concomitant infection is present.
  4. Plasmapheresis or plasma exchange may be considered in critical situations: First-line therapy in Guillain-Barré syndrome, TTP, second line for SLE-related hemolytic anemia, cerebritis, and DAH. Infectious complications are common.
- Therapy targeting B cells:
  1. Rituximab: Anti-CD 20 monoclonal antibody. Randomized controlled trials for rituximab as an adjunct induction agent were negative in terms of both renal and nonrenal outcomes but were felt to be limited by study design. Some observational studies have shown efficacy in those who have failed other regimens.
  2. Epratuzumab: An anti-CD 22 agent. Studies initially showed positive data, but in July 2015 both phase III trials for SLE failed to meet their primary endpoint and this medication is no longer studied.
  3. Belimumab: Decreases activation of B cells. When used in addition to standard therapy, patients on belimumab showed improvement in cutaneous and musculoskeletal disease. Belimumab-treated patients had decreased SLE activity, a reduced time to disease flare, and lower glucocorticoid exposure. Safety data were good. Patients with central nervous system or serious kidney disease were excluded. There is interest in adding belimumab to standard lupus nephritis regimen, but data from BLISS-LN are not yet available.
  4. Abatacept: Downregulates T cell activation. Data is limited regarding improvement in arthritis, fatigue, sleep if added to routine therapy. Negative data as adjunct agent for lupus arthritis when added to MMF or CYC. Abatacept data provided evidence that low-dose cyclophosphomide may be as effective as high-dose cyclophosphomide in Blacks (ACCESS trial).
  5. Interferon therapy: Interferon α (INFα) has been linked to increased disease activity in SLE. INFα blocking therapies are in phase II clinical trials. Sifalimumab, a monoclonal antibody against INFα, reduced moderate to severe mucocutaneous involvement in SLE and decreased active joint count and fatigue scores in preliminary data analysis. Development of sifalimumab has been terminated in favor of anifrolumab, a similar INFα blocking agent. The TULIP-1 study of that molecule did not meet response criteria based on score used in BLISS trial. TULIP-2 used BICLA as response measure and showed statistically significant improvement compared to placebo. The phase III trial is ongoing.
  6. There is continuous interest in studying B cell- and interferon-based treatment, but no FDA approved treatment, other than above, is currently used clinically.
  7. Novel potential targeted treatment approaches may include blocking IL17, IL12/23, and JAK inhibitors (early data for 4-mg baricitinib showed positive results). Research remains very active and ongoing to find new therapeutic targets.
- Recommended assessment and monitoring of patients with SLE with nonrenal, non–central nervous system manifestations are summarized in Box 1.

TABLE 6 General Management of Cutaneous Lesions in Systemic Lupus Erythematosus

	Acute	SCLE	DLE
Nonpharmacologic Measures			
	Photoprotection Avoidance of photosensitizing drugs Smoking cessation	Photoprotection Avoidance of photosensitizing drugs Smoking cessation	Photoprotection Avoidance of photosensitizing drugs Smoking cessation
Topical Treatment			
	Topical calcineurin inhibitors	Topical glucocorticoids Topical calcineurin inhibitors Intralesional glucocorticoids	Topical corticosteroids Topical calcineurin inhibitors Intralesional glucocorticoids R-salbutamol
Systemic Treatment			
First line	Antimalarials Glucocorticoids	Antimalarials	Antimalarials Glucocorticoids
Second line		Systemic retinoids	MTX Systemic retinoids Antimalarial combination
Refractory Cases			
	According to systemic involvement RTX Belimumab	Thalidomide Leflunomide MMF IVIGs RTX Belimumab	Dapsone Thalidomide Belimumab RTX Lenalidomide
Therapies Under Investigation			
	Abatacept	Abatacept Sifalimumab Apremilast	Abatacept Sifalimumab Apremilast

DLE, Discoid lupus erythematosus; *IVIG,* intravenous immunoglobulin; *MMF,* mycophenolate mofetil; *MTX,* methotrexate; *RTX,* rituximab; *SCLE,* subacute cutaneous lupus erythematosus; *SLE,* systemic lupus erythematosus.
From Hochberg MC: *Rheumatology,* ed 7, Philadelphia, 2019, Elsevier.

DISPOSITION

- Most patients with SLE experience remissions and exacerbations.
- 5-yr survival rate has improved to more than 90% in patients with newly diagnosed SLE since the advent of potent immunosuppressive therapy. The 15-yr survival rate is now 85%.
- Early death related to SLE activity and infections; late death due to CVD.
- Lupus nephritis progression rate to ESRD in 10% to 30% within 15 yr.
- African Americans, Asian Americans, and Hispanic Americans in general have a worse prognosis. The leading cause of death in SLE patients in developed countries is premature atherosclerosis. The quality of life for many SLE patients is poor due to fatigue, chronic pain, and cognitive impairment.

REFERRAL

- Rheumatology consultation for all patients with SLE
- Hematology consultation for patients with significant hematologic abnormalities (e.g., severe hemolytic anemia or thrombocytopenia)
- Nephrology consultation in patients with proteinuria and/or suspected renal involvement
- Dermatology consultation for patients with unexplained or unusual skin rash
- Cardiology consultation for patients with lupus carditis, arrhythmias
- Ophthalmology referral for all patients on hydroxychloroquine and chloroquine

PEARLS & CONSIDERATIONS

- Arthritis in SLE often has no prolonged morning stiffness and is not erosive on x-rays; reversible joint deformities in lupus are termed Jaccoud arthropathy.
- Myocardial infarction is 50 times more common in young female patients than in age-matched control group.
- Prevent adverse effects of medications: Consider prophylaxis for infections and appropriate vaccinations, ensure yearly Pap and other cancer screening as clinically indicated; for patients taking CYC, intervention to preserve bladder and fertility should be considered; manage bone health.
- Based on small clinical data, a vitamin D level >40 may have modest reduction in disease activity; in addition, vitamin D may reduce risk of thrombosis, based on oncology research.

SUGGESTED READINGS

Available at ExpertConsult.com

RELATED CONTENT

Systemic Lupus Erythematosus (Patient Information)
Discoid Lupus (Related Key Topic)
Renal Lupus (Related Key Topic)

AUTHOR: **Katarzyna Gilek-Seibert, MD, RhMUS**

BOX 1 Recommended Assessment and Monitoring of Patients with Systemic Lupus Erythematosus with Nonrenal, Non–Central Nervous System Manifestations

Patient general assessment

In addition to the standard care of patients without lupus of the same age and sex, the assessment of patients with SLE must include the evaluation of:

- Disease activity by a validated index at each visit
- Organ damage annually
- General quality of life by patient history and/or by a 0-10 VAS (patient global score) at each visit
- Comorbidities
- Drug toxicity

Cardiovascular risk factors

At baseline and during follow-up at least once a year:

- Assess smoking, vascular events (cerebral and cardiovascular), physical activity, oral contraceptives, hormonal therapies, and family history of cardiovascular disease
- Perform blood tests: Blood cholesterol, glucose
- Examine for blood pressure and BMI (and/or waist circumference)
- NB: Some patients may need more frequent follow-up (e.g., those taking glucocorticoids).

Osteoporosis risk

All patients with SLE:

- Should be assessed for adequate calcium and vitamin D intake, regular exercise, and smoking habits
- Should be screened and followed for osteoporosis according to existing guidelines (1) for postmenopausal women and (2) for patients taking glucocorticoids or on any other medication that may reduce BMD

Cancer risk

Cancer screening is recommended according to the guidelines for the general population, including cervical smear tests.

Infection risk

Screening: Patients with SLE should be screened for:

- HIV based on the patient's risk factors
- HCV and HBV based on the patient's risk factors, particularly before IS drugs including high-dose glucocorticoids are given
- Tuberculosis, according to local guidelines, especially before IS drugs including high-dose glucocorticoids are given
- CMV testing should be considered during treatment in selected patients.

Vaccination: Patients with SLE are at high risk of infections, and prevention should be recommended. The administration of inactivated vaccines (especially flu and pneumococcus), following CDC guidelines for patients who are immunosuppressed, should be encouraged strongly in patients with SLE who take IS drugs, preferably administered when the SLE is inactive. For other vaccinations, an individual risk–benefit analysis is recommended.

Monitoring: At follow-up visits, continuous assessment of the risk of infection by taking into consideration the presence of:

- Severe neutropenia (<500 cells/mm^3)
- Severe lymphopenia (<500 cells/mm^3)
- Low IgG (<500 mg/dl)

Frequency of assessments

In patients with no activity, no damage, and no comorbidity, assessments are recommended every 6-12 mo. During these visits, preventive measures should be emphasized.

Laboratory assessment

It is recommended to monitor the following autoantibodies and complement:

- At baseline: ANA, anti-dsDNA, anti-Ro, anti-La, anti-RNP, anti-Sm, antiphospholipid, C3, C4
- Reevaluation of aPLs in previously negative patients before pregnancy, surgery, transplant, and use of estrogen-containing treatments or in the presence of a new neurologic or vascular event; anti-Ro and anti-La antibodies before pregnancy; anti-dsDNA/C3 C4 may support evidence of disease activity or remission

Other laboratory assessments. At 6- to 12-mo intervals, patients with inactive disease should have:

- CBC
- ESR
- CRP
- Serum albumin
- Serum creatinine (or eGFR)
- Urinalysis and urine protein-to-creatinine ratio

NB: If a patient is on a specific drug treatment, monitoring for that drug is required as well.

Mucocutaneous involvement

Mucocutaneous lesions should be characterized, according to existing classification systems, as to whether they may be:

- LE specific
- LE nonspecific
- LE mimickers
- Drug-related

Lesions should be assessed for activity and damage using validated indices (e.g., CLASI).

Eye assessment

In patients treated with glucocorticoids or antimalarials, a baseline eye examination is recommended according to standard guidelines. An eye examination during follow-up is recommended:

- In selected patients taking glucocorticoids (high risk of glaucoma or cataracts)
- In patients on antimalarial drugs. (Low risk: HCQ: No further testing is required until after 5 yr of baseline, and after the first 5 yr of treatment, eye assessment is recommended yearly; High risk: Eye assessment is recommended yearly, especially when using CQ.)

ANA, Antinuclear antibodies; *aPL,* antiphospholipid antibody; *BMD,* bone mineral density; *BMI,* body mass index; *CBC,* complete blood count; *CDC,* Centers for Disease Control and Prevention; *CLASI,* Cutaneous Lupus Erythematosus Disease Area and Severity Index; *CMV,* cytomegalovirus; *CQ,* chloroquine; *CRP,* C-reactive protein; *eGFR,* estimated glomerular filtration rate; *ESR,* erythrocyte sedimentation rate; *HBV,* hepatitis B virus; *HCQ,* hydroxychloroquine; *HCV,* hepatitis C virus; *IgG,* immunoglobulin G; *IS,* immunosuppressors; *LE,* lupus erythematosus; *NB,* nota bene; *SLE,* systemic lupus erythematosus; *VAS,* visual analog scale.

From Hochberg MC: *Rheumatology,* ed 7, Philadelphia, 2019, Elsevier.

BASIC INFORMATION

DEFINITION

Takotsubo cardiomyopathy, also known as stress cardiomyopathy (SC), is a syndrome characterized by transient systolic and diastolic dysfunction with a characteristic ballooning of the apical and/or mid segments of the left ventricle (LV). It mimics acute myocardial infarction (MI) but without evidence of obstruction of an epicardial coronary artery. Typically, but not always, it is preceded by severe illness or intense emotional, physical, or psychological stress. Initially described in the 1990s in Japan, the systolic LV on left angiogram has a distinctive shape similar to a *tako-tsubo* pot with a narrow neck and round bottom, used by fishermen to trap octopi. The variants of SC include apical (81.7%), midventricular (14.6%), basal/reverse takotsubo (2.2%), and focal (1.5%).

SYNONYMS

Stress cardiomyopathy (SC)
Left ventricular apical ballooning syndrome (LVABS)
Ampulla cardiomyopathy
Broken heart syndrome

ICD-10CM CODE

I51.81 Takotsubo syndrome

EPIDEMIOLOGY & DEMOGRAPHICS

INCIDENCE: An estimated 15 to 30 new cases per 100,000 per yr

PREVALENCE: About 1% to 2% of patients presenting with troponin-positive acute coronary syndrome (ACS) have SC.

PREDOMINANT SEX & AGE: On presentation, 90% are females, and 80% are females >50 yr of age. Mean age of presentation is 68.8 yr.

RISK FACTORS: SC can be triggered by physical stress (severe medical illness like acute respiratory failure, neurological conditions, malignancy, infection, postsurgery or physical trauma), or intense emotional psychosocial stress (death of loved ones, domestic abuse, fierce arguments, financial hardships, severe pain, natural disasters, etc.). A positive life event (happy heart syndrome) also can cause SC. Takotsubo cardiomyopathy associated with physical stress has a higher mortality rate than SC triggered by emotional stress. Familial case series have raised the possibility of a genetic predisposition.

PHYSICAL FINDINGS & CLINICAL PRESENTATION

- Acute substernal chest pain, dyspnea, and syncope are the most common presenting complaints (International Takotsubo Registry study).
- On physical examination, a systolic ejection murmur (due to left ventricular outflow tract obstruction and mitral regurgitation) may be present. The following could be present: S3 gallop, rales, jugular venous distension, hypotension, or narrow pulse pressure.
- SC can manifest as heart failure (30%), ventricular arrhythmias, cardiogenic shock (10%), or sudden cardiac death.

ETIOLOGY

The proposed mechanisms for SC include the following:

- In postmenopausal women, estrogen deficiency leads to endothelial vasomotor dysfunction. Lack of endothelial-dependent vasodilation causes excessive coronary vasoconstriction.
- Increased catecholamine from an acute event can be directly toxic to the myocardium. The increased density of beta-adrenoreceptors in the apex makes it more sensitive to catecholamine and accounts for the apical ballooning.
- Impaired microvascular perfusion resulting in ischemic stunning.
- Fig. 1 depicts the interplay among triggers, pathogenic factors, and predisposing factors in SC.

DIAGNOSIS

Mayo Clinic proposed criteria (2008) for diagnosis of SC: All four criteria are required to make diagnosis.

- Transient wall motion abnormalities that extend beyond a single epicardial vascular distribution (Fig. 2). A stressful trigger is often, but not always, present
- Absence of obstructive coronary disease or angiographic evidence of acute plaque rupture
- New ECG abnormalities (ST-segment elevation and/or T-wave inversion) or modest elevation in cardiac troponins
- Absence of pheochromocytoma or myocarditis

DIFFERENTIAL DIAGNOSIS

- Acute coronary syndrome
- Cardiac syndrome X/microvascular angina
- Prinzmetal angina
- Acute myocarditis
- Cocaine cardiomyopathy
- Cardiomyopathy associated with pheochromocytoma

WORKUP

- A high index of suspicion is required when a postmenopausal woman presents with ACS after intense stress.
- Cardiology consult should be immediately obtained.
- Obstructive coronary artery disease needs to be ruled out.

LABORATORY TESTS

- Cardiac biomarkers (troponin, CK-MB) are often modestly elevated.
- Cardiac natriuretic peptide (brain natriuretic peptide [BNP] and pro-BNP) levels are also commonly elevated.

IMAGING STUDIES

- ECG: ST elevation in precordial leads (reciprocal changes typically absent), T-wave inversions (which may be dramatic) in the anterior or lateral leads, QT prolongation, and abnormal Q waves.
- Echocardiography (ECHO) typically shows the characteristic apical ballooning. Contrast ECHO is quite useful to exclude apical thrombus.
- Obstructive coronary artery disease should be excluded with a coronary angiogram.
- Cardiac magnetic resonance imaging (Fig. 3) can show the absence of late gadolinium enhancement (seen in MI).
- Coronary computed tomography angiography may help evaluate for stenosis in epicardial coronary arteries in specific clinical settings (e.g., poor MRI acoustic windows).

COMPLICATIONS

- Approximately 20% have in-hospital complications including heart failure, cardiogenic shock requiring mechanical support, life-threatening arrhythmias, acute mitral regurgitation, LV outflow tract (LVOT) obstruction, free wall rupture, and death.
- Due to the Venturi effect, mitral valve systolic anterior motion could cause LVOT obstruction and mitral regurgitation (14% to 45% of patients).

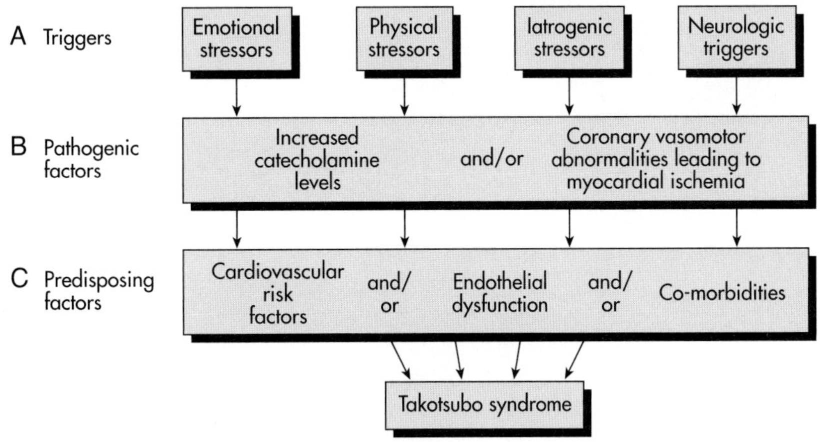

FIG. 1 The interplay among triggers, pathogenic factors, and predisposing factors in Takotsubo disease. (From Pelliccia F et al: Takotsubo syndrome [stress cardiomyopathy]: an intriguing clinical condition in search of its identity, *Am J Med* 127:699-704, 2014.)

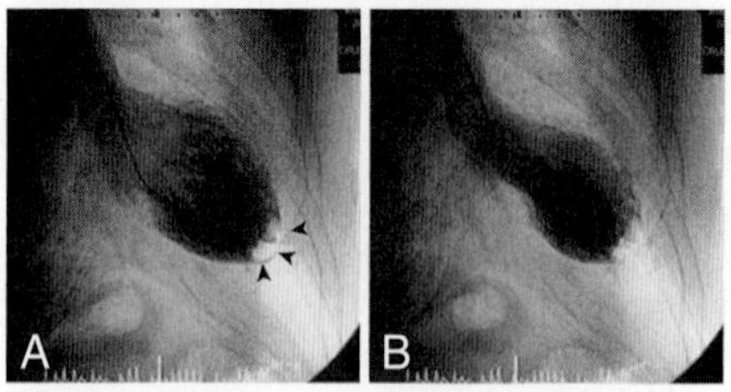

FIG. 2 A and **B,** Left ventriculogram showing apical ballooning characteristic of stress-induced cardiomyopathy. (From Mitsuma W et al: *JACC* 51[1]: cover, 2008.)

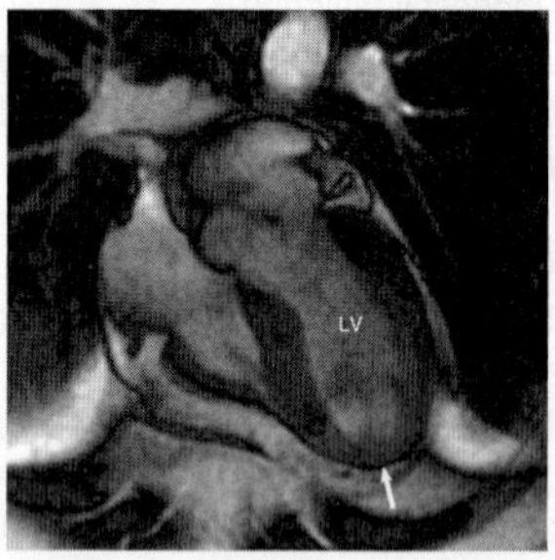

FIG. 3 Takotsubo cardiomyopathy. The patient was a 58-yr-old woman who was referred for cardiovascular magnetic resonance (CMR) after a coronary angiogram revealed no obstructive disease despite the presence of ST-segment elevations on electrocardiogram and positive biomarker assays. A diagnosis of Takotsubo cardiomyopathy was made on the basis of the CMR image, which shows LV apical akinesis and ballooning (*arrow*). *LV,* Left ventricle. (From Mann DL et al: *Braunwald's heart disease,* ed 10, Philadelphia, 2015, Elsevier.)

- Arrhythmias (25%) include supraventricular tachycardia and ventricular arrhythmias.
- Systemic thromboembolism and increased risk of stroke.
- Intramyocardial hemorrhage and rupture.

Rx TREATMENT

Initially, patients should be treated for presumptive acute coronary syndrome until this is excluded.

NONPHARMACOLOGIC THERAPY

Supportive care such as the elimination of the physical or emotional trigger is important.

ACUTE GENERAL Rx

- Hemodynamically stable: Treat with diuretics, vasodilators, and venodilators (nitroglycerin, nitroprusside).
- Cardiogenic shock *without* LVOT obstruction: Vasopressors and inotropes may be required. When treatment is refractory to medical therapy, percutaneous and surgical mechanical circulatory support will be required.

Cardiogenic shock *with* LVOT obstruction: Avoid inotropes as they can worsen outflow obstruction. Consider fluid resuscitation if no pulmonary congestion. Vasopressors can be used, but phenylephrine should be used cautiously because it could increase afterload and thus increase the LVOT gradient. Beta-blockers can improve the obstruction.

CHRONIC Rx

- Guideline-directed medical therapy for systolic heart failure (beta-blockers, ACE inhibitors, angiotensin II receptor blocker, aldosterone antagonist, angiotensin receptor-neprilysin inhibitor) until resolution of LV dysfunction. Consider long-term use if no contraindication and if tolerated.
- Repeat ECHO (in 4 to 6 wk) to ensure normalization of systolic function.
- 3 mo of anticoagulation is suggested if an intraventricular thrombus is detected.

DISPOSITION

- Carries a favorable prognosis compared to STEMI or NSTEMI; in-hospital mortality is up to 5%. The recurrence rate is around 2% to 4% per yr.
- In a Medicare cohort, patients ≥85 yr of age had higher in-hospital, 30-day, 1-yr mortality, and 30-day readmission rates; hence, the need for good discharge planning is key.
- In the International Takotsubo registry, a substantial number of SC patients show an association with malignancy. History of malignancy might increase the risk for TTS, and therefore, appropriate screening for malignancy should be considered in these patients.

REFERRAL

Follow up with a cardiologist

PEARLS & CONSIDERATIONS

COMMENTS

- The term *takotsubo* is the Japanese name for an octopus trap (*tako-tsubo*), which has a similar shape of the LV in systole during a left ventriculogram (see Fig. 2).
- Patients with takotsubo cardiomyopathy have a higher prevalence of neurologic or psychiatric disorders than those with an acute coronary syndrome.

PREVENTION

Minimizing stress may reduce incidence but no data to support this.

SUGGESTED READINGS

Available at ExpertConsult.com

AUTHORS: **Mostafa Ghanim, MD,** and **Maxwell Eyram Afari, MD**

BASIC INFORMATION

DEFINITION

Tardive dyskinesia (TD) is a neurological disorder of involuntary movements associated with the long-term use of antipsychotic medication, particularly first-generation antipsychotics. Patients exhibit rapid, repetitive, stereotypic movements that mostly involve the oral, lingual, trunk, and limb areas.

SYNONYMS

Orofacial dyskinesia
Tardive syndrome
TD

ICD-10CM CODE
G24.01 Drug induced subacute dyskinesia
DSM-5 CODE
335.85

EPIDEMIOLOGY & DEMOGRAPHICS

- The disorder is caused by dopamine-blocking antipsychotics (e.g., haloperidol) and antiemetics (e.g., metoclopramide, prochlorperazine, and promethazine).
- With first-generation antipsychotics, at least 20% of patients are affected with TD, and ~5% are expected to develop TD with each year of antipsychotic treatment.
- The incidence of TD with second-generation antipsychotics is reduced only by about one third. With the increasing use of these medications, TD remains a serious problem.
- Risk increases with the duration of antipsychotic treatment, in female and in elderly patients, in patients with brain damage or dementia, with concurrent anticholinergic use, and in patients with nonschizophrenia diagnoses.

PHYSICAL FINDINGS & CLINICAL PRESENTATION

- TD is classically described as a chronic condition of insidious onset, but symptoms are variable over time and may even improve despite continued antipsychotic therapy.
- The condition typically appears with the reduction or withdrawal of the antipsychotic medications.
- TD classically involves stereotypic movements of the mouth and tongue, including lip smacking and puckering, tongue twisting and protrusion, and facial grimacing.
- TD may also involve slow, writhing movements of the trunk or choreoathetoid movements of the fingers and toes.
- The involuntary mouth movements associated with TD may be suppressed by voluntary actions (e.g., putting food in the mouth, talking).
- Variants of TD with similar treatment include tardive dystonia (e.g., torticollis, blepharospasm), tardive myoclonus, tardive akathisia, and tardive tics.

ETIOLOGY

TD is caused by chronic exposure to dopamine receptor antagonists that is thought to result in the upregulation of dopamine receptors in the basal ganglia as well as damage to striatal cholinergic neurons. Dysfunction of striatal GABAergic interneurons has also been implicated. It has been proposed that dopamine receptor hypersensitivity and neurodegenerative changes might cause altered synaptic plasticity of excitatory synapses onto striatal interneurons, resulting in an imbalance between the direct and indirect basal ganglia pathways.

Dx DIAGNOSIS

DIFFERENTIAL DIAGNOSIS

- Acute extrapyramidal symptoms (e.g., short-term withdrawal dyskinesias, Parkinsonism, akathisia)
- Basal ganglia movement disorders (e.g., Huntington chorea, Tourette syndrome, levodopa-induced dyskinesia in Parkinson disease, Wilson disease)
- Autoimmune diseases (Sydenham chorea, multiple sclerosis)
- Other causes of neurologic damage (e.g., lead or mercury toxicity, HIV, neurosyphilis, head injury, neurodegeneration from illicit substances)
- Mannerisms associated with disorganized type or catatonic type schizophrenia or catatonic syndrome associated with mood disorder or medical illness
- Hyperthyroidism-induced choreoathetosis
- Edentulous dyskinesias and improperly fitted dentures
- Rabbit syndrome (a rare variant of extrapyramidal symptoms with rapid vertical orofacial movements without tongue involvement); may respond to anticholinergic agents

WORKUP

TD is a diagnosis of exclusion, with emphasis on a complete neuropsychiatric and medication history and a thorough physical examination. Abnormal Involuntary Movement Scale (AIMS) can be used to evaluate and monitor the severity of TD.

IMAGING STUDIES

Standard brain imaging is normal in patients with TD.

Rx TREATMENT

ACUTE GENERAL Rx

- Treatment is predicated on prevention: Limit the indications for antipsychotics; use the lowest effective dose; discontinue the drugs, when feasible; and monitor patients frequently. Anticholinergic medications may worsen symptoms.
- Switch to second-generation antipsychotics, if possible.

CHRONIC Rx

- If continued antipsychotic treatment is needed, switching to clozapine or quetiapine remains the preferred initial treatment if feasible, though evidence is insufficient.
- Valbenazine and deutetrabenazine, inhibitors of the vesicular monoamine transporter 2 (VMAT2), are centrally acting synaptic dopamine depleters that are the first FDA-approved treatments for TD and are recommended as first-line treatment options when discontinuation of antipsychotic not indicated. The older version, tetrabenazine, may also improve TD and might be considered.
- Clonazepam, botulinum toxin, amantadine, and ginkgo have limited evidence to improve TD.
- For treatment-resistant, disabling TD, deep brain stimulation of internal globus pallidus seems to provide significant symptom reduction without exacerbation of psychiatric symptoms.
- TD is potentially irreversible in nearly two thirds of patients; thus, patients undergoing long-term treatment with dopamine receptor blocking agents require frequent monitoring and aggressive management at the onset of TD symptoms.

REFERRAL

Movement disorder specialist consultation if symptoms are severe

PEARLS & CONSIDERATIONS

- After removal of the causative medication, symptoms of tardive dyskinesia can take months to resolve or may become permanent (higher risk in elderly, female sex, prolonged use, and higher dose of causative medication).
- First-generation antipsychotics should be resumed to treat TD in the absence of active psychosis only as a last resort for persistent, disabling, and treatment-resistant TD.
- Avoid anticholinergic medications (e.g., benztropine), which may exacerbate TD symptoms.
- Recent evidence suggests increased overall mortality among patients with TD, which highlights the need for referral for more aggressive specialized interventions.

SUGGESTED READINGS

Available at ExpertConsult.com

RELATED CONTENT

Tardive Dyskinesia (Patient Information)

AUTHORS: **Shreedhar Paudel, MD, MPH,** and **John A. Gray, MD, PhD**

BASIC INFORMATION

DEFINITION

Temporomandibular joint (TMJ) syndrome refers to a group of disorders leading to symptoms of the TMJ. Box 1 describes a classification of temporomandibular joint disorder (TMD), which also can be classified as intraarticular (within the joint) or extraarticular (involving the surrounding musculature). The TMJ is a diarthrotic joint, meaning neither joint can move independently of the other because each is hinged at both ends. The joint is a true synovial joint capable of two actions of movement: Translational and rotational. The articulating surfaces are the glenoid fossa of the temporal bone and the condylar process of the mandible, with the articular disk interposed between the two.

SYNONYMS

Temporomandibular dysfunction
Painful temporomandibular joint
TMJ
Temporomandibular disorders (TMD)

ICD-10CM CODE
N26.60 Temporomandibular joint disorder, unspecified

EPIDEMIOLOGY & DEMOGRAPHICS

- 15% to 25% of the population have symptoms of TMJ disorders at some point in their lives.
- Females are affected more often than males (up to 4:1 ratio).
- Occurs between the second and fourth decades of life.
- Usually unilateral, affecting either side with equal frequency.

PHYSICAL FINDINGS & CLINICAL PRESENTATION

- Symptoms may appear or be worse during stressful life events.
  1. Often unilateral pain in the muscles of mastication, usually described as a "dull" ache
  2. Otalgia
  3. Odontalgia
  4. Headaches (frontal, temporal, retroorbital)
  5. Tinnitus
  6. Dizziness
  7. Clicking or popping sounds with movement of the TMJ
  8. Joint locking
- Fig. E1 illustrates the clinical examination of the temporomandibular joint, range of mandibular motion, and muscle palpation.
- Physical exam findings:
  1. Tender to palpation over TMJ in external auditory meatus or preauricular region anterior to tragus
  2. Limited jaw opening or trismus
  3. Clicking or popping of TMJs with joint mobility
  4. Lateral deviation of mandible
  5. TMJ crepitus

ETIOLOGY:

- Myofascial pain-dysfunction syndrome: The most common cause of TMJ syndrome and results from teeth grinding and clenching the jaw (bruxism)
- Internal TMJ derangement: Abnormal connection of the articular disk to the mandibular condyle as a result of disk displacement or chronic dislocations
- Degenerative joint disease
- Rheumatoid arthritis
- Gouty arthritis
- Pseudogout
- Ankylosing spondylitis
- Trauma (i.e., fractures)
- Congenital defects (i.e., aplasia, hypoplasia)
- Prior surgery (orthodontic, intraarticular steroid injection)
- Tumors

Dx DIAGNOSIS

Can be made based on history and physical examination in most cases.

DIFFERENTIAL DIAGNOSIS

Includes the list provided earlier. Myofascial pain-dysfunction syndrome, internal TMJ derangement, and degenerative joint disease represent >90% of all causes of TMJ syndrome. Others not mentioned include dental problems such as dental caries, loss of posterior teeth support, and Eagle syndrome (stylohyoid syndrome, carotidynia, and trigeminal neuralgia). Alternative diagnoses such as otitis, mastoiditis, salivary gland disorders, migraine headache, sinusitis, postherpetic neuralgia, trigeminal neuralgia, glossopharyngeal neuralgia, and giant cell arteritis should always be excluded.

WORKUP

The diagnosis is based largely on history and physical examination findings. Radiographic imaging evaluation is used to exclude anatomic or systemic causes of disease when conservative management has failed.

LABORATORY TESTS

Laboratory examination is often not needed but may be helpful in ruling out certain conditions. CBC if infection is suspected. Rheumatoid factor if rheumatoid arthritis is suspected.

IMAGING STUDIES

- Plain radiographs: The most common views are the panoramic, transorbital, and transpharyngeal in both opened and closed positions.
- CT scan is highly accurate in diagnosing osseous derangements of the TMJ.
- MRI is the procedure of choice and has replaced arthrography in cases of disabling pain or if locking occurs. It is used to determine disk position and morphology along with degenerative bony changes.
- Arthrography is helpful in looking for meniscus involvement but is seldom performed anymore, as it is more invasive and less accurate than MRI for TMJ imaging.

Rx TREATMENT

NONPHARMACOLOGIC THERAPY

- Soft diet to rest the muscles of mastication
- Heat 15 to 20 min 4 to 6 times per day
- Massage of the masseter and temporalis muscles
- Formed splints or bite appliances to reduce compression of retrodiscal tissue (Fig. 2)
- Range-of-motion exercises
- Cognitive-behavioral therapy and biofeedback have been shown to reduce pain.
- Acupuncture

ACUTE GENERAL Rx

- NSAIDs: Ibuprofen 800 PO mg tid prn or naproxen 500 mg PO bid prn, titrated to relieve symptoms

BOX 1 Classification of Temporomandibular Joint Disorder

Myofascial pain disorder and dysfunction
Most common; primarily of muscular origin
Characterized by myogenous pain and limited mandibular function
May be associated with parafunctional habits, stress, anxiety, depression, or trauma

Temporomandibular joint internal displacement (disk displacement)
Reducing or nonreducing (closed lock) with joint sounds and deviation with opening
Most common is anteromedial displacement of the disk
Results in a mechanical interference, leading to moderate to severe restriction in range of motion

Systemic diseases (arthritides, e.g., rheumatoid arthritis, psoriatic arthritis, osteoarthritis)
Affect the joint through inflammation or degenerative processes
May result in condylar remodeling and degenerative joint disease
Also may be related to infectious processes triggering joint inflammation

Congenital and developmental diseases (including trauma and neoplasms)
Hemifacial microsomia or condylar hyperplasia
Idiopathic condylar resorption
Ankylosis
Tumors (e.g., osteochondroma)

From Hochberg MC: *Rheumatology,* ed 7, Philadelphia, 2019, Elsevier.

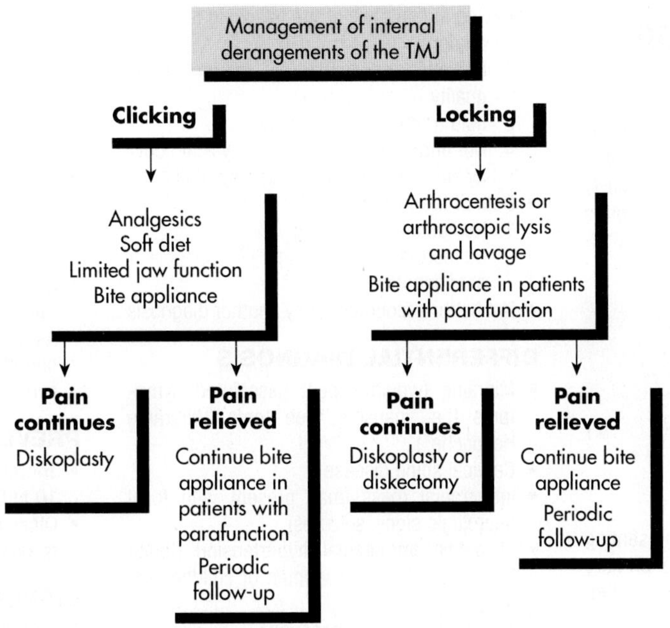

FIG. 2 Management of internal derangements of the temporomandibular joint *(TMJ).* Patients with painful clicking or locking are treated medically initially, whereas those with locking require surgical intervention. (From Firestein GS et al: *Kelley's textbook of rheumatology,* ed 9, Philadelphia, 2013, Saunders.)

- Muscle relaxants or benzodiazepines at bedtime: Diazepam 2.5 to 5 mg PO tid prn or amitriptyline 5 to 100 mg PO qd prn
- In degenerative joint disease of the TMJ, intraarticular steroid injection can be tried
- Botulism toxin injections into the masticatory muscles
- Arthrocentesis with joint lavage and lysis of adhesions (Fig. E3)
- In patients with pain and clicking in the TMJ that is unresponsive to nonsurgical treatment, the disc should be repositioned arthroscopically or by open surgery (discoplasty) (see "Chronic Rx")

CHRONIC Rx

- Most of the above treatments are used for myofascial pain-dysfunction syndrome; however, they can be applied to other causes of TMJ syndrome. Surgery is usually a measure of last resort in patients who do not respond to nonpharmacologic and acute general treatment. Absolute indications for surgical therapy include neoplasms, growth abnormalities, and joint ankylosis.
- Surgical procedures include:
  1. Meniscoplasty
  2. Meniscectomy
  3. Subcondylar osteotomy
  4. TMJ reconstruction

DISPOSITION

The course depends on the underlying etiology; however, less than 5% of adults with temporomandibular symptoms develop chronic symptoms.

REFERRAL

All patients with TMJ syndrome refractory to conservative nonpharmacologic and acute therapy should be referred to a periodontist, oral maxillofacial surgeon, or ear-nose-throat surgeon.

PEARLS & CONSIDERATIONS

Patients with rheumatoid arthritis involving the TMJ usually have bilateral involvement.

COMMENTS

Frequently, emotional stress initiates the myofascial pain-dysfunction, which accounts for 85% of all cases of TMJ syndrome.

RELATED CONTENT

Temporomandibular Joint (TMJ) Syndrome (Patient Information)

SUGGESTED READING

Available at ExpertConsult.com

AUTHOR: **Louis F. Insalaco, MD**

Tension-Type Headache (PTG)

BASIC INFORMATION

DEFINITION

Tension-type headache (TTH) is a highly prevalent primary headache disorder not associated with nausea or vomiting. Although previously thought to be caused by psychological factors and muscle contraction, current thinking implicates neurobiological mechanisms.

ICD-10CM CODES

G44.201	Tension-type headache, unspecified, intractable
G44.209	Tension-type headache, unspecified, not intractable

EPIDEMIOLOGY & DEMOGRAPHICS

Most common type of headache, representing 70% of all headaches presenting to primary care physicians. Women are affected more often than men.

PHYSICAL FINDINGS & CLINICAL PRESENTATION

Headaches have an insidious progression, ranging from infrequent (<1 day per mo) to chronic. Although considered a "featureless" headache disorder, either photophobia or phonophobia may still be present. Concurrent problems, such as anxiety, depression, and analgesic overuse, may aggravate the headaches. Patients may have pericranial tenderness to palpation on exam. The rest of the examination should be normal.

PATHOPHYSIOLOGY

- TTH is no longer thought to be due to either a psychological problem or abnormal muscle contraction. Similar to migraine, TTH is likely a heterogeneous disorder with several possible pathophysiologic mechanisms.
- In episodic TTH, peripheral mechanisms may predominate, whereas in chronic TTH, central mechanisms are involved.

DIAGNOSIS

The International Headache Society criteria for tension-type headache are as follows:

- At least 10 headaches
- Lasting from 30 min to 7 days
- Having at least two of the following features:
  1. Bilateral
  2. Pressure or tightening (nonpulsating) quality
  3. Mild or moderate intensity
  4. Not aggravated by routine physical activity such as walking or climbing stairs
- Both of the following:
  1. No nausea or vomiting
  2. No more than one of either photophobia or phonophobia
- Not better accounted for by another diagnosis

DIFFERENTIAL DIAGNOSIS

- Migraine (would expect associated symptoms [i.e., nausea]; see topic "Migraine Headache")
- Cervical spine disease
- Intracranial mass (may present with focal neurologic signs, seizures)
- Idiopathic intracranial hypertension (found more often in obese women of childbearing age)
- Medication overuse headache
- Secondary headache (e.g., obstructive sleep apnea, temporomandibular joint syndrome, hypo- or hyperthyroidism, drug side effects)
- Section II describes the differential diagnosis of headaches

WORKUP

- Routine testing is not needed; the diagnosis may be established clinically.
- Thorough history to identify any red flag features (see topic "Migraine Headache," SSNOOP5 mnemonic in Differential Diagnosis) and physical examination (looking for papilledema) for all patients being evaluated for headache.
- Neuroimaging, preferably with contrast-enhanced MRI, should be performed only when red flag features are identified by history or unexplained neurologic findings are present on examination.
- Erythrocyte sedimentation rate and C-reactive protein in patients 50 yr of age and older to screen for giant cell arteritis.

TREATMENT

Current evidence supports synergistic benefits of combined nonpharmacologic and pharmacologic interventions. Nonpharmacologic therapy may include behavioral sleep modification, acupuncture, cognitive-behavioral therapy, relaxation training, and biofeedback.

ACUTE Rx

- Simple analgesics (i.e., NSAID, acetaminophen).
- Combination analgesics containing caffeine may be used as second-line treatment, although use on more than 10 days per mo may lead to medication overuse headache.
- As with migraine headaches, narcotic- and barbiturate-containing analgesics should be avoided in tension-type headaches.

PREVENTIVE Rx

- Tricyclic antidepressants (e.g., amitriptyline 10 to 50 mg qhs) (first choice)
- Other options: Mirtazapine, venlafaxine, and tizanidine

DISPOSITION

The headache prognosis is generally favorable. Some patients will not respond to treatment.

REFERRAL

If red flags are present on history or exam or if the patient is not improving with treatment

PEARLS & CONSIDERATIONS

It is imperative to avoid overuse of caffeine as well as narcotic-, and barbiturate-containing medications because of the risk of rebound headaches.

SUGGESTED READINGS

Available at ExpertConsult.com

RELATED CONTENT

Tension Headache (Patient Information)

AUTHOR: **Jonathan H. Smith, MD**

BASIC INFORMATION

DEFINITION

Testicular cancers are primary germ cell cancers originating in the testis. They are the most common cancers in men between the ages of 15 and 44 yr, and incidence has been increasing gradually since 1975.

SYNONYMS

Testis tumor
Testicular neoplasms

ICD-10CM CODES

C62.00	Malignant neoplasm of unspecified undescended testis
C62.01	Malignant neoplasm of undescended right testis
C62.02	Malignant neoplasm of undescended left testis
C62.10	Malignant neoplasm of unspecified descended testis
C62.11	Malignant neoplasm of descended right testis
C62.12	Malignant neoplasm of descended left testis
D40.10	Neoplasm of uncertain behavior of unspecified testis
D40.11	Neoplasm of uncertain behavior of right testis
D40.12	Neoplasm of uncertain behavior of left testis

EPIDEMIOLOGY & DEMOGRAPHICS

INCIDENCE: There were an estimated 9610 new cases and 440 deaths associated with testicular cancer in the U.S. in 2020. The incidence is 5.4 cases per 100,000 men annually. White men have the highest incidence, whereas black men have the lowest incidence.

PREVALENCE: It accounts for 1% to 2% of all cancers in males.

PHYSICAL FINDINGS & CLINICAL PRESENTATION

- Testicular cancer typically presents as a painless mass in the testis. Any mass within the testicle should be considered cancer until proven otherwise. It may be found by the patient, who brings it to the attention of a physician, or it may be found by a physician on a routine examination.
- Symptoms other than scrotal or testicular swelling are typically absent unless the cancer has metastasized (10% of patients at diagnosis). Occasionally a patient may report scrotal fullness or heaviness. About 10% of patients present with acute pain. Back pain secondary to enlarged retroperitoneal lymph nodes can occur. Gynecomastia from tumors that secrete beta-human chorionic gonadotropin (hCG) is found in 5% of men with testicular cancer.
- Testicular palpation should be performed with two hands. Transillumination may distinguish a solid mass (e.g., cancer) and a fluid-filled lesion (e.g., hydrocele or spermatocele). The mass is nontender; indeed, it is less sensitive than a normal testicle.

ETIOLOGY, CLASSIFICATION, & PATHOLOGY

- Cryptorchidism (undescended testes) is a major risk factor even if corrected by orchiopexy; however, treatment of undescended testis before puberty decreases the risk of testicular cancer from fivefold to twofold.
- Family history is an important risk factor (risk is four to eight times as high in a brother of a person with testicular cancer and four to six times higher in sons of a father with testicular cancer).
- Other risk factors include genetic disorders (Down syndrome, testicular dysgenesis syndrome), Klinefelter syndrome, infertility, tobacco use, and white race (risk is highest among whites and lowest among blacks).
- Classification: Testicular cancers can be classified as pure seminomas or nonseminomatous germ cell tumors (embryonal carcinoma, choriocarcinoma, yolk sac carcinoma, teratoma, or mixed germ cell tumors).
- Germ-cell tumors appear to develop as a result of a tumorigenic event in utero that leads to a precursor lesion classified as intratubular germ-cell neoplasia. Approximately 90% of germ-cell tumors are associated with adjacent intratubular germ-cell neoplasia, which carries a 50% risk of testicular cancer within 5 yr. Table 1 summarizes germ cell tumors and serum markers.
- A genetic locus that confers a predisposition to testicular cancer is at 12q21, the location of the genes encoding the proteins involved in KITLG–KIT signaling. The development of intratubular germ-cell neoplasia may involve aberrantly activated KITLG–KIT in utero, which induces arrest of embryonic germ cells at the gonocyte stage; subsequently, overexpression of embryonic transcription factors leads to suppression of apoptosis, increased proliferation, and accumulation of mutations in gonocytes.
- The incidence of various subtypes of testicular cancers is as below:

Cell Type	Frequency (%)
Seminoma	42
Embryonal cell carcinoma	26
Teratocarcinoma	26
Teratoma	5
Choriocarcinoma	1

- Other rare types:
  1. Yolk sac carcinoma
  2. Mixed germ cell tumors
  3. Carcinoid tumor
  4. Sertoli cell tumors
  5. Leydig cell tumors
  6. Lymphoma
  7. Metastatic cancer to the testes

STAGING

- TNM staging system for testicular cancer is described in Table 2 and Table 3.
- The clinical stages consist of stage I, with tumor confined to the testis; stage II, with positive regional lymph nodes; and stage III, with metastases. Fig. 1 shows the clinical staging of testicular cancer.

Dx DIAGNOSIS

DIFFERENTIAL DIAGNOSIS

- Spermatocele
- Varicocele
- Hydrocele
- Epididymitis/orchitis
- Epidermoid cyst of the testicle
- Epididymis tumors
- Inguinal hernia
- Hematocele or testicular rupture
- Torsion of testicular appendage
- Skin cancer

WORKUP

Physical examination, laboratory tests, and imaging studies (Fig. 2). A radical inguinal orchiectomy is diagnostic and therapeutic. Immunohistochemical analysis is used to determine the histologic composition of the tumor. Staging involves CT of chest, abdomen, and pelvis

TABLE 1 Germ Cell Tumors and Serum Markers

Histology	Marker Negative (%)	Elevated hCG Alone (%)	Elevated AFP Alone (%)
Seminoma	90	10 (usually <100 IU/ml)	0 (if +, by definition, NSGCT)
All NSGCTs	15	50-60	40
Embryonal		0	10-40
Yolk sac tumors		Rare	80-90 (alone or with elevated hCG)
Choriocarcinoma (or syncytiotrophoblast elements)		>90 (level can be very high)	0

AFP, α-Fetoprotein; *hCG,* human chorionic gonadotropin; *NSGCT,* nonseminoma germ cell tumor.
From Niederhuber JE: *Abeloff's clinical oncology,* ed 6, Philadelphia, 2020, Elsevier.

TABLE 2 TNM Staging for Testicular Cancer *(AJCC 8th Edition Staging Cancer Manual)*

pT Stage	Primary Tumor
pT_X	Primary tumor cannot be assessed
pT_0	No evidence of primary tumor
pT_{is}	Germ cell neoplasia *in situ*
pT_1	Tumor limited to testis (including rete testis invasion) without lymphovascular invasion pT_{1a}: Tumor smaller than 3 cm in size (seminoma only) pT_{1b}: Tumor 3 cm or larger in size (seminoma only)
pT_2	Tumor limited to testis (including rete testis invasion) with lymphovascular invasion OR tumor invading hilar soft tissue or epididymis or penetrating visceral mesothelial layer covering the external surface of tunica albuginea with or without lymphovascular invasion
pT_3	Tumor directly invades spermatic cord soft tissue with or without lymphovascular invasion
pT_4	Tumor invades scrotum with or without lymphovascular invasion
N Stage	**Regional Lymph Nodes**
N_x	Regional lymph nodes cannot be assessed
N_0	No regional lymph node metastasis
N_1	Metastasis with a lymph node mass 2 cm or smaller in greatest dimension OR multiple lymph nodes, none larger than 2 cm in greatest dimension
N_2	Metastasis with a lymph node mass larger than 2 cm but not larger than 5 cm in greatest dimension OR multiple lymph nodes, any one mass larger than 2 cm but not larger than 5 cm in greatest dimension
N_3	Metastasis with a lymph node mass larger than 5 cm in greatest dimension
M Stage	**Distant Metastasis**
M_0	No distant metastasis
M_1	Distant metastasis present M_{1a}: Nonretroperitoneal nodal or pulmonary metastases M_{1b}: Nonpulmonary visceral metastases
S	**Serum Tumor Markers**
S_X	Not available
S_0	Markers within normal levels
S_1	LDH $<1.5 \times$ N *and* hCG (mIU/ml) <5000 *and* AFP (ng/ml) <1000
S_2	LDH 1.5-10 $\times$ N *or* hCG (mIU/ml) 5000-50,000 *or* AFP (ng/ml) 1000-10,000
S_3	LDH $>10 \times$ N *or* hCG (mIU/ml) >50,000 *or* AFP (ng/ml) >10,000

AJCC, American Joint Committee on Cancer; *TNM,* tumor, necrosis, metastases.

TABLE 3 AJCC Prognostic Stage Groupings

Stage	T	N	M	S
0	pT_{is}	N_0	M_0	S_0
I	pT_{1-4}	N_0	M_0	S_X
I_A	pT_1	N_0	M_0	S_0
I_B	pT_{2-4}	N_0	M_0	S_0
I_S	Any T	N_0	M_0	S_{1-3}
II	Any T	N_{1-3}	M_0	S_X
II_A	Any T	N_1	M_0	S_0-S_1
II_B	Any T	N_2	M_0	S_0-S_1
II_C	Any T	N_3	M_0	S_0-S_1
III	Any T	Any N	M_1	S_X
III_A	Any T	Any N	M_{1a}	S_0-S_1
III_B	Any T	Any N	M_0-M_{1a}	S_2
III_C	Any T	Any N	M_0-M_{1a}	S_3
	Any T	Any N	M_{1b}	Any S

AJCC, American Joint Committee on Cancer.

and measurement of beta subunit of human chorionic gonadotropins (β-hCG), alpha-fetoprotein (AFP), and lactate dehydrogenase (LDH).

LABORATORY TESTS

- Serum β-hCG is elevated in approximately 20% of patients with pure seminomas.
- Serum AFP is elevated in nonseminoma tumors, never elevated in patients with pure seminomas. One or both of these tumor markers will be elevated in 70% of cases of testicular cancer.
- Serum lactate LDH level is elevated with rapid turnover of malignant cells.
- Testicular biopsy is contraindicated.

IMAGING STUDIES

- Testicular ultrasound
- CT scan of chest, pelvis, and abdomen
- MRI of the brain in patients with neurologic symptoms
- PET scan is not recommended (frequent false positives)

Rx TREATMENT

- Fertility preservation is an important consideration that is often underutilized in the management of these patients. Serum cryopreservation is the most cost-effective procedure for fertility preservation and should be offered to all patients before the start of therapy.
- Box E1 summarizes a treatment algorithm for testicular cancer.
- Seminoma:
    1. Stage I: Most patients (80%-85%) are cured with orchiectomy. The addition of adjuvant chemotherapy (one cycle of single-agent carboplatin) or radiation therapy (to the paraaortic lymph nodes) is a standard treatment option that increases cure rates to >95%. In most instances, though, active postorchiectomy surveillance is routine in clinical practice. Long-term survival approaches 100% irrespective of the initial option chosen.[1]
    2. Stage II_A or II_B: Radiotherapy or combination chemotherapy (e.g., bleomycin, etoposide, and cisplatin [BEP] regimen).
- Nonseminoma:
    1. Stage I_A: Radical orchiectomy plus nerve-sparing retroperitoneal lymph node dissection (RPLND)
    2. Stage I_B: Same as stage I_A plus two cycles of chemotherapy (bleomycin, etoposide, and cisplatin [BEP])
    3. Stages II-III: Multiagent cisplatin-based chemotherapy regimens for three or four cycles depending on risk stratification (low/intermediate or high). RPLND is offered for residual lymph nodal disease after chemotherapy
- Relapsed disease:
    1. Salvage chemotherapy using multiagent regimens is offered. Active chemotherapy regimens include TIP (paclitaxel, ifosfamide, cisplatin) and VIP (vinblastine, ifosfamide, cisplatin) regimens.
    2. Chemotherapy-sensitive patients can be successfully treated with high-dose chemotherapy followed by autologous stem cell transplantation (ASCT).
- Posttreatment surveillance for testicular cancer survivors (annually):
    1. Fertility assessment
    2. Physical examination and skin examination (increased risk of dysplastic nevi)
    3. Testicular examination (3% to 4% risk of second testicular cancer)
    4. Serum tumor markers (hCG, AFP)

[1] Hanna NH, Einhorn LH: Testicular cancer, discoveries and updates, *N Engl J Med* 371:2005-2016, 2014.

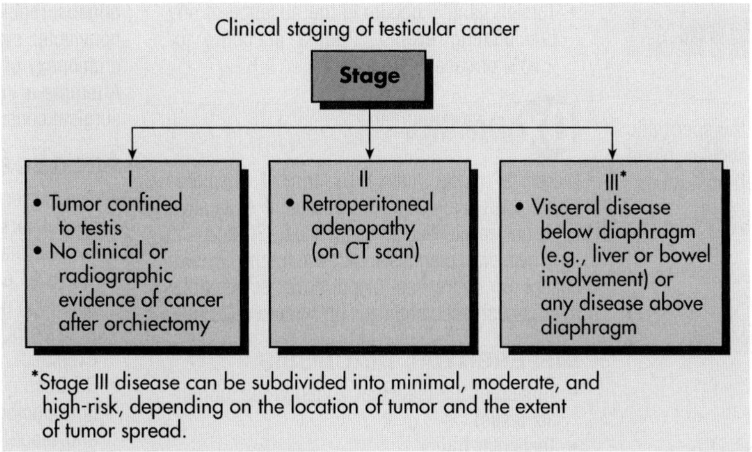

FIG. 1 Clinical staging of testicular cancer. The American Joint Committee on Cancer TNM staging system is less commonly used, because it is based upon histologic evaluation of the orchidectomy specimen and retroperitoneal periaortic lymph node dissection. Because the latter may not be performed in every patient, the clinical staging system is generally more practical. (From Skarin AT: *Atlas of diagnostic oncology,* ed 4, St Louis, 2010, Mosby.)

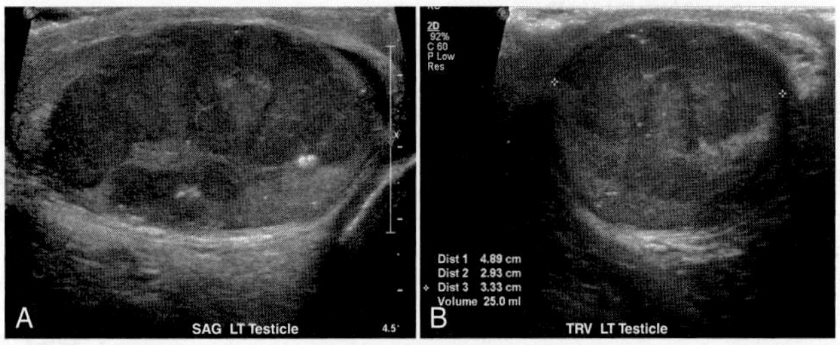

FIG. 2 Seminoma in an 18-year-old patient with painless left scrotal mass. A and **B,** Sagittal and transverse sonograms of the left testis demonstrate a testicular volume of 25 ml, with a lobulated, heterogeneous, relatively hypoechoic mass occupying most of the testis with a thin rim of normal testis and a few tiny clusters of calcification, as well as multiple, tiny, brightly echoic speckles both inside and outside the mass. The tiny speckles represent microlithiasis. (From Rumack CM et al: *Diagnostic ultrasound,* ed 4, Philadelphia, 2011, Elsevier.)

5. Abdominal and pelvic CT every 3 to 4 mo for 2 yr, every 6 to 12 mo in third and fourth yr, and annually thereafter

DISPOSITION

- The overall cure for testicular cancer is >95% (80% for metastatic disease). Patients with pure seminomas have a better prognosis. Prognosis can be determined by criteria established by the International Germ Cell Consensus Criteria (Table E4). Given these favorable outcomes, the U.S. Preventive Services Task Force recommends against screening asymptomatic men for testicular cancer.
- There is an increased risk for metabolic syndrome (insulin resistance, hypertension, dyslipidemia, abdominal obesity) after radiation or chemotherapy. Additionally, effects on long-term reproductive health, lower fertility, hearing impairment, neuropathy, and Raynaud phenomenon are long-term toxicities seen with chemotherapy use.
- Therapeutic radiation and chemotherapy are both risk factors for the development of solid and hematologic second malignant neoplasms (SMNs) in survivors. In a recent SEER analysis of 29,400 patients, the 30-yr cumulative incidences of solid-SMN after radiotherapy, chemotherapy, and surgery alone were 16.9%, 10.1% , and 8.8%, respectively. Increased leukemia risks after chemotherapy were driven by statistically significant sevenfold excesses of acute myeloid leukemia 1 to 10 yr after testicular cancer diagnosis. Risks for lymphoma and plasma cell dyscrasias were not elevated. Common reported cancers include those of the thyroid, kidney, pancreas, and stomach, as well as leukemia.

SUGGESTED READINGS

Available at ExpertConsult.com

RELATED CONTENT

Testicular Cancer (Patient Information)

AUTHOR: **Bharti Rathore, MD**

Testicular Torsion (PTG)

BASIC INFORMATION

DEFINITION

Testicular torsion is a twisting of the spermatic cord leading to cessation of testicular blood flow, ischemia, and infarction if left untreated.

SYNONYM

Spermatic cord torsion

ICD-10CM CODE

N44.03 Torsion of testis, unspecified

EPIDEMIOLOGY & DEMOGRAPHICS

INCIDENCE: Affects 1 in 4000 males <25 yr

PREDOMINANT AGE: Two thirds of all cases occur between the ages of 12 and 18 yr but may occur at any age, including antenatally.

PHYSICAL FINDINGS & CLINICAL PRESENTATION

- Typical sequence is sudden onset of hemiscrotal pain, then swelling, nausea, and vomiting without fever or urinary symptoms.
- Physical examination may reveal a tender firm testis, high-riding testis, horizontal lie of testis, absent cremasteric reflex, and no pain with elevation of testis. Absence of the cremasteric reflex (stroking or pinching the medial thigh causing contraction of cremaster muscle and elevation of testis) is the most sensitive physical finding.
- Painless testicular swelling occurs in 10%.
- One out of three patients reports previous episodes of spontaneously remitting scrotal pain.
- In the neonate, testicular torsion should be presumed in patients with a painless, discolored hemiscrotal swelling.
- In rare cases, torsion may involve an undescended testicle. In such situations an empty hemiscrotum is palpated with a tender lump in the inguinal area.

ETIOLOGY

- There are three types of testicular torsion: Extravaginal, caused by nonadherence of the tunica vaginalis to the dartos layer; intravaginal torsion, caused by malrotation of the spermatic cord with the tunica vaginalis; and torsion of the testis below the epididymis (Fig. 1). Intravaginal torsion accounts for 90% of cases.
- Torsion usually occurs in the absence of any precipitating events. Trauma accounts for <10% of cases.

Dx DIAGNOSIS

Diagnosis made mainly by clinical suspicion (Table E1). Color Doppler ultrasound evaluation or a nuclear testicular scan (Figs. E1 and E2) may help with diagnosis. Ultrasonography shows absent or decreased blood flow; scintigraphy reveals decreased perfusion on symptomatic side.

DIFFERENTIAL DIAGNOSIS

- Torsion of the testicular appendages (appendix testis)
- Testicular tumor
- Epididymitis
- Incarcerated inguinoscrotal hernia
- Orchitis
- Spermatocele
- Hydrocele, varicocele

WORKUP

The diagnosis is usually based on history and physical examination.

IMAGING STUDIES

- Doppler ultrasonic stethoscope (Doppler flowmetry) (Fig. E2)
- Radionuclide scrotal scanning (technetium-99m): Cold testicle (Fig. E1)

Rx TREATMENT

Surgical derotation of the spermatic cord followed by bilateral testicular fixation with nonabsorbable sutures. If affected testis is nonviable, orchiectomy of affected testis and orchiopexy of contralateral side are performed. Attempts at manual detorsion should not delay surgical consultation.

PROGNOSIS

- The degree of ischemia depends on the duration of torsion and the degree of rotation of the spermatic cord.
- There is an 80% testicular salvage rate if detorsion occurs within 12 hr of onset.
- After 24 hr, irreversible testicular infarction is expected.
- Because contralateral testes can be affected (immunologic process), if treatment delayed and blood flow does not return after detorsion, some recommend orchiectomy of the infarcted testicle.

PEARLS & CONSIDERATIONS

- Manual detorsion by external rotation of the testis toward the thigh can be attempted for adolescent intravaginal torsion if an operating facility is not readily available.
- Extravaginal torsion is diagnosed in the newborn. Intravaginal torsion can occur at any age but is usually diagnosed in males ages 12 to 18 yr.

RELATED CONTENT

Testicular Torsion (Patient Information)

AUTHOR: **Fred F. Ferri, MD**

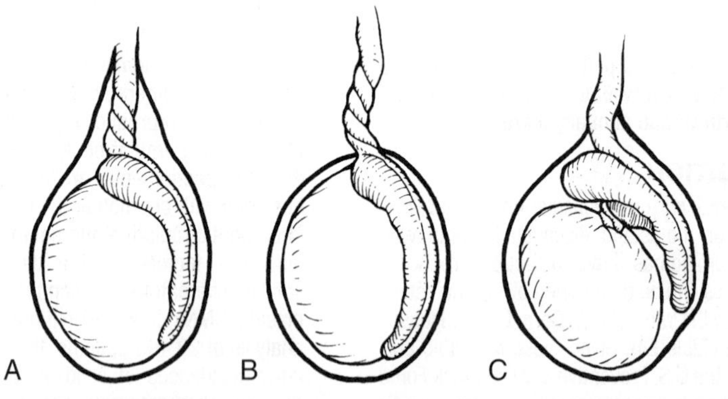

FIG. 1 Types of testicular torsion. A, Intravaginal torsion above the epididymis. **B,** Extravaginal torsion. **C,** Torsion of the testis below the epididymis. (From Rumack CM et al: *Diagnostic ultrasound,* ed 4, Philadelphia, 2011, Elsevier.)

BASIC INFORMATION

DEFINITION

Thoracic outlet syndrome (TOS) describes a condition producing upper extremity symptoms believed to result from neurovascular compression at the thoracic outlet (Fig. E1, Table 1). Three types are described on the basis of point of compression: (1) cervical rib and scalenus syndrome, in which abnormal scalene muscles or the presence of a cervical rib may cause compression; (2) costoclavicular syndrome, in which compression may occur under the clavicle; and (3) subcoracoid pectoralis minor syndrome, in which compression may occur in the subcoracoid area or retropectoralis minor area. The compression occurs in three anatomic structures: Arteries, veins, and nerves, and specific terminology is used to describe TOS depending on the predominantly affected structure: Arterial TOS, venous TOS, and neurogenic TOS. TOS usually is caused by a combination of two factors: (1) having abnormal anatomy that creates compression in the thoracic outlet, (2) having some environmental factor such as injury at the thoracic outlet or excessive repetitive motion that predisposes to compression.

- Neurogenic TOS (nTOS): Caused by compression of brachial nerve plexus
- Arterial TOS (aTOS): Caused by subclavian artery compression and almost always associated with complete cervical rib or anomalous first rib
- Venous TOS (vTOS): Caused by compression of subclavian vein and may also occur in patients with chronic indwelling intravenous catheters

SYNONYM

TOS

ICD-10CM CODE
G54.0 Brachial plexus disorders

EPIDEMIOLOGY & DEMOGRAPHICS

PREVALENCE: TOS is an uncommon disorder. Varies from source to source; presence of cervical ribs in 0.5% to 1% of population (50% bilateral), but most are asymptomatic. Approximately 90% of all TOS disorders are neurogenic, and the remaining 10% are arterial or venous.

PREDOMINANT SEX: Females affected more often than males (ratio of 3.5:1)

PREDOMINANT AGE: Rare in those age <20 yr

PHYSICAL FINDINGS & CLINICAL PRESENTATION

- Symptoms and signs are related to the degree of involvement of each of the various structures at the level of the first rib.
- True venous or arterial involvement is not common.
- Diagnosis is most often used in the consideration of neural pain affecting the arm, which suggests involvement of the brachial plexus.
  1. Arterial compression: Pallor, pain, paresthesias, diminished pulses, coolness, Raynaud phenomenon, digital gangrene, digital ischemia, supraclavicular bruit or mass, and stroke
  2. Venous compression: Edema, cyanosis and pain, thrombosis causing superficial venous dilation in the shoulder area
  3. Neurologic compression: Pain and/or paresthesia of neck, shoulder region, arm or hand, depending on the root involved with difficulty; intrinsic weakness and diminished sensation on examination; occipital headache
  4. Possible supraclavicular tenderness
  5. Provocative tests: Adson (Fig. E2), Wright (hyperabduction test where the strength of the radial pulse weakens as the arm is passively abducted and externally rotated), elevated arm stress test or EAST (Roos), upper limb tension test or ULTT (Elvey). May reproduce pain but are of disputed usefulness.

ETIOLOGY

- Congenital cervical rib or fibrous extension of cervical rib
- Abnormal scalene muscle insertion
- Drooping of shoulder girdle from generalized hypotonia or trauma
- Narrowed costoclavicular interval as a result of downward and backward pressure on shoulder (sometimes seen in individuals who carry heavy backpacks), poor posturing, pregnancy
- Acute venous thrombosis with exercise (effort thrombosis or Paget-Schroetter syndrome)
- Bony abnormalities of first rib
- Abnormal fibromuscular bands
- Malunion of clavicle fracture

Dx DIAGNOSIS

DIFFERENTIAL DIAGNOSIS

- Carpal tunnel syndrome
- Cervical radiculopathy
- Brachial neuritis
- Ulnar nerve compression (cubital tunnel syndrome)
- Complex regional pain syndrome
- Superior sulcus tumor
- Intrinsic shoulder dysfunction

WORKUP

Fig. 3 describes a diagnostic algorithm for thoracic outlet syndrome. Preliminary criteria for the clinical diagnosis of neurogenic thoracic outlet syndrome are summarized in Table 2. Except for venous or arterial pathology, no ancillary diagnostic tests are reliable for diagnostic confirmation.

IMAGING STUDIES

- Electromyography, nerve conduction velocity studies to rule out carpal tunnel syndrome, cervical radiculopathy
- Doppler ultrasound for initial evaluation for arterial or venous thoracic outlet syndrome with provocative maneuvers
- Cervical spine radiographs to rule out cervical disk disease
- Chest radiograph to rule out lung tumor
- Computed tomography (CT) with IV contrast for detailed anatomic relationship of vascular structure to surrounding muscles and bones
- Computed tomography angiography (CTA) or contrast-enhanced magnetic resonance angiography (MRA) can be very useful in assessing vessel imaging while using provocative arm positions
- Magnetic resonance imaging (MRI) with and without IV contrast for evaluation of neurogenic thoracic outlet syndrome
- Arteriography or venography (Fig. E4) can be used for dynamic studies while performing upper extremity maneuvers and also performing thrombolysis, if needed

TABLE 1 Sites and Structures Compressed in Thoracic Outlet Syndrome

Site	Description	Abnormalities	Structures Compressed
Sternal-costovertebral circle	This aperture can be narrowed by bony variations	• Cervical first rib • First rib • Long transverse process	• Subclavian artery • Subclavian vein • Brachial plexus
Scalene muscle triangle	The scalenus anterior and middle muscle insert on the first rib, creating a tunnel	Scalenus anterior and middle	• Subclavian artery • Brachial plexus
First rib, clavicular space	The neurovascular structures lie above the rib and below the clavicle	• Costoclavicular ligament • Clavicle • First rib	• Subclavian vein • Subclavian artery • Brachial plexus
Behind the pectoralis minor muscle	The neurovascular structures travel to and from the arm behind this muscle	• Pectoralis minor • Costocoracoid ligament	• Subclavian vein • Subclavian artery • Brachial plexus

From Sellke FW et al: *Sabiston & Spencer surgery of the chest,* ed 9, Philadelphia, 2016, Elsevier.

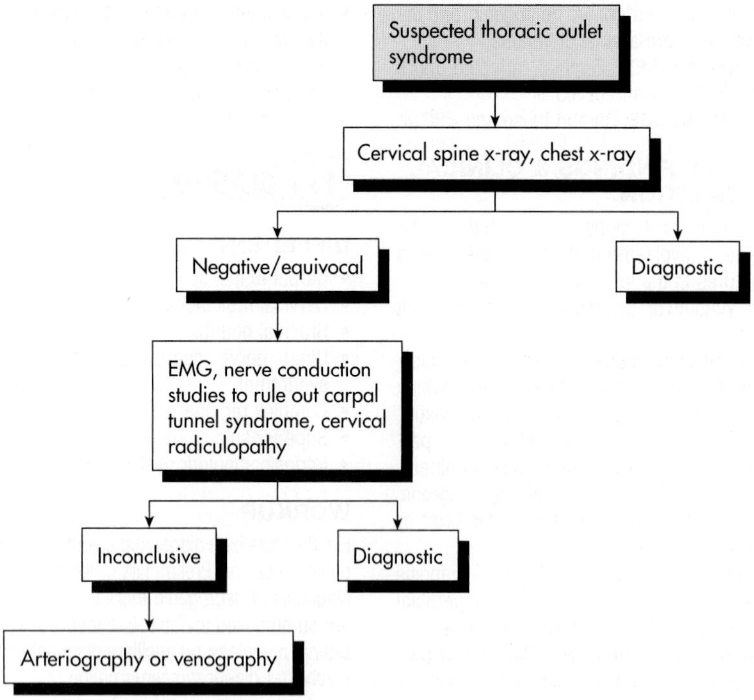

FIG. 3 Thoracic outlet syndrome. *EMG,* Electromyogram.

TABLE 2 Preliminary Criteria for the Clinical Diagnosis of Neurogenic Thoracic Outlet Syndrome

Unilateral or bilateral upper extremity symptoms that:

(1) Extend beyond the distribution of a single cervical nerve root or peripheral nerve
(2) Have been present for at least 12 wk
(3) Have not been explained satisfactorily by another condition
(4) Meet at least one criterion in at least four of the following five categories:

1. Principal symptoms	1A. Pain in the neck, upper back, shoulder, arm, or hand
	1B. Numbness; paresthesias; or weakness in the arm, hand, or digits
2. Symptom characteristics	2A. Pain, paresthesias, or weakness exacerbated with elevated arm positions
	2B. Pain, paresthesias, or weakness exacerbated by prolonged or repetitive arm or hand use or by prolonged work on a keyboard or other repetitive strain
	2C. Pain or paresthesias radiate down the arm from the supraclavicular or infraclavicular space
3. Clinical history	3A. Symptoms began after occupational, recreational, or accidental injury of the head, neck, or upper extremity, including repetitive upper extremity strain or overuse activity
	3B. Previous clavicle or first rib fracture or known cervical rib(s)
	3C. Previous cervical spine or peripheral nerve surgery without sustained improvement
	3D. Previous conservative or surgical treatment for thoracic outlet syndrome
4. Physical examination	4A. Local tenderness on palpation over scalene triangle or subcoracoid space
	4B. Arm, hand, or digit paresthesias on palpation over scalene triangle or subcoracoid space
	4C. Weak handgrip, intrinsic muscles, or digit 5 or thenar or hypothenar atrophy
5. Provocative maneuvers	5A. Positive upper limb tension test (ULTT)
	5B. Positive 1- or 3-min elevated arm stress test (EAST)
	5C. Positive Adson test
	5D. Positive Wright test (or hyperabduction)

From Cameron JL, Cameron AM: *Current surgical therapy,* ed 12, Philadelphia, 2017, Elsevier.

Rx TREATMENT

ACUTE GENERAL Rx

- Avoid weight gain
- Sling for pain relief
- Physical therapy modalities plus shoulder girdle–strengthening exercises
- Postural reeducation
- Nonsteroidal antiinflammatory drugs
- Muscle relaxants
- Muscle block with injection of local anesthetic agent or botulinum toxin A in anterior scalene (for diagnostic and therapeutic reasons, e.g., predicting response to surgical intervention)

CHRONIC Rx

Surgical treatment is indicated:
- After failure of physical therapy
- With complications such as thrombosis, aneurysms
- With neurologic compressions
- With sympathetic cervical rib

Surgical options:
- Thoracic outlet decompression including cervical rib resection and anterior scalenectomy
- Thoracic sympathetectomy
- Vascular reconstruction
- Catheter-directed thrombolysis or aspiration mechanical thrombectomy, followed by thoracic outlet decompression and anticoagulation for deep vein thrombosis due to venous TOS

DISPOSITION

- Nonsurgical treatment is often successful for patients with pain as the primary symptom.
- Nonsurgical management is initially recommended in neurogenic TOS. Operative management is often required in arterial TOS and venous TOS.
- Complications of surgical treatment include transient dysesthesia, hematoma, pneumothorax, hemothorax, venous injury, arterial injuries, or brachial plexus injuries.

REFERRAL

For vascular surgery consultation when venous or arterial impairment is present

PEARLS & CONSIDERATIONS

COMMENTS

- True thoracic outlet syndrome is probably an uncommon condition.
- Diagnosis is often used to describe a wide variety of clinical symptoms.
- Considerable disagreement exists regarding the frequency of this disorder.

SUGGESTED READINGS

Available at ExpertConsult.com

RELATED CONTENT

Thoracic Outlet Syndrome (Patient Information)

AUTHORS: **Erica Lin, MD,** and **Philippe Montgrain, MD**

BASIC INFORMATION

DEFINITION

Thrombocytosis is defined by an elevated platelet count (>450,000/ml) in peripheral blood. It is caused by overproduction of platelets (reactive thrombocytosis) or clonal expansion of megakaryocytes (clonal thrombocytosis). Reactive thrombocytosis is driven by excessive cytokines induced by various stimuli, such as trauma or inflammation. Clonal thrombocytosis is defined as chronic myeloproliferative neoplasms (MPNs), of which four subgroups are well characterized: Chronic myelogenous leukemia (CML), polycythemia vera (PV), primary myelofibrosis (PMF), and essential thrombocythemia (ET). In addition, platelet count can be spuriously elevated in some conditions (see "Differential Diagnosis"). Extreme thrombocytosis is defined as platelet count >1 million/ml.

SYNONYMS

Thrombocythemia
Essential thrombocythemia
ET

ICD-10CM CODES	
D47.3	Essential (hemorrhagic) thrombocythemia
D75.89	Other specified diseases of blood and blood-forming organs
D75.9	Disease of blood and blood-forming organs, unspecified
D77	Other disorders of blood and blood-forming organs in diseases classified elsewhere

EPIDEMIOLOGY & DEMOGRAPHICS

Reactive thrombocytosis is much more frequent than clonal thrombocytosis (70% vs. 22% in one series).

Epidemiology for essential thrombocythemia:

INCIDENCE: 1.2 to 3.0 per 100,000 population/yr

PREVALENCE: Estimated at 24 cases/100,000 population

PREDOMINANT SEX & AGE: The median age at diagnosis is 58 yr. Female:male ratio is 2:1.

PHYSICAL FINDINGS & CLINICAL PRESENTATION

- Regardless of the cause, a high platelet count may be associated with vasomotor symptoms such as headache, visual disturbances, dizziness, atypical chest pain, acral dysesthesia, and erythromelalgia.
- Thrombotic and bleeding complications can occur. Thrombosis at unusual sites (hepatic vein, IVC, portal vein, splenic vein) are especially concerning.
- Symptoms and complications are much more likely to occur in association with clonal thrombocytosis than reactive thrombocytosis.
- The degree of thrombocytosis does not predict the likelihood of clonal thrombocytosis and does not generally correlate to the risk of thrombosis.
- Splenomegaly is common with MPNs.
- Coexistent leukocytosis and erythrocytosis are common with CML and PV.
- Disease transformation from ET to PV, PMF, and acute myeloid leukemia (AML) is uncommon. In patients with ET, the 20-yr rate of leukemic transformation is estimated at 5%.

ETIOLOGY

- Essential thrombocytosis, a myeloproliferative neoplasm, is a clonal disorder of a multipotent hematopoietic progenitor cell.
- Abnormality in JAK2-STAT pathway (including *JAK2, CALR*, and *MPL* gene mutations) may play a role in pathogenesis of MPN.

Dx DIAGNOSIS

DIFFERENTIAL DIAGNOSIS

- Spurious thrombocytosis:
  1. Mixed cryoglobulinemia—precipitated cryoglobulin particles are counted as platelets by automatic counters; generally occurs at low temperatures.
  2. Circulating cytoplasmic fragments miscounted as platelets—seen mainly in patients with leukemia, lymphoma, severe hemolysis, or burns
- Reactive thrombocytosis:
  1. Benign hematologic disorders
  2. Acute hemorrhage, iron deficiency anemia, hemolytic anemia
  3. Chronic infection, such as tuberculosis
  4. Acute and chronic inflammatory disorders
  5. Rheumatologic disorders
  6. Inflammatory bowel disease
  7. Celiac disease
  8. Functional and surgical asplenia
  9. Tissue damage
  10. Trauma, thermal burn
  11. Myocardial infarction
  12. Acute pancreatitis
  13. Recent surgery
  14. Renal failure, nephrotic syndrome
  15. Exercise
  16. Medications, such as vincristine, epinephrine
- Clonal thrombocytosis:
  1. CML
  2. PV
  3. PMF
  4. Myelodysplastic syndrome (5q-syndrome)
  5. AML with inv(3), t(3;3)
  6. Essential thrombocytosis (Box 1)

WORKUP

- Comprehensive history and physical examination to exclude many of the common causes of reactive thrombocytosis: History and physical examination suggestive of acute blood loss, iron deficiency, acute or chronic infection/inflammation, medication use, asplenia, malignancy, and trauma should be evaluated. Fig. E1 describes a diagnostic algorithm for thrombocytosis. The diagnosis of ET requires platelet counts >450 × 10^3/ml on two separate occasions >4 wk apart, absence of Philadelphia chromosome, and exclusion of secondary causes of thrombocytosis.
- Repeat CBC with peripheral blood smear and bone marrow biopsy (Figs. E2 and E3) to exclude spurious thrombocytosis.

LABORATORY TESTS

- CBC with peripheral blood smear: Howell-Jolly bodies and target cells are present in patients with asplenia; nucleated RBC, teardrop RBC and WBC precursors in patients with PMF.
- Serum ferritin level: Low ferritin level suggests iron deficiency.

BOX 1 World Health Organization Diagnostic Criteria for Essential Thrombocythemia

Diagnosis requires that all of the following criteria be met:
- Sustained platelet count ≥450 × 10^9/L*
- Bone marrow biopsy specimen showing proliferation mainly of the megakaryocytic lineage, with increased numbers of enlarged, mature megakaryocytes; no significant increase or left shift of neutrophil granulopoiesis or erythropoiesis
- Failure to meet the WHO criteria for polycythemia vera,‡,† primary myelofibrosis, ‡ BCR-ABL1–positive chronic myelogenous leukemia,§ myelodysplastic syndrome,¶ or other myeloid neoplasms
- Demonstration of *JAK2 V617F* or other clonal marker; or, in the absence of *JAK2 V617F*, no evidence of reactive thrombocytosis¶

WHO, World Health Organization.

*Sustained during the workup process.

‡Requires the absence of relevant reticulin fibrosis, collagen fibrosis, peripheral blood leukoerythroblastosis, or markedly hypercellular marrow accompanied by megakaryocyte morphology typical for primary myelofibrosis—small to large megakaryocytes with an aberrant nuclear-to-cytoplasmic ratio and hyperchromatic, bulbous, or irregularly folded nuclei and dense clustering.

†Requires the failure of iron replacement therapy to increase the hemoglobin level to the polycythemia vera range in the presence of decreased serum ferritin. Exclusion of polycythemia vera is based on hemoglobin and hematocrit levels; red cell mass measurement is not required.

§Requires the absence of BCR-ABL1.

¶Causes of reactive thrombocytosis include iron deficiency, splenectomy, surgery, infection, inflammation, connective tissue disease, metastatic cancer, and lymphoproliferative disorders. Requires the absence of dyserythropoiesis and dysgranulopoiesis.

From Swerdlow SH et al (eds): *WHO classification of tumours of haematopoietic and lymphoid tissues,* Lyon, France, 2008, IARC Press.

TABLE 1 Choice of Drugs for Treatment of Patients with High-Risk Essential Thrombocythemia

Age (yr)	Treatment of Choice	Second Line
<50	Interferon	Anagrelide Hydroxyurea
50-75	Hydroxyurea	Interferon Anagrelide
>75	Hydroxyurea	Anagrelide

From Hoffman R et al: *Hematology: basic principles and practice*, ed 7, Philadelphia, 2018, Elsevier.

- Serum C-reactive protein (CRP), ESR, and plasma fibrinogen: Nonspecific markers of infection or inflammation.
- Philadelphia chromosome or BCR-ABL rearrangement: Positive in CML.
- Serum erythropoietin assay: Low to normal in PV and ET.
- *JAK2* mutation analysis: PV and ET; *JAK2* mutation is found in 95% to 99% of patient with PV, in 40% to 60% of patients with PMF, and in about 50% to 55% of patients with ET.
- *MPL, THPO, TET2,* and *CALR* mutation analysis: Frequency is reported as 4% and 15% to 36%, respectively, in ET:
    1. These mutations are associated with differences in prognosis and risk of thrombosis.
    2. *JAK2, CALR, THPO, TET2,* and *MPL* mutations are mutually exclusive. They are not confined to a particular myeloproliferative neoplasm, and their absence does not exclude any of the MPNs.
    3. About 17% of patients with ET will be negative for *JAK2, CALR,* and *MPL* mutations.
- Bone marrow chromosome analysis: 5q-syndrome and other myelodysplastic syndrome, CML.
- Bone marrow exam in ET may show clusters of abnormal megakaryocytes and increased reticulin fibrosis (see Fig. E3).

Rx TREATMENT

No therapies are known to alter survival or leukemic transformation in ET. Reactive thrombocytosis has been rarely associated with thrombosis or bleeding and generally does not require specific therapy.

ACUTE GENERAL Rx

- Vasomotor symptoms easily manageable with low-dose aspirin (<100 mg/day).
- Bleeding:
    1. Discontinue any platelet antiaggregating agent, such as aspirin or nonsteroidal antiinflammatory agents.
    2. Evaluate for disseminated intravascular coagulopathy and coagulation factor deficiency. Acquired factor V deficiency is occasionally present in association with clonal thrombocytosis. In that case, treat with fresh frozen plasma infusion.
    3. In case of extreme thrombocytosis (platelet count generally >1,000,000/uL [1000×10^9/L]), acquired von Willebrand disease may occur. Immediate definitive therapy with a platelet-lowering agent is essential in this instance. Platelet pheresis should be reserved for cases of acute thrombosis or bleeding.
- Thrombosis:
    1. Arterial or venous thrombosis occurs in 20% to 30% of patients.
    2. If the platelet count is >800,000/ml, platelet apheresis coupled with a platelet-lowering agent should be considered with the goal of platelet count <400,000/mm^3.
    3. Anticoagulant therapy for 3 mo to indefinite based on the presence or absence of additional thrombophilic defects.

CHRONIC Rx

Treatment strategies for ET are based on the presence or absence of risk factors for thrombosis. Objective risk stratification is done by calculating IPSET-thrombosis score with age, history of thrombosis, cardiac risk factor, and presence of JAK2 mutation. Smoking cessation and obesity management should be discussed with all patients with ET. In low-risk patients (age <60 yr, no history of thrombosis or hemorrhage, platelet count <1 million/ml), observation may be adequate. Treatment with low-dose aspirin is indicated in low-risk patients with vasomotor symptoms or with other indications for aspirin use. The cytoreductive therapy along with low-dose aspirin therapy is indicated in high-risk patients (age >60 yr and/or with previous history of thrombosis) regardless of vasomotor symptoms. Exception is if a high-risk patient has no history of arterial thrombosis but has history of venous thrombosis, in which case systemic anticoagulation instead of low-dose aspirin is recommended.

- Low-dose aspirin (81 mg/day) may be safe and effective in preventing vascular events. It is also effective in preventing recurrent vascular events in high-risk patients and in treating the vasomotor symptoms.
- Cytoreductive therapy (Table 1):
    1. First-line therapies typically include hydroxyurea and interferon in the majority of cases. Anagrelide and interferon (if not used previously) generally are considered second line.
    2. Hydroxyurea (HU) versus anagrelide: HU plus aspirin is suggested to be safer and more effective than anagrelide plus aspirin in regard to thrombosis, bleeding, and transformation to PMF at 5 yr in a randomized trial. Monitor liver function tests and the degree of neutropenia or anemia with HU therapy.
    3. The incidence of leukemic conversion in patients with ET treated with HU alone is reported as <1%. Interferon alpha may be effective for controlling platelet count in patients failing treatment with HU.

DISPOSITION

- Although long survival is expected in patients with ET, it is inferior to the sex- and age-matched U.S. population.
- An International Prognostic Score for Essential Thrombocythemia (IPSET) was proposed by International Working Group on Myelofibrosis Research and Treatment based on age, WBC count, and history of thromboembolism at diagnosis.

REFERRAL

Refer to hematologist/oncologist when platelet count is consistently elevated >450,000/mm^3 without causes for reactive thrombocytosis.

PEARLS & CONSIDERATION

COMMENTS

- Some patients with clinically apparent ET have Philadelphia chromosome or BCR-ABL rearrangement, even in the absence of other features of CML. It is suggested that it should be tested in all ET patients due to its potential therapeutic implications.
- The risk of bleeding with aspirin use in patients with ET paradoxically increases when the platelet count is >1 million/ml, likely due to acquired von Willebrand disease.

PATIENT & FAMILY EDUCATION

Smoking cessation is encouraged in both patients with ET and reactive thrombocytosis.

SUGGESTED READINGS

Available at ExpertConsult.com

AUTHORS: **Hyun Lee, MD,** and **John L. Reagan, MD**

BASIC INFORMATION

DEFINITION

Superficial venous thrombophlebitis (SVT) is an inflammation of a vein with subsequent secondary thrombus formation. SVT most frequently involves superficial veins of the leg, but any superficial vein can be affected. SVT has been reported to occur in 125,000 people in the U.S. per yr; however, the actual incidence is likely far greater. SVT is not always a benign condition. SVT should be regarded as the superficial venous manifestation of a systemic process known as venous thromboembolism (DVT, PE).

SYNONYMS

SVT
Superficial phlebitis
Superficial suppurative thrombophlebitis
Suppurative thrombophlebitis

ICD-10CM CODES

I80.00	Phlebitis and thrombophlebitis of superficial vessels of unspecified lower extremity
I80.8	Phlebitis and thrombophlebitis of other sites
I80.9	Phlebitis and thrombophlebitis of unspecified site

EPIDEMIOLOGY & DEMOGRAPHICS

- Approximately 30% to 45% of patients diagnosed with SVT are men with an average age of 54 yr.
- Approximately 55% to 70% of patients diagnosed with SVT are women with an average age of 58 yr.
- The overall recurrence of SVT is 18% over an average observation period of 15 mo, equally involving varicose and nonvaricose veins.
- The lifetime incidence of SVT in those with untreated varicose veins has been estimated at 25% to 50%.

PHYSICAL FINDINGS & CLINICAL PRESENTATION

- Subcutaneous vein is palpable as a tender cord or "wormlike" mass with increased warmth and erythema.
- Induration, redness, and tenderness are localized along the course of the vein. This linear appearance rather than circular appearance is useful to distinguish thrombophlebitis from other conditions (cellulitis, erythema nodosum).
- There is some swelling of the overlying skin and subcutaneous tissue but without generalized edema of the limb.
- Low-grade fever may be present.

ETIOLOGY

- In the lower extremity, 70% of SVT occurs in patients with varicose veins, with the great saphenous vein being most commonly involved (60% to 80%)
- Intravenous catheters and infusion of caustic drugs are the most common cause of upper-extremity SVT
- Malignancy
- Pregnancy/puerperium
- Hypercoagulable states
- Previous DVT/SVT
- OCP (oral contraceptive pill)/HRT (hormone replacement therapy)

Dx DIAGNOSIS

DIFFERENTIAL DIAGNOSIS

- Lymphangitis
- Cellulitis
- Erythema nodosum
- Panniculitis
- Acute lipodermatosclerosis

WORKUP

The clinical investigation includes not only the local findings but also the presence of varicose veins with or without the stigmata of chronic venous insufficiency. Today, duplex ultrasound is the most important additional diagnostic tool.

IMAGING STUDIES

- Duplex ultrasound offers the advantage of being inexpensive, noninvasive, and repeatable for follow-up examination.
- Ultrasonography confirms the diagnosis, shows the location of the thrombus and its location regarding the saphenofemoral and/or saphenopopliteal junctions.
- Ultrasound examination of patients with SVT has revealed that a concomitant DVT can exist in 15% to 20%.
- In up to 25% of these patients, the DVT may not be contiguous with the SVT and may be found in the contralateral leg.
- Therefore, bilateral duplex exam is recommended in all cases of SVT that involve the main trunk of the great saphenous vein (GSV) or small saphenous vein (SSV).

Rx TREATMENT

NONPHARMACOLOGIC THERAPY

- Warm, moist compresses
- Do not restrict activity. Immediate mobilization with walking exercises

ACUTE GENERAL Rx

- Treatment guidelines for SVT are not well established because of the lack of controlled clinical trials. In general, the primary goal of management should be to prevent thrombus extension and the risk of venous thromboembolism. All other therapy is directed at patient comfort with analgesics and NSAIDs (in patients not receiving anticoagulants).
- In patients with migratory SVT, recurrent SVT, or SVT without varicose veins, the underlying condition should be investigated, and treatment directed accordingly.
- The most common cause of upper-extremity SVT is an intravenous catheter. Treatment starts with removal of the cannula and application of warm compresses. The resultant lump may persist for mos. No anticoagulant therapy is required.
- In patients with lower-extremity SVT in a varicose vein branch, control of pain with analgesics and the use of gradient compression stockings are usually sufficient. Patients are encouraged to continue their usual daily activities.
- Many investigators favor systemic anticoagulation when there is superficial thrombosis of 5 cm or more in length, the thrombus is within 1 cm of the saphenous junctions, or more than 5 cm of the saphenous trunk is involved, as shown by duplex ultrasonography. Anticoagulation is also reasonable for patients with SVT and cancer or previous DVT.
- The American College of Chest Physicians guidelines recommend anticoagulation for 45 days over no anticoagulation in patients with lower-extremity SVT within 1 cm of the saphenofemoral or saphenopopliteal junction.
- In the case of patients with varicose veins secondary to saphenous vein reflux, a catheter vein ablation procedure should be performed only after the acute SVT episode is over in order to avoid the thromboembolic complications induced by such procedures.

PEARLS & CONSIDERATIONS

SUPERFICIAL SUPPURATIVE THROMBOPHLEBITIS

- Superficial suppurative thrombophlebitis is associated with an intravenous catheter or multiple puncture sites secondary to IV drug abuse and is located primarily in the upper extremity.
- Clinical presentation is similar to that of nonsuppurative SVT but with associated fever, leukocytosis, and/or septicemia.
- Most cases of intravenous catheter sepsis are not complicated by suppurative thrombophlebitis; local IV catheter site infections occur in about 7% of cases and septicemia is found in only 1 of every 400 IV catheterizations.
- The incidence of peripheral vein suppurative thrombophlebitis is highest in patients with specific risk factors such as burns, steroids, and IV drug abuse.
- Treatment consists of antibiotics with adequate coverage of gram-negative rods and *Staphylococcus aureus,* including MRSA. Initial empirical treatment is with IV vancomycin 1 g q12h *plus* ceftriaxone 1 g IV q24h. Alternative regimen consists of daptomycin 6 mg/kg IV q 12h *plus* ceftriaxone 1 g IV q24h.

SUGGESTED READINGS

Available at ExpertConsult.com

RELATED CONTENT

Thrombophlebitis (Patient Information)
Deep Vein Thrombosis (Related Key Topic)

AUTHOR: **Frank G. Fort, MD, FACS, RPHS**

Thrombotic Thrombocytopenic Purpura ALG

BASIC INFORMATION

DEFINITION

Thrombotic thrombocytopenic purpura (TTP) is a rare autoimmune disorder characterized by thrombocytopenia and microangiopathic hemolytic anemia that can be associated commonly with other hallmarks such as neurologic impairment, renal dysfunction, and fever. The laboratory hallmark of TTP is a severe deficiency of the *ADAMTS13* factor (activity <10%).

SYNONYMS

Immune mediated thrombocytopenic purpura
iTTP
TTP
Upshaw-Schulman Syndrome

ICD-10CM CODE
M31.1 Thrombotic microangiopathy

EPIDEMIOLOGY & DEMOGRAPHICS

- About 90% of new TTP cases are seen in adults (mostly females between 18 and 50 yr).
- The incidence of new TTP is 3 to 11 cases per million population per yr. The prevalence is ~10 cases per million population.
- There is increased incidence in HIV/AIDS and during pregnancy.

PHYSICAL FINDINGS & CLINICAL PRESENTATION

- The disease often begins as a flulike illness ultimately followed by clinical and laboratory abnormalities.
- Most patients present with nonspecific constitutional symptoms (weakness, nausea, abdominal pain, vomiting).
- Purpura (secondary to thrombocytopenia).
- Jaundice, pallor (from hemolysis).
- Mucosal bleeding.
- Fever.
- Fluctuating levels of consciousness (caused by thrombotic occlusion of the cerebral vessels). However, one third of patients have no neurologic abnormalities.
- Renal failure and neurologic events are usually end-stage features.

ETIOLOGY

- Acquired TTP is an autoimmune disorder caused by autoantibody inhibition of *ADAMTS13* activity. Hereditary TTP (also called Upshaw-Schulman syndrome) is caused by homozygous or compound heterozygous *ADAMTS13* mutations (Table 1).
- Many drugs, including clopidogrel, ticlopidine, penicillin, antineoplastic agents (gemcitabine, mitomycin C), calcineurin inhibitors (cyclosporine), oral contraceptives, and quinine, have been associated with TTP.
- Other precipitating causes include infectious agents, pregnancy, malignancies, allogeneic stem cell transplantation, and neurologic disorders.

Dx DIAGNOSIS

DIFFERENTIAL DIAGNOSIS

It is challenging to differentiate TTP from other thrombotic microangiopathies given the significant overlap in clinical presentation, but this distinction is critical in selecting an appropriate therapy for patients.

- Disseminated intravascular coagulation (DIC)
- Malignant hypertension
- Vasculitis
- Eclampsia or preeclampsia
- Hemolytic-uremic syndrome (HUS) and atypical HUS
- Gastroenteritis as a result of a serotoxin-producing serotype of *Escherichia coli*

WORKUP

A comprehensive history, physical examination, and laboratory evaluation usually confirm the diagnosis (Fig. 1).

LABORATORY TESTS

- Severe anemia and thrombocytopenia (platelet count <50,000 or >50% reduction from previous counts)
- Peripheral blood smear (Fig. E2, Fig. E3) reveals numerous red cell fragments (schistocytes)
- Elevated blood urea nitrogen and creatinine
- Evidence of hemolysis: Elevated reticulocyte count, indirect bilirubin, lactate dehydrogenase, decreased haptoglobin
- Urinalysis: Hematuria (red blood cells [RBCs] and RBC casts in urine sediment) and proteinuria
- Peripheral smear: Severely fragmented RBCs (schistocytes). More than 4% RBC fragments in the peripheral blood
- No laboratory evidence of DIC (normal fibrin degradation product, fibrinogen)
- The diagnosis of hereditary TTP requires documentation of *ADAMTS13* deficiency and an absence of *ADAMTS13* autoantibody inhibitor, and confirmation requires documentation of *ADAMTS13* mutations. Diagnostic criteria for acquired TTP are the presence of microangiopathic hemolytic anemia and thrombocytopenia without another apparent cause. An *ADAMTS13* level indicating less than 10% of normal activity supports the clinical diagnosis of acquired TTP while moderately decreased levels of >20% suggest the presence of other diagnoses.

Rx TREATMENT

ACUTE GENERAL Rx

- Discontinue potential offending agents. Initiate *ADAMTS13* replacement by plasma infusion in patients with hereditary TTP.
- Current therapy for TTP is built on two complementary pillars: Therapeutic plasma exchange (TPE) and immunosuppression.
- In 1991, TPE was established as a modality that reduced mortality rates from >90% to <20%. Daily TPE with replacement of 1.0 to 1.5 times the predicted plasma volume of the patient is standard therapy for TTP. TPE should be continued for a minimum of 2 days after the platelet count returns to normal (>150,000 cells/m^3).
- High-dose plasma infusion (25 ml/kg/day) may be useful only if TPE cannot be promptly started and for patients with very severe or refractory disease between plasma exchange sessions. High-dose plasma infusions can cause volume overload in patients with renal insufficiency.
- Patients with hereditary TTP who experience severe plasma allergic reactions have been effectively treated with plasma-derived factor VIII concentrate that contains *ADAMTS13*.

TABLE 1 Etiology, Epidemiology, and Pathogenesis of TTP, HUS, and *ADAMTS13*-Related Parameters

	Congenital TTP	Acquired TTP	HUS
Etiology	*ADAMTS13* mutation	Antibody to *ADAMTS13*, endothelial cell activation	*Escherichia coli* or other microorganisms
Epidemiology	5-10 cases per yr per million	≤1 case per yr per million	1-5 cases per yr per million, mainly in children
Pathogenesis	Defective cleavage of vWF multimers, massive secretion of ultra-large vWF multimers, increased platelet deposition under shear condition, occlusion of blood vessels in microcirculation		Intoxication with Shiga-like toxin, damage of endothelial cells, enterohemorrhagic colitis, renal disorder
ADAMTS13 antigen	Very low or absent	Low or variable	Normal or moderately decreased
ADAMTS13 activity	≤5%-10%	≤5%-10% or variable	30%-100%
Inhibitor against *ADAMTS13*	No	Mostly yes	No

ADAMTS13, A disintegrin and metalloproteinase with a thrombospondin type 1 motif, member 13; *HUS,* hemolytic uremic syndrome; *TTS,* thrombotic thrombocytopenic purpura; *vWF,* von Willebrand factor.
From McPherson RA, Pincus MR: *Henry's clinical diagnosis and management by laboratory methods,* ed 23, Philadelphia, 2017, Elsevier.

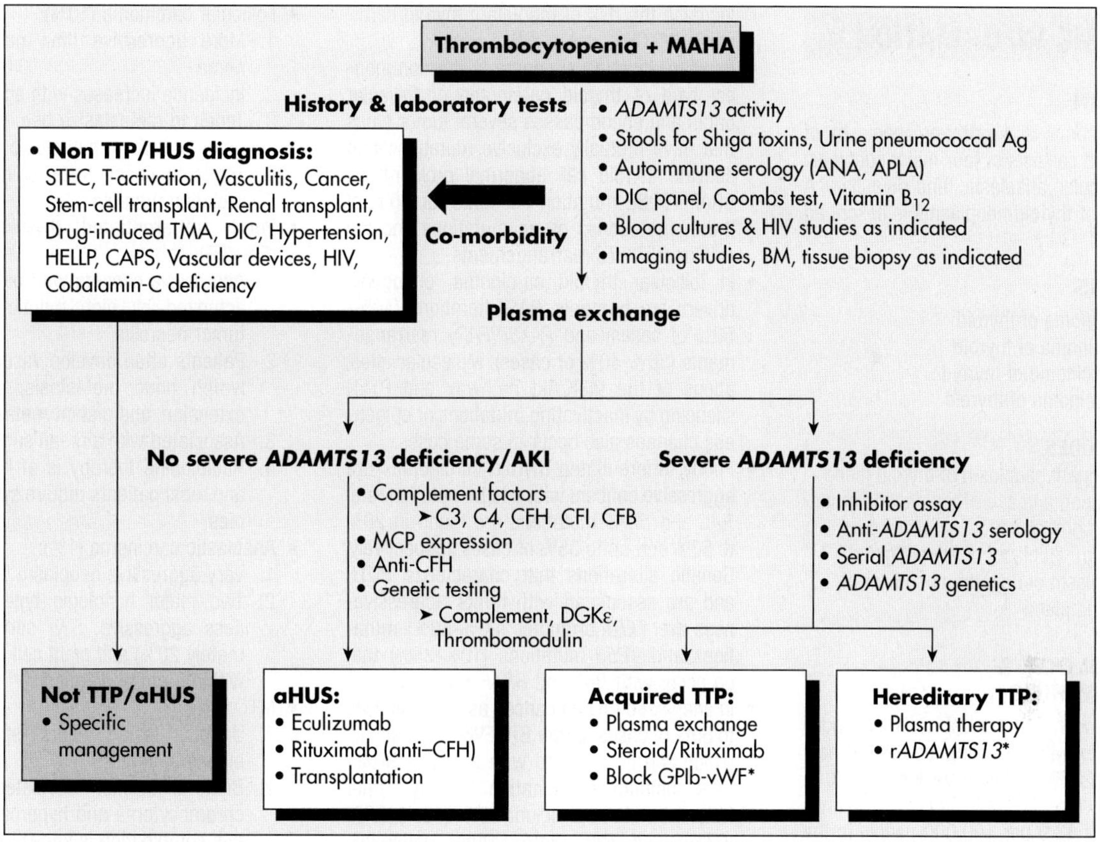

FIG. 1 An approach to diagnosis and management of thrombotic microangiopathies. *ADAMTS13,* A disintegrin and metalloproteinase with thrombospondin type 1 motifs, member 13; *Ag,* antigen; *aHUS,* atypical hemolytic uremic syndrome; *AKI,* acute kidney injury; *ANA,* antinuclear antibody; *APLA,* antiphospholipid antibodies; *BM,* bone marrow; *CAPS,* catastrophic antiphospholipid syndrome; *CFB,* complement factor B; *CFH,* complement factor H; *CFI,* complement factor I; *DGKE,* diacyl glycerol kinase ε; *DIC,* disseminated intravascular coagulation; *GP,* glycoprotein; *HELLP,* hemolysis, elevated liver enzymes, and low platelet count; *HIV,* human immunodeficiency virus; *HUS,* hemolytic uremic syndrome; *MAHA,* macroangiopathic hemolytic anemia; *MCP,* membrane cofactor protein; *rADAMTS13,* recombinant *ADAMTS13; STEC,* Shiga toxin-producing *E. coli*; *TMA,* thrombotic microangiopathy; *TTP,* thrombotic thrombocytopenic purpura; *vWF,* von Willebrand factor. *Bullet points* are diagnoses or therapies. *Indicates therapies under investigation. (From Hoffman R et al: *Hematology: basic principles and practice,* ed 7, Philadelphia, 2018, Elsevier.)

- Immunosuppression with the use of corticosteroids (prednisone 1 to 2 mg/kg/day) typically is administered concomitantly with TPE and tapered over a period of 3 to 4 wk after stable platelet counts are achieved.
- The monoclonal anti-CD20 antibody rituximab is traditionally used for treatment of suboptimally responsive TTP (inadequate platelet recovery after 3 to 5 days of TPE) and results in remissions in the majority of patients. Frontline use of rituximab results in shorter hospitalization with fewer relapses but results in overtreatment in many cases.
- Caplacizumab, an anti–von Willebrand factor humanized, bivalent, variable-domain-only immunoglobulin fragment, inhibits interaction between von Willebrand factor multimers and platelets. In a randomized trial,[1] treatment with caplacizumab and plasma exchange was associated with faster normalization of the platelet count and lower incidence of a composite of TTP-related death, recurrence of TTP, or a thromboembolic event during the treatment period than placebo. It has been FDA approved for use in combination with plasma exchange and immunosuppressive therapy for treatment of immune mediated thrombotic thrombocytopenic purpura.
- Recombinant *ADAMTS13* is being evaluated, and early data have demonstrated its efficacy in increasing *ADAMTS13* activity in congenital TTP and potential efficacy as an adjunct to TPE.
- Platelet transfusions are contraindicated except in severely thrombocytopenic patients with documented bleeding or those who are facing surgery or other invasive procedures in the setting of severe thrombocytopenia.
- Use of antiplatelet agents (acetylsalicylic acid, dipyridamole) is controversial.
- Splenectomy is performed in refractory cases.
- Dialysis is rarely required.

CHRONIC Rx

- Relapsing TTP may be initially retreated with TPE.
- TTP unresponsive to conventional therapy is usually effectively treated with rituximab and occasionally with chemotherapy agents (vincristine, cyclophosphamide, bortezomib).
- Splenectomy done while patients are in remission has been used historically to decrease the frequency of relapses.

DISPOSITION

- Survival of patients with TTP currently exceeds 80% with TPE.
- Relapse occurs in 20% to 40% of patients who have achieved initial remission.

PEARLS & CONSIDERATIONS

COMMENTS

- TTP should be considered in pregnant women with vague neurologic, gastrointestinal, or renal symptoms in either the obstetric triage or emergency department areas.
- TTP is fatal in 90% of patients without therapy.

SUGGESTED READINGS

Available at ExpertConsult.com

RELATED CONTENT

Hemolytic-Uremic Syndrome (Related Key Topic)

AUTHOR: **Bharti Rathore, MD**

[1]Scully M et al: Caplacizumab Treatment for Acquired Thrombotic Thrombocytopenic Purpura, *N Engl J Med* 380:335-346, 2019.

BASIC INFORMATION

DEFINITION

Thyroid carcinoma is a primary neoplasm of the thyroid and consists of four major subtypes: Papillary, follicular, anaplastic, and medullary. A classification of thyroid neoplasms is described in Table E1.

SYNONYMS

Papillary carcinoma of thyroid
Follicular carcinoma of thyroid
Anaplastic carcinoma of thyroid
Medullary carcinoma of thyroid

ICD-10CM CODES

C73	Malignant neoplasm of thyroid gland
D09.3	Carcinoma in situ of thyroid and other endocrine glands
D34	Benign neoplasm of thyroid gland
D44.0	Neoplasm of uncertain behavior of thyroid gland

EPIDEMIOLOGY & DEMOGRAPHICS

- Thyroid cancer is the most common endocrine cancer, with an estimated 52,890 new cases and 2180 deaths occurring in 2020 in the U.S.
- Incidence is 13.9 per 100,000 people in the U.S. and increasing over last 4 decades.
- Female:male ratio is 3:1.
- Median age at diagnosis: 45 to 50 yr.
- Occult thyroid cancer is identified in 20% of autopsy specimens.

PHYSICAL FINDINGS & CLINICAL PRESENTATION

- Thyroid cancer is often identified incidentally.
- Physical exam may reveal:
  - Presence of thyroid nodule
  - Hoarseness and cervical lymphadenopathy
  - Painless swelling in the region of the thyroid

ETIOLOGY

- Risk factors: Prior neck irradiation.
- Multiple endocrine neoplasia II (medullary carcinoma).
- Inherited syndromes associated with thyroid cancer are described in Table 2.
- GLP-1 receptor agonists for the treatment of type 2 DM (e.g., exenatide, albiglutide) can increase the risk of medullary thyroid carcinoma (MTC).
- Papillary thyroid carcinoma is the commonest type of thyroid carcinoma of follicular origin and encompasses several tumor types that have mutually exclusive mutations that activate thyroid cell abnormal proliferation. BRAF V600E mutation accounts for 60% of these mutations; other mutations include *RAS* or *RET/PTC* rearrangements.
- In follicular thyroid carcinoma, oncogenic drivers are primarily *RAS* alterations (40%-50% of cases) and *PAX8/PPARγ* rearrangements (30%-40% of cases). Molecular alterations of the PI3K/Akt pathway and PTEN silencing by inactivating mutations or epigenetic changes also occur in some cases.
- Poorly differentiated thyroid carcinomas are aggressive cancers with a high mutation rate. *RAS* and *BRAF* mutations are found in 20% to 50% and up to 35% of cases, respectively. Genetic alterations that characterize PDTC and are associated with tumor aggressiveness are *TERT* promoter (20%-50%) mutations and *TP53* mutations (10%-35%) that co-occur with *RAS* and *BRAF* mutations.
- In anaplastic thyroid cancer, as many as 25% to 50% of cases harbor BRAFV600 mutations, which can be targeted with available BRAF/MEK inhibitor combination therapy. Other frequent mutations include *TERT* (75%), *TP53* (63%), and *RAS* (24%). Other actionable molecular drivers with available targeted therapies include *RET* rearrangements, *ALK* rearrangements, *NTRK* fusions, and *TSC2* mutations, suggesting the need for broad molecular profiling.
- Pathways in the development of thyroid cancer are depicted in Fig. E1.

TABLE 2 Inherited Syndromes Associated with Thyroid Cancer

Multiple endocrine neoplasia (MEN) 2A and 2B
Isolated familial medullary thyroid cancer
Gardner syndrome
Familial adenomatous polyposis
Carney complex
Cowden syndrome
Familial nonmedullary thyroid cancer

From Cameron JL, Cameron AM: *Current surgical therapy*, ed 10, Philadelphia, 2011, Saunders.

DIAGNOSIS

DIFFERENTIAL DIAGNOSIS

- Multinodular goiter
- Lymphocytic thyroiditis
- Ectopic thyroid

WORKUP

The workup of thyroid carcinoma includes laboratory evaluation and diagnostic imaging. Key features of thyroid malignancies are summarized in Table 3. Diagnosis is confirmed with fine-needle aspiration or surgical biopsy. At diagnosis, the vast majority of thyroid cancers are well differentiated, with excellent prognosis. The characteristics of thyroid carcinoma vary with the type:

- Papillary carcinoma (80%):
  1. Most frequently occurs in women during second or third decades
  2. Histologically, psammoma bodies (calcific bodies present in papillary projections) are pathognomonic; found in 35% to 45% of papillary thyroid carcinomas
  3. Majority are not papillary lesions but mixed papillary follicular carcinomas
  4. Spread is by lymphatics and by local invasion
- Follicular carcinoma (10%):
  1. More aggressive than papillary carcinoma
  2. Incidence increases with age
  3. Tends to metastasize hematogenously to bone, producing pathologic fractures
  4. Tends to concentrate iodine (useful for radiation therapy)
- Poorly differentiated thyroid carcinoma (5%-6%):
  1. Aggressive cancers with pathology characterized by high mitotic activity and tumor necrosis.
  2. Patients often develop vascular invasion, lymph node metastasis, extrathyroidal extension, and distant metastases.
  3. Associated with a mean survival of 3.2 yr.
  4. Radioiodine therapy is of limited benefit and most patients require systemic therapies.
- Anaplastic carcinoma (1%):
  1. Very aggressive neoplasm
  2. Two major histologic types: Small cell (less aggressive, 5-yr survival approximately 20%) and giant cell (death usually within 6 mo of diagnosis)
- MTC (4%):
  1. Unifocal lesion: Found sporadically in elderly patients
  2. Bilateral lesions: Associated with pheochromocytoma and hyperparathyroidism; this combination is known as MEN-II and is inherited as an autosomal-dominant disorder

LABORATORY TESTS

- Thyroid function studies are generally normal. Thyroid-stimulating hormone (TSH), T4, and serum thyroglobulin levels should be obtained before thyroidectomy in patients with confirmed thyroid carcinoma. Serum thyroglobulin levels can be useful postoperatively to monitor recurrence of thyroid carcinoma (Fig. E2).
- Increased plasma calcitonin assay in patients with medullary carcinoma (tumors produce thyrocalcitonin). RET proto-oncogene sequencing and measurement of plasma free metanephrine and normetanephrine levels to rule out coexistent pheochromocytoma are recommended in all patients with medullary thyroid cancer.
- Fine-needle aspiration biopsy is the best method to assess a thyroid nodule (see "Thyroid Nodule" in Section I). Table 4 describes the Bethesda system for thyroid cytopathology.

IMAGING STUDIES (FIG. E3)

- Thyroid ultrasound can detect solitary solid nodules that have a high risk of malignancy. However, a negative ultrasound does not exclude diagnosis of thyroid carcinoma.
- Thyroid scanning with iodine-123 or technetium-99m can identify hypofunctioning (cold) nodules, which are more likely to be malignant. However, warm nodules can also be malignant.

TABLE 3 Thyroid Malignancies—Key Features

	Description	Pattern of Spread
Papillary carcinoma (70%-80%)	Low-grade tumors with a good prognosis (histologically multicentric) ▸ Tumors concentrate radio-iodine	Early lymph node spread (metastatic lymph nodes may be normal in size, cystic, calcified, hemorrhagic, or contain colloid) ▸ Distant metastases are rare (and usually to the lungs)
Follicular carcinoma (10%-20%)	Slow growing ▸ Tumors concentrate radio-iodine	It rarely metastasizes to the regional lymph nodes ▸ The tendency is to spread via the bloodstream and disseminate to the lungs, bones, or liver
Anaplastic carcinoma (1%-2%)	Undifferentiated malignant tumors that do not concentrate radio-iodine ▸ There is a poor prognosis ▸ They tend to occur in older patients ▸ Punctate calcification and necrosis frequently are present	Lymphatic metastases occur in the majority of patients
Medullary carcinoma (5%-10%)	This originates from the parafollicular C cells ▸ It does not concentrate radio-iodine ▸ It may be sporadic or familial (and associated with the MEN type II syndrome or other endocrine neoplasms) ▸ It is usually a unilateral, solitary lesion ▸ Calcification is seen in 10% ▸ ^{123}I-MIBG and somatostatin analogs (e.g., octreotide) can be used for evaluation ▸ Circulating calcitonin levels are usually elevated	It may invade locally, spread to the regional nodes, or demonstrate hematogenous spread to the lungs, bones, or liver
Lymphoma (10%)	It is usually a non-Hodgkin lymphoma ▸ It occurs in one third of patients with Hashimoto thyroiditis (a MALT-type lymphoma) ▸ It presents as a rapidly enlarging, solitary nodule (80%) or as multiple nodules (imaging cannot distinguish between a lymphoma and thyroiditis) ▸ Necrosis and calcification are uncommon	It can involve the nodes with spread to the GI tract
Metastases (<1%)	The most common primary is renal cell carcinoma	

From Grant LA: *Grainger & Allison's diagnostic radiology essentials,* ed 2, Philadelphia, 2019, Elsevier.

TABLE 4 The Bethesda System for Thyroid Cytopathology

Category	Risk of Malignancy (%)	Recommended Management
Nondiagnostic or unsatisfactory	1-4	Repeat FNA with ultrasound guidance
Benign	0-3	Clinical follow-up
Atypia of undetermined significance (AUS) or follicular lesion of undetermined significance (FLUS)	5-15	Repeat FNA*
Follicular neoplasm or suspicious for follicular neoplasm	15-30	Lobectomy
Suspicious for malignancy	60-75	Lobectomy with or without frozen section or total thyroidectomy
Malignant	97-99	Total thyroidectomy

FNA, Fine-needle aspiration.
*Lobectomy also can be considered depending on clinical or sonographic characteristics.
From Niederhuber JE: *Abeloff's clinical oncology,* ed 6, Philadelphia, 2020, Elsevier.

STAGING (TABLE E5)

- Stage I: Thyroid cancer of any size without distal spread in patient <45 yr. In patients >45 yr, tumor size ≤2 cm without local invasion or positive cervical lymph nodes
- Stage II: Distal spread in patient <45 yr. In patients >45 yr, tumors >2 cm but <4 cm without local invasion or positive cervical lymph nodes
- Stage III: Tumors >4 cm in patient >45 yr of age
- Stage IV: Distal spread in patient >45 yr of age

Rx TREATMENT

ACUTE GENERAL Rx

- Papillary carcinoma:
  1. Total thyroidectomy is indicated if the patient has:
     a. Extrapyramidal extension of carcinoma
     b. Papillary carcinoma limited to thyroid but a positive history of irradiation to the neck
     c. Lesion >2 cm
  2. Lobectomy with isthmectomy may be considered in patients with intra-thyroid papillary carcinoma <2 cm and no history of neck or head irradiation; surgery should be followed with suppressive therapy with thyroid hormone because these tumors are TSH responsive. The accepted practice is to suppress serum TSH concentrations to <0.1 microunit/ml in patients with persistent disease, suppression to 0.1 to 0.5 microunit/ml in patients who are disease free but are at high risk of recurrence, and a goal TSH level of 0.3 to 2.0 microunits/ml in patients who are disease free and have a low risk of recurrence.
  3. Radioiodine ablation reduces rates of death and recurrence (Table 6). Radioiodine is administered for stages III and IV disease.
  4. In cases that have progressed after radioiodine therapy, oral targeted inhibitors (lenvatinib, sorafenib) have significant survival benefit.
- Follicular carcinoma:
  1. Total thyroidectomy followed by TSH suppression, as previously noted.
  2. Radiotherapy with iodine-131 followed by thyroid suppression therapy with triiodothyronine is useful in patients with metastasis (see Table 6).
  3. In cases that have progressed after radioiodine therapy, oral targeted inhibitors (lenvatinib, sorafenib) have significant survival benefit.
- Anaplastic carcinoma:
  1. At diagnosis, this neoplasm is rarely operable; palliative surgery is indicated for extremely large tumor compressing the trachea.
  2. Management is usually restricted to radiation therapy or chemotherapy (combination of doxorubicin, cisplatin, and other antineoplastic agents) (see Table 6); these measures rarely provide significant palliation.
- Medullary carcinoma:
  1. Thyroidectomy should be performed, followed by TSH suppression.
  2. Vandetanib and cabozantinib are oral tyrosine kinase inhibitors that are FDA-approved for treatment of symptomatic or progressive, unresectable, locally advanced or metastatic medullary thyroid cancer.

TABLE 6 Indications for Iodine-131 Treatment in Patients with Papillary, Follicular, or Hürthle Cell Thyroid Carcinoma after Initial Definitive Near-Total Thyroidectomy

No Indication
Adult patients at very low risk for cause-specific mortality or relapse: Complete surgical resection, favorable histology, and limited extent of disease (e.g., PTC patients with MACIS scores <6; patients with tumor size <1 cm, N0, and M0).
Definite Indications
Distant metastasis at diagnosis
Incomplete tumor resection
Complete tumor resection but high risk for mortality or recurrence (e.g., PTC patients with MACIS scores ≥6 and pTNM stage II/III FTC or HCC)
Probable Indications
Incomplete surgery (less than near-total thyroidectomy, no lymph node dissection)
PTC or FTC in a child younger than 16 yr
If PTC, tall cell or columnar cell variant and diffuse sclerosing variant
If FTC, widely invasive or poorly differentiated tumor
Bulky nodal metastases

FTC, Follicular thyroid carcinoma; *HCC,* Hürthle cell carcinoma; *MACIS,* scoring system based on metastasis, age, completeness of resection, invasion, and size; *PTC,* papillary thyroid carcinoma; *pTNM,* pathologic tumor-node-metastasis classification.
From Melmed S et al (eds): *Williams textbook of endocrinology,* ed 12, Philadelphia, 2011, Saunders.

TABLE 7 Characteristics of Thyroid Cancers

Type of Cancer	Percentage of Thyroid Cancers	Age of Onset (yr)	Treatment	Prognosis
Papillary	88	40-80	Thyroidectomy, followed by radioactive iodine ablation and TSH suppression	Good
Follicular	10	45-80	Thyroidectomy, followed by radioactive iodine ablation and TSH suppression	Fair to good
Medullary	3-4	20-50	Thyroidectomy and central compartment lymph node dissection and TSH suppression	Fair
Anaplastic	1	50-80	Isthmusectomy followed by palliative x-ray treatment	Poor
Lymphoma	<1	25-70	X-ray therapy and/or chemotherapy	Fair

From Andreoli TE et al: *Andreoli and Carpenter's Cecil essentials of medicine,* ed 8, Philadelphia, 2010, Saunders.

3. Patients and their families should be screened for pheochromocytoma and hyperparathyroidism.

DISPOSITION

Overall 5 yr survival rate is 98.17, but prognosis varies with the type of thyroid carcinoma: 5-yr survival is over 80% for follicular carcinoma and is approximately 5% with anaplastic carcinoma (Table 7).

PEARLS & CONSIDERATIONS

COMMENTS

- Follow-up surveillance (Table E8) involves neck ultrasound 6 to 12 mo after initial treatment and periodically and lab evaluation with TSH, serum thyroglobulin (T8), and thyroglobulin antibody (T8 Ab).
- Family members of patients with medullary carcinoma should be screened; DNA analysis for the detection of mutations in the *RET* gene structure permits the identification of *MEN IIA* gene carriers.
- While there is little controversy regarding the benefit of radioactive iodine in iodine-avid advanced-stage well-differentiated thyroid cancer, the indications for radioactive iodine following total thyroidectomy in patients with very low risk disease is controversial. Proponents argue that its use may destroy microscopic metastases, while opponents counter that the risk of secondary cancer due to radioactive iodine is not warranted in patients whose prognosis is typically excellent.
- Metastatic thyroid cancers that are refractory to radioiodine (iodine-131) are associated with a poor prognosis.
- Small-molecule tyrosine kinase inhibitors, including vandetanib, cabozantinib, sorafenib, and lenvatinib, are now FDA-approved and have shown clinical benefit with improved survival in advanced differentiated and medullary thyroid cancer.
- Targeted therapy with a combined regimen of BRAF/MEK inhibitors (dabrafenib plus trametinib) is efficacious and approved in patients with metastatic BRAFV600E-mutated anaplastic thyroid cancer.
- In a subset of patients with anaplastic thyroid cancer, the immune checkpoint inhibitor pembrolizumab may be an effective salvage therapy when added to kinase inhibitors at the time of progression on these drugs. In patients with advanced, differentiated thyroid cancer, pembrolizumab has a manageable safety profile and demonstrates evidence of antitumor activity in a minority of treated patients.

SUGGESTED READINGS

Available at ExpertConsult.com

RELATED CONTENT

Thyroid Cancer (Patient Information)
Thyroid Nodule (Related Key Topic)
Multiple Endocrine Neoplasia (Related Key Topic)

AUTHOR: **Bharti Rathore, MD**

BASIC INFORMATION

DEFINITION

An abnormal growth of thyroid tissue detected on either physical examination or radiographic imaging.

ICD-10CM CODES

E04.1	Nontoxic single thyroid nodule or cyst
E04.9	Nontoxic goiter
E05.1	Thyrotoxicosis with toxic single thyroid nodule
E05.2	Thyrotoxicosis with toxic multinodular goiter
E05.11	Thyrotoxicosis with toxic single thyroid nodule with thyrotoxic crisis or storm

EPIDEMIOLOGY & DEMOGRAPHICS

- Thyroid nodules are present in up to 50% of the population.
- Only 5% of the population has a palpable nodule.
- Incidence of thyroid nodules increases after 45 yr. They are more common in women by a ratio of 4:1.
- The vast majority of nodules (approximately 95%), regardless of size, are benign.

PHYSICAL FINDINGS & CLINICAL PRESENTATION

- Anatomic: Characteristics of the nodule include size, firmness (ranges from soft to rock hard), mobility, presence of single or multiple nodules, and presence of enlarged cervical lymph nodes. Additional physical findings to look for include exophthalmos, which would suggest Graves disease, and hoarseness suggestive of recurrent laryngeal nerve dysfunction usually associated with advanced malignancy.
- Physiologic: Symptoms of thyrotoxicosis that can be seen with a toxic nodule or toxic multinodular goiter include palpitations, anxiety, insomnia, weight loss, and heat intolerance. The signs of thyrotoxicosis include tremor, lid lag, tachycardia, pressured speech, and restlessness.

ETIOLOGY

- Most nodules are benign. They can be solitary or multiple. Positive family history is common. Iodine deficiency is rarely a cause of nodule formation in developed countries, where salt is iodized.
- Malignancy risks include family history of thyroid cancer and prior head and neck irradiation. Indicators of malignancy: Nodule significantly increasing in size, regional lymphadenopathy, fixation to adjacent tissues, very young or very old age at onset, symptoms of local invasion (dysphagia, hoarseness, neck pain), male sex.
- Inherited syndromes: MEN II predisposes to medullary thyroid cancer and Cowden's predisposes to follicular neoplasms. Other syndromic causes include Carney complex, Gardner syndrome, and familial adenomatous polyposis.

Dx DIAGNOSIS

DIFFERENTIAL DIAGNOSIS

- Benign functioning or nonfunctioning thyroid adenoma
- Benign thyroid cyst
- Thyroid carcinoma
- Multinodular goiter
- Thyroglossal duct cyst (midline neck mass at level of hyoid)
- Epidermoid cyst (subcutaneous firm mobile mass)
- Laryngocele (superior lateral neck mass)
- Nonthyroid neck neoplasm (lymphoma or lymph node metastases)
- Branchial cleft cyst (lateral neck mass, often with a draining fistula tract)

WORKUP

Physical exam is helpful if there are overt signs of hyperthyroidism or malignancy, but these are uncommon. Diagnosis usually relies on laboratory tests, radiographic studies, and cytology. The first step is always ruling out hyperthyroidism, because functional nodules are almost never cancers, and therefore should not be biopsied. If blood work diagnoses hyperthyroidism, a radioiodine uptake scan should be ordered to determine if the nodule in question is functional. If it is, biopsy should be avoided, and treatment of a benign toxic nodule should be initiated. Otherwise, consideration of fine-needle aspiration (FNA) biopsy is necessary.

LABORATORY TESTS

- Serum TSH should be obtained in all patients with thyroid nodules. If suppressed, obtain free T4 and free T3 and thyroid scan to rule out "hot nodule," indicative of a hyperfunctioning adenoma. If the TSH is normal or elevated, consider biopsy based on ultrasonographic characteristics.
- Serum calcitonin is only recommended when suspecting medullary carcinoma (MTC), such as a patient with a family history of MEN II or familial MTC, or history of pheochromocytoma or hyperparathyroidism.
- If the patient may have Hashimoto's thyroiditis, check an antimicrosomal or antithyroid peroxidase antibody level to confirm (see "Thyroiditis" in Section I). These patients often have marked heterogeneity of the thyroid parenchyma on ultrasound, which can be mistaken for nodule disease.
- Molecular analysis of thyroid tissue is now commercially available, and it may be useful when FNA biopsy results are indeterminate. Several companies offer the testing, and in general they are beneficial as rule-out tests. They can be used to identify a subpopulation of patients with a low likelihood of cancer, thereby avoiding unnecessary thyroid lobectomy in patients with indeterminate FNA. These tests have a high negative predictive value for cytologically indeterminate nodules (95% for an atypia or follicular lesion of undetermined significance, 94% for a follicular neoplasm). It is less common to find a gene that is highly predictive of cancer, such as *BRAF, RET/PTC,* and *PAX8-PPAR* gamma. The presence of *RAS* mutations is not as helpful, as it is commonly found in benign follicular adenomas, noninvasive follicular thyroid neoplasms with papillary-like nuclear features, and follicular cancers.

BIOPSY

- Fine-needle aspiration (FNA) biopsy is the best means of distinguishing benign from malignant nodules, but it requires the availability of an expert cytopathologist.
- Decision to perform ultrasound-guided biopsy is based on size and ultrasound features. The American Thyroid Association guidelines for thyroid nodules tallies the number of benign or suspicious ultrasound features and then recommends biopsy or observation based on nodule size. The American College of Radiology has published a thyroid nodule scoring system called TI-RADS (thyroid imaging reporting and data system [Table 1]), which is used in a similar way. If the likelihood of malignancy is low, a 1-yr follow-up ultrasound should be performed.
- FNA is discouraged for thyroid nodules <1 cm in diameter unless there are highly concerning features, such as concern for tracheal or nerve involvement, or suspicion of metastatic disease.

TABLE 1 American College of Radiology Thyroid Nodule Scoring System: TI-RADS

Scoring and Classification	Recommendations
TR1: 0 points	TR1: No FNA required (0.3% risk)
TR2: 2 points	TR2: No FNA required (1.5% risk)
TR3: 3 points	TR3: ≥1.5 cm follow-up at 1, 3, 5 yr, ≥2.5 cm FNA (4.8% risk)
TR4: 4-6 points	TR4: ≥1.0 cm follow-up at 1, 2, 3, 5 yr ≥1.5 cm FNA (9.1% risk)
TR5: ≥7 points	TR5: ≥0.5 cm follow-up each year, ≥1.0 cm FNA (35% risk)

ACR TI-RADS is a reporting system for thyroid nodules on ultrasound proposed by the American College of Radiology (ACR) and is based on composition, echogenicity, shape, margin, and echogenic foci.
From Tessler FN et al: ACR Thyroid Imaging, Reporting and Data System (TI-RADS): white paper of the ACR TI-RADS committee, *J Am Coll Radiol* 14:587-595, 2017.

TABLE 2 Bethesda Classification System for Thyroid Nodules

Diagnostic Category Bethesda Classification	Risk of Malignancy	Action
I Nondiagnostic	1-4	Repeat biopsy after 4 wk; if very low risk, follow with ultrasound
II Benign	1-3	1-yr follow-up ultrasound
III Atypia (follicular lesion) of undetermined significance (AUS/FLUS)	5-15	Repeat biopsy in 3 mo; consider genetic testing
IV Follicular neoplasm	15-30	Thyroid lobectomy Consider genetic testing if nodule appears low risk or patient wishes to avoid surgery
V Suspicious	60-75	Thyroid lobectomy or total thyroidectomy
VI Malignant	97-99	Thyroid lobectomy or total thyroidectomy

Adapted from Cibas ES, Ali SZ: The Bethesda system for reporting thyroid cytopathology, *Am J Clin Pathol* 132:658-665, 2009.

- FNA biopsy is very low yield for thyroid cystic lesions because of a paucity of cellular material. Most asymptomatic simple cysts can be observed. Large compressive cysts, or those with a significant solid component, should be considered for resection.
- Previous endocrine, surgery, and radiology algorithms recommended biopsy of all solid thyroid nodules over 1 cm. Over the last 5 yr, there has been a marked shift toward risk stratifying nodules by their ultrasound characteristics using the TI-RADS scoring system or the American Thyroid Association risk assessment. Lower-risk nodules can be followed with ultrasound unless they cross certain size thresholds. Higher-risk nodules still follow the 1-cm cutoff for FNA biopsy.
- FNA biopsy results at most tertiary care institutions are now reported using the Bethesda classification system. The Bethesda Classification system (Table 2) estimates the probability of malignancy at histology based on FNA biopsy cytology and treatment recommendation.

IMAGING STUDIES

- Iodine uptake scanning is only indicated in patients with suppressed TSH levels to determine if the nodule is toxic or not.
- Ultrasonography is an inexpensive and effective modality to stratify malignancy risk.
- Ultrasound (Fig. E1) is useful to evaluate the size of the thyroid and the number of nodules, as well as their dimensions and characteristics. These include whether it is solid or cystic, echogenicity relative to normal thyroid tissue, irregular versus smooth borders, presence of calcifications, shape, and vascularity.

Table E3 summarizes ultrasound features of benign and malignant thyroid nodules. The three ultrasound characteristics most predictive of malignancy in solid thyroid nodules are shape taller than wide, microcalcifications, and hypoechogenicity, in that order. The positive predictive value for malignancy steadily rises as the number of suspicious ultrasound findings mounts. However, FNA biopsy remains necessary for a definitive diagnosis. Very low risk ultrasound features include simple cystic lesions and spongiform nodules (sponge-like in appearance with layers of solid and cystic contents). Ultrasound follow-up is reasonable in such cases without biopsy, although it is acceptable to biopsy spongiform nodules over 2 cm based on practitioner and patient preference.

Rx TREATMENT

GENERAL Rx

- Evaluation of results of FNA:
  1. Regardless of biopsy result, symptomatic compressive nodules, substernal nodules, and those causing tracheal deviation are all indications for thyroidectomy.
  2. Table 1 contains the guidelines for management of each of the possible results after FNA biopsy. Nondiagnostic biopsies contain insufficient cells and require repeat, unless they are obviously benign cystic lesions.
  3. Benign nodules carry a 5% false-negative biopsy rate and should be reassessed at 1 yr for growth. If they have grown more than 3 mm, repeat biopsy should be considered.
  4. AUS/FLUS carries a 15% risk of malignancy. Usually a repeat biopsy is performed at 3 mo in hopes of obtaining a definitive result. Genetic testing is a consideration.
  5. Follicular neoplasms are higher risk and usually warrant lobectomy.
  6. Suspected malignancy and papillary thyroid cancer are treated similarly with lobectomy or total thyroidectomy.

DISPOSITION

Variable with results of FNA biopsy. Once patients have had a benign biopsy and a 1-yr follow-up ultrasound shows no significant growth, they do *not* require annual thyroid ultrasound exams. They can be followed with an annual neck exam. If growth is detected or symptoms develop, repeat ultrasound is indicated.

REFERRAL

Surgical referral for possible FNA biopsy if nodule is solid and over 1 cm

PEARLS & CONSIDERATIONS

COMMENTS

- Most solid, benign nodules grow; therefore, an increase in nodule volume alone is not a reliable predictor of malignancy.
- Thyroid nodules incidentally identified on fluorodeoxyglucose-PET (FDG-PET) scan done for other disorders has a much higher malignancy rate (30% to 50%).
- Surgery is indicated in hard or fixed nodule, presence of dysphagia or hoarseness, and rapidly growing solid masses regardless of "benign" results on FNA.
- Suppressive therapy of malignant thyroid nodules postoperatively with thyroxine is indicated. The use of suppressive therapy for benign solitary nodules is controversial.

SUGGESTED READINGS

Available at ExpertConsult.com

RELATED CONTENT

Thyroid Nodule (Patient Information)
Thyroiditis (Related Key Topic)
Thyroid Carcinoma (Related Key Topic)

AUTHOR: **Peter J. Mazzaglia, MD**

BASIC INFORMATION

DEFINITION

Thyroiditis is an inflammatory disease of the thyroid. It is a multifaceted disease with various etiologies, different clinical characteristics (depending on the stage), and distinct histopathology. Thyroiditis can be subdivided into three common types (Hashimoto, painful, and painless) and two rare forms (suppurative and Riedel). To add to the confusion, there are various synonyms for each form, and there is no internationally accepted classification of autoimmune thyroid disease.

SYNONYMS

Hashimoto thyroiditis: Chronic lymphocytic thyroiditis, chronic autoimmune thyroiditis, lymphadenoid goiter

Painful subacute thyroiditis: Subacute thyroiditis, giant cell thyroiditis, de Quervain thyroiditis, subacute granulomatous thyroiditis, pseudogranulomatous thyroiditis

Painless postpartum thyroiditis: Subacute lymphocytic thyroiditis, postpartum thyroiditis

Painless sporadic thyroiditis: Silent sporadic thyroiditis, subacute lymphocytic thyroiditis

Infectious thyroiditis: Acute suppurative thyroiditis, bacterial thyroiditis, microbial inflammatory thyroiditis, pyogenic thyroiditis

Riedel thyroiditis: Fibrous thyroiditis

ICD-10CM CODES

E06.3	Autoimmune thyroiditis
E06.1	Subacute thyroiditis
E06.9	Thyroiditis, unspecified
E06.0	Acute thyroiditis
E06.5	Other chronic thyroiditis

PHYSICAL FINDINGS & CLINICAL PRESENTATION

- Thyroiditis typically has three phases: Thyrotoxic and hypothyroid (each lasting approximately 3 mo) and return to euthyroidism.
- Hashimoto: Patients may have signs of hyperthyroidism (tachycardia, diaphoresis, palpitations, weight loss) or hypothyroidism (fatigue, weight gain, delayed reflexes) depending on the stage of the disease. Usually there is diffuse, firm enlargement of the thyroid gland; the gland may also be of normal size (atrophic form with clinically manifested hypothyroidism).
- Painful subacute: Exquisitely tender, enlarged thyroid, fever; signs of hyperthyroidism are initially present; signs of hypothyroidism can subsequently develop.
- Painless thyroiditis: Clinical features are similar to subacute thyroiditis except for the absence of tenderness of the thyroid gland.
- Suppurative: Patient is febrile with severe neck pain, focal tenderness of the involved portion of the thyroid, erythema of the overlying skin.
- Riedel: Slowly enlarging hard mass in the anterior neck; often mistaken for thyroid cancer; signs of hypothyroidism occur in advanced stages.

ETIOLOGY

- Hashimoto: Autoimmune disorder that begins with the activation of CD4 T-helper lymphocytes specific for thyroid antigens. The etiologic factor for the activation of these cells is unknown
- Painful subacute: Possibly postviral; usually follows a respiratory illness not considered to be a form of autoimmune thyroiditis
- Painless thyroiditis: Frequently occurs postpartum
- Infectious (suppurative): Infectious etiology, generally bacterial, although fungi and parasites have also been implicated; often occurs in immunocompromised hosts or after a penetrating neck injury
- Riedel: Fibrous infiltration of the thyroid; etiology unknown
- Drug induced: Typically painless due to lithium, interferon-alfa, amiodarone, interleukin-2
- Radiation thyroiditis: Occurs 5 to 10 days after treatment with radioactive iodine; it is painful and may result in transient exacerbation of hyperthyroidism

DIAGNOSIS

DIFFERENTIAL DIAGNOSIS

- The hyperthyroid phase of Hashimoto, subacute, and silent thyroiditis can be mistaken for Graves disease.
- Riedel thyroiditis can be mistaken for carcinoma of the thyroid.
- Painful subacute thyroiditis can be mistaken for infections of the oropharynx and trachea or for suppurative thyroiditis.
- Factitious hyperthyroidism can mimic silent thyroiditis.

WORKUP

- The diagnostic workup includes laboratory and radiologic evaluation to rule out other conditions that may mimic thyroiditis (see previously) and differentiate the various forms of thyroiditis.
- The patient's medical history may be helpful in differentiating the various types of thyroiditis (e.g., presentation after childbirth is suggestive of silent [postpartum, painless] thyroiditis; occurrence after a viral respiratory infection suggests subacute thyroiditis; history of penetrating injury to the neck indicates suppurative thyroiditis).

LABORATORY TESTS

- Thyroid-stimulating hormone, free T4: May be normal or indicative of hypothyroidism or hyperthyroidism depending on the stage of the thyroiditis.
- White blood cell (WBC) with differential: Increased WBC with left shift occurs with subacute and suppurative thyroiditis.
- Antimicrosomal antibodies: Detected in >90% of patients with Hashimoto thyroiditis and 50% to 80% of patients with silent thyroiditis.
- Serum thyroglobulin levels are elevated in patients with subacute and silent thyroiditis; this test is nonspecific but may be useful in monitoring the course of subacute thyroiditis and distinguishing silent thyroiditis from factitious hyperthyroidism (low or absent serum thyroglobulin level).

IMAGING STUDIES (FIGS. E1 and E2)

24-hr radioactive iodine uptake (RAIU) is useful to distinguish Graves disease (increased RAIU) from thyroiditis (normal or low RAIU). Table E1 summarizes factors that influence 24-hr thyroid iodide uptake.

TREATMENT

ACUTE GENERAL Rx

- The duration of the thyrotoxic phase of thyroiditis is usually 10 to 12 wk. This phase is followed by a hypothyroid phase typically lasting up to 12 wk.
- Treat hypothyroid phase in symptomatic patients somatic with levothyroxine 25 to 50 mcg/day initially and monitor serum thyroid-stimulating hormone initially every 6 to 8 wk.
- Control symptoms of hyperthyroidism with beta-blockers (e.g., propranolol 20 to 40 mg PO q6h or atenolol).
- Control pain in patients with subacute thyroiditis with nonsteroidal antiinflammatory drugs. Prednisone 20 to 40 mg qd may be used if nonsteroidals are insufficient, but it should be gradually tapered off over several weeks.
- Use IV antibiotics and drain abscess (if present) in patients with suppurative thyroiditis.

DISPOSITION

- Hashimoto thyroiditis: Long-term prognosis is favorable; most patients recover their thyroid function.
- Painful subacute thyroiditis: Permanent hypothyroidism occurs in 10% of patients.
- Painless thyroiditis: 6% of patients have permanent hypothyroidism.
- Infectious thyroiditis: There is usually full recovery after treatment.
- Riedel thyroiditis: Hypothyroidism occurs when fibrous infiltration involves the entire thyroid.

REFERRAL

- Surgical referral in patients with compression of adjacent neck structures and in some patients with infectious (suppurative) thyroiditis
- Total thyroidectomy has been shown to improve symptoms in patients with Hashimoto thyroiditis who still have symptoms despite having normal thyroid gland function while receiving medical therapy.[1]

RELATED CONTENT

Thyroiditis (Patient Information)
Hyperthyroidism (Related Key Topic)
Hypothyroidism (Related Key Topic)

AUTHOR: **Fred F. Ferri, MD**

[1]Guldvog I et al: Thyroidectomy versus medical management for euthyroid patients with Hashimoto disease and persisting symptoms: a randomized trial, *Ann Int Med* 170:453-464, 2019.

Tinea Capitis

BASIC INFORMATION

DEFINITION

Tinea capitis is a dermatophyte infection of hair shaft and follicles of the scalp, eyebrows, and eyelashes. It is a form of superficial mycosis. Etiologic agents are fungal species of the genera *Microsporum* and *Trichophyton.*

SYNONYMS

Ringworm of the scalp
Ringworm of the head
Gray patch tinea capitis
Black dot tinea capitis
Tinea tonsurans
Herpes tonsurans
Kerion
Favus

ICD-10CM CODE

B35.0 Tinea barbae and tinea capitis

EPIDEMIOLOGY & DEMOGRAPHICS

- Tinea capitis primarily affects prepubertal children with peak age between 3 and 7 yr old. Adult cases are rare, possibly because of the fungistatic effect of the sebum found in older persons. Urban living, large family size, low socioeconomic status, and crowded living conditions may contribute to an increased incidence of tinea capitis. The elderly and immunocompromised individuals have an increased risk of infection. The incidence of the disease varies worldwide; however, it is relatively low in the U.S. It is reportedly widespread in parts of Central and South America, India, and Africa.
- In the U.S., peak incidence occurs in school-aged children of low socioeconomic status, with African American male children accounting for the greatest proportion of cases. About 3% to 8% of American children are affected, and 34% of household contacts are asymptomatic carriers.

PHYSICAL FINDINGS & CLINICAL PRESENTATION

- Classic triad of scalp scaling, alopecia, and cervical adenopathy. Table 1 summarizes clinical manifestations of tinea capitis in children.
- Most forms of tinea capitis begin with one or few round patches of scale (Fig. E1) or alopecia (Fig. E2).
- Primary lesions include plaques, papules, pustules, or nodules on the scalp (usually occipital region).
- Secondary lesions include scales, alopecia (usually reversible), erythema, exudates, and edema.
- Scalp pruritus may be present.
- Fever, pain, and lymphadenopathy (commonly postcervical) may occur with inflammatory lesions.
- Different clinical patterns of tinea capitis have been described:
  1. Gray patch: Lesions are scaly and well demarcated. The hairs within the patch break off a few millimeters above the scalp. One or several lesions may be present; sometimes the lesions join to form larger ones.
  2. Black dot: Early lesions with erythema and scaling patch are easily overlooked until areas of alopecia develop. Hairs within the patches break at the surface of the scalp, leaving behind a pattern of swollen black dots.
  3. Kerion (Fig. E3): Inflamed, exudative, pustular, boggy, tender nodules exhibiting marked edema, and hair loss seen in severe tinea capitis. Caused by immune response to the fungus. May lead to some scarring.
  4. Favus: Production of scutula (hair matted together with dermatophyte hyphae and keratin debris), characterized by yellow cup-shaped crusts around hair shafts. A fetid odor may be present.

TABLE 1 Clinical Manifestations of Tinea Capitis in Children

Clinical Feature	Comment
Scalp	
Alopecia	One or multiple patches; may simulate alopecia areata
Scaling	May be minimally inflammatory; may mimic seborrheic dermatitis
Erythema	Localized or widespread
Pustules	Differential diagnosis includes sterile folliculitis or bacterial folliculitis
"Black dots"	Alopecia with hair shafts broken off at surface of skin; may simulate trichotillomania
Kerion	Boggy, tender plaque with pustules and purulent discharge; represents a vigorous host immune response
Scarring	Rarely seen when untreated; usually follows kerion
Favus	Yellow, cup-shaped crusts around the hair
Other	
Lymphadenopathy	Common; cervical or occipital
Id reaction	Widespread, papular or papulovesicular eruption; extremity-predominant; usually seen after initiation of therapy; must be recognized as distinct from true drug reaction

From Paller AS, Mancini AJ: *Hurwitz clinical pediatric dermatology: a textbook of skin disorders of childhood and adolescence,* ed 5, 2016, Elsevier.

ETIOLOGY

Although fungi of the *Microsporum* or *Trichophyton* genera cause most cases of tinea capitis, causative species vary between geographic areas and across time. *T. tonsurans* is the predominant cause of tinea capitis, present in more than 90% of cases in North and Central America. *Microsporum canis, M. audouinii,* and *Trichophyton mentagrophytes* are less common. The most common causative species for black dot tinea capitis is *T. tonsurans,* while gray patch tinea capitis tends to be caused by *M. audouinii* and *M. canis.* Infection of the hair shaft is preceded by invasion of the stratum corneum of the scalp. Transmission of *T. tonsurans* occurs from person-to-person via infected persons or asymptomatic carriers, fallen infected hairs, animal vectors, and fomites. *M. audouinii* is commonly spread by dogs and cats. Infectious fungal particles may remain viable for many months. Even though the organism remains viable on combs, hairbrushes, and other fomites for long periods of time, the role of fomites in spreading the infection may vary in different geographic areas.

DIAGNOSIS

DIFFERENTIAL DIAGNOSIS

Seborrheic dermatitis and psoriasis may be confused with tinea capitis. Other conditions that resemble tinea capitis include alopecia areata, impetigo, pediculosis, trichotillomania, traction alopecia, folliculitis, pseudopelade, seborrhea/atopic dermatitis, psoriasis, carbuncles, pyoderma, lichen ruber planus, and lupus erythematosus; these should also be considered in the differential. Table 2 highlights distinctive features of conditions that may be confused for tinea capitis.

WORKUP

- KOH testing of hair shaft extracted from the lesion, not the scale, because the *T. tonsurans* spores attach to or reside inside hair shafts and will rarely be found in the scales.
- Wood's ultraviolet light fluoresces blue-green on hair shafts for *Microsporum* infections but will fail to identify *T. tonsurans.*
- Fungal culture of hairs and scales on fungal medium such as Sabouraud agar may be used to confirm the diagnosis, especially if uncertain.
- Histology of biopsies with fungal staining in cases where mycology tests are negative because of treatment initiation.

TREATMENT

- Griseofulvin is the gold standard FDA-approved treatment. Published studies show mean efficacy for griseofulvin treatment of about 68% for *Trichophyton* species and 88% for *Microsporum.* It is less costly than other drug options and has an excellent long-term safety profile. Micronized and ultramicronized preparations are absorbed better, and side effects are infrequent, especially when administered with fatty meals. Periodic monitoring of hematologic, liver, and renal function may be indicated, especially in prolonged treatment over 8 wk.
  1. **Children:** Griseofulvin is approved for children older than 2 yr of age: Microsize griseofulvin 10 to 25 mg/kg PO per day in one single dose or two divided doses (maximum, 1 g/day; for tinea capitis, higher doses [20-25 mg/kg/day] have been recommended) or ultramicrosize griseofulvin, 5 to 15 mg/kg PO per day

TABLE 2 Differential Diagnosis of Tinea Capitis

Disorder	Differentiating Features
Psoriasis	Red skin with thick, uniform, silvery scale, sharply demarcated; often psoriasis at other body sites also.
Dermatitis	Main possibility is seborrheic dermatitis: Usually more diffuse and has uniform fine scaling, rather than localized areas; doesn't typically cause alopecia or significant inflammation. May also be present on the face, especially the nasolabial fold, or as otitis externa. Atopic dermatitis is generally diffuse on scalp and almost inevitably present at other sites, but may coexist with tinea capitis, especially in children.
Pityriasis amiantacea	Thick sheets of asbestos-like scale, very adherent, generally a solitary patch. This may occur in various dermatoses.
Lichen simplex	Usually nape of neck; cobblestoned or lichenified skin thickening, with broken hairs that are not coated with scale.
Alopecia areata	Usually not inflamed (may be mildly so), not scaly, usually sharply defined. "Exclamation mark" hairs occur but are not coated with fungus; "cadaverized" hairs especially cause difficulty, as they mimic black dot alopecia.
Scarring alopecias	Examples: Discoid lupus erythematosus, lichen planus of scalp; cause perifollicular inflammation around intact hairs; usually associated with lesions at other sites also. Dissecting cellulitis of scalp is also in this differential.
Bacterial infections	Impetigo causes crusting but little inflammation, and hairs are intact; carbuncle is deeper and very tender but may be in the differential of kerion.
Trichotillomania	Broken hairs of unequal length, but hair shafts themselves and the scalp are normal.
Damage from hairdressing processes	Usually clear from the timescale.
Neoplasm	May be in the differential of kerion; usually slower-growing and mainly on elderly, balding scalp, whereas kerion is in children or young adults with previously intact hair.

From White GM, Cox NH (eds): *Diseases of the skin: a color atlas and text*, ed 2, St Louis, 2006, Mosby.

(maximum, 750 mg/day), in one single dose or two divided doses. Optimally, griseofulvin is given after a meal containing fat (e.g., peanut butter or ice cream). Recommended treatment length is 6 to 8 wk and should be continued 2 wk beyond clinical resolution (until hair regrowth occurs). Some children may require higher doses to achieve clinical cure.

2. **Adults and elderly persons:** Microsize griseofulvin 500 mg PO per day in one single dose or divided doses. The other option is ultramicrosize griseofulvin 375 mg PO per day in one single dose or divided doses. Recommended treatment length is 4 to 6 wk.

- Newer alternative treatments: Oral terbinafine, itraconazole, or fluconazole are comparable in efficacy and safety to griseofulvin, with possibly shorter treatment and better patient compliance. Preferred when resistant or when an allergy to griseofulvin is of concern. Monitoring of CBC, liver function tests, and renal function may be indicated.
  1. Terbinafine—4-wk course of therapy as effective as with griseofulvin. Dosages are 67.5 mg/day for patients weighing <20 kg; 125 mg/day for patients weighing 20 to 40 kg; and 250 mg for patients weighing >40 kg
  2. Itraconazole—3.5 mg/kg daily for 4 to 6 wk or pulse therapy of 5 mg/kg daily for 1 wk each mo for 2 to 3 mo (not approved for children)
  3. Fluconazole—the only oral antifungal agent approved for children <2 yr, 6 mg/kg/day for 6 wk in children (3-6 wk in adults) or 8 mg/kg weekly for 8 to 12 wk (cap at 150 mg weekly for adults)
- The adjuvant use of antifungal shampoos may be recommended for all patients and household contacts. Shampoo like selenium sulfide 2.5% used for 5 min or ketoconazole shampoo used 2 to 3 times/wk can help prevent infection or eradicate asymptomatic carrier state by inhibiting fungal growth.
- Severe inflammatory kerion can be managed with additional prednisone 40 mg daily (1 mg/kg/day in children) and tapering over 2 wk.
- Prompt treatment is indicated, as is examination of siblings and other household contacts for evidence of tinea capitis.
- Recommend follow-up visit every 2 to 4 wk with Wood's light, microscopic study, and fungal culture. A mycologic documented cure is the goal of treatment.
- Pets that are infected or asymptomatic carriers should be treated.
- Children receiving treatment for tinea capitis may attend school once they start therapy with griseofulvin or other effective systemic agent.

PEARLS & CONSIDERATIONS

- Systemic antifungal therapy is required for tinea capitis because topical antifungal medications are not effective.
- Shaving of the head, haircuts, or wearing a cap or scarf during treatment is unnecessary.
- Sharing of combs, hair ribbons, and hairbrushes should be discouraged.

COMMENTS

- Confirming the diagnosis of tinea capitis with a laboratory specimen is important because misdiagnosis will result in delay or improper treatment.
- Patients and their families should look for sources of infections and disinfect contaminated objects such as combs, brushes, towels, and headgear. Avoid sharing personal hygiene utensils.
- Culture of hairs and scalp dander facilitates carrier identification and prevention.

SUGGESTED READING

Available at ExpertConsult.com

RELATED CONTENT

Tinea Capitis (Patient Information)

AUTHORS: **Priya Sarin Gupta, MD, MPH, Nadine Mbuyi, MD,** and **Alvaro M. Rivera, MD**

Tinea Corporis (PTG)

BASIC INFORMATION

DEFINITION

Tinea corporis is a dermatophyte fungal infection caused by the genera *Trichophyton* or *Microsporum.* Tinea corporis includes all superficial dermatophyte infections of the skin other than those involving the scalp, beard, face, hands, feet, and groin.

SYNONYMS

Ringworm
Body ringworm
Tinea circinata

ICD-10CM CODE
B35.4 Tinea corporis

EPIDEMIOLOGY & DEMOGRAPHICS

- The disease is more common in warm climates.
- There is no predominant age or sex.

PHYSICAL FINDINGS & CLINICAL PRESENTATION

- Typically appears as single (Fig. E1) or multiple annular lesions with an advancing scaly border (Fig. E2); the margin is slightly raised, reddened (Fig. E3), and may be pustular.
- The central area becomes hypopigmented and less scaly as the active border progresses outward, thus the name "ringworm."
- The trunk and legs are primarily involved.
- Pruritus is variable.
- It is important to remember that recent topical corticosteroid use can significantly alter the appearance of the lesions.
- Tinea gladiatorum is a common problem for wrestlers.

ETIOLOGY

Trichophyton rubrum is the most common pathogen. Other common causes in the U.S. are *M. canis* and *T. mentagrophytes.* Table 1 summarizes common dermatophytes that cause tinea corporis.

DIAGNOSIS

DIFFERENTIAL DIAGNOSIS

- Pityriasis rosea
- Erythema multiforme
- Psoriasis
- Cutaneous systemic lupus erythematosus
- Secondary syphilis
- Nummular eczema
- Eczema
- Granuloma annulare
- Lyme disease
- Tinea versicolor
- Contact dermatitis

WORKUP

Diagnosis is usually made on clinical grounds. It can be confirmed by direct visualization under the microscope of a small fragment of the scale using wet mount preparation and potassium hydroxide solution; dermatophytes appear as translucent branching filaments (hyphae) with lines of separation appearing at irregular intervals.

LABORATORY TESTS

- Microscopic examination of hyphae.
- Mycotic culture is usually not necessary.
- Biopsy is indicated only when the diagnosis is uncertain and the patient has not responded to treatment.
- HIV (widespread tinea corporis may be a presenting sign of AIDS).

TREATMENT

NONPHARMACOLOGIC THERAPY

Affected areas should be kept clean and dry.

ACUTE GENERAL Rx

- Various creams are effective; the application area should include normal skin approximately 2 cm beyond the affected area:
  1. Butenafine cream applied qd for 14 days
  2. Terbinafine cream applied bid for 7 to 14 days
  3. Other effective topical agents are sulconazole, miconazole, clotrimazole, ketoconazole, naftifine, ciclopirox olamine, and efinaconazole
- Systemic therapy is reserved for severe cases and is usually given up to 4 wk; commonly used agents:
  1. Fluconazole, 150 mg once a week for 4 wk
  2. Terbinafine, 250 mg qd for 7 to 14 days
  3. Itraconazole, 200 mg/day for 1 wk

DISPOSITION

Majority of cases resolve without sequelae within 3 to 4 wk of therapy.

REFERRAL

Dermatology referral in patients with persistent or recurrent infections

RELATED CONTENT

Ringworm (Patient Information)
Tinea Capitis (Related Key Topic)
Tinea Cruris (Related Key Topic)

AUTHOR: **Fred F. Ferri, MD**

TABLE 1 Common Dermatophytes that Cause Tinea Corporis

Dermatophyte	Clinical Features
Anthropophilic	
Trichophyton rubrum	Commonly harbored by hair follicles; may produce concentric rings; can recur; causative organism in nodular perifolliculitis (Majocchi granuloma) and most common cause of tinea corporis
T. tonsurans	Commonly seen in adults who care for children with tinea capitis caused by this organism
Epidermophyton floccosum	Generally restricted to groin or feet; responsible for eczema marginatum
T. concentricum	Responsible for tinea imbricata; infections typically chronic
T. interdigitale (previously *T. mentagrophytes* var. *interdigitale*)	Causes interdigital tinea pedis, tinea cruris, and onychomycosis
Zoophilic	
T. mentagrophytes (previously *T. mentagrophytes* var. *mentagrophytes*)	May be associated with dermatophytid reaction; causes inflammatory tinea pedis and tinea barbae; associated with exposure to small mammals
Microsporum canis	Associated with pet exposure (cat or dog)
T. verrucosum	May mimic bacterial furunculosis; associated with exposure to cattle
Geophilic	
M. gypseum	Frequently associated with outdoor/occupational exposure; lesions may be inflammatory or bullous

From Bolognia J et al: *Dermatology,* ed 4, Philadelphia, 2018, Elsevier.

BASIC INFORMATION

DEFINITION

Tinea cruris is a dermatophyte infection of the groin.

SYNONYMS

Jock itch
Groin ringworm
Crotch itch

ICD-10CM CODE

B35.6 Tinea cruris

EPIDEMIOLOGY & DEMOGRAPHICS

- Most common during the summer in adolescent and young adult males.
- Males are affected more frequently than females; however, it has become more common in postpubertal females who are overweight or who often wear tight jeans or pantyhose.
- The infection often coexists with tinea pedis.

PHYSICAL FINDINGS & CLINICAL PRESENTATION

- It begins as a small erythematous, and scaling or crusted patch that spreads peripherally.
- Erythematous plaques have a half-moon shape and a scaling border.
- The acute inflammation tends to move down the inner thigh (Fig. E1) and usually spares the scrotum; in severe cases the fungus may spread onto the buttocks.
- Itching may be severe.
- Red papules, vesicles, and pustules may be present.
- An important diagnostic sign is the advancing well-defined border with a tendency toward central clearing.

ETIOLOGY

- Dermatophytes of the genera *Trichophyton, Epidermophyton,* and *Microsporum. T. rubrum* and *E. floccosum* are the most common infecting agents. Table 1 summarizes common causative agents of tinea cruris.
- Transmission from direct contact (e.g., infected persons, animals). The patient's feet should be evaluated as a source of infection because tinea cruris is often associated with tinea pedis.

DIAGNOSIS

DIFFERENTIAL DIAGNOSIS

- Candidal intertrigo
- Psoriasis
- Seborrheic dermatitis
- Erythrasma
- Contact dermatitis
- Tinea versicolor

WORKUP

Diagnosis is based on clinical presentation and demonstration of hyphae microscopically using potassium hydroxide.

LABORATORY TESTS

- Microscopic examination.
- Cultures are generally not necessary.

TREATMENT

NONPHARMACOLOGIC THERAPY

- Keep infected area clean and dry.
- Boxer shorts are preferred to briefs. The reduction of perspiration and enhancement of evaporation from the crural area are necessary prophylactic measures.

ACUTE GENERAL Rx

- Various topical antifungal agents are available:
  1. Butenafine cream, applied qd × 14 days
  2. Terbinafine cream, applied bid × 14 days
- Drying powders (e.g., miconazole nitrate) may be useful in patients with excessive perspiration.
- Oral antifungal therapy is generally reserved for cases unresponsive to topical agents or can be used along with topical agents in severe cases. Effective medications are fluconazole 200 mg qd × 7 days or 150 mg once a wk for 4 wk, terbinafine 250 mg qd × 14 days, or itraconazole 200 mg/day for 7 days.

DISPOSITION

Most cases respond promptly to therapy with complete resolution within 2 to 3 wk.

RELATED CONTENT

Tinea Cruris (Patient Information)
Tinea Capitis (Related Key Topic)
Tinea Corporis (Related Key Topic)

AUTHOR: **Fred F. Ferri, MD**

TABLE 1 Tinea Cruris: Common Causative Pathogens

Dermatophyte	Clinical features
Trichophyton rubrum	• Most common cause of tinea cruris • Infection tends to be chronic • Fungus not viable in scale (e.g., on furniture, rugs, linens) for long periods of time • Frequent extension to buttocks, waist, and thighs
Epidermophyton floccosum	• Commonly associated with "epidemics" of tinea cruris in locker rooms or dormitories • Infection is acute (rarely chronic) • Arthroconidia are viable in scale (e.g., on furniture, rugs, linens) for long periods of time • Infection rarely extends beyond groin region • Causative agent of "eczema marginatum" (well demarcated borders with multiple small vesicles or, sometimes, vesiculopustules)
T. mentagrophytes (previously *T. mentagrophytes* var. *mentagrophytes*)	• Infection tends to be more severe and acute, with intense inflammation and pustule formation • May rapidly spread to the trunk and lower extremities, causing a severe inflammatory condition • Often acquired from animal dander

From Bolognia J et al: *Dermatology,* ed 4, Philadelphia, 2018, Elsevier.

BASIC INFORMATION

DEFINITION

Tinea pedis is a dermatophyte infection of the feet.

SYNONYM

Athlete's foot

ICD-10CM CODE
B35.3 Tinea pedis

EPIDEMIOLOGY & DEMOGRAPHICS

- Most common dermatophyte infection
- Increased incidence in hot humid weather; occlusive footwear is a contributing factor
- Occurrence is rare before adolescence
- More common in adult males

PHYSICAL FINDINGS & CLINICAL PRESENTATION

- Typical presentation is variable and ranges from erythematous scaling plaques and isolated blisters to interdigital maceration (Fig. E1). The four major types of tinea pedis are summarized in Fig. E2.
- The infection usually starts in the interdigital spaces of the foot. Most infections are found in the toe webs or on the soles.
- Fourth or fifth toes are most commonly involved.
- Pruritus is common and is most intense after removal of shoes and socks.
- Infection with *Trichophyton rubrum* often manifests with a "moccasin" distribution affecting the soles and lateral feet.

Tinea pedis caused by *Trichophyton mentagrophytes* (interdigitale) can present with:

- Erythema and desquamation between the toes
- Multilocular bullae involving the thin skin of the plantar arch and along the sides of the feet and heel
- White superficial onychomycosis

ETIOLOGY

- Dermatophyte infection caused by *T. rubrum, Trichophyton mentagrophytes*, or less commonly *Epidermophyton floccosum.*
- There may be an autosomal dominant predisposition to this form of infection.

DIAGNOSIS

DIFFERENTIAL DIAGNOSIS

- Contact dermatitis
- Toe web infection (bacterial or candidal infection)
- Eczema
- Psoriasis
- Keratolysis exfoliativa
- Juvenile plantar dermatosis

WORKUP

- Diagnosis is usually made by clinical observation.
- Laboratory testing, when performed, generally consists of a simple potassium hydroxide preparation with mycologic examination under a light microscope to confirm the presence of dermatophytes.

LABORATORY TESTS

- Microscopic examination of a scale or the roof of a blister with 10% KOH under low or medium power will reveal hyphae.
- Mycologic culture is rarely indicated in the diagnosis of tinea pedis.
- Biopsy is reserved for when the diagnosis remains in question after testing or failure to respond to treatment.

TREATMENT

NONPHARMACOLOGIC THERAPY

- Hyperhidrosis is a predisposing factor for tinea pedis. Keep infected area clean and dry. Aerate feet by using sandals when possible.
- Use 100% cotton socks rather than nylon socks to reduce moisture.
- Areas likely to become infected should be dried completely before being covered with clothes.

ACUTE GENERAL Rx

- Benzylamines: Butenafine HCl 1% cream applied bid for 1 wk or qd for 4 wk is effective in interdigital tinea pedis.
- Allylamines: Terbinafine cream applied bid × 14 days, or naftifine 1% cream applied qd or naftifine gel applied bid for 4 wk produces a significantly high cure rate.
- Imidazoles: Econazole, ketoconazole, miconazole, luliconazole, and clotrimazole cream are also effective agents. Clotrimazole 1% cream is an over-the-counter treatment. It should be applied to affected and surrounding area bid for up to 4 wk.
- Ciclopirox and tolnaftate are other antifungal agents available in cream, suspension, or gel. Tolnaftate is also available as a lotion, spray, or powder.
- When using topical preparations, the application area should include normal skin approximately 2 cm beyond the affected area.
- Areas of maceration can be treated with Burow solution soaks for 10 to 20 min bid followed by foot elevation.
- Oral agents (fluconazole 150 mg once per wk for 4 wk, terbinafine 250 mg/day for 14 days, itraconazole 200 mg bid × 7 days, or griseofulvin 500 to 1000 mg/day for 14 days) can be used in combination with topical agents in resistant cases.

PEARLS & CONSIDERATIONS

- Use of tolnaftate powder (Tinactin) or Zeasorb medicated powder on the feet after bathing may be helpful in preventing recurrent tinea pedis in susceptible persons.
- Combination therapy of antifungal and corticosteroid (clotrimazole/betamethasone [Lotrisone]) should only be used when the diagnosis of fungal infection is confirmed and inflammation is a significant issue.
- Nystatin is not effective and should not be used.

RELATED CONTENT

Athlete's Foot (Patient Information)

AUTHOR: **Fred F. Ferri, MD**

BASIC INFORMATION

DEFINITION

Tinea unguium is defined as a persistent fungal infection affecting the toenails and fingernails.

SYNONYMS

Onychomycosis
Ringworm of the nails

ICD-10CM CODE

B35.1 Tinea unguium

EPIDEMIOLOGY & DEMOGRAPHICS

- Tinea unguium is most commonly found in people between the ages of 40 and 60 yr.
- Tinea unguium rarely occurs before puberty.
- Incidence: 20 to 100 cases/1000 population.
- Toenail infection is 4 to 6 times more common than fingernail infection.
- Tinea unguium affects men more often than women.
- Occurs more frequently in patients with diabetes, peripheral vascular disease, and any conditions resulting in the suppression of the immune system.
- Occlusive footwear, physical exercise followed by communal showering, and incompletely drying the feet predispose the individual to developing tinea unguium.

PHYSICAL FINDINGS & CLINICAL PRESENTATION

- Tinea unguium causes nails to become thick, brittle, hard, distorted, and discolored (yellow to brown color) (Fig. E1). Eventually, the nail may loosen, separate from the nail bed, and fall off (Fig. E2).
- Tinea unguium is frequently associated with tinea pedis (athlete foot).

ETIOLOGY

- The most common causes of tinea unguium are dermatophyte, yeast, and nondermatophyte molds.
- The dermatophyte *Trichophyton rubrum* accounts for 80% of all nail infections caused by fungus.
- *Trichophyton interdigitale* and *Trichophyton mentagrophytes* are other fungi causing tinea unguium.
- The yeast *Candida albicans* is responsible for 5% of the cases of tinea unguium and tends to involve fingernails more than toenails.
- Nondermatophyte molds *Scopulariopsis brevicaulis* and *Aspergillus niger,* although rare, can also cause tinea unguium.
- Tinea unguium is classified according to the clinical pattern of nail bed involvement. The main types are:
  1. Distal and lateral subungual tinea unguium (DLSO)
  2. Superficial tinea unguium
  3. Proximal subungual tinea unguium
  4. Endonyx tinea unguium
  5. Total dystrophic tinea unguium

DIAGNOSIS

The diagnosis of tinea unguium is based on the clinical nail findings and confirmed by direct microscopy and culture.

DIFFERENTIAL DIAGNOSIS

- Psoriasis
- Contact dermatitis
- Lichen planus
- Subungual keratosis
- Paronychia
- Infection (e.g., *Pseudomonas*)
- Trauma
- Peripheral vascular disease
- Yellow nail syndrome

WORKUP

The workup of suspected tinea unguium is directed at confirming the diagnosis of tinea unguium by visualizing hyphae under the microscope by KOH prep or by culturing the organism. Although the standard for the diagnosis of fungal nail disease is a positive result on microscopic examination and culture of nail clippings with subungual debris or from surface debris in superficial white tinea unguium, treatment is often prescribed in the absence of confirmatory findings.

LABORATORY TESTS

- KOH prep: Specificity is high, but sensitivity is variable.
- Fungal cultures on Sabouraud medium: Culture may take 4 to 6 wk.
- Dermatophyte test medium (DTM): An alternative to Sabouraud that takes only 3 to 7 days and can be done in office setting. A color change indicates dermatophyte growth.
- Nail plate biopsy with periodic acid–Schiff (PAS) stain.
- Blood tests are not specific in the diagnosis of tinea unguium and therefore not useful.

IMAGING STUDIES

- Imaging studies are not very specific in making the diagnosis of tinea unguium and not useful.
- If an infection is present and osteomyelitis is a consideration, an x-ray of the specific area and a bone scan may help establish the diagnosis.

CLASSIFICATION

- The Onychomycosis Severity Index (OSI) is a new classification system for grading the severity of tinea unguium.
- The OSI score is obtained by multiplying the score for the area of involvement (range, 0 to 5) by the score for the proximity of the disease to the matrix (range, 1-5). Ten points are added for the presence of a longitudinal streak or a patch (dermatophytoma) or for >2 mm of subungual hyperkeratosis.
- Mild tinea unguium corresponds to a score of 1 to 5; moderate to a score of 6 to 15; severe to a score of 16 to 35.
- Indicators of more severe onychomycosis are summarized in Table 1.

TREATMENT

NONPHARMACOLOGIC THERAPY

- Surgical removal of the nail plate is a treatment option; however, the relapse rate is high.
- Prevent reinfection by wearing properly fitted shoes, avoiding public showers, and keeping feet and nails clean and dry.
- Short-pulse laser therapy is fungicidal and is a newer treatment modality for tinea unguium. Most patients will require two to four treatments, each lasting 15 to 30 min. Laser therapy is useful in patients with contraindications to oral agents. It is, however, expensive ($250 to $1000 per treatment) and not covered by most insurance plans.

ACUTE GENERAL Rx

- Topical antifungal creams are used for early superficial nail infections:
  1. Miconazole 2% cream applied over the nail plate bid
  2. Clotrimazole 1% cream bid
  3. Ciclopirox: Topical antifungal nail lacquer can be used for moderate tinea unguium that spares the lunula. Success rate <10%
  4. Efinaconazole 10% topical solution (Jublia) is modestly effective in treating toenail tinea unguium due to *Trichophyton rubrum* and/or *Trichophyton mentagrophytes.* Dosage is 1 drop (2 drops for big toenail) once daily for 48 wk. Cost and formulary are limiting factors with this agent

TABLE 1 Indicators of More Severe Onychomycosis with a Poor Response to Treatment

Nail factors	• Subungual hyperkeratosis >2 mm thick • Significant lateral involvement • Dermatophytoma • >50% involvement of nail bed • Slow nail growth rate • Total dystrophic onychomycosis • Matrix involvement
Patient factors	• Immunosuppression • Peripheral arterial disease • Poorly controlled diabetes mellitus

Adapted from Carney C et al: A new classification system for grading the severity of onychomycosis: onychomycosis severity index, *Arch Dermatol* 147:1277-1282, 2011. From Bolognia J et al: *Dermatology,* ed 4, Philadelphia, 2018, Elsevier.

5. Tavaborole 5% solution (Kerydin) is an oxaborole antifungal drug approved by the U.S. FDA for topical treatment of toenail tinea unguium due to *T. rubrum* or *T. mentagrophytes.* It is applied to affected toenails once daily for 48 wk. It is modestly effective but much more expensive than topical ciclopirox 8% nail lacquer.

- Oral agents:
  1. Terbinafine:
     a. For toenails: 250 mg/day for 3 mo
     b. For fingernails: 250 mg/day for 6 wk
  2. Itraconazole:
     a. For toenails: 200 mg PO daily for 3 mo
     b. For fingernails: 200 mg PO daily for 6 wk
  3. Fluconazole: Not as effective as terbinafine or itraconazole:
     a. For toenails: 150 to 300 mg once weekly for 18 to 26 wk
     b. For fingernails: 150 to 300 mg once weekly for 12 to 16 wk
- All oral agents used for tinea unguium require periodic monitoring of liver function blood tests. Patients should be advised to watch for symptoms of drug-induced hepatitis (anorexia, fatigue, nausea, right upper quadrant pain) while taking these oral antifungal agents. They should stop their medication and contact their physician immediately if symptoms occur.
- Itraconazole is contraindicated in patients taking cisapride, astemizole, triazolam, midazolam, and terfenadine. Statins should be discontinued during itraconazole therapy. Itraconazole requires gastric acidity for absorption; patients should be advised not to take oral antacids, H_2 blockers, or proton pump inhibitors while taking itraconazole.
- Fluconazole is contraindicated in patients taking cisapride and terfenadine.
- Oral antifungal agents should not be initiated during pregnancy.

DISPOSITION

- Spontaneous remission of tinea unguium is rare.
- A disease-free toenail is reported to occur in approximately 25% to 50% of patients treated with the oral antifungal agents mentioned previously.

REFERRAL

- Podiatry consultation is indicated in diabetic patients for proper instruction in foot care, footwear, and nail debridement or surgical removal of the toenail.
- Dermatology consultation is indicated in patients refractory to treatment or if another diagnosis is considered (e.g., psoriasis).

PEARLS & CONSIDERATIONS

COMMENTS

- The growth of fungus on an infected nail typically begins at the end of the nail and spreads under the nail plate to infect the nail bed as well.
- Carefully consider the informational insert regarding drug-drug interactions and contraindications before initiating oral antifungal agents.
- Meta-analysis showed cure rates with the oral agents as follows: Terbinafine (about 75%), itraconazole (60%-65%), and fluconazole (about 50%).

SUGGESTED READINGS

Available at ExpertConsult.com

RELATED CONTENT

Nail Fungus (Patient Information)
Ringworm (Patient Information)

AUTHOR: **Glenn G. Fort, MD, MPH**

BASIC INFORMATION

DEFINITION

Tinea versicolor is a fungal infection of the skin caused by the yeast *Pityrosporum orbiculare (Malassezia furfur),* a commensal lipophilic fungus that lives in the hair follicles and stratum corneum.

SYNONYM

Pityriasis versicolor

ICD-10CM CODE

B36.0 Pityriasis versicolor

EPIDEMIOLOGY & DEMOGRAPHICS

- Increased incidence in adolescence and young adulthood
- More common during the summer (hypopigmented lesions are more evident when the skin is tanned)

PHYSICAL FINDINGS & CLINICAL PRESENTATION

- Most lesions begin as multiple small, circular macules of various colors (Fig. E1) on the trunk and upper arms.
- The macules may be darker (Fig. E2) or lighter (Fig. E3) than the surrounding normal skin and will scale with scraping.
- Most frequent site of distribution is trunk.
- Facial lesions are more common in children (forehead is most common facial site).
- Eruption is generally of insidious onset and asymptomatic.
- Lesions may be hyperpigmented in blacks.
- Lesions may be inconspicuous in fair-complexioned individuals, especially during the winter.
- Most patients become aware of the eruption when the involved areas do not tan.
- Mild itching and inflammation around the patches may be present.
- Facial lesions may occur in infants and immunocompromised patients.

ETIOLOGY

The infection is caused by *Malassezia* species (*M. globosa, M. restricta, M. sympodialis, M. furfur, M. obtusa,* and *M. slooffiae*). Factors that favor proliferation are pregnancy, malnutrition, immunosuppression, oral contraceptives, and excess heat and humidity.

Dx DIAGNOSIS

DIFFERENTIAL DIAGNOSIS

- Vitiligo
- Pityriasis alba
- Secondary syphilis
- Pityriasis rosea
- Seborrheic dermatitis
- Postinflammatory hyperpigmentation or hypopigmentation
- Pityriasis rubra pilaris
- Syphilis
- Hansen disease

WORKUP

Diagnosis is based on clinical appearance. The *Malassezia* fungus is easily demonstrated in scraping of the profuse scales that cover the lesions. Identification of hyphae and budding spores ("spaghetti and meatballs" appearance) with microscopy confirms diagnosis.

LABORATORY TESTS

Microscopic examination with potassium hydroxide confirms diagnosis.

Rx TREATMENT

NONPHARMACOLOGIC THERAPY

Sunlight accelerates repigmentation of hypopigmented areas.

ACUTE GENERAL Rx

- Topical treatment: Selenium sulfide 2.5% suspension (Selsun or Exsel) applied daily for 30 min for 7 consecutive days results in a cure rate of 80% to 90%. The scalp can be shampooed monthly with selenium sulfide to reduce scalp colonization.
- Antifungal topical agents (e.g., miconazole, ciclopirox, clotrimazole) are also effective.
- Oral treatment can be given along with topical agents but is generally reserved for resistant cases. Effective agents are fluconazole and itraconazole. Table 1 summarizes treatment options for tinea versicolor.

DISPOSITION

The prognosis is good, with eradication of the fungus usually occurring within 3 to 4 wk of treatment; however, recurrence is common. After initial therapy, use of monthly application of selenium sulfide may lower risk of recurrence.

PEARLS & CONSIDERATIONS

COMMENTS

Patients should be informed that the hypopigmented areas will not disappear immediately after treatment and that several months may be necessary for the hypopigmented areas to regain their pigmentation.

RELATED CONTENT

Tinea Versicolor (Patient Information)

AUTHOR: **Fred F. Ferri, MD**

TABLE 1 Treatment of Tinea (Pityriasis) Versicolor

Initial therapy (often combination)	*Topical** • Antifungal shampoo applied as a body cleanser for 10-15 min before rinsing, twice weekly for 2-4 wk 1. Selenium sulfide shampoo, 1% (OTC) or 2.5% 2. Ketoconazole shampoo, 1% (OTC) or 2% 3. Zinc pyrithione shampoo 4. Ciclopirox olamine shampoo, 1% • Antifungal cream applied several hand-widths beyond clinically visible lesions, daily to twice daily for 2 wk 1. Imidazole, e.g., ketoconazole 2% cream 2. Ciclopirox olamine 0.77% cream, gel, or lotion *Oral†* • Fluconazole: 200 mg PO daily × 5-7 days‡; 200-300 mg weekly × 2-3 wk; or 400 mg once • Itraconazole: 200 mg PO daily × 5-7 days
Maintenance therapy to prevent recurrence	• Treat previously affected sites with topical imidazole daily for 2 wk prior to anticipated sun exposure • Apply antifungal shampoo (see earlier) 1-2 times weekly

Oral ketoconazole is no longer indicated for treatment of superficial fungal infections due to risks of severe hepatotoxicity, QT prolongation, and serious drug interactions.
OTC, Over-the-counter; *PO,* by mouth.
*Treatment of all the skin from the neck down to the knees may lead to higher success rates.
†Although there are few comparative studies of oral antifungal medications, cure rates of 98% to 100% have been reported in several randomized controlled trials of itraconazole 200 mg daily × 5 days and an open-label study of fluconazole 300 mg weekly × 2 wk.
‡Based on authors' personal experience.
From Bolognia J et al: *Dermatology,* ed 4, Philadelphia, 2018, Elsevier.

BASIC INFORMATION

DEFINITION

Tinnitus is a perceived sound in the absence of acoustic stimulus external to the head. It may be unilateral, bilateral, or lateral dominant. It is commonly described as a ringing, buzzing, roaring, hissing, whistling, humming, cricket-like, or pulsing sound. It is frequently a symptom associated with hearing loss, Ménière disease, acoustic neuroma, drug toxicity, depression, or an autoimmune inner ear disease. The sound may be internal and perceived only by the patient, called subjective or tonal tinnitus, or it may be heard by both the patient and the examiner, called objective or nontonal tinnitus.

ICD-10CM CODES

H93.1	Tinnitus
H93.2	Other abnormal auditory perceptions
H93.11	Tinnitus, right ear
H93.12	Tinnitus, left ear
H93.13	Tinnitus, bilateral
H93.19	Tinnitus, unspecified ear

EPIDEMIOLOGY & DEMOGRAPHICS

PREVALENCE:

- The American Tinnitus Association reports 50 to 60 million Americans have tinnitus for >6 mo.
- Prevalence increases steadily with age, peaking for persons aged 60 to 69 yr.
- Prevalence in the U.S. based on National Health Interview Survey (NHIS) in 1996:
  1. 2.98% all ages
  2. 0.26% for persons <18 yr old
  3. 1.6% for persons aged 18 to 44 yr
  4. 5.96% for persons aged 45 to 64 yr: 7.7% males, 4.3% females
  5. 9.6% for persons aged 65 to 74 yr: 12% males, 7.7% females
  6. 7.6% for persons >75 yr: 11.4% males, 5.3% females
  7. 2:1 South/Northeast regions
- Up to 18% of people in industrialized societies are mildly affected by chronic tinnitus, and 0.5% report tinnitus having a severe effect on their daily life.
- Only 20% of patients with persistent tinnitus ever seek medical evaluation.

PREDOMINANT SEX & AGE: Persons most affected are male, Caucasian, elderly, persons with hearing impairment, persons living in southern U.S. For military veterans, tinnitus is the third most common service-related disability.

RISK FACTORS: Any condition causing hearing loss or damage to the auditory system can produce tinnitus. Cochlear damage from exposure to noise is the most common cause. Exposure to ototoxic drugs is also important.

PHYSICAL FINDINGS & CLINICAL PRESENTATION

- History should focus on exposure to loud noises, evidence of hearing loss, and ototoxic drugs.
- Patient should be screened for depression.
- Patient who complains of sound in ear may also complain of ear pain or fullness.
- Objective tinnitus is pulsatile and coincides with patient's pulse.
- Physical examination should focus on HEENT, neck, and neurologic exam.
- There may be no significant physical findings.

ETIOLOGY

- The mechanism behind tinnitus is poorly understood. It may originate at any point along the auditory pathway. Causes of tinnitus include injured cochlear hair cells, spontaneous activity in auditory nerve fibers, hyperactivity in the auditory nuclei in the brain stem, or a reduction in the suppressive activity of the central auditory cortex.
- Medications implicated in causing tinnitus include salicylates, NSAIDs, aminoglycosides, loop diuretics, valproate, quinine, chemotherapeutic agents, cisplatin, vincristine, and heavy metals such as lead.

DIAGNOSIS

DIFFERENTIAL DIAGNOSIS

- Subjective/tonal tinnitus:
  1. Otologic: Tympanic membrane disorder, inner ear disorder (hair cells, organ of Corti), Ménière disease
  2. Ototoxic medications
  3. Neurologic: Multiple sclerosis, head trauma, cochlear nerve lesion, acoustic schwannoma, neurofibroma, meningioma
  4. Metabolic: Thyroid disorder, hyperlipidemia (leading to plaque formation), vitamin B_{12} deficiency
  5. Psychogenic: Depression, anxiety, fibromyalgia
  6. Infectious: Otitis media, Lyme disease, meningitis, syphilis
- Objective/nontonal tinnitus:
  1. Vascular: Arterial bruit, venous hum, arteriovenous malformation, vascular tumors
  2. Neurologic: Contraction of muscles of the eustachian tube, contraction of the stapedius muscle, contraction of the tensor tympani muscles, or a palatal myoclonus, glomus jugulare tumor
  3. Conductive: Patulous (wide-open) eustachian tube

WORKUP

- Audiometry.
- Tympanometry.
- Electronystagmography is used to evaluate for Ménière disease.
- An algorithm for tinnitus evaluation is described in Fig. E1 and Fig. E2.

LABORATORY TESTS

Evaluate for metabolic abnormalities: TSH, CBC, B_{12}, and lipid panel.

IMAGING STUDIES

- CT/MRI: To evaluate for subjective tinnitus
- MRI/MRA: To evaluate objective tinnitus
- Imaging should not be part of routine management. Clinicians must distinguish patients with bothersome tinnitus from patients with nonbothersome tinnitus. For patients without persistent and bothersome tinnitus, audiometric testing is optional.

TREATMENT

NONPHARMACOLOGIC THERAPY

- It is best to avoid exposure to excessive noise, ototoxic agents, and to wear protective equipment in noisy environments, or mask the tinnitus through amplification of normal sounds with a hearing aid. Habituation techniques such as tinnitus retraining therapy may help. Cognitive-behavioral therapy helps patients cope with tinnitus distress through biofeedback.
- Recent trials involving brain stimulation in the form of repetitive transcranial magnetic stimulation (rTMS have shown reduction in the perception or severity of tinnitus).[1]

ACUTE GENERAL Rx

- If the tinnitus is severe enough to cause suicidal symptoms, immediate referral to a psychiatrist and an otolaryngologist is recommended to minimize the time to diagnosis and optimize treatment.
- Patients with persistent symptoms or tinnitus accompanied by visual changes or headache should be evaluated for tumors such as acoustic neuroma.
- Clinicians should not routinely recommend anxiolytics, anticonvulsants, or intratympanic medications.

CHRONIC Rx

There is insufficient evidence to support the use of any medication, vitamin, or nutritional supplement to treat tinnitus. Empirical use of over-the-counter supplements or prescription medications should be discouraged.

DISPOSITION

Clinical course is variable. About 20% to 25% of patients with chronic tinnitus consider it a significant problem. Individualized tinnitus management programs can be beneficial in most patients.

PEARLS & CONSIDERATIONS

PREVENTION

- Avoid loud, chronic noise and ototoxic drugs.
- Higher caffeine intake is associated with a lower risk of incidence of tinnitus in women.

RELATED CONTENT

Tinnitus (Patient Information)

AUTHORS: **Vicky H. Bhagat, MD, MPH,** and **Dawn Hogan, MD**

[1] Folmer RL et al: Repetitive transcranial magnetic stimulation treatment for chronic tinnitus: a randomized clinical trial, *JAMA Otolaryngol Head Neck Surg* 141(8):716-722, 2015.

BASIC INFORMATION

DEFINITION

The term *Torsade de Pointes* (TdP) refers to a polymorphic ventricular tachycardia (VT) associated with a prolonged QT interval and electrocardiographically characterized by QRS complexes of changing amplitude that appear to twist around the isoelectric line, hence the name *Torsade de Pointes,* or "twisting of the points" (Fig. 1).

Torsade is typically initiated by a short-long-short sequence of ventricular beats but can also be initiated by a short-coupled variant. Typically, TdP occurs in the setting of a markedly prolonged QT interval (>500 msec); the QTc prolongs even further during the long diastolic interval of a compensatory pause after an early beat, followed by an early PVC on the T wave, leading to a polymorphic VT with a ventricular rate of 160 to 250 beats per min, irregular RR intervals, and a cycling of the QRS axis through 180 degrees every 5 to 20 beats. It may be repetitive, nonsustained, or sustained and may degenerate into ventricular fibrillation. In some cases, the result is sudden cardiac death.

SYNONYMS

Torsades
TdP

ICD-10CM CODE
I47.2 Ventricular tachycardia

EPIDEMIOLOGY & DEMOGRAPHICS

INCIDENCE: The precise incidence of TdP is unclear but accounts for fewer than 5% of all sudden cardiac arrests. In congenital long QT syndromes (LQTS), TdP may occur in up to 6% of cases at rest and 9% of cases during an exercise test. Among drug-induced causes of TdP, the incidence may vary between <1% in cases of antibiotics and antipsychotics to 2% to 4% when caused by class III antiarrhythmics such as sotalol, ibutilide, and dofetilide.

PREDOMINANT SEX & AGE: Because testosterone shortens the QT interval, women have a longer baseline QT interval, which is believed to be the reason for a two- to threefold increased incidence of TdP in women.

GENETICS:

- Of the congenital LQTS channelopathies, long QT syndromes 1, 2, and 3 account for >70% of all cases. In general, the risk of TdP increases as the QT lengthens; however, there are also genotype-phenotype relationships that help define risk; for example, LQTS3 carries a higher risk of TdP than LQTS1. Similarly, the Jervell and Lange-Nielsen syndrome and Romano-Ward syndrome may lead to TdP.
- It is also likely that genetic factors are at play in acquired LQT and in the development of TdP. For example, in large populations, the QT interval prolongs very little with the administration of QT-prolonging drugs such as fluoroquinolones; however, certain individuals will have markedly exaggerated QT prolongation that leads to TdP; this is likely due to some underlying genetic factor.

RISK FACTORS:

- TdP in patients with congenital LQTS is often initiated by an external trigger (Table 1). Triggers can include exercise, noise, emotion, sudden waking from sleep by an alarm clock, telephone ringing, thunder, swimming, or diving. TdP in LQT1 patients is classically triggered by vigorous exercise or swimming; in LQT2 by emotion, pregnancy, or noise; and in LQT3 when at rest or asleep. Risk factors for drug-induced TdP are outlined in Table 2.
- The risk factors for developing TdP in patients with acquired long QT are extensive and are outlined in Table 3.

PATHOPHYSIOLOGY

- Changes in the balance of transmembrane ionic currents lead to lengthening of the QT interval and to abnormal action potentials called early afterdepolarizations (EADs). An EAD, in the setting of electrical instability induced by the prolonged QT, initiates the torsades. Perpetuation may be caused by transmural entry, triggered activity, or abnormal automaticity. A distinct group of cells called the M cells, located in the mid-myocardium, has a less rapid delayed rectifier potassium current (IKr), and these cells are central to the genesis of TdP.
- Drugs with the potential to cause TdP most frequently inhibit the rapid potassium channels and result in prolongation of the action potential duration, producing a prolonged QT on ECG.

PHYSICAL FINDINGS & CLINICAL PRESENTATION

- Clinical features depend on whether the TdP is caused by acquired or congenital long QT syndrome. Congenital LQTS patients may have certain specific triggers, such as noise, exercise, and emotions (see "Risk Factors").
- Symptoms of the tachycardia itself include palpitations, pre-syncope, syncope (sometimes with jerking movements from myoclonus, often misinterpreted as seizures), and sudden cardiac death (SCD).
- Patients resuscitated from SCD have an especially ominous prognosis, with a relative risk of 12.9% of experiencing another cardiac arrest.

ETIOLOGY

The etiology or triggers of TdP may be congenital or acquired causes of QT prolongation (see Table 1). For a comprehensive list of drugs that can cause or have the potential to cause TdP, see "Patient/Family Education."

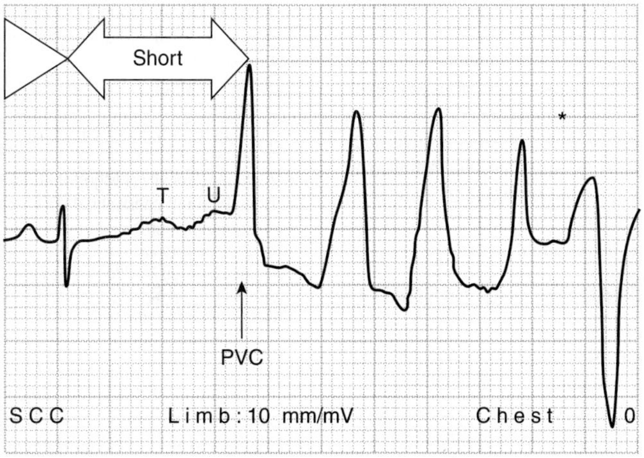

FIG. 1 Onset of Torsade de Pointes during the recording of a standard 12-lead electrocardiogram (ECG) in a young male with a history of drug addiction treated with chronic methadone therapy who presented to a hospital emergency department after ingesting an overdose of prescription and over-the-counter drugs from his parent's drug cabinet. Classic ECG features evident in this rhythm strip include a prolonged QT interval with distorted T-U complex, initiation of the arrhythmia after a short-long-short cycle sequence by a PVC that falls near the peak of the distorted T-U complex, "warm-up" phenomenon with initial R-R cycles longer than subsequent cycles, and abrupt switching of QRS morphology from predominantly positive to predominantly negative complexes *(asterisk).* (From Drew BJ et al: Prevention of Torsade de Pointes in hospital settings: a scientific statement from the American Heart Association and the American College of Cardiology Foundation, *J Am Coll Cardiol* 55:934-947, 2010.)

DIAGNOSIS

DIFFERENTIAL DIAGNOSIS

Other causes of syncope:

- Other causes of broad complex tachycardia such as:
  1. Polymorphic VT
  2. Wolff-Parkinson-White (WPW) syndrome with rapid atrial fibrillation
  3. ECG artifact

WORKUP

- ECG (Fig. 2) and telemetry are the mainstays of diagnosing TdP as they detect the arrhythmia, the preceding prolonged QT interval, and the long-short cycles that trigger it.
- Determination and treatment of the etiology of TdP (see Table 1) is key.

TABLE 1 Causes and Triggers of Torsade de Pointes

Congenital	• Romano-Ward syndrome (autosomal dominant) • Jervell and Lange-Nielsen syndrome (autosomal recessive) • LQTS channelopathies
Acquired	
Metabolic syndromes	• Hypokalemia • Hypocalcemia • Hypomagnesemia • Starvation • Anorexia nervosa • Liquid protein diets • Hypothyroidism
Bradyarrhythmias	• Sinus node dysfunction • Second- or third-degree AV block
Antiarrhythmic drugs	• Quinidine • Procainamide • Disopyramide • Amiodarone and dronedarone • Sotalol • Dofetilide, ibutilide, azimilide
Antimicrobial drugs	• Erythromycin, clarithromycin, azithromycin • Pentamidine • Azole antifungals like voriconazole • Fluoroquinolones such as levofloxacin and moxifloxacin • Chloroquine
Antihistaminics	• Terfenadine • Astemizole
Psychiatric drugs	• Phenothiazines • Thioridazine • Tricyclic antidepressants • Haloperidol • Risperidone • Selective serotonin reuptake inhibitors
Antineoplastic agents	• Tyrosine kinase inhibitors such as sunitinib, dasatinib • Vorinostat • Arsenic
Gastric motility agents	• Cisapride, domperidone
Opioid dependence drugs	• Methadone
Other factors	• Myocardial ischemia • Hypothermia • Intracranial disease • HIV infection • Connective tissue disease with anti-Ro/SSA antibodies • Periodic paralysis (Andersen syndrome) • Cocaine

TABLE 2 Risk Factors for Drug-Induced Torsade de Pointes

- Congenital long QT
- Female gender
- Electrolyte abnormalities (hypokalemia, hypomagnesemia, hypocalcemia)
- Diuretic use
- Bradycardia
- Cardiac hypertrophy
- Myocardial fibrosis
- Congestive heart failure
- Renal and liver insufficiency
- Coadministration of drugs blocking P450 isoenzyme CYP3A4
- High doses or rapid intravenous infusion of the drug
- Baseline electrocardiographic abnormalities (prolonged QT, T-wave lability)

From Gowda RM et al: Torsades de Pointes: the clinical considerations, *Int J Cardiol* 96(1):1-6, 2004.

TABLE 3 Risk Factors for Torsade de Pointes in Hospitalized Patients

- Clinically recognizable risk factors
- QTc >500 msec
- LQT2-type repolarization: Notched or "bifid" T-wave
- Use of QT-prolonging drugs
- Concurrent use of more than one QT-prolonging drug
- Rapid infusion by intravenous route
- Structural heart disease
- Congestive heart failure
- Myocardial infarction
- Advanced age
- Female sex
- Hypokalemia
- Hypomagnesemia
- Hypocalcemia
- Treatment with diuretics
- Impaired hepatic drug metabolism
- Bradycardia
- Sinus bradycardia, heart block, incomplete heart block with pauses
- Premature QRS complexes leading to short-long-short cycles
- Multiple clinically recognizable risk factors
- Occult (latent) congenital LQTS
- Genetic polymorphisms

From Drew BJ et al: Prevention of Torsade de Pointes in hospital settings: a scientific statement from the American Heart Association and the American College of Cardiology Foundation, *Circulation* 121(8):1047, 2010.

LABORATORY TESTS

- Electrolytes: Assess for hypokalemia, hypocalcemia, and hypomagnesemia
- Thyroid function tests
- Genetic studies if suspicion of congenital LQT syndrome

IMAGING STUDIES

- Echocardiography to rule out structural heart disease as a cause of VT
- Stress test to rule out myocardial ischemia. Stress ECG with dynamic assessment of the QT interval during varying heart rates may be diagnostic of long QT syndromes and related TdP
- CT scan of the head if intracranial disease is suspected

Rx TREATMENT

The cornerstone of treatment comprises intravenous magnesium and acceleration of the heart rate, either by mechanical overdrive pacing or by infusion of isoproterenol. Withdrawal of causative drugs and correction of underlying causes such as electrolyte imbalances, hypothermia, and ischemia are also important.

NONPHARMACOLOGIC THERAPY

- Withdrawal of any offending drugs and correction of electrolyte abnormalities are recommended in patients presenting with TdP (Class I recommendation).
- Temporary atrial or ventricular overdrive pacing is a Class I recommendation for all causes of TdP if intravenous magnesium fails.
- Acute and long-term pacing is recommended for patients presenting with TdP due to heart block and symptomatic bradycardia (Class 1) or those with recurrent pause-dependent torsades (Class IIa).
- Active internal and external rewarming if hypothermia is the etiology.
- If TdP degenerates into ventricular fibrillation, defibrillation and advanced cardiac life support protocol should be followed.

ACUTE GENERAL Rx

- Intravenous magnesium sulfate 1 to 2 g given over 1 to 2 min is first-line therapy for patients who present with LQTS and few episodes of TdP (Class IIa). Magnesium is not likely to be effective in patients with a normal QT interval.
- Isoproterenol is reasonable as temporary treatment in patients with acute disease who

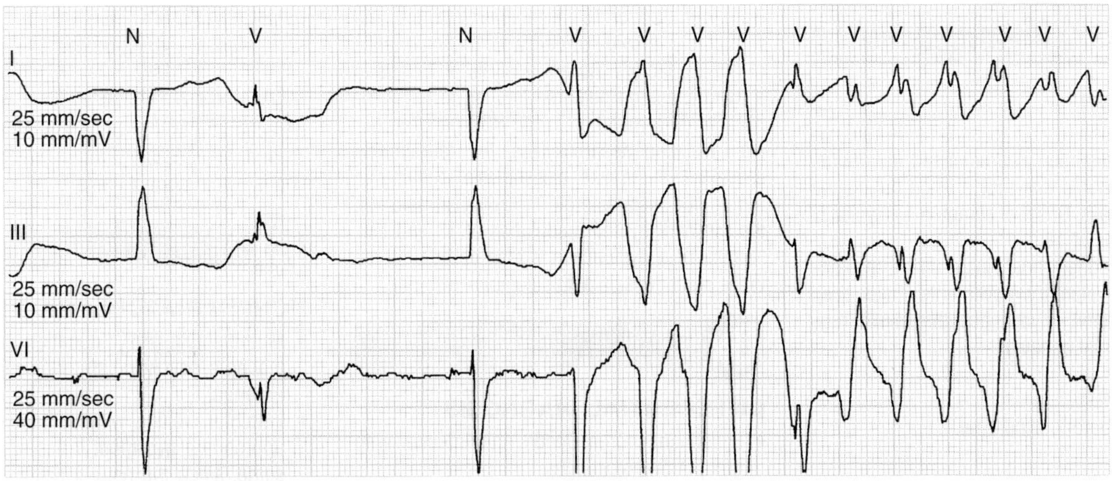

FIG. 2 Torsade de Pointes. This lead I, III, and V_1 rhythm strip shows sinus bradycardia with left bundle branch block and marked QT prolongation with premature ventricular contractions (R-on-T) that initiates a very rapid polymorphic ventricular tachycardia with the characteristic twisting of the QRS complex around the isoelectric baseline. Torsade de Pointes literally means "twisting of the points." (From Olshansky B et al: *Arrhythmia essentials,* ed 2, Philadelphia, 2017, Elsevier.)

present with recurrent pause-dependent TdP and who do not have congenital LQTS (Class IIa).
- Beta-blockade combined with pacing is reasonable acute therapy for patients who present with TdP and sinus bradycardia (Class IIa).
- Potassium repletion to 4.5 to 5 mmol/L may be considered for patients who present with TdP and hypokalemia (Class IIb).
- Intravenous lidocaine, oral mexiletine, or phenytoin may be considered in patients who present with LQT3 and TdP (Class IIb).
- TdP is usually self-limited, and cardioversion should be performed only as a last resort in the setting of pulseless VF because of the high likelihood of immediate recurrence of the TdP after cardioversion.

CHRONIC Rx

- TdP resulting from congenital LQTS is treated with beta-blockade (propranolol or nadolol are preferred), pacing, and implantable cardioverter-defibrillator (ICD) in high-risk cases. For patients who continue to have syncope despite maximal drug therapy, cervical-thoracic sympathectomy may be considered.
- Long-term pacing is recommended for patients presenting with TdP due to heart block and symptomatic bradycardia.
- Avoid use of QT-prolonging drugs.
- Lifestyle modification in case of congenital LQTS.
- In patients with eating disorders, nutritional rehabilitation will correct the QT prolongation over the long term (3-18 mo).
- Psychiatric evaluation of patients with drug overdose and eating disorders.

DISPOSITION

Patients with TdP should be monitored in an intensive care setting.

REFERRAL

Patients should have an urgent cardiology consultation.

PEARLS & CONSIDERATIONS

COMMENTS

- Identification of the etiology for TdP is key in diagnosis, management, and prognosis of this condition.
- Drugs associated with TdP vary greatly in their risk for arrhythmia; an updated list can be found at https://crediblemeds.org. The risk-benefit ratio should be assessed for each individual to determine whether the potential therapeutic benefit of a drug outweighs the risk for TdP.
- Risk factors for drug-induced TdP include older age, female sex, heart disease, electrolyte disorders (especially hypokalemia and hypomagnesemia), renal or hepatic dysfunction, bradycardia or rhythms with long pauses, treatment with more than one QT-prolonging drug, and genetic predisposition.
- After initiation of a drug associated with TdP, ECG signs indicative of risk for arrhythmia include an increase in QTc from predrug baseline of >60 msec, marked QTc interval prolongation >500 msec, T-U wave distortion that becomes more exaggerated in the beat after a pause, visible T-wave alternans, new-onset ventricular ectopy, and couplets and nonsustained polymorphic ventricular tachycardia initiated in the beat after a pause.

PREVENTION

The 2011 AHA/ACC scientific statement on prevention of TdP suggests a strategy of documenting the QTc interval before and at least every 8 to 12 hr after the initiation, increased dose, or overdose of QT-prolonging drugs. If QTc prolongation is observed, documentation of more frequent measurements is recommended. The duration of QTc monitoring depends upon the duration of treatment with the QT-prolonging drug and the drug half-life.

PATIENT & FAMILY EDUCATION

- Patients should be educated about avoiding use of QT-prolonging drugs. A complete list of these drugs can be found at https://crediblemeds.org.
- First-degree relatives of all patients with congenital LQTS should undergo genetic testing.
- Congenital LQTS patients should avoid certain specific triggers (e.g., swimming and exercise in LQTS 1 and LQTS 2 and acoustic stimuli in LQTS 2).
- It is recommended that all patients affected by LQTS avoid competitive sports activity.

RELATED CONTENT

Long QT Syndrome (Related Key Topic)

AUTHOR: **John Wylie, MD, FACC**

BASIC INFORMATION

DEFINITION

Tourette syndrome (TS) is an inherited neuropsychiatric disorder characterized by motor, vocal, and phonic tics that change during the course of illness. Onset of symptoms is typically before the age of 18.

Tics are sudden, brief, intermittent, involuntary or semi-voluntary movements (motor tics), or sounds (phonic or vocal tics) that mimic fragments of normal behavior.

SYNONYMS

Gilles de la Tourette syndrome
TS
Tourette disorder

ICD-10CM CODE
F95.2 Combined vocal and multiple motor tic disorder [de la Tourette]

EPIDEMIOLOGY & DEMOGRAPHICS

PREVALENCE (IN U.S.): Unknown; estimates range from 0.3% to 0.9% in children

PREDOMINANT SEX: Approximate male:female ratio of 4:1

PREDOMINANT AGE: Typical age of onset is between 2 and 15 yr (mean 5-7 yr).

PHYSICAL FINDINGS & CLINICAL PRESENTATION

- Neurologic examination is normal.
- Vocal and phonic tics are characterized as simple (e.g., clearing of throat, sniffing, grunting, sucking) or complex (e.g., repetition of short phrases, swearing [coprolalia]).
- Motor tics can be simple (e.g., blinking, grimacing, head jerking [Fig. 1]) or complex (e.g., gesturing [Fig. 2]). Tics wax, wane, change over time, and are often suppressed for short periods. Commonly, they are preceded by an urge to perform the tic.
- TS is often associated with a variety of behavioral symptoms, most commonly attention deficit hyperactivity disorder (ADHD) and obsessive-compulsive disorder (OCD).
- TS can be diagnosed using the DSM-5 criteria as follows:
  1. Both multiple motor and one or more vocal tics must be present at some time during the illness, although not necessarily concurrently.
  2. The tics may wax and wane in frequency but have persisted for more than 1 yr since first tic onset.
  3. Age at onset is less than 18 yr.
  4. Disturbance is not attributable to the direct physiologic effects of a substance (e.g., stimulants) or another medical condition (e.g., Huntington disease or postviral encephalitis).

ETIOLOGY

The exact pathogenesis is unknown. Genetic predisposition is likely as there is a strong family history of OCD or TS in patients with tics, and twin studies provide evidence for the importance of genetic factors. Recent analysis of linkage in a two-generation pedigree has led to the identification of a mutation in the HDC gene encoding l-histidine decarboxylase, the rate-limiting enzyme in histamine biosynthesis, pointing to a role for histaminergic neurotransmission in the mechanism and modulation of TS and tics. Immunologic dysfunction is also being explored in the pathogenesis of this complex disorder.

DIAGNOSIS

DIFFERENTIAL DIAGNOSIS

- Sydenham chorea: Occurs after infection with group A *Streptococcus.*
- Pediatric autoimmune neuropsychiatric disorder associated with group A streptococci (PANDAS).
- Sporadic tic disorders: Tics tend to be motor or vocal but not both.
- Head trauma.
- Drug intoxication: Many drugs are known to induce or exacerbate tic disorders, including methylphenidate, amphetamines, anticholinergics, antiepileptics, and antihistamines.
- Postinfectious encephalitis.
- Inherited disorders: Huntington disease, neurodegeneration with brain iron accumulation, and neuroacanthocytosis. These conditions should have other observed abnormalities on neurologic examination.

WORKUP

Clinical observation and history to confirm diagnosis

LABORATORY TESTS

No definitive laboratory tests

IMAGING STUDIES

CT scan and MRI of brain are unremarkable in TS and unnecessary if the neurologic examination is within normal limits.

TREATMENT

NONPHARMACOLOGIC THERAPY

- Multidisciplinary: Education of parents, teachers, psychologists, and school nurses is essential.
- Watchful waiting without intervention is an appropriate treatment if tics are not bothersome, since the natural history of tics is to improve with time. 60% of patients have minimal or no tics 6 yr after initial diagnosis.
- Cognitive behavioral therapy, termed habit-reversal treatment or Comprehensive Behavioral Intervention for Tics (CBIT), is efficacious in suppressing tics and is the first-line treatment.
- Screening for ADHD, OCD, and depression on a regular basis is important.

ACUTE GENERAL Rx

Dopamine-blocking agents may be used to acutely reduce the severity of tics. However, these agents carry a risk of side effects, such as acute dystonic reactions.

CHRONIC Rx

Tics only require long-term treatment when they interfere with an individual's psychosocial, educational, and occupational function.

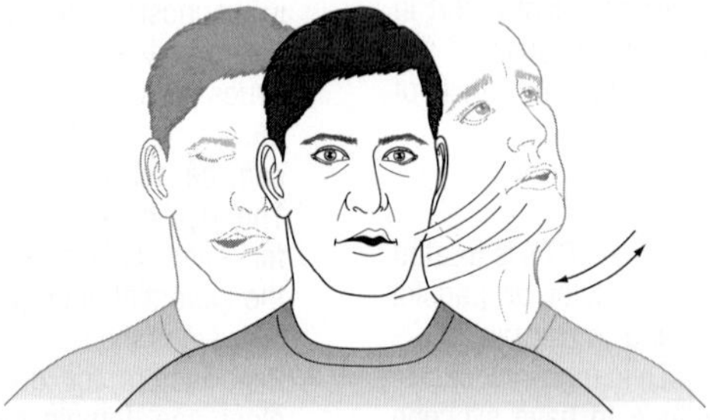

FIG. 1 This young man with Tourette disorder has multiple motor tics, including head jerking (head toss), grimacing of the right side of his mouth (half-smile), and depression of his forehead (frowning). Vocal tics of throat clearing and a short blowing sound accompany his motor tics. All of his tics continue throughout the day and briefly during sleep. Conversation, eating, and social situations have little influence, but with effort he can suppress his tics for several minutes. (From Kaufman DM et al: *Kaufman's clinical neurology for psychiatrists,* ed 8, Philadelphia, 2017, Elsevier.)

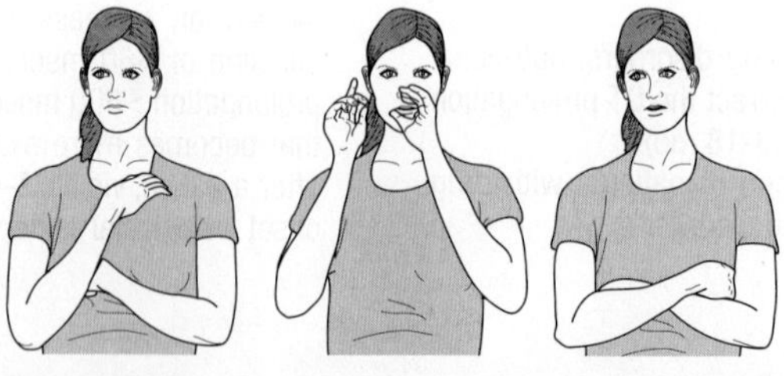

FIG. 2 This woman has compulsive obscene gestures—copropraxia. Similar to coprolalia, they have no affective or sexual content. (From Kaufman DM et al: *Kaufman's clinical neurology for psychiatrists,* ed 8, Philadelphia, 2017, Elsevier.)

TICS:

- Alpha-2 agonists, such as clonidine and guanfacine, are used for treatment of motor tics and are considered by some experts as first-line medications after behavioral therapy because of their favorable adverse effect profile. However, they are more beneficial for treatment of behavioral symptoms and are preferred for patients with predominant psychiatric disorders.
- Haloperidol, aripiprazole, and pimozide are the only U.S. Food and Drug Administration–approved neuroleptics for the treatment of tics in TS. Pimozide is started at a dose of 0.5 to 1.0 mg at night and increased every 5 to 7 days to a therapeutic dose of 2 to 8 mg. Haloperidol is started at a dose of 0.25 to 0.5 mg and can be increased to 1 to 4 mg depending on response and side effects. Use of neuroleptics carries a small but significant risk of tardive dyskinesia.
- Tetrabenazine, deutetrabenazine, and valbenazine are dopamine-depleting agents (VMAT2) that can be used effectively in TS patients to control tics.
- Topiramate is an antiepileptic used off-label to treat tics.
- Botulinum toxin (local injection) is effective for focal tics like eye blinking and neck and shoulder tics. The benefits are temporary, lasting 3 to 6 mo.
- Surgical treatment with deep brain stimulation is effective in some patients with disabling tics that are refractory to medications.

ADHD: Stimulants are useful for symptoms of ADHD but may exacerbate tics in 25% of patients. These medications should be used if troublesome behavioral symptoms persist.

OCD: Selective serotonin reuptake inhibitors, such as fluoxetine, are the most effective treatment for OCD.

DISPOSITION

- The intensity and frequency of tics typically diminishes during the later teenage years.
- One third of patients will achieve significant remission, although complete, lifelong remission is rare.
- One third will have mild, persistent, but "non-impairing" tics.

REFERRAL

Neurologist to confirm the initial diagnosis and for treatment in difficult cases

PEARLS & CONSIDERATIONS

- Tics do not need treatment unless they interfere with an individual's ability to function.
- Greater improvement in symptom severity among children with TS and chronic tic disorder has been reported with a comprehensive behavioral intervention compared with supportive therapy and education.
- An important part of treatment is appropriate evaluation and therapy of coexisting conditions (e.g., ADHD, OCD), as these conditions often cause more disability than the tics themselves.
- Deep brain stimulation has shown promising results as an alternative therapy in patients with medically refractory disease.

COMMENTS

Patient education may be obtained from the Tourette Syndrome Association, 4240 Bell Blvd., Bayside, NY 11361-2864; 800-237-0717 or 718-224-2999; http://www.tsa-usa.org.

SUGGESTED READINGS

Available at ExpertConsult.com

RELATED CONTENT

Tourette Syndrome (Patient Information)

AUTHORS: **Corey Goldsmith, MD,** and **Fariha Jamal, MD**

BASIC INFORMATION

DEFINITION

Toxic megacolon is a rare but severe complication of colonic inflammation, usually inflammatory bowel disease (IBD). It is characterized by total or segmental nonobstructive colonic distension (>6 cm) associated with systemic toxicity of inflammatory or infectious etiology.

SYNONYM

Toxic dilation of the colon

ICD-10CM CODES	
A04.7	Megacolon due to *Clostridium difficile*
K59.3	Megacolon, not elsewhere classified

EPIDEMIOLOGY & DEMOGRAPHICS

INCIDENCE: Varies depending on etiology. Incidence in patients with ulcerative colitis (UC) is approximately 10% and nearly 5% in patients with Crohn disease. *Clostridium difficile* infections may be complicated by toxic megacolon in up to 3% of cases.

PREDOMINANT SEX & AGE: With increasing rates of *Clostridium difficile (C. diff)* infections, patients ages 65 and older are at higher risk for developing toxic megacolon as a result of *C. diff* infection.

GENETICS: There are no known genetic factors that predispose patients to developing toxic megacolon associated with an inflammatory or infectious etiology.

RISK FACTORS: Major risk factors include inflammatory, infectious, and ischemic conditions of the colon, especially in individuals who are immunocompromised. Other risk factors include hypokalemia, use of narcotics or antidiarrheal agents, pregnancy, and recent instrumentation (such as colonoscopy).

PHYSICAL FINDINGS & CLINICAL PRESENTATION

- Patients with toxic megacolon usually appear severely ill. Clinical symptoms are similar to those of IBD and acute colitis and may include abdominal pain, diarrhea (usually bloody) and vomiting.
- Physical exam findings may include a distended, tender, and tympanic abdomen with reduced or absent bowel sounds. The patient may also present with signs of shock such as fever, tachycardia, mental status changes, and hypovolemia. Older patients are less likely to demonstrate a peritoneal abdominal examination.
- Laboratory findings may include leukocytosis, lactic acidosis, anemia, and electrolyte abnormalities such as hypokalemia and hypoalbuminemia.

ETIOLOGY

- Most common etiologies are inflammatory conditions such as UC, Crohn disease, and Behçet disease.
- Infections such as *C. diff, Salmonella, Shigella, E. coli,* cytomegalovirus, and *Entamoeba* can also be complicated by toxic megacolon.
- Other less common etiologies include ischemic colitis, malignancy such as lymphoma, and Kaposi sarcoma. In general, toxic megacolon is more likely to be associated with pancolitis than segmental colitis (Box 1).

DIAGNOSIS

DIFFERENTIAL DIAGNOSIS

Ischemic colitis, Crohn disease, ulcerative colitis

WORKUP

- General principles of workup include physical examination to evaluate for an acute abdomen, laboratory testing and radiography to evaluate for colonic dilation.
- Clinical criteria for toxic megacolon, proposed by Jalan et al in 1969, are still used. A diagnosis can be made if radiographic evidence of colonic distension >6 cm is present with at least three of the following: Fever >38° C (100.4° F), heart rate >120, leukocytosis >10.5, or anemia. In addition, at least one of the following must also be present: Dehydration, altered level of consciousness, electrolyte abnormalities, or hypotension.
- Patients with suspected toxic megacolon should be triaged emergently to an emergent care setting to facilitate rapid diagnosis and treatment.

LABORATORY TESTS

Initial testing should include a CBC, full chemistry panel, lactic acid, coagulation panel, liver function panel, and a type and screen.

IMAGING STUDIES

- All patients should initially receive a plain abdominal radiograph (Fig. 1) to assess for colonic dilation. Common findings include mucosal irregularity, loss of haustrations, "thumb printing" due to bowel wall edema, and thickening of the colonic wall with a continuous segment of air-filled colon >6 cm in diameter. The transverse or right colon is usually the most dilated segment seen.
- Computed tomography (CT) has been increasingly used to assess disease extent and for surgical planning (Fig. 2). It can also be helpful when differentiating between the various etiologies of toxic megacolon and to assess for complications such as intraabdominal hemorrhage or abscess.

BOX 1 Disorders Associated with Toxic Megacolon

- Inflammatory bowel disease
  1. Ulcerative colitis
  2. Crohn disease
- Infectious colitis
  1. *Salmonella, Shigella*, amoebic colitis
  2. *Clostridium difficile*
  3. Cytomegalovirus colitis
  4. HIV infection
- Cancer chemotherapy
- Ischemia

HIV, Human immunodeficiency virus.

From Vincent JL et al: *Textbook of critical care,* ed 6, Philadelphia, 2011, WB Saunders.

TREATMENT

Treatment includes both medical and surgical options. Principles of initial management include treating the underlying cause, managing shock, analgesia, and early surgical and gastroenterology consultation.

NONPHARMACOLOGIC THERAPY

- Surgery may be required in up to 50% of patients with toxic megacolon who do not show clinical improvement within 24 to 48 hr. The preferred first-line surgical treatment is subtotal colectomy with an end ileostomy. Other options include total proctocolectomy or colon decompression via the Turnbull method.
- Timing of surgical treatment is still controversial, with many advocating for aggressive medical treatment and observation before surgical intervention. Definitive indications for early surgical treatment include perforation, persistent colonic hemorrhage, or rapid clinical deterioration.

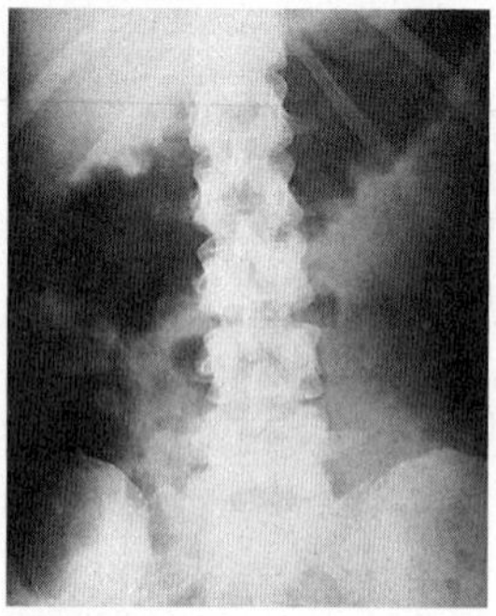

FIG. 1 Toxic megacolon secondary to ulcerative colitis. The smooth indentations seen along the margin of the colon represent pseudopolyps. (From Marx JA et al [eds]: *Rosen's emergency medicine: concepts and clinical practice,* ed 7, Philadelphia, 2010, Elsevier.)

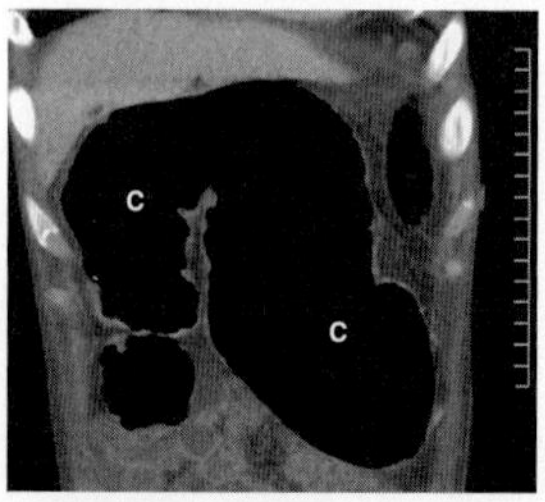

FIG. 2 Toxic megacolon. In a young patient with severe ulcerative colitis, coronal computed tomography demonstrates marked dilation of the colon *(c)* with thinning of its walls. The diameter of the lumen of the colon exceeds 7 cm. This finding places the patient at high risk of colon perforation. (From Webb WR et al: *Fundamentals of body CT,* ed 4, Philadelphia, 2015, Saunders.)

ACUTE GENERAL Rx

- Medications that impact colonic motility such as anticholinergics, opioids, and antidiarrheal agents should be discontinued and avoided.
- Electrolyte abnormalities, dehydration, and anemia are common clinical findings and should be addressed early. Fluid resuscitation with an isotonic solution and correction of electrolyte disturbances (especially hypokalemia) can help prevent worsening atony of the colonic wall. Patients with anemia from colonic hemorrhage should receive blood transfusion(s).
- Patients with toxic megacolon should receive broad-spectrum antibiotics as soon as possible. Infections due to *C. diff* should be treated with vancomycin (oral or rectal) or metronidazole (oral or IV). Toxic megacolon due to cytomegalovirus should be treated with ganciclovir IV.
- Patients with inflammatory etiologies such as UC or Crohn should receive high-dose IV steroids, either hydrocortisone 100 mg IV or methylprednisolone 60 mg IV. Steroids should not be used in patients with a confirmed infectious etiology.
- There are currently no data to support empiric treatment of toxic megacolon due to IBD with cyclosporine or infliximab. These treatment options should be reserved for patients who are not steroid responsive and should be limited to one attempt at clinical improvement so as not to delay surgical intervention.
- A management algorithm for toxic megacolon is outlined in Fig. 3.

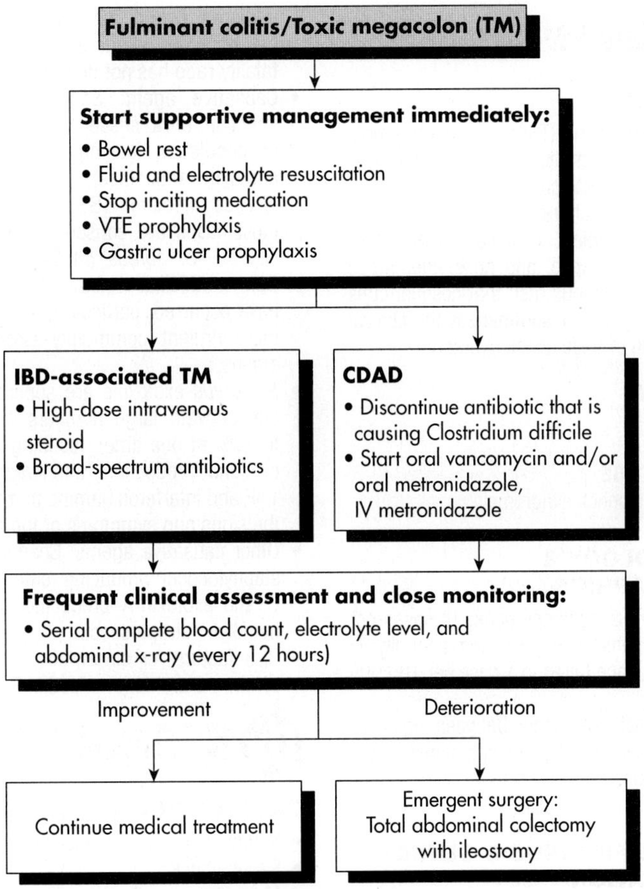

FIG. 3 Management algorithm for toxic megacolon. *CDAD, C. difficile*-associated disease; *IBD,* inflammatory bowel disease; *VTE,* venous thromboembolism. (From Cameron JL, Cameron AM: *Current surgical therapy,* ed 12, Philadelphia, 2017, Elsevier.)

CHRONIC Rx

Patients with IBD will need continued treatment for the underlying disease process once the acute processes associated with toxic megacolon have resolved.

DISPOSITION

All patients with toxic megacolon will require admission, possibly to the intensive care unit, depending on their clinical presentation.

REFERRAL

- Patients with suspected toxic megacolon presenting outside an emergency department should be referred there immediately.
- Surgical consultation in all cases.
- All patients with toxic megacolon due to newly diagnosed IBD who are discharged from the hospital should be referred to a gastroenterologist for continued treatment.

PEARLS & CONSIDERATIONS

COMMENTS

- Early recognition and treatment of toxic megacolon is critical given the associated high morbidity and mortality.
- Anticholinergic medications, antidiarrheal agents, and opioids can precipitate or worsen toxic megacolon.
- Management includes medical and surgical treatment with inpatient hospitalization and treatment of the underlying cause.

PREVENTION

Prevention focuses on treatment of underlying causes of colitis to prevent complications such as toxic megacolon.

SUGGESTED READINGS

Available at ExpertConsult.com

RELATED CONTENT

Clostridium difficile Infection (Related Key Topic)
Crohn Disease (Related Key Topic)
Small Bowel Obstruction (Related Key Topic)
Ulcerative Colitis (Related Key Topic)

AUTHOR: **Rory Merritt, MD, MEHP**

BASIC INFORMATION

DEFINITION

Toxic shock syndrome (TSS) is an acute febrile illness resulting in multiple organ system dysfunction caused most commonly by a bacterial exotoxin. Disease characteristics also include hypotension, vomiting, myalgia, watery diarrhea, vascular collapse, and an erythematous sunburn-like cutaneous rash that desquamates during recovery. Box 1 summarizes the clinical case definition of toxic shock syndrome.

SYNONYM

TSS

ICD-10CM CODE
A48.3 Toxic shock syndrome

EPIDEMIOLOGY & DEMOGRAPHICS

- Case reported incidence peak: 14 cases per 100,000 menstruating women annually in 1980; has since fallen to 1 case per 100,000 persons
- Occurs most commonly between ages 10 and 30 yr in healthy, young, menstruating white females
- Case fatality ratio of 3%

PHYSICAL FINDINGS & CLINICAL PRESENTATION

- Fever (>38.0° C; 100.4° F)
- Diffuse macular erythrodermatous rash that involves both skin and mucous membranes, resembles sunburn, and also involves the palms and soles. The rash then desquamates 1 to 2 wk after disease onset in survivors
- Orthostatic hypotension
- Gastrointestinal symptoms: Vomiting, diarrhea, abdominal tenderness
- Constitutional symptoms: Myalgia, headache, photophobia, rigors, altered sensorium, conjunctivitis, arthralgia
- Respiratory symptoms: Dysphagia, pharyngeal hyperemia, strawberry tongue
- Genitourinary symptoms: Vaginal discharge, vaginal hyperemia, adnexal tenderness
- End-organ failure
- Severe hypotension and acute renal failure
- Hepatic failure
- Cardiovascular symptoms: Disseminated intravascular coagulation, pulmonary edema, acute respiratory distress syndrome (ARDS), endomyocarditis, heart block

ETIOLOGY

- Menstruation-associated TSS: 45% of cases associated with tampons, diaphragm, or vaginal sponge use. There has been a decline in these cases and in the case-fatality ratio.
- Non–menstruation-associated TSS: 55% of cases associated with puerperal sepsis, post-cesarean section endometritis, mastitis, sinusitis, wound or skin infection, septorhinoplasty (nasal packings), pelvic inflammatory disease, respiratory infections following influenza, enterocolitis, and burns. The number of cases is increasing and the case-fatality ratio has not declined.
- Causative agent: *Staphylococcus aureus* infection of a susceptible individual (10% of population lacking sufficient levels of antitoxin antibodies), which liberates the disease mediator TSST-1 (exotoxin). While most cases are caused by methicillin-susceptible *S. aureus* (MSSA), cases of TSS from methicillin-resistant *S. aureus* (MRSA) have occurred, particularly those due to the more virulent, community-associated MRSA strains.
- *S. aureus* exotoxins are superantigens that can activate large numbers of T cells (up to 20% at one time), resulting in a massive cytokine production: Interleukin (Il-1), Il-2, TNF, and interferon gamma that then mediate the signs and symptoms of the disease.
- Other causative agents: Coagulase-negative staphylococci producing enterotoxins B or C, and exotoxin A–producing group A beta-hemolytic streptococci.
- Risk factors for staphylococcal toxic shock syndrome are summarized in Box 2.

Dx DIAGNOSIS

DIFFERENTIAL DIAGNOSIS

- Staphylococcal food poisoning
- Septic shock
- Mucocutaneous lymph node syndrome
- Scarlet fever
- Rocky Mountain spotted fever
- Meningococcemia
- Toxic epidermal necrolysis
- Kawasaki syndrome
- Leptospirosis
- Legionnaires' disease
- Hemolytic-uremic syndrome
- Stevens-Johnson syndrome
- Scalded skin syndrome
- Erythema multiforme
- Acute rheumatic fever

WORKUP

Broad-spectrum syndrome with multiorgan system involvement and variable but acute clinical presentation, including the following diagnostic criteria for staphylococcal toxic shock syndrome:

- Fever (>38° C; 100.4° F)
- Classic desquamating rash (1 to 2 wk)
- Hypotension/orthostatic systolic blood pressure ≤90 mm Hg
- Syncope
- Negative throat and cerebrospinal fluid cultures
- Negative serologic test for Rocky Mountain spotted fever, rubeola, and leptospirosis
- Clinical involvement of three or more of the following:
  1. Cardiopulmonary: ARDS, pulmonary edema, endomyocarditis, second- or third-degree atrioventricular block
  2. Central nervous system: Altered sensorium without focal neurologic findings
  3. Hematologic: Thrombocytopenia (platelets <100,000)
  4. Liver: Elevated liver function test results

BOX 1 Clinical Case Definition of Toxic Shock Syndrome

Clinical Findings

- Fever: Temperature of ≥38.9° C (102° F)
- Rash: Diffuse macular erythroderma
- Desquamation: 1 to 2 wk after onset of illness, particularly on palms, soles, fingers, and toes
- Hypotension: Systolic blood pressure ≤90 mm Hg for adults; <5th percentile by age for children <16 yr; orthostatic drop in diastolic blood pressure of ≥15 mm Hg from lying to sitting; orthostatic syncope or orthostatic dizziness
- Involvement of three or more of the following organ systems:
  - Gastrointestinal: Vomiting or diarrhea at onset of illness
  - Muscular: Severe myalgia or creatinine phosphokinase level greater than twice the upper limit of normal for the laboratory
  - Mucous membrane: Vaginal, oropharyngeal, or conjunctival hyperemia
  - Renal: Blood urea nitrogen or serum creatinine greater than twice the upper limit of normal, or five or more white blood cells per high-power field in the absence of a urinary tract infection
  - Hepatic: Total bilirubin, aspartate transaminase, or alanine transaminase greater than twice the upper limit of normal for the laboratory
  - Hematologic: Platelets <100,000/mm^2
  - Central nervous system: Disorientation or alterations in consciousness without focal neurologic signs when fever and hypotension are absent
- Negative results on the following tests, if obtained:
  - Blood, throat, or cerebrospinal fluid cultures; blood culture may be positive for *Staphylococcus aureus*
  - Serologic tests for Rocky Mountain spotted fever, leptospirosis, or measles

Case Classification

- *Probable:* A case with five of the six clinical findings above
- *Confirmed:* A case with all six of the clinical findings above, including desquamation, unless the patient dies before desquamation can occur

From Wharton M et al: Case definitions for public health surveillance, *MMWR Recomm Rep* 39[RR-13]:1-43, 1990. In Cherry JD et al: *Feigin and Cherry's pediatric infectious diseases,* ed 8, Philadelphia, 2019, Elsevier.

BOX 2 Risk Factors for Staphylococcal Toxic Shock Syndrome

I. Colonization of infection with toxin-producing *Staphylococcus aureus*
II. Absence of protective antitoxin antibody
III. Infected site
   A. Primary *S. aureus* infection:
      - Carbuncle
      - Cellulitis
      - Dental abscess
      - Empyema
      - Endocarditis
      - Folliculitis
      - Mastitis
      - Osteomyelitis
      - Peritonitis
      - Peritonsillar abscess
      - Pneumonia
      - Pyarthrosis
      - Pyomyositis
      - Sinusitis
      - Tracheitis
   B. Postsurgical wound infection:
      - Abdominal
      - Breast
      - Cesarean section
      - Dermatologic
      - Ear, nose, and throat
      - Genitourinary
      - Neurosurgery
      - Orthopedic
   C. Skin or mucous membrane disruption:
      - Burns (chemical, scald, etc.)
      - Dermatitis
      - Influenza
      - Pharyngitis
      - Postpartum (vaginal delivery)
      - Superficial/penetrating trauma (insect bite, needle stick)
      - Viral infection
      - Varicella
   D. Foreign body placement:
      - Augmentation mammoplasty
      - Catheters
      - Contraceptive sponge
      - Diaphragm
      - Surgical prostheses, stents, packing material, sutures
      - Tampons
   E. No obvious focus of infection (vaginal or pharyngeal colonization)

Cherry JD et al: *Feigin and Cherry's pediatric infectious diseases,* ed 8, Philadelphia, 2019, Elsevier.

5. Renal: >5 cells/high-power field, negative urine cultures, azotemia, and increased creatinine (double normal)
6. Mucous membrane involvement: Vagina, oropharynx, conjunctiva
7. Musculoskeletal: Myalgia, creatine phosphokinase twice normal
8. Gastrointestinal: Vomiting, diarrhea

For streptococcal toxic shock syndrome the diagnostic criteria is as follows:

- Definite case: Isolation of group A β-hemolytic streptococci (GABHS) from a sterile site
- Probable case: Isolation of GABHS from a nonsterile site
- Hypotension: Presence of two of the following findings:
  1. Acute kidney injury or failure
  2. Elevated aminotransferase
  3. Erythematous macular rash, soft tissue necrosis
  4. Coagulopathy, including thrombocytopenia and disseminated intravascular coagulation
  5. Acute respiratory distress syndrome

TABLE 1 Staphylococcal Versus Streptococcal Toxic Shock Syndrome

Feature	Staphylococcal	Streptococcal
Age	Primarily 15-35 yr	Primarily 20-50 yr
Gender	Higher frequency in women	Men and women equally affected
Severe pain	Rare	Common
Hypotension	100%	100%
Erythroderma rash	Very common	Less common
Renal failure	Common	Common
Bacteremia	Low frequency	60%
Tissue necrosis	Rare	Common
Predisposing factors	Tampons, surgery	Cuts, burns, varicella
Thrombocytopenia	Common	Common
Mortality rate	<3%	30%-70%

From Mandell GL et al: *Principles and practice in infectious diseases,* ed 7, Philadelphia, 2008, Churchill Livingstone.

BOX 3 Therapeutic Principles for Management of Toxic Shock Syndrome

1. Identify the focus of infection; debride and irrigate extensively and remove any foreign material
2. Isolate the organism for antimicrobial susceptibility studies
3. Administer parenteral antimicrobial therapy to stop toxin production and eradicate the organism
4. Manage systemic multiorgan actions of toxins or mediators
5. Administer fluid therapy to maintain adequate venous return and cardiac filling pressure and prevent end-organ damage
6. Consider intravenous immunoglobulin for the following:
   - Disease refractory to initial fluid replacement and vasopressor support
   - A focus of infection that cannot be drained

Cherry JD et al: *Feigin and Cherry's pediatric infectious diseases,* ed 8, Philadelphia, 2019, Elsevier.

LABORATORY TESTS

- Pan culture (cervix and vagina, throat, nasal passages, urine, blood, cerebrospinal fluid, wound) for *Staphylococcus, Streptococcus* (Table 1), and other pathogenic organisms
- Electrolytes to detect hypokalemia, hyponatremia
- Complete blood count with differential and clotting profile for anemia (normocytic or normochromic), thrombocytopenia, leukocytosis, coagulopathy, and bacteremia
- Chemistry profile to detect decreased protein, increased aspartate aminotransferase, increased alanine aminotransferase, hypocalcemia, elevated blood urea nitrogen and creatinine, hypophosphatemia, increased lactate dehydrogenase, increased creatine phosphokinase
- Urinalysis to detect white blood cells (>5 cells/high-power field), proteinemia, microhematuria
- Arterial blood gases to assess respiratory function and acid-base status
- Serologic tests considered for Rocky Mountain spotted fever, rubeola, and leptospirosis

IMAGING STUDIES

- Chest x-ray to evaluate pulmonary edema
- ECG to evaluate arrhythmia
- Sonography, CT scan, or MRI considered if pelvic abscess or tuboovarian abscess suspected

Rx TREATMENT

NONPHARMACOLOGIC THERAPY

- Therapeutic principles for management of toxic shock syndrome are outlined in Box 3.
- For optimal outcome: High index of suspicion and early and aggressive supportive management in an ICU setting
- Aggressive fluid resuscitation (maintenance of circulating volume, cardiac output, systolic blood pressure)
- Thorough search for a localized infection or nidus: Incision and drainage, debridement, removal of tampon or vaginal sponge
- Central hemodynamic monitoring, Swan-Ganz catheter, and arterial line for surveillance of hemodynamic status and response to therapy
- Foley catheter to monitor hourly urine output
- Possible military antishock trousers as temporary measure

- Acute ventilator management if severe respiratory compromise
- Renal dialysis for severe renal impairment
- Surgical intervention for indicated conditions (i.e., ruptured tubo-ovarian abscess, wound abscess, mastitis)
- Hyperbaric oxygen treatment can be used adjunctively

ACUTE GENERAL Rx

- Isotonic crystalloid (normal saline solution) for volume replacement following "7-3" rule (refers to the response in millimeters of mercury [mm Hg] of the pulmonary artery wedge pressure to volume replacement).
- Electrolyte replacement (K^+, C^+).
- Packed red blood cells, coagulation factor replacement, fresh frozen plasma to treat anemia or dilation and curettage.
- Vasopressor therapy for hypotension refractory to fluid volume replacement (e.g., dopamine beginning at 2 to 5 μg/kg/min).
- Steroids have been used but are not generally recommended due to lack of evidence of benefit.
- It is not clear whether antibiotics alter the course of acute TSS. Most authors recommend that patients receive 10 to 14 days of combination antibiotic therapy. In staphylococcal TSS, effective agents are clindamycin (900 mg IV every 8 hr in adults or 25 to 40 mg/kg per day in children) plus vancomycin (adults: 30 mg/kg per day IV in two divided doses; children: 40 mg/kg per day IV in four divided doses). Oxacillin or nafcillin sodium (2 g IV every 4 hr in adults; children: 100 to 150 mg/kg per 24 hr divided in four doses) can be used instead of vancomycin if TSS is due to MSSA. An alternative to vancomycin is linezolid.
- In streptococcal TSS, effective agents are penicillin G 24 million units/day in divided doses *plus* clindamycin 900 mg IV q8h. Alternative agents are ceftriaxone 2 g IV q24h *plus* clindamycin 900 mg IV q8h.
- Broad-spectrum antibiotic including gram-negative coverage added if concurrent sepsis suspected with TSS.
- Intravenous immune globulin (IVIG): While no controlled trials exist, most authors recommend IVIG (400 mg/kg in a single dose administered over several hours) in severe cases of TSS that are not responding to fluids or vasopressors. It may neutralize superantigen and decrease tissue damage.
- Tetracycline added if considering Rocky Mountain spotted fever.

CHRONIC Rx

- Severely ill patient: May require prolonged hospitalization and supportive management with gradual recovery and/or sequelae from severe end-organ involvement (ARDS or renal failure requiring dialysis)
- Majority of patients: Complete recovery
- Early-onset complications (within 2 wk):
  1. Skin desquamation
  2. Impaired digit sensation
  3. Denuded tongue
  4. Vocal cord paralysis
  5. Acute tubular necrosis
  6. ARDS
- Late-onset complications (after 8 wk):
  1. Nail splitting and loss
  2. Alopecia
  3. Central nervous system sequelae
  4. Renal impairment
  5. Cardiac dysfunction
- Recurrent TSS:
  1. More common in menstruation-related cases.
  2. Less common in patients treated with beta-lactamase–resistant antistaphylococcal antibiotics.
  3. Patients with history of TSS: If suspect signs and symptoms occur, have high index of suspicion and low threshold for evaluation and treatment.
  4. Screen for nasal carriage of *S. aureus* in patients with *S. aureus* TSS and treat with mupirocin in those with positive cultures.

PREVENTION

- Avoidance of tampons or use of low-absorbency tampons only (<4 hr in situ) and alternate with napkins
- Education for patients concerning signs and symptoms of TSS
- Avoidance of tampons for patients with history of TSS

DISPOSITION

- Complete recovery for most patients
- Long-term management of early- and late-onset complications for minority of patients

REFERRAL

- For multidisciplinary management, involving primary physician, gynecologist, internist, infectious disease specialist, and other supportive care specialists
- To tertiary-level hospital

PEARLS & CONSIDERATIONS

COMMENTS

Antibiotic prophylaxis against invasive group A streptococcal infection with benzathine penicillin G plus rifampin, clindamycin, or azithromycin is recommended for immunocompromised household contacts of patients with streptococcal TSS-like syndrome.

SUGGESTED READINGS

Available at ExpertConsult.com

RELATED CONTENT

Toxic Shock Syndrome (Patient Information)

AUTHOR: **Glenn G. Fort, MD, MPH**

BASIC INFORMATION

DEFINITION

Toxoplasmosis is an infection caused by the protozoal parasite *Toxoplasma gondii* transmitted through ingestion of undercooked meat, undercooked shellfish, or cat feces.

ICD-10CM CODES

B58.9	Toxoplasmosis, unspecified
B58.3	Pulmonary toxoplasmosis
B58.89	Toxoplasmosis with other organ involvement
P37.1	Congenital toxoplasmosis

EPIDEMIOLOGY & DEMOGRAPHICS

INCIDENCE (IN U.S.):

- Seroprevalence varies widely between different geographic locations, increasing with age, prevalence of cats in the area, and certain activities such as working in slaughterhouses or owning cats.
- Seroprevalence among women of childbearing age was 9.1% between 2009 and 2010.
- 0.23 cases of congenital toxoplasmosis per 10,000 live births between 2006 and 2014.
- Among patients with HIV, seroprevalence is approximately 11% in the U.S.

PREDOMINANT SEX: Equal gender distribution

PREDOMINANT AGE:

- Infancy (congenital infection)
- Prevalence increases with age

PEAK INCIDENCE: Seroprevalence is much higher in Latin America, Africa, and other temperate climates than in the U.S.

GENETICS: Congenital infection:

- Incidence and severity vary with the trimester of gestation during which the mother acquired infection.
  1. 10% to 25% (first trimester)
  2. 30% to 54% (second trimester)
  3. 60% to 65% (third trimester)
- Congenital infection occurring in the first trimester is the most severe.
- 89% to 100% of infections in the third trimester are asymptomatic.
- Risk to the fetus is not correlated with symptoms in the mother.

PHYSICAL FINDINGS & CLINICAL PRESENTATION

- Acquired (immunocompetent host): Usually subclinical, though may develop adenopathy, fatigue, and other constitutional symptoms that, while generally mild, can take weeks to resolve.
- Acquired (in patients with AIDS especially with CD4 count <100, hematopoietic stem cell transplant recipients): Most common presentation is encephalitis with headache, confusion, and fever. May have motor weakness or other focal neurologic abnormalities and seizures. Can also present as pneumonitis, chorioretinitis, or other end-organ involvement.
- Acquired (immunocompromised patients):
  1. Encephalitis
  2. Myocarditis (especially in heart transplant patients)
  3. Pneumonitis
- Ocular infection in the immunocompetent host: If not congenital, then presents in second or third decade of life as a focal necrotizing retinitis with photophobia, blurred vision, pain, and potentially loss of central vision if the macula is involved.
- Congenital: Results from acute infection acquired by the mother within 6 to 8 wk before conception or during gestation and is usually asymptomatic in the mother. In the infant, symptomatic disease is estimated at 40%. Ocular disease can include chorioretinitis and blindness, while central nervous system (CNS) manifestations can include intracranial calcifications resulting in epilepsy, hydrocephalus, microcephaly, psychomotor or mental retardation, and encephalitis.

ETIOLOGY

- *Toxoplasma gondii:*
  1. Ubiquitous intracellular protozoan
  2. Present worldwide
  3. Cat is the definitive host (Fig. E1)
  4. Oocysts can remain viable up to a year in moist soil, despite freezing temperatures.
- Human infection:
  1. Ingestion of oocysts shed by cats in soil, litter boxes, vegetables
  2. Ingestion of inadequately cooked meat or shellfish containing tissue cysts
  3. Vertical transmission

Dx DIAGNOSIS

DIFFERENTIAL DIAGNOSIS

- Lymphadenopathy:
  1. Infectious mononucleosis
  2. Cytomegalovirus (CMV) mononucleosis
  3. Cat-scratch disease
  4. Sarcoidosis
  5. Tuberculosis
  6. Lymphoma
  7. Metastatic cancer
- Cerebral mass lesions in immunocompromised host:
  1. Lymphoma
  2. Tuberculosis
  3. Bacterial abscess
- Pneumonitis in immunocompromised host:
  1. *Pneumocystis jiroveci (carinii)* pneumonia
  2. Tuberculosis
  3. Fungal infection
- Chorioretinitis:
  1. Syphilis
  2. Tuberculosis
  3. Histoplasmosis (competent host)
  4. CMV
  5. Herpes simplex
  6. Fungal infection
  7. Tuberculosis
- Myocarditis:
  1. Organ rejection in heart transplant recipients
- Congenital infection:
  1. Rubella
  2. CMV
  3. Herpes simplex
  4. Syphilis
  5. Listeriosis
  6. Erythroblastosis fetalis
  7. Sepsis

WORKUP

- Acute infection, immunocompetent host:
  1. Complete blood count
  2. *Toxoplasma* serology (immunoglobulin [Ig]G, IgM) in serial blood specimens 3 wk apart
  3. Lymph node biopsy if diagnosis uncertain
  4. Bone marrow exam (Fig. E2) in suspected bone marrow involvement
- Immunocompromised host:
  1. CNS symptoms:
     a. Cerebral computed tomography (CT) scan or MRI if CNS symptoms present
     b. Spinal tap, if safe
     c. Brain biopsy (Fig. E3) if no response to empiric therapy
  2. Ocular symptoms:
     a. Funduscopic examination (Fig. E4)
     b. Serologic studies
     c. Rarely, vitreous tap
  3. Pulmonary symptoms:
     a. Chest x-ray examination
     b. Bronchoalveolar lavage
     c. Transbronchial or open-lung biopsy
  4. Myocarditis:
     a. Cardiac enzymes
     b. Electrocardiogram
     c. Endomyocardial biopsy for definitive diagnosis
- Toxoplasmosis in pregnancy (Fig. 5):
  1. Initial maternal screening with IgM and IgG
     a. If negative, mother at risk of acute infection and should be retested monthly
     b. If both IgG and IgM positive, obtain IgA and IgE ELISA, AC/HS test
     c. IgA and IgE ELISA, AC/HS test elevated in acute infection
     d. Ig high for 1 yr or more
     e. IgG repeated 3 to 4 wk later to determine if titer is stable
  2. Acute maternal infection not excluded or documented:
     a. Fetal blood sampling (for culture, Ig, IgA, IgE)
     b. Amniotic fluid polymerase chain reaction (PCR)
  3. Fetal ultrasound every other week if maternal infection documented to look for ventriculomegaly, calcifications in the brain, and enlarged liver and spleen
- Congenital toxoplasmosis (Fig. 6):
  1. Placental histology
  2. Specific IgM or IgA in infant's blood

LABORATORY TESTS

- Antibody studies:
  1. More than one test necessary to establish diagnosis of acute toxoplasmosis (look for seroconversion or 4x increase)

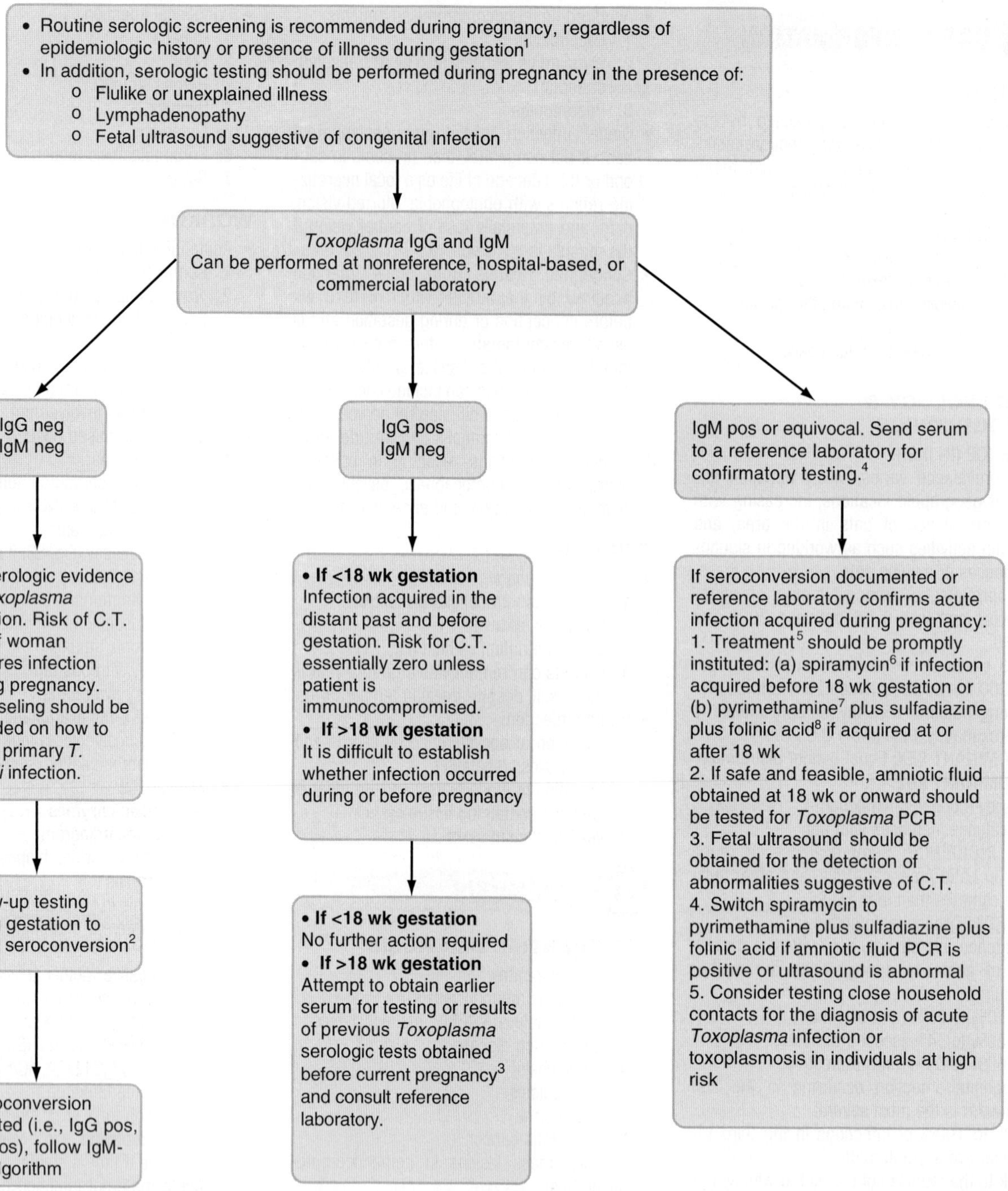

FIG. 5 Diagnostic approach and management algorithm of toxoplasmosis during pregnancy. Most of the initial serologic screening can be accomplished by nonreference or commercial laboratories. Only positive immunoglobulin M results should be considered for additional testing and consultation with medical experts at a reference laboratory. *CT,* Congenital toxoplasmosis; *IgG,* immunoglobulin G; *IgM,* immunoglobulin M; *neg,* negative test result; *pos,* positive test result. [1]Up to 50% of women who acquire *Toxoplasma* infection during gestation do not have a known risk factor for acute infection or an illness suggestive of toxoplasmosis. Thus to identify all women at risk, serologic screening should be performed in all pregnant women, along with other routine screening tests. [2]In a recent study from Lyon, France, monthly screening of seronegative pregnant women was reported to significantly decrease the risk of vertical transmission and of clinical signs at 3 yr of age. Consider consultation with a physician expert in management of toxoplasmosis during pregnancy (e.g., in the U.S., Palo Alto Medical Foundation–*Toxoplasma* Serology Laboratory [PAMF-TSL], http://www.pamf.org/serology/; 650-853-4828; e-mail, toxolab@pamf.org; or U.S. [Chicago] National Collaborative Treatment Trial Study [NCCTS]; 773-834-4152). [4]Consider sending serum sample to a reference laboratory (e.g., PAMF-TSL). [5]Treatment regimens vary by country. The pyrimethamine-sulfadiazine-folinic acid regimen should not be offered to any pregnant woman before 12 wk of gestation because of potential teratogenicity. In some centers in Europe, this regimen is offered at 14 wk of gestation or later; in the U.S., it is recommended at 18 wk or later. [6]Spiramycin is not commercially available in the U.S. It can be obtained at no cost and after consultation (with PAMF-TSL or the NCCTS through the U.S. Food and Drug Administration). [7]When using pyrimethamine, folic acid should be discontinued from the prenatal multivitamins. Folic acid can potentially counteract the antiparasitic effect of the drug. [8]Folic acid should not be erroneously used instead of folinic acid. (From Bennett JE et al: *Mandell, Douglas, and Bennett's principles and practice of infectious diseases,* ed 8, Philadelphia, 2015, Saunders.)

- Screen all newborns born to mothers suspected or confirmed to have acquired *T. gondii* infection during gestation
- Consider neonatal serologic screening in newborns born to mothers who were not screened during gestation[1]
- In addition, laboratory testing should be performed at birth in the presence of:
  - Visual abnormalities (e.g., strabismus, blindness, chorioretinitis)
  - Encephalitis, seizures, hydrocephaly, or microcephaly
  - Brain or hepatic calcifications
  - Unexplained sepsis
  - Hepatosplenomegaly
  - Pneumonitis
  - Anemia, jaundice, petechiae, thrombocytopenia
  - Skin rash, diarrhea, hypothermia

↓

- *Toxoplasma* IgG, IgM, IgA
  - Can be performed at nonreference, hospital-based, or commercial laboratories
  - However, recommend IgG, IgM-ISAGA, and IgA at reference laboratory[2]
- If clinical suspicion is high:
  - *Toxoplasma* PCR in peripheral blood, urine, and CSF[3]
  - Ophthalmologic evaluation by pediatric retinal specialist
  - Hearing evaluation
  - Ultrasound or CT (preferred) scan of the brain
  - Lumbar puncture for CSF[3] examination[4]

Initial treatment indicated[5]

- Positive results for IgG plus positive results for:
  - IgM in serum sample obtained after 5 days of life and/or
  - IgA in serum sample obtained after 10 days of life and/or
  - PCR in peripheral blood, urine, or CSF
- Positive results for IgG plus
  - Major clinical signs[6] present plus
  - Newborn was born to a mother who was infected during gestation

Initial treatment not indicated; serologic follow-up indicated

- Positive results for IgG in the absence of major clinical signs plus negative results for:
  - IgM and
  - IgA and, if performed:
  - PCR in peripheral blood, urine, and CSF
- Follow-up of serum IgG every 4 to 8 wk, IgG of maternal origin typically falls by half every month[7]
- Serologic test results in the mother can aid in the interpretation of newborn's serologies

Treatment and serologic follow-up not indicated

- Newborn:
  - Negative IgG and
  - Negative IgM and
  - Negative IgA

and

- Mother
  - Negative IgG and
  - Negative IgM

FIG. 6 Diagnostic approach and management algorithm of the newborn whose mother has been suspected or confirmed to have acquired toxoplasmosis during gestation. *CSF,* Cerebrospinal fluid; *CT,* computed tomography; *IgG, IgM,* and *IgA,* immunoglobulins G, M, and A, respectively; *ISAGA,* immunosorbent agglutination assay; *PCR,* polymerase chain reaction. [1]Consider consultation with a physician expert in management of toxoplasmosis during pregnancy (e.g., in the U.S., Palo Alto Medical Foundation–*Toxoplasma* Serology Laboratory [PAMF-TSL], http://www.pamf.org/serology/; 650-853-4828; e-mail, toxolab@pamf.org; or U.S. [Chicago] National Collaborative Treatment Trial Study, 773-834-4152). [2]Consider sending serum sample to a reference laboratory (e.g., PAMF-TSL). [3]If lumbar puncture is clinically indicated, deemed safe, and feasible. [4]In an attempt to confirm the diagnosis of congenital toxoplasmosis, CSF should be sent for cell count and differential (congenital toxoplasmosis is one of the few causes of eosinophilic meningitis), protein (congenital toxoplasmosis is one of the few causes of extreme elevation of CSF protein), glucose, and *T. gondii* PCR. [5]The recommended regimen is pyrimethamine plus sulfadiazine plus folinic acid (see text). [6]Major clinical signs are referred here: Chorioretinitis, brain calcifications, and hydrocephalus. [7]Maternally transferred IgG antibodies usually decline and disappear within 6 to 12 mo of life. (From Bennett JE et al: *Mandell, Douglas, and Bennett's principles and practice of infectious diseases,* ed 8, Philadelphia, 2015, Saunders.)

TABLE 1 Guidelines for Interpretation of Serologic Tests for Toxoplasmosis

IgG	IgM	IgG Avidity	Interpretation
Positive	Negative	—	Remote infection, immune. IgG avidity testing is best used when both IgG and IgM are positive and timing of infection is crucial, as in pregnancy (see below). False-negative IgM results occur in approximately 25% of cases when evaluating infection in the newborn. If infection is suspected in this setting, further testing (dye test, IgM EIA, IgA EIA, IgE EIA/ISAGA, PCRs, ideally with paired maternal serology tests—see text) is necessary in a reference laboratory (*Toxoplasma* Serology Laboratory, PAMF Research Institute, 795 El Camino Real, Ames Building Palo Alto, CA, 94301; 650-853-4828).
Positive	Positive or equivocal	High	Infection within the past 18 mo but likely >12 wk ago. If pregnant and beyond first trimester, consider sending specimen to reference laboratory for dye test, repeat IgG avidity and IgM EIA, IgA EIA, IgE EIA/ISAGA, and AC/HS testing (see above).
Positive	Positive or equivocal	Low	Infection within the past 12 wk. Consider sending specimen to a reference laboratory (see above) to time infection more accurately (dye test, repeat IgG avidity and IgM EIA, IgA EIA, IgE EIA/ISAGA, and AC/HS) in the setting of pregnancy.
Equivocal	Negative	—	Indeterminate. Test a new specimen or consider a different assay (IFA or ELISA).
Equivocal	Equivocal	—	Indeterminate. Test a new specimen or consider a different assay (IFA or ELISA).
Equivocal	Positive	—	Acute infection or false-positive IgM result. Test a second specimen; if IgG becomes positive or remains equivocal, consider sending specimen to a reference laboratory to time infection more accurately (dye test, IgG avidity, IgM EIA, IgA EIA, IgE EIA/ISAGA, AC/HS—see text) in the setting of pregnancy.
Negative	Negative	—	No evidence of *Toxoplasma* infection; not immune.
Negative	Equivocal	—	Either false-positive IgM result or possible recent infection. Obtain a new specimen and retest. If infection is recent, IgM and IgG should become positive, with low IgG avidity. If repeated testing is still IgG negative and IgM equivocal, patient is likely uninfected. Consider IgM ISAGA.
Negative	Positive	—	Acute infection or false-positive IgM result. Repeat testing on new specimen. If the result is the same, it is likely a false-positive IgM result. Consider IgM ISAGA.

AC/HS, Differential agglutination test; *EIA*, enzyme immunoassay; *ELISA*, enzyme-linked immunosorbent assay; *IFA*, immunofluorescence assay; *Ig*, immunoglobulin; *ISAGA*, immunosorbent agglutination assay; *PCR*, polymerase chain reaction.
From Cherry JD et al: *Feigin and Cherry's pediatric infectious diseases*, ed 8, Philadelphia, 2019, Elsevier.

2. IgM antibody:
    a. Appears 5 days into infection
    b. Peaks at 2 wk
    c. Falls to low level or disappears within 2 mo
    d. May persist at low levels for 1 yr or more
3. Antibody not measurable:
    a. Ocular toxoplasmosis
    b. Reactivation
    c. Immunocompromised hosts
4. IgG antibody:
    a. Appears 1 to 2 wk after infection
    b. Peaks at 6 to 8 wk
    c. Gradually declines over mo to yr
5. Guidelines for interpretation of serologic tests for toxoplasmosis are summarized in Table 1

IMAGING STUDIES

- Chest x-ray if pulmonary involvement suspected
- Cerebral CT scan (Fig. E7) or MRI if encephalitis suspected

Rx TREATMENT

NONPHARMACOLOGIC THERAPY

- Selected cases of ocular infection:
    1. Photocoagulation
    2. Vitrectomy
    3. Lentectomy
- Selected cases of congenital cerebral infection:
    1. Ventricular shunting

ACUTE GENERAL Rx

- Acute infection, immunocompetent, nonpregnant host:
    1. Usually requires no treatment, unless severe and persistent symptoms or vital organ damage
- Acute infection, immunocompromised host, non-AIDS:
    1. Treat even if asymptomatic
    2. Duration:
        a. Until 4 to 6 wk after resolution of all signs and symptoms
        b. Usually 6 mo or longer
- Reactivated infection, immunocompromised host, non-AIDS:
    1. Treat if symptomatic
- Acute or reactivated infection, AIDS:
    1. Treat in all cases
    2. Induction course:
        a. 3 to 6 wk
        b. Maintenance therapy continued for life; consider discontinuation of suppressive therapy if the patient has a good response to antiretroviral therapy and if the CD4 count remains >200 cells/mm^3 for more than 3 mo
    3. Empiric therapy:
        a. AIDS with positive IgG
        b. Multiple ring-enhancing lesions on cerebral CT scan or MRI
        c. Response seen by day 7 in 71% and day 14 in 91%
- Ocular infection:
    1. Treat in all cases
    2. Therapy continued for 1 mo or longer if needed
    3. Response seen in 70% within 10 days
    4. Retreat as needed
    5. Steroids may be indicated in patients with signs or symptoms of increased intracranial pressure
    6. Surgical treatment in selected cases
- Treatment regimens (Table 2):
    1. Pyrimethamine 200 mg loading dose once PO, then 50 mg (<60 kg) to 75 mg (>60 kg) q day; *plus*
    2. Leucovorin 10 to 20 mg PO qid; *plus*
    3. Sulfadiazine 1 (<60 kg) to 1.5 g (>60 kg) PO q6h

    Other treatment options (if sulfa hypersensitivity or allergy is present): Pyrimethamine 50 to 75 mg/day PO with leucovorin 10 to 20 mg/day PO and either (1) clindamycin 600 mg q6h PO or IV (up to 1200 mg IV) q6h, or (2) clarithromycin 1 g PO bid, or (3) dapsone 100 mg/day PO, or (4) atovaquone 750 mg PO q6h.
- Acute infection in pregnancy:
    1. Treat immediately
    2. Risk of fetal infection reduced by 60% with treatment
        a. Seroconversion in the first trimester
            (1) Spiramycin 1 g every 8 hr
        b. Seroconversion beyond the first trimester or positive amniotic fluid PCR/ultrasound findings consistent with congenital toxoplasmosis:
            (1) Sulfadiazine 75 mg/kg/day in two divided doses ×2 days, then 50 mg/kg twice daily, *plus*
            (2) Pyrimethamine 50 mg bid ×2 days, then 50 mg PO daily, *plus*
            (3) Leucovorin 10 to 20 mg PO daily
- Postnatal treatment of congenital infection:
    1. Sulfadiazine 50 mg/kg PO bid, *plus*

TABLE 2 Treatment of Toxoplasmosis

Disease	Medication	Dosage	Length of Therapy
Acute acquired—generally not treated unless severe or persistent symptoms, vital organ damage, or host immunosuppression[a]	Pyrimethamine *plus*	2 mg/kg/day for 2 days, then 1 mg/kg/day	4-6 wk or 2 wk after symptoms resolve for normal host; 4–6 wk beyond resolution for immunosuppressed hosts. In AIDS patients, treat until $CD4^+$ count >200
	Sulfadiazine *plus*	75-100 mg/kg/day divided twice daily (maximum 4 g/day); consider the lower dose in children >20 kg (see text)	
	Folinic acid	5-20 mg 3 times weekly; use higher doses if marrow suppression	
Ocular, older child	Pyrimethamine *plus*	2 mg/kg/day for 2 days, then 1 mg/kg/day (maximum 50 mg/day)	4-6 wk or 2 wk after symptoms resolve
	Sulfadiazine *plus*	75-100 mg/kg/day divided twice daily (maximum 4 g/day); consider the lower dose in children >20 kg (see text)	Prednisone should be continued until resolution of sight-threatening active chorioretinitis
	Folinic acid *plus*	5-20 mg 3 times weekly	
	Prednisone	1 mg/kg/day divided twice daily	
Congenital	Pyrimethamine *plus*	2 mg/kg per day for 2 days, then 1 mg/kg/day for 6 mo, then 3 times weekly (M-W-F) for 6 mo	1 yr
	Sulfadiazine *plus*	100 mg/kg per day divided twice daily	
	Folinic acid *plus*	5-10 mg 3 times weekly	
	Prednisone	1 mg/kg/day divided twice daily	Until resolution of elevated CSF protein level or sight-threatening active chorioretinitis
Pregnant women—acute infection first 21 wk of gestation	Spiramycin	3 g/day divided twice daily without food	Until fetal infection documented or excluded at 21 wk of gestation; if fetus infected, change to pyrimethamine plus sulfadiazine plus folinic acid until delivery
Pregnant women—fetal infection confirmed (amniotic fluid PCR positive)	Pyrimethamine *plus*	100 mg/day divided twice daily for 2 days, then 50 mg/day	Until delivery
	Sulfadiazine *plus*	3 g/day divided twice daily	
	Folinic acid	5-20 mg/day	

AIDS, Acquired immunodeficiency syndrome; *CSF,* cerebrospinal fluid; *PCR,* polymerase chain reaction.
[a]For more detailed recommendations for patients with human immunodeficiency virus infection/AIDS, see http://aidsinfo.nih.gov/guidelines.
From Cherry JD et al: *Feigin and Cherry's pediatric infectious diseases,* ed 8, Philadelphia, 2019, Elsevier.

2. Pyrimethamine 2 mg/kg PO for 2 days, then 1 mg/kg PO daily for the first 2 to 6 mo, then three times weekly, *plus*
3. Leucovorin 5 to 20 mg PO three times weekly
4. Minimum duration of treatment: 12 mo

CHRONIC Rx

Maintenance therapy in AIDS patients because of the high risk (80%) of relapse:
- Pyrimethamine 25 mg PO qid
- Sulfadiazine 500 mg PO qid
- Leucovorin 10 to 20 mg PO qid

DISPOSITION

- Prognosis:
  1. Excellent in the immunocompetent host
  2. Good in ocular infection (although relapses are common)
- Treatment of acute infection in pregnancy:
  1. Reduces incidence and severity of congenital toxoplasmosis
- Treatment of congenital infection:
  1. Improvement in intellectual function
  2. Regression of retinal lesions
- AIDS:
  1. 70% to 95% response to therapy

REFERRAL

- To infectious disease expert:
  1. Immunocompromised hosts
  2. Pregnant women
  3. Difficulty in making a diagnosis or deciding on treatment
- To pediatric infectious disease expert:
  1. Congenital infection
- To obstetrician:
  1. Pregnant seronegative mother
  2. Acute seroconversion
- To ophthalmologist:
  1. Congenital infection
  2. Any case of ocular infection

PEARLS & CONSIDERATIONS

COMMENTS

- Prevention of toxoplasmosis is most important in seronegative pregnant women and immunocompromised hosts.
- Patient instructions:
  1. Cook meat to 66° C (150.8° F).
  2. Cook eggs.
  3. Do not drink unpasteurized milk.
  4. Wash hands thoroughly after handling raw meat.
  5. Wash kitchen surfaces that come in contact with raw meat.
  6. Wash fruits and vegetables.
  7. Avoid contact with materials potentially contaminated with cat feces.

SUGGESTED READINGS

Available at ExpertConsult.com

RELATED CONTENT

Toxoplasmosis (Patient Information)

AUTHORS: **Tara C. Bouton, MD, MPH, TM, Philip A. Chan, MD, MS,** and **Glenn G. Fort, MD, MPH**

BASIC INFORMATION

DEFINITION

Hemolytic transfusion reactions may be acute (occurring during or immediately after the transfusion) or delayed (occurring more than 24 hr after the transfusion). Acute hemolytic transfusion reaction (AHTR) is in vivo hemolysis most commonly caused by an alloantibody in a recipient's plasma to a cognate antigen on the donor red cells. The most commonly involved alloantibodies are to ABO antigens, but alloantibodies to minor blood group antigens have also been implicated. Typically the alloantibodies are of the IgM class, but complement fixing IgGs may also cause such a reaction. The clinical features vary, but usually there are high fever, chills, nausea, and backache. Red or brown urine may be passed due to hemoglobinuria. The plasma may show hemoglobinemia, and the direct Coombs test can be either positive or negative. Delayed hemolytic reactions are usually caused by an anamnestic alloantibody response upon re-exposure to cognate erythrocyte antigen. They are typically IgG and usually noncomplement fixing. They occur 1 to 10 days after transfusion. In delayed transfusion reactions, hemoglobinemia is unusual, and the only clinical manifestations may be fever, the serologic finding of a newly positive indirect antiglobulin (indirect Coombs test), and/or the presence of a positive direct Coombs test. Delayed reactions can be clinically silent (called delayed serologic hemolytic reactions) or manifest with fever, chills, nausea, vomiting, unexplained anemia, or jaundice. There is no specific treatment other than supportive care.

SYNONYMS

AHTR
DSTR
DHTR
Acute hemolytic transfusion reaction

ICD-10CM CODES

T80.3	ABO incompatibility reaction
T80.4	Rh incompatibility reaction
T80.8	Other complications following infusion, transfusion, and therapeutic injection
T80.9	Unspecified complication following infusion, transfusion, and therapeutic injection

EPIDEMIOLOGY & DEMOGRAPHICS

- Approximately 1% of transfused products result in serious adverse reactions; hemolytic transfusion reactions account for up to 5% of these serious adverse reactions.
- Acute intravascular hemolysis occurs in one to five per 50,000 transfusions.
- Delayed reactions occur about 1:1500 red cell transfusions.

PHYSICAL FINDINGS & CLINICAL PRESENTATION

- Fever, chills, nausea, tachycardia, chest pain, dyspnea, dizziness, bronchospasm.
- Lower back pain due to ischemic muscle pain or vasospasm hypotension.
- Severe reactions may occur in surgical patients under anesthesia who are unable to give any warning signs.
- Patients with delayed hemolytic transfusion reactions typically do not present as a clinical emergency. In most cases, presentation is with a low-grade fever from the generation of IL-1 or other proinflammatory cytokines. Hemoglobinuria and hemoglobinemia are rarely present. Unexplained anemia and jaundice are other possible presentations.
- Tables 1 and 2 summarize signs and symptoms of acute adverse reactions to blood transfusion. In the differential diagnosis of hemolysis.

ETIOLOGY

Most fatal hemolytic reactions are caused by clerical errors and mislabeled specimens.

DIAGNOSIS

DIFFERENTIAL DIAGNOSIS

- Septic reaction
- Transfusion-related acute lung injury

MANAGEMENT

The transfusion must be stopped immediately. The blood bank must be notified, and the donor transfusion bag must be returned to the blood bank along with a freshly drawn posttransfusion specimen. Table 3 summarizes immediate investigations in the case of an acute transfusion reaction.

LABORATORY TESTS

- The direct antiglobulin test (DAT) is usually positive in a delayed reaction, and preparation of an eluate will help identify the offending antibody.
- In some delayed reactions, the only finding is a positive indirect Coombs test, and the implicated alloantibody can be identified in an antibody panel.
- In acute reactions, the urine may show hemoglobinuria (wine-colored urine) and the plasma hemoglobinemia (pink plasma).
- Labs (Table 4): Decreased hematocrit and serum haptoglobin (haptoglobin low to 0 mg/dl). Elevated LDH, indirect bilirubin and creatinine, if acute.
- In acute cases, monitor coagulation status (PT, aPTT, fibrinogen) for disseminated intravascular coagulation.

TREATMENT

NONPHARMACOLOGIC THERAPY

- Stop transfusion immediately. Test anticoagulated blood from the recipient for the presence of free hemoglobin in the plasma.
- Monitor vital signs closely and maintain IV access with a suitable crystalloid or colloid solution.
- Maintain an adequate airway.

TABLE 1 Signs and Symptoms of Acute Adverse Reactions to Blood Transfusion

Reaction	Fever	Chills/ Rigors	Nausea/ Vomiting	Chest Discomfort/Pain	Facial Flushing	Wheezing/ Dyspnea	Back/Lumbar Pain	Discomfort at Infusion Site	Hypotension
Acute hemolytic	X	X	X	X	X	X	X	X	X
Febrile nonhemolytic	X	X		X	X				
Nonimmune hemolysis									
Acute lung injury	X			X		X			X
Allergic									
Massive transfusion complications									
Anaphylaxis	X	X	X	X	X	X	X	X	X
Passive cytokine infusion	X	X	X			X			
Hypervolemia						X			
Bacterial sepsis	X	X	X				X	X	X
Air embolus				X		X			

From Goldman L, Bennett JC (eds): *Cecil's textbook of medicine*, ed 22, Philadelphia, 2004, Saunders.

TABLE 2 Types of Acute Transfusion Reactions

Reaction Type	Presenting Signs and Symptoms
Acute hemolytic	Fever, chills, dyspnea, vomiting, hypotension, tachycardia, infusion site pain, back pain, hemoglobinuria, hemoglobinemia, indirect hyperbilirubinemia, renal failure, DIC
Febrile reaction	Fever, chills, rigors
Allergic	Urticaria, pruritus, flushing, angioedema, dyspnea, bronchospasm stridor, hypotension, tachycardia, abdominal cramping
Hypervolemic	Dyspnea, tachycardia, hypertension, headache, jugular venous distention
Septic	Fever, chills, hypotension, tachycardia, vomiting
Transfusion-related acute lung injury	Dyspnea, hypoxemia, fever, hypotension

DIC, Disseminated intravascular coagulation.
From Hoffman R et al: *Hematology: basic principles and practice,* ed 7, Philadelphia, 2018, Elsevier.

TABLE 3 Immediate Investigations in the Case of an Acute Transfusion Reaction

Check for hemolysis.
Perform visual examination of patient's plasma and urine (plasma and urine hemoglobin can be checked, but this is not essential).
Blood film may show spherocytosis.
Bilirubin and lactate dehydrogenase (LDH) levels will be raised.
Check for incompatibility.
Check the documentation and the patient's identity.
Repeat ABO group of patient on pretransfusion and posttransfusion samples and of the donor unit(s).
Screen the patient for red cell antibodies pretransfusion and posttransfusion.
Repeat crossmatch with pretransfusion and posttransfusion samples.
Direct antiglobulin test (DAT) on pretransfusion and posttransfusion samples.
Eluate from patient's red cells.
Check for disseminated intravascular coagulation.
Perform blood count and film, coagulation screen, and fibrin degradation products (or D-dimers).
Check for renal dysfunction.
Check blood urea, creatinine, and electrolytes.
Check for bacterial infection.
Take blood cultures from the patient and donor unit including immediate Gram stain.

From Bain BJ et al: *Dacie and Lewis practical haematology,* ed 12, Philadelphia, 2017, Elsevier.

TABLE 4 Hemolytic Transfusion Reactions: Serologic Presentation

Type	Antibody Detectable Initially	Primary Antibody Type	Degree of Complement Binding	Example
Acute intravascular	Yes	IgM	Full (C1-9)	ABO system
Acute extravascular	Yes	IgG	None/partial	Rh system
Delayed intravascular	No	IgG	Full (C1-9)	Kidd system
Delayed extravascular	No	IgG	None/partial	Duffy system

From Hoffman R et al: *Hematology: basic principles and practice,* ed 7, Philadelphia, 2018, Elsevier.

ACUTE GENERAL Rx

- Treatment is supportive and consists of fluid resuscitation, vasopressor support, and mannitol.
- Vigorous IV hydration (0.9% NaCl or some other suitable crystalloid solution) to maintain urine flow at >100 ml/hr until hypotension is corrected and hemoglobinuria clears. IV furosemide may be necessary to maintain adequate renal flow.
- The addition of mannitol may prevent renal damage (controversial). Mannitol, if chosen, must be used with caution; if acute tubular necrosis occurs before mannitol infusion, pulmonary edema may occur as a result of the acute increase in intravascular volume secondary to fluid expansion.
- Monitor for the presence of disseminated intravascular coagulation. PT, aPTT, and fibrinogen levels should be closely monitored.
- If sepsis is suspected, culture as appropriate.

DISPOSITION

Mortality rate is 3% to 10% in severe transfusion reactions.

PEARLS & CONSIDERATIONS

COMMENTS

Hemolysis caused by minor antigen systems is generally less severe and may be delayed 1 to 10 days after transfusion.

SUGGESTED READINGS

Available at ExpertConsult.com

AUTHOR: **Joseph Sweeney, MD, FACP, FRCPath**

Transient Global Amnesia

BASIC INFORMATION

DEFINITION

A clinical syndrome lasting up to 24 hr of sudden onset, severe anterograde and variable retrograde amnesia without loss of other neurologic function.

SYNONYM

TGA

ICD-10CM CODE

G45.4 Transient global amnesia

EPIDEMIOLOGY & DEMOGRAPHICS

INCIDENCE (IN U.S.): 3.4 to 10.4 per 100,000 people.

PEAK INCIDENCE: Most between ages 50 to 70 and equally common in men and women. In population older than 50 the incidence increases to 23.5 per 100,000 per year. TGA is also more common in individuals with migraine.[1]

RECURRENCE RATE: 2.9% to 23.8%

RISK FACTORS

Earlier age at first episode and personal or family history of migraine are associated with greater risk for recurrent transient global amnesia.[2]

PHYSICAL FINDINGS & CLINICAL PRESENTATION[3]

- Cannot recall novel episodic information, repeatedly asking the same questions
- No impairment in consciousness or nonmemory cognitive domains, no focal neurologic deficit
- Complex procedural memory is often preserved (i.e., driving)
- Triggers include Valsalva maneuver, immersion in cold or hot, sexual intercourse, emotional stress
- Typically a single attack that is self-limited, with amnestic gap of the duration of episode
- Those with recent head injury or epilepsy diagnosis are excluded[3]

[1]Arena JE et al: Transient global amnesia, *Mayo Clin Proc* 90(2):264-272, 2015.

[2]Morris KA et al: Factors associated with risk of recurrent transient global amnesia, *JAMA Neurol* 77(12):1-8, 2020.

[3]Arena JE et al: Long-term outcome in patients with transient global amnesia: a population-based study, *Mayo Clin Proc* 92(3):399-405, 2017.

ETIOLOGY

- Several proposed mechanisms of patho-physiology:
  1. Hypoperfusion or arterial ischemia of the hippocampi
  2. Internal jugular venous flow reversal causing venous hypertension to the medial temporal lobe
  3. Migraine phenomena with cortical spreading depression

DIAGNOSIS

DIFFERENTIAL DIAGNOSIS

- Posterior cerebral artery transient ischemic attack: Can be associated with confusion or memory loss. Commonly with vascular risk factors and other focal neurologic signs (homonymous hemianopsia, aphasia, hemiparesis, hemisensory loss, hemi-body pain, oculomotor nerve palsy or vertical gaze palsy).
- Transient epileptic amnesia: Epilepsy syndrome, consisting of atypical TGA or recurrent attacks of amnesia, often less than 1 hour and upon waking, responsive to antiepileptic medications. Associated with olfactory hallucinations or oral automatisms. Interictal EEG may be abnormal. Hippocampal atrophy on MRI may be seen.
- Dissociative fugue, or transient dissociative amnesia: Extensive retrograde amnesia, loss of personal identity may occur, unlike in TGA where such is preserved.
- Hypoglycemia: Metabolic dysfunction can cause impairment in consciousness, focal signs, or prolonged cognitive impairment unlike TGA.

WORKUP

- Largely a clinical diagnosis, workup should focus on exclusion of vascular or epileptic source of symptoms.
- Collateral history of witnessed event and exclusion of prior event.
- Cognitive examination with evaluation of registration, delayed recall, and orientation.
- Careful cranial nerve examination to exclude posterior circulation stroke.

LABORATORY TESTS

- Complete blood count with erythrocyte sedimentation rate and C-reactive protein
- Serum chemistries, including lipid profile
- Troponins and electrocardiogram

DIAGNOSTIC STUDIES

- MRI of the brain may show reversible T2 hyperintensity or diffusion restriction exclusive to the hippocampi.
- Electroencephalogram (EEG) to exclude epileptiform activity.

TREATMENT

NONPHARMACOLOGIC THERAPY

Self-limited, not requiring specific pharmacologic or nonpharmacologic treatment

ACUTE GENERAL Rx

Investigate as an emergency.

CHRONIC Rx

- Does not lead to long-term sequela of memory loss. Complete recovery of cognitive function has been reported 5 days to 6 mo after the episode.
- Low risk of subsequent ischemic cerebral stroke or seizures though possible increased risk of future dementia.

DISPOSITION

Due to the benign nature of transient global amnesia, rarely is continued follow-up necessary.

REFERRAL

Referral to a neurologist is necessary when the diagnosis is uncertain or with atypical features of the clinical presentation.

SUGGESTED READINGS

Available at ExpertConsult.com

AUTHOR: **Rituparna Das, MD**

BASIC INFORMATION

DEFINITION

Transient ischemic attack (TIA) is a transient episode of neurologic dysfunction caused by focal brain, spinal cord, or retinal ischemia without acute infarction on MRI. TIA symptoms typically resolve within 60 min and by definition within 24 hr. Despite complete symptom resolution, 20% to 50% of patients clinically suspected to have suffered a TIA have evidence of acute tissue infarction on MRI.

SYNONYMS

TIA
Amaurosis fugax
Ophthalmologic TIA
"Mini-stroke"
Pre-stroke

ICD-10CM CODES

G45.9	Transient cerebral ischemic attack, unspecified
G45.8	Other transient cerebral ischemic attacks and related syndromes
Z86.73	Personal history of transient ischemic attack (TIA), and cerebral infarction without residual deficits

EPIDEMIOLOGY & DEMOGRAPHICS

INCIDENCE: 70 to 101 cases per 100,000 persons annually
PEAK INCIDENCE: After age 60 yr
PREVALENCE: 200,000 to 500,000 persons in the United States. The annual risk of stroke after either a TIA or minor stroke is approximately 3% to 4%.
PREDOMINANT SEX & RACE: Males > females; African American > Caucasian
RISK FACTORS: Same as for ischemic stroke

PHYSICAL FINDINGS & CLINICAL PRESENTATION

- TIAs often present with transient neurologic symptoms including ipsilateral transient monocular blindness (amaurosis fugax), contralateral numbness or weakness, contralateral homonymous hemianopsia, and/or aphasia.
- Box 1 summarizes carotid artery TIAs.
- Vertebrobasilar artery TIAs are described in Box 2.

ETIOLOGY

Embolic (cardioembolism in 10%-15%), large vessel atherothrombotic disease (20%-25%), lacunar disease, hypoperfusion, hypercoagulable state, arteritis

DIAGNOSIS

DIFFERENTIAL DIAGNOSIS

Seizures, hypoglycemia, hemiplegic migraine, intracranial hemorrhage, mass lesion, vestibular disease, Bell palsy, meningitis, multiple sclerosis, subdural hematoma, brain abscess, cervical or lumbar spine disease, conversion disorder

WORKUP

Given the high risk of stroke within the first 48 hr following TIA (up to 10%), hospital admission for workup is advised. Most of the immediate risk of stroke is secondary to carotid disease.

The American Heart Association recommends that the ABCD2 score be used in the evaluation of TIA. It consists of 1 point for age ≥60 yr, 1 point for BP ≥140 mm Hg systolic or ≥90 mm Hg diastolic, clinical features (2 points for unilateral weakness, 1 point for speech impairment), duration of TIA (2 points for duration ≥60 min, 1 point for duration 10-59 min), presence of diabetes mellitus (1 point). According to the guidelines, it is reasonable to hospitalize patients with TIA if they present within 72 hr and have an ABCD2 score ≥3. There is some debate about the usefulness of this scale since it fails to account for changes seen on echocardiogram, carotid Dopplers, or ECG that may place the patient at more imminent risk of stroke (carotid stenosis, Afib, cardiac thrombus, etc.). Alternatives to this scoring system are being investigated.

LABORATORY TESTS

Complete blood count, basic metabolic panel, prothrombin time, activated partial thromboplastin time, sedimentation rate, fasting lipid panel, serum glucose and hemoglobin A_{1c} (to detect latent diabetes mellitus), and TSH.

IMAGING STUDIES

- CT scan should be obtained to exclude hemorrhage; MRI with diffusion-weighted images if immediately available to determine whether infarction occurred.
- Imaging of the vessels should be obtained via magnetic resonance angiography (MRA) head and neck, computed tomography angiography (CTA) head and neck, or carotid Doppler/transcranial Doppler (CD/TCD). If symptoms are localizable to the posterior circulation, MRA or CTA should be obtained in lieu of CD/TCD.
- Transthoracic echocardiogram should be obtained.
- An echocardiogram with bubble should be obtained in all patients younger than 50 yr with TIA symptoms.

BOX 1 Carotid Artery Transient Ischemic Attacks

Symptoms
  Contralateral hemiparesis, hemianopsia, hemisensory loss
  Aphasia, if dominant hemisphere
  Neglect and hemi-inattention, if nondominant hemisphere
  Ipsilateral amaurosis fugax
Associated findings
  Carotid bruit
  Retinal artery emboli
Tests
  Ultrasonography (carotid Doppler studies)
  Magnetic resonance imaging angiography (MRA)
  Cerebral arteriography
Therapy
  Medical: Platelet inhibitors (e.g., aspirin)
  Risk-reduction measures (e.g., control blood pressure, glucose levels, cholesterol)
  Surgical: Carotid endarterectomy, if stenosis >70% and symptomatic
  Endovascular: Placement of stent

From Kaufman DM et al: *Kaufman's clinical neurology for psychiatrists,* ed 8, Philadelphia, 2017, Elsevier.

BOX 2 Vertebrobasilar Artery Transient Ischemic Attacks

Symptoms
  Vertigo, vomiting, tinnitus
  Circumoral paresthesias or numbness
  Dysarthria, dysphagia
  Drop attacks
Associated findings
  Nystagmus
  Ataxia
  Cranial nerve abnormalities
Tests
  Ultrasonography (transcranial Doppler studies)
  Magnetic resonance imaging angiography (MRA)
  Cerebral arteriography
Therapy
  Medical: Platelet inhibitors (see Box 1)
  Risk-reduction measures
  Surgical: None

From Kaufman DM et al: *Kaufman's clinical neurology for psychiatrists,* ed 8, Philadelphia, 2017, Elsevier.

- Electrocardiogram should be obtained to exclude the presence of arrhythmias, namely atrial fibrillation.
- At least 24 hr of heart rhythm monitoring should be accomplished to screen for arrhythmia. Many stroke centers now utilize prolonged ambulatory cardiac rhythm monitoring over several weeks to months to identify paroxysmal atrial fibrillation in select patients when there is a high index of clinical suspicion.
- Paroxysmal atrial fibrillation is common in patients with TIA. A recent study found that noninvasive ambulatory ECG monitoring for 30 days significantly improved the detection of atrial fibrillation by a factor of more than five and nearly doubled the rate of anticoagulant treatment as compared with the standard practice of short-duration ECG monitoring.

Rx TREATMENT

NONPHARMACOLOGIC THERAPY

- Carotid endarterectomy or carotid stenting should be considered for patients found to have carotid stenosis of ≥50% as the cause for TIA. Efficacy is greatest in the 2 wk immediately following a TIA or ischemic stroke. Please refer to the "Carotid Artery Stenosis" chapter for more information.
- The practice of intracranial angioplasty and stenting has largely declined following the publication of negative results from clinical trials and is only used in select patients who fail maximal medical management with aggressive platelet inhibition, strict risk factor control such as hyperlipidemia, hypertension, diabetes mellitus, weight loss, treatment of sleep apnea, and smoking cessation among others.

ACUTE GENERAL Rx

- In the absence of contraindications, patients with atrial fibrillation should be considered for anticoagulation. Choices for anticoagulants include the direct oral anticoagulants (such as dabigatran, rivaroxaban, apixaban, edoxaban, betrixaban) and/or warfarin. In patients with TIA and atrial fibrillation or a cardiac thrombus, therapeutic anticoagulation should be achieved rapidly. Those who are not candidates for a direct oral anticoagulation and who will need chronic warfarin should first be started on either intravenous heparin or therapeutic anticoagulant doses of Lovenox, along with warfarin, until target INR between 2.0 and 3.0 is achieved, at which point warfarin should be continued as monotherapy.
- Although no compelling evidence exists for the use of heparin in the acute treatment of TIAs without cardioembolic source, patients who develop recurrent symptoms within the same vascular territory that increase in duration, severity, and/or frequency (crescendo TIA/stuttering TIA) may benefit from its use pending cardiac and vascular imaging and identification of a possible source.
- Patients with high-risk TIA (ABCD2 score >3) or minor stroke may be started on dual antiplatelet therapy of clopidrogel 600 mg on day 1 followed by 75 mg daily and aspirin for 21 to 30 days based on the POINT trial.

CHRONIC Rx

- Chronic therapy includes single antiplatelet (after 21-30 days) or anticoagulation therapy and modifying the four major risk factors: Hypertension, dyslipidemia, diabetes mellitus, and smoking cessation.
- Antiplatelet therapy should be used to reduce the risk of recurrent TIAs or subsequent stroke. Three antiplatelet agents are commonly used in stroke prevention: Aspirin, aspirin/dipyridamole, and clopidogrel. All are reasonable choices, but practitioners should consider their individual patient's comorbidities when selecting an antiplatelet agent. Chronic long-term dual antiplatelet therapy is not recommended as this increases the risk of hemorrhagic complications.
- Warfarin (INR 2.0-3.0) or use of direct oral anticoagulants instead of an antiplatelet is indicated for prevention of future strokes in atrial fibrillation patients.

PEARLS & CONSIDERATIONS

- All cause mortality in 1 yr is 25% in patients diagnosed TIA.
- Approximately 20% to 30% of ischemic strokes are heralded by transient ischemic symptoms.[1]
- Previous studies conducted between 1987 and 2003 estimated the risk of stroke or an acute coronary syndrome was 12% to 20% during the first 3 mo after a TIA. New data estimate the 1-yr risk to be 6.2%. Multiple infarctions on brain imaging, large-artery atherosclerosis, and an $ABCD^2$ score of 6 or 7 were each associated with more than a doubling of the risk of stroke.[3]

PREVENTION

- A healthy lifestyle and management of cardiovascular risk factors should be encouraged.
- Antiplatelet therapy has not been proven efficacious in primary prevention of TIA or stroke but is very beneficial in secondary prevention.

PATIENT & FAMILY EDUCATION

Patients should be counseled on the early signs of stroke symptoms and instructed to promptly seek medical attention if they develop symptoms concerning for stroke. Patients should be encouraged to pursue a healthy lifestyle to include exercise and smoking cessation. In addition, patients should take an active role in controlling blood pressure and blood glucose. Further educational materials can be found online at www.strokecenter.org/.

SUGGESTED READINGS

Available at ExpertConsult.com

RELATED CONTENT

Transient Ischemic Attack (TIA) (Patient Information)
Carotid Artery Stenosis (Related Key Topic)
Atrial Fibrillation (Related Key Topic)
Stroke, Acute Ischemic (Related Key Topic)
Stroke, Secondary Prevention (Related Key Topic)

AUTHORS: **Corey Goldsmith, MD,** and **Joseph S. Kass, MD, JD, FAAN**

[1] Amarenco P: Transient ischemic attack, *N Engl J Med* 382:1933-1941, 2020.
[2] Amarenco P et al: One-year risk of stroke after transient ischemic attack or minor stroke, *N Engl J Med* 374:1533-1542, 2016.
[3] Kernan WN et al: Pioglitazone after ischemic stroke or transient ischemic attack, *N Engl J Med* 374:1321-1331, 2016.

BASIC INFORMATION

DEFINITION

Demyelination in a transverse region of the spinal cord due to an inflammatory process that leads to sensory and motor changes below the lesion as well as autonomic dysfunction. The term "transverse myelitis" of late refers to any cause of inflammatory myelopathy, irrespective of severity or degree of structural or functional interruption of pathways through a transverse spinal cord section. Transverse myelitis that extends across three or more segments of the cord is referred to as longitudinally extensive transverse myelitis. The pathologic hallmark of transverse myelitis is the presence of focal collections of lymphocytes and monocytes with varying degrees of demyelination, axonal injury, and astroglial and microglial activation within the spinal cord.

SYNONYMS

Idiopathic transverse myelitis (ITM)
TM
ITM

ICD-10CM CODES	
G37.3	Acute transverse myelitis in demyelinating disease of central nervous system
G04.89	Other myelitis

EPIDEMIOLOGY & DEMOGRAPHICS

INCIDENCE: Annual incidence ranges from 1.3 to 8 cases per million. The incidence increases to 24.6 cases per million annually if causes of acquired demyelination such as multiple sclerosis (MS) or neuromyelitis optic spectrum disorder are included.
PREVALENCE: Unknown
PREDOMINANT SEX: None, but female preponderance seen in cases associated with multiple sclerosis and neuromyelitis optica spectrum disorder.
GENETICS: No genetic predisposition has been shown.
PEAK INCIDENCE: Can occur at any age. Bimodal peak in the incidence between 10 to 19 yr and 30 to 39 yr. 20% of cases occur in children with a bimodal peak of incidence between 0 to 2 yr and 5 to 17 yr.
RISK FACTORS: Infection, vaccination

PHYSICAL FINDINGS & CLINICAL PRESENTATION

- Rapid onset of symmetric or asymmetric paraparesis or paraplegia of the lower extremities over a few days, ascending paresthesia, sensory level at the trunk, back pain, sphincter dysfunction, and positive Babinski, which can be bilateral. The arms may also be involved if the cervical cord is involved, but cervical involvement is less common than thoracic involvement. In the acute phase the weakness is flaccid, with diminished deep tendon reflexes mimicking a peripheral neuropathy such as Guillain-Barré syndrome.
- One third to one half of patients present with localizing back pain or a bandlike area of altered sensation, usually at the dermatomal level corresponding to the lesion within the cord.
- There is progression to nadir of clinical deficits between 4 hr and 21 days after symptom onset.
- Urinary incontinence or retention, GI disturbances (incontinence or constipation), and sexual dysfunction are common.
- Acute flaccid myelitis is a subtype of myelitis in which patients present with acute limb weakness and have primarily involvement of gray matter on spinal cord imaging.

ETIOLOGY

- The clinical signs are caused by an interruption in ascending and descending sensory, motor, and autonomic pathways in the transverse plane of the spinal cord, resulting in sensory-level weakness and autonomic dysfunction at and below the level of the lesion due to demyelination or inflammation of the spinal cord.
- Can be idiopathic demyelination (15% to 30%) that is a monophasic one-time event or demyelination secondary to neurologic or systemic conditions (Box 1).
- Secondary causes include postinfection, postvaccination, acute demyelinating encephalomyelitis (where transverse myelitis tends to be monophasic), and others such as multiple sclerosis, neuromyelitis optica spectrum disorder (NMOSD), connective tissue disorders such as systemic lupus, Sjögren syndrome, antiphospholipid antibody syndrome, sarcoidosis, and paraneoplastic conditions, which can be progressive or relapsing.
- Infectious causes of myelitis include HIV, syphilis, varicella zoster (associated with shingles), HTLV-1, Lyme disease, arboviruses such as West Nile virus (typically causing a poliomyelitis-type acute flaccid paralysis), or enteroviruses (typically causing acute flaccid paralysis mainly in children).
- About 50% of patients have had a recent upper respiratory infection.

DIAGNOSIS

DIFFERENTIAL DIAGNOSIS

- MS (Table 1)
- Neuromyelitis optica spectrum disorder (NMOSD)
- Metastatic disease
- Spinal cord tumors
- Herniated or slipped disks
- Spinal stenosis
- Spinal epidural abscess
- Vascular malformation
  1. Spinal dural arteriovenous fistula (most common)
  2. Arteriovenous malformation of the spinal cord

BOX 1 Central Nervous System and Systemic Autoimmune Disorders Associated with Acute Transverse Myelitis

Central Nervous System Disorders
Acute disseminated encephalomyelitis
Multiple sclerosis
Neuromyelitis optica

Systemic Autoimmune Disorders
Antiphospholipid antibody syndrome
Behçet disease
Mixed connective tissue disorder
Neurosarcoidosis
Sjögren syndrome
Systemic lupus erythematosus

From Cherry JD et al: *Feigin and Cherry's textbook of pediatric infectious diseases,* ed 8, Philadelphia, 2019, Elsevier.

TABLE 1 Distinguishing Acute Transverse Myelitis from Other Central Nervous System Demyelinating Disorders

Finding	ATM	ADEM	MS	NMO
Myelitis	+	+/−	+/− (partial)	+
Acute mental status changes	−	+	−	+/−
Optic neuritis	−	+/−	+/−	+/−
Abnormal brain MRI	−	+	+	+/−
CSF oligoclonal bands	−	+/−	+	+/−
Serum AQP4-IgG	−	−	−	+/−
Recurrences	+/−	+/−	+	+

+, Always present; +/−, variably present; −, usually absent.
ADEM, Acute disseminated encephalomyelitis; *AQP,* aquaporin 4; *ATM,* acute transverse myelitis; *CSF,* cerebrospinal fluid; *MRI,* magnetic resonance imaging; *MS,* multiple sclerosis; *NMO,* neuromyelitis optica.
From Cherry JD et al: *Feigin and Cherry's textbook of pediatric infectious diseases,* ed 8, Philadelphia, 2019, Elsevier.

TABLE 2 Suggested Diagnostic Workup for Recurrent Central Nervous System Demyelinating Disorders and Systemic Autoimmune Disorders Associated with Acute Transverse Myelitis

All Patients	Suggestive of Neuromyelitis Optica	Also Consider
Brain MRI with gadolinium	Ophthalmology consultation	Angiotensin-converting enzyme (serum, CSF)
CSF oligoclonal bands	Visual evoked potentials	Other autoantibodies
Antinuclear antibodies	Formal visual field testing	Anti-dsDNA
Antiphospholipid antibodies		Anti-La
Serum AQP4-IgG		Anti-Ro
		Anti-Smith

CSF, Cerebrospinal fluid; *MRI,* magnetic resonance imaging; *NMO,* neuromyelitis optica.
From Cherry JD et al: *Feigin and Cherry's textbook of pediatric infectious diseases,* ed 8, Philadelphia, 2019, Elsevier.

TABLE 3 Suggested Diagnostic Workup for Infections Associated with Acute Transverse Myelitis

Blood	Cerebrospinal Fluid	Other
• Blood cultures • Acute and convalescent titers to *Borrelia burgdorferi*, EBV, *Mycoplasma pneumoniae*	• Bacterial culture • Viral culture • PCR testing for CMV, EBV, Enterovirus, HSV, *M. pneumoniae*, VZV	• Viral culture of stool and respiratory secretions • Consider stool ova and parasite testing and serum titers if parasitic infection is suspected

CMV, Cytomegalovirus; *EBV,* Epstein-Barr virus; *HSV,* herpes simplex virus; *PCR,* polymerase chain reaction; *VZV,* varicella zoster virus.
From Cherry JD et al: *Feigin and Cherry's textbook of pediatric infectious diseases,* ed 8, Philadelphia, 2019, Elsevier.

- Spinal cord infarction due to either anterior spinal artery or posterior spinal artery occlusion

WORKUP

Transverse myelitis (TM) should be suspected in patients with a history of rapid (hours to days) onset of motor weakness and sensory abnormalities with bladder or bowel dysfunction that is referable to the spinal cord. The dysfunction is bilateral (not necessarily symmetric), and there is often a clearly defined sensory (dermatomal) level. It is important to distinguish idiopathic TM from TM due to MS or neuromyelitis optica spectrum disorder because idiopathic TM does not relapse and does not require long-term immunomodulatory therapy. A suggested diagnostic workup for recurrent CNS demyelinating disorders and systemic autoimmune disorders associated with acute transverse myelitis is summarized in Table 2.

LABORATORY TESTS

- Lumbar puncture looking for CSF pleocytosis, oligoclonal bands for MS, or serology and PCR looking for infection (Table 3) such as varicella zoster virus and enterovirus PCR.
- ANA, hepatitis B serology, Lyme disease serology, VDRL, SSA, SSB, anticardiolipin antibody, lupus anticoagulant, copper, ceruloplasmin, vitamin B_{12}, RPR.
- Serum NMO-IgG and myelin oligodendrocyte glycoprotein (MOG) antibodies to evaluate for neuromyelitis optica spectrum disorder.
- If a paraneoplastic etiology is suspected, then appropriate antibodies should be ordered and appropriate cancer screening undertaken.

IMAGING STUDIES

- Gadolinium-enhanced magnetic resonance imaging (MRI) of brain and MRI of the entire spine (Fig. E1, Fig. E2). This will show demyelinating lesion on T_2 with contrast enhancement. In MS there is usually a short segment lesion (less than three vertebral segments) that is dorsally located. Longitudinally extensive transverse myelitis that spans more than three or more segments of the cord is more typical of NMOSD, postinfectious, vascular, or other inflammatory causes.
- Computed tomography (CT) of the spine with and without contrast should be obtained if MRI is unavailable, but CT does not allow for visualization of the spinal cord itself.
- CT myelogram may also be obtained if MRI is unavailable to evaluate for compression; however, this does not image the parenchyma of the cord directly.
- Chest CT with and without contrast if sarcoidosis is suspected.

Rx TREATMENT

Corticosteroids (IV methylprednisolone 1 g/day for 3 to 7 days) are the first-line treatment for transverse myelitis.

NONPHARMACOLOGIC THERAPY

- Physical therapy
- Respiratory and oropharyngeal support

ACUTE GENERAL Rx

- High-dose IV corticosteroid (e.g., methylprednisolone 1000 mg/day for 3 to 7 days) to stop inflammatory damage to the spinal cord.
- Rescue therapy with plasma exchange may be helpful in patients who do not respond to corticosteroids.
- Combination therapy with plasmapheresis and corticosteroids or other immunosuppressive agents (e.g., rituximab or cyclophosphamide) may also be effective.
- Analgesia for pain.

CHRONIC Rx

- Baclofen or tizanidine for muscle spasms
- Gabapentin or pregabalin for neuropathic pain
- Low-molecular-weight heparin for DVT prophylaxis in patients with immobility
- Need for chronic immunosuppression will depend on underlying etiology

DISPOSITION

- One third of patients with transverse myelitis will have complete recovery, one third will have fair recovery, and one third have permanent disability and do not recover. Recurrence or relapse is possible, especially if the patient has MS, NMOSD, or sarcoidosis.
- Patients who need further care, including those with urinary retention, may need home nursing assistance. Some patients may benefit from rehabilitation, either inpatient or outpatient.

REFERRAL

- Referral to a neurologist to evaluate need for long-term therapy.
- Referral for physical and occupational therapy.
- Consider psychiatric consultation (high incidence of long-term mood and anxiety disorders).

SUGGESTED READINGS

Available at ExpertConsult.com

AUTHORS: **Padmaja Sudhakar, MBBS,** and **Corey Goldsmith, MD**

BASIC INFORMATION

DEFINITION

- Impact to the head resulting in varying levels of cellular and macroscopic changes, detected with clinical examination supplemented by imaging stuikdies.
- Mild traumatic brain injury (TBI) is defined as loss of consciousness <30 minutes, a Glasgow Coma Scale (GCS) of 13 to 15, and normal imaging.
- Moderate TBI is defined as loss of consciousness for 30 minutes to 24 hours with even longer alteration in consciousness, a GCS of 9 to 12, and may or may not have abnormal imaging.
- Severe TBI is defined as >24 hours of loss of consciousness with a GCS of 3 to 8 and prolonged posttraumatic amnesia with normal or abnormal imaging.

SYNONYMS

TBI
Head injury
Concussion
Intracranial contusion

ICD-10CM CODES

S06.9 X0A	Intracranial injury
S06.1X7A	Traumatic cerebral edema with loss of consciousness of any duration with death due to brain injury prior to regaining consciousness, initial encounter
S06.2X9A	Diffuse traumatic brain injury with loss of consciousness of unspecified duration, initial encounter
S06.300A	Unspecified focal traumatic brain injury without loss of consciousness, initial encounter
S06.305A	Unspecified focal traumatic brain injury with loss of consciousness greater than 24 hours with return to pre-existing conscious level, initial encounter
S06.309A	Unspecified focal traumatic brain injury with loss of consciousness of unspecified duration, initial encounter

EPIDEMIOLOGY & DEMOGRAPHICS

Traumatic brain injury (TBI) is a worldwide leading cause of mortality in young individuals. Urbanization and increasing use of motor vehicles has led to an overall increase in TBI, especially in high-income and developing countries.

INCIDENCE: Globally, more than 10 million people suffer TBI resulting in mortality or requiring hospitalization each yr. By 2020, it is projected that TBI will surpass many diseases as the major cause of death and disability worldwide. TBI likely accounts for 9% of global mortality and is a threat to health in every country in the world. The financial burden of TBI has been estimated to be greater than $80 billion per yr in the United States alone. According to estimates from the CDC, about 2.87 million emergency department visits, including deaths and hospitalizations, were associated with TBI in 2014.

PREVALENCE: The prevalence of TBI in the United States has been estimated at approximately 5.3 million. In the European Union with 330 million inhabitants, approximately 7,775,000 new TBI cases occur each yr. According to the CDC, combined rates of TBI-related hospitalizations, emergency department visits, and deaths have risen from 521/100,000 in 2000 to 823.7/100,000 in 2010.

PEAK INCIDENCE: Approximate incidence in the US per CDC data is 103/100,000 population. In the European Union, this is estimated to be at 235/100,000.

PREDOMINANT SEX & AGE: TBI occurs more frequently in young adults, particularly males 15 to 25 yr of age, and has a high cost to society because of life years lost. Hospitalizations and deaths are the highest in older adults >75 yr of age.

GENETICS: TBI and Apo E ε4 synergistically are also associated with a tenfold increased risk for Alzheimer disease as well as larger intracerebral hematomas and greater ischemia after TBI.

RISK FACTORS: N/A.

PHYSICAL FINDINGS & CLINICAL PRESENTATION

TBI patients can present with a spectrum of clinical symptoms including nausea, vomiting, headache, seizures, altered mental status, and/or coma. Stigmata of trauma, including bruises, scalp lacerations, and periorbital or mastoid ecchymosis suggesting skull base fractures, are telltale signs of possible underlying traumatic brain injury. Box 1 describes risk stratification in patients with minor head trauma. The spectrum of TBI is most commonly assessed using the GCS, which ranges from 3 to 15 and utilizes eye, motor, and verbal exams (Table 1).

ETIOLOGY

- Mechanical falls (35%), motor vehicle accidents (17%), and assaults resulting in direct or indirect trauma to the head are the most common etiologies. The most deaths occur from motor vehicle accidents.
- An estimated 283,000 children seek care in U.S. emergency departments each yr for a sport- or recreation-related TBI. TBIs sustained in contact sports account for approximately 45% of these visits. Football, bicycling, basketball, playground activities, and soccer account for the highest number of emergency department visits.[1]

DIAGNOSIS

DIFFERENTIAL DIAGNOSIS

Differential diagnosis of TBI is quite limited; however, there are several considerations and diagnoses considered as a possibility within the realm of TBI. These are enumerated in the imaging section.

WORKUP

TBI workup is always a part of the advanced trauma life support (ATLS) protocol. Primary and secondary survey followed by imaging studies constitutes the standardized approach to TBI. Focused TBI workup includes:

- History: Including timing of injury, duration of loss of consciousness if applicable, seizures (if any), comorbidities, use of anticoagulants and antiplatelet agents (requires reversal in the event of intracranial blood on imaging).
- Neurological examination: Glasgow Coma Scale, cranial nerves, motor/sensory exam. Assess for scalp lacerations, specifically overlying a skull fracture as well as CSF otorrhea or rhinorrhea.

BOX 1 Risk Stratification in Patients with Minor Head Trauma

High Risk
- Focal neurologic findings
- Asymmetrical pupils
- Skull fracture on clinical examination
- Multiple trauma
- Serious, painful, distracting injuries
- External signs of trauma above the clavicles
- Initial Glasgow Coma Scale score of 14 or 15
- Loss of consciousness
- Posttraumatic confusion or amnesia
- Progressively worsening headache
- Vomiting
- Posttraumatic seizure
- History of bleeding disorder or anticoagulation
- Recent ingestion of intoxicants
- Unreliable or unknown history of injury
- Previous neurologic diagnosis
- Previous epilepsy
- Suspected child abuse
- Age above 60 yr or below 2 yr

Medium Risk
- Initial Glasgow Coma Scale score of 15
- Brief loss of consciousness
- Posttraumatic amnesia
- Vomiting
- Headache
- Intoxication

Low Risk
- Currently asymptomatic
- No other injuries
- No focality on examination
- Normal pupils
- No change in consciousness
- Intact orientation and memory
- Initial Glasgow Coma Scale score of 15
- Accurate history
- Trivial mechanism
- Injury less than 24 hours ago
- No or mild headache
- No vomiting
- No preexisting high-risk factors

[1]Sarmiento K et al: Emergency Department Visits for Sports- and Recreation-Related Traumatic Brain Injuries Among Children—United States, 2010–2016, *MMWR* 68;241, 2019.

TABLE 1 Useful Criteria to Assess the Severity of Head Injury[a]

Quantifying the Degree of Head Injury	Glasgow Coma Scale (GCS)	Score
• Moderate TBI (GCS 9-13)	**Eye Opening**	
• Severe TBI (GCS <8)	Spontaneous	4
• Significant head CT:	To speech	3
• Cerebral edema	To pain	2
• Midline shift	None	1
• Subdural/epidural bleeding	**Verbal Response**	
• Open head injury with intracranial air	Orientated	5
	Confused conversation	4
	Inappropriate words	3
	Incomprehensible sounds	2
	None	1
	Best Motor Response	
	Obeys commands	6
	Localizes pain	5
	Flexion withdrawal to pain	4
	Abnormal flexion (decorticate)	3
	Extension (decerebrate)	2
	None (flaccid)	1

[a]Consultation with other specialists (i.e., neurosurgeon) may be valuable for the orthopedic surgeon unfamiliar with the process of "clearing" the patient's head injury for IMN fixation.

From Browner B et al: *Skeletal trauma: basic science, management, and reconstruction,* ed 6, Philadelphia, 2019, Elsevier.

BOX 2 American College of Emergency Physicians Clinical Policy Regarding Neuroimaging in Adults with Mild Traumatic Brain Injury

A noncontrast head CT is indicated (level-1 recommendation) in adults with LOC or posttraumatic amnesia only if one or more of the following is present:
- Headache
- Vomiting
- Age >60 yr
- Drug or alcohol intoxication
- Deficits in short-term memory
- Physical evidence of trauma above the clavicle
- Posttraumatic seizure
- GCS score <15
- Focal neurologic deficit
- Coagulopathy

A noncontrast head CT should be considered (level-2 recommendation) in head trauma patients with no LOC or posttraumatic amnesia if there is:
- Focal neurologic deficit
- Vomiting
- Severe headache
- Age ≥ 65 yr
- Physical signs of a basilar skull fracture
- GCS score <15
- Coagulopathy
- A dangerous mechanism (e.g., ejection from motor vehicle, pedestrian struck, fall of more than 3 feet or 5 stairs)

CT, Computed tomography; *GCS,* Glasgow Coma Scale; *LOC,* loss of consciousness.

From Marx JA et al: *Rosen's emergency medicine,* ed 8, Philadelphia, 2014, Elsevier.

- CT imaging of the head if there is a significant history of impact to the head, polytrauma, positive loss of consciousness, or stigmata of trauma to the head. The American College of Emergency Physicians Clinical Policy Regarding Neuroimaging in adults with mild TBI is summarized in Box 2.

LABORATORY TESTS

- Basic labs including CBC, basic metabolic panel, prothrombin time, activated partial thromboplastin time, urine drug screen, and ethanol blood level.
- Consider tests for platelet function analysis for unknown antiplatelet use.
- No blood biomarker currently exists. (Figs. 1 and E2)

IMAGING STUDIES (TABLE 2)

CT imaging forms the current cornerstone of imaging modalities for head trauma. Usually, in addition to a plain CT of the head (Fig. 3), CTA head/neck and CT of the spine is helpful if arterial or C-spine injury is suspected, respectively. Other imaging modalities such as MRI can be helpful in certain situations but are typically adjuncts in the acute setting to CT-guided management. Canadian CT head rules are a useful guide in determining utility of obtaining a CT scan. These are based on risk factors:

HIGH RISK:
- Failure to reach GCS of 15 within 2 hours
- Suspected open or any signs of basal skull fracture
- More than two episodes of vomiting
- Age older than 65

LOW RISK:
- Dangerous mechanism of injury or polytrauma
- Loss of consciousness lasting >30 minutes

Pathologies that can be identified with imaging are noted in the following:
- Primary extraaxial: Epidural, subdural, subarachnoid hemorrhage
- Primary intraaxial: Axonal injury, cortical contusion, intracerebral or intraventricular hemorrhage, encephalomalacia (from prior TBI or vascular insult)
- Skull fracture: Linear, depressed, open, involving frontal sinus or skull base
- Penetrating brain injury: Gunshot wounds, sharp objects resulting in parenchymal and vascular injury
- Vascular injury: Dissection, traumatic carotid-cavernous fistula (CCF), dural arteriovenous fistula (dAVF), pseudoaneurysm formation
- Secondary acute injury: Diffuse cerebral swelling/dysautoregulation (seen more commonly in children from posttraumatic hyperemia), infarction, infection from penetrating trauma, brain herniation from mass lesion or cerebral edema
- Secondary chronic injury: Hydrocephalus (posttraumatic due to disruption of normal CSF absorption pathways), encephalomalacia, CSF leak (from skull base fractures, manifests as otorrhea or rhinorrhea, leptomeningeal cyst (seen most commonly in infants, skull fracture resulting in underlying dural injury)

Rx TREATMENT

Prevention of secondary injury is the primary goal of prehospital and early in-hospital management. Most common mechanisms of secondary injury are either intracranial (ICP, hematoma) or systemic (hypoxia, hypovolemia, hypotension). Early categorization of head trauma patients according to the severity (based on GCS) and transport to facilities equipped with personnel and technology to deal with issues pertaining to head trauma has improved the overall management of head injury patients and prevention of secondary injury. Assessment and treatment recommendations for mild TBI are summarized in Table 3. Airway, breathing, and circulation, however, still remain the most important parameters to be stabilized and both directly and indirectly affect GCS and overall outcome. Trauma guidelines suggest intubation should be performed in any patient with a GCS

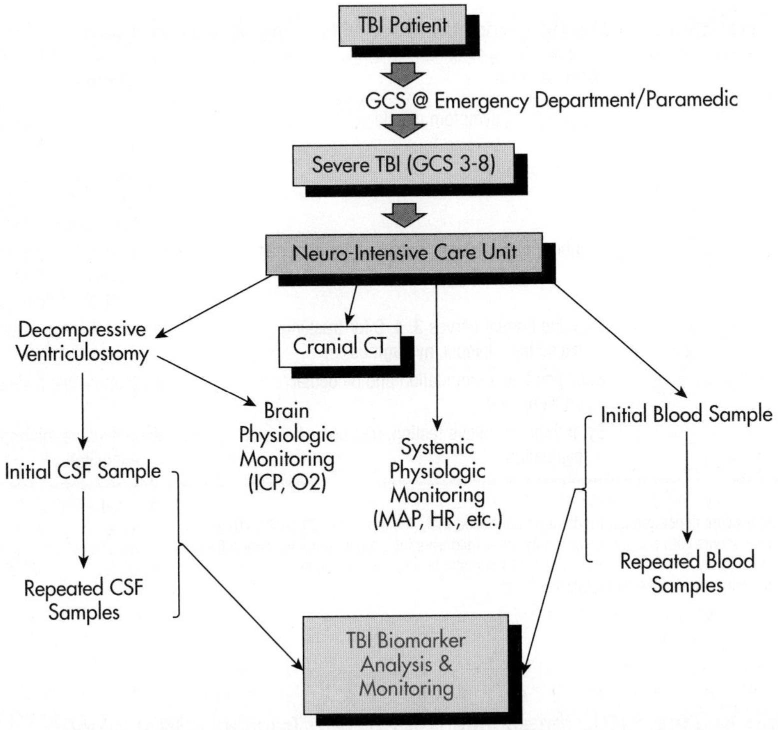

FIG. 1 Envisioned uses of brain biomarkers for severe traumatic brain injury (TBI) patient management. *CSF,* Cerebrospinal fluid; *CT,* computed tomography; *GCS,* Glasgow Coma Scale; *HR,* heart rate; *ICP,* intracranial pressure; *MAP,* mean arterial blood pressure. (From Vincent JL et al: *Textbook of critical care,* ed 7, Philadelphia, 2017, Elsevier.)

TABLE 2 Comparison of Head Imaging Modalities

	Computed Tomography Scans	Magnetic Resonance Imaging	Angiography	Skull Radiography
Advantages	Fast Patient accessible for monitoring Defines acute hemorrhages, mass effects, bone injuries, hydrocephalus, intraventricular blood, edema	Defines contusions and pericontusion edema, posttraumatic ischemic infarction, brainstem injuries	Helps localize acute traumatic lesions Defines vascular injuries, injuries to venous sinuses Detects mass effects	Readily available May help screen some patients for further imaging studies
Disadvantages	Artifacts arise from patient's movement, foreign bodies Streak artifacts may obscure brainstem or posterior fossa	Slow Patients not easily accessible for monitoring Does not define most acute hemorrhagic lesions Not useful for bone injuries	Does not define nature of acute lesion Does not detect infratentorial masses	Does not indicate presence or absence of intracranial injury
Indications	Acute severe head trauma Acute moderate head trauma Suspected depressed skull fracture High-risk minor head trauma Suspected child abuse in minor head trauma Deteriorating neurologic status	Persistent symptoms with postconcussive syndrome Suspected posttraumatic ischemic infarction Suspected contusions not seen on CT scan	Suspected vascular injury CT scan not available	CT scan may not be done Penetrating head trauma

CT, Computed tomography.
From Marx JA et al: *Rosen's emergency medicine: concepts and clinical practice,* ed 7, 2010, Elsevier.

of 8 or less to prevent hypoxemia and hypercapnia. Intravenous fluid resuscitation should also be started early to prevent hypovolemia resulting in hypotension, shown to double mortality. Transfer to and care in a Level I trauma center are associated with better outcomes. Monitoring and treatment recommendations for severe TBI are summarized in Table 4.

Details of in-hospital management including critical care and surgical intervention is beyond the scope of this text. Some important points are summarized below.

- ATLS protocol (airway, breathing, circulation, disability, exposure).
- Ventilatory support.
- Optimization of oxygenation, ventilation, and fluid status.
- CT head (Fig. E4) to evaluate for mass lesion (hematoma) or cerebral edema. These findings may necessitate either surgical intervention or ICP monitor placement. ATLS guidelines recommend maximum 30 minutes between initial assessment and CT head.
- In case of either a severe TBI (GCS 8 or less) or a moderate TBI (GCS 8 to 13) with an unreliable neurological exam, patients

TABLE 3 Assessment and Treatment Recommendations for Mild Traumatic Brain Injury

Function	Assessment	Treatment
Overall recovery	Standardized symptom checklist	Physical rest 1-2 days[1] followed by subsymptomatic aerobic exercise[2]
Headache	Determine the type	HA persisting more than 3-4 days may require abortive treatment tailored to phenotype (migraine, tension-type, occipital neuralgia, etc.)
Vertigo	Romberg test, dynamic standing, tandem gait	If Hallpike Dix is normal, or if Epley maneuver does not relieve symptoms, consider physical therapy for vestibular rehabilitation
Eye movements	Examine cranial nerves 3, 4, 6 for tracking, saccades, diplopia, nystagmus	Physical therapy evaluation for vestibular rehabilitation
Near-vision	Near-point accommodation and binocular convergence	Ophthalmologic evaluation for vision therapy
Cognitive function	Symptoms, cognitive testing, neuropsychologist evaluation	Sleep hygiene, neuropsychology evaluation for cognitive rehabilitation[3]

HA, Headache.
[1]Thomas DG et al: Benefits of strict rest after acute concussion: a randomized controlled trial, *Pediatrics* 135:213-223, 2015.
[2]Kurowski BG et al: Aerobic exercise for adolescents with prolonged symptoms after mild traumatic brain injury: an exploratory randomized clinical trial, *J Head Trauma Rehabil* 32:79-89, 2017.
[3]Cooper DB et al: Cognitive rehabilitation for military service members with mild traumatic brain injury: a randomized clinical trial, *J Head Trauma Rehabil* 32:E1-E15, 2017.
From Goldman L, Schafer AI: *Goldman-Cecil medicine,* ed 26, 2019, Elsevier.

TABLE 4 Monitoring and Treatment Recommendations for Severe Traumatic Brain Injury*

Monitoring	Indication and/or Recommendation
Intracranial pressure (ICP)	GCS ≤8 *AND* abnormal head CT† *OR* any 2 of the following: Age >40, motor posturing, SBP <90 mm Hg. Treatments should aim to keep ICP ≤22 mg Hg.
Cerebral perfusion pressure (CPP)	Treatments should aim for a CPP of 60-70 mm Hg.
Advanced cerebral monitoring	Jugular bulb monitoring of AV oxygen difference. Treatments should aim to keep venous saturation ≥50%.
SBP	Treatments should aim to keep SBP ≥110 mm Hg in those 18-49 and >70 yr old, ≥100 mm Hg in those 50-69 yr old.
Treatment	
Decompressive craniectomy	Not recommended to improve outcome, but may shorten ICU stay and result in less ICP-targeting interventions.
Prophylactic hypothermia	Does not improve outcome.[1]
Hyperosmolar therapy	Mannitol for signs of herniation or progressive neurologic deterioration.
CSF drainage	Within first 12 hours in those with GCS <6. Continuous drainage is better than intermittent.
Ventilation	Short-term hyperventilation can be used to reduce elevated ICP, but avoid in the first 24 hours after injury. Prolonged hyperventilation with Pa_{CO_2} ≤25 mm Hg is not recommended; if used, monitor jugular venous saturation.
Sedation	Propofol to control ICP. High-dose barbiturate administration is restricted to ICP refractory to standard surgical and medical treatments.
Corticosteroids	Not recommended (high-dose methylprednisolone is associated with increased mortality risk).
Nutrition	Achieving basic caloric replacement by postinjury day 5-7 to reduce mortality risk. Transgastric jejunal feeding tube reduces ventilator-associated pneumonia.
Prophylactic antibiotics	Povidone-iodine oral care does not reduce ventilator-associated pneumonia. Antimicrobial-impregnated catheters may prevent catheter-related infections during external ventricular drainage.
DVT prophylaxis	LMWH or low-dose unfractionated heparin may be used (in combination with compression stockings) if the traumatic brain injury is stable and the benefit outweighs the increased risk of intracranial hemorrhage expansion.
Seizure prophylaxis	Phenytoin to prevent early post-traumatic seizures (within 1 wk of injury), although early seizures are not associated with worse outcome; antiepileptic drugs are not recommended to prevent late seizures.

AV, Arteriovenous; *CSF,* cerebrospinal fluid; *CT,* computed tomography; *DVT,* deep venous thrombosis; *GCS,* Glasgow Coma Scale; *ICU,* intensive care unit; *LMWH,* low-molecular-weight heparin; *SBP,* systolic blood pressure.
*Brain Trauma Foundation Guidelines.
†Hematoma, contusion, swelling, herniation, or compressed basal cisterns.
[1]Lewis SR et al: Hypothermia for traumatic brain injury, *Cochrane Database Syst Rev* 9:CD001048, 2017.
From Goldman L, Schafer AI: *Goldman-Cecil medicine,* ed 26, 2019, Elsevier.

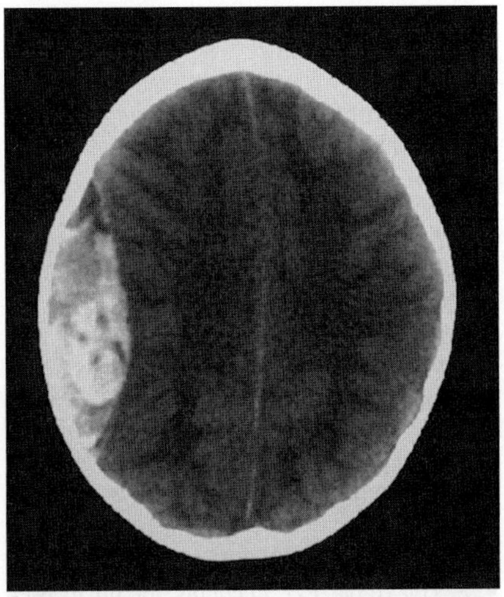

FIG. 3 Noncontrast-enhanced computed tomography scan of acute epidural hematoma at the level of right midconvexity. There is an associated mass effect and moderate midline shift. (From Marx JA et al: *Rosen's emergency medicine: concepts and clinical practice*, ed 7, 2010, Elsevier.)

should be admitted to the intensive care unit for frequent neurological checks. TBI guidelines suggest ICP monitor placement for GCS 8 or less to monitor intracranial pressure closely. ICP monitors are of various kinds, and the most commonly used include external ventricular drain, intraparenchymal pressure monitor, and a bolt device with brain tissue oxygen pressure monitoring with fiberoptic pressure monitor. Recent research has also supported the use of brain tissue oxygen monitoring for severe TBI patients. Surgical decompression may involve evacuation of hematoma (epidural, subdural intraparenchymal contusion) through craniotomy alone (replacement of bone after completion of operation) versus decompressive craniectomy (complete removal of bone without replacement) in certain cases where cerebral edema is out of proportion to the presence of mass lesion. Skull fractures are treated depending on the morphology of the fracture. Open, depressed fractures require surgical debridement and elevation in most cases, in addition to broad-spectrum antibiotics.

- Avoid electrolyte imbalance, especially hyponatremia and hyperglycemia, which may contribute to cerebral edema and increase intracranial pressure.
- Elevation of head of bed to allow better venous drainage to reduce intracranial pressure.
- ICP management, which may include the following: Drainage of cerebrospinal fluid via external ventricular drain, surgical hematoma evacuation, administration of hyperosmotic fluids to reduce edema, pharmacologic sedation and paralysis, pentobarbital-induced coma, and surgical decompression of the brain. Decompressive craniectomy in patients with TBI and refractory intracranial hypertension results in lower mortality and higher rates of vegetative state, lower severe disability, and upper severe disability than medical care.[2] In patients with traumatic brain injury, hypothermia can reduce intracranial hypertension, but recent trials in patients with an intracranial pressure of more than 20 mm Hg after TBI, therapeutic hypothermia, plus standard care to reduce intracranial pressure did not result in outcomes better than those with standard care alone. The new TBI guidelines do not recommend hypothermia.[3]
- Prevention of seizures in the acute setting. The most commonly used and studied drug is phenytoin. Indications for acute seizure prophylaxis in severe head trauma are described in Box 3. Levetiracetam is also a beneficial antiepileptic now commonly used in the TBI setting. Seizure prophylaxis, however, has not shown to prevent long-term development of traumatic epilepsy.
- DVT prophylaxis is recommended in almost all patients on hospital day 1 in addition to sequential compression devices (SCDs) for immobile or bedbound patients to prevent DVTs.
- Early initiation of parenteral nutrition.
- Early tracheostomy for ventilator-dependent patients is recommended to reduce mechanical ventilation days.

BOX 3 Indications for Acute Seizure Prophylaxis in Severe Head Trauma

- Depressed skull fracture
- Paralyzed and intubated patient
- Seizure at the time of injury
- Seizure at emergency department presentation
- Penetrating brain injury
- Severe head injury (Glasgow Coma Scale score ≤8)
- Acute subdural hematoma
- Acute epidural hematoma
- Acute intracranial hemorrhage
- Prior history of seizures

CHRONIC Rx

- TBI can lead to short- or long-term emotional, physiologic, and cognitive sequelae. Patients suffering from TBI are shown to benefit from neurocognitive, occupational, and physical therapy. The Glasgow Outcome Scale is a comprehensive measure of severity and eventual outcome of brain injury. Posttraumatic amnesia, age, length of coma, GCS score within the first 24 hours, and imaging study scales are some of the factors affecting outcome and dictating long-term prognosis.
- Chronic treatment addresses several sequelae of TBI, including, but not limited to, the following: Dysautonomia, agitation, sleep disturbance, posttraumatic epilepsy, spasticity, dysphagia, syndrome of the trephined, posttraumatic hydrocephalus, apathy, fecal/urinary incontinence, headache, and neuropathic pain syndromes.
- Neurostimulants such as amantadine, zolpidem, bromocriptine, amphetamine, and methylphenidate are used in the rehabilitation phase with anecdotal data, but good RCTs are lacking in this area.

DISPOSITION

Depending on severity of head injury, patients may require admission to a rehabilitation facility or discharge to home with outpatient neurocognitive therapy.

REFERRAL

Early transfer to a Level 1 Trauma Center with neurosurgical personnel if high-risk findings are noted on clinical exam or CT head, and is associated with better outcomes.

PEARLS & CONSIDERATIONS

TBI is major healthcare issue. Guidelines have been developed to address TBI in a timely and effective fashion. Clinical acumen and judgment, however, is irreplaceable and should be exercised for better patient care and outcomes. Early recognition of high-risk patients and early imaging and early evaluation at a Level 1 Trauma Center by a specialist are associated with improved outcomes. The goal of healthcare providers in the field or in the community is to identify patients who need this attention.

PATIENT & FAMILY EDUCATION

- Brain Injury Association of America www.biausa.org/
- Brain Injury Resource Center www.headinjury.com/linktbisup.htm

SUGGESTED READING

Available at ExpertConsult.com

RELATED CONTENT

Concussion (Related Key Topic)
Postconcussion Syndrome (Related Key Topic)

AUTHORS: **Farhan A. Mirza, MD,** and **Justin F. Fraser, MD**

[2]Andrews PJD et al: Hypothermia for intracranial hypertension after traumatic brain injury, *N Engl J Med* 373:2103-2112, 2015.

[3]Hutchinson PJ: Trial of decompressive craniectomy for traumatic intracranial hypertension, *N Engl J Med* 379:1119-1130, 2016.

BASIC INFORMATION

DEFINITION

Traveler diarrhea (TD) is defined as three or more loose-to-watery stools, with or without associated fever, abdominal cramps, and vomiting, within a 24-hr period. It develops during or within 10 days of traveling to developing areas of the world.

SYNONYMS

TD
Enterotoxigenic *E. coli*
Enteroaggregative *E. coli*
Infectious diarrhea
Postinfectious irritable bowel syndrome

ICD-10CM CODE

A09 Infectious diarrhea

EPIDEMIOLOGY & DEMOGRAPHICS

- Traveler diarrhea is mostly caused by bacteria and other pathogens in food and water.
- At least one episode of diarrhea occurs in 40% to 50% of travelers during their stay abroad. Table 1 describes pathogens and epidemiologic features associated with traveler diarrhea.

INCIDENCE:
- **High risk (>20%):** South and Southeast Asia, Africa (except South Africa), South and Central America, and Mexico
- **Moderate risk (10% to 20%):** Caribbean Islands, South Africa, Central and East Asia (including Russia and China), Eastern Europe, and the Middle East, including Israel
- **Low risk (<10%):** Northern and Western Europe, Australia, New Zealand, United States, Canada, Singapore, Japan

PEAK INCIDENCE:
- Peak incidence occurs during the first week of travel and progressively declines after that
- Seasonal variation does exist for TD, with lower rates in the winter months

PREVALENCE: Acute and chronic diarrhea account for a third of medical visits by returned travelers as per the GeoSentinel database.

PREDOMINANT SEX & AGE:
- Travelers in their 30s are at highest risk, possibly secondary to more adventurous travel.
- Gender does not seem to influence the risk for TD.
- Infants and toddlers are more likely to have a more severe form of TD and are more likely to need hospitalization.

GENETICS: Travelers with the O blood group are at higher risk for diarrhea caused by Norovirus and *Shigella*.

RISK FACTORS:
- Gastric acid protects against enteropathogens, so medications that reduce gastric acid secretion (i.e., PPI or H2-receptor blockers) are known to increase risk for TD by a factor of 12.
- Immunocompromised travelers such as those with HIV/AIDS are at higher risk for parasitic infections.
- Backpackers are at higher risk than those staying at a resort.
- Food bought from street vendors or prepared by persons not wearing gloves carries a higher risk.

PHYSICAL FINDINGS & CLINICAL PRESENTATION

- The clinical presentation does not allow determination of infectious cause.
- Ninety percent of cases occur within 2 wk of stay.
- Acute watery diarrhea predominates in 90% of patients.
- Signs of invasive infection, including fever and bloody/mucoid diarrhea, occur in 3% to 30%.
- Most patients report three to five bowel movements a day, but in 20% a higher frequency of up to 20 daily bowel movements occurs.
- Nausea (10% to 70%), vomiting (4% to 36%), abdominal cramps/tenesmus (80%), urgency (90%).
- Other: Myalgia, arthralgia, headache.
- Average episode resolves in 3 to 5 days.
- Prolonged symptoms lasting more than 1 wk: 8% to 15%; chronic diarrhea >30 days: 1% to 3%.
- Severe episodes may result in electrolyte imbalance (K+ loss).
- Fifty percent of all travelers are incapacitated for at least 24 hr, but up to 20% are ill in bed for 1 to 2 days.

ETIOLOGY

- *E. coli* (Table E2): Accounts for up to 60% of all cases of TD and is most prevalent in Central and South America, South Asia, and Africa. Table E3 summarizes etiology of traveler diarrhea in Latin America, Africa, and Asia.
  1. Enterotoxigenic *E. coli* (ETEC): Produce heat labile and heat stable toxin and are the most common cause, accounting for 10% to 45% of cases. Frequently seen in Latin America, Africa, and South Asia.
  2. Enteroaggregative *E. coli* (EAEC): More commonly seen in Latin America.
  3. Other *E. coli* (enteropathogenic [EPEC], enteroinvasive [EIEC], enterohemorrhagic [EHEC]): Shiga toxin-producing or diffuse adhering *E. coli* are much less common.
- *Campylobacter:* 2% to 32% of cases. More common in Southeast Asia, where it is more frequent than ETEC.
- Shigella: 2% to 9%. More common in Africa.
- Salmonella: <5% of cases except in Asia, where it is seen in up to 10% of cases.

TABLE 1 Pathogens and Epidemiologic Features Associated with Traveler Diarrhea

Organism	Approximate Percentage of Cases (%)	Epidemiologic Features
Enterotoxigenic *Escherichia coli*	15-50	Most important causative agent of traveler diarrhea overall; not diagnosed by routine microbiologic methods
Enteroaggregative *E. coli*	20-35	Not diagnosed by routine microbiologic methods
Shigella spp. and enteroinvasive *E. coli*	10-25	Most important causes of dysentery; enteroinvasive *E. coli* not diagnosed by routine microbiologic methods
Nontyphoidal *Salmonella* spp.	5-10	
Campylobacter jejuni	3-15	More common in Asia; antimicrobial resistance a concern
Aeromonas	5	
Plesiomonas	5	
Giardia lamblia	<2	Affects hikers and campers who drink from contaminated freshwater streams
Cryptosporidium hominis/parvum	<2	Occasional large-scale waterborne outbreaks
Cyclospora cayetanensis	<2	
Vibrio cholerae		Ongoing outbreaks in Haiti and Zimbabwe, and endemic in many countries in Asia; rare cause of disease in travelers
Norovirus		Outbreaks on cruise ships
Entamoeba histolytica		May cause liver abscess

From Bennett JE et al: *Mandell, Douglas, and Bennett's principles and practice of infectious diseases*, ed 8, Philadelphia, 2015, Saunders.

- Other bacteria: *Aeromonas, Arcobacter, Plesiomonas,* enterotoxigenic *Bacteroides fragilis, Vibrio cholera,* noncholera vibrios.
- Viral pathogens:
  1. Norovirus: Up to 17% of cases from Caribbean and Africa
  2. Rotavirus: 4% to 7% of cases
- Protozoans:
  1. *Entamoeba histolytica:* More common in South and Southeast Asia
  2. *Giardia lamblia:* More common in South and Southeast Asia, especially Nepal
  3. *Cryptosporidium, Cyclospora, Isospora*

Dx DIAGNOSIS

DIFFERENTIAL DIAGNOSIS

- Malaria
- Dengue fever
- Influenza
- Rocky Mountain spotted fever
- Irritable bowel syndrome
- Inflammatory bowel disease
- Shellfish poisoning
- Mushroom poisoning

WORKUP

- Most cases of TD are self-limiting, do not require workup, and are treated symptomatically without regard to etiologic agent.
- In patients with diarrhea, fever, and colitic symptoms (bloody stools, cramping), a stool culture should be obtained to look for specific bacterial pathogens.

LABORATORY TESTS

- Stool culture ×3 for bacterial pathogens.
- Stool for ova and parasites to help identify protozoans. Special stains such as modified acid fast or trichrome stain may be necessary for *Cryptosporidium, Cyclospora,* and *Isospora.*
- Blood cultures in patients with systemic illness to rule out *Salmonella* species.

Rx TREATMENT

NONPHARMACOLOGIC THERAPY

- Fluid replacement to treat volume depletion of diarrhea is important.
- Mild cases: Alternate fluids that contain salts and fluids that contain sugars, such as broths or fruit juices. Pedialyte is effective as an over-the-counter product.
- Severe cases: Oral rehydration solution (ORS) packets are available in most pharmacies. They should be mixed with clean water to replace lost electrolytes and are used until patient is urinating regularly. An alternative home-based solution can be made with: ½ teaspoon of salt, ½ teaspoon of baking soda, and 4 tablespoons of sugar in 1 liter of clean water.

ACUTE GENERAL Rx

- Antisecretory agents may reduce symptoms but do not treat underlying cause:
  1. Bismuth subsalicylate: 1 dose of 525 mg (2 tablets of Pepto-Bismol) PO every 30 min up to 8 doses a day. Can reduce number of bowel movements by 50%. Dosages are available for children based on weight, and the product is available in liquid or chewable tablet form.
  2. Loperamide: 4 mg PO, then 2 mg after each loose bowel movement, not to exceed 16 mg per day. Use for up to 48 hr. Has antisecretory and antimotility effect. Antimotility drugs should not be used in cases of bloody diarrhea or dysentery (increased risk of colitis and colonic perforation). When used, they should be given only in conjunction with antimicrobial therapy.
- Antibiotics are warranted only for moderate to severe diarrhea (i.e., >four bowel movements a day, fever, or blood, pus, or mucus in stool. Antibiotics can reduce duration of diarrhea by 1 to 2 days.
  1. Azithromycin: The preferred antibiotic for empiric treatment of moderate to severe TD. It is also the preferred agent for children and pregnant women. Dose of 1 gram PO is the single dose for women. Children: 10 mg/kg/day single dose or for 3 days. Particularly effective against quinolone-resistant *Campylobacter* infections in Southeast Asia. Another option for children: Ceftriaxone 50 mg/kg/day IV once daily ×3 days.
     a. Ciprofloxacin: 500 mg twice a day for 1 to 3 days
     b. Levaquin: 500 mg a day for 1 to 3 days
  2. Fluoroquinolones are also effective agents for bacterial causes of TD, but resistance to fluoroquinolones is increasing. Cannot be used in children under 15 and in pregnant women.
  3. Rifaximin: 200 mg PO tid for 3 days for children age >12 and adults is effective for afebrile, noncolitic diarrhea such as ETEC. Does not treat *Salmonella, Shigella,* or *Campylobacter.*
  4. Rifamycin is now FDA approved for TD caused by noninvasive strains of *E. coli.* It is not recommended for TD complicated by fever and/or bloody stools. Dosage is 388 mg (2 tablets) bid ×3 days.
- Concerns of use of antibiotics:
  1. Widespread use of antibiotics has led to resistance. Tetracycline and sulfa agents such as Bactrim are no longer used due to widespread resistance.
  2. Antibiotic treatment may lead to prolonged colonization in infections with *Salmonella* and nontyphoid *Salmonella.*
  3. In cases of EHEC (Shiga toxin production) treatment with quinolones, but not rifaximin, may increase risk of complications such as hemolytic uremic syndrome.
  4. *Clostridia difficile* infection can occur with use of antibiotics.

PREVENTION BY ANTIBIOTICS AND NONANTIBIOTIC AGENTS

- Antibiotic prophylaxis can be considered for certain groups, such as persons with underlying illness, athletes, and politicians for up to 2 to 3 wk. Ciprofloxacin 250 to 500 mg a day is effective in preventing 90% of TD. Rifaximin dosed daily has been shown to help prevent TD for U.S. travelers to Mexico, but not as effectively as Ciprofloxacin.
- Bismuth subsalicylate can be used. It must be given 4× daily and can cause black tongue and stools. As it contains salicylates, it can interact with anticoagulants and lead to toxicity in patients on long-term salicylate therapy.
- Probiotics are being studied for their potential use but evidence of their effectiveness is limited.

REFERRAL

Infectious diseases physician for more difficult cases lasting more than 72 hr

PEARLS & CONSIDERATIONS

- Travelers on cruises have lower incidence of TD than land-based trips, but cruise ship passengers and staff are at higher risk of large outbreaks of Norovirus that are difficult to contain. Norovirus infection needs only a low inoculum of virus to cause illness, and the virus is relatively resistant to cleaning.
- In up to 40% of cases of TD, no pathogen is identified.
- *Giardia* is the most frequent cause of long-lasting TD.

PREVENTION

- There are oral and injectable vaccines against *Salmonella typhi* available in the U.S.
- Dukoral oral vaccine is available in some countries such as Canada and Australia and in Europe to help prevent cholera and ETEC.

PATIENT & FAMILY EDUCATION

Food hygiene education: Wash hands often, especially after going to bathroom and before eating. Avoid raw fruits and vegetables (unless peeled and washed in clean water). Avoid undercooked meats, fish, and seafood. Avoid tap water and ice. Choose beverages in factory-sealed containers (such as bottled water and carbonated soft drinks). Try to avoid buffet-style foods.

SUGGESTED READINGS

Available at ExpertConsult.com

RELATED CONTENT

Traveler Diarrhea (Patient Information)

AUTHOR: **Glenn G. Fort, MD, MPH**

BASIC INFORMATION

DEFINITION

Trigeminal neuralgia is an intense, usually unilateral, paroxysmal, stabbing pain in the sensory distribution of the trigeminal (cranial nerve V) nerve.

SYNONYM

Tic douloureux ("painful tics/spasms")

ICD-10CM CODE
G50.0 Trigeminal neuralgia

EPIDEMIOLOGY & DEMOGRAPHICS

INCIDENCE: 4 per 100,000
PEAK INCIDENCE: Incidence increases with age and peaks at 67 yr of age; onset in 90% of patients is after age 40.
PREVALENCE: 155 in 1 million
PREDOMINANT SEX & AGE: Male:female ratio is 1:1.5.
RISK FACTORS: Most cases are idiopathic; age and multiple sclerosis are risk factors.

PHYSICAL FINDINGS & CLINICAL PRESENTATION

- Patients present with paroxysmal, unilateral facial pain that is usually described as shock-like, stabbing, or electric (Fig. 1). Right side of the face is affected more often than the left side.[1]
- Pain can be spontaneous or triggered by touch, an air current, or activities such as shaving, eating, or brushing teeth. Triggered paroxysmal pain is particular to trigeminal neuralgia and is reported by 91% to 99% of patients indicating that this feature may be pathognomonic of trigeminal neuralgia.[1]
- In severe cases, facial spasms can accompany the pain.
- Pain is usually described in distribution of the second (V2-maxillary) and third (V3-mandibular) divisions of the trigeminal nerve.

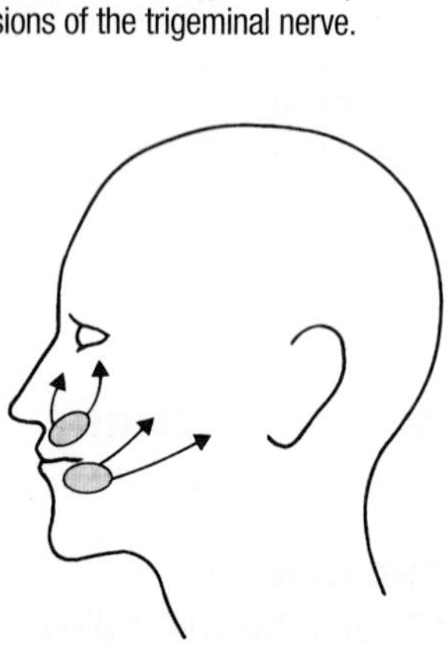

FIG. 1 Trigeminal neuralgia. The two most common sites of origin and radiation of pain are shown: mouth-ear and nose-orbit. Pain usually starts in the region of the encircled area and radiates in the directions shown.

[1]Cruccu G et al: Trigeminal neuralgia, *N Engl J Med* 383:754-762, 2020.

- The pain seldom lasts more than a few seconds to a minute.
- There is usually no sensory or motor loss.

ETIOLOGY

- Idiopathic or "classical": Cause usually unknown, likely an aberrant artery or vein compressing cranial nerve V at or near the pons. Neurovascular contact is also commonly found incidentally on imaging in asymptomatic individuals.
- Secondary: Accounts for up to 15% of cases; caused by nonvascular lesions such as a demyelinating plaque from multiple sclerosis or compression from a tumor near the pons.
- Box 1 summarizes causes of trigeminal neuralgia.

DIAGNOSIS

DIFFERENTIAL DIAGNOSIS

- Trigeminal neuropathy
- Primary stabbing headache
- Short-lasting unilateral neuralgiform headache with conjunctival injection and tearing (SUNCT)
- Postherpetic neuralgia
- Glossopharyngeal neuralgia
- Dental pain

WORKUP

Trigeminal neuralgia is a clinical diagnosis (see previously); however, if any neurologic deficits or atypical features are present, strongly consider secondary causes of facial pain.

IMAGING STUDIES

Neuroimaging (contrast-enhancing brain MRI) should be considered in young patients (<40 yr) with atypical symptoms (sensory loss, bilateral symptoms). MRI is useful to identify potential compressors or demyelinating causes. It detects nonvascular structure pathology in 15% of patients. Brain MRI is useful to identify neurovascular contact between trigeminal nerve and superior cerebellar artery.

BOX 1 Causes of Trigeminal Neuralgia

Classical
Neurovascular compression by an artery or vein
Symptomatic
Saccular aneurysm
Arteriovenous malformation
Tumors/mass-lesions at cerebellopontine angle:
- Vestibular schwannoma
- Meningioma
- Epidermoid

Primary demyelinating disorders:
- Multiple sclerosis
- Charcot-Marie-Tooth disease (rare)

Infiltrative disorders:
- Trigeminal amyloidoma

Nondemyelinating lesions:
- Small infarct or angioma in the brainstem

Familial

Modified from Adams JG et al: *Emergency medicine: clinical essentials,* ed 2, Philadelphia, 2013, Elsevier.

TREATMENT

PHARMACOLOGIC Rx

- Carbamazepine 400 to 800 mg, 2 to 3 times daily divided dosing is the recommended initial treatment. This can be titrated to pain relief by 100 to 200 mg every 3 days to a maximum of 1200 mg divided bid or tid. HLA phenotype must be sent prior to starting in patients of East Asian ancestry due to high association with risk of Stevens-Johnson syndrome with carbamazepine.
- Oxcarbazepine can be used if carbamazepine is not tolerated due to side effects. Other medications include botulinum toxin type A, lidocaine, baclofen, phenytoin, gabapentin, clonazepam, lamotrigine, and levetiracetam.
- Drug combinations can be tried when one medication is partially effective before proceeding with secondary intervention.
- Spontaneous remissions may be seen in trigeminal neuralgia, and therefore periodic medication tapers should be considered if the patient is pain free.
- In the elderly population, caution should be used when initiating and titrating the above medications. Caution and extensive counseling should also be used in women of childbearing age when initiating treatment with anti-seizure medications.

NONPHARMACOLOGIC THERAPY

Patients with refractory pain eventually need secondary intervention such as microvascular decompression, selective nerve fiber destruction (rhizotomy), glycerol injection, thermal lesioning, chemical ablation, or gamma knife radiosurgery. Microvascular decompression is the only available nondestructive procedure and is effective in 75% of patients, and possesses observed long-term benefits.

DISPOSITION

- Most patients are responsive to initial pharmacologic treatment. Spontaneous remission is possible.
- Medical management is eventually ineffective in 30% to 50% of patients.

REFERRAL

Referral to a neurologist is appropriate if there is uncertainty about diagnosis or if symptoms are refractory to conservative management.

PEARLS & CONSIDERATIONS

In a young patient with trigeminal neuralgia, secondary causes such as multiple sclerosis should be considered, and an MRI of the head obtained. In secondary disease, initial therapy should address underlying secondary causes.

SUGGESTED READINGS

Available at ExpertConsult.com

RELATED CONTENT

Trigeminal Neuralgia (Patient Information)

AUTHORS: **Jonathan H. Smith, MD,** and **Corey Goldsmith, MD**

BASIC INFORMATION

DEFINITION

Pulmonary tuberculosis (TB) is an infection of the lung and, occasionally, surrounding structures, caused by the bacterium *Mycobacterium tuberculosis* (Mtb). Multidrug-resistant (MDR) TB is defined as disease caused by strains of Mtb that are at least resistant to treatment with isoniazid and rifampin (two of the most effective first-line drugs); extensively drug-resistant (XDR) TB refers to disease caused by MDR strains that are also resistant to treatment with any fluoroquinolone and any of the injectable drugs used in second-line anti-TB treatment regimens.

SYNONYM

TB

ICD-10CM CODES	
A15.0	Tuberculosis of lung
A15.7	Primary respiratory tuberculosis

EPIDEMIOLOGY & DEMOGRAPHICS

INCIDENCE (WORLDWIDE):

- One fourth of the world's population is infected with TB, and it is still one of the deadliest diseases known to humans.
- In 2017, there were an estimated 10 million new cases of active tuberculosis; 9% involved coinfection with HIV; 1.3 million deaths from TB, including 300,000 among HIV-infected patients; 457,560 incident cases of multidrug-resistant TB worldwide.

INCIDENCE (IN U.S.):

- In 2018, a total of 9,029 new TB cases were reported in the U.S., representing a 0.7% decrease from 2017. The U.S. TB incidence in 2018 was 2.8 per 100,000 persons.
- The rate among non–U.S.-born persons was >14 times that in the U.S.-born persons.[1] Since 1993, TB case counts and rates have declined in the U.S (Fig. E1). As the number of cases decreases overall, an increasing percentage of cases occurs among non-U.S. born persons.
- More than 90% of new cases each yr from reactivated prior infections, while 9% represent new infections.
- Only 10% of patients with purified protein derivative (PPD) conversions will develop TB, most within 1 to 2 yr, though this is higher in HIV-positive patients (8%/yr).
- Two thirds of all new cases in racial and ethnic minorities and 80% of new cases in children occur in racial and ethnic minorities.
- Occurs most frequently in geographic areas and among populations with highest AIDS prevalence.
  1. Urban blacks and Hispanics between 25 and 45 yr old.
  2. Poor, crowded urban communities.

[1] Colangeli R et al: Bacterial factors that predict relapse after tuberculosis therapy, *N Engl J Med* 379:823-833, 2018.

- Two thirds of new TB cases in 2018 occurred in non–U.S.-born persons, where the top five countries of birth were Mexico, the Philippines, India, Vietnam, and China.
- In 2017 in the U.S., 1.9% of cases were MDR TB, which is a decline from 8.2% in 2008. There were three cases of XDR TB in the U.S. in 2017.

PREVALENCE (IN U.S.):

- Between 3.1% and 5.0% of the U.S. population is estimated to be infected with latent TB infection
- Varies widely among population groups

PREDOMINANT SEX:

- Globally, in 2017, 6 million men contracted TB compared to 3.2 million women
- Male predominance in AIDS, shelters, and prisons reflected in disproportionate male incidence (Box 1)

PREDOMINANT AGE:

- Ages 24 to 45
- Childhood cases common among minorities
- Nursing home outbreaks among elderly

PEAK INCIDENCE:

- Infancy
- Teenage yr
- Pregnancy
- Elderly
- HIV-positive patients at highest risk regardless of age

BOX 1 High-risk Groups for Tuberculosis Infection and Disease

Groups at High Risk for Exposure or Infection

Close contacts of persons with tuberculosis
Foreign-born persons from high-risk regions (Asia, Africa, Latin America, Russia, eastern Europe)
Residents and employees of high-risk congregate settings (correctional institutions, nursing homes, homeless shelters, hospitals serving high-risk populations, drug treatment centers)
Medically underserved, low-income populations
High-risk racial or ethnic minority populations
Injectable drug users
Children exposed to adults in high-risk categories

Groups at Higher Risk for Disease Once Infected

Immunosuppressed patients, including those with HIV
Patients with recent tuberculosis infection (within past 2 yr)
Persons with certain medical conditions (diabetes mellitus, silicosis, cancer, end-stage renal disease, gastrectomy, body weight ≤90% of ideal)
Injectable drug users
History of inadequately treated tuberculosis
Children age ≤4 yr, especially infants

From Cherry JD et al: *Feigin and Cherry's textbook of pediatric infectious diseases,* ed 8, Philadelphia, 2019, Elsevier.

GENETICS:

- Populations with widespread low native resistance have been intensely infected when initially exposed to TB.
- Following elimination of those with least native resistance, incidence and prevalence of TB tends to decline.

PHYSICAL FINDINGS & CLINICAL PRESENTATION

- See "Etiology"
- Primary pulmonary TB infection generally asymptomatic
- Reactivation pulmonary TB:
  1. Fever
  2. Night sweats
  3. Cough
  4. Hemoptysis
  5. Scanty nonpurulent sputum
  6. Weight loss
  7. Chest pain
- Progressive primary pulmonary TB disease: Same as reactivation pulmonary TB
- TB pleurisy:
  1. Pleuritic chest pain
  2. Fever
  3. Shortness of breath
- Rare massive, suffocating, fatal hemoptysis secondary to erosion of pulmonary artery within a cavity (Rasmussen aneurysm)
- Chest examination:
  1. Not specific
  2. Usually underestimates extent of disease
  3. Rales accentuated following a cough (posttussive rales)

ETIOLOGY

- Mtb, a slow-growing, aerobic, non-spore-forming, nonmotile bacillus, with a lipid-rich cell wall:
  1. Lacks pigment
  2. Produces niacin
  3. Reduces nitrate
  4. Produces heat-labile catalase
  5. Mtb staining, acid-fast and acid-alcohol fast by Ziehl-Neelsen method, appearing as red, slightly bent, beaded rods 2 to 4 microns long (acid-fast bacilli [AFB]), against a blue background
  6. Polymerase chain reaction (PCR) to detect <10 organisms/ml in sputum (compared with the requisite 10,000 organisms/ml for AFB smear detection)
  7. Culture:
     a. Growth on solid media (Löwenstein-Jensen; Middlebrook 7H11) in 2 to 6 wk
     b. Growth in liquid media (BACTEC, using a radioactive carbon source for early growth detection) often in 9 to 16 days
     c. Enhanced in a 5% to 10% carbon dioxide atmosphere
  8. Genome sequencing:
     a. Facilitates immediate identification of MTB strains and resistance in early growing cultures
     b. False negatives possible if growth suboptimal

9. Humans are the only reservoir for Mtb
10. Transmission:
    a. Aerosolized droplets containing AFB generated through cough, speaking, singing, bronchoscopy, or autopsy are inhaled directly into alveoli
    b. Facilitated by close exposure to high-velocity cough (unprotected by proper mask or respirators) from patients with AFB-positive sputum and cavitary lesions
    c. Locations of increased TB transmission risk include hospitals, homeless shelters, correctional facilities, nursing homes, and residential homes for those with HIV

- Pathogenesis:
  1. Mtb are ingested by macrophages in alveoli, then transported to regional lymph nodes, where spread is contained
  2. Some Mtb may reach bloodstream and disseminate widely
  3. Primary TB (often asymptomatic, minimal pneumonitis in lower or midlung fields, with hilar lymphadenopathy) is essentially an intracellular infection, with multiplication of organisms continuing 2 to 12 wk after primary exposure, until cell-mediated hypersensitivity (detected by positive skin test reaction to tuberculin PPD) matures, and results in subsequent containment of infection
  4. Local and disseminated Mtb are thus contained by the following T-cell–mediated immune responses:
     a. Recruitment of monocytes
     b. Transformation of lymphocytes with secretion of lymphokines
     c. Activation of macrophages and histiocytes
     d. Organization into granulomas, where Mtb may survive within macrophages (Langhans giant cells), but within which multiplication essentially ceases (95%) and from which spread is prohibited
  5. Progressive primary pulmonary disease:
     a. May immediately follow the asymptomatic phase:
     b. Necrotizing pulmonary infiltrates
     c. Tuberculous bronchopneumonia
     d. Endobronchial TB
     e. Interstitial TB
     f. Widespread miliary lung lesions
  6. Postprimary TB pleurisy with pleural effusion:
     a. Develops after early primary infection, although often before conversion to positive PPD
     b. Results from pleural seeding from a peripheral lung lesion or rupture of lymph node into pleural space
     c. May produce a large (sometimes hemorrhagic) exudative effusion (with polymorphonuclear cells early, rapidly replaced by lymphocytes), frequently without pulmonary infiltrates
     d. Generally resolves without treatment
     e. Portends a high risk of subsequent clinical disease, and therefore must be diagnosed and treated early (pleural biopsy and culture) to prevent future catastrophic TB illness
     f. May result in disseminated extrapulmonary infection
  7. Reactivation pulmonary TB:
     a. Occurs mo to yr following primary TB
     b. Preferentially involves the apical posterior segments of the upper lobes and superior segments of the lower lobes
     c. Associated with necrosis and cavitation of involved lung, hemoptysis, chronic fever, night sweats, weight loss
     d. Spread within lung occurs via cough and inhalation
  8. Reinfection TB:
     a. May mimic reactivation TB
     b. Ruptured caseous foci and cavities, which may produce endobronchial spread
  9. Mtb in both progressive primary and reactivation pulmonary TB:
     a. Intracellular (macrophage) lesions (undergoing slow multiplication)
     b. Closed caseous lesions (undergoing slow multiplication)
     c. Extracellular, open cavities (undergoing rapid multiplication)
     d. INH and rifampin are bactericidal in all three sites
     e. Pyrazinamide (PZA) especially active within acidic macrophage environment
     f. Extrapulmonary reactivation disease also possible
  10. Rapid local progression and dissemination in infants with devastating illness before PPD conversion occurs
  11. Most symptoms (fever, weight loss, anorexia) and tissue destruction (caseous necrosis) from cytokines and cell-mediated immune responses
  12. Mtb has no important endotoxins or exotoxins
  13. Granuloma formation related to tumor necrosis factor (TNF) secreted by activated macrophages

Dx DIAGNOSIS

DIFFERENTIAL DIAGNOSIS

- Necrotizing pneumonia (anaerobic, gram-negative)
- Histoplasmosis
- Coccidioidomycosis
- Melioidosis
- Interstitial lung diseases (rarely)
- Cancer
- Sarcoidosis
- Silicosis
- Rare pneumonias:
  1. *Rhodococcus equi* (cavitation)
  2. *Bacillus cereus* (50% hemoptysis)
  3. *Eikenella corrodens* (cavitation)

WORKUP

- Sputum for AFB stains and Mtb culture.
- Chest x-ray (Fig. E2).
- PPD (tuberculin skin test [TST]) or interferon gamma release assays (IGRA) can be used for screening of latent TB infection (LTBI):
  1. Recent conversion from negative to positive within 3 mo of exposure is highly suggestive of recent infection.
  2. Negative PPD never rules out acute TB.
  3. Prior positive PPD may become negative after several yr and return to positive only after second repeated PPD; repeat second PPD within 1 wk, which thus may mimic skin test conversion.
  4. Positive PPD reaction is determined as follows:
     a. Induration after 72 hours of intradermal injection of 0.1 ml of 5 TU-PPD.
     b. 5-mm induration if HIV-positive (or other severe immunosuppressed state affecting cellular immune function), close contact of active TB, fibrotic chest lesions.
     c. 10-mm induration if in high–medical risk groups (immunosuppressive disease or therapy, renal failure, gastrectomy, silicosis, diabetes), foreign-born high-risk group (Southeast Asia, Latin America, Africa, India), low socioeconomic groups, IV drug addict, prisoner, health care worker.
     d. 15-mm induration if low risk.
  5. PPD cannot distinguish between TB disease and TB infection.
- Interferon gamma release assays (IGRAs): Diagnostic test for latent TB infection, known as the QuantiFERON TB Gold test (QFT-G) and T-SPOT.TB Assay. These blood tests measure interferon response to specific Mtb antigens. The test may assist in distinguishing true positive reactions from individuals with latent TB, from PPD reactions related to nontuberculous mycobacteria; prior BCG vaccination; or difficult-to-interpret skin-test results from people with dermatologic conditions or immediate allergic reactions to PPD. IGRAs have a specificity >95% for diagnosis of latent TB. The sensitivity of the T-SPOT assay (90%) appears to be higher than the QFT-G test (80%). It should be noted that IGRA sensitivity is diminished by HIV infection. As with PPD, negative tests do not rule out active TB disease, and positive tests cannot distinguish between TB infection and disease.
- The Xpert MTB/RIF is an automated molecular test for Mtb and resistance to rifampin (RIF) that provides sensitive detection of TB and rifampin resistance directly from untreated sputum in less than 2 hr with minimal hands-on time.

LABORATORY TESTS

- Sputum for AFB stains and culture:
  1. Induced sputum if patient not coughing productively
- Sputum from bronchoscopy if high suspicion of TB in patients unable to produce expectorated induced sputum for AFB:
  1. Positive AFB smear is essential before or shortly after treatment to ensure subsequent growth for definitive diagnosis and sensitivity testing
  2. Consider lung biopsy if sputum negative, especially if infiltrates are predominantly interstitial
- AFB stain-negative sputum may grow Mtb subsequently (especially in HIV)
- Gastric aspirates may be helpful, especially in children
- CBC:
  1. Variable values:
     a. WBCs: Low, normal, or elevated (including leukemoid reaction: >50,000)
     b. Normocytic, normochromic anemia often
  2. Rarely helpful diagnostically
- ESR usually elevated
- Thoracentesis:
  1. Exudative effusion:
     a. Elevated protein and adenosine deaminase
     b. Decreased glucose
     c. Elevated WBCs (polymorphonuclear leukocytes early, replaced later by lymphocytes)
     d. May be hemorrhagic
  2. Pleural fluid usually AFB-negative
  3. Pleural biopsy often diagnostic—may need to be repeated for diagnosis
  4. Culture pleural biopsy tissue for AFB
- Bone marrow biopsy is often diagnostic in difficult-to-diagnose cases, especially miliary TB

IMAGING STUDIES

- Chest x-ray:
  1. Primary infection reflected by calcified peripheral lung nodule with calcified hilar lymph node
  2. Reactivation pulmonary TB:
     a. Necrosis
     b. Cavitation (especially on apical lordotic views)
     c. Fibrosis and hilar retraction
     d. Bronchopneumonia
     e. Interstitial infiltrates
     f. Miliary pattern
     g. Many of the previous findings may also accompany progressive primary TB
  3. TB pleurisy:
     a. Pleural effusion, often rapidly accumulating and massive
  4. TB activity not established by single chest x-ray examination
  5. Serial chest x-ray examinations are excellent indicators of progression or regression

Rx TREATMENT

NONPHARMACOLOGIC THERAPY

- Increased rest during acute phase of treatment
- High-calorie, high-protein diet to reverse malnutrition and enhance immune response to TB
- Isolation in negative-pressure rooms with high-volume air replacement and circulation, with health care provider wearing proper protective 0.5- to 1-micron filter respirators, until three consecutive sputum AFB smears are negative during workup (taken in 8- to 24-hr intervals, with at least one being an early morning specimen) or a diagnosed case has been on standard multidrug treatment for at least 2 wk and is clinically improving

ACUTE GENERAL Rx

- Generally, treatment of active tuberculosis consists of two phases: an intensive phase, followed by a continuation phase
- Compliance (rigid adherence to treatment regimen) chief determinant of success:
  1. Supervised directly observed therapy (DOT) recommended for all patients and mandatory for patients with high likelihood of loss to follow-up
- Adult initial regimen:
  1. Isoniazid 5 mg/kg (INH; max 300 mg), rifampin 10 mg/kg (RIF; max 600 mg), ethambutol by weight increments (EMB; 40-55 kg, 800 mg; 56-75 kg,1200 mg; 76-90 kg, 1600 mg), and pyrazinamide by weight increments (PZA; 40-55 kg, 1000 mg; 56-75 kg, 1500 mg; 76-90kg, 2000 mg) dosed daily
  2. Pyridoxine (vitamin B_6, 25 mg/day) should be given with INH to prevent peripheral neuropathy
  3. Usually decreased to INH and RIF after 8 wk depending on susceptibilities, with ultimate duration of therapy dependent on HIV treatment status, extent of disease, regimen used, and treatment response, but generally at least 6 mo
  4. Alternative, more complicated DOT regimens
- Monitor for clinical toxicity (especially hepatitis)
  1. Patient and physician awareness that anorexia, nausea, right upper quadrant pain, and unexplained malaise require immediate cessation of treatment
  2. Evaluation of liver function testing:
     a. Minimal SGOT/SGPT elevations without symptoms generally transient and not clinically significant
- Drug resistance (often multiple drug resistance TB [MDRTB]) increased by:
  1. Prior treatment
  2. Acquisition of TB in high-TB-burden countries
  3. Known contact with MDRTB
  4. Other factors associated with increased risk: Homelessness, incarceration, AIDS, intravenous drug use
- Other medications used in MDR or XDR TB include levofloxacin, moxifloxacin, cycloserine, aminoglycosides such as amikacin or kanamycin, PAS, clofazimine, bedaquiline, delamanid, pretomanid, linezolid, and ethionamide. A recent trial[2] with the combination of bedaquiline, pretomanid, and linezolid revealed a favorable outcome at 6 mo after the end of therapy in a high percentage of patients with highly drug-resistant forms of TB
- Drug-resistant TB should be treated in consultation with a TB expert
- Preventive treatment for PPD conversion only (infection without disease):
  1. Must be certain that chest x-ray examination is negative and patient has no symptoms of TB
  2. Most important groups:
     a. HIV-positive and other severely immunocompromised patients
     b. Close contact with active TB
     c. Recent converter
     d. Old TB on chest x-ray examination
     e. IV drug addict
     f. Medical risk factor
     g. High-risk foreign country
     h. Homeless
     i. Box 2 summarizes persons in whom preventive therapy should be initiated to prevent progression to tuberculosis
  3. Treatment of **latent *M. tuberculosis*** (Tables 1 and 2)
- Infants generally given prophylaxis immediately if recent contact with active TB (even if infant PPD negative), then retested with PPD in 3 mo (continuing INH if PPD becomes positive and stopping preventive treatment if PPD remains negative)

CHRONIC Rx

Generally not indicated beyond treatment described previously

DISPOSITION

- Monthly follow-up by physician experienced in TB treatment.
- Confirm sensitivity testing and alter treatment appropriately.
- Frequent sputum samples until culture is negative.
- Confirm chest x-ray regression at 2 to 3 mo.
- Approximately 5% of patients with drug-susceptible TB have a relapse after 6 mo of first-line therapy. Higher MIC values of isoniazid or rifampin in predominant isolates of *M. tuberculosis* are associated with a greater risk of relapse.[3]

REFERRAL

- To infectious disease expert for:
  1. HIV-positive patient
  2. Patient with suspected drug-resistant TB
  3. Patients previously treated for TB

[2] Conradie F et al: Treatment of highly drug-resistant pulmonary tuberculosis, *N Engl J Med* 382:893-902, 2020.

BOX 2 Persons in Whom Treatment Should Be Initiated to Prevent Progression to Tuberculosis

Household members and other close associates of persons with potentially infectious tuberculosis
- Contacts of any age with a Mantoux tuberculin skin test reading of 5 mm or greater and no documented history of reaction in the past, or with a positive interferon gamma release assay (IGRA), should be considered recently infected and receive therapy if they have not been treated previously
- Newly infected people, regardless of age, who have had a tuberculin skin test or IGRA conversion within the past 2 yr
- People with HIV infection who have a reaction of 5 mm or greater to a Mantoux test or positive IGRA
- People of any age with past tuberculosis infection who received inadequate treatment
- People of any age with a positive tuberculin skin test or positive IGRA and an abnormal but stable chest radiograph
- People with significant tuberculin reactions or positive IGRAs who have special clinical situations, including silicosis, diabetes mellitus, prolonged corticosteroid therapy, immunosuppressive therapy, hematologic malignant disease, or end-stage renal disease
- All children and adolescents with a positive tuberculin skin test reaction or interferon release assay result

Adapted from Cherry JD et al: *Feigin and Cherry's textbook of pediatric infectious diseases,* ed 8, Philadelphia, 2019, Elsevier.

TABLE 1 Recommendations for Regimens to Treat Latent Tuberculosis Infection

Priority Rank*	Regimen	Recommendation (strong or conditional)	Evidence (high, moderate, low, or very low)
Preferred	3 mos isoniazid plus rifapentine given once weekly	Strong	Moderate
Preferred	4 mos rifampin given daily	Strong	Moderate (HIV negative)†
Preferred	3 mos isoniazid plus rifampin given daily	Conditional Conditional	Very low (HIV negative) Low (HIV positive)
Alternative	6 mos isoniazid given daily	Strong§ Conditional	Moderate (HIV negative) Moderate (HIV positive)
Alternative	9 mos isoniazid given daily	Conditional	Moderate

HIV, Human immunodeficiency virus.
**Preferred:* excellent tolerability and efficacy, shorter treatment duration, higher completion rates than longer regimens and therefore higher effectiveness; *alternative:* excellent efficacy but concerns regarding longer treatment duration, lower completion rates, and therefore lower effectiveness.
†No evidence reported in HIV-positive persons.
§Strong recommendation for those persons unable to take a preferred regimen (e.g., due to drug intolerability or drug-drug interactions).
From Sterling TR et al: Guidelines for the treatment of latent tuberculosis infection: recommendations from the National Tuberculosis Controllers Association and CDC, 2020, *Morbidity and Mortality Weekly Report* 69(1), Feb. 14, 2020, Table 3.

4. Patients whose fever has not decreased and sputum has not converted to negative in 2 to 4 wk
5. Patients with overwhelming pulmonary or extrapulmonary TB

- To pulmonologist for bronchoscopy or pleural biopsy, if necessary for diagnosis

PEARLS & CONSIDERATIONS

COMMENTS

- All contacts (especially close household contacts and infants) should be properly tested for PPD conversions during 3 mo following exposure.
- Those with positive PPD should be evaluated for active TB and properly treated or given prophylaxis.
- Previous treatment is a common risk factor for XDR and MDR TB.
- In treatment of latent TB infections, evidence exists for the efficacy and safety of 6-mo isoniazid monotherapy, rifampicin monotherapy, and combination therapies with 3 to 4 mo of isoniazid and rifampicin.[4]
- Left untreated, 5% to 10% of patients with latent TB develop active TB. Updated guidelines from the CDC and the National Tuberculosis Controllers Association for latent TB treatment include any of the following regimines:[5]

1. Once-weekly isoniazid plus rifapentine for 3 mo administered under direct observation. The guideline recommends this regimen for adults and children (age <2 yr), including patients who are HIV-positive.
2. Daily rifampin for 4 mo is also recommended strongly, especially for HIV-negative people, and perhaps has the lowest toxicity.
3. Daily rifampin plus isoniazid for 3 mo is another alternative.

SUGGESTED READINGS

Available at ExpertConsult.com

AUTHORS: **Tara C. Bouton, MD, MPH, TM,** and **Glenn G. Fort, MD, MPH**

[4] Zenner D et al: Treatment of latent tuberculosis infection, *Ann Intern Med* 167:248–255, 2017.
[5] Sterling TR et al: Guidelines for the treatment of latent tuberculosis infection: recommendations from the National Tuberculosis Controllers Association and CDC, 2020, *MMWR Recomm Rep* 69(1):1-11, 2020.

TABLE 2 Dosages for Recommended Latent Tuberculosis Infection Treatment Regimens

Drug	Duration	Dose and age group	Frequency	Total doses
Isoniazid* and rifapentine†	3 mos	**Adults and children aged ≥12 yrs** Isoniazid: 15 mg/kg rounded up to the nearest 50 or 100 mg; 900 mg maximum Rifapentine: 10-14.0 kg, 300 mg 14.1-25.0 kg, 450 mg 25.1-32.0 kg, 600 mg 32.1-49.9 kg, 750 mg ≥50.0 kg, 900 mg maximum **Children aged 2-11 yrs** Isoniazid*: 25 mg/kg; 900 mg maximum Rifapentine†: See above	Once weekly	12
Rifampin¶	4 mos	**Adults:** 10 mg/kg **Children:** 15-20 mg/kg** **Maximum dose:** 600 mg	Daily	120
Isoniazid* and rifampin¶	3 mos	**Adults** Isoniazid*: 5 mg/kg; 300 mg maximum Rifampin¶: 10 mg/kg; 600 mg maximum **Children** Isoniazid*: 10-20 mg/kg††; 300 mg maximum Rifampin¶: 15-20 mg/kg; 600 mg maximum	Daily	90
Isoniazid*	6 mos	**Adults:** 5 mg/kg **Children:** 10-20 mg/kg†† **Maximum dose:** 300 mg	Daily	180
		Adults: 15 mg/kg **Children:** 20-40 mg/kg†† **Maximum dose:** 900 mg	Twice weekly§	52
	9 mos	**Adults:** 5 mg/kg **Children:** 10-20 mg/kg†† **Maximum dose:** 300 mg	Daily	270
		Adults: 15 mg/kg **Children:** 20–40 mg/kg†† **Maximum dose:** 900 mg	Twice weekly§	76

*Isoniazid is formulated as 100-mg and 300-mg tablets.
†Rifapentine is formulated as 150-mg tablets in blister packs that should be kept sealed until use.
§Intermittent regimens must be provided via directly observed therapy (i.e., a health care worker observes the ingestion of medication).
¶Rifampin (rifampicin) is formulated as 150-mg and 300-mg capsules.
The American Academy of Pediatrics acknowledges that some experts use rifampin at 20-30 mg/kg for the daily regimen when prescribing for infants and toddlers (Source:** American Academy of Pediatrics: Tuberculosis. In Kimberlin DW et al [eds]: *Red book: 2018 report of the Committee on Infectious Diseases,* ed 31, Itasca, IL: 2018, American Academy of Pediatrics, pp. 829-853).
††The American Academy of Pediatrics recommends an isoniazid dosage of 10-15 mg/kg for the daily regimen and 20-30 mg/kg for the twice-weekly regimen.
From Sterling TR et al: Guidelines for the treatment of latent tuberculosis infection: recommendations from the National Tuberculosis Controllers Association and CDC, 2020, *Morbidity and Mortality Weekly Report* 69(1), Feb. 14, 2020, Table 4.

BASIC INFORMATION

DEFINITION

- Tumor lysis syndrome (TLS) is an oncologic emergency referring to the acute release of potentially injurious intracellular contents into the systemic circulation from tumor cell breakdown.
- TLS is a constellation of metabolic disturbances that occurs typically in the setting of rapid tumor cell lysis induced by cancer-targeted treatment (chemotherapy and/or other interventions such as embolization or radiation). However, spontaneous tumor cell turnover has produced TLS (i.e., no chemotherapy administration).
- TLS is characterized by hyperuricemia, hyperphosphatemia, hypocalcemia, hyperkalemia, and acute kidney injury (AKI), often with progressive oliguria.
- In the current classification system by Cairo and Bishop, TLS may be defined by laboratory or clinical parameters (Table 1). Grading of clinical tumor lysis syndrome is summarized in Table 2.
  1. **Laboratory TLS:** Clinically silent; defined by at least two of the following biochemical variables within 3 days before or 7 days after initiation of chemotherapy despite adequate volume status and uric acid–lowering agents.
     a. Hyperuricemia:
        (1) Results from the rapid release and catabolism of intracellular nucleic acids.
        (2) Purine nucleic acids are metabolized to hypoxanthine, xanthine, and, last, uric acid.
        (3) In an acidic environment, uric acid can precipitate in renal tubules and produce intrarenal obstruction.
     b. Hyperkalemia
     c. Hyperphosphatemia: Phosphate may precipitate with calcium to form calcium phosphate stones in renal tubules
     d. Hypocalcemia: Occurs secondary to precipitation with phosphorus
  2. **Clinical TLS** occurs when laboratory TLS is complicated by at least one of the following clinical complications that is not attributed to the chemotherapeutic regimen: Severe renal impairment, cardiac arrhythmias, central nervous system toxicity, and/or death.

SYNONYM

TLS

ICD-10CM CODE

E88.3 Tumor lysis syndrome

EPIDEMIOLOGY & DEMOGRAPHICS

INCIDENCE: The frequency of TLS is unknown, but it is the most common disease-related emergency encountered by physicians who treat children or adults with hematologic cancers. Incidence depends on cancer mass, patient characteristics (e.g., preexisting chronic kidney disease, volume depletion, hypotension), and supportive care. Tumor bulk, proliferation rate, and treatment sensitivity are associated with greater frequency of TLS.

PREVALENCE: Variable

PREDOMINANT SEX & AGE:

- No sex predilection.
- Occurs in all age groups. Older adults are more susceptible to TLS due to a decline in glomerular filtration rate with age.

GENETICS: No racial predilection

RISK FACTORS:

- Large tumor burden:
  1. Large tumor size
  2. LDH >1500 IU/L
  3. WBC >25,000/mm^3
  4. Risk of TLS is further stratified by tumor type:
     a. High risk:
        (1) Burkitt lymphoma
        (2) High-grade non-Hodgkin lymphoma
        (3) Lymphoblastic lymphoma
        (4) Acute T-cell leukemia
        (5) Other acute leukemias
     b. Moderate risk:
        (1) Low-grade lymphoma treated with chemotherapy/radiation/corticosteroids
        (2) Multiple myeloma
        (3) Breast carcinoma treated with chemotherapy/hormonal therapy
        (4) Small cell lung carcinoma
        (5) Germ cell tumors (e.g., seminoma, ovarian)
     c. Low risk:
        (1) Low-grade lymphoma treated with interferon
        (2) Merkel cell carcinoma
        (3) Adenocarcinoma of the gastrointestinal tract
- Administration of certain agents:
  1. Paclitaxel
  2. Hydroxyurea
  3. Etoposide
  4. Fludarabine
  5. Sorafenib
- Extensive bone marrow involvement
- Elevated pretreatment uric acid, potassium, or phosphorus levels
- Tumor that is highly sensitive to treatment
- Volume depletion
- Chronic kidney disease
- Decreased urine output
- Acidic urine
- Tumor involvement of the renal vasculature
- Advanced age
- Posttranscatheter arterial chemoembolization (TACE), radiofrequency thermal ablation
- Chimeric antigen receptor T-cells therapy (CAR-T cell)

ETIOLOGY

Most commonly occurs in patients with acute leukemias; bulky, solid tumors; or high-grade lymphomas. The pathophysiology of tumor lysis syndrome is illustrated in Fig. E1.

- Can occur spontaneously or after antitumor intervention (chemotherapy, radiation, etc.)
- Associated with administration of certain chemotherapeutic agents (whether intravenous, intrathecal, etc.):
  1. Paclitaxel
  2. Hydroxyurea
  3. Etoposide
  4. Fludarabine
- Spontaneous TLS
  1. Rare
  2. Lysis of tumor cells without chemotherapy or in setting of minimal chemotherapy (e.g., steroid monotherapy lymphoma)
  3. Related to rapidity of cell turnover
  4. Associations with pregnancy, fever, and, rarely, general anesthesia in predisposed individuals
  5. Hyperphosphatemia may not recur because of the reutilization of released

TABLE 1 Classification of Tumor Lysis Syndrome

Laboratory tumor lysis syndrome	Two or more of the metabolic abnormalities in the next column present on the same day Occurring within 3 days before initiation of therapy or 7 days after initiation of therapy Assumes the patient receives adequate hydration and a hypouricemic agent	Uric acid ≥476 µmol/L (8 mg/dl) in adults or the upper limits of normal in children Potassium ≥6.0 mmol/L Phosphorus ≥1.5 mmol/L (4.5 mg/dl) in adults or ≥2.1 mmol/L (6.5 mg/dl) in children Calcium ≤1.75 mmol/L (7 mg/dl) or ionized calcium <1.2 mmol/L (4.5 mg/dl)
Clinical tumor lysis syndrome	Laboratory tumor lysis syndrome plus any of the criteria in the next column (not attributable to other causes)	Acute kidney injury, defined as an increase in creatinine of 26.5 µmol /L (0.3 mg/dl) or when no baseline creatinine is documented, a single value ≥1.5 times the upper limits of normal for the patient's age and sex Symptomatic hypocalcemia (e.g., tetany or paresthesias), seizure, cardiac dysrhythmia, or sudden death attributed to hypocalcemia or hyperkalemia

From Niederhuber JE: *Abeloff's clinical oncology,* ed 6, Philadelphia, 2020, Elsevier.

TABLE 2 Grading of Clinical Tumor Lysis Syndrome

Stage I	Stage II	Stage III	Stage IV	Stage V
Renal failure	Serum creatinine = 1.5 UNL or creatinine clearance 30-45 ml/min	Serum creatinine = 1.5-3 UNL or creatinine clearance 20-30 ml/min	Serum creatinine = 3-6 UNL or creatinine clearance 10-20 ml/min	Serum creatinine >6 UNL or creatinine clearance <10 ml/min
Cardiac arrhythmia	Intervention not indicated	Nonurgent intervention indicated	Symptomatic and incompletely controlled or controlled with device (e.g., defibrillator)	Life-threatening (e.g., arrhythmia associated with heart failure, hypotension, syncope, shock)
Seizures	None	One brief, generalized seizure; seizure(s) well controlled by anticonvulsant, or infrequent focal motor seizures	Seizure in which consciousness is altered; poorly controlled seizure disorder, with generalized breakthrough seizures despite medical intervention	Seizure of any kind that is prolonged, repetitive, or difficult to control (e.g., status epilepticus, intractable epilepsy)

From Ronco C et al: *Critical care nephrology*, ed 3, Philadelphia, 2019, Elsevier.

phosphorus for resynthesis of newer tumor cells

PHYSICAL FINDINGS & CLINICAL PRESENTATION

CLINICAL PRESENTATION: Patients may present with a number of symptoms before starting chemotherapy or commonly within 3 days after initiating cytotoxic treatment. Common symptoms include any of the following:
- Nausea
- Vomiting
- Edema
- Shortness of breath (from fluid overload or congestive heart failure)
- Lethargy or weakness
- Seizure
- Syncope
- Muscle cramp
- Tetany

PHYSICAL FINDINGS

- Associated with specific metabolic abnormalities, including hyperkalemia, hyperphosphatemia, hyperuricemia, and hypocalcemia
- Metabolic derangements often overlap
  1. Hyperkalemia:
     a. Generalized weakness
     b. Paresthesias
     c. Paralysis
     d. ECG abnormalities:
        (1) Peaked T waves
        (2) Flattened P waves
        (3) Widened QRS complexes
        (4) Bradycardia
     e. Cardiac arrhythmias, including:
        (1) Ventricular tachycardia
        (2) Ventricular fibrillation
        (3) Asystole
        (4) Pulseless electrical activity
     f. Cardiac arrest
  2. Hyperphosphatemia:
     a. Oliguric or anuric AKI
     b. Cardiac arrhythmias
  3. Hypocalcemia:
     a. Paresthesias
     b. Tetany
     c. Neuromuscular irritability: Twitching, Chvostek sign (nonspecific), and carpopedal spasm
     d. Bronchospasm
     e. ECG abnormalities, including:
        (1) Inverted T waves
        (2) Prolonged QTc interval from ionized hypocalcemia
        (3) Ventricular arrhythmias
        (4) Heart block
     f. Cardiac arrest

ETIOLOGY

- TLS is caused by massive release of intracellular contents into the bloodstream at the time of death of neoplastic cells.
- Can occur spontaneously or after initiation of therapy in patients with:
  1. Acute leukemias
  2. Bulky solid tumors
  3. High-grade lymphomas
- Administration of certain agents:
  1. Paclitaxel
  2. Hydroxyurea
  3. Etoposide
  4. Fludarabine

  1. Reported in some cancer patients who received intrathecal chemotherapy
  2. Rare causes: Pregnancy, fever, and rarely, general anesthesia in predisposed individuals

Dx DIAGNOSIS

DIFFERENTIAL DIAGNOSIS

See "Acute Kidney Injury" topic in Section I.

LABORATORY TESTS

- Early identification of abnormal laboratory values may prevent or reduce complications of TLS
- Laboratory TLS is defined by the presence of at least two of the following biochemical criteria within 3 days before or 7 days after initiation of chemotherapy despite adequate volume repletion or use of uric acid-lowering agents:
  1. Uric acid: >8.0 mg/dl in adults or above the upper limit of the normal range for age in children
  2. Phosphorus: >4.5 mg/dl in adults or >6.5 mg/dl in children
  3. Potassium: >6.0 mmol/L
  4. Calcium: Corrected calcium <7.0 mg/dl or ionized calcium <1.12 mg/dl (0.66 mmol/L)
- Patients should undergo careful and frequent laboratory and clinic monitoring
  1. Perform frequent ECGs or continuous cardiac monitoring for arrhythmia detection
  2. Monitor renal status closely and follow daily weights and fluid intakes and outputs
  3. Monitor BUN, creatinine, phosphorus, potassium, calcium, uric acid, and LDH in high-risk patients before and up to 72 hr after initiating therapy:
     a. If evidence of TLS develops, laboratory parameters should be checked twice daily

IMAGING STUDIES

- Consider abdominal/renal ultrasound if kidney failure present.
- Consider computed tomography chest/abdominal/pelvis to evaluate for underlying malignancies.

Rx TREATMENT

GENERAL PRINCIPLES

- Prevention is mainstay of therapy.
- Identify high-risk patients (evaluate extent of tumor burden, kidney function, and pathologic findings) to initiate prophylactic measures in a timely fashion. Delayed treatment may lead to life-threatening complications.
- Optimal treatment involves preservation of renal function and prevention of cardiac dysrhythmias and neuromuscular irritability.
- Metabolic derangements should be corrected before starting cancer therapy.
- Prevention for high-risk patients without TLS:
  1. Prompt, vigorous volume repletion and administration of uricosuric agent are mainstays of therapy. Box 1 summarizes treatment recommendations for tumor lysis syndrome.
     a. Volume repletion:
        (1) Prevents volume depletion and corrects electrolyte derangement.

(2) Fluid intake (whether oral or intravenous) should be maintained at 2 to 3 L/m^2 per day.
(3) Begin 24 to 48 hr before initiating cancer treatment and continue for up to 72 hr after treatment.
(4) If intravenous fluids are required, isotonic solutions are appropriate (e.g., 0.9% saline or 1 L D_5W plus 3, 50-ml ampules of 1 M $NaHCO_3$).
(5) Maintain urine output at 80 to 100 ml/m^2 per hr.
(6) Patients with underlying cardiac or kidney dysfunction should be monitored for volume overload and necessity for loop diuretics.
(7) Hypouricemic agents (e.g., allopurinol, rasburicase, and febuxostat). Uric acid is freely filtered at the glomerulus, and handling in the renal proximal tubule is a combination of reabsorption and secretion mediated by luminal urate/anion exchanger urate transporter 1 (URAT-1) and the basolateral organic anion transporter (OAT). When the capacity to transport luminal uric acid is overwhelmed, there is potential for uric acid to crystallize within the tubular lumen. An acidic urine pH favors this process. Uric acid crystals can cause direct tubular injury by obstruction. Furthermore, intratubular and parenchymatous uric acid precipitations causes renal injury by a granulomatous reaction and necrosis of the distal tubule epithelium through induction of chemokine-mediated inflammation from monocyte chemoattractant protein-1 (MCP-1) and macrophage migration inhibition factor (MIF). There are also crystal-independent mechanisms, which target hemodynamics: these include increased peritubular capillary pressures, increased vasoconstriction, and decreased blood flow. Uric acid also may prevent recovery from AKI in TLS because it inhibits proximal tubule cell proliferation. These diverse mechanisms are united in their propensity to cause AKI, as reported in Fig. 2.[1]
(8) Allopurinol:
  (a) Xanthine oxidase inhibitor prevents conversion of xanthine and hypoxanthine to uric acid.
  (b) Prophylactic dose is 200 to 400 mg/m^2 daily in 1 to 3 divided doses, up to a maximum of 800 mg daily. The treatment dose is 300 to 900 mg/day.
  (c) In patients with high-grade liquid tumors, Allopurinol prophylaxis may cause xanthine nephropathy/nephrolithiasis:
    - Low serum uric acid levels and high urinary xanthine levels aid in diagnosis.
    - Consideration for reduction/cessation of allopurinol therapy should then be considered.
(9) Rasburicase:
  (a) Recombinant urate oxidase is used when uric acid levels cannot be lowered by standard measures
  (b) Given by intravenous or intramuscular route in dosages from 50 to 100 units/kg per day for 1 to 5 days
  (c) Should not be administered simultaneously with allopurinol, because allopurinol reduces uric acid levels and may reduce rasburicase efficacy
  (d) Contraindicated in pregnancy and glucose-6-phosphate dehydrogenase deficiency due to hemolytic concerns
  (e) Cost is a limiting factor
(10) Febuxostat dosage is 120 mg by mouth daily. It has fewer drug-drug interactions than allopurinol. Dose requirement required in patients with mild-to-moderate renal impairment. Cost is a limiting factor.

b. Urinary alkalinization:
  (1) Uric acid is more soluble at urinary alkaline pH
  (2) Remains controversial and has fallen out of favor
  (3) Contraindicated with hyperphosphatemia because of risk of calcium phosphate deposition leading to stones/nephrocalcinosis

BOX 1 Tumor Lysis Syndrome: Treatment Recommendations

When no metabolic aberration exists:
- Allopurinol 300 mg/day; reduce to 100 mg/day after 3 days of chemotherapy

  OR
- Rasburicase 0.2 mg/kg IV daily × 5 days
- Hydration: 0.45% saline 3000 ml/day
- Initiate chemotherapy within 24– every 12-24 hours

When metabolic aberration exists:
- Allopurinol or rasburicase as above; reduce dose if hyperuricemia is controlled or for renal insufficiency.
- Hydration with D_5W with 2 ampules/L of $NaCO_3$, add nonthiazide diuretics as needed.
- Urinary alkalization to keep urine pH >7.0; may discontinue when serum uric acid level is normal.
- Postpone chemotherapy until uric acid has decreased and electrolytes are stable.
- Monitor serum chemistries every 6-8 hours.
- Replace calcium with slow intravenous infusion of calcium gluconate (if symptomatic or for ECG changes).
- Treat hyperkalemia and hyperphosphatemia with exchange resins and phosphate binders, respectively.

Criteria for hemodialysis in patients unresponsive to the measures listed above:
- Serum potassium >6.0 mEq/L
- Serum uric acid >20 mg/dl
- Serum phosphorus >10 mg/dl
- Fluid overload unresponsive to diuretics

Symptomatic hypercalcemia

D_5W, 5% dextrose in water; *ECG*, electrocardiogram; *$NaCO_3$*, sodium carbonate.

From Parrillo JE, Dellinger RP: *Critical care medicine: principles of diagnosis and management in the adult,* ed 4, Philadelphia, 2014, Elsevier. From Brudno JN et al: Toxicities of chimeric antigen receptor T cells: recognition and management, *Blood,* May 20, 2016.

TREATMENT OF PATIENTS WITH TUMOR LYSIS SYNDROME

- Principles:
  1. Early consultations for nephrology and critical care teams
  2. Preventive measures as indicated previously
  3. Aggressive treatment of electrolyte disturbances to prevent cardiac arrhythmias and neuromuscular irritability
     a. Arrhythmias tend to be resistant to conventional therapy
     b. Arrhythmias are a leading cause of death in patients with severe TLS
  4. Treatment of kidney failure
- Management of electrolyte disturbances:
  1. Multiple, coexisting electrolyte abnormalities may make conservative management strategies difficult
     a. Systemic alkalinization may be required for concurrent hyperphosphatemia, hyperuricemia, and acidemia. Alkalinization may worsen hypocalcemia
  2. Hyperuricemia:
     a. Uric acid–lowering agents including allopurinol or rasburicase
  3. Hyperkalemia:
     a. Low-potassium diet
     b. Intravenous calcium chloride/gluconate for ECG changes of hyperkalemia

[1] Ronco C: *Critical care nephrology,* 3rd ed, Philadelphia, 2019, Elsevier.

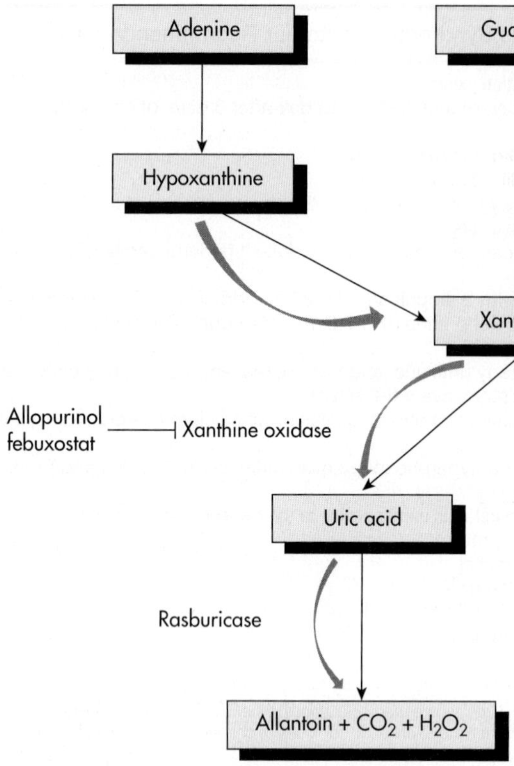

FIG. 2 Principles of therapy for the prevention and treatment of tumor lysis syndrome. (From Ronco C et al: *Critical care nephrology,* ed 3, Philadelphia, 2019, Elsevier.)

   c. Intravenous infusions of glucose and insulin to shift potassium into intracellular compartments
   d. Oral potassium-exchange resins (not for acute management)
   e. Hemodialysis
4. Hyperphosphatemia:
   a. Low phosphorus diet
   b. Intravenous infusion of glucose and insulin to shift phosphorus into cells
   c. Oral phosphate binders
5. Hypocalcemia:
   a. Treat only if neuromuscular irritability is present
   b. Intravenous calcium chloride/gluconate
   c. Calcitriol can be used if the serum phosphorus level is normal, but is a relatively slow form of therapy

- Management of kidney failure:
  1. Perform standard workup for kidney failure, including urinalysis, urine microscopy, urinary electrolytes, kidney ultrasound, etc.
  2. Supportive care with intravenous fluids and diuretics (if required).
  3. Consider early dialysis if above methods fail (especially if cardiac abnormalities present).

REFERRAL

- Nephrology
- Critical care

PEARLS & CONSIDERATIONS

COMMENTS

- TLS is an oncologic emergency, which can occur spontaneously, or, more commonly, during chemotherapy-related tumor cell lysis.
- TLS is associated with the release of several intracellular contents, including potassium, phosphorus, and uric acid. With concomitant renal failure, these products are retained to pathological levels, leading to cardiac and neurologic abnormalities.
- Common risk factors for TLS include highly proliferative tumors and large tumor burdens (e.g., high-grade lymphomas and acute leukemias), and preexisting metabolic derangements and renal failure.
- High-risk patients should undergo prophylactic measures initiated 24 to 48 hr before initiation of cytotoxic agents.
- Prophylactic measures include aggressive intravenous volume repletion and administration of urate–lowering drugs.
- Frequent laboratory testing and monitoring of vital signs, intakes and outputs, and cardiac/neurologic abnormalities are recommended.
- Complications may include continued electrolyte disturbances, renal failure, uremic complications, cardiac arrhythmias, and pulmonary edema from aggressive volume repletion.

SUGGESTED READINGS

Available at ExpertConsult.com

AUTHOR: **Hesham Shaban, MD**

BASIC INFORMATION

DEFINITION

Ulcerative colitis (UC) is an idiopathic, remitting and relapsing, chronic inflammatory bowel disease that starts in the rectum and extends proximally.

SYNONYMS

UC
Inflammatory bowel disease (IBD)
Idiopathic proctocolitis
Pancolitis

ICD-10CM CODES

K51.0	Ulcerative pancolitis
K51.2	Ulcerative proctitis
K51.3	Ulcerative rectosigmoiditis
K51.5	Left-sided colitis
K51.90	Ulcerative colitis, unspecified, without complications
K51.80	Other ulcerative colitis without complications
K51.811	Other ulcerative colitis with rectal bleeding
K51.812	Other ulcerative colitis with intestinal obstruction
K51.813	Other ulcerative colitis with fistula
K51.814	Other ulcerative colitis with abscess
K51.818	Other ulcerative colitis with other complication
K51.819	Other ulcerative colitis with unspecified complications
K51.911	Ulcerative colitis, unspecified with rectal bleeding
K51.912	Ulcerative colitis, unspecified with intestinal obstruction
K51.913	Ulcerative colitis, unspecified with fistula
K51.914	Ulcerative colitis, unspecified with abscess
K51.918	Ulcerative colitis, unspecified with other complication
K51.919	Ulcerative colitis, unspecified with unspecified complications

EPIDEMIOLOGY & DEMOGRAPHICS

INCIDENCE: The incidence of UC is 9 to 12 cases per 100,000 persons per yr in the U.S.; worldwide, the estimated incidence ranges from 1.2 to 20.3 cases per 100,000 person-yrs and its prevalence ranges from 7.6 to 246.0 per 100,000 persons. It is most common between ages 15 and 40 yr, with a second peak between 50 and 80 yr. The disease affects men and women at similar rates. Infection with nontyphoid salmonella or campylobacter is associated with an 8 to 10 times higher risk of developing ulcerative colitis in the following yr. Worldwide UC is more common than Crohn disease.

PREVALENCE: The prevalence of UC is 7.6 to 246.0 cases per 100,000 per yr. Higher prevalence in Ashkenazi Jewish descendants.

GEOGRAPHIC DISTRIBUTION: The highest incidence and prevalence of IBD are seen in northern Europe and North America, and the lowest in continental Asia.

GENETICS:

- Both specific and nonspecific gene variants are associated with UC.
- There are 47 loci associated with UC, of which 19 are specific for UC and 28 are shared with Crohn disease.
- Abnormalities in humoral and cellular adaptive immunity are also found in UC.

ETIOLOGY & PATHOGENESIS

Accumulating evidence suggests that it may result from an inappropriate inflammatory response to environmental triggers and immune dysregulation involving CD4+ T-cell Th2 response in a genetically susceptible host.

PHYSICAL FINDINGS & CLINICAL PRESENTATION

- Patients with UC often present with acute onset of bloody diarrhea accompanied by tenesmus, fever, and dehydration. At presentation 40% of adults have proctitis, 40% have left-sided colitis, and 20% have pancolitis. Diarrhea is not always present in UC patients with proctosigmoiditis and proctitis, and patients may have constipation.
- Abdominal pain is not usually a prominent symptom. Abdominal distention and tenderness may indicate the presence of complications such as toxic megacolon.
- The onset of symptoms is typically acute and is generally followed by periods of spontaneous remission and frequent relapses.
- Fever, evidence of dehydration may be present during the acute flare-up.
- Evidence of extraintestinal manifestations may be present in nearly 25% of patients: Liver disease, sclerosing cholangitis, iritis, uveitis, episcleritis, arthritis, erythema nodosum, pyoderma gangrenosum, aphthous stomatitis. Box 1 summarizes common extraintestinal manifestations of UC.

DIAGNOSIS

DIFFERENTIAL DIAGNOSIS (TABLE 1, BOX 2)

- Crohn disease
- Bacterial infections:
  1. Acute: *Campylobacter, Yersinia, Salmonella, Shigella, Chlamydia, Escherichia coli, Clostridium difficile,* gonococcal proctitis
  2. Chronic: Whipple disease, tuberculosis, enterocolitis
- Irritable bowel syndrome
- Protozoal and parasitic infections (amebiasis, giardiasis, cryptosporidiosis)
- Neoplasm (intestinal lymphoma, carcinoma of colon)
- Ischemic bowel disease
- Diverticulitis
- Celiac sprue, lymphocytic or collagenous colitis, radiation enteritis, endometriosis
- Solitary rectal ulcer
- Acute self-limited colitis
- Medication (NSAIDs, chemotherapy)

WORKUP

An accurate diagnosis of UC should define the extent and severity of inflammation. Diagnostic workup includes:

- Comprehensive history, physical examination
- Laboratory tests (see "Laboratory Tests")
- Colonoscopy to establish the presence of mucosal inflammation; typical endoscopic findings in UC are areas of continuous friable mucosa; diffuse, uniform erythema replacing the usual mucosal vascular pattern (Table 2); and pseudopolyps. The transition from abnormal to normal tissue tends to be abrupt. Rectal involvement is invariably present if the disease is active. Pathologic findings suggestive of UC include crypt abscesses and atrophy, mucin depletion, basal plasmacytosis, basal lymphoid aggregates, increased lamina propria cellularity, and Paneth cell metaplasia

LABORATORY TESTS

- Anemia and high erythrocyte sedimentation rate (in severe colitis) are common, but normal levels do not rule out the disorder.

BOX 1 Common Extraintestinal Manifestations of Ulcerative Colitis

Cutaneous/Oral
Angular stomatitis
Aphthous stomatitis
Erythema nodosum
Oral ulcerations
Psoriasis
Pyoderma gangrenosum
Pyostomatitis vegetans
Sweet syndrome (acute febrile neutrophilic dermatosis)

Ophthalmologic
Conjunctivitis
Episcleritis
Retinal vascular disease
Scleritis
Uveitis, iritis

Musculoskeletal
Ankylosing spondylitis
Osteomalacia
Osteonecrosis
Osteopenia
Osteoporosis
Peripheral arthropathy
Sacroiliitis

Hepatobiliary
Autoimmune hepatitis
Cholangiocarcinoma
Pericholangitis
PSC
Hepatic steatosis

Hematologic
Anemia of chronic disease
Autoimmune hemolytic anemia
Hypercoagulable state
Iron deficiency anemia
Leukocytosis or thrombocytosis
Leukopenia or thrombocytopenia

PSC, Primary sclerosing cholangitis.

From Feldman M et al: *Sleisenger and Fordtran's gastrointestinal and liver disease,* ed 10, Philadelphia, 2016, Elsevier.

TABLE 1 Features That Distinguish Ulcerative Colitis from Other Diagnoses

Diagnosis	Clinical Features	Radiologic and Colonoscopic Features	Histologic Features
UC	Bloody diarrhea	Extends proximally from rectum; fine mucosal ulceration	Distortion of crypts; acute and chronic diffuse inflammatory cell infiltrate; goblet cell depletion; crypt abscesses; lymphoid aggregates
Crohn colitis	Perianal lesions are common; may be associated with ileitis; frank bleeding is less common than in UC	Segmental disease; rectal sparing; strictures, fissures, ulcers, fistulas; small bowel involvement	Focal inflammation; submucosal involvement; granulomas; goblet cell preservation; transmural inflammation; fissuring
Ischemic colitis	Occurs in older adults; sudden onset, often painful; usually resolves spontaneously in several days	Segmental splenic flexure and sigmoid involvement are most common, with thumbprinting early and ulceration after 24-72 hr; rectal involvement is rare	Mucosal necrosis with ghost cells; congestion with red blood cells; hemosiderin-laden macrophages and fibrosis (when disease is chronic)
Microscopic colitis	Watery diarrhea; normal-appearing mucosa at colonoscopy	Usually normal	Chronic inflammatory infiltrate; increased intraepithelial lymphocytes (lymphocytic colitis) and/or subepithelial collagen band (collagenous colitis)
Infectious colitis	Sudden onset; identifiable source in some cases (e.g., *Salmonella* spp.); pain may predominate (e.g., *Campylobacter* spp.); pathogens are present in stool	Nonspecific findings	Crypt architecture is usually normal; edema, superficial neutrophilic infiltrate, crypt abscesses
Amebic colitis	History of travel to endemic area; amebae may be detected in a fresh stool specimen, but ELISA for amebic lectin antigen is the preferable diagnostic test	Discrete ulcers; ameboma or strictures	Similar to UC; amebae present in lamina propria or in flask-shaped ulcers, identified by periodic acid–Schiff stain
Gonococcal proctitis	Rectal pain; pus	Granular changes in rectum	Intense polymorphonuclear neutrophil infiltration; purulent exudate; gram-negative diplococci
Pseudomembranous colitis	Often a history of antibiotic use; characteristic pseudomembranes may be seen on sigmoidoscopy; *Clostridium difficile* toxin is detectable in stools	Edematous; shaggy outline of colon; pseudomembranes may be identified radiologically or seen at colonoscopy	May resemble acute ischemic colitis; summit lesions of fibrinopurulent exudate

ELISA, Enzyme-linked immunosorbent assay; *UC,* ulcerative colitis.
From Feldman M et al: *Sleisenger and Fordtran's gastrointestinal and liver disease,* ed 10, Philadelphia, 2016, Elsevier.

- Potassium, magnesium, calcium, and albumin may be decreased.
- Antineutrophil cytoplasmic antibodies (ANCA) with a perinuclear staining pattern (pANCA) can be found in >45% of patients; there is an increased frequency in treatment-resistant left-sided colitis, suggesting a possible association between these antibodies and a relative resistance to medical therapy in patients with UC.
- Calprotectin is a protein that is measured in feces as a marker of intestinal mucosa leukocyte activity that may be useful for screening of patients with suspected IBD. Trials have shown that based on a pretest probability of IBD of 32% in adults, an abnormal fecal calprotectin test would increase the posttest probability to 91% and a normal result would reduce the probability to 3%.
- Fecal lactoferrin is also a sensitive marker of intestinal inflammation.
- Stool examinations for ova and parasites, stool culture, and testing for *Clostridium difficile* toxin and *E. coli* 0157:H7 may be useful to eliminate other causes of diarrhea in selected patients with risk factors.

IMAGING STUDIES

Image studies (plain radiography, computed tomography [CT] scan [Fig. E1]) are generally reserved for suspected complications such as perforation of bowel or toxic megacolon.

Rx TREATMENT

NONPHARMACOLOGIC THERAPY

- Correct nutritional deficiencies; total parenteral nutrition with bowel rest may be necessary in severe cases. Folate supplementation may reduce the incidence of dysplasia and cancer in chronic UC.
- Avoid oral feedings during acute exacerbation to decrease colonic activity; a low-roughage diet may be helpful in early relapse.
- Psychotherapy is useful in most patients. Referral to self-help groups is also important because of the chronicity of the disease and the young age of the patients.

ACUTE GENERAL Rx

The therapeutic options vary with the degree of disease (mild, severe, fulminant) and areas of involvement (distal, extensive).

- Mild disease can be treated with 5-aminosalicylate agents (mesalamine, olsalazine, balsalazide, sulfasalazine). It can be administered as an enema (40 mg once daily at bedtime for 3 to 6 wk) or suppository (500 mg bid) for patients with distal colonic disease. Oral forms in which the 5-acetyl salicylic acid is in a slow-release or pH-dependent matrix (Pentasa 1 g qid, Asacol 800 mg PO tid) can deliver therapeutic concentrations to the more proximal small bowel or distal ileum. Olsalazine can be useful for maintenance of remission of UC in patients intolerant to sulfasalazine. Usual dose is 500 mg bid taken with food. Balsalazide is indicated for mild to moderately active UC. Usual dose is three 750-mg capsules tid. Probiotics may also be helpful in inducing remission in mild-to-moderate UC.
- Mild-to-moderate UC is often treated with a combination of rectal and oral 5-aminosalicylate. Refractory patients are candidates for oral glucocorticoids or immunosuppressive agents (e.g., cyclosporine). An algorithm for the management of mildly to moderately active UC is illustrated in Fig. 2.
- Severe disease usually responds to oral corticosteroids (e.g., prednisone 40 to 60 mg/day); the FDA has recently approved an extended-release formulation of the corticosteroid budesonide for induction of remission in mild to moderate ulcerative colitis. Corticosteroid suppositories or enemas are also useful for distal colitis. The immunosuppressant azathioprine or mercaptopurine also provides effective long-term treatment for Crohn disease. Fig. 3 describes an algorithm for the management of severely active UC.
- Biologic agents are emerging treatment options for the management of ulcerative

BOX 2 Differential Diagnosis of Ulcerative Colitis

Infectious Causes
Aeromonas hydrophila
Campylobacter jejuni
Chlamydia spp.
Clostridium difficile
Cytomegalovirus
Entamoeba histolytica
Escherichia coli O157:H7, other EHEC
HSV
Listeria monocytogenes
Neisseria gonorrhoeae
Salmonella spp.
Schistosomiasis
Shigella spp.
Yersinia enterocolitica

Noninfectious Causes
Acute self-limited colitis
Behçet disease
Crohn disease
Diversion colitis
Diverticulitis
Drugs and toxins
  Chemotherapy
  Gold
  Penicillamine
Eosinophilic colitis
Graft-versus-host disease
Ischemic colitis
Microscopic colitis
  Collagenous
  Lymphocytic
Neutropenic colitis (typhlitis)
NSAIDs
Radiation colitis
SCAD
Solitary rectal ulcer syndrome

EHEC, Enterohemorrhagic *Escherichia coli; HSV,* herpes simplex virus; *SCAD,* segmental colitis associated with diverticulosis.

From Feldman M et al: *Sleisenger and Fordtran's gastrointestinal and liver disease,* ed 10, Philadelphia, 2016, Elsevier.

colitis. Infliximab, a chimeric monoclonal antibody, has been shown to be effective in patients who have not responded to corticosteroid therapy. Newer tumor necrosis factor inhibitors include adalimumab (ADA), golimumab, and vedolizumab for treatment of moderate-to-severe ulcerative colitis. These agents can be used for induction and maintenance of remission in patients that have not responded to other therapies or are corticosteroid-dependent. Head-to-head trials of these biologic agents are necessary to establish the best therapeutic option.

- Fulminant disease generally requires hospital admission and parenteral corticosteroids (e.g., intravenous [IV] hydrocortisone 100 mg q6h). When bowel movements have returned to normal and the patient is able to eat normally, oral prednisone is resumed. IV cyclosporine can also be used in severe refractory cases; renal toxicity is a potential complication.
- Surgery is indicated in patients who do not respond to intensive medical therapy. Fig. 4 illustrates the surgical management of chronic UC.
- Proctocolectomy is usually curative in these patients and also eliminates the high risk of developing adenocarcinoma of the colon (10% to 20% of patients develop it after 10 yr with the disease). Total proctocolectomy with ileal pouch-anal anastomosis (IPAA) is the procedure of choice for most patients who require elective surgery, since it preserves anal sphincter function. Continent ileostomy is an alternative procedure.

TABLE 2 Endoscopic Differentiation of Ulcerative Colitis and Crohn Disease

Feature	Ulcerative Colitis	Crohn Disease
Distribution	Diffuse inflammation that extends proximally from the anorectal junction	Rectal sparing, frequent skip lesions
Inflammation	Diffuse erythema, early loss of vascular markings with mucosal granularity or friability	Focal and asymmetric, cobblestoning; granularity and friability less commonly seen
Ulceration	Small ulcers in a diffusely inflamed mucosa; deep, ragged ulcers in severe disease	Aphthoid ulcers, linear or serpiginous ulceration; intervening mucosa is often normal
Colonic lumen	Often narrowed in long-standing chronic disease; tubular colon; strictures are rare	Strictures are common

From Feldman M et al: *Sleisenger and Fordtran's gastrointestinal and liver disease,* ed 10, Philadelphia, 2016, Elsevier.

CHRONIC Rx

- Colonoscopic surveillance and multiple biopsies should be instituted approximately 10 yr after diagnosis because of the increased risk of colon carcinoma.
- Erythropoietin is useful in patients with anemia refractory to treatment with iron and vitamins.
- In patients on long-term steroid therapy, periodic bone density scans are recommended to screen for glucocorticoid-induced osteoporosis.

DISPOSITION

- The natural history of the disease is one of remission and episodic flares.
- The clinical course is variable. ~66% of patients will achieve clinical remission with medical therapy, and nearly 80% of treatment-compliant patients maintain remission. Fifteen percent to 20% of patients eventually require colectomy. Pouchitis is the most common long-term complication of IPAA (up to 40% of patients). >75% of patients treated medically will experience relapse.

REFERRAL

- Gastrointestinal consultation for initial diagnostic sigmoidoscopy/colonoscopy in suspected cases.
- Surgical referral for patients with severe disease unresponsive to medical therapy. Indications for surgery in patients with UC are summarized in Box 3.

SUGGESTED READINGS

Available at ExpertConsult.com

RELATED CONTENT

Ulcerative Colitis (Patient Information)

AUTHOR: **Fred F. Ferri, MD**

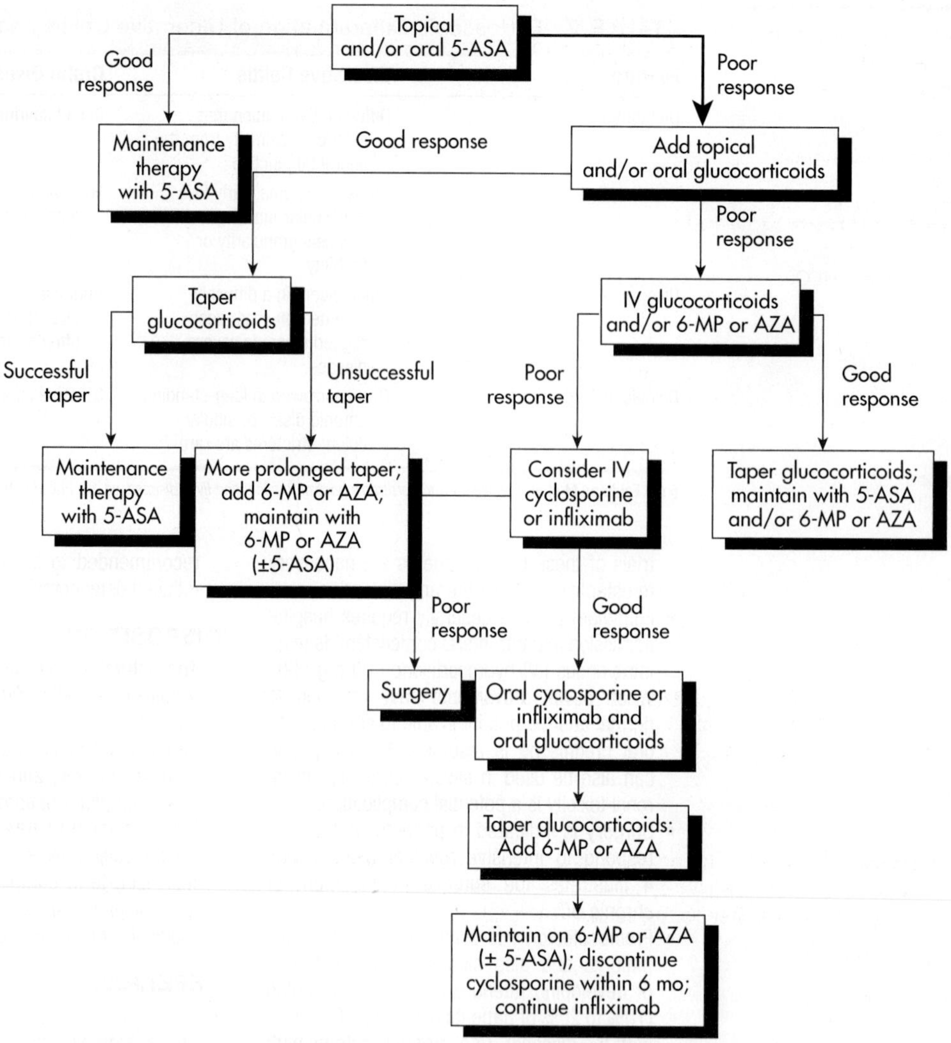

FIG. 2 Algorithm for the management of mildly to moderately active ulcerative colitis. *5-ASA,* 5-Aminosalicylate; *AZA,* azathioprine; *IV,* intravenous; *6-MP,* 6-mercaptopurine. (From Feldman M et al: *Sleisenger and Fordtran's gastrointestinal and liver disease,* ed 10, Philadelphia, 2016, Elsevier.)

BOX 3 Indications for Surgery in Patients with Ulcerative Colitis

Colonic dysplasia or carcinoma
Colonic perforation
Growth retardation
Intolerable or unacceptable side effects of medical therapy
Medically refractory disease
Systemic complications that are recurrent or unmanageable
Toxic megacolon
Uncontrollable colonic hemorrhage

From Feldman M et al: *Sleisenger and Fordtran's gastrointestinal and liver disease,* ed 10, Philadelphia, 2016, Elsevier.

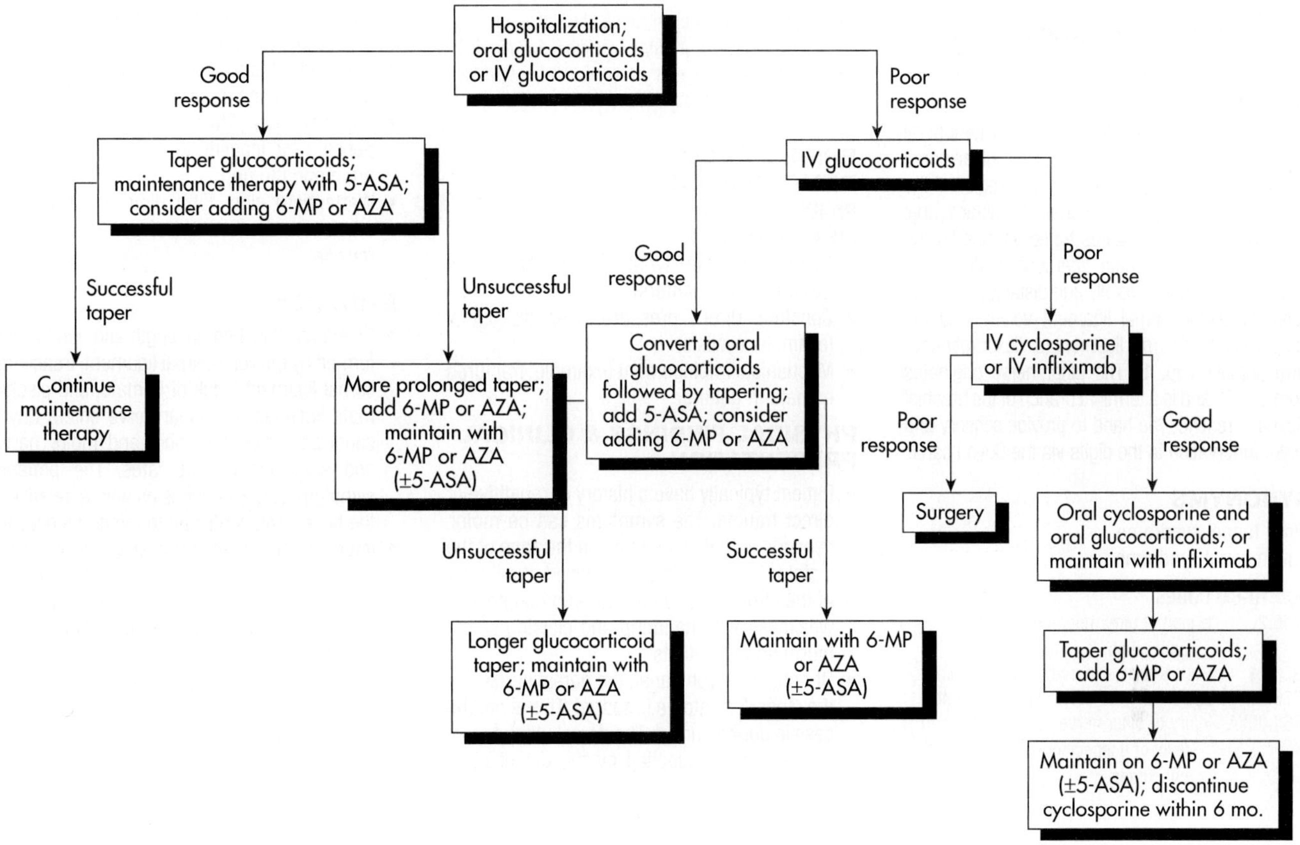

FIG. 3 Algorithm for the management of severely active ulcerative colitis. *5-ASA,* 5-Aminosalicylate; *AZA,* azathioprine; *IV,* intravenous; *6-MP,* 6-mercaptopurine. (From Feldman M et al: *Sleisenger and Fordtran's gastrointestinal and liver disease,* ed 10, Philadelphia, 2016, Elsevier.)

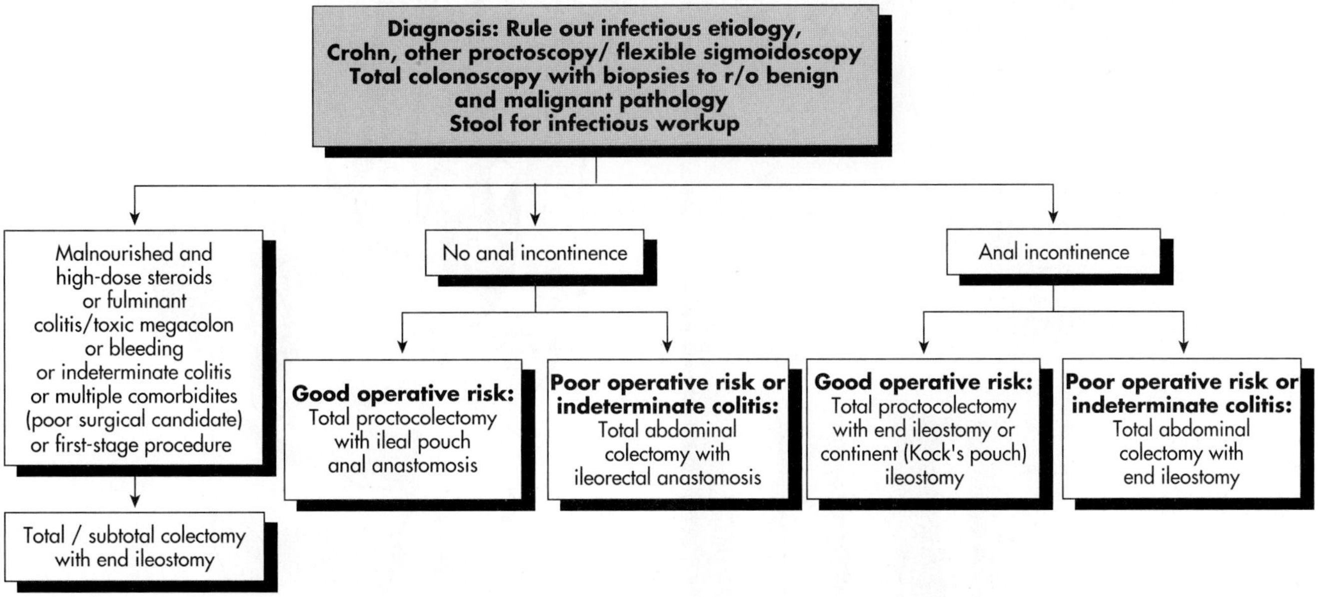

FIG. 4 Surgical management of chronic ulcerative colitis. (From Cameron JL, Cameron AM: *Current surgical therapy,* ed 12, Philadelphia, 2017, Elsevier.)

BASIC INFORMATION

DEFINITION

Ulnar tunnel syndrome syndrome is a peripheral neuropathy that involves injury to the ulnar nerve as it passes through narrow anatomic region of the wrist referred to as Guyon canal. The ulnar tunnel is a triangular fibro-osseous tunnel formed by the pisiform and pisohamate ligament medially, the hook of the hamate laterally and distally, the superficial transverse carpal ligament volarly, and the deep transverse carpal ligament (or flexor retinaculum) dorsally (Fig. 1). The ulnar nerve originates from C8–T1 and is a terminal branch of the brachial plexus. It reaches the hand to provide sensory and motor innervation to the digits via the Guyon canal.

SYNONYMS

Ulnar tunnel syndrome
Guyon canal syndrome

ICD 10-CM CODES

G56.20	Lesion of ulnar nerve, unspecified upper limb
G56.21	Lesion of ulnar nerve, right upper limb
G56.22	Lesion of ulnar nerve, left upper limb
S64.00XA	Injury of ulnar nerve at wrist and hand level of unspecified arm, initial encounter
S64.01XA	Injury of ulnar nerve at wrist and hand level of right arm, initial encounter
S64.02XA	Injury of ulnar nerve at wrist and hand level of left arm, initial encounter

EPIDEMIOLOGY & DEMOGRAPHICS

INCIDENCE: Rare

RISK FACTORS:

- Overuse of the wrist, especially flexion (example: weightlifters)
- Constant direct pressure over the canal (example: cyclists)
- Mechanical impingement (example: fractured hamate in golfers)

PHYSICAL FINDINGS & CLINICAL PRESENTATION

- Patient typically have a history of repetitive or direct trauma. The symptoms can be motor, sensory, or both depending on the zone of the distal ulnar nerve that is involved. Weakness of the intrinsic hand muscles can manifest as weakness with handgrip and clawing of the fourth and fifth digits.
- Of note, in Guyon canal, the dorsal surface of the ulnar dermatome is spared. This is not the case in cubital tunnel. The dorsal ulnar aspect of the hand is supplied by the dorsal ulnar cutaneous branch of the ulnar nerve, which comes of 5 cm proximal to Guyon canal.
- Tinel sign: Reproduce symptoms by tapping the suspect site of compression.
- Froment sign: Thumb IP flexion to compensate for inability to adduct thumb when attempting to grip.
- Wartenberg sign: Fifth digit is overabducted due to denervation of palmar interossei muscle.

ETIOLOGY

- Guyon canal is 4 cm in length and had borders formed by the volar carpal ligament, transverse carpal ligament, hook of hamate, and pisohamate ligament. The ulnar nerve enters Guyon canal as a mixed sensory and motor nerve, and subsequently bifurcates. The patient's symptomatology depends on where, relative to the bifurcation, the insult to the nerve occurs.
- Injury to the ulnar nerve at the level of the Guyon canal can occur due to compression, inflammation, or trauma, particularly fractures of the hook of the hamate (Fig. 2).
  1. Ganglion cyst
  2. Hook of hamate fracture
  3. Tumors
  4. Aberrant muscle, fat tissue

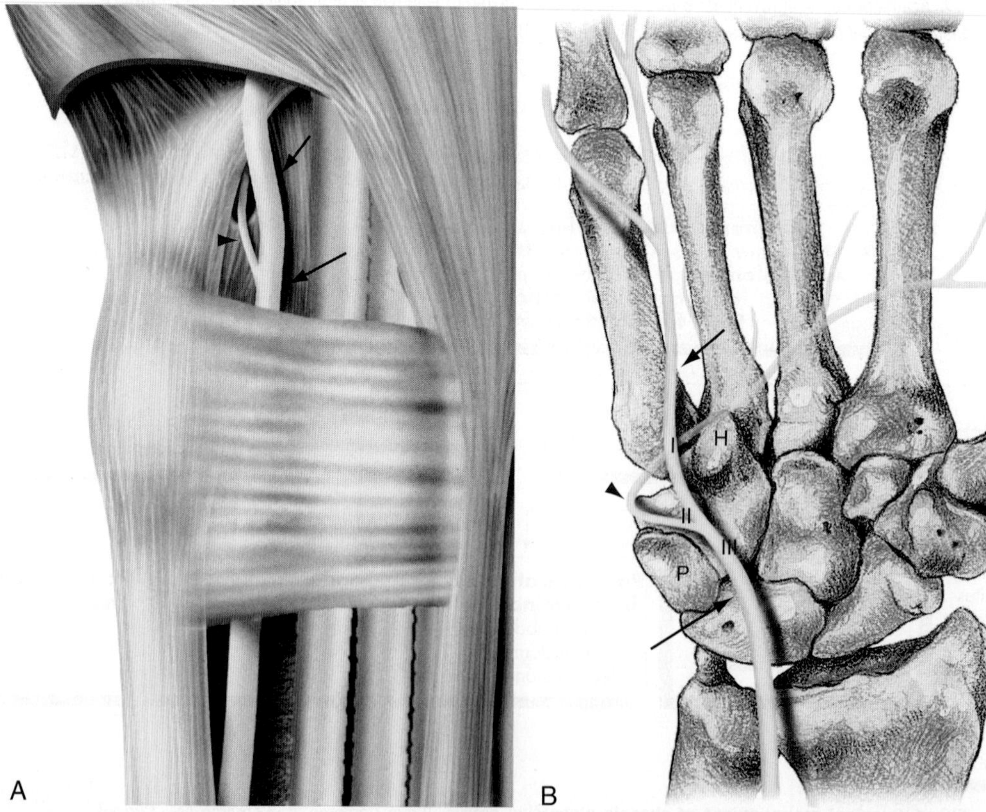

FIG. 1 Guyon canal and ulnar nerve. A and B, Drawings demonstrating the normal anatomy of the Guyon canal. Note the ulnar nerve as it enters into the Guyon canal under the transverse carpal ligament, between the pisiform *(P)* and the hook of the hamate *(H)*. The ulnar nerve (*long arrow*) branches into the deep motor branch (*arrowhead*) and the superficial sensory branch (*short arrow*). The ulnar nerve or its branches can be compressed at zone I, adjacent to the hook of the hamate, affecting the superficial sensory branch, or in zone II, adjacent to the superior pole of the pisiform, affecting the deep motor branch, or more proximally, before the nerve bifurcates (zone III), in which case both motor and sensory deficit will be present. (From Pope TL et al. *Musculoskeletal imaging*, ed 2, Philadelphia, 2015, Elsevier.)

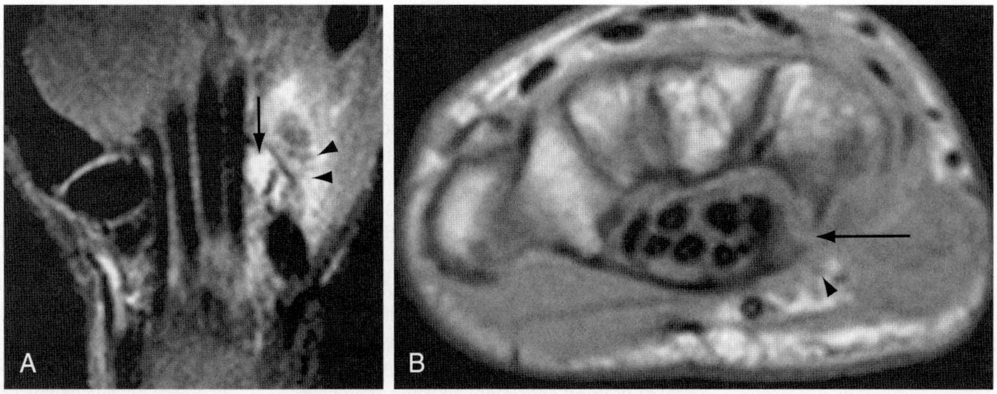

FIG. 2 Guyon canal syndrome due to fracture of the hook of the hamate. Coronal short tau inversion recovery **(A)** and axial T1-weighted **(B)** magnetic resonance images demonstrate the fracture of the hook of the hamate (*arrow* in **A** and **B**) with extensive bone marrow and surrounding soft tissue edema (*arrowheads* in **A**), producing compression of the superficial sensory branch of the ulnar nerve (*arrowhead* in **B**) at zone I. (From Pope TL et al. *Musculoskeletal imaging*, ed 2, Philadelphia, 2015, Elsevier.)

Dx DIAGNOSIS

DIFFERENTIAL DIAGNOSIS

- Cubital tunnel syndrome
- C8 nerve root impingement
- Brachial plexus injury

WORKUP/IMAGING STUDIES

- Detailed history and physical
- Radiographs (include carpal tunnel view): Evaluate for hook of hamate fracture
- Nerve conduction study (NCS)/Electromyography (EMG)
- MRI: Can detect ganglion cysts and/or ulnar artery aneurysms
- Doppler ultrasound: To evaluate for ulnar artery aneurysm

Rx TREATMENT

Management of ulnar tunnel syndrome ranges from conservative treatment with observation and symptomatic management to surgical treatment involving decompression of the ulnar tunnel with possible additional interventions based upon severity of accompanying deformity in the hand.

NONPHARMACOLOGIC THERAPY

- Conservative management is the first line of treatment for patients with mild symptoms.
- Activity modification: Avoiding activities that worsen symptoms (activities involving repetitive motions of the wrist and hand).
- Splinting: Immobilizing the wrist can provide support during activity while limiting continued motion of the wrist, therefore allowing inflammation to dissipate.

ACUTE GENERAL Rx

Combination of NSAIDs and acetaminophen taken as an alternating regimen can provide effective symptomatic relief of symptoms.

SURGICAL MANAGEMENT

- Local decompression of the ulnar nerve at the level of the ulnar tunnel can definitively release the nerve and can be effective in severe cases where conservative management has failed.
- In severe cases involving clawed fingers and loss of finger strength as a result of chronic compression of the ulnar nerve, more complex surgical procedures, such as tendon transfers, may be indicated.
- In patients with compression of both the ulnar tunnel and the carpal tunnel that is refractory to conservative management, surgical release of both tunnels may be indicated.

DISPOSITION

- For patients with mild symptoms, conservative therapy can be effective in allowing patients to perform activities with symptomatic control.
- Surgical decompression of the ulnar tunnel is the definitive management of the pathology and is effective in cases refractory to conservative management.
- Patients should be advised that it may take a minimum of several months for resolution of symptoms after surgical decompression in severe cases due to the significant time required for an injured nerve to heal.

REFERRAL

Patients should be referred to orthopedic hand or upper extremity surgeons for evaluation, diagnosis, and discussion of treatment options with initiation of management.

COMMENTS

Early diagnosis and initiation of treatment is essential, as early conservative management can either improve symptoms or prevent their progression. Early referral to an upper extremity specialist is recommended.

RELATED CONTENT

Cubital tunnel syndrome (Related Key Topic)
Carpal tunnel syndrome (Related Key Topic)

AUTHORS: **Zainab Ibrahim, MD, Stephen E. Marcaccio, MD, Christopher McDonald, MD,** and **Joseph Gil, MD**

BASIC INFORMATION

DEFINITION

Urethritis is a well-defined clinical syndrome manifested by dysuria, a urethral discharge, or both.

SYNONYMS

Gonococcal urethritis
GCU

ICD-10CM CODE
A54.00 Gonococcal infection of lower genitourinary tract, unspecified

EPIDEMIOLOGY & DEMOGRAPHICS

- Urethritis commonly is divided into two major categories based on etiology: Gonococcal urethritis (GCU, *Neisseria gonorrhoeae* species) and nongonococcal urethritis (NGU, all other pathogens, most commonly *Chlamydia trachomatis*).
- This differentiation is based historically on *N. gonorrhoeae*'s easy visualization on Gram stain as gram-negative, kidney-shaped diplococci.
- In the U.S., rates of gonorrheal urethritis are rising; however, the incidence varies greatly based on race and geography; the prevalence of GCU is disproportionately higher in the South and among black, non-Hispanic men. The urethra is the most common site of infection in all men.

PHYSICAL FINDINGS & CLINICAL PRESENTATION

- Symptoms of GCU: Dysuria is the most common chief complaint in patients with GCU, which is often accompanied by discharge and pruritus. Acute-onset purulent discharge is a hallmark of this infection. Additionally, meatal edema and urethral tenderness to palpation may occur. Approximately 5% to 10% of patients with GCU remain asymptomatic.
- GCU may spread to other parts of the GU system. Prostatic involvement can cause urinary frequency, urgency, and nocturia and may present with mucopurulent discharge. Epididymal involvement can result in unilateral testicular pain and edema.
- Time frame: The incubation period of GCU is variable but is commonly 4 to 7 days. Without treatment, urethritis will persist for 3 to 7 wk, with 95% of men becoming asymptomatic after 3 mo.
- Complications: Periurethritis leading to urethral stenosis can occur. Additionally, disseminated infection can lead to tenosynovitis and arthritis. Rarely, hepatitis, myocarditis, endocarditis, and meningitis can occur.

DIAGNOSIS

DIFFERENTIAL DIAGNOSIS

- NGU
- Herpes simplex virus

LABORATORY TESTS

- Urethritis is diagnosed when a symptomatic male has any of the following characteristics: Positive leukocyte esterase and WBC on first-void urine dipstick, purulent discharge on exam, or >2 WBCs per field of Gram stain or urethral swab.
- If Gram staining is available, it is indicated and should be performed first, with modified Thayer-Martin media.
- Nucleic acid amplification tests (NAATs) have largely replaced culture in many health care settings. They are not more sensitive than culture for detecting *N. gonorrhoeae* in cervical or urethral specimen; however, they have specificities of >99% and retain sensitivity when used to test first-catch urine or self-collected vaginal swabs. The performance of NAATs with respect to overall sensitivity, specificity, and ease of specimen transport is better than that of any of the other tests available for the diagnosis of chlamydial and gonococcal infections. NAATs should be used to detect chlamydia and gonorrhea except in cases of child sexual assault, rectal and oropharyngeal infections in prepubescent girls, and when evaluating a potential gonorrhea treatment failure in which case culture and susceptibility testing might be required.
- For culture and susceptibility testing: Rayon, Dacron, or calcium alginate tips with plastic or wire shafts should be used (not cotton-tipped swabs, which are bactericidal). A swab of the urethra should be performed within 2 to 4 hr after voiding to prevent bacterial washout with urination. Collect cultures of the pharynx and rectum when indicated for concomitant *Chlamydia* testing on all patients.
- Concomitant serologic testing for syphilis and HIV infections should be offered to all patients.

TREATMENT

Regimen for uncomplicated gonococcal infections of the cervix, urethra, or rectum:[1]

- Ceftriaxone 500 mg IM as a single dose for persons weighing <150 kg (300 lb)
- For persons weighing ≥ 150 kg (300 lb), 1 g of IM ceftriaxone should be administered.
- If chlamydial infection has not been excluded, providers should treat for chlamydia with doxycycline 100 mg orally twice daily for 7 days. During pregnancy, azithromycin 1 g as a single dose is recommended to treat chlamydia.
- It is imperative to appropriately counsel patients on the avoidance of intercourse or use of barrier protection until a cure has been obtained and sexual partners have been evaluated. Once treated, patients should be advised to abstain from sex for 7 days.

[1] St Cyr S et al. Update to CDC's treatment guidelines for gonococcal infection, 2020, *MMWR Morb Mortal Wkly Rep* 69:1911-1916, 2020. http://doi.org/10.15585/mmwr.mm6950a6

- A test of cure is not necessary for men treated with these first-line agents.

Alternative regimens for uncomplicated gonococcal infections of the cervix, urethra, or rectum if ceftriaxone is not available:

- Gentamicin 240 mg IM as a single dose plus azithromycin 2 g orally as a single dose.
- Cefixime 800 mg orally as a single dose. If treating with cefixime, and chlamydial infection has not been excluded, providers should treat for chlamydia with doxycycline 100 mg orally twice daily for 7 days. During pregnancy, azithromycin 1 g as a single dose is recommended to treat chlamydia.

In cases of suspected cephalosporin treatment failure, clinicians should obtain relevant clinical specimens for culture and antimicrobial susceptibility testing, consult an infectious disease specialist or STD clinical expert (http:// www.stdccn.org/) for guidance in clinical management, and report the case to CDC through state and local public health authorities within 24 hr. Health departments should prioritize notification and culture evaluation for the patient's sex partner(s) from the preceding 60 days for those with suspected cephalosporin treatment failure or persons whose gonococcal isolates demonstrate reduced susceptibility to cephalosporins.

A test of cure is unnecessary for persons with uncomplicated urogenital or rectal gonorrhea who are treated with any of the recommended or alternative regimens; however, for persons with pharyngeal gonorrhea, a test of cure is recommended, using culture or nucleic acid amplification tests 7 to 14 days after initial treatment, regardless of the treatment regimen. Because reinfection within 12 mo ranges from 7% to 12% among persons previously treated for gonorrhea, persons who have been treated for gonorrhea should be retested 3 mo after treatment regardless of whether they believe their sex partners were treated. If retesting at 3 mo is not possible, clinicians should retest within 12 mo after initial treatment.

CHRONIC INFECTION

- Reinfection is the most common cause of recurrence
- Repeat swab and culture of the urethra, pharynx, and rectum (where applicable) are mandatory.
- Persistence of *N. gonorrhoeae* by smear or culture requires treatment for *N. gonorrhoeae.*
- Postgonococcal urethritis (PGU): Persistence of polymorphonuclear cells (PMNs) in the absence of gram-negative intracellular diplococci. This occurs when GCU is treated with a regimen that is ineffective against coincident nongonococcal infection; it represents NGU after GCU and should be treated as such.

PEARLS & CONSIDERATIONS

COMMENTS

- Partner notification: The names and contact information of sexual partners should be gathered at the time of diagnosis and referred to the health department, or the patient can notify the contact directly.

- Expedited partner treatment is recommended by the Centers for Disease Control and Prevention (CDC) and is approved in most states. This consists of giving prescriptions to the infected patient for their partner(s) who has not been evaluated by a physician and is unlikely to seek medical care.
- On examination of the urethral smear, the presence of small numbers of PMNs provides objective evidence of urethritis. The complete absence of PMNs on a urethral smear argues against urethritis. If in addition to the PMNs there are gram-negative, intracellular diplococci, the diagnosis of gonorrhea is established.

SUGGESTED READINGS

Available at ExpertConsult.com

RELATED CONTENT

Gonococcal Urethritis (Patient Information)
Gonorrhea (Related Key Topic)

AUTHORS: **Robin Metcalfe-Klaw, MD,** and **Rachel Wright Heinle, MD, FACOG**

BASIC INFORMATION

DEFINITION

Nongonococcal urethritis (NGU) is urethral inflammation caused by any of several organisms (see "Etiology").

SYNONYMS

NGU
Nongonococcal urethritis

ICD-10CM CODES

A56.0 Chlamydial infection of lower genitourinary tract
N34.1 Nonspecific urethritis

EPIDEMIOLOGY & DEMOGRAPHICS

- The occurrence is 50% in sexually transmitted disease clinics. *Chlamydia trachomatis* is the most common notifiable disease in the U.S., with >1.5 million infections reported to the Centers for Disease Control and Prevention (CDC) in 2016.
- NGU most commonly affects men in a higher socioeconomic class, affecting heterosexual men more frequently than men who have sex with men.
- NGU carries a greater morbidity rate than gonococcal urethritis (GCU).

PHYSICAL FINDINGS & CLINICAL PRESENTATION

- Incubation period: 2 to 35 days.
- Symptoms: Dysuria, whitish-clear urethral discharge, and urethral itching. The onset of symptoms in NGU is less acute than GCU. The majority of persons with *C. trachomatis* infection are not aware of their infection because they do not have symptoms that would prompt them to seek medical care.
- Signs: Whitish-clear urethral discharge, meatal edema, and erythema. Infected women manifest pyuria, and the disease can present as acute urethral syndrome.

COMPLICATIONS

- Epididymitis in men may be linked to nonbacterial prostatitis, proctitis in men who have sex with men, or Reiter syndrome.
- Urethritis complications are more common in women and can be associated with ectopic pregnancy, pelvic inflammatory disease, or infertility.

ETIOLOGY

- Most common agent is *Chlamydia* spp., an obligate intracellular parasite possessing both DNA and RNA, which replicates by binary fission. It causes 20% to 50% of NGU cases. Two species exist:
  1. *Chlamydia psittaci*
  2. *Chlamydia trachomatis* with its 15 serotypes:
     a. Serotypes A through C cause hyperendemic-blinding trachoma.
     b. Serotypes D through K cause genital tract infection.
     c. Serotypes L1 through L3 cause lymphogranuloma venereum.
- Other causes of NGU: *Mycoplasma genitalium* (found in 44% of treatment failures with double infection with *C. trachomatis* in up to 15% of cases); *Ureaplasma urealyticum*, causing 15% to 30% of the cases of NGU; *Trichomonas vaginalis*; herpes simplex virus; and Adenovirus. The cause of 20% of the cases of NGU has not been identified.
- Asymptomatic infection occurs in 28% of the contacts of women with chlamydial cervical infection.

DIAGNOSIS

DIFFERENTIAL DIAGNOSIS

- GCU
- Herpes simplex virus
- Trichomoniasis

LABORATORY TESTS

- Requires demonstration of urethritis and exclusion of infection with *N. gonorrhoeae.*
- Nucleic acid amplification tests (NAATs): These tests have replaced culture in many settings where persons are screened for asymptomatic genital infection. The performance of NAATs with respect to overall sensitivity, specificity, and ease of specimen transport is better than that of any of the other tests available for the diagnosis of chlamydial and gonococcal infections. NAATs should be used to detect chlamydia and gonorrhea except in cases of child sexual assault involving boys, rectal and oropharyngeal infections in prepubescent girls, and when evaluating a potential gonorrhea treatment failure, in which case culture and susceptibility testing might be required.
- *Chlamydia* culture: The appearance of PMNs on urethral smear confirms the diagnosis of urethritis. Because *Chlamydia* is an intracellular parasite of the columnar epithelium, the best specimen for culture is an endourethral swab taken from an area 2 to 4 cm inside the urethra. For culture, a Dacron-tipped swab is used; avoid calcium alginate or cotton swabs. The organism can only be grown in tissue culture, which is expensive.

TREATMENT

- Because it is impossible to differentiate among the common etiologies of NGU, the condition is treated syndromically, including in the initial treatment regimen those drugs effective against the common causative agents.
- In patients with isolated uncomplicated NGU, recommended regimens are azithromycin 1 g orally single dose or doxycycline 100 mg bid × 7 days. Recommended regimen in pregnancy is azithromycin, 1 g orally as a single dose.
- In patients with confirmed urethritis and unclear etiology, concurrent treatment for gonorrhea and *Chlamydia* is recommended. In these patients, uncomplicated infections of the urethra can be treated with combination of a single 1-g dose of oral azithromycin or 100 mg doxycycline bid × 7 days *plus* ceftriaxone 250 mg × 1 dose.
- In areas where *T. vaginitis* is prevalent, men who have sex with women and have persistent or recurrent urethritis should be presumably treated with metronidazole 2 g orally or a single dose of tinidazole 2 g orally
- Recurrent NGU in patients initially treated with doxycycline should be treated with a single dose of azithromycin 1 g. If azithromycin was used for initial treatment, patients with recurrent NGU should be retreated with moxifloxacin 400 mg daily × 6 days.

PEARLS & CONSIDERATIONS

COMMENTS

- Partner notification: The names and contact information of all sexual partners within preceding 60 days should be gathered at the time of the visit and referred to the health department, or the patient notifies the contacts directly. Expedited partner treatment is recommended by the CDC and approved in several states. This consists of giving prescriptions to the infected patient for their partner(s) who have not been evaluated by a physician and are unlikely to seek medical care.
- Patients should abstain from intercourse for 7 days after therapy completion.

RELATED CONTENT

Nongonococcal Urethritis (Patient Information)
Cervicitis (Related Key Topic)
Chlamydia Genital Infections (Related Key Topic)

SUGGESTED READINGS

Available at ExpertConsult.com

AUTHORS: **Rachel Wright Heinle, MD, FACOG,** and **Christine Burke, MD**

BASIC INFORMATION

DEFINITION

Urinary tract infection (UTI) is a term that encompasses a broad range of clinical entities that have in common a positive urine culture. Most cases are caused by bacteria ascending from the urethra into the bladder. A conventional threshold is growth of >100,000 colony-forming units per milliliter from a midstream-catch urine sample with no more than two species of organisms and at least one sign or symptom of UTI (urgency, frequency, dysuria, suprapubic tenderness, fever >38.0° C [100.4° F]). In symptomatic patients, using a lower threshold of between 100 and 10,000 colony-forming units per milliliter increases diagnostic sensitivity without significantly compromising specificity.

ICD-10CM CODES

N39.0	Urinary tract infection, site not specified
N99.521	Infection of other external stoma of urinary tract
N99.531	Infection of other stoma of urinary tract
N30.00	Acute cystitis without hematuria
N30.30	Trigonitis without hematuria
N30.20	Other chronic cystitis without hematuria

CLASSIFICATION

- Uncomplicated UTI: Occurs in a normal urinary tract and resolves rapidly with conventional antimicrobials. These patients have a low risk of upper UTI.
- Complicated UTI: Occurs in patients with coexisting pathology (strictures, stones, comorbidities [diabetes mellitus, multiple sclerosis, spinal cord injuries]). These patients are considered at high risk for upper UTI.
- First infection: The first documented UTI; tends to be uncomplicated and is easily treated.
- Unresolved bacteriuria: UTI in which the urinary tract is not sterilized during therapy. Main causes are bacterial resistance, patient noncompliance with treatment, mixed bacterial infection, rapid reinfection, azotemia, infected stones, Munchausen syndrome, and papillary necrosis.
- Bacterial persistence: UTI in which the urine cultures become sterile during therapy, but a persistent source of infection gives rise to reinfection by the same organism. Causes include infected stone, chronic bacterial prostatitis, atrophic infected kidney, vesicovaginal or enterovesical fistulas, obstructive uropathy, infected pyelocaliceal diverticula, infected ureteral stump after nephrectomy, infected necrotic papillae from papillary necrosis, infected urachal cysts, infected medullary sponge kidney, urethral diverticula, and foreign bodies.
- Reinfection: UTI in which a new infection occurs with new pathogens at variable intervals after a previous infection has been eradicated.
- Relapse: A less common form of recurrent infection; occurs within 2 wk of treatment when the same organism reappears in the same site as the previous infection. Relapsing infections of the urinary tract most commonly occur in pyelonephritis, kidney obstruction from a stone, foreign body, and prostatitis.

EPIDEMIOLOGY & DEMOGRAPHICS

INCIDENCE:

- UTI is the most common bacterial infection encountered in the ambulatory care setting in the U.S. The self-reported annual incidence of UTI in women is 12%, and half of all women report having had at least one UTI by 32 yr of age.
- UTIs account for 8 million health care visits per yr and 15% of all outpatient prescriptions.
- Incidence by age group:
  1. In neonates: More common in boys as a result of anatomic abnormalities such as the posterior urethral valves.
  2. In preschool children: More common in girls than in boys (4.5% vs. 0.5%).
  3. In adulthood: More common in women, with a 1% to 3% prevalence in nonpregnant women. Table 1 describes risk factors for acute uncomplicated UTIs in women.
  4. In pregnancy: At 12 wk the incidence of asymptomatic bacteriuria is similar to nonpregnant women (2% to 10%). However, 25% to 30% of pregnant women with untreated asymptomatic bacteriuria develop acute pyelonephritis, especially in the second and third trimesters, and pregnant women have a pyelonephritic recurrence rate of 10%.
  5. In adults aged ≥65: At least 10% of men and 20% of women have bacteriuria.

PHYSICAL FINDINGS & CLINICAL PRESENTATION

- Typical symptoms of UTI include:
  1. Urinary frequency and/or urgency
  2. Dysuria
  3. Suprapubic pain
  4. Gross or microscopic hematuria
- The probability of cystitis is greater than 50% in women with any symptom of UTI and greater than 90% in women who have dysuria and frequency without vaginal symptoms.
- Clinical symptoms alone can be used to make the diagnosis of uncomplicated UTI in women without a urine culture.
- When negative cultures are associated with significant pyuria, vaginal discharge, or hematuria, infections with *Chlamydia trachomatis, Neisseria gonorrhoeae*, and *Trichomonas vaginalis* should be considered.
- Acute pyelonephritis presents with fever, flank or abdominal pain, chills, malaise, and vomiting. It is these systemic symptoms that distinguish pyelonephritis from cystitis. Complications of acute pyelonephritis are renal abscess, perinephric abscess, emphysematous pyelonephritis, and pyonephrosis.

ETIOLOGY & PATHOGENESIS

- Most UTIs are caused by fecal flora, which can colonize the vaginal and periurethral tissues and ascend into the bladder.
- Other risk factors include incomplete bladder emptying due to neurologic disease, bladder outlet obstruction or urethral stricture, renal failure, diabetes, vesicoureteral reflux, fistula, urinary diversion, infected stones, advanced age, pregnancy, recent sexual activity, and instrumentation.
- Catheters: Patients who require a long-term Foley catheter will eventually develop significant levels of bacteriuria. Treatment is reserved for individuals who become symptomatic (leukocytosis, fever, chills, malaise, loss of appetite, etc). Using prophylactic antibiotics to treat patients who have chronic catheters is not indicated because of the risk of acquiring bacteria resistant to antibiotic therapy.
- Once bacteria reach the urinary tract, three factors determine whether symptomatic infection occurs (Box 1). These factors also determine the anatomic level of the UTI:
  1. Virulence of the microorganism
  2. Inoculum size
  3. Adequacy of the host defense mechanisms
- Urinary pathogens: In 90% of UTIs the infecting organism is gram-negative bacilli. *Escherichia coli* is the most common pathogen, causing 85% of UTI cases (predominantly O, K, and H antigen serotypes). *Staphylococcus saprophyticus* causes 10% of infections, especially in young, sexually active women. Other less common urinary pathogens include *Klebsiella, Enterobacter, Serratia, Proteus,* and *Pseudomonas.*
- In contrast, the organisms that commonly colonize the distal urethra and skin of both

TABLE 1 Factors Modulating Risk for Acute Uncomplicated Urinary Tract Infections in Women

Host Determinants	Uropathogen Determinants
Behavioral: Sexual intercourse, use of spermicidal products, recent antimicrobial use, suboptimal voiding habits	*Escherichia coli* virulence determinants: P, S, Dr, and type I fimbriae; hemolysin; aerobactin; serum resistance
Genetic: Innate and adaptive immune response, enhanced epithelial cell adherence, antibacterial factors in urine and bladder mucosa, nonsecretor of ABO blood group antigens, P_1 blood group phenotype, reduced *CXCR1* expression, previous history of recurrent cystitis	
Biologic: Estrogen deficiency in postmenopausal women, micturition	

From Floege J et al: *Comprehensive clinical nephrology,* ed 4, Philadelphia, 2010, Saunders.

BOX 1 Bacterial Factors

- The size of the inoculum
- The virulence of the infecting organism
  1. Virulence factors
     a. P-fimbriae facilitate the adherence of bacteria to biologic surfaces.
     b. K-antigens facilitate adherence and protect the organisms from the host-immune response.
     c. O-antigens are an important source of systemic reactions such as fever and shock that occur with bacterial infections.
     d. H-antigens are associated with flagella and are related to bacterial locomotion.
     e. Hemolysin may potentiate tissue damage and facilitate local bacterial growth.
     f. Urease alkalinizes the urine and facilitates stone formation, thus potentiating infection.
  2. Biofilms harbor bacteria on prosthetic devices and may be a source of recurrent infections.
  3. The presence of sialosyl galactosyl globoside on the surface of kidney cells. This compound is a highly powerful receptor for *Escherichia coli* bacteria.
  4. Women with a deficiency in human beta-defensin-1 are at greater risk for urinary tract infection.
- Adequacy of host defense mechanisms

men and women and the vagina of women are *Staphylococcus epidermidis*, diphtheroids, lactobacilli, *Gardnerella vaginalis*, and a variety of anaerobes that rarely cause UTIs. In general, the isolation of two or more bacterial species from a urine culture signifies a contaminated specimen unless the patient is being managed with an indwelling catheter or urinary diversion, or has a chronic complicated infection.

- Innate defense mechanisms against cystitis include low urine pH and high urine osmolarity, mucopolysaccharide glycosaminoglycan (GAG) protective layer, complete bladder emptying, and low vaginal pH due to the presence of estrogen and resulting colonization of the genital tract by lactobacillus. At the level of the kidney, uromodulin (also known as Tamm-Horsfall protein) is secreted by renal tubular epithelial cells to inhibit adherence of bacteria to urothelial cells.

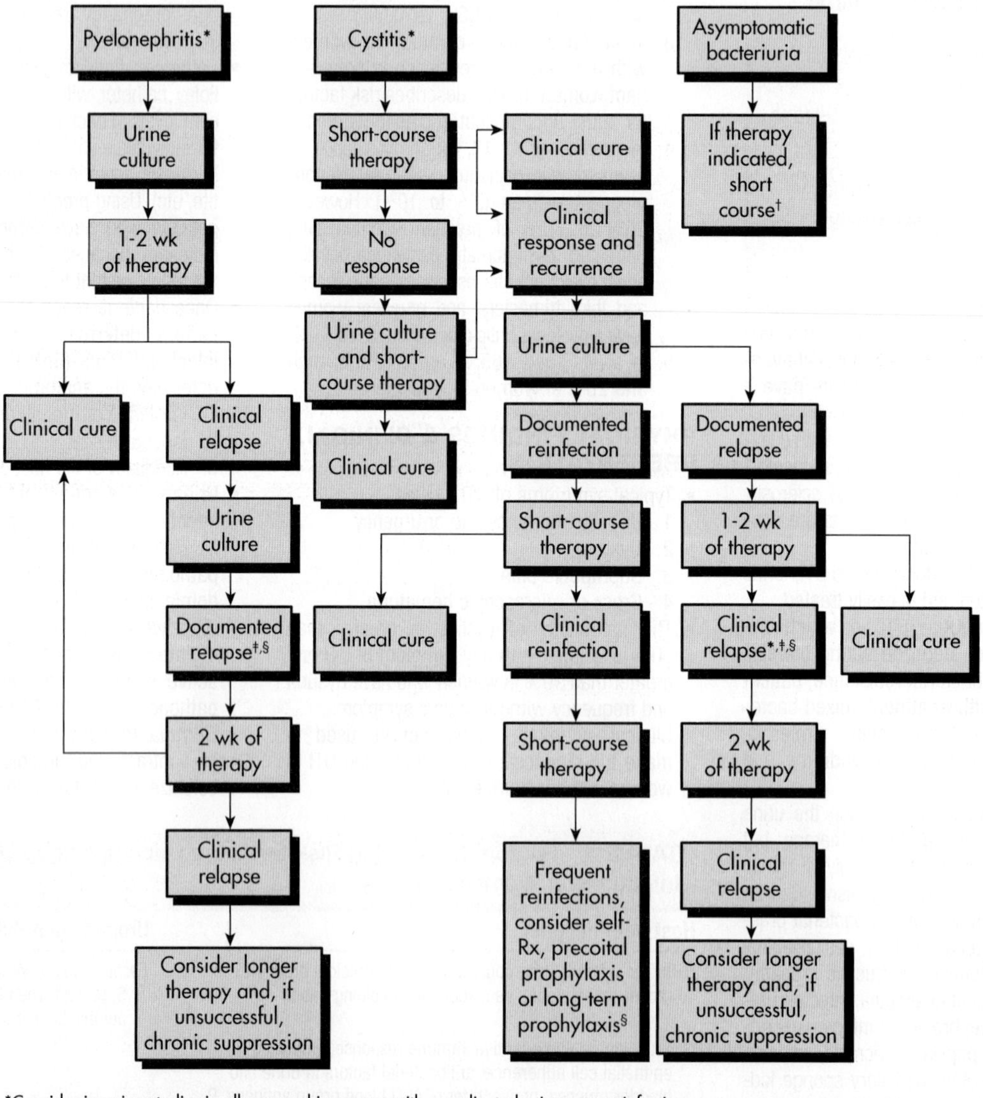

*Consider imaging studies in all men and in women with complicated urinary tract infection.
†No therapy except for renal transplant patients or prior to urologic procedures. Follow-up culture only in transplant patients.
‡Evaluate men for chronic bacterial prostatitis.
§Consider imaging studies in women.

FIG. 1 Approach to the management of urinary tract infection in nonpregnant adults. (From Bennett JE et al: *Mandell, Douglas, and Bennett's principles and practice of infectious diseases*, ed 8, Philadelphia, 2015, Saunders.)

- In uncomplicated, nonpregnant patients, cystitis rarely progresses to pyelonephritis or other serious infections such as bacteremia.

Dx DIAGNOSIS (FIG. 1)

DIFFERENTIAL DIAGNOSIS

- Vaginitis
- Urethritis (gonococcal, nongonococcal, *Trichomonas*)
- Interstitial cystitis (painful bladder syndrome)
- Pelvic inflammatory disease
- Nephrolithiasis
- Structural urethral abnormalities such as diverticulum or stricture

LABORATORY TESTS

- Microscopic urinalysis of clean-catch urine for bacteria and pyuria. The presence of $\geq$10 leukocytes/μl of unspun urine from a midstream catch indicates possible UTI. The absence of pyuria should call into question the diagnosis of UTI.
- Dipstick urinalysis with the presence of nitrites or leukocyte esterase is indicative of UTI. However, dipstick urinalysis may not be useful in symptomatic patients, as a negative dipstick urinalysis does not exclude the diagnosis of UTI. Additionally, dipsticks may be falsely positive when the urine is contaminated. Overall, a dipstick positive for nitrites and leukocyte esterase has a sensitivity of 75% and specificity of 82% in patients with >100,000 CFU/ml.
- Urine culture and sensitivity are useful in complicated UTIs and to help guide therapy in patients who fail initial therapy. They are generally not needed in uncomplicated UTIs.

IMAGING STUDIES

- Warranted only if renal infection or genitourinary abnormality is suspected
- CT urogram, voiding cystourethrogram, renal ultrasound, and intravenous pyelogram
- Specialty examination: Cystoscopy and retrograde pyelography to rule out obstructive uropathy, urethral diverticulum, mesh obstruction, or malignancy.

Rx TREATMENT

NONPHARMACOLOGIC THERAPY

Urinary analgesics such as phenazopyridine and aggressive hydration

ACUTE GENERAL Rx

- First-line antimicrobials for uncomplicated UTI recommended by the Infectious Disease Society of North America, the American Urologic Society, and the American College of Obstetricians and Gynecologists include nitrofurantoin bid for 5 days, trimethoprim plus sulfamethoxazole (TMP-SMX) bid for 3 days, or fosfomycin 3-g sachet in a single dose.
- Antimicrobial stewardship and drug resistance needs to be considered when choosing antibiotic therapy. Nitrofurantoin continues to have the lowest rates of antimicrobial resistance. Empiric treatment with TMP-SMX is considered appropriate when resistance rates are below 20%. Beta lactam antibiotics may be appropriate in cases of known patient intolerance or allergy to conventional first-line agents.
- Nitrofurantoin may have lower rates of bioavailability in patients >65 yr old due to decline in renal function. If Cr Cl is < 30 ml/min, Nitrofurantoin should be avoided, as it may not reach therapeutic concentration in the urine.
- Many women with a history of UTIs are aware of symptom onset. Patient-initiated therapy, in which a patient is given a prescription for the treatment of an uncomplicated UTI and instructed to start therapy when symptoms develop, has been found to be safe, effective, and less costly.
- High rates of resistance and the potential for serious side effects should limit the use of fluoroquinolone antimicrobials. The U.S. FDA has warned against the use of fluoroquinolone antibiotics for routine infections when suitable alternatives are available.
- Pyelonephritis may be treated as an outpatient in stable, well-hydrated patients with close follow-up. Antimicrobial selection is ideally based on urine culture results. Empiric treatment with fluoroquinolone antimicrobials or TMP-SMX is acceptable. Initiation of treatment in the emergency room setting with a single parenteral dose of a long-acting beta lactam or aminoglycoside antibiotic followed by oral treatment with fluoroquinolones or TMP-SMX is an acceptable regimen. Patients should be assessed for a proper response to treatment within 48 hr. Nitrofurantoin and fosfomycin are not indicated for the treatment of pyelonephritis due to inadequate renal tissue levels.
- Inpatient management of pyelonephritis should begin with parenteral antimicrobials followed by transition to oral agents based on clinical response and culture results.
- Pyelonephritis requires a total duration of 10 to 14 days of therapy, although evidence exists that 7 to 10 days may be equally effective in low-risk patients. See Table 2.

PEARLS & CONSIDERATIONS

COMMENTS

- Asymptomatic bacteriuria occurs commonly in postmenopausal women. Treatment of asymptomatic bacteriuria with antimicrobials is discouraged because it seldom resolves and can result in the development of drug-resistant organisms. Patients with cloudy or foul-smelling urine should be encouraged to aggressively hydrate to eliminate these symptoms. Postmenopausal women with vaginal atrophy can be treated with vaginal estrogen to reduce the incidence of bacteriuria. Exceptions include immunocompromised patients, patients with structural urinary tract abnormalities, and pregnant patients.
- Pregnancy: 25% to 30% of pregnant women with untreated asymptomatic bacteriuria develop pyelonephritis. All pregnant women should be screened for asymptomatic bacteriuria and treated. Nitrofurantoin, TMP-SMX, and beta lactam antibiotics are appropriate first-line choices in pregnancy.

TABLE 2 Dosage and Toxicity of Antibiotics Commonly Used to Treat Urinary Tract Infections

Drug	Oral Dose and Frequency	Minor Toxicity	Major Toxicity
Trimethoprim-sulfamethoxazole	160 mg/800 mg, q12h	Allergic	Serious skin reactions, blood dyscrasia
Nitrofurantoin macrocrystals	100 mg, q12h	GI upset	Peripheral neuropathy, pneumonitis
Ampicillin	250-500 mg, q6h	Allergic, candidal overgrowth	Allergic reactions, pseudomembranous colitis
Tetracycline	250-500 mg, q6h	GI upset, skin rash, candidal overgrowth	Hepatic dysfunction, nephrotoxicity
Cephalexin	250-500 mg, q6h	Allergic	Hepatic dysfunction
Ciprofloxacin	250 mg, q12h	Nausea, vomiting, diarrhea, abdominal pain, headache, skin rash	Arrhythmias, angina, convulsions, gastrointestinal bleeding, nephritis

GI, Gastrointestinal.
From Walters M, Karram M: *Urogynecology and reconstructive pelvic surgery, ed 4*, Philadelphia, 2015, Elsevier.

TABLE 3 Spectrum of Antimicrobial Activity against Common Lower Urinary Tract Pathogens

Organism	Nitrofurantoin	TMP-SMX	Ciprofloxacin	Levofloxacin	Cephalexin	Ampicillin	Fosfomycin
Escherichia coli	+	±	+	+	+	±	+
Pseudomonas	–	–	+	±	–	–	+
Klebsiella	–	±	+	+	+	–	+
Proteus	±	±	+	+	±	+	±
Enterobacter	±	±	+	+	–	–	±
Enterococcus	+	–	–	±	–	+	±
Staphylococcus	+	+	±	±	±	+	+
Serratia marcescens	–	±	+	+	–	–	±

From Walters M, Karram M: *Urogynecology and reconstructive pelvic surgery, ed 4,* Philadelphia, 2015, Elsevier.

- Recurrent UTI: Two or more symptomatic UTIs over a 6-mo period or three or more episodes over a 12-mo period. Causes include unresolved infection, abnormal vaginal colonization by the originally infecting organism, or reinfection with a new strain. Management of recurrent UTI includes antibiotic prophylaxis for 6 mo or longer, intermittent self-treatment, and postcoital prophylaxis depending on the circumstances. Patients with recurrent UTIs can be considered for an anatomic evaluation including office cystoscopy and upper urinary tract imaging (renal ultrasound or CT urography).
- Nonantimicrobial strategies to prevent UTI have shown mixed results. Nonantimicrobial agents with antiseptic effects on the lower urinary tract include cranberry supplements with vitamin C, d-mannose, and methenamine. Studies demonstrating clinical effectiveness of these agents show modest effects with few side effects. Topical estrogen has been shown to normalize the vaginal flora and may increase the thickness of the urothelium over time and should be used as an adjunct in postmenopausal women with recurrent UTI. Oral probiotics may also be beneficial by decreasing the vaginal pH.

ANTIMICROBIAL RESISTANCE:

- Because of the overuse of antibiotics, organisms once sensitive to a number of antimicrobial agents are now increasingly resistant, making effective treatment of UTI and pyelonephritis more challenging. Most important has been the increasing resistance to trimethoprim plus sulfamethoxazole (TMP-SMX), the current primary care provider drug of choice for acute uncomplicated UTI in women.
- Fluoroquinolone use for the treatment of acute cystitis in women should be avoided when suitable alternatives exist. The U.S. FDA has changed the labeling of quinolone antibiotics to reflect this recommendation.
- When choosing a treatment regimen, physicians should consider such factors as:
  1. In vitro susceptibility
  2. Adverse effects on individual patients
  3. Adverse effects on the population (stewardship)
  4. Cost-effectiveness
  5. Resistance rates in their respective communities
- Meropenem (1 g IV every 8 hr) or IV plazomicin (15 mg/kg BW once daily) are effective for the treatment of complicated UTIs and acute pyelonephritis caused by Enterobacteriaceae, including multidrug-resistant strains. See Table 3.

SUGGESTED READINGS

Available at ExpertConsult.com

RELATED CONTENT

Urinary Tract Infection (Patient Information)
Urinary Tract Infection (Child) (Patient Information)
Pyelonephritis (Related Key Topic)

AUTHORS: **Sydney Ford, MD, MPH,** and **Kelly McNamara, MD**

BASIC INFORMATION

DEFINITION

Urolithiasis is the presence of calculi within the urinary tract. The five major types of urinary stones are calcium oxalate (60%-70%), calcium phosphate (20%), uric acid (7%), struvite (7%), and cystine (1%) (Table 1).

SYNONYMS

Kidney stones
Kidney calculi
Renal stones
Renal calculi
Ureteral stones
Ureteral calculi
Nephrolithiasis
Ureterolithiasis

ICD-10CM CODES

N20.0	Calculus of kidney
N20.1	Calculus of ureter
N20.2	Calculus of kidney with calculus of ureter
N20.9	Urinary calculus, unspecified
N21.0	Calculus in bladder
N21.1	Calculus in urethra
N21.8	Other lower urinary tract calculus
N21.9	Calculus of lower urinary tract, unspecified

EPIDEMIOLOGY & DEMOGRAPHICS

- Urinary stones affect approximately 1 in 11 persons in the U.S., with a lifetime prevalence of approximately 10% in males and 7% in females.
- Peak incidence is in the fourth to sixth decade of life.
- Urolithiasis appears to be more common among whites than Hispanics, Asians, or African Americans.
- The incidence of urinary stone disease is increasing, likely due to increased use of cross-sectional imaging and changing dietary and lifestyle factors.
- The incidence of symptomatic urolithiasis is greatest during the summer presumably from increased temperature with resulting dehydration and urinary concentration.
- Annually, between 1 and 2 million emergency department visits are due to kidney stones and renal colic.
- First-time stone-formers have up to an estimated 50% risk for recurrence over the next 10 yr.
- Approximately 90% of all urinary stones are radio-opaque. Cystine stones are faintly radio-opaque. Uric acid stones are radiolucent.

PHYSICAL FINDINGS & CLINICAL PRESENTATION

Stones may be asymptomatic or cause the following signs and symptoms, often from urinary tract obstruction:

- Acute, often severe, flank pain (renal colic)
- Pain radiating from the flank downward and anteriorly, with referred pain to the groin and genitalia (common as stone progresses down ureter)
- Low back and lower abdominal pain, often ipsilateral to the stone
- Nausea and vomiting
- Hematuria, gross or microscopic
- Inability to find a comfortable position
- Urinary urgency and frequency with distal ureteral stones mimicking a urinary tract infection
- Fever and chills accompanying acute renal colic from superimposed infection
- Elderly patients, children, and patients with neurologic deficits may present with nonspecific and vague abdominal discomfort and pain

ETIOLOGY

- Urine composition: Supersaturation of various solutes and stone constituents is the driving force in kidney stone formation. Various metabolic abnormalities such as low or high urine pH, idiopathic hypercalciuria, hypocitraturia, hyperoxaluria, and hyperuricosuria predispose patients to urinary stone formation.
- Low urine volume is the most common cause in many stone-formers.
- Dietary factors: Diets high in sodium and animal protein increase the risk of urinary stone formation. Remarkably high dietary oxalate consumption and heavy intake of phosphoric acid-containing carbonated drinks likely increase the risk of stone formation. Foods with high potential renal acid load such as cheese and meats increase the risk of urinary stone formation. Fruits and vegetables with low potential renal acid load may reduce the risk.
- Anatomic factors predisposing patients to urinary stasis: Malrotated, horseshoe, or ectopic kidney; ureteropelvic junction obstruction; vesicoureteral reflux in young children; bladder outlet obstruction; and strictures affecting the urinary tract.
- Disease states:
  1. Hyperparathyroidism with hypercalcemia and hypercalciuria
  2. Sarcoidosis with hypercalcemia
  3. Malabsorption (e.g., inflammatory bowel disease) with increased oxalate absorption
  4. Chronic diarrheal states
  5. Gastric bypass surgery with enteric hyperoxaluria
  6. Metabolic syndrome (e.g., diabetes, overweight) produces acidic urine predisposing patients to uric acid stones. It has also been suggested that metabolic syndrome increases calcium oxalate stone formation by increasing the excretion of promoters of stone formation
  7. Gouty diathesis
  8. Primary hyperoxaluria: Genetic, rare, and usually presenting as a childhood disorder
  9. Medullary sponge kidney
  10. Hyperuricosuria (e.g., metabolic defects, dietary excess) (Box 1)
  11. Type I (distal) renal tubular acidosis (>1% of calcium phosphate stones)
  12. Cystinuria: Autosomal recessive disorder produces 1% of stones

BOX 1 Uric Acid Stones

Low urine pH (≤5.5)
High animal protein diet
Diarrhea
Insulin resistance (high body mass index, metabolic syndrome, type 2 diabetes)

Low Urine Volume
Inadequate fluid intake
Excessive extrarenal fluid losses
Diarrhea
Insensible losses (e.g., perspiration)

Hyperuricosuria
Excessive dietary purine intake
Hyperuricemia
  Gout
  Intracellular-to-extracellular uric acid shift
  Myeloproliferative disorders
  Tumor lysis syndrome
Inborn errors of metabolism
  Lesch-Nyhan syndrome
  Glucose-6-phosphatase deficiency

From Floege J et al: *Comprehensive clinical nephrology*, ed 4, Philadelphia, 2010, Saunders.

TABLE 1 Types of Urinary Tract Stones and Their Etiology

Composition	Etiological Factors	Percentage of All Stones
Calcium oxalate/calcium oxalate mixed with calcium phosphate	An underlying metabolic disorder (e.g., idiopathic hypercalciuria or hyperoxaluria) ▸ in 25% no metabolic abnormality is identified	75
Struvite or matrix calculi (composed of magnesium ammonium phosphate)	Renal infection	10-15
Uric acid	Hyperuricemia or hyperuricosuria ▸ it is idiopathic in 50%	6
Cysteine	A renal tubular defect	1-2

Other stones (e.g., xanthine stones, which may be related to a metabolic abnormality, or indinavir stones, which are drug related) are uncommon and account for <5% of all renal stones.
From Grant LA: *Grainger & Allison's diagnostic radiology essentials*, ed 2, Philadelphia, 2019, Elsevier.

BOX 2 Factors Associated with Struvite Stone Formation

- Urease-producing bacteria:
  1. *Proteus*
  2. *Klebsiella*
  3. *Providencia*
  4. *Pseudomonas*
  5. *Staphylococcus epidermidis*
  6. *Haemophilus*
  7. *Yersinia species*
  8. *Serratia*
  9. *Citrobacter*
  10. *Ureaplasma*
- Elevated urinary pH

Modified from Floege J et al: *Comprehensive clinical nephrology*, ed 4, Philadelphia, 2010, Saunders.

- Chronic infections: Urease-producing organisms (e.g., *Proteus* [most common], *Providencia, Pseudomonas, Klebsiella, Staphylococcus*) produce alkaline urine favoring struvite or magnesium ammonium phosphate crystal formation (Box 2).
- Medications: Protease inhibitors (e.g., indinavir, ritonavir), topiramate, and chronic laxative overuse.

Dx DIAGNOSIS

DIFFERENTIAL DIAGNOSIS

- Urinary tract infection (e.g., cystitis)
- Pyelonephritis
- Diverticulitis
- Appendicitis
- Pelvic inflammatory disease
- Ovarian pathology, including torsion
- Dysmenorrhea
- Ectopic pregnancy
- Small bowel obstruction
- Constipation
- Malignancy (primary urinary tract or retroperitoneal lymphadenopathy causing ureteral/kidney obstruction)
- Ureteropelvic junction obstruction
- Testicular torsion in children and teenagers
- Musculoskeletal back pain
- Renal infarction and renal bleeds
- Factitious (illicit substance-seeking behavior), often with recurrent stone formers

The differential diagnosis of obstructive uropathy is described in Section II.

WORKUP

- Stone composition of recovered stones should be determined by infrared spectroscopy or x-ray crystallography. Box 3 summarizes indications for a metabolic stone evaluation.
- Box 4 describes events in the medical history that may be significant with regard to urolithiasis.

LABORATORY TESTS

- Urinalysis: Hematuria is often present, but the absence of hematuria does not exclude stones. Urine pH may help identify stone type: pH >7.5 is associated with struvite stones; pH <5.5 is generally associated with uric acid stones; and low serum bicarbonate concentration with urine pH ≥6 is consistent with a renal tubular acidosis.
- Urine culture and sensitivity results should be obtained selectively in patients who may have superimposed infections, based on clinical symptoms of dysuria, fever, chills, urinalysis suggestive of infection, or when surgical intervention is planned.
- Serum chemistries include electrolytes, blood urea nitrogen (BUN), creatinine, calcium, phosphate, uric acid, and parathyroid hormone.
- Additional tests: 24-hr urine collection for volume, creatinine, calcium, uric acid, phosphate, oxalate, urea nitrogen reflecting protein intake, and citrate excretion is generally reserved for patients with recurrent stones, young patients, bilateral stones, and large stone burden. A 24-hr urine collection may be appropriate for motivated, first-time stone patients interested in preventing recurrent stones. An abbreviated evaluation of single-stone formers is described in Box 5. Table 2 summarizes diagnostic criteria for various disorders associated with urolithiasis.

BOX 3 Indications for a Metabolic Stone Evaluation

Recurrent stone formers
Strong family history of stones
Intestinal disease (particularly chronic diarrhea)
Pathologic skeletal fractures
Osteoporosis
History of urinary tract infection with calculi
Personal history of gout
Infirm health (unable to tolerate repeat stone episodes)
Solitary kidney
Anatomic abnormalities
Chronic kidney disease
Stones composed of cystine, uric acid, struvite

From Partin AW et al: *Campbell-Walsh-Wein urology*, ed 12, Philadelphia, 2021, Elsevier.

IMAGING STUDIES

- Common diagnostic modalities for renal colic are summarized in Table 3.
- Noncontrast computed tomography (CT) scanning ("low-dose") is rapid and accurate, has the greatest sensitivity (nearly 100%) and specificity (94%-96%), and can identify almost all stone types in essentially all locations. This modality provides additional anatomic detail such as hydronephrosis. CT scan is the best test upon which to base stone treatment recommendations, evaluate stone persistence or passage, and plan for surgery. Protease inhibitor stones and pure matrix stones are typically radiolucent and poorly visualized by noncontrast CT and usually require contrast-enhanced CT for visualization. A high index of suspicion is required for diagnosis.
- CT scans may be ordered by urologists planning surgical intervention because a CT yields information on adjacent organs and stone density that ultrasound and plain film radiography cannot reveal.
- Ultralow-dose CT protocols are becoming more widely available and preserve most of the diagnostic accuracy of regular stone protocol CT scans and deliver lower radiation exposures (<3 mSv versus 10 mSv).
- Ultrasonography (Fig. 1) may be an adequate initial study to detect stone presence (i.e., hydronephrosis), especially in patients known to have a history of stones and in patients where radiation should be avoided (e.g., pregnancy and children). Ultrasonography is 50% to 70% sensitive in detecting stones within the kidneys, and approximately 90% sensitive in detecting hydronephrosis.
- Point-of-care ultrasound use is increasing in emergency departments and some clinical settings.
- Initial ultrasonography may be associated with lower cumulative radiation exposure than initial CT, without significant differences in missing, serious, or alternative diagnoses; adverse events; pain scores; return emergency department visits; or hospitalizations. It is reasonable to use ultrasonography as the initial imaging modality in suspected nephrolithiasis and to monitor known stones.
- Accuracy of sonography in detecting distal ureteral stones is heterogeneous due to variable stone size, body habitus, and operator expertise. The absence of an ipsilateral ureteral jet suggests the possibility of renal tract obstruction, but this sign is not pathognomonic.
- Abdominal radiography or a kidney-ureter-bladder x-ray (KUB) can identify radio-opaque stones (e.g., calcium-containing) but not radiolucent stones (uric acid stones). However, the KUB has much lower detections rates than CT, with an estimated sensitivity of 57% and specificity of 76%. Major limitations include inability to visualize all stone types (uric acid) and potential overlying structures, including bowel gas or bone.

Rx TREATMENT

ACUTE GENERAL Rx

- Diagnosis with labs, imaging, and patient history.
- Pain control: NSAIDs are excellent for managing renal colic (e.g., ketorolac, ibuprofen) and are preferred first-line agents. Opiates may be required for severe pain. Initial pain control with NSAIDs can reduce overall opiate dosing for renal colic. Fig. 2 illustrates a guideline algorithm for the evaluation, treatment, and disposition of patients with presumed renal colic.
- Intravenous fluids and antiemetics may be required.
- Patients with suspected urinary tract infections and obstructing stones require urgent kidney drainage (ureteral stent by a urologist

BOX 4 Components of the Medical History that Are Significant for Urolithiasis

- Diseases associated with disturbances of calcium metabolism: Primary hyperparathyroidism, medullary sponge kidney, osteoporosis, immobilization, sarcoidosis, osteolytic metastases, plasmacytoma, neuroendocrine tumors, and Paget disease
- Dietary history: Purine intake, calcium excess, calcium and alkali intake, oxalate excess, sodium excess, and low citrus fruit intake
- Medications: Uricosurics, diuretics, analgesics, vitamins C and D, antacids (especially phosphorus-binding agents), acetazolamide, calcium channel blockers, triamterene, estrogens, theophylline, protease inhibitors (indinavir), and sulfonamides
- Diseases associated with disturbances of oxalate metabolism: Types 1 and 2 primary hyperoxaluria, Crohn disease, ulcerative colitis, intestinal bypass surgery (e.g., jejunoileal bypass), and ileal resection
- Genetic disorders associated with disturbances of purine metabolism (e.g., Lesch Nyhan, hypoxanthine phosphoribosyl transferase deficiency, and adenine phosphoribosyl transferase deficiency)
- Intrinsic metabolic disorders: Anemias and neoplastic disorders with rapid purine turnover (e.g., leukemias), intoxication, myocardial infarction, irradiation, and cytotoxic chemotherapy
- Altered urate excretion: Chronic kidney disease, metabolic acidosis
- Infectious history: Organisms (particularly *Proteus* and *Klebsiella*), febrile, upper tract involvement, and dates (if hospitalized)

Modified from Nseyo UO et al (eds): *Urology for primary care physicians,* Philadelphia, 1999, Saunders.

BOX 5 Abbreviated Evaluation of Single-Stone Formers

History
- Underlying predisposing conditions (see Box 3 and Etiology section in text)
- Medications (calcium, vitamin C, vitamin D, acetazolamide, steroids)
- Dietary excesses, inadequate fluid intake, excessive fluid loss

Multichannel blood screen
- Basic metabolic panel (sodium, potassium, chloride, carbon dioxide, blood urea nitrogen, creatinine)
- Calcium
- Intact parathyroid hormone
- Uric acid

Urine
- Urinalysis
  - pH >7.5: Infection-related lithiasis
  - pH <5.5: Uric acid lithiasis
  - Sediment for crystalluria
- Urine culture
  - Urea-splitting organisms: Suggestive of infection lithiasis
- Quantitative cystine assay

Radiography
- Radiopaque stones: Calcium oxalate, calcium phosphate, magnesium ammonium phosphate (struvite), cystine
- Radiolucent stones: Uric acid, xanthine, triamterene
- CT scan, renal ultrasound or intravenous pyelogram: Radiolucent stones, anatomic abnormalities

Stone analysis

CT, Computed tomography.
From Partin AW et al: *Campbell-Walsh-Wein urology,* ed 12, Philadelphia, 2021, Elsevier.

TABLE 2 Diagnostic Criteria

	SERUM			URINARY							
	Ca	P	PTH	Ca Fasting	Ca Load	Ca Restricted	UA	Ox	Cit	pH	Mg
Absorptive hypercalciuria type I	N	N	N	N	↑	↑	N	N	N	N	N
Absorptive hypercalciuria type II	N	N	N	↑	N	N	N	N	N	N	N
Renal hypercalciuria	N	N	↑	↑	↑	↑	N	N	N	N	N
Primary hyperparathyroidism	↑	↓	↑	↑	↑	↑	N	N	N	N	N
Unclassified hypercalciuria	N	N/↓	N	↑	↑	↑	N	N	N	N	N
Hyperuricosuria	N	N	N	N	N	N	↑	N	N	N	N
Enteric hyperoxaluria	N/↓	N/↓	N/↓	↓	↓	↓	↓	↑	↓	N	N
Hypocitraturia	N	N	N	N	N	N	N	N	↓	N	N
Renal tubular acidosis	N	N	N/↑	↑	N	N/↑	N	N	↓	N/↑	N
Hypomagnesuria	N	N	N	N	N	N	N/↓	N	↓	N	↓
Gouty diathesis	N	N	N	N	N	N	N/↑	N	N/↓	↓	N
Infection lithiasis	N	N	N	N	N	N	N	N	↓	↑	N

Fasting samples represent 2-hr collections obtained in morning after an overnight fast. Calcium load samples were obtained over a 4-hr period subsequent to oral ingestion of 1 g calcium. ↑, High; ↓, low; *Cit,* citrate; *Mg,* magnesium; *N,* normal; *Ox,* oxalate; *PTH,* immunoreactive parathyroid hormone; *UA,* uric acid.
From Wein AJ et al: *Campbell–Walsh urology,* ed 11, Philadelphia, 2016, Elsevier.

TABLE 3 Common Diagnostic Imaging Modalities for Renal Colic

Modality	Information Provided	Radiation Dose	Contrast	Approximate Cost	Time
CT	Renal and ureteral stones, stone size, location, number, evidence of obstruction Alternative diagnoses, such as AAA, appendicitis, and free air	4-10 mSv	No	$750-$1000	Less than 5 min to perform, 30 min for interpretation
CT with IV contrast	Same as noncontrast CT Delineation of renal masses Additional information about vascular dissections and mesenteric ischemia	4-10 mSv	Yes	$750-$1000	Less than 5 min, after delay to measure creatinine
CT with IV and oral contrast	Same as CT with IV contrast Potentially improved diagnosis of bowel abnormalities	4-10 mSv	Yes	$750-$1000	Less than 5 min, after delay of approximately 2 hr to ingest oral contrast
Intravenous urogram	Structural and functional information about obstruction Rarely, identification of other pathology, such as AAA	1.5 mSv	Yes	$350	Approximately 75 min
X-ray	Possible identification of stone, but cannot assess for hydronephrosis or most other pathology	0.5-1 mSv	No	$250	Less than 5 min
Ultrasound	Identification of hydronephrosis or hydroureter Possible identification of stone Used to assess for AAA or biliary disease	No	No	$150	Approximately 15-30 min—bedside ultrasound is quicker

AAA, Abdominal aortic aneurysm; *CT,* computed tomography; *IV,* intravenous.
From Lipshultz LI et al: *Urology and the primary care practitioner,* ed 3, Philadelphia, 2008, Elsevier.

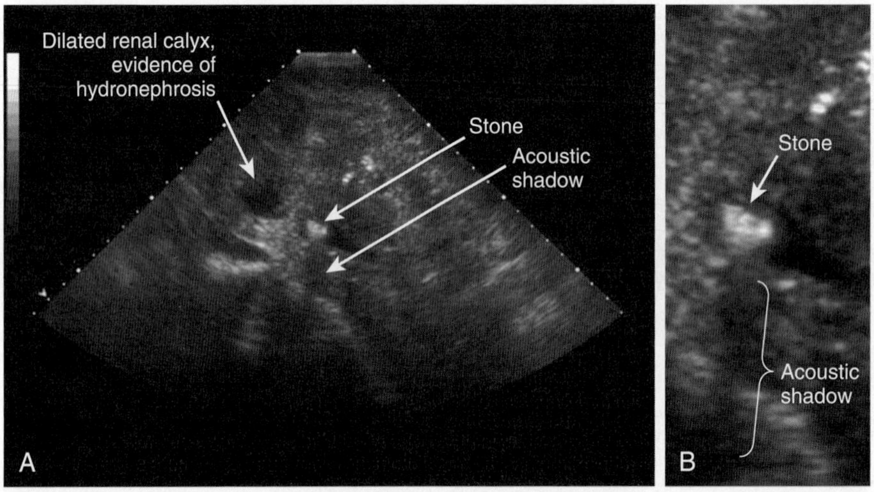

FIG. 1 Ultrasound of renal stone. Ultrasound can be used to assess for renal stones and complications such as hydronephrosis. Stones can be difficult to detect, whereas hydronephrosis is usually readily identified. Because stones are dense, they reflect sound and prevent its transmission. As a result, stones are echogenic *(bright)* on ultrasound and generate an acoustic shadow *(black).* **A,** Short-axis view of kidney. **B,** Close-up view. (From Broder JS: *Diagnostic imaging for the emergency physician,* Philadelphia, 2011, Saunders.)

or nephrostomy tube placement) and antibiotics. Patients with acute kidney injury or electrolyte derangements or those whose pain cannot be controlled may also require urgent kidney drainage.
- For patients who have a stone with a high probability of passage (i.e., small stone, especially distal ureter), medical expulsive therapy with α-blockers or calcium channel blockers (used less often due to side effects) may be helpful. New Level 1 evidence suggests that medical expulsive treatment may not be superior to placebo when considering all stone sizes; however, contemporary and numerous older studies have shown benefit to passage of distal stones ≥5 mm in size with the use of medical expulsive therapy.

PREVENTION

- Generally, patients at increased risk for stones should increase fluid intake to maintain a urine volume of at least 2.5 L per day.
- Recommended daily allowance of dietary calcium is 1000 to 1200 mg/day. However, calcium restriction has been shown to paradoxically increase the risk for stone formation. Lower calcium consumption results in less intestinal calcium-oxalate binding and consequently, greater colonic oxalate absorption, which in turn increases urinary oxalate excretion and risk for calcium-based stones.
- Limiting nondairy animal protein is recommended.
- Increasing fruit and vegetable intake increases urinary excretion of citrate (stone inhibitor).
- Dietary sodium restriction with intake of <2 g sodium daily reduces renal calcium excretion. High dietary loads of sodium lead to hypercalciuria.
- Dietary oxalate restriction in patients with hyperoxaluria may be beneficial. However,

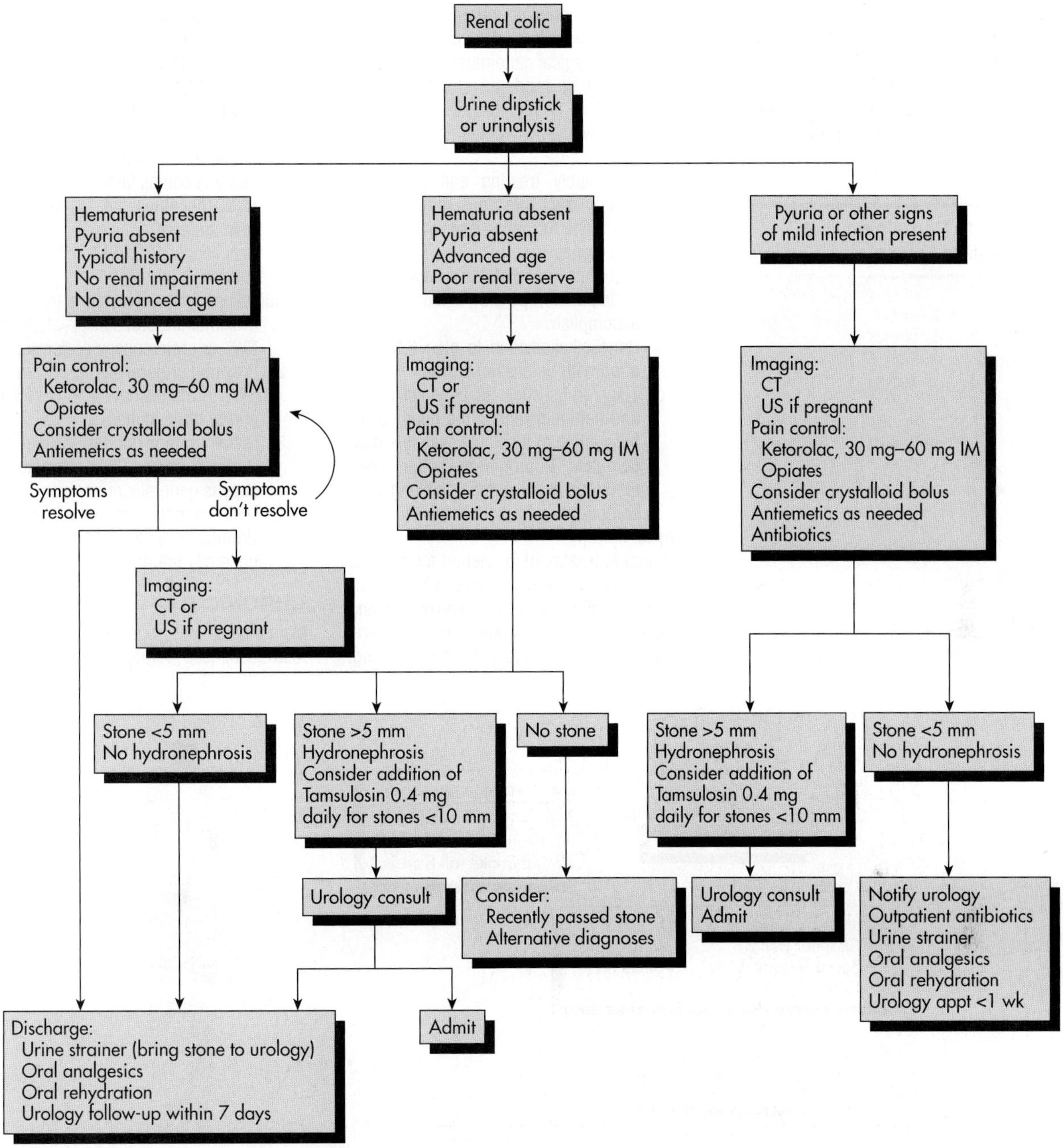

FIG. 2 Guideline algorithm for the evaluation, treatment, and disposition of patients with presumed renal colic. *CT,* Computed tomography; *IV,* intravenously; *US,* ultrasonography. (Modified from Adams JG et al: *Emergency medicine, clinical essentials,* ed 2, Philadelphia, 2013, Elsevier.)

adherence to a low-oxalate diets may be challenging. Box 6 describes foods containing high oxalate concentrations.

- There is conflicting evidence regarding the association between vitamin C consumption and urinary oxalate excretion. Nevertheless, we do not recommend ingestion of 2 g of vitamin C daily.
- Increase dietary citrate (e.g., lemons, limes, oranges). For citrus juices and drinks, encourage low-calorie, low-sugar options.
- Stone specific therapy (Fig. 3):
  1. Uric acid stones:
     a. Major goal in the management of uric acid stones is alkalinization of urine pH to >5.5. The ideal morning urine pH is between 6.0 and 6.5. This can dissolve existing uric acid stones and prevent the formation of new ones.
     b. Often accomplished with potassium citrate or sodium bicarbonate taken two or three times daily with food.
     c. Alkalinizing the urine to a pH >7.0 should be avoided because of an increased risk for development of calcium phosphate stones.
     d. Reduction of nondairy animal protein and correction of metabolic syndrome, obesity, and diabetes reduce the frequency of uric acid stones.
  2. Calcium stones:
     a. In general, cannot be dissolved and either persist, pass, or are removed.
     b. With hypercalciuria, thiazide diuretics and low-sodium diet are appropriate. Potassium citrate supplementation for patients with calcium stones and a low 24-hr urine citrate excretion. Potassium citrate may also be effective with calcium stones even when urine citrate excretion is not low. Potassium citrate can treat the hypokalemia induced by thiazide diuretics.
     c. Urate-lowering treatment for patients with hyperuricosuria but not hypercalciuria.

3. Struvite stones:
   a. Surgical interventions are usually required. Percutaneous nephrolithotomy (PCNL) and/or ureteroscopy are preferred, while shock wave lithotripsy (SWL) is an alternative.

BOX 6 Foods Containing High Oxalate Levels

Tea (black)
Cocoa
Spinach
Mustard greens
Pokeweed
Swiss chard
Beets
Rhubarb
Okra
Berries (some)
Chocolate
Nuts
Wheat germ
Soy crackers
Pepper

From Partin AW et al: *Campbell-Walsh-Wein urology,* ed 12, Philadelphia, 2021, Elsevier.

   b. Urease inhibitor treatment by acetohydroxamic acid is considered for poor surgical candidates or if patients cannot be rendered stone free. This agent is poorly tolerated and infrequently used in contemporary practice.
   c. Adequately treating and preventing urinary tract infections reduces struvite stone formation and recurrence.
4. Cystine stones:
   a. High fluid intake of 3 to 4 L daily is the principal therapy, although it is hard to accomplish.
   b. Urine alkalinization to pH >6.5 to 7, often with potassium citrate.
   c. Thiol drugs such as D-penicillamine and tiopronin reduce the poorly soluble cystine to a soluble cysteine–drug complex. Tiopronin is better tolerated than penicillamine, but long-term compliance with both is infrequent.

- Surgical therapy
  1. Surgical treatment is needed for patients with severe pain unresponsive to medication, possible infection from an obstructing stone, acute kidney injury from ureteral obstruction, refractory nausea/vomiting, and prolonged kidney obstruction (i.e., risk of irreversible renal damage).
  2. Ureteral stones can often be managed with ureteroscopy or SWL.
  3. Stones in the kidney can be managed with ureteroscopy or SWL if <1 to 2 cm in diameter and in a favorable location. As a stone becomes larger and more complex, PCNL becomes the preferred means of management.
  4. Indications for PCNL are described in Table 4.
- Guidelines for ureteral stone treatment:
  1. Proximal ureteral stones <1 cm diameter: SWL or ureteroscopy preferred.
  2. Proximal ureteral stones >1 cm diameter: SWL, ureteroscopy or PCNL for complex and/or large stones.
  3. Distal ureteral stones <1 cm diameter: Ureteroscopy or SWL, although ureteroscopy is generally preferred.
  4. Distal ureteral stones >1 cm diameter: Ureteroscopy or SWL; ureteroscopy is generally preferred.

CHRONIC Rx

Maintenance of proper hydration and dietary restrictions (see "Acute General Rx")

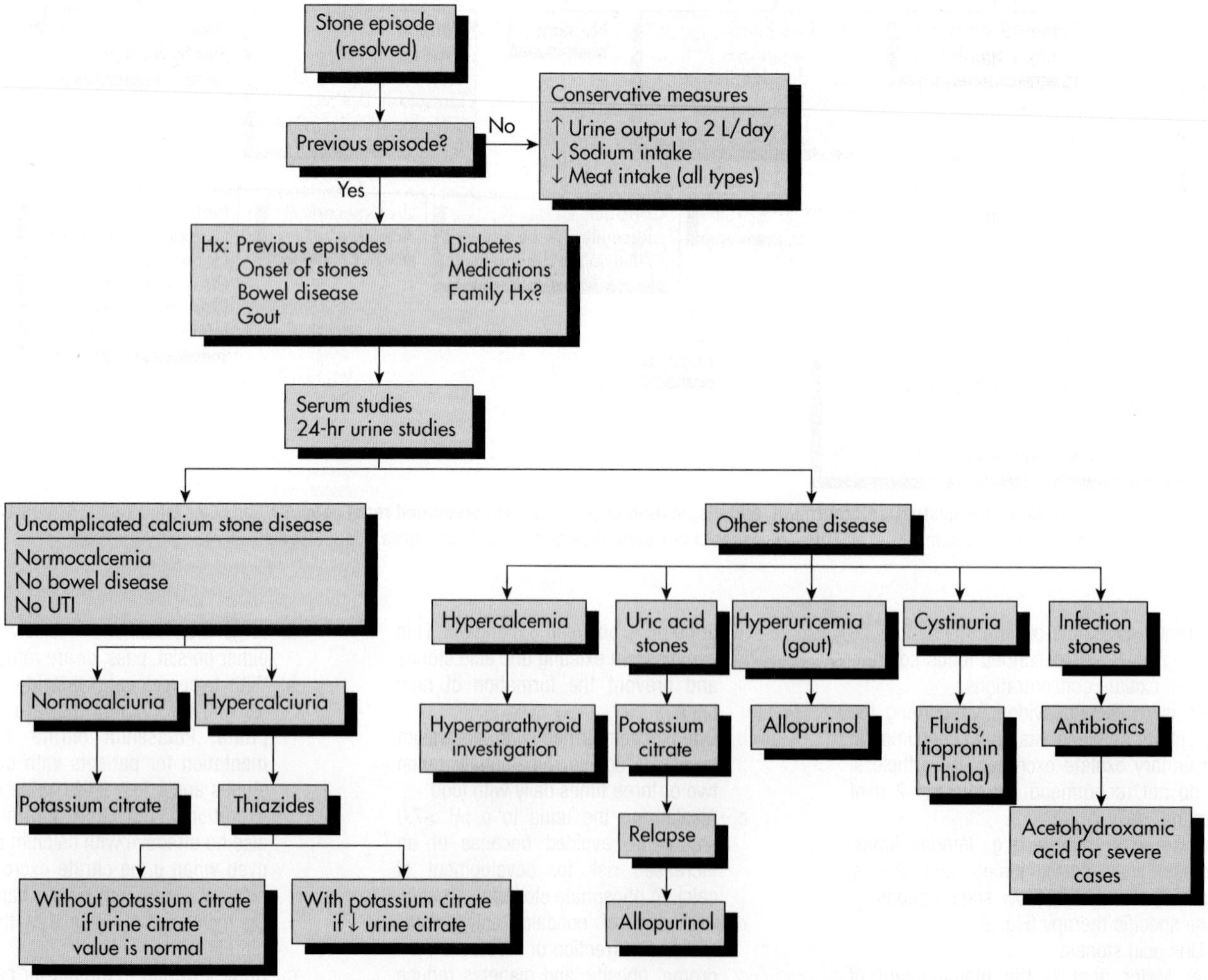

FIG. 3 Simplified treatment algorithm for the evaluation and medical management of urinary lithiasis. *Hx,* History; *UTI,* urinary tract infection. (Modified from CY Pak. From Wein AJ et al: *Campbell-Walsh urology,* ed 11, Philadelphia, 2016, Elsevier.)

TABLE 4 Indications for Percutaneous Nephrolithotomy

Indicator	Description	Treatment
Stone size	≥1.5-2 cm or staghorn	
Composition*,**	Struvite stones	Complete removal necessary to reduce infection and minimize stone recurrence
	Calcium oxalate monohydrate and brushite stones	Difficult to pulverize by SWL
	Cystine stones	Difficult to pulverize by SWL
Stone position	Lower pole stones	Fragments less easily evacuated from dependent lower pole calyces; may not be accessible with ureteroscopy
Anatomic abnormalities	UPJ obstruction; calyceal diverticula; urinary diversion	Prevent passage of fragments after SWL; not always accessible with ureteroscopy
Patient characteristics	Morbid obesity; ureteral obstruction	Stone cannot be placed in focal point of SWL machine; not always accessible with ureteroscopy

SWL or ureteroscopy is the first choice for stone intervention, except in those circumstances that may favor PCNL. *SWL,* Extracorporeal shock wave lithotripsy; *PCNL,* percutaneous nephrolithotomy; *UPJ,* ureteropelvic junction.

*Stone composition can be defined with certainty only by direct stone analysis, but advances in imaging may ultimately provide a means to accurately assess stone composition in situ before treatment, thus allowing the urologist to select the treatment most likely to be successful.

**Ureteroscopy and laser lithotripsy also may be used to treat all stone types, including those listed in this table. Thus, stone size and location ultimately influence PCNL versus ureteroscopy decision.

Modified from Floege J et al: *Comprehensive clinical nephrology,* ed 4, Philadelphia, 2010, Saunders.

DISPOSITION

- More than 50% to 80% of patients will pass a ureteral stone within 4 to 6 wk of presentation. Remember the “10 minus size of the stone in mm × 100% rule.” For example, a 3-mm stone has an approximately 70% probability of spontaneous passage while an 8-mm stone has only a 20% chance.
- Lifetime stone recurrence is as high as 50% and depends on stone factors (composition, size, location, and number of stones) and patient factors (anatomic, genetic, race, comorbidities, hydration status, diet, climate, and occupation).

REFERRAL

Urology referral is appropriate for any urinary stone patient, especially when spontaneous passage is unlikely; if a patient cannot be directly discharged from an emergency department; when there is an obstructing kidney stone and presumed or associated urinary tract infection; when there are large or recurrent stones; and when patients have solitary kidneys or complex anatomy that may predispose them to stones.

PEARLS & CONSIDERATIONS

COMMENTS

- Approximately 60% to 80% of ureteral stones will pass spontaneously within 4 to 6 wk. Similarly, approximately 60% to 80% of patients will not require admission or surgery for a ureteral stone.
- Imaging is key to diagnosing urolithiases. Ultrasound or KUB is a suitable screening test, while CT scan is most accurate and often determines treatment recommendations.
- Consider NSAIDs as first-line therapy for pain control with kidney stones, unless there are contraindications (e.g., allergy or acute kidney injury).
- Patients should be referred to a urologist if they have large stones unlikely to pass spontaneously, multiple or bilateral stones at presentation, complex stones, or recurrent stones.
- An obstructing urinary stone in the setting of presumed urinary tract infection should be treated with prompt urinary tract drainage via insertion of a ureteral stent or percutaneous nephrostomy tube and with antibiotics. Delay in renal drainage can lead to rapid and life-threatening sepsis.
- Patients with nephrolithiasis and elevated serum calcium level should be evaluated for primary hyperparathyroidism.[1]

SUGGESTED READINGS

Available at ExpertConsult.com

RELATED CONTENT

Kidney Stones (Patient Information)
Urinary Tract Infection (Patient Information)

AUTHORS: **Jeffrey Budzyn, MD,** and **David A. Leavitt, MD**

[1]Ganesan C et al: Analysis of primary hyperparathyroidism screening among U.S. veterans with kidney stones, *JAMA Surg* 155:861-868, 2020.

BASIC INFORMATION

DEFINITION

Urticaria is a pruritic rash involving the epidermis and the upper portions of the dermis caused by localized capillary vasodilation and the release of histamine and other vasoactive mediators. It is followed by transudation of protein-rich fluid in the surrounding tissue and manifests clinically with the presence of raised erythematous, circumscribed lesions with central pallor. Urticaria is classified according to its chronicity into acute (<6-wk duration) and chronic (>6-wk duration).

SYNONYMS

Hives
Wheals

ICD-10CM CODES	
L50.0	Allergic urticaria
L50.1	Idiopathic urticaria
L50.2	Urticaria due to cold and heat
L50.8	Other urticaria
L50.9	Urticaria, unspecified
L50.6	Contact urticaria

EPIDEMIOLOGY & DEMOGRAPHICS

- Between 15% and 25% of the population will have at least one episode of urticaria during their lifetime.
- The incidence of chronic urticaria is thought to be around 1.4% annually. It is more common in adults, with the average age of occurrence between the third and fifth decades of life. Females are twice as likely to be affected as males.
- Incidence is increased in atopic patients.

PHYSICAL FINDINGS & CLINICAL PRESENTATION

- Presence of elevated, erythematous or white circumscribed lesions that change in size and shape over time (Fig. E1) in no specific distribution; they are characterized by extreme pruritus and are evanescent in nature, with individual lesions generally lasting <24 hr in duration and disappearing without scarring. If the patient has persistent symptoms, new lesions typically have a novel distribution.
- Stroking of the skin can lead to urticarial reaction (dermatographism) (Fig. E2).
- Angioedema occurs in approximately 40% of cases of urticaria and is caused by mast cell mediator release in the subcutaneous tissue and deep dermis.
- Although not yet well understood, patients with chronic urticaria may have a range of concurrent systemic symptoms such as fatigue, rhinorrhea, dyspnea, gastritis, joint pain, and hypertension. These patients also tend to have higher rates of depression and anxiety.

ETIOLOGY

Acute urticaria (Table 1):

- Food allergies (e.g., shellfish [Fig. E3], tree nuts, legumes, milk, eggs)
- Medication allergies (e.g., penicillin, aspirin, sulfonamides, hormone therapy)
- Insect sting allergies (e.g., honey bee, Hymenoptera, fire ant)
- Systemic diseases (e.g., systemic lupus erythematosus, serum sickness, autoimmune thyroid disease, cutaneous mastocytosis)
- Infections (viral infections such as hepatitis B and C, fungal infections, chronic bacterial infections, helminthic); viral upper respiratory infections are the predominant cause
- Contact (nonimmunologic) urticaria (e.g., caterpillars, plants)
- Other: Pregnancy, cryoglobulinemia, hair bleaches, chemicals, saliva, cosmetics, perfumes, pemphigoid, emotional stress, malignancy (lymphomas, endocrine tumors)
- Idiopathic urticaria is diagnosed in approximately 50% of patients with acute urticaria

Chronic urticaria:

- Chronic urticaria (CU) is classified as either chronic spontaneous urticaria (CSU) or chronic inducible urticaria (CIndU), depending on whether the skin lesions appear spontaneously or can be induced.
- Physical stimuli (e.g., pressure, cholinergic, solar, cold/heat, aquagenic, or vibration) are found in approximately 20% of patients.
- CSU results from the pathogenic activation of mast cells and basophils, which leads to the release of proinflammatory mediators, such as histamine, leukotrienes, and prostaglandins.
- Up to 50% of CSU patients may have an autoimmune component with contributions from immunoglobulin G [IgG]- and IgE-specific autoantibodies (most commonly to interleukin-24 [IL-24] and FcεR1, with the latter found on the surface of dermal mast cells and basophils). CSU patients also tend to have higher levels of proinflammatory cytokines: IL-17, IL-31, and IL-33. The clinical significance of these antibodies and inflammatory markers is currently being studied and reviewed as potential therapeutic targets.

DIAGNOSIS

DIFFERENTIAL DIAGNOSIS

- Erythema multiforme
- Erythema marginatum
- Erythema infectiosum
- Urticarial vasculitis
- Herpes gestationis
- Drug eruption
- Multiple insect bites
- Bullous pemphigoid
- Mastocytosis
- Mast cell activation syndrome
- Viral exanthema
- Pityriasis rosea
- Atopic dermatitis
- Contact dermatitis
- Henoch-Schönlein purpura

WORKUP

- It is useful to determine whether hives are acute or chronic; a medical history focused on various etiologic factors is necessary before embarking on additional laboratory testing.
- Most cases of acute urticaria resolve spontaneously and diagnostic testing is not required. However, in patients with acute urticaria, it is crucial to consider anaphylaxis before further workup of urticaria because this may require urgent management.
- The etiology of chronic urticaria (CU) is often never determined, and no diagnostic testing may be necessary based on a detailed history and physical examination. Targeted laboratory testing based on clinical findings is appropriate.

LABORATORY TESTS

- If the history is consistent with allergen-induced contact urticaria, skin testing with allergen extracts and screening for dermatographism by attempting to elicit a wheal after application of linear skin pressure should be performed only after withholding antihistamines for 36 to 72 hr to prevent false-negative results.
- CBC with differential, ESR, TSH, and liver function tests should be considered only in patients with a history or physical exam concerning for an underlying systemic condition. Routine testing is not indicated. Even with extensive testing, the cause of chronic urticaria is rarely established.
- Measurement of C4, C1 inhibitor antigenic level and function, and C1q may be helpful in patients who present with angioedema alone. In these patients, C1-inhibitor deficiency should be considered.
- Skin biopsy is helpful in patients with fever, arthralgias, and elevated erythrocyte sedimentation rate. Histologic evidence of leukocytoclasia (neutrophilic infiltration with fragmentation of nuclei) is indicative of urticarial vasculitis.
- When food or contact allergy is suspected in acute urticaria, testing can be performed using skin prick or ImmunoCAP testing.

TREATMENT

NONPHARMACOLOGIC THERAPY

Remove all suspected etiologic agents (e.g., stop aspirin and all nonessential drugs) and avoid any triggers that may have been observed to precipitate an attack.

ACUTE URTICARIA Rx

- Oral antihistamines: Use of second-generation H_1 antihistamines (e.g., cetirizine 10 mg/day, levocetirizine 5 mg/day, loratadine 10 mg/day, fexofenadine 180 mg/day) is preferred over first-generation sedating antihistamines (e.g., hydroxyzine, diphenhydramine). Higher doses of second-generation antihistamines up to 4 times the FDA-approved dose may be required to achieve adequate control of symptoms.
- Leukotriene receptor antagonists (e.g., montelukast) can be added to H_1 antagonists in

TABLE 1 Some Causes of Urticaria*

Infections	Eggs†
Bacterial infections	Cheese
Dental abscess	Inhalants
Sinusitis	Animal danders
Otitis	Pollen
Pneumonitis	Contactants
Gastritis	Wool
Hepatitis	Silk
Cholecystitis	Occupational exposure
Cystitis	Potatoes
Vaginitis	Antibiotics
Fungal infections	Cosmetics
Dermatophytes	Dyes
Candida	Hairspray
Other infections/infestations	Nail polish
Scabies	Mouthwash
Helminth	Toothpaste
Protozoa	Perfumes
Trichomonas	Hand cream
Drugs and Chemicals	Soap
Salicylates	Insect repellent
Indomethacin and other, newer nonsteroidal antiinflammatory agents†	Physical stimuli
Opiates†	Light
Radiocontrast material†	Pressure
Penicillin (medication, milk, blue cheese)	Heat
Sulfonamides	Cold
Sodium benzoate	Water
Douches	Vibration
Ear drops or eye drops	Endocrinopathies
Insulin	Thyroid disease
Menthol (cigarettes, toothpaste, iced tea, hand cream, lozenges, candy)	Diabetes mellitus
Tartrazine (vitamins, birth control pills, antibiotics, FDC yellow #5)	Pregnancy
Foods	Menstruation
Nuts	Menopause
Berries†	Systemic diseases
Fish	Rheumatic fever
Seafood	Connective tissue diseases (lupus erythematosus, Sjögren syndrome, rheumatoid arthritis, Still disease, dermatomyositis, polymyositis, other)
Shellfish†	Leukemia
Bananas	Lymphoma
Grapes	Acquired immunodeficiency disease
Tomatoes	Ovarian tumors

*Partial list of most frequently described causes in each category.
†May be mediated by nonimmunologic mechanisms independent of immunoglobulin E.
From Callen JP et al: *Dermatological signs of systemic disease*, ed 5, Philadelphia, 2017, Elsevier.

refractory cases, although the utility of this has not been consistently shown.
- Oral corticosteroids are not beneficial for acute urticaria[1] and should be reserved for refractory cases and prescribed for a very limited course (e.g., prednisone 20 mg daily or 20 mg twice daily for 5 days).

[1]Palungwachira P et al: A randomized controlled trial of adding intravenous corticosteroids to H1 antihistamines in patients with acute urticaria, *Am J Emerg Med* 19;S0735-6757(20)30098-X, 2020. Epub ahead of print.

CHRONIC URTICARIA Rx

Stepwise approach for management of chronic urticaria is described in Fig. E4.

- Step 1: Monotherapy with second-generation H_1 antihistamines. Avoidance of triggers (e.g., NSAIDs, alcohol, opiates, physical triggers).
- Step 2: Dose advancement of second-generation antihistamine (up to 4× the daily recommended dose). Consider addition of leukotriene receptor antagonist (e.g., montelukast) or first-generation H_1 antihistamine (hydroxyzine or doxepin) to be taken at bedtime.
- Step 3: Referral to allergy specialist for evaluation and management. Add omalizumab (monoclonal anti-IgE antibody that downregulates surface IgE receptors) to antihistamine therapy. Ligelizumab is a newer high-affinity humanized monoclonal anti-IgE antibody that in recent trials has shown a higher percentage of patients with chronic spontaneous urticaria achieving compliance control of symptoms than omalizumab.
- Step 4: If adequate control is not reached by 18 wk, alternative agents should be considered, including antiinflammatory (dapsone, hydroxychloroquine, sulfasalazine, methotrexate) or immunosuppressive agents (cyclosporine A, mycophenolate, tacrolimus, sirolimus).
- Step 5: Consider addition of immunomodulatory biologic agents (tumor necrosis factor-α [TNF-α] inhibitor, IL-1) or alternative therapies such as ultraviolet light therapy, intravenous immunoglobulin, or plasmapheresis.
- Patients should be evaluated at each visit and, if symptoms are well managed, should be considered for step down in treatment.

DISPOSITION

- Most cases of urticaria resolve within 6 wk.
- More than 50% of patients may not achieve satisfactory control of chronic urticaria with antihistamines alone and may require additional therapies. The median duration of CU is between 3 to 5 yr, but it can often be present for much longer durations.

PEARLS & CONSIDERATIONS

COMMENTS

- Topical treatment (e.g., starch baths or oatmeal baths) may be temporarily soothing in selected patients; however, they are not recommended for long-term control of CU.
- If individual urticarial lesions leave residual ecchymoses, pigmentation and/or lesions that typically last >24 hr at a single location, consider skin biopsy to evaluate for urticarial vasculitis.
- Be judicious when prescribing NSAIDs in CU patients, as up to 30% of these patients will experience an exacerbation of urticaria and/or angioedema.

SUGGESTED READINGS

Available at ExpertConsult.com

RELATED CONTENT

Hives (Patient Information)
Chronic Urticaria (Related Key Topic)

AUTHORS: **Quan Phung, MD,** and **Shyam Joshi, MD**

BASIC INFORMATION

DEFINITION

Uterine fibroids, also called leiomyomas or uterine myomas, are benign tumors of muscle cells of the myometrium and connective tissue. The incidence of malignancy is less than 1 in 350 to 1000. They are typically discrete nodular tumors that vary in size and number.

Fibroids are classified by location in the uterus relative to the myometrium.

- Subserosal: Located directly underneath the uterine serosa
- Intramural: Located in the myometrium proper
- Submucosal: Also known as intracavitary as they are located adjacent to the endometrium and protrude into the uterine cavity
- Pedunculated: Located on a pedicle or stalk, either from the serosa or in the cavity

Fibroids can occur singly but are often multiple. They can be located within the cervix, broad ligament, adnexa, and vagina or vulva. Less commonly, fibroids can develop diffusely in the body, such as within the abdomen on peritoneum, lungs, cardiac chambers, or within skin. Parasitic fibroids attach to nearby pelvic structures and acquire a blood supply from a nonuterine source (Fig. 1).

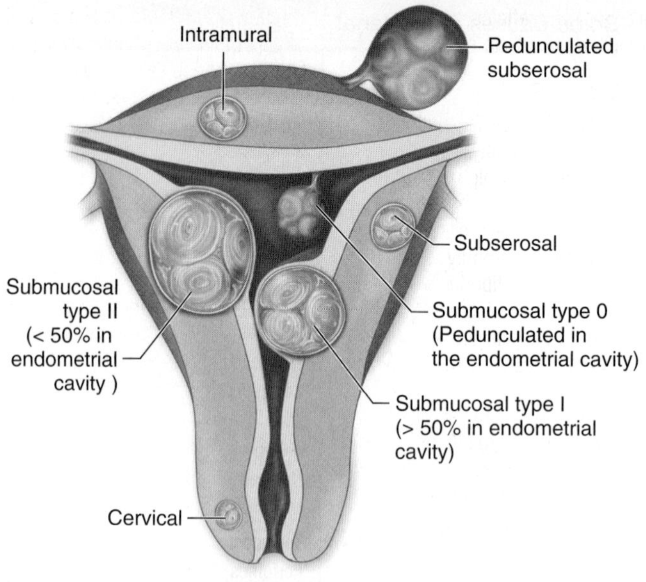

FIG. 1 Drawing of uterus in the coronal plane, illustrating possible location of uterine leiomyomas. (From Fielding JR et al: *Gynecologic imaging,* Philadelphia, 2011, Saunders.)

SYNONYMS

Uterine leiomyomas
Uterine myomas
Fibroids
Leiomyomas

ICD-10CM CODES	
D25.0	Submucous leiomyoma of uterus
D25.1	Intramural leiomyoma of uterus
D25.2	Subserosal leiomyoma of uterus
D25.9	Leiomyoma of uterus, unspecified

EPIDEMIOLOGY & DEMOGRAPHICS

- Estimated cumulative incidence of 70% to 80% in women by age 50.
- The most common benign solid pelvic tumor diagnosed in women and the most common reason for benign hysterectomy.
- Risk factors include age, African American race, early menarche, exposure to DES, obesity, hypertension, PCOS, and no history of pregnancy.
- There is increased familial incidence.
- Approximately 50% of all fibroids are estimated to produce symptoms that impact women including restriction of social, physical, and work activities.
- Frequently diagnosed incidentally on pelvic examination.
- Potential to enlarge during pregnancy as well as regress after menopause.
- Approximately 200,000 hysterectomies, 30,000 myomectomies, and thousands of selective uterine-artery embolizations and high-intensity focused ultrasound procedures are performed annually in the U.S. to remove or destroy uterine fibroids.[1]

PHYSICAL FINDINGS & CLINICAL PRESENTATION

- Enlarged, irregular uterus on pelvic examination
- Uterine fibroids are asymptomatic in up to 50% of affected women
- Presenting symptoms (when present):
  1. Abnormal uterine bleeding (most common)
  2. Chronic pelvic pain (dysmenorrhea, dyspareunia, pelvic pressure)
  3. Bulk symptoms (bloating, increase in abdominal girth)
  4. Anemia
  5. Acute pain (torsion of pedunculated fibroid, infarction, and degeneration)
  6. Urinary symptoms (frequency from bladder pressure, partial ureteral obstruction, complete ureteral obstruction, incontinence in setting of prolapse)
  7. GI symptoms (rectosigmoid compression with constipation or intestinal obstruction, pain with defecation)
  8. Prolapse through cervix of pedunculated submucosal fibroid
  9. Infertility
  10. Pregnancy complications including preterm birth, small fetus for gestational age, malpresentation, and potentially recurrent miscarriage

ETIOLOGY

Not well understood. It is suggested that fibroids arise from an original single smooth muscle cell in the myometrium. Each individual fibroid is monoclonal (all the cells are derived from one progenitor myocyte) and sensitive to estrogen and progesterone hormones, primarily developing during the reproductive years. Malignant degeneration of preexisting leiomyoma is extremely uncommon (<0.5%). There is a racial disparity in the prevalence, suggesting a genetic component, with most fibroids having a normal chromosomal makeup. A small group of women have an autosomal dominant disorder, hereditary leiomyomatosis, and renal cell carcinoma syndrome, in which there is a genetic mutation in the fumarate hydratase gene, causing diminished suppressor function in fibroid formation.

[1]Bulun SE: Uterine fibroids. *N Engl J Med* 369:1344-1355, 2013.

Dx DIAGNOSIS

DIFFERENTIAL DIAGNOSIS

- Ovarian mass (neoplastic, nonneoplastic, endometrioma)
- Adenomyosis
- Endometriosis
- Endometrial polyp
- Endometrial carcinoma
- Leiomyosarcoma/uterine carcinosarcoma
- Inflammatory mass (reproductive organ or GI origin)
- Pregnancy

WORKUP

- Complete pelvic examination, including speculum exam as well as bimanual exam
- Estimation of size of uterus/mass and location of fibroids via imaging
- Endometrial sampling may be indicated (biopsy or dilation and curettage) when abnormal bleeding and pelvic mass are present
- If significant urinary symptoms are prominent, intravenous pyelogram to rule out impingement on urinary system

LABORATORY TESTS

- Pregnancy test
- Complete blood count

- Blood urea nitrogen/creatinine
- Thyroid stimulating hormone

IMAGING STUDIES

- Pelvic ultrasound (Fig. 2) is useful as a primary diagnostic modality. Transvaginal ultrasound commonly has higher diagnostic accuracy.
- MRI scan (Fig. E3) is helpful in planning treatment if malignancy is strongly suspected. Also important to localize fibroids, especially if myomectomy is contemplated. Size, number, and location of fibroids are also important if a minimally invasive myomectomy is considered.
- Diagnostic hysteroscopy can be performed in the office and may provide direct evidence of intrauterine pathology or submucosal leiomyoma that distorts uterine cavity.
- Saline infusion sonography can be helpful in determining location and degree of intrusion into uterine cavity.

Rx TREATMENT

Management (Fig. 4) should be based on primary symptoms and may include observation with close follow-up, medical management, temporizing surgical therapies, embolization, or definitive surgical procedures. Treatment is generally indicated if bleeding is requiring blood transfusions, renal function is affected by size of the enlarged fibroid uterus, or when symptoms are present and are severe enough to be unacceptable to the patient.

NONSURGICAL Rx

- Patient observation and follow-up with periodic repeat pelvic examinations to ensure that tumors are not growing rapidly.

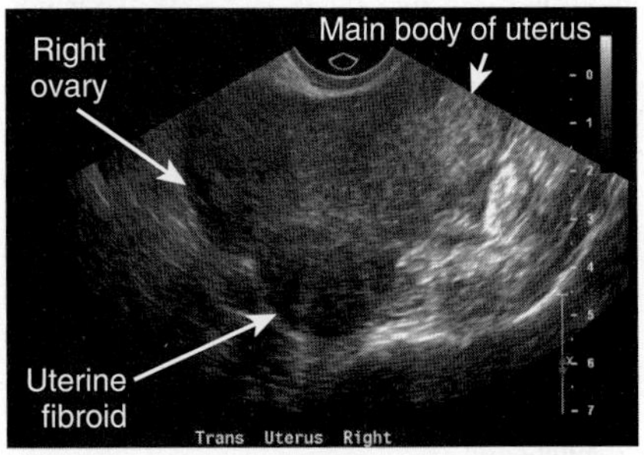

FIG. 2 Fibroid uterus: Endovaginal ultrasound. Ultrasound is the primary modality used for evaluation of uterine fibroids (leiomyomas). Typical features include a well-circumscribed appearance. Fibroids may be hypoechoic or hyperechoic relative to the uterus. They may be exophytic or intramural, or they may project into the uterine cavity. Whereas malignant uterine tumors may invade adjacent structures, a fibroid is contained within the uterine serosa. Uterine tumors, both benign and malignant, can show central necrosis, which usually appears hypoechoic with ultrasound. In this 38-yr-old woman, the fibroid is exophytic. The right ovary lies adjacent and is difficult to distinguish in this case. (From Broder JS: *Diagnostic imaging for the emergency physician,* Philadelphia, 2011, Saunders.)

- Hormonal therapies can reduce bleeding symptoms, and many have the added benefit of contraception. There is no evidence that exogenous estrogen or progestin increases risk of myomas.
  1. Combined hormonal methods with estrogen and progestin, including combined oral contraceptives, contraceptive patch, contraceptive vaginal ring.
  2. Progestin-only agents including oral progestins, intramuscular progestin injection, subcutaneous progestin implant, levonorgestrel intrauterine device (IUD).
  3. Progesterone IUD can be used to treat menorrhagia, but intracavitary fibroids may be a relative contraindication.
  4. Ulipristal acetate, not yet available in the U.S. for treatment of fibroids, is a selective progesterone-receptor modulator (SPRM) that acts on progesterone receptors in myometrial and endometrial tissue and inhibits ovulation without significant effects on estradiol levels or antiglucocorticoid activity.

A combination of gonadotropin-releasing hormone antagonist (Elagolix), estrogen, and norethindrone acetate was approved by the FDA in May 2020 for management of menorrhagia due to fibroids in premenopausal women. Bone mineral density is preserved with relugolix combination therapy with relugolix monotherapy.[2]

- Gonadotropin-releasing hormone (GnRH) agonist use results in 40% to 60% reduction in uterine volume within 3 mo of initiating treatment. Hypoestrogenism, reversible bone loss, and hot flushes are associated with use. Consider low-dose progesterone replacement to minimize hypoestrogenic effects. GnRH agonist therapy is not recommended to be used longer than 6 mo without add-back therapy due to these effects.
  1. Regrowth and return of bleeding symptoms occurs in approximately 50% of women treated within a few months after cessation.
  2. Indications for GnRH agonist:
     a. Anemia treatment to normalize hemoglobin before surgery
     b. Women approaching menopause to avoid surgery
     c. Preoperative for large myomas to make vaginal hysterectomy, hysteroscopic resection/ablation, or laparoscopic destruction more feasible
     d. Women with medical contraindications for surgery
  3. Use of GnRH agonists may alter the consistency of the fibroid, making myomectomy more challenging.
- Nonhormonal medical therapies:
  1. Nonsteroidal antiinflammatory drugs.
  2. Tranexamic acid, an oral antifibrinolytic agent that prevents fibrinolysis of menstrual fluid, can decrease menorrhagia by 40% to 65%. Side effects include abdominal cramps, headaches, fatigue, and increase risk of venous thromboembolism.
- Other drugs used and under investigation:
  1. Danazol: Androgen and multienzyme inhibitor of steroidogenesis
  2. Mifepristone: Antiprogesterone shown to reduce the fibroid volume by 40% to 50% with amenorrhea
  3. Raloxifene: Selective estrogen receptor modulator, either alone or with a GnRH agonist, shown to reduce the fibroid volume 70% up to 1 yr but only in postmenopausal women
  4. Fadrozole: Aromatase inhibitor reported to have produced a 71% reduction in volume that is not yet available in the U.S.
  5. Vilaprisan: Selective progesterone receptor modulator (SPRM) currently in phase 3 trials showing decreasing amenorrhea rates and reduction in fibroid size

SURGICAL Rx

- Indications:
  1. Abnormal uterine bleeding with anemia refractory to hormonal therapy
  2. Chronic pain with severe dysmenorrhea, dyspareunia, or lower abdominal pressure/pain
  3. Acute pain, torsion, or prolapsing submucosal fibroid
  4. Urinary symptoms or signs such as hydronephrosis
  5. Rapid uterine enlargement premenopausal or any growth after menopause
  6. Infertility or recurrent pregnancy loss with submucous leiomyoma as only finding
  7. Enlarged uterus with compression symptoms or discomfort
- Procedures:
  1. Hysterectomy (definitive procedure): Vaginal, laparoscopic, robotic, or abdominal approach, dependent on surgical preference/expertise and uterine size.
  2. Myomectomy (to preserve fertility or due to patient preference): May be performed via abdominal, laparoscopic, or robotic approach.
  3. Vaginal myomectomy for prolapsed pedunculated submucous fibroid.
  4. Hysteroscopic resection: Typically at least 50% of the fibroid must be intracavitary for a hysteroscopic approach to be successful.
  5. Radiofrequency volumetric thermal ablation: FDA-approved uterine-sparing procedure in which laparoscopic or transcervical ultrasound-guided ablation of individual fibroids is performed. This causes myolysis (necrosis of the tissue) resulting in the fibroid shrinking.
  6. Uterine artery embolization (UAE): Safe and effective short-term alternative to surgery, but its less invasive nature should be balanced against a higher rate for treatment failure or complications at 5 yr (32%) versus the surgery group

[2]Al-Hendy A et al: Treatment of Uterine Fibroid Symptoms with Relugolix Combination Therapy, *N Engl J Med* 384:630-642, 2021.

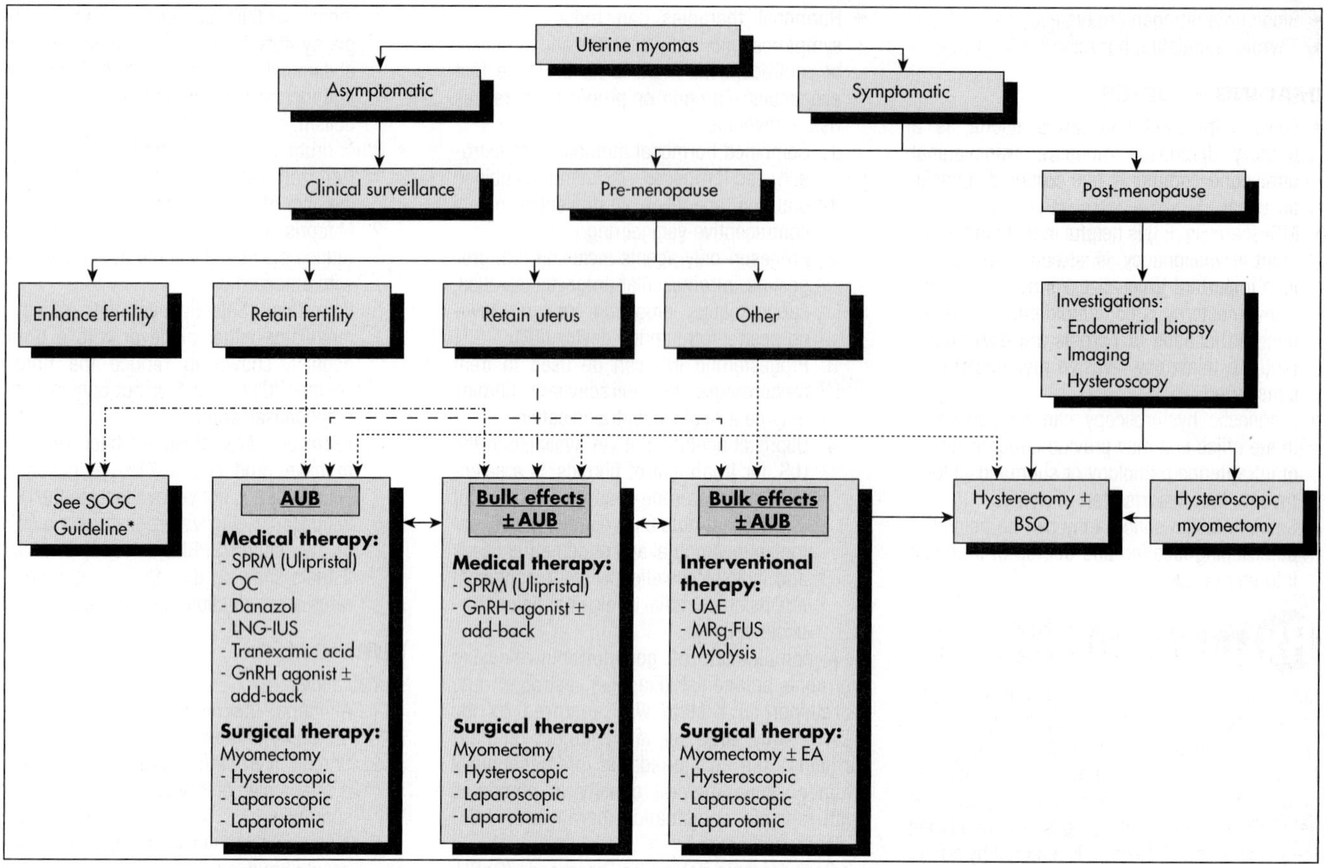

BSO, Bilateral salpingo-oophorectomy; *MRg-FUS*, magnetic resonance-guided focused ultrasound; *OC*, oral contraceptives

FIG. 4 Algorithm for the management of uterine fibroids. *GnRH*, Gonadotropin-releasing hormone; *UAE*, uterine artery embolization. (From Vilos GA et al: The management of uterine leiomyomas. *J Obstet Gynaecol Can* 37(2):163, 2015. Carranza-Mamane B et al; Society of Obstetrics and Gynaecology Canada Reproductive Endocrinology and Infertility Committee: The management of uterine fibroids in women with otherwise unexplained infertility. SOGC Clinical Practice Guidelines. *J Obstet Gynaecol Can* 37(3):277-285, 2015.)

(4%). Age 40 yr and under at embolization and history of previous myomectomy are significant predictors of embolization failure. If the patient wishes to preserve future fertility, UAE should not be performed. A trial comparing uterine-artery embolization and myomectomy among women with symptomatic uterine fibroids revealed that those who underwent myomectomy had a better fibroid-related quality of life at 2 yr than those who underwent uterine-artery embolization.[3]

7. Endometrial ablation: Performed specifically to decrease menorrhagia.
8. MRI-guided focus ultrasound surgery for fibroids is a noninvasive thermoablative procedure that allows high-energy ultrasound waves to converge on a fibroid localized by MRI. Note, there is limited availability of this procedure.

[3]Manyonda I et al: Uterine-Artery Embolization or Myomectomy for Uterine Fibroids, *N Engl J Med* 383:440-451, 2020.

COMPLICATIONS

- Red degeneration occurs when the fibroid outgrows its blood supply leading to hemorrhage in the center of the fibroid. This is typically seen in the second trimester of pregnancy but is a rare occurrence.
- Leiomyosarcoma (<0.1%). Recent concern has been voiced by the U.S. FDA regarding the use of morcellation in minimally invasive surgery because of the possibility of spreading occult malignancy in the peritoneal cavity.

REFERRAL

Consultation with gynecologic oncologist if suspicious of malignancy

SUGGESTED READINGS

Available at ExpertConsult.com

RELATED CONTENT

Uterine Fibroids (Patient Information)
Dysfunctional Uterine Bleeding (Related Key Topic)

AUTHORS: **Shivani Parikh, MD,** and **Nima R. Patel, MD, MS**

BASIC INFORMATION

DEFINITION

Cancers of the uterine corpus include tumors originating from the endometrium (endometrial stromal cancers). The most common type of endometrial cancer is adenocarcinoma, which includes endometrioid, clear cell, mucinous, and papillary serous subtypes (see "Endometrial cancer"). Uterine cancer also includes tumors that result from abnormal proliferation of cells originating from the connective, muscular, vascular, or fibrous tissue elements of the uterine wall (myometrium).

SYNONYMS

Leiomyosarcomas
Endometrial stromal sarcoma
Malignant mixed Müllerian tumors
Adenosarcomas

ICD-10CM CODES

C54.1	Malignant neoplasm of endometrium
C54.2	Malignant neoplasm of the myometrium
C54.0	Malignant neoplasm of isthmus uteri
C54.8	Malignant neoplasm of overlapping sites of corpus uteri

EPIDEMIOLOGY & DEMOGRAPHICS

INCIDENCE: Incidence of uterine cancer (including endometrial) is 27 per 100,000 women per yr, with 5 deaths per 100,000 women as of 2016. Endometrial cancer remains the most common gynecologic malignancy in the U.S. Uterine cancer is one of the few cancers with increasing incidence and mortality in the U.S., reflecting in part increases in the prevalence of obesity since the 1980s. It is the fourth most common cancer diagnosed and the sixth most common cause of cancer death among U.S. women.[1]

PREVALENCE: Uterine sarcoma accounts for approximately 8% of all cancers of the uterine corpus and is associated with poor prognosis.

MEAN AGE AT DIAGNOSIS: 60 yr

RISK FACTORS: Box 1 describes risk factors for uterine sarcoma.

PHYSICAL FINDINGS & CLINICAL PRESENTATION

- Abnormal vaginal bleeding is the most common symptom (90% of women with diagnosis)
- Vaginal discharge also may be a presenting symptom (10% of these patients have nonbloody discharge)
- May also present as pelvic pain or pressure and pelvic mass on examination (10% of women with uterine sarcoma)
- Urinary symptoms
- Abdominal pain or distension
- Weight loss

[1] Henley SJ et al: Uterine cancer incidence and mortality—United States, 1999-2016, *MMWR* 67(48): 1333-1338, 2018.

ETIOLOGY

- The exact etiology is unknown.
- Endometrial cancer is possibly related to the balance between progesterone and estrogen in the body.

DIAGNOSIS

- Endometrial cancer: Endometrial biopsy or dilation and curettage with histologic evidence of malignancy
- Uterine sarcoma: Postsurgical histologic examination of uterine tissue

DIFFERENTIAL DIAGNOSIS

- Endometrial hyperplasia
- Leiomyoma

WORKUP

Diagnosis is made histologically by biopsy for abnormal bleeding. Workup includes biopsy (in the office or operating room, in conjunction with hysteroscopy) and imaging (see below). Histologic criteria include mitotic index, cellular atypia, and coagulative necrosis.

LABORATORY TESTS

- CBC depending on level of bleeding
- CA-125 (high levels can be a sign of metastasis, not diagnostic, not always elevated)

IMAGING STUDIES

- Pelvic ultrasound is a lower-cost method of detecting uterine corpus mass or thickened endometrial lining. Features concerning for uterine sarcoma: Heterogeneous texture, central necrosis, irregular vessel distribution.
- Chest x-ray is usually done as routine preoperative testing.
- Computed tomography (CT) scans (Fig. 1), MRI, and PET are useful for assessing tumor spread once diagnosis is made.

STAGING

Staging of endometrial carcinoma and uterine adenosarcoma is summarized in Tables 1 and 2.

TREATMENT (TABLE 3)

NONPHARMACOLOGIC THERAPY

- Surgical excision is the mainstay of treatment, with or without lymph node mapping and with or without peritoneal lavage or peritoneal biopsies. Degree of removal and exploration depends on grading, staging, and type of cancer.

BOX 1 Risk Factors for Uterine Sarcoma

- Nulliparity
- Obesity
- History of pelvic radiation
- Exposure to tamoxifen

From Fielding JR et al: *Gynecologic imaging,* Philadelphia, 2011, Saunders.

- Endometrial stromal sarcoma: Stage 1 disease is usually followed up by surveillance. Stage 2 or higher can be offered endocrine therapy or radiation therapy.
- Leiomyosarcoma: Usually followed with surveillance. Chemotherapeutic agents can be considered for stage 3 or higher; they have produced only partial and short-term responses

DISPOSITION

- Survival varies with each type of sarcoma but is generally very poor. Box 2 describes uterine prognostic factors.
- Five-yr survival for grade I endometrial stromal sarcoma is 91% and drops to 42% for grade III.

TABLE 1 International Federation of Gynecology and Obstetrics 2009 Staging for Endometrial Carcinoma (Including Carcinosarcoma)

Stage	
I_A	Tumor confined to uterine corpus, <50% myometrial invasion
I_B	Tumor confined to uterine corpus, ≥50% myometrial invasion
II	Tumor invades cervical stroma but confined to uterus
III_A	Tumor invades uterine serosa or adnexa
III_B	Involvement of vagina or parametrium
III_{C1}	Metastasis to pelvic lymph nodes
III_{C2}	Metastasis to paraaortic lymph nodes
IV_A	Invasion of bladder or bowel mucosa
IV_B	Distant metastases including intraabdominal metastasis, inguinal lymph nodes, or both

From Niederhuber JE: *Abeloff's clinical oncology,* ed 6, Philadelphia, 2020, Elsevier.

TABLE 2 International Federation of Gynecology and Obstetrics 2009 Staging for Uterine Adenosarcoma

Stage	
I_A	Tumor limited to endometrium
I_B	Tumor limited to uterus, <50% myometrial invasion
I_C	Tumor limited to uterus, ≥50% myometrial invasion
II_A	Adnexal involvement
II_B	Extrauterine pelvic tissue involvement
III	Involvement of abdominal tissues
III_A	1 site
III_B	>1 site
III_C	Metastases to pelvic, paraaortic lymph nodes, or both
IV_A	Tumor invades bladder or rectum
IV_B	Distant metastases

From Niederhuber JE: *Abeloff's clinical oncology,* ed 6, Philadelphia, 2020, Elsevier.

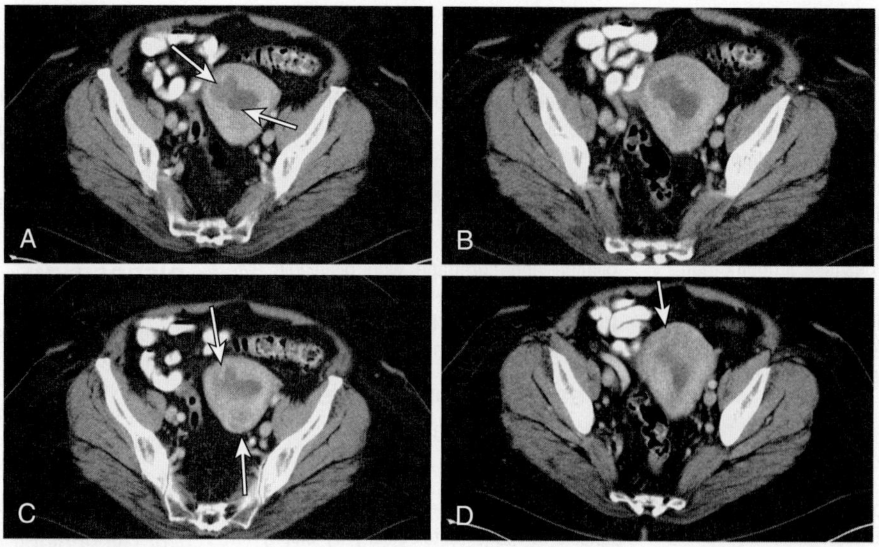

FIG. 1 A 50-yr-old patient with uterine sarcoma. A, Axial contrast-enhanced computed tomographic (CT) image. Low-attenuation lobulated and infiltrating soft tissue fills the endometrial canal *(arrows),* extending into the myometrium. **B,** Axial contrast-enhanced CT image showing same as **A.** Low-attenuation, lobulated, and infiltrating soft tissue fills the endometrial canal, extending into the myometrium. **C,** Axial contrast-enhanced CT image. Low-attenuation lobulated and infiltrating soft tissue fills the endometrial canal. Subtle myometrial invasion is seen anterior and posterior *(arrows).* **D,** Axial contrast-enhanced CT image. Low-attenuation lobulated and infiltrating soft tissue fills the endometrial canal *(arrow),* showing same. Subtle myometrial invasion is seen fundally. (From Fielding JR et al: *Gynecologic imaging,* Philadelphia, 2011, Saunders.)

TABLE 3 National Comprehensive Cancer Network Guidelines for Treatment of Uterine Serous, Clear Cell Endometrial Carcinoma, and Carcinosarcoma

Stage	Adjuvant Treatment
I_A without myometrial invasion	Observe, or chemotherapy, or VBT, or combination therapy
I_A with myometrial invasion, I_B, II	Chemotherapy ± tumor-directed RT, or whole abdominopelvic RT ± VBT
III, IV (adequately debulked)	Chemotherapy ± tumor-directed RT, or whole abdominopelvic RT ± VBT
III, IV (inadequately debulked)	Chemotherapy

RT, Radiation therapy; *VBT,* vaginal brachytherapy.
From Niederhuber JE: *Abeloff's clinical oncology,* ed 6, Philadelphia, 2020, Elsevier.

BOX 2 Uterine Sarcoma Prognostic Factors

- Tumor stage
- Tumor grade
- Tumor size
- Patient age
- Vascular space involvement
- Mitotic count
- Residual disease at surgery
- Adjuvant chemotherapy

From Fielding JR et al: *Gynecologic imaging,* Philadelphia, 2011, Saunders.

BOX 3 Uterine Sarcoma: Key Points

- The disease mainly affects postmenopausal women.
- Most patients present early with postmenopausal bleeding.
- The primary treatment is hysterectomy.
- Adjuvant radiotherapy to the pelvis is used if poor prognosis features in stage 1 or if spread has occurred beyond the corpus.

From Greer IA et al: *Mosby's color atlas and text of obstetrics and gynecology,* London, 2001, Harcourt.

- Five-yr survival for leiomyosarcoma ranges from 76% for stage 1 to 29% for stage 4.
- Five-yr survival for undifferentiated sarcoma ranges from 70% for stage 1 to 23% for stage 4.

REFERRAL

Uterine sarcoma should be managed by a gynecologic oncologist and radiation oncologist. Key points in the management of uterine sarcoma are described in Box 3.

SUGGESTED READINGS

Available at ExpertConsult.com

RELATED CONTENT

Uterine Cancer (Patient Information)
Endometrial Cancer (Related Key Topic)

AUTHORS: **Ashwini U. Dhokte, MD,** and **Rachel Wright Heinle, MD, FACOG**

BASIC INFORMATION

DEFINITION

Prepubescent vulvovaginitis is an inflammatory condition of the vulva and vagina.

SYNONYM

Vulvovaginitis

ICD-10CM CODES
N76.0 Acute vaginitis
N76.1 Subacute and chronic vaginitis

EPIDEMIOLOGY & DEMOGRAPHICS

- Most common gynecologic problem of premenarchal girls.
- Prepubertal girls are susceptible to irritation and trauma because of the absence of protective hair and labial fat pads, as well as a lack of estrogenization leading to atrophic vaginal mucosa.
- Symptoms of vulvovaginitis and introital irritation and discharge account for 80% to 90% of gynecologic visits.
- Nonspecific etiology in approximately 75% of children with vulvovaginitis.
- Majority of vulvovaginitis in girls involves a primary irritation of the vulva with secondary involvement of the lower third of the vagina.

PHYSICAL FINDINGS & CLINICAL PRESENTATION

- Vulvar pain, dysuria, pruritus.
- Discharge is not a primary symptom but can occur.
- If present, vaginal discharge may be foul smelling or bloody.

ETIOLOGY

- Most commonly attributed to poor hygiene or nonspecific irritants. Etiologic factors in premenarcheal vulvovaginitis are summarized in Box 1.
- Hypoestrogenic state increases risk of infection or irritation due to:
    1. Higher vaginal pH (more hospitable to infectious agents)
    2. Underdeveloped labia minora and lack of significant adipose and hair of labia majora (less intrinsic protection of the vagina from trauma, irritants, infectious agents)
- Infections:
    1. Bacterial: Often respiratory or enteric organisms
    2. Protozoal/parasitic
    3. Mycotic
    4. Viral
- Endocrine disorders
- Labial adhesions
- Skin disorders
- Sexual abuse
- Allergic substance
- Trauma
- Foreign body
- Masturbation
- Constipation

DIAGNOSIS

DIFFERENTIAL DIAGNOSIS

- Physiologic leukorrhea
- Foreign body
- Bacterial vaginosis
- Fungal vulvovaginitis
- Precocious puberty
- Sexual abuse and possibly an associated sexually transmitted infection such as gonorrhea, *Chlamydia*, or *Trichomonas*
- Pinworms

WORKUP

- History regarding symptoms, hygiene practices, exposures to known irritants
- Examination, including Tanner staging, pelvic/genital examination; possibly speculum examination
    - May need rectal examination.
    - Knee-chest position for examination may be easier for the child to tolerate. May need to consider exam under anesthesia for more thorough evaluation or for intolerance of exam, if necessary.
- KOH and normal saline preparation of discharge
- Vaginoscopy if considering a foreign body

LABORATORY TESTS

- Urinalysis to rule out urinary tract infection and diabetes
- Cultures including sexually transmitted diseases

TREATMENT

NONPHARMACOLOGIC THERAPY

- Avoid tight clothing
- Appropriate hygiene education
- Avoid chemical irritants
- If foreign body, removal via irrigation or exam under anesthesia
- If vulva is irritated, can use a topical over-the-counter emollient
- Reassurance

ACUTE GENERAL Rx

- *Streptococcal* and *staphylococcal* spp., *Haemophilus influenzae*: For children <20 kg, ampicillin 25 mg/kg q6h or amoxicillin 20 mg/kg q12h for 5 to 10 days; for children >20 kg, ampicillin 500 mg q6h or amoxicillin 20 mg/kg q12h for 5 to 10 days.
- *Escherichia coli*: Azithromycin PO, 10 mg/kg on day 1 and then 5 mg/kg for 4 days.
- *Proteus vulgaris*: TMP-SMX 5 mg/kg q12h for 5 to 10 days.
- *Chlamydia trachomatis*: For children <45 kg, treat with erythromycin base or ethylsuccinate 50 mg/kg/day PO qid ×14 days. For children ≥45 kg but younger than 8 yr, treat with azithromycin 1g PO single dose. If older than 8 yr, also can consider doxycycline 100 mg PO bid for 7 days.
- *Neisseria gonorrhoeae*: For children ≤45 kg, treat with ceftriaxone 25 to 50 mg/kg IV or IM in a single dose, not to exceed 125 mg IM. Children >45 kg should be treated with ceftriaxone 250 mg IM plus azithromycin 1 g PO once.
- *Trichomonas*: Metronidazole 15 mg/kg/day (divided into two doses per day) ×7 days or a single dose of 40 mg/kg.
- Pinworms: Mebendazole 100-mg chewable tablet, repeat in 2 to 3 wk.
- Labial agglutination: Spontaneous resolution or topical estrogen cream for 7 to 10 days. High degree of efficacy with topical estrogen.

CHRONIC Rx

See "Referral."

DISPOSITION

Further education:

- Discuss appropriate hygiene.
- If sexually active, discuss pregnancy prevention and safe sexual practices. Have a high suspicion of sexual abuse and report to child protective services with any concerns for abuse.

REFERRAL

- To obstetrician/gynecologist, preferably a physician with specialized training in pediatric and adolescent gynecology if available
- To pediatrician

SUGGESTED READINGS

Available at ExpertConsult.com

RELATED CONTENT

Chlamydia Genital Infections (Related Key Topic)
Pruritus Vulvae (Related Key Topic)
Vaginitis, Fungal (Related Key Topic)
Vaginitis, *Trichomonas* (Related Key Topic)
Vaginosis, Bacterial (Related Key Topic)

AUTHOR: **Margaret R. Hines, MD**

BOX 1 Etiologic Factors in Premenarcheal Vulvovaginitis

Bacterial Infections
Nonspecific mixed infections secondary to:
Poor perineal hygiene
Foreign body in vagina
Respiratory tract infections
Skin infections (impetigo)
Urinary tract infection
Specific nonvenereal infection:
Hemolytic streptococci (groups A, B, F)
Escherichia coli
Shigella flexneri, Shigella sonnei
Neisseria meningitidis, Neisseria sicca
Haemophilus influenzae type b, *nontypeable strains*
Streptococcus pneumoniae
Corynebacterium diphtheriae
Yersinia enterocolitica
Mycobacterium tuberculosis
Moraxella (Branhamella) catarrhalis
Staphylococcus aureus
Specific venereal infections:
Neisseria gonorrhoeae
Treponema pallidum
Chlamydia trachomatis
Chancroid (*Haemophilus ducreyi*)
Granuloma inguinale
Bacterial vaginosis:
Gardnerella vaginalis
Mobiluncus species

Fungal infections
Candida albicans
Other yeasts
Dermatophytes

Protozoan and parasitic infections
Trichomoniasis
Amebiasis
Enterobius vermicularis
Hirudiniasis
Schistosomiasis
Other parasitic infections (ascariasis, trichuriasis)

Viral infections
Venereal:
- Herpes simplex
- Condyloma acuminatum (papillomavirus)
- Molluscum contagiosum

Involvement as part of systemic infection:
- Measles
- Varicella
- Mononucleosis (Epstein-Barr virus)
- Coxsackievirus
- Smallpox

Infestations
Pediculosis
Scabies

Contact irritation or allergic reactions
Bubble bath preparations
Hair shampoos
Vulvar deodorant sprays
Soaps, laundry detergents
Other medications

Vulvar or perineal skin diseases
Local:
- Seborrhea
- Lichen sclerosus et atrophicus
- Lichen planus
- Lichen simplex chronicus
- Premalignant leukoplakia
- Erythrasma (*Corynebacterium minutissimum*)
- Bartholinitis
- Skenitis

Involvement as part of a systemic disorder:
- Psoriasis
- Bullous pemphigoid
- Atopic dermatitis
- Drug eruption
- Generalized pruritus with excoriation
- Chronic liver disease
- Chronic renal disease
- Metabolic errors
- Psychosomatic
- Crohn disease
- Sjögren syndrome
- Henoch-Schönlein purpura
- Histiocytosis
- Kawasaki disease
- Stevens-Johnson syndrome
- Typhoid
- Zinc deficiency

Physical factors
Sand (sandbox)
Chemical or thermal trauma
Physical trauma (accidents, abuse, masturbation)
Nylon, rayon underclothing
Tight garments (maceration in warm climates)
Anatomic abnormalities:
- Neoplasms (sarcoma botryoides)
- Polyps
- Labial agglutination, adhesion
- Prolapsed urethra
- Ectopic ureter
- Rectal fistula
- Draining pelvic abscess via fistula

From Cherry JD et al: *Feigin and Cherry's textbook of pediatric infectious diseases,* ed 8, Philadelphia, 2019, Elsevier.

BASIC INFORMATION

DEFINITION

Trichomonas vulvovaginitis is the inflammation of vulva and vagina caused by *Trichomonas vaginalis.*

SYNONYMS

Trichomonas vaginalis
Trichomoniasis
TV

ICD-10CM CODE

A59.01 Trichomonal vulvovaginitis

EPIDEMIOLOGY & DEMOGRAPHICS

- Acquired through sexual contact
- Diagnosed in:
  1. 50% to 75% of sex workers
  2. 5% to 15% of women visiting gynecology clinics
  3. 7% to 32% of women in sexually transmitted disease (STD) clinics
  4. 5% of women in family planning clinics
  5. 8% to 13% of black women, 0.8% to 1.8% of non-Hispanic white women
  6. More than 11% of women ≥40 yr old
- Most prevalent nonviral sexually transmitted infection in the U.S.

PHYSICAL FINDINGS & CLINICAL PRESENTATION

These symptoms and physical findings may or may not be present depending on the case:

- Yellow-green, malodorous vaginal discharge
- Vaginal and/or vulvar pruritus
- Dysuria
- Dyspareunia
- Intense erythema of the vaginal mucosa
- Cervical petechiae ("strawberry cervix")
- Infected men may have symptoms of urethritis, epididymitis, or prostatitis
- Asymptomatic in ~50% of women and 90% of men

ETIOLOGY

Single-cell protozoan *Trichomonas vaginalis*

RISK FACTORS

- Multiple sexual partners
- History of previous STDs
- HIV infection

DIAGNOSIS

DIFFERENTIAL DIAGNOSIS (TABLE 1)

- Bacterial vaginosis
- Fungal vulvovaginitis
- Atrophic vulvovaginitis
- Vaginal or cervical infection with other sexually transmitted infections such as gonorrhea or chlamydia

WORKUP

- Pelvic examination
- Speculum examination
- Evaluation for mobile trichomonads seen on normal saline preparation (Fig. E1): 30% to 70% sensitivity; sensitivity decreases if there is a delay in evaluating slides
- Assessment of vaginal pH: Trichomonas is associated with elevated pH (>5) of vaginal discharge
- Laboratory testing (see below)

LABORATORY TESTS

Nucleic acid amplification tests (NAATs) have been developed that combine excellent performance characteristics (sensitivity and specificity >95%) with a more rapid turnaround time compared with culture. Thus, they are now considered better laboratory tests than culture. There are now multiple FDA-approved tests available in the U.S.

- Rapid tests are also available:
  1. The OSOM Trichomonas Rapid test (Sekisui Diagnostics, Framingham, MA) is an antigen detection test on vaginal secretions. It provides results in 10 min and can be done as a point-of-care test. It has a sensitivity of 82% to 95% and a specificity of 97% to 100%.
  2. The Affirm VP III (Becton Dickinson, Sparks, MD) is a DNA hybridization probe test; results are available within 45 min. Sensitivity is 63% and specificity >99%.
- Culture, when available, is considered the traditional gold standard laboratory test for diagnosis of trichomonas, with sensitivity 75% to 96% and specificity approaching 100%.

TREATMENT

NONPHARMACOLOGIC THERAPY

Condom use: The best way to prevent trichomoniasis is through consistent and correct use of condoms during all penile-vaginal sexual encounters

ACUTE GENERAL Rx

- Preferred initial treatment: Metronidazole 2 g PO × 1 *or* tinidazole single 2-g oral dose in both sexes. Treatment of the sexual partner is essential to prevent reinfection.
- Alternative regimen: Metronidazole 500 mg PO bid × 7 days.
- Alcohol consumption should be avoided during treatment with metronidazole (at least 24 hr after completion of therapy) and tinidazole (at least 72 hr after completion of therapy) to reduce possibility of disulfiram-like reaction.
- CDC recommends retesting sexually active women within 3 mo of treatment to assess for possible reinfection.

CHRONIC Rx

- For persistent infections, the CDC recommends first trying metronidazole 500 mg PO bid × 7 days.
- If treatment is still unsuccessful, proceed with metronidazole or tinidazole 2 g PO daily × 7 days.
- Allergy, intolerance, or adverse reactions: Alternatives to metronidazole or tinidazole are not recommended. Patients who are allergic to nitroimidazoles can be managed by desensitization.

TABLE 1 Typical Features of Trichomoniasis and Differentials

	Trichomoniasis	Vulvovaginal Candidiasis	Bacterial Vaginosis
Symptoms			
Vulvar irritation	4+	4+	0-1+
Dysuria	20%	External	0
Odor	0-2+	0	1+-4+
Signs			
Labial erythema	1+-4+	1+-4+	0
Satellite lesions	0	Frequent	0
Discharge			
Consistency	Frothy (25%)	Minimal to curdy	Homogeneous, often frothy
Color	Yellow-green (25%)	White	Gray, white
Adherence to vaginal walls	0	Often	Usually
Whiff test	60%-90%	0	70%-90%
Alkalinity	≥4.7 (70%-90%)	≤4.5	≥4.7 (90%)
Bimanual Examination			
Adnexal tenderness	Occasional	0	0
Vaginal wall tenderness	0-2+	0-2+	0
Wet Mount			
Epithelial cells	Normal	Normal	Clue cells (90%)
PMN/epithelial cell	≥1	Variable	≤1
Bacteria	Rods or coccobacilli	Rods	Coccobacilli and motile rods
Pathogens	Trichomonads (60%)	Yeasts and pseudohyphae (50%)	Nonspecific

PMN, Polymorphonuclear neutrophils.

- Pregnancy:
  1. Associated with adverse outcomes (i.e., premature rupture of membranes, preterm delivery), although it is unclear whether treatment decreases the incidence of these outcomes.
  2. Treat with metronidazole 2 g PO × 1 day; avoid tinidazole as there is little known about tinidazole in pregnancy.

DISPOSITION

- *Trichomonas* infection is considered an STD; therefore, treatment of the sexual partner is necessary.
- *T. vaginalis* infection is associated with two- to threefold increased risk for HIV acquisition.
- *T. vaginalis* infection in pregnancy is associated with premature rupture of membranes, preterm birth, and delivery of low birth weight infants.

REFERRAL

To obstetrician/gynecologist for recurrence and pregnancy

SUGGESTED READINGS

Available at ExpertConsult.com

RELATED CONTENT

Trichomoniasis (Patient Information)
Pruritus Vulvae (Related Key Topic)

AUTHOR: **Margaret R. Hines, MD**

BASIC INFORMATION

DEFINITION

Bacterial vaginosis (BV) is a polymicrobial infection in which anaerobic bacteria overgrow and replace the normal hydrogen peroxide-producing lactobacilli, resulting in thin, gray, and malodorous vaginal discharge.

SYNONYMS

Bacterial vaginosis
BV
Nonspecific vaginitis
Gardnerella vaginalis vaginitis

ICD-10CM CODES	
N76.0	Acute vaginitis
N77.1	Vaginitis, vulvitis and vulvovaginitis in diseases classified elsewhere

EPIDEMIOLOGY & DEMOGRAPHICS

- Most common cause of vaginal discharge in women of reproductive age.
- Most common organisms include *Gardnerella vaginalis*, *Porphyromonas* species, *Mycoplasma hominis, Bacteroides* species, *Peptostreptococcus* species, *Ureaplasma urealyticum, Fusobacterium* species, *Prevotella* species, and *Atopobium vaginae*, and other facultative anaerobes.
- Women with BV are at increased risk for acquiring other sexually transmitted diseases (STDs) such as HIV, *N. gonorrhoeae, C. trachomatis,* and HSV-2. BV may contribute to persistent HPV infection. Also associated with pelvic inflammatory disease (PID) and complications after gynecologic surgery. Preoperative evaluation and treatment before planned hysterectomy or abortion decreases the infection complication rate.
- May be associated with low birth weight, premature rupture of membranes (PROM), and prematurity.
- BV may recur in 30% within the first 3 mo after treatment, which may be due to:
  1. Persistence of pathogenic bacteria
  2. Reinfection from exogenous sources including sexual partners
  3. Failure of the normal lactobacillus-dominant flora to reestablish
- Risk factors: Multiple female or male sexual partners, sexually transmitted infections, douching, tobacco use, lack of condom use, and lack of vaginal lactobacilli.

PHYSICAL FINDINGS & CLINICAL PRESENTATION

- 50% to 75% of patients are asymptomatic.
- A thin, dull, and gray homogeneous discharge (Fig. E1)
- Characterized by a "fishy" odor from the vagina
- Vaginal pH >4.5
- BV alone does not typically cause dysuria or dyspareunia, and presence may suggest concomitant infection with another pathogen
- Clue cells on microscopic examination (Fig. E2)

ETIOLOGY

- *Gardnerella vaginalis* detected in 40% to 50% of vaginal secretions.
- Increase in vaginal pH secondary to decrease in hydrogen peroxide producing lactobacilli allows predominance of anaerobes that produce amines.
- It is unclear how the vaginal floral imbalance occurs and the role sexual activity plays in the pathogenesis of BV.
- *G. vaginalis* may be important in epithelial biofilm formation.
- Ethnicity and age may contribute to the vaginal microbial environment.

DIAGNOSIS

WORKUP

At least three of the Amsel clinical diagnostic criteria must be present for diagnosis:

- Sensitivity of 92% and specificity of 77%:
  1. Thin, gray, and homogeneous, malodorous discharge that adheres to the vaginal walls.
  2. Vaginal pH >4.5.
  3. Positive whiff-amine test:
     a. Conducted by placing wet mount specimen and adding 10% potassium hydroxide, which creates a fishy odor.
  4. More than 20% of the epithelial cells are clue cells on microscopy.
- Gram staining: Considered the gold-standard laboratory method to determine the concentration of lactobacilli and gram-negative and gram-positive bacteria.
- If microscopy is unavailable, other diagnostic tests include Affirm VPIII (Becton Dickinson, Sparks, MD), which is a DNA-hybridization probe test for high concentrations of *G. vaginalis*, and the OSOM BV Blue test (Sekisui Diagnostics, Framingham, MA), which detects vaginal fluid sialidase activity. A molecular test for the vaginal microbiome for BV, candidiasis, and trichomonas (BD MAX Vaginal Panel) has also shown promising results in early studies.
- Cultures are unnecessary.
- Pap smear is not a reliable test for BV.
- Rule out other causes such as vulvar diseases, STDs, and atrophic vaginitis.

TREATMENT

ACUTE GENERAL Rx

- Recommended regimens (similar efficacy):
  1. Metronidazole 500 mg PO bid for 7 days *or*
  2. Metronidazole 0.75% gel, one full applicator (5 gm) intravaginally daily for 5 days *or*
  3. Clindamycin 2% cream, one full applicator (5 gm) intravaginally at bedtime for 7 days
- Alternate regimens:
  1. Clindamycin 300 mg PO bid for 7 days or clindamycin 100 mg ovules intravaginally once at bedtime for 3 days. May be associated with antimicrobial resistance.
  2. Tinidazole 1g PO once daily for 5 days. Longer half-life than metronidazole (~12-14 hr vs. ~6-7 hr)
  3. Secnidazole 2g PO once. Longer half-life than metronidazole (~17 hr vs. ~8 hr). Shown to be superior to placebo in phase 3 trial and at least as effective as metronidazole 500 mg PO bid in noninferiority trial. Single 1-g oral dose appears to be effective also. Single dose improves compliance, but more expensive than multidose metronidazole therapy.
- Disulfiram-type reactions may occur while taking oral or topical metronidazole and patients should be advised to avoid alcohol while undergoing treatment.
- Sexual partners: It is not necessary to treat male partners of affected females; however, females who partner with females need to be aware of the signs and symptoms of BV, and treatment is indicated in this population if symptoms occur.
- Follow-up visits after treatment and resolution of symptoms are unnecessary, but patients are advised to return if symptoms recur.
- Not enough evidence for or against probiotic use for treatment and prevention.
- Clindamycin cream may weaken latex condoms if used together. Avoid treatment of asymptomatic patients.
- Treatment in pregnancy:
  1. Symptomatic pregnant patients with BV should be treated to relieve bothersome symptoms.
  2. Insufficient evidence to recommend routine screening for BV in asymptomatic pregnant women at high or low risk of preterm delivery.
  3. Can use oral or topical therapy for symptomatic pregnant women with same regimen as nonpregnant women.
  4. There is no evidence that metronidazole or clindamycin have any teratogenic effect during pregnancy. Tinidazole should be avoided in pregnancy.
- Recurrent BV:
  1. Condom use may help reduce the risk of recurrence.
  2. Chronic suppressive therapy has been proven to reduce the development or recurrence of BV.

PEARLS & CONSIDERATIONS

- BV is the most common cause of vaginitis in reproductive women.
- BV has been associated with PID, postprocedural gynecologic complications, and other STDs. It is reasonable to treat asymptomatic women who are to undergo gynecologic surgery and screen for other STDs.
- ACOG, USPSTF, and CDC all agree to not routinely screen and treat all pregnant women with asymptomatic BV to prevent preterm birth.

SUGGESTED READINGS

Available at ExpertConsult.com

RELATED CONTENT

Bacterial Vaginal Infections (Patient Information)

AUTHOR: **Emily Saks, MD, MSCE**

Vancomycin-Resistant *Enterococcus* (VRE)

BASIC INFORMATION

DEFINITION

Enterococci are gram-positive, facultative anaerobic organisms usually oval in shape and can be seen as single cells, pairs, or chains. Vancomycin-resistant *Enterococcus* (VRE) are enterococci that have become resistant to vancomycin and several antibiotics normally used to treat enterococcal infections.

SYNONYM

VRE

ICD-10CM CODE
Z16.39 Resistance to other specified antimicrobial drug

EPIDEMIOLOGY & DEMOGRAPHICS

INCIDENCE:
- VRE may be associated with the use or overuse of specific classes of antibiotics.
- VRE can spread within hospital units, causing widespread colonization or clinical outbreaks, and is generally considered hospital acquired or nursing home acquired

PEAK INCIDENCE: VRE was first reported in Europe in 1986, and there has been a steady rise in the incidence of enterococcal strains resistant to vancomycin. In 2007, 80% of *E. faecium* isolates and 7% of *E. faecalis* isolates were resistant to vancomycin.

OUTCOMES: VRE infections are associated with adverse outcomes, with mortality rates significantly higher in patients with VRE infections versus vancomycin-susceptible enterococcal infections

RISK FACTORS:
- Prior antimicrobial therapy, especially vancomycin
- Prolonged hospitalization
- Chronic medical conditions, renal failure
- Invasive devices
- ICU stay
- Colonization: VRE colonize the gastrointestinal tract; can be found on skin or perirectal swab culture or stool culture

PHYSICAL FINDINGS & CLINICAL PRESENTATION

Patients may be asymptomatic and have gastrointestinal colonization; it can be associated with diarrhea. In hospitalized patients, infection is associated with colonization and can cause wound infections, bacteremia, abscesses (intraabdominal), and, rarely, pneumonia, urinary tract infections, and endocarditis.

ETIOLOGY

- The Clinical and Laboratory Standards Institute uses the following MIC definitions for vancomycin susceptibility and resistance in enterococci:
  1. Vancomycin susceptible: ≤4 mcg/ml
  2. Vancomycin resistant: ≥32 mcg/ml
  3. Vancomycin intermediate: 8 to 16 mcg/ml (vancomycin not recommended)
- Enterococci are primarily found in the human digestive tract and female genital tract, where they make up a significant portion of the normal bacterial population in healthy people. Enterococci can cause urinary tract, wound, bloodstream, heart valve, and brain infections. In the great majority of cases, VRE infections occur in hospitalized patients who have compromised immune systems. Most cases of VRE are caused by the *E. faecium* strains that have acquired resistance when they came in contact with other bacteria and shared genetic information.
- VRE is most commonly transmitted from one patient to another by health care workers whose hands have become contaminated inadvertently with feces or fluids of a person carrying the organism. VRE are not airborne but can survive on surfaces for several weeks.

DIAGNOSIS

DIFFERENTIAL DIAGNOSIS

- Other bacterial pathogens in blood, wounds, or urine.
- Once colonized, increased incidence to become infected

LABORATORY TESTS

- VRE rectal swab culture
- VRE stool culture
- Blood, urine, and wound cultures

TREATMENT

- For rectal or stool colonization, therapy is not recommended.
- Therapy is complicated by the fact that strains exhibit inherent resistance to many commonly used antibiotics.
- More than 80% of vancomycin-resistant *E. faecium* strains are also resistant to ampicillin.
- In symptomatic patients, if VRE strains are known to be susceptible, potential therapeutic agents include:
  1. Linezolid: 600 mg IV or PO q12h
  2. Daptomycin: 4 mg/kg/day IV for nonbacteremia infections and 6 mg/kg/day IV for bacteremias
  3. Tigecycline: 100 mg IV load dose, then 50 mg IV q12h. Although not specifically FDA approved for VRE strains, it offers an option for patients intolerant to other agents
  4. Quinupristin-dalfopristin (Synercid) only effective for *E. faecium* strains with no activity for *E. faecalis* strains: 7.5 mg/kg q8 to 12h. Can cause severe myalgias and arthralgias and venous irritation that often requires use of a central line, which has limited the use of this antibiotic
  5. Salvage regimens for severe VRE infections include:
     a. Daptomycin plus gentamicin and/or ampicillin or ceftaroline
     b. Daptomycin plus tigecycline
  6. The Healthcare Infection Control Practices Advisory Committee recommends that between one and three negative stool/rectal cultures be obtained at weekly intervals to remove a patient from contact precautions.

REFERRAL

To infectious disease specialist

PEARLS & CONSIDERATIONS

COMMENTS

- Patients who are colonized with VRE have about an 8% rate of developing a true VRE infection in hospital or after discharge. The rate is higher in immunocompromised and severely ill patients.
- Incidence increases with comorbidity and hospitalization.
- The number of patients already colonized with VRE in a defined geographic area (colonization pressure) is the most significant factor for predicting new acquisition of VRE.
- An association between VRE colonization and *Clostridium difficile* infection has been reported in patients with hematologic malignancies.

PREVENTION

- Hand hygiene: Most important and practical method of preventing spread in hospital environment. Soap and water (used as a 30-sec wash) and alcohol-based hand rubs are effective, as is chlorhexidine.
- Cohorting and isolation (contact precautions) techniques: Use of private rooms and use of gowns and gloves has been shown to decrease the risk of spread of multidrug-resistant bacteria. In 2018 the Society of Healthcare Epidemiology of America (SHEA) published guidelines that suggested isolation could be discontinued after between one and three negative stool swabs except for immunocompromised patients, patients in burn units, or patients in units with high VRE colonization rates.
- Cleaning contaminated objects or surfaces with standard hospital disinfectants, antibiotic management (prudent vancomycin use and antibiotic stewardship), and surveillance also help prevent spread.

SUGGESTED READINGS

Available at ExpertConsult.com

RELATED CONTENT

Health Care-Related Infections (Related Key Topic)

AUTHOR: **Glenn G. Fort, MD, MPH**

BASIC INFORMATION

DEFINITION

Vasculitis refers generically to inflammation occurring within the walls of blood vessels. Blood vessel inflammation can result in either perforation of affected vessels with hemorrhage into adjacent structures or thrombosis with subsequent ischemia and infarction of supplied tissues. Vasculitis can occur as a primary process or secondary to another connective tissue disease, infection, or drug exposure. The systemic vasculitides are a heterogeneous group of disorders (Table 1) characterized by blood vessel inflammation affecting vessels of varying size and location resulting in a wide range of clinical manifestations dictated largely by which vessels are affected (Fig. 1 and Fig. E2). Vasculitis is traditionally classified according to the size of the blood vessels predominantly affected (Table 2). Antineutrophilic cytoplasmic autoantibody (ANCA)–associated vasculitis (AAV) includes granulomatosis with polyangiitis (GPA); microscopic polyangiitis (MPA), including renal-limited vasculitis (RLV); and eosinophilic granulomatosis with polyangiitis (EGPA). All are associated with ANCA and have similar features on renal histology (e.g., a focal necrotizing, and often crescentic, pauciimmune glomerulonephritis). Several of these are covered in individual topics, including topics on ANCA-associated vasculitis, giant cell arteritis (GCA), Takayasu arteritis, and Henoch-Schönlein purpura (HSP). Severity varies between and within specific vasculitides from a relatively benign, self-limited process to severe, life-threatening multisystem organ involvement with significant morbidity and mortality.

ICD-10CM CODES

M30.0	Polyarteritis nodosa
M30.3	Mucocutaneous lymph node syndrome [Kawasaki]
M31.30 31	Wegener granulomatosis without renal involvement
M31.5	Giant cell arteritis with polymyalgia rheumatica
M31.6	Other giant cell arteritis
M31.4	Aortic arch syndrome [Takayasu]
D 69.0	Allergic purpura
L95.9	Vasculitis limited to the skin, unspecified

EPIDEMIOLOGY & DEMOGRAPHICS

- The epidemiology and demographics of the various vasculitides vary by the individual disease and, where applicable, are covered under the relevant vasculitis disease chapters.
- The most common form of systemic vasculitis in the U.S. is giant cell arteritis, with an approximate incidence of 170 cases per 1 million per yr in individuals older than 50 yr.
- ANCA-associated vasculitis is significantly less common with aggregate incidence

TABLE 1 Comparing the Vasculitides

Disease	Pathophysiology	Classic Features	Testing	Treatment
Giant cell arteritis	Mononuclear cell infiltration and giant cell formation	Headache, scalp tenderness, visual disturbance	ESR, CRP biopsy	Prednisone and aspirin, may need tocilizumab or sarilumab
Takayasu arteritis	Mononuclear cell infiltration and giant cell formation	Visual disturbance, chest pain, abdominal pain, differences in extremity blood pressure and pulses	Angiography	Prednisone Surgical or angiographic intervention
Polyarteritis nodosa	Polymorphonuclear infiltration	Fever, hypertension, myalgias, abdominal pain, hematuria, CHF, GI bleeding, orchitis	ESR, CRP biopsy Angiography	Prednisone (mild disease) plus cyclophosphamide (moderate-severe disease) Antiviral therapy if concurrent hepatitis B or C Azathioprine or methotrexate for maintenance of remission
Kawasaki disease	Polymorphonuclear infiltration	5-day fever, conjunctivitis, oral lesions, rash, red palms and soles, edema, cervical lymphadenopathy	ESR, CRP leukocytosis Thrombocytosis Echocardiography	Aspirin plus IV gamma globulin
Granulomatosis with polyangiitis (Wegener granulomatosis)	Granuloma formation secondary to aggregating neutrophils	Upper and lower respiratory symptoms, renal insufficiency, skin lesions, visual disturbance	ESR, CRP c-ANCA/PR3	Prednisone and methotrexate (mild disease) Cyclophosphamide or rituximab plus prednisone (moderate to severe disease)
Eosinophilic granulomatosis with polyangiitis (Churg-Strauss syndrome)	Eosinophilic infiltration Allergic granulomas	Allergic rhinitis, nasal polyps, asthma	Leukocytosis Eosinophilia ESR, CRP biopsy	Prednisone with or without cyclophosphamide, mepolizumab
Henoch-Schönlein purpura	IgA complex deposition	Palpable purpura, arthralgias, GI disturbances, glomerulonephritis	Leukocytosis Eosinophilia Ig A elevation, skin biopsy	Usually self-limited NSAIDs Prednisone if necessary Rituximab (refractory cases)
Cryoglobulinemic vasculitis	Cold precipitable monoclonal or polyclonal immunoglobulins	Palpable purpura, glomerulonephritis, myalgias, weakness, peripheral neuropathy	Low complement levels, hepatitis C Renal biopsy	Rituximab with or without prednisone Peg interferon plus ribavirin (HCV infection)
Cutaneous leukocytoclastic vasculitis	Neutrophilic infiltration Mononuclear and eosinophilic infiltration	Palpable purpura, macules, vesicles, bullae, urticaria	Skin biopsy	Prednisone Colchicine Dapsone
Behçet syndrome	Polymorphonuclear infiltration	Recurrent oral aphthous ulcers, genital ulcers, skin lesions, visual disturbance	ESR, CRP leukocytosis Oral mucosa autoantibodies	Topical corticosteroids Prednisone with azathioprine (end-organ disease) Colchicine (aphthous ulcer and arthritis) Apremilast Infliximab (refractory disease)

c-ANCA, Cytoplasmic antineutrophil cytoplasmic antibody; *CHF,* congestive heart failure; *CRP,* C-reactive protein; *ESR,* erythrocyte sedimentation rate; *GI,* gastrointestinal; *IgA,* immunoglobulin A; *IV,* intravenous.
From Adams JG et al: *Emergency medicine, clinical essentials,* ed 2, Philadelphia, 2013, Elsevier.

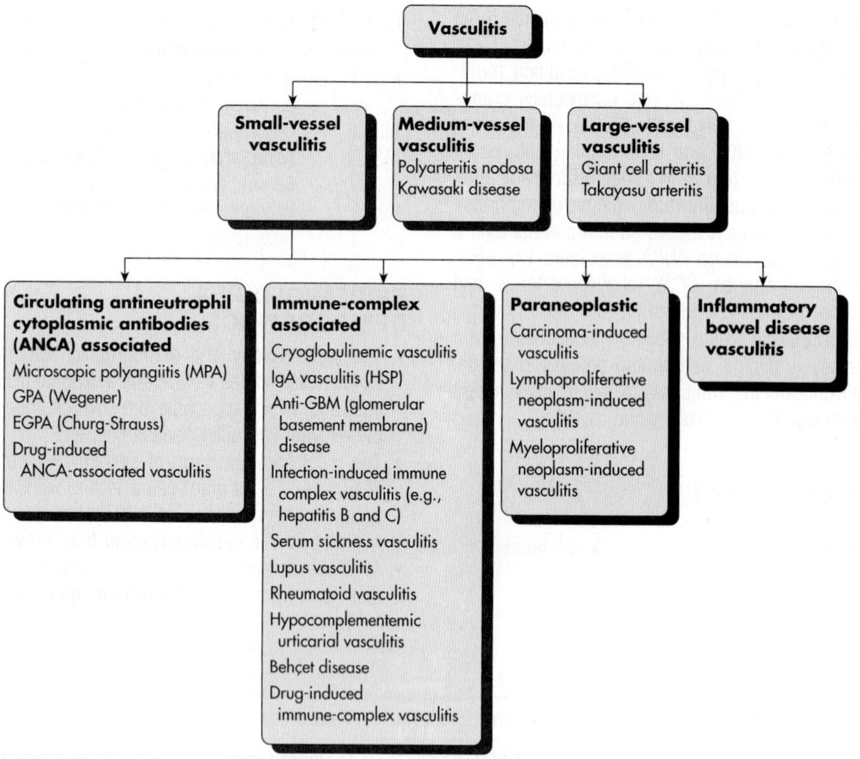

FIG. 1 Major categories of noninfectious vasculitis. Not included are vasculitides that are known to be caused by direct invasion of vessel walls by infectious pathogens, such as rickettsial vasculitis and neisserial vasculitis. *EGPA,* Eosinophilic granulomatous polyangiitis; *GPA,* granulomatous polyangiitis; *HSP,* Henoch-Schönlein purpura. (From Freehally J et al: *Comprehensive clinical nephrology,* ed 6, Philadelphia, 2019, Saunders.)

estimated at approximately 20 per million in the U.S.

- Polyarteritis nodosa (PAN) has an annual incidence of 1 per 100,000 persons but has a higher incidence in patients with existing hepatitis B or C infections.
- Age distribution can demonstrate significant variability between the vasculitides as shown by the fact that GCA generally does not occur before age 50, while 90% of cases of HSP occur in the pediatric population, and 80% of patients with Kawasaki disease are under age 5.
- Although genetic factors clearly play a role in disease susceptibility, familial cases of vasculitis are rare.

PHYSICAL FINDINGS & CLINICAL PRESENTATION

- Clinical presentation often includes nonspecific constitutional symptoms including fever, malaise, headache, and weight loss.
- Signs and symptoms are generally dictated by the tropism of involved vessels.
- Skin manifestations of vasculitis include petechiae, palpable purpura (Fig. E3), subcutaneous nodules, livedo reticularis, ulcerations, and digital ischemia.
- Kidney involvement of medium-sized and large vessel vasculitis is often in the form of renovascular hypertension. Glomerulonephritis may be seen in small vessel vasculitis.
- Pulmonary small vessel involvement can cause alveolar hemorrhage, which can present with cough, dyspnea, and alveolar hemorrhage.
- Mononeuritis multiplex is the characteristic finding of vasculitis affecting the vasa nervorum of the peripheral nervous system.
- Gastrointestinal involvement of the mesenteric vasculature can cause postprandial pain, bleeding, and perforation.
- Testicular pain or tenderness can be seen with hepatitis B infection in PAN.
- Cardiac involvement can include chest pain secondary to ischemic infarcts in the coronary arteries, pericarditis, cardiomyopathy, and arrhythmias.
- Arthritis, while nonspecific, can be present.
- Significant clinical variability exists between the various vasculitides, although overlapping symptoms may be seen.

ETIOLOGY

Most forms of systemic vasculitis are of unknown etiology. Cryoglobulinemia vasculitis is often secondary to hepatitis C infection, and cutaneous leukocytoclastic vasculitis is often related to a drug exposure.

Dx DIAGNOSIS

DIFFERENTIAL DIAGNOSIS

- Infective endocarditis
- Atrial myxoma
- Cholesterol emboli
- Malignancy
- Hypercoagulopathy
- Congenital collagen vascular disorder

WORKUP

- The diagnosis of most forms of systemic vasculitis relies on the history and physical examination as well as supportive laboratory testing. Table 3 describes differential diagnostic features of selected forms of small vessel vasculitis.
- Tissue biopsy is important in establishing an accurate diagnosis; biopsy sites should target affected tissues.
- Electromyography and nerve conduction studies can evaluate for site of nerve or muscle involvement for biopsy in patients with neuropathy or myopathy.
- Imaging such as mesenteric angiography can be supportive and may obviate the need for tissue biopsy.

LABORATORY TESTS

- Laboratory markers of systemic inflammation include elevated erythrocyte sedimentation rate (ESR), C-reactive protein (CRP), and anemia of chronic disease.
- ANCA targeting myeloperoxidase (MPO) and proteinase 3 (PR3) are frequently found in several small vessel vasculitides, including GPA (Wegener), microscopic polyangiitis (MPA), and EGPA (Churg-Strauss).
- Hepatitis C antibodies and rheumatoid factor are often present in cryoglobulinemic vasculitis.
- Positive hepatitis B serologies are commonly found in PAN.
- Urinalysis in patients with glomerulonephritis due to small vessel ANCA-associated vasculitis will generally demonstrate hematuria with active urinary sediment, with red blood cell casts and proteinuria.

IMAGING STUDIES

- Computed tomographic angiography, magnetic resonance angiography, and angiography can demonstrate vascular narrowing and aneurysm formation in suspected medium-size and large-vessel vasculitis.
- Pulmonary and sinus computed tomography scans can demonstrate active pulmonary and upper airway disease in ANCA-associated vasculitis.

Rx TREATMENT

Treatment of vasculitis depends on the specific type of vasculitis and is tailored to the severity of disease activity. Novel treatments are covered under the relevant vasculitis disease chapters.

ACUTE GENERAL Rx

- Systemic corticosteroids are generally required to gain initial control of active vasculitis, although mild cases of drug-induced cutaneous leukocytoclastic vasculitis often require cessation of the offending medication and at times, low-dose corticosteroid use.
- HSP and vasculitis limited to the skin, including cutaneous PAN, can often be managed without further immunosuppression.
- Major organ-threatening disease in systemic vasculitis has traditionally required pulse steroids and oral or intravenous cyclophosphamide for induction of remission.

TABLE 2 Classification Scheme of Vasculitides According to Size of Predominant Blood Vessels Involved

- Primary vasculitides
- Predominantly large vessel vasculitides
- Takayasu arteritis
- Giant cell arteritis (temporal arteritis)
- Cogan syndrome
- Behçet disease*
- Predominantly medium-sized vessel vasculitides
- Polyarteritis nodosa
- Cutaneous polyarteritis nodosa
- Buerger disease
- Kawasaki disease
- Primary angiitis of the central nervous system
- Predominantly small vessel vasculitides
- Immune complex mediated
- Goodpasture disease (anti–glomerular basement membrane disease)†
  1. Cutaneous leukocytoclastic angiitis ("hypersensitivity vasculitis")
  2. Henoch-Schönlein purpura
  3. Hypocomplementemic urticarial vasculitis
  4. Essential cryoglobulinemia‡
  5. Erythema elevatum diutinum
- ANCA-associated disorders§
  1. Granulomatosis with polyangiitis (GPA, Wegener granulomatosis)‡
  2. Microscopic polyangiitis (MPA)‡
  3. Eosinophilic granulomatosis with polyangiitis (EGPA, Churg-Strauss syndrome)‡
  4. Renal-limited vasculitis (RLV)
- Secondary forms of vasculitis
- Miscellaneous small vessel vasculitides
- Connective tissue disorders‡ (rheumatoid vasculitis, lupus erythematosus, Sjögren syndrome, inflammatory myopathy)
- Inflammatory bowel disease
- Paraneoplastic
- Infection
- Drug-induced vasculitis: ANCA-associated, other

ANCA, Antineutrophil cytoplasmic antibody.
*May involve small, medium-sized, and large blood vessels.
†Immune complexes formed in situ, in contrast to other forms of immune complex–mediated vasculitis.
‡Frequent overlap of small and medium-sized blood vessel involvement.
§Not all forms of these disorders are always associated with ANCA.
From Firestein G et al: *Kelley's textbook of rheumatology,* ed 8, Philadelphia, 2008, Saunders.

- Studies have demonstrated noninferiority of rituximab compared to cyclophosphamide in ANCA-associated vasculitis with major organ involvement, and it is approved for this use.
- Rituximab with prednisone has also been shown to be effective in the treatment of relapsing flares of disease activity in ANCA-associated vasculitis.
- Less severe disease such as granulomatosis with polyangiitis limited to the upper airways can be managed with methotrexate rather than cyclophosphamide.
- Trimethoprim/sulfamethoxazole should be used to prevent *Pneumocystis carinii* infection with concurrent immunosuppressive therapy.
- The goal of acute therapy is to induce remission of disease activity and is generally continued for 1 to 2 mo once this is achieved, at which point chronic therapy is used.

CHRONIC Rx

- The goal of chronic therapy is to prevent disease relapse and minimize medication side effects.
- Steroids are gradually tapered as allowed by disease activity.
- Immunomodulatory agents such as methotrexate or azathioprine are commonly used for maintenance therapy in place of cyclophosphamide to reduce side effects.
- Cryoglobulinemic vasculitis due to chronic hepatitis C will often improve with treatment of the underlying viral infection.
- In PAN with concurrent hepatitis B infection, appropriate antiviral treatment (interferon alpha-2b or lamivudine with or without plasma exchange) is indicated.
- Rituximab may also be an appropriate remission maintenance agent in ANCA-associated vasculitis. For GPA or MPA, scheduled redosing of rituximab every 4 to 6 mo is conditionally recommended over redosing based on ANCA titers or CD19 B-cell counts.

DISPOSITION

Varies widely among the various vasculitides

REFERRAL

Systemic vasculitis care is generally coordinated by a rheumatologist. Renal, pulmonary, neurology, and gastrointestinal consultations are often needed when vasculitis involves these organ systems. Isolated cutaneous leukocytoclastic vasculitis is often managed by dermatology.

SUGGESTED READINGS

Available at ExpertConsult.com

RELATED CONTENT

Cogan Syndrome (Related Key Topic)
Cryoglobulinemia (Related Key Topic)
Giant Cell Arteritis (Related Key Topic)
ANCA-Associated Vasculitis (Related Key Topic)
IgA Vasculitis (Related Key Topic)
Kawasaki Disease (Related Key Topic)
Takayasu Arteritis (Related Key Topic)

AUTHORS: **Nicole B. Yang, MD, Anthony M. Reginato, PhD, MD, Sarah Aziz, DO,** and **Syeda M. Sayeed, MD**

TABLE 3 Differential Diagnostic Features of Selected Forms of Small Vessel Vasculitis

Features	Microscopic Polyangiitis (MPA)	Granulomatosis with Polyangiitis (GPA)	Eosinophilic Granulomatosis with Polyangiitis	Henoch-Schönlein Purpura (HSP)	Cryoglobulinemic Vasculitis
Vasculitic signs and symptoms	+	+	+	+	+
ImmunoglobulinA-dominant immune deposits	–	–	–	+	–
Cryoglobulins in blood and vessels	–	–	–	–	+
Antineutrophil cytoplasmic antibodies in blood	+	+	+	–	–
Necrotizing granulomas	–	+	+	–	–
Asthma and eosinophils	–	–	+	–	–

From Freehally J et al: *Comprehensive clinical nephrology,* ed 6, Philadelphia, 2019, Saunders.

Venous Insufficiency, Chronic

BASIC INFORMATION

DEFINITION

The spectrum of chronic venous disease (CVD) ranges from varicose veins to leg edema and skin manifestations consisting of hyperpigmentation, eczema, lipodermatosclerosis, and venous ulcer. These latter venous-specific skin changes constitute an advanced form of CVD known as chronic venous insufficiency (CVI).

SYNONYMS

Stasis dermatitis
Postthrombotic syndrome (PTS)
Chronic venous disease

ICD-10CM CODES

I87.2	Venous insufficiency (chronic) (peripheral)
I87.8	Other specified disorders of veins
I87.9	Disorder of vein, unspecified
I83.10	Varicose veins of unspecified lower extremity with inflammation

EPIDEMIOLOGY & DEMOGRAPHICS

- From 10% to 35% of adults in the United States have some form of CVI.
- Venous ulcers are the complication of CVI that results in the greatest morbidity and affects 4% of people over the age of 65.
- The population-based costs to the U.S. government for CVI treatment and venous ulcer care have been estimated at >$1 billion/yr.
- In addition, 4.6 million workdays/yr are lost to chronic venous-related diseases.

PHYSICAL FINDINGS & CLINICAL PRESENTATION

The manifestations of CVI can be viewed using the internationally accepted classification system, CEAP (clinical, etiology, anatomy, and pathophysiology) (Table 1). The spectrum of cutaneous changes of CVI in the affected leg include:

- Varicose eczema: The most common and earliest sign, this involves the skin above the medial ankle and consists of pruritic, red, and scaly eczematous patches and plaques.
- Hyperpigmentation: Caused by the breakdown of red blood cells and leads to hemosiderin deposition and dark staining of the skin (Fig. E1).
- Atrophie blanche: Usually presents as hypopigmented white patches with focal red punctate dots or telangiectasia surrounded by hyperpigmentation. Skin in this condition is avascular and prone to ulceration (Fig. E2).
- Lipodermatosclerosis: A chronic, brawny induration of the skin and underlying fat that usually involves the skin from medial malleolus up to the lower border of the calf. Progression of the disease leads to an "inverted champagne bottle" appearance. The induration and lack of perfusion of the skin in this area make it susceptible to ulcer formation.

TABLE 1 CEAP Classification

Clinical Classification	
C_0	No visible or palpable signs of venous disease
C_1	Telangiectasias or reticular veins
C_2	Varicose veins; diameter >3 mm
C_3	Edema
C_4	Changes in skin and subcutaneous tissue: Pigmentation, eczema, lipodermatosclerosis, or atrophie blanche
C_5	Healed venous ulcer
C_6	Active venous ulcer
	Each limb is further classified as asymptomatic (A) or symptomatic (S)
Etiologic Classification	
E_C	Congenital
E_P	Primary
E_S	Secondary (postthrombotic)
E_N	No venous cause identified
Anatomic Classification	
A_S	Superficial veins
A_P	Perforator veins
A_O	Deep veins
A_N	No venous location identified
Pathophysiologic Classification	
P_R	Reflux
P_R	Obstruction
$P_{R,O}$	Reflux and obstruction
P_N	No venous pathophysiology identifiable

CEAP, Clinical-Etiological-Anatomical-Pathophysiological.
From Fillit HM: *Brocklehurst's textbook of geriatric medicine and gerontology,* ed 8, 2017, Elsevier.

ETIOLOGY

- CVI occurs as a result of sustained venous hypertension in the leg, which can be caused by the following:
  1. Primary: Vein valve failure with reflux in the superficial venous system or perforating veins (most common cause of CVI)
  2. Secondary: Postthrombotic syndrome in which a deep vein thrombosis causes outflow obstruction *or*
  3. Combination of the two previous processes
- This sustained elevation in venous pressure or venous hypertension results in pathologic effects in the skin and subcutaneous tissues such as edema, eczema, hyperpigmentation, fibrosis, and ultimately venous ulceration.

DIAGNOSIS

The diagnosis and evaluation of CVI are directed primarily by a detailed history and physical examination.

DIFFERENTIAL DIAGNOSIS

- Contact dermatitis
- Atopic dermatitis
- Cellulitis
- Dermatophyte infection
- Pretibial myxedema
- Nummular eczema
- Xerosis
- Asteatotic eczema

WORKUP

The primary goal is to identify the cause of sustained venous hypertension. Fig. 3 describes the evaluation and management of chronic venous insufficiency.

LABORATORY TESTS

Generally not indicated

IMAGING STUDIES

- Evaluation of the patient is performed in the standing position with duplex ultrasonography to identify reflux in the superficial, deep, and perforating veins as well as obstruction of the deep veins.
- No exam of a leg with CVI is complete without palpation of pulses and/or determination of ankle-brachial index (ABI).

TREATMENT

NONPHARMACOLOGIC THERAPY

- Leg elevation above heart level for 30 min three to four times a day
- Weight reduction because obesity is a risk factor for deep vein thrombosis and CVI
- Walking exercises to improve calf function
- Physical therapy to improve ankle joint mobility
- For weeping skin lesions, wet-to-dry dressing changes

ACUTE GENERAL Rx

- The fundamental role of compression in the treatment of CVI is well recognized and has been validated by randomized controlled trials (RCTs).
- The beneficial effects of gradient compression stockings (decrease in edema and control of discomfort) are due to their effect on microvascular hemodynamics and Starling forces.
- Below-knee compression stocking with a gradient of at least 20 to 30 mm Hg will control edema, alleviate pain, and improve the quality of life in CVI patients.
- Compression stockings are contraindicated in patients with an ABI of <0.6.
- Some patients (acute lipodermatosclerosis) may benefit from nonelastic compression with the Unna gel paste gauze boot to alleviate their symptoms and acute increase in their swelling. The Unna boot is changed once a week.
- Topical corticosteroid creams or ointments (e.g., triamcinolone 0.12% bid) may be used to help reduce inflammation and itching. Steroids should never be applied to ulcer.
- Antibiotics should only be used when treating a clinically apparent, culture-proved infection. Most secondary infections are the result of *Staphylococcus* or *Streptococcus* organisms.
- Diuretics have no role in the treatment of CVI-related edema.

CHRONIC Rx

- While conservative care is fundamental, patients with CVI should be considered for correction of their underlying venous hypertension.

APPROACH TO THE EVALUATION AND TREATMENT OF CHRONIC VENOUS ULCERS

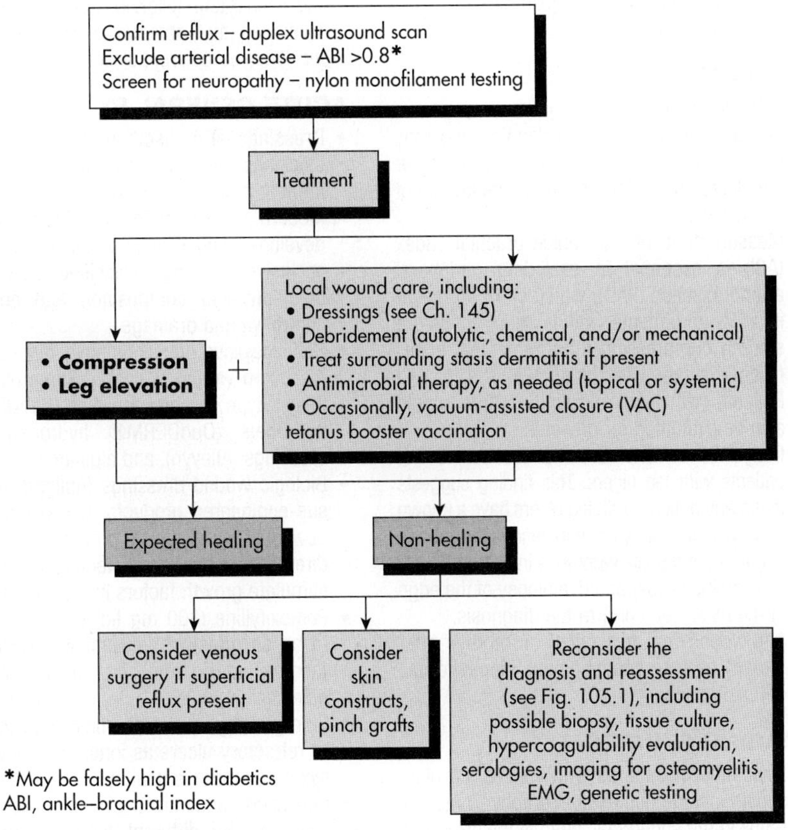

FIG. 3 Approach to the evaluation and treatment of chronic venous ulcers. (From Bolognia JL et al: *Dermatology*, ed 4, Philadelphia, 2018, Elsevier.)

- The majority of patients with CVI have superficial vein or perforator vein reflux as their underlying pathology and would benefit from the newer vein ablation procedures listed below.
  1. Endovenous ablation of superficial (saphenous) or perforator vein reflux.
  2. RF ablation with VNUS closure.
  3. Endovenous laser therapy (EVLT).
  4. Ultrasound-guided foam sclerotherapy.

COMPLEMENTARY & ALTERNATIVE MEDICINE

Several groups of drugs have been evaluated in the treatment of CVI, including coumarins, flavonoids, and saponosides (horse chestnut extracts). These drugs have venoactive properties and are widely used in Europe but are not approved for use in the U.S. The precise mechanism of action is not known. Horse chestnut seed extract has been found, in the short term, to be as effective as compression stockings in reducing pain and edema, but long-term efficacy has not been established.

REFERRAL

- Phlebology
- Vascular surgery
- Indications for referral:
  1. Skin and subcutaneous changes consistent with CVI
  2. Associated peripheral arterial insufficiency (PAD)
  3. Longstanding varicose vein disease
  4. Consideration for vein ablation procedure

PEARLS & CONSIDERATIONS

COMMENTS

- Inflammatory skin changes from CVI are irreversible. The goal of therapy is to eliminate venous hypertension and prevent progression.
- Venous ulcers are often an end-stage manifestation of CVI. Refer to "Venous Ulcers" for more information.

SUGGESTED READINGS

Available at ExpertConsult.com

RELATED CONTENT

Stasis Dermatitis (Patient Information)
Varicose Veins (Related Key Topic)
Venous Ulcers (Related Key Topic)

AUTHOR: **Frank G. Fort, MD, FACS, RPHS**

Venous Ulcers

BASIC INFORMATION

DEFINITION

Venous ulcers are defined as chronic defects of the skin that fail to heal spontaneously and persist for longer than 4 wk. Venous ulcers account for about 70% of all lower-extremity ulcerations. They are usually located in the "gaiter" region and can be accompanied by varicose veins, edema, hyperpigmentation, and lipodermatosclerosis. Venous ulceration develops in patients as a result of sustained venous hypertension.

SYNONYM

Stasis ulcers

ICD-10CM CODES

I87.2	Venous insufficiency (chronic) (peripheral)
L97.909	Non-pressure chronic ulcer of unspecified part of unspecified lower leg with unspecified severity

EPIDEMIOLOGY & DEMOGRAPHICS

In industrialized nations, up to 1.5% of the population will suffer from venous ulcers. In patients ≥65 yr, the incidence increases to 4%. In the U.S., >500,000 people suffer from stasis ulcers.

RISK FACTORS:
- Obesity
- Increasing age
- Family history of chronic venous insufficiency
- History of deep venous thromboembolism

PHYSICAL FINDINGS & CLINICAL PRESENTATION

Venous ulcers are most commonly located in the lower leg just above the ankle (gaiter region). They are a partial-thickness, irregularly shaped wound with well-defined borders with granulation tissue and fibrin present in the ulcer base (Fig. E1). Venous ulcers are relatively painless and are surrounded by brown-stained skin and/or dry, itchy, and reddened skin. In about 50% of patients, there are visible varicose veins in an aching, swollen leg.

ETIOLOGY

The exact mechanism of the role of venous hypertension in the etiology of venous ulcers is not certain. Hemodynamic forces such as venous hypertension, circulatory stasis, and modified conditions of shear stress appear to play an important role in an inflammatory reaction accompanied by leukocyte activation that clinically leads to fibrosclerotic remodeling of the skin and then to ulceration.

DIAGNOSIS

DIFFERENTIAL DIAGNOSIS

- Arterial ulcer
- Neurotrophic ulcers (located predominantly in the foot)
- Vasculitis
- Pyoderma gangrenosum
- Ulcerated skin tumors like basal cell or squamous cell carcinoma (Marjolin ulcer)
- Rheumatoid arthritis

WORKUP

- The history and clinical signs and symptoms of leg ulcers are often misleading and may not differentiate venous ulcers from other leg ulcers; about 30% of leg ulcers are not of venous origin.
- Measurement of the ankle-brachial index (ABI) is essential in excluding peripheral arterial disease (PAD), which can be present in 20% of patients and is required before starting compression therapy. Arterial insufficiency is suggested by an ABI <0.9.
- Patients with lower-extremity ulcers should also be evaluated for diabetes.
- Coagulation defects have been found in 40% of patients with leg ulcers. This finding suggests that many patients with leg ulcers have a known or suspected history of deep venous thrombosis and a thrombophilia workup is indicated.
- If vasculitis is suspected, a biopsy of the edge of the ulcer can confirm the diagnosis.
- Any wound that has failed to improve after therapy of 4 wk should have a biopsy to rule out malignancy.

IMAGING STUDIES

- Evaluation of patients with venous leg ulcer should include duplex sonography to identify reflux in the superficial, deep, and perforating veins as well as possible obstruction of the deep veins.
- If the ulcer appears to be infected, consider tissue for culture, plain x-ray films, and bone scan to evaluate for osteomyelitis.

TREATMENT

NONPHARMACOLOGIC THERAPY

- Fig. 2 describes an algorithm for the treatment of venous ulcers.
- Surgical debridement to remove all nonviable material can be accomplished in the office setting with the use of a topical xylocaine gel. Debridement produces the release of growth factors that allow the development of healthy granulation tissue and the initiation of the healing process.
- The first-line treatment of ulcers includes below-knee compression stockings to improve venous return to the heart, thereby decreasing edema, inflammation, and tissue ischemia (used only if the ABI is between 0.6 and 0.85 because compression can cause limb ischemia).
- There is Level A evidence that graduated compression stockings alone can lead to healing of a venous ulcer. The stockings should be worn during the day and removed at night.
- Regular, brisk walking 30 min a day, five times a week is recommended.
- Elevate leg above heart level and raise the foot of bed with 3-in. blocks to reduce edema.
- Role of surgery: In a randomized controlled trial, endovenous catheter ablation of superficial reflux showed no improvement in the healing rate of ulcers but did demonstrate a reduction of ulcer recurrence from 28% to 12% at 12 mo. Longer term follow-up (median 3-5 yr) also confirmed that abrasive procedures lowered incidence of recurrent ulcers.[1]

ACUTE GENERAL Rx

- Dressings are used under compression stockings to provide a clean, moist environment to promote healing.
- Modern, more complex dressings have been developed and include occlusive and semiocclusive dressings, classified according to their physical composition and ability to control wound drainage.
- Semiocclusive dressings have varying ability to absorb wound drainage. Some examples of this type are hydrocolloids (DuoDERM®), hydrogels (DuoDERM® hydrogel), foam dressings (Allevyn), and alginates.
- Biologic wound dressings (Apligraf) and tissue-engineered products (Oasis) have been developed, and these products can either directly provide growth factors or indirectly stimulate growth factors in the ulcer bed.
- Pentoxifylline (800 mg tid) has been shown to be an effective adjuvant to compression therapy as reported in a meta-analysis of nine clinical trials.
- Skin grafting should be considered for large or refractory ulcers as long as the wound is clean and there is healthy granulation tissue.
- Published randomized clinical trials on the value of the different types of dressings in the management of leg ulcers have not shown effects on ulcer healing. Despite the lack of evidence to support their use, modern dressings remain a part of the standard of care. Decisions regarding their use should be based on local cost of the dressings and the physician's clinical experience.
- Trials involving the use of weekly, low-dose, high-frequency ultrasound for hard-to-heal venous leg ulcers do not support adding therapeutic ultrasound to standard care for venous leg ulcers.

DISPOSITION

The overall prognosis for this condition is poor; the healing rate depends on the initial size of the ulcer. Although 65% to 70% of venous ulcers are healed within 6 mo, the 5-yr recurrence rate of healed venous ulcers can be as high as 40%. Maintenance of lifelong compression therapy is recommended.

REFERRAL

All patients should be evaluated weekly during the first month of therapy. Nonhealing ulcers with little to no improvement should also be referred to a wound care clinic.

SUGGESTED READINGS

Available at ExpertConsult.com

AUTHOR: **Frank G. Fort, MD, FACS, RPHS**

[1]Gohel MS et al: Long-term clinical and cost-effectiveness of early endovenous ablation in venous ulceration: a randomized clinical trial, *JAMA Surg* 155:1113, 2020.

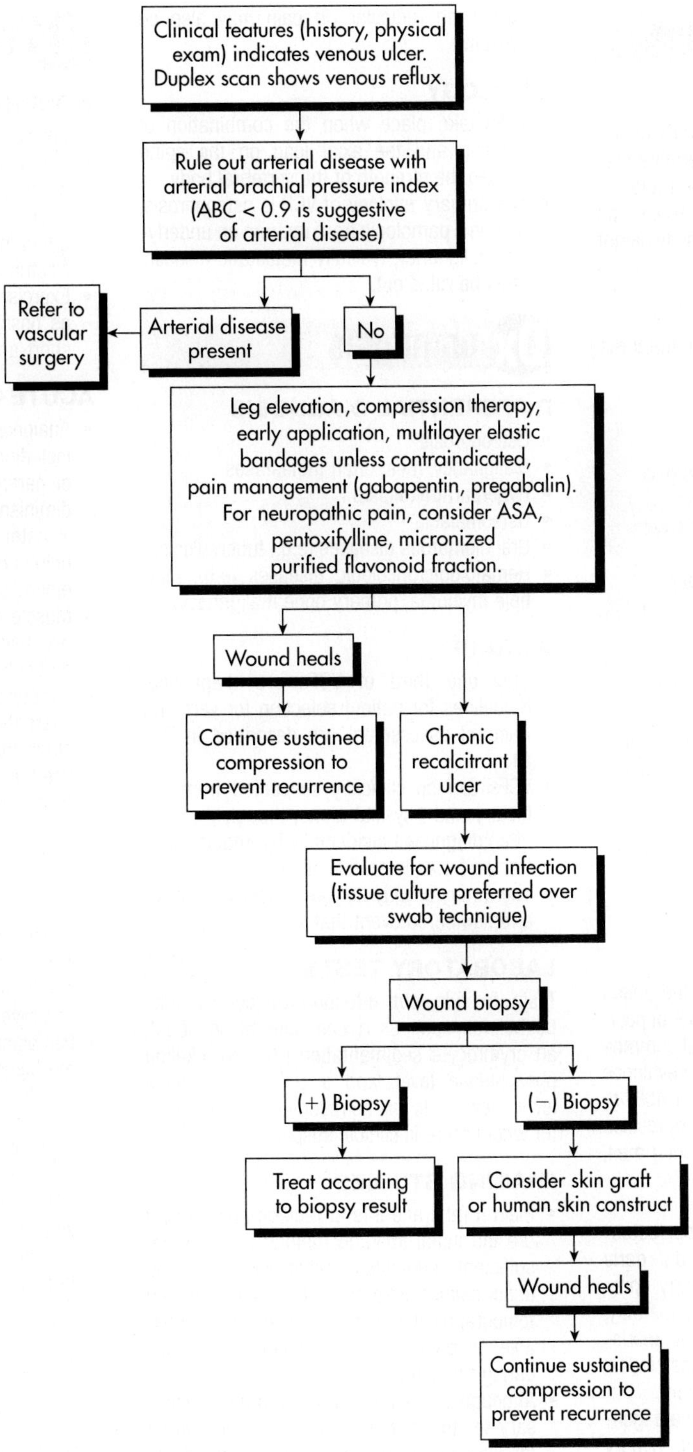

FIG. 2 Algorithm for the care of a patient with a venous leg ulcer.

BASIC INFORMATION

DEFINITION

Vertebral compression fractures (VCFs) are defined as fractures of spinal vertebrae in which a bony surface is driven toward another bony surface. These fractures are classified as radiographic reductions in vertebral body height of more than 15%.

SYNONYMS

Thoracolumbar vertebral compression fractures
Osteoporotic fractures
VCF

ICD-10CM CODES	
M80.0	Post-menopausal osteoporosis with pathologic fracture
M80.4	Drug-induced osteoporosis with pathological fracture
M80.5	Idiopathic osteoporosis with pathological fracture
M80.8	Other osteoporosis with pathological fracture
M80.9	Unspecified osteoporosis with pathological fracture
S32.009A	Unspecified fracture of unspecified lumbar vertebra, initial encounter for closed fracture
S22.009A	Unspecified fracture of unspecified thoracic vertebra, initial encounter for closed fracture

EPIDEMIOLOGY & DEMOGRAPHICS

Approximately 700,000 VCFs occur in the United States each yr, and they affect up to 25% of postmenopausal women. They are the most common complication of osteoporosis. The prevalence increases with age, reaching a peak of 40% to 50% among women aged >80 yr. Compression fractures are also a major concern among men, although their rates of VCF are lower.

RISK FACTORS:

- Modifiable: Tobacco or alcohol use, osteoporosis, estrogen deficiency (i.e., early menopause, bilateral oophorectomy, premenopausal amenorrhea for >1 yr), frailty, impaired vision, abusive situations, inadequate physical activity, low body mass index, and deficiency of vitamin D or calcium.
- Nonmodifiable: Advanced age, female gender, dementia, Caucasian descent, history of fractures in adulthood and among first-degree relatives, and falls.

PHYSICAL FINDINGS & CLINICAL PRESENTATION

- Asymptomatic: Most VCFs are asymptomatic, except for height loss or kyphosis (i.e., dowager's hump [Fig. E1]), which is often a sign of multiple VCFs and height loss of >6 cm has a sensitivity/specificity of 94% and 30%, respectively, for VCF.
- Symptomatic: When symptomatic, VCFs usually present as acute back pain after activity (e.g., bending, lifting) or coughing; neck strain and radicular rib pain may also be present.

ETIOLOGY

- VCFs take place when the combination of bending and the axial load on the spine exceed the strength of the vertebral body.
- The primary etiology of VCF is osteoporosis, though a pathologic fracture from an underlying malignancy, typically metastatic disease, must be ruled out.

DIAGNOSIS

DIFFERENTIAL DIAGNOSIS

- Osteoporosis
- Malignancy, most often metastases
- Hyperparathyroidism
- Osteomalacia
- Granulomatous diseases (e.g., tuberculosis)
- Hematologic/oncologic diseases (e.g., multiple myeloma, primary bone malignancy)

WORKUP

- Only one third of VCFs are diagnosed. Guidelines for patient selection for vertebral fractural assessment are described in Box E1.
- VCFs can be clinically suspected from the history and physical alone, though they are often diagnosed incidentally by imaging performed for another indication.
- There may or may not be a specific injury or a remembered event that led to the VCF.

LABORATORY TESTS

Tests to rule out infection or cancer may be helpful, such as a complete blood count, an erythrocyte sedimentation rate, an alkaline phosphatase level, and a C-reactive protein level; these tests can be reserved for individuals for whom there is clinical suspicion.

IMAGING STUDIES

- Plain frontal and lateral radiographs (x-rays) are the initial imaging method and may be sufficient, particularly when no neurologic abnormalities are present. MRI and computed tomography (CT) scans may be uncomfortable or painful for the patient, especially during the acute phase.
- Although CT scans are not routinely necessary for the diagnosis, they can be helpful for visualizing fractures that are not seen on plain films, for evaluating the integrity of the posterior vertebral wall, for ruling out other causes of back pain, for detecting spinal canal narrowing, and for assessing instability.
- MRI may be useful when spinal cord compression is suspected, if neurologic symptoms are present, or to distinguish malignancy from osteoporosis (e.g., in patients <55 yr with VCF after minimal or no trauma).
- Bone density studies may be helpful to determine the severity of osteoporosis, which is a key risk factor for future fractures.

TREATMENT (FIG. 2)

NONPHARMACOLOGIC THERAPY

- Physical therapy.
- External back braces: Frequently recommended to relieve pain and improve mobility, however, controlled trials have not shown any effect in patients with vertebral compression fractures.
- Exercise programs: Getting active as soon as possible is extremely important for both short-and long-term recovery.

ACUTE GENERAL Rx

- Analgesics are first line for pain control, including acetaminophen and opioids (oral or parenteral), and pain can be expected to diminish over 4 to 6 wk.
- Nonsteroidal antiinflammatory drugs are helpful but must be used with caution among elderly patients or when contraindicated.
- Muscle relaxants should be used judiciously because they have significant side effects, particularly in the elderly.
- Intranasal calcitonin (200 units once daily, alternating nostrils) has been shown in some small trials to hasten relief from pain when used as an adjunct to oral analgesics, and a 2- to 4-wk course may be useful for patients who do not achieve adequate control with oral analgesics alone.
- Early mobilization with physical therapy is important for recovery and prevention of subsequent fractures.
- The efficacy of vertebroplasty versus kyphoplasty versus conservative treatment remains controversial.
- Percutaneous vertebroplasty (Fig. E3) involves the injection of acrylic bone cement into the affected vertebral body in an effort to stabilize the fracture and reduce pain, whereas in kyphoplasty, a high-pressure inflatable bone tamp or balloon is expanded within the body of the affected vertebra to restore pre-fracture vertebral height before the injection of bone cement. These two procedures were thought to be helpful in patients who did not respond to conservative therapy; however, further studies showed them to be no more effective than sham procedures. Nonetheless, Klazen et al (2010) demonstrated in an open-label prospective randomized trial that for the subgroup of patients with acute osteoporotic VCFs and persistent pain, percutaneous vertebroplasty may provide immediate pain relief, sustained for at least a yr, which may be significantly greater than that achieved with conservative treatment. Zampini (2010) showed in a nonrandomized cohort study that elderly patients who underwent kyphoplasty were more likely to be discharged home. Analysis of Medicare claims of patients with VCF treated with kyphoplasty or vertebroplasty compared with medical management revealed no difference in mortality or major medical outcomes but decreased health care utilization in the conservatively managed group. These procedures are

still in their infancy, and more answers should be forthcoming as to their efficacy, as well as questions regarding the amount of time that conservative therapy alone should be pursued and which procedure, if any, should be advised. Most current guidelines recommend 4 to 6 wk of medical therapy before pursuing surgical intervention in neurologically intact VCF.

CHRONIC Rx

Osteoporosis should be treated with the reduction of risk factors (e.g., smoking, alcohol), diet, exercise, calcium and vitamin D supplements, and with medications used to treat osteoporosis (e.g., bisphosphonates).

REFERRAL

Referral is indicated for neurologic abnormalities, unremitting pain, instability, continued disability, or when the investigation of the cause of the fracture reveals serious underlying pathology.

PEARLS & CONSIDERATIONS

Prevention of osteoporosis and conservative therapy remain the mainstay of treatment.

COMMENTS

- VCFs should be suspected in anyone aged >50 yr with the acute onset of low back pain. There are many opportunities for diagnosis and treatment that are easy to miss, especially for males.
- Solitary vertebral fractures higher than T7 are unusual and should raise suspicion for other pathologic causes.
- Diagnosing and treating osteoporosis reduce the incidence of VCFs.
- Getting people with VCF physically active as soon as possible will be efficacious both acutely and in the long term.
- In general, VCF will be best managed through a partnership of the patient, the primary care physician, an orthopedist, a physical therapist, a dietitian, and a social worker.

PREVENTION

Reducing the effects of modifiable risk factors is key.

SUGGESTED READINGS

Available at ExpertConsult.com

AUTHOR: **Fred F. Ferri, MD**

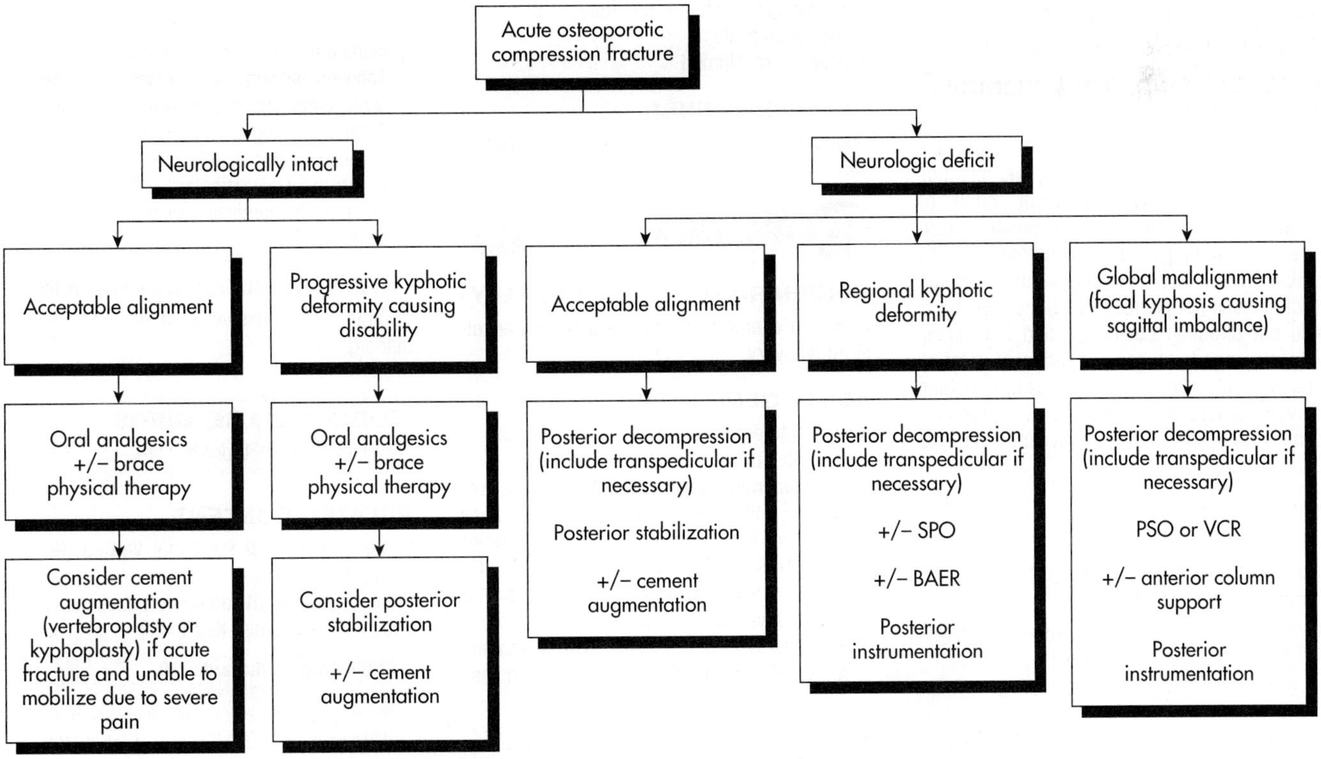

FIG. 2 A generalized treatment algorithm for osteoporotic spine fractures. *BAER*, Balloon-assisted endplate reduction; *PSO*, pedicle subtraction osteotomy; *SPO*, Smith–Petersen osteotomy; *VCR*, vertebral column resection. (From Browner BD et al: *Skeletal trauma: basic science, management, and reconstruction*, ed 6, Philadelphia, 2020, Elsevier.)

BASIC INFORMATION

DEFINITION

Vestibular neuronitis is a syndrome of sudden-onset dysfunction of the peripheral vestibular system, often severe, with prolonged vertigo, nausea, and vomiting.

SYNONYMS

Vestibular neuritis
Acute neuritis
Neurolabyrinthitis
Vestibular neuropathy

ICD-10CM CODES	
H81.2	Vestibular neuronitis
H81.23	Vestibular neuronitis, bilateral
H81.20	Vestibular neuronitis, unspecified ear
H81.21	Vestibular neuronitis, right ear
H81.22	Vestibular neuronitis, left ear

EPIDEMIOLOGY & DEMOGRAPHICS

Vestibular neuritis is the second most common cause of peripheral vestibular vertigo with an incidence of about 3.5:100,000 population. Although etiology remains uncertain, it is thought to result from viral infection causing selective inflammation of the vestibular nerve. Infectious origin is supported by the fact that it occurs in epidemics, may affect several family members, and occurs more commonly in spring and early summer. The male:female ratio is nearly 1:1. There is selective damage to the superior part of the vestibular labyrinth, supplied by the superior vestibular portion of the eighth cranial nerve.

PHYSICAL FINDINGS & CLINICAL PRESENTATION

Develops acutely over a period of hr and resolves over periods of days or wk, although long-term sequelae may occur, such as residual imbalance and nonspecific dizziness persisting for mos. Symptoms include sudden-onset, spontaneous, isolated vertigo; spontaneous peripheral nystagmus (horizontal and not direction changing); and imbalance. Patients report intense sensation of rotation and difficulty standing and walking and tend to veer toward the affected side; autonomic symptoms occur with pallor, sweating, nausea, and vomiting.

ETIOLOGY

Etiology remains uncertain but viral and postviral inflammatory disorders are suspected. Herpes zoster, reactivation of herpes simplex type I, and other viruses have been implicated, but evidence is circumstantial.

Dx DIAGNOSIS

DIFFERENTIAL DIAGNOSIS

- Cerebellar infarction
- Labyrinthitis: Similar symptoms of vertigo, with the addition of unilateral hearing loss
- Labyrinthine infarction
- Acoustic neuroma
- Perilymph fistula
- Migraine-associated vertigo
- Ménière disease
- Multiple sclerosis

WORKUP

- Patient may fall toward affected side when attempting ambulation or during Romberg tests.
- Hallpike maneuver: Checking for nystagmus and asking about re-creation of vertigo symptoms.
- Head-impulse test: Grasp patient's head, apply brief small-amplitude rapid head turn, first to one side and then the other; patient fixates on examiner's nose: Positive test is lack of or slowing of corrective eye movements ("saccades") on affected side. A positive test supports the diagnosis of vestibular neuronitis.
- Laboratory testing and imaging are generally not indicated but may help rule out other etiologies.

LABORATORY TESTS

- Electronystagmography (ENG): A battery of eye movement tests that may provide an objective assessment of the vestibular and oculomotor systems and may help localize the lesion's site
- Audiogram: Normal

IMAGING STUDIES

Brain imaging: Computed tomography or MRI—normal

Rx TREATMENT

NONPHARMACOLOGIC THERAPY

Vestibular exercises, when tolerated, will accelerate recovery.

ACUTE GENERAL Rx

Most treatments are empirical and related to symptoms. Further studies are needed.

- Corticosteroids: Corticosteroids are often prescribed, although a Cochrane review finds that there is insufficient evidence for administration. Some studies have shown that glucocorticoids administered within 3 days after onset of vestibular neuronitis may improve long-time recovery of vestibular function and reduce the length of hospital stay and may improve the caloric extent and recovery of canal paresis while others show no significant difference
- Antihistamines: Meclizine, dimenhydrinate, promethazine
- Anticholinergics: Scopolamine
- Antiemetics: Droperidol, prochlorperazine
- Benzodiazepines: Diazepam, valium, lorazepam
- Valacyclovir, either alone or in combination, is likely ineffective in treating vestibular neuronitis

CHRONIC Rx

- Vestibular rehabilitation exercises
- Anti-GABA agents
- Antihistamines

DISPOSITION

Most patients can be treated as outpatients, but inpatient care may be required in cases where vomiting is uncontrollable. If dehydrated because of severe vomiting, sufferers may require brief parenteral therapy.

REFERRAL

- ENT: If diagnosis uncertain, and if these patients are at risk for benign paroxysmal positional vertigo (BPPV) subsequently; also if symptoms linger
- Neurology: If question of central origin or migraine

PEARLS & CONSIDERATIONS

COMMENTS

- Diagnosis unlikely to be vestibular neuronitis if hearing is impaired or other neurologic signs and symptoms are present.
- Although patients may recover from dramatic acute symptoms, subtle vestibular deficits may linger for prolonged period, if not indefinitely (i.e., residual imbalance and nonspecific dizziness).
- Program of vestibular habituation head movement exercises can reduce imbalance symptoms.

PATIENT & FAMILY EDUCATION

Vestibular Disorders Association: https://vestibular.org/

SUGGESTED READINGS

Available at ExpertConsult.com

RELATED CONTENT

Benign Paroxysmal Positional Vertigo (Related Key Topic)
Ménière Disease (Related Key Topic)
Labyrinthitis (Related Key Topic)

AUTHOR: **Rocco J. Richards, MD**

BASIC INFORMATION

- Vitamin D is a hormone and a steroid and, by definition, not a vitamin. There are two forms of vitamin D: Vitamin D_2 and vitamin D_3.
- Vitamin D_2 (ergocalciferol) is mainly found in some plant foods.
- Vitamin D_3 (cholecalciferol) is produced in skin exposed to ultraviolet (UV) B radiation from sunlight (Fig. E1). Gloson, Whistler, and DeBoot independently described rickets in the mid-seventeenth century. Sniadecki first reported the association of rickets with inadequate exposure to sunlight in 1822.
- The major functions of vitamin D include:
  1. Increasing calcium and phosphorus absorption from the small intestines
  2. Promoting the maturation of osteoclast to resorb calcium from bones

DEFINITION

Vitamin D deficiency is characterized by hypocalcemia and/or hypophosphatemia leading to impaired bone mineralization. It is classified as a serum 25-hydroxyvitamin D (25[OH]D) level of <20 ng/ml (50 nmol/L).This standard definition of vitamin D deficiency has been recently challenged, and some endocrinologists recommend a cutoff of 12 mg/ml for vitamin D deficiency.[1] Vitamin D insufficiency is defined as a 25(OH)D between 12 and 20 ng/ml.

The consequences of vitamin D deficiency include:

- Bone disease (rickets, osteoporosis, low bone mass)
- May impair reproductive success
- Decrease the ability to combat infection (especially tuberculosis, influenza, viral infection)
- May induce or worsen autoimmune disorders
- May increase the incidence of death due to heart disease, inflammatory bowel disease, fracture, and cancer of the breast, colon, and prostate
- Subclinical vitamin D deficiency may occur in developed countries and be associated with increased fall risk, possible fractures, and osteoporosis

SYNONYMS

The sunshine vitamin
The antirachitic factor
Cholecalciferol

ICD-10CM CODE
E55.9 Vitamin D deficiency, unspecified

EPIDEMIOLOGY & DEMOGRAPHICS

INCIDENCE:

- Vitamin D insufficiency is very high among older adults and hospitalized and institutionalized people.
- Worldwide deficiency and insufficiency affect about 1 billion people.
- Children and young adults: 40% to 50% of preadolescent Caucasian girls, and Hispanic and African American adolescents, are vitamin D deficient.

PREVALENCE: 41.6% of adults (at least 20 yr old) have 25(OH)D levels <20 ng/dl.

PREDOMINANT SEX & AGE:

- Decreased skin production of vitamin D with age
- Increased prevalence among darker-skinned individuals

PEAK INCIDENCE: In the U.S., 40% to 100% of the elderly are vitamin D deficient.

Sixty percent of nursing home residents may be vitamin D deficient.

RISK FACTORS:

- Age (due to decreased ability to produce D_3)
- Sunshine-deficient areas (geographic location, living in higher latitudes)
- Dark-skinned individuals (melanin competes with vitamin D_3 precursors for UV photons and thus decreases pre-D_3 formation)
- Obese individuals
- Institutionalized individuals
- Pregnant and lactating women
- Use of sunscreen (sun radiation that causes skin cancer also produces pre-vitamin D_3 in skin)
- Patients on certain medications that antagonize vitamin D action (phenobarbital, phenytoin)
- Intestinal resection
- Severe chronic liver diseases (such as cirrhosis)
- Kidney disease (e.g., nephritic syndrome)
- Sarcoidosis and lymphomas (increased catabolism of 25[OH]D to 1,25[OH]2D)
- Intestinal malabsorption disease (caused by celiac sprue, cystic fibrosis, Whipple disease)

PHYSICAL FINDINGS & CLINICAL PRESENTATION

- Clinical presentation of vitamin D deficiency is dependent on the duration and severity of deficiency
- Most patients with mild to moderate vitamin D deficiency are asymptomatic
- Severe deficiency may lead to rickets (in children), osteomalacia (in adults), bone demineralization, hypokalemia, and phosphaturia
- Rickets: seen in children; caused by defective mineralization in the skeleton (Fig. E2)
  1. Bowing of the legs
  2. Leg bone pain
  3. Delayed growth
  4. Seizure due to hypocalcemia
- Osteomalacia: seen in adults with severe and prolonged vitamin D deficiency
  1. Periosteal bone pain (best detected by putting firm pressure on tibia or sternal bones)
  2. Proximal muscle weakness
  3. Chronic muscle aches/pain
- Fracture with very minimal trauma (brittle and easily broken bones)
- Severe hypocalcemia: especially in late vitamin D deficiency leading to seizure tetany
- Hypophosphatemia
- Paresthesia
- Tetany
- Muscle cramps

ETIOLOGY

- Inadequate exposure to sunlight, such as:
  1. During winter
  2. In nursing home and health care institution residents
  3. With excessive use of sunscreen
- Medications: Individuals on certain medications, such as phenobarbital, phenytoin, and rifampin (antagonize vitamin D action/increase vitamin D catabolism)
- Diseases and disease states:
  1. Diseases causing vitamin D malabsorption:
     a. Cystic fibrosis
     b. Whipple disease
     c. Celiac sprue
  2. Diseases increasing vitamin D catabolism:
     a. Lymphoma
     b. Sarcoidosis
  3. Intestinal resection
  4. Decreased 25(OH)D production:
     a. Kidney disease
     b. Liver cirrhosis

Dx DIAGNOSIS

DIFFERENTIAL DIAGNOSIS

- Arthritis
- Fibromyalgia

WORKUP

- Population-wide screening for vitamin D deficiency is not recommended because evidence to support this practice is lacking. Appropriate to screen high-risk individuals.
- Screening is needed for individuals at risk (osteoporosis, history of falls, obese persons, pregnant and lactating women, diseases causing vitamin D malabsorption, African Americans). Workup involves blood and urine tests as well as radiography, as outlined in the next section.

LABORATORY TESTS (TABLE 1)

- Serum 25(OH)D: This is the best test to determine vitamin D status.
- Parathyroid hormone (PTH): Increased levels in vitamin D insufficiency. It is a marker of vitamin D insufficiency.
- Increased (serum or bone) alkaline phosphatase.
- Decreased 24-hr urine calcium (patient should not be on a thiazide).
- In patients at risk for osteomalacia [s-25(OH) D is less than 10 ng/ml], check Ca, Ph, alkaline phosphatase, PTH, basic metabolic panel, and tissue transglutaminase antibodies.

IMAGING STUDIES

- Radiographs may show:
  1. Pseudofractures of the pelvis, femur, metatarsals
  2. Nontraumatic fractures

[1] Shah S et al: Serum 25-hydroxyvitamin D insufficiency in search of a bone disease. *J Clin Endocrinol Metab* 102:2321-2328, 2017.

TABLE 1 Laboratory Tests

	SERUM			URINE
	Calcium	Phosphorus	Alkaline phosphatase	Calcium
Osteoporosis	N	N	N	N
Hyperparathyroidism				
Primary	↑		N or ↑	N or ↑
Secondary	N or ↑	↑	↑	↓
Tertiary	↑	N or ↓	N or ↑	N or ↑
Hypoparathyroidism	↓	↑	N	↓
Pseudohypoparathyroidism	↓	↑	N	↓
Rickets/osteomalacia				
Vit D deficient	↓	↓	↑	
Vit D refractory	N	↓	↑	↓
Hypophosphatasia	N or ↑	N	↓	N or ↑

Vit, Vitamin.
From Grant LA: *Grainger & Allison's diagnostic radiology essentials*, ed 2, Philadelphia, 2019, Elsevier.

- Bone density:
  1. Decreased bone mineral density (osteopenia or osteoporosis). Note that bone mineral density is not routinely performed in patients whose only risk factor is decreased Vitamin D levels.

Rx TREATMENT

NONPHARMACOLOGIC THERAPY

- Natural sources of vitamin D. These include:
  1. Exposure to sunlight. A mild sunburn is equivalent to consuming 10,000 to 25,000 IU of dietary vitamin D.
  2. Dietary sources are not enough to meet daily requirements. Oily fish such as salmon, cod, and mackerel are rich sources of vitamin D_3.
- Foods fortified with vitamin D.
  1. Mainly fortified dairy products.
  2. Fortified orange juice.

ACUTE GENERAL Rx

- Treating deficiency (general population): Cholecalciferol (vitamin D_3), when available, is preferred for vitamin D supplementation.
  1. 50,000 IU of vitamin D every wk for 8 wk, *or*
  2. 6000 IU daily to achieve a serum level of 25(OH)D of at least 30 ng/ml
- Maintenance measures after treatment (general population): 1500 to 2000 IU daily.
- Treating deficiency (obese patients, patients with malabsorption syndromes, or those taking certain medications, as indicated earlier).
  1. 6000 to 10,000 IU daily
- Maintenance measures after treatment (obese patients, patients with malabsorption syndromes, or those taking certain medications, as indicated earlier):
  1. 3000 to 6000 IU daily
- After treating deficiency, recheck 25(OH)D in 12 to 16 wk.

If deficiency persists after several attempts at treatment, try UV B light therapy.

REFERRAL

Referral to an endocrinologist is recommended if there is no response to treatment.

PREVENTION

- Food fortification with vitamin D_2 or vitamin D_3.
- Adequate sun exposure, for example, exposure in the middle of the day (between 10:00 am and 3:00 pm).
- Use vitamin D_3 for supplementation when available.
- Vitamin D supplementation (per the Endocrine Society):
  1. Infants (age range 1-12 mo) require at least 400 IU/day of vitamin D
  2. Children (age range 1-18 yr) require 600 IU/day of vitamin D
  3. Adult supplementation (adults 19-70 yr): 600 IU of vitamin D daily
  4. Adult supplementation (persons ≥70 yr): 800 IU of vitamin D daily
  5. Exceptions: Pregnant or lactating women, obese persons, and patients on antiseizure medications, steroids, antifungals, and AIDS medications should be given 2× to 3× more vitamin D
  6. To reduce the risk of fracture and falls, the American Geriatric Society recommends a daily intake of at least 1000 IU and the National Osteoporosis Foundation 800 to 1000 IU in adults 65 yr or older

SCREENING: Routine screening for low-risk adults is not recommended. Screening is recommended only for individuals at high risk for vitamin D deficiency such as blacks and Hispanics, obese individuals (BMI >30 kg/m^2), patients with osteoporosis, the elderly, and patients with certain chronic diseases (see "Risk Factors"). According to the U.S. Preventive Services Task Force (USPSTF), current evidence is insufficient to assess the balance of benefits and harms of screening for vitamin D deficiency in asymptomatic adults.

PEARLS & CONSIDERATIONS

- In the U.S., vitamin D supplements are available by prescription as vitamin D_2 (ergocalciferol) or over the counter as vitamin D_3 (cholecalciferol, usually in 400- to 1000-IU doses). Both vitamin D_2 and vitamin D_3 are acceptable as supplements. On average, oral vitamin D_3 raises blood levels more than does vitamin D_2.
- Upper limit of maintenance tolerability in healthy adults is 4000 IU a day. More than 4000 IU of vitamin D daily in nondeficient individuals increases the risk of harm. High-level supplements (>10,000 IU daily) are associated with kidney and tissue damage.
- Vitamin D supplementation is recommended for fall prevention. High-dose vitamin D supplementation (≥800 IU daily) has been shown to be favorable in the prevention of hip fracture and any nonvertebral fracture in persons 65 yr of age or older.
- Prescribing more than the recommended daily amount to improve quality of life or prevent cardiovascular disease or death is not advised.
- Trials have shown that low vitamin D levels are associated with depressive symptoms, especially in persons with a history of depression. These findings suggest that measuring vitamin D levels may be useful in patients with a history of depression.
- A recent trial revealed that Vitamin D supplementation at doses of 1,000 IU daily or higher did not prevent falls in older adults, and fall risk increased with higher doses.[2]
- Recent data suggest that vitamin D deficiency is associated with the risk of developing certain cancers (including breast, colon, and prostate).
- Vitamin D deficiency is associated with some autoimmune diseases (types 1 and 2 diabetes, metabolic syndrome, multiple sclerosis).

SUGGESTED READINGS

Available at ExpertConsult.com

RELATED CONTENT

Vitamin D Deficiency (Patient Information)
Osteomalacia and Rickets (Related Key Topic)
Vitamin Deficiency (Related Key Topic)

AUTHOR: **Daniel K. Asiedu, MD, PhD, FACP**

[2]Appel LJ et al: The effects of four doses of vitamin D supplements on falls in older adults: a responsive-adaptive, randomized clinical trial. *Ann Intern Med* Dec 8, 2020.

BASIC INFORMATION

DEFINITION

Vitamins are organic compounds that cannot be synthesized by humans but are required as nutrients in minute amounts for normal metabolism. Vitamins have several different functions: They may regulate cell growth and differentiation, as catalysts, as antioxidants, and as co-enzymes. Vitamins are classified as either fat soluble (vitamins A, D, E, K) or water soluble (B group of vitamins and C). Deficiency of most vitamins is rare in Western countries. Certain groups may be prone to vitamin deficiency, and these are discussed here. Vitamin D deficiency is discussed in a separate topic.

SYNONYMS

Hypovitaminosis
Vitamin A: Retinol
Vitamin E: Alpha tocopherol
Vitamin K: Phytonadione or menadiol
Vitamin B_1: Thiamine
Vitamin B_2: Riboflavin
Niacin: Vitamin B_3; nicotinic acid
Vitamin B_5: Pantothenic acid
Vitamin B_6: Pyridoxine; pyridoxal phosphate
Folic acid: Vitamin B_9; folate
Vitamin B_{12}: Cyanocobalamin
Vitamin C: Ascorbic acid

ICD-10CM CODES	
E50	Vitamin A deficiency
E51	Thiamine deficiency
E53	Deficiency of other B group vitamins
E55	Vitamin D deficiency
E56	Other vitamin deficiencies
E56.0	Deficiency of vitamin E
E56.1	Deficiency of vitamin K
E53.0	Riboflavin deficiency
E52	Niacin deficiency [pellagra]
E53.1	Pyridoxine deficiency
E53.8	Deficiency of other specified B group vitamins
E54	Ascorbic acid deficiency

EPIDEMIOLOGY & DEMOGRAPHICS

Deficiency can occur in all age groups but is most common in the elderly.

- Vitamin A deficiency: Affects 250 million preschool children worldwide.
- Vitamin K deficiency: Varies by geographic regions; no race predilection; affects both sexes equally. Encountered often in infants.
- Vitamin B_1 (thiamine) deficiency: Incidence is unknown; no sex, race, or age predilection.
- Vitamin B_2 (riboflavin): More common than previously appreciated. Deficiency is referred to as ariboflavinosis.
- Vitamin B_5 (pantothenic acid) deficiency: Rare, as it is present in all foods.
- Vitamin B_{12} (cobalamin) deficiency: Relatively common. Occurs in all age groups but more common in the elderly.
- Vitamin B_9 (folic acid) deficiency: Mandatory fortification started in 1998. Prevalence before fortification 16% and after 0.5%. Neural tube defect associated with low maternal folate status during pregnancy. Pregnant women and the elderly are at greatest risk of folic acid deficiency.
- Vitamin C (ascorbic acid) deficiency: Smokers and low-income persons are at increased risk.

Fig. 1 shows environmental and nutritional factors in disease.

PHYSICAL FINDINGS & CLINICAL PRESENTATION

- Vitamin A: Xerophthalmia, xerosis of the cornea, keratomalacia, Bitot spots (abnormal squamous cell proliferation and keratinization of the conjunctiva), nyctalopia (poor adaptation to darkness)/night blindness, poor bone growth, dry skin and hair, follicular hyperkeratosis (caused by blockage of hair follicles by keratin), pruritus, broken fingernails
- Vitamin K: Clinical manifestation usually occurs if hypoprothrombinemia is present. Major symptom is bleeding to minor trauma. Also can show easy bruisability, epistaxis, hematoma, or gum bleeding
- Vitamin E: Nerve dysfunction (ataxia; hyporeflexia, peripheral neuropathy); bone weakness
- Vitamin B_1 (thiamine): Beriberi, which has two subtypes (infantile and adult). Adult type is described below:
  1. Dry beriberi (affecting the nervous system): Symmetrical peripheral neuropathy (with sensory and motor impairments), Wernicke encephalopathy (nystagmus, ataxia, ophthalmoplegia, and confusion), Korsakoff syndrome (impaired short-term memory loss and confabulation but normal cognition)
  2. Wet beriberi (affecting the cardiovascular system): Cardiomegaly, cardiomyopathy, heart failure, tachycardia, hypotension, chest pain, peripheral edema
  3. Gastrointestinal (GI): Anorexia; constipation
- Vitamin B_2 (riboflavin):
  1. Cheilosis (chapping and fissure of the lip)
  2. Glossitis (sore red tongue)
  3. Oily, scaly rashes on nasolabial folds, eyelids, scrotum, labia majora
  4. Red itchy eyes
  5. Normocytic or normochromic anemia
  6. Peripheral neuropathy
- Vitamin B_3 (niacin):
  1. Pellagra (4 *Ds*—diarrhea, dermatitis, dementia, and ultimately death)
  2. Hyperpigmentation of sun-exposed skin
  3. "Raw beef" swollen and painful tongue
  4. Deficiency can be seen in prolonged use of Isoniazid, in carcinoid syndrome, and in Hartnup syndrome
- Vitamin B_5 (pantothenic acid):
  1. Deficiency is rare
  2. Deficiency leads to "burning feet syndrome" (distal paresthesia and dysesthesia)
  3. Anemia
  4. GI symptoms
- Vitamin B_6 (Pyridoxine): Rare to see overt deficiency.
  1. Mild deficiency—glossitis, cheilosis, impaired proprioception; sensory ataxia, confusion, depression
  2. Severe deficiency—seborrheic dermatitis, seizure, microcytic
- Vitamin B_{12} (cyanocobalamin):
  1. Megaloblastic anemia (pernicious anemia)
  2. Neurologic symptoms including peripheral neuropathy, ataxia (shuffling gait), paresthesia; subacute degeneration of the spinal cord (demyelination of the dorsal column), visual disturbances due to optic atrophy
  3. Glossitis and GI symptoms such as nausea, vomiting, and anorexia are also common
  4. Patients may also have dementia/mental sluggishness, depression, and weakness
- Vitamin B_9 (folic acid):
  1. Patchy hyperpigmentation of skin (especially between fingers and toes) and mucous membranes
  2. Moderate fever (temp <102° F; 38.9° C) despite the absence of infection
  3. Neural tube defect
  4. Angular stomatitis
  5. Red, beefy, smooth, and shiny tongue
  6. Megaloblastic anemia
- Vitamin C: Scurvy (bruising, petechiae, follicular hyperkeratosis, perifollicular hemorrhage), poor wound healing, fatigue, gingivitis/bleeding gums, weight loss, bone abnormalities (Fig. E2)

ETIOLOGY

- Fat-soluble vitamins (vitamins A, D, E, K):
  1. Decreased ingestion, malnutrition, eating disorders
  2. Diseases that affect fat absorption decrease the absorption of fat-soluble vitamins—for example, cystic fibrosis, celiac sprue, inflammatory bowel disease, cholestasis, hepatobiliary disease, small bowel surgery
  3. Change in vitamin metabolism:
     a. Alcoholism
     b. Drugs such as cholestyramine, warfarin, anticonvulsants, antibiotics (e.g., cephalosporins)
     c. Chronic kidney disease
- Increased risk in:
  1. Vegans
  2. Recent immigrants
  3. Refugees
  4. Toddlers/preschoolers living below the poverty line
- Water-soluble vitamins (the B group of vitamins and vitamin C)—there are several etiologic factors, including:
  1. Inadequate intake
  2. Decreased absorption
  3. Alcoholism
  4. Pregnancy/lactation
  5. Peritoneal dialysis
  6. Medications (e.g., isoniazid, phenothiazines, tricyclic antidepressants, metformin [vit B_{12}])
  7. Malabsorption
  8. Low income
  9. Advanced age

Vitamin	Function	Consequences of deficiency
A	Retinal function, epithelial growth control	Night blindness, keratomalacia, xerophthalmia
B_1 (thiamine)	Co-enzyme	Beriberi, Wernicke's encephalopathy
B_2 (riboflavin)	Co-enzyme	Dermatitis, glossitis, keratitis, neuropathy, confusion
B_6 (pyridoxine)	Co-enzyme	Neuropathy
B_{12} (cobalamin)	Nucleic acid synthesis	Megaloblastic anemia Subacute combined degeneration of spinal cord
Niacin	Co-enzyme NAD, NADP	Pellagra (diarrhea, dermatitis, and dementia)
Folate	Co-enzyme in nucleic acid synthesis	Megaloblastic anemia, villous atrophy of gut
Vitamin C	Co-factor in hydroxylation	Scurvy
Vitamin D	Calcium and phosphate absorption	Rickets (childhood) Osteomalacia (adults)
Vitamin E	Antioxidant	Spinocerebellar degeneration
Vitamin K	Co-factor for coagulation factor synthesis	Bleeding due to coagulation defects

FIG. 1 Environmental and nutritional factors in disease. (From Stevens A: *Core pathology,* St Louis, 2009, Elsevier.)

- Vitamin B_{12} deficiency—caused by:
  1. Insufficient dietary intake, as in strict vegans
  2. Decreased absorption secondary to intrinsic factor deficiency, decreased intrinsic factor secretion, gastric atrophy, gastrectomy/gastric bypass
  3. Terminal ileum disease such as celiac disease, enteritis, tropical sprue
- Folic acid deficiency:
  1. Increased needs can lead to deficiency (e.g., pregnancy, lactation, malignancy)
  2. Derangement of folate metabolism by:
     a. Medication (e.g., methotrexate)
     b. Disease (e.g., hypothyroidism)
     c. Increased excretion: As seen in alcoholics

Dx DIAGNOSIS

LABORATORY TESTS

General initial laboratory tests include:
- Complete blood cell count (CBC)
- Liver function tests (LFTs)
- Basic metabolic panel (BMP)
- Albumin
- Measurement of serum levels of the specific vitamin in question

Specific tests may be considered in the following cases:
- Vitamin A:
  1. Serum retinol level (best test, a direct measure, expensive)
  2. Retinol binding protein (easier to perform, less expensive)
  3. Dark-adaptation threshold test
- Vitamin K:
  1. Prothrombin time/partial thromboplastin time (PT/PTT)
  2. Prothrombin
  3. Des-gamma-carboxyprothrombin (most sensitive test).
  4. Niacin: Urine-*N*-methylnicotinamide (level <0.8 mg/day indicates niacin deficiency)
- Vitamin B_1 (thiamine):
  1. Blood thiamine levels
  2. Thiamine pyrophosphate levels in blood
  3. Erythrocyte thiamine transketolase activity (ETKA)
  4. Urinary thiamine excretion
- Vitamin B_3 (niacin): Check urinary N-methylnicotinamide or erythrocyte NAD/NADP ratio (tests are not readily available)
- Vitamin B_2: Check plasma riboflavin concentration
- Vitamin B_{12}:
  1. Serum vitamin B_{12} <190 pg/ml is diagnostic of vitamin B_{12} deficiency
  2. Serum methylmalonic acid, which is elevated in B_{12} deficiency
  3. Antiparietal antibody
  4. Intrinsic factor antibody is decreased
  5. Blood smear shows macrocytosis and hypersegmentation of megaloblasts
  6. CBC shows increased mean corpuscle volume (MCV)
  7. Megaloblastic anemia
- Folic acid:
  1. Check serum folate level.
  2. Additional testing includes checking for serum homocysteine level, which will be elevated.
  3. Red cell folate level shows chronic folate status.

Rx TREATMENT

Most of the vitamins are available over the counter individually or in different multivitamin formulations.

- Vitamin A deficiency: Treat with oral supplementation 10,000 IU daily.
  1. Consume vitamin A–rich foods such as liver, beef, carrots, oranges, mangoes.
  2. Five servings of fruit and vegetables give enough carotenoids for a day.
- Vitamin K deficiency: Treatment depends on the severity of bleeding, administered subcutaneously (SQ) or intramuscularly (IM).
- Vitamin B_1 (thiamine) deficiency: Give intramuscular thiamine 50 mg for several days.
  1. If B_1 deficiency is suspected and patient needs intravenous glucose, give thiamine first before intravenous glucose. This prevents the development of Korsakoff psychosis.
- Vitamin B_{12} deficiency: Give 1000 mcg IM daily for 7 days, then once a wk for 1 mo, then once a mo indefinitely.
  1. A potential option is oral supplementation.
- Folic acid deficiency: Daily requirement is 400 to 1000 mcg (1 mg) daily.
  1. Centers for Disease Control and Prevention (CDC) recommend that women of childbearing age take 400 mcg of folic acid daily.

SUGGESTED READING

Available at ExpertConsult.com

RELATED CONTENT

Anemia, Pernicious (Related Key Topic)
Osteomalacia and Rickets (Related Key Topic)
Vitamin D Deficiency (Related Key Topic)
Wernicke Syndrome (Related Key Topic)
Vitamins and Their Functions (Appendix IIb)

AUTHOR: **Daniel K. Asiedu, MD, PhD, FACP**

BASIC INFORMATION

DEFINITION

von Willebrand disease is an inherited disorder of hemostasis characterized by a quantitative or qualitative deficiency in von Willebrand factor (vWF), a protein product of a gene located on the short arm of chromosome 12. The vWF factor is mostly synthesized in endothelial cells. von Willebrand disease results from a failure to synthesize or secrete vWF or an accelerated clearance of vWF. vWF is the carrier protein for clotting factor VIII (FVIII:C). vWF binds to denuded subendothelial collagen or glycosaminoglycans and causes platelets to adhere by acting as a ligand for glycoprotein IB on the platelet surface. This latter activity is measured in the laboratory by a test called the ristocetin cofactor (RCF). vWF circulates in plasma as a multimeric protein consisting of protomers attached by disulfide bonds. By definition, vWD is present if the level RCF is <30% of normal. A clinical entity known as low vWF exists when the level is between 30% and 60%. Such patients may exhibit a bleeding phenotype. Previously, this was considered mild vWD. There are several subtypes of von Willebrand disease. The most common type (80% of cases) is type I, where levels of vWF, FVIII:C, and RCF are reduced but concordant. Within type 1, there is type 1 mild, which is common; type 1 severe (T1S), which is rare; and type 1 C, in which the low vWF is due to accelerated clearance. There are four type 2 subtypes: Type 2A, type 2B, type 2N, and type 2M. All the type 2 variants are due to a qualitative defect in vWF and show a discordancy between levels of RCF and FVIII:C. The type 2 vWD variants are characterized by low levels of RCF. Type 3 is rare and either an autosomal recessive disorder or double heterozygote and characterized by a near-complete quantitative deficiency of vWF and very low FVIII:C. Acquired vWD disease is a rare disorder that presents with mucocutaneous bleeding abnormalities and no clinical family history. It is seen often in association with hematoproliferative or autoimmune disorder or may occur in hypothyroidism. Successful treatment of the associated illness can reverse the clinical and laboratory manifestations.

SYNONYMS

Pseudohemophilia
vWD

ICD-10CM CODE

D68.0 von Willebrand disease

EPIDEMIOLOGY & DEMOGRAPHICS

- Autosomal-dominant disorder predominantly; rarely recessive or double-heterozygotic.
- Most common inherited bleeding disorder.
- Prevalence is 0.6% to 1.3% in general population, according to screening studies; estimates based on referral for symptoms of bleeding suggest a prevalence of 1 case per 10,000 persons.

PHYSICAL FINDINGS & CLINICAL PRESENTATION

- Generally normal physical examination
- Mucosal bleeding (gingival bleeding, epistaxis) and gastrointestinal bleeding may occur
- Easy bruising
- Bleeding after surgery or dental extraction, menorrhagia
- Rarely, muscle or joint bleeding in type 3

ETIOLOGY

Quantitative or qualitative deficiency of vWF (see "Definition")

DIAGNOSIS

The diagnosis of von Willebrand disease generally requires two criteria: (1) a personal history, family history, or physical evidence of mucocutaneous bleeding and (2) a qualitative or quantitative decrease in functional activity of von Willebrand disease. The American Society of Hematology states that a definitive diagnosis of vWD may be made if RCF levels are <30 IU/dl.

DIFFERENTIAL DIAGNOSIS

Platelet function disorders, clotting factor deficiencies

WORKUP (FIG. 1)

SCREENING LABORATORY TESTS:

- Laboratory evaluation (Table 1).

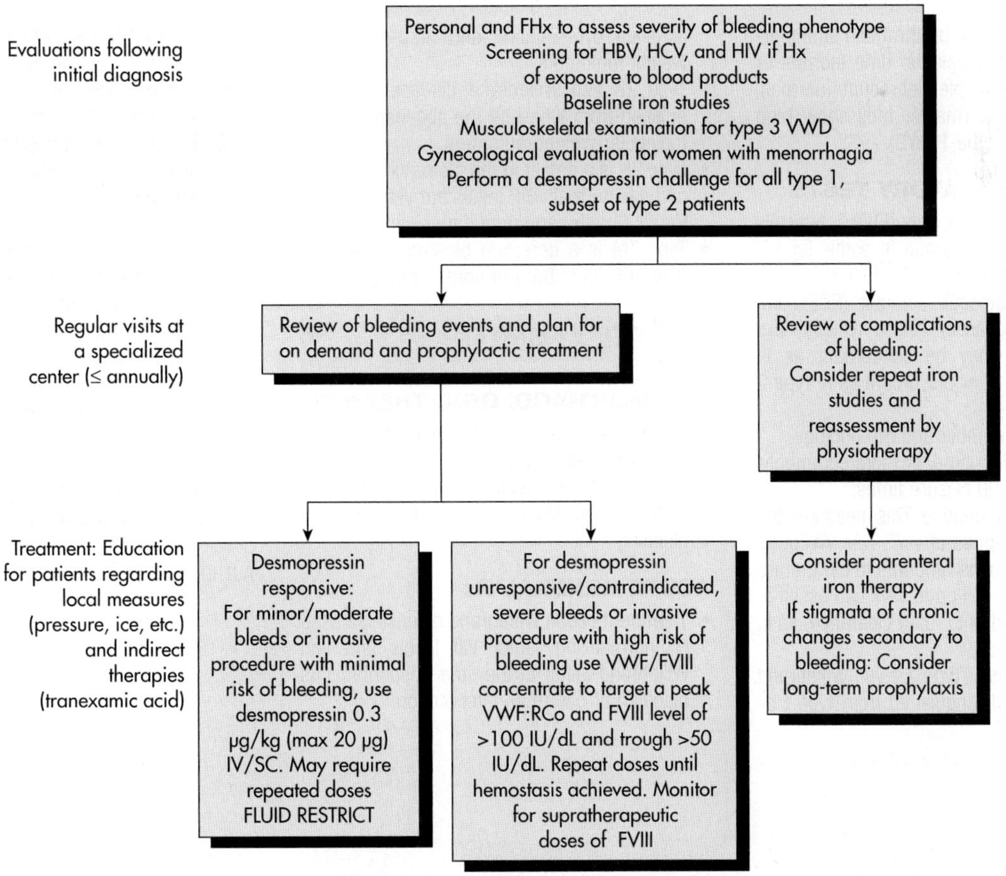

FIG. 1 Approach to the management of von Willebrand disease. *FHx,* Family history; *FVIII,* factor VIII; *HBV,* hepatitis B virus; *HCV,* hepatitis C virus; *HIV,* human immunodeficiency virus; *Hx,* history; *IV,* intravenous; *RCo,* ristocetin cofactor; *SC,* subcutaneous; *VWD,* von Willebrand disease; *VWF,* von Willebrand factor. (From Hoffman R: *Hematology, basic principles and practice*, ed 7, Philadelphia, 2018, Elsevier.)

TABLE 1 Table of Investigations

vWD Type	vWF:RCo IU/dl[a]	vWF:Ag IU/dl[a]	RCo/Ag IU/dl[a]	FVIII:C IU/dl[a]	Multimer Pattern[b]	Other
1	Low	Low	Equivalent	~1.5× vWF:Ag	Normal	
2A	Low	Low	vWF:RCo <vWF:Ag	Low or normal	Abnormal ↓ HMWM	
2B	Low	Low	vWF:RCo <vWF:Ag	Low or normal	Abnormal ↓ HMWM	↑ RIPA[c](↓ platelet count)
2M	Low	Low	vWF:RCo <vWF:Ag	Low or normal	Normal	
2N	Normal/low	Normal/low	Equivalent	<30	Normal	↓ vWF:FVIIIB[d]
3	Absent	Absent	NA	<10	Absent	

Ag, Antigen; *FVIII:C*, FVIII level; *NA*, not applicable; *RCo*, ristocetin cofactor; *RIPA*, ristocetin-induced platelet aggregation; *vWD*, von Willebrand disease; *vWF:FVIIIB*, FVIII-binding assay.
[a]Relative to the reference range (approximate values); vWF:RCo (50-200 IU/dl); vWF:Ag (50-200 IU/dl); FVIII:C (50-150 IU/dl).
[b]HMWM, High-molecular-weight multimers.
[c]Increased agglutination at low concentrations of ristocetin.
[d]The ability of vWF to bind and protect FVIII is reduced. vWF and FVIII levels can look exactly like those in males with mild hemophilia A or in symptomatic hemophilia A carrier females.
From Hoffman R: *Hematology, basic principles and practice*, ed 7, Philadelphia, 2018, Elsevier.

TABLE 2 Desmopressin Responsiveness in the Various Subtypes of von Willebrand Disease

vWD Type	vWF:RCo	vWF:Ag	RCo/Ag	FVIII:C IU/dl	vWF:CB	vWF:CB/vWF:Ag
1	Increase	Increase	Remains >0.7	Increase	Increase	Remains >0.7
2A	No/little change	Increase	Remains <0.7	Increase	No/little change	Remains <0.7
2M (GP1B-binding dysfunction)	No/little change	Increase	Remains <0.7	Increase	Increase	Remains >0.7
3	No/little change	No/little change		No/little change	No/little change	

Ag, Antigen; *FVIII:C*, factor VIII level; *GP1B*, glycoprotein 1B; *RCo*, ristocetin cofactor; *vWD*, von Willebrand disease; *vWF*, von Willebrand factor; *CB*, collagen assays-binding.
Modified from Favaloro EJ: Rethinking the diagnosis of von Willebrand disease. *Thromb Res* 127(Suppl 2):17, 2011; In Hoffman R: *Hematology, basic principles and practice*, ed 7, Philadelphia, 2018, Elsevier.

- Initial testing includes prothrombin time (normal), partial thromboplastin time (normal or slightly increased), platelet count (normal), and PFA-100 (abnormal or may show high normal values in type 1 vWD).

SPECIFIC LABORATORY TESTS

- Factor VIII coagulant activity (FVIII:C, typically decreased, may be normal in some Type 2 variants).
- vWF antigen, ristocetin cofactor (RCF), and collagen binding assay (these typically are decreased and may be concordant as in type 1 and type 3, or discordant as in type 2 variants).
- Normal platelet number and morphology.
- Prolonged bleeding time, or more commonly, prolonged PFA-100 closure times.
- von Willebrand propeptide. This measures the N-terminal propeptide of vWF. This vWFpp is secreted in equimolar amounts to the mature vWF. The ratio of vWFpp to vWF can assist in identifying vWD due to rapid clearance, as in type 1C.
- Multimeric analysis: Type 2A von Willebrand disease can be distinguished from type I by absence of medium- and high-molecular-weight multimers.
- Type 2B von Willebrand disease is distinguished from type I by the absence of high-molecular-weight multimers.
- Type 2N is a defect in the factor VIII:C binding and has normal vWF levels but very low factor VIII:C with normal multimer pattern.
- Type 2M is a defect in binding to platelets (low RCF, low CBA) but normal multimers.

Rx TREATMENT

NONPHARMACOLOGIC THERAPY

- Avoidance of aspirin and other nonsteroidal antiinflammatory drugs
- Use of antifibrinolytics such as tranexamic acid, especially for menorrhagia or oral bleeding

ACUTE GENERAL Rx

- Treatment of von Willebrand disease is based on normalizing factor VIII levels and von Willebrand factor at the time of spontaneous bleeding or before an intervention.
- Use of DDAVP (Table 2): DDAVP binds to V2 receptors in certain endothelial cells and causes the release of vWF. This is suitable for the management of the milder forms of vWD. Dose is 0.3 mcg/kg in 50 to 100 ml of normal saline solution IV infused over 20 min. DDAVP is also available as a nasal spray (dose of 150 mcg spray administered to each nostril) as a preparation for minor surgery and management of minor bleeding episodes.
- When a patient undergoes surgery or receives repeated therapeutic doses of concentrates, use of a plasma-derived vWF concentrate such as Humate-P or a new recombinant vWF (Vonvendi) may need to be administered.

SUGGESTED READINGS

Available at ExpertConsult.com

AUTHOR: **Joseph Sweeney, MD, FACP, FRCPath**

BASIC INFORMATION

DEFINITION

Waldenström macroglobulinemia (WM) is an indolent B-cell lymphoplasmacytic lymphoma (LPL) characterized by lymphoplasmacytic infiltration in the bone marrow (BM) and other organs, and a monoclonal immunoglobulin M (IgM) paraprotein in the serum. Less than 5% of LPL secrete IgG, IgA, or light chains. Rare nonsecretory cases exist.

SYNONYMS

WM
Monoclonal macroglobulinemia
Lymphoplasmacytic lymphoma

ICD-10CM CODE

C88.0 Waldenström macroglobulinemia

EPIDEMIOLOGY & DEMOGRAPHICS

- Accounts for 2% of all hematologic cancers
- A reported 1500 to 2000 new cases diagnosed every yr in the U.S.
- Overall incidence: 3.4 per million person-yr in men, 1.7 per million person-yr in women
- Median age at diagnosis: 69 yr
- More common among men than women and among whites than blacks

PHYSICAL FINDINGS & CLINICAL PRESENTATION

- 30% to 50% of patients can be asymptomatic at presentation
- Weakness, fatigue, and pallor, usually associated with anemia (50%)
- Fever, night sweats, and weight loss (30%)
- Demyelinating peripheral sensory neuropathy, slowly progressive and usually affecting the feet symmetrically, associated with anti-MAG antibodies in half of the cases (20%)
- Lymphadenopathy (15%)
- Hepatosplenomegaly (15%)
- Hyperviscosity syndrome (10%), characterized by headaches, recurrent nosebleeds, blurry vision due to retinal hemorrhages (Fig. E1); retinal vein link: Sausage shaped
- Acquired von Willebrand disease (5%-10%)
- Acrocyanosis, livedo reticularis, purpura, and/or peripheral ulcerations usually associated with symptomatic cryoglobulinemia (5%-10%)
- Hemolytic anemia caused by cold agglutinin disease (5%)
- Amyloidosis causing renal dysfunction, neuropathy, and/or cardiac dysfunction (<5%)
- Meningeal signs caused by CNS involvement by WM (Bing Neel syndrome; 1%)

ETIOLOGY

- The main risk factor for development of WM is having IgM monoclonal gammopathy of unknown significance (MGUS).
- Other risk factors are older age and male sex.
- Multiple reports suggest familial clustering in about 20% of the patients, which may indicate a genetic predisposition to WM and other blood cancers.
- Approximately 20% of the patients have an Ashkenazi Jewish ancestry.
- There is an increased risk of WM in people with a personal history of autoimmune diseases.
- Radiation exposure, occupational chemicals, viral infection (hepatitis C), and chronic inflammatory stimulation have been suggested, but there is insufficient evidence to substantiate these hypotheses.

DIAGNOSIS

The diagnosis of WM is usually established by laboratory blood tests and by bone marrow (BM) biopsy. Diagnosis requires demonstration of LPL involving the BM space and the presence of an IgM monoclonal paraprotein (Table 1). *MYD88 L265P* is a commonly recurring mutation in WM seen in >90% of the patients with WM and 50% to 60% of patients with IgM MGUS and can be useful in differentiating WM from other IgM-secreting B-cell disorders such as marginal zone lymphoma, IgM multiple myeloma, and atypical forms of chronic lymphocytic. Non-*L265P MYD88* mutations rarely have been described (<5%) and should be excluded in patients who test negative for *MYD88 L265P* by PCR-based assays. Mutations in the *CXCR4* gene have been described in 40% of patients, and may impact clinical presentation and response to ibrutinib treatment.

DIFFERENTIAL DIAGNOSIS

- IgM MGUS
- IgM multiple myeloma
- Marginal zone lymphoma
- Atypical chronic lymphocytic leukemia

WORKUP

In any patient suspected of having WM, specific blood tests (CBC, serum or urine protein electrophoresis [SPEP or UPEP, respectively], serum IgM level, beta 2-microglobulin, serum viscosity) should be ordered. BM biopsy confirms the diagnosis. *MYD88* mutation testing can be helpful in supporting the diagnosis of WM.

LABORATORY TESTS

- CBC with differential:
  1. Anemia is a common finding, with a median hemoglobin value of approximately 10 g/dl. WBC count is usually normal; thrombocytopenia can occur.
  2. Peripheral smear may reveal "stacked coin" rouleaux formations and malignant lymphoid cells in some patients.
- SPEP: Homogeneous M spike (monoclonal gammopathy).
- Immunoelectrophoresis: Confirms IgM responsible for the M spike.
- Serum IgM levels are elevated.
- High serum beta 2-microglobulin levels are associated with poor prognosis.
- Serum viscosity. Hyperviscosity usually occurs when the serum viscosity is four times the viscosity of normal serum; classic feature although presents in only 10% of cases.
- Cryoglobulins or cold agglutinins may be present.
- BM biopsy: BM reveals infiltration by a lymphoplasmacytic cell population constituted

TABLE 1 Physicochemical and Immunologic Properties of the Monoclonal Immunoglobulin M Protein in Waldenström Macroglobulinemia

Properties of IgM Monoclonal Protein	Diagnostic Condition	Clinical Manifestations
Pentameric structure	Hyperviscosity	Headaches, blurred vision, epistaxis, retinal hemorrhages, leg cramps, impaired mentation, intracranial hemorrhage
Precipitation on cooling	Cryoglobulinemia (type I)	Raynaud phenomenon, acrocyanosis, ulcers, purpura, cold urticaria
Autoantibody activity to myelin-associated glycoprotein, ganglioside M_1, sulfatide moieties on peripheral nerve sheaths	Peripheral neuropathies	Sensorimotor neuropathies, painful neuropathies, ataxic gait, bilateral foot drop
Autoantibody activity to IgG	Cryoglobulinemia (type II)	Purpura, arthralgia, renal failure, sensorimotor neuropathies
Autoantibody activity to red blood cell antigens	Cold agglutinins	Hemolytic anemia, Raynaud phenomenon, acrocyanosis, livedo reticularis
Tissue deposition as amorphous aggregates	Organ dysfunction	Skin: Bullous skin disease, papules, Schnitzler syndrome Gastrointestinal: Diarrhea, malabsorption, bleeding Kidney: Proteinuria, renal failure (light-chain component)
Tissue deposition as amyloid fibrils (light-chain component most commonly)	Organ dysfunction	Fatigue, weight loss, edema, hepatomegaly, macroglossia, organ dysfunction of involved organs (heart, kidney, liver, peripheral sensory and autonomic nerves)

IgM, Immunoglobulin M.
From Hoffman R: *Hematology, basic principles and practice,* ed 7, Philadelphia, 2018, Elsevier.

TABLE 2 Summary of Consensus Response Criteria for Waldenström Macroglobulinemia

Response Type	Abbreviation	Criteria
Complete response	CR	Absence of serum monoclonal IgM protein by immunofixation Normal serum IgM level Complete resolution of extramedullary disease (i.e., lymphadenopathy/splenomegaly if present at baseline) Morphologically normal bone marrow aspirate and trephine biopsy
Very good partial response	VGPR	Monoclonal IgM protein is detectable 90% reduction in serum IgM level from baseline or normalization of serum IgM level Complete resolution of extramedullary disease (i.e., lymphadenopathy/splenomegaly if present at baseline) No new signs or symptoms of active disease
Partial response	PR	Monoclonal IgM protein is detectable ≥50% but <90% reduction in serum IgM level from baseline Reduction in extramedullary disease (i.e., lymphadenopathy/splenomegaly if present at baseline) No new signs or symptoms of active disease
Minor response	MR	Monoclonal IgM protein is detectable ≥25% but <50% reduction in serum IgM level from baseline No new signs or symptoms of active disease
Stable disease	SD	Monoclonal IgM protein is detectable <25% reduction and <25% increase in serum IgM level from baseline No progression in extramedullary disease (i.e., lymphadenopathy/splenomegaly) No new signs or symptoms of active disease
Progressive disease	PD	>25% increase in serum IgM level from lowest nadir (requires confirmation) and/or progression in clinical features attributable to the disease

IgM, Immunoglobulin M.

From Owen RG et al: Response assessment in Waldenström macroglobulinemia. *Br J Haematol* 160:171, 2013. In Hoffman R et al: *Hematology, basic principles and practice,* ed 7, Philadelphia, 2018, Elsevier.

by small lymphocytes with evidence of plasmacytoid and plasma cell differentiation. The BM infiltration should be confirmed by immunophenotypic studies (flow cytometry and immunohistochemistry) showing the following profile: sIgM+ CD19+ CD20+ CD22+ CD79+.

IMAGING STUDIES

CT of the chest, abdomen, and pelvis may show lymphadenopathy, hepatosplenomegaly, and rarely, extralymphatic/extramedullary areas of disease.

Rx TREATMENT

- Because of the incurable nature of WM, the aim of treatment is to relieve symptoms and reduce the risk of organ damage. Initiation of therapy should not be based on the IgM levels alone because this may not correlate with either disease burden or symptomatic status. Patients with smoldering or asymptomatic WM and preserved hematologic function should be observed without therapy.
- Initiation of therapy is appropriate for patients with constitutional symptoms. Considerations for the initiation of treatment include the following: Significant adenopathy or organomegaly, symptomatic hyperviscosity, moderate to severe neuropathy, amyloidosis, symptomatic cryoglobulinemia or cold agglutinin disease, hemoglobin concentration <10 g/dl, or evidence of disease transformation.
- Treatment is directed at both hyperviscosity and the lymphoproliferative disorder itself.

NONPHARMACOLOGIC THERAPY

Asymptomatic patients do not require treatment, and these patients should be monitored periodically for the onset of symptoms or changes in blood tests (e.g., worsening anemia, thrombocytopenia, rising IgM levels, and serum viscosity). Plasmapheresis should be the initial treatment in patients with symptoms of hyperviscosity or cryoglobulinemia followed immediately by more definitive therapy. Serum IgM level, percentage of bone marrow involvement, serum albumin level, and serum beta 2-microglobuline level can be used to estimate the risk of requiring therapy (https://awmrisk.com).

INITIAL Rx

- Treatment of the lymphoproliferative disorder includes single or combination therapy. There is no universally agreed upon standard of care:
  1. Combination regimens include alkylating agents (cyclophosphamide and bendamustine) or proteasome inhibitors (bortezomib, carfilzomib, and ixazomib) in combination with rituximab. These should be used in patients with severe constitutional symptoms, symptomatic bulky disease, hyperviscosity, or profound hematologic compromise. Response rates are 80% to 90% with any of these regimens.
  2. Rituximab, a monoclonal anti-CD20 antibody, can be used in symptomatic patients who are not candidates for combination therapy. Response rates are 40% to 50%. Rituximab can be used as maintenance therapy after rituximab-containing combination regimens.
  3. In April 2015, the FDA granted approval for the oral Bruton tyrosine kinase (BTK) inhibitor ibrutinib to be used in patients with symptomatic WM. The response rate to ibrutinib is 90%, with a median time to response of 4 wk. Major responses were absent in patients who do not carry the *MYD88* mutation. The response was delayed in patients who carry any *CXCR4* mutation.
  4. In August 2018, the FDA approved the combination of ibrutinib and rituximab for the treatment of symptomatic WM patients. The combination was associated with higher response rate and longer median progression-free survival than rituximab and placebo.
  5. Treatment with BTK inhibitors should continue until disease progression or unacceptable toxicity.

RX ON RELAPSED/REFRACTORY DISEASE

- Previously treated patients can be retried on original therapy if length of response from initial therapy was substantial. If the response from the initial therapy was short, alternative first-line agents can be used.
- Other treatment options: Fludarabine, ofatumumab, thalidomide, everolimus, and clinical trials. Autologous stem cell transplantation should be considered in heavily pretreated patients.
- Acalabrutinib and zanubrutinib are new BTK inhibitors that have shown to be safe and effective in WM patients. These agents have higher affinity for BTK, fewer off-target effects, and might be associated with lower rates of atrial fibrillation than ibrutinib.

DISPOSITION

- The progression of WM is slow and insidious, with median survival from time of diagnosis of about 10 yr. Table 2 summarizes

TABLE 3 Prognostic Scoring Systems in Waldenström Macroglobulinemia

Study	Adverse Prognostic Factors	Number of Groups	Survival
Gobbi et al[1]	Hgb <9 g/dl Age >70 yr Weight loss Cryoglobulinemia	0-1 prognostic factors 2-4 prognostic factors	Median: 48 mo Median: 80 mo
Morel et al[2]	Age ≥65 yr Albumin <4 g/dl Number of cytopenias: Hgb <12 g/dl Platelets <150 × 10^9/L WBC <4 × 10^9/L	0-1 prognostic factors 2 prognostic factors 3-4 prognostic factors	5-yr: 87% of patients 5-yr: 62% 5-yr: 25%
Dhodapkar et al[3]	β_2M ≥3 g/dl Hgb <12 g/dl IgM <4 g/dl	β_2M <3 mg/dl + Hgb ≥12 g/dl β_2M <3 mg/dl + Hgb <12 g/dl β_2M ≥3 mg/dl + IgM ≥4 g/dl β_2M ≥3 mg/dl + IgM <4 g/dl	5-yr: 87% of patients 5-yr: 63% 5-yr: 53% 5-yr: 21%
Dimopoulos et al[4]	Albumin ≤3.5 g/dl β_2M ≥3.5 mg/L	Albumin ≥3.5 g/dl + β_2M <3.5 mg/dl Albumin ≤3.5 g/dl + β_2M <3.5 or β_2M 3.5-5.5 mg/dl β_2M >5.5 mg/dl	Median: NR Median: 116 mo Median: 54 mo
Morel et al[5]	Age >65 yr Hgb <11.5 g/dl Platelets <100 × 10^9/L β_2M >3 mg/L IgM >7 g/dl	0-1 prognostic factors (excluding age) 2 prognostic factors (or age >65 yr) 3-5 prognostic factors	5 yr: 87% of patients 5 yr: 68% 5 yr: 36%

β_2M, β_2-microglobulin; *Hgb,* hemoglobulin; *IgM,* immunoglobulin M; *NR,* not reported; *WBC,* white blood cell count.
[1]Gobbi PG et al: Study of prognosis in Waldenström's macroglobulinemia: a proposal for a simple binary classification with clinical and investigational utility. *Blood* 83:2939, 1994.
[2]Morel P et al: Prognostic factors in Waldenström macroglobulinemia: a report on 232 patients with the description of a new scoring system and its validation on 253 other patients. *Blood* 96:852, 2000.
[3]Dhodapkar MV et al: Prognostic factors and response to fludarabine therapy in patients with Waldenström macroglobulinemia: results of United States intergroup trial (Southwest Oncology Group S9003). *Blood* 98:41, 2001.
[4]Dimopoulos M et al: The international staging system for multiple myeloma is applicable in symptomatic Waldenström's macroglobulinemia. *Leuk Lymphoma* 45:1809, 2004.
[5]Morel P et al: International prognostic scoring system for Waldenström macroglobulinemia. *Blood* 113:4163, 2009.
From Hoffman R et al: *Hematology, basic principles and practice,* ed 7, Philadelphia, 2018, Elsevier.

consensus response criteria for Waldenström macroglobulinemia.
- Younger patients tend to have more prolonged survival.
- About 10% to 20% of patients die from progression of the disease.
- Some patients develop acute myelogenous leukemia, usually secondary to exposure to chemotherapy, and some patients can develop more aggressive lymphomas.
- The risk of thyroid cancer, kidney cancer, and melanoma is increased in patients with WM.
- A staging system using age, serum beta 2-microglobulin level, hemoglobin level, platelet count and serum IgM concentration before treatment provide insight into prognosis and survival. Prognostic scoring systems in Waldenström macroglobulinemia are summarized in Table 3.

REFERRAL

A hematology consultation is helpful in guiding future workup, treatment, and monitoring. Participation in clinical trials is highly encouraged in patients with WM.

PEARLS & CONSIDERATIONS

COMMENTS

WM was first described in 1944 by the Swedish physician Jan Gösta Waldenström, who also described the X-linked Bruton agammaglobulinemia.

SUGGESTED READINGS

Available at ExpertConsult.com

AUTHOR: **Jorge J. Castillo, MD**

BASIC INFORMATION

DEFINITION

Warts are benign epidermal lesions caused by human papillomavirus (HPV).

SYNONYMS

Verruca vulgaris (common warts)
Verruca plana (flat warts)
Condyloma acuminatum (venereal warts)
Verruca plantaris (plantar warts)
Mosaic warts (cluster of many warts)
HPV infection

ICD-10CM CODES

B07.9	Viral wart, unspecified
B07.8	Other viral warts
A63.0	Anogenital (venereal) warts
B07.0	Plantar wart

EPIDEMIOLOGY & DEMOGRAPHICS

- Risk factors include use of communal showers, occupational handling of meat, and immunosuppression. Common warts occur most frequently in children and young adults.
- Anogenital warts are most common in young, sexually active patients. Genital warts are the most common viral sexually transmitted disease in the U.S., with up to 79 million Americans carrying the causative virus, and 14 million persons are newly infected each yr in the U.S.
- Persistent infection with oncogenic HPV types can cause cervical cancer in women as well as other anogenital and oropharyngeal cancers in women and men. 66% of cervical cancers, 55% of vaginal cancers, 79% of anal cancers, and 62% of oropharyngeal cancers are attributable to HPV types 16 or 18.
- Common warts are longer lasting and more frequent in immunocompromised patients (e.g., lymphoma, AIDS, immunosuppressive drugs).
- Plantar warts occur most frequently at points of maximal pressure (over the heads of the metatarsal bones or on the heels).

PHYSICAL FINDINGS & CLINICAL PRESENTATION

- Common warts (Fig. E1) have an initial appearance of a flesh-colored papule with a rough surface; they subsequently develop a hyperkeratotic appearance with black dots on the surface (thrombosed capillaries). They may be single or multiple and are most common on the hands.
- Warts obscure normal skin lines (important diagnostic feature). Cylindrical projections from the wart may become fused, forming a mosaic pattern.
- Flat warts (Fig. E2) generally are pink or light yellow, slightly elevated, and often found on the forehead, back of hands, mouth, and beard area. They often occur in lines corresponding to trauma (e.g., a scratch), are often misdiagnosed (particularly when present on the face), and are inappropriately treated with topical corticosteroids.
- Filiform warts have a fingerlike appearance with various projections; they are generally found near the mouth, beard, or periorbital and paranasal regions.
- Plantar warts (Fig. E3) are slightly raised and have a roughened surface; they may cause pain when walking; as they involute, small hemorrhages (caused by thrombosed capillaries) may be noted.
- Genital warts (Fig. E4) are generally pale pink with several projections and a broad base. They may coalesce in the perineal area to form masses with a cauliflower-like appearance. Intraanal warts occur predominantly in patients who have had receptive anal intercourse, in contrast with perianal warts, which may occur in men and women without a history of anal sex.
- Genital warts on the cervical epithelium can produce subclinical changes that may be noted on Pap smear or colposcopy.

ETIOLOGY

- HPV infection; >150 types of viral DNA have been identified. Transmission of warts is by direct contact. Approximately 40 different types of HPV are transmitted through sexual contact.
- Genital warts: 90% are caused by HPV types 6 or 11. HPV types 16, 18, 31, 33, and 35 are found occasionally in visible genital warts (usually as coinfections with HPV 6 or 11) and can be associated with foci of high-grade, intraepithelial neoplasia, particularly in persons who are infected with HIV infection. In addition to warts on genital areas, HPV types 6 and 11 have been associated with conjunctival, nasal, oral, and laryngeal warts.

DIAGNOSIS

DIFFERENTIAL DIAGNOSIS

- Molluscum contagiosum
- Condyloma latum
- Acrochordon (skin tags) or seborrheic keratosis
- Epidermal nevi
- Hypertrophic actinic keratosis
- Squamous cell carcinomas
- Acquired digital fibrokeratoma
- Varicella-zoster virus in patients with AIDS
- Recurrent infantile digital fibroma
- Plantar corns (may be mistaken for plantar warts)

WORKUP

- Diagnosis is generally based on clinical findings.
- Suspect lesions should be biopsied.
- The application of 3% to 5% acetic acid, which causes skin color to turn white, has been used by some providers to detect HPV-infected genital mucosa. However, acetic acid application is not a specific test for HPV infection. Therefore, the routine use of this procedure for screening to detect mucosal changes attributed to HPV infection is not recommended.

LABORATORY TESTS

- Screening for cervical cancer with cytology, which is performed by either Pap smear or liquid-based cytology. Screening guidelines recommend starting screening at age 21. Annual cytology is recommended until at least three normal cytology results are obtained.
- Colposcopy with biopsy is recommended in patients with cervical squamous cell changes.

TREATMENT

NONPHARMACOLOGIC THERAPY

- Importance of use of condoms to reduce transmission of genital warts should be emphasized.
- Watchful waiting is an acceptable option in the treatment of nongenital cutaneous warts because many warts will disappear without intervention over time. However, many patients often request treatment because of social stigma or discomfort.
- Plantar warts that are not painful do not need treatment.
- Factors that influence selection of treatment include wart size, wart number, anatomic site of the wart, wart morphology, patient preference, cost of treatment, convenience, adverse effects, and provider experience. Factors that might affect response to therapy include the presence of immunosuppression and compliance with therapy.

GENERAL Rx

- Common warts (Fig. 5):
  1. Application of topical salicylic acid 17%. Soak area for 5 min in warm water and dry. Apply thin layer once or twice daily for up to 12 wk, avoiding normal skin. Bandage.
  2. Liquid nitrogen and electrocautery are also common methods of removal. Cure rates for cryotherapy are 50% to 70% after three to four treatments.
  3. Blunt dissection can be used in large lesions or resistant lesions.
  4. Duct tape occlusion is also effective for treating common warts. It is cut to cover warts and left in place for 6 days. It is removed after 6 days and the warts are soaked in water and then filed with pumice stones. New tape is applied 12 hr later. This treatment can be repeated until warts resolve.
  5. Recalcitrant warts can be treated with injection of *Candida* or mumps skin antigen into the wart every 3 to 4 wk for up to three treatments, photodynamic therapy with aminolevulinic acid, pulsed dye laser, and intralesional bleomycin.
- Filiform warts: Surgical removal is necessary.
- Flat warts: Generally more difficult to treat.

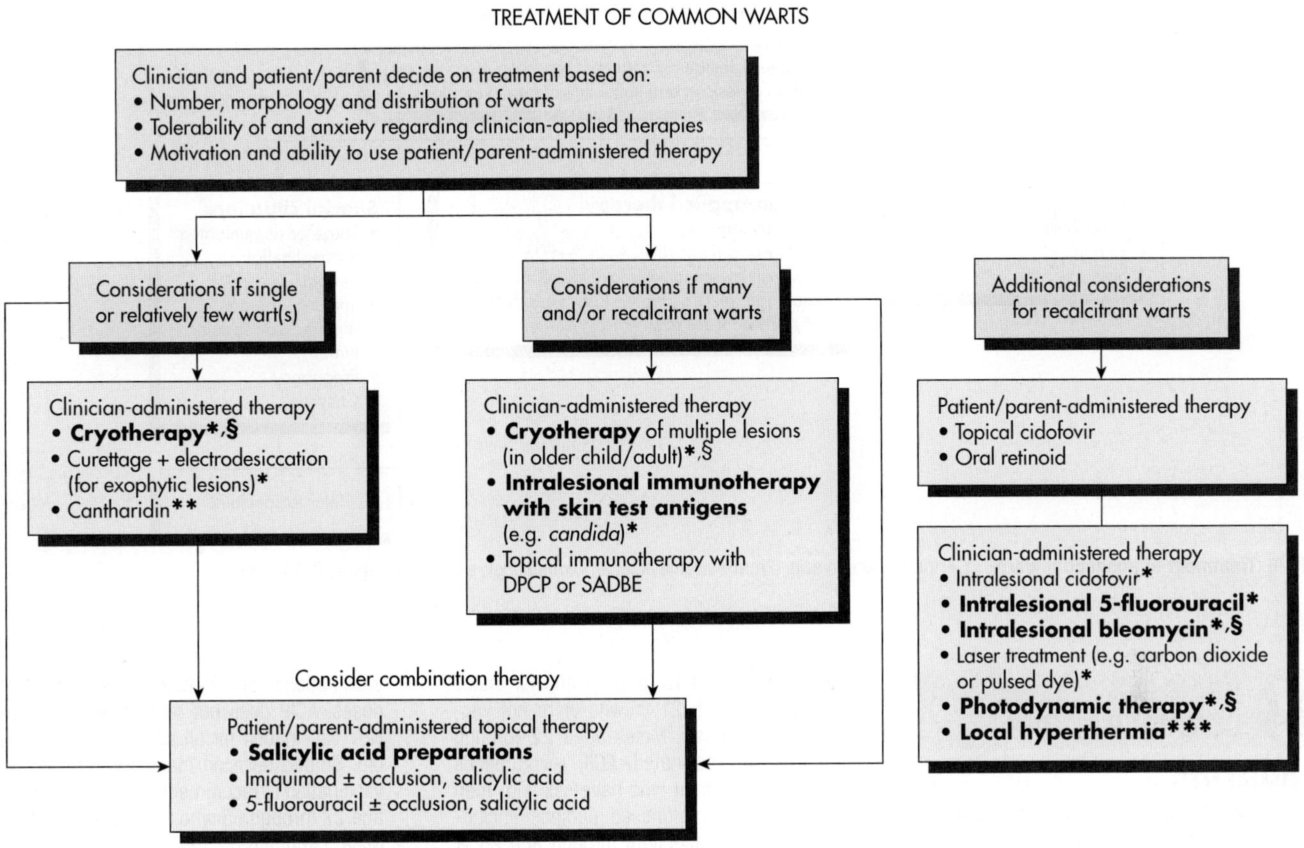

* Treatment-related discomfort/anxiety may be difficult for young children to tolerate
** Higher likelihood of "doughnut" wart formation; may be combined with podophyllotoxin and salicylic acid
§ Results in controlled trials have been inconsistent
*** 44°C/111°F for 30 minutes on days 1, 2, 3, 17 and 18

FIG. 5 Treatment of common warts. Therapies found to be effective in controlled trials are in bold . While still employed by some clinicians, three double-blind, placebo-controlled trials failed to confirm efficacy of cimetidine therapy for recalcitrant common warts. *DPCP,* diphenylcyclopropenone; *SADBE,* squaric acid dibutyl ester. (From Bolognia JL et al: *Dermatology,* ed 4, 2018, Philadelphia, Elsevier.)

1. Tretinoin cream applied at bedtime over the involved area for several weeks may be effective.
2. Application of liquid nitrogen.
3. Electrocautery.
4. 5-Fluorouracil cream applied once or twice a day for 3 to 5 wk is also effective. Persistent hyperpigmentation may occur after Efudex use.

- Plantar warts:
  1. Salicylic acid therapy (e.g., Occlusal-HP). Soak wart in warm water for 5 min, remove loose tissue, dry. Apply to area, allow to dry, reapply. Use once or twice daily; maximum 12 wk. Use of 40% salicylic acid plasters (Mediplast) is also a safe, nonscarring treatment; it is particularly useful in treating mosaic warts covering a large area.
  2. Blunt dissection is also a fast and effective treatment modality.
  3. Laser therapy can be used for plantar warts and recurrent warts; however, it leaves open wounds that require 4 to 6 wk to fill with granulation tissue.
  4. Interlesional bleomycin is also effective but generally used when all other treatments fail.
- Genital warts (Fig. 6):
  1. Can be effectively treated with 20% podophyllin resin in compound tincture of benzoin applied with a cotton tip applicator by the treating physician and allowed to air dry. The treatment can be repeated weekly if necessary.
  2. Podofilox (Condylox 0.5% gel) is available for application by the patient. Local adverse effects include pain, burning, and inflammation at the site.
  3. Cryosurgery with liquid nitrogen delivered with a probe or as a spray is effective for treating smaller genital warts.
  4. Carbon dioxide laser can also be used for treating primary or recurrent genital warts (cure rate >90%).
  5. Imiquimod cream, 5%, is a patient-applied immune response modifier effective in the treatment of external genital and perianal warts (complete clearing of genital warts in >70% of females and >30% of males in 4-16 wk). Sexual contact should be avoided while the cream is on the skin. It is applied 3 times per wk before normal sleeping hours and is left on the skin for 6 to 10 hr.
  6. Sinecatechins (Veregen), a botanical drug product, is also effective for treatment of external genital and perianal warts. Formulation is a 15% ointment applied to affected area tid for up to 16 wk.
- Application of trichloroacetic acid or bichloroacetic acid 80% to 90% is also effective for external genital warts. A small amount should be applied only to warts and allowed to dry, at which time a white "frosting" develops. This treatment can be repeated weekly if necessary.

DISPOSITION

- Warts can be effectively treated with the previous modalities with complete resolution in the majority of patients; however, the recurrence rate is high.
- Cervical carcinomas and precancerous lesions in women are associated with genital papillomavirus infection.
- Squamous cell anal cancer is also associated with a history of genital warts.

REFERRAL

- Dermatology referral for warts resistant to conservative therapy
- Surgical referral in selected cases
- Sexually transmitted disease counseling for patients with anogenital warts

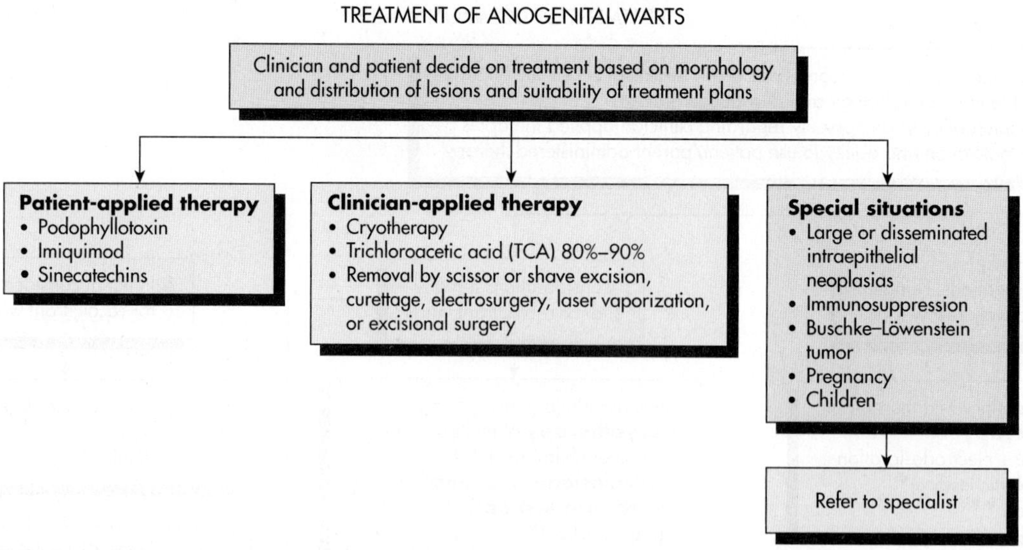

FIG. 6 Treatment of anogenital warts. *TCA*, trichloroacetic acid. (From Bolognia JL et al: *Dermatology*, ed 4, Philadelphia, 2018, Elsevier.)

PEARLS & CONSIDERATIONS

COMMENTS

- Subungual and periungual warts are generally more resistant to treatment. Dermatology referral for cryosurgery is recommended in resistant cases.
- Examination of sex partners is not necessary for the management of genital warts because no data indicate that reinfection plays a role.

PREVENTION

- Two HPV vaccines (Gardasil, Gardasil-9, Cervarix) have been licensed in the U.S. Advisory Committee on Immunization Practices (ACIP) recommends routine vaccination with HPV4 or HPV2 for females aged 11 to 12 yr and HPV4 for males aged 11 to 12 yr. Vaccination is also recommended for females aged 13 to 26 yr and for males aged 13 through 21 yr who were not vaccinated previously. Males aged 22 through 26 may be vaccinated. ACIP recommends vaccination of men who have sex with men and immunocompromised persons (including those with infection) through age 26 yr if not previously vaccinated. The 9-valent HPV vaccine (Gardasil-9) is approved for use in girls and women 9 to 26 yr old and boys 9 to 15 yr old. It is indicated to prevent diseases associated with HPV infection with types 6, 11, 16, 18, 31, 33, 45, 52, and 58. It appears to be more effective than the other 2 currently available vaccines. It consists of two doses. The first dose is administered at 11 to 12 yr of age, and the second dose 6 to 12 mo later. However, if the second dose is given less than 5 mo apart, a third dose will be needed at age 9 to 14. Patients with a weak immune system and in those starting vaccination at age 15 to 26 yr will need three doses. ACIP does not recommend catch-up HPV vaccination for all adults over 26 years old. Shared decision making regarding HPV vaccination is recommended for some adults age 27 through 65 who are unvaccinated.
- Male circumcision decreases heterosexual transmission of HPV.

SUGGESTED READINGS

Available at ExpertConsult.com

RELATED CONTENT

Human Papillomavirus Infection (Patient Information)
Warts (Patient Information)
Condyloma Acuminatum (Related Key Topic)

AUTHOR: **Fred F. Ferri, MD**

BASIC INFORMATION

DEFINITION

Wolff-Parkinson-White (WPW) syndrome is a congenital heart condition in which, in addition to the normal electrical conduction through the atrioventricular (AV) node, there is an accessory pathway (AP) that connects the atria to the ventricles. Consequently, a portion of the ventricular myocardium is depolarized via the AP earlier than the normal AV nodal conduction, resulting in ventricular preexcitation. The terms "WPW syndrome" and "WPW pattern" often are used in describing patients with ventricular preexcitation. Patients with WPW syndrome have ECG findings of preexcitation, including short PR and slurring of the initial segment of the QRS complex known as the delta wave together with symptoms suggestive of arrhythmia or documented arrhythmia, which may be atrioventricular (AV) reentrant tachycardia, atrial fibrillation (AF), or both. Patients with the WPW pattern have characteristic ECG findings of preexcitation without evidence of symptoms or arrhythmia.

SYNONYMS

Preexcitation syndrome
WPW

ICD-10CM CODE

I45.6 Preexcitation syndrome

EPIDEMIOLOGY & DEMOGRAPHICS

- The prevalence of a WPW pattern on the surface ECG is 0.1% to 0.3% in the general population. The prevalence is increased to 0.55% in first-degree relatives of affected patients. It is estimated that approximately 65% of adolescents and 40% of individuals older than 30 yr with WPW pattern on a resting ECG are asymptomatic.
- The prevalence of WPW is higher among males and decreases with age.
- Most patients with WPW have structurally normal hearts, but it may also occur in patients with congenital heart disease, most notably in patients with Ebstein anomaly, which is associated with right-side AP and often multiple and slowly conducting APs.

PHYSICAL FINDINGS & CLINICAL PRESENTATION

- The physical examination is usually unremarkable.
- Symptoms are typically related to tachyarrhythmias, including the following:
  1. Palpitations, lightheadedness, anxiety, dyspnea, or chest pain
  2. Syncope or near syncope
  3. Sudden cardiac death
- The common arrhythmias in WPW syndrome are:
  1. Supraventricular tachycardia: AV reciprocating tachycardia (AVRT). This is the most common arrhythmia, further classified as orthodromic AVRT (narrow complex tachycardia, with antegrade conduction through the AV node and retrograde conduction via the AP that occurs in 70% of symptomatic patients) or antidromic AVRT (wide complex tachycardia with antegrade conduction via the AP and retrogradely through the AV node, which occurs in 4% to 5% of patients).
  2. AF (~10%-38%), the second most common tachycardia, can be complicated by a very rapid ventricular response due to conduction over the AP, which can lead to ventricular fibrillation (VF) and sudden death. This risk is dependent on the antegrade refractory period of AP during AF.
  3. The risk of sudden death in symptomatic patients with WPW syndrome is estimated to be approximately 0.25% per yr or 3% to 4% over a lifetime.
- In a meta-analysis including approximately 2000 subjects with asymptomatic WPW, children had a sudden death rate of 1.9 compared with 0.9 in adults per 1000 patient-yrs of follow-up. This incidence is comparable with the estimated 0.1% per yr risk of death in the general population in Europe, Japan, and the U.S.

ETIOLOGY & PATHOGENESIS

- APs are thought to be an embryologic remnant, as substantiated by reports of SVT in uterus and by a greater prevalence of WPW in newborns and infants.
- Left free wall APs are most common followed by posteroseptal, right free wall, and anteroseptal locations.
- Some patients with WPW syndrome (~5%-10%) have multiple APs.
- In subjects with WPW, two parallel routes of AV conduction are present: One is subject to delay through the AV node, and the other occurs without delay through the AP and results in preexcitation of the ventricles. The resulting QRS complex is a fusion beat, as a portion of the ventricle is preexcited and activated via the AP giving rise to the delta wave, and the remainder of the ventricle is activated by the normal activation pathway (Fig. 1).
- Reciprocating tachycardias occur when conduction is anterograde in one pathway (usually the AV node, i.e., orthodromic AVRT) and retrograde in the other (usually the AP) as a result of different refractory periods. This is usually initiated by a premature atrial or ventricular depolarization.

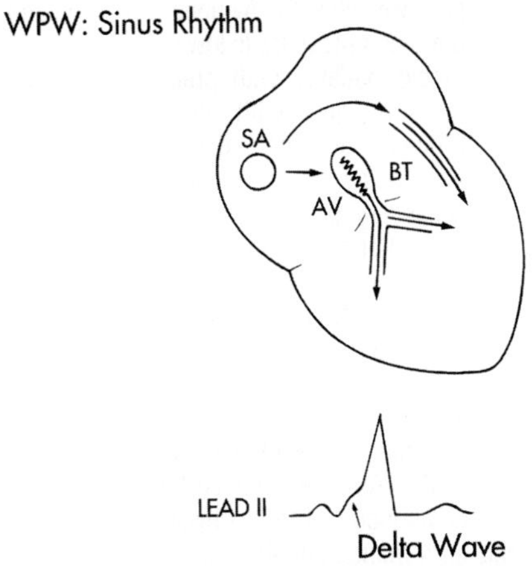

FIG. 1 With Wolff-Parkinson-White (WPW) syndrome, an abnormal accessory pathway called a bypass tract connects the atria and the ventricles.

DIAGNOSIS

- Three basic features characterize the ECG abnormalities associated with WPW pattern:
  1. PR interval <120 ms.
  2. QRS complex can be >120 ms with a slurred, slowly rising onset of QRS in some leads (delta wave) and a normal terminal QRS portion. The width of the QRS complex depends on the amount of preexcited ventricular tissue.
  3. Secondary ST-T wave changes directed in an opposite direction to the major delta and QRS vectors may be present.
- ECG patterns with abnormal QRS complexes and ST and T changes can mask or mimic myocardial infarction (in particular posteroseptal AP with negative delta waves in the inferior wall, which mimics old inferior wall myocardial infarction), bundle branch block (Fig. 2), or ventricular hypertrophy.
- Most commonly seen tachycardia (orthodromic AVRT) is characterized by a normal QRS with a regular rate of 150 to 250 bpm. Onset and termination are abrupt.
- Variants of preexcitation:
  1. Lown-Ganong-Levine syndrome is characterized by a short PR interval, a narrow QRS complex without a delta wave, and a clinical syndrome of paroxysmal SVTs. Postulated mechanisms to the short PR interval include a variant of the normal, enhanced sympathetic tone or specialized intra-nodal fibers with enhanced AV nodal conduction.
  2. Atriofascicular accessory pathway (Mahaim fiber): A slowly conducting AP with AV-nodal like properties that conducts only in antegrade direction and connects the right atrium with the right bundle branch or the apical myocardium. In the baseline state, minimal or no preexcitation may be present. During preexcitation the QRS appears like a typical LBBB pattern. The typical arrhythmia in patients with atriofascicular accessory pathway is antidromic tachycardia with LBBB morphology.
  3. Nodoventricular or nodofascicular APs: Rare variants that connect the AV node and the ventricle or the bundle branch appropriately.
- An electrophysiology study is the gold standard to confirm the diagnosis, determine the location, and assess the conduction properties of the AP.

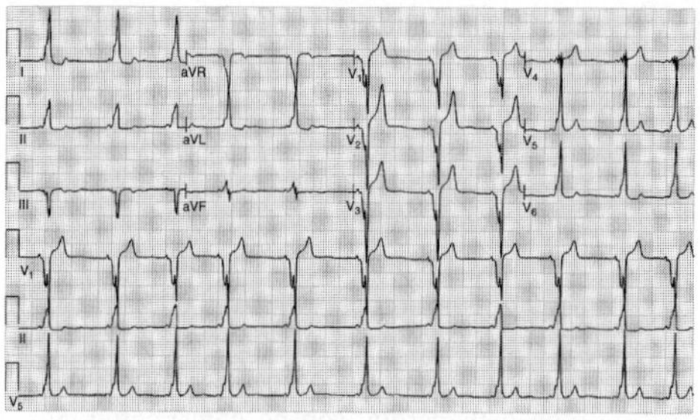

FIG. 2 Wolff-Parkinson-White (WPW) syndrome. This 12-lead electrocardiogram with rhythm strips shows preexcitation with an accessory pathway connecting the right atrium to the right ventricle. This gives rise to a pattern like left bundle branch block because the ventricles are activated over the right-sided accessory pathway. The tracing shows the typical characteristics of WPW syndrome, including a short PR interval, a wide QRS complex, and a delta wave. (From Olshansky B et al: *Arrhythmia essentials*, ed 2, Philadelphia, 2017, Elsevier.)

BOX 1 Goals of Electrophysiologic Evaluation in Patients with Wolff-Parkinson-White Syndrome

- Confirmation of the presence of an accessory pathway (AP)
- Evaluation for the presence of multiple APs
- Localization of the AP(s)
- Evaluation of the refractory period of the AP and its implications for life-threatening arrhythmias
- Induction and evaluation of tachycardias
- Demonstration of the AP role in the tachycardia
- Evaluation of other tachycardias not dependent on the presence of the AP
- Ablation of the AP, when indicated.

From Issa Z et al: *Clinical arrhythmology and electrophysiology*, ed 2, Philadelphia, 2012, WB Saunders.

RISK STRATIFICATION

- Intermittent and abrupt loss of preexcitation on a beat-to-beat basis is usually indicative of lower risk, assessed with Holter monitoring or with an exercise stress test. The loss of preexcitation after administration of the antiarrhythmic drug procainamide has also been used to indicate a low-risk subgroup. More recent evidence, however, has begun to demonstrate that intermittent preexcitation is not 100% specific for identification of a "low-risk" AP. In a study of 295 children at a single institution, "high-risk" EPS characteristics were identified in 5% of patients with intermittent preexcitation and 31% with abrupt loss of preexcitation on exercise test.
- In patients with a persistent preexcitation pattern, electrophysiology study is the procedure of choice for risk stratification.

Rx TREATMENT

Goals of electrophysiologic evaluation in patients with WPW syndrome are described in Box 1.

ACUTE MANAGEMENT

- Urgent cardioversion, for an acute tachycardia episode with hemodynamic instability.
- Narrow QRS tachycardia (c/w orthodromic AVRT):
  1. Vagal maneuvers and/or IV adenosine.
  2. IV beta-blockers, diltiazem, or verapamil can be administered for regular and **narrow** QRS tachycardia, implying antegrade conduction via the AV node, when the patient is hemodynamically stable and IV adenosine is ineffective.
- Wide QRS complex tachycardias (WCTs):
  1. Most commonly caused by atrial fibrillation with antegrade conduction via the AP and the AV node. AV nodal blocking therapies (i.e., beta-blockers, calcium channel blockers, digoxin, and adenosine) are potentially dangerous and should be avoided in these cases because of the risk of causing VF by enhancement of the ventricular response through the accessory pathway when the AV node is blocked and the blood pressure is lowered.
  2. Stable patients with preexcited AF can be managed with IV procainamide. Procainamide can decrease ventricular rate by slowing conduction over the accessory pathway and have the additional benefit of possibly terminating AF. Electrical cardioversion should be performed if the patient is hemodynamically unstable.
  3. In a patient with WCT due to antidromic tachycardia, drug treatment may be directed at the AP (IV procainamide) or at the AV node because both are critical components of the tachycardia circuit.

Long-term management:

- Asymptomatic:
  1. In low-risk patients with AP effective refractory period (APERP) ≥250 ms, or shortest preexcited RR interval (SPERRI) ≥250 ms, no therapy is required. An electrophysiology study may be considered in asymptomatic patients with intermittent loss of preexcitation for further risk stratification in order to assess the APERP and SPERRI.
  2. In high-risk patients with APERP ≤250 ms or SPERRI≤ 250 ms, competitive athletes, or high-risk occupation (i.e., pilots), ablation should be considered.
- Symptomatic:
  1. Patients who presented with aborted sudden cardiac death, preexcited tachycardia (i.e., atrial fibrillation, flutter, atrial tachycardia), or syncope suggestive of cardiac origin should undergo an electrophysiology study for further characterization and ablation of the AP accordingly.
  2. Patients with symptomatic palpitations or documented AVRT should be offered an electrophysiology study and ablation of the AP to prevent recurrence and to allow the patient to avoid long-term medical therapy. Ongoing management for stable patients with history of orthodromic AVRT who are not candidates for, or prefer not to undergo, catheter ablation:
     - Class IC antiarrhythmics (flecainide, propafenone), in the absence of structural heart disease.
     - Class III antiarrhythmics (amiodarone, sotalol or dofetilide).
     - Oral beta blockers, diltiazem, or verapamil.

SUGGESTED READINGS

Available at ExpertConsult.com

RELATED CONTENT

Wolff-Parkinson-White Syndrome (Patient Information)

AUTHOR: **Yuval Konstantino, MD**

SECTION II

Differential Diagnosis

ABDOMINAL DISTENTION

ICD-10CM # R14.0 Abdominal distension (gaseous)

NONMECHANICAL OBSTRUCTION

Excessive intraluminal gas.
Intraabdominal infection.
Trauma.
Retroperitoneal irritation (renal colic, neoplasms, infections, hemorrhage).
Vascular insufficiency (thrombosis, embolism).
Mechanical ventilation.
Extraabdominal infection (sepsis, pneumonia, empyema, osteomyelitis of spine).
Metabolic/toxic abnormalities (hypokalemia, uremia, lead poisoning).
Chemical irritation (perforated ulcer, bile, pancreatitis).
Peritoneal inflammation.
Severe pain, pain medications.

MECHANICAL OBSTRUCTION

Neoplasm (intraluminal, extraluminal).
Adhesions, endometriosis.
Infection (intraabdominal abscess, diverticulitis).
Gallstones.
Foreign body, bezoars.
Pregnancy.
Hernias.
Volvulus.
Stenosis at surgical anastomosis, radiation stenosis.
Fecaliths.
Inflammatory bowel disease.
Gastric outlet obstruction.
Hematoma.
Other: parasites, superior mesenteric artery (SMA) syndrome, pneumatosis intestinalis, annular pancreas, Hirschsprung disease, intussusception, meconium.

ABDOMINAL PAIN, ADOLESCENCE[63]

ICD-10CM # R10.817 Generalized abdominal tenderness
R10.827 Generalized rebound abdominal tenderness

Acute gastroenteritis.
Irritable bowel syndrome (IBS).
Anxiety.
Mittelschmerz.
Appendicitis.
Inflammatory bowel disease.
Peptic ulcer disease (PUD).
Cholecystitis.
Neoplasm.
Diabetic ketoacidosis.
Functional abdominal pain.
Pelvic inflammatory disease (PID).
Pregnancy.
Pyelonephritis.
Renal stone.
Trauma.

ABDOMINAL PAIN, CHILDHOOD[63]

ICD-10CM # R10.817 Generalized abdominal tenderness
R10.827 Generalized rebound abdominal tenderness

Acute gastroenteritis.
Appendicitis.
Constipation.
Cholecystitis, acute.
Intestinal obstruction.
Pancreatitis.
Neoplasm.
Inflammatory bowel disease.
Other:
- Functional abdominal pain.
- Pyelonephritis.
- Pneumonia.
- Diabetic ketoacidosis.
- Heavy metal poisoning.
- Sickle cell crisis.
- Trauma.
- Anxiety.
- Sexual abuse.

ABDOMINAL PAIN, CHRONIC LOWER[95]

ICD-10CM # R10.814 Left lower quadrant abdominal tenderness
R10.824 Left lower quadrant rebound abdominal tenderness
R10.813 Right lower quadrant abdominal tenderness
R10.823 Right lower quadrant rebound abdominal tenderness
R10.30 Lower abdominal pain, unspecified

ORGANIC DISORDERS

Common
Gynecologic disease.
Lactase deficiency.
Diverticulitis/diverticulosis.
Crohn disease.
Intestinal obstruction.
Uncommon
Chronic intestinal pseudoobstruction.
Mesenteric ischemia.
Malignancy (e.g., ovarian carcinoma).
Abdominal wall pain.
Spinal disease.
Testicular disease.
Metabolic diseases (e.g., diabetes mellitus, familial Mediterranean fever, C1 esterase deficiency [angioneurotic edema], porphyria, lead poisoning, tabes dorsalis, renal failure).

FUNCTIONAL DISORDERS

Common
Irritable bowel syndrome.
Functional abdominal bloating.
Uncommon
Functional abdominal pain.

ABDOMINAL PAIN, DIFFUSE

ICD-10CM # R10.817 Generalized abdominal tenderness
R10.827 Generalized rebound abdominal tenderness

Early appendicitis.
Aortic aneurysm.
Gastroenteritis.
Intestinal obstruction.
Diverticulitis.
Peritonitis.
Mesenteric insufficiency or infarction.
Pancreatitis.
Inflammatory bowel disease.
Irritable bowel.
Mesenteric adenitis.
Metabolic: toxins, lead poisoning, uremia, drug overdose, diabetic ketoacidosis (DKA), heavy metal poisoning.
Sickle cell crisis.
Pneumonia (rare).
Trauma.
Urinary tract infection, PID.
Other: anxiety, acute intermittent porphyria, tabes dorsalis, periarteritis nodosa, Henoch-Schönlein purpura, adrenal insufficiency.

ABDOMINAL PAIN, EPIGASTRIC

ICD-10CM # R10.816 Epigastric abdominal tenderness
R10.826 Epigastric rebound abdominal tenderness

Gastric: PUD, gastric outlet obstruction, gastric ulcer.
Duodenal: PUD, duodenitis.
Biliary: cholecystitis, cholangitis, biliary dyskinesia.
Hepatic: hepatitis.
Pancreatic: pancreatitis.
Intestinal: high small bowel obstruction, early appendicitis.
Cardiac: angina, MI, pericarditis.
Pulmonary: pneumonia, pleurisy, pneumothorax.
Subphrenic abscess.
Vascular: dissecting aneurysm, mesenteric ischemia.
Psychiatric: anxiety.

ABDOMINAL PAIN, EXTRAABDOMINAL AND SYSTEMIC CAUSES[30]

ICD-10CM # R10.817 Generalized abdominal tenderness

EXTRAABDOMINAL AND SYSTEMIC CAUSES OF ACUTE ABDOMINAL PAIN

Cardiac
Endocarditis.
Heart failure.
Myocardial ischemia and infarction.
Myocarditis.

Thoracic
Empyema.
Esophageal rupture (Boerhaave syndrome).
Esophageal spasm.
Esophagitis.
Pleurodynia (Bornholm disease).
Pneumonitis.
Pneumothorax.
Pulmonary embolism and infarction.

Hematologic
Acute leukemia.
Hemolytic anemia.
Henoch-Schönlein purpura.
Sickle cell disease.

Metabolic
Acute adrenal insufficiency (Addison disease).
Diabetes mellitus (especially with ketoacidosis).
Hyperlipidemia.
Hyperparathyroidism.
Hypersensitivity reactions (e.g., to insect bites, reptile venoms).
Lead poisoning.
Porphyria.
Toxins.
Uremia.

Infections
Herpes zoster.
Osteomyelitis.
Typhoid fever.

Neurologic
Abdominal epilepsy.
Radiculopathy, spinal cord or peripheral nerve tumors, degenerative arthritis of spine, herniated vertebral disk.
Tabes dorsalis.

Miscellaneous
Angioedema.
Familial Mediterranean fever.
Heat stroke.
Muscle contusion, hematoma, tumor.
Narcotic withdrawal.
Psychiatric disorders.

ABDOMINAL PAIN, INFANCY[63]

ICD-10CM #	R10.817	Generalized abdominal tenderness
	R10.827	Generalized rebound abdominal tenderness

Acute gastroenteritis.
Appendicitis.
Intussusception.
Volvulus.
Meckel diverticulum.
Other: colic, trauma.

ABDOMINAL PAIN, LEFT LOWER QUADRANT

ICD-10CM #	R10.814	Left lower quadrant abdominal tenderness
	R10.824	Left lower quadrant rebound abdominal tenderness

Intestinal: diverticulitis, diverticulosis, intestinal obstruction, perforated ulcer, inflammatory bowel disease, perforated descending colon, inguinal hernia, neoplasm, appendicitis.
Reproductive: ectopic pregnancy, ovarian cyst, torsion of ovarian cyst, tuboovarian abscess, mittelschmerz, endometriosis, seminal vesiculitis.
Renal: renal or ureteral calculi, pyelonephritis, neoplasm.
Vascular: leaking aortic aneurysm.
Psoas abscess.
Trauma.

ABDOMINAL PAIN, LEFT UPPER QUADRANT

ICD-10CM #	R19.02	Left upper quadrant abdominal swelling, mass, and lump

Gastric: PUD, gastritis, pyloric stenosis, hiatal hernia.
Pancreatic: pancreatitis, neoplasm, stone in pancreatic duct or ampulla.
Cardiac: MI, angina pectoris.
Splenic: splenomegaly, ruptured spleen, splenic abscess, splenic infarction.
Renal: calculi, pyelonephritis, neoplasm.
Pulmonary: pneumonia, empyema, pulmonary infarction.
Vascular: ruptured aortic aneurysm.
Cutaneous: herpes zoster.
Trauma.
Intestinal: high fecal impaction, perforated colon, diverticulitis.

ABDOMINAL PAIN, NONSURGICAL CAUSES

ICD-10CM #	R19.8	Other specified symptoms and signs involving the digestive system and abdomen
	R10.817	Generalized abdominal tenderness

Irritable bowel syndrome.
Urinary tract infection, pyelonephritis, salpingitis, PID.
Gastroenteritis, gastritis, peptic ulcer.
Diverticular spasm.
Hepatitis, mononucleosis.
Pancreatitis.
Inferior wall myocardial infarction.
Basilar pneumonia, pulmonary embolism.
Diabetic ketoacidosis.
Strain or hematoma of rectus muscle.
Ruptured Graafian follicle.
Herpes zoster.
Nerve root compression.
Sickle cell crisis.
Acute adrenal insufficiency.
Other: acute porphyria, familial Mediterranean fever, tabes dorsalis, anxiety, sexual abuse.

ABDOMINAL PAIN, PERIUMBILICAL

ICD-10CM #	R10.815	Periumbilic abdominal tenderness
	R10.825	Periumbilic rebound abdominal tenderness

Intestinal: small bowel obstruction or gangrene, early appendicitis.
Vascular: mesenteric thrombosis, dissecting aortic aneurysm.
Pancreatic: pancreatitis.
Metabolic: uremia, DKA.
Trauma.

ABDOMINAL PAIN, POORLY LOCALIZED[63]

ICD-10CM #	R10.819	Abdominal tenderness, unspecified site

EXTRAABDOMINAL

Metabolic
DKA, acute intermittent porphyria, hyperthyroidism, hypothyroidism, hypercalcemia, hypokalemia, uremia, hyperlipidemia, hyperparathyroidism.

Hematologic
Sickle cell crisis, leukemia or lymphoma, Henoch-Schönlein purpura.

Infectious
Infectious mononucleosis, Rocky Mountain spotted fever, acquired immunodeficiency syndrome (AIDS), streptococcal pharyngitis (in children), herpes zoster.

Drugs and Toxins
Heavy metal poisoning, black widow spider bites, withdrawal syndromes, mushroom ingestion.

Referred Pain
Pulmonary: pneumonia, pulmonary embolism, pneumothorax.
Cardiac: angina, MI, pericarditis, myocarditis.
Genitourinary: prostatitis, epididymitis, orchitis, testicular torsion.
Musculoskeletal: rectus sheath hematoma.

Functional
Somatization disorder, malingering, hypochondriasis, Munchausen syndrome.

INTRAABDOMINAL

Early appendicitis, gastroenteritis, peritonitis, pancreatitis, abdominal aortic aneurysm, mesenteric insufficiency or infarction, intestinal obstruction, volvulus, ulcerative colitis.

ABDOMINAL PAIN, POST-CHOLECYSTECTOMY[30]

ICD-10CM # R10.817 Generalized abdominal tenderness

CAUSES OF ABDOMINAL PAIN AFTER CHOLECYSTECTOMY

Biliary Causes

Biliary stricture.
Biliary tract malignancy.
Choledocholithiasis.
Choledochocele.
Cystic duct remnant.
SOD.

Pancreatic Causes

Pancreatitis.
Pseudocyst.
Malignancy.

Other GI Disorders

Esophageal motor disorders.
GERD.
Intestinal malignancy.
Intraabdominal adhesions.
IBS.
Mesenteric ischemia.
PUD.

Extraintestinal Disorders

Coronary artery disease.
Intercostal neuritis.
Neurologic disorders.
Psychiatric disorders.
Wound neuroma.

ABDOMINAL PAIN, PREGNANCY

ICD-10CM # R10.817 Generalized abdominal tenderness
R10.827 Generalized rebound abdominal tenderness

GYNECOLOGIC (GESTATIONAL AGE IN PARENTHESES)

Miscarriage	(<20 wk; 80% <12 wk)
Septic abortion	(<20 wk)
Ectopic pregnancy	(<14 wk)
Corpus luteum cyst rupture	(<12 wk)
Ovarian torsion	(especially <24 wk)
Pelvic inflammatory disease	(<12 wk)
Chorioamnionitis	(>16 wk)
Abruptio placentae	(>16 wk)

NONGYNECOLOGIC

Appendicitis	(Throughout)
Cholecystitis	(Throughout)
Hepatitis	(Throughout)
Pyelonephritis	(Throughout)
Preeclampsia	(>20 wk)

ABDOMINAL PAIN, RIGHT LOWER QUADRANT

ICD-10CM # R10.813 Right lower quadrant abdominal tenderness
R10.823 Right lower quadrant rebound abdominal tenderness

Intestinal: acute appendicitis, regional enteritis, incarcerated hernia, cecal diverticulitis, intestinal obstruction, perforated ulcer, perforated cecum, Meckel diverticulitis.
Reproductive: ectopic pregnancy, ovarian cyst, torsion of ovarian cyst, salpingitis, tuboovarian abscess, mittelschmerz, endometriosis, seminal vesiculitis.
Renal: renal and ureteral calculi, neoplasms, pyelonephritis.
Vascular: leaking aortic aneurysm.
Cutaneous: herpes zoster.
Psoas abscess.
Trauma.
Cholecystitis.

ABDOMINAL PAIN, RIGHT UPPER QUADRANT

ICD-10CM # R10.811 Right upper quadrant abdominal tenderness
R10.821 Right upper quadrant rebound abdominal tenderness

Biliary: calculi, infection, inflammation, neoplasm.
Hepatic: hepatitis, abscess, hepatic congestion, neoplasm, trauma.
Gastric: PUD, pyloric stenosis, neoplasm, alcoholic gastritis, hiatal hernia.
Pancreatic: pancreatitis, neoplasm, stone in pancreatic duct or ampulla.
Renal: calculi, infection, inflammation, neoplasm, rupture of kidney.
Pulmonary: pneumonia, pulmonary infarction, right-sided pleurisy.
Intestinal: retrocecal appendicitis, intestinal obstruction, high fecal impaction, diverticulitis.
Cardiac: myocardial ischemia (particularly involving the inferior wall), pericarditis.
Cutaneous: herpes zoster.
Trauma.
Fitz-Hugh-Curtis syndrome (perihepatitis).

ABDOMINAL PAIN, RIGHT UPPER QUADRANT, DIFFERENTIAL DIAGNOSIS IN PREGNANCY[34]

ICD-10CM # R10.811 Right upper quadrant abdominal tenderness
R10.821 Right upper quadrant rebound abdominal tenderness

DIFFERENTIAL DIAGNOSIS OF RIGHT UPPER QUADRANT ABDOMINAL PAIN DURING PREGNANCY

Hepatic Disorders:
Hepatitis.
Hepatic vascular engorgement.
Hepatic hematoma.
Hepatic malignancy.

Biliary Tract Disease:
Biliary colic.
Choledocholithiasis.
Cholangitis.
Cholecystitis.

Diseases Related to Pregnancy:
Preeclampsia or eclampsia.
Hemolysis, elevated liver enzymes, and low platelet count (HELLP) syndrome.
Acute fatty liver of pregnancy.
Hepatic hemorrhage or rupture.

Renal Disorders:
Pyelonephritis.
Nephrolithiasis.

Gastrointestinal Disorders:
Peptic ulcer disease.
Perforated duodenal ulcer.

Other Conditions in RUQ:
Rib fracture.
Shingles.

Referred Pain from Other Organ Disease:
Pneumonia.
Pulmonary embolus or infarct.
Pleural effusion.
Radiculopathy.
Inferior wall myocardial infarction.
Colon cancer.

ABDOMINAL PAIN, SUPRAPUBIC

ICD-10CM # R10.30 Lower abdominal pain, unspecified

Intestinal: colon obstruction or gangrene, diverticulitis, appendicitis.
Reproductive system: ectopic pregnancy, mittelschmerz, torsion of ovarian cyst, PID, salpingitis, endometriosis, rupture of endometrioma.
Cystitis, rupture of urinary bladder.

ABDOMINAL WALL MASSES[95]

ICD-10CM # R19.00 Intraabdominal and pelvic swelling, mass and lump, unspecified site

LUMPS ARISING IN THE SKIN AND SUBCUTANEOUS FAT (THAT COULD OCCUR ANYWHERE ON THE BODY)

Lipoma.
Sebaceous cyst.

LUMPS ARISING IN THE SKIN AND SUBCUTANEOUS FAT (SPECIFIC TO THE ANTERIOR ABDOMINAL WALL)

Tumor nodule of the umbilicus (secondary to the intraperitoneal malignancy, also called *Sister Mary Joseph nodule*).

LUMPS ARISING IN THE FASCIA AND MUSCLE

Rectus sheath hematoma (usually painful).
Desmoid tumor (associated with Gardner syndrome).

HERNIA

Incisional:	It has an overlying scar. The sac may be very much larger than the neck of the hernia.
Umbilical:	The hernia is through the umbilical scar. Those presenting at birth commonly resolve in the first years of life.
Paraumbilical:	The neck is just lateral to the umbilical scar. Patients usually present later in life.
Epigastric:	It occurs in the midline between the xiphoid process and the umbilicus. They are usually small (<2 cm). They result when a knuckle of extraperitoneal fat extrudes through a small defect in the linea alba. Commonly irreducible and without an expansile cough impulse.
Spigelian:	A rare hernia found along the linea semilunaris at the lateral edge of the rectus sheath, most commonly a third of the way between the umbilicus and the pubis.

DIVARICATION OF THE RECTI

Supraumbilical elliptical swelling of the attenuated linea alba (no cough impulse).

ABORTION, RECURRENT

ICD-10CM # P01.8 Newborn (suspected to be) affected by other maternal complications of pregnancy

Congenital anatomic abnormalities.
Adhesions (uterine synechiae).
Uterine fibroids.
Endometriosis.
Endocrine abnormalities (luteal phase insufficiency, hypothyroidism, uncontrolled diabetes mellitus [DM]).
Parenteral chromosome abnormalities.
Maternal infections (cervical mycoplasma, ureaplasma, chlamydia).
DES exposure, heavy metal exposure.
Thrombocytosis.
Allogenic immunity, autoimmunity, lupus anticoagulant.

ACALCULOUS GALLBLADDER DISEASE[23]

ICD-10CM # K82.9 Other diseases of gallbladder

Biliary tract anomaly (e.g., choledochal cyst).
Bone marrow transplant.
Burns.
Chemotherapy in oncology patients.
Critical illness in intensive care unit patients.
Crohn disease, Henoch-Schönlein purpura, Kawasaki disease, systemic lupus erythematosus.
Infectious agents (atypical microbes).
Microlithiasis.
Postoperative state (e.g., cardiac surgery).
Sepsis.
Sludge.
Systemic inflammatory states.
Total parenteral nutrition.
Traumatic spinal cord injury.

ACHES AND PAINS, DIFFUSE[55]

ICD-10CM # M25.50 Pain in unspecified joint

Postviral arthralgias/myalgias.
Bilateral soft tissue rheumatism.
Overuse syndromes.
Fibrositis.
Hypothyroidism.
Metabolic bone disease.
Paraneoplastic syndrome.
Myopathy (polymyositis, dermatomyositis).
Rheumatoid arthritis (RA).
Sjögren syndrome.
Polymyalgia rheumatica.
Hypermobility.
Benign arthralgias/myalgias.
Chronic fatigue syndrome.
Hypophosphatemia.

ACIDOSIS, HYPERCHLORIC METABOLIC[97]

ICD-10CM # E87.2 Acidosis

GASTROINTESTINAL BICARBONATE LOSS

Diarrhea.
External pancreatic or small bowel drainage.
Ureterosigmoidostomy, jejunal loop.
Drugs:
- Calcium chloride (acidifying agent).
- Magnesium sulfate (diarrhea).
- Cholestyramine (bile acid diarrhea).

RENAL ACIDOSIS

Hypokalemic:
- Proximal RTA (type 2).
- Distal (classic) RTA (type 1).
- Drug-induced hypokalemia:
  - Acetazolamide (proximal RTA).
  - Amphotericin B (distal RTA).

Hyperkalemic:
- Generalized distal nephron dysfunction (type 4 RTA).
  - Mineralocorticoid deficiency or resistance (pseudohypoaldosteronism type 1) PHA-I, PHA-II.
  - ↓ Na^+ delivery to distal nephron.
  - Tubulointerstitial disease.
  - Ammonium excretion defect.
  - Drug-induced hyperkalemia:
    - Potassium-sparing diuretics (amiloride, triamterene, spironolactone).
    - Trimethoprim.
    - Pentamidine.
    - Angiotensin-converting enzyme inhibitors and angiotensin II receptor blockers.
    - Nonsteroidal antiinflammatory drugs.
    - Cyclosporine, tacrolimus.

Normokalemic:
Early renal insufficiency.

OTHER

Acid loads (ammonium chloride, hyperalimentation).
Loss of potential bicarbonate: ketosis with ketone excretion.
Dilution acidosis (rapid saline administration).
Hippurate.
Cation-exchange resins.

ACIDOSIS, LACTIC[97]

ICD-10CM # E87.2 Acidosis

CAUSES OF LACTIC ACIDOSIS

L-Lactic Acidosis

Conditions associated with type A lactic acidosis:
- Poor tissue perfusion.
- Shock:
  - Cardiogenic.
  - Hemorrhagic.
  - Septic.

Profound hypoxemia:
- Severe asthma.
- Carbon monoxide poisoning.

Conditions associated with type B lactic acidosis:
- Liver disease.
- Metformin.
- Inborn errors of metabolism.
- Pyroglutamic acidosis.
- Kombucha tea.

d-Lactic Acidosis

Short bowel syndrome.
Ischemic bowel.
Small bowel obstruction.

ACIDOSIS, METABOLIC

ICD-10CM # E87.2 Acidosis

METABOLIC ACIDOSIS WITH INCREASED ANION GAP (AG ACIDOSIS)

Lactic acidosis.
Ketoacidosis (DM, alcoholic ketoacidosis).
Uremia (chronic renal failure).
Ingestion of toxins (paraldehyde, methanol, salicylate, ethylene glycol).
High-fat diet (mild acidosis).

METABOLIC ACIDOSIS WITH NORMAL AG (HYPERCHLOREMIC ACIDOSIS)

Renal tubular acidosis (including acidosis of aldosterone deficiency).
Intestinal loss of HCO_3^- (diarrhea, pancreatic fistula).
Carbonic anhydrase inhibitors (e.g., acetazolamide).
Dilutional acidosis (as a result of rapid infusion of bicarbonate-free isotonic saline).
Ingestion of exogenous acids (ammonium chloride, methionine, cystine, calcium chloride).
Ileostomy.
Ureterosigmoidostomy.
Drugs: amiloride, triamterene, spironolactone, β-blockers.

ACIDOSIS, RESPIRATORY

ICD-10CM # E87.2 Acidosis

Pulmonary disease (COPD, severe pneumonia, pulmonary edema, interstitial fibrosis).
Airway obstruction (foreign body, severe bronchospasm, laryngospasm).
Thoracic cage disorders (pneumothorax, flail chest, kyphoscoliosis).
Defects in muscles of respiration (myasthenia gravis, hypokalemia, muscular dystrophy).
Defects in peripheral nervous system (amyotrophic lateral sclerosis, poliomyelitis, Guillain-Barré syndrome, botulism, tetanus, organophosphate poisoning, spinal cord injury).
Depression of respiratory center (anesthesia, narcotics, sedatives, vertebral artery embolism or thrombosis, increased intracranial pressure).
Failure of mechanical ventilator.

ACUTE KIDNEY INJURY AND LIVER DISEASE, CAUSES[31,32]

ICD-10CM #	S37.009A	Unspecified injury of unspecified kidney, initial encounter
	K76.89	Other specified diseases of liver

Prerenal uremia:	Diuretic use, GI loss, peritoneal aspiration, hypoalbuminemia.
Hepatorenal syndrome	
Acute tubular necrosis:	Hyperbilirubinemia, sepsis, toxic shock syndrome.
Drugs:	Acetaminophen (paracetamol), NSAIDs, tetracycline, rifampicin, isoniazid, anesthetic agents, sulfonamides, allopurinol, methotrexate.
Infections:	Hepatitis C and cryoglobulinemia, hepatitis B and polyarteritis nodosa, leptospirosis, hantavirus, Epstein-Barr virus, gram-negative sepsis, spontaneous bacterial peritonitis.
Other:	Papillary necrosis and obstruction, inhalation of chlorinated hydrocarbons, mushroom poisoning *(Amanita phalloides).*

ACUTE KIDNEY INJURY DUE TO INTRINSIC RENAL DISEASES[65]

ICD-10CM # Varies with specific diagnosis

INTRINSIC RENAL DISEASES THAT CAUSE ACUTE KIDNEY INJURY

Vascular Diseases
Large-Vessel Diseases
Renal artery thrombosis or stenosis.
Renal vein thrombosis.
Atheroembolic disease.
Small- and Medium-Vessel Diseases
Scleroderma.
Malignant hypertension.
Hemolytic uremic syndrome.
Thrombotic thrombocytopenic purpura.
HIV-associated microangiopathy.
Glomerular Diseases
Systemic Diseases
Systemic lupus erythematosus.
Infective endocarditis.
Systemic vasculitis (e.g., periarteritis nodosa, granulomatosis with polyangiitis).
Henoch-Schönlein purpura.
HIV-associated nephropathy.
Essential mixed cryoglobulinemia.
Goodpasture syndrome.
Primary Renal Diseases
Poststreptococcal glomerulonephritis.
Other postinfectious glomerulonephritis.
Rapidly progressive glomerulonephritis.
Tubulointerstitial Diseases and Conditions
Drugs (many).
Toxins (e.g., heavy metals, ethylene glycol).
Infections.
Multiple myeloma.
Acute Tubular Necrosis
Ischemia
Shock.
Sepsis.
Severe prerenal azotemia.
Nephrotoxins
Antibiotics.
Radiographic contrast agents.
Myoglobinuria.
Hemoglobinuria.
Other Diseases and Conditions
Severe liver disease.
Allergic reactions.
NSAIDs.

ACUTE KIDNEY INJURY, HIV PATIENT, CAUSES[31,32]

ICD-10CM # S37.009A Unspecified injury of unspecified kidney, initial encounter with B20 human immunodeficiency virus (HIV) disease

Prerenal:	Diarrhea, nausea and vomiting, cirrhosis and hepatorenal syndrome, sepsis.
Vascular:	Thrombotic microangiopathy.
Glomerular:	Immune complex glomerulonephritis (MPGN secondary to hepatitis C virus, postinfectious glomerulonephritis), HIVAN.
Acute tubular necrosis:	Sepsis, hypotension, nephrotoxins (aminoglycosides, amphotericin, acyclovir, cidofovir, tenofovir, pentamidine).
Acute interstitial nephritis:	Drug-induced (co-trimoxazole), rifampicin, foscarnet, nevirapine), CMV infection, DILS.
Drug-induced intratubular obstruction:	Sulfadiazine, indinavir, foscarnet, acyclovir.
Postrenal obstruction:	Stones, tuberculosis, fungal ball, tumor.
Associated with IV drug use:	Sepsis, endocarditis, heroin-associated nephropathy (FSGS), rhabdomyolysis.

CMV, Cytomegalovirus; *DILS,* diffusive infiltrative lymphocytosis syndrome; *FSGS,* focal segmental glomerulosclerosis; *HIVAN,* HIV-associated nephropathy; *MPGN,* membranoproliferative glomerulonephritis.

ACUTE KIDNEY INJURY IN SPECIFIC CLINICAL SETTINGS[87]

ICD-10CM # N17.9 Acute kidney failure, unspecified

MAJOR CAUSES OF ACUTE KIDNEY INJURY IN SPECIFIC CLINICAL SETTINGS

AKI in the Cancer Patient
Prerenal azotemia:
- Hypovolemia (e.g., poor intake, vomiting, diarrhea).

Intrinsic AKI:
- Exogenous nephrotoxins: chemotherapy, antibiotics, contrast media.
- Endogenous toxins: hyperuricemia, hypercalcemia, tumor lysis, paraproteins.
- Other: radiation, HUS/TTP, glomerulonephritis, amyloid, malignant infiltration.

Postrenal AKI:
- Ureteric or bladder neck obstruction.

AKI after Cardiac Surgery
Prerenal azotemia:
- Hypovolemia (surgical losses, diuretics), cardiac failure, vasodilators.

Intrinsic AKI:
- Ischemic ATN (even in absence of hypotension).
- Atheroembolic disease after aortic manipulation/intraaortic balloon pump.
- Preoperative or perioperative administration of contrast medium.
- Allergic interstitial nephritis induced by perioperative antibiotics.

Postrenal AKI:
- Obstructed urinary catheter, exacerbation of voiding dysfunction.

AKI in Pregnancy
Prerenal azotemia:
Acute fatty liver of pregnancy with fulminant hepatic failure.
Intrinsic AKI:
Preeclampsia or eclampsia.
Postpartum HUS/TTP.
HELLP syndrome.
Ischemia: postpartum hemorrhage, abruptio placentae, amniotic fluid embolus.
Direct toxicity of illegal abortifacients.
Postrenal AKI:
Obstruction with pyelonephritis.

AKI after Solid Organ or Bone Marrow Transplantation
Prerenal azotemia:
Intravascular volume depletion (e.g., diuretic therapy).
Vasoactive drugs (e.g., calcineurin inhibitors, amphotericin B).
Hepatorenal syndrome, venoocclusive disease of liver (BMT).
Intrinsic AKI:
Postoperative ischemic ATN (even in absence of hypotension).
Sepsis.
Exogenous nephrotoxins: aminoglycosides, amphotericin B, radiocontrast media.
HUS/TTP (e.g., cyclosporine or myeloablative radiotherapy related).
Allergic tubulointerstitial nephritis.
Postrenal AKI:
Obstructed urinary catheter.

AKI and Pulmonary Disease (Pulmonary Renal Syndrome)
Prerenal azotemia:
Diminished cardiac output complicating pulmonary embolism, severe pulmonary hypertension, or positive-pressure mechanical ventilation.
Intrinsic AKI:
Vasculitis.
Goodpasture syndrome, ANCA-associated vasculitis, SLE, eosinophilic granulomatosis with polyangiitis, polyarteritis nodosa, cryoglobulinemia, right-sided endocarditis, lymphomatoid granulomatosis, sarcoidosis, scleroderma.
Toxins:
Ingestion of paraquat or diquat.
Infections:
Legionnaires disease, *Mycoplasma* infection, tuberculosis, disseminated viral or fungal infection.
AKI from any cause with hypervolemia and pulmonary edema.
Lung cancer with hypercalcemia, tumor lysis, or glomerulonephritis.

AKI and Liver Disease
Prerenal azotemia:
Reduced true (GI hemorrhage, GI losses from lactulose, diuretics, large-volume paracentesis) circulatory volume or effective (hypoalbuminemia, splanchnic vasodilation).
Hepatorenal syndrome type 1 or 2.
Tense ascites with abdominal compartment syndrome.
Intrinsic AKI:
Ischemic (severe hypoperfusion—see earlier) or direct nephrotoxicity and hepatotoxicity of drugs or toxins (e.g., carbon tetrachloride, acetaminophen, tetracyclines, methoxyflurane).
Tubulointerstitial nephritis plus hepatitis caused by drugs (e.g., sulfonamides, rifampin, phenytoin, allopurinol, phenindione), infections (leptospirosis, brucellosis, Epstein-Barr virus infection, cytomegalovirus infection), malignant infiltration (leukemia, lymphoma), or sarcoidosis.
Glomerulonephritis or vasculitis (e.g., polyarteritis nodosa, ANCA-associated glomerulonephritis, cryoglobulinemia, SLE, postinfectious hepatitis or liver abscess.

AKI and Nephrotic Syndrome
Prerenal azotemia:
Intravascular volume depletion (diuretic therapy, hypoalbuminemia).
Intrinsic AKI:
Manifestation of primary glomerular disease.
Collapsing glomerulopathy (e.g., HIV, pamidronate).
Associated ATN (older hypertensive males).
Associated interstitial nephritis (NSAIDs, rifampin, interferon alfa).
Other: amyloid or light-chain deposition disease, renal vein thrombosis, severe interstitial edema.

AKI, Acute kidney injury; *ANCA,* antineutrophil cytoplasmic antibody; *ATN,* acute tubular necrosis; *BMT,* bone marrow transplantation; *GI,* gastrointestinal; *HELLP, h*emolysis, *e*levated *l*iver enzymes, *l*ow *p*latelets; *HIV,* human immunodeficiency virus; *HUS,* hemolytic uremic syndrome; *NSAID,* nonsteroidal antiinflammatory drug; *SLE,* systemic lupus erythematosus; *TTP,* thrombotic thrombocytopenic purpura.

ACUTE KIDNEY INJURY, PIGMENT INDUCED[65]

ICD-10CM # Varies with specific diagnosis

CAUSES OF PIGMENT-INDUCED ACUTE KIDNEY INJURY

Rhabdomyolysis and myoglobinuria.
Vigorous exercise.
Arterial embolization.
Status epilepticus.
Status asthmaticus.
Coma-induced and pressure-induced myonecrosis.
Heat stress.
Diabetic ketoacidosis.
Myopathy.
Alcoholism.
Hypokalemia.
Hypophosphatemia.
Hemoglobinuria.
Transfusion reactions.
Snake envenomation.
Malaria.
Mechanical destruction of RBCs by prosthetic valves.
G6PD deficiency.

G6PD, Glucose-6-phosphate dehydrogenase.

ACUTE LIVER FAILURE[19]

ICD-10CM # K71.01 Toxic liver disease with hepatic necrosis

DIFFERENTIAL DIAGNOSIS OF ACUTE LIVER FAILURE

Viruses	Hepatitis A and B viruses (typical viruses causing viral hepatitis). Hepatitis C virus (rare). Hepatitis D virus. Hepatitis E virus (often in pregnant women in endemic areas). Cytomegalovirus. Hemorrhagic fever viruses. Herpes simplex virus. Paramyxovirus. Epstein-Barr virus.
Drugs	Paracetamol hepatotoxicity. Idiosyncratic hypersensitivity reactions (e.g., isoniazid, statins, halothane). Illicit drugs (e.g., Ecstasy, cocaine). Alternative medicines (e.g., chaparral and *Teucrium polium*), traditional Chinese medicine.
Toxins	Mushroom poisoning (usually *Amanita phalloides*). *Bacillus cereus* toxin. Cyanobacteria toxin. Organic solvents (e.g., carbon tetrachloride). Yellow phosphorus.
Vasculopathy	Ischemic hepatitis. Hepatic vein thrombosis (Budd-Chiari syndrome). Hepatic veno-occlusive disease. Portal vein thrombosis. Hepatic arterial thrombosis.
Metabolic	Acute fatty liver of pregnancy/hemolysis, elevated liver enzymes, low platelet count (HELLP) syndrome. α_1-antitrypsin deficiency. Fructose intolerance. Galactosemia. Lecithin-cholesterol acyltransferase deficiency. Reye syndrome. Tyrosinemia. Wilson disease.
Autoimmune	Autoimmune hepatitis.
Malignancy	Primary liver malignancy (hepatocellular carcinoma or cholangiocarcinoma). Secondary (e.g., extensive hepatic metastases or infiltration of adenocarcinoma).
Miscellaneous	Adult-onset Still disease. Heat stroke. Primary graft nonfunction (in liver transplant recipients). Indeterminate etiology (approximately 20% of acute liver failure cases).

ACUTE LUNG INJURY, DISEASE AND DISORDER ASSOCIATIONS[66]

ICD-10CM # S27.3 Injury, lung

CLINICAL DISORDERS ASSOCIATED WITH ACUTE LUNG INJURY

Infectious Causes

Gram-negative or gram-positive sepsis.
Bacterial pneumonia.
Viral pneumonia.
Fungal pneumonia
Parasitic infections.
Mycobacterial disease.

Aspiration

Gastric acid.
Food and other particulate matter.
Fresh or sea water (near drowning).
Hydrocarbon fluids.

Trauma

Lung contusion.
Fat emboli.
Nonthoracic trauma.
Thermal injury (burns).
Blast injury (explosion, lightning).
Overdistention (mechanical ventilation).
Inhaled gases (phosgene, ammonia).

Hemodynamic Disturbances

Shock of any etiology.
Anaphylaxis.
High-altitude pulmonary edema.
Reperfusion.
Air embolism.
Amniotic fluid embolism.

Drugs

Heroin.
Methadone.
Propoxyphene.
Naloxone.
Cocaine.
Barbiturates.
Colchicine.
Salicylates.
Ethchlorvynol.
Interleukin-2.
Protamine.
Hydrochlorothiazide.

Hematologic Disorders

Disseminated intravascular coagulation.
Incompatible blood transfusion.
Rh incompatibility.
Antileukocyte antibodies.
Leucoagglutinin reactions.
Post–cardiopulmonary bypass, pump oxygenator.

Metabolic Disorders

Pancreatitis.
Diabetic ketoacidosis.

Neurologic Disorders

Head trauma.
Grand mal seizures.
Increased intracranial pressure (any cause).
Subarachnoid or intracerebral hemorrhage.

Miscellaneous Disorders

Lung reexpansion.
Upper airway obstruction.

ACUTE RESPIRATORY DISTRESS IN PREGNANCY[77]

ICD-10CM # J96.00 Acute respiratory failure

Disorder	Distinguishing Features
Pregnancy-Specific	
Amniotic fluid embolism.	Cardiorespiratory collapse, seizures, DIC.
Pulmonary edema secondary to preeclampsia.	Hypertension, proteinuria.
ARDS secondary to obstetric sepsis.	Evidence of obstetric sepsis, shock.
Tocolytic pulmonary edema.	Tocolytic administration, rapid improvement.
Peripartum cardiomyopathy.	Gradual onset, cardiac gallop, cardiomegaly.
Trophoblastic embolism.	Nodular infiltrate, molar pregnancy.
Risk Increased by Pregnancy	
Aspiration pneumonitis.	Vomiting, aspiration.
Venous thromboembolism.	Evidence of DVT, positive $\dot{V}/\dot{Q}$ scan, leg Doppler, CT angiogram.
Pneumomediastinum.	Occurs during delivery, subcutaneous emphysema.
Valvular heart disease.	Pulmonary edema, cardiac murmur, cardiomegaly.
ARDS secondary to sepsis.	Evidence of sepsis (e.g., pyelonephritis).
Unrelated to Pregnancy	
Asthma.	Features similar to nonpregnant patient.
Pneumonia.	Features similar to nonpregnant patient.

ARDS, Acute respiratory distress syndrome; *CT,* computed tomography; *DIC,* disseminated intravascular coagulopathy; *DVT,* deep venous thrombosis; $\dot{V}/\dot{Q}$, ventilation-perfusion.

ACUTE SCROTUM

ICD-10CM # R10.2 Pelvic and perineal pain

Testicular torsion.
Epididymitis.
Testicular neoplasm.
Orchitis.
Trauma.

ADNEXAL MASS[63]

ICD-10CM # R19.00 Intraabdominal and pelvic swelling, mass and lump, unspecified site

Ovary (neoplasm, endometriosis, functional cyst).
Fallopian tube (ectopic pregnancy, neoplasm, tubo-ovarian abscess, hydrosalpinx, paratubal cyst).
Uterus (fibroid, neoplasm).
Retroperitoneum (neoplasm, abdominal wall hematoma or abscess).
Urinary tract (pelvic kidney, distended bladder, urachal cyst).
Inflammatory bowel disease.
GI tract neoplasm.
Diverticular disease.
Appendicitis.
Bowel loop with feces.

ADRENAL CALCIFICATIONS[81]

ICD-10CM # E27.8 Other specified disorder of adrenal gland

CAUSES OF ADRENAL CALCIFICATION

Infection:
- Tuberculosis.
- Histoplasmosis.
- *Echinococcus.*

Prior hemorrhage.
Neoplasm:
- Adrenocortical carcinoma.
- Myelolipoma.
- Pheochromocytoma.

Hemangioma (rare).

ADRENAL CYSTIC LESIONS[81]

ICD-10CM # E27.8 Other specified disorder of adrenal gland

CYSTIC ADRENAL LESIONS

Pseudocyst.
Endothelial cyst.
Epithelial cyst.
Infection (*Echinococcus,* abscess).
Necrotic neoplasm.
Cystic pheochromocytoma.
Lymphangioma.

ADRENAL INSUFFICIENCY, CRITICALLY ILL PATIENT[80]

ICD-10CM # E27.40 Unspecified adrenocortical insufficiency

CAUSES OF ADRENAL INSUFFICIENCY IN CRITICALLY ILL PATIENTS

Reversible Dysfunction of the HPA Axis

Sepsis/septic shock.
Acute lung injury.
Burns.
Pancreatitis.
Liver failure.
Hypothermia.
Drugs:
- Etomidate (primary AI).
- Corticosteroids (secondary AI).
- Ketoconazole (primary AI).
- Megestrol acetate (secondary AI).
- Rifampin (increased cortisol metabolism).
- Phenytoin (increased cortisol metabolism).
- Metyrapone (primary AI).
- Mitotane (primary AI).

Primary Adrenal Insufficiency (Adrenal Failure)

Autoimmune adrenalitis.
HIV infection:
- HART therapy.
- HIV virus.
- CMV.

Metastatic carcinoma:

- Lung.
- Breast.
- Kidney.

Systemic fungal infection:
- Histoplasmosis.
- Cryptococcus.
- Blastomycosis.

Tuberculosis.

Adrenal hemorrhage/infarction:
- DIC.
- Meningococcemia.
- Anticoagulation.
- Antiphospholipid syndrome.
- HIT.
- Trauma.

AI, Adrenal insufficiency; *CMV*, cytomegalovirus; *DIC*, disseminated intravascular coagulation; *HIT*, heparin-induced thrombocytopenia; *HPA*, hypothalamic-pituitary axis.

ADRENAL MASSES[91]

ICD-10CM #	C74.90	Malignant neoplasm of unspecified part of unspecified adrenal gland
	E27.8	Other specified disorders of adrenal gland

UNILATERAL ADRENAL MASSES

Functional Lesions

Adrenal adenoma.
Adrenal carcinoma.
Pheochromocytoma.
Primary aldosteronism, adenomatous type.

Nonfunctional Lesions

Incidentaloma of adrenal.
Ganglioneuroma.
Myelolipoma.
Hematoma.
Adenolipoma.
Metastasis.

BILATERAL ADRENAL MASSES

Functional Lesions

ACTH-dependent Cushing syndrome.
Congenital adrenal hyperplasia.
Pheochromocytoma.
Conn syndrome, hyperplastic variety.
Micronodular adrenal disease.
Idiopathic bilateral adrenal hypertrophy.

Nonfunctional Lesions

Infection (tuberculosis, fungi).
Infiltration (leukemia, lymphoma).
Replacement (amyloidosis).
Hemorrhage.
Bilateral metastases.

ADRENAL PSEUDOMASSES[81]

ICD-10CM #	E27.8	Other specified disorder of adrenal gland

Thickened diaphragmatic crus.
Accessory spleen.
Gastric fundus.
Gastric diverticulum.
Renal vein.
Retrocrural and retroperitoneal adenopathy.
Upper-pole renal cysts and tumors.
Pancreatic tumors.
Hypertrophied caudate lobe of liver.
Fluid-filled colon interposed between stomach and kidney.

ADRENERGIC TOXIDROME[80]

ICD-10CM #	T44.8X1S	Poisoning by centrally acting and adrenergic-neuron-blocking agents, accidental (unintentional), sequela

COMMON CAUSES OF THE ADRENERGIC TOXIDROME

Recreational drugs:
Cocaine.
Amphetamines and other "designer drugs"[a]; "ecstasy" (3,4-methylenedioxymethamphetamine [MDMA]); 3,4-methylenedioxyamphetamine (MDA); 3,4-methylenedioxyethylamphetamine (MDEA); paramethoxyamphetamine (PMA); methamphetamine.

β_1-Adrenergic agents:
- Salbutamol.
- Theophylline.

Inotropic agents:
- Norepinephrine.
- Epinephrine.
- Isoproterenol.

Over-the-counter cough and cold preparations and nasal decongestants:
- Phenylpropanolamine.
- Pseudoephedrine.

Amphetamine-like agents prescribed for ADD or weight loss:
- Methylphenidate.
- Dextroamphetamine.

Psychostimulants.

ADD, Attention deficit disorder.

[a] Up to 80% of ecstasy tablets sold in Australia are actually methamphetamine.

ADRENOCORTICAL HYPERFUNCTION[3]

ICD-10CM #	E26.9	Hyperaldosteronism, unspecified

SYNDROMES OF ADRENOCORTICAL HYPERFUNCTION

States of Glucocorticoid Excess

Physiologic States

Stress.
Strenuous exercise.
Last trimester of pregnancy.

Pathologic States

Psychiatric conditions (pseudo-Cushing disorders):
- Depression.
- Alcoholism.
- Anorexia nervosa.
- Panic disorders.
- Alcohol and drug withdrawal.

ACTH-dependent states:
- Pituitary adenoma (Cushing disease).
- Ectopic ACTH syndrome.
- Bronchial carcinoid.
- Thymic carcinoid.
- Islet cell tumor.
- Small cell lung carcinoma.
- Ectopic CRH secretion.

ACTH-independent states:
- Adrenal adenoma.
- Adrenal carcinoma.
- Micronodular adrenal disease.

Exogenous Sources

Glucocorticoid intake.
ACTH intake.

States of Mineralocorticoid Excess

Primary Aldosteronism

Aldosterone-secreting adenoma.
Bilateral adrenal hyperplasia.
Aldosterone-secreting carcinoma.
Glucocorticoid-suppressible hyperaldosteronism.

Adrenal Enzyme Deficiencies

11b-Hydroxylase deficiency.
17a-Hydroxylase deficiency.
11b-Hydroxysteroid dehydrogenase, type II.

Exogenous Mineralocorticoids

Licorice.
Carbenoxolone.
Fludrocortisone.

Secondary Hyperaldosteronism

Associated with hypertension:
- Accelerated hypertension.
- Renovascular hypertension.
- Estrogen administration.
- Renin-secreting tumors.

Without hypertension:
- Bartter syndrome.
- Sodium-wasting nephropathy.
- Renal tubular acidosis.
- Diuretic and laxative abuse.
- Edematous states (cirrhosis, nephrosis, congestive heart failure).

ACTH, Adrenocorticotropin hormone; *CRH*, corticotropin-releasing hormone.

ADRENOCORTICAL HYPOFUNCTION

ICD-10CM #	E27.49	Other adrenocortical insufficiency

SYNDROMES OF ADRENOCORTICAL HYPOFUNCTION

Primary Adrenal Disorders

Combined Glucocorticoid and Mineralocorticoid Deficiency

Autoimmune:
- Isolated autoimmune disease (Addison disease).
- Polyglandular autoimmune syndrome, type I.
- Polyglandular autoimmune syndrome, type II.

Infectious:
- Tuberculosis.
- Fungal.
- Cytomegalovirus.
- Human immunodeficiency virus.

Vascular:
- Bilateral adrenal hemorrhage.
- Sepsis.
- Coagulopathy.
- Thrombosis; embolism.
- Adrenal infarction.

Infiltration:
- Metastatic carcinoma and lymphoma.
- Sarcoidosis.
- Amyloidosis.
- Hemochromatosis.

Congenital:
- Congenital adrenal hyperplasia.
  - 21-Hydroxylase deficiency.
  - 3b-o1 Dehydrogenase deficiency.
  - 20,22-Desmolase deficiency.

Adrenal unresponsiveness to ACTH.
Congenital adrenal hypoplasia.
Adrenoleukodystrophy.
Adrenomyeloneuropathy.

Iatrogenic

Bilateral adrenalectomy.
Drugs:
- Metyrapone, aminoglutethimide, trilostane, ketoconazole, o,p'-DDD, mifepristone.

Mineralocorticoid deficiency without glucocorticoid deficiency

Corticosterone methyl oxidase deficiency.
Isolated zona glomerulosa defect.
Heparin therapy.
Critical illness.
Converting-enzyme inhibitors.

Secondary Adrenal Disorders

Secondary Adrenal Insufficiency

Hypothalamic-pituitary dysfunction.
Exogenous glucocorticoids.
After removal of an ACTH-secreting tumor.

Hyporeninemic Hypoaldosteronism

Diabetic nephropathy.
Tubulointerstitial diseases.
Obstructive uropathy.
Autonomic neuropathy.
Nonsteroidal antiinflammatory drugs.
β-Adrenergic drugs.

ACTH, Adrenocorticotropic hormone.

ADVERSE FOOD REACTIONS, DIFFERENTIAL DIAGNOSIS[58]

ICD-10CM #	T78.1XXA	Other adverse food reactions, not elsewhere classified, initial encounter

GASTROINTESTINAL DISORDERS (WITH VOMITING AND/OR DIARRHEA)

Structural abnormalities (pyloric stenosis, Hirschsprung disease).
Enzyme deficiencies (primary or secondary):
- Disaccharidase deficiency: lactase, fructose, sucrase-isomaltase.
- Galactosemia.

Other: pancreatic insufficiency (cystic fibrosis), peptic disease.

CONTAMINANTS AND ADDITIVES

Flavorings and preservatives—rarely cause symptoms: sodium metabisulfite, monosodium glutamate, nitrites.
Dyes and colorings—very rarely cause symptoms (urticaria, eczema): tartrazine.
Toxins: bacterial, fungal (aflatoxin), fish-related (scombroid, ciguatera).
Infectious organisms:
- Bacteria *(Salmonella, Escherichia coli, Shigella).*
- Virus (rotavirus, enterovirus).
- Parasites *(Giardia,* Akis simplex [in fish]).

Accidental contaminants: heavy metals, pesticides.
Pharmacologic agents: caffeine, glycosidal alkaloid solanine (potato spuds), histamine (fish), serotonin (banana, tomato), tryptamine (tomato), tyramine (cheese).

PSYCHOLOGIC REACTIONS

Food phobias.

ADYNAMIC ILEUS[63]

ICD-10CM #	K56.0	Paralytic ileus
	K56.7	Ileus, unspecified

Abdominal trauma.
Infection (retroperitoneal, pelvic, intrathoracic).
Laparotomy.
Metabolic disease (hypokalemia).
Renal colic.
Skeletal injury (rib fracture, vertebral fracture).
Medications (e.g., narcotics).

AEROPHAGIA (BELCHING, ERUCTATION)

ICD-10CM #	R14.0	Abdominal distention (gaseous)
	R14.1	Gas pain
	R14.2	Eructation
	R14.3	Flatulence

Anxiety disorders.
Rapid food ingestion.
Carbonated beverages.
Nursing infants (especially when nursing in horizontal position).
Eating or drinking in supine position.
Gum chewing.
Poorly fitting dentures, orthodontic appliances.
Hiatal hernia, gastritis, nonnuclear dyspepsia.
Cholelithiasis, cholecystitis.
Ingestion of legumes, onions, peppers.

AIR-SPACE OPACIFICATION ON X-RAY[41]

ICD-10CM #	R91.8	Other nonspecific abnormal finding of lung field

CAUSES OF AIR-SPACE OPACIFICATION

Edema

Cardiogenic.
Non-cardiogenic.

Inflammation/Infection

Granulomatosis with polyangiitis.
Cryptogenic organizing pneumonia.

Blood

Idiopathic pulmonary hemosiderosis.
Antibasement membrane antibody disease.
Systemic lupus erythematosus.

Miscellaneous Causes

Eosinophilic pneumonia.
Alveolar proteinosis.
Alveolar cell carcinoma.
Alveolar microlithiasis.
Lymphoma (MALToma).
Sarcoidosis.

AIRWAY OBSTRUCTION, PEDIATRIC AGE[48]

ICD-10CM #	J44.9	Chronic obstructive pulmonary disease, unspecified
	T17.900A	Unspecified foreign body in respiratory tract, part unspecified causing asphyxiation, initial encounter
	T17.908A	Unspecified foreign body in respiratory tract, part unspecified causing other injury, initial encounter
	T17.910A	Gastric contents in respiratory tract, part unspecified causing asphyxiation, initial encounter
	T17.918A	Gastric contents in respiratory tract, part unspecified causing other injury, initial encounter
	T17.920A	Food in respiratory tract, part unspecified causing asphyxiation, initial encounter
	T17.928A	Food in respiratory tract, part unspecified causing other injury, initial encounter
	T17.990A	Other foreign object in respiratory tract, part unspecified in causing asphyxiation, initial encounter
	T17.998A	Other foreign object in respiratory tract, part unspecified causing other injury, initial encounter
	J38.5	Laryngeal spasm
	J68.9	Unspecified respiratory condition due to chemicals, gases, fumes, and vapors

CONGENITAL CAUSES

Craniofacial dysmorphism.
Hemangioma.
Laryngeal cleft/web.
Laryngoceles, cysts.

Laryngomalacia.
Macroglossia.
Tracheal stenosis.
Vascular ring.
Vocal cord paralysis.

ACQUIRED INFECTIOUS CAUSES

Acute laryngotracheobronchitis.
Epiglottitis.
Laryngeal papillomatosis.
Membranous croup (bacterial tracheitis).
Mononucleosis.
Retropharyngeal abscess.
Spasmodic croup.
Diphtheria.

ACQUIRED NONINFECTIOUS CAUSES

Anaphylaxis.
Foreign body aspiration.
Supraglottic hypotonia.
Thermal/chemical burn.
Trauma.
Vocal cord paralysis.
Angioneurotic edema.

AKINETIC/RIGID SYNDROME[3]

ICD-10CM # R29.8 Akinesis

Parkinsonism (idiopathic, drug-induced).
Catatonia (psychosis).
Progressive supranuclear palsy.
Multisystem atrophy (Shy-Drager syndrome, olivopontocerebellar atrophy).
Diffuse Lewy-body disease.
Toxins (MPTP, manganese, carbon monoxide).
Huntington disease and other hereditary neurodegenerative disorders.

ALCOHOL-RELATED SEIZURES[65]

ICD-10CM # F10.232 Alcohol dependence with withdrawal with perceptual disturbance

DIFFERENTIAL DIAGNOSIS OF ALCOHOL-RELATED SEIZURES

Withdrawal (alcohol or drugs).
Exacerbation of idiopathic or posttraumatic seizures.
Acute intoxication (amphetamines, anticholinergics, cocaine, isoniazid, organophosphates, phenothiazines, tricyclic antidepressants, salicylates, lithium).
Metabolic (hypoglycemia, hyponatremia, hypernatremia, hypocalcemia, hepatic failure).
Infectious (meningitis, encephalitis, brain abscess).
Trauma (intracranial hemorrhage).
Cerebrovascular accident.
Sleep deprivation.
Noncompliance with anticonvulsants.

ALKALOSIS, METABOLIC

ICD-10CM # E87.3 Alkalosis

CAUSES OF METABOLIC ALKALOSIS

Exogenous HCO_3^- loads.
Acute alkali administration.
Milk-alkali syndrome.

Effective Extracellular Volume Contraction, Normotension, Hypokalemia, and Secondary Hyperreninemic Hyperaldosteronism

GI origin:
- Vomiting.
- Gastric aspiration.
- Congenital chloridorrhea.
- Villous adenoma.
- Combined administration of sodium polystyrene sulfonate (Kayexalate and aluminum hydroxide).

Renal origin:
- Diuretics (especially thiazides and loop diuretics).
- Acute.
- Chronic.
- Edematous states.
- Posthypercapnic state.
- Hypercalcemia-hypoparathyroidism.
- Recovery from lactic acidosis or ketoacidosis.
- Nonreabsorbable anions such as penicillin, carbenicillin.
- Mg++ deficiency.
- K^+ depletion.
- Bartter syndrome (loss-of-function mutation of Cl– transport in thick ascending limb of Henle loop).
- Gitelman syndrome (loss-of-function mutation in Na^+/Cl^- cotransporter).
- Carbohydrate refeeding after starvation.

Extracellular Volume Expansion, Hypertension, K^+ Deficiency, and Hypermineralocorticoidism

Associated with high renin:
- Renal artery stenosis.
- Accelerated hypertension.
- Renin-secreting tumor.
- Estrogen therapy.

Associated with low renin:
- Primary aldosteronism.
- Adenoma.
- Hyperplasia.
- Carcinoma.
- Glucocorticoid suppressible.

Adrenal enzymatic defects:
- 11β-Hydroxylase deficiency.
- 17α-Hydroxylase deficiency.

Cushing syndrome or disease:
- Ectopic corticotropin.
- Adrenal carcinoma.
- Adrenal adenoma.
- Primary pituitary.

Other:
- Licorice.
- Carbenoxolone.
- Chewer's tobacco.
- Lydia Pinkham tablets.

Gain-of-Function Mutation of ENaC with Extracellular Fluid Volume Expansion, Hypertension, K^+ Deficiency, and Hyporeninemic Hypoaldosteronism

Liddle syndrome.

ALKALOSIS, RESPIRATORY

ICD-10CM # E87.3 Alkalosis

Hypoxemia (pneumonia, pulmonary embolism, atelectasis, high-altitude living).
Drugs (salicylates, xanthenes, progesterone, epinephrine, thyroxine, nicotine).
Central nervous system (CNS) disorders (tumor, cerebrovascular accident [CVA], trauma, infections).
Psychogenic hyperventilation (anxiety, hysteria).
Hepatic encephalopathy.
Gram-negative sepsis.
Hyponatremia.
Sudden recovery from metabolic acidosis.
Assisted ventilation.

ALOPECIA[36,66]

ICD-10CM #		
	L65.9	Nonscarring hair loss, unspecified
	L63.2	Ophiasis
	L63.8	Other alopecia areata
	Q84.0	Congenital alopecia
	Q84.1	Congenital morphological disturbances of hair, not elsewhere classified
	Q84.2	Other congenital malformations of hair
	F54	Psychological and behavioral factors associated with disorders or diseases classified elsewhere

SCARRING ALOPECIA

Congenital (aplasia cutis).
Tinea capitis with inflammation (kerion).
Bacterial folliculitis.
Discoid lupus erythematosus.
Lichen planopilaris.
Folliculitis decalvans.
Neoplasm.
Trauma.

NONSCARRING ALOPECIA

Cosmetic treatment.
Tinea capitis.
Structural hair shaft disease.
Trichotillomania (hair pulling).
Anagen arrest.
Telogen arrest.
Alopecia areata.
Androgenetic alopecia.

ALOPECIA AND HYPOTRICHOSIS, IN CHILDREN AND ADOLESCENTS

ICD-10CM #		
	L65.9	Nonscarring hair loss, unspecified
	L63.2	Ophiasis
	L63.8	Other alopecia areata
	Q84.0	Congenital alopecia
	Q84.1	Congenital morphological disturbances of hair, not elsewhere classified
	Q84.2	Other congenital malformations of hair

Congenital total alopecia: atrichia with papules, Moynahan alopecia syndrome.
Congenital localized alopecia: aplasia cutis, triangular alopecia, sebaceous nevus.
Hereditary hypotrichosis: Marie-Unna syndrome, hypotrichosis with juvenile macular dystrophy, hypotrichosis–Mari type, ichthyosis with hypotrichosis, cartilage-hair hypoplasia, Hallermann-Streiff syndrome, trichorhinophalangeal syndrome, ectodermal dysplasia ("pure" hair and nail and other ectodermal dysplasias).
Diffuse alopecia of endocrine origin: hypopituitarism, hypothyroidism, hypoparathyroidism, hyperthyroidism.
Alopecia of nutritional origin: marasmus, kwashiorkor, iron deficiency, zinc deficiency (acrodermatitis enteropathica), gluten-sensitive enteropathy, essential fatty acid deficiency, biotinidase deficiency.
Disturbances of the hair cycle: telogen effluvium.
Toxic alopecia: anagen effluvium.
Autoimmune alopecia: alopecia areata.
Traumatic alopecia: traction alopecia, trichotillomania.
Cicatricial alopecia: lupus erythematosus, lichen planopilaris, pseudopelade, morphea (en coup de saber), dermatomyositis, infection (kerion, favus, tuberculosis, syphilis, folliculitis, leishmaniasis, herpes zoster, varicella), acne keloidalis, follicular mucinosis, sarcoidosis.
Hair shaft abnormalities: monilethrix, pili annulati, pili torti, trichorrhexis invaginata, trichorrhexis nodosa, woolly hair syndrome, Menkes disease, trichothiodystrophy, tricho-dento-osseous syndrome, uncombable hair syndrome (spun-glass hair, pili trianguli et canaliculi).

ALOPECIA, DRUG-INDUCED

ICD-10CM #	L65.9	Nonscarring hair loss, unspecified
	L63.8	Alopecia areata

DRUGS REPORTED TO INDUCE HAIR LOSS

ACE inhibitors (captopril, enalapril, moexipril, ramipril).
Allopurinol.
Amiodarone.
Amphetamines.[1,2]
Analgesics, antiinflammatories (ibuprofen, indomethacin, naproxen).
Androgens.[3]
Anticoagulants (coumarin, dextran, heparin/heparinoids).
Antiepileptics (carbamazepine, hydantoins, lamotrigine, troxidone, valproic acid, vigabatrin).
Antipsychotics (flupenthixol decanoate, fluphenazine decanoate).
Antithyroid drugs (carbimazole, iodine, thiouracil).
Appetite suppressants.
Aromatase inhibitors (fadrozole, 4-OHA, vorozole).
Benzimidazoles (albendazole, mebendazole)
β-Blockers (levobunolol, metoprolol, nadolol, propranolol, timolol).
Bromocriptine.
Buspirone.
Butyrophenones.
Cantharidin.
Chloramphenicol.
Cholestyramine.
Cidofovir.
Cimetidine.
Clonazepam.
Clotrimazole.
Colchicine.
Contraceptives (oral).[4]
Danazol.
Diazoxide.
Diclofenac.
Dixyrazine.
Ethambutol.
Ethionamide.
Fibrates (clofibrate, fenofibrate).
G-CSF (granulocyte-colony stimulating factor)
Gefitinib.[5]
Gentamicin.
Glatiramer acetate.
Glibenclamide.
Gold salts.
Haloperidol.
Immunoglobulins.
Indanediones.
Indinavir.
Interferons.
Isonicotinic acid hydrazide.[6]
Leflunomide.
Levodopa.
Lithium.
Maprotiline.
Mesalazine.
Methyldopa.
Methysergide.
Metyrapone.
Minoxidil.
Nicotinic acid.
Nitrofurantoin.
Octreotide.
Olanzapine.
Pentosan polysulfate.
Phenindione.
Potassium thiocyanate.
Pyridostigmine.
Radiation (<700 Gy).
Retinoids (acitretin, etretinate, isotretinoin).
Retinol (vitamin A).
Risperidone.
Salicylates.
Serotonin reuptake inhibitors (fluoxetine, fluvoxamine, paroxetine, sertraline).
Sorafenib.
Spironolactone.
Strontium ranelate.
Sulfasalazine.
Tamoxifen.
Terbinafine.
Terfenadine.
Thiamphenicol.
Thyroxine.
Tocopherol (vitamin E).
Trazodone.
Triazoles (fluconazole, itraconazole).
Tricyclic antidepressants (amitriptyline, desipramine, doxepin, imipramine, maprotiline).
Trimethadione.
Triparanol.
Vasopressin.[†]

[1] Denotes causes of painful' jaundice.
[2] More frequent cause.
[3] Absent in disseminated infection in compromised hosts.
[4] Genetic transmission.
[5] Not listed as a syndrome by ILAE but instead recognized under absence seizures with special features.
[6] Includes schizophrenia, schizophreniform disorder, brief reactive psychosis.
[†] Hair loss usually severe.

ALVEOLAR CONSOLIDATION

ICD-10CM #	J18.2	Hypostatic pneumonia, unspecified organism
	J81.1	Hypostatic pneumonia, unspecified organism

Infection.
Neoplasm (bronchoalveolar carcinoma, lymphoma).
Aspiration.
Trauma.
Hemorrhage (granulomatosis with polyangiitis, Goodpasture, bleeding diathesis).
ARDS.
CHF.
Renal failure.
Eosinophilic pneumonia.
Bronchiolitis obliterans.
Pulmonary alveolar proteinosis.

ALVEOLAR HEMORRHAGE[71]

ICD-10CM #	P26.1	Massive pulmonary hemorrhage originating in the perinatal period
	K08.8	Alveolar hemorrhage
	P26.8	Other pulmonary hemorrhages originating in the perinatal period

Hematologic disorders (coagulopathies, thrombocytopenia).
Goodpasture syndrome (anti-basement membrane antibody disease).
Granulomatosis with polyangiitis.
Immune complex-mediated vasculitis.
Idiopathic pulmonary hemosiderosis.
Drugs (penicillamine).
Lymphangiogram contrast.
Mitral stenosis.

AMENORRHEA

ICD-10CM #	N91.2	Amenorrhea, unspecified

PREGNANCY

Early Menopause

Hypothalamic Dysfunction

Defective synthesis or release of LHRH, anorexia nervosa, stress, exercise.

Pituitary Dysfunction

Neoplasm, postpartum hemorrhage, surgery, radiotherapy.

Ovarian Dysfunction

Gonadal dysgenesis, 17a-hydroxylase deficiency, premature ovarian failure, polycystic ovarian disease, gonadal stromal tumors.

UTEROVAGINAL ABNORMALITIES

Congenital: imperforate hymen, imperforate cervix, imperforate or absent vagina, Müllerian agenesis.

Acquired: destruction of endometrium with curettage (Asherman syndrome), closure of cervix or vagina caused by traumatic injury, hysterectomy.

OTHER

Metabolic diseases (liver, kidney), malnutrition, rapid weight loss, exogenous obesity, endocrine abnormalities (Cushing syndrome, Graves disease, hypothyroidism).

AMNESIA

ICD-10CM #	F19.96	Other psychoactive substance use, unspecified with psychoactive substance-induced persisting amnestic disorder
	F44.0	Dissociative amnesia
	R41.2	Retrograde amnesia
	G45.4	Transient global amnesia

Degenerative diseases (e.g., Alzheimer, Huntington disease).
CVA (especially when involving thalamus, basal forebrain, and hippocampus).
Head trauma.
Postsurgical (e.g., mammillary body surgery, bilateral temporal lobectomy).
Infections (herpes simplex encephalitis, meningitis).
Wernicke-Korsakoff syndrome.
Cerebral hypoxia.
Hypoglycemia.
CNS neoplasms.
Creutzfeldt-Jakob disease.
Medications (e.g., midazolam and other benzodiazepines).
Psychosis.
Malingering.

AMNIOTIC FLUID α-FETOPROTEIN ELEVATION[41]

ICD-10CM #	Z36	Encounter for antenatal screening of mother

CAUSES OF ELEVATED AMNIOTIC FLUID α-FETOPROTEIN

Craniospinal defect (open neural tube defect).
Omphalocele.
Gastroschisis.
Duodenal atresia.
Congenital nephrosis.
Cystic hygroma.
Unbalanced D/G dislocation.
Down, Tay-Sachs, Klinefelter, Turner syndromes.
Fetal tumors.
Epidermolysis bullosa.
Pilonidal sinus.
Rhesus disease.
Fetal demise.
Incorrect dates.
Multiple pregnancies.

ANAL ABSCESS AND FISTULA[95]

ICD-10CM #	K61.0	Anal abscess
	K61.1	Rectal abscess
	K61.3	Ischiorectal abscess
	K60.3	Anal fistula

Primary anal gland infection.
Secondary abscess:
  Inflammatory bowel disease:
    Crohn disease.
    Ulcerative colitis.
Infection:
  Tuberculosis.
  Actinomycosis.
  Threadworm.
Trauma.
Leukopenia.
Immunosuppression:
  HIV.
  Drugs.
Rectal cancer.
Diabetes mellitus.

ANAL INCONTINENCE[63]

ICD-10CM #	R15.9	Full incontinence of feces

TRAUMATIC

Nerve injured in surgery.
Spinal cord injury.
Obstetric trauma.
Sphincter injury.

NEUROLOGIC

Spinal cord lesions.
Dementia.
Autonomic neuropathy (e.g., DM).
Obstetrics: pudendal nerve stretched during surgery.
Hirschsprung disease.

MASS EFFECT

Carcinoma of anal canal.
Carcinoma of rectum.
Foreign body.
Fecal impaction.
Hemorrhoids.

MEDICAL

Procidentia.
Inflammatory disease.
Diarrhea.
Laxative abuse.

PEDIATRIC

Congenital.
Meningocele.
Myelomeningocele.
Spina bifida.
After corrective surgery for imperforate anus.
Sexual abuse.
Encopresis.

ANAPHYLAXIS[54]

ICD-10CM #	T78.2	Anaphylactic shock, unspecified, initial encounter

PULMONARY

Laryngeal edema.
Epiglottitis.
Foreign body aspiration.
Pulmonary embolus.
Asphyxiation.
Hyperventilation.

CARDIOVASCULAR

Myocardial infarction.
Arrhythmia.
Hypovolemic shock.
Cardiac arrest.

CNS

Vasovagal reaction.
CVA.
Seizure disorder.
Drug overdose.

ENDOCRINE

Hypoglycemia.
Pheochromocytoma.
Carcinoid syndrome.
Catamenial (progesterone-induced anaphylaxis).

PSYCHIATRIC

Vocal cord dysfunction syndrome.
Munchausen syndrome.
Panic attack/globus hystericus.

OTHER

Hereditary angioedema.
Cord urticaria.
Idiopathic urticaria.
Mastocytosis.
Serum sickness.
Idiopathic capillary leak syndrome.
Sulfite exposure.
Scombroid poisoning (tuna, blue fish, mackerel).

ANAPHYLAXIS MIMICS[76]

ICD-10CM #	Varies with specific diagnosis

CONDITIONS THAT MIMIC ANAPHYLAXIS

Vasovagal episodes.
Acute pulmonary events:
  Acute asthmatic attacks.
  Acute pulmonary edema.
  Pulmonary embolus.
  Spontaneous pneumothorax.
  Foreign body aspiration.
Acute cardiac events:
  Supraventricular tachycardias.
  Acute myocardial infarction/ischemia.
Drug overdoses.
Insulin shock.
Carcinoid attacks.

ANAPHYLAXIS, PATHOPHYSIOLOGIC CLASSIFICATION[2]

ICD-10CM # T78.2 Anaphylactic shock, unspecified, initial encounter

PATHOPHYSIOLOGIC CLASSIFICATION OF ANAPHYLAXIS

IgE Dependent, Immunologic

Foods.
Drugs.
Insect stings and bites.
Exercise (food dependent).
Other causes.

IgE Independent, Immunologic

Immune aggregates.
IgG anti-IgA.
Cytotoxic.
Disturbance of arachidonic acid metabolism:
- Aspirin.
- Other nonsteroidal antiinflammatory drugs.

Activation of kallikrein-kinin contact system:
- Dialysis membranes.
- Radiocontrast media.

Multimediator recruitment:
- Complement.
- Clotting.
- Clot lysis.
- Kallikrein-kinin contact system.

Other causes.

Nonimmunologic

Direct mediator release from mast cells and basophils:
- Drugs, e.g., opiates.
- Physical factors, e.g., cold and sunlight.

Exercise.
c-kit Mutation (D816V).
Other causes.

Idiopathic

ANAPHYLACTOID SYNDROME OF PREGNANCY[1]

ICD-10CM # 088.113

CARDIOVASCULAR COLLAPSE, HYPOTENSION

Acute coronary syndromes, myocardial infarction.
Cardiomyopathy.
Pulmonary embolism.
Anesthesia complications, transfusion reaction.
Sepsis, systemic inflammatory response syndrome.

RESPIRATORY ARREST

Pulmonary embolism, air embolism.
Anesthesia complications, transfusion reaction.
Aspiration.

ALTERED MENTAL STATUS, SEIZURE

Eclampsia.
Cerebrovascular accident.
Hypoglycemia.

COAGULOPATHY

Disseminated intravascular coagulation.
Consumptive coagulopathy from hemorrhage.

ANDROGEN EXCESS, REPRODUCTIVE-AGE WOMAN

ICD-10CM # E28.1 Androgen excess

Polycystic ovary syndrome.
Idiopathic.
Medications (e.g., anabolizing agents, testosterone, danazol).
Pregnancy (luteoma, hyperreaction luteinalis).
Sertoli-Leydig ovarian neoplasm.
Adrenal adenoma or hyperplasia.
Cushing syndrome.
Glucocorticoid resistance.
Hypothyroidism.
Hyperprolactinemia.

ANDROGEN RESISTANCE[67]

ICD-10CM # E34.5 Androgen resistance syndrome

CONGENITAL OR DEVELOPMENTAL DISORDERS

Uncommon causes:
- Kennedy disease (spinal and bulbar muscular atrophy).
- Partial androgen insensitivity syndrome (AR mutations).
- 5α-reductase type 2 deficiency.
- Complete androgen insensitivity syndrome (female phenotype).

ACQUIRED DISORDERS

Common causes:
- AR antagonists (bicalutamide, nilutamide).
- Drugs (spironolactone, cyproterone acetate, marijuana, histamine 2 receptor antagonists).

Uncommon causes:
- Celiac disease.

ANEMIA, APLASTIC[50]

ICD-10CM # D61.09 Other constitutional aplastic anemia

ACQUIRED APLASTIC ANEMIA

Secondary aplastic anemia.
Irradiation.
Drugs and chemicals.
Regular effects.
Cytotoxic agents.
Benzene.
Idiosyncratic reactions.
Chloramphenicol.
Nonsteroidal antiinflammatory drugs.
Antiepileptics.
Gold.
Other drugs and chemicals.
Viruses.
Epstein-Barr virus (infectious mononucleosis).
Hepatitis virus (non-A, non-B, non-C, non-G hepatitis).
Parvovirus (transient aplastic crisis, some pure red cell aplasia).
Human immunodeficiency virus (acquired immunodeficiency syndrome).
Immune diseases.
Eosinophilic fasciitis.
Hyperimmunoglobulinemia.
Thymoma and thymic carcinoma.
Graft-versus-host disease in immunodeficiency.
Paroxysmal nocturnal hemoglobinuria.
Pregnancy.
Idiopathic aplastic anemia.

INHERITED APLASTIC ANEMIA

Fanconi anemia.
Dyskeratosis congenita.
Shwachman-Diamond syndrome.
Reticular dysgenesis.
Amegakaryocytic thrombocytopenia.
Familial aplastic anemias.
Preleukemia (e.g., monosomy 7).
Nonhematologic syndromes (e.g., Down, Dubowitz, Seckel).

ANEMIA, APLASTIC, DUE TO DRUGS AND CHEMICALS[1]

ICD-10CM #	D61.1	Drug-induced aplastic anemia
	D61.2	Aplastic anemia due to other external agents
	D61.89	Other specified aplastic anemias and other bone marrow failure syndromes

Agents that regularly produce marrow depression as a major toxic effect when used in commonly employed doses or normal exposures:
- Cytotoxic drugs used in cancer chemotherapy.
- Alkylating agents (busulfan, melphalan, cyclophosphamide).
- Antimetabolites (antifolic compounds, nucleotide analogs), antimitotics (vincristine, vinblastine, colchicine).
- Some antibiotics (daunorubicin, doxorubicin [Adriamycin]).
- Benzene (and less often benzene-containing chemicals; kerosene, carbon tetrachloride, Stoddard solvent, chlorophenols).

Agents probably associated with aplastic anemia but with a relatively low probability relative to their use:
- Chloramphenicol.
- Insecticides.
- Antiprotozoals (quinacrine and chloroquine).
- NSAIDs (including phenylbutazone, indomethacin, ibuprofen, sulindac, diclofenac, naproxen, piroxicam, fenoprofen, fenbufen, aspirin).
- Anticonvulsants (hydantoins, carbamazepine, phenacemide, ethosuximide).
- Gold, arsenic, and other heavy metals such as bismuth and mercury.
- Sulfonamides as a class.

- Antithyroid medications (methimazole, methylthiouracil, propylthiouracil).
- Antidiabetes drugs (tolbutamide, carbutamide, chlorpropamide).
- Carbonic anhydrase inhibitors (acetazolamide, methazolamide, mesalazine).
- D-Penicillamine.
- 2-Chlorodeoxyadenosine.

Agents more rarely associated with aplastic anemia:

- Antibiotics (streptomycin, tetracycline, methicillin, ampicillin, mebendazole and albendazole, sulfonamides, flucytosine, mefloquine, dapsone).
- Antihistamines (cimetidine, ranitidine, chlorpheniramine).
- Sedatives and tranquilizers (chlorpromazine, prochlorperazine, piperacetazine, chlordiazepoxide, meprobamate, methyprylon, remoxipride).
- Antiarrhythmics (tocainide, amiodarone).
- Allopurinol (can potentiate marrow suppression by cytotoxic drugs).
- Ticlopidine.
- Methyldopa.
- Quinidine.
- Lithium.
- Guanidine.
- Canthaxanthin.
- Thiocyanate.
- Carbimazole.
- Cyanamide.
- Deferoxamine.
- Amphetamines.

ANEMIA, CAUSES IN PREGNANCY[34]

ICD-10CM #	D50.8	Other iron deficiency anemias
	D50.9	Iron deficiency anemia, unspecified
	D51.0	Vitamin B_{12} deficiency anemia due to intrinsic factor deficiency
	D51.1	Vitamin B_{12} deficiency anemia due to selective vitamin B_{12} malabsorption with proteinuria
	D51.3	Other dietary vitamin B_{12} deficiency anemia
	D51.8	Other vitamin B_{12} deficiency anemias
	D52.0	Dietary folate deficiency anemia
	D52.1	Drug-induced folate deficiency anemia
	D52.8	Other folate deficiency anemias
	D52.9	Folate deficiency anemia, unspecified
	D53.1	Other megaloblastic anemias, not elsewhere classified
	D53.0	Protein deficiency anemia
	D53.2	Scorbutic anemia
	D53.8	Other specified nutritional anemias
	D53.9	Nutritional anemia, unspecified
	D64.0	Hereditary sideroblastic anemia
	D64.1	Secondary sideroblastic anemia due to disease
	D64.2	Secondary sideroblastic anemia due to drugs and toxins
	D64.3	Other sideroblastic anemias

CAUSES OF ANEMIA DURING PREGNANCY

Common causes—85% of anemia:
- Physiologic anemia.
- Iron deficiency.

Uncommon causes:
- Folic acid deficiency.
- Vitamin B_{12} deficiency (due to the rapid increase in bariatric surgery).
- Hemoglobinopathies:
  - Sickle cell disease.
  - Hemoglobin SC.
  - β-Thalassemia minor.
- Bariatric surgery.
- GI bleeding.

Rare causes:
- Hemoglobinopathies.
  - β-Thalassemia major.
  - α-Thalassemia.

Syndromes of chronic hemolysis:
- Hereditary spherocytosis.
- Paroxysmal nocturnal hemoglobinuria.

Hematologic malignancy.

ANEMIA, DRUG-INDUCED[44]

ICD-10CM #	D61.1	Drug-induced aplastic anemia

DRUGS THAT MAY INTERFERE WITH RED CELL PRODUCTION BY INDUCING MARROW SUPPRESSION OR APLASIA

- Alcohol.
- Antineoplastic drugs.
- Antithyroid drugs.
- Antibiotics.
- Oral hypoglycemic agents.
- Phenylbutazone.
- Azidothymidine (AZT).

DRUGS THAT INTERFERE WITH VITAMIN B_{12}, FOLATE, OR IRON ABSORPTION OR UTILIZATION

- Nitrous oxide.
- Anticonvulsant drugs.
- Antineoplastic drugs.
- Isoniazid.
- Cycloserine A.

DRUGS CAPABLE OF PROMOTING HEMOLYSIS

Immune Mediated
- Penicillins.
- Quinine.
- α-methyldopa.
- Procainamide.
- Mitomycin C.

Oxidative Stress
- Antimalarials.
- Sulfonamide drugs.
- Nalidixic acid.

DRUGS THAT MAY PRODUCE OR PROMOTE BLOOD LOSS

- Aspirin.
- Alcohol.
- Nonsteroidal antiinflammatory agents.
- Corticosteroids.
- Anticoagulants.

ANEMIA, HYPOCHROMIC[50]

ICD-10CM #	D50.8	Other Iron deficiency anemias
	D50.9	Iron deficiency anemia, unspecified
	D64.0	Hereditary sideroblastic anemia
	D64.1	Secondary sideroblastic anemia due to disease
	D64.2	Secondary sideroblastic anemia due to drugs and toxins
	D64.3	Other sideroblastic anemias

DECREASED BODY IRON STORES

Iron deficiency anemia.

NORMAL OR INCREASED BODY IRON STORES

- Impaired iron metabolism.
- Anemia of chronic disease.
- Defective absorption, transport, or use of iron.
- Disorders of globin synthesis:
  - Thalassemia.
  - Other microcytic hemoglobinopathies.
- Disorders of heme synthesis: sideroblastic anemias:
  - Hereditary.
  - Acquired.

ANEMIA, LOW RETICULOCYTE COUNT[3]

ICD-10CM #	D64.9	Anemia, unspecified

MICROCYTIC ANEMIA (MCV <80)

- Iron deficiency.
- Thalassemia minor.
- Sideroblastic anemia.
- Lead poisoning.

MACROCYTIC ANEMIA (MCV >100)

- Megaloblastic anemias.
- Folate deficiency.
- Vitamin B_{12} deficiency.
- Drug-induced megaloblastic anemia.
- Nonmegaloblastic macrocytosis.
- Liver disease.
- Hypothyroidism.

NORMOCYTIC ANEMIA (MCV 80-100)

Early iron deficiency.
Aplastic anemia.
Myelophthisic disorders.
Endocrinopathies.
Anemia of chronic disease.
Uremia.
Mixed nutritional deficiency.

ANEMIA, MEGALOBLASTIC[91]

ICD-10CM #	D51.0	Vitamin B_{12} deficiency anemia due to intrinsic factor deficiency
	D51.1	Vitamin B_{12} deficiency anemia due to selective vitamin B_{12} malabsorption with proteinuria
	D51.3	Other dietary vitamin B_{12} deficiency anemia
	D51.8	Other vitamin B_{12} deficiency anemias
	D52.0	Dietary folate deficiency anemia
	D52.1	Drug-induced folate deficiency anemia
	D52.8	Other folate deficiency anemias
	D52.9	Folate deficiency anemia, unspecified
	D53.1	Other megaloblastic anemias, not elsewhere classified
	D53.0	Protein deficiency anemia
	D53.2	Scorbutic anemia
	D53.8	Other specified nutritional anemias
	D53.9	Nutritional anemia, unspecified

COBALAMIN (CBL) DEFICIENCY

Nutritional CBL Deficiency (Insufficient CBL Intake)

Vegetarians, vegans, breastfed infants of mothers with pernicious anemia.

Abnormal Intragastric Events (Inadequate Proteolysis of Food CBL)

Atrophic gastritis, partial gastrectomy with hypochlorhydria.

Loss/Atrophy of Gastric Oxyntic Mucosa (Deficient Intrinsic Factor [If] Molecules)

Total or partial gastrectomy, pernicious anemia (PA), caustic destruction (lye).

Abnormal Events in Small Bowel Lumen

Inadequate pancreatic protease (R-CBL not degraded, CBL not transferred to IF).
 Insufficiency of pancreatic protease—pancreatic insufficiency.
 Inactivation of pancreatic protease—Zollinger-Ellison syndrome.
Usurping of luminal CBL (inadequate CBL binding to IF).
 By bacteria—stasis syndromes (blind loops, pouches of diverticulosis, strictures, fistulas, anastomoses); impaired bowel motility (scleroderma, pseudoobstruction), hypogammaglobulinemia.
 By *Diphyllobothrium latum.*

Disorders of Ileal Mucosa/IF Receptors (IF-CBL not Bound to IF Receptors)

Diminished or absent IF receptors—ileal bypass/resection/fistula.
Abnormal mucosal architecture/function—tropical/nontropical sprue, Crohn disease, TB ileitis, infiltration by lymphomas, amyloidosis.
IF-/post IF-receptor defects—Imerslund-Gräsbeck syndrome, TC II deficiency.
Drug-induced effects (slow K, biguanides, cholestyramine, colchicine, neomycin, PAS).

DISORDERS OF PLASMA CBL TRANSPORT (TC II-CBL NOT DELIVERED TO TC II RECEPTORS)

Congenital TC II deficiency, defective binding of TC II-CBL to TC II receptors (rare).

METABOLIC DISORDERS (CBL NOT UTILIZED BY CELL)

Inborn enzyme errors (rare).
Acquired disorders: (CBL oxidized to cob[III]alamin)—N_2O inhalation.

FOLATE DEFICIENCY

Nutritional Causes

Decreased dietary intake—poverty and famine (associated with kwashiorkor, marasmus), institutionalized individuals (psychiatric/nursing homes), chronic debilitating disease/goats' milk (low in folate), special diets (slimming), cultural/ethnic cooking techniques (food folate destroyed) or habits (folate-rich foods not consumed).
Decreased diet and increased requirements:
 Physiologic: pregnancy and lactation, prematurity, infancy.
 Pathologic: intrinsic hematologic disease (autoimmune hemolytic disease), drugs, malaria; hemoglobinopathies (SS, thalassemia), RBC membrane defects (hereditary spherocytosis, paroxysmal nocturnal hemoglobinopathy); abnormal hematopoiesis (leukemia/lymphoma, myelodysplastic syndrome, agnogenic myeloid metaplasia with myelofibrosis); infiltration with malignant disease; dermatologic (psoriasis).

Folate Malabsorption

With normal intestinal mucosa:
 Some drugs (controversial).
 Congenital folate malabsorption (rare).
 With mucosal abnormalities—tropical and nontropical sprue, regional enteritis.

Defective Cellular Folate Uptake—Familial Aplastic Anemia (Rare), Inadequate Cellular Utilization

Folate antagonists (methotrexate).
Hereditary enzyme deficiencies involving folate.

Drugs (Multiple Effects on Folate Metabolism)

Alcohol, sulfasalazine, triamterene, pyrimethamine, trimethoprim-sulfamethoxazole, diphenylhydantoin, barbiturates.

MISCELLANEOUS MEGALOBLASTIC ANEMIAS (NOT CAUSED BY CBL OR FOLATE DEFICIENCY)

Congenital Disorders of DNA Synthesis (Rare)

Orotic aciduria, Lesch-Nyhan syndrome, congenital dyserythropoietic anemia.

Acquired Disorders of DNA Synthesis

Thiamine-responsive megaloblastosis (rare).
 Malignancy—erythroleukemia—refractory sideroblastic anemias—all antineoplastic drugs that inhibit DNA synthesis.
 Toxins: alcohol.

ANEMIA, MICROCYTIC, HYPOCHROMIC, DIFFERENTIAL DIAGNOSIS[49]

ICD-10CM #	D50.8	Other iron deficiency anemias
	D50.9	Iron deficiency anemia, unspecified
	D64.0	Hereditary sideroblastic anemia
	D64.1	Secondary sideroblastic anemia due to disease
	D64.2	Secondary sideroblastic anemia due to drugs and toxins
	D64.3	Other sideroblastic anemias

DIFFERENTIAL DIAGNOSIS OF MICROCYTIC HYPOCHROMIC ANEMIA

Decreased Body Iron Stores

Iron deficiency anemia.

Normal or Increased Body Iron Stores

Anemia of chronic disease.
Defective absorption, transport, or use of iron.
Iron-refractory, iron deficiency anemia after parenteral iron.
Atransferrinemia.
Aceruloplasminemia.
Divalent metal transporter 1 (DMT1 or SLC11A2) deficiency.
Ferroportin-associated hemochromatosis with impaired iron export (type 4A).
Heme oxygenase 1 deficiency.
Disorders of globin synthesis.

Decreased Body Iron Stores

Thalassemia.
 Other microcytic hemoglobinopathies.
 Disorders of heme synthesis.
Sideroblastic anemias.
 Hereditary.
 Acquired.

ANERGY, CUTANEOUS[91]

ICD-10CM #	D89.9	Disorder involving the immune mechanism, unspecified

IMMUNOLOGIC

Acquired (AIDS, acute leukemia, carcinoma, CLL, Hodgkin lymphoma, NHL).

Congenital (ataxia-telangiectasia, Di George syndrome, severe combined immunodeficiency, Wiskott-Aldrich syndrome).

INFECTIONS

Bacterial (bacterial pneumonia, brucellosis).
Disseminated mycotic infections.
Mycobacterial (lepromatous leprosy, TB).
Viral (varicella, hepatitis, influenza, mononucleosis, measles, mumps).

IMMUNOSUPPRESSIVE MEDICATIONS

Systemic corticosteroids.
Methotrexate, cyclophosphamide.
Rifampin.

OTHER

Alcoholic cirrhosis, biliary cirrhosis, sarcoidosis, rheumatic disease.
Diabetes, Crohn disease, uremia.
Anemia, pyridoxine deficiency, sickle cell anemia.
Burns, malnutrition, pregnancy, old age, surgery.

ANEURYSMS, THORACIC AORTA

ICD-10CM #	I71.2	Thoracic aortic aneurysm, without rupture

Trauma.
Infection.
Inflammatory (syphilis, Takayasu disease).
Collagen vascular disease (RA, ankylosing spondylitis).
Annuloaortic ectasia (Marfan syndrome, Ehlers-Danlos syndrome).
Congenital.
Coarctation.
Cystic medial necrosis.

ANHIDROSIS

ICD-10CM #	L74.0	Miliaria rubra
	L74.1	Miliaria crystallina
	L74.2	Miliaria profunda

Drugs (anticholinergics).
Dehydration.
Hysteria.
Obstruction of sweat ducts (e.g., inflammation, miliaria).
Local radiant heat or pressure.
CNS lesions (medulla, hypothalamus, pons).
Spinal cord lesions.
Lesions of sympathetic nerves.
Congenital sweat gland disturbances.

ANION GAP ACIDOSIS[97]

ICD-10CM #	E87.2	Acidosis

CLINICAL CAUSES OF HIGH ANION GAP AND NORMAL ANION GAP ACIDOSIS

High Anion Gap

Ketoacidosis:
- Diabetic ketoacidosis (acetoacetate).
- Alcoholic (β-hydroxybutyrate).
- Starvation.

Lactic acid acidosis:
- L-Lactic acid acidosis (types A and B).
- D-Lactic acid acidosis.
- Renal failure: sulfate, phosphate, urate, hippurate.

Ingestions (toxins and their metabolites):
- Ethylene glycol → glycolate, oxalate.
- Methyl alcohol → formate.
- Salicylate → ketones, lactate, salicylate.
- Paraldehyde → organic anions.
- Toluene → hippurate (commonly presents with normal anion gap).
- Propylene glycol → lactate.
- Pyroglutamic acidosis (acetaminophen use) → 5-oxoproline.

Normal Anion Gap

GI loss of HCO_3^- (negative urine anion gap):
- Diarrhea.
- Fistula, external.

Renal loss of HCO_3^- or failure to excrete NH_4^+ (positive urine anion gap):
- Proximal renal tubular acidosis (RTA type 2).
- Acetazolamide.
- Classic distal renal tubular acidosis (low serum K^+) RTA type 1.
- Generalized distal renal tubular defect (high serum K^+) RTA type 4.

Miscellaneous:
- NH_4Cl ingestion.
- Sulfur ingestion.
- Dilutional acidosis.
- Late stages in treatment of diabetic ketoacidosis.

ANION GAP INCREASE

ICD-10CM #	E87.8	Other disorders of electrolyte and fluid balance, not elsewhere classified

Uremia.
Ketoacidosis (diabetic, starvation, alcoholic).
Lactic acidosis.
Ethylene glycol poisoning.
Salicylate overdose.
Methanol poisoning.

ANISOCORIA

ICD-10CM #	H57.02	Anisocoria

Mydriatic or miotic drugs.
Prosthetic eye.
Inflammation (keratitis, iridocyclitis).
Infections (herpes zoster, syphilis, meningitis, encephalitis, TB, diphtheria, botulism).
Subdural hemorrhage.
Cavernous sinus thrombosis.
Intracranial neoplasm.
Cerebral aneurysm.
Glaucoma.
CNS degenerative diseases.
Internal carotid ischemia.
Toxic polyneuritis (alcohol, lead).
Adie syndrome.
Horner syndrome.
DM.
Trauma.
Congenital.

ANKLE AND FOOT PAIN[47]

ICD-10CM #	M25.579	Pain in unspecified ankle and joint pain in unspecified foot

Anterior ankle	Anterior impingement. Ankle arthritis or synovitis. Osteochondral defect or lesion (cartilage injury). Loose body within the joint. Talar avascular necrosis. Talar stress fracture. Tenosynovitis of the extensor hallucis longus, extensor digitorum longus. Deep (central) or superficial (anterolateral) peroneal nerve injury. Saphenous (anteromedial) nerve injury.
Posterior ankle	Os trigonum (accessory ossicle involving the posterior lateral tubercle of the talus). Posterior impingement. Retrocalcaneal bursitis. Achilles tendinopathy. Flexor hallucis longus tendinopathy or stenosis.
Posterolateral ankle	Peroneal tendinopathy. Subfibular impingement caused by flatfoot and impingement. Fibular stress fracture. Sural nerve injury. Lateral ligament injury (sprain).
Posteromedial ankle	Posterior tibial tendinopathy. Flexor digitorum longus or flexor hallucis longus tendinopathy. Tibial stress fracture. Medial malleolar stress fracture. Tarsal tunnel syndrome. Tibial nerve injury. Deltoid ligament injury.
Heel	Achilles insertional tendinopathy. Inflammatory enthesitis. Plantar fasciitis. Haglund disease (pump bump). Calcaneal stress fracture.
Hindfoot	Subtalar, talonavicular, or calcaneocuboid arthritis or synovitis. Posterior tibial tendon dysfunction or tendinopathy (medial) or peroneal tendon dysfunction (lateral). Occult fracture of the talus, calcaneus cuboid, or navicular Accessory navicular.
Midfoot	Insertional tendinopathy (peroneal, posterior tibial, tibialis anterior). Arthritis or synovitis (navicular–cuneiform, cuneiform–metatarsal, cuboid–metatarsal). Navicular stress fracture. Spring ligament strain.

Forefoot

First ray, first MTP joint, hallux	Arthritis or synovitis MTP (hallux limitus/rigidus) and IP joints.
	Hallux valgus.
	Hallux varus.
	Sesamoiditis.
	Gouty monoarthritis.
Second to fifth rays, MTP joints, lesser toes	Arthritis or synovitis (MTP, proximal and distal IP joints).
	Lesser toe deformities (hammer and claw toes).
	Metatarsalgia.
	MTP instability.
	MTP dislocations.
	Morton neuroma (interdigital neuralgia).
	Stress fracture of the metatarsals.
	Bunionette (fifth metatarsal phalangeal deviation).
	Rheumatoid nodules.
	Bursitis (intermetatarsal or adventitious).
	Ulcer.
	Infection.

IP, Interphalangeal; *MTP*, metatarsophalangeal.

ANORECTAL DISEASE, AIDS PATIENT[30]

ICD-10CM # Varies with specific diagnosis

DIFFERENTIAL DIAGNOSIS OF ANORECTAL DISEASE IN PATIENTS WITH AIDS

Infections

Bacteria

*Chlamydia trachomatis.**
Lymphogranuloma venereum.
*Neisseria gonorrhoeae.**
Shigella flexneri.
Mycobacterium tuberculosis.

Protozoa

Entamoeba histolytica.
Leishmania donovani.

Viruses

HSV.*
Cytomegalovirus.*

Fungi

Candida albicans.
Histoplasma capsulatum.

Neoplasms

Lymphoma.*
Kaposi sarcoma.
Squamous cell carcinoma.
Cloacogenic carcinoma.
Condyloma acuminatum.

Other

Idiopathic ulcers.*
Perirectal abscess, fistula.*

*More frequent diagnosis.

ANOREXIA[95]

ICD-10CM # R63.0 Anorexia

SELECTED CAUSES OF ANOREXIA

Gastrointestinal Tract/Liver

Gastric outlet obstruction or small bowel obstruction.
Gastric cancer.
Hepatic metastases.
Acute viral hepatitis.

Metabolic

Addison disease.
Hypopituitarism.
Hyperparathyroidism.

Functional

Extremely unpleasant sight/smell.

Systemic

Chronic pain.
Renal failure.
Severe congestive heart failure.
Respiratory failure.

Psychiatric

Depression.
Anorexia nervosa.

Medications

Digoxin.
Narcotic analgesics.
Diuretics.
Antihypertensives.
Chemotherapeutic agents.
Amphetamines.

Miscellaneous

Excessive smoking.
Excessive alcohol intake.
Oral cavity disease.
Thiamine deficiency.
Early pregnancy.
Hypogeusia or dysgeusia.

ANOVULATION

ICD-10CM # N97.0 Female infertility associated with anovulation

Anorexia and bulimia.
Strenuous exercise.
Weight loss/malnutrition.
Empty sella syndrome.
Pituitary disorders (infarction, infection, trauma, irradiation, surgery, microadenomas, macroadenomas).
Idiopathic hypopituitarism.
Drug induced.
Thyroid dysfunction (hypothyroidism, hyperthyroidism).
Systemic diseases (e.g., liver disease).
Adrenal hyperfunction (Cushing syndrome, congenital adrenal hyperplasia).
Polycystic ovarian syndrome.
Isolated gonadotropin deficiency.

ANOVULATION, HYPOTHALAMIC PITUITARY CAUSES[68]

ICD-10CM # N97.0 Female infertility associated with anovulation

CLASSIFICATION OF ANOVULATION CAUSED BY DISORDERS OF THE HYPOTHALAMIC-PITUITARY UNIT

Functional hypothalamic anovulation (amenorrhea):
- Stress (psychogenic or physical).
- Dieting.
- Vigorous exercise.
- Chronic illness (e.g., chronic liver or renal insufficiency, AIDS).

Psychiatric-medical emergencies:
- Anorexia nervosa.

Medications:
- Antipsychotics (e.g., olanzapine, risperidone, amisulpride, clozapine).
- Opiates.

Hypothyroidism.

ANATOMICALLY OR GENETICALLY DEFINED PATHOLOGIC CONDITIONS OF THE HYPOTHALAMIC-PITUITARY UNIT

Pituitary tumors.
Prolactinoma.
Clinically nonfunctioning adenoma.
GH-secreting adenoma (acromegaly).
ACTH-secreting adenoma (Cushing disease).
Other pituitary tumors (e.g., metastasis, meningioma).
Pituitary stalk section.
Hemorrhagic pituitary destruction, including pituitary apoplexy and Sheehan syndrome.
Pituitary aneurysm.
Infiltrative disease of the pituitary (e.g., lymphocytic hypophysitis, sarcoidosis, histiocytosis X, tuberculosis).
Empty sella syndrome.
Tumors that affect hypothalamic function (e.g., metastasis, craniopharyngioma).
Infiltrative granulomatous disease of the hypothalamus (e.g., sarcoidosis, histiocytosis X, tuberculosis).
Head trauma.
Irradiation to the head.
CNS infection.
Isolated gonadotropin deficiency (including Kallmann syndrome).
Other.

ACTH, Adrenocorticotropic hormone; *AIDS*, acquired immunodeficiency syndrome; *CNS*, central nervous system; *GH*, growth hormone.

AORTIC ARCH SEGMENT ABNORMALITIES[14]

ICD-10CM # Q25.49 Other congenital malformations of aorta

DIFFERENTIAL DIAGNOSIS OF AORTIC ARCH SEGMENT ABNORMALITIES

Dilated aortic arch:
- Aortic aneurysm.
- Aortic dissection.
- Aortic pseudoaneurysm.
- Mass silhouetting aortic arch.

Small or inapparent arch:
- Right-sided aortic arch.
- Coarctation of the aorta.
- Interruption of the aortic arch.
- Double aortic arch.

APPENDICITIS, DIFFERENTIAL DIAGNOSIS IN PREGNANCY[34]

ICD-10CM # Varies with specific diagnosis

DIFFERENTIAL DIAGNOSIS OF APPENDICITIS DURING PREGNANCY

Gynecologic Conditions
Ruptured ovarian cyst.
Adnexal torsion.
Pelvic inflammatory disease or salpingitis.
Endometriosis.
Ovarian cancer.
Obstetrical Causes
Abruptio placentae.
Chorioamnionitis.
Endometritis.
Uterine fibroid degeneration.
Labor (preterm or term).
Viscus perforation after abortion.
Ruptured ectopic pregnancy.
Gastrointestinal Causes
Crohn disease.
Colonic diverticulitis (right side).
Cholecystitis.
Pancreatitis.
Mesenteric lymphadenitis.
Gastroenteritis.
Colon cancer.
Intestinal obstruction.
Hernia (incarcerated inguinal or internal).
Colonic intussusception.
Ruptured Meckel diverticulum.
Colonic perforation.
Acute mesenteric ischemia.
Other Causes
Pyelonephritis.
Urolithiasis.

APPETITE LOSS IN INFANTS AND CHILDREN[48]

ICD-10CM #	R63.0	Anorexia
	F50.8	Other eating disorders
	F98.29	Other feeding disorders of infancy and early childhood

ORGANIC DISEASE

Infection (Acute or Chronic) Neurologic
Congenital degenerative disease.
Hypothalamic lesion.
Increased intracranial pressure (including a brain tumor).
Swallowing disorders (neuromuscular).
Gastrointestinal
Oral lesions (e.g., thrush or herpes simplex).
Gastroesophageal reflux.
Obstruction (especially with gastric or intestinal distention).
Inflammatory bowel disease.
Celiac disease.
Constipation.
Cardiac
Congestive heart failure (especially associated with cyanotic lesions).
Metabolic
Renal failure and/or renal tubule acidosis.
Liver failure.
Congenital metabolic disease.
Lead poisoning.
Nutritional
Marasmus.
Iron deficiency.
Zinc deficiency.
Fever
RA.
Rheumatic fever.
Drugs
Morphine.
Digitalis.
Antimetabolites.
Methylphenidate.
Amphetamines.
Miscellaneous
Prolonged restriction of oral feedings, beginning in the neonatal period.
Systemic lupus erythematosus (SLE).
Tumor.

PSYCHOLOGIC FACTORS

Anxiety, fear, depression, mania (limbic influence on the hypothalamus).
Avoidance of symptoms associated with meals (abdominal pain, diarrhea, bloating, urgency, dumping syndrome).
Anorexia nervosa.
Excessive weight loss and food aversion in athletes, simulating anorexia nervosa.

ARTERIAL OCCLUSION[37]

ICD-10CM #	I74.3	Embolism and thrombosis of arteries of the lower extremities
	I74.2	Embolism and thrombosis of arteries of the upper extremities

Thromboembolism (post-MI, mitral stenosis, rheumatic valve disease, atrial fibrillation, atrial myxoma, marantic endocarditis, bacterial endocarditis, Libman-Sacks endocarditis).
Atheroembolism (microemboli composed of cholesterol, calcium, and platelets from proximal atherosclerotic plaques).
Arterial thrombosis (endothelial injury, altered arterial blood flow, trauma, severe atherosclerosis, acute vasculitis).
Vasospasm.
Trauma.
Hypercoagulable states.
Miscellaneous (irradiation, drugs, infections, necrotizing).

ARTHRITIS AND ABDOMINAL PAIN

ICD-10CM #	M00.9	Pyogenic arthritis, unspecified
	R10.817	Generalized abdominal tenderness
	M02.9	Reactive arthropathy

Viral syndrome.
Inflammatory bowel disease.
Celiac disease.
Vasculitis.
SLE.
RA.
Scleroderma.
Amyloidosis.
Chronic hepatitis C.
Whipple disease.
Polyarteritis nodosa.
Behçet disease.
Familial Mediterranean fever.
Blind loop syndrome.
Babesiosis.
Lyme disease.
Ehrlichiosis.

ARTHRITIS AND DIARRHEA

ICD-10CM #	M00.9	Pyogenic arthritis, unspecified
	R19.7	Diarrhea, unspecified

Viral syndrome.
Inflammatory bowel disease.
Celiac disease.
Whipple disease.
Enterogenic (bacterial) reactive arthritis.
Collagenous colitis.
Behçet disease.
Hyperthyroidism.
Spondyloarthropathy.
Blind loop syndrome.

ARTHRITIS AND EYE LESIONS[20]

ICD-10CM #	M00.9	Pyogenic arthritis, unspecified
	M02.3	Reiter disease
	M02.9	Reactive arthropathy

SLE.
Sjögren syndrome.
Behçet syndrome.
Sarcoidosis.
Subacute bacterial endocarditis (SBE).
Lyme disease.
Granulomatosis with polyangiitis.
Giant cell arteritis.
Takayasu arteritis.
RA, JRA.
Scleroderma.
Inflammatory bowel disease.
Whipple disease.
Ankylosing spondylitis.
Reactive arthritis.
Psoriatic arthritis.

ARTHRITIS AND HEART MURMUR[20]

ICD-10CM #	M00.9	Pyogenic arthritis, unspecified
	I01.8	Other acute rheumatic heart disease
	M02.9	Reactive arthropathy

SBE.
Cardiac myxoma.
Ankylosing spondylitis.
Reactive arthritis.

Acute rheumatic fever.
RA.
SLE with Libman-Sacks endocarditis.
Relapsing polychondritis.

ARTHRITIS AND MUSCLE WEAKNESS[22]

ICD-10CM #	M00.9	Pyogenic arthritis, unspecified
	M62.9	Disorder of muscle, unspecified
	M02.9	Reactive arthropathy

RA.
Ankylosing spondylitis.
Polymyositis.
Dermatomyositis.
SLE, scleroderma, mixed connective tissue disease.
Sarcoidosis.
HIV-associated arthritis.
Whipple disease.

ARTHRITIS AND RASH[20]

ICD-10CM #	M00.9	Pyogenic arthritis, unspecified
	R21	Rash and other non-specific skin eruption
	M02.9	Reactive arthropathy

Chronic urticaria.
Vasculitic urticaria.
SLE.
Dermatomyositis.
Polymyositis.
Psoriatic arthritis.
Reactive arthritis.
Chronic sarcoidosis.
Serum sickness.
Sweet syndrome.
Leprosy.

ARTHRITIS AND SUBCUTANEOUS NODULES[20]

ICD-10CM #	M00.9	Pyogenic arthritis, unspecified
	A18.4	Tuberculosis of skin and subcutaneous tissue
	M02.9	Reactive arthropathy

RA.
Gout.
Pseudogout (rare).
Sarcoidosis.
Light chain (LA) amyloidosis (primary, multiple myeloma).
Acute rheumatic fever (ARF).
Hemochromatosis.
Whipple disease.
Multicentric reticulohistiocytosis.

ARTHRITIS AND WEIGHT LOSS[20]

ICD-10CM #	M00.9	Pyogenic arthritis, unspecified
	R63.4	Abnormal weight loss
	M02.9	Reactive arthropathy

Severe RA.
RA with vasculitis.
Reactive arthritis.
RA or psoriatic arthritis or ankylosing spondylitis with amyloidosis.
Cancer.
Enteropathic arthritis (Crohn, ulcerative colitis).
HIV infection.
Whipple disease.
Blind loop syndrome.
Scleroderma with intestinal bacterial overgrowth.

ARTHRITIS OR EXTREMITY PAIN, IN CHILDREN AND ADOLESCENTS[58]

ICD-10CM #	M02.9	Reactive arthropathy

CAUSES OF ARTHRITIS OR EXTREMITY PAIN IN CHILDREN AND ADOLESCENTS

Rheumatic and Inflammatory Diseases
Juvenile idiopathic arthritis.
Systemic lupus erythematosus.
Juvenile dermatomyositis.
Polyarteritis.
Vasculitis.
Scleroderma.
Sjögren syndrome.
Behçet disease.
Overlap syndromes.
Granulomatosis with polyangiitis (Wegener granulomatosis).
Sarcoidosis.
Kawasaki syndrome.
Henoch-Schönlein purpura.
Chronic recurrent multifocal osteomyelitis.

Seronegative Spondyloarthropathies
Juvenile ankylosing spondylitis.
Inflammatory bowel disease.
Psoriatic arthritis.
Reactive arthritis associated with urethritis, iridocyclitis, and mucocutaneous lesions.

Infectious Illnesses
Bacterial arthritis (septic arthritis, *Staphylococcus aureus,* pneumococcus, gonococcus, *Haemophilus influenzae*).
Lyme disease.
Viral illness (parvovirus, rubella, mumps, Epstein-Barr virus, hepatitis B).
Fungal arthritis.
Mycobacterial infection.
Spirochetal infection.
Endocarditis.

Reactive Arthritis
Acute rheumatic fever.
Reactive arthritis (postinfectious due to *Shigella, Salmonella, Yersinia, Chlamydia,* or meningococcus).
Serum sickness.
Toxic synovitis of the hip.
Postimmunization.

Immunodeficiencies
Hypogammaglobulinemia.
Immunoglobulin A deficiency.
Human immunodeficiency virus.

Congenital and Metabolic Disorders
Gout.
Pseudogout.
Mucopolysaccharidoses.
Thyroid disease (hypothyroidism, hyperthyroidism).
Hyperparathyroidism.
Vitamin C deficiency (scurvy).
Hereditary connective tissue disease (Marfan syndrome, Ehlers-Danlos syndrome).
Fabry disease.
Farber disease.
Amyloidosis (familial Mediterranean fever).

Bone and Cartilage Disorders
Trauma.
Patellofemoral syndrome.
Hypermobility syndrome.
Osteochondritis dissecans.
Avascular necrosis (including Legg-Calvé-Perthes disease).
Hypertrophic osteoarthropathy.
Slipped capital femoral epiphysis.
Osteolysis.
Benign bone tumors (including osteoid osteoma).
Histiocytosis.
Rickets.

Neuropathic Disorders
Peripheral neuropathies.
Carpal tunnel syndrome.
Charcot joints.

Neoplastic Disorders
Leukemia.
Neuroblastoma.
Lymphoma.
Bone tumors (osteosarcoma, Ewing sarcoma).
Histiocytic syndromes.
Synovial tumors.

Hematologic Disorders
Hemophilia.
Hemoglobinopathies (including sickle cell disease).

Miscellaneous Disorders
Pigmented villonodular synovitis.
Plant-thorn synovitis (foreign body arthritis).
Myositis ossificans.
Eosinophilic fasciitis.
Tendinitis (overuse injury).
Raynaud phenomenon.

Pain Syndromes
Fibromyalgia.
Growing pains.
Depression (with somatization).
Reflex sympathetic dystrophy.
Regional myofascial pain syndromes.

ARTHRITIS, AXIAL SKELETON

ICD-10CM #	M45.9	Ankylosing spondylitis of unspecified sites in spine
	L40.54	Psoriatic juvenile arthropathy
	L40.59	Other psoriatic arthropathy
	M15.9	Polyosteoarthritis, unspecified
	M45.9	Ankylosing spondylitis of unspecified sites in spine

RA.
Psoriatic arthritis.
Reiter syndrome (reactive arthritis).
Ankylosing spondylitis.
Juvenile RA.
Degenerative disease of the nucleus pulposus.
Spondylosis deformans.
Diffuse idiopathic skeletal hyperostosis (DISH).
Alkaptonuria.
Infection.

ARTHRITIS, CHRONIC, MONOARTICULAR OR OLIGOARTICULAR, INFECTIOUS CAUSES[10]

ICD-10CM # Varies with specific diagnosis

INFECTIOUS CAUSES OF CHRONIC MONOARTICULAR OR OLIGOARTICULAR ARTHRITIS

Bacterial
Borrelia burgdorferi.
Tropheryma whipplei.
Treponema pallidum.
Nocardia spp.
Fungi
Candida spp.
Cryptococcus neoformans.
Blastomyces dermatitidis.
Coccidioides spp.
Paracoccidioides brasiliensis.
Sporothrix schenckii.
Aspergillus spp. and other molds, including *Rhizopus, Scedosporium,* and *Fusarium.*
Mycobacteria
Mycobacterium tuberculosis.
M. kansasii.
M. marinum.
M. avium-intracellulare complex.
M. terrae.
M. fortuitum, M. chelonae, M. abscessus.
M. haemophilum.
M. leprae.
Parasites
Helminths.
Filariae.

ARTHRITIS, FEVER, AND RASH[20]

ICD-10CM #	M00.9	Pyogenic arthritis, unspecified
	M02.9	Reactive arthropathy
	R21	Rash and other nonspecific skin eruption
	R50.9	Fever, unspecified

Rubella, parvovirus B19.
Gonococcemia, meningococcemia.
Secondary syphilis, Lyme borreliosis.
Adult acute rheumatic fever, adult Still disease, adult Kawasaki disease.
Vasculitic urticaria.
Acute sarcoidosis.
Familial Mediterranean fever.
Hyperimmunoglobulinemia D and periodic fever syndrome.

ARTHRITIS, MONOARTICULAR AND OLIGOARTICULAR[7]

ICD-10CM #	M19.90	Unspecified osteoarthritis, unspecified site
	M01.X0	Direct infection of unspecified joint in infectious and parasitic diseases classified elsewhere
	M13.10	Monoarthritis, not elsewhere classified, unspecified site

Septic arthritis (*S. aureus, Neisseria gonorrhoeae,* meningococci, streptococci, *Streptococcus pneumoniae,* enteric gram-negative bacilli).
Crystalline-induced arthritis (gout, pseudogout, calcium oxalate, hydroxyapatite and other basic calcium/phosphate crystals).
Traumatic joint injury.
Hemarthrosis.
Monoarticular or oligoarticular flare of an inflammatory polyarticular rheumatic disease (RA, psoriatic arthritis, Reiter syndrome [reactive arthritis], SLE).

ARTHRITIS, PEDIATRIC AGE[48]

ICD-10CM #	M01.X0	Direct infection of unspecified joint in infectious and parasitic diseases classified elsewhere
	M08.00	Unspecified juvenile rheumatoid arthritis of unspecified site
	M08.3	Juvenile rheumatoid polyarthritis (seronegative)
	M08.40	Pauciarticular juvenile rheumatoid arthritis, unspecified site

RHEUMATIC DISEASES OF CHILDHOOD

Acute rheumatic fever.
SLE.
Juvenile ankylosing spondylitis.
Polymyositis and dermatomyositis.
Vasculitis.
Scleroderma.
Psoriatic arthritis.
Mixed connective tissue disease and overlap syndromes.
Kawasaki disease.
Behçet syndrome.
Familial Mediterranean fever.
Reiter syndrome (reactive arthritis).
Reflex sympathetic dystrophy.
Fibromyalgia (fibrositis).

INFECTIOUS DISEASES

Bacterial arthritis.
Viral or postviral arthritis.
Fungal arthritis.
Osteomyelitis.
Reactive arthritis.

NEOPLASTIC DISEASES

Leukemia.
Lymphoma.
Neuroblastoma.
Primary bone tumors.

NONINFLAMMATORY DISORDERS

Trauma.
Avascular necrosis syndromes.
Osteochondroses.
Slipped capital femoral epiphysis.
Diskitis.
Patellofemoral dysfunction (chondromalacia patellae).
Toxic synovitis of the hip.
Overuse syndromes.

GENETIC OR CONGENITAL SYNDROMES

Hematologic Disorders
Sickle cell disease.
Hemophilia.

INFLAMMATORY BOWEL DISEASE

Miscellaneous
Growing pains.
Psychogenic arthralgias (conversion reactions).
Hypermobility syndrome.
Villonodular synovitis.
Foreign body arthritis.

ARTHRITIS, POLYARTICULAR

ICD-10CM #	M15.0	Primary generalized (osteo)arthritis
	M12.89	Other specific arthropathies, not elsewhere classified, multiple sites
	M08.3	Juvenile rheumatoid polyarthritis (seronegative)

RA, juvenile (rheumatoid) polyarthritis.
SLE, other connective tissue diseases, erythema nodosum, palindromic rheumatism, relapsing polychondritis.
Psoriatic arthritis, ankylosing spondylitis.
Sarcoidosis.
Lyme arthritis, bacterial endocarditis, *Neisseria gonorrhoeae* infection, rheumatic fever, Reiter disease (reactive arthritis).
Crystal deposition disease.
Hypersensitivity to serum or drugs.
Hepatitis B, HIV, rubella, mumps.
Other: serum sickness, leukemias, lymphomas, enteropathic arthropathy, Whipple disease, Behçet syndrome, Henoch-Schönlein purpura, familial Mediterranean fever, hypertrophic pulmonary osteoarthropathy.

ASCENDING AORTA, ABNORMAL SEGMENT[13]

ICD-10CM #	Q25.49	Other congenital malformations of aorta

DIFFERENTIAL DIAGNOSIS OF AN ABNORMAL ASCENDING AORTA SEGMENT

Aortic aneurysm.
Aortic dissection.
Poststenotic dilation in aortic stenosis.
Aortic dilation in aortic insufficiency.

ASCITES

ICD-10CM #	R18.0	Malignant ascites
	C78.6	Secondary malignant neoplasm of retroperitoneum and peritoneum
	I89.8	Other specified noninfective disorders of lymphatic vessels and lymph nodes

Hypoalbuminemia: nephrotic syndrome, protein-losing gastroenteropathy, starvation.
Cirrhosis.
Hepatic congestion: CHF, constrictive pericarditis, tricuspid insufficiency, hepatic vein obstruction (Budd-Chiari syndrome), inferior vena cava or portal vein obstruction.
Peritoneal infections: TB and other bacterial infections, fungal diseases, parasites.
Neoplasms: primary hepatic neoplasms, metastases to liver or peritoneum, lymphomas, leukemias, myeloid metaplasia.
Lymphatic obstruction: mediastinal tumors, trauma to the thoracic duct, filariasis.
Ovarian disease: Meigs syndrome, struma ovarii.
Chronic pancreatitis or pseudocyst: pancreatic ascites.
Leakage of bile: bile ascites.
Urinary obstruction or trauma: urine ascites.
Myxedema.
Chylous ascites.

ASPIRATION LUNG INJURY, CHILDREN[58]

ICD-10CM #	P24.8	Neonatal aspiration syndromes

CONDITIONS PREDISPOSING TO ASPIRATION LUNG INJURY IN CHILDREN

Anatomic and Mechanical
Tracheoesophageal fistula.
Laryngeal cleft.
Vascular ring.
Cleft palate.
Micrognathia.
Macroglossia.
Achalasia.
Esophageal foreign body.
Tracheostomy.
Endotracheal tube.
Nasoenteric tube.
Collagen vascular disease (scleroderma, dermatomyositis).
Gastroesophageal reflux disease.
Obesity.
Neuromuscular
Altered consciousness.
Immaturity of swallowing/prematurity.
Dysautonomia.
Increased intracranial pressure.
Hydrocephalus.
Vocal cord paralysis.
Cerebral palsy.
Muscular dystrophy.
Myasthenia gravis.
Guillain-Barré syndrome.
Werdnig-Hoffmann disease.
Ataxia-telangiectasia.
Cerebral vascular accident.
Miscellaneous
Poor oral hygiene.
Gingivitis.
Prolonged hospitalization.
Gastric outlet or intestinal obstruction.
Poor feeding techniques (bottle propping, overfeeding, inappropriate foods for toddlers).
Bronchopulmonary dysplasia.
Viral infection.

ASTHENIA

ICD-10CM #	G93.3	Postviral fatigue syndrome
	R53.1	Weakness
	R53.81	Other malaise
	R53.83	Other fatigue

Depression.
Chronic fatigue syndrome.
Sleep disorders.
Anemia.
Hypothyroidism.
Sedentary lifestyle.
Medications (e.g., narcotics, sedatives).
Infections.
Dehydration/electrolyte disorders.
COPD and other pulmonary disorders.
Renal failure.
CHF.
Diabetes.
Addison disease.
Paraneoplastic syndrome.

ASTHMA, CHILDHOOD[9]

ICD-10CM #	J45.20	Mild intermittent asthma, uncomplicated
	J45.22	Mild intermittent asthma with status asthmaticus

INFECTIONS

Bronchiolitis (RSV).
Pneumonia.
Croup.
Tuberculosis, histoplasmosis.
Bronchiectasis.
Bronchiolitis obliterans.
Bronchitis.
Sinusitis.

ANATOMIC, CONGENITAL

Cystic fibrosis.
Vascular rings.
Ciliary dyskinesia.
B-lymphocyte immune defect.
Congestive heart failure.
Laryngotracheomalacia.
Tumor, lymphoma.
H-type tracheoesophageal fistula.
Repaired tracheoesophageal fistula.
Gastroesophageal reflux.

VASCULITIS, HYPERSENSITIVITY

Allergic bronchopulmonary aspergillosis.
Allergic alveolitis, hypersensitivity pneumonitis.
Churg-Strauss syndrome.
Periarteritis nodosa.

OTHER

Foreign body aspiration.
Pulmonary thromboembolism.
Psychogenic cough.
Sarcoidosis.
Bronchopulmonary dysplasia.
Vocal cord dysfunction.

ATAXIA

ICD-10CM #	R27.0	Ataxia, unspecified
	R27.8	Other lack of coordination
	R27.9	Unspecified lack of coordination
	F10.229	Alcohol dependence with intoxication, unspecified
	F10.20	Alcohol dependence, uncomplicated
	G11.1	Early-onset cerebellar ataxia
	G31.89	Other specified degenerative diseases of nervous system
	F44.4	Conversion disorder with motor symptom or deficit
	F44.6	Conversion disorder with sensory symptom or deficit

Vertebral-basilar artery ischemia.
Diabetic neuropathy.
Tabes dorsalis.
Vitamin B_{12} deficiency.
Multiple sclerosis and other demyelinating diseases.
Meningomyelopathy.
Cerebellar neoplasms, hemorrhage, abscess, infarct.
Nutritional (Wernicke encephalopathy).
Paraneoplastic syndromes.
Parainfectious: Guillain-Barré syndrome, acute ataxia of childhood and young adults.
Toxins: phenytoin, alcohol, sedatives, organophosphates.
Wilson disease (hepatolenticular degeneration).
Hypothyroidism.
Myopathy.
Cerebellar and spinocerebellar degeneration: ataxia/telangiectasia, Friedreich ataxia.
Frontal lobe lesions: tumors, thrombosis of anterior cerebral artery, hydrocephalus.
Labyrinthine destruction: neoplasm, injury, inflammation, compression.
Hysteria.
AIDS.

ATAXIA, ACUTE OR RECURRENT[27]

ICD-10CM #	R27.0	Ataxia, unspecified
	R27.8	Other lack of coordination
	R27.9	Unspecified lack of coordination
	F10.229	Alcohol dependence with Intoxication, unspecified
	F10.20	Alcohol dependence, uncomplicated
	G11.1	Early-onset cerebellar ataxia
	G31.89	Other specified degenerative diseases of nervous system
	F44.4	Conversion disorder with motor symptom or deficit
	F44.6	Conversion disorder with sensory symptom or deficit

Drug ingestion (e.g., phenytoin, carbamazepine, sedatives, hypnotics, and phencyclidine) or intoxication (e.g., alcohol, ethylene glycol, hydrocarbon fumes, lead, mercury, or thallium).
Postinfectious (cerebellitis [e.g., varicella], acute disseminated encephalomyelitis).
Head trauma.
Basilar migraine.
Benign paroxysmal vertigo (migraine equivalent).
Brain tumor or neuroblastoma (if accompanied by opsoclonus or myoclonus [i.e., "dancing eyes, dancing feet"]).
Hydrocephalus.
Infection (e.g., labyrinthitis, abscess).
Seizure (ictal or postictal).
Vascular events (e.g., cerebellar hemorrhage or stroke).
Miller-Fisher variant of Guillain-Barré syndrome (ataxia, ophthalmoplegia, and areflexia). Warning: If bulbar signs present, disease is likely progressive; patient may lose ability to protect airway and/or ability to breathe.
Inherited ataxias.
Inborn errors of metabolism (e.g., mitochondrial disorders, amino-acidopathies, urea cycle defects).
Conversion reaction.
Multiple sclerosis.

ATAXIA, CEREBELLAR, ADULT ONSET[88]

ICD-10CM #	G11.0	Congenital nonprogressive ataxia
	G11.2	Late-onset cerebellar ataxia

CAUSES OF ADULT ONSET CEREBELLAR ATAXIA

Inherited
Later onset SCA syndromes.
Rarely Friedreich ataxia.
Congenital
Arnold–Chiari malformation (cerebellar ectopia).
Inflammatory
Multiple sclerosis.
Sarcoidosis.
Infections (TB, viral).
Neoplastic
Often metastatic in adults.
Meningioma, neurofibroma.
Hemangioblastoma.
Paraneoplastic
Usually with small cell bronchial carcinoma.
Vascular
Infarction, hemorrhage.
Arteriovenous malformations.
Trauma
Head injury.
Postsurgical.
Toxic
Alcohol, phenytoin, solvent abuse.
Endocrine
Hypothyroidism (very rare).
Degenerative
Multiple system atrophy (MSA).

ATAXIA, CEREBELLAR, CHILDREN[88]

ICD-10CM #	G11.0	Congenital nonprogressive ataxia
	G11.2	Late-onset cerebellar ataxia

CAUSES OF CEREBELLAR ATAXIA IN CHILDREN

Congenital Malformations
Cerebellar agenesis/hypoplasia.
Dandy–Walker syndrome.
Arnold–Chiari malformation.
Hereditary Ataxias
Friedreich ataxia.
Trauma
Birth trauma.
Head injury in childhood.
Infectious
Secondary to bacterial meningitis.
Secondary to encephalitis.
Hydrocephalus
Tumors
Medulloblastoma.
Astrocytoma.
Hemangioblastoma.

ATAXIA, CHRONIC OR PROGRESSIVE[27]

ICD-10CM #	R27.0	Ataxia, unspecified
	R27.8	Other lack of coordination
	R27.9	Unspecified lack of coordination
	G11.1	Early-onset cerebellar ataxia
	G11.0	Congenital nonprogressive ataxia
	G11.2	Late-onset cerebellar ataxia
	G11.3	Cerebellar ataxia with defective DNA repair
	G11.8	Other hereditary ataxia

Hydrocephalus.
Hypothyroidism.
Tumor or paraneoplastic syndrome.
Low vitamin E levels (e.g., cystic fibrosis).
Wilson disease.
Inborn errors of metabolism.
Inherited ataxias (e.g., ataxia-telangiectasia, Friedreich ataxia).

ATAXIA IN CHILDHOOD[98]

ICD-10CM #	G11.1	Early-onset cerebellar ataxia

SELECTED CAUSES OF ATAXIA IN CHILDHOOD

Congenital:
- Agenesis of vermis of the cerebellum.
- Aplasia or dysplasia of the cerebellum.
- Basilar impression.
- Cerebellar dysplasia with microgyria, macrogyria, or agyria.
- Cervical spinal bifida with herniation of the cerebellum (Chiari malformation, type 3).
- Chiari malformation.
- Dandy-Walker syndrome.
- Encephalocele.
- Hydrocephalus (progressive).
- Hypoplasia of the cerebellum.

Degenerative and/or genetic:
- Acute intermittent cerebellar ataxia.
- Ataxia, retinitis pigmentosa, deafness, vestibular abnormality, and intellectual deterioration.
- Ataxia-telangiectasia.
- Biemond posterior column ataxia.
- Cerebellar ataxia with deafness, anosmia, absent caloric responses, nonreactive pupils, and hyporeflexia.
- Cockayne syndrome.
- Dentate cerebellar ataxia (dyssynergia cerebellaris progressiva).
- Familial ataxia with macular degeneration.
- Friedreich ataxia.
- Hereditary cerebellar ataxia, intellectual retardation, choreoathetosis, and eunuchoidism.
- Hereditary cerebellar ataxia with myotonia and cataracts.
- Hypertrophic interstitial neuritis.
- Marie ataxia.
- Marinesco-Sjögren syndrome.
- Pelizaeus-Merzbacher disease.
- Periodic attacks of vertigo, diplopia, and ataxia—autosomal dominant inheritance.
- Posterior and lateral column difficulties, nystagmus, and muscle atrophy.
- Progressive cerebellar ataxia and epilepsy.
- Ramsay Hunt syndrome (myoclonic seizures and ataxia).
- Roussy-Lévy syndrome.
- Spinocerebellar ataxia (SCAs); olivopontocerebellar ataxias.

Endocrinologic:
- Cretinism.
- Hypothyroidism.

Infectious or postinfectious:
- Acute cerebellar ataxia.
- Acute disseminated encephalomyelitis.
- Cerebellar abscess.

- Coxsackievirus.
- Diphtheria.
- Echovirus.
- Fisher syndrome.
- Infectious mononucleosis (Epstein-Barr virus infection).
- Infectious polyneuropathy.
- Japanese B encephalitis.
- Mumps encephalitis.
- *Mycoplasma pneumoniae.*
- Pertussis.
- Polio.
- Postbacterial meningitis.
- Rubeola.
- Tuberculosis.
- Typhoid.
- Varicella.

Metabolic:
- Abetalipoproteinemia.
- Argininosuccinic aciduria.
- Ataxia with vitamin E deficiency (AVED).
- GM2 gangliosidosis (late).
- Hartnup disease.
- Hyperalaninemia.
- Hyperammonemia I and II.
- Hypoglycemia.
- Kearns-Sayre syndrome.
- Leigh disease.
- Maple syrup urine disease (intermittent).
- MERRF (Myoclonic epilepsy with ragged red fibers).
- Metachromatic leukodystrophy.
- Mitochondrial complex defects (I, III, IV).
- Multiple carboxylase deficiency (biotinidase deficiency).
- Neuronal ceroid-lipofuscinosis.
- Neuropathy, ataxia, retinitis pigmentosa (NARP).
- Niemann-Pick disease (late infantile).
- 5-Oxoprolinuria.
- Pyruvate decarboxylase deficiency.
- Refsum disease.
- Sialidosis.
- Triose-phosphate isomerase deficiency.
- Tryptophanuria.
- Wernicke encephalopathy (thiamine or B_1 deficiency).

Neoplastic:
- Frontal lobe tumors.
- Hemispheric cerebellar tumors.
- Midline cerebellar tumors.
- Neuroblastoma.
- Pontine tumors (primarily gliomas).
- Spinal cord tumors.

Primary psychogenic:
- Conversion reaction.

Toxic:
- Alcohol.
- Benzodiazepines.
- Carbamazepine.
- Clonazepam.
- Lead encephalopathy.
- Phenobarbital.
- Phenytoin.
- Primidone.
- Tick paralysis poisoning.

Traumatic:
- Acute cerebellar edema.
- Acute frontal lobe edema.

Vascular:
- Angioblastoma of cerebellum.
- Basilar migraine.
- Cerebellar embolism.
- Cerebellar hemorrhage.
- Cerebellar thrombosis.
- Posterior cerebellar artery disease.
- Vasculitis.
- von Hippel-Lindau disease.

ATAXIA, TOXIC CAUSES[93]

ICD-10CM # R27.0 Early-onset cerebellar ataxia

SELECTED TOXIC CAUSES OF ATAXIA

Medications:
- Acetohexamide.
- Amiodarone.
- Anticholinergic agents.
- Antidepressants, including selective serotonin reuptake inhibitors.
- Antiepileptic drugs.
- Antihistamines.
- Antimicrobials, antifungals.
- Antineoplastics.
- Antiparasitics.
- Baclofen.
- Buspirone.
- Dextromethorphan.
- Disulfiram.
- Ethanol.
- Fenfluramine.
- Lithium.
- Lysergic acid diethylamide (LSD), phencyclidine palmitate (PCP).
- Mexiletine.
- Sedatives, narcotics.

Industrial toxins:
- Aluminum compounds.
- Butyl alcohol.
- Carbon monoxide.
- Carbon tetrachloride.
- Ethylene glycol.
- Formaldehyde.
- Gasoline.
- Manganese.
- Metaldehyde (snail bait, fire starters).
- Paradichlorobenzene (moth repellent, diaper pail deodorant).
- Rodenticides: aluminum phosphide, sodium monofluoroacetate.
- Solvents.

Biologic toxins:
- Belladonna, hyoscyamine.
- Buckeye (*Aesculus* spp.).
- Mayapple (*Podophyllum peltatum*).
- Mescaline, peyote.
- Podophyllum (ingested).
- Poison hemlock (*Conium maculatum*).

ATELECTASIS

ICD-10CM # J98.11 Atelectasis

- Lung neoplasm (primary or metastatic).
- Infection (pneumonia, TB, fungal, histoplasmosis).
- Postoperative (lower lobes).
- Sarcoidosis.
- Mucoid impaction.
- Foreign body.
- Postinflammatory (middle lobe syndrome).
- Pneumothorax.
- Pleural effusion.
- Pneumoconiosis.
- Interstitial fibrosis.
- Bulla.
- Mediastinal or adjacent mass.

ATRIAL ENLARGEMENT, LEFT ATRIUM[41]

ICD-10CM # I51.7 Cardiomegaly

CAUSES OF LARGE LEFT ATRIUM

Causes Due to Volume Overload
- Mitral regurgitation (often with left ventricular failure).
- Ventricular septal defect.
- Patent ductus arteriosus.
- Atrial septal defect with shunt reversal (i.e., pulmonary hypertension).
- ASD with tricuspid atresia (obligatory shunt reversal).
- Aortopulmonary window.

Causes Due to Pressure Overload
- Mitral stenosis.
- Noncompliant left ventricle: hypertension, hypertrophic cardiomyopathy, aortic stenosis.
- Left ventricular failure (often with secondary mitral regurgitation).
- Left atrial myxoma.

Other Causes (Both Rare)
- Atrial fibrillation.
- Isolated/idiopathic.

ATRIAL ENLARGEMENT, RIGHT ATRIUM

ICD-10CM # I51.7 Cardiomegaly

- Right ventricular failure.
- Atrial septal defect.
- Tricuspid regurgitation.
- Tricuspid stenosis.
- Pulmonary hypertension.
- Restrictive cardiomyopathy.
- Right atrial myxoma.
- Ebstein anomaly.
- Anomalous pulmonary venous drainage to the right atrium.
- Endomyocardial fibrosis.
- Sinus of Valsalva fistula.
- Arrhythmogenic right ventricular dysplasia.

ATYPICAL LYMPHOCYTOSIS, HETEROPHIL NEGATIVE, INFECTIOUS CAUSES[3]

ICD-10CM # D72.820 Lymphocytosis (symptomatic)

MOST COMMON INFECTIOUS CAUSES OF HETEROPHIL-NEGATIVE ATYPICAL LYMPHOCYTOSIS

- Babesiosis.
- Cytomegalovirus.

Epstein-Barr virus (particularly in children).
Human herpesvirus 6.
Human immunodeficiency virus (especially during acute seroconversion).
Infectious mononucleosis.
Malaria.
Measles.
Toxoplasmosis.
Varicella.
Infectious hepatitis.

AV NODAL BLOCK[37]

ICD-10CM #	I44.30	Unspecified atrioventricular block
	I44.2	Atrioventricular block, complete

Idiopathic fibrosis (Lenègre disease).
Sclerodegenerative processes (e.g., Lev disease with calcification of the mitral and aortic annuli).
AV node radiofrequency ablation procedure.
Medications (e.g., digoxin, beta-blockers, calcium channel blockers, class III antiarrhythmics).
Acute inferior wall MI.
Myocarditis.
Infections (endocarditis, Lyme disease).
Infiltrative diseases (e.g., hemochromatosis, sarcoidosis, amyloidosis).
Trauma (including cardiac surgical procedures).
Collagen vascular diseases.
Aortic root diseases (e.g., spondylitis).
Electrolyte abnormalities (e.g., hyperkalemia).

BACK PAIN

ICD-10CM #	M54.89	Other dorsalgia
	M54.9	Dorsalgia, unspecified
	M54.5	Low back pain
	F45.42	Pain disorder with related psychological factors
	M54.08	Panniculitis affecting regions of neck and back, sacral and sacrococcygeal region
	S23.9XXA	Sprain of unspecified parts of thorax, initial encounter
	M43.27	Fusion of spine, lumbosacral region
	M43.28	Fusion of spine, sacral and sacrococcygeal region
	M53.2X7	Spinal instabilities, lumbosacral region
	M53.3	Sacrococcygeal disorders, not elsewhere classified

Trauma: injury to bone, joint, or ligament.
Mechanical: pregnancy, obesity, fatigue, scoliosis.
Degenerative: osteoarthritis.
Infections: osteomyelitis, subarachnoid or spinal abscess, TB, meningitis, basilar pneumonia.
Metabolic: osteoporosis, osteomalacia.
Vascular: leaking aortic aneurysm, subarachnoid or spinal hemorrhage/infarction.
Neoplastic: myeloma, Hodgkin disease, carcinoma of pancreas, metastatic neoplasm from breast, prostate, lung.
GI: penetrating ulcer, pancreatitis, cholelithiasis, inflammatory bowel disease.
Renal: hydronephrosis, calculus, neoplasm, renal infarction, pyelonephritis.
Hematologic: sickle cell crisis, acute hemolysis.
Gynecologic: neoplasm of uterus or ovary, dysmenorrhea, salpingitis, uterine prolapse.
Inflammatory: ankylosing spondylitis, psoriatic arthritis, Reiter syndrome (reactive arthritis).
Lumbosacral strain.
Psychogenic: malingering, hysteria, anxiety.
Endocrine: adrenal hemorrhage or infarction.

BACK PAIN, CHILDREN AND ADOLESCENTS[58]

ICD-10CM #	M54.5	Low back pain
	M54.9	Dorsalgia

INFLAMMATORY OR INFECTIOUS

Diskitis.
Vertebral osteomyelitis (pyogenic, tuberculous).
Spinal epidural abscess.
Pyelonephritis.
Pancreatitis.

RHEUMATOLOGIC

Pauciarticular juvenile rheumatoid arthritis.
Reiter syndrome (reactive arthritis).
Ankylosing spondylitis.
Psoriatic arthritis.

DEVELOPMENTAL

Spondylolysis.
Spondylolisthesis.
Scheuermann disease.
Scoliosis.

TRAUMATIC (ACUTE VERSUS REPETITIVE)

Hip-pelvis anomalies.
Herniated disk.
Overuse syndromes.
Vertebral stress fractures.
Upper cervical spine instability.

NEOPLASTIC

Vertebral Tumors

Benign

Eosinophilic granuloma.
Aneurysmal bone cyst.
Osteoid osteoma.
Osteoblastoma.

Malignant

Osteogenic sarcoma.
Leukemia.
Lymphoma.
Metastatic tumors.

Spinal Cord, Ganglia, and Nerve Roots

Intramedullary spinal cord tumor.
Sympathetic chain.
Ganglioneuroma.
Ganglioneuroblastoma.
Neuroblastoma.

OTHER

Intraabdominal or pelvic pathology.
Following lumbar puncture.
Conversion reaction.
Juvenile osteoporosis.

BACK PAIN, LOW, ACUTE[7]

ICD-10CM #	M54.5	Low back pain

DIFFERENTIAL CONSIDERATIONS IN ACUTE LOW BACK PAIN

Emergent

Aortic dissection.
Cauda equina syndrome.
Epidural abscess or hematoma.
Meningitis.
Ruptured/expanding aortic aneurysm.
Spinal fracture or subluxation with cord or root impingement.

Urgent

Back pain with neurologic deficits.
Disk herniation causing neurologic compromise.
Malignancy.
Sciatica with motor nerve root compression.
Spinal fractures without cord impingement.
Spinal stenosis.
Transverse myelitis.
Vertebral osteomyelitis.

Common or Stable

Acute ligamentous injury.
Acute muscle strain.
Ankylosing spondylitis.
Degenerative joint disease.
Intervertebral disk disease without impingement.
Pathologic fracture without impingement.
Seropositive arthritis.
Spondylolisthesis.

Referred or Visceral

Cholecystitis.
Esophageal disease.
Nephrolithiasis.
Ovarian torsion, mass, or tumor.
Pancreatitis.
Peptic ulcer disease.
Pleural effusion.
Pneumonia.
Pulmonary embolism.
Pyelonephritis.
Retroperitoneal hemorrhage or mass.

BACK PAIN, VISCEROGENIC ORIGIN

ICD-10CM #	F45.41	Pain disorder exclusively related to psychological factors
	M54	Dorsalgia
	M54.5	Low back pain

Urolithiasis.
Aortic aneurysm.
Colorectal carcinoma.
Endometriosis.
Tubal pregnancy.
Prostatitis.
Peptic ulcer.

Pancreatitis.
Diverticular spasm.
Metastatic neoplasm (e.g., bladder, uterus, ovary, kidney).

BACTERIAL OVERGROWTH, SMALL INTESTINE[95]

ICD-10CM # A04.9 Bacterial Intestinal Infection, Unspecified

Gastric surgery—Billroth II.
Small bowel diverticula.
Small bowel stricture:
- Crohn disease.
- Radiation enteritis.

Impaired small intestinal motility:
- Scleroderma.
- Diabetes mellitus.
- Chronic intestinal pseudoobstruction.

Miscellaneous/multifactorial:
- Elderly.
- Immune deficiency syndromes.
- Chronic pancreatitis.
- Cirrhosis.

BALLISM[7]

ICD-10CM # G25.4 Drug-induced chorea
G25.5 Other chorea

Cerebral infarction or hemorrhage.
Medications (e.g., dopamine agonists, phenytoin).
CNS neoplasm (primary or metastatic).
Nonketotic hyperosmolar state.

BILE DUCT, DILATED[95]

ICD-10CM # K83.1 Obstruction of bile duct

Normal variant.
Post-cholecystectomy.
Unsuspected bile duct stone.
Sphincter of Oddi stenosis.
Occult bile duct stricture.
Previous bile duct injury.
Early carcinoma of the pancreas, carcinoma of the bile duct, or carcinoma of the ampulla.
Extrinsic compression of the bile duct by a primary or secondary neoplasm.

BILIARY OBSTRUCTION[81]

ICD-10CM # Varies with specific diagnosis

CAUSES OF BILIARY OBSTRUCTION

Benign Miscellaneous
Choledocholithiasis.[7]
Hemobilia.[8]
Congenital biliary diseases.[9]
Caroli disease.[10]
Choledochal cysts.
Cholangitis.
Infectious.
Acute pyogenic cholangitis.[11]
Biliary parasites.[12]
Recurrent pyogenic cholangitis.[13]
HIV cholangiopathy.
Sclerosing cholangitis.
Neoplasms
Cholangiocarcinoma.
Gallbladder carcinoma.
Locally invasive tumors (esp. pancreatic adenocarcinoma).
Ampullary tumors.
Metastases.
Extrinsic compression
Mirizzi syndrome.
Pancreatitis.
Adenopathy.

BILIARY TREE, REFLUX OF GAS OR BOWEL[98]

ICD-10CM # Varies with specific diagnosis

CAUSES OF REFLUX OF GAS OR BOWEL CONTRAST INTO THE BILIARY TREE

Iatrogenic.
Sphincterotomy.
Choledochojejunostomy.
Gallstone fistula.
Cholecystoduodenal fistula.
Perforated ulcer.
Choledochoduodenal fistula.
Carcinoma.
Choledochoenteric fistula.

BLADDER (URINARY) WALL THICKENING[81]

ICD-10CM # Varies with specific diagnosis

CAUSES OF BLADDER WALL THICKENING

Focal
Neoplasm
Transitional cell carcinoma.
Squamous cell carcinoma.
Adenocarcinoma.
Lymphoma.
Metastases.
Infectious/Inflammatory.
Tuberculosis (acute).
Schistosomiasis (acute).
Cystitis.
Malakoplakia.
Cystitis cystica.
Cystitis glandularis.
Fistula.
Medical Diseases
Endometriosis.
Amyloidosis.
Trauma
Hematoma.
Diffuse
Neoplasm
Transitional cell carcinoma.
Squamous cell carcinoma.
Adenocarcinoma.
Infectious/Inflammatory
Cystitis.
Tuberculosis (chronic).
Schistosomiasis (chronic).
Medical Diseases
Interstitial cystitis.
Amyloidosis.
Neurogenic Bladder
Detrusor hyperreflexia.
Bladder Outlet Obstruction
With muscular hypertrophy.

BLEEDING, GI IN PATIENTS WITH AIDS[30]

ICD-10CM # K92.2 Gastrointestinal bleeding, unspecified

(EXCLUDING NON-AIDS-SPECIFIC DIAGNOSES)

Esophagus
Candida spp.*
Cytomegalovirus.[14]
HSV.
Idiopathic ulcer.
Stomach
Cytomegalovirus.*
Kaposi sarcoma.*
Cryptosporidiosis.
Lymphoma.
Small Intestine
Kaposi sarcoma.
Lymphoma.
Cytomegalovirus.
Salmonella spp.
Cryptosporidium.
Colon
Cytomegalovirus.*
Kaposi sarcoma.*
Entamoeba histolytica.
Campylobacter jejuni.
Clostridium difficile.
Shigella spp.
Idiopathic ulcerations.
Lymphoma.

---

[7] Diagnoses for which particular symptoms are indicative are in *italics*. Exposure to regions of the world that are most likely to be significant to the diagnosis are presented in (parentheses). Vectors, risk behaviors, and sources associated with acquisition are presented in [brackets]. Special clinical characteristics are listed within {braces}.

[8] Most frequent parasitic causes of massive eosinophilia (>5000/mm^3).

[9] Although visual hallucinations are likely to complicate almost any form of dementia, they are characteristic of dementia with Lewy bodies disease.

[10] Denotes causes of painful jaundice.

[11] Despite incapacitating movements, many choreoathetosis patients have no mental retardation.

[12] Denotes causes of painful jaundice.

[13] Includes hypnotics, glucocorticoids, marijuana, phencyclidine, atropine, dopaminergic agents (e.g., amantadine, bromocriptine, L-dopa), immunosuppressants.

*More frequent diagnosis.

[14] Includes digitalis, theophylline, cimetidine, anticholinergics, glucocorticoids, catecholaminergic agents.

BLEEDING, LOWER GI

ICD-10CM # K92.2 Gastrointestinal hemorrhage, unspecified

(ORIGINATING BELOW THE LIGAMENT OF TREITZ)

Small Intestine

Ischemic bowel disease (mesenteric thrombosis, embolism, vasculitis, trauma).
Small bowel neoplasm: leiomyomas, carcinoids.
Hereditary hemorrhagic telangiectasia (Rendu-Osler-Weber syndrome).
Meckel diverticulum and other small intestine diverticula.
Aortoenteric fistula.
Intestinal hemangiomas: blue rubber-bleb nevi, intestinal hemangiomas, cutaneous vascular nevi.
Hamartomatous polyps: Peutz-Jeghers syndrome (intestinal polyps, mucocutaneous pigmentation).
Infections of small bowel: tuberculous enteritis, enteritis necroticans.
Volvulus.
Intussusception.
Lymphoma of small bowel, sarcoma, Kaposi sarcoma.
Irradiation ileitis.
AV malformation of small intestine.
Inflammatory bowel disease.
Polyarteritis nodosa.
Other: pancreatoenteric fistulas, Henoch-Schönlein purpura, Ehlers-Danlos syndrome, SLE, amyloidosis, metastatic melanoma.

Colon

Carcinoma (particularly left colon).
Diverticular disease.
Inflammatory bowel disease.
Ischemic colitis.
Colonic polyps.
Vascular abnormalities: angiodysplasia, vascular ectasia.
Radiation colitis.
Infectious colitis.
Uremic colitis.
Aortoenteric fistula.
Lymphoma of large bowel.
Hemorrhoids.
Anal fissure.
Trauma, foreign body.
Solitary rectal/cecal ulcers.
Long-distance running.

BLEEDING, LOWER GI, PEDIATRIC[7]

ICD-10CM # K92.2 Gastrointestinal hemorrhage, unspecified

<3 MO

Swallowed maternal blood.
Infectious colitis.
Milk allergy.
Bleeding diathesis.
Intussusception.
Midgut volvulus.
Meckel diverticulum.
Necrotizing enterocolitis.

<2 YR

Anal fissure.
Infectious colitis.
Milk allergy.
Colitis.
Intussusception.
Meckel diverticulum.
Polyp.
Duplication.
Hemolytic-uremic syndrome.
Inflammatory bowel disease.
Pseudomembranous enterocolitis.

<5 YR

Infectious colitis.
Anal fissure.
Polyp.
Intussusception.
Meckel diverticulum.
Henoch-Schönlein purpura.
Hemolytic-uremic syndrome.
Inflammatory bowel disease.
Pseudomembranous enterocolitis.

5 TO 18 YR

Infectious colitis.
Inflammatory bowel disease.
Pseudomembranous enterocolitis.
Polyp.
Hemolytic-uremic syndrome.
Hemorrhoids.

BLEEDING, RECTAL[95]

ICD-10CM # K92.2 Gastrointestinal hemorrhage, unspecified

IN PATIENTS <40 YR

Very Common

Hemorrhoids.
Anal fissure.
Inflammatory bowel disease (mainly proctitis).

Less Common

Polyps (hamartomatous or adenomatous).
Infective colitis.
Meckel diverticulum.
Intussusception.

Rare

Colorectal cancer.

IN PATIENTS >40 YR

Hemorrhoids.
Anal fissure.
Colorectal cancer.
Colorectal polyps (mostly adenomas).
Angiodysplasia.
Diverticular disease.
Inflammatory bowel disease.
Ischemic colitis.
Infective colitis.

BLEEDING, THIRD TRIMESTER[1]

ICD-10CM # N93.9 Abnormal uterine and vaginal bleeding, unspecified

Placental abruption.
Placenta previa.
Bloody show (extrusion of cervical mucus).
Vasa previa.
Disseminated intravascular coagulopathy.
Uterine rupture.
Cervicitis, cervical cancer, or other cervical abnormality.
Vaginal laceration.

BLEEDING, UPPER GI

ICD-10CM # K92.2 Gastrointestinal hemorrhage, unspecified

(ORIGINATING ABOVE THE LIGAMENT OF TREITZ)

Swallowed Hemoptysis

Oral or pharyngeal lesions: swallowed blood from nose or oropharynx.
Esophageal: varices, ulceration, esophagitis, Mallory-Weiss tear, carcinoma, trauma.
Gastric: peptic ulcer (including Cushing and Curling ulcers), gastritis, angiodysplasia, gastric neoplasms, hiatal hernia, gastric diverticulum, pseudoxanthoma elasticum, Rendu-Osler-Weber syndrome.
Duodenal: peptic ulcer, duodenitis, angiodysplasia, aortoduodenal fistula, duodenal diverticulum, duodenal tumors, carcinoma of ampulla of Vater, parasites (e.g., hookworm), Crohn disease.
Biliary: hematobilia (e.g., penetrating injury to liver, hepatobiliary malignancy, endoscopic papillotomy).

BLEEDING, UPPER GI, PEDIATRIC[7]

ICD-10CM # K92.2 Gastrointestinal hemorrhage, unspecified

<3 MO

Swallowed maternal blood.
Gastritis.
Ulcer, stress.
Bleeding diathesis.
Foreign body (NG tube).
Vascular malformation.
Duplication.

<2 YR

Esophagitis.
Gastritis.
Ulcer.
Pyloric stenosis.
Mallory-Weiss syndrome.
Vascular malformation.
Duplication.

<5 YR

Esophagitis.
Gastritis.
Ulcer.
Esophageal varices.
Foreign body.
Mallory-Weiss syndrome.
Hemophilia.
Vascular malformations.

5 TO 18 YR

Esophagitis.
Gastritis.
Ulcer.
Esophageal varices.
Mallory-Weiss syndrome.
Inflammatory bowel disease.
Hemophilia.
Vascular malformation.

BLEEDING, VAGINAL, NON-PREGNANT FEMALE[1]

ICD-10CM #	N93.9	Abnormal uterine and vaginal bleeding, unspecified

TRAUMA

Blunt force.
Penetrating force.
Foreign bodies.

INFECTIOUS

Vaginitis.
Cervicitis.
Endometritis.

DYSFUNCTIONAL UTERINE BLEEDING

Ovulatory.
Anovulatory.
Adenomyosis.

BENIGN GROWTHS

Uterine leiomyomas.
Cervical polyps.

MALIGNANCY

Vulvar.
Cervical.
Uterine.
Ovarian.

SYSTEMIC DISEASE

Medications

Anticoagulation (warfarin [Coumadin], low-molecular-weight heparin, clopidogrel [Plavix]).
Antipsychotics.
Corticosteroids.
Tamoxifen.
Selective serotonin reuptake inhibitors.
Contraceptives (oral, intrauterine devices, intramuscular).

BLINDNESS, GERIATRIC AGE

ICD-10CM #	H54.8	Legal blindness, as defined in USA

Cataracts.
Glaucoma.
Diabetic retinopathy.
Macular degeneration.
Trauma.
CVA.
Corneal scarring.
Giant cell arteritis.
Ocular herpes zoster.

BLINDNESS, MONOCULAR, TRANSIENT

ICD-10CM #	H54.41	Blindness, right eye, normal vision left eye
	H54.42	Blindness, left eye, normal vision right eye

Migraine (vasospasm).
Embolic cerebrovascular disease.
Intermittent angle-closure glaucoma.
Partial retinal vein occlusion.
Hyphema.
Optic disc edema.
Giant cell arteritis.
Psychogenic.
Hypotension.
Hypercoagulopathy disorders.
Multiple sclerosis.

BLINDNESS, PEDIATRIC AGE[60]

ICD-10CM #	H54.41	Blindness, right eye, normal vision left eye
	H54.42	Blindness, left eye, normal vision right eye

CONGENITAL

Optic nerve hypoplasia or aplasia.
Optic coloboma.
Congenital hydrocephalus.
Hydranencephaly.
Porencephaly.
Microencephaly.
Encephalocele, particularly occipital type.
Morning glory disc.
Aniridia.
Anterior microphthalmia.
Peter anomaly.
Persistent pupillary membrane.
Glaucoma.
Cataracts.
Persistent hyperplastic primary vitreous.

PHAKOMATOSES

Tuberous sclerosis.
Neurofibromatosis (special association with optic glioma).
Sturge-Weber syndrome.
von Hippel–Lindau disease.

TUMORS

Retinoblastoma.
Optic glioma.
Perioptic meningioma.
Craniopharyngioma.
Cerebral glioma.
Posterior and intraventricular tumors when complicated by hydrocephalus.
Pseudotumor cerebri.

NEURODEGENERATIVE DISEASES

Cerebral storage disease.
Gangliosidoses, particularly Tay-Sachs disease (infantile amaurotic familial idiocy), Sandhoff variant, generalized gangliosidosis.
Other lipidoses and ceroid lipofuscinoses, particularly the late-onset amaurotic familial idiocies such as those of Jansky-Bielschowsky and of Batten-Mayou-Spielmeyer-Vogt.
Mucopolysaccharidoses, particularly Hurler syndrome and Hunter syndrome.
Leukodystrophies (dysmyelination disorders), particularly metachromatic leukodystrophy and Canavan disease.
Demyelinating sclerosis (myelinoclastic diseases), especially Schilder disease and Devic neuromyelitis optica.
Special types: Dawson disease, Leigh disease, Bassen-Kornzweig syndrome, Refsum disease.
Retinal degenerations: retinitis pigmentosa and its variants, Leber congenital type.
Optic atrophies: congenital autosomal recessive type, infantile and congenital autosomal dominant types, Leber disease, and atrophies associated with hereditary ataxias—the types of Behr, of Marie, and of Sanger-Brown.

INFECTIOUS PROCESSES

Encephalitis, especially in the prenatal infection syndromes caused by *Toxoplasma gondii*, cytomegalovirus, rubella virus, *Treponema pallidum*, herpes simplex.
Meningitis, arachnoiditis.
Chorioretinitis.
Endophthalmitis.
Keratitis.

HEMATOLOGIC DISORDERS

Leukemia with CNS involvement.

VASCULAR AND CIRCULATORY DISORDERS

Collagen vascular diseases.
Arteriovenous malformations: intracerebral hemorrhage, subarachnoid hemorrhage.
Central retinal occlusion.

TRAUMA

Contusion or avulsion of optic nerves, chiasm, globe, cornea.
Cerebral contusion or laceration.
Intracerebral, subarachnoid, or subdural hemorrhage.

DRUGS AND TOXINS OTHER

Retinopathy of prematurity.
Sclerocornea.
Conversion reaction.
Optic neuritis.
Osteopetrosis.

BLISTERS, SUBEPIDERMAL

ICD-10CM #	T07	Unspecified multiple injuries

Burns.
Porphyria cutanea tarda.
Bullous pemphigoid.
Bullous drug reaction.
Arthropod bite reaction.
Toxic epidermal necrosis.
Dermatitis herpetiformis.
Polymorphous light eruption.
Variegate porphyria.
SLE.
Epidermolysis bullosa.
Pseudoporphyria.
Acute graft-versus-host reaction.
Linear IgA disease.
Leukocytoclastic vasculitis.
Pressure necrosis.
Urticaria pigmentosa.
Amyloidosis.

BONE AND/OR SOFT TISSUE HYPERTROPHY[78]

ICD-10CM #	M85.80	Other specified disorders of bone density and structure, unspecified site

DISORDERS ASSOCIATED WITH BONE AND/OR SOFT TISSUE HYPERTROPHY

Conditions Associated with Generalized Overgrowth

Pituitary gigantism and acromegaly.
Other endocrine disorders.
Cerebral gigantism (Sotos).

Conditions Associated with Limb Hemihypertrophy

Lipomatosis.
Idiopathic congenital hemihypertrophy (associated with tumors, e.g., Wilms tumor, adrenocortical tumors, hepatoblastoma).
Proteus syndrome (capillary port-wine hemangiomas, lymphangiomas, lipomas, epidermal nevi, hypertrophy hands and feet, macrocephaly).
Maffucci syndrome (enchondromas, exostosis, lymphangiomas, venous angiomas).
Klippel-Trenaunay syndrome (capillary port-wine hemangiomas, varicosities, lymphangiomas).
Parkes Weber syndrome (capillary port-wine hemangiomas, varicosities, arteriovenous fistula).
Blue rubber bleb nevus syndrome (cavernous hemangiomas of skin, GI tract).
Other angiodysplasias (e.g., Servelle-Martorell syndrome; venous arterial malformations with limb hypertrophy and bony hypoplasia).
Beckwith-Wiedemann syndrome (macroglossia, visceromegaly, omphaloceles, hemihypertrophy, etc.).

Conditions Associated with Macrodactyly

Neurofibromatosis.
Macrodystrophia lipomatosa.
Proteus syndrome.
Bannayan-Zonana syndrome (lipomatosis, angiomatosis, macrocephaly).
Hemangiomatosis and other vascular malformations (Klippel-Trenaunay and Parkes Weber).
Lymphangiomatosis.
Arteriovenous malformation.
Maffucci syndrome, Ollier disease.
Epidermal nevus syndrome.

BONE DENSITY, DECREASED, GENERALIZED[41]

ICD-10CM #	M85.80	Other specified disorders of bone density and structure, unspecified site

DISORDERS ASSOCIATED WITH GENERALIZED LOSS OF BONE DENSITY

Disorders of Multiple or Uncertain Cause

Senile osteoporosis.[15]
Juvenile osteoporosis.
Osteogenesis imperfecta.[16]

Secondary Bone Disorders

Endocrine

Adrenal cortex:
- Cushing disease.
- Addison disease.

Gonadal disorders:
- Postmenopausal osteoporosis.
- Hypogonadism.

Pituitary:
- Acromegaly.
- Hypopituitarism.

Pancreas:
- Diabetes mellitus.

Thyroid:
- Hyperthyroidism.
- Hypothyroidism.

Parathyroid:
- Hyperparathyroidism.

Marrow Replacement and Expansion

Myeloma.
Leukemia.
Lymphoma.
Metastatic disease.
Gaucher disease.
Anemias (sickle cell, thalassemia, hemophilia).

Drugs and Other Substances

Steroids.
Heparin (osteoporosis).
Anticonvulsants (osteomalacia).
Immunosuppressants.
Alcohol.

Chronic Disease

Chronic renal disease.
Hepatic insufficiency.
GI malabsorption syndromes.
Chronic inflammatory polyarthropathies.
Chronic debility or immobilization.

[15] Patients who cannot synthesize Lewis blood group antigens (~5% of the population) do not produce CA-19-9 antigen.
[16] Common cause of decrease in bone density in children.

BONE DENSITY, DECREASED, LOCALIZED[41]

ICD-10CM #	Z82.62	Family history of osteoporosis
	M85.80	Other specified disorders of bone density and structure, unspecified site

DISORDERS ASSOCIATED WITH LOCALIZED LOSS OF BONE DENSITY

Disuse osteoporosis.[17]
Reflex sympathetic dystrophy (Sudeck).
Osteolytic syndromes:
- Acro-osteolysis, primary and secondary.
- Massive osteolysis of Gorham.
- Carpotarsal osteolysis.

Transient regional osteoporosis.
Neuromuscular disorders.
Infection.
Arthropathies.
Tumors, primary and secondary, myelomatosis.

[17] Common causes.

BONE LESIONS, PREFERENTIAL SITE OF ORIGIN[90]

ICD-10CM #	C41.0	Malignant neoplasm of bones of skull and face
	C41.1	Malignant neoplasm of mandible
	C41.2	Malignant neoplasm of vertebral column
	C41.3	Malignant neoplasm of ribs, sternum and clavicle
	C40.00	Malignant neoplasm of scapula and long bones of unspecified upper limb
	C40.10	Malignant neoplasm of short bones of unspecified upper limb
	C41.4	Malignant neoplasm of pelvic bones, sacrum and coccyx
	C40.20	Malignant neoplasm of long bones of unspecified lower limb
	C40.30	Malignant neoplasm of short bones of unspecified lower limb
	C41.9	Malignant neoplasm of bone and articular cartilage, unspecified
	C79.51	Secondary malignant neoplasm of bone
	C79.52	Secondary malignant neoplasm of bone marrow

EPIPHYSIS

Chondroblastoma.
Giant cell tumor—after fusion of growth plate.
Langerhans cell histiocytosis.
Clear cell chondrosarcoma.
Osteosarcoma.

METAPHYSIS

Parosteal sarcoma.
Chondrosarcoma.
Fibrosarcoma.
Nonossifying fibroma.
Giant cell tumor—before fusion of growth plate.
Unicameral bone cyst.
Aneurysmal bone cyst.

DIAPHYSIS

Myeloma.
Ewing tumor.
Reticulum cell sarcoma.

METADIAPHYSEAL

Fibrosarcoma.
Fibrous dysplasia.
Enchondroma.
Osteoid osteoma.
Chondromyofibroma.

BONE MARROW FAILURE SYNDROMES, INHERITED[50]

ICD-10CM #	D61.89	Other specified aplastic anemias and other bone marrow failure syndromes

BI-LINEAGE AND TRI-LINEAGE CYTOPENIAS

Fanconi anemia.
Shwachman-Diamond syndrome.
Dyskeratosis congenita.
Amegakaryocytic thrombocytopenia:
- Other inherited thrombocytopenia disorders.

Other genetic syndromes:
- Down syndrome.
- Dubowitz syndrome.
- Seckel syndrome.
- Reticular dysgenesis.
- Schimke immunoosseous dysplasia.
- Noonan syndrome.
- Cartilage-hair hypoplasia.
- Familial marrow failure (non-Fanconi).

UNI-LINEAGE CYTOPENIA

Diamond-Blackfan anemia.
Kostmann syndrome/Congenital neutropenia:
- *ELA2* mutations.
- *HAX1* mutations.
- *GFI1* mutations.
- *WASP* mutations.
- Constitutive cell surface G-CSF-R mutations.

Other inherited neutropenia syndromes:
- Barth syndrome.
- Glycogen storage disease 1b.
- Miscellaneous.

Thrombocytopenia with absent radii.
Congenital dyserythropoietic anemias (CDAs):
- Types I, II, III, IV.
- Variants.
- Nonclassifiable CDAs.
- Groups IV, V, VI, VII.

BONE MARROW FIBROSIS[36]

ICD-10CM #	D75.9	Disease of blood and blood-forming organs, unspecified

MYELOID DISORDERS

Myelofibrosis with myeloid metaplasia.
Metastatic cancer.
Chronic myeloid leukemia.
Myelodysplastic syndrome.
Atypical myeloid disorder.
Acute megakaryocytic leukemia.
Other acute myeloid leukemias.
Gray platelet syndrome.

LYMPHOID DISORDERS

Hairy cell leukemia.
Multiple myeloma.
Lymphoma.

NONHEMATOLOGIC DISORDERS

Connective tissue disorder.
Infections (tuberculosis, kala-azar).
Vitamin D deficiency (rickets).
Renal osteodystrophy.

BONE MASS, LOW[3]

ICD-10CM #	M85.80	Other specified disorders of bone density and structure, unspecified site

SECONDARY CAUSES OF LOW BONE MASS

Endocrine Diseases
Female hypogonadism.
Hyperprolactinemia.
Hypothalamic amenorrhea.
Anorexia nervosa.
Premature and primary ovarian failure.
Female athlete triad.
Male hypogonadism.
Primary gonadal failure (e.g., Klinefelter syndrome).
Secondary gonadal failure (e.g., idiopathic hypogonadotropic hypogonadism, androgen deprivation therapy for prostate cancer).
Hyperthyroidism.
Hyperparathyroidism.
Hypercortisolism.
Vitamin D insufficiency or deficiency.
Gastrointestinal Diseases
Subtotal gastrectomy.
Gastric bypass surgery.
Malabsorption syndromes.
Chronic obstructive jaundice.
Primary biliary cirrhosis and other cirrhoses.
Bone Marrow Disorders
Multiple myeloma.
Monoclonal gammopathy of unknown significance (MGUS).
Lymphoma.
Leukemia.
Hemolytic anemias.
Systemic mastocytosis.
Disseminated carcinoma.
Connective Tissue Diseases
Osteogenesis imperfecta.
Ehlers-Danlos syndrome.
Marfan syndrome.
Homocystinuria.
Drugs
Alcohol.
Antiseizure medications.
Aromatase inhibitors.
Chemotherapy.
Cyclosporine.
Depo-medroxyprogesterone.
Excess thyroid hormone.
Glucocorticoids.
Gonadotropin-releasing hormone agonists.
Heparin.
Miscellaneous Causes
Immobilization.
Rheumatoid arthritis.
Chronic obstructive pulmonary disease.
Weight loss.

BONE MINERAL DENSITY, INCREASED

ICD-10CM #	M89.30	Hypertrophy of bone, unspecified site
	M89.8X9	Other specified disorders of bone, unspecified site
	M94.8X9	Other specified disorders of cartilage, unspecified sites

Paget disease of bone.
Skeletal metastases.
DISH.
Osteonecrosis.
Sarcoidosis.
Hypoparathyroidism, pseudohypoparathyroidism.
Milk-alkali syndrome.
Osteopetrosis.
Hypervitaminosis A or D.
Dysplasias (craniodiaphyseal, craniometaphyseal, frontometaphyseal).
Endosteal hyperostosis.
Fluorosis.
Heavy metal poisoning.
Ionizing radiation.
Other: lymphoma, leukemia, mastocytosis, multiple myeloma, polycythemia vera.

BONE PAIN

ICD-10CM #	M89.8	Pain, bone

Trauma.
Neoplasm (primary or metastatic).
Osteoporosis with compression fracture.
Paget disease of bone.
Infection (osteomyelitis, septic arthritis).
Osteomalacia.
Viral syndrome.
Sickle cell disease.
Anxiety.

BONE RESORPTION[90]

ICD-10CM #	M89.9	Disorder of bone, unspecified
	M94.9	Disorder of cartilage, unspecified

DISTAL CLAVICLE

Hyperparathyroidism.
RA.
Scleroderma.
Posttraumatic osteolysis.
Progeria.
Pycnodysostosis.
Cleidocranial dysplasia.

INFERIOR ASPECT OF RIBS

Vascular impression associated with but not limited to coarctation of the aorta.
Hyperparathyroidism.
Neurofibromatosis.

TERMINAL PHALANGEAL TUFTS

Scleroderma.
Raynaud phenomenon.
Vascular disease.
Frostbite, electrical burns.
Psoriasis.
Tabes dorsalis.
Hyperparathyroidism.

GENERALIZED RESORPTION

Paraplegia.
Myositis ossificans.
Osteoporosis.

BOWEL WALL THICKENING[98]

ICD-10CM # Varies with specific diagnosis

BENIGN VERSUS MALIGNANT BOWEL WALL THICKENING

Benign
Homogeneous attenuation.
Symmetrical.
Circumferential.
Thickening <1 cm.
Segmental or diffuse involvement.
Double halo sign.
Dark inner ring.
Bright outer ring.
Target sign.
Bright inner ring.
Dark middle ring.
Bright outer ring.
Malignant
Heterogeneous attenuation.
Asymmetrical.
Eccentric.
Thickening >1 to 2 cm.
Focal mass.
Abrupt transition.
Lobulated contour.
Spiculated contour.
Narrowed bowel lumen.
Enlarged lymph nodes.
Liver metastases.

BOW LEGS (GENU VARUM), CLASSIFICATION[58]

ICD-10CM #	E64.3	Genu varum, acquired
	Q74.1	Congenital malformation of knee

PHYSIOLOGIC

Asymmetric Growth
Tibia vara (Blount disease):
Infantile.
Juvenile.
Adolescent.
Focal fibrocartilaginous dysplasia.
Physeal injury.
Trauma.
Infection.
Tumor.

METABOLIC DISORDERS

Vitamin D deficiency (nutritional rickets).
Vitamin D–resistant rickets.
Hypophosphatasia.

SKELETAL DYSPLASIA

Metaphyseal dysplasia.
Achondroplasia.
Enchondromatosis.

BRACHYCARDIA, ICU PATIENT[97]

ICD-10CM #	R00.1	Bradycardia, unspecified

COMMON CAUSES OF BRADYCARDIA IN THE ICU

Medications: antiarrhythmics, β-blockers, calcium channel blockers, clonidine, dexmedetomidine, digoxin, lithium, opioids, phenytoin, and propofol.
Age-related degeneration.
Cardiac ischemia.
Electrolyte abnormalities.
Elevated intracranial pressure.
Elevated vagal tone.
Endotracheal intubation.
Hypertension.
Hypothermia.
Hypothyroidism.
Hypoxia.
Inflammatory disease.
Obstructive sleep apnea.
Post-cardiac surgery.

BRADYCARDIA, SINUS[37]

ICD-10CM #	I49.8	Other specified cardiac arrhythmias
	R00.1	Bradycardia, unspecified

Idiopathic.
Degenerative processes (e.g., Lev disease, Lenègre disease).
Medications
β-Blockers.
Some calcium channel blockers (diltiazem, verapamil).
Digoxin (when vagal tone is high).
Class I antiarrhythmic agents (e.g., procainamide).
Class III antiarrhythmic agents (amiodarone, sotalol).
Clonidine.
Lithium carbonate.

ACUTE MYOCARDIAL ISCHEMIA AND INFARCTION

Right or left circumflex coronary artery occlusion or spasm.
High vagal tone (e.g., athletes).

BRAIN MASS[1]

ICD-10CM #	C71	Malignant neoplasm of brain
	D33	Benign neoplasm of brain
	I61.9	Intracranial hemorrhage, unspecified

METASTATIC BRAIN TUMOR

Primary Brain Tumor
Meningioma.
Glioma.
Pituitary adenoma.
Vestibular schwannoma.
Primary or secondary CNS lymphoma.
Infections
Abscess.
Toxoplasmosis.
Neurocysticercosis.
Tuberculoma.
Progressive multifocal leukoencephalopathy.

VASCULAR DISEASE

Hemorrhage
Anomalies (arteriovenous malformation).
Intratumoral.
Hypertensive.
Infarct
Embolism.
Thrombosis (sinus venous).
Inflammatory
Multiple sclerosis.
Encephalomyelitis.

BREAST INFLAMMATORY LESION[28]

ICD-10CM #	N61	Inflammatory disorders of breast
	N60.19	Diffuse cystic mastopathy of unspecified breast
	P39.0	Neonatal infective mastitis
	P83.4	Breast engorgement of newborn

Mastitis (*S. aureus*, β-hemolytic *Streptococcus*).
Trauma.
Foreign body (sutures, breast implants).
Granuloma (TB, fungal).

Fat necrosis post biopsy.
Necrosis or infarction (anticoagulant therapy, pregnancy).
Breast malignancy.

BREAST MASS

ICD-10CM #	N63	Unspecified lump in breast

Fibrocystic breasts.
Benign tumors (fibroadenoma, papilloma).
Mastitis (acute bacterial mastitis, chronic mastitis).
Malignant neoplasm.
Fat necrosis.
Hematoma.
Duct ectasia.
Mammary adenosis.

BREATH ODOR[86]

ICD-10CM #	R19.6	Halitosis

Sweet, fruity: DKA, starvation ketosis.
Fishy, stale: uremia (trimethylamines).
Ammonia-like: uremia (ammonia).
Musty fish, clover: fetor hepaticus (hepatic failure).
Foul, feculent: intestinal obstruction/diverticulum.
Foul, putrid: nasal/sinus pathology (infection, foreign body, cancer), respiratory infections (empyema, lung abscess, bronchiectasis).
Halitosis: tonsillitis, gingivitis, respiratory infections, Vincent angina, gastroesophageal reflux, achalasia, certain foods (garlic, onions, protein drinks, etc.)
Cinnamon: pulmonary TB.

BREATHING, NOISY[86]

ICD-10CM #	R06.00	Dyspnea, unspecified
	R06.09	Other forms of dyspnea
	R06.3	Periodic breathing
	R06.83	Snoring
	R06.89	Other abnormalities of breathing
	R06.1	Stridor

Infection: upper respiratory infection, peritonsillar abscess, retropharyngeal abscess, epiglottitis, laryngitis, tracheitis, bronchitis, bronchiolitis.
Irritants and allergens: hyperactive airway, asthma (reactive airway disease), rhinitis, angioneurotic edema.
Compression from outside of the airway: esophageal cysts or foreign body, neoplasms, lymphadenopathy.
Congenital malformation and abnormality: vascular rings, laryngeal webs, laryngomalacia, tracheomalacia, hemangiomas within the upper airway, stenoses within the upper airway, cystic fibrosis.
Acquired abnormality (at every level of the airway): nasal polyps, hypertrophied adenoids and/or tonsils, foreign body, intraluminal tumors, bronchiectasis.
Neurogenic disorder: vocal cord paralysis.

BRONCHIAL OBSTRUCTION[41]

ICD-10CM #	J98.0	Tracheobronchial collapse

CAUSES OF BRONCHIAL OBSTRUCTION

Outside the Bronchus
Lymph nodes and other masses.
In the Wall of the Bronchus
Tumors
Lung carcinoma (commonly squamous cell).
Bronchial carcinoid.
Metastasis.
Hamartoma.
Inflammation
Tuberculosis.
Sarcoidosis.
Granulomatosis with polyangiitis.
Inflammatory bowel disease.
Bronchomalacia
Broncholith.
Inside the Bronchus
Mucous plug.
Inhaled foreign body.

BRONCHOPLEURAL FISTULA[41]

ICD-10CM #	J86.0	Bronchopleural fistula

CAUSES OF BRONCHOPLEURAL FISTULA

Trauma
Penetrating.
Iatrogenic (especially post-pneumonectomy, post-lobectomy, post-biopsy).
Infection
Necrotizing pneumonia.
Empyema.
Tuberculosis.
Septic embolus.
Infected pulmonary infarct.

BROWN URINE

ICD-10CM #	R82	Other abnormal findings in urine

Bile pigments.
Myoglobin.
Concentrated urine.
Use of multivitamin supplements.
Medications (antimalarials, metronidazole, nitrofurantoin, levodopa, methyldopa, phenazopyridine).
Diet rich in fava beans.
Urinary tract infection.

BRUISING

ICD-10CM #	I99.8	Other disorder of circulatory system

Medication-induced (warfarin, aspirin, NSAIDs, prednisone).
Alcohol abuse.
Senile purpura.
Purpura simplex.
Physical abuse.
Vasculitis.
Platelet disorders.
Coagulation factor deficiencies.
Cushing disease.
Vitamin C deficiency.
Marfan syndrome.
Ehlers-Danlos syndrome.
Disseminated intravascular coagulation.
Leukemia.
Hereditary hemorrhagic telangiectasia.

BULLOUS DISEASES

ICD-10CM #	L13.9	Bullous disorder, unspecified
	L12.0	Bullous pemphigoid
	L12.8	Other pemphigoid
	L10.0	Pemphigus vulgaris
	L10.1	Pemphigus vegetans
	L10.2	Pemphigus foliaceous
	L10.4	Pemphigus erythematosus
	L10.9	Pemphigus, unspecified

Bullous pemphigoid.
Pemphigus vulgaris.
Pemphigus foliaceus.
Paraneoplastic pemphigus.
Cicatricial pemphigoid.
Erythema multiforme.
Dermatitis herpetiformis.
Herpes gestationis.
Impetigo.
Erosive lichen planus.
Linear IgA bullous dermatosis.
Epidermolysis bullosa acquisita.

CAFÉ-AU-LAIT SPOTS[58]

ICD-10CM #	L81.3	Cafe au lait spots

Neurofibromatosis types 1 and 2.
McCune-Albright syndrome.
Russell-Silver syndrome.
Ataxia-telangiectasia.
Fanconi anemia.
Tuberous sclerosis.
Bloom syndrome.
Basal cell nevus syndrome.
Gaucher disease.
Chédiak-Higashi syndrome.
Hunter syndrome.
Maffucci syndrome.
Multiple mucosal neuroma syndrome.
Watson syndrome.
Proteus syndrome.
Turner syndrome.
Ring chromosome syndrome.
Jaffe-Campanacci syndrome.

CALCIFICATION ON CHEST X-RAY

ICD-10CM #	J98.4	Calcification of lung
	M51.84	Other intervertebral disc disorders, thoracic region
	M51.85	Other intervertebral disc disorders, thoracolumbar region

Lung neoplasm (primary or metastatic).
Silicosis.
Idiopathic pulmonary fibrosis.
Tuberculosis.
Histoplasmosis.

Disseminated varicella infection.
Mitral stenosis (end-stage).
Secondary hyperparathyroidism.

CALCIFICATIONS, ABDOMINAL, NONVISCERAL ON X-RAY[41]

ICD-10CM #	M61.9	Calcification and ossification of muscle, unspecified

NONVISCERAL ABDOMINAL CALCIFICATION

Common
Atherosclerosis.
Mesenteric lymph nodes.
Phleboliths.
Aneurysm.
Dermoid cyst.
Differentiate
Rib cartilage.
Injections in the buttocks.
Uncommon
Infestations:
- *Armillifer armillatus.*
- Cysticercosis.
- Guinea worm.
- Hydatid.

Tumors:
- Lipoma.
- Hemangioma.
- Neuroblastoma.
- Osteo/chondrosarcoma of soft tissues.
- Retroperitoneal sarcoma of soft tissues.
- Peritoneal metastases.
- Pheochromocytoma.

Tuberculosis:
- Peritonitis.
- Psoas abscess.

Meconium peritonitis.
Pseudomyxoma Peritonei
Mesenteric cyst.
Pancreatitis with saponification.
Lithopedion.
Appendices Epiploicae
Ligaments.
Foreign bodies.
Posttraumatic buttock cysts.

CALCIFICATIONS, ADRENAL GLAND ON X-RAY[41]

ICD-10CM #	E27.4	Calcification, adrenal gland

ADRENAL GLAND CALCIFICATION

Common
Idiopathic.
Hemorrhage.
Tuberculosis.
Neuroblastoma/ganglioneuroma.
Pheochromocytoma.
Uncommon
Other tumors:
- Adenoma.
- Carcinoma.
- Dermoid.

Addison disease.
Cyst.
Histoplasmosis.

CALCIFICATIONS, CARDIAC ON X-RAY[41]

ICD-10CM #	I51.5	Calcification, myocardium
	I25.1	Calcification, arteriosclerotic

CAUSES OF VISIBLE CALCIFICATION WITHIN THE HEART

Coronary Artery
Atherosclerosis.
Aortic Root
Atherosclerotic aorta.
Thrombus.
Syphilis.
Ankylosing spondylitis.
Homograft calcification.
Pericardium
Chronic pericarditis, tuberculosis, hemopericardium, pyogenic or viral pericarditis.
Posttraumatic.
Postoperative.
Uremic pericarditis.
Asbestosis (may be pleural calcification applied to pericardium).
Myocardium
Ventricular aneurysm (may mimic pericardial calcification).
Calcified myocardial infarction.
Postmyocarditis.
Endocardium
Endomyocardial fibrosis.
Thrombus.
Valve Cusps
Calcified valves (particularly mitral and aortic valves).
Mitral annulus calcification.
Homograft calcification.
Old vegetation.
Valve Annulus
Submitral.
Mitral.
Aortic.
Left Atrium
Wall.
Thrombus.
Atrial myxoma.
Pulmonary Artery
Pulmonary hypertension.
Postoperative:
- Postoperative serumoma calcified hydatid cyst.

CALCIFICATIONS, CUTANEOUS

ICD-10CM #	L94.2	Calcinosis cutis
	L98.8	Other specified disorders of the skin and subcutaneous tissue

Calcification, Raynaud phenomenon, esophageal dysmotility, sclerodactyly, and telangiectasia (CREST) syndrome.
Trauma.
Pancreatitis or pancreatic cancer.
Chronic renal failure.
Sarcoidosis.
Hyperparathyroidism.
Milk-alkali syndrome.
Hypervitaminosis D.
Panniculitis.
Idiopathic.
Iatrogenic (e.g., application of calcium alginate dressing to skin).
Multiple myeloma.
Dermatomyositis.
Parasitic infections.
Leukemia.
Lymphoma.

CALCIFICATIONS, GENITAL TRACT, FEMALE ON X-RAY[41]

ICD-10CM #	E83.59	Other disorders of calcium metabolism

FEMALE GENITAL TRACT CALCIFICATION

Uterus
Leiomyomas.
Squamous cell carcinoma.
Adenocarcinoma of endometrium.
Leiomyosarcoma.
Lithopedion.
Fallopian Tubes
Ovary.
Dermoid cyst.
Serous cystadenoma/carcinoma.
Tuberculosis.
Cysts.
Autoamputation.

CALCIFICATIONS, LIVER ON X-RAY[41]

ICD-10CM #	K76.89	Other specified diseases of liver
	NEC K75.3	Granuloma, hepatic

LIVER CALCIFICATION

Common
Granuloma (tuberculosis, histoplasmosis, brucellosis).
- Multiple scattered round densities.

Hydatid cyst:
- Fine curvilinear in wall, or dense and irregular if contracted.

Primary liver tumor (hemangioma, hepatoblastoma, hepatoma, cholangiocarcinoma).
- Irregular patterns or multiple nodules.

Metastases (mucinous primary of colon or breast, cystadenocarcinoma of ovary).
- Finely stippled, may be extensive.

Uncommon
Hepatic artery aneurysm.
Armillifer armillatus infestation.
Chronic granulomatous disease of childhood.
Cyst (congenital or acquired).
Hematoma.
Intrahepatic gallstones.
Old liver abscess.
Portal vein thrombosis.

Differentiate
Hemochromatosis.
Thorotrast, thallium, iron.

CALCIFICATIONS, PANCREAS ON X-RAY[41]

ICD-10CM #	K86.8	Calcification, pancreas

PANCREATIC CALCIFICATION

Common
Chronic pancreatitis.
Uncommon
Acute pancreatitis (saponification).
Tumors:
- Cystadenoma.
- Cystadenocarcinoma.
- Islet cell tumor.
- Metastases.

Hereditary pancreatitis (large clumps).
Hemorrhage.
Hyperparathyroidism.
Pseudocyst.
Cavernous lymphangioma.
Mucoviscidosis.
Kwashiorkor.

CALCIFICATIONS, SPLEEN ON X-RAY[41]

ICD-10CM #	D73.8	Calcification, spleen

SPLENIC CALCIFICATION

Larger than 10 mm
Splenic artery aneurysm.
Splenic artery atheroma.
Cyst:
- Posttraumatic.
- Dermoid.
- Epidermoid.
- Hydatid.

Hematoma.
Infarct.
Abscess.
Tuberculosis.
Smaller than 10 mm
Histoplasmosis.
Tuberculosis.
Phleboliths.
Armillifer armillatus infestation.
Brucellosis.
Infarcts.

CALCIFICATIONS, VALVULAR ON X-RAY[41]

ICD-10CM #	I51.5	Calcification, heart

CAUSES OF RADIOGRAPHICALLY VISIBLE VALVE CALCIFICATION

Aortic Valve
Rheumatic aortic valve disease.
Bicuspid aortic valve.
Age/degenerate aortic valve.
Syphilis.
Ankylosing spondylitis.
Homograft calcification.
Mitral Valve
Rheumatic mitral valve disease.
Mitral annulus calcification.
Old vegetation (may only be visible on CT).
Homograft calcification.
Pulmonary Valve
Congenital pulmonary valve stenosis.
Rheumatic pulmonary valve disease (rare).
Fallot tetralogy (usually after repair).
Pulmonary hypertension.
Homograft calcification.
Tricuspid Valve
Rheumatic tricuspid valve disease.
Old vegetation (may only be visible on ultrafast CT).

CALCIUM STONES

ICD-10CM #	N20.9	Urinary calculus, unspecified

Medications (e.g., antacids, loop diuretics, vitamin D, acetazolamide, glucocorticoids).
Primary hyperparathyroidism.
Hypercalcemia from malignancy.
Sarcoidosis.
Prolonged immobilization.
Hyperoxaluria (e.g., Crohn disease, celiac disease, chronic pancreatitis).
Hyperuricosuria (e.g., hyperuricemia, excessive dietary purine, allopurinol, probenecid).
Renal tubular acidosis.
Milk-alkali syndrome.
Thyrotoxicosis.
Hypocitraturia (e.g., metabolic acidosis, hypomagnesemia, hypokalemia).

CARDIAC ARREST, NONTRAUMATIC[63]

ICD-10CM #	I46.9	Cardiac arrest, cause unspecified

Cardiac (coronary artery disease, cardiomyopathies, structural abnormalities, valve dysfunction, arrhythmias).
Respiratory (upper airway obstruction, hypoventilation, pulmonary embolism, asthma, COPD exacerbation, pulmonary edema).
Circulatory (tension pneumothorax, pericardial tamponade, PE, hemorrhage, sepsis).
Electrolyte abnormalities (hypokalemia or hyperkalemia, hypomagnesemia or hypermagnesemia, hypocalcemia).
Medications (tricyclic antidepressants, digoxin, theophylline, calcium channel blockers).
Drug abuse (cocaine, heroin, amphetamines).
Toxins (carbon monoxide, cyanide).
Environmental (drowning/near-drowning, electrocution, lightning, hypothermia or hyperthermia, venomous snakes).

CARDIAC DEATH, SUDDEN[3]

ICD-10CM #	Z86.74	Personal history of sudden cardiac arrest

Ventricular tachycardia.
Bradyarrhythmia, sick sinus syndrome.
Aortic stenosis.
Tetralogy of Fallot.
Pericardial tamponade.
Cardiac tumors.
Complications of infective endocarditis.
Hypertrophic cardiomyopathy (arrhythmia or obstruction).
Myocardial ischemia.
Atherosclerosis.
Prinzmetal angina.
Kawasaki arteritis.

CARDIAC ENLARGEMENT[37]

ICD-10CM #	I51.7	Cardiomegaly
	Q23.8	Other congenital malformations of aortic and mitral valves
	Q24.8	Other specified congenital malformations of heart
	I11.9	Hypertensive heart disease without heart failure

CHAMBER ENLARGEMENT

Chronic Volume Overload
Mitral or aortic regurgitation.
Left-to-right shunt (PDA, VSD, AV fistula).
Cardiomyopathy
Ischemic.
Nonischemic.
Decompensated Pressure Overload
Aortic stenosis.
Hypertension.
High-Output States
Severe anemia.
Thyrotoxicosis.
Bradycardia
Severe sinus bradycardia.
Complete heart block.

LEFT ATRIUM

LV failure of any cause.
Mitral valve disease.
Myxoma.

RIGHT VENTRICLE

Chronic volume overload.
Tricuspid or pulmonic regurgitation.
Left-to-right shunt (ASD).
Decompensated pressure overload:
- Pulmonic stenosis.
- Pulmonary artery hypertension:
  - Primary.
  - Secondary (PE, COPD).
  - Pulmonary venoocclusive disease.

RIGHT ATRIUM

RV failure of any cause.
Tricuspid valve disease.
Myxoma.
Ebstein anomaly.

MULTICHAMBER ENLARGEMENT

Hypertrophic cardiomyopathy.
Acromegaly.
Severe obesity.

PERICARDIAL DISEASE

Pericardial effusion with or without tamponade.
Effusive constrictive disease.
Pericardial cyst, loculated effusion.

PSEUDOCARDIOMEGALY

Epicardial fat.
Chest wall deformity (pectus excavatum, straight back syndrome).
Low lung volumes.
AP chest x-ray.
Mediastinal tumor, cyst.

CARDIAC MASSES[104]

ICD-10CM #	C38.0	Malignant neoplasm of heart
	D15.1	Benign neoplasm of heart

Intracardiac thrombus.
Focal myocardial hypertrophy.
Left ventricular noncompaction.
Infectious disease (abscess).
Primary cardiac tumor.
Secondary cardiac tumor (metastasis).
Lipomatous hypertrophy of septum.
Cyst.
Imaging artifact.

CARDIAC MURMURS

ICD-10CM #	R01.0	Benign and innocent cardiac murmurs
	R01.1	Cardiac murmur, unspecified

SYSTOLIC

Mitral regurgitation (MR).
Tricuspid regurgitation (TR).
Ventricular septal defect (VSD).
Aortic stenosis (AS).
Idiopathic hypertrophic subaortic stenosis (IHSS).
Pulmonic stenosis (PS).
Innocent murmur of childhood.
Coarctation of aorta.
Mitral valve prolapse (MVP).

DIASTOLIC

Aortic regurgitation (AR).
Atrial myxoma.
Mitral stenosis (MS).
Pulmonary artery branch stenosis.
Tricuspid stenosis (TS).
Graham Steell murmur (diastolic decrescendo murmur heard in severe pulmonary hypertension).
Pulmonic regurgitation (PR).
Severe mitral regurgitation (MR).
Austin Flint murmur (diastolic rumble heard in severe AR).
Severe VSD and patent ductus arteriosus.

CONTINUOUS

Patent ductus arteriosus.
Pulmonary AV fistula.

CARDIAC TUMORS[38]

ICD-10CM #	C38.0	Malignant neoplasm of heart
	D15.1	Benign neoplasm of heart

PRIMARY

Benign:
- Myxoma.
- Lipoma.
- Fibroma.
- Rhabdomyoma.
- Fibroelastoma.

Malignant:
- Sarcoma.
- Mesothelioma.
- Lymphoma.

SECONDARY

Direct Extension
Lung cancer.
Breast cancer.
Mediastinal tumors.
Metastatic Tumors
Malignant melanoma.
Leukemia.
Lymphoma.
Venous Extension
Renal cell cancer.
Adrenal cancer.
Liver cancer.

CARDIOEMBOLISM

ICD-10CM #	I21.3 ST	Elevation (STEMI) myocardial infarction of unspecified site
	I21.9	Acute myocardial infarction, unspecified

Acute MI.
Atrial fibrillation.
Left ventricular aneurysm.
Valvular heart disease (e.g., rheumatic mitral valve disease, mitral valve prolapse).
Dilated cardiomyopathy.
Atrial septal defect.
Patent foramen ovale.
Cardioversion for atrial fibrillation.
Infective endocarditis.
Atrial septal aneurysm.
Sick sinus syndrome and cardiac arrhythmias.
Nonbacterial thrombotic endocarditis.
Prosthetic heart valves.
Atrial myxoma and other intracardiac tumors.
Cyanotic heart disease.
Balloon angioplasty.
Coronary artery bypass grafting.
Aneurysms of sinus of Valsalva.
Other: VVI pacing, ventricular support devices, heart transplantation, intracardiac defects with paradoxical embolism.

CARDIOGENIC SHOCK

ICD-10CM #	R57.0	Cardiogenic shock

Myocardial infarction.
Arrhythmias.
Pericardial effusion/tamponade.
Chest trauma.
Valvular heart disease.
Myocarditis.
Cardiomyopathy.
CHF, end-stage.

CATARACTS, PEDIATRIC AGE

ICD-10CM #	H26.0	Infantile, juvenile, and presenile cataracts

DEVELOPMENTAL VARIANTS

Prematurity (Y-suture vacuoles) with or without retinopathy of prematurity.

GENETIC DISORDERS

Simple Mendelian Inheritance
Autosomal dominant (most common).
Autosomal recessive.
X-linked.
Major Chromosomal Defects
Trisomy disorders (13, 18, 21).
Turner syndrome (45X).
Deletion syndromes (11p13, 18p, 18q).
Duplication syndromes (3q, 20p, 10q).
Multisystem Genetic Disorders
Alport syndrome (hearing loss, renal disease).
Alström syndrome (nerve deafness, diabetes mellitus).
Apert disease (craniosynostosis, syndactyly).
Cockayne syndrome (premature senility, skin photosensitivity).
Conradi disease (chondrodysplasia punctata).
Crouzon disease (dysostosis craniofacialis).
Hallermann-Streiff syndrome (microphthalmia, small pinched nose, skin atrophy, hypotrichosis).
Hypohidrotic ectodermal dysplasia (anomalous dentition, hypohidrosis, hypotrichosis).
Ichthyosis (keratinizing disorder with thick, scaly skin).
Incontinentia pigmenti (dental anomalies, mental retardation, cutaneous lesions).
Lowe syndrome (oculocerebrorenal syndrome: hypotonia, renal disease).
Marfan syndrome.
Marinesco-Sjögren syndrome (cerebellar ataxia, hypotonia).
Meckel-Gruber syndrome (renal dysplasia, encephalocele).
Myotonic dystrophy.
Nail-patella syndrome (renal dysfunction, dysplastic nails, hypoplastic patella).
Nevoid basal cell carcinoma syndrome (autosomal dominant, basal cell carcinoma erupts in childhood).
Peters anomaly (corneal opacifications with iris-corneal dysgenesis).
Reiger syndrome (iris dysplasia, myotonic dystrophy).
Rothmund-Thomson syndrome (poikiloderma: skin atrophy).
Rubinstein-Taybi syndrome (broad great toe, mental retardation).
Smith-Lemli-Opitz syndrome (toe syndactyly, hypospadias, mental retardation).
Sotos syndrome (cerebral gigantism).
Spondyloepiphyseal dysplasia (dwarfism, short trunk).
Werner syndrome (premature aging in 2nd decade of life).
Inborn Errors of Metabolism
Abetalipoproteinemia (absent chylomicrons, retinal degeneration).
Fabry disease (α-galactosidase A deficiency).

Galactokinase deficiency.
Galactosemia (galactose-1-phosphate uridyl transferase deficiency).
Homocystinemia (subluxation of lens, mental retardation).
Mannosidosis (acid α-mannosidase deficiency).
Niemann-Pick disease (sphingomyelinase deficiency).
Refsum disease (phytanic acid α-hydrolase deficiency).
Wilson disease (accumulation of copper leads to cirrhosis and neurologic symptoms).

ENDOCRINOPATHIES

Hypocalcemia (hypoparathyroidism).
Hypoglycemia.
Diabetes mellitus.

CONGENITAL INFECTIONS

Toxoplasmosis.
Cytomegalovirus infection.
Syphilis.
Rubella.
Perinatal herpes simplex infection.
Measles (rubeola).
Poliomyelitis.
Influenza.
Varicella-zoster.

OCULAR ANOMALIES

Microphthalmia.
Coloboma.
Aniridia.
Mesodermal dysgenesis.
Persistent papillary membrane.
Posterior lenticonus.
Persistent hyperplastic primary vitreous.
Primitive hyaloid vascular system.

MISCELLANEOUS DISORDERS

Atopic dermatitis.
Drugs (corticosteroids).
Radiation.
Trauma.
Idiopathic

CAVITARY LESION ON CHEST X-RAY[40]

ICD-10CM # R91.8 Other nonspecific abnormal finding of lung field

NECROTIZING INFECTIONS

Bacteria: anaerobes, *Staphylococcus aureus,* enteric gram-negative bacteria, *Pseudomonas aeruginosa, Legionella* spp., *Haemophilus influenzae, Streptococcus pyogenes, Streptococcus pneumoniae, Rhodococcus, Actinomyces.*
Mycobacteria: *Mycobacterium tuberculosis, Mycobacterium kansasii,* MAI.
Bacteria-like: *Nocardia* spp.
Fungi: *Coccidioides immitis, Histoplasma capsulatum, Blastomyces hominis, Aspergillus* spp., *Mucor* spp.
Parasitic: *Entamoeba histolytica, Echinococcus, Paragonimus westermani.*

CAVITARY INFARCTION

Bland infarction (with or without superimposed infection).
Lung contusion.

SEPTIC EMBOLISM

S. aureus, anaerobes, others.

VASCULITIS

Granulomatosis with polyangiitis, periarteritis.

NEOPLASMS

Bronchogenic carcinoma, metastatic carcinoma, lymphoma.

MISCELLANEOUS LESIONS

Cysts, blebs, bullae, or pneumatocele with or without fluid collections.
Sequestration.
Empyema with air-fluid level.
Bronchiectasis.

CEREBRAL INFARCTION SECONDARY TO INHERITED DISORDERS

ICD-10CM # I63.50 Cerebral infarction due to unspecified occlusion or stenosis of unspecified cerebral artery

Homocystinuria.
Marfan syndrome.
Ehlers-Danlos syndrome.
Rendu-Osler-Weber syndrome.
Pseudoxanthoma elasticum.
Fabry disease.

CEREBRAL VASCULITIS, CAUSES[33]

ICD-10CM # Varies with specific diagnosis

PRIMARY CEREBRAL VASCULITIDES

Takayasu arteritis.
Primary cerebral vasculitis.
Polyarteritis nodosa.

SECONDARY VASCULITIDES

Immune Disorders

Systemic lupus erythematosus.
Wegner granulomatosis.
Kawasaki syndrome.
Sarcoidosis.
Henoch-Schönlein purpura.

Primary Intracranial Infections

Bacterial meningitis (especially *Diplococcus pneumoniae*).
Tuberculous meningitis.
Mycotic infections.
Cat-scratch disease.
Human immunodeficiency virus/acquired immunodeficiency syndrome.
Malaria.
Lyme disease.
Rickettsial infections.
Brucellosis.

CEREBROVASCULAR DISEASE, ISCHEMIC[102]

ICD-10CM # I67.9 Cerebrovascular disease, unspecified

VASCULAR DISORDERS

Large-vessel atherothrombotic disease.
Lacunar disease.
Arterial-to-arterial embolization.
Carotid or vertebral artery dissection.
Fibromuscular dysplasia.
Migraine.
Venous thrombosis.
Radiation.
Complications of arteriography.
Multiple, progressive intracranial arterial occlusions.

INFLAMMATORY DISORDERS

Giant cell arteritis.
Polyarteritis nodosa.
SLE.
Granulomatous angiitis.
Takayasu disease.
Arteritis associated with amphetamine, cocaine, or phenylpropanolamine.
Syphilis, mucormycosis.
Sjögren syndrome.
Behçet syndrome.

CARDIAC DISORDERS

Rheumatic heart disease.
Mural thrombus.
Arrhythmias.
Mitral valve prolapse.
Prosthetic heart valve.
Endocarditis.
Myxoma.
Paradoxical embolus.

HEMATOLOGIC DISORDERS

Thrombotic thrombocytopenic purpura.
Sickle cell disease.
Hypercoagulable states.
Polycythemia.
Thrombocytosis.
Leukocytosis.
Lupus anticoagulant.

CERVICAL INSTABILITY, PEDIATRIC

ICD-10CM # M50 Cervical disc disorders

CONGENITAL

Vertebral (Bony Anomalies)

Cranioocipital defects (occipital vertebrae, basilar impression, occipital dysplasias, condylar hypoplasia, occipitalized atlas).
Atlantoaxial defects (aplasia of atlas arch, aplasia of odontoid process).
Subaxial anomalies (failure of segmentation and/or fusion, spina bifida, spondylolisthesis).

Ligamentous or Combined Anomalies

Found at birth as an element of somatogenic aberration.

Syndromic Disorders
Down syndrome.
Klippel-Feil syndrome.
22q11.2 deletion syndrome.
Larsen syndrome.
Marfan syndrome.
Ehlers-Danlos syndrome.

ACQUIRED

Trauma.
Infection (pyogenic, granulomatous).
Tumor (including neurofibromatosis).
Inflammatory conditions (e.g., juvenile rheumatoid arthritis).
Osteochondrodysplasias (e.g., achondroplasia, diastrophic dysplasia, metatropic dysplasia, spondyloepiphyseal dysplasia).
Storage disorders (e.g., mucopolysaccharidoses).
Metabolic disorders (rickets).
Miscellaneous (including osteogenesis imperfecta, sequela of surgery).

CHEST PAIN, CHILDREN[9]

ICD-10CM #		
	R07.9	Chest pain, unspecified
	R07.82	Intercostal pain
	R07.89	Other chest pain
	R07.1	Chest pain on breathing
	R07.81	Pleurodynia

MUSCULOSKELETAL (COMMON)

Trauma (accidental, abuse).
Exercise, overuse injury (strain, bursitis).
Costochondritis (Tietze syndrome).
Herpes zoster (cutaneous).
Pleurodynia.
Fibrositis.
Slipping rib.
Sickle cell anemia vasoocclusive crisis.
Osteomyelitis (rare).
Primary or metastatic tumor (rare).

PULMONARY (COMMON)

Pneumonia.
Pleurisy.
Asthma.
Chronic cough.
Pneumothorax.
Infarction (sickle cell anemia).
Foreign body.
Embolism (rare).
Pulmonary hypertension (rare).
Tumor (rare).

GASTROINTESTINAL (LESS COMMON)

Esophagitis (gastroesophageal reflux).
Esophageal foreign body.
Esophageal spasm.
Cholecystitis.
Subdiaphragmatic abscess.
Perihepatitis (Fitz-Hugh-Curtis syndrome).
Peptic ulcer disease.

CARDIAC (LESS COMMON)

Pericarditis.
Postpericardiotomy syndrome.
Endocarditis.
Mitral valve prolapse.
Aortic or subaortic stenosis.
Arrhythmias.
Marfan syndrome (dissecting aortic aneurysm).
Anomalous coronary artery.
Kawasaki disease.
Cocaine, sympathomimetic ingestion.
Angina (familial hypercholesterolemia).

IDIOPATHIC (COMMON)

Anxiety, hyperventilation.
Panic disorder.

OTHER (LESS COMMON)

Spinal cord or nerve root compression.
Breast-related pathologic condition.
Castleman disease (lymph node neoplasm).

CHEST PAIN, NONPLEURITIC[24]

ICD-10CM #		
	R07.9	Chest pain, unspecified
	R07.82	Intercostal pain
	R07.89	Other chest pain

Cardiac: myocardial ischemia/infarction, myocarditis.
Esophageal: spasm, esophagitis, ulceration, neoplasm, achalasia, diverticula, foreign body.
Referred pain from subdiaphragmatic GI structures.
Gastric and duodenal: hiatal hernia, neoplasm, PUD.
Gallbladder and biliary: cholecystitis, cholelithiasis, impacted stone, neoplasm.
Pancreatic: pancreatitis, neoplasm.
Dissecting aortic aneurysm.
Pain originating from skin, breasts, and musculoskeletal structures: herpes zoster, mastitis, cervical spondylosis.
Mediastinal tumors: lymphoma, thymoma.
Pulmonary: neoplasm, pneumonia, pulmonary embolism/infarction.
Psychoneurosis.
Chest pain associated with mitral valve prolapse.

CHEST PAIN, PLEURITIC

ICD-10CM #		
	R07.1	Chest pain on breathing
	R07.81	Pleurodynia

Cardiac: pericarditis, postpericardiotomy/Dressler syndrome.
Pulmonary: pneumothorax, hemothorax, embolism/infarction, pneumonia, empyema, neoplasm, bronchiectasis, pneumomediastinum, TB, carcinomatous effusion.
GI: liver abscess, pancreatitis, esophageal rupture, Whipple disease with associated pericarditis or pleuritis.
Subdiaphragmatic abscess.
Pain originating from skin and musculoskeletal tissues: costochondritis, chest wall trauma, fractured rib, interstitial fibrositis, myositis, strain of pectoralis muscle, herpes zoster, soft tissue and bone tumors.
Collagen vascular diseases with pleuritis.
Psychoneurosis.
Familial Mediterranean fever.

CHEST WALL TUMORS, PRIMARY[17]

ICD-10CM # Varies with specific diagnosis

SOFT TISSUE

Benign
Lipoma.
Hemangioma.
Lymphangioma.
Fibroma.
Rhabdomyoma.
Neurofibroma.
Desmoid tumor.
Malignant
Malignant fibrous histiocytoma.
Rhabdosarcoma.
Liposarcoma.
Neurofibrosarcoma.
Leiomyosarcoma.

BONY AND CARTILAGINOUS

Benign
Fibrous dysplasia.
Osteochondroma.
Chondroma.
Askin tumor.
Plasmacytoma.
Malignant
Chondrosarcoma.
Osteogenic sarcoma.
Ewing sarcoma.

CHIASMAL DISEASE[13]

ICD-10CM # Varies with specific diagnosis

CAUSES OF CHIASMAL DISEASE

Tumors
Pituitary adenomas.
Craniopharyngioma.
Meningioma.
Glioma.
Chordoma.
Dysgerminoma.
Nasopharyngeal tumors.
Metastases.
Non-neoplastic masses
Aneurysm.
Rathke pouch cysts.
Fibrous dysplasia.
Sphenoidal sinus mucocele.
Arachnoid cysts.
Miscellaneous
Demyelination.
Inflammation (e.g., sarcoidosis).
Trauma.
Radiation-induced necrosis.
Toxicity (e.g., ethambutol).
Vasculitis.

CHILDHOOD EOSINOPHILIA

ICD-10CM #		
	D72.1	Eosinophilia

PHYSIOLOGIC

Prematurity.
Infants receiving hyperalimentation.
Familial.

INFECTIOUS

Parasitic (with tissue-invasive helminths, e.g., trichinosis, strongyloidiasis, pneumocystosis, filariasis, cysticercosis, cutaneous and visceral larva migrans, echinococcosis).
Bacterial (brucellosis, tularemia, cat-scratch disease, *Chlamydia*).
Fungal (histoplasmosis, blastomycosis, coccidioidomycosis, allergic bronchopulmonary aspergillosis).
Mycobacterial (tuberculosis, leprosy).
Viral (hepatitis A, hepatitis B, hepatitis C, Epstein-Barr virus).

PULMONARY

Allergic (rhinitis, asthma).
Loeffler syndrome.
Hypersensitivity pneumonitis.
Eosinophilic pneumonia.
Pulmonary interstitial eosinophilia.

DERMATOLOGIC

Atopic dermatitis.
Pemphigus.
Dermatitis herpetiformis.
Infantile eosinophilic pustular folliculitis.
Episodic angioedema and urticaria.
Eosinophilic fasciitis (Schulman syndrome).
Eosinophilic cellulitis (Wells syndrome).
Kimura disease.

ONCOLOGIC

Neoplasm (lung, GI, uterine).
Hodgkin disease.
Leukemia.
Myelofibrosis.

IMMUNOLOGIC

T-cell immunodeficiencies.
Hyperimmunoglobulin E (Job) syndrome.
Wiskott-Aldrich syndrome.
Graft-versus-host disease.
Drug hypersensitivity.
Post-irradiation.
Post-splenectomy.

ENDOCRINE

Post-adrenalectomy.
Addison disease.
Panhypopituitarism.

CARDIOVASCULAR

Loeffler disease (fibroplastic endocarditis).
Congenital heart disease.
Hypersensitivity vasculitis.

GASTROINTESTINAL

Milk protein allergy.
Inflammatory bowel disease.
Eosinophilic esophagitis.
Eosinophilic gastroenteritis.

CHOLANGITIS, ACUTE[17]

ICD-10CM # K83.0 Cholangitis

NONIATROGENIC

Benign Conditions

Choledocholithiasis.
- Primary.
- Secondary.

Pancreatitis (chronic/acute), including pancreatic pseudocyst.
Papillary stenosis.
Mirizzi syndrome.
Choledochal cysts (type V, Caroli disease).
Primary sclerosing cholangitis.

Malignancies

Pancreatic cancer.
Cholangiocarcinoma.
Porta hepatis tumor/metastasis.

IATROGENIC

Obstructed biliary endoprosthesis.
Iatrogenic biliary stricture.
Direct surgical trauma.
Ischemia-induced stricture.
Anastomotic stricture (biliobiliary/bilioenteric anastomosis).

CHOLESTASIS[36]

ICD-10CM # K80.65 Calculus of gallbladder and bile duct with chronic cholecystitis with obstruction

EXTRAHEPATIC

Choledocholithiasis.
Bile duct stricture.
Cholangiocarcinoma.
Pancreatic carcinoma.
Chronic pancreatitis.
Papillary stenosis.
Ampullary cancer.
Primary sclerosing cholangitis.
Choledochal cysts.
Parasites (e.g., ascaris, clonorchis).
AIDS.
Cholangiography.
Biliary atresia.
Portal lymphadenopathy.
Mirizzi syndrome.

INTRAHEPATIC

Viral hepatitis.
Alcoholic hepatitis.
Drug induced.
Ductopenia syndromes.
Primary biliary cirrhosis.
Benign recurrent intrahepatic cholestasis.
Byler disease.
Primary sclerosing cholangitis.
Alagille syndrome.
Sarcoid.
Lymphoma.
Postoperative.
Total parenteral nutrition.
α-1-antitrypsin deficiency.

CHOLESTASIS, NEONATAL AND INFANTILE, DIFFERENTIAL DIAGNOSIS[58]

ICD-10CM # 026.6 Liver disorders in pregnancy, childbirth and the puerperium

INFECTIOUS

Generalized bacterial sepsis.
Viral hepatitis:
- Hepatitis A, B, C, D.
- Cytomegalovirus.
- Rubella virus.
- Herpesvirus: herpes simplex, human herpesvirus 6 and 7.
- Varicella virus.
- Coxsackievirus.
- Echovirus.
- Reovirus type 3.
- Parvovirus B19.
- HIV.
- Adenovirus.

Others:
- Toxoplasmosis.
- Syphilis.
- Tuberculosis.
- Listeriosis.
- Urinary tract infection.

TOXIC

Sepsis.
Parenteral nutrition related.
Drug related.

METABOLIC

Disorders of amino acid metabolism:
- Tyrosinemia.

Disorders of lipid metabolism:
- Wolman disease.
- Niemann-Pick disease (type C).
- Gaucher disease.

Cholesterol ester storage disease.
Disorders of carbohydrate metabolism:
- Galactosemia.
- Fructosemia.
- Glycogenosis IV.

Disorders of bile acid biosynthesis.
Other metabolic defects:
- α1-Antitrypsin deficiency.
- Cystic fibrosis.
- Hypopituitarism.
- Hypothyroidism.
- Zellweger (cerebrohepatorenal) syndrome.
- Neonatal iron storage disease.
- Indian childhood cirrhosis/infantile copper overload.
- Congenital disorders of glycosylation.
- Mitochondrial hepatopathies.
- Citrin deficiency.

GENETIC OR CHROMOSOMAL

Trisomy 17, 18, 21.
Donahue syndrome.

INTRAHEPATIC CHOLESTASIS SYNDROMES

"Idiopathic" neonatal hepatitis.
Alagille syndrome (arteriohepatic dysplasia).
Nonsyndromic bile duct paucity syndrome.
Intrahepatic cholestasis (PFIC):
- FIC-1 deficiency.
- BSEP deficiency.
- MDR3 deficiency.

Familial benign recurrent cholestasis associated with lymphedema (Aagenaes).
Congenital hepatic fibrosis.
Caroli disease (cystic dilatation of intrahepatic ducts).

Differential Diagnosis II

EXTRAHEPATIC DISEASES

Biliary atresia.
Sclerosing cholangitis.
Bile duct stricture/stenosis.
Choledochal-pancreaticoductal junction anomaly.
Spontaneous perforation of the bile duct.
Choledochal cyst.
Mass (neoplasia, stone).
Bile/mucous plug ("inspissated bile").

MISCELLANEOUS

Shock and hypoperfusion.
Associated with enteritis.
Associated with intestinal obstruction.
Neonatal lupus erythematosus.
Myeloproliferative disease (trisomy 21).
Hemophagocytic lymphohistiocytosis.
Arthrogryposis cholestatic pigmentary syndrome.

CHOLESTATIC LIVER ENZYME ELEVATION, EXTRAHEPATIC CAUSES[30]

ICD-10CM # Varies with specific diagnosis

EXTRAHEPATIC CAUSES OF CHOLESTATIC LIVER ENZYMES IN ADULTS

Intrinsic

Choledocholithiasis.
Immune-mediated duct injury:
  Autoimmune pancreatitis.
  PSC.
Malignancy:
  Ampullary cancer.
  Cholangiocarcinoma.
Infections:
  AIDS cholangiopathy:
    Cytomegalovirus.
    Cryptosporidiosis.
    Microsporidiosis.
  Parasitic infections:
    Ascariasis.

Extrinsic

Malignancy:
  Gallbladder cancer.
  Metastases, including portal adenopathy from metastases.
  Pancreatic cancer.
Mirizzi syndrome.
Pancreatitis.
Pancreatic pseudocyst.

CHOLESTATIC LIVER ENZYME ELEVATION, INTRAHEPATIC CAUSES[30]

ICD-10CM # Varies with specific causes

INTRAHEPATIC CAUSES OF CHOLESTATIC LIVER ENZYME ELEVATIONS IN ADULTS

Drugs*

Bland cholestasis:
  Anabolic steroids.
  Estrogens.
Cholestatic hepatitis:
  Angiotensin-converting enzyme inhibitors: captopril, enalapril.
  Antimicrobials: amoxicillin-clavulanic acid, ketoconazole.
  Azathioprine.
  Chlorpromazine.
  NSAIDs: sulindac, piroxicam.
Granulomatous hepatitis:
  Allopurinol.
  Antibiotics: sulfonamides.
  Antiepileptics: carbamazepine, phenytoin.
  Cardiovascular agents: hydralazine, procainamide, quinidine.
  Phenylbutazone.
Vanishing bile duct syndrome:
  Amoxicillin-clavulanic acid.
  Chlorpromazine.
  Dicloxacillin.
  Flucloxacillin.
  Macrolides.

PBC

PSC

Granulomatous Liver Disease

Infections:
  Brucellosis.
  Fungal: histoplasmosis, coccidioidomycosis.
  Leprosy.
  Q fever.
  Schistosomiasis.
  TB, *Mycobacterium avium* complex, bacillus Calmette-Guérin.
Sarcoidosis.
Idiopathic granulomatous hepatitis.
Other:
  Crohn disease.
  Heavy metal exposure: beryllium, copper.
  Hodgkin disease.

Viral Hepatitis

HAV and HEV.
HBV and HCV, including fibrosing cholestatic hepatitis.
EBV.
Cytomegalovirus.

Idiopathic Adulthood Ductopenia

Genetic Conditions

Progressive familial intrahepatic cholestasis:
  Type 1 (formerly Byler disease).
  Type 2.
  Type 3.
Benign recurrent intrahepatic cholestasis:
  Type 1.
  Type 2.
CF.

Malignancy

Hepatocellular carcinoma.
Metastatic disease.
Paraneoplastic syndrome:
  Non-Hodgkin lymphoma.
  Prostate cancer.
  Renal cell cancer.

Infiltrative Liver Disease

Amyloidosis.
Lymphoma.

Intrahepatic Cholestasis of Pregnancy

TPN:
  Graft-versus-host disease
  Sepsis

*Diffuse, uniform loss, but many hairs left randomly distributed in area of loss.

CHOREA

ICD-10CM # G25.4 Drug-induced chorea
G25.5 Other chorea

Medications (e.g., neuroleptics, tricyclics, antiparkinsonian drugs).
Cerebral palsy.
Huntington disease.
Benign hereditary chorea.
Thyroid disorder (hyperthyroidism, hypothyroidism).
Friedreich ataxia.
Ataxia-telangiectasia.
Hypoglycemia, hyperglycemia.
Electrolyte abnormalities (hyponatremia, hypocalcemia, hypomagnesemia, hypernatremia).
Vitamin B_{12} deficiency.
SLE.
Wilson disease.
Alcohol.
Cocaine.
Carbon monoxide poisoning.
Mercury poisoning.

CHOREA, PEDIATRIC PATIENT[93]

ICD-10CM # G25.5 Other chorea

CAUSES OF CHOREA IN CHILDHOOD

Static Injury/Structural Disorders

Cerebral palsy.
Stroke.
Trauma.
Moyamoya disease.
Vasculitis.
Tumors.
Congenital malformations.
Joubert syndrome.

Hereditary/Degenerative Disorders

Ataxia-telangiectasia (A-T), and Ataxia-telangiectasia-like disorder (ATLD).
Ataxia oculomotor apraxia (AOA) (includes AOA-1, AOA-2, and early onset cerebellar ataxia and hypoalbuminemia [EOCA-HA]).
Fahr disease.
Pantothenate kinase-associated neurodegeneration (PKAN, associated with mutations in the pantothenate kinase-2 [*PANK-2*] gene), and other causes of neuronal brain iron accumulation (NBIA).

Metabolic Disorders

Acyl-CoA dehydrogenase deficiencies.
Mitochondrial disorders, including Leigh syndrome.
GM_1 gangliosidosis.
Lesch-Nyhan disease.
Niemann-Pick type C.
Methylmalonic aciduria.
Nonketotic hyperglycemia.
Kernicterus.
Hypoparathyroidism.
Propionic acidemia.
Hypernatremia.
Hypomagnesemia.
Hypocalcemia.
Hypo- or hyperglycemia.
Vitamin E deficiency or malabsorption.
Bassen-Kornzweig disease.
Complications of cardiac bypass.

Infectious/Parainfectious Disease
Encephalitis/postencephalitis.
Immune-Mediated/Demyelinating Disorders
Sydenham chorea.
Lupus erythematosus.
Henoch-Schönlein purpura.
Anticardiolipin or antiphospholipid antibody syndrome.
Anti-NMDA antibody syndrome.
Drugs/Toxins
Neuroleptic medications, and neuroleptic-like antiemetics (haloperidol, chlorpromazine, pimozide, prochlorperazine, metoclopramide).
Calcium channel blockers (flunarizine, cinnarizine).
Antiseizure medications (phenytoin, carbamazepine, valproate, phenobarbital).
Anticholinergic medications (trihexyphenidyl, benztropine).
Antihistamines.
Tricyclic antidepressants.
Clomipramine.
Stimulants (including methylphenidate, dexamphetamine, pemoline, and bronchodilators).
Clonidine.
L-dopa.
Cocaine.
Bismuth.
Lithium.
Manganese.
Ethanol.
Carbon monoxide.
Oral contraceptives.
General anesthesia (including propofol)—during induction or emergence.
Paroxysmal Disorders
Complex migraine.
Alternating hemiplegia of childhood.
Paroxysmal kinesigenic dyskinesia (PKD).
Paroxysmal nonkinesigenic dyskinesia (PNKD).
Paroxysmal exercise-induced dyskinesia (PED).
Endocrine Disorders
Hyperthyroidism.
Pheochromocytoma.

CHOREOATHETOSIS[71]

ICD-10CM # G25.5 Choreoathetosis

SYSTEMIC DISEASES

SLE.
Polycythemia.
Thyrotoxicosis.
Rheumatic fever.
Cirrhosis of the liver (acquired hepatocerebral degeneration).
DM.
Wilson disease.

PRIMARY DEGENERATIVE BRAIN DISEASES

Huntington chorea.
Olivopontocerebellar atrophies.
Neuroacanthocytosis.

FOCAL BRAIN DISEASES

Hemichorea.
Stroke.
Tumor.
Arteriovenous malformation.

DRUG-INDUCED CHOREOATHETOSIS

Parkinson Disease Drugs
Levodopa.

EPILEPSY DRUGS

Phenytoin.
Carbamazepine.
Phenobarbital.
Gabapentin.
Valproate.
Psychostimulant Drugs
Cocaine.
Amphetamine.
Methamphetamine.
Dextroamphetamine.
Methylphenidate.
Pemoline.
Psychotropic Drugs
Lithium.
Tricyclic antidepressant drugs.
Oral Contraceptive Drugs
Cimetidine

CHRONIC PNEUMONIA[89]

ICD-10CM # J17 Pneumonia in diseases classified elsewhere

CAUSES OF CHRONIC PNEUMONIA

Infectious
Bacteria.
Mixed aerobic and anaerobic bacteria.
Actinomyces spp.
Burkholderia pseudomallei.
Nocardia spp.
Rhodococcus equi.
Mycobacteria.
Mycobacterium abscessus.
Mycobacterium avium complex.
Mycobacterium kansasii.
Mycobacterium tuberculosis.
Parasites.
Dirofilaria.
Echinococcus granulosus.
Filaria.
Paragonimus westermani.
Fungi.
Aspergillus spp.
Blastomyces dermatitidis.
Coccidioides spp.
Cryptococcus spp.
Histoplasma capsulatum.
Scedosporium spp.
Sporothrix schenckii.
Noninfectious
Neoplasia.
Cystic fibrosis.
Sarcoidosis.
Amyloidosis.
Vasculitis.
Drugs.
Radiation.
Recurrent pulmonary emboli.
Bronchial obstruction.
Pulmonary infiltration with eosinophilia syndrome.
Pneumoconiosis.

CHYLOTHORAX

ICD-10CM # I89.8 Other specified noninfective disorders of lymphatic vessels and lymph nodes

Post-lymph node dissection of neck or chest.
Subclavian venous catheterization.
Thoracic aneurysm repair.
Trauma to chest and neck.
Mediastinal tumor resection.
Esophagectomy, pneumonectomy.
Lymphangitis, mediastinitis.
Neoplasms (lymphoma, carcinoma of esophagus, lung, mediastinal malignancies).
Sympathectomy.
Venous thrombosis.
Congenital.

CLOUDY URINE

ICD-10CM # R82 Other abnormal findings in urine

Concentrated urine.
Use of multivitamin supplements.
Diet high in purine-rich foods.
Pyuria.
Phosphaturia.
Urinary tract infection.
Lipiduria.
Chyluria.
Hyperoxaluria.

CLUBBING

ICD-10CM # R68.3 Clubbing of fingers

Pulmonary neoplasm (lung, pleura).
Other neoplasm (GI, liver, Hodgkin, thymus, osteogenic sarcoma).
Pulmonary infectious process (empyema, abscess, bronchiectasis, TB, chronic pneumonitis).
Extrapulmonary infectious process (subacute bacterial endocarditis, intestinal TB, bacterial or amebic dysentery, arterial graft sepsis).
Pneumoconiosis.
Cystic fibrosis.
Sarcoidosis.
Cyanotic congenital heart disease.
Endocrine (Graves disease, hyperparathyroidism).
Inflammatory bowel disease.
Celiac disease.
Chronic liver disease, cirrhosis (particularly biliary and juvenile).
Pulmonary AV malformations.
Idiopathic.
Thyroid acropachy.
Hereditary (pachydermoperiostosis).
Chronic trauma (jackhammer operators, machine workers).

COBALAMIN DEFICIENCY[50]

ICD-10CM # E53.8 Deficiency of other specified B group vitamins

ETIOPATHOPHYSIOLOGIC CLASSIFICATION OF COBALAMIN DEFICIENCY

Nutritional cobalamin deficiency (i.e., insufficient cobalamin intake):
- Vegetarians, poverty-imposed near-vegetarians, breastfed infants of mothers with pernicious anemia.

Abnormal intragastric events (i.e., inadequate proteolysis of food cobalamin):
- Atrophic gastritis, partial gastritis with hypochlorhydria, proton-pump inhibitors, H_2 blockers.

Loss or atrophy of gastric oxyntic mucosa (i.e., deficient intrinsic factor [IF] molecules):
- Total or partial gastrectomy, pernicious anemia, caustic destruction (lye).

Abnormal events in small bowel lumen:
- Inadequate pancreatic protease (e.g., R-cobalamin not degraded, cobalamin not transferred to IF):
  - Insufficient pancreatic protease (i.e., pancreatic insufficiency).
  - Inactivation of pancreatic protease (i.e., Zollinger–Ellison syndrome).
- Usurping of luminal cobalamin (i.e., inadequate cobalamin binding to IF):
- By bacteria, during stasis syndromes (e.g., blind loops, pouches of diverticulosis, strictures, fistulas, anastomosis), impaired bowel motility (e.g., scleroderma), hypogammaglobulinemia.
- By *Diphyllobothrium latum* (fish tapeworm).

Disorders of ileal mucosa/IF–cobalamin receptors (i.e., IF–cobalamin not bound to IF–cobalamin receptors):
- Diminished or absent IF–cobalamin receptors (e.g., ileal bypass, resection, fistula).
- Abnormal mucosal architecture/function (e.g., tropical or nontropical sprue, Crohn disease, tuberculosis ileitis, infiltration by lymphomas, amyloidosis).
- IF-/post-IF–cobalamin receptor defects (e.g., Imerslund–Gräsbeck syndrome, transcobalamin II [TC II] deficiency).
- Drug effects (e.g., slow K, metformin, cholestyramine, colchicine, neomycin).

Disorders of plasma cobalamin transport (i.e., TC II–cobalamin not delivered to TC II receptors):
- Congenital TC II deficiency, defective binding of TC II–cobalamin to TC II receptors (rare).

Metabolic disorders (i.e., cobalamin not used by cells):
- Inborn enzyme errors (rare).
- Acquired disorders (e.g., cobalamin functionally inactivated by irreversible oxidation, N_2O inhalation).

COGNITIVE IMPAIRMENT[92]

ICD-10CM # G31.84 Mild cognitive impairment, so stated

CAUSES OF COGNITIVE IMPAIRMENT: DIAGNOSES BY CATEGORIES WITH REPRESENTATIVE EXAMPLES

Degenerative:
Alzheimer disease.
Frontotemporal dementias.
Dementia with Lewy bodies.
Corticobasal degeneration.
Huntington disease.
Wilson disease.
Parkinson disease.
Multiple system atrophy.
Progressive supranuclear palsy.

Psychiatric:
Depression.
Schizophrenia.

Vascular:
Vascular dementia.
Binswanger encephalopathy.
Amyloid dementia.
Diffuse hypoxic/ischemic injury.

Obstructive:
Normal-pressure hydrocephalus.
Obstructive hydrocephalus.

Traumatic:
Chronic subdural hematoma.
Chronic traumatic encephalopathy.
Post-concussion syndrome.

Neoplastic:
Tumor: malignant, primary and secondary.
Tumor: benign (e.g., frontal meningioma).
Paraneoplastic limbic encephalitis.

Infections:
Chronic meningitis.
Post-herpes encephalitis.
Focal cerebritis/abscesses.
HIV dementia.
HIV-associated infection.
Syphilis.
Lyme encephalopathy.
Subacute sclerosing panencephalitis.
Creutzfeldt–Jakob disease.
Progressive multifocal leukoencephalopathy.
Parenchymal sarcoidosis.
Chronic systemic infection.

Demyelinating:
Multiple sclerosis.
Adrenoleukodystrophy.
Metachromatic leukodystrophy.

Autoimmune:
Systemic lupus erythematosus.
Polyarteritis nodosa.

Drugs/Toxins
Medications:
- Anticholinergics.
- Antihistamines.
- Anticonvulsants.
- β-blockers.
- Sedative–hypnotics.

Substance abuse:
Alcohol.
Inhalants.
Phencyclidine (PCP).

Toxins
Arsenic.
Bromide.
Carbon monoxide.
Lead.
Mercury.
Organophosphates.

COLIC, ACUTE ABDOMINAL[95]

ICD-10CM # R10.0 Acute abdomen

Acute gastroenteritis.
Food poisoning.
Nonspecific causes.
Constipation.
Gastric outlet obstruction:
- Chronic peptic ulceration.
- Gastric cancer.

Small bowel obstruction:
- Adhesions:
  - Postsurgical.
  - Inflammatory (e.g., diverticular).
  - Radiation.
  - Meckel diverticulum.
  - Metastatic.
- Stricture:
  - Ischemic.
  - Radiation.
  - Inflammatory (e.g., Crohn disease).
- Volvulus intussusception:
  - Tumor (e.g., Peutz-Jeghers syndrome).
  - Superior mesenteric artery syndrome.
- Intraluminal bolus:
  - Gallstone.
  - Bezoar.
- Hernia:
  - Abdominal wall.
  - Internal.
- Neoplasm:
  - Benign (e.g., leiomyoma).
  - Malignant (e.g., carcinoid tumor, adenocarcinoma).

Large bowel obstruction:
- Colon cancer.
- Diverticular disease.
- Volvulus.

Uterine:
- Missed abortion.
- Parturition.
- Period pain.

COLON ISCHEMIA[30]

ICD-10CM # Varies with specific diagnosis

CAUSES OF COLON ISCHEMIA

Acute pancreatitis.
Allergy.
Amyloidosis.
Heart failure or cardiac arrhythmias.
Hematologic disorders and coagulopathies:
- Activated protein C resistance.
- Antithrombin deficiency.
- Factor V Leiden mutation.
- Paroxysmal nocturnal hemoglobinuria.
- Polycythemia vera.
- Protein C and S deficiencies.
- Prothrombin G20210A mutation.
- Sickle cell disease.

Infection:
- Bacteria (*Escherichia coli* 0157:H7).
- Parasites (*Angiostrongylus costaricensis*).
- Viruses (HBV, HCV, cytomegalovirus).

Inferior mesenteric artery thrombosis.
Long-distance running.
Medications and toxins:
- Alosetron.
- Cocaine.
- Danazol.
- Digitalis compounds.
- Ergots.
- Estrogens.
- Flutamide.

Glycerin enema.
Gold salts.
Immunosuppressive agents.
Interferon-α.
Methamphetamine.
NSAIDs.
Penicillin.
Phenylephrine.
Polyethylene glycol 3350 colon lavage solutions.
Pit viper toxin.
Progestins.
Pseudoephedrine.
Psychotropic drugs.
Saline laxatives.
Sumatriptan.
Tegaserod.
Vasopressin.
Pheochromocytoma.
Ruptured ectopic pregnancy.
Shock.
Strangulated hernia.
Surgery/procedures:
Aortic aneurysmectomy.
Aortoiliac reconstruction.
Barium enema.
Colectomy with inferior mesenteric artery ligation.
Colon bypass.
Colonoscopy.
Exchange transfusions.
Gynecologic operations.
Lumbar aortography.
Thromboembolism:
Cholesterol (atheroembolism).
Myxoma (left atrial).
Trauma (blunt or penetrating).
Vasculitis and vasculopathy:
Buerger disease.
Eosinophilic granulomatosis with angiitis.
Fibromuscular dysplasia.
Kawasaki disease.
Polyarteritis nodosa.
Rheumatoid vasculitis.
SLE.
Takayasu arteritis.
Volvulus.

COLOR CHANGES, CUTANEOUS[86]

ICD-10CM # L81.9 Disorder of pigmentation, unspecified

BROWN

Generalized: pituitary, adrenal, liver disease, ACTH-producing tumor (e.g., oat cell lung carcinoma).
Localized: nevi, neurofibromatosis.

WHITE

Generalized: albinism.
Localized: vitiligo, Raynaud phenomenon.

RED (ERYTHEMA)

Generalized: fever, polycythemia, urticaria, viral exanthems.
Localized: inflammation, infection, Raynaud phenomenon.

YELLOW

Generalized: liver disease, chronic renal disease, anemia.
Generalized (except sclera): hypothyroidism, increased intake of vegetables containing carotene.
Localized: resolving hematoma, infection, peripheral vascular insufficiency.

BLUE

Lips, mouth, nail beds: cardiovascular and pulmonary diseases, Raynaud phenomenon.

COMA

ICD-10CM # R40.20 Unspecified coma

Vascular: hemorrhage, thrombosis, embolism.
CNS infections: meningitis, encephalitis, cerebral abscess.
Cerebral neoplasms with herniation.
Head injury: subdural hematoma, cerebral concussion, cerebral contusion.
Drugs: narcotics, sedatives, hypnotics.
Ingestion or inhalation of toxins: CO, alcohol, lead.
Metabolic disturbances.
Hypoxia.
Acid-base disorders.
Hypoglycemia, hyperglycemia.
Hepatic failure.
Electrolyte disorders.
Uremia.
Hypothyroidism.
Hypothermia, hyperthermia.
Hypotension, malignant hypertension.
Postictal.

COMA, NORMAL COMPUTED TOMOGRAPHY[3]

ICD-10CM # R40.20 Unspecified coma

MENINGEAL DISORDERS

Subarachnoid hemorrhage (uncommon).
Bacterial meningitis.
Encephalitis.
Subdural empyema.

EXOGENOUS TOXINS

Sedative drugs and barbiturates.
Anesthetics and γ-hydroxybutyrate.[18]
Alcohols.
Stimulants:
Phencyclidines.[19]
Cocaine and amphetamines.[20]
Psychotropic drugs:
Cyclic antidepressants.
Phenothiazines.
Lithium.
Anticonvulsants.
Opioids.
Clonidine.[21]
Penicillins.
Salicylates.
Anticholinergics.
Carbon monoxide, cyanide, and methemoglobinemia.

ENDOGENOUS TOXINS/ DEFICIENCIES/DERANGEMENTS

Hypoxia and ischemia.
Hypoglycemia.
Hypercalcemia.
Osmolar:
Hyperglycemia.
Hyponatremia.
Hypernatremia.
Organ system failure:
Hepatic encephalopathy.
Uremic encephalopathy.
Pulmonary insufficiency (carbon dioxide narcosis).

SEIZURES

Prolonged postictal state.
Spike-wave stupor.

HYPOTHERMIA OR HYPERTHERMIA

Brain stem ischemia.
Basilar artery stroke.
Brain stem or cerebellar hemorrhage.
Conversion or malingering.

[18] Involvement principally of cancellous bone
[19] Involvement of cancellous and cortical bone
[20] Coma after seizures or status (i.e., a prolonged postictal state).
[21] An antihypertensive agent active through the opiate receptor system; frequent overdose when used to treat narcotic withdrawal.

COMA, PEDIATRIC POPULATION[79]

ICD-10CM # R40.20 Unspecified coma

ANOXIA

Birth asphyxia.
Carbon monoxide poisoning.
Croup/epiglottitis.
Meconium aspiration.

INFECTION

Hemolysis.
Blood loss.
Hydrops fetalis.
Infection.
Meningoencephalitis.
Sepsis.
Postimmunization encephalitis.

INCREASED INTRACRANIAL PRESSURE

Anoxia.
Inborn metabolic errors.
Toxic encephalopathy.
Reye syndrome.
Head trauma/intracranial bleed.
Hydrocephalus.
Posterior fossa tumors.

HYPERTENSIVE ENCEPHALOPATHY
Coarctation of aorta.
Nephritis.
Vasculitis.
Pheochromocytoma.

ISCHEMIA
Hypoplastic left heart.
Shunting lesions.
Aortic stenosis.
Cardiovascular collapse (any cause).

PURPURIC CAUSES
Disseminated intravascular coagulation.
Hemolytic-uremic syndrome.
Leukemia.
Thrombotic purpura.

HYPERCAPNIA
Cystic fibrosis.
Bronchopulmonary dysplasia.
Congenital lung anomalies.

NEOPLASM
Medulloblastoma.
Glioma of brain stem.
Posterior fossa tumors.

DRUGS/TOXINS
Maternal sedation.
Alcohol.
Any drug.
Lead.
Salicylism.
Arsenic.
Pesticides.

ELECTROLYTE ABNORMALITIES
Hypernatremia (diarrhea, dehydration, salt poisoning).
Hyponatremia (SIADH, androgenital syndrome, gastroenteritis).
Hyperkalemia (renal failure, salicylism, androgenitalism).
Hypokalemia (diarrhea, hyperaldosteronism, salicylism, DKA).
Hypocalcemia (vitamin D deficiency, hyperparathyroidism).
Severe acidosis (sepsis, cold injury, salicylism, DKA).

HYPOGLYCEMIA
Birth injury or stress.
Diabetes.
Alcohol.
Salicylism.
Hyperinsulinemia.
Iatrogenic.

POSTSEIZURE
Renal Causes
Nephritis.
Hypoplastic kidneys.
Hepatic Causes
Acute hepatitis.
Fulminant hepatic failure.
Inborn metabolic errors.
Bile duct atresia.

COMPRESSION SYNDROMES, NEUROVASCULAR CAUSES[76]

ICD-10CM #	M47.016	Anterior spinal artery compression syndromes, lumbar region
	M47.019	Anterior spinal artery compression syndromes, site unspecified
	M47.013	Anterior spinal artery compression syndromes, cervicothoracic region
	M47.021	Vertebral artery compression syndromes, occipito-atlanto-axial region
	M47.022	Vertebral artery compression syndromes, cervical region

Anatomic
Potential sites of neurovascular compression:
- Interscalene triangle.
- Costoclavicular space.
- Subcoracoid area.

Congenital
Cervical rib and its fascial remnants.
Rudimentary first thoracic rib.
Scalene muscles:
- Anterior.
- Middle.
- Minimus.

Adventitious fibrous bands.
Bifid clavicle or first rib.
Exostosis of first thoracic rib.
Enlarged transverse process of C7.
Omohyoid muscle.
Anomalous course of transverse cervical artery.
Abnormal lateral insertion of costoclavicular ligament.
Flat clavicle.
Traumatic
Fracture of clavicle.
Dislocation of head of humerus.
Crushing injury to upper thorax.
Sudden, unaccustomed muscular efforts involving shoulder girdle muscles.
Cervical spondylosis and injuries to cervical spine.
Atherosclerosis.

CONGESTIVE HEART FAILURE AND CARDIOMYOPATHY[3]

ICD-10CM #	I50.9	Heart failure, unspecified
	I42.7	Cardiomyopathy due to drug and external agent

CAUSES OF CONGESTIVE HEART FAILURE AND CARDIOMYOPATHY
Coronary Artery Disease
Acute ischemia.
Myocardial infarction.
Ischemic cardiomyopathy with hibernating myocardium.
Idiopathic
Idiopathic dilated cardiomyopathy.
Idiopathic restrictive cardiomyopathy.
Peripartum.
Pressure Overload
Hypertension.
Aortic stenosis.
Volume Overload
Mitral regurgitation.
Aortic insufficiency.
Anemia.
Atrioventricular fistula.
Toxins
Ethanol.
Cocaine.
Doxorubicin (Adriamycin).
Methamphetamine.
Metabolic-Endocrine
Thiamine deficiency.
Diabetes.
Hemochromatosis.
Thyrotoxicosis.
Obesity.
Infiltrative
Amyloidosis.
Inflammatory
Viral myocarditis.
Hereditary
Hypertrophic.
Dilated.

Genetic bases for these cardiomyopathies have been identified in a large number of individual patients and families. Most of the mutations have been found in cardiac contractile or structural proteins.

CONGESTIVE HEART FAILURE, INFANT[1]

ICD-10CM #	I05.9	Heart failure, unspecified

Critical coarctation of the aorta.
Interrupted aortic arch.
Congenital aortic stenosis.
Hypoplastic left heart syndrome.
Large ventricular septal defect.
Truncus arteriosus.
Unrecognized supraventricular tachycardia.
Cardiac tamponade.
Myocarditis.

CONJUNCTIVAL NEOPLASM

ICD-10CM # Varies with specific diagnosis

MALIGNANT
Squamous cell carcinoma.
Melanoma.
Sebaceous carcinoma.
Kaposi sarcoma.
Metastatic neoplasms.

BENIGN
Melanocytic nevus.
Squamous papilloma.
Hemangioma.
Lymphangioma.
Myxoma.

CONSCIOUSNESS IMPAIRMENT, ACUTE, IN CRITICALLY ILL PATIENT

ICD-10CM # F05.9 Delirium, unspecified

GENERAL CAUSES OF ACUTELY IMPAIRED CONSCIOUSNESS IN THE CRITICALLY ILL

Infection
Sepsis encephalopathy.
CNS infection.

Drugs
Narcotics.
Benzodiazepines.
Anticholinergics.
Anticonvulsants.
Tricyclic antidepressants.
Selective serotonin uptake inhibitors.
Phenothiazines.
Steroids.
Immunosuppressants (cyclosporine, FK-506, OKT3).
Anesthetics.

Electrolyte and Acid-Base Disturbances
Hyponatremia.
Hypernatremia.
Hypercalcemia.
Hypermagnesemia.
Severe acidemia and alkalemia.

Organ System Failure
Shock.
Renal failure.
Hepatic failure.
Pancreatitis.
Respiratory failure (hypoxia, hypercapnia).

Endocrine Disorders
Hypoglycemia.
Hyperglycemia.
Hypothyroidism.
Hyperthyroidism.
Pituitary apoplexy.

Drug Withdrawal
Alcohol.
Opiates.
Barbiturates.
Benzodiazepines.

Vascular Causes
Shock.
Hypotension.
Hypertensive encephalopathy.
CNS vasculitis.
Cerebral venous sinus thrombosis.

Central Nervous System Disorders
Hemorrhage.
Stroke.
Brain edema.
Hydrocephalus.
Increased intracranial pressure.
Meningitis.
Ventriculitis.
Brain abscess.
Subdural empyema.
Seizures.
Vasculitis.

Seizures
Convulsive and nonconvulsive status epilepticus.

Miscellaneous
Fat embolism syndrome.
Neuroleptic malignant syndrome.
Thiamine deficiency (Wernicke encephalopathy).
Psychogenic unresponsiveness.

CONSTIPATION

ICD-10CM # K59.00 Constipation, unspecified

Intestinal obstruction.
Fecal impaction.
Diverticular disease.
GI neoplasm.
Strangulated femoral hernia.
Gallstone ileus.
Tuberculous stricture.
Adhesions.
Ameboma.
Volvulus.
Intussusception.
Inflammatory bowel disease.
Hematoma of bowel wall, secondary to trauma or anticoagulants.
Poor dietary habits: insufficient bulk in diet, inadequate fluid intake.
Change from daily routine: travel, hospital admission, physical inactivity.
Acute abdominal conditions: renal colic, salpingitis, biliary colic, appendicitis, ischemia.
Hypercalcemia or hypokalemia, uremia.
Irritable bowel syndrome, pregnancy, anorexia nervosa, depression.
Painful anal conditions: hemorrhoids, fissure, stricture.
Decreased intestinal peristalsis: old age, spinal cord injuries, myxedema, diabetes, multiple sclerosis, Parkinsonism and other neurologic diseases.
Drugs: codeine, morphine, antacids with aluminum, verapamil, anticonvulsants, anticholinergics, disopyramide, cholestyramine, alosetron, iron supplements.
Hirschsprung disease, meconium ileus, congenital atresia in infants.

CONSTIPATION, ADULT PATIENT[95]

ICD-10CM # K59.00 Constipation, unspecified

NO GROSS STRUCTURAL ABNORMALITY

Inadequate fiber intake.
Irritable bowel syndrome (associated with abdominal pain) or functional constipation.
Idiopathic slow-transit constipation.
"Obstructed defecation" pelvic floor dysfunction (or dyssynergia).

STRUCTURAL DISORDERS

Anal fissure, infection, or stenosis.
Colon cancer or stricture.
Aganglionosis and/or abnormal myenteric plexus:
- Hirschsprung disease.
- Chagas disease.
- Neuropathic pseudoobstruction.

Abnormal colonic muscle:
- Myopathy.
- Dystrophia myotonica.
- Systemic sclerosis.
- Idiopathic megarectum and/or megacolon.
- Proximal megacolon.

NEUROLOGIC CAUSES

Diabetic autonomic neuropathy.
Damage to the sacral parasympathetic outflow.
Spinal cord damage or disease (e.g., multiple sclerosis).
Parkinson disease.
Blunting of consciousness, mental retardation, psychosis.
Pain induced by straining (e.g., sciatic nerve compression).

ENDOCRINE OR METABOLIC CAUSES

Hypothyroidism.
Hypercalcemia.
Porphyria.
Pregnancy.

PSYCHOLOGIC DISORDERS

Depression.
Anorexia nervosa.
Denied bowel habit.
- Drug side effects.

CONSTIPATION, PEDIATRIC PATIENT[59]

ICD-10CM # K59.00 Constipation

Nonorganic (Functional)—Retentive

Anatomic
Anal stenosis, atresia with fistula.
Imperforate anus.
Anteriorly displaced anus.
Intestinal stricture (postnecrotizing enterocolitis).
Anal stricture.

Abnormal Musculature
Prune-belly syndrome.
Gastroschisis.
Down syndrome.
Muscular dystrophy.

Intestinal Nerve or Muscle Abnormalities
Hirschsprung disease.
Pseudoobstruction (visceral myopathy or neuropathy).
Intestinal neuronal dysplasia.
Spinal cord lesions.
Tethered cord.
Autonomic neuropathy.
Spinal cord trauma.
Spina bifida.
Chagas disease.

Drugs
Anticholinergics.
Narcotics.
Methylphenidate.
Phenytoin.
Antidepressants.
Chemotherapeutic agents (vincristine).
Pancreatic enzymes (fibrosing colonopathy).
Lead, arsenic, mercury.
Vitamin D intoxication.
Calcium channel blocking agents.

Metabolic Disorders
Hypokalemia.
Hypercalcemia.
Hypothyroidism.
Diabetes mellitus, diabetes insipidus.
Porphyria.
Intestinal Disorders
Celiac disease.
Cow's milk protein intolerance.
Cystic fibrosis (meconium ileus equivalent).
Inflammatory bowel disease (stricture).
Tumor.
Connective tissue disorders.
Systemic lupus erythematosus.
Scleroderma.
Psychiatric Diagnosis
Anorexia nervosa.

COPD DECOMPENSATION[65]

ICD-10CM # J44.1 Chronic obstructive pulmonary distress with acute exacerbation

CAUSES OF ACUTE DECOMPENSATION IN THE PATIENT WITH CHRONIC OBSTRUCTIVE PULMONARY DISEASE

Acute Exacerbations
Infectious
Viral.
Rhinovirus, respiratory syncytial virus, coronavirus, influenza virus.
Bacterial.
Haemophilus influenzae, Streptococcus pneumoniae, Moraxella (Branhamella) catarrhalis, Pseudomonas aeruginosa.
Atypical bacteria.
Chlamydia pneumoniae, Legionella.
Air Pollution
Nitrogen dioxide.
Ozone.
Particulates, dust.
Other Critical Events
Pneumothorax.
Pulmonary embolism.
Lobar atelectasis.
Congestive heart failure.
Pneumonia.
Pulmonary compression (e.g., obesity, ascites, gastric distention, pleural effusion).
Trauma (e.g., rib fractures, pulmonary contusion).
Neuromuscular and metabolic disorders.
Unrelated treatable chronic pulmonary disease (bronchiectasis, tuberculosis, sarcoidosis).
Noncompliance with prescribed treatment regimens.
Iatrogenic:
Inadequate therapy.
Inappropriate therapy (e.g., deleterious drugs).

CORNEAL SENSATION, DECREASED

ICD-10CM # H18.899 Other specified disorders of cornea, unspecified eye

Herpes (simplex, zoster).
Contact lens wear.
Topical agents (NSAIDs, anesthetics, beta-blockers).
Diabetes.
Eye trauma.
Postsurgery.

COUGH

ICD-10CM # R05 Cough

Infectious process (viral, bacterial).
Postinfectious.
"Smoker's cough."
Rhinitis (allergic, vasomotor, postinfectious).
Asthma.
Exposure to irritants (noxious fumes, smoke, cold air).
Drug-induced (especially ACE inhibitors, beta-blockers).
GERD.
Interstitial lung disease.
Lung neoplasms.
Lymphomas, mediastinal neoplasms.
Bronchiectasis.
Cardiac (CHF, pulmonary edema, mitral stenosis, pericardial inflammation).
Recurrent aspiration.
Inflammation of larynx, pleura, diaphragm, mediastinum.
Cystic fibrosis.
Anxiety.
Other: pulmonary embolism, foreign body inhalation, aortic aneurysm, Zenker diverticulum, osteophytes, substernal thyroid, thyroiditis, PMR.

COUGH, CHRONIC, ADULT PATIENT[2]

ICD-10CM # R05 Cough

CAUSES OF CHRONIC COUGH IN ADULTS

Intrathoracic Causes
Lungs and Airways
Asthma.
Nonasthmatic eosinophilic bronchitis.
Chronic bronchitis.
Bronchiectasis.
ACEIs.
Inhaled medications.
Chronic exposure to environmental and occupational irritants.
Bronchogenic and metastatic carcinoma.
Bronchial carcinoid.
Foreign body or endobronchial suture.
Broncholith.
Infectious and noninfectious bronchiolitis.
Chronic infectious pneumonias (e.g., bacterial, tuberculous, fungal, parasitic).
Chronic infectious tracheobronchitis (as in tuberculosis or aspergillosis).
Chronic interstitial lung disease (e.g., sarcoidosis, HSP, IPF, asbestosis).
Pulmonary vasculitis (as in granulomatosis with polyangiitis).
Sjögren syndrome with xerotrachea.
Relapsing polychondritis.
Pleura
Chronic effusion.
Diaphragm
Transvenous pacemaker stimulation.
Mediastinum
Neural tumors.
Thymoma.
Teratoma.
Lymphoma.
Metastatic lymphadenopathy.
Intrathoracic goiter.
Bronchogenic cyst.
Cardiovascular
Mitral stenosis.
Left ventricular failure.
Pulmonary thromboembolism.
Enlarged left atrium.
Vascular ring.
Aberrant innominate artery.
Aortic aneurysm.
Pericardial stimulation by transvenous pacemaker.
Extrathoracic Causes
Head and Neck
Rhinitis and sinusitis.
Nasal polyps.
Rhinolith.
Oropharyngeal dysphagia.
Laryngeal disorders (e.g., vocal fold dysfunction, laryngomalacia).
Postviral vagal neuropathy.
Recurrent aspiration.
Elongated uvula.
Chronically infected tonsils.
Neurilemmoma of vagus nerve.
Neuroma of internal laryngeal nerve.
Ascending palatine artery aneurysm.
Osteophytes of cervical spine.
Mammomanogamus (Syngamus) laryngeus infection.
Thyroiditis.
Upper Gastrointestinal
Gastroesophageal reflux disease.
Esophageal cyst or diverticulum.
Tracheoesophageal fistula.
Central Nervous System
Psychogenic or habit cough.
Tic disorders.
Gilles de la Tourette syndrome.

ACEI, Angiotensin-converting enzyme inhibitor; *HSP,* hypersensitivity pneumonitis; *IPF,* idiopathic pulmonary fibrosis.

COUGH, CHRONIC, PEDIATRIC PATIENT[59]

ICD-10CM # R05 Cough

DIFFERENTIAL DIAGNOSIS OF RECURRENT AND PERSISTENT COUGH IN CHILDREN

Recurrent Cough
Reactive airway disease (asthma).
Drainage from upper airways.
Aspiration.
Frequently recurring respiratory tract infections in immunocompetent or immunodeficient patients.
Symptomatic Chiari malformation.
Idiopathic pulmonary hemosiderosis.
Hypersensitivity (allergic) pneumonitis.

Persistent Cough

Hypersensitivity of cough receptors after infection.
Reactive airway disease (asthma).
Chronic sinusitis.
Chronic rhinitis (allergic or nonallergic).
Bronchitis or tracheitis caused by infection or smoke exposure.
Bronchiectasis, including cystic fibrosis, primary ciliary dyskinesia, immunodeficiency.
Habit cough.
Foreign-body aspiration.
Recurrent aspiration owing to pharyngeal incompetence, tracheolaryngoesophageal cleft or tracheoesophageal fistula.
Gastroesophageal reflux, with or without aspiration.
Pertussis.
Extrinsic compression of the tracheobronchial tract (vascular ring, neoplasm, lymph node, lung cyst).
Tracheomalacia, bronchomalacia.
Endobronchial or endotracheal tumors.
Endobronchial tuberculosis.
Hypersensitivity pneumonitis.
Fungal infections.
Inhaled irritants, including tobacco smoke.
Irritation of external auditory canal.
Angiotensin-converting enzyme inhibitors.

CREEPING ERUPTION, TRAVELERS[82]

ICD-10CM # Varies with specific diagnosis

CAUSES OF CREEPING ERUPTION IN TRAVELERS

Nematode larvae

Animal hookworms (HrCLM)*, *Pelodera strongyloides*, zoonotic *Strongyloides* spp.
Gnathostomiasis (*Gnathostoma* spp.).
Larva currens (*Strongyloides stercoralis*).

Adult nematodes

Loiasis (*Loa loa*).
Dracunculiasis (*Dracunculus medinensis*).
Dirofilariasis (*Dirofilaria immitis*).

Trematode larvae

Fascioliasis (*Fasciola gigantica*).

Fly maggots

Migratory myiasis (*Gasterophilus* spp.).

Mites

Scabies *(Sarcoptes scabiei)*.*
Pyemotes dermatitis *(Pyemotes ventricosus)*.
HrCLM, Hookworm-related cutaneous larva migrans.

* Common cause.

CUTANEOUS CALCIFICATIONS[11]

ICD-10CM # Varies with specific diagnosis

Disorders of Cutaneous Calcification

Dystrophic

Autoimmune connective tissue diseases, especially dermatomyositis, CREST.
Cutaneous tumors or cysts (e.g., pilomatricomas, pilar cysts).
Infections, especially parasitic.
Trauma, including "heel sticks" in neonates, injection sites, surgical scars.
Panniculitis.
Genetic disorders (e.g., pseudoxanthoma elasticum, Ehlers–Danlos syndrome).

Metastatic

Advanced chronic kidney disease.
Calciphylaxis.*
Benign nodular calcification of renal disease.
Hypervitaminosis D.
Milk-alkali syndrome.
Sarcoidosis.
Tumoral calcinosis (familial).
Hyperparathyroidism.
Neoplasms (e.g., multiple myeloma, adult T-cell leukemia/lymphoma, SCC of the lung or head and neck).

Idiopathic

Idiopathic calcified nodules of the scrotum.
Subepidermal calcified nodule.
Tumoral calcinosis (sporadic).
Milia-like calcinosis.

Iatrogenic

Extravasation of intravenous solutions containing calcium or phosphate
Application of calcium-containing electrode paste for EMGs and EEGs
Application of calcium alginate dressings to denuded skin
Organ transplantation, especially liver
Gadolinium (nephrogenic systemic fibrosis).

CREST, *C*alcification, *R*aynaud phenomenon, *e*sophageal dysmotility, *s*clerodactyly and *t*elangiectasia; EEG, electroencephalogram; EMG, electromyography; SCC, squamous cell carcinoma.

CUTANEOUS INFECTIONS, ATHLETES

ICD-10CM #	L08.9	Local infection of the skin and subcutaneous tissue, unspecified

Tinea pedis.
Tinea cruris.
Molluscum contagiosum.
Herpes simplex.
Verruca vulgaris.
Folliculitis.
Impetigo.
Furuncles.
Otitis externa.
Erythrasma.

CUTANEOUS ULCERS, TRAVELERS[82]

ICD-10CM # Varies with specific diagnosis

CAUSES OF CUTANEOUS ULCER IN TRAVELERS

Noninfectious Causes

Spider bite.
Cupping.

Bacterial Infection

Ecthyma.*
Tick eschar* (rickettsiosis).
Anthrax.
Mycobacterial infection (*M. ulcerans*).
Melioidosis.
Glanders.
Tularemia.
Cutaneous diphtheria.
Plague.

Parasitic Infection

Leishmaniasis.*
Trypanosomal chancre (African trypanosomiasis).
Chagoma (American trypanosomiasis).
Cutaneous amebiasis.

Fungal Infection

Sporotrichosis.
Mycetomas.
West African histoplasmosis.
North American blastomycosis.
Paracoccidioidomycosis.
Chromomycosis.

Viral Infection

Herpes simplex infection.

*Common cause.

CYANOSIS[7]

ICD-10CM #	R23.0	Cyanosis

DIFFERENTIAL DIAGNOSIS OF CYANOSIS

Peripheral Cyanosis

Low cardiac output states

Shock.
Left ventricular failure.
Hypovolemia.

Environmental exposure (cold)

Air or water.

Arterial occlusion

Thrombosis.
Embolism.
Vasospasm (Raynaud phenomenon).
Peripheral vascular disease.

Venous obstruction

Redistribution of blood flow from extremities

Central Cyanosis

Decreased arterial oxygen saturation

High altitude (>8000 ft).
Impaired pulmonary function:
- Hypoventilation.
- Impaired oxygen diffusion.
- Ventilation-perfusion mismatching:
  - Pulmonary embolism.
  - Acute respiratory distress syndrome.
  - Pulmonary hypertension.
- Respiratory compromise:
  - Upper airway obstruction.
  - Pneumonia.
  - Diaphragmatic hernia.
  - Tension pneumothorax.
  - Polycythemia.

Anatomic Shunts

Pulmonary arteriovenous fistulae and intrapulmonary shunts.
Cerebral, hepatic, peripheral arteriovenous fistulae.
Cyanotic congenital heart disease:
- Endocardial cushion defects.
- Ventricular septal defects.
- Coarctation of aorta.
- Tetralogy of Fallot.
- Total anomalous pulmonary venous drainage.
- Hypoplastic left ventricle.
- Pulmonary vein stenosis.
- Tricuspid atresia and anomalies.
- Premature closure of foramen ovale.
- Dextrocardia.
- Pulmonary stenosis of atrial septal defect.
- Patent ductus arteriosus with reversed shunt.

Abnormal Hemoglobin

Methemoglobinemia:
- Hereditary.
- Acquired.

Sulfhemoglobinemia.
Mutant hemoglobin with low oxygen affinity (e.g., hemoglobin Kansas).

CYANOSIS, CENTRAL, SECONDARY TO CARDIAC DEFECT[104]

ICD-10CM # R23.0 Cyanosis

Transposition of the great arteries.	Ebstein anomaly.
Tetralogy of Fallot.	Eisenmenger physiology.
Tricuspid atresia.	Critical pulmonary stenosis or atresia.
Truncus arteriosus.	Functionally single ventricle.
Total anomalous pulmonary venous return.	

Note 5 Ts and 2 Es.

CYANOSIS, NEONATAL[1]

ICD-10CM # R23.0 Cyanosis

RESPIRATORY

Upper Airway
Choanal atresia.
Macroglossia.
Glossoptosis (secondary to micrognathia).
Laryngomalacia.
Laryngeal web or cyst.
Vascular anomalies (e.g., cystic hygromas, rings).
Subglottic stenosis (commonly secondary to intubation).
Foreign body.
Lower Airway
Pneumonia.
Bronchiolitis.
Pulmonary edema.
Atelectasis.
Bronchopulmonary dysplasia.

SYSTEMIC

Sepsis.
Trauma.
Poisons.

CARDIAC

Cyanotic congenital heart diseases.
Transposition of the great vessels (most common neonatal).
Tetralogy of Fallot.
Truncus arteriosus.
Tricuspid atresia.
Total anomalous pulmonary venous return.
Ebstein anomaly.
GI.
Gastroesophageal reflux.

NEUROLOGIC

Seizures.
Central hypoventilation syndrome (Ondine curse).
Spinal muscular atrophy type I (Werdnig-Hoffmann).
Botulism.
Congenital myopathies.

HEMATOLOGIC

Methemoglobinemia.

CYTOPENIAS, OLDER ADULTS[51]

ICD-10CM # D46.A Refractory cytopenia with multilineage dysplasia

Cytopenia of one or more lineages.
Hematologic neoplasm.
Vitamin B_{12} deficiency.
Autoimmune disorder.
Consumptive coagulopathy.
Systemic inflammation.
Alcohol.
Splenomegaly.
Thyroid dysfunction.
Human immunodeficiency virus.

DAYTIME SLEEPINESS

ICD-10CM # R53.82 Chronic fatigue, unspecified

Sleep deprivation.
Medication induced (e.g., benzodiazepines, beta-blockers, narcotics, sedative antidepressants, gabapentin).
Depression.
Obstructive sleep apnea.
Medical illness (e.g., severe anemia, hypothyroidism, COPD, hepatic failure, renal insufficiency, CHF, electrolyte disturbances).
Circadian rhythm abnormalities (e.g., jet lag, shift work sleep disorder).
Restless legs syndrome.
Posttrauma.
Narcolepsy.
Neurologic disorders (e.g., neurodegenerative disorders; parkinsonism; multiple sclerosis; lesions affecting thalamus, hypothalamus, or brain stem).

DEAFNESS, ACQUIRED

ICD-10CM #		
	H91.93	Unspecified hearing loss, bilateral
	H91.92	Unspecified hearing loss, left ear
	H91.91	Unspecified hearing loss, right ear
	H91.90	Unspecified hearing loss, unspecified ear
	H91.9	Unspecified hearing loss
	H91	Other and unspecified hearing loss
	H90.5	Unspecified sensorineural hearing loss
	H91.09	Ototoxic hearing loss, unspecified ear
	H90.2	Conductive hearing loss, unspecified
	H91.8X9	Other specified hearing loss, unspecified ear

COMMON CAUSES OF ACQUIRED DEAFNESS

Conductive Hearing Loss
Acute otitis media, otitis media with effusion, chronic otitis media.
Sensorineural Hearing Loss
Severe hypoxia.
Lassa fever.
Sepsis neonatorum.
Bacterial meningitis.
Viral infections (e.g., mumps).
Hyperbilirubinemia.
Noise-induced damage.
Autoimmune sensorineural hearing loss.
Presbycusis.
Head trauma.
Ménière's disease.
Scrub typhus.
Sudden idiopathic sensorineural hearing loss.
HIV/AIDS, tuberculosis.
Ototoxicity.
Tumors, hydatid cyst in the cerebellopontine angle.

DELAYED PASSAGE OF MECONIUM[41]

ICD-10CM # P76.0 Meconium plug syndrome

Ileal atresia.
Meconium ileus.
Functional immaturity of the colon.
Colon atresia.
Anorectal malformations.
Hirschsprung disease.
Megacystis-microcolon-intestinal hypoperistalsis syndrome.
Extrinsic compression of the distal bowel by a mass lesion.
Mesenteric cyst.
Enteric duplication cyst.
Paralytic ileus, sepsis, drugs, and metabolic upset.

DELIRIUM[63]

ICD-10CM #		
	R40.0	Somnolence
	R40.1	Stupor
	F05	Delirium due to known physiological condition

PHARMACOLOGIC AGENTS

Anxiolytics (benzodiazepines).
Antidepressants (e.g., amitriptyline, doxepin, imipramine).
Cardiovascular agents (e.g., methyldopa, digitalis, reserpine, propranolol, procainamide, captopril, disopyramide).
Antihistamine.
Cimetidine.
Corticosteroids.
Antineoplastics.
Drugs of abuse (alcohol, cannabis, amphetamines, cocaine, hallucinogens, opioids, sedative-hypnotics, phencyclidine).

METABOLIC DISORDERS

Hypercalcemia.
Hypercarbia.

Hypoglycemia.
Hyponatremia.
Hypoxia.

INFLAMMATORY DISORDERS

Sarcoidosis.
SLE.
Giant cell arteritis.

ORGAN FAILURE

Hepatic encephalopathy.
Uremia.

NEUROLOGIC DISORDERS

Alzheimer disease.
CVA.
Encephalitis (including HIV).
Encephalopathies.
Epilepsy.
Huntington disease.
Multiple sclerosis.
Neoplasms.
Normal-pressure hydrocephalus.
Parkinson disease.
Pick disease.
Wilson disease.

ENDOCRINE DISORDERS

Addison disease.
Cushing syndrome.
Panhypopituitarism.
Parathyroid disease.
Postpartum psychosis.
Recurrent menstrual psychosis.
Sydenham chorea.
Thyroid disease.

DEFICIENCY STATES

Niacin.
Thiamine, vitamin B_{12}, and folate.

DELIRIUM AND AGITATION, DRUG-INDUCED

ICD-10CM # F05.9 Delirium, unspecified

COMMONLY USED DRUGS ASSOCIATED WITH DELIRIUM AND AGITATION

Benzodiazepines.
Opiates (especially meperidine).
Anticholinergics.
Antihistamines.
H_2 blockers.
Antibiotics.
Corticosteroids.
Metoclopramide.

DELIRIUM, AGITATED[7]

ICD-10CM # F05 Delirium due to known physiological condition

Metabolic causes:
- Electrolyte abnormalities.
- Hypoglycemia.
- Hypoxia.
- Uremia/hyperammonemia.

Structural lesions of the CNS:
- Trauma.
- Stroke.
- Hemorrhage.
- Mass.

Endocrine disease:
- Thyrotoxicosis.

Infections:
- Bacterial/viral meningitis/encephalitis.

Toxicologic causes:
- Sympathomimetic/stimulants.
- Cocaine.
- Amphetamines and derivatives.
- Caffeine.
- Phencyclidine/ketamine.
- Anticholinergics.
- Serotonin syndrome.
- Sedative-hypnotic withdrawal.

Heatstroke.
Postictal state.

CNS, Central nervous system.

DELIRIUM, DIALYSIS PATIENT[63]

ICD-10CM # F05 Delirium due to known physiological condition
F06.8 Other specified mental disorders due to known physiological condition

STRUCTURAL

Cerebrovascular accident (particularly hemorrhage).
Subdural hematoma.
Intracerebral abscess.
Brain tumor.

METABOLIC

Disequilibrium syndrome.
Uremia.
Drug effects.
Meningitis.
Hypertensive encephalopathy.
Hypotension.
Postictal state.
Hypernatremia or hyponatremia.
Hypercalcemia.
Hypermagnesemia.
Hypoglycemia.
Severe hyperglycemia.
Hypoxemia.
Dialysis dementia.

DEMENTIA, ADOLESCENT PATIENT[56]

ICD-10CM # F03 Unspecified dementia
F03.90 Unspecified dementia without behavioral disturbance

CAUSES OF DEMENTIA IN ADOLESCENTS

Autoimmune or inflammatory diseases:
- Paraneoplastic syndromes, including NMDA antibody encephalitis.
- Vasculitis.

Cerebral and noncerebral neoplasms:
- Chemotherapy (intrathecal).
- Radiotherapy treatment.

Drug, inhalant, and alcohol abuse, including overdose.
Head trauma, including child abuse.
Infections:
- HIV-associated dementia.
- Variant Creutzfeldt–Jakob disease (vCJD).
- Subacute sclerosing panencephalitis (SSPE).

Metabolic abnormalities:
- Adrenoleukodystrophy.
- Wilson disease.

Neurodegenerative illnesses:
- Huntington disease.
- Metachromatic leukodystrophy.
- Other rare, usually genetically transmitted, illnesses.

DEMYELINATING DISEASES[102]

ICD-10CM # G37.9 Demyelinating disease of central nervous system, unspecified

MULTIPLE SCLEROSIS

Relapsing and chronic progressive forms.
Acute multiple sclerosis.
Neuromyelitis optica (Devic disease).

DIFFUSE CEREBRAL SCLEROSIS

Schilder encephalitis periaxialis diffusa.
Baló concentric sclerosis.

ACUTE DISSEMINATED ENCEPHALOMYELITIS

After measles, chickenpox, rubella, influenza, mumps.
After rabies or smallpox vaccination.

NECROTIZING HEMORRHAGIC ENCEPHALITIS

Hemorrhagic leukoencephalitis.

LEUKODYSTROPHIES

Krabbe globoid leukodystrophy.
Metachromatic leukodystrophy.
Adrenoleukodystrophy.
Adrenomyeloneuropathy.
Pelizaeus-Merzbacher leukodystrophy.
Canavan disease.
Alexander disease.

DEXTROCARDIA[14]

ICD-10CM # Q24.0 Dextrocardia

TYPES OF DEXTROCARDIA

Primary Dextrocardia

Dextroversion: The left ventricle is to the left of the right ventricle, as it is in the normal heart.
Mirror-image dextrocardia: The left ventricle is to the right of the right ventricle.

Secondary Dextrocardia

Skeletal causes:
- Scoliosis.
- Sternal or rib deformity.

Lung causes:
- Pneumonectomy.
- Collapse.
- Pneumothorax.
- Unilateral airtrapping.

Pleural causes:
- Diaphragmatic hernia with displacement of the gut into left thorax.

DIAPER DERMATITIS[74]

ICD-10CM #	L22	Diaper dermatitis

DIFFERENTIAL DIAGNOSIS OF DIAPER DERMATITIS

Chafing dermatitis.
Irritant contact dermatitis.
Diaper candidiasis.
Seborrheic dermatitis.
Psoriasis.
Intertrigo.
Jacquet dermatitis.
Perianal pseudoverrucous papules and nodules.
Miliaria.
Folliculitis.
Impetigo.
Scabies.
Nutritional deficiency (i.e., acrodermatitis enteropathica, cystic fibrosis, biotin deficiency).
Allergic contact dermatitis.
Atopic dermatitis.
Granuloma gluteale infantum.
Langerhans cell histiocytosis.
Burns.
Child abuse.
Epidermolysis bullosa.
Congenital syphilis.
Varicella/herpes.
Tinea cruris.
Chronic bullous dermatosis of childhood.
Bullous mastocytosis.

DIAPHRAGM ELEVATION, BILATERAL, SYMMETRICAL[41]

ICD-10CM #	J98.6	Disorders of diaphragm

CAUSES OF BILATERAL SYMMETRICAL ELEVATION OF THE DIAPHRAGM

Supine position.
Poor inspiration.
Obesity.
Pregnancy.
Abdominal distention (ascites, intestinal obstruction, abdominal mass).
Diffuse pulmonary fibrosis.
Lymphangitis carcinomatosa.
Disseminated lupus erythematosus.
Bilateral basal pulmonary emboli.
Painful conditions (after abdominal surgery).
Bilateral diaphragmatic paralysis.

DIAPHRAGM ELEVATION, UNILATERAL[41]

ICD-10CM #	J98.6	Disorders of diaphragm

CAUSES OF UNILATERAL ELEVATION OF THE DIAPHRAGM

Posture—lateral decubitus position (dependent side).
Gaseous distention of stomach or colon.
Dorsal scoliosis.
Pulmonary hypoplasia.
Pulmonary collapse.
Phrenic nerve palsy.
Eventration.
Pneumonia or pleurisy.
Pulmonary thromboembolism.
Rib fracture and other painful conditions.
Subphrenic infection.
Subphrenic mass.

DIARRHEA, ACUTE WATERY AND BLOODY[95]

ICD-10CM #	Code	Description
	K52.2	Allergic and dietetic gastroenteritis and colitis
	K52.89	Other specified noninfective gastroenteritis and colitis
	R19.7	Diarrhea, unspecified

ACUTE WATERY DIARRHEA

GI infections:
- Protozoal (e.g., *Giardia*).
- Bacterial (e.g., enterotoxigenic *Escherichia coli*, cholera).
- Viral (e.g., rotavirus, Norwalk virus).

Drugs.
Toxins.
Dietary constituents (e.g., lactose intolerance).
Onset of chronic diarrheal illness.

ACUTE BLOODY DIARRHEA

Infectious colitis:
- Confluent proctocolitis (e.g., *Shigella, Campylobacter, Salmonella, Entamoeba histolytica*).
- Segmental colitis (e.g., *Campylobacter, Salmonella*, enteroinvasive *E. coli, Aeromonas, E. histolytica*).
- Drug-induced colitis (e.g., NSAIDs).
- Inflammatory bowel disease.
- Ischemic colitis (usually elderly patient with underlying heart disease or arrhythmias).
- Antibiotic-associated colitis.

DIARRHEA, CRITICALLY ILL PATIENT[87]

ICD-10CM #	R19.7	Diarrhea, unspecified

COMMON CAUSES OF DIARRHEA IN CRITICALLY ILL PATIENTS

Medication
Antibiotics.
H2-recepter antagonists, antacids.
Drugs: significant amounts of sorbitol, magnesium, or hypertonic medications.
Laxative use (unintended).

Gastrointestinal Dysfunction
Gastric or small bowel resection.
Inflammatory bowel disease.
Pancreatic insufficiency.
Radiation enteritis.
Sprue.
Protein-losing gastroenteropathies.
Bowel impaction (paradoxic).

Malnutrition
Hypoproteinemia.
Micronutrient deficiencies.

Enteral Nutrition–Associated
Excessive feeding rate, concentration, volume, or osmolality.
Adaptation in malnourished patients or those whose GI tract has not been used recently.
Intolerance or allergy to feeding formula.

Infection
Clostridium difficile enterocolitis.
Opportunistic GI infection.
Significant amounts of contaminated feeding formula.
Altered GI flora.

Endocrine Dysfunction
Diabetes mellitus.
Hyperthyroidism.
Hypocortisolism.

DIARRHEA, INFECTIOUS[7]

ICD-10CM #	A09	Infectious gastroenteritis and colitis, unspecified

ETIOLOGIC AGENTS OF INFECTIOUS DIARRHEA

Viral (60% of Cases)
Astrovirus.
Calicivirus.
Coronavirus.
Cytomegalovirus.[22]
Enteric adenovirus.
Hepatitis A through G.
Herpes simplex virus.
HIV enteropathy.
Norwalk-like agents.
Pararotavirus.
Norwalk virus.
Picornavirus.
Rotavirus.
Small round viruses.

Bacterial (20% of Cases)

Invasive
Aeromonas spp.
Campylobacter spp.
Clostridium difficile.
Enteroinvasive *E. coli.*
Mycobacterium spp.
Plesiomonas shigelloides.
Salmonella spp.
Shigella spp.
Vibrio fluvialis.
Vibrio parahaemolyticus.
Vibrio vulnificus.
Yersinia enterocolitica.
Yersinia pseudotuberculosis.

Toxigenic
Food poisoning with preformed toxins:
- *Bacillus cereus.*

[22] All of these disorders may cause localized low back pain.

Clostridium botulinum.
Staphylococcus aureus.
Toxin formation after colonization:
Aeromonas hydrophila.
Clostridium perfringens.
Enterohemorrhagic *E. coli* 0157:H7.
Enterotoxigenic *E. coli.*
Klebsiella pneumoniae.
Shigella spp.
Vibrio cholerae.
Other bacteria
Parasitic (5% of Cases)
Protozoa
Balantidium coli.
Blastocystis hominis.
Cryptosporidium.
Cyclospora.
Dientamoeba fragilis.
Entamoeba histolytica.
Entamoeba polecki.
Enteromonas hominis.
Giardia lamblia.
Isospora belli.
Microsporidia.
Sarcocystis hominis.
Helminths
Angiostrongylus costaricense.
Anisakiasis.
Ascaris lumbricoides.
Diphyllobothrium latum.
Enterobius vermicularis.
Hookworms.
Schistosoma spp.
Strongyloides stercoralis.
Taenia spp.
Trichinella spiralis.
Trichuris trichiura.

DIARRHEA, NONINFECTIOUS[7]

ICD-10CM # K59.1 Functional diarrhea

CAUSES OF NONINFECTIOUS DIARRHEA

Toxins
Drugs
ACE inhibitors.
Alprazolam.
Antacids (Mg).
Antibiotics.
Antidepressants.
Antiepileptic drugs.
Antihypertensives.
Antiparkinson drugs.
Beta-blockers.
Caffeine.
Cardiac antiarrhythmics.
Chemotherapy agents.
Cholesterol-lowering drugs.
Cholinergic agents.
Cholinesterase inhibitors.
Colchicine.
Digitalis.
Diuretics.
Flurouracil.
Fluoxetine.
Histamine H_2-receptor antagonists.
Hydralazine.
Lactulose.
Laxatives/cathartics.
Levodopa.
Lithium.
NSAIDs.
Neomycin.
Podophyllin.
Procainamide.
Prostaglandins.
Quinidine.
Ricinoleic acid.
Theophylline.
Thyroid hormone.
Valproic acid.
Dietetic foods
Mannitol.
Sorbitol.
Xylitol.
Fish-associated toxins
Amnestic shellfish poisoning.
Ciguatera.
Echinoderms.
Neurotoxic shellfish poisoning.
Paralytic shellfish poisoning.
Scombroid.
Tetroton.
Plant-associated toxins
Herbal preparations.
Horse chestnut.
Mushrooms—*Amanita* spp.
Nicotine.
Other plant toxins:
Pesticides—organophosphates.
Pokeweed.
Rhubarb.
Miscellaneous:
Allergic reactions.
Carbon monoxide poisoning.
Ethanol.
Heavy metals.
Monosodium glutamate (MSG).
Opiate withdrawal.
Gastrointestinal Pathology
Appendicitis.
Autonomic dysfunction.
Bile acid malabsorption.
Blind loop.
Bowel obstruction.
Celiac disease.
Cirrhosis.
Defects in amino acid transport.
Diverticular disease.
Familial dysautonomia.
Fecal impaction.
Fecal incontinence.
GI bleed.
GI cancer.
Hirschsprung disease.
Inflammatory bowel disease (ulcerative colitis, Crohn disease).
Intussusception.
Irritable bowel syndrome.
Ischemic bowel.
Lactose/fructose intolerance.
Malabsorption syndromes.
Malrotation.
Postsurgical.
Postvagotomy.
Radiation therapy.
Short gut syndrome.
Small bowel resection.
Strictures.
Toxic megacolon.
Tropical sprue.
Volvulus.
Whipple disease.
Endocrine Related
Carcinoid syndrome (serotonin).
Hormonal hypersecretion.
Hyperthyroidism (thyroid hormone).
Medullary carcinoma of the thyroid (calcitonin).
Pancreatic cholera (VIP).
Somatostatinoma (somatostatin).
Systemic mastocytosis (histamine).
Zollinger-Ellison syndrome (gastrin).
Endocrine pathology
Adrenal insufficiency.
Diabetes enteropathy.
Hypoparathyroidism.
Pancreatic insufficiency.
Systemic Illness/Other
Alcoholism.
Amyloidosis.
Connective tissue disease.
Cystic fibrosis.
Ectopic pregnancy.
Hemolytic-uremic syndrome.
Henoch-Schönlein purpura.
Lymphoma.
Otitis media—infants.
Pelvic inflammatory disease.
Pneumonia/sepsis.
Pyelonephritis.
Scleroderma/SLE.
Severe malnutrition.
Stevens-Johnson syndrome.
Toxic shock syndrome.
Wilson disease.
Miscellaneous:
Factitious diarrhea.
Runner's diarrhea.

ACE, Angiotensin-converting enzyme; *GI,* gastrointestinal; *NSAIDs,* nonsteroidal antiinflammatory drugs; *SLE,* systemic lupus erythematosus; *VIP,* vasoactive intestinal polypeptide.

DIARRHEA IN PATIENTS WITH AIDS[30]

ICD-10CM # R19.7 Diarrhea, unspecified

PROTOZOA

*Microsporidium.**
Cryptosporidium spp.*
Isospora belli.
Toxoplasma spp.
Giardia lamblia.
Entamoeba histolytica.
Leishmania donovani.
Blastocystis hominis.
Cyclospora spp.
Pneumocystis jiroveci.

BACTERIA

Clostridium difficile.
Salmonella spp.

*More frequent cause.

Shigella spp.
Campylobacter jejuni
Mycobacterium avium complex.
Mycobacterium tuberculosis.
SIBO.
Vibrio spp.

VIRUSES
CMV.
HSV.
Adenoviruses.
Rotavirus spp.
Norovirus.
HIV?

FUNGI
Histoplasmosis.
Coccidioidomycosis.
Cryptococcosis.
Candidiasis.
Penicillium marneffei.

NEOPLASMS
Lymphoma.
Kaposi sarcoma.

IDIOPATHIC
"AIDS enteropathy."

DRUG INDUCED
HIV protease inhibitors.

PANCREATIC DISEASE
Pancreatic insufficiency.
Chronic pancreatitis.
Infectious pancreatitis (CMV, MAC).
Drug-induced pancreatitis (e.g., pentamidine).

CMV, Cytomegalovirus.

DIARRHEA, PEDIATRIC PATIENT[59]

ICD-10CM # R19.7 Diarrhea, unspecified

Acute
Common
Gastroenteritis (viral > bacterial > protozoal).
Systemic infection.
Antibiotic associated.
Overfeeding.
Rare
Primary disaccharidase deficiency.
Hirschsprung toxic colitis.
Adrenogenital syndrome.
Neonatal opiate withdrawal.
Chronic
Common
Postinfectious secondary lactase deficiency.
Cow's milk or soy protein intolerance (allergy).
Chronic nonspecific diarrhea of infancy.
Excessive fruit juice (sorbitol) ingestion.
Celiac disease.
Cystic fibrosis.
AIDS enteropathy.
Rare:
Primary immune defects.
Autoimmune enteropathy.
IPEX and IPEX-like syndromes.
Glucose-galactose malabsorption.
Microvillus inclusion disease (microvillus atrophy).
Congenital transport defects (chloride, sodium).
Primary bile acid malabsorption.
Factitious syndrome by proxy.
Hirschsprung disease.
Shwachman syndrome.
Secretory tumors.
Acrodermatitis enteropathica.
Lymphangiectasia.
Abetalipoproteinemia.
Eosinophilic gastroenteritis.
Short bowel syndrome.

CHILD
Acute
Common
Gastroenteritis (viral > bacterial > protozoal).
Food poisoning.
Systemic infection.
Antibiotic associated.
Rare
Toxic ingestion.
Hemolytic uremic syndrome.
Intussusception.
Chronic
Common
Postinfectious secondary. lactase deficiency.
Irritable bowel syndrome.
Celiac disease.
Cystic fibrosis.
Lactose intolerance.
Excessive fruit juice (sorbitol) ingestion.
Giardiasis.
Inflammatory bowel disease.
AIDS enteropathy.
Rare
Primary and acquired immune defects.
Secretory tumors.
Pseudoobstruction.
Sucrase-isomaltase deficiency.
Eosinophilic gastroenteritis.
Secretory tumors.

ADOLESCENT
Acute
Common
Gastroenteritis (viral > bacterial > protozoal).
Food poisoning.
Antibiotic associated.
Rare
Hyperthyroidism.
Appendicitis.
Chronic
Common
Irritable bowel syndrome.
Inflammatory bowel disease.
Lactose intolerance.
Giardiasis.
Laxative abuse (anorexia nervosa).
Constipation with encopresis.
Rare
Secretory tumor.
Primary bowel tumor.
Parasitic infections and venereal diseases.
Appendiceal abscess.
Addison disease.

IPEX, Immunodysregulation polyendocrinopathy enteropathy X-linked.

DIARRHEA, TUBE-FED PATIENT[36]

ICD-10CM # K91.89 Other postprocedural complications and disorders of digestive system

COMMON CAUSES UNRELATED TO TUBE FEEDING
Elixir medications containing sorbitol.
Magnesium-containing antacids.
Antibiotic-induced sterile gut.
Pseudomembranous colitis.

POSSIBLE CAUSES RELATED TO TUBE FEEDING
Inadequate fiber to form stool bulk.
High fat content of formula (in the presence of fat malabsorption syndrome).
Bacterial contamination of enteral products and delivery systems (causal association with diarrhea not documented).
Rapid advancement in rate (after the GI tract is unused for prolonged periods).

UNLIKELY CAUSES RELATED TO TUBE FEEDING
Formula hyperosmolality (proven not to be the cause of diarrhea).
Lactose (absent from nearly all enteral feeding formulas).

DIFFUSE PARENCHYMAL LUNG DISEASE, DRUG-INDUCED[101]

ICD-10CM # J84.89 Other specified interstitial pulmonary diseases

CYTOTOXIC CHEMOTHERAPY
Bleomycin.
Busulfan.
Cyclophosphamide.
Gemcitabine.
Nitrosoureas.
Taxanes (e.g., paclitaxel, docetaxel).

ANTIMETABOLITES
Methotrexate.

TARGETED BIOLOGIC AGENTS
Tumor necrosis factor (TNF)-α inhibitors or soluble receptors:
- Infliximab.
- Adalimumab.
- Certolizumab pegol.
- Etanercept.

Tyrosine kinase inhibitors:
- Afatinib.
- Erlotinib.
- Gefitinib.
- Idelalisib.
- Imatinib.
- Osimertinib.
- Trametinib.

Checkpoint inhibitors (antibodies against PD-1, PD-1 ligand, or CTLA-4):
- Ipilimumab.
- Nivolumab.
- Pembrolizumab.

Inhibitors of anaplastic lymphoma kinase (ALK):
- Alectinib.
- Ceritinib.
- Crizotinib.

MISCELLANEOUS

Trastuzumab (monoclonal antibody against HER2).
Rituximab (monoclonal antibody against CD20).
Inhibitors of mechanistic target of rapamycin (mTOR, e.g., everolimus).

MISCELLANEOUS OTHER DRUGS

Nitrofurantoin.
Amiodarone.

DRUG-INDUCED SYNDROMES

Drug-induced lupus (e.g., procainamide, hydralazine).
Drug-induced pulmonary infiltrates with eosinophilia (e.g., sulfa-containing drugs).

DIPLOPIA, BINOCULAR

ICD-10CM # H53.2 Diplopia

Cranial nerve palsy (3rd, 4th, 6th).
Thyroid eye disease.
Myasthenia gravis.
Decompensated strabismus.
Orbital trauma with blowout fracture.
Orbital pseudotumor.
Cavernous sinus thrombosis.

DIPLOPIA, MONOCULAR

ICD-10CM # H53.2 Diplopia

Postoperative corrected long-standing tropia.
Defective contact lenses.
Poorly fitting bifocals.
Trauma to iris.
Corneal disorder (e.g., dry eye, astigmatism).
Cataracts.
Lens subluxation.
Nystagmus.
Eyelid twitching.
Foreign body in aqueous or vitreous media.
Migraine.
Lesions of occipital cortex.
Psychogenic.

DIPLOPIA, VERTICAL

ICD-10CM # H53.2 Diplopia

Myasthenia.
Superior oblique palsy.
Myositis or pseudotumor with orbital involvement.
Lymphoma or metastases affecting the orbits.
Brain stem or cerebellar lesions.
Hydrocephalus.
Third nerve palsy.
Botulism.
Wernicke encephalopathy.
Dysthyroid orbitopathy (muscle infiltration).

DIZZINESS

ICD-10CM # R42 Dizziness and giddiness

Viral syndrome.
Anxiety, hyperventilation.
Benign positional paroxysmal vertigo.
Medications (e.g., sedatives, antihypertensives, analgesics).
Withdrawal from medications (e.g., benzodiazepines, SSRIs).
Alcohol or drug abuse.
Postural hypotension.
Hypoglycemia, hyperglycemia.
Hematologic disorders (e.g., anemia, polycythemia, leukemia).
Head trauma.
Menière disease.
Vertebrobasilar ischemia.
Cervical osteoarthritis.
Cardiac abnormalities (arrhythmias, cardiomyopathy, CHF, pericarditis).
Multiple sclerosis.
Peripheral vestibulopathy.
Air or sea travel.
Electrolyte abnormalities.
Eye problems (cornea, lens, retina).
Migraine.
Brain stem infarct.
Autonomic neuropathy.
Chronic otomastoiditis.
Complex partial seizures.
Ramsey Hunt syndrome.
Arteritis.
Syncope and presyncope.
Perilymph fistula.
Cerebellopontine tumor.
Hepatic or renal disease.

DRUG-INDUCED LUPUS[47]

ICD-10CM # M32.0 Drug-induced lupus

DRY EYE

ICD-10CM # H04.129 Dry eye syndrome of unspecified lacrimal gland

Contacts.
Medications (antihistamines, clonidine, beta-blockers, ibuprofen, scopolamine).
Keratoconjunctivitis sicca.
Trauma.
Environmental causes (air conditioning in patient with contacts).

DYSENTERY AND INFLAMMATORY ENTEROCOLITIS[10]

ICD-10CM # Varies with specific diagnosis

DIFFERENTIAL DIAGNOSIS OF ACUTE BACTERIAL DYSENTERY AND INFLAMMATORY ENTEROCOLITIS

Specific Infectious Processes

Bacillary dysentery (*Shigella dysenteriae, Shigella flexneri, Shigella sonnei, Shigella boydii;* invasive *Escherichia coli*).
Campylobacteriosis (*Campylobacter jejuni*).
Amebic dysentery (*Entamoeba histolytica*).
Ciliary dysentery (*Balantidium coli*).
Vibriosis (*Vibrio parahaemolyticus*).
Salmonellosis (*Salmonella typhimurium*).
Typhoid fever (*Salmonella typhi*).
Enteric fever (*Salmonella choleraesuis, Salmonella paratyphi*).
Yersiniosis (*Yersinia enterocolitica*).

Proctitis

Gonococcal (*Neisseria gonorrhoeae*).
Herpetic (herpes simplex virus).
Chlamydial (*Chlamydia trachomatis*).
Syphilitic (*Treponema pallidum*).

Other Syndromes

Necrotizing enterocolitis of the newborn.
Enteritis necroticans.
Pseudomembranous enterocolitis or *Clostridium difficile* colitis without overt pseudomembranes (*C. difficile*).
Diverticulitis.
Typhlitis.

Chronic Inflammatory Processes

Enteropathogenic and enteroaggregative *E. coli.*
Syphilis.
GI tuberculosis.
GI mycosis (including *Basidiobolus ranarum*).
Parasitic enteritis.

Syndromes without Known Infectious Cause

Idiopathic ulcerative colitis.
Crohn disease.
Radiation enteritis.
Ischemic colitis.
Allergic enteritis.
Brainerd diarrhea.

DYSLIPOPROTEINEMIAS, SECONDARY CAUSES[104]

ICD-10CM # E78.4 Other hyperlipidemia

Cause	Disorder
Metabolic	Diabetes. Lipodystrophy. Glycogen storage disorders.
Renal	Chronic renal failure. Glomerulonephritis with nephritic syndrome.
Hepatic	Cirrhosis. Biliary obstruction. Porphyria. Primary biliary cirrhosis (with secondary LCAT deficiency).
Hormonal	Estrogens. Progesterones. Growth hormone. Thyroid disorders (hypothyroidism). Corticosteroids.
Lifestyle	Physical inactivity. Obesity. Diet rich in fats, saturated fats. Alcohol intake. Smoking.
Medications	Retinoic acid derivatives. Glucocorticoids. Exogenous estrogens. Thiazide diuretics. Beta-adrenergic blockers (selective). Testosterone and other anabolizing steroids. Immunosuppressive medications (cyclosporine). Antiviral medications (HIV protease inhibitors). Antischizophrenic medications.

HIV, Human immunodeficiency virus; *LCAT,* lecithin-cholesterol acyltransferase.

DYSPAREUNIA[28]

ICD-10CM #	N94.1	Dyspareunia
	N44.8	Other noninflammatory disorders of the testis
	N50.8	Other specified disorders of male genital organs
	N53.12	Painful ejaculation
	F52.6	Dyspareunia not due to a substance or known physiological condition

INTROITAL

Vaginismus.
Intact or rigid hymen.
Clitoral problems.
Vulvovaginitis.
Vaginal atrophy: hypoestrogen.
Vulvar dystrophy.
Bartholin or Skene gland infection.
Inadequate lubrication.
Operative scarring.

MIDVAGINAL

Urethritis.
Trigonitis.
Cystitis.
Short vagina.
Operative scarring.
Inadequate lubrication.

DEEP

Endometriosis.
Pelvic infection.
Uterine retroversion.
Ovarian pathology.
GI.
Orthopedic.
Abnormal penile size or shape.

DYSPEPSIA AND PYROSIS, DIFFERENTIAL DIAGNOSIS DURING PREGNANCY[34]

ICD-10CM #	K30	Dyspepsia, atonic
	F45.3	Dyspepsia, psychogenic

DIFFERENTIAL DIAGNOSIS OF DYSPEPSIA OR PYROSIS DURING PREGNANCY

Gastroesophageal reflux disease.
Peptic ulcer disease.
Nausea and vomiting of pregnancy.
Hyperemesis gravidarum.
Pancreatitis.
Biliary colic.
Acute cholecystitis.
Viral hepatitis.
Appendicitis.
Acute fatty liver of pregnancy (in late pregnancy).
Irritable bowel syndrome/nonulcer dyspepsia.

DYSPHAGIA

ICD-10CM #	R13.10	Dysphagia, unspecified

Esophageal obstruction: neoplasm, foreign body, achalasia, stricture, spasm, esophageal web, diverticulum, Schatzki ring.
Peptic esophagitis with stricture, Barrett stricture.
External esophageal compression: neoplasms (thyroid neoplasm, lymphoma, mediastinal tumors), thyroid enlargement, aortic aneurysm, vertebral spurs, aberrant right subclavian artery (dysphagia lusoria).
Hiatal hernia, GERD.
Oropharyngeal lesions: pharyngitis, glossitis, stomatitis, neoplasms.
Hysteria: globus hystericus.
Neurologic and/or neuromuscular disturbances: bulbar paralysis, myasthenia gravis, ALS, multiple sclerosis, Parkinsonism, CVA, diabetic neuropathy.
Toxins: poisoning, botulism, tetanus, postdiphtheritic dysphagia.
Systemic diseases: scleroderma, amyloidosis, dermatomyositis.
Candida and herpes esophagitis.
Presbyesophagus.

DYSPHAGIA, ESOPHAGEAL[30]

ICD-10CM #	R13-14	Dysphagia, pharyngoesophageal phase

COMMON CAUSES OF ESOPHAGEAL DYSPHAGIA

Motility (Neuromuscular) Disorders

Primary

Achalasia.
Distal esophageal spasm.
Hypercontractile (jackhammer) esophagus.
Hypertensive LES.
Nutcracker (high-pressure) esophagus.
Other peristaltic abnormalities.[23]

Secondary

Chagas disease.
Reflux-related dysmotility.
Scleroderma and other rheumatologic disorders.

Structural (Mechanical) Disorders

Intrinsic

Carcinoma and benign tumors.
Diverticula.
Eosinophilic esophagitis.
Esophageal rings and webs (other than Schatzki ring).
Foreign body.
Lower esophageal (Schatzki) ring.
Medication-induced stricture.
Peptic stricture.

Extrinsic

Mediastinal mass.
Spinal osteophytes.
Vascular compression.

LES, Lower esophageal sphincter.
[23] Peristaltic abnormalities include absent peristalsis and weak peristalsis, as well as hypertensive peristalsis (nutcracker esophagus).

DYSPHAGIA, OROPHARYNGEAL[95]

ICD-10CM #	R13.12	Dysphagia, oropharyngeal phase

FUNCTIONAL DISORDERS

Central Nervous System

Stroke.
Head injury.
Parkinson disease.
Motor neuron disease.
Multiple sclerosis.
Tumor.
Drugs (e.g., phenothiazines).
Malformations (e.g., syrinx, Arnold–Chiari).

Neural

Motor neuron disease.
Myasthenia gravis.
Radiotherapy.
Poliomyelitis.
Familial dysautonomia.

Muscle

Autoimmune myopathy (polymyositis, dermatomyositis, systemic lupus erythematosus).
Thyrotoxic myopathy.
Guillain-Barré motor neuropathy.
Muscular dystrophies.

STRUCTURAL DISORDERS

Head/neck surgery.
Stricture.
Radiotherapy.
Tumor.
Pharyngeal pouch.
Web.
Extrinsic (e.g., osteophytes).

MISCELLANEOUS

Xerostomia.

DYSPNEA

ICD-10CM #	R06.9	Unspecified abnormalities of breathing

Upper airway obstruction: trauma, neoplasm, epiglottitis, laryngeal edema, tongue retraction, laryngospasm, abductor paralysis of vocal cords, aspiration of foreign body.
Lower airway obstruction: neoplasm, COPD, asthma, aspiration of foreign body.
Pulmonary infection: pneumonia, abscess, empyema, TB, bronchiectasis.
Pulmonary hypertension.
Pulmonary embolism/infarction.
Parenchymal lung disease.
Pulmonary vascular congestion.
Cardiac disease: ASHD, valvular lesions, cardiac dysrhythmias, cardiomyopathy, pericardial effusion, cardiac shunts.
Space-occupying lesions: neoplasm, large hiatal hernia, pleural effusions.
Disease of chest wall: severe kyphoscoliosis, fractured ribs, sternal compression, morbid obesity.

Neurologic dysfunction: Guillain-Barré syndrome, botulism, polio, spinal cord injury.
Interstitial pulmonary disease: sarcoidosis, collagen vascular diseases, DIP, Hamman-Rich pneumonitis, etc.
Pneumoconioses: silicosis, berylliosis, etc.
Mesothelioma.
Pneumothorax, hemothorax, pleural effusion.
Inhalation of toxins.
Cholinergic drug intoxication.
Carcinoid syndrome.
Hematologic: anemia, polycythemia, hemoglobinopathies.
Thyrotoxicosis, myxedema.
Diaphragmatic compression caused by abdominal distention, subphrenic abscess, ascites.
Lung resection.
Metabolic abnormalities: uremia, hepatic coma, DKA.
Sepsis.
Atelectasis.
Psychoneurosis.
Diaphragmatic paralysis.
Pregnancy.

DYSTONIA, PEDIATRIC PATIENT[93]

ICD-10CM #	G24.9	Dystonia, unspecified
	G24.2	Idiopathic nonfamilial dystonia
	G24.1	Genetic torsion dystonia

CAUSES OF DYSTONIA IN CHILDHOOD

Static Injury/Structural Disorders

Cerebral palsy.
Hypoxic-ischemic injury.
Kernicterus.
Head trauma.
Encephalitis.
Tumors.
Stroke in the basal ganglia (which may be due to vascular abnormalities or varicella).
Congenital malformations affecting basal ganglia.

Hereditary/Degenerative Disorders

DYT1 (autosomal dominant, Torsin A).
DYT2 (autosomal-recessive, Hippocalcin).
DYT4 (autosomal dominant, β-tubulin 4a).
DYT5 (autosomal dominant, GTP cyclohydrolase 1).
DYT6 (autosomal dominant, THAP1).
DYT8 (autosomal dominant, Myofibrillogenesis regulator 1).
DYT9 (autosomal dominant, GLUT1).
DYT10 (autosomal dominant, PRRT2).
DYT11 (autosomal dominant [maternal imprinting], ε-Sarcoglycan).
DYT12 (autosomal dominant, Na^+/K^+ATPase α3 subunit).
DYT15 (autosomal dominant, unknown).
DYT16 (autosomal recessive, Protein kinase activator PRKRA).
Pantothenate kinase-associated neurodegeneration (PKAN; neuronal brain iron accumulation type 1, due to mutations in *PANK2*).
PLA2G6-associated neurodegeneration (PLAN).
Huntington disease (Westphal variant, IT15–4p16.3).
Spinocerebellar ataxias (SCAs, particularly SCA3/Machado-Joseph disease).
Striatal necrosis.
Leigh syndrome.
Neuroacanthocytosis.
HARP syndrome (hypoprebetalipoproteinemia, acanthocytosis, retinitis pigmentosa, and pallidal degeneration).
Tay-Sachs disease.
Sandhoff disease.
Niemann-Pick type C.

Metabolic Disease

Glutaric aciduria types 1 and 2.
Acyl-CoA dehydrogenase deficiencies.
Neurotransmitter disorders.
Mitochondrial disorders.
GM_1 gangliosidosis.
Lesch-Nyhan disease.
Wilson disease.
Vitamin E deficiency.
Methylmalonic aciduria.
Tyrosinemia.

Drugs/Toxins

Neuroleptic and neuroleptic-like antiemetic medications (haloperidol, chlorpromazine, olanzapine, risperidone, prochlorperazine).
Calcium channel blockers.
Stimulants (amphetamine, cocaine, ergot alkaloids).
Anticonvulsants (carbamazepine, phenytoin).
Thallium.
Manganese.
Carbon monoxide.
Ethylene glycol.
Cyanide.
Methanol.

Paroxysmal Disorders

Paroxysmal kinesigenic dyskinesia (PKD).
Paroxysmal nonkinesigenic dyskinesia (PNKD).
Exercise-induced dyskinesia (PED).

DYSURIA

ICD-10CM #	R30.0	Dysuria
	R30.9	Painful micturition, unspecified

Urinary tract infection.
Estrogen deficiency (in postmenopausal female).
Vaginitis.
Genital infection (e.g., herpes, condyloma).
Interstitial cystitis.
Chemical irritation (e.g., deodorant aerosols, douches).
Meatal stenosis or stricture.
Reiter syndrome.
Bladder neoplasm.
GI etiology (diverticulitis, Crohn disease).
Impaired bladder or sphincter action.
Urethral carbuncle.
Chronic fibrosis posttrauma.
Radiation therapy.
Prostatitis.
Urethritis (gonococcal, *Chlamydia*).
Behçet syndrome.
Stevens-Johnson syndrome.

EARACHE[84]

ICD-10CM #	H92.09	Otalgia, unspecified ear

Otitis media.
Serous otitis media.
Eustachitis.
Otitis externa.
Otitic barotrauma.
Mastoiditis.
Foreign body.
Impacted cerumen.
Referred otalgia, as with TMJ dysfunction, dental problems, and tumors.

ECTOPIC ACTH SECRETION[36]

ICD-10CM #	E34.2	Ectopic hormone secretion, not elsewhere classified

Small cell carcinoma of lung.
Endocrine tumors of foregut origin.
- Thymic carcinoid.
- Islet cell tumor.
- Medullary carcinoid, thyroid.
- Bronchial carcinoid.

Pheochromocytoma.
Ovarian tumors.

EDEMA, CHILDREN[48]

ICD-10CM #	R60.0	Localized edema
	R60.1	Generalized edema
	R60.9	Edema, unspecified

CARDIOVASCULAR

Congestive heart failure.
Acute thrombi or emboli.
Vasculitis of many types.

RENAL

Nephrotic syndrome.
Glomerulonephritis of many types.
End-stage renal failure.

ENDOCRINE OR METABOLIC

Thyroid disease.
Starvation.
Hereditary angioedema.

IATROGENIC

Drugs (diuretics and steroids).
Water or salt overload.

HEMATOLOGIC

Hemolytic disease of the newborn.

GASTROINTESTINAL

Hepatic cirrhosis.
Protein-losing enteritis.
Lymphangiectasis.
Cystic fibrosis.
Celiac disease.
Enteritis of many types.

LYMPHATIC ABNORMALITIES

Congenital (gonadal dysgenesis).
Acquired.

EDEMA, GENERALIZED

ICD-10CM #	R60.0	Localized edema
	R60.1	Generalized edema
	R60.9	Edema, unspecified

Congestive heart failure (CHF).
Cirrhosis.
Nephrotic syndrome.
Pregnancy.
Idiopathic.
Acute nephritic syndrome.
Myxedema.
Medications (NSAIDs, estrogens, vasodilators).

EDEMA, LEG, UNILATERAL[63]

ICD-10CM #	R60.0	Localized edema
	R60.9	Edema, unspecified

WITH PAIN

DVT.
Postphlebitic syndrome.
Popliteal cyst rupture.
Gastrocnemius rupture.
Cellulitis.
Psoas or other abscess.

WITHOUT PAIN

DVT.
Postphlebitic syndrome.
Other venous insufficiency (after saphenous vein harvest, varicosities).
Lymphatic obstruction/lymphedema (carcinoma, lymphoma, sarcoidosis, filariasis, retroperitoneal fibrosis).

EDEMA OF LOWER EXTREMITIES

ICD-10CM #	R60.0	Localized edema
	R60.9	Edema, unspecified

CHF (right-sided).
Hepatic cirrhosis.
Nephrosis.
Myxedema.
Lymphedema.
Pregnancy.
Abdominal mass: neoplasm, cyst.
Venous compression from abdominal aneurysm.
Varicose veins.
Bilateral cellulitis.
Bilateral thrombophlebitis.
Vena cava thrombosis, venous thrombosis.
Retroperitoneal fibrosis.

EJECTION SOUND OR CLICK

ICD-10CM #	R01.2	Other cardiac sounds

Aortic regurgitation.
Aortic root dilatation.
Systemic hypertension.
Chronic pulmonary hypertension.
Tetralogy of Fallot.
Atrial septal defect.
Pulmonary valve stenosis.
Aortic aneurysm.

ELBOW PAIN

ICD-10CM #	M25.529	Pain in unspecified elbow

Trauma.
Infection.
Inflammatory arthritis.
Lateral or medial epicondylitis.
Entrapment neuropathy.
Olecranon bursitis.
Osteoarthritis.
Gout.
Cervical disease (referred pain).
Shoulder disease (referred pain).
Partial subluxation.
Synovial osteochondromatosis.
Loose body.

ELEVATED HEMIDIAPHRAGM

ICD-10CM #	J98.6	Disorders of diaphragm
	Q79.0	Congenital diaphragmatic hernia
	Q79.1	Other congenital malformations of diaphragm

Neoplasm (bronchogenic carcinoma, mediastinal neoplasm, intrahepatic lesion).
Substernal thyroid.
Infectious process (pneumonia, empyema, TB, subphrenic abscess, hepatic abscess).
Atelectasis.
Idiopathic.
Eventration.
Phrenic nerve dysfunction (myelitis, myotonia, herpes zoster).
Trauma to phrenic nerve or diaphragm (e.g., surgery).
Aortic aneurysm.
Intraabdominal mass.
Pulmonary infarction.
Pleurisy.
Radiation therapy.
Rib fracture.

EMBOLI, ARTERIAL[63]

ICD-10CM #	I74.3	Embolism and thrombosis of arteries of the lower extremities
	I74.2	Embolism and thrombosis of arteries of the upper extremities

Myocardial infarction with mural thrombi.
Atrial fibrillation.
Cardiomyopathies.
Prosthetic heart valves.
CHF.
Endocarditis.
Left ventricular aneurysm.
Left atrial myxoma.
Sick sinus syndrome.
Paradoxical embolus from venous thrombosis.
Aneurysms of large blood vessels.
Atheromatous ulcers of large blood vessels.

EMESIS, PEDIATRIC AGE[48]

ICD-10CM #	R11.10	Vomiting, unspecified
	R11.11	Vomiting without nausea
	R11.12	Projectile vomiting

INFANCY

Gastrointestinal Tract

Congenital

Regurgitation: chalasia, gastroesophageal reflux.
Atresia: stenosis (tracheoesophageal fistula, prepyloric diaphragm, intestinal atresia).
Duplication.
Volvulus (errors in rotation and fixation, Meckel diverticulum).
Congenital bands.
Hirschsprung disease.
Meconium ileus (cystic fibrosis), meconium plug.

Acquired

Acute infectious gastroenteritis, food poisoning (staphylococcal, clostridial).
Pyloric stenosis.
Gastritis, duodenitis.
Intussusception.
Incarcerated hernia—inguinal, internal secondary to old adhesions.
Cow's milk protein intolerance, food allergy, eosinophilic gastroenteritis.
Disaccharidase deficiency.
Celiac disease—presents after introduction of gluten in diet; inherited risk.
Adynamic ileus—the mediator for many nongastrointestinal causes.
Neonatal necrotizing enterocolitis.
Chronic granulomatous disease with gastric outlet obstruction.

Nongastrointestinal Tract

Infectious: otitis, urinary tract infection, pneumonia, upper respiratory tract infection, sepsis, meningitis.
Metabolic: aminoaciduria and organic aciduria, galactosemia, fructosemia, adrenogenital syndrome, renal tubular acidosis, diabetic ketoacidosis, Reye syndrome.
CNS: trauma, tumor, infection, diencephalic syndrome, rumination, autonomic responses (pain, shock).
Medications: anticholinergics, aspirin, alcohol, idiosyncratic reaction (e.g., codeine).

CHILDHOOD

Gastrointestinal Tract

Peptic ulcer—vomiting is a common presentation in children younger than 6 yr old.
Trauma: duodenal hematoma, traumatic pancreatitis, perforated bowel.
Pancreatitis: mumps, trauma, cystic fibrosis, hyperparathyroidism, hyperlipidemia, organic acidemias.
Crohn disease.
Idiopathic intestinal pseudoobstruction.
Superior mesenteric artery syndrome.

Nongastrointestinal Tract

CNS: cyclic vomiting, migraine, anorexia nervosa, bulimia.

ENCEPHALOMYELITIS, NONVIRAL CAUSES[63]

ICD-10CM #	G04.81	Other encephalitis and encephalomyelitis

Subacute bacterial endocarditis.
Rocky Mountain spotted fever.
Typhus.
Ehrlichia.
Q fever.
Chlamydia.
Mycoplasma.
Legionella.
Brucellosis.
Listeria.
Whipple disease.
Cat-scratch disease.
Syphilis (meningovascular).
Relapsing fever.
Lyme disease.
Leptospirosis.
Nocardia.
Actinomycosis.
Tuberculosis.
Cryptococcus.
Histoplasma.
Toxoplasma.
Plasmodium falciparum.
Trypanosomiasis.
Behçet disease.
Vasculitis.
Carcinoma.
Drug reactions.

ENCEPHALOPATHY, HYPERTENSIVE[97]

ICD-10CM # Varies with specific diagnosis

Cerebral infarction.
Subarachnoid hemorrhage.
Intracerebral hemorrhage.
Subdural or epidural hematoma.
Brain tumor or other mass lesion.
Seizure disorder.
CNS vasculitis.
Encephalitis/meningitis.
Drug ingestion.
Drug withdrawal.

ENCEPHALOPATHY, METABOLIC[91]

ICD-10CM #	F10.27	Alcohol dependence with alcohol-induced persisting dementia
	K72.90	Hepatic failure, unspecified without coma
	K72.91	Hepatic failure, unspecified with coma
	G92	Toxic encephalopathy
	T56.0X1A	Toxic effect of lead and its compounds, accidental (unintentional), initial encounter
	T56.0X2A	Toxic effect of lead and its compounds, intentional self-harm, initial encounter

Substrate deficiency: hypoxia/ischemia, carbon monoxide poisoning, hypoglycemia.
Cofactor deficiency: thiamine, vitamin B_{12}, pyridoxine (INH administration).
Electrolyte disorders: hyponatremia, hypercalcemia, carbon dioxide narcosis, dialysis, hypermagnesemia, disequilibrium syndrome.
Endocrinopathies: DKA, hyperosmolar coma, hypothyroidism, hyperadrenocorticism, hyperparathyroidism.
Endogenous toxins: liver disease, uremia, porphyria.
Exogenous toxins: drug overdose (sedative/hypnotics, ethanol, narcotics, salicylates, tricyclic antidepressants), drug withdrawal, toxicity of therapeutic medications, industrial toxins (e.g., organophosphates, heavy metals), sepsis.
Heat stroke.
Epilepsy (postictal).

ENDOMETRIAL THICKENING[81]

ICD-10CM # Varies with specific diagnosis

CAUSES OF ENDOMETRIAL THICKENING

Early intrauterine pregnancy.
Incomplete abortion.
Ectopic pregnancy.
Retained products of conception.
Trophoblastic disease.
Endometritis.
Adhesions.
Hyperplasia.
Polyps.
Carcinoma.

ENTERIC FEVER[23]

ICD-10CM #	**A01.00**	Typhoid fever, unspecified
	A01.3	Paratyphoid fever
	R50.9	Fever, unspecified

Epstein-Barr infection.
Dengue.
Tuberculosis.
Brucellosis.
Bartonella henselae.
Leptospirosis.
Tularemia.
Ehrlichiosis.
Plague.
Typhus.
Malaria.
Disseminated histoplasmosis.

ENTHESOPATHY

ICD-10CM #	M46.00	Spinal enthesopathy, site unspecified

Viremia or bacteremia.
Ankylosing spondylitis.
Psoriatic arthritis.
Drug-induced (quinolones, etretinate).
Reactive arthritis.
DISH.
Reiter syndrome.

EOSINOPHILIA, DISEASE ASSOCIATIONS[62]

ICD-10CM #	D72.1	Eosinophilia
	NEC J82	Eosinophilia, pulmonary

DISEASES, SYNDROMES, AND CONDITIONS COMMONLY ASSOCIATED WITH PERIPHERAL BLOOD EOSINOPHILIA AND/OR TISSUE EOSINOPHILIA

Infectious Agents

Parasitic Infections

Tropical eosinophilia.
Visceral larval migrans (VLM, toxocariasis).
Helminth infections.
Filariasis (*Wuchereria bancrofti, Brugia malayi*).
Onchocerciasis.
Schistosomiasis.
Fascioliasis.
Paragonimiasis.
Strongyloidiasis.
Trichinosis.
Hookworm.
Ascariasis.
Echinococcosis/hydatid disease.

Fungal Infections

Coccidioidomycosis.
Cryptococcosis (CSF eosinophilia) in HIV.

Allergic Diseases

Asthma (atopic and intrinsic, nasal polyps, aspirin intolerance syndromes).
Bronchopulmonary aspergillosis.
Allergic rhinitis.
Urticarias (acute allergic and chronic idiopathic).
Atopic dermatitis.
Acute drug (hypersensitivity) reactions (interstitial nephritis, cholestatic hepatitis, exfoliative dermatitis).

Respiratory Tract Disorders

Hypersensitivity pneumonitis (rare).
Allergic bronchopulmonary aspergillosis.
Eosinophilic pneumonia.
Transient pulmonary infiltrates (Löeffler syndrome).
Prolonged pulmonary infiltrates with eosinophilia (PIE syndrome).
Tropical pulmonary eosinophilia (TPE).
Bronchiectasis.
Cystic fibrosis.

Endocrinologic Disorders

Addison disease.

Gastrointestinal Diseases

Inflammatory bowel disease (IBD).
Eosinophilic gastroenteritis, eosinophilic esophagitis (EE).
Allergic gastroenteritis (young children).
Celiac disease (when associated with EE).

Toxic Reactions to Ingested Agents
Eosinophil myalgia syndrome (L-tryptophan).
Toxic oil syndrome.
Reactions to Cytokine Therapies
IL-2 and IL-2 plus lymphokine activated killer (LAK) cells.
GM-CSF therapy.
Cutaneous Disorders
Atopic dermatitis.
Immunologic skin diseases.
Scabies.
Myiasis.
Chlamydial pneumonia of infancy.
Scarlet fever and pneumococcal pneumonia (convalescent phase).
Cat scratch disease.
Eosinophilic cellulitis (Wells syndrome).
Episodic angioedema with eosinophilia.
Chronic idiopathic urticaria.
Bullous pemphigoid.
Herpes gestationis.
Angioblastic lymphoid hyperplasia (Kimura disease).
Immunodeficiency Syndromes
Wiskott-Aldrich syndrome.
Selective IgA deficiency with atopy.
Hyper-IgE recurrent infection syndrome (Job syndrome).
Swiss-type and sex-linked combined immunodeficiency.
Nezelof syndrome.
Graft-versus-host-disease (GVHD).
Connective Tissue Diseases
Vasculitis/Collagen Vascular Disorders
- Hypersensitivity vasculitis.
- Allergic granulomatosis with angiitis (Churg-Strauss syndrome).
- Serum sickness.
- Eosinophilic fasciitis.
- Sjögren syndrome.
- Rheumatoid arthritis (severe).

Neoplastic, Myeloproliferative, and Lymphoproliferative Neoplasms and Syndromes
Neoplastic
- Ovarian carcinoma.
- Solid tumors (mucin-secreting, epithelial cell origin).

Chronic eosinophil leukemia.
Idiopathic hypereosinophilic syndromes (HES).
Systemic mastocytosis.
Myeloproliferative
- Chronic myelogenous leukemia (CML) acute myelogenous leukemia (AML) and myelodysplastic syndrome (MDS).
- Myelomonocytic leukemia with bone marrow eosinophilia (M4Eo, inversion 16).

Lymphoproliferative
- T-cell lymphocytic leukemia.
- Lymphomas (T cell, Hodgkin disease).
- Angioimmunoblastic lymphadenopathy.

Rare Causes
Chronic active hepatitis.
Chronic dialysis.
Acute pancreatitis.
Postirradiation.
Hypopituitarism.

EOSINOPHILIA, GI[30]

ICD-10CM # D72.1 Eosinophilia

CAUSES OF GI EOSINOPHILIA

GERD
Eosinophilic GI disorders:
- Eosinophilic esophagitis:
  - Connective tissue disease-associated eosinophilic esophagitis.
  - Familial eosinophilic esophagitis.
- Eosinophilic gastritis.
- Eosinophilic enteritis.
- Eosinophilic gastroenteritis.

Infections:
- Schistosomiasis.
- Anisakiasis.
- GI basidiobolomycosis.
- Toxocariasis.

Celiac disease.
Hypereosinophilic syndrome.
Drug hypersensitivity response.
IBD.
Transplant-associated eosinophilic enteritis.
Eosinophilic granulomatosis with polyangiitis.
Toxic injury.
Graft-versus-host disease.

EOSINOPHILIC LUNG DISEASE[41]

ICD-10CM # NEC J82 Eosinophilia, pulmonary

IDIOPATHIC

Simple pulmonary eosinophilia (Löffler syndrome).
Acute eosinophilic pneumonia.
Chronic eosinophilic pneumonia.
Hypereosinophilic syndrome.

DRUG-INDUCED

Aminosalicylic acid.
Para-aminosalicylic acid.
NSAIDs.
Captopril.
Cocaine.
Minocycline.
Nitrofurantoin.
Phenytoin.

INFECTION

Parasitic (ascariasis, paragonimiasis. tropical eosinophilia).
Fungal (aspergillus).
Bacterial (TB, atypical mycobacterial infection, brucella).
Viral (respiratory syncytial virus).

IMMUNOLOGIC DISEASES

Granulomatosis with polyangiitis.
Churg–Strauss syndrome.
Rheumatoid disease.
Sarcoidosis.

NEOPLASMS

Bronchogenic carcinoma.
Bronchial carcinoid.
Lymphoma (Hodgkin, non-Hodgkin).

EOSINOPHILIA, PARASITIC CAUSES[10]

ICD-10CM # Varies with specific diagnosis

PARASITIC CAUSES OF EOSINOPHILIA

Widespread Geographic Distribution
Ascariasis (migratory phase).
Hookworm.†
Strongyloidiasis.*‡
Tropical pulmonary eosinophilia.
Lymphatic filariasis.
Schistosomiasis.
Toxocariasis.
Cysticercosis (*Taenia solium*).
Echinococcosis (cyst rupture).
Trichinosis.
Trichuriasis.
Aberrant helminthiasis from animals.
Limited Geographic Distribution
Clonorchiasis.
Paragonimiasis.
Fascioliasis.
Angiostrongyliasis.
Opisthorchiasis.
Onchocerciasis, loiasis, and other nonlymphatic filariases.
Gnathostomiasis.
Capillariasis.
Trichostrongyliasis.

EPIGASTRIC PAIN[95]

ICD-10CM #	R10.816	Epigastric abdominal tenderness
	R10.826	Epigastric rebound abdominal tenderness

Peptic ulceration (uncomplicated).[24]
Peptic ulceration (perforated).
Biliary colic.
Acute pancreatitis.
Abdominal aortic aneurysm.
Anxiety.
Inferior wall MI.

EPILEPSY

ICD-10CM # G40.909 Epilepsy, unspecified, not intractable, without status epilepticus

Psychogenic spells.
Transient ischemic attack.
Hypoglycemia.
Syncope.
Narcolepsy.
Migraine.

---

†Although these are most common neoplastic lesions of the lumbosacral spine, most occur infrequently.
*Most frequent parasitic causes of massive eosinophilia (>5000/mm³).
‡Absent in disseminated infection in compromised hosts.
[24] Conditions that also cause right upper quadrant pain

Paroxysmal vertigo.
Arrhythmias.
Drug reaction.

EPILEPSY MIMICS, PEDIATRIC PATIENT[93]

ICD-10CM # Varies with specific diagnosis

DISORDERS THAT MAY MIMIC CHILDHOOD EPILEPSY

Confused with Generalized Tonic–Clonic Seizures

Pallid syncope (reflex anoxic seizure).
Vasodepressor syncope (reflex anoxic seizure).
Cyanotic breath-holding attacks.
Collapsing attacks with cardiac dysrhythmias.
Cataplexy.

Confused with Generalized Absence Seizures

Behavioral staring attacks.
Complex partial (dyscognitive) seizures.
Tic disorder.

Confused with Complex Partial (Dyscognitive) Seizures

Self-stimulatory behavior, especially in children with autistic spectrum disorders.
Sleep walking.
Night terrors.
Temper tantrums with amnesia for the rage event.
Benign paroxysmal vertigo.
Migraine-related disorders.

Confused with Epileptic Myoclonus

Physiologic hypnagogic myoclonus.
Benign infantile sleep myoclonus.
Startle disease.

EPILEPSY SYNDROMES, AGE SPECIFIC[23]

ICD-10CM #	G40.90	Epilepsy, unspecified, not intractable
	G40.301	Generalized idiopathic epilepsy and epileptic syndromes, not intractable, with status epilepticus
	G40.40	Other generalized epilepsy and epileptic syndromes, not intractable

EPILEPSY SYNDROMES BY AGE OF ONSET

Neonatal

Benign familial neonatal epilepsy.
Early myoclonic encephalopathy.
Ohtahara syndrome.

Infancy

Epilepsy of infancy with migrating focal seizures.
West syndrome (infantile spasms, hypsarrhythmia; to be distinguished from benign myoclonus of early infancy, a nonepilepsy).
Myoclonic epilepsy in infancy (benign Dravet variant).
Benign infantile epilepsy.
Benign familial infantile epilepsy.
Severe myoclonic epilepsy of infancy (classic Dravet syndrome).
Myoclonic encephalopathy in nonprogressive disorders.

Childhood

Genetic epilepsy with febrile seizures plus (GEFS +; can begin in infancy).
Panayiotopoulos syndrome.
Epilepsy with myoclonic atonic (previously astatic) seizures (Doose syndrome).
Benign epilepsy with centrotemporal spikes (BECTS, or benign rolandic epilepsy).
Autosomal-dominant nocturnal frontal lobe epilepsy (ADNFLE).
Late-onset childhood occipital epilepsy (Gastaut syndrome).
Epilepsy with myoclonic absences (Tassinari syndrome).
Lennox–Gastaut syndrome.
Epileptic encephalopathy with continuous spike-and-wave during sleep (CSWS).
Landau–Kleffner syndrome (LKS).
Childhood absence epilepsy (pyknolepsy).
Generalized epilepsy with eyelid myoclonia (Jeavons syndrome).*

Adolescence–Adult

Juvenile absence epilepsy (JAE).
Juvenile myoclonic epilepsy (JME).
Epilepsy with generalized tonic-clonic seizures alone.
Progressive myoclonus epilepsies (PME).
Autosomal-dominant epilepsy with auditory features.
Other familial temporal lobe epilepsies.

Less Specific Age Relationship

Familial focal epilepsy with variable foci (childhood to adult).
Reflex epilepsies (e.g., photosensitive, audiogenic, or reading-induced seizures; may or may not coexist with spontaneous seizures).

EPISTAXIS

ICD-10CM # R04.0 Epistaxis

Trauma.
Medications (nasal sprays, NSAIDs, anticoagulants, antiplatelets).
Nasal polyps.
Cocaine use.
Coagulopathy (hemophilia, liver disease, DIC, thrombocytopenia).
Systemic disorders (hypertension, uremia).
Infections.
Anatomic malformations.
Rhinitis.
Nasal polyps.
Local neoplasms (benign and malignant).
Desiccation.
Foreign body.

ERECTILE DYSFUNCTION, ORGANIC[79]

ICD-10CM # N52.9 Male erectile dysfunction, unspecified

*Not listed as a syndrome by ILAE but instead recognized under absence seizures with special features.

Neurogenic abnormalities: somatic nerve neuropathy, CNS abnormalities.
Psychogenic causes: depression, performance anxiety, marital conflict.
Endocrine causes: hyperprolactinemia, hypogonadotropic hypogonadism, testicular failure, estrogen excess.
Trauma: pelvic fracture, prostate surgery, penile fracture.
Systemic disease: DM, renal failure, hepatic cirrhosis.
Medications: diuretics, antidepressants, H_2 blockers, exogenous hormones, alcohol, antihypertensives, nicotine abuse, finasteride, etc.
Structural abnormalities: Peyronie disease.

EROSIONS, GENITALIA

ICD-10CM # N36.8 Other specified disorders of urethra

Candidiasis.
Intraepithelial neoplasia.
Squamous cell carcinoma.
Lichen planus.
Pemphigus vulgaris.
Erythema multiforme.
Lichen sclerosus.
Bullous pemphigoid.
Extramammary Paget disease.
Impetigo.

ERYTHEMATOUS ANNULAR SKIN LESIONS

ICD-10CM # L53.8 Other specified erythematous conditions

Tinea corporis.
Warfarin plaques.
Erythema multiforme.
Erythema annulare.
Cutaneous lupus.
Cutaneous sarcoidosis.
Trauma.
Acute febrile neutrophilic dermatosis (Sweet syndrome).

ERYTHROCYTOSIS[50]

ICD-10CM # D75.0 Familial erythrocytosis

CAUSES OF ERYTHROCYTOSIS

Relative or Spurious Erythrocytosis (Normal Red Cell Mass)

Hemoconcentration secondary to dehydration (diarrhea, diaphoresis, diuretics, water deprivation, emesis, ethanol, hypertension, preeclampsia, pheochromocytoma, carbon monoxide intoxication).

True or Absolute Erythrocytosis

Polycythemia vera.
Primary congenital polycythemia.
Secondary erythrocytosis caused by:
- Congenital causes (e.g., activating mutation of erythropoietin receptor).
- Hypoxia caused by carbon monoxide poisoning, high oxygen affinity hemoglobin, high-alti-

tude residence, chronic pulmonary disease, hypoventilation syndromes such as sleep apnea, right to left cardiac shunt, neurologic defects involving the respiratory center.

Nonhypoxic causes with pathologic erythropoietin production.

Renal disease (cysts, hydronephrosis, renal artery stenosis, focal glomerulonephritis, renal transplantation).

Tumors (renal cell cancer, hepatocellular carcinoma, cerebellar hemangioblastoma, uterine fibromyoma, adrenal tumors, meningioma, pheochromocytoma).

Drug-associated causes:

Androgen therapy.

Exogenous erythropoietin growth factor therapy.

ERYTHRODERMA

ICD-10CM #	L53.9	Erythematous condition, unspecified

Drug reaction (e.g., allopurinol, ampicillin, phenytoin, vancomycin, dapsone, omeprazole, carbamazepine).
Atopic dermatitis.
Psoriasis.
Contact dermatitis.
Idiopathic.
Pityriasis rubra.
Chronic actinic dermatitis.
Bullous pemphigoid.
Paraneoplastic.
Cutaneous T-cell lymphoma.
Connective tissue disease.
Hypereosinophilia syndrome.

ESOPHAGEAL PERFORATION[63]

ICD-10CM #	K22.3	Perforation of esophagus
	S27.819A	Unspecified injury of esophagus (thoracic part), initial encounter

Trauma.
Caustic burns.
Iatrogenic.
Foreign bodies.
Spontaneous rupture (Boerhaave syndrome).
Postoperative breakdown of anastomosis.

ESOPHAGEAL STRICTURES[85]

ICD-10CM # Varies with specific diagnosis

BENIGN

Congenital
Esophageal atresia.
Tracheoesophageal fistula.
Web.

ACQUIRED

Peptic:
- Gastroesophageal reflux.
- Scleroderma.

Schatzki ring.
Caustic ingestion.
Drug-induced:
- Anticholinergic medications.
- Aspirin.
- Ferrous sulfate.
- Fosamax.
- Nonsteroidal antiinflammatory.
- Quinidine.
- Potassium supplements.
- Tetracycline.
- Vitamin C.

Eosinophilic esophagitis.
Iatrogenic:
- Variceal ligation/injection.
- Endoscopic mucosal resection.
- Ablation therapy (cryotherapy/radiofrequency).
- Postoperative (anastomotic).
- Radiation.
- Instrumentation.
- Nasogastric tube.

Infections:
- Fungal: moniliasis.
- Bacterial: syphilis.
- Mycobacterial: tuberculosis.

Granulomatous:
- Crohn disease.

Dermatosis:
- Epidermolysis bullosa dystrophica.
- Pemphigoid.
- Behçet syndrome.

MALIGNANT

Primary.
Secondary.

ESOPHAGEAL TUMORS, BENIGN[85]

ICD-10CM # Varies with specific diagnosis

CLASSIFICATION OF BENIGN ESOPHAGEAL TUMORS

Mucosa (First and Second Esophageal Ultrasound [EUS] Layers)
Squamous papilloma.
Fibrovascular polyp.
Retention cyst.

Submucosa (Third EUS Layer)
Lipoma.
Fibroma.
Neurofibroma.
Granular cell tumor.
Hemangiomas.
Salivary gland–type tumor.

Muscularis Propria (Fourth EUS Layer)
Leiomyoma.
Duplication cyst.

Periesophageal Tissue (Fifth EUS Layer)
Foregut cyst.

ESOPHAGITIS[63]

ICD-10CM #	K20.9	Esophagitis, unspecified

INFECTIOUS

Candidiasis.
Cytomegalovirus.
Herpes simplex virus.
HIV infection, acute.

NONINFECTIOUS

Gastroesophageal reflux.
Mucositis from cancer chemotherapy.
Mucositis from radiation therapy.
Aphthous ulcers.

ESOPHAGUS, SYSTEMIC DISEASES[85]

ICD-10CM # Varies with specific diagnosis

SYSTEMIC DISEASES OF THE ESOPHAGUS

Connective Tissue Disorders
Scleroderma.
Systemic lupus erythematosus.
Polymyositis.
Dermatomyositis.
Mixed connective tissue disorder.
Raynaud phenomenon.

Allergic Disease
Eosinophilic esophagitis.

Metabolic Diseases
Amyloidosis.
Diabetes mellitus.
Hypothyroidism.
Hyperthyroidism.

Dermatologic Diseases
Epidermolysis bullosa.
Pemphigus vulgaris.
Pemphigoid.
Erythema multiforme.
Lichen planus.
Behçet disease.

Infectious Diseases
Histoplasmosis.
Tuberculosis.
Actinomycosis.
Immunocompromised host:
- Fungal: *Candida* spp.
- Viral: herpes simplex, cytomegalovirus.
- Mycobacterial.
- Bacterial: *Streptococcus viridans, Staphylococcus,* bacilli, *Treponema pallidum.*
- Protozoal.

Miscellaneous Disorders
Sarcoidosis.
Crohn disease.

ESOTROPIA

ICD-10CM #	H50.00	Unspecified esotropia
	H50.43	Accommodative component in esotropia
	H50.05	Alternating esotropia

Congenital.
Accommodative esotropia.
Myasthenia gravis.
Abducens palsy.
Pseudo-sixth nerve palsy.
Medial rectus entrapment (e.g., blowout fracture).
Posterior internuclear ophthalmoplegia.
Wernicke encephalopathy.
Thyroid myopathy.
Chiari malformation.

EXANTHEMS[71]

ICD-10CM # R21 Rash and other nonspecific skin eruption

Measles.
Rubella.
Erythema infectiosum (fifth disease).
Roseola exanthema.
Varicella.
Enterovirus.
Adenovirus.
Epstein-Barr virus.
Kawasaki disease.
Staphylococcal scalded skin.
Scarlet fever.
Meningococcemia.
Rocky Mountain spotted fever.

EYELID NEOPLASM

ICD-10CM # C44.101 Unspecified malignant neoplasm of skin of unspecified eyelid, including canthus

MALIGNANT

Melanoma.
Basal cell carcinoma.
Squamous cell carcinoma.
Bowen disease.
Sebaceous cell carcinoma.
Metastatic lymphoma/leukemia.

BENIGN

Melanocytic nevus.
Pilar, eccrine, or apocrine tumor.
Neurofibroma.
Keratosis.
Squamous papilloma.
Keratoacanthoma.

EYELID RETRACTION

ICD-10CM # H02.89 Other specified disorders of eyelid

Congenital.
Graves ophthalmopathy.
Myasthenia gravis.
Postsurgical.
Guillain-Barré syndrome.
Cerebellar disease.
Horizontal gaze palsy.
Partial palsy of superior rectus muscle.
Encephalitis.
Closed head injury.
Disseminated sclerosis.
Eye trauma.
Contact lens wear.
Proptosis.
Eyelid neoplasm.
Atopic dermatitis.
Herpes zoster ophthalmicus.
Botulinum toxin injection.
Cyclic oculomotor paralysis.
Spheroid wing meningioma.
Hepatic cirrhosis.
Down syndrome.
Essential hypertension.
Meningitis.
Paget disease of bone.

EYE PAIN

ICD-10CM # H57.13 Ocular pain, bilateral

Foreign body.
Herpes zoster.
Trauma.
Conjunctivitis.
Iritis.
Iridocyclitis.
Uveitis.
Blepharitis.
Ingrown lashes.
Orbital or periorbital cellulitis/abscess.
Sinusitis.
Headache.
Glaucoma.
Inflammation of lacrimal gland.
Tic douloureux.
Cerebral aneurysm.
Cerebral neoplasm.
Entropion.
Retrobulbar neuritis.
UV light.
Dry eyes.
Irritation or inflammation from eye drops, dust, cosmetics, etc.

FACIAL PAIN

ICD-10CM # G50.1 Atypical facial pain

Infection, abscess.
Postherpetic neuralgia.
Trauma, posttraumatic neuralgia.
Tic douloureux.
Cluster headache, "lower-half headache."
Geniculate neuralgia.
Anxiety, somatization syndrome.
Glossopharyngeal neuralgia.
Carotidynia.

FACIAL PARALYSIS[71]

ICD-10CM # G51.0 Bell palsy

INFECTION

Bacterial: otitis media, mastoiditis, meningitis, Lyme disease.
Viral: herpes zoster, mononucleosis, varicella, rubella, mumps, Bell palsy.
Mycobacterial: TB, meningitis, leprosy.
Miscellaneous: syphilis, malaria.

TRAUMA

Temporal bone fracture, facial laceration.
Surgery.

NEOPLASM

Malignant: squamous cell carcinoma, basal cell and adenocystic tumors, leukemia, parotid neoplasms, metastatic tumors.
Benign: facial nerve neuroma, vestibular schwannoma, congenital cholesteatoma.

IMMUNOLOGIC

Guillain-Barré syndrome, periarteritis nodosa.
Reaction to tetanus antiserum.

METABOLIC

Pregnancy.
Hypothyroidism.
DM.

FAILURE TO THRIVE

ICD-10CM # R62.50 Unspecified lack of expected normal physiological development in childhood

PSYCHOSOCIAL/BEHAVIORAL

Inadequate diet because of poverty/food insufficiency, errors in food preparation.
Poor parenting skills (lack of knowledge of sufficient diet).
Child/parent interaction problems (autonomy struggles, coercive feeding, maternal depression).
Food refusal.
Rumination.
Parental cognitive or mental health problems.
Child abuse or neglect; emotional deprivation.

NEUROLOGIC

Cerebral palsy.
Hypothalamic and other CNS tumors (diencephalic syndrome).
Neuromuscular disorders.
Neurodegenerative disorders.

RENAL

Recurrent urinary tract infection.
Renal tubular acidosis.
Renal failure.

ENDOCRINE

Diabetes mellitus.
Diabetes insipidus.
Hypothyroidism/hyperthyroidism.
Growth hormone deficiency.
Adrenal insufficiency.

GENETIC/METABOLIC/CONGENITAL

Sickle cell disease.
Inborn errors of metabolism (organic acidosis, hyperammonemia, storage disease).
Fetal alcohol syndrome.
Skeletal dysplasias.
Chromosomal disorders.
Multiple congenital anomaly syndromes (VATER [vertebral defects, imperforate anus, tracheoesophageal fistula, radial and renal dysplasia], CHARGE [coloboma, heart disease, atresia choanae, retarded growth and retarded development and/or CNS anomalies, genital hypoplasia, ear anomalies and/or deafness]).

GASTROINTESTINAL

Pyloric stenosis.
Gastroesophageal reflux.
Repair of tracheoesophageal fistula.
Malrotation.
Malabsorption syndromes.
Celiac disease.
Milk intolerance: lactose, protein.
Pancreatic insufficiency syndromes (cystic fibrosis).

Chronic cholestasis.
Inflammatory bowel disease.
Chronic congenital diarrhea states.
Short bowel syndrome.
Pseudoobstruction.
Hirschsprung disease.
Food allergy.

CARDIAC

Cyanotic heart lesions.
Congestive heart failure.
Vascular rings.

PULMONARY/RESPIRATORY

Severe asthma.
Cystic fibrosis; bronchiectasis.
Chronic respiratory failure.
Bronchopulmonary dysplasia.
Adenoid/tonsillar hypertrophy.
Obstructive sleep apnea.

MISCELLANEOUS

Collagen vascular disease.
Malignancy.
Primary immunodeficiency.
Transplantation.

INFECTIONS

Perinatal infection (TORCHES [toxoplasma, other, rubella, cytomegalovirus, herpes simplex]).
Occult/chronic infections.
Parasitic infestation.
Tuberculosis.
HIV.

FATIGUE

ICD-10CM #		
	R53.83	Other fatigue
	F48.0	Neurasthenia

Depression.
Anxiety, emotional stress.
Inadequate sleep.
Chronic fatigue syndrome.
Prolonged physical activity.
Pregnancy and postpartum period.
Anemia.
Hypothyroidism.
Medications (β-blockers, anxiolytics, antidepressants, sedating antihistamines, clonidine, methyldopa).
Viral or bacterial infections.
Sleep apnea syndrome.
Dieting.
Renal failure, CHF, COPD, liver disease.

FATIGUE, CHRONIC

ICD-10CM #		
	R53.83	Other fatigue
	F48.0	Neurasthenia

CHRONIC INFECTIONS

Hepatitis C.
Lyme disease.
Parasitic and fungal infections.
Tuberculosis.
Human immunodeficiency virus.
Xenotropic murine leukemia retrovirus.

SLEEP DISORDERS

Obstructive sleep apnea.
Restless leg syndrome.
Circadian rhythm disorder.
Upper airway resistance syndrome.
Narcolepsy/parasomnias.
Alpha-delta sleep disorder.

ENDOCRINE/METABOLIC DISORDERS

Addison disease.
Cushing syndrome.
Poorly controlled diabetes.
Thyroid disorders.
Hemochromatosis.
Hypopituitarism.
Diabetes insipidus.

GENERAL MEDICAL DISORDERS

Anemia (any cause).
Chronic renal/hepatic failure.
Malnutrition.
Medication side effects.
Chronic pain disorders.

PSYCHOLOGICAL

Mood disorders (depression, anxiety, bipolar).
Schizophrenia.
Posttraumatic stress disorder.
Anorexia nervosa/bulimia.
Childhood abuse and/or neglect.

CHRONIC INFLAMMATION

Rheumatoid arthritis.
Systemic lupus erythematosus.
Sjögren syndrome.
Polymyositis/dermatomyositis.
Vasculitis.
Sarcoidosis.

CARDIOPULMONARY

Congestive heart failure.
Neurally mediated hypotension.
Postural orthostatic tachycardia syndrome.
Pulmonary hypertension.
Chronic obstructive pulmonary disease.
Mitral valve prolapse.

GASTROINTESTINAL

Celiac disease.
Inflammatory bowel disease.
Autoimmune hepatitis.
Hepatic cirrhosis.

MALIGNANCY

Lymphoma and occult malignancies.
Postchemotherapy syndrome.

NEUROLOGIC DISORDERS

Multiple sclerosis.
Myasthenia gravis.
Muscular dystrophies.
Parkinson disease.
Early dementia.

LIFESTYLE FACTORS

Chronic overwork.
Persistent unresolved stress.
Inadequate exercise.
Morbid obesity (body mass index >40).
Alcoholism/drug abuse.

FATTY LIVER

ICD-10CM #		
	K76.0	Fatty (change of) liver, not elsewhere classified
	K76.89	Other specified diseases of liver

Obesity.
Alcohol abuse.
DM.
Acute fatty liver of pregnancy.
Medications (tetracycline, valproic acid, glucocorticoids, amiodarone, estrogen, methotrexate).
Reye syndrome.
Wilson disease.
Nonalcoholic steatosis.

FEVER, ABDOMINAL PAIN, JAUNDICE IN PEDIATRIC PATIENT[23]

ICD-10CM #		
	R50.9	Fever, unspecified

Cholangitis.
Cholecystitis.
Cholelithiasis.
Sepsis.
Hepatitis.
Choledochal cyst.
Pancreatitis.
Urinary tract infection.
Leptospirosis and other systemic infections with hepatic involvement.
Spontaneous perforation of common bile duct.
Biliary cyst.
Appendicitis.

FEVER AND CARDIOPULMONARY FAILURE[29]

ICD-10CM #		
	R50.9	Fever, unspecified

DIFFERENTIAL DIAGNOSIS OF FEVER AND RAPIDLY PROGRESSIVE CARDIOPULMONARY FAILURE

Bacterial Infection

Severe community-acquired pneumonia.
Meningitis, endocarditis.
Rickettsial disease (babesiosis, ehrlichiosis, Rocky Mountain spotted fever, scrub typhus, Mediterranean spotted fever).
Q-Fever (*Coxiella burnetii*).
Brucellosis.
Plague (*Yersinia pestis*).
Tularemia (*Francisella tularensis*).
Typhoid fever/salmonellosis.
Leptospirosis (*Leptospira interrogans*).
Anthrax.
Mycobacterial infections.

Viral Infections
Viral pneumonia (influenza, CMV, EBV, VZV, SARS).
Hantavirus.
Dengue fever and yellow fever.
Hemorrhagic fever (Lassa, Marburg, or Ebola viruses).
Fungal Infections
Coccidiomycosis.
Cryptococcus.
Histoplasmosis.
Blastomycosis.
Parasitic Infections
Malaria.
Leishmaniasis.
Schistosomiasis.
Strongyloides.
Noninfectious Causes
Inflammatory:
- Rapid-onset interstitial pneumonia (acute interstitial pneumonia, acute hypersensitivity pneumonitis).
- Acute eosinophilic pneumonia.
- ARDS due to other causes (inhalation injury, drug overdose, trauma).

Rheumatologic disorders:
- Wegener granulomatosis, Churg-Strauss disease, Goodpasture syndrome.
- Systemic lupus erythematosus, antiphospholipid syndrome.

Other:
- Malignancy, lymphoma, lymphoproliferative disease, leukemia.
- Pulmonary embolism, aortic dissection, acute myocardial infarction.
- Adrenal insufficiency, thyroid storm.

ARDS, Acute respiratory distress syndrome; *CMV,* Cytomegalovirus; *EBV,* Epstein-Barr virus; *SARS,* severe acute respiratory syndrome; *VZV,* varicella zoster virus.

FEVER AND JAUNDICE

ICD-10CM #	R50.9	Fever, unspecified
	R17	Unspecified jaundice

Bacterial sepsis.
Cholangitis.
Hepatic abscess.
Leptospirosis.
Malaria.
Viral hepatitis.
Yellow fever.

FEVER AND LYMPHADENOPATHY

ICD-10CM #	R59.9	Enlarged lymph nodes, unspecified
	R50.9	Fever, unspecified

REGIONAL
Cervical
Streptococci.
Tuberculosis.
Viral upper respiratory infection.
Peripheral
Bartonella henselae.
Herpesviruses.
Lymphoma.
Metastatic cancer.
Sporotrichosis.
Streptococci.
Inguinal
Chancroid.
Herpes.
Lymphogranuloma venereum.
Syphilis (primary).

GENERALIZED
Cytomegalovirus.
Epstein-Barr virus.
HIV.
Lymphoma.
Sarcoidosis.
Syphilis (secondary).
Toxoplasmosis.
Viral hepatitis.

FEVER AND RASH

ICD-10CM #	R21	Rash and other nonspecific skin eruption
	R21	Rash and other nonspecific skin eruption
	R50.9	Fever, unspecified

Drug hypersensitivity: penicillin, sulfonamides, thiazides, anticonvulsants, allopurinol.
Viral infection: measles, rubella, varicella, erythema infectiosum, roseola, enterovirus infection, viral hepatitis, infectious mononucleosis, acute HIV.
Other infections: meningococcemia, staphylococcemia, scarlet fever, typhoid fever, *Pseudomonas* bacteremia, Rocky Mountain spotted fever, Lyme disease, secondary syphilis, bacterial endocarditis, babesiosis, brucellosis, listeriosis.
Serum sickness.
Erythema multiforme.
Erythema marginatum.
Erythema nodosum.
SLE.
Dermatomyositis.
Allergic vasculitis.
Pityriasis rosea.
Herpes zoster.

FEVER AND RASH IN ICU[95]

ICD-10CM #	R21	Rash and other nonspecific skin eruption
	R50.9	Fever, unspecified

DIFFERENTIAL DIAGNOSTIC CLINICAL FEATURES OF FEVER AND RASH IN THE ICU
Rash with Shock
Infectious causes: toxic shock syndrome, meningococcemia, postsplenectomy sepsis, overwhelming *Staphylococcus aureus* bacteremia/acute bacterial endocarditis, arboviral hemorrhagic fevers, hemorrhagic smallpox, *Vibrio vulnificus*, gas gangrene, dengue fever.
Noninfectious cause: systemic lupus erythematosus (on steroids).

RASH WITH MENTAL CHANGES
Infectious causes: Rocky Mountain spotted fever, meningococcemia (with meningitis), *S. aureus* acute bacterial endocarditis, Chikungunya fever, typhus.
Noninfectious cause: systemic lupus erythematosus.

RASH WITH CONJUNCTIVAL SUFFUSION
Infectious causes: Rocky Mountain spotted fever, dengue fever, arboviral hemorrhagic fevers, toxic shock syndrome.
Noninfectious cause: adult Kawasaki disease.

RASH WITH RELATIVE BRADYCARDIA
Infectious causes: Rocky Mountain spotted fever, typhus, dengue fever, typhoid, arboviral hemorrhagic fevers.
Noninfectious cause: drug rash.

RASH WITH ABDOMINAL PAIN
Infectious causes: *V. vulnificus,* gas gangrene, *Clostridium sordelli,* scarlet fever.
Noninfectious causes: cholesterol emboli syndrome, systemic lupus erythematosus.

RASH ON PALMS AND SOLES
Infectious causes: Rocky Mountain spotted fever, toxic shock syndrome, chickenpox, smallpox, monkeypox, scarlet fever.
Noninfectious cause: drug rash.

RASH WITH DIARRHEA
Infectious causes: *V. vulnificus,* gas gangrene, toxic shock syndrome, dengue fever, arboviral hemorrhagic fevers.
Noninfectious cause: none.

RASH WITH EDEMA OF DORSUM OF HANDS/FEET
Infectious causes: Rocky Mountain spotted fever, toxic shock syndrome.
Noninfectious cause: adult Kawasaki disease.

RASH WITH BULLAE
Infectious causes: *V. vulnificus, S. aureus* complicated skin/skin structure infection, gas gangrene.
Noninfectious cause: none.

RASH WITH HEART MURMUR
Infectious cause: acute bacterial endocarditis.
Noninfectious cause: systemic lupus erythematosus.
Rash with gangrene of nose tip
Infectious cause: *S. aureus* acute bacterial endocarditis.
Noninfectious causes: systemic lupus erythematosus, vasculitis.

RASH WITH CEREBROVASCULAR ACCIDENT
Infectious causes: cholesterol emboli syndrome, *S. aureus* acute bacterial endocarditis.
Noninfectious cause: none.

RASH WITH SPLENOMEGALY

Infectious causes: Rocky Mountain spotted fever, typhus.
Noninfectious causes: systemic lupus erythematosus, adult Kawasaki disease.

RASH WITH DEAFNESS

Infectious causes: Rocky Mountain spotted fever, typhus, meningococcal meningitis.
Noninfectious cause: none.

RASH WITH HEPATOSPLENOMEGALY

Infectious causes: Rocky Mountain spotted fever, typhus.
Noninfectious cause: atypical measles.

RASH WITH HEPATOMEGALY

Infectious cause: typhus.
Noninfectious cause: none.

FEVER, AFTER TRAVEL TO THE TROPICS[3]

ICD-10CM #	R50.81	Fever presenting with conditions classified elsewhere

CAUSES OF FEVER AFTER TRAVEL TO THE TROPICS

80% of Specific Infections Causing Fever (Includes Respiratory and Urinary Tract Infection)

Malaria.
Viral hepatitis.
Febrile illness unrelated to foreign travel.
Dengue fever.
Enteric fever (typhoid and paratyphoid fevers).

Other Causes

Gastroenteritis.
Rickettsia.
Leptospirosis.
Schistosomiasis.
Amebic liver abscess.
Tuberculosis.
Acute HIV infection.
Others.

FEVER, COMMON INFECTIOUS CAUSES[97]

ICD-10CM #	R50.9	Fever, unspecified

CENTRAL NERVOUS SYSTEM

Meningitis:
- Encephalitis.
- Brain abscess.
- Epidural abscess.

HEAD AND NECK

Acute suppurative parotitis:
- Acute sinusitis.
- Parapharyngeal and retropharyngeal space infections.
- Acute suppurative otitis media.

CARDIOVASCULAR

Catheter-related infection:
- Endocarditis.

PULMONARY AND MEDIASTINAL

Pneumonia:
- Empyema.
- Mediastinitis.

HEPATOBILIARY AND GASTROINTESTINAL

Diverticulitis:
- Appendicitis.
- Peritonitis (spontaneous or secondary).
- Intraperitoneal abscess.
- Perirectal abscess.
- Infected pancreatitis.
- Acute cholecystitis.
- Cholangitis.
- Hepatic abscess.
- Acute viral hepatitis.

GENITOURINARY

Bacterial or fungal cystitis:
- Pyelonephritis.
- Perinephric abscess.
- Tubo-ovarian abscess.
- Endometritis.
- Prostatitis.

BREAST

Mastitis:
- Breast abscess.

CUTANEOUS AND MUSCULAR

Cellulitis:
- Suppurative wound infection.
- Necrotizing fasciitis.
- Bacterial myositis or myonecrosis.
- Herpes zoster.

OSSEOUS

Osteomyelitis.

FEVER, DRUG-INDUCED[38]

ICD-10CM #	R50.2	Drug induced fever

SELECTED AGENTS ASSOCIATED WITH DRUG-INDUCED FEVER

Common

Antimicrobial:
- Amphotericin B.
- β-Lactams.
- Sulfonamides.

Cardiovascular:
- Procainamide.
- Quinidine.

CNS:
- Carbamazepine.
- Phenytoin.

Miscellaneous:
- Bleomycin.
- Interferon-α.
- Interleukin-2.

Less Common

Antimicrobial:
- Clindamycin.
- Fluoroquinolones.
- Rifampin.

Cardiovascular:
- Diltiazem.
- Hydralazine.

CNS:
- Haloperidol.
- Serotonin reuptake inhibitors.

Miscellaneous:
- Allopurinol.
- Cimetidine.
- Tacrolimus.

FEVER, HOSPITAL ASSOCIATED[38]

ICD-10CM #	R50.2	Drug induced fever
	R50.9	Fever, unspecified

SELECTED CAUSES OF HOSPITAL-ASSOCIATED FEVER

Common

Infectious:
- *Clostridium difficile* enterocolitis.
- Pneumonia.
- Surgical wound.
- Urinary tract.
- Vascular catheter.

Noninfectious:
- Drug-induced fever.
- Hematoma.
- Immediate postoperative state.
- Transfusion reaction.
- Venous thromboembolism.

Less Common

Infectious:
- Biliary tract disease.
- Endometritis.
- Intraabdominal abscess.
- Mediastinitis.
- Sinusitis.

Noninfectious:
- Adrenal insufficiency.
- Gout.
- Myocardial infarction.
- Organ infarction.
- Pancreatitis.

FEVER IN RETURNING TRAVELERS AND IMMIGRANTS[71]

ICD-10CM #	R50.81	Fever presenting with conditions classified elsewhere

COMMON*

Acute respiratory tract infection (worldwide).
Gastroenteritis (worldwide) [foodborne, waterborne, fecal-oral].

*A vegetative state may not necessarily begin with coma but can also develop as the end stage of neurodegenerative diseases (e.g., Alzheimer disease) of adults or children and can accompany severe congenital developmental abnormalities of the brain such as anencephaly.

Enteric fever, including typhoid (worldwide) [food, water].
Urinary tract infection (worldwide) [sexual contact].
Drug reactions [antibiotics, prophylactic agents, other] {rash frequent}.
Malaria (tropics, limited areas of temperate zones) [mosquitoes].
Arboviruses (Africa; tropics) [mosquitoes, ticks, mites].
Dengue (Asia, Caribbean, Africa) [mosquitoes].
Viral hepatitis (worldwide).
Hepatitis A (worldwide) [food, fecal-oral].
Hepatitis B (worldwide, especially Asia, sub-Saharan Africa) [sexual contact] {long incubation period}.
Hepatitis C (worldwide) [blood or sexual contact].
Hepatitis E (Asia, North Africa, Mexico, others) [food, water].
Tuberculosis (worldwide) [airborne, milk] {long period to symptomatic infection}.
Sexually transmitted diseases (worldwide) [sexual contact].

LESS COMMON*

Filariasis (Asia, Africa, South America) [biting insects] {long incubation period, eosinophilia}.
Measles (developing world) [airborne] {in susceptible individual}.
Amebic abscess (worldwide) [food].
Brucellosis (worldwide) [milk, cheese, food, animal contact].
Listeriosis (worldwide) [foodborne] {meningitis}.
Leptospirosis (worldwide) [animal contact, open fresh water] {jaundice, meningitis}.
Strongyloidiasis (warm and tropical areas) [soil contact] {eosinophilia}.
Toxoplasmosis (worldwide) [undercooked meat].

RARE

Relapsing fever (western Americas, Asia, northern Africa) [ticks, lice].
Hemorrhagic fevers (worldwide) [arthropod and nonarthropod transmitted].
Yellow fever (tropics) [mosquitoes] {hepatitis}.
Hemorrhagic fever with renal syndrome (Europe, Asia, North America) [rodent urine] {renal impairment}.
Hantavirus pulmonary syndrome (western North America, other) [rodent urine] {respiratory distress syndrome}.
Lassa fever (Africa) [rodent excreta, person to person] {high mortality rate}.
Other: chikungunya, Rift Valley, Ebola-Marburg, etc. (various) [insect bites, rodent excreta, aerosols, person to person] {often severe}.
Rickettsial infections {rashes and eschars}.
Leishmaniasis, visceral (Middle East, Mediterranean, Africa, Asia, South America) [biting flies] {long incubation period}.

*Diagnoses for which particular symptoms are indicative are in *italics*. Exposure to regions of the world that are most likely to be significant to the diagnosis are presented in (parentheses). Vectors, risk behaviors, and sources associated with acquisition are presented in [brackets]. Special clinical characteristics are listed within {braces}.

Acute schistosomiasis (Africa, Asia, South America, Caribbean) [fresh water].
Chagas disease (South and Central America) [reduviid bug bites] {often asymptomatic}.
African trypanosomiasis (Africa) [tsetse fly bite] {neurologic syndromes, sleeping sickness}.
Bartonellosis (South America) [sandfly bite] {skin nodules}.
HIV infection/AIDS (worldwide) [sexual and blood contact].
Trichinosis (worldwide) [undercooked meat] {eosinophilia}.
Plague (temperate and tropical plains) [animal exposures and fleas].
Tularemia (worldwide) [animal contact, fleas, aerosols] {ulcers, lymph nodes}.
Anthrax (worldwide) [animal, animal product contact] {ulcers}.
Lyme disease (North America, Europe) [tick bites] {arthritis, meningitis, cardiac abnormalities}.

FEVER, NONINFECTIOUS CAUSES[7]

ICD-10CM # R50.9 Fever, unspecified

DIFFERENTIAL DIAGNOSIS—NONINFECTIOUS CAUSES OF FEVER

Critical Diagnoses
Acute myocardial infarction.
Pulmonary embolism/infarction.
Intracranial hemorrhage.
Cerebrovascular accident.
Neuroleptic-malignant syndrome.
Thyroid storm.
Acute adrenal insufficiency.
Transfusion reaction.
Pulmonary edema.
Emergent Diagnoses
Congestive heart failure.
Dehydration.
Recent seizure.
Sickle cell disease.
Transplant rejection.
Pancreatitis.
Deep vein thrombosis.
Nonemergent Diagnoses
Drug fever.
Malignancy.
Gout.
Sarcoidosis.
Crohn disease.
Postmyocardiotomy syndrome.

FEVER OF UNKNOWN ORIGIN, PEDIATRIC PATIENT[23]

ICD-10CM # R50.9 Fever, unspecified

INFECTIOUS DISEASES

Bacterial
Bacterial endocarditis.
Brucellosis.
Cat-scratch disease.
Leptospirosis.
Liver abscess.
Mastoiditis (chronic).
Osteomyelitis.
Pelvic abscess.
Perinephric abscess.
Pyelonephritis.
Salmonellosis.
Sinusitis.
Subdiaphragmatic abscess.
Tuberculosis.
Tularemia.
Viral
Adenovirus.
Arboviruses.
Cytomegalovirus.
Epstein-Barr virus (infectious mononucleosis).
Hepatitis viruses.
Chlamydial
Lymphogranuloma venereum.
Psittacosis.
Rickettsial
Q fever.
Rocky Mountain spotted fever.
Fungal
Blastomycosis (nonpulmonary).
Histoplasmosis (disseminated).
Parasitic
Malaria.
Toxoplasmosis.
Visceral larva migrans.
Unclassified
Sarcoidosis.
Collagen Vascular Diseases
Juvenile rheumatoid arthritis.
Polyarteritis nodosa.
Systemic lupus erythematosus.
Malignancies
Hodgkin disease.
Leukemia and lymphoma.
Neuroblastoma.
Miscellaneous
Central diabetes insipidus.
Drug fever.
Ectodermal dysplasia.
Factitious fever.
Familial dysautonomia.
Granulomatous colitis.
Hemophagocytic lymphohistiocytosis.
Infantile cortical hyperostosis.
Kikuchi-Fujimoto disease.
Nephrogenic diabetes insipidus.
Pancreatitis.
Periodic fever.
Serum sickness.
Thyrotoxicosis.
Ulcerative colitis.

FEVER, POSTPARTUM[1]

ICD-10CM # R50.9 Fever, unspecified

MOST COMMON

Metritis.
Urinary tract infection.
Pneumonia.
Wound infection.

Mastitis.
Superficial or deep vein thrombosis.

MOST THREATENING

Toxic shock syndrome.
Necrotizing fasciitis.
Pelvic phlegmon.
Pelvic abscess.
Peritonitis.
Septic pelvic thrombosis.
Breast abscess.

FEVER, PERIODIC[33]

ICD-10CM # R50.9 Fever, unspecified

HEREDITARY

Nonhereditary

Infectious

Hidden infectious focus (e.g., aortoenteric fistula, Caroli disease).
Recurrent reinfection (e.g., chronic meningococcemia, host defense defect).
Specific infection (e.g., Whipple disease, malaria).
Noninfectious inflammatory disorder, e.g.:
- Adult-onset Still disease.
- Juvenile chronic rheumatoid arthritis.
- Periodic fever, aphthous stomatitis, pharyngitis, and adenitis.
- Schnitzler syndrome.
- Behçet syndrome.
- Crohn disease.
- Sarcoidosis.
- Extrinsic alveolitis.
- Humidifier lung, polymer fume fever.
- Neoplastic.

Lymphoma (e.g., Hodgkin disease, angioimmunoblastic lymphoma).
Solid tumor (e.g., pheochromocytoma, myxoma, colon carcinoma).

Vascular (e.g., recurrent pulmonary embolism)

Hypothalamic

Psychogenic periodic fever.
Factitious or fraudulent.

FEVER, PEDIATRIC, ACUTE[1]

ICD-10CM # R50.9 Fever, unspecified

COMMON VIRAL INFECTIONS

Central Nervous System

Meningitis.
Encephalitis.
Tumor.
Brain abscess.

Head, Ears, Eyes, Nose, and Throat

Otitis media.
Pharyngitis.
Retropharyngeal abscess.
Peritonsillar abscess.
Lateral pharyngeal wall abscess.
Stomatitis.
Influenza.
Sinusitis.
Parotitis.
Cervical adenitis.
Periorbital cellulitis.
Orbital cellulitis or abscess.

Respiratory System

Bronchiolitis.
Croup.
Epiglottitis.
Pneumonia.
Upper respiratory infection.

Cardiovascular System

Myocarditis.
Pericarditis.
Endocarditis.

Genitourinary System

Urinary tract infection.
Tuboovarian abscess.

Gastrointestinal Tract

Acute viral gastroenteritis.
Bacterial enteritis.
Appendicitis.

Focal Soft Tissue Infections

Cellulitis.

Musculoskeletal System

Osteomyelitis.
Septic arthritis.

Rheumatologic Disorders

Acute rheumatic fever.
Juvenile rheumatoid arthritis.
Henoch-Schönlein purpura.

Vasculitis

Behçet syndrome.

Malignancy

Leukemia.
Lymphoma.
Sarcoma.

Systemic Illness

Bacteremia.
Viremia.
Sepsis.
Kawasaki disease.
Toxic shock syndrome.
Rocky Mountain spotted fever.
Meningococcemia.

MISCELLANEOUS DISORDERS

Toxicologic

Anticholinergic toxidromes.
Salicylate overdose.
Amphetamine.
Cocaine.

Endocrine

Thyrotoxicosis.

FEVER, RECURRENT OR PERIODIC, IN CHILDREN[58]

ICD-10CM # R50.2 Drug induced fever
R50.9 Fever, unspecified

INFECTIOUS DISEASES

Brucellosis.
Rat-bite fever.
Relapsing fever.

RHEUMATIC DISEASES

Juvenile idiopathic arthritis (systemic onset).
Behçet disease.
Systemic lupus erythematosus.
Relapsing polychondritis.
Crohn disease.

HEREDITARY AUTOINFLAMMATORY SYNDROMES

Familial Mediterranean fever (FMF).
Cryopyrinopathies:
- Familial cold autoinflammatory syndrome (FCAS).
- Muckle-Wells syndrome (MWS).
- Chronic infantile neurologic cutaneous and articular (CINCA) syndrome, also called neonatal-onset multisystem inflammatory disease (NOMID).

Tumor necrosis factor receptor–associated periodic syndrome (TRAPS).
Hyperimmunoglobulinemia D with periodic fever syndrome (HIDS).

CYCLIC HEMATOPOIESIS

Hereditary form.
Acquired form.

IDIOPATHIC CONDITIONS

Periodic fever with aphthous stomatitis, pharyngitis, and adenitis (PFAPA).

FEVER WITH MACULOPAPULAR OR PETECHIAL RASH[76]

ICD-10CM # R21 Rash and nonspecific skin eruption
ICD-10CM # R50.9 Fever, unspecified

DIFFERENTIAL DIAGNOSIS OF FEVER WITH MACULOPAPULAR OR PETECHIAL RASH

Rocky Mountain spotted fever.
Meningococcal disease.
Enteroviral infection (echovirus and coxsackievirus).
Human herpesvirus 6 infection (roseola).
Human parvovirus B19 infection (fifth disease).
Epstein-Barr virus infection.
Disseminated gonococcal infection.
Murine typhus.
Ehrlichiosis.
Group A streptococcal pharyngitis.
Mycoplasma pneumoniae Infection.
Leptospirosis.
Secondary syphilis.
Kawasaki disease.
Thrombotic thrombocytopenic purpura (TTP).
Drug reactions.
Immune complex–mediated illness.
Toxic shock syndrome.
Erythema multiforme.
Stevens-Johnson syndrome.

FEVERS PRONE TO RELAPSE[47]

ICD-10CM # R50.9 Fever, unspecified

Infectious Causes

Relapsing fever (*Borrelia recurrentis*).
Q fever (*Coxiella burnetii*).
Typhoid fever (*Salmonella typhi*).
Syphilis (*Treponema pallidum*).
Tuberculosis.
Histoplasmosis.
Coccidioidomycosis.
Blastomycosis.
Melioidosis (*Pseudomonas pseudomallei*).
Lymphocytic choriomeningitis (LCM) infection.
Dengue fever.
Yellow fever.
Chronic meningococcemia.
Colorado tick fever.
Leptospirosis.
Brucellosis.
Oroya fever (*Bartonella bacilliformis*).
Acute rheumatic fever.
Rat-bite fever (*Spirillum minus*).
Visceral leishmaniasis.
Lyme disease (*Borrelia burgdorferi*).
Malaria.
Babesiosis.
Noninfluenza respiratory viral infection.
Epstein-Barr virus infection.

Noninfectious Causes

Behçet disease.
Crohn disease.
Weber-Christian disease (panniculitis).
Leukoclastic angiitis syndromes.
Sweet syndrome.
Systemic lupus erythematosus and other autoimmune disorders.

Periodic Fever Syndromes

Familial Mediterranean fever.
Cyclic neutropenia.
Periodic fever, aphthous stomatitis, pharyngitis, and adenopathy (PFAPA).
Hyper–immunoglobulin D syndrome.
Hibernian fever (tumor necrosis factor superfamily immunoglobulin A–associated syndrome [TRAPS]).
Muckle-Wells syndrome.
Others.

FINGER LESIONS, INFLAMMATORY

ICD-10CM #	B08.8	Other specified viral infections characterized by skin and mucous membrane lesions
	L03.0	Cellulitis of finger 6

Paronychia.
Herpes simplex type 1 (herpetic whitlow).
Dyshidrotic eczema (pompholyx).
Herpes zoster.
Bacterial endocarditis (Osler nodes).
Psoriatic arthritis.

FLACCID PARALYSIS, ACUTE, DIFFERENTIAL DIAGNOSIS[58]

ICD-10CM #	G83.9	Paralytic syndrome, unspecified

Brain stem stroke.
Brain stem encephalitis.
Acute anterior poliomyelitis.
 Caused by poliovirus.
 Caused by other neurotropic viruses.
Acute myelopathy.
 Space-occupying lesions.
 Acute transverse myelitis.
Peripheral neuropathy.
 Guillain-Barré syndrome.
 Post-rabies vaccine neuropathy.
 Diphtheritic neuropathy.
 Heavy metals, biologic toxins, or drug intoxication.
 Acute intermittent porphyria.
 Vasculitic neuropathy.
 Critical illness neuropathy.
 Lymphomatous neuropathy.
Disorders of neuromuscular transmission.
 Myasthenia gravis.
 Biologic or industrial toxins.
 Tic paralysis.
Disorders of muscle.
 Hypokalemia.
 Hypophosphatemia.
 Inflammatory myopathy.
 Acute rhabdomyolysis.
 Trichinosis.
 Periodic paralyses.

FLATULENCE AND BLOATING[84]

ICD-10CM #	R14.0	Abdominal distension (gaseous)
	R14.1	Gas pain
	R14.2	Eructation
	R14.3	Flatulence

Ingestion of nonabsorbable carbohydrates.
Ingestion of carbonated beverages.
Malabsorption: pancreatic insufficiency, biliary disease, celiac disease, bacterial overgrowth in small intestine.
Lactase deficiency.
Irritable bowel syndrome.
Anxiety disorders.
Food poisoning, giardiasis.

FLUSHING[69]

ICD-10CM #	R23.2	Flushing

Physiologic flushing: menopause, ingestion of monosodium glutamate (Chinese restaurant syndrome), ingestion of hot drinks.
Drugs: alcohol (with or without disulfiram, metronidazole, or chlorpropamide), nicotinic acid, diltiazem, nifedipine, levodopa, bromocriptine, vancomycin, amyl nitrate.
Neoplastic disorders: carcinoid syndrome, VIPoma syndrome, medullary carcinoma of thyroid, systemic mastocytosis, basophilic chronic myelocytic leukemia, renal cell carcinoma.
Anxiety.
Agnogenic flushing.

FOLATE DEFICIENCY[50]

ICD-10CM #	D52.0	Dietary folate deficiency anemia
	D52.1	Drug-induced folate deficiency anemia
	D52.8	Other folate deficiency anemias
	D52.9	Folate deficiency anemia, unspecified

ETIOPATHOPHYSIOLOGIC CLASSIFICATION OF FOLATE DEFICIENCY

Nutritional causes:
 Decreased dietary intake:
  Poverty and famine.
  Institutionalized individuals (e.g., psychiatric, nursing homes), chronic debilitating disease.
  Prolonged feeding of infants with goat's milk, special slimming diets or food fads (i.e., folate-rich foods not consumed), cultural or ethnic cooking techniques (i.e., food folate destroyed).
 Decreased diet and increased requirements:
  Physiologic (e.g., pregnancy and lactation, prematurity, hyperemesis gravidarum, infancy).
  Pathologic (e.g., intrinsic hematologic diseases involving hemolysis with compensatory erythropoiesis, abnormal hematopoiesis, or bone marrow infiltration with malignant disease and dermatologic disease such as psoriasis).
Folate malabsorption:
 With normal intestinal mucosa:
  Some drugs (controversial).
  Congenital folate malabsorption (rare).
  With mucosal abnormalities (e.g., tropical and nontropical sprue, regional enteritis).
Defective cellular folate uptake:
 Familial aplastic anemia (rare).
 Acute cerebral folate deficiency.
Inadequate cellular use:
 Folate antagonists (e.g., methotrexate).
 Hereditary enzyme deficiencies involving folate.
Drugs:
 Multiple effects on folate metabolism (e.g., alcohol, sulfasalazine, triamterene, pyrimethamine, trimethoprim-sulfamethoxazole, diphenylhydantoin, barbiturates).
Acute folate deficiency:
 Intensive care unit setting.
 Uncertain origin.

FOOT AND ANKLE PAIN[31]

ICD-10CM #	M25.5	Pain in joint
	M25.9	Joint disorder, unspecified

TENDON, LIGAMENT, AND MUSCLE

Gastrocnemius-soleus strain.
Plantaris rupture.
Anterior talofibular ligament tear.
Calcaneofibular ligament tear.
Deltoid ligament tear.
Anterolateral impingement due to complete tear of anterior talofibular ligament and anterior inferior tibiofibular ligament.
Syndesmotic impingement due to tear of syndesmosis.

Sinus tarsi syndrome (lateral hindfoot pain and instability due to injury of contents of the sinus and tarsal tunnel).
Achilles tendinitis.
Achilles rupture.
Plantar fasciitis.
Posterior tibial tendon dysfunction.
Flexor hallucis longus dysfunction.
Tibialis anterior tendon tear.
Peroneus brevis tendon tear.

BONE

Fracture of talus.
Calcaneal fracture.
Navicular fractures.
Lisfranc fracture-dislocation (fracture of the first metatarsal base with dislocation of medial cuneiform).
Metatarsal stress fracture.
Freiberg infraction (sclerosis and flattening of the second metatarsal head due to trauma or microtrauma).
Avascular necrosis of the talus.
Fracture of the phalanges.
Fracture of the sesamoids.
Sesamoiditis.
Metatarsalgia.

JOINT

Osteoarthritis.
Gout.
Rheumatoid arthritis.
Other inflammatory arthritides.
Charcot joint.
Osteochondral lesion of the talus.

PERIARTICULAR STRUCTURES

Shin splint (periosteal avulsion and periostitis at the insertion of the medial soleus due to repetitive overuse, such as in running and hiking).
Hallux rigidus.
Hallux valgus.
Ingrown toenail.
Toe deformities.
Turf toe (sprain of the first metatarsophalangeal joint due to hyperextension forces).
Plantar fasciitis.
Plantar fibromatosis.

NERVES

Anterior tarsal tunnel syndrome (involvement of deep peroneal nerve under the superficial fascia of the ankle).
Morton neuroma.

VESSELS

Atherosclerosis.
Compartment syndrome.

REFERRED PAIN

Complex regional pain syndrome.

FOOT AND ANKLE PAIN, IN DIFFERENT AGE GROUPS[22]

ICD-10CM #	M25.579	Pain in unspecified ankle and joints of unspecified foot

COMMON CAUSES OF FOOT AND ANKLE PAIN IN DIFFERENT AGE GROUPS

Childhood (2-10 yr)
Intraarticular
Club foot.
Congenital midfoot and forefoot deformities.
Septic arthritis.
Periarticular
Osteomyelitis.
Adolescence (10-18 yr)
Intraarticular
Arch disorders (pes cavus, pes planus).
Periarticular
Osteomyelitis.
Tumors.
Early Adulthood (18-30 yr)
Intraarticular
Metatarsalgia.
Hallux valgus.
Hallux rigidus.
Osteochondritis.
Accessory ossicles.
Periarticular
Achilles tendonitis.
Achilles tendon rupture.
Fasciitis.
Referred
Lumbar spine.
Knee.
Adulthood (30-50 yr)
Intraarticular
Osteoarthritis.
Inflammatory arthritis.
Gout.
Metatarsalgia.
Hallux valgus.
Hallux rigidus.
Osteochondritis.
Accessory ossicles.
Periarticular
Ischemic foot pain.
Diabetes.
Bursitis.
Tendonitis.
Plantar fasciitis.
Corns.
Referred
Lumbar spine.
Knee.
Old Age (>50 yr)
Intraarticular
Osteoarthritis.
Inflammatory arthritis.
Gout.
Metatarsalgia.
Hallux valgus.
Hallux rigidus.
Periarticular
Ischemic foot pain.
Diabetes.
Bursitis.
Tendonitis.
Plantar fasciitis.
Corns.
Referred
Lumbar spine.
Knee.

FOOT DERMATITIS

ICD-10CM #	B35.3	Tinea pedis
	K25	Unspecified contact dermatitis

Tinea pedis.
Dyshidrotic eczema.
Tylosis (mechanically induced hyperkeratosis, fissuring, and dryness).
Allergic contact dermatitis.
Psoriasis.
Peripheral vascular insufficiency.
Neuropathic foot ulcers (DM, poorly fitting shoes).
Acquired plantar keratoderma.
Sézary syndrome.

FOOTDROP

ICD-10CM #	M21.379	Foot drop, unspecified foot

Peripheral neuropathy.
L5 radiculopathy.
Peroneal nerve compression.
Sciatic nerve palsy.
Scapuloperoneal syndromes.
Spasticity.
Peroneal nerve compression.
Myopathy.
Dystonia.

FOOT LESION, ULCERATING

ICD-10CM #	S90.929A	Unspecified superficial injury of unspecified foot, initial encounter
	S90.933A	Unspecified superficial injury of unspecified great toe, initial encounter
	S90.936A	Unspecified superficial injury of unspecified lesser toe(s), initial encounter
	L08.89	Other specified local infections of the skin and subcutaneous tissue

Cellulitis.
Plantar wart.
Squamous cell carcinoma.
Actinomycosis (Madura foot).
Plantar fibromatosis.
Pseudoepitheliomatous hyperplasia.

FOOT PAIN

ICD-10CM #	M25.579	Pain in unspecified ankle and joints of unspecified foot

Trauma (fractures, musculoskeletal and ligamentous strain).
Inflammation (plantar fasciitis, Achilles tendonitis or bursitis, calcaneal apophysitis).
Arterial insufficiency, Raynaud phenomenon, thromboangiitis obliterans.
Gout, pseudogout.

Calcaneal spur.
Infection (cellulitis, abscess, lymphangitis, gangrene).
Decubitus ulcer.
Paronychia, ingrown toenail.
Thrombophlebitis, postphlebitic syndrome.

FOOT PAIN BY AGE[58]

ICD-10CM # M25.579 Pain in unspecified ankle and joints of unspecified foot

0 TO 6 YEARS

Poorly fitting shoes.
Foreign body.
Fracture.
Osteomyelitis.
Leukemia.
Puncture wound.
Drawing of blood.
Dactylitis.
Juvenile rheumatoid arthritis (JRA).

6 TO 12 YEARS

Poorly fitting shoes.
Sever disease.
Enthesopathy (JRA).
Foreign body.
Accessory navicular.
Tarsal coalition.
Ewing sarcoma.
Hypermobile flatfoot.
Trauma (sprains, fractures).
Puncture wound.

12 TO 20 YEARS

Poorly fitting shoes.
Stress fracture.
Foreign body.
Ingrown toenail.
Metatarsalgia.
Plantar fasciitis.
Osteochondroses (avascular necrosis).
Freiberg infarction.
Köhler disease.
Achilles tendinitis.
Trauma (sprains).
Plantar warts.
Tarsal coalition.

FOREARM AND HAND PAIN

ICD-10CM #		
	S59.809A	Other specified injuries of unspecified elbow, initial encounter
	S59.919A	Unspecified injury of unspecified forearm, initial encounter
	S69.80XA	Other specified injuries of unspecified wrist, hand and finger(s), initial encounter
	S69.90XA	Unspecified injury of unspecified wrist, hand and finger(s), initial encounter

Epicondylitis.
Tenosynovitis.
Osteoarthritis.
Cubital tunnel syndrome.
Carpal tunnel syndrome.
Trauma.
Herpes zoster.
Peripheral vascular insufficiency.
Infection (cellulitis, abscess).

FOREARM FRACTURES[3]

ICD-10CM # S52 Fracture of forearm

TRAUMATIC

Wrist sprain, elbow sprain.
Ligamentous injuries, forearm contusions, hematomas.
Dislocations of the elbow or wrist (including nursemaid's elbow).

INFECTIOUS

Cellulitis of the forearm, abscesses.
Necrotizing fasciitis.

VASCULAR

Acute arterial occlusion.
Venous thrombosis.

NEUROLOGIC

Neurapraxias, carpal tunnel syndrome.
Systemic neurologic syndromes involving the nerves of the upper extremities.

ARTHRITIS

Septic joint, gonococcal arthritis, rheumatoid arthritis, osteoarthritis.
Pseudogout, gout.
Systemic lupus erythematosus, rheumatic fever, viral syndrome.
Reiter syndrome, Lyme disease, serum sickness.

OTHER

Olecranon bursitis, soft tissue masses.
Normal growth plates, nutrient vessels.

GAIT ABNORMALITY

ICD-10CM #		
	R26.0	Ataxic gait
	R26.1	Paralytic gait
	R26.89	Other abnormalities of gait and mobility
	R26.9	Unspecified abnormalities of gait and mobility

Parkinsonism.
Degenerative joint disease (hips, back, knees).
Multiple sclerosis.
Trauma, foot pain.
CVA.
Cerebellar lesions.
Infections (tabes, encephalitis, meningitis).
Sensory ataxia.
Dystonia, cerebral palsy, neuromuscular disorders.
Metabolic abnormalities.

GALACTORRHEA[71]

ICD-10CM # N64.3 Galactorrhea not associated with childbirth

Prolonged suckling.
Drugs (INH, phenothiazines, reserpine derivatives, amphetamines, spironolactone and tricyclic antidepressants).
Major stressors (surgery, trauma).
Hypothyroidism.
Pituitary tumors.

GALLBLADDER SONOGRAPHIC NONVISUALIZATION[81]

ICD-10CM # Varies with specific diagnosis

CAUSES OF SONOGRAPHIC NONVISUALIZATION OF GALLBLADDER

Previous cholecystectomy.
Physiologic contraction.
Fibrosed gallbladder duct—chronic cholecystitis.
Air-filled gallbladder or emphysematous cholecystitis.
Tumefactive sludge.
Agenesis of gallbladder.
Ectopic location.

GALLBLADDER WALL THICKENING[81]

ICD-10CM # Varies with specific diagnosis

CAUSES OF GALLBLADDER WALL THICKENING

Generalized Edematous States
Congestive heart failure.
Renal failure.
End-stage cirrhosis.
Hypoalbuminemia.
Inflammatory Conditions
Primary:
- Acute cholecystitis.
- Cholangitis.
- Chronic cholecystitis.

Secondary:
- Acute hepatitis.
- Perforated duodenal ulcer.
- Pancreatitis.
- Diverticulitis/colitis.

Neoplastic Conditions
Gallbladder adenocarcinoma.
Metastases.
Miscellaneous
Adenomyomatosis.
Mural varicosities.

GALLSTONE DISEASE, PEDIATRIC PATIENT[23]

ICD-10CM # K80.20 Calculus of gallbladder without cholecystitis without obstruction

Biliary tract anomaly (e.g., choledochal cyst).
Cephalosporin use.
Crohn disease.
Cystic fibrosis.
Genetic predisposition (e.g., ABCB4, UGT1A1 mutations).
Hemolytic disorders (e.g., sickle-cell anemia, hereditary spherocytosis).
Hispanic or Latino ancestry.
Malabsorption.
Metabolic syndrome.
Obesity.
Parasitic disease (*Ascaris lumbricoides*).
Pregnancy.
Rapid weight loss.
Solid organ and hematologic transplant (e.g., liver, kidney, heart, bone marrow).
Total parenteral nutrition.

GASTRIC DILATION[41]

ICD-10CM # K31.0 Acute dilatation of stomach

CAUSES OF A MASSIVELY DILATED STOMACH

Mechanical Gastric Outlet Obstruction
Duodenal or pyloric canal ulceration.
Carcinoma of pyloric antrum.
Extrinsic compression.
Paralytic Ileus
Surgery.
Trauma.
Peritonitis.
Pancreatitis.
Cholecystitis.
Diabetes mellitus.
Hepatic coma.
Drugs.
Gastric Volvulus
Intubation.
Air swallowing.

GASTRIC EMPTYING, DELAYED[3]

ICD-10CM # K30 Functional dyspepsia

CAUSES OF DELAYED GASTRIC EMPTYING

Mechanical Causes
Peptic ulcer disease, scarred pylorus.
Malignancy: gastric cancer, gastric lymphoma, pancreatic cancer.
Gastric surgery: vagotomy, gastric resection, Roux-en-Y anastomosis.
Crohn disease.
Endocrine and Metabolic Causes
Diabetes mellitus.
Hypothyroidism.
Hypoadrenal states.
Electrolyte abnormalities.
Chronic renal failure.
Medications.
Anticholinergics.
Opiates.
Dopamine agonists.
Tricyclic antidepressants.
Abnormalities of Gastric Smooth Muscle
Scleroderma.
Polymyositis, dermatomyositis.
Amyloidosis.
Pseudoobstruction.
Myotonic dystrophy.
Neuropathy.
Scleroderma.
Amyloidosis.
Autonomic neuropathy.
Central Nervous System or Psychiatric Disorders
Brain stem tumors.
Spinal cord injury.
Anorexia nervosa.
Stress.
Miscellaneous
Idiopathic gastroparesis.
Gastroesophageal reflux disease.
Nonulcer (functional) dyspepsia.
Cancer cachexia or anorexia.

GASTRIC EMPTYING, RAPID

ICD-10CM # K30 Functional dyspepsia

Pancreatic insufficiency.
Dumping syndrome.
Peptic ulcer.
Celiac disease.
Promotility agents.
Zollinger-Ellison disease.

GASTROINTESTINAL BLEEDING, PEDIATRIC PATIENT[59]

ICD-10CM # K92.2 Gastrointestinal hemorrhage, unspecified

INFANT

Common
Bacterial enteritis.
Milk protein allergy intolerance.
Intussusception.
Swallowed maternal blood.
Anal fissure.
Lymphonodular hyperplasia

Rare
Volvulus.
Necrotizing enterocolitis.
Meckel diverticulum.
Stress ulcer, gastritis.
Coagulation disorder (hemorrhagic disease of newborn).
Esophagitis.

CHILD

Common
Bacterial enteritis.
Anal fissure.
Colonic polyps.
Intussusception.
Peptic ulcer/gastritis.
Swallowed epistaxis.
Prolapse (traumatic) gastropathy secondary to emesis.
Mallory-Weiss syndrome.
Rare
Esophageal varices.
Esophagitis.
Meckel diverticulum.
Lymphonodular hyperplasia.
Henoch-Schönlein purpura.
Foreign body.
Hemangioma, arteriovenous malformation.
Sexual abuse.
Hemolytic-uremic syndrome.
Inflammatory bowel disease.
Coagulopathy.
Duplication cyst:
Angiodysplasia.
Angiodysplasia with von Willebrand disease.
Blue rubber bleb nevus syndrome.

ADOLESCENT

Common
Bacterial enteritis.
Inflammatory bowel disease.
Peptic ulcer/gastritis.
Prolapse (traumatic) gastropathy secondary to emesis.
Mallory-Weiss syndrome.
Colonic polyps.
Anal fissure.
Rare
Hemorrhoids.
Esophageal varices.
Esophagitis.
Pill ulcer.
Telangiectasia-angiodysplasia.
Graft versus host disease.
Duplication cyst:
Angiodysplasia.
Angiodysplasia with von Willebrand disease.
Blue rubber bleb nevus syndrome.

GASTROINTESTINAL OBSTRUCTION, PEDIATRIC PATIENT[59]

ICD-10CM #	K56.2	Volvulus
	K5.1	Intussusception
	K56.9	Ileus unspecified
	K56.6	Other and unspecified intestinal obstruction

Esophagus

Congenital
Esophageal atresia.
Vascular rings.
Schatzki ring.
Tracheobronchial remnant.
Acquired
Esophageal stricture.
Foreign body.
Achalasia.
Chagas disease.
Collagen vascular disease.

Stomach

Congenital
Antral webs.
Pyloric stenosis.

Acquired
Bezoar, foreign body.
Pyloric stricture (ulcer).
Chronic granulomatous disease of childhood.
Eosinophilic gastroenteritis.
Crohn disease.
Epidermolysis bullosa.

Small Intestine
Congenital
Duodenal atresia.
Annular pancreas.
Malrotation/volvulus.
Malrotation/Ladd bands.
Ileal atresia.
Meconium ileus.
Meckel diverticulum with volvulus or intussusception.
Inguinal hernia.
Internal hernia.
Intestinal duplication.
Pseudoobstruction.

Acquired
Postsurgical adhesions.
Crohn disease.
Intussusception.
Distal ileal obstruction syndrome (cystic fibrosis).
Duodenal hematoma.
Superior mesenteric artery syndrome.

Colon
Congenital
Meconium plug.
Hirschsprung disease.
Colonic atresia, stenosis.
Imperforate anus.
Rectal stenosis.
Pseudoobstruction.
Volvulus.
Colonic duplication.

Acquired
Ulcerative colitis (toxic megacolon).
Chagas disease.
Crohn disease.
Fibrosing colonopathy (cystic fibrosis).

GASTROINTESTINAL SYMPTOMS IN CHILDREN, NONDIGESTIVE CAUSES[59]

ICD-10CM # Varies with specific diagnosis

Anorexia
Systemic disease: inflammatory, neoplastic.
Cardiorespiratory compromise.
Iatrogenic: drug therapy, unpalatable therapeutic diets.
Depression.
Anorexia nervosa.

Vomiting
Inborn errors of metabolism.
Medications: erythromycin, chemotherapy, nonsteroidal antiinflammatory drugs, marijuana.
Increased intracranial pressure.
Brain tumor.
Infection of the urinary tract.
Labyrinthitis.
Adrenal insufficiency.
Pregnancy.
Psychogenic.
Abdominal migraine.
Poisoning/toxins.
Renal disease.

Diarrhea
Infection: otitis media, urinary tract infection.
Uremia.
Medications: antibiotics, cisapride.
Tumors: neuroblastoma.
Pericarditis.
Adrenal insufficiency.

Constipation
Hypothyroidism.
Spina bifida.
Developmental delay.
Dehydration: diabetes insipidus, renal tubular lesions.
Medications: narcotics.
Lead poisoning.
Infant botulism.

Abdominal Pain
Pyelonephritis, hydronephrosis, renal colic.
Pneumonia (lower lobe).
Pelvic inflammatory disease.
Porphyria.
Fabry disease.
Angioedema.
Endocarditis.
Abdominal migraine.
Familial Mediterranean fever.
Sexual or physical abuse.
Systemic lupus erythematosus.
School phobia.
Sickle cell crisis.
Vertebral disk inflammation.
Psoas abscess.
Pelvic osteomyelitis or myositis.
Medications.

Abdominal Distention Or Mass
Ascites: nephrotic syndrome, neoplasm, heart failure.
Discrete mass: Wilms tumor, hydronephrosis, neuroblastoma, mesenteric cyst, hepatoblastoma, lymphoma.
Pregnancy.

Jaundice
Hemolytic disease.
Urinary tract infection.
Sepsis.
Hypothyroidism.
Panhypopituitarism.

GENITAL DISCHARGE, FEMALE[28]

ICD-10CM #	N94.9	Unspecified condition associated with female genital organs and menstrual cycle

Physiologic discharge: cervical mucus, vaginal transudation, bacteria, squamous epithelial cells.
Individual variation.
Pregnancy.
Sexual response.
Menstrual cycle variation.
Infection.
Foreign body: tampon, cervical cap, other.
Neoplasm.
Fistula.
IUD.
Cervical ectropion.
Spermicide.
Nongenital causes: urinary incontinence, urinary tract fistula, Crohn disease, rectovaginal fistula.

GENITAL LESIONS, INFECTIOUS CAUSES[10]

ICD-10CM # Varies with specific diagnosis

INFECTIOUS CAUSES OF GENITAL LESIONS
Sexually Transmitted Infections
Syphilis:
  Primary (chancre).
  Secondary (condyloma latum).
Herpes simplex virus types 1 and 2.
Chancroid *(Haemophilus ducreyi).*
Lymphogranuloma venereum.
Granuloma inguinale (donovanosis).
Human papillomavirus.
Sarcoptes scabiei.
Molluscum contagiosum.

Nonsexually Transmitted Infections
Folliculitis.
Tuberculosis.
Tularemia.
Histoplasmosis.
Candida (balanitis or vaginitis).
Amebiasis.

GENITAL LESIONS, NONINFECTIOUS CAUSES[10]

ICD-10CM # Varies with specific diagnosis

NONVENEREAL CAUSES OF GENITAL LESIONS
Trauma.
Malignancies (e.g., squamous cell carcinoma).
Behçet syndrome.
Lipschütz vulvar ulcers.
Peyronie disease.
Fixed-drug eruption.
Eczema.
Psoriasis.
Inflammatory bowel disease.
Contact dermatitis.
Lichen planus.
Hidradenitis suppurativa.
Postinflammatory hypopigmentation.
Aphthous ulcers (associated with human immunodeficiency virus).

GENITAL SORES[3]

ICD-10CM #	A60.9	Anogenital herpesviral infection, unspecified
	A51.0	Primary genital syphilis
	A63.0	Anogenital (venereal) warts
	A57	Chancroid
	A58	Granuloma inguinale
	A55	Chlamydial lymphogranuloma (venereum)
	N94.89	Other specified conditions associated with female genital organs and menstrual cycle
	N50.8	Other specified disorders of male genital organs

Herpes genitalis.
Syphilis.
Chancroid.
Lymphogranuloma venereum.
Granuloma inguinale.
Condyloma acuminatum.
Neoplastic lesion.
Trauma.

GLOMERULONEPHRITIS ASSOCIATED WITH MALIGNANCY[87]

ICD-10CM # N00.9 Acute nephritic syndrome with unspecified morphologic changes

Membranous glomerulonephritis:
Breast cancer.
Lung cancer.
Colon cancer.
Prostate cancer.
Graft-versus-host disease.
Minimal change disease:
Hodgkin lymphoma.
Non-Hodgkin lymphoma.
Graft-versus-host disease.
Case reports.
Immunoglobulin A nephritis.
Antineutrophil cytoplasmic antibody vasculitis.
Focal segmental glomerulosclerosis.

GLOMERULONEPHRITIS, RAPIDLY PROGRESSIVE[3]

ICD-10CM # N05.9 Unspecified nephritic syndrome with unspecified morphologic changes

DIFFERENTIAL DIAGNOSIS OF RAPIDLY PROGRESSIVE GLOMERULONEPHRITIS

Linear Immune Staining
Anti-GBM disease.
Goodpasture syndrome.
Rarely membranous glomerulonephritis.
Granular Immune Staining
Subacute bacterial endocarditis (past infectious).
Lupus nephritis.
Cryoglobulinemia.
Membranoproliferative glomerulonephritis (type II more than type I).
Immunoglobulin A nephropathy, Henoch-Schönlein purpura.
Idiopathic.
No Immune Staining (Pauci-immune)
Antineutrophil cytoplasmic antibody-associated vasculitis (Wegener granulomatosis, microscopic polyangiitis, Churg-Strauss syndrome).
Idiopathic.

GLOMERULOPATHIES, THROMBOTIC, MICROANGIOPATHIC[3]

ICD-10CM # M31.1 Thrombotic microangiopathy

THROMBOTIC MICROANGIOPATHIC GLOMERULOPATHIES

Thrombotic thrombocytopenic purpura.
Hemolytic-uremic syndrome.
Malignant hypertension.
Scleroderma renal crisis.
Preeclampsia, eclampsia.
HELLP syndrome (hemolysis, elevated liver enzymes, low platelets).
Antiphospholipid antibody syndrome.
Drugs: oral contraceptives, quinine, cyclosporine, tacrolimus, ticlopidine, clopidogrel.

GLOMERULOSCLEROSIS, FOCAL SEGMENTAL[3]

ICD-10CM # N03.3 Chronic nephritic syndrome with diffuse mesangial proliferative glomerulonephritis

ETIOLOGY OF FOCAL SEGMENTAL GLOMERULOSCLEROSIS (FSGS)

Primary idiopathic FSGS.
Secondary FSGS.
HIV (usually collapsing variant).
Reflux nephropathy.
Heroin abuse.
Sickle cell disease.
Oligomeganephronia.
Renal dysgenesis or agenesis (low nephron mass).
Radiation nephritis.
Familial podocytopathies.
NPHS1 (nephrin) mutation.
NPHS2 (podocin) mutation.
TRPC6 (cation channel) mutation.
ACTN4 (a-actinin 4 mutation).

GLOSSODYNIA[95]

ICD-10CM # K14.6 Glossodynia

DENTURE-RELATED

Dentures (ill-fitting, monomer from denture base).
Dental plaque.
Oral parafunction.

INFECTIVE/DERMATOLOGIC

Candidiasis.
Lichen planus.

DEFICIENCY STATES

Iron, vitamin B_{12}, folate, B_2 (riboflavin), B_6 (pyridoxine), zinc.

ENDOCRINE

Diabetes.
Myxedema.
Hormonal changes occurring during menopause.

NEUROLOGICALLY MEDIATED

Referred from tonsils, teeth.
Lingual nerve neuropathy.
Glossopharyngeal neuralgia.
Esophageal reflux.

IATROGENIC

Mouthwash.

XEROSTOMIA

PSYCHOGENIC DIOPATHIC

GLUCOCORTICOID DEFICIENCY[36]

ICD-10CM # E27.1 Primary adrenocortical insufficiency
E27.3 Drug-induced adrenocortical insufficiency

ACTH-independent causes.
TB.
Autoimmune (idiopathic).
Other rare causes:
- Fungal infection.
- Adrenal hemorrhage.
- Metastases.
- Sarcoidosis.
- Amyloidosis.
- Adrenoleukodystrophy.
- Adrenomyeloneuropathy.
- HIV infection.
- Congenital adrenal hyperplasia.
- Medications (e.g., ketoconazole).

ACTH-dependent causes:
- Hypothalamic-pituitary-adrenal suppression.
- Exogenous.
- Glucocorticoid.
- ACTH.
- Endogenous—cure of Cushing syndrome.

Hypothalamic-pituitary lesions.
- Neoplasm:
  - Primary pituitary tumor.
  - Metastatic tumor.
  - Craniopharyngioma.
- Infection:
  - Tuberculosis.
  - Actinomycosis.
  - Nocardiosis.
- Sarcoid.
- Head trauma.
- Isolated ACTH deficiency.

GOITER

ICD-10CM # E01.2 Iodine-deficiency related (endemic) goiter, unspecified
E04.9 Nontoxic goiter, unspecified
E04.9 Nontoxic goiter, unspecified
E07.1 Dyshormogenetic goiter
E01.2 Iodine-deficiency related (endemic) goiter, unspecified
E04.9 Nontoxic goiter, unspecified
E04.2 Nontoxic multinodular goiter

	E04.0	Nontoxic diffuse goiter
	E05.10	Thyrotoxicosis with toxic single thyroid nodule without thyrotoxic crisis or storm

Thyroiditis.
Toxic multinodular goiter.
Graves disease.
Medications (PTU, methimazole, sulfonamides, sulfonylureas, ethionamide, amiodarone, lithium, etc.).
Iodine deficiency.
Sarcoidosis, amyloidosis.
Defective thyroid hormone synthesis.
Resistance to thyroid hormone.

GRANULOMATOUS DERMATITIDES

ICD-10CM #	L92.9	Granulomatous disorder of the skin and subcutaneous tissue, unspecified

Granuloma annulare.
Sarcoidosis.
Necrobiosis lipoidica diabeticorum.
Cutaneous Crohn disease.
Rheumatoid nodules.
Annular elastolytic giant cell granuloma (actinic granuloma).
Foreign body granuloma.

GRANULOMATOUS DISORDERS[83]

ICD-10CM #	M31.30	Granulomatosis with polyangiitis without renal involvement
	K75.3	Granulomatous hepatitis
	L92.9	Granulomatous disorder of skin and subcutaneous tissue, unspecified

INFECTIONS

Fungi
Histoplasma.
Coccidioides.
Blastomyces.
Sporothrix.
Aspergillus.
Cryptococcus.
Protozoa
Toxoplasma.
Leishmania.
Metazoa
Toxocara.
Schistosoma.
Spirochetes
Treponema pallidum.
T. pertenue.
T. carateum.
Mycobacteria
M. tuberculosis.
M. leprae.
M. kansasii.
M. marinum.
M. avian.
Bacille Calmette-Guérin (BCG) vaccine.
Bacteria
Brucella.
Yersinia.
Other Infections
Cat-scratch disease.
Lymphogranuloma.

NEOPLASIA

Carcinoma.
Reticulosis.
Pinealoma.
Dysgerminoma.
Seminoma.
Reticulum cell sarcoma.
Malignant nasal granuloma.

CHEMICALS

Beryllium.
Zirconium.
Silica.
Starch.

IMMUNOLOGIC ABERRATIONS

Sarcoidosis.
Crohn disease.
Primary biliary cirrhosis.
Granulomatosis with polyangiitis.
Giant cell arteritis.
Peyronie disease.
Hypogammaglobulinemia.
SLE.
Lymphomatoid granulomatosis.
Histiocytosis X.
Hepatic granulomatous disease.
Immune complex disease.
Rosenthal-Melkersson syndrome.
Churg-Strauss allergic granulomatosis.

LEUKOCYTE OXIDASE DEFECT

Chronic granulomatous disease of childhood.

EXTRINSIC ALLERGIC ALVEOLITIS

Farmer's lung.
Bird fancier's.
Mushroom worker's.
Suberosis (cork dust).
Bagassosis.
Maple bark stripper's.
Paprika splitter's.
Coffee bean.
Spatlese lung.

OTHER DISORDERS

Whipple disease.
Pyrexia of unknown origin.
Radiotherapy.
Cancer chemotherapy.
Panniculitis.
Chalazion.
Sebaceous cyst.
Dermoid.
Sea urchin spine injury.

GRANULOMATOUS LIVER DISEASE

ICD-10CM #	K75.3	Granulomatous hepatitis

Sarcoidosis.
Granulomatosis with polyangiitis.
Vasculitis.
Inflammatory bowel disease.
Allergic granulomatosis.
Erythema nodosum.
Infections (fungal, viral, parasitic).
Primary biliary cirrhosis.
Lymphoma.
Hodgkin disease.
Drugs (e.g., allopurinol, hydralazine, sulfonamides, penicillins).
Toxins (copper sulfate, beryllium).

GREEN OR BLUE URINE

ICD-10CM #	R82	Other abnormal findings in urine

Pseudomonal urinary tract infection
Medications: triamterene, amitriptyline, IV cimetidine, IV promethazine.
Biliverdin.
Dyes (methylene blue, indigo carmine).

GROIN LUMP[95]

ICD-10CM #	R19.09	Other intraabdominal and pelvic swelling, mass and lump
	R22.9	Localized swelling, mass and lump, unspecified

COMMON CAUSES

Inguinal hernia.
Femoral hernia.
Lymph node.

OTHER CAUSES

Saphena varix.
Femoral artery aneurysm/pseudoaneurysm.
Psoas abscess.
Lipoma of the cord.
Encysted hydrocele of the cord (male).
Testicular maldescent (male).
Hydrocele of canal of Nuck (female).

GROIN MASSES

ICD-10CM #	R22.9	Localized swelling, mass and lump, unspecified
	S39.848A	Other specified injuries of external genitals, initial encounter

Hernia (inguinal, femoral).
Hydrocele.
Varicocele.
Sebaceous cyst.
Hidradenitis of inguinal apocrine glands.
Neoplasm: lymphoma, metastases.

Lipoma.
Hematoma.
Reactive inguinal adenopathy, femoral adenitis.
Folliculitis, psoas abscess.
Epididymitis, testicular torsion, ectopic testes.
Aneurysm or pseudoaneurysm of femoral artery.

GROIN PAIN[17]

ICD-10CM # R52 Pain, unspecified

DIFFERENTIAL DIAGNOSIS OF GROIN PAIN

Surgery
Workers' Compensation.
Hernia.
Recurrent hernia.
Posthernia.
Orthopedic
Hip disorders:
- Acetabular labral tears.
- Avascular necrosis.
- Chondritis dissecans.
- Legg-Calvé-Perthes disease.
- Osteoarthritis.
- Pelvic stress fractures.
- Slipped femoral capital epiphysis.
- Synovitis.

Urology
Cystitis.
Epididymitis.
Nephrolithiasis.
Prostate cancer.
Prostatitis.
Torsion of testes.
Urethral extravasation.
Urinary tract infection.
Vas granuloma/fibrosis.
Dermatology
Lymphadenitis.
Psoriasis/burn.
Sebaceous cyst/hidradenitis.
Thrombophlebitis/cellulitis.
Neurosurgery
Disk disease.
Spinal injuries, inflammation, tumors.
Spondylolisthesis.
Spondylolysis.
Rheumatology
Connective tissue disorders.
Iliopsoas bursitis.
Osteitis pubis.
Systemic lupus erythematosus.
Neurology
Lumbosacral disorders.
Neurofibromatosis.
Infectious Disease
Herpes zoster.
HIV/tuberculosis.
Lyme disease.
Psoas abscess.
Sports Medicine
"Sports hernia" (adductor strains).
Gilmore groin.
Vascular
Abscess hematoma.
Post-vein stripping.
Pseudoaneurysm.
Vascular graft.
Gastroenterology
Appendicitis/adhesions.
Diverticulitis.
Inflammatory retroperitoneal phlegmon (pancreatitis).
Meckel diverticulum.
Granulomatous colitis.
Gynecology
Cesarean section.
Cervical cancer.
Endometriosis.
Tubal/ovarian disorders.

GROIN PAIN, ACTIVE PATIENT[94]

ICD-10CM #	S39.848A	Other specified injuries of external genitals, initial encounter
	R52	Pain, unspecified

MUSCULOSKELETAL

Avascular necrosis of the femoral head.
Avulsion fracture (lesser trochanter, anterior superior iliac spine, anterior inferior iliac spine).
Bursitis (iliopectineal, trochanteric).
Entrapment of the ilioinguinal or iliofemoral nerve.
Gracilis syndrome.
Muscle tear (adductors, iliopsoas, rectus abdominis, gracilis, sartorius, rectus femoris).
Myositis ossificans of the hip muscles.
Osteitis pubis.
Osteoarthritis of the femoral head.
Slipped capital femoral epiphysis.
Stress fracture of the femoral head or neck and pubis.
Synovitis.

HERNIA-RELATED

Avulsion of the internal oblique muscle in the conjoined tendon.
Defect at the insertion of the rectus abdominis muscle.
Direct inguinal hernia.
Femoral ring hernia.
Indirect inguinal hernia.
Inguinal canal weakness.

UROLOGIC

Epididymitis.
Fracture of the testis.
Hydrocele.
Kidney stone.
Posterior urethritis.
Prostatitis.
Testicular cancer.
Torsion of the testis.
Urinary tract infection.
Varicocele.

GYNECOLOGIC

Ectopic pregnancy.
Ovarian cyst.
Pelvic inflammatory disease.
Torsion of the ovary.
Vaginitis.

LYMPHATIC ENLARGEMENT IN GROIN

GROIN PAIN, ATHLETES[18]

ICD-10CM # R52 Pain, unspecified

DIFFERENTIAL DIAGNOSIS OF GROIN PAIN IN ATHLETES

Hip-Associated Causes
- Acetabular labral tear and femoroacetabular impingement.
- Osteoarthritis.
- Snapping hip syndrome and iliopsoas tendonitis.
- Avascular necrosis.
- Iliotibial band syndrome.

Visceral Causes
- Inguinal hernia.
- Other abdominal hernias.
- Testicular torsion.

Infectious Causes
- Septic arthritis.
- Osteomyelitis.
- Pelvic inflammatory disease.
- Prostatitis.
- Epididymitis and orchitis.
- Herpes infection.

Inflammatory Causes
- Endometriosis.
- Inflammatory bowel disease.
- Pelvic inflammatory disease.
- Primary osteitis pubis.

Traumatic Causes
- Stress fracture.
- Tendon avulsion.
- Muscle contusion.
- Baseball pitcher–hockey goalie syndrome.

Developmental Causes
- Apophysitis.
- Growth plate stress injury or fracture.
- Legg-Calvé-Perthes disease.
- Developmental dysplasia.
- Slipped capital femoral epiphysis.

Neurologic Causes
- Nerve entrapment syndromes.
- Referred pain.
- Sacroiliitis.
- Sciatic entrapment (piriformis syndrome).
- Hamstring strain.
- Knee pain.

Neoplastic Causes
- Testicular carcinoma.
- Osteoid osteoma.

GYNECOMASTIA

ICD-10CM # N62 Hypertrophy of breast

Physiologic (puberty, newborns, aging).
Drugs (estrogen and estrogen precursors, 5-a reductase inhibitors, digitalis, testosterone and exogenous androgens, clomiphene, cimetidine, spironolactone, ketoconazole, amiodarone, ACE inhibitors, isoniazid, phenytoin, methyldopa, metoclopramide, phenothiazine).
Increased prolactin level (prolactinoma).
Liver disease.
Adrenal disease.

Thyrotoxicosis.
Increased estrogen production (hCG-producing tumor, testicular tumor, bronchogenic carcinoma).
Secondary hypogonadism.
Primary gonadal failure (trauma, castration, viral orchitis, granulomatous disease).
Defects in androgen synthesis.
Testosterone deficiency.
Klinefelter syndrome.

HAIR LOSS[43]

ICD-10CM #	L63.8	Other alopecia areata
	L63.9	Alopecia areata, unspecified
	L64.0	Drug-induced androgenic alopecia
	L64.8	Other androgenic alopecia

GENERALIZED

Acute blood loss.*
Childbirth.
Crash diets (inadequate protein).
Drugs:
  Coumarin.
  Heparin.
  Propranolol.
  Vitamin A.
  High fever.
Hypothyroidism and hyperthyroidisms.
Physical stress (e.g., surgery).
Physiologic stress (e.g., neonate).
Psychologic stress.
Severe illness (e.g., systemic lupus erythematosis).
Cancer chemotherapeutic agents.
Poisoning:
  Thallium (rat poison).
  Arsenic.
Radiation therapy.
Secondary syphilis: "moth eaten" alopecia.

LOCALIZED

Androgenetic alopecia:†
  Male pattern.
  Female pattern.
Hirsutism.
Alopecia areata.
Trichotillomania.
Traction alopecia.
Scarring alopecia:
  Developmental defects: aplasia cutis.
Physical injury: burns, pressure.
Infection:
  Fungal: kerion.
  Bacterial: folliculitis, furuncle.
  Viral: herpes zoster.
Neoplasms:
  Metastatic carcinoma.
  Sclerosing basal cell carcinoma.
Lupus erythematosus.
Lichen planus.

*Diffuse, uniform loss, but many hairs left randomly distributed in area of loss.
†Most or all hair missing from involved area.

Cicatricial pemphigoid.
Scleroderma.

HALITOSIS

ICD-10CM #	R19.6	Halitosis

Tobacco use.
Alcohol use.
Dry mouth (mouth breathing, inadequate fluid intake).
Foods (onion, garlic, meats, nuts, protein drinks).
Disease of mouth or nose (infections, cancer, inflammation).
Medications (antihistamines, antidepressants).
Systemic disorders (diabetes, uremia).
GI disorders (esophageal diverticula, hiatal hernia, GERD, achalasia).
Sinusitis.
Pulmonary disorders (bronchiectasis, pneumonia, neoplasms, TB).

HALLUCINATIONS, VISUAL, NEUROLOGIC CAUSES[56]

ICD-10CM #	R44.1	Visual hallucinations

Blindness/sensory deprivation—Charles Bonnet syndrome.
Palinopsia.
Dementia-producing diseases:
  Alzheimer.
  Dementia with Lewy bodies.*
  Parkinson.†
Intoxications:
  Alcoholic hallucinosis.
    Delirium tremens (DTs).
Hallucinogens:
  Amphetamines.
  Cocaine.
  Lysergic acid diethylamide (LSD).
  Phencyclidine (PCP).
Medicines:
  Atropine, scopolamine.
  Levodopa and dopamine agonists.
  Steroids.
Migraine with aura (classic migraine).
Narcolepsy: hypnopompic (awakening) and hypnagogic (falling asleep) hallucinations.
Seizures.
Peduncular hallucinations.

HAND PAIN AND SWELLING[20]

ICD-10CM #	729.5	Pain in limb

Trauma.
Gout.
Pseudogout.
Cellulitis.
Lymphangitis.
DVT of upper extremity.
Thrombophlebitis.

*Although visual hallucinations are likely to complicate almost any form of dementia, they are characteristic of dementia with Lewy bodies disease.
†Dopaminergic medications such as levodopa-carbidopa (Sinemet) are more likely than Parkinson disease itself to produce hallucinations.

RA.
Remitting seronegative symmetrical synovitis with pitting edema (RS3PE).
Polymyalgia rheumatica.
Mixed connective tissue disease.
Scleroderma.
Rupture of the olecranon bursa.
Metzger syndrome (neoplasia).
The puffy hand of drug addiction.
Reflex sympathetic dystrophy.
Eosinophilic fasciitis.
Sickle cell (hand-foot syndrome).
Leprosy.
Factitial (the rubber band syndrome).

HEADACHE[35]

ICD-10CM #	G44.1	Vascular headache, not elsewhere classified
	R51	Headache
	G44.209	Tension-type headache, unspecified, not intractable
	G44.009	Cluster headache syndrome, unspecified, not intractable
	G43.909	Migraine, unspecified, not intractable, without status migrainosus
	G44.1	Vascular headache, not elsewhere classified

Vascular: migraine, cluster headaches, temporal arteritis, hypertension, cavernous sinus thrombosis.
Musculoskeletal: neck and shoulder muscle contraction, strain of extraocular and/or intraocular muscles, cervical spondylosis, temporomandibular arthritis.
Infections: meningitis, encephalitis, brain abscess, sepsis, sinusitis, osteomyelitis, parotitis, mastoiditis.
Cerebral neoplasm.
Subdural hematoma.
Cerebral hemorrhage/infarct.
Pseudotumor cerebri.
Normal-pressure hydrocephalus (NPH).
Postlumbar puncture.
Cerebral aneurysm, arteriovenous malformations.
Posttrauma.
Dental problems: abscess, periodontitis, poorly fitting dentures.
Trigeminal neuralgia, glossopharyngeal neuralgia.
Otitis and other ear diseases.
Glaucoma and other eye diseases.
Metabolic: uremia, carbon monoxide inhalation, hypoxia.
Pheochromocytoma, hypoglycemia, hypothyroidism.
Effort induced: benign exertional headache, cough, headache, coital cephalalgia.
Drugs: alcohol, nitrates, histamine antagonists.
Paget disease of the skull.
Emotional, psychiatric.

HEADACHE, ACUTE[27]

ICD-10CM # R51 Headache

DIFFERENTIAL DIAGNOSIS OF ACUTE HEADACHE

Evaluation of the first acute headache should exclude pathologic causes listed here before consideration of more common etiologies.
Increased intracranial pressure (ICP): trauma, hemorrhage, tumor, hydrocephalus, pseudotumor cerebri, abscess, arachnoid cyst, cerebral edema.
Decreased ICP: after ventriculoperitoneal shunt, lumbar puncture, cerebrospinal fluid leak from basilar skull fracture.
Meningeal inflammation: meningitis, leukemia, subarachnoid or subdural hemorrhage.
Vascular: Vasculitis, arteriovenous malformation, hypertension, cerebrovascular accident.
Bone, soft tissue: referred pain from scalp, eyes, ears, sinuses, nose, teeth, pharynx, cervical spine, temporomandibular joint.
Infection: systemic infection, encephalitis, sinusitis, etc.
First migraine.

HEADACHE AND FACIAL PAIN[91]

ICD-10CM #		
	R51	Headache
	G44.1	Vascular headache, not elsewhere classified

VASCULAR HEADACHES

Migraine

Migraine with headaches and inconspicuous neurologic features:
Migraine without aura ("common migraine").
Migraine with headaches and conspicuous neurologic features:
With transient neurologic symptoms:
Migraine with typical aura ("classic migraine").
Sensory, basilar, and hemiplegic migraine.
With prolonged or permanent neurologic features ("complicated migraine"):
Ophthalmoplegic migraine.
Migrainous infarction.
Migraine without headaches but with conspicuous neurologic features ("migraine equivalents"):
Abdominal migraine.
Benign paroxysmal vertigo of childhood.
Migraine aura without headache ("isolated auras," transient migrainous accompaniments).

Cluster Headaches

Episodic cluster headache ("cyclic cluster headaches").
Chronic cluster headaches.
Chronic paroxysmal hemicrania.

Other Vascular Headaches

Headaches of reactive vasodilation (fever, drug-induced, postictal, hypoglycemia, hypoxia, hypercarbia, hyperthyroidism).
Headaches associated with arterial hypertension:
Chronic severe hypertension (diastolic 120 mm Hg).
Paroxysmal severe hypertension (pheochromocytoma, some coital headaches).
Headaches caused by cranial arteritis:
Giant cell arteritis ("temporal arteritis").
Other vasculitides.

HEADACHES ASSOCIATED WITH DEMONSTRABLE MUSCLE SPASM

Headache caused by posturally induced or perilesional muscle spasm:
Headaches of sustained or impaired posture (e.g., prolonged close work, driving).
Headaches associated with cervical spondylosis and other diseases of cervical spine.
Myofascial pain dysfunction syndrome (headache or facial pain associated with disorders of teeth, jaws, and related structures, or "TMJ syndrome").
Headaches caused by psychophysiologic muscular contraction ("muscle contraction headaches," or tension-type headache associated with disorder of pericranial muscles).

HEADACHES AND FACIAL PAIN WITHOUT DEMONSTRABLE PHYSICAL SUBSTRATE

Headaches of uncertain etiology:
"Tension headaches" (tension-type headache unassociated with disorder of pericranial muscles).
Some forms of posttraumatic headache.
Psychogenic headaches (e.g., hypochondriacal, conversional, delusional, malingered).
Facial pain of uncertain etiology ("atypical facial pain").

COMBINED TENSION-MIGRAINE HEADACHES

Episodic migraine superimposed on chronic tension headaches.
Chronic daily headaches:
Associated with analgesic and/or ergotamine overuse ("rebound headaches").
Not associated with drug overuse.

HEADACHES AND HEAD PAINS CAUSED BY DISEASES OF EYES, EARS, NOSE, SINUSES, TEETH, OR SKULL

Headaches Caused by Meningeal Inflammation

Subarachnoid hemorrhage.
Meningitis and meningoencephalitis.
Others (e.g., meningeal carcinomatosis).

HEADACHES ASSOCIATED WITH ALTERED INTRACRANIAL PRESSURE ("TRACTION HEADACHES")

Increased Intracranial Pressure

Intracranial mass lesions (neoplasm, hematoma, abscess, etc.).
Hydrocephalus.
Benign intracranial hypertension.
Venous sinus thrombosis.

Decreased Intracranial Pressure

Post-lumbar puncture headaches.
Spontaneous hypoliquorrheic headaches.

HEADACHES AND HEAD PAINS CAUSED BY CRANIAL NEURALGIAS

Presumed Irritation of Superficial Nerves

Occipital neuralgia.
Supraorbital neuralgia.

Presumed Irritation of Intracranial Nerves

Trigeminal neuralgia ("tic douloureux").
Glossopharyngeal neuralgia.

HEADACHE, CHRONIC[27]

ICD-10CM # R51 Headache

DIFFERENTIAL DIAGNOSIS OF RECURRENT OR CHRONIC HEADACHES

Migraine (with or without aura).
Tension.
Analgesic rebound.
Caffeine withdrawal.
Sleep deprivation (e.g., in children with sleep apnea) or chronic hypoxia.
Tumor.
Psychogenic: conversion disorder, malingering.
Cluster headache.

HEAD AND NECK, SOFT TISSUE MASSES

ICD-10CM #		
	R22.0	Localized swelling, mass and lump, head
	R22.1	Localized swelling, mass and lump, neck

Lipoma.
Pilar cyst.
Epidermal inclusion cyst.
Dermoid cyst.
Bone cyst.
Hemangioma.
Eosinophilic granuloma.
Other: facial nerve neuroma, teratoma, rhabdomyoma, rhabdomyosarcoma, branchial cleft cyst.

HEARING LOSS, ACUTE[63]

ICD-10CM # H91.23 Sudden idiopathic hearing loss, bilateral

Infectious: mumps, measles, influenza, herpes simplex, herpes zoster, CMV, mononucleosis, syphilis.
Vascular: macroglobulinemia, sickle cell disease, Berger disease, leukemia, polycythemia, fat emboli, hypercoagulable states.
Metabolic: diabetes, pregnancy, hyperlipoproteinemia.
Conductive: cerumen impaction, foreign bodies, otitis media, otitis externa, barotrauma, trauma.
Medications: aminoglycosides, loop diuretics, antineoplastics, salicylates, vancomycin.
Neoplasm: acoustic neuroma, metastatic neoplasm.

HEARTBURN AND INDIGESTION[84]

ICD-10CM # R12 Heartburn
K30 Functional dyspepsia

Reflux esophagitis.
Gastritis.
Nonulcer dyspepsia.
Functional GI disorder (anxiety disorder, social/environmental stresses).
Excessive intestinal gas (ingestion of flatulogenic foods, GI stasis, constipation).
Gas entrapment (hepatitis or splenic flexure syndrome).
Neoplasm (adenocarcinoma of stomach or esophagus, lymphoma).
Gallbladder disease.

HEART DISEASE, TRAUMATIC CAUSES[64]

ICD-10CM # S26.020 Mild laceration of heart with hemopericardium
S26.021 Moderate laceration of heart with hemopericardium
S26.022 Major laceration of heart with hemopericardium

Penetrating:
- Stab wounds: knives, swords, ice picks, fence posts, wire, sports.
- Projectile wounds: handguns, rifles, nail guns, lawnmower projectiles.
- Shotgun wounds: pellets, close-range versus distant.

Nonpenetrating (blunt):
- Motor vehicle accident:
  - Seat belt.
  - Air bag.
  - Dashboard/steering wheel.

Vehicular-pedestrian accident.
Falls from a height.
Crushing: industrial accident.
Blasts: improvised explosive devices, grenades, fragments (combined blunt/penetrating).
Assault.
Sternal or rib fractures.
Recreational: sporting events (e.g., rodeo, baseball).

HEART FAILURE WITH PRESERVED LEFT VENTRICULAR EJECTION FRACTION[38]

ICD-10CM # I50.9 Heart failure, unspecified

CAUSES OF (AND ALTERNATIVE EXPLANATIONS FOR) HEART FAILURE WITH PRESERVED LEFT VENTRICULAR EJECTION FRACTION (>45% TO 50%)

Inaccurate diagnosis of heart failure (e.g., pulmonary disease, obesity).
Inaccurate measurements of ejection fraction.
Systolic function overestimated by ejection fraction (e.g., mitral regurgitation).
Episodic, unrecognized systolic dysfunction.
Intermittent ischemia.
Arrhythmia.
Severe hypertension.
Alcohol abuse.
Diastolic dysfunction.
Abnormalities of myocardial relaxation:
- Ischemia.
- Hypertrophy.

Abnormalities of myocardial compliance:
- Hypertrophy.
- Aging.
- Fibrosis.
- Diabetes mellitus.
- Infiltrative disease (amyloidosis, sarcoidosis).
- Storage disease (hemochromatosis).
- Endomyocardial disease (endomyocardial fibrosis, radiation, anthracyclines).

Pericardial disease (constriction, tamponade).

HEART FAILURE, ACUTE[7]

ICD-10CM # I50.9 Heart failure, unspecified

COMMON PRECIPITATING CAUSES OF ACUTE HF

Systemic hypertension.
Myocardial infarction or ischemia.
Dysrhythmia.
Systemic infection.
Anemia.
Dietary, physical, environmental, and emotional excesses.
Pregnancy.
Thyrotoxicosis or hypothyroidism.
Acute myocarditis.
Acute valvular dysfunction.
Pulmonary embolus.
Pharmacologic complications.

HEART FAILURE, CHRONIC[12]

ICD-10CM # I50.9 Heart failure, unspecified

Myocardial disease.
Coronary artery disease:
- Myocardial infarction.[25]
- Myocardial ischemia.

Chronic pressure overload:
- Hypertension.
- Obstructive valvular disease.

Chronic volume overload:
- Regurgitant valvular disease.
- Intracardiac (left-to-right) shunting.
- Extracardiac shunting.

Nonischemic dilated cardiomyopathy:
- Familial or genetic disorders.
- Infiltrative disorders.
- Toxic or drug-induced damage.
- Metabolic disorder.
- Viral or other infectious agents.

Disorders of rate and rhythm:
- Chronic bradyarrhythmias.
- Chronic tachyarrhythmias.

Pulmonary heart disease
- Cor pulmonale.
- Pulmonary vascular disorders.

High-output states.
Metabolic disorders:
- Thyrotoxicosis.
- Nutritional disorders (beriberi).

Excessive blood flow requirements:
- Systemic arteriovenous shunting.
- Chronic anemia.

[25] Indicates conditions that can also lead to HF with a preserved EF.

HEART FAILURE, CONGENITAL HEART DISEASE CAUSES[75]

ICD-10CM # I50.9 Heart failure, unspecified

CAUSES OF CONGESTIVE HEART FAILURE RESULTING FROM CONGENITAL HEART DISEASE

Age of Onset	Cause
At birth:	HLHS. Volume overload lesions:Severe tricuspid or pulmonary insufficiency. Large systemic arteriovenous fistula.
First week	TGA. PDA in small premature infants. HLHS (with more favorable anatomy). TAPVR, particularly those with pulmonary venous obstruction. Others. Systemic arteriovenous fistula. Critical AS or PS.
1-4 wk	COA with associated anomalies. Critical AS. Large left-to-right shunt lesions (VSD, PDA) in premature infants. All other lesions previously listed.
4-6 wk	Some left-to-right shunt lesions such as ECD.
6 wk-4 mo	Large VSD. Large PDA. Others, such as anomalous left coronary artery from the PA.

AS, Aortic stenosis; *COA,* coarctation of the aorta; *ECD,* endocardial cushion defect; *HLHS,* hypoplastic left heart syndrome; *PA,* pulmonary artery; *PDA,* patent ductus arteriosus; *PS,* pulmonary stenosis; *TAPVR,* total anomalous pulmonary venous return; *TGA,* transposition of the great arteries; *VSD,* ventricular septal defect.

HEART FAILURE, PATHOGENIC CAUSES[38]

ICD-10CM # I50.9 Heart failure, unspecified

IMPAIRED SYSTOLIC (CONTRACTILE) FUNCTION

Ischemic damage or dysfunction:
- Myocardial infarction.
- Persistent or intermittent myocardial ischemia.
- Hypoperfusion (shock).

Chronic pressure overloading:
- Hypertension.
- Obstructive valvular disease.

Chronic volume overload:
- Regurgitant valvular disease.
- Intracardiac left-to-right shunting.
- Extracardiac shunting.

Nonischemic dilated cardiomyopathy:
- Familial/genetic disorders.
- Toxic/drug-induced damage
- Immunologically mediated necrosis.
- Infectious agents.
- Metabolic disorders.
- Infiltrative processes.
- Idiopathic conditions.

IMPAIRED DIASTOLIC FUNCTION (RESTRICTED FILLING, INCREASED STIFFNESS)

Pathologic myocardial hypertrophy:
- Primary (hypertrophic cardiomyopathies).
- Secondary (hypertension).
- Aging.
- Ischemic fibrosis.
- Restrictive cardiomyopathy:
  - Infiltrative disorders (amyloidosis, sarcoidosis).
  - Storage diseases (hemochromatosis, genetic abnormalities).

Endomyocardial disorders.

MECHANICAL ABNORMALITIES

Intracardiac:
- Obstructive valvular disease.
- Regurgitant valvular disease.
- Intracardiac shunts.
- Other congenital abnormalities.

Extracardiac:
- Obstructive (coarctation, supravalvular aortic stenosis).
- Left-to-right shunting (patent ductus arteriosus).

DISORDERS OF RATE AND RHYTHM

Bradyarrhythmias (sinus node dysfunction, conduction abnormalities).
Tachyarrhythmias (ineffective rhythms, chronic tachycardia).

PULMONARY HEART DISEASE

Cor pulmonale.
Pulmonary vascular disorders.

HIGH-OUTPUT STATES

Metabolic disorders:
- Thyrotoxicosis.
- Nutritional disorders (beriberi).
- Excessive blood flow requirements:
  - Chronic anemia.
  - Systemic arteriovenous shunting.

HEART FAILURE, PREGNANCY

ICD-10CM # I50.9 Heart failure, unspecified

Congenital valvular heart disease exacerbated by pregnancy.
Peripartum cardiomyopathy.
Untreated thyrotoxicosis.
Hypothyroidism.
Pulmonary hypertension.
Myocardial infarction.

HEAT STROKE[1]

ICD-10CM # T67.0 Heatstroke and sunstroke

Sepsis.
Encephalitis.
Meningitis.
Brain abscess.
Malaria (cerebral falciparum).
Typhoid fever.
Tetanus.
Alcohol withdrawal syndrome.
Neuroleptic malignant syndrome.
Anticholinergic toxicity.
Salicylate toxicity.
Phencyclidine hydrochloride (PCP), cocaine, or amphetamine toxicity.
Status epilepticus.
Cerebral hemorrhage.
Diabetic ketoacidosis.
Thyroid storm.

HEEL PAIN

ICD-10CM # M25.50 Pain in unspecified joint

Achilles tendonitis/tendinopathy (insertional, noninsertional).
Retrocalcaneal bursitis (superficial, deep).
Plantar fasciopathy.
Neuropathy (tarsal tunnel, posterior tibial nerve [medial calcaneal branch], abductor digiti quinti).
Calcaneal stress fracture.
Puncture wound, foreign body.
Cellulitis.
Spondyloarthropathy.
Fat pad atrophy.
Soft tissue tumor.
S1 radiculopathy.
Paget disease of bone.
Haglund deformity.
Primary or metastatic bone tumor.

HEEL PAIN, PLANTAR[55]

ICD-10CM # M79.609 Pain in unspecified limb

SKIN

Keratoses.
Verruca.
Ulcer.
Fissure.

CONNECTIVE TISSUE

Fat

Atrophy.
Panniculitis.

Dense Connective Tissue

Inflammatory fasciitis.
Fibromatosis.
Enthesopathy.
Bursitis.

Bone (Calcaneus)

Stress fracture.
Paget disease.
Benign bone cyst/tumor.
Malignant bone tumor.
Metabolic bone disease (osteopenia).

Nerve

Tarsal tunnel.
Plantar nerve entrapment.
S1 nerve root radiculopathy.
Painful peripheral neuropathy.

INFECTION

Dermatomycoses.
Acute osteomyelitis.
Plantar abscess.

MISCELLANEOUS

Foreign body.
Nonunion calcaneus fracture.
Psychogenic.
Idiopathic.

HEMARTHROSIS

ICD-10CM # T14.90 Injury, unspecified

Trauma.
Anticoagulant therapy.
Thrombocytopenia, thrombocytosis.
Bleeding disorders (e.g., von Willebrand disease).
Charcot joint.
Idiopathic.
Other: pigmented villonodular synovitis, hemangioma, synovioma, AV fistula, ruptured aneurysm.

HEMATEMESIS[95]

ICD-10CM # K92.0 Hematemesis

CAUSES OF HEMATEMESIS

Very Common

Gastric or duodenal ulcer or erosions.

Common

Mallory-Weiss tear (a laceration at the gastroesophageal junction).
Ulcerative esophagitis.
Esophageal varices.

Uncommon

Vascular malformations.
Ulcerated GI stromal tumor.
Carcinoma of esophagus or stomach.
Aortoenteric fistula.

HEMATURIA

ICD-10CM # R31.9 Hematuria, unspecified

Use the mnemonic TICS:

T (Trauma): blow to kidney, insertion of Foley catheter or foreign body in urethra, prolonged and severe exercise, very rapid emptying of overdistended bladder. (Tumor): hypernephroma, Wilms tumor, papillary carcinoma of the bladder, prostatic and urethral neoplasms.(Toxins): turpentine, phenols, sulfonamides and other antibiotics, cyclophosphamide, NSAIDs.

I (Infections): glomerulonephritis, TB, cystitis, prostatitis, urethritis, *Schistosoma haematobium,* yellow fever, blackwater fever. (Inflammatory processes): Goodpasture syndrome, periarteritis, postirradiation.

C (Calculi): renal, ureteral, bladder, urethra. (Cysts): simple cysts, polycystic disease. (Congenital anomalies): hemangiomas, aneurysms, AVM.

S (Surgery): invasive procedures, prostatic resection, cystoscopy.(Sickle cell disease and other hematologic disturbances): hemophilia, thrombocytopenia, anticoagulants.(Somewhere else): bleeding genitals, factitious (drug addicts).

HEMATURIA, DIFFERENTIAL BASED ON AGE AND SEX

ICD-10CM #	R31.9	Hematuria, unspecified

0 TO 20 YR

Acute urinary tract infections.
Acute glomerulonephritis.
Congenital urinary tract anomalies with obstruction.
Trauma to genitals.

20 TO 40 YR

Acute urinary tract infection.
Trauma to genitals.
Urolithiasis.
Bladder cancer.

40 TO 60 YR (WOMEN)

Acute urinary tract infection.
Bladder cancer.
Urolithiasis.

40 TO 60 YR (MEN)

Acute urinary tract infection.
Bladder cancer.
Urolithiasis.

60 YR AND OLDER (WOMEN)

Acute urinary tract infection.
Bladder cancer.
Vaginal trauma or irritation.
Urolithiasis.

60 YR AND OLDER (MEN)

Acute urinary tract infection.
Benign prostatic hyperplasia.
Bladder cancer.
Urolithiasis.
Trauma.

HEMATURIA, IN CHILDREN[7]

ICD-10CM #	R31.9	Hematuria, unspecified

EXTRARENAL

Trauma.
Meatal stenosis or posterior urethral valves.
Exercise.
Menstruation or rectal bleeding.
Foreign bodies.
Cystitis, urethritis, or epididymitis.

INTRARENAL

Pyelonephritis.
Renal or bladder stones or tumors.
Poststreptococcal or idiopathic glomerulonephritis.
Acute interstitial nephritis.
Acute tubular necrosis.
Basement membrane glomerular disease.
Renal vein or arterial thrombosis.
Recurrent familial hematuria.
Polycystic kidney disease.

SYSTEMIC

Henoch-Schönlein purpura.
Systemic lupus erythematosus.
Hemolytic-uremic syndrome.
Infectious mononucleosis.
Sickle cell disease or other hemoglobinopathies.
Bacterial endocarditis or artificial cardiac valves.
Bleeding disorders, warfarin, or aspirin.
Medications such as amitriptyline or chlorpromazine, radiocontrast dyes.
Munchausen syndrome or factitious.

HEMIPARESIS/HEMIPLEGIA

ICD-10CM #	G81.00	Flaccid hemiplegia affecting unspecified side
	G81.10	Spastic hemiplegia affecting unspecified side

CVA.
Transient ischemic attack.
Cerebral neoplasm.
Multiple sclerosis or other demyelinating disorder.
CNS infection.
Migraine.
Hypoglycemia
Subdural hematoma.
Vasculitis.
Todd paralysis.
Epidural hematoma.
Metabolic (hyperosmolar state, electrolyte imbalance).
Psychiatric disorders.
Congenital disorders.
Leukodystrophies.

HEMOLYSIS AND HEMOGLOBINURIA

ICD-10CM #	P55.8	Other hemolytic diseases of newborn
	P55.9	Hemolytic disease of newborn, unspecified
	R82.3	Hemoglobinuria

Erythrocyte trauma (prosthetic cardiac valves, marching and severe trauma, extensive burns).
Infections (malaria, *Bartonella, Clostridium welchii*).
Brown recluse spider bite.
Incompatible blood transfusions.
Hemolytic-uremic syndrome.
Thrombotic thrombocytopenic purpura (TTP).
Paroxysmal nocturnal hemoglobinuria (PNH).
Drugs (penicillins, quinidine, methyldopa, sulfonamides, nitrofurantoin).
Erythrocyte enzyme deficiencies (e.g., exposure to fava beans in patients with glucose-6-phosphate dehydrogenase deficiency).

HEMOLYSIS, INTRAVASCULAR

ICD-10CM #	D59.6	Hemoglobinuria due to hemolysis from other external causes
	D59.8	Other acquired hemolytic anemias

Infections.
Exertional hemolysis (e.g., prolonged march).
Valve hemolysis.
Microangiopathic hemolytic anemia.
Osmotic and chemical agents.
Thermal injury.
Cold agglutinins.
Venoms (snakes, spiders).
Paroxysmal nocturnal hemoglobinuria (PNH).

HEMOLYSIS, MECHANICAL

ICD-10CM #	D59.4	Other nonautoimmune hemolytic anemias

Prosthetic heart valves.
Aortic stenosis.
Malignant hypertension.
Metastatic adenocarcinoma.
Traumatic exercise.
Renal transplants.
Renal cortical necrosis.
Glomerulonephritis.
Thrombotic thrombocytopenic purpura (TTP), hemolytic-uremic syndrome (HUS).
Renal vasculitis.
Scleroderma.
Diabetes mellitus.

HEMOLYSIS, OXIDATIVE, DRUG-INDUCED[51]

ICD-10CM #	D59	Acquired hemolytic anemia
	D59.1	Other autoimmune hemolytic anemias

AGENTS THAT CAUSE OXIDATIVE HEMOLYSIS

Therapeutic Agents
Nitrofurantoin (Furadantin).
Sulfasalazine (Azulfidine).
p-Aminosalicylic acid.
Phenazopyridine (Pyridium).
Clotrimoxazole.
Quinolones.
Phenacetin.
Rasburicase.
Dapsone and other sulfones.
Primaquine.
Recreational Drugs
Isobutyl nitrate.
Amyl nitrite.
Miscellaneous Agents
Naphthalene mothballs.
Methylene blue.
Paraquat.
Hydrogen peroxide.

HEMOPERITONEUM

ICD-10CM # K66.1 Hemoperitoneum

Ruptured Graafian follicle.
Ruptured spleen.
Ectopic pregnancy.
Traumatic laceration of liver.
Ruptured aneurysm.
Ruptured bladder.
Traumatic laceration of bowel, pancreas, uterus.

HEMOPTYSIS

ICD-10CM # R04.2 Hemoptysis

CARDIOVASCULAR

Pulmonary embolism/infarction.
Left ventricular failure.
Mitral stenosis.
AV fistula.
Severe hypertension.
Erosion of aortic aneurysm.

PULMONARY

Neoplasm (primary or metastatic).
Infection.
Pneumonia: *Streptococcus pneumoniae, Klebsiella pneumoniae, Staphylococcus aureus, Legionella pneumophila.*
Bronchiectasis.
Abscess.
TB.
Bronchitis.
Fungal infections (aspergillosis, coccidioidomycosis).
Parasitic infections (amebiasis, ascariasis, paragonimiasis).
Vasculitis: granulomatosis with polyangiitis, Churg-Strauss syndrome, Henoch-Schönlein purpura.
Goodpasture syndrome.
Trauma (needle biopsy, foreign body, right-sided heart catheterization, prolonged and severe cough).
Cystic fibrosis, bullous emphysema.
Pulmonary sequestration.
Pulmonary AV fistula.
SLE.
Idiopathic pulmonary hemosiderosis.
Drugs: aspirin, anticoagulants, penicillamine.
Pulmonary hypertension.
Mediastinal fibrosis.

OTHER

Epistaxis, trauma.
Laryngeal bleeding (laryngitis, laryngeal neoplasm).
Hematologic disorders (clotting abnormalities, DIC, thrombocytopenia).

HEMORRHAGIC CYSTITIS[99]

ICD-10CM # N39.0 Urinary tract infection

DIFFERENTIAL DIAGNOSIS FOR HEMORRHAGIC CYSTITIS[26]

Infectious:
- Bacterial.
- Viral (especially BK virus, adenovirus).
- Fungal.
- Parasitic.

Trauma:
- External.
- Postsurgical (e.g., transurethral resection of the bladder).

Malignancy:
- Bladder primary.
- Bladder invasion from local/distant primary.

Vascular malformation.
Chemical exposure:
- Cyclophosphamide.
- Ifosfamide.
- Busulfan.
- Thiotepa.
- Temozolomide.
- Aniline dye.
- Ether.
- Nonoxynol-9 (accidental urethral insertion of vaginal contraceptive).

Radiation therapy history (e.g., prostate cancer, cervical cancer).
Medication induced:
- Penicillin and derivatives (via immune reaction).
- Bleomycin.
- Danazol.
- Tiaprofenic.
- Allopurinol.
- Phensuximide.
- Methenamine mandelate.
- Acetic acid.

Manifestation of systemic disease:
- Amyloidosis.
- Rheumatoid arthritis.
- Crohn disease.

HEPATIC CYSTS[91]

ICD-10CM #	Q44.6	Cystic disease of liver
	B67.8	Echinococcosis, unspecified, of liver

[26] Bleeding localized to bladder after diagnostic workup for gross hematuria with cystoscopy, urine cytology, and upper tract imaging is without clear cause of alternative bleeding source.

CONGENITAL HEPATIC CYSTS

Parenchymal: solitary cyst, polycystic disease.
Ductal: localized dilatation, multiple cystic dilatations of intrahepatic ducts (Caroli disease).

ACQUIRED HEPATIC CYSTS

Inflammatory cysts: retention cysts, echinococcal cyst, amebic cyst.
Neoplastic cyst.
Peliosis hepatis.

HEPATIC DYSFUNCTION, POSTOPERATIVE[30]

ICD-10CM # K91.82 Postprocedural hepatic failure

CAUSES OF POSTOPERATIVE HEPATIC DYSFUNCTION

Hepatocellular Injury (predominant serum ALT elevation, with or without hyperbilirubinemia)
Acute transfusion-associated viral hepatitis.
Hepatic allograft rejection.
Hepatic artery thrombosis.
Inhalational anesthetics: halothane, others.
Ischemic hepatitis (shock liver).
Other drugs: antihypertensives (e.g., labetalol), heparin.
Unrecognized chronic liver disease: NASH, hepatitis C, other disorders.
Cholestatic Jaundice (elevated serum alkaline phosphatase ± ALT; direct hyperbilirubinemia)
Acalculous cholecystitis.
Benign postoperative cholestasis.
Bile duct injury: after cholecystectomy or liver transplantation.
Bile duct obstruction: gallstones, pancreatitis.
Cardiac bypass of prolonged duration.
Cholangitis.
Drugs: amoxicillin-clavulanic acid, chlorpromazine, erythromycin, telithromycin, trimethoprim/sulfamethoxazole, warfarin, others.
Hemobilia.
Microlithiasis (biliary sludge).
Prolonged TPN.
Sepsis.
Indirect Hyperbilirubinemia (serum alkaline phosphatase and ALT often normal)
Gilbert syndrome.
Hemolytic anemia (G6PD deficiency, other causes).
Multiple transfusions.
Resorbing hematoma.

G6PD, Glucose-6-phosphate dehydrogenase; *NASH,* nonalcoholic steatohepatitis.

HEPATIC GRANULOMAS[3]

ICD-10CM # K75.3 Granulomatous hepatitis

INFECTIONS

Bacterial, spirochetal: TB and atypical mycobacterial infections, tularemia, brucellosis, leprosy, syphilis, Whipple disease, listeriosis.
Viral: mononucleosis, CMV.
Rickettsial: Q fever.

Fungal: coccidioidomycosis, histoplasmosis, cryptococcal infections, actinomycosis, aspergillosis, nocardiosis.
Parasitic: schistosomiasis, clonorchiasis, toxocariasis, ascariasis, toxoplasmosis, amebiasis.

HEPATOBILIARY DISORDERS

Primary biliary cirrhosis, granulomatous hepatitis, jejunoileal bypass.

SYSTEMIC DISORDERS

Sarcoidosis, granulomatosis with polyangiitis, inflammatory bowel disease, Hodgkin disease, lymphoma.

DRUGS/TOXINS

Beryllium, parenteral foreign material (starch, talc, silicone, etc.), phenylbutazone, α-methyldopa, procainamide, allopurinol, phenytoin, nitrofurantoin, hydralazine.

HEPATITIS, ACUTE[63]

ICD-10CM #	B17.8	Acute viral hepatitis, unspecified
	B15	Acute hepatitis A
	B16	Acute hepatitis B
	B17.1	Acute hepatitis C
	B17.2	Acute hepatitis E

Infectious:
- Hepatitis A, B, C, D, E.
- Epstein-Barr virus.
- Cytomegalovirus.
- Herpes simplex virus.
- Yellow fever.
- Leptospirosis.
- Q fever.
- HIV.
- Brucellosis.
- Lyme disease.
- Syphilis.

Noninfectious:
- Drug induced.
- Autoimmune.
- Ischemic.
- Acute fatty liver of pregnancy.
- Acute Budd-Chiari syndrome.
- Wilson disease.

HEPATITIS, CHRONIC[63]

ICD-10CM #	K73.9	Chronic hepatitis, unspecified
	B18.0	Chronic viral hepatitis B with δ-agent
	B18.2	Chronic viral hepatitis C

Chronic viral hepatitis:
- Hepatitis B.
- Hepatitis C.
- Hepatitis D.

Autoimmune hepatitis and variant syndromes.
Hereditary hemochromatosis.
Wilson disease.
α_1-Antitrypsin deficiency.
Fatty liver and nonalcoholic steatohepatitis.
Alcoholic liver disease.
Drug-induced liver disease.
Hepatic granulomas:
- Infectious.
- Drug induced.
- Neoplastic.
- Idiopathic.

HEPATITIS, IN CHILDREN[58]

ICD-10CM #	B17.9	Acute viral hepatitis, unspecified
	K73.9	Chronic hepatitis, unspecified

CAUSES AND DIFFERENTIAL DIAGNOSIS OF HEPATITIS IN CHILDREN

Infectious

Hepatotropic viruses:
- HAV.
- HBV.
- HCV.
- HDV.
- HEV.
- Hepatitis non–A-E viruses.

Systemic infection that can include hepatitis:
- Adenovirus.
- Arbovirus.
- Coxsackievirus.
- Cytomegalovirus.
- Enterovirus.
- Epstein-Barr virus.
- "Exotic" viruses (e.g., yellow fever).
- Herpes simplex virus.
- Human immunodeficiency virus.
- Paramyxovirus.
- Rubella.
- Varicella zoster.

Other.

Nonviral liver infections

Abscess.
Amebiasis.
Bacterial sepsis.
Brucellosis.
Fitz-Hugh-Curtis syndrome.
Histoplasmosis.
Leptospirosis.
Tuberculosis.
Other.

Autoimmune

Autoimmune hepatitis.
Sclerosing cholangitis.
Other (e.g., systemic lupus erythematosus, juvenile rheumatoid arthritis).

Metabolic

α1-Antitrypsin deficiency.
Tyrosinemia.
Wilson disease.
Other.

Toxic

Iatrogenic or drug induced (e.g., acetaminophen).
Environmental (e.g., pesticides).

Anatomic

Choledochal cyst.
Biliary atresia.
Other.

Hemodynamic

Shock.
Congestive heart failure.
Budd-Chiari syndrome.
Other.

Nonalcoholic Fatty Liver Disease

Idiopathic.
Reye syndrome.
Other.

HEPATOMEGALY

ICD-10CM #	R16.0	Hepatomegaly, not elsewhere classified

FREQUENT JAUNDICE

Infectious hepatitis.
Toxic hepatitis.
Carcinoma: liver, pancreas, bile ducts, metastatic neoplasm to liver.
Cirrhosis.
Obstruction of common bile duct.
Alcoholic hepatitis.
Biliary cirrhosis.
Cholangitis.
Hemochromatosis with cirrhosis.

INFREQUENT JAUNDICE

CHF.
Amyloidosis.
Liver abscess.
Sarcoidosis.
Infectious mononucleosis.
Alcoholic fatty infiltration.
Nonalcoholic steatohepatitis.
Lymphoma.
Leukemia.
Budd-Chiari syndrome.
Myelofibrosis with myeloid metaplasia.
Familial hyperlipoproteinemia type 1.
Other: amebiasis, hydatid disease of liver, schistosomiasis, kala-azar *(Leishmania donovani),* Hurler syndrome, Gaucher disease, kwashiorkor.

HEPATOMEGALY, BY SHAPE OF LIVER[95]

ICD-10CM #	R16.0	Hepatomegaly, not elsewhere classified

DIFFUSELY ENLARGED AND SMOOTH

Massive

Metastatic disease.
Alcoholic liver disease with fatty infiltration.
Myeloproliferative diseases (e.g., polycythemia rubra vera, myelofibrosis).

Moderate

The above causes.
Hemochromatosis.
Hematologic disease (e.g., chronic myeloid leukemia, lymphoma).
Fatty liver (e.g., diabetes mellitus, obesity).
Infiltrative disorders (e.g., amyloid).

Mild

The above causes.
Hepatitis (viral, drugs).
Cirrhosis.
Biliary obstruction.

Granulomatous disorders (e.g., sarcoid).
HIV infection.

DIFFUSELY ENLARGED AND IRREGULAR

Metastatic disease.
Cirrhosis.
Hydatid disease.
Polycystic liver disease.

LOCALIZED SWELLINGS

Riedel lobe (a normal variant—the lobe may be palpable in the right lumbar region).
Metastasis.
Large simple hepatic cyst.
Hydatid cyst.
Hepatoma.
Liver abscess (e.g., amebic abscess).

HERMAPHRODITISM[9]

ICD-10CM #	Q56.3	Pseudohermaphroditism, unspecified
	Q56.4	Indeterminate sex, unspecified

Female Pseudohermaphroditism
- Androgen exposure:
  - Fetal source:
    - 21-Hydroxylase (P450 c21) deficiency.
    - 11β-Hydroxylase (P450 c11) deficiency.
    - 3β-Hydroxysteroid dehydrogenase II (3β-HSD II) deficiency.
    - Aromatase (P450arom) deficiency.
    - Maternal source.
    - Virilizing ovarian tumor.
    - Virilizing adrenal tumor.
    - Androgenic drugs.
- Undetermined origin:
  - Associated with genitourinary and GI tract defects.

MALE PSEUDOHERMAPHRODITISM

Defects in testicular differentiation:
- Denys-Drash syndrome (mutation in WT1 gene).
- WAGR syndrome (*W*ilms tumor, *a*niridia, *g*enitourinary malformation, *r*etardation).
- Deletion of 11p13.
- Camptomelic syndrome (autosomal gene at 17q24.3-q25.1) and SOX 9 mutation.
- XY pure gonadal dysgenesis (Swyer syndrome).
- Mutation in SRY gene.
- Unknown cause.
- XY gonadal agenesis.

Deficiency of testicular hormones:
- Leydig cell aplasia.
- Mutation in LH receptor.
- Lipoid adrenal hyperplasia (P450 scc) deficiency; mutation in StAR (steroidogenic acute regulatory protein).
- 3α-HSD II deficiency.
- 17-Hydroxylase/17, 20-lyase (P450 c17) deficiency.
- Persistent Müllerian duct syndrome.
- Gene mutations, Müllerian-inhibiting substance (MIS).
- Receptor defects for MIS.

Defect in androgen action:
- 5α-Reductase II mutations.
- Androgen receptor defects:
  - Complete androgen insensitivity syndrome.
  - Partial androgen insensitivity syndrome.
  - Reifenstein and other syndromes.
  - Smith-Lemli-Opitz syndrome.

Defect in conversion of 7-dehydrocholesterol to cholesterol.

TRUE HERMAPHRODITISM

XX.
XY.
XX/XY chimeras.

HICCUPS[54]

ICD-10CM #	R06.6	Hiccough

TRANSIENT HICCUPS

Sudden excitement, emotion.
Gastric distention.
Esophageal obstruction.
Alcohol ingestion.
Sudden change in temperature.

PERSISTENT OR CHRONIC HICCUPS

Toxic/metabolic: uremia, DM, hyperventilation, hypocalcemia, hypokalemia, hyponatremia, gout, fever.
Drugs: benzodiazepines, steroids, α-methyldopa, barbiturates.
Surgery/general anesthesia.
Thoracic/diaphragmatic disorders: pneumonia, lung cancer, asthma, pleuritis, pericarditis, myocardial infarction, aortic aneurysm, esophagitis, esophageal obstruction, diaphragmatic hernia or irritation.
Abdominal disorders: gastric ulcer or cancer, hepatobiliary or pancreatic disease, IBD, bowel obstruction, intraabdominal or subphrenic abscess, prostatic infection or cancer.
CNS disorders: traumatic, infectious, vascular, structural.
Ear, nose, and throat disorders: pharyngitis, laryngitis, tumor, irritation of auditory canal.
Psychogenic disorders.
Idiopathic disorders.

HILAR AND MEDIASTINAL LYMPH NODE ENLARGEMENT[38]

ICD-10CM #	R59.0	Mediastinal adenopathy

DISORDERS ASSOCIATED WITH HILAR AND MEDIASTINAL LYMPH NODE ENLARGEMENT

Sarcoidosis.
Lymphoma.
Fungal disease.
Tuberculosis.
Metastatic cancer.
Silicosis, coal worker's pneumoconiosis, beryllium lung.

HIP PAIN, CHILDREN[63]

ICD-10CM #	S79.819A	Other specified injuries of unspecified hip, initial encounter
	S79.829A	Other specified injuries of unspecified thigh, initial encounter
	S79.919A	Unspecified injury of unspecified hip, initial encounter

TRAUMA

Hip or pelvis fractures.
Overuse injuries.

INFECTION

Septic arthritis.
Osteomyelitis.

INFLAMMATION

Transient synovitis.
Juvenile RA.
Rheumatic fever.

NEOPLASM

Leukemia.
Osteogenic or Ewing sarcoma.
Metastatic disease.

HEMATOLOGIC DISORDERS

Hemophilia.
Sickle cell anemia.

MISCELLANEOUS

Legg-Calvé-Perthes disease.
Slipped capital femoral epiphysis.

HIP PAIN, DIFFERENTIAL DIAGNOSIS[46]

ICD-10CM #	M25.559	Pain in unspecified hip

ARTICULAR

Inflammatory joint disease
Rheumatoid arthritis.
Spondyloarthropathies.
Polymyalgia rheumatica.
Degenerative joint disease
Primary osteoarthritis.
Secondary osteoarthritis.
Metabolic joint diseases
Gout.
Pseudogout.
Ochronosis.
Hemochromatosis.
Wilson disease.
Acromegaly.
Femoroacetabular impingement
Acetabular labral tear
Infections
Tumors

Benign:
- Pigmented villonodular sclerosis.
- Osteochondromatosis.

Malignant:
- Synovial sarcoma.
- Synovial metastasis.

Hemarthrosis

In children:

Toxic synovitis.
Juvenile chronic arthritis.

REFERRED PAIN

Thoracolumbar spine:
- Intraabdominal structures.
- Retroperitoneal structures.

PERIARTICULAR

Bursitis:
- Trochanteric.
- Iliopsoas.
- Ischiogluteal.

Tendinitis:
- Trochanteric.
- Adductor.

Acute calcific periarthritis.
Heterotropic ossification.

OSSEOUS

Bone lesions.
Fractures.
Neoplasms.
Infection.
Osteonecrosis of the femoral head.
Paget disease.
Metabolic bone disease.
Stress fracture.
Transient osteoporosis.
In children:
- Congenital dislocation of the hip.
- Acetabular dysplasia.
- Coxa vara.
- Slipped capital femoral epiphysis.
- Legg-Calvé-Perthes disease.
- Rickets.

NEUROLOGIC

Entrapment neuropathies.
Lateral femoral cutaneous nerve (meralgia paresthetica).
Lumbar nerve root compression.
L2, L3, and L4.

VASCULAR

Atherosclerosis of aorta, iliac vessels.

HIP PAIN, IN DIFFERENT AGE GROUPS[22]

ICD-10CM #	M25.559	Pain in unspecified hip

COMMON CAUSES OF HIP PAIN IN DIFFERENT AGE GROUPS

Childhood (2 to 10 yr)

Intraarticular

Developmental dislocation of the hip.
Perthes disease.
Irritable hip.
Rickets.

Periarticular

Osteomyelitis.

Referred

Abdominal.

Adolescence (10 to 18 yr)

Intraarticular

Slipped upper femoral epiphysis.
Torn labrum.

Periarticular

Trochanteric bursitis.
Snapping hip.
Osteomyelitis.
Tumors.

Referred

Abdominal.
Lumbar spine.

Early Adulthood (18 to 30 yr)

Intraarticular

Inflammatory arthritis.
Torn labrum.

Periarticular

Bursitis.

Referred

Abdominal.
Lumbar spine.

Adulthood (30 to 50 yr)

Intraarticular

Osteoarthritis.
Inflammatory arthritis.
Osteonecrosis.
Transient osteoporosis.

Periarticular

Bursitis.

Referred

Abdominal.
Lumbar spine.

Old Age (>50 yr)

Intraarticular

Osteoarthritis.
Inflammatory arthritis.

Referred

Abdominal.
Lumbar spine.

HIP PAIN WITHOUT OBVIOUS FRACTURE[7]

ICD-10CM #	R52	Pain, unspecified
	M25.559	Pain in unspecified hip

DIFFERENTIAL DIAGNOSIS OF A PAINFUL HIP WITHOUT OBVIOUS FRACTURE

Referred pain (lumbar spine, hip, or knee).
Avascular necrosis of the femoral head.
Degenerative joint disease or osteoarthritis.
Herniation of a lumbar disk.
Diskitis.
Toxic synovitis of the hip.
Septic arthritis.
Bursitis.
Tendonitis.
Ligamentous injuries of the knee or hip.
Occult fracture.
Slipped capital femoral epiphysis.
Perthes disease.
Tumor (lymphoma).
Deep venous thrombosis.
Arterial insufficiency.
Osteomyelitis.
Iliopsoas abscess.
Retroperitoneal hematoma.
Inguinal hernia.
Inguinal lymphadenopathy.
Genitourinary complaints.
Sports-related hernia.

HIRSUTISM

ICD-10CM #	L68.0	Hirsutism

Idiopathic: familial, possibly increased sensitivity to androgens.
Menopause.
Polycystic ovarian syndrome.
Drugs: androgens, anabolic steroids, methyltestosterone, minoxidil, diazoxide, phenytoin, glucocorticoids, cyclosporine.
Congenital adrenal hyperplasia.
Adrenal virilizing tumor.
Ovarian virilizing tumor: arrhenoblastoma, hilus cell tumor.
Pituitary adenoma.
Cushing syndrome.
Hypothyroidism (congenital and juvenile).
Acromegaly.
Testicular feminization.

HIV INFECTION, ANORECTAL LESIONS[63]

ICD-10CM #	B20	Human immunodeficiency virus [HIV] disease
	Z21	Asymptomatic human immunodeficiency virus [HIV] infection status

COMMON CONDITIONS

Anal fissure.
Abscess and fistula.
Hemorrhoids.
Pruritus ani.
Pilonidal disease.

COMMON STDS

Gonorrhea.
Chlamydia.
Herpes.
Chancroid.
Syphilis.
Condylomata acuminata.

ATYPICAL CONDITIONS

Infectious: TB, CMV, actinomycosis, cryptococcus.
Neoplastic: lymphoma, Kaposi sarcoma, squamous cell carcinoma.
Other: idiopathic and ulcer.

HIV INFECTION, CHEST RADIOGRAPHIC ABNORMALITIES[63]

ICD-10CM #	B20	Human immunodeficiency virus [HIV] disease
	Z21	Asymptomatic human immunodeficiency virus [HIV] infection status

DIFFUSE INTERSTITIAL INFILTRATION

Pneumocystis jiroveci.
Cytomegalovirus.
Mycobacterium tuberculosis.
Mycobacterium avium complex.
Histoplasmosis.
Coccidioidomycosis.
Lymphoid interstitial pneumonitis.

FOCAL CONSOLIDATION

Bacterial pneumonia.
Mycoplasma pneumoniae.
Pneumocystis jiroveci.
Mycobacterium tuberculosis.
Mycobacterium avium complex.

NODULAR LESIONS

Kaposi sarcoma.
Mycobacterium tuberculosis.
Mycobacterium avium complex.
Fungal lesions.
Toxoplasmosis.

CAVITARY LESIONS

Pneumocystis jiroveci.
Mycobacterium tuberculosis.
Bacterial infection.

PLEURAL EFFUSION

Kaposi sarcoma.
(Small effusion may be associated with any infection).

ADENOPATHY

Kaposi sarcoma.
Lymphoma.
Mycobacterium tuberculosis.
Cryptococcus.

PNEUMOTHORAX

Kaposi sarcoma.

HIV INFECTION, COGNITIVE IMPAIRMENT[63]

ICD-10CM #	B20	Human immunodeficiency virus [HIV] disease

EARLY TO MID-STAGE HIV DISEASE

Depression.
Alcohol and substance abuse.
Medication-induced cognitive impairment.
Metabolic encephalopathies.
HIV-related cognitive impairment.

ADVANCED HIV DISEASE (CD4+ <100/MM^3)

Opportunistic infection of CNS.
Neurosyphilis.
CNS lymphoma.
Progressive multifocal leukoencephalopathy.
Depression.
Metabolic encephalopathies.
Medication-induced cognitive impairment.
Stroke.
HIV dementia.

HIV INFECTION, CUTANEOUS MANIFESTATIONS[54]

ICD-10CM #	B20	Human immunodeficiency virus [HIV] disease
	Z21	Asymptomatic human immunodeficiency virus [HIV] infection status

BACTERIAL INFECTION

Bacillary angiomatosis: numerous angiomatous nodules associated with fever, chills, weight loss.
Staphylococcus aureus: folliculitis, ecthyma, impetigo, bullous impetigo, furuncles, carbuncles.
Syphilis: may occur in different forms (primary, secondary, tertiary); chancre may become painful because of secondary infection.

FUNGAL INFECTION

Candidiasis: mucous membranes (oral, vulvovaginal), less commonly candida intertrigo or paronychia.
Cryptococcoses: papules or nodules that strongly resemble molluscum contagiosum; other forms include pustules, purpuric papules, and vegetating plaques.
Seborrheic dermatitis: scaling and erythema in the hair-bearing areas (eyebrows, scalp, chest, and pubic area).

ARTHROPOD INFESTATIONS

Scabies: pruritus with or without rash, usually generalized but can be limited to a single digit.

VIRAL INFECTION

Herpes simplex: vesicular lesion in clusters; perianal, genital, orofacial, or digital; can be disseminated.
Herpes zoster: painful dermatomal vesicles that may ulcerate or disseminate.
HIV: discrete erythematous macules and papules on the upper trunk, palms, and soles are the most characteristic cutaneous finding of acute HIV infection.
Human papillomavirus: genital warts (may become unusually extensive).
Kaposi sarcoma (herpesvirus): erythematous macules or papules; enlarge at varying rates; violaceous nodules or plaques; occasionally painful.
Molluscum contagiosum: discrete umbilicated papules commonly on the face, neck, and intertriginous sites (axilla, groin, or buttocks).

NONINFECTIOUS

Drug reactions: more frequent and severe in HIV patients.
Nutritional deficiencies: mainly seen in children and patients with chronic diarrhea; diffuse skin manifestations, depending upon the deficiency.
Psoriasis: scaly lesions; diffuse or localized; can be associated with arthritis.
Vasculitis: palpable purpuric eruption (can resemble septic emboli).

HIV INFECTION, ESOPHAGEAL DISEASE

ICD-10CM #	B20	Human immunodeficiency virus [HIV] disease
	K21.9	Gastro-esophageal reflux disease without esophagitis

Candida infection.
Cytomegalovirus infection.
Aphthous ulcer.
Herpes simplex.

HIV INFECTION, HEPATIC DISEASE[63]

ICD-10CM #	B20	Human immunodeficiency virus [HIV] disease

VIRUSES

Hepatitis A.
Hepatitis B.
Hepatitis C.
Hepatitis D (with HBV).
Epstein-Barr virus.
Cytomegalovirus.
Herpes simplex virus.
Adenovirus.
Varicella-zoster virus.

MYCOBACTERIA

Mycobacterium avium complex.
Mycobacterium tuberculosis.

FUNGI

Histoplasma capsulatum.
Cryptococcus neoformans.
Coccidioides immitis.
Candida albicans.
Pneumocystis jiroveci.
Penicillium marneffei.

PROTOZOA

Toxoplasma gondii.
Cryptosporidium parvum.
Microsporida.
Schistosoma.

BACTERIA

Bartonella henselae (peliosis hepatis).

MALIGNANCY

Kaposi sarcoma (HHV-8).
Non-Hodgkin lymphoma.
Hepatocellular carcinoma.

MEDICATIONS

Zidovudine.
Didanosine.
Ritonavir.
Other HIV-1 protease inhibitors.
Fluconazole.
Macrolide antibiotics.
Isoniazid.
Rifampin.
Trimethoprim-sulfamethoxazole.

HIV INFECTION, LOWER GI TRACT DISEASE[63]

ICD-10CM # B20 Human immunodeficiency virus [HIV] disease

CAUSES OF ENTEROCOLITIS

Bacteria
Campylobacter jejuni and other spp.
Salmonella spp.
Shigella flexneri.
Aeromonas hydrophila.
Plesiomonas shigelloides.
Yersinia enterocolitica.
Vibrio spp.
Mycobacterium avium complex.
Mycobacterium tuberculosis.
Escherichia coli (enterotoxigenic, enteroadherent).
Bacterial overgrowth.
Clostridium difficile (toxin).
Parasites
Cryptosporidium parvum.
Microsporida (*Enterocytozoon bieneusi, Septata intestinalis*).
Isospora belli.
Entamoeba histolytica.
Giardia lamblia.
Cyclospora cayetanensis.
Viruses
Cytomegalovirus.
Adenovirus.
Calicivirus.
Astrovirus.
Picobirnavirus.
Human immunodeficiency virus.
Fungi
Histoplasma capsulatum.

CAUSES OF PROCTITIS

Bacteria
Chlamydia trachomatis.
Neisseria gonorrhoeae.
Treponema pallidum.
Viruses
Herpes simplex.
Cytomegalovirus.

HIV INFECTION, MUSCULOSKELETAL DISORDERS[78]

ICD-10CM # B20 Human immunodeficiency virus [HIV] disease

MUSCULOSKELETAL DISORDERS ASSOCIATED WITH HIV INFECTION

Joints, Ligaments, and Soft Tissues
Painful articular syndrome.
HIV-associated arthritis.
Reactive arthritis.
Septic arthritis.
Psoriatic arthritis.
Diffuse infiltrative lymphocytosis syndrome.
Systemic lupus erythematosus.
Rheumatoid arthritis.
Vasculitis (polyarteritis nodosa, drug induced).
Immune reconstitution inflammatory syndrome.
Cellulitis and soft tissue abscesses.
Fasciitis (including necrotizing fasciitis).
Bursitis and tenosynovitis.
Muscles
HIV myopathy.
Nucleoside reverse transcriptase inhibitor (NRTI) myopathy.
Muscle infections (pyomyositis, toxoplasmosis).
Other (rhabdomyolysis, non-Hodgkin lymphoma, myasthenia gravis, nemaline [rod] myopathy, and inclusion body myositis).
Bones
Osteomyelitis.
Osteopenia and osteoporosis.
Osteonecrosis.
Hypertrophic osteoarthropathy.
Opportunistic Infections, HIV/AIDS-Defining Neoplastic Disorders, and Other Disorders Affecting Any Part of the Musculoskeletal System in HIV Infection
Neoplasia:
- Kaposi sarcoma.
- Non-Hodgkin lymphoma.
- Hodgkin lymphoma.
- Leiomyosarcoma.
- Ewing sarcoma.

Infection:
- Tuberculosis.
- Disseminated *Mycobacterium avium* complex infection.
- Coccidioidomycosis.
- Toxoplasmosis.
- Bacillary angiomatosis.

Other:
- HIV-related lipodystrophy.
  - HIV wasting syndrome.

HIV INFECTION, OCULAR MANIFESTATIONS[91]

ICD-10CM # B20 Human immunodeficiency virus [HIV] disease
Z21 Asymptomatic human immunodeficiency virus [HIV] infection status

EYELIDS

Molluscum contagiosum.
Kaposi sarcoma.

CORNEA/CONJUNCTIVA

Keratoconjunctivitis sicca.
Bacterial/fungal ulcerative keratitis.
Herpes simplex.
Herpes zoster ophthalmicus.
Conjunctival microvasculopathy.
Kaposi sarcoma.

RETINA, CHOROID, AND VITREOUS

Microvasculopathy.
Endophthalmitis.
Cytomegalovirus retinitis.
Acute retinal necrosis.
Syphilis.
Toxoplasmosis.
Pneumocystis choroidopathy.
Cryptococcosis.
Mycobacterial infection.
Intraocular lymphoma.
Candidiasis.
Histoplasmosis.

DRUGS ASSOCIATED WITH OCULAR TOXICITY

Rifabutin.
Didanosine.

NEUROOPHTHALMIC

Disc edema.
Primary or secondary optic neuropathy.
Cranial nerve palsies.

ORBITAL

Lymphoma.
Infection.
Pseudotumor.

HIV INFECTION, PULMONARY DISEASE[10,63]

ICD-10CM # B20 Human immunodeficiency virus [HIV] disease
I28.8 Other diseases of pulmonary vessels

RADIOGRAPHIC APPEARANCE

Diffuse Interstitial Infiltrates
Pneumocystis jiroveci.
Mycobacterium tuberculosis, especially with advanced human immunodeficiency virus disease.
Histoplasma capsulatum.
Coccidioides spp.
Cryptococcus neoformans.
Toxoplasma gondii.
Cytomegalovirus.
Influenza.
Lymphocytic interstitial pneumonitis.
Abacavir hypersensitivity.
Focal Consolidation
Pyogenic bacterial pneumonia from *Streptococcus pneumoniae, Haemophilus influenzae.*
M. tuberculosis.
Legionella spp.
Rhodococcus equi.
Hilar Adenopathy
M. tuberculosis.
H. capsulatum.
Coccidioides spp.
Non-Hodgkin or Hodgkin lymphoma.
Mycobacterium avium complex.
Cavitary Disease
Pyogenic bacterial pneumonia from *Pseudomonas aeruginosa, Staphylococcus aureus*, Enterobacteriaceae.
M. tuberculosis.
C. neoformans.
R. equi.
Aspergillus spp.
Nocardia spp.
Mycobacterium avium complex.
P. jiroveci.

Nodules or Masses
M. tuberculosis.
C. neoformans.
Aspergillus spp.
H. capsulatum.
Nocardia spp.
Non-Hodgkin lymphoma.
Kaposi sarcoma.
Lung cancer.
Normal Radiograph
P. jiroveci.
M. tuberculosis.

CAUSES

Mycobacterial
M. tuberculosis.
M. kansasii.
M. avium complex.
Other nontuberculous mycobacteria.
Other Bacterial
Streptococcus pneumoniae.
Staphylococcus aureus.
Haemophilus influenzae.
Enterobacteriaceae.
Pseudomonas aeruginosa.
Moraxella catarrhalis.
Group A *Streptococcus.*
Nocardia spp.
Rhodococcus equi.
Chlamydia pneumoniae.
Fungal
Pneumocystis carinii.
Cryptococcus neoformans.
Histoplasma capsulatum.
Coccidioides immitis.
Aspergillus spp.
Blastomyces dermatitidis.
Penicillium marneffei.
Viral
Cytomegalovirus.
Herpes simplex virus.
Adenovirus.
Respiratory syncytial virus.
Influenza viruses.
Parainfluenza virus.
Other
Toxoplasma gondii.
Strongyloides stercoralis.
Kaposi sarcoma.
Lymphoma.
Lung cancer.
Lymphocytic interstitial pneumonitis.
Nonspecific interstitial pneumonitis.
Bronchiolitis obliterans with organizing pneumonia.
Pulmonary hypertension.
Emphysema-like or bullous disease.
Pneumothorax.
Congestive heart failure.
Diffuse alveolar damage.
Pulmonary embolus.

HOARSENESS

ICD-10CM # R49.8 Other voice and resonance disorders

Allergic rhinitis.
Infections (laryngitis, epiglottitis, tracheitis, croup).
Vocal cord polyps.
Voice strain.
Irritants (tobacco smoke).
Vocal cord trauma (intubation, surgery).
Neoplastic involvement of vocal cord (primary or metastatic).
Neurologic abnormalities (multiple sclerosis, ALS, parkinsonism).
Endocrine abnormalities (puberty, menopause, hypothyroidism).
Other (laryngeal webs or cysts, psychogenic, muscle tension abnormalities).

HYDROCEPHALUS

ICD-10CM # G91.1 Obstructive hydrocephalus

Head trauma.
Brain neoplasm (primary or metastatic).
Spinal cord tumor.
Cerebellar infarction.
Exudative or granulomatous meningitis.
Cerebellar hemorrhage.
Subarachnoid hemorrhage.
Aqueductal stenosis.
Third ventricle colloid cyst.
Hindbrain malformation.
Viral encephalitis.
Metastases to leptomeninges.

HYPERCALCEMIA

ICD-10CM # E83.52 Hypercalcemia

Malignancy: increased bone resorption via osteoclast-activating factors, secretion of PTH-like substances, prostaglandin E2, direct erosion by tumor cells, transforming growth factors, colony-stimulating activity. Hypercalcemia is common in the following neoplasms:
- Solid tumors: breast, lung, pancreas, kidneys, ovary.
- Hematologic cancers: myeloma, lymphosarcoma, adult T-cell lymphoma, Burkitt lymphoma.

Hyperparathyroidism: increased bone resorption, GI absorption, and renal absorption; etiology:
- Parathyroid hyperplasia, adenoma.
- Hyperparathyroidism or renal failure with secondary hyperparathyroidism.

Granulomatous disorders: increased GI absorption (e.g., sarcoidosis).
Paget disease: increased bone resorption, seen only during periods of immobilization.
Vitamin D intoxication, milk-alkali syndrome; increased GI absorption.
Thiazides: increased renal absorption.
Other causes: familial hypocalciuric hypercalcemia, thyrotoxicosis, adrenal insufficiency, prolonged immobilization, vitamin A intoxication, recovery from acute renal failure, lithium administration, pheochromocytoma, disseminated SLE.

HYPERCALCEMIA, MALIGNANCY-INDUCED

ICD-10CM # E83.52 Hypercalcemia

Lung carcinoma	(6% frequency, 35% of hypercalcemic cases)
Breast carcinoma	(10% frequency, 25% of hypercalcemic cases)
Multiple myeloma	(33% frequency, 10% of hypercalcemic cases)
Lymphoma	(4% of hypercalcemic cases)
Genitourinary cancer	(6% of hypercalcemic cases)

HYPERCAPNIA, PERSISTENT[91]

ICD-10CM # R06.00 Dyspnea, unspecified
R06.09 Other forms of dyspnea
R06.89 Other abnormalities of breathing

Hypercapnia with normal lungs: CNS disturbances (CVA, parkinsonism, encephalitis), metabolic alkalosis, myxedema, primary alveolar hypoventilation, spinal cord lesions.
Diseases of the chest wall (e.g., kyphoscoliosis, ankylosing spondylitis).
Neuromuscular disorders (e.g., myasthenia gravis, Guillain-Barré syndrome, amyotrophic lateral sclerosis, muscular dystrophy, poliomyelitis).
COPD.

HYPERCOAGULABLE STATE, ASSOCIATED DISORDERS[50]

ICD-10CM # D68.69 Other thrombophilia

Systemic lupus erythematosus in association with the presence of a lupus anticoagulant or antiphospholipid antibodies.

MALIGNANCY

Disease-related: includes migratory superficial thrombophlebitis (Trousseau syndrome), nonbacterial thrombotic endocarditis, thrombosis associated with chronic DIC, thrombotic microangiopathy.
Treatment-related: associated with the administration of various chemotherapeutic agents (L-asparaginase, mitomycin, some adjuvant chemotherapeutic agents for treatment of breast cancer, thalidomide or lenalidomide in conjunction with high doses of dexamethasone).
Infusion of prothrombin complex concentrates.
Nephrotic syndrome.
Heparin-induced thrombocytopenia.
Myeloproliferative disorders.
Paroxysmal nocturnal hemoglobinuria.

DIC, Disseminated intravascular coagulopathy.

HYPERGASTRINEMIA

ICD-10CM # E16.4 Abnormal secretion of gastrin

Decreased gastrin release inhibition from medications (proton pump inhibitors [PPIs], H_2 receptor antagonists), vagotomy.

Chronic renal failure.
Hypochlorhydria due to atrophic gastritis, gastric carcinoma, pernicious anemia.
Gastrinoma (Zollinger-Ellison syndrome).
Pyloric obstruction.
Hyperplasia of antral G cells.
RA.

HYPERHIDROSIS[9]

ICD-10CM # R61 Generalized hyperhidrosis

CORTICAL

Emotional.
Familial dysautonomia.
Congenital ichthyosiform erythroderma.
Epidermolysis bullosa.
Nail-patella syndrome.
Jadassohn-Lewandowsky syndrome.
Pachyonychia congenita.
Palmoplantar keratoderma.

HYPOTHALAMIC

Drugs
Antipyretics.
Emetics.
Insulin.
Meperidine.
Exercise Infection
Defervescence.
Chronic illness.
Metabolic
Debility.
DM.
Hyperpituitarism.
Hyperthyroidism.
Hypoglycemia.
Obesity.
Porphyria.
Pregnancy.
Rickets.
Infantile scurvy.
Cardiovascular
Heart failure.
Shock.
Vasomotor
Cold injury.
Raynaud phenomenon.
RA.
Neurologic
Abscess.
Familial dysautonomia.
Postencephalitic.
Tumor.
Miscellaneous
Chédiak-Higashi syndrome.
Compensatory.
Phenylketonuria.
Pheochromocytoma.
Vitiligo.
Medullary
Physiologic gustatory sweating.
Encephalitis.
Granulosis rubra nasi.
Syringomyelia.
Thoracic sympathetic trunk injury.
Spinal
Cord transection.
Syringomyelia.
Changes in Blood Flow
Mallucci syndrome.
Arteriovenous fistula.
Klippel-Trenaunay syndrome.
Glomus tumor.
Blue rubber bleb nevus syndrome.

HYPERKALEMIA

ICD-10CM # E87.5 Hyperkalemia

Pseudohyperkalemia.
- Hemolyzed specimen.
- Severe thrombocytosis (platelet count 0.106 ml).
- Severe leukocytosis (white blood cell count 0.105 ml).
- Fist clenching during phlebotomy.

Excessive potassium intake (often in setting of impaired excretion).
- Potassium replacement therapy.
- High-potassium diet.
- Salt substitutes with potassium.
- Potassium salts of antibiotics.

Decreased renal excretion.
- Potassium-sparing diuretics (e.g., spironolactone, triamterene, amiloride).
- Renal insufficiency.
- Mineralocorticoid deficiency.
- Hyporeninemic hypoaldosteronism.
- Tubular unresponsiveness to aldosterone (e.g., SLE, multiple myeloma, sickle cell disease).
- Type 4 RTA.
- ACE inhibitors.
- Heparin administration.
- NSAIDs.
- Trimethoprim-sulfamethoxazole.
- Beta-blockers.
- Pentamidine.

Redistribution (excessive cellular release):
- Acidemia (each 0.1 decrease in pH increases the serum potassium by 0.4 to 0.6 mEq/L). Lactic acidosis and ketoacidosis cause minimal redistribution.
- Insulin deficiency.
- Drugs (e.g., succinylcholine, markedly increased digitalis level, arginine, beta-adrenergic blockers).
- Hypertonicity.
- Hemolysis.
- Tissue necrosis, rhabdomyolysis, burns.
- Hyperkalemic periodic paralysis.

HYPERKALEMIA, DRUG-INDUCED[97]

ICD-10CM # E87.5 Hyperkalemia

IMPAIRED RENIN-ALDOSTERONE ELABORATION/FUNCTION

Cyclooxygenase inhibitors (NSAIDs).
β-Adrenergic antagonists.
Spironolactone.
Angiotensin-converting enzyme inhibitors and angiotensin II receptor blockers.
Heparin.

INHIBITORS OF RENAL POTASSIUM SECRETION

Potassium-sparing diuretics (amiloride, triamterene).
Trimethoprim.
Pentamidine.
Cyclosporine.
Digitalis overdose.
Lithium.

ALTERED POTASSIUM DISTRIBUTION

Insulin antagonists (somatostatin, diazoxide).
β-Adrenergic antagonists.
α-Adrenergic agonists.
Hypertonic solutions.
Digitalis.
Succinylcholine.
Arginine hydrochloride, lysine hydrochloride.

HYPERKALEMIA IN CHILDREN[87]

ICD-10CM # E87.5 Hyperkalemia

MOST RELEVANT CAUSES OF HYPERKALEMIA IN PEDIATRIC PATIENTS

Pseudohyperkalemia
Improper collection of blood.
Hematologic disorders: leukocytosis, thrombocytosis, spherocytosis.
Transcellular Shift of Potassium
Acidosis.
Insulin deficiency.
Hyperosmolality.
Exercise with nonselective β-blockers.
Familial hyperkalemic periodic paralysis.
Increased Potassium Load
From exogenous origin: pharmacologic supplements.
From endogenous origin (cellular lysis): burns, trauma, intravascular hemolysis, rhabdomyolysis, tumor mass destruction.
Decreased Urinary Excretion
Renal failure.
Mineralocorticoid deficiency.
Addison disease.
Hypoaldosteronism.
Mineralocorticoid resistance.
Type 1 and type 2 pseudohypoaldosteronism.
Renal tubular acidosis: type 4 and hyperkalemic form of type 1.
"Hyperkalemic" drugs: potassium-sparing diuretics, trimethoprim, calcineurin inhibitors, blockers of the renin angiotensin aldosterone system.

HYPERKINETIC MOVEMENT DISORDERS[73]

ICD-10CM #	F90.8	Attention-deficit hyperactivity disorder, other type
	E83.00	Disorder of copper metabolism, unspecified
	E83.01	Wilson disease

	E83.09	Other disorders of copper metabolism
	G24.02	Drug induced acute dystonia
	G24.1	Genetic torsion dystonia

Chorea, choreoathetosis: drug-induced, Huntington chorea, Sydenham chorea.
Tardive dyskinesia (e.g., phenothiazines).
Hemiballismus (lacunar CVA near subthalamic nuclei in basal ganglia, metastatic lesions, toxoplasmosis [in AIDS]).
Dystonia (idiopathic, familial, drug-induced [prochlorperazine, metoclopramide]), Wilson disease.
Liver failure.
Thyrotoxicosis.
SLE, polycythemia.

HYPERMAGNESEMIA

ICD-10CM #	E83.40	Disorders of magnesium metabolism, unspecified
	E83.41	Hypermagnesemia

Renal failure (decreased GFR).
Decreased renal excretion secondary to salt depletion.
Abuse of antacids and laxatives containing magnesium in patients with renal insufficiency.
Endocrinopathies (deficiency of mineralocorticoid or thyroid hormone).
Increased tissue breakdown (rhabdomyolysis).
Redistribution: acute DKA, pheochromocytoma.
Other: lithium, volume depletion, familial hypocalciuric hypercalcemia.

HYPEROSTOSIS, CORTICAL BONE[41]

ICD-10CM #	M48.19	Ankylosing hyperostosis [Forestier], multiple sites in spine

DISORDERS ASSOCIATED WITH HYPEROSTOSIS OF CORTICAL BONE

Progressive diaphyseal dysplasia.
Endosteal hyperostosis.
Pachydermoperiostosis.
Hypertrophic osteoarthropathy.
Thyroid acropachy.
Hypervitaminosis A.
Paget disease.
Infantile cortical hyperostosis.

HYPERPHOSPHATEMIA

ICD-10CM #	E83.30	Disorder of phosphorus metabolism, unspecified

Excessive phosphate administration.
Excessive oral intake or IV administration.
Laxatives containing phosphate (phosphate tablets, phosphate enemas).
Decreased renal phosphate excretion.
Acute or chronic renal failure.
Hypoparathyroidism or pseudohypoparathyroidism.
Acromegaly, thyrotoxicosis.
Bisphosphonate therapy.
Tumor calcinosis.
Sickle cell anemia.
Transcellular shift out of cells.
Chemotherapy of lymphoma or leukemia, tumor lysis syndrome, hemolysis.
Acidosis.
Rhabdomyolysis, malignant hyperthermia.
Artifact: in vitro hemolysis.
Pseudohyperphosphatemia: hyperlipidemia, paraproteinemia, hyperbilirubinemia.

HYPERPHOSPHATEMIA IN CHILDREN[87]

ICD-10CM #	E83.30	Disorder of phosphorus metabolism, unspecified

CAUSES OF HYPERPHOSPHATEMIA

Impaired Renal Excretion of Phosphate
Renal insufficiency.
Hypoparathyroidism, pseudohypoparathyroidism.
Transient parathyroid resistance of infancy.
Acromegaly.
Tumoral calcinosis.
Hyperthyroidism.
Juvenile hypogonadism.
High ambient temperature.
Heparin.
Bisphosphonate etidronate.
Increased Phosphate Intake
Exogenous Loads
Phosphate salts: laxatives and enemas.
Vitamin D intoxication.
Blood transfusion.
White phosphorus burns.
Liposomal amphotericin B.
Fosphenytoin.
Parenteral phosphate.
Endogenous Loads
Crush injury.
Rhabdomyolysis.
Cytotoxic therapy of neoplasms: tumor lysis.
Hemolysis.
Malignant hyperthermia.
Catabolic states.
Lactic acidosis.
Fulminant hepatitis.
Transcellular Shift of Phosphate
Cellular shift in diabetes ketoacidosis.
Metabolic acidosis.
Respiratory acidosis.
Miscellaneous
Hyperostosis.

HYPERPIGMENTATION[16]

ICD-10CM #	L81.4	Other melanin hyperpigmentation

Addison disease.[27]
Arsenic ingestion.
ACTH- or MSH-producing tumors (e.g., oat cell carcinoma of the lung).
Drug induced (e.g., antimalarials, some cytotoxic agents).
Hemochromatosis ("bronze" diabetes).
Malabsorption syndrome (Whipple disease and celiac sprue).
Melanoma.
Melanotropic hormone injection.
Pheochromocytoma.
Porphyrias (porphyria cutanea tarda and variegate porphyria).
Pregnancy.
Progressive systemic sclerosis and related conditions.
PUVA therapy (psoralen administration) for psoriasis and vitiligo.

---

[27] Accentuation on sun-exposed surfaces.

ACTH, Adrenocorticotropic hormone; *MSH,* melanocyte-stimulating hormone; *PUVA,* psoralen plus ultraviolet A.

HYPERPROLACTINEMIA[67]

ICD-10CM #	E22.1	Hyperprolactinemia

PHYSIOLOGIC

Pregnancy.
Lactation.
Stress.
Sleep.
Coitus.
Exercise.

PATHOLOGIC

Hypothalamic-Pituitary Stalk Damage
Tumors: craniopharyngioma, suprasellar pituitary mass extension, meningioma, dysgerminoma, hypothalamic metastases.
Granulomas.
Infiltrations.
Rathke cyst.
Irradiation.
Trauma: pituitary stalk section, sellar surgery, head trauma.
Pituitary
Prolactinoma.
Acromegaly.
Macroadenoma (compressive).
Idiopathic.
Plurihormonal adenoma.
Lymphocytic hypophysitis or parasellar mass.
Macroprolactinemia.
Systemic Disorders
Chronic renal failure.
Polycystic ovary syndrome.
Cirrhosis.
Pseudocyesis.
Epileptic seizures.
Cranial irradiation.
Chest: neurogenic chest wall trauma, surgery, herpes zoster.

PHARMACOLOGIC

Neuropeptide
Thyrotropin-releasing hormone.

Drug-Induced Hypersecretion
Dopamine receptor blockers:
Phenothiazines: chlorpromazine, perphenazine.
Butyrophenones: haloperidol.
Thioxanthenes.
Metoclopramide.
Dopamine synthesis inhibitors:
α-Methyldopa.
Catecholamine depleters:
Reserpine.
Cholinergic Agonist
Physostigmine.
Antihypertensives
Labetalol.
Reserpine.
Verapamil.
H_2 Antihistamines
Cimetidine.
Ranitidine.
Estrogens
Oral contraceptives.
Oral contraceptive withdrawal.
Anticonvulsant
Phenytoin.
Anesthetics
Neuroleptics
Chlorpromazine.
Risperidone.
Promazine.
Promethazine.
Trifluoperazine.
Fluphenazine.
Butaperazine.
Perphenazine.
Thiethylperazine.
Thioridazine.
Haloperidol.
Pimozide.
Thiothixene.
Molindone.
Opiates and Opiate Antagonists
Heroin.
Methadone.
Apomorphine.
Morphine.
Antidepressants
Tricyclic antidepressants: chlorimipramine, amitriptyline.
Selective serotonin reuptake inhibitors: fluoxetine.

HYPERSPLENISM, ASSOCIATED CONDITIONS

ICD-10CM # D73.1 Hypersplenism

Cirrhosis.
Portal vein thrombosis.
Myeloproliferative diseases.
Lymphomas.
Leukemias.
Splenic vein thrombosis.
Autoimmune disease.
Sickle cell disease.
Thalassemias.
Gaucher disease.
Niemann-Pick disease.

HYPERTENSION, ADRENOCORTICAL CAUSES[67]

ICD-10CM # I15.8 Other secondary hypertension

LOW RENIN AND HIGH ALDOSTERONE

Primary Aldosteronism

Aldosterone-producing adenoma (APA)	35% of cases
Bilateral idiopathic hyperplasia (IHA)	60% of cases
Primary (unilateral) adrenal hyperplasia	2% of cases
Aldosterone-producing adrenocortical carcinoma	<1% of cases
Familial hyperaldosteronism (FH)	
Glucocorticoid-remediable aldosteronism (FH type I)	<1% of cases
FH type II (APA or IHA)	<2% of cases
Ectopic aldosterone-producing adenoma or carcinoma	<0.1% of cases

LOW RENIN AND LOW ALDOSTERONE

Hyperdeoxycorticosteronism
Congenital adrenal hyperplasia:
11β-Hydroxylase deficiency.
17α-Hydroxylase deficiency.
Deoxycorticosterone-producing tumor.
Primary cortisol resistance.
Apparent mineralocorticoid excess (AME)/11β-HSD[28] deficiency.
Genetic: Type 1 AME.
Acquired: licorice or carbenoxolone ingestion (type 1 AME), Cushing syndrome (type 2 AME).
Cushing Syndrome
Exogenous glucocorticoid administration—most common cause.
Endogenous:
ACTH[29] -dependent—85% of cases: pituitary, ectopic.
ACTH-independent—15% of cases: unilateral adrenal disease (adenoma or carcinoma), bilateral adrenal disease (massive macronodular hyperplasia [rare], primary pigmented nodular adrenal disease [rare]).

[28] Includes alcohol, barbiturates, benzodiazepines.
[29] ACTH, corticotropin

HYPERTENSION, ENDOCRINE CAUSES[67]

ICD-10CM # I15.8 Other secondary hypertension

ADRENAL-DEPENDENT CAUSES

Pheochromocytoma.
Primary aldosteronism.
Hyperdeoxycorticosteronism:
Congenital adrenal hyperplasia: 11β-hydroxylase deficiency, 17α-hydroxylase deficiency.
Deoxycorticosterone-producing tumor.
Primary cortisol resistance.
Cushing syndrome.

AME/11β-HSD (HYDROXYSTEROID DEHYDROGENASE) DEFICIENCY

Genetic:
Type 1 apparent mineralocorticoid excess (AME).
Acquired:
Licorice or carbenoxolone ingestion (type 1 AME).
Cushing syndrome (type 2 AME).

THYROID-DEPENDENT CAUSES

Hypothyroidism.
Hyperthyroidism.

PARATHYROID-DEPENDENT CAUSES

Hyperparathyroidism.

PITUITARY-DEPENDENT CAUSES

Acromegaly.
Cushing syndrome.

HYPERTENSION, IN CHILDREN[7]

ICD-10CM # I10 Essential (primary) hypertension

PRIMARY

Essential hypertension.

SECONDARY

Renal
Glomerulonephritis.
Henoch-Schönlein purpura.
Pyelonephritis.
Obstruction of reflux.
Polycystic kidney disease.
Diabetic nephropathy.
Trauma.
Renal transplant or hemodialysis.
Tuberous sclerosis.
Systemic lupus nephritis.
Endocrine
Pheochromocytoma.
Cushing syndrome.
Congenital adrenal hyperplasia.
Corticosteroid treatment.
Hyperthyroidism.
Neuroblastoma.
Ovarian tumor.
Cardiac
Congestive heart failure.
Coarctation of the aorta.
Vascular
Hemolytic-uremic syndrome.

Kawasaki syndrome.
Renal artery thrombosis or stenosis.
Neurologic
CNS tumor or infection.
CNS trauma or abuse.
Increased intracranial pressure.
Guillain-Barré syndrome.
Neoplastic
Neuroblastoma.
Wilms tumor.
Pheochromocytoma.
Adrenal carcinoma.
Drugs
Corticosteroids.
Cocaine.
Sympathomimetics.
Oral contraceptives.
Phencyclidine.
Beta-blocker or clonidine withdrawal.
Lead, mercury.
Others
Iatrogenic fluid overload.
Volume overload from end-stage renal disease.

HYPERTENSION, RESISTANT[87]

ICD-10CM #	I10	Essential (primary) hypertension
ICD-10CM #	I15	Secondary hypertension

CAUSES OF RESISTANT HYPERTENSION

Pseudoresistance:
- White coat hypertension or office elevations.
- Pseudohypertension in older patients.
- Use of small cuff on very obese arm.

Nonadherence to therapeutic regimen.
Volume overload.
Drug-related causes:
- Antihypertensive drug dosage too low.
- Wrong type of diuretic.
- Inappropriate combinations of antihypertensive drugs.

Drug actions and interactions:
- Sympathomimetics.
- Nasal decongestants.
- Appetite suppressants.
- Cocaine.
- Caffeine.
- Oral contraceptives.
- Adrenal steroids.
- Licorice (may be found in chewing tobacco).
- Cyclosporine, tacrolimus.
- Erythropoiesis-stimulating agents (ESAs) and erythropoietin.
- Antidepressants.
- Nonsteroidal antiinflammatory drugs.

Concomitant conditions:
- Obesity.
- Sleep apnea.
- Ethanol intake >1 oz (30 ml)/day.
- Anxiety, hyperventilation.

Secondary causes of hypertension:
- Renovascular hypertension.
- Primary aldosteronism.
- Pheochromocytoma.
- Hypothyroidism.
- Hyperthyroidism.
- Hyperparathyroidism.
- Aortic coarctation.
- Renal disease.

HYPERTENSIVE CRISIS SYNDROMES[97]

ICD-10CM #	I13	Hypertensive heart and renal disease
	I15	Secondary hypertension

Malignant hypertension.
Nonmalignant hypertension with target organ disorders:
- Patient requiring emergency surgery with poorly controlled hypertension.
- Hyperviscosity syndrome.
- Postoperative patient.
- Renal transplant patient: acute rejection, transplant renal artery stenosis.
- Quadriplegic patient with autonomic hyperreflexia.
- Severe burns.
- Acute aortic dissection.
- Intracranial hemorrhage, ischemic stroke, or subarachnoid hemorrhage.
- Hypertensive encephalopathy.
- Myocardial ischemia/acute left ventricular failure.
- Preeclampsia/eclampsia.
- Antiphospholipid antibody syndrome.
- Acute renal failure:
  - Scleroderma renal crisis.
  - Chronic glomerulonephritis.
  - Reflux nephropathy.
  - Analgesic nephropathy.
  - Acute glomerulonephritis.
  - Radiation nephritis.
  - Ask-Upmark kidney.
  - Chronic lead intoxication.
- Renovascular hypertension:
  - Fibromuscular dysplasia.
  - Atherosclerosis.
- Endocrine hypertension:
  - Congenital adrenal hyperplasia.
  - Pheochromocytoma.
  - Oral contraceptives.
  - Aldosteronism.
  - Cushing disease.
  - Systemic vasculitis.
  - Atheroembolic renal crisis.
- Drugs:
  - Oral contraceptives.
  - Nonsteroidal antiinflammatory agents.
  - Atropine.
  - Corticosteroids.
  - Sympathomimetics.
  - Cyclosporine.
  - Erythropoietin.
- Lead intoxication.
- Catecholamine excess states:
  - Pheochromocytoma.
  - MAO/tyramine interaction.
  - Antihypertensive withdrawal.
  - Cocaine intoxication, sympathomimetic overdose.

HYPERTENSIVE ENCEPHALOPATHY[77]

ICD-10CM #	I67.4	Hypertensive encephalopathy

Ischemic stroke.
Intracerebral hemorrhage.
Subarachnoid hemorrhage.
Subdural hematoma.
Epidural hematoma.
Central nervous vasculitis.
Brain mass.
Seizure disorder.
Central nervous system infection.
Drug toxicity.
Withdrawal syndrome.

HYPERTRICHOSIS[21]

ICD-10CM #	L68.0	Hirsutism
	L68.1	Acquired hypertrichosis lanuginosa
	L68.3	Polytrichia
	L68.9	Hypertrichosis, unspecified
	Q84.1	Congenital morphological disturbances of hair, not elsewhere classified

DRUGS

Dilantin.
Streptomycin.
Hexachlorobenzene.
Penicillamine.
Diazoxide.
Minoxidil.
Cyclosporine.

SYSTEMIC ILLNESS

Hypothyroidism.
Anorexia nervosa.
Malnutrition.
Porphyria.
Dermatomyositis.

IDIOPATHIC

HYPERTRICHOSIS, CONGENITAL, GENERALIZED[74]

ICD-10CM #	L68.9	Hypertrichosis, unspecified

Congenital Syndromes Associated with Generalized Hypertrichosis
- Barber-Say syndrome.
- Cantú syndrome (hypertrichosis with osteochondrodysplasia).
- Coffin-Siris syndrome.
- Cornelia de Lange (Brachmann–de Lange) syndrome.
- Craniofacial dysostosis.
- Hemimaxillofacial dysplasia.
- Lipodystrophies:
  - Berardinelli-Seip syndrome.
  - Donohue syndrome (leprechaunism).

Mitochondrial encephalopathy, lactic acidosis, and stroke-like episodes (MELAS) syndrome.
Mucopolysaccharidoses:
Hunter syndrome.
Hurler syndrome.
Sanfilippo syndrome.
Rubinstein-Taybi syndrome.
Schinzel-Giedion syndrome.
Porphyrias:
Erythropoietic porphyria (Gunther disease).
Familial porphyria cutanea tarda.
Hepatoerythropoietic porphyria.
Stiff skin syndrome.
Toxin exposure:
Fetal alcohol syndrome.
Fetal hydantoin syndrome.
Winchester syndrome.

HYPERTROPHIC OSTEOARTHROPATHY

ICD-10CM # M89.40 Other hypertrophic osteoarthropathy, unspecified site

Idiopathic.
Pulmonary disease (e.g., pulmonary fibrosis, cystic fibrosis, sarcoidosis).
Bronchogenic carcinoma.
AIDS.
GI neoplasm (e.g., esophagus, colon).
Hepatic neoplasm, cirrhosis.
Cardiovascular diseases, aortic aneurysm, aortic prosthesis.
Congenital cyanotic heart disease, patent ductus arteriosus.
Pulmonary infections, bacterial endocarditis, amebic dysentery.
Inflammatory bowel disease.
Connective tissue diseases.
Lymphomas.
Thyroid acropachy.

HYPERVENTILATION, PERSISTENT[91]

ICD-10CM # R06.4 Hyperventilation

Fibrotic lung disease.
Metabolic acidosis (e.g., diabetes, uremia).
CNS disorders (midbrain and pontine lesions).
Hepatic coma.
Salicylate intoxication.
Fever.
Sepsis.
Psychogenic (e.g., anxiety).

HYPOCALCEMIA

ICD-10CM # E83.51 Hypocalcemia

Renal insufficiency: hypocalcemia caused by:
Increased calcium deposits in bone and soft tissue secondary to increased serum phosphate level.
Decreased production of 1,25-dihydroxyvitamin D.
Excessive loss of 25-OHD (nephrotic syndrome).
Hypoalbuminemia: each decrease in serum albumin (g/L) will decrease serum calcium by 0.8 mg/dl but will not change free (ionized) calcium.
Vitamin D deficiency:
Malabsorption (most common cause).
Inadequate intake.
Decreased production of 1,25-dihydroxyvitamin D (vitamin D–dependent rickets, renal failure).
Decreased production of 25-OHD (parenchymal liver disease).
Accelerated 25-OHD catabolism (phenytoin, phenobarbital).
End-organ resistance to 1,25-dihydroxyvitamin D.
Hypomagnesemia: hypocalcemia caused by:
Decreased PTH secretion.
Inhibition of PTH effect on bone.
Pancreatitis, hyperphosphatemia, osteoblastic metastases: hypocalcemia is secondary to increased calcium deposits (bone, abdomen).
Pseudohypoparathyroidism (PHP): autosomal recessive disorder characterized by short stature, shortening of metacarpal bones, obesity, and mental retardation; the hypocalcemia is secondary to congenital end-organ resistance to PTH.
Idiopathic hypoparathyroidism, surgical removal of parathyroids (e.g., neck surgery).
"Hungry bones syndrome": rapid transfer of calcium from plasma into bones after removal of a parathyroid tumor.
Sepsis.
Massive blood transfusion (as a result of EDTA in blood).

HYPOCALCEMIA IN PEDIATRIC PATIENTS[87]

ICD-10CM # E83.51 Hypocalcemia

CAUSES OF HYPOCALCEMIA

Neonatal Hypocalcemia

Early neonatal hypocalcemia (first few days of life)
Maternal hyperparathyroidism.
Maternal diabetes mellitus.
Toxemia of pregnancy.
Sepsis.
SGA, IUGR, prematurity.
Asphyxia.
Transfusion (citrated blood products).
Congenital rubella.
Hypomagnesemia.
Respiratory or metabolic alkalosis.

Late neonatal hypocalcemia (fourth to tenth day of life)
Vitamin D deficiency: nutritional deficiency; VDR loss-of-function mutation; deficient 1α-hydroxylase activity.
Phosphate overload: excessive intake of evaporated/whole milk.
Nutritional calcium deficiency.
Hypomagnesemia.
Hypoalbuminemia (nephrotic syndrome).
Transfusion (citrated blood products).
Acute/chronic kidney insufficiency.
Diuretics (furosemide).
Organic acidemia.
Primary hypoparathyroidism: DiGeorge syndrome; familial hypoparathyroidism; pseudohypoparathyroidism; Kenny-Caffey syndrome; partial deletion of GCMB; retardation dysmorphism syndrome; Pearson mitochondriopathy; Kerns-Sayre mitochondriopathy; PTH gene defects; CaSR-activating gene mutation.

Hypocalcemia in Childhood

Parathyroid-related hypocalcemia
Primary hypoparathyroidism: DiGeorge syndrome; familial hypoparathyroidism; pseudohypoparathyroidism; Kenny-Caffey syndrome; Sanjad-Sakati syndrome; partial deletion of GCMB; retardation dysmorphism syndrome; Pearson mitochondropathy; Kerns-Sayre mitochondropathy; PTH gene defects; CaSR-activating gene mutation; Bartter syndrome type 5.
Secondary hypoparathyroidism: radiation; surgery; infiltration (hemochromatosis, thalassemia, Wilson disease).
Autoimmune polyglandular syndrome type 1.

Vitamin D–related hypocalcemia
Nutritional vitamin D deficiency.
Defective 1α-hydroxylase activity.
VDR loss-of-function mutation.

Nutritional calcium deficiencyHypomagnesemia
Hyperphosphatemia: kidney failure, rhabdomyolysis, tumor lysis
Hypoalbuminemia (nephrotic syndrome)
Medications: diuretics, chemotherapy, transfusion (citrated blood)
Organic acidemia (IVA, MMA, PPA)

CaSR, Calcium-sensing receptor; *GCMB,* glial cell missing homolog B (a parathyroid-specific transcription factor); *IUGR,* intrauterine growth retardation; *IVA,* isovaleric acidemia; *MMA,* methylmalonic acidemia; *PPA,* propionic acidemia; *PTH,* parathyroid hormone; *SGA,* small for gestational age; *VDR,* vitamin D receptor.

HYPOCAPNIA

ICD-10CM # R06.8 Hypoventilation

Hyperventilation.
Pneumonia, pneumonitis.
Fever, sepsis.
Medications (salicylates, beta-adrenergic agonists, progesterone, methylxanthines).
Pulmonary disease (asthma, interstitial fibrosis).
Pulmonary embolism.
Hepatic failure.
Metabolic acidosis.
High altitude.
CHF.
Pregnancy.
Pain.
CNS lesions.

HYPOGLYCEMIA

ICD-10CM # E16.2 Hypoglycemia, unspecified
E10.65 Type 1 diabetes mellitus with hyperglycemia

	E15	Nondiabetic hypoglycemic coma
	K91.2	Postsurgical malabsorption, not elsewhere classified
	E16.2	Hypoglycemia, unspecified

Oral hypoglycemics (therapeutic, factitious).
Exogenous insulin (therapeutic, factitious).
Postoperative gastric emptying (alimentary hyperinsulinism).
Severe malnutrition.
Liver disease.
Hypermetabolic state (sepsis).
Ketotic hypoglycemia.
Insulinoma.
Antibodies to endogenous insulin.
Hormone deficiencies (glucagon, growth hormone, hypoadrenalism).
Enzyme disorders in metabolism of glycogen, hexose, glycolysis, and Krebs cycle.
Idiopathic.

HYPOGLYCEMIA, IN INFANTS AND CHILDREN[58]

ICD-10CM #	E16.2	Hypoglycemia, unspecified

CLASSIFICATION OF HYPOGLYCEMIA IN INFANTS AND CHILDREN

Neonatal Transient Hypoglycemia

Associated with Inadequate Substrate or Immature Enzyme Function in Otherwise Normal Neonates

Prematurity.
Small for gestational age.
Normal newborn.

Transient Neonatal Hyperinsulinism Also Present in

Infant of diabetic mother.
Discordant twin.
Birth asphyxia.
Infant of toxemic mother.

NEONATAL, INFANTILE, OR CHILDHOOD PERSISTENT HYPOGLYCEMIAS

Hormonal Disorders

Hyperinsulinism.
Recessive KATP channel HI.
Recessive HADH (hydroxyl acyl CoA dehydrogenase) mutation HI.
Recessive UCP2 (mitochondrial uncoupling protein 2) mutation HI.
Focal KATP channel HI.
Dominant KATP channel HI.
Dominant glucokinase HI.
Dominant glutamate dehydrogenase HI (hyperinsulinism/hyperammonemia syndrome).
Dominant mutation in HNF4A (hepatic nuclear factor 4 alpha) HI with MODY later in life.
Dominant mutation in SLC16A1 (the pyruvate transporter)-exercise-induced hypoglycemia.
Acquired islet adenoma.
Beckwith-Wiedemann syndrome.
Insulin administration (Munchausen syndrome by proxy).
Oral sulfonylurea drugs.
Congenital disorders of glycosylation.

Counter-Regulatory Hormone Deficiency

Panhypopituitarism.
Isolated growth hormone deficiency.
Addison disease.
Epinephrine deficiency.

Glycogenolysis and Gluconeogenesis Disorders

Glucose-6-phosphatase deficiency (GSD 1a).
Glucose-6-phosphate translocase deficiency (GSD 1b).
Amylo-1,6-glucosidase (debranching enzyme) deficiency (GSD 3).
Liver phosphorylase deficiency (GSD 6).
Phosphorylase kinase deficiency (GSD 9).
Glycogen synthetase deficiency (GSD 0).
Fructose-1,6-diphosphatase deficiency.
Pyruvate carboxylase deficiency.
Galactosemia.
Hereditary fructose intolerance.

Lipolysis Disorders

Fatty Acid Oxidation Disorders

Carnitine transporter deficiency (primary carnitine deficiency).
Carnitine palmitoyltransferase-1 deficiency.
Carnitine translocase deficiency.
Carnitine palmitoyltransferase-2 deficiency.
Secondary carnitine deficiencies.
Very long-, long-, medium-, short-chain acyl-CoA dehydrogenase deficiency.

OTHER ETIOLOGIES

Substrate-Limited

Ketotic hypoglycemia.
Poisoning: drugs.
Salicylates.
Alcohol.
Oral hypoglycemic agents.
Insulin.
Propranolol.
Pentamidine.
Quinine.
Disopyramide.
Ackee fruit (unripe): hypoglycin.
Vacor (rat poison).
Trimethoprim-sulfamethoxazole (with renal failure).

Liver Disease

Reye syndrome.
Hepatitis.
Cirrhosis.
Hepatoma.

Amino Acid and Organic Acid Disorders

Maple syrup urine disease.
Propionic acidemia.
Methylmalonic acidemia.
Tyrosinosis.
Glutaric aciduria.
3-Hydroxy-3-methylglutaric aciduria.

Systemic Disorders

Sepsis.
Carcinoma/sarcoma (secreting—insulin-like growth factor II).
Heart failure.
Malnutrition.
Malabsorption.
Anti-insulin receptor antibodies.
Anti-insulin antibodies.
Neonatal hyperviscosity.
Renal failure.
Diarrhea.
Burns.
Shock.
Postsurgical.
Pseudohypoglycemia (leukocytosis, polycythemia).
Excessive insulin therapy of insulin-dependent diabetes mellitus.
Factitious.
Nissen fundoplication (dumping syndrome).
Falciparum malaria.

GSD, Glycogen storage disease; *HI,* hyperinsulinemia; *KATP,* regulated potassium channel.

HYPOGONADISM

ICD-10CM #	E28.310	Symptomatic premature menopause
	E29.1	Testicular hypofunction
	E28.39	Other primary ovarian failure
	E23.6	Other disorders of pituitary gland

HYPERGONADOTROPIC HYPOGONADISM

Hormone resistance (androgen, LH insensitivity).
Gonadal defects (e.g., Klinefelter syndrome, myotonic dystrophy).
Drug-induced (e.g., spironolactone, cytotoxins).
Alcoholism, radiation-induced.
Mumps orchitis.
Anatomic defects, castration.

HYPOGONADOTROPIC HYPOGONADISM

Pituitary lesions (neoplasms, granulomas, infarction, hemochromatosis, vasculitis).
Drug-induced (e.g., glucocorticoids).
Hyperprolactinemia.
Genetic disorders (Laurence-Moon-Biedl syndrome, Prader-Willi).
Delayed puberty.
Other: chronic disease, nutritional deficiency, Kallmann syndrome, idiopathic isolated LH or FSH deficiency.

HYPOKALEMIA

ICD-10CM #	E87.6	Hypokalemia

Cellular shift (redistribution) and undetermined mechanisms.
Alkalosis (each 0.1 increase in pH decreases serum potassium by 0.4 to 0.6 mEq/L).
Insulin administration.
Vitamin B_{12} therapy for megaloblastic anemias, acute leukemias.
Hypokalemic periodic paralysis: rare familial disorder manifested by recurrent attacks of flaccid paralysis and hypokalemia.
Beta-adrenergic agonists (e.g., terbutaline), decongestants, bronchodilators, theophylline, caffeine.

Barium poisoning, toluene intoxication, verapamil intoxication, chloroquine intoxication.
Correction of digoxin intoxication with digoxin antibody fragments (Digibind).
Increased renal excretion.
Drugs:
- Diuretics, including carbonic anhydrase inhibitors (e.g., acetazolamide).
- Amphotericin B.
- High-dose sodium penicillin, nafcillin, ampicillin, or carbenicillin.
- Cisplatin.
- Aminoglycosides.
- Corticosteroids, mineralocorticoids.
- Foscarnet sodium.

RTA: distal (type 1) or proximal (type 2).
Diabetic ketoacidosis (DKA), ureteroenterostomy.
Magnesium deficiency.
Postobstruction diuresis, diuretic phase of ATN.
Osmotic diuresis (e.g., mannitol).
Bartter syndrome: hyperplasia of juxtaglomerular cells leading to increased renin and aldosterone, metabolic alkalosis, hypokalemia, muscle weakness, and tetany (seen in young adults).
Increased mineralocorticoid activity (primary or secondary aldosteronism), Cushing syndrome.
Chronic metabolic alkalosis from loss of gastric fluid (increased renal potassium secretion).
GI loss:
- Vomiting, nasogastric suction.
- Diarrhea.
- Laxative abuse.
- Villous adenoma.
- Fistulas.
- Inadequate dietary intake (e.g., anorexia nervosa).
- Cutaneous loss (excessive sweating).
- High dietary sodium intake, excessive use of licorice.

HYPOKALEMIA IN PEDIATRIC PATIENTS[87]

ICD-10CM # E87.6 Hypokalemia

MOST RELEVANT CAUSES OF HYPOKALEMIA IN PEDIATRIC PATIENTS

Acute Redistribution of Potassium to the Intracellular Compartment

Metabolic alkalosis.
Insulin administration.
Hypokalemic periodic paralysis.

Prolonged Lack of Intake

Increased Renal Loss

Drugs: diuretics, antibiotics, aminoglycosides, penicillin, amphotericin B, capreomycin.
Metabolic acidosis and diabetic ketoacidosis.
Increased mineralocorticoid activity.
Cushing syndrome.
Congenital adrenal hyperplasia.
Primary or secondary hyperaldosteronism.
Primary tubulopathies.
Bartter syndrome.
Gitelman syndrome.
Liddle syndrome.
Types 1 and 2 renal tubular acidosis.
Epilepsy, ataxia, sensorineural deafness, and tubulopathy (EAST) syndrome.
Fanconi syndrome.

Increased Gastrointestinal Loss

Vomiting (hypertrophic pyloric stenosis).
Diarrhea.

HYPOMAGNESEMIA

ICD-10CM #	E83.40	Disorders of magnesium metabolism, unspecified
	E83.42	Hypomagnesemia

GASTROINTESTINAL AND NUTRITIONAL

Defective GI absorption (malabsorption).
Inadequate dietary intake (e.g., alcoholics).
Parenteral therapy without magnesium.
Chronic diarrhea, villous adenoma, prolonged nasogastric suction, fistulas (small bowel, biliary).

EXCESSIVE RENAL LOSSES

Diuretics.
RTA.
Diuretic phase of ATN.
Endocrine disturbances (DKA, hyperaldosteronism, hyperthyroidism, hyperparathyroidism), SIADH, Bartter syndrome, hypercalciuria, hypokalemia.
Cisplatin, alcohol, cyclosporine, digoxin, pentamidine, mannitol, amphotericin B, foscarnet, methotrexate.
Antibiotics (gentamicin, ticarcillin, carbenicillin).
Redistribution: hypoalbuminemia, cirrhosis, administration of insulin and glucose, theophylline, epinephrine, acute pancreatitis, cardiopulmonary bypass.
Miscellaneous: sweating, burns, prolonged exercise, lactation, "hungry-bones" syndrome.

HYPOMAGNESEMIA IN PEDIATRIC PATIENTS[87]

ICD-10CM # E83.42 Hypomagnesemia

MAIN CAUSES OF HYPOMAGNESEMIA IN CHILDREN

Primary Inherited Disorders

Familial hypomagnesemia with hypercalciuria and nephrocalcinosis.
Hypomagnesemia with secondary hypocalcemia.
Autosomal dominant hypomagnesemia.
Isolated autosomal recessive hypomagnesemia with normocalciuria.
Activating mutations of calcium-sensing receptor.
Gitelman syndrome.
Bartter syndrome.

Secondary Disorders

Decreased GI absorption:
- Malabsorptive syndromes.
- Vomiting and diarrhea.

Increased urinary excretion:
- Extracellular volume expansion.
- Polyuric states: obstructive uropathy, kidney transplant.

Drugs:
- Diuretics.
- Calcineurin antagonists.
- Others: cisplatinum, aminoglycosides, amphotericin B.
- Metabolic acidosis.

Miscellaneous: "hungry bone," low-birth-weight newborn, infant of diabetic mother.

HYPONATREMIA

ICD-10CM # E87.1 Hypo-osmolality and hyponatremia

Renal loss from renal disease, diuretics.
GI loss (diarrhea, vomiting, suction).
Hypertonic hyponatremia (e.g., increased serum osmolality from hyperglycemia).
Transcutaneous loss (extensive burns, excessive sweating).
Fluid sequestration (e.g., ascites).
Osmotic diuresis (e.g., mannitol, glucose).
Dilutional (psychogenic polydipsia, iatrogenic).
Syndrome of inappropriate antidiuretic hormone secretion.
Edema with water and sodium retention.
Artifact (e.g., severe hyperlipidemia).
Laboratory error.
Adrenal insufficiency.

HYPOPHOSPHATEMIA

ICD-10CM #	E83.30	Disorder of phosphorus metabolism, unspecified
	E83.31	Familial hypophosphatemia

Decreased intake (prolonged starvation [alcoholics], hyperalimentation, or IV infusion without phosphate).
Malabsorption.
Phosphate-binding antacids.
Renal loss:
- RTA.
- Fanconi syndrome, vitamin D–resistant rickets.
- ATN (diuretic phase).
- Hyperparathyroidism (primary or secondary).
- Familial hypophosphatemia.
- Hypokalemia, hypomagnesemia.
- Acute volume expansion.
- Glycosuria, idiopathic hypercalciuria.
- Acetazolamide.

Transcellular shift into cells:
- Alcohol withdrawal.
- DKA (recovery phase).
- Glucose-insulin or catecholamine infusion.
- Anabolic steroids.
- Total parenteral nutrition.
- Theophylline overdose.
- Severe hyperthermia; recovery from hypothermia.
- "Hungry bones" syndrome.

HYPOPHOSPHATEMIA IN PEDIATRIC PATIENTS[87]

ICD-10CM # E83.30 Disorder of phosphorus metabolism, unspecified

CAUSES OF HYPOPHOSPHATEMIA

Decreased Phosphate Intake

Starvation, inadequate phosphate intake, chronic diarrhea, chronic alcoholism.
Total parenteral nutrition with insufficient phosphate content.

Increased Loss of Phosphate

Increased renal phosphate excretion:
- Primary hyperparathyroidism.
- Secondary hyperparathyroidism: vitamin D deficiency or resistance (including 1α-hydroxylase deficiency, VDR mutations, VDDR); imatinib.
- Excess FGF-23 or phosphatonins: X-linked hypophosphatemia, AD hypophosphatemic rickets, tumor-induced osteomalacia, epidermal nevus, McCune-Albright syndrome.
- Fanconi syndrome, cystinosis, Wilson disease, Dent disease, Lowe syndrome, multiple myeloma, amyloidosis, heavy-metal toxicity, rewarming of hyperthermia, Na/Pi-IIa and Na/Pi-IIc mutation (HHRH).
- PTHrP-dependent hypercalcemia of malignancy.
- Hypomagnesemia.

Decreased intestinal absorption:
- Vitamin D deficiency or resistance (VDDR I and II).
- Malabsorption.

Increased intestinal loss:
- Phosphate binding antacids used in treating peptic ulcers.

Increased loss from other routes:
- Skin: severe burns.
- Vomiting.

Phosphate Shifting from Extracellular Compartment to Cells and Bones

Diabetic ketoacidosis.
Alcohol intoxication.
Acute respiratory alkalosis, salicylate intoxication, gram-negative sepsis, toxic shock syndrome, acute gout.
Refeeding syndromes from starvation, anorexia nervosa, hepatic failure: acute intravenous glucose, fructose, glycerol.
Rapid cellular proliferation: intensive erythropoietin therapy, GM-CSF therapy, leukemic blast crisis.
Recovery from hypothermia.
Heat stroke.
Post parathyroidectomy; "hungry bone" disease: osteoblastic metastases, antiresorptive treatment of severe Paget disease.
Catecholamine (albuterol, dopamine, terbutaline, epinephrine).
Thyrotoxic periodic paralysis.
Hypocalcemic periodic paralysis.

Miscellaneous

Hyperaldosteronism.
Oncogenic hypophosphatemia.
Post kidney transplantation.
Post partial hepatectomy.
High-dose corticosteroids, estrogens.
Medications: ifosfamide, toluene, calcitonin, bisphosphonate, tenofovir, paraquat, cisplatin, acetazolamide and other diuretics.
Post obstructive diuresis.

AD, Autosomal dominant; *FGF-23,* fibroblast growth factor 23; *GM-CSF,* granulocyte-macrophage colony-stimulating factor; *HHRH,* hereditary hypophosphatemic rickets with hypercalciuria; *Na/Pi-II,* type II sodium-dependent phosphate cotransporter; *PTHrP,* parathyroid hormone–related peptide; *VDR,* vitamin D receptor; *VDDR,* vitamin D–dependent rickets.

HYPOPIGMENTATION

ICD-10CM # L81.9 Disorder of pigmentation, unspecified

Vitiligo.
Tinea versicolor.
Atopic dermatitis.
Chemical leukoderma.
Idiopathic hypomelanosis.
Sarcoidosis.
SLE.
Scleroderma.
Oculocutaneous albinism.
Phenylketonuria.
Nevoid hypopigmentation.

HYPOTENSION, POSTURAL

ICD-10CM # I95.89 Other hypotension

Antihypertensive medications (especially a-blockers, diuretics, ACE inhibitors).
Volume depletion (hemorrhage, dehydration).
Impaired cardiac output (constrictive pericarditis, aortic stenosis).
Peripheral autonomic dysfunction (DM, Guillain-Barré).
Idiopathic orthostatic hypotension.
Central autonomic dysfunction (Shy-Drager syndrome).
Peripheral venous disease.
Adrenal insufficiency.

HYPOTHYROIDISM, CONGENITAL[58]

ICD-10CM # E03.0 Congenital hypothyroidism with diffuse goiter
E03.1 Congenital hypothyroidism without goiter

ETIOLOGIC CLASSIFICATION OF CONGENITAL HYPOTHYROIDISM

Primary Hypothyroidism

Defect of fetal thyroid development (dysgenesis):
- Aplasia.
- Hypoplasia.
- Ectopia.

Defect in thyroid hormone synthesis (dyshormonogenesis):
- Iodide transport defect: mutation in thyroglobulin gene.
- Thyroid organification, or coupling defect: mutation in thyroid peroxidase gene.
- Defects in H_2O_2 generation: mutations in DUOXA2 maturation factor or *DUOX2* gene.
- Thyroglobulin synthesis defect: mutation in thyroglobulin gene.
- Deiodination defect: mutation in *DEHAL1* gene.

TSH unresponsiveness:
- $G_s\alpha$ mutation (e.g., type 1A pseudohypothyroidism).
- Mutation in TSH receptor.

Defect in thyroid hormone transport: mutation in monocarboxylate transporter 8 *(MCT8)* gene.
Iodine deficiency (endemic goiter).
Maternal antibodies: thyrotropin receptor–blocking antibody (TRBAb, also termed *thyrotropin-binding inhibitor immunoglobulin*).
Maternal medications:
- Iodides, amiodarone.
- Propylthiouracil, methimazole.
- Radioiodine.

CENTRAL (HYPOPITUITARY) HYPOTHYROIDISM

PIT-1 mutations:
- Deficiency of thyroid-stimulating hormone (TSH).
- Deficiency of growth hormone.
- Deficiency of prolactin.

PROP-1 mutations:
- Deficiency of TSH.
- Deficiency of growth hormone.
- Deficiency of prolactin.
- Deficiency of luteinizing hormone.
- Deficiency of follicle-stimulating hormone.
- ±Deficiency of adrenocorticotropic hormone.

TSH deficiency: mutation in TSH β subunit gene (manifests as primary hypothyroidism with elevated TSH level).
Multiple pituitary deficiencies (e.g., craniopharyngioma).
Thyroid-releasing hormone (TRH) deficiency:
- Isolated.
- Multiple hypothalamic deficiencies (e.g., septooptic dysplasia).

TRH unresponsiveness.
Mutations in TRH receptor.

HYPOTONIA, INFANTILE, DIFFERENTIAL DIAGNOSIS[58]

ICD-10CM # H44.40 Unspecified hypotony of eye

Cerebral hypotonia:
- Benign congenital hypotonia.
- Chromosome disorders.
- Prader-Willi syndrome.
- Trisomy.
- Chronic nonprogressive encephalopathy.
- Cerebral malformation.
- Perinatal distress.
- Postnatal disorders.
- Peroxisomal disorders.
- Cerebrohepatorenal syndrome (Zellweger syndrome).

Neonatal adrenoleukodystrophy.
Other genetic defects.
Familial dysautonomia.
Oculocerebrorenal syndrome (Lowe syndrome).
Other metabolic defects.
Acid maltase deficiency (see "Metabolic Myopathies").
Infantile GM, gangliosidosis.
Spinal cord disorders.
Spinal muscular atrophies:
Acute infantile.
Autosomal dominant.
Autosomal recessive.
Cytochrome-*c* oxidase deficiency.
X-linked.
Chronic infantile:
Autosomal dominant.
Autosomal recessive.
Congenital cervical spinal muscular atrophy.
Infantile neuronal degeneration.
Neurogenic arthrogryposis.
Polyneuropathies:
Congenital hypomyelinating neuropathy.
Giant axonal neuropathy.
Hereditary motor-sensory neuropathies.
Disorders of neuromuscular transmission:
Familial infantile myasthenia.
Infantile botulism.
Transitory myasthenia gravis.
Fiber-type disproportion myopathies.
Central core disease.
Congenital fiber-type disproportion myopathy.
Myotubular (centronuclear) myopathy.
Acute.
Chronic.
Nemaline (rod) myopathy.
Autosomal dominant.
Autosomal recessive.
Metabolic myopathies:
Acid maltase deficiency.
Cytochrome-*c* oxidase deficiency.
Muscular dystrophies:
Bethlem myopathy.
Congenital dystrophinopathy.
Congenital muscular dystrophy.
Merosin deficiency, primary.
Merosin deficiency, secondary.
Merosin positive.
Congenital myotonic dystrophy.

HYPOTONIC POLYURIA[87]

ICD-10CM # Varies with specific diagnosis

CAUSES OF HYPOTONIC POLYURIA

Central (Neurogenic) Diabetes Insipidus

Congenital (congenital malformations, autosomal dominant, arginine vasopressin [AVP] neurophysin gene mutations).
Drug- or toxin-induced (ethanol, diphenylhydantoin, snake venom).
Granulomatous (histiocytosis, sarcoidosis).
Neoplastic (craniopharyngioma, germinoma, lymphoma, leukemia, meningioma, pituitary tumor; metastases).
Infectious (meningitis, tuberculosis, encephalitis).
Inflammatory, autoimmune (lymphocytic infundibuloneurohypophysitis).
Trauma (neurosurgery, deceleration injury).
Vascular (cerebral hemorrhage or infarction, brain death).
Idiopathic.

Osmoreceptor Dysfunction

Granulomatous (histiocytosis, sarcoidosis).
Neoplastic (craniopharyngioma, pinealoma, meningioma, metastases).
Vascular (anterior communicating artery aneurysm or ligation, intrahypothalamic hemorrhage).
Other (hydrocephalus, ventricular or suprasellar cyst, trauma, degenerative diseases).
Idiopathic.

Increased AVP Metabolism

Pregnancy

Nephrogenic Diabetes Insipidus

Congenital (X-linked recessive, AVP V2 receptor gene mutations, autosomal recessive or dominant, aquaporin-2 water channel gene mutations).
Drug-induced (demeclocycline, lithium, cisplatin, methoxyflurane).
Hypercalcemia.
Hypokalemia.
Infiltrating lesions (sarcoidosis, amyloidosis).
Vascular (sickle cell anemia).
Mechanical (polycystic kidney disease, bilateral ureteral obstruction).
Solute diuresis (glucose, mannitol, sodium, radiocontrast dyes).
Idiopathic.

Primary Polydipsia

Psychogenic (schizophrenia, obsessive-compulsive behaviors).
Dipsogenic (downward resetting of thirst threshold, idiopathic or similar lesions, as with central DI).

HYPOVOLEMIA[87]

ICD-10CM # Varies with specific diagnosis

CAUSES OF ABSOLUTE AND RELATIVE HYPOVOLEMIA

Absolute

Extrarenal

GI fluid loss.
Bleeding.
Skin fluid loss.
Respiratory fluid loss.
Extracorporeal ultrafiltration.

Renal

Diuretics.
Obstructive uropathy/postobstructive diuresis.
Hormone deficiency.
Hypoaldosteronism.
Adrenal insufficiency.
Na^+ wasting tubulopathies.
Genetic.
Acquired tubulointerstitial disease.

Relative

Extrarenal

Edematous states.
Heart failure.
Cirrhosis.
Generalized vasodilation.
Sepsis.
Drugs.
Pregnancy.
Third-space loss.

Renal

Severe nephrotic syndrome.

HYPOVOLEMIC SHOCK, PEDIATRIC POPULATION[33]

ICD-10CM # R57.1 Hypovolemic shock
R57.8 Other shock

ETIOLOGIES OF HYPOVOLEMIC SHOCK

Whole blood loss.
Absolute loss: hemorrhage.
External bleeding.
Internal bleeding:
GI.
Intraabdominal (spleen, liver).
Major vessel injury.
Intracranial (in infants).
Fractures.
Relative loss:
Pharmacologic (barbiturates, vasodilators).
Positive pressure ventilation.
Spinal cord injury.
Sepsis.
Anaphylaxis.
Plasma loss.
Burns.
Capillary leak syndromes:
Inflammation, sepsis.
Anaphylaxis.
Protein-losing syndromes.
Fluid and electrolyte loss.
Vomiting and diarrhea.
Excessive diuretic use.
Endocrine:
Adrenal insufficiency.
Diabetes insipidus.
Diabetes mellitus.

HYPOXEMIA AND HYPERCAPNIC RESPIRATORY FAILURE[76]

ICD-10CM # Varies with specific diagnosis

COMMON CAUSES OF HYPOXEMIC AND HYPERCAPNIC RESPIRATORY FAILURE

Brain

Bulbar poliomyelitis.
Central alveolar hypoventilation.
Cerebrovascular accident.
Cerebral malignancy.
Drug overdose (e.g., narcotic, sedative/hypnotic).
Elevated intracranial pressure.
Encephalitis and meningitis.
Pontine herniation.
Postoperative anesthetic depression.

Spinal Cord

Amyotrophic lateral sclerosis.

Cervical cordotomy.
Guillain-Barré syndrome.
Poliomyelitis.
Spinal cord trauma.

Neuromuscular System

Acute intermittent porphyria.
Botulism.
Cholinergic crisis.
Curariform drugs.
Electrolyte disorders (e.g., hypophosphatemia, hypomagnesemia).
Hypokalemic periodic paralysis.
Multiple sclerosis.
Myasthenia gravis.
Myxedema.
Neuromuscular blocking antibiotics (e.g., polymyxin, streptomycin).
Organophosphate insecticides.
Peripheral neuritis.
Polymyositis.
Respiratory muscle fatigue—critical illness polyneuropathy/polymyopathy.
Tetanus.

Upper Airway

Epiglottitis and laryngotracheitis.
Large tonsils and adenoids.
Obstructive sleep apnea.
Postintubation laryngeal edema.
Tracheal obstruction.
Vocal cord paralysis.

Thorax and Pleura

Chest wall burn with eschar formation.
Chest wall trauma—flail chest.
Kyphoscoliosis.
Massive abdominal distention.
Massive obesity.
Muscular dystrophy.
Large pleural effusion/pleural fibrosis.
Pneumothorax.
Rheumatoid spondylitis.
Thoracoplasty.

Cardiovascular System

Cardiogenic pulmonary edema.
Left ventricular failure.
Mitral stenosis.
Biventricular failure.
Fat embolism.
Snake bite.
Uremia.
Volume overload.
Pulmonary veno-occlusive disease.

Lower Airway and Alveoli

Acute respiratory distress syndrome (ARDS).
Aspiration.
Asthma.
Atelectasis.
Bronchiectasis.
Bronchiolitis.
Chronic obstructive pulmonary disease.
Cystic fibrosis.
Interstitial lung disease.
Massive bilateral pneumonia.
Near-drowning.
Pancreatitis.
Pulmonary contusion.
Radiation lung injury.
Sepsis.
Smoke inhalation.
Surgical resection of lung parenchym.

ILIAC FOSSA PAIN, LEFT SIDED[95]

ICD-10CM # M25.5 Pain in joint

GASTROINTESTINAL CAUSES OF ACUTE LEFT ILIAC FOSSA PAIN

Nonspecific left iliac fossa pain including constipation.
Acute gastroenteritis.
Acute diverticulitis.
Colonic carcinoma.
Colonic ischemia.
Localized small bowel perforation.

ILIAC FOSSA PAIN, RIGHT SIDED[95]

ICD-10CM # M25.5 Pain in joint

DIFFERENTIAL DIAGNOSIS OF RIGHT ILIAC FOSSA PAIN

Gastrointestinal Causes

Nonspecific right iliac fossa pain.
Acute appendicitis.
Mesenteric adenitis.
Terminal ileitis.
Acute inflammation of Meckel diverticulum.
Crohn disease of the terminal ileum.
Cecal carcinoma.
Inflammatory cecal lesion (e.g., diverticulitis in a solitary cecal diverticulum).
Inflammatory lesion of the terminal ileum (e.g., foreign body perforation).

Non-Gastrointestinal Causes

Ruptured ovarian follicle (mittelschmerz).
Acute salpingitis (pelvic inflammatory disease).
Rupture/torsion or hemorrhage of an ovarian cyst.
Endometriosis.
Ectopic pregnancy.
Urinary tract infection.

IMMUNODEFICIENCY, CONGENITAL (PRIMARY)

ICD-10CM #	D80.0	Hereditary hypogammaglobulinemia
	D80.1	Nonfamilial hypogammaglobulinemia
	D80.2	Selective deficiency of IgA
	D80.3	Selective deficiency of IgG
	D80.4	Selective deficiency of IgM

CONGENITAL (PRIMARY) CAUSES OF IMMUNODEFICIENCY

T-lymphocyte Deficiencies

DiGeorge syndrome (thymic aplasia with reduced CD4 and CD3 cells).
Purine nucleoside phosphorylase deficiency (marked T-cell depletion).

B-lymphocyte Deficiencies

Bruton X-linked agammaglobulinemia (absence of B cells, plasma cells, and antibody).
Selective immunoglobulin G (IgG) subclass deficiencies.
Selective IgA deficiency.
Hyper-IgM immunodeficiency (elevated IgM but reduced IgG and IgA).

Mixed T- and B-lymphocyte Deficiencies

Common variable immunodeficiency (leads to various B-cell activation or differentiation defects and gradual deterioration of T-cell number and function).
Severe combined immunodeficiency (severe reduction in IgG and absence of T cells).
Wiskott-Aldrich syndrome (decreased T-cell number and function, low IgM, occasionally low IgG).
Ataxia-telangiectasia (decreased T-cell number and function; IgA, IgE, IgG_2, and IgG_4 deficiency).

Disorders of Complement

C3 deficiency (congenital absence of C3 or consumption of C3 due to deficiency of C3b inactivator).

Phagocyte Defects

Chronic granulomatous disease (defect in nicotinamide adenine dinucleotide phosphate oxidase in phagocytic cells).
Chédiak-Higashi syndrome (impaired microbicidal activity of phagocytes).
Kostmann syndrome, Shwachman-Diamond syndrome, cyclic neutropenia (low neutrophil count).

IMPAIRED CONSCIOUSNESS AND COMA[93]

ICD-10CM # R40.20 Unspecified coma

INFECTIOUS OR INFLAMMATORY

Infectious

Bacterial meningitis.
Viral encephalitis.
Rickettsial infection.
Protozoan infection.
Helminth infestation.

Inflammatory

Sepsis-associated encephalopathy.
Vasculitis, collagen vascular disorders.
Demyelination.
Acute disseminated encephalomyelitis.
Multiple sclerosis.

STRUCTURAL

Traumatic

Concussion.
Cerebral contusion.
Epidural hematoma or effusion.
Intracerebral hematoma.
Diffuse axonal injury.
Abusive head trauma.

Neoplasms

Vascular Disease

Cerebral infarction:
- Thrombosis.
- Embolism.
- Venous sinus thrombosis.

Cerebral hemorrhage:
- Subarachnoid hemorrhage.
- Arteriovenous malformation.

Aneurysm.
Congenital abnormality or dysplasia of vascular supply
Trauma to carotid or vertebral arteries in the neck

Focal Infection

Abscess.
Cerebritis.

Hydrocephalus

METABOLIC, NUTRITIONAL, OR TOXIC

Hypoxic-Ischemic Encephalopathy

Shock.
Cardiac or pulmonary failure.
Near-drowning.
Carbon monoxide poisoning.
Cyanide poisoning.
Strangulation.

Metabolic Disorders

Sarcoidosis.
Hypoglycemia.
Fluid and electrolyte imbalance.
Endocrine disorders:
With acidosis:
- Diabetic ketoacidosis.
- Aminoacidemias.
- Organic acidemias.

With hyperammonemia:
- Hepatic encephalopathy.
- Urea cycle disorders.
- Disorders of fatty acid metabolism.
- Reye syndrome.
- Valproic acid encephalopathy.

Uremia.
Porphyria.
Mitochondrial disorders.
Leigh syndrome.

Nutritional

Thiamine deficiency.
Niacin or nicotinic acid deficiency.
Pyridoxine dependency.
Folate and vitamin B_{12} deficiency.

Exogenous Toxins and Poisons

Alcohol intoxication.
Over-the-counter medications.
Prescription medications (oral and ophthalmic).
Herbal treatments.
Heavy-metal poisoning.
Mushroom and plant intoxication.
Illegal drugs.
Industrial agents.

Hypertensive Encephalopathy

Burn Encephalopathy

IMPOTENCE[69]

ICD-10CM #	F52.21	Male erectile disorder
	F52.8	Other sexual dysfunction not due to a substance or known physiological condition
	N52.9	Male erectile dysfunction, unspecified

Psychogenic.
Endocrine: hyperprolactinemia, DM, Cushing syndrome, hypothyroidism or hyperthyroidism, abnormality of hypothalamic-pituitary-testicular axis.
Vascular: arterial insufficiency, venous leakage, AV malformation, local trauma.
Medications.
Neurogenic: autonomic or sensory neuropathy, spinal cord trauma or tumor, CVA, multiple sclerosis, temporal lobe epilepsy.
Systemic illness: renal failure, COPD, cirrhosis of liver, myotonic dystrophy.
Peyronie disease.
Prostatectomy.

INCONTINENCE, FECAL[95]

ICD-10CM # R15.9 Full incontinence of feces

NORMAL SPHINCTER

Diarrhea.
Anorectal conditions:
- Rectal carcinoma.
- Inflammatory bowel disease.
- Hemorrhoids.
- Mucosal prolapse.
- Fissure-in-ano.
- Abnormal rectal sensation.

ABNORMAL SPHINCTER

Congenital abnormalities.
Anal sepsis.
Neurologic conditions.
Rectal prolapse.
Sphincter trauma.
Neurogenic (idiopathic) incontinence.

INFECTIOUS DIARRHEA IN TROPICS[30]

ICD-10CM # R19.7 Diarrhea, unspecified

CAUSES OF INFECTIOUS DIARRHEA IN THE TROPICS

Bacteria

Aeromonas hydrophila.
Arcobacter butzleri.
Bacteroides fragilis, enterotoxigenic.
Campylobacter jejuni.
Escherichia coli: enterotoxigenic, enteroaggregative, enteroinvasive, enterohemorrhagic.
Laribacter hongkongensis.
Plesiomonas shigelloides.
Salmonella, non-typhoidal.
Shigella spp.: *S. dysenteriae, S. flexneri, S. sonnei, S. boydii.*
Vibrio cholerae 01, 0139, non-01 non-0139.
Vibrio parahaemolyticus.
Yersinia enterocolitica.

Helminths

Paracapillaria philippinensis.
Fasciolopsis buski.
Heterophyiasis (Metagonimus yokogawai, Haplorchis taichui).
Schistosoma mansoni.
Strongyloides stercoralis.

Protozoa

Blastocystis hominis.
Cryptosporidium parvum.
Cyclospora cayetanensis.
Encephalitozoon intestinalis.
Enterocytozoon bieneusi.
Giardia lamblia.
Isospora belli.
Leishmania donovani.

Viruses

Astroviruses.
Caliciviruses: norovirus and sapovirus.
Enteric adenoviruses.
HIV.
Picornaviruses.
Rotavirus.

INFERTILITY, FEMALE[36]

ICD-10CM # N97.9 Female infertility, unspecified

FALLOPIAN TUBE PATHOLOGY

PID or puerperal infection.
Congenital anomalies.
Endometriosis.
Secondary to past peritonitis of nongenital origin.
Amenorrhea and anovulation.
Minor anovulatory disturbances.

CERVICAL AND UTERINE FACTORS

Leiomyomas and polyps.
Uterine anomalies.
Intrauterine synechiae (Asherman syndrome).
Destroyed endocervical glands (postsurgery or postinfection).

VAGINAL FACTORS

Congenital absence of vagina.
Imperforate hymen.
Vaginismus.
Vaginitis.

IMMUNOLOGIC FACTORS

Sperm-immobilizing antibodies.
Sperm-agglutinating antibodies.

NUTRITIONAL AND METABOLIC FACTORS

Thyroid disorders.
DM.
Severe nutritional disturbances.

INFERTILITY, MALE[36]

ICD-10CM # N46.9 Male infertility, unspecified

DECREASED PRODUCTION OF SPERMATOZOA

Varicocele.
Testicular failure.
Endocrine disorders.
Cryptorchidism.
Stress, smoking, caffeine, nicotine, recreational drugs.

DUCTAL OBSTRUCTION

Epididymal (postinfection).
Congenital absence of vas deferens.
Ejaculatory duct (postinfection).
Postvasectomy.

INABILITY TO DELIVER SPERM INTO VAGINA

Ejaculatory disturbances.
Hypospadias.
Sexual problems (i.e., impotence), medical or psychological.

ABNORMAL SEMEN

Infection.
Abnormal volume.
Abnormal viscosity.
Abnormal sperm motion.

IMMUNOLOGIC FACTORS

Sperm-immobilizing antibodies.
Sperm-agglutinating antibodies.

INSOMNIA[84]

ICD-10CM #	780.51	Insomnia with sleep apnea
	G47.00	Insomnia, unspecified
	F51.01	Primary insomnia
	F51.03	Paradoxical insomnia
	F51.09	Other insomnia not due to a substance or known physiological condition

Anxiety disorder, psychophysiologic insomnia.
Depression.
Drugs (e.g., caffeine, amphetamines, cocaine), hypnotic-dependent sleep disorder.
Pain, fibromyalgia.
Inadequate sleep hygiene.
Restless leg syndrome.
Obstructive sleep apnea.
Sleep bruxism.
Medical illness (e.g., GERD, sleep-related asthma, parkinsonism and movement disorders).
Narcolepsy.
Other: periodic leg movement of sleep, central sleep apnea, REM behavioral disorder.

INTESTINAL PSEUDOOBSTRUCTION[59,91]

ICD-10CM #	K56.0	Paralytic ileus
	K56.9	Ileus, unspecified
	K59.9	Functional intestinal disorder, unspecified

"PRIMARY" (IDIOPATHIC INTESTINAL PSEUDOOBSTRUCTION)

Hollow visceral myopathy:
- Familial.
- Sporadic.

Neuropathic:
- Abnormal myenteric plexus.
- Normal myenteric plexus.

SECONDARY

Scleroderma.
Myxedema.
Amyloidosis.
Muscular dystrophy.
Hypokalemia.
Chronic renal failure.
DM.
Drug toxicity caused by:
- Anticholinergics.
- Opiate narcotics.

Ogilvie syndrome.

Causes of Secondary Chronic Intestinal Pseudoobstruction in Children

Autoimmune
Autoimmune myositis.
Autoimmune ganglionitis.
Scleroderma.
Endocrine
Diabetes mellitus.
Hypoparathyroidism.
Hypothyroidism.
Gastrointestinal
Celiac disease.
Eosinophilic gastroenteritis.
Inflammatory bowel disease.
Hematology/oncology
Multiple myeloma.
Paraneoplastic syndromes.
Pheochromocytoma.
Sickle cell disease.
Infection
Chagas disease.
Cytomegalovirus.
Epstein-Barr virus.
Herpes zoster.
JC virus.
Kawasaki disease.
Postviral neuropathy.
Medications and toxins
Chemotherapy.
Cyclopentolate and phenylephrine eye drops.
Diltiazem and nifedipine.
Fetal alcohol syndrome.
Jellyfish envenomation.
Opioid medications.
Postanesthesia.
Radiation injury.
Mitochondrial disorders
Mitochondrial neurogastrointestinal encephalomyopathy.
Musculoskeletal disorders
Ehlers-Danlos syndrome.
Myotonic dystrophy.
Duchenne muscular dystrophy.
Rheumatology
Amyloidosis.
Dermatomyositis.
Polymyositis.
Systemic lupus erythematous.

From Wyllie R, Hyams JS, Kay M, editors: *Pediatric gastrointestinal and liver disease,* 5th ed, Elsevier, 2016, Philadelphia, Box. 44.3, p. 548.

INTRAABDOMINAL MASS LESION, NEONATAL[41]

ICD-10CM #	R19.00	Intraabdominal and pelvic swelling, mass and lump, unspecified site

CAUSES OF A NEONATAL INTRA-ABDOMINAL MASS LESION

Complicated meconium ileus.
Dilated bowel proximal to an obstruction.
Mesenteric or duplication cyst.
Abscess.
GU causes:
- Hydronephrosis.
- Renal cystic disease.
- Mesoblastic nephroma.
- Wilms tumor.
- Adrenal hemorrhage.
- Neuroblastoma.
- Retroperitoneal teratoma.
- Ovarian cyst.
- Hydrometrocolpos.

Hemangioendothelioma.
Hepatoblastoma.
Choledochal, hepatic, or splenic cysts.

INTRACEREBRAL HEMORRHAGE, NONHYPERTENSIVE CAUSES

ICD-10CM #	I61.9	Nontraumatic intracerebral hemorrhage, unspecified

Trauma.
Anticoagulation.
Intracranial tumors.
Vascular malformations.
Bleeding disorders.
Vasculitides (e.g., polyarteritis nodosa, granulomatous angiitis).
Cocaine and other sympathomimetic agents.
Cerebral amyloid angiopathy.

INTRACRANIAL LESION

ICD-10CM #	G93.89	Other specified disorders of brain

Tumor (primary or metastatic).
Abscess.
Stroke.
Intracranial hemorrhage.
Angioma.
Multiple sclerosis (initial single lesion).
Granuloma.
Herpes encephalitis.
Artifact.

INTRACRANIAL TUMORS[39]

ICD-10CM #	D33.2	Benign neoplasm of brain, unspecified
	C71.9	Malignant neoplasm of brain, unspecified

Differential Diagnosis of Intracranial Tumors

- Infection.
- Brain abscess.
- Bacterial.
- Fungal.
- Parasitic (e.g., cysticercosis).
- Herpes encephalitis.
- Vascular disease.
- Stroke.
- Intracranial hemorrhage.
- Inflammatory conditions.
- Granuloma (sarcoid).
- Multiple sclerosis: tumefactive single large lesion.
- Vascular malformations.

Cavernous angiomas.
Venous angiomas.
Congenital abnormalities.
Cortical dysplasia.
Heterotopia.

INTRAOCULAR NEOPLASM

ICD-10CM #	C69.9	Malignant disorder of eye, unspecified

MALIGNANT

Retinoblastoma.
Melanoma.
Reticulum cell sarcoma.
Metastatic tumor.

BENIGN

Melanocytic nevus.
Hemangioma.
Reactive lymphoid hyperplasia.

IRON METABOLISM DISORDERS[5]

ICD-10CM #	E83.10	Disorder of iron metabolism, unspecified

IRON DEFICIENCY

Deficient Iron Intake

Diet of low bioavailability.
Increased physiological requirements due to rapid growth in early childhood and in adolescence.
Blood loss.
Physiological (e.g., menstruation).
Pathological (e.g., GI).

Malabsorption of Iron

Reduced or absent gastric acid secretion (e.g., after partial or total gastrectomy or with atrophic gastritis).
Reduced duodenal absorption (e.g., in coeliac disease).
Bypass of stomach and duodenum (bariatric surgery).
Rare, inherited iron-refractory iron deficiency anemia (e.g., deficiency of TMPRSS6 [transmembrane protease, serine 6], also known as matriptase-2).

Redistribution of Iron

Macrophage iron accumulation in reticuloendothelial system in inflammatory, infectious, or malignant diseases (anemia of chronic disease, also known as anemia of inflammation).
Macrophage iron accumulation within the lungs in idiopathic pulmonary hemosiderosis.

IRON OVERLOAD

Due to Increased Iron Absorption

Hereditary hemochromatosis—commonly (among Northern Europeans) homozygosity for *HFE* C282Y but sometimes involving non-C282Y *HFE* or other genes (*HAMP, HFE2* [encoding hemojuvelin], *TFR2, SLC40A1*).
Substantial ineffective erythropoiesis (e.g., β thalassemia intermedia and major, some types of sideroblastic anemia, congenital dyserythropoietic anemia).
Sub-Saharan iron overload ("Bantu siderosis")—only in combination with increased dietary iron.
Other rare inherited disorders (e.g., congenital atransferrinemia, DMT1 deficiency, aceruloplasminemia).
Inappropriate iron therapy (rare).

DUE TO MULTIPLE BLOOD TRANSFUSIONS FOR REFRACTORY ANEMIAS OR FOR OTHER REASONS

Thalassemia major.
Aplastic anemia.
Myelodysplastic syndromes.
Sickle cell disease (when regularly transfused).

IRON OVERLOAD[50]

ICD-10CM #	E83.10	Disorder of iron metabolism, unspecified

HEREDITARY IRON OVERLOAD

Hereditary hemochromatosis:
- HFE-associated (type 1).
- Non–HFE-associated:
  - Transferrin receptor 2–associated (type 3).

Juvenile hemochromatosis (type 2):
- Hemojuvelin-associated (type 2A).
- Hepcidin-associated (type 2B).

Autosomal dominant hemochromatosis:
- Ferroportin-associated (type 4).
- DMT1-associated hemochromatosis.
- Atransferrinemia.
- Aceruloplasminemia.

ACQUIRED IRON OVERLOAD

Iron-loading anemias (refractory anemias with hypercellular erythroid marrow).
Chronic liver disease.
Porphyria cutanea tarda.
Insulin resistance–associated hepatic iron overload.
African dietary iron overload.[30]
Medical iron ingestion.
Parenteral iron overload:
- Transfusional iron overload.
- Inadvertent iron overload from therapeutic injections.

PERINATAL IRON OVERLOAD

Neonatal hemochromatosis.
Trichohepatoenteric syndrome.
Cerebrohepatorenal syndrome.
GRACILE (Fellman) syndrome.[31]

FOCAL SEQUESTRATION OF IRON

Idiopathic pulmonary hemosiderosis.
Renal hemosiderosis.
Associated with neurologic abnormalities:
- Pantothenate kinase–associated neurodegeneration (formerly called Hallervorden-Spatz syndrome).
- Neuroferritinopathy.
- Friedreich ataxia.

[30] May have a genetic component.
[31] GRACILE, Growth retardation, aminoaciduria, cholestasis, iron overload, lactic acidosis, and early death.

ISCHEMIA, UPPER EXTREMITY, CAUSES[17]

ICD-10CM #	S45.809A	Unspecified injury of other specified blood vessels at shoulder and upper arm level, unspecified arm, initial encounter

VASOSPASM

Raynaud disease.
Medication induced: vasopressors, β-blockers.
Ergot poisoning.

INTRINSIC ARTERIAL DISEASE

Atherosclerosis.
Radiation arteritis.
Azotemic arteriopathy.
Spontaneous dissection.
Fibromuscular dysplasia.

INFLAMMATORY DISEASES

Connective tissue disorders.
Buerger disease.
Takayasu arteritis.
Temporal (giant cell) arteritis.
Hypersensitivity angiitis.

NONINFLAMMATORY MEDICAL DISEASE

Thrombophilic states.
Myeloproliferative disorders.
Cold injury.
Hepatitis-associated vasculitis.
Cryoglobulinemia.
Vinyl chloride exposure.

EMBOLISM

Cardiac (most common).
Proximal aneurysm.
Arterial thoracic outlet syndrome.
Atheroembolism.
Paradoxic embolus (with accompanying septal defect).

TRAUMA

Iatrogenic.
Blunt arterial injury.
Penetrating arterial injury.
Hypothenar hammer syndrome.
Vibration.

ISCHEMIC BOWEL DISEASE[1]

ICD-10CM #	K55.1	Vascular disorder of intestine
	I99	Other and unspecified disorders of circulatory system

Abdominal aortic aneurysm: rupture or expansion.
Perforated ulcer or viscus.
Ruptured ectopic pregnancy (woman of childbearing age).
Incarcerated or strangulated hernia.

Septic shock.
Intussusception.
Volvulus.
Salpingitis or tuboovarian abscess.
Torsion of the ovary or testicle.
Appendicitis.
Pelvic mass or torsion.
Pancreatitis.
Diverticulitis.
Ruptured ovarian cyst.
Renal colic.
Biliary colic.
Also consider atypical manifestations of:
- Inferior wall myocardial infarction.
- Pulmonary embolism.
- Pneumonia.
- Diabetic ketoacidosis.
- Acute glaucoma.

Differential diagnoses are listed in order of urgency.

ISCHEMIC COLITIS, NONOCCLUSIVE[54]

ICD-10CM #	K55.1	Chronic vascular disorders of intestine

ACUTE DIMINUTION OF COLONIC INTRAMURAL BLOOD FLOW

Small Vessel Obstruction

Collagen-vascular disease.
Vasculitis, diabetes.
Oral contraceptives.

Nonocclusive Hypoperfusion

Hemorrhage.
CHF, MI, arrhythmias.
Sepsis.
Vasoconstricting agents: vasopressin, ergot.
Increased viscosity: polycythemia, sickle cell disease, thrombocytosis.

INCREASED DEMAND ON MARGINAL BLOOD FLOW

Increased Motility

Mass lesion, stricture.
Constipation.

Increased Intraluminal Pressure

Bowel obstruction.
Colonoscopy.
Barium enema.

ISCHEMIC NECROSIS OF CARTILAGE AND BONE[36]

ICD-10CM #	M89.9	Disorder of bone, unspecified
	M94.9	Disorder of cartilage, unspecified

ENDOCRINE/METABOLIC

Ethanol abuse.
Glucocorticoid therapy.
Cushing disease.
DM.
Hyperuricemia.
Osteomalacia.
Hyperlipidemia.

STORAGE DISEASES (E.G., GAUCHER DISEASE)

Hemoglobinopathies (e.g., sickle cell disease).
Trauma (e.g., dislocation, fracture).
HIV infection.
Dysbaric conditions (e.g., caisson disease).
Collagen-vascular disorders.
Irradiation.
Pancreatitis.
Organ transplantation.
Hemodialysis.
Burns.
Intravascular coagulation.
Idiopathic, familial.

JAUNDICE

ICD-10CM #	R17	Unspecified jaundice
	K83.8	Other specified diseases of biliary tract
	E80.7	Disorder of bilirubin metabolism, unspecified

PREDOMINANCE OF DIRECT (CONJUGATED) BILIRUBIN

Extrahepatic obstruction.
Common duct abnormalities: calculi, neoplasm, stricture, cyst, sclerosing cholangitis.
Metastatic carcinoma.
Pancreatic carcinoma, pseudocyst.
Ampullary carcinoma.
Hepatocellular disease: hepatitis, cirrhosis.
Drugs: estrogens, phenothiazines, captopril, methyltestosterone, labetalol.
Cholestatic jaundice of pregnancy.
Hereditary disorders: Dubin-Johnson syndrome, Rotor syndrome.
Recurrent benign intrahepatic cholestasis.

PREDOMINANCE OF INDIRECT (UNCONJUGATED) BILIRUBIN

Hemolysis: hereditary and acquired hemolytic anemias.
Inefficient marrow production.
Impaired hepatic conjugation: chloramphenicol.
Neonatal jaundice.
Hereditary disorders: Gilbert syndrome, Crigler-Najjar syndrome.

JAUNDICE, CLASSIFICATION[3]

ICD-10CM #	R17	Unspecified jaundice

PREHEPATIC (PREDOMINANTLY UNCONJUGATED HYPERBILIRUBINEMIA)

Overproduction

Hemolysis (e.g., spherocytosis, sickle cell disease, hemolysis of the newborn, autoimmune disorders).
Ineffective erythropoiesis (e.g., megaloblastic anemias).
Hematomas.
Pulmonary emboli.

HEPATIC (UNCONJUGATED HYPERBILIRUBINEMIA)

Decreased Hepatic Uptake

Gilbert syndrome.
Drugs (e.g., rifampin, radiographic contrast agents).
Neonatal jaundice.
Posthepatitis.
Decreased cystolic binding proteins (e.g., newborn or premature infants).
Portacaval shunt.
Prolonged fasting.

Decreased Conjugation Due to Limited Glucuronyl Transferase Activity

Gilbert disease.
Crigler-Najjar syndrome, types I and II.
Neonatal jaundice.
Breast-milk jaundice.
Chronic persistent hepatitis.
Wilson disease.
Noncirrhotic portal fibrosis.
Drug inhibition (e.g., chloramphenicol).

PREDOMINANTLY CONJUGATED HYPERBILIRUBINEMIA

Impaired Hepatic Excretion

Familial disorders (Dubin-Johnson syndrome, Rotor syndrome, benign recurrent cholestasis, cholestasis of pregnancy).
Hepatocellular infiltrative disorders.
Liver metastasis.
Liver cirrhosis.
Hepatitis (viral, bacterial, parasitic, autoimmune, ethanol, and drug-induced).
Drug-induced cholestasis (especially chlorpromazine, erythromycin estolate, isoniazid, halothane).
Primary biliary cirrhosis.
Primary sclerosing cholangitis.
Pericholangitis.
Congestive heart failure.
Shock.
Toxemia of pregnancy.
Sarcoidosis.
Hepatic trauma.
Amyloidosis.
Autoimmune cholangiopathy.
Vanishing bile duct syndrome.
Sepsis.
Postoperative complications.

EXTRAHEPATIC

Extrahepatic Biliary Obstruction

Gallstones, choledocholithiasis.
Cholecystitis.
Tumors of the head of the pancreas (adenocarcinoma, mucinous duct ectasia, neuroendocrine tumors, metastasis).
Tumors of bile ducts (cholangiocarcinoma, Klatskin tumor: cholangiocarcinoma at the bifurcation).
Gallbladder cancer.
Tumors of the ampulla of Vater (adenoma, adenocarcinoma).
Tumors of the duodenum (adenocarcinoma, lymphoma).
Hemobilia (blood in the biliary tree).

Biliary strictures (postcholecystectomy, post-liver transplantation, primary sclerosing cholangitis).
Congenital disorders (biliary atresia, idiopathic dilation of common bile duct, cystic fibrosis).
Metastasis to the hepatic hilum.
Primary bile duct lymphoma.
Cholangiopathy of acquired immunodeficiency syndrome.
Choledochal cysts.
Infectious cholangiopathy *(Clonorchis sinensis, Ascaris lumbricoides, Fasciola hepatica).*
Chronic pancreatitis (fibrosis of the head of the pancreas).

JAUNDICE, NEONATAL[3]

ICD-10CM #		
ICD-10CM #	P59.9	Neonatal jaundice, unspecified

PREHEPATIC

Hereditary spherocytosis.
Nonspherocytic hemolytic anemia (glucose-6-phosphate dehydrogenase deficiency, α-thalassemia, vitamin K_3–induced hemolysis, pyruvate kinase deficiency).

HEPATIC

Crigler-Najjar syndrome, types I and II.
α_1-Antitrypsin deficiency.
Sepsis.
Drug-induced.
Hypothyroidism.
Breast-milk jaundice.
Fetomaternal blood group incompatibility (Rhesus, Landsteiner groups ABO).

POSTHEPATIC

Extrahepatic biliary obstruction.
Biliary atresia.
Bile duct paucity.
Alagille syndrome.

JOINT AND PERIARTICULAR PAIN, ACUTE[31]

ICD-10CM #	M25.50	Joint pain

COMMON ACUTE MONOARTHRITIS

Septic arthritis (nongonococcal, gonococcal).
Crystal arthritis (gout, pseudogout).
Reactive arthritides.
Lyme disease.
Plant thorn synovitis.
Other infections (mycobacterial, viral, soft tissue).

TRAUMA OR INTERNAL DERANGEMENT

Loose bodies.
Stress fractures.
Ischemic necrosis.
Hemarthrosis.

ACUTE MONOARTHRITIS OR POLYARTHRITIS

Psoriatic arthritis.
Enteropathic arthritis.
Rheumatoid arthritis/palindromic rheumatism.
Juvenile inflammatory arthritides.

MONOARTHROPATHIES FROM NONINFLAMMATORY DISEASE

Osteoarthritis.
Charcot joints.
Storage diseases (hemochromatosis, ochronosis).

SYNOVIAL DISEASES

Pigmented villonodular synovitis.
Lipoma arborescens.
Synovial osteochondromatosis.
Reflex sympathetic dystrophy.
Sarcoidosis.
Amyloid.

ACUTE MONOARTHRITIS OF SYSTEMIC DISEASE

Systemic lupus erythematosus.
Vasculitides (antineutrophil cytoplasmic antibody positive and negative).
Henoch-Schönlein purpura.
Behçet disease.
Bacterial endocarditis.
Familial Mediterranean fever.
Relapsing polychondritis.

SOFT TISSUE LESIONS

Bone Diseases

Paget disease.
Osteomyelitis (Brodie abscess).
Osteogenic/osteoid tumors.
Metastatic disease.
Pulmonary hypertrophic osteoarthropathy.

This table shows the causes of inflammation in any one joint (monoarthritis) and pain around the joint that presents without inflammation (monoarthropathy).

JOINT PAIN, ANTERIOR HIP, MEDIAL THIGH, KNEE[71]

ICD-10CM #	M25.50	Pain in unspecified joint
	M25.559	Pain in unspecified hip
	M25.569	Pain in unspecified knee

ACUTE

Acute rheumatic fever.
Adductor muscle strain.
Avascular necrosis.
Crystal arthritis.
Femoral artery (pseudo) aneurysm.
Fracture (femoral neck or intertrochanteric).
Hemarthrosis.
Hernia.
Herpes zoster.
Iliopectineal bursitis.
Iliopsoas tendinitis.
Inguinal lymphadenitis.
Osteomalacia.
Painful transient osteoporosis of hip.
Septic arthritis.

SUBACUTE AND CHRONIC

Adductory muscle strain.
Amyloidosis.
Acute rheumatic fever.
Femoral artery aneurysm.
Hernia (inguinal or femoral).
Iliopectineal bursitis.
Iliopsoas tendinitis.
Inguinal lymphadenopathy.
Osteochondromatosis.
Osteomyelitis.
Osteitis deformans (Paget disease).
Osteomalacia (pseudofracture).
Postherpetic neuralgia.
Sterile synovitis (e.g., RA, psoriatic, SLE).

JOINT PAIN, HIP, LATERAL THIGH[71]

ICD-10CM #	S79.919A	Unspecified injury of unspecified hip, initial encounter
	S79.929A	Unspecified injury of unspecified thigh, initial encounter
	M25.9	Joint disorder, unspecified

ACUTE

Herpes zoster.
Iliotibial tendinitis.
Impacted fracture of femoral neck.
Lateral femoral cutaneous neuropathy (meralgia paresthetica).
Radiculopathy: L4-5.
Trochanteric avulsion fracture (greater trochanter).
Trochanteric bursitis.
Trochanteric fracture.

SUBACUTE AND CHRONIC

Lateral femoral cutaneous neuropathy (meralgia paresthetica).
Osteomyelitis.
Postherpetic neuralgia.
Radiculopathy: L4-5.
Tumors.

JOINT PAIN, POLYARTICULAR

ICD-10CM #	M25.50	Pain in unspecified joint

Osteoarthritis.
RA.
Fibromyalgia.
Viral syndrome (e.g., human parvovirus B19 infection).
SLE.
Psoriatic arthritis.
Ankylosing spondylitis.

JOINT PAIN, POSTERIOR HIPS, THIGH, BUTTOCKS[71]

ICD-10CM #	M25.50	Pain in unspecified joint
	M25.559	Pain in unspecified hip
	M25.569	Pain in unspecified knee

ACUTE
Gluteal muscle strain.
Herpes zoster.
Ischial bursitis.
Ischial or sacral fracture.
Osteomalacia (pseudofracture).
Sciatic neuropathy.
Radiculopathy: L5-S1.

SUBACUTE AND CHRONIC
Gluteal muscle strain.
Ischial bursitis.
Lumbar spinal stenosis.
Osteoarthritis of hip.
Osteitis deformans (Paget disease).
Osteomyelitis.
Osteochondromatosis.
Osteomalacia (pseudofracture).
Postherpetic neuralgia.
Radiculopathy: L5-S1.
Tumors.

JOINT SWELLING

ICD-10CM #	M25.40	Effusion, unspecified joint

Trauma.
Osteoarthritis.
Gout.
Pyogenic arthritis.
Pseudogout.
RA.
Viral syndrome.

JUGULAR VENOUS DISTENTION

ICD-10CM #	I99.8	Other disorder of circulatory system

Right-sided heart failure.
Cardiac tamponade.
Constrictive pericarditis.
Goiter.
Tension pneumothorax.
Pulmonary hypertension.
Cardiomyopathy (restrictive).
Superior vena cava syndrome.
Valsalva maneuver.
Right atrial myxoma.
COPD.

KERATITIS, NONINFECTIOUS

ICD-10CM #	H16.9	Unspecified keratitis

Collagen vascular disease.
Atopic keratoconjunctivitis.
Chemical injury.
Thermal injury.
Ectropion/entropion.
Lid defects.
Exophthalmos.
Keratoconjunctivitis sicca.
Erythema multiforme.
Mucous membrane pemphigoid.
DM (delayed epithelial healing).
Neuroparalytic (cranial nerve VII).
Neurotrophic (diabetes, cranial nerve V).

KIDNEY CYSTIC DISEASE[99]

ICD-10CM # Varies with specific diagnosis

CYSTIC DISEASES OF THE KIDNEY
Inheritable
Autosomal recessive (infantile) polycystic kidney disease.
Autosomal dominant (adult) polycystic kidney disease.
Juvenile nephronophthisis and medullary cystic disease complex.
Juvenile nephronophthisis (autosomal recessive).
Medullary cystic disease (autosomal dominant).
Congenital nephrosis (familial nephrotic syndrome) (autosomal recessive).
Familial hypoplastic glomerulocystic disease (autosomal dominant).
Multiple malformation syndromes with renal cysts (e.g., tuberous sclerosis, von Hippel-Lindau disease).
Nonheritable
Multicystic kidney (multicystic dysplastic kidney).
Benign multilocular cyst (cystic nephroma).
Simple cysts.
Medullary sponge kidney.
Sporadic glomerulocystic kidney disease.
Acquired renal cystic disease.
Calyceal diverticulum (pyelogenic cyst).

KIDNEY ENLARGEMENT, UNILATERAL[95]

ICD-10CM #	N13.30	Unspecified hydronephrosis

Hydronephrosis (may be bilateral).
Polycystic kidney (may be bilateral).
Simple cyst of kidney.
Renal cell carcinoma.
Pyonephrosis (may be bilateral).
Acute renal vein thrombosis.

KIDNEY INJURY, CANCER PATIENTS[87]

ICD-10CM # Varies with specific diagnosis

CAUSES OF ACUTE KIDNEY INJURY IN CANCER PATIENTS
Prerenal
Sepsis
Volume depletion (vomiting, diarrhea, mucositis).
Hepatorenal syndrome (venoocclusive disease of the liver).
Capillary leak syndrome (interleukin-2 administration).
Hypercalcemia.
Intrinsic
Acute tubular necrosis
Ischemia (sepsis/shock).
Nephrotoxic (aminoglycosides, amphotericin B, chemotherapy).
Tubulointerstitial nephritis
Tumor lysis syndrome (urate and phosphate nephropathy).
Allergic reaction.
Pyelonephritis.
Opportunistic infections.
Infiltration (lymphoma/leukemia).
Vascular
Thrombotic microangiopathy.
Cancer treated.
Drug induced.
Bone marrow transplantation.
Radiation injury.
Amyloidosis
Light-chain deposition disease
Paraneoplastic syndromes (membranous, antineutrophil cytoplasmic antibody associated, focal segmental glomerulosclerosis)
Postrenal
Intrarenal (urate, acyclovir, methotrexate)
Extrarenal (retroperitoneal fibrosis, lymphadenopathy, direct invasion)

KNEE PAIN[71]

ICD-10CM #	S83.419A	Sprain of medial collateral ligament of unspecified knee, initial encounter
	S83.509A	Sprain of unspecified cruciate ligament of unspecified knee, initial encounter
	M23.50	Chronic instability of knee, unspecified knee
	M23.8X9	Other internal derangements of unspecified knee
	S83.289A	Other tear of lateral meniscus, current injury, unspecified knee, initial encounter
	S83.249A	Other tear of medial meniscus, current injury, unspecified knee, initial encounter
	M25.669	Stiffness of unspecified knee, not elsewhere classified

DIFFUSE
Articular.
Anterior.
Prepatellar bursitis.
Patellar tendon enthesopathy.
Chondromalacia patellae.
Patellofemoral osteoarthritis.
Cruciate ligament injury.
Medial plica syndrome.

MEDIAL
Anserine bursitis.
Spontaneous osteonecrosis.

Osteoarthritis.
Medial meniscal tear.
Medial collateral ligament bursitis.
Referred pain from hip and L3.
Fibromyalgia.

LATERAL

Iliotibial band syndrome.
Meniscal cyst.
Lateral meniscal tear.
Collateral ligament.
Peroneal tenosynovitis.

POSTERIOR

Popliteal cyst (Baker cyst).
Tendinitis.
Aneurysms, ganglions, sarcoma.

KNEE PAIN, IN DIFFERENT AGE GROUPS[22]

ICD-10CM #	M25.569	Pain in unspecified knee

COMMON CAUSES OF KNEE PAIN IN DIFFERENT AGE GROUPS

Childhood (2 to 10 yr)
Intraarticular
Juvenile arthritis.
Osteochondritis dissecans.
Infection.
Torn discoid meniscus.
Periarticular
Osteomyelitis.
Referred
Perthes disease.
Irritable hip.
Adolescence (10 to 18 yr)
Intraarticular
Osteochondritis dissecans.
Torn meniscus.
Anterior knee pain syndrome.
Patellar instability.
Periarticular
Osgood–Schlatter disease.
Sinding–Larsen–Johansson syndrome.
Osteomyelitis.
Bone tumors.
Referred
Slipped upper femoral epiphysis.
Early Adulthood (18 to 30 yr)
Intraarticular
Torn meniscus.
Patellar instability.
Anterior knee pain syndrome.
Inflammatory arthritis.
Periarticular
Ligament injuries.
Bursitis.
Adulthood (30 to 50 yr)
Intraarticular
Degenerate meniscal tears.
Osteoarthritis.
Inflammatory arthritis.
Periarticular
Bursitis.
Referred
Osteoarthritis of hip.
Spinal disorders.
Old Age (>50 yr)
Intraarticular
Osteoarthritis.
Inflammatory arthritis.
Periarticular
Bursitis.
Referred
Osteoarthritis of hip.
Spinal disorders.

LARGE BOWEL STRICTURE[41]

ICD-10CM #	S36.5	Injury of colon

CAUSES OF LARGE BOWEL STRICTURES

Physiologic:
- Spasm.
- Distended bladder.

Malignant:
- Annular carcinoma.
- Scirrhous carcinoma.
- Lymphoma.

Diverticular disease:
- Muscle thickening.
- Pericolic abscess.
- Superimposed malignancy.

Ischemia.
Radiation colitis.
Inflammatory bowel disease:
- Ulcerative colitis.
- Crohn disease.
- Tuberculosis.
- Lymphogranuloma venereum.
- Amebiasis.

Extrinsic disease:
- Intraabdominal masses.
- Metastatic carcinoma.
- Endometriosis.
- Pelvic lipomatosis.
- Cholecystitis.
- Pancreatitis.

Miscellaneous:
- Postoperative anastomosis.
- Trauma.
- Hirschsprung disease.

LEFT AXIS DEVIATION[57]

ICD-10CM #	I44.7	Left bundle-branch block, unspecified
	I44.4	Left anterior fascicular block
	I44.5	Left posterior fascicular block
	I44.60	Unspecified fascicular block
	I44.69	Other fascicular block

Normal variation.
Left anterior fascicular block (hemiblock).
Left bundle branch block.
Left ventricular hypertrophy.
Mechanical shifts causing a horizontal heart, high diaphragm, pregnancy, ascites.
Some forms of ventricular tachycardia.
Endocardial cushion defects and other congenital heart disease.

LEFT BUNDLE BRANCH BLOCK

ICD-10CM #	I44.7	Left bundle-branch block, unspecified

Ischemic heart disease.
Electrolyte abnormalities (e.g., hyperkalemia).
Cardiomyopathy.
Idiopathic.
LVH.
Pulmonary embolism.
Cardiac trauma.
Bacterial endocarditis.

LEG CRAMPS, NOCTURNAL

ICD-10CM #	R25.2	Cramp and spasm

Diabetic neuropathy.
Medications.
Electrolyte abnormalities (hypokalemia, hyponatremia, hypocalcemia, hyperkalemia, hypophosphatemia).
Respiratory alkalosis.
Uremia.
Hemodialysis.
Peripheral nerve injury.
ALS.
Alcohol use.
Heat cramps.
Vitamin B_{12} deficiency.
Hyperthyroidism.
Contractures.
DVT.
Hypoglycemia.
Peripheral vascular insufficiency.
Baker cyst.

LEG LENGTH DISCREPANCIES[60]

ICD-10CM #	M21.759	Unequal limb length (acquired), unspecified femur
	M21.769	Unequal limb length (acquired), unspecified tibia and fibula
	Q72.899	Other reduction defects of unspecified lower limb

CONGENITAL

Proximal femoral local deficiency.
Coxa vara.
Hemiatrophy-hemihypertrophy (anisomelia).
Developmental dysplasia of the hip.

DEVELOPMENTAL

Legg-Calvé-Perthes disease.

NEUROMUSCULAR

Polio.
Cerebral palsy (hemiplegia).

INFECTIOUS

Pyogenic osteomyelitis with physeal damage.

TRAUMA

Physeal injury with premature closure.
Overgrowth.
Malunion (shortening).

TUMOR

Physeal destruction.
Radiation-induced physeal injury.
Overgrowth.

LEG MOVEMENT WHEN STANDING, INVOLUNTARY

ICD-10CM # R25.8 Other abnormal involuntary movements

Benign essential tremor.
Orthostatic tremor.
Spastic ataxia.
Cerebellar truncal tremor.
Postanoxic myoclonus.

LEG PAIN, EXERTIONAL[104]

ICD-10CM # R25.2 Cramp and spasm

Vascular Causes

Atherosclerosis.
Thrombosis.
Embolism.
Vasculitis:
- Thromboangiitis obliterans.
- Takayasu arteritis.
- Giant cell arteritis.

Aortic coarctation.
Fibromuscular dysplasia.
Irradiation.
Endofibrosis of the external iliac artery.
Extravascular compression:
- Arterial entrapment (e.g., popliteal artery entrapment, thoracic outlet syndrome).

Adventitial cysts.

Nonvascular Causes

Lumbosacral radiculopathy:
- Degenerative arthritis.
- Spinal stenosis.
- Herniated disc.

Arthritis:
- Hips, knees.

Venous insufficiency.
Myositis.
Glycogen storage disease type V (McArdle syndrome).

LEG PAIN WITH EXERCISE

ICD-10CM # R25.2 Cramp and spasm

Shin splints.
Arteriosclerosis obliterans.
Neurogenic (spinal cord compression or ischemia).
Venous claudication.
Popliteal cyst.
DVT.
Thromboangiitis obliterans.
Adventitial cysts.
Popliteal artery entrapment syndrome.
McArdle syndrome.

LEG SWELLING[1]

ICD-10CM # R60.0 Localized edema

Deep vein thrombosis.
Cellulitis.
Baker cyst rupture or inflammation.
Congestive heart failure.
Renal failure.
Liver failure.
Inferior vena cava compression.
Musculoskeletal trauma.
Polyarteritis nodosa.
Erythema nodosum.
Myositis.
Tendinitis.
Lymphedema.
Superficial thrombophlebitis.
Compartment syndrome.

LEG ULCERS[71]

ICD-10CM # I70.25 Atherosclerosis of native arteries of other extremities with ulceration
L97.909 Non-pressure chronic ulcer of unspecified part of unspecified lower leg with unspecified severity

VASCULAR

Arterial: arteriosclerosis, thromboangiitis obliterans, AV malformation, cholesterol emboli.
Venous: superficial varicosities, incompetent perforators, DVT, lymphatic abnormalities.

VASCULITIS HEMATOLOGIC

Sickle cell anemia, thalassemia, polycythemia vera, leukemia, cold agglutinin disease.
Macroglobulinemia, protein C and protein S deficiency, cryoglobulinemia, lupus anticoagulant, antiphospholipid syndrome.

INFECTIOUS

Fungal: blastomycosis, coccidioidomycosis, histoplasmosis, sporotrichosis.
Bacterial: Furuncle, ecthyma, septic emboli.
Protozoal: leishmaniasis.

METABOLIC

Necrobiosis lipoidica diabeticorum.
Localized bullous pemphigoid.
Gout, calcinosis cutis, Gaucher disease.

TUMORS

Basal cell carcinoma, squamous cell carcinoma, melanoma.
Mycosis fungoides, Kaposi sarcoma, metastatic neoplasms.

TRAUMA

Burns, cold injury, radiation dermatitis.
Insect bites.
Factitial, excessive pressure.

NEUROPATHIC

Diabetic trophic ulcers.
Tabes dorsalis, syringomyelia.

DRUGS

Warfarin, IV colchicine extravasation, methotrexate, halogens, ergotism, hydroxyurea.

PANNICULITIS

Weber-Christian disease.
Pancreatic fat necrosis, alpha-antitrypsinase deficiency.

LEPTOMENINGEAL LESIONS

ICD-10CM # G03.9 Leptomeningitis

Metastases.
Multiple sclerosis.
Bacterial or viral meningitis.
Vasculitis.
Lyme disease.
Tuberculosis.
Fungal infections (e.g., *Cryptococcus*).
Sarcoidosis.
Granulomatosis with polyangiitis.
Neurocysticercosis.
Rheumatoid nodules.
Histiocytosis.

LEUKOCORIA

ICD-10CM # H57.9 Unspecified disorder of eye and adnexa

Cataract.
Retinal detachment.
Retinoblastoma.
Retinal telangiectasia.
Retrolenticular vascularized membrane.
Familial exudative vitreoretinopathy.

LID RETRACTION, CAUSES[53]

ICD-10CM # H02.539 Eyelid retraction unspecified eye, unspecified lid

Thyroid eye disease.
Neurogenic:
- Contralateral unilateral ptosis.
- Unopposed levator action due to facial palsy.
- 3rd nerve misdirection.
- Marcus Gunn jaw-winking syndrome.
- Collier sign of the dorsal midbrain (Parinaud syndrome).
- Infantile hydrocephalus (setting sun sign).
- Parkinsonism.
- Sympathomimetic drops.

Mechanical:
- Surgical over-correction of ptosis.
- Scarring of upper lid skin.

Congenital:
- Isolated.
- Duane retraction syndrome.
- Down syndrome.
- Transient "eye popping" reflex in normal infants.

Miscellaneous:
- Prominent globe (pseudo-lid retraction).
- Uremia (Summerskill sign).
- Idiopathic.

LIGHT-NEAR DISSOCIATION[13]

ICD-10CM # Varies with specific diagnosis

CAUSES OF LIGHT-NEAR DISSOCIATION

Unilateral

Afferent conduction defect.
Adie pupil.
Herpes zoster ophthalmicus.
Aberrant regeneration of the third cranial nerve.

Bilateral

Neurosyphilis.
Type 1 diabetes mellitus.
Myotonic dystrophy.
Parinaud (dorsal midbrain) syndrome.
Familial amyloidosis.
Encephalitis.
Chronic alcoholism.

LIMB ISCHEMIA, ACUTE, NONTRAUMATIC[17]

ICD-10CM #	I70.2	Atherosclerosis of arteries of extremities

CAUSES OF NONTRAUMATIC ACUTE LIMB ISCHEMIA

Atherosclerotic

In situ thrombosis.
Atheroembolism from thoracic aortic aneurysm/abdominal aortic aneurysm.
Femoral/popliteal aneurysm with or without compression.
Dissection.

Nonatherosclerotic

Embolism from cardiac thrombosis (atrial fibrillation, post–myocardial infarction akinesis).
Graft thrombosis, graft aneurysm.
Mycotic emboli.
Raynaud phenomenon.
Arteritis with thrombosis.
Inherited and acquired hypercoagulable states.
Drug-induced vasospasm.
External compression (Baker cyst, popliteal entrapment).

Mimics

Phlegmasia cerulea dolens.
Acute neuropathy.
Hypovolemia.
Systemic shock.

LIMP

ICD-10CM #	R26.0	Ataxic gait
	R26.1	Paralytic gait
	R26.89	Other abnormalities of gait and mobility
	R26.9	Unspecified abnormalities of gait and mobility
	M25.80	Other specified joint disorders, unspecified joint
	F44.4	Conversion disorder with motor symptom or deficit
	F44.6	Conversion disorder with sensory symptom or deficit

Degenerative joint disease, osteochondritis dissecans, chondromalacia patellae.
Trauma to extremities, vertebral disk, hips.
Poorly fitting shoes, foreign body in shoe, unequal leg length.
Splinter in foot.
Joint infection (septic arthritis, osteomyelitis), viral arthritis.
Abdominal pain (e.g., appendicitis, incarcerated hernia), testicular torsion.
Polio, neuromuscular disorders, Guillain-Barré syndrome, multiple sclerosis.
Osgood-Schlatter disease.
Legg-Calvé-Perthes disease.
Factitious, somatization syndrome.
Neoplasm (local or metastatic).
Other: diskitis, periostitis, sickle cell disease, hemophilia.

LIMPING, PEDIATRIC AGE[60]

ICD-10CM #	R26.0	Ataxic gait
	R26.1	Paralytic gait
	R26.89	Other abnormalities of gait and mobility
	R26.9	Unspecified abnormalities of gait and mobility

TODDLER (1 TO 3 YR)

Infection:
- Septic arthritis:
  - Hip.
  - Knee.
- Osteomyelitis.
- Diskitis.

Occult trauma:
- Toddler's fracture.

Neoplasia.

CHILDHOOD (4 TO 10 YR)

Infection:
- Septic arthritis:
  - Hip.
  - Knee.
- Osteomyelitis.
- Diskitis.
- Transient synovitis, hip.

LCPD.
Tarsal coalition.
Rheumatologic disorder:
- JRA.

Trauma.
Neoplasia.

ADOLESCENCE (11+ YR)

SCFE.
Rheumatologic disorder:
- JRA.
- Trauma.
- Tarsal coalition.
- Hip dislocation (DDH).
- Neoplasia.

DDH, Developmental dysplasia of the hip; *JRA,* juvenile RA; *LCPD,* Legg-Calvé-Perthes disease; *SCFE,* slipped capital femoral epiphysis.

LIVEDO RETICULARIS

ICD-10CM #	L95.0	Livedoid vasculitis

Emboli (SBE, left atrial myxoma, cholesterol emboli).
Thrombocythemia or polycythemia.
Antiphospholipid antibody syndrome.
Cryoglobulinemia, cryofibrinogenemia.
Leukocytoclastic vasculitis.
SLE, RA, dermatomyositis.
Pancreatitis.
Drugs (quinine, quinidine, amantadine, catecholamines).
Physiologic (cutis marmorata).
Congenital.

LIVER DISEASE, PREGNANCY[95]

ICD-10CM #	K75.89	Other specified inflammatory liver diseases

INCIDENTAL TO PREGNANCY

Viral hepatitis.
Alcohol related.
Autoimmune chronic active hepatitis.

RELATED TO PREGNANCY (POSSIBLY INFLUENCED BY HORMONES PRESENT IN PREGNANCY)

Complicated gallstone disease.
Hepatic adenoma.
Focal nodular hyperplasia.
Budd-Chiari syndrome.

SPECIFIC TO PREGNANCY

Severe hyperemesis gravidarum.
Benign intrahepatic cholestasis.
Acute fatty liver of pregnancy.
Preeclampsia (HELLP).

LIVER LESIONS, BENIGN, OFTEN CONFUSED WITH MALIGNANCY

ICD-10CM #	K76.1	Chronic passive congestion of liver
	K76.89	Other specified diseases of liver

Fatty infiltration.
Adenoma.
Hemangioma.
Cysts.
Flow artifacts.
Focal nodular hyperplasia.
Nonenhanced vessels.

LOWER GI ULCERATIVE LESIONS[26]

ICD-10CM # Varies with specific diagnosis

INFECTIOUS

Epstein-Barr virus.
Human immunodeficiency virus.
Cytomegalovirus.
Herpes simplex.
Herpes zoster.
Syphilis.

Erosive candidiasis.
Mycobacterial infection.
Chancroid.
Lymphogranuloma venereum.

NOT INFECTIOUS

Behçet disease.
Excoriation.
Aphthous (idiopathic) ulcer.
Erythema multiforme.
Carcinoma.

LOW-VOLTAGE ECG

ICD-10CM # R94.31 Abnormal electrocardiogram [ECG] [EKG]

Hypothyroidism.
Obesity.
Pericardial effusion.
Anasarca.
Pleural effusion.
Pneumothorax.
Amyloidosis.
Aortic stenosis.

LUMBAR SPINE, VISCEROGENIC PAIN REFERRED TO LUMBAR SPINE[47]*

ICD-10CM # M54.5 Low back pain

Vascular
Expanding aortic aneurysm.
Genitourinary
Endometriosis.
Tubal pregnancy.
Kidney stone.
Prostatitis.
Gastrointestinal
Pancreatitis.
Peptic ulcers.
Colon cancer.

LUNG CANCER, OCCUPATIONAL CAUSES[41]

ICD-10CM # C34.90 Malignant neoplasm of unspecified part of unspecified bronchus or lung

CAUSES OF OCCUPATIONAL LUNG CANCER

Asbestos	Lagging, insulation
Arsenic	Metal smelting, pesticide manufacture
Beryllium	Electronics, dental prosthetic manufacture
Chromium	Coloring pigment production, electroplating
Nickel	Electroplating
Silica	Grinding, quarrying, sandblasting
Radon	Mining
Uranium	Mining

*All of these disorders may cause localized low back pain.

LUNG DISEASE AND GASTROINTESTINAL AND LIVER INVOLVEMENT[66]

ICD-10CM # Varies with specific diagnosis

ESOPHAGEAL REFLUX

Aspiration pneumonia.
Asthma.
Scleroderma.
Bronchitis.
Bronchiectasis.
Cough.
Pulmonary fibrosis.
Mycobacterial disease.

INFLAMMATORY BOWEL DISEASE

Bronchitis.
Bronchiectasis.
Bronchiolitis.
Colobronchial fistula.
Desquamative interstitial lung disease.
Drug reactions for agents that treat inflammatory bowel disease.
Eosinophilic lung disease.
Interstitial lung disease.
Necrobiotic nodules.
Obstructive lung disease.
Organizing pneumonia.
Reduced diffusing capacity.
Sarcoidosis.
Serositis affecting pleura or pericarditis.
Tracheal stenosis.

LIVER

Alpha1-antitrypsin deficiency.
Chronic active hepatitis.
Hepatopulmonary syndrome.
Portapulmonary hypertension.
Primary biliary cirrhosis.
Hepatosplenomegaly.
- Amyloidosis.
- Collagen vascular disease.
- Eosinophilic granulomatosis.
- Lymphatic interstitial pneumonia.
- Sarcoidosis.

LUNG DISEASE AND RENAL INVOLVEMENT[66]

ICD-10CM # Varies with specific diagnosis

LUNG DISEASE WITH RENAL INVOLVEMENT

Glomerulonephritis
Systemic vasculitis.
Collagen vascular disease.
Antibasement membrane.
Sarcoidosis.
Nephrotic Syndrome
Amyloidosis.
Disseminated Langerhans cell histiocytosis.
Drug-induced lung disease.
Paraneoplastic syndrome.
Post transplantation.
Pulmonary hydatid disease.
Systemic lupus erythematosus.
Vasculitis.
Venous thrombosis.
Renal Mass
Lymphangioleiomyomatosis.
Metastasis neoplasm.
Renal carcinoid.
Tuberous sclerosis.
Granulomatosis with polyangiitis.
Nephrolithiasis
Alveolar proteinosis.
Cystic fibrosis.
Hypercalcemic syndromes.
Osteolysis from mycobacteria or fungi.
Sarcoidosis.
Systemic Hypertension
Collagen vascular disease.
Diffuse alveolar hemorrhage.
Pulmonary renal syndromes.
Neurofibromatosis.
Sleep apnea.

LUNG DISEASE AND SKIN AND SUBCUTANEOUS LESIONS[66]

ICD-10CM # Varies with specific diagnosis

SKIN AND SUBCUTANEOUS LESIONS ASSOCIATED WITH LUNG DISEASE

Skin Lesions
Diffuse pigment change:
- Acanthosis nigricans—lung neoplasm.
- Albinism—Hermansky-Pudlak syndrome.
- Bronze pigmentation—hemosiderosis.
- Gray-brown—Whipple disease.

Cutaneous draining sinus:
- Fungal infections (especially histoplasmosis).
- Mycobacterial infections (especially tuberculosis).
- Neoplasms (especially mesothelial tumors).
- Necrotizing vasculitis.
- Other bacterial infections (especially actinomycosis).

Cutaneous ulcers:
- Beryllium disease.
- Chronic venous insufficiency.
- Fungal infections (especially histoplasmosis).
- Mycobacterial disease.
- Necrotizing vasculitis.
- Parasitic disease.
- Polycythemia.
- Sickle cell disease.
- Tularemia.

Cutaneous vasculitis:
- Behçet syndrome.
- Churg-Strauss syndrome.
- Collagen vascular disease.
- Sarcoidosis.
- Granulomatosis with polyangiitis.

Erythema multiforme:
- Drug reactions.
- Fungi (especially coccidiomycosis).
- Mycoplasma and other infectious agents.
- Neoplasms.
- Exfoliative dermatitis.
- Adverse drug reactions.
- Chemotherapy.

Disseminated malignancy.
Graft-versus-host disease.
Radiation therapy.

Flushing:
- Bronchial carcinoid, pheochromocytoma, other neoplasms.
- Carbon dioxide, cyanide, and other toxins.
- Drugs.
- Foods and vasodilatory substances.
- Hormones.
- Mastocytosis.
- Metabolic states (e.g., hyperthyroidism, fever).

Macular rash:
- Anti-basement membrane disease.
- Café-au-lait spots (neurofibromatosis).
- Coal miner's scars.
- Collagen vascular disease.
- Idiopathic pulmonary fibrosis.
- Rose spots (psittacosis).
- Sarcoidosis.
- Syphilis.
- Viral pneumonia.

Maculopapular rash:
- Amyloidosis.
- Drug-induced lung disease.
- Collagen vascular disease.
- Gaucher disease.
- Kaposi sarcoma.
- Lung neoplasm.
- Lymphomatoid granulomatosis.
- Lymphoma.
- Parasites.
- Sarcoidosis.
- Syphilis.
- Vasculitis.
- Viral pneumonia

Telangiectasia:
- Arteriovenous malformation.
- Ataxia-telangiectasia.
- Carcinoid syndrome.
- Cushing disease.
- Hepatopulmonary syndrome and other chronic liver diseases.
- Hereditary hemorrhagic telangiectasia (Osler-Weber-Rendu).
- Mastocytosis.
- Systemic sclerosis and other collagen vascular diseases.

Urticaria:
- Asthma.
- Drug reactions.
- Cystic fibrosis.
- Exercise-induced urticaria.
- Food allergy.
- Hereditary angioneurotic edema.
- Inhaled antigens.
- Insect bites and stings.
- Infectious agents, such as mycoplasma and helicobacter.
- Mastocytosis.
- Occupational sensitization.
- Parasites.
- Vasculitis.

Nail Changes with Lung Disease

Color changes:
- Cigarette smoking discoloration.
- Splinter hemorrhages.
- Yellow nail syndrome.

Beau lines (any severe illness):
- Dermatomyositis.
- Sarcoidosis.
- Seronegative arthropathies.
- Systemic sclerosis.

Lung Disease with Subcutaneous Involvement

Adenopathy:
- Environmental mycobacteria.
- Fungal infections.
- Human immunodeficiency virus infections.
- Metastatic neoplasm.
- Leukemia.
- Lymphoma.
- Sarcoidosis.
- Tuberculosis.

Calcinosis:
- Dermatomyositis.
- Metastatic osteosarcoma.
- Mixed connective tissue disease.
- Scleroderma.
- Tuberculosis.
- Uremic metastatic calcification.

Erythema induratum (Bazin disease):
- Aortic stenosis.
- Cryoglobulinemia.
- Nodular vasculitis.
- Panniculitis.
- Peripheral neuropathy.
- Takayasu disease.
- Streptococcus infection.
- Tuberculosis and other mycobacterial disease.
- Weber-Christian disease.

Erythema nodosa:
- Neoplasm.
- Other infectious and inflammatory diseases.
- Primary coccidiomycosis, histoplasmosis.
- Primary tuberculosis.
- Psittacosis.
- Sarcoidosis.

Subcutaneous nodules:
- Amyloidosis.
- Neoplasm.
- Neurofibromatosis.
- Rheumatoid arthritis.
- Tuberous sclerosis (angiofibromas).
- von Recklinghausen.
- Weber-Christian disease.

Lung Disease with Salivary Gland Enlargement

Bulimia and aspiration.
Gaucher disease.
Lymphoid interstitial pneumonitis.
Lymphatic carcinoma.
Lymphoma.
Other causes of lymphadenopathy.
Sarcoidosis.
Sjögren disease.

LUNG DISEASE WITH BONE, JOINT, NERVE, AND MUSCLE INVOLVEMENT[66]

ICD-10CM # Varies with specific diagnosis

ARTHRITIS

Ankylosing spondylitis.
Collagen vascular diseases.
Reactive arthritis.
Sarcoidosis.
Systemic vasculitis.
Tuberculosis.

BONE LESIONS

Ankylosing spondylitis.
Blastomycosis and other fungal disease.
Collagen vascular diseases.
Eosinophilic granulomatosis.
Fibrous histiocytoma.
Gaucher disease.
Neoplasm.
Sarcoidosis.
Tuberculosis.

MUSCLE DISEASE

Collagen vascular disease.
L-Tryptophan.
Diabetes insipidus.
Eosinophilic granulomatosis.
Polymyositis.
Sarcoidosis.

NEUROLOGIC DISEASE

Acute inflammatory polyneuropathy.
Amyotrophic lateral sclerosis.
Aspiration.
Botulism.
Lambert-Eaton syndrome.
Myasthenia gravis.
Organophosphate poisoning.
Polio and postpolio syndrome.
Sarcoidosis.
Churg-Strauss syndrome.
Granulomatosis with polyangiitis.

LUNG TUMORS, BENIGN[85]

ICD-10CM # Varies with specific disorder

COMMON BENIGN TUMORS OF THE LUNG BASED ON CELLS OF ORIGIN

Tumors of Epithelial Origin

Mucous gland adenoma.
Clara cell adenoma.
Mucous cystadenoma.
Pleomorphic adenoma.

Tumors of Mesenchymal Origin

Hamartoma.
Inflammatory pseudotumor.
Chondroma.
Fibroma.
Benign endobronchial fibrous histiocytoma.
Leiomyoma.
Lipoma.
Lymphatic lesions.

Tumors of Miscellaneous Origin

Nodular pulmonary amyloidosis.
Clear cell tumor (sugar tumor).
Thymoma.
Granular cell tumor.
Teratoma.
Pulmonary paraganglioma.

LUNG VOLUMES IN DIFFUSE LUNG DISEASE[38]

ICD-10CM # Varies with specific disorder

LARGE LUNG VOLUMES

Emphysema.
Chronic asthma.
Diffuse bronchiolitis obliterans.
Highly trained athletes.
Lymphangioleiomyomatosis.

SMALL LUNG VOLUMES

End-stage lung fibrosis.
Bilateral diaphragmatic paralysis.
Massive ascites.

NORMAL LUNG VOLUMES

Sarcoidosis.
Langerhans cell histiocytosis.
Neurofibromatosis.
Emphysema with pulmonary fibrosis.

LYMPHADENOPATHY[36]

ICD-10CM #	R59.9	Enlarged lymph nodes, unspecified

GENERALIZED

AIDS.
Lymphoma: Hodgkin disease, non-Hodgkin lymphoma.
Leukemias, reticuloendotheliosis.
Infectious mononucleosis, CMV, and other viral infections.
Diffuse skin infection: generalized furunculosis, multiple tick bites.
Parasitic infections: toxoplasmosis, filariasis, leishmaniasis, Chagas disease.
Serum sickness.
Collagen vascular diseases (RA, SLE).
Dengue (arbovirus infection).
Sarcoidosis and other granulomatous diseases.
Drugs: INH, hydantoin derivatives, antithyroid and antileprosy drugs.
Secondary syphilis.
Hyperthyroidism, lipid-storage diseases.

LOCALIZED

Cervical Nodes
Infections of the head, neck, ears, sinuses, scalp, pharynx.
Mononucleosis.
Lymphoma.
TB.
Malignancy of head and neck.
Rubella.
Scalene/Supraclavicular Nodes
Lymphoma.
Lung neoplasm.
Bacterial or fungal infection of thorax or retroperitoneum.
GI malignancy.
Axillary Nodes
Infections of hands and arms.
Cat-scratch disease.
Neoplasm (lymphoma, melanoma, breast carcinoma).
Brucellosis.
Epitrochlear Nodes
Infections of the hand.
Lymphoma.
Tularemia.
Sarcoidosis, secondary syphilis (usually bilateral).
Inguinal Nodes
Infections of leg or foot, folliculitis (pubic hair).
LGV, syphilis.
Lymphoma.
Pelvic malignancy.
Pasteurella pestis.
Hilar Nodes
Sarcoidosis.
TB.
Lung carcinoma.
Fungal infections, systemic.
Mediastinal Nodes
Sarcoidosis.
Lymphoma.
Lung neoplasm.
TB.
Mononucleosis.
Histoplasmosis.
Abdominal/Retroperitoneal Nodes
Lymphoma.
TB.
Neoplasm (ovary, testes, prostate, and other malignancies).

LYMPHANGITIS[63]

ICD-10CM #	I89.1	Lymphangitis

Acute:
- Group A streptococci.
- *Staphylococcus aureus.*
- *Pasteurella multocida.*

Chronic:
- *Sporothrix schenckii* (sporotrichosis).
- *Mycobacterium marinum* (swimming pool granuloma).
- *Mycobacterium kansasii.*
- *Nocardia brasiliensis.*
- *W. bancrofti.*

LYMPHEDEMA[52]

ICD-10CM #	I89.0	Lymphedema, not elsewhere classified
	I97.2	Postmastectomy lymphedema syndrome
	Q82.0	Hereditary lymphedema

CLASSIFICATION OF LYMPHEDEMA

Primary lymphedema
Congenital lymphedema (Milroy disease).
Lymphedema praecox.
Lymphedema tarda.
Syndromes associated with primary lymphedema
Yellow nail syndrome.
Turner syndrome.
Noonan syndrome.
Pes cavus.
Phakomatosis pigmentovascularis.
Distichiasis-lymphedema.
Emberger syndrome.
WILD syndrome.
Hypotrichosis-telangiectasia-lymphedema syndrome.
Cutaneous disorders sometimes associated with primary lymphedema
Yellow nails.
Hemangiomas.
Xanthomatosis and chylous lymphedema.
Congenital absence of nails.
Secondary lymphedema
Postmastectomy lymphedema.
Melphalan isolated limb perfusion.
Malignant occlusion with obstruction.
Extrinsic pressure.
Factitial lymphedema.
Postradiation therapy.
Following recurrent lymphangitis/cellulitis.
Lymphedema of upper limb in recurrent eczema.
Granulomatous disease.
Rosaceous lymphedema.
Primary amyloidosis.
Complications of lymphedema
Cellulitis of lymphedema.
Elephantiasis nostra verrucosa.
Ulceration.
Lymphangiosarcoma.

LYMPHOCYTOSIS, ATYPICAL[63]

ICD-10CM #	D72.89	Other specified disorders of white blood cells

Epstein-Barr virus primary infection (infectious mononucleosis).
Cytomegalovirus primary infection (heterophile-negative mono).
Human herpesvirus 6 primary infection (roseola).
Primary HIV infection.
Toxoplasmosis.
Acute viral hepatitis.
Rubella, mumps.
Drug reactions (e.g., phenytoin, sulfa).

MACROTHROMBOCYTOPENIA, INHERITED[50]

ICD-10CM # Varies with specific disorder

Bernard-Soulier syndrome.
MHY9-related disorders:
- May-Hegglin anomaly.
- Sebastian syndrome.
- Fechtner syndrome.
- Epstein syndrome.

Gray platelet syndrome.
Montreal platelet syndrome.
Mediterranean macrothrombocytopenia.
Mediterranean stomatocytosis/macrothrombocytemia.
GATA1 mutations.
Sialyl-Lewis-S antigen deficiency.
Paris-Trousseau syndrome.
Platelet-type von Willebrand disease.

MACULAR CRYSTALS[13]

ICD-10CM # Varies with specific diagnosis

OTHER CAUSES OF MACULAR CRYSTALS

Primary hyperoxaluria.

Bietti corneoretinal crystalline dystrophy.
Cystinosis.
Sjögren–Larsson syndrome.
Gyrate atrophy.
Acquired parafoveal telangiectasis.
Talc-corn starch emboli.
West African crystalline maculopathy.

MADAROSIS[13]

ICD-10CM # H02.729 Madarosis of unspecified eye, unspecified eyelid and periocular area

CAUSES OF MADAROSIS

Local
Chronic anterior lid margin disease.
Infiltrating lid tumors.
Burns.
Radiotherapy or cryotherapy of lid tumors.
Skin disorders
Generalized alopecia.
Psoriasis.
Systemic diseases.
Myxoedema.
Systemic lupus erythematosus.
Acquired syphilis.
Lepromatous leprosy.
Following removal
Procedures for trichiasis.
Trichotillomania (psychiatric disorder of hair removal).

MALABSORPTION[95]

ICD-10CM # K90.89 Other intestinal malabsorption

CAUSES OF MALABSORPTION

More Common
Celiac disease.
Chronic pancreatitis.
Post gastrectomy.
Crohn disease.
Small bowel resection.
Small intestinal bacterial overgrowth.
Lactase deficiency.
Less Common
AIDS (*Mycobacterium avium intracellulare,* AIDS enteropathy).
Whipple disease.
Intestinal lymphoma.
Immunoproliferative small intestinal disease (alpha heavy chain disease).
Radiation enteritis.
Collagenous sprue.
Tropical sprue.
Non-granulomatous ulcerative jejunoileitis.
Eosinophilic gastroenteritis.
Amyloidosis.
Zollinger-Ellison syndrome.
Intestinal lymphangiectasia.
Systemic mastocytosis.
Chronic mesenteric ischemia.
Abetalipoproteinemia (autosomal recessive).

MALABSORPTION SYNDROME IN TROPICS[30]

ICD-10CM # K90.89 Other intestinal malabsorption

CAUSES OF MALABSORPTION SYNDROME IN THE TROPICS

SIBO
Following ulcer surgery.
Secondary to intestinal TB and Crohn disease.
Infections
Bacteria
Mycobacterium avium intracellulare complex.
Mycobacterium tuberculosis.
Helminths
Paracapillaria philippinensis.
Strongyloides stercoralis.
Protozoa
Cryptosporidium parvum.
Cyclospora cayetanensis.
Encephalitozoon intestinalis.
Enterocytozoon bieneusi.
Giardia lamblia.
Isospora belli.
Leishmania donovani.
Lymphatic Obstruction
Intestinal lymphangiectasia.
Mucosal Diseases
Autoimmune enteropathy.
Celiac disease.
Eosinophilic gastroenteritis.
HIV enteropathy.
Immunoproliferative small intestinal disease.
Intestinal lymphoma.
Primary immunodeficiencies.
Tropical sprue.
Neonatal Diseases
Microvillus inclusion disease.
Tufting enteropathy.
Pancreatic Insufficiency
Alcoholic pancreatitis.
CF.
Tropical pancreatitis.
Specific Transport Disorders
Abetalipoproteinemia.
Fructose malabsorption.
Glucose-galactose malabsorption.
Hypolactasia.
Sucrose intolerance.

MALNUTRITION, CAUSES IN EARLY LIFE[58]

ICD-10CM # E46 Unspecified protein-energy malnutrition

0 TO 6 MO

Breastfeeding difficulties.
Improper formula preparation.
Impaired parent/child interaction.
Congenital syndromes.
Prenatal infections or teratogenic exposures.
Poor feeding (sucking, swallowing) or feeding refusal (aversion).
Maternal psychological disorder (depression or attachment disorder).
Congenital heart disease.
Cystic fibrosis.
Neurologic abnormalities.
Child neglect.
Recurrent infections.

6 TO 12 MO

Celiac disease.
Food intolerance.
Child neglect.
Delayed introduction of age-appropriate foods or poor transition to food.
Recurrent infections.
Food allergy.

AFTER INFANCY

Acquired chronic diseases.
Highly distractible child.
Inappropriate mealtime environment.
Inappropriate diet (e.g., excessive juice consumption, avoidance of high-calorie foods).
Recurrent infections.

MEDIASTINAL COMPARTMENTS, ANATOMY AND PATHOLOGY[100]

ICD-10CM # Varies with specific disorder

ANTERIOR

Normal Structures
Lymph nodes.
Connective tissue.
Thymus (remnant in adults).
Masses
Thymoma.
Germ cell neoplasm.
Lymphoma.
Thyroid enlargement (intrathoracic goiter).
Other tumors.

MIDDLE

Normal Structures
Pericardium.
Heart.
Vessels: ascending aorta, venae cavae, main pulmonary arteries.
Trachea.
Lymph nodes.
Nerves: phrenic, upper vagus.
Masses
Carcinoma.
Lymphoma.
Pericardial cyst.
Bronchogenic cyst.
Benign lymph node enlargement (granulomatous disease).

POSTERIOR

Normal Structures
Vessels: descending aorta.
Esophagus.
Vertebral column.
Nerves: sympathetic chain, lower vagus.
Lymph nodes.
Connective tissue.
Masses
Neurogenic tumor.
Diaphragmatic hernia.

MEDIASTINAL MASSES OR WIDENING ON CHEST X-RAY

ICD-10CM # R59.9 Enlarged lymph nodes, unspecified
J98.5 Diseases of mediastinum, not elsewhere classified

Lymphoma: Hodgkin disease and non-Hodgkin lymphoma.
Sarcoidosis.
Vascular: aortic aneurysm, ectasia, or tortuosity of aorta or bronchocephalic vessels.
Carcinoma: lungs, esophagus.
Esophageal diverticula.
Hiatal hernia.
Achalasia.
Prominent pulmonary outflow tract: pulmonary hypertension, pulmonary embolism, right-to-left shunts.
Trauma: mediastinal hemorrhage.
Pneumomediastinum.
Lymphadenopathy caused by silicosis and other pneumoconioses.
Leukemias.
Infections: TB, viral (rare), *Mycoplasma* (rare), fungal, tularemia.
Substernal thyroid.
Thymoma.
Teratoma.
Bronchogenic cyst.
Pericardial cyst.
Neurofibroma, neurosarcoma, ganglioneuroma.

MEDIASTINAL MASSES, SITES OF ORIGIN[98]

ICD-10CM # Varies with specific diagnosis

DIFFERENTIAL DIAGNOSIS OF MEDIASTINAL MASSES BASED ON COMMON SITES OF ORIGIN

Prevascular space (anterior mediastinum)
Thymic masses.
Thymoma.
Thymic carcinoma.
Thymic neuroendocrine tumor.
Thymolipoma.
Thymic cyst.
Thymic hyperplasia.
Thymic lymphoma.
Germ cell tumors.
Teratoma and dermoid cyst.
Seminoma.
Nonseminomatous germ cell tumors.
Thyroid abnormalities (goiter and neoplasm).
Parathyroid tumor or hyperplasia.
Lymph node masses (particularly Hodgkin lymphoma).
Vascular abnormalities (aorta and great vessels).
Mesenchymal abnormalities (e.g., lipomatosis, lipoma).
Foregut cyst.
Lymphangioma.
Hemangioma.
Retrosternal space (anterior mediastinum)
Lymph node masses.
Pretracheal space (middle mediastinum)
Lymph node masses.
Lung carcinoma.
Sarcoidosis.
Lymphoma (particularly Hodgkin disease).
Metastases.
Infections (e.g., tuberculosis).
Foregut cyst.
Tracheal tumor.
Mesenchymal masses (e.g., lipomatosis, lipoma).
Thyroid abnormalities.
Vascular abnormalities (aorta and great vessels).
Lymphangioma and hemangioma.
Aortopulmonary window (middle mediastinum)
Lymph node masses.
Lung carcinoma.
Sarcoidosis.
Lymphoma.
Metastases.
Infections (e.g., tuberculosis).
Mesenchymal masses (e.g., lipomatosis, lipoma).
Vascular abnormalities (aorta or pulmonary artery).
Chemodectoma.
Foregut cyst.
Subcarinal space and azygoesophageal recess (middle mediastinum)
Lymph node masses.
Lung carcinoma.
Sarcoidosis.
Lymphoma.
Metastases.
Infections (e.g., tuberculosis).
Foregut cyst.
Dilated azygos vein.
Esophageal masses.
Varices.
Hernia.
Paravertebral masses (posterior mediastinum)
Neurogenic tumor.
Nerve sheath tumors.
Sympathetic ganglia tumors.
Paraganglioma.
Meningocele.
Foregut cyst.
Neurenteric cyst.
Thoracic spine abnormalities.
Extramedullary hematopoiesis.
Fluid collections and pseudocyst.
Vascular abnormalities.
Hernias.
Esophageal masses.
Varices.
Mesenchymal masses (e.g., lipomatosis, lipoma).
Lymph node masses.
Lymphoma (particularly non-Hodgkin).
Metastases.
Dilated azygos or hemiazygos vein.
Hernia.
Lymphangioma and hemangioma.
Thymic mass or germ cell tumor.
Anterior cardiophrenic angle masses.
Lymph node masses (particularly lymphoma and metastases).
Pericardial cyst.
Fat pad.
Morgagni hernia.
Thymic masses.
Germ cell tumors.

MEDIASTINITIS, ACUTE[63]

ICD-10CM # J98.5 Diseases of mediastinum, not elsewhere classified

Esophageal perforation.
Iatrogenic.
EGD, esophageal dilation, esophageal variceal sclerotherapy, nasogastric tube, Sengstaken-Blackmore tube, endotracheal intubation, esophageal surgery, paraesophageal surgery, transesophageal echocardiography, anterior stabilization of cervical vertebral bodies.
Swallowed foreign bodies.
Trauma.
Spontaneous perforation (e.g., emesis, carcinoma).
Head and neck infections (e.g., tonsillitis, pharyngitis, parotitis, epiglottitis, odontogenic).
Infections originating at another site (e.g., TB, pneumonia, pancreatitis, osteomyelitis of sternum, clavicle, ribs).
Cardiothoracic surgery (median sternotomy) (e.g., CABG, valve replacement, other types of cardiothoracic surgery).

MELANONYCHIA

ICD-10CM # NEC L81.4 Melanin hyperpigmentation

Pregnancy.
Trauma.
Medications (e.g., AZT, 5-fluorouracil, doxorubicin, psoralens).
Nail matrix nevus.
HIV infection.
Onychomycosis.
Melanocyte hyperplasia.
Verrucae.
Pustular psoriasis.
Lichen planus.
Basal cell carcinoma.
Nail matrix melanoma.
Subungual keratosis.
Addison disease.
Bowen disease.

MEMORY LOSS SYMPTOMS, ELDERLY PATIENTS

ICD-10CM # R41.2 Retrograde amnesia

Age-related mild cognitive impairment.
Depression (pseudodementia).
Medications (e.g., anticholinergics, sedatives).
Hypothyroidism.
Chronic hypoxia.
Cerebrovascular infarcts.
Alzheimer disease.
Hepatic disease.
Chronic renal failure.
Hyperthyroidism.
Frontotemporal dementia.
Lewy body dementia.

MENINGITIS, CHRONIC[63]

ICD-10CM # G03.1 Chronic meningitis

TB.
Fungal CNS infection.
Tertiary syphilis.
CNS neoplasm.
Metabolic encephalopathies.
Multiple sclerosis.
Chronic subdural hematoma.
SLE cerebritis.
Encephalitides.
Sarcoidosis.
NSAIDs.
Behçet syndrome.
Anatomic defects (traumatic, congenital, postoperative).
Granulomatous angiitis.

MENINGITIS, RECURRENT[63]

ICD-10CM # G03.2 Benign recurrent meningitis [Mollaret]

Drug induced (with rechallenge).
Parameningeal focus:
- Infection (sinusitis, mastoiditis, osteomyelitis, brain abscess).
- Tumor (epidermoid cyst, craniopharyngioma).

Posttraumatic (bacterial).
Mollaret meningitis.
SLE.
Herpes simplex virus.

MENTAL STATUS CHANGES AND COMA[7]

ICD-10CM # R41.82 Altered mental status, unspecified

METABOLIC/SYSTEMIC ETIOLOGY OF ALTERED MENTAL STATUS AND COMA

Hypoxia

Severe pulmonary disease (hypoventilation).
Severe anemia.
Environmental/toxin:
Methemoglobinemia:
- Cyanide.
- Carbon monoxide.
- Decreased atmospheric oxygen (high altitude).
- Near-drowning.

Disorders of Glucose

Hypoglycemia:
- Chronic alcohol abuse and liver disease.
- Excessive use of insulin or other hypoglycemic agents.
- Insulinoma.

Hyperglycemia:
- Diabetic ketoacidosis.
- Nonketotic hyperosmolar coma.

Decreased Cerebral Blood Flow

Hypovolemic shock.
Cardiac:
- Vasovagal syncope.
- Arrhythmias.
- Myocardial infarction.
- Valvular disorders.
- Congestive heart failure.
- Pericardial effusion/tamponade.
- Myocarditis.

Infectious:
- Septic shock.
- Bacterial meningitis.

Vascular/hematologic:
- Hypertensive encephalopathy.
- Pseudotumor cerebri.
- Hyperviscosity (sickle cell, polycythemia).
- Hyperventilation.
- Cerebral lupus vasculitis.
- Thrombotic thrombocytopenic purpura.
- Disseminated intravascular coagulation.

Metabolic Cofactor Deficiency

Thiamine (Wernicke-Korsakoff syndrome).
Pyridoxine (isoniazid overdose).
Folic acid (chronic alcohol abuse).
Cyanocobalamin.
Niacin.

Electrolyte/pH Disturbances

Acidosis/alkalosis.
Hypernatremia/hyponatremia.[32]
Hypercalcemia/hypocalcemia.
Hypophosphatemia.
Hypermagnesemia/hypomagnesemia.

Endocrine Disorders

Myxedema coma, thyrotoxicosis.
Hypopituitarism.
Addison disease (primary or secondary).
Cushing disease.
Pheochromocytoma.
Hyperparathyroidism/hypoparathyroidism.

Endogenous Toxins

Hyperammonemia (liver failure).
Uremia (renal disease).
Carbon dioxide narcosis (pulmonary disease).
Porphyria.

Exogenous Toxins

Alcohols:
- Ethanol, isopropyl alcohol, methanol, ethylene glycol.

Acid poisons:
- Salicylates.
- Paraldehyde.
- Ammonium chloride.

Antidepressant medications:
- Lithium.
- Tricyclic antidepressants (TCAs).
- Selective serotonin reuptake inhibitors (SSRIs).
- Monamine oxidase inhibitors (MAOIs).

Stimulants:
- Amphetamines/methamphetamines.
- Cocaine.
- Over-the-counter sympathomimetics.

Narcotics/opiates:
- Morphine.
- Heroin.
- Codeine, oxycodone, meperidine, hydrocodone.
- Methadone.
- Fentanyl.
- Propoxyphene.

Sedative-hypnotics:
- Benzodiazepines.
- Barbiturates.
- Rohypnol.
- Bromide.

[32] Can be associated with dilution of formula in infant feeding.

Hallucinogens:
- Lysergic acid diethylamide (LSD).
- Marijuana.
- Mescaline, peyote.
- Mushrooms.
- Phencyclidine (PCP).

Herbs/plants:
- Aconite.
- Jimson weed.
- Morning glory.

Volatile substances:
- Hydrocarbons (gasoline, butane, toluene, benzene, chloroform).
- Nitrites.
- Anesthetic agents (nitrous oxide, ether).

Other:
- γ-Hydroxybutyrate (GHB).
- Ketamine.
- Penicillin.
- Cardiac glycosides.
- Anticonvulsants.
- Steroids.
- Heavy metals.
- Cimetidine.
- Organophosphates.

Disorders of Temperature Regulation/Environmental

Hypothermia.
Heat stroke.
Malignant hyperthermia.
Neuroleptic malignant syndrome.
High-altitude cerebral edema (HACE).
Dysbarism.

Primary Glial or Neuronal Disorders

Adrenoleukodystrophy.
Creutzfeldt-Jakob disease.
Progressive multifocal leukoencephalopathy.
Marchiafava-Bignami disease.
Gliomatosis cerebri.
Central pontine myelinolysis.

Other Disorders of Unknown Etiology

Seizures.
Postictal states.
Reye syndrome.[33]
Intussusception.

MENTAL STATUS CHANGES AND COMA, STRUCTURAL CAUSES[1]

ICD-10CM # R40.1 Stupor

COMMON AGE-RELATED CAUSES OF ALTERED MENTAL STATUS AND COMA

Infant

Infection.
Trauma, abuse.
Metabolic.

Child

Toxic ingestion.

Adolescent, Young Adult

Toxic ingestion.
Recreational drug use.
Trauma.

[33] Prominent in the pediatric population

Elderly
Medication changes.
Over-the-counter medications.
Infection.
Alterations in living environment.
Stroke.
Trauma.

MENTAL STATUS CHANGES AND COMA, METABOLIC AND SYSTEMIC CAUSES

ICD-10CM # F05.9 Delirium, unspecified

METABOLIC AND SYSTEMIC CAUSES OF ALTERED MENTAL STATUS AND COMA

Hypoxia, Hypercapnia
Severe pulmonary disease (hypoventilation).
Severe anemia.
Environmental, toxic.
Methemoglobinemia.
Cyanide.
Carbon monoxide.
Decreased atmospheric oxygen (high altitude).
Near-drowning.

Glucose Disorders
Hypoglycemia:
- Chronic alcohol abuse and liver disease.
- Excessive dosage of insulin or other hypoglycemic agents.
- Insulinoma.

Hyperglycemia:
- Diabetic ketoacidosis.
- Nonketotic hyperosmolar coma.

Decreased Cerebral Blood Flow
Hypovolemic shock.
Cardiac:
- Vasovagal syncope.
- Arrhythmias.
- Myocardial infarction.
- Valvular disorders.
- Congestive heart failure.
- Pericardial effusion, tamponade.
- Myocarditis.

Infectious:
- Septic shock.
- Bacterial meningitis.

Vascular, hematologic
- Hypertensive encephalopathy.
- Pseudotumor cerebri.
- Hyperviscosity (sickle cell, polycythemia).
- Hyperventilation.
- Cerebral vasculitis as a manifestation of systemic lupus erythematosus.
- Thrombotic thrombocytopenic purpura.
- Disseminated intravascular coagulation.

Metabolic Cofactor Deficiency
Thiamine (Wernicke-Korsakoff syndrome).
Pyridoxine (isoniazid overdose).
Folic acid (chronic alcohol abuse).
Cyanocobalamin.
Niacin.

Electrolyte, pH Disturbances
Acidosis, alkalosis.
Hypernatremia, hyponatremia.[34]
Hypercalcemia, hypocalcemia.
Hypophosphatemia.
Hypermagnesemia, hypomagnesemia.

Endocrine Disorders
Myxedema coma, thyrotoxicosis.
Hypopituitarism.
Addison disease (primary or secondary).
Cushing disease.
Pheochromocytoma.
Hyperparathyroidism, hypoparathyroidism.

Endogenous Toxins
Hyperammonemia (liver failure).
Uremia (renal disease).
Carbon dioxide narcosis (pulmonary disease).
Porphyria.

Exogenous Toxins
Alcohols:
- Ethanol, isopropyl alcohol, methanol, ethylene glycol.

Acid poisons:
- Salicylates.
- Paraldehyde.
- Ammonium chloride.

Antidepressant medications:
- Lithium.
- Tricyclic antidepressants.
- Selective serotonin reuptake inhibitors.
- Monoamine oxidase inhibitors.

Stimulants:
- Amphetamines, methamphetamines.
- Cocaine.
- Over-the-counter sympathomimetics.

Narcotics, opiates:
- Morphine.
- Heroin.
- Codeine, oxycodone, meperidine, hydrocodone.
- Methadone.
- Fentanyl.
- Propoxyphene.

Sedative-hypnotics:
- Benzodiazepines.
- Barbiturates.
- Rohypnol.
- Bromide.

Hallucinogens:
- Lysergic acid diethylamide.
- Marijuana.
- Mescaline, peyote.
- Mushrooms.
- Phencyclidine.

Herbs, plants:
- Aconite.
- Jimsonweed.
- Morning glory.

Volatile substances:
- Hydrocarbons (gasoline, butane, toluene, benzene, chloroform).
- Nitrites.
- Anesthetic agents (nitrous oxide, ether).

Other:
- γ-Hydroxybutyrate.
- Ketamine.
- Penicillin.
- Cardiac glycosides.
- Anticonvulsants.
- Steroids.
- Heavy metals.
- Cimetidine.
- Organophosphates.

Disorders of Temperature Regulation, Environmental
Hypothermia.
Heat stroke.
Malignant hyperthermia.
Neuroleptic malignant syndrome.
High-altitude cerebral edema.
Dysbarism.

Primary Glial or Neuronal Disorders
Adrenoleukodystrophy.
Creutzfeldt-Jakob disease.
Progressive multifocal leukoencephalopathy.
Marchiafava-Bignami disease.
Gliomatosis cerebri.
Central pontine myelinolysis.

Other Disorders with Unknown Etiology
Seizures.
Postictal states.
Reye syndrome.
Intussusception.

[34] Can be associated with dilution of formula in infant feeding.

MESENTERIC ARTERIAL EMBOLISM, ASSOCIATED FACTORS[7]

ICD-10CM # I74.09 Other arterial embolism and thrombosis of abdominal aorta

FACTORS ASSOCIATED WITH MESENTERIC ARTERIAL EMBOLISM

Coronary artery disease:
- Post-myocardial infarction mural thrombi.
- Congestive heart failure.

Valvular heart disease:
- Rheumatic mitral valve disease.
- Nonbacterial endocarditis.

Arrhythmias:
- Chronic atrial fibrillation.

Aortic aneurysms or dissections.
Coronary angiography.

MESENTERIC ISCHEMIA, NONOCCLUSIVE[63]

ICD-10CM #	K55.0	Acute vascular disorders of intestine
	K55.1	Chronic vascular disorders of intestine
	S35.8X9A	Unspecified injury of other blood vessels at abdomen, lower back and pelvis level, initial encounter

Cardiovascular disease resulting in low-flow states (CHF, cardiogenic shock, post cardiopulmonary bypass, dysrhythmias).
Septic shock.
Drug induced (cocaine, vasopressors, ergot alkaloid poisoning).

MESENTERIC VENOUS THROMBOSIS[63]

ICD-10CM # I82.91 Chronic embolism and thrombosis of unspecified vein

Hypercoagulable states (protein C or S deficiency, antithrombin III deficiency, Factor V Leyden, malignancy, polycythemia vera, sickle cell disease, homocystinemia, lupus anticoagulant, cardiolipin antibody).
Trauma (operative venous injury, abdominal trauma, postsplenectomy).
Inflammatory conditions (pancreatitis, diverticulitis, appendicitis, cholangitis).
Other: CHF, renal failure, portal hypertension, decompression sickness.

METASTATIC NEOPLASMS

ICD-10CM #	C79.51	Secondary malignant neoplasm of bone
	C79.52	Secondary malignant neoplasm of bone marrow
	C79.31	Secondary malignant neoplasm of brain
	C78.7	Secondary malignant neoplasm of liver and intrahepatic bile duct
	C78.00	Secondary malignant neoplasm of unspecified lung

To Bone	To Brain
Breast.	Lung.
Lung.	Breast.
Prostate.	Melanoma.
Thyroid.	GU tract.
Kidney.	Colon.
Bladder.	Sinuses.
Endometrium.	Sarcoma.
Cervix.	Skin.
Melanoma.	Thyroid.

To Liver	To Lung
Colon.	Breast.
Stomach.	Colon.
Pancreas.	Kidney.
Breast.	Testis.
Lymphomas.	Stomach.
Bronchus.	Thyroid.
Lung.	Melanoma.
Sarcoma.	
Choriocarcinoma.	
Kidney.	

METHAEMOGLOBINAEMIA, DRUG-INDUCED[49]

ICD-10CM # D74 Methaemoglobinaemia

SUBSTANCES ASSOCIATED WITH METHAEMOGLOBINAEMIA

Acetaminophen (nitrobenzene derivative).
Acetanilide.
Local anesthetics:
- Benzocaine.
- Lidocaine.
- Prilocaine.

Aniline dyes.
Celecoxib.
Dapsone.
Flutamide.
Ifosfamide.
Metoclopramide.
Nitric oxide.
Nitrites:
- Amyl nitrite.
- Isobutyl nitrite.
- Sodium nitrite.
- Nitrates (bacterial conversion to nitrites).

Nitrobenzenes/nitrobenzoates.
Nitroethane (nail polish remover).
Nitrofurans.
Nitroglycerin.
Paraquat/monolinuron.
Phenacetin.
Phenazopyridine (pyridium).
Primaquine.
Rasburicase.
Sulfamethoxazole.

MICROCEPHALY[9]

ICD-10CM # Q02 Microcephaly

PRIMARY (GENETIC)

Familial (autosomal recessive).
Autosomal dominant.
Syndromes:
- Down (21-trisomy).
- Edward (18-trisomy).
- Cri-du-chat (5 p-).
- Cornelia de Lange.
- Rubinstein-Taybi.
- Smith-Lemli-Opitz.

SECONDARY (NONGENETIC)

Radiation.
Congenital infections:
- Cytomegalovirus.
- Rubella.
- Toxoplasmosis.

Drugs:
- Fetal alcohol.
- Fetal hydantoin.
- Meningitis/encephalitis.
- Malnutrition.
- Metabolic.
- Hyperthermia.
- Hypoxic-ischemic encephalopathy.

MICROPENIS[69]

ICD-10CM #	N48.89	Other specified disorders of penis
	Q55.62	Hypoplasia of penis

HYPOGONADOTROPIC HYPOGONADISM (HYPOTHALAMIC OR PITUITARY DEFICIENCIES)

Kallmann syndrome: autosomal dominant; associated with hyposmia.
Prader-Willi syndrome: hypotonia, mental retardation, obesity, small hands and feet.
Rud syndrome: hyposomia, ichthyosis, mental retardation.
De Morsier syndrome (septooptic dysplasia): hypopituitarism, hypoplastic optic discs, absent septum pellucidum.

HYPERGONADOTROPIC HYPOGONADISM

Primary testicular defect: disorders of testicular differentiation or inborn errors of testosterone synthesis.
Klinefelter syndrome.
Other X polysomies (i.e., XXXXY, XXXY).
Robinow syndrome: brachymesomelic dwarfism, dysmorphic facies.

PARTIAL ANDROGEN INSENSITIVITY

Idiopathic
Defective morphogenesis of the penis.

MIOSIS

ICD-10CM # H57.03 Miosis

Medications (e.g., morphine, pilocarpine).
Neurosyphilis.
Congenital.
Iritis.
CNS pontine lesion.
CNS infections.
Cavernous sinus thrombosis.
Inflammation/irritation of cornea or conjunctiva.

MONOARTHRITIS, ACUTE

ICD-10CM # M13.10 Monoarthritis, not elsewhere classified, unspecified site

Overuse.
Trauma.
Gout.
Pseudogout.
Osteoarthritis.
Infectious arthritis (e.g., gonococcal, Lyme disease, viral, mycobacteria, fungi).
Osteomyelitis.
Avascular necrosis of bone.
Hemarthrosis.
Bowel disease–associated arthritis.
Bone malignancy.
Psoriatic arthritis.
Juvenile RA.
Sarcoidosis.
Hemoglobinopathies.
Vasculitic syndromes.
Behçet syndrome.
Foreign body synovitis.
Hypertrophic pulmonary osteoarthropathy.
Amyloidosis, familial Mediterranean fever.

MONOCYTOSIS[50]

ICD-10CM # D72.821 Monocytosis (symptomatic)

Inflammatory diseases:
- Autoimmune/granulomatous.
- Systemic lupus erythematosus.
- Rheumatoid arthritis.
- Giant cell arteritis.
- Myositis.
- Polyarteritis.
- Ulcerative colitis.
- Regional enteritis.
- Sarcoidosis.

Infectious diseases:
- Tuberculosis.
- Syphilis.
- Subacute bacterial endocarditis.

Malignant disorders:
- Preleukemia.
- Nonlymphocytic leukemia.
- Histiocytoses.
- Hodgkin disease.
- Non-Hodgkin lymphoma.
- Carcinomas.

Miscellaneous:
- Chronic neutropenia.
- Post splenectomy.

MONONEUROPATHY

ICD-10CM # G58.9 Mononeuropathy, unspecified

Herpes zoster.
Herpes simplex.
Vasculitis.
Trauma, compression.
Diabetes.
Postinfectious or inflammatory.

MONONEUROPATHY, ISOLATED[7]

ICD-10CM # G56.90 Unspecified mononeuropathy of unspecified upper limb

UPPER EXTREMITY

Radial nerve:
- Axilla.
- Humerus.
- Elbow (posterior interosseous neuropathy).
- Wrist (superficial cutaneous radial neuropathy).

Ulnar nerve:
- Axilla.
- Humerus.
- Elbow.
- Condylar groove.
- Cubital tunnel.

Wrist (Guyon canal):

Hand:
- Superficial terminal ulnar neuropathy.
- Deep terminal ulnar neuropathy:
  - Proximal hypothenar.
  - Distal hypothenar.

Median nerve.

Axilla.

Humerus (musculocutaneous mononeuropathy).

Forearm:
- Anterior interosseus.
- Pronator syndrome.

Wrist (carpal tunnel).

Hand (recurrent motor branch).

Suprascapular mononeuropathy:
- Axillary mononeuropathy.

LOWER EXTREMITY

Sciatic nerve.

Femoral nerve:
- Iliacus compartment (proximal).
- Saphenous mononeuropathy (distal).

Lateral femoral cutaneous (meralgia paresthetica).

Peroneal nerve:
- Common peroneal mononeuropathy (fibular head, popliteal fossa).
- Deep peroneal mononeuropathy (anterior compartment).

Tibial nerve:
- Popliteal fossa (proximal).
- Tarsal tunnel (distal).

Sural nerve:
- Popliteal fossa, calf (proximal).
- Fifth metatarsal base (distal).

Plantar nerve:
- Distal to tarsal tunnel.
- Interdigital neuropathies (Morton neuroma).

Obturator mononeuropathy.

MONONEUROPATHY MULTIPLEX[65]

ICD-10CM # G58.9 Mononeuropathy, unspecified

MONONEUROPATHY MULTIPLEX

Vasculitis

Systemic vasculitis:
- Polyarteritis nodosa.
- Rheumatoid arthritis.
- Systemic lupus erythematosus.
- Sjögren syndrome (keratoconjunctivitis sicca).

Nonsystemic vasculitis

Diabetes mellitus

Neoplastic

Paraneoplastic.
Direct infiltration.

Infectious

Lyme disease.
HIV infection.

Sarcoid

Toxic (lead)

Transient (polycythemia vera)

Cryoglobulinemia (hepatitis C)

MONONUCLEOSIS, MONOSPOT NEGATIVE[3]

ICD-10CM # B27.90 Infectious mononucleosis, unspecified without complication

DIFFERENTIAL DIAGNOSIS OF MONOSPOT-NEGATIVE MONONUCLEOSIS

Acute HIV infection.
EBV mononucleosis (particularly in children).
Cytomegalovirus.
Acute toxoplasmosis.
Streptococcal pharyngitis.
Acute hepatitis B infection.

EBV, Epstein-Barr virus; *HIV,* human immunodeficiency virus.

MOVEMENT DISORDER, HYPERKINETIC[39]

ICD-10CM # G25.9 Extrapyramidal and movement disorder, unspecified

Hyperkinetic Movement Disorders

Tremor.
Chorea.
Ballism.
Dystonia.
Athetosis.
Tics.
Myoclonus.
Startle.
Stereotypies.
Miscellaneous.

MOVEMENT DISORDER, PEDIATRIC PATIENT[56]

ICD-10CM # G25.9 Extrapyramidal and movement disorder, unspecified

COMMONLY CITED MOVEMENT DISORDERS THAT MAY BEGIN IN CHILDHOOD OR ADOLESCENCE

Early Childhood

Athetosis or choreoathetosis.
Lesch–Nyhan syndrome.*

Childhood

Dopa-responsive dystonia.*
Dystonia associated with *DYT1* gene.*
Myoclonus from subacute sclerosing panencephalitis (SSPE).
Parkinson disease.
Sydenham chorea.
Tourette disorder.*
Withdrawal-emergent dyskinesia.

Adolescence

Essential tremor.*
Huntington disease (juvenile Huntington disease).*
Medication- and drug-induced movements.
Tardive dyskinesias.
Wilson disease.*

MOVEMENT DISORDERS AND COGNITIVE IMPAIRMENT[56]

ICD-10CM # G25.9 Extrapyramidal and movement disorder, unspecified

MOVEMENT DISORDERS ASSOCIATED WITH COGNITIVE IMPAIRMENT

Young Children

Athetosis or choreoathetosis.*
Lesch–Nyhan syndrome.
Rett syndrome.

Older Children and Adolescents

Huntington disease.
Subacute sclerosing panencephalitis.
Wilson disease.

Adults

Creutzfeldt-Jakob disease.†
Huntington disease.
Parkinson disease.

*Despite incapacitating movements, many choreoathetosis patients have no mental retardation.
*Genetic transmission.
†Myoclonus.

MOVEMENT DISORDERS, NEUROLEPTIC-INDUCED[56]

ICD-10CM # G25.70 Drug-induced movement disorder, unspecified

Acute dyskinesias:
- Akathisia.
- Neuroleptic-malignant syndrome.
- Oculogyric crisis and other dystonias.

Tardive dyskinesias:
- Akathisia.
- Dystonia.
- Oral-buccal-lingual dyskinesia.*
- Tics.
- Tremor.
- Stereotypies.

Dose-dependent dyskinesia:
- Parkinsonism.

Withdrawal-emergent dyskinesias.

*Commonly referred to as "tardive dyskinesia

MULTIVALVULAR HEART DISEASE[104]

ICD-10CM # Varies with specific diagnosis

Acquired

Systemic diseases:
- Infective endocarditis.
- Carcinoid heart disease.
- Systemic lupus erythematosus.

Cardiac diseases:
- Infective endocarditis.
- Rheumatic heart disease.

Degenerative:
- Calcific diseases, increased with age, prior radiation, chronic kidney disease.

Iatrogenic:
- Adverse drug effects: ergot-related antagonists.
- Radiation therapy.

Functional (annulus dilatation), caused by:
- Ischemic heart disease.
- Hypertensive heart disease.
- Chronic arrhythmia.
- Pulmonary hypertension.
- Cardiomyopathy.

Congenital

Connective tissue disorders:
- Marfan syndrome.
- Ehlers-Danlos syndrome.

Other:
- Trisomy 18, 13, and 15.
- Shone syndrome.
- Ochronosis.

Mixed

Multiple conditions may contribute to valve dysfunction, such as:
- Degenerative diseases may lead to associated functional disease.
- Congenital heart disease may predispose to infective endocarditis or degenerative disease.

MUSCLE DISEASE[88]

ICD-10CM # M60.009 Infective myositis, unspecified site

CLASSIFICATION OF MUSCLE DISEASE

Muscular Dystrophies

Duchenne.
Becker.
Limb girdle.
Childhood.
Facioscapulohumeral.

Myotonic Disorders

Dystrophia myotonica.
Myotonica congenita.

Inflammatory

Infective: bacterial, viral, parasitic.
Unknown cause: polymyositis, dermatomyositis, sarcoidosis.

Endocrine

Thyroid disease—hyper- and hypothyroidism.
Cushing disease.
Addison disease.
Hyperparathyroidism.

Metabolic

Glycogen storage diseases.
Periodic paralyses.
Mitochondrial diseases.

Drug-induced

Corticosteroids.
Chloroquine.
Amiodarone.
Penicillamine.
Alcohol.
Zidovudine.
Clofibrate.

Other

Inclusion body myositis.

MUSCLE WEAKNESS

ICD-10CM # M62.9 Disorder of muscle, unspecified

Physical deconditioning.
Impaired cardiac output (e.g., mitral stenosis, mitral regurgitation).
Uremia, liver failure.
Electrolyte abnormalities (hypokalemia, hyperkalemia, hypophosphatemia, hypercalcemia), hypoglycemia.
Drug induced (e.g., statin myopathy).
Muscular dystrophies.
Steroid myopathy.
Alcoholic myopathy.
Myasthenia gravis, Lambert-Eaton syndrome.
Infections (polio, botulism, HIV, hepatitis, diphtheria, tick paralysis, neurosyphilis, brucellosis, TB, trichinosis).
Pernicious anemia, other anemias, beriberi.
Psychiatric illness (depression, somatization syndrome).
Organophosphate or arsenic poisoning.
Inflammatory myopathies (e.g., collagen vascular disease, RA, sarcoidosis).
Endocrinopathies (e.g., adrenal insufficiency, hypothyroidism), diabetic neuropathy.
Other: motor neuron disease, mitochondrial myopathy, L-tryptophan (eosinophilia-myalgia), rhabdomyolysis, glycogen storage disease, lipid storage disease.

MUSCLE WEAKNESS, LOWER MOTOR NEURON VERSUS UPPER MOTOR NEURON

ICD-10CM # M62.9 Disorder of muscle, unspecified

LOWER MOTOR NEURON

Weakness, usually severe.
Marked muscle atrophy.
Fasciculations.
Decreased muscle stretch reflexes.
Clonus not present.
Flaccidity.
No Babinski sign.
Asymmetric and may involve one limb only in the beginning to become generalized as the disease progresses.

UPPER MOTOR NEURON

Weakness, usually less severe.
Minimal disuse muscle atrophy.
No fasciculations.
Increased muscle stretch reflexes.
Clonus may be present.
Spasticity.
Babinski sign.
Often initial impairment of only skilled movements.
In the limbs the following muscles may be the only ones weak or weaker than the others: triceps; wrist and finger extensors; interossei; iliopsoas; hamstrings; and foot dorsiflexors, inverters, and extroverters.

MUSCULOSKELETAL BENIGN TUMORS AND TUMOR-LIKE LESIONS[78]

ICD-10CM # Varies with specific diagnosis

Fibrous dysplasia.
Enchondromatosis.
Osteochondromatosis.
Synovial cysts.
Brown tumors in hyperparathyroidism.
Langerhans cell histiocytosis (eosinophilic granuloma).
Hemangiomatosis.
Bone islands, osteoma (Gardner syndrome).
Fibrous cortical defect, nonossifying fibroma.
Giant cell tumor.
Neurofibromatosis.
Amyloidosis.
Mastocytosis.
SAPHO, chronic multifocal osteomyelitis.

SAPHO, Synovitis, acne, pustulosis, hyperostosis, osteitis.

MUSCULOSKELETAL MALIGNANT TUMORS AND TUMOR-LIKE LESIONS[78]

ICD-10CM # Varies with specific diagnosis

Metastases.
Myeloma.
Angiosarcoma.

Leukemia.
Neuroblastoma.
Ewing sarcoma.
Osteosarcomatosis.
Lymphoma.

MYDRIASIS

ICD-10CM # H57.04 Mydriasis

Coma.
Medications (cocaine, atropine, epinephrine, etc.).
Glaucoma.
Cerebral aneurysm.
Ocular trauma.
Head trauma.
Optic atrophy.
Cerebral neoplasm.
Iridocyclitis.

MYELIN DISORDERS

ICD-10CM # Varies with specific diagnosis

Multiple sclerosis.
Vitamin B_{12} deficiency.
Radiation.
Hypoxia.
Toxicity from carbon monoxide, alcohol, mercury.
Progressive multifocal encephalopathy.
Acute disseminated encephalomyelitis.
Acute hemorrhagic leukoencephalopathy.
Phenylketonuria.
Adrenoleukodystrophy.
Krabbe disease.

MYELITIS[97]

ICD-10CM #	G04.91	Myelitis, unspecified
	G04.89	Other myelitis

Viral
HIV.
HSV-1 and HSV-2.
VZV.
CMV.
EBV.
WNV.
HTLV.
Bacterial
Mycoplasma pneumoniae.
Borrelia burgdorferi.
Treponema pallidum.
Pyogenic bacteria.
Mycobacterium tuberculosis.
Fungal
Coccidioides immitis.
Actinomyces.
Aspergillus.
Blastomyces dermatitidis.
Histoplasmosis.
Immune-Mediated
Multiple sclerosis.
Neuromyelitis optica.
Connective tissue disorders (neuro-lupus, neuro-Sjögren).
Neurosarcoidosis.
Paraneoplastic.
Noninflammatory Myelopathies
Vitamin B_{12} deficiency.
Folic acid deficiency.
Copper deficiency.
Vitamin E deficiency.
Nitrous oxide toxicity.
Heroin.
Radiation myelopathy.
Traumatic/compressive myelopathy.
Vascular myelopathy.

MYELOPATHY AND MYELITIS[91]

ICD-10CM #	M51.9	Unspecified thoracic, thoracolumbar and lumbosacral intervertebral disc disorder
	G95.9	Disease of spinal cord, unspecified

INFLAMMATORY

Infectious: spirochetal TB, zoster, rabies, HIV, polio, rickettsial, fungal, parasitic.
Noninfectious: idiopathic transverse myelitis, multiple sclerosis.

TOXIC/METABOLIC

DM, pernicious anemia, chronic liver disease, pellagra, arsenic.

TRAUMA COMPRESSION

Spinal neoplasm, cervical spondylosis, epidural abscess, epidural hematoma.

VASCULAR

AV malformation, SLE, periarteritis nodosa, dissecting aortic aneurysm.
Physical Agents
Electrical injury, irradiation.
Neoplastic
Spinal cord tumors, paraneoplastic myelopathy.

MYOCARDIAL ISCHEMIA[91]

ICD-10CM #	I25.5	Ischemic cardiomyopathy
	I25.89	Other forms of chronic ischemic heart disease
	I25.9	Chronic ischemic heart disease, unspecified
	I24.8	Other forms of acute ischemic heart disease

Atherosclerotic obstructive coronary artery disease.
Nonatherosclerotic coronary artery disease:
- Coronary artery spasm.
- Congenital coronary artery anomalies:
  - Anomalous origin of coronary artery from pulmonary artery.
  - Aberrant origin of coronary artery from aorta or another coronary artery.
  - Coronary arteriovenous fistula.
  - Coronary artery aneurysm.

Acquired disorders of coronary arteries:
- Coronary artery embolism.
- Dissection:
  - Surgical.
  - During percutaneous coronary angioplasty.
  - Aortic dissection.
  - Spontaneous (e.g., during pregnancy).
- Extrinsic compression:
  - Tumors.
  - Granulomas.
  - Amyloidosis.
- Collagen-vascular disease:
  - Polyarteritis nodosa.
  - Temporal arteritis.
  - RA.
  - SLE.
  - Scleroderma.
- Miscellaneous disorders:
  - Irradiation.
  - Trauma.
  - Kawasaki disease.
- Syphilis.
- Hereditary disorders:
  - Pseudoxanthoma elasticum.
  - Gargoylism.
  - Progeria.
  - Homocystinuria.
  - Primary oxaluria.

"Functional" causes of myocardial ischemia in absence of anatomic coronary artery disease:
- Syndrome X.
- Hypertrophic cardiomyopathy.
- Dilated cardiomyopathy.
- Muscle bridge.
- Hypertensive heart disease.
- Pulmonary hypertension.
- Valvular heart disease; aortic stenosis, aortic regurgitation.

MYOCLONUS

ICD-10CM # G25.3 Myoclonus

Physiologic (e.g., exercise or anxiety induced).
Renal failure.
Hepatic failure.
Hyponatremia.
Hypoglycemia or severe hyperglycemia.
Postdialysis.
Epileptic myoclonus.
Postencephalitis.
CNS lesion (stroke, neoplasm).
CNS trauma.
Parkinson disease.
Medications (e.g., tricyclics, L-dopa).
Friedreich ataxia.
Ataxia-telangiectasia.
Wilson disease.
Huntington disease.
Progressive supranuclear palsy.
Heavy metal poisoning.
Benign familial.

MYOCLONUS, DRUG-INDUCED[93]

ICD-10CM # G25.79 Other drug-induced movement disorders

SELECTED AGENTS ASSOCIATED WITH MYOCLONUS

Medications
Antibiotics (β-lactams).
Antidepressants.

Antineoplastics: busulfan, chlorambucil.
Carbamazepine, vigabatrin.
Clozapine.
L-dopa.
Lidocaine.
Lithium.
Lorazepam (preterm infants).
Methaqualone.
Morphine.
Nitroprusside.
Piperazine.

Industrial Toxins

Camphor.
Chlorophenoxy herbicides.
Gasoline.

Biological Toxins

Buckeye (*Aesculus* spp.).
Lupine.
Shellfish (domoic acid poisoning).

MYOCLONUS, PEDIATRIC PATIENT[59]

ICD-10CM # G25.3 Myoclonus

SELECTED CAUSES OF MYOCLONUS IN CHILDREN

Physiologic Causes

Hiccups.
Hypnic jerks (sleep starts).
Nocturnal (sleep) myoclonus.

Developmental Causes

Benign neonatal sleep myoclonus.
Benign myoclonus of early infancy.
Myoclonus with fever.

Storage Diseases

Juvenile Gaucher disease (type III).
Sialidosis type 1 (cherry-red spot–myoclonus).
GM_1 gangliosidosis.
Neuronal ceroid-lipofuscinosis (late infantile).

Inherited Degenerative Diseases

Dentatorubral-pallidoluysian atrophy (DRPLA).
Huntington disease.
Progressive myoclonus ataxia.
Ramsay Hunt syndrome.
Early myoclonic encephalopathy.
Rasmussen encephalitis.

Infectious and Postinfectious Diseases

Meningitis (viral or bacterial).
Encephalitis.
Epstein-Barr virus (EBV).
Coxsackievirus.
Influenza.
Human immunodeficiency virus (HIV).
Acute disseminated encephalomyelitis (ADEM).

Metabolic Causes

Uremia.
Hepatic failure.
Electrolyte disturbances.
Hypoglycemia or hyperglycemia.
Aminoacidurias.
Organic acidurias.
Urea cycle disorders.
POLG1 mutations.
Myoclonic epilepsy with ragged red fibers (MERRF).
Mitochondrial encephalomyopathy, lactic acidosis, and stroke-like episodes (MELAS).
Biotinidase deficiency (usually epileptic).
Cobalamin deficiency (infantile).
Leigh syndrome.

Toxic Causes

Psychotropic medications (tricyclic antidepressants, lithium, selective serotonin reuptake inhibitors, monoamine oxidase inhibitors, neuroleptics).
Antibiotics (penicillin, cephalosporins, quinolones).
Antiepileptics (phenytoin, carbamazepine, lamotrigine, gabapentin, benzodiazepines [in infants], vigabatrin).
Opioids.
General anesthetics.
Antineoplastic drugs.
Strychnine, toluene, lead, carbon monoxide, mercury.

Hypoxia

Lance-Adams syndrome.

Functional (Psychogenic) Causes

MYOPATHIC SYNDROMES, DRUG-INDUCED[46]

ICD-10CM # G72.9 Myopathy, unspecified

TYPE OF MYOPATHY

Necrotizing myopathy.
Inflammatory myopathy.
Mitochondrial myopathy.
Hypokalemic myopathy.
Antimicrotubular myopathy.
Lysosomal storage myopathy.
Corticosteroid myopathy.
Others.

DRUGS

HMG-CoA reductase inhibitors (statins), fibrates, alcohol.
Penicillamine, interferon-a, procainamide.
Zidovudine.
Diuretics, laxatives, licorice, amphotericin B, alcohol.
Colchicine, vincristine.
Chloroquine, hydroxychloroquine, quinacrine, amiodarone, perhexiline.
Corticosteroids, especially fluorinated.
Ipecac syrup, emetine.

MYOPATHIES ASSOCIATED WITH REST PAIN[46]

ICD-10CM # G72.9 Myopathy, unspecified

Childhood dermatomyositis.
Hypothyroid myopathy.
Acute alcoholic myopathy.
Drug-induced myopathies.
Infectious myopathies.
Myopathies associated with metabolic bone disease.
Carnitine palmitoyl transferase deficiency.
Rhabdomyolysis from any cause.

MYOPATHIES, HIV ASSOCIATED[31]

ICD-10CM # G72.9 Myopathy, unspecified

HIV-Associated Myopathies	Myopathies Secondary to Antiretrovirals	Others
HIV polymyositis.	Zidovudine myopathy.	Opportunistic infections involving muscle (toxoplasmosis).
Inclusion body myositis.	Toxic mitochondrial myopathies related to other NRTIs.	Tumor infiltrations of skeletal muscle.
Nemaline myopathy.		
Diffuse infiltrative lymphocytosis syndrome.	HIV-associated lipodystrophy syndrome.	Rhabdomyolysis.
HIV wasting syndrome.	Immune reconstitution syndrome related to ART.	
Vasculitic processes.		
Myasthenia gravis and other myasthenic syndromes.		
Chronic fatigue and fibromyalgia.		

ART, Antiretroviral therapy; *NRTIs,* nucleoside reverse transcriptase inhibitors.

MYOPATHIES, INFECTIOUS

ICD-10CM # G72.9 Myopathy, unspecified

HIV.
Viral myositis.
Trichinosis.
Toxoplasmosis.
Cysticercosis.

MYOPATHIES, INFLAMMATORY

ICD-10CM # G72.9 Myopathy, unspecified

SLE, RA.
Sarcoidosis.
Paraneoplastic syndrome.
Polymyositis, dermatomyositis.
Polyarteritis nodosa.
Mixed connective tissue disease.
Scleroderma.
Inclusion body myositis.
Sjögren syndrome.
Cimetidine, d-penicillamine.

MYOPATHIES, METABOLIC[46]

ICD-10CM # G72.9 Myopathy, unspecified

DISORDERED GLYCOGEN METABOLISM

Myophosphorylase deficiency (McArdle disease).
Phosphorylase b kinase deficiency.
Phosphofructokinase deficiency.
Debrancher enzyme deficiency.
Brancher enzyme deficiency.
Phosphoglycerate kinase deficiency.
Phosphoglycerate mutase deficiency.
Lactate dehydrogenase deficiency.
Acid maltase deficiency.
Aldolase deficiency.
β-Enolase deficiency.

DISORDERED LIPID METABOLISM

Carnitine deficiencies.
Carnitine palmitoyltransferase deficiency.
Fatty acid acyl-CoA dehydrogenase deficiencies.

MITOCHONDRIAL MYOPATHIES

Coenzyme Q10 deficiency.
Respiratory chain complex deficiencies.

ENDOCRINE

Acromegaly.
Hypothyroidism.
Hyperthyroidism.
Hyperparathyroidism.
Cushing disease.
Addison disease.
Hyperaldosteronism.

METABOLIC-NUTRITIONAL

Uremia.
Hepatic failure.
Malabsorption.
Periodic paralysis.
Vitamin D deficiency.
Vitamin E deficiency.

ELECTROLYTE DISORDERS

Sodium: hypernatremia and hyponatremia.
Potassium: hyperkalemia and hypokalemia.
Calcium: hypercalcemia and hypocalcemia.
Phosphate: hypophosphatemia.
Magnesium: hypomagnesemia.

MYOPATHIES, TOXIC[3]

ICD-10CM # G72.2 Myopathy due to other toxic agents

Inflammatory: cimetidine, d-penicillamine.
Noninflammatory necrotizing or vacuolar: cholesterol-lowering agents, chloroquine, colchicine.
Acute muscle necrosis and myoglobinuria: cholesterol-lowering drugs, alcohol, cocaine.
Malignant hyperthermia: halothane, ethylene, others; succinylcholine.
Mitochondrial: zidovudine.
Myosin loss: nondepolarizing neuromuscular blocking agents; glucocorticoids.

MYOPATHY, DRUG-INDUCED[47]

ICD-10CM # G72.9 Myopathy, unspecified

DRUGS AND TOXINS THAT MAY INDUCE MYOPATHY

Example	Comments
Cimetidine.	
Chloroquine.	Vacuolar myopathy.
Colchicine.	Vacuolar myopathy.
Emetine.	
Ethanol.	Acute rhabdomyolysis and chronic myopathy.
Glucocorticoids.	Type II fiber atrophy.
Heroin.	
IFN-α.	Dermatomyositis and polymyositis reported.
Penicillamine.	Typical polymyositis. Mitochondrial myopathy.
Statins and fibrates.	Cases of autoimmune necrotizing myopathy, polymyositis, rhabdomyolysis, and noninflammatory myopathies reported.
AntiTNF.	In RA patients existing reports of polymyositis, dermatomyositis and anti–Jo-1–positive myositis during TNF blockade.
Zidovudine (AZT).	
(Many others reported at the case level.)	

AZT, Zidovudine; *IFN,* interferon; *RA,* rheumatoid arthritis; *TNF,* tumor necrosis factor.

MYOSITIS, INFECTIOUS CAUSES[46]

ICD-10CM # M60.009 Infective myositis, unspecified site

VIRAL

Influenza A and B viruses.
Enteroviruses (coxsackieviruses, echoviruses).
Human immunodeficiency virus.
Human T-cell lymphotrophic virus type 1.
Hepatitis B and C viruses.
Cytomegalovirus.
Epstein-Barr virus.
Adenovirus.
Varicella-zoster virus.
Parainfluenza.

PARASITIC

Trichinella spp.
Echinococcus spp.
Schistosoma spp.
Toxoplasma gondii.
Trypanosoma cruzi.
Sarcocystis spp.

BACTERIAL

Staphylococcus aureus.
Streptococcus, groups A and B.
Aeromonas hydrophila.
Borrelia burgdorferi.
Clostridium perfringens.
Anaerobic streptococci.
Mycobacterium spp.
Rickettsia spp.

FUNGAL

Candida spp.
Cryptococcus neoformans.
Microsporida.

MYOSITIS, INFLAMMATORY[3]

ICD-10CM # M60.009 Infective myositis, unspecified site
M60.9 Myositis, unspecified
M60.10 Interstitial myositis of unspecified site

INFECTIOUS

Viral myositis:
- Retroviruses (HIV, HTLV-I).
- Enteroviruses (echovirus, Coxsackievirus).
- Other viruses (influenza, hepatitis A and B, Epstein-Barr virus).

Bacterial: pyomyositis.
Parasites: trichinosis, cysticercosis.
Fungi: candidiasis.

IDIOPATHIC

Granulomatous myositis (sarcoid, giant cell).
Eosinophilic myositis.
Eosinophilia-myalgia syndrome.

ENDOCRINE/METABOLIC DISORDERS

Hypothyroidism.
Hyperthyroidism.
Hypercortisolism.
Hyperparathyroidism.
Hypoparathyroidism.
Hypocalcemia.
Hypokalemia.

METABOLIC MYOPATHIES

Myophosphorylase deficiency (McArdle disease).
Phosphofructokinase deficiency.
Myoadenylate deaminase deficiency.
Acid maltase deficiency.
Lipid storage diseases.
Acute rhabdomyolysis.

DRUG-INDUCED MYOPATHIES

Alcohol.
d-Penicillamine.
Zidovudine.
Colchicine.
Chloroquine, hydroxychloroquine.
Lipid-lowering agents.
Cyclosporine.
Cocaine, heroin, barbiturates.
Corticosteroids.

NEUROLOGIC DISORDERS

Muscular dystrophies.
Congenital myopathies.
Motor neuron disease.
Guillain-Barré syndrome.
Myasthenia gravis.

NAIL CLUBBING

ICD-10CM # R68.3 Clubbing of nails

COPD.
Pulmonary malignancy.
Cirrhosis.
Inflammatory bowel disease.
Chronic bronchitis.
Congenital heart disease.
Endocarditis.
AV malformations.
Asbestosis.
Trauma.
Idiopathic.

NAIL, HORIZONTAL WHITE LINES (BEAU LINES)

ICD-10CM # L60.4 Beau lines

Malnutrition.
Idiopathic.
Trauma.
Prolonged systemic illnesses.
Pemphigus.
Raynaud phenomenon.

NAIL KOILONYCHIA

ICD-10CM # L60.8 Other nail disorders

Trauma.
Iron deficiency.
SLE.
Hemochromatosis.
Raynaud phenomenon.
Nail-patella syndrome.
Idiopathic.

NAIL ONYCHOLYSIS

ICD-10CM # L60.1 Onycholysis

Infection.
Trauma.
Psoriasis.
Connective tissue disorders.
Sarcoidosis.
Hyperthyroidism.
Amyloidosis.
Nutritional deficiencies.

NAIL PITTING

ICD-10CM # L60.8 Other nail disorders

Psoriasis.
Alopecia areata.
Reiter syndrome.
Trauma.
Idiopathic.

NAIL SPLINTER HEMORRHAGE

ICD-10CM # L60.8 Other nail disorders

SBE.
Trauma.
Malignancies.
Oral contraceptives.
Pregnancy.
SLE.
Antiphospholipid syndrome.
Psoriasis.
RA.
Peptic ulcer disease.

NAIL STRIATIONS

ICD-10CM # L60.8 Other nail disorders

Psoriasis.
Alopecia areata.
Trauma.
Atopic dermatitis.
Vitiligo.

NAIL TELANGIECTASIA

ICD-10CM # L60.8 Other nail disorders

RA.
Scleroderma.
Trauma.
SLE.
Dermatomyositis.

NAIL WHITENING (TERRY NAILS)

ICD-10CM # L60.8 Other nail disorders

Malnutrition.
Trauma.
Liver disease (cirrhosis, hepatic failure).
DM.
Hyperthyroidism.
Idiopathic.

NAIL YELLOWING

ICD-10CM # L60.8 Other nail disorders

Tobacco abuse.
Nephrotic syndrome.
Chronic infections (TB, sinusitis).
Bronchiectasis.
Lymphedema.
Raynaud phenomenon.
RA.
Pleural effusions.
Thyroiditis.
Immunodeficiency.

NASAL AND PARANASAL SINUS TUMORS[41]

ICD-10CM # C30.0 Malignant neoplasm of nasal cavity

BENIGN AND MALIGNANT NASAL AND PARANASAL SINUS TUMORS

Epithelial Tumors

BENIGN

Papilloma.
Adenoma.
Inverting papilloma.

MALIGNANT

Squamous carcinoma.
Adenocarcinoma.
Melanoma.
Adenoid cystic carcinoma.
Malignant salivary tumors.

MESENCHYMAL TUMORS

Benign

Osteoma.
Ossifying fibroma complex.
Angiofibroma.
Chondroma.

Malignant

Osteogenic sarcoma.
Fibrosarcoma.
Angiosarcoma.
Chondrosarcoma.
Lymphoma.
Rhabdomyosarcoma.

NASAL MASSES, CONGENITAL[41]

ICD-10CM # J34.1 Cyst and mucocele of nose and nasal sinus
J34.89 Other specified disorders of nose and nasal sinuses

Dermoid.
Nasal cerebral heterotopia (glioma).
Frontal meningoencephalocele.
Nasolacrimal duct mucocele.
Nasal hamartoma.
Nasal hemangioma.

NAUSEA AND VOMITING

ICD-10CM # R11.2 Nausea with vomiting, unspecified

Infections (viral, bacterial).
Intestinal obstruction.
Metabolic (uremia, electrolyte abnormalities, DKA, acidosis, etc.).
Severe pain.
Anxiety, fear.
Psychiatric disorders (bulimia, anorexia nervosa).
Pregnancy.
Medications (NSAIDs, erythromycin, morphine, codeine, aminophylline, chemotherapeutic agents, etc.).
Withdrawal from substance abuse (drugs, alcohol).
Head trauma.
Vestibular or middle ear disease.
Migraine headache.
CNS neoplasms.
Radiation sickness.
PUD.
Carcinoma of GI tract.
Reye syndrome.
Eye disorders.
Abdominal trauma.

NAUSEA AND VOMITING, CAUSES DURING PREGNANCY[34]

ICD-10CM # R11.2 Nausea with vomiting, unspecified

DIFFERENTIAL DIAGNOSIS OF NAUSEA AND VOMITING DURING PREGNANCY

Nausea and vomiting of pregnancy.
Hyperemesis gravidarum.
Pancreatitis.
Symptomatic cholelithiasis.
Viral hepatitis.
Peptic ulcer disease.
Gastric cancer.
Intestinal obstruction.
Intestinal pseudoobstruction.
Gastroparesis diabeticorum.
Gastritis.
Gastroesophageal reflux disease.
Acute pyelonephritis.
Drug toxicity.
Vagotomy.
Preeclampsia/eclampsia.
Acute fatty liver of pregnancy.
Hemolysis, elevated liver enzymes, and low platelets (HELLP) syndrome.
Anorexia nervosa/bulimia.
Other neuropsychiatric disorders.

NAUSEA AND VOMITING, CHRONIC[30]

ICD-10CM # R11.2 Nausea with vomiting, unspecified

DIFFERENTIAL DIAGNOSIS OF CHRONIC NAUSEA AND VOMITING

Mechanical GI tract obstruction (pylorus, bile duct, small intestine, colon).
Mucosal inflammation.
Peritoneal irritation.
Carcinomas (e.g., gastric, ovarian, renal, bronchogenic).
Metabolic/endocrine disorders (diabetic mellitus, hypothyroidism, hyperthyroidism, adrenal insufficiency, uremia).
Medications (anticholinergics, narcotics, L-dopa, progesterone, calcium channel blockers, digitalis, NSAIDs, antidysrhythmic agents, lubiprostone, cannabis, metformin, amylin analogs).
Gastroparesis.
Gastric dysrhythmias (tachygastria, bradygastria, mixed).
CNS disorders (tumors, migraine, seizures, stroke, orthostatic intolerance).
Psychogenic disorders (anorexia nervosa, bulimia nervosa).

NECK AND ARM PAIN

ICD-10CM # M54.2 Cervicalgia
S46.919A Strain of unspecified muscle, fascia and tendon at shoulder and upper arm level, unspecified arm, initial encounter

Cervical disk syndrome.
Trauma, musculoskeletal strain.
Rotator cuff syndrome.
Bicipital tendonitis.
Glenohumeral arthritis.
Acromioclavicular arthritis.
Thoracic outlet syndrome.
Pancoast tumor.
Infection (cellulitis, abscess).
Angina pectoris.

NECK MASS[71]

ICD-10CM # R22.1 Localized swelling, mass and lump, neck

CONGENITAL ANOMALIES

Thyroglossal duct cyst.
Bronchial apparatus anomalies.
Teratomas.
Ranula.
Dermoid cysts.
Hemangioma.
Laryngoceles.
Cystic hygroma.

NONNEOPLASTIC INFLAMMATORY ETIOLOGIES

Folliculitis.
Adenopathy secondary to peritonsillar abscess.
Retropharyngeal or parapharyngeal abscess.
Salivary gland infections.
Viral infections (mononucleosis, HIV, CMV).
TB.
Cat-scratch disease.
Toxoplasmosis.
Actinomyces.
Atypical mycobacterium.
Jugular vein thrombus.

NEOPLASM (PRIMARY OR METASTATIC)

LIPOMA

NECK PAIN[71]

ICD-10CM # M54.2 Cervicalgia

INFLAMMATORY DISEASES

RA.
Spondyloarthropathies.
Juvenile RA.

NONINFLAMMATORY DISEASE

Cervical osteoarthritis.
Diskogenic neck pain.
Diffuse idiopathic skeletal hyperostosis.
Fibromyalgia or myofascial pain.

INFECTIOUS CAUSES

Meningitis.
Osteomyelitis.
Infectious diskitis.

NEOPLASMS

Primary.
Metastatic.

REFERRED PAIN

Temporomandibular joint pain.
Cardiac pain.
Diaphragmatic irritation.
GI sources (gastric ulcer, gallbladder, pancreas).

NECK PAIN FROM RHEUMATOLOGIC DISORDERS[31]

ICD-10CM # M54.2 Cervicalgia

Rheumatoid arthritis:
- Without disease of the C1-C2 joint.
- With structural cervical abnormalities: C1-C2 subluxation, C1-C2 facet involvement.

Spondyloarthropathies.
Reactive arthritis.
Psoriatic arthritis.
Enteropathic arthritis.
Polymyalgia rheumatica.
Osteoarthritis.
Fibromyalgia.
Nonspecific musculoskeletal pain.
Miscellaneous spondyloarthropathies.
- Whipple disease.
- Behçet disease.
- Paget disease.
- Acromegaly.
- Ossification of the posterior longitudinal ligament.
- Diffuse idiopathic skeletal hyperostosis.

NECK PAIN, NONMUSCULAR CAUSES[47]

ICD-10CM # M54.2 Cervicalgia

Structure	Condition
Pharynx.	Pharyngitis.
Larynx.	Laryngitis. Carcinoma.
Trachea.	Tracheitis.
Thyroid.	Thyroiditis.
Lymph nodes.	Lymphadenitis.
Carotid arteries.	Carotidynia. Dissection. Inflammation.
Aorta.	Aneurysm. Dissection.
Heart.	Angina. Infarction.
Pericardium.	Pericarditis.
Diaphragm.	Inflammation by blood, infection.

NECROTIZING PNEUMONIAS[3]

ICD-10CM # J15.8 Pneumonia due to other specified bacteria

COMMON

Tuberculosis.
Staphylococcus.
Gram-negative bacilli.
Anaerobes.
Fungi.
Pneumocystis jirovecii.

RARE

Streptococcus pneumoniae.
Legionella.
Viruses.
Mycoplasma pneumoniae.

NEOPLASTIC LESIONS, LUMBOSACRAL SPINE[47,*]

ICD-10CM # M54.5 Low back pain

BENIGN

Osteoid osteoma.
Osteoblastoma.
Osteochondroma.
Giant cell tumor.
Aneurysmal bone cyst.
Hemangioma.
Eosinophilic granuloma.
Sacroiliac lipoma.

MALIGNANT

Multiple myeloma.
Chondrosarcoma.
Chordoma.
Lymphoma.
Skeletal metastases.

SPINAL CORD TUMORS

Extradural metastases.
Intradural–extramedullary:
  Neurofibroma.
  Meningioma.
Intramedullary:
  Ependymoma.
  Astrocytoma.

NEPHRITIC SYNDROME, ACUTE[3]

ICD-10CM # N00.8 Acute nephritic syndrome with other morphologic changes

LOW SERUM COMPLEMENT LEVEL

Acute postinfectious glomerulonephritis.
Membranoproliferative glomerulonephritis.
SLE.
Subacute bacterial endocarditis.
Visceral abscess "shunt" nephritis.
Cryoglobulinemia.

NORMAL SERUM COMPLEMENT LEVEL

IgA nephropathy.
Antiglomerular basement membrane disease.
Polyarteritis nodosa.
Granulomatosis with polyangiitis.
Henoch-Schönlein purpura.
Goodpasture syndrome.

NEPHROCALCINOSIS

ICD-10CM # E83.59 Other disorders of calcium metabolism

Sarcoidosis.
Hyperparathyroidism.
Chronic glomerulonephritis.
Milk-alkali syndrome.
Distal renal tubular acidosis.
Medullary sponge kidney.
Bartter syndrome.
Hypervitaminosis D.
Idiopathic hypercalciuria.
Hyperoxaluria.
Cortical necrosis.
Tuberculosis.
Idiopathic hypercalciuria.
Rapidly progressive osteoporosis.

*Although these are most common neoplastic lesions of the lumbosacral spine, most occur infrequently.

NEPHROPATHY, OBSTRUCTIVE[99]

ICD-10CM # Varies with specific diagnosis

POSSIBLE CAUSES OF OBSTRUCTIVE NEPHROPATHY

Renal
Congenital
Polycystic kidney.
Renal cyst.
Peripelvic cyst.
Ureteropelvic junction obstruction.
Neoplastic
Wilms tumor.
Renal cell carcinoma.
Transitional cell carcinoma of the collecting system.
Multiple myeloma.
Inflammatory
Tuberculosis.
Echinococcus infection.
Metabolic
Calculi.
Miscellaneous
Sloughed papillae.
Trauma.
Renal artery aneurysm.
Ureter
Congenital
Stricture.
Ureterocele.
Obstructing megaureter.
Retrocaval ureter.
Prune belly syndrome.
Neoplastic
Primary carcinoma of ureter.
Metastatic carcinoma.
Inflammatory
Tuberculosis.
Amyloidosis.
Schistosomiasis.
Abscess.
Ureteritis cystica.
Endometriosis.
Miscellaneous
Retroperitoneal fibrosis.
Pelvic lipomatosis.
Aortic aneurysm.
Radiation therapy.
Lymphocele.
Trauma.
Urinoma.
Pregnancy.
Radiofrequency ablation.
Bladder and Urethra
Congenital
Posterior urethral valve.
Phimosis.
Hydrocolpos.
Neoplastic
Bladder carcinoma.
Prostate carcinoma.
Carcinoma of urethra.
Carcinoma of penis.
Inflammatory
Prostatitis.
Paraurethral abscess.
Miscellaneous
Benign prostatic hypertrophy.
Neurogenic bladder.
Urethral stricture.

NEUROGENIC BLADDER[72]

ICD-10CM # N31.9 Neuromuscular dysfunction of bladder, unspecified

SUPRATENTORIAL

CVA.
Parkinson disease.
Alzheimer disease.
Cerebral palsy.

SPINAL CORD

Spinal cord injury.
Spinal stenosis.
Central cord syndrome.
ALS.
Multiple sclerosis.
Myelodysplasia.

PERIPHERAL NEUROPATHY

Diabetes.
Alcohol.
Shingles.
Syphilis.

NEUROLOGIC DEFICIT, FOCAL[63]

ICD-10CM #	G45.9	Transient cerebral ischemic attack, unspecified
	I67.848	Other cerebrovascular vasospasm and vasoconstriction

TRAUMATIC: INTRACRANIAL, INTRASPINAL

Subdural hematoma.
Intraparenchymal hemorrhage.
Epidural hematoma.
Traumatic hemorrhagic necrosis.

INFECTIOUS

Brain abscess.
Epidural and subdural abscesses.
Meningitis.

NEOPLASTIC

Primary CNS tumors.
Metastatic tumors.
Syringomyelia.

Vascular.
Thrombosis.
Embolism.
Spontaneous hemorrhage: arteriovenous malformation, aneurysm, hypertensive.

METABOLIC

Hypoglycemia.
Vitamin B_{12} deficiency.
Postseizure.
Hyperosmolar nonketotic.

OTHER

Migraine.
Bell palsy.
Psychogenic.

NEUROLOGIC DEFICIT, MULTIFOCAL[63]

ICD-10CM #	I67.89	Other cerebrovascular disease
	G45.9	Transient cerebral ischemic attack, unspecified
	I67.848	Other cerebrovascular vasospasm and vasoconstriction

Acute disseminated encephalomyelitis: postviral or postimmunization.
Infectious encephalomyelitis: poliovirus, enteroviruses, arbovirus, herpes zoster, Epstein-Barr virus.
Granulomatous encephalomyelitis: sarcoid.
Autoimmune: SLE.
Other: familial spinocerebellar degenerations.

NEUROMUSCULAR JUNCTION DYSFUNCTION[3]

ICD-10CM #	N31.9	Neuromuscular dysfunction of bladder, unspecified

DISORDERS OF THE NEUROMUSCULAR JUNCTION

Autoimmune
Myasthenia gravis.
Lambert-Eaton myasthenic syndrome.
Congenital
Presynaptic defects in ACh resynthesis, packaging, or release.
Synaptic defect: congenital end plate AChE deficiency.
Postsynaptic defects: slow-channel syndromes.
Postsynaptic defects: decreased response to ACh.
Fast-channel syndromes.
AChR deficiency without kinetic abnormality.
Familial limb-girdle myasthenia.
Toxic
Botulism.
Drug-induced disorders.
Organophosphate intoxication.

Ach, Acetylcholine; *AChE*, acetylcholinesterase; *AChR*, acetylcholine receptor.

NEURONOPATHIES, SENSORY (GANGLIONOPATHIES)[7]

ICD-10CM #	G60.0	Hereditary motor and sensory neuropathy

Herpes:
Herpes simplex I and II.
Varicella zoster (shingles).
Inflammatory sensory polyganglionopathy (ISP).
Paraneoplastic.
Primary biliary cirrhosis.
Sjögren syndrome (keratoconjunctivitis sicca).
Toxin-induced:
Pyridoxine (vitamin B_6) overdose.
Metals:
Platinum (cisplatin).
Methyl mercury.
Vitamin E deficiency.

NEUROPATHIC BLADDER

ICD-10CM #	N31.9	Neuromuscular dysfunction of bladder, unspecified

Diabetes.
Stroke.
Multiple sclerosis.
Parkinson disease.
Dementia.
Encephalopathy.
Brain trauma.
Spinal cord trauma.
Pelvic surgery.
Spina bifida.

NEUROPATHIES WITH FACIAL NERVE INVOLVEMENT

ICD-10CM #	G51.8	Other disorders of facial nerve

Sarcoidosis.
HIV.
Lyme disease.
Guillain-Barré.
Others: chronic inflammatory polyneuropathy, Tangier disease, amyloidosis.

NEUROPATHIES, AUTONOMIC[58]

ICD-10CM #	G63	Polyneuropathy in diseases classified elsewhere

GUILLAIN-BARRÉ SYNDROME

Non–Guillain-Barré syndrome autoimmunity.
Paraneoplastic (type I antineuronal nuclear antibody).
Lambert-Eaton syndrome.
Antibodies to neuronal nicotinic acetylcholine receptors.
Antibodies to P/Q type calcium channels.
Other autoantibodies.
Systemic lupus erythematosus.

HEREDITARY

Type I autosomal dominant.
Type II autosomal recessive (Morvan disease).
Type III autosomal recessive (Riley-Day).
Type IV autosomal recessive (congenital insensitivity to pain with anhidrosis).
Type V absence of pain.

METABOLIC

Fabry disease.
Diabetes mellitus.
Tangier disease.
Porphyria.

INFECTIOUS

HIV.
Chagas disease.
Botulism.
Leprosy.
Diphtheria.

OTHER

Triple A (Allgrove) syndrome.
Navajo Indian neuropathy.
Multiple endocrine neoplasia type 2b.
TOXINS

NEUROPATHIES, AUTONOMIC, PERIPHERAL, CAUSES[38]

ICD-10CM #	G90.09	Other idiopathic peripheral autonomic neuropathy

METABOLIC

Diabetes mellitus.
Alcohol.
Acute intermittent porphyria.
Uremia.

AUTOIMMUNE

Autoimmune autonomic ganglionopathy.
Guillain-Barré syndrome.
Morvan syndrome.
Lambert-Eaton myasthenic syndrome.
Chronic inflammatory demyelinating polyradiculoneuropathy.
Sjögren syndrome.
Systemic lupus erythematosus.
Mixed connective tissue diseases.

PARAPROTEINEMIC

Amyloidosis.

NUTRITIONAL

Cyanocobalamin deficiency.
Thiamine deficiency.
Gluten-sensitive neuropathy.

TOXIC

Heavy metals.
Organic solvents.
Organophosphates.
Vacor.
Acrylamide.

DRUG INDUCED

Cisplatin.
Vincristine.
Amiodarone.

Metronidazole.
Perhexiline.
Paclitaxel.

INFECTIOUS

HIV.
Leprosy.
Chagas disease.
Botulism.
Diphtheria.
Lyme disease.

GENETIC

Hereditary sensory and autonomic neuropathies:
- Types I and II.
- Type III (familial dysautonomia).
- Type IV (congenital insensitivity to pain).
- Type V.

Fabry disease.

IDIOPATHIC

Adie syndrome.
Ross syndrome.
Acute cholinergic neuropathy.
Chronic idiopathic anhidrosis.
Amyotrophic lateral sclerosis.

NEUROPATHIES, PAINFUL[102]

ICD-10CM #	G58.9	Mononeuropathy, unspecified
	G62.1	Alcoholic polyneuropathy
	G61.89	Other inflammatory polyneuropathies
	G60.0	Hereditary motor and sensory neuropathy
	G60.0	Hereditary motor and sensory neuropathy
	E11.42	Type 2 diabetes mellitus with diabetic polyneuropathy
	E10.42	Type 1 diabetes mellitus with diabetic polyneuropathy

MONONEUROPATHIES

Compressive neuropathy (carpal tunnel, meralgia paresthetica).
Trigeminal neuralgia.
Ischemic neuropathy.
Polyarteritis nodosa.
Diabetic mononeuropathy.
Herpes zoster.
Idiopathic and familial brachial plexopathy.

POLYNEUROPATHIES

DM.
Paraneoplastic sensory neuropathy.
Nutritional neuropathy.
Multiple myeloma.
Amyloid.
Dominantly inherited sensory neuropathy.
Toxic (arsenic, thallium, metronidazole).
AIDS-associated neuropathy.
Tangier disease.
Fabry disease.

NEUROPATHIES, PERIPHERAL, ASYMMETRICAL PROXIMAL/DISTAL[7]

ICD-10CM #	G99.0	Autonomic neuropathy in diseases classified elsewhere

BRACHIAL PLEXOPATHY

Open

Direct plexus injury (knife or gunshot wound).
Neurovascular (plexus ischemia).
Iatrogenic (central line insertion).

Closed

Traction injuries:
- "Stingers."
- Traction neurapraxia.
- Partial or complete nerve root avulsion.

Radiation.
Neoplastic.
Idiopathic brachial plexitis.
Thoracic outlet.

LUMBOSACRAL PLEXOPATHIES

Open

Closed

Traction injuries:
- Pelvic double vertical shearing fracture.
- Posterior hip dislocation.
- Retroperitoneal hemorrhage.

Vasospastic (deep buttock injection).
Neoplastic.
Radiation.
Idiopathic lumbosacral plexitis.
Infectious:
- Herpesvirus (sacrococcygeal).
- Herpes simplex II.
- Herpes zoster.

Cytomegalovirus (CMV) polyradiculopathy (HIV).

NEUROPATHIES, TOXIC AND METABOLIC[58]

ICD-10CM #	NEC G62.2	Toxic neuropathy

METALS

Arsenic (insecticide, herbicide).
Lead (paint, batteries, pottery).
Mercury (metallic, vapor).
Thallium (rodenticides).
Gold.

OCCUPATIONAL OR INDUSTRIAL CHEMICALS

Acrylamide (grouting, flocculation).
Carbon disulfide (solvent).
Cyanide.
Dichlorophenoxyacetate.
Dimethylaminopropionitrite.
Ethylene oxide (gas sterilization).
Hexacarbons (glue, solvents).
Organophosphates (insecticides, petroleum additive).
Polychlorinated biphenyls.
Tetrachlorbiphenyl.
Trichloroethylene.

DRUGS

Amiodarone.
Chloramphenicol.
Chloroquine.
Cisplatin.
Colchicine.
Dapsone.
Ethambutol.
Ethanol.
Gold.
Hydralazine.
Isoniazid.
Metronidazole.
Nitrofurantoin.
Nitrous oxide.
Nucleosides (antiretroviral agents ddC, ddI, d4T, others).
Penicillamine.
Pentamidine.
Phenytoin.
Pyridoxine (excessive).
Statins.
Stilbamidine.
Suramin.
Taxanes (paclitaxel, docetaxel).
Thalidomide.
Tryptophan (eosinophilia-myalgia syndrome).
Vincristine.

METABOLIC DISORDER

Fabry disease.
Krabbe disease.
Leukodystrophies.
Porphyria.
Tangier disease.
Tyrosinemia.
Uremia.

NEUTROPENIA, DRUG-INDUCED[49]

ICD-10CM #	D70.9	Other neutropenia

DRUGS COMMONLY ASSOCIATED WITH NEUTROPENIA

Antibiotics:
- Vancomycin.
- Semisynthetic penicillins.
- Chloramphenicol.
- Sulfa.
- Linezolid.

Antithyroid drugs:
- Methimazole.
- Propylthiouracil.

Cardiovascular:
- Ticlopidine.
- Procainamide.

Antipsychotics:
- Clozapine.
- Olanzapine.
- Chlorpromazine.

Anticonvulsants:
- Phenytoin.
- Carbamazepine
- Valproic acid.

Antiinflammatory agents:
- Indomethacin.
- Sulfasalazine.

Phenylbutazone.
H2 blockers:
Cimetidine.
Ranitidine.
Analgesics:
Dipyrone.
Antineoplastic:
Rituximab.
Anthelminthic:
Levamisole.

NEUTROPENIA WITH DECREASED MARROW RESERVE[50]

ICD-10CM # D70.8 Other neutropenia

PRIMARY

Severe congenital neutropenia.
Shwachman–Diamond syndrome.
Cyclic neutropenia.

SECONDARY

Lymphoproliferative disorder of granular lymphocytes.
Chemotherapy.
Drug induced (nonimmune).
Nutritional.
Viral infection (varicella, EBV, measles, CMV, hepatitis, HIV).

NEUTROPENIA WITH NORMAL MARROW RESERVE[50]

ICD-10CM # D70.9 Neutropenia, unspecified

Chronic benign neutropenia of infancy and childhood.
Ethnic or benign familial neutropenia.
Autoimmune neutropenia.
Alloimmune neutropenia.
Drug-induced neutropenia.
Infection-related neutropenia.
Hypersplenism.

NEUTROPENIA, IN CHILDHOOD[96]

ICD-10CM # D70.8 Other neutropenia
D70.9 Neutropenia unspecified

ACQUIRED

Infection.
Immune mediated.
Hypersplenism.
Vitamin B_{12}, folate, copper deficiency.
Drugs or toxic substances.
Aplastic anemia.
Malignancies or preleukemic disorders.
Ionizing radiation.

CONGENITAL

Cyclic neutropenia.
Severe congenital neutropenia (Kostmann syndrome).
Chronic benign neutropenia of childhood.
Shwachman-Diamond syndrome.
Fanconi anemia.
Metabolic disorders (amino acidopathies, Barth syndrome, glycogen storage disorders).
Osteopetrosis.
Neutropenia with pigmentation abnormalities, e.g., Chédiak-Higashi.

NEUTROPHILIA[50]

ICD-10CM # D72.0 Neutrophilia, hereditary giant
D71 Functional disorders of polymorphonuclear neutrophils

CLASSIFICATION OF NEUTROPHILIA

Primary (No Other Evident Associated Disease)
Hereditary neutrophilia.
Chronic idiopathic neutrophilia.
Chronic myelogenous leukemia (CML) and other myeloproliferative diseases.
Familial myeloproliferative disease.
Congenital anomalies and leukemoid reaction.
Leukocyte adhesion factor deficiency (LAD).
Familial cold urticaria and leukocytosis.
Secondary
Infection.
Stress neutrophilia.
Chronic inflammation.
Drug induced.
Nonhematologic malignancy.
Generalized marrow stimulation as in hemolysis.
Asplenia and hyposplenism.

NIPPLE DISCHARGE[59]

ICD-10CM # Varies with specific diagnosis

Pregnancy.
Hormones (oral contraceptives, estrogen, progesterone).
Blood pressure drugs (methyldopa, verapamil).
Tricyclic antidepressants.
Tranquilizers (antipsychotics).
Antinausea drugs (metoclopramide).
Herbs (nettle, fennel, blessed thistle, anise, fenugreek seed).
Illicit drugs (marijuana, opiates).
Stimulation of the breast (sexual or from exercise).
Thyroid abnormalities.
Chronic emotional stress.
Hypothalamic tumors.
Chest wall conditions.
Herpes zoster.
Trauma.
Burns.
Tumors.
Breast conditions:
Mammary duct ectasia.
Chronic cystic mastitis.
Intraductal cysts.
Intraductal papillomas.

NIPPLE LESIONS

ICD-10CM # Varies with specific diagnosis

Contact dermatitis.
Trauma.
Paget disease.
Sebaceous hyperplasia.
Neurofibroma.
Accessory nipple.
Papillary adenoma.
Nevoid hyperkeratosis.
Cellulitis.

NODULAR LESIONS, SKIN

ICD-10CM # R22.9 Localized swelling, mass and lump, unspecified

Lipoma.
Cherry angioma.
Angiokeratoma.
Hemangioma.
Classic Kaposi sarcoma.
Nodular melanoma.
Pyogenic granuloma.
Angiosarcoma.
Eccrine poroma.

NODULES, PAINFUL

ICD-10CM # R22.9 Localized swelling, mass and lump, unspecified

Arthropod bite or sting.
Erythema nodosum.
Glomus tumor.
Neuroma.
Leiomyoma.
Angiolipoma.
Dermatofibroma.
Osler node.
Blue rubber bleb nevus.
Vasculitis.
Sweet syndrome.

NYSTAGMUS

ICD-10CM # H55.00 Unspecified nystagmus
H55.89 Other irregular eye movements

Medications (meperidine, barbiturates, phenytoin, phenothiazines, etc.).
Multiple sclerosis.
Congenital.
Neoplasm (cerebellar, brain stem, cerebral).
Labyrinthine or vestibular lesions.
CNS infections.
Optic atrophy.
Other: Arnold–Chiari malformation, syringobulbia, chorioretinitis, meningeal cysts.

NYSTAGMUS, MONOCULAR

ICD-10CM # H55.09 Other forms of nystagmus
H55.00 Unspecified nystagmus

Amblyopia.
Strabismus.
Multiple sclerosis.
Monocular blindness.
Internuclear ophthalmoplegia.
Lid fasciculations.
Brain stem infarct.

ODYNOPHAGIA[95]

ICD-10CM # Varies with specific diagnosis

CAUSES OF ODYNOPHAGIA

Infections
Herpes simplex virus.
Cytomegalovirus.
Candidiasis.
Chemical, Inflammatory
Gastroesophageal reflux.
Drug induced (Slow-K, tetracyclines, quinidine).
Radiation.
Graft-versus-host disease.
Crohn disease.
Dermatologic diseases (pemphigus and pemphigoid).

OPACIFICATION OF HEMIDIAPHRAGM ON X-RAY[41]

ICD-10CM # Varies with specific diagnosis

CAUSES OF OPACIFICATION OF A HEMITHORAX

Pleural effusion.
Consolidation.
Collapse.
Massive tumor.
Fibrothorax.
Combination of above lesions.
Pneumonectomy.
Lung agenesis.

OPHTHALMOPLEGIA[3]

ICD-10CM #	H51.9	Unspecified disorder of binocular movement
	H49.00	Third [oculomotor] nerve palsy, unspecified eye

BILATERAL

Botulism.
Myasthenia gravis.
Wernicke encephalopathy.
Acute cranial polyneuropathy.
Brain stem stroke.

UNILATERAL

Carotid-posterior (3rd cranial nerve, pupil involved communicating aneurysm).
Diabetic-idiopathic (3rd or 6th cranial nerve, pupil spared).
Myasthenia gravis.
Brain stem stroke.[35]

[35] Spontaneous, multivector, chaotic eye movement

OPSOCLONUS[33]

ICD-10CM #	H55.89	Other irregular eye movements

Multiple sclerosis.
Encephalitis.
CNS lymphoma.
Hydrocephalus.
Pontine hemorrhage.
Thalamic disorder (glioma, hemorrhage).
Hyperosmolar coma.
Carcinoma, paraneoplastic.
Cocaine.
Medications (e.g., phenytoin, haloperidol, amitriptyline, diazepam, vidarabine).

OPTIC ATROPHY[88]

ICD-10CM #	H47.20	Unspecified optic atrophy

CAUSES OF OPTIC ATROPHY

Optic Nerve Compression
Pituitary tumor.
Carotid aneurysm.
Glaucoma.
Optic nerve tumor.
Sphenoid meningioma.
Olfactory groove meningioma.
Optic Neuritis Following Long-standing Papilledema Central Retinal Artery Occlusion Toxic/Metabolic
Diabetes.
Methyl alcohol.
Tobacco.
Quinine.
Ethambutol.
Lead and arsenic.
Anemia.
Secondary to Retinal Disease
Senile macular degeneration.
Retinitis pigmentosa.
Severe chorioretinitis.
Secondary to Trauma
Orbital fracture.
Hereditary
Leber optic atrophy.
Hereditary ataxias.
Spinocerebellar degeneration.

OPTIC DISC ELEVATION[13]

ICD-10CM # Varies with specific diagnosis

CAUSES OF OPTIC DISC ELEVATION

Papilloedema.
Accelerated hypertension.
Anterior optic neuropathy.
Ischemic.
Inflammatory.
Infiltrative.
Compressive, including orbital disease.
Pseudopapilloedema.
Disc drusen.
Tilted optic disc.
Peripapillary myelinated nerve fibers.
Crowded disc in hypermetropia.
Mitochondrial optic neuropathies.
Leber hereditary optic neuropathy.
Methanol poisoning.
Intraocular disease.
Central retinal vein occlusion.
Uveitis.
Posterior scleritis.
Hypotony.

ORAL MUCOSA, ERYTHEMATOUS LESIONS[24]

ICD-10CM #	K12.2	Cellulitis and abscess of mouth
	K13.70	Unspecified lesions of oral mucosa
	K13.79	Other lesions of oral mucosa

Allergy.
Erythroplakia.
Candidiasis.
Geographic tongue.
Stomatitis areata migrans.
Plasma cell gingivitis.
Pemphigus vulgaris.

ORAL MUCOSA, PIGMENTED LESIONS[24]

ICD-10CM #	K12.2	Cellulitis and abscess of mouth
	K13.70	Unspecified lesions of oral mucosa
	K13.79	Other lesions of oral mucosa
	K13.5	Oral submucous fibrosis

Racial pigmentation.
Oral melanotic macule.
Peutz-Jeghers syndrome.
Neurofibromatosis.
Albright syndrome.
Addison disease.
Chloasma.
Drug reaction: quinacrine, Minocin, chlorpromazine, Myleran.
Amalgam tattoo.
Lead line.
Smoker's melanosis.
Nevi.
Melanoma.

ORAL MUCOSA, PUNCTATE EROSIVE LESIONS[24]

ICD-10CM #	K12.2	Cellulitis and abscess of mouth
	K13.70	Unspecified lesions of oral mucosa
	K13.79	Other lesions of oral mucosa

Viral lesion: herpes simplex, coxsackievirus (A, B, A16), herpes zoster.
Aphthous stomatitis.

Sutton disease (giant aphthae).
Behçet syndrome.
Reiter syndrome.
Neutropenia.
Acute necrotizing ulcerative gingivostomatitis (ANUG).
Drug reaction.
Inflammatory bowel disease.
Contact allergy.

ORAL MUCOSA, WHITE LESIONS[24]

ICD-10CM #	K12.2	Cellulitis and abscess of mouth
	K13.70	Unspecified lesions of oral mucosa
	K13.79	Other lesions of oral mucosa
	K13.5	Oral submucous fibrosis

Leukoplakia.
White, hairy leukoplakia.
Squamous cell carcinoma.
Lichen planus.
Stomatitis nicotinica.
Benign intraepithelial dyskeratosis.
White spongy nevus.
Leukoedema.
Darier-White disease.
Pachyonychia congenital.
Candidiasis.
Allergy.
SLE.

ORAL SOFT TISSUE TUMORS[39]

ICD-10CM #	Varies with specific diagnosis

Connective Tissue Hyperplasia (Normal-Appearing Overlying Mucosa)
- Irritation fibroma.
- Denture-associated hyperplasia.
- Palatal papillomatosis (papillary hyperplasia).
- Generalized gingival hyperplasias.
- Drug-induced (phenytoin, nifedipine, cyclosporine).
- Hereditary.

Reactive Hyperplasia (Erythematous Overlying Mucosa)
- Pyogenic granuloma/pregnancy tumor.
- Peripheral giant cell granuloma.
- Inflammatory gingival hyperplasia.
- Hyperplastic lingual tonsil.

Epithelial Masses (Usually Irregular White Surface)
- Papilloma/oral wart.
- Squamous cell carcinoma.
- Verrucous carcinoma.
- Focal epithelial hyperplasia (Heck disease).
- Condyloma acuminatum (venereal wart).
- Keratoacanthoma (on lips).

Salivary Duct Obstruction (Minor Salivary Glands)
- Mucocele/ranula (usually fluctuant).
- Salivary stone (sialolith).

Subepithelial Neoplasms
- Primary connective tissue or salivary gland tumors.
- Metastatic lesions (especially in the mandible).
- Lymphoma (especially in the palate or posterior mandible).
- Focal or generalized leukemic infiltrates in the gingiva (especially with acute monocytic leukemia).

ORAL ULCERS, ACUTE

ICD-10CM #	K13.70	Unspecified lesions of oral mucosa
	K13.79	Other lesions of oral mucosa

Trauma (including thermal trauma).
Aphthous stomatitis.
Syphilis.
Herpes simplex infection.
Herpes zoster.

ORAL VESICLES AND ULCERS[3]

ICD-10CM #	K13.70	Unspecified lesions of oral mucosa
	K13.79	Other lesions of oral mucosa

Aphthous stomatitis.
Primary herpes simplex infection.
Vincent stomatitis.
Syphilis.
Coxsackievirus A (herpangina).
Fungi (histoplasmosis).
Behçet syndrome.
SLE.
Reiter syndrome.
Crohn disease.
Erythema multiforme.
Pemphigus.
Pemphigoid.

ORBITAL INFLAMMATION[13]

ICD-10CM #	H05.019	Cellulitis of unspecified orbit
	C69.10	Malignant neoplasm of unspecified orbit
	D31.60	Benign neoplasm of unspecified orbit
	H05.029	Osteomyelitis of unspecified orbit
	H05.049	Tendonitis of unspecified orbit
	H05.229	Edema of unspecified orbit
	H05.239	Hemorrhage of unspecified orbit

DIFFERENTIAL DIAGNOSIS OF AN ACUTELY INFLAMED ORBIT

Infection
Bacterial orbital cellulitis.
Fungal orbital infection.
Dacryocystitis.
Infective dacryoadenitis.

Vascular lesions
Acute orbital hemorrhage,
Cavernous sinus thrombosis.
Carotid–cavernous fistula.

Neoplasia
Rapidly progressive retinoblastoma.
Lacrimal gland tumor.
Other neoplasms (e.g., metastatic lesion with inflammation, lymphoma, Waldenström macroglobulinemia).
Rhabdomyosarcoma, leukemia, lymphangioma, or neuroblastoma in children

Endocrine
Thyroid eye disease of rapid onset.

Non-neoplastic inflammation
Idiopathic orbital inflammatory disease.
Tolosa–Hunt syndrome.
Orbital myositis.
Acute allergic conjunctivitis with lid swelling.
Herpes zoster ophthalmicus.
Herpes simplex skin rash.
Sarcoidosis.
Vasculitides: Wegener granulomatosis, polyarteritis nodosa.
Scleritis, including posterior scleritis.
Ruptured dermoid cyst.

ORBITAL LESIONS, CALCIFIED

ICD-10CM #	H05.89	Other disorders of orbit

Chronic inflammation.
Phlebolith.
Dermoid cyst.
Mucocele walls.
Tumors (lacrimal gland, fibro-osseous).
Meningioma (optic sheath).
Lymphangioma.
Orbital varix.

ORBITAL LESIONS, CYSTIC

ICD-10CM #	H05.9	Unspecified disorder of orbit

Sweat gland cyst.
Dermoid cyst.
Lacrimal gland cyst.
Abscess.
Conjunctival cyst.
Lymphangioma.
Schwannoma.

ORBITAL NEOPLASMS, MALIGNANT[70]

ICD-10CM #	C69.10	Malignant neoplasm of unspecified orbit

LESIONS WITH CLINICALLY MALIGNANT BEHAVIOR

Langerhans cell tumors.[36]
Non-Langerhans cell tumors.
Atypical lymphoid hyperplasia.
Meningioma of optic nerve.

[36]Relatively common tumor

PRIMARY MALIGNANT TUMORS OF ORBIT

Lymphoma.
Lacrimal gland carcinomas.
Rhabdomyosarcoma.
Primitive neuroectodermal tumors.
Malignant peripheral nerve sheath tumor.
Alveolar soft part sarcoma.
Melanoma.
Osteosarcoma.
Fibrosarcoma.
Leiomyosarcoma.
Chondrosarcoma.
Liposarcoma.
Glioma of optic nerve.

SECONDARY MALIGNANT TUMORS OF ORBIT

Eyelid malignancies.
Conjunctival malignancies.
Uveal melanoma.
Retinoblastoma.
Lacrimal drainage system malignancies.
Paranasal sinus and nasal carcinoma.
Brain tumors.

METASTATIC TUMORS OF ORBIT

Distant carcinomas (e.g., breast, lung, gastrointestinal tract).
Neuroblastoma.
Leukemia (granulocytic sarcoma).
Carcinoid tumor.
Metastatic melanoma.

ORGASM DYSFUNCTION[28]

ICD-10CM #	F52.31	Female orgasmic disorder
	F52.32	Male orgasmic disorder

Anorgasmia: inadequate stimulation or learning.
Spinal cord lesion or injury.
Multiple sclerosis.
Alcoholic neuropathy.
Amyotrophic lateral sclerosis.
Spinal cord accident.
Spinal cord trauma.
Peripheral nerve damage.
Radical pelvic surgery.
Herniated lumbar disk.
Hypothyroidism.
Addison disease.
Cushing disease.
Acromegaly.
Hypopituitarism.
Pharmacologic agents (e.g., SSRIs, beta-blockers).
Psychogenic.

OROFACIAL PAIN

ICD-10CM # R51 Facial pain

Dental abscess.
Sinusitis.
Otitis media.
Otitis externa.
Wisdom tooth eruption.
Sialoadenitis.
Herpes zoster.
Trigeminal neuralgia.
Parotitis.
Anxiety disorder.
Malingering.

OSTEOLYTIC BENIGN BONE LESIONS, MULTIPLE[78]

ICD-10CM # Varies with specific diagnosis

COMMON MULTIPLE OSTEOLYTIC BENIGN LESIONS

Cystic lesions in joint disease.
Amyloidosis.
Brown tumors in hyperparathyroidism.
Enchondromatosis.
Fibrous dysplasia.
Osteomyelitis (including tuberculosis, hydatid, sarcoid, etc.).
Massive osteolysis (Gorham disease).
Mastocytosis.
Neurofibromatosis.
Langerhans cell histiocytosis (histiocytosis X).

OSTEOMYELITIS, PEDIATRIC PATIENT[23]

ICD-10CM # M86 Osteomyelitis

Fractures.
Thrombophlebitis.
Scurvy.
Septicemia.
Cellulitis.
Septic bursitis.
Myositis.
Pyomyositis.
Rheumatic fever.
Toxic synovitis.
Reactive arthritis.
Complex regional pain syndrome.
Chronic recurrent multifocal osteomyelitis.
Osteoid osteoma.
Langerhans cell histiocytosis.
Leukemia.
Ewing sarcoma.
Malignant primary bone tumors.
Bone infarction (sickle-cell or Gaucher disease).

OSTEOPOROSIS IN CHILDREN[78]

ICD-10CM # M81.8 Other osteoporosis without current pathological fracture

CAUSES OF OSTEOPOROSIS IN CHILDREN

Systemic long-term oral glucocorticoid therapy.
Chronic inflammatory disease (e.g., juvenile inflammatory arthritis).
Hypogonadism—primary or secondary.
Prolonged immobilization.
Osteogenesis imperfecta.
Idiopathic juvenile osteoporosis.

OSTEOPOROSIS, SECONDARY CAUSES

ICD-10CM # M81.0 Age-related osteoporosis without current pathological fracture

Medication induced (e.g., glucocorticoids, anticonvulsants, heparin, LHRH agonists or antagonists).
Hyperparathyroidism.
Hyperthyroidism.
Prolonged immobilization.
Chronic renal failure.
Sickle cell disease.
Multiple myeloma.
Myeloproliferative diseases.
Leukemias and lymphomas.
Acromegaly.
Prolactinoma.
DM.
Total parenteral nutrition.
Malabsorption.
Chronic hypophosphatemia.
Connective tissue disorders (e.g., osteogenesis imperfecta, Marfan syndrome, Ehlers-Danlos).
Hepatobiliary disease.
Postgastrectomy.
Aluminum-containing antacids.
Systemic mastocytosis.
Homocystinuria.[37]

OSTEOSCLEROSIS, DIFFUSE[41]

ICD-10CM # Q77.4 Congenital osteosclerosis

DISORDERS ASSOCIATED WITH DIFFUSE OSTEOSCLEROSIS

Neoplastic Causes[37]
Prostate carcinoma, breast carcinoma, GI adenocarcinoma, carcinoid tumors, transitional cell carcinoma of the bladder, myeloma, lymphoma, leukemia.
Hematologic Causes
Sickle cell disorders, mastocytosis, myelofibrosis, polycythemia vera.
Metabolic Causes
Renal osteodystrophy, primary hyperparathyoidism, familial hypophosphatemic osteomalacia, hypervitaminosis D, fluorosis, hypoparathyroidism, pseudohypoparathyroidism.[38]
Primary Osseous Disorders[38]
Osteoporosis.
Pyknodysostosis.
Paget disease.

[37]Involvement principally of cancellous bone
[38]Involvement of cancellous and cortical bone

OSTEOSCLEROTIC BENIGN BONE LESIONS, MULTIPLE[78]

ICD-10CM # Q78.2 Osteosclerosis

COMMON MULTIPLE OSTEOSCLEROTIC BENIGN LESIONS

Bone infarcts.
Bone islands.
Callus.
Osteomyelitis (chronic, multifocal).
Paget disease.
Fibrous dysplasia.
Enchondromatosis.
Mastocytosis.
Matured benign lesions (e.g., nonossifying fibromas).
Osteomas (Gardner syndrome).
Osteopathia striata.
Osteopoikilosis.

OVARIAN ENLARGEMENT, NONNEOPLASTIC[26]

ICD-10CM #	N83.209	Unspecified ovarian cyst, unspecified side
	N83.29	Other ovarian cysts
	N80.1	Endometriosis of ovary
	O00.209	Unspecified ovarian pregnancy without intrauterine pregnancy

NON-NEOPLASTIC CAUSES OF OVARIAN ENLARGEMENT IN THE NONPREGNANT PATIENT

Functional

Hemorrhagic corpus luteum.
Follicle cyst.
Cortical stromal hyperplasia (hyperthecosis).
Polycystic ovarian syndrome (PCOS).
Mesothelial/müllerian.
Endometriotic cyst.
Xanthomatous pseudotumor.
Cystic adhesions/cystic mesothelioma.
Simple cyst.

Vascular

Ovarian torsion/infarction.
Massive ovarian edema.

OVULATORY DYSFUNCTION[54]

ICD-10CM #	N97.0	Female infertility associated with anovulation
	N92.3	Ovulation bleeding

HYPERANDROGENIC ANOVULATION

Polycystic ovarian syndrome.
Late-onset congenital adrenal hyperplasias.
Ovarian hyperthecosis.
Androgen-producing ovarian tumors.
Androgen-producing adrenal tumors.
Cushing syndrome.

HYPOESTROGENIC ANOVULATION (HYPOTHALAMIC OR PITUITARY ETIOLOGY)

Hypogonadotropic Hypoestrogenic States

Reversible:
- Functional hypothalamic amenorrheas:
  - Eating disorders (anorexia nervosa, excessive weight loss).
  - Excessive athletic training.

Neoplastic:
- Craniopharyngioma.
- Pituitary stalk compression.

Infiltrative diseases:
- Histiocytosis-X.
- Sarcoidosis.

Hypophysitis.
Pituitary adenomas:
- Hyperprolactinemia.
- Euprolactinemic galactorrhea.

Endocrinopathies:
- Hypothyroidism/hyperthyroidism.
- Cushing disease.

Irreversible:
- Kallmann syndrome.
- Isolated gonadotropin deficiency (hypothalamic or pituitary origin).
- Panhypopituitarism/pituitary insufficiency:
  - Sheehan syndrome, pituitary apoplexy.
  - Pituitary irradiation or ablation.

Hypergonadotropic Hypoestrogenic States

Physiologic states:
- Menopause.
- Perimenopause.

Premature ovarian failure.
Immune-related:
- Radiation/chemotherapy-induced.

Ovarian dysgenesis.
Turner syndrome.
46XX with mutations of X.
Androgen insensitivity syndrome.

MISCELLANEOUS

Endometriosis.
Luteal phase defect.

PAIN, MIDFOOT

ICD-10CM #	M25.579	Pain in unspecified ankle and joints of unspecified foot

MEDIAL ASPECT

Tendonitis of posterior tibialis.
Tendonitis of flexor digitorum longus.
Tendonitis of flexor hallucis longus.
Infection (osteomyelitis, septic arthritis, cellulitis) of foot.
Peripheral vascular insufficiency.
Fracture.
Osteoarthritis.
Gout, pseudogout.
Neuropathy.
Tumor.

LATERAL ASPECT

Peroneus longus tendonitis.
Peroneus brevis tendonitis.
Infection (osteomyelitis, septic arthritis, cellulitis) of foot.
Peripheral vascular insufficiency.
Fracture.
Osteoarthritis.
Gout, pseudogout.
Neuropathy.
Tumor.

PAIN, PLANTAR ASPECT, HEEL

ICD-10CM #	M25.579	Pain in unspecified ankle and joints of unspecified foot

Plantar fasciitis.
Tarsal tunnel syndrome.
Neuroma.
Infection (osteomyelitis, septic arthritis, cellulitis) of foot.
Peripheral vascular insufficiency.
Fracture.
Bone cyst.
Osteoarthritis.
Gout, pseudogout.
Neuropathy.
Tumor.
Heel pad atrophy.
Plantar fascia rupture.

PAIN, POSTERIOR HEEL

ICD-10CM #	M79.609	Pain in unspecified limb

Achilles tendonitis.
Retrocalcaneal bursitis.
Retroachilles bursitis.
Infection (osteomyelitis, septic arthritis, cellulitis) of foot.
Peripheral vascular insufficiency.
Fracture.
Osteoarthritis.
Gout, pseudogout.
Neuropathy.
Tumor.

PALINDROMIC RHEUMATISM[20]

ICD-10CM #	M12.30	Palindromic rheumatism, unspecified site
	M12.319	Palindromic rheumatism, unspecified shoulder
	M12.329	Palindromic rheumatism, unspecified elbow
	M12.339	Palindromic rheumatism, unspecified wrist
	M12.349	Palindromic rheumatism, unspecified hand
	M12.359	Palindromic rheumatism, unspecified hip
	M12.369	Palindromic rheumatism, unspecified knee
	M12.379	Palindromic rheumatism, unspecified ankle and foot
	M12.38	Palindromic rheumatism, vertebrae
	M12.39	Palindromic rheumatism, multiple sites

Palindromic RA.
Essential palindromic rheumatism.
Crystal synovitis (gout, CPPD, pseudogout, calcific periarthritis).
Lyme borreliosis, stages 2 and 3.
Sarcoidosis.
Whipple disease.
Acute rheumatic fever.
Reactive arthritis (rare).

PALMOPLANTAR HYPERKERATOSIS

ICD-10CM #	L85.1	Acquired keratosis [keratoderma] palmaris et plantaris
	L85.2	Keratosis punctata (palmaris et plantaris)
	L87.0	Keratosis follicularis et parafollicularis in cutem penetrans

Superficial skin infection.
Chronic eczema.
Repeated trauma.
Psoriasis.
Reiter syndrome.
Paraneoplastic acrokeratosis.

PALPITATIONS[84]

ICD-10CM #	R00.2	Palpitations

Anxiety.
Electrolyte abnormalities (hypokalemia, hypomagnesemia).
Exercise.
Hyperthyroidism.
Ischemic heart disease.
Ingestion of stimulant drugs (cocaine, amphetamines, caffeine).
Medications (digoxin, beta-blockers, calcium channel antagonists, hydralazines, diuretics, minoxidil).
Hypoglycemia in type 1 DM.
Mitral valve prolapse.
Wolff-Parkinson-White (WPW) syndrome.
Sick sinus syndrome.

PANCOAST SYNDROME[77]

ICD-10CM #	Varies with specific diagnosis

CAUSES OF PANCOAST SYNDROME

Neoplasms

Primary bronchogenic carcinomas.
Other primary thoracic neoplasms: adenoid cystic carcinomas.
Hemangiopericytoma.
Mesothelioma.
Metastatic neoplasms: carcinoma of the larynx, cervix, urinary bladder, and thyroid gland.
Hematologic neoplasms: plasmacytoma, lymphoid granulomatosis, lymphoma.

Infectious Processes

Bacterial: staphylococcal and pseudomonal pneumonia, thoracic actinomycosis.
Fungal: aspergillosis, allescheriasis, cryptococcosis.
Tuberculosis.
Parasitic: echinococcosis (hydatid cyst).

PANCREATIC CALCIFICATIONS

ICD-10CM #	K86.1	Other chronic pancreatitis
	K86.8	Other specified diseases of pancreas

Chronic pancreatitis.
Hyperparathyroidism.
Metastatic neoplasm.
Pseudocyst.
Hereditary pancreatitis.
Cystoadenoma.
Cystoadenocarcinoma.
Cavernous lymphangioma.
Hemorrhage.
Acute pancreatitis (saponification).

PANCREATIC CYSTIC LESIONS[98]

ICD-10CM #	K86.2	Cyst of pancreas
	K86.3	Pseudocyst of pancreas

Pseudocyst.
Serous cystadenoma.
Mucinous cystic neoplasm.
Intraductal papillary mucinous neoplasm.
Solid and papillary epithelial neoplasm.
True epithelial cyst.
Duodenal diverticulum.
Cystic neuroendocrine tumors.
Ductal adenocarcinoma with cystic degeneration.
Cystic metastases.
Cystic degeneration in sarcoma, hemangioma, and paraganglioma.

PANCREATIC SOLID LESIONS[98]

ICD-10CM #	C25.9	Malignant neoplasm of pancreas, unspecified
	D13.6	Benign neoplasm of pancreas

Neoplastic solid tumors.
Ductal adenocarcinoma.
Pancreatic neuroendocrine tumor.
Pancreatic lymphoma.
Metastases to the pancreas.
Solid pseudopapillary tumor.
Pancreaticoblastoma.
Acinar cell carcinoma.
Mesenchymal tumors (sarcoma, fibrous histiocytoma, etc.).
Nonneoplastic solid lesions.
Focal chronic pancreatitis.
Autoimmune pancreatitis.
Groove pancreatitis.
Focal sparing of diffuse pancreatic fatty infiltration.
Intrapancreatic accessory spleen.
Developmental pancreas lobulation.
Sarcoidosis of the pancreas.

PANCREATITIS, ACUTE, IN CHILDREN[58]

ICD-10CM #	K85	Acute pancreatitis

CAUSES OF ACUTE PANCREATITIS IN CHILDREN

Drugs and Toxins

Acetaminophen overdose.
Alcohol.
L-Asparaginase.
Azathioprine.
Carbamazepine.
Cimetidine.
Corticosteroids.
Enalapril.
Erythromycin.
Estrogen.
Furosemide.
Isoniazid.
Lisinopril.
6-Mercaptopurine.
Methyldopa.
Metronidazole.
Organophosphate poisoning.
Pentamidine.
Retrovirals: DDC, DDI, tenofovir.
Sulfonamides: mesalamine, 5-aminosalicylates, sulfasalazine, trimethoprim/sulfamethoxazole.
Sulindac.
Tetracycline.
Thiazides.
Valproic acid.
Venom (spider, scorpion, Gila monster lizard).
Vincristine.

Genetic

Cationic trypsinogen gene *(PRSS1)*.
Chymotrypsin C gene *(CTRC)*.
Cystic fibrosis gene *(CFTR)*.
Trypsin inhibitor gene *(SPINK1)*.

Infectious

Ascariasis.
Coxsackie B virus.
Epstein-Barr virus.
Hepatitis A, B.
Influenza A, B.
Leptospirosis.
Malaria.
Measles.
Mumps.
Mycoplasma.
Reye syndrome: varicella, influenza B.
Rubella.
Rubeola.
Septic shock.

Obstructive

Ampullary disease.
Ascariasis.
Biliary tract malformations.
Choledochal cyst.
Choledochocele.
Cholelithiasis, microlithiasis, and choledocholithiasis (stones or sludge).
Duplication cyst.
Endoscopic retrograde cholangiopancreatography (ERCP) complication.
Pancreas divisum.
Pancreatic ductal abnormalities.
Postoperative.

Sphincter of Oddi dysfunction.
Tumor.
Systemic Disease
Autoimmune pancreatitis.
Brain tumor.
Collagen vascular diseases.
Crohn disease.
Diabetes mellitus.
Head trauma.
Hemochromatosis.
Hemolytic-uremic syndrome.
Hyperlipidemia: type I, IV, V.
Hyperparathyroidism/hypercalcemia.
Kawasaki disease.
Malnutrition.
Organic acidemia.
Peptic ulcer.
Periarteritis nodosa.
Renal failure.
Systemic lupus erythematosus.
Transplantation: bone marrow, heart, liver, kidney, pancreas.
Vasculitis.
Traumatic
Blunt injury.
Burns.
Child abuse.
Hypothermia.
Surgical trauma.
Total body cast.

PANCREATITIS, DRUG-INDUCED[7]

ICD-10CM # K85.3 Drug induced acute pancreatitis

DEFINITE

Acetaminophen.
Azathioprine.
Cimetidine.
Cisplatin.
Corticosteroids.
Didanosine.
Erythromycin.
Estrogens.
Ethyl alcohol.
Furosemide.
L-Asparaginase.
Mercaptopurine.
Metronidazole.
Methyldopa.
Nitrofurantoin.
Octreotide.
Organophosphates.
Pentamidine.
Ranitidine.
Tetracycline.
Salicylates.
Sulfonamides, trimethoprim-sulfamethoxazole, sulfasalazine.
Sulindac.
Valproic acid.

POSSIBLE

Bumetanide.
Carbamazepine.
Chlorthalidone.
Clonidine.
Colchicine.
Cyclosporine.
Cytarabine.
Diazoxide.
Enalapril.
Ergotamine.
Ethacrynic acid.
Indomethacin.
Isoniazid.
Isotretinoin.
Mefenamic acid.
Opiates.
Phenformin.
Piroxicam.
Procainamide.
Rifampin.
Thiazides.

PANCYTOPENIA[50]

ICD-10CM # D61.818 Other pancytopenia

PANCYTOPENIA WITH HYPOCELLULAR BONE MARROW

Acquired aplastic anemia.
Inherited aplastic anemia (Fanconi anemia and others).
Some myelodysplasia syndromes.
Rare aleukemic leukemia (acute myelogenous leukemia).
Some acute lymphoblastic leukemias.
Some lymphomas of bone marrow.

PANCYTOPENIA WITH CELLULAR BONE MARROW

Primary bone marrow diseases.
Myelodysplasia syndromes.
Paroxysmal nocturnal hemoglobinuria.
Myelofibrosis.
Some aleukemic leukemias.
Myelophthisis.
Bone marrow lymphoma.
Hairy cell leukemia.
Secondary to systemic diseases.
Systemic lupus erythematosus, Sjögren syndrome.
Hypersplenism.
Vitamin B_{12}, folate deficiency (familial defect).
Overwhelming infection.
Alcohol.
Brucellosis.
Ehrlichiosis.
Sarcoidosis.
Tuberculosis and atypical mycobacteria.

HYPOCELLULAR BONE MARROW ± CYTOPENIA

Q fever.
Legionnaires disease.
Mycobacteria.
Tuberculosis.[39]
Anorexia nervosa, starvation.
Hypothyroidism.

[39] Pancytopenia in tuberculosis only rarely is associated with a hypocellular bone marrow at biopsy or autopsy. Marrow failure in the setting of tuberculosis is almost always fatal; exceptional patients probably had underlying myelodysplasia or acute leukemia.

PANCYTOPENIA SYNDROME, INHERITED[58]

ICD-10CM # D61.818 Other pancytopenia

Fanconi anemia.
Shwachman-Diamond syndrome.
Dyskeratosis congenita.
Congenital amegakaryocytic thrombocytopenia.
Unclassified inherited bone marrow failure syndromes.
Other genetic syndromes:
- Down syndrome.
- Dubowitz syndrome.
- Seckel syndrome.
- Reticular dysgenesis.
- Schimke immunoosseous dysplasia.
- Familial aplastic anemia (non-Fanconi).
- Cartilage-hair hypoplasia.
- Noonan syndrome.

PAPILLEDEMA

ICD-10CM # H47.10 Unspecified papilledema

CNS infections (viral, bacterial, fungal).
Medications (lithium, cisplatin, corticosteroids, tetracycline, etc.).
Head trauma.
CNS neoplasm (primary or metastatic).
Pseudotumor cerebri.
Cavernous sinus thrombosis.
SLE.
Sarcoidosis.
Subarachnoid hemorrhage.
Carbon dioxide retention.
Arnold–Chiari malformation and other developmental or congenital malformations.
Orbital lesions.
Central retinal vein occlusion.
Hypertensive encephalopathy.
Metabolic abnormalities.

PAPULOSQUAMOUS DISEASES[36]

ICD-10CM # L98.8 Other specified disorders of the skin and subcutaneous tissue

Psoriasis.
Pityriasis rubra pilaris.
Pityriasis rosea.
Lichen planus.
Lichen nitidus.
Secondary syphilis.
Pityriasis lichenoides.
Parapsoriasis.
Mycosis fungoides.
Dermatophytosis.
Tinea versicolor.

PARALYSIS AND MUSCULAR RIGIDITY, DRUG-INDUCED[93]

ICD-10CM # G83 Other paralytic syndromes
R29.818 Other symptoms and signs involving the nervous system

SELECTED AGENTS ASSOCIATED WITH PARALYSIS AND MUSCULAR RIGIDITY

Paralysis

Medications and Industrial Toxins

Aminoglycoside antibiotics.
Beta-blockers.
Chloroquine (with color vision shift).
Cholinesterase inhibitors: neostigmine, pyridostigmine.
d-Penicillamine.
Pesticides: organophosphates, carbamates.
Pyrithioxine.
Trimethadione.

Biologic Toxins

Cobra venom.
Poison hemlock (*Conium maculatum*).
Scorpion fish (Scorpaenidae).
Snake venom, ticks, botulinum toxin.
Star of Bethlehem (*Hippobroma longiflora*).
Sweet pea (*Lathyrus odoratus*).
Tetrodotoxin (puffer fish, blue-ringed octopus, others).

Muscular Rigidity

Black widow spider venom (*Latrodectus mactans*).
Strychnine (*Strychnos nux vomica,* "slang nut").
Tetanus toxin.

PARALYTIC ILEUS[42]

ICD-10CM # K56 Paralytic ileus and intestinal obstruction

CAUSES OF A PARALYTIC ILEUS

Peritonitis.	Congestive heart failure.
Surgery.	Pneumonia.
Trauma:	Renal colic.
Spine.	Renal failure.
Ribs.	Leaking abdominal aortic aneurysm.
Hip.	Low serum potassium.
Retroperitoneum.	Drugs (e.g., morphine).
Inflammation:	Spinal lesions.
Appendicitis.	General debility or infection.
Pancreatitis.	Vascular occlusion.
Cholecystitis.	
Salpingitis.	

PARANEOPLASTIC NEUROLOGIC SYNDROMES

ICD-10CM # G13.0 Paraneoplastic neuromyopathy and neuropathy

Lambert-Eaton myasthenic syndrome.
Myasthenia gravis.
Guillain-Barré syndrome.
Amyotrophic lateral sclerosis.
Dermatomyositis.
Carcinoid myopathy.
Cerebellar degeneration.
Encephalomyelitis.
Optic neuritis, uveitis, retinopathy.
Stiff-man syndrome.
Autonomic neuropathy.
Brachial neuritis.
Sensory neuropathy.
Progressive multifocal leukoencephalopathy.

PARANEOPLASTIC SYNDROMES, ENDOCRINE[91]

ICD-10CM # G13.0 Paraneoplastic neuromyopathy and neuropathy

Hypercalcemia.
Syndrome of inappropriate secretion of antidiuretic hormone.
Hypoglycemia.
Zollinger-Ellison syndrome.
Ectopic secretion of human chorionic gonadotropin.
Cushing syndrome.

PARANEOPLASTIC SYNDROMES, NONENDOCRINE[91]

ICD-10CM # G13.0 Paraneoplastic neuromyopathy and neuropathy

CUTANEOUS

Dermatomyositis.
Acanthosis nigricans.
Sweet syndrome.
Erythema gyratum repens.
Systemic nodular panniculitis (Weber-Christian disease).

RENAL

Nephrotic syndrome.
Nephrogenic diabetes insipidus.

NEUROLOGIC

Subacute cerebellar degeneration.
Progressive multifocal leukoencephalopathy.
Subacute motor neuropathy.
Sensory neuropathy.
Ascending acute polyneuropathy (Guillain-Barré syndrome).
Myasthenic syndrome (Eaton-Lambert syndrome).

HEMATOLOGIC

Microangiopathic hemolytic anemia.
Migratory thrombophlebitis (Trousseau syndrome).
Anemia of chronic disease.

RHEUMATOLOGIC

Polymyalgia rheumatica.
Hypertrophic pulmonary osteoarthropathy.

PARAPARESIS, ACUTE OR SUBACUTE[88]

ICD-10CM # G82.2 Paraparesis

CAUSES OF ACUTE OR SUBACUTE PARAPARESIS

Trauma to a Previously Normal Spine

Vertebral Disease

Metastatic carcinoma.
Cervical spondylosis.
Dorsal disk prolapse.
Paget disease.
Rheumatoid arthritis.
Pott disease of spine.

Tumors

Extradural or intradural carcinoma, lymphoma, myeloma, leukemia.
Dorsal meningioma.
Neurofibroma.

Hematologic Disease

Any cause of thrombocytopenia.
Other clotting disorders.
Leukemia.
Anticoagulant treatment.
Epidural or intramedullary hemorrhage.

Infection

Epidural abscess.
TB abscess.
Syphilitic myelitis.
HIV infection.
Vascular myelopathy.

Vascular

Anterior spinal artery occlusion.
Infarction secondary to hypotension.
Embolic infarction.
Infarction secondary to aortic dissection.
Arteriovenous malformation: infarction or hemorrhage.
Primary intramedullary hemorrhage.
Vasculitis—polyarteritis nodosa (PAN).

Inflammatory

Myelitis of unknown cause.
Multiple sclerosis.
Systemic lupus erythematosus.
Sarcoidosis.

Metabolic

Subacute degeneration of the cord.

PARAPARESIS, CHRONIC PROGRESSIVE[88]

ICD-10CM # G82.2 Paraparesis

CAUSES OF CHRONIC PROGRESSIVE PARAPARESIS

Vertebral Disease

Cervical spondylosis.
Dorsal disk prolapse.
Rheumatoid arthritis.
Pott disease of spine.
Ankylosing spondylitis.

Tumors

Meningioma.
Neurofibroma.
Glioma.
Ependymoma.
Chordoma.
Lipoma.

Syringomyelia

With Arnold–Chiari malformation.
With tumor.
Posttraumatic.

Infection

Tropical spastic paraparesis (HTLV-1 infection).
Syphilitic myelitis.

Vascular

Arteriovenous malformation.

Inflammatory

Multiple sclerosis.

Sarcoidosis.
Radiation myelopathy.
Arachnoiditis.
Metabolic
Subacute combined degeneration of the cord.
Paget disease.
Degenerative
Motor neuron disease.
Hereditary
Hereditary spastic paraplegia.

PARAPARESIS, PAINLESS[56]

ICD-10CM #	G82	Paraplegia (paraparesis) and quadriplegia (quadriparesis)

FREQUENTLY OCCURRING CAUSES OF PAINLESS PARAPARESIS

Inflammatory CNS diseases:
  Multiple sclerosis (MS).
  Neuromyelitis optica (NMO).
Genetic disorders:
  Spinal cerebellar ataxias (SCAs).
  Hereditary spastic paraparesis (HSP).
Infectious illnesses:
  Human T-lymphotropic virus type 1 (HTLV-1) myelopathy.
Compressive lesions*:
  Cervical spondylosis.
  Spinal meningiomas.
  Metastatic tumors.
Neurodegenerative illnesses:
  ALS.
Nutritional deficiencies:
  Copper deficiency.
  Vitamin B_{12} deficiency (combined system disease).

*May be associated with spine pain.

PARAPLEGIA

ICD-10CM #	G82.20	Paraplegia, unspecified
	G80.1	Spastic diplegic cerebral palsy
	I69.969	Other paralytic syndrome following unspecified cerebrovascular disease affecting unspecified side

Trauma: penetrating wounds to motor cortex, fracture-dislocation of vertebral column with compression of spinal cord or cauda equina, prolapsed disk, electrical injuries.
Neoplasm: parasagittal region, vertebrae, meninges, spinal cord, cauda equina, Hodgkin disease, NHL, leukemic deposits, pelvic neoplasms.
Multiple sclerosis and other demyelinating disorders.
Mechanical compression of spinal cord, cauda equina, or lumbosacral plexus: Paget disease, kyphoscoliosis, herniation of intervertebral disk, spondylosis, ankylosing spondylitis, RA, aortic aneurysm.
Infections: spinal abscess, syphilis, TB, poliomyelitis, leprosy.
Thrombosis of superior sagittal sinus.
Polyneuritis: Guillain-Barré syndrome, diabetes, alcohol, beriberi, heavy metals.
Heredofamilial muscular dystrophies.
ALS.
Congenital and familial conditions: syringomyelia, myelomeningocele, myelodysplasia.
Hysteria.

PARASELLAR MASSES[67]

ICD-10CM # Varies with specific diagnosis

GENETIC

Transcription factor mutations (e.g., PROP1[40]).

CYSTS

Rathke.
Arachnoid.
Epidermoid.
Dermoid.

TUMORS

Hormone-secreting or nonfunctional pituitary adenoma.
Granular cell tumor.
Craniopharyngioma (cystic components).
Chordoma.
Meningioma.
Sarcoma.
Glioma.
Schwannoma.
Germ cell tumor.
Vascular tumor.
Solid or hematological metastasis.

MALFORMATION AND HAMARTOMAS

Ectopic pituitary, neurohypophyseal, or salivary tissue.
Hypothalamic hamartoma.
Gangliocytoma.

MISCELLANEOUS LESIONS

Aneurysms.
Hypophysitis.
Infections.
Sarcoidosis.
Giant cell granuloma.
Histiocytosis X.

PARESTHESIAS

ICD-10CM #	R20.2	Paresthesia of skin
	G54.8	Other nerve root and plexus disorders

Multiple sclerosis.
Nutritional deficiencies (thiamin, vitamin B_{12}, folic acid).
Compression of spinal cord or peripheral nerves.
Medications (e.g., INH, lithium, nitrofurantoin, gold, cisplatin, hydralazine, amitriptyline, sulfonamides, amiodarone, metronidazole, dapsone, disulfiram, chloramphenicol).

[40] PROP1, prophet of Pit1 (paired-like homeodomain transcription factor).

Toxic chemicals (e.g., lead, arsenic, cyanide, mercury, organophosphates).
DM.
Myxedema.
Alcohol.
Sarcoidosis.
Neoplasms.
Infections (HIV, Lyme disease, herpes zoster, leprosy, diphtheria).
Charcot-Marie-Tooth syndrome and other hereditary neuropathies.
Guillain-Barré neuropathy.

PARKINSONISM[93]

ICD-10CM #	G20	Parkinson disease
	G21	Secondary parkinsonism
	G21.9	Secondary parkinsonism, unspecified
	G21.19	Other drug-induced Secondary parkinsonism
	G21.4	Vascular parkinsonism
	G21.2	Secondary parkinsonism due to other external agents

CAUSES OF PARKINSONISM

Static Injury/Structural Disorders
Basal ganglia infarcts.
Brain tumor.
Hydrocephalus.
Hereditary/Degenerative Disorders
Juvenile Parkinson disease.
Spinocerebellar ataxia.
Huntington disease (Westphal variant).
Pallidal-pyramidal disorder.
Neurodegeneration with brain iron accumulation (NBIA).
Pantothenate kinase-associated neurodegeneration (PKAN).
Rett syndrome.
Pelizaeus-Merzbacher disease.
Machado-Joseph disease (spinocerebellar ataxia type 3).
Neuronal ceroid lipofuscinoses.
Neuronal intranuclear inclusion body disease.
Metabolic Disorders
Dopa-responsive dystonia.
Tyrosine hydroxylase deficiency and other abnormalities of bioamine metabolism.
Abnormalities of folate metabolism.
Wilson disease.
Basal ganglia calcification (Fahr syndrome, hypoparathyroidism).
Infectious/Para-Infectious Disorders
Encephalitis lethargica (Von Economo disease).
Autoimmune encephalitides, including anti-NMDA receptor associated encephalitis.
Viral encephalitis.
Acute demyelinating encephalomyelitis.
Drugs/Toxins
1-methyl-4-phenyl-1,2,3,6-tetrahydropyridine (MPTP) poisoning.
Rotenone.
Tetrabenazine.

Reserpine.
Methyldopa.
Sedatives.
Neuroleptics.
Antiemetics.
Calcium channel blockers.
Isoniazid.
Serotonin reuptake inhibitors (sertraline, fluoxetine).
Meperidine.

Disorders That Mimic Parkinsonism

Catatonia.
Spasticity.
Hypothyroidism.
Depression (with psychomotor retardation).

PARKINSONISM AND OTHER ACUTE EXTRAPYRAMIDAL REACTIONS, DRUG-INDUCED[93]

ICD-10CM #	G21.19	Other drug-induced secondary parkinsonism

SELECTED AGENTS ASSOCIATED WITH PARKINSONISM AND OTHER ACUTE EXTRAPYRAMIDAL REACTIONS

Medications

Amiodarone.
Anticholinergic agents: benztropine.
Antidepressants (including selective serotonin reuptake inhibitors).
Antiepileptic drugs.
Antifungal agents.
Antihistamines.
Antipsychotics and related drugs (including "novel" agents).
Bethanechol.
Bupropion (acute).
Buspirone.
Captopril (acute).
Clonazepam.
Diazoxide.
Digoxin (chorea).
Estrogen (chorea).
Heroin.
Ketamine.
L-dopa.
Lithium (chorea).
I-Methyl-4-phenyl-1,2,3,6,-tetrahydropyridine (MPTP).
Metronidazole (oculogyric crisis).
Ofloxacin (Tourette-like syndrome).
Opiates/opioids.
Reserpine.
Stimulants.
Sulfasalazine (chorea).
Vinblastine.

Industrial Toxins

Carbon monoxide.
Metals: manganese, thallium, aluminum.
Methanol.
Trichloroethylene.

Biologic Toxins

Arthrinium mycotoxin.

PARKINSONISM-PLUS SYNDROMES

ICD-10CM #	G21.8	Other secondary parkinsonism

Parkinson disease.
Shy-Drager syndrome.
Corticobasal degeneration.
Olivo-ponto-cerebellar atrophy.
Dementia with Lewy bodies.
Progressive supranuclear palsy.
Striatonigral degeneration.

PAROTID SWELLING[8]

ICD-10CM #	K11.20	Sialoadenitis, unspecified
	B26.9	Mumps without complication
	K11.8	Other diseases of salivary glands
	K11.5	Sialolithiasis
	K11.3	Abscess of salivary gland

INFECTIOUS

Mumps.
Parainfluenza.
Influenza.
Cytomegalovirus infection.
Coxsackievirus infection.
Lymphocytic choriomeningitis.
Echovirus infection.
Suppuration (bacterial).
Actinomyces infection.
Mycobacterial infection.
Cat-scratch disease.

NONINFECTIOUS

Drug hypersensitivity (thiouracil, phenothiazines, thiocyanate, iodides, copper, isoprenaline, lead, mercury, phenylbutazone).
Sarcoidosis.
Tumors, mixed.
Hemangioma, lymphangioma.
Sialectasis.
Sjögren syndrome.
Mikulicz syndrome (scleroderma, mixed connective tissue disease, SLE).
Recurrent idiopathic parotitis.
Pneumoparotitis.
Trauma.
Sialolithiasis.
Foreign body.
Cystic fibrosis.
Malnutrition (marasmus, alcohol cirrhosis).
Dehydration.
DM.
Waldenström macroglobulinemia.
Reiter syndrome (reactive arthritis).
Amyloidosis.

NONPAROTID SWELLING

Hypertrophy of masseter muscle.
Lymphadenopathy.
Rheumatoid mandibular joint swelling.
Tumors of jaw.
Infantile cortical hyperostosis.

PELVIC AVULSION FRACTURES[78]

ICD-10CM #	M84.350A	Stress fracture pelvis, initial encounter
	M84.454A	Pathological fracture pelvis, initial encounter

ACUTE AVULSION FRACTURE

Nontraumatic avulsion fracture	Bone metastasis, prior graft harvesting.
Soft tissue injury	Tendon tear, muscle strain.
Aggressive-looking appearance	Osteomyelitis, tumor.
Incidental normal variant	Accessory bone.

CHRONIC AVULSION FRACTURE

Apophyseal avulsion injury	Apophysitis, traction periostitis.
Soft tissue injury	Bursitis, degenerative tendinopathy, calcific tendinitis.

PELVIC MASS

ICD-10CM #	R19.09	Other intraabdominal and pelvic swelling, mass and lump

Hemorrhagic ovarian cyst.
Simple ovarian cyst (follicle or corpus luteum).
Ovarian carcinoma, carcinoma of fallopian tube, colorectal carcinoma, metastatic carcinoma, prostate carcinoma, bladder carcinoma, lymphoma, Hodgkin disease.
Cystadenoma, teratoma, endometrioma.
Leiomyoma.
Leiomyosarcoma.
Diverticulitis, diverticular abscess.
Appendiceal abscess, tuboovarian abscess.
Ectopic pregnancy, intrauterine pregnancy.
Paraovarian cyst.
Hydrosalpinx.

PELVIC PAIN, CAUSES IN WOMEN[7]

ICD-10CM #	N94	Pain and other conditions associated with female genital organs and menstrual cycle
	G10.2	Pelvic and perineal pain
	G89.4	Chronic pain syndrome

POTENTIAL CAUSES OF PELVIC PAIN IN WOMEN

Reproductive Tract

Ovarian torsion.
Ovarian cyst.
Salpingitis/tubo-ovarian abscess.
Septic pelvic thrombophlebitis.
Endometritis.
Endometriosis.
Uterine perforation.

Uterine fibroids.
Dysmenorrhea.
Pregnancy-related
First Trimester
Ectopic pregnancy.
Threatened abortion.
Nonviable pregnancy.
Ovarian hyperstimulation syndrome.
Second and Third Trimesters
Placenta previa.
Placental abruption.
Round ligament pain.
Intestinal Tract
Appendicitis.
Diverticulitis.
Ischemic bowel.
Perforated viscus.
Bowel obstruction.
Incarcerated/strangulated hernia.
Inflammatory bowel disease.
Gastroenteritis.
Urinary Tract
Pyelonephritis.
Cystitis.
Ureteral stone.

PELVIC PAIN, CHRONIC[21]

ICD-10CM #	N94.89	Other specified conditions associated with female genital organs and menstrual cycle
	R10.2	Pelvic and perineal pain
	R10.10	Upper abdominal pain, unspecified
	R10.2	Pelvic and perineal pain
	R10.30	Lower abdominal pain, unspecified

GYNECOLOGIC DISORDERS

Primary dysmenorrhea.
Endometriosis.
Adenomyosis.
Adhesions.
Fibroids.
Retained ovary syndrome after hysterectomy.
Previous tubal ligation.
Chronic pelvic infection.

MUSCULOSKELETAL DISORDERS

Myofascial pain syndrome.

GASTROINTESTINAL DISORDERS

Irritable bowel syndrome.
Inflammatory bowel disease.

URINARY TRACT DISORDERS

Interstitial cystitis.
Nonbacterial urethritis.

PELVIC PAIN, CYCLIC AND ACYCLIC[19]

ICD-10CM #	R10.10	Abdominal and pelvic pain

CAUSES OF CYCLIC AND ACYCLIC PELVIC PAIN

Cyclic
Mittelschmerz.
Endometriosis.[41]
Adenomyosis.
Cervical stenosis.[41]
Leiomyoma (fibroid).
Primary dysmenorrhea.
Acyclic
Chronic PID.
Pelvic adhesions.
Uterine prolapse.
Chronic urethritis.
Diverticulitis.
Irritable bowel syndrome.
Levator syndrome.
Detrusor instability.
Interstitial cystitis.
Abdominal hernia.
Abdominal wall myofascial pain.
Abuse syndromes: physical and sexual.
Depression.

PID, Pelvic inflammatory disease.
[41] May become acyclic.

PELVIC PAIN, GENITAL ORIGIN[63]

ICD-10CM #	N94.89	Other specified conditions associated with female genital organs and menstrual cycle
	R10.2	Pelvic and perineal pain
	R10.10	Upper abdominal pain, unspecified
	R10.2	Pelvic and perineal pain
	R10.30	Lower abdominal pain, unspecified

PERITONEAL IRRITATION

Ruptured ectopic pregnancy.
Ovarian cyst rupture.
Ruptured tuboovarian abscess.
Uterine perforation.

TORSION

Ovarian cyst or tumor.
Pedunculated fibroid.

INTRATUMOR HEMORRHAGE OR INFARCTION

Ovarian cyst.
Solid ovarian tumor.
Uterine leiomyoma.

INFECTION

Endometritis.
Pelvic inflammatory disease.
Trichomonas cervicitis or vaginitis.
Tuboovarian abscess.

PREGNANCY-RELATED

First Trimester
Ectopic pregnancy.
Abortion.
Corpus luteum hematoma.
Late Pregnancy
Placental problems.
Preeclampsia.
Premature labor.

MISCELLANEOUS

Endometriosis.
Foreign objects.
Pelvic adhesions.
Pelvic neoplasm.
Primary dysmenorrhea.

PELVIC PAIN, NON-PREGNANT FEMALE[1]

ICD-10CM #	N94.89	Other specified conditions associated with female genital organs and menstrual cycle
	R10.2	Pelvic and perineal pain
	R10.10	Upper abdominal pain, unspecified
	R10.30	Lower abdominal pain, unspecified

DIFFERENTIAL DIAGNOSIS OF PELVIC PAIN IN NONPREGNANT FEMALES

Gynecologic Diagnoses
Infectious:
- Vaginitis.
- Cervicitis.
- Endometritis.
- Tuboovarian abscess.
- Pelvic inflammatory disease.

Ovarian:
- Ovarian torsion.
- Ruptured ovarian cyst.
- Ovarian tumor.
- Degenerating ovarian tumor.
- Mittelschmerz.

Cervical:
- Cervical polyps.
- Cervical stenosis.
- Cervical cancer.

Uterine:
- Uterine fibroids.
- Degenerating uterine fibroids.
- Adenomyosis.
- Endometrial carcinoma.

Extrauterine:
- Endometriosis.
- Adhesions.
- Residual accessory ovary.

Nongynecologic Diagnoses
GI:
- Acute appendicitis.
- Mesenteric lymphadenitis.
- Diverticulitis.
- Inflammatory bowel disease.
- Irritable bowel syndrome.
- Bowel obstruction.
- Intraabdominal abscess.
- Colorectal carcinoma.

Urinary:
- Cystitis.
- Renal colic.
- Bladder cancer.

Musculoskeletal:
- Abdominal wall pain.
- Lumbar back pain.
- Fibromyalgia.
- Muscular strain.
- Piriformis syndrome.

Neurologic:
- Lumbar radiculopathy.
- Shingles.
- Spondylosis.

Psychologic:
- Personality disorders.
- Major depressive disorder.

PENILE RASH

ICD-10CM #	R21	Rash and other nonspecific skin eruption

Herpes simplex 2.
Balanitis (*Candida*).
Condyloma acuminatum.
Molluscum contagiosum.
Scabies.
Pediculosis pubis.
Pearly penile papules.
Lichen nitidus.
Fox-Fordyce disease (follicular papules).
Trauma.

PERIANAL PAIN[95]

ICD-10CM #	K62.89	Other specified diseases of anus and rectum

Fissure-in-ano.

Anal sepsis:
- Anal abscess.
- Anal fistula.

Hemorrhoids:
- Internal hemorrhoids.
- External hemorrhoids.

Pruritus ani.
Proctalgia fugax.

Chronic perianal pain syndromes:
- Coccygodynia.
- Descending perineum syndrome.
- Levator ani syndrome.
- Idiopathic perineal pain.

PERICARDIAL EFFUSION

ICD-10CM #	I30.9	Acute pericarditis, unspecified
	I31.3	Pericardial effusion

Pericarditis.
Uremia.
Myxedema.
Neoplasm (leukemia, lymphoma, metastatic).
Hemorrhage (trauma, leakage of thoracic aneurysm).
SLE, rheumatoid disease.
Myocardial infarction.

PERIPHERAL ARTERIAL DISEASE, NONATHEROSCLEROTIC CAUSES[51]

ICD-10CM #	I73.9	Peripheral vascular disease, unspecified
	I73.8	Other specified peripheral vascular diseases
	I79.8	Other disorders of arteries, arterioles, and capillaries in diseases classified elsewhere

NONATHEROSCLEROTIC CAUSES OF PERIPHERAL ARTERY DISEASE

Thromboembolism.
Atheroembolism.
Vasculitides:
Large vessel vasculitides, such as giant cell arteritis and Takayasu arteritis.
Small vessel vasculitides, such as thromboangiitis obliterans (Buerger disease).
Trauma.
Popliteal artery entrapment.
Cystic adventitial disease.
- Fibromuscular dysplasia.

Iliac artery endofibrosis.

PERIODIC PARALYSIS, HYPERKALEMIC

ICD-10CM #	G83.9	Paralytic syndrome, unspecified

Chronic renal failure.
Renal insufficiency with excessive potassium supplementation.
Potassium-sparing diuretics.
Endocrinopathies (hypoaldosteronism, adrenal insufficiency).

PERIODIC PARALYSIS, HYPOKALEMIC

ICD-10CM #	G83.9	Paralytic syndrome, unspecified

Chronic diarrhea (laxative abuse, sprue, villous adenoma).
Potassium-depleting diuretics.
Medications (amphotericin B, corticosteroids).
Chronic licorice ingestion.
Thyrotoxicosis.
Renal tubular acidosis.
Conn syndrome.
Barter syndrome.
Barium intoxication.

PERITONEAL CARCINOMATOSIS[36]

ICD-10CM #	C78.6	Secondary malignant neoplasm of retroperitoneum and peritoneum

PRIMARY DISORDERS OF THE PERITONEUM: MESOTHELIOMA

Metastatic spread from:
Stomach.
Colon.
Pancreas.
Carcinoid.
Other Intraabdominal Organs
Ovary.
Pseudomyxoma peritonei.
Extraabdominal Primary Tumors
Breast.
Lung.
Hematologic Malignancy
Lymphoma.

PERITONEAL EFFUSION[45]

ICD-10CM #	R18	Ascites
	R85.9	Unspecified abnormal finding in specimens from digestive organs and abdominal cavity
	R88.8	Abnormal findings in other body fluids and substances

TRANSUDATES

Increased hydrostatic pressure or decreased plasma oncotic pressure.
Congestive heart failure.
Hepatic cirrhosis.
Hypoproteinemia.

EXUDATES

Increased capillary permeability or decreased lymphatic resorption.
Infections (TB, spontaneous bacterial peritonitis, secondary bacterial peritonitis).
Neoplasms (hepatoma, metastatic carcinoma, lymphoma, mesothelioma).
Trauma.
Pancreatitis.
Bile peritonitis (e.g., ruptured gallbladder).

CHYLOUS EFFUSION

Damage or obstruction to thoracic duct.
Trauma.
Lymphoma.
Carcinoma.
Tuberculosis.
Parasitic infection.

PERIUMBILICAL SWELLING

ICD-10CM #	R19.00	Intraabdominal and pelvic swelling, mass and lump, unspecified site

Umbilical hernia.
Lipoma.
Epigastric hernia.
Umbilical granuloma.
Omphalocele.
Gastroschisis.
Caput medusae.

PHARYNGEAL OBSTRUCTION, CAUSES[66]

ICD-10CM # Varies with specific diagnosis

CAUSES OF PHARYNGEAL OBSTRUCTION

Malignant or benign tumors (e.g., papillomas, polyps).
Infection (e.g., croup, epiglottitis, tonsillar abscess).
Edema or hypertrophy (e.g., angioneurotic edema, anaphylactic reactions, postradiation therapy, obstructive sleep apnea).
Trauma (e.g., cricoid fracture, cervical subluxation, precervical hematoma).
Burn injury.
Extrinsic compression (e.g., goiter or pregnancy-related thyroid enlargement).
Foreign body.
Congenital web (infants).
Sarcoidosis and other granulomatous diseases.
Amyloid.

PHEOCHROMOCYTOMA-TYPE SPELLS[67]

ICD-10CM #	I15.2	Hypertension due to pheochromocytoma

DIFFERENTIAL DIAGNOSIS OF PHEOCHROMOCYTOMA-TYPE SPELLS

Endocrine Causes
Carbohydrate intolerance.
Hyperadrenergic spells.
Hypoglycemia.
Pancreatic tumors (e.g., insulinoma).
Pheochromocytoma.
Primary hypogonadism (menopausal syndrome).
Thyrotoxicosis.
Cardiovascular Causes
Angina.
Cardiovascular deconditioning.
Labile essential hypertension.
Orthostatic hypotension.
Paroxysmal cardiac arrhythmia.
Pulmonary edema.
Renovascular disease.
Syncope (e.g., vasovagal reaction).
Psychologic Causes
Factitious (e.g., drugs, Valsalva).
Hyperventilation.
Severe anxiety and panic disorders.
Somatization disorder.
Pharmacologic Causes
Chlorpropamide-alcohol flush.
Combination of a monoamine oxidase inhibitor and a decongestant.
Illegal drug ingestion (cocaine, phencyclidine, lysergic acid diethylamide).
Sympathomimetic drug ingestion.
Vancomycin ("red man syndrome").
Withdrawal of adrenergic-inhibitor.
Neurologic Causes
Autonomic neuropathy.
Cerebrovascular insufficiency.
Diencephalic epilepsy (autonomic seizures).
Migraine headache.
Postural orthostatic tachycardia syndrome.
Stroke.
Other Causes
Carcinoid syndrome:
- Mast cell disease.
- Recurrent idiopathic anaphylaxis.
- Unexplained flushing spells.

PHOTODERMATOSES[36]

ICD-10CM #	L56.0	Drug phototoxic response
	L56.1	Drug photoallergic response
	L56.2	Photocontact dermatitis [berloque dermatitis]

Polymorphous light eruption.
Chronic actinic dermatitis.
Solar urticaria.
Phototoxicity and photoallergy.
Porphyrias.

PHOTOSENSITIVITY

ICD-10CM #	L56.0	Drug phototoxic response
	L56.1	Drug photoallergic response
	L56.2	Photocontact dermatitis [berloque dermatitis]

Solar urticaria.
Photoallergic reaction.
Phototoxic reaction.
Polymorphous light eruption.
Porphyria cutanea tarda.
SLE.
Drug induced (e.g., tetracyclines).

PIGMENTURIA[7]

ICD-10CM #	R82	Other abnormal findings in urine

HEMOGLOBINURIA

Hemolysis.

HEMATURIA

Renal causes.
Trauma.

ACUTE INTERMITTENT PORPHYRIA

Bilirubinuria
Food
Beets.
Drugs
Vitamin B_{12}.
Rifampin.
Phenytoin.
Laxatives.

PITUITARY INSUFFICIENCY, ACQUIRED[68]

ICD-10CM #	E23.0	Hypopituitarism
	E89.3	Postprocedural hypopituitarism
	E23.1	Drug-induced hypopituitarism

CAUSES OF ACQUIRED PITUITARY INSUFFICIENCY

Traumatic
- Surgical resection.
- Radiation damage.
- Traumatic brain injury.

Infiltrative/Inflammatory
Primary Hypophysitis
- Lymphocytic.
- Granulomatous.
- Xanthomatous.

Secondary Hypophysitis
- Sarcoidosis.
- Histiocytosis X.
- Infections.
- Wegener granulomatosis.
- Takayasu disease.
- Hemochromatosis.

Infections
- Tuberculosis.
- *Pneumocystis jirovecii* infection.
- Fungal (histoplasmosis, aspergillosis).
- Parasites (toxoplasmosis).
- Viral (cytomegalovirus).

Vascular
- Pregnancy related.
- Aneurysm.
- Apoplexy.
- Diabetes.
- Hypotension.
- Arteritis.
- Sickle cell disease.

Neoplastic
- Pituitary adenoma.
- Parasellar mass:
  - Rathke cyst.
  - Dermoid cyst.
  - Meningioma.
- Germinoma.
  - Ependymoma.
  - Glioma.
- Craniopharyngioma.
- Hypothalamic harmatoma, gangliocytoma.
- Pituitary metastatic deposits.
- Hematologic malignancy:
  - Leukemia.
  - Lymphoma.

PITUITARY REGION TUMORS[41]

ICD-10CM # Varies with specific diagnosis

PRIMARY TUMORS IN THE SELLAR AND PARASELLAR REGION

Pituitary macroadenoma.
Meningioma.
Schwannoma (e.g., of fifth nerve).
Chordoma.
Chondrosarcoma.
Craniopharyngioma.
Rathke cleft cyst.
Dermoid.
Epidermoid.
Tuber cinereum hamartoma.
Optic glioma.
Germ cell tumors.

PLATELET DYSFUNCTION, DRUG-INDUCED[51]

ICD-10CM #	D69.1	Qualitative platelet defects

Anti-Platelet Drugs

COX inhibitors: aspirin.
ADP receptor antagonists:
- Thienopyridines: clopidogrel, ticlopidine, prasugrel.
- Nonthienopyridines: ticagrelor, cangrelor.

$\alpha_{IIb}\beta_3$ inhibitors: abciximab, eptifibatide, tirofiban.
PDE inhibitors:
- Nonselective PDE inhibitors: pentoxifylline, caffeine, theophylline.
- PDE3 inhibitors: cilostazol, milrinone, anagrelide.
- PDE5 inhibitors: dipyridamole, sildenafil.

Adenyl cyclase stimulators: epoprostenol, iloprost, beraprost.
Drugs that adversely affect platelet function.
NSAIDs: ibuprofen, naproxen, indomethacin.
Cardiovascular agents:
- Calcium channel blockers: nifedipine, diltiazem, verapamil.
- β-Blockers: propranolol.
- Vasodilators: nitrates, nitroprusside.
- Diuretics: furosemide.
- Angiotensin II receptor antagonist: losartan, valsartan, and olmesartan.

Antibiotics: β-lactams, amphotericin, hydroxychloroquine, nitrofurantoin.
Antifungal drugs: Miconazole, amphotericin B:
- Psychiatric drugs: TCAs, fluoxetine, chlorpromazine, promethazine, trifluoperazine.
- Oncologic drugs: mithramycin, daunorubicin, BCNU, asparaginase, vincristine, dasatinib, ibrutinib.
- Anesthetics: dibucaine, procaine, halothane, sevoflurane, propofol.
- Plasma expanders: dextran, hydroxyl ethyl starch.
- Heparins and thrombolytic agents.
- Miscellaneous: clofibrate, statins, cocaine, ketanserin, radiographic contrast agents, antihistamines, immunosuppressive drugs.

ADP, Adenosine diphosphate; *BCNU,* carmustine; *COX,* cyclooxygenase; *NSAID,* nonsteroidal antiinflammatory drug; *PDE,* phosphodiesterase; *TCA,* tricyclic antidepressant.

PLEURAL EFFUSIONS

ICD-10CM # J91.8 Pleural effusion in other conditions classified elsewhere

EXUDATIVE

Neoplasm: bronchogenic carcinoma, breast carcinoma, mesothelioma, lymphoma, ovarian carcinoma, multiple myeloma, leukemia, Meigs syndrome.
Infections: viral pneumonia, bacterial pneumonia, *Mycoplasma,* TB, fungal and parasitic diseases, extension from subphrenic abscess.
Trauma.
Collagen vascular diseases: SLE, RA, scleroderma, polyarteritis, granulomatosis with polyangiitis.
Pulmonary infarction.
Pancreatitis.
Postcardiotomy/Dressler syndrome.
Drug-induced SLE (hydralazine, procainamide).
Postabdominal surgery.
Ruptured esophagus.
Chronic effusion secondary to congestive failure.

TRANSUDATIVE

CHF.
Hepatic cirrhosis.
Nephrotic syndrome.
Hypoproteinemia from any cause.
Meigs syndrome.

PLEURAL EFFUSIONS, MALIGNANCY-ASSOCIATED

ICD-10CM # C78.2 Secondary malignant neoplasm of pleura

Lung cancer	(30% to 40%)
Breast cancer	(20% to 25%)
Lymphoma	(10% to 15%)
Leukemia	(5% to 10%)
GI tract	(5%)
GU tract	(5%)
Reproductive	(3%)

PLEURAL HYPERPLASIA[85]

ICD-10CM # Varies with specific diagnosis

BENIGN CAUSES OF PLEURAL HYPERPLASIA

Pleural infections.
Radiation.
Surgery.
Trauma.
Intracavitary treatments (chemotherapy or sclerosing agents).
Collagen vascular diseases.
Systemic immune diseases (systemic lupus erythematosus, rheumatoid arthritis, Sjögren syndrome, Wegener granulomatosis).
Subpleural pulmonary abnormalities (infarction, infection, neoplasia).
Pneumothorax.
Drug reactions (nitrofurantoin, bromocriptine, methysergide, procarbazine).
Pancreatitis, uremia.
Pneumoconiosis (asbestosis).

PLEURAL MASSES[85]

ICD-10CM # Varies with specific diagnosis

CAUSES OF PLEURAL MASSES

Inflammatory pleural reactions:
- Reactive mesothelial hyperplasia or organizing pleuritis versus atypical mesothelial hyperplasia.
- Nodular pleural plaques.

Pulmonary tumors that may resemble pleural tumors:
- Inflammatory pseudotumor of the lung.

Benign pleural tumors:
- Solitary fibrous tumor.
- Lipomas and lipoblastomas.
- Adenomatous tumors.
- Calcifying fibrous tumors.
- Mesothelial cysts.
- Multicystic mesothelioma.
- Schwannoma.

Pleural tumors with low malignant potential:
- Desmoid tumors.
- Well-differentiated papillary mesothelioma.
- Pleural thymoma.

Primary malignant pleural tumors that may look like benign tumors:
- Malignant solitary fibrous tumor.
- Pleuropulmonary blastoma.
- Localized malignant mesothelioma.
- Vascular sarcoma.
- Liposarcoma.
- Pleuropulmonary synovial sarcoma.
- Askin tumor or primitive neuroectodermal tumor (PNET).
- Desmoplastic small round cell tumor.

Malignant pleural tumors:
- Metastatic malignancies to the pleura.
- Malignant mesothelioma.

PNEUMATOSIS INTESTINALIS IN NEONATE AND OLDER CHILD[41]

ICD-10CM # Varies with specific diagnosis

CAUSES OF PNEUMATOSIS INTESTINALIS IN THE NEONATE AND THE OLDER CHILD

Necrotizing enterocolitis.
Bowel ischemia, inflammation, and obstruction.
Cyanotic congenital heart disease.
Hirschsprung disease.
Gastroschisis.
Anorectal atresia.
Inflammatory bowel disease.
Lymphoma.
Leukemia.
CMV and rotavirus gastroenteritis.
Colonoscopy.
Caustic ingestion.
Short bowel syndrome.
Congenital immune deficiency states.
Clostridium infection.
Chronic steroid use.
Posthepatic, renal, or bone marrow transplant.
Collagen vascular disease.
Graft-versus-host disease.
AIDS.

PNEUMONIA, CHRONIC[10]

ICD-10CM #	J15.9	Unspecified bacterial pneumonia
	J12.9	Viral pneumonia, unspecified
	B25.0	Cytomegaloviral pneumonitis
	J18.0	Bronchopneumonia, unspecified organism

INFECTIOUS AGENTS THAT TYPICALLY CAUSE CHRONIC PNEUMONIA

Bacteria

Mixed aerobic and anaerobic bacteria.
Actinomyces spp.
Nocardia spp.
Rhodococcus equi.
Burkholderia pseudomallei.

Mycobacteria

Mycobacterium tuberculosis.
Mycobacterium kansasii.
Mycobacterium avium complex.

Mycobacterium abscessus.
Mycobacterium terrae.
Fungi
Aspergillus spp.
Blastomyces dermatitidis.
Coccidioides spp.
Cryptococcus neoformans.
Cryptococcus gattii.
Dark-walled molds.
Emmonsia parvum var. crescens.
Histoplasma capsulatum.
Sporothrix schenckii complex.
Paracoccidioides brasiliensis.
Penicillium marneffei.
Scedosporium apiospermum.
Parasites
Dirofilaria:
Echinococcus granulosus.
Filaria (tropical pulmonary eosinophilia).
Paragonimus westermani.

NONINFECTIOUS CAUSES OF CHRONIC PNEUMONIA

Neoplasia
Carcinoma (primary or metastatic).
Hodgkin disease and non-Hodgkin lymphoma.
Other lymphoproliferative disorders.
Cystic Fibrosis
Sarcoidosis
Amyloidosis
Vasculitis (autoimmune diseases)
Systemic lupus erythematosus.
Polyarteritis nodosa.
Granulomatosis with polyangiitis.
Allergic angiitis and granulomatosis (Churg-Strauss syndrome).
Goodpasture syndrome.
Microscopic polyangiitis.
Lymphomatoid granulomatosis.
Progressive systemic sclerosis.
Rheumatoid arthritis.
Mixed connective tissue syndrome (overlap syndrome).
Chemicals, Drugs
Radiation
Recurrent pulmonary emboli
Bronchial obstruction with atelectasis (e.g., tumor, foreign body)
Pulmonary sequestration
Pulmonary infiltration with eosinophilia syndrome (Löffler syndrome—usually transient.)
Pneumonia plus asthma (e.g., allergic bronchopulmonary aspergillosis).
Bronchocentric granulomatosis.
Chronic eosinophilic pneumonia.
Pneumoconiosis
Asbestosis.
Berylliosis.
Silicosis.
Anthracosilicosis.
Chronic Form of Extrinsic Allergic Alveolitis (Hypersensitivity Pneumonitis)

OTHER LUNG DISEASES: CAUSE UNKNOWN

Chronic Organizing Pneumonia
Chronic Interstitial Pneumonia (Fibrosing Alveolitis, Idiopathic Pulmonary Fibrosis)
Usual interstitial pneumonia (UIP).
Desquamative interstitial pneumonia (DIP).
Lymphocytic interstitial pneumonia (LIP).
Giant cell interstitial pneumonia (GIP).
Eosinophilic granuloma (histiocytosis X).
Lymphangioleiomyomatosis.
Pulmonary alveolar proteinosis.
Pulmonary alveolar microlithiasis.
Idiopathic pulmonary hemosiderosis.
Angiocentric immunoproliferative lesions.

PNEUMONIA MIMICS[15]

ICD-10CM # Varies with specific diagnosis

NONINFECTIOUS CAUSES THAT MAY PRESENT AS PNEUMONIA

Radiologic Technique
Inadequate inspiration.
Breast shadow.
Thymus.
Uneven grid on film.
Underpenetrated film.
Primary Pulmonary
Asthma.
Bronchiectasis.
Atelectasis.
Bronchopulmonary dysplasia.
Cystic fibrosis.
Pulmonary sequestration.
Congenital cystic adenomatoid malformation.
α_1-Antitrypsin deficiency.
Aspiration
Foreign body.
Chemical.
Recurrent caused by anatomic or physiologic disorders.
Primary Cardiac
Congenital heart disease.
CHF
Pulmonary Infarction
Sickle cell vasoocclusive crisis.
Pulmonary embolism.
Collagen Vascular Disorders
Acute Respiratory Distress Syndrome
Pleural effusion
Neoplasm.

PNEUMONIA, NONRESPONDING, CAUSES[66]

ICD-10CM #	J15.9	Unspecified bacterial pneumonia
	J12.9	Viral pneumonia, unspecified
	B25.0	Cytomegaloviral pneumonitis
	J18.0	Bronchopneumonia, unspecified organism

CAUSES OF NONRESPONDING PNEUMONIA

Infectious Pneumonia
Resistant microorganisms:
Community-acquired pneumonia (e.g., *Streptococcus pneumoniae, Staphylococcus aureus*).
Nosocomial pneumonia (e.g., *Acinetobacter*, methicillin-resistant *Staphylococcus aureus* (MRSA), *Pseudomonas aeruginosa*).
Uncommon microorganisms (e.g., *Mycobacterium tuberculosis, Nocardia* spp., fungi, *Pneumocystis jirovecii*).
Complications of pneumonia:
Empyema.
Abscess or necrotizing pneumonia.
Metastatic infection.
Noninfectious Pneumonia
Neoplasms.
Pulmonary hemorrhage.
Pulmonary embolism.
Sarcoidosis.
Eosinophilic pneumonia.
Pulmonary edema.
Acute respiratory distress syndrome.
Bronchiolitis obliterans with organizing pneumonia.
Drug-induced pulmonary disease.
Pulmonary vasculitis.

PNEUMONIA, RECURRENT

ICD-10CM #	J15.9	Unspecified bacterial pneumonia
	J12.9	Viral pneumonia, unspecified
	B25.0	Cytomegaloviral pneumonitis
	J18.0	Bronchopneumonia, unspecified organism

Mechanical obstruction from neoplasm.
Chronic aspiration (tube feeding, alcoholism, CVA, neuromuscular disorders, seizure disorder, inability to cough).
Bronchiectasis.
Kyphoscoliosis.
COPD, CHF, asthma, silicosis, pulmonary fibrosis, cystic fibrosis.
Pulmonary TB, chronic sinusitis.
Immunosuppression (HIV, corticosteroids, leukemia, chemotherapy, splenectomy).

PNEUMOPERITONEUM, NEONATAL[41]

ICD-10CM # Varies with specific diagnosis

CAUSES OF NEONATAL PNEUMOPERITONEUM

Necrotizing enterocolitis.
Spontaneous perforation of a hollow viscus:
Stomach.
Duodenum.
Ileum.
Colon.
Malrotation and volvulus.
Distal obstruction.
Perforation of Meckel diverticulum.
Anterior abdominal wall defects:
Pentalogy of Cantrell.
Omphalocele.
Gastroschisis.
Cloacal exstrophy.
Stress and peptic ulcers.
Mechanical ventilation (air leak) or resuscitation ("bagging").
Post-laparotomy.
Iatrogenic gastric perforation with an orogastric tube.

Iatrogenic colon perforation:
- Thermometer.
- During an enema.

Indomethacin.
Dexamethasone treatment.

PNEUMOTHORAX, IN CHILDREN[58]

ICD-10CM #	J93.0	Spontaneous tension pneumothorax
	J93	Pneumothorax
	J93.9	Pneumothorax unspecified

SPONTANEOUS

Primary idiopathic—usually resulting from ruptured subpleural blebs.
Secondary blebs.
Congenital lung disease:
- Congenital cystic adenomatoid malformation.
- Bronchogenic cysts.
- Pulmonary hypoplasia.

Conditions associated with increased intrathoracic pressure:
- Asthma.
- Bronchiolitis.
- Air-block syndrome in neonates.
- Cystic fibrosis.
- Airway foreign body.

Infection:
- Pneumatocele.
- Lung abscess.
- Bronchopleural fistula.

Diffuse lung disease:
- Langerhans cell histiocytosis.
- Tuberous sclerosis.
- Marfan syndrome.
- Ehlers-Danlos syndrome.

Metastatic neoplasm—usually osteosarcoma (rare).

TRAUMATIC

Noniatrogenic:
- Penetrating trauma.
- Blunt trauma.
- Loud music (air pressure).

Iatrogenic:
- Thoracotomy.
- Thoracoscopy, thoracentesis.
- Tracheostomy.
- Tube or needle puncture.

Mechanical ventilation.

POLIOSIS[13]

ICD-10CM # Varies with specific diagnosis

CAUSES OF POLIOSIS

Ocular

Chronic anterior blepharitis.
Sympathetic ophthalmitis.
Idiopathic uveitis.

Systemic

Vogt–Koyanagi–Harada syndrome.
Waardenburg syndrome.
Vitiligo.
Marfan syndrome.
Tuberous sclerosis.

POLYCYTHEMIA

ICD-10CM #	D45	Polycythemia primary
	D75.1	Polycythemia secondary

Tobacco abuse.
Chronic lung disease.
High altitude.
Sleep apnea.
Right-to-left cardiac shunts.
Erythropoietin administration.
Androgens/anabolic steroids.
Polycystic kidney disease.
Renal cell carcinoma.
Hepatocellular carcinoma.
Polycythemia vera.
Carbon monoxide exposure.
Primary familial and congenital polycythemia.
High-oxygen–affinity hemoglobins.
Uterine leiomyoma, meningioma, pheochromocytoma, parathyroid carcinoma.
Cobalt exposure.

POLYCYTHEMIAS, DIFFERENTIAL DIAGNOSIS[49]

ICD-10CM #	D45	Polycythemia primary
	D75.1	Polycythemia secondary

DIFFERENTIAL DIAGNOSIS OF THE POLYCYTHEMIAS

Relative or Spurious Polycythemia

Decreased plasma volume—reduced fluid intake, marked loss of body fluids (diaphoresis, vomiting, diarrhea, "third spacing").
Gaisböck syndrome.
Overfilling of blood in collection vacuum tubes.
Absolute polycythemia
Secondary polycythemia.
Acquired.
Hypoxia:
- Pulmonary disease.
- Cyanotic congenital heart disease.
- Hypoventilation syndromes:
  - Sleep apnea.
  - Pickwickian syndrome.
  - High altitude.
  - Smokers' polycythemia, hookah polycythemia, carbon monoxide intoxication caused by industrial exposure.

Postrenal transplantation erythrocytosis.
Aberrant erythropoietin production.
Tumors:
- Renal cell carcinoma.
- Wilms tumor.
- Hepatic carcinoma.
- Uterine leiomyomata.

Virilizing ovarian tumors.
Vascular cerebellar tumors.
Miscellaneous renal and hepatic disorders:
- Solitary renal cysts.
- Polycystic kidney disease.
- Renal artery stenosis hydronephrosis.
- Viral hepatitis.
- Endocrine disorders:
- Cushing syndrome.
- Primary aldosteronism.
- Androgen use.
- Erythropoietin use.

Congenital polycythemias:
- Abnormal high-affinity hemoglobin variants.
- Bisphosphoglycerate deficiency.
- Congenital methemoglobinemia.
- Chuvash polycythemia (von Hippel Lindau mutations).
- Prolyl hydroxylase mutations.
- Hypoxia-inducible factor gene mutations.

Primary polycythemias:
- Primary congenital and familial polycythemia.
- Polycythemia vera.

POLYCYTHEMIA, RELATIVE VERSUS ABSOLUTE[50]

ICD-10CM #	D75.1	Secondary polycythemia

RELATIVE OR SPURIOUS POLYCYTHEMIA

Decreased plasma volume—reduced fluid intake, marked loss of body fluids (diaphoresis, vomiting, diarrhea, "third-spacing").
Gaisböck syndrome.
Overfilling of blood in collection vacuum tubes.

ABSOLUTE POLYCYTHEMIA

Primary Congenital and Familial Polycythemia

Secondary Polycythemia Acquired

Hypoxia:
- Pulmonary disease.
- Cyanotic congenital heart disease.
- Hypoventilation syndromes: sleep apnea, Pickwickian syndrome.

High altitude.
Smokers' polycythemia, carbon monoxide intoxication due to industrial exposure.
Postrenal transplantation erythrocytosis.
Aberrant erythropoietin production.
Tumors: renal cell carcinoma, Wilms tumor, hepatic carcinoma, uterine leiomyomata, virilizing ovarian tumors, vascular cerebellar tumors.
Miscellaneous renal and hepatic disorders: solitary renal cysts, polycystic kidney disease, renal artery stenosis, hydronephrosis, viral hepatitis.
Endocrine disorders: Cushing syndrome, primary aldosteronism.
Androgen use.
Erythropoietin use.
Congenital:
- Abnormal high-affinity hemoglobin variants.
- Bisphosphoglycerate deficiency.
- Congenital methemoglobinemia.
- Chuvash polycythemia (von Hippel–Lindau mutations).
- Prolyl hydroxylase mutations.
- Polycythemia Vera.

POLYMYALGIAS[46]

ICD-10CM #	M35.3	Polymyalgia rheumatica

DISEASE ENTITIES WITH POLYMYALGIAS

Rheumatoid arthritis.
Rotator cuff syndrome.

Osteoarthritis of shoulder and hip joints.
Fibromyalgia.
Polymyositis/dermatomyositis.
Spondyloarthritis.
Systemic lupus erythematosus.
Vasculitides.
Paraneoplastic myalgias.
Infection-associated myalgias.
Statin therapy.
RS3PE (remitting seronegative symmetric synovitis and pitting edema).
Parkinson disease.
Hypothyroidism.

POLYNEUROPATHY[102]

ICD-10CM # G61.9 Inflammatory polyneuropathy, unspecified

PREDOMINANTLY MOTOR

Guillain-Barré syndrome.
Porphyria.
Diphtheria.
Lead.
Hereditary sensorimotor neuropathy, types I and II.
Paraneoplastic neuropathy.

PREDOMINANTLY SENSORY

Diabetes.
Amyloidosis.
Leprosy.
Lyme disease.
Paraneoplastic neuropathy.
Vitamin B_{12} deficiency.
Hereditary sensory neuropathy, types I-IV.

PREDOMINANTLY AUTONOMIC

Diabetes.
Amyloidosis.
Alcoholic neuropathy.
Familial dysautonomias.

MIXED SENSORIMOTOR

Systemic diseases: renal failure, hypothyroidism, acromegaly, RA, periarteritis nodosa, SLE, multiple myeloma, macroglobulinemia, remote effect of malignancy.
Medications: isoniazid, nitrofurantoin, ethambutol, chloramphenicol, chloroquine, vincristine, vinblastine, dapsone, disulfiram, diphenylhydantoin, cisplatin, 1-tryptophan.
Environmental toxins: *N*-hexane, methyl *N*-butyl ketone, acrylamide, carbon disulfide, carbon monoxide, hexachlorophene, organophosphates.
Deficiency disorders: malabsorption, alcoholism, vitamin B_1 deficiency, Refsum disease, metachromatic leukodystrophy.

POLYNEUROPATHY, DEMYELINATING[7]

ICD-10CM # G37.9 Demyelinating disease of central nervous system, unspecified

Guillain-Barré syndrome:
- Acute inflammatory demyelinating polyradiculoneuropathy (AIDP).
- Acute motor axonal neuropathy (AMAN).
- Acute motor and sensory axonal neuropathy (AMSAN).
- Miller Fisher syndrome.

Chronic inflammatory demyelinating polyradiculoplexo-neuropathy.
Malignancy.
HIV.
Hepatitis B.
Buckthorn.
Diphtheria.

POLYNEUROPATHY, DISTAL SENSORIMOTOR[7]

ICD-10CM # G63 Polyneuropathy in diseases classified elsewhere

Diabetes mellitus.
Alcoholism.
Neoplastic or paraneoplastic.
Hereditary motor and sensory neuropathies (Charcot-Marie-Tooth).
Cryptogenic sensorimotor polyneuropathies (CSPN).
HIV.
Toxins:
- Organic or industrial agents:
  - Acrylamide.
  - Allyl chloride.
  - Carbon disulfide.
  - Ethylene oxide.
  - Hexacarbons.
  - Methyl bromide.
  - Organophosphate-induced delayed polyneuropathy (OPIDP).
  - Polychlorinated biphenyls (PCBs).
  - Trichloroethylene.
  - Vacor.

Metals:
- Arsenic.
- Gold.
- Mercury (inorganic).
- Thallium.

Therapeutic agents:
- Amiodarone.
- Antiretrovirals.
- Dapsone.
- Disulfiram.
- Isoniazid.
- Metronidazole.
- Nitrofurantoin.
- Paclitaxel (Taxol).
- Phenytoin.
- Statins (HMG-CoA reductase inhibitors).
- Thalidomide.
- Vinca alkaloids (vincristine, vinblastine).

Nutritional:
- Beriberi (thiamine or vitamin B_1).
- Pellagra (niacin, B vitamins).
- Pernicious anemia (vitamin B_{12}).
- Pyridoxine deficiency (vitamin B_6).

End-organ dysfunction
- Acromegaly.
- Chronic pulmonary disease.
- Hypothyroidism.
- Renal failure (uremic neuropathy).

Paraproteinemias:
- Amyloidosis.
- Monoclonal gammopathy of unknown significance (MGUS).
- Multiple myeloma.
- Waldenström macroglobulinemia.

Porphyria.

HMG-CoA, Hydroxymethylglutaryl coenzyme A.

POLYNEUROPATHY, DRUG-INDUCED[102]

ICD-10CM # G62.0 Drug-induced polyneuropathy

DRUGS IN ONCOLOGY

Vincristine.
Procarbazine.
Cisplatin.
Misonidazole.
Metronidazole
Taxol.

DRUGS IN INFECTIOUS DISEASES

Isoniazid.
Nitrofurantoin.
Dapsone.
ddC (dideoxycytidine).
ddI (dideoxyinosine).

DRUGS IN CARDIOLOGY

Hydralazine.
Perhexiline maleate.
Procainamide.
Disopyramide.

DRUGS IN RHEUMATOLOGY

Gold salts.
Chloroquine.

DRUGS IN NEUROLOGY AND PSYCHIATRY

Diphenylhydantoin.
Glutethimide.
Methaqualone.

MISCELLANEOUS

Disulfiram (Antabuse).
Vitamin: (pyridoxine in megadoses).

POLYNEUROPATHY, SYMMETRIC[102]

ICD-10CM # G61.9 Inflammatory polyneuropathy, unspecified

ACQUIRED NEUROPATHIES

Toxic:
- Drugs.
- Industrial toxins.
- Heavy metals.
- Abused substances.

Metabolic/endocrine:
- Diabetes.
- Chronic renal failure.
- Hypothyroidism.
- Polyneuropathy of critical illness.

Nutritional deficiency:
- Vitamin B_{12} deficiency.
- Alcoholism.
- Vitamin E deficiency.

Paraneoplastic:
- Carcinoma.
- Lymphoma.

Plasma cell dyscrasia:
- Myeloma, typical, atypical, and solitary forms.
- Primary systemic amyloidosis.

Idiopathic chronic inflammatory demyelinating polyneuropathies.
Polyneuropathies associated with peripheral nerve autoantibodies.
AIDS.

INHERITED NEUROPATHIES

Neuropathies with Biochemical Markers
Refsum disease.
Bassen-Kornzweig disease.
Tangier disease.
Metachromatic leukodystrophy.
Krabbe disease.
Adrenomyeloneuropathy.
Fabry disease.

Neuropathies without Biochemical Markers or Systemic Involvement
Hereditary motor neuropathy.
Hereditary sensory neuropathy.
Hereditary sensorimotor neuropathy.

POLYURIA

ICD-10CM # R35.8 Other polyuria

DM.
Diabetes insipidus.
Primary polydipsia (compulsive water drinking).
Hypercalcemia.
Hypokalemia.
Postobstructive uropathy.
Diuretic phase of renal failure.
Drugs: diuretics, caffeine, alcohol, lithium.
Sickle cell trait or disease, chronic pyelonephritis (failure to concentrate urine).
Anxiety, cold weather.

POPLITEAL SWELLING

ICD-10CM#	I87.1	Compression of vein
	I72.4	Aneurysm of artery of lower extremity
	S85.009A	Unspecified injury of popliteal artery, unspecified leg, initial encounter
	I77.3	Arterial fibromuscular dysplasia
	M71.20	Synovial cyst of popliteal space [Baker], unspecified knee
	I80.3	Phlebitis and thrombophlebitis of lower extremities, unspecified
	M66.369	Spontaneous rupture of flexor tendons, unspecified lower leg

Phlebitis (superficial).
Lymphadenitis.
Trauma: fractured tibia or fibula, contusion, traumatic neuroma.
DVT.
Ruptured varicose vein.
Baker cyst.
Popliteal abscess.
Osteomyelitis.
Ruptured tendon.
Aneurysm of popliteal artery.
Neoplasm: lipoma, osteogenic sarcoma, neurofibroma, fibrosarcoma.

PORTAL HYPERTENSION[3]

ICD-10CM # K76.6 Portal hypertension

INCREASED RESISTANCE TO FLOW

Presinusoidal
Portal or splenic vein occlusion (thrombosis, tumor).
Schistosomiasis.
Congenital hepatic fibrosis.
Sarcoidosis.

Sinusoidal
Cirrhosis (all causes).
Alcoholic hepatitis.

Postsinusoidal
Venoocclusive disease.
Budd-Chiari syndrome.
Constrictive pericarditis.

INCREASED PORTAL BLOOD FLOW

Splenomegaly not caused by liver disease.
Arterioportal fistula.

POSTMENOPAUSAL BLEEDING

ICD-10CM # N95.0 Postmenopausal bleeding

Hormone replacement therapy.
Neoplasm (uterine, ovarian, cervical, vaginal, vulvar).
Atrophic vaginitis.
Vaginal infection.
Polyp.
Extragenital (GI, urinary).
Tamoxifen.
Trauma.

POSTURAL HYPOTENSION, NONNEUROLOGIC CAUSES

ICD-10CM # I95.1 Orthostatic hypotension

Diuretics and hypertensive agents.
GI hemorrhage.
Alcohol.
Excessive heat.
Rapid volume loss from diarrhea, vomiting.
Hemodialysis.
Extensive burns.
Pyrexia.
Aortic stenosis (impaired output).
Constrictive pericarditis, atrial myxoma (impaired cardiac filling).
Adrenal insufficiency.
Diabetes insipidus.
Vasodilatory agents (e.g., nitrates).

PREMATURE GRAYING, SCALP HAIR

ICD-10CM # Varies with specific diagnosis

Chemical exposure (e.g., phenol/catechol derivatives, sulfhydryls, arsenic).
Physical agents (e.g., ionizing radiation, lasers).
Hyperthyroidism.
Vitamin B_{12} deficiency.
Down syndrome.
Chronic and severe protein deficiency.
Vitiligo.
Idiopathic.
Myotonic dystrophy.
Ataxia-telangiectasia.
Progeria.
Werner syndrome.

PREMATURE VENTRICULAR CONTRACTIONS AND VENTRICULAR TACHYCARDIA[7]

ICD-10CM #	I49.40	Unspecified premature depolarization
	I47.2	Ventricular tachycardia

CAUSES OF PREMATURE VENTRICULAR CONTRACTIONS AND VENTRICULAR TACHYCARDIA

Acute or previous myocardial infarction/ischemia.
Hypokalemia.
Hypoxemia.
Ischemic heart disease.
Valvular disease.
Catecholamine excess.[42]
Other drug intoxications (especially cyclic antidepressants).
Idiopathic causes.[43]
Digitalis toxicity.
Hypomagnesemia.
Hypercapnia.
Class I antidysrhythymic agents.
Ethanol.
Myocardial contusion.
Cardiomyopathy.
Acidosis.
Alkalosis.
Methylxanthine toxicity.

[42] Relative increase in sympathetic tone from drugs (direct or indirect) or conditions that augment catecholamine release or decrease parasympathetic tone.
[43] Isolated premature ventricular contractions (PVCs) can occur in up to 50% of young subjects without obvious cardiac or noncardiac disease; however, multiform and repetitive PVCs and ventricular tachycardia are rarely seen in this population.

PRESACRAL MASSES IN CHILDREN[81]

ICD-10CM # Varies with specific diagnosis

PRESACRAL MASSES IN CHILDREN

Solid

Sacrococcygeal teratoma.
Neuroblastoma.
Rhabdomyosarcoma.
Fibroma.
Lipoma.
Leiomyoma.
Lymphoma.
Hemangioendothelioma.
Sacral bone tumors.

Cystic

Abscess.
Rectal duplication.
Hematoma.
Lymphocele.
Neurenteric cyst.
Sacral osteomyelitis.
Ulcerative colitis.
Anterior meningocele.

PROLONGED QT SYNDROMES[65]

ICD-10CM # I45.81 Long QT syndrome

CLASSIFICATION AND CAUSES OF PROLONGED QT SYNDROMES THAT PRODUCE TORSADES DE POINTES

Pause Dependent (Acquired)

Drug induced: class IA and IC antidysrhythmics; many phenothiazines and butyrophenones (notably haloperidol and droperidol), cyclic antidepressants, antibiotics (especially macrolides), organophosphates, antihistamines, antifungals, antiseizure and antiemetic agents.
Electrolyte abnormalities: hypokalemia, hypomagnesemia, hypocalcemia (rarely).
Diet related: starvation, low protein.
Severe bradycardia or atrioventricular block.
Hypothyroidism.
Contrast injection.
Cerebrovascular accident (especially intraparenchymal).
Myocardial ischemia.

Adrenergic Dependent (Tachycardia Prompted)

Congenital:
- Jervell and Lange-Nielsen syndrome (deafness, autosomal recessive).
- Romano-Ward syndrome (normal hearing, autosomal dominant).
- Sporadic (normal hearing, no familial tendency).
- Mitral valve prolapse.

Acquired (Rare):
- Cerebrovascular disease (especially subarachnoid hemorrhage).
- Autonomic surgery: radical neck dissection, carotid endarterectomy, truncal vagotomy.

PROPTOSIS[73]

ICD-10CM #	H05.20	Unspecified exophthalmos
	H05.2	Ocular proptosis

Thyrotoxicosis.
Orbital pseudotumor.
Optic nerve tumor.
Cavernous sinus AV fistula, cavernous sinus thrombosis.
Cellulitis.
Metastatic tumor to orbit.

PROPTOSIS AND PALATAL NECROTIC ULCERS

ICD-10CM #	K13.70	Unspecified lesions of oral mucosa
	K13.79	Other lesions of oral mucosa
	H05.20	Unspecified exophthalmos

Cavernous sinus thrombosis.
Bacterial orbital cellulitis.
Metastatic neoplasm.
Rhinocerebral mucormycosis.
Ecthyma gangrenosum.
CNS aspergillosis.

PROTEIN-LOSING ENTEROPATHY, PEDIATRIC AGE[58]

ICD-10CM # E44.0 Moderate protein-energy malnutrition

CAUSES OF PROTEIN-LOSING ENTEROPATHY

Mucosal inflammation:
Infection:
- Cytomegalovirus.
- Bacterial overgrowth.
- Invasive bacterial infection.

Gastric inflammation:
- Ménétrier disease.
- Eosinophilic gastroenteropathy.

Intestinal inflammation:
- Celiac disease.
- Crohn disease.

Eosinophilic gastroenteropathy:
- Tropical sprue.
- Radiation enteritis.

Primary intestinal lymphangiectasia.
Secondary intestinal lymphangiectasia:
- Constrictive pericarditis.
- Congestive heart failure.
- Post–Fontan procedure.
- Malrotation.
- Lymphoma.
- Sarcoidosis.
- Radiation therapy.

Colonic inflammation:
- Inflammatory bowel diseases.
- Necrotizing enterocolitis.

Congenital disorders of glycosylation.

PROTEINURIA

ICD-10CM # R80.9 Proteinuria, unspecified

Nephrotic syndrome as a result of primary renal diseases.
Malignant hypertension.
Malignancies: multiple myeloma, leukemias, Hodgkin disease.
CHF.
DM.
SLE, RA.
Sickle cell disease.
Goodpasture syndrome.
Malaria.
Amyloidosis, sarcoidosis.
Tubular lesions: cystinosis.
Functional (after heavy exercise).
Pyelonephritis.
Pregnancy.
Constrictive pericarditis.
Renal vein thrombosis.
Toxic nephropathies: heavy metals, drugs.
Radiation nephritis.
Orthostatic (postural) proteinuria.
Benign proteinuria: fever, heat, or cold exposure.

PRURITUS

ICD-10CM #	L29.9	Pruritus, unspecified
	L29.3	Anogenital pruritus, unspecified

Dry skin.
Drug-induced eruption, fiberglass exposure.
Scabies.
Skin diseases.
Myeloproliferative disorders: mycosis fungoides, Hodgkin lymphoma, multiple myeloma, polycythemia vera.
Cholestatic liver disease.
Endocrine disorders: DM, thyroid disease, carcinoid, pregnancy.
Carcinoma: breast, lung, gastric.
Chronic renal failure.
Iron deficiency.
AIDS.
Neurosis.
Sjögren syndrome.

PRURITUS ANI[65]

ICD-10CM # L29.0 Pruritus ani

FECAL IRRITATION

Poor hygiene.
Anorectal conditions (fissure, fistula, hemorrhoids, skin tags, perianal clefts).
Spicy foods, citrus foods, caffeine, colchicine, quinidine.

CONTACT DERMATITIS

Anesthetic agents, topical corticosteroids, perfumed soap.

DERMATOLOGIC DISORDERS

Psoriasis, seborrhea, lichen simplex or sclerosus.

SYSTEMIC DISORDERS

Chronic renal failure, myxedema, DM, thyrotoxicosis, polycythemia vera, Hodgkin disease.

SEXUALLY TRANSMITTED DISEASES

Syphilis, herpes simplex virus, human papillomavirus.

OTHER INFECTIOUS AGENTS

Pinworms.
Scabies.
Bacterial infection, viral infection.

PRURITUS VULVAE[88]

ICD-10CM # L29.3 Anogenital pruritus, unspecified

CAUSES OF PRURITUS VULVAE

Diseases Special to Vulval Skin

Lichen sclerosus et atrophicus.
Leukoplakia.
Carcinoma.

Skin Disease

Psoriasis.
Atopic dermatitis.
Irritant and allergic contact dermatitis (especially medicaments).

Infection

Candidiasis.
Trichomonas.

Infestation

Pediculosis.

Psychogenic

Anxiety.
Depression.
Unknown

PSEUDOCELLULITIS[11]

ICD-10CM # Varies with specific diagnosis

CAUSES OF PSEUDOCELLULITIS

Infections and Bites

Arthropod bite reactions (e.g., insect, spider).
Erythema migrans.
Herpes zoster.
Toxin-mediated erythema (e.g., recurrent toxin-mediated perineal erythema).

Neutrophilic Dermatoses

Sweet syndrome, neutrophilic panniculitis.
Familial Mediterranean fever, other autoinflammatory syndromes.

Drug Reactions

Fixed drug eruptions (especially nonpigmenting).
Vaccine/injection site reactions.
Toxic erythema of chemotherapy (e.g. due to gemcitabine), neutrophilic eccrine hidradenitis.*

Other Inflammatory Disorders

Allergic contact dermatitis (including airborne and dermal), stasis dermatitis.
Phytophotodermatitis.
Well syndrome.
Panniculitis (e.g., lipodermatosclerosis, erythema nodosum).
Thrombophlebitis.
Angioedema.
Interstitial granulomatous dermatitis, patch type granuloma annulare.
Inflammatory morphea.
Acute inflammatory edema of the ICU.

Metabolic Disorders

Gout.

Malignancy

Erysipeloid skin metastases (especially breast carcinoma).

ICU, Intensive care unit.

*Occasionally develops before onset of leukemia or due to infection.

PSEUDOCYANOSIS, ETIOLOGY

ICD-10CM # Varies with etiology

Medications: amiodarone, minocycline, chlorpromazine.
Heavy metals:
- Gold (systemic absorption).
- Silver (systemic absorption).

Local contact with color dyes, gold, silver.

PSEUDOHERMAPHRODITISM, FEMALE

ICD-10CM #		
	E25.0	Congenital adrenogenital disorders associated with enzyme deficiency
	E25.8	Other adrenogenital disorders
	E25.9	Adrenogenital disorder, unspecified
	Q56.3	Pseudohermaphroditism, unspecified
	Q56.4	Indeterminate sex, unspecified

Congenital adrenal hyperplasia.
Maternal use of testosterone or related steroids.
Virilizing ovarian or adrenal tumor.
Virilizing luteoma of pregnancy.
Disturbances in differentiation of urogenital structures, non-androgen related.
Maternal virilizing adrenal hyperplasia.
Fetal P450 aromatase deficiency.

PSEUDOHERMAPHRODITISM, MALE

ICD-10CM#		
	E25.0	Congenital adrenogenital disorders associated with enzyme deficiency
	E25.8	Other adrenogenital disorders
	E25.9	Adrenogenital disorder, unspecified
	Q56.3	Pseudohermaphroditism, unspecified
	Q56.4	Indeterminate sex, unspecified

Maternal ingestion of progestogens.
End-organ resistance to androgenic hormones.
5-α-reductase-2 deficiency.
XY gonadal dysgenesis.
Testicular regression syndrome.
Defects in testosterone metabolism by peripheral tissues.
Testosterone biosynthesis defects.

PSEUDOINFARCTION[57]

ICD-10CM # Varies with specific diagnosis

Cardiac tumors, primary and secondary.
Cardiomyopathy (particularly hypertrophic and dilated).
Chagas disease.
Chest deformity.
COPD (particularly emphysema).
HIV infection.
Hyperkalemia.
Left anterior fascicular block.
Left bundle branch block.
Left ventricular hypertrophy.
Myocarditis and pericarditis.
Normal variant.
Pneumothorax.
Poor R wave progression, rotational changes, and lead placement.
Pulmonary embolism.
Trauma to chest (nonpenetrating).
Wolff-Parkinson-White syndrome.
Rare causes: pancreatitis, amyloidosis, sarcoidosis, scleroderma.

PSYCHOSIS[71]

ICD-10CM #		
	F29	Unspecified psychosis not due to a substance or known physiological condition
	F29	Unspecified psychosis not due to a substance or known physiological condition
	F10.231	Alcohol dependence with withdrawal delirium
	F01.51	Vascular dementia with behavioral disturbance

Differential Diagnosis II

PRIMARY

Schizophrenia-related.[44]
Major depression.
Dementia.
Bipolar disorder.

SECONDARY

Drug use.[45]
Drug withdrawal. [46]
Drug toxicity.[47]
Charles Bonnet syndrome.
Infections (pneumonia).
Electrolyte imbalance.
Syphilis.
Congestive heart failure.
Parkinson disease.
Trauma to temporal lobe.
Postpartum psychosis.
Hypothyroidism/hyperthyroidism.
Hypomagnesemia.
Epilepsy.
Meningitis.
Encephalitis.
Brain abscess.
Herpes encephalopathy.
Hypoxia.
Hypercarbia.
Hypoglycemia.
Thiamine deficiency.
Postoperative states.

PSYCHOSIS, MEDICAL DISORDERS-INDUCED[65]

ICD-10CM #	F29	Unspecified psychosis not due to a substance or known physiological condition
	F53	Puerperal psychosis

MEDICAL DISORDERS THAT MAY CAUSE ACUTE PSYCHOSIS

Metabolic Disorders
Hypercalcemia.
Hypercarbia.
Hypoglycemia.
Hyponatremia.
Hypoxia.
Inflammatory Disorders
Sarcoidosis.
Systemic lupus erythematosus.
Temporal (giant cell) arteritis.
Organ Failure
Hepatic encephalopathy.
Uremia.
Neurologic Disorders
Alzheimer disease.
Cerebrovascular disease.
Encephalitis (including HIV infection).
Encephalopathies.
Epilepsy.
Huntington disease.
Multiple sclerosis.
Neoplasms.
Normal-pressure hydrocephalus.
Parkinson disease.
Pick disease.
Wilson disease.
Endocrine disorders
Addison disease.
Cushing disease.
Panhypopituitarism.
Parathyroid disease.
Postpartum psychosis.
Recurrent menstrual psychosis.
Sydenham chorea.
Thyroid disease.
Deficiency States
Niacin.
Thiamine.
Vitamin B_{12} and folate.

[44] Includes schizophrenia, schizophreniform disorder, brief reactive psychosis.
[45] Includes hypnotics, glucocorticoids, marijuana, phencyclidine, atropine, dopaminergic agents (e.g., amantadine, bromocriptine, L-dopa), immunosuppressants.
[46] Includes alcohol, barbiturates, benzodiazepines.
[47] Includes digitalis, theophylline, cimetidine, anticholinergics, glucocorticoids, catecholaminergic agents.

PSYCHOSIS, MEDICATION-INDUCED[65]

ICD-10CM #	F10.5	Psychotic disorder due to psychoactive substance use

PHARMACOLOGIC AGENTS THAT MAY CAUSE ACUTE PSYCHOSIS

Antianxiety Agents
Alprazolam.
Chlordiazepoxide.
Clonazepam.
Clorazepate.
Diazepam.
Ethchlorvynol.
Antibiotics
Isoniazid.
Rifampin.
Anticonvulsants
Ethosuximide.
Phenobarbital.
Phenytoin.
Primidone.
Antidepressants
Amitriptyline.
Doxepin.
Imipramine.
Protriptyline.
Trimipramine.
Cardiovascular Drugs
Captopril.
Digitalis.
Disopyramide.
Methyldopa.
Procainamide.
Propranolol.
Reserpine.
Drugs of Abuse
Alcohol.
Amphetamines.
Cannabis.
Cocaine.
Hallucinogens.
Opioids.
Phencyclidine.
Sedative-hypnotics.
Miscellaneous Drugs
Antihistamines.
Antineoplastics.
Bromides.
Cimetidine.
Corticosteroids.
Disulfiram.
Heavy metals.

PTOSIS

ICD-10CM #	H02.409	Unspecified ptosis of unspecified eyelid
	Q10.0	Congenital ptosis
	H02.419	Mechanical ptosis of unspecified eyelid
	H02.429	Myogenic ptosis of unspecified eyelid
	H02.439	Paralytic ptosis unspecified eyelid

Third nerve palsy.
Myasthenia gravis.
Horner syndrome.
Senile ptosis.

PUBERTY, DELAYED[69]

ICD-10CM #	E30.0	Delayed puberty

NORMAL OR LOW SERUM GONADOTROPIN LEVELS

Constitutional delay in growth and development.
Hypothalamic and/or pituitary disorders:
- Isolated deficiency of growth hormone.
- Isolated deficiency of Gn-RH.
- Isolated deficiency of LH and/or FSH.
- Multiple anterior pituitary hormone deficiencies.
- Associated with congenital anomalies: Kallmann syndrome; Prader-Willi syndrome; Laurence-Moon-Biedl syndrome; Friedreich ataxia.
- Trauma.
- Postinfection.
- Hyperprolactinemia.
- Postirradiation.
- Infiltrative disease (histiocytosis).
- Tumor.
- Autoimmune hypophysitis.
- Idiopathic.

Functional:
- Chronic endocrinologic or systemic disorders.
- Emotional disorders.
- Drugs: cannabis.

INCREASED SERUM GONADOTROPIN LEVELS

Gonadal abnormalities:
- Congenital:
  - Gonadal dysgenesis.
  - Klinefelter syndrome.
  - Bilateral anorchism.
  - Resistant ovary syndrome.
  - Myotonic dystrophy in males.
  - 17-Hydroxylase deficiency in females.
  - Galactosemia.
- Acquired:
  - Bilateral gonadal failure resulting from trauma or infection or after surgery, irradiation, or chemotherapy.
  - Oophoritis: isolated or with other autoimmune disorders.
- Uterine or vaginal disorders:
  - Absence of uterus and/or vagina.
  - Testicular feminization: complete or incomplete androgen insensitivity.

PUBERTY, PRECOCIOUS

ICD-10CM #	E25.0	Congenital adrenogenital disorders associated with enzyme deficiency
	E25.8	Other adrenogenital disorders
	E25.9	Adrenogenital disorder, unspecified

Idiopathic.
Congenital virilizing adrenal hyperplasia.
Hypothalamic tumors.
Head trauma.
Hydrocephalus.
Degenerative CNS disease.
Arachnoid cyst.
Sex chromosome abnormalities (e.g., 47, XXY, 48, XXXY).
Perinatal asphyxia.
CNS infection (e.g., meningitis, encephalitis).

PULMONARY ARTERY SEGMENT ABNORMALITIES[14]

ICD-10CM #	Q25.72	Congenital pulmonary arteriovenous malformation

Differential Diagnosis of the Main Pulmonary Artery Segment

DILATED MPA SEGMENT

- Increased pulmonary artery volume (shunt):
  - VSD.
  - ASD.
  - PDA.
- Increased pulmonary artery pressure (pulmonary hypertensio'n):
  - Mitral stenosis.
  - COPD/emphysema.
  - Interstitial pulmonary fibrosis.
  - Cystic fibrosis.
  - Chronic thromboembolism.
  - Primary PH.
- Increased pulmonary artery volume and pressure:
  - ASD with PH.
- Normal pulmonary artery pressure and flow:
  - Valvular pulmonic stenosis.

FLAT OR CONCAVE MPA SEGMENT

- Tetralogy of Fallot.
- Tetralogy variants.
- Tetralogy with pulmonary atresia.
- Pulmonary atresia with VSD.
- Double-chamber RV.
- Double-outlet RV.
- Tricuspid atresia.
- Ebstein malformation.

NO MPA SEGMENT PRESENT

- Persistent truncus arteriosus.
- D-transposition of the great arteries.

ASD, Atrial septal defect; *COPD,* chronic obstructive pulmonary disease; *MPA,* main pulmonary artery; *PDA,* patent ductus arteriosus; *PH,* pulmonary hypertension; *RV,* right ventricle; *VSD,* ventricular septal defect.

PULMONARY CRACKLES

ICD-10CM #	R09.8	Friction sounds, chest

Pneumonia.
Left ventricular failure.
Asbestosis, silicosis, interstitial lung disease.
Chronic bronchitis.
Alveolitis (allergic, fibrosing).
Neoplasm.

PULMONARY CYSTS ON X-RAY[41]

ICD-10CM #	Q33.0	Polycystic lungs, congenital
	J98.4	Pulmonary manifestations

CAUSES OF CYSTS IN THE LUNG ON CHEST RADIOGRAPH

Cystic fibrosis.
Cystic bronchiectasis.
Bronchopulmonary dysplasia (neonate and older).
Tuberculosis (apical thick walled).
Pulmonary abscess (thick wall, fluid level).
Empyema.
Streptococcal pneumatocele (thin wall, postinfective).
Cavitating pneumonia.
Mycetoma (apical cyst with contents).
Cystic congenital adenomatoid malformation (basal cysts of varying size).
Diaphragmatic hernia (cysts of similar size).
Hiatal hernia (posterior).
Morgagni hernia (midline anterior).
Bronchopulmonary sequestration (basal).
Congenital lobar emphysema.
Hydatid disease (in endemic areas).
Kerosene inhalation (pneumatocele).
Histiocytosis and other causes of interstitial disease.

PULMONARY EDEMA, NONCARDIOGENIC[41]

ICD-10CM #	J81.0	Acute pulmonary edema

CAUSES OF NONCARDIOGENIC PULMONARY EDEMA

Adult respiratory distress syndrome.
Drowning.
Asphyxia.
Upper airway obstruction (usually with cardiomegaly).
High altitude.
Increased intracranial pressure.
Postictal.
Noxious gases:
- Smoke.
- Nitrous dioxide (silo filler's disease).
- Sulfur dioxide.
- Nitrogen mustard.

Drugs:
- Aspirin.
- Diazepam, chlordiazepoxide, barbiturates.
- Narcotics (heroin, methadone, morphine).
- β-adrenergic drugs (terbutaline).
- Contrast media.
- Colchicine.
- Fluorescein.
- Hydrochlorothiazide.
- Nitrofurantoin.
- Propoxyphene.

Poisons:
- Parathion.

Transfusion reactions.
Renal failure: transplantation.
Bone marrow transplantation.
Fat embolism.
Pancreatitis.

PULMONARY EOSINOPHILIA[2]

ICD-10CM #	NEC J82	Eosinophilia, pulmonary

TYPES AND CAUSES OF PULMONARY EOSINOPHILIA

- Drug- and toxin-induced eosinophilic lung diseases.
- Helminth and fungal infection-related eosinophilic lung diseases:
  - Transpulmonary passage of larvae (i.e., Löffler syndrome): Ascaris, hookworm, Strongyloides.
  - Pulmonary parenchymal invasion: mostly helminths, paragonimiasis.
  - Heavy hematogenous seeding with helminths: trichinellosis, disseminated strongyloidiasis, cutaneous and visceral larva migrans, schistosomiasis.
  - Tropical pulmonary eosinophilia: filaria.
  - Allergic bronchopulmonary aspergillosis.

Chronic eosinophilic pneumonia.
Acute eosinophilic pneumonia.
Churg-Strauss syndrome (vasculitis).
Other: neoplasia, idiopathic hypereosinophilic syndrome, bronchocentric granulomatosis.

PULMONARY HEMORRHAGE, DIFFUSE, ALVEOLAR[77]

ICD-10CM # R04.8 Pulmonary hemorrhage

IMMUNOLOGIC DISEASES

Anti–glomerular basement membrane antibody disease (Goodpasture syndrome).
Vasculitides associated with circulating or in situ immune complexes:
- Systemic lupus erythematosus.
- Mixed connective tissue disease.
- Schönlein-Henoch purpura.
- Essential mixed cryoglobulinemia.
- Tumor-related vasculitis.
- Endocarditis-related vasculitis.
- Polyarteritis nodosa.
- Systemic necrotizing vasculitis.

Vasculitides associated with antineutrophil cytoplasmic antibodies:
- Wegener granulomatosis.
- Microscopic polyangiitis.
- Idiopathic necrotizing crescentic glomerulonephritis.

Rapidly progressive glomerulonephritis.
Associated with other connective tissue diseases, pathophysiology unknown:
- Rheumatoid arthritis.
- Progressive systemic sclerosis.
- Behçet disease.

Associated with other renal diseases.
Immunoglobulin A nephropathy.
Diabetic nephropathy.
Associated with precipitating antibodies to milk (Heiner syndrome).
Idiopathic pulmonary hemosiderosis.
Primary antiphospholipid antibody syndrome.

CHEMICAL OR DRUG-RELATED CAUSES

Amiodarone.
D-Penicillamine.
Isocyanates.
Nitrofurantoin.
Retinoic acid.
Trimellitic anhydride.
"Crack" cocaine.
Sirolimus.
Everolimus.
Propylthiouracil-induced vasculitis.
Erlotinib.
Bevacizumab.
Gemcitabine.
Infliximab.

TRANSPLANT-RELATED CAUSES

Bone marrow transplant.
Renal transplant.
Lung transplant.

BLEEDING DIATHESIS

Thrombocytopenia.
Leukemia with diffuse alveolar damage.
Viral pneumonia.
Bacterial or fungal sepsis.
Radiation.
Chemotherapy toxic to lung.
Blast counts >80,000/μL.
Extrinsic anticoagulants/thrombolytics.
Warfarin overdose.
Tissue plasminogen activator.
Platelet glycoprotein IIb/IIIa inhibitors.
Coagulopathies.
Cirrhosis.
Disseminated intravascular coagulation.

INFECTIONS

Adenovirus.
Aspergillosis (invasive).
Cytomegalovirus.
Dengue.
Hantavirus.
Influenza.
Legionella.
Leptospirosis.
Malaria.
Mycoplasma.
Staphylococcus aureus.

PULMONARY VENOUS HYPERTENSION

Mitral stenosis.
Mitral regurgitation.
Pulmonary capillary hemangiomatosis.
Pulmonary veno-occlusive disease.
Fibrosing mediastinitis.
Congenital heart disease.

DIFFUSE LUNG INJURY

Negative-pressure pulmonary hemorrhage.
Breath-hold diving.
Postictal neurogenic pulmonary edema.

PULMONARY HEMORRHAGE, FOCAL[76]

ICD-10CM # R04.8 Pulmonary hemorrhage

CAUSES OF FOCAL PULMONARY HEMORRHAGE

Iatrogenic Disorders

Bronchoscopy.
Lung biopsy.
Pulmonary artery catheterization.
Transtracheal aspiration.
Radiofrequency ablation.
Brachytherapy.

Infectious Disorders

Lung abscess.
Mycetoma.
Necrotizing pneumonia (*Staphylococcus aureus,* gram-negative aerobes, *Legionella,* Actinomyces spp., *Stenotrophomonas, Kytococcus sedentarius,* Leptospira spp., *Yersinia pestis, Francisella tularensis*).
Parasitic infection (paragonimiasis, amebiasis, ascariasis, clonorchiasis, echinococcosis, hookworm infestation, strongyloidiasis, trichinosis, schistosomiasis).
Parenchymal fungal infection (aspergillosis, mucormycosis, coccidioidomycosis, histoplasmosis, maduromycosis, botryomycosis).
Tuberculosis (active or inactive).
Viral tracheitis.
Herpetic tracheobronchitis.

Interstitial Lung Diseases

Lymphangioleiomyomatosis.
Sarcoidosis.
Tuberous sclerosis.
Pneumoconiosis.
Langerhans cell granulomatosis.

Miscellaneous Disorders

Amyloidosis.
Bronchogenic cyst.
Broncholithiasis.
Bronchopleural fistula.
Thoracic endometriosis.
Foreign body.
Tracheopathia osteoplastica.
Lipoid pneumonia.
Organophosphate aspiration.
Chronic pancreatitis.

Neoplastic Disorders

Bronchial adenoma.
Lung cancer.
Tracheal tumors (mucoepidermoid, squamous cell, adenoid cystic, glomus).
Pulmonary blastoma.
Pleuropulmonary angiosarcoma.
Sarcoma (synovial, myofibroblastic).
Clear cell tumor.
Metastatic disease (prostate, renal, breast, ovarian).
Tracheobronchial schwannoma.

Pulmonary Airway Diseases

Bronchiectasis.
Bronchitis.
Granulomatous tracheobronchitis (ulcerative colitis, Crohn disease, granulomatosis with polyangiitis).
Cystic fibrosis.
Bullous emphysema.

Traumatic Injury

Blunt chest trauma.
Penetrating injury.
Ruptured bronchus.
Lightning injury.
Thoracic splenosis.

Vascular Disorders

Pulmonary embolism, infarction.
Systemic cholesterol emboli.
Intralobar sequestration.
Pulmonary artery aneurysms.
Behçet disease, Hughes-Stovin syndrome, traumatic pseudoaneurysms.
Acquired arteriovenous malformations.
Osler-Weber-Rendu syndrome (hereditary hemorrhagic telangiectasia).
Takayasu arteritis.
Aortic aneurysms.
Trachea–innominate artery fistulas.
Scimitar syndrome.
Vena cava-bronchial.
Dieulafoy disease of bronchus.
Ventriculopulmonary fistulas.
Hemangioma (sclerosing, cavernous, tracheal).

PULMONARY HEMORRHAGE, PEDIATRIC AGE

ICD-10CM # P26.9 Pulmonary hemorrhage newborn

CAUSES OF PULMONARY HEMORRHAGE (HEMOPTYSIS)

Focal Hemorrhage

Bronchitis and bronchiectasis (especially cystic fibrosis related).
Infection (acute or chronic), pneumonia, abscess.
Tuberculosis.
Trauma.
Pulmonary arteriovenous malformation.
Foreign body (chronic).
Neoplasm including hemangioma.
Pulmonary embolus with or without infarction.
Bronchogenic cysts.
Diffuse hemorrhage
Idiopathic of infancy.
Congenital heart disease (including pulmonary hypertension, venoocclusive disease, congestive heart failure).
Prematurity.
Cow's milk hyperreactivity (Heiner syndrome).
Goodpasture syndrome.
Collagen vascular diseases (systemic lupus erythematosus, rheumatoid arthritis).
Henoch-Schönlein purpura and vasculitic disorders.
Granulomatous disease (Wegener granulomatosis).
Celiac disease.
Coagulopathy (congenital or acquired).
Malignancy.
Immunodeficiency.
Exogenous toxins.
Hyperammonemia.
Pulmonary hypertension.
Pulmonary alveolar hemosiderosis.
Tuberous sclerosis.
Lymphangiomyomatosis or lymphangioleiomyomatosis.
Physical injury or abuse.

PULMONARY HEMORRHAGIC SYNDROMES, DIFFUSE[41]

ICD-10CM # P26.1 Massive pulmonary hemorrhage originating in the perinatal period
R04.8 Pulmonary hemorrhage

CLASSIFICATION OF DIFFUSE PULMONARY HEMORRHAGE SYNDROMES

Non-immunocompromised patients

Antibasement membrane antibody disease/Goodpasture syndrome.
Diseases of presumed immune etiology, with or without nephropathy:
- Systemic lupus erythematosus.
- Rheumatoid arthritis.
- Systemic sclerosis.
- Systemic necrotizing vasculitis.
- Granulomatosis with polyangiitis.
- Microscopic polyarteritis.

Diseases with no known immune etiology:
- Idiopathic pulmonary hemosiderosis.
- Rapidly progressive glomerulonephritis without immune complexes.
- Fibrillary glomerulonephritis.
- Drug-induced (anticoagulants, trimellitic anhydride, cocaine, lymphangiography).
- Valvular heart disease.
- Disseminated intravascular coagulation.
- Acute lung injury.
- Tumors.

Immunocompromised Patients

Blood dyscrasias.
Infection.
Tumors.

PULMONARY INFILTRATES ASSOCIATIONS[70]

ICD-10CM # Varies with specific diagnosis

PULMONARY INFILTRATES AND THEIR ASSOCIATION WITH SPECIFIC INFECTIOUS AND NONINFECTIOUS DISORDERS

Radiologic Sign	Potential Etiologic Disorder(s)
Interstitial infiltrates.	Pulmonary edema.
Diffuse alveolar damage.	Idiopathic pneumonia syndrome. Respiratory virus infection: RSV, parainfluenza virus, influenza virus, adenovirus, enterovirus. Herpesvirus infection: CMV, HSV, VZV, HHV-6. *Pneumocystis* pneumonia.
Focal airspace disease.	Bacterial pneumonia. Fungal pneumonia.
Nodules.	Fungal pneumonia (aspergillosis). *Nocardia* infection. *Legionella* infection. Septic bacterial emboli. Mycobacterial infection (with cavitation). EBV lymphoproliferative disorder. Relapsed malignancy. Pulmonary embolism (pleura based).
Halo sign or air-crescent sign.	Aspergillosis.

CMV, Cytomegalovirus; *EBV,* Epstein-Barr virus; *HHV,* human herpesvirus; *HSV,* herpes simplex virus; *RSV,* respiratory syncytial virus; *VZV,* varicella-zoster virus.

PULMONARY INFILTRATES, IMMUNOCOMPROMISED HOST[100]

ICD-10CM # J82 Pulmonary eosinophilia, not elsewhere classified
J98.4 Other disorders of lung

CAUSES OF PULMONARY INFILTRATES IN THE IMMUNOCOMPROMISED HOST

Infections:
- Bacteria:
  - Gram-positive cocci, especially *Staphylococcus.*
  - Gram-negative bacilli.
  - Mycobacterium tuberculosis.
  - Nontuberculous mycobacteria.
  - Nocardia.
- Viruses:

Cytomegalovirus.
Herpesvirus.
- Fungi:
  - *Aspergillus.*
  - *Cryptococcus.*
  - *Candida.*
  - *Mucor.*
  - *Pneumocystis jiroveci.*
- Protozoa:
  - Toxoplasma gondii (rare).
- Pulmonary effects of therapy:
  - Chemotherapeutic agents.
  - Radiation therapy.
  - Pulmonary hemorrhage.
  - Congestive heart failure.
  - Disseminated malignancy.
  - Nonspecified interstitial pneumonitis (no defined etiology).

PULMONARY LESIONS

ICD-10CM# J98.4 Other disorders of lung
J70.9 Respiratory conditions due to unspecified external agent
S27.309A Unspecified injury of lung, unspecified, initial encounter

TB.
Legionella pneumonia.
Mycoplasma pneumonia.
Viral pneumonia.
Pneumocystis carinii.
Hypersensitivity pneumonitis.
Aspiration pneumonia.
Fungal disease (aspergillosis, histoplasmosis).
ARDS associated with pneumonia.
Psittacosis.
Sarcoidosis.
Septic emboli.
Metastatic cancer.
Multiple pulmonary emboli.
Rheumatoid nodules.

PULMONARY MASS, SOLITARY, CAUSES[41]

ICD-10CM # R91.1 Solitary pulmonary nodule

CAUSES OF A SOLITARY PULMONARY MASS

Bronchial carcinoma.
Bronchial carcinoid.
Granuloma.
Hamartoma.
Metastasis.
Chronic pneumonia or abscess.
Hydatid cyst.
Pulmonary hematoma.
Bronchocele.
Fungus ball.

Massive fibrosis in coal workers.
Bronchogenic cyst.
Sequestration.
Arteriovenous malformation.
Pulmonary infarct.
Round atelectasis.

PULMONARY MASS, SOLITARY, MIMICS[41]

ICD-10CM # Varies with specific diagnosis

SIMULANTS OF A SOLITARY PULMONARY MASS

Extrathoracic artifacts.
Cutaneous masses.
Bony lesions.
Pleural tumors or plaques.
Encysted pleural fluid.
Pulmonary vessels.

PULMONARY NODULE, SOLITARY

ICD-10CM # J98.4 Other disorders of lung

Bronchogenic carcinoma.
Granuloma from histoplasmosis.
TB granuloma.
Granuloma from coccidioidomycosis.
Metastatic carcinoma.
Bronchial adenoma.
Bronchogenic cyst.
Hamartoma.
AV malformation.
Other: fibroma, intrapulmonary lymph node, sclerosing hemangioma, bronchopulmonary sequestration.

PULMONARY OPACITIES[39]

ICD-10CM # Varies with specific diagnosis

CLASSIFICATION OF LARGE PULMONARY OPACITIES

Diffuse homogeneous.
Multifocal patchy.
Lobar without atelectasis.
Lobar with atelectasis.
Perihilar.
Peripheral.

PULMONARY–RENAL SYNDROMES, CAUSES[32]

ICD-10CM # Varies with specific diagnosis

Systemic vasculitis	Anti-GBM disease (Goodpasture). ANCA associated: Granulomatosis with polyangiitis. Microscopic polyarteritis. Churg-Strauss syndrome. Drugs (penicillamine, hydralazine, propylthiouracil). Immune complex disease. Lupus erythematosus. Henoch-Schönlein purpura. Mixed cryoglobulinemia. Rheumatoid vasculitis.
Infection	Severe bacterial pneumonia, postinfectious glomerulonephritis, *Legionella,* hantavirus, opportunistic infection in immunocompromised patients, infective endocarditis.
Pulmonary edema and AKI	Volume overload, severe left ventricular failure.
Multiorgan failure	Acute respiratory distress syndrome and AKI.
Other	Paraquat poisoning, renal vein or IVC thrombosis with pulmonary emboli.

AKI, Acute kidney injury; *ANCA,* anti-neutrophil cytoplasmic antibody; *GBM,* glomerular basement membrane; *IVC,* inferior vena cava.

PULSELESS ELECTRICAL ACTIVITY

ICD-10CM # I46.9 Cardiac arrest, cause unspecified

Hypovolemia.
Hypoxia.
Hyperkalemia.
Acidosis.
Cardiac tamponade.
Tension pneumothorax.
Pulmonary embolus.
Drug overdose.
Hypothermia.

PUPILLARY DILATATION, POOR RESPONSE TO DARKNESS

ICD-10CM # H21.569 Pupillary abnormality, unspecified eye

Drugs (narcotics, general anesthetics, cholinergics).
Acute trauma (spasm from prostaglandin release).
Inflammation, infection (interruption of inhibitory fibers to the Edinger-Westphal nucleus).
Old age (loss of inhibition at midbrain from reticular activating formation).
Horner syndrome (sympathetic neuron interruption).
Adie syndrome tonic pupil.
Lymphoma.
Congenital miosis.

PURPURA

ICD-10CM #		
	D69.2	Other nonthrombocytopenic purpura
	D69.0	Allergic purpura
	D69.49	Other primary thrombocytopenia
	M31.1	Thrombotic microangiopathy

THROMBOTIC

Trauma.
Septic emboli, atheromatous emboli.
DIC.
Thrombocytopenia.
Meningococcemia.
Rocky Mountain spotted fever.
Hemolytic-uremic syndrome.
Viral infection: echo, coxsackie.
Scurvy.
Other: left atrial myxoma, cryoglobulinemia, vasculitis, hyperglobulinemic purpura.

PURPURA, NONPALPABLE[50]

ICD-10CM # D69.2 Other nonthrombocytopenic purpura

INCREASED TRANSMURAL PRESSURE GRADIENT

Acute (Valsalva, coughing, vomiting, high altitude, weight lifting).
Chronic—venous stasis.

DECREASED MECHANICAL INTEGRITY OF MICROCIRCULATION AND SUPPORTING TISSUES

Age related (infancy and actinic purpura).
Glucocorticoid excess—Cushing syndrome and glucocorticoid therapy.
Vitamin C deficiency (scurvy).
Abnormal connective tissue—Ehlers-Danlos syndrome.
Amyloid infiltration of blood vessels.
Colloid milium.
Hormonal—female easy bruising syndrome (purpura simplex).
Lorenzo oil.
MELAS syndrome.

TRAUMA TO BLOOD VESSELS

Physical:
- Injuries.
- Child abuse.
- Factitial purpura.

Ultraviolet purpura:
- Purpuric sunburn.
- Solar purpura.

Infectious:
- Bacterial.
- Rickettsial.
- Fungal.
- Viral.
- Parasitic.

Embolic:
- Infectious organisms.
- Atheroemboli (cholesterol crystal emboli).
- Fat emboli.

Allergic and/or inflammatory:
- Serum sickness.
- Pigmented purpuric eruptions.
- Pyoderma gangrenosum.
- Contact dermatitis.
- Familial Mediterranean fever.

Neoplastic.
Metabolic:
- Erythropoietic porphyria.
- Calciphylaxis.

Immunoglobulin related (hyperglobulinemic purpura of Waldenström and light-chain vasculitis).
Drug related.

Thrombotic:
- Disseminated intravascular coagulation.
- Warfarin (Coumadin)-induced skin necrosis.
- Protein C or protein S deficiency, factor V Leiden, prothrombin G20201A.
- Purpura fulminans.
- Paroxysmal nocturnal hemoglobinuria.
- Antiphospholipid antibody syndrome.
- Hemangioma with thrombocytopenia and consumptive coagulopathy (Kasabach-Merritt syndrome).

UNKNOWN CAUSE—PSYCHOGENIC PURPURA

PURPURA, NONPURPURIC DISORDERS SIMULATING PURPURA[3]

ICD-10CM # Varies with specific diagnosis

Disorders with telangiectasias:
- Cherry angiomas.
- Hereditary hemorrhagic telangiectasia.
- Chronic actinic telangiectasia.
- Scleroderma.
- CREST syndrome.
- Ataxia-telangiectasia.
- Chronic liver disease.
- Pregnancy-related telangiectasia.

Kaposi sarcoma and other vascular sarcomas.
Fabry disease.
Neonatal extramedullary hematopoiesis.
Angioma serpiginosum.

PURPURA, PALPABLE[50]

ICD-10CM #	D69.2	Other nonthrombocytopenic purpura

Cutaneous vasculitis:
- Systemic vasculitides.
- Paraneoplastic vasculitis.
- Henoch-Schönlein purpura.
- Acute hemorrhagic edema of infancy.
- Livedoid vasculitis.
- Idiopathic.
- Urticarial.

Cryoglobulinemia.
Cryofibrinogenemia.
Primary cutaneous diseases

QT INTERVAL PROLONGATION[57]

ICD-10CM #	R94.31	Abnormal electrocardiogram [ECG] [EKG]
	I45.81	Long QT syndrome

Drugs:
- Class I antiarrhythmics (e.g., disopyramide, procainamide, quinidine).
- Class III antiarrhythmics.
- Tricyclic antidepressants.
- Phenothiazines.
- Astemizole.
- Terfenadine.
- Adenosine.
- Antibiotics (e.g., erythromycin and other macrolides):
  - Antifungal agents.
  - Pentamidine, chloroquine.

Ischemic heart disease.
Cerebrovascular disease.
Rheumatic fever.
Myocarditis.
Mitral valve prolapse.
Electrolyte abnormalities.
Hypocalcemia.
Hypothyroidism.
Liquid protein diets.
Organophosphate insecticides.
Congenital prolonged QT syndrome.

RADIATION-INDUCED NEOPLASMS[90]

ICD-10CM # Varies with specific diagnosis

RADIATION-INDUCED NEOPLASMS

Osteochondroma
Benign.
Exclusively with childhood irradiation.
Histologically identical to spontaneous osteochondroma.

Sarcoma
Malignant.
Latent period of 4 years or more.
Histologically identical to spontaneous sarcoma.
Commonly malignant fibrous histiocytoma or osteosarcoma.
Occurs in either bone or soft tissue.

Tumors in Other Organ Systems
Squamous cell cancer of the skin.
Breast cancer.
Leukemia, with shorter latent period than sarcoma.

RECTAL MASS, PALPABLE[95]

ICD-10CM #	R22.9	Localized swelling, mass and lump, unspecified

Rectal carcinoma.
Rectal polyp.
Hypertrophied anal papilla.
Diverticular phlegmon (prolapsing into the pouch of Douglas).
Sigmoid colon carcinoma (prolapsing into the pouch of Douglas).
Metastatic deposits at the pelvic reflection (Blumer shelf).
Primary pelvic malignancy (uterine, ovarian, prostatic, or cervical).
Mesorectal lymph nodes.
Endometriosis.
Solitary rectal ulcer syndrome.
Foreign body.
Feces.
Presacral cyst.
Amebic granuloma.
Vaginal tampon and even the pubic bone may be mistaken for a rectal mass.

RECTAL PAIN

ICD-10CM #	K62.89	Other specified diseases of anus and rectum

Anal fissure.
Thrombosed hemorrhoid.
Anorectal abscess.
Foreign bodies.
Fecal impaction.
Endometriosis.
Neoplasms (primary or metastatic).
Pelvic inflammatory disease.
Inflammation of sacral nerves.
Compression of sacral nerves.
Prostatitis.
Other: proctalgia fugax, uterine abnormalities, myopathies, coccygodynia.

RED BLOOD CELL APLASIA, ACQUIRED, ETIOLOGY

ICD-10CM #	D61.01	Constitutional (pure) red blood cell aplasia

Idiopathic (>50% of cases).
Medications (most frequent with phenytoin).
Non-Hodgkin lymphoma.
Viral infections (parvovirus B19, EB virus, mumps, hepatitis).
Myelodysplastic syndromes.
Thymoma.
Autoimmune diseases.
Allogenic bone marrow transplant from ABO incompatible donor.
Pregnancy.

RED BLOOD CELL FRAGMENTATION HEMOLYSIS, CAUSES[49]

ICD-10CM # Varies with specific disorder

CAUSES OF RED BLOOD CELL FRAGMENTATION HEMOLYSIS

Damaged microvasculature.
Thrombotic thrombocytopenic purpura–hemolytic uremic syndrome (TTP–HUS).
Associated with pregnancy: preeclampsia or eclampsia; hemolysis plus elevated liver enzymes plus low platelets (HELLP syndrome).
Associated with malignancy, with or without mitomycin C treatment.
Vasculitis: polyarteritis, Wegener granulomatosis, acute glomerulonephritis, or *Rickettsia*-like infections.
Systemic lupus erythematosus.
Abnormalities of renal vasculature: malignant hypertension, acute glomerulonephritis, scleroderma, or allograft rejection with or without cyclosporine treatment.
Disseminated intravascular coagulation.
Malignant hypertension.
Catastrophic antiphospholipid antibody syndrome.
Atrioventricular malformations.
Kasabach-Merritt syndrome.
Hemangioendotheliomas.
Atrioventricular shunts for congenital and acquired conditions (e.g., stents, coils, transjugular intrahepatic portosystemic shunt, Levine shunts).

Cardiac abnormalities:
- Replaced valve, prosthesis, graft, or patch.
- Aortic stenosis or regurgitant jets (e.g., in ruptured sinus of Valsalva).

Drugs:
- Cyclosporine.
- Mitomycin.
- Ticlopidine.
- Clopidogrel.
- Tacrolimus.
- Cocaine.

Systemic infection:
- Bacterial endocarditis.
- Brucellosis.
- Cytomegalovirus.
- Human immunodeficiency virus.
- Ehrlichiosis.
- Rocky Mountain spotted fever

RED EYE

ICD-10CM # H57.8 Other specified disorders of eye and adnexa

Infectious conjunctivitis (bacterial, viral).
Allergic conjunctivitis.
Acute glaucoma.
Keratitis (bacterial, viral).
Iritis.
Trauma.

RED EYE, ACUTE[4]

ICD-10CM # H57.8 Other specified disorders of eye and adnexa

Obvious open globe.
Corneal abrasion.
Corneal ulcer.
Subconjunctival hemorrhage.
Hyphema.
Occult open globe.
Herpes simplex virus glaucoma.
Iritis, traumatic iritis.
Scleritis.
Conjunctivitis.
Blepharitis.
Ultraviolet keratitis.
Episcleritis.
Conjunctival foreign body.
Dry eye.
Contact lens overwear syndrome.

RED HOT JOINT

ICD-10CM # Varies with specific diagnosis

Trauma.
Gout.
Infection (septic joint).
Pseudogout (calcium pyrophosphate dehydrate crystal deposition).
Psoriatic arthropathy.
Reactive arthritis.
Palindromic rheumatism.

RED URINE

ICD-10CM # R39.19 Other difficulties with micturition

Hematuria.
Porphyrins.
Hemoglobinuria.
Myoglobinuria.
Medications (phenazopyridine, aminosalicylic acid, deferoxamine, phenazopyridine, phenolphthalein, NSAIDs, rifampin, phenytoin, methyldopa, doxorubicin, phenacetin).
Foods (beets, berries, maize).
Urate crystalluria.

RENAL ALLOGRAFT DYSFUNCTION[38]

ICD-10CM # T86.1 Complications of renal allograft

IMMEDIATE/DELAYED GRAFT FUNCTION (1 TO 3 DAYS)

Acute tubular necrosis.
Hyperacute humoral rejection.
Urinary leak or obstruction.
Renal artery or vein thrombosis.
Recurrence of disease (e.g., focal segmental glomerulosclerosis).

EARLY POSTTRANSPLANTATION PERIOD (FIRST MONTH)

Acute cellular rejection.
Acute humoral rejection.
Calcineurin inhibitor toxicity.
Urinary tract obstruction.
Volume depletion.
Recurrence of disease.

Late Acute Dysfunction

Acute rejection.
Cyclosporine or tacrolimus toxicity.
Recurrence of primary disease.
Tubulointerstitial nephritis, drug-induced.
Renal artery stenosis.
Infection (bacterial urinary tract infection [UTI], cytomegalovirus, BK virus).
Hemodynamic (volume; use of angiotensin-converting enzyme inhibitor, angiotensin II receptor blocker).

Chronic Dysfunction

Chronic rejection.
Cyclosporine or tacrolimus toxicity.
Recurrent renal disease.
De novo renal disease.
Urinary tract obstruction.
Bacterial UTI.
Hypertensive nephrosclerosis.

RENAL ARTERY OCCLUSION, CAUSES

ICD-10CM # N28.0 Ischemia and infarction of kidney

Atrial fibrillation.
Angiography or stent placement.
Abdominal aortic surgery.
Trauma.
Renal artery aneurysm/dissection.
Vasculitis.
Thrombosis in patient with fibromuscular dysplasia.
Atherosclerosis.
Septic embolism.
Mural thrombus thromboembolism.
Atrial myxoma thromboembolism.
Mitral stenosis thromboembolism.
Prosthetic valve thromboembolism.
Renal cell carcinoma.

RENAL COLIC[4]

ICD-10CM # N23 Unspecified renal colic

Vascular:
- Abdominal aortic aneurysm.
- Aortic dissection.
- Renal artery dissection.
- Renal artery stenosis.
- Renal vein thrombosis.
- Renal infarct.
- Mesenteric ischemia.
- Retroperitoneal hemorrhage.

GI:
- Incarcerated hernia.
- Appendicitis.
- Cholecystitis.
- Biliary colic.
- Pancreatitis.
- Bowel obstruction.
- Diverticulitis.

Gynecologic:
- Ectopic pregnancy.
- Ovarian torsion.
- Tuboovarian abscess.
- Pelvic inflammatory disease.
- Endometriosis.

Genitourinary:
- Testicular torsion.
- Pyelonephritis.
- Perinephric abscess.
- Urinary tract tumor.
- Renal papillary necrosis.
- Upper urinary tract hemorrhage.

Musculoskeletal:
- Lumbar strain.
- Radiculopathy.
- Disk herniation.
- Vertebral compression fracture.

Dermatologic:
- Herpes zoster.

Miscellaneous:
- Factitious.

RENAL CYSTIC DISORDERS

ICD-10CM # Q61.01 Congenital single renal cyst

Simple cysts.
Acquired cystic kidney disease.
Autosomal dominant polycystic kidney disease.
Autosomal recessive polycystic kidney disease.
Medullary cystic disease.
Medullary sponge kidney.

RENAL DISEASE, SKIN MANIFESTATIONS[87]

ICD-10CM # Varies with specific diagnosis

SKIN MANIFESTATIONS SECONDARY TO RENAL DISEASE

Nonspecific

Pruritus.
Xerosis.
Acquired ichthyosis.
Pigmentary alteration:
- Pallor (secondary to anemia).
- Hyperpigmentation.
- Dyspigmentation (yellow tint).

Infections (fungal, bacterial, viral).
Purpura.

Somewhat Specific

Acquired perforating dermatosis.
Calciphylaxis.
Metastatic calcification.
Blistering disorders:
- Porphyria cutanea tarda.
- Pseudoporphyria.

Eruptive xanthomas.
Pseudo–Kaposi sarcoma.

Specific

Nephrogenic systemic fibrosis.
Dialysis-associated steal syndrome.
Metastatic renal cell carcinoma.
Dialysis-related amyloidosis.
Arteriovenous shunt dermatitis.
Uremic frost.

RENAL FAILURE, ACUTE, PIGMENT-INDUCED[7]

ICD-10CM #	N19	Unspecified kidney failure

CAUSES OF PIGMENT-INDUCED ACUTE RENAL FAILURE

Rhabdomyolysis and myoglobinuria.
Vigorous exercise.
Arterial embolization.
Status epilepticus.
Status asthmaticus.
Coma-induced and pressure-induced myonecrosis.
Heat stress.
Diabetic ketoacidosis.
Myopathy.
Alcoholism.
Hypokalemia.
Hypophosphatemia.
Hemoglobinuria.
Transfusion reactions.
Snake envenomation.
Malaria.
Mechanical destruction of RBCs by prosthetic valves.
G6PD deficiency.

G6PD, Glucose-6-phosphate dehydrogenase; *RBCs,* red blood cells.

RENAL FAILURE, CHRONIC[38]

ICD-10CM #	N18.9	Chronic kidney disease, unspecified

CAUSES OF CHRONIC RENAL FAILURE

Diabetic glomerulosclerosis (systemic disease involving the kidney).
Hypertensive nephrosclerosis.
Glomerular disease:
- Glomerulonephritis.
- Amyloidosis, light chain disease (systemic disease involving the kidney).
- Systemic lupus erythematosus, Wegener granulomatosis (systemic disease involving the kidney).

Tubulointerstitial disease:
- Reflux nephropathy (chronic pyelonephritis).
- Analgesic nephropathy.
- Obstructive nephropathy (stones, benign prostatic hypertrophy).
- Myeloma kidney (systemic disease involving the kidney).

Vascular disease:
- Scleroderma (systemic disease involving the kidney).
- Vasculitis (systemic disease involving the kidney).
- Renovascular renal failure (ischemic nephropathy).
- Atheroembolic renal disease (systemic disease involving the kidney).

Cystic disease:
- Autosomal dominant polycystic kidney disease.
- Medullary cystic kidney disease.

RENAL FAILURE, INTRINSIC OR PARENCHYMAL CAUSES[91]

ICD-10CM #	N17.0	Acute kidney failure with tubular necrosis
	N17.1	Acute kidney failure with acute cortical necrosis
	N17.2	Acute kidney failure with medullary necrosis
	N17.8	Other acute kidney failure
	N17.9	Acute kidney failure, unspecified
	N18.9	Chronic kidney disease, unspecified

ABNORMALITIES OF THE VASCULATURE

Renal arteries: atherosclerosis, thromboembolism, arteritis.
Renal veins: thrombosis.
Microvasculature: vasculitis, thrombotic microangiopathy.

ABNORMALITIES OF GLOMERULI (ACUTE GLOMERULONEPHRITIS)

Antiglomerular membrane disease (Goodpasture syndrome).
Immune complex glomerulonephritis: SLE, postinfectious, idiopathic, membranoproliferative.

ABNORMALITIES OF INTERSTITIUM (ACUTE INTERSTITIAL NEPHRITIS)

Drugs (e.g., antibiotics, NSAIDs, diuretics, anticonvulsants, allopurinol).
Infectious pyelonephritis.
Infiltrative: lymphoma, leukemia, sarcoidosis.

ABNORMALITIES OF TUBULES

Physical obstruction (uric acid, oxalate, light chains).
Acute tubular necrosis:
- Ischemic.
- Toxic (antibiotics, chemotherapy, immunosuppressives, radiocontrast dyes, heavy metals, myoglobin, hemolyzed RBCs).

RENAL FAILURE, POSTRENAL CAUSES[91]

ICD-10CM #	N17.0	Acute kidney failure with tubular necrosis
	N17.1	Acute kidney failure with acute cortical necrosis
	N17.2	Acute kidney failure with medullary necrosis
	N17.8	Other acute kidney failure
	N17.9	Acute kidney failure, unspecified
	N18.9	Chronic kidney disease, unspecified

URETER AND RENAL PELVIS

Intrinsic obstruction:
- Blood clots.
- Stones.
- Sloughed papillae: diabetes, sickle cell disease, analgesic nephropathy.
- Inflammatory: fungus ball.

Extrinsic obstruction:
- Malignancy.
- Retroperitoneal fibrosis.
- Iatrogenic: inadvertent ligation of ureters.

BLADDER

Prostatic hypertrophy or malignancy.
Neuropathic bladder.
Blood clots.
Bladder cancer.
Stones.

URETHRAL

Strictures.
Congenital valves.

RENAL FAILURE, PRERENAL CAUSES[91]

ICD-10CM #	N17.0	Acute kidney failure with tubular necrosis
	N17.1	Acute kidney failure with acute cortical necrosis
	N17.2	Acute kidney failure with medullary necrosis
	N17.8	Other acute kidney failure
	N17.9	Acute kidney failure, unspecified
	N18.9	Chronic kidney disease, unspecified

DECREASED CARDIAC OUTPUT

CHF.
Arrhythmias.
Pericardial constriction or tamponade.
Pulmonary embolism.

HYPOVOLEMIA

GI tract loss (vomiting, diarrhea, nasogastric suction).
Blood losses (trauma, GI tract surgery).
Renal losses (diuretics, mineralocorticoid deficiency, postobstructive diuresis).
Skin losses (burns).

VOLUME REDISTRIBUTION (DECREASE IN EFFECTIVE BLOOD VOLUME)

Hypoalbuminemic states (cirrhosis, nephrosis).
Sequestration of fluid in "third" space (ischemic bowel, peritonitis, pancreatitis).
Peripheral vasodilation (sepsis, vasodilators, anaphylaxis).

ALTERED RENAL VASCULAR RESISTANCE

Increase in afferent vascular resistance (NSAIDs, liver disease, sepsis, hypercalcemia, cyclosporine).
Decrease in efferent arteriolar tone (ACE inhibitors).

RENAL INFARCTION[32]

ICD-10CM #	N28.0	Ischemia and infarction of kidney

CAUSES OF RENAL INFARCTION

Thrombosis: Spontaneous
Atherosclerotic disease of aorta and renal artery.
Fibromuscular dysplasia of renal artery.
Aneurysms of aorta or renal artery.
Dissection of aorta or renal artery:
- Marfan syndrome.
- Ehlers-Danlos syndrome.

Vasculitis involving renal artery:
- Polyarteritis nodosa.
- Takayasu arteritis.
- Kawasaki disease.
- Thromboangiitis obliterans.
- Other necrotizing vasculitides.

Inflammatory disease of the aorta or renal artery:
- Syphilis.
- Tuberculosis.
- Mycoses.

Hypercoagulable states:
- Nephrotic syndrome.
- Antiphospholipid syndrome.
- Antithrombin III deficiency.
- Homocystinuria.

Thrombotic microangiopathies:
- Hemolytic-uremic syndrome.
- Thrombotic thrombocytopenic purpura.
- Antiphospholipid syndrome.
- Malignant hypertension.
- Scleroderma.
- Sickle cell nephropathy.
- Polycythemia vera.
- Postpartum hemolytic-uremic syndrome.
- Hyperacute vascular allograft rejection.

Thrombosis: Induced
Traumatic.
Following endovascular intervention.
Post renal transplantation.

Embolism
Cardiac source:
- Atrial fibrillation or other arrhythmias.
- Native and prosthetic valvular heart disease.
- Infective endocarditis.
- Marantic endocarditis.

Myocardial infarction with mural thrombi.
Left atrial myxoma or other tumor.
Noncardiac sources:
- Atheromatous embolic disease.
- Paradoxical emboli.
- Fat emboli.
- Tumor emboli.

Therapeutic renal embolization.
Segmental renal infarction of childhood.
Cisplatinum and gemcitabine.
Sickle cell disease or sickle cell trait.

RENAL PARENCHYMAL DISEASE, CHRONIC[41]

ICD-10CM #	N28.9	Disorder of kidney and ureter, unspecified

DIFFERENTIAL DIAGNOSIS OF CHRONIC RENAL PARENCHYMAL DISEASE

No Papillary/Caliceal Abnormality
Diffuse Parenchymal Loss
Bilateral:
- Chronic glomerulonephritis.
- Diffuse small-vessel disease.
- Hereditary nephropathies.

Unilateral:
- Renal artery stenosis.
- Postirradiation.
- Rare:
  - Hypoplastic kidney.
  - Postobstructive atrophy.

FOCAL PARENCHYMAL LOSS

Infarct.
Previous trauma.

Papillary/Caliceal Abnormality
Diffuse Parenchymal Loss
Obstructive nephropathy.
Generalized reflux nephropathy.

No Parenchymal Loss
Papillary necrosis.
TB.
Medullary sponge kidney.
Megacalices.
Pelvicaliceal cyst.

Focal Parenchymal Loss
Focal reflux nephropathy (chronic atrophic pyelonephritis).
TB.
Calculus disease.

RENAL VEIN THROMBOSIS, CAUSES

ICD-10CM #	I82.3	Embolism and thrombosis of renal vein

Nephrotic syndrome.
Renal cell carcinoma.
Aortic aneurysm causing compression.
Lymphadenopathy.
Retroperitoneal fibrosis.
Estrogen therapy.
Pregnancy.
Renal cell carcinoma with vein invasion.
Severe dehydration.

RESPIRATORY DISTRESS IN THE NEWBORN, CAUSES[34]

ICD-10CM #	J96.00	Acute respiratory failure

RESPIRATORY DISTRESS IN THE NEWBORN

Noncardiopulmonary
Hypothermia or hyperthermia.
Hypoglycemia.
Metabolic acidosis.
Drug intoxications; withdrawal.
Polycythemia.
CNS insult.
Asphyxia.
Hemorrhage.
Neuromuscular disease.
Werdnig-Hoffman disease.
Myopathies.
Phrenic nerve injury.
Skeletal abnormalities.
Asphyxiating thoracic dystrophy.

Cardiovascular
Left-sided outflow obstruction.
Hypoplastic left heart.
Aortic stenosis.
Coarctation of the aorta.
Cyanotic lesions.
Transposition of the great vessels.
Total anomalous pulmonary venous return.
Tricuspid atresia.
Right-sided outflow obstruction.

Pulmonary
Upper airway obstruction.
Choanal atresia.
Vocal cord paralysis.
Meconium aspiration.
Clear fluid aspiration.
Transient tachypnea.
Pneumonia.
Pulmonary hypoplasia.
Primary.
Secondary.
Hyaline membrane disease.
Pneumothorax.
Pleural effusions.
Mass lesions.
Lobar emphysema.
Cystic adenomatoid malformation.

RESPIRATORY FAILURE, HYPOVENTILATORY[71]

ICD-10CM #	J96.00	Acute respiratory failure, unspecified whether with hypoxia or hypercapnia

J96.90	Respiratory failure, unspecified, unspecified whether with hypoxia or hypercapnia

ABNORMAL RESPIRATORY CAPACITY (NORMAL RESPIRATORY WORKLOADS)

Acute depression of CNS:
- Various causes.

Chronic central hypoventilation syndromes:
- Obesity-hypoventilation syndrome.
- Sleep apnea syndrome.
- Hypothyroidism.
- Shy-Drager syndrome (multisystem atrophy syndrome).

Acute toxic paralysis syndromes:
- Botulism.
- Tetanus.
- Toxic ingestion or bites.
- Organophosphate poisoning.

Neuromuscular disorders (acute and chronic):
- Myasthenia gravis.
- Guillain-Barré syndrome.
- Drugs.
- Amyotrophic lateral sclerosis.
- Muscular dystrophies.
- Polymyositis.
- Spinal cord injury.
- Traumatic phrenic nerve paralysis.

ABNORMAL PULMONARY WORKLOADS

Chronic obstructive pulmonary disease:
- Chronic bronchitis.
- Asthmatic bronchitis.
- Emphysema.

Asthma and acute bronchial hyperreactivity syndromes.
Upper airway obstruction.
Interstitial lung diseases.

ABNORMAL EXTRAPULMONARY WORKLOADS

Chronic thoracic cage disorders:
- Severe kyphoscoliosis.
- After thoracoplasty.
- After thoracic cage injury.

Acute thoracic cage trauma and burns.
Pneumothorax.
Pleural fibrosis and effusions.
Abdominal processes.

RESPIRATORY MUSCLE WEAKNESS[76]

ICD-10CM # Varies with specific diagnosis

CAUSES OF DECREASED RESPIRATORY MUSCLE STRENGTH OR ENDURANCE

Disorders of the phrenic nerve:
- Guillain-Barré syndrome.
- Poliomyelitis.

Respiratory muscle atrophy.
Disorders of neuromuscular transmission:
- Myasthenia gravis.
- Ventilator dependence.
- Malnutrition.
- Myopathy.
- Critical illness polyneuropathy/myopathy.

Altered diaphragmatic force-length relationship:
- Dynamic hyperinflation and diaphragmatic flattening.

RETINOPATHY, HYPERTENSIVE

ICD-10CM #	H35.039	Hypertensive retinopathy, unspecified eye

Retinal venous obstruction.
Diabetic retinopathy.
Ocular ischemic syndrome.
Hyperviscosity.
Tortuosity of retinal artery.

RHINITIS

ICD-10CM #	J31.0	Chronic rhinitis
	J30.0	Vasomotor rhinitis
	J30.1	Allergic rhinitis due to pollen
	J30.2	Other seasonal allergic rhinitis
	J30.5	Allergic rhinitis due to food
	J30.89	Other allergic rhinitis
	J30.9	Allergic rhinitis, unspecified

Allergic rhinitis.
Infectious rhinitis.
Vasomotor rhinitis.
Exercise-induced rhinitis.
Emotional rhinitis.
Rhinitis medicamentosa.
Hormone-mediated rhinitis (menses, pregnancy, oral contraceptives, hypothyroidism).
GERD.
Chemical- or irritant-induced rhinitis.
Rhinitis mimics:
- Deviated septum.
- Enlarged adenoids.
- Nasal polyps/tumors.
- Foreign bodies.
- CSF rhinorrhea.
- Sarcoidosis.
- Midline granuloma.
- Granulomatosis with polyangiitis.
- SLE.
- Sjögren syndrome.

RHINITIS, CHRONIC[2]

ICD-10CM #	J31.0	Chronic rhinitis

CLASSIFICATION OF CHRONIC RHINITIS

Allergic
Systemic.
Local (entopy).
Work-Related
Irritant.
Corrosive.
Immunologic.
Infectious (Rhinosinusitis)
Allergic.
Nonallergic.
Nonallergic
Idiopathic.
Nonallergic with eosinophilia.
Atrophic.
Primary.
Secondary.
Medication-related.
Topical vasoconstrictors (rhinitis medicamentosa).
Oral medications.
Exercise-induced.
Cold air-induced.
Gustatory.
Hormonal.
Aging.
Systemic diseases.

RHINOSINUSITIS, DIFFERENTIAL DIAGNOSIS[66]

ICD-10CM # Varies with specific diagnosis

DIFFERENTIAL DIAGNOSIS OF RHINOSINUSITIS

Allergic Rhinitis
Seasonal.
Perennial.
Combined seasonal and perennial.
Allergic fungal rhinosinusitis.
Nonallergic Rhinitis
Nonallergic, noninflammatory idiopathic rhinopathy (vasomotor rhinitis).
Nonallergic rhinitis with eosinophilia syndrome (NARES).
Cold dry air-induced rhinitis.
Gustatory rhinitis.
Infectious Rhinosinusitis
Bacterial.
Viral.
Fungal.
Granulomatous.
Drug-Induced Rhinitis
Oral contraceptives.
Various antihypertensives and ocular β-blockers.
Topical decongestants (rhinitis medicamentosa).
Phosphodiesterase-5 antagonists.
Mechanical Causes of Rhinosinusitis
Septal deviation.
Nasal foreign body.
Choanal atresia or stenosis.
Adenoid hypertrophy.
Encephalocele.
Glioma.
Dermoid.
Innate and Acquired Immunity Disorders
Congenital or acquired immunodeficiencies.
Cystic fibrosis.
Immotile cilia syndrome.
Systemic Inflammatory Disorders
Sarcoidosis.
Granulomatosis with polyangiitis.
Vasculitis.
Neoplastic Causes
Benign:
- Polyps.

Nasopharyngeal angiofibroma.
Inverting papilloma.
Malignant:
Adenocarcinoma.
Squamous cell carcinoma.
Esthesioneuroblastoma.
Lymphoma.
Rhabdomyosarcoma.

RIB DEFECTS ON X-RAY[41]

ICD-10CM # Varies with specific diagnosis

CAUSES OF SUPERIOR MARGINAL RIB DEFECTS

Normal
Isolated defects.
Projectional artifacts (due to lordosis).
Neurologic
Paralytic poliomyelitis.
Quadriparesis.
Collagen Vascular Disease
Rheumatoid arthritis.
SLE.
Systemic sclerosis.
Local Pressure
Chest drainage tube.
Osteochondroma.
Neural tumor.
Coarctation of aorta.
Hyperparathyroidism Miscellaneous
Osteogenesis imperfecta.
Marfan syndrome.

RIB NOTCHING ON X-RAY[41]

ICD-10CM # Varies with specific diagnosis

CAUSES OF INFERIOR RIB NOTCHING

ARTERIAL

AORTIC OBSTRUCTION

Aortic coarctation.
Aortic thrombosis.
Aortitis.

SUBCLAVIAN ARTERY OBSTRUCTION

Blalock-Taussig operation.
Arteritis.
Atherosclerotic occlusion.

PULMONARY OLIGEMIA

Pulmonary atresia.
Tetralogy of Fallot.
Multiple pulmonary arterial stenoses.
Venous

CHRONIC SUPERIOR VENA CAVAL OBSTRUCTION

Arteriovenous
Arteriovenous Malformation
Pulmonary.
Chest wall.
Neural
Neurofibromas

RIGHT AXIS DEVIATION[57]

ICD-10CM # Varies with specific diagnosis

Normal variation.
Right ventricular hypertrophy.
Left posterior fascicular block.
Lateral myocardial infarction.
Pulmonary embolism.
Dextrocardia.
Mechanical shifts or emphysema causing a vertical heart.

SALIVARY GLAND ENLARGEMENT

ICD-10CM #	K11.1	Hypertrophy of salivary gland

Neoplasm.
Sialolithiasis.
Infection (mumps, bacterial infection, HIV, TB).
Sarcoidosis.
Idiopathic.
Acromegaly.
Anorexia/bulimia.
Chronic pancreatitis.
Medications (e.g., phenylbutazone).
Cirrhosis.
DM.

SALIVARY GLAND SECRETION, DECREASED

ICD-10CM #	K11.7	Disturbances of salivary secretion
	R68.2	Dry mouth, unspecified

Medications (antihistamines, antidepressants, neuroleptics, antihypertensives).
Dehydration.
Anxiety.
Sjögren syndrome.
Sarcoidosis.
Mumps.
Amyloidosis.
CNS disorders.
Head and neck radiation.

SCLERODERMA-LIKE SYNDROMES[3]

ICD-10CM # Varies with specific diagnosis

OTHER DISEASES

Morphea.
Eosinophilic fasciitis.
Scleredema (of Buschke).
Scleromyxedema.
Graft-versus-host disease.
Nephrogenic-fibrosing dermopathy.

ENVIRONMENTAL AGENTS AND DRUGS

Bleomycin.
L-Tryptophan.
Organic solvents.
Pentazocine.
Toxic oil syndrome.
Vinyl chloride disease.
Gadolinium.

SCROTAL CALCIFICATIONS[81]

ICD-10CM # Varies with specific diagnosis

SCROTAL CALCIFICATIONS

Testicular
Solitary, postinflammatory granulomatous, vascular.
Microlithiasis.
"Burned-out" germ cell tumor.
Large-cell calcifying Sertoli cell tumor.
Teratoma.
Mixed germ cell tumor.
Sarcoid.
TB.
Chronic infarct
Extratesticular
Tunica vaginalis "scrotal pearls"
Chronic epididymitis
Schistosomiasis

SCROTAL MASSES, BOYS AND ADOLESCENTS[58]

ICD-10CM #	R22.9	Localized swelling, mass and lump, unspecified

PAINFUL

Testicular torsion.
Torsion of appendix testis.
Epididymitis.
Trauma: ruptured testis, hematocele.
Inguinal hernia (incarcerated).
Mumps orchitis.

PAINLESS

Hydrocele.
Inguinal hernia.[48]
Varicocele.
Spermatocele.
Testicular tumor.
Henoch-Schönlein purpura.
Idiopathic scrotal edema.

SCROTAL PAIN[71]

ICD-10CM#	S31.30XA	Unspecified open wound of scrotum and testes, initial encounter
	N50.9	Disorder of male genital organs, unspecified
	R10.2	Pelvic and perineal pain
	N49.9	Inflammatory disorder of unspecified male genital organ
	N50.1	Vascular disorders of male genital organs
	N49.9	Inflammatory disorder of unspecified male genital organ

[48] May be associated with discomfort.

Torsion:
- Appendages.
- Spermatic cord.

Infection:
- Orchitis.
- Abscess.
- Epididymitis.

Neoplasia:
- Benign.
- Malignant.

Incarcerated hernia.
Trauma.
Hydrocele.
Spermatocele.
Varicocele.

SCROTAL PAIN, ADOLESCENT OR PEDIATRIC PATIENT[99]

ICD-10CM # Varies with specific diagnosis

DIFFERENTIAL DIAGNOSIS OF PEDIATRIC ADOLESCENT ACUTE SCROTAL PAIN

Appendage torsion:
- Appendix testis.
- Other appendage (epididymis, paradidymis, vas aberrans).

Spermatic cord torsion:
- Intravaginal, acute or intermittent.
- Extravaginal.

Epididymitis:
- Infectious:
  - Urinary tract infection.
  - Sexually transmitted disease.
  - Viral.
- Sterile or traumatic.

Scrotal edema or erythema:
- Diaper dermatitis, insect bite, or other skin lesions.
- Idiopathic scrotal edema.

Orchitis:
- Associated with epididymitis with or without abscess.
- Vasculitis (e.g., Henoch-Schönlein purpura).
- Viral illness (mumps).

Trauma:
- Hematocele or scrotal contusion or testis rupture.

Hernia or hydrocele:
- Inguinal hernia with or without incarceration.
- Communicating hydrocele.
- Encysted hydrocele with or without torsion.
- Associated with acute abdominal pathology (e.g., appendicitis, peritonitis).

Varicocele.

Intrascrotal mass:
- Cystic dysplasia or tumor of testis.
- Epididymal cyst, spermatocele or tumor.
- Other paratesticular tumors.

Musculoskeletal pain from inguinal tendonitis or muscle strain.
Referred pain (e.g., ureteral calculus or anomaly).

SCROTAL SWELLING

ICD-10CM # N50.8 Other specified disorders of male genital organs

Hydrocele.
Varicocele.
Neoplasm.
Acute epididymitis.
Orchitis.
Trauma.
Hernia.
Torsion of spermatic cord.
Torsion of epididymis.
Torsion of testis.
Insect bite.
Folliculitis.
Sebaceous cyst.
Thrombosis of spermatic vein.
Other: lymphedema, dermatitis, fat necrosis, Henoch-Schönlein purpura, idiopathic scrotal edema.

SEIZURE

ICD-10CM # R56.9 Unspecified convulsions

Syncope.
Alcohol abuse/withdrawal.
TIA.
Hemiparetic migraine.
Psychiatric disorders.
Carotid sinus hypersensitivity.
Hyperventilation, prolonged breath holding.
Hypoglycemia.
Narcolepsy.
Movement disorders (tics, hemiballismus).
Hyponatremia.
Brain tumor (primary or metastatic).
Tetanus.
Strychnine, phencyclidine poisoning.

SEIZURE, PEDIATRIC[7]

ICD-10CM # R56.9 Unspecified convulsions
P90 Convulsions of newborn

FIRST MONTH OF LIFE

First Day

Hypoxia.
Drugs.
Trauma.
Infection.
Hyperglycemia.
Hypoglycemia.
Pyridoxine deficiency.

Day 2 to 3

Infection.
Drug withdrawal.
Hypoglycemia.
Hypocalcemia.
Developmental malformation.
Intracranial hemorrhage.
Inborn error of metabolism.
Hyponatremia or hypernatremia.

Day >4

Infection.
Hypocalcemia.
Hyperphosphatemia.
Hyponatremia.
Developmental malformation.
Drug withdrawal.
Inborn error of metabolism.

1 TO 6 MO

As above.

6 MO TO 3 YR

Febrile seizures.
Birth injury.
Infection.
Toxin.
Trauma.
Metabolic disorder.
Cerebral degenerative disease.

>3 YR

Idiopathic.
Infection.
Trauma.
Cerebral degenerative disease.

SEIZURE MIMICS[3]

ICD-10CM # Varies with specific diagnosis

NON-EPILEPTIC EPISODIC DISORDERS THAT MAY RESEMBLE SEIZURES

Movement disorders: myoclonus, paroxysmal choreoathetosis, episodic ataxias, hyperexplexia (startle disease).
Migraine: confusional, vertebrobasilar, visual auras.
Syncope.
Behavioral and psychiatric: psychogenic nonepileptic attacks (pseudoseizures), hyperventilation syndrome, panic or anxiety disorder, dissociative states.
Cataplexy (usually associated with narcolepsy).
Transient ischemic attack.
Alcoholic blackouts.
Hypoglycemia.

SEXUAL DIFFERENTIATION ABNORMALITIES[99]

ICD-10CM # Varies with specific diagnosis

ABNORMAL SEXUAL DIFFERENTIATION

Disorders of gonadal differentiation.
- Seminiferous tubule dysgenesis.
- Klinefelter syndrome.
- 46,XX male.
- Syndromes of gonadal dysgenesis:
  - Turner syndrome.
  - Pure gonadal dysgenesis.
  - Mixed gonadal dysgenesis.
  - Partial gonadal dysgenesis (dysgenetic male pseudohermaphroditism).
  - Bilateral vanishing testis, testicular regression syndromes.

Ovotesticular DSD (true hermaphroditism).

46,XX DSD (masculinized female):
- Congenital adrenal hyperplasia (21-hydroxylase, 11β-hydroxylase, 3β-hydroxysteroid dehydrogenase deficiencies).
- Maternal androgens.

46,XY DSD (undermasculinized male).
- Leydig cell agenesis, unresponsiveness.
- Disorders of testosterone biosynthesis.

Variants of congenital adrenal hyperplasia affecting corticosteroid and testosterone synthesis:
StAR deficiency (congenital lipoid adrenal hyperplasia).
Cytochrome P450 oxidoreductase (POR) deficiency.
3β-Hydroxysteroid dehydrogenase deficiency.
17β-Hydroxylase deficiency.
Disorders of testosterone biosynthesis:
17, 20-Lyase deficiency.
17β-Hydroxysteroid oxidoreductase deficiency.
Disorders of androgen-dependent target tissue:
Androgen receptor and postreceptor defects.
Syndrome of complete (severe) androgen insensitivity.
Syndrome of partial androgen insensitivity.
Mild androgen insensitivity syndrome (MAIS).
Disorders of testosterone metabolism by peripheral tissues:
5α-Reductase deficiency.
Disorders of synthesis, secretion, or response to müllerian-inhibiting substance.
Persistent müllerian duct syndrome.
Unclassified forms:
In females: Mayer-Rokitansky-Küster-Hauser syndrome.
Disorder of sex development (DSD).

SEXUAL DYSFUNCTION, FEMALE[3]

ICD-10CM #	R37	Sexual dysfunction, unspecified

FACTORS THAT MAY INFLUENCE SEXUAL FUNCTIONING IN WOMEN

Biological
Medications (e.g., antidepressants, antihypertensives).
Vaginal atrophy, pain with intercourse.
Low testosterone levels (e.g., bilateral oophorectomy).
Illness (e.g., diabetes, hypothyroidism, cerebrovascular accident).
Sleep disturbances, fatigue.
Disability or pain from illness (e.g., arthritis).
Incontinence.
Psychological
Depression.
Body image.
Interpersonal
Marital issues.
Poor communication.
Partner's sexual problems (e.g., erectile dysfunction).
Partner's health problems (e.g., myocardial infarction).
Sociocultural
Ageism ("too old" to want sex).
Multiple other obligations and commitments.
Lack of partner.

SEXUALLY TRANSMITTED DISEASES, ANORECTAL REGION[65]

ICD-10CM #	K62.89	Other specified diseases of anus and rectum

ULCERATIVE

Lymphogranuloma venereum.
Herpes simplex virus.
Early (primary) syphilis.
Chancroid (*Haemophilus ducreyi*).
Cytomegalovirus.
Idiopathic (usually HIV positive).

NONULCERATIVE

Condyloma acuminatum.
Gonorrhea.
Chlamydia (*Chlamydia trachomatis*).
Syphilis.

SEXUAL PRECOCITY[103]

ICD-10CM #	E30.1	Precocious puberty
	E30.8	Other disorders of puberty

TRUE PRECOCIOUS PUBERTY

Premature reactivation of LHRH pulse generator.

INCOMPLETE SEXUAL PRECOCITY

(Pituitary gonadotropin independent).
Males
Chorionic gonadotropin-secreting tumor.
Leydig cell tumor.
Familial testotoxicosis.
Virilizing congenital adrenal hyperplasia.
Virilizing adrenal tumor.
Premature adrenarche.
Females
Granulosa cell tumor (follicular cysts may be manifested similarly).
Follicular cyst.
Feminizing adrenal tumor.
Premature thelarche.
Premature adrenarche.
Late-onset virilizing congenital adrenal hyperplasia.
In Both Sexes
McCune-Albright syndrome.
Primary hypothyroidism.

SHOULDER PAIN

ICD-10CM #	M24.819	Other specific joint derangements of unspecified shoulder, not elsewhere classified
	M75.80	Other shoulder lesions, unspecified shoulder
	S43.409A	Unspecified sprain of unspecified shoulder joint, initial encounter
	S46.919A	Strain of unspecified muscle, fascia and tendon at shoulder and upper arm level, unspecified arm, initial encounter

WITH LOCAL FINDINGS IN SHOULDER

Trauma: contusion, fracture, muscle strain, trauma to spinal cord.
Arthrosis, arthritis, RA, ankylosing spondylitis.
Bursitis, synovitis, tendinitis, tenosynovitis.
Aseptic (avascular) necrosis.
Local infection: septic arthritis, osteomyelitis, abscess, herpes zoster, TB.

WITHOUT LOCAL FINDINGS IN SHOULDER

Cardiovascular disorders: ischemic heart disease, pericarditis, aortic aneurysm.
Subdiaphragmatic abscess, liver abscess.
Cholclithiasis, cholecystitis.
Pulmonary lesions: apical bronchial carcinoma, pleurisy, pneumothorax, pneumonia.
GI lesions: PUD, gastric neoplasm, peptic esophagitis.
Pancreatic lesions: carcinoma, calculi, pancreatitis.
CNS abnormalities: neoplasm, vascular abnormalities.
Multiple sclerosis.
Syringomyelia.
Polymyositis/dermatomyositis.
Psychogenic.
Polymyalgia rheumatica.
Ectopic pregnancy.

SHOULDER PAIN BY LOCATION

ICD-10CM #	M75.80	Other shoulder lesions, unspecified shoulder
	S43.499A	Other sprain of unspecified shoulder joint, initial encounter
	S46.019A	Strain of muscle(s) and tendon(s) of the rotator cuff of unspecified shoulder, initial encounter
	S46.819A	Strain of other muscles, fascia and tendons at shoulder and upper arm level, unspecified arm, initial encounter

TOP OF SHOULDER (C4)

Cervical source.
Acromioclavicular.
Sternoclavicular.
Diaphragmatic.

SUPEROLATERAL (C5)
Rotator cuff tendinitis.
Impingement.
Adhesive capsulitis.
Glenohumeral arthritis.

ANTERIOR
Bicipital tendinitis and rupture.
Glenoid labral tear.
Adhesive capsulitis.
Glenohumeral arthritis.
Osteonecrosis.

AXILLARY
Neoplasm (Pancoast, mediastinal).
Herpes zoster.

SHOULDER PAIN, IN DIFFERENT AGE GROUPS[22]

ICD-10CM # M25.519 Pain in unspecified shoulder

COMMON CAUSES OF SHOULDER PAIN IN DIFFERENT AGE GROUPS

Childhood (2 to 10 yr)
Intraarticular
Instability.
Periarticular
Osteochondromas.
Adolescence (10 to 18 yr)
Intraarticular
Instability.
Early Adulthood (18 to 30 yr)
Intraarticular
Instability.
Acromioclavicular joint sprain.
Periarticular
Calcific tendonitis.
Impingement.
Referred
Cervical.
Adulthood (30 to 60 yr)
Intraarticular
Osteochondritis.
Osteoarthritis.
Frozen shoulder.
Inflammatory arthritis.
Periarticular
Calcific tendonitis.
Impingement.
Rotator cuff tear.
Bicipital tendonitis.
Referred
Cervical.
Old Age (>60 yr)
Intraarticular
Osteochondritis.
Osteoarthritis.
Frozen shoulder.
Inflammatory arthritis.
Periarticular
Impingement.
Rotator cuff tear.
Referred
Cervical.

SINUS NODE DYSFUNCTION[38]

ICD-10CM # Varies with specific diagnosis

CAUSES OF SINUS NODE DYSFUNCTION

Intrinsic
Hypothyroidism.
Fibrocalcific degeneration.
Increased vagal tone, especially in sleep apnea.
Congenital mutations.
Scleroderma.
Amyloidosis.
Chagas disease.
Extrinsic
Trauma, including cardiac surgery.
Drugs:
- Calcium-channel blockers.
- β-Blockers.
- Digoxin.
- Antiarrhythmic medications (amiodarone, dronedarone, sotalol, flecainide, propafenone).
- Lithium.

SINUS OF VALSALVA ANEURYSMS[14]

ICD-10CM # Varies with specific diagnosis

Congenital: single cusp involved with normal aorta.
- Localized deficiency of the tissue in the aortic annulus.
- Retraction of a cusp into a closing ventricular septal defect.

Inherited: all cusps involved with annuloaortic ectasia.
- Marfan syndrome.
- Ehlers-Danlos syndrome.

Acquired: saccular false aneurysms.
- Aortic root abscess with endocarditis.
- Luetic aortitis.
- Aortic dissection.

SINUS OSTIAL OBSTRUCTION[10]

ICD-10CM # Varies with specific diagnosis

FACTORS THAT PREDISPOSE TO SINUS OSTIAL OBSTRUCTION

Mucosal Swelling
Systemic factors:
- Viral upper respiratory infection.
- Allergic inflammation.
- Cystic fibrosis.
- Immune disorders.
- Ciliary dyskinesia.
- Tobacco smoke.

Local insult:
- Facial trauma.
- Swimming, diving.
- Rhinitis medicamentosa.
- Nasal intubation.

Mechanical Obstruction
Choanal atresia.
Deviated septum.
Nasal polyps.
Foreign body.
Tumor.
Ethmoid bullae.

SINUS TACHYCARDIA[76]

ICD-10CM # R00.0 Tachycardia, unspecified

DIFFERENTIAL DIAGNOSIS OF SINUS TACHYCARDIA

Etiologic Category
Specific Disorders
Hemodynamic:
- Heart failure: systolic and diastolic heart failure caused by ischemic, valvular, or nonischemic myopathy.
- Loss of circulating blood volume: GI bleeding, anemia, shifts of intravascular fluid due to changes in colloidal osmotic pressure or inflammation.
- Septic shock: dehydration.
- Vascular shunts: intracardiac as well as aortovenous malformations, fistulas.
- Pulmonary embolism.

Metabolic and neurohumoral:
- Sepsis: infections and inflammatory conditions.
- Hyperthyroidism.
- Paget disease of the bone.
- Pheochromocytoma.
- Carcinoid syndrome.
- Beriberi heart disease.
- Carcinoma.
- Hyperpyrexia.
- Acidosis.
- Exercise.

Pharmacologic:
- Sympathomimetic agents: isoproterenol, epinephrine, or dopamine.
- Vagolytic agents, atropine, scopolamine.
- Vasodilators: nitrates, angiotensin-converting enzyme inhibitors, angiotensin receptor blockers, hydrazine, as well as centrally acting vasodilators.
- Thyroid preparations, caffeine and nicotine.
- Bronchodilators, including theophylline and terbutaline.
- Anesthetic agents, including spinal anesthetics, causing peripheral vasodilation.
- Drugs of abuse: amphetamines, cocaine, "ecstasy," cannabis.

Neurologic/psychological:
- Pain.
- Fear, anxiety, and hysteria.
- Hyper-beta adrenergic phase of neurocardiogenic syncope.
- Autonomic dysfunction such as with diabetes.

SKIN AND RENAL[87]

ICD-10CM # Varies with specific diagnosis

SELECTED CONDITIONS WITH CONCURRENT SKIN AND RENAL INVOLVEMENT

More Common
Lupus erythematosus.
Leukocytoclastic vasculitis.

Henoch-Schönlein purpura.
Mixed cryoglobulinemia.
Diabetes mellitus.
Systemic vasculitis.

Less Common

Nail-patella syndrome.
Hemolytic-uremic syndrome.
Toxic shock syndrome.
Mixed connective tissue disease.
Dermatomyositis.
Rheumatoid arthritis.
Sjögren syndrome.
Dermatitis herpetiformis.
Sarcoidosis.
Systemic sclerosis.
Ulcerative colitis.
Amyloidosis.
Toxic epidermolysis.
Hypothyroidism.
Graves disease.
Fabry disease.
Neurofibromatosis.
Hurler syndrome.
Castleman disease.
Infectious endocarditis.
Staphylococcal scalded skin syndrome (in adults).

SKIN INDURATION, CHRONIC[46]

ICD-10CM # Varies with specific diagnosis

CONDITIONS ASSOCIATED WITH CHRONIC SKIN INDURATION

Systemic sclerosis.
Localized scleroderma.
Scleroderma variants.
Scleredema:
- Scleredema adultorum of Buschke.
- Scleredema diabeticorum.
- Scleredema neonatorum.

Scleromyxedema.
Nephrogenic fibrosing dermopathy.
Eosinophilic syndromes:
- Eosinophilic fasciitis (diffuse fasciitis with eosinophilia, Schulman disease).
- Eosinophilia-myalgia syndrome.
- Toxic oil syndrome.

Chronic graft-versus-host disease.
Pseudoscleroderma (local injection of vitamin K, bleomycin, pentazocine).
Metabolic diseases:
- Porphyria cutanea tarda.
- Phenylketonuria.
- Werner syndrome.
- Acromegaly.

Pachydermoperiostitis.
Polyneuropathy, organomegaly, endocrinopathy, monoclonal gammopathy (POEMS).
Stiff skin syndrome.
Reflex sympathetic dystrophy.
Hemiplegia.

SMALL BOWEL MASSES[95]

ICD-10CM # Varies with specific diagnosis

Cyst:
- Mesenteric cyst.

Tumor:
- Benign.
- Malignant.

Intussusception.
Inflammation:
- Crohn disease.

SMALL BOWEL OBSTRUCTION[65]

ICD-10CM #	K56.5	Intestinal adhesions [bands] with obstruction (postprocedural) (postinfection)
	Q41.9	Congenital absence, atresia and stenosis of small intestine, part unspecified

INTRINSIC

Congenital (atresia, stenosis).
Inflammatory (Crohn, radiation enteritis).
Neoplasms (metastatic or primary).
Intussusception.
Traumatic (hematoma).

EXTRINSIC

Hernias (internal and external).
Adhesions.
Volvulus.
Compressing masses (tumors, abscesses, hematomas).

INTRALUMINAL

Foreign body.
Gallstones.
Bezoars.
Barium.
Ascaris infestation.

SMALL INTESTINE ULCERATION

ICD-10CM # K63.3 Ulcer of intestine

Inflammatory bowel disease.
Celiac disease.
Vasculitis, SLE, Behçet syndrome.
Uremia.
Infections (*Campylobacter,* TB, *Yersinia,* parasites, typhoid, cytomegalovirus [CMV], *Clostridium).*
Mesenteric insufficiency.
Neoplasms.
Radiation.
Drugs (salicylates, potassium, indomethacin, antimetabolites).
Meckel diverticulum.
Zollinger-Ellison syndrome.
Lymphocytic enterocolitis.
Stomal ulceration.

SMELL DISTURBANCE

ICD-10CM # R43.8 Other disturbances of smell and taste

Upper respiratory tract infection.
Nasal or paranasal sinus disease.
Exposure to noxious vapors.
Head trauma.
Idiopathic.
Dental caries, periodontal disease.
Medications.

SODIUM RETENTION, RENAL CAUSES[87]

ICD-10CM # Varies with specific diagnosis

CAUSES OF RENAL SODIUM RETENTION

Primary

Oliguric acute kidney injury.
Chronic kidney disease.
Glomerular disease.
Severe bilateral renal artery stenosis.
Na+-retaining tubulopathies (genetic).
Mineralocorticoid excess.

Secondary

Heart failure.
Cirrhosis.
Idiopathic edema.

SOFT TISSUE MASS MIMICKING MALIGNANCY[78]

ICD-10CM # Varies with specific diagnosis

OVERVIEW OF DISEASES THAT CAN PRESENT AS A SOFT TISSUE MASS MIMICKING MALIGNANCY

Etiology	Disease Entity
Trauma:	Muscle contusion. Hematoma. Muscle herniation. Calcific myonecrosis. Hypothenar hammer syndrome. Myositis ossificans.
Metabolic:	Diabetic myopathy. Gout. Pseudogout. Calcific tendinosis.
Congenital:	Accessory muscle.
Infectious:	Necrotizing fasciitis. Abscess. Pyomyositis. Hydatid cystic disease. Cat-scratch disease. Actinomycosis.
Inflammation:	Bursitis. Sarcoidosis. Foreign body reaction. Injection granuloma. Granuloma annulare. Epidermal inclusion cyst.
Vascular:	Adventitial cystic disease. Pseudoaneurysm. Thrombosed vein. Arteriovenous vascular malformation.
Miscellaneous:	Focal myositis. Amyloid tumor of soft tissue.

SOFT TISSUE TUMORS, PEDIATRIC PATIENTS[78]

ICD-10CM # Varies with specific diagnosis

PEDIATRIC SOFT TISSUE TUMORS

Vascular lesions:
- Hemangioma of infancy.*
- Congenital hemangioma.
- Hemangioendothelioma (Kasabach-Merritt syndrome).
- Arteriovenous malformation.
- Venous malformations.
- Lymphatic malformation (lymphangioma, cystic hygroma).
- Capillary malformation.

Adipocytic tumors:
- Lipoma.
- Lipoblastoma.
- Liposarcoma.

Fibrohistiocytic tumors:
- Pigmented villonodular synovitis.
- Giant cell tumor of tendon sheath.

Fibroblastic and myofibroblastic tumors:
- Nodular fasciitis.
- Fibrous hamartoma of infancy.
- Myofibroma, myofibromatosis.
- Infantile fibrosarcoma.
- Fibromatosis colli.

Neurogenic tumors:
- Schwannoma.
- Neurofibroma.
- Malignant nerve sheath tumor.

Leiomyoma

Rhabdomyosarcoma

Tumors of uncertain differentiation
- Synovial cell sarcoma.
- Primitive neuroectodermal tumor (Ewing sarcoma).

Pilomatricoma

SORE THROAT[7]

ICD-10CM # J02 Acute pharyngitis

DIFFERENTIAL DIAGNOSIS FOR SORE THROAT

Infectious Causes

Aerobes

Common:
- *Streptococcus pyogenes* (GABHS).
- *Peptostreptococcus* spp.
- Non–group A streptococcus.
- *Neisseria gonorrhoeae.*
- *Neisseria meningitides.*
- *Mycoplasma pneumoniae.*
- *Arcanobacterium hemolyticum.*
- *Chlamydia trachomatis.*
- *Staphylococcus aureus.*

Uncommon:
- *Haemophilus influenzae.*
- *Haemophilus parainfluenzae.*
- *Coccidioides* spp.
- *Corynebacterium diphtheriae.*
- *Streptococcus pneumoniae.*
- *Yersinia enterocolitica.*
- *Treponema pallidum.*
- *Francisella tularensis.*
- *Legionella pneumophila.*
- *Mycobacterium* spp.

ANAEROBES

Bacteroides spp.
Peptococcus spp.
Clostridium spp.
Fusobacterium spp.
Prevotella spp.

OTHER

Candida spp.

VIRAL

Rhinovirus.
Adenovirus.
Coronavirus.
Herpes simplex 1, 2.
Influenza A, B.
Parainfluenza.
Cytomegalovirus.
Epstein-Barr.
Varicella-zoster.
Hepatitis virus.

Noninfectious Causes

SYSTEMIC

Kawasaki disease.
Stevens-Johnson syndrome.
Cyclic neutropenia.
Thyroiditis.
Connective tissue disease.

TRAUMA, MISCELLANEOUS

Penetrating injury.
Angioneurotic edema.
Retained foreign body.
Anomalous aortic arch.
Laryngeal fracture.
Calcific retropharyngeal tendinitis.
Retropharyngeal hematoma.
Caustic exposure.

TUMOR

Tongue.
Larynx.
Thyroid.
Leukemia.

SPASTIC PARAPLEGIAS

ICD-10CM # G82.20 Paraplegia, unspecified

Cervical spondylosis.
Friedreich ataxia.
Multiple sclerosis.
Spinal cord tumor.
HIV.
Tertiary syphilis.
Vitamin B_{12} deficiency.
Spinocerebellar ataxias.
Syringomyelia.
Spinal cord AV malformations.
Adrenoleukodystrophy.

SPINAL CORD COMPRESSION, EPIDURAL

ICD-10CM # Varies with specific diagnosis

Osteoarthritis.
Meningioma.
Spinal epidural abscess.
Spinal epidural hematoma.
Spinal epidural vascular malformations.
RA.
Metastatic cancer (vertebral, intramedullary, leptomeninges).
Radiation myelopathy.
Neurofibroma.
Sarcoidosis.
Paraneoplastic myelopathy.
Histiocytosis.

SPINAL CORD DYSFUNCTION

ICD-10CM #	G95.9	Disease of spinal cord, unspecified
	Q07.9	Congenital malformation of nervous system, unspecified
	D51.1	Vitamin B_{12} deficiency anemia due to selective vitamin B_{12} malabsorption with proteinuria
	D51.3	Other dietary vitamin B_{12} deficiency anemia
	D51.8	Other vitamin B_{12} deficiency anemias
	G95.89	Other specified diseases of spinal cord
	G95.19	Other vascular myelopathies

Trauma.
Multiple sclerosis.
Transverse myelitis.
Neoplasm (primary, metastatic).
Syringomyelia.
Spinal epidural abscess.
HIV myelopathy.
Diskitis.
Spinal epidural hematoma.
Spinal cord infarction.
Spinal AV malformation.
Subarachnoid hemorrhage.

SPINAL CORD DYSFUNCTION, NONTRAUMATIC[7]

ICD-10CM # Q07.9 Congenital malformation of nervous system, unspecified

NONTRAUMATIC ETIOLOGIES OF SPINAL CORD DYSFUNCTION

Processes Affecting the Spinal Cord or Blood Supply Directly

Multiple sclerosis.
Transverse myelitis.

*Lesions with MR-specific features.

Spinal arteriovenous malformation/subarachnoid hemorrhage.
Syringomyelia.
HIV myelopathy.
Other myelopathies.
Spinal cord infarction.

Compressive Lesions Affecting the Spinal Cord

Spinal epidural abscess.
Spinal epidural hematoma.
Diskitis.
Neoplasm.
Metastatic.
Primary CNS.

CNS, Central nervous system; *HIV,* human immunodeficiency virus.

SPINAL CORD ISCHEMIC SYNDROMES

ICD-10CM # Varies with specific diagnosis

Systemic hypotension.
Venous or arterial occlusion.
Arterial dissection.
Thromboembolism.
Endovascular procedures.
Vasculitis.
Fibrocartilaginous embolism.
Regional hemodynamic compromise.

SPINAL TUMORS[36]

ICD-10CM # Varies with specific diagnosis

EXTRADURAL

Metastases.
Primary bone tumors arising in spine.

INTRADURAL EXTRAMEDULLARY

Meningiomas.
Neurofibromas.
Schwannomas.
Lipomas.
Arachnoid cysts.
Epidermoid cysts.
Metastasis.

INTRAMEDULLARY

Ependymoma.
Glioma.
Hemangioblastoma.
Lipoma.
Metastases.

SPLENIC CYSTS, CLASSIFICATION[17]

ICD-10CM # D73.4 Cyst of spleen

Primary (true).
Parasitic.
Nonparasitic.
Congenital.
Epidermoid.
Dermoid.
Mesothelial (serous).
Transitional.
Neoplastic.
Secondary (false): pseudocysts.
Traumatic.
Degenerative.
Inflammatory.
Hemorrhagic.

SPLENIC MASSES, FOCAL SOLID[81]

ICD-10CM # Varies with specific diagnosis

FOCAL SOLID SPLENIC MASSES

Benign

Hemangioma.
Hamartoma.
Littoral cell angioma.
Lymphangioma.
Sclerosing angiomatoid nodular transformation (SANT).
Inflammatory pseudotumor.

Malignant

Lymphoma.
Metastases.
Angiosarcoma.
Hemangiopericytoma.

Other

Infarct.

SPLENIC NODULES[81]

ICD-10CM # Varies with specific diagnosis

CAUSES OF SPLENIC NODULES

Infectious

Tuberculosis/*Mycobacterium avium*-intracellulare complex.
Pyogenic abscesses.
Histoplasmosis.
Candida abscesses.
Cat-scratch disease.
Pneumocystis jiroveci (formerly *P. carinii* pneumonia).

Inflammatory

Sarcoidosis.

Malignant

Lymphoma.
Metastases.

Other

Gamna-Gandy bodies.
Gaucher disease.

SPLENIC TUMORS, CLASSIFICATION[17]

ICD-10CM # C26.1 Malignant neoplasm of spleen

Malignant.
Lymphoproliferative disease.
Non-Hodgkin lymphoma.
Hodgkin disease.
Hairy cell leukemia.
Chronic lymphocytic leukemia.
Myeloproliferative disease.
Chronic myelogenous leukemia.
Myelofibrosis.
Primary tumors.
Angiosarcoma.
Metastatic tumors.
Benign.
Hemangiomas.
Hamartomas.
Lymphangiomas.
Sclerosing angiomatoid nodular transformation (SANT).

SPLENOMEGALY

ICD-10CM #	R16.1	Splenomegaly, not elsewhere classified
	D73.2	Chronic congestive splenomegaly
	R16.1	Splenomegaly, not elsewhere classified

Hepatic cirrhosis.
Neoplastic involvement: CML, CLL, lymphoma, multiple myeloma.
Bacterial infections: TB, infectious endocarditis, typhoid fever, splenic abscess.
Viral infections: infectious mononucleosis, viral hepatitis, HIV.
Gaucher disease and other lipid storage diseases.
Sarcoidosis.
Parasitic infections (malaria, kala-azar, histoplasmosis).
Hereditary and acquired hemolytic anemias.
Idiopathic thrombocytopenic purpura (ITP).
Collagen vascular disorders: SLE, RA (Felty syndrome), polyarteritis nodosa.
Serum sickness, drug hypersensitivity reaction.
Splenic cysts and benign tumors: hemangioma, lymphangioma.
Thrombosis of splenic or portal vein.
Polycythemia vera, myeloid metaplasia.

SPLENOMEGALY AND HEPATOMEGALY[95]

ICD-10CM #	R16.1	Splenomegaly, not elsewhere classified
	R16.0	Hepatomegaly, not elsewhere classified

CAUSES OF SPLENOMEGALY AND HEPATOSPLENOMEGALY

Massive Splenomegaly

Hematologic disease (e.g., chronic myeloid leukemia, myelofibrosis).

Moderate Splenomegaly

The above causes.
Portal hypertension.
Hematologic disease (e.g., lymphoma, leukemia, thalassemia).
Storage disease (e.g., Gaucher disease).

Small Splenomegaly

The above causes.
Infective (hepatitis, leptospirosis, malaria, bacterial endocarditis).
Hematologic disease (e.g., hemolytic anemias, essential thrombocythemia, polycythemia rubra vera).
Connective tissue diseases or vasculitis (e.g., rheumatoid arthritis, systemic lupus erythematosus, polyarteritis nodosa).
Solitary cyst, polycystic syndrome, hydatid cyst.

Infiltration (amyloid, sarcoid).

Hepatosplenomegaly

Chronic liver disease with portal hypertension.

Hematologic disease (e.g., myeloproliferative disease, lymphoma).

Infection (e.g., amyloid, sarcoid).

Connective tissue disease (e.g., systemic lupus erythematosus).

SPLENOMEGALY AND HYPERSPLENISM[51]

ICD-10CM #	R16.1	Splenomegaly, not elsewhere classified
	D73.1	Hypersplenism
	D73.81	Neutropenic splenomegaly

DIFFERENTIAL DIAGNOSIS OF SPLENOMEGALY AND HYPERSPLENISM

Infections

Acute

Viral (viral hepatitis, infectious mononucleosis, CMV infection).

Bacterial (septicemia, salmonellosis, brucellosis, splenic abscess).

Parasite (toxoplasmosis).

Subacute and Chronic

Subacute bacterial endocarditis.

Tuberculosis.

Malaria.

Kala-azar.

Fungal disease.

Inflammation

Felty syndrome.

SLE.

Serum sickness.

Rheumatic fever.

Sarcoidosis.

ALPS.

Congestive Splenomegaly

Intrahepatic

Cirrhosis.

Extrahepatic

Portal vein obstruction.

Splenic vein obstruction.

Hepatic vein occlusion (Budd-Chiari syndrome).

Chronic Passive Congestion

Heart failure.

Hematologic Disorders

RBC disorders: hemolytic anemias, thalassemia, sickle cell disorders.

Neoplasia

Malignant

MPDs.

Myeloid metaplasia.

Polycythemia rubra vera.

Essential thrombocythemia.

Chronic leukemia.

Chronic myeloid leukemia.

Chronic lymphocytic leukemia.

Hairy cell leukemia.

Lymphoma.

Acute leukemia.

Malignant histiocytosis.

Benign

Hamartoma.

Hemangioma.

Lymphangioma.

Fibroma.

Storage Diseases

Gaucher disease.

Niemann-Pick disease.

Miscellaneous

Amyloidosis.

Cysts.

ALPS, Autoimmune lymphoproliferative syndrome; *CMV,* cytomegalovirus; *MPD,* myeloproliferative disorder; *RBC,* red blood cell; *SLE,* systemic lupus erythematosus.

SPLENOMEGALY, CHILDREN[50]

ICD-10CM #	R16.1	Splenomegaly, not elsewhere classified

DISORDERS OF THE BLOOD

Hemolytic anemia: congenital/acquired.

Thalassemia.

Sickle cell disease.

Leukemia.

Osteopetrosis.

Myelofibrosis/myeloid metaplasia/thrombocythemia.

INFECTIONS: ACUTE AND CHRONIC

Viral:
- Congenital (e.g., TORCH association).
- Mononucleosis (e.g., EBV, CMV infection).
- Virus-associated hemophagocytic syndrome.
- HIV.

Bacterial:
- Sepsis/abscess.
- Brucellosis.
- Salmonellosis.
- Tularemia.
- Tuberculosis.
- Subacute bacterial endocarditis.
- Syphilis.
- Lyme disease.

Fungal:
- Histoplasmosis (disseminated).

Rickettsial:
- Rocky Mountain spotted fever.
- Cat-scratch disease.

Parasitic:
- Toxoplasmosis.
- Malaria.
- Leishmaniasis (kala-azar).
- Schistosomiasis.
- Echinococcosis.

HEPATIC/PORTAL SYSTEM DISORDERS

Acute/chronic active hepatitis.

Cirrhosis/hepatic fibrosis/biliary atresia.

Portal or splenic venous obstruction (Banti syndrome).

AUTOIMMUNE DISEASE

Juvenile rheumatoid arthritis.

Systemic lupus erythematosus.

Autoimmune lymphoproliferative syndrome (Canale–Smith syndrome).

NEOPLASMS/CYSTS

Lymphomas (Hodgkin and non-Hodgkin).

Hemangiomas/lymphangiomas.

Hamartomas.

Congenital or acquired (posttraumatic) cysts.

STORAGE DISEASES/INBORN ERRORS OF METABOLISM

Lipidoses: Gaucher disease, Niemann–Pick disease, others.

Mucopolysaccharidoses.

Defects in carbohydrate metabolism: galactosemia, fructose intolerance.

Sea-blue histiocyte syndrome.

MISCELLANEOUS DISORDERS

Histiocytoses:
- Reactive.
- Langerhans cell.
- Malignant.

Sarcoidosis.

Congestive heart failure.

Familial Mediterranean fever.

CMV, Cytomegalovirus; *EBV,* Epstein-Barr virus; *TORCH,* toxoplasmosis, other infections, rubella, cytomegalovirus infection, herpes simplex.

SPONTANEOUS PNEUMOTHORAX[65]

ICD-10CM #	J93.0	Spontaneous tension pneumothorax
	J93.11	Primary spontaneous pneumothorax
	J93.12	Secondary spontaneous pneumothorax

CAUSES OF SECONDARY SPONTANEOUS PNEUMOTHORAX

Airway Disease

Chronic obstructive pulmonary disease.

Asthma.

Cystic fibrosis.

Infections

Necrotizing bacterial pneumonia, lung abscess.

Pneumocystis jiroveci pneumonia.

Tuberculosis.

Interstitial Lung Disease

Sarcoidosis.

Idiopathic pulmonary fibrosis.

Lymphangiomyomatosis.

Tuberous sclerosis.

Pneumoconioses.

Neoplasms

Primary lung cancers.

Pulmonary or pleural metastases.

Miscellaneous

Connective tissue diseases.

Pulmonary infarction.

Endometriosis, catamenial pneumothorax.

STATURAL OVERGROWTH[67]

ICD-10CM #	E34.4	Constitutional tall stature

FETAL OVERGROWTH

Maternal diabetes mellitus.
Cerebral gigantism (Sotos syndrome).
Weaver syndrome.
Beckwith-Wiedemann syndrome.
Other insulin-like growth factor 2 (IGF2) excess syndromes.

POSTNATAL OVERGROWTH LEADING TO CHILDHOOD TALL STATURE

Familial (constitutional) tall stature.
Cerebral gigantism.
Beckwith-Wiedemann syndrome.
Exogenous obesity.
Excess growth hormone (GH) secretion (pituitary gigantism).
McCune-Albright syndrome or multiple endocrine neoplasia (MEN) associated with excess GH secretion.
Precocious puberty.
Marfan syndrome.
Klinefelter syndrome (XXY).
Weaver syndrome.
Fragile X syndrome.
Homocystinuria.
XYY.
Hyperthyroidism.

POSTNATAL OVERGROWTH LEADING TO ADULT TALL STATURE

Familial (constitutional) tall stature.
Androgen or estrogen deficiency/estrogen resistance (in males).
Testicular feminization.
Excess GH secretion.
Marfan syndrome.
Klinefelter syndrome (XXY).
XYY.

STEATOHEPATITIS

ICD-10CM #	K76.0	Fatty (change of) liver, not elsewhere classified
	K76.89	Other specified diseases of liver

Alcohol abuse.
Obesity.
DM.
Parenteral nutrition.
Medications (high-dose estrogen, amiodarone, corticosteroids, methotrexate, nifedipine).
Jejunoileal bypass.
Abetalipoproteinemia.
Wilson disease, Weber-Christian disease.

STEATOSIS, MACROVESICULAR AND MICROVESICULAR[39]

ICD-10CM #	K75.81	Nonalcoholic steatohepatitis (NASH)
	K70.9	Alcoholic liver disease, unspecified

Common Causes of Macrovesicular and Microvesicular Steatosis

Macrovesicular Steatosis	Microvesicular Steatosis
Obesity, type 2 diabetes, metabolic syndrome, and dyslipidemia (nonalcoholic fatty liver disease).	Reye syndrome. Medications (valproate, antiretroviral medicines, intravenous tetracycline).
Excessive alcohol consumption.	Heat stroke.
Hepatitis C (genotype 3).	Acute fatty liver of pregnancy.
Wilson disease.	HELLP syndrome.
Lipodystrophy starvation.	Inborn errors of metabolism (lecithin–cholesterol acyltransferase deficiency, cholesterol ester storage disease, Wolman disease).
Jejunoileal bypass.	
Parenteral nutrition.	
Medications (amiodarone, methotrexate, tamoxifen, corticosteroids, antipsychotics).	

HELLP = *H*emolysis, *el*evated *l*iver enzymes, and *l*ow *p*latelets.

STERILE PYURIA[19]

ICD-10CM #	R82.998	Other abnormal findings in urine

Common Causes of Sterile Pyuria
- Nonspecific urethritis in males.
- Prostatitis.
- Renal tract neoplasm.
- Renal calculi.
- Catheterization.
- Renal tuberculosis.
- Previous antibiotic treatment.

STOMATITIS, BULLOUS

ICD-10CM #	K12.30	Oral mucositis (ulcerative), unspecified

Erythema multiforme.
Erosive lichen planus.
Bullous pemphigoid.
SLE.
Pemphigus vulgaris.
Mucous membrane pemphigoid.

STRIDOR IN NEONATES[1]

ICD-10CM #	R06.1	Stridor

INTRINSIC LESIONS

Larynx

Laryngomalacia.
Infection (laryngitis).
Vocal cord paralysis.
Laryngeal web.
Laryngocele or laryngeal cyst.
Laryngotracheal esophageal cleft.
Foreign body.

Trachea

Tracheomalacia.
Tracheal stenosis.
Tracheoesophageal fistula.
Subglottic hemangioma.
Tracheal web.

Extrinsic Compression

Vascular ring.
Anomalous innominate artery.
Mediastinal mass.
Esophageal foreign body.

Other

Macroglossia.
Gastroesophageal reflux.

STRIDOR, PEDIATRIC AGE[9]

ICD-10CM #	R06.1	Stridor

RECURRENT

Allergic (spasmodic) croup.
Respiratory infections in a child with otherwise asymptomatic anatomic narrowing of the large airways.
Laryngomalacia.

PERSISTENT

Laryngeal obstruction:
- Laryngomalacia.
- Papillomas, other tumors.
- Cysts and laryngoceles.
- Laryngeal webs.
- Bilateral abductor paralysis of the cords.
- Foreign body.

Tracheobronchial disease:
- Tracheomalacia.
- Subglottic tracheal webs.

Endotracheal, endobronchial tumors.
Subglottic tracheal stenosis.
Congenital.
Acquired.
Extrinsic masses.
Mediastinal masses.
Vascular ring.
Lobar emphysema.
Bronchogenic cysts.
Thyroid enlargement.
Esophageal foreign body.
Tracheoesophageal fistulas.
Other.
Gastroesophageal reflux.
Macroglossia, Pierre Robin syndrome.
Cri-du-chat syndrome.
Hysterical stridor.
Hypocalcemia.

STROKE[91]

ICD-10CM #	Varies with specific diagnosis

STROKE "MIMICS"

Hypoglycemia.
Drug overdose or intoxication.
Hysterical conversion reaction.
Hyperventilation.
Metabolic encephalopathy.
Migraine.
Syncope.
Transient global amnesia.

Seizures.
Vestibular vertigo.

STROKE, PEDIATRIC AGE[57]

ICD-10CM #	I67.89	Other cerebrovascular disease

CARDIAC DISEASE

Congenital:
- Aortic stenosis.
- Mitral stenosis; mitral prolapse.
- Ventricular septal defects.
- Patent ductus arteriosus.
- Cyanotic congenital heart disease involving right-to-left shunt.

Acquired:
- Endocarditis (bacterial, SLE).
- Kawasaki disease.
- Cardiomyopathy.
- Atrial myxoma.
- Arrhythmia.
- Paradoxical emboli through patent foramen ovale.
- Rheumatic fever.
- Prosthetic heart valve.

HEMATOLOGIC ABNORMALITIES

Hemoglobinopathies:
- Sickle cell (SS) disease.
- Sickle (SC) disease.

Polycythemia.
Leukemia/lymphoma.
Thrombocytopenia.
Thrombocytosis.
Disorders of coagulation:
- Protein C deficiency.
- Protein S deficiency.
- Factor V Leiden.
- Antithrombin III deficiency.
- Lupus anticoagulant.

Oral contraceptive pill use.
Pregnancy and the postpartum state.
Disseminated intravascular coagulation.
Paroxysmal nocturnal hemoglobinuria.
Inflammatory bowel disease (thrombosis).

INFLAMMATORY DISORDERS

Meningitis:
- Viral.
- Bacterial.
- Tuberculosis.

Systemic infection:
- Viremia.
- Bacteremia.
- Local head and neck infections.

Drug-induced inflammation:
- Amphetamine.
- Cocaine.

Autoimmune disease:
- SLE.
- Juvenile RA.
- Takayasu arteritis.
- Mixed connective tissue disease.
- Polyarteritis nodosum.
- Primary CNS vasculitis.
- Sarcoidosis.
- Behçet syndrome.
- Granulomatosis with polyangiitis.

METABOLIC DISEASE ASSOCIATED WITH STROKE

Homocystinuria.
Pseudoxanthoma elasticum.
Fabry disease.
Sulfite oxidase deficiency.
Mitochondrial disorders:
- MELAS.
- Leigh syndrome.

Ornithine transcarbamylase deficiency.

INTRACEREBRAL VASCULAR PROCESSES

Ruptured aneurysm.
Arteriovenous malformation.
Fibromuscular dysplasia.
Moyamoya disease.
Migraine headache.
Postsubarachnoid hemorrhage vasospasm.
Hereditary hemorrhagic telangiectasia.
Sturge-Weber syndrome.
Carotid artery dissection.
Postvaricella.

TRAUMA AND OTHER EXTERNAL CAUSES

Child abuse.
Head trauma/neck trauma.
Oral trauma.
Placental embolism.
ECMO therapy.

CNS, Central nervous system; *ECMO,* extracorporeal membrane oxygenation; *MELAS,* mitochondrial encephalomyopathy, lactic acidosis, and stroke.

STROKE, YOUNG ADULT, CAUSES[3]

ICD-10CM #	I64	Stroke
	I67.89	Other cerebrovascular disease

Cardiac factors (ASD, MVP, patent foramen ovale).
Inflammatory factors (SLE, polyarteritis nodosa).
Infections (endocarditis, neurosyphilis).
Drugs (cocaine, heroin, oral contraceptives, decongestants).
Arterial dissection.
Hematolic factors (DIC, TTP, deficiency of protein S, protein C, antithrombin III).
Migraine.
Postpartum angiopathy.
Other: premature atherosclerosis, fibromuscular dysplasia.

ST-SEGMENT DEPRESSION, NONCORONARY CAUSES[12]

ICD-10CM #	R94.31	Abnormal electrocardiogram

NONCORONARY CAUSES OF ST-SEGMENT DEPRESSION

Anemia.
Cardiomyopathy.
Digitalis use.
Glucose load.
Hyperventilation.
Hypokalemia.
Intraventricular conduction disturbance.
Left ventricular hypertrophy.
Mitral valve prolapse.
Preexcitation syndrome.
Severe aortic stenosis.
Severe hypertension.
Severe hypoxia.
Severe volume overload (aortic, mitral regurgitation).
Sudden excessive exercise.
Supraventricular tachyarrhythmias.

ST-SEGMENT ELEVATION[1]

ICD-10CM #	R94.31	Abnormal electrocardiogram [ECG] [EKG]

DIFFERENTIAL DIAGNOSIS OF ST-SEGMENT ELEVATION ON ELECTROCARDIOGRAPHY

ST-segment elevation myocardial infarction.
Pericarditis.
Benign early repolarization.
Left bundle branch block.
Left ventricular hypertrophy.
Left ventricular aneurysm.
Paced ventricular rhythms.
Prinzmetal angina.
Hyperkalemia.
Hypothermia with Osborne waves.
Intracranial hemorrhage.
Brugada syndrome.
Normal variant.

ST SEGMENT ELEVATIONS, NONISCHEMIC

ICD-10CM #	R94.31	Abnormal electrocardiogram [ECG] [EKG]

Early repolarization.
Acute pericarditis.
LVH.
Normal pattern variant.
LBBB.
Pulmonary embolism.
Hyperkalemia.
Postcardioversion.

SUDDEN CARDIAC DEATH[64]

ICD-10CM #	**Z86.74**	Personal history of sudden cardiac arrest
	Z82.41	Family history of sudden cardiac death

CAUSES OF AND CONTRIBUTING FACTORS IN SUDDEN CARDIAC DEATH

Coronary Artery Abnormalities

Coronary atherosclerosis:
- Chronic coronary atherosclerosis with acute or transient myocardial ischemia—thrombosis, spasm, physical stress.

Acute myocardial infarction, onset and early phase.
Chronic atherosclerosis with a change in myocardial substrate, including previous myocardial infarction.
Congenital abnormalities of coronary arteries:
Anomalous origin from the pulmonary artery.
Other coronary arteriovenous fistula.
Origin of a left coronary branch from the right or noncoronary sinus of Valsalva.
Origin of the right coronary artery from the left sinus of Valsalva.
Hypoplastic or aplastic coronary arteries.
Coronary-intracardiac shunt.
Coronary artery embolism:
Aortic or mitral endocarditis.
Prosthetic aortic or mitral valves.
Abnormal native valves or left ventricular mural thrombus.
Platelet embolism.
Coronary arteritis:
Polyarteritis nodosa, progressive systemic sclerosis, giant cell arteritis.
Mucocutaneous lymph node syndrome (Kawasaki disease).
Syphilitic coronary ostial stenosis.
Miscellaneous mechanical obstruction of the coronary arteries:
Coronary artery dissection in Marfan syndrome.
Coronary artery dissection in pregnancy.
Prolapse of aortic valve myxomatous polyps into the coronary ostia.
Dissection or rupture of the sinus of Valsalva.
Functional obstruction of the coronary arteries:
Coronary artery spasm with or without atherosclerosis.
Myocardial bridges.

Hypertrophy of the Ventricular Myocardium

Left ventricular hypertrophy associated with coronary heart disease.
Hypertensive heart disease without significant coronary atherosclerosis.
Hypertrophic myocardium secondary to valvular heart disease.
Hypertrophic cardiomyopathy:
Obstructive.
Nonobstructive.
Primary or secondary pulmonary hypertension:
Advanced chronic right ventricular overload.
Pulmonary hypertension in pregnancy (highest risk peripartum).

Myocardial Diseases and Dysfunction, With or Without Heart Failure

Chronic congestive heart failure:
Ischemic cardiomyopathy.
Idiopathic dilated cardiomyopathy, acquired.
Hereditary dilated cardiomyopathy.
Alcoholic cardiomyopathy.
Hypertensive cardiomyopathy.
Postmyocarditis cardiomyopathy.
Peripartum cardiomyopathy.
Idiopathic fibrosis.
Acute and subacute cardiac failure:
Massive acute myocardial infarction.
Myocarditis, acute or fulminant.
Acute alcoholic cardiac dysfunction.
Takotsubo syndrome (uncertain risk for sudden death).
Ball valve embolism in aortic stenosis or prosthesis.
Mechanical disruptions of cardiac structures:
Rupture of the ventricular free wall.
Disruption of the mitral apparatus:
Papillary muscle.
Chordae tendineae.
Leaflet.
Rupture of the interventricular septum.
Acute pulmonary edema in noncompliant ventricles.

Inflammatory, Infiltrative, Neoplastic, and Degenerative Processes

Viral myocarditis, with or without ventricular dysfunction:
Acute phase.
Postmyocarditis interstitial fibrosis.
Myocarditis associated with the vasculitides.
Sarcoidosis.
Progressive systemic sclerosis.
Amyloidosis.
Hemochromatosis.
Idiopathic giant cell myocarditis.
Chagas disease.
Cardiac ganglionitis.
Arrhythmogenic right ventricular dysplasia, right ventricular cardiomyopathy.
Neuromuscular diseases (e.g., muscular dystrophy, Friedreich ataxia, myotonic dystrophy).
Intramural tumors:
Primary.
Metastatic.
Obstructive intracavitary tumors:
Neoplastic.
Thrombotic.

Diseases of the Cardiac Valves

Valvular aortic stenosis/insufficiency.
Mitral valve disruption.
Mitral valve prolapse.
Endocarditis.
Prosthetic valve dysfunction.

Congenital Heart Disease

Congenital aortic (potentially high risk) or pulmonic (low risk) valve stenosis.
Congenital septal defects with Eisenmenger physiology:
Advanced disease.
During labor and delivery.
Late after surgical repair of congenital lesions (e.g., tetralogy of Fallot).

Electrophysiologic Abnormalities

Abnormalities of the conducting system:
Fibrosis of the His-Purkinje system:
Primary degeneration (Lenègre disease).
Secondary to fibrosis and calcification of the "cardiac skeleton" (Lev disease).
Postviral conducting system fibrosis.
Hereditary conducting system disease.
Anomalous pathways of conduction (Wolff-Parkinson-White syndrome, short refractory period bypass).
Abnormalities of repolarization:
Congenital abnormalities in duration of the QT interval:
Congenital long–QT interval syndromes:
Romano-Ward syndrome (without deafness).
Jervell and Lange-Nielsen syndrome (with deafness).
Congenital short–QT interval syndrome.
Acquired (or provoked) long–QT interval syndromes:
Drug effect (with genetic predisposition?):
Cardiac, antiarrhythmic.
Noncardiac.
Drug interactions.
Electrolyte abnormality (response modified by genetic predisposition?).
Toxic substances.
Hypothermia.
CNS injury, subarachnoid hemorrhage.
Brugada syndrome—right bundle branch block and ST-segment elevations in the absence of ischemia:
Early repolarization syndrome.
Ventricular fibrillation of unknown or uncertain cause:
Absence of identifiable structural or functional causes:
"Idiopathic" ventricular fibrillation.
Short-coupled torsades de pointes, polymorphic ventricular tachycardia.
Nonspecific fibrofatty infiltration in a previously healthy victim (variation of right ventricular dysplasia?).
Sleep-death in Southeast Asians (see VIIB3, Brugada syndrome):
Bangungut.
Pokkuri.
Lai-tai.

Electrical Instability Related to Neurohumoral and Central Nervous System Influences

Catecholaminergic polymorphic ventricular tachycardia.
Other catecholamine-dependent arrhythmias.
CNS related:
Psychic stress, emotional extremes (Takotsubo syndrome).
Auditory related:
"Voodoo death" in primitive cultures.
Diseases of the cardiac nerves.
Arrhythmia expression in congenital long–QT interval syndrome.

Sudden Infant Death Syndrome and Sudden Death in Children

Sudden infant death syndrome:
Immature respiratory control function.
Long–QT interval syndrome.
Congenital heart disease.
Myocarditis.
Sudden death in children:
Eisenmenger syndrome, aortic stenosis, hypertrophic cardiomyopathy, pulmonary atresia.
After corrective surgery for congenital heart disease.
Myocarditis.
Genetic disorders of electrical function (e.g., long–QT interval syndrome).
No identified structural or functional cause.

Miscellaneous

Sudden death during extreme physical activity (seek predisposing causes).
Commotio cordis—blunt chest trauma.
Mechanical interference with venous return:
Acute cardiac tamponade.
Massive pulmonary embolism.

Acute intracardiac thrombosis.
Dissecting aneurysm of the aorta.
Toxic and metabolic disturbances (other than the QT interval effects listed above):
Electrolyte disturbances.
Metabolic disturbances.
Proarrhythmic effects of antiarrhythmic drugs.
Proarrhythmic effects of noncardiac drugs.
Mimics sudden cardiac death:
"Café coronary."
Acute alcoholic states ("holiday heart").
Acute asthmatic attacks.
Air or amniotic fluid embolism.

SUDDEN DEATH, PEDIATRIC AGE[9]

ICD-10CM # R99 Ill-defined and unknown cause of mortality

SIDS AND SIDS "MIMICS"

SIDS.
Long QT syndromes.
Inborn errors of metabolism.
Child abuse.
Myocarditis.
Duct-dependent congenital heart disease.

CORRECTED OR UNOPERATED CONGENITAL HEART DISEASE

Aortic stenosis.
Tetralogy of Fallot.
Transposition of great vessels (postoperative atrial switch).
Mitral valve prolapse.
Hematologic left heart syndrome.
Eisenmenger syndrome.

CORONARY ARTERIAL DISEASE

Anomalous origin.
Anomalous tract.
Kawasaki disease.
Periarteritis.
Arterial dissection.
Marfan syndrome.
Myocardial infarction.

MYOCARDIAL DISEASE

Myocarditis.
Hypertrophic cardiomyopathy.
Dilated cardiomyopathy.
Arrhythmogenic right ventricular dysplasia.

CONDUCTION SYSTEM ABNORMALITY/ARRHYTHMIA

Long QT syndromes.
Proarrhythmic drugs.
Preexcitation syndromes.
Heart block.
Commotio cordis.
Idiopathic ventricular fibrillation.
Heart tumor.

MISCELLANEOUS

Pulmonary hypertension.
Pulmonary embolism.
Heat stroke.
Cocaine.
Anorexia nervosa.
Electrolyte disturbances.

SIDS, Sudden infant death syndrome.

SUDDEN DEATH, YOUNG ATHLETE

ICD-10CM # R99 Ill-defined and unknown cause of mortality

Hypertrophic cardiomyopathy.
Coronary artery anomalies.
Myocarditis.
Ruptured aortic aneurysm (Marfan syndrome).
Arrhythmias.
Aortic valve stenosis.
Asthma.
Trauma (cerebral, cardiac).
Drug and alcohol abuse.
Heat stroke.
Cardiac sarcoidosis.
Atherosclerotic coronary artery disease.
Dilated cardiomyopathy.

SUPERIOR VENA CAVA SEGMENT ABNORMALITIES[14]

ICD-10CM # Q26.8 Other congenital malformations of great veins

Differential Diagnosis of an Abnormal Superior Vena Cava Segment
Increased SVC Pressure
SVC obstruction:
Lung cancer.
Stricture resulting from long-term cannulation.
Right-sided heart failure.
Increased SVC Volume
Vein of Galen aneurysm.
Upper extremity AVM.
Partial anomalous pulmonary venous connection.
Interruption of the IVC with azygos continuation.
AVM, Arteriovenous malformation; *IVC,* inferior vena cava; *SVC,* superior vena cava.

SWOLLEN LIMB

ICD-10CM # M79.89 Other specified soft tissue disorders

Trauma.
Insect bite.
Abscess.
Lymphedema.
Thrombophlebitis.
Lipoma.
Neurofibroma.
Postphlebitic syndrome.
Myositis ossificans.
Nephrosis, cirrhosis, CHF.
Hypoalbuminemia.
Varicose veins.

SYMPATHOMIMETIC TOXICITY[19]

ICD-10CM # Varies with specific diagnosis

Substances that can Cause Sympathomimetic Toxicity
Methamphetamines (ice [crystals]); speed (powder), pills, base (oily powder).
3, 4-methylenedioxymethamphetamine (MDMA or Ecstasy).
Phenylethylamines (bath salts).
Cocaine.
Ma huang (herbal ecstasy).
Paramethoxyamphetamine (PMA or "death").
Mephedrone (4-MMC).
Pseudoephedrine.
Methylphenidate.
Imidazolines: decongestants (naphazoline, oxymetazoline, tetrahydrozoline).
Clonidine withdrawal.[49]
Dexamphetamine.
Caffeine.
Yohimbe-containing supplements (used in combinations with stimulants).

[49] Clonidine is a central α_2 agonist; it does not cause acute sympathomimetic syndrome except in abrupt withdrawals.

TALL STATURE[69]

ICD-10CM # E22.0 Acromegaly and pituitary gigantism

CONSTITUTIONAL (FAMILIAL OR GENETIC)—MOST COMMON CAUSE

Endocrine Causes
Growth hormone excess—gigantism.
Sexual precocity (tall as children, short as adults):
True sexual precocity.
Pseudosexual precocity.
Androgen deficiency:
Klinefelter syndrome.
Bilateral anorchism.

GENETIC CAUSES

Klinefelter syndrome.
Syndromes of XYY, XXYY.

MISCELLANEOUS SYNDROMES AND DISORDERS

Cerebral gigantism or Sotos syndrome: prominent forehead, hypertelorism, high arched palate, dolichocephaly, mental retardation, large hands and feet, and premature eruption of teeth. Large at birth, with most rapid growth in first 4 yr of life.
Marfan syndrome: disorder of mesodermal tissues, subluxation of the lenses, arachnodactyly, and aortic aneurysm.
Homocystinuria: same phenotype as Marfan syndrome.
Obesity: tall as infants, children, and adolescents.

Total lipodystrophy: large hands and feet, generalized loss of subcutaneous fat, insulin-resistant DM, and hepatomegaly.
Beckwith-Wiedemann syndrome: neonatal tallness, omphalocele, macroglossia, and neonatal hypoglycemia.
Weaver-Smith syndrome: excessive intrauterine growth, mental retardation, megalocephaly, widened bifrontal diameter, hypertelorism, large ears, micrognathia, camptodactyly, broad thumbs, and limited extension of elbows and knees.
Marshall-Smith syndrome: excessive intrauterine growth, mental retardation, blue sclerae, failure to thrive, and early death.

TARDIVE DYSKINESIA[35]

ICD-10CM #	R27.9	Unspecified lack of coordination
	F44.4	Conversion disorder with motor symptom or deficit
	F44.6	Conversion disorder with sensory symptom or deficit
	G24.4	Idiopathic orofacial dystonia

DIFFERENTIAL DIAGNOSIS

Medications (antidepressants, anticholinergics, amphetamines, lithium, L-dopa, phenytoin).
Brain neoplasms.
Ill-fitting dentures.
Huntington disease.
Idiopathic dystonias (tics, blepharospasm, aging).
Wilson disease.
Extrapyramidal syndrome (postanoxic or postencephalitic).
Torsion dystonia.

TASTE AND SMELL LOSS[3]

ICD-10CM #	R43.0	Anosmia
	R43.1	Parosmia
	R43.2	Parageusia

TASTE

Local: radiation therapy.
Systemic: cancer, renal failure, hepatic failure, nutritional deficiency (vitamin B_{12}, zinc), Cushing syndrome, hypothyroidism, DM, infection (influenza), drugs (antirheumatic and antiproliferative).
Neurologic: Bell palsy, familial dysautonomia, multiple sclerosis.

SMELL

Local: allergic rhinitis, sinusitis, nasal polyposis, bronchial asthma.
Systemic: renal failure, hepatic failure, nutritional deficiency (vitamin B_{12}), Cushing syndrome, hypothyroidism, DM, infection (viral hepatitis, influenza), drugs (nasal sprays, antibiotics).
Neurologic: head trauma, multiple sclerosis, Parkinson disease, frontal brain tumor.

TELANGIECTASIA

ICD-10CM #	I78.8	Other diseases of capillaries
	I78.9	Disease of capillaries, unspecified

Oral contraceptive agents.
Pregnancy.
Rosacea.
Varicose veins.
Trauma.
Drug induced (corticosteroids, systemic or topical).
Spider telangiectases.
Hepatic cirrhosis.
Mastocytosis.
SLE, dermatomyositis, systemic sclerosis.

TENDINOPATHY[65]

ICD-10CM #	M67.90	Unspecified disorder of synovium and tendon, unspecified site
	M71.9	Bursopathy, unspecified

INTRINSIC FACTORS

Anatomic Factors
Malalignment.
Muscle weakness or imbalance.
Muscle inflexibility.
Decreased vascularity.
Systemic Factors
Inflammatory conditions (e.g., SLE).
Pregnancy.
Quinolone-induced tendinopathy.
Age-Related Factors
Tendon degeneration.
Increased tendon stiffness.
Tendon calcification.
Decreased vascularity.

EXTRINSIC FACTORS

Repetitive Mechanical Load
Excessive duration.
Excessive frequency.
Excessive intensity.
Poor technique.
Workplace factors.
Equipment Problems
Footwear.
Athletic field surface.
Equipment factors (e.g., racquet size).
Protective gear.

TESTICULAR CYSTIC LESIONS[81]

ICD-10CM # Varies with specific diagnosis

Benign
Tunica albuginea cysts.
Tunica vaginalis cysts.
Intratesticular cysts.
Tubular ectasia of rete testis.
Cystic dysplasia.
Epidermoid cysts.
Abscess.

Malignant
Nonseminomatous germ cell tumor.
Necrosis or hemorrhage in tumor.
Tubular obstruction by tumor.
Lymphoma.

TESTICULAR FAILURE[25]

ICD-10CM # E29 Testicular dysfunction

PRIMARY

Klinefelter syndrome (XXY).
XYY.
Vanishing testes syndrome (in utero or early postnatal torsion).
Noonan syndrome.
Varicocele.
Myotonic dystrophy.
Orchitis (mumps, gonorrhea).
Cryptorchidism.
Chemical exposure.
Irradiation to testes.
Spinal cord injury.
Polyglandular failure.
Idiopathic oligospermia or azoospermia.
Germinal cell aplasia (Sertoli cell-only syndrome).
Idiopathic testicular failure.
Testicular torsion.
Testicular trauma.
Diethylstilbestrol (maternal use during pregnancy leading to in utero estrogen exposure).
Testicular tumor with subsequent irradiation therapy, chemotherapy, or surgery (retroperitoneal lymph node dissection or orchiectomy).

SECONDARY

Delayed puberty.
Kallmann syndrome.
Isolated gonadotropin deficiency.
Prader-Labhart-Willi syndrome.
Lawrence-Moon-Biedl syndrome.
CNS irradiation.
Prepubertal panhypopituitarism.
Postpubertal panhypopituitarism.
Hypogonadism secondary to hyperprolactinemia.
Adrenogenital syndrome.
Chronic liver disease.
Chronic renal failure/uremia.
Hemochromatosis.
Cushing syndrome.
Malnutrition.
Massive obesity.
Sickle cell anemia.
Hyper/hypothyroidism.
Anabolic steroid use.

TESTICULAR PAIN

ICD-10CM #	N50.9	Disorder of male genital organs, unspecified
	R10.2	Pelvic and perineal pain

Testicular torsion.
Trauma.
Epididymitis.

Orchitis.
Neoplasm.
Urolithiasis.
Inguinal hernia.
Infection (cellulitis, abscess, folliculitis).
Anxiety.

TESTICULAR SIZE VARIATIONS[25]

ICD-10CM #	N50.0	Atrophy of testis
	N44.2	Benign cyst of testis
	N44.8	Other noninflammatory disorders of the testis
	N50.3	Cyst of epididymis
	N50.8	Other specified disorders of male genital organs
	N53.12	Painful ejaculation
	E29.1	Testicular hypofunction

SMALL TESTES

Hypothalamic-pituitary dysfunction.
Gonadotropin deficiency.
Growth hormone deficiency.
Normal variant.
Primary hypogonadism.
Autoimmune destruction.
Chemotherapy.
Cryptorchidism.
Irradiation.
Klinefelter syndrome.
Orchiditis.
Testicular regression syndrome.
Torsion.
Trauma.

LARGE TESTES

Adrenal rest tissue.
Compensatory.
Fragile X syndrome.
Idiopathic.
Tumor.

TETANUS[65]

ICD-10CM #	A35	Other tetanus

TETANUS "MIMICS"

Acute abdomen.
Black widow spider bite.
Dental abscess.
Dislocated mandible.
Dystonic reaction.
Encephalitis.
Head trauma.
Hyperventilation syndrome.
Hypocalcemia.
Meningitis.
Peritonsillar abscess.
Progressive fluctuating muscular rigidity (stiff-man syndrome).
Psychogenic.
Rabies.
Sepsis.
Subarachnoid hemorrhage.
Status epilepticus.
Strychnine poisoning.
Temporomandibular joint syndrome.

THORACIC AORTIC ANEURYSMS[14]

ICD-10CM #	I71.2	Thoracic aortic aneurysm, without rupture

ANEURYSMS OF THE THORACIC AORTA

By Location

Sinuses of Valsalva:
- Infected.
- Congenital.
- Trauma.
- Annuloaortic ectasia.

Ascending aorta:
- Aortitis.
- Takayasu disease.
- Syphilis.
- Trauma.
- Annuloaortic ectasia.
- Marfan syndrome.
- Ehlers-Danlos syndrome.

Aortic arch:
- Trauma.
- Infected.
- Syphilis.
- Of patent ductus arteriosus.
- Coarctation.
- Takayasu disease.
- Duct of Kommerell from aberrant right subclavian artery.

Descending aorta:
- Atherosclerosis.
- Infected.
- Inflammatory.
- Syphilis.
- Takayasu disease.

By Shape

Saccular:
- Trauma.
- Infected.
- Of ductus arteriosus.
- Syphilis.
- Penetrating ulcer.

Fusiform:
- Cystic medial necrosis.
- Atherosclerosis.

By Integrity of the Aortic Wall

True:
- Cystic medial necrosis.
- Atherosclerosis.
- Collagen vascular disease.
- Rheumatoid arthritis.
- Ankylosing spondylitis.
- Aortitis.

False:
- Trauma.
- Infected.
- Penetrating ulcer.
- Rupture.
- After aortotomy.

THROMBOCYTOPENIA

ICD-10CM #	D47.3	Essential (hemorrhagic) thrombocythemia
	D69.59	Other secondary thrombocytopenia
	D69.6	Thrombocytopenia, unspecified

INCREASED DESTRUCTION

Immunologic

Drugs: quinine, quinidine, digitalis, procainamide, thiazide diuretics, sulfonamides, phenytoin, aspirin, penicillin, heparin, gold, meprobamate, sulfa drugs, phenylbutazone, NSAIDs, methyldopa, cimetidine, furosemide, INH, cephalosporins, chlorpropamide, organic arsenicals, chloroquine, platelet glycoprotein IIb/IIIa receptor inhibitors, ranitidine, indomethacin, carboplatin, ticlopidine, clopidogrel.
Idiopathic thrombocytopenic purpura (ITP).
Transfusion reaction: transfusion of platelets with plasminogen activator (PLA) in recipients without PLA-1.
Fetal/maternal incompatibility.
Collagen vascular diseases (e.g., SLE).
Autoimmune hemolytic anemia.
Lymphoreticular disorders (e.g., CLL).

Nonimmunologic

Prosthetic heart valves.
Thrombotic thrombocytopenic purpura (TTP).
Sepsis.
DIC.
Hemolytic-uremic syndrome (HUS).
Giant cavernous hemangioma.

DECREASED PRODUCTION

Abnormal marrow.
Marrow infiltration (e.g., leukemia, lymphoma, fibrosis).
Marrow suppression (e.g., chemotherapy, alcohol, radiation).
Hereditary disorders.
Wiskott-Aldrich syndrome: X-linked disorder characterized by thrombocytopenia, eczema, and repeated infections.
May-Hegglin anomaly: increased megakaryocytes but ineffective thrombopoiesis.
Vitamin deficiencies (e.g., vitamin B_{12}, folic acid).

SPLENIC SEQUESTRATION, HYPERSPLENISM

Dilutional, as a result of massive transfusion.

THROMBOCYTOPENIA, IN PREGNANCY[50]

ICD-10CM #	D69.59	Other secondary thrombocytopenia

Incidental thrombocytopenia of pregnancy (gestational thrombocytopenia).
Preeclampsia/eclampsia.
- Peripartum/postpartum thrombotic microangiopathy.

Disseminated intravascular coagulation (DIC) secondary to:
- Abruptio placentae.
- Endometritis.
- Amniotic fluid embolism.
- Retained fetus.

Thrombotic thrombocytopenic purpura.
Hemolytic-uremic syndrome.

THROMBOCYTOPENIA, INHERITED DISORDERS[3]

ICD-10CM # D47.3 Essential (hemorrhagic) thrombocythemia

Amegakaryocytic thrombocytopenia.
Thrombocytopenia–absent radii.
MYH9-related thrombocytopenia:
May-Hegglin anomaly.
Fechtner syndrome.
Epstein syndrome.
Sebastian syndrome.
X-linked macrothrombocytopenia.
Wiskott-Aldrich syndrome.
X-linked thrombocytopenia.
Thrombocytopenia and radioulnar synostosis.
Familial platelet disorder—AML.
Familial dominant thrombocytopenia.
Paris-Trousseau thrombocytopenia.
Bernard-Soulier syndrome.
Bernard-Soulier carrier/Mediterranean macrothrombocytopenia.

THROMBOCYTOPENIA IN NEWBORNS, DIFFERENTIAL DIAGNOSIS[49]

ICD-10CM #	D47.3	Essential (hemorrhagic) thrombocythemia
	D69.59	Other secondary thrombocytopenia
	D69.6	Thrombocytopenia, unspecified

DIFFERENTIAL DIAGNOSIS OF THROMBOCYTOPENIA IN NEWBORNS

Perinatal hypoxemia
Placental insufficiency
Congenital infection
- Sepsis.
- Toxoplasmosis.
- Rubella.
- Cytomegalovirus.

Autoimmune:
- Maternal immune thrombocytopenia.
- Maternal systemic lupus erythematosus.

Disseminated intravascular coagulation
Maternal drug exposure
Congenital heart disease
Hereditary thrombocytopenia
- MYH9 macrothrombocytopenia (including May-Hegglin anomaly).
- Thrombocytopenia absent radii syndrome.
- Amegakaryocytic thrombocytopenia.
- Wiskott-Aldrich syndrome.
- Fanconi anemia.

Hemangioma with thrombocytopenia
- Kasabach-Merritt syndrome.

Bone marrow infiltration
- Congenital leukemia.

THROMBOCYTOSIS

ICD-10CM # D75.9 Disease of blood and blood-forming organs, unspecified

Iron deficiency.
Posthemorrhage.
Neoplasms (GI tract).
CML.
Polycythemia vera.
Myelofibrosis with myeloid metaplasia.
Infections.
After splenectomy.
Postpartum.
Hemophilia.
Pancreatitis.
Cirrhosis.
Idiopathic.

THROMBOSIS OR THROMBOTIC DIATHESIS[3]

ICD-10CM # I74.09 Other arterial embolism and thrombosis of abdominal aorta

DIFFERENTIAL DIAGNOSIS OF THE PATIENT PRESENTING WITH THROMBOSIS OR THROMBOTIC DIATHESIS

Inherited (Primary) Hypercoagulable States

Activated protein C resistance caused by factor V Leiden mutation.
Prothrombin gene mutation (G to A transition at position 20210 in the 3-untranslated region).
Antithrombin III deficiency.
Protein C deficiency.
Protein S deficiency.
Dysfibrinogenemias (rare).

Acquired (Secondary) Hypercoagulable States

In association with physiologic or thrombogenic stimuli:
- Pregnancy (especially the postpartum period).
- Estrogen use (oral contraceptives, hormone replacement therapy).
- Immobilization.
- Trauma.
- Postoperative state.

Advancing age.
Obesity.
Prolonged air travel.
Lupus anticoagulant or antiphospholipid antibody syndrome.
In association with other clinical disorders.

Mixed/Unknown

Activated protein C resistance in the absence of factor V Leiden.
Elevated factor VIII level.
Elevated factor XI level.
Elevated factor IX level.
Elevated thrombin activatable fibrinolysis inhibitor (TAFI) level.
Decreased free tissue factor pathway inhibitor (TFPI) level.
Decreased plasma fibrinolytic activity.

THYMIC MASSES[85]

ICD-10CM # Varies with specific diagnosis

THYMIC MASSES

Thymic hyperplasia.
Thymoma.
Thymic carcinoma.
Thymic neuroendocrine tumors.
- Carcinoid.
- Small-cell carcinoma.

Thymic cysts (not rhizomatous).
Thymolipoma.
Metastases to the thymus.

THYMOMA, DISEASES ASSOCIATIONS[85]

ICD-10CM # Varies with specific diagnosis

SYSTEMIC DISEASES MOST COMMONLY ASSOCIATED WITH THYMOMA

Myasthenia gravis.
Cytopenias (most commonly red cell hypoplasia).
Nonthymic malignancies.
Hypogammaglobulinemia.
Systemic lupus erythematosus.
Polymyositis.
Rheumatoid arthritis.
Thyroiditis.
Sjögren syndrome.
Ulcerative colitis.

THYROMEGALY

ICD-10CM # Varies with specific diagnosis

Goiter.
Graves disease.
Thyroiditis (lymphocytic, granulomatous, suppurative).
Toxic adenoma.
Neoplasm (primary, metastatic).

THYROTOXICOSIS[67]

ICD-10CM # E05.80

CAUSES OF THYROTOXICOSIS

Sustained Hormone Overproduction (Hyperthyroidism)

Low TSH, high RAIU:
- Graves disease (von Basedow disease).
- Toxic multinodular goiter.
- Toxic adenoma.
- Chorionic gonadotropin-induced:
  - Gestational hyperthyroidism: physiologic hyperthyroidism of pregnancy, familial gestational hyperthyroidism due to TSH receptor mutations.
  - Trophoblastic tumors.

Inherited nonimmune hyperthyroidism associated with TSH receptor or G protein mutations.
Low TSH, low RAIU:
- Iodide-induced hyperthyroidism (Jod-Basedow effect).
- Amiodarone-associated hyperthyroidism due to iodide release.

Struma ovarii:
- Metastatic functioning thyroid carcinoma.

Normal or elevated TSH:
- TSH-secreting pituitary tumors.
- Thyroid hormone resistance with pituitary predominance.

TRANSIENT HORMONE EXCESS (THYROTOXICOSIS)

Low TSH, low RAIU
- Thyroiditis:
  - Autoimmune: lymphocytic thyroiditis (silent thyroiditis, painless thyroiditis, postpartum thyroiditis), acute exacerbation of Hashimoto disease.

Viral or postviral:
- Subacute (granulomatous, painful, postviral) thyroiditis.

Drug-induced or associated thyroiditis:
- Amiodarone.
- Lithium, interferon-α, interleukin-2, GM-CSF.

Infectious thyroiditis.
Exogenous thyroid hormone:
- Iatrogenic overreplacement.
- Thyrotoxicosis factitia.
- Ingestion of natural products containing thyroid hormone:
  - "Hamburger" thyrotoxicosis.
  - Natural foodstuffs.
  - Thyromimetic compounds (e.g., tiratricol PLB).
  - Occupational exposure to thyroid hormone (e.g., pill manufacturing, veterinary occupations).

GM-CSF, granulocyte-macrophage colony-stimulating factor; *RAIU,* radioactive iodine uptake; *TSH,* thyroid-stimulating hormone.

TICK-RELATED INFECTIONS

ICD-10CM #		
	A77.0	Spotted fever due to Rickettsia rickettsii
	A93.2	Colorado tick fever
	B60.0	Babesiosis
	A77.8	Other spotted fevers
	A69.20	Lyme disease, unspecified

Lyme disease.
Rocky Mountain spotted fever.
Babesiosis.
Tularemia.
Q fever.
Colorado tick fever.
Ehrlichiosis.
Relapsing fever.

TICS

ICD-10CM # F95.9 Tic disorder, unspecified

Tourette syndrome.
Physiologic tic.
Anxiety disorder.
Huntington disease.
Medications (e.g., antipsychotics, carbamazepine, phenytoin, phenobarbital).
Encephalitis.
Head trauma.
Schizophrenia.
Carbon monoxide poisoning.
Stroke.
Sydenham chorea.
Creutzfeldt-Jakob disease.

TORSADES DE POINTES[57]

ICD-10CM # I47.2 Ventricular tachycardia

Antiarrhythmics known to increase the QT interval (e.g., quinidine, procainamide, amiodarone, disopyramide, sotalol).
Tricyclic antidepressants and phenothiazines.
Histamine (H_1) antagonists (e.g., astemizole, terfenadine).
Antiviral and antifungal agents and antibiotics.
Hypokinemia.
Hypomagnesemia.
Insecticide poisoning.
Bradyarrhythmias.
Congenital long QT syndrome.
Subarachnoid hemorrhage.
Chloroquinine, pentamidine.
Cocaine abuse.

TOXIC MEGACOLON, CAUSES[17]

ICD-10CM # K59.3 Megacolon, not elsewhere classified

INFLAMMATORY

Ulcerative colitis.
Crohn disease.

INFECTIOUS

Bacterial:
- *Clostridium difficile* pseudomembranous colitis.
- *Salmonella* (typhoid and nontyphoid).
- *Shigella.*
- *Campylobacter.*
- *Yersinia.*

Parasitic:
- *Entamoeba histolytica.*
- *Cryptosporidium.*

Viral:
- Cytomegalovirus colitis.

OTHER

Ischemia.
Kaposi sarcoma.

TRACHEOBRONCHIAL NARROWING ON X-RAY[41]

ICD-10CM # Varies with specific diagnosis

CAUSES OF TRACHEOBRONCHIAL NARROWING

Long-Segment/Diffuse Narrowing

Sarcoidosis.
Amyloidosis.
Granulomatosis with polyangiitis.
Relapsing polychondritis.
Tracheobronchopathia osteochondroplastica.
Pemphigoid.

Short-Segment Narrowing

Previous intubation or tracheostomy.
Congenital stenosis or web.
Extrinsic compression (from thyroid).
Adenoid cystic carcinoma.
Squamous carcinoma.

TREMOR

ICD-10CM #		
	R25.0	Abnormal head movements
	R25.1	Tremor, unspecified
	R25.2	Cramp and spasm
	R25.3	Fasciculation
	R25.9	Unspecified abnormal involuntary movements
	G25.0	Essential tremor
	G25.1	Drug-induced tremor
	G25.2	Other specified forms of tremor

REST TREMORS

Parkinson disease.
Other parkinsonian syndromes (less commonly).
Midbrain (rubral) tremor: rest <postural <kinetic.
Wilson disease (also acquired hepatocerebral degeneration).
Essential tremor—only if severe: rest <postural and action.

POSTURAL AND ACTION (TERMINAL) TREMORS

Physiologic tremor.
Exaggerated physiologic tremor (these factors can also aggravate other forms of tremor).
- Stress, fatigue, anxiety, emotion.
- Endocrine: hypoglycemia, thyrotoxicosis, pheochromocytoma, adrenocorticosteroids.
- Drugs and toxins: beta-agonists, dopamine agonists, amphetamines, lithium, tricyclic antidepressants, neuroleptics, theophylline, caffeine, valproic acid, alcohol withdrawal, mercury (Hatter shakes), lead, arsenic, others.

Essential tremor (familial or sporadic)
Primary writing tremor.
With other CNS disorders:
- Parkinson disease.
- Other akinetic-rigid syndromes.
- Idiopathic dystonia, including focal dystonias.

With peripheral neuropathy:
- Charcot-Marie-Tooth syndrome (controversial whether to call this the Roussy-Levy syndrome).
- Variety of other peripheral neuropathies (especially dysgammaglobulinemia).

Cerebellar tremor.

KINETIC (INTENTION) TREMOR

Disease of cerebellar outflow (dentate nucleus and superior cerebellar peduncle): multiple sclerosis, trauma, tumor, vascular disease, Wilson acquired hepatocerebral degeneration, drugs, toxins (e.g., mercury), others.

MISCELLANEOUS RHYTHMICAL MOVEMENT DISORDERS

Psychogenic tremor.
Orthostatic tremor.
Rhythmical movements in dystonia (dystonic tremor).
Rhythmical myoclonus (segmental myoclonus—e.g., palatal or branchial myoclonus, spinal myoclonus, limb myorhythmia).
Oscillatory myoclonus.
Asterixis.
Clonus.
Epilepsia partialis continua.
Hereditary chin quivering.
Spasmus nutans.
Head bobbing with third ventricular cysts.
Nystagmus.

TREMOR, IN CHILDREN, CAUSES[58]

ICD-10CM #	R25.0	Abnormal head movements
	R25.1	Tremor, unspecified
	R25.2	Cramp and spasm
	R25.3	Fasciculation
	R25.9	Unspecified abnormal involuntary movements

BENIGN

Enhanced physiologic tremor.
Shuddering attacks.
Jitteriness.
Spasmus nutans.

STATIC INJURY/STRUCTURAL

Cerebellar malformation.
Stroke (particularly in the midbrain or cerebellum).
Multiple sclerosis.

HEREDITARY/DEGENERATIVE

Familial essential tremor.
Fragile X premutation.
Wilson disease.
Huntington disease.
Juvenile parkinsonism (tremor is rare).
Pallidonigral degeneration.

METABOLIC

Hyperthyroidism.
Hyperadrenergic state (including pheochromocytoma and neuroblastoma).
Hypomagnesemia.
Hypocalcemia.
Hypoglycemia.
Hepatic encephalopathy.
Vitamin B_{12} deficiency.
Inborn errors of metabolism.
Mitochondrial disorders.

DRUGS/TOXINS

Valproate, phenytoin, carbamazepine, lamotrigine, gabapentin, lithium, tricyclic antidepressants, stimulants (cocaine, amphetamine, caffeine, thyroxine, bronchodilators), neuroleptics, cyclosporin, toluene, mercury, thallium, amiodarone, nicotine, lead, manganese, arsenic, cyanide, naphthalene, ethanol, lindane, serotonin reuptake inhibitors.

PERIPHERAL NEUROPATHIES

PSYCHOGENIC

TRICHOMEGALY[13]

ICD-10CM # Not available

CAUSES OF TRICHOMEGALY

Drug-induced: topical prostaglandin analogues, phenytoin and cyclosporine.
Malnutrition.
AIDS.
Porphyria.
Hypothyroidism.
Familial.
Congenital: Oliver–McFarlane, Cornelia de Lange, Goldstein–Hutt, Hermansky–Pudlak syndromes.

TUBULOINTERSTITIAL DISEASE, ACUTE[36]

ICD-10CM # N17.0 Acute kidney failure with tubular necrosis

DRUGS

Antibiotics, penicillins, cephalosporins, rifampin.
Sulfonamides: cotrimoxazole, sulfamethoxazole.
NSAIDs: propionic acid derivatives.
Miscellaneous: phenytoin, thiazides, allopurinol, cimetidine, ifosfamide.

INFECTIONS

Invasion of renal parenchyma.
Reaction to systemic infections: streptococcal, diphtheria, hantavirus.

SYSTEMIC DISEASES

Immune mediated: SLE, transplanted kidney, cryoglobulinemias.
Metabolic: urate, oxalate.
Neoplastic: lymphoproliferative diseases.

IDIOPATHIC

TUBULOINTERSTITIAL KIDNEY DISEASE[36]

ICD-10CM # N17.0 Acute kidney failure with tubular necrosis

Ischemic and toxic acute tubular necrosis.
Allergic interstitial nephritis.
Interstitial nephritis secondary to immune complex-related collagen vascular disease (e.g., SLE, Sjögren).
Granulomatous diseases (sarcoidosis, uveitis).
Pigment-related tubular injury (myoglobinuria, hemoglobinuria).
Hypercalcemia with nephrocalcinosis.
Tubular obstruction (drugs such as indinavir, uric acid in tumor lysis syndrome).
Myeloma kidney or cast nephropathy.
Infection-related interstitial nephritis: *Legionella, Leptospira.*
Infiltrative diseases (e.g., lymphoma).

TUMOR MARKERS ELEVATION[95]

ICD-10CM # R97.8 Other abnormal tumor markers

CAUSES OF ELEVATED LEVELS OF TUMOR MARKERS

Carcinoembryonic Antigen (CEA)

Colonic cancer (higher levels if the tumor is more differentiated or is extensive or has spread to the liver).
Lung or breast cancer; seminoma.
Cigarette smokers.
Cirrhosis, inflammatory bowel disease, rectal polyps, pancreatitis.
Advanced age.

Alpha-Fetoprotein

Hepatocellular cancer: very high titers or a rising titer is strongly suggestive, but >10% of patients do not have an elevated level.
Hepatic regeneration (e.g., cirrhosis, alcoholic or viral hepatitis).
Cancer of the stomach, colon, pancreas, or lung.
Teratocarcinoma or embryonal cell carcinoma (testis, ovary, extragonadal).
Pregnancy.
Ataxia-telangiectasia.
Normal variant.

Prostate-Specific Antigen

Prostate carcinoma (localized disease).
Prostatic hyperplasia.
Prostatitis.
Prostatic infarction.

Cancer-Associated Antigen (CA-19-9)

Pancreatic carcinoma (80% with advanced, well-differentiated cancer have an elevated level).
Other GI cancers: colon, stomach, bile duct.
Acute or chronic pancreatitis.
Chronic liver disease.
Biliary tract disease.

UPPER AIRWAY OBSTRUCTION[19]

ICD-10CM # Varies with specific diagnosis

CAUSES OF UPPER AIRWAY OBSTRUCTION

Altered conscious state:
- Head injury.
- Cerebrovascular accident.
- Drugs and toxins.
- Metabolic—hypoglycemia, hyponatremia.

Foreign bodies.
Infections:
- Tonsillitis.
- Peritonsillar abscess (quinsy).
- Epiglottitis.
- Ludwig angina.
- Other abscesses and infections.

Trauma:
- Blunt or penetrating trauma resulting in edema or hematoma formation.
- Uncontrolled hemorrhage.
- Thermal injuries.
- Inhalation burns.

Neoplasms:
- Larynx, trachea, thyroid.

Allergic reactions:
- Anaphylaxis.
- Angioedema.

Anatomic:
- Tracheomalacia—congenital or acquired (secondary to prolonged intubation).
- Other congenital malformations.

Functional upper airway obstruction syndrome.

Acute-on-chronic causes.

Patients with chronic narrowing of the airway (e.g., due to tracheomalacia) may present with worsening obstruction from an acute upper respiratory tract illness or injury.

UREMIC ENCEPHALOPATHY, DIFFERENTIAL DIAGNOSIS[32]

ICD-10CM # G93.40 Encephalopathy, unspecified

Differential Diagnosis	Comment
Hypertensive encephalopathy	
Systemic inflammatory response syndrome (SIRS):	Observed in septic patients.
Systemic vasculitis:	Vasculitis or lupus with cerebral involvement.
Drug-induced neurotoxicity	
Analgesics:	Meperidine, codeine, morphine, gabapentin.
Antibiotics:	High-dose penicillins (may cause seizures), acyclovir, ethambutol (optic nerve damage), erythromycin and aminoglycosides (may cause ototoxicity), nitrofurantoin and isoniazid (peripheral neuropathy).
Psychotropics:	Lithium, haloperidol, clonazepam, diazepam, chlorpromazine.
Immunosuppressants:	Cyclosporine, tacrolimus.
Chemotherapeutics:	Cisplatinum, ifosfamide.
Others:	High doses of loop diuretics (ototoxic), ephedrine, methyldopa, aluminum.
Cerebral atheroembolic disease:	Follows recent aortic or cardiac angiography; associated with peripheral manifestations, including lower extremity cyanosis, livedo reticularis, and eosinophilia.
Subdural hematoma	
Posterior leukoencephalopathy:	Observed particularly following renal transplantation due to reversible, abnormal permeability of the blood-brain barrier Often manifests as headache followed by mental depression, visual loss, and seizures in the context of volume expansion, acute hypertension, and often treatment with corticosteroids or calcineurin inhibitors Lesions in the parietal, temporal, and occipital lobes may be seen on imaging studies.

URETERAL COLIC[61]

ICD-10CM #		
	R33.8	Other retention of urine
	N13.8	Other obstructive and reflux uropathy

DIAGNOSTIC DIFFERENTIALS OF RENAL OR URETERAL COLIC

Acute cholecystitis, acute cholelithiasis.
Acute appendicitis.
Pelvic inflammatory disease.
Diverticulosis and/or diverticulitis.
Intestinal obstruction.
Leaking abdominal aortic aneurysm.
Musculoskeletal sprains.
Herniated disk.
Herpes zoster (shingles).
GI dysfunction with ileus and/or toxic colonic dilatation.

URETERAL STRICTURE[99]

ICD-10CM # Varies with specific diagnosis

ETIOLOGY OF URETERAL STRICTURE

Malignancy (e.g., transitional cell carcinoma, cervical cancer).
Ureteral calculus.
Radiation.
Ischemia or trauma caused by surgical dissection.
Periureteral fibrosis caused by abdominal aortic aneurysm or endometriosis.
Endoscopic instrumentation.
Renal ablation injury.
Infection (tuberculosis).
Idiopathic condition.

URETERIC OBSTRUCTION, CONGENITAL[41]

ICD-10CM #		
	N13.8	Other obstructive and reflux uropathy
	N20.9	Urolithiasis

CONGENITAL CAUSES OF URETERIC OBSTRUCTION

Primary megaureter.
Ureterocele (ectopic and orthotopic).
Ureteric valve.
Distal ureteric stenosis.
Ureteric atresia.
Circumcaval ureter and variants.
Bladder diverticulum.

URETHRAL BLEEDING[99]

ICD-10CM # Varies with specific diagnosis

DIFFERENTIAL DIAGNOSIS FOR URETHRAL BLEEDING

Male

Trauma:
- Blunt (straddle injury, kick to perineum).
- Penetrating (foreign body insertion, failed urethral catheterization).
- Intercourse related (penile fracture, masturbation).

Urethritis:
- Bacterial (gonococcal, nongonococcal).
- Viral.
- Chemical.
- Autoimmune (Reiter syndrome).

Malignancy:
- Urothelial carcinoma.
- Squamous cell carcinoma (meatus/glans).

Condyloma.
Calculus disease.

Female

Trauma:
- Blunt (pelvic fracture).
- Penetrating (foreign body).

Urethral diverticulum.
Urethral caruncle.
Urethritis.
Malignancy.
Calculus disease.

URETHRAL DISCHARGE AND DYSURIA

ICD-10CM #		
	R36.0	Urethral discharge without blood
	R36.9	Urethral discharge, unspecified
	N36.9	Urethral disorder, unspecified
	N39.9	Disorder of urinary system, unspecified
	R30.0	Dysuria
	R30.9	Painful micturition, unspecified

Urethritis (gonococcal, chlamydial, trichomonal).
Cystitis.
Prostatitis.
Vaginitis (candidiasis, chemical).
Meatal stenosis.
Interstitial cystitis.
Trauma (foreign body, masturbation, horseback or bike riding).

URETHRAL OBSTRUCTION, CHILDREN[41]

ICD-10CM # N13.8 Other obstructive and reflux uropathy

CAUSES OF URETHRAL OBSTRUCTION IN CHILDREN

Intrinsic Lesions

Valve (posterior, anterior, saccular diverticulum).
Stenosis, atresia.
Inflammatory stricture.
Traumatic stricture:
- External trauma (saddle injury, and so on).
- Iatrogenic trauma (catheter, cystoscopy, surgery).

Urethral "tumors":
- Girls: leiomyoma.
- Boys: polyp, rhabdomyosarcoma.

Miscellaneous (epidermolysis bullosa).

Extrinsic Lesions

Presacral mass dissecting inferiorly (tumor, cyst).
Fecal impaction (Hirschsprung, postrepair anal atresia, habitual constipation, neuropathy).
Mass originating in genital organs:
- Boys: utricle cyst, prostate rhabdomyosarcoma, seminal vesicle cyst, Cowper duct cyst.
- Girls: hydrometrocolpos, hydrocolpos, fused labia.

URETHRITIS, PEDIATRIC PATIENT[23]

ICD-10CM # N34.1 Nonspecific urethritis
N34.2 Other urethritis

ETIOLOGY OF URETHRITIS

Infectious	Noninfectious
Sexually Transmitted Infections	**Vasculitides**
Neisseria gonorrhoeae.	Reiter syndrome.
	Erythema multiforme.
Chlamydia trachomatis.	Kawasaki disease.
	Mechanical
Trichomonas vaginalis.	Masturbation.
	Foreign body.
Herpes simplex virus type 2.	Trauma.
	Dysfunctional elimination.
Mycoplasma spp.	
Non–Sexually Transmitted Infections	**Chemical**
	Soaps.
	Detergents.
Staphylococcus saprophyticus.	Drugs.
Enterobacteriaceae.	
Gardnerella vaginalis.	
Streptococcus spp.	
Enterobius vermicularis.	

URIC ACID STONES

ICD-10CM # N20.9 Urolithiasis

Hyperuricemia.
Excessive dietary purine.
Medications (salicylates, allopurinol, probenecid).
Urine pH <5.5 (e.g., diarrhea, high animal protein diet).
Decreased urine output (dehydration, malabsorption, diarrhea, inadequate fluid intake).
Tumor lysis.
Hemolytic anemia.
Myeloproliferative disorders.

URINARY INCONTINENCE, CHILDREN[58]

ICD-10CM # R32 Unspecified urinary incontinence

CAUSES OF URINARY INCONTINENCE IN CHILDHOOD

Overactive bladder.
Infrequent voiding.
Detrusor-sphincter dyssynergia.
Non-neurogenic neurogenic bladder (Hinman syndrome).
Vaginal voiding.
Giggle incontinence.
Cystitis.
Bladder outlet obstruction (posterior urethral valves).
Ectopic ureter and fistula.
Sphincter abnormality (epispadias, exstrophy; urogenital sinus abnormality).
Neuropathic.
Overflow incontinence.
Traumatic.
Iatrogenic.
Behavioral.
Combination.

URINARY RETENTION[61]

ICD-10CM # R33.9 Retention of urine, unspecified

COMMON CAUSES OF URINARY RETENTION

Obstructive Cause

Urethral stricture.
Enlarged prostate.
Lower genitourinary tract malignancy.
Pelvic malignancy.
Bladder stones.
Foreign body.
Blood clot.
Posterior urethral valves.
Ureterocele.

Primary Detrusor Insufficiency

Detrusor areflexia.
Multiple sclerosis.
Iatrogenic injury during abdominal or back surgery.
Spinal cord injury.
Myelomeningocele.

URINARY RETENTION, ACUTE

ICD-10CM # R33.9 Retention of urine, unspecified

Mechanical obstruction: urethral stone, foreign body, urethral stricture, BPH, prostate carcinoma, prostatitis, trauma with hematoma formation.
Neurogenic bladder.
Neurologic disease (MS, parkinsonism, tabes dorsalis, CVA).
Spinal cord injury.
CNS neoplasm (primary or metastatic).
Spinal anesthesia.
Lower urinary tract instrumentation.
Medications (antihistamines, antidepressants, narcotics, anticholinergics).
Abdominal or pelvic surgery.
Alcohol toxicity.
Pregnancy.
Anxiety.
Encephalitis.
Postoperative pain.
Spina bifida occulta.

URINARY TRACT BLEEDING, UPPER[99]

ICD-10CM # Varies with specific diagnosis

DIFFERENTIAL DIAGNOSIS FOR UPPER URINARY TRACT BLEEDING

Renal glomerular diseases:
- IgA nephropathy (Berger disease).
- Thin basement membrane disease.
- Acute glomerulonephritis (e.g., poststreptococcal).
- Lupus nephritis.
- Hereditary nephritis (e.g., Alport syndrome).

Renal tubulointerstitial diseases:
- Papillary necrosis.
- Sickle cell nephropathy.
- Analgesic nephropathy.
- Polycystic kidney disease.
- Medullary sponge kidney.

Vasculitis:
- Henoch-Schönlein purpura.
- Wegener granulomatosis.

Infection:
- Pyelonephritis.
- Xanthogranulomatous pyelonephritis.
- Renal tuberculosis.
- Fungal infection.

Obstruction:
- Ureteropelvic junction obstruction.
- Ureteral stricture.

Nephrolithiasis.
Malignancy:
- Renal cortical tumors (renal cell carcinoma, benign tumors).
- Upper tract urothelial carcinoma.

Fibroepithelial polyp.
Vascular diseases:
- Renal arteriovenous malformations (congenital, acquired).
- Iliac arterio-ureteral fistula.
- Renal artery aneurysm (especially ruptured).
- Renal artery pseudoaneurysm.
- Renal artery and/or vein thrombosis.
- Hemangioma.
- Atheroembolic disease.
- Nutcracker syndrome.
- Loin-pain hematuria syndrome.

Trauma:
- Blunt.
- Penetrating.

Lateralizing essential hematuria.

URINARY TRACT OBSTRUCTION[38]

ICD-10CM #	N21.8	Other lower urinary tract calculus
	N20.9	Urolithiasis

INTRARENAL

Uric acid nephropathy.
Sulfonamide precipitates.
Acyclovir, indinavir precipitates.
Multiple myeloma.

URETERAL

Intrinsic

Intraluminal:
- Nephrolithiasis.
- Papillary necrosis.
- Blood clots.
- Fungus balls.

Intramural:
- Ureteropelvic junction dysfunction.
- Ureterovesical junction dysfunction.
- Ureteral valve, polyp, or tumor.
- Ureteral stricture.
  - Schistosomiasis.
  - Tuberculosis.
  - Scarring from instrumentation.
  - Drugs (e.g., NSAIDs).

Extrinsic

Vascular system:
- Aneurysm: abdominal aorta or iliac vessels.
- Aberrant vessels: ureteropelvic junction.
- Venous: retrocaval ureter.

GI tract:
- Crohn disease.
- Diverticulitis.
- Appendiceal abscess.
- Colon cancer.
- Pancreatic tumor, abscess, or cyst.

Reproductive system:
- Uterus: pregnancy, prolapse, tumor, endometriosis.
- Ovary: abscess, tumor, ovarian remnants.
- Gartner duct cyst, tuboovarian abscess.

Retroperitoneal disease:
- Retroperitoneal fibrosis: radiation, drugs, idiopathic.
- Inflammatory: tuberculosis, sarcoidosis.
- Hematoma.
- Primary tumor (e.g., lymphoma, sarcoma).
- Metastatic tumor (e.g., cervix, ovarian, bladder, colon).
- Lymphocele.
- Pelvic lipomatosis.

BLADDER

Neurogenic bladder:
- Diabetes mellitus.
- Spinal cord defect.
- Trauma.
- Multiple sclerosis.
- Stroke.
- Parkinson disease.
- Spinal anesthesia.
- Anticholinergics.

Bladder neck dysfunction.
Bladder calculus.
Bladder cancer.

URETHRA

Urethral stricture.
Prostate hypertrophy or cancer.
Obstruction from instrumentation.

URINARY TRACT OBSTRUCTION, CONGENITAL CAUSES[87]

ICD-10CM # Varies with specific diagnosis

CONGENITAL CAUSES OF URINARY TRACT OBSTRUCTION

Ureteropelvic Junction

Ureteropelvic junction obstruction.

Proximal and Middle Ureter

Ureteral folds.
Ureteral valves.
Strictures.
Benign fibroepithelial polyps.
Retrocaval ureter.

Distal Ureter

Ureterovesical junction obstruction.
Vesicoureteral reflux.
Prune-belly syndrome.
Ureteroceles.

Bladder

Bladder diverticula.
Neurologic conditions (e.g., spina bifida).

Urethra

Posterior urethral valves.
Urethral diverticula.
Anterior urethral valves.
Urethral atresia.
Labial fusion.

URINE CASTS

ICD-10CM #	R82.99	Other abnormal findings in urine

Normal finding.
Pyelonephritis.
Chronic renal disease.
Nephrotic syndrome.
Acute tubular necrosis.
Interstitial nephritis.
Nephritic syndrome.
Glomerulonephritis.
Eclampsia.
Heavy metal ingestion.
Allograft rejection.
Hypothyroidism.

URINE COLOR ABNORMALITIES[61]

ICD-10CM #	R82.5	Elevated urine levels of drugs, medicaments and biological substances
	R82.99	Other abnormal findings in urine

COMMON CAUSES OF ABNORMAL URINE COLOR

Colorless.

DISEASE

Diabetes mellitus.
Diabetes insipidus.

DRUG

Ethyl alcohol.
Diuretics.

MISCELLANEOUS

Overhydration.
Yellow-orange

DRUG

Tetracycline.
Flutamide.
Pyridium.
Azo Gantrisin (Roche Labs, Nutley, NJ).
Sulfasalazine.
Vitamin B.

MISCELLANEOUS

Dehydration.

Milky White

DISEASE

Urinary tract infection/pyuria.

Blue-green

DISEASE

Pseudomonas urinary tract infection.

DRUG

Methylene blue.
Urised (Polymedica Pharmaceuticals, Woburn, MA).
Indigo carmine.
Doan's pills (Novartis Consumer Health, Parsippany, NJ).
Clorets (Cadbury Adams, Parsippany, NJ).
Amitriptyline.

Red-brown

DISEASE

Hematuria.
Hemolytic anemia.
Hemoglobinuria.
Lead poisoning.
Mercury poisoning.
Porphyria.

DRUG

Rifampin.
Ex-Lax (Novartis Consumer Health, Parsippany, NJ).
Phenolphthalein.
Phenothiazines.
Nitrofurantoin.
Doxorubicin.

MISCELLANEOUS

Beets.
Blackberries.
Rhubarb.

Brown-black

DISEASE

Fecaluria.
Methemoglobinuria.
Melaninuria.

DRUG

Metronidazole.
Methyldopa.
Methocarbamol.

MISCELLANEOUS

Fava beans.
Aloe.

URINE, RED[72]

ICD-10CM # Varies with specific diagnosis

WITH A POSITIVE DIPSTICK

Hematuria.
Hemoglobinuria: negative urinalysis.
Myoglobinuria: negative urinalysis.

WITH A NEGATIVE DIPSTICK

Drugs

Aminosalicylic acid.
Deferoxamine mesylate.
Ibuprofen.
Phenacetin.
Phenolphthalein.
Phensuximide.
Rifampin.
Anthraquinone laxatives.
Doxorubicin.
Methyldopa.
Phenazopyridine.
Phenothiazine.
Phenytoin.

Dyes

Azo dyes.
Eosin.

Foods

Beets, berries, maize.
Rhodamine B.

Metabolic

Porphyrins.
Serratia marcescens (red diaper syndrome).
Urate crystalluria.

UROLITHIASIS-LIKE PAIN[87]

ICD-10CM # Varies with specific diagnosis

DIFFERENTIAL DIAGNOSIS OF UROLITHIASIS-LIKE PAIN

Category
Disorders

Renal:
- Pyelonephritis.
- Blood clot.
- Renal infarction.
- Tumor (kidney or pelvis).
- Papillary necrosis.

Ureteral:
- Tumor.
- Blood clot.
- Stricture.

Bladder:
- Tumor.
- Blood clot.
- Urinary retention.

Intraabdominal:
- Peritonitis.
- Appendicitis.
- Biliary disease.
- Bowel obstruction.
- Vascular disorder.
- Aortic aneurysm.
- Mesenteric insufficiency.

Retroperitoneal:
- Lymphadenopathy.
- Fibrosis.
- Tumor.

Gynecologic:
- Ectopic or tubal pregnancy.
- Ovarian torsion, cyst rupture.
- Pelvic inflammatory disease.
- Cervical cancer.
- Endometriosis.
- Ovarian vein syndrome.

Neuromuscular:
- Muscle pain.
- Rib fracture.
- Radiculitis.

Infectious:
- Herpes zoster.
- Pleuritis, pneumonia.
- Fungal bezoar.

UROPATHY, OBSTRUCTIVE[91]

ICD-10CM #	N13.9	Obstructive and reflux uropathy, unspecified
	N20.9	Urolithiasis

INTRINSIC CAUSES

Intraluminal

Intratubular deposition of crystals (uric acid, sulfas).
Stones.
Papillary tissue.
Blood clots.

Intramural

Functional.
Ureter (ureteropelvic or ureterovesical dysfunction).
Bladder (neurogenic): spinal cord defect or trauma, diabetes, multiple sclerosis, Parkinson disease, cerebrovascular accidents.
Bladder neck dysfunction.

Anatomic

Tumors.
Infection, granuloma.
Strictures.

EXTRINSIC CAUSES

Originating in the Reproductive System

Prostate: benign hypertrophy or cancer.
Uterus: pregnancy, tumors, prolapse, endometriosis.
Ovary: abscess, tumor, cysts.

Originating in the Vascular System

Aneurysms (aorta, iliac vessels).
Aberrant arteries (ureteropelvic junction).
Venous (ovarian veins, retrocaval ureter).

Originating in the Gastrointestinal Tract

Crohn disease.
Pancreatitis.
Appendicitis.
Tumors.

Originating in the Retroperitoneal Space

Inflammations.
Fibrosis.
Tumor, hematomas.

UROSEPSIS[61]

ICD-10CM # A41.9 Sepsis, unspecified organism

COMMON CAUSES OF UROSEPSIS

Obstructing ureteral stone with pyonephrosis.
Staghorn calculus with urinary tract infection.
Ureteral obstruction with proximal urinary tract infection.
Urinary retention with urinary tract infection.
Acute prostatitis with prostatic abscess.
Perinephric abscess or renal carbuncle.
Urethral stricture with periurethral abscess.
Fournier gangrene.
Foreign body within urinary tract (e.g., Foley catheter).

URTICARIA IN TRAVELERS[82]

ICD-10CM # L50.9 Urticaria, unspecified

CAUSES OF URTICARIA IN TRAVELERS

Noninfectious causes: adverse drug reaction.*
Viral infection: hepatitis A infection.
Parasitic infection: invasive phase of helminthic diseases (ascariasis, hookworm, strongyloidiasis, anisakiasis, gnathostomiasis, schistosomiasis,* fascioliasis), chronic helminthic infections where humans are dead-end host (trichinellosis, toxocariasis), and rupture of cyst during hydatid disease.

UTERINE BLEEDING, ABNORMAL[28]

ICD-10CM #	N92.6	Irregular menstruation, unspecified
	N93.9	Abnormal uterine and vaginal bleeding, unspecified

PREGNANCY

Threatened abortion.
Incomplete abortion.
Complete abortion.
Molar pregnancy.
Ectopic pregnancy.
Retained products of conception.

OVULATORY

Vulva: infection, laceration, tumor.
Vagina: infection, laceration, tumor, foreign body.
Cervix: polyps, cervical erosion, cervicitis, carcinoma.
Uterus: fibroids (submucous fibroids most likely to cause abnormal bleeding), polyps, adenomyosis, endometritis, intrauterine device, atrophic endometrium.

*Common cause.

Pregnancy complications: ectopic pregnancy; threatened, incomplete, complete abortion; retained products of conception.
Abnormality of clotting system.
Midcycle bleeding.
Halban disease (persistent corpus luteum).
Menorrhagia.
Pelvic inflammatory disease.

ANOVULATORY

Physiologic causes:
Puberty.
Perimenopausal.
Pathologic causes:
Ovarian failure (FSH over 40 IU/ml).
Hyperandrogenism.
Hyperprolactinemia.
Obesity.
Hypothalamic dysfunction (polycystic ovaries); LH/FSH ratio greater than 2:1.
Hyperplasia.
Endometrial carcinoma.
Estrogen-producing tumors.
Hypothyroidism.

UVEITIS, PEDIATRIC AGE

ICD-10CM # H20.9 Anterior uveitis

ANTERIOR UVEITIS

Juvenile rheumatoid arthritis (pauciarticular).
Sarcoidosis.
Trauma.
Tuberculosis.
Kawasaki disease.
Ulcerative colitis.
Postinfectious (enteric or genital) with arthritis and rash.
Spirochetal (syphilis, leptospiral).
Heterochromic iridocyclitis (Fuchs).
Viral (herpes simplex, herpes zoster).
Ankylosing spondylitis.
Stevens-Johnson syndrome.
Idiopathic.
Drugs.

POSTERIOR UVEITIS (CHOROIDITIS—MAY INVOLVE RETINA)

Toxoplasmosis.
Parasites (toxocariasis).
Sarcoidosis.
Tuberculosis.
Viral (rubella, herpes simplex, HIV, cytomegalovirus).
Subacute sclerosing panencephalitis.
Idiopathic.

ANTERIOR AND/OR POSTERIOR UVEITIS

Sympathetic ophthalmia (trauma to other eye).
Vogt-Koyanagi-Harada syndrome (uveo-otocutaneous syndrome: poliosis, vitiligo, deafness, tinnitus, uveitis, aseptic meningitis, retinitis).
Behçet syndrome.
Lyme disease.

VAGINAL BLEEDING, ABNORMAL[19]

ICD-10CM # N93.9 Abnormal uterine and vaginal bleeding, unspecified

DIFFERENTIAL DIAGNOSIS OF ABNORMAL VAGINAL BLEEDING

Ovulatory bleeding—menorrhagia.
Anovulatory bleeding—sometimes known as dysfunctional uterine bleeding (DUB).
Uterine and ovarian pathology:
Uterine fibroids (pelvic pain, dysmenorrhea).
Endometriosis; adenomyosis (dysmenorrhea, dyspareunia, pelvic pain, infertility).
Pelvic inflammatory disease and pelvic infection (fever, vaginal discharge, pelvic pain, intermenstrual and postcoital bleeding).
Endometrial polyps (intermenstrual bleeding).
Endometrial hyperplasia; endometrial carcinoma (pelvic pain, abnormal bleeding, postcoital bleeding).
Polycystic ovary syndrome (irregular bleeding, infertility, and hirsutism)
Systemic disease:
Coagulation disorder; bleeding diathesis such as von Willebrand disease.
Liver or renal disease.
Hypothyroidism (fatigue, constipation, coarse features, alopecia).
Iatrogenic cause:
Anticoagulation.
Intrauterine device.
Chemotherapy.
Sex steroids.

VAGINAL BLEEDING, PREGNANCY[21]

ICD-10CM # N93.9 Abnormal uterine and vaginal bleeding, unspecified

FIRST TRIMESTER

Implantation bleeding.
Abortion:
Threatened.
Complete.
Incomplete.
Missed.
Ectopic pregnancy.
Neoplasia.
Hydatidiform mole.
Cervix.

THIRD TRIMESTER

Placenta previa.
Placental abruption.
Premature labor.
Choriocarcinoma.

VAGINAL DISCHARGE, PREPUBERTAL GIRLS[48]

ICD-10CM # N89.8 Other specified noninflammatory disorders of vagina

Irritative (bubble baths, sand):
Poor perineal hygiene.
Foreign body.
Associated systemic illness (group A streptococci, chickenpox).
Infections.
Escherichia coli with foreign body.
Shigella organisms.
Yersinia organisms.
Infections (consider sexual abuse):
Chlamydia trachomatis.
Neisseria gonorrhoeae.
Trichomonas vaginalis.
Tumor (rare).

VALVULAR HEART DISEASE[3]

ICD-10CM # Varies with specific diagnosis

MAJOR CAUSES OF VALVULAR HEART DISEASE IN ADULTS

Aortic Stenosis
Bicuspid aortic valve.
Rheumatic fever.
Degenerative stenosis.
Aortic Regurgitation
Bicuspid aortic valve.
Aortic dissection.
Endocarditis.
Rheumatic fever.
Aortic root dilation.
Mitral Stenosis
Rheumatic fever.
Mitral Regurgitation

CHRONIC

Mitral valve prolapse.
Left ventricular dilation.
Posterior wall myocardial infarction.
Rheumatic fever.
Endocarditis.

ACUTE

Posterior wall or papillary muscle ischemia.
Papillary muscle or chordal rupture.
Endocarditis.
Prosthetic valve dysfunction.
Systolic anterior motion of mitral valve.

TRICUSPID REGURGITATION

Functional (annular) dilation.
Tricuspid valve prolapse.
Endocarditis.
Carcinoid heart disease.

VASCULAR LESIONS OF GI TRACT[30]

ICD-10CM # Varies with specific diagnosis

Primary Vascular Lesions
Aneurysms of the aorta and its branches.
Angioectasia (angiodysplasia, vascular ectasia).
Arteriovenous malformation.
Blue rubber bleb nevus.
Capillary phlebectasia.
Dieulafoy lesion.
Glomus tumor.
Hemangioma.

Hemangiomatosis.
Hemangioendothelioma.
Hemangiopericytoma.
Hemangiosarcoma.
Hemorrhoids.
Kaposi sarcoma.
Diseases and Syndromes with Vascular Lesions
Blue rubber bleb nevus syndrome.
Ehlers-Danlos syndrome.
Hereditary hemorrhagic telangiectasia (Osler-Weber-Rendu disease).
Klippel-Trenaunay or Parkes Weber syndrome.
Kohlmeier-Degos syndrome.
Marfan syndrome.
Pseudoxanthoma elasticum.
PSS (scleroderma, CREST).
Scurvy.
Turner syndrome.
von Willebrand disease.
Systemic Disorders Associated with Vascular Lesions
Portal hypertension:
  Congestive gastropathy and colopathy.
  GAVE (watermelon stomach).
  Spider telangiectasias.
  Varices.
Renal failure:
  GI telangiectasias.
  GAVE (watermelon stomach).
Vasculitis (e.g., polyarteritis nodosa).
Iatrogenic lesions:
  Radiation telangiectasia.

CREST, Calcinosis, Raynaud phenomenon, esophageal dysmotility, sclerodactyly, telangiectasia; *GAVE,* gastric antral vascular ectasia

VASCULITIS, CLASSIFICATION[65]

ICD-10CM # I77.6 Arteritis, unspecified

LARGE VESSEL DISEASE

Arteritis
Giant cell arteritis.
Takayasu arteritis.
Arteritis associated with Reiter syndrome (reactive arthritis), ankylosing spondylitis.

MEDIUM AND SMALL VESSEL DISEASE

Polyarteritis Nodosa
Primary (idiopathic).
Associated with viruses (hepatitis B or C, CMV, HIV, herpes zoster).
Associated with malignancy (hairy cell leukemia).
Familial Mediterranean fever.
Granulomatous Vasculitis
Granulomatosis with polyangiitis.
Lymphomatoid granulomatosis.
Behçet Disease
Kawasaki Disease (Mucocutaneous Lymph Node Syndrome)

PREDOMINANTLY SMALL VESSEL DISEASE

Hypersensitivity Vasculitis (Leukocytoclastic Vasculitis)
Henoch-Schönlein purpura.
Mixed cryoglobulinemia.
Serum sickness.
Vasculitis associated with connective tissue diseases (SLE, Sjögren syndrome).
Vasculitis associated with specific syndromes:
  Primary biliary cirrhosis.
  Lyme disease.
  Chronic active hepatitis.
  Drug-induced vasculitis.
Churg-Strauss Syndrome
Goodpasture Syndrome
Erythema Nodosum
Panniculitis. Buerger Disease (Thrombophlebitis Obliterans)

VASCULITIS (DISEASES THAT MIMIC VASCULITIS)[71]

ICD-10CM # Varies with specific diagnosis

EMBOLIC DISEASE

Infectious or marantic endocarditis.
Cardiac mural thrombus.
Atrial myxoma.
Cholesterol embolization syndrome.

NONINFLAMMATORY VESSEL WALL DISRUPTION

Atherosclerosis.
Arterial fibromuscular dysplasia.
Drug effects (vasoconstrictors, anticoagulants).
Radiation.
Genetic disease (neurofibromatosis, Ehlers-Danlos syndrome).
Amyloidosis.
Intravascular malignant lymphoma.

DIFFUSE COAGULATION

Disseminated intravascular coagulation.
Thrombotic thrombocytopenic purpura.
Hemolytic-uremic syndrome.
Protein C and S deficiencies, factor V/Leiden mutation.
Antiphospholipid syndrome.

VEGETATIVE STATE, PERSISTENT[3]

ICD-10CM # R40.3 Persistent vegetative state

PERSISTENT VEGETATIVE STATE: COMMON CAUSES[50]

Trauma (diffuse axonal injury).
Cardiac arrest and hypoperfusion (laminar necrosis of cortical mantle and/or thalamic necrosis).
Bihemispheric infarctions.
Purulent meningitis or encephalitis (cortical injury).
Carbon monoxide.
Prolonged hypoglycemic coma.

[50]A vegetative state may not necessarily begin with coma but can also develop as the end stage of neurodegenerative diseases (e.g., Alzheimer disease) of adults or children and can accompany severe congenital developmental abnormalities of the brain such as anencephaly.

VENTILATION–PERFUSION MISMATCH ON LUNG SCAN

ICD-10CM # Varies with specific diagnosis

Pulmonary embolism.
Emphysema.
Irradiation.
Pulmonary hypertension.
AV malformations.
Pulmonary thrombosis.
External compression of pulmonary artery (neoplasm, cysts, fibrosing mediastinitis).
Vasculitis.
Tuberculosis.
Pulmonary thrombosis.
Congenital (pulmonary artery hypoplasia, congenital heart disease with upper lobe diversion).
Sequestered segment.
Parasitic lung disease.
Intraluminal obstruction from catheter fragments.

VENTRICULAR FAILURE

ICD-10CM # I51.9 Heart disease, unspecified

LEFT VENTRICULAR FAILURE

Systemic hypertension.
Valvular heart disease (AS, AR, MR).
Cardiomyopathy, myocarditis.
Bacterial endocarditis.
Myocardial infarction.
Idiopathic hypertrophic subaortic stenosis.

RIGHT VENTRICULAR FAILURE

Valvular heart disease (mitral stenosis).
Pulmonary hypertension.
Bacterial endocarditis (right-sided).
Right ventricular infarction.

BIVENTRICULAR FAILURE

Left ventricular failure.
Cardiomyopathy.
Myocarditis
Arrhythmias.
Anemia.
Thyrotoxicosis.
Arteriovenous fistula.
Paget disease.
Beriberi.

VERRUCOUS LESIONS

ICD-10CM # Varies with specific diagnosis

Warts.
Seborrheic keratosis.
Lichen simplex.
Acanthosis nigricans.
Scabies (Norwegian, crusted).
Verrucous carcinoma.
Nevus sebaceous.
Deep fungal infection.

VERTEBRAL LESIONS[70]

ICD-10CM # Varies with specific diagnosis

Anatomic Distribution of Vertebral Lesions

Anterior Elements of the Spine	Posterior Elements of the Spine	Both Anterior and Posterior Elements of the Spine
Multiple myeloma.	Osteoid osteoma.	Metastasis (spares disc end plates).
Hemangioma.	Osteoblastoma.	Infection (involves disc end plates).
Paget disease of bone.	Aneurysmal bone cyst.	Classic osteosarcoma.
Histiocytosis X (vertebra plana).		Postradiation sarcoma.
Giant cell tumor of bone.		Malignant histiocytoid variety.
Reparative granuloma.		Osteosarcoma.
Ewing sarcoma (primitive neuroectodermal tumor).		Osteochondroma.
Lymphoma of bone.		Primary chondrosarcoma.
Malignant fibrous histiocytoma.		Secondary chondrosarcoma.
Chordoma.		

VERTIGO

ICD-10CM #		
	R42	Dizziness and giddiness
	H81.13	Benign paroxysmal vertigo, bilateral
	H81.49	Vertigo of central origin, unspecified ear
	H81.399	Other peripheral vertigo, unspecified ear
	H81.23	Vestibular neuronitis, bilateral

PERIPHERAL

Otitis media.
Acute labyrinthitis.
Vestibular neuronitis.
Benign positional vertigo.
Meniere disease.
Ototoxic drugs: streptomycin, gentamicin.
Lesions of the eighth nerve: acoustic neuroma, meningioma, mononeuropathy, metastatic carcinoma.
Mastoiditis.

CNS OR SYSTEMIC

Vertebrobasilar artery insufficiency.
Posterior fossa tumor or other brain tumors.
Infarction/hemorrhage of cerebral cortex, cerebellum, or brain stem.
Basilar migraine.
Metabolic: drugs, hypoxia, anemia, fever.
Hypotension/severe hypertension.
Multiple sclerosis.
CNS infections: viral, bacterial.
Temporal lobe epilepsy.
Arnold–Chiari malformation, syringobulbia.
Psychogenic: ventilation, hysteria.

VERTIGO, CENTRAL[1]

ICD-10CM # R42

MAJOR CAUSES OF CENTRAL VERTIGO

Demyelination:
- Acquired.
- Leukodystrophies.
- Multiple sclerosis.

Familial disorders:
- Friedreich ataxia.
- Spinocerebellar ataxia.
- Familial episodic ataxia (type 1 and type 2).
- Olivopontocerebellar atrophy.

CNS infections:
- Lyme neuroborreliosis.
- Meningitis.
- Tuberculosis.

Intrinsic brainstem lesion:
- Tumor.
- Arteriovenous malformation.
- Trauma.

Migraine:
- Basilar.
- Benign paroxysmal positional vertigo of childhood.

Toxins:
- Drugs, alcohol.
- Analgesics.
- Anticonvulsants.
- Antihypertensives.
- Hypnotics.
- Tranquilizers.

Metabolic and endocrine disorders:
- Hyperinsulinism.
- Impaired glucose tolerance.
- Diabetes mellitus.
- Hypertriglyceridemia.
- Hypothyroidism.

Systemic conditions:
- Paget disease.

Stroke/ischemia:
- Vertebrobasilar.
- Cerebellar.
- Posterior inferior cerebellar artery syndrome.
- Lateral medullary syndrome.
- Medial medullary infarct.
- Basilar artery syndrome.
- Anterior inferior cerebellar artery.

Other causes of posterior ischemia:
- Subclavian steal syndrome.
- Rotational vertebral artery occlusion syndrome.
- Vertebral artery dissection.
- Vertebral or basilar artery dolichoectasia.
- Neoplasm of the fourth ventricle.
- Chiari malformation.
- Superficial siderosis of the CNS.
- Vestibular epilepsy.

VESICULAR OR BULLOUS SKIN RASH[19]

ICD-10CM # R21 Rash and other nonspecific skin eruption

CAUSES OF A VESICULAR OR BULLOUS SKIN RASH

Most Common

Viral:
- Herpes zoster
- Herpes simplex

Impetigo
Scabies
Insect bites and papular urticaria
Bullous eczema and pompholyx
Drugs:
- Sulphonamides
- Penicillin
- Barbiturates

Less Common

Erythema multiforme major ("target lesions" rash, plus one mucous membrane involved) or erythema multiforme minor (1–2 cm "target lesions" only):
- Mycoplasma pneumonia
- Herpes simplex
- Drugs such as sulphur, penicillins
- Idiopathic (50%)

SJS and TEN with epidermal detachment and mucosal erosions:
- Drugs such as anticonvulsants, sulphonamides, NSAIDs, and penicillins

Staphylococcal scalded-skin syndrome (children)
Dermatitis herpetiformis (gluten sensitivity)
Pemphigus and pemphigoid

Rare

Porphyria cutanea tarda
Epidermolysis bullosa

NSAIDs, Nonsteroidal anti-inflammatory drugs; *SJS,* Stevens–Johnson syndrome; *TEN,* toxic epidermal necrolysis.

VESICULOBULLOUS DISEASES[36]

ICD-10CM #		
	L94.2	Calcinosis cutis
	L98.8	Other specified disorders of the skin and subcutaneous tissue

IMMUNOLOGICALLY MEDIATED DISEASES

Bullous pemphigoid.
Herpes gestationis.
Mucous membrane pemphigoid.
Epidermolysis bullosa acquisita.
Dermatitis herpetiformis.
Pemphigus (vulgaris, foliaceus, paraneoplastic).

HYPERSENSITIVITY DISEASES

Erythema multiforme minor.
Erythema multiforme major (Stevens-Johnson syndrome).
Toxic epidermal necrolysis.

METABOLIC DISEASES

Porphyria cutanea tarda.
Pseudoporphyria.
Diabetic blisters.

INHERITED GENETIC DISORDERS

Epidermolysis bullosa:
- Simplex.
- Junctional.
- Dystrophic.

INFECTIOUS DISEASES

Impetigo.
Staphylococcal scalded skin syndrome.
Herpes simplex.
Varicella.
Herpes zoster.

VIRAL ENCEPHALITIS, COMMON CAUSES[39]

ICD-10CM #	A86	Unspecified viral encephalitis
	A85.2	Arthropod-borne viral encephalitis, unspecified
	A84.9	Tick-borne viral encephalitis, unspecified
	A83.9	Mosquito-borne viral encephalitis, unspecified
	A85.8	Other specified viral encephalitis
	A85	Other viral encephalitis, not elsewhere classified

COMMON CAUSES OF VIRAL ENCEPHALITIS

Causes of Viral Encephalitis

Nonseasonal:
- Herpes simplex virus type 1 (herpes simplex encephalitis).
- Herpes simplex virus type 2 (neonatal encephalitis or adult meningoencephalitis).

Seasonal—summer and fall—arboviruses (arthropod borne):
- West Nile virus.
- St. Louis encephalitis virus.
- Eastern equine encephalitis virus.
- Western equine encephalitis virus.
- La Crosse/California encephalitis virus.
- Powassan encephalitis virus.
- Chikungunya virus.

Seasonal—non–arthropod borne:
- Summer and fall: enteroviruses (including coxsackieviruses, echoviruses, polioviruses, and enterovirus 71).
- Winter: influenza virus.

Immunosuppressed patients:
- Human immunodeficiency virus (chronic HIV encephalitis).
- Varicella-zoster virus (subacute encephalitis).
- JC virus (progressive multifocal leukoencephalopathy).
- Cytomegalovirus (ventriculitis or encephalitis).
- Human herpesvirus 6 (subacute encephalitis).
- Epstein-Barr virus (subacute encephalitis).

Uncommon Causes in the U.S.

Powassan encephalitis virus.
Zika virus.
Chikungunya virus.
Variegated squirrel bornavirus.
Lymphotropic choriomeningitis virus.
Rabies.
Measles (subacute sclerosing panencephalitis).
Mumps.
Adenovirus.
Herpes B virus (of monkeys).
Rubella (progressive rubella panencephalitis).

Causes Outside the United States

Zika virus (Africa, Asia, Caribbean, Central America, Pacific Islands, South America).
Chikungunya virus (Africa, Asia, Central America, Pacific Islands, South America, Western Europe).
Tick-borne encephalitis virus (Russia, Asia).
Japanese encephalitis virus (Japan, Southeast Asia, Malaysia).
Venezuelan equine encephalitis virus (Central and South America).
Dengue virus (Southern Asia, Africa, South America).
Rift Valley fever virus (east central Africa).
Murray Valley encephalitis virus (Australia).
Powassan encephalitis virus (Canada).
Nipah virus (Malaysia and Bangladesh).

VISION LOSS, ACUTE, PAINFUL

ICD-10CM #	H53.139	Sudden visual loss, unspecified eye

Acute angle-closure glaucoma.
Corneal ulcer.
Uveitis.
Endophthalmitis.
Factitious.
Somatization syndrome.
Trauma.

VISION LOSS, ACUTE, PAINLESS

ICD-10CM #	H53.139	Sudden visual loss, unspecified eye

Retinal artery occlusion.
Optic neuritis.
Retinal vein occlusion.
Vitreous hemorrhage.
Retinal detachment.
Exudative macular degeneration.
CVA.
Ischemic optic neuropathy.
Factitious.
Somatization syndrome, anxiety reaction.

VISION LOSS AFTER DIVING[4]

ICD-10CM #	H53.139

DIFFERENTIAL DIAGNOSIS OF DECREASED VISION AFTER DIVING

Decompression sickness.
Arterial gas embolism.
Bubbles under contact lenses.
Displaced contact lens.
Antifog agent keratopathy.
Contact lens adherence syndrome.
Transdermal scopolamine
Hyperoxic myopia.
Oxymetazoline optic neuropathy.
Diving-induced migraine phenomena.
Eye disorders not related to diving.

VISION LOSS, CHILDREN

ICD-10CM #	H53.9	Unspecified visual disturbance

Craniopharyngioma.
Hereditary optic atrophy.
Optic nerve glioma.
Glioma of chiasm.
Albinism.
Optic nerve hypoplasia.

VISION LOSS, CHRONIC, PROGRESSIVE

ICD-10CM #	H54.7	Unspecified visual loss

Cataract.
Macular degeneration.
Cerebral neoplasm.
Refractive error.
Open-angle glaucoma.

VISION LOSS, MONOCULAR, TRANSIENT

ICD-10CM #	H54.7	Unspecified visual loss

Thromboembolism.
Vasculitis.
Migraine (vasospasm).
Anxiety reaction.
CNS tumor.
Temporal arteritis.
Multiple sclerosis.

VITREOUS HEMORRHAGE[53]

ICD-10CM #	H43.13	Vitreous hemorrhage, bilateral

CAUSES OF VITREOUS HEMORRHAGE

Acute posterior vitreous detachment associated either with a retinal tear or avulsion of a peripheral vessel.

Proliferative retinopathies:
- Diabetic.
- Following retinal vein occlusion.
- Sickle cell disease.
- Eales disease.
- Vasculitis.

Miscellaneous retinal disorders:
- Macroaneurysm.
- Telangiectasis.
- Capillary hemangioma.

Trauma:
- Blunt.

Penetrating.
Iatrogenic.
Systemic:
Bleeding disorders.
Terson syndrome.

VOCAL CORD PARALYSIS

ICD-10CM #	J38.00	Paralysis of vocal cords and larynx, unspecified
	J38.01	Paralysis of vocal cords and larynx, unilateral
	J38.02	Paralysis of vocal cords and larynx, bilateral

Neoplasm: primary or metastatic (e.g., lung, thyroid, parathyroid, mediastinum).
Neck surgery (parathyroid, thyroid, carotid endarterectomy, cervical spine).
Idiopathic.
Viral, bacterial, or fungal infection.
Trauma (intubation, penetrating neck injury).
Cardiac surgery.
RA.
Multiple sclerosis.
Parkinsonism.
Toxic neuropathy.
CVA.
CNS abnormalities: hydrocephalus, Arnold–Chiari malformation, meningomyelocele.

VOLUME DEPLETION[3]

ICD-10CM #	E86.9	Volume depletion, unspecified

GI losses:
Upper: bleeding, nasogastric suction, vomiting.
Lower: bleeding, diarrhea, enteric or pancreatic fistula, tube drainage.
Renal losses:
Salt and water: diuretics, osmotic diuresis, postobstructive diuresis, acute tubular necrosis (recovery phase), salt-losing nephropathy, adrenal insufficiency, renal tubular acidosis.
Water loss: diabetes insipidus.
Skin and respiratory losses:
Sweat, burns, insensible losses.
Sequestration without external fluid loss:
Intestinal obstruction, peritonitis, pancreatitis, rhabdomyolysis, internal bleeding.

VOLUME EXCESS[3]

ICD-10CM #	Varies with specific diagnosis

Primary Renal Sodium Retention (Increased Effective Circulating Volume)
Renal failure, nephritic syndrome, acute glomerulonephritis.
Primary hyperaldosteronism.
Cushing syndrome.
Liver disease.

Secondary Renal Sodium Retention (Decreased Effective Circulating Volume)
Heart failure.
Liver disease.
Nephrotic syndrome (minimal change disease).
Pregnancy.

VOMITING

ICD-10CM #	R11.10	Vomiting, unspecified
	R11.11	Vomiting without nausea
	R11.12	Projectile vomiting

GI disturbances:
Obstruction: esophageal, pyloric, intestinal.
Infections: viral or bacterial enteritis, viral hepatitis, food poisoning, gastroenteritis.
Pancreatitis.
Appendicitis.
Biliary colic.
Peritonitis.
Perforated bowel.
Diabetic gastroparesis.
Other: gastritis, PUD, IBD, GI tract neoplasms.
Drugs: morphine, digitalis, cytotoxic agents, bromocriptine.
Severe pain: MI, renal colic.
Metabolic disorders: uremia, acidosis/alkalosis, hyperglycemia, DKA, thyrotoxicosis.
Trauma: blows to the testicles, epigastrium.
Vertigo.
Reye syndrome.
Increased intracranial pressure.
CNS disturbances: trauma, hemorrhage, infarction, neoplasm, infection, hypertensive encephalopathy, migraine.
Radiation sickness.
Nausea and vomiting of pregnancy, hyperemesis gravidarum.
Motion sickness.
Bulimia, anorexia nervosa.
Psychogenic: emotional disturbances, offensive sights or smells.
Severe coughing.
Pyelonephritis.
Boerhaave syndrome.
Carbon monoxide poisoning.

VOMITING, NEONATAL[1]

ICD-10CM #	R11.10	Vomiting, unspecified

CAUSES OF NEONATAL VOMITING

Anatomic Causes
Esophagus, trachea, great vessels:
Stricture.
Web.
Tracheoesophageal fistula.
Laryngeal cleft.
Double aortic arch.
Stomach and duodenum:
Pyloric stenosis.
Duodenal atresia (usually noted on the first day of life)
Small and large intestine:
Volvulus secondary to malrotation.
Incarcerated hernia.
Hirschsprung disease (secondary to obstipation).
Necrotizing enterocolitis.
Genitourinary:
Testicular torsion.

Nonanatomic Causes
Infection:
Septicemia.
Meningitis.
Urinary tract infection.
Gastroenteritis.
Otitis media
Increased intracranial pressure:
Cerebral edema.
Subdural hematoma.
Hydrocephalus.
Brain tumor.
Congenital adrenal hyperplasia (salt-losing variety).
Inborn errors of metabolism.
Renal disease.

VULVAR LESIONS[28]

ICD-10CM #	N77.0	Ulceration of vulva in diseases classified elsewhere
	N90.7	Vulvar cyst
	N90.89	Other specified noninflammatory disorders of vulva and perineum
	D07.1	Carcinoma in situ of vulva
	N90.89	Other specified noninflammatory disorders of vulva and perineum
	N90.5	Atrophy of vulva

RED LESION

Infection/Infestation
Fungal infection:
Candida.
Tinea cruris.
Intertrigo.
Pityriasis versicolor.
Sarcoptes scabiei.
Erythrasma: *Corynebacterium minutissimum.*
Granuloma inguinale: Calymmatobacterium granulomatis.
Folliculitis: *Staphylococcus aureus.*
Hidradenitis suppurativa.
Behçet syndrome.

Inflammation
Reactive vulvitis.
Chemical irritation:
Detergent.
Dyes.
Perfume.
Spermicide.
Lubricants.
Hygiene sprays.
Podophyllum.
Topical 5-FU.
Saliva.
Gentian violet.
Semen.
Mechanical trauma: scratching.
Vestibular adenitis.
Essential vulvodynia.

Psoriasis.
Seborrheic dermatitis.
Neoplasm
Vulvar intraepithelial neoplasia (VIN):
- Mild dysplasia.
- Moderate dysplasia.
- Severe dysplasia.
- Carcinoma-in-situ.

Vulvar dystrophy.
Bowen disease.
Invasive cancer:
- Squamous cell carcinoma.
- Malignant melanoma.
- Sarcoma.
- Basal cell carcinoma.
- Adenocarcinoma.
- Paget disease.
- Undifferentiated.

WHITE LESION

Vulvar dystrophy:
- Lichen sclerosus.
- Vulvar dystrophy.
- Vulvar hyperplasia.
- Mixed dystrophy.

VIN.
Vitiligo.
Partial albinism.
Intertrigo.
Radiation treatment.

DARK LESION

Lentigo.
Nevi (mole).
Neoplasm (see "Neoplasm, Vulvar," below).
Reactive hyperpigmentation.
Seborrheic keratosis.
Pubic lice.

ULCERATIVE LESION

Infection
Herpes simplex.
Vaccinia.
Treponema pallidum.
Granuloma inguinale.
Pyoderma.
Tuberculosis.
Noninfectious
Behçet disease.
Crohn disease.
Pemphigus.
Pemphigoid.
Hidradenitis suppurativa (see "Neoplasm, Vulvar," below).
Neoplasm
Basal cell carcinoma.
Squamous cell carcinoma.
Vulvar tumor <1 cm:
- Condyloma acuminatum.
- Molluscum contagiosum.
- Epidermal inclusion.
- Vestibular cyst.
- Mesonephric duct.
- VIN.
- Hemangioma.
- Hidradenoma.
- Neurofibroma.
- Syringoma.
- Accessory breast tissue.
- Acrochordon.
- Endometriosis.
- Fox-Fordyce disease.
- Pilonidal sinus.

Vulvar tumor >1 cm:
- Bartholin cyst or abscess.
- Lymphogranuloma venereum.
- Fibroma.
- Lipoma.
- Verrucous carcinoma.
- Squamous cell carcinoma.
- Hernia.
- Edema.
- Hematoma.
- Acrochordon.
- Epidermal cysts.
- Neurofibromatosis.
- Accessory breast tissue.

VULVAR PAIN[26]

ICD-10CM #	N94.81	Vulvodynia
	R10.2	Pelvic and perineal pain

DISEASES ASSOCIATED WITH VULVAR PAIN, NOT QUALIFYING FOR THE DIAGNOSIS OF VULVODYNIA

Podophyllin overdose.
Condylox (podofilox) overdose.
Behçet disease.
Aphthous ulcers.
Herpes (simplex and zoster).
Candidiasis.
Trichomonas.
Chancroid.
Sjögren disease.
Contact dermatitis.
Endometriosis.
Pemphigus.
Pemphigoid.
Atrophy.
Lichen sclerosus.
Lichen planus.
Crohn disease.
Bartholin abscess.
Trauma.
Imperforate hymen.
Prolapsed urethra.
Vulvar intraepithelial neoplasia.
Carcinoma.

VULVITIS, GRANULOMATOUS

ICD-10CM #	N76.2	Acute vulvitis
	N76.3	Subacute and chronic vulvitis

Differential diagnosis of granulomatous vulvitis
Syphilis.
Lymphogranuloma venereum.
Mycobacteria.
Fungus.
Bacillary angiomatosis.
Folliculitis.
Ruptured pilosebaceous unit.
Ruptured cyst.
Crohn disease.
Vulvitis granulomatosa.
Hydradenitis suppurativa.

WEAKNESS, ACUTE, EMERGENT[65]

ICD-10CM #	M62.81	Muscle weakness (generalized)

Demyelinating disorders (Guillain-Barré, chronic inflammatory demyelinating polyneuropathy [CIDP]).
Myasthenia gravis.
Infectious (poliomyelitis, diphtheria).
Toxic (botulism, tick paralysis, paralytic shellfish toxin, puffer fish, newts).
Metabolic (acquired or familial hypokalemia, hypophosphatemia, hypermagnesemia).
Metal poisoning (arsenic, thallium).
Porphyria.

WEAKNESS, GRADUAL ONSET

ICD-10CM #	M62.81	Muscle weakness (generalized)

Depression.
Malingering.
Anemia.
Hypothyroidism.
Medications (e.g., sedatives, antidepressants, narcotics).
CHF.
Renal failure.
Liver failure.
Respiratory insufficiency.
Alcoholism.
Nutritional deficiencies.
Disorders of motor unit.
Basal ganglia disorders.
Upper motor neuron lesions.

WEAKNESS, NONNEUROMUSCULAR CAUSES

ICD-10CM #	G93.3	Postviral fatigue syndrome
	R53.1	Weakness
	R53.81	Other malaise
	R53.83	Other fatigue

Anxiety disorder.
Infectious process.
Anemia.
Renal insufficiency.
Hyperventilation.
Malignancy.
Hypothyroidism.
Hypotension.
Hypercapnia.
Hypoglycemia.
Cardiac arrhythmias.
Hepatic insufficiency.
Electrolyte imbalance.
Malnutrition.
Cerebrovascular insufficiency.

WEIGHT GAIN

ICD-10CM #	R63.5	Abnormal weight gain
	E66.9	Obesity, unspecified

Sedentary lifestyle.
Fluid overload.
Discontinuation of tobacco abuse.
Endocrine disorders (hypothyroidism, hyperinsulinism associated with maturity-onset DM, Cushing syndrome, hypogonadism, insulinoma, hyperprolactinemia, acromegaly).
Medications (nutritional supplements, oral contraceptives, glucocorticoids, etc.).
Anxiety disorders with compulsive eating.
Laurence-Moon-Biedl syndrome, Prader-Willi syndrome, other congenital diseases.
Hypothalamic injury (rare; <100 cases reported in medical literature).

WEIGHT LOSS

ICD-10CM # R63.4 Abnormal weight loss

Malignancy.
Psychiatric disorders (depression, anorexia nervosa).
New-onset DM.
Malabsorption.
COPD.
AIDS.
Uremia, liver disease.
Thyrotoxicosis, pheochromocytoma, carcinoid syndrome.
Addison disease.
Intestinal parasites.
Peptic ulcer disease.
Inflammatory bowel disease.
Food faddism.
Postgastrectomy syndrome.

WHEEZING

ICD-10CM # R06.2 Wheezing

Asthma.
COPD.
Interstitial lung disease.
Infections (pneumonia, bronchitis, bronchiolitis, epiglottitis).
Cardiac asthma.
GERD with aspiration.
Foreign body aspiration.
Pulmonary embolism.
Anaphylaxis.
Obstruction of airway (neoplasm, goiter, edema or hemorrhage from trauma, aneurysm, congenital abnormalities, strictures, spasm).
Carcinoid syndrome.

WHEEZING, PEDIATRIC AGE[9]

ICD-10CM # R06.2 Wheezing

Reactive airways disease.
Atopic asthma.
Infection-associated airway reactivity.
Exercise-induced asthma.
Salicylate-induced asthma and nasal polyposis.
Asthmatic bronchitis.
Other hypersensitivity reactions:
- Hypersensitivity pneumonitis.
- Tropical eosinophilia.
- Visceral larva migrans.
- Allergic bronchopulmonary aspergillosis.

Aspiration:
- Foreign body.
- Food, saliva, gastric contents.
- Laryngotracheoesophageal cleft.
- Tracheoesophageal fistula, H-type.
- Pharyngeal incoordination or neuromuscular weakness.

Cystic fibrosis.
Primary ciliary dyskinesia.
Cardiac failure.
Bronchiolitis obliterans.
Extrinsic compression of airways:
- Vascular ring.
- Enlarged lymph node.
- Mediastinal tumor.
- Lung cysts.

Tracheobronchomalacia.
Endobronchial masses.
Gastroesophageal reflux.
Pulmonary hemosiderosis.
Sequelae of bronchopulmonary dysplasia.
"Hysterical" glottic closure.
Cigarette smoke, other environmental insults.

WRIST AND HAND PAIN[47]

ICD-10CM # S69.90XA Unspecified injury of unspecified wrist, hand and finger(s), initial encounter

Articular	
Arthritis of the wrist, MCP, PIP, or DIP as a result of:	Trauma, hypermobility, sprain. RA (wrist, MCP, PIP joints). Osteoarthritis (first CMC, PIP, and DIP joints). Other forms of arthritis: gout, psoriatic arthritis, infection. Joint neoplasm.
Periarticular	
Subcutaneous.	RA nodules, gouty tophi, painful subcutaneous calcific nodules in scleroderma, glomus tumor of the nail bed.
Palmar fascia.	Dupuytren contracture.
Tendon sheath.	Wrist extensor tenosynovitis, including de Quervain tenosynovitis and extensor carpi radialis tenosynovitis. Wrist volar flexor tenosynovitis (including carpal tunnel syndrome). Thumb flexor tenosynovitis (trigger or snapping thumb). Finger flexor tenosynovitis (trigger finger). Pigmented villonodular tenosynovitis (giant cell tumor of the tendon sheath).
Acute calcific periarthritis ganglion.	Wrist, MCP, and rarely the PIP and DIP joints.
Osseous	
Bone lesions.	Fractures; neoplasm; infection; osteonecrosis, including Kienböck disease (lunate) and Preiser disease (scaphoid).
Neurologic	
Nerve entrapment syndromes	
Median nerve.	Carpal tunnel syndrome (at the wrist). Pronator teres syndrome (at the pronator teres). Anterior interosseous nerve syndrome.
Ulnar nerve.	Cubital tunnel syndrome (at the elbow). Guyon canal (at the wrist).
Posterior interosseous nerve syndrome.	Radial nerve palsy (spiral groove syndrome).
Lower brachial plexus.	Thoracic outlet syndrome, Pancoast tumor.
Cervical nerve roots.	Herniated cervical disk, tumors.
Spinal cord lesion	
Spinal tumors, syringomyelia.	
Vascular	
Vasoplastic disorders with Raynaud phenomenon.	Scleroderma, occupational vibration syndrome.
Small- or large-vessel vasculitis.	With digital ischemia, ischemic ulcers (e.g., SLE, RA, and Takayasu arthritis).
Referred pain	
Cervical spine disorders. Reflex sympathetic dystrophy syndrome.	Shoulder–hand syndrome and causalgia.
Cardiac.	Angina pectoris.

CMC, Carpometacarpal; *DIP,* distal interphalangeal; *MCP,* metacarpophalangeal; *PIP,* proximal interphalangeal; *RA,* rheumatoid arthritis; *SLE,* systemic lupus erythematosus.

WRIST AND HAND PAIN, IN DIFFERENT AGE GROUPS[22]

ICD-10CM # S69.80XA Other specified injuries of unspecified wrist, hand and finger(s), initial encounter
S69.90XA Unspecified injury of unspecified wrist, hand and finger(s), initial encounter

COMMON CAUSES OF WRIST AND HAND PAIN IN DIFFERENT AGE GROUPS

Childhood (2 to 10 yr)
Intraarticular
Infection.
Periarticular
Fracture.
Osteomyelitis.
Adolescence (10 to 18 yr)
Intraarticular
Infection.
Periarticular
Trauma.
Osteomyelitis.
Tumors.
Ganglion.
Idiopathic wrist pain.
Early Adulthood (18 to 30 yr)
Intraarticular
Inflammatory arthritis.
Infection.
Osteoarthritis.
Periarticular
Peripheral nerve entrapment.
Tendonitis.
Referred
Cervical.
Adulthood (30 to 50 yr)
Intraarticular
Inflammatory arthritis.
Infection.
Osteoarthritis.
Periarticular
Peripheral nerve entrapment.
Tendonitis.
Referred
Cervical.
Chest.
Cardiac.
Old age (>50 yr)
Intraarticular
Inflammatory arthritis.
Osteoarthritis.
Periarticular
Peripheral nerve entrapment.
Tendonitis.
Referred
Cervical.
Chest.
Cardiac.

WRIST PAIN

ICD-10CM #	S69.80XA	Other specified injuries of unspecified wrist, hand and finger(s), initial encounter
	S69.90XA	Unspecified injury of unspecified wrist, hand and finger(s), initial encounter

MECHANICAL

Osteoarthritis.
Ligament tear.
Fracture.
Ganglion.
De Quervain tenosynovitis.
Avascular necrosis (scaphoid, lunate).
Nonunion of scaphoid or lunate.
Neoplasm.

METABOLIC

Pregnancy.
Diabetes.
Gout.
Pseudogout.
Paget disease.
Acromegaly.
Hypothyroidism.
Hyperparathyroidism.

INFECTIOUS

Osteomyelitis.
Septic arthritis.
Cat-scratch disease.
Tick bite (Lyme disease, babesiosis).
Tuberculosis.

NEUROLOGIC

Peripheral neuropathy.
Nerve injury (median, ulnar, radial nerve).
Thoracic outlet compression syndrome.
Distal posterior interosseous nerve syndrome.

RHEUMATOLOGIC

Psoriasis.
RA.
SLE, mixed connective tissue disorder (MCTD).
Scleroderma.

MISCELLANEOUS

Granulomatous (sarcoidosis).
Amyloidosis.
Multiple myeloma.
Leukemia.

XANTHOMAS[11]

ICD-10CM #	L99	Other disorders of skin and subcutaneous tissue in diseases classified elsewhere

Differential Diagnosis of Xanthomas

Eruptive xanthomas:
- Non-Langerhans cell histiocytosis.

Xanthoma disseminatum.
Papular xanthoma.
Generalized eruptive histiocytomas.
Indeterminate cell histiocytosis.
Rosai-Dorfman disease.
Juvenile xanthogranuloma (micronodular form).
Xanthomatous lesions of Langerhans cell histiocytosis.
Disseminated granuloma annulare.
Tuberous xanthomas:
- Erythema elevatum diutinum.
- Multicentric reticulohistiocytosis.

Tendinous xanthomas:
- Giant cell tumor of the tendon sheath.
- Rheumatoid nodule.
- Subcutaneous granuloma annulare.
- Erythema elevatum diutinum.

Xanthelasma:
- Syringomas.
- Necrobiotic xanthogranuloma.
- *A*dult-onset *a*sthma and *peri*o*c*ular *x*anthogranuloma (AAPOX).
- Sebaceous hyperplasia.
- Palpebral sarcoidosis.

XEROPHTHALMIA[71]

ICD-10CM #	H11.149	Conjunctival xerosis, unspecified, unspecified eye

MEDICATIONS

Tricyclic antidepressants: amitriptyline, doxepin.
Antihistamines: diphenhydramine, chlorpheniramine, promethazine, and many cold and decongestant preparations.
Anticholinergic agents: antiemetics such as scopolamine, antispasmodic agents such as oxybutynin chloride.

ABNORMALITIES OF EYELID FUNCTION

Neuromuscular disorders.
Aging.
Thyrotoxicosis.

ABNORMALITIES OF TEAR PRODUCTION

Hypovitaminosis A.
Stevens-Johnson syndrome.
Familial diseases affecting sebaceous secretions.

ABNORMALITIES OF CORNEAL SURFACES

Scarring from past injuries and herpes simplex infection.

XEROSTOMIA[71]

ICD-10CM #	K11.7	Disturbances of salivary secretion
	R68.2	Dry mouth, unspecified

MEDICATIONS

Tricyclic antidepressants: amitriptyline, doxepin.
Antihistamines: diphenhydramine, chlorpheniramine, promethazine, and many cold and decongestant preparations.
Anticholinergic agents: antiemetics such as scopolamine, antispasmodic agents such as oxybutynin chloride.

DEHYDRATION

Debility.
Fever.

POLYURIA

Alcohol intake.
Arrhythmia.
Diabetes.

PREVIOUS HEAD AND NECK IRRADIATION SYSTEMIC DISEASES

Sjögren syndrome.
Sarcoidosis.
Amyloidosis.
HIV infection.
Graft-versus-host disease.

YELLOW URINE

ICD-10CM # R82 Other abnormal findings in urine

Normal coloration
Concentrated urine
Use of multivitamin supplements
Diet rich in carrots
Use of Cascara
Urinary tract infection

REFERENCES

1. Adams JG et al: *Emergency medicine, clinical essentials*, ed 2, Philadelphia, 2013, Elsevier.
2. Adkinson NF et al: *Middleton's allergy principles and practice*, ed 8, Philadelphia, 2014, Saunders.
3. Andreoli TE et al: *Cecil essentials of medicine*, ed 5, Philadelphia, Saunders.
4. Auerbach P: *Wilderness medicine*, Philadelphia, Saunders.
5. Bain BJ, Bates I, Laffan MA: *Dacie and Lewis practical haematology*, ed 12, Philadelphia, 2017, Elsevier.
6. Ballinger A: *Kumar & Clark's essentials of clinical medicine*, ed 6, Edinburgh, Saunders.
7. Barkin RM, Rosen P: *Emergency pediatrics: a guide to ambulatory care*, ed 5, St Louis, Mosby.
8. Baude AI: *Infectious diseases and medical microbiology*, ed 2, Philadelphia, Saunders.
9. Behrman RE: *Nelson textbook of pediatrics*, ed 16, Philadelphia, Saunders.
10. Bennett JE, Dolin R, Blaser MJ: *Mandell, Douglas, and Bennett's principles and practice of infectious diseases*, ed 8, Philadelphia, 2015, Saunders.
11. Bolognia JL, Schaffer JV, Cerroni L: *Dermatology*, ed 4, 2018, Elsevier.
12. Bonow RO et al: *Braunwauld's heart disease*, ed 9, Philadelphia, Elsevier.
13. Bowling B: *Kanski's clinical ophthalmology*, ed 8, Philadelphia, 2016, Elsevier.
14. Boxt LM, Abbara S: *Cardiac imaging: The requisites*, ed 4, Philadelphia, 2016, Elsevier.
15. Boyer KM: Nonbacterial pneumonia. In Feigin RD, Cherry JD, editors: *Textbook of pediatric infectious diseases*, ed 4, Philadelphia, 1998, WB Saunders, pp 260-273.
16. Callen JP: *Color atlas of dermatology*, ed 2, Philadelphia, WB Saunders.
17. Cameron JL, Cameron AM: *Current surgical therapy*, ed 10, Philadelphia, Saunders.
18. Cameron JL, Cameron AM: *Current surgical therapy*, ed 12, Philadelphia, 2017, Elsevier.
19. Cameron P, Little M, Mitra B, Deasy C: *Textbook of adult emergency medicine*, ed 5, 2020, Elsevier.
20. Canoso J: *Rheumatology in primary care*, Philadelphia, Saunders.
21. Carlson KJ: *Primary care of women*, ed 2, St Louis, Mosby.
22. Carr A, Hamilton W: *Orthopedics in primary care*, ed 2, Philadelphia, Saunders.
23. Cherry JD: *Feigin and Cherry's pediatric infectious diseases*, ed 8, Philadelphia, 2019, Elsevier.
24. Conn R: *Current diagnosis*, ed 9, Philadelphia, Saunders.
25. Copeland LJ: *Textbook of gynecology*, ed 2, Philadelphia, Saunders.
26. Crum CP: *Diagnostic gynecologic and obstetric pathology*, ed 3, Philadelphia, 2018, Elsevier.
27. Custer JW, Rau RE: *The Harriet Lane handbook*, ed 18, St Louis, Mosby.
28. Danakas G: *Practical guide to the care of the gynecologic/obstetric patient*, St Louis, Mosby.
29. Eberlein M: A fall in Ghana, *Am J Med* 122:1091, 2009.
30. Feldman M, Friedman LS, Brandt LJ: *Sleisenger and Fordtran's gastrointestinal and liver disease*, ed 10, Philadelphia, 2016, Elsevier.
31. Firestein GS, Budd RC, Gabriel SE et al: *Kelly's textbook of rheumatology*, ed 9, Philadelphia, Saunders.
32. Floege J et al: *Comprehensive clinical nephrology*, ed 4, Philadelphia, Saunders.
33. Fuhrman BP et al: *Pediatric critical care*, ed 4, Philadelphia, Saunders.
34. Gabbe SG: *Obstetrics*, ed 6, Philadelphia, Saunders.
35. Goldberg RJ: *The care of the psychiatric patient*, ed 3, St Louis, Mosby.
36. Goldman L, Ausiello D: *Cecil textbook of medicine*, ed 21, Philadelphia, Saunders.
37. Goldman L, Braunwald E: *Braunwauld primary cardiology*, Philadelphia, Saunders.
38. Goldman L, Schafer AI: *Goldman Cecil medicine*, ed 24, Philadelphia, Saunders.
39. Goldman L, Schafer AI: *Goldman-Cecil medicine*, ed 26, Philadelphia, 2020, Elsevier.
40. Gorbach SL: *Infectious diseases*, ed 2, Philadelphia, Saunders.
41. Grainger RG, Allison D: *Grainger & Allison's diagnostic radiology, a textbook of medical imaging*, ed 4, London, Churchill Livingstone.
42. Grant LA, Griffin N: *Grainger & Allison's diagnostic radiology essentials*, ed 2, Philadelphia, 2019, Elsevier.
43. Habif TP: *Clinical dermatology*, ed 6, Philadelphia, 2016, Elsevier.
44. Harrington J: *Consultation in internal medicine*, ed 2, St Louis, Mosby.
45. Henry JB: *Clinical diagnosis and management by laboratory methods*, ed 20, Philadelphia, Saunders.
46. Hochberg MC et al: *Rheumatology*, ed 5, Mosby: St. Louis.
47. Hochberg MC: *Rheumatology*, ed 7, Philadelphia, 2019, Elsevier.
48. Hoekelman R: *Primary pediatric care*, ed 3, St Louis, Mosby.
49. Hoffman R et al: *Hematology: basic principles and practice*, ed 6, Philadelphia, Saunders.
50. Hoffmann R et al: *Hematology: basic principles and practice*, ed 5, Philadelphia, Churchill Livingstone.
51. Hoffman R: *Hematology, basic principles and practice*, ed 7, Philadelphia, 2018, Elsevier.
52. James WD: *Andrews' diseases of the skin*, ed 12, Philadelphia, 2016, Saunders.
53. Kanski JJ, Bowling B: *Clinical ophthalmology, a systematic approach*, ed 7, Philadelphia, Saunders.
54. Kassirer J: *Current therapy in adult medicine*, ed 4, St Louis, Mosby.
55. Kassirer J: *Practical rheumatology*, London, Mosby.
56. Kaufman DM, Geyer HL, Milstein MJ: *Kaufman's clinical neurology for psychiatrists*, ed 8, Philadelphia, 2017, Elsevier.
57. Khan MG: *Rapid ECG interpretation*, Philadelphia, Saunders.
58. Kliegman RM et al: *Nelson textbook of pediatrics*, ed 19, Philadelphia, Saunders.
59. Kliegman RM: *Nelson textbook of pediatrics*, ed 21, Philadelphia, 2020, Elsevier.
60. Kliegman R: *Practical strategies in pediatric diagnosis and therapy*, Philadelphia, Saunders.
61. Lipshultz LI, Khera M, Atwal DT: *Urology and the primary care practitioner*, ed 3, Philadelphia, Elsevier.
62. Mahanty S, Nutman TB: Eosinophilia and eosinophil-related disorders. In Middleton EJ, Reed CE, Ellis EF et al [eds]: *Allergy: principles and practice*, ed 4, Mosby-Year Book: St Louis, p. 1077.
63. Mandell GL: *Mandell, Douglas, and Bennett's principles and practice of infectious diseases*, ed 6, New York, Churchill Livingstone.
64. Mann DL, Zipes DP, Libby P, Bonow RO: *Braunwald's heart disease*, ed 10, Philadelphia, 2015, Elsevier.
65. Marx JA: *Rosen's emergency medicine*, ed 8, Philadelphia, 2014, Saunders.
66. Mason RJ: *Murray & Nadel's textbook of respiratory medicine*, ed 5, Philadelphia, Saunders.
67. Melmed S, Polonsky KS, Larsen PR, Kronenberg HM: *Williams textbook of endocrinology*, ed 12, Philadelphia, Saunders.
68. Melmed S et al: *Williams textbook of endocrinology*, ed 14, Philadelphia, 2020, Elsevier.
69. Moore WT, Eastman RC: *Diagnostic endocrinology*, ed 2, St Louis, Mosby.
70. Niederhuber JE et al: *Abeloff's clinical oncology*, ed 6, Philadelphia, 2020, Elsevier.
71. Noble J: *Primary care medicine*, ed 3, St Louis, Mosby.
72. Nseyo UO: *Urology for primary care physicians*, Philadelphia, Saunders.
73. Palay D: *Ophthalmology for the primary care physician*, St Louis, Mosby.
74. Paller AS, Mancini AJ: *Hurwitz clinical pediatric dermatology*, ed 5, 2016, Elsevier.
75. Park MK: *Park's Pediatric cardiology for practitioners*, ed 6, Philadelphia, 2014, Saunders.
76. Parrillo JE, Dellinger RP: *Critical care medicine, principles of diagnosis and management in the adult*, ed 4, Philadelphia, 2014, Elsevier.
77. Parrillo JE, Dellinger RP: *Critical care medicine, principles of diagnosis and management in the adult*, ed 5, Philadelphia, 2019, Elsevier.
78. Pope TL, Bloem HL, Beltran J, Morrison WB, Wilson DJ: *Musculoskeletal imaging*, ed 2, Philadelphia, 2014, Saunders.
79. Rakel RE: *Principles of family practice*, ed 6, Philadelphia, Saunders.
80. Ronco C: *Critical care nephrology*, ed 3, Philadelphia, 2019, Elsevier.
81. Rumack CM: *Diagnostic ultrasound*, ed 4, Philadelphia, 2011, Elsevier.
82. Ryan ET et al: *Hunter's tropical medicine and emerging infectious diseases*, ed 10, 2020, Elsevier.
83. Schwarz MI: *Interstitial lung disease*, ed 2, St Louis, Mosby.

84. Seller RH: *Differential diagnosis of common complaints*, ed 4, Philadelphia, Saunders.
85. Sellke FW, del Nido PJ, Swanson SJ: *Sabiston & Spencer surgery of the chest*, ed 9, Philadelphia, 2016, Elsevier.
86. Siedel HM: *Mosby's guide to physical examination*, ed 4, St Louis, Mosby.
87. Skorecki K: *Brenner & Rector's the kidney*, ed 10, Philadelphia, 2016, Elsevier.
88. Souhami RL, Moxham J: *Textbook of medicine*, ed 4, London, Churchill Livingstone.
89. Spec A et al: *Comprehensive review of infectious diseases*, 2020, Elsevier.
90. Specht N: *Practical guide to diagnostic imaging*, St Louis, Mosby.
91. Stein JH: *Internal medicine*, ed 5, St Louis, Mosby.
92. Stern TA: *Massachusetts General Hospital handbook of general hospital psychiatry*, ed 7, Philadelphia, 2018, Elsevier.
93. Swaiman KF et al: *Swaiman's pediatric neurology, principles and practice*, ed 6, Philadelphia, 2017, Elsevier.
94. Swain R, Snodgrass JG: Managing groin pain, *Phys Sportmed* 23(56), 1995.
95. Talley NJ, Martin CJ: *Clinical gastroenterology*, ed 2, Sydney, Churchill Livingstone.
96. Tschudy MM, Arcara KM: *The Harriet Lane handbook*, ed 19, Philadelphia, Mosby.
97. Vincent JL et al: *Textbook of critical care*, ed 6, Philadelphia, Saunders.
98. Webb WR, Brant WE, Major NM: *Fundamentals of body CT*, ed 4, Philadelphia, 2015, Saunders.
99. Wein AJ: *Campbell-Walsh urology*, ed 11, Philadelphia, 2016, Elsevier.
100. Weinberger SE et al: *Principles of pulmonary medicine*, ed 5, Philadelphia, Saunders.
101. Weinberger SE et al: *Principles of pulmonary medicine*, ed 7, Philadelphia, 2019, Elsevier.
102. Wiederholt WC: *Neurology for non-neurologists*, ed 4, Philadelphia, Saunders.
103. Wilson JD: *Williams textbook of endocrinology*, ed 9, Philadelphia, Saunders.
104. Zipes DP: *Braunwald's heart disease, a textbook of cardiovascular medicine*, ed 11, Philadelphia, 2019, Elsevier.

SECTION III

Clinical Algorithms

PLEASE NOTE: These algorithms are designed to assist clinicians in the evaluation and treatment of patients. They may not apply to all patients with a particular disorder and are not intended to replace the clinician's individual judgment.

Additional algorithms content available at ExpertConsult.com

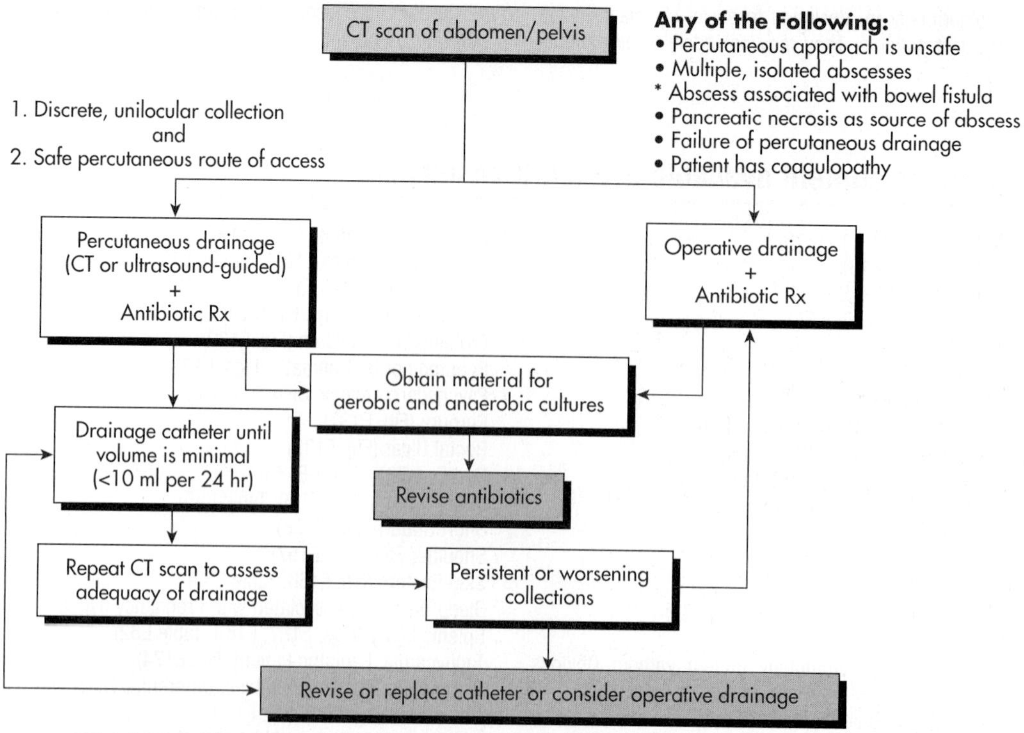

FIG. 1 Approach to management of intraabdominal abscesses including indications for consideration of percutaneous versus operative drainage. *CT,* Computed tomography; *Rx,* treatment. (From Parrillo JE, Dellinger RP: *Critical care medicine, principles of diagnosis and management in the adult,* ed 5, Philadelphia, 2019, Elsevier.)

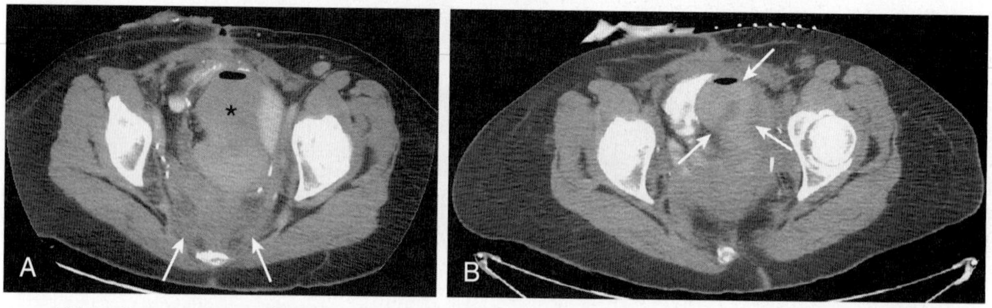

FIG. 2 A, Axial computed tomography (CT) image shows an apparently rim-enhancing structure containing gas (*asterisk*) in the deep pelvis adjacent to tethered bowel loops in a patient with prior pelvic irradiation. The structure could represent an abscess or a dilated loop of small bowel. The presacral inflammation *(arrows)* is related to radiation change. **B,** CT image obtained 2 hr later shows ingested oral contrast in this structure *(arrows)* confirming that this is a bowel loop rather than an abscess. (From Feldman M et al: *Sleisenger and Fortran's gastrointestinal and liver disease,* ed 10, Philadelphia, 2016, Elsevier.)

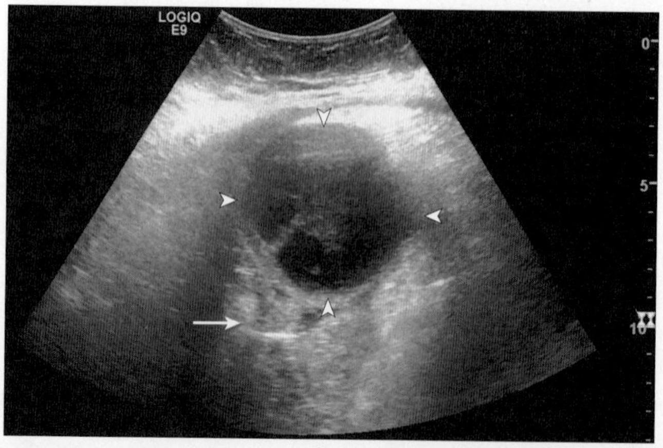

FIG. 3 Abdominal ultrasound of a typical abscess *(arrowheads)* demonstrating central decreased echogenicity, thickened wall, and debris arising anterior to the descending colon *(arrow)* in a patient with diverticulosis compatible with a diverticular abscess. (From Feldman M et al: *Sleisenger and Fortran's gastrointestinal and liver disease,* ed 10, Philadelphia, 2016, Elsevier.)

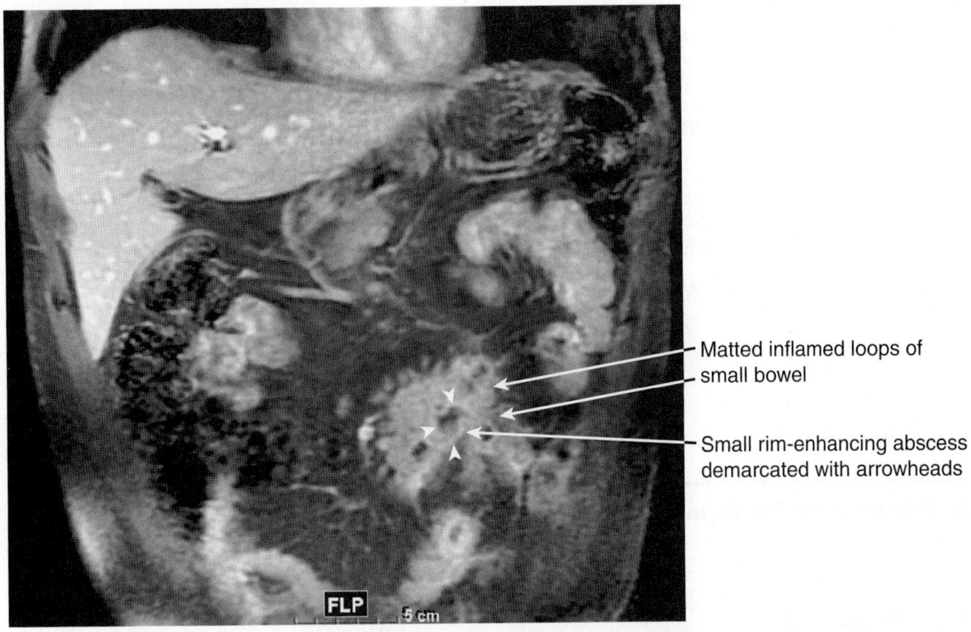

FIG. 4 Coronal magnetic resonance image with gadolinium contrast of a patient with Crohn disease showing a small rim-enhancing collection *(arrowheads)* interposed between several loops of inflamed bowel *(arrows)* compatible with an interloop abscess. Interloop abscesses are not amenable to percutaneous drain placement. (From Feldman M et al: *Sleisenger and Fortran's gastrointestinal and liver disease*, ed 10, Philadelphia, 2016, Elsevier.)

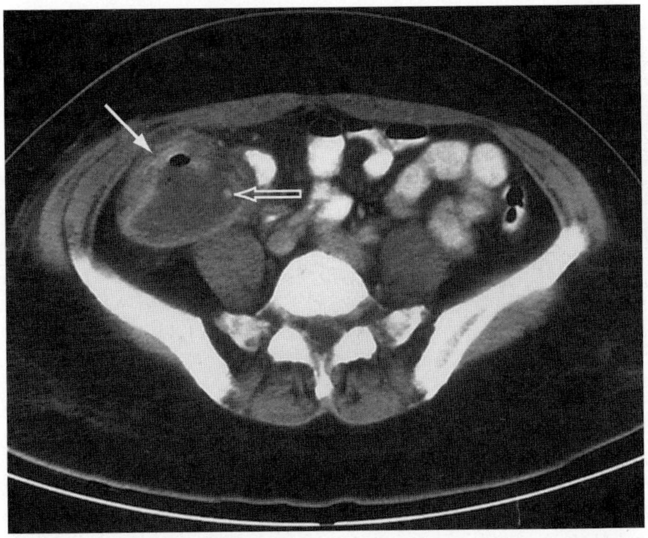

FIG. 5 Axial computed tomography demonstrating a right lower quadrant abscess *(closed arrow)* with an appendicolith *(open arrow).* Such extraluminal appendicoliths may predict clinical failure with percutaneous drainage. (From Feldman M et al: *Sleisenger and Fortran's gastrointestinal and liver disease*, ed 10, Philadelphia, 2016, Elsevier.)

BOX 1 Causes of Intraabdominal Abscesses

Abdominal trauma
Appendicitis
Cholecystectomy and other operations or invasive procedures
Crohn disease
Diverticulitis
Neoplastic disease
Pancreatitis
Perforated hollow viscus (e.g., duodenal or gastric ulcer)

From Feldman M et al: *Sleisenger and Fortran's gastrointestinal and liver disease*, ed 10, Philadelphia, 2016, Elsevier.

BOX 2 Clinical Risk Factors for Intraabdominal Abscess

Chronic glucocorticoid use
Increasing age
Malnutrition
Preexisting organ dysfunction
Transfusion
Underlying malignancy

From Feldman M et al: *Sleisenger and Fortran's gastrointestinal and liver disease*, ed 10, Philadelphia, 2016, Elsevier.

BOX 3 Antibiotic Choices in the Treatment of Intraabdominal Infections

Single-Agent Therapy
Second-Generation Cephalosporins
Cefoxitin

Carbapenems
Imipenem-cilastatin
Meropenem
Doripenem
Ertapenem (no *Pseudomonas* coverage)

Extended-Spectrum Penicillin–β-Lactamase Inhibitor Combinations
Piperacillin sodium-tazobactam
Ticarcillin disodium-clavulanate

Glycylcyclines
Tigecycline

Combination Therapy (Antiaerobe[a] + Antianaerobe)
Third- or Fourth-Generation Cephalosporins
Ceftriaxone + metronidazole
Cefotaxime + metronidazole
Ceftazidime (*Pseudomonas* coverage) + metronidazole
Cefepime (*Pseudomonas* coverage) + metronidazole

Fluoroquinolones
Ciprofloxacin + metronidazole
Levofloxacin + metronidazole
Moxifloxacin[b]

[a]Aminoglycoside therapy as an antiaerobic drug should not be used in routine practice owing to an increase in nephrotoxicity and possible worsened patient outcomes with its use.
[b]Moxifloxacin has adequate anaerobic coverage, making metronidazole unnecessary.
From Feldman M et al: *Sleisenger and Fortran's gastrointestinal and liver disease*, ed 10, Philadelphia, 2016, Elsevier.

TABLE 1 Comparison of Common Causes of Acute Abdominal Pain

Cause	Onset	Location	Character	Descriptor	Radiation	Intensity
Appendicitis	Gradual	Periumbilical area early; RLQ late	Diffuse early; localized later	Aching	None	++
Cholecystitis	Acute	RUQ	Localized	Constricting	Scapula	++
Pancreatitis	Acute	Epigastrium, back	Localized	Boring	Midback	++ to +++
Diverticulitis	Gradual	LLQ	Localized	Aching	None	++ to +++
Perforated peptic ulcer	Sudden	Epigastrium	Localized early, diffuse later	Burning	None	+++
Small bowel obstruction	Gradual	Periumbilical area	Diffuse	Cramping	None	++
Mesenteric ischemia, infarction	Sudden	Periumbilical area	Diffuse	Agonizing	None	+++
Ruptured abdominal aortic aneurysm	Sudden	Abdomen, back, flank	Diffuse	Tearing	None	+++
Gastroenteritis	Gradual	Periumbilical area	Diffuse	Spasmodic	None	+ to ++
Pelvic inflammatory disease	Gradual	Either LQ, pelvis	Localized	Aching	Upper thigh	++
Ruptured ectopic pregnancy	Sudden	Either LQ, pelvis	Localized	Sharp	None	++

+, Mild; ++, moderate; +++, severe; *LLQ*, left lower quadrant; *LQ*, lower quadrant; *RLQ*, right lower quadrant; *RUQ*, right upper quadrant.
From Feldman M et al: *Sleisenger and Fortran's gastrointestinal and liver disease*, ed 10, 2016, Elsevier.

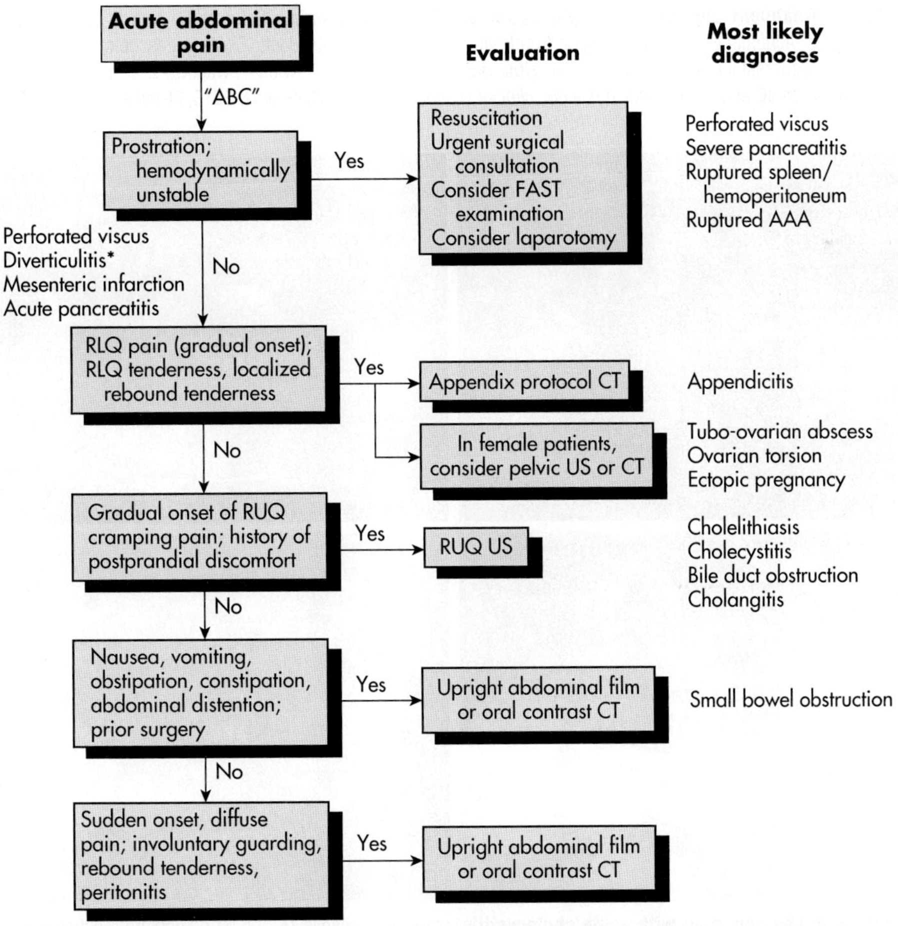

FIG. 6 An approach to the urgent evaluation of abdominal pain. Specific complaints and physical examination findings are coupled with appropriate radiologic imaging. *For left lower quadrant pain, the most likely diagnosis is diverticulitis. *AAA*, Abdominal aortic aneurysm; *ABC*, airway, breathing, circulation; *CT*, computed tomography; *FAST*, focused abdominal sonogram for trauma; *RLQ*, right lower quadrant; *RUQ*, right upper quadrant; *US*, ultrasound. (From Feldman M et al: *Sleisenger and Fortran's gastrointestinal and liver disease*, ed 10, 2016, Elsevier.)

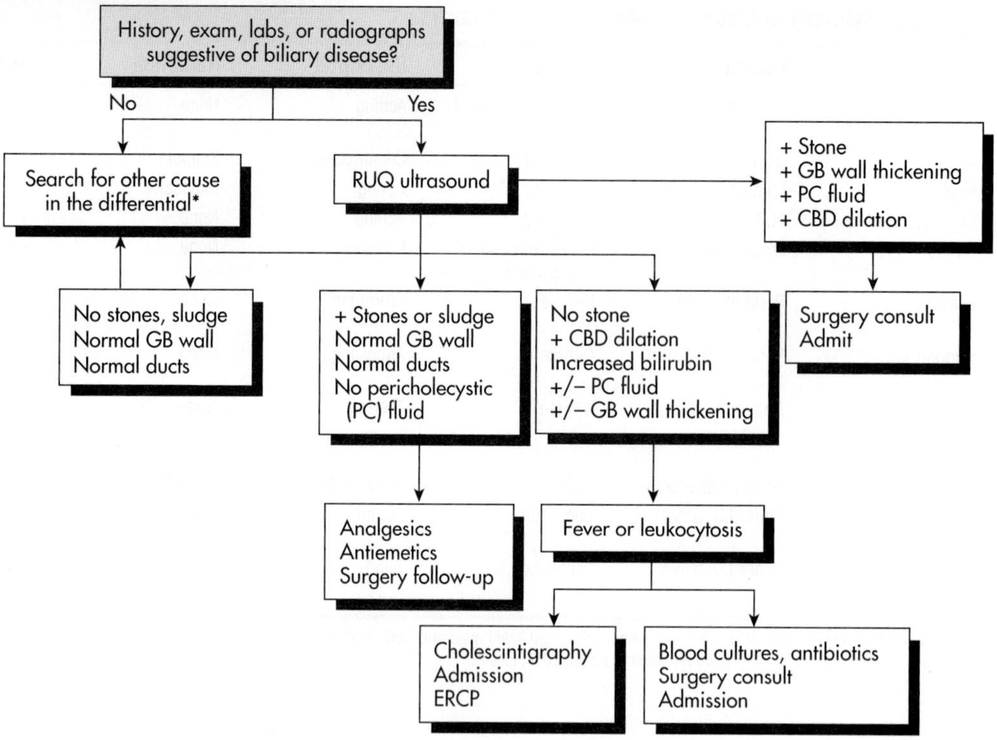

FIG. 7 Treatment algorithm for right upper quadrant *(RUQ)* pain. *Refer to Section II, Differential Diagnosis: Abdominal Pain, Right Upper Quadrant. *CBD,* Common bile duct; *ERCP,* endoscopic retrograde cholangiopancreatography; *GB,* gallbladder; *RUQ,* right upper quadrant; +, with; –, without; ±, with or without. (From Adams JG et al: *Emergency medicine, clinical essentials,* ed 2, Philadelphia, 2013, Elsevier.)

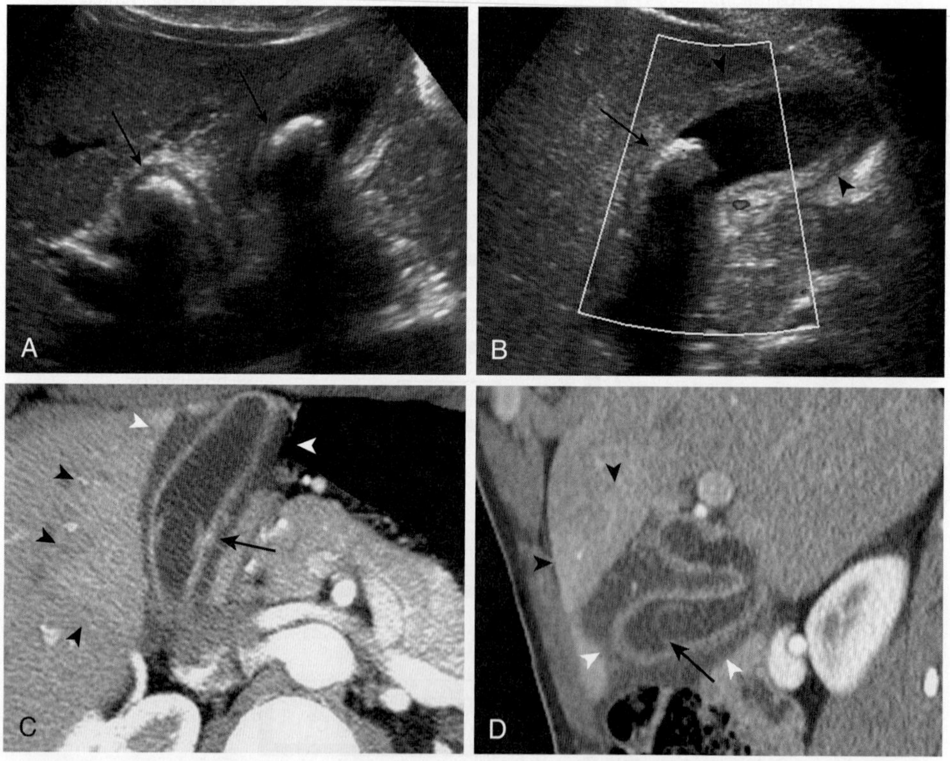

FIG. 8 A 43-yr-old man with acute cholecystitis. Ultrasound images **(A** and **B)** demonstrate echogenic, shadowing gallstones *(arrows)* with gallbladder wall thickening *(arrowheads)* in a patient in whom a sonographic Murphy sign was elicited. Axial **(C)** and sagittal **(D)** portal venous phase computed tomography images reveal a gallstone *(arrows)*, as well as a thickened gallbladder wall *(white arrowheads)*. Although not acquired in the arterial phase of contrast, hepatic hyperenhancement consistent with secondary inflammation is nevertheless seen *(black arrowheads)*. These findings are specific for this life-threatening complication and should be recognized and treated urgently. (From Soto JA, Lucey BC: *Emergency radiology, the requisites,* ed 2, 2017, Elsevier.)

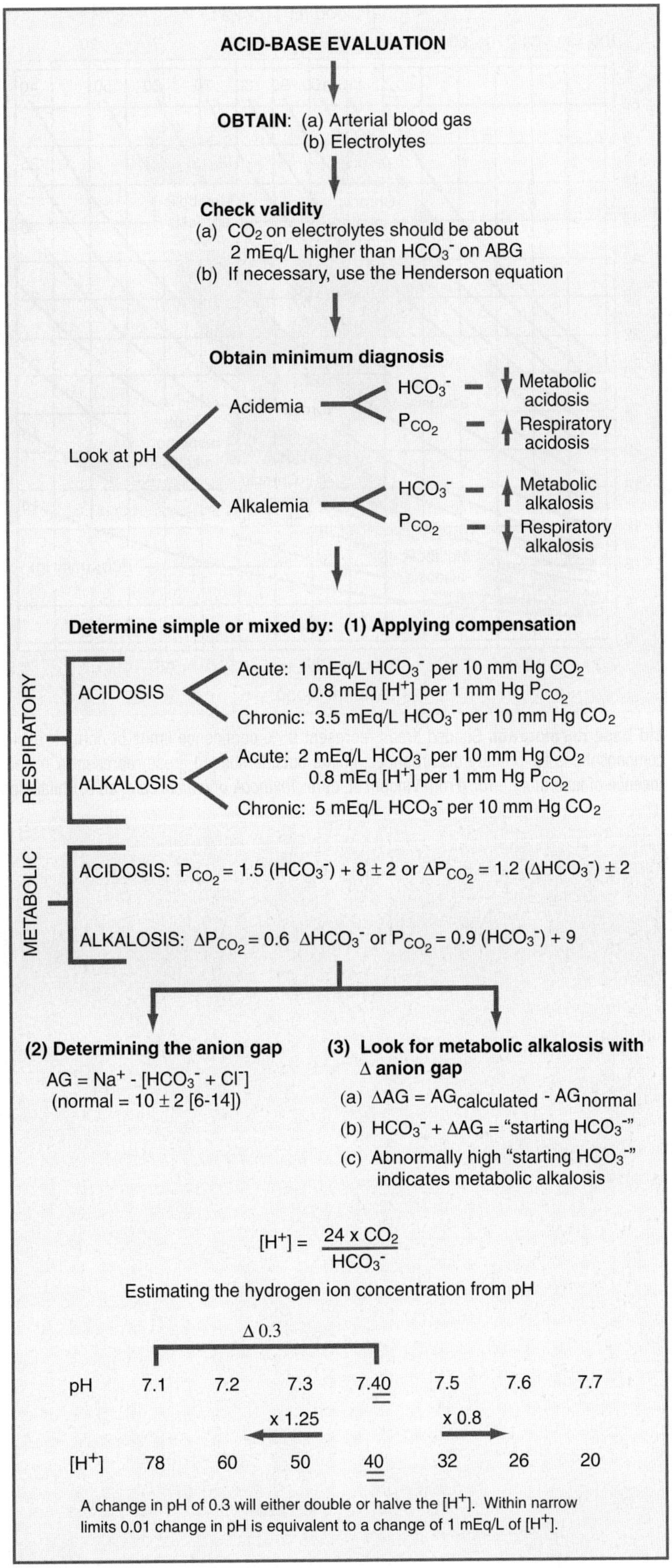

FIG. 9 Scheme for assessing acid-base homeostasis. *ABG,* Arterial blood gases; *AG,* anion gap; *PCO_2,* partial pressure of carbon dioxide. (Modified from Andreoli TE [ed]: *Cecil essentials of medicine,* ed 7, Philadelphia, 2008, Saunders.)

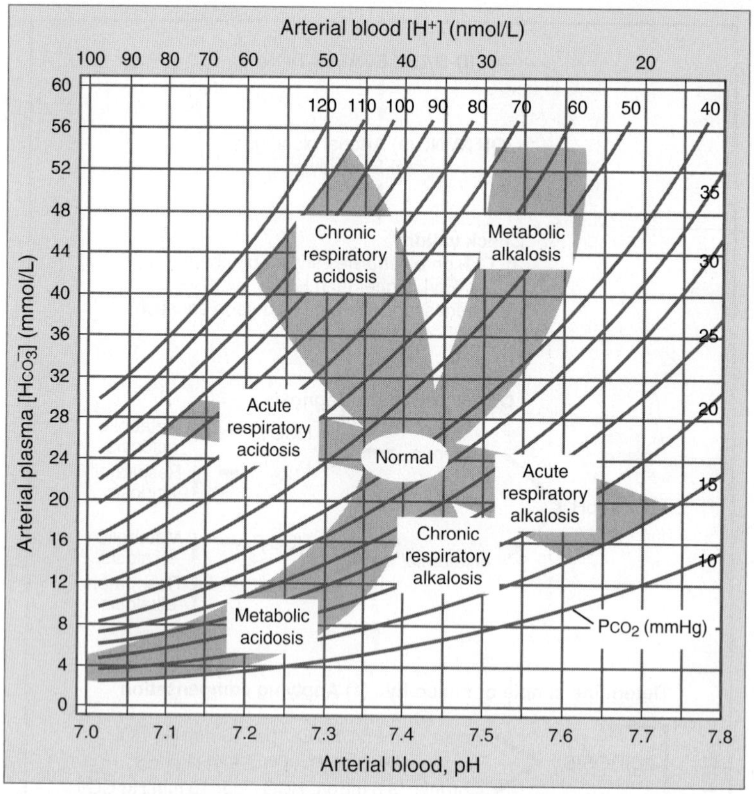

FIG. 10 Acid base normogram. Shaded areas represent 95% confidence limits of normal respiratory and metabolic compensations for primary disturbances. Points outside shaded areas represent a mixed disorder, assuming absence of laboratory error. (From Vincent JL et al: *Textbook of critical care*, ed 6, Philadelphia, 2011, Saunders.)

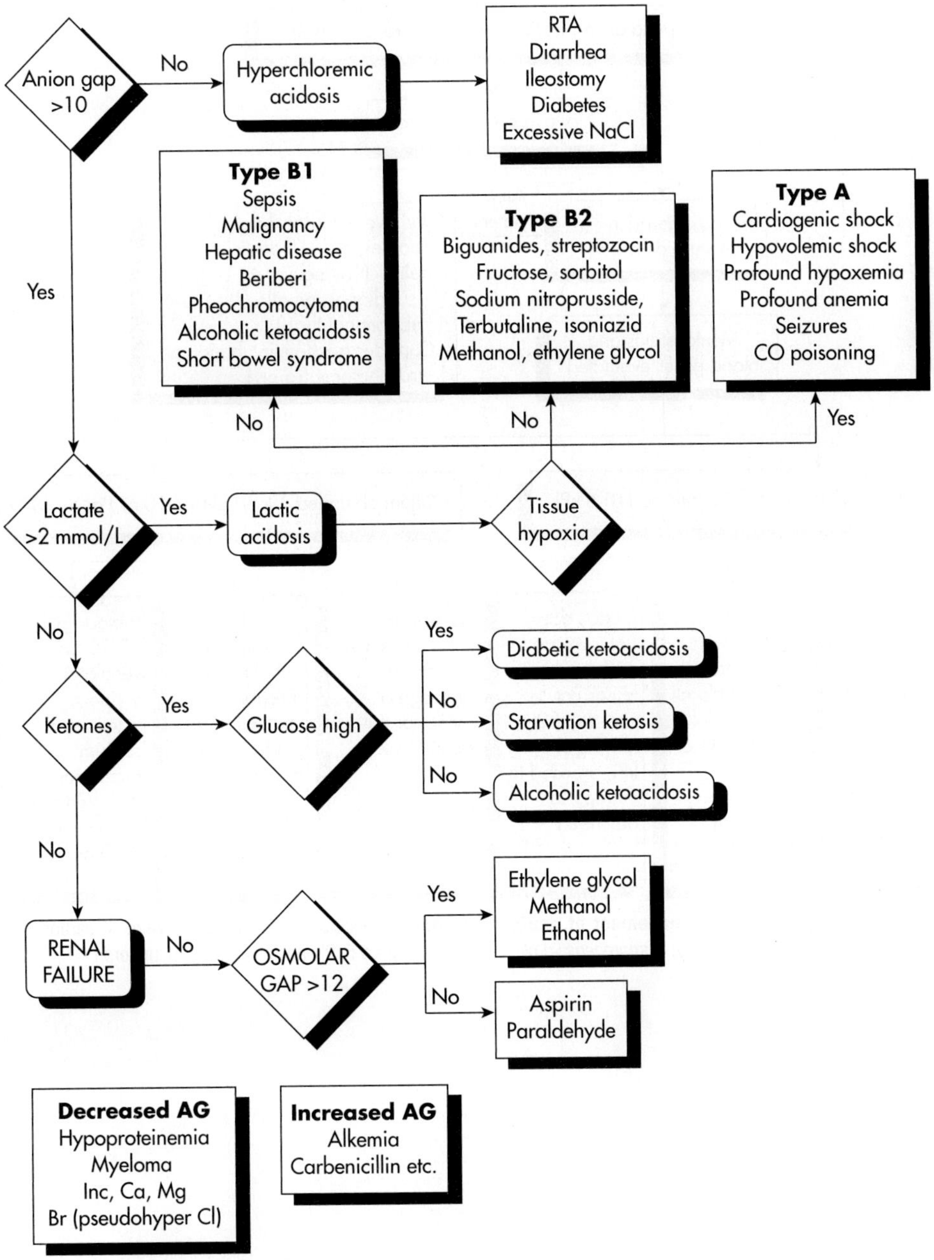

FIG. 11 Diagnostic approach to metabolic acidosis. *AG,* Anion gap; *CO,* carbon monoxide; *RTA,* renal tubular acidosis. (From Vincent JL et al: *Textbook of critical care,* ed 7, Philadelphia, 2017, Elsevier.)

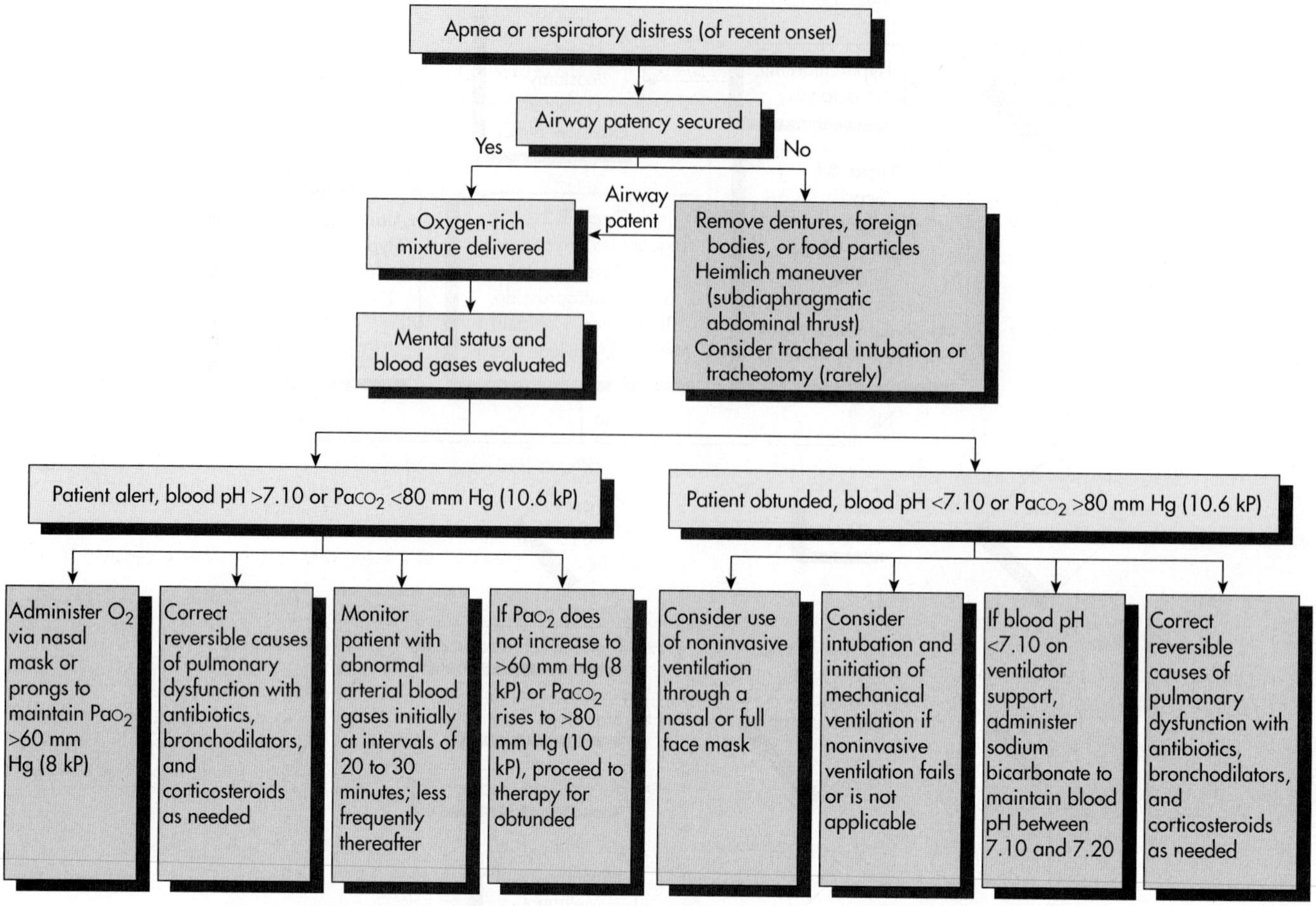

FIG. 12 Algorithm for management of acute respiratory acidosis. *PCO_2*, Partial pressure of carbon dioxide. (From Johnson R et al: *Comprehensive clinical nephrology*, ed 5, Philadelphia, 2015, Saunders.)

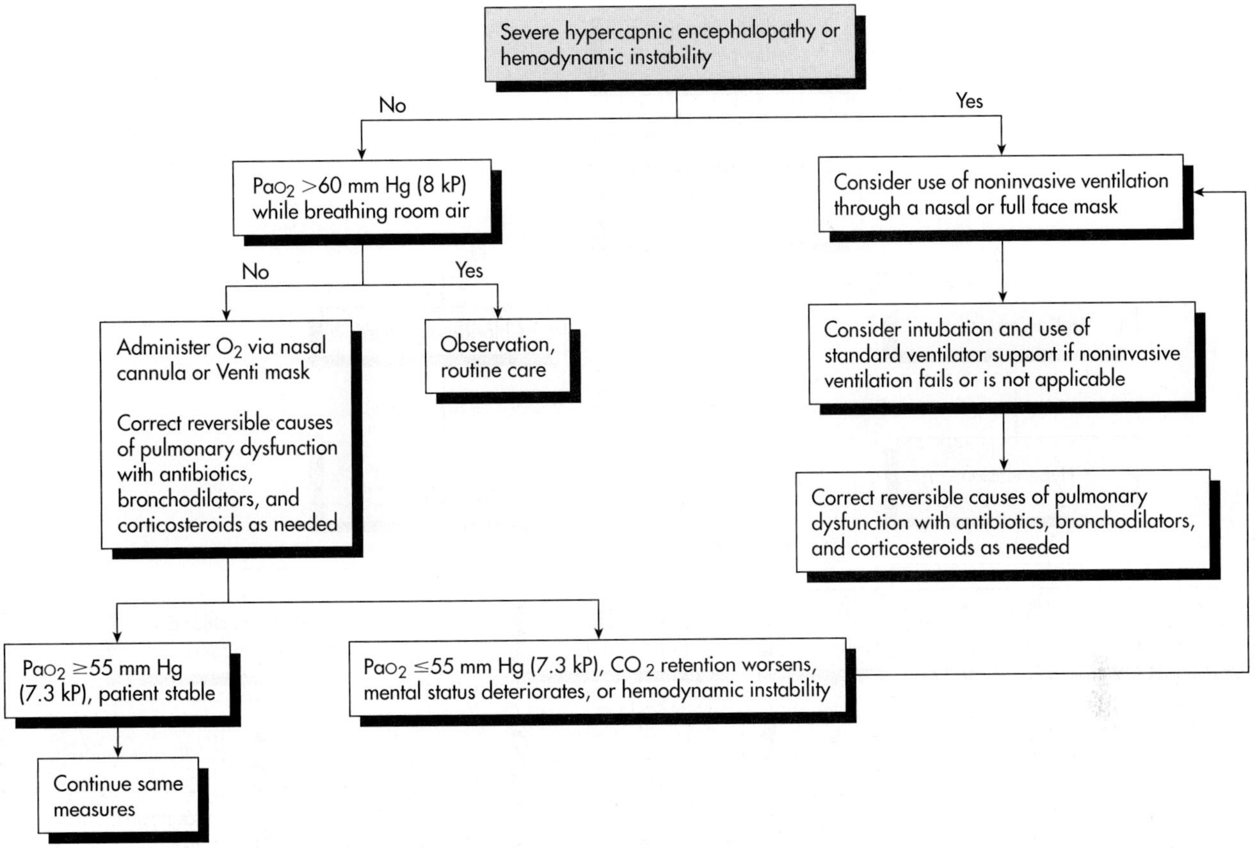

FIG. 13 Algorithm for management of chronic respiratory acidosis. *PaO_2*, Partial pressure of oxygen. (From Johnson R et al: *Comprehensive clinical nephrology*, ed 5, Philadelphia, 2015, Saunders.)

TABLE 2 Causes of Chronic Alveolar Hypoventilation/Respiratory Acidosis

	Site of Defect	Condition
Defects in respiratory drive	Central and peripheral chemoreceptors	Brainstem lesions Primary alveolar hypoventilation syndrome (Ondine's curse), extreme obesity (Pickwickian syndrome) Spinal cord lesions
Neuromuscular defects	*Neuromuscular*	*Motor neuron disease:* Critical illness polyneuropathy, multiple sclerosis, amyotrophic lateral sclerosis
	Muscular disease	Myasthenia gravis, critical illness myopathy
Defects in respiratory mechanics and gas exchange	*Lung*	*Increased dead space:* Chronic obstructive pulmonary disease, chronic pulmonary embolism *Increased lung elastance*: Pulmonary fibrosis *Increased chest wall elastance*: Extreme obesity, fibrothorax, kyphoscoliosis *Increased respiratory resistance*: Airway stenosis, chronic obstructive pulmonary disease

From Ronco C: *Critical care nephrology*, ed 3, Philadelphia, 2019, Elsevier.

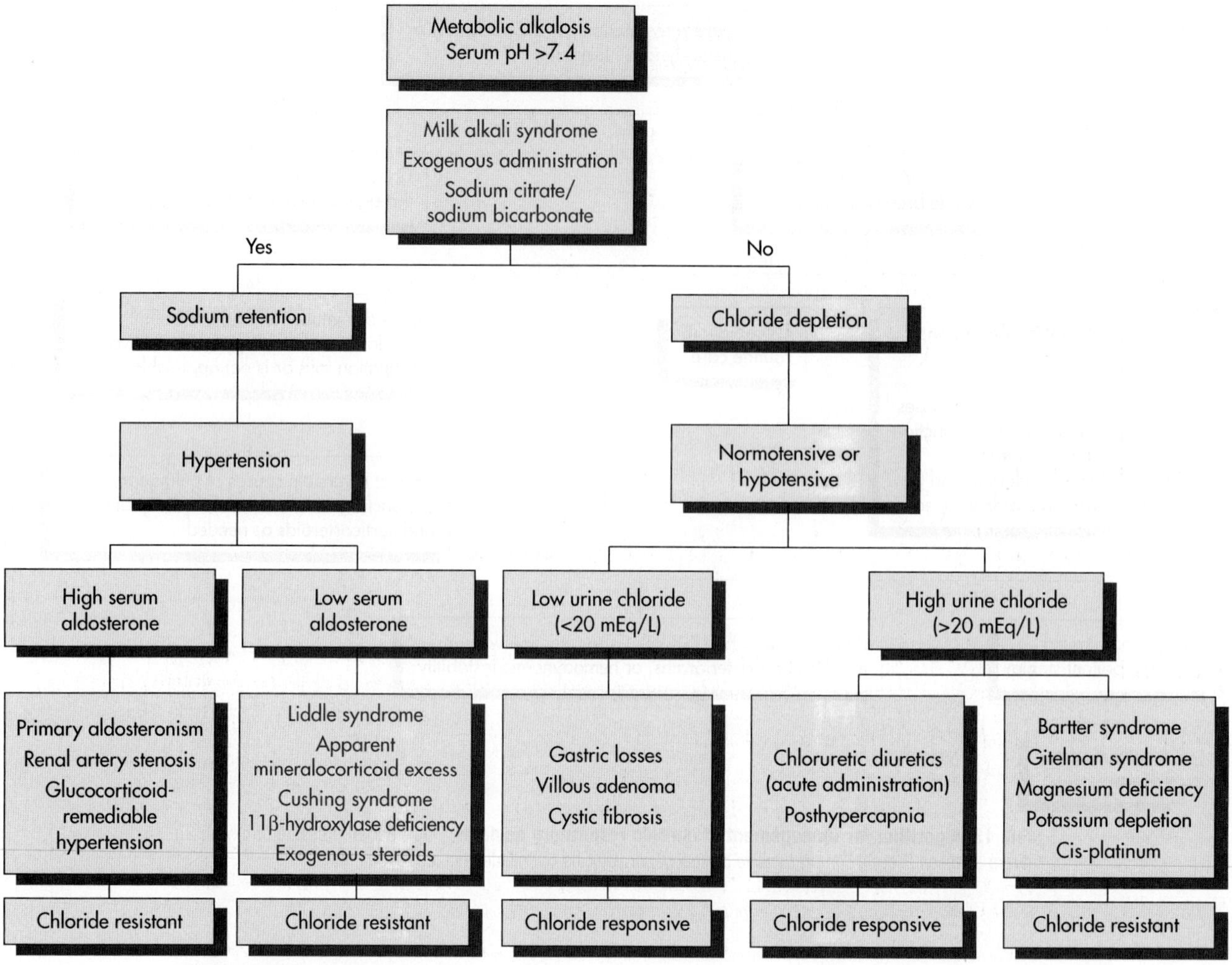

FIG. 16 Differential diagnosis of metabolic alkalosis. (From Ronco C: *Critical care nephrology,* ed 3, Philadelphia, 2019, Elsevier.)

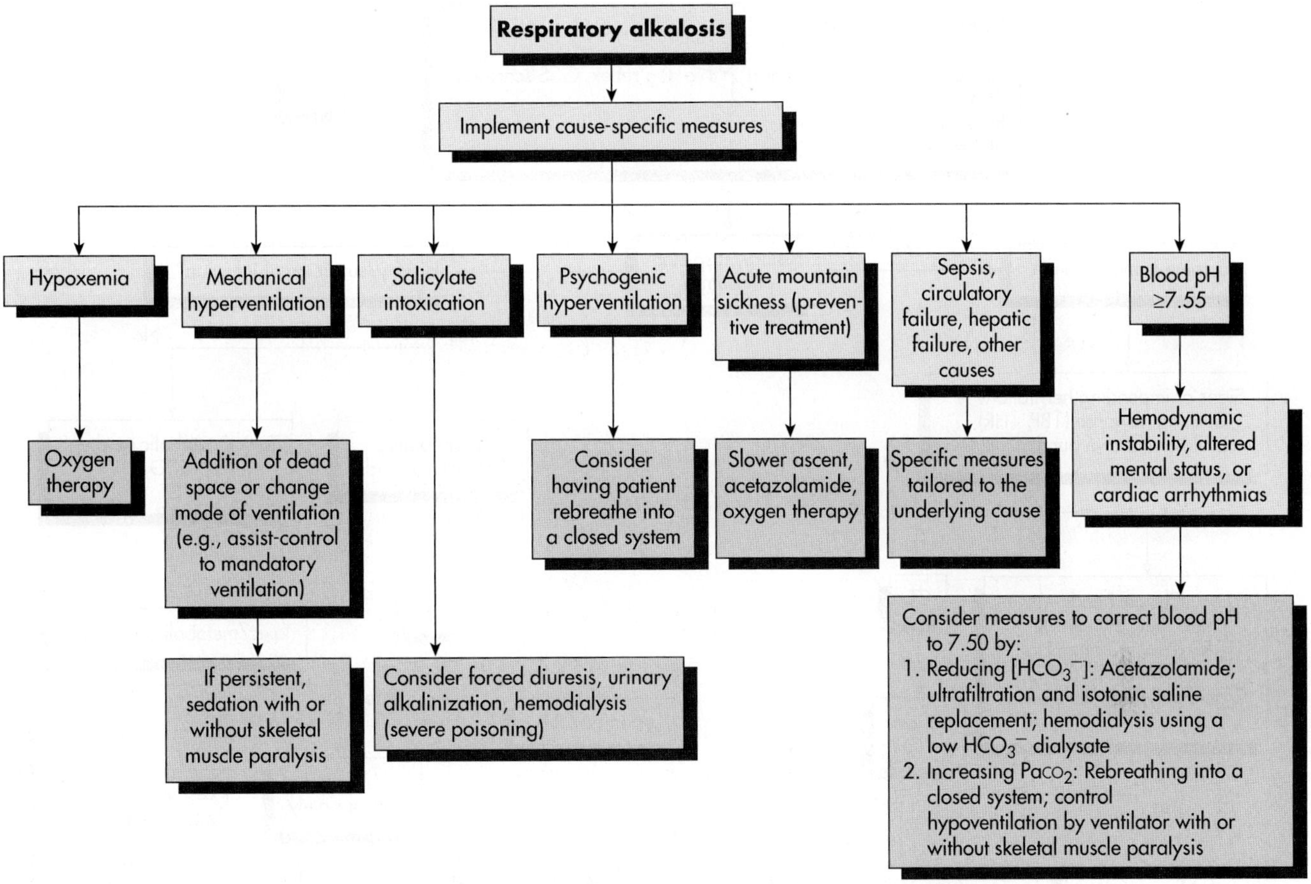

FIG. 17 Recommended treatment of respiratory alkalosis. *PCO_2,* Partial pressure of carbon dioxide. (From Johnson R et al: *Comprehensive clinical nephrology*, ed 5, Philadelphia, 2015, Saunders.)

TABLE 3 Causes of Alveolar Hyperventilation/Respiratory Alkalosis

	Site of Defect	Condition
Defects in respiratory drive	Central chemoreceptors	*Voluntary hyperventilation psychogenic:* Pain, panic attack *Central neurogenic hyperventilation:* Brainstem injuries, brain tumors *Hormonal:* Increased progesterone levels in pregnancy and liver cirrhosis *Infectious:* Meningitis, encephalitis *Thermal hyperpnea:* Fever, hyperthermia *Intoxication:* Salicylate, topiramate *Therapeutic:* Doxapram
	Peripheral chemoreceptors	*Increased activity of peripheral chemoreceptors:* Hypoxic pulmonary disease, high altitude *Increased activity of lung receptors*, e.g., pulmonary edema, pneumonia, pulmonary embolism, interstitial fibrosis
Iatrogenic		*Mechanical ventilation:* Excessive mechanical ventilation (accidental, or therapeutic for traumatic brain injury) *Extracorporeal gas exchange:* Excessive extracorporeal CO_2 removal

From Ronco C: *Critical care nephrology*, ed 3, Philadelphia, 2019, Elsevier.

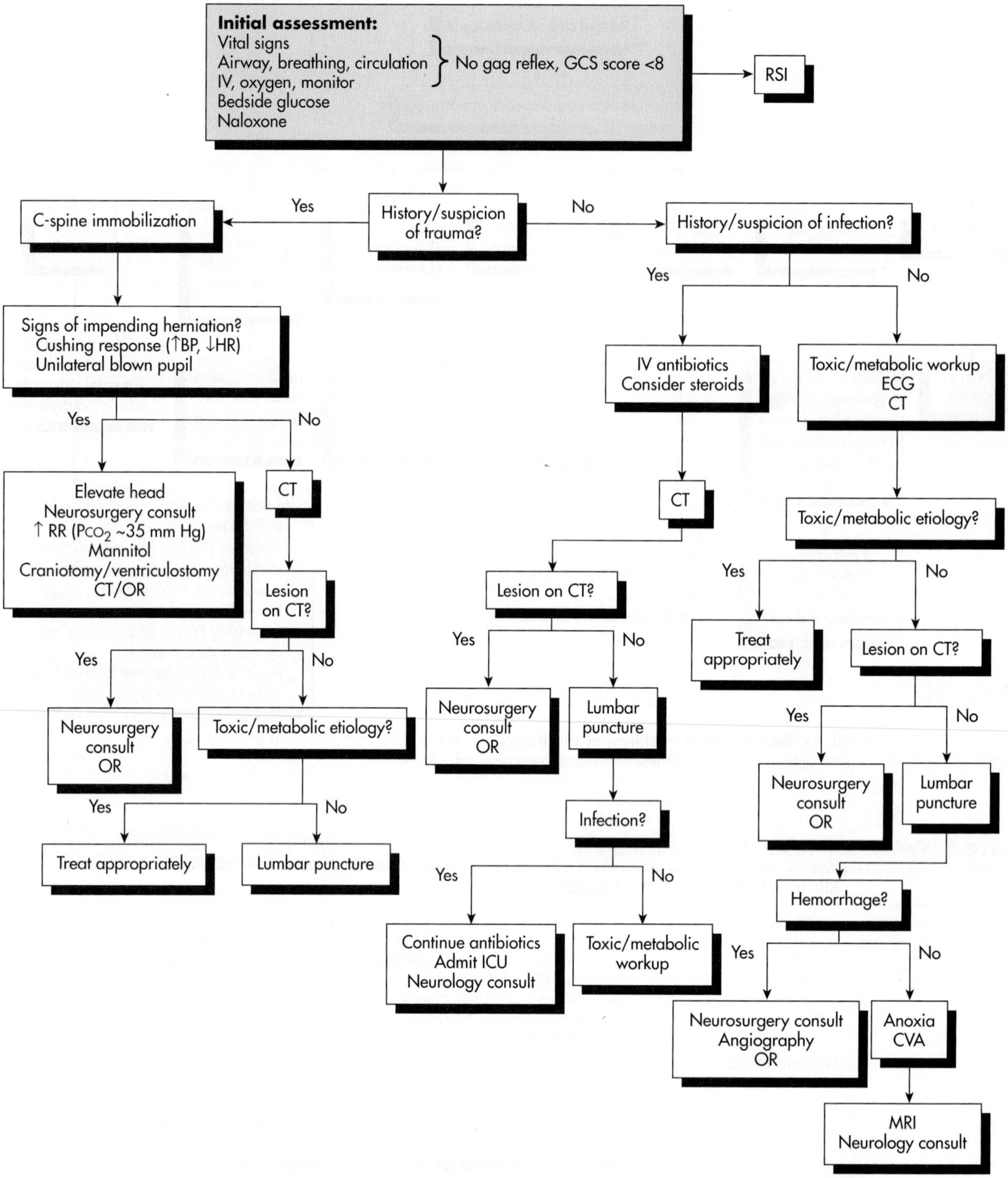

FIG. 19 Diagnostic approach to altered mental status and coma. *BP,* Blood pressure; *C-spine,* cervical spine; *CT,* computed tomography; *CVA,* cerebrovascular accident; *ECG,* electrocardiography; *GCS,* Glasgow Coma Scale; *HR,* heart rate; *ICU,* intensive care unit; *IV,* intravenous; *MRI,* magnetic resonance imaging; *OR,* operating room; *PCO_2,* Partial pressure of carbon dioxide; *RR,* respiratory rate; *RSI,* rapid-sequence intubation. (From Adams JG et al: *Emergency medicine, clinical essentials,* ed 2, Philadelphia, 2013, Elsevier.)

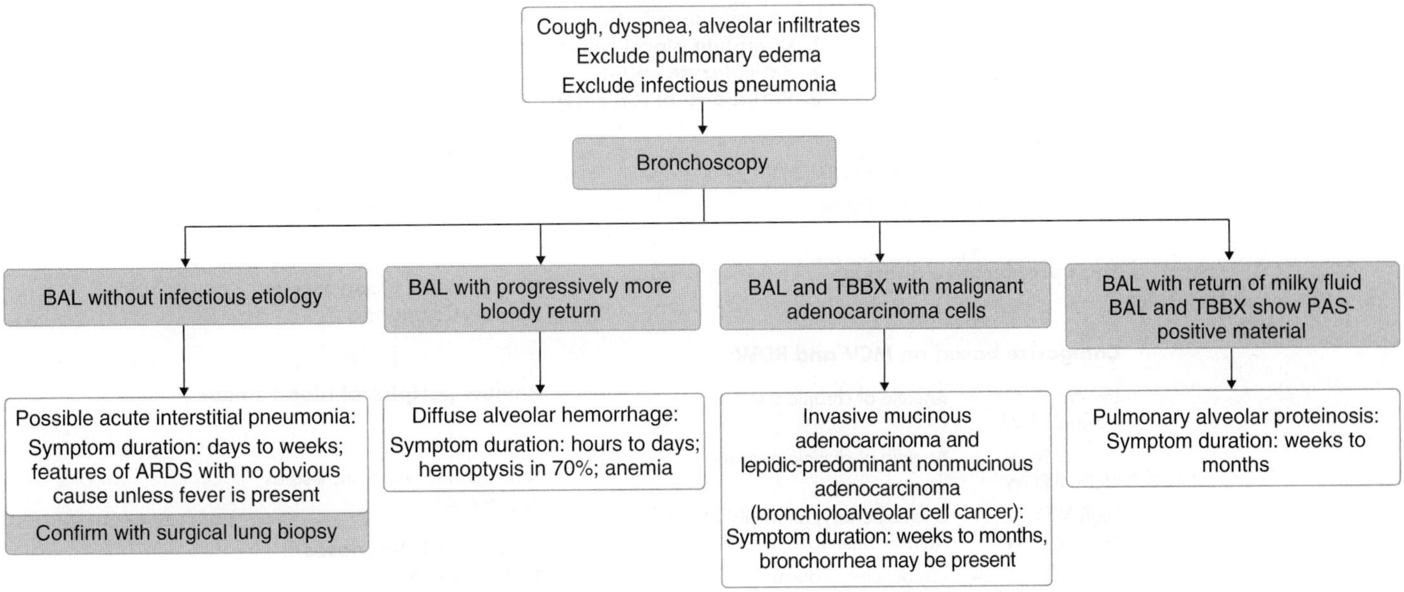

FIG. 20 A general approach to the alveolar filling disorders. *ARDS,* Acute respiratory distress syndrome; *BAL,* bronchoalveolar lavage; *PAS,* periodic acid-Schiff; *TBBX,* transbronchial biopsy. (From Goldman L, Shafer AI: *Goldman-Cecil medicine*, ed 26, Philadelphia, 2020, Elsevier. Fig. 85-1.)

TABLE 4 Alveolar Filling Disorders

Diseases	Pathophysiology	Radiographic Findings
Pulmonary alveolar proteinosis	Impaired processing of surfactant by alveolar macrophages caused by defects in GM-CSF signaling	Bilateral alveolar opacities with "crazy paving" and diffuse areas of ground-glass attenuation on CT scan
Acute interstitial pneumonia	Diffuse alveolar damage with temporal uniformity	Diffuse alveolar filling process similar to the acute respiratory distress syndrome
Diffuse alveolar hemorrhage	Bleeding from the pulmonary microcirculation, usually from the capillaries	Acute development of bilateral alveolar opacities
Invasive mucinous adenocarcinoma and lepidic predominant nonmucinous adenocarcinoma (formerly called bronchioloalveolar cell carcinoma)	Cancer cells growing along the alveolar septa	Pneumonic opacities, consolidation with air bronchograms, ground-glass opacities (either solitary or multiple)

CT, Computed tomography; *GM-CSF*, granulocyte-macrophage colony-stimulating factor.
From Goldman L, Shafer AI: *Goldman-Cecil medicine*, ed 26, Philadelphia, 2020, Elsevier. Table 85-1.

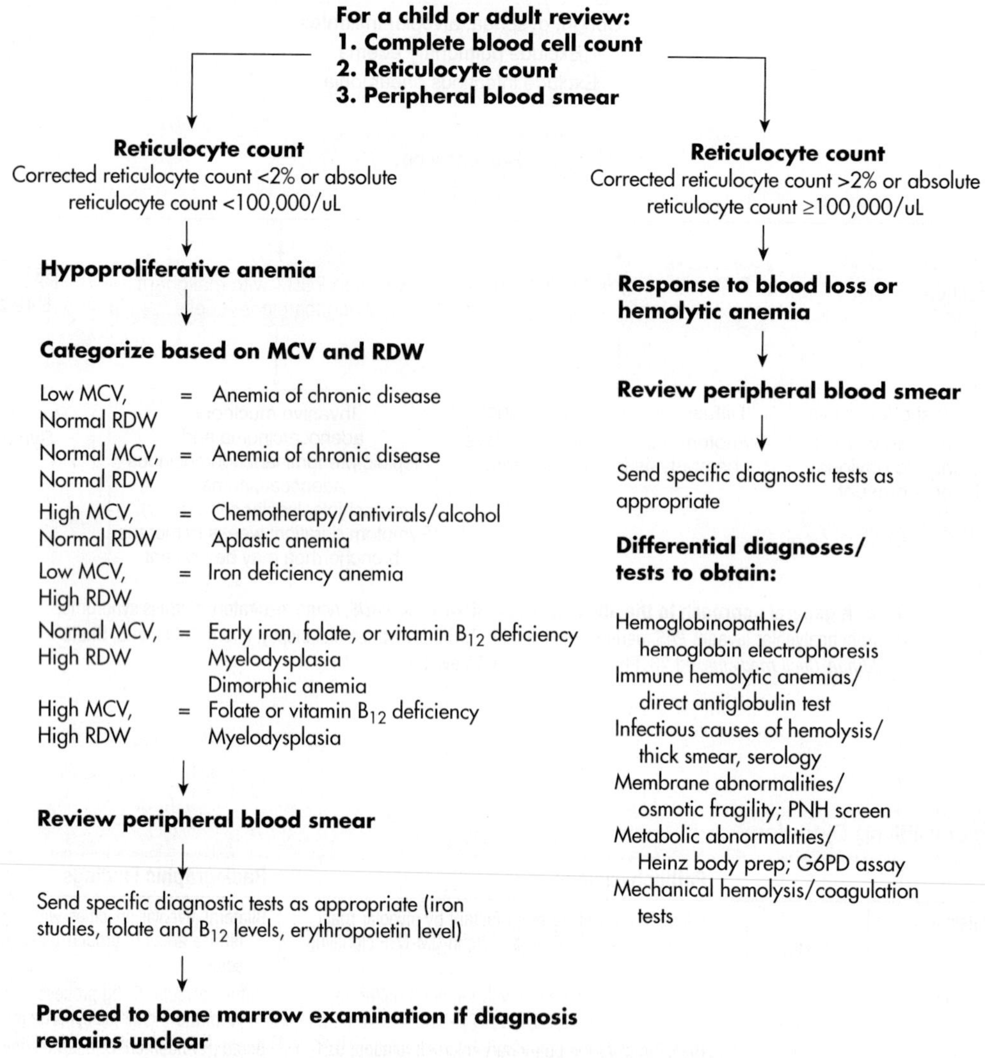

FIG. 25 Approach to the differential diagnosis of anemia in adults and children. *G6PD,* Glucose-6-phosphate dehydrogenase; *MCV,* mean corpuscular volume; *PNH,* paroxysmal nocturnal hemoglobinuria; *RDW,* red blood cell distribution width. (From Hoffman R: *Hematology, basic principles and practice,* ed 7, Philadelphia, 2018, Elsevier.)

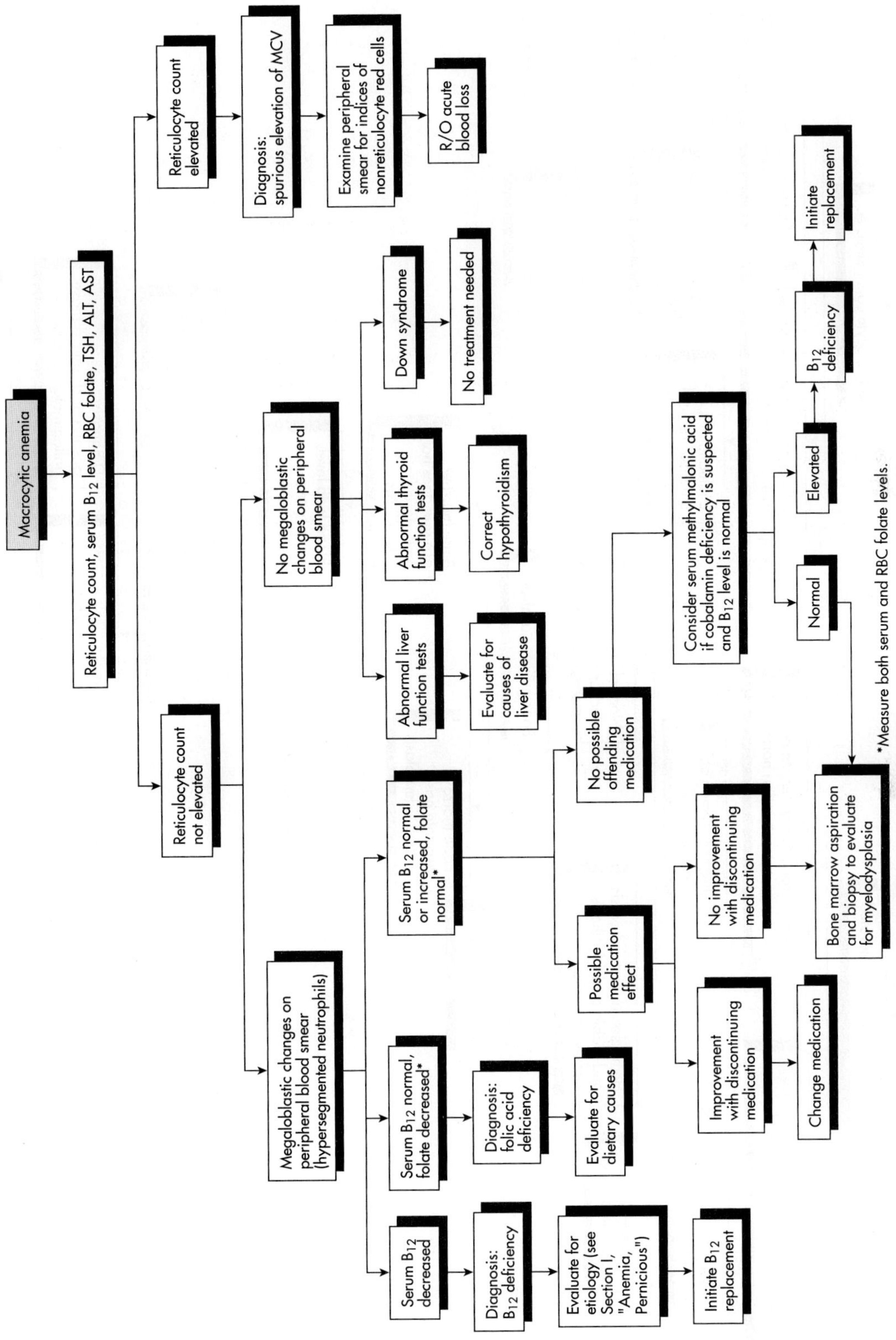

FIG. 26 Differential diagnosis of macrocytic anemia. *ALT,* Alanine tranaminase; *AST,* aspartate aminotransferase; *MCV,* mean corpuscular volume; *RBC,* red blood cell; *R/O,* rule out; *TSH,* thyroid-stimulating hormone. (Modified and updated from Rakel RE [ed]: *Principles of family practice,* ed 7, Philadelphia, 2007, Saunders.)

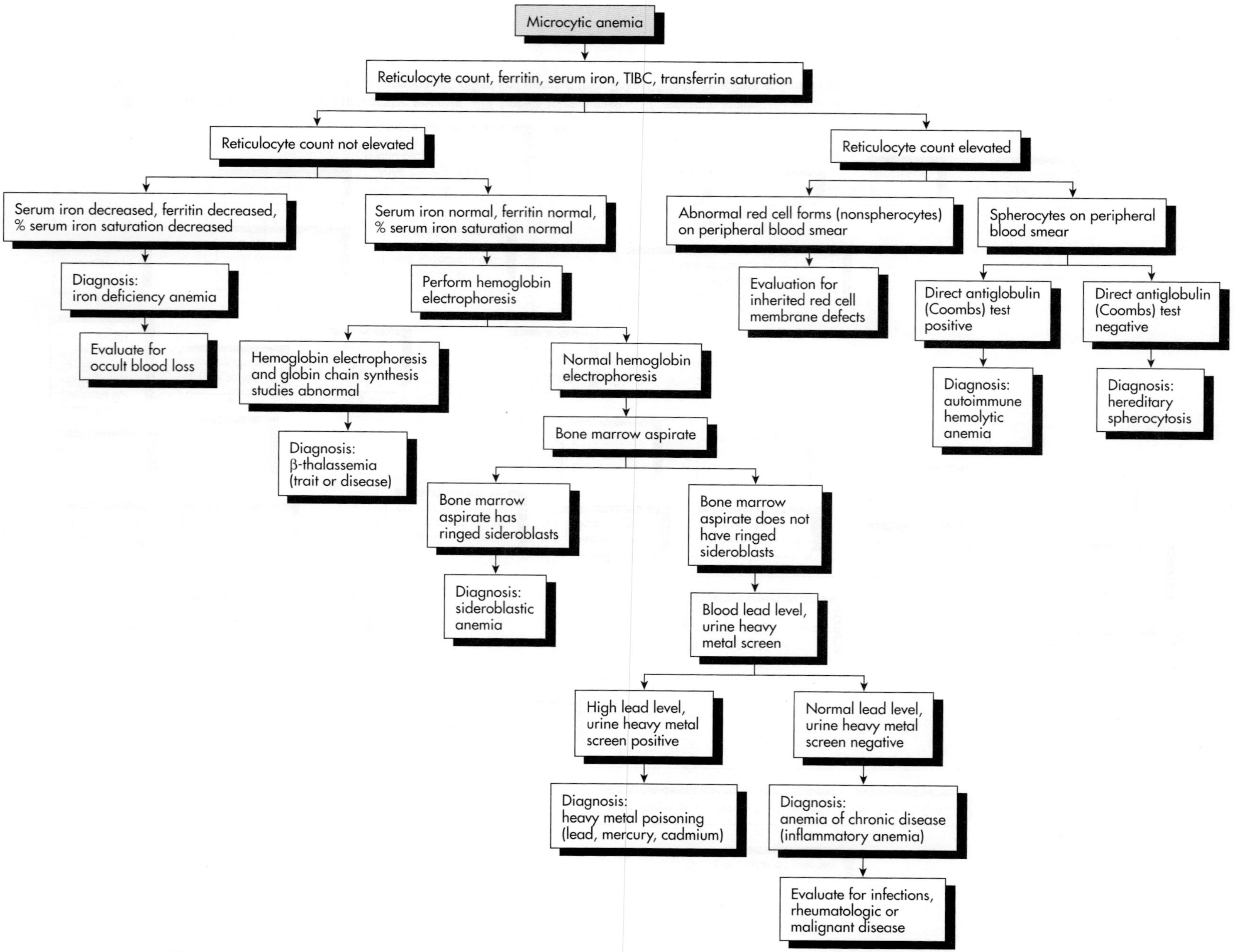

FIG. 27 Differential diagnosis of microcytic anemia. *TIBC,* Total iron binding capacity. (Modified and updated from Rakel RE [ed]: *Principles of family practice*, ed 7, Philadelphia, 2007, Saunders.)

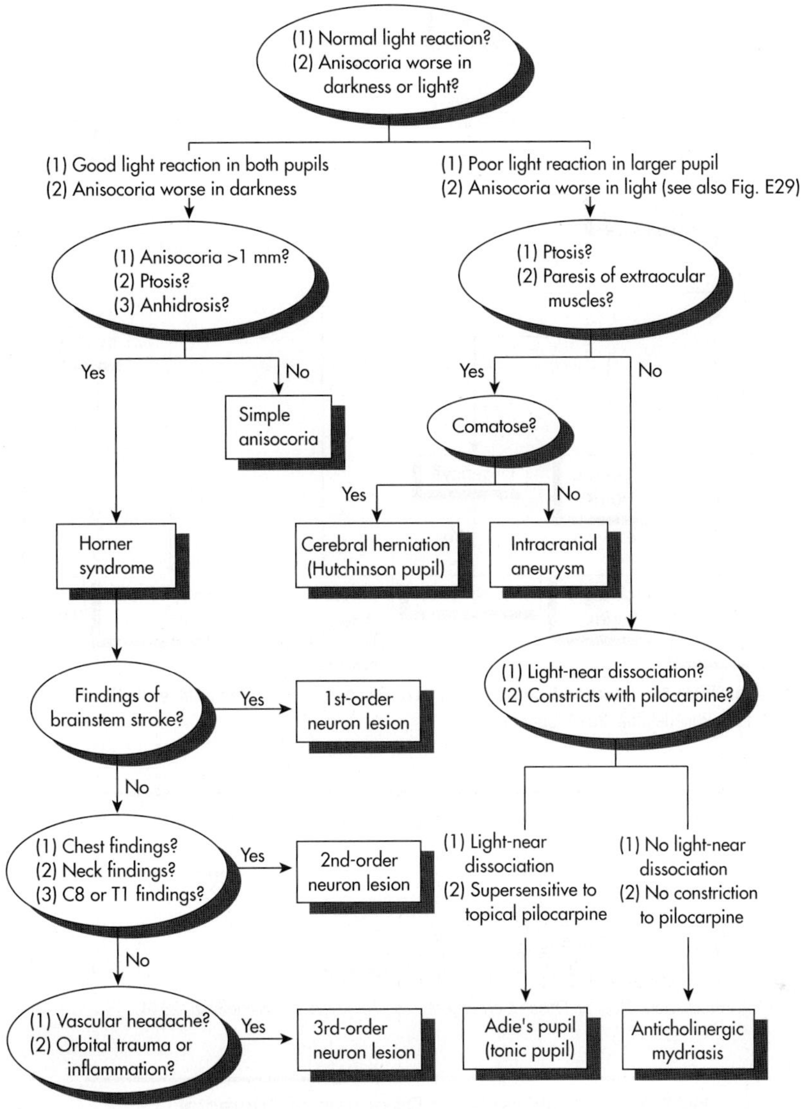

FIG. 28 Summary of approach to anisocoria. The first two questions (Is there a normal light reaction? and Is anisocoria worse in darkness or light?) distinguish problems with the pupillary dilator muscle (i.e., Horner syndrome, simple anisocoria; *left side* of the figure) from problems with the pupillary constrictor muscle (i.e., third cranial nerve, iris; *right side* of the figure). Two other tests distinguish Horner syndrome from simple anisocoria: The cocaine or apraclonidine eyedrop tests and pupillary dilator lag (i.e., the pupil dilates slowly in darkness, as documented by photographs). (From McGee S: *Evidence-based physical diagnosis,* ed 4, Philadelphia, 2018, Elsevier.)

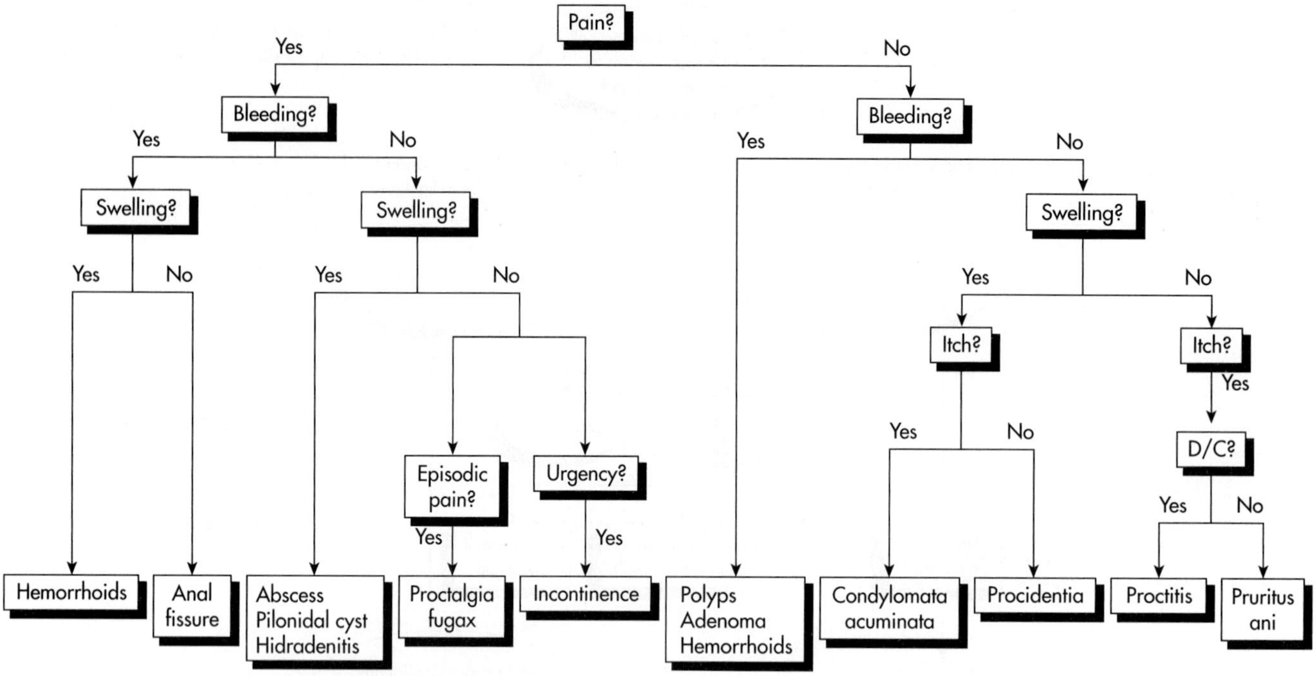

FIG. 30 Algorithm for anorectal complaints. *D/C,* Discharge. (From Marx JA et al: *Rosen's emergency medicine*, ed 8, Philadelphia, 2014, Saunders.)

BOX 6 The WASH Regimen for Management of Hemorrhoids

- *W*arm water
- *A*nalgesic agents
- *S*tool softeners
- *H*igh-fiber diet

From Marx JA et al: *Rosen's emergency medicine,* ed 8, Philadelphia, 2014, Saunders.

BOX 7 Medical History in Diagnosis of Anorectal Disorders

Anorectal History
- Pain
- Bleeding
- Swelling
- Itching
- Discharge
- Urgency

Gastrointestinal History
- Change in bowel habits (straining, flatus, color, consistency, frequency)
- Nausea or vomiting
- Incontinence of stool
- Underlying GI disease (Crohn disease, cancer, polyps)

Systemic Disease History
- Diabetes mellitus
- Coagulopathy
- Cancer
- HIV infection

Sexual History of the Anus
- Penetration
- Known STDs
- Assault

GI, Gastrointestinal; *HIV,* human immunodeficiency virus; *STD,* sexually transmitted disease.
From Marx JA et al: *Rosen's emergency medicine,* ed 8, Philadelphia, 2014, Saunders.

ICD-10CM #		
	M54.5	Low back pain
	L29	Pruritus
	M54.89	Other dorsalgia
	M54.9	Dorsalgia, unspecified
	F45.42	Pain disorder with related psychological factors
	M54.08	Panniculitis affecting regions of neck and back, sacral and sacrococcygeal region
	S23.9XXA	Sprain of unspecified parts of thorax, initial encounter
	M43.27	Fusion of spine, lumbosacral region
	M43.28	Fusion of spine, sacral and sacrococcygeal region
	M53.2X7	Spinal instabilities, lumbosacral region
	M53.3	Sacrococcygeal disorders, not elsewhere classified

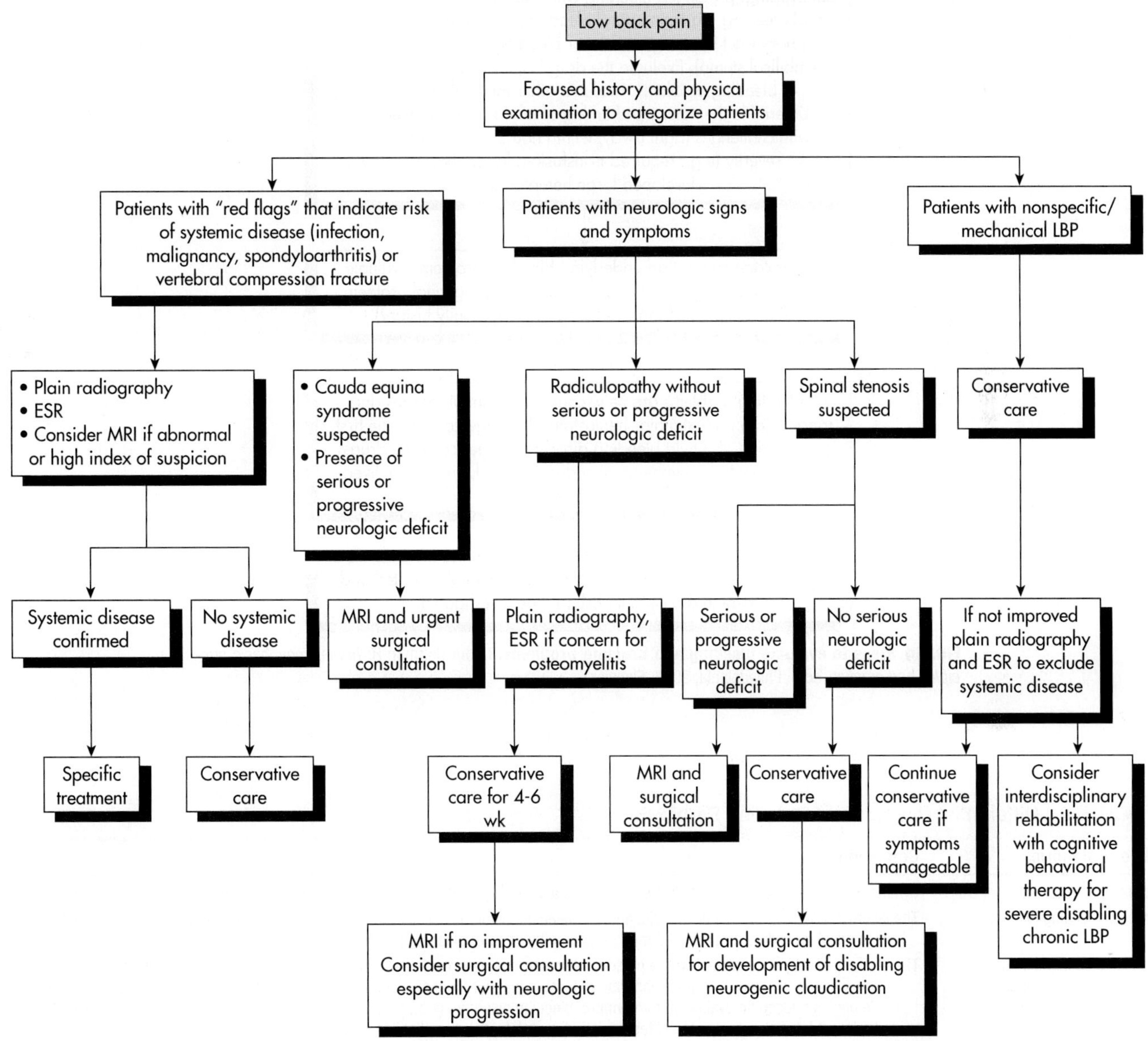

FIG. 33 Algorithm for the differential diagnosis and treatment of low back pain. *ESR*, Erythrocyte sedimentation rate; *LBP*, low back pain; *MRI*, magnetic resonance imaging. (From Firestein GS et al: *Kelley and Firestein's textbook of rheumatology,* ed 10, Philadelphia, 2017, Elsevier.)

TABLE 5 Red Flags for Potentially Serious Conditions

Possible Fracture	Possible Tumor or Infection	Possible Cauda Equina Syndrome
From Medical History		
Major trauma, such as vehicle accident or fall from height Minor trauma or even strenuous lifting (in older or potentially osteoporotic patient)	Age over 50 or under 20 yr History of cancer Constitutional symptoms, such as recent fever or chills or unexplained weight loss Risk factors for spinal infection: Recent bacterial infection (e.g., urinary tract infection), intravenous drug abuse, or immune suppression (from steroids, transplant, or human immunodeficiency virus) Pain that worsens when supine; severe nighttime pain	Saddle anesthesia Recent onset of bladder dysfunction, such as urinary retention, increased frequency, or overflow incontinence Severe or progressive neurologic deficit in the lower extremity

BLEEDING AND BRUISING PROBLEMS

ICD-10CM # D68.9 Coagulation defect, unspecified
D68.8 Other specified coagulation defects

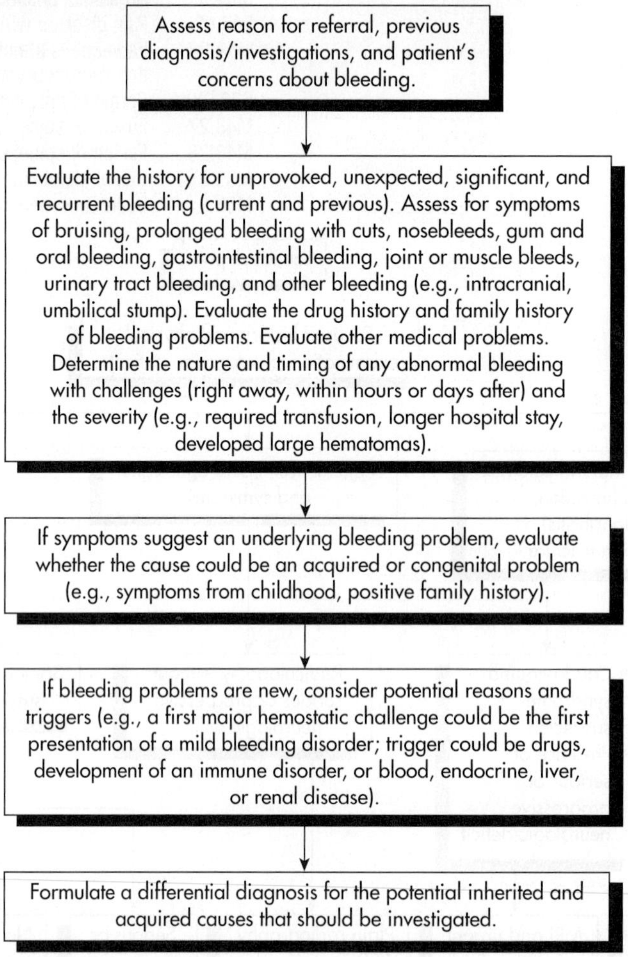

FIG. 34 Steps to evaluate bleeding and bruising problems. (From Hoffman R: *Hematology, basic principles and practice*, ed 7, Philadelphia, 2018, Elsevier.)

TABLE 6 Differential Diagnosis of Bleeding Problems

Major Categories	Comments
No bleeding disorder	Symptoms do not reflect a bleeding disorder and have another explanation (e.g., a surgical bleed, not caused by a bleeding disorder).
Possible bleeding disorder	The laboratory findings are nondiagnostic, and the bleeding history is considered equivocal (e.g., unexplained serious bleed with one surgical procedure; unexplained menorrhagia without other bleeding problems).
Definite bleeding disorder, undefined or indeterminate type	The bleeding history is consistent with a bleeding disorder; however, the laboratory findings are nondiagnostic. Commonly the bleeding history resembles mild to moderate defects in platelet function or von Willebrand factor. The diagnosis should only be made once an adequate evaluation for common bleeding disorders (e.g., for von Willebrand disease and platelet aggregation and release defects) is completed. If testing is not complete, the classification should indicate the types of conditions excluded or not excluded, for example mild mucocutaneous bleeding problem, von Willebrand disease excluded, mild mucocutaneous bleeding problem, platelet release defects not yet excluded.
Definite bleeding disorder with cause	The symptoms and laboratory findings are considered diagnostic of a bleeding disorder. Tables 7 and 8 summarize many of a define the potential inherited and acquired causes.

From Hoffman R: *Hematology, basic principles and practice*, ed 7, Philadelphia, 2018, Elsevier.

TABLE 7 Differential Diagnosis of Congenital Bleeding Disorders

Disorder	Comments
Fibrinogen deficiency or dysfunction	Deficiencies can be mild-moderate hypofibrinogenemia or severe afibrinogenemia. Fibrinogen function is abnormal in dysfibrinogenemias, which can present with bleeding, thrombosis, or both. Fibrinogen levels can be reduced in some dysfibrinogenemias.
X-linked coagulation factor deficiencies—hemophilia	Presentation is influenced by the degree of deficiency. Factor VIII deficiency is more common than factor IX deficiency. If factor VIII is low, von Willebrand disease needs to be excluded as the cause.
Rarer, coagulation factor deficiencies	Deficiencies can affect factors XI, V, II, VII, or X, and the presentation is dependent on the severity of the deficiency. Hereditary deficiencies of multiple coagulation factors are rare (e.g., of factors V and VIII, or multiple vitamin K-dependent coagulation factors for congenital defects impairing γ-carboxylation) and can easily be excluded by measuring multiple factors.
Fibrinolytic defects	Causes include disorders caused by loss of function, such as α2-antiplasmin or PAI-1 deficiency, and by gain-of-function defects, such as Quebec platelet disorder (overexpression of urokinase plasminogen activator in megakaryocytes).
von Willebrand disease	Causes include quantitative (partial type 1 to severe type 3) and qualitative defects (loss of function in type 2M and 2A, gain of function in type 2B and platelet-type). Type 1 von Willebrand disease can be confused with low von Willebrand factor levels (e.g., because of blood group O).
Platelet disorders	These conditions can affect platelet number, function, or both. The most common type of platelet function disorder is a platelet secretion defect, which may or may not also impair aggregation responses. Disorders of platelet function are commonly subclassified by the nature of the defect, such as the following: Defects of membrane receptors for adhesive proteins (e.g., Glanzmann thrombasthenia and Bernard-Soulier syndrome) or agonists (e.g., $P2Y_{12}$ deficiency) Defects of signaling or secretion (the largest subcategory) Cytoskeletal defects (e.g., MYH9-related disorders) Storage pool disorders (e.g., gray platelet syndrome, dense granule deficiency, $\alpha\gamma$-storage pool deficiency, Quebec platelet disorder) Defects of procoagulant function (e.g., Scott syndrome)
Vascular disorders	Congenital vascular malformation, including hereditary hemorrhagic telangiectasia, Ehlers-Danlos syndrome

MYH9, Myosin heavy polypeptide 9; *PAI-1,* plasminogen activator inhibitor 1.
From Hoffman R: *Hematology, basic principles and practice,* ed 7, Philadelphia, 2018, Elsevier.

TABLE 8 Differential Diagnosis of Acquired Bleeding Problems

Disorder	Comments
Drug induced	Aspirin, NSAIDs, other platelet function inhibitors (e.g., $P2Y_{12}$ $\alpha_{IIb}\beta_3$ inhibitors), anticoagulants, fibrinolytic drugs, and antidepressants are common causes.
Acquired factor deficiencies	The causes can be immune (e.g., acquired factor VIII deficiency, acquired factor V deficiency) or nonimmune. Reductions in multiple factors can result from vitamin K deficiency, treatment with vitamin K antagonists, liver disease, hemodilution, and rarely snakebites. Severe acquired hypofibrinogenemia is commonly caused by a postpartum coagulopathy or severe liver disease. Prothrombin deficiency occurs with some lupus anticoagulants. Amyloidosis can cause an acquired factor X deficiency, which may be associated with reductions in other coagulation factors synthesized in the liver if the liver is involved.
Disseminated intravascular coagulation	The manifestations can include thrombocytopenia, consumption of coagulation factors, including fibrinogen, and impairment of hemostatic mechanisms from the fibrin/fibrinogen degradation products. Causes are wide ranging and include postpartum consumptive states, prostate and other cancers, and snakebites.
Acquired von Willebrand disease	The cause can be immune (often in association with an IgG paraprotein) or nonimmune (e.g., increased proteolysis of von Willebrand factor with stenotic aortic valvular disease).
Immune thrombocytopenia	Bleeding is usually influenced by the extent of the thrombocytopenia. Some autoantibodies interfere with platelet membrane receptor function, causing bleeding disproportionate to the thrombocytopenia.
Non–drug-induced, acquired platelet function disorders	The cause can be immune (see earlier) or nonimmune, typically from bone marrow disorders, although secretion defects can be secondary to Cushing syndrome or hypothyroidism.
Liver disease	Liver disease can cause thrombocytopenia, deficiencies of coagulation factors, hypofibrinogenemia and dysfibrinogenemia, and increased fibrinolysis. In mild liver disease, factor VII and sometimes factors XI and XII are low. Fibrinogen is often increased in early liver disease, and if low, the finding suggests severe liver disease.
Renal disease	Anemia is an important predictor of uremic bleeding. Uremic bleeding is typically associated with severe renal impairment.
Hypothyroidism	Hypothyroidism can cause an acquired von Willebrand disease and acquired defects in platelet function.
Cushing syndrome	This syndrome should be suspected when there are symptoms and findings suggestive of Cushing syndrome or treatment with systemic or topical glucocorticoids.
Surgical bleeding	This is often a diagnosis of exclusion, although the procedural notes sometimes document that a technical problem was encountered that led to abnormal bleeding.
Vitamin K deficiency	Newborns are at risk, as are individuals with malabsorption and/or receiving broad-spectrum antibiotics that reduce vitamin K production by reducing gut bacteria. Older adults are also at greater risk for developing vitamin K deficiency because of reduced stores from poorer intake of vitamin K. If the patient does not respond to parenteral vitamin K, other causes should be considered.
Vitamin C deficiency (scurvy)	This diagnosis should be considered when there is lethargy with skin and gum bleeding (perifollicular hemorrhages, gum bleeding with swelling). The condition is rare in developed countries. The cause is usually a very poor diet or malabsorption.

IgG, Immunoglobulin G; *NSAID,* nonsteroidal antiinflammatory drug.
From Hoffman R: *Hematology, basic principles and practice,* ed 7, Philadelphia, 2018, Elsevier.

BOX 8 The Laboratory Manifestations of Bleeding Disorders

The laboratory manifestations of bleeding disorders can include abnormalities from the following:

1. The underlying hemostatic defect
2. Bleeding complications (e.g., anemia, iron deficiency, coagulopathy secondary to hemodilution after resuscitation for a massive bleed, development of red cell antibodies after transfusion)
3. False-positive abnormalities (e.g., prolonged aPTT caused by incidental mild factor XII deficiency, which is found in about 1 of 200 patients, or a lupus anticoagulant, which can be a transient finding in about 5% of hospitalized patients)
4. Extremes of normal variation (e.g., mildly low von Willebrand factor levels in an individual who is blood group O, absent secondary aggregation with epinephrine in adjusted platelet-rich plasma aggregation studies)

aPTT, Activated partial thromboplastin time.
From Hoffman R: *Hematology, basic principles and practice,* ed 7, Philadelphia, 2018, Elsevier.

BOX 9 Influences on Presenting Problems

When evaluating a bleeding history, it is important to recognize that the presenting problems are influenced by the following factors:

- The nature and severity of the defect, and the presence of single or multiple risk factors for bleeding
- Whether the bleeding problem is congenital or acquired
- Antecedent exposure to hemostatic challenges (such as surgery, dental extraction, menses, and childbirth) and the risk for bleeding with each of these challenges
- The presence of other medical problems (e.g., renal, hepatic, or thyroid disease), including anemia
- Variability in the bleeding symptoms experienced by individuals without bleeding disorders (e.g., nosebleeds, bruising) and by individuals with known bleeding disorders, even within families with the same defect
- Local factors (e.g., sun-damage to the skin, vascular lesions, diverticular disease, or cancerous lesions in the gastrointestinal tract) and the possibility of nonaccidental trauma
- Treatments that increase the risk for bleeding (e.g., antiplatelet drugs, such as aspirin and nonsteroidal antiinflammatory drugs used for pain control, anticoagulant therapy, etc.)
- Whether treatments were used to prevent or control bleeding
- Whether treatments prescribed for other reasons may have reduced bleeding (e.g., reduced menstrual bleeding while on oral contraceptives to prevent pregnancy)

From Hoffman R: *Hematology, basic principles and practice,* ed 7, Philadelphia, 2018, Elsevier.

BOX 10 Case 1: Illustration of a Mild, Inherited Bleeding Problem

A 77-yr-old man who is starting treatment for multiple myeloma was discovered to have a prolonged activated partial thromboplastin time. Review of his records indicated that the abnormality was present on a previous admission for spinal cord compression, which was treated with surgery. He required 4 units of packed red blood cells several days after this surgery because of delayed postoperative bleeding. There was no other bleeding history. He was found to have mild factor IX deficiency, unrelated to the myeloma, and his daughter proved to be a carrier of this defect.

From Hoffman R: *Hematology, basic principles and practice,* ed 7, Philadelphia, 2018, Elsevier.

BOX 11 Case 2: Illustration of the Importance of Assessing Both Personal and Familial Bleeding Problems

A 22-yr-old woman was referred for evaluation of a possible platelet disorder. She had a history of menorrhagia (4 days out of 7 days of menstrual flow were heavy when not on treatment), prolonged nosebleeds in childhood, and hematuria with urinary tract infections. She did not have thrombocytopenia, and she had no exposure to major hemostatic challenges. Her father, uncle, and grandfather had a striking bleeding history, and two of them had thrombocytopenia. The bleeding in her relatives included joint bleeds with trauma and severe, delayed-onset bleeding after trauma and surgery (usually more than a day later), which continued for weeks despite platelet transfusions. One of these relatives reported no bleeding when he had a tooth extracted while receiving fibrinolytic inhibitor therapy. Although menorrhagia is not specific to any one type of bleeding disorder, the delayed bleeding in affected relatives suggests a possible autosomal dominant disorder and either a fibrinolytic defect of a factor defect or deficiency (e.g., affected relatives). Because of the family history of thrombocytopenia, joint bleeds, and delayed bleeding, which did not respond well to platelet transfusions, testing was done for the Quebec platelet disorder. Genetic testing for duplication mutation of the urokinase plasminogen activator gene confirmed this diagnosis in the patient and her relatives. The case illustrates the importance of evaluating both the personal and family bleeding history and highlights the fact that bleeding-symptom severity can vary among affected family members, in part because of their different exposures to challenges and treatments.

From Hoffman R: *Hematology, basic principles and practice,* ed 7, Philadelphia, 2018, Elsevier.

BOX 12 Case 3: Illustration of the Importance of Assessing Bleeding Problems Over Time

A 72-yr-old man was referred for evaluation of a severe bleed after receiving a single dose of low–molecular-weight heparin for unconfirmed deep vein thrombosis. He had a history of a similar bleeding episode several years previously while on warfarin treatment for atrial fibrillation. There was no other bleeding history, and the patient subsequently developed a spontaneous iliopsoas bleed. He had undergone numerous surgeries earlier in life without any bleeding problems, and there was no family history of bleeding. The bleeding history suggested the possibility of an acquired bleeding problem, possibly acquired von Willebrand disease or an acquired factor XIII deficiency. Diagnostic testing indicated that he had acquired factor XIII deficiency. This case illustrates the fact that there may be more than one risk factor for bleeding: In this case, several exposures to anticoagulants triggered bleeding in a patient with an acquired factor deficiency. On initial treatment of his iliopsoas bleed with factor XIII concentrate, there was partial neutralization of the infused factor followed by accelerated clearance, consistent with acquired factor XIII deficiency secondary to an autoantibody.

From Hoffman R: *Hematology, basic principles and practice,* ed 7, Philadelphia, 2018, Elsevier.

BLEEDING DISORDERS

ICD-10CM # D68.8 Other specified coagulation defects
D68.9 Coagulation defect, unspecified

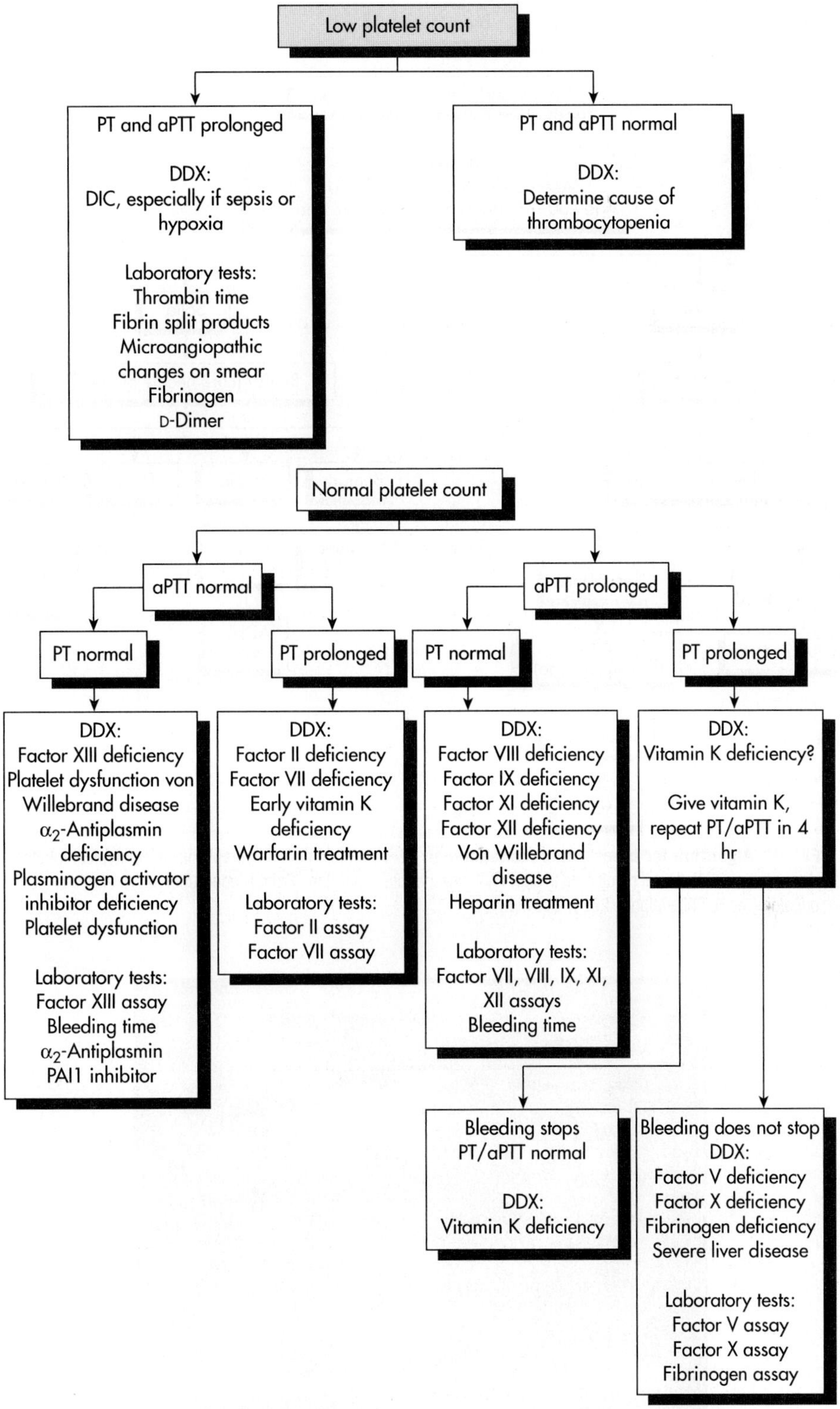

FIG. 35 Differential diagnosis *(DDx)* of bleeding disorders. *aPTT,* Activated partial thromboplastin time; *DIC,* disseminated intravascular coagulation; *PT,* prothrombin time. (From Hughes HK, Kahl LK: *The Harriet Lane handbook,* ed 21, St Louis, 2018, Mosby)

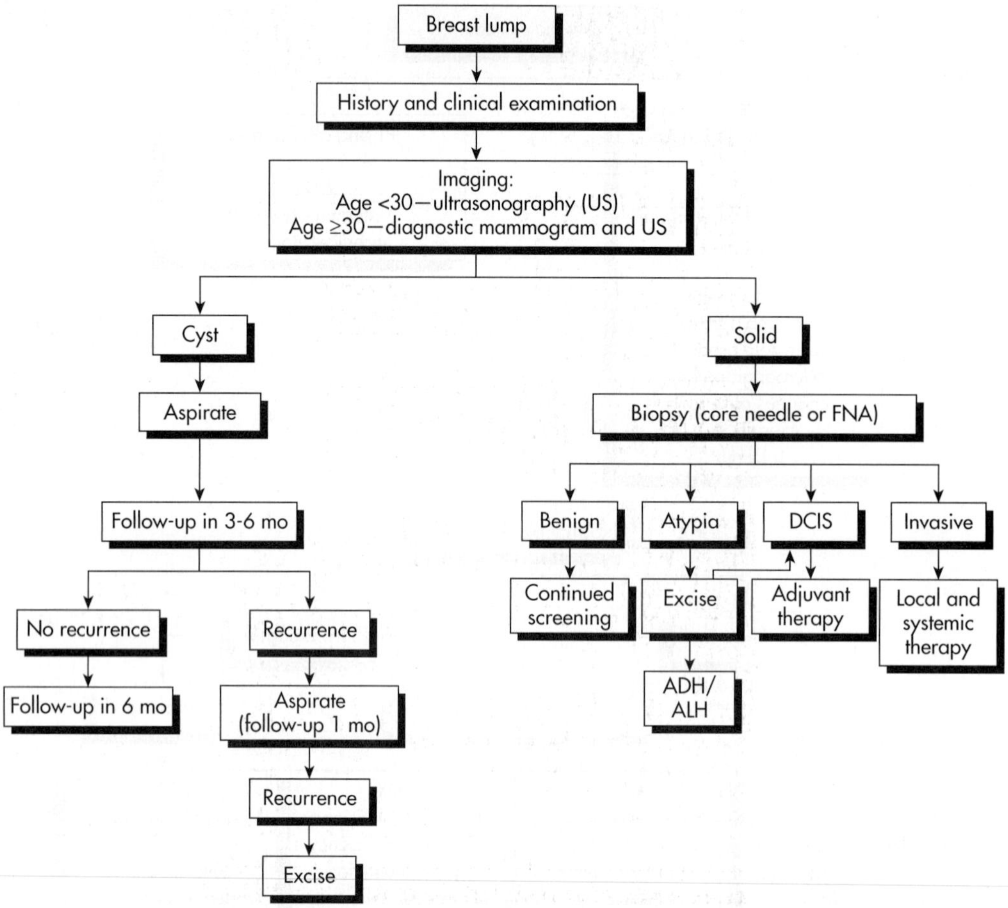

FIG. 40 Algorithm for breast lump management. *ADH,* Atypical ductal hyperplasia; *ALH,* atypical lobular hyperplasia; *DCIS,* ductal carcinoma in situ; *FNA,* fine-needle aspiration. (From Niederhuber JE: *Abeloff's clinical oncology,* ed 6, Philadelphia, 2020, Elsevier.)

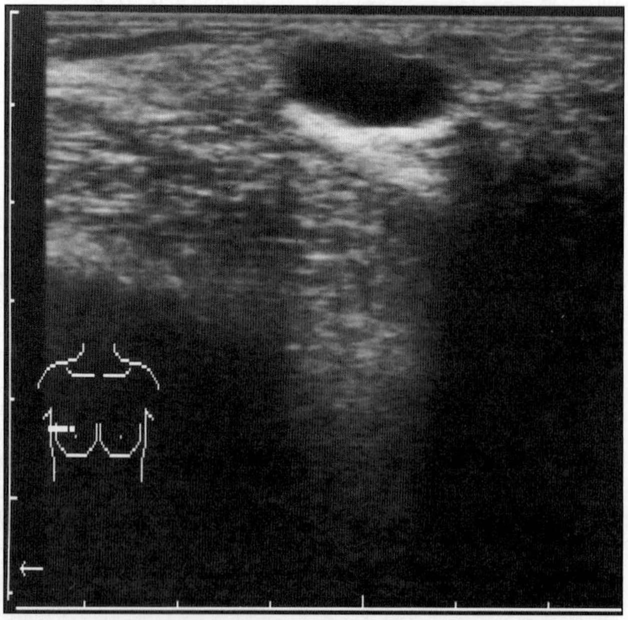

FIG. 41 Ultrasound image of the breast showing the palpable lump to be cystic. Cystic lesions have a characteristic hypoechoic pattern, with prominent acoustic shadowing. (From Niederhuber JE: *Abeloff's clinical oncology,* ed 6, Philadelphia, 2020, Elsevier.)

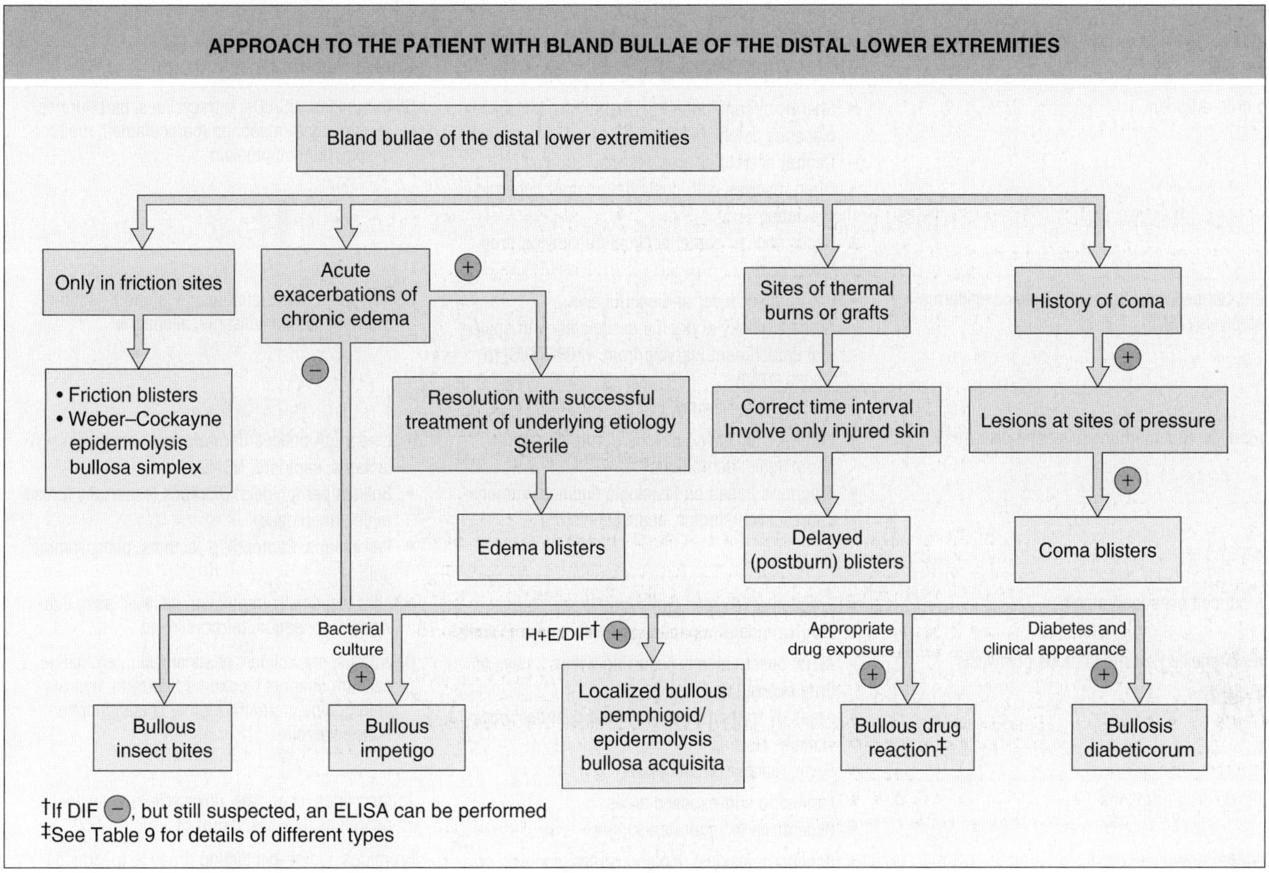

FIG. 42 Approach to the patient with bland bullae of the distal lower extremities. (From Bolognia JL: *Dermatology*, ed 4, Philadelphia, 2018, Elsevier.)

TABLE 9 Bullous Drug Eruptions

Disease	Characteristic Features	Commonly Implicated Drugs
Fixed drug eruption	• Sharply circumscribed erythematous to dusky violaceous patches • Central blisters or erosions may appear • Often resolves with postinflammatory hyperpigmentation • Recurrence at same location(s) following drug reexposure	Sulfonamides, NSAIDs, tetracyclines, barbiturates, aspirin, acetaminophen (paracetamol), metronidazole, phenolphthalein
Stevens-Johnson syndrome (SJS), toxic epidermal necrolysis (TEN)	• Prodrome of fever and painful skin • Areas of dusky erythema associated with epidermal detachment (varying from <10% [SJS] to >30% [TEN]) • Mucosal involvement	NSAIDs, antibiotics (sulfonamides and β-lactams), aromatic anticonvulsants, allopurinol
Drug-induced autoimmune blistering diseases	• Primarily, linear IgA bullous dermatosis, bullous pemphigoid, pemphigus • Diagnosis based on histologic findings, immunofluorescence studies, and drug history	• Linear IgA bullous dermatosis: Vancomycin > β-lactams, captopril, NSAIDs • Bullous pemphigoid: Diuretics (especially furosemide), antibiotics • Pemphigus: Captopril, β-lactams, penicillamine, gold
Drug-induced pseudoporphyria	• Eruption resembles porphyria cutanea tarda • Porphyrin determinations are within normal limits	NSAIDs (especially naproxen), nalidixic acid, thiazides, furosemide, tetracyclines
Acute generalized exanthematous pustulosis	• Acute onset, usually occurring within 2 days of drug exposure • Areas of erythema studded with pustules; occasionally vesicles • Fever, malaise, leukocytosis	β-lactams, macrolides, pristinamycin, terbinafine, calcium channel blockers (diltiazem), hydroxychloroquine, carbamazepine, acetaminophen, metronidazole
Phototoxic drug eruptions	• Limited to sun-exposed areas • Resembles exaggerated sunburn	Tetracyclines (especially doxycycline), quinolones, psoralens, NSAIDs, diuretics
Bromoderma and iododerma	• Acneiform lesions, papulopustules, nodules, or even vegetating lesions simulating pemphigus vegetans • Clear or hemorrhagic blisters can develop (more common in iododerma)	Bromides, iodine-containing drugs (e.g., amiodarone), radiographic contrast media
Palmoplantar erythrodysesthesia (acral variant of toxic erythema of chemotherapy	• Painful erythema develops primarily on the palms, soles and digits following chemotherapy administration • The skin becomes edematous, its color changes to dark red or violet, and blisters and erosions may develop	Cytarabine, doxorubicin, capecitabine, 5-fluorouracil (especially prolonged infusions), multikinase inhibitors (e.g. sorafenib, sunitinib), busulfan, taxanes, clofarabine, pralatrexate

Occasionally, eczematous drug reactions (e.g., secondary to warfarin, calcium channel blockers) and systemic contact dermatitis can be papulovesicular; patients with drug reaction with eosinophilia and systemic symptoms (DRESS)/drug-induced hypersensitivity syndrome (DIHS) can also develop vesicles. Coma blisters and bullous small vessel vasculitis are discussed in the text. *NSAIDs,* nonsteroidal antiinflammatory drugs.

From Bolognia JL: *Dermatology*, ed 4, Philadelphia, 2018, Elsevier.

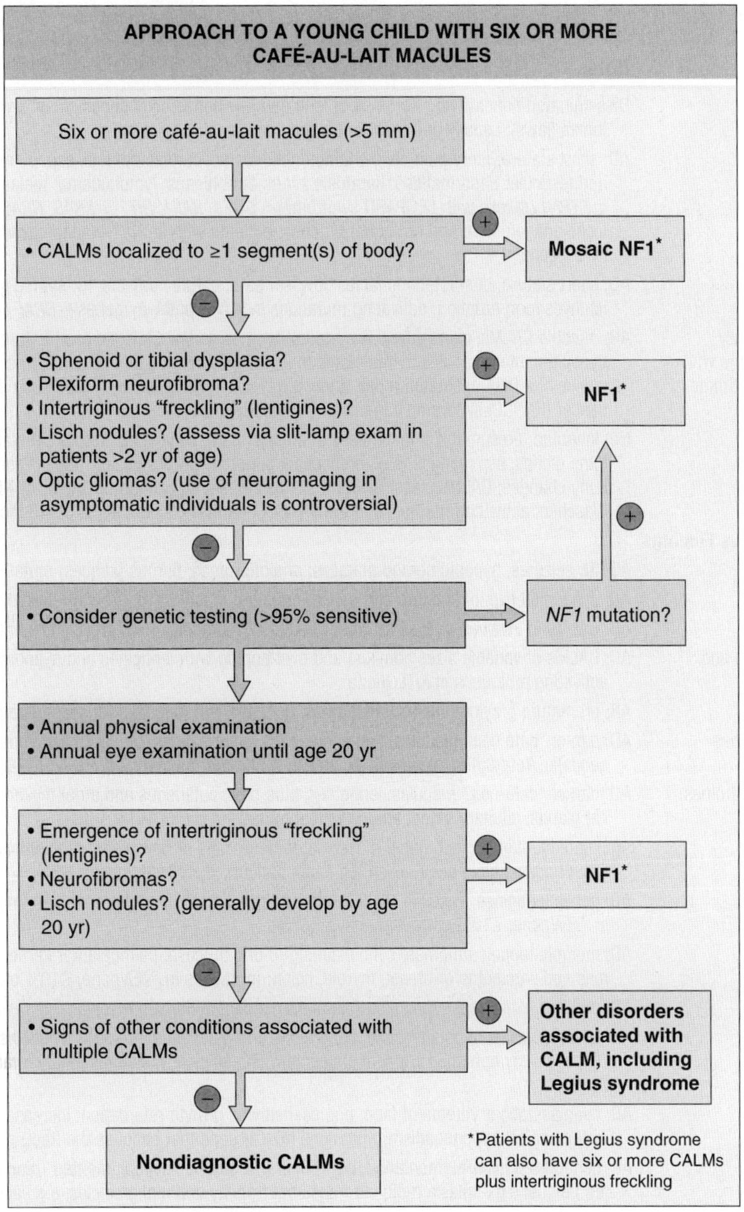

FIG. 43 Approach to a young child with six or more café-au-lait macules. More than half of these patients will eventually prove to have NF1 or, less often, one of the other CALM-associated syndromes (see Table 10). Although uncommon, the latter should be considered if other NF1 signs do not develop. Genetic testing for NF1 is commercially available. *CALMs,* Café-au-lait macules. (From Bolognia JL: *Dermatology*, ed 4, Philadelphia, 2018, Elsevier.)

TABLE 10 Disorders Associated with Multiple Café-au-Lait Macules (CALMs)

Disorder	Notes
Neurofibromatosis and Related Disorders	
Neurofibromatosis 1 (NF1)	AD; six or more CALMs in >90% of patients; mutations in *NF1* gene
Neurofibromatosis 2	AD; six or more CALMs in minority of patients; mutations in *NF2* gene
Mosaic (segmental) NF1 (formerly neurofibromatosis 5)	Neurofibromas alone or CALMs ± "freckling" in a block-like or other mosaic pattern; due to a postzygotic *NF1* mutation, which may involve the gonads in some patients
Legius (NF1-like) syndrome	AD; six or more CALMs in >80% and intertriginous "freckling" in ~50% of patients; lack neurofibromas, Lisch nodules, optic gliomas, and typical osseous lesions of NF1; macrocephaly and learning disabilities are common; lipomas, hypopigmented macules, and vascular anomalies in minority; loss-of-function mutations in *SPRED1* gene, the protein product of which inhibits MAPK signaling
Watson syndrome	AD; short stature; pulmonic stenosis; ID; may also have Lisch nodules, axillary/inguinal freckling, and neurofibromas; allelic with NF1; 60/100*

Continued

TABLE 10 Disorders Associated with Multiple Café-au-Lait Macules (CALMs)—cont'd

Disorder	Notes
Jaffe-Campanacci syndrome	Disseminated nonossifying fibromas of long and jaw bones; hypogonadism or cryptorchidism; D; giant cell granulomas (jaws); usually due to *NF1* mutation
Noonan syndrome	AD; short stature; pterygium colli; characteristic facies; cardiac defects, esp. pulmonic valve stenosis; skeletal and testicular abnormalities; keratosis pilaris atrophicans; lymphedema; melanocytic nevi; activating mutations in *PTPN11* (allelic with LEOPARD syndrome) > *SOS1, RAF1, RIT1* > *KRAS, NRAS, MAP2K1, CBL, SHOC2* (with loose anagen hair), and rarely other genes; patients with an NF1–Noonan overlap phenotype have mutations in *NF1* gene
Cardio-facio-cutaneous syndrome	AD; short stature; characteristic facies; low-set ears; cardiac defects; ID; sparse curly hair; dry skin to generalized ichthyosiform eruption; activating mutations in MAPK pathway genes—*BRAF* > *MEK1, MEK2* > *KRAS*
Constitutional mismatch repair deficiency syndrome (childhood tumor syndrome with NF1 phenotype; formerly Turcot syndrome type 1)	AR; multiple CALMs, axillary freckling, neurofibromas and/or CNS gliomas (features similar to NF1) as well as hypopigmented macules, hematologic malignancies, and colorectal carcinoma; patients have mutations in both copies of a DNA mismatch repair gene, e.g., *MLH1, MSH2, MSH6, PMS2*; hereditary nonpolyposis colorectal cancer (HNPCC) syndrome can occur in heterozygotes
McCune–Albright syndrome	Not inherited; presumably lethal unless in mosaic state; polyostotic fibrous dysplasia; hyperfunction of endocrine glands, esp. gonads (e.g., precocious puberty); CALMs usually appear during infancy and can overlie bony changes; CALMs classically end at midline, but so can larger CALMs of NF; CALMs may follow lines of Blaschko; activating mutations in the *GNAS1* gene that encodes $G_s\alpha$; 35/100*
Disorders With Additional Cutaneous Findings	
Tuberous sclerosis complex (TSC)	AD; ID; seizures; hypopigmented macules; angiofibromas; fibrous plaques; mutations in *TSC1* and *TSC2* genes
Westerhof syndrome	AD; congenital hypopigmented and hyperpigmented macules; ID; growth retardation
Piebaldism	AD; CALMs in involved as well as uninvolved skin; mutations in *KIT* proto-oncogene
Familial progressive hyperpigmentation and hypopigmentation	AD; CALMs of variable sizes admixed and overlapping with lentigines and hypopigmented macules and patches; activating mutations in *KITLG* gene
Mukamel syndrome	AR; premature graying (infancy); lentigines; depigmented macules; ID; spastic paraparesis, microcephaly, scoliosis
Noonan syndrome with multiple lentigines (LEOPARD syndrome)	AD; darker "café noir" macules; *L*entigines, *E*CG abnormalities, *O*cular hypertelorism, *P*ulmonic stenosis, *A*bnormal genitalia, *R*etardation of growth, *D*eafness syndrome; mutations in *PTPN11*; 38/100*
Carney complex (NAME and LAMB syndromes)	AD; darker "café-noir" macules, lentigines, blue nevi; cutaneous and atrial myxomas; endocrine neoplasia of adrenal glands, pituitary gland, and/or testes; mutations in *PRKAR1A*
Partial unilateral lentiginosis	Agminated lentigines; debatable if associated neurologic or psychiatric problems; unilateral axillary freckling and Lisch nodules have been described (such patients likely have mosaic NF1)
Bannayan-Riley-Ruvalcaba syndrome‡	AD; penile lentigines; vascular malformations; lipomas; intestinal hamartomas; macrocephaly; mutations in *PTEN* gene; ≤10% of patients have CALMs
Cowden syndrome‡	AD; multiple tricholemmomas; cobblestoning of oral mucosa; palmoplantar keratoses; sclerotic fibromas, hamartomas and carcinoma of breast, thyroid, colon; mutations in *PTEN* gene; ≤10% of patients have CALMs
Gastrocutaneous syndrome†	AD; multiple lentigines; peptic ulcer/hiatal hernia; hypertelorism; myopia
Ataxia-telangiectasia	AR; telangiectasias of conjunctivae, head/neck, and acral sites; premature canities; cerebellar ataxia; abnormal DNA repair; lymphomas and leukemias; immunodeficiency; sinopulmonary infections; mutations in *ATM* gene; 20/100*
Bloom syndrome	AR; telangiectatic erythema of face; photosensitivity; growth retardation; increased sister chromatid exchanges; malignancies; hypogonadism; mutations in *BLM* gene that encodes the RecQ protein-like-3 DNA helicase
Fanconi anemia	AR; generalized hyperpigmentation, esp. flexural ± guttate "hypopigmented" macules; pancytopenia; skeletal malformations, e.g., aplasia radii; chromosomal fragility and malignancies, e.g., acute myelogenous leukemia
Chromosomal anomalies/mosaicism	In particular, ring chromosomes (7, 11, 12, 15, 17); rearrangements of 7 and 14; ring 7 also associated with vascular lesions (hemangiomas and capillary malformations) and congenital melanocytic nevi
Extensive epidermal and sebaceous nevi	Mosaic; "syndrome" includes seizures, ID, musculoskeletal and ocular abnormalities; hypophosphatemic vitamin D–resistant rickets
Multiple endocrine neoplasia 1	AD; tumors of the pituitary, parathyroid, and pancreatic islet cells; multiple facial angiofibromas, collagenomas, gingival papules, confetti-like hypomelanotic macules, lipomas; *MEN1* gene
Multiple endocrine neoplasia 2B	AD; mucosal neuromas; marfanoid habitus; medullary thyroid carcinoma; intestinal ganglioneuromatosis; pheochromocytoma; mutations in *RET* proto-oncogene
Johnson-McMillin syndrome	Probable AD; alopecia; anosmia; deafness; hypogonadism; microtia
Tricho-hepato-enteric syndrome	AR; CALM and lentigines on hips and legs; diffuse pigmentary dilution (skin and hair), woolly hair; dysmorphic facies with hypertelorism; intractable diarrhea, liver disease; immune deficiency; mutations in *TTC37* or *SKIV2L*
Tay syndrome†	?AR; growth retardation; ID; triangular face; cirrhosis; trident hands; premature canities; vitiligo
Other Disorders§	
Russell-Silver syndrome	Growth retardation; triangular face; clinodactyly 5th finger; hemihypertrophy; epigenetic changes on chromosome 15p13 or maternal uniparental disomy of chromosome 7; 45/100*

*Estimates of prevalence of CALMs [Source: Gutmann DH et al: The diagnostic evaluation and multidisciplinary management of neurofibromatosis 1 and neurofibromatosis 2. *JAMA* 1997;278:51-57.]
†To date, observed in a single family.
‡Overlapping conditions collectively referred to as PTEN hamartoma tumor syndrome.
§Single case reports of multiple CALMs in association with X-linked hypohidrotic ectodermal dysplasia, woolly hair, and osteoma cutis.
Multiple CALMs may also be seen in patients with segmental pigmentation disorder.
AD, Autosomal dominant; *AR,* autosomal recessive; *DNA,* deoxyribonucleic acid; *ID,* intellectual disability; *KITLG,* KIT ligand; *MAPK,* mitogen-activated protein kinase.
From Bolognia JL: *Dermatology,* ed 4, 2018, Elsevier.

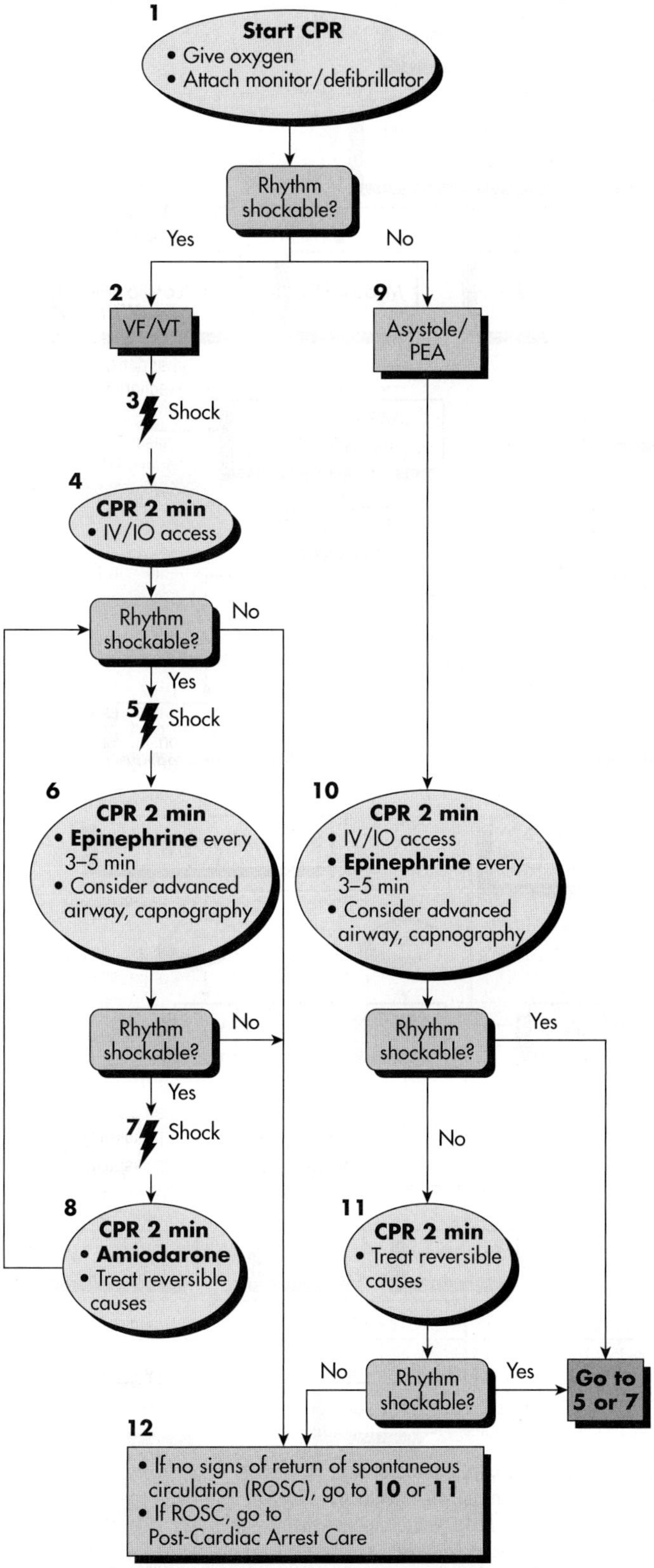

CPR Quality
- Push hard (2 in [5 cm]) and fast (100–120/min) and allow complete chest recoil
- Minimize interruptions in compressions
- Avoid excessive ventilation
- Rotate compressor every 2 min or sooner if fatigued
- If no advanced airway, 30:2 compression-ventilation ratio
- Quantitative waveform capnography
  - If P_{ETCO_2} <10 mm Hg, attempt to improve CPR quality
- Intraarterial pressure
  - If relaxation phase (diastolic) pressure <20 mm Hg, attempt to improve CPR quality

Shock Energy for Defibrillation
- **Biphasic:** Manufacturer recommendation (e.g., initial dose of 120–200 J); if unknown, use maximum available. Second and subsequent doses should be equivalent, and higher doses may be considered
- **Monophasic:** 360 J

Drug Therapy
- **Epinephrine IV/IO Dose:** 1 mg every 3–5 min
- **Amiodarone IV/IO Dose:** First dose: 300 mg bolus Second dose: 150 mg

Advanced Airway
- Endotracheal intubation or supraglottic advanced airway
- Waveform capnography or capnometry to confirm and monitor ET tube placement
- Once advanced airway in place, give 1 breath every 6 s (10 breaths/min) with continuous chest compressions

Return of Spontaneous Circulation (ROSC)
- Pulse and blood pressure
- Abrupt sustained increase in P_{ETCO_2} (typically ≥40 mm Hg)
- Spontaneous arterial pressure waves with intraarterial monitoring

Reversible Causes
- **H**ypovolemia
- **H**ypoxia
- **H**ydrogen ion (acidosis)
- **H**ypo-/hyperkalemia
- **H**ypothermia
- **T**ension pneumothorax
- **T**amponade, cardiac
- **T**oxins
- **T**hrombosis, pulmonary
- **T**hrombosis, coronary

FIG. 44 American Heart Association Advanced Cardiac Life Support (ACLS) algorithm. *CPR,* Cardiopulmonary resuscitation; *ET,* endotracheal; *IO,* intraosseous; *IV,* intravenous; *PEA,* pulseless electrical activity; *P_{ETCO_2},* partial pressure of end tidal carbon dioxide; *pVT,* pulseless ventricular tachycardia; *ROSC,* return of spontaneous circulation; *VF,* ventricular fibrillation; *VT,* ventricular tachycardia. (From Link MS et al: Part 7: adult advanced cardiovascular life support: 2015 American Heart Association guidelines update for cardiopulmonary resuscitation and emergency cardiovascular care, *Circulation* 132[18 suppl 2]:S444-S464, 2015. In Parrillo JE, Dellinger RP: *Critical care medicine, principles of diagnosis and management in the adult,* ed 5, Philadelphia, 2019, Elsevier.)

Clinical Algorithms III

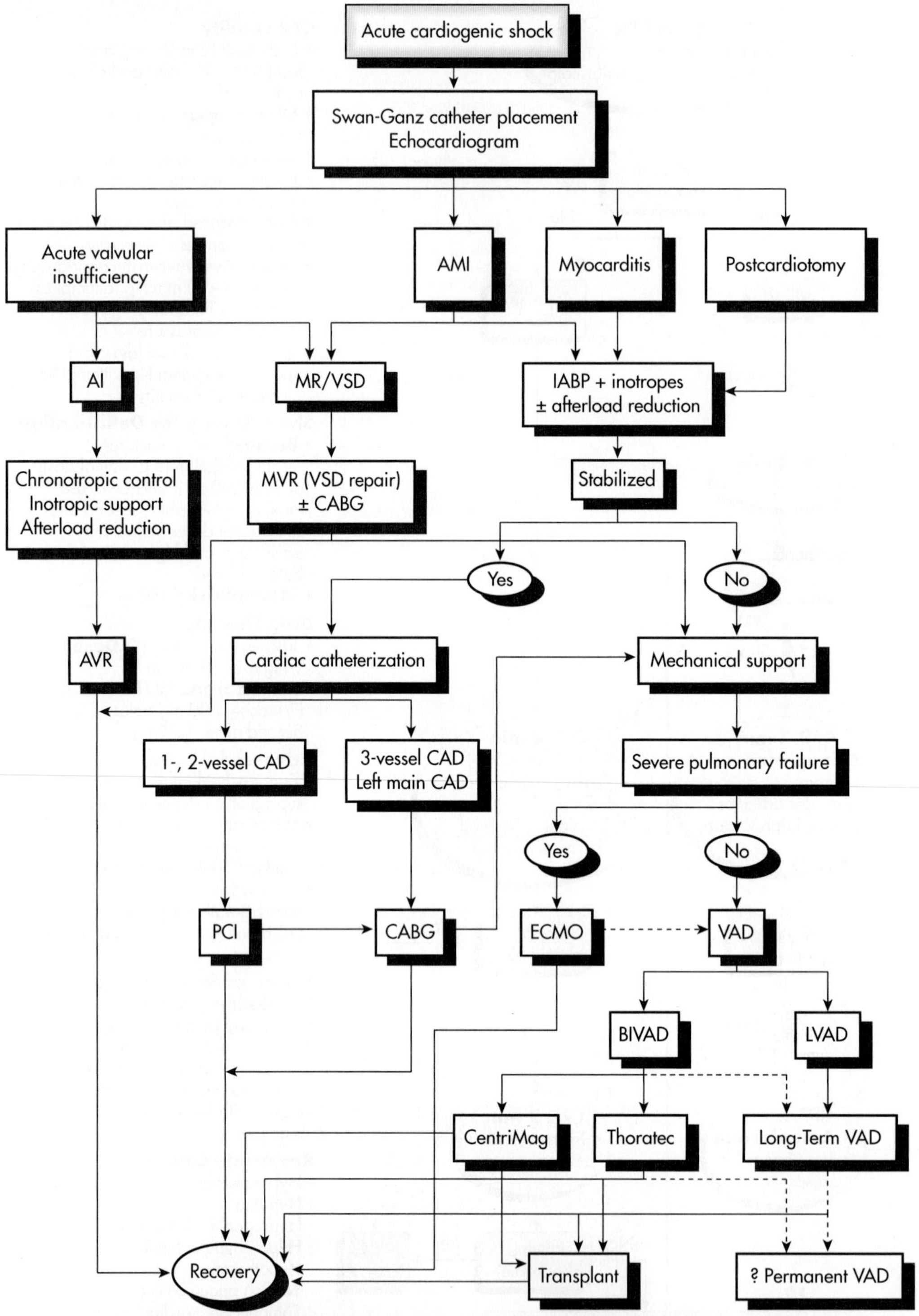

FIG. 45 Algorithm for the management of acute cardiogenic shock. *AI,* Adrenal insufficiency; *AMI,* acute myocardial infarction; *AVR,* aortic valve replacement; *BIVAD,* biventricular assist device; *CABP,* coronary artery bypass procedure; *CAD,* coronary artery disease; *ECMO,* extracorporeal membrane oxygenation; *IABP,* intra-aortic balloon pump; *LVAD,* left ventricular assist device; *MR,* mitral regurgitation; *PCI,* percutaneous coronary intervention; *VAD,* ventricular assist device; *VSD,* ventricular septal defect. (From Vincent JL et al: *Textbook of critical case,* ed 7, Philadelphia, 2017, Elsevier.)

ICD-10CM # I51.7 Cardiomegaly
Q24.8 Other specified congenital malformations of heart
I11.9 Hypertensive heart disease without heart failure
I11.0 Hypertensive heart disease with heart failure
Q23.8 Other congenital malformations of aortic and mitral valves

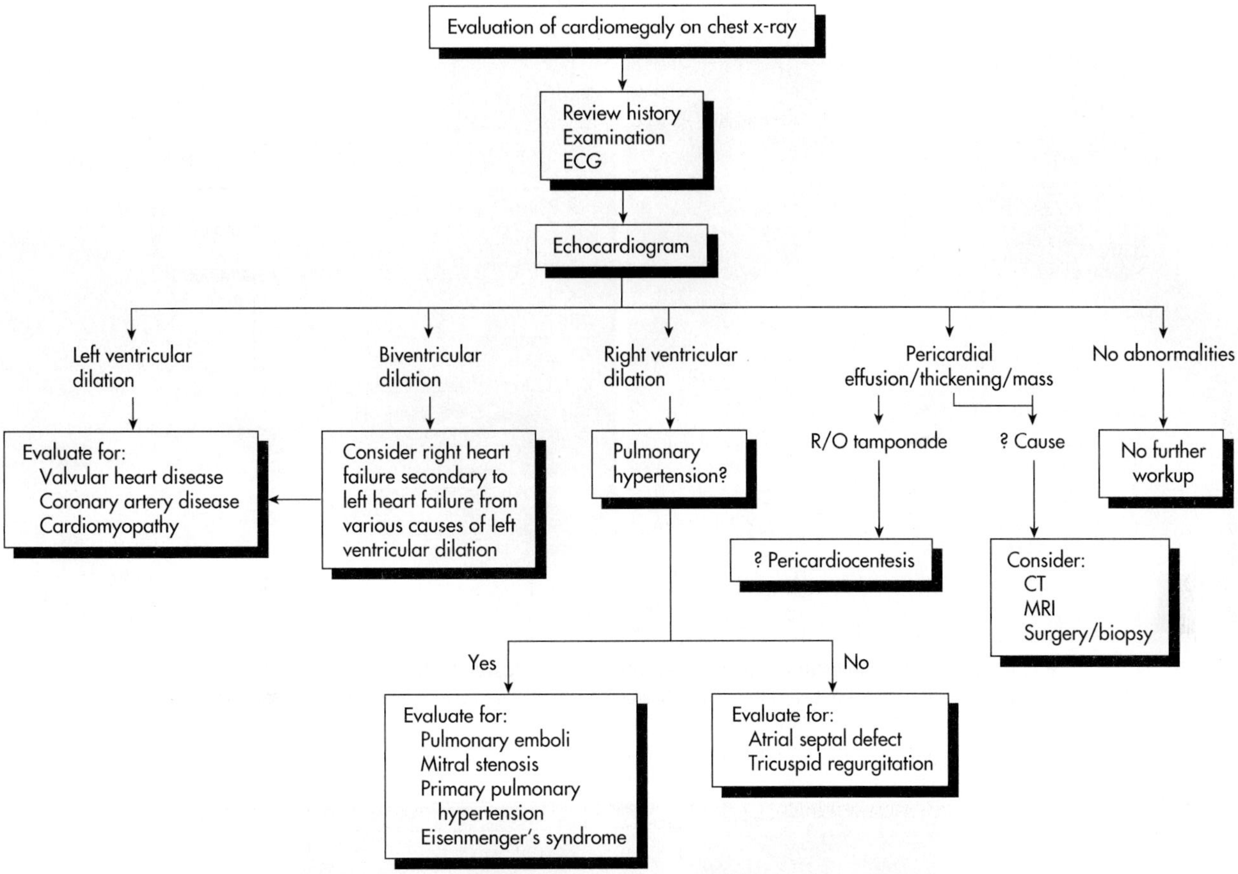

FIG. 46 Approach to the patient with cardiomegaly. When cardiomegaly is found on the chest radiograph, the history and physical examination should be reviewed and an electrocardiogram *(ECG)* performed before obtaining a two-dimensional Doppler echocardiographic study. Cardiomegaly may be explained by left ventricular dilation, biventricular dilation, right ventricular dilation, or pericardial abnormalities, or it may be found to be spurious on the echocardiogram. Rarely, isolated abnormalities of the atrium, particularly the left atrium, may cause abnormalities on the chest radiograph but will not cause true cardiomegaly. Depending on the echocardiographic findings, further tests can help elucidate the cause of echocardiographically confirmed cardiomegaly. *CT,* Computed tomography; *MRI,* magnetic resonance imaging; *R/O,* rule out. (From Goldman L, Braunwald E [eds]: *Primary cardiology,* ed 2, Philadelphia, 2003, Saunders.)

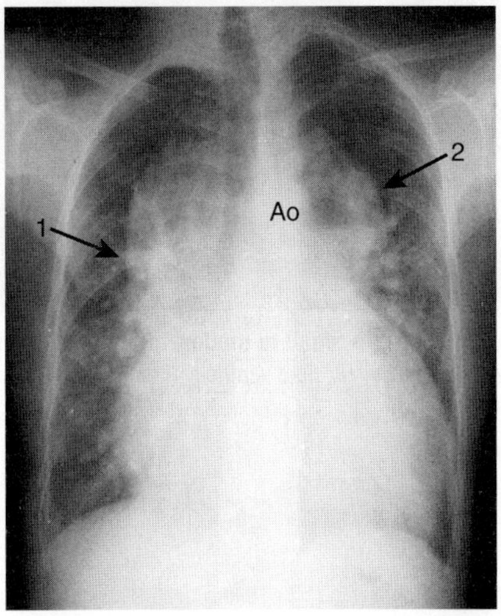

FIG. 47 "Snowman" heart in a 36-yr-old man with increasing shortness of breath. Posteroanterior chest film examination shows cardiomegaly and increased pulmonary blood flow. The superior mediastinum is widened, the result of dilation of the left vertical vein *(arrow 2)* and the right-sided superior vena cava *(arrow 1).* The trachea is displaced by a normal left-sided aortic arch *(Ao).* (From Boxt LM, Abbara S: *Cardiac imaging: the requisites,* ed 4, Philadelphia, 2016, Elsevier.)

Clinical Algorithms III

ICD-10CM # I51.7 Cardiomegaly
Q24.8 Other specified congenital malformations of heart
I11.9 Hypertensive heart disease without heart failure
I11.0 Hypertensive heart disease with heart failure
Q23.8 Other congenital malformations of aortic and mitral valves

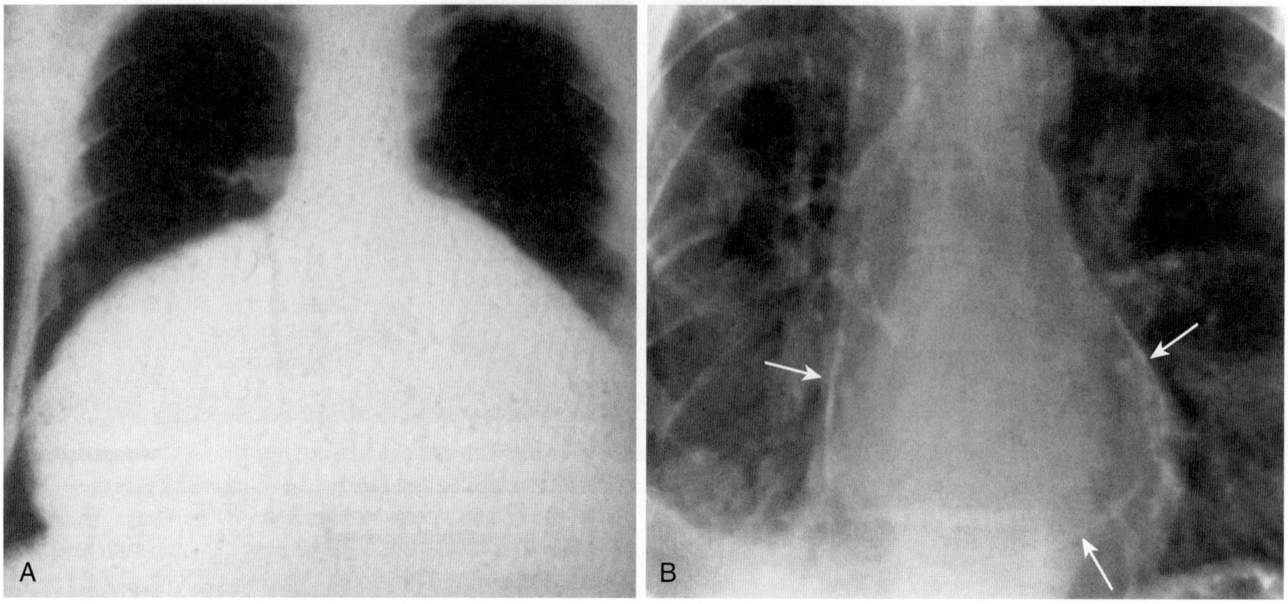

FIG. 48 Chest radiographs in a patient with a very large pericardial effusion. A, "Water bottle" sign. **B,** A patient with constrictive pericarditis and pericardial calcifications (*white arrows*). (From Vincent JL et al: *Textbook of critical care,* ed 7, Philadelphia, 2017, Elsevier.)

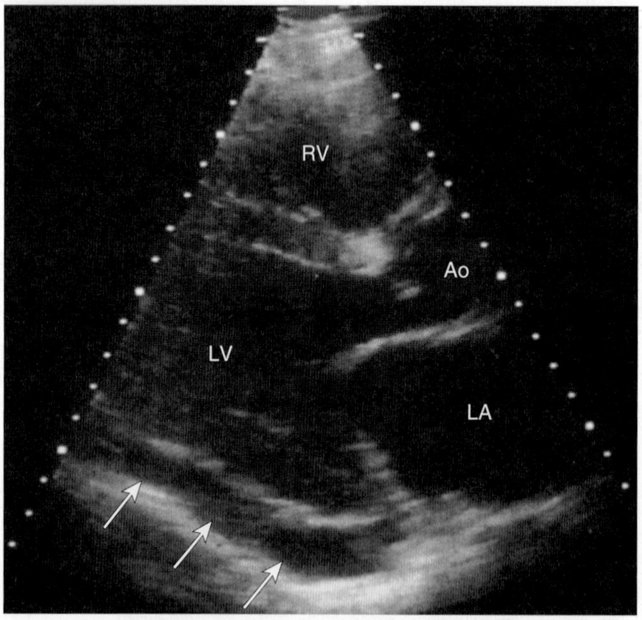

FIG. 49 Echocardiographic findings in a small to moderate pericardial effusion *(white arrows). Ao,* Aortic root; *LA,* left atrium; *LV,* left ventricle; *RV,* right ventricle. (From Vincent JL et al: *Textbook of critical care,* ed 7, Philadelphia, 2017, Elsevier.)

ICD-10CM # I51.7 Cardiomegaly
Q24.8 Other specified congenital malformations of heart
I11.9 Hypertensive heart disease without heart failure
I11.0 Hypertensive heart disease with heart failure
Q23.8 Other congenital malformations of aortic and mitral valves

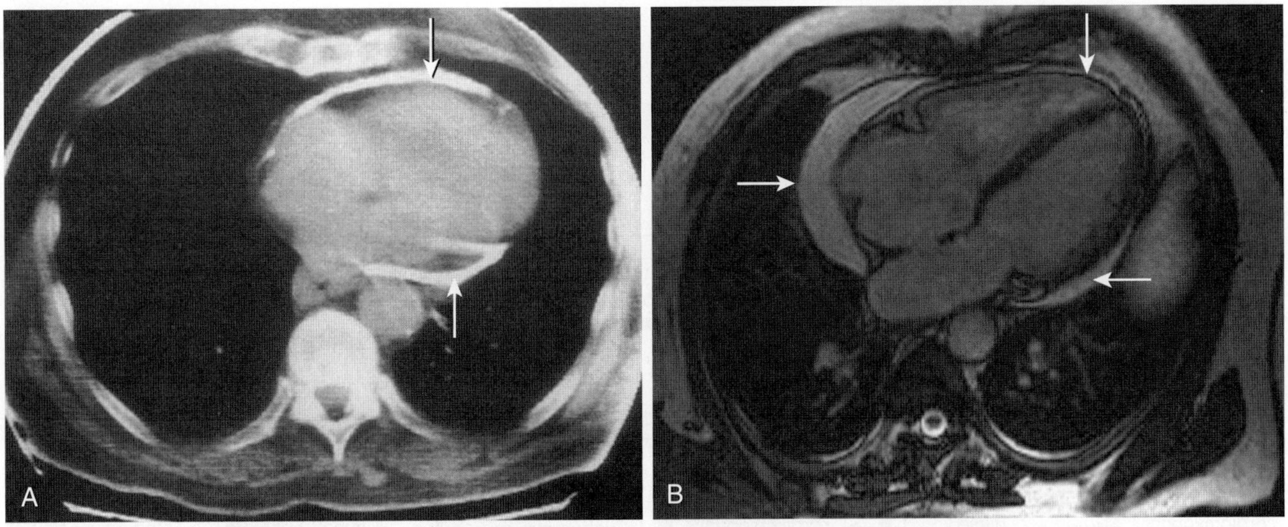

FIG. 50 A, Computed tomography findings in constrictive pericarditis. White vertical arrows are depicting thickened pericardium and pericardial calcification. **B,** The magnetic resonance imaging results of a patient with effusive-constrictive pericarditis are shown in the right image. Horizontal arrows show a loculated pericardial effusion, and the vertical arrow shows thickened pericardium. (From Vincent JL et al: *Textbook of critical care,* ed 7, Philadelphia, 2017, Elsevier.)

TABLE 11 Diagnosis of Cardiac Tamponade

Clinical presentation	Elevated systemic venous pressure,* hypotension,† pulsus paradoxus,‡ tachycardia,§ dyspnea, or tachypnea with clear lungs
Precipitating factors	Drugs (cyclosporine, anticoagulants, thrombolytics), recent cardiac surgery, indwelling instrumentation, blunt chest trauma, malignancies, connective tissue disease, renal failure, septicemia‖
ECG	Can be normal or nonspecifically changed (ST-T wave), electrical alternans (QRS, rarely T), bradycardia (end stage), electromechanical dissociation (agonal phase)
Chest radiograph	Enlarged cardiac silhouette with clear lungs
M-mode/two-dimensional echocardiogram	Diastolic collapse of the anterior RV free wall,¶ RA collapse, LA and rarely LV collapse, increased LV diastolic wall thickness "pseudohypertrophy," IVC dilation (no collapse in inspiration), "swinging heart"
Doppler	Tricuspid flow increases and mitral flow decreases during inspiration (reverse in expiration)
	Systolic and diastolic flows are reduced in systemic veins in expiration and reverse flow with atrial contraction is increased
M-mode color Doppler	Large respiratory fluctuations in mitral/tricuspid flows
Cardiac catheterization	Confirmation of the diagnosis and quantification of the hemodynamic compromise
	RA pressure is elevated (preserved systolic x descent and absent or diminished diastolic y descent)
	Intrapericardial pressure is also elevated and virtually identical to RA pressure (both pressures fall in inspiration)
	RV mid-diastolic pressure is elevated and equal to the RA and pericardial pressures (no dip-and-plateau configuration)
	Pulmonary artery diastolic pressure is slightly elevated and may correspond to the RV pressure
	Pulmonary capillary wedge pressure is also elevated and nearly equal to intrapericardial and right atrial pressure
	LV systolic and aortic pressures may be normal or reduced
	Documenting that pericardial aspiration is followed by hemodynamic improvement**
	Detection of coexisting hemodynamic abnormalities (LV failure, constriction, pulmonary hypertension)
	Detection of associated cardiovascular diseases (cardiomyopathy, coronary artery disease)
RV/LV angiography	Atrial collapse and small hyperactive ventricular chambers
Coronary angiography	Coronary compression in diastole

ECG, electrocardiogram; *IVC,* inferior vena cava; *LA,* left atrium; *LV,* left ventricle; *QRS,* Q wave, R wave, S wave; *RA,* right atrium; *RV,* right ventricle.

*Jugular venous distention is less notable in hypovolemic patients or in "surgical tamponade." An inspiratory increase or lack of fall of pressure in the neck veins (Kussmaul sign), when verified by tamponade or after pericardial drainage, indicates effusive-constrictive disease.

†Heart rate is usually greater than 100 beats per minute but may be lower in patients with hypothyroidism or uremia.

‡Pulsus paradoxus is defined as a drop in systolic blood pressure greater than 10 mm Hg during inspiration, while diastolic blood pressure remains unchanged. It is easily detected by simply feeling the pulse, which diminishes significantly during inspiration. Clinically significant pulsus paradoxus is apparent when the patient is breathing normally. When this sign is present only in deep inspiration, it should be interpreted with caution. The magnitude of pulsus paradoxus is evaluated by sphygmomanometry. If pulsus paradoxus is present, the first Korotkoff sound is not heard equally well throughout the respiratory cycle but only during expiration at a given blood pressure. The blood pressure cuff is therefore inflated above the patient's systolic pressure. Then it is slowly deflated, while the clinician observes the phase of respiration. During deflation, the first Korotkoff sound is intermittent. Correlation with the patient's respiratory cycle identifies a point at which the sound is audible during expiration but disappears when the patient breathes in. As the cuff pressure drops further, another point is reached when the first blood pressure sound is audible throughout the respiratory cycle. The difference in systolic pressure between these two points is the clinical measure of pulsus paradoxus. Pulsus paradoxus is absent in tamponade complicating an atrial septal defect and in patients with significant aortic regurgitation.

§Occasional patients are hypertensive, especially if they have preexisting hypertension.

‖Febrile tamponade may be misdiagnosed as septic shock.

¶Right ventricular collapse can be absent in elevated right ventricular pressure and right ventricular hypertrophy or in right ventricular infarction.

**If after drainage of the pericardial effusion, the intrapericardial pressure does not fall below atrial pressure, effusive-constrictive disease should be considered.

From Vincent JL et al: *Textbook of critical care,* ed 7, Philadelphia, 2017, Elsevier.

ICD-10CM # I42.5 Other restrictive cardiomyopathy
I42.8 Other cardiomyopathies

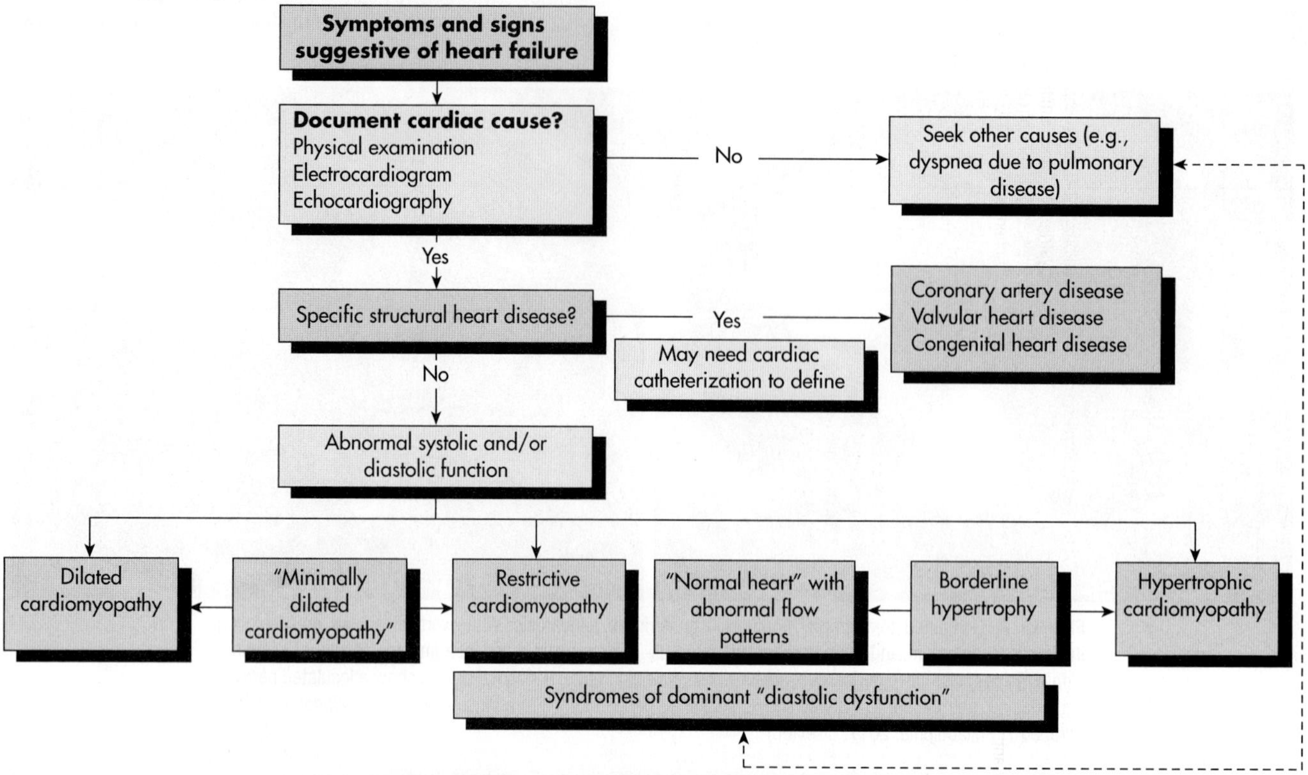

FIG. 51 Initial approach to classification of cardiomyopathy. The evaluation of symptoms or signs consistent with heart failure first includes confirmation that they can be attributed to a cardiac cause. Although this conclusion is often apparent from routine physical examination and electrocardiography, echocardiography serves to confirm cardiac disease and provides clues to the presence of other cardiac diseases, such as focal abnormalities suggesting primary valve disease or congenital heart disease. Having excluded these conditions, cardiomyopathy is generally considered to be dilated, restrictive, or hypertrophic, as shown in the figure. Patients with apparently normal cardiac structure and contraction are occasionally found to demonstrate abnormal intracardiac flow patterns consistent with diastolic dysfunction but should also be evaluated carefully for other causes of their symptoms. Most patients with so-called diastolic dysfunction also demonstrate at least borderline criteria for left ventricular hypertrophy, frequently in the setting of chronic hypertension and diabetes. A moderately decreased ejection fraction without marked dilation or a pattern of restrictive cardiomyopathy is sometimes referred to as minimally dilated cardiomyopathy, which may represent either a distinct entity or a transition between acute and chronic disease. (From Goldman L, Schafer AI: *Goldman Cecil medicine,* ed 25, Philadelphia, 2016, Saunders.)

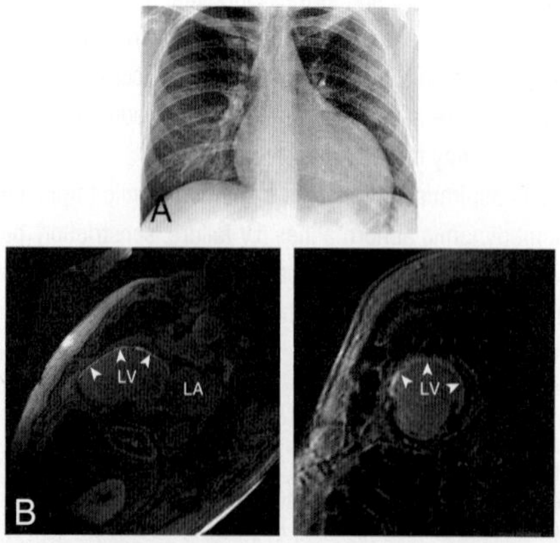

FIG. 52 Dilated cardiomyopathy. A, The heart shows enlargement of all four chambers. The azygos vein and superior vena cava are slightly dilated, reflecting high central venous pressure. **B,** Delayed enhanced magnetic resonance images demonstrate ischemic dilated cardiomyopathy. Extensive subendocardial delayed hyperenhancement *(arrowheads)* demonstrates features of old myocardial infarction—it follows a vascular territory (the left anterior descending), it is based on the subendocardium, and there is thinning of the affected myocardium. *LA,* Left atrium; *LV,* left ventricle. (Boxt LM, Abbara S: *Cardiac imaging: the requisites,* ed 4, Philadelphia, 2016, Elsevier.)

TABLE 12 Classification of the Cardiomyopathies by Phenome and Genome

	PHENOME			GENOME		
Type	**Morphology**	**Physiology**	**Pathology**	**Systemic Conditions or Diseases, Clinically Relevant Features, Classic Risk Factors, Associations**	**Nonsyndromic, Usually Single Gene**	**Syndromic**
Dilated (DCM)	LV/RV dilation with minimal or no wall thickening	Reduced contractility is the primary defect; variable degree of diastolic dysfunction	Myocyte hypertrophy; scattered fibrosis	Hypertension; alcohol use; thyrotoxicosis, myxedema; persistent tachycardia; toxins, e.g., chemotherapy, especially anthracyclines; radiation; pregnancy	Diverse gene ontology with >30 genes implicated	Diverse array of associated conditions, especially muscular dystrophies (MDs): Emery-Dreifuss MD, limb-girdle MD, Duchenne/Becker MD; Laing distal myopathy; Barth syndrome; Kearns-Sayre; others
Restrictive (RCM)	Usually normal chamber sizes; minimal wall thickening	Contractility normal or near-normal with a marked increase in end-diastolic filling pressure	Specific to type, diagnosis: Amyloid, iron, glycogen storage disease, others	Endomyocardial fibrosis, amyloid, sarcoid, scleroderma, Churg-Strauss syndrome, cystinosis, lymphoma, pseudoxanthoma elasticum, hypereosinophilic syndrome, carcinoid	If not associated with a systemic genetic disease (e.g., hemochromatosis), genetic cause found most commonly to result from sarcomeric gene mutations	Gaucher disease, hemochromatosis, Fabry disease, familial amyloidosis. Mucopolysaccharidoses, Noonan syndrome
Hypertrophic (HCM)	Usually normal or reduced internal chamber dimension; wall thickening pronounced, especially septal hypertrophy	Systolic function increased or normal	Myocyte hypertrophy, classically with disarray	Severe hypertension can confound clinical, morphologic diagnosis	Mutations of genes encoding sarcomeric proteins	Noonan/Leopard, Danon, Fabry, WPW, Friedrich ataxia, MERRF, MELAS
Arrhythmogenic cardiomyopathy (ACM)	Scattered fibrofatty infiltration, classically of the right ventricle but also commonly involving the left ventricle; RV dilation, LV dilation, or both are common although not universal	Ventricular arrhythmias (VT, VF) early or late, reduced contractility with progressive disease; can mimic DCM	Islands of fatty replacement; fibrosis	Palmoplantar keratoderma, wooly hair in Naxos syndrome	Mutations of genes encoding proteins of the desmosome	Naxos syndrome
Left ventricular noncompaction (LVNC)	Ratio of noncompacted to compacted myocardium increased; normal chamber dimensions varying to a DCM phenotype	Normal to reduced systolic function	Myocardium normal and ranging to findings consistent with other coexisting cardiomyopathy	Phenotype has been observed in the setting of other types of cardiomyopathy	Various cardiomyopathy genes associated but uncertain whether genetic cause or developmental defect during organogenesis; see text	
Infiltrative	Usually thickened walls; occasional dilation	Restrictive physiology; systolic function usually mildly reduced	Specific to type, diagnosis: Amyloid, iron, glycogen storage disease, others		See "RCM" above	See "RCM" above
Inflammatory	Normal or dilated without hypertrophy	Reduced systolic function	Inflammatory infiltrates	Hypereosinophilic syndrome (see text), acute myocarditis		
Ischemic	Normal or dilated without hypertrophy	Reduced systolic function	Areas of infarcted myocardium	Hypercholesterolemia, hypertension, diabetes, cigarette smoking, family history	Familial hypercholesterolemia; other heritable lipid disorders	Familial hypercholesterolemia
Infectious		Normal or dilated without hypertrophy	Reduced systolic function	Specific to infection	Viral (especially acute myocarditis); protozoal (e.g., Chagas); bacterial, direct infection (e.g., Lyme disease), or from acute cellular toxicity as a result of systemic toxins (*Streptococcus*, gram-negatives, etc.)	Genetic predisposition to infection and/or variable response to infective agent

LV, Left ventricle; *MELAS*, mitochondrial encephalopathy, lactic acidosis, and stroke-like symptoms; *MERRF*, myoclonic epilepsy associated with ragged red fibers; *RV*, right ventricle; *VF*, ventricular fibrillation; *VT*, ventricular tachycardia; *WPW*, Wolff-Parkinson-White syndrome.
From Mann DL et al: *Braunwald's heart disease*, ed 10, Philadelphia, 2015, Elsevier.

ICD-10CM # R07.4 Pain(s) chest
R07.2 Pain(s) heart
R07.3 Pain(s) chest anterior wall

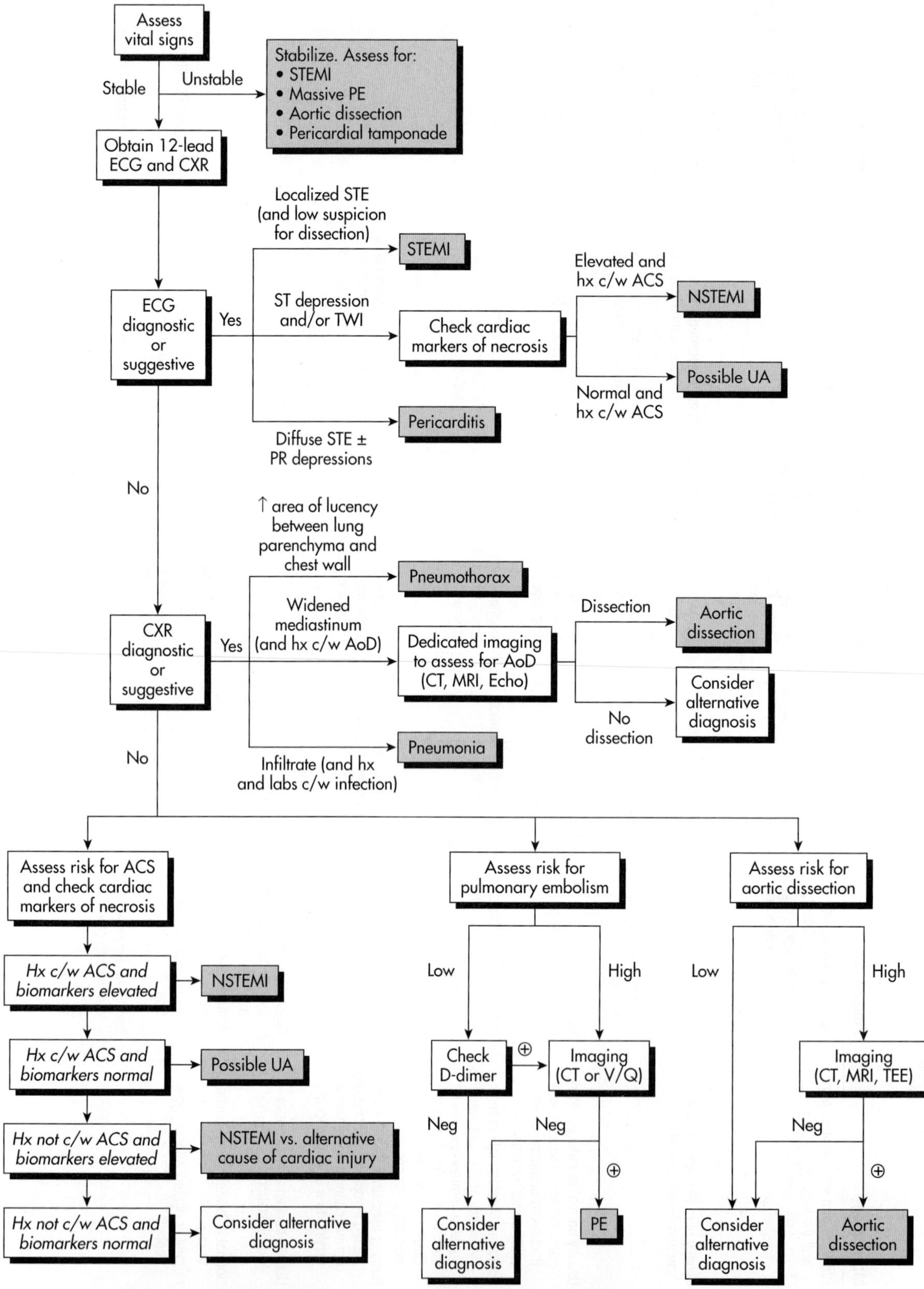

FIG. 53 Algorithm for the initial diagnostic approach to a patient with chest pain. *ACS,* Acute coronary syndrome; *AoD,* aortic dissection; *c/w,* consistent with; *CT,* computed tomography; *CXR,* chest x-ray film; *ECG,* electrocardiogram; *Echo,* echocardiography; *hx,* history; *MRI,* magnetic resonance imaging; *NSTEMI,* non–ST-segment elevation myocardial infarction; *PE,* pulmonary embolism; *STE,* ST-segment elevation; *STEMI,* ST-segment elevation myocardial infarction; *TEE,* transesophageal echocardiography; *UA,* unstable angina; *TWI,* T wave inversion; *V/Q,* ventilation-perfusion scan. (From Zipes DP: *Braunwald's heart disease, a textbook of cardiovascular medicine,* ed 11, Philadelphia, 2019, Elsevier.)

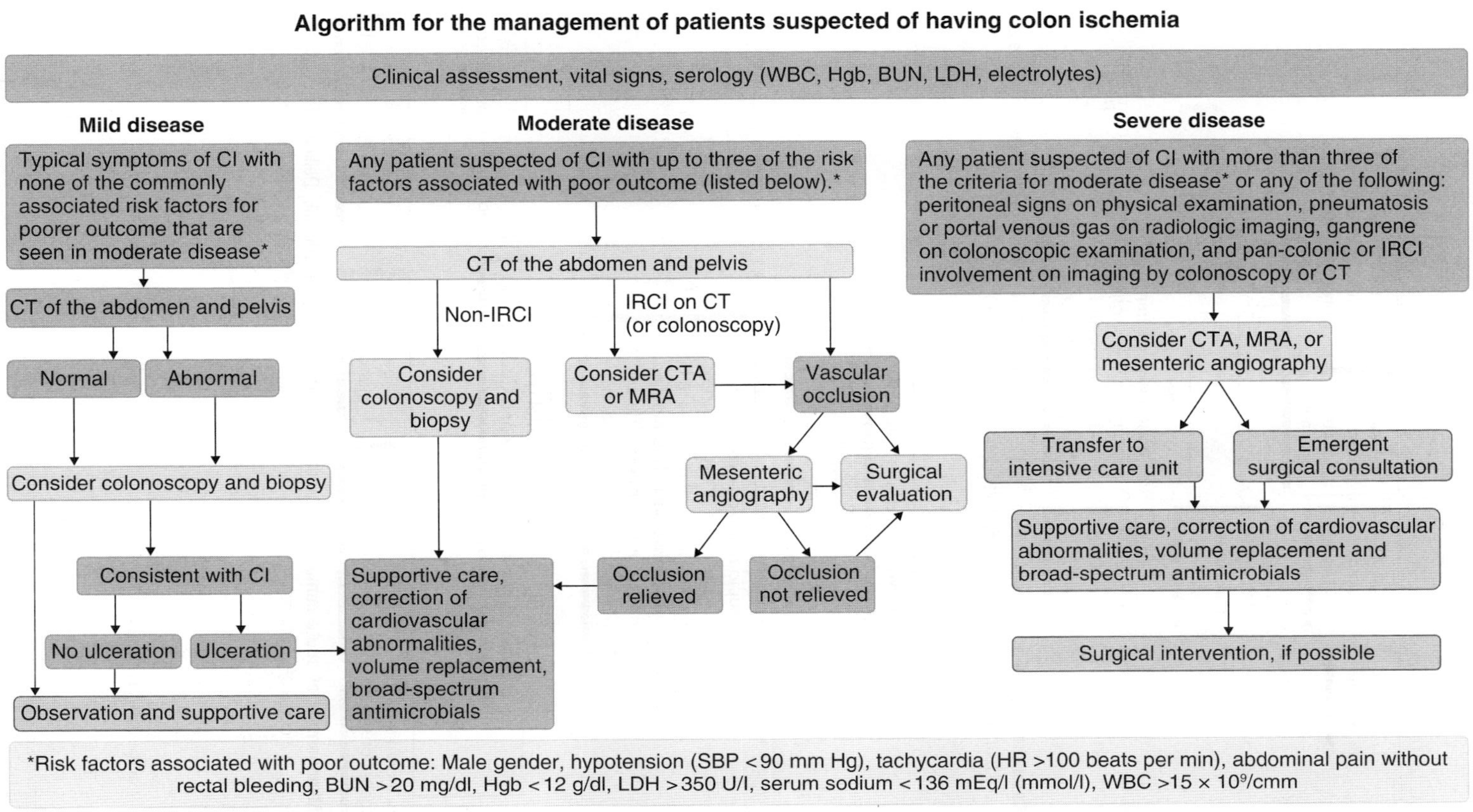

FIG. 54 Colon ischemia algorithm. Diagnosis and treatment of colon ischemia (CI) based on disease severity. *BUN,* Blood urea nitrogen; *CT,* computed tomography; *CTA,* computed tomography angiography; *Hgb,* hemoglobin; *IRCI,* isolated right-colon ischemia; *LDH,* lactate dehydrogenase; *MRA,* magnetic resonance angiography; *MRI,* magnetic resonance imaging; *WBC,* white blood cell count. (From Brandt LJ et al: ACG clinical guideline: epidemiology, risk factors, patterns of presentation, diagnosis, and management of colon ischemia [CI], *Am J Gastroenterol* 2015;110:18-44. In: Goldman L, Shafer AI: *Goldman-Cecil medicine,* ed 26, Philadelphia, 2020, Elsevier. Fig. 134-7.)

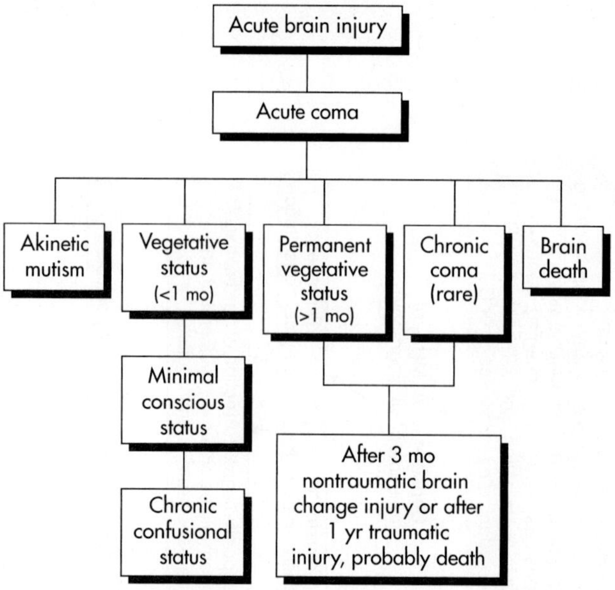

FIG. 55 Natural course of acute coma. (From Parrillo JE, Dellinger RP: *Critical care medicine, principles of diagnosis and management in the adult,* ed 5, Philadelphia, 2019, Elsevier.)

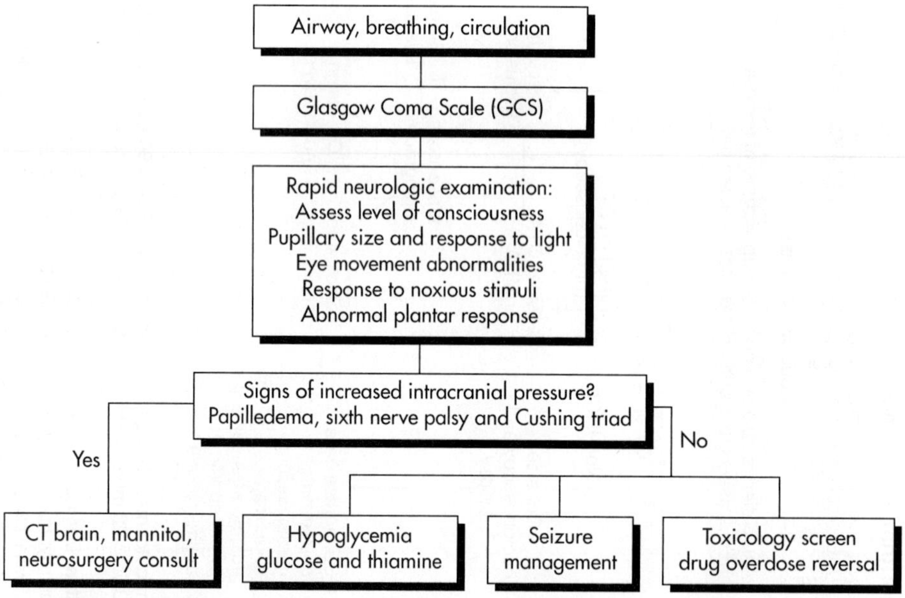

FIG. 56 Management of acute coma. *CT,* Computed tomography. (From Parrillo JE, Dellinger RP: *Critical care medicine, principles of diagnosis and management in the adult,* ed 5, Philadelphia, 2019, Elsevier.)

TABLE 13 Characteristic Clinical Features of Disorders of Consciousness and Locked-In Syndrome

Disorder	Consciousness	Cognition	Receptive Language	Expressive Language	Visual Perception	Motor Function	Structure Injured
Coma	No sleep-wake cycles	None	None	None	None	Primitive reflexes only	RAS *OR* Diffuse brain damage
Vegetative state	Intermittent periods of wakefulness	None	None	None	Variable visual startle responses	Involuntary movements only	Cerebral cortex Thalamocortical pathway ± RAS
Minimally conscious state	Intermittent periods of wakefulness	Inconsistent but clear behavioral signs of self or environmental awareness	Inconsistently one-step command following	Aspontaneous and ranging from single words or short phrases	Visual pursuit Object recognition	Localize to noxious stimuli Object manipulation Automatic movement sequences	Normal to variable lesion in RAS
Akinetic mutismAbulia	Normal or depressed	Normal or depressed	Normal or depressed	Normal or depressed	Normal	Delayed, slow responses	Hypothalamic Basal forebrain
Acute confusional state	Extended period of wakefulness	Confusion and disorientation	Consistent one-step command following	Yes-no responses Perseverative Short sentences Confused	Object recognition	No functional deficit	Normal to variable lesions in RAS
Brain death	Absent	Absent	None	None	None	Preserved postural and motor reflex	Global brain damage
Locked-in syndrome	Normal sleep-wake cycles	Normal to near-normal	Normal	Aphonic	Normal	Quadriplegia	Bilateral ventral pons

RAS, Reticular activating system.
From Parrillo JE, Dellinger RP: *Critical care medicine, principles of diagnosis and management in the adult,* ed 5, Philadelphia, 2019, Elsevier.

TABLE 14 Etiologies and Clinical Features of Different Causes of Impaired Consciousness

	Etiology	Clinical Features for Differential Diagnosis
Supratentorial lesion	• Destructive: Ischemic infarct, hemorrhage (SAH, SDH, ICH) • Compressive lesion: Ischemic infarct, hemorrhage, aneurysm, vascular malformation, tumor, venous thrombosis, abscess • Head injury, concussion	• Initial focal cerebral dysfunction • Dysfunction progresses rostral to caudal • Signs reflect cortical dysfunction, often multifocal • Often asymmetric cortical involvement and presentation
Infratentorial lesion	• Destructive: Ischemic infarct, hemorrhage (SAH, ICH) • Compressive lesion: Ischemic infarct, hemorrhage, aneurysm, vascular malformation, tumor, venous thrombosis	• Symptoms of brainstem dysfunction or sudden onset coma (posturing) • Brainstem signs precede/accompany coma • Cranial nerve and oculovestibular dysfunction: Ocular bobbing, vertical pendular oscillation (pons), monocular movement (midbrain) • Early onset of abnormal respiratory pattern
Diffuse brain lesion	• Traumatic brain injury • Anoxic injury • Toxic encephalopathy • Seizure, nonconvulsive, postictal • Primary neuronal disorder • Infectious encephalitis (prion disease, progressive leukoencephalopathy) • Inflammatory encephalitis (ADEM) • Vasculitis	• Often asymmetric in presentation • Focal signs depending on main brain lesion

Continued on next page

TABLE 11 Etiologies and Clinical Features of Different Causes of Impaired Consciousness—cont'd

	Etiology	Clinical Features for Differential Diagnosis
Metabolic coma	• Hypoglycemia • Nutritional (thiamine, niacin, pyridoxine, cyanocobalamin, folic acid), Wernicke encephalopathy • Hepatic encephalopathy • Uremia and dialysis • CO_2 narcosis • Exocrine pancreatic encephalopathy • Endocrine: Addison disease, pheochromocytoma, diabetes • Paraneoplastic • Drug poisoning • Thermal injury • Electrolyte/acid-base imbalance	• Confusion/stupor precede motor signs • Motor signs usually symmetric • Pupil responses generally preserved • Myoclonus, asterixis, tremulousness, and generalized seizures common • Acid-base imbalance common with compensatory ventilator changes • Periodic alternating gaze deviation • Systemic: Altered mental state with normal brainstem function (especially normal pupils). Possible triphasic waves on EEG • Stimulant-induced coma (cocaine, amphetamine, phencyclidine, tricyclic antidepressant) • Fever, mydriasis (except miosis with phencyclidine), and seizure • Sedatives (alcohol, benzodiazepine, barbiturates, antiepileptics) • Ataxia, impaired eye movements but normal pupils • Opiate-induced miosis
Psychiatric	• Conversion disorder • Depression • Psychosis—catatonia	• Forced eye closure • Pupils reactive or dilated, nonreactive • Unpredictable oculocephalic reflex: Nystagmus on caloric test • Normal or inconsistent motor tone • No pathologic reflexes • Awake-pattern EEG

ADEM, Acute disseminated encephalomyelitis; *CO_2,* carbon dioxide; *EEG,* electroencephalogram; *ICH,* intracranial hematoma; *SAH,* subarachnoid hemorrhage; *SDH,* subdural hematoma.
From Parrillo JE, Dellinger RP: *Critical care medicine, principles of diagnosis and management in the adult,* ed 5, Philadelphia, 2019, Elsevier.

TABLE 15 Types of Brain Herniation Syndromes

Syndrome	Mechanism	Imaging Findings	Clinical Presentation
Uncal	• Downward displacement of medial temporal lobe into the posterior fossa through the incisural opening • Seen in patients with unilateral hemispheric mass lesions	• Contralateral temporal horn widening • Ipsilateral ambient and prepontine cistern widening • Uncus extending into the suprasellar cistern	• Ipsilateral pupil dilation and ophthalmoplegia • Contralateral or ipsilateral hemiparesis • Decerebrate posturing
Central (transtentorial)	• Downward displacement of cerebral hemispheres and basal nuclei compressing and displacing diencephalon and midbrain rostrocaudally through the tentorial notch	• Effacement of the sulci • Obliteration of the suprasellar cistern • Compression and posterior displacement of the quadrigeminal cistern	• Medium-sized, fixed pupils • Early coma • Decorticate posturing • Cheyne-Stokes respiration • Diabetes insipidus
Cingulate (subfalcine)	• Lateral displacement of the cingulate gyrus under the anterior falx	• Attenuation of ipsilateral aspect of frontal horn • Asymmetric anterior falx • Obliteration of ipsilateral atrium of lateral ventricle • Septum pellucidum shift	• Small reactive pupils • Headache • Contralateral leg paralysis
Ascending	• Infratentorial mass effect protruding through the tentorial opening compressing the midbrain and cerebellar structures at the tentorial edges	• Spinning top appearance of midbrain • Narrowing of bilateral ambient and quadrigeminal cisterns	• Progressive stupor • Nausea and vomiting
Tonsillar	• Cerebellar tonsils protruding into the foramen magnum compressing adjacent medulla and upper cervical cord	• Cerebellar tonsils at the level of the dens on axial view and 5 mm below foramen magnum on sagittal view (7 mm in children)	• Cushing triad • Coma • Bilateral arm dysesthesia

From Parrillo JE, Dellinger RP: *Critical care medicine, principles of diagnosis and management in the adult,* ed 5, Philadelphia, 2019, Elsevier.

TABLE 16 Neuroimaging and Electrophysiologic Techniques and Findings in Disorders of Consciousness

Technique	Measurement	Strengths	Limitations	Vegetative State	Minimally Conscious State	Comatose
FDG-PET	Metabolic	Relatively direct measure of neuronal energy use (glucose uptake)	Ionizing (limited repeated measures)	Voxel-based: Hypometabolism in lateral and medial frontoparietal cortices	Metabolic dysfunction in left hemisphere	
Functional MRI	CBF	High-resolution structural imaging of grey-white matter (DTI) and functional imaging (spectroscopy, resting, passive, and active CBF paradigms)	• Sensitive to movement artifacts requiring sedation/anesthesia • Incompatible with ferromagnetic material (deprivation, pumps, electrodes)	Activation fMRI: Low-level cortical activation DMN—partially preserved	Activation fMRI: Near-normal high-level cortical activation	
EEG/ERPs	Electrical	Repeatable, portable, and inexpensive	Muscle, eye, and dysautonomia artifacts Challenging source reconstruction		EEG: Slow-wave activity through night and periods of REM sleep	ERP-poor outcome with absence of a cortical response to electrical stimulation of median nerves
EEG-TMS	Electrical	Stereotaxic stimulation connectivity studies	Stimulation areas are limited by muscle artifacts	TMS triggers a simple, local EEG response similar to deep sleep/anesthesia	Complex activations in distant cortical areas	

CBF, Cerebral blood flow; *DMN,* default model network; *DTI,* diffuse tensor imaging; *EEG,* electroencephalogram; *ERPs,* event-related potentials; *FDG,* ^{18}F-fluorodeoxyglucose; *fMRI,* functional magnetic resonance imaging; *PET,* positron emission tomography; *REM,* rapid eye movement; *TMS,* transcranial magnetic stimulation.

From Parrillo JE, Dellinger RP: *Critical care medicine, principles of diagnosis and management in the adult,* ed 5, Philadelphia, 2019, Elsevier.

ICD-10CM # M35.9 Syndrome, connective tissue

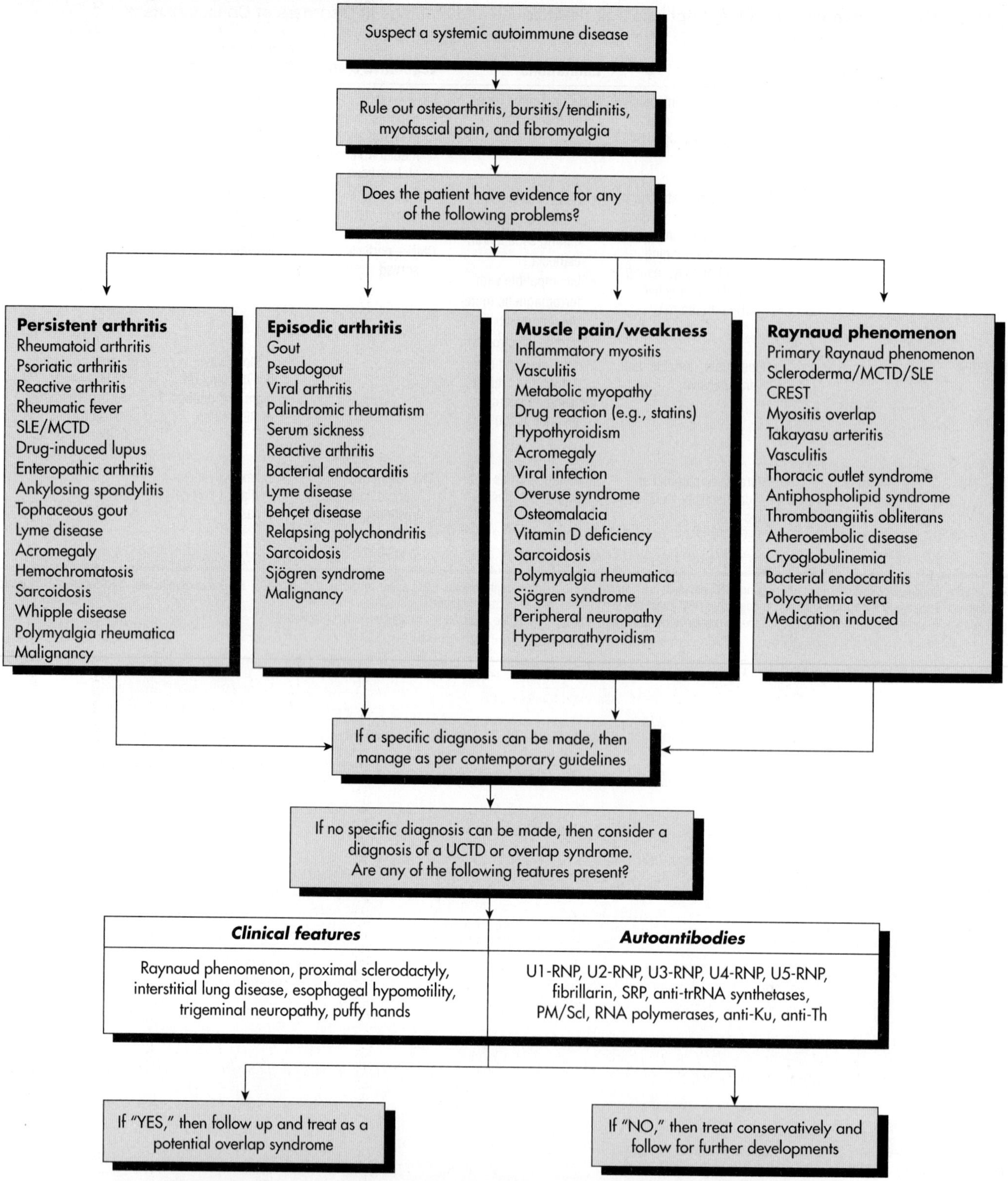

FIG. 57 Algorithm for evaluating patients with undifferentiated connective tissue disease (UCTD). *CREST,* Calcinosis, Raynaud phenomenon, esophageal dysmotility, sclerodactyly, and telangiectasia; *MCTD,* mixed connective tissue disease; *PM/Scl,* polymyositis/scleroderma; *RNA,* ribonucleic acid; *SLE,* systemic lupus erythematosus; *SRP,* signal recognition particle; *trRNA,* transfer ribonucleic acid; *UCTD,* undifferentiated connective tissue disease. (From Firestein GS, Budd RC, Gabriel SE et al: *Kelley and Firestein's textbook of rheumatology,* ed 10, Philadelphia, 2017, Elsevier.)

CONNECTIVE TISSUE LABORATORY SCREENING TESTS

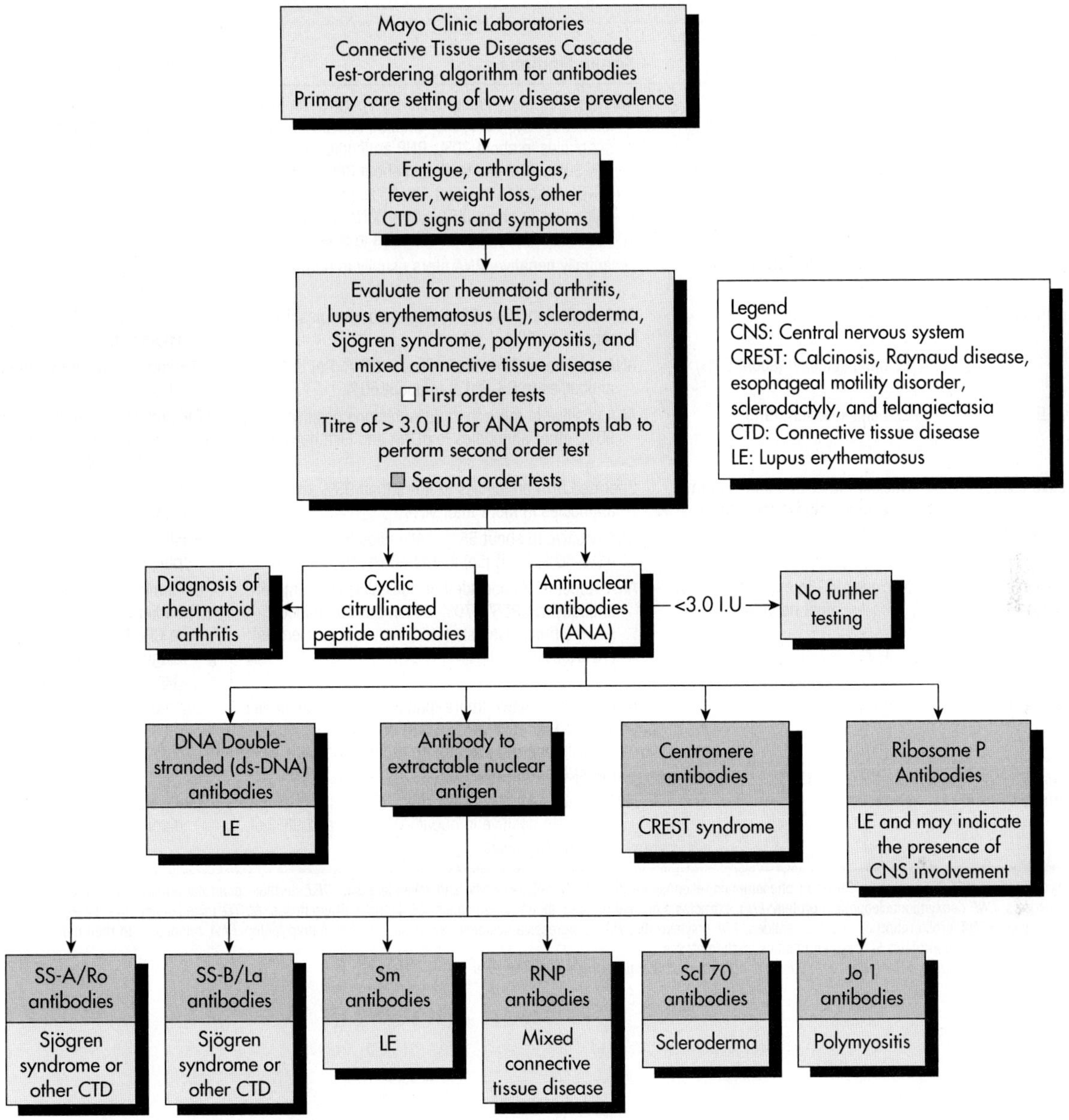

FIG. 58 Subacute cutaneous lupus erythematosus. Papulosquamous pattern. Lesions are confined to exposed areas on the upper half of the body. *DNA,* Deoxyribonucleic acid; RNP, ribonucleoprotein. (From Habif TP: *Clinical dermatology, a color guide to diagnosis and therapy,* ed 6, Philadelphia, 2016, Elsevier.)

TABLE 17 Autoantibody Tests for Connective Tissue Diseases

Antibody	Clinical Significance
Antinuclear antibodies	Screening for SLE and PSS
Centromere antibodies	Marker for CREST
Histone antibodies	To exclude drug-induced LE
ENA: Sm antibodies	Marker for SLE
RNP antibodies	SLE, MCTD, scleroderma
SS-A (Ro)/SS-B (La) antibodies	SLE, Sjögren syndrome, SCLE, and others
Scl-70 antibodies	Marker for scleroderma
Jo-1 antibodies	Marker for polymyositis
Ku (Ki) antibodies	Polymyositis/scleroderma overlap, SLE
Phospholipid antibodies (lupus anticoagulant)	Marker for SLE subset with thrombosis: Frequent aborters

CREST, Calcinosis, Raynaud phenomenon, esophageal dysmotility, sclerodactyly, and telangiectasia; *ENA,* extractable nuclear antigen; *LE,* lupus erythematosus; *MCTD,* mixed connective tissue disease; *PSS,* progressive systemic sclerosis; *RNP,* ribonucleoprotein; *SCLE,* subacute cutaneous lupus erythematosus; *SLE,* systemic lupus erythematosus.
From Habif TP: *Clinical dermatology, a color guide to diagnosis and therapy,* ed 6, Philadelphia, 2016, Elsevier.

TABLE 18 Diagnostic Significance of Immunologic Findings in Serum and Skin Biopsies in Connective Tissue Diseases

Disease	Biopsy Findings: Direct Immunofluorescence	Serum Findings	Relevance
Systemic LE	LE band (granular immune deposits, IgG, and/or IgM) IgA, C3 at DEJ in lesional and/or normal skin (over 90% in sun-exposed skin)	ANA elevated titers (about 95%-99%); nDNA antibodies about 50%-75%; DNP antibodies <50%; Sm antibodies in about 20%; RNP antibodies in about 5%-30%; SS-A antibodies in about 30%-40%; SS-B antibodies in about 1%-15%; phospholipid antibodies in about 30%-50%; PCNA antibodies in about 2%-10%; Ku(Ki) antibodies in about 10%	DIF, ANA, and ENA usually diagnostic; nDNA and Sm antibodies are diagnostic markers
Discoid LE	LE band, mostly IgG and C in lesion ONLY	Essentially negative; ANA titers usually in normal range	LE band highly characteristic
Subacute, cutaneous LE	LE band in lesion	ANA positive in 70%; SS-A (Ro) antibodies positive in more than 60%	DIF and anti–SS-A (Ro) highly characteristic
Neonatal LE	LE band in lesion (about 50%)	ANA positive in 30%; antibodies to SS-A (Ro) in 100%; antibodies to SS-B (La) in about 60%	DIF and anti–SS-A (Ro) highly characteristic
Drug-induced LE	LE band in lesion (rare)	ANA positive in more than 90%; histone positive about 90%; other antibodies to nDNA and ENA negative	DIF and histone antibodies in absence of other nuclear antibodies highly characteristic
Mixed connective tissue disease	Nuclear IgG or LE band in normal and/or lesional epidermis	Speckled ANA antibodies in more than 95% and RNP antibodies in more than 90%	Serology and/or DIF of nuclei diagnostic for MCTD, SLE, or PSS
Sjögren syndrome	Negative	ANA positive in about 55%; antibodies to SS-A (Ro) in 43%-88%; SS-B (La) in 14%-60%; RF positive	Positive serum results support diagnosis
Progressive systemic sclerosis (scleroderma)	Nucleolar IgG in epidermis in few cases; most negative	ANA (about 85%) speckled or nucleolar; centromere antibody in CREST (70%-90%); Scl-70 antibodies in diffuse sclerosis (45%) and in acrosclerosis (15%-20%)	DIF limited value; centromere antibodies are diagnostic marker in CREST; Scl-70 antibodies are diagnostic marker in scleroderma
Polymyositis/dermatomyositis	Negative	ANA usually positive (more than 80%); Jo-1 antibodies in 30% PM, 10% DM; SS-A (Ro) antibodies in 55% PM/scleroderma overlap; Ku (Ki) antibodies in 10% PM/scleroderma overlap	Limited value, but positive serum results support diagnosis
Rheumatoid arthritis	Negative	ANA usually negative or low titer; RF positive in about 90%; RNA positive in about 70%-90% and 95% of RF-negative cases	Positive serum results support diagnosis

ANA, Antinuclear antibodies; *CREST,* calcinosis, Raynaud phenomenon, esophageal dysmotility, sclerodactyly, and telangiectasia; *DEJ,* dermal-epidermal junction; *DIF,* direct immunofluorescence; *DM,* dermatomyositis; *DNP,* deoxyribonucleoprotein protein; *ENA,* extractable nuclear antigen; *Ig,* immunoglobulin; *LE,* lupus erythematosus; *MCTD,* mixed connective tissue disease; *nDNA,* nuclear deoxyribonuceic acid; *PCNA,* proliferating cell nuclear antigen; *PM,* polymyositis; *PSS,* progressive systemic sclerosis; *RF,* rheumatoid factor; *RNA,* antibodies to rheumatoid arthritis-associated nuclear antigen; *RNP,* ribonucleoprotein; *SLE,* systemic lupus erythematosus.

From Habif TP: *Clinical dermatology, a color guide to diagnosis and therapy,* ed 6, Philadelphia, 2016, Elsevier.

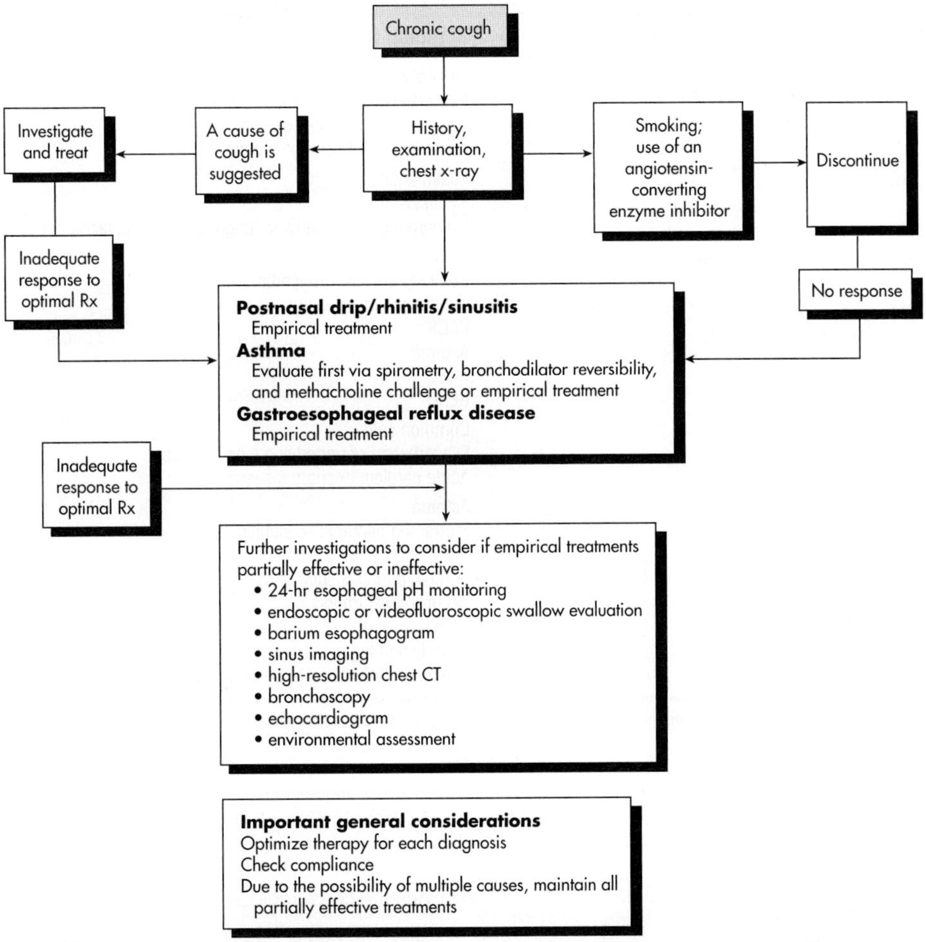

FIG. 60 Algorithm for the management of chronic cough lasting >8 wk. *CT,* Computed tomography; *Rx,* prescription. (From Goldman L, Schafer AI: *Goldman's Cecil medicine,* ed 24, Philadelphia, 2012, Saunders.)

TABLE 19 Testing Characteristics of Diagnostic Protocol for Evaluation of Chronic Cough

Tests	Diagnosis	Positive Predictive Value (%)	Negative Predictive Value (%)
Sinus radiograph	Sinusitis	57-81	95-100
Methacholine inhalation challenge	Asthma	60-82	100
Modified barium esophagography	GERD, esophageal stricture	38-63	63-93
Esophageal pH*	GERD	89-100	>100
Bronchoscopy	Endobronchial mass/lesion	50-89	100

*24-hr esophageal pH monitoring. *GERD,* Gastroesophageal reflux disease.
From Goldman L, Schafer AI (eds): *Goldman's Cecil medicine,* ed 24, Philadelphia, 2012, Saunders.

TABLE 20 Definitions and Common Causes of Cough in Adults and Children

Age Group	Type of Cough	Duration (wk)	Common Causes
Adults	Acute	<3	Common cold Exacerbation of lung disease (e.g., asthma) Acute environmental exposure Acute cardiopulmonary disease
	Subacute	3-8	Postinfectious cough Pertussis infection Exacerbation of underlying lung disease (e.g., asthma, COPD, bronchiectasis)
	Chronic	>8	ACEI therapy Smoking/chronic bronchitis Underlying lung disease UACS Asthma NAEB GERD
Children	Acute	<4	Common cold Exacerbation of underlying lung disease Acute cardiopulmonary disease
	Chronic	>4	Asthma Protracted bacterial bronchitis Tracheobronchomalacia Chronic rhinosinusitis Recurrent aspiration GERD Underlying lung disease (e.g., bronchiectasis) Pulmonary infections (e.g., pertussis)

ACEI, Angiotensin-converting enzyme inhibitor; *COPD,* chronic obstructive pulmonary disease; *GERD,* gastroesophageal reflux disease; *NAEB,* nonasthmatic eosinophilic bronchitis; *UACS,* upper airway cough syndrome.
From Adkinson NF et al: *Middleton's allergy principles and practice*, ed 8, Philadelphia, 2014, Saunders.

BOX 13 Pitfalls and Errors in the Diagnosis and Management of Chronic Cough in Adults

General Considerations
- Failing to consider that UACS, asthma/NAEB, and/or GERD are likely when the chest radiograph is normal or near-normal in appearance and the patient is a nonsmoker and is not taking an ACEI
- Failing to include UACS, asthma/NAEB, and/or GERD in the differential diagnosis because clinical or radiographic evidence confirms the presence of an "obvious" cause of the patient's cough (e.g., solitary pulmonary nodule, idiopathic pulmonary fibrosis)
- Not recognizing multiple simultaneous causes of cough
- Failing to continue treatment trials long enough to accurately assess their effectiveness
- Prematurely diagnosing "unexplained" cough before a bronchoscopy has been performed to assess for unsuspected airway disease
- Mistakenly diagnosing "unexplained" cough or diagnosing psychogenic cough before a complete evaluation for cough has been performed

Upper Airway Cough Syndrome
- Failing to realize that UACS can manifest as cough productive of phlegm
- Not recognizing that chronic cough can be the sole manifestation of UACS in at least 20% of the cases
- Failing to consider sinusitis as a cause of UACS
- Mistakenly assuming that selective histamine H_1 receptor antagonists are effective in treating nonallergic causes of UACS
- Missing allergic rhinitis because symptoms are perennial
- Missing aspirin-exacerbated disease in a patient with nasal polyps

Asthma/NAEB
- Failing to realize that these conditions can sometimes manifest as cough productive of phlegm
- Not recognizing that chronic cough can sometimes be the sole manifestation of asthma (so-called cough variant asthma)
- Mistakenly assuming that a positive result on bronchial challenge (e.g., methacholine challenge) is diagnostic of asthma when it is merely *consistent* with the diagnosis
- Failing to consider NAEB when the bronchial challenge test yields a negative result
- Not recognizing that inhaled medications can sometimes provoke cough
- Failing to consider occupational and environmental causes of asthma/NAEB

Gastroesophageal Reflux Disease
- Failing to realize that GERD can sometimes manifest as cough productive of phlegm
- Not recognizing that chronic cough can sometimes be the sole manifestation of GERD (so-called silent GERD)
- Mistakenly concluding that cough cannot be due to GERD simply because cough does not resolve with relief of gastrointestinal symptoms
- Not considering nonacid reflux and mistakenly assuming that cough will always respond to acid suppression
- Failing to assess the adequacy of GERD treatment by using 24-hr monitoring of esophageal pH and impedance
- Not recognizing coexisting diseases (e.g., sleep apnea) and medications (e.g., nitrates, progesterone) that may impair the effectiveness of GERD treatment
- Failing to recognize that surgery may help when intensive medical therapy has failed

Angiotensin-Converting Enzyme Inhibitor
- Failing to consider ACEI therapy as a cause of chronic cough simply because the cough predated initiation of the ACEI
- Mistakenly concluding that ACEI therapy is not the cause of chronic cough because the cough did not resolve within 1-3 wk of stopping the ACEI

ACEI, Angiotensin-converting enzyme inhibitor; *GERD,* gastroesophageal reflux disease; *NAEB,* nonasthmatic eosinophilic bronchitis; *UACS,* upper airway cough syndrome.
From Adkinson NF et al: *Middleton's allergy principles and practice*, ed 8, Philadelphia, 2014, Saunders.

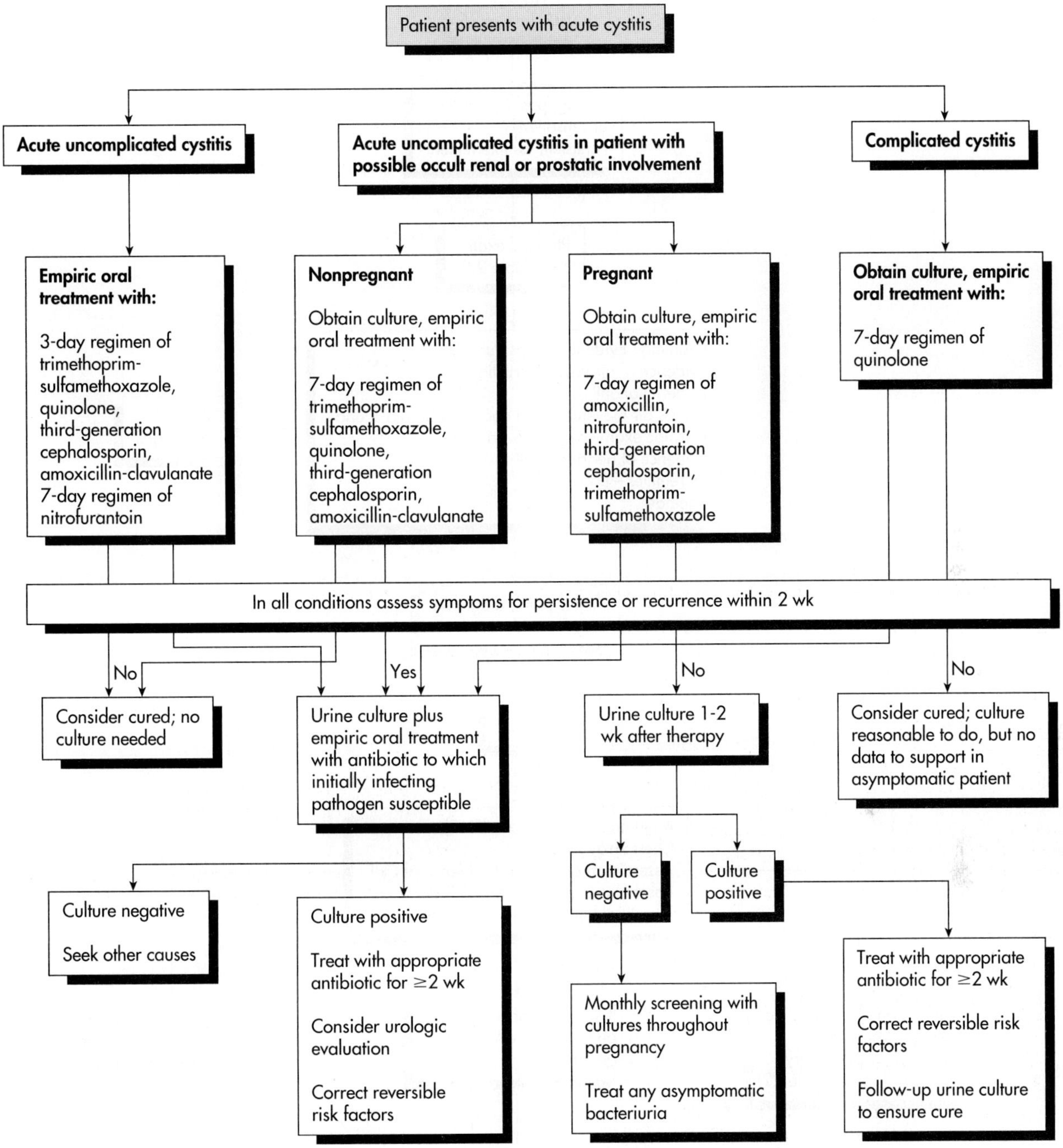

FIG. 61 Algorithm for management of acute cystitis based on severity and complicating factors.
(From Johnson R et al: *Comprehensive clinical nephrology*, ed 5, Philadelphia, 2015, Saunders.)

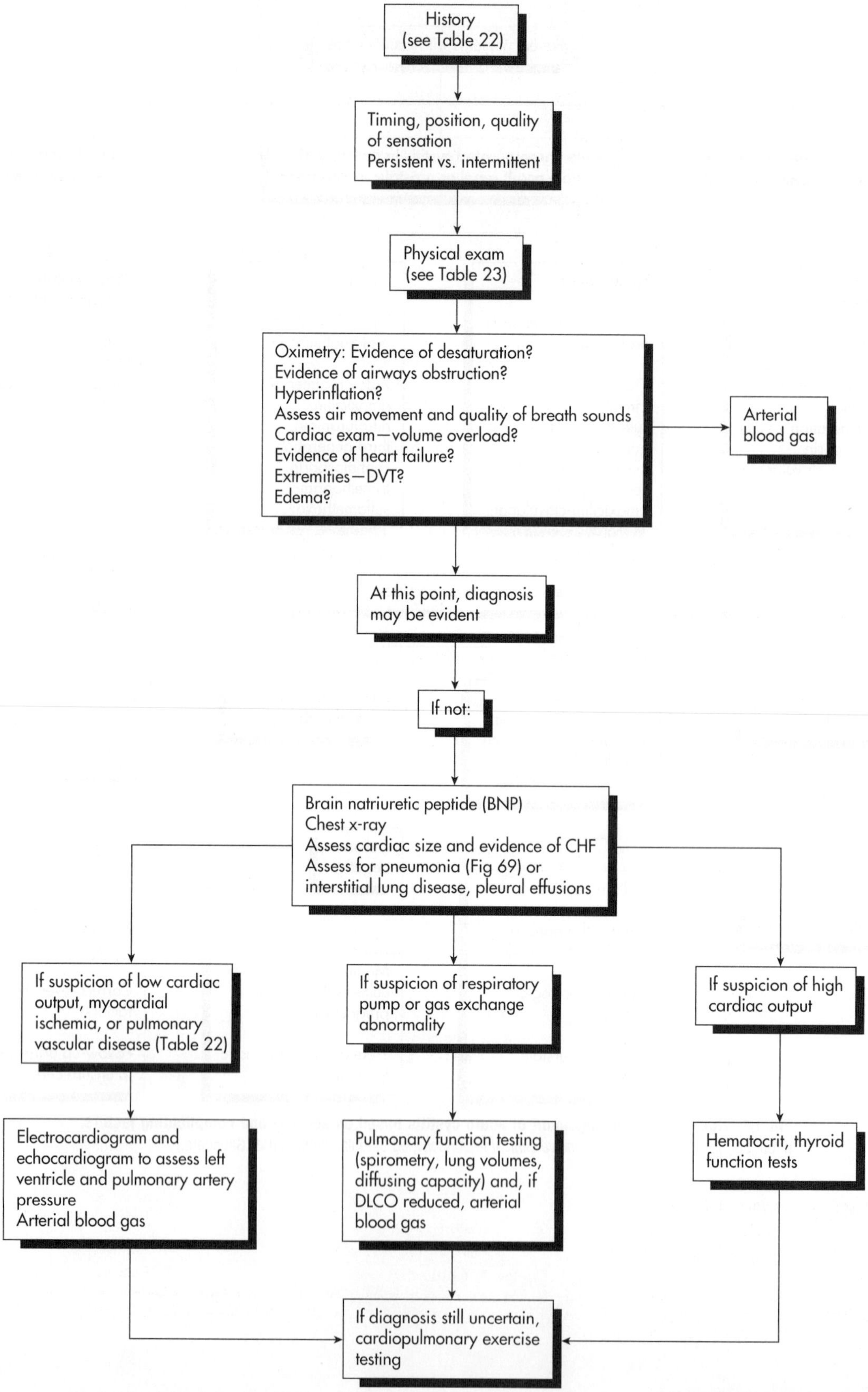

FIG. 68 Algorithm for the evaluation of the patient with dyspnea. The pace and completeness with which one approaches this framework depends on the intensity and acuity of the patient's symptoms. In a patient with severe, acute dyspnea, for example, an arterial blood gas measurement may be one of the first laboratory evaluations, whereas this measurement might not be obtained until much later in the workup in a patient with chronic breathlessness of unclear cause. A therapeutic trial of a medication, for example, a bronchodilator, may be instituted at any point if one is fairly confident of the diagnosis based on the data available at that time. *CHF,* Congestive heart failure; *DLCO,* diffusing capacity of the lung for carbon monoxide; *DVT,* deep venous thrombosis. (Modified from Schwartzstein RM, Feller-Kopman D: Approach to the patient with dyspnea. In Braunwald E, Goldman L [eds]: *Primary cardiology,* ed 2, Philadelphia, 2003, Saunders.)

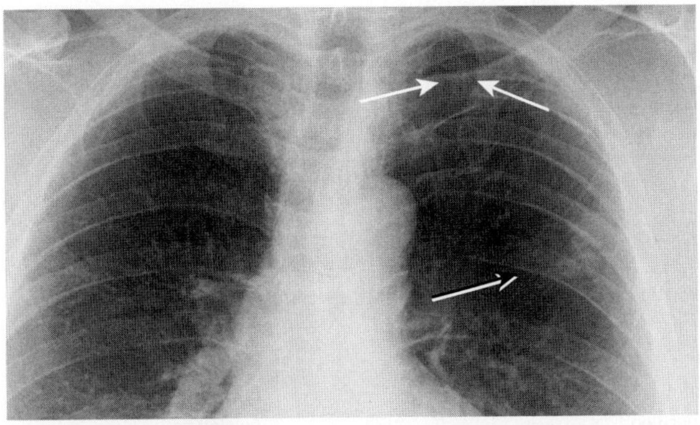

FIG. 69 Chest radiograph of a patient presenting with cough and fever. A faint area of opacification within the left midlung proved to be pneumonia *(black arrow)*. Additionally, a small left apical carcinoma was detected *(white arrows)*. Because of multiple overlying structures, including the first ribs and the clavicles, the pulmonary apices are a "danger" area in terms of risk of missed findings on chest radiographs. Close inspection of the apices is warranted on every chest radiograph. (From Soto JA, Lucey BC: *Emergency radiology: the requisites,* ed 2, Philadelphia, 2017, Elsevier.)

TABLE 22 Differential Diagnoses for Acute Dyspnea

Organ System	Critical Diagnoses	Emergent Diagnoses	Nonemergent Diagnoses
Pulmonary	Airway obstruction Pulmonary embolus Noncardiogenic edema Anaphylaxis Ventilatory failure	Spontaneous pneumothorax Asthma Cor pulmonale Aspiration Pneumonia (CAP score >70)	Pleural effusion Neoplasm Pneumonia (CAP score ≤70) COPD
Cardiac	Pulmonary edema Myocardial infarction Cardiac tamponade	Pericarditis	Congenital heart disease Valvular heart disease Cardiomyopathy
Primarily Associated with Normal or Increased Respiratory Effort			
Abdominal		Mechanical interference Hypotension, sepsis from ruptured viscus, bowel obstruction, inflammatory or infectious process	Pregnancy Ascites obesity
Psychogenic			Hyperventilation syndrome Somatization disorder Panic attack
Metabolic or endocrine	Toxic ingestion DKA	Renal failure Electrolyte abnormalities Metabolic acidosis	Fever Thyroid disease
Infectious	Epiglottitis	Pneumonia (CAP score >70)	Pneumonia (CAP score ≤70)
Traumatic	Tension pneumothorax Cardiac tamponade Flail chest	Simple pneumothorax, hemothorax Diaphragmatic rupture	Rib fractures
Hematologic	Carbon monoxide poisoning Acute chest syndrome	Anemia	
Primarily Associated with Decreased Respiratory Effort			
Neuromuscular	CVA, intracranial insult Organophosphate poisoning	Multiple sclerosis Guillain-Barré syndrome Tick paralysis	ALS Polymyositis Porphyria

ALS, Amyotrophic lateral sclerosis; *CAP,* community-acquired pneumonia; *COPD,* chronic obstructive pulmonary disease; *CVA,* cerebrovascular accident; *DKA,* diabetic ketoacidosis.
From Marx JA et al: *Rosen's emergency medicine,* ed 8, Philadelphia, 2014, Saunders.

TABLE 23 Pivotal Findings in Physical Examination

Sign	Physical Finding	Diagnoses to Consider
Vital signs	Tachypnea	Pneumonia, pneumothorax
	Hypopnea	Intracranial insult, drug or toxin ingestion
	Tachycardia	PE, traumatic chest injury
	Hypotension	Tension pneumothorax
	Fever	Pneumonia, PE
General appearance	Cachexia, weight loss	Malignancy, acquired immune disorder, mycobacterial infection
	Obesity	Hypoventilation, sleep apnea, PE
	Pregnancy	PE
	Barrel chest	COPD
	"Sniffing" position	Epiglottitis
	"Tripoding" position	COPD or asthma with severe distress
	Traumatic injury	Pneumothorax (simple, tension), rib fractures, flail chest, hemothorax, pulmonary contusion
Skin and nails	Tobacco stains or odor	COPD, malignancy, infection
	Clubbing	Chronic hypoxia, intracardiac shunts, or pulmonary vascular anomalies
	Pallid skin or conjunctivae	Anemia
	Muscle wasting	Neuromuscular disease
	Bruising	Chest wall: Rib fractures, pneumothorax
		Diffuse: Thrombocytopenia, chronic steroid use, anticoagulation
	Subcutaneous emphysema	Rib fractures, pneumothorax, tracheobronchial disruption
	Hives, rash	Allergic reaction, infection, tick-borne illness
Neck	Stridor	Upper airway edema or infection, foreign body, traumatic injury, anaphylaxis
	JVD	Tension pneumothorax, COPD or asthma exacerbation, fluid overload or CHF, PE
Lung examination	Wheezes	CHF, anaphylaxis
		Bronchospasm
	Rales	CHF, pneumonia, PE
	Unilateral decrease	Pneumothorax, pleural effusion, consolidation, rib fractures or contusion, pulmonary contusion
	Hemoptysis	Malignancy, infection, bleeding disorder, CHF
	Sputum production	Infection (viral, bacterial)
	Friction rub	Pleurisy
	Abnormal respiratory pattern (e.g., Cheyne-Stokes)	Intracranial insult
Chest examination	Crepitance or pain on palpation	Rib or sternal fractures
	Subcutaneous emphysema	Pneumothorax, tracheobronchial rupture
	Thoracoabdominal desynchrony	Diaphragmatic injury with herniation; cervical spinal cord trauma
	Flail segment	Flail chest, pulmonary contusion
Cardiac examination	Murmur	PE
	S_3 or S_4 gallop	PE
	S_2 accentuation	PE
	Muffled heart sounds	Cardiac tamponade
Extremities	Calf tenderness, Homans sign	PE
	Edema	CHF
Neurologic examination	Focal deficits (motor, sensory, cognitive)	Stroke, intracranial hemorrhage causing central abnormal respiratory drive; if long-standing, risk of aspiration pneumonia
	Symmetrical deficits	Neuromuscular disease
	Diffuse weakness	Metabolic or electrolyte abnormality (hypocalcemia, hypomagnesemia, hypophosphatemia), anemia
	Hyporeflexia	Hypermagnesemia
	Ascending weakness	Guillain-Barré syndrome

CHF, Congestive heart failure; *COPD,* chronic obstructive pulmonary disease; *JVD,* jugular venous distention; *PE,* pulmonary embolism.
From Marx JA et al: *Rosen's emergency medicine,* ed 8, Philadelphia, 2014, Saunders.

TABLE 24 Diagnostic Table: Patterns of Diseases Often Resulting in Dyspnea

Disease	History (Dyspnea)	Associated Symptoms	Signs and Physical Findings	Tests
Pulmonary embolism	HPI: Abrupt onset, pleuritic pain, immobility (travel, recent surgery) PMH: Malignancy, DVT, PE, hypercoagulability, oral contraception, obesity	Diaphoresis, exertional dyspnea	Tachycardia, tachypnea, low-grade fever	• Pulse oximetry, ABG (A-a gradient), D-dimer • ECG (dysrhythmia, right-sided heart strain) • CXR (Westermark sign, Hampton hump), spiral CT, MRV • Pulmonary angiogram • Ultrasound positive for DVT
Pneumonia	Fever, productive cough, chest pain	Anorexia, chills, nausea, vomiting, exertional dyspnea, cough	Fever, tachycardia, tachypnea, rales, or decreased breath sounds	CXR, CBC, sputum and blood cultures
Bacterial	SH: Tobacco use			Pulse oximetry Waveform capnography if altered mental status, ABG if capnography unavailable and acid-base derangement or hypercarbia suspected
Viral	Exposure (e.g., influenza, varicella)			
Opportunistic	Immune disorder, chemotherapy			
Fungal or parasitic	Exposure (e.g., birds), indolent onset	Episodic fever, nonproductive cough		
Pneumothorax	Abrupt onset: Trauma, chest pain, thin males more likely to have spontaneous pneumothorax	Localized chest pain	Decreased breath sounds, subcutaneous emphysema, chest wall wounds or instability	• CXR: Pneumothorax, rib fractures, hemothorax • Ultrasound: Pneumothorax, pleural effusion
Simple				Ultrasound positive for pneumothorax
Tension	Decompensation of simple pneumothorax	Diaphoresis	JVD, tracheal deviation, muffled heart sounds, cardiovascular collapse	Clinical diagnosis: Requires immediate decompression. May verify via bedside ultrasound
COPD or asthma	Tobacco use, medication noncompliance, URI symptoms, sudden weather change	Air hunger, diaphoresis	• Retractions, accessory muscle use, tripoding, cyanosis • "Shark fin" capnograph	• CXR: Rule out infiltrate, pneumothorax, atelectasis (mucus plug) • Ultrasound: Distinguish from heart failure
	PMH: Environmental allergies FH: Asthma			Waveform capnography
Malignancy	Weight loss, tobacco, or other occupational exposure	Dysphagia	Hemoptysis	CXR, chest CT: Mass, hilar adenopathy, focal atelectasis
Fluid overload	• Gradual onset, dietary indiscretion or medication noncompliance, chest pain • PMH: Recent MI, diabetes, CHF	Worsening orthopnea, PND	JVD, peripheral edema, S_3 or S_4 gallop, new cardiac dysrhythmia, hepatojugular reflux	• CXR and/or ultrasound: Pleural effusion, interstitial edema, Kerley B lines, cardiomegaly • ECG: Ischemia, dysrhythmia • NT-proBNP
Anaphylaxis	Abrupt onset, exposure to allergen	Dysphagia	Oral swelling, stridor, wheezing, hives	

A-a, Alveolar-arterial; *ABG,* arterial blood gas; *CBC,* complete blood count; *CHF,* congestive heart failure; *COPD,* chronic obstructive pulmonary disease; *CT,* computed tomography; *CXR,* chest x-ray examination; *DVT,* deep vein thrombosis; *ECG,* electrocardiogram; *FH,* family history; *HPI,* history of present illness; *JVD,* jugular venous distention; *MI,* myocardial infarction; *MRV,* magnetic resonance venography; *NT-proBNP,* amino-terminal pro–B-type natriuretic peptide; *PE,* pulmonary embolism; *PMH,* past medical history; *PND,* paroxysmal nocturnal dyspnea; *SH,* social history; *URI,* upper respiratory infection.
From Marx JA et al: *Rosen's emergency medicine,* ed 8, Philadelphia, 2014, Saunders.

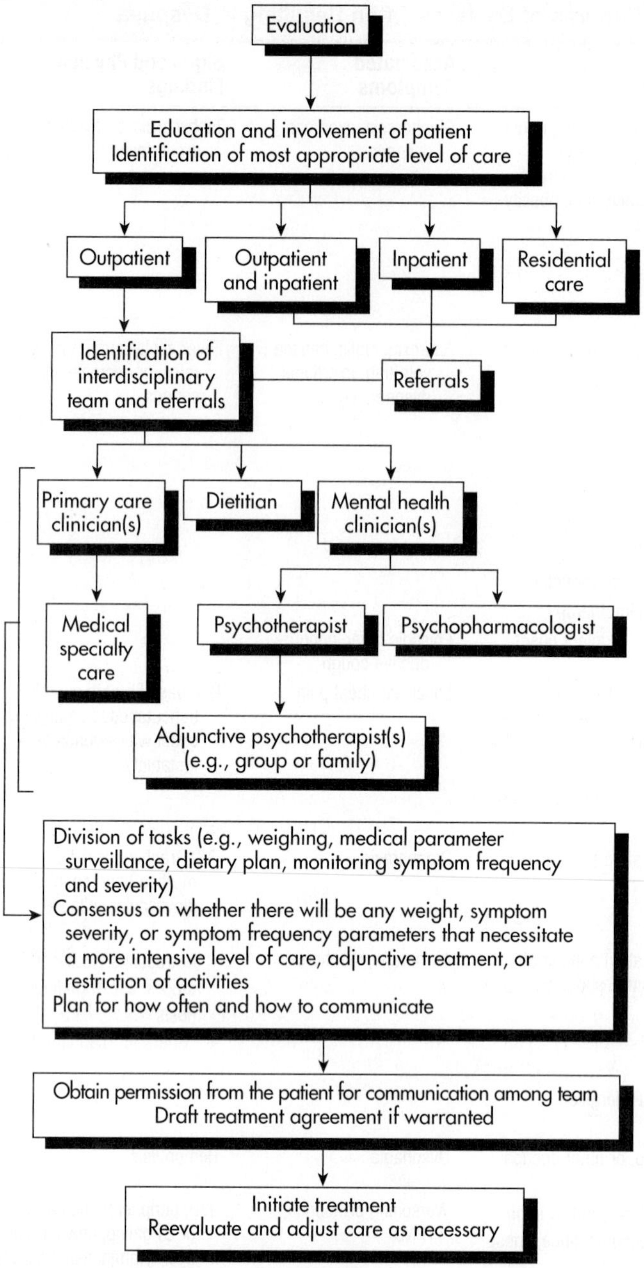

FIG. 70 Algorithm for team management of adult patients with an eating disorder. (From Feldman M et al: *Sleisenger and Fortran's gastrointestinal and liver disease*, ed 10, Philadelphia, 2016, Elsevier.)

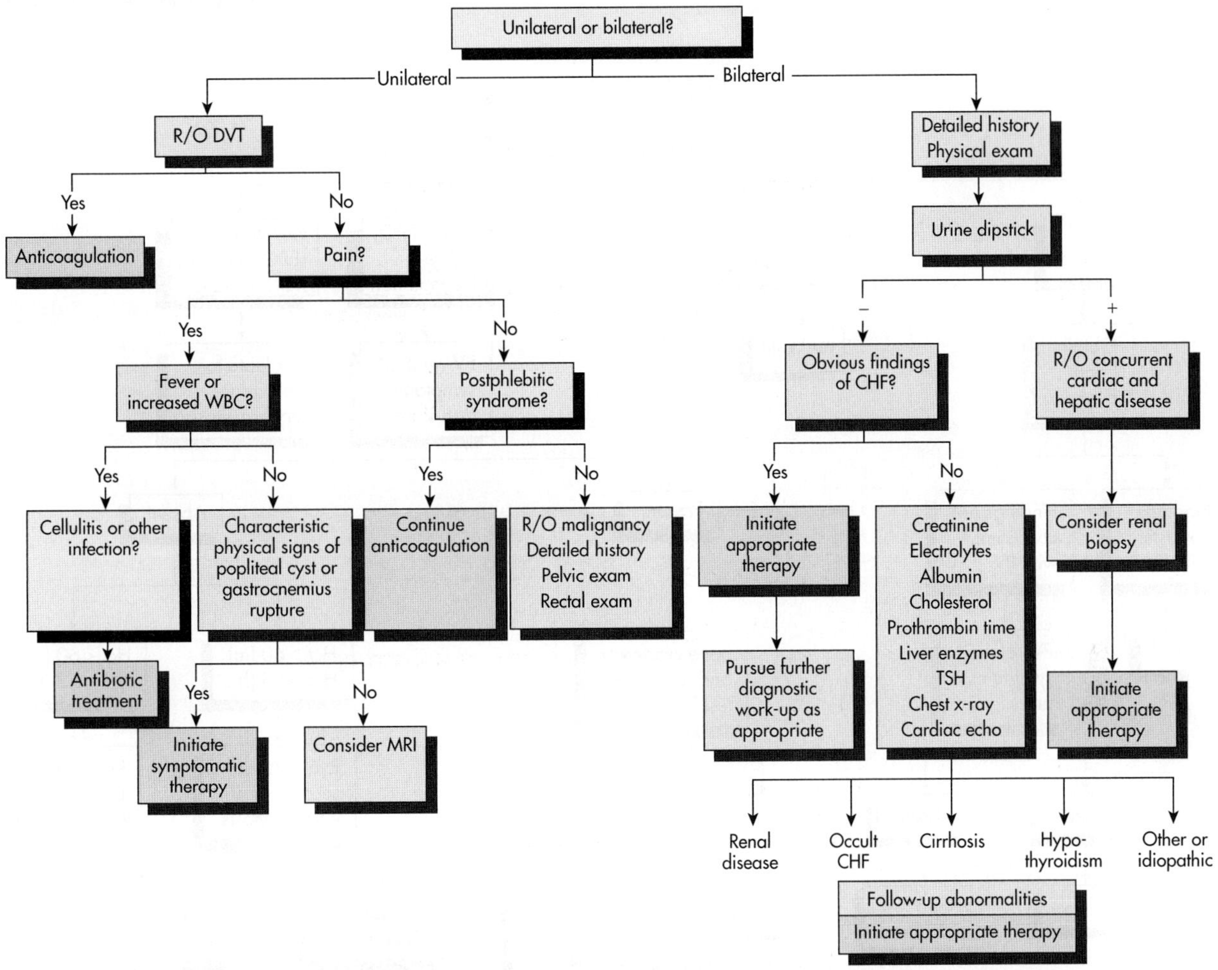

FIG. 71 Diagnostic approach to patients with edema. *CHF,* Congestive heart failure; *DVT,* deep vein thrombosis; *MRI,* magnetic resonance imaging; *R/O,* rule out; *TSH,* thyroid-stimulating hormone; *WBC,* white blood cell count. (From Chertow G: Approach to the patient with edema. In: Braunwald E, Goldman L [eds]: *Primary cardiology,* ed 2, Philadelphia, 2003, Saunders.)

ICD-10CM # D75.0 Familial erythrocytosis
D75.1 Secondary polycythemia
D45 Polycythemia vera
P61.1 Polycythemia neonatorum

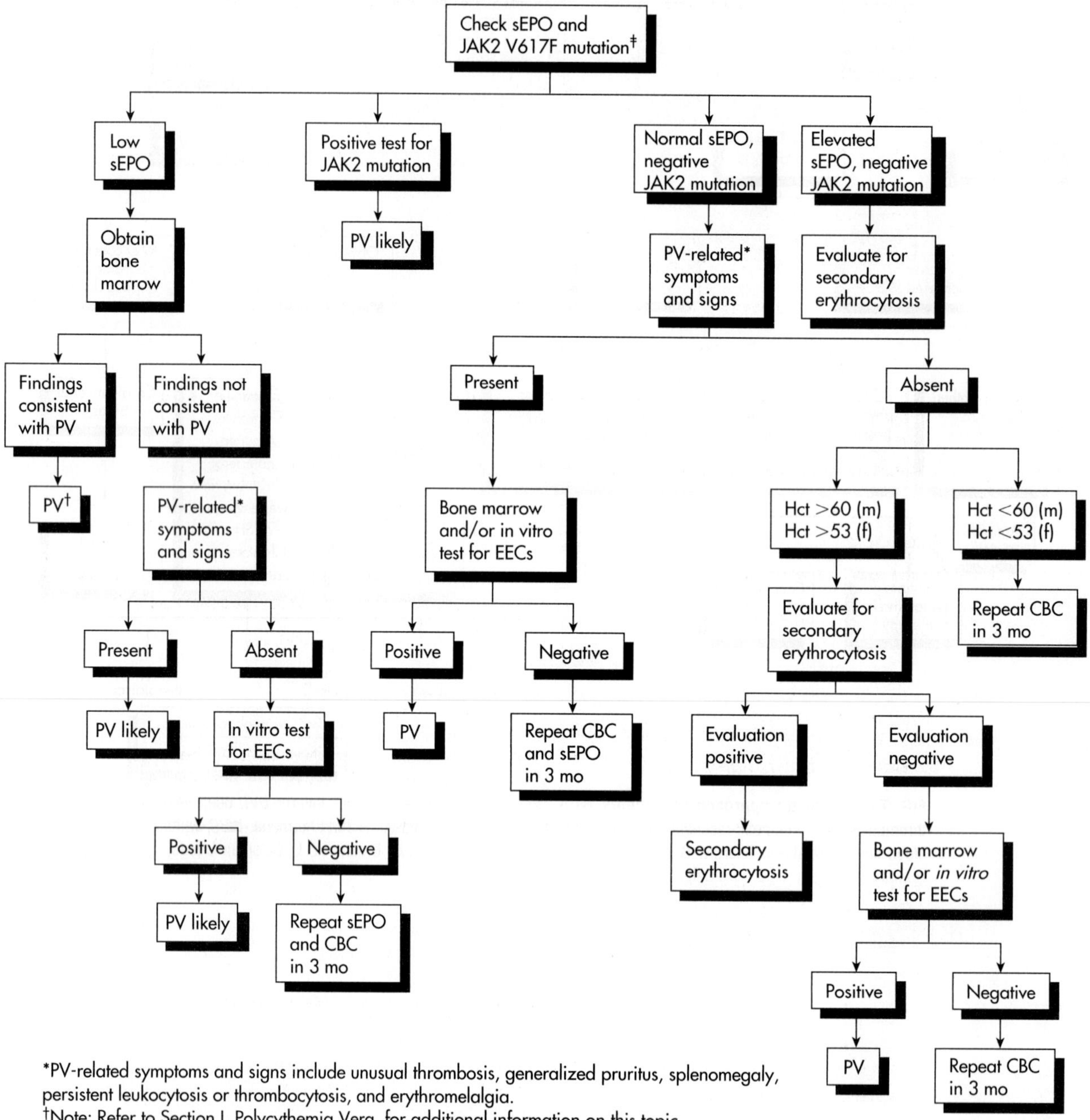

*PV-related symptoms and signs include unusual thrombosis, generalized pruritus, splenomegaly, persistent leukocytosis or thrombocytosis, and erythromelalgia.
†Note: Refer to Section I, Polycythemia Vera, for additional information on this topic.
‡The JAK2 mutation is found in >95% of patients with PV and can be used for diagnostic purposes.

FIG. 72 A diagnostic approach to acquired erythrocytosis. *CBC,* Complete blood cell count; *EEC,* endogenous (spontaneous) erythroid colonies; *f,* female; *Hct,* hematocrit; *m,* male; *PV,* polycythemia vera; *sEPO,* serum erythropoietin level. (Modified from Goldman L, Schafer AL [eds]: *Cecil textbook of medicine,* ed 24, Philadelphia, 2012, Saunders.)

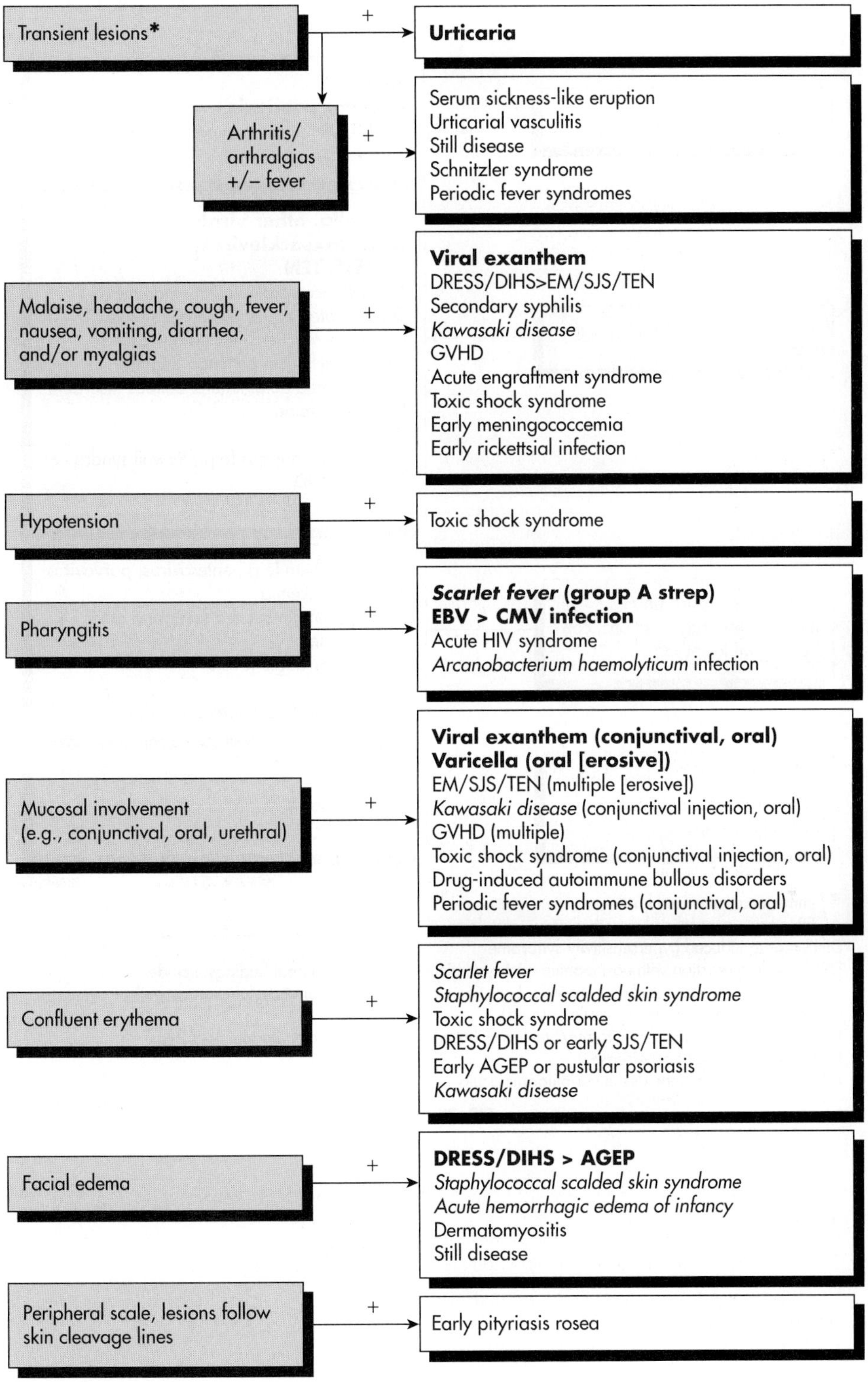

*Individual lesions last <24 hr, which can be documented by outlining them with ink; exceptions include urticarial vasculitis and, occasionally, Schnitzler or periodic fever syndromes

FIG. 79 Approach to the differential diagnosis of an exanthematous drug reaction. With a few exceptions (e.g., pityriasis rosea, drug-induced autoimmune bullous disorders), patients with these entities may be febrile. Entities in italics occur primarily in children. Toxic shock syndrome can be staphylococcal or streptococcal. Drug-induced autoimmune bullous disorders: Bullous pemphigoid or linear IgA bullous dermatosis > drug-induced pemphigus. *AGEP,* Acute generalized exanthematous pustulosis; *CMV,* cytomegalovirus; *DIHS,* drug-induced hypersensitivity syndrome; *DRESS,* drug reaction with eosinophilia and systemic symptoms; *EBV,* Epstein-Barr virus; *EM,* erythema multiforme; *Ig,* immunoglobulin; *GVHD,* graft versus host disease; *SJS,* Stevens-Johnson syndrome; *TEN,* toxic epidermal necrolysis. (From Bolognia JL: *Dermatology*, ed 4, Philadelphia, 2018, Elsevier.)

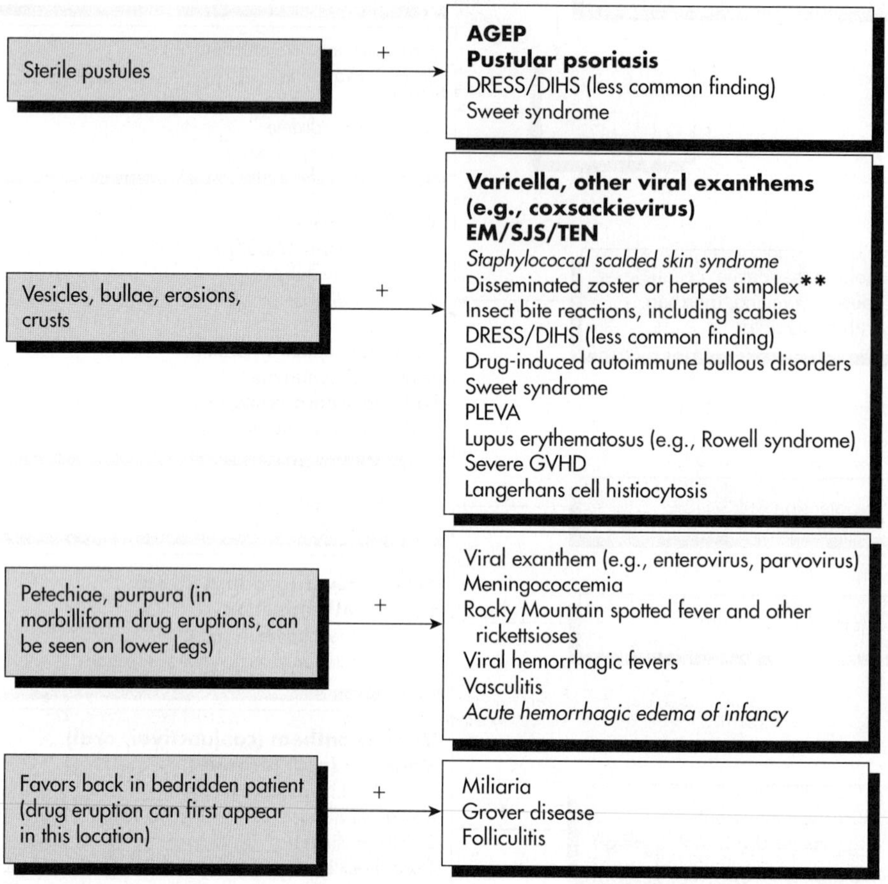

**Immunocompromised host
AGEP = acute generalized exanthematous pustulosis
DIHS = drug-induced hypersensitivity syndrome
DRESS = drug reaction with eosinophilia and systemic symptoms (additional findings include lymphadenopathy, atypical lymphocytosis, hepatitis, myocarditis and renal dysfunction as well as facial swelling > vesicles or sterile pustules)
EM/SJS/TEN = erythema multiforme/Stevens–Johnson syndrome/toxic epidermal necrolysis
GVHD = graft-versus-host disease
PLEVA = pityriasis lichenoides et varioliformis acuta

FIG. 79, cont'd

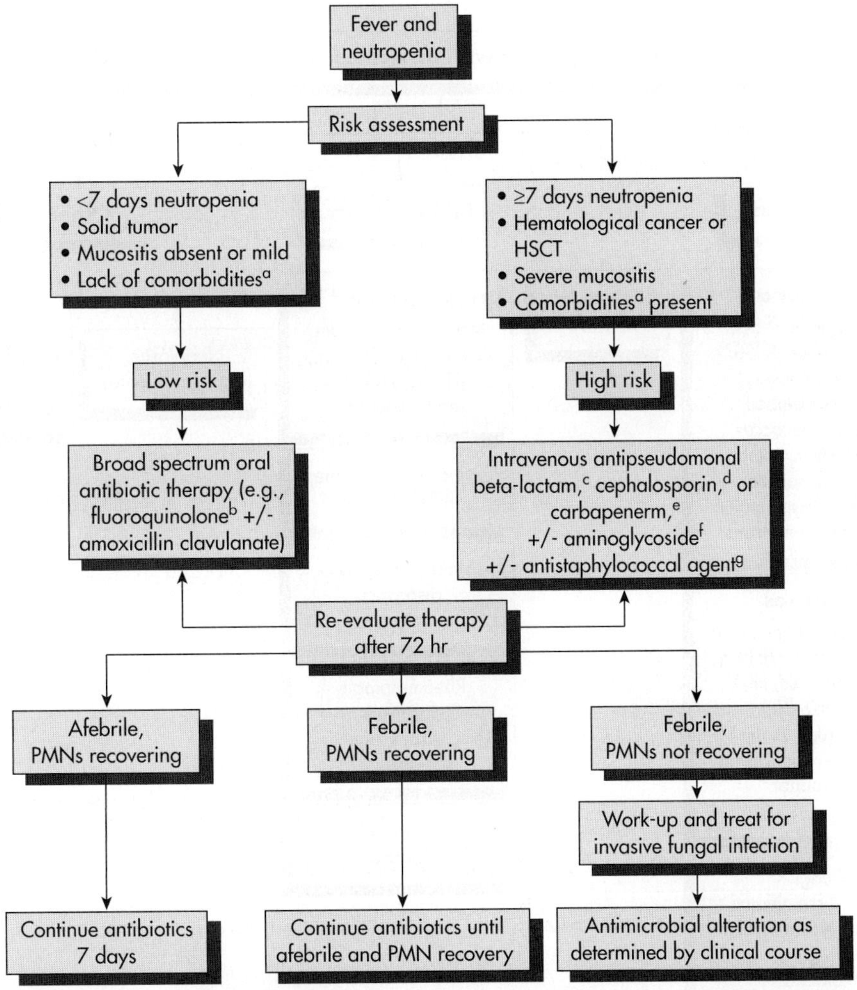

a Hypotension, altered mental status, neurologic changes, respiratory failure, abdominal pain, hemorrhage, cardiac compromise or new arrhythmia, catheter tunnel infection, extensive cellulitis, acute renal or liver failure
b Institution sensitivity dependent, ciprofloxacin, levofloxacin, moxifloxacin
c Drug selection and dosing institution-specific: Piperacillin tazobactam, ticarcillin/clavulanate
d Drug selection and dosing institution-specific: Ceftazidime
e imipenem, cefepime/cilastatin, meropenem, doripenem
f Gentamicin, tobramycin, or amikacin
g Drug selection and institution institution-specific: Vancomycin, linezolid, daptomycin, ceftaroline

FIG. 81 Approach to patient with fever and neutropenia. *HSCT*, Hematopoietic stem cell transplant; *PMN*, polymorphonuclear neutrophil. (From Hoffman R: *Hematology: basic principles and practice*, ed 7, Philadelphia, 2018, Elsevier.)

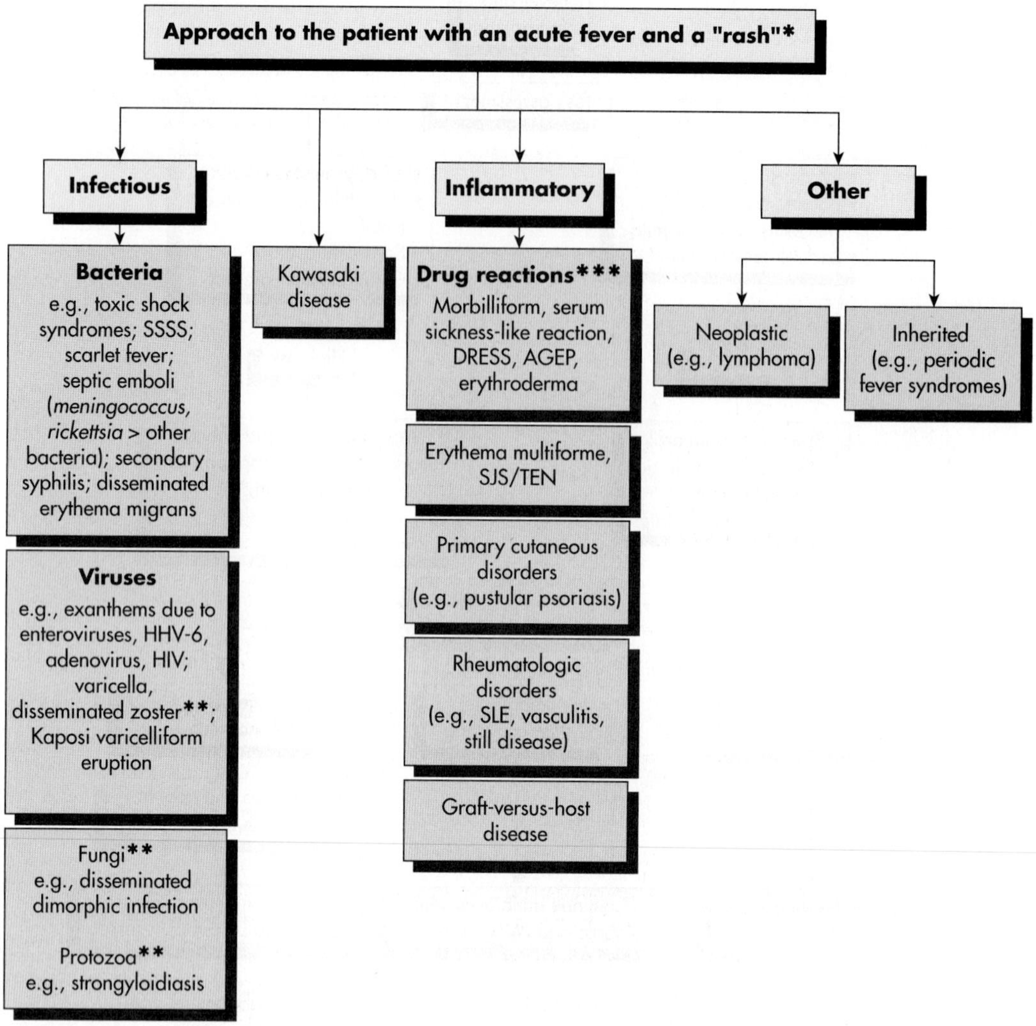

* Not a single site as in cellulitis, necrotizing fasciitis
** More likely in immunocompromised patient
*** Early on, more serious drug reactions, e.g., DRESS, may resemble a morbilliform eruption

FIG. 83 Approach to the patient with an acute fever and a "rash." *AGEP,* Acute generalized exanthematous pustulosis; *DRESS,* drug reaction with eosinophilia and systemic symptoms (also referred to as drug-induced hypersensitivity syndrome [DIHS]); *HHV,* human herpes virus; *HIV,* human immunodeficiency virus; *SJS,* Stevens-Johnson syndrome; *SLE,* systemic lupus erythematosus; *SSSS,* staphylococcal scalded skin syndrome; *TEN,* toxic epidermal necrolysis. (From Bolognia J: *Dermatology,* ed 4, Philadelphia, 2018, Elsevier.)

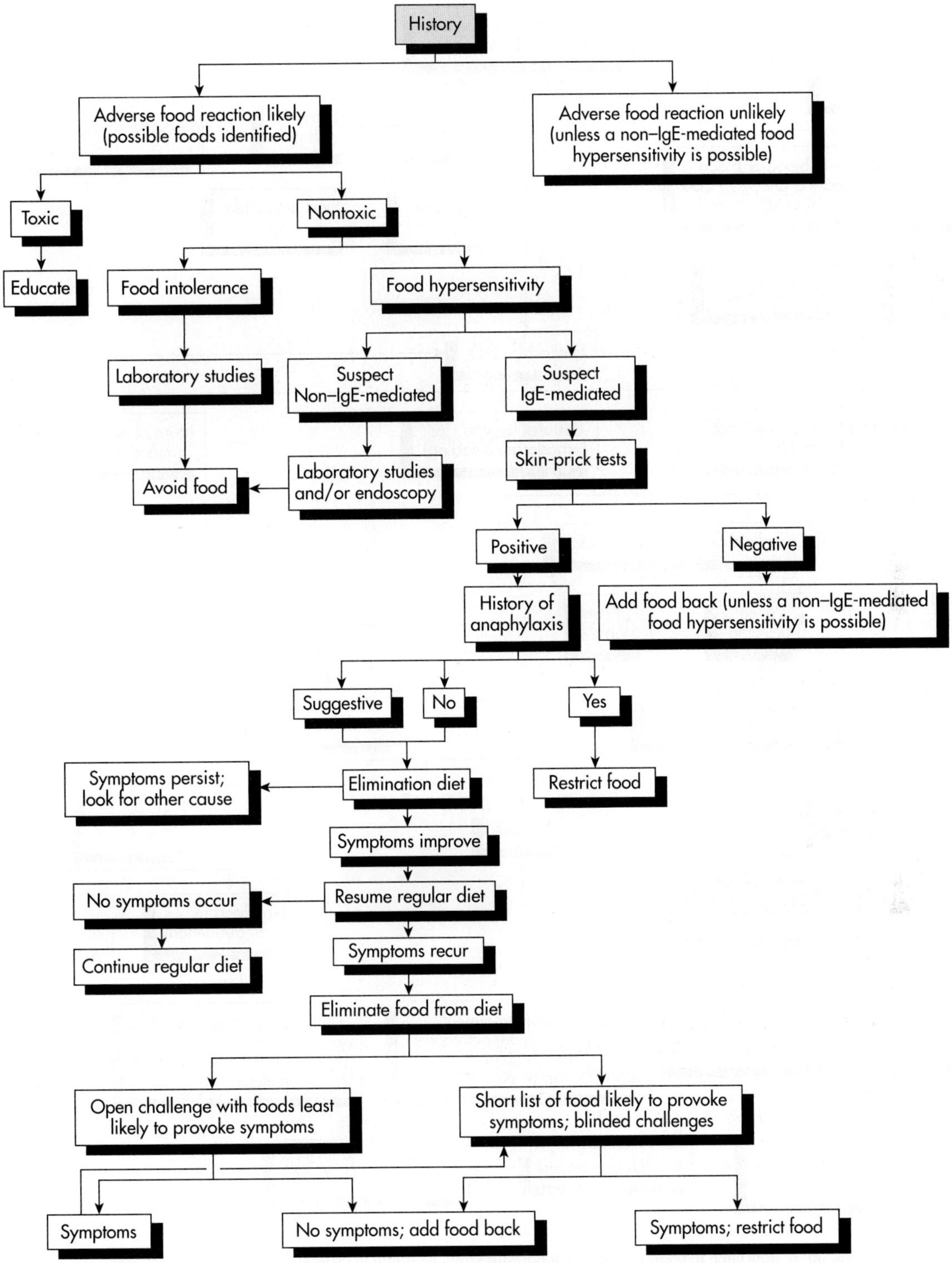

FIG. 84 Algorithm for the evaluation and management of adverse food reactions. *Ig,* Immunoglobulin. (From Feldman M et al: *Sleisenger and Fortran's gastrointestinal and liver disease,* ed 10, Philadelphia, 2016, Elsevier.)

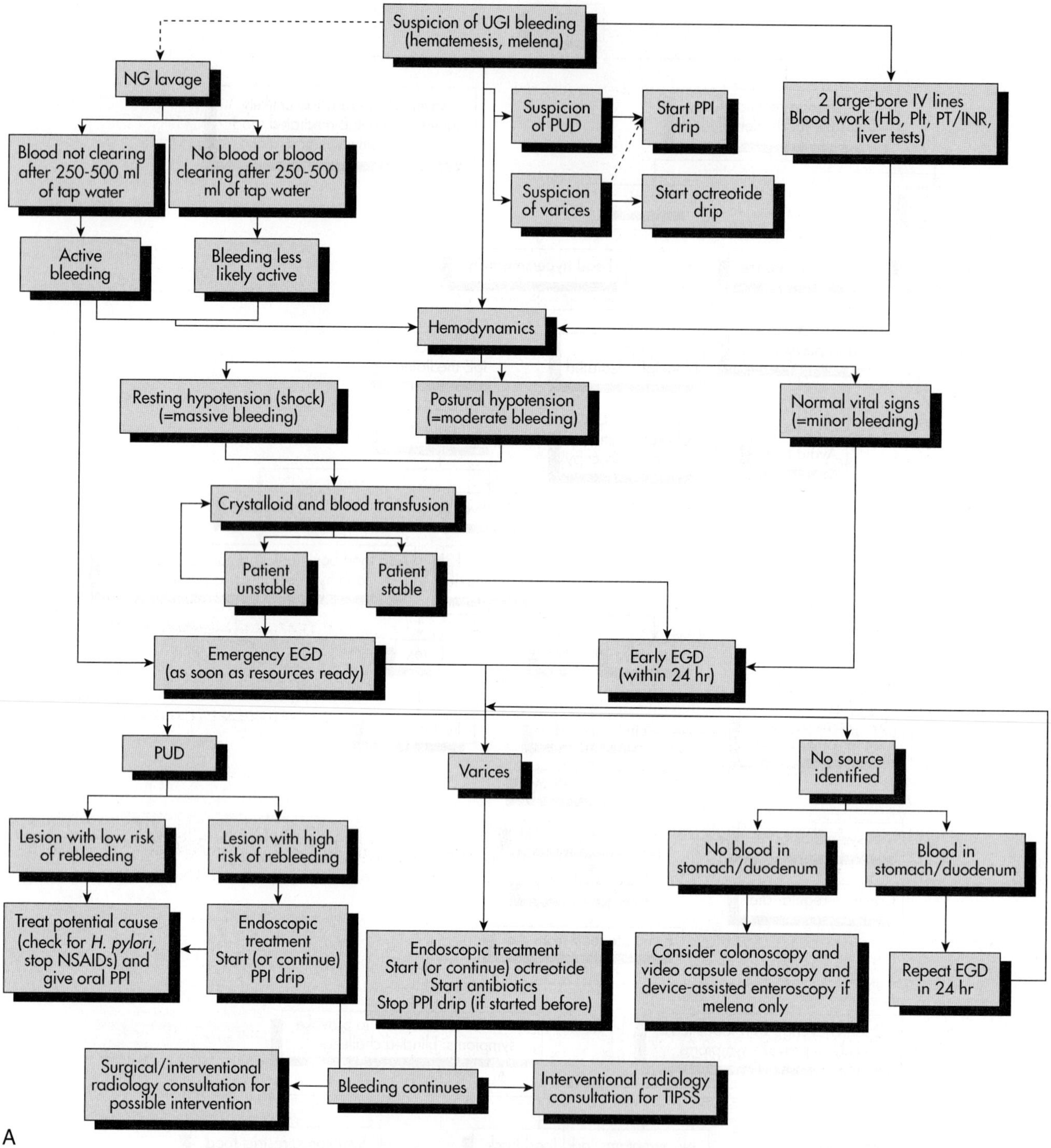

A

FIG. 85 A, Approach to managing upper gastrointestinal bleeding in critical care patients. B, Approach to managing lower gastrointestinal bleeding in critical care patients. *AVM,* Arteriovenous malformation; *EGD,* esophagogastroduodenoscopy; *Hb,* hemoglobin; *INR,* international normalized ratio; *IV,* intravenous; *LGI,* lower gastrointestinal; *NG,* nasogastric; *NSAIDs,* nonsteroidal antiinflammatory drugs; *Plt,* platelets; *PPI,* proton pump inhibitor; *PT,* prothrombin time; *PUD,* peptic ulcer disease; *RBC,* red blood cell; *TIPSS,* transjugular intrahepatic portosystemic stent shunt; *UGI,* upper gastrointestinal. (From Parrillo JE, Dellinger RP: *Critical care medicine, principles of diagnosis and management in the adult,* ed 4, 2014, Elsevier.)

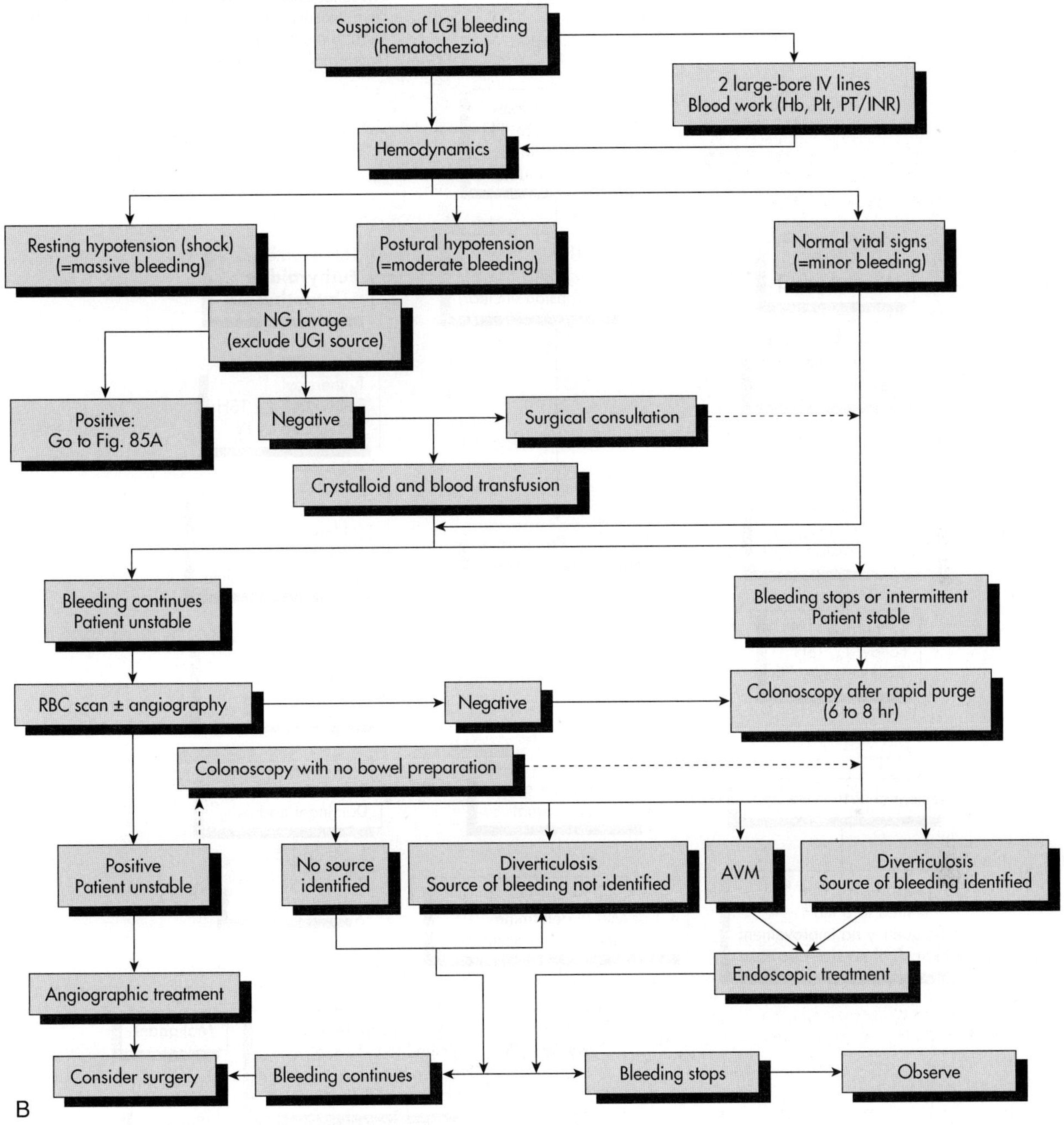

FIG. 85 (Continued)

GOITER EVALUATION AND MANAGEMENT

ICD-10CM #		
	E04.9	Nontoxic goiter, unspecified
	E01.2	Iodine-deficiency related (endemic) goiter, unspecified
	E04.0	Nontoxic diffuse goiter
	E05.10	Thyrotoxicosis with toxic single thyroid nodule without thyrotoxic crisis or storm
	E05.20	Thyrotoxicosis with toxic multinodular goiter without thyrotoxic crisis or storm
	E07.1	Dyshormogenetic goiter

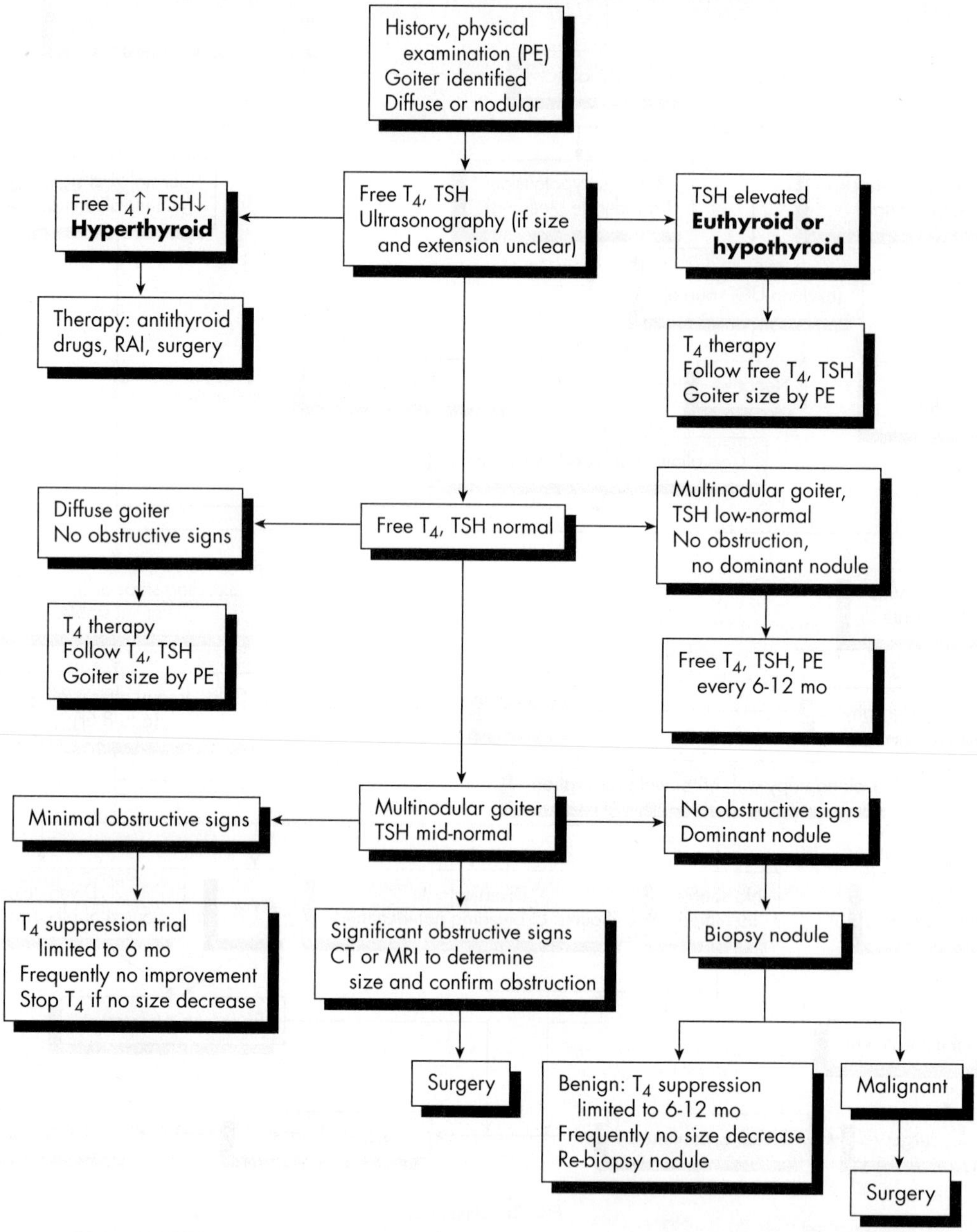

FIG. 87 Evaluation and management of patients with nontoxic diffuse and nodular goiter and undetermined thyroid status. *CT,* Computed tomography; *MRI,* magnetic resonance imaging; *RAI,* radioactive iodine; *TSH,* thyroid-stimulating hormone. (From Goldman L, Schafer AL [eds]: *Cecil textbook of medicine,* ed 24, Philadelphia, 2012, Saunders.)

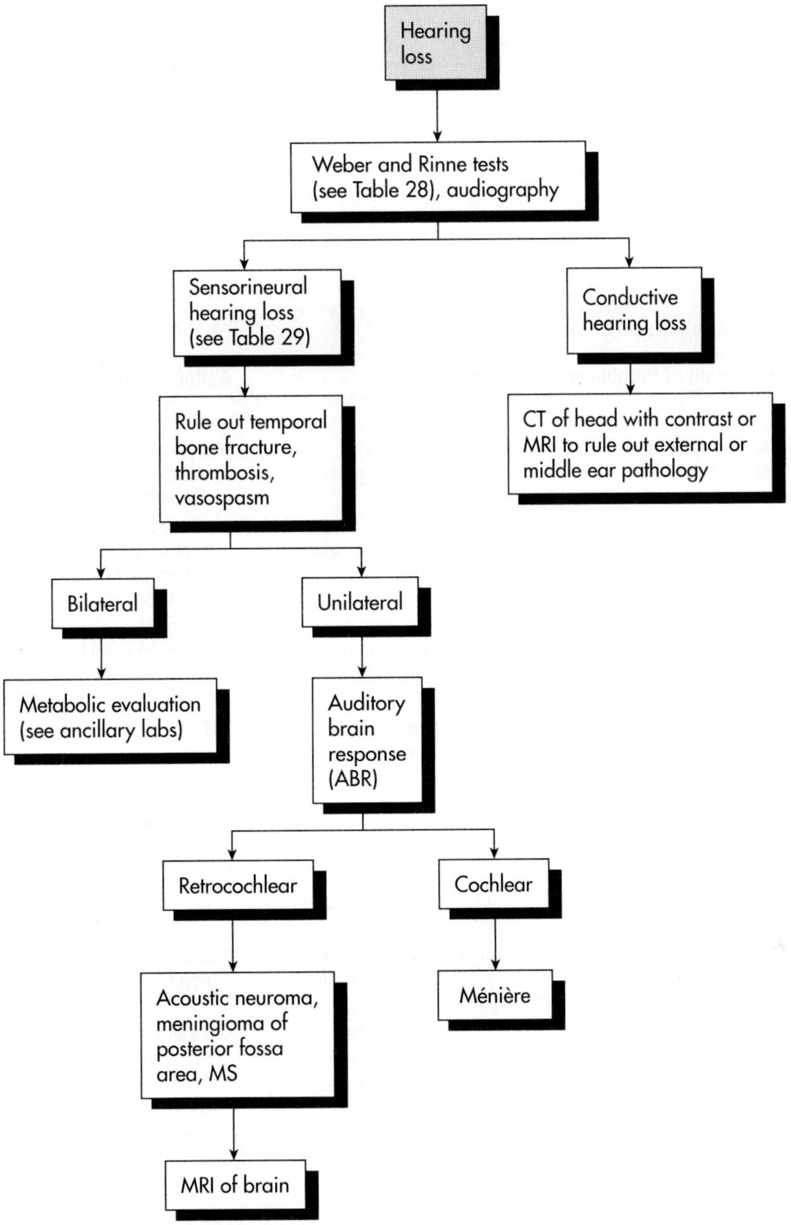

FIG. 89 Evaluation of hearing loss. *CT*, Computed tomography; *MRI*, magnetic resonance imaging; *MS*, multiple sclerosis. (From Ferri FF: *Ferri's best test: a practical guide to clinical laboratory medicine and dig*, ed 4, Philadelphia, 2018, Mosby.)

BOX 14 Hearing Loss

Diagnostic imaging

Best test

None

Ancillary tests

- CT of head with contrast or MRI with contrast
- CT of temporal bone without contrast

Lab evaluation

Best test

- None

Ancillary tests

- CBC
- ALT, AST
- ANA, VDRL
- TSH

ALT, Alanine aminotransferase; *ANA*, antibody to nuclear antigens; *AST*, angiotensin sensitivity test; *CBC*, complete blood count; *CT*, computed tomography; *TSH*, thyroid-stimulating hormone; *VDRL*, Venereal Disease Research Laboratory.

From Ferri FF: *Ferri's best test: a practical guide to clinical laboratory medicine and diagnostic imaging*, ed 4, Philadelphia, 2018, Mosby.

TABLE 28 Interpretation of the Weber and Rinne Tests

	Weber without Lateralization	Weber Lateralizes Right	Weber Lateralizes Left
Rinne both ears: AC >BC	Normal	S/N loss in the left ear	S/N loss in the right ear
Rinne left ear: BC >AC	–	Combined loss: Conduction and S/N loss in the left ear	Conduction loss in the left ear
Rinne right ear: BC >AC	–	Conduction loss in the right ear	Combined loss: Conduction and S/N loss in the right ear

AC, Air conduction; *BC,* bone conduction; *S/N,* sensorineural.
From Adams JG et al: *Emergency medicine, clinical essentials*, ed 2, Philadelphia, 2013, Elsevier.

TABLE 29 Lesions That Cause Hearing Loss

	Description of Pathology	Onset/Course	Actions or Treatment	Prognosis
Conductive Lesion				
Foreign body	Mass in external canal blocks sound conduction	Acute onset associated or not with pain, drainage, or odor	Removal. Evaluate for infection. Evaluate for TM perforation	Excellent
Otitis externa	Edema and detritus obstruct external canal	Rapid onset. Pain, edema, swelling. Drainage, odor often present	Aural toilet to remove debris. Topical (±oral) antibiotics. Evaluate for necrotizing otitis	Excellent if treated appropriately
Exostosis	Bony growths obstruct canal. Often seen with prolonged exposure to cold water (divers)	Slow insidious onset. No pain or drainage unless causes complete obstruction	Evaluate for infection. Reassure patient. Refer to ENT	Good
Tympanosclerosis	TM scarring from perforations or infections. Decreased mobility impairs sound conduction	Slow onset following perforations, trauma, or infections	ENT referral. Reassurance	Variable
Perforated TM	Disruption of TM integrity results in impaired transmission of sound to ossicle	Acute onset. May follow direct trauma or sudden barotrauma. May have sudden relief from pain if caused by otitis media	Treat infectious causes. Counsel on importance of keeping water out of ear canal. ENT referral	Good
Sterile effusion (barotrauma)	Fluid in middle ear dampens conduction through ossicles	Often following flight, diving, or URI. Bubbles can cause intermittent pain	Decongestants. Evaluate for infection. Follow-up	Excellent
Acute otitis media	Pus (or fluid) in middle ear dampens conduction through ossicles	Acute to subacute onset, often following URI. Often associated with pain ± fever	Antibiotics (unless viral cause suspected), decongestants, pain control	Excellent if treated appropriately
Cholesteatoma	Trapped stratified squamous epithelial mass in middle ear. Interferes with ossicle conduction	Slow onset. Often history of previous perforations or chronic infections	ENT referral	Variable. May destroy ossicles or erode into surrounding structures
Glomus tumor	Vascular tumor occupies middle ear space. Interferes with ossicle conduction	Slow onset. May be associated with rushing pulsatile sensation	ENT referral	Variable
Cancer	Squamous cell most common. Obstructs external canal	Slow onset. Often noticed first by others. Painless unless occlusion causes otitis externa	ENT referral. Evaluate for secondary infection	Variable
Sensorineural Lesion				
Perilymph fistula (inner ear barotrauma)	Disruption of round or oval window allows leakage of perilymph into middle ear	Sudden onset of hearing loss often with tinnitus and vertigo. Frequently follows straining or abrupt change in pressure. Turning in direction of fistula exacerbates symptoms	Complete bed rest. Elevate head of bed and avoid increases in CSF pressure. Severe symptoms or noncompliance may require hospitalization. ENT consultation for possible oval or round window patch	Variable
Viral cochleitis	Cochlear inflammation. Often following URI	Rapid onset. Often following URI	Steroids often used (no good data)	Variable
Presbycusis	Age-related hearing loss. May be related to previous chronic noise exposure	Slow onset. Usually symmetric. High frequencies most affected. Tinnitus may occur	Hearing aid may help with both hearing loss and tinnitus	Variable

TABLE 29 Lesions That Cause Hearing Loss—cont'd

	Description of Pathology	Onset/Course	Actions or Treatment	Prognosis
Acoustic neuroma	Benign schwannoma of 8th cranial nerve	Slow onset. Usually unilateral. May exhibit tinnitus, vertigo. May exhibit facial hyperesthesias or twitching	May require surgical excision if symptoms debilitating	Variable
Ototoxic agents	Direct toxicity to inner ear structures	Variable onset. High frequency most affected. Exposure to ototoxic drugs. May have associated tinnitus	Stop use of offending agent	Variable. Hearing loss at time of stopping offending agent is usually permanent
Multiple sclerosis	Multiple demyelinating lesions interfere with nerve conduction	Often other associated neurologic findings. May wax and wane	Standard multiple sclerosis treatment (steroids, cytotoxic agents)	Variable
Stroke/CVA	Focal ischemic lesion of auditory nerve or auditory cortex	Sudden onset. Often associated with other neurologic deficits	Treat CVA risk factors (ASA, anticoagulants, glycemic control, BP control)	Variable
Meningitis	Infection enters inner ear through CNS-perilymph connection. Damages organ of Corti	Follows clinical picture of meningitis	Treat infection. Steroids may limit inflammation and damage	Variable
Ménière disease (endolymphatic hydrops)	Abnormal homeostasis of inner ear fluids (clinical diagnosis; definitive diagnosis made histologically)	Episodic spells of vertigo. Associated sensation of fullness, tinnitus, and SNHL or auditory distortion. Low-frequency ranges most affected	Reduce salt, caffeine, nicotine (vasoconstrictors) intake. Consider diuretics, antihistamines, anticholinergics. ENT referral	Variable
Chronic noise exposure	Direct mechanical damage to cochlear structures and hair cells	Slow onset. Usually high frequency most affected	Prevention measures (earplugs). Stop exposure	Usually permanent
Skull trauma	Interruption of cranial nerve VIII, ossicle disruption, or shearing effects on organ of Corti	Sudden onset after trauma	ENT consultation for possible surgical repair	Variable: Ossicle disruption has better prognosis than nerve or organ of Corti damage
Autoimmune causes	Vascular or neuronal inflammatory changes	Bilateral asymmetric SNHL. May be fluctuating or progressive. Often other systemic autoimmune findings	Outpatient autoimmune evaluation. Steroids and cytotoxic agents may slow progression	Variable

ASA, Acetylsalicylic acid; *BP,* blood pressure; CNS, central nervous system; *CSF,* cerebrospinal fluid; *CVA,* cerebrovascular accident; *ENT,* ear, nose, and throat; SNHL, sensorineural hearing loss; *TM,* tympanic membrane; *URI,* upper respiratory infection.

From Adams JG et al: *Emergency medicine, clinical essentials*, ed 2, Philadelphia, 2013, Elsevier.

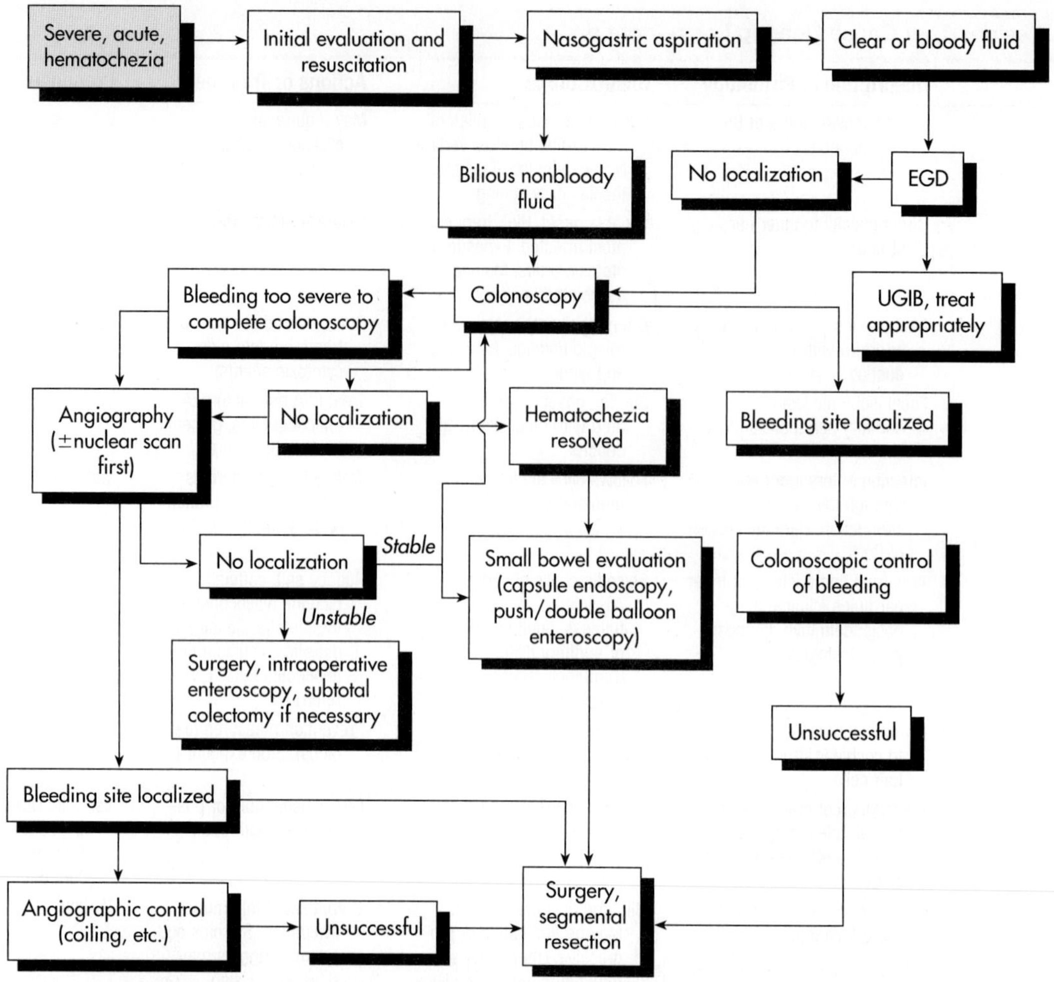

FIG. 90 Management algorithm for hematochezia. *EGD,* Esophagogastroduodenoscopy; *UGIB,* upper gastrointestinal biopsy. (From Cameron JL, Cameron AM: *Current surgical therapy,* ed 10, Philadelphia, 2011, Saunders.)

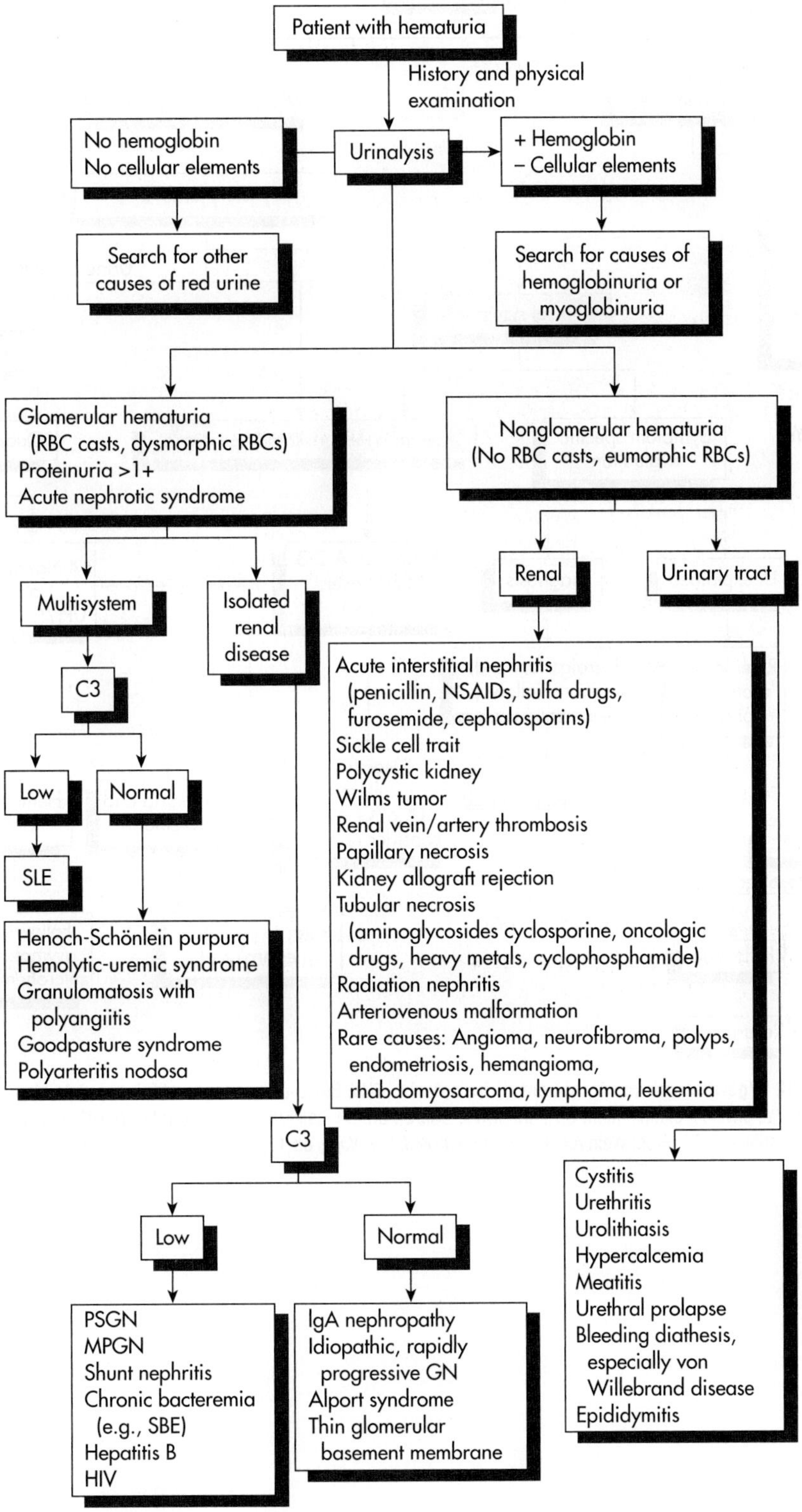

FIG. 91 Diagnostic strategy for hematuria. *GN,* Glomerulonephritis; *HIV,* human immunodeficiency virus; *Ig,* immunoglobulin; *MPGN,* membranoproliferative glomerulonephritis; *NSAIDs,* nonsteroidal antiinflammatory drugs; *PSGN,* poststreptococcal glomerulonephritis; *RBC,* red blood cell; *SBE,* subacute bacterial endocarditis; *SLE,* systemic lupus erythematosus. (From The Johns Hopkins Hospital et al: *The Harriet Lane handbook,* ed 21, St Louis, 2018, Elsevier.)

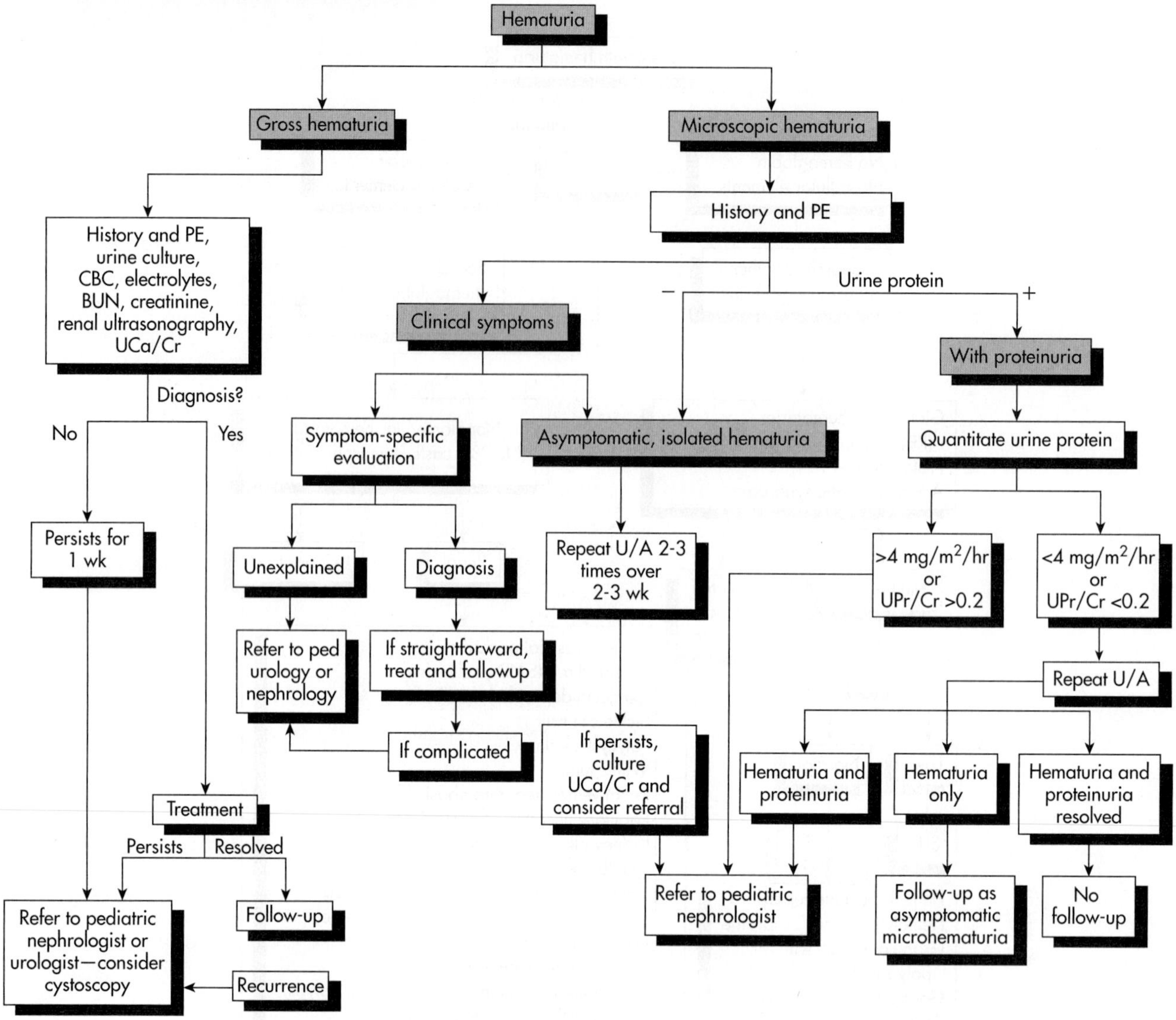

FIG. 92 Algorithm for the treatment of hematuria. *BUN,* Blood urea nitrogen; *CBC,* complete blood cell count; *PE,* physical examination; *U/A,* urinalysis; *UCa/Cr,* urinary calcium/creatinine ratio; *UPr/Cr,* urinary protein/creatinine ratio. (From Wein AJ et al: *Campbell-Walsh urology,* ed 11, Philadelphia, 2016, Elsevier.)

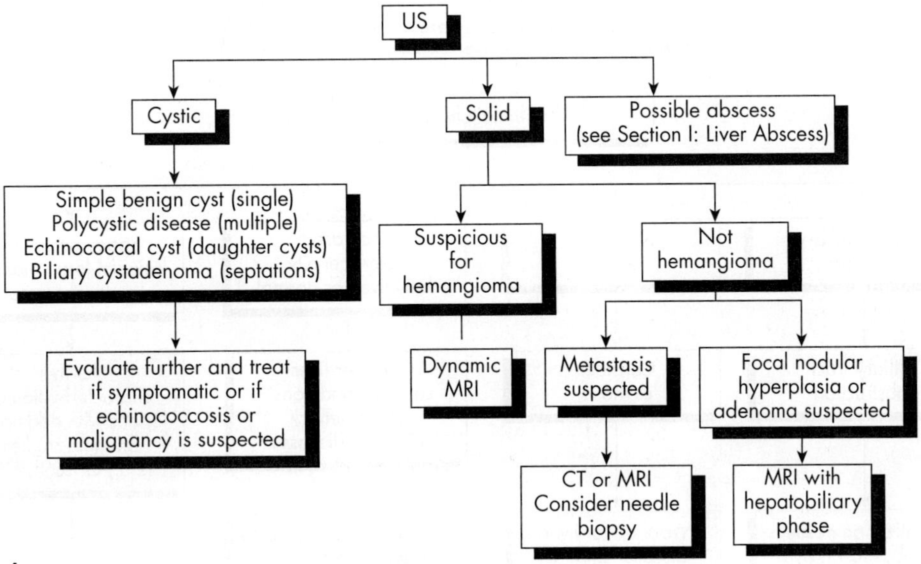

A

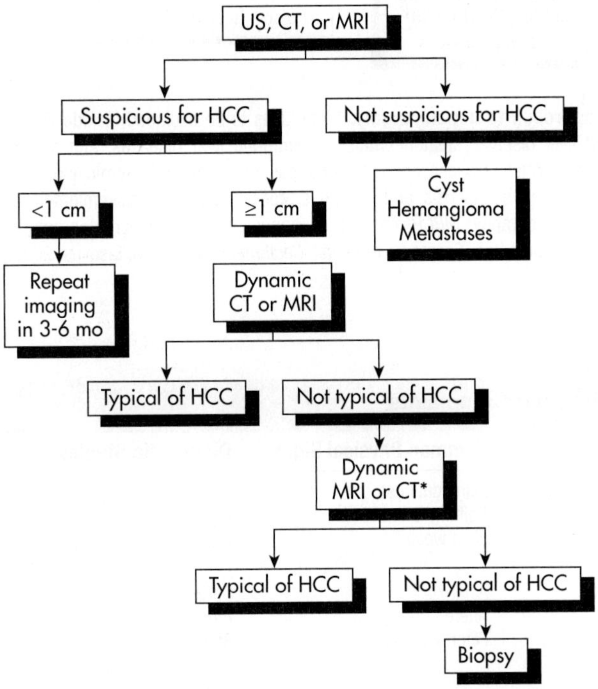

B

FIG. 93 A, Algorithm for the approach to the management of a patient, not known to have cirrhosis, with a hepatic mass (often incidental, possibly symptomatic). B, Algorithm for the approach to the management of a patient with known or suspected cirrhosis and a hepatic mass (found on routine surveillance, because of symptoms, or because of an increasing alpha-fetoprotein level). *Perform imaging modality not previously performed. *CT,* Computed tomography; *HCC,* hepatocellular carcinoma; *MRI;* magnetic resonance imaging; *US,* ultrasound. (From Feldman M et al: *Sleisenger and Fortran's gastrointestinal and liver disease,* ed 10, Philadelphia, 2016, Elsevier.)

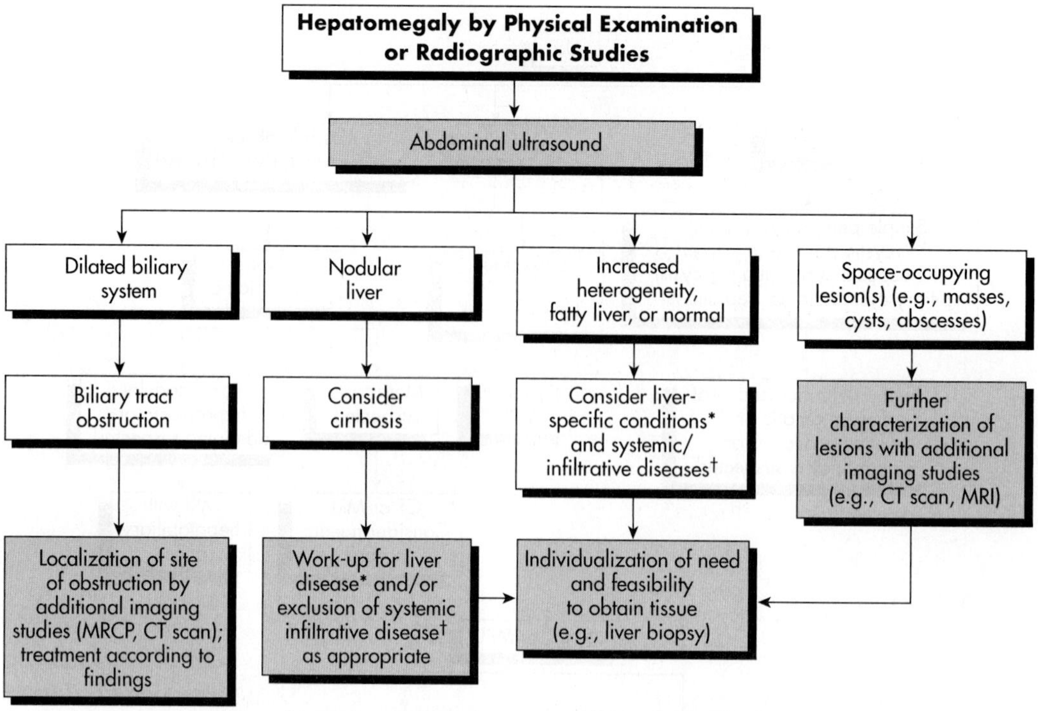

FIG. 94 Diagnostic approach to hepatomegaly. *Conditions to be excluded include viral hepatitis; alcohol- and drug-induced liver disease; steatohepatitis; autoimmune liver diseases; and metabolic disorders, including hemochromatosis, Wilson disease, and α 1 -antitrypsin deficiency. † Systemic and infiltrative diseases include amyloidosis, lymphoma, sarcoidosis, and infectious processes such as disseminated tuberculosis and fungemia. *CT,* Computed tomography; *MRCP,* magnetic resonance cholangiopancreatography; *MRI,* magnetic resonance imaging. (From Goldman L, Shafer AI: *Goldman-Cecil medicine*, ed 26, Elsevier, 2020.)

TABLE 30 Approach to Common Hepatic Complaints

Presentation	Common Symptoms	Common Physical Signs	Diagnostic Studies	Common Diagnoses
Ascites	Abdominal distention and pain, ankle edema	Flank dullness Shifting dullness Fluid wave	Ultrasound with Doppler Diagnostic paracentesis Urinalysis	Cirrhosis Budd-Chiari syndrome Heart failure Nephrotic syndrome
Hepatic encephalopathy	Sleep disorientation, confusion, coma	Asterixis Altered mentation Fetor hepaticus	Serum ammonia Blood cultures Stool Hemoccult Serum creatinine and electrolytes	Decompensated cirrhosis Acute liver failure Other metabolic encephalopathies (renal, respiratory)
Hepatic mass	None or abdominal pain	Hepatic bruit or rub	α-Fetoprotein Ultrasound CT scan MRI Biopsy	Benign lesions: Hemangioma, adenoma, focal nodular hyperplasia Malignant lesions: Hepatocellular carcinoma, cholangiocarcinoma, metastases
Abdominal pain	Nausea, vomiting, fever	Right upper quadrant tenderness Palpable gallbladder Murphy sign	Ultrasound HIDA scan Paracentesis for ascites if present	Biliary colic Acute cholecystitis Hepatic congestion Hepatic metastases

CT, Computed tomography; *HIDA,* hepatobiliary iminodiacetic acid; *MRI,* magnetic resonance imaging.
From Goldman L, Shafer AI: *Goldman-Cecil medicine*, ed 26, Philadelphia, 2020, Elsevier.

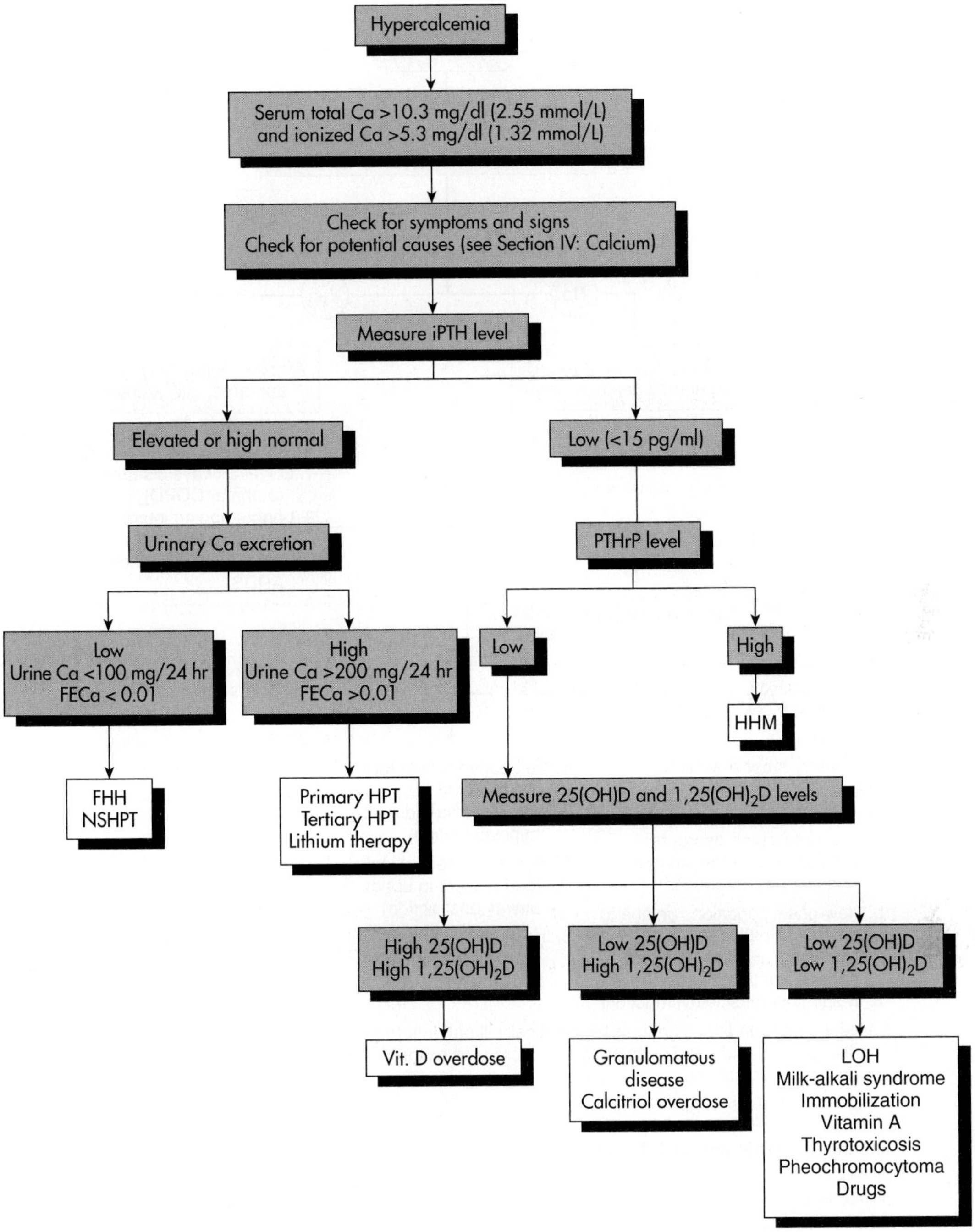

FIG. 95 Algorithm for evaluation of hypercalcemia. *FECa,* Fractional excretion of calcium; *FHH,* familial hypocalciuric hypercalcemia; *HHM,* humoral hypercalcemia of malignancy; *HPT,* hyperparathyroidism; *iPTH,* intact parathyroid hormone; *LOH,* localized osteolytic hypercalcemia; *NSHPT,* neonatal severe hyperparathyroidism; *PTHrP,* parathyroid hormone-related peptide. (From Skorecki K et al: *Brenner & Rector's the kidney,* ed 10, Philadelphia, 2016, Elsevier.)

Diagnostic Imaging

Best Test(s)

- None

Ancillary Tests

- Radiograph of painful bones (r/o bone neoplasm, multiple myeloma)
- Tc-99m parathyroid scan (r/o parathyroid adenoma)
- Ultrasound of parathyroid glands
- Ultrasound of kidneys (r/o renal cell carcinoma)

Lab Evaluation

Best Test(s)

- Serum calcium level
- PTH level

Ancillary Tests

- Serum phosphate, magnesium, alkaline phosphatase, albumin
- Electrolytes, BUN, creatinine
- 24-hr urine collection for calcium
- Urinary cyclic AMP
- PSA (if prostate carcinoma is suspected)
- Serum and urine protein immunoelectrophoresis (if multiple myeloma suspected)

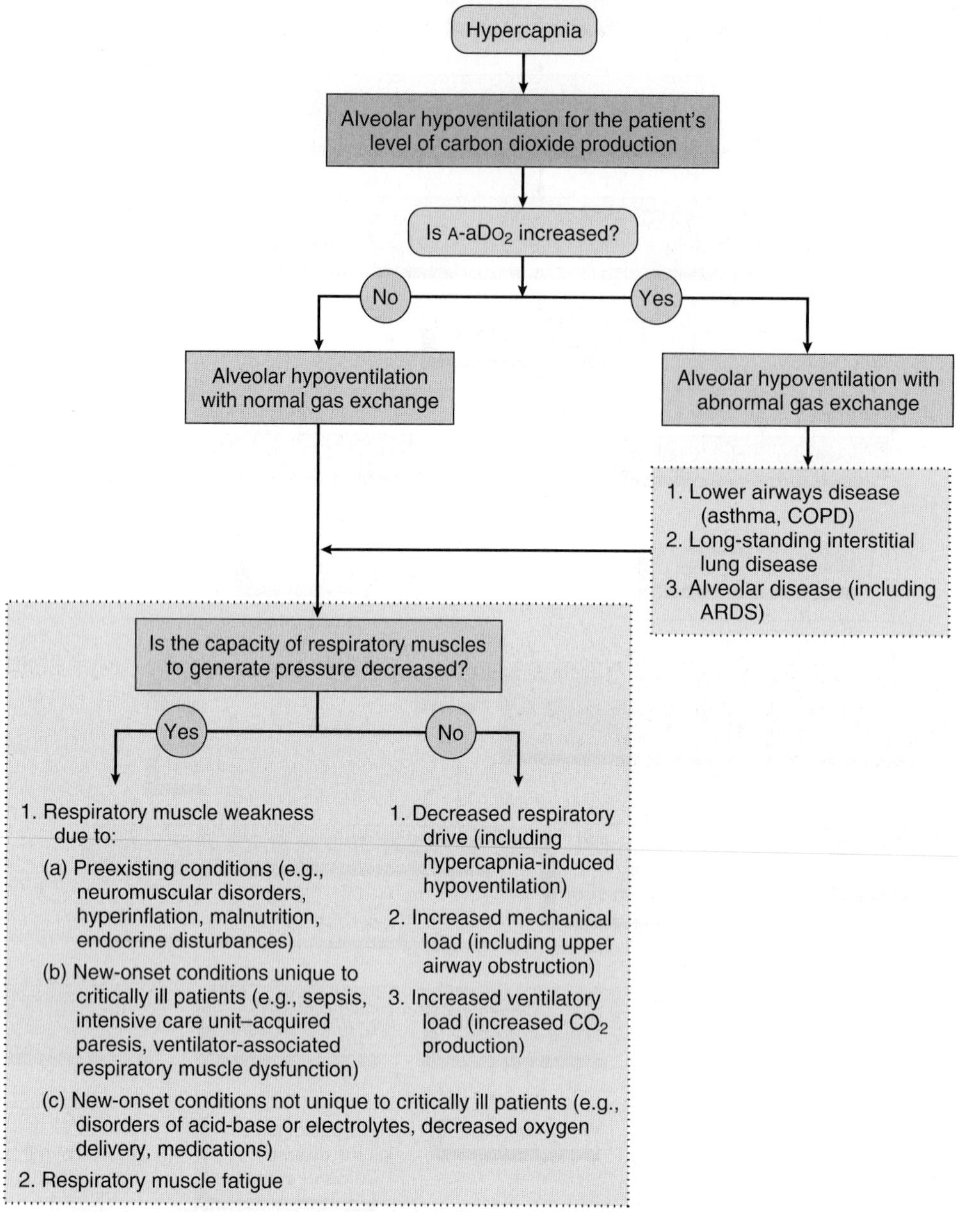

FIG. 96 Diagnostic approach to critically ill patient with hypercapnia. *A-aDo$_2$,* Alveolar-arterial difference in partial pressure of oxygen; *ARDS,* acute respiratory distress syndrome; *COPD,* chronic obstructive pulmonary disease. (From Parrillo JE, Dellinger RP: *Critical care medicine, principles of diagnosis and management in the adult,* ed 5, Philadelphia, 2019, Elsevier.)

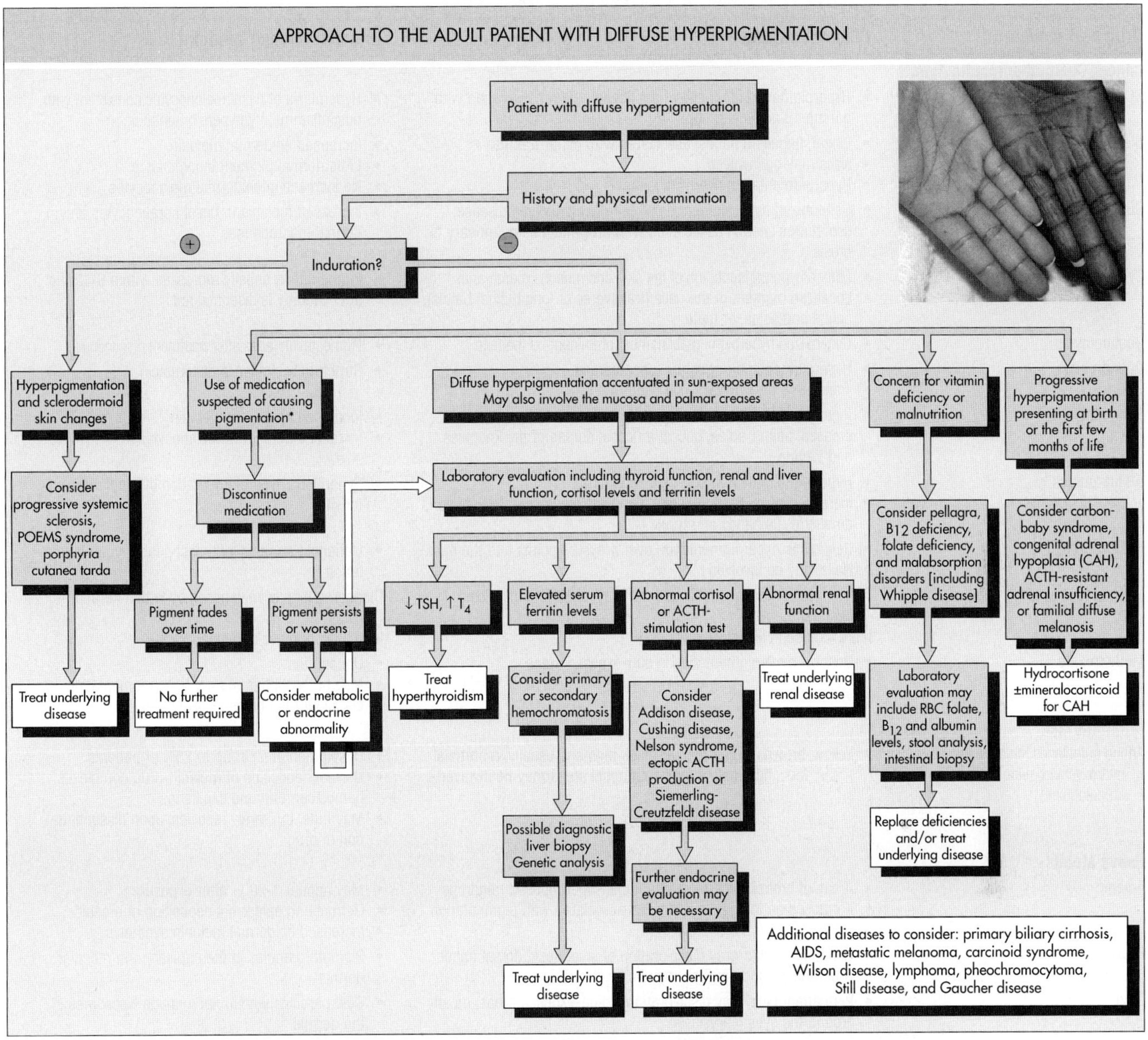

FIG. 97 Approach to the adult patient with diffuse hyperpigmentation. The palm on the right in the inset photograph shows diffuse hyperpigmentation in a patient with POEMS syndrome (*p*olyneuropathy, *o*rganomegaly, *e*ndocrinopathy, *m*onoclonal gammopathy, and *s*kin lesions). *ACTH,* Adrenocorticotropic hormone; *RBC,* red blood cell; T_4, thyroxine; *TSH,* thyroid-stimulating hormone. *See Table 31 for a list of drugs and chemicals associated with diffuse hyperpigmentation. (From Bolognia JL et al: *Dermatology,* ed 3, St Louis, 2012, Elsevier.)

TABLE 31 Drugs and Chemicals Associated with Hyperpigmentation

Drug or Chemical	Clinical Features	Histopathology/Comment
Cancer Chemotherapeutic Agents		
BCNU (Topical)	• Hyperpigmentation at site of application (no reaction seen with parenteral administration)	• Hyperplasia of basal melanocytes consistent with postinflammatory hyperpigmentation
Bleomycin	• Linear, flagellate bands, associated with minor trauma • Nails may be involved • Hyperpigmentation overlying joints	• Increased epidermal melanin • Little dermal pigment incontinence • No increase in epidermal melanocytes
Busulfan	• Generalized hyperpigmentation resembling Addison disease; sometimes seen in association with drug-induced pulmonary fibrosis	• Increased melanin in basal keratinocytes and in dermal macrophages
Cyclophosphamide	• Diffuse hyperpigmentation of the skin and mucous membranes • Localized pigment of the nails (transverse or longitudinal bands), palms and soles, or teeth	• Pigmentation usually regresses within 6-12 mo after therapy is discontinued
Dactinomycin	• Generalized hyperpigmentation, most prominent on the face	• Pigmentation fades after treatment discontinued
Daunorubicin	• Hyperpigmentation of light-exposed areas • Transverse brown-black nail bands	• Structurally similar to doxorubicin
Doxorubicin	• Pigmentation of the nails; hyperpigmentation of the palmar creases, palms, soles, buccal mucosa, dorsae of the knuckles and tongue	• Increased epidermal melanin • Increased number of melanocytes
5-Fluorouracil	• Hyperpigmentation in sun-exposed areas • Increased pigmentation of skin overlying veins used for infusion, dorsae of the hands and trunk	• Synergistic hyperpigmentation of irradiation portal sites
Hydroxyurea	• Reversible hyperpigmentation over pressure points and the back • Nails may be involved	• Lichenoid eruption with secondary hyperpigmentation
Mechlorethamine (nitrogen mustard)	Topical use for cutaneous lymphoma may result in generalized hyperpigmentation More intense in lesional skin	Disaggregation of melanosomes within keratinocytes Increased number of melanocytes
Methotrexate	• Uniform hyperpigmentation in sun-exposed areas	• Uncommon • May be postinflammatory hyperpigmentation secondary to photosensitivity reaction
Antimalarials		
Amino quinolones (chloroquine, hydroxychloroquine, amodiaquine)	• Yellow-brown or gray to blue-black pigment, usually in pretibial areas; face, hard palate, and subungual areas may be involved	• Dyspigmentation in up to 25% of patients • Dermal deposition of melanin-drug complexes; hemosiderin around capillaries • May fade, but rarely resolves, upon discontinuation of drug
Heavy Metals		
Arsenic	• Areas of bronze hyperpigmentation ± superimposed raindrops • Keratoses on the palms and soles associated with pigmentation	• May appear 1-20 yr after exposure • Dermal and epidermal deposition of arsenic • Increased epidermal melanin synthesis
Bismuth	• Generalized blue-gray discoloration of face, neck, dorsal hands • Oral mucosa and gingivae may be involved	• Bismuth granules in the papillary and reticular dermis
Gold	• Permanent blue-gray discoloration in sun-exposed areas, mostly around the eyes (chrysiasis)	• Gold particles within macrophage lysosomes in the dermis
Iron	• Permanent brown pigment at injection or application sites	• Pigment coats collagen fibers and is deposited in dermal macrophages
Lead	• "Lead line" in gingival margin • Nail pigmentation	• Lead line is due to subepithelial deposition of lead granules
Mercury	• Slate-gray pigmentation, particularly in skin folds	• Brown-black granules free in dermis, in association with elastic fibers, and within macrophages
Silver	• Generalized slate-gray pigmentation, increased in sun-exposed areas • Nails and sclerae may also be involved • Localized at sites of application	• Silver granules in the basement membrane and on the membrana propria of eccrine glands
Hormones		
Oral contraceptives	• Melasma; increased pigment of nipples and nevi	• Increased melanocytes and increased melanin synthesis
ACTH/MSH	• Diffuse brown or bronze pigmentation; seen in Addison disease and Cushing syndrome	• Increased melanin synthesis
Miscellaneous Compounds		
Amiodarone	• Slate-gray to violaceous discoloration of sun-exposed skin	• Yellow-brown granules in dermis, mostly perivascular • Lysosomal inclusions with a lipid-like substance
Azidothymidine (zidovudine, AZT)	• Nail and mucocutaneous hyperpigmentation	• Skin biopsy shows increased epidermal and dermal melanin
Clofazimine	• Diffuse red to red-brown discoloration of skin • Violet-brown to bluish discoloration, especially lesional skin	• Redness secondary to drug in fat • Phagolysosomes with lipofuscin material

TABLE 31 Drugs and Chemicals Associated with Hyperpigmentation—cont'd

Drug or Chemical	Clinical Features	Histopathology/Comment
Dioxins	• Chloracne most common skin finding • Hyperpigmentation may occur in sun-exposed areas	• Rare, except in accidental exposure
Hydroquinone	• Hyperpigmentation in areas of application due to exogenous ochronosis	• Yellow-brown banana-shaped fibers in papillary dermis
Minocycline	• Blue-black discoloration in old acne scars or sites of inflammation as well as lower extremities • May also involve nails, sclerae, oral mucosa, bones, and teeth • Generalized "muddy brown" pigmentation pattern in some patients	• Iron-containing granules and/or increased melanin, depending on clinical type
Psoralens	• Increased pigmentation after exposure to UVA light (PUVA)	• Proliferation of follicular melanocytes • Increased synthesis and transfer of melanin
Psychotropic drugs (phenothiazine, chlorpromazine, imipramine, desipramine)	• Slate-gray discoloration in sun-exposed areas	• Golden-brown granules in the upper dermis • Electron-dense inclusion bodies

ACTH, Adrenocorticotropic hormone; *AZT,* azidothymidine, now renamed zidovudine; *BCNU,* carmustine; *MSH,* melanocyte-stimulating hormone; *PUVA,* psoralen + ultraviolet light A; *UVA,* ultraviolet light A.
From Bolognia JL et al (eds): *Dermatology,* ed 2, St Louis, 2008, Mosby.

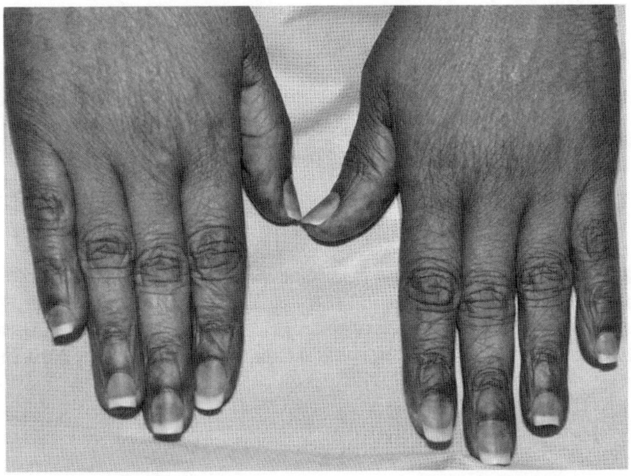

FIG. 98 Hyperpigmentation of the nails in a 61-yr-old woman receiving paclitaxel for breast cancer. (From Callen JP et al: *Dermatologic signs of systemic disease,* ed 5, 2017, Elsevier.)

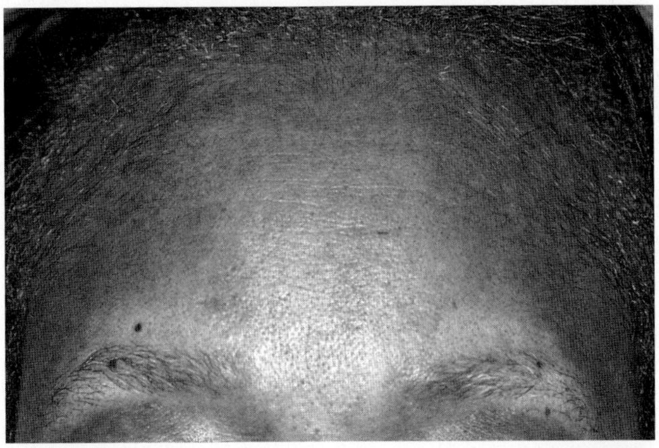

FIG. 99 Grade 1 skin (facial) hyperpigmentation in a 62-yr-old woman, during treatment with imatinib for a gastrointestinal stromal tumor. (From Callen JP et al: *Dermatologic signs of systemic disease,* ed 5, 2017, Elsevier.)

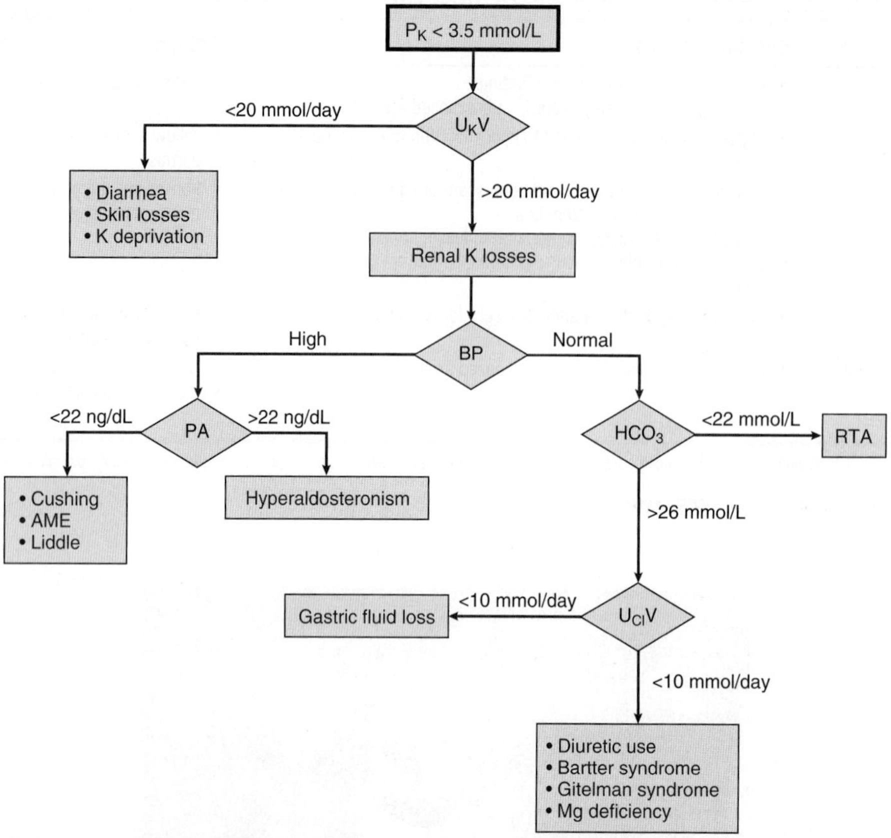

FIG. 100 Diagnostic evaluation of chronic hypokalemia. *AME,* Syndrome of apparent mineralocorticoid excess; *BP,* blood pressure; *HCO_3^-*, bicarbonate; *PA,* stimulated plasma aldosterone (see text); *RTA,* renal tubular acidosis; *$U_{Cl}V$,* urinary chloride excretion; *U_KV,* urinary potassium excretion. (From Parrillo JE, Dellinger RP: *Critical care medicine, principles of diagnosis and management in the adult*, ed 5, Philadelphia, 2019, Elsevier.)

BOX 15 Causes of Acute Hypokalemia

- Treatment of diabetic ketoacidosis
- Refeeding syndrome
- Rapid cell production
  Vitamin B_{12} treatment of pernicious anemia
  GM-CSF treatment of leukopenia
- Pharmacologic agents
  β_2-Adrenoceptor agonists
  Epinephrine
  Soluble barium salts
- Hypokalemic periodic paralysis
  Familial
  Sporadic
  Thyrotoxic
- Pseudohypokalemia

GM-CSF, Granulocyte-macrophage colony-stimulating factor.
From Parrillo JE, Dellinger RP: *Critical care medicine, principles of diagnosis and management in the adult*, ed 5, Philadelphia, 2019, Elsevier.

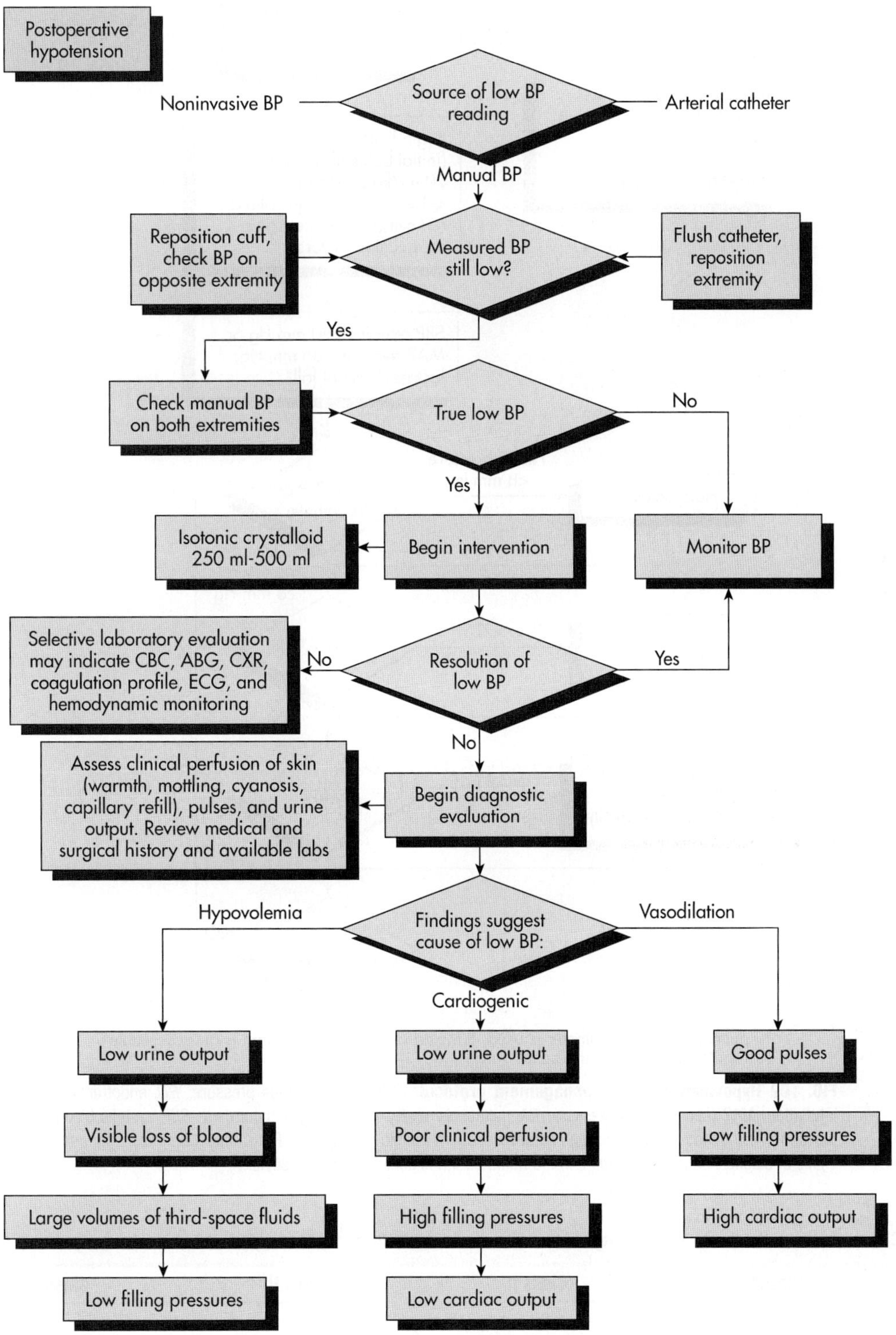

FIG. 101 Approach to managing postoperative hypotension. *ABG,* Arterial blood gases; *BP,* blood pressure; *CBC,* complete blood count; *CXR,* chest x-ray study; *ECG,* electrocardiogram. (From Parrillo JE, Dellinger RP: *Critical care medicine: principles of diagnosis and management in the adult,* ed 4, Philadelphia, 2014, Elsevier.)

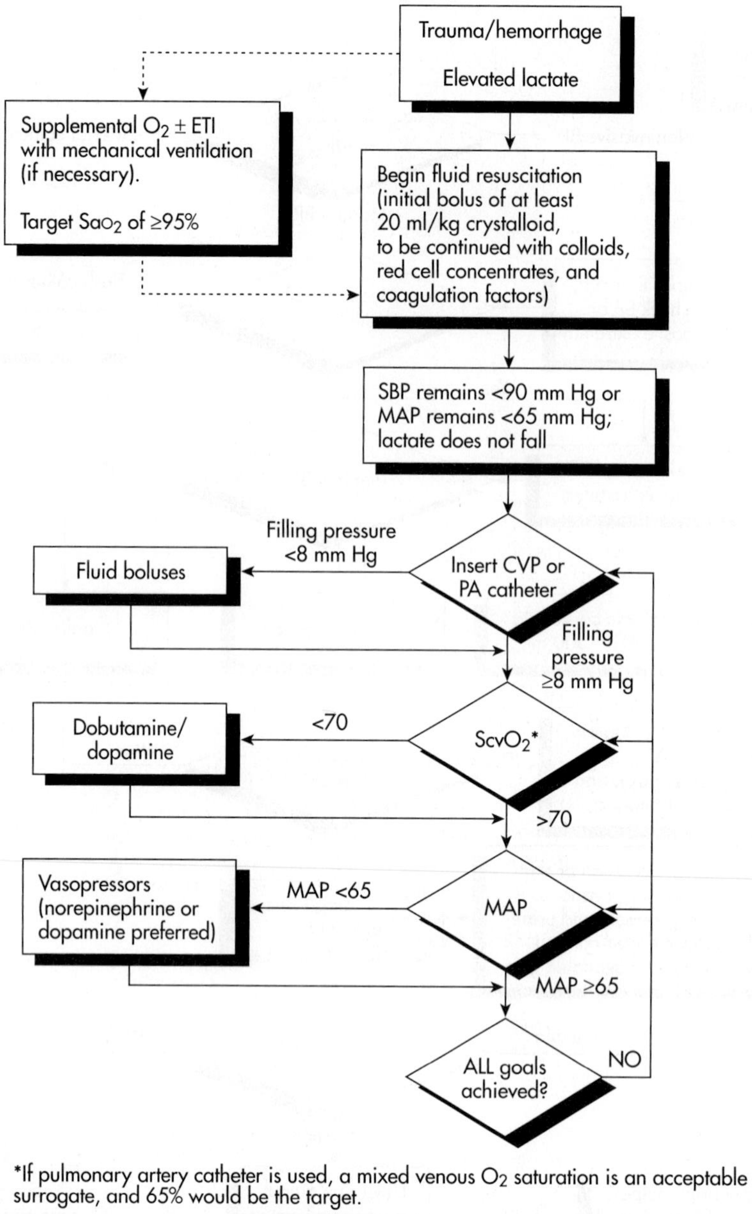

FIG. 102 Hypovolemic shock management protocol. *CVP,* Central venous pressure; *ETI,* endotracheal intubation; *MAP,* mean arterial pressure; *PA,* pulmonary artery; *Sao_2,* oxygen saturation; *SBP,* systolic blood pressure; *$Scvo_2$,* central venous oxygen saturation. (From Parrillo JE, Dellinger RP: *Critical care medicine: principles of diagnosis and management in the adult,* ed 4, Philadelphia, 2014, Elsevier.)

TABLE 32 Clinical Classification of Severity of Posthemorrhagic Hypovolemic Shock

Feature	Class I	Class II	Class III	Class IV
Blood loss				
Ml	<750	750-1500	>1500-2000	>2000
%	<15	15-30	>30-40	>40
Heart rate (beats/min)	<100	>100	>120	>140
Blood pressure	Normal	Normal	Decreased	Decreased
Pulse pressure	Normal	Decreased	Decreased	Decreased
Respiratory rate	14-20	20-30	30-40	>40
Urinary output (ml/hr)	>30	20-30	5-15	Negligible
Mental status	Slightly anxious	Mildly anxious	Anxious, confused	Confused, lethargic
Fluid replacement (ml/hr)	Crystalloid	Crystalloid/colloid	Crystalloid and blood	Crystalloid and blood

MI, Myocardial infarction.
From Parrillo JE, Dellinger RP: *Critical care medicine: principles of diagnosis and management in the adult,* ed 4, Philadelphia, 2014, Elsevier.

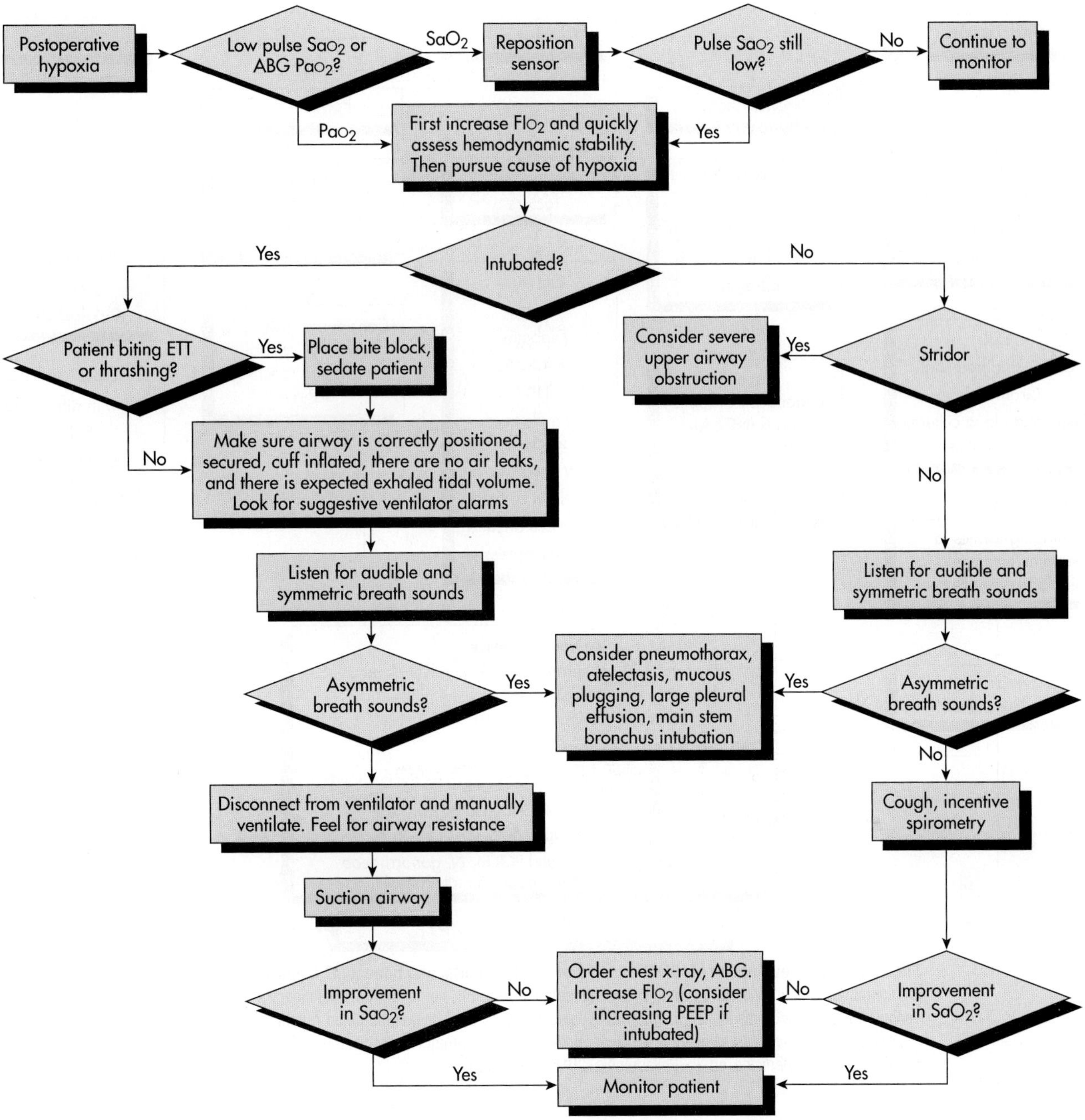

FIG. 103 Approach to managing postoperative hypoxemia. *ABG,* Arterial blood gas; *ETT,* endotracheal tube; *FIO_2,* fraction of inspired oxygen; *PaO_2,* arterial oxygen tension; *PEEP,* positive end-expiratory pressure; *SaO_2,* arterial oxygen saturation. (From Parrillo JE, Dellinger RP: *Critical care medicine: principles of diagnosis and management in the adult,* ed 4, Philadelphia, 2014, Elsevier.)

ICD-10CM # T84.3 Infection and inflammatory reaction
M00.9 Pyogenic arthritis, unspecified
M86.9 Osteomyelitis unspecified
M79.9 Soft tissue disorder, unspecified

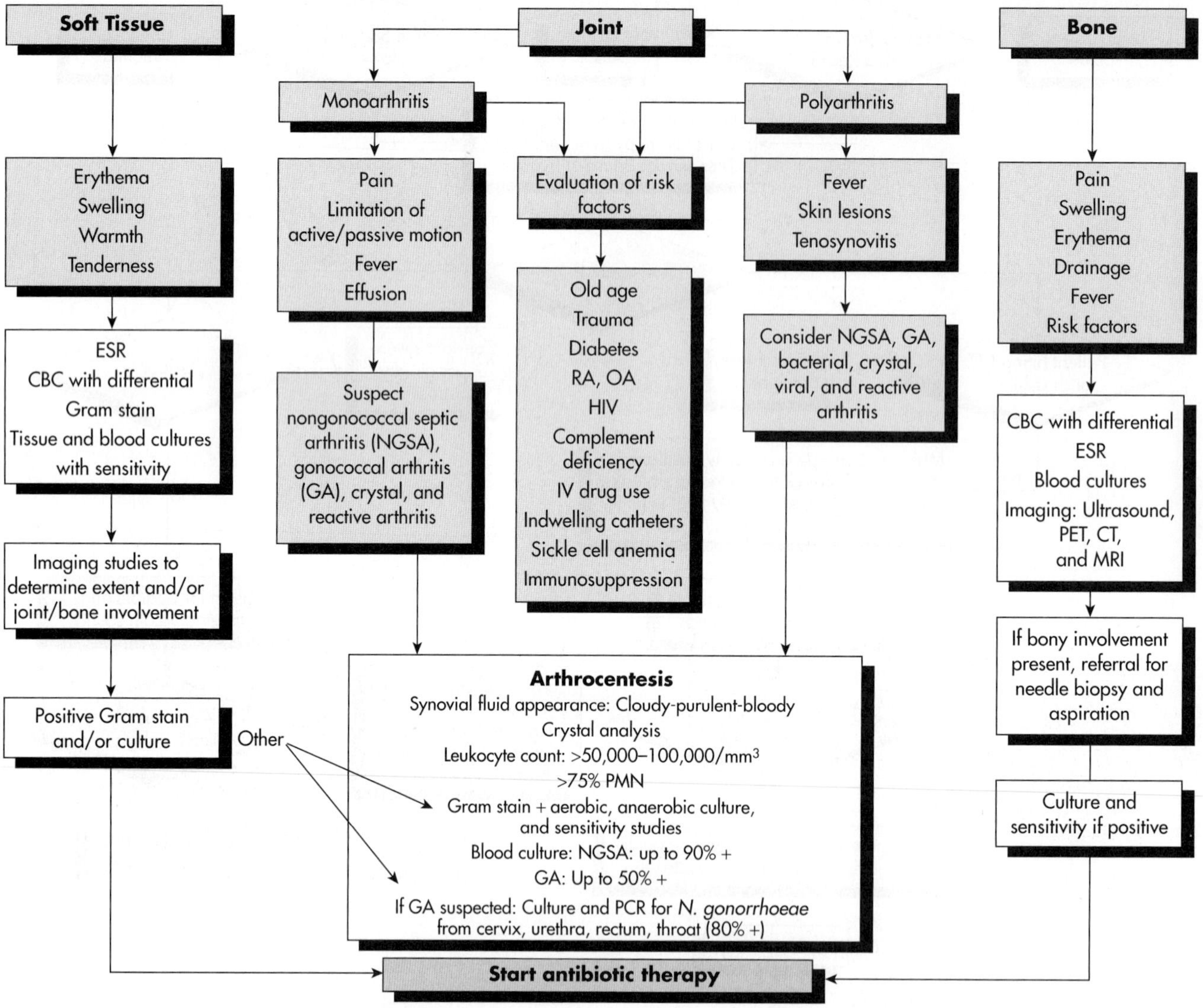

FIG. 104 Clinical evaluation of infections of soft tissues, joints, and bone. *CBC,* Complete blood count; *CT,* computed tomography; *ESR,* erythrocyte sedimentation rate; *HIV,* human immunodeficiency virus; *IV,* intravenous; *MRI,* magnetic resonance imaging; *OA,* osteoarthritis; *PCR,* polymerase chain reaction; *PET,* positron emission tomography; *PMN,* polymorphonuclear leukocyte; *RA,* rheumatoid arthritis. (From Goldman L, Schafer AI: *Goldman Cecil medicine,* ed 25, Philadelphia, 2016, Saunders.)

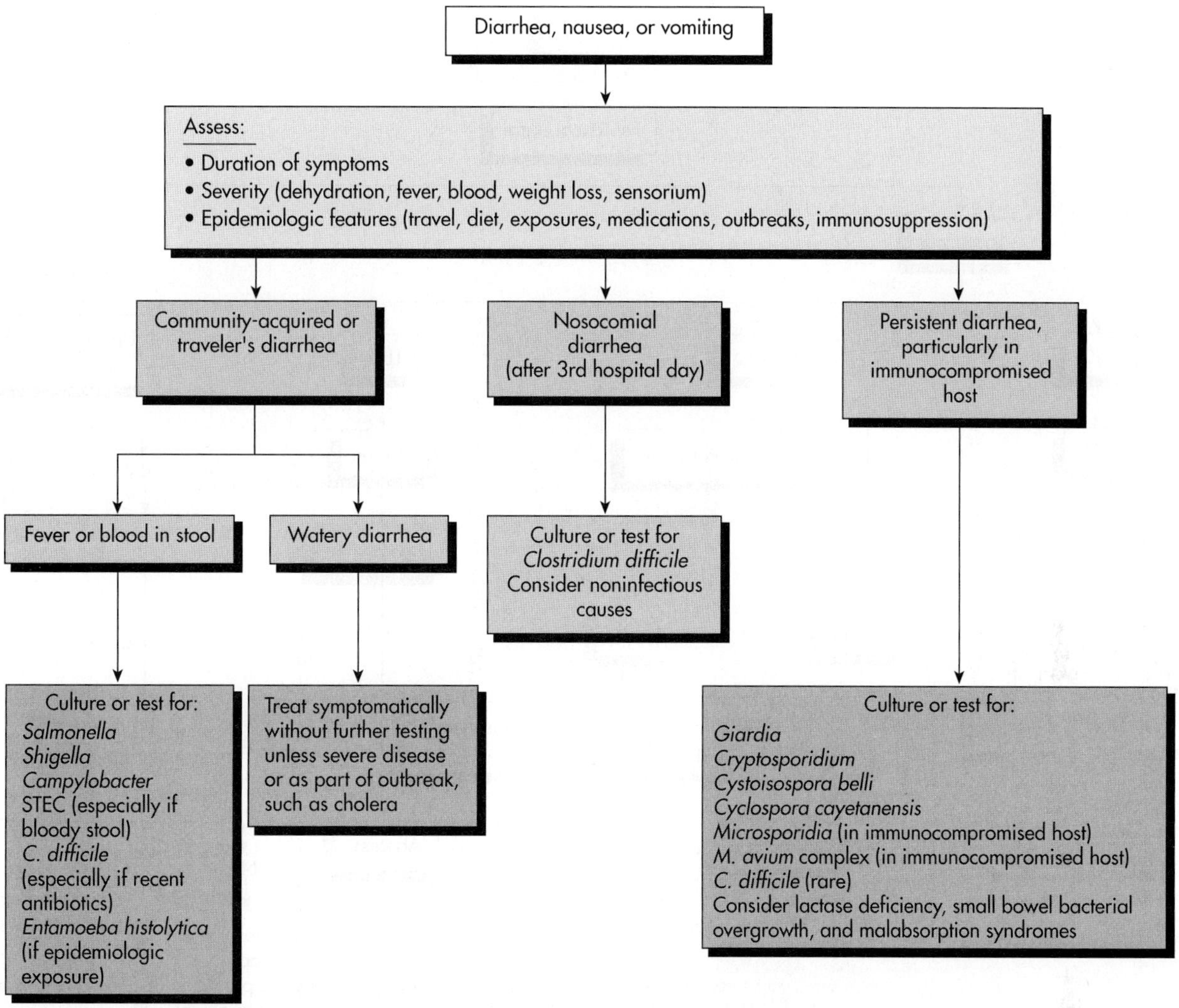

FIG. 105 Approach to diagnosis of infectious diarrhea. *STEC,* Shiga toxin-producing *Escherichia coli.* (From Bennett JE et al: *Mandell, Douglas, and Bennett's principles and practice of infectious diseases*, ed 8, Philadelphia, 2015, Saunders.)

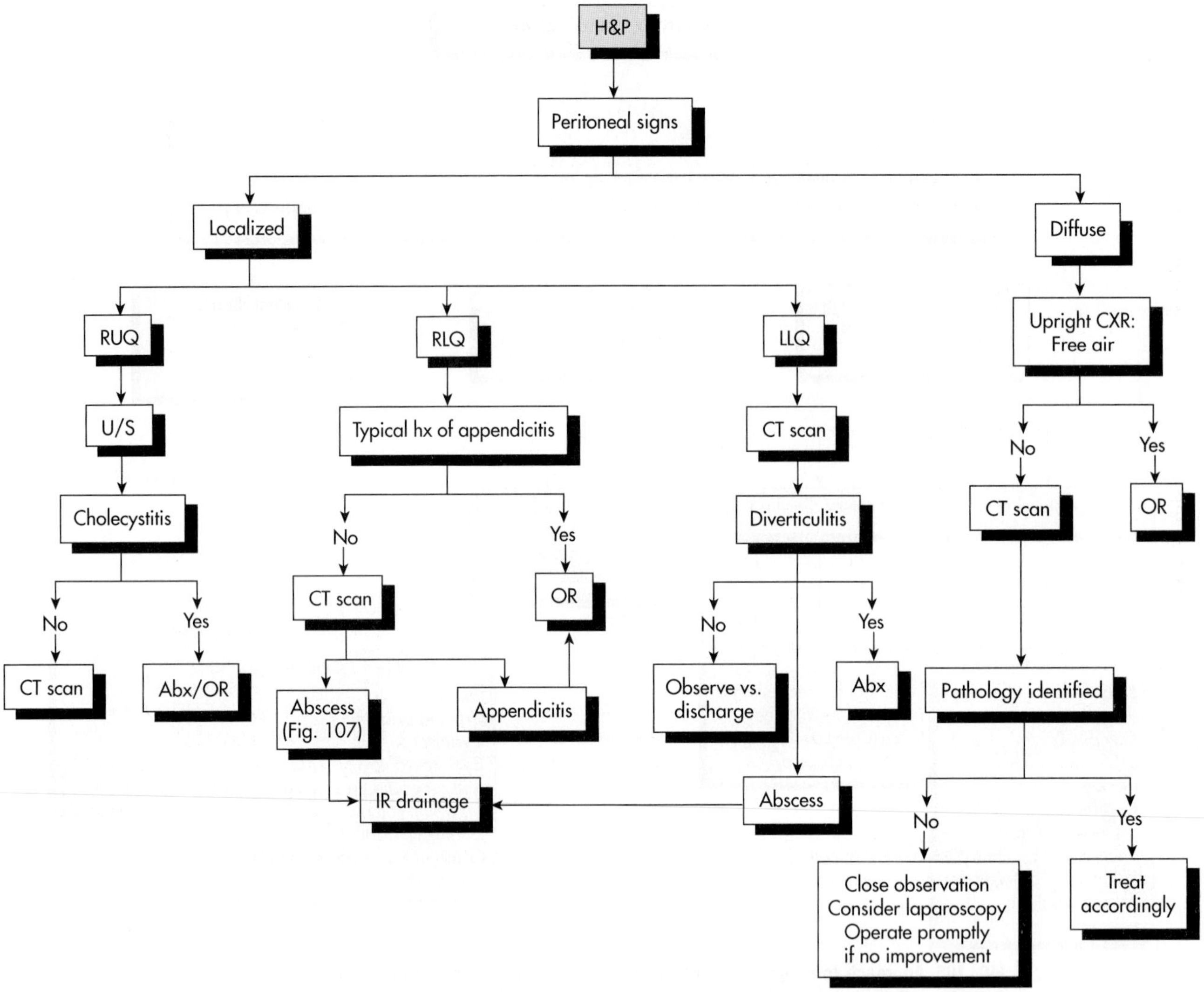

FIG. 106 Algorithm for the diagnosis and management of patients with suspected intraabdominal infection. *Abx,* Antibiotics; *CT,* computed tomography; *CXR,* chest radiograph; *H&P,* History and physical exam; *hx,* history; *IR,* interventional radiology; *LLQ,* left lower quadrant; *OR,* operating room; *RLQ,* right lower quadrant; *RUQ,* right upper quadrant; *U/S,* ultrasound. (From Cameron JL, Cameron AM: *Current surgical therapy,* ed 10, Philadelphia, 2011, Saunders.)

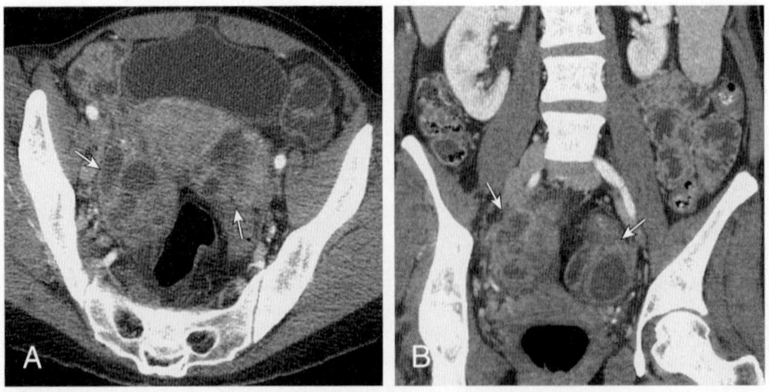

FIG. 107 Axial **(A)** and coronal **(B)** postcontrast computed tomographic images showing bilateral tuboovarian abscesses *(arrows).* (From Fielding JR et al: *Gynecologic imaging,* Philadelphia, 2011, Saunders.)

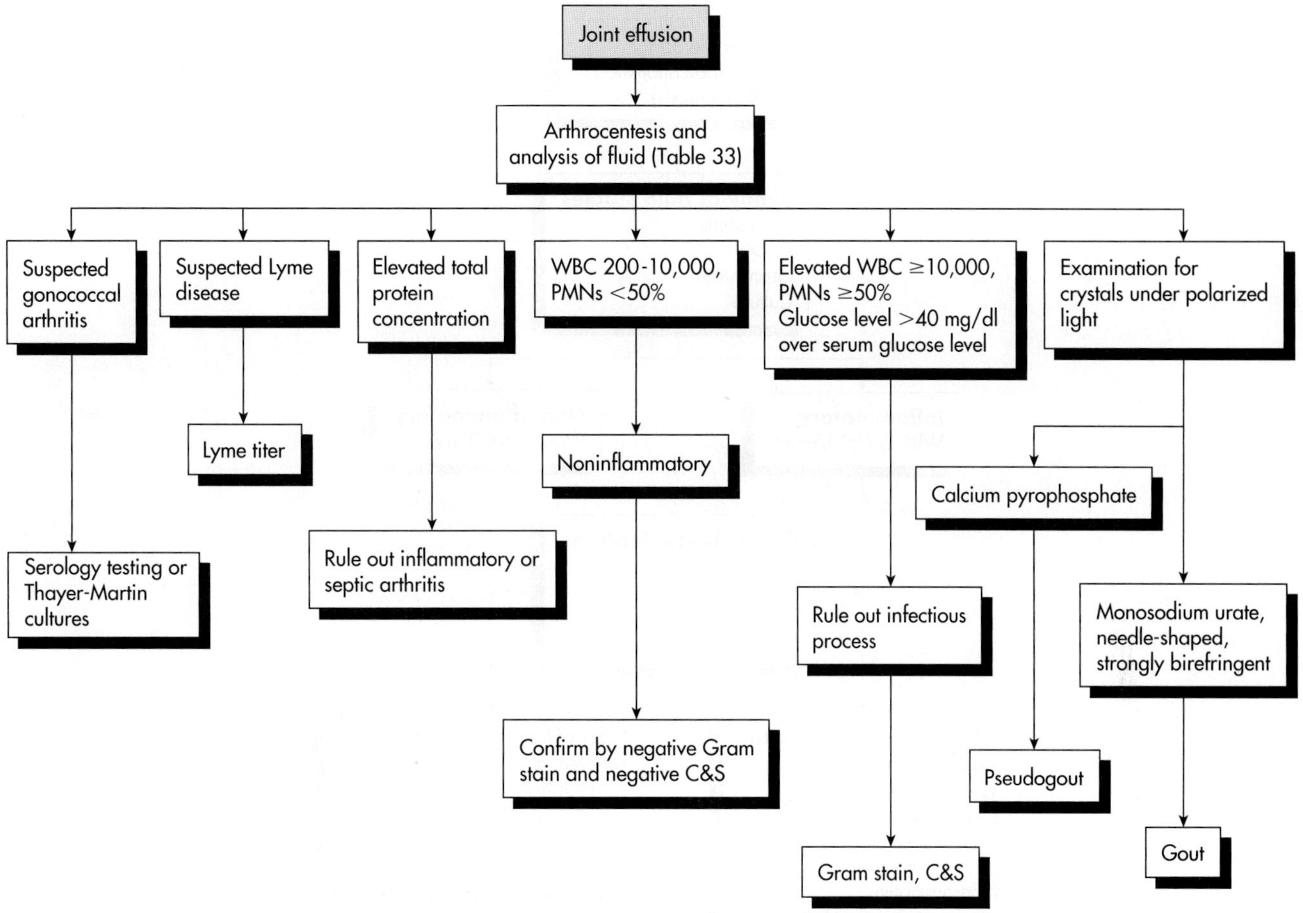

FIG. 108 Joint effusion. See also "Section IV," "Arthrocentesis Fluid." *C&S,* Culture and sensitivity; *PMNs,* polymorphonuclear leukocytes; *WBC,* white blood cell count.

TABLE 33 Indications for Arthrocentesis

Undiagnosed Arthritis with Effusion
Characterize type of arthritis
Noninflammatory (WBC <2000/mm^3)
Inflammatory (WBC >2000/mm^3)
Septic (WBC >50,000/mm^3)
Definitive diagnosis
Gout (urate crystals)
Pseudogout (calcium pyrophosphate dihydrate crystals)
Septic arthritis (Gram stain [rare] or culture)
Undiagnosed Arthritis without Effusion
May be definitive in gout (knee, first metatarsophalangeal joint)
Patient with Known Diagnosis
Septic arthritis (repeated taps for adequate drainage)
Other types of arthritis for symptomatic relief (with or without injection)*

WBC, White blood cells.
*Most studies show improved effect if fluid is aspirated before injection.
From Firestein GS et al: *Kelley's textbook of rheumatology,* ed 9, Philadelphia, 2013, Saunders.

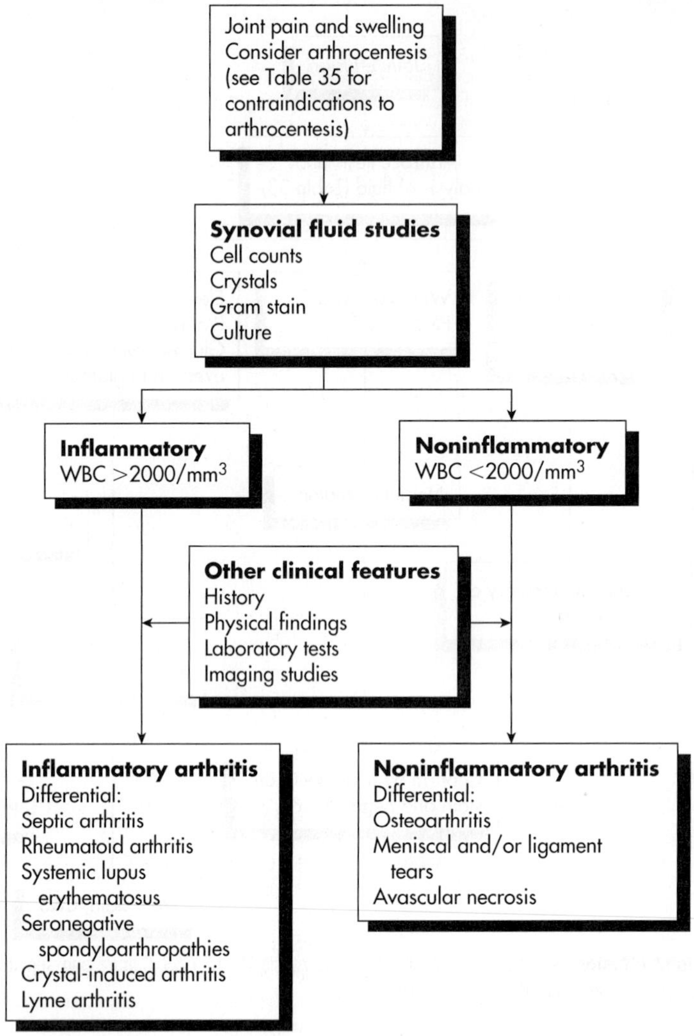

FIG. 109 Diagnostic approach for swollen joints. *WBC,* White blood cell count. (From Goldman L, Schafer AL [eds]: *Cecil textbook of medicine,* ed 24, Philadelphia, 2012, Saunders.)

TABLE 34 Clinical and Radiological Findings in Joint Disease

Condition	Site of Involvement	Discriminatory Findings
Primary osteoarthritis (F>M • >45 yr)	Hands	PIP and DIP joint involvement (Heberden and Bouchard nodes) • no osteopenia
	Large joints (e.g., hip, knee)	Joint space narrowing • subchondral sclerosis • subchondral cysts • marginal osteophytes
	Spine	Degenerative disc disease • spondylosis deformans • apophyseal joint involvement • spinal stenosis • foraminal stenosis
Erosive osteoarthritis (affects middle-aged females)	Hands	PIP and DIP joint involvement • joint ankylosis • 'gull-wing' deformities (central erosions and marginal osteophytes)
Rheumatoid arthritis (F>M • Rh factor positive)	Hand and wrist	Symmetrical arthritis • MCP and PIP joint involvement • periarticular (early) and diffuse (late) osteopenia • marginal erosions • subluxation (swan neck and boutonnière deformities) • periostitis is uncommon
	Large joints	Joint space narrowing • marginal erosions • synovial cysts • protrusio acetabulae
	Spine	Atlantoaxial subluxation

TABLE 34 Clinical and Radiological Findings in Joint Disease—cont'd

Condition	Site of Involvement	Discriminatory Findings
Juvenile idiopathic arthritis (M = F • affects children)	Hands	Joint ankylosis • florid periosteal reaction • osteopenia
	Large joints (e.g., knee)	Abnormalities of growth and maturation • epiphyseal overgrowth and premature closure of the physis • widened intercondylar notch
	Cervical spine	Apophyseal joint fusion • atlantoaxial subluxation
Psoriatic arthritis (M>F • nail changes • HLA-B27 +ve)	Upper extremities (e.g., hands)	"Sausage" digit • DIP joint involvement • terminal tuft erosion • pencil-in-cup deformity • joint ankylosis • arthritis mutilans • periosteal reaction • no osteopenia
	SI joints	Asymmetric or unilateral sacroiliitis
	Spine	Coarse syndesmophytes
Reites syndrome (affects young male adults)	Lower extremities (e.g., foot)	Hallux involvement • periosteal reaction • calcaneal erosions • osteopenia not prominent
	Spine	Coarse syndesmophytes
	SI joints	Asymmetric or unilateral sacroiliitis
Ankylosing spondylitis (M>F • affects young adults • HLA-B27 +ve in 95%)	SI joints	Bilateral symmetrical sacroiliitis • ankylosis
	Spine	Anterior vertebral body squaring • syndesmophytes • paravertebral ossification • bamboo spine
	Pelvis	"Whiskering" of the iliac crests and ischial tuberosities
Enteropathic arthropathies	SI joints	Symmetrical sacroiliitis
Gout (M>F)	Hands and feet (especially the great toe)	MTP joint of the great toe • juxta-articular erosions • punched-out lesions with an overhanging margin • no periarticular osteopenia • tophi
CPPD crystal deposition disease (M = F)	Any peripheral joint • predilection for the knee	Degenerative changes • chondrocalcinosis • paucity of subchondral sclerosis
HA crystal deposition disease (M = F)	Predilection for the shoulder (supraspinatus tendon)	Periarticular calcification
Hemochromatosis (M>F)	Hands	2nd and 3rd MCP joint involvement ("squared" metacarpal heads) • joint space narrowing • "hooklike" osteophytes • numerous subchondral cysts
Alkaptonuria (ochronosis) (M = F)	Intervertebral discs • SI joints • large joints	Degenerative changes: Disc calcification • joint space narrowing • periarticular sclerosis
Systemic lupus erythematosus (F>M • affects young adults)	Hands	Reversible MCP joint subluxation
Scleroderma (F>M • affects adults)	Hands	IP joint arthritis • acroosteolysis • soft tissue calcifications
Mixed connective tissue disease (overlap syndrome)	Hands	PIP joint, MCP joint, mid-carpal involvement • soft tissue swelling, calcifications, or atrophy
Multicentric reticulohistiocytosis (F>M)	Hands and feet	DIP joint and carpal involvement • soft tissue swelling • articular erosions • no osteopenia
Polymyositis/dermatomyositis	Proximal extremities	Soft tissue calcification
	Hands	DIP joint erosions

Continued

TABLE 34 Clinical and Radiological Findings in Joint Disease—cont'd

Condition	Site of Involvement	Discriminatory Findings
Sarcoidosis	Distal and middle phalanges of the hands and feet	Punched-out cystlike lesions • "lacelike" appearance
Hemophilic arthropathy (affecting males—but with female carriers)	Predilection for large joints (e.g., knee)	Epiphyseal overgrowth • juxtaarticular osteopenia • erosion and cartilage destruction • widened intercondylar and trochlear notches • squared patella
Neuropathic arthropathy	Any joint	5 "Ds": Normal bone **D**ensity • joint **D**istension • bony **D**ebris • joint **D**isorganization • **D**islocation
Hypertrophic osteoarthropathy	Tubular bones (radius and ulna > tibia and fibula)	Diaphyseal and metaphyseal painful periostitis

CPPD, Calcium pyrophosphate deposition disease; *DIP,* distal interphalangeal; *F,* female; *HA,* hydroxyapatite; *HLA,* human leukocyte antigen; *IP,* interphalangeal; *M,* male; *MCP,* metacarpophalangeal; *MTP,* metatarsophalangeal; *PIP,* proximal interphalangeal; *Rh,* Rhesus; *SI,* sacroiliac.
From Grant LA, Griffin N: *Grainger & Allison's diagnostic radiology essentials,* ed 2, Philadelphia, 2019, Elsevier.

TABLE 35 Contraindications to Arthrocentesis and Joint Injection

Contraindication	Comment
Established infection in nearby structures (e.g., cellulitis, septic bursitis)	Sometimes gout mimics cellulitis, creating a confusing picture
Septicemia (theoretic risk of introducing organism into joint)	Need to tap suspected septic joints in septic patients
Disrupted skin barrier (e.g., psoriasis)	Do not tap through lesions
Bleeding disorder (not absolute, but use more care)	Risk of bleeding very low, even in patients taking warfarin
Septic joint	Steroid injection contraindicated
Prior lack of response	Relative contraindication
Difficult-to-access joint	Relative contraindication without imaging aid

From Firestein GS et al: *Kelley's textbook of rheumatology,* ed 9, Philadelphia, 2013, Saunders.

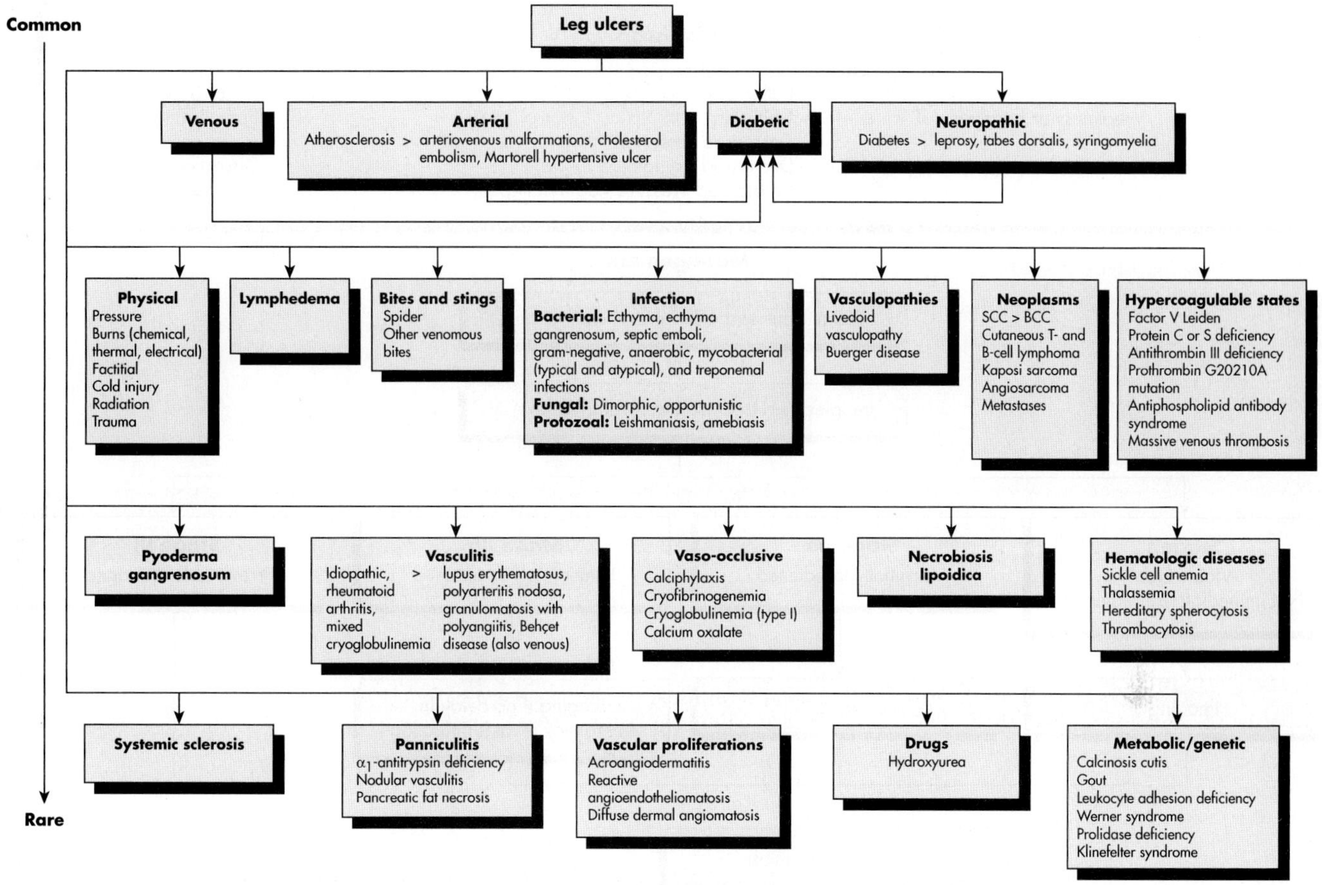

FIG. 110 Causes of leg ulcers. Patients with Behçet disease also develop lower extremity ulcers due to vasculitis and/or venous insufficiency related to deep vein thromboses, and, occasionally, erosive pustular dermatosis is a cause of leg ulcers. Hydroxyurea-induced leg ulcers are often on the malleolus or tibial crest, exceedingly painful, and surrounded by atrophic skin. (From Bolognia J: *Dermatology,* ed 4, Philadelphia, 2018, Elsevier.)

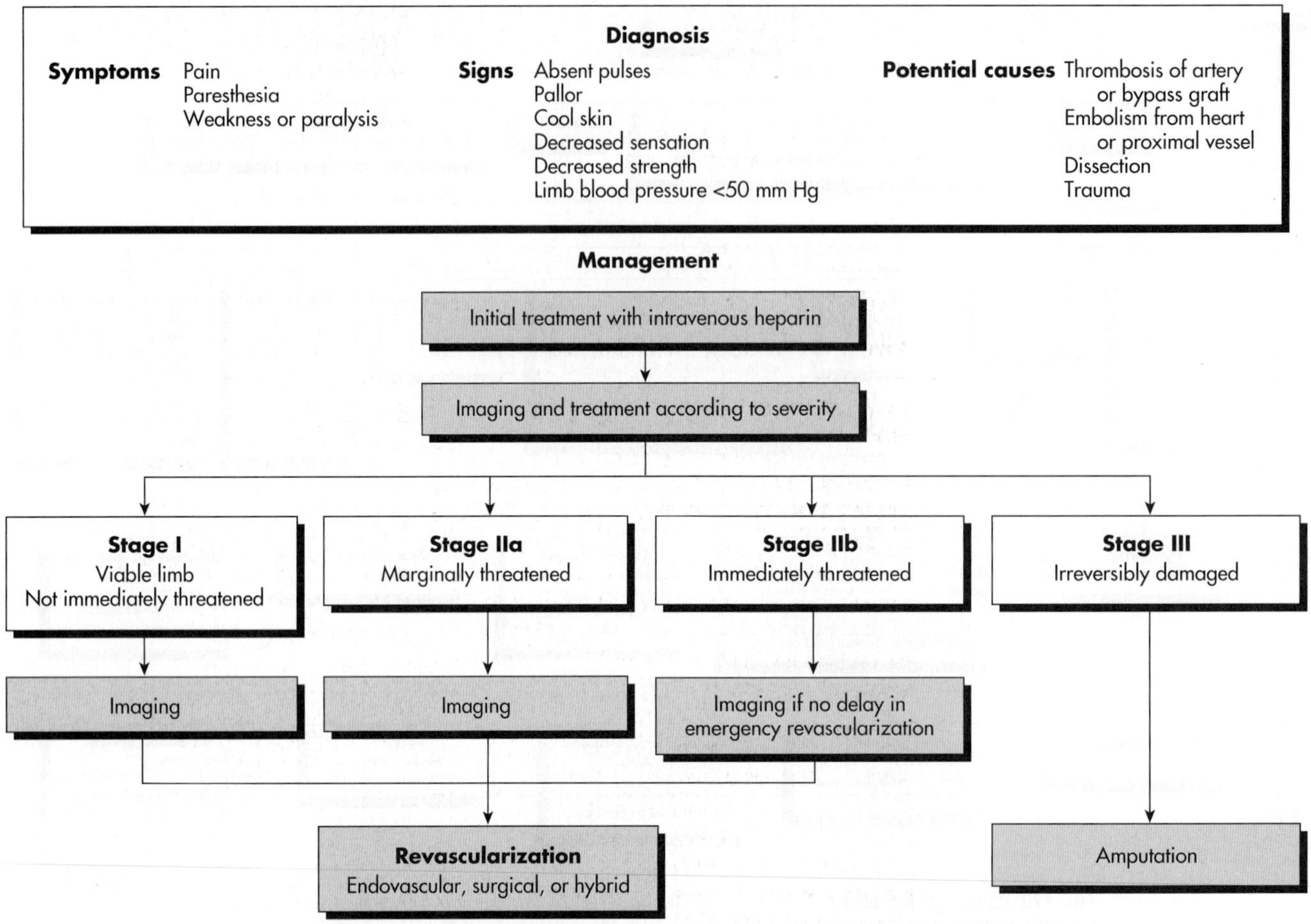

FIG. 111 Diagnostic and treatment approach for patients presenting with acute limb ischemia. (From Zipes DP: *Braunwald's heart disease, a textbook of cardiovascular medicine*, ed 11, Philadelphia, 2019, Elsevier.)

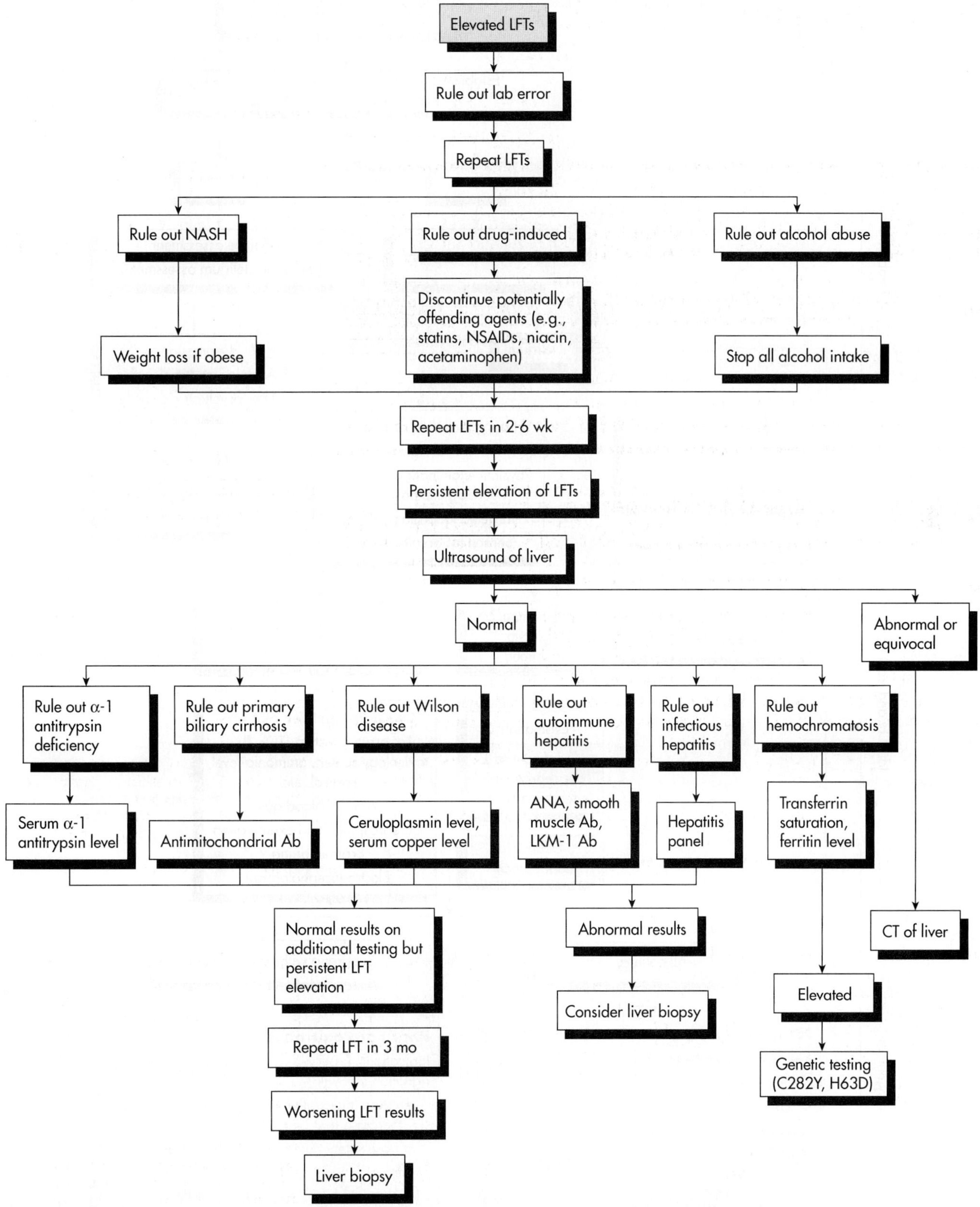

FIG. 112 Liver function test elevations. *Ab,* Antibody; *ANA,* antibody to nuclear antigens; *CT,* computed tomography; *LFTs,* liver function tests; *LKM,* liver-kidney microsome; *NASH,* nonalcoholic steatohepatitis; *NSAIDs,* nonsteroidal antiinflammatory drugs.

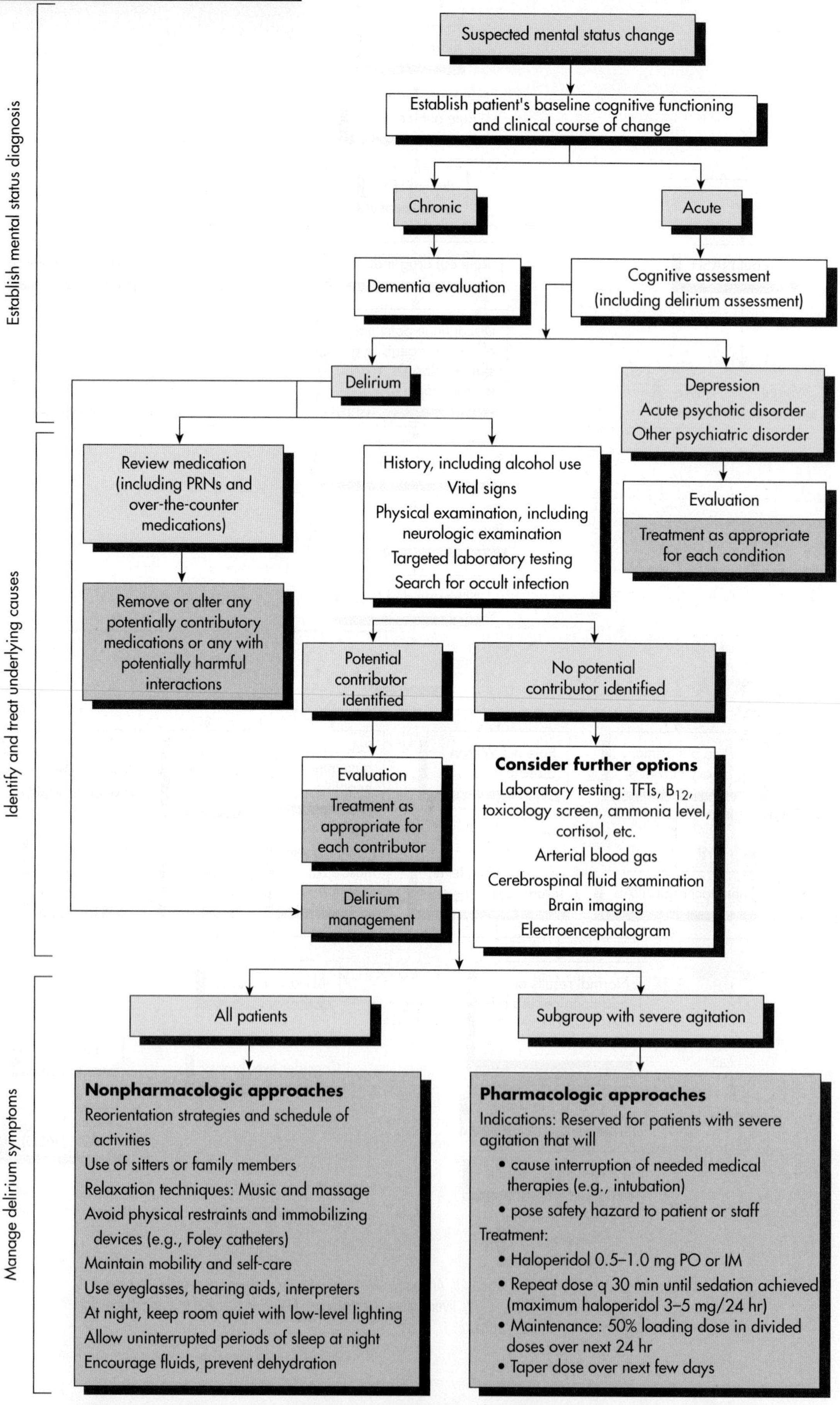

FIG. 113 Algorithm for the evaluation of suspected mental status change in older patients. *IM,* Intramuscular; *PO,* by mouth; *PRN,* as needed; *TFTs,* thyroid function tests. (From Goldman L, Schafer AI: *Goldman Cecil medicine*, ed 25, Philadelphia, 2016, Saunders.)

ICD-10CM # M25.50 Pain(s) joint
Arthralgia (allergic)
Arthrodynia
Polyarthralgia

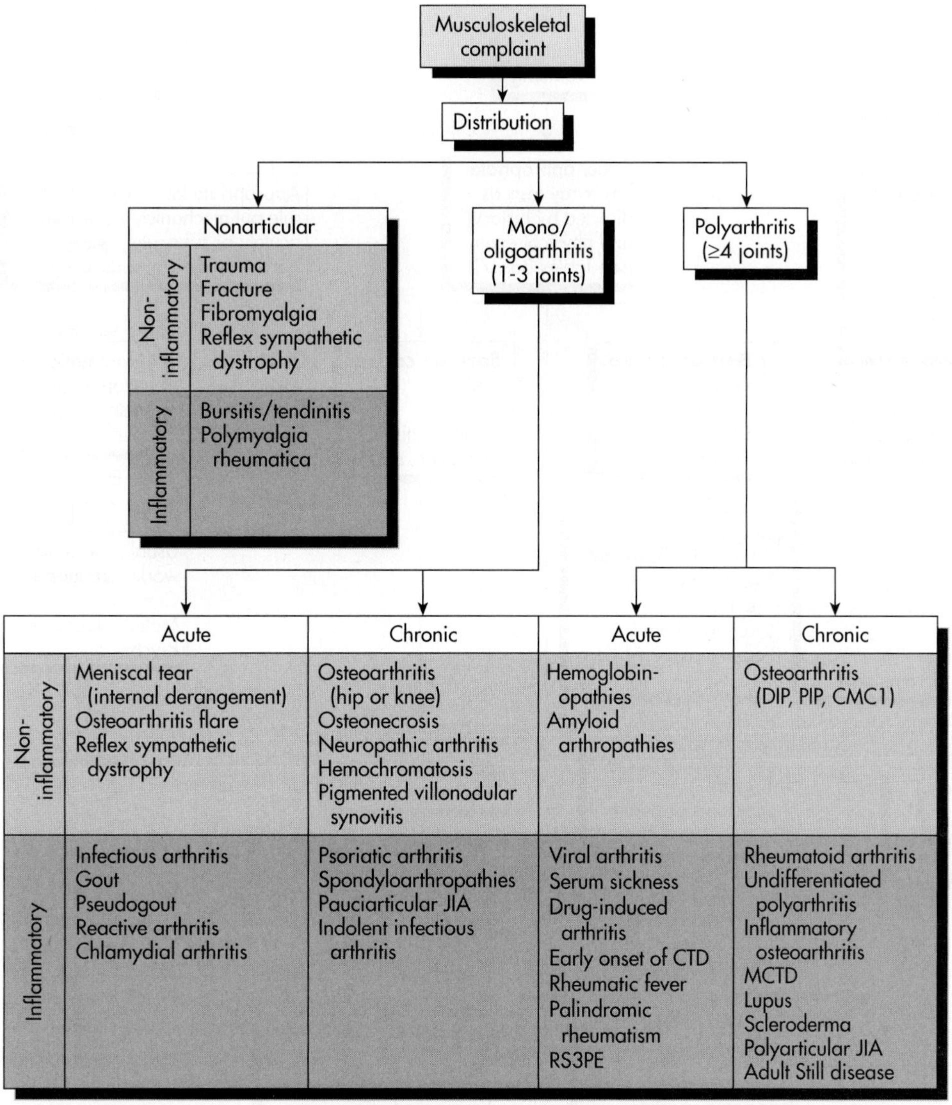

FIG. 114 Algorithm for assessing initial history and examination. *CMC,* Carpometacarpal; *CTD,* connective tissue disease; *DIP,* distal interphalangeal; *JIA,* juvenile idiopathic arthritis; *MCTD,* mixed connective tissue disease; *PIP,* proximal interphalangeal. (From Firestein GS et al: *Kelley's textbook of rheumatology*, ed 9, Philadelphia, 2013, Saunders.)

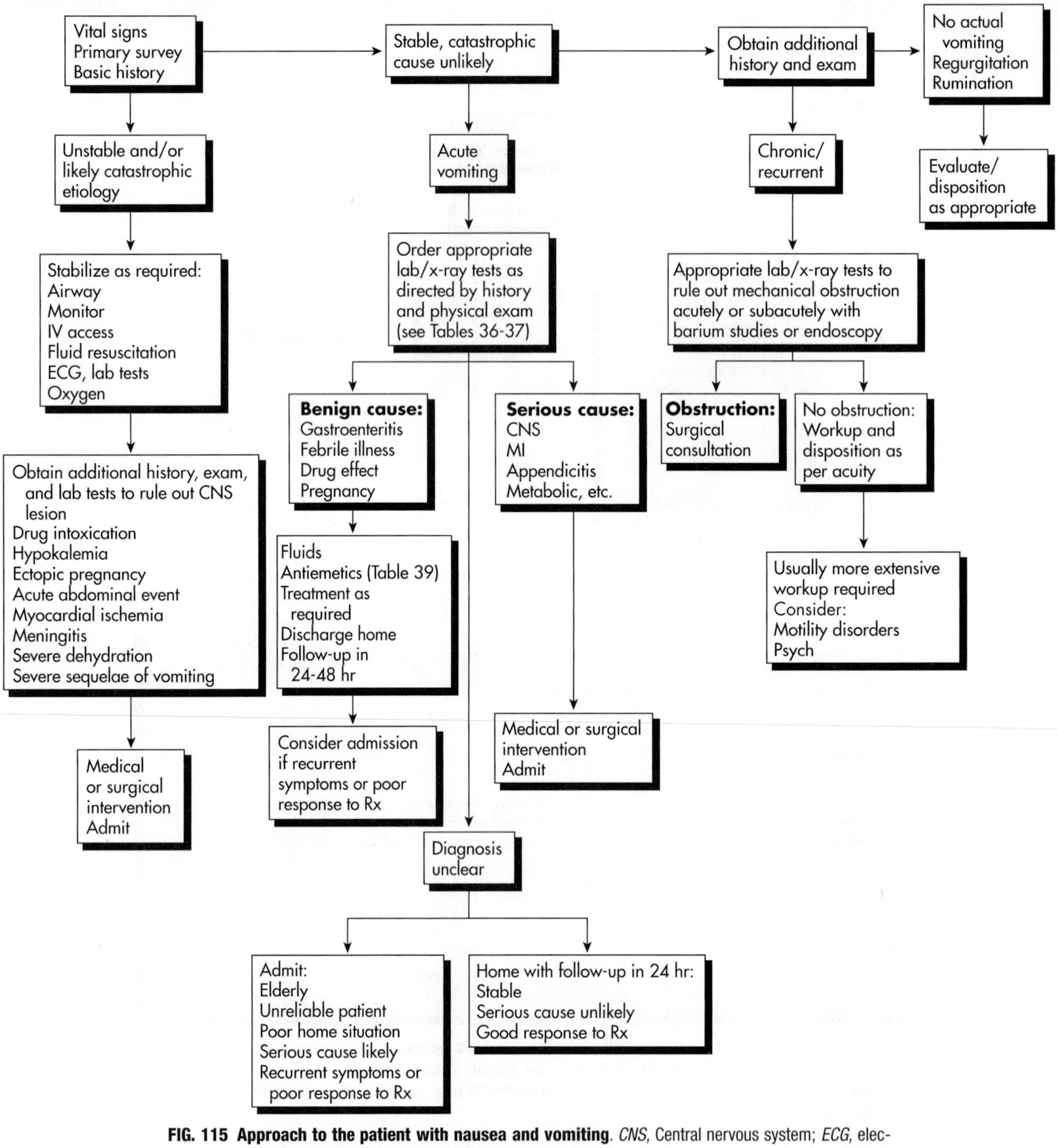

FIG. 115 Approach to the patient with nausea and vomiting. *CNS,* Central nervous system; *ECG,* electrocardiogram; *IV,* intravenous; *MI,* myocardial infarction; *Psych,* psychogenic; *Rx,* treatment. (From Marx JA et al: *Rosen's emergency medicine*, ed 8, Philadelphia, 2014, Saunders.)

TABLE 36 Differential Diagnosis of Nausea and Vomiting

Etiologic Category	Critical Diagnoses	Emergent Diagnoses	Nonemergent Diagnoses
Gastrointestinal (GI)	• Boerhaave syndrome • Ischemic bowel • GI bleeding	• Gastric outlet obstruction • Pancreatitis • Cholecystitis or cholangitis • Bowel obstruction or ileus • Ruptured viscus • Appendicitis • Peritonitis • Spontaneous bacterial peritonitis	• Gastritis • Gastroparesis • Peptic ulcer disease • Inflammatory bowel disease • Biliary colic • Hepatitis • Gastroenteritis
Neurologic	• Intracerebral bleed • Meningitis	• Migraine • CNS tumor • Raised ICP	
Endocrine	• DKA	• Adrenal insufficiency • Uremia	• Thyroid
Pregnancy		• Hyperemesis gravidarum	• Nausea and vomiting of pregnancy
Drug toxicity		• Acetaminophen • Digoxin • Aspirin • Theophylline	
Therapeutic drug use			• Aspirin • Antibiotics • Erythromycin • Ibuprofen • Chemotherapy
Drugs of abuse			• Narcotics • Narcotic withdrawal • Alcohol
Genitourinary		• Gonadal torsion	Urinary tract infection Poisoning Nephrolithiasis
Miscellaneous	• Myocardial infarction • Sepsis	• Carbon monoxide • Electrolyte disorders • Organophosphate poisoning	• Motion sickness • Labyrinthitis

CNS, Central nervous system; *DKA,* diabetic ketoacidosis; *ICP,* intracranial pressure.
From Marx JA et al: *Rosen's emergency medicine,* ed 8, Philadelphia, 2014, Saunders.

TABLE 37 Disorders Commonly Associated with Vomiting

Disorder	History	Prevalence	Physical Examination	Useful Tests	Comments
Nausea and vomiting of pregnancy (NVP)	Vomiting occurs predominantly in the morning. Associated breast tenderness. NVP typically starts in weeks 4-7, peaks in weeks 10-16, and disappears by week 20. Vomiting that begins after week 12 or continues past week 20 should prompt a search for another cause.	Very common Affects 75% of all pregnancies	Benign abdomen	Urine pregnancy test Serum electrolytes, urine ketones to exclude hyperemesis gravidarum	Consider NVP in all females of childbearing age. Prognosis for mother and infant is excellent. NVP is associated with a decreased risk of miscarriage, fetal growth retardation, and fetal mortality.
Hyperemesis gravidarum	Severe, protracted form of NVP. No universally accepted definition of the disease. Generally accepted hallmarks include 5% weight loss, ketonuria, and electrolyte disturbance. Hyperemesis is associated with multiple gestation, molar pregnancy, and nulliparity.	Uncommon Affects <1% of pregnancies	Signs of dehydration Benign abdomen	β-hCG Urinalysis for ketones Serum electrolytes Ultrasound examination to exclude molar pregnancy or multiple gestation	Most studies have found no adverse outcomes for the fetus. A few studies, however, have shown a correlation with fetal growth retardation.

TABLE 37 Disorders Commonly Associated with Vomiting—cont'd

Disorder	History	Prevalence	Physical Examination	Useful Tests	Comments
Gastroenteritis	Fever, diarrhea, and crampy abdominal pain. Vomiting and pain occur early, usually followed by diarrhea within 24 hr.	Very common	Benign abdomen	Usually not necessary	Early gastroenteritis, when only vomiting and periumbilical pain are present, may be confused with early appendicitis. Diarrhea is usually in the diagnosis of gastroenteritis.
Gastritis	Epigastric pain, belching, bloating, fullness, heartburn, and food intolerance. Use of NSAIDs or ETOH common.	Very common	Mild epigastric tenderness may be present.	Lipase and pregnancy test may be necessary to exclude other diagnoses.	Removal of inciting agent along with antacid therapy will resolve symptoms in most patients.
Peptic ulcer disease (PUD)	Epigastric pain present in 90% of cases. Classically, duodenal ulcer pain is relieved by food whereas gastric ulcer pain is made worse. Presence of severe pain should raise suspicion of perforation.	Very common	Mild epigastric tenderness	Hemoglobin if bleeding is suspected Heme-positive stool Upright abdominal film if perforation is suspected	Three major causes of PUD are NSAIDs, *Helicobacter pylori* infection, and hypersecretory states.
Biliary disease	Abdominal pain may be midepigastric or right upper quadrant (RUQ). Onset frequently after a fatty meal. May have history of similar episodes in the past.	Very common	RUQ tenderness present in most cases. If instructed to breathe deeply during palpation in the RUQ, the patient experiences heightened tenderness and inspiratory arrest (Murphy sign).	WBCs Lipase Serum bilirubin Alkaline phosphatase RUQ ultrasound examination ERCP	Normal temperature, WBCs, and spontaneous resolution of symptoms suggest biliary colic. Fever, Murphy sign, elevated WBCs, and suggestive ultrasound indicate cholecystitis.
Myocardial infarction (MI)	Patients typically have substernal chest pain that may radiate to left arm or jaw. Often associated with dyspnea, diaphoresis, or dizziness.	Common	Patients often are anxious and in distress from pain. No diagnostic examination findings.	ECG (new Q waves, ST segment changes, or T wave inversions) troponin	Not all patients have chest pain. A subset of patients, particularly diabetics and elders, may have only nausea, vomiting, and epigastric discomfort.
Diabetic ketoacidosis (DKA)	Polydipsia and polyuria occur early Without treatment, altered mental status and coma may develop. In patients with long-standing diabetes, DKA may be triggered by infection, trauma, MI, or surgery.	Common	"Fruity" breath odor results from serum acetone. Tachypnea occurs with attempts to "blow off" carbon dioxide to compensate for metabolic acidosis. Signs of dehydration may be present. Severe cases often manifest with altered mental status or coma.	Serum glucose, urine ketones, ABGs	DKA may be the first manifestation of diabetes in some patients. These patients often do not recognize the importance of polydipsia and polyuria. They often report only nausea, vomiting, and epigastric pain.
Pancreatitis	Presenting symptom is epigastric pain, which often radiates to the back. Most cases are caused by gallstones or alcoholism. Other causes include hypercalcemia, hyperlipidemia, drugs (sulfas and thiazides), ERCP.	Common	Epigastric tenderness is present. Associated paralytic ileus may cause abdominal distention and decreased bowel sounds. Frank shock may be present in severe cases.	Lipase WBCs, serum glucose, LDH, AST Hematocrit, BUN, calcium, ABGs	Criteria correlating with higher mortality: *At admission*—age >55 yr, WBCs >16,000/mm^3, glucose >200 dl, base deficit >4, LDH >350 IU/L, AST >250 U/L *Within 48 hr*—Hct drop of 10%, BUN >2 mg/dl, Po_2 <60 mm Hg, calcium <8 mg, fluid sequestration >4 L
Appendicitis	Abdominal pain classically begins in periumbilical region and later moves to right lower quadrant. Anorexia is common.	Common	Localized tenderness over right lower quadrant. Low-grade fever may be present.	WBCs Ultrasound Abdominal CT	Early appendicitis can be a difficult diagnosis to make. It is still frequently missed on the first physician encounter.
Bowel obstruction	Classically, abdominal pain consists of intermittent cramps occurring at regular intervals. The frequency of the cramps varies with the level of the obstruction; the higher the level, the more frequent the cramps. The location of the pain also varies with the level of the obstruction; high obstruction causes epigastric pain, midlevel obstruction causes periumbilical pain, colonic obstruction causes hypogastric pain.	Common	Abdominal distention, mild diffuse tenderness, and high-pitched "tinkling" bowel sounds may be present. Thorough search for hernias should be performed.	Supine and upright plain abdominal films Abdominal CT	Adhesions, hernias, and tumors account for 90% of bowel obstructions. Other causes include intussusception, volvulus, foreign bodies, gallstone ileus, inflammatory bowel disease, stricture, cystic fibrosis, and hematoma.

TABLE 37 Disorders Commonly Associated with Vomiting—cont'd

Disorder	History	Prevalence	Physical Examination	Useful Tests	Comments
Carbon monoxide (CO) poisoning	Headache is usually present. CO poisoning often occurs during winter months when furnaces are turned on. Family members may have similar symptoms if they also have been exposed.	Uncommon	No reliable signs of early CO poisoning	CO level	Because CO is a tasteless, odorless gas, patients may not realize they have been exposed. It is important to keep a high index of suspicion during the cold months.
Boerhaave syndrome	Patients may have neck, chest, or epigastric pain. Forceful, protracted vomiting usually causes the tear. Most cases follow a bout of heavy eating and drinking. Other reported causes include childbirth, defecation, seizures, and heavy lifting.	Uncommon	Tachypnea, tachycardia, and hypotension may be present. Escaped air from the esophagus may produce subcutaneous emphysema. Air in the mediastinum produces a "crunching" sound as the heart beats (Hamman sign).	CXR may show pleural effusion, widened mediastinum, pneumothorax, or pneumomediastinum. Esophagogram with water-soluble contrast is definitive.	The classic presentation includes forceful vomiting, severe chest pain, subcutaneous emphysema, and multiple CXR findings. There is a growing body of evidence that most cases do not have this "classic" picture. In more subtle presentations, the diagnosis can be difficult to make.

ABGs, Arterial blood gases; *AST,* aspartate aminotransferase; *β-hCG,* β-human chorionic gonadotropin; *BUN,* blood urea nitrogen; *CT,* computed tomography; *CXR,* chest radiography; *ECG,* electrocardiogram; *ERCP,* endoscopic retrograde cholangiopancreatography; *ETOH,* ethyl alcohol; *Hct,* hematocrit; *LDH,* lactate dehydrogenase; *NSAID,* nonsteroidal antiinflammatory drug; Po_2, partial pressure of oxygen; *RUQ,* right upper quadrant; *WBC,* white blood cell.
From Marx JA et al: *Rosen's emergency medicine,* ed 8, Philadelphia, 2014, Saunders.

TABLE 38 Etiology of Nausea and Vomiting in Pediatric Age Groups

Etiologic Category	Newborn	Infant	Child	Adolescent
Infectious	Sepsis, meningitis, UTI, thrush	Pneumonia, otitis media, thrush	Gastroenteritis	Gastroenteritis, URI
Anatomic	Atresia and webs, malrotation, stenosis, meconium ileus, Hirschsprung disease	Pyloric stenosis, intussusception, Hirschsprung disease	Bezoars, chronic granulomatous disease	PUD, superior mesenteric syndrome
Gastrointestinal	Reflux, overfeeding, gastric outlet obstruction, volvulus	Reflux, gastritis, milk intolerance	Appendicitis, pancreatic, hepatitis, other food intolerance	Achalasia, hepatitis
Neurologic	Subdural hematoma, hydrocephalus	Subdural hematoma	Neoplasia, migraine, Reye syndrome, motion sickness, hypertension	Neoplasia, migraine, motion sickness, hypertension
Metabolic	Organic or amino acidemias, urea cycle defects, galactosemia, hypercalcemia, phenylketonuria, kernicterus	Hereditary fructose intolerance, disorders of fatty acid metabolism, uremia, adrenal hyperplasia, kernicterus	Diabetes, vitamin A excess	Diabetes, pregnancy, acute intermittent porphyria
Other	Idiopathic, cardiac failure	Rumination, cardiac failure	Cyclic vomiting syndrome, toxins, food poisoning, Munchausen syndrome by proxy	Psychogenic, anorexia

PUD, Peptic ulcer disease; *URI,* upper respiratory infection; *UTI,* urinary tract infection.
Adapted from Li HK, Sunku BK: Vomiting and nausea. In Wyllie R, Hyams JS (eds): *Pediatric gastrointestinal and liver disease: pathophysiology, diagnosis, management,* Philadelphia, 2005, Saunders; 127-149. From Marx JA et al: *Rosen's emergency medicine,* ed 8, Philadelphia, 2014, Saunders.

TABLE 39 Commonly Used Medications for the Treatment of Nausea and Vomiting

Medication	Dose	Comments
Promethazine (Phenergan)	*Adult:* 12.5-25 mg IV, IM, PO, or by rectum *Pediatric:* 0.25-1 mg/kg/dose q4-6h prn IV, IM, PO, or by rectum; max 25 mg/dose	May be repeated every 4-6 hr until cessation of vomiting. May cause dry mouth, dizziness, blurred vision. Boxed warning for use under 2 yr old.
Prochlorperazine (Compazine)	*Adult:* 5-10 mg IM or PO; 2.5-10 mg IV; 25 mg by rectum *Pediatric:* 0.4 mg/kg/24 hr tid-qid PO or by rectum; 0.1-0.15 mg/kg/dose tid-qid IM; max 40 mg/24 hr	May be repeated every 4 hr IV or IM or every 12 hr by rectum until cessation of vomiting. May cause lethargy, hypotension, extrapyramidal effects.
Metoclopramide (Reglan)	*Adult:* 10 mg IM or IV, may repeat q6h *Pediatric:* 1-2 mg/kg/dose q2-6h IV q2-3h	May cause dystonic reactions, tardive dyskinesia, neuroleptic malignant syndrome.
Ondansetron (Zofran)	*Adult:* 4 mg IV single dose *Pediatric:* Up to 40 kg: 0.1 mg/kg; >40 kg: 4 mg/dose IV single dose	May cause headache, dizziness, and musculoskeletal pain.

IM, Intramuscularly; *IV,* intravenously; *PO,* orally; *prn,* as needed; *q,* every.
From Marx JA et al: *Rosen's emergency medicine,* ed 8, Philadelphia, 2014, Saunders.

ICD-10CM # R22.1 Localized swelling, mass and lump, neck
R22.0 Localized swelling, mass and lump, head

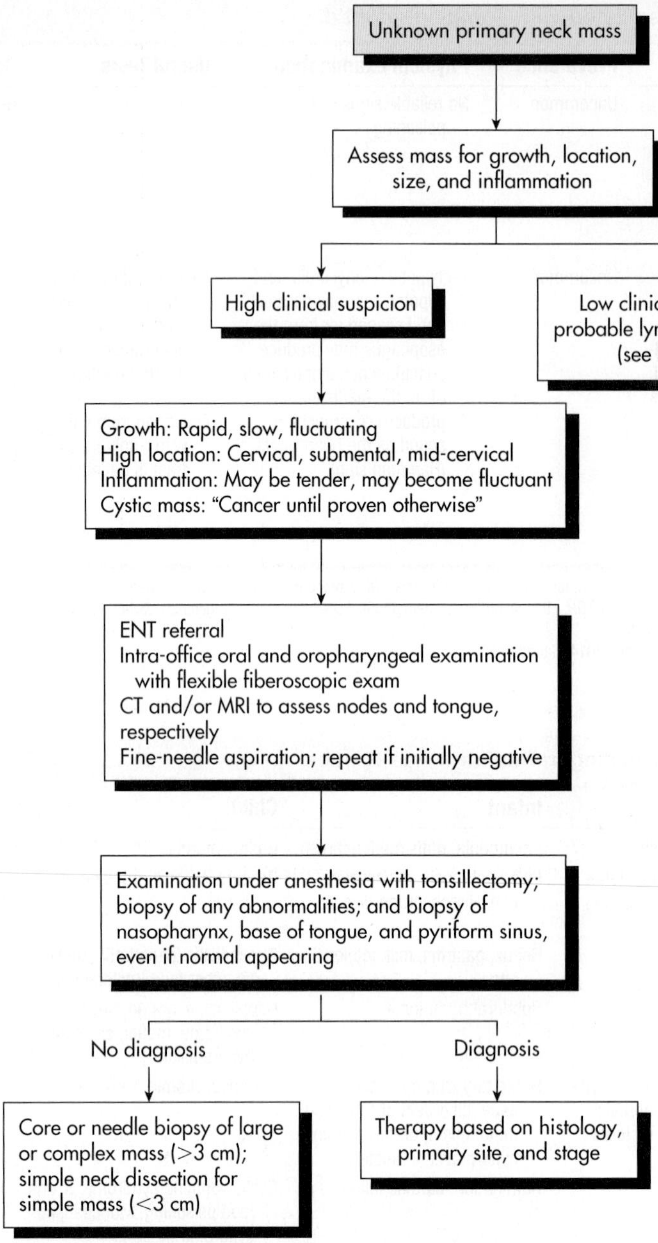

FIG. 116 Evaluation of an unknown primary neck mass. *CT,* Computed tomography; *ENT,* ear, nose, and throat; *MRI,* magnetic resonance imaging. (From Goldman L, Schafer AL [eds]: *Cecil textbook of medicine,* ed 24, Philadelphia, 2012, Saunders.)

BOX 16 An Approach to the Patient with Lymphadenopathy

- Does the patient have a known illness that causes lymphadenopathy? Treat and monitor for resolution.
- Is there an obvious infection to explain the lymphadenopathy (e.g., infectious mononucleosis)? Treat and monitor for resolution.
- Are the nodes very large and/or very firm and thus suggestive of malignancy? Perform a biopsy.
- Is the patient very concerned about malignancy and unable to be reassured that malignancy is unlikely? Perform a biopsy.
- If none of the preceding are true, perform a complete blood cell count, and if it is unrevealing, monitor for a predetermined period (usually 2-6 wk). If the nodes do not regress or if they increase in size, perform a biopsy.

From Goldman L, Ausiello D (eds): *Cecil textbook of medicine*, ed 23, Philadelphia, 2008, Saunders.

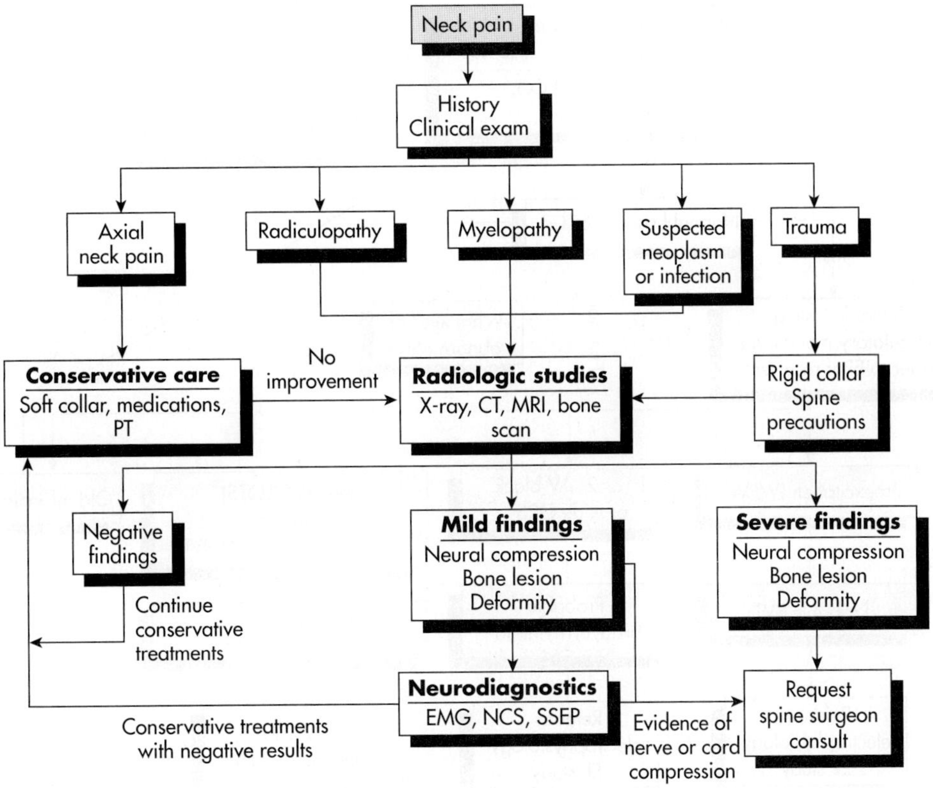

FIG. 117 Algorithm of neck pain. *CT,* Computed tomography; *EMG,* electromyogram; *MRI,* magnetic resonance imaging; *NCS,* nerve conduction study; *PT,* physical therapy; *SSEP,* somatosensory evoked potentials. (From Firestein GS et al: *Kelley's textbook of rheumatology,* ed 9, Philadelphia, 2013, Saunders.)

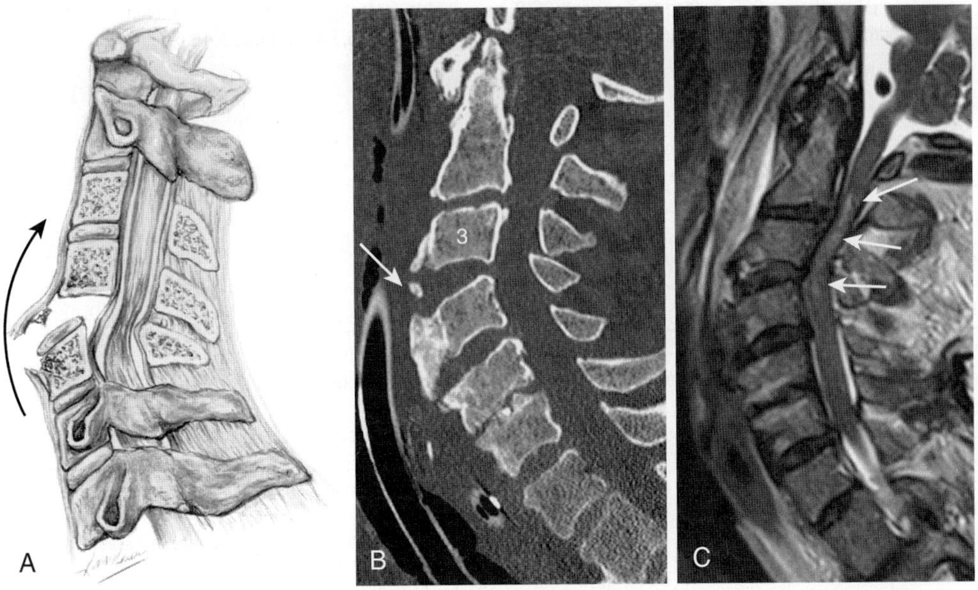

FIG. 118 Extension injury. A, Drawing shows mechanism and injury. There is a small avulsion from the anterosuperior margin of the vertebra immediately below the affected level. Note the wide disk space and retrolisthesis, hallmarks of this injury. The spinal cord is frequently injured in this setting. **B,** Sagittal reconstructed computed tomography image shows widening of the C3 disk space with an avulsed fragment of bone *(arrow)* and retrolisthesis. **C,** T2-weighted magnetic resonance image shows cord hemorrhage *(arrows).* The patient is quadriplegic. (From Pope TL et al: *Musculoskeletal imaging,* ed 2, Philadelphia, 2015, Elsevier.)

ICD-10CM # R42 Dizziness and giddiness
R55 Syncope and collapse

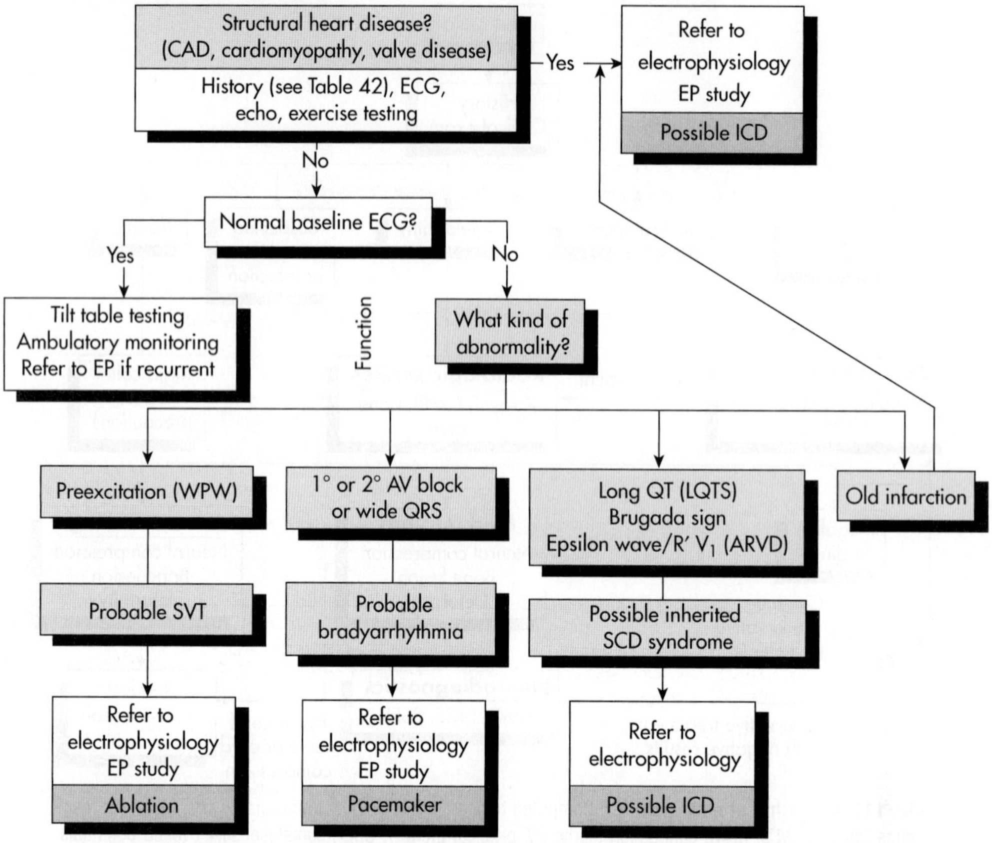

FIG. 121 Algorithm for evaluating patients with symptoms of palpitation, dizziness, or syncope. *ARVD,* Arrhythmogenic right ventricular dysplasia; *AV,* atrioventricular; *CAD,* coronary artery disease; *ECG,* electrocardiogram; *echo,* echocardiogram; *EP,* electrophysiology; *ICD,* implantable cardioverter-defibrillator; *LQTS,* long QT syndrome; *SCD,* sudden cardiac death; *SVT,* supraventricular tachycardia; *WPW,* Wolff-Parkinson-White syndrome. (From Goldman L, Schafer AI: *Goldman Cecil medicine,* ed 25, Philadelphia, 2016, Saunders.)

TABLE 42 Items to Be Covered in History of Patient with Palpitation

Does the Palpitation Occur:	If So, Suspect:
As isolated "jumps" or "skips"?	Extrasystoles
In attacks known to be of abrupt beginning, with a heart rate of 120 beats/min or over, with regular or irregular rhythm?	Paroxysmal rapid heart action
Independent of exercise or excitement adequate to account for the symptom?	Atrial fibrillation, atrial flutter, thyrotoxicosis, anemia, febrile states, hypoglycemia, anxiety state
In attacks developing rapidly, though not absolutely abruptly, unrelated to exertion or excitement?	Hemorrhage, hypoglycemia, tumor of the adrenal medulla
In conjunction with the taking of drugs?	Tobacco, coffee, tea, alcohol, epinephrine, ephedrine, aminophylline, atropine, thyroid extract, monoamine oxidase inhibitors
On standing?	Postural hypotension
In middle-aged women, in conjunction with flushes and sweats?	Menopausal syndrome
When the rate is known to be normal and the rhythm regular?	Anxiety state

From Goldman L, Braunwald E: Chest discomfort and palpitation. In Isselbacher KJ, Braunwald E et al (eds): *Harrison's principles of internal medicine,* ed 13, New York, 1994, McGraw-Hill.

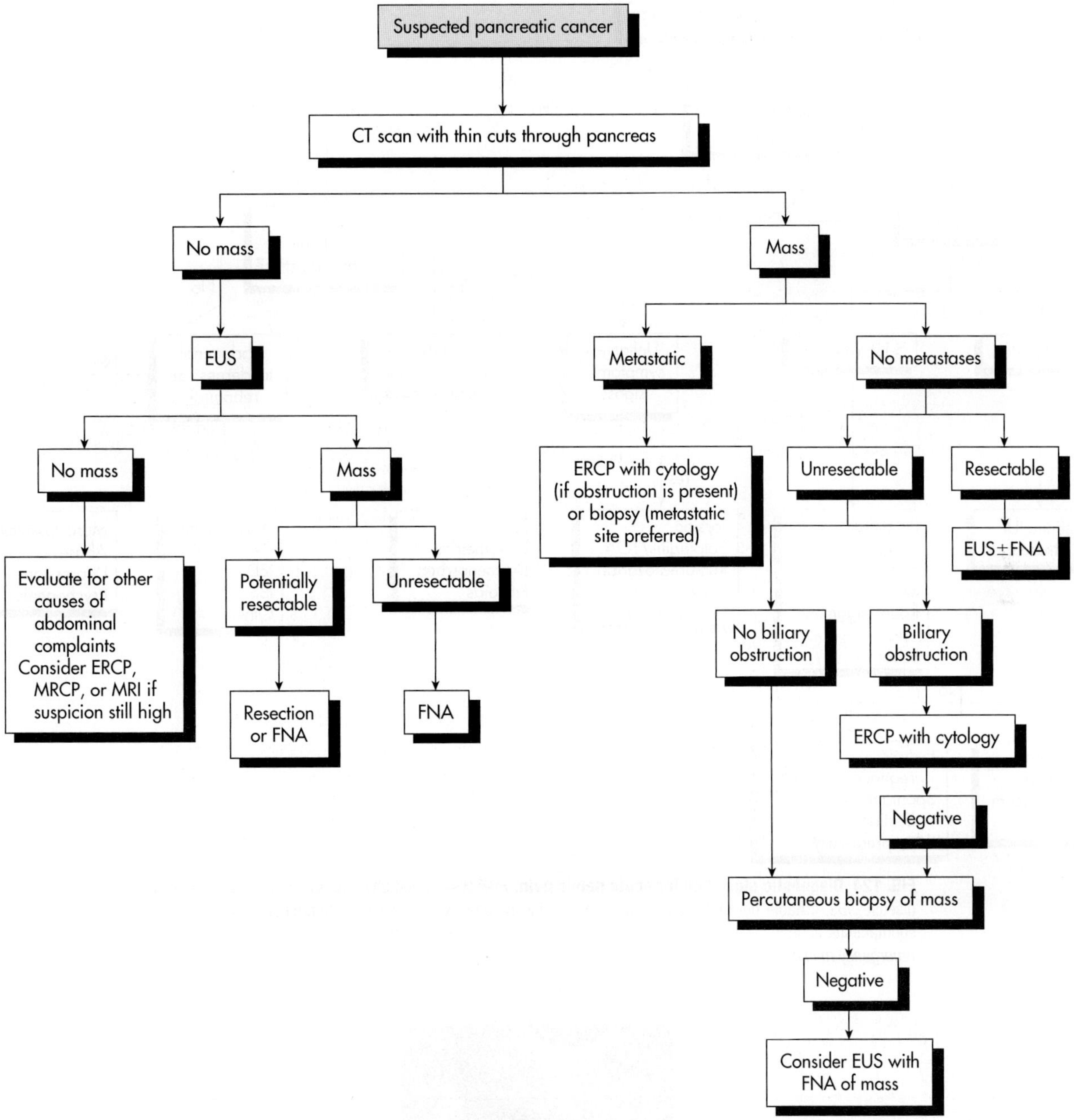

FIG. 123 Diagnostic algorithm for pancreatic cancer. Intraoperative fine-needle aspiration (FNA) if found inoperable during surgery. *CT,* Computed tomography; *ERCP,* endoscopic retrograde cholangiopancreatography; *EUS,* endoscopic ultrasonography; *MRCP,* magnetic resonance cholangiopancreatography; *MRI,* magnetic resonance imaging. (From Goldman L, Schafer AL [eds]: *Cecil textbook of medicine,* ed 24, Philadelphia, 2012, Saunders.)

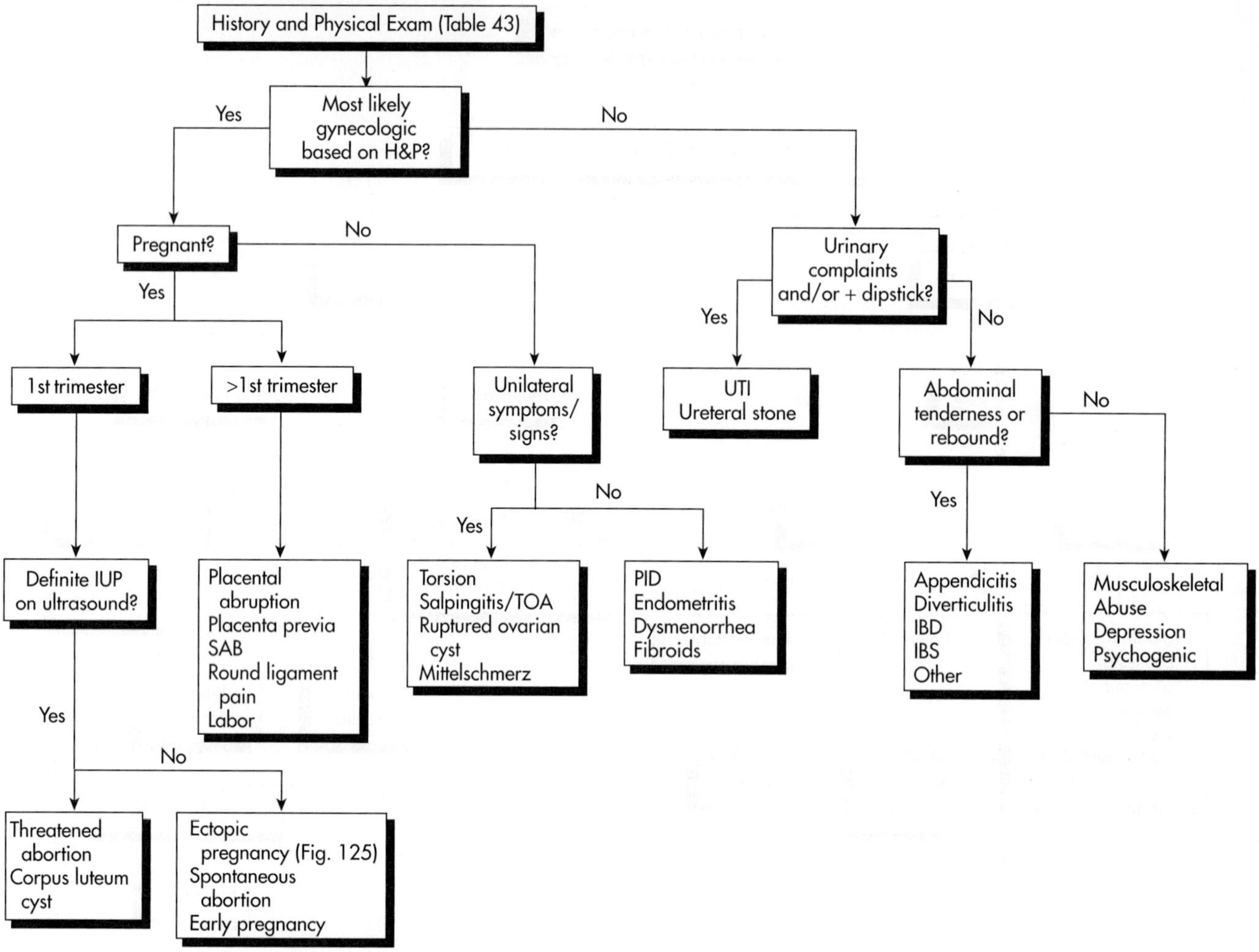

FIG. 124 Diagnostic algorithm for acute pelvic pain. *H&P,* History and physical; *IBD,* inflammatory bowel disease; *IBS,* irritable bowel syndrome; *IUP,* intrauterine pregnancy; *PID,* pelvic inflammatory disease; *SAB,* spontaneous abortion; *TOA,* tubo-ovarian abscess; *UTI,* urinary tract infection. (From Marx JA et al: *Rosen's emergency medicine*, ed 8, Philadelphia, 2014, Saunders.)

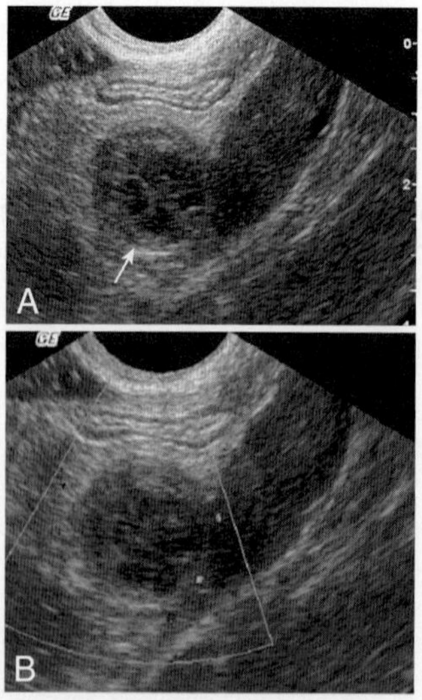

FIG. 125 Ectopic pregnancy seen as mixed-echogenicity mass. A 30-yr-old woman presented with left lower quadrant pain at 7 wk gestation and β-hCG of 500 mIU/ml and falling over a 3-day period. **A,** In the left adnexa, medial to the left ovary, there was a 2-cm mass *(arrow)* with mixed echogenicity, and **B,** only minimal peripheral vascularity. A left ectopic pregnancy was confirmed and, based on a falling β-hCG, was treated expectantly and resolved without complication. (From Rumack CM et al: *Diagnostic ultrasound,* ed 4, Philadelphia, 2011, Elsevier.)

TABLE 43 Differentiation of Common or Potentially Catastrophic Causes of Pelvic Pain

Causative Disorder or Condition	Pain History	Associated Symptoms	Supporting History	Prevalence in ED	Physical Examination	Useful Tests	Atypical or Additional Aspects
Ectopic pregnancy (critical if ruptured)	Classically severe, sharp, lateral pelvic pain, but severity, location, and quality highly variable	Vaginal bleeding (often mild, can be absent)	Missed period; history of previous ectopic pregnancy, infertility, pelvic surgery, PID, or IUD use	Common	Classically unilateral adnexal tenderness, adnexal mass, and CMT	Pelvic US, quantitative β-hCG, T&C, laparoscopy	Cannot reliably exclude diagnosis based on history and physical examination. Severe pain, hypotension, or peritonitis suggests rupture
Ruptured ovarian cyst (emergent—critical with significant hemorrhage; otherwise, urgent)	Abrupt moderate to severe lateral pain	Light-headedness if bleeding is severe; rectal pain arises from fluid in cul-de-sac		Uncommon	Hypotension and tachycardia if blood loss is significant; possible peritonitis	Pelvic US, CBC, T&C	Physical examination findings often do not correlate with volume of blood in pelvis at US
Ovarian torsion (emergent)	Acute onset of moderate to severe lateral pain	Nausea and vomiting	History of ovarian mass or cyst	Uncommon	Adnexal mass and tenderness, possible peritonitis	US with Doppler flow studies, laparoscopy	Torsion can be intermittent
Appendicitis (emergent)	Duration often <48 hr, generalized followed by localized RLQ pain	Low-grade fever, nausea, anorexia	Migration of pain to RLQ from center, abdominal pain before vomiting	Common	RLQ tenderness, possible peritonitis	US or CT in unclear cases	Early in course, tenderness may be minimal or poorly localized
PID, TOA (TOA: Emergent; PID: Urgent-emergent)	Without TOA, pain usually bilateral. May manifest acutely within 48 hr or subacutely with up to 3 wk of pain	Fever, vaginal discharge	Vaginal discharge, history of PID, history of unprotected intercourse or multiple partners	PID: Common TOA: Uncommon	Pus from cervical os, CMT, adnexal tenderness. Peritonitis suggests severe PID or TOA	CBC, ESR, CRP, pelvic US, laparoscopy, cervical cultures, cervical smear for WBCs	History and physical examination may be inaccurate for diagnosis, particularly in patients with subacute presentation
UTI (urgent)	Pain with urination. Patient may have flank pain from associated pyelonephritis	Urinary urgency and frequency; fever and vomiting if patient has associated pyelonephritis	Recent urologic procedure, prior history of UTI	Common	Suprapubic tenderness, flank tenderness and fever with pyelonephritis	Urinalysis, urine culture (if recurrent or complicated)	WBCs can be present in urine with PID and appendicitis. RBCs present in urine with hemorrhagic cystitis
Ureteral colic (urgent)	Acute onset, manifests within hours. Pain is lateral, usually moderate to severe. Often radiates into the groin or costovertebral angle or flank	Nausea and vomiting	Prior history of stones	Common	Patient often appears uncomfortable, but physical examination can be otherwise unremarkable	Urinalysis: Hematuria present in approximately 80% of cases. Renal ultrasound for hydronephrosis. Abdominal CT	If stone is at ureterovesicular junction, patient can have localized pain that can mimic appendicitis or other acute pelvic pathology
Unruptured ovarian cyst or tumor	Lateral ache, gradual onset	Often minimal	Prior history of similar pain	Common	Lateral pelvic tenderness, with or without a mass	Pelvic US	
Endometriosis	Unilateral or bilateral pelvic pain, often recurrent	Dysmenorrhea, dyspareunia	Prior history of same type of pain in association with menstrual cycle	Common	Unilateral or bilateral adnexal tenderness, occasionally pelvic mass present, peritoneal findings uncommon	Pelvic US, laparoscopy	Symptoms can mimic other types of pelvic pathology; laparoscopy often is needed for confirmation

β-*hCG*, β-Human chorionic gonadotropin; *CBC*, complete blood count; *CMT*, cervical motion tenderness; *CRP*, C-reactive protein; *CT*, computed tomography; *ED*, emergency department; *ESR*, erythrocyte sedimentation rate; *IUD*, intrauterine device; *PID*, pelvic inflammatory disease; *RBC*, red blood cell; *RLQ*, right lower quadrant; *T&C*, type and crossmatch; *TOA*, tubo-ovarian abscess; *US*, ultrasonography; *UTI*, urinary tract infection; *WBC*, white blood cell.

From Marx JA et al: *Rosen's emergency medicine*, ed 8, Philadelphia, 2014, Saunders.

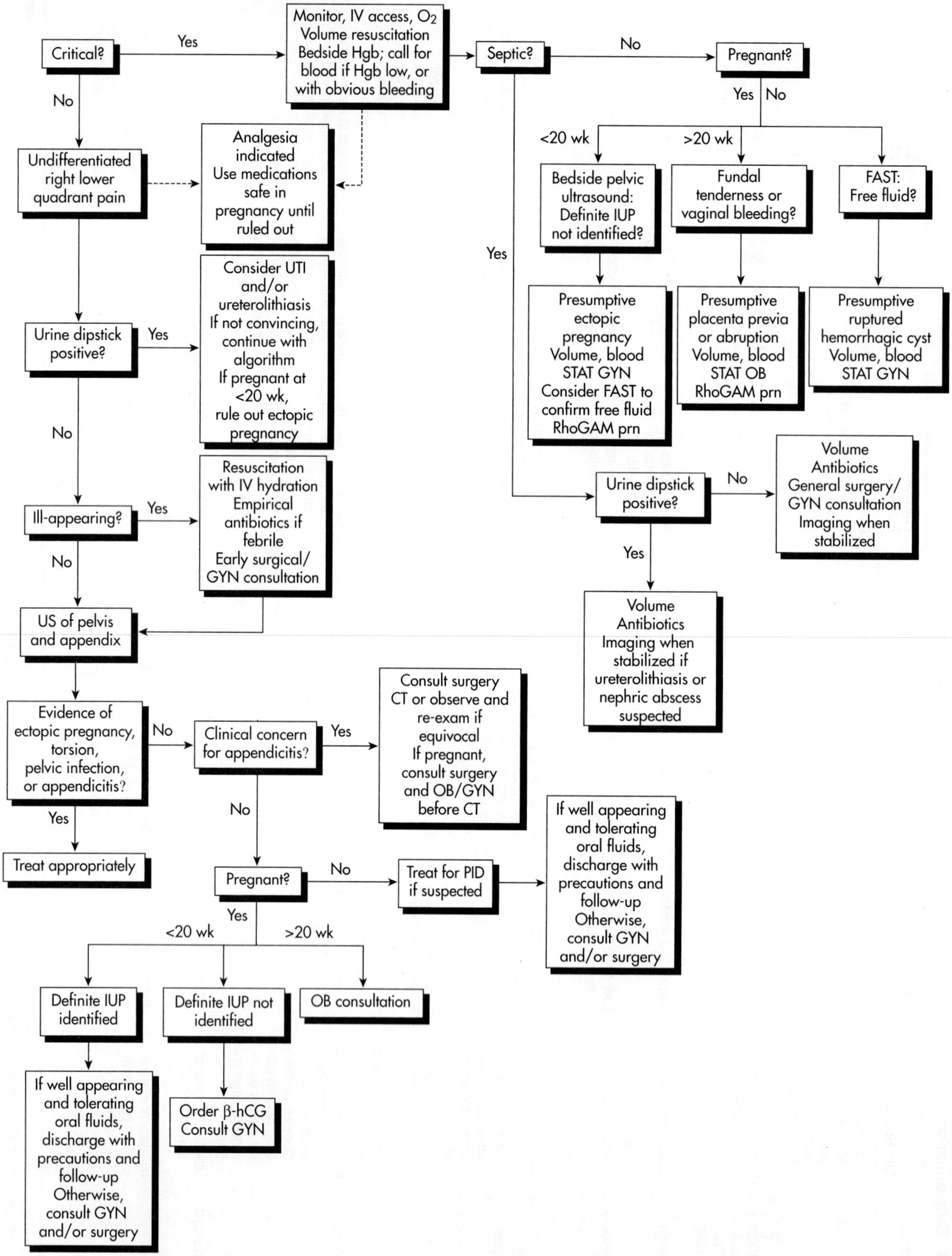

FIG. 126 Management algorithm for acute pelvic pain: Critical patients and right lower quadrant pain presentations. β-*hCG*, β-Human chorionic gonadotropin; *CT*, computed tomography; *FAST*, focused assessment with sonography for trauma; *GYN*, gynecology; *Hgb*, hemoglobin; *IUP*, intrauterine pregnancy; *IV*, intravenous; *OB*, obstetrics; *PID*, pelvic inflammatory disease; *prn*, as needed; *STAT*, immediately; *US*, ultrasound; *UTI*, urinary tract infection. (From Marx JA et al: *Rosen's emergency medicine*, ed 8, Philadelphia, 2014, Saunders.)

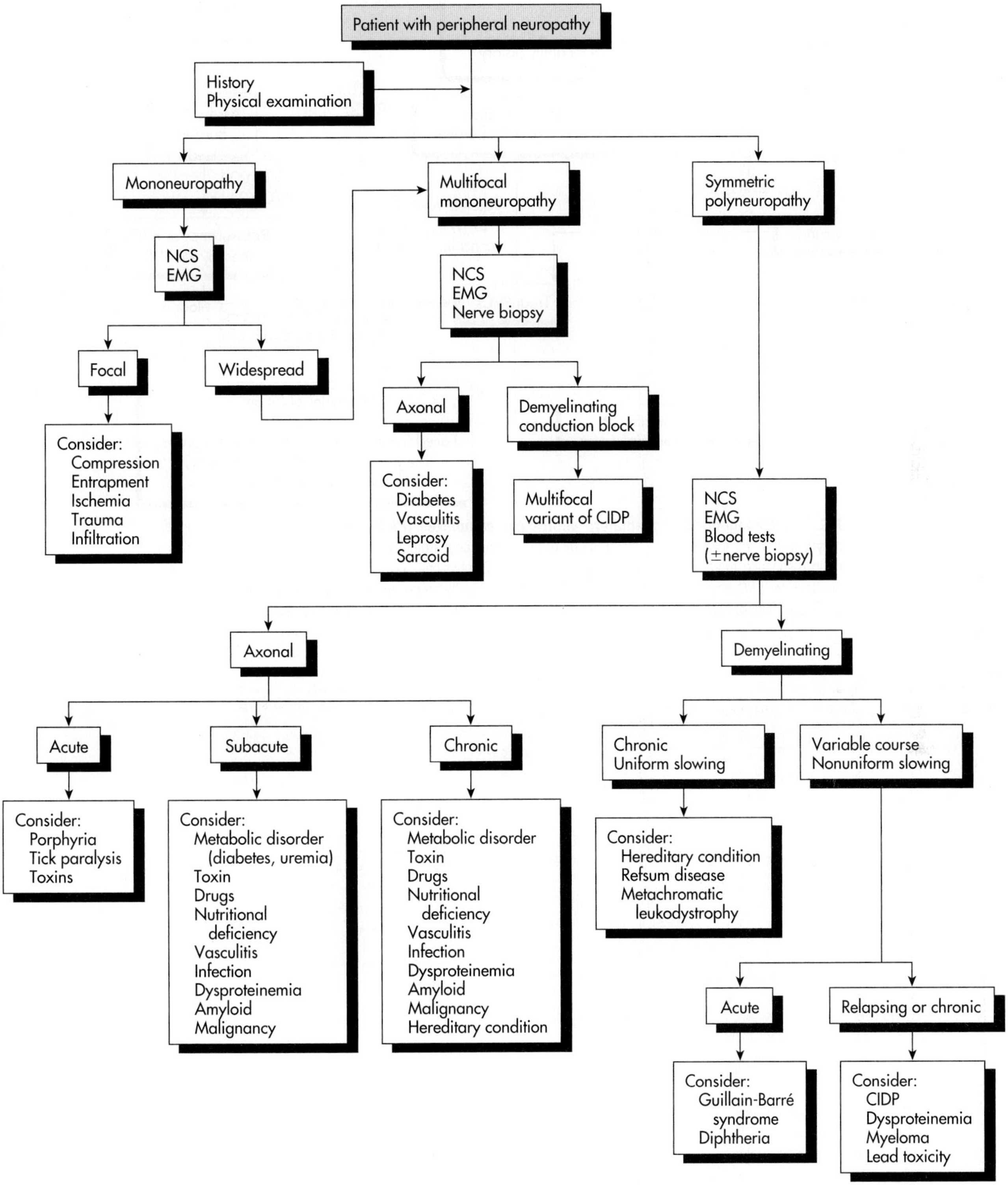

FIG. 127 Approach to the patient with peripheral neuropathy. *CIDP,* Chronic inflammatory demyelinating polyradiculopathy; *EMG,* electromyogram; *NCS,* nerve conduction studies. (Modified from Greene HL et al: *Decision making in medicine*, ed 2, St Louis, 1988, Mosby.)

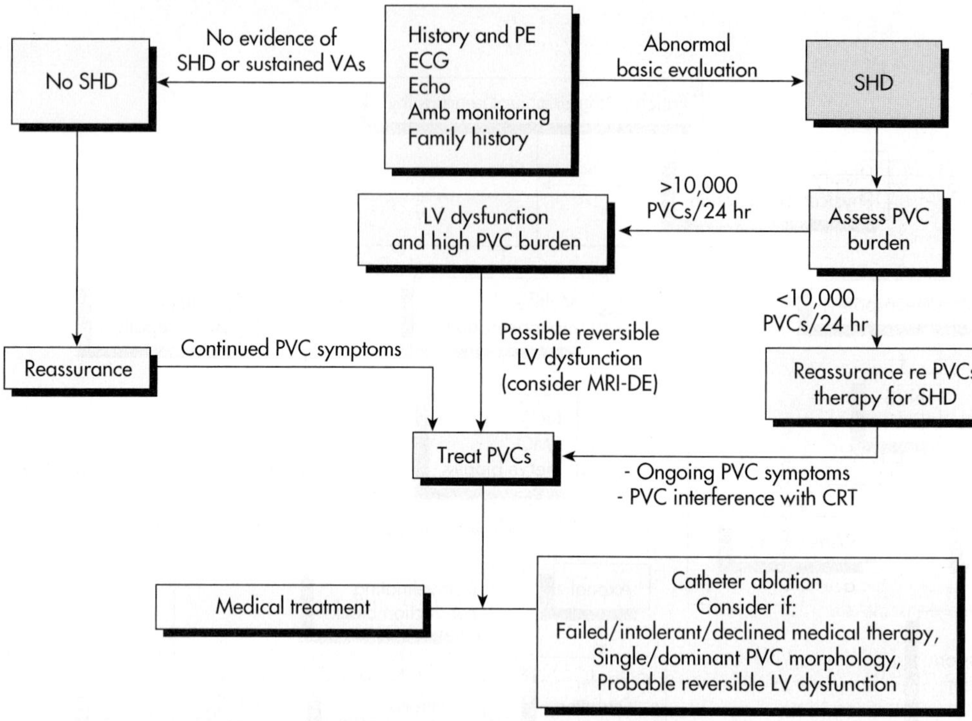

FIG. 131 Management of premature ventricular complexes *(PVCs)*. *Amb,* Ambulatory; *CRT,* cardiac resynchronization therapy; *ECG,* electrocardiogram; *Echo,* echocardiogram; *LV,* left ventricular; *MRI-DE,* magnetic resonance imaging with delayed enhancement; *PE,* physical examination; *PVC,* premature ventricular contraction; *SHD,* structural heart disease; *VAs,* ventricular arrhythmias. (From Parrillo JE, Dellinger RP: *Critical care medicine, principles of diagnosis and management in the adult,* ed 5, Philadelphia, 2019, Elsevier.)

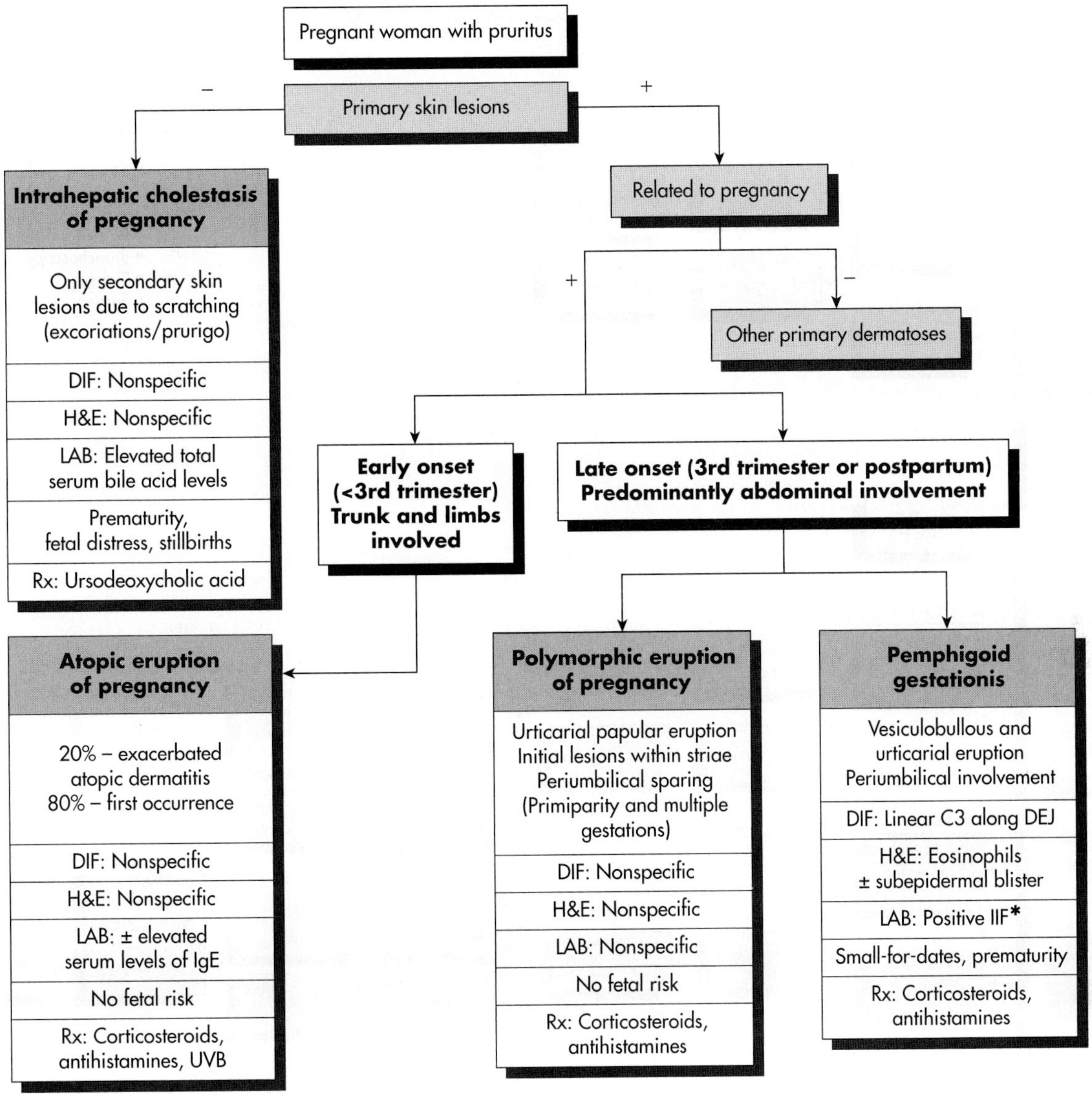

DEJ, Dermal – epidermal junction; *DIF*, direct immunofluorescence; *H&E*, hematoxylin and eosin-stained histologic sections; *IIF*, indirect immunofluorescence; *LAB*, laboratory findings; *Rx*, treatment.

*Conventional – 30%; complement-added – nearly all.

FIG. 133 Approach to the pregnant woman with pruritus. Patients with refractory pemphigoid gestationis may benefit from plasmapheresis during pregnancy. (From Ambros-Rudolph CM, Müllegger RR, Vaughan-Jones SA, et al: The specific dermatoses of pregnancy revisited and reclassified. Results of a retrospective two-center study on 505 pregnant patients. *J Am Acad Dermatol* 2006; 54: pp. 395-404.)

BOX 17 Causes of Pruritus with and without Skin Disease

With Skin Disease

Drugs, scabies, pediculosis, insect bites, parasites (roundworm)
Eczema
Contact dermatitis
Urticaria
Lichen planus
Pityriasis rosea ("Herald" patch)
Dermatitis herpetiformis (gluten sensitivity)

Without Skin Disease

Hepatobiliary—jaundice, including primary biliary cirrhosis
Chronic renal failure
Hematologic:
- Lymphoma
- Polycythaemia rubra vera

Endocrine:
- Myxoedema
- Thyrotoxicosis

Carcinoma:
- Lung
- Stomach

Drugs

From Cameron P et al: *Textbook of adult emergency medicine*, ed 5, Philadelphia, 2020, Elsevier.

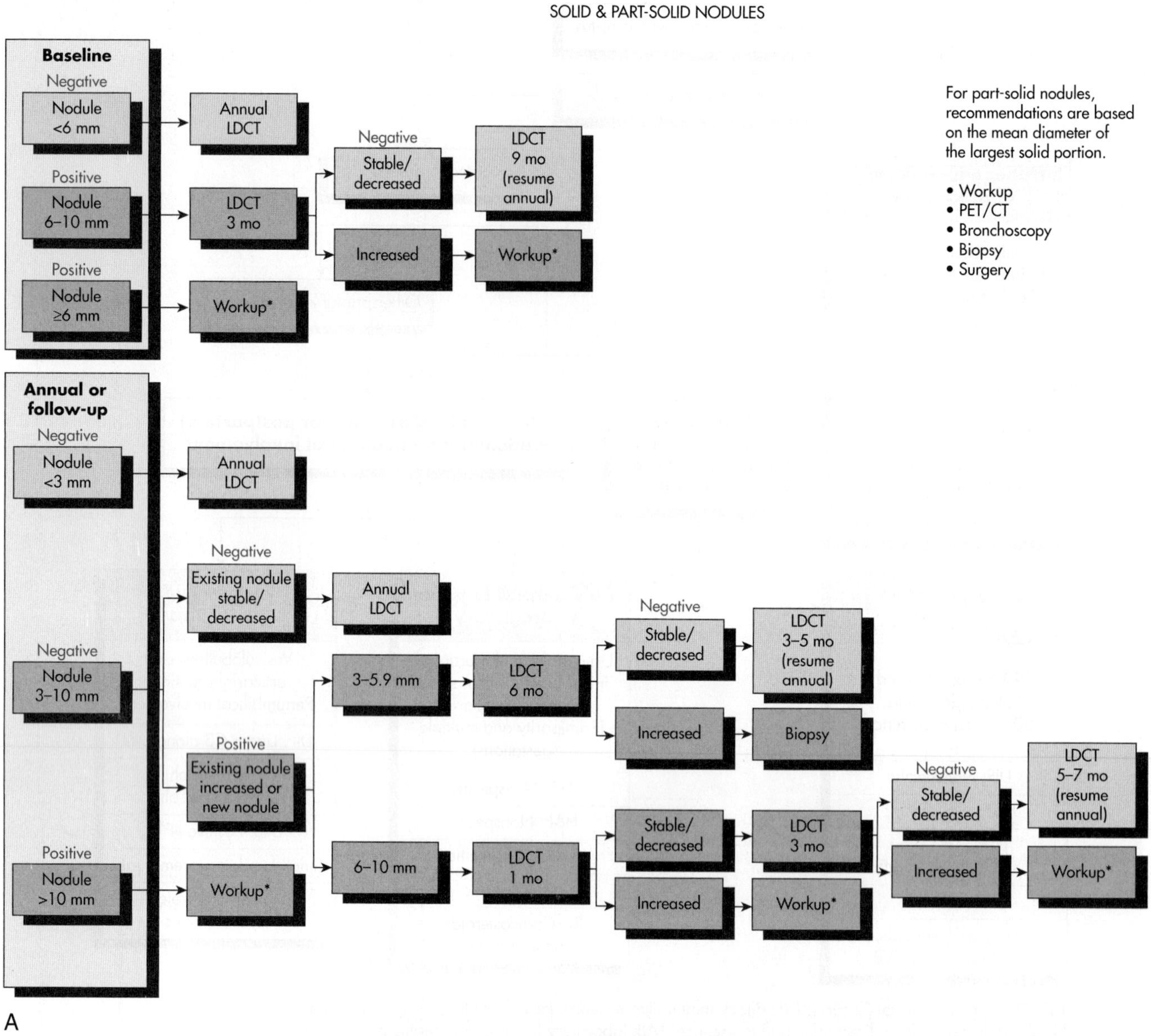

FIG. 135 The diagnostic algorithm for (A) solid or part-solid nodules and (B) nonsolid nodules. This algorithm was created through discussion by a multidisciplinary group composed of thoracic surgeons, radiologists, pulmonologists, oncologists, and pathologists. *Workup is at the discretion of the treating physicians but typically consists of a PET/CT and tissue diagnosis, either by bronchoscopy, CT-guided biopsy, or for highly suspicious nodules, minimally invasive surgery. *CT,* Computed tomography; *LDCT,* low-dose computed tomography; *PET,* positron emission tomography. (From Sellke FW: *Sabiston & Spencer surgery of the chest,* ed 9, Philadelphia, 2016, Elsevier. The Fleishner Society recommendations for computed tomography follow-up of pulmonary nodules are summarized in Tables 46-48.)

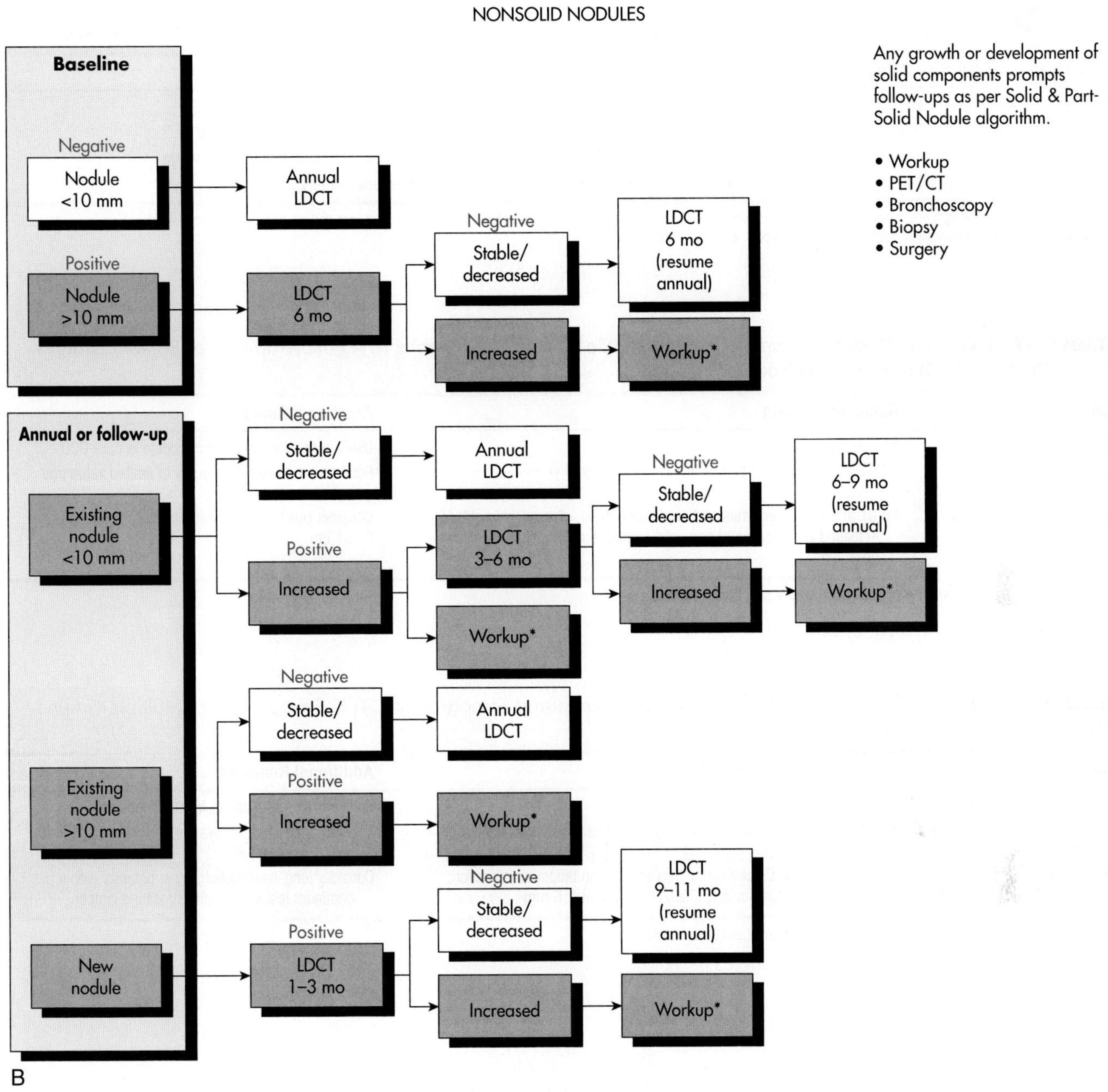

FIG. 135 (Continued)

TABLE 46 Fleischner Society Recommendations for Computed Tomography (CT) Follow-up (FU) of Solid Nodules*

Nodule Size	Low-Risk Patient	High-Risk Patient
≤4 mm	No FU CT needed (FU is optional)	FU CT at 12 mo; if unchanged, no further FU
>4-6 mm	FU CT at 12 mo; if unchanged, no further FU	FU CT at 6-12 mo, then at 18-24 mo if no change
>6-8 mm	FU CT at 6-12 mo, then at 18-24 mo if no change	FU CT at 3-6 mo, then at 9-12 and 24 mo if no change
>8 mm	Options: FU CT at 3, 9, and 24 mo; positron emission tomography; biopsy; video-assisted thoracic surgery	

*Nodule size is average of length and width. Low-risk patient, minimal or absent history of smoking or other known risk factors; high-risk patient, history of smoking or other known risk factors.
From Webb WR et al: *Fundamentals of body CT*, ed 4, Philadelphia, 2015, Saunders.

TABLE 47 Fleischner Society Recommendations for Computed Tomography (CT) Follow-up (FU) of Solitary Ground-Glass Opacity (GGO) or Part-GGO Nodules

Nodule Type	Recommendation	Additional Remarks
Solitary pure GGO ≤5 mm	No FU CT required	Use 1-mm slices to confirm nodule is pure GGO
Solitary pure GGO >5 mm	FU CT at 3 mo; if persistent, yearly FU for at least 3 yr	Positron emission tomography of limited value and not recommended
Solitary part-solid nodules	FU CT at 3 mo; if persistent and solid component <5 mm, yearly FU for at least 3 yr; if persistent and solid component ≥5 mm, then biopsy or resection	Consider positron emission tomography if nodule >1 cm

From Webb WR et al: *Fundamentals of body CT*, ed 4, Philadelphia, 2015, Saunders.

TABLE 48 Fleischner Society Recommendations for Computed Tomography (CT) Follow-up (FU) of Multiple Ground-Glass Opacity (GGO) or Part-GGO Nodules

Nodule Type	Recommendation	Additional Remarks
Multiple pure GGO ≤5 mm	FU CT at 2 and 4 yr	Consider alternate cause for GGO nodules
Multiple pure GGO >5 mm; no dominant lesion	FU CT at 3 mo; if persistent, yearly FU for at least 3 yr	Positron emission tomography of limited value and not recommended
Dominant part-solid nodule(s)	FU CT at 3 mo; if persistent, then biopsy or resection, particularly if solid component ≥ 5 mm	Consider lung-sparing surgery in patients with a dominant lesion suspicious for lung cancer

From Webb WR et al: *Fundamentals of body CT*, ed 4, Philadelphia, 2015, Saunders.

ICD-10CM # D69.0 Allergic purpura
D69.2 Other nonthrombocytopenic purpura
D69.49 Other primary thrombocytopenia
M31.1 Thrombotic microangiopathy

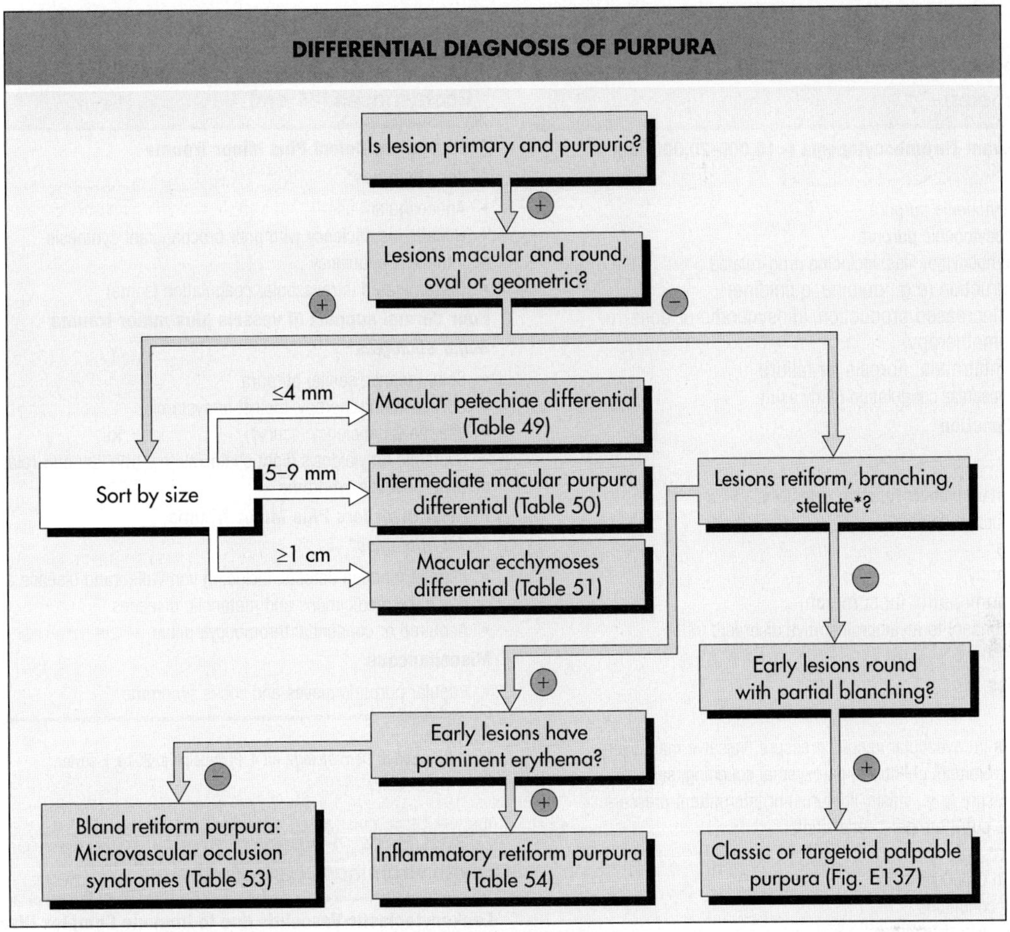

FIG. 136 Differential diagnosis of purpura. *Very few lesions are truly stellate, that is, characterized by a central area of necrosis or hemorrhage with radiating extensions, but some authors continue to use this term to describe these lesions. (From Bolognia J: *Dermatology,* ed 4, Philadelphia, 2018, Elsevier.)

ICD-10CM # D69.0 Allergic purpura
D69.2 Other nonthrombocytopenic purpura
D69.49 Other primary thrombocytopenia
M31.1 Thrombotic microangiopathy

TABLE 49 Differential Diagnosis of Macular Petechiae (≤4 mm in diameter)

Hemostatically Relevant Thrombocytopenia (<10,000-20,000/mm³)*

Major etiologies†

- Idiopathic thrombocytopenic purpura
- Thrombotic thrombocytopenic purpura
- Other acquired thrombocytopenias, including drug-related
  - Peripheral destruction (e.g., quinine, quinidine)
  - Drug-induced decreased production, idiosyncratic or dose-related (e.g., chemotherapy)
  - Bone marrow infiltration, fibrosis, or failure
- Disseminated intravascular coagulation (early sign)

Abnormal Platelet Function

Major etiologies†

- Congenital or hereditary platelet function defects
- Acquired platelet function defects
  - Aspirin, NSAIDs
  - Renal insufficiency
  - Monoclonal gammopathy (uncommon)
- Thrombocytosis secondary to myeloproliferative disorders (often >1,000,000/mm³)

Nonplatelet Etiologies

major etiologies†

- Spiking elevations of intravascular venous pressure (Valsalva maneuver-like, e.g., repetitive vomiting, childbirth, paroxysmal coughing, seizure)
- Fixed increased pressure (e.g., stasis, ligatures) or intermittent pressure (e.g., blood pressure cuff [Rumpel-Leede sign])
- Trauma (often linear)
- Perifollicular (vitamin C deficiency)
- Mildly inflammatory conditions
  - Pigmented purpuric eruptions
  - Hypergammaglobulinemic purpura of Waldenström

NSAID, Nonsteroidal antiinflammatory drug.
*Platelets provide factors necessary for hemostasis of endothelial cell junctions. When counts fall below 10,000-20,000/mm³, inadequate platelet support leads to degradation of junction function, increased permeability, and hemorrhage.[3]
†Partial list.
From Bolognia J: *Dermatology,* ed 4, Philadelphia, 2018, Elsevier.

TABLE 50 Differential Diagnosis of Intermediate Macular Purpura (5-9 mm)

Major Etiologies*

- Hypergammaglobulinemic purpura of Waldenström
- Infection/inflammation in patients with thrombocytopenia
- Rarely, minimally inflamed cutaneous small vessel vasculitis (usually dependent distribution)

*Partial list.
From Bolognia J: *Dermatology,* ed 4, Philadelphia, 2018, Elsevier.

TABLE 51 Differential Diagnosis of Macular Ecchymoses (≥1 cm)

Procoagulant Defect Plus Minor Trauma

Major etiologies*

- Anticoagulant use
- Hepatic insufficiency with poor procoagulant synthesis
- Vitamin K deficiency
- Disseminated intravascular coagulation (some)

Poor dermal support of vessels plus minor trauma

Major etiologies*

- Solar (actinic, senile) purpura
- Corticosteroid therapy, topical or systemic
- Vitamin C deficiency (scurvy)
- Systemic amyloidosis (light chain-related, transthyretin-related
- Ehlers-Danlos syndrome

Platelet Disorders Plus Minor Trauma

Major etiologies*

- Platelet function defects, including von Willebrand disease and those induced by medications and metabolic diseases
- Acquired or congenital thrombocytopenia

Miscellaneous

- Papular purpuric gloves and socks syndrome

*Partial list.
From Bolognia J: *Dermatology,* ed 4, Philadelphia, 2018, Elsevier.

TABLE 52 Palpable Purpura: Inflammatory Purpura with Prominent Early Erythema

Leukocytoclastic Vasculitis due to Immune Complex Disease

Small vessels only

- Idiopathic, infection- or drug-associated IgG or IgM complexes
- Idiopathic IgA complexes (HSP), or IgA complexes associated with drugs or infection
- Hypergammaglobulinemic purpura of Waldenström
- Urticarial vasculitis: Often minimally purpuric
- Pustular vasculitis (e.g., bowel bypass syndrome)

Small- and medium-sized (macroscopic) vessels may be involved

- Mixed cryoglobulinemia
- Rheumatic vasculitides (LE, RA, Sjögren syndrome)

Pauci-immune leukocytoclastic vasculitis

ANCA-associated

- Granulomatosis with polyangiitis
- Microscopic polyangiitis
- Eosinophilic granulomatosis with polyangiitis (Churg-Strauss syndrome)

Other

- Erythema elevatum diutinum
- Sweet syndrome (vasculitis unusual)

Not leukocytoclastic vasculitis

Small vessels only

- Erythema multiforme
- Pityriasis lichenoides et varioliformis acuta (PLEVA)
- Pigmented purpuric eruptions
- Hypergammaglobulinemic purpura of Waldenström (although some lesions have histologic evidence of leukocytoclastic vasculitis)

Classic target lesion—usually erythema multiforme, but can be small vessel vasculitis, especially IgA-associated

ANCA, Antineutrophil cytoplasmic antibodies; *IgG,* immunoglobin G; *IgM,* immunoglobin M; *HSP,* Henoch-Schönlein purpura; *LE,* lupus erythematosus; *RA,* rheumatoid arthritis.
Modified from Bolognia J: *Dermatology,* ed 4, Philadelphia, 2018, Elsevier.

TABLE 53 Differential Diagnosis of Noninflammatory Retiform Purpura

Occlusion Primarily due to Platelet-Related Thrombopathy

Major etiologies*

- Heparin-induced thrombocytopenia syndrome (HITS)
- Thrombocytosis secondary to myeloproliferative disorders
- Paroxysmal nocturnal hemoglobinuria
- Thrombotic thrombocytopenic purpura (though platelet plugs form primarily in visceral vessels, and skin hemorrhage is due more often to thrombocytopenia)

Cold-related precipitation or agglutination

Major etiologies*

- Cryoglobulinemia, usually monoclonal (early lesions of mixed cryoglobulinemia are more often inflammatory and leukocytoclastic due to immune complex deposition)
- Cryofibrinogenemia (though most cryofibrinogens are incidental findings in hospitalized patients)
- Cold agglutinins (rarely cause occlusion; usually cause hemolysis or are asymptomatic)

Occlusion due to organisms growing in vessels

Major etiologies*

- Vessel-invasive fungi (e.g., *Mucor* spp., *Aspergillus* spp.; usually in immunocompromised patients)
- Ecthyma gangrenosum (often *Pseudomonas* spp. or other gram-negative bacilli proliferating in adventitia of subcutaneous arterioles)
- Disseminated strongyloidiasis
- Lucio phenomenon of Hansen disease
- Rocky Mountain spotted fever, other rickettsial spotted fevers

Systemic alteration in control of coagulation

Major etiologies*

- Protein C- and S-related
  - Homozygous protein C or protein S deficiency
  - Acquired protein C deficiency (some patients with sepsis-associated DIC)
  - Warfarin necrosis** (protein C dysfunction)
  - Postinfectious purpura fulminans (protein S dysfunction)
  - Antiphospholipid antibody, lupus anticoagulant
  - Levamisole-adulterated cocaine^

Vascular coagulopathy

- Livedoid vasculopathy/atrophie blanche (may also have a systemic prothrombotic component)
- Malignant atrophic papulosis/Degos disease (antiphospholipid antibody syndrome can mimic this disease)
- Sneddon syndrome (can be related to antiphospholipid antibody syndrome)
- Deficiency of adenosine deaminase 2 (ADA2)

Embolization or crystal deposition

Major etiologies*

- Cholesterol emboli
- Oxalate crystal deposition (rare)
- Marantic endocarditis, atrial myxoma, crystal globulins, hypereosinophilic syndrome (all rare)

Reticulocyte, red blood cell occlusion

- Sickle cell disease
- Severe malaria (usually *Plasmodium falciparum*)

Miscellaneous

- Cutaneous calciphylaxis
- Brown recluse (*Loxosceles*) spider bite reaction
- Intravascular B-cell lymphoma
- Hydroxyurea (rare)

DIC, Disseminated intravascular coagulation.
*Partial list.
**Also referred to as Coumadin® necrosis.
^Early lesions primarily thrombotic, but vasculitis can also occur.
From Bolognia J: *Dermatology,* ed 4, Philadelphia, 2018, Elsevier.

TABLE 54 Differential Diagnosis of Inflammatory Retiform Purpura

Vasculitis

Primarily dermal vessels

- IgA vasculitis

Dermal and Subcutaneous Vessels Usually Involved

- Mixed cryoglobulinemia
- Rheumatic vasculitides (LE, RA)
- Polyarteritis nodosa
- Microscopic polyangiitis
- Granulomatosis with polyangiitis
- Eosinophilic granulomatosis with polyangiitis (Churg-Strauss syndrome)

Dermal Vessel Inflammation/Occlusion/Constriction

- Livedoid vasculopathy
- Septic vasculitis
- Chilblains (pernio)
- Pyoderma gangrenosum

IgA, Immunoglobin A; *LE,* Lupus erythematosus; *RA,* rheumatoid arthritis.
From Bolognia J: *Dermatology,* ed 4, Philadelphia, 2018, Elsevier.

RASH, ACUTE GENERALIZED SKIN ERUPTION

ICD-10CM # R21 Rash and other nonspecific skin eruption

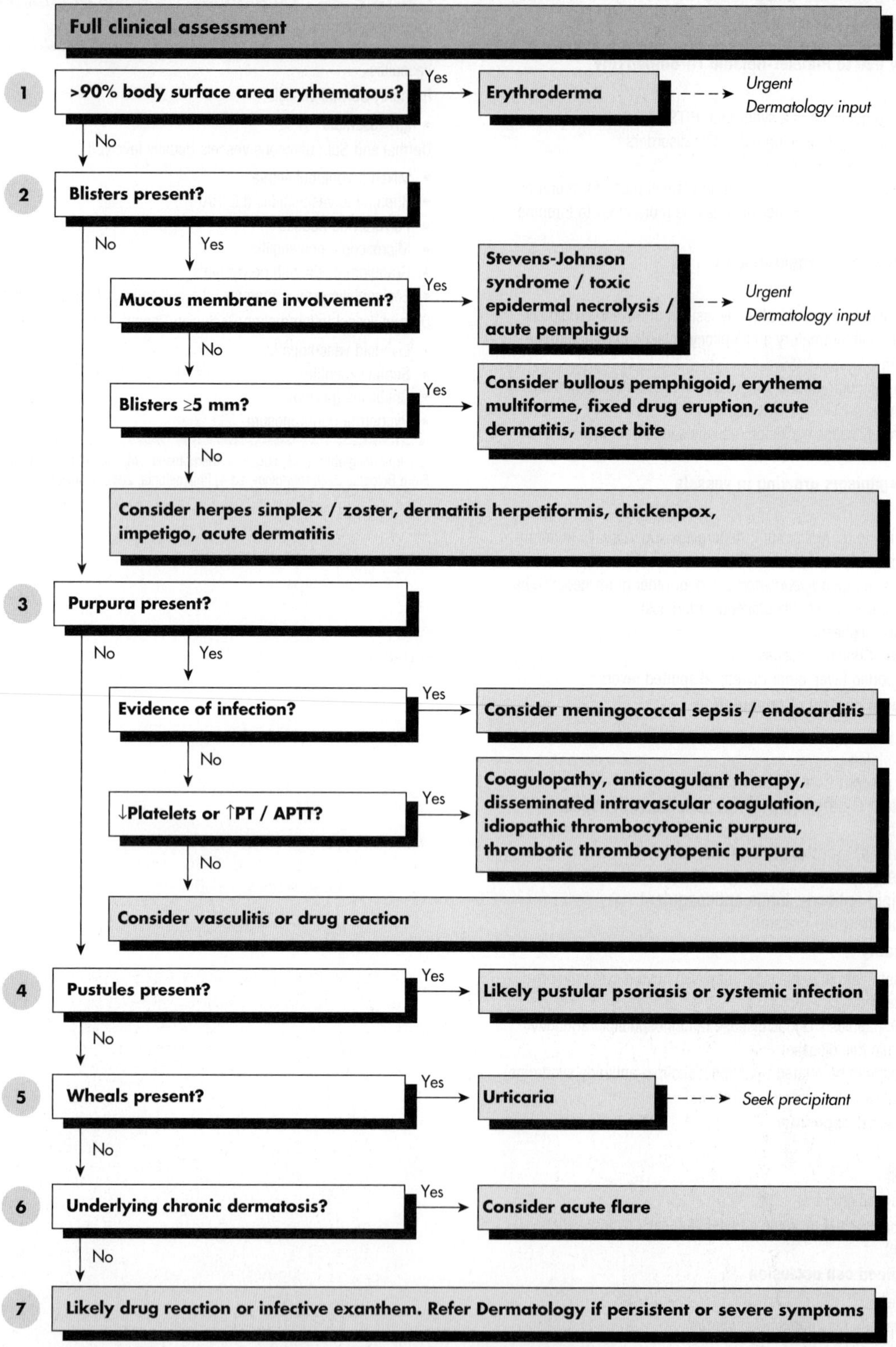

FIG. 138 Rash: Acute generalized skin eruption. *APTT,* Activated partial thromboplastin time; *PT,* prothrombin time. (From Gawkrodger DJ: *Dermatology ICT,* ed 4, Edinburgh, 2008, Churchill Livingstone; Japp AG, Robertson C: *Macleod's clinical diagnosis,* ed 2, Philadelphia, 2018, Elsevier.)

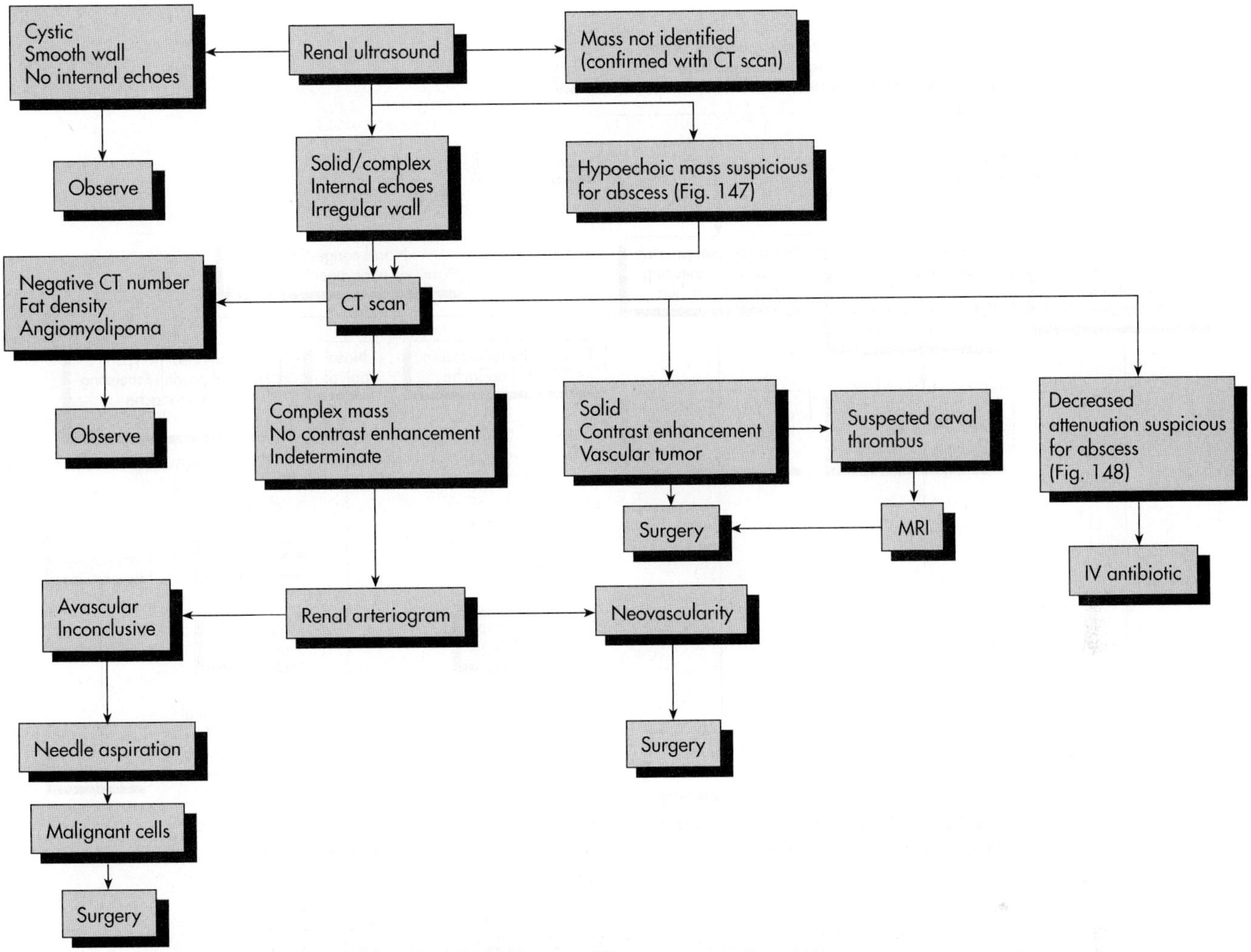

FIG. 146 Evaluation of a patient with a renal mass on renal ultrasound. *CT,* Computed tomography; *MRI,* magnetic resonance imaging. (Modified from Williams RD: Tumors of the kidney, ureter, and bladder. In Goldman L, Schafer AL [eds]: *Cecil textbook of medicine,* ed 23, Philadelphia, 2008, Saunders.)

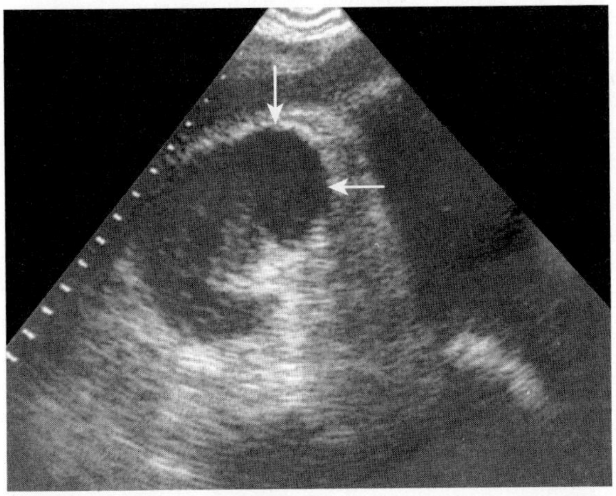

FIG. 147 Acute renal abscess. Transverse ultrasound image of the right kidney demonstrates a poorly marginated rounded focal hypoechoic mass *(arrows)* in the anterior portion of the kidney. (From Wein AJ et al: *Campbell-Walsh urology,* ed 11, Philadelphia, 2016, Elsevier.)

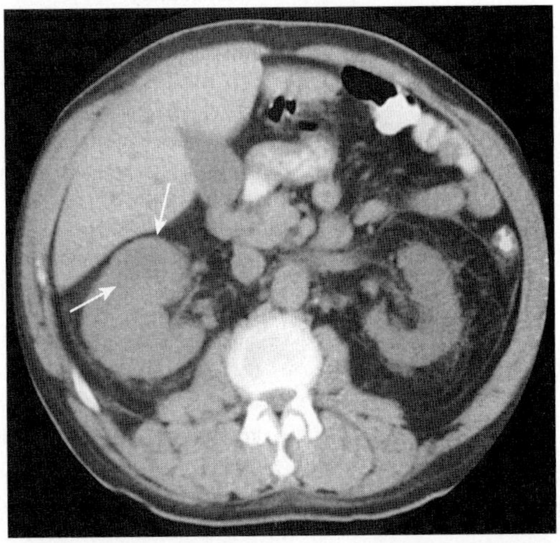

FIG. 148 Acute renal abscess. Nonenhanced computed tomography scan through the mid-pole of the right kidney demonstrates right renal enlargement and an area of decreased attenuation *(arrows)*. After antimicrobial therapy, a follow-up scan showed complete regression of these findings. (From Wein AJ et al: *Campbell-Walsh urology,* ed 11, Philadelphia, 2016, Elsevier.)

ICD-10CM # J31.0 Chronic rhinitis
J30.0 Vasomotor rhinitis
J30 Vasomotor and allergic rhinitis

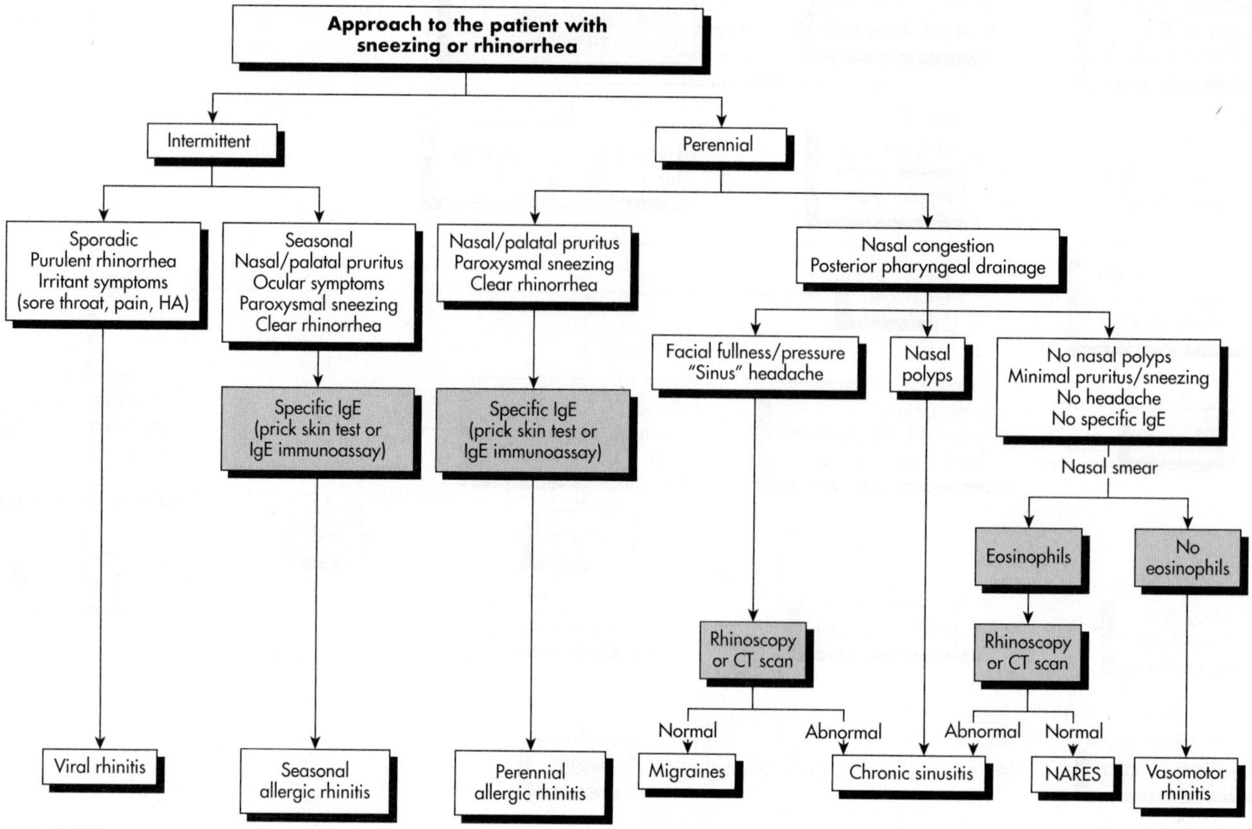

FIG. 150 Approach to the patient with rhinitis symptoms. *CT,* Computed tomography; *HA,* headache; *IgE,* immunoglobulin E; *NARES,* nonallergic rhinitis with eosinophilia syndrome. (From Goldman L, Shafer AI: *Goldman-Cecil medicine,* ed 26, Philadelphia, 2020, Elsevier.)

TABLE 56 Differential Diagnosis of Rhinitis

Allergic
Seasonal allergic rhinitis
Perennial allergic rhinitis
Inflammatory
Infectious rhinitis (viral)
Nonallergic rhinitis with eosinophilia syndrome
Chronic sinusitis with or without nasal polyposis
Laryngopharyngeal reflux
Hormonal
Pregnancy, oral contraceptives, perimenopause
Hypothyroidism
Hyperthyroidism
Rhinitis Medicamentosa
Topical or, less commonly, oral decongestants
Antihypertensives
Antidepressants
Cocaine
Vasomotor
Irritant induced (pollution, cigarette smoke)
Cold air induced
Gustatory (food induced)
Anatomic
Nasal septal deviation
Tumor, neoplasm
Foreign body
Cerebrospinal fluid leak
Atrophic (postsurgical or trauma)

From Goldman L, Shafer AI: *Goldman-Cecil medicine*, ed 26, Philadelphia, 2020, Elsevier.

SCROTAL MASS

ICD-10CM # N44.2 Benign cyst of testis
N44.8 Other noninflammatory disorders of the testis
N50.3 Cyst of epididymis
N50.8 Other specified disorders of male genital organs

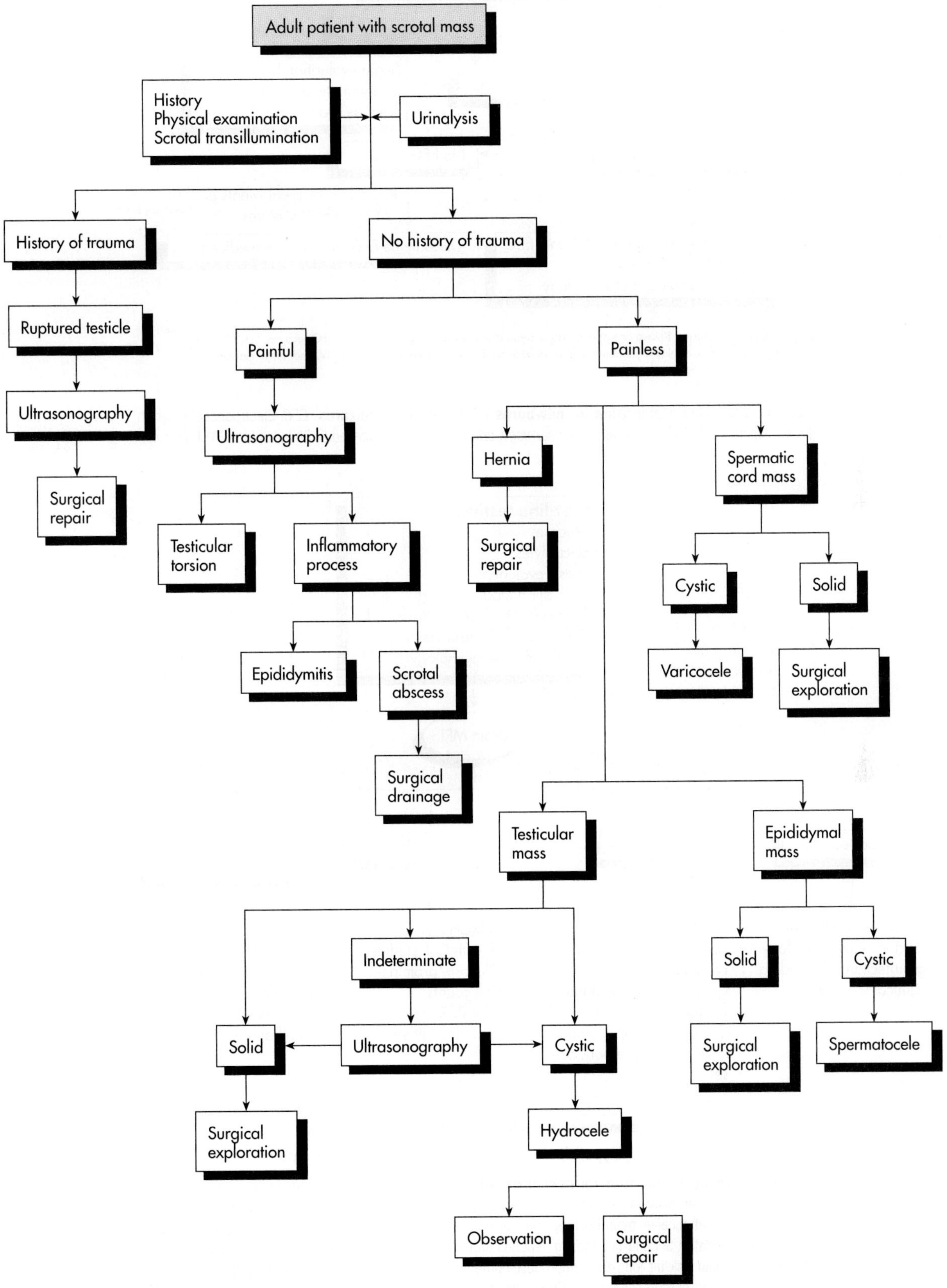

FIG. 151 Evaluation of scrotal mass. (Modified from Greene HL et al [eds]: *Decision making in medicine*, ed 2, St Louis, 1998, Mosby.)

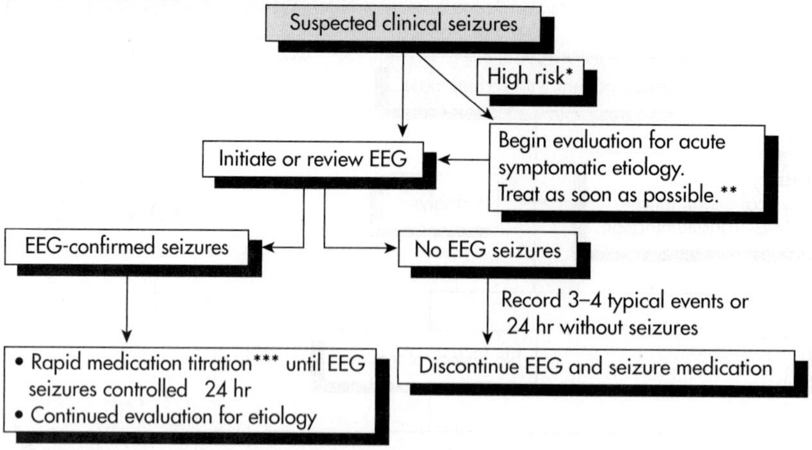

* High-risk scenarios: Known or suspected acute brain injury, encephalopathy, previous EEG seizures, first 72 hr of life

** Reverse glucose or electrolyte abnormalities, and/or administer lorazepam 0.1 mg/kg IV, and/or administer phenobarbital loading dose.

*** Refer to Fig. 154

FIG. 152 Assessment algorithm for newborns with suspected seizures. *EEG,* Electroencephalogram. (From Swaiman KF: *Swaiman's pediatric neurology, principles and practice*, ed 6, Philadelphia, 2017, Elsevier.)

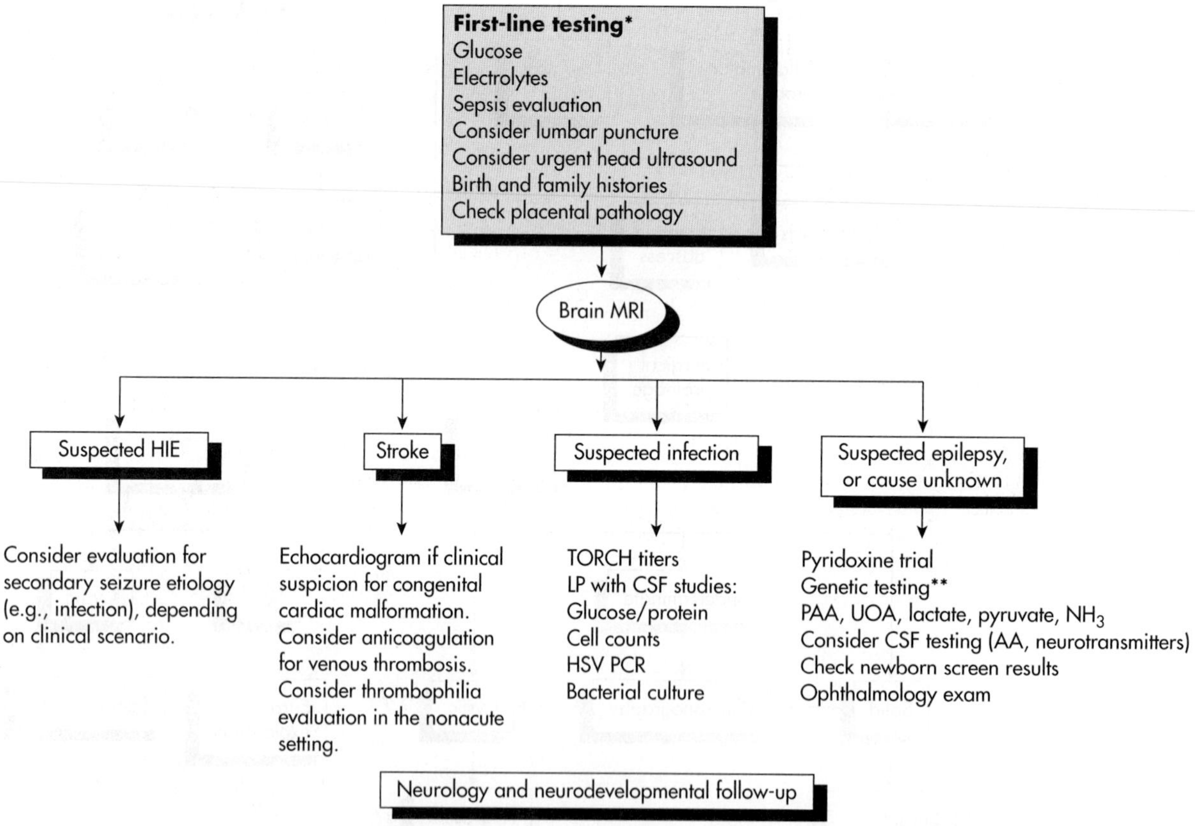

**Genetic testing can include karyotype, chromosomal microarray, epilepsy gene panel, or single gene testing.

FIG. 153 Assessment algorithm for newborns with seizures. *First-line testing should occur simultaneously with initiation of electroencephalography (and empiric seizure treatment in high-risk clinical scenarios). Most infants should receive neuroimaging, and brain magnetic resonance imaging *(MRI)* is the preferred neuroimaging modality. Second-line testing depends on the clinical scenario and MRI findings. Newborns with seizures are at high risk for long-term neurodevelopmental disability and epilepsy, and so they require careful follow-up by appropriate clinicians. *CSF,* Cerebrospinal fluid; *HIE,* hypoxic ischemic encephalopathy; *HSV,* herpes simplex virus; *LP,* lumbar puncture; *PCR,* polymerase chain reaction; *TORCH,* Toxoplasma gondii, other viruses, rubella, cytomegalovirus, and herpes simplex. (From Swaiman KF: *Swaiman's pediatric neurology: principles and practice*, ed 6, Philadelphia, 2017, Elsevier.)

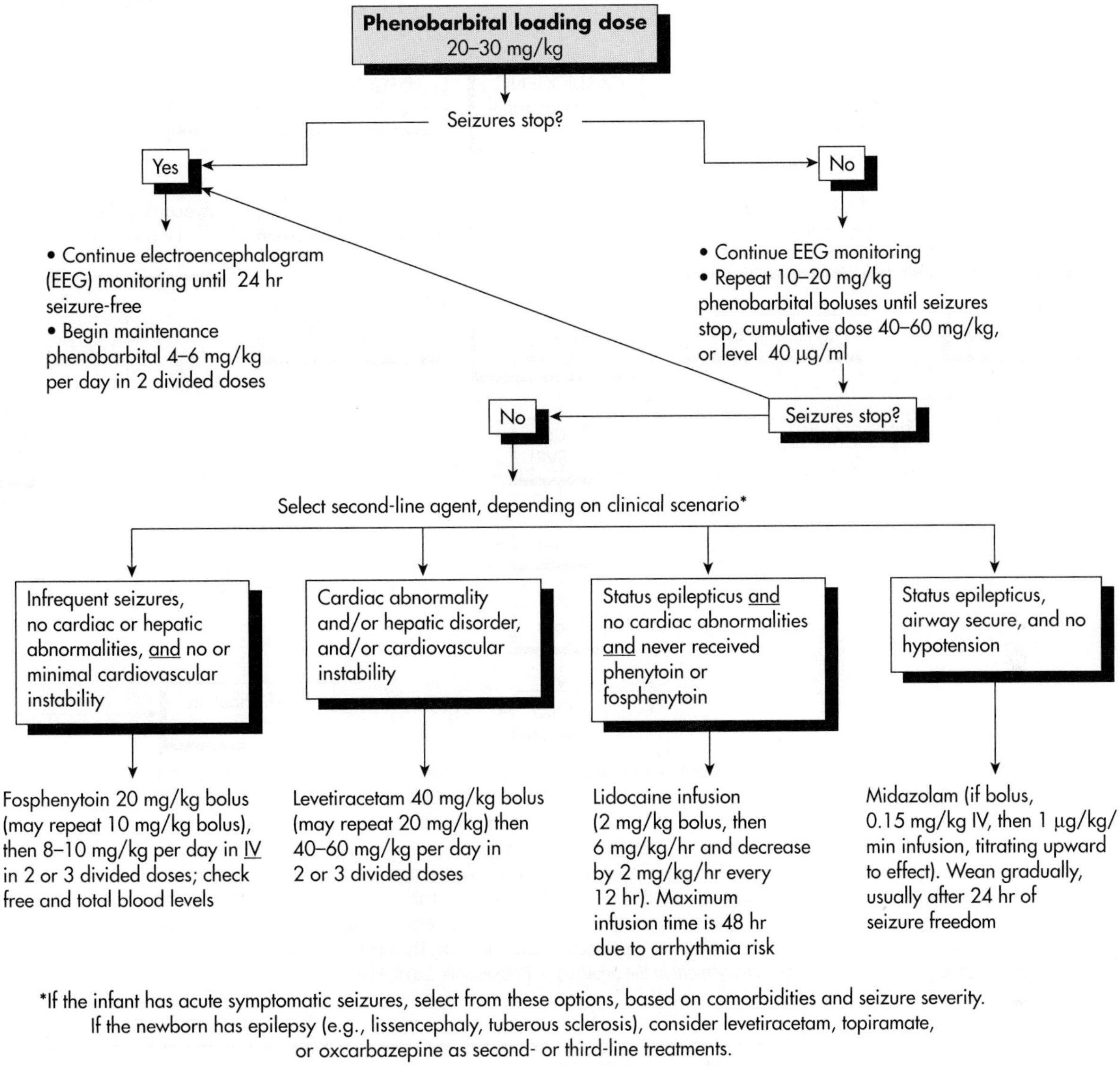

FIG. 154 Suggested treatment algorithm for neonatal seizures. The rapidity of medication administration will depend on local guidelines and resources. Frequent assessment of treatment response is recommended. *IV,* Intravenous. (From Swaiman KF: *Swaiman's pediatric neurology: principles and practice*, ed 6, Philadelphia, 2017, Elsevier.)

SHOCK

ICD-10CM # R57.9 Shock, unspecified
R57.0 Cardiogenic shock
R57.1 Hypovolemic shock
R57.8 Other shock

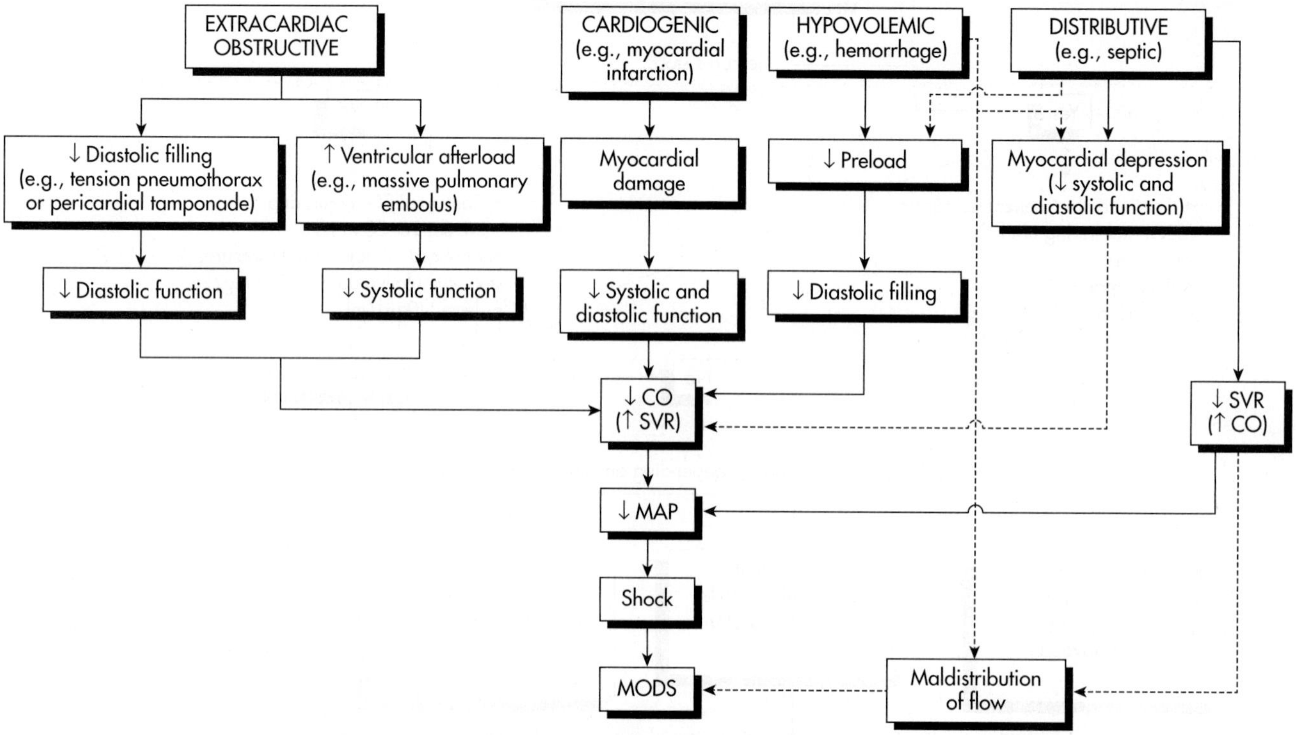

FIG. 155 The interrelationships between different forms of shock. For cardiogenic, hypovolemic, and obstructive shock, hypotension is primarily due to decreased cardiac output with systemic vascular resistance rising secondarily. With distributive (and particularly, septic) shock, hypotension is primarily due to a decrease in systemic vascular resistance with a secondary increase of cardiac output. In many forms of shock, the hemodynamic characteristics are influenced by elements of hypovolemia, myocardial depression (ischemic or otherwise), and vascular dysfunction (which may affect afterload). Dominant pathophysiologic pathways are denoted by *heavier lines. CO,* Cardiac output; *MAP,* mean arterial blood pressure; *MODS,* multiple organ dysfunction syndrome; *SVR,* systemic vascular resistance. (From Parrillo JE, Dellinger RP: *Critical care medicine, principles of diagnosis and management in the adult*, ed 5, Philadelphia, 2019, Elsevier.)

BOX 18 Determinants of Effective Tissue Perfusion in Shock

1. Cardiovascular performance (total systemic perfusion/cardiac output)
   - Cardiac function
     - Preload
     - Afterload
     - Contractility
     - Heart rate
   - Venous return
     - Right atrial pressure (dependent on cardiac function)
     - Mean circulatory pressure
     - Stressed vascular volume
     - Mean vascular compliance
     - Venous vascular resistance
     - Distribution of blood flow
2. Distribution of cardiac output
   - Intrinsic regulatory systems (local tissue factors)
   - Extrinsic regulatory systems (sympathetic/adrenal activity)
   - Anatomic vascular disease
   - Exogenous vasoactive agents (inotropes, vasopressors, vasodilators)
3. Microvascular function
   - Precapillary and postcapillary sphincter function
   - Capillary endothelial integrity
   - Microvascular obstruction (fibrin, platelets, WBC, RBC)
4. Local oxygen unloading and diffusion
   - Oxyhemoglobin affinity
   - RBC 2,3-DPG
   - Blood pH
   - Temperature
5. Cellular energy generation/utilization capability
   - Citric acid (Kreb) cycle
   - Oxidative phosphorylation pathway
   - Other energy metabolism pathways (e.g., ATP utilization)

2,3-DPG, 2,3-Diphosphoglycerate; *ATP,* adenosine triphosphate; *RBC,* red blood cell; *WBC,* white blood cell.

From Parrillo JE, Dellinger RP: *Critical care medicine, principles of diagnosis and management in the adult*, ed 5, Philadelphia, 2019, Elsevier.

BOX 19 Classification of Shock

1. Hypovolemic (Oligemic)
    - Hemorrhagic
        - Trauma
        - Gastrointestinal
        - Retroperitoneal
    - Intravascular fluid depletion (nonhemorrhagic)
        - External fluid loss
            - Dehydration
            - Vomiting
            - Diarrhea
            - Polyurea
        - Interstitial fluid redistribution
            - Thermal injury
            - Trauma
            - Anaphylaxis
    - Increased vascular capacitance (venodilation)
        - Sepsis
        - Anaphylaxis
        - Toxins/Drugs
2. Cardiogenic
    - Myopathic
        - Myocardial infarction
            - Left ventricle
            - Right ventricle
        - Myocardial contusion (trauma)
        - Myocarditis
        - Cardiomyopathy
        - Postischemic myocardial stunning
        - Septic myocardial depression
        - Drug toxicity
            - Anthracycline cardiotoxicity
            - Calcium channel blockers
        - Mechanical
            - Valvular failure (stenotic or regurgitant)
            - Hypertrophic cardiomyopathy
            - Ventricular septal defect
        - Arrhythmic
            - Bradycardia
            - Sinus (e.g., vagal syncope)
            - Atrioventricular blocks
            - Tachycardia
            - Supraventricular
            - Ventricular
3. Extracardiac Obstructive
    - Impaired diastolic filling (decreased ventricular preload)
        - Direct venous obstruction (vena cava)
            - Intrathoracic obstructive tumors
        - Increased intrathoracic pressure (decreased transmural pressure gradient)
            - Tension pneumothorax
            - Mechanical ventilation (with positive end-expiratory pressure [PEEP] or volume depletion)
        - Decreased cardiac compliance
            - Constrictive pericarditis
            - Cardiac tamponade
                - Acute
                    - Post MI free wall rupture
                    - Traumatic
                    - Hemorrhagic (anticoagulation)
                - Chronic
                    - Malignant
                    - Uremic
                    - Idiopathic
    - Impaired systolic contraction (increased ventricular afterload)
        - Right ventricle
            - Pulmonary embolus (massive)
            - Acute pulmonary hypertension
        - Left ventricle
            - Saddle embolus
            - Aortic dissection
4. Distributive
    - Septic (bacterial, fungal, viral, rickettsial)
    - Toxic shock syndrome
    - Anaphylactic, anaphylactoid
    - Neurogenic (spinal shock)
    - Endocrinologic
        - Adrenal crisis
        - Thyroid storm
    - Toxic (e.g., nitroprusside, bretylium)

MI, Myocardial infarction.
From Parrillo JE, Dellinger RP: *Critical care medicine, principles of diagnosis and management in the adult*, ed 5, Philadelphia, 2019, Elsevier.

ICD-10CM # R57.9 Shock, unspecified
R57.0 Cardiogenic shock
R57.1 Hypovolemic shock
R57.8 Other shock

BOX 20 Cardiovascular/Metabolic Compensatory Responses to Shock

1. Maintain mean circulatory pressure (venous pressure)
   Volume
      Fluid redistribution to vascular space (increased total vascular volume) from interstitium (Starling effect) from intracellular space (osmotic)
      Decreased renal fluid losses
      Decreased glomerular filtration rate
      Increased aldosterone
      Increased vasopressin
   Pressure
      Decreased venous capacitance (increased stressed volume) increased sympathetic activity
      Increased circulating (adrenal) epinephrine
      Increased angiotensin
      Increased vasopressin
2. Maximize cardiac performance
   Increase contractility
   Sympathetic stimulation
   Adrenal stimulation
3. Redistribute perfusion
   Extrinsic regulation of systemic arterial tone
   Dominant autoregulation of vital organs (heart, brain)
4. Optimize oxygen unloading
   Increased RBC 2,3-DPG
   Tissue acidosis
   Pyrexia
   Decreased tissue Po_2

2,3-DPG, 2,3-Diphosphoglycerate; *Po_2,* partial pressure of oxygen; *RBC,* red blood cell.

From Parrillo JE, Dellinger RP: *Critical care medicine, principles of diagnosis and management in the adult,* ed 5, Philadelphia, 2019, Elsevier.

BOX 21 General Approach to Shock: Immediate Goals

General
   Find cause of shock and apply specific treatment (examples: Antibiotics for sepsis or pericardiocentesis for tamponade)
Hemodynamic
   MAP >65 mm Hg (higher in the presence of coronary artery disease or chronic hypertension)
   CVP = 8-12 mm Hg/PAOP = 12-15 mm Hg (may be higher for cardiogenic shock)[a]
   CI >2.1 L/min per m^2a
Optimization of oxygen delivery
   Hemoglobin >7-9 g/dl; >7 g/L after shock is sufficient
   Arterial saturation >92%
   Mvo_2 >60%, $scvO_2$ >70%
   Normalization of serum lactate (to <2.2 mM/L)
Reverse organ system dysfunction
   Reverse encephalopathy
   Maintain urine output >0.5 ml/kg per hr

CI, Cardiac index; *CVP,* central venous pressure; *MAP,* mean arterial pressure; *Mvo_2,* mixed venous oxygen saturation; *PAOP,* pulmonary artery occlusion pressure.
[a]Optional.
From Parrillo JE, Dellinger RP: *Critical care medicine, principles of diagnosis and management in the adult*, ed 5, Philadelphia, 2019, Elsevier.

TABLE 57 Organ System Dysfunction in Shock

Central nervous system	Encephalopathy (ischemic or septic)
	Cortical necrosis
Heart	Tachycardia, bradycardia
	Supraventricular tachycardia
	Ventricular ectopy
	Myocardial ischemia
	Myocardial depression
Pulmonary system	Acute respiratory failure
	Acute respiratory distress syndrome
Kidney	Prerenal failure
	Acute tubular necrosis
Gastrointestinal system	Ileus
	Erosive gastritis
	Pancreatitis
	Acalculous cholecystitis
	Colonic submucosal hemorrhage
	Transluminal translocation of bacteria/antigens
Liver	Ischemic hepatitis
	"Shock" liver
	Intrahepatic cholestasis
Hematologic system	Disseminated intravascular coagulation
	Dilutional thrombocytopenia
Metabolic	Hyperglycemia
	Glycogenolysis
	Gluconeogenesis
	Hypoglycemia (late)
	Hypertriglyceridemia
Immune system	Gut barrier function depression
	Cellular immune depression
	Humoral immune depression

From Parrillo JE, Dellinger RP: *Critical care medicine, principles of diagnosis and management in the adult,* ed 5, Philadelphia, 2019, Elsevier.

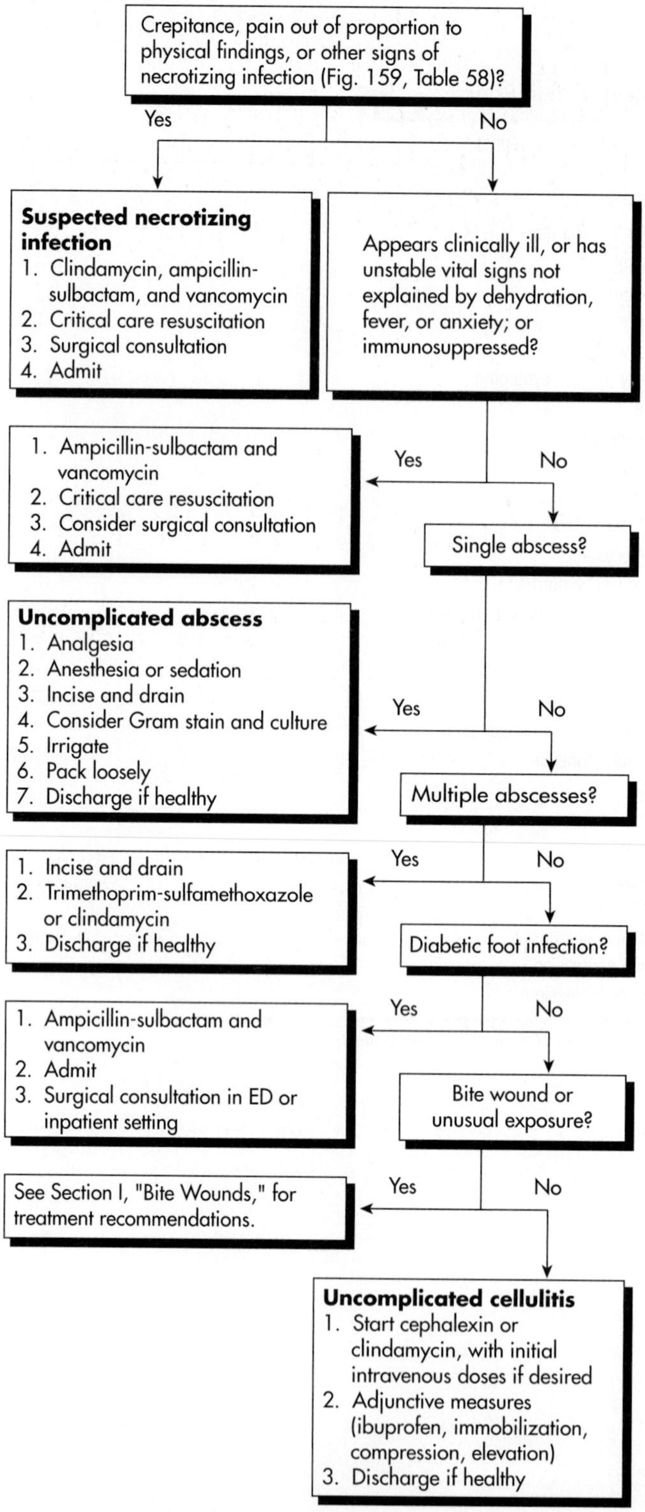

FIG. 158 Universal algorithm for skin and soft tissue infections (assuming no prior treatment). *ED*, Emergency department. (From Marx JA et al: *Rosen's emergency medicine*, ed 8, Philadelphia, 2014, Saunders.)

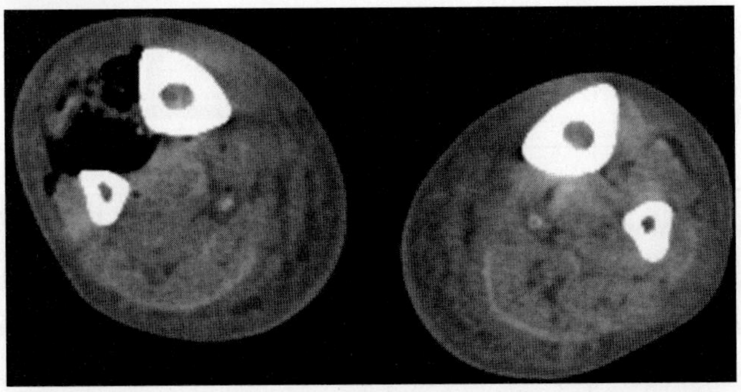

FIG. 159 Necrotizing fasciitis. Axial computed tomography through the lower extremities demonstrates gas in the anterior soft tissues. Necrotizing fasciitis is a clinical diagnosis. Imaging may lead to a delay in treatment. (From Webb WR et al: *Fundamentals of body CT,* ed 4, Philadelphia, 2015, Elsevier.)

TABLE 58 Differentiating Features of Necrotizing Skin and Soft Tissue Infections

Feature	Progressive Bacterial Synergistic Gangrene	Nonclostridial Anaerobic Cellulitis	Clostridial Myonecrosis (Gas Gangrene)	Necrotizing Fasciitis Type 1	Necrotizing Fasciitis Type 2
Risk factors	Surgery, ileostomy, colostomy, chronic ulceration	Diabetes mellitus	Trauma, surgery	Diabetes mellitus, surgery, perineal infection	Trauma, surgery, none
Microbiology	Microaerophilic streptococci plus *Staphylococcus aureus*	Non–spore-forming anaerobes ± coliforms, streptococci, *S. aureus*	*Clostridium* spp.	Polymicrobial (Enterobacteriaceae plus anaerobes)	Group A streptococci
Course	Slow	Slow or rapid	Very rapid	Rapid	Very rapid
Pain	++++	++/+++	++++	+++/++++	++++
Gas formation	–	++++	++	++	–
Appearance	Central necrotic ulcer, erythematous periphery	Erythematous skin necrosis	Bullae, necrosis	Bullae, skin	Bullae, necrotic skin and tissue
Drainage	Purulent if present	Purulent	Serosanguineous	"Dishwater," seropurulent	Serous if present
Depth of involvement	Skin, soft tissue	Skin, soft tissue	Muscle	Fascia	Fascia
Systemic toxicity	±	+++/++++	++++	+++/++++	++++

–, Absent; ±, occasionally present; +, minimal; ++, mild; +++, moderate; ++++, marked or severe.
From Parrillo JE, Dellinger RP: *Critical care medicine, principles of diagnosis and management in the adult,* ed 5, Philadelphia, 2019, Elsevier.

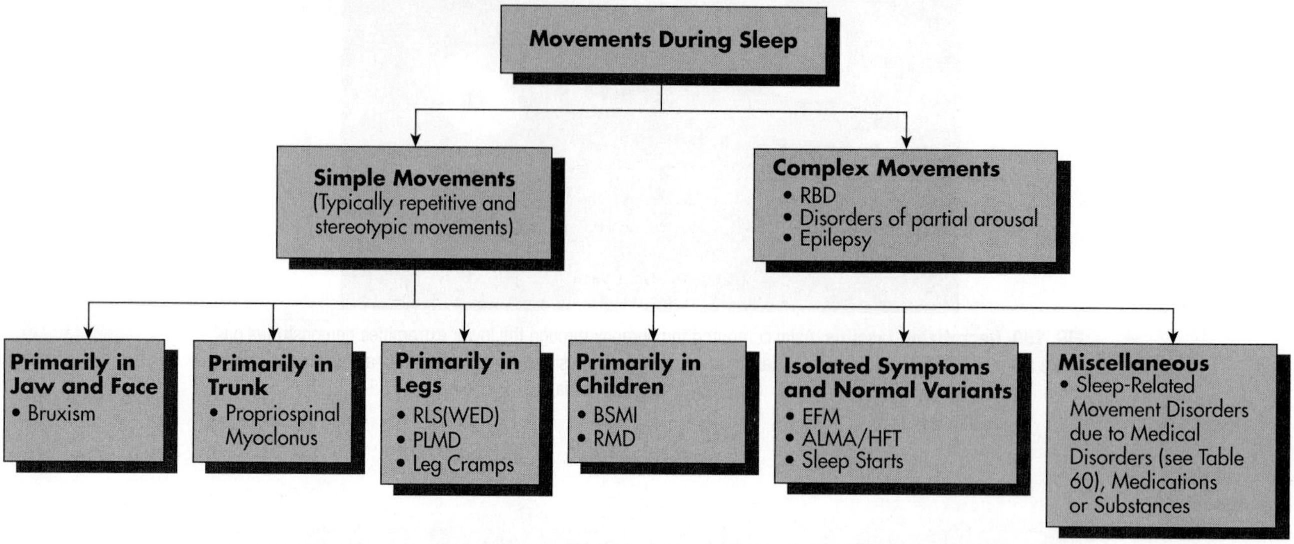

FIG. 162 Flow chart for the approach to the differential diagnosis of sleep-related movement disorders. *ALMA,* Alternating leg muscle activation; *BSMI,* benign sleep myoclonus of infancy; *EFM,* excessive fragmentary myoclonus; *HFT,* hypnagogic foot tremor; *PLMD,* periodic limb movement disorder; *RBD,* rapid eye movement (REM) sleep behavior disorder; *RLS (WED),* restless legs syndrome (Willis-Ekbom disease); *RMD,* rhythmic movement disorder. (From Kryger M et al: *Principles and practice of sleep medicine,* ed 6, Philadelphia, 2017, Elsevier.)

TABLE 60 Distinguishing Features of Nocturnal Events

Feature	Disorders of Arousal	Sleep-Related Eating Disorder	REM Behavior Disorder	Recurrent Isolated Sleep Paralysis	Exploding Head Syndrome	Psychogenic Events	Nocturnal Seizures
Behavior	Confused; semi-purposeful movement with eyes open	Eating typically high-calorie foods; eyes open	Sometimes combative with eyes closed	Episodes of inability to move	Painless sensation of explosion inside the head	Variable	Dependent on the portion of brain involved
Age of onset	Childhood and adolescence	Variable	Older adult	Variable	Adult	Adolescence to adulthood	Variable
Time of occurrence	First third of night	First half of night	During REM	Typically on awakening	Usually near sleep onset but can be variable	Anytime	Anytime
Frequency of events	Less than one per night	Variable	Multiple per night	Variable less than weekly	Rare	Variable	Frontal seizures—multiple per night
Duration	Minutes	Minutes	Seconds to minute	Seconds to minutes	Seconds	Variable minutes or longer	Usually under 3 minutes
Memory of event	Usually none	Usually none or limited	Dream recall	Yes	Yes	None	Usually none
Stereotypical movements	No	No	No	No	Similar sensation	No	Yes
Polysomnogram findings	Arousals from slow wave sleep	Arousal from NREM sleep	Excessive electromyogram tone during REM sleep	Arousal from REM sleep	Usually occurs in light sleep	Occur from awake state	Potentially epileptiform activity

REM, Rapid eye movement; *NREM,* nonrapid eye movement.
From Kryger M et al: *Principles and practice of sleep medicine,* ed 6, Philadelphia, 2017, Elsevier.

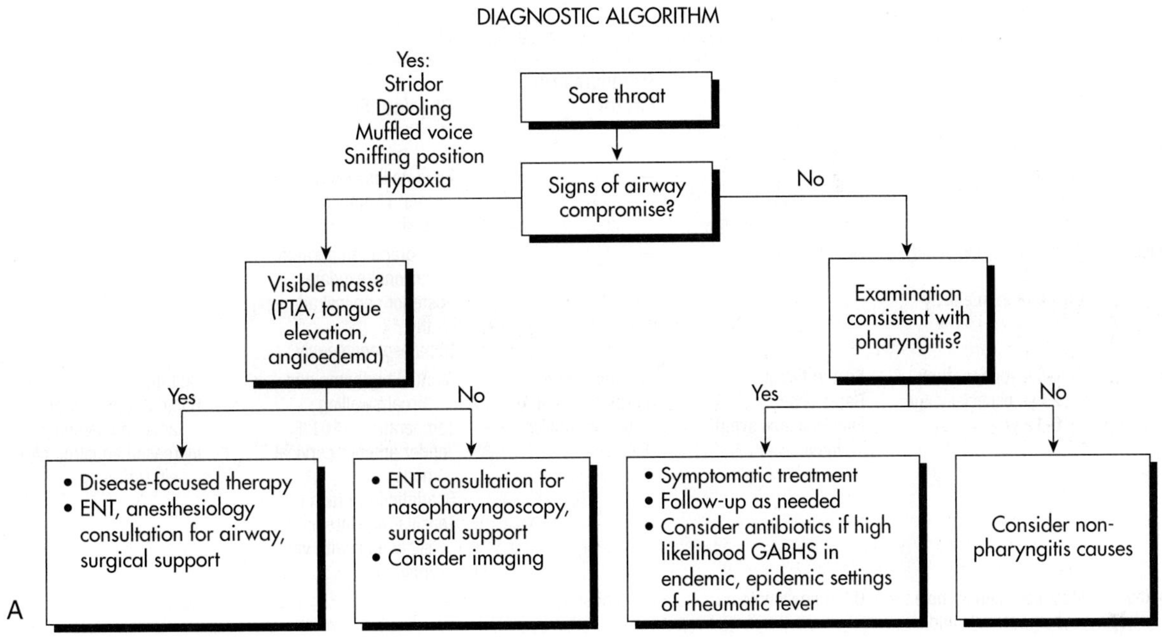

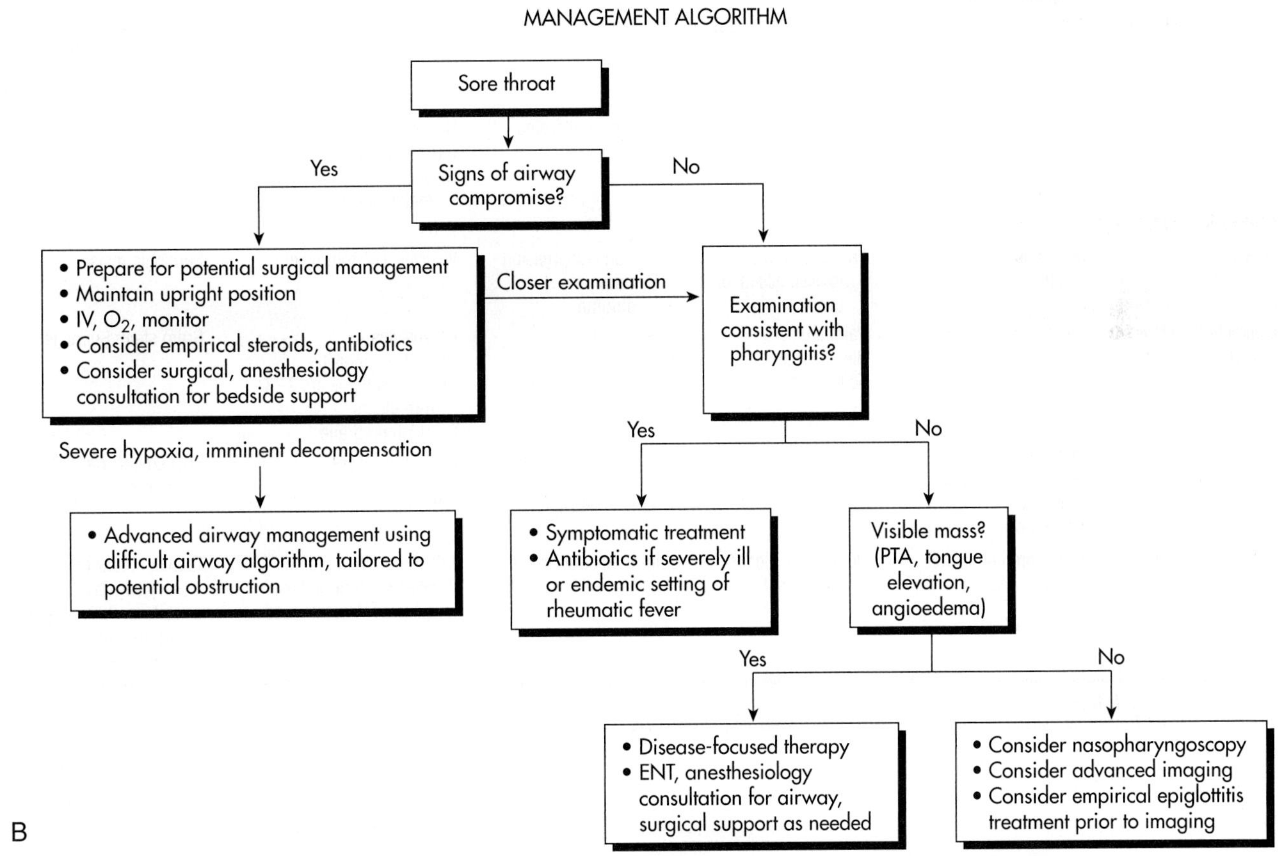

FIG. 163 Clinical approach to the patient with sore throat—diagnosis **(A)** and management **(B)**. Refer to Section I topics Pharyngitis/Tonsillitis and Epiglottitis for additional information. *ENT,* Ear-nose-throat; *GABHS,* group A beta-hemolytic streptococcus; *IV,* intravenous; *PTA,* peritonsillar abscess. (From Marx JA et al: *Rosen's emergency medicine*, ed 8, Philadelphia, 2014, Saunders.)

ICD-10CM # J02.9 Acute pharyngitis, unspecified
J31.2 Chronic pharyngitis
J02.0 Streptococcal pharyngitis

TABLE 61 Differential Diagnosis of Sore Throat

Type of Pharyngitis	Nature of Patient	Nature of Symptoms	Predisposing Factors	Physical Findings	Diagnostic Studies
Without Pharyngeal Ulcers					
Viral	All ages	Pain in throat Rapid onset Systemic symptoms	—	Exudate less likely than with streptococcal infections	—
Infectious mononucleosis	Adolescents and young adults Uncommon in elderly	Gradual onset	—	Low-grade temperature Occasional exudate Posterior cervical adenopathy Hepatosplenomegaly	Monospot test
Streptococcal pharyngitis	Patients younger than 25 yr, especially age 6-12 yr	Pain in throat Rapid onset Few systemic symptoms	Fall and winter Streptococcal infection in family Diabetes	Marked erythema and throat swelling Temperature >101°F Tender anterior cervical nodes Scarlatiniform rash Tonsillar exudate more likely than with viral infection	Culture Rapid streptococcal antigen screening Increased antistreptolysin O titer
Gonococcal pharyngitis	Most common in male homosexuals and people with anogenital gonorrhea	Often no symptoms	Orogenital sex	—	Culture
Sinusitis with postnasal drip	Adults	Mild throat soreness Symptoms often worse with recumbency	—	Evidence of sinusitis Postnasal drip	CT/flexible rhinoscopy (in recalcitrant cases)
Allergic pharyngitis	—	—	Seasonal allergies	No fever Intermittent postnasal drip Swollen pharynx with minimal injection	Allergy testing
With Pharyngeal Ulcers					
Herpangina	More common in children	Painful ulcers on tonsils, pillars, or uvula	Immunosuppression Summer and autumn	Vesicles 1-2-mm ulcers	Serologic tests
Fusospirochetal infection (Vincent angina)	Children and people with poor oral hygiene	Painful ulcers Bleeding gums Foul breath	—	No vesicles Ulcerative gingivitis Gray, necrotic ulcers 2-30-mm ulcers Pseudomembrane	Gram stain: Spirochetes
Candidiasis	Children Immunosuppressed patients Those taking antibiotics	—	Immunosuppression Antibiotics Inhaled steroids	3-11-mm ulcers No vesicles	KOH smear: *Candida* culture
Herpes simplex	Most common in children	Not usually a cause of sore throat	Immunosuppression	1-2-mm painful ulcers Vesicles present on lips, gingivae, buccal mucosa, or tongue	Tzanck smear (not very sensitive) viral culture, PCR, herpes simplex virus antibody assay

CT, Computed tomography; *PCR,* polymerase chain reaction.
Modified from Seller RH, Symons AB: *Differential diagnosis of common complaints,* ed 7, Philadelphia, 2018, Elsevier.

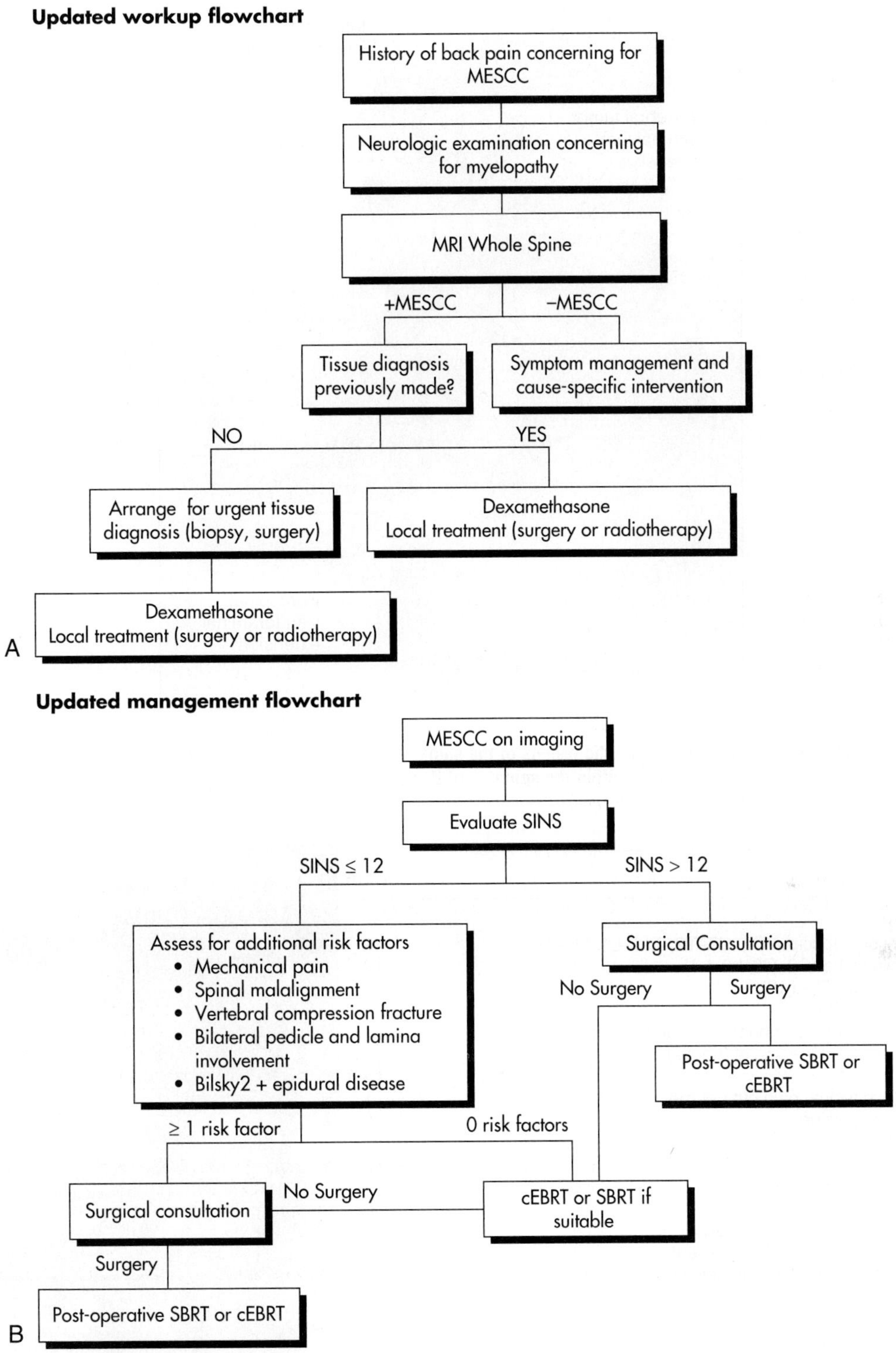

FIG. 164 (A) Flowchart for the initial workup of a patient with suspected spinal metastatic disease. **(B)** Flowchart for the management of metastatic epidural spinal cord compression *(MESCC)*. *cEBRT,* Conventional external beam radiotherapy; *MRI,* magnetic resonance imaging; *SBRT,* stereotactic body radiation therapy; *SINS,* Spine Instability Neoplastic Score. (From Niederhuber JE: *Abeloff's clinical oncology*, ed 6, Philadelphia, 2020, Elsevier.)

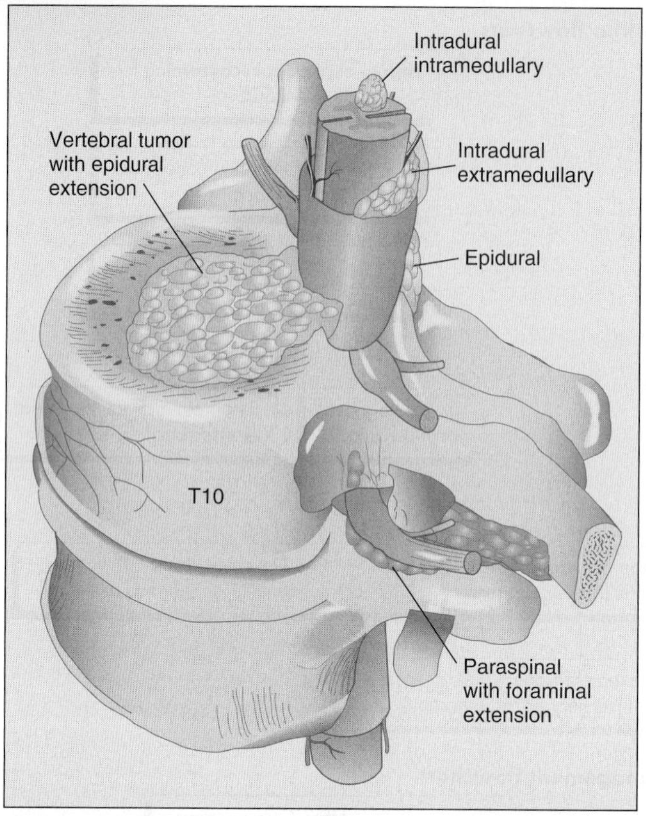

FIG. 165 Locations of metastatic lesions of the spine: Vertebral body, epidural space, neural foramen, intradural space, and within the spinal cord itself. (From Niederhuber JE: *Abeloff's clinical oncology*, ed 6, Philadelphia, 2020, Elsevier.)

Element of SINS	Score
Location	
Junctional (occiput-C2, C7–T2, T11–L1, L5–S1)	3
Mobile spine (C3–C6, L2–L4)	2
Semi-rigid (T3–T10)	1
Rigid (S2–S5)	0
Pain relief with recumbency and/or pain with movement/loading of the spine	
Yes	3
No (occasional pain but not mechanical)	1
Pain free lesion	0
Bone lesion	
Lytic	2
Mixed (lytic/blastic)	1
Blastic	0
Radiographic spinal alignment	
Subluxation/translation present	4
De novo deformity (kyphosis/scoliosis)	2
Normal alignment	0
Vertebral body collapse	
>50% collapse	3
<50% collapse	2
No collapse with >50% body involved	1
None of the above	0
Posterolateral involvement of the spinal elements (facet, pedicle or CV joint fracture or replacement with tumor)	
Bilateral	3
Unilateral	1
None of the above	0

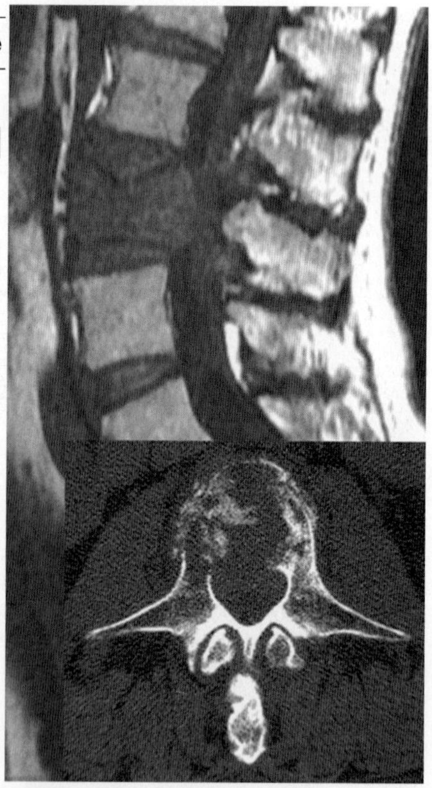

FIG. 166 Spinal Instability Neoplastic Score *(SINS)* elements with axial and sagittal computed tomography *(CT)* example of an L3 metastasis. In this case, the overall SINS was 11 (2 for location, 3 for pain, 1 for bone lesion, 0 for radiographic spinal alignment, 2 for vertebral body collapse, and 3 for posterolateral involvement of the spinal elements). (From Niederhuber JE: *Abeloff's clinical oncology*, ed 6, Philadelphia, 2020, Elsevier.)

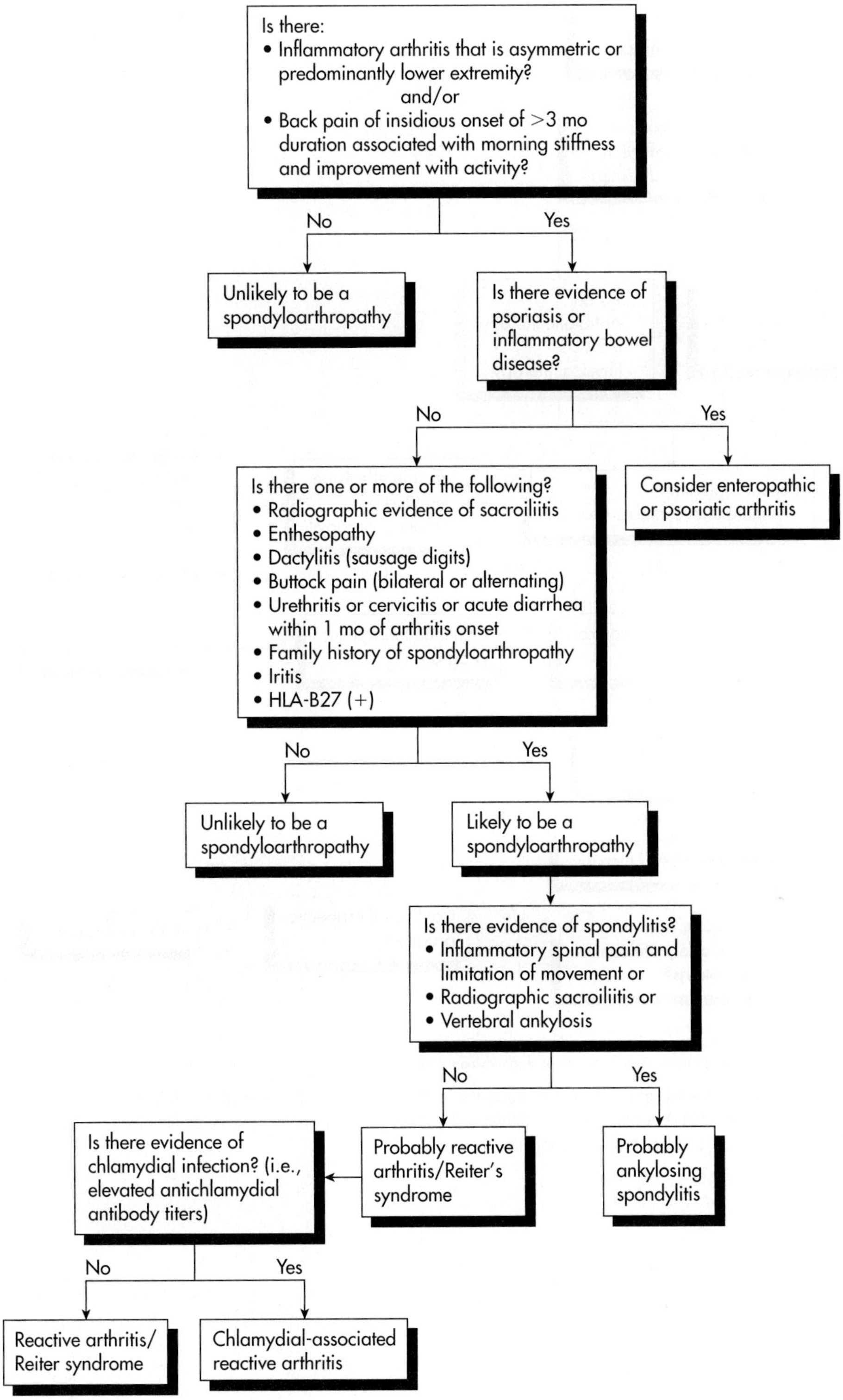

FIG. 169 Algorithm for diagnosis of the spondyloarthropathies. *HLA,* Human leukocyte antigen. (From Goldman L, Schafer AL: *Cecil textbook of medicine,* ed 24, Philadelphia, 2012, Saunders.)

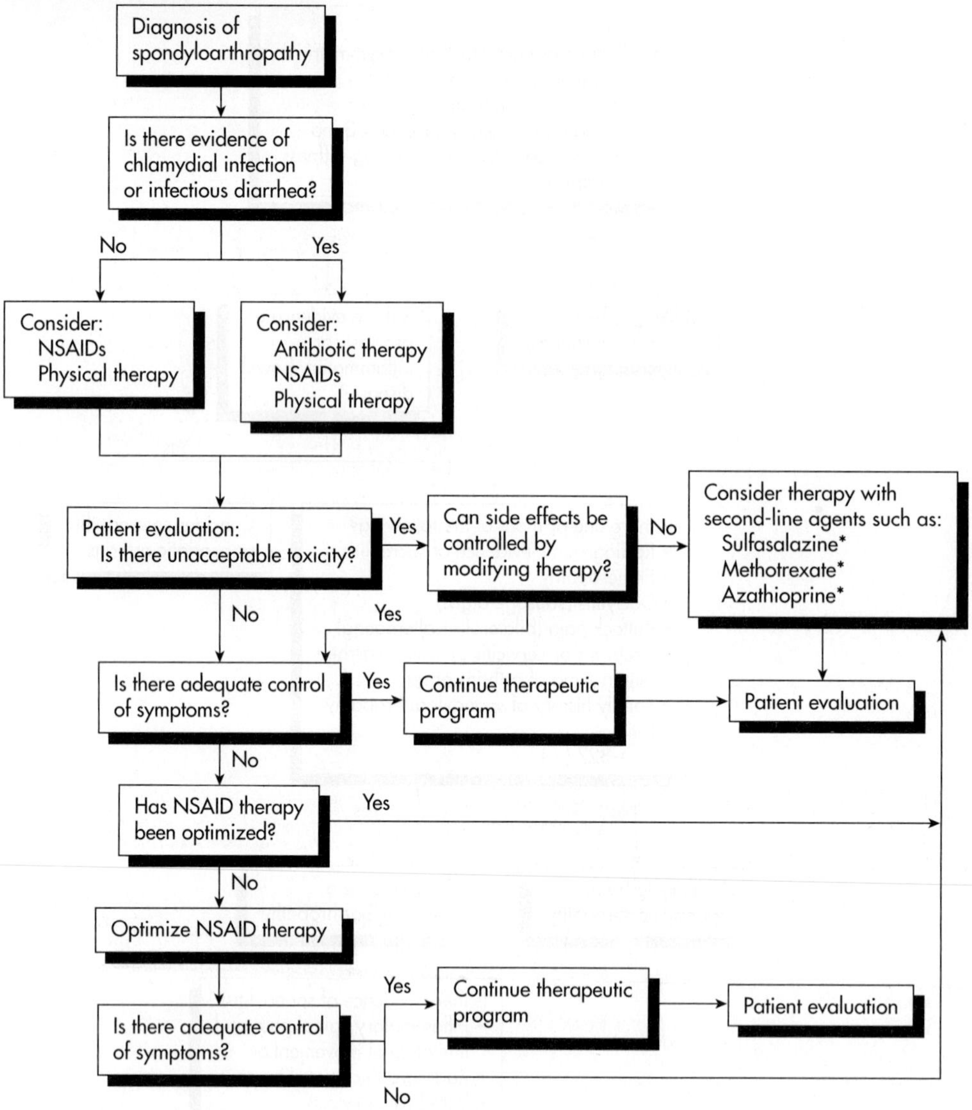

* Not approved by the FDA for treatment of spondyloarthropathies.

FIG. 170 Treatment algorithm for patients with a spondyloarthropathy. *FDA,* Food and Drug Administration; *NSAID,* nonsteroidal antiinflammatory drug. (From Goldman L, Schafer AL: *Cecil textbook of medicine,* ed 24, Philadelphia, 2012, Saunders.)

TACHYCARDIA, DIAGNOSTIC APPROACH

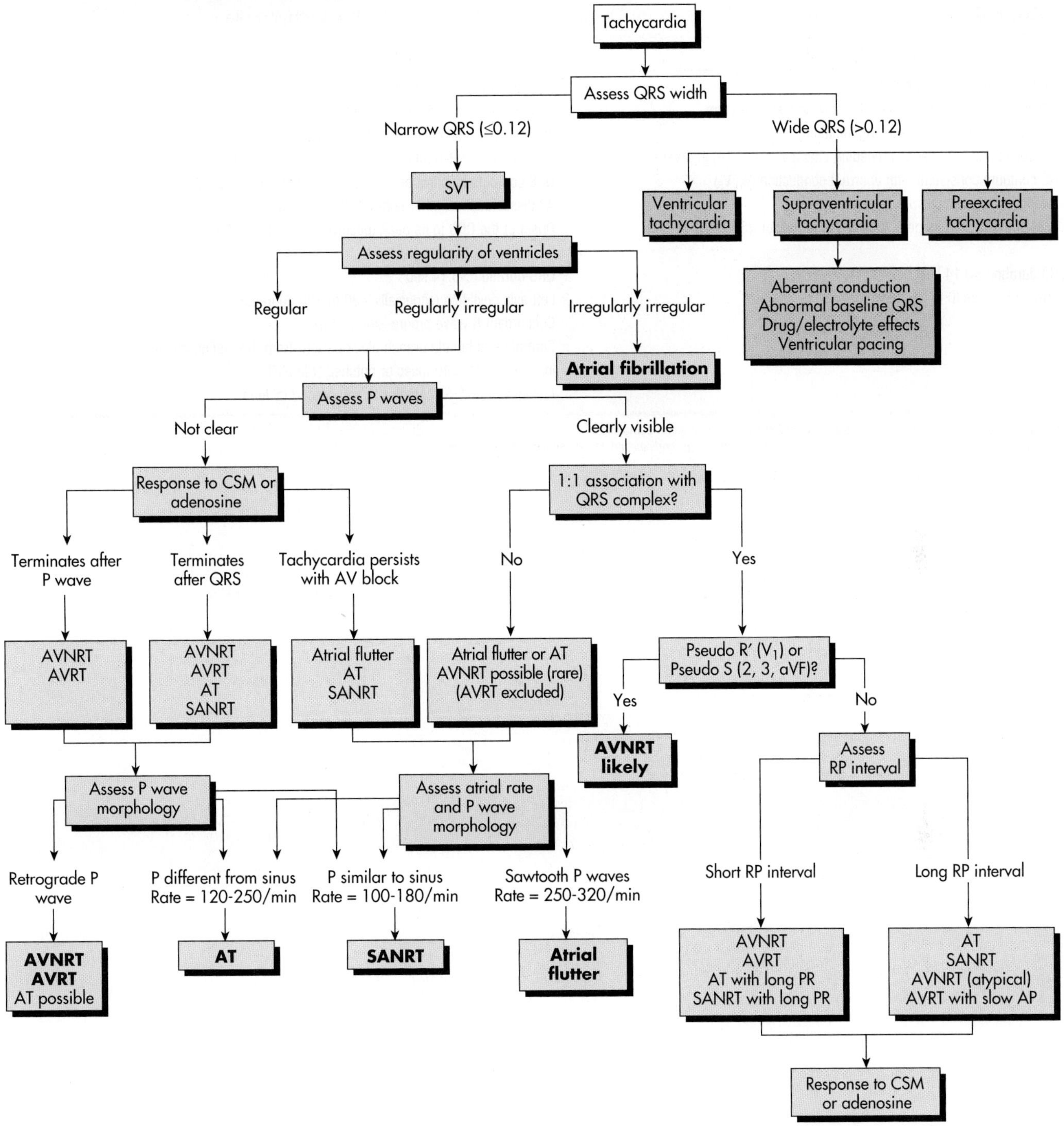

FIG. 171 Stepwise approach to diagnosis of the type of tachycardia based on a 12-lead electrocardiogram during the episode. The initial step is to determine whether the tachycardia has a wide or narrow QRS complex. For wide-complex tachycardia, see Table 63; the remainder of the algorithm is helpful in diagnosis of the type of narrow-complex tachycardia. *AP,* Accessory pathway; *AT,* atrial tachycardia; *AV,* atrioventricular; *AVNRT,* atrioventricular nodal reentrant tachycardia; *AVRT,* atrioventricular reciprocating tachycardia; *CSM,* carotid sinus massage; *SANRT,* sinoatrial nodal reentry tachycardia; *SVT,* supraventricular tachycardia. (From Zipes DP: *Braunwald's heart disease, a textbook of cardiovascular medicine*, ed 11, Philadelphia, 2019, Elsevier.)

TABLE 63 Electrocardiographic Distinctions for Diagnosis of Wide-QRS Complex Tachycardia

Favor Supraventricular Tachycardia	Favor Ventricular Tachycardia
Initiation with a premature P wave	Initiation with a premature QRS complex
Tachycardia complexes identical to those in resting rhythm	Tachycardia beats identical to PVCs during sinus rhythm
"Long-short" sequence preceding initiation	"Short-long" sequence preceding initiation
Changes in the P-P interval preceding changes in the R-R interval	Changes in the R-R interval preceding changes in the P-P interval
QRS contours consistent with aberrant conduction (V_1, V_6)	QRS contours inconsistent with aberrant conduction (V_1, V_6)
Slowing or termination with vagal maneuvers	AV dissociation or other non-1:1 AV relationship
Onset of the QRS to its peak (positive or negative) <50 msec	Onset of the QRS to its peak (positive or negative) ≥50 msec
	Fusion beats, capture beats
QRS duration ≤0.14 sec	QRS duration >0.14 sec
Normal QRS axis (0 to +90 degrees)	Left axis deviation (especially −90 to 180 degrees)
	Concordant R wave progression pattern
	Contralateral bundle branch block pattern from the resting rhythm
	Initial R, q, or r >40 msec or notched Q in aVR
	Absence of an "rS" complex in any precordial lead

AV, Atrioventricular; *aVR,* augmented vector right; *PVC,* premature ventricular complexes.
From Zipes DP: *Braunwald's heart disease, a textbook of cardiovascular medicine*, ed 11, Philadelphia, 2019, Elsevier.

ICD-10CM # I49.02 Ventricular flutter
I49.8 Other specified cardiac arrhythmias
R00.1 Bradycardia, unspecified

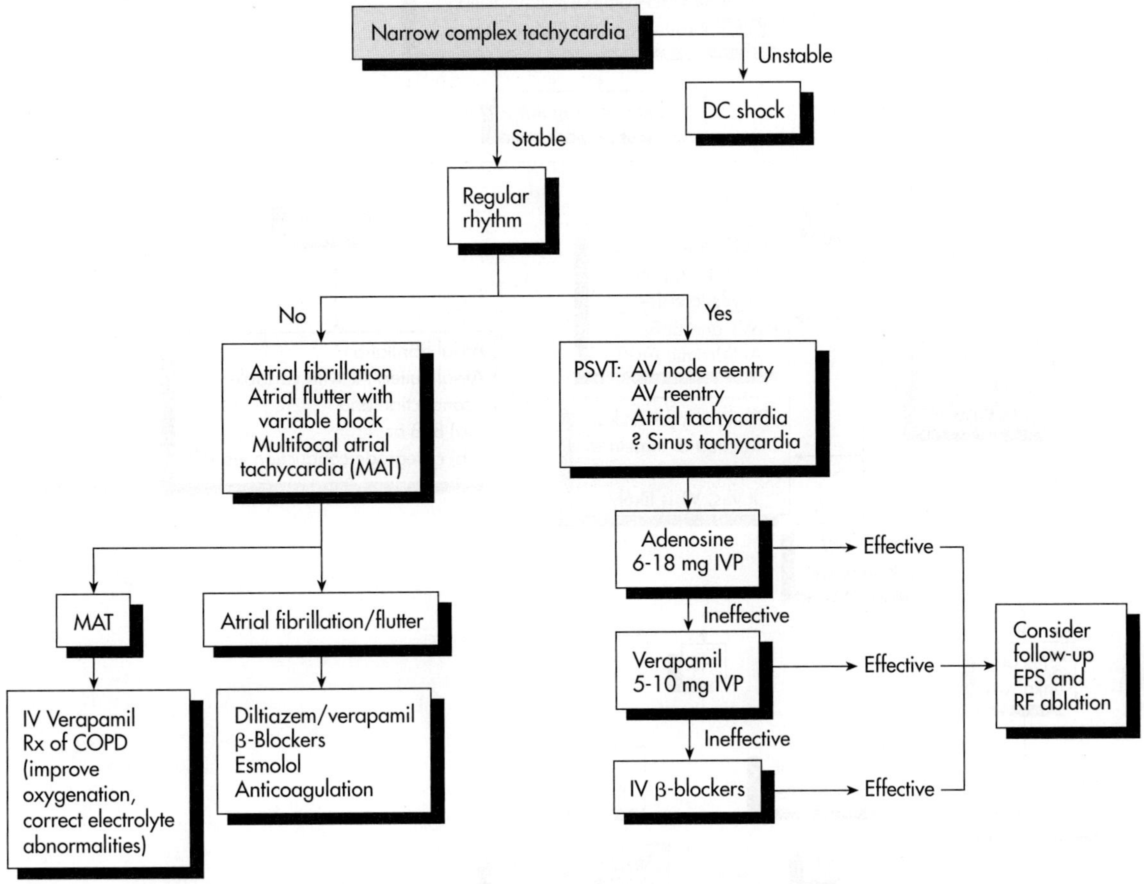

FIG. 172 Evaluation and management of narrow complex tachycardia. *AV,* Atrioventricular; *COPD,* chronic obstructive pulmonary disease; *DC,* direct current; *EPS,* electrophysiologic studies; *IV,* intravenous; *IVP,* intravenous push; *PSVT,* paroxysmal supraventricular tachycardia; *RF,* radiofrequency; *Rx,* treatment.

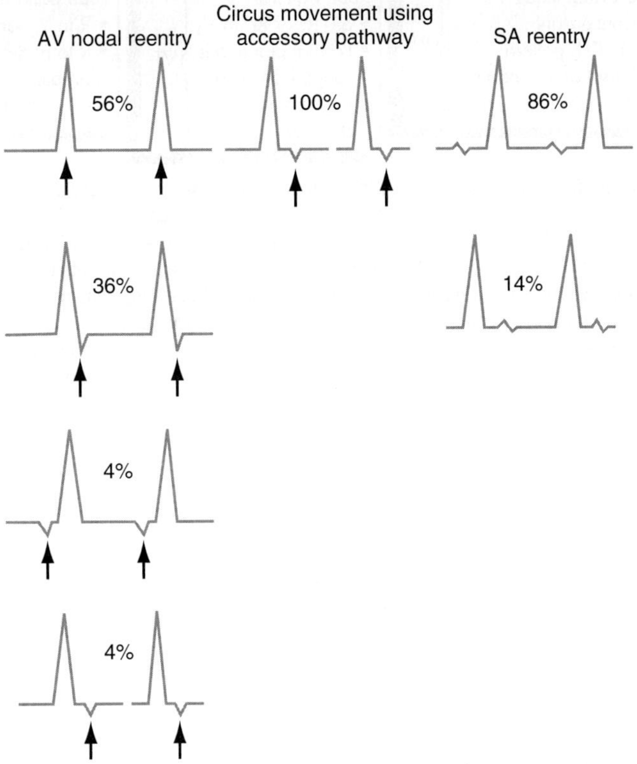

FIG. 173 Location of P waves in common causes of regular narrow-complex tachycardia. *AV,* Atrioventricular; *SA,* sinoatrial. (From Marriott HJL, Conover MB: *Advanced concepts in dysrhythmias,* 2nd ed. St Louis, Mosby, 1989. In Marx JA et al: *Rosen's emergency medicine,* ed 8, Philadelphia, 2014, Saunders.)

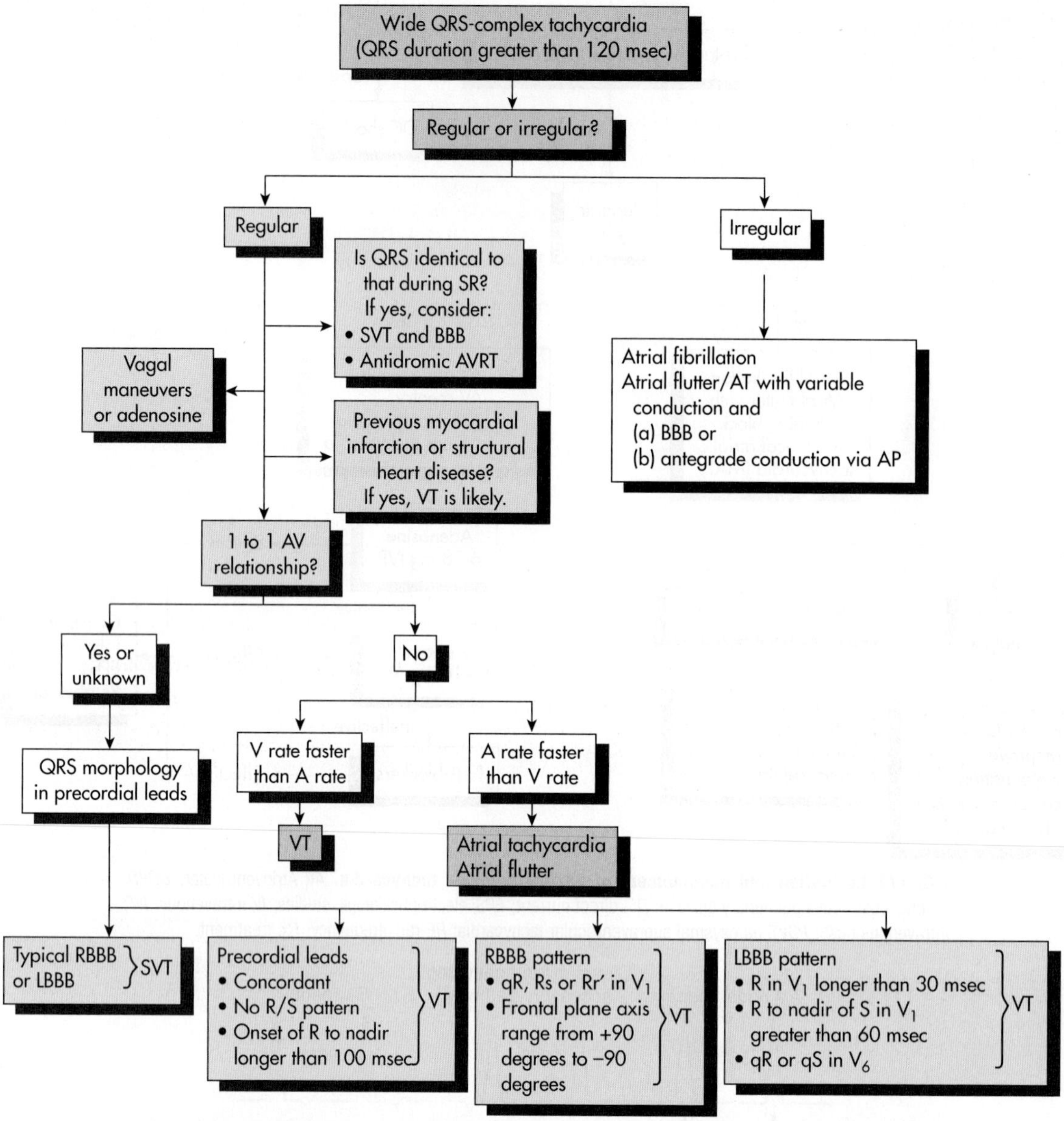

FIG. 175 Algorithm for diagnosis of wide-QRS tachycardia. *AP,* Accessory pathway; *AT,* atrial tachycardia; *AV,* atrioventricular; *AVRT,* AV reentrant tachycardia; *BBB,* bundle branch block; *LBBB,* left bundle branch block; *RBBB,* right bundle branch block; *SVT,* supraventricular tachycardia; *VT,* ventricular tachycardia. (From Bloomstrom-Lundqvist C et al: ACC/AHA/ESC guidelines for the management of patients with supraventricular arrhythmias—executive summary: a report of the American College of Cardiology/American Heart Association Task Force on Practice Guidelines and the European Society of Cardiology Committee for Practice Guidelines [Writing Committee to Develop Guidelines for the Management of Patients with Supraventricular Arrhythmias], *Circulation* 108:1871, 2003; Mann DL et al: *Braunwald's heart disease*, ed 10, Philadelphia, 2015, Elsevier.)

TABLE 64 Stepwise Criteria Favoring Ventricular Tachycardia Patients with Wide-Complex Tachycardias Using Different Algorithms

ACC/AHA/ESC Algorithm*	Kindwall Criteria†	Wellens Criteria‡	Brugada Criteria§	Miller criteria§
See Fig. 175	R >30 ms in V_1 or V_2→ VT	AV dissociation → VT	Absence of RS complex in all precordial leads → VT	Initial R wave in aVR → VT
	Any Q in V_6→ VT	QRS width >140 ms →VT	Longest R/S interval >100 ms in any precordial lead → VT	aVR with initial r or q >40 sec in duration → VT
	>60 ms to S wave nadir in V_1 or V_2→ VT	Left axis deviation >–30° → VT	AV dissociation → VT	aVR with a notch on the descending limb of a negative-onset and predominantly negative QRS in aVR → VT
	Notched downstroke S wave in V_1 or V_2→ VT	If RBBB morphology, monophasic or biphasic QRS in V_1→ SVT or R-to-S ratio of <1 in V_6→ VT	If RBBB morphology, monophasic R or qR in V_1→ VT R taller than R′→ VT rS in V_6→ VT	In aVR, mV of initial 40 msec divided by terminal 40 msec ($v/v_t \leq 1$) → VT
		If LBBB morphology, S in V_1-V_2→ VT	If LBBB morphology, initial R >40 ms in duration →VT Slurred or notched S in V_1 or V_2→ VT Beginning Q or QS in V_6→ VT	

ACC, American College of Cardiology; *AHA,* American Heart Association; *AV,* atrioventricular; *aVR,* augmented vector right; *ESC,* European Society of Cardiology; *LBBB,* left bundle branch block; *RBBB,* right bundle branch block; *VT,* ventricular tachycardia. ‖Vereckei A et al: New algorithm using only lead aVR for differential diagnosis of wide QRS complex tachycardia. *Heart Rhythm* 5:89, 2008.

*Blomström-Lundqvist C et al: ACC/AHA/ESC guidelines for the management of patients with supraventricular arrhythmias—executive summary: a report of the American College of Cardiology/American Heart Association Task Force on Practice Guidelines and the European Society of Cardiology Committee for Practice Guidelines (Writing Committee to Develop Guidelines for the Management of Patients With Supraventricular Arrhythmias). *Circulation* 108:1871, 2003.

†Kindwall KE et al: Electrocardiographic criteria for ventricular tachycardia in wide complex left bundle branch block morphology tachycardias. *Am J Cardiol* 61:1279, 1988.

‡Wellens HJ et al: The value of the electrocardiogram in the differential diagnosis of a tachycardia with a widened QRS complex. *Am J Med* 64:27, 1978.

§Brugada P et al: A new approach to the differential diagnosis of a regular tachycardia with a wide QRS complex. *Circulation* 83:1649, 1991.

From Bloomstrom-Lundqvist C et al: ACC/AHA/ESC guidelines for the management of patients with supraventricular arrhythmias—executive summary: a report of the American College of Cardiology/American Heart Association Task Force on Practice Guidelines and the European Society of Cardiology Committee for Practice Guidelines [Writing Committee to Develop Guidelines for the Management of Patients with Supraventricular Arrhythmias], *Circulation* 108:1871, 2003; Mann DL et al: *Braunwald's heart disease*, ed 10, Philadelphia, 2015, Elsevier.

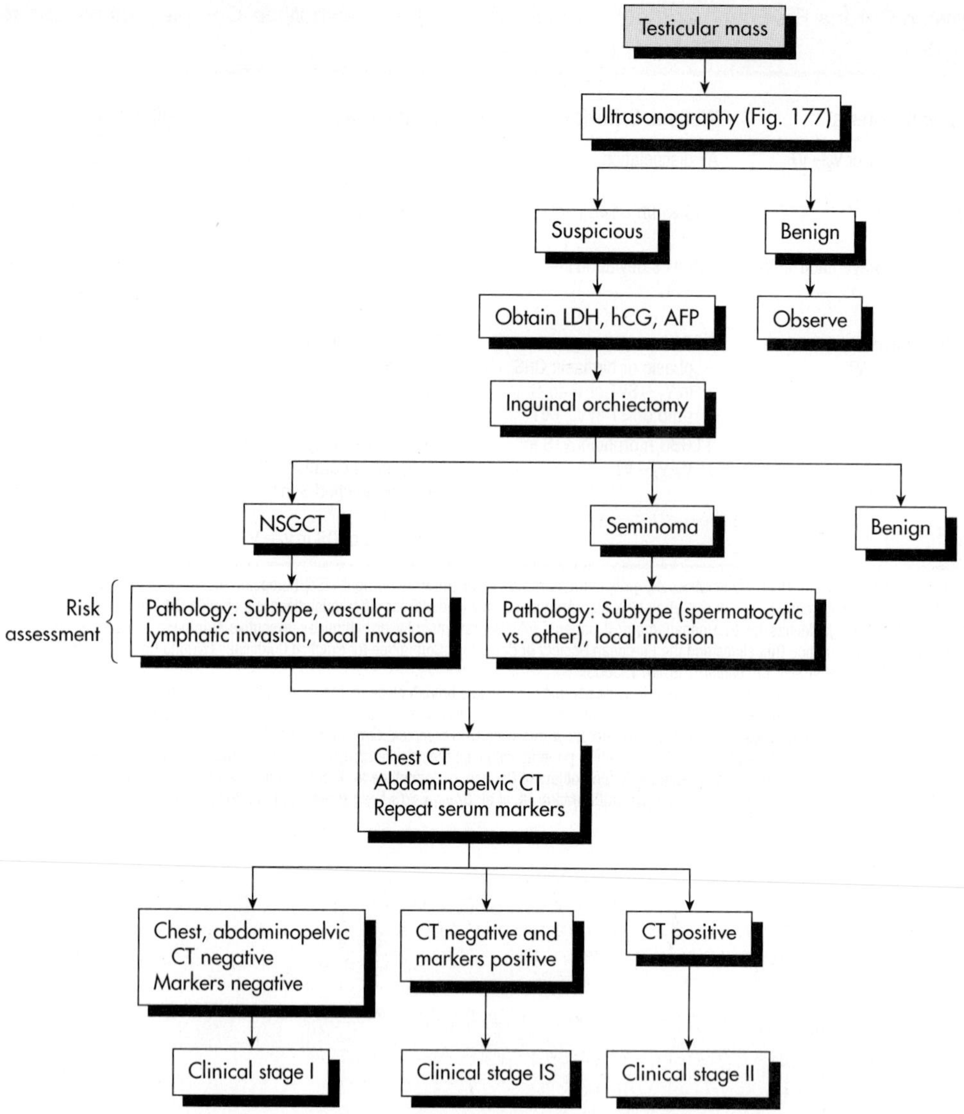

FIG. 176 Diagnosis, staging, and risk assessment of patients with testicular germ cell tumor. See "Section I topic Testicular Cancer" for additional information. *AFP,* α-Fetoprotein; *CT,* computed tomography; *hCG,* human chorionic gonadotropin; *LDH,* lactic dehydrogenase; *NSGCT,* nonseminoma germ cell tumor. (From Abeloff MD: *Clinical oncology,* ed 4, New York, 2007, Churchill Livingstone.)

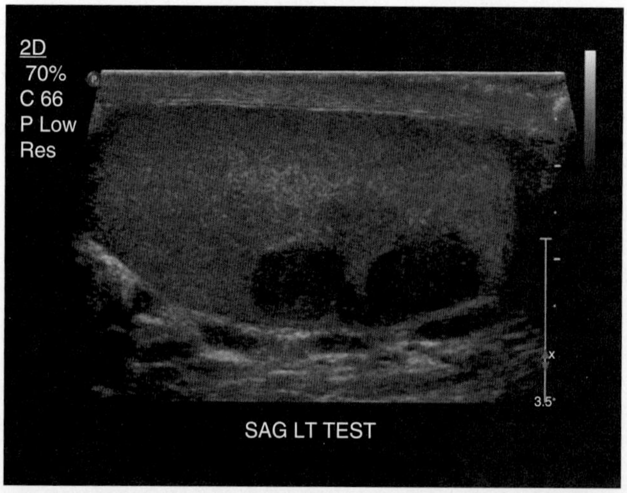

FIG. 177 Sagittal view of ultrasound of left testis showing multinodular hypoechoic intratesticular lesion confirmed to be pure seminoma at orchiectomy. (From Wein AJ et al: *Campbell-Walsh urology,* ed 11, Philadelphia, 2016, Elsevier.)

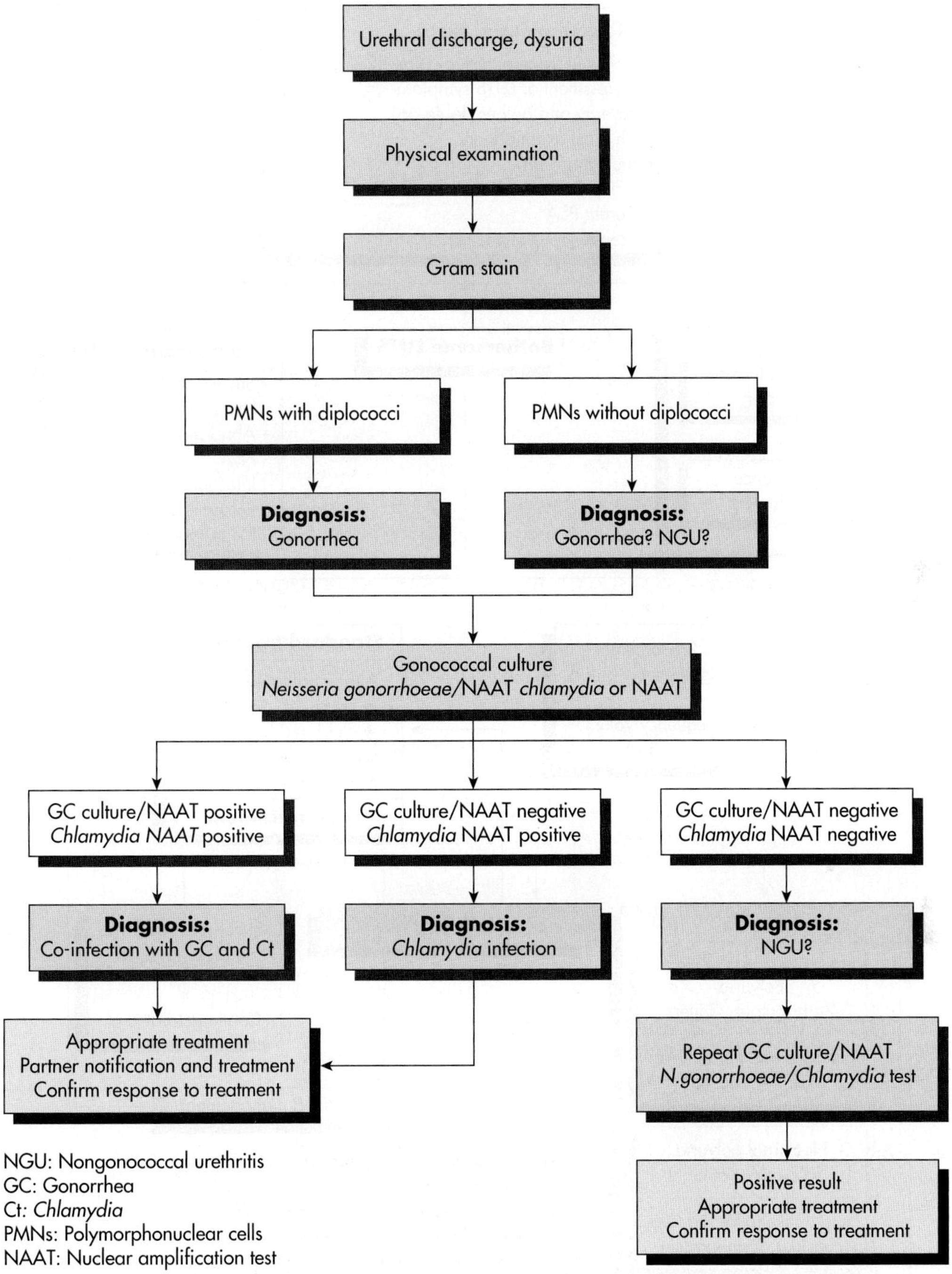

FIG. 181 Diagnostic algorithm for evaluation of urethral discharge or dysuria. (From Bolognia J: *Dermatology,* ed 4, Philadelphia, 2018, Elsevier.)

ICD-10CM # R33.9 Retention of urine, unspecified
N21.8 Other lower urinary tract calculus
R32 Unspecified urinary incontinence

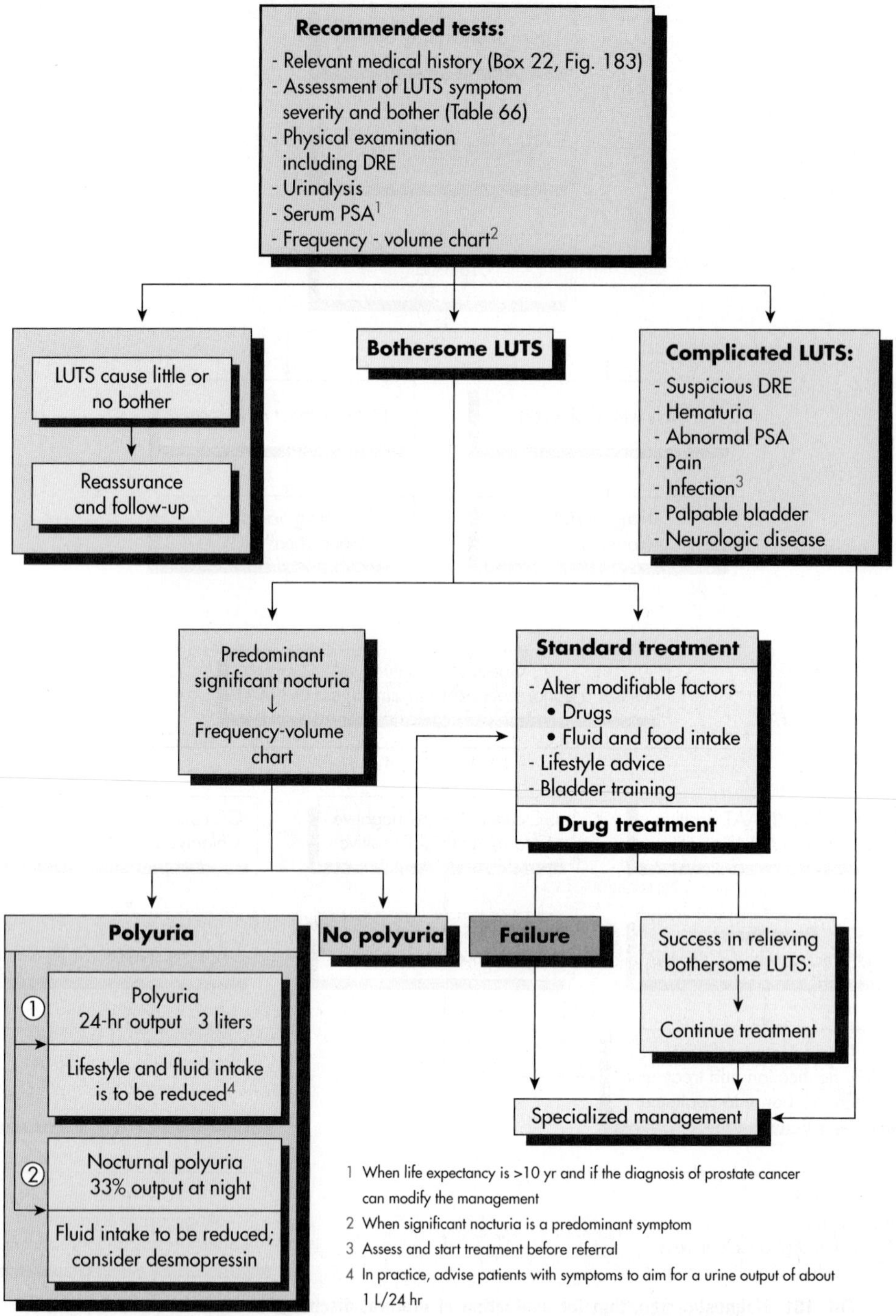

1 When life expectancy is >10 yr and if the diagnosis of prostate cancer can modify the management
2 When significant nocturia is a predominant symptom
3 Assess and start treatment before referral
4 In practice, advise patients with symptoms to aim for a urine output of about 1 L/24 hr

FIG. 182 Basic management of lower urinary tract symptoms *(LUTS)* in men. *DRE,* Digital rectal examination; *PSA,* prostate-specific antigen. (From Fillit HM: *Brocklehurst's textbook of geriatric medicine and gerontology*, ed 8, Philadelphia, 2017, Elsevier.)

BOX 23 Causes of Male Lower Urinary Tract Symptoms

Benign prostatic enlargement (secondary to benign prostatic hyperplasia)
Urinary tract infection
Prostatitis
Overactive bladder
Neurogenic bladder dysfunction
Urethral stricture
Bladder neck contracture
Phimosis
Urinary tract stones
Bladder tumor
Advanced prostate cancer
Foreign body in the bladder
Medications, illicit drugs, and dietary factors (including caffeine, alcohol, ketamine, and decongestants)
Diabetes mellitus

From Fillit HM: *Brocklehurst's textbook of geriatric medicine and gerontology,* ed 8, Philadelphia, 2017, Elsevier.

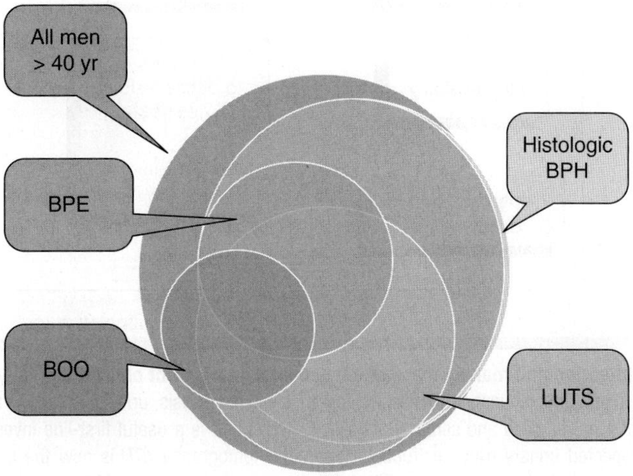

FIG. 183 Occurrence of LUTS with and without BOO, BPE, or BPH. *BOO,* Bladder outflow obstruction; *BPH,* benign prostate hyperplasia; *BPE,* benign prostate enlargement; *LUTS,* lower urinary tract symptoms. (From Fillit HM: *Brocklehurst's textbook of geriatric medicine and gerontology,* ed 8, Philadelphia, 2017, Elsevier.)

TABLE 65 International Continence Society Definitions of Lower Urinary Tract Symptoms

Voiding symptoms	• *Hesitancy* is difficulty in initiating micturition, resulting in a delay in the onset of voiding after being ready to pass urine. • *Slow stream* is the perception of reduced urine flow, usually compared to previous performance or in comparison to others. • *Splitting or spraying* of the urine stream. • *Intermittent stream* (intermittency) is the term used to describe urine flow that stops and starts, on one or more occasions, during micturition. • *Straining* to void describes the muscular effort used to initiate, maintain, or improve the urinary stream. • *Terminal dribble* is the term used to describe a prolonged final part of micturition, when the flow has slowed to a trickle or dribble.
Storage symptoms	• *Increased daytime frequency* is the complaint by the patient who considers that he voids too often during the day. • *Nocturia* is the complaint that the man has to wake at night one or more times to void. • *Urgency* is the complaint of a sudden compelling desire to pass urine that is difficult to defer. • *Urinary incontinence* is the complaint of any involuntary leakage of urine.
Postmicturition symptoms	• *Feeling of incomplete emptying* is a self-explanatory term for a feeling experienced by the individual after passing urine. • *Postmicturition dribble* is the term used to describe the involuntary loss of urine immediately after finishing passing urine, usually after leaving the toilet.

From Fillit HM: *Brocklehurst's textbook of geriatric medicine and gerontology,* ed 8, Philadelphia, 2017, Elsevier.

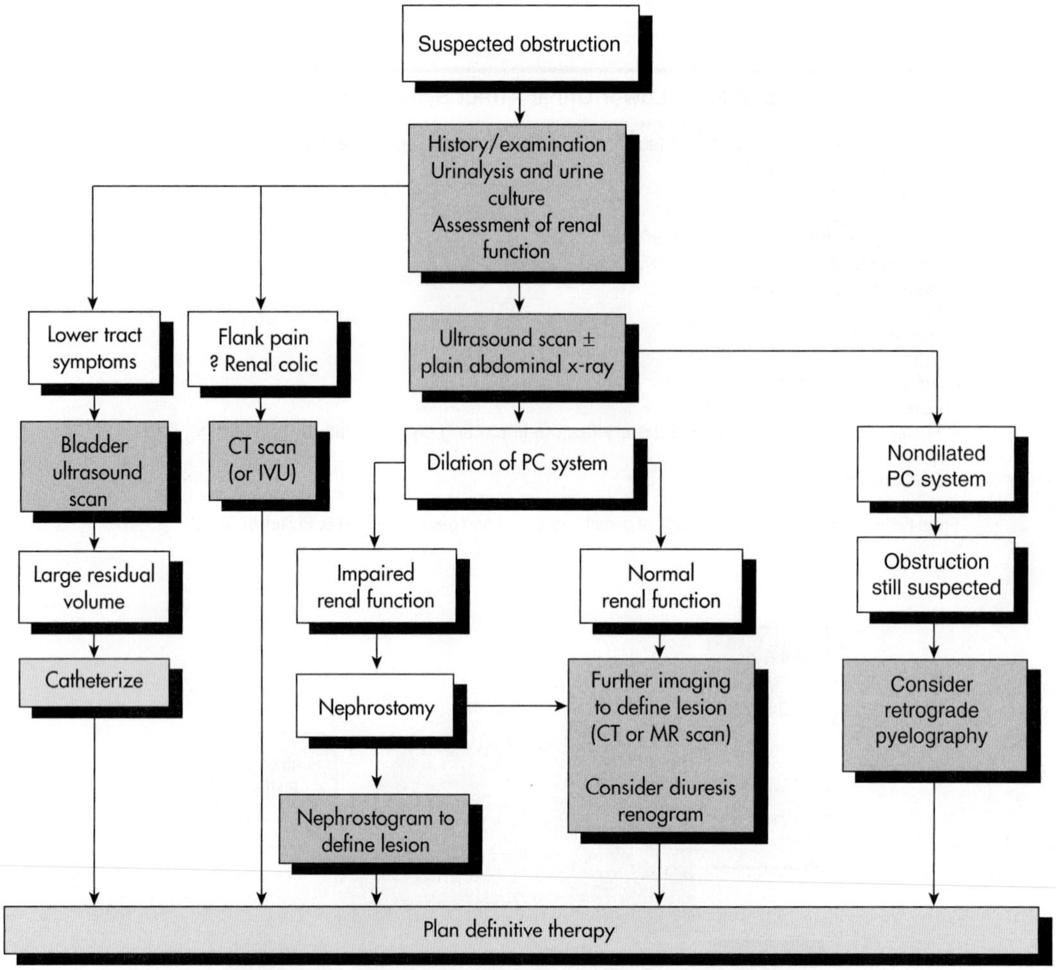

FIG. 184 Investigation and management of suspected urinary tract obstruction. A full history should be taken and a thorough examination performed, together with urinalysis, urine microscopy and culture, and measurement of renal function and serum electrolytes. Ultrasound is a useful first-line investigation for any patient with suspected urinary tract obstruction. Computed tomography *(CT)* is now the preferred imaging technique when renal calculi are suspected. Either CT or magnetic resonance *(MR)* urography can accurately diagnose both the site and cause of obstruction in most cases. If there is renal impairment, a nephrostomy allows the effective relief of the obstruction and time for renal function to recover while definitive therapy is planned. *IVU,* Intravenous urography; *PC,* pelvicalyceal. (From Johnson R et al: *Comprehensive clinical nephrology*, ed 5, Philadelphia, 2015, Saunders.)

BOX 24 Diagnostic Tests Used in Obstructive Uropathy

Upper Urinary Tract Obstruction
- Sonography (ultrasound)
- Plain films of the abdomen (KUB)
- Excretory or intravenous pyelography (very rarely needed)
- Retrograde pyelography
- Isotopic renography
- Computed tomography (helical CT)
- Magnetic resonance imaging
- Pressure flow studies (the Whitaker test)

Lower Urinary Tract Obstruction
- Some of the tests listed at left
- Cystoscopy
- Voiding cystourethrogram
- Retrograde urethrography
- Urodynamic tests
- Debimetry
- Cystometrography
- Electromyography
- Urethral pressure profile

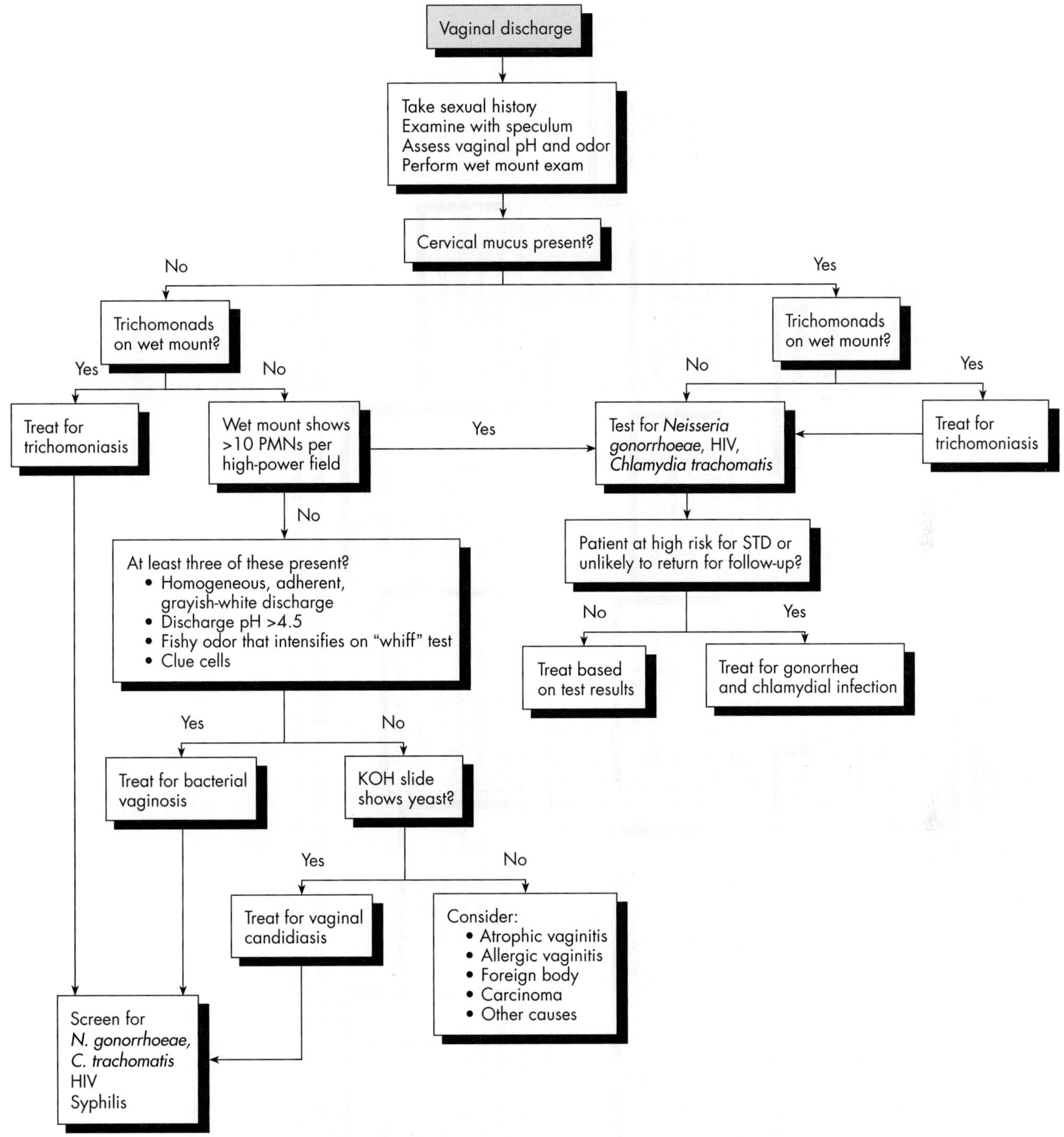

FIG. 185 Evaluation of vaginal discharge. See "Section I" topics "Vaginitis," "Fungal and Vaginitis," "Trichomonas" for additional information. *HIV,* Human immunodeficiency virus; *KOH,* potassium hydroxide; *PMN,* polymorphonuclear leukocyte; *STD,* sexually transmitted disease.

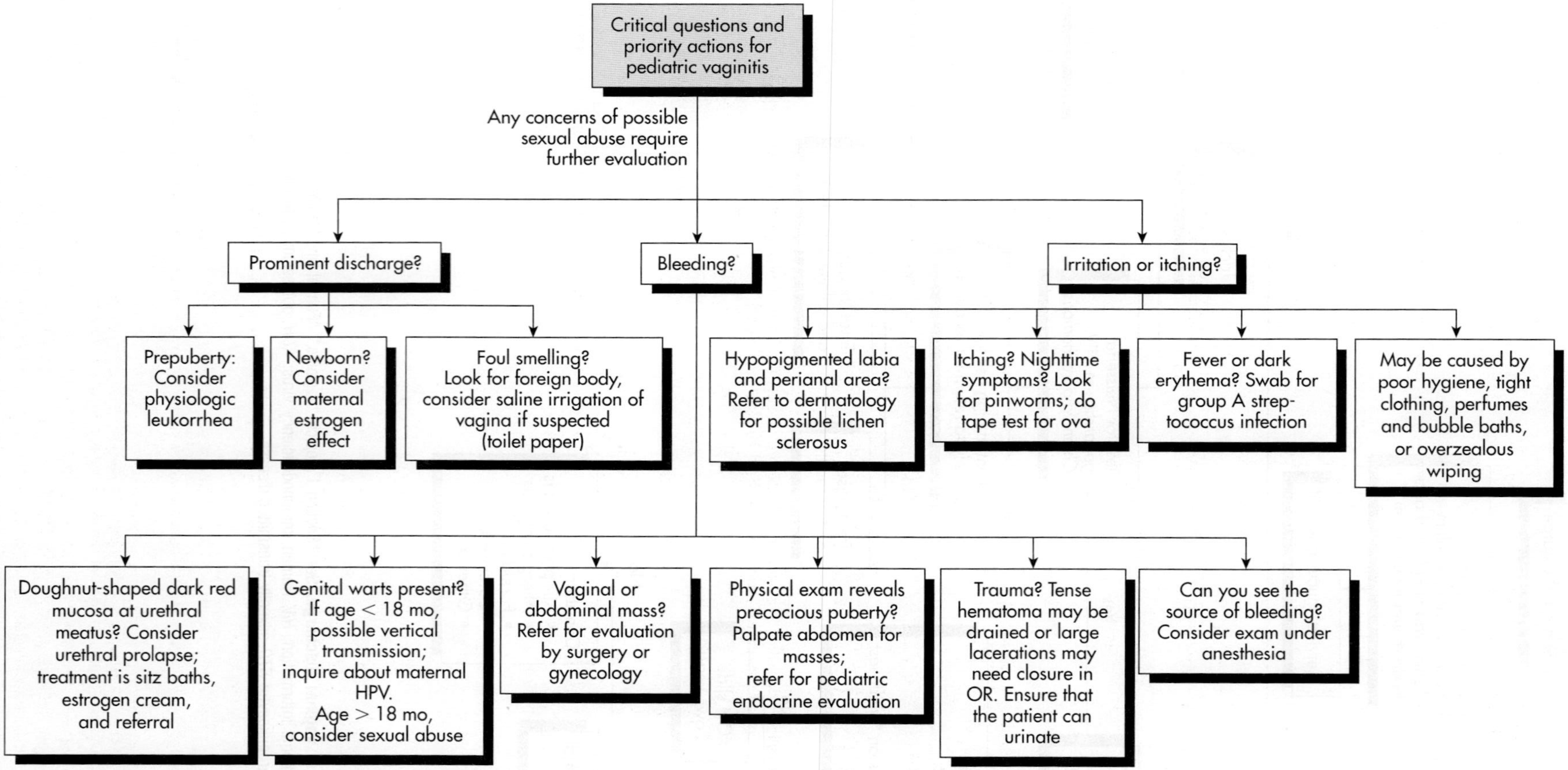

FIG. 186 Algorithm showing critical questions and priority actions for pediatric vaginitis. Additional information available in Section I topic Vaginitis, Prepubescent. *HPV,* Human papillomavirus; *OR,* operating room. (From Adams JG et al: *Emergency medicine: clinical essentials*, ed 2, Philadelphia, 2013, Elsevier.)

VENTILATOR-ASSOCIATED PNEUMONIA

ICD-10CM # J15.9 Unspecified bacterial pneumonia
J15.1 Pneumonia due to pseudomonas
J15.6 Pneumonia due to other aerobic gram-negative bacteria
J15.212 Pneumonia due to methicillin-resistant *Staphylococcus aureus*

Patient has a baseline period of stability or Improvement on the ventilator, defined by ≥ 2 calendar days of stable or decreasing daily minimum* FiO_2 or PEEP values. The baseline period is defined as the 2 calendar days immediately preceding the first day of increased daily minimum PEEP or FiO_2.

*Daily minimum defined bv lowest value of FiO_2 or PEEP during a calendar day that is maintained for >1 hr.

↓

After a period of stability or Improvement on the ventilator, the patient has at least one of the following Indicators of worsening oxygenation:
(1) Increase in daily minimum* FiO_2 of ≥ 0.20 (20 points) over the daily minimum FiO_2 of the first day in the baseline period, sustained for ≥ 2 calendar days.
(2) Increase In daily minimum· PEEP values of ~ 3 cm H_2O over the daily minimum PEEP of the first day in the baseline period†, sustained for ≥ 2 calendar days.

*Daily minimum defined by lowest value of FiO_2 or PEEP during a calendar day that is maintained for >1 hr.
†Daily minimum PEEP values of 0-5 cm H_2O are considered equivalent for the purposes of VAE surveillance.

↓

Ventilator-Associated Condition (VAC)

↓

On or after calendar day 3 of mechanical ventilation and within 2 calendar days before or after the onset of worsening oxygenation, the patient meets both of the following criteria:
(1) Temperature > 38 °C or > 38 °C **OR** white blood cell count ≥12,000 cells/mm^3 or ≤4,000 cells/mm^3.
AND
(2) A new antimicrobial agent(s) (see Appendix for eligible antimicrobial agents) is started, and is continued for ≥ 4 qualifying antimicrobial days (QAD).

↓

Infection-related Ventilator-Associated Complication (IVAC)

↓

On or after calendar day 3 of mechanical ventilation and within 2 calendar days before or after the onset of worsening oxygenation, ONE of the following criteria is met (**taking Into account organism exclusions specified in the protocol**):

(1) Criterion 1: Positive culture of one of the following specimens, meeting quantitative or semi-quantitative thresholds† as outlined in protocol, without requirement for purulent respiratory secretions:
- Endotracheal aspirate, ≥ 10^5 CFU/ml or corresponding semi-quantitative result
- Bronchoalveolar lavage, ≥ 10^4 CFU/ml or corresponding semi-quantltatlve result
- Lung tissue, ≥ 10^4 CFU/g or corresponding semi-quantitative result
- Protected specimen brush, ≥ 10^3 CFU/ml or corresponding semi-quantitative result

(2) Criterion 2: Purulent respiratory secretions (defined as secretions from the lungs, bronchi, or trachea that contain ≥25 neutrophils and ≤10 squamous epithelial cells per low power field [lpf, x100])† **PLUS** organism identified from one of the following specimens (to include qualitative culture, or quantitative/semi-quantitative culture without sufficient growth to meet criterion #1):
- Sputum
- Endotracheal aspirate
- Bronchoalveolar lavage
- Lung tissue
- Protected specimen brush

(3) Criterion 3: One of the following positive tests:
- Organism Identified from pleural fluid (where specimen was obtained during thoracentesis or initial placement of chest tube and NOT from an indwelling chest tube)
- Lung histopathology, defined as: (1) abscess formation or foci of consolidation with intense neutrophil accumulation in bronchioles and alveoli; (2) evidence of lung parenchyma Invasion by fungi (hyphae, pseudohyphae or yeast forms); (3) evidence of infection with the viral pathogens listed below based on results of immunohistochemical assays, cytology, or microscopy performed on lung tissue
- Diagnostic test for *Legionella* species
- Diagnostic test on respiratory secretions for influenza virus, respiratory syncytial virus, adenovirus, parainfluenza virus, rhinovirus, human metapneumovirus, coronavirus

† If the laboratory reports semi-quantitative results, those results must correspond to the quantitative thresholds. Refer to Table 2 and 3.

↓

Possible Ventilator-Associated Pneumonia (PVAP)

FIG. 187 Ventilator-associated events surveillance algorithm. *CFU*, Colony-forming unit; *FiO_2*, fraction of inspired oxygen; *PEEP*, positive end-expiratory pressure; *VAE*, ventilator-associated events. (From Centers for Disease Control and Prevention: Ventilator-associated event [VAE], device-associated module, *NHSN Patient Safety Component Manual*, pp 10-1-10-46, January 2015 [modified April 2015]. Available at www.cdc.gov/nhsn/pdfs/pscmanual/pcsmanual_current.pdf)

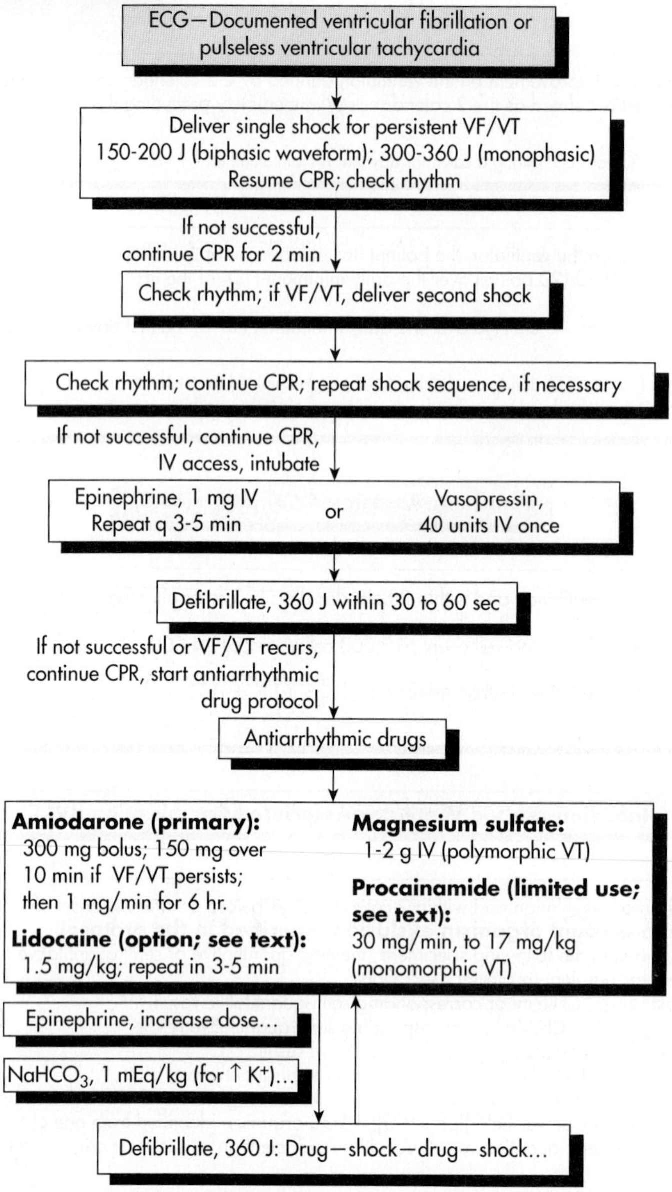

FIG. 188 General algorithm for advanced cardiac life support *(ACLS)* response to ventricular fibrillation *(VF)* or pulseless ventricular tachycardia *(VT)*. NOTE: In a 2008 advisory, 200 compression-only sequences were suggested as an alternative to standard CPR cycles between shocks, and this approach is under consideration for future guidelines. *CPR*, Cardiopulmonary resuscitation; *ECG*, electrocardiogram; *IV*, intravenous. (From Goldman L, Schafer AI: *Goldman Cecil medicine*, ed 25, Philadelphia, 2016, Saunders.)

ICD-10CM # H81.13 Benign paroxysmal vertigo, bilateral
R42 Dizziness and giddiness
H81.49 Vertigo of central origin, unspecified ear
H81.399 Other peripheral vertigo, unspecified ear
H81.23 Vestibular neuronitis, bilateral

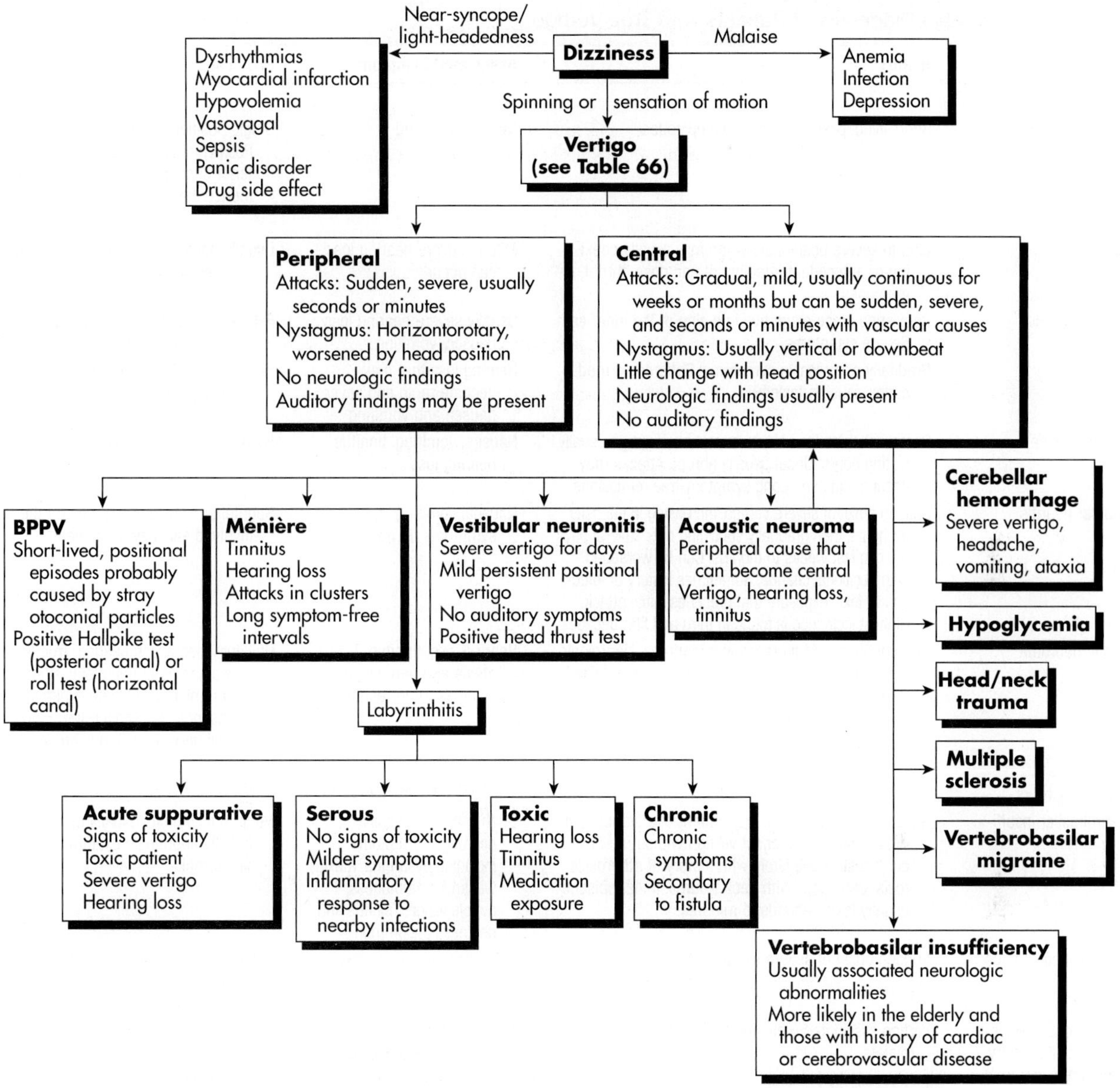

FIG. 189 Diagnostic algorithm for dizziness and vertigo. Also see "Section I" topics "Vestibular Neuronitis," "Acoustic Neuroma," "Labyrinthitis," "Ménière Disease," and "Benign Paroxysmal Positional Vertigo." *BPPV,* Benign paroxysmal positional vertigo. (From Marx JA et al: *Rosen's emergency medicine*, ed 8, Philadelphia, 2014, Saunders.)

ICD-10CM #		
	H81.13	Benign paroxysmal vertigo, bilateral
	R42	Dizziness and giddiness
	H81.49	Vertigo of central origin, unspecified ear
	H81.399	Other peripheral vertigo, unspecified ear
	H81.23	Vestibular neuronitis, bilateral

TABLE 66 Differential Diagnosis of Patients with True Vertigo

Cause	History	Associated Symptoms	Physical
Peripheral			
• Benign paroxysmal positional vertigo	Short-lived, positional, fatigable episodes	Nausea, vomiting	Single position can precipitate vertigo. Positive result on Hallpike test (posterior semicircular canal) or Roll test (horizontal canal).
• Labyrinthitis			
• Serous	Mild to severe positional symptoms. Usually coexisting or antecedent infection of ear, nose, throat, or meninges.	Mild to severe hearing loss can occur	Usually nontoxic patient with minimal fever elevation
• Acute suppurative	Coexisting acute exudative infection of the inner ear. Severe symptoms.	Usually severe hearing loss, nausea, vomiting	Febrile patient showing signs of toxicity. Acute otitis media.
• Toxic	Gradually progressive symptoms: Patients on medication causing toxicity.	Hearing loss that may become rapid and severe, nausea and vomiting	Hearing loss. Ataxia common feature in chronic phase.
• Ménière disease	Recurrent episodes of severe rotational vertigo usually lasting hours. Onset usually abrupt. Attacks may occur in clusters. Long symptom-free remissions.	Nausea, vomiting, tinnitus, hearing loss	Positional nystagmus not present
• Vestibular neuritis	Sudden onset of severe vertigo, increasing in intensity for hours, then gradually subsiding over several days but can last weeks to months. Can be worsened with positional change. Sometimes history of infection or toxic exposure that precedes initial attack. Highest incidence is found in third and fifth decades.	Nausea, vomiting. Auditory symptoms do not occur.	Spontaneous nystagmus toward the involved ear may be present.
• Acoustic neuroma	Gradual onset and increase in symptoms. Neurologic signs in later stages. Most occur in women aged 30-60.	Hearing loss, tinnitus. True ataxia and neurologic signs as tumor enlarges.	Unilateral decreased hearing. True truncal ataxia and other neurologic signs when tumor enlarges. May have diminution or absence of corneal reflex. Eighth cranial nerve deficit may be present.
Central			
• Vascular disorders			
• Vertebrobasilar insufficiency	Should be considered in any patient of advanced age with isolated new-onset vertigo without an obvious cause. More likely with history of atherosclerosis. Can occur with neck trauma. Initial episode usually lasts seconds to minutes.	Often headache. Usually neurologic symptoms including dysarthria, ataxia, weakness, numbness, double vision. Tinnitus and deafness uncommon.	Neurologic deficits usually present, but initially neurologic examination can be normal.
• Cerebellar hemorrhage	Sudden onset of severe symptoms	Headache, vomiting, ataxia	Signs of toxicity. Dysmetria, true ataxia. Ipsilateral sixth cranial nerve palsy may be present.
• Occlusion of posterior inferior cerebellar artery (Wallenberg syndrome)	Vertigo associated with significant neurologic complaints	Nausea, vomiting, loss of pain and temperature sensation, ataxia, hoarseness	Loss of pain and temperature sensation on the side of the face ipsilateral to the lesion and on the opposite side of the body, paralysis of the palate, pharynx, and larynx. Horner syndrome (ipsilateral ptosis, miosis, and decreased facial sweating).
• Head trauma	Symptoms begin with or shortly after head trauma. Positional symptoms most common type after trauma. Self-limited symptoms that can persist weeks to months.	Usually mild nausea	Occasionally, basilar skull fracture
• Vertebrobasilar migraine	Vertigo almost always followed by headache. Patient has usually had similar episodes in past. Most patients have a family history of migraine. Syndrome usually begins in adolescence.	Dysarthria, ataxia, visual disturbances, or paresthesias usually precede headache	No residual neurologic or otologic signs are present after attack
• Multiple sclerosis	Vertigo presenting symptom in 7%-10% and appears in the course of the disease in a third. Onset may be severe and suggest labyrinth disease. Disease onset usually between ages 20 and 40. Often history of other attacks with varying neurologic signs or symptoms.	Nausea and vomiting, which may be severe	May have horizontal, rotary, or vertical nystagmus. Nystagmus may persist after the vertiginous symptoms have subsided. Bilateral internuclear ophthalmoplegia and ataxic eye movements suggest multiple sclerosis.
• Temporal lobe epilepsy	Can be initial or prominent symptom in some patients with the disorder	Memory impairment, hallucinations, trancelike states, seizures	May have aphasia or convulsions
• Hypoglycemia	Should be considered in diabetics and any other patient with unexplained symptoms	Sweating, anxiety	Tachycardia, mental status change may be present

From Marx JA et al: *Rosen's emergency medicine,* ed 8, Philadelphia, 2014, Saunders.

VIRAL EXANTHEM

ICD-10CM # B09 Unspecified viral infection characterized by skin and mucous membrane lesions
B08.8 Other specified viral infections characterized by skin and mucous membrane lesions

1. Exclude other causes →
- Drug reaction
- Kawasaki disease
- Bacterial infections, e.g., group A β-hemolytic streptococcal, *Arcanobacterium haemolyticum**, meningococcemia (if petechiae), ehrlichiosis, leptospirosis, rickettsioses, syphilis
- Other viral exanthems, e.g., due to HIV seroconversion, chikungunya fever, dengue, and infections with Zika, Barmah forest, and Ross River viruses

↓

2. Specific features

↓

Clinical signs and symptoms		Viruses: Measles (rubeola)	Rubella	Parvovirus B19	HHV-6 or-7	Epstein–Barr virus	Adenovirus	Enterovirus	Cytomegalo-virus†	West Nile virus
Exanthem	Cephalocaudad spread	✓	✓							
	Rose-pink macules		✓		✓	✓	✓	✓	✓	
	Red cheeks; reticulate or lacy			✓						
	Punctate lesions on extremities									✓
	Rash starts as fever subsides				✓					
	Most prominent following antibiotics					✓			✓	
	Petechiae	✓		✓		✓	✓	✓	✓	
Enanthem	Gray–white papules, buccal mucosa (koplik)	✓								
	Red macules, soft palate (forschheimer)		✓							
	Red papules, soft palate/uvula (nagayama)				✓					
	Uvulo-palatoglossal junctional ulcers				✓					
	Painful erosions, esp. of posterior pharynx			✓				✓		
	Pharyngitis					✓	✓	✓		
Lymph-adenopathy	Generalized	✓				✓				✓
	Localized: Occipital, posterior auricular		✓							
	Localized: Cervical					✓		✓	✓	
Musculoskeletal	Arthralgias/arthritis		✓	✓		✓		✓	✓	✓
	Muscle weakness									✓
Eye	Conjunctivitis	✓	✓				✓	✓		✓
Liver/spleen	Hepatosplenomegaly	✓				✓			✓	
CNS	Encephalitis (E) ± Meningitis (M)	✓(E)	✓(E)		✓(E**)		✓(E,M)	✓(E,M)	✓(E)	✓(E,M)
Lungs	Pneumonia	✓					✓	✓		
Heart	Myocarditis	✓	✓					✓		
3. Laboratory tests		Serology; Virus isolation NP; xxxxxx	Serology; Virus isolation NP/U/CSF; xxxxxx	Serology; xxxxxx	Serology; xxxxxx	Heterophile antibody; Serology; Atypical lymphocytosis; xxxxxx	Antigen detection T/S; Virus isolation NP; Serology; xxxxxx	Virus isolation T/S/V; Serology; xxxxxx	Antigen detection, xxxxxx Blood[ab]; Virus isolation U[b]; Serology	Serology also CSF; xxxxxx

Key:
- Serology
- Virus isolation
- xxxxxx Polymerase chain reaction assay
- Antigen detection
- Heterophile antibody
- Atypical lympho-cytosis

CSF=Cerebrospinal fluid
NP = Nasopharyngeal
V = Vesicle fluid
U = Urine
T = Throat
S = Stool

Notes: [a]Immunocompromised host [b]Immunocompetent host

FIG. 190 Approach to the patient with a presumed morbilliform or macular/papular viral exanthem. *Gram-positive rod; may result in severe pharyngitis and scarlatiniform exanthem in adolescents and young adults. **Usually febrile seizures. †Intracellular inclusions within endothelial cells represent an additional finding. (From Bolognia J: *Dermatology,* ed 4, Philadelphia, 2018, Elsevier.)

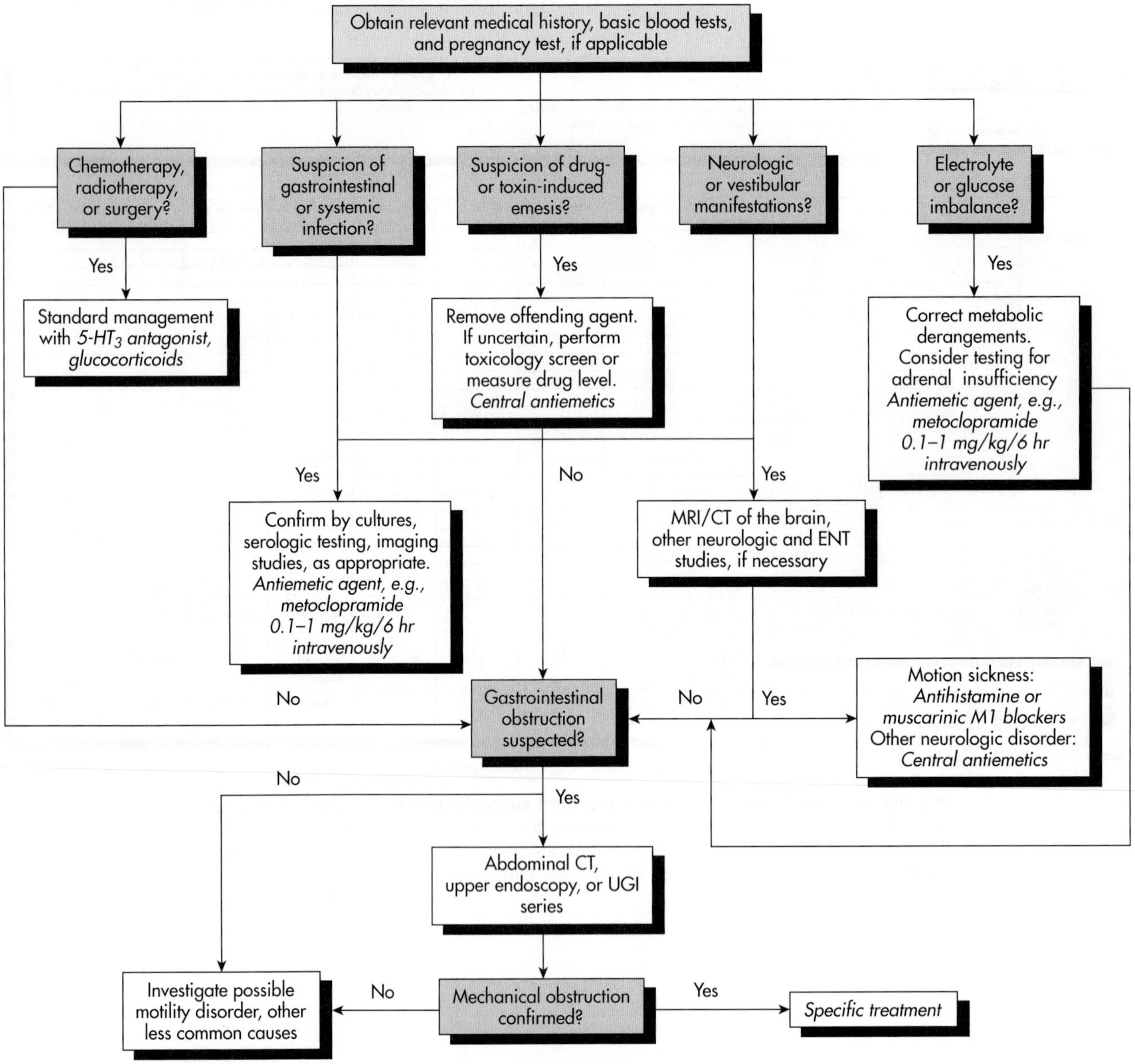

FIG. 191 Algorithm for management of a patient with acute vomiting. Possible treatments are italicized. *CT,* Computed tomography; *ENT,* ear, nose, and throat; *5-HT,* 5-hydroxytryptamine; *MRI,* magnetic resonance imaging; *UGI,* upper GI. Potential treatments are shown in italics. (From Feldman M et al: *Sleisenger and Fortran's gastrointestinal and liver disease*, ed 10, Philadelphia, 2016, Elsevier.)

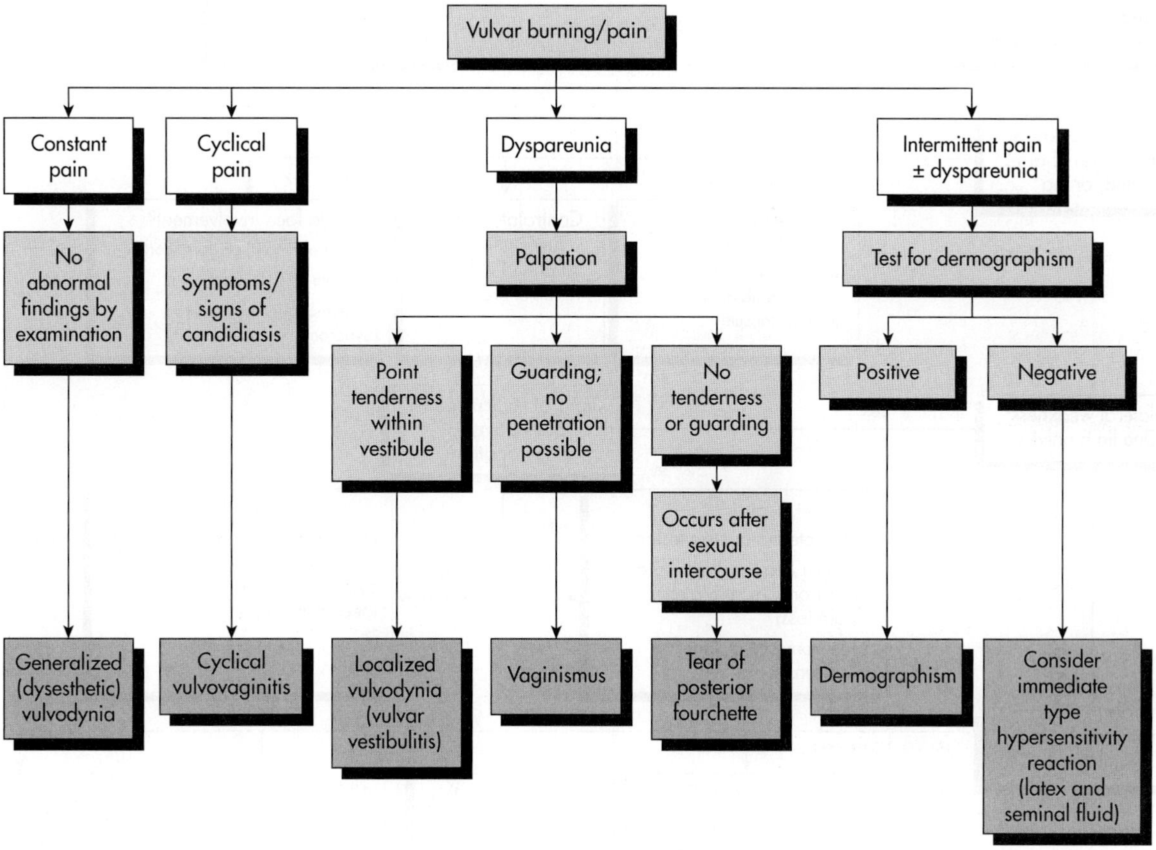

FIG. 192 Diagnosis of vulvar burning/pain in the setting of a normal-appearing vulva. (From Bolognia J: *Dermatology,* ed 4, Philadelphia, 2018, Elsevier.)

ICD-10CM # R53.1 Weakness
M62.81 Muscle weakness (generalized)

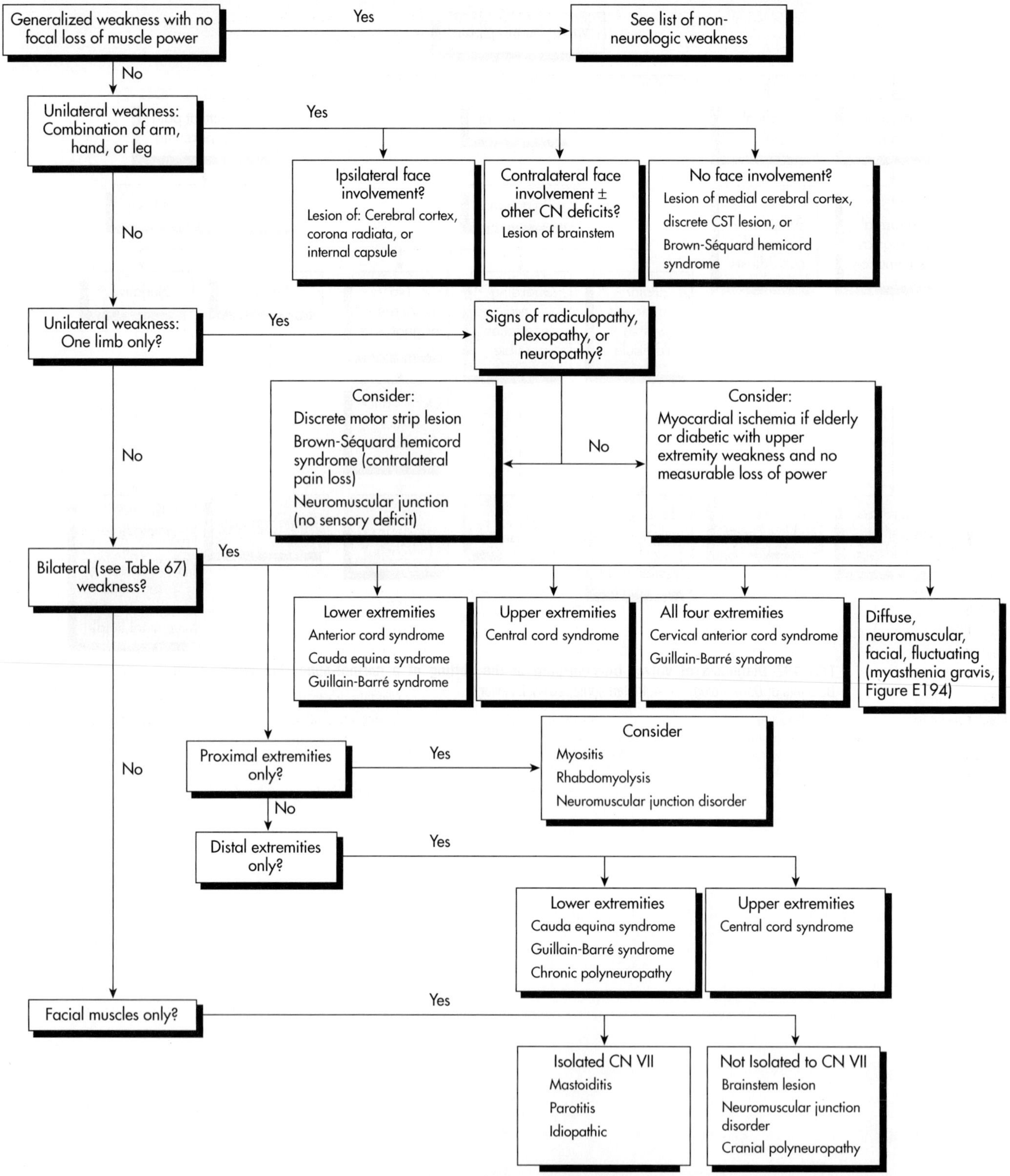

FIG. 193 Common clinical patterns of weakness, classified and assessed. *CN,* Cranial nerve; *CST,* corticospinal tract. (Modified from Marx JA et al: *Rosen's emergency medicine,* ed 8, Philadelphia, 2014, Saunders.)

TABLE 67 Critical and Emergent Causes of Neuromuscular Weakness

Critical Diagnoses	
Cerebral cortex or subcortical	Ischemic or hemorrhagic cerebrovascular accident (CVA)
Brainstem	Ischemic or hemorrhagic CVA
Spinal cord	Ischemia, compression (disk, abscess, or hematoma)
Peripheral nerve	Acute demyelination (Guillain-Barré syndrome)
Neuromuscular junction	Myasthenic or cholinergic crisis Botulism Tick paralysis Organophosphate poisoning
Muscle	Rhabdomyolysis
Emergent Diagnoses	
Cerebral cortex or subcortical	Tumor, abscess, demyelination
Brainstem	Demyelination
Spinal cord	Demyelination (transverse myelitis) Compression (disk, spondylosis)
Peripheral nerve	Compressive plexopathy (hematoma, aneurysm) Paraneoplastic vasculitis uremia
Muscle	Inflammatory myositis

From Marx JA et al: *Rosen's emergency medicine*, ed 8, Philadelphia, 2014, Saunders.

TABLE 68 Clinical Signs That Point to the Origin of Neuromuscular Weakness

Sign	UMNs	LMNs	NMJ	Myopathy
Atrophy	None	Severe	Mild	Mild
Fasciculation	None	Common	None	None
Deep tendon reflexes	Hyperreflexic	Areflexic/hyporeflexic	Normal/hyporeflexic	Normal/hyporeflexic
Distribution of weakness	Pyramidal/regional	Distal/segmental	Variable/fatigable weakness	Proximal > distal
Tone	Spastic	Decreased/flaccid	Decreased/flaccid	Normal/decreased
Plantar response	Upgoing	Downgoing or absent	Downgoing or absent	Downgoing or absent

LMNs, Lower motor neurons; *NMJ,* neuromuscular junction; *UMNs,* upper motor neurons.
From Cameron P et al: *Textbook of adult emergency medicine,* ed 5, Edinburgh, 2019, Elsevier.

TABLE 69 Nonneuromuscular Conditions Associated with Weakness

Condition	Manifestations
Anemia	Breathlessness and fatigue usually worse with acute-onset anemia
Cardiac failure	Fatigue and weakness are common symptoms of heart failure in elderly patients, especially weakness in females over 50 yr
Malignancy	Paraneoplastic syndromes (e.g., generalized wasting)
Psychological disorders	Depression/anxiety, psychosis, medication side effects, malingering
Malnutrition	Institutionalized patients, impoverished elderly, anorexia nervosa
Chronic fatigue syndrome	Possibly postviral syndrome
Rheumatologic disorders	Rheumatoid arthritis, systemic lupus erythematosus, fibromyalgia
Medications	Many medications have been associated with weakness; the commonly encountered ones include glucocorticoids, statins, antiretrovirals, alcohol, colchicine, and polypharmacy, especially in the elderly
Acute electrolyte derangement (e.g., hypokalemia and hyperkalemia, hypocalcemia)	Acute-onset weakness and/or tetany with hypocalcemia
Sepsis	Acidosis, deranged metabolic state
Dehydration	Lethargy/fatigue
Hypothyroidism	Lethargy, cold intolerance, weight gain, weakness
Chronic disease	Respiratory, renal, hepatic failure

From Cameron P et al: *Textbook of adult emergency medicine,* ed 5, Edinburgh, 2019, Elsevier.

TABLE 70 Key Features of Conditions Associated with the Symptom of Weakness

Disease	Pathophysiology	Assessment	ED Management
Primary Neurological			
Guillain-Barré syndrome, most common cause of acute symmetric weakness	Immune-mediated polyradiculopathy Postinfective (15%-40%), esp. due to *Campylobacter* or viral infection; >50% are idiopathic	Suggestive history (e.g., diarrhea) Symmetric ascending flaccid weakness; loss of DTRs; early facial palsy common; ± autonomic dysfunction Serial assessment of respiratory function crucial to predict need for intubation/ventilation CSF high protein with normal glucose and cell count	Supportive care; early intubation for respiratory failure Early neurology and ICU consultation Early administration of IVIG ± plasmapheresis beneficial Corticosteroids *not* indicated
Myasthenia gravis, localized variant more common Myasthenic crises/respiratory decompensation (rare) are main ED issues	Immune-mediated Ach receptor dysfunction; may be precipitated by thymic disorders	Fluctuating, fatigable weakness of voluntary muscles, especially ocular muscles or proximal limbs. Cranial nerve involvement with ptosis in >25% cases; ± dysphagia, weakness of masticatory muscles; normal sensation; normal reflexes Improves with rest Serial respiratory assessment if severe Ice-pack test if there is ptosis	Supportive care Avoid potential precipitants including corticosteroids Anticholinesterase treatment as directed by neurologist
Multiple sclerosis, relapsing/remitting course most common	Immune-mediated scattered neuron demyelination; affects motor, sensory, visual, and cerebellar function Classically ≥2 separate episodes of neurologic dysfunction indicating white matter or spinal cord lesions at distinct locations	Acute exacerbations, acute worsening of clinical signs; variable weakness, hypertonicity, spasticity, clonus, altered pain/temp/vibration and proprioceptive senses Lhermitte sign Optic neuritis in up to 30% with acute central vision loss, afferent papillary defect, red desaturation lung puncture, MRI, evoked potentials in consultation with neurologist	Pulse methylprednisolone therapy for exacerbations Supportive care for generalized weakness Neurology consultation Long-term disease modification and lifestyle strategies (e.g., vitamin D)
Cord compression	Spinal stenosis ± malignancy or infection	Thorough neurologic examination Red flags (e.g., fever, malignancy, IVDU warrant MRI)	Neurosurgical consultation Decompression, antibiotics, targeted radiotherapy as indicated
Myopathies			
Congenital Dystrophin disorders, Duchenne muscular dystrophy (DMD); Becker muscular dystrophy (BMB) DMD/BMD, mitochondrial disorders	X-linked dystrophin gene dysfunction Males affected more severely by DMD; life expectancy to early 20s; BMD of later onset less severe	Generalized weakness Usual ED presentation is acute deterioration with respiratory compromise Spirometry/respiratory assessment Mitochondrial disorders—variable episodic weakness and fluctuating consciousness	Supportive care Discussion with patient, advocates, neurologists regarding appropriateness of intensive intervention Consider advance care directives Ventilatory support as appropriate

TABLE 70 Key Features of Conditions Associated with the Symptom of Weakness—cont'd

Disease	Pathophysiology	Assessment	ED Management
Acquired Metabolic/electrolyte disorders Hypokalemic periodic paralysis Endocrine Cushing disease Addison disease Thyrotoxicosis Toxic Statins, corticosteroids	Variable weakness; may be acute episodic weakness with hypokalaemia ± thyrotoxicosis Drug-induced or history of endocrine myopathies suggestive	Periodic paralysis; may be preceded by vomiting/diarrheal illness; may have family history Check electrolytes, especially K^+ ECG if K^+ deranged Endocrine—assess for other stigmata of endocrinopathy (e.g., cushingoid, addisonian)	Electrolyte (K^+) reconstitution Supportive care Correct endocrine abnormalities Discontinue offending medications
Intoxications			
Botulism due to *Clostridium botulinum* toxin	Deranged neurotransmission Ingested botulinum toxin prevents Ach release at NMJ	History of ingestion GI symptoms in 50% Descending flaccid paralysis Postural hypotension, diplopia, blurred vision, ptosis, dysphagia, respiratory compromise, progressing to limb weakness Ileus common	Supportive care ICU admission for ventilatory support as needed Specific antiserum in consultation with toxicology/neurology
Tetanus due to *Clostridium tetani* tetanospasmin toxin Endemic in developing countries	Impaired inhibitory neurotransmission causing skeletal muscle spasm and rigidity Classically infected deep wounds in nonimmunized patients	Suggestive history—recent wound, vulnerable patient (e.g., elderly, nonimmune) Trismus/dysphagia common early; progressive to painful skeletal muscle spasms; exacerbated by minor stimuli (e.g., touch) May be a localized form Clinical diagnosis	Supportive care, ICU for ventilatory support and sedation Tetanus antitoxin Tetanus immunization is protective Antibiotics (penicillin) to treat clostridial infection
Tick paralysis due to tick toxin, ascending flaccid paralysis mimics Guillain-Barré syndrome	Impaired neurotransmission *Ixodes holocyclus* (Australian paralysis tick) Death from respiratory paralysis	Mostly children in tick-endemic area ± tick found on patient; ataxia, weakness ± extraocular palsy/dysphagia May progress after tick removal to generalized/respiratory paralysis	Tick removal/observation sufficient in most cases If severe, ventilatory support Antiserum administration as directed by toxicology/neurology
Marine intoxications Ciguatera Puffer fish Blue-ringed octopus	Ciguatera toxin (from reef fish) Tetrodotoxin (puffer fish, blue-ringed octopus) block sodium channels and impair neurotransmission Tetrodotoxin also acts on CTZ and impairs ventilation	History of tropical fish ingestion; onset of symptoms within a few hours Ciguatera—paresthesias, electrical sensations in response to hot/cold Tetrodotoxin—progressive flaccid weakness with respiratory compromise	Supportive treatment esp. ventilatory support

CSF, Cerebrospinal fluid; *CTZ,* chemoreceptor trigger zone; *DTRs,* deep tendon reflexes; *ECG,* electrocardiogram; *ED,* emergency department; *GI,* gastrointestinal; *ICU,* intensive care unit; *IVDU,* intravenous drug user; *IVIG,* intravenous immunoglobulin; *MRI,* magnetic resonance imaging; *NMJ,* neuromuscular junction.
From Cameron P et al: *Textbook of adult emergency medicine*, ed 5, Edinburgh, 2019, Elsevier.

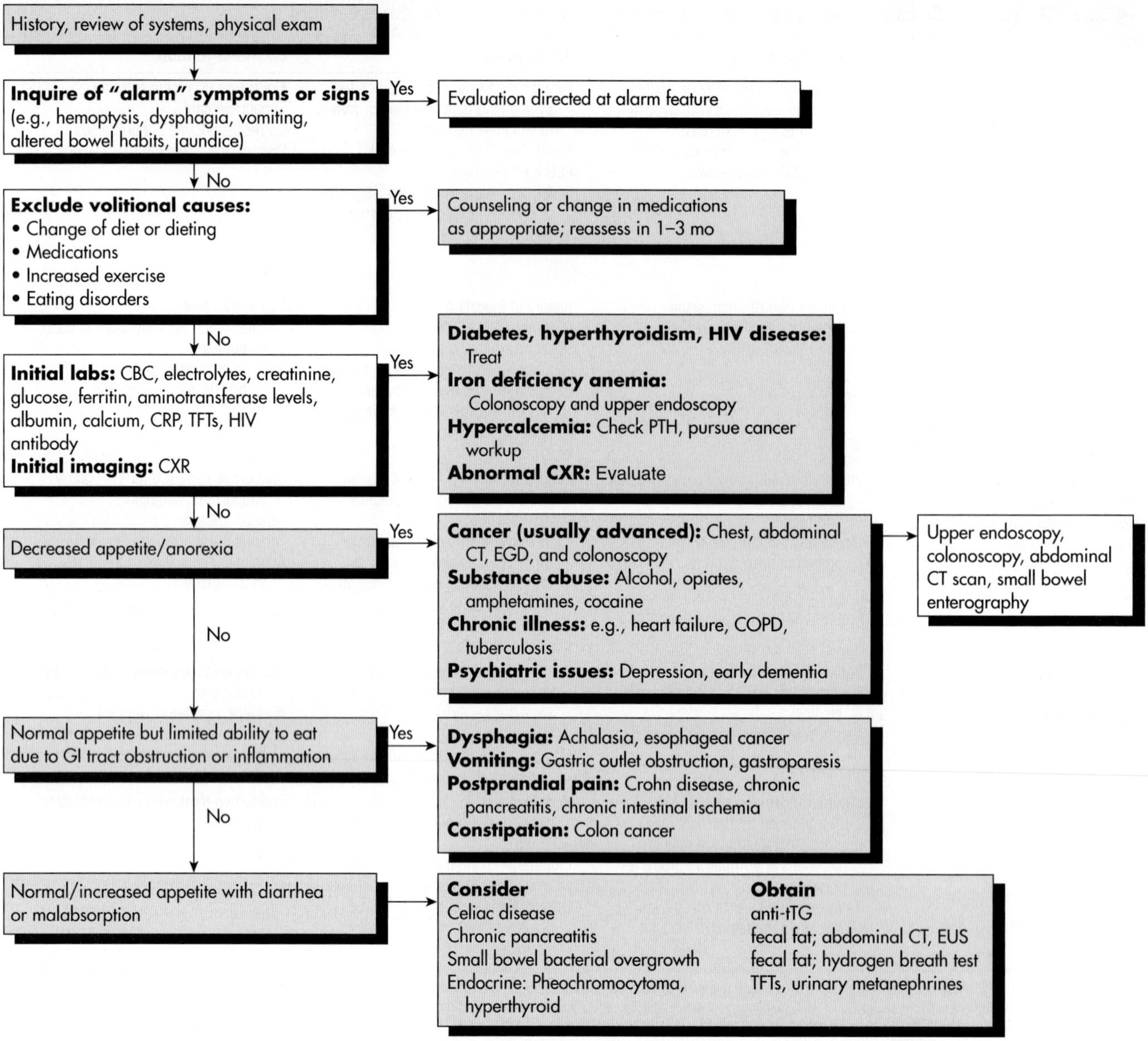

FIG. 195 Approach to the patient with unintentional weight loss of more than 5%. *CBC,* Complete blood count; *COPD,* chronic obstructive pulmonary disease; *CRP,* C-reactive protein; *CT,* computed tomography; *CXR,* chest radiograph; *EGD,* esophagogastroduodenoscopy; *EUS,* endoscopic ultrasound; *GI,* gastrointestinal; *HIV,* human immunodeficiency virus; *PTH,* parathyroid hormone; *TFTs,* thyroid function tests; *tTG,* tissue transglutaminase. (From Goldman L, Schafer AI: *Goldman Cecil medicine,* ed 25, Philadelphia, 2016, Saunders.)

TABLE 71 Causes of Involuntary Weight Loss

Condition	Quality	Duration	Aggravating or Relieving Factors	Associated Symptoms or Signs	Diagnostic Studies
Weight Loss Secondary to Gastrointestinal Causes					
GI, pancreatic, or hepatobiliary malignant disease	Progressive, fast	Months	Better with cancer therapy (e.g., surgery, XRT, chemotherapy)	Dysphagia (esophageal); anorexia, nausea, vomiting (gastric, small or large bowel obstruction); visible or occult blood in stool; altered bowel habits; jaundice or hepatomegaly (biliary obstruction, hepatic tumor, metastatic disease); iron deficiency anemia	CBC, FOBT, ferritin, CEA, CA19-9, AFP, EGD, colonoscopy, abdominal CT, PET
Malabsorption (poor absorption of nutrients due to pancreatic insufficiency, small intestinal mucosal disorders, or bacterial overgrowth)	Progressive, slow	Months to years	Diarrhea or steatorrhea, excessive flatulence; worse with eating and resolves with NPO status	Usually associated with increased appetite; may have anemia (iron, B_{12}, folate), osteoporosis, or osteomalacia (vitamin D, calcium, phosphorus); easy bruising (vitamin K), night blindness (vitamin A)	72-hr stool for fecal fat; fecal elastase; vitamins A and D and INR; calcium, ferritin, B_{12}, albumin; celiac disease antibodies (e.g., anti-tTG, antiendomysial antibodies); EGD with small bowel biopsy; breath test for bacterial overgrowth
Inflammatory bowel disease (especially Crohn disease)	Progressive, slow	Months	Eating causes pain, cramps, increased diarrhea and urgency; improved by low-residue diet or NPO status	Bloody stools, abdominal cramps and pain, perianal disease, extraintestinal manifestations (e.g., oral ulcers, uveitis, erythema nodosum, arthralgias)	CBC, albumin, ESR, CRP, colonoscopy with biopsies, CT or MR enterography, wireless capsule study
GI motility disorders	Intermittent, slow	Years	Worse with eating	Nausea, vomiting, distention, diarrhea, or constipation may be present	EGD and colonoscopy, gastric emptying study, CT or MR enterography, surgical full-thickness intestinal biopsies
Cirrhosis	Muscle wasting with edema, so weight may increase	Months to years	Worse with salt or fluid intake	Ascites, peripheral edema	Liver biopsy
Chronic intestinal ischemia	Progressive	Months to years	Worse with eating	Afraid to eat; postprandial abdominal pain, nausea; associated atherosclerotic disease	CT or MR angiography
Weight Loss Secondary to Nongastrointestinal Causes					
Poor or inadequate calorie intake due to social factors	Intermittent or progressive, acute (hospitalized) or chronic	Days to months to years	Common in elderly, teenagers; exacerbated by poor dentition or poorly fitting dentures	Will eat if food is made available	Review dietary log and how food is obtained and prepared
Medications	Intermittent or progressive	Months	Worse with medication; resolves with discontinuation of offending drug	Anorexia, nausea, vomiting	Review drug profile
Non-GI malignant disease	Progressive	Months	Better with cancer therapy (e.g., surgery, XRT, chemotherapy)	Anorexia, nausea, vomiting; pain; metastatic disease	Calcium, cortisol; CT for underlying disease, PET

TABLE 71 Causes of Involuntary Weight Loss—cont'd

Condition	Quality	Duration	Aggravating or Relieving Factors	Associated Symptoms or Signs	Diagnostic Studies
Endocrine disorders: DM, hyperthyroidism, adrenal insufficiency	DM—appetite increased or decreased, early satiety; hyperthyroidism—increased appetite	Months to years	Worse with disease chronicity	DM: Gastroparesis, neuropathy, retinopathy, nephropathy Adrenal insufficiency: Nausea, vomiting, diarrhea, abdominal pain	Serum glucose, TFT, cortisol
Chronic infections, including HIV and TB	Progressive, fast	Months	Better with directed therapy, megestrol acetate (Megace)	Nausea, anorexia, other infections	HIV test, PPD, cultures, biopsies if necessary
Systemic inflammatory disorders	Progressive, moderate	Months to years	Better with directed therapy, megestrol acetate (Megace)	Arthritis, rash, vasculitis	ANA, RF, ESR, CRP
Chronic renal failure	Progressive, slow; edema may increase weight	Months to years	Better with dialysis, megestrol acetate (Megace)	Nausea, anorexia, weight gain	BUN, Cr, 24-hr creatinine clearance
Advanced COPD or heart failure	Progressive, slow	Months to years	Better with oxygen and specific treatment	Fatigue, dyspnea, edema, wasting	Pulmonary function testing or two-dimensional echocardiography
Psychiatric illness: Depression, manic-depressive illness	Progressive, slow	Months to years	Depression common in elderly; flat affect; manic phase associated with hyperactivity and decreased intake	Psychological testing	
Psychogenic eating disorders—anorexia nervosa, bulimia	Intermittent or progressive	Months to years	Worse with stressors	Refusal to eat, loss of tooth enamel, calluses and healing ulcerations of hand	Psychiatric testing
Substance abuse (alcohol, opiates, CNS stimulants)	Intermittent or progressive	Months	Resolves with discontinuation	Anorexia, nausea, vomiting	Careful interview; patients may deny or minimize

AFP, α-fetoprotein; *ANA,* antinuclear antibody; *BUN,* blood urea nitrogen; *CBC,* complete blood count; *CEA,* carcinoembryonic antigen; *CNS,* central nervous system; *COPD,* chronic obstructive pulmonary disease; *Cr,* creatinine; *CRP,* C-reactive protein; *CT,* computed tomography; *DM,* diabetes mellitus; *EGD,* esophagogastroduodenoscopy; *ESR,* erythrocyte sedimentation rate; *FOBT,* fecal occult blood test; *GI,* gastrointestinal; *HIV,* human immunodeficiency virus; *INR,* international normalized ratio; *MR,* magnetic resonance; *NPO,* nothing orally; *PET,* positron emission tomography; *PPD,* purified protein derivative; *RF,* rheumatoid factor; *TB,* tuberculosis; *TFT,* thyroid function test; *tTG,* tissue transglutaminase; *XRT,* x-ray therapy.

From Goldman L, Shafer AI: *Goldman-Cecil medicine*, ed 26, Philadelphia, 2020, Elsevier.

SECTION IV

Laboratory Tests and Interpretation of Results

This section contains over 300 commonly performed laboratory tests. In general, the tests are discussed in the following format:

1. Laboratory test.
2. Normal range in adult patients. Normal values are given using the present (traditional) reference interval, followed by the Système Internationale (SI) reference interval, the conversion factor (CF), and the suggested minimum increment (SMI).
3. Common abnormalities, such as positive test, increased, or decreased value.
4. Causes of abnormal result.
5. The normal ranges may differ slightly, depending on the laboratory. The reader should be aware of the "normal range" of the particular laboratory performing the test. Every attempt has been made to present current laboratory test data with emphasis on practical considerations.

ACE LEVEL

See "ANGIOTENSIN-CONVERTING ENZYME"

ACETONE (serum or plasma)

Normal: Negative
Elevated in: Diabetic ketoacidosis (DKA), starvation, isopropanol ingestion

ACETYLCHOLINE RECEPTOR (AChR) ANTIBODY

Normal: <0.03 nmol/L
Elevated in: Myasthenia gravis. Changes in AChR concentration correlate with the clinical severity of myasthenia gravis following therapy and during therapy with prednisone and immunosuppressants. False-positive AChR antibody results may be found in patients with Eaton-Lambert syndrome.

ACID-BASE REFERENCE VALUES

See Tables 1, 2, and 3.

ACID PHOSPHATASE (serum)

Normal range: 0-5.5 U/L (0-90 nkat/L [CF: 16.67; SMI: 2 nkat/L])
Elevated in: Carcinoma of prostate, other neoplasms (breast, bone), Paget disease, osteogenesis imperfecta, malignant invasion of bone, Gaucher disease, multiple myeloma, myeloproliferative disorders, benign prostatic hypertrophy, prostatic palpation or surgery, hyperparathyroidism, liver disease, chronic renal failure, idiopathic thrombocytopenic purpura, bronchitis

ACID SERUM TEST

See "HAM TEST"

ACTIVATED CLOTTING TIME (ACT)

Normal: This test is used to determine the dose of protamine sulfate to reverse the effect of heparin as an anticoagulant during angioplasty, cardiac surgery, and hemodialysis. The accepted goal during cardiopulmonary bypass surgery is usually 400-500 sec.

ACTIVATED PARTIAL THROMBOPLASTIN TIME (APTT, aPTT)

See "PARTIAL THROMBOPLASTIN TIME"

ADRENOCORTICOTROPIC HORMONE (ACTH)

Normal: 9-52 pg/ml. Table 4 describes patterns of serum levels of ACTH and cortisol in different adrenal gland disorders.
Elevated in: Addison disease, ectopic ACTH-producing tumors, congenital adrenal hyperplasia, Nelson syndrome, pituitary-dependent Cushing disease
Decreased in: Secondary adrenocortical insufficiency, hypopituitarism, adrenal adenoma or adrenal carcinoma

ALANINE AMINOPEPTIDASE

Normal
Male: 1.11-1.71 mcg/ml
Female: 0.96-1.52 mcg/ml
Elevated in: Liver or pancreatic disease, ethanol use, oral contraceptives use, malignancy, tobacco use, pregnancy
Decreased in: Abortion

ALANINE AMINOTRANSFERASE (ALT, SGPT)

See Fig. 1, an algorithm for evaluation of elevated ALT. Table 5 describes patterns of liver function tests in liver disorders.
Normal range: 0-35 U/L (0.058 μkat/L [CF: 0.02 μkat/L])
Elevated in: Liver disease (hepatitis, cirrhosis, Reye syndrome), hepatic congestion, infectious mononucleosis, myocardial infarction, myocarditis, severe muscle trauma, dermatomyositis/polymyositis, muscular dystrophy, drugs (antibiotics, narcotics, antihypertensive agents, heparin, labetalol, statins, NSAIDs, amiodarone, chlorpromazine, phenytoin), malignancy, renal and pulmonary infarction, seizures, eclampsia, shock liver

TABLE 1 Commonly Used Acid-Base Reference Values for Arterial and Venous Plasma or Serum (Averaged from Various Sources)

	ARTERIAL		VENOUS	
	Conventional Units	SI Units*	Conventional Units	SI Units*
pH	7.40 (7.35-7.45)	7.40 (7.35-7.45)	7.37 (7.32-7.42)	7.37 (7.32-7.42)
Pco_2	40 mm Hg (35-45)	5.33 kPa (4.67-6.10)	45 mm Hg (45-50)	6.10 kPa (5.33-6.67)
Po_2	80-100 mm Hg	10.66-13.33 kPa	40 mm Hg (37-43)	5.33 kPa (4.93-5.73)
HCO_3^- (CO_2 combining power)	24 mEq/L (20-28)	24 mmol/L (20-28)	26 mEq/L (22-30)	26 mmol/L (22-30)
CO_2 content	25 mEq/L (22-28)	25 mmol/L (22-28)	27 mEq/L (24-30)	27 mmol/L(24-30)

*International system.
From Ravel R: *Clinical laboratory medicine*, ed 6, St Louis, 1995, Mosby.

TABLE 2 Summary of Laboratory Findings in Primary Uncomplicated Respiratory and Metabolic Acid-Base Disorders*

Disorder	Pco_2	pH	Base Excess
Acute primary respiratory hypoactivity (respiratory acidosis)	Increase	Decrease	Normal/positive
Acute primary respiratory hyperactivity (respiratory alkalosis)	Decrease	Increase	Normal/negative
Uncompensated metabolic acidosis	Normal	Decrease	Negative
Uncompensated metabolic alkalosis	Normal	Increase	Positive
Partially compensated metabolic acidosis	Decrease	Decrease	Negative
Partially compensated metabolic alkalosis	Increase	Increase	Positive
Chronic primary respiratory hypoactivity (compensated respiratory acidosis)	Increase	Normal	Positive
Fully compensated metabolic alkalosis	Increase	Normal	Positive
Chronic primary respiratory hyperactivity (compensated respiratory alkalosis)	Decrease	Normal	Negative
Fully compensated metabolic acidosis	Decrease	Normal	Negative

*Base excess results refer to negative (–) values more than 22 and positive (+) values more than 12.
From Ravel R: *Clinical laboratory medicine*, ed 6, St Louis, 1995, Mosby.

TABLE 3 Acid-Base Abnormalities and Appropriate Compensatory Responses for Simple Disorders

Primary Acid-Base Disorders	Primary Defect	Effect on pH	Compensatory Response	Expected Range of Compensation	Limits of Compensation
Respiratory acidosis	Alveolar hypoventilation (↑ P_{CO_2})	↓	↑ Renal HCO_3^- reabsorption (HCO_3^-↑)	Acute: $\Delta[HCO_3^-] = +1$ mEq/L for each ↑ΔP_{CO_2} of 10 mm Hg	$[HCO_3^-] = 38$ mEq/L
				Chronic: $\Delta[HCO_3^-] = +4$ mEq/L for each ↑ΔP_{CO_2} of 10 mm Hg	$[HCO_3^-] = 45$ mEq/L
Respiratory alkalosis	Alveolar hyperventilation (↓ P_{CO_2})	↑	↓ Renal HCO_3^- reabsorption (HCO_3^-↓)	Acute: $\Delta[HCO_3^-] = -2$ mEq/L for each ↓ΔP_{CO_2} of 10 mm Hg	$[HCO_3^-] = 18$ mEq/L
				Chronic: $\Delta[HCO_3^-] = -5$ mEq/L for each ↓ΔP_{CO_2} of 10 mm Hg	$[HCO_3^-] = 15$ mEq/L
Metabolic acidosis	Loss of HCO_3^- or gain of H^+ (↓ HCO_3^-)	↓	Alveolar hyperventilation to ↑ pulmonary CO_2 excretion (↓ P_{CO_2})	$P_{CO_2} = 1.5[HCO_3^-] + 8 \pm 2$ P_{CO_2} = last 2 digits of pH × 100 $P_{CO_2} = 15 + [HCO_3^-]$	$P_{CO_2} = 15$ mm Hg
Metabolic alkalosis	Gain of HCO_3^- or loss of H^+ (↑ HCO_3^-)	↑	Alveolar hypoventilation to ↓ pulmonary CO_2 excretion (↑ P_{CO_2})	$P_{CO_2} = +0.6$ mm Hg for $\Delta[HCO_3^-]$ of 1 mEq/L. $P_{CO_2} = 15 + [HCO_3^-]$	$P_{CO_2} = 55$ mm Hg

From Vincent JL et al: *Textbook of critical care*, ed 7, Philadelphia, 2017, Elsevier. Adapted and updated from Bidani A, Tauzon DM, Heming TA: Regulation of whole body acid-base balance. In DuBose TD, Hamm LL (eds): *Acid base and electrolytes disorders: a companion to Brenner and Rector's the kidney,* Philadelphia, 2002, Saunders, p. 1-21.

TABLE 4 Patterns of Serum Levels of Adrenocorticotropic Hormone (ACTH) and Cortisol in Different Adrenal Gland Conditions

Condition	Cortisol	ACTH	Dexamethasone Suppression, Low Dose	Dexamethasone Suppression, High Dose	Site of Disease
Normal adrenal	Normal	Normal	N/A	N/A	None
Primary hypoadrenalism	Low	High	N/A	N/A	Adrenal gland
Secondary hypoadrenalism	Low	Low	N/A	N/A	Pituitary
Primary hyperadrenalism—high cortisol, low ACTH	High	Low	N/A	N/A	Adrenal
Primary hyperadrenalism—high cortisol, borderline low ACTH	High	Borderline low	Positive	N/A	Adrenal
Primary hyperadrenalism due to adrenal hyperplasia—high cortisol, borderline low ACTH	High	Borderline low	Negative	Positive	Adrenal
Primary hyperadrenalism due to adrenal adenoma/carcinoma—high cortisol, borderline low ACTH	High	Borderline low	Negative	Negative	Adrenal
Secondary hyperadrenalism	High	High	N/A	N/A	Pituitary

From McPherson RA, Pincus MR: *Henry's clinical diagnosis and management by laboratory methods*, ed 23, St Louis, 2017, Elsevier.

ALBUMIN (serum)

Normal range: 4-6 g/dl (40-60 g/L [CF:10; SMI: 1 g/L])
Elevated in: Dehydration (relative increase)
Decreased in: Liver disease, nephrotic syndrome, poor nutritional status, rapid IV hydration, protein-losing enteropathies (e.g., inflammatory bowel disease), severe burns, neoplasia, chronic inflammatory diseases, pregnancy, oral contraceptives, prolonged immobilization, lymphomas, hypervitaminosis A, chronic glomerulonephritis

ALCOHOL DEHYDROGENASE

Normal: 0-7 U/L
Elevated in: Drug-induced hepatocellular damage, obstructive jaundice, malignancy, inflammation, infection

ALDOLASE (serum)

Normal range: 0-6 U/L (0-100 nkat/L [CF: 16.67; SMI: 20 nkat/L])
Elevated in: Muscular dystrophy, rhabdomyolysis, dermatomyositis/polymyositis, trichinosis, acute hepatitis and other liver diseases, myocardial infarction, prostatic carcinoma, hemorrhagic pancreatitis, gangrene, delirium tremens, burns
Decreased in: Loss of muscle mass, late stages of muscular dystrophy

ALDOSTERONE

Normal range:
Recumbent: 50-150 ng/L
Upright: 150-300 ng/L
(Highest levels in neonates, decreasing over time to adult levels). The normal renin-angiotensin-aldosterone axis is illustrated in Fig. 2.
Elevated in: Primary aldosteronism, secondary aldosteronism, pseudoprimary aldosteronism. Table 6 differentiates the various causes of hyperaldosteronism.
Decreased in: Patient with hypertension: Diabetes mellitus, Turner syndrome, acute alcohol intoxication, excess secretion of deoxycorticosterone, corticosterone, and 18-hydroxycorticosterone

Patient without hypertension: Addison disease, hypoaldosteronism resulting from renin deficiency, isolated aldosterone deficiency. Table 7 differentiates the various causes of hypoaldosteronism.

ALKALINE PHOSPHATASE (ALP) (serum)

See Fig. 3 for investigating a raised ALP in general practice.
See Fig. E4 for approach to elevated ALP.

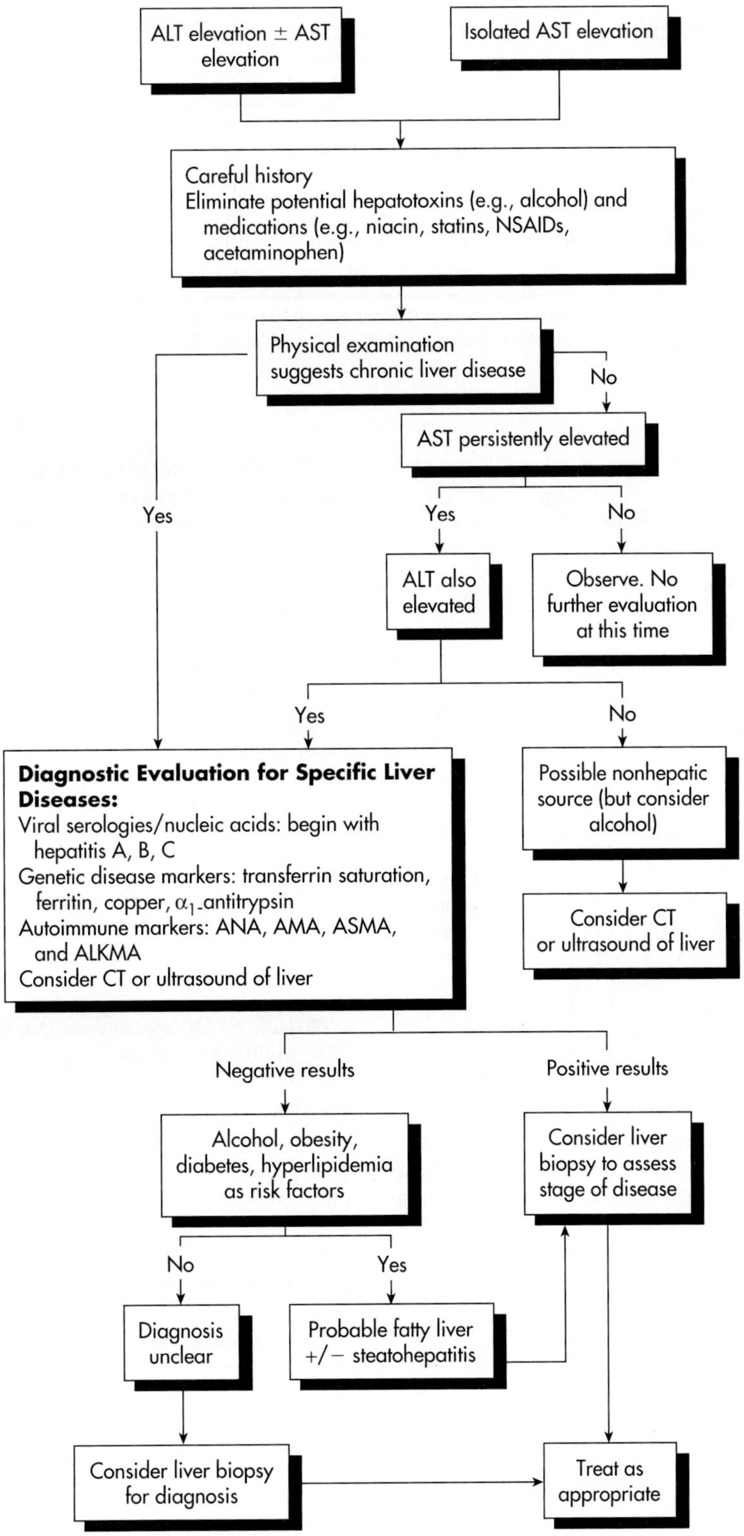

FIG. 1 Approach to the evaluation of isolated elevated levels of serum alanine aminotransferase *(ALT)* and/or aspartate aminotransferase *(AST)* in the asymptomatic patient. *ALKMA,* Anti-liver/kidney microsomal antibody; *AMA,* antimitochondrial antibody; *ANA,* antinuclear antibody; *ASMA,* antismooth muscle antibody; *CT,* computed tomography; *NSAIDs,* nonsteroidal antiinflammatory drugs. (Modified from Goldman L, Ausiello D [eds]: *Cecil textbook of medicine,* ed 24, Philadelphia, 2012, Saunders.)

TABLE 5 Six Fundamental Patterns of Liver Function Tests

Condition	AST	ALT	LD	AP	TP	Albumin	Bilirubin	Ammonia
1. Hepatitis	H	H	H	H	N	N	H	N
2. Cirrhosis	N	N	N	N-sl H	L	L	H	H
3. Biliary obstruction	N	N	N	H	N	N	H	N
4. Space-occupying lesion	N or H	N or H	H	H	N	N	N-H	N
5. Passive congestion	sl H	sl H	sl H	N-sl H	N	N	N-sl H	N
6. Fulminant failure	Very H	H	H	H	L	L	H	H

ALT, Alanine aminotransferase; *AP,* alkaline phosphatase; *AST,* aspartate aminotransferase; *H,* high; *L,* low; *LD,* lactate dehydrogenase; *N,* normal; *sl,* slightly; *TP,* total protein.
From McPherson RA, Pincus MR: *Henry's clinical diagnosis and management by laboratory methods,* ed 23, St Louis, 2017, Elsevier.

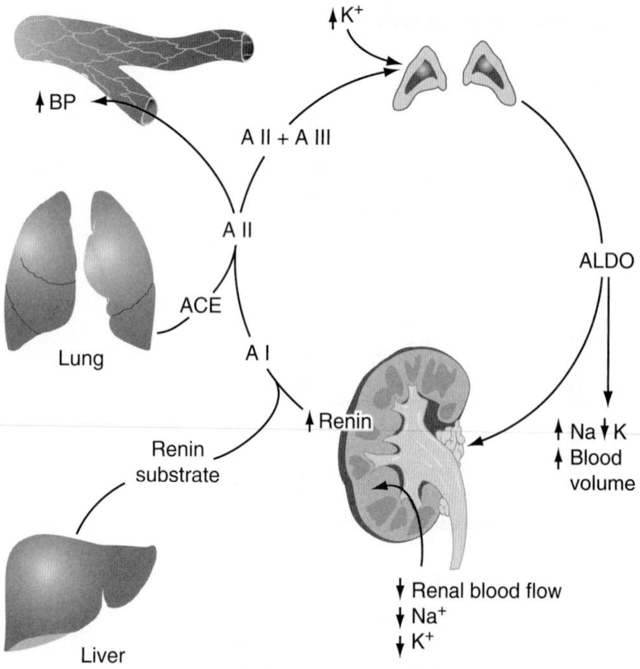

FIG. 2 The normal renin-angiotensin-aldosterone axis. Renin, secreted by the kidney, cleaves angiotensin I from renin substrate (angiotensinogen) produced by the liver. Angiotensin I is converted to angiotensin II by angiotensin-converting enzyme *(ACE)* mainly in the lung. Angiotensin II increases peripheral vascular resistance and, together with angiotensin III, stimulates aldosterone *(ALDO)* secretion, which results in sodium retention and increased plasma volume. (Adapted from Stewart PM: The adrenal cortex. In Larsen PR et al [eds]: *Williams textbook of endocrinology,* ed 10, Philadelphia, 2003, Saunders, p 499. McPherson RA, Pincus MR: *Henry's clinical diagnosis and management by laboratory methods,* ed 23, St Louis, 2017, Elsevier.)

TABLE 6 Differentiating the Various Causes of Hyperaldosteronism

Disorder	Aldosterone	Renin	Serum K^+
Primary hyperaldosteronism	↑	↓	↓
Renin-secreting tumor	↑	↑	↓—N
Dexamethasone-suppressible hyperaldosteronism	↑	↓	↓
Renovascular hypertension	N—↑	N—↑	↓—N
Bartter syndrome	↑	↑	↓
Diuretics, congestive heart failure, cirrhosis, nephrotic syndrome	↑	↑	N—↓

N, Normal.
From McPherson RA, Pincus MR: *Henry's clinical diagnosis and management by laboratory methods,* ed 23, St Louis, 2017, Elsevier.

TABLE 7 Differentiating the Various Causes of Hypoaldosteronism

Disorder	Aldosterone	Renin	Serum K^+
Addison disease	↓	↑	↑
Cushing syndrome	↓	↓	N or ↓
Liddle syndrome	↓	↓	↓
Hyporeninemic hypoaldosteronism	↓	↓	↑
Apparent mineralocorticoid excess	↓	↓	↓
Isolated hypoaldosteronism	↓	↑	↑

N, Normal.
From McPherson RA, Pincus MR: *Henry's clinical diagnosis and management by laboratory methods,* ed 23, St Louis, 2017, Elsevier.

Normal range: 30-120 U/L (0.5-2 μkat/L [CF:0.01667; SMI: 0.1 μkat/L])

Elevated in

LIVER AND BILIARY TRACT ORIGIN
Extrahepatic bile duct obstruction
Intrahepatic biliary obstruction
Liver cell acute injury
Liver passive congestion
Drug-induced liver cell dysfunction
Space-occupying lesions
Primary biliary cirrhosis
Sepsis

BONE ORIGIN (OSTEOBLAST HYPERACTIVITY)
Physiologic (rapid) bone growth (childhood and adolescence)
Metastatic tumor with osteoblastic reaction
Fracture healing
Paget disease of bone

CAPILLARY ENDOTHELIAL ORIGIN
Granulation tissue formation (active)

PLACENTAL ORIGIN
Pregnancy
Some parenteral albumin preparations

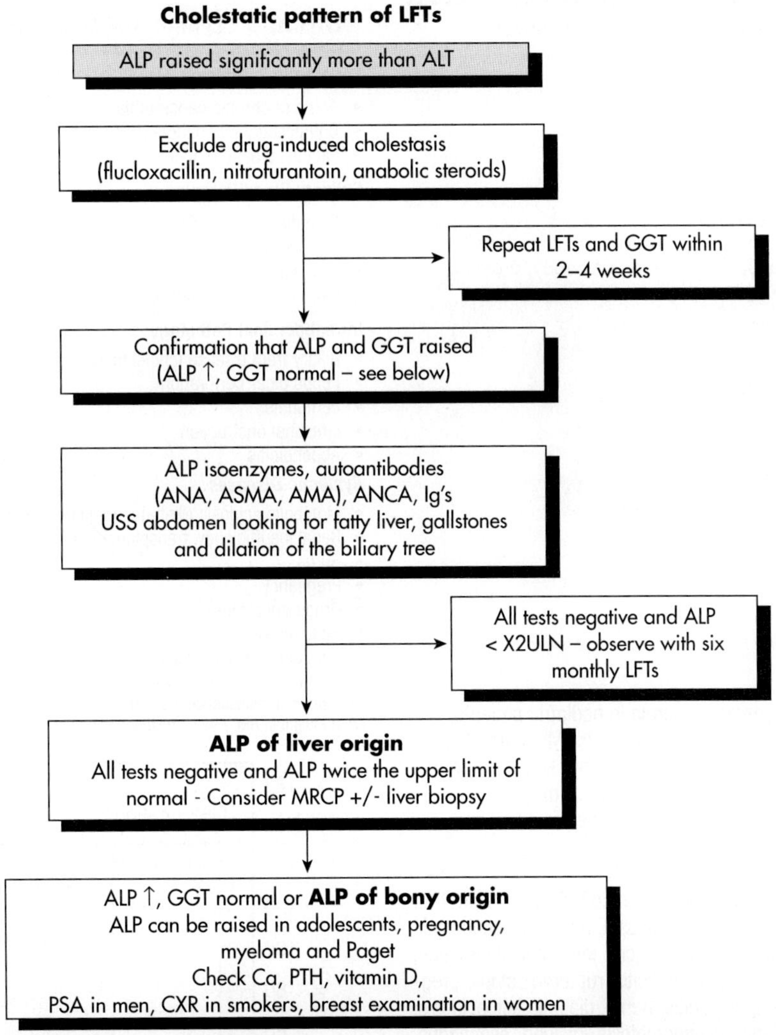

FIG. 3 Investigating a raised ALP in general practice. *ALP,* Alkaline phosphatase; *ALT,* alanine transaminase; *AMA,* antimitochondrial antibody; *ANA,* antinuclear antibody; *ANCA,* antineutrophil cytoplasmic antibody; *ASMA,* antismooth muscle antibody; *CXR,* chest x-ray; *GGT,* γ-glutamyl transpeptidase; *Ig,* immunoglobulin; *LFT,* liver function test; *MRCP,* magnetic resonance cholangiopancreatography; *PSA,* prostate-specific antigen; *PTH,* parathyroid hormone; *USS,* ultrasound scan. (From Fillit HM: *Brocklehurst's textbook of geriatric medicine and gerontology,* ed 8, Philadelphia, 2017, Elsevier.)

OTHER
Thyrotoxicosis
Benign transient hyperphosphatasemia
Primary hyperparathyroidism
Decreased in: Hypothyroidism, pernicious anemia, hypophosphatemia, hypervitaminosis D, malnutrition

ALPHA-1-ANTITRYPSIN (serum)

Normal range: 110-140 mg/dl
Decreased in: Homozygous or heterozygous deficiency

ALPHA-1-FETOPROTEIN (serum)

See "α-1 FETOPROTEIN"

ALT

See "ALANINE AMINOTRANSFERASE"

ALUMINUM (serum)

Normal range: 0-6 ng/ml
Elevated in: Chronic renal failure on dialysis, parenteral nutrition, industrial exposure

AMA

See "ANTIMITOCHONDRIAL ANTIBODY"

AMEBIASIS SEROLOGIC TEST

Test description: Test is used to support diagnosis of amebiasis caused by *Entamoeba histolytica.* Serum acute and convalescent titers are drawn 1-3 wk apart. A fourfold increase in titer is the most indicative result.

AMINOLEVULINIC ACID (δ-ALA) (24-hr urine collection)

Normal: 1.5-7.5 mg/day
Elevated in: Acute porphyrias, lead poisoning, DKA, pregnancy, anticonvulsant drugs, hereditary tyrosinemia
Decreased in: Alcoholic liver disease

AMMONIA (serum)

See Box 1 for differential diagnosis of hyperammonemia.

BOX 1 Differential Diagnosis of Hyperammonemia

- Acute liver failure
- Chronic kidney disease
- Cigarette smoking
- Cirrhosis
- GI bleeding
- Inborn errors of metabolism
  - Proline metabolism disorders
  - Urea cycle defects (e.g., carbamoyl phosphate synthetase I deficiency, ornithine transcarbamylase deficiency, argininosuccinate lyase deficiency, *N*-acetylglutamate synthetase deficiency)
- Medications/toxins
  - Alcohol
  - Diuretics (e.g., acetazolamide)
  - Narcotics
  - Valproic acid
- Muscle exertion and ischemia
- Portosystemic shunts
- Technique and conditions of blood sampling
  - High body temperature
  - High-protein diet
- Tourniquet use

GI, Gastrointestinal.
From Feldman M et al: *Sleisenger and Fordtran's gastrointestinal and liver disease*, ed 10, Philadelphia, 2016, Elsevier.

See Fig. E5 for approach to hyperammonemia in pediatric patients.
Normal range: 10-80 μg/dl (5-50 μmol/L [CF: 0.5872; SMI: 5 μmol/L])
Elevated in: Hepatic failure, hepatic encephalopathy, Reye syndrome, portacaval shunt, drugs (diuretics, polymyxin B, methicillin)
Decreased in: Drugs (neomycin, lactulose, tetracycline), renal failure

AMYLASE (serum)

Normal range: 0-130 U/L (0-2.17 μkat/L [CF: 0.01667; SMI: 0.01 μkat/L])
Elevated in: Acute pancreatitis, pancreatic neoplasm, abscess, pseudocyst, ascites, macroamylasemia, perforated peptic ulcer, intestinal obstruction, intestinal infarction, acute cholecystitis, appendicitis, ruptured ectopic pregnancy, salivary gland inflammation, peritonitis, burns, diabetic ketoacidosis, renal insufficiency, drugs (morphine), carcinomatosis (of lung, esophagus, ovary), acute ethanol ingestion, mumps, prostate tumors, postendoscopic retrograde cholangiopancreatography, bulimia, anorexia nervosa (Table 8)
Decreased in: Advanced chronic pancreatitis, hepatic necrosis, cystic fibrosis

AMYLASE, URINE

See "URINE AMYLASE"

AMYLOID A PROTEIN (serum)

Normal: <10 mcg/ml
Elevated in: Inflammatory disorders (acute phase-reacting protein), infections, acute coronary syndrome, malignancies

ANA

See "ANTINUCLEAR ANTIBODY"

ANCA

See "ANTINEUTROPHIL CYTOPLASMIC ANTIBODY"

ANDROSTENEDIONE (serum)

Normal
Male: 75-205 ng/dl
Female: 85-275 ng/dl
Elevated in: Congenital adrenal hyperplasia, polycystic ovary syndrome, ectopic ACTH-producing tumor, Cushing syndrome, hirsutism, hyperplasia of ovarian stroma, ovarian neoplasm
Decreased in: Ovarian failure, adrenal failure, sickle cell anemia

ANGIOTENSIN II

Normal: 10-60 pg/ml

TABLE 8 Differential Diagnosis of Hyperamylasemia

Pancreatic Pathology
- Acute or chronic pancreatitis
- Complications of pancreatitis (pseudocyst, ascites, abscess)
- Factitious pancreatitis

Salivary Gland Pathology
- Parotitis (mumps, *Staphylococcus aureus*, cytomegalovirus, HIV, Epstein-Barr virus)
- Sialadenitis (calculus, radiation)
- Eating disorders (anorexia nervosa, bulimia)

Intraabdominal Pathology
- Biliary tract disease (cholelithiasis)
- Peptic ulcer perforation
- Peritonitis
- Intestinal obstruction
- Appendicitis

Systemic Diseases
- Metabolic acidosis (diabetes mellitus, shock)
- Renal insufficiency, transplantation
- Burns
- Pregnancy
- Drugs (morphine)
- Head injury
- Cardiopulmonary bypass

HIV, Human immunodeficiency virus.
From Kliegman RM: *Nelson textbook of pediatrics*, ed 21, Philadelphia, 2020, Elsevier.

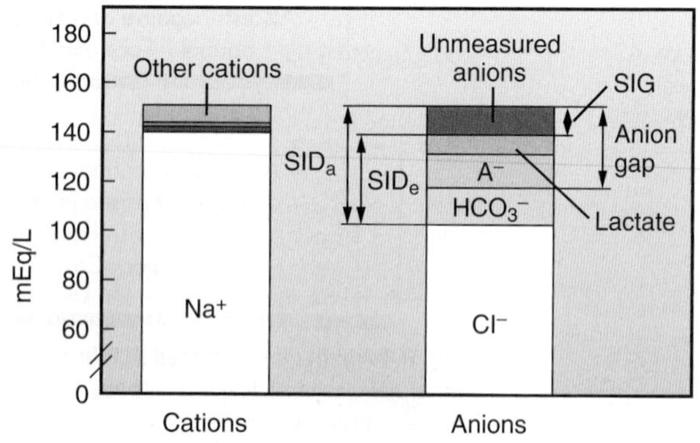

FIG. 6 Charge balance in blood plasma. "Other cations" include Ca^{2+} and Mg^{2+}. The strong ion difference (SID) is always positive (in plasma) and SID minus effective SID *(SIDe)* must equal 0. Any difference between SID apparent *(SIDa)* and SIDe is the strong ion gap *(SIG)* and must represent unmeasured anions. *A–*, Concentration of dissociated weak acids; *HCO_3^-*, bicarbonate. (From Ronco C: *Critical care nephrology*, ed 3, Philadelphia, 2019, Elsevier.)

Elevated in: Hypertension, congestive heart failure (CHF), cirrhosis, renin-secreting renal tumor, volume depletion
Decreased in: ACE inhibitor drugs, angiotensin-converting enzyme inhibitor (ARB) drugs, primary aldosteronism, Cushing syndrome

ANGIOTENSIN-CONVERTING ENZYME (ACE level)

Normal range: <40 nmol/ml/min (<670 nkat/L [CF: 16.67; SMI: 10 nkat/L])
Elevated in: Sarcoidosis, primary biliary cirrhosis, alcoholic liver disease, hyperthyroidism, hyperparathyroidism, diabetes mellitus, amyloidosis, multiple myeloma, lung disease (asbestosis, silicosis, berylliosis, allergic alveolitis, coccidioidomycosis), Gaucher disease, leprosy

ANH

See "ATRIAL NATRIURETIC HORMONE"

ANION GAP (AG)

The AG is the net change difference between the cations Na^+, K^+, and the anions Cl– and HCO_3^-
See Fig. 6 for charge balance in blood plasma.
See Tables 9, 10, 11.

TABLE 9 Equations Used to Estimate the Quantity of Unmeasured Ions

Anion gap (AG)	$(Na^+ + K^+) - (Cl^- + HCO_3^-)$	Normal values: 12 ± mEq/L (with K^+) 8 ± 4 mEq/L (without K^+)
Connected anion gap (cAG)	$(Na^+ + K^+) - (Cl^- + HCO_3^- +$ 2[albumin g/dl] + 0.5[phosphate mg/dl] + lactate) SI (all units mEq/L): $(Na^+ + K^+) - (Cl^- + HCO_3^- +$ 0.2[albumin g/L] + 1.5[phosphate mmol/L] + lactate)	Normal values: 0 ± 5 mEq/L
Apparent strong ion difference (SID_a)	$(Na^+ + K^+ + Ca^{2+} + Mg^{2+}) - (Cl^- +$ lactate)	The difference between measured strong cations and anions. Concentrations should be expressed in mEq/L (Ca^{2+} and Mg^{2+} multiplied by 2 from mmol/L).
Effective strong ion difference (SID_e)	$(HCO_3^-$ + [albumin g/dl] × (0.123 × pH − 0.631) + $[PO^{2}-_{4}]$ × (0.39 × pH− 0.469)	
Strong ion gap (SIG)	$SID_a - SID_e$	Should theoretically approach 0, but is normally 5 (±5) in critically ill patients
$\Delta AG/\Delta HCO-_3$ (delta ratio)	$(cAG - cAG_{normal})/(24 - HCO_3^-)$	Normal values 0.8-1.6
Osmolar gap	Measured osmolality− ([1.86 × Na^+] + glucose mg/dl/18 + BUN mg/dl/2.8 + ethanol mg/dl/4.6) SI (all units mmol/L): Measured osmolality− ([1.86 × Na^+] + glucose + urea + 1.25 × ethanol)	Normally ≤ 19 mmol/L

BUN, Blood urea nitrogen; *SI,* strong ion.
From Ronco C et al: *Critical care nephrology*, ed 3, Philadelphia, 2019, Elsevier.

Normal range: 9-14 mEq/L
Elevated in: Lactic acidosis, ketoacidosis (diabetes, alcoholic starvation), uremia (chronic renal failure), ingestion of toxins (paraldehyde, methanol, salicylates, ethylene glycol), hyperosmolar nonketotic coma, antibiotics (carbenicillin)
Decreased in: Hypoalbuminemia, severe hypermagnesemia, IgG myeloma, lithium toxicity, laboratory error (falsely decreased sodium or overestimation of bicarbonate or chloride), hypercalcemia of parathyroid origin, antibiotics (e.g., polymyxin)

ANTICARDIOLIPIN ANTIBODY (ACA)

Normal range: Negative. Test includes detection of IgG, IgM, and IgA antibodies to phospholipid, cardiolipin
Present in: Antiphospholipid antibody syndrome, chronic hepatitis C

ANTICOAGULANT

See "CIRCULATING ANTICOAGULANT"

ANTIDIURETIC HORMONE

Normal range: mOsm/kg 295-300 (4-12 pg/ml)
Elevated in: SIADH, antipsychotic medications, ectopic ADH from systemic neoplasm, Guillain-Barré syndrome, CNS infections, brain tumors, nephrogenic diabetes insipidus

TABLE 10 Causes of Increased Anion Gap or Strong Ion Gap

Common causes	Lactic acidosis*
	L-lactate (hypoxic and nonhypoxic)
	D-lactate (in short bowel syndrome)
	Renal failure
	Ketoacidosis
	Diabetic
	Alcoholic
	Starvation
	Metabolic errors
	Toxins
	Methanol
	Ethylene and propylene glycol
	Salicylates
	5-oxoproline (pyroglutamic acid)
	Sepsis
Rare causes	Severe liver disease
	Sodium salts
	Sodium lactate
	Sodium citrate
	Sodium acetate
	Sodium penicillin (>50 million units/day)
	Carbenicillin (>30 g/day)
	Decreased unmeasured cations
	Hypomagnesemia
	Hypocalcemia
	Massive rhabdomyolysis
	Alkalemia

*Lactate, Mg^{2+}, and Ca^{2+} are accounted for in the strong ion gap.
From Ronco C: *Critical care nephrology*, ed 3, Philadelphia, 2019, Elsevier.

TABLE 11 Causes of Normal Anion Gap or Strong Ion Gap Acidosis

Nonrenal causes: Urine SID (Na + K − Cl) < 0	Low SID infusions (e.g., normal saline)
	Strong cation (or HCO_3^-) losses though diarrhea
	Ureteral diversions
	Biliary or pancreatic fistulas
Renal causes: Urine SID (Na + K − Cl) >0	Type 1 (distal) RTA
	Type 2 (proximal) RTA
	Type 4 (hypoaldosteronism) RTA

RTA, Renal tubular acidosis; *SID,* strong ion difference.
From Ronco C: *Critical care nephrology*, ed 3, Philadelphia, 2019, Elsevier.

Decreased in: Central diabetes insipidus, nephritic syndrome, psychogenic polydipsias, demeclocycline, lithium, phenytoin, alcohol. Table 12 describes the water deprivation test used for diagnosing and classifying diabetes insipidus. Table 13 summarizes tests in the differential diagnosis of water homeostasis. Causes of polyuria due to water diuresis are described in Box 2.

ANTI-DNA

Normal range: Absent
Present in: Systemic lupus erythematosus, chronic active hepatitis, infectious mononucleosis, biliary cirrhosis

ANTI-DS DNA

Normal: <25 U
Elevated in: Systemic lupus erythematosus

ANTIGLOBULIN TEST

See "DIRECT ANTIGLOBULIN (COOMBS DIRECT)"
See "INDIRECT ANTIGLOBULIN (COOMBS INDIRECT)"

ANTIGLOMERULAR BASEMENT ANTIBODY

See "GLOMERULAR BASEMENT MEMBRANE ANTIBODY"

ANTIHISTONE

Normal: <1 U
Elevated in: Drug-induced lupus erythematosus

TABLE 12 Water Deprivation Test for Diagnosing and Classifying Diabetes Insipidus

Patients with mild polyuria may be instructed to withhold all fluid intake from 10 P.M. onward. For those with more severe polyuria (8-10 L/day), water deprivation should be started early in the morning under close observation.

1. During testing, the patient is forbidden to take in anything by mouth.
2. Obtain the following baseline parameters: Urine volume (Uvol) and urinary osmolality (Uosm), plasma osmolality (Posm), and plasma sodium (PNa). Also record the weight and blood pressure (BP)/pulse (P) seated and standing.
3. Urine and plasma are collected hourly for Uvol, Uosm, and Posm. Weight, BP, and P are also recorded. Record requests for fluid.
4. When the Uosm has plateaued (e.g., hourly increase <30 mOsm/kg for 3 consecutive hours), or when body weight has decreased by 3%-5%, or the patient develops a >20-mm Hg drop in systolic BP, obtain samples for Uvol, Uosm, Posm, PNa, and AVP (plasma).
5. Administer 1 mcg of desmopressin IV or IM, or 5 mcg of AVP SC Uosm; urine output and Posm are recorded at 30, 60, and 120 min after the injection. The highest Uosm value is used to evaluate the patient's response to AVP.

Precautions

When possible, discontinue any medications that can influence ADH secretion. Observe for hypotension and nausea, which may stimulate ADH secretion. The patient should not be permitted to smoke during the test.

Interpretation

Normal	Final Uosm before AVP challenge is higher than Posm. Following AVP challenge, the Uosm is less than 10% higher than the maximal Uosm achieved with water restriction alone.
Neurogenic DI	Final Uosm before AVP challenge is less than Posm. Following AVP administration, there is a greater than 50% increase in Uosm.
Nephrogenic DI	Final Uosm before AVP challenge is less than Posm. Following AVP administration, there is a less than 10% increase in Uosm.
Partial central DI	Uosm may be higher than Posm following dehydration; however, there is only a 10%-50% increase in Uosm following administration of AVP.
Partial nephrogenic DI	Uosm may be higher than Posm following dehydration; however, there is a greater than 10% increase in Uosm following administration of AVP.

Plotting basal and postdehydration Uosm and plasma ADH on the nomograms from Zerbe and Robertson will permit further distinction between partial nephrogenic DI, partial central DI, and primary polydipsia

ADH, Antidiuretic hormone; *AVP,* arginine vasopressin; *DI,* diabetes insipidus; *IM,* intramuscular; *IV,* intravenous; *SC,* subcutaneous.
From McPherson RA, Pincus MR: *Henry's clinical diagnosis and management by laboratory methods*, ed 23, St Louis, 2017, Elsevier.

TABLE 13 Tests in the Differential Diagnosis of Disorders of Water Homeostasis

	BASELINE			AFTER 12-HOUR FLUID RESTRICTION			
Disorder	**Serum Na+ and Osmolality**	**Urine Na+ and Osmolality**	**Serum ADH**	**Serum Na+ and Osmolality**	**Urine Na+ and Osmolality**	**Serum ADH**	**Urine Osmolality Post-AVP Challenge**
Normal control	N	N	N	N	High	High	Same
SIADH	Low	N-High	High	Low-N	High	High	—
Neurogenic DI	N-High	Low	Low	High	Low-N	Low	Increased
Nephrogenic DI	N-High	Low	N-High	High	Low-N	High	Same
Psychogenic polydipsia	Low-N	Low	Low	N	N-High	N-High	Same

ADH, Antidiuretic hormone; *AVP,* arginine vasopressin; *DI,* diabetes insipidus; *N,* normal; *SIADH,* syndrome of inappropriate secretion of ADH.
From McPherson RA, Pincus MR: *Henry's clinical diagnosis and management by laboratory methods,* ed 23, St Louis, 2017, Elsevier.

ANTIMITOCHONDRIAL ANTIBODY (AMA, Mitochondrial antibody)

Normal range: <1:20 titer
Elevated in: Primary biliary cirrhosis (85%-95%), chronic active hepatitis (25%-30%), cryptogenic cirrhosis (25%-30%)

ANTINEUTROPHIL CYTOPLASMIC ANTIBODY (ANCA)

Positive test: Cytoplasmic pattern (c-ANCA): Positive in granulomatosis with polyangiitis (see Fig. E7 and Table E14 for approach to patient with positive c-ANCA)

Perinuclear pattern (p-ANCA): Positive in inflammatory bowel disease, primary biliary cirrhosis, primary sclerosing cholangitis, autoimmune chronic active hepatitis, crescentic glomerulonephritis (see Table E14 for approach to patient with positive p-ANCA)

BOX 2 Causes of Polyuria Due to Water Diuresis

Lack of ADH
Central diabetes insipidus (DI): Congenital or acquired (idiopathic cell degeneration, tumors and granulomas, surgery, trauma, infarction, and infection of the pituitary gland or hypothalamus)
Dipsogenic: Psychogenic, organic brain disease, iatrogenic
Gestational DI: Excess vasopressinase

Failure of the Kidney to Respond to ADH (Nephrogenic DI)
Congenital nephrogenic DI: A defect in ADH receptor, a defect in aquaporin expression.
Chronic renal failure.
Acquired nephrogenic DI: Lithium toxicity, demeclocycline toxicity, methoxyflurane toxicity, amyloidosis, light chain nephropathy, hypercalcemia, hypokalemia, obstructive uropathy

ADH, Antidiuretic hormone.
From McPherson RA, Pincus MR: *Henry's clinical diagnosis and management by laboratory methods*, ed 23, St Louis, 2017, Elsevier.

TABLE 15 Frequency of Antinuclear Antibodies in Autoimmune and Nonrheumatic Diseases

	Sensitivity (%)
Autoimmune disease	
Systemic lupus erythematosus	95-100
Systemic sclerosis	60-80
Mixed connective tissue disease	100
Polymyositis or dermatomyositis	60
Rheumatoid arthritis	50
Rheumatoid vasculitis	30-50
Sjögren syndrome	40-70
Drug-induced lupus	90
Discoid lupus	15
Pauciarticular juvenile chronic arthritis	70
Nonrheumatic diseases	
Hashimoto thyroiditis	45
Graves disease	50
Autoimmune hepatitis	50
Primary pulmonary hypertension	40

From Hochberg MC: *Rheumatology*, ed 7, Philadelphia, 2019, Elsevier.

ANTINUCLEAR ANTIBODY (ANA)

Fig. E8 describes an algorithm for the use of antinuclear antibodies in the diagnosis of connective tissue disorders. See Fig. E9 for approach to positive ANA pattern. Table 15 shows the frequency of antinuclear antibodies in autoimmune and nonrheumatic diseases.

Normal range: <1:20 titer

Positive test: Systemic lupus erythematosus (more significant if titer >1:160), drugs (phenytoin, ethosuximide, primidone, methyldopa, hydralazine, carbamazepine, penicillin, procainamide, chlorpromazine, griseofulvin, thiazides), chronic active hepatitis, autoimmune thyroid disease (positive ANA is found in up to 45% of patients), idiopathic thrombocytopenic purpura, multiple sclerosis, rheumatoid arthritis, scleroderma, mixed connective tissue disease, necrotizing vasculitis, Sjögren syndrome, tuberculosis, pulmonary interstitial fibrosis. Positive ANA results are nonspecific and can be found in healthy individuals (13.8% of the adult general population). Table 16 describes diseases associated with ANA subtypes. Fig. 10 illustrates various fluorescent ANA test patterns.

ANTI-RNP ANTIBODY

See "EXTRACTABLE NUCLEAR ANTIGEN"

ANTI-SCL-70

Normal: Absent

Elevated in: Scleroderma

ANTI-SM (anti-Smith) ANTIBODY

See "EXTRACTABLE NUCLEAR ANTIGEN"

ANTI-SMOOTH MUSCLE ANTIBODY

See "SMOOTH MUSCLE ANTIBODY"

ANTISTREPTOLYSIN O TITER (Streptozyme, ASLO titer)

Normal range for adults: <160 Todd units

Elevated in: Streptococcal upper airway infection, acute rheumatic fever, acute glomerulonephritis, increased levels of β-lipoprotein

NOTE: A fourfold increase in titer between acute and convalescent specimens is diagnostic of streptococcal upper airway infection regardless of the initial titer.

ANTITHROMBIN III

See Table 17.

Normal range: 81%-120% of normal activity; 17-30 mg/dl

TABLE 16 Disease-Associated Antinuclear Antibody Subtypes

Nuclear Location	Disease(s)
"Native" DNA (dsDNA, or dsDNA/ssDNA complex)	SLE (60%-70%; range, 35%-75%) Also PSS (5%-55%), MCTD (11%-25%), RA (5%-40%), DM (5%-25%), SS (5%)
sNP	SLE (50%) Also other collagen diseases
DNP (DNA-histone complex)	SLE (52%) Also MCTD (8%), RA (3%)
Histones	Drug-induced SLE (95%) Also SLE (30%), RA (15%-24%)
ENA Sm	SLE (30%-40%; range, 28%-40%) Also MCTD (0%-8%); RNP (U1-RNP) MCTD (in high titer without any other ANA subtype present: 95%-100%) Also SLE (26%-50%), PSS (11%-22%), RA (10%), SS (3%)
SS-A (Ro)*	SS without RA (60%-70%) Also SLE (26%-50%), neonatal SLE (over 95%), PSS (30%), MCTD (50%), SS with RA (9%), PBC (15%-19%)
SS-B (La)	SS without RA (40%-60%) Also SLE (5%-15%), SS with RA (5%)
Scl-70*	PSS (15%-43%)
Centromere*	CREST syndrome (70%-90%; range, 57%-96%) Also PSS (4%-20%), PBC (12%)
Nucleolar	PSS (scleroderma) (54%-90%) Also SLE (25%-26%), RA (9%)
RAP (RANA)	SS with RA (60%-76%) Also SS without RA (5%)
Jo-1	Polymyositis (30%)
PM-1	Polymyositis or PMS/PSS overlap syndrome (60%-90%) Also DM (17%)
ssDNA	SLE (60%-70%) Also CAH, infectious mononucleosis, RA, chronic GN, chronic infections, PBC
Cytoplasmic Location	Disease(s)
Mitochondrial	PBC (90%-100%) Also CAH (7%-30%), cryptogenic cirrhosis (30%), acute hepatitis, viral hepatitis (3%), other liver diseases (0%-20%), SLE (5%), SS and PSS (8%)
Microsomal†	Chronic active hepatitis (60%-80%), Hashimoto thyroiditis (97%)
Ribosomal	SLE (5%-12%)
Smooth muscle‡	Chronic active hepatitis (60%-91%)

ANA, Antinuclear antibody; *CAH,* chronic active hepatitis; *CREST,* calcinosis, Raynaud phenomenon, esophageal dysfunction, sclerodactyly, and telangiectasia; *DM,* dermatomyositis; *GN,* glomerulonephritis; *MCTD,* mixed connective tissue disease; *MS,* multiple sclerosis; *PBC,* primary biliary cirrhosis; *PMS,* premenstrual syndrome; *PSS,* progressive systemic sclerosis; *RA,* rheumatoid arthritis; *RNP,* ribonucleoprotein; *SLE,* systemic lupus erythematosus; *SS,* Sjögren syndrome; *ssDNA,* single-stranded DNA.

*Not detected using rat or mouse liver or kidney tissue method.

†Not detected by cultured cell method.

‡Detected by cultured cells but better with rat or mouse tissue.

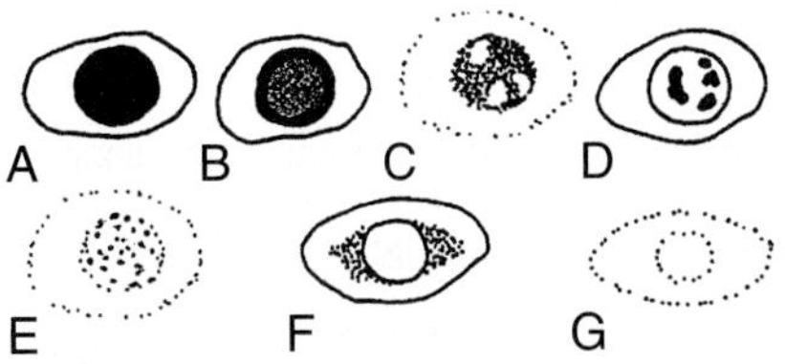

FIG. 10 Fluorescent antinuclear antibody test patterns (HEP-2 cells). **A,** Solid (homogeneous). **B,** Peripheral (rim). **C,** Speckled. **D,** Nucleolar. **E,** Anticentromere. **F,** Antimitochondrial. **G,** Normal (nonreactive).

TABLE 17 Assay Measurements in Heterozygous Antithrombin (ATIII) Deficiency for Diagnosis

	ACTIVITY		
Type	**Antigen**	**Heparin Cofactor**	**Progressive ATIII**
I	Low	Low	Low
II			
Active site defect	Normal	Low	Low
Heparin-binding site defect	Normal	Low	Normal

Decreased in: Hereditary deficiency of antithrombin III, disseminated intravascular coagulation, pulmonary embolism, cirrhosis, thrombolytic therapy, chronic liver failure, postsurgery, third trimester of pregnancy, oral contraceptives, nephrotic syndrome, IV heparin >3 days, sepsis, acute leukemia, carcinoma, thrombophlebitis
Elevated in: Warfarin drugs, postmyocardial infarction

APOLIPOPROTEIN A-1 (Apo A-1)

Normal: Desirable >120 mg/dl
Elevated in: Familial hyperalphalipoproteinemia, statins, niacin, estrogens, weight loss, familial cholesteryl ester transfer protein (CETP) deficiency
Decreased in: Familial hypoalphalipoproteinemia, Tangier disease, diuretics, androgens, cigarette smoking, hepatocellular disorders, chronic renal failure, nephritic syndrome, coronary heart disease, cholestasis

APOLIPOPROTEIN B (Apo B)

Normal: Desirable <100 mg/dl; high risk >120 mg/dl
Elevated in: High saturated fat diet, high-cholesterol diet, hyperapobetalipoproteinemia, familial combined hyperlipidemia, anabolic steroids, diuretics, beta-blockers, corticosteroids, progestins, diabetes, hypothyroidism, chronic renal failure, liver disease, Cushing syndrome, coronary heart disease
Decreased in: Statins, niacin, low-cholesterol diet, malnutrition, abetalipoproteinemia, hypobetalipoproteinemia, hyperthyroidism

ARTERIAL BLOOD GASES

Normal range
Po_2: 75-100 mm Hg
Pco_2: 35-45 mm Hg
HCO_3^-: 24-28 mEq/L
pH: 7.35-7.45
Abnormal values: Acid-base disturbances (see the following)
METABOLIC ACIDOSIS
Causes of metabolic acidosis by net acid excretion are summarized in Box 3.
Metabolic acidosis with increased AG (AG acidosis)
Lactic acidosis (see Box 4)
Ketoacidosis (diabetes mellitus, alcoholic ketoacidosis)
Uremia (chronic renal failure)
Ingestion of toxins (paraldehyde, methanol, salicylate, ethylene glycol)
High-fat diet (mild acidosis)

EXTRARENAL ACIDOSIS: INCREASE IN NET ACID EXCRETION

Gastrointestinal loss of bicarbonate
Ingestion of acids or acid precursors: Ammonium chloride, sulfur-containing compounds
Acid precursors or toxins: Salicylate, ethylene glycol, methanol, toluene, acetaminophen, paraldehyde
Organic acidosis:
- L-lactic acidosis
- D-lactic acidosis
- Ketoacidosis
- Pyroglutamic acidosis

BOX 3 Causes of Metabolic Acidosis by Net Acid Excretion

Renal Acidosis: Absolute or Relative Reduction in Net Acid Excretion
Uremic acidosis
Renal tubular acidosis
- Distal renal tubular acidosis (type I)
- Proximal renal tubular acidosis (type II)
- Aldosterone deficiency or unresponsiveness (type IV)

From McPherson RA, Pincus MR: *Henry's clinical diagnosis and management by laboratory methods*, ed 23, St Louis, 2017, Elsevier.

BOX 4 Causes of L-Lactic Acidosis

Type A Lactic Acidosis Due to Tissue Hypoxia
Circulatory shock
Severe hypoxemia
Heart failure
Severe anemia
Grand mal seizure

Type B Lactic Acidosis, No Tissue Hypoxia
Acute alcoholism
Drugs and toxins (e.g., metformin, antiretroviral drugs, salicylate intoxication)
Diabetes mellitus
Leukemia
Deficiency of thiamin or riboflavin
Idiopathic

From McPherson RA, Pincus MR: *Henry's clinical diagnosis and management by laboratory methods,* ed 23, St Louis, 2017, Elsevier.

Metabolic acidosis with normal AG (hyperchloremic acidosis)
Renal tubular acidosis (including acidosis of aldosterone deficiency)
Intestinal loss of HCO_3^- (diarrhea, pancreatic fistula)
Carbonic anhydrase inhibitors (e.g., acetazolamide)
Dilutional acidosis (as a result of rapid infusion of bicarbonate-free isotonic saline)
Ingestion of exogenous acids (ammonium chloride, methionine, cystine, calcium chloride)
Ileostomy
Ureterosigmoidostomy
Drugs: Amiloride, triamterene, spironolactone, β-blockers
RESPIRATORY ACIDOSIS
Pulmonary disease (chronic obstructive pulmonary disease (COPD), severe pneumonia, pulmonary edema, interstitial fibrosis)
Airway obstruction (foreign body, severe bronchospasm, laryngospasm)
Thoracic cage disorders (pneumothorax, flail chest, kyphoscoliosis)
Defects in muscles of respiration (myasthenia gravis, hypokalemia, muscular dystrophy)
Defects in peripheral nervous system (amyotrophic lateral sclerosis, poliomyelitis, Guillain-Barré syndrome, botulism, tetanus, organophosphate poisoning, spinal cord injury)
Depression of respiratory center (anesthesia, narcotics, sedatives, vertebral artery embolism or thrombosis, increased intracranial pressure)
Failure of mechanical ventilator
METABOLIC ALKALOSIS
Divided into chloride-responsive (urinary chloride <15 mEq/l) and chloride-resistant forms (urinary chloride level >15 mEq/l)
Chloride-responsive
Vomiting
Nasogastric (NG) suction
Diuretics
Posthypercapnic alkalosis
Stool losses (laxative abuse, cystic fibrosis, villous adenoma)

Massive blood transfusion
Exogenous alkali administration
Chloride-resistant
Hyperadrenocorticoid states (Cushing syndrome, primary hyperaldosteronism, secondary mineralocorticoidism [licorice, chewing tobacco])
Hypomagnesemia
Hypokalemia
Bartter syndrome
RESPIRATORY ALKALOSIS
Hypoxemia (pneumonia, pulmonary embolism, atelectasis, high-altitude living)
Drugs (salicylates, xanthines, progesterone, epinephrine, thyroxine, nicotine)
Central nervous system (CNS) disorders (tumor, cerebrovascular accident [CVA], trauma, infections)
Psychogenic hyperventilation (anxiety, hysteria)
Hepatic encephalopathy
Gram-negative sepsis
Hyponatremia
Sudden recovery from metabolic acidosis
Assisted ventilation

TABLE 18 Reference Intervals for Synovial Fluid Constituents

Constituent	Synovial Fluid	Plasma
Total protein	1-3 g/dl	6-8 g/dl
Albumin	55%-70%	50%-65%
α1-Globulin	6%-8%	3%-5%
α2-Globulin	5%-7%	7%-13%
β-Globulin	8%-10%	8%-14%
γ-Globulin	10%-14%	12%-22%
Hyaluronic acid	0.3-0.4 g/dl	
Glucose	70-110 mg/dl	70-110 mg/dl
Uric acid	2-8 mg/dl	2-8 mg/dl
Lactate	9-29 mg/dl	9-29 mg/dl

McPherson RA, Pincus MR: *Henry's clinical diagnosis and management by laboratory methods*, ed 23, 2017, Elsevier.

ARTHROCENTESIS FLUID

Reference intervals for synovial fluid constituents are described in Table 18. Also see Fig. 11.

Interpretation of results

1. **Color:** Normally it is clear or pale yellow; cloudiness indicates inflammatory process or presence of crystals, cell debris, fibrin, or triglycerides.
2. **Viscosity:** Normally it has a high viscosity because of hyaluronate; when fluid is placed on a slide, it can be stretched to a string >2 cm in length before separating (low viscosity indicates breakdown of hyaluronate [lysosomal enzymes from leukocytes] or the presence of edema fluid).
3. **Mucin clot:** Add 1 ml of fluid to 5 ml of a 5% acetic acid solution and allow 1 minute for the clot to form; a firm clot (does not fragment on shaking) is normal and indicates the presence of large molecules of hyaluronic acid (this test is nonspecific and infrequently done).
4. **Glucose:** Normally it approximately equals serum glucose level; a difference of more than 40 mg/dl is suggestive of infection.
5. **Protein:** Total protein concentration is <2.5 g/dl in the normal synovial fluid; it is elevated in inflammatory and septic arthritis.
6. Microscopic examination for crystals
   a. **Gout:** Monosodium urate crystals
   b. **Pseudogout:** Calcium pyrophosphate dihydrate crystals

ASLO TITER

See "ANTISTREPTOLYSIN O TITER"

ASPARTATE AMINOTRANSFERASE (AST, SGOT)

Normal range: 0-35 U/L (0-0.58 μkat/L [CF: 0.01667, SMI: 0.01 μkat/L])
Elevated in:
HEART
Acute myocardial infarction
Pericarditis (active—some cases)
LIVER
Hepatitis virus, Epstein-Barr, or cytomegalovirus infection
Active cirrhosis
Liver passive congestion or hypoxia
Alcohol- or drug-induced liver dysfunction
Space-occupying lesions (active)
Fatty liver (severe)
Extrahepatic biliary obstruction (early)
Drug-induced
SKELETAL MUSCLE
Acute skeletal muscle injury
Muscle inflammation (infectious or noninfectious)

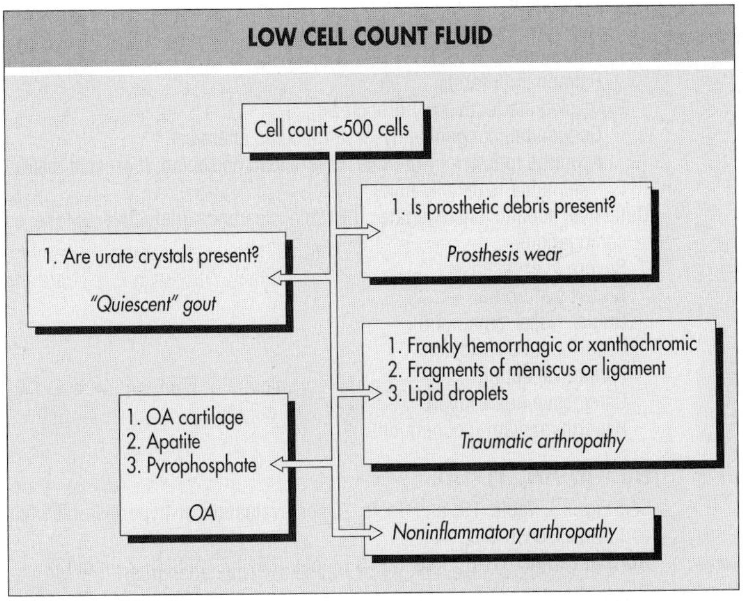

FIG. 11 Low cell count fluid. *OA*, Osteoarthritis. (From Hochberg MC: *Rheumatology*, ed 7, Philadelphia, 2019, Elsevier.)

Muscular dystrophy (active)
Recent surgery
Delirium tremens
KIDNEY
Acute injury or damage
Renal infarct
OTHER
Intestinal infarction
Shock
Cholecystitis
Acute pancreatitis
Hypothyroidism
Heparin therapy (60%-80% of cases)
Fig. 1 describes an approach to the evaluation of AST elevation.
Box 5 describes causes of elevated serum aminotransferase levels.

ATRIAL NATRIURETIC HORMONE (ANH)

Normal: 20-77 pg/ml
Elevated in: CHF, volume overload, cardiovascular disease with high filling pressure
Decreased with: Prazosin and other alpha blockers

BOX 5 Causes of Elevated Serum Aminotransferase Levels*

Chronic, Mild Elevations, ALT > AST (<150 U/L or 5 × normal)
Hepatic Causes
α_1-Antitrypsin deficiency
Autoimmune hepatitis
Chronic viral hepatitis (B, C, and D)
Hemochromatosis
Medications and toxins
Steatosis and steatohepatitis
Wilson disease
Nonhepatic Causes
Celiac disease
Hyperthyroidism
Severe, Acute Elevations, ALT > AST (>1000 U/L or >20 to 25 × normal)
Hepatic Causes
Acute bile duct obstruction
Acute Budd-Chiari syndrome
Acute viral hepatitis
Autoimmune hepatitis
Drugs and toxins
Hepatic artery ligation
Ischemic hepatitis
Wilson disease
Severe, Acute Elevations, AST > ALT (>1000 U/L or >20 to 25 × normal)
Hepatic Cause
Medications or toxins in a patient with underlying alcoholic liver injury
Nonhepatic Cause
Acute rhabdomyolysis
Chronic, Mild Elevations, AST > ALT (<150 U/L, <5 × normal)
Hepatic Causes
Alcohol-related liver injury (AST/ALT > 2:1, AST nearly always <300 U/L)
Cirrhosis
Nonhepatic Causes
Hypothyroidism
Macro-AST
Myopathy
Strenuous exercise

*To detect colorectal cancer, the sensitivity of CEA ranges from 68% for a threshold of 10 mcg/L to 82% for a threshold of 2.5 mcg/L, and the specificity ranges from 97% for a threshold of 10 mcg/L to 80% for a threshold of 2.6 mcg/L.
ALT, alanine aminotransferase; *AST*, aspartate aminotransferase.
From Feldman M, Friedman LS, Brandt LJ: *Sleisenger and Fortran's gastrointestinal and liver disease*, ed 10, Philadelphia, 2016, Elsevier.

B-TYPE NATRIURETIC PEPTIDE (BNP)

Normal range: Up to 100 mcg/L. Natriuretic peptides are secreted to regulate fluid volume, blood pressure, and electrolyte balance. They have activity in both the central and peripheral nervous systems. In humans the main source of circulatory BNP is the heart ventricles.
Elevated in: Heart failure. This test is useful to differentiate heart failure patients from those with chronic obstructive pulmonary disease presenting with dyspnea. Levels are also increased in asymptomatic left ventricular dysfunction, arterial and pulmonary hypertension, cardiac hypertrophy, valvular heart disease, arrhythmia, and acute coronary syndrome. See Fig. 12.

BASOPHIL COUNT

Key causes of basophilia are summarized in Box 6.
Normal range
a. 0.4%-1% of total white blood cells (WBCs); 40-100/mm^3
Elevated in: Leukemia, inflammatory processes, polycythemia vera, Hodgkin lymphoma, hemolytic anemia, after splenectomy, myeloid metaplasia, myxedema
Decreased in: Stress, hypersensitivity reaction, steroids, pregnancy, hyperthyroidism, postirradiation

BICARBONATE

Normal
Arterial: 21-28 mEq/L
Venous: 22-29 mEq/L
Elevated in: Metabolic alkalosis, compensated respiratory acidosis, diuretics, corticosteroids, laxative abuse
Decreased in: Metabolic acidosis, compensated respiratory alkalosis, acetazolamide, cyclosporine, cholestyramine, methanol or ethylene glycol poisoning

BILE, URINE

See "URINE BILE"

BILIRUBIN, DIRECT (conjugated bilirubin)

Normal range: 0-0.2 mg/dl (0-4 μmol/L [CF: 17.10; SMI: 2 μmol/L])
Elevated in: Hepatocellular disease, biliary obstruction, drug-induced cholestasis, hereditary disorders (Dubin-Johnson syndrome, Rotor syndrome)

BILIRUBIN, INDIRECT (unconjugated bilirubin)

Normal range: 0-1.0 mg/dl (2-18 μmol/L [CF: 17.10; SMI: 2 μmol/L])
Elevated in: Increased bilirubin production (if normal liver, serum unconjugated bilirubin is usually less than 4 mg/100 ml)
Hemolytic anemia
Acquired
Congenital
Resorption from extravascular sources
Hematomas
Pulmonary infarcts
Excessive ineffective erythropoiesis
Congenital (congenital dyserythropoietic anemias)
Acquired (pernicious anemia, severe lead poisoning; if present, bilirubinemia is usually mild)
Defective hepatic unconjugated bilirubin clearance (defective uptake or conjugation)
Severe liver disease
Gilbert syndrome
Crigler-Najjar type I or II
Drug-induced inhibition
Portacaval shunt
Congestive heart failure
Hyperthyroidism (uncommon)

BILIRUBIN, TOTAL

See Fig. 13, Table 19, and Table 20 for evaluation of hyperbilirubinemia and liver disease.
Normal range: 0-1.0 mg/dl (2-18 μmol/L [CF: 17.10, SMI: 2 μmol/L])

Elevated in: Liver disease (hepatitis, cirrhosis, cholangitis, neoplasm, biliary obstruction, infectious mononucleosis), hereditary disorders (Gilbert disease, Dubin-Johnson syndrome), drugs (steroids, statins, niacin, acetaminophen, diphenylhydantoin, phenothiazines, penicillin, erythromycin, clindamycin, captopril, amphotericin B, sulfonamides, azathioprine, isoniazid, 5-aminosalicylic acid, allopurinol, methyldopa, indomethacin, halothane, oral contraceptives, procainamide, tolbutamide, labetalol), hemolysis, pulmonary embolism or infarct, hepatic congestion secondary to congestive heart failure

BOX 6 Key Causes of Basophilia

- Myeloproliferative disease
- Allergic—food, drugs, foreign proteins
- Infectious—variola, varicella
- Chronic hemolytic anemia—especially postsplenectomy
- Inflammatory—collagen vascular disease, ulcerative colitis

From McPherson RA, Pincus MR: *Henry's clinical diagnosis and management by laboratory methods,* ed 23, St Louis, 2017, Elsevier.

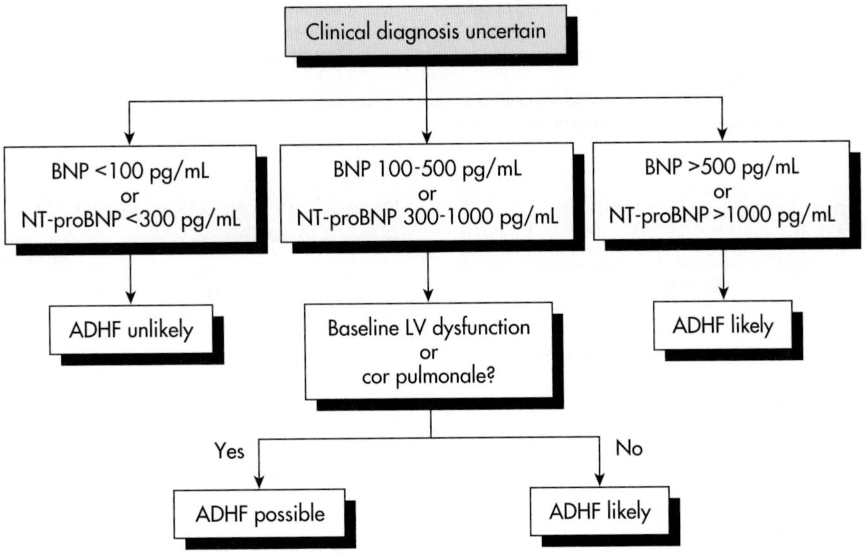

FIG. 12 Interpretation of natriuretic peptide levels. *ADHF,* Acute decompensated heart failure; *BNP,* B-type natriuretic peptide; *LV,* left ventricle; *NT-proBNP,* inactive N-terminal fragment of BNP. (From Adams JG et al: *Emergency medicine, clinical essentials,* ed 2, Philadelphia, 2013, Elsevier.)

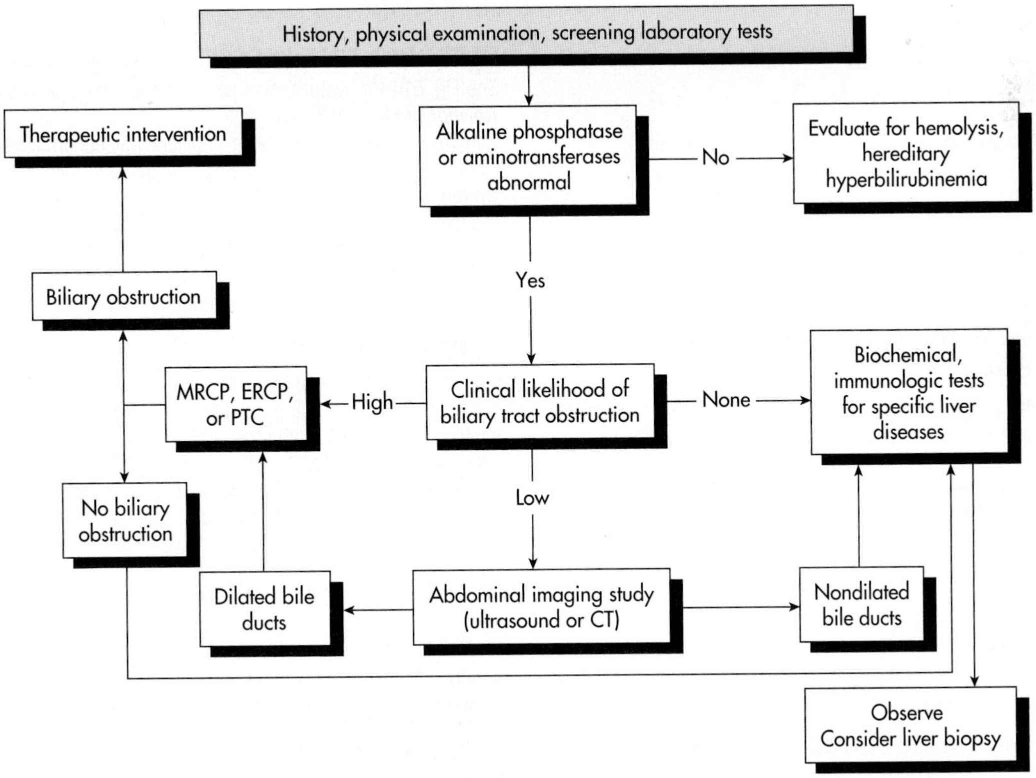

FIG. 13 Diagnosis algorithm for the evaluation of hyperbilirubinemia and other liver test abnormalities and/or signs and symptoms suggestive of liver disease. *CT,* Computed tomography; *ERCP,* endoscopic retrograde cholangiopancreatography; *MRCP,* magnetic resonance cholangiopancreatography; *PTC,* percutaneous cholangiogram. (From Goldman L, Ausiello D [eds]: *Cecil textbook of medicine,* ed 24, Philadelphia, 2012, Saunders.)

TABLE 19 Obstructive Jaundice vs. Cholestatic Liver Disease

Feature	Suggests Obstructive Jaundice	Suggests Parenchymal Liver Disease
History	Abdominal pain; fever, rigors; prior biliary surgery; older age; acholic stools	Anorexia, malaise, myalgias, suggestive of viral prodrome; known infectious exposure; receipt of blood products, use of intravenous drugs; exposure to known hepatotoxin; family history of jaundice
Physical examination	High fever; abdominal tenderness; palpable abdominal mass; abdominal scar	Ascites; other stigmata of liver disease (e.g., prominent abdominal veins, gynecomastia, spider angiomata, asterixis, encephalopathy, Kayser-Fleischer rings)
Laboratory studies	Predominant elevation of serum bilirubin and alkaline phosphatase; prothrombin time that is normal or normalizes with vitamin K administration; elevated serum amylase	Predominant elevation of serum aminotransferases; prolonged prothrombin time that does not correct with vitamin K administration; blood tests indicative of specific liver disease

From Goldman L, Ausiello D (eds): *Cecil textbook of medicine,* ed 24, Philadelphia, 2012, Saunders.

TABLE 20 Causes and Mechanisms of Isolated Hyperbilirubinemia in Adults

Cause	Mechanism
Indirect Hyperbilirubinemia	
Hemolytic Disorders	Overproduction of bilirubin
Inherited	
Red cell enzyme defects (e.g., glucose-6-phosphate dehydrogenase deficiency)	
Sickle cell disease	
Spherocytosis and elliptocytosis	
Acquired	
Drugs and toxins	
Hypersplenism	
Immune mediated	
Paroxysmal nocturnal hemoglobinuria	
Traumatic: Macro- or microvascular injury	
Ineffective Erythropoiesis	Overproduction of bilirubin
Cobalamin deficiency	
Folate deficiency	
Profound iron deficiency	
Thalassemia	
Drugs: Rifampin, Probenecid	Impaired hepatocellular uptake of bilirubin
Inherited Conditions	Impaired conjugation of bilirubin
Crigler-Najjar syndrome types I and II	
Gilbert syndrome	
Other	
Hematoma and massive blood transfusion	Overproduction of bilirubin
Direct Hyperbilirubinemia	
Inherited Conditions	
Dubin-Johnson syndrome	Impaired excretion of conjugated bilirubin
Rotor syndrome	

From Feldman M et al: *Sleisenger and Fordtran's gastrointestinal and liver disease,* ed 10, Philadelphia, 2016, Elsevier.

BILIRUBIN, URINE

See "URINE BILE"

BLADDER TUMOR ASSOCIATED ANTIGEN

Normal

≤14 U/ml. Test is used to detect bladder cancer recurrence. Sensitivity 57%-83% and specificity 68%-72%.

Elevated in: Bladder cancer, renal stones, nephritis, UTI, hematuria, renal cancer, cystitis, recent bladder or urinary tract trauma

TABLE 21 ABO Compatibility

	RECIPIENT TYPE			
Donor Type	**0**	**A**	**B**	**AB**
0	R P	R	R	R
A	P	R P		R
B			R P	R
AB	P	P	P	R P

P, Plasma-containing components (platelets, fresh frozen plasma) are compatible; *R,* red cells are compatible.

From McPherson RA, Pincus MR: *Henry's clinical diagnosis and management by laboratory methods,* ed 23, St Louis, 2017, Elsevier.

BLEEDING TIME (MODIFIED IVY METHOD)

See Fig. E14 for evaluation of patients with prolonged bleeding time.

Normal range: 2-9.5 min

Elevated in: Thrombocytopenia, capillary wall abnormalities, platelet abnormalities (Bernard-Soulier disease, Glanzmann disease), drugs (aspirin, warfarin, antiinflammatory medications, streptokinase, urokinase, dextran, β-lactam antibiotics, moxalactam), disseminated intravascular coagulation, cirrhosis, uremia, myeloproliferative disorders, von Willebrand disease

Bleeding time tests are no longer performed at many hospitals and have been replaced by the platelet function analyzer (PFA-100) assay.

BLOOD TYPE

Blood components must be serologically compatible with the recipient. ABO compatibility is the primary consideration. Transfused red cells must be compatible with recipient antibodies, and transfused plasma must be compatible with recipient red cells. Therefore, whole blood must be of identical ABO type to the recipient. Red blood cells contain a limited amount of plasma and need to be compatible but not necessarily identical to the ABO type of the recipient. Similarly, plasma and platelet concentrates contain few, if any, red cells. ABO-compatible blood component selection is summarized in Table 21. Red blood cells must also be negative for clinically significant antigens when transfused to alloimmunized recipients. It is highly desirable to transfuse only Rh-negative red cells to Rh-negative recipients because there is approximately a 30% risk for immunization to Rh(D). This is particularly important for women of childbearing potential because of the risk for hemolytic disease of the newborn in subsequent pregnancies. Special considerations apply to recipients of ABO-incompatible hematopoietic progenitor cell transplants. During the course of transplantation, such individuals will change their blood type. Transfused red cells should be compatible with both donor and recipient isohemagglutinins, and transfused plasma–containing components should be compatible with both donor and recipient red cells. Thus, the optimal choice for such a patient will depend on current and expected future typing results.

BLOOD VOLUME, TOTAL

Normal range: 60-80 ml/kg
Elevated in: Polycythemia vera, pulmonary disease, CHF, renal insufficiency, pregnancy, acidosis, thyrotoxicosis
Decreased in: Anemia, hemorrhage, vomiting, diarrhea, dehydration, burns, starvation

BNP

See "B-TYPE NATRIURETIC PEPTIDE"

BORDETELLA PERTUSSIS SEROLOGY

Test description: Polymerase chain reaction (PCR) of nasopharyngeal aspirates or secretions is used to identify *Bordetella pertussis,* the organism responsible for whooping cough.

BRCA ANALYSIS

DESCRIPTION OF ANALYSIS

Comprehensive BRCA analysis

BRCA1: Full sequence determination in both forward and reverse directions of approximately 5500 base pairs comprising 22 coding exons and one noncoding exon (exon 4) and approximately 800 adjacent base pairs in the noncoding intervening sequence (intron). Exon 1, which is noncoding, is not analyzed. The wild-type *BRCA1* gene encodes a protein comprising 1863 amino acids.

BRCA2: Full sequence determination in both forward and reverse directions of approximately 10,200 base pairs comprising 26 coding exons and approximately 900 adjacent base pairs in the noncoding intervening sequence (intron). Exon 1, which is noncoding, is not analyzed. The wild-type *BRCA2* gene encodes a protein comprising 3418 amino acids.

The noncoding intronic regions of *BRCA1* and *BRCA2* that are analyzed do not extend more than 20 base pairs proximal to the 5' end and 10 base pairs distal to the 3' end of each exon.

Single-site BRCA analysis: DNA sequence analysis for a specified mutation in *BRCA1* and/or *BRCA2.*

Multisite 3 BRCA analysis: DNA sequence analysis of specific portions of *BRCA1* exon 2, *BRCA1* exon 20, and *BRCA2* exon 11 designed to detect only mutations 187delAG and 5385insC in *BRCA1* and 6174delT in *BRCA2.*

Interpretive Criteria:

"**Positive for a deleterious mutation**": Includes all mutations (nonsense, insertions, deletions) that prematurely terminate ("truncate") the protein product of *BRCA1* at least 10 amino acids from the C-terminus, or the protein product of *BRCA2* at least 110 amino acids from the C-terminus (based on documentation of deleterious mutations in *BRCA1* and *BRCA2*).

In addition, specific missense mutations and noncoding intervening sequence (IVS) mutations are recognized as deleterious on the basis of data derived from linkage analysis of high-risk families, functional assays, biochemical evidence, and/or demonstration of abnormal messenger ribonucleic acid (mRNA) transcript processing.

"**Genetic variant, suspected deleterious**": Includes genetic variants for which the available evidence indicates a likelihood, but not proof, that the mutation is deleterious. The specific evidence supporting such an interpretation will be summarized for individual variants on each such report.

"**Genetic variant, favor polymorphism**": Includes genetic variants for which available evidence indicates that the variant is highly unlikely to contribute substantially to cancer risk. The specific evidence supporting such an interpretation will be summarized for individual variants on each such report.

"**Genetic variant of uncertain significance**": Includes missense mutations and mutations that occur in analyzed intronic regions whose clinical significance has not yet been determined, as well as chain-terminating mutations that truncate *BRCA1* and *BRCA2* distal to amino acid positions 1853 and 3308, respectively.

"**No deleterious mutation detected**": Includes nontruncating genetic variants observed at an allele frequency of approximately 1% of a suitable control population (providing that no data suggest clinical significance), as well as all genetic variants for which published data demonstrate absence of substantial clinical significance. Also includes mutations in the protein-coding region that neither alter the amino acid sequence nor are predicted to significantly affect exon splicing, and base pair alterations in noncoding portions of the gene that have been demonstrated to have no deleterious effect on the length or stability of the mRNA transcript.

There may be uncommon genetic abnormalities in *BRCA1* and *BRCA2* that will not be detected by *BRCA* analysis. This analysis, however, is believed to rule out the majority of abnormalities in these genes, which are believed responsible for most hereditary susceptibility to breast and ovarian cancer.

"**Specific variant/mutation not identified**": Specific and designated deleterious mutations or variants of uncertain clinical significance are not present in the individual being tested. If one (or rarely two) specific deleterious mutations have been identified in a family member, a negative analysis for the specific mutation(s) indicates that the tested individual is at the general population risk of developing breast or ovarian cancer.

BREATH HYDROGEN TEST (hydrogen breath test)

Normal: This test is for bacterial overgrowth. H_2 excretion fasting: 4.6 ± 5.1, after lactulose, early increase <12. Lactulose usually results in a colonic response >30 min after ingestion.
Elevated in: A high fasting breath H_2 level and an increase of at least 12 ppm within 30 min after lactulose challenge are indicative of bacterial overgrowth in the small intestine. The increase must precede the colonic response.
False positives in: Accelerated gastric emptying, laxative use
False negatives in: Use of antibiotics and patients who are nonhydrogen producers

BUN

See "UREA NITROGEN, BLOOD"

C282Y AND H63D MUTATION ANALYSIS

Procedure: Detection of the C282Y and H63D mutations is accomplished by amplification of exons 2 and 4 of the *HFE* gene on chromosome 6 by polymerase chain reaction (PCR) followed by allele-specific hybridization and chemiluminescent detection of hybridized probes. H63D is viewed by some as a polymorphism rather than a mutation because of its prevalence in the population, because 15% of the individuals affected with hereditary hemochromatosis (HH) are compound heterozygotes for C282Y and H63D and about 1% of patients are H63D homozygotes, which suggests that H63D may be causative in the development of the disorder at reduced penetrance.
Interpretation of results: Homozygosity for the C282Y mutation has been associated with an increased risk of being affected with HH compared with the general population. The genotype is observed in 60% to 90% of individuals affected with HH and occurs in less than 1% of the general population. However, approximately 25% of asymptomatic individuals with this genotype do not develop the disorder.

C3

See "COMPLEMENT"

C4

See "COMPLEMENT"

CALCITONIN (serum)

Normal range: <100 pg/ml (<100 ng/L [CF: 1; SMI: 10 ng/L])
Elevated in: Medullary carcinoma of the thyroid (particularly if level >1500 pg/ml), carcinoma of the breast, apudomas, carcinoids, renal failure, thyroiditis

CALCIUM (serum)

Laboratory values in various altered states of calcium metabolism are summarized in Table 22.
See Figs. 15 and 16.
Normal range: 8.8-10.3 mg/dl (2.2-2.58 μmol/L [CF: 0.2495; SMI: 0.02 μmol/L])
ELEVATED
Relatively common:
Neoplasia
Bone primary

TABLE 22 Laboratory Values in Various Altered States of Calcium Metabolism

	Primary Hyperparathyroidism	Humoral Hypercalcemia of Malignancy	Secondary Hyperparathyroidism	Tertiary Hyperparathyroidism	Familial Hypocalciuric Hypercalcemia
Urine calcium	High	High	Normal, high	Normal, high	Low
Serum phosphate	Low	Low	Low, normal, high	Low, normal, high	Low
Urine phosphate	High	High	High	High	High
1,25(OH)D	Normal, high	Low, normal	Low, normal, high	Low, normal, high	Normal, high
PTH intact	High	Low	High	High	High
PTH-r protein	Normal	High	Normal	Normal	Normal

PTH, Parathyroid hormone; *PTH-r,* parathyroid hormone-related.
From McPherson RA, Pincus MR: *Henry's clinical diagnosis and management by laboratory methods,* ed 23, St Louis, 2017, Elsevier.

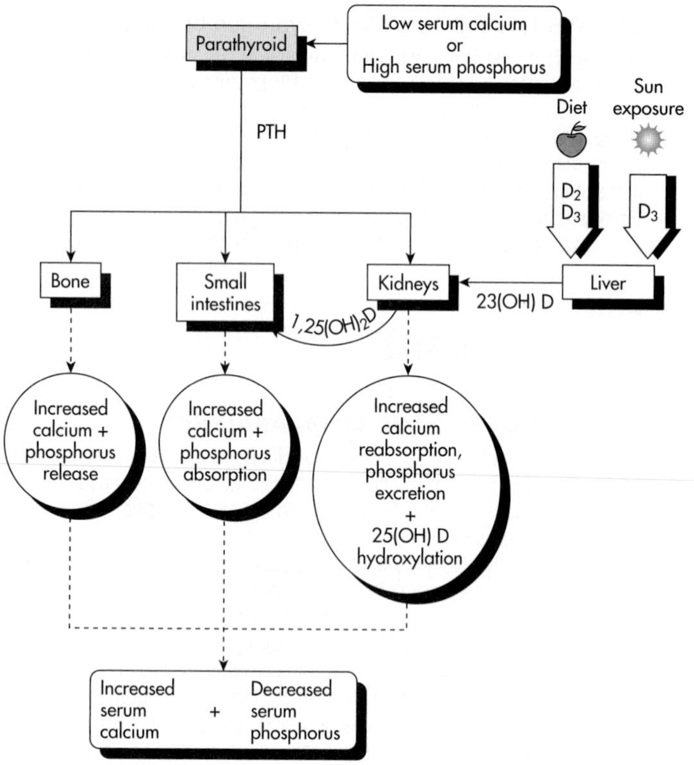

FIG. 15 Calcium homeostasis. Parathyroid hormone *(PTH)* is released from the parathyroid glands in response to hypocalcemia and hyperphosphatemia. PTH acts on bone, the small intestines, and the kidneys to effect a rise in serum calcium and a net decrease in serum phosphorus. Hydroxylation of inactive forms of vitamin D occurs in the liver and kidneys. 1,25(OH)2D facilitates intestinal absorption of calcium and phosphorus. *D_2,* vitamin D_2; *D_3,* vitamin D_3. (From Adams JG et al: *Emergency medicine, clinical essentials,* ed 2, Philadelphia, 2013, Elsevier.)

Myeloma
Acute leukemia
Nonbone solid tumors
Breast
Lung
Squamous nonpulmonary
Kidney
Neoplasm secretion of parathyroid hormone-related protein (PTHrP, "ectopic PTH")
Primary hyperparathyroidism
Thiazide diuretics
Tertiary (renal) hyperparathyroidism
Idiopathic
Spurious (artifactual) hypercalcemia
Dehydration
Serum protein elevation
Laboratory technical problem (lab error)
Relatively uncommon
Sarcoidosis
Hyperthyroidism
Immobilization (mostly seen in children and adolescents)
Diuretic phase of acute renal tubular necrosis
Vitamin D intoxication
Milk-alkali syndrome
Addison disease
Lithium therapy
Idiopathic hypercalcemia of infancy
Acromegaly
Theophylline toxicity

Table 23 describes the laboratory differential diagnosis of hypercalcemia.

Box 7 describes the differential diagnosis of hypercalcemia in older adults.

DECREASED
Artifactual
Hypoalbuminemia
Hemodilution
Primary hypoparathyroidism
Pseudohypoparathyroidism
Vitamin D related
Vitamin D deficiency
Malabsorption
Renal failure
Magnesium deficiency
Sepsis
Chronic alcoholism
Tumor lysis syndrome
Rhabdomyolysis
Alkalosis (respiratory or metabolic)

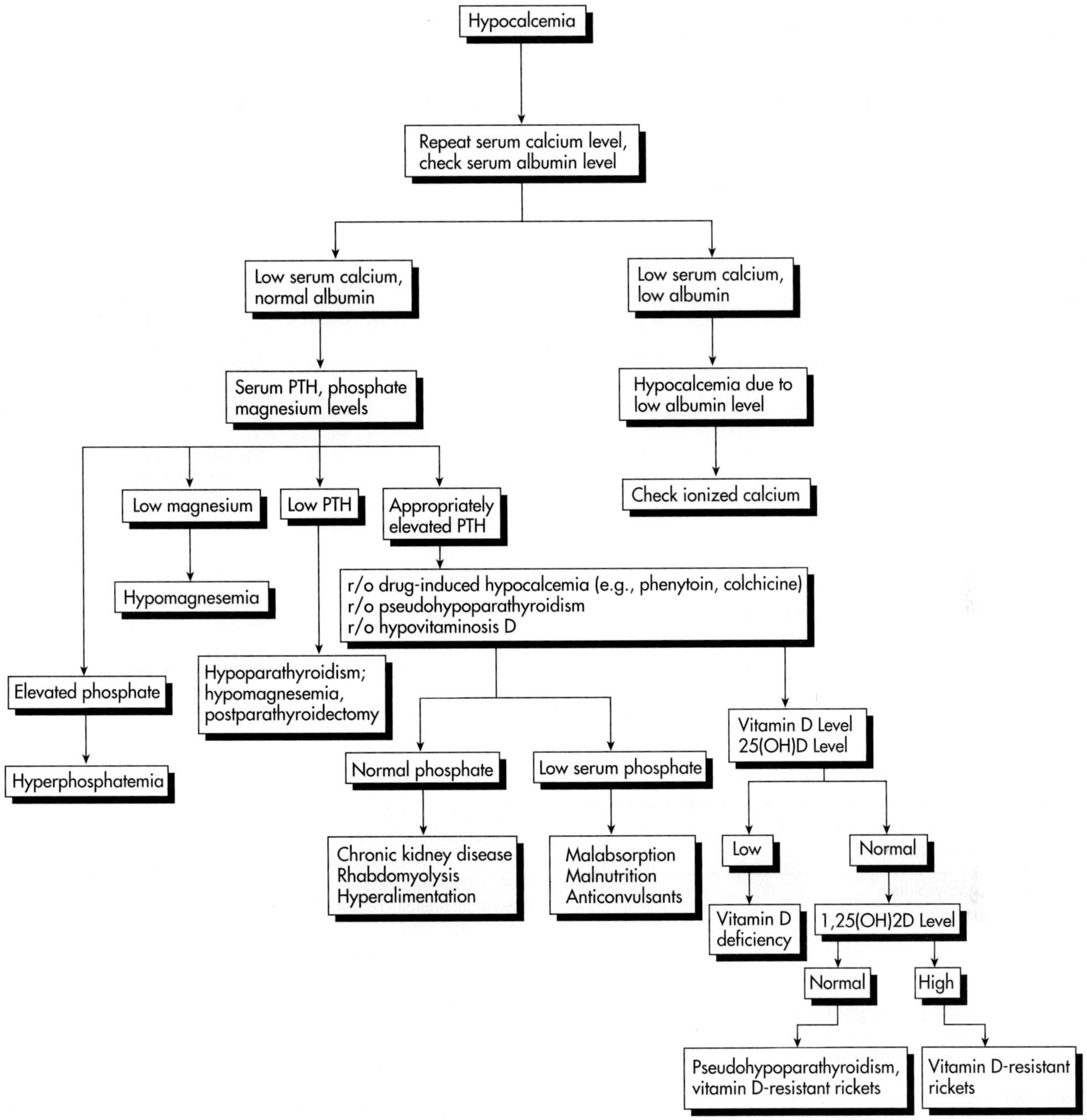

FIG. 16 Diagnostic algorithm. *PTH,* Parathyroid hormone. (From Ferri F: *Ferri's best test: a practical guide to clinical laboratory medicine and diagnostic imaging,* ed 3, Philadelphia, 2014, Saunders.)

Acute pancreatitis
Drug-induced hypocalcemia
Large doses of magnesium sulfate
Anticonvulsants
Mithramycin
Gentamicin
Cimetidine

Table 24 describes the laboratory differential diagnosis of hypocalcemia.

CALCIUM, URINE

See "URINE CALCIUM"

CANCER ANTIGEN 15-3 (CA 15-3)

Normal: <30 U/ml
Elevated in: Approximately 80% of women with metastatic breast cancer. Clinical sensitivity is 0.60, specificity 0.87, positive predictive value 0.91. This test is generally used to predict recurrence of breast cancer and evaluate response to therapy. May also be elevated in liver cancer, pancreatic cancer, ovarian cancer, colorectal cancer. Elevations can also occur with benign breast and liver disease.

CANCER ANTIGEN 27-29 (CA 27-29)

Normal: <38 U/ml
Elevated in: Approximately 75% of women with metastatic breast cancer. Clinical sensitivity is 0.57, specificity 0.97, positive predictive value 0.83, negative predictive value 0.92. This test is generally used to predict recurrence of breast cancer and evaluate response to therapy. May also be elevated in liver cancer, pancreatic cancer, ovarian cancer, colorectal cancer. Elevations can also occur with benign breast and liver disease.

CANCER ANTIGEN 72-4 (CA 72-4)

Normal: <4.0 ng/ml
Elevated in: Gastric cancer (elevated in >50% of patients). Often used in combination with CA 72-4, CA 19-9, and CEA to monitor gastric cancer after treatment.

TABLE 23 Laboratory Differential Diagnosis of Hypercalcemia

	Plasma Tests					Urine Tests			
Diagnosis	**Ca**	**PO_4**	**PTH**	**25(OH)D**	**$1,25(OH)_2D$**	**cAMP**	**TmP/GFR**	**Ca**	**Comments**
Primary hyperparathyroidism	↑	N/↓	↑	N	N/↑	↑	↓	↑	Parathyroid adenoma most common
MEN I									Parathyroid hyperplasia; also includes pituitary and pancreatic neoplasms
MEN IIa									Parathyroid hyperplasia; also includes medullary thyroid carcinoma and pheochromocytoma
MEN IIb									Parathyroid disease uncommon, primarily medullary thyroid carcinoma and pheochromocytoma
FHH	↑	N	N/↑	N	N	N/↑	N/↓	↓↓	Autosomal dominant inheritance; hypercalcemia present within first decade; benign
Malignancy									
Solid tumor, humoral	↑	N/↓	↓	N	N	↑	↓	↑↑	Primarily epidermoid tumors; PTH-related protein(s) is mediator
Solid tumor, osteolytic	↑	N/↑	↓	N	N	↓	↑	↑↑	
Lymphoma	↑	N/↑	↓	N/↓	↑	↓	↑	↑↑	
Granulomatous disease	↑	N/↑	↓	N/↓	↑↑	↓	↑	↑↑	Sarcoid most common etiology
Vitamin D intoxication	↑	N/↑	↓	↑↑	N	↓	↑	↑↑	
Hyperthyroidism	↑	N	↓	N	N	N	N	↑↑	Plasma concentrations of T_4 and/or T_3 are elevated

Ca, Calcium; *cAMP,* cyclic adenosine monophosphate; *FHH,* familial hypocalciuric hypercalcemia; *GFR,* glomerular filtration rate; *MEN,* multiple endocrine neoplasia; *25(OH)D,* 25 hydroxyvitamin D; *PO_4,* phosphate; *PTH,* parathyroid hormone; *T_3,* triiodothyronine; *T_4,* thyroxine; *TmP,* renal threshold for phosphorus.

BOX 7 Differential Diagnosis of Hypercalcemia in Older Adults

Primary hyperparathyroidism
Malignancy
Renal failure
Addison disease
Hyperthyroidism
Immobilization
Medications: Thiazide diuretics, calcium supplements, lithium
Milk alkali syndrome
Paget disease (when immobilized)
Sarcoidosis
Tuberculosis
Vitamin D or vitamin A intoxication

Symptoms of Acute Hypercalcemia
Neurologic: Drowsiness, confusion, irritability hypotonia, coma
Gastrointestinal: Anorexia, nausea, vomiting, acute pancreatitis
Cardiovascular: Arrhythmias
Renal: Polyuria, polydipsia, dehydration

From Fillit HM: *Brocklehurst's textbook of geriatric medicine and gerontology*, ed 8, Philadelphia, 2017, Elsevier.

CANCER ANTIGEN 125 (CA 125)

Normal range: <1.4%

This test uses an antibody against antigen from tissue culture of an ovarian tumor cell line. Various published evaluations report sensitivity of about 75%-80% in patients with ovarian carcinoma. There is also an appreciable incidence of elevated values in nonovarian malignancies and in certain benign conditions (see later). Test values may transiently increase during chemotherapy.

MALIGNANT

Epithelial ovarian carcinoma, 75%-80% (range, 25%-92%; better in serous than mucinous cystadenocarcinoma)
Endometrial carcinoma, 25%-48% (2%-90%)
Pancreatic carcinoma, 59%
Colorectal carcinoma, 20% (15%-56%)
Endocervical adenocarcinoma, 83%
Squamous cervical or vaginal carcinoma, 7%-14%
Lung carcinoma, 32%
Breast carcinoma, 12%-40%
Lymphoma, 35%

BENIGN

Cirrhosis, 40%-80%
Acute pancreatitis, 38%
Acute peritonitis, 75%
Endometriosis, 88%
Acute pelvic inflammatory disease, 33%
Pregnancy first trimester, 2%-24%
During menstruation (occasionally)
Renal failure (?frequency)
Normal persons, 0.6%-1.4%

CAPTOPRIL STIMULATION TEST

Normal: Test performed by giving 25 mg captopril orally after overnight fast. Patient should be seated during test. After captopril, aldosterone <15 ng/dl, renin >2 ng angiotensin L/ml/hr.

Interpretation of results: In patients with primary aldosteronism, plasma aldosterone remains high and plasma renin activity remains low after captopril.

CARBAMAZEPINE LEVEL

Therapeutic range and general information are summarized in Table 25.

CARBAMAZEPINE (Tegretol)

Normal therapeutic range: 4-12 mcg/ml

CARBOHYDRATE ANTIGEN 19-9

Normal: <37.0 U/ml

Elevated in: GI cancer, most frequently pancreatic cancer. Amount of elevation has no relation to tumor mass. Elevations can also occur with cirrhosis, cholangitis, and chronic or acute pancreatitis.

TABLE 24 Laboratory Differential Diagnosis of Hypocalcemia

	Plasma Tests					Urine Tests					
Diagnosis	**Ca**	**PO_4**	**PTH**	**25(OH) D**	**1,25 $(OH)_2D$**	**cAMP**	**cAMP after PTH**	**TmP/ GFR**	**TmP/GFR after PTH**	**Ca**	**Comments**
Hypoparathyroidism	↓	↑	N/↓	N	↓	↓	↑↑	↑	↓↓	N/↓	Deficiency of PTH
Pseudohypoparathyroidism											
Type I	↓	↑	↑↑	N	↓	↓	NC	↑	↑	N/↓	Resistance to PTH; patients may have Albright hereditary osteodystrophy and resistance to multiple hormones
Type II	↓	N	↑↑	N	↓	↓	↑	↑	↑	N/↓	Renal resistance to cAMP
Vitamin D deficiency	↓	N/↓	↑↑	↓↓	N/↓	↑	↑	↓	↓	↓↓	Deficient supply (e.g., nutrition) or absorption (e.g., pancreatic insufficiency) of vitamin D
Vitamin D-dependent Rickets											
Type I	↓	N/↓	↑↑	N	↓	↑↑		↓		↓↓	Deficient activity of renal 25(OH)D-1α-hydroxylase
Type II	↓	N/↓	↑↑	N	↑↑	↑		↓		↓↓	Resistance to $1,25(OH)_2D$

Ca, Calcium; *cAMP,* cyclic adenosine monophosphate; *FHH,* familial hypocalciuric hypercalcemia; *GFR,* glomerular filtration rate; *MEN,* multiple endocrine neoplasia; *NC,* no change or small increase; *(OH)D,* hydroxycalciferol D; *PO_4,* phosphate; *PTH,* parathyroid hormone; *T_3,* triiodothyronine; *T_4,* thyroxine; *TmP,* renal threshold for phosphorus.

TABLE 25 Carbamazepine (Tegretol)

Purpose	**Treatment of Generalized Tonic-Clonic Seizures, Simple Partial Seizures, Complex Partial Seizures, Trigeminal Neuralgia, and Glossopharyngeal Neuralgia**
General adult dose	Oral: 0.8-1.2 g/day maintenance for seizure control; 0.2-1.2 g/day for neuralgia
Usual bioavailability	70%
Half-life	Initially approximately 35 hours; approximately 8-20 hours after 3-4 weeks of administration
General therapeutic range	4-12 mcg/ml
General toxic level	>12 mcg/ml
Transport	60%-70% plasma protein bound
Metabolism	Hepatic: Carbamazepine-10,11-epoxide (active); carbamazepine-10,11-transdihydrodiol (inactive)
Elimination	1%-2% unchanged in urine
Steady state	3-7 days
Mechanism of action	Decreases sodium and calcium ion influx into repeatedly depolarizing CNS neurons; reduces excitatory synaptic transmission in the spinal trigeminal nucleus
Toxic effects	Drowsiness, ataxia, dizziness, nausea, vomiting, involuntary movements, abnormal reflexes, irregular pulse

From McPherson RA, Pincus MR: *Henry's clinical diagnosis and management by laboratory methods,* ed 23, St Louis, 2017, Elsevier.

CARBON DIOXIDE, PARTIAL PRESSURE

Normal
Male: 35-48 mm Hg
Female: 32-45 mm Hg
Elevated in: Respiratory acidosis
Decreased in: Respiratory alkalosis

CARBON MONOXIDE

See "CARBOXYHEMOGLOBIN"

CARBOXYHEMOGLOBIN

Normal range: Saturation of hemoglobin <2%; smokers <9%
Elevated in: Smoking, exposure to smoking, exposure to automobile exhaust fumes, malfunctioning gas-burning appliances

CARCINOEMBRYONIC ANTIGEN (CEA)

Normal range
Nonsmokers: 0-2.5 ng/ml (0-2.5 μg/L [CF: 1; SMI: 0.1 μg/L])
Smokers: 0-5 ng/ml (0-5 μg/L [CF: 1; SMI: 0.1 μg/L])
Elevated in
Colorectal carcinomas*, pancreatic carcinomas, and metastatic disease (usually produce higher elevations: >20 ng/ml)
Carcinomas of the esophagus, stomach, small intestine, liver, breast, ovary, lung, and thyroid (usually produce lesser elevations)
Benign conditions (smoking, inflammatory bowel disease, hypothyroidism, cirrhosis, pancreatitis, infections) (usually produce levels <10 ng/ml)

CAROTENE (serum)

Normal range: 50-250 μg/dl (0.9-4.6 μmol/L [CF: 0.01863; SMI: 0.1 μmol/L])
Elevated in: Carotenemia, chronic nephritis, diabetes mellitus, hypothyroidism, nephrotic syndrome, hyperlipidemia
Decreased in: Fat malabsorption, steatorrhea, pancreatic insufficiency, lack of carotenoids in diet, high fever, liver disease

CATECHOLAMINES, URINE

See "URINE CATECHOLAMINES"

CBC

See "COMPLETE BLOOD COUNT"

CD40 LIGAND

Normal: <5 mcg/L. CD40 ligand is a soluble protein that is shed from activated leukocytes and platelets and used in risk stratification for acute coronary syndrome.
Elevated in: Acute coronary syndrome. Increased CD40 ligand is associated with higher incidence of death or nonfatal myocardial infarction (MI).

*To detect colorectal cancer, the sensitivity of CEA ranges from 68% for a threshold of 10 mcg/L to 82% for a threshold of 2.5 mcg/L, and the specificity ranges from 97% for a threshold of 10 mcg/L to 80% for a threshold of 2.6 mcg/L.

TABLE 26 Relation of CD4 Lymphocyte Counts to the Onset of Certain HIV-Associated Infections and Neoplasms in North America

CD4 Count (Cells/ mm^3)*	Opportunistic Infection or Neoplasm	Frequency (%)†
>500	Herpes zoster, polydermatomal	5-10
200-500	*Mycobacterium tuberculosis* infection, pulmonary and extrapulmonary	2-20
	Oral hairy leukoplakia	40-70
	Candida pharyngitis (thrush)	40-70
	Recurrent *Candida* vaginitis	15-30 (F)
	Kaposi sarcoma, mucocutaneous	15-30 (M)
	Bacterial pneumonia, recurrent	15-20
	Cervical neoplasia	1-2 (F)
100-200	*Pneumocystis carinii* pneumonia	15-60
	Herpes simplex, chronic, ulcerative	5-10
	Histoplasma capsulatum infection, disseminated	0-20
	Kaposi sarcoma, visceral	3-8 (M)
	Progressive multifocal leukoencephalopathy	2-3
	Lymphoma, non-Hodgkin	2-5
<100	*Candida* esophagitis	15-20
	Mycobacterium avium-intracellulare, disseminated	25-40
	Toxoplasma gondii encephalitis	5-25
	Cryptosporidium enteritis	2-10
	CMV retinitis	20-35
	Cryptococcus neoformans encephalitis	2-5
	CMV esophagitis or colitis	6-12
	Lymphoma, central nervous system	4-8

CMV, Cytomegalovirus; *F,* exclusively in women; *HIV,* human immunodeficiency virus; *M,* almost exclusively in men.
*Table indicates CD4 count at which specific infections or neoplasms generally begin to appear. Each infection may recur or progress during the subsequent course of HIV disease.
†Even within the United States, great regional differences in the incidence of specific opportunistic infections are apparent. For example, disseminated histoplasmosis is common in the Mississippi River drainage area but very rare in individuals who have lived exclusively on the East or West Coast.

CD4+ T-LYMPHOCYTE COUNT (CD4+ T cells)

Calculated as total WBC × % lymphocytes × % lymphocytes stained with CD4.

This test is used primarily to evaluate immune dysfunction in HIV infection. It is useful as a prognostic indicator and as a criterion for initiating prophylaxis for several opportunistic infections that are sequelae of HIV infection. Progressive depletion of CD4+ T lymphocytes is associated with an increased likelihood of clinical complications (Table 26).

CEA

See "CARCINOEMBRYONIC ANTIGEN"

CEREBROSPINAL FLUID (CSF)

Adult lumbar CSF reference values are summarized in Table 27. CSF proteins in various central nervous system diseases are described in Table 28.

Interpretation of results

Appearance of the fluid

Clear: Normal.

Yellow color (xanthochromia) in the supernatant of centrifuged CSF within 1 hour or less after collection is usually the result of previous bleeding (subarachnoid hemorrhage); it may also be caused by increased CSF protein, melanin from meningeal melanosarcomas, or carotenoids.

TABLE 27 Adult Lumbar CSF Reference Values

Analyte	Conventional Units	SI Units
Protein	15-60 mg/dL	0.15-0.60 g/L
Prealbumin	2%-7%	
Albumin	56%-76%	
α_1-Globulin	2%-7%	
α_2-Globulin	4%-12%	
β-Globulin	8%-18%	
γ-Globulin	3%-12%	
Electrolytes		
Osmolality	280-300 mOsm/L	280-300 mmol/L
Sodium	135-150 mEq/L	135-150 mmol/L
Potassium	2.6-3.0 mEq/L	2.6-3.0 mmol/L
Chloride	115-130 mEq/L	115-130 mmol/L
Carbon dioxide	20-25 mEq/L	20-25 mmol/L
Calcium	2.0-2.8 mEq/L	1.0-1.4 mmol/L
Magnesium	2.4-3.0 mEq/L	1.2-1.5 mmol/L
Lactate	10-22 mg/dL	1.1-2.4 mmol/L
pH		
Lumbar fluid	7.28-7.32	
Cisternal fluid	7.32-7.34	
pCO_2		
Lumbar fluid	44-50 mm Hg	
Cisternal fluid	40-46 mm Hg	
pO_2	40-44 mm Hg	
Other Constituents		
Ammonia	10-35 μg/dL	6-20 μmol/L
Glutamine	5-20 mg/dL	0.3-1.4 mmol/L
Creatinine	0.6-1.2 mg/dL	45-92 μmol/L
Glucose	50-80 mg/dL	2.8-4.4 mmol/L
Iron	1-2 μg/dL	0.2-0.4 μmol/L
Phosphorus	1.2-2.0 mg/dL	0.4-0.7 mmol/L
Total lipid	1-2 mg/dL	0.01-0.02 g/L
Urea	6-16 mg/dL	2.0-5.7 mmol/L
Urate	0.5-3.0 mg/dL	30-180 μmol/L
Zinc	2-6 μg/dL	0.3-0.9 μmol/L

CSF, Cerebrospinal fluid; *pCO_2*, partial pressure of carbon dioxide; *pO_2*, partial pressure of oxygen.
From McPherson RA, Pincus MR: *Henry's clinical diagnosis and management by laboratory methods,* ed 23, St Louis, 2017, Elsevier.

TABLE 28 CSF Proteins and Central Nervous System Diseases

Protein	Major Diseases/Disorders
α_2-Macroglobulin	Subdural hemorrhage, bacterial meningitis
β-Amyloid and τ proteins	Alzheimer's disease
β_2-Microglobulin	Leukemia/lymphoma, Behçet's syndrome
C-reactive protein	Bacterial and viral meningitis
Fibronectin	Lymphoblastic leukemia, AIDS, meningitis
Methemoglobin	Mild subarachnoid/subdural hemorrhage
Myelin basic protein	Multiple sclerosis, tumors, others
Protein 14-3-3	Creutzfeldt-Jakob disease
Transferrin	CSF leakage (otorrhea, rhinorrhea)

AIDS, Acquired immunodeficiency syndrome; *CSF,* cerebrospinal fluid.
From McPherson RA, Pincus MR: *Henry's clinical diagnosis and management by laboratory methods,* ed 23, St Louis, 2017, Elsevier.

Pinkish color is usually the result of a bloody tap; the color generally clears progressively from tubes 1-4 (the supernatant is usually crystal clear in traumatic taps).

Turbidity usually indicates the presence of leukocytes (bleeding introduces approximately 1 WBC/500 RBCs into the CSF).

CSF pressure: Elevated pressure can be seen with meningitis, meningoencephalitis, pseudotumor cerebri, mass lesions, and intracerebral bleeding.

Cell count: In the adult the CSF is normally free of cells (although up to five mononuclear cells/mm^3 is considered normal); the presence of granulocytes is never normal.

Neutrophils: Seen in bacterial meningitis, early viral meningoencephalitis, and early tuberculosis (TB) meningitis. Box 8 summarizes causes of increased CSF neutrophils.

Increased lymphocytes: TB meningitis, viral meningoencephalitis, syphilitic meningoencephalitis, fungal meningitis. Causes of CSF lymphocytosis are summarized in Box 9.

CSF plasmacytosis: Box 10 describes inflammatory and infectious causes of CSF plasmacytosis.

CSF eosinophilia: Causes of CSF eosinophilic pleocytosis are summarized in Box 11.

Protein: Serum proteins are generally too large to cross the normal blood-CSF barrier; however, increased CSF protein is seen with meningeal inflammation, traumatic tap, increased CNS synthesis, tissue degeneration, obstruction to CSF circulation, and Guillain-Barré syndrome. Mean concentrations of plasma and CSF proteins are summarized in Table 29. Conditions associated with increased CSF total protein are summarized in Box 12.

BOX 8 Causes of Increased CSF Neutrophils

- Meningitis
  - Bacterial meningitis
  - Early viral meningoencephalitis
  - Early tuberculous meningitis
  - Early mycotic meningitis
  - Amebic encephalomyelitis
- Other infections
  - Cerebral abscess
  - Subdural empyema
  - AIDS-related CMV radiculopathy
- Following seizures
- Following CNS hemorrhage
  - Subarachnoid
  - Intracerebral
- Following CNS infarct
- Reaction to repeated lumbar punctures
- Injection of foreign material in subarachnoid space (e.g., methotrexate, contrast media)
- Metastatic tumor in contact with CSF

AIDS, Acquired immunodeficiency syndrome; *CMV*, cytomegalovirus; *CNS*, central nervous system; *CSF*, cerebrospinal fluid.
From McPherson RA, Pincus MR: *Henry's clinical diagnosis and management by laboratory methods*, ed 23, St Louis, 2017, Elsevier.

BOX 9 Causes of CSF Lymphocytosis

Meningitis
- Viral meningitis
- Tuberculous meningitis
- Fungal meningitis
- Syphilitic meningoencephalitis
- Leptospiral meningitis
- Bacterial due to uncommon organisms
- Early bacterial meningitis where leukocyte counts are relatively low
- Parasitic infestations (e.g., cysticercosis, trichinosis, toxoplasmosis)
- Aseptic meningitis due to septic focus adjacent to meninges

Degenerative Disorders
- Subacute sclerosing panencephalitis
- Multiple sclerosis
- Drug abuse encephalopathy
- Guillain-Barré syndrome
- Acute disseminated encephalomyelitis

Other Inflammatory Disorders
- HaNDL syndrome (headache with neurologic deficits and CSF lymphocytosis)
- Sarcoidosis
- Polyneuritis
- CNS periarteritis

CNS, Central nervous system; *CSF*, cerebrospinal fluid.
From McPherson RA, Pincus MR: *Henry's clinical diagnosis and management by laboratory methods*, ed 23, St Louis, 2017, Elsevier.

BOX 10 Inflammatory and Infectious Causes of CSF Plasmacytosis

- Acute viral infections
- Guillain-Barré syndrome
- Multiple sclerosis
- Parasitic CNS infestations
- Sarcoidosis
- Subacute sclerosing panencephalitis
- Syphilitic meningoencephalitis
- Tuberculous meningitis

CNS, Central nervous system; *CSF*, cerebrospinal fluid.
From McPherson RA, Pincus MR: *Henry's clinical diagnosis and management by laboratory methods*, ed 23, St Louis, 2017, Elsevier.

BOX 11 Causes of CSF Eosinophilic Pleocytosis

Commonly Associated with
- Acute polyneuritis
- CNS reaction to foreign material (drugs, shunts)
- Fungal infections
- Idiopathic eosinophilic meningitis
- Idiopathic hypereosinophilic syndrome
- Parasitic infections

Infrequently Associated with
- Bacterial meningitis
- Leukemia/lymphoma
- Myeloproliferative disorders
- Neurosarcoidosis
- Primary brain tumors
- Tuberculous meningoencephalitis
- Viral meningitis

CNS, Central nervous system; *CSF*, cerebrospinal fluid.
Modified from Kjeldsberg CR, Knight JA: *Body fluids: laboratory examination of amniotic, cerebrospinal, seminal, serous and synovial fluids*, ed 3, Chicago, 1993, American Society for Clinical Pathology, with permission. In McPherson RA, Pincus MR: *Henry's clinical diagnosis and management by laboratory methods*, ed 23, St Louis, 2017, Elsevier.

TABLE 29 Mean Concentrations of Plasma and CSF Proteins

Protein	CSF, mg/L	Plasma/CSF Ratio
Prealbumin	17.3	14
Albumin	155.0	236
Transferrin	14.4	142
Ceruloplasmin	1.0	366
Immunoglobulin (Ig)G	12.3	802
IgA	1.3	1346
α_2-Microglobulin	2.0	1111
Fibrinogen	0.6	4940
IgM	0.6	1167
β-Lipoprotein	0.6	6213

CSF, Cerebrospinal fluid.
Adapted and updated from Felgenhauer K: Protein size and cerebrospinal fluid composition, *Klin Wochenschr* 52:1158, 1974, with permission. (McPherson RA, Pincus MR: *Henry's clinical diagnosis and management by laboratory methods*, ed 23, St Louis, 2017, Elsevier.)

BOX 12 Conditions Associated with Increased CSF Total Protein

Traumatic Spinal Puncture
Increased blood-CSF permeability
Arachnoiditis (e.g., following methotrexate therapy)
Meningitis (bacterial, viral, fungal, tuberculous)
Hemorrhage (subarachnoid, intracerebral)
Endocrine/metabolic disorders
- Milk-alkali syndrome with hypercalcemia
- Diabetic neuropathy
- Hereditary neuropathies and myelopathies
- Decreased endocrine function (thyroid, parathyroid)
- Other disorders (uremia, dehydration)

Drug Toxicity
Ethanol, phenothiazines, phenytoin

CSF Circulation Defects
Mechanical obstruction (tumor, abscess, herniated disk)
Loculated CSF effusion

Increased Immunoglobulin (Ig)G Synthesis
Multiple sclerosis

Neurosyphilis
Subacute sclerosing panencephalitis

Increased IgG Synthesis and Blood-CSF Permeability
Guillain-Barré syndrome
Collagen vascular diseases (e.g., lupus, periarteritis)
Chronic inflammatory demyelinating polyradiculopathy

From McPherson RA, Pincus MR: *Henry's clinical diagnosis and management by laboratory methods*, ed 23, St Louis, 2017, Elsevier.

Glucose

Decreased glucose is seen with bacterial meningitis, TB meningitis, fungal meningitis, subarachnoid hemorrhage, and some cases of viral meningitis.

A mild increase in CSF glucose can be seen in patients with very elevated serum glucose levels.

Table 30 describes CSF findings in infectious and inflammatory diseases of the central nervous system and meninges.

Causes of xanthochromia are summarized in Table 31.

CERULOPLASMIN (serum)

Normal range: 20-35 mg/dl (200-350 mg/L [CF: 10; SMI: 10 mg/L])
Elevated in: Pregnancy, estrogens, oral contraceptives, neoplastic diseases (leukemias, Hodgkin lymphoma, carcinomas), inflammatory states, systemic lupus erythematosus, primary biliary cirrhosis, rheumatoid arthritis
Decreased in: Wilson disease (values often <10 mg/dl), nephrotic syndrome, advanced liver disease, malabsorption, total parenteral nutrition, Menkes syndrome

CHLAMYDIA GROUP ANTIBODY SEROLOGIC TEST

Test description: Acute and convalescent sera is drawn 2-4 wk apart. A fourfold increase in titer between acute and convalescent sera is necessary for confirmation. A single titer ≥1:64 is considered indicative of psittacosis or lymphogranuloma venereum (LGV).

CHLAMYDIA TRACHOMATIS PCR

Test description: Test is performed on endocervical swab, urine, and intraurethral swab (Table 32).
Normal: Negative

CHLORIDE (serum)

Normal range: 95-105 mEq/L (95-105 mmol/L [CF: 1; SMI: 1 mmol/L])
Elevated in: Dehydration, excessive infusion of normal saline solution, cystic fibrosis (sweat test), hyperparathyroidism, renal tubular disease, metabolic acidosis, prolonged diarrhea, drugs (ammonium chloride administration, acetazolamide, boric acid, triamterene)
Decreased in: Congestive heart failure, syndrome of inappropriate antidiuretic hormone secretion, Addison disease, vomiting, gastric suction, salt-losing nephritis, continuous infusion of D_5W, thiazide diuretic administration, diaphoresis, diarrhea, burns, diabetic ketoacidosis

CHLORIDE (sweat)

Normal: 0-40 mmol/L
Borderline/indeterminate: 41-60 mmol/L
Consistent with cystic fibrosis: >60 mmol/L

False low results can occur with edema, excessive sweating, and hypoproteinemia.

CHLORIDE, URINE

See "URINE CHLORIDE"

CHOLECYSTOKININ-PANCREOZYMIN (CCK, CCK-PZ)

Normal: <80 pg/ml
Elevated in: Pancreatic disease, celiac disease, gastric ulcer, postgastrectomy, irritable bowel syndrome (IBS), fatty food intolerance

CHOLESTEROL, HIGH-DENSITY LIPOPROTEIN

See "HIGH-DENSITY LIPOPROTEIN CHOLESTEROL"

CHOLESTEROL, LOW-DENSITY LIPOPROTEIN

See "LOW-DENSITY LIPOPROTEIN CHOLESTEROL"

CHOLESTEROL, TOTAL

Normal range: Varies with age

Generally <200 mg/dl (<5.20 mmol/L [CF: 0.02586; SMI: 0.05 mmol/L])

Elevated in: Primary hypercholesterolemia, biliary obstruction, diabetes mellitus, nephrotic syndrome, hypothyroidism, primary biliary cirrhosis, high-cholesterol diet, pregnancy third trimester, myocardial infarction, drugs (steroids, phenothiazines, oral contraceptives). Classic hyperlipidemia phenotypes are summarized in Table 33.
Decreased in: Medications (statins, niacin), starvation, malabsorption, sideroblastic anemia, thalassemia, abetalipoproteinemia, hyperthyroidism, Cushing syndrome, hepatic failure, multiple myeloma, polycythemia vera, chronic myelocytic leukemia, myeloid metaplasia, Waldenström macroglobulinemia, myelofibrosis

CHORIONIC GONADOTROPINS, HUMAN (serum) (hCG)

Normal range, serum
- Female, premenopausal: <0.8 IU/L; postmenopausal <3.3 IU/L
- Male: <0.7 IU/L

Elevated in

Pregnancy, choriocarcinoma, gestational trophoblastic neoplasia (including molar gestations), placental site trophoblastic tumors; human antimouse antibodies (HAMA) can produce false serum assay for hCG.

The principal use of this test is to diagnose pregnancy. The concentration of hCG increases significantly during the initial 6 wk of pregnancy.

Normal range: Varies with gestational stage:
1 wk: 5-50 mU/ml
1-2 wk: 50-550 mU/ml
2-3 wk: Up to 5000 mU/ml
3-4 wk: Up to 10,000 mU/ml
4-5 wk: Up to 50,000 mU/ml
2-3 mo: 10,000-100,000 mU/ml

Peak values approaching 100,000 IU/L occur 60-70 days following implantation.

hCG levels generally double every 1-3 days. In patients with concentration <2000 IU/L, an increase of serum hCG <66% after 2 days is suggestive of spontaneous abortion or ruptured ectopic gestation.

CHYMOTRYPSIN

Normal: <10 mcg/L
Elevated in: Acute pancreatitis, chronic renal failure, oral enzyme preparations, gastric cancer, pancreatic cancer
Decreased in: Chronic pancreatitis, late cystic fibrosis

CIRCULATING ANTICOAGULANT (lupus anticoagulant)

Normal: Negative

TABLE 30 Cerebrospinal Fluid Findings in Infectious and Inflammatory Diseases of the Central Nervous System

Condition	Pressure (mm H_2O)	Leukocytes/µL	Protein (mg/dl)	Sugar (mg/dl)	Specific Findings
Acute bacterial meningitis	Usually elevated; average 300	Several hundred to >10,000; usually a few thousand; occasionally <100 (especially meningococcal or early in disease); PMLs predominate	Usually 100-500, occasionally >1000	<40 in more than half the cases	Organism usually seen on smear or recovered on culture in >90% of cases
Subdural empyema	Usually elevated; average 300	<100 to a few thousand; PMLs predominate	Usually 100-500	Normal	No organisms on smear or by culture unless concurrent meningitis
Brain abscess	Usually elevated	Usually 10-200; fluid rarely is acellular; lymphocytes predominate	Usually 75-400	Normal	No organisms on smear or by culture
Ventricular empyema (rupture of brain abscess)	Elevated	Several thousand to 100,000; usually >90% PMLs	Usually several hundred	Usually <40	Organisms may be seen on smear or cultured
Cerebral epidural abscess	Slight to modest elevation	Few to several hundred or more cells; lymphocytes predominate	Usually 50-200	Normal	No organisms on smear or by culture
Spinal epidural abscess	Usually reduced with spinal block	Usually 10-100; lymphocytes predominate	Usually several hundred	Normal	No organisms on smear or by culture
Thrombophlebitis (often associated with subdural empyema)	Often elevated	Few to several hundred; PMLs and lymphocytes	Slightly to moderately elevated	Normal	No organisms on smear or by culture
Bacterial endocarditis (with embolism)	Normal or slightly elevated	Few to <100; lymphocytes and PMLs	Slightly elevated	Normal	No organisms on smear or by culture
Acute hemorrhagic encephalitis	Usually elevated	Few to >1000; PMLs predominate	Moderately elevated	Normal	No organisms on smear or by culture
Tuberculous infection	Usually elevated	Usually 25-100, rarely >500; lymphocytes predominate except in early stages when PMLs may account for 80% of cells	Nearly always elevated; usually 100-200; may be much higher if block in CSF flow	Usually reduced; <50 in 75% of cases	Acid-fast organisms may be seen on smear of protein coagulum (pellicle) or recovered from inoculated guinea pig or by culture
Cryptococcal infection	Usually elevated	Average 50 (0-800); lymphocytes predominate	Average 100; usually 20-500	Reduced in more than half of cases; often higher in patients with concomitant diabetes mellitus	Organisms may be seen in India ink preparation and on culture (Sabouraud medium); usually grow on blood agar; may produce alcohol in CSF from fermentation of glucose
Syphilis (acute)	Usually elevated	Average 500; usually lymphocytes; rarely PMLs	Average, 100; γ-globulin often high, with abnormal colloidal gold curve	Normal (rarely reduced)	Positive reagin test result for syphilis; spirochete not demonstrable by usual techniques of smear or by culture
Sarcoidosis	Normal to considerably elevated	0 to <100 mononuclear cells	Slight to moderate elevation	Normal	No specific findings

CSF, Cerebrospinal fluid; *PMLs*, polymorphonuclear leukocytes.
From Cherry JD: *Feigin and Cherry's pediatric infectious diseases*, ed 8, Philadelphia, 2019, Elsevier.

TABLE 31 Xanthochromia and Associated Diseases/Disorders

CSF Supernatant Color	Associated Diseases/Disorders
Pink	RBC lysis/hemoglobin breakdown products
Yellow	RBC lysis/hemoglobin breakdown products Hyperbilirubinemia CSF protein >150 mg/dl (1.5 g/L)
Orange	RBC lysis/hemoglobin breakdown products Hypervitaminosis A (carotenoids)
Yellow-green	Hyperbilirubinemia (biliverdin)
Brown	Meningeal metastatic melanoma

CSF, Cerebrospinal fluid; *RBC*, red blood cell.
From McPherson RA, Pincus MR: *Henry's clinical diagnosis and management by laboratory methods*, ed 23, St Louis, 2017, Elsevier.

Detected in: Systemic lupus erythematosus, drug-induced lupus, long-term phenothiazine therapy, multiple myeloma, ulcerative colitis, rheumatoid arthritis, postpartum, hemophilia, neoplasms, chronic inflammatory states, AIDS, nephrotic syndrome

NOTE: The name is a misnomer because these patients are prone to hypercoagulability and thrombosis.

CK

See "CREATINE KINASE"

CLONIDINE SUPPRESSION TEST

Interpretation of results: Clonidine inhibits neurogenic catecholamine release and will cause a decrease in plasma norepinephrine into the reference interval in hypertensive subjects without pheochromocytoma. Test is performed by giving 4.3 mcg clonidine/kg orally after overnight fast. Norepinephrine is measured at 3 hr. Result should be within established

Laboratory Tests

IV

reference range and decrease to <50% of baseline concentration. Lack of decrease in norepinephrine is suggestive of pheochromocytoma.

CLOSTRIDIUM DIFFICILE TOXIN ASSAY (stool)

Normal: Negative

Detected in: Antibiotic-associated diarrhea and pseudomembranous colitis

CO

See "CARBOXYHEMOGLOBIN"

COAGULATION FACTORS

A differential diagnosis of abnormal coagulation screening tests is described in Table 34.

See Table 35 for characteristics of coagulation factors.

See Table 36 for differential diagnosis of low factor VIII.

Factor reference ranges

V: >10%

VII: >10%

VIII: 50%-170%

IX: 60%-136%

X: >10%

XI: 50%-150%

XII: >30%

Table 37 describes screening laboratory results in coagulation factor deficiencies. Characterization of coagulation factors and their deficiencies is summarized in Table 38.

COBALAMIN, SERUM

See VITAMIN B_{12}

COLD AGGLUTININS TITER

Normal range: <1:32

Elevated in

Primary atypical pneumonia (*Mycoplasma* pneumonia), infectious mononucleosis, CMV infection

Others: Hepatic cirrhosis, acquired hemolytic anemia, frostbite, multiple myeloma, lymphoma, malaria

COMPLEMENT

Inherited deficiencies in complement and complement-related proteins are summarized in Table 39.

Normal range

1. C3: 70-160 mg/dl (0.7-1.6 g/L [CF: 0.01; SMI: 0.1 g/L])
2. C4: 20-40 mg/dl (0.2-0.4 g/L [CF: 0.01; SMI: 0.1 g/L])

TABLE 32 Specimens for Detection of *Chlamydia trachomatis**

Disease	Specimen
Mucopurulent cervicitis	Endocervical swab, urine
Acute urethral syndrome (women)	Urethral swab, urine
Acute endometritis	Endometrial aspirate
Acute salpingitis	Fallopian tube biopsy
Nongonococcal urethritis (men)	Urethral swab, urine
Inclusion conjunctivitis	Conjunctival scrapings/swab
Trachoma	Conjunctival scrapings/swab
Lymphogranuloma venereum	Lymph node aspirate, biopsy of ulcerated lesion, serum
Pneumonitis (infants)	Serum, tracheobronchial aspirate, nasopharyngeal swab

*Urine is acceptable for some enzyme-linked immunoassays and for the commercial nucleic acid amplification tests.

From McPherson RA, Pincus MR: *Henry's clinical diagnosis and management by laboratory methods*, ed 23, St Louis, 2017, Elsevier.

TABLE 34 Differential Diagnosis of Abnormal Coagulation Screening Tests

Abnormal Activated Partial Thromboplastin Time (APTT) Alone

Associated with bleeding: VIII, IX, and XI defects

Not associated with bleeding: XII, prekallikrein (PK), high molecular weight kininogen, lupus anticoagulants

Abnormal Prothrombin Time (PT) Alone

Factor VII defects

Combined Abnormal APTT and PT

Medical conditions: Anticoagulants, disseminated intravascular coagulation (DIC), liver disease, vitamin K deficiency, massive transfusion

Rarely dysfibrinogenemia; factor X, V, and II defects

From McPherson RA, Pincus MR: *Henry's clinical diagnosis and management by laboratory methods*, ed 23, St Louis, 2017, Elsevier.

TABLE 33 Classic Hyperlipidemia Phenotypes

WHO ICD and OMIM Numbers	Type	Particle	Triglycerides	Cholesterol	Comments
E78.3 238600	1 (familial chylomicronemia or LPL deficiency)	CM	High	Normal	Low cardiac risk; hereditary, found mostly in pediatric patients and young adults; autosomal recessive mutation in *LPL* or *APOC2; APOA5, LMF-1,* and *GPIHBP1* mutations are linked to this phenotype
E78.0 143890	2A (heterozygous and homozygous familial hypercholesterolemia)	LDL	Normal	High	High cardiac risk; mostly polygenic disease; about 10% are monogenic; heterozygous form is due to mutations in *LDLR, APOB,* or *PCSK9*; homozygous form is due to mutations in *LDLR* or *LDLRAP1* (ARH)
E78.4 144250	2B (combined hyperlipoproteinemia)	VLDL, LDL	High	High	High cardiac risk; polygenic disease; links to mutations in *USF1, APOB,* and *LPL*
E78.2 107741	3 (dysbetalipoproteinemia)	IDL	High	High	High cardiac risk; mutations in *APOE* gene or homozygous for E2 allele of *APOE*
E78.1 144600, 145750	4 (primary hypertriglyceridemia)	VLDL	High	Normal	Lower cardiac risk than type 2 or 3; polygenic disease
E78.3 144650	5 (mixed hyperlipidemia)	VLDL, CM	High	High	Low cardiac risk; polygenic disease; 10% of patients have mutations in *LPL, APOC2,* and *APOA5*; mutations in *APOE, TRIB1, CHREBP, GALNT2, GCKR,* and *ANGPTL3* are thought to contribute to this disease

ANGPTL3, Angiopoietin-like 3; *APOA5,* apolipoprotein A-V; *APOB,* apolipoprotein B; *APOC2,* apolipoprotein C-II; *APOE,* apolipoprotein E; *CHREBP,* carbohydrate response element binding protein (or *MLXIPL*); *CM,* chylomicron; *GALNT2,* UDP-N′-acetyl-alpha-D-galactosamine-polypeptide *N*-acetylgalactosaminyltransferase 2; *GCKR,* glucokinase regulator; *ICD,* International Classification of Diseases; *IDL,* intermediate-density lipoprotein; *LDL,* low-density lipoprotein; *LDLRAP1,* LDLR adaptor protein 1 (also known as ARH); *LPL,* lipoprotein lipase; *OMIM,* Online Mendelian Inheritance in Man; *TRIB1,* tribbles homologue 1; *USF1,* upstream transcription factor 1; *VLDL,* very-low-density lipoprotein; *WHO,* World Health Organization.

From McPherson RA, Pincus MR: *Henry's clinical diagnosis and management by laboratory methods*, ed 23, St Louis, 2017, Elsevier.

TABLE 35 Characteristics of Coagulation Factors

Factor	Descriptive Name	Source	Approximate Half-Life (hr)	Function
I	Fibrinogen	Liver	120	Substrate for fibrin clot (CP)
II	Prothrombin	Liver (VKD)	60	Serine protease (CP)
V	Proaccelerin, labile factor	Liver	12-36	Cofactor (CP)
VII	Serum prothrombin conversion accelerator, proconvertin	Liver (VKD)	6	(?) Serine protease (EP)
VIII	Antihemophilic factor or globulin	Endothelial cells and (?) elsewhere	12	Cofactor (IP)
IX	Plasma thromboplastin component, Christmas factor	Liver (VKD)	24	Serine protease (IP)
X	Stuart-Prower factor	Liver (VKD)	36	Serine protease (CP)
XI	Plasma thromboplastin antecedent	(?) Liver	40-84	Serine protease (IP)
XII	Hageman factor	(?) Liver	50	Serine protease contact activation (IP)
XIII	Fibrin-stabilizing factor	(?) Liver	96-180	Transglutaminase (CP)
Prekallikrein	Fletcher factor	(?) Liver	?	Serine protease contact activation (IP)
High-molecular-weight kininogen	Fitzgerald factor, Flaujeac or Williams factor	(?) Liver	?	Cofactor, contact activation (IP)

CP, Common pathway; *EP,* extrinsic pathway; *IP,* intrinsic pathway; *VKD,* vitamin K dependent.

TABLE 36 Differential Diagnosis of a Low Factor VIII Level

6. FVIII <10%
   1. Severe or moderately severe hemophilia A
   2. Severe type 1 vWD
   3. Type 3 vWD
   4. Type 2N vWD
   5. Acquired hemophilia A
   6. Acquired vWD
7. FVIII: 10%-50%
   - Mild hemophilia A
   - Type 1 vWD
   - Type 2N vWD
   - Combined FVIII and FV deficiency

FV, Factor V; *FVIII,* factor VIII; *vWD,* von Willebrand disease.
From Hoffman R: *Hematology: basic principles and practice,* ed 6, Philadelphia, 2013, Saunders.

TABLE 37 Screening Laboratory Results in Coagulation Factor Deficiencies

Deficient Factor	Frequency	PT	PTT	TT
I (fibrinogen)	Rare	↑	↑	↑
II (prothrombin)	Very rare	↑	↑	↑
V 1:1,000,000	↑	↑	NL	
VII	1:500,000	↑	NL	NL
VIII	1:5000 (male)	NL	↑	NL
IX	1:30,000 (male)	NL	↑	NL
X 1:500,000	↑	↑	NL	
XI	Rare*	NL	↑	NL
XII or HMWK or PK†	Rare	NL	↑	NL
XIII	Rare	NL	NL	↑

↑, Increased over normal range; *HMWK,* high-molecular-weight kininogen; *NL,* normal; *PK,* prekallikrein; *PT,* prothrombin time; *PTT,* partial thromboplastin time; *TT,* thrombin time.
*Except in those of Ashkenazi Jewish descent (approximately 4% are heterozygous for factor XI deficiency).
†Not associated with clinical bleeding.

Abnormal values
Decreased C3: Active SLE, immune complex disease, acute glomerulonephritis, inborn C3 deficiency, membranoproliferative glomerulonephritis, infective endocarditis, serum sickness, autoimmune/chronic active hepatitis
Decreased C4: Immune complex disease, active SLE, infective endocarditis, inborn C4 deficiency, hereditary angioedema, hypergammaglobulinemic states, cryoglobulinemic vasculitis.
NOTE: The complement system has daunting nomenclature; accordingly, some basic definitions are given in Box 13.

COMPLETE BLOOD COUNT (CBC)

Common types of anemias and their diagnostic workups are summarized in Table 40.
See Fig. 17, which describes an algorithm for the evaluation of patients with neutropenia.
White blood cells 3200 to 9800/mm^3 (3.2 to 9.8 × 10^9/L [CF: 0.001; SMI: 0.1 × 10^9/L])
Red blood cells
  Male: 4.3 to 5.9 × 10^6/mm^3 (4.3 to 5.9 × 10^{12}/L [CF: 0.001; SMI: 0.1 × 10^{12}/L])
  Female: 3.5 to 5 × 10^6/mm^3 (3.5 to 5 × 10^{12}/L [CF: 0.001; SMI: 0.1 × 10^{12}/L])
Hemoglobin
  Male: 13.6-17.7 g/dl (136-172 g/L [CF: 10; SMI: 1 g/L])
  Female: 12-15 g/dl (120-150 g/L [CF: 10; SMI: 1 g/L])
Hematocrit
  Male: 39%-49% (0.39-0.49 [CF: 0.01; SMI: 0.01])
  Female: 33%-43% (0.33-0.43 [CF: 0.01; SMI: 0.01])
Mean corpuscular volume (MCV): 76-100 μm^3 (76-100 fL [CF: 1; SMI: 1 fL])
Mean corpuscular hemoglobin (MCH): 27-33 pg (27-33 pg [CF: 1; SMI: 1 pg])
Mean corpuscular hemoglobin concentration (MCHC): 33-37 g/dl (330-370 g/L [CF: 10; SMI: 10 g/L])
Red blood cell distribution width index (RDW): 11.5%-14.5%
Platelet count: 130 to 400 × 10^3/mm^3 (130-400 × 10^9/L [CF: 1; SMI: 5 × 10^9/L])
Differential:
  2-6 stabs (bands, early mature neutrophils)
  60-70 segs (mature neutrophils)
  1-4 eosinophils
  0-1 basophils
  2-8 monocytes
  25-40 lymphocytes

CONJUGATED BILIRUBIN

See "BILIRUBIN, DIRECT"

TABLE 38 Characterization of Coagulation Factors and Their Deficiencies

Factor	Molecular Weight, kDa	Gene Location	Normal Circulating Half-Life	Incidence	Inheritance	Bleeding Severity
Fibrinogen	330	4q31.3-q32.1	2-4 days	1:1 million	Recessive	Mild-severe*
II	72	11p11.2	3-4 days	Very rare	Recessive	Mild-moderate
V	330	1q24.2	36 hours	1:1 million	Recessive	Moderate
V and VIII combined	—	LMAN1:18q21.32 MCFD2:2p21	36 hours for FV; 10-14 hours for FVIII	1:2 million	Recessive	Mild-moderate
VII	50	13q34	3-6 hours	1:500,000	Recessive	Mild-severe
VIII	330	Xq28	10-14 hours	1:10,000	Sex-linked	Mild-severe
IX	56	Xq27	18-24 hours	1:30,000	Sex-linked	Mild-severe
X	58	13q34	40-60 hours	1:500,000	Recessive	Mild-severe
XI	160	4q35.2	40-70 hours	Rare†	Recessive	Mild-moderate
XII	80	5q33-qter	50-70 days	Rare	Recessive	No bleeding
PK	88	4q33-q35	Not known	Very rare	Recessive	No bleeding
HK	120	3q27	9-10 hours	Extremely rare	Recessive	No bleeding
XIII	320	A:6p25.1 B:1q31.3	11-14 days	<1:1 million	Recessive	Moderate-severe

HK, High molecular weight kininogen; *PK,* prekallikrein.
*May be associated with thrombosis.
†Rare except in those of Ashkenazi Jewish descent.
From McPherson RA, Pincus MR: *Henry's clinical diagnosis and management by laboratory methods*, ed 23, St Louis, 2017, Elsevier.

TABLE 39 Inherited Deficiencies in Complement and Complement-Related Proteins

Protein	Pattern of Inheritance	Major Clinical Correlate(s)*
Common to All Pathways		
C3	Autosomal recessive	Recurrent pyogenic infections, glomerulonephritis
Classical Pathway		
C1q	Autosomal recessive	Glomerulonephritis, SLE
C1r	Autosomal recessive	Glomerulonephritis, SLE
C1s	Autosomal recessive	Glomerulonephritis, SLE
C4†	Autosomal recessive	SLE, scleroderma, IgA nephropathy, membranous glomerulonephritis
C2†	Autosomal recessive	SLE, DLE, juvenile rheumatoid arthritis, glomerulonephritis
Alternative Pathway		
Factor B	Autosomal recessive	*Neisseria meningitidis* infection
Factor D	Autosomal recessive	Recurrent pyogenic infections
Properdin	X-linked	Recurrent pyogenic infections, fulminant meningococcemia
MBLectin Pathway		
MBL	Autosomal dominant	Recurrent infections
Membrane Attack Complex		
C5	Autosomal recessive	Recurrent disseminated neisserial infections, SLE
C6	Autosomal recessive	Recurrent disseminated neisserial infections
C7	Autosomal recessive	Recurrent disseminated neisserial infections, Raynaud's disease
C8 (β or α-γ chains)	Autosomal recessive	Recurrent disseminated neisserial infections
C9	Autosomal recessive	None
Fluid-Phase Control Proteins		
C1-Inh	Autosomal dominant or acquired	Hereditary angioedema, autoimmune diseases‡
C4bp	Autosomal recessive	Angioedema, Behçet-like syndrome
Factor I	Autosomal recessive	Recurrent pyogenic infections
Factor H	Autosomal recessive	Recurrent pyogenic infections, glomerulonephritis, age-related macular degeneration
Cell-Bound Proteins		
CR1	Autosomal recessive§	Association between low erythrocyte expression and SLE
CR3	Autosomal recessive	Leukocyte adhesion deficiency-1 (LAD-1), recurrent pyogenic infections, leukocytosis
DAF/CD59/HRF	Acquired	Paroxysmal nocturnal hemoglobinuria

dAF, Decay-accelerating factor; *DLE,* disseminated lupus erythematosus; *MBL,* mannan-binding lectin; *SLE,* systemic lupus erythematosus.
*Note that some people with complement deficiencies, especially C2 and components of the membrane attack complex, are clinically well. A substantial number of patients with defects in C5 to C9 have had autoimmune disease. Deficiencies of C1 to C9 are associated with a CH50 of 0. Deficiencies of C1, C4, and C2 are associated with SLE, and patients often have negative LE preps. Deficiencies of C3 to C9 are associated with absent or low bactericidal activity in serum. Deficiency of C3 or C5 is associated with absent or diminished chemotactic activity of serum and may be associated with absent leukocyte response to infection.
†Deficiency in C4 genes (*C4A* and *C4B*) is referred to as "q0," for quantity zero. Such deficiency is designated C4Aq0 or C4Bq0. Patients with such deficiencies have a higher than normal incidence of autoimmune disease. Heterozygous C2-deficient individuals also have an increased incidence of autoimmune disease.
‡Approximately 85% of cases involve silent alleles, and 15% involve alleles encoding for acquired dysfunctional variant C1 inhibitor protein. In hereditary angioedema, the C1 level is normal or depressed, the C3 level is always normal, and the C4 level is depressed. In the acquired disease, C1 and C4 levels are depressed, the antigenic C1 inhibitor level usually is normal or high, and the functional C1 inhibitor level is very low.
§Homozygosity for low (not absent) numeric expression of CR1 on erythrocytes is detectable in vitro and may be associated with SLE. An acquired defect in the number of CR1 may also be operative. Low, but not absent, levels of leukocyte CR3 are detectable in both parents of most CR3-deficient children.
From McPherson RA, Pincus MR: *Henry's clinical diagnosis and management by laboratory methods*, ed 23, St Louis, 2017, Elsevier.

BOX 13 Definitions

Classical pathway: C1, C4, C2, C3, and the terminal components.
Alternative pathway: Factor B, factor D, properdin, and the terminal components.
Lectin activation pathway: MBL, MASP1, MASP2, C3, and the terminal components.
Anaphylatoxins: C3a, C4a, C5a. These are mediators of smooth muscle contraction, degranulation of mast cells, enhanced neutrophil aggregation, increased vascular permeability.
Opsonization: Renders a particle more easily phagocytosed
C3 tickover: This term occasionally is used to describe spontaneous C3 hydrolysis.
Membrane attack complex (terminal components): C5, C6, C7, C8, C9
CH50: Used to define the dilution of serum capable of lysing 50% of sensitized sheep red cells. This assay measures the intactness of the classical pathway through the terminal components.
AH50: Used to define the dilution of serum capable of lysing 50% of nonsensitized rabbit red cells. This assay measures the intactness of the alternative pathway through the terminal components.

From Adkinson NF et al: *Middleton's allergy principles and practice*, ed 8, Philadelphia, 2014, Saunders.

TABLE 40 Common Types of Anemias and Their Diagnostic Workups*

Anemia	Cause	Common Analyte Abnormality
1. Hypoproliferative, microcytic	Iron deficiency	Low ferritin Increased IBC Decreased serum iron Reduced Fe/TIBC ratio Generally increased RDW
2. Hypoproliferative, microcytic	Anemia of chronic disease	Generally high ferritin Normal IBC Decreased serum iron Normal Fe/TIBC ratio Generally normal RDW
3. Hyperproliferative, normocytic	Hemolytic anemia	Schistocytosis Increased reticulocytes Low haptoglobin Elevated carboxyhemoglobin Elevated LD and potassium Elevated indirect bilirubin Generally increased RDW
4. Hypoproliferative, normocytic	Aplastic anemia	Leukopenia Thrombocytopenia Hypocellular bone marrow Generally normal RDW
5. Hypoproliferative, normocytic	Renal failure	Elevated BUN and creatinine Low erythropoietin Burr cells may be present Generally normal RDW
6. Hypoproliferative, macrocytic		
A. Megaloblastic	Vitamin B_{12} and/or folate deficiency	Low vitamin B_{12} and/or folate Hyperlobulated polymorphonuclear leukocytes Macro-ovalocytes Increased RDW
B. Nonmegaloblastic	Hypothyroidism	• Elevated TSH • Normal RDW

IBC, Iron-binding capacity; *TIBC,* total IBC; *RDW,* red cell distribution width; *Fe,* iron; *LD,* lactate dehydrogenase; *BUN,* blood urea nitrogen; *TSH,* thyroid-stimulating hormone.
*Low is equivalent to depressed, and high is equivalent to elevated. Ferritin, haptoglobin, LD, bilirubin, BUN, creatinine, erythropoietin, TSH, and T4 are all expressed as concentrations. All of these analytes are measured in serum.
From McPherson RA, Pincus MR: *Henry's clinical diagnosis and management by laboratory methods,* ed 23, St Louis, 2017, Elsevier.

COPPER (serum)

Normal range: 70-140 μg/dl (11-22 μmol/L [CF: 0.1574, SMI: 0.2 μmol/L])
Decreased in: Wilson disease, Menkes syndrome, malabsorption, malnutrition, nephrosis, total parenteral nutrition, acute leukemia in remission
Elevated in: Aplastic anemia, biliary cirrhosis, systemic lupus erythematosus, hemochromatosis, hyperthyroidism, hypothyroidism, infection, iron deficiency anemia, leukemia, lymphoma, oral contraceptives, pernicious anemia, rheumatoid arthritis

COPPER, URINE

See "URINE COPPER"

CORTICOTROPIN RELEASING HORMONE (CRH) STIMULATION TEST

Normal: A dose of 0.5 mg of dexamethasone is given every 6 hours for 2 days; 2 hours after last dose 1 mcg/kg CRH is given IV. Samples are drawn after 15 min. Normally there is a twofold to fourfold increase in mean baseline concentration of ACTH or cortisol. Cortisol >1.4 mcg/L is virtually 100% specific and 100% diagnostic.
Interpretation of results
Normal or exaggerated response: Pituitary Cushing disease
No response: Ectopic ACTH-secreting tumor
A positive response to CRH or a suppressed response to high-dose dexamethasone has a 97% positive predictive value for Cushing disease. However, a lack of response to either test excludes Cushing disease in only 64%-78% of patients. When the tests are considered together, negative responses from both have a 100% predictive value for ectopic ACTH secretion.

CORTISOL, PLASMA

Normal range
Varies with time of collection (circadian variation):
1. 8 A.M: 4-19 μg/dl (110-520 nmol/L [CF: 27.59; SMI: 10 nmol/L])
2. 4 P.M: 2-15 μg/dl (50-410 nmol/L [CF: 27.59; SMI: 10 nmol/L])

Elevated in: Ectopic adrenocorticotropic hormone production (i.e., oat cell carcinoma of lung), loss of normal diurnal variation, pregnancy, chronic renal failure, iatrogenic, stress, adrenal or pituitary hyperplasia, or adenomas
Decreased in: Primary adrenocortical insufficiency, anterior pituitary hypofunction, secondary adrenocortical insufficiency, adrenogenital syndromes

COOMBS DIRECT

See "DIRECT ANTIGLOBULIN"

COOMBS INDIRECT

See "INDIRECT ANTIGLOBULIN"

COVID-19

Name: Coronavirus
Value: Not detected
Reference range: Not detected

A Not Detected (negative) test result for this test means that SARS-CoV-2 RNA was not present in the specimen above the limit of detection. A negative test does not rule out the possibility of COVID-19 and should not be used as the sole basis for treatment or patient management decisions. If COVID-19 is still suspected, based on exposure history together with other clinical findings, re-testing should be considered in consultation with public health authorities.

Laboratory test results should always be considered in the context of clinical observations and epidemiological data in making a final diagnosis and patient management decisions.

C-PEPTIDE

Elevated in: Insulinoma, sulfonylurea administration
Decreased in: Insulin-dependent diabetes mellitus, factitious insulin administration

CPK

See "CREATINE KINASE"

C-REACTIVE PROTEIN

Normal range: 6.8-820 μg/dl (68-8200 μg/L [CF: 10; SMI: 10 μg/L])

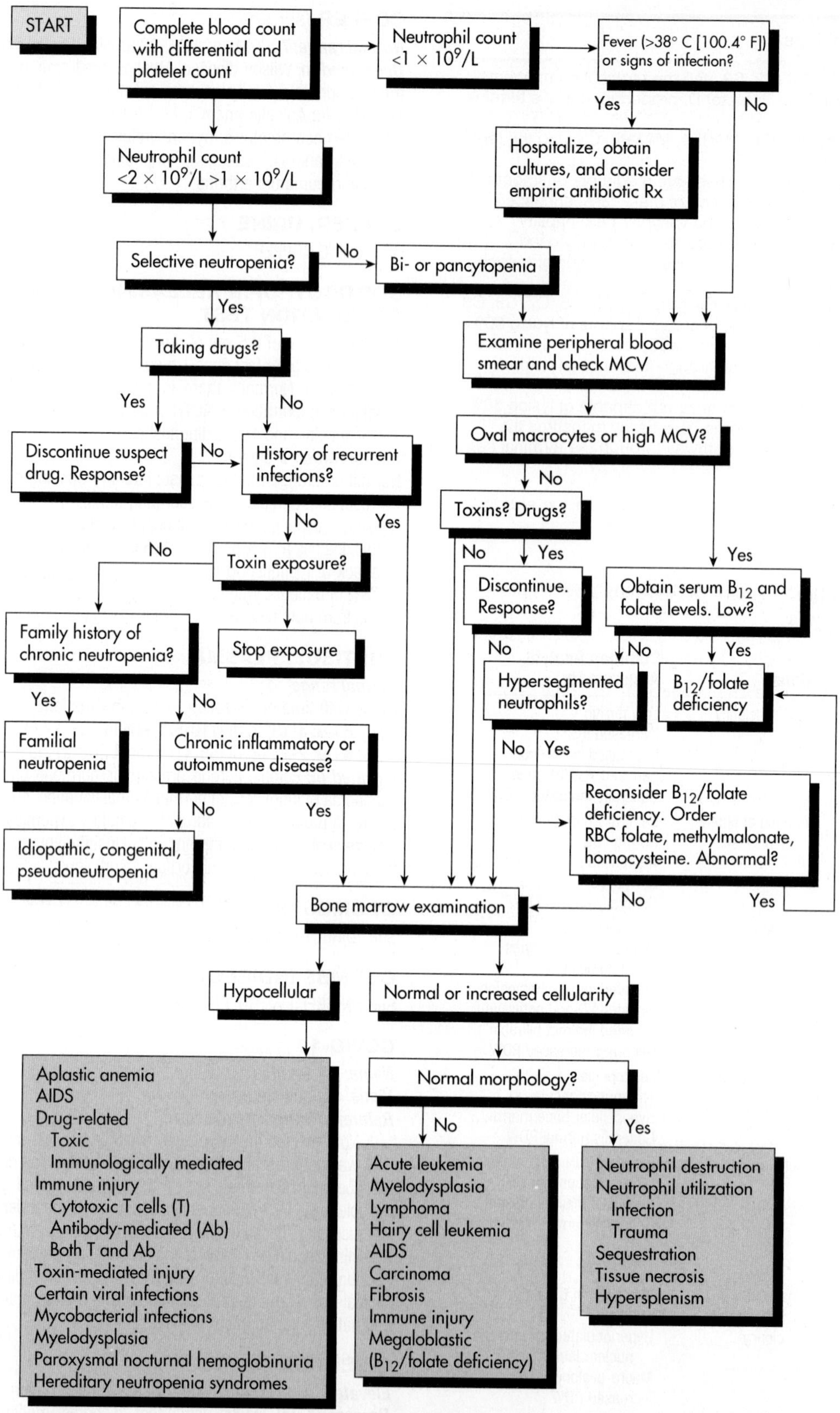

FIG. 17 A practical algorithm for the evaluation of patients with neutropenia. The fundamental diagnostic principle is that for patients with severe neutropenia or for those with bicytopenia or pancytopenia, bone marrow examination will likely be necessary unless the following diagnoses are made: (1) a nutritional (folate or vitamin B_{12}) deficiency or (2) drug- or toxin-induced neutropenia in a patient whose neutropenia resolves after discontinuation of the offending agent. *AIDS*, Acquired immunodeficiency syndrome; *MCV*, mean corpuscular volume; *RBC*, red blood cell. (From Goldman L, Ausiello D [eds]: *Cecil textbook of medicine*, ed 24, Philadelphia, 2012, Saunders.)

TABLE 41 Comparison of Erythrocyte Sedimentation Rate and C-Reactive Protein

	Erythrocyte Sedimentation Rate	C-Reactive Protein
Advantages	Much clinical information in the literature. May reflect overall health status	Rapid response to inflammatory stimuli. Wide range of clinically relevant values are detectable Unaffected by age and gender Reflects value of a single acute phase protein Can be measured on stored sera Quantitation is precise and reproducible
Disadvantages	Affected by age and gender Affected by red blood cell morphology Affected by anemia and polycythemia Reflects levels of many plasma proteins, not all of which are acute phase proteins Responds slowly to inflammatory stimuli Requires fresh sample May be affected by drugs	None

From Firestein GS et al: *Kelley's textbook of rheumatology*, ed 9, Philadelphia, 2013, Saunders.

TABLE 42 Conditions Associated with Elevated C-Reactive Protein Levels

Normal or Minor Elevation (<1 mg/dl)	Moderate Elevation (1-10 mg/dl)	Marked Elevation (>10 mg/dl)
Vigorous exercise Common cold Pregnancy Gingivitis Seizures Depression Insulin resistance and diabetes Several genetic polymorphisms Obesity	Myocardial infarction Malignancies Pancreatitis Mucosal infection (bronchitis, cystitis) Most connective tissue diseases Rheumatoid arthritis	Acute bacterial infection (80%-85%) Major trauma Systemic vasculitis

From Firestein GS et al: *Kelley's textbook of rheumatology*, ed 9, Philadelphia, 2013, Saunders.

Elevated in: Rheumatoid arthritis, rheumatic fever, inflammatory bowel disease, bacterial infections, myocardial infarction, oral contraceptives, third trimester of pregnancy (acute phase reactant), inflammatory and neoplastic diseases. Table 41 shows a comparison of erythrocyte sedimentation rate and C-reactive protein, and Table 42 shows conditions associated with elevated C-reactive protein levels.

C-REACTIVE PROTEIN, HIGH SENSITIVITY (hs-CRP, cardio-CRP)

This is a cardiac risk marker. It is increased in patients with silent atherosclerosis years before a cardiovascular event and is independent of cholesterol level and other lipoproteins. It can be used to help stratify cardiac risk.

Interpretation of Results

Cardio-CRP result (mg/L)	Risk
0.6	Lowest risk
0.7-1.1	Low risk
1.2-1.9	Moderate risk
2.0-3.8	High risk
3.9-4.9	Highest risk
≥5.0	Results may be confounded by acute inflammatory disease. If clinically indicated, a repeat test should be performed in 2 or more wk

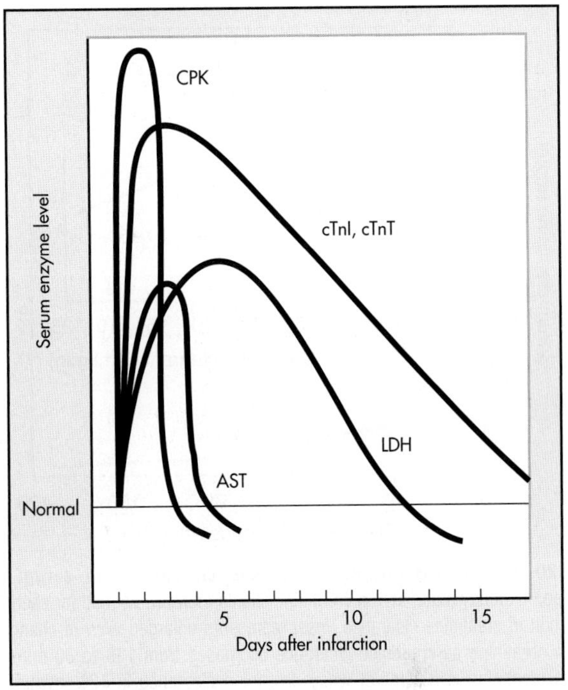

FIG. 19 Enzyme levels postmyocardial infarction. *AST,* Aspartate aminotransferase; *CPK,* creatine kinase; *cTnI,* cardiac troponin I; *cTnT,* cardiac troponin T; *LDH,* lactate dehydrogenase.

CREATINE KINASE (CK, CPK)

Fig. E18 describes a diagnostic approach to creatine kinase elevation.

Normal range: 0-130 U/L (0-2.16 μkat/L [CF: 0.01667; SMI: 0.01 μkat/L])

Elevated in: Myocardial infarction, myocarditis, rhabdomyolysis, myositis, crush injury/trauma, polymyositis, dermatomyositis, vigorous exercise, muscular dystrophy, myxedema, seizures, malignant hyperthermia syndrome, intramuscular (IM) injections, cerebrovascular accident, pulmonary embolism and infarction, acute dissection of aorta

Decreased in: Corticosteroid use, decreased muscle mass, connective tissue disorders, alcoholic liver disease, metastatic neoplasms

CREATINE KINASE ISOENZYMES

CK-BB

Elevated in: Cerebrovascular accident, subarachnoid hemorrhage, neoplasms (prostate, gastrointestinal tract, brain, ovary, breast, lung), severe shock, bowel infarction, hypothermia, meningitis

CK-MB

Elevated in: Myocardial infarction (MI), myocarditis, pericarditis, muscular dystrophy, cardiac defibrillation, cardiac surgery, extensive rhabdomyolysis, strenuous exercise (marathon runners), mixed connective tissue disease, cardiomyopathy, hypothermia

NOTE: CK-MB exists in the blood in two subforms. MB_2 is released from cardiac cells and converted in the blood to MB_1. Rapid assay of CK-MB subforms can detect MI ($CK\text{-}MB_2 \geq 1.0$ U/L, with a ratio of $CK\text{-}MB_2/CK\text{-}MB_1 \geq 1.5$) within 6 hours of onset of symptoms.

Fig. 19 illustrates the time course of CK, AST, troponins, and lactate dehydrogenase (LDH) activity after acute MI.

CK-MM

Elevated in: Crush injury, seizures, malignant hyperthermia syndrome, rhabdomyolysis, myositis, polymyositis, dermatomyositis, vigorous exercise, muscular dystrophy, IM injections, acute dissection of aorta

CREATININE (serum)

Normal range: 0.6-1.2 mg/dl (50-110 μmol/L [CF: 88.4; SMI: 10 μmol/L]). Fig. 20 illustrates the relationship between creatinine clearance and serum creatinine. Factors that may alter serum creatinine level are described in Box 14.

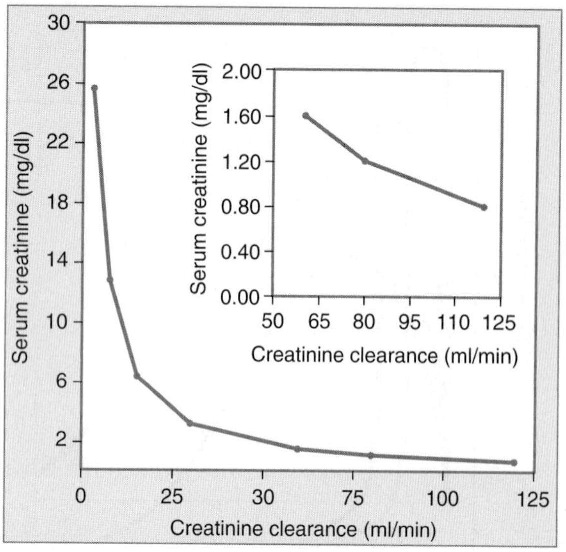

FIG. 20 Relationship between creatinine clearance and serum creatinine. In steady state, serum creatinine should increase twofold for each 50% reduction in creatinine clearance. *Inset* represents enlarged view of changes in serum creatinine as creatinine clearance decreases from 120 to 60 ml/min. If serum creatinine is 0.8 mg/dl when creatinine clearance is 120 ml/min, creatinine clearance can decrease by 33% such that increased serum creatinine is still within normal range. (From Vincent JL et al: *Textbook of critical care,* ed 6, Philadelphia, 2011, Saunders.)

BOX 14 Factors That May Alter Serum Creatinine (Cr) Level

Endogenous
Reduced muscle mass: ↓
Hyperbilirubinemia: ↓

Exogenous
Medications inhibiting tubular secretion (trimethoprim, cimetidine): ↑

Medications Interfering with Laboratory Assays*
Flucytosine and cefoxitin: ↑
Catecholamines: ↓

*Varies by assay type used.
From Parrillo JE, Dellinger RP: *Critical care medicine, principles of diagnosis and management in the adult*, ed 4, Philadelphia, 2014, Elsevier.

Elevated in: Renal insufficiency (acute and chronic), decreased renal perfusion (hypotension, dehydration, congestive heart failure), urinary tract infection, rhabdomyolysis, ketonemia

Drugs (antibiotics [aminoglycosides, cephalosporins], hydantoin, diuretics, methyldopa)

The RIFLE criteria for acute kidney injury is summarized in Table 43. A classification of acute kidney injury (AKI) is described in Table 44.

Falsely elevated in: Diabetic ketoacidosis, administration of some cephalosporins (e.g., cefoxitin, cephalothin)

Decreased in: Decreased muscle mass (including amputees and older persons), pregnancy, prolonged debilitation

CREATININE CLEARANCE

Normal range

3. 75-124 ml/min (1.24-2.08 ml/sec [CF: 0.01667; SMI: 0.02 ml/sec])
4. Table 45 shows equations commonly used to estimate renal clearance.
5. The Cockcroft-Gault formula to calculate creatinine clearance is described in Box 15.

TABLE 43 RIFLE Criteria for Acute Kidney Injury

	GFR and Serum Creatinine Changes	Urine Volume Changes
R (Risk)	Increase in SCreat >1.5×	Urine volume <0.5 ml/kg/hr >6 hr
	Decrease in GFR >25%	
I (Injury)	Increase in SCreat >2×	Urine volume <0.5 ml/kg/hr >12 hr
	Decrease in GFR >50%	
F (Failure)	Increase in SCreat >3×	Urine volume <0.3 ml/kg/hr >24 hr
	Decrease in GFR >75%	Anuria >12 hr
	SCreat >4 mg/dl	
L (Loss)	Complete loss of kidney function >4 wk	
E (ESRD)	End-stage kidney disease >3 mo	

GFR, Glomerular filtration rate; *SCreat,* serum creatinine.
From McPherson RA, Pincus MR: *Henry's clinical diagnosis and management by laboratory methods*, ed 23, St Louis, 2017, Elsevier.

TABLE 44 New Classification for Acute Kidney Injury (AKI) Criteria

Stage	Serum Creatinine Criteria	Urine Output Criteria
1	>0.3 mg/dl (26.4 μmol/L) or >150%-200%	<0.5 ml/kg for >6 hr
2	>200%-300%	<0.5 ml/kg for >12 hr
3	>300%, 4 mg/dl (354 μmol/L) or acute increase of >0.5 mg/dl	<0.3 ml/kg for >24 hr or anuria >12 hr

From McPherson RA, Pincus MR: *Henry's clinical diagnosis and management by laboratory methods*, ed 23, St Louis, 2017, Elsevier.

Elevated in

4. Pregnancy, exercise

Decreased in

5. Renal insufficiency, drugs (cimetidine, procainamide, antibiotics, quinidine)

CREATININE, URINE

See "URINE CREATININE"

CRYOGLOBULINS (serum)

Normal range: Not detectable
Present in: Collagen vascular diseases, chronic lymphocytic leukemia, hemolytic anemias, multiple myeloma, Waldenström macroglobulinemia, chronic active hepatitis, Hodgkin disease

CRYPTOSPORIDIUM ANTIGEN BY EIA (stool)

Normal range: Not detected
Present in: Cryptosporidiosis

CSF

See "CEREBROSPINAL FLUID"

CYSTATIN C

Normal: Cystatin C is a cysteine protease inhibitor that is produced at a constant rate by all nucleated cells. It is freely filtered by the glomerulus and reabsorbed (but not secreted) by the renal tubules with no extrarenal excretion. Its concentration is not affected by diet, muscle mass, or acute inflammation. Normal range when measured by particle-enhanced nephelometric immunoassay (PENIA) is <0.28 mg/L.

TABLE 45 Equations Commonly Used to Estimate Renal Clearance[1,2,3,4,5]

Equation	Measure	Equation	Considerations
Cockcroft-Gault	CrCl (ml/min)	(140 − age) BW/(SCr × 72) (0.85 if female)	• Inaccurate in patients with acutely changing renal function • Weight parameter is controversial in obese patients
Reexpressed MDRD (4 variable)	GFR (ml/min/1.73 m^2)	175 × $SCr^{-1.154}$ × $age^{-0.203}$ × (0.742 if female) × (1.21 if AA)	• Inaccurate in patients with acutely changing renal function • Must be individualized for BSA by multiplying estimated GFR × (estimated BSA/1.73 m^2) • Little information available in obese, elderly, or hepatic disease patients
Obesity 1 (Winter et al[2])	CrCl (ml/min)	(140 − age) BW/(S_{Cr} × 72) × (0.85 if female)Use various weights	• Underweight use actual weight • Normal weight use ideal weight • If BMI 26-50, use adjusted weight using 40% factor = [(actual − ideal weight) × 0.40] + ideal weight
Obesity 2 (Demirovic et al[5])	CrCl (ml/min)	(140 − age) LBW/(S_{Cr} × 72) × (0.85 if female)	6. For BMI >40 kg/m^2 7. LBW_{male} = (9270 × TBW)/(6680 + 216 × BMI) 8. LBW_{female} = (9270 × TBW)/(8780 + 244 × BMI)
Cystatin C	eGFR (ml/min)	135 × min(S_{Cr}/κ, 1)α × max(S_{Cr}/κ, $1)^{-0.601}$ × min(S_{cys}/0.8, $1)^{-0.375}$ × max(S_{cys}/0.8, $1)^{-0.711}$ × 0.995^{Age} × 0.969 [if female] × 1.08 [if AA] κ = −0.7 (if female), 0.9 (if male) α = −0.248 (if female), 0.207 (if male) min (S_{Cr}/κ or 1) = minimum of S_{Cr}/κ or 1max (S_{Cr}/κ or 1) = maximum of S_{Cr}/κ or 1min (S_{cys}/0.8, 1) = minimum of S_{cys}/0.8 or 1max (S_{cys}/0.8, 1) = maximum of S_{cys}/0.8 or 1	

AA, African American; *BMI*, body mass index; *BSA*, body surface area; *BW*, body weight in kg; *CrCl*, creatinine clearance; *eGFR*, estimated glomerular filtration rate; *LBW*, lean body weight; *GFR*, glomerular filtration rate; *MDRD*, Modification of Diet in Renal Disease equation; S_{Cr}, serum creatinine; S_{cys}, serum cystatin C; *TBW*, total body weight. Ideal weight = (height in inches − 60) × 2.3 + 50 kg for males or 45.5 kg for females.

[1]Cockcroft DW, Gault MH: Prediction of creatinine clearance from serum creatinine, *Nephron* 16:31-41, 1976.

[2]Winter MA, Guhr KN, Berg GM: Impact of various body weights and serum creatinine concentrations on the bias and accuracy of the Cockcroft-Gault equation, *Pharmacotherapy* 32:604-612, 2012.

[3]Inker LA, Schmid CH, Tighiourt H et al: Estimating glomerular filtration rate from serum creatinine and cystatin C, *N Engl J Med* 367:20-29, 2012.

[4]Levey AS, Coresh J, Greene T et al: Expressing the Modification of Diet in Renal Disease Study equation for estimating glomerular filtration rate with standardized serum creatinine values, *Clin Chem* 53:766-772, 2007.

[5]Demirovic JA, Pai AB, Pai MJ: Estimation of creatinine clearance in morbidly obese patients, *Am J Health Syst Pharm* 66:642-648, 2009.

From Parrillo JE, Dellinger RP: *Critical care medicine, principles of diagnosis and management in the adult,* ed 5, Philadelphia, 2019, Elsevier.

BOX 15 Cockcroft-Gault Formula to Calculate Creatinine Clearance (C_{cr})

$$C_{cr} = \frac{(140 - \text{age in year}) \times (\text{lean body weight in kg})}{S_{cr}\text{ in mg/dl} - 72}$$

Elevated in: Renal disorders. Good predictor of the severity of acute tubular necrosis. Cystatin C increases more rapidly than creatinine in the early stages of GFR impairment. The cystatin C concentration is an independent risk factor for heart failure in older adults and appears to provide a better measure of risk assessment than the serum creatinine concentration.

CYSTIC FIBROSIS PCR

Test description: Test can be performed on whole blood or tissue. Common mutations in the cystic fibrosis transmembrane regulator (CFTR) gene can be used to detect 75%-80% of mutant alleles.

CYTOMEGALOVIRUS BY PCR

Test description: Test can be performed on whole blood, plasma, or tissue. Qualitative PCR is highly sensitive but may not be able to differentiate between latent and active infection.

D-DIMER

Normal range: <0.5 mcg/ml

Elevated in

6. DVT, pulmonary embolism, high levels of rheumatoid factor, activation of coagulation and fibrolytic system from any cause
7. D-dimer assay by enzyme-linked immunosorbent assay (ELISA) assists in the diagnosis of DVT and pulmonary embolism. This test has significant limitations because it can be elevated whenever the coagulation and fibrinolytic systems are activated and can also be falsely elevated with high rheumatoid factor levels.
8. A positive D-dimer is suggestive but not diagnostic for pulmonary embolism (PE). Patients with positive D-dimer and clinical suspicion for PE need additional tests such as chest CT to confirm diagnosis.
9. PE might be ruled out in patients with negative D-dimer and low pretest probability for PE.

DEHYDROEPIANDROSTERONE SULFATE

Normal:

Males:

Ages 19-30:	125-619 mcg/dl
31-50:	59-452 mcg/dl
51-60:	20-413 mcg/dl
61-83:	10-285 mcg/dl

Females:

Ages 19-30:	29-781 mcg/dl
31-50:	12-379 mcg/dl
Postmenopausal:	30-260 mcg/dl

Elevated in: Hirsutism, congenital adrenal hyperplasia, adrenal carcinomas, adrenal adenomas, polycystic ovary syndrome, ectopic ACTH-producing tumors, Cushing disease, spironolactone

DEHYDROTESTOSTERONE (serum, urine)

Normal

Serum: Males: 30-85 ng/dl; females: 4-22 ng/dl

Urine, 24 h: Males: 20-50 mcg/day; females: <8 mcg/day

Elevated in: Hirsutism

Decreased in: 5-α-reductase deficiency, hypogonadism

TABLE 46 Applications for Direct and Indirect Antiglobulin Techniques

	Applications	Purpose	What Is Detected
Direct antiglobulin test (DAT)	Investigation of HTR	To detect circulating donor red cells that are sensitized with recipient antibody. A positive DAT is the first immunohematologic evidence of a hemolytic reaction after transfusion	DAT positive owing to IgG and/or C3d depending on the antibodies responsible
	Diagnosis of HDFN	To detect maternal antibodies that have crossed the placenta to sensitize fetal red cells	DAT almost always positive as a result of IgG; occasionally C3d if ABO antibodies involved
	Diagnosis of AIHA	To detect autoantibody sensitizing a patient's own red cells	Warm autoantibodies: DAT almost always positive owing to IgG Cold autoantibodies: DAT may be due to C3d only
	Investigation of drug-induced hemolysis	To detect antidrug/red cell antibodies and/or subsequent activation of the complement system	DAT may be positive owing to IgG, C3d, or both, depending on the mechanism involved
	Antibody detection (or antibody screen)	To detect clinically significant IgG alloantibodies in the recipient	Recipient IgG antibodies bound to reagent screening cells*
	Antibody identification	To specifically identify those antibodies detected by reagent screening cells or by donor red cells	Recipient IgG antibodies bound to reagent cells from a panel of 10-12 donors*
	Crossmatching	To detect antibodies that may have been missed by the antibody screen because of absence of the corresponding antigen or presence of a dosing antibody	Recipient IgG antibodies bound to donor red cells*
	Red cell antigen typing	To type patient or donor red cells for antigens that can be detected by IgG antisera reactive only by the AGT. A common example of this would be the weak D test	Specific binding of reagent IgG antibodies to red cells positive for the corresponding antigen

AGT, Antihuman globulin test; *AIHA*, autoimmune hemolytic anemia; *C3*, complement component 3; *HDFN*, hemolytic disease of the fetus and newborn; *HTR*, hemolytic transfusion reaction; *Ig*, immunoglobulin.
*If complement is fixed in vitro, it may be detected if polyspecific antiglobulin is used.
From McPherson RA, Pincus MR: *Henry's clinical diagnosis and management by laboratory methods*, ed 23, St Louis, 2017, Elsevier.

DEOXYCORTICOSTERONE (11-deoxycorticosterone, DOC) (serum)

Normal: 2-19 ng/dl. Normal secretion depends on ACTH and is suppressible by dexamethasone.
Elevated in: Adrenogenital syndromes due to 17- and 11-hydroxylase deficiencies, pregnancy
Decreased in: Preeclampsia

DEXAMETHASONE SUPPRESSION TEST, OVERNIGHT

Normal: Test is performed by giving 1 mg dexamethasone orally at 11 PM and measuring serum cortisol at 8 AM the following morning. Normal response is cortisol suppression to <3 mcg/dl; if dose of 4 mg dexamethasone is given, cortisol suppression will be to <50% of baseline.
Interpretation of results: Cushing syndrome (<10 mcg/dl), endogenous depression (half of patients suppress test values <5 mcg/dl). Most patients with pituitary Cushing disease demonstrate suppression, whereas patients with adrenal adenoma, carcinoma, and ectopic ACTH-producing tumors do not.

DIGOXIN

Normal therapeutic range: 0.5-2 ng/ml
Elevated in: Impaired renal function, excessive dosing, concomitant use of quinidine, amiodarone, verapamil, fluoxetine, nifedipine. Toxicity may occur at a lower blood concentration in the presence of hypokalemia, hypomagnesemia, and hypercalcemia. See Table 46.

DIGOXIN LEVEL

Therapeutic range and general information are summarized in Table 47.

DILANTIN

See "PHENYTOIN"

DIRECT ANTIGLOBULIN (Coombs Direct)

Normal: Negative
Positive: Autoimmune hemolytic anemia, erythroblastosis fetalis, transfusion reactions, drugs (α-methyldopa, penicillins, tetracycline, sulfonamides, levodopa, cephalosporins, quinidine, insulin)
False positive: May be seen with cold agglutinins

TABLE 47 Digoxin

Purpose	Treatment of Congestive Heart Failure and Atrial Fibrillation-Flutter
General adult dose	Oral: 0.75-1.5 mg for digitalization, 0.125-0.5 mg/day for maintenance
Usual bioavailability	Approximately 60%-85% for tablet or elixir; 90%-100% for liquid-filled capsules
Half-life	Approximately 35-40 hours; however, prolonged in patients with decreased renal function
General therapeutic range	0.5-2 ng/ml
General toxic level	>2 ng/ml, but somewhat variable
Transport	Approximately 20%-25% plasma protein bound
Metabolism	Generally, only small amounts are metabolized (liver, lumen of large intestine)
Elimination	Approximately 50%-75% unchanged in urine
Steady state	Approximately 7 days in undigitalized patients with normal renal function
Mechanism of action	Causes release of calcium ions in T-system of myocardium; slows AV node conduction
Toxic effects	Gastric disturbances, nausea, vomiting, atrial and ventricular arrhythmias, irregular pulse

AV, Atrioventricular.
From McPherson RA, Pincus MR: *Henry's clinical diagnosis and management by laboratory methods*, ed 23, St Louis, 2017, Elsevier.

DISACCHARIDE ABSORPTION TESTS

Normal: Test is used to diagnose malabsorption due to disaccharide deficiency. It is performed by giving disaccharide orally 1 g/kg body weight to a total of 25 g. Blood is drawn at 0, 30, 60, 90, and 120 min. Normal response is a change in glucose from fasting value >30 mg/dl, inconclusive when increase is 20-30 mg/dl, abnormal when increase is >20 mg/dl. Test can also be performed by measuring air at 0, 30, 60, 90, and 120 min. Normal is H_2>20 ppm above baseline level before a colonic response.

Decreased in: Disaccharide deficiency (lactose, fructose, sorbitol), celiac disease, sprue, acute gastroenteritis

DOC

See "DEOXYCORTICOSTERONE"

DONATH-LANDSTEINER (D-L) TEST FOR PAROXYSMAL COLD HEMOGLOBINURIA

Normal: No hemolysis
Interpretation of results: Hemolysis indicates presence of bithermic cold hemolysins or Donath-Landsteiner antibodies (D-L Ab)

DOPAMINE

Normal range: 175 pg/ml
Elevated in: Pheochromocytomas, neuroblastomas, stress, vigorous exercise, certain foods (bananas, chocolate, coffee, tea, vanilla)

D-XYLOSE ABSORPTION

Normal range: 21%-31% excreted in 5 hours
Decreased in: Malabsorption syndrome

D-XYLOSE ABSORPTION TEST

Normal range
a. URINE: ≥4 g/5 hours (5-hour urine collection in adults >12 yr [25-g dose])
b. SERUM: ≥25 mg/dl (adult, 1 hour, 25-g dose, normal renal function)
Normal results: In patients with malabsorption, normal results suggest pancreatic disease as an etiology of the malabsorption.
Abnormal results: Celiac disease, Crohn disease, tropical sprue, surgical bowel resection, AIDS. False positives can occur with decreased renal function, dehydration/hypovolemia, surgical blind loops, decreased gastric emptying, vomiting.

ELECTROPHORESIS, HEMOGLOBIN

See "Hemoglobin Electrophoresis"

ELECTROPHORESIS, PROTEIN

See Protein Electrophoresis

ENA COMPLEX

See "Extractable Nuclear Antigen"

ENDOMYSIAL ANTIBODIES

Normal: Not detected
Present in: Celiac disease, dermatitis herpetiformis

EOSINOPHIL COUNT

Normal range: 1%-4% eosinophils (0-440/mm^3)
Elevated in
HELMINTHIC PARASITE
Ascaris lumbricoides (invasive larval stage)
Hookworms (invasive larval stage)
Strongyloides stercoralis (initial infection and autoinfection)
Trichinosis
Filariasis
Echinococcus granulosus and *E. multilocularis*
Toxocara species
Animal hookworms
Angiostrongylus cantonensis and *A. costaricensis*
Schistosomiasis
Liver flukes
Fasciolopsis buski
Anisakiasis
Capillaria philippinensis
Paragonimus westermani
"Tropical eosinophilia" (unidentified microfilariae)
NOTE: Table 48 describes an approach to investigation of eosinophilia in returning travelers.

TABLE 48 Eosinophilia Investigation in Returning Travelers

History	Allergies Drugs and vitamins (L-tryptophan) Regions, localities, and duration of exposure
Physical examination	Skin, subcutaneous tissues Liver/spleen Signs of other systemic disease
Initial investigations	Full blood count and differential white blood cell count Stool examination for ova and parasites (×3) Urine analysis Examination of midday urine for ova and parasites (×3) (in those who have traveled to Africa or the Middle East)
Further investigations as suggested by travel and exposure from history	*Strongyloides* culture and serologic testing; duodenal aspirate (strongyloidiasis, hookworm) Serologic testing (schistosomiasis, filariasis); day/night blood films (filariasis)
Further studies if suggested by history and physical examination	Skin snips (onchocerciasis) Chest x-ray examination (hydatid cyst, tropical pulmonary eosinophilia, paragonimiasis) Soft tissue x-ray examination (cysticercosis); sputum examination for ova and parasites (paragonimiasis) Abdominal ultrasound examination (hydatid cyst) Cystoscopy with or without biopsy (schistosomiasis) Rectal snips (schistosomiasis)

From Hoffman R: *Hematology: basic principles and practice*, ed 6, Philadelphia, 2013, Saunders.

OTHER INFECTIONS/INFESTATIONS
d. Pulmonary aspergillosis
e. Severe scabies
ALLERGIES
Asthma
Hay fever
Drug reactions
Atopic dermatitis
AUTOIMMUNE AND RELATED DISORDERS
Polyarteritis nodosa
Necrotizing vasculitis
Eosinophilic fasciitis
Pemphigus
NEOPLASTIC DISEASES
Hodgkin disease
Mycosis fungoides
Chronic myelocytic leukemia
Eosinophilic leukemia
Polycythemia vera
Mucin-secreting adenocarcinomas
IMMUNODEFICIENCY STATES
Hyperimmunoglobulin E with recurrent infection
Wiskott-Aldrich syndrome
OTHER
Addison disease
Inflammatory bowel disease
Dermatitis herpetiformis
Toxic/chemical syndrome
Eosinophilic myalgia syndrome, tryptophan, toxic oil syndrome
Hypereosinophilic syndrome (unknown etiology)

Fig. 21 describes an algorithm for patients with eosinophil disorders.

Table 49 describes hematopoietic neoplasms accompanied by eosinophilia.

Table 50 describes the differential diagnosis of childhood eosinophilia.

EPINEPHRINE, PLASMA

Normal range: 0-90 pg/ml
Elevated in: Pheochromocytomas, neuroblastomas, stress, vigorous exercise, certain foods (bananas, chocolate, coffee, tea, vanilla), hypoglycemia (Box 16)

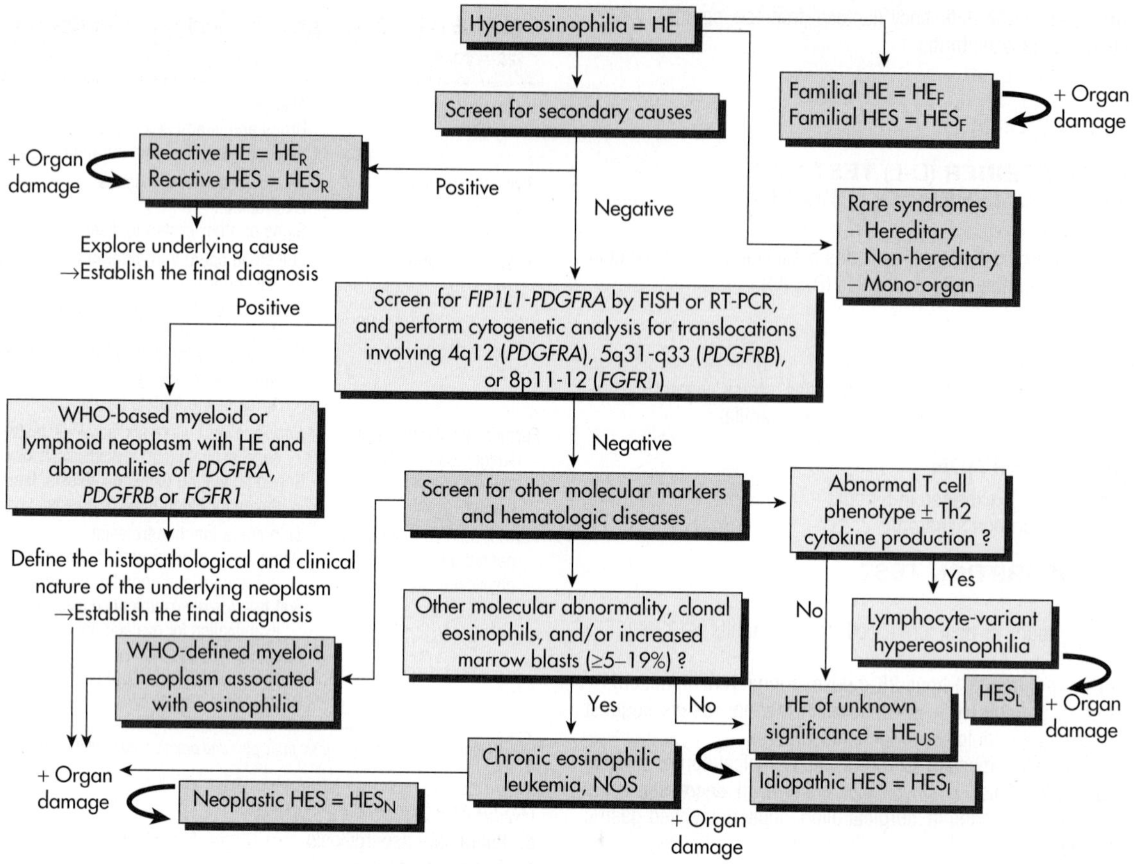

FIG. 21 Diagnostic algorithm for patients with eosinophil disorders. The first important step in the algorithm is to confirm the presence of hypereosinophilia *(HE)*, defined by a persistent (>4 weeks) increase in eosinophils above 1500/μL blood. The next important question is whether HE is reactive (HE_R) or neoplastic (clonal = HE_N) in nature. In patients with HE_N, WHO criteria should be applied in order to define the underlying molecular lesion. In addition, morphologic and histopathologic criteria are used to arrive at a final diagnosis regarding the underlying disease. In patients with HE_R, an underlying disease must also be defined. In both groups of patients, the next important question is whether (or not) HE-related organ damage is present. If such organopathy is found, it is appropriate to diagnose the (additional) presence of HES. According to the underlying etiology (disease), HES is classified again into HES_R and HES_N. In some patients with HES, a clonal T-cell population, but no lymphoproliferative disease, is detected. In these patients, the HES_L variant is diagnosed. If no clonal T cells and no underlying reactive or neoplastic condition is detected in a patient with HES, the (provisional) diagnosis of an HES_I is established. If no underlying disease and no HES are detected, the patient has HE_{US} by definition. Familial cases of HE or HES are very rare, and the same holds true for hereditary syndromes and mono-organ syndromes accompanied by HE. *FISH,* Fluorescence in situ hybridization; *HES,* hypereosinophilic syndrome; *NOS,* not otherwise specified; *RT-PCR,* reverse transcription polymerase chain reaction; *WHO,* World Health Organisation. (From Hoffman R: *Hematology: basic principles and practice*, ed 7, Philadelphia, 2018, Elsevier.)

EPSTEIN-BARR VIRUS SEROLOGY

Normal range: IgG anti-viral capsid antigen (VCA) <1:10 or negative>

Abnormal

IgG anti-VCA >1:10 or positive indicates either current or previous infection.

IgM anti-VCA >1:10 or positive indicates current or recent infection.

Anti-Epstein-Barr virus nuclear antigen (EBNA) ≥1.5 or positive indicates previous infection.

Table 51 and Fig. 22 describe test interpretation.

ERYTHROCYTE SEDIMENTATION RATE (ESR, sed rate, sedimentation rate)

See Table 52 for erythrocyte sedimentation rate ranges in health.

Normal range

Male: 0-15 mm/hr

Female: 0-20 mm/hr

Elevated in: Collagen vascular diseases, infections, myocardial infarction, neoplasms, inflammatory states (acute phase reactant), hyperthyroidism, hypothyroidism, rouleaux formation

Decreased in: Sickle cell disease, polycythemia, corticosteroids, spherocytosis, anisocytosis, hypofibrinogenemia, increased serum viscosity

ERYTHROPOIETIN (EP)

Normal: 3.7-16.0 IU/L by radioimmunoassay

Erythropoietin is a glycoprotein secreted by the kidneys that stimulates RBC production by acting on erythroid-committed stem cells.

Increased in

Extremely high: Generally seen in patients with severe anemia (Hct, <25; Hb<7) such as in cases of aplastic anemia, severe hemolytic anemia, hematologic cancers

Very high: Patients with mild to moderate anemia (Hct, 25-35; Hb, 7-10)

High: Patients with mild anemia (e.g., AIDS, myelodysplasia)

Erythropoietin can be inappropriately elevated in patients with malignant neoplasms, renal cysts, postrenal transplant, meningioma, hemangioblastoma, and leiomyoma.

Decreased in: Renal failure, polycythemia vera, autonomic neuropathy

TABLE 49 Hematopoietic Neoplasms Accompanied by Eosinophilia

Neoplasms in Which Eosinophils Are Likely to Be Clonal Cells

Acute eosinophilic leukemia (AEL)
Chronic eosinophilic leukemia (CEL)
Acute myeloid leukemia with inv(16) (FAB AML M4eo)
Chronic myeloid leukemia (CML –*BCR-ABL1*+)
Myeloid neoplasms with *PDGFR* abnormalities (WHO types)
Hematopoietic neoplasms with *FGFR1* abnormalities (WHO types)
Smoldering systemic mastocytosis
Aggressive systemic mastocytosis (ASM)
Mast cell leukemia (MCL)
SM-AHN (SM-CEL)

Neoplasms in Which Eosinophils May or May Not Be Part of the Malignant Clone

Other myeloproliferative neoplasms (MPN) with eosinophiliaa
Myelodysplastic syndromes (MDS) with eosinophilia
Other MDS/MPN overlap syndromes with eosinophilia[a]
Indolent systemic mastocytosis

Neoplasms in Which Eosinophils Usually Are Not Part of the Malignant Clone

Hodgkin disease
B- or T-cell non-Hodgkin lymphoma
Acute lymphoblastic leukemia (ALL)
Chronic lymphocytic leukemia (CLL)
Langerhans cell histiocytosis

AHN, Associated hematologic neoplasm; *FAB,* French–American–British Cooperative Study Group; *SM,* systemic mastocytosis; *WHO,* World Health Organization.
[a]Other MPN or MPN/MDS: Neoplasms where no abnormalities in the *PDGFR* or *FGFR1* genes are detectable.
From Hoffman R: *Hematology: basic principles and practice*, ed 7, Philadelphia, 2018, Elsevier.

ESTRADIOL (serum)

Normal range:
Female, premenopausal: 30-400 pg/ml, depending on phase of menstrual cycle
Female, postmenopausal: 0-30 pg/ml
Male, adult: 10-50 pg/ml
Decreased in: Ovarian failure
Elevated in: Tumors of ovary, testis, adrenal, or nonendocrine sites (rare)

ESTROGEN

Normal range (serum):

Males:	20-80 pg/ml
Females:	
Follicular:	60-200 pg/ml
Luteal:	160-400 pg/ml
Postmenopausal:	<130 pg/ml

Normal range (urine):

Males:	4-23 μg/g creatinine
Females:	
Follicular:	7-65 μg/g creatinine
Midcycle:	32-104 μg/g creatinine
Luteal:	8-135 μg/g creatinine

Elevated in: Hyperplasia of adrenal cortex, ovarian tumors producing estrogen, granulosa and thecal cell tumors, testicular tumors
Decreased in: Menopause, hypopituitarism, primary ovarian malfunction, anorexia nervosa, hypofunction of adrenal cortex, ovarian agenesis, psychogenic stress, gonadotropin-releasing hormone deficiency

TABLE 50 Differential Diagnosis of Childhood Eosinophilia

Physiologic

Prematurity
Infants receiving hyperalimentation
Hereditary

Infectious

1. Parasitic (with tissue-invasive helminths, e.g., trichinosis, strongyloidiasis, pneumocystosis, filariasis, cysticercosis, cutaneous and visceral larva migrans, echinococcosis)
2. Bacterial (brucellosis, tularemia, cat-scratch disease, *Chlamydia*)
3. Fungal (histoplasmosis, blastomycosis, coccidioidomycosis, allergic bronchopulmonary aspergillosis)
4. Mycobacterial (tuberculosis, leprosy)
5. Viral (HIV-1, HTLV-1, hepatitis A, hepatitis B, hepatitis C, Epstein-Barr virus)

Pulmonary

1. Allergic (rhinitis, asthma)
2. Eosinophilic granulomatosis with polyangiitis (Churg-Strauss syndrome)
3. Loeffler syndrome
4. Hypersensitivity pneumonitis
5. Eosinophilic pneumonia (chronic, acute)
6. Pulmonary interstitial eosinophilia

Dermatologic

Atopic dermatitis
Pemphigus
Dermatitis herpetiformis
Infantile eosinophilic pustular folliculitis
Eosinophilic fasciitis (Schulman syndrome)
Eosinophilic cellulitis (Wells syndrome)
Kimura disease (angiolymphoid hyperplasia with eosinophilia)

Hematologic/Oncologic

Neoplasm (lung, gastrointestinal, uterine)
Leukemia/lymphoma
Myelofibrosis
Myeloproliferative (FIP1L1–PDGFRA-positive) hypereosinophilic syndrome
Lymphatic hypereosinophilic syndrome
Systemic mastocytosis

Immunologic

T-cell immunodeficiencies
Hyper-IgE (Job) syndrome
Wiskott-Aldrich syndrome
Graft-versus-host disease
Drug hypersensitivity
Postirradiation
Postsplenectomy

Endocrine

Addison disease
Hypopituitarism

Cardiovascular

Loeffler disease (fibroplastic endocarditis)
Congenital heart disease
Hypersensitivity vasculitis
Eosinophilic myocarditis

Gastrointestinal

Benign proctocolitis
Inflammatory bowel disease
Eosinophilic gastrointestinal diseases (EGID)

FIP1L1-PDGFRA, FIP1-like 1–platelet-derived growth factor receptor α.

Ig, Immunoglobulin.
From Kliegman RM: *Nelson textbook of pediatrics*, ed 21, Philadelphia, 2020, Elsevier.

BOX 16 Epstein-Barr Virus–Associated Malignancies

Malignancy	Epstein-Barr Virus Frequency
Hodgkin disease	≈40%
Non-Hodgkin lymphomas	
Burkitt lymphoma	20%-95%
Diffuse large B-cell lymphoma and CD30+ Ki-1+ anaplastic large cell lymphoma	10%-35%
Lymphomatoid granulomatosis	80%-95%
T cell-rich B-cell lymphoma	20%
Angioimmunoblastic lymphoma	>80%
T-cell, NK cell, and T/NK-cell lymphomas	30%-90%
Nasopharyngeal carcinoma	>95%
Gastric adenocarcinoma	5%-10%
Pyothorax-associated lymphoma	>95%
Leiomyosarcoma in immunocompromised patients	>95%

NK, Natural killer.
From Hoffman R: *Hematology: basic principles and practice*, ed 6, Philadelphia, Saunders, 2013.

TABLE 51 Antibody Tests in Epstein-Barr Viral Infection

	Appearance	Peak	Disappears
Heterophil Ab	3-5 days after onset of Sx (range, 0-21 days)	During second wk after onset of Sx (1-4 wk)	2-3 mo after onset of Sx (still found at 1 yr in 20% of cases)
VCA-IgM	Beginning of Sx (1 wk before to 1 wk after Sx begin)	During first wk after onset of Sx (0-21 days)	2-3 mo after onset of Sx (1-6 mo)
VCA-IgG	3 days after onset of Sx (0-2 wk)	During second wk after onset of Sx (1-3 wk)	Decline to lower level, then persists for life
EBNA-IgG	3 wk after onset of Sx (1-4 wk)	8 mo after appearance (3-12 mo)	Lifelong
EA-D	5 days after onset of Sx (during first 1-2 wk after onset of Sx)	14-21 days after onset of Sx (1-4 wk)	9 wk after appearance (2-6 mo)
EBNA-IgM	Same as VCA-IgM	Same as VCA-IgM	Same as VCA-IgM

Ab, Antibody; *EA*, early antigen; *EBNA*, Epstein-Barr virus nuclear antigen; *Ig*, immunoglobulin; *Sx*, symptoms; *VCA*, viral capsid antigen.

ETHANOL (blood)

Normal range

Negative (values <10 mg/dl are considered negative)

Ethanol is metabolized at 10-25 mg/dl/hr. Levels ≥80 mg/dl are considered evidence of impairment for driving. Fatal blood concentration is considered to be >400 mg/dl. Table 53 summarizes the influence of acute ethanol ingestion on ethanol levels and behavior.

EXTRACTABLE NUCLEAR ANTIGEN (ENA complex, anti-RNP antibody, anti-sm, anti-Smith)

Normal: Negative

Present in

- Systemic lupus erythematosus, rheumatoid arthritis, Sjögren syndrome, mixed connective tissue disease

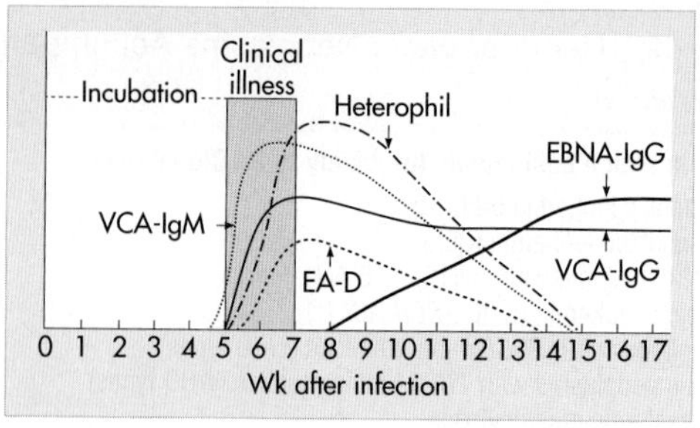

FIG. 22 Tests in Epstein-Barr viral infection. See Table 51 for abbreviations.

TABLE 52 Erythrocyte Sedimentation Ranges in Health

Age Range (Yr)	ESR Mean (mm in 1 h)
10-19	8
20-29	10.8
30-39	10.4
40-49	13.6
50-59	14.2
60-69	16
70-79	16.5
80-91	15.8
Pregnancy	
Early gestation	48 (62 if anaemic)
Later gestation	70 (95 if anaemic)

ESR, Erythrocyte sedimentation range.
From Bain BJ et al: *Dacie and Lewis practical haematology*, ed 12, Philadelphia, 2017, Elsevier.

TABLE 53 Influence of Acute Ethanol Ingestion on Ethanol Levels and Behavior

Ounces	Blood Concentration	Influence
1-2	10-50 mg/dl (2.2-10.9 mmol/L)	None to mild euphoria
3-4	50-100 mg/dl (10.9-21.7 mmol/L or greater)	Mild influence on stereoscopic vision and dark adaptation
	100 mg/dl (21.7 mmol/L)	Legally intoxicated
4-6	100-150 mg/dl (21.7-32.6 mmol/L)	Euphoria; disappearance of inhibition; prolonged reaction time
6-7	150-200 mg/dl (32.6-43.4 mmol/L)	Moderately severe poisoning; reaction time greatly prolonged; loss of inhibition and slight disturbances in equilibrium and coordination
8-9	200-250 mg/dl (43.4-54.3 mmol/L)	Severe degree of poisoning; disturbances of equilibrium and coordination; retardation of the thought processes and clouding of consciousness
10-15	250-400 mg/dl (54.3-86.8 mmol/L)	Deep, possibly fatal, coma

From McPherson RA, Pincus MR: *Henry's clinical diagnosis and management by laboratory methods*, ed 23, St Louis, 2017, Elsevier.

FACTOR V LEIDEN

Test description: PCR test performed on whole blood or tissue. This single mutation, found in 2%-8% of the general Caucasian population, is the single most common cause of hereditary thrombophilia.

FASTING BLOOD SUGAR

See "GLUCOSE, FASTING"

FBS

See "GLUCOSE, FASTING"

FDP

See "FIBRIN DEGRADATION PRODUCT"

FECAL FAT, QUANTITATIVE (72-hr collection)

Normal range: 2-6 g/24 hr (7-21 mmol/dl [CF: 3.515; SMI: 1 mmol/dl])
Elevated in: f. Malabsorption syndrome

FECAL GLOBIN IMMUNOCHEMICAL TEST

Normal: Negative. This test is performed by immunochromatography on a cellulose strip that has been impregnated with various antibodies. The test uses a small amount of toilet water as the specimen and is placed onto absorbent pads of card similar to traditional occult blood (OB) card. There is no direct handling of stool. This test is specific for the globin portion of the hemoglobin molecule, which confers lower GI bleeding specificity. It specifically detects blood from the lower GI tract; guaiac tests are not lower GI specific. It is more sensitive than typical Hemoccult test (detection limit 50 mcg Hb/g feces versus >500 mcg Hb/g feces for Hemoccult). It has no dietary restrictions and gives no false-positives due to plant peroxidases and red meats. It has no medication restrictions. Iron supplements and NSAIDs do not cause false positives. Vitamin C does not cause false-negatives.
Positive in: Lower GI bleeding

FERRITIN (serum)

Normal range: 18-300 ng/ml (18-300 µg/L [CF: 1; SMI: 10 µg/L])
Elevated in: Hyperthyroidism, inflammatory states, liver disease (ferritin elevated from necrotic hepatocytes), neoplasms (neuroblastomas, lymphomas, leukemia, breast carcinoma), iron replacement therapy, hemochromatosis, hemosiderosis. Table 54 summarizes hereditary iron overload disorders.
Decreased in: Iron deficiency anemia

TABLE 54 Hereditary Iron Overload Disorders

Disorder	Gene, Chromosome Location	Inheritance	Plasma Transferrin Saturation	Plasma Ferritin	Iron Deposition Sites	Clinical Manifestations
Hereditary hemochromatosis, *HFE*-associated (type 1; OMIM 235200)	*HFE*, 6p21	Autosomal recessive	Early increase; >45%	Later increase after third decade	Parenchymal iron overload affecting hepatocytes, heart, pancreas, other organs	Liver and heart disease, diabetes, gonadal failure, arthritis, skin pigmentation
Hereditary hemochromatosis, TfR2-associated (type 3; OMIM 604250)	*TFR2*, 7q22	Autosomal recessive	Early increase; >45%	Later increase after third decade	Parenchymal iron overload affecting hepatocytes, heart, pancreas, other organs	Liver and heart disease, diabetes, gonadal failure, arthritis, skin pigmentation
Juvenile hemochromatosis, hemojuvelin-associated (type 2A; OMIM 602390)	*HJV*, 1q21	Autosomal recessive	Early increase; >45%	Increased by second decade	Parenchymal iron overload affecting hepatocytes, heart, pancreas, other organs	As for hereditary hemochromatosis, but liver involvement less prominent
Juvenile hemochromatosis, hepcidin-associated (type 2B; OMIM 613313)	*HAMP*, 19q13	Autosomal recessive	Early increase; >45%	Increased by second decade	Parenchymal iron overload affecting hepatocytes, heart, pancreas, other organs	As for hereditary hemochromatosis, but liver involvement less prominent
Hemochromatosis, DMT1-associated (OMIM 206100)	*SCL11A2*, 12q13	Autosomal recessive	Early increase; >45%	Normal to moderately elevated	Hepatic iron overload, predominantly in hepatocytes	Severe microcytic anemia, liver dysfunction
Atransferrinemia (OMIM 209300)	*TF*, 3q22	Autosomal recessive	No plasma transferrin	Increased	Parenchymal iron overload affecting hepatocytes, heart, pancreas; no iron in bone marrow or spleen	Transfusion-dependent iron deficiency anemia, growth retardation, poor survival
Aceruloplasminemia (OMIM 604290)	*CP*, 3q24-q25	Autosomal recessive	Decreased	Increased	Marked iron accumulation in basal ganglia, liver, pancreas	Diabetes, progressive neurologic disease, retinal degeneration
Hemochromatosis, ferroportin-associated, with impaired iron export (type 4A; OMIM 606069)	*SLC40A1*, 2q32	Autosomal dominant	Remains normal or low	Early increase	Predominantly macrophage iron deposition	None
Hemochromatosis, ferroportin-associated, with hepcidin resistance (type 4B; OMIM 606069)	*SLC40A1*, 2q32	Autosomal dominant	Early increase; >45%	Early increase	Parenchymal iron overload affecting hepatocytes, heart, pancreas, other organs	Similar to HFE-associated hemochromatosis

OMIM, Online Mendelian Inheritance in Man.
From Hoffman R et al: *Hematology: basic principles and practice*, ed 6, Philadelphia, 2013, Saunders.

BOX 17 Etiopathophysiologic Classification of Folate Deficiency

Nutritional causes
Decreased dietary intake: Poverty and famine, institutionalized individuals (psychiatric/nursing homes)/chronic debilitating disease, prolonged feeding of infants with goat's milk, special slimming diets or food fads (folate-rich foods not consumed), cultural/ethnic cooking techniques (food folate destroyed)
Decreased diet and increased requirements
Physiologic: Pregnancy and lactation, prematurity, hyperemesis gravidarum, infancy
Pathologic
Intrinsic hematologic diseases involving hemolysis with compensatory erythropoiesis, abnormal hematopoiesis, or bone marrow infiltration with malignant disease
Dermatologic disease: Psoriasis
Folate malabsorption
With normal intestinal mucosa
Drugs: Sulfasalazine, pyrimethamine, proton pump inhibitors (via inhibition of proton-coupled folate transporter [PCFT])
Hereditary folate malabsorption (mutations in PCFTs) (rare)
With mucosal abnormalities: Tropical and nontropical sprue, regional enteritis
Defective cerebral spinal fluid folate transport: Cerebral folate deficiency (mutation or autoantibodies to folate receptors) (rare)
Inadequate cellular utilization
1. Folate antagonists (methotrexate)
2. Hereditary enzyme deficiencies involving folate
Drugs (multiple effects on folate metabolism): Alcohol, sulfasalazine, triamterene, pyrimethamine, trimethoprim-sulfamethoxazole, diphenylhydantoin, barbiturates

From Hoffman R: *Hematology: basic principles and practice,* ed 6, Philadelphia, 2013, Saunders.

α-1 FETOPROTEIN

Normal range: 0-20 ng/ml (0-20 μg/L [CF: 1; SMI: 1 μg/L])
Elevated in: Hepatocellular carcinoma (usually values >1000 ng/ml), germinal neoplasms (testis, ovary, mediastinum, retroperitoneum), liver disease (alcoholic cirrhosis, acute hepatitis, chronic active hepatitis), fetal anencephaly, spina bifida, basal cell carcinoma, breast carcinoma, pancreatic carcinoma, gastric carcinoma, retinoblastoma, esophageal atresia

FIBRIN DEGRADATION PRODUCT (FDP)

Normal range: <10 μg/ml
Elevated in: Disseminated intravascular coagulation, primary fibrinolysis, pulmonary embolism, severe liver disease
NOTE: The presence of rheumatoid factor may cause falsely elevated FDP.

FIBRINOGEN

Normal range: 200-400 mg/dl (2-4 g/L [CF: 0.01; SMI: 0.1 g/L])
Elevated in: Tissue inflammation or damage (acute phase protein reactant), oral contraceptives, pregnancy, acute infection, myocardial infarction
Decreased in: Disseminated intravascular coagulation, hereditary afibrinogenemia, liver disease, primary or secondary fibrinolysis, cachexia

FOLATE (folic acid)

Normal range: Plasma: 2-10 ng/ml (4-22 nmol/L [CF: 2.266; SMI: 2 nmol/L])
Red blood cells: 140-960 ng/ml (550-2200 nmol/L [CF: 2.266; SMI: 10 nmol/L])
Decreased in: Folic acid deficiency (inadequate intake, malabsorption), alcoholism, drugs (methotrexate, trimethoprim, phenytoin, oral contraceptives, Azulfidine), vitamin B_{12} deficiency (defective red cell folate absorption), hemolytic anemia. Box 17 summarizes an etiophysiologic classification of folate deficiency.
Elevated in: Folic acid therapy

FOLLICLE-STIMULATING HORMONE (FSH)

Normal range: 5-20 mIU/ml
Elevated in: Menopause, primary gonadal failure, alcoholism, castration, Klinefelter syndrome, gonadotropin-secreting pituitary hormones
Decreased in: Pregnancy, polycystic ovary disease, anorexia nervosa, anterior pituitary hypofunction

FREE T_4

See "T_4, FREE"

FREE THYROXINE INDEX

Normal range: 1.1-4.3
INCREASED THYROXINE OR FREE THYROXINE VALUES
Laboratory error
Primary hyperthyroidism (T4/T3 type)
Severe thyroxine-binding globulin elevation
Excess therapy of hypothyroidism
Excessive dose of levothyroxine
Active thyroiditis (subacute, painless, early active Hashimoto disease)
Familial dysalbuminemic hyperthyroxinemia (some FT4 kits, especially analog types)
Peripheral resistance to T4 syndrome
Amiodarone or propranolol
Postpartum transient toxicosis
Factitious hyperthyroidism
Jod-Basedow (iodine-induced) hyperthyroidism
Severe nonthyroid illness
Acute psychosis (especially paranoid schizophrenia)
T4 sample drawn 2-4 hr after levothyroxine dose
Struma ovarii
Pituitary thyroid-stimulating hormone-secreting tumor
Certain x-ray contrast media (Telepaque and Oragrafin)
Acute porphyria
Heparin effect (some T4 and FT4 kits)
Amphetamine, heroin, methadone, and phencyclidine abuse
Perphenazine or 5-fluorouracil
Antithyroid or anti-IgG heterophil (HAMA) autoantibodies
"T4" hyperthyroidism
Hyperemesis gravidarum; about 50% of patients
High altitudes
DECREASED THYROXINE OR FREE THYROXINE VALUES
Laboratory error
Primary hypothyroidism
Severe nonthyroid illness
Lithium therapy
Severe thyroxine-binding globulin decrease (congenital, disease, or drug-induced) or severe albumin decrease
Dilantin, Depakene, or high-dose salicylate drugs
Pituitary insufficiency
Large doses of inorganic iodide (e.g., saturated solution of potassium iodide)
Moderate or severe iodine deficiency
Cushing syndrome
High-dose glucocorticoid drugs
Pregnancy, third trimester (low normal or small decrease)
Addison disease; some patients (30%)
Heparin effect (a few FT4 kits)
Desipramine or amiodarone drugs
Acute psychiatric illness

FTA-ABS (serum)

Normal: Nonreactive
Reactive in:
- Syphilis, other treponemal diseases (yaws, pinta, bejel), SLE, pregnancy

FUROSEMIDE STIMULATION TEST

Normal: Test is performed by giving 60 mg furosemide orally after overnight fast. Patient should be on a normal diet without medications the wk before the test. Normal results: Renin 1-6 ng angiotensin L/ml/hr.
Elevated in: Renovascular hypertension, Bartter syndrome, high-renin essential hypertension, pheochromocytoma
No response in
Primary aldosteronism, low-renin essential hypertension, hyporeninemic hypoaldosteronism

GAMMA-GLUTAMYL TRANSFERASE (GGT)

See "γ-GLUTAMYL TRANSFERASE"

GASTRIN (serum)

Normal range: 0-180 pg/ml (0-180 ng/L [CF: 1; SMI: 10 ng/L])
Elevated in: Zollinger-Ellison syndrome (gastrinoma), pernicious anemia, hyperparathyroidism, retained gastric antrum, chronic renal failure, gastric ulcer, chronic atrophic gastritis, pyloric obstruction, malignant neoplasms of the stomach, H_2-blockers, omeprazole, calcium therapy, ulcerative colitis, rheumatoid arthritis

GASTRIN STIMULATION TEST

Normal: Gastrin stimulation test after calcium infusion is performed by giving a calcium infusion (15 mg/kg in 500 ml normal saline over 4 hours). Serum is drawn in fasting state before infusion and at 1, 2, 3, and 4 hr. Normal response is little or no increase over baseline gastrin level.
Elevated in: Gastrinoma (gastrin >400 pg/ml), duodenal ulcer (gastrin level increase <400 ng/L)
Decreased in: Pernicious anemia, atrophic gastritis

GLIADIN ANTIBODIES, IGA AND IGG

Normal: <25 U, equivocal 20-25 U, positive >25 U. Test is useful to monitor compliance with gluten-free diet in patients with celiac disease.
Elevated in: Celiac disease with dietary noncompliance

GLOMERULAR BASEMENT MEMBRANE (GBM) ANTIBODY

Normal: Negative
Present in: Goodpasture syndrome

GLOMERULAR FILTRATION RATE

See Box 18 for a summary of common equations for calculating GFR or creatinine clearance. Chronic kidney disease stages based on GFR are summarized in Table 55.
Normal:

Ages 20-29	116 ml/min/1.73 m^2
Ages 30-39	107 ml/min/1.73 m^2
Ages 40-49	99 ml/min/1.73 m^2
Ages 50-59	93 ml/min/1.73 m^2
Ages 60-69	85 ml/min/1.73 m^2
Ages >75	75 ml/min/1.73 m^2

Decreased in: Renal insufficiency, decreased renal blood flow

GLUCAGON

Normal: 20-100 pg/ml
Elevated in: Glucagonoma (900-7800 pg/ml), chronic renal failure, diabetes mellitus, glucocorticoids, insulin, nifedipine, danazol, sympathomimetic amines
Decreased in: Hyperlipoproteinemia (types III, IV), beta-blockers, secretin

GLUCOSE, FASTING (FBS, fasting blood sugar)

Fig. E23 describes the approach to hypoglycemia. An algorithm for evaluation of hypoglycemia in children is described in Fig. E24.

BOX 18 Common Equations for Estimating Glomerular Filtration Rate or Creatinine Clearance

Cockcroft-Gault (C_{Cr} · BSA/1.73 m^2)
For men: C_{Cr} = [(140 – age) · weight (kg)]/S_{Cr} · 72
For women: C_{Cr} = ([(140 – age) · weight (kg)]/S_{Cr} · 72) · 0.85

MDRD (1)
g. GFR = 170 · $[S_{Cr}]^{-0.999}$ · $[age]^{-0.176}$ · [0.762 if patient is female] · [1.18 if patient is black] · $[BUN]^{-0170}$ · $[Alb]^{0.318}$

MDRD (2)
GFR = 186 · $[S_{Cr.}]^{-1.154}$ · $[age]^{-0.203}$ · [0.742 if patient is female] · [1.212 if patient is black]

Jellife (1) (C_{Cr} · BSA/1.73 m^2)
For men: (98 – [0.8 · (age – 20)])/S_{Cr}
For women: (98 – [0.8 · (age – 20)])S_{Cr} · 0.90

Jellife (2)
For men: $(100/S_{Cr})^{-12}$
For women: $(80/S_{Cr})^{-7}$

Mawer
For men: weight · [29.3 – (0.203 · age)] · [1 – (0.03 · SCr)]
For women: weight · [25.3 – (0.175 · age)] · [1 – (0.03 · SC_r)]

Bjornsson
For men: [27 – (0.173 · age)] · weight · 0/S_{Cr}
For women: [25 – (0.175 · age)] · weight · 0.07/S_{Cr}

Gates
For men: (89.4 · $S_{Cr}^{-1.2}$) + (55 – age) · (0.447 · $S_{Cr}^{-1.1}$)
For women: (89.4 · $S_{Cr}^{-1.2}$) + (55 – age) · (0.447 · $S_{Cr}^{-1.1}$)

Salazar-Corcoran
For men: [137 – age] · [(0.285 · weight) + (12.1 · $height^2$)]/(51 · S_{Cr})
For women: [146 – age] · [(0.287 · weight) + (9.74 · $height^2$)]/(60 · S_{Cr})

Alb, Albumin; *BSA*, body surface area; *BUN*, blood urea nitrogen; C_{cr}, creatinine clearance; *MDRD*, Modification of Diet in Renal Disease; S_{cr}, serum creatinine.
From Vincent JL et al: *Textbook of critical care,* ed 6, Philadelphia, 2011, Saunders.

TABLE 55 Chronic Kidney Disease Stages

Stage	eGFR (ml/min/1.73 m^2)	Urinalysis Findings
1	≥90	Hematuria, proteinuria, or imaging abnormalities at >3 mo
2	60-89	Hematuria, proteinuria, or imaging abnormalities at >3 mo
3	30-59	↑ or normal
4	15-29	↑ or normal
5	0-14	↑ or normal

eGFR, Estimated glomerular filtration rate.
From Parrillo JE, Dellinger RP: *Critical care medicine, principles of diagnosis and management in the adult,* ed 4, Philadelphia, 2014, Elsevier.

Normal range: 60-99 mg/dl (3.8-6.0 mmol/L [CF: 0.05551; SMI: 0.1 mmol/L])
Elevated in: Diabetes mellitus, stress, infections, myocardial infarction, cerebrovascular accident, Cushing syndrome, acromegaly, acute pancreatitis, glucagonoma, hemochromatosis, drugs (glucocorticoids, diuretics [thiazides, loop diuretics]), glucose intolerance, impaired fasting glucose
Decreased in: Sulfonylurea therapy, insulin therapy, reactive hypoglycemia (e.g., subtotal gastrectomy), starvation, insulinoma, glycogen storage disorders, severe liver disease or renal disease, ethanol-induced hypoglycemia, mesenchymal tumors that secrete insulin-like hormones

GLUCOSE, POSTPRANDIAL

Normal range: <140 mg/dl (<7.8 mmol/L [CF: 0.05551; SMI: 0.1 mmol/L])
Elevated in: Diabetes mellitus, glucose intolerance

TABLE 56 Glycemic Goals in Adults*

	Hemoglobin A_{1c} (%)	Preprandial Glucose mg/dl	Preprandial Glucose mmol/L	Postprandial Glucose** mg/dl	Postprandial Glucose** mmol/L
ADA†: Adults	<7.0‡	80-130	4.4-7.2	<180	<10.0
Pregnant adults	<6.0	60-99	3.3-5.5	100-129	5.6-7.2
Older adults:					
Healthy	<7.5	90-130	5.0-7.2	90-150	5.0-8.3
Intermediate	<8.0	90-150	5.0-8.3	100-180	5.6-10.0
Poor health	<8.5	100-180	5.6-10.0	110-200	6.1-11.1
AACE§¶	≤6.5	≤110	≤6.1	≤140	<7.8

AACE, American Association of Clinical Endocrinologists; *ADA,* American Diabetes Association.
*Youth <18 years of age: Goal hemoglobin A_{1c}<7.5%.
**1-2 hours after beginning a meal for adults, except bedtime for older adults.
†American Diabetes Association (2015); Chiang et al (2014).
‡Lower goals may be appropriate for selected individuals if this can be accomplished safely (without significant hypoglycemia). Higher goals may be appropriate in some individuals (e.g., with a history of severe hypoglycemia, limited life expectancy, advanced complications, extensive comorbid conditions, or long-standing diabetes in whom the goal is difficult to achieve with appropriate education, monitoring, and therapies, including insulin).
§AACE, American Association of Clinical Endocrinologists, 2015.
¶For patients without concurrent serious illness and at low hypoglycemia risk.
From McPherson RA, Pincus MR: *Henry's clinical diagnosis and management by laboratory methods,* ed 23, St Louis, 2017, Elsevier.

Decreased in: Post gastrointestinal resection, reactive hypoglycemia, hereditary fructose intolerance, galactosemia, leucine sensitivity

GLUCOSE TOLERANCE TEST

Normal values above fasting

11. 30 min: 30-60 mg/dl (1.65-3.3 mmol/L [CF: 0.05551; SMI: 0.1 mmol/L])
12. 60 min: 20-50 mg/dl (1.1-2.75 mmol/L [CF: 0.05551; SMI: 0.1 mmol/L])
13. 120 min: 5-15 mg/dl (0.28-0.83 mmol/L [CF: 0.05551; SMI: 0.1 mmol/L])
14. 180 min: Fasting level or below

Abnormal in: Glucose intolerance, diabetes mellitus, Cushing syndrome, acromegaly, pheochromocytoma, gestational diabetes

GLUCOSE-6-PHOSPHATE DEHYDROGENASE (G6PD) Screen (blood)

Normal: G6PD enzyme activity detected
Abnormal: If a deficiency is detected, quantitation of G6PD is necessary; a G6PD screen may be falsely interpreted as "normal" after an episode of hemolysis because most G6PD-deficient cells have been destroyed.

γ-GLUTAMYL TRANSFERASE (GGT)

Normal range: 0-30 U/L (0.050 μkat/L [CF: 0.01667; SMI: 0.01 μkat/L])
Elevated in: Chronic alcoholic liver disease, neoplasms (hepatoma, metastatic disease to the liver, carcinoma of the pancreas), systemic lupus erythematosus, congestive heart failure, trauma, nephrotic syndrome, sepsis, cholestasis, drugs (phenytoin, barbiturates)

GLYCOHEMOGLOBIN (glycated glycosylated hemoglobin), (HbA1c)

Normal range: 4.0%-5.9%. Glycemic goals in adults are summarized in Table 56.
Elevated in: Uncontrolled diabetes mellitus (glycated hemoglobin levels reflect the level of glucose control over the preceding 120 days), lead toxicity, alcoholism, iron deficiency anemia, hypertriglyceridemia
Decreased in: Hemolytic anemias, decreased red blood cell survival, pregnancy, acute or chronic blood loss, chronic renal failure, insulinoma, congenital spherocytosis, hemoglobin S, C, and D diseases

GROWTH HORMONE

Normal: Male: 1-9 ng/ml; female: 1-16 ng/ml
Elevated in: Pituitary gigantism, acromegaly, ectopic GH secretion, cirrhosis, renal failure, anorexia nervosa, stress, exercise, prolonged fasting, amphetamines, beta-blockers, insulin, levodopa, metoclopramide, clonidine, vasopressin, human growth hormone (HGH) supplementation
Decreased in: Hypopituitarism, pituitary dwarfism, adrenocortical hyperfunction, bromocriptine, corticosteroids, glucose

GROWTH HORMONE RELEASING HORMONE (GHRH)

Normal: <50 pg/ml
Elevated in: Acromegaly caused by GHRH secretion by neoplasms

GROWTH HORMONE SUPPRESSION TEST (after glucose)

Normal: Test is done by giving 1.75 g glucose/kg orally after overnight fast. Blood is drawn at baseline, after 60 min, and after 120 min of glucose load. Normal response is growth hormone suppression to <2 ng/ml or undetectable levels.
Abnormal: There is no or incomplete suppression from the high basal level in gigantism or acromegaly.

HAM TEST (acid serum test)

Normal: Negative
Positive in: Paroxysmal nocturnal hemoglobinuria
False-positive in: Hereditary or acquired spherocytosis, recent transfusion with aged red blood cells, aplastic anemia, myeloproliferative syndromes, leukemia, hereditary dyserythropoietic anemia type II

HAPTOGLOBIN (serum)

Normal range: 50-220 mg/dl (0.50-2.2 g/L [CF: 0.01; SMI: 0.01 g/L])
Elevated in: Inflammation (acute phase reactant), collagen vascular diseases, infections (acute phase reactant), drugs (androgens), obstructive liver disease
Decreased in: Hemolysis (intravascular more than extravascular), megaloblastic anemia, severe liver disease, large tissue hematomas, infectious mononucleosis, drugs (oral contraceptives)

HBA_{1C}

See "GLYCOHEMOGLOBIN"

HDL

See "HIGH-DENSITY LIPOPROTEIN CHOLESTEROL"

HELICOBACTER PYLORI (serology, stool antigen)

Normal range: Not detected
Detected in: *H. pylori* infection. Positive serology can indicate current or past infection. Positive stool antigen test indicates acute infection (sensitivity and specificity >90%). Stool testing should be delayed at least 4 wk after eradication therapy.

HEMATOCRIT

Normal range
1. Male: 39%-49% (0.39-0.49 [CF: 0.01; SMI: 0.01])
2. Female: 33%-43% (0.33-0.43 [CF: 0.01; SMI: 0.01])

Elevated in: Polycythemia vera, smoking, chronic obstructive pulmonary disease, high altitudes, dehydration, hypovolemia
Decreased in: Blood loss (gastrointestinal, genitourinary) anemia

HEMOGLOBIN

Normal range
Male: 13.6-17.7 g/dl (136-172 g/L [CF: 10; SMI: 1 g/L])
Female: 12.0-15.0 g/dl (120-150 g/L [CF: 10; SMI: 1 g/L])
Elevated in: Hemoconcentration, dehydration, polycythemia vera, chronic obstructive pulmonary disease, high altitudes, false elevations (hyperlipemic plasma, white blood cells >50,000/mm^3), stress
Decreased in: Hemorrhagic (gastrointestinal, genitourinary) anemia

HEMOGLOBIN A_{1C}

See "GLYCOHEMOGLOBIN"

HEMOGLOBIN ELECTROPHORESIS

Table 57 describes neonatal hemoglobin electrophoresis patterns, Table 58 summarizes types of hemoglobin, and Table 59 describes classifications of hemoglobinopathies.

Normal range
- **a.** HbA_1: 95%-98%
- **b.** HbA_2: 1.5%-3.5%
- **c.** HbF: <2%
- **d.** HbC: Absent
- **e.** HbS: Absent

HEMOGLOBIN, GLYCATED

See "GLYCOHEMOGLOBIN"

HEMOGLOBIN, GLYCOSYLATED

See "GLYCOHEMOGLOBIN"

HEMOGLOBIN H

See Table 58.

TABLE 57 Neonatal Hemoglobin (Hb) Electrophoresis Patterns*

FA	Fetal Hb and adult normal Hb; the normal newborn pattern.
FAV	Indicates the presence of both HbF and HbA. However, an anomalous band (V) is present, which does not appear to be any of the common Hb variants.
FAS	Indicates fetal Hb, adult normal HbA, and HbS, consistent with benign sickle cell trait.
FS	Fetal and sickle HbS without detectable adult normal HbA. Consistent with clinically significant homozygous sickle Hb genotype (S/S) or sickle β-thalassemia, with manifestations of sickle cell anemia during childhood.
FC†	Designates the presence of HbC without adult normal HbA. Consistent with clinically significant homozygous HbC genotype (C/C), resulting in a mild hematologic disorder presenting during childhood.
FSC	HbS and HbC present. This heterozygous condition could lead to the manifestations of sickle cell disease during childhood.
FAC	HbC and adult normal HbA present, consistent with benign HbC trait.
FSA	Heterozygous HbS/β-thalassemia, a clinically significant sickling disorder.
F†	Fetal HbF is present without adult normal HbA. Although this may indicate a delayed appearance of HbA, it is also consistent with homozygous β-thalassemia major, or homozygous hereditary persistence of fetal HbF.
FV†	Fetal HbF and an anomalous Hb variant (V) are present.
AF	May indicate prior blood transfusion. Submit another filter paper blood specimen when the infant is 4 mo of age, at which time the transfused blood cells should have been cleared.

NOTE: HbA: $\alpha 2\beta 2$; HbF: $\alpha 2\gamma 2$; HbA2: $\alpha 2\delta 2$.
*Hemoglobin variants are reported in order of decreasing abundance; for example, FA indicates more fetal than adult hemoglobin.
†Repeat blood specimen should be submitted to confirm the original interpretation.
From Tschudy MM, Arcara KM: *The Harriet Lane handbook,* ed 19, Philadelphia, 2012, Mosby.

TABLE 58 Types of Hemoglobin

	Hemoglobin	Structure	Comment
Normal	A	$\alpha_2\beta_2$	97% of adult hemoglobin
	A_2	$\alpha_2\delta_2$	2% of adult Hb; elevated in β-thalassemia
	F	$\alpha_2\gamma_2$	Normal Hb in fetus from 3rd-9th mo; increased in β-thalassemia
Abnormal chain production	H	β_4	Found in α-thalassemia, biologically useless
	Barts	γ_4	Found in α-thalassemia, biologically useless
Abnormal chain structure	S	$\alpha_2\beta_2$	Substitution of valine for glutamic acid in position 6 of β chain
	C	$\alpha_2\beta_2$	Substitution of lysine for glutamic acid in position 6 of β chain

From Ballinger A: *Kumar & Clark's essentials of clinical medicine,* ed 6, Edinburgh, 2012, Saunders.

Normal: Negative
Present in: Hemoglobin H disease, alpha-thalassemia trait, unstable hemoglobin disorders

HEMOGLOBIN, URINE

See "URINE HEMOGLOBIN, FREE"

HEMOSIDERIN, URINE

See "URINE HEMOGLOBIN, FREE"

HEPARIN-INDUCED THROMBOCYTOPENIA ANTIBODIES

Normal: Antigen assay: Negative, <0.45; weak, 0.45-1.0; strong, >1.0
Elevated in: Heparin-induced thrombocytopenia

TABLE 59 Classification of Hemoglobinopathies

Structural hemoglobinopathies—hemoglobins with altered amino acid sequences that result in deranged function or altered physical or chemical properties
Abnormal hemoglobin polymerization—HBS
Altered oxygen affinity
High affinity—polycythemia
Low affinity—cyanosis, pseudoanemia
Hemoglobins that oxidize readily
Unstable hemoglobins, hemolytic anemia, jaundice
M hemoglobins—methemoglobinemia, cyanosis
Thalassemias—defective production of globin chains
α-Thalassemias
β-Thalassemias
δβ-, γδβ-, αβ-Thalassemias
Structural hemoglobinopathies—structurally abnormal Hb associated with coinherited thalassemia phenotype
HbE
Hb constant spring
Hb lepore
Hereditary persistence of fetal hemoglobin—persistence of high levels of HbF into adult life
Pancellular—all red blood cells contain elevated HbF levels
Nondeletion forms
Deletion forms
Hb Kenya
Heterocellular—only specific subpopulation of red blood cells contain elevated levels of HbF
Acquired hemoglobinopathies
Methemoglobin due to toxic exposures
Sulfhemoglobin due to toxic exposures
Carboxyhemoglobin
HbH in erythroleukemia
Elevated HbF in states of erythroid stress and bone marrow dysplasia, usually heterocellular

Hb, Hemoglobin.
From Hoffman R: *Hematology: basic principles and practice*, ed 6, Philadelphia, 2013, Saunders.

HEPATITIS A ANTIBODY

Normal: Negative
Present in: Viral hepatitis A; can be IgM or IgG (if IgM, acute hepatitis A; if IgG, previous infection with hepatitis A)

See Fig. 25 for serologic tests in HAV infection.

See Table 60 for serologic and virologic tests for hepatitis viruses.

HEPATITIS A VIRUS-IGM ANTIBODY

Appearance: About the same time as clinical symptoms (3-4 wk after exposure; range, 14-60 days), or just before beginning of AST/ALT elevation (range, 10 days before to 7 days after)
Peak: About 3-4 wk after onset of symptoms (1-6 wk)
Becomes nondetectable: 3-4 mo after onset of symptoms (1-6 mo). In a few cases HAV-IgM antibody can persist as long as 12-14 mo.

HAV TOTAL ANTIBODY

Appearance: About 3 wk after IgM becomes detectable (therefore about the middle of clinical symptom period to early convalescence)
Peak: About 1-2 mo after onset
Becomes nondetectable: Remains elevated for life but can somewhat slowly fall

HEPATITIS A VIRAL INFECTION

Best all-purpose test(s) to diagnose acute HAV infection = HAV-Ab (IgM)
Best all-purpose test(s) to demonstrate past HAV infection/immunity = HAV-Ab (total)

HEPATITIS B SURFACE ANTIGEN (HBsAg)

Normal: Not detected
Detected in: Acute viral hepatitis type B, chronic hepatitis B
Appearance: 2-6 wk after exposure (range, 6 days to 6 mo); 5%-15% of patients are negative at onset of jaundice
Peak: 1-2 wk before to 1-2 wk after onset of symptoms
Becomes nondetectable: 1-3 mo after peak (range, 1 wk to 5 mo)

HEPATITIS B VIRAL INFECTION

See Table 61

Figs. 26, 27, and 28 illustrate antigens and antibodies in hepatitis B infection.

HB_S

-Ag

HB_SAg: Shows current active hepatitis B virus (HBV) infection
Persistence over 6 mo indicates carrier/chronic HBV infection
HBV nucleic acid probe: Present before and longer than HB_SAg
More reliable marker for increased infectivity than HB_SAg and/or HB_eAg

-Ab

HB_SAb-total: Shows previous healed HBV infection and evidence of immunity

HB_C

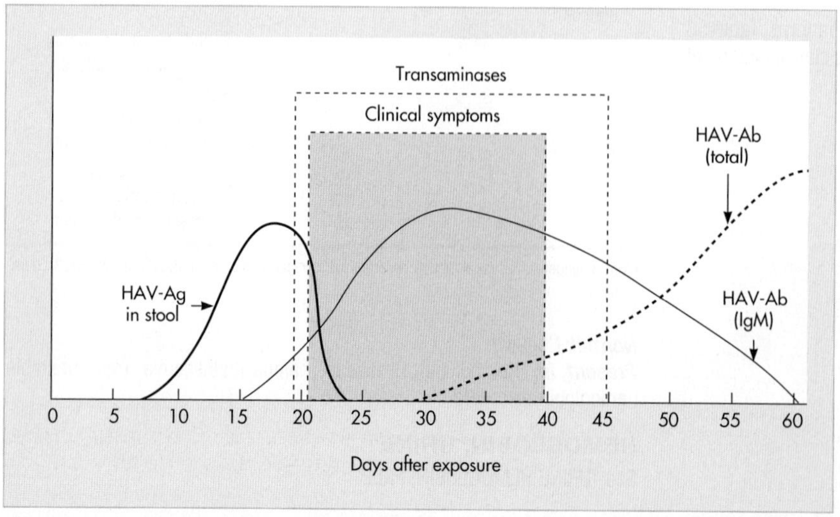

FIG. 25 Serologic tests in hepatitis A viral infection. *HAV,* Hepatitis A virus; *HAV-Ab,* hepatitis A virus antibodies test; *HAV-Ag,* hepatitis A virus antigen test; *Ig,* immunoglobulin.

TABLE 60 Serologic and Virologic Tests for Hepatitis Viruses

	IgM Anti-HAV	IgG Anti-HAV	HBsAg	Anti-HBs	IgM Anti-HBVc	HBeAg	Anti-HBe	HBV DNA	Anti-HCV Screen	HCV RNA	Anti-HDV	Anti-HEV
HAV:												
Acute	+	+										
Remote	+	+										
HBV:												
Early			+	−	+	+	−	+				
Window			−	−	+	−	−	+				
Resolving			−/+	+	−	−/+	+	−/+				
Chronic			+	−/+	−	+	+/−	+				
TX monitoring								+				
Remote			−	+	−	−/+	+/−	−/+				
HCV:												
Screen									+	+		
Acute									+/−	+		
Chronic									+	+		
TX monitoring										+		
Remote									+	−/+		
HDV:												
Superinfection			+	−	+/−	+	−/+	+/−			+	
HEV												+

DNA, Deoxyribonucleic acid; *HAV*, hepatitis A virus; *HBeAg*, hepatitis E antigen; *HBsAg*, hepatitis B surface antigen; *HBV*, hepatitis B virus; *HCV*, hepatitis C virus; *HDV*, hepatitis D virus; *HEV*, hepatitis E virus; *Ig*, immunoglobulin; *RNA*, ribonucleic acid; *TX*, Texas; +, positive; −, negative.
Data from CDC: Surveillance for acute hepatitis, United States, 2007, *MMWR* 58(SS-3), 2009. From McPherson RA, Pincus MR: *Henry's clinical diagnosis and management by laboratory methods*, ed 23, Philadelphia, 2017, Elsevier.

TABLE 61 Serologic Markers of Hepatitis B Infection

	HBsAg	anti-HBc	anti-HBs	IgM anti-HBc
Susceptible to infection	Negative	Negative	Negative	Negative
Immune due to natural infection	Negative	Positive	Positive	Negative
Immune due to hepatitis B vaccination	Negative	Negative	Positive	Negative
Acutely infected	Positive	Positive	Negative	Positive
Chronically infected	Positive	Positive	Negative	Negative

HBsAg, Hepatitis B surface antigen; *Ig*, immunoglobulin.
From Ballinger A: *Kumar & Clark's essentials of clinical medicine*, ed 6, Edinburgh, 2012, Saunders.

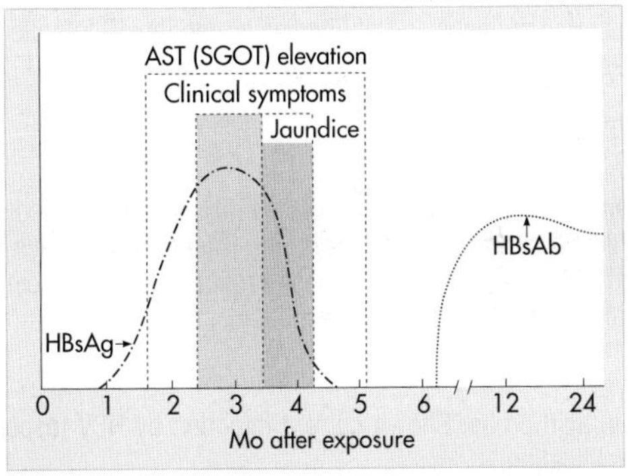

FIG. 27 Hepatitis B virus surface antigen and antibody (HB_SAg and HB_SAb-total). *AST*, Aspartate aminotransferase; *SGOT*, serum glutamic-oxaloacetic transaminase.

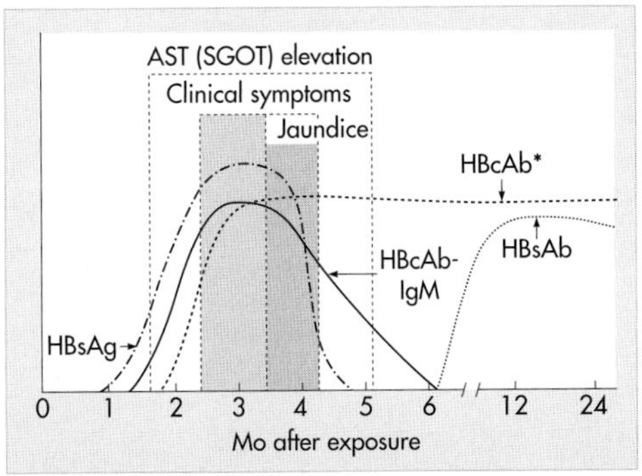

FIG. 26 Hepatitis B virus surface antigen-antibody and core antibodies. Note "core window." *HB_CAb = HB_CAb-IgM + HBCAb-IgG (combined). *AST*, Aspartate aminotransferase; *HBcAb*, hepatitis B core antibody; *HBsAb*, hepatitis B surface antibody; *HBsAg*, hepatitis B surface antigen; *Ig*, immunoglobulin; *SGOT*, serum glutamic-oxaloacetic transaminase.

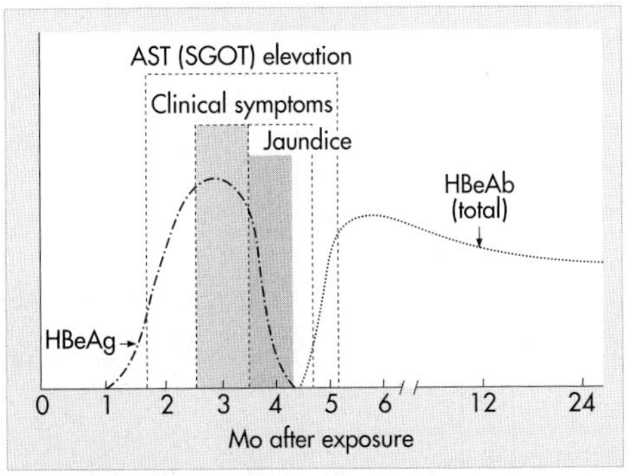

FIG. 28 HBVe antigen and antibody. *AST*, Aspartate aminotransferase; *HBeAb*, hepatitis B e-antibody; *SGOT*, serum glutamic-oxaloacetic transaminase.

-Ab

HB_CAb-IgM: Shows either acute or very recent infection by HBV

In convalescent phase of acute HBV, may be elevated when HB_SAg has disappeared (core window)

Negative HB_CAb-IgM with positive HB_SAg suggests either very early acute HBV or carrier/chronic HBV

HB_CAb-total: Only useful to show past HBV infection if HB_SAg and HB_cAb-IgM are both negative

HB_E

-Ag

HB_e-AbAg: When present, especially without HB_eAb, suggests increased patient infectivity

HB_eAb-total: When present, suggests less patient infectivity

- HB_SAg positive, HB_CAb negative
  - About 5% (range, 0%-17%) of patients with early-stage HBV acute infection (HB_CAb rises later)
- HB_SAg positive, HB_CAb positive, HB_SAb negative
  - Most of the clinical symptom stage
  - Chronic HBV carriers without evidence of liver disease ("asymptomatic carriers")
  - Chronic HBV hepatitis (chronic persistent type or chronic active type)
- HB_SAg negative, HB_CAb positive, HB_SAb negative
  - Late clinical symptom stage or early convalescence stage (core window)
  - Chronic HBV infection with HB_SAg below detection levels with current tests
  - Old previous HBV infection
- HB_SAg negative, HB_CAb positive, HB_SAb positive
  - Late convalescence to complete recovery
  - Old infection

HEPATITIS C VIRAL INFECTION

Fig. 29 illustrates antigens and antibodies in hepatitis C infection. Table 62 summarizes interpretation of patterns of HCV markers.

HEPATITIS C RNA

Normal: Negative

Elevated in: Hepatitis C. Detection of hepatitis C-RNA is used to confirm current infection and to monitor treatment. Quantitative assays (viral load) are needed before treatment to assess response (<2 log decrease after 12-wk treatment indicates lack of response).

HCV

-Ag

HCV nucleic acid probe: Shows current infection by HCV (especially with PCR amplification).

-Ab

HCV-Ab (IgG): Current, convalescent, or old HCV infection.

HAV

-Ag

HAV-Ag by EM: Shows presence of virus in stool early in infection.

-Ab

HAV-Ab (IgM): Current or recent HAV infection.

HAV-Ab (total): Convalescent or old HAV infection.

HEPATITIS D VIRAL INFECTION

Fig. 30 illustrates antigens and antibodies in hepatitis D infection.

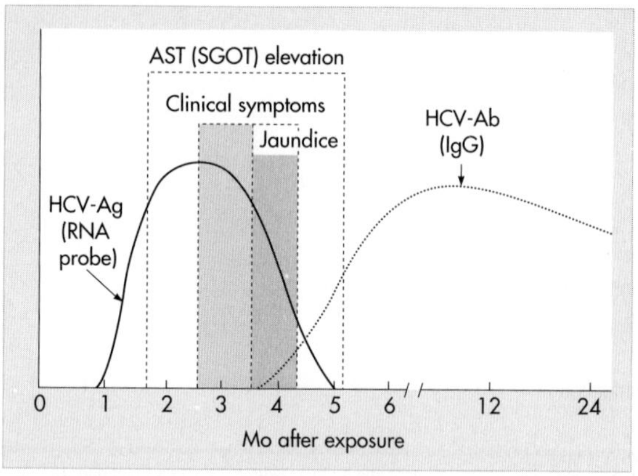

FIG. 29 Hepatitis C virus antigen and antibody. *AST,* Aspartate aminotransferase; *HCV-Ab,* hepatitis C virus antibody; *HCV-Ag,* hepatitis C virus core antigen; *Ig,* immunoglobulin; *RNA,* ribonucleic acid; *SGOT,* serum glutamic-oxaloacetic transaminase.

TABLE 62 Interpretation of Patterns of HCV Markers

Interpretation	Anti-HCV	RIBA	HCV RNA
Acute HCV infection	–	–	+
Active HCV infection	+	+	+
Possible HCV clearance	+	+	–
False-positive HCV test	+	–	–
Requires further study	+	Indeterminate*	–

HCV, Hepatitis C; *RIBA,* recombinant immunoassay.; *RNA,* ribonucleic acid

*Indeterminate result: Only one band positive, or more than one band and nonspecific reactivity.

From McPherson RA, Pincus MR: *Henry's clinical diagnosis and management by laboratory methods,* ed 23, St Louis, 2017, Elsevier.

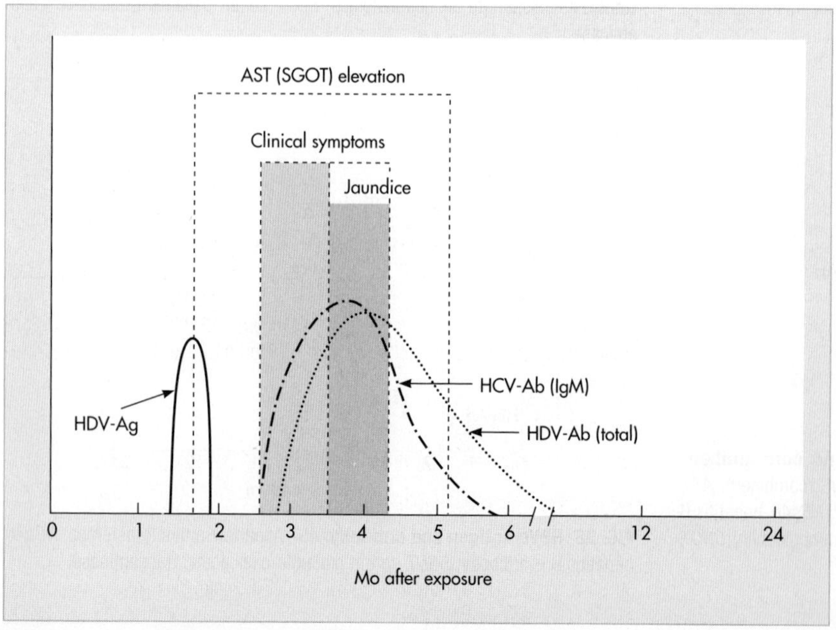

FIG. 30 Hepatitis D virus antigen and antibodies. *AST,* Aspartate aminotransferase; *HCV-Ab,* hepatitis C virus antibody; *HDV-Ab,* hepatitis D virus antibody; *HDV-Ag,* hepatitis D virus antigen; *Ig,* immunoglobulin; *SGOT,* serum glutamic-oxaloacetic transaminase.

TABLE 63 Significant Human Apolipoproteins

					PLASMA CONCENTRATION	
Apolipoprotein	Major Lipoproteins	Mr* (kDa)	Amino Acids	Chromosome	mmol/L	mg/dl
A-I	HDL	29	243-245	11	32-46	90-130
A-II	HDL	17.4	154	1	18-29	30-50
A-IV	HDL, LDL	44.5	396	11		
(a)	Lp(a)	350-700	Variable	6		
B-100	VLDL, IDL, LDL	512.7	4536	2	1.5-1.8	80-100
B-48	CM	240.8	2152	2	<0.2	<5
C-I	CM, LDL	6.6	57	19	6.1-10.8	4-7
C-II	CM, LDL	8.9	78 or 79	19	3.4-9.1	3-8
C-III	CM	8.8	79	11	9.1-17.1	8-15
D	HDL	19	169	3		
E	CM, LDL, IDL	34.1	299	19	0.8-1.6	3-6
F	HDL, LDL, VLDL	29	162	12		8.35
H	VLDL	50	326	17		20
J	HDL	80	449	8		
L	HDL	39-42	383	22	Not present in plasma	
M	HDL, LDL, VLDL, CM	26	188	6		2-15
0	HDL, LDL, VLDL	22.3	198	X		

CM, Chylomicron; *HDL,* high-density lipoprotein; *IDL,* intermediate-density lipoprotein; *LDL,* low-density lipoprotein; *Lp(a),* lipoprotein A; *VLDL,* very-low-density lipoprotein.
*Relative molecular mass.
From McPherson RA, Pincus MR: *Henry's clinical diagnosis and management by laboratory methods,* ed 23, St Louis, 2017, Elsevier.

Best current all-purpose screening test = HDV-Ab (total)
Best test to differentiate acute from chronic infection = HDV-Ab (IgM)

DELTA HEPATITIS COINFECTION (acute HDV1 acute HBV) or Superinfection (acute HDV1 chronic HBV)

HDV

-Ag

HDV-Ag: Shows current infection (acute or chronic) by HDV.
HDV nucleic acid probe: Detects antigen before and longer than HDV-Ag by EIA.

-Ab

HDV-Ab (IgM): High elevation in acute HDV; does not persist
Low or moderate elevation in convalescent HDV; does not persist
Low to high persistent elevation in chronic HDV (depends on degree of cell injury and sensitivity of the assay)
HDV-Ab (total): High elevation in acute HDV; does not persist
High persistent elevation in chronic HDV

HDV-AG

1. Detected by DNA probe, less often by immunoassay
Appearance: Prodromal stage (before symptoms); just at or after initial rise in ALT (about a wk after appearance of HB_SAg and about the time HB_CAb-IgM level begins to rise)
Peak: 2-3 days after onset
Becomes nondetectable: 1-4 days (may persist until shortly after symptoms appear)

HDV-AB (IgM)

Appearance: About 10 days after symptoms begin (range, 1-28 days)
Peak: About 2 wk after first detection
Becomes nondetectable: About 35 days (range, 10-80 days) after first detection (most other IgM antibodies take 3-6 months to become nondetectable)

HDV-AB (total)

Appearance: About 50 days after symptoms begin (range, 14-80 days); about 5 wk after HDV-Ag (range, 3-11 wk)
Peak: About 2 wk after first detection
Becomes nondetectable: About 7 months after first detection (range, 4-14 mo)

HER-2/*NEU*

Normal: Negative
Present in: 25%-30% of primary breast cancers. It can also be found in other epithelial tumors, including lung, hepatocellular, pancreatic, colon, stomach, ovarian, cervical, and bladder cancer. Trastuzumab (Herceptin) is a humanized monoclonal antibody against Her-2/*neu.* This test is useful to identify patients with metastatic; recurrent; and/or treatment-refractory, unresectable, locally advanced breast cancer for trastuzumab treatment.

HERPES SIMPLEX VIRUS (HSV)

Test description: The PCR test can be performed on serum biopsy samples, CSF, vitreous humor.

HFE SCREEN FOR HEREDITARY HEMOCHROMATOSIS

Test description: PCR test can be performed on whole blood or tissue. One mutation (C282Y) and two polymorphisms (H63D, S65C) account for the majority of alleles associated with this disease.

HETEROPHIL ANTIBODY

Normal: Negative
Positive in: Infectious mononucleosis

HIGH-DENSITY LIPOPROTEIN (HDL) CHOLESTEROL

Normal range
a. Male: 40-70 mg/dl (0.8-1.8 mmol/L [CF: 0.02586; SMI: 0.05 mmol/L])
b. Female: 50-90 mg/dl (1.1-2.35 mmol/L [CF: 0.02586; SMI: 0.05 mmol/L])
Increased in: Use of gemfibrozil, statins, fenofibrate, nicotinic acid, estrogens, regular aerobic exercise, small (1 oz) daily alcohol intake
Decreased in: Deficiency of apoproteins, liver disease, probucol ingestion, Tangier disease

NOTE: A cholesterol/HDL ratio >4.0 is associated with increased risk of coronary artery disease. Table 63 summarizes significant human apolipoproteins.

HLA ANTIGENS

Associated disorders: See Table 64.

HOMOCYSTEINE (plasma)

Normal range:

0-30 yr:	4.6-8.1 mcmol/L
30-59 yr:	6.3-11.2 mcmol/L (males), 4.5-7.9 mcmol/L (females)
>59 yr:	5.8-11.9 mcmol/L

TABLE 64 HLA Antigens Associated with Specific Diseases

Antigen	Condition	Antigen	Condition
HLA-B27	Ankylosing spondylitis	HLA-B8, Dw3	Celiac disease
	Reiter syndrome	HLA-B8, Dw3	Dermatitis herpetiformis
	Psoriatic arthritis	HLA-B8	Myasthenia gravis
HLA-A10, B18, Dw2	C2 deficiency	HLA-B8	Chronic active hepatitis in children
HLA-A2, B40, Cw3	C4 deficiency	HLA-Drw4	Active chronic hepatitis in adults
HLA-B7, Dw2	Multiple sclerosis	HLA-B13, Bw17	Psoriasis
HLA-A3	Hemochromatosis		

HLA, Human leukocyte antigen.
From Cerra FB: *Manual of critical care,* St Louis, 1987, Mosby.

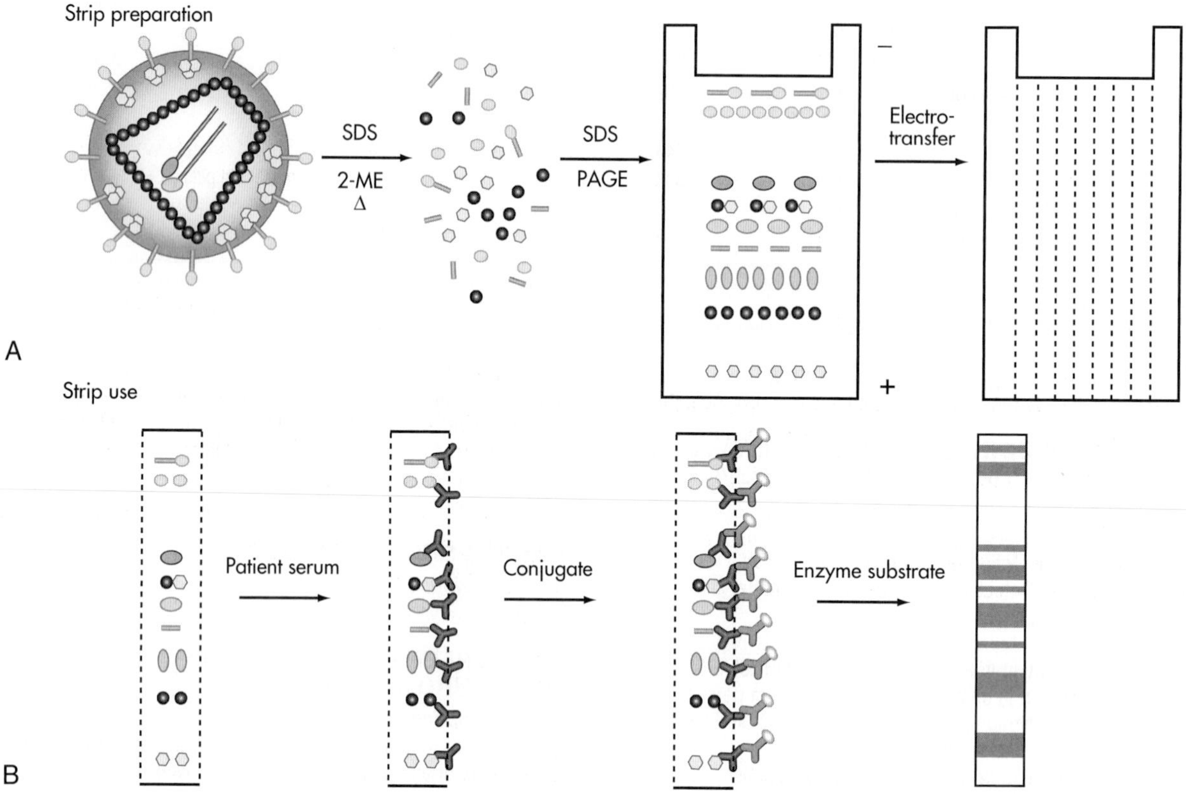

FIG. 31 Human immunodeficiency virus *(HIV)* Western blot. A, Western blot strips are prepared with purified HIV virions that are disrupted with ionic detergent and reducing agent, subjected to sodium dodecyl sulfate-polyacrylamide gel electrophoresis *(SDS-PAGE),* and electrotransferred to solid strips, typically of nitrocellulose. **B,** Strips are sequentially incubated with patient sample (serum, plasma, saliva, or urine); enzyme-conjugated antihuman IgG; and enzyme substrate. The positions of enzymes bound identify the presence of antibody to individual HIV proteins. (From Bennett JE et al: *Mandell, Douglas, and Bennett's principles and practice of infectious diseases*, ed 8, Philadelphia, 2015, Saunders.)

Increased: Thrombophilic states, B_6, B_{12}, folic acid, riboflavin deficiency, pregnancy, homocystinuria

NOTE: An increased homocysteine level is an independent risk factor for atherosclerosis.

HUMAN CHORIONIC GONADOTROPIN (hCG)

Normal range: Varies with gestational stage:

1 wk:	5-50 mU/ml
1-2 wk:	50-550 mU/ml
2-3 wk:	up to 5000 mU/ml
3-4 wk:	up to 10,000 mU/ml
4-5 wk:	up to 50,000 mU/ml
2-3 mo:	10,000-100,000 mU/ml

Elevated in: Normal pregnancy, hydatidiform mole, choriocarcinoma, germ cell tumors of testicle, some nontrophoblastic neoplasms (e.g., neoplasms of cervix, gastrointestinal tract, ovary, lung, breast)

HUMAN HERPES VIRUS 8 (HHV8)

Test description: PCR test can be performed on whole blood, tissue, bone marrow, and urine. HHV8 is found in all forms of Kaposi sarcoma.

HUMAN IMMUNODEFICIENCY VIRUS ANTIBODY, TYPE 1 (HIV-1)

Normal range: Not detected
Abnormal result: HIV antibodies usually appear in the blood 1-4 mo after infection.
Testing sequence:
ELISA is the recommended initial screening test. Sensitivity and specificity are >99%. False-positive ELISA may occur with autoimmune disorders, administration of immune globulin manufactured before 1985, within 6 wk of testing, in the presence of rheumatoid factor, in the presence of DLA-DR antibodies in multigravida female, with administration of influenza vaccine within 3 mo of testing, with hemodialysis, with positive

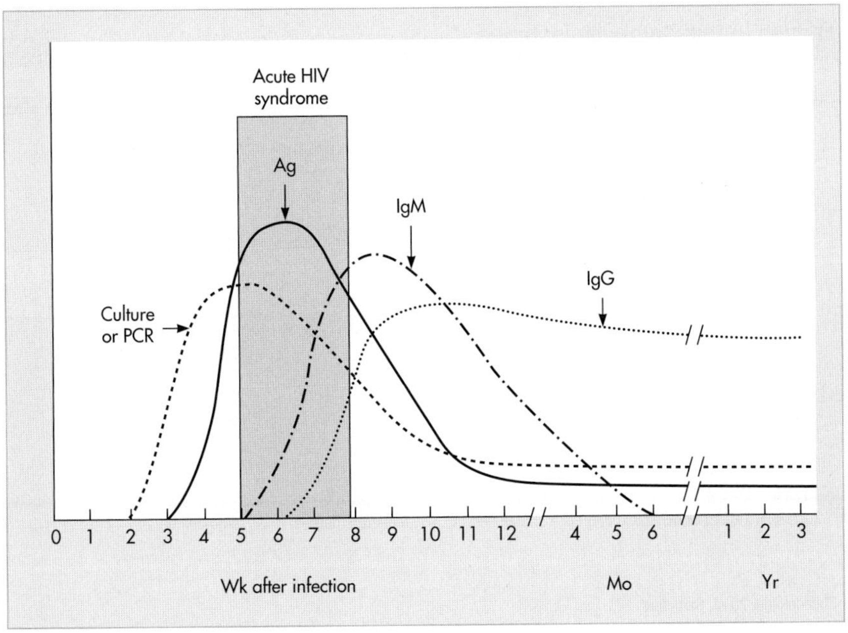

FIG. 32 Tests in human immunodeficiency virus (*HIV*)-1 infection. *Ag,* Antigen; *Ig,* immunoglobulin; *PCR,* polymerase chain reaction. (From Ravel R [ed]: *Clinical laboratory medicine,* ed 6, St Louis, 1995, Mosby.)

plasma reagin test, and with certain medical disorders (hemophilia, hypergammaglobulinemia, alcoholic hepatitis).

A positive ELISA is confirmed with Western blot (Fig. 31). False-positive Western blot may result from connective tissue disorders, human leukocyte antigen antibodies, polyclonal gammopathies, hyperbilirubinemia, presence of antibody to another human retrovirus, or cross-reaction with other non–virus-derived proteins in healthy persons. Undetermined Western blot may occur in AIDS patients with advanced immunodeficiency (caused by loss of antibodies) and in recent HIV infections.

PCR is used to confirm indeterminate Western blot results or negative results in persons with suspected HIV infection.

Fig. 32 describes tests in HIV infection; indications for plasma HIV RNA testing are described in Table 65.

HUMAN IMMUNODEFICIENCY VIRUS TYPE 1 (HIV-1) Antigen (p24), Qualitative (p24 antigen)

Normal range: Negative. This test detects uncomplexed HIV-1 p24 antigen. The core protein p24 is the first detectable protein encoded by the group-specific antigen *(gag)* gene. This protein is a marker for viremia. This test should not be used in place of HIV-1 antibody testing as a screen for HIV-1 infection. HIV-1 p24 may be detectable in the first mo of acute HIV-1 infection and generally falls to undetectable levels during the asymptomatic stage of HIV-1 infection. A negative result does not exclude the possibility of infection or exposure to HIV-1. It is recommended that a negative result be followed with repeat testing at least 8 wk after the original test. This test is used primarily for screening of donated blood and plasma and as an aid for the prognosis of HIV-1 infection.

HUMAN IMMUNODEFICIENCY VIRUS TYPE 1 (HIV-1) VIRAL LOAD

Normal range: HIV-1 RNA, quant. bDNA 3: Less than 50 copies/ml or less than 1.7 log copies/ml

This test should be used only in individuals with documented HIV-1 infection for monitoring the progression of infection, response to antiretroviral therapy, and disease prognosis. It is not indicated for diagnosis of HIV infection.

HUMAN PAPILLOMA VIRUS (HPV)

Test description: PCR test can be performed on cervical smears, biopsies, scrapings, liquid cytology specimen, and anogenital tissues.

HUNTINGTON DISEASE PCR

Test description: PCR can be performed on whole blood. Huntington disease is caused by the expansion of the trinucleotide repeat cytosine-adenine-guanine (CAG) within IT 15 (huntingtin). Pre- and posttest counseling should be performed when ordering this test.

TABLE 65 Indications for Plasma HIV RNA Testing*

Clinical Indication	Information	Use
Syndrome consistent with acute HIV infection	Establishes diagnosis when HIV antibody test is negative or indeterminate	Diagnosis†
Initial evaluation of newly diagnosed HIV infection	Baseline viral load set point	Decision to start or defer therapy
Every 3-4 mo in patients not on therapy	Changes in viral load	Decision to start therapy
4-8 wk after initiation of antiretroviral therapy	Initial assessment of drug efficacy	Decision to continue or change therapy
3-4 mo after start of therapy	Maximal effect of therapy	Decision to continue or change therapy
Every 3-4 mo in patients on therapy	Durability of antiretroviral effect	Decision to continue or change therapy
Clinical event or significant decline in CD4+ T cells	Association with changing or stable	Decision to continue, initiate, or change

HIV, Human immunodeficiency virus; *RNA,* ribonucleic acid.

*Acute illness (e.g., bacterial pneumonia, tuberculosis, herpes simplex virus [HSV], *Pneumocystis carinii* pneumonia [PCP]) and immunizations can cause increase in plasma HIV RNA for 2-4 wk; viral load testing should not be performed during this time. Plasma HIV RNA results should usually be verified with a repeat determination before starting or making changes in therapy. HIV RNA should be measured using the same laboratory and the same assay.

†Diagnosis of HIV infection determined by HIV RNA testing should be confirmed by standard methods (e.g., Western blot serology) performed 2-4 mo after the initial indeterminate or negative test.

HYDROGEN BREATH TEST

See "BREATH HYDROGEN TEST"

5-HYDROXYINDOLE-ACETIC ACID, URINE

See "URINE 5-HYDROXYINDOLE-ACETIC ACID"

TABLE 66 Selected Biologic Properties of Human Immunoglobulin Isotypes

Characteristics	IgG1	IgG2	IgG3	IgG4	IgM	IgA1	IgA2	IgD	IgE
Physical Properties									
Molecular weight (kD)	146	146	165	146	970*	160	160	170	190
Serum half-life (days)	29	27	7	16	5	6	6	–	2
Anatomic Distribution									
Mean serum level (mg/ml)	5-12	2-6	0.5-1.0	0.2-1.0	0.5-1.5	0.5-2.0	0-0.2	0-0.4	0-0.002
Transport across placenta	+++	+	++	±	–	–	–	–	–
Transport across epithelium	–	–	–	–	+	+++†	+++†	–	–
Extravascular diffusion	+++	+++	+++	+++	±	++‡	++‡	+	+
Functional Activity									
Antigen neutralization	++	++	++	++	++	++	++	–	–
Complement fixation	++	+	++	–	+++	+	+	–	–
ADCC	+	+	+	±	–	–	–	–	+
Immediate hypersensitivity	–	–	–	–	–	–	–	–	+++

ADCC, Antibody-dependent cellular cytotoxicity; *Ig*, immunoglobulin; –, no effect; ±, no effect or negligible degree; +, small degree; ++, moderate degree; +++, large degree.
*Pentameric IgM plus J chain.
†Dimer.
‡Monomer.
From Adkinson NF et al: *Middleton's allergy principles and practice*, ed 8, Philadelphia, 2014, Saunders.

IMMUNE COMPLEX ASSAY

Normal: Negative
Detected in: Collagen vascular disorders, glomerulonephritis, neoplastic diseases, malaria, primary biliary cirrhosis, chronic acute hepatitis, bacterial endocarditis, vasculitis

IMMUNOGLOBULINS

Normal range:
IgA: 50-350 mg/dl (0.5-3.5 g/L [CF: 0.01; SMI: 0.01 g/L])
IgD: <6 mg/dl (<60 mg/L [CF: 0.01; SMI: 0.01 g/L])
IgE: <25 μg/dl (<0.00025 g/L [CF: 0.01; SMI: 0.01 g/L])
IgG: 800-1500 mg/dl (8-15 g/L [CF: 0.01; SMI: 0.01 g/L])
IgM: 45-150 mg/dl (0.45-1.5 g/L [CF: 0.01; SMI: 0.01 g/L])

Table 66 summarizes biologic properties of human immunoglobulin isotopes. Box 19 summarizes selected conditions associated with monoclonal immunoglobulins. Disease states associated with polyclonal hyperimmunoglobulinemia are described in Table 67.
Elevated in
17. **IgA:** Lymphoproliferative disorders, Berger nephropathy, chronic infections, autoimmune disorders, liver disease
18. **IgE:** Allergic disorders, parasitic infections, immunologic disorders, IgE myeloma (see Box 20 for summary of nonallergic diseases associated with high levels of IgE. Box 21 summarizes conditions with very high IgE levels)
19. **IgG:** Chronic granulomatous infections, infectious diseases, inflammation, myeloma, liver disease
20. **IgM:** Primary biliary cirrhosis, infectious diseases (brucellosis, malaria), Waldenström macroglobulinemia, liver disease

Decreased in
IgA: Nephrotic syndrome, protein-losing enteropathy, congenital deficiency, lymphocytic leukemia, ataxia-telangiectasia, chronic sinopulmonary disease
IgE: Hypogammaglobulinemia, neoplasms (breast, bronchial, cervical), ataxia-telangiectasia, primary biliary cirrhosis (see Box 20)
IgG: Congenital or acquired deficiency, lymphocytic leukemia, phenytoin, methylprednisolone, nephrotic syndrome, protein-losing enteropathy
IgM: Congenital deficiency, lymphocytic leukemia, nephrotic syndrome

INDIRECT ANTIGLOBULIN (Coombs Indirect)

Normal: Negative

BOX 19 Selected Conditions Associated with Monoclonal Immunoglobulins

Multiple myeloma
Macroglobulinemia of Waldenström
Chronic lymphocytic leukemia
Other leukemias
Lymphomas
"Benign" monoclonal gammopathy
Systemic capillary leak syndrome
Amyloidosis
Chronic liver disease such as chronic active hepatitis, primary biliary cirrhosis
Autoimmune disorders, including rheumatoid arthritis, systemic lupus erythematosus, thyroiditis, pernicious anemia, polyarteritis nodosa, Sjögren syndrome
Gaucher disease
Malignancies of various types
Hereditary spherocytosis
HIV infection, including AIDS

AIDS, Acquired immune deficiency syndrome; *HIV*, human immunodeficiency virus.
From McPherson RA, Pincus MR: *Henry's clinical diagnosis and management by laboratory methods*, ed 23, St Louis, 2017, Elsevier.

Positive: Acquired hemolytic anemia, incompatible cross-matched blood, anti-Rh antibodies, drugs (methyldopa, mefenamic acid, levodopa)
Fig. 33 illustrates the mechanism of Coombs test.

INFLUENZA A AND B TESTS

Test description: PCR can be performed on nasopharyngeal swab, wash, or aspirate.
Normal: Negative

INSULIN AUTOANTIBODIES

Normal: Negative
Present in: Exogenous insulin from insulin therapy. The presence of islet cell antibodies indicates ongoing beta cell destruction. This test is useful in the early diagnosis of type 1a diabetes mellitus and in the identification of patients at high risk for type 1a diabetes.

INSULIN, FREE

Normal: <17 mcU/ml
Elevated in: Insulin overdose, insulin resistance syndromes, endogenous hyperinsulinemia

TABLE 67 Polyclonal Hyperimmunoglobulinemias: Some Associated Disease States

Condition	Immunoglobulin (Ig) Classes
Immunodeficiency Diseases	
Hyperimmunoglobulin E and recurrent infections	IgE
Wiskott-Aldrich syndrome	IgA, IgE
"Dysgammaglobulinemia type I"	IgM
Hyperimmunoglobulin A and recurrent infections	IgA
Acquired immune deficiency syndrome (AIDS)	All classes
Infections	
Congenital infections (syphilis, toxoplasmosis, rubella, cytomegalovirus)	IgM
Infectious mononucleosis	IgM or all
Trypanosomiasis	IgM or all
Intestinal parasitism	All classes
Several helminthic infections	IgE
Visceral larva migrans	All classes
Chronic granulomatous disease of childhood	All classes
Leprosy	All classes
Chronic infection in general	All classes, with a preference for IgG
Liver Diseases	
Chronic active hepatitis	IgG predominates
Acute hepatitis	IgG predominates
Biliary cirrhosis	IgM predominates
Lupoid hepatitis	All classes
Pulmonary Disorders	
Pulmonary hypersensitivity syndrome	All classes
Sarcoidosis	All classes
Berylliosis	All classes
"Autoimmune" Disorders	
Systemic lupus erythematosus	All classes
Rheumatoid arthritis	IgA or all
Many "autoimmune" states such as thyroiditis	All classes
Scleroderma	All classes
Cold agglutinin disease	IgM
Anaphylactoid purpura	IgA
Miscellaneous	
Down syndrome	All classes
Amyloidosis	All classes
Narcotic addiction	IgM
Renal tubular disease	All classes

From McPherson RA, Pincus MR: *Henry's clinical diagnosis and management by laboratory methods*, ed 23, St Louis, 2017, Elsevier.

Decreased in: Inadequately treated type 1 diabetes mellitus

INSULIN-LIKE GROWTH FACTOR-1 (IGF-1) (Serum)

Normal range:

Ages 16-24:	182-780 ng/ml
Ages 25-39:	114-492 ng/ml
Ages 40-54:	90-360 ng/ml
Ages >55:	71-290 ng/ml

BOX 20 Nonallergic Diseases Associated with Altered Total Serum Immunoglobulin E Levels

Increased Levels (≥500 IU/ml)

Parasitic Diseases
Ascariasis
Visceral larva migrans
Capillariasis
Paragonimiasis
Fascioliasis
Schistosomiasis
Hookworm
Trichinosis
Filariasis
Strongyloidiasis
Echinococcosis
Onchocerciasis
Malaria

Infections
Allergic bronchopulmonary mycosis
Systemic candidiasis
Coccidioidomycosis
Leprosy
Epstein-Barr virus mononucleosis
Cytomegalovirus mononucleosis
Viral respiratory infections
Human immunodeficiency virus (HIV) type 1 infections
Pertussis

Cutaneous Diseases
Alopecia areata
Bullous pemphigoid
Chronic acral dermatitis
Streptococcal erythema nodosum

Other Diseases and Disorders
Nephrotic syndrome
Drug-induced interstitial nephritis
Liver disease
Cystic fibrosis
Kawasaki disease
Infantile polyarteritis nodosa
Primary pulmonary hemosiderosis
Guillain-Barré syndrome
Burns
Rheumatoid arthritis
Bone marrow transplantation
Cigarette smoking
Alcoholism

Neoplastic Diseases
Hodgkin disease
Immunoglobulin E (IgE) myeloma
Bronchial carcinoma

Immunodeficiency Diseases
Wiskott-Aldrich syndrome
Hyper-IgE syndrome
Thymic hypoplasia (DiGeorge syndrome)
Cellular immunodeficiency with immunoglobulins (Nezelof syndrome)
Selective IgA deficiency

Medications
Enfuvirtide
Pholcodine

Decreased Levels (<5 IU/ml)
Familial IgE deficiency and recurrent sinopulmonary infections
Human T cell lymphotropic virus type 1 infections
Primary biliary cirrhosis

From Adkinson NF et al: *Middleton's allergy principles and practice*, ed 8, Philadelphia, 2014, Saunders.

Elevated in: Adolescence, acromegaly, pregnancy, precocious puberty, obesity
Decreased in: Malnutrition, delayed puberty, diabetes mellitus, hypopituitarism, cirrhosis, old age

INSULIN-LIKE GROWTH FACTOR-II

Normal range: 288-736 ng/ml
Elevated in: Hypoglycemia associated with non-islet cell tumors, hepatoma, and Wilms tumor
Decreased in: Growth hormone deficiency

INTERNATIONAL NORMALIZED RATIO (INR)

The INR is a comparative rating of prothrombin time (PT) ratios. The INR represents the observed PT ratio adjusted by the International Reference Thromboplastin. It provides a universal result indicative of what the patient's PT result would have been if measured using the primary World Health Organization International Reference reagent. For proper interpretation of INR values, the patient should be on stable anticoagulant therapy.

BOX 21 Conditions Associated with Unusually High Serum Immunoglobulin E Concentrations (≥500 IU/ml)

Allergic bronchopulmonary mycosis
Allergic fungal sinusitis
Atopic dermatitis
Human immunodeficiency virus (HIV) infection
Hyperimmunoglobulin E (hyper-IgE) syndrome
Immunoglobulin E myeloma
Kimura disease
Lymphoma
Netherton syndrome
Systemic helminthic parasitosis
Tuberculosis

From Adkinson NF et al: *Middleton's allergy principles and practice*, ed 8, Philadelphia, 2014, Saunders.

RECOMMENDED INR RANGES

Proximal deep vein thrombosis:	2-3
Pulmonary embolism:	2-3
Transient ischemic attacks:	2-3
Atrial fibrillation:	2-3
Mechanical prosthetic valves:	2.5-3.5
Recurrent venous thromboembolic disease:	2.5-3.5

INTRINSIC FACTOR ANTIBODIES

Normal: Negative
Present in: Pernicious anemia (>50% of patients). Cyanocobalamin may give false-positive results.

IRON (Serum)

Normal: Male: 65-175 mcg/dl; female: 50-1170 mcg/dl
Elevated in: Hemochromatosis, excessive iron therapy, repeated transfusions, lead poisoning, hemolytic anemia, aplastic anemia, pernicious anemia
Decreased in: Iron deficiency anemia, hypothyroidism, chronic infection

IRON-BINDING CAPACITY, TOTAL (TIBC)

Normal range: 250-460 μg/dl (45-82 μmol/L [CF: 0.1791; SMI: 1 μmol/L])
Elevated in: Iron deficiency anemia, pregnancy, polycythemia, hepatitis, weight loss
Decreased in: Anemia of chronic disease, hemochromatosis, chronic liver disease, hemolytic anemias, malnutrition (protein depletion)
Table 68 describes TIBC and serum iron abnormalities.

IRON SATURATION (% Transferrin Saturation)

Normal
m. Male: 20%-50%
n. Female: 15%-50%
Elevated in: Hemochromatosis, excessive iron intake, aplastic anemia, thalassemia, vitamin B_6 deficiency
Decreased in: Hypochromic anemias, GI malignancyLactate (blood)
Normal range: 0.5-2.0 mEq/L

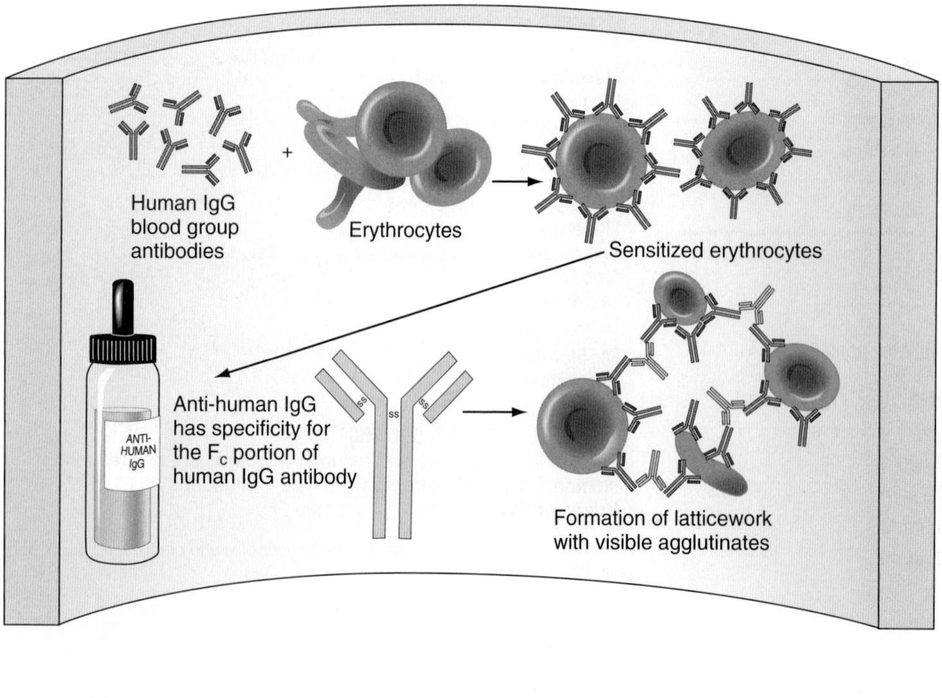

FIG. 33 Antihuman globulin antibodies form a bridge between adjacent erythrocytes sensitized with human immunoglobulin *(Ig)*G or complement components. (From McPherson RA, Pincus MR: *Henry's clinical diagnosis and management by laboratory methods*, ed 23, St Louis, 2017, Elsevier.)

TABLE 68 Serum Iron and Total Iron-Binding Capacity Patterns

SI↓	TIBC↓	Chronic diseases; uremia
SI↓	TIBC↑	Chronic iron deficiency anemia; pregnancy in third trimester
SI↑	TIBC↓	Hemochromatosis iron therapy overload (TIBC may be normal); hemolytic anemia; thalassemia; lead poisoning; megaloblastic anemia; aplastic, pyridoxine deficiency, or other sideroblastic anemias
SI↑	TIBC↑	Oral contraceptives; acute hepatitis (some report TIBC is low normal); chronic hepatitis (some patients)
SI↑	TIBCNL	B_{12} or folate deficiency
SI↓	TIBCNL	Chronic iron deficiency (some patients); acute infection, surgery, tissue damage
SI NL	TIBC↑	B_{12}/folate deficiency plus iron deficiency

NL, Normal; *SI,* serum iron; *TIBC,* total iron-binding capacity.

Elevated in: Tissue hypoxia (shock, respiratory failure, severe CHF, severe anemia, carbon monoxide or cyanide poisoning), systemic disorders (liver or renal failure, seizures), abnormal intestinal flora (d-lactic acidosis), drugs or toxins (salicylates, ethanol, methanol, ethylene glycol), G6PD deficiency

LACTATE DEHYDROGENASE (LDH)

Normal range: 50-150 U/L (0.82-2.66 μkat/L [CF: 0.01667; SMI: 0.02 μkat/L])
Elevated in: Infarction of myocardium, lung, kidney
Diseases of cardiopulmonary system, liver, collagen, central nervous system
Hemolytic anemias, megaloblastic anemias, transfusions, seizures, muscle trauma, muscular dystrophy, acute pancreatitis, hypotension, shock, infectious mononucleosis, inflammation, neoplasia, intestinal obstruction, hypothyroidism

LACTATE DEHYDROGENASE ISOENZYMES

Normal range:

LDH_1: 22%-36% (cardiac, red blood cell) (0.22-0.36 [CF: 0.01, SMI: 0.01])
LDH_2: 35%-46% (cardiac, red blood cell) (0.35-0.46)
LDH_3: 13%-26% (pulmonary) (0.15-0.26)
LDH_4: 3%-10% (striated muscle, liver) (0.03-0.1)
LDH_5: 2%-9% (striated muscle, liver) (0.02-0.09)

Normal ratios
o. $LDH_1 < LDH_2$
p. $LDH_5 < LDH_4$
Abnormal values
LDH1 >LDH2: Myocardial infarction (can also be seen with hemolytic anemias, pernicious anemia, folate deficiency, renal infarct)
LDH5 >LDH4: Liver disease (cirrhosis, hepatitis, hepatic congestion)

LACTOSE TOLERANCE TEST (serum)

Normal: Test is performed by giving 2 g/kg body weight lactose orally and drawing glucose level at 0, 30, 45, 60, and 90 min. Normal response is change in glucose from fasting value to >30 mg/dl. Inconclusive response is increase of 20-30 mg/dl, abnormal response is increase <20 mg/dl. Table 69 summarizes laboratory tests in the differential diagnosis of diarrhea.
Abnormal in: Lactase deficiency

LAP SCORE

See "LEUKOCYTE ALKALINE PHOSPHATASE"

LEAD

Normal: Child, <10 mcg/dl; adult, <25 mcg/dl; acceptable for industrial exposure, <50 mcg/dl
Elevated in: Lead exposure, lead poisoning

LDH

See "LACTATE DEHYDROGENASE"

LDL

See "LOW-DENSITY LIPOPROTEIN CHOLESTEROL"

LEGIONELLA PNEUMOPHILA PCR

Test description: PCR can be performed on lung tissue, water sputum, bronchoalveolar lavage, and other respiratory fluids.

LEGIONELLA TITER

Normal: Negative
Positive in: Legionnaires disease (presumptive: ≥1:256 titer; definitive: fourfold titer increase to ≥1:128)

LEUKOCYTE ALKALINE PHOSPHATASE (LAP)

Normal range: 13-100 (33-188 U)
Elevated in: Leukemoid reactions, neutrophilia secondary to infections (except in sickle cell crisis—no significant increase in LAP score), Hodgkin disease, polycythemia vera, hairy cell leukemia, aplastic anemia, Down syndrome, myelofibrosis
Decreased in: Acute and chronic granulocytic leukemia, thrombocytopenic purpura, paroxysmal nocturnal hemoglobinuria, hypophosphatemia, collagen disorders

LEUKOCYTE COUNT

See "COMPLETE BLOOD COUNT"

LIPASE

Normal range: 0-160 U/L (0-2.66 μkat/L [CF: 0.01667; SMI: 0.02 μkat/L])
Elevated in: Acute pancreatitis, perforated peptic ulcer, carcinoma of pancreas (early stage), pancreatic duct obstruction, bowel infarction, intestinal obstruction

LIPOPROTEIN(a)

Normal: Male: 1.35-19.6 mg/dl; female: 1.24-20.1 mg/dl. Fig. 34 illustrates lipoprotein structure. Table 70 summarizes the major classes of human plasma lipoproteins. The chemical composition of major classes of plasma lipoproteins is described in Table 71.
Elevated in: Coronary artery disease, uncontrolled diabetes, hypothyroidism, chronic renal failure, pregnancy, tobacco use, infections, nephritic syndrome
Decreased in: Niacin, omega-3 fatty acids, estrogens, tamoxifen, statins

LIPOPROTEIN CHOLESTEROL, HIGH-DENSITY

See "HIGH-DENSITY LIPOPROTEIN CHOLESTEROL"

LIPOPROTEIN CHOLESTEROL, LOW-DENSITY

See "LOW-DENSITY LIPOPROTEIN CHOLESTEROL"

LIVER KIDNEY MICROSOME TYPE 1 ANTIBODIES (LKM1)

Normal: <20 U
Elevated in: Autoimmune hepatitis type 2

TABLE 69 Laboratory Tests in the Differential Diagnosis of Diarrhea

Test	Method	Use
Initial Screening Tests		
Fecal leukocytes	Wright stain or methylene blue	Identify inflammatory diarrhea
Fecal occult blood test	Immunochemical	Detect blood
Fecal osmotic gap	290 − 2 × (fecal Na^+ + K^+)	Distinguish secretory vs. osmotic diarrhea
Stool alkalinization	Color change after adding NaOH to stool/urine	Phenolphthalein laxative ingestion
Infectious Causes		
Stool bacterial culture	Routine culture and sensitivity	Identify *Shigella, Salmonella*
Stool special culture	Specialized culture and serotyping	Identify *E. coli* 0157:H7, *Yersinia, Campylobacter*
Stool *C. difficile* toxin assay	EIA for toxins A and B	Pseudomembranous colitis
HIV serology	EIA, Western blot	HIV enteritis
Stool rotavirus screen	EIA for antigen	Rotavirus enteritis
Stool ova and parasites	Concentration and stains	Enteric parasitic infection
Stool mycobacteria	Acid-fast stain, culture and sensitivity, PCR	*Mycobacterium*, antibiotic selection
Stool *E. histolytica* Ag	EIA for antigen	*Entamoeba histolytica*
Stool *Giardia* Ag	EIA for antigen	*Giardia lamblia*
Stool *Cryptosporidium* Ag	EIA for antigen	*Cryptosporidium parvum*
Endocrine Causes		
Urine 5-HIAA or blood serotonin	HPLC	Carcinoid syndrome
Serum VIP	RIA	VIPoma
Serum TSH, free T4	Immunoassay	Hyperthyroidism
Serum gastrin	RIA	Zollinger-Ellison syndrome
Serum calcitonin	RIA	Hypocalcemia-related diarrhea
Serum somatostatin	RIA	Somatostatinoma
Malabsorption		
Lactose tolerance test	See text	Lactase deficiency
Stool reducing sugars	Clinitest tablets	Carbohydrate intolerance
Sweat chloride	See text	Cystic fibrosis
D-Xylose absorption test	See text	Evaluate pancreatic and jejunal function
Fecal fat stain	Fat stain	Lipid malabsorption
Serum carotene	Spectrophotometry	Lipid malabsorption
^{14}C-glyceryl trioleate test malabsorption	See text	Lipid malabsorption
Serum IgA	Nephelometry	Rule out IgA deficiency
Antitissue transglutaminase antibody	EIA	Celiac disease
Hydrogen breath test	Electrochemical hydrogen monitorinomatography g	Carbohydrate malabsorption
Bacterial colony count	Small bowel aspirate and quantitative culture	Bacterial overgrowth
Other		
Serum ionized calcium	Ion-specific electrode	Hypocalcemia-related diarrhea
Serum protein and albumin	Nephelometry, photometry	IBD, protein-losing enteropathy
Stool alpha-1-antitrypsin	Nephelometry	Protein-losing enteropathy
Quantitative immunoglobulins	Nephelometry	Agammaglobulinemia
7α-Hydroxy-4-cholestin-3-one	HPLC	Bile salt malabsorption
Fecal elastase or pancreolauryl test	EIA	Pancreatic insufficiency
Intestinal biopsy	Endoscopic or open biopsy	Whipple disease, MAI, abetalipoproteinemia, neoplasia, lymphoma, amyloidosis, eosinophilic gastroenteritis, agammaglobulinemia, intestinal lymphangiectasia, Crohn disease, tuberculosis, graft-versus-host disease, *Giardia*, other parasitic infections, collagenous colitis, microscopic colitis
Extraintestinal causes	See text	Hyperthyroidism, diabetes, hypoparathyroidism, adrenal cortical insufficiency, hormone-secreting tumors

5-HIAA, 5-Hydroxyindoleacetic acid; *Ab,* antibody; *Ag,* antigen; *EIA,* enzyme immunoassay; *HIV,* human immunodeficiency virus; *HPLC,* high-performance liquid chromatography; *IBD,* inflammatory bowel disease; *Ig,* immunoglobulin; *MAI, Mycobacterium avium-intracellulare*; *PCR,* polymerase chain reaction; *RIA,* radioimmunoassay; *T4,* thyroxine; *TSH,* thyroid-stimulating hormone; *VIP,* vasoactive intestinal peptide; *VIPoma,* vasoactive intestinal peptide tumor.

From McPherson RA, Pincus MR: *Henry's clinical diagnosis and management by laboratory methods*, ed 23, St Louis, 2017, Elsevier.

LKM1

See "LIVER KIDNEY MICROSOME TYPE 1 ANTIBODIES"

LOW-DENSITY LIPOPROTEIN (LDL) CHOLESTEROL

Normal range: 50-130 mg/dl (1.30-1.68 mmol/L [CF: 0.02586; SMI: 0.05 mmol/L]). Fig. 35 illustrates the LDL receptor pathway and regulation of cholesterol metabolism.

<70	Optimal in diabetics, prior MI, and patients with cardiac risk factors
100-129	Near or above optimal
130-159	Borderline high
160-189	High
≥190	Very high

LUPUS ANTICOAGULANT

See "CIRCULATING ANTICOAGULANT"

LUTEINIZING HORMONE

Luteinizing hormone (LH) changes during the menstrual cycle are illustrated in Fig. 36. LH changes in different disease states are summarized in Table 72.

Normal range: 5-25 mIU/ml

Elevated in: Postmenopause, pituitary adenoma, primary gonadal dysfunction, polycystic ovary syndrome

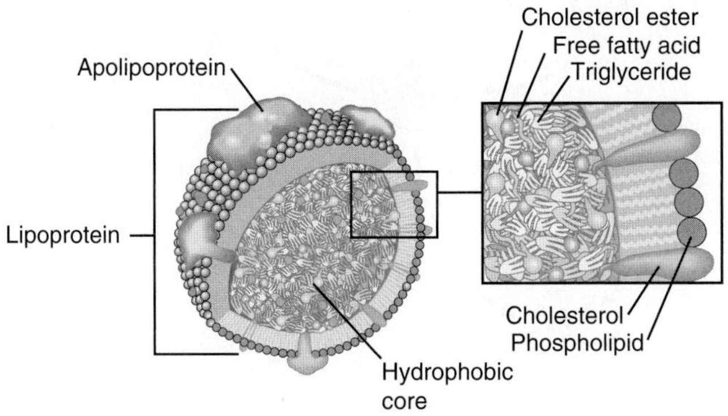

FIG. 34 Lipoprotein structure. Lipoproteins are spherical particles with a hydrophobic core and an amphiphilic surface. The surface consists of a single layer of phospholipids. This surface layer also contains proteins and free cholesterol. The hydrophobic core mainly contains triglycerides and cholesterol esters. (From McPherson RA, Pincus MR: *Henry's clinical diagnosis and management by laboratory methods*, ed 23, St Louis, 2017, Elsevier.)

Decreased in: Severe illness, anorexia nervosa, malnutrition, pituitary or hypothalamic impairment, severe stress

LYME DISEASE ANTIBODY TITER

Normal range: Negative

Positive result: Fig. 37 illustrates the usual serologic response in Lyme disease.

A serologic test is not necessary or helpful for several days after a tick bite because it is only 40%-50% sensitive in this stage, and a negative test does not rule out the diagnosis.

LYMPHOCYTES

Normal range

15%-40%

Total lymphocyte count = 800-2600/mm^3

Total T lymphocyte = 800-2200/mm^3

CD4 lymphocytes = ≥ 400/mm^3

CD8 lymphocytes = 200-800/mm^3

Normal CD4/CD8 ratio is 2.0.

Elevated in: Chronic infections, infectious mononucleosis and other viral infections, chronic lymphocytic leukemia, Hodgkin disease, ulcerative colitis, hypoadrenalism, idiopathic thrombocytopenia

Decreased in

AIDS, bone marrow suppression from chemotherapeutic agents or chemotherapy, aplastic anemia, neoplasms, steroids, adrenocortical hyperfunction, neurologic disorders (multiple sclerosis, myasthenia gravis, Guillain-Barré syndrome)

CD4 lymphocytes are calculated as total white blood cells × % lymphocytes × % lymphocytes stained with CD4. They are decreased in AIDS and other immune dysfunction.

Table 73 describes various lymphocyte abnormalities in peripheral blood.

Box 22 summarizes key causes of lymphocytopenia.

TABLE 70 Major Classes of Human Plasma Lipoproteins: Physicochemical Characteristics

Particle	Electrophoretic Mobility*	Major Apolipoproteins	Diameter (Å)	Density (kg/L)	Sf†
Chylomicrons	Origin	ApoA-I, A-IV, B-48, C-I, C-II, C-III, E	750-12,000	<0.95	>400
VLDL	Pre-β	ApoB-100, C-I, C-II, C-III, E	300-700	0.95-1.006	20-400
IDL	β or pre-β	ApoB-100, E1.006-1.019	12-20		
LDL	B	ApoB-100	180-300	1.019-1.063	0-12
HDL_2	A	ApoA-I, A-II, E	50-120	1.063-1.125	
HDL_3	A	ApoA-II, A-I, E	50-120	1.125-1.210	
Lp(a)	Pre-β	ApoB-100, Apo(a)		1.045-1.080	

HDL_2, Ultracentrifugation subclass of high-density lipoprotein; *HDL_3*, ultracentrifugation subclass of high-density lipoprotein; *IDL*, intermediate-density lipoprotein; *LDL*, low-density lipoprotein; *Lp(a)*, lipoprotein A; *VLDL*, very-low-density lipoprotein.
*Agarose gel electrophoresis.
†Svedberg flotation rate.
From McPherson RA, Pincus MR: *Henry's clinical diagnosis and management by laboratory methods*, ed 23, St Louis, 2017, Elsevier.

TABLE 71 Chemical Composition of Major Classes of Plasma Lipoproteins

	Protein (%)*	Free Cholesterol (%)	Cholesterol Esters (%)	Triglyceride (%)	Phospholipid (%)
Chylomicrons	1-2	1-3	2-4	80-95	3-6
VLDL	6-10	4-8	16-22	45-65	15-20
IDL	Intermediate between VLDL and LDL				
LDL	18-22	6-8	45-50	4-8	18-24
HDL	45-55	3-5	15-20	2-7	26-32

HDL, High-density lipoprotein; *IDL*, intermediate-density lipoprotein; *LDL*, low-density lipoprotein; *VLDL*, very-low-density lipoprotein.
*Percentage of dry weight.
From McPherson RA, Pincus MR: *Henry's clinical diagnosis and management by laboratory methods*, ed 23, St Louis, 2017, Elsevier.
Data from Albers (1974), Gaubatz et al (1983), Fless et al (1984), Gotto et al (1986), Gries et al (1988), and Hegele (2009).

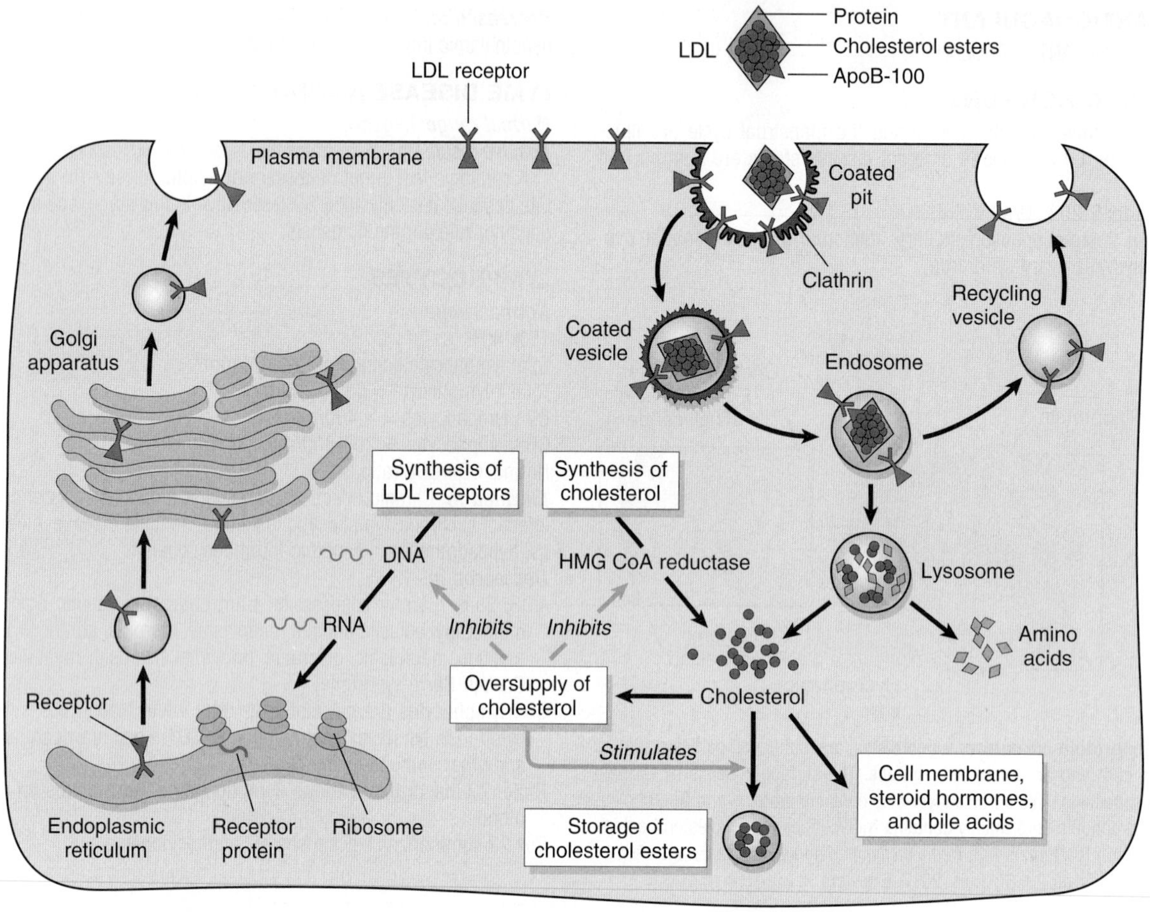

FIG. 35 The low-density lipoprotein *(LDL)* receptor pathway and regulation of cholesterol metabolism. *Apo,* Apolipoprotein; *DNA,* deoxyribonucleic acid; *HMG CoA,* 3-hydroxy-3-methylglutaryl coenzyme A; *RNA,* ribonucleic acid. (From McPherson RA, Pincus MR: *Henry's clinical diagnosis and management by laboratory methods*, ed 23, St Louis, 2017, Elsevier.)

MAGNESIUM (serum)

See Figs. 38 and 39.

Normal range: 1.8-3.0 mg/dl (0.80-1.20 mmol/L [CF: 0.4114; SMI: 0.02 mmol/L])

CAUSES OF HYPERMAGNESEMIA

Decreased renal excretion
Renal failure—glomerular filtration rate less than 30 ml/min
Hyperparathyroidism
Hypothyroidism
Addison disease
Lithium intoxication
Familial hypocalciuric hypercalcemia
Other causes: Usually in association with decrease in glomerular filtration rate
Endogenous loads
Diabetic ketoacidosis
Severe tissue injury: Burns
Exogenous loads
Gastrointestinal
- Magnesium-containing laxatives and antacids
- High-dose vitamin D analogs

Parenteral: Management of toxemia of pregnancy

CAUSES OF HYPOMAGNESEMIA

Alcohol abuse
Diuretic use
Renal losses
Acute and chronic renal failure
Postobstructive diuresis
Acute tubular necrosis
Chronic glomerulonephritis
Chronic pyelonephritis
Interstitial nephropathy
Renal transplantation
Gastrointestinal losses
Chronic diarrhea
Nasogastric suctioning
Short bowel syndrome
Protein-calorie malnutrition
Bowel fistula
Total parenteral nutrition
Acute pancreatitis
Endocrine
Diabetes mellitus
Hyperaldosteronism
Hyperthyroidism
Hyperparathyroidism
Acute intermittent porphyria
Pregnancy
Drugs
Aminoglycosides

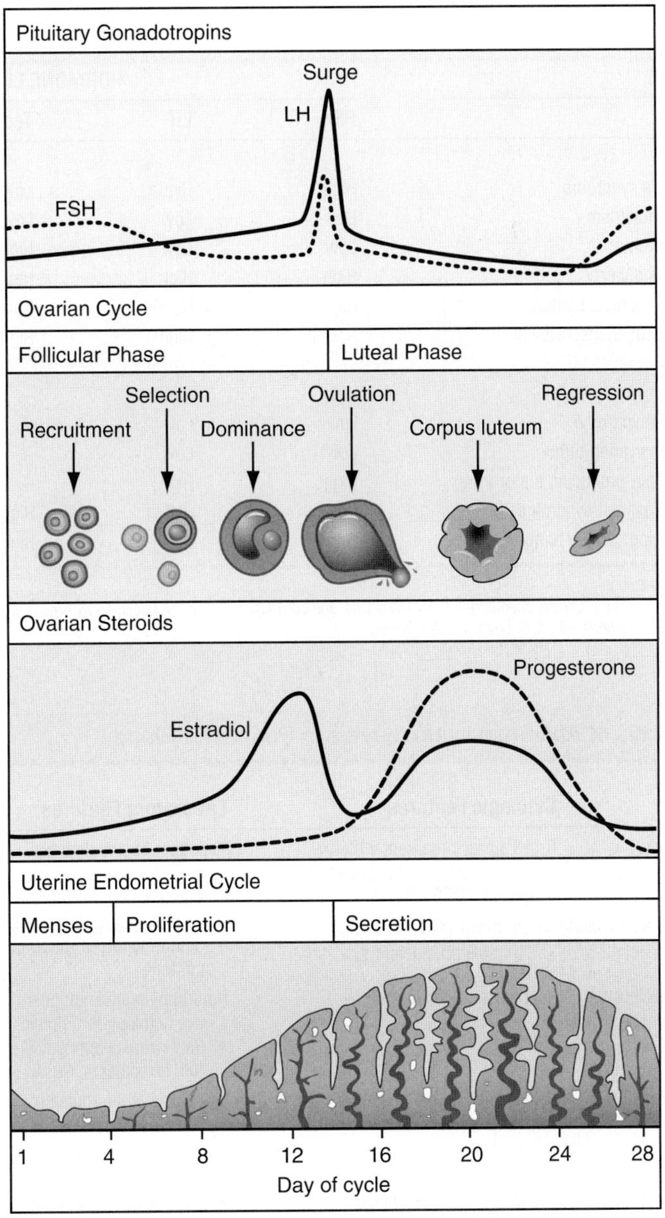

FIG. 36 Pituitary, ovarian, and uterine changes during the human menstrual cycle. *FSH,* Follicle-stimulating hormone; *LH,* luteinizing hormone. (From McPherson RA, Pincus MR: *Henry's clinical diagnosis and management by laboratory methods*, ed 23, St Louis, 2017, Elsevier.)

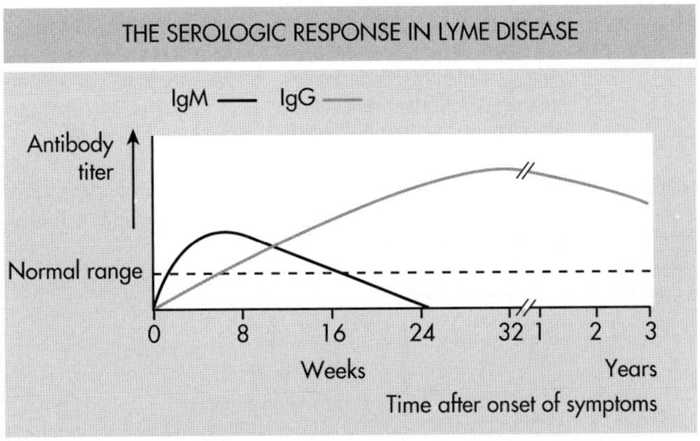

FIG. 37 Immunoglobulin (Ig)M and IgG responses in Lyme disease.

TABLE 72 Changes in Reproductive Hormone Levels in Different Disease States

DISEASE STATE		HORMONE LEVEL			
Classification	**Example**	**FSH**	**LH**	**Testosterone**	**Estradiol**
Male					
Primary deficiency	Klinefelter's syndrome	High	High	Low	–
Secondary deficiency	Panhypopituitarism	Low	Low	Low	–
Primary excess	Testicular tumor	Low	Low	High	–
Secondary excess	Precocious puberty	High	High	High	–
Other	Seminiferous tubule failure	High	Normal	Normal	–
Other	Partial androgen insensitivity	Normal	High	High	–
Female					
Primary deficiency	Menopause	High	High	–	Low
Secondary deficiency	Sheehan's syndrome	Low	Low	–	Low
Primary excess	Feminizing ovarian tumor	Low	Low	–	High
Secondary excess	Gonadotropin-producing tumor (rare)	High	High	–	High
Other	Polycystic ovarian syndrome	Normal	High	High	–
Other	Masculinizing ovarian tumor	Low	Low	High	–

FSH, Follicle-stimulating hormone; *LH,* luteinizing hormone.
From Nickel KL: The gonads. In Kaplan LA, Pesce AJ, editors: *Clinical chemistry—theory, analysis, and correlation,* 3rd ed. St Louis, 1996, Mosby, pp 892–911. In: McPherson RA, Pincus MR: *Henry's clinical diagnosis and management by laboratory methods*, ed 23, St Louis, 2017, Elsevier.

TABLE 73 Differential Diagnosis of Abnormal Lymphocytes in Peripheral Blood

Lymphocyte Type	Usual Disease Association	Cytologic Features	Laboratory Features	Clinical Features
Small lymphocyte	Chronic lymphocytic leukemia	B-cell surface markers with low concentration of surface immunoglobulin, CD5 antigen	Hypogammaglobulinemia in 50%; positive direct Coombs test in 15%; on node biopsy, diffuse, well-differentiated lymphocytic infiltrate	Elderly adults; presentation runs gamut from asymptomatic with lymphocytosis only to bulky disease with adenopathy, splenomegaly, and "packed" bone marrow
Atypical lymphocyte	Infectious mononucleosis, other viral illnesses	Suppressor T-cell markers	Heterophil agglutinin; positive serology for Epstein-Barr virus, cytomegalovirus, toxoplasma, HBsAg	Pharyngitis, fever, adenopathy, rash, splenomegaly, palatal petechiae, jaundice
Plasmacytoid lymphocyte	Waldenström macroglobulin anemia	Cytoplasmic IgM, periodic acid-Schiff positivity	IgM paraprotein, rouleaux, cryoglobulins	Adenopathy, splenomegaly, absence of bone lesions, hyperviscosity syndrome, cryopathic phenomena
Lymphoblast	ALL	Terminal transferase positivity, common ALL antigen, B- or T-precursor markers	Anemia, granulocytopenia, thrombocytopenia, hyperuricemia, diffuse bone marrow infiltration	Peak incidence in childhood, acute onset, bone pain frequent
Lymphosarcoma cell	Lymphocytic lymphoma	B-cell surface markers with high concentration of monoclonal surface immunoglobulin	Nodular or diffuse, poorly differentiated lymphocytic lymphoma on node biopsy, patchy, peritrabecular bone marrow involvement	Middle-aged to older adults, generalized adenopathy, constitutional symptoms
Sézary cell	Cutaneous lymphomas	T-lymphocyte surface markers	Skin biopsy is diagnostic	Exfoliative erythroderma, cutaneous plaques or tumors
Hairy cell	Hairy cell leukemia	B-lymphocyte markers, cytoplasmic projections, tartrate-resistant acid phosphatase, interleukin-2 receptors, CD11 antigen	Pancytopenia	Middle-aged males, moderate to marked splenomegaly without adenopathy
Prolymphocyte	Prolymphocytic leukemia	B-cell surface markers with high concentration of surface immunoglobulin, CD5 negative	Marked lymphocytosis (frequently $>100 \times 10^9$/L)	Elderly adults, massive splenomegaly, minimum adenopathy, poor response to therapy

ALL, Acute lymphoblastic leukemia; *HBsAg,* Hepatitis B surface antigen; *Ig,* immunoglobulin.

Amphotericin
β-agonists
Cisplatin
Cyclosporine
Diuretics
Foscarnet
Pentamidine
Theophylline
Congenital disorders
Familial hypomagnesemia
Maternal diabetes
Maternal hypothyroidism
Maternal hyperparathyroidism

BOX 22 Key Causes of Lymphocytopenia

Destructive: Radiation, chemotherapy, corticosteroids
Debilitative: Starvation, aplastic anemia, terminal cancer, collagen vascular disease, renal failure
Infectious: Viral hepatitis, influenza, typhoid fever, TB
AIDS-associated: HIV cytopathic effect, nutritional imbalance, drug effect
Congenital immunodeficiency: Wiskott-Aldrich syndrome
Abnormal lymphatic circulation: Intestinal lymphangiectasia, obstruction, thoracic duct drainage/rupture, CHF

AIDS, Acquired immunodeficiency syndrome; *CHF,* congestive heart failure; *HIV,* human immunodeficiency virus; *TB,* tuberculosis.
From McPherson RA, Pincus MR: *Henry's clinical diagnosis and management by laboratory methods,* ed 23, St Louis, 2017, Elsevier.

MEAN CORPUSCULAR VOLUME (MCV)

Laboratory features in microcytic hypochromic anemias are summarized in Table 74.
Normal range: 76-100 μm^3 (76-100 fL) (76-100 fL [CF: 1; SMI: 1 fL])
Table 75 summarizes clinical conditions not to be confused with megaloblastosis. See Tables 76 and 77 for descriptions of MCV abnormalities. Table 78 describes the usefulness of the MCV and RBC distribution width in the diagnosis of anemia. Table 79 describes peripheral blood film evaluation in a patient with red cell membrane disorder.

METANEPHRINES, URINE

See "URINE METANEPHRINES"

METHYLMALONIC ACID (Serum)

Normal: <0.2 μmol/L
Elevated in: Vitamin B_{12} deficiency, pregnancy, methylmalonic acidemia

MITOCHONDRIAL ANTIBODY (AMA)

Normal: Negative
Present in: Primary biliary cirrhosis (>90% of patients)

MONOCYTE COUNT

Normal range: 2%-8%
Elevated in: Viral diseases, parasites, infections, neoplasms, inflammatory bowel disease, monocytic leukemia, lymphomas, myeloma, sarcoidosis
Decreased in: Aplastic anemia, lymphocytic leukemia, glucocorticoid administration
See Table 80 for changes in monocyte number.

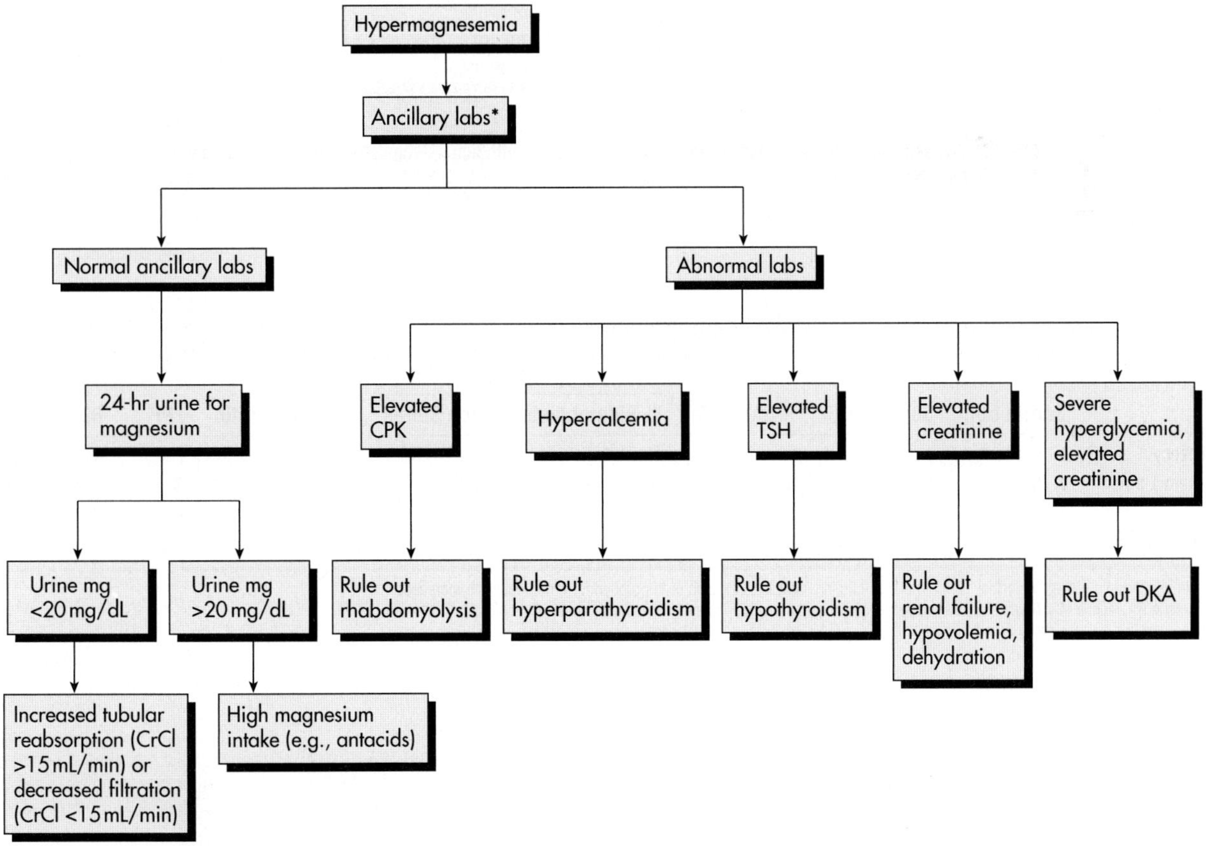

FIG. 38 Diagnostic algorithm for hypermagnesemia. *Serum electrolytes, calcium, blood urea nitrogen (BUN), creatinine, glucose, thyroid stimulating hormone (TSH), creatine phosphokinase (CPK). *CrCl,* Creatinine clearance; *DKA,* diabetic ketoacidosis. (From Ferri F: *Ferri's best test: a practical guide to clinical laboratory medicine and diagnostic imaging,* ed 3, Philadelphia, 2014, Saunders.)

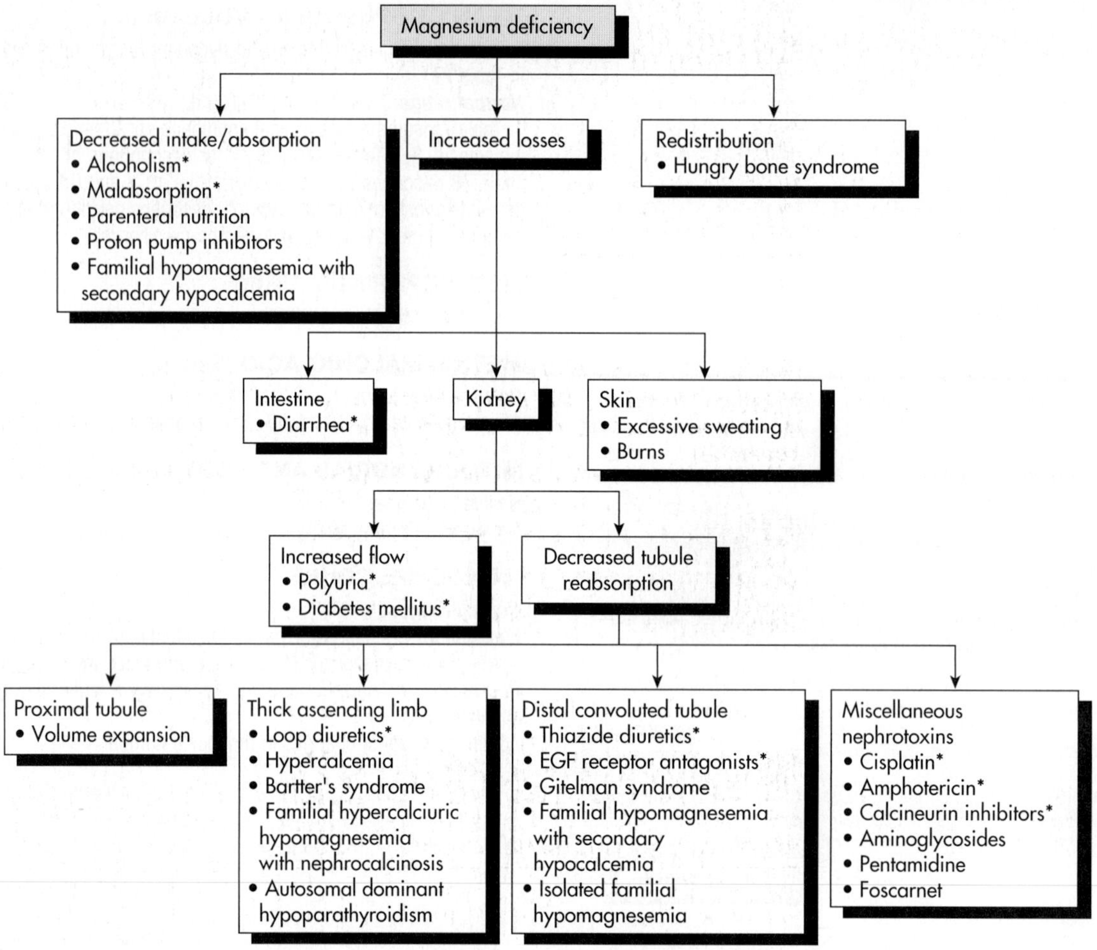

*Common causes.

FIG. 39 Causes of magnesium deficiency. *EGF,* Epidermal growth factor. (From Skorecki K et al: *Brenner & Rector's the kidney*, ed 10, Philadelphia, 2016, Elsevier.)

TABLE 74 Laboratory Features in Microcytic Hypochromic Anemias

				MARROW					
	Serum Iron	**Serum TIBC**	**% Saturation**	**% Sideroblasts**	**Iron Stores**	**Serum Ferritin**	**ZPP**	**Hb A_2**	**Hb F**
Iron deficiency	↓	↑	↓	↓	↓	↓	↑	N-↓	N
β-Thalassemia trait	N (↑)	N	N	N	N-↑	N-↑	N	↑	N-↑
ACD	↓	N-↓	↓	↓	N-↑	N-↑	↑	N	N
Sideroblastic anemia	↑	↓	↑	↑	↑	↑	↑ (↓)	N	N-↑

ACD, Anemia of chronic disease; *N,* normal; *TIBC,* total iron-binding capacity; *ZPP,* zinc protoporphyrins; ↓, decreased; ↑, increased.
From McPherson RA, Pincus MR: *Henry's clinical diagnosis and management by laboratory methods,* ed 23, St Louis, 2017, Elsevier.

TABLE 75 Clinical Conditions Not to Be Confused with Megaloblastosis

Macrocytosis* without Megaloblastosis†
Reticulocytosis
Liver disease
Aplastic anemia
Myelodysplastic syndromes (especially 5q-)
Multiple myeloma
Hypoxemia
Smokers

Spurious Increases in MCV without Macro-Ovalocytosis‡
Cold agglutinin disease
Marked hyperglycemia
Leukocytosis
Older individuals

MCV, Mean corpuscular volume.
*The central pallor that normally occupies about one third of the normal red blood cell is decreased in macro-ovalocytes. This contrasts with the finding of thin macrocytes, in which the central pallor is increased.
†Although megaloblastosis implies that a bone marrow test has been performed, with the addition of highly sensitive tests for the specific diagnosis of cobalamin and folate deficiency, the need for a bone marrow test is often dictated by the urgency to make the diagnosis.
‡When the Coulter counter readings of a high MCV are not confirmed by looking at the peripheral smear.
From Hoffman R: *Hematology: basic principles and practice,* ed 6, Philadelphia, 2013, Saunders.

TABLE 77 Some Causes of Decreased Mean Corpuscular Volume (Microcytosis)

Common	Less Common
Chronic iron deficiency	Some cases of polycythemia
α- or β-thalassemia (minor)	Some cases of lead poisoning
Anemia of chronic disease	Some cases of congenital spherocytosis Some cases of sideroblastic anemia. Certain abnormal hemoglobins (HbE, Hb Lepore)

Hb, Hemoglobin.

MYCOPLASMA PNEUMONIAE PCR

Test description: PCR can be performed on sputum, bronchoalveolar lavage, nasopharyngeal and throat swabs, other respiratory fluids, and lung tissue.

MYELIN BASIC PROTEIN, CEREBROSPINAL FLUID

Normal: <2.5 ng/ml
Elevated in: Multiple sclerosis, CNS trauma, stroke, encephalitis

MYOGLOBIN, URINE

See "URINE MYOGLOBIN"

TABLE 76 Some Causes of Increased Mean Corpuscular Volume (Macrocytosis)

Causes	% of All Macrocytosis Patients*	% of Macrocytosis in Each Disease†
Common		
Folate or B_{12} deficiency	20-30 (5-50)‡	80-90 (4-100)
Chronic liver disease	15-20 (6-28)	25-30 (8-65)
Chronic alcoholism	10-12 (3-15)	60 (26-90)
Cytotoxic chemotherapy	10-15 (2-20)	30-40 (13-82)
Cardiorespiratory abnormality	8 (7-9.5)	?
Reticulocytosis	6-7 (0-15)	Depends on severity
Myelodysplastic syndromes	Frequent over age 40 yr	>60 in RAEB and RARS
Unexplained	25 (22.5-27)	—
Normal newborn		
Less Common	**<4**	
Noncytotoxic drugs		
> Zidovudine		
Phenytoin		30 (14-50)
Azathioprine		
Hypothyroidism		20-30 (8-55)
Chronic leukemia/myelofibrosis		
Radiotherapy for malignancy		
Chronic renal disease (occasional patients)		
Distance-runner macrocytosis (some persons)		
Down syndrome		
Artifactual (e.g., cold agglutinins)		

RAEB, Refractory anemia with excessive blasts; *RARS,* refractory anemia with ring sideroblasts (formerly called "IASA," or idiopathic acquired sideroblastic anemia).
*Percentage of all patients with macrocytosis.
†Percentage of patients with each condition listed who have macrocytosis.
‡Numbers in parentheses are literature range.

TABLE 78 Usefulness of the Mean Corpuscular Value and Red Blood Cell Distribution Width in the Diagnosis of Anemia

	Low MCV (<80fL)	Normal MCV (80-99fL)	High MCV (≥100fL)
Normal RDW	Anemia of chronic disease α- or β-thalassemia trait Hemoglobin E trait	Acute blood loss Anemia of chronic disease Anemia of renal disease	Aplastic anemia Chronic liver disease Chemotherapy, antivirals, or alcohol
Elevated RDW	Iron deficiency Sickle cell–β-thalassemia	Early iron, folate, or vitamin B_{12} deficiency Dimorphic anemia (for example, iron + folate deficiency) Sickle cell anemia Sickle cell disease Chronic liver disease Myelodysplasia	Folate or vitamin B_{12} deficiency Immune hemolytic anemia Cytotoxic chemotherapy Chronic liver disease Myelodysplasia Hereditary spherocytosis, hereditary elliptocytosis, congenital hemoglobinopathies, and RBC enzymopathies

MCV, mean corpuscular value; *RBC,* red blood cell; *RDW,* red blood cell distribution width.
From Hoffman R: *Hematology: basic principles and practice,* ed 7, Philadelphia, 2018, Elsevier.

TABLE 79 Peripheral Blood Film Evaluation in a Patient with Red Cell Membrane Disorder

Shape	Pathobiology	Diagnosis
Microspherocytes	Loss of membrane lipids leading to a reduction of surface area resulting from deficiencies of spectrin, ankyrin, or band 3 and protein 4.2 Removal of membrane material from antibody-coated red cells by macrophages Removal of membrane-associated Heinz bodies, with the adjacent membrane lipids, by the spleen	HS Immunohemolytic anemias Heinz body hemolytic anemias
Elliptocytes	Permanent red cell deformation resulting from a weakening of skeletal protein interactions (such as the spectrin dimer-dimer contact). This facilitates disruption of existing protein contacts during shear-stress-induced elliptical deformation. Subsequently, new protein contacts are formed that stabilize elliptical shape Unknown	Mild common HE Iron deficiency, megaloblastic anemias, myelofibrosis, myelophthisic anemias, myelodysplastic syndrome, thalassemias
Poikilocytes/fragments	Weakening of skeletal protein contacts resulting from skeletal protein mutations Unknown	Hemolytic HE/HPP Iron deficiency, megaloblastic anemias, myelofibrosis, myelophthisic anemias, myelodysplastic syndrome, thalassemias
Schistocytes, fragmented red cells	Red cells “torn” by mechanical trauma (fibrin strands, turbulent flow)	“Microangiopathic” hemolytic anemia associated with disseminated intravascular coagulation, thrombotic thrombocytopenic purpura, vasculitis, heart valve prostheses
Acanthocytes	Uptake of cholesterol and its preferential accumulation in the outer leaflet of the lipid bilayer Selective accumulation of sphingomyelin in the outer lipid leaflet Unknown	Spur cell hemolytic anemia in severe liver disease Abetalipoproteinemia Chorea-acanthocytosis syndrome, malnutrition, hypothyroidism, McLeod phenotype
Echinocytes	Expansion of the surface area of the outer hemileaflet of lipid bilayer relative to the inner hemileaflet Unknown	Hemolytic anemia associated with hypomagnesemia and hypophosphatemia in malnourished patients, pyruvate kinase deficiency; in vitro artifact of low blood storage (ATP depletion), contact with glass or elevated pH Hemolysis in long-distance runners, renal failure
Stomatocytes	Expansion of the surface area of the inner hemileaflet of the bilayer relative to the outer leaflet Unknown	Exposure of red cells to cationic anesthetics in vitro; in vivo the drug concentrations may not be sufficient to produce similar effect Alcoholism, inherited disorders of membrane permeability (hereditary stomatocytosis)
Target cells	Absolute excess of membrane lipids (both cholesterol and phospholipids: “Symmetric” lipid gain), followed by an increase of cell surface area Relative excess of surface area because of a decrease in cell volume	Obstructive jaundice, liver disease with intrahepatic cholestasis Thalassemias and some hemoglobinopathies (C, D, E)

ATP, Adenosine triphosphate; *HE,* hereditary elliptocytosis; *HPP,* hereditary pyropoikilocytosis; *HS,* hereditary spherocytosis.
From Hoffman R: *Hematology: basic principles and practice,* ed 7, Philadelphia, 2018, Elsevier.

TABLE 80 Changes in Monocyte Number

Monocytosis
Infections: Tuberculosis, granulomatous infection, brucellosis, subacute bacterial endocarditis
Connective tissue disorder
Recovery from myelosuppression
Hematologic malignancies
MDS, MPD, MDS-MPD overlap, CMML
Acute and chronic monocytic leukemia, myelomonocytic leukemia
Hodgkin and non-Hodgkin lymphomas
Monocytopenia
Hairy cell leukemia
MonoMAC syndrome
Aplastic anemia
Drugs: Chemotherapy, IFN-α, glucocorticoids (transient)
Radiation therapy

CMML, Chronic myelomonocytic leukemia; *IFN,* interferon; *MDS,* myelodysplastic syndrome; *monoMAC,* monocytopenia and mycobacterium avium complex syndrome; *MPD,* myeloproliferative disorder.
From Hoffman R: *Hematology: basic principles and practice,* ed 6, Philadelphia, 2013, Saunders.

BOX 23 Drugs That Cause Neutropenia

Antiarrhythmics: Tocainide, procainamide, propranolol, quinidine
Antibiotics: Chloramphenicol, penicillins, sulfonamides, *p*-aminosalicylic acid (PAS), rifampin, vancomycin, isoniazid, nitrofurantoin
Antimalarials: Dapsone, quinine, pyrimethamine
Anticonvulsants: Phenytoin, mephenytoin, trimethadione, ethosuximide, carbamazepine
Hypoglycemic agents: Tolbutamide, chlorpropamide
Antihistamines: Cimetidine, brompheniramine, tripelennamine
Antihypertensives: Methyldopa, captopril
Antiinflammatory agents: Aminopyrine, phenylbutazone, gold salts, ibuprofen, indomethacin
Antithyroid agents: Propylthiouracil, methimazole, thiouracil
Diuretics: Acetazolamide, hydrochlorothiazide, chlorthalidone
Phenothiazines: Chlorpromazine, promazine, prochlorperazine
Immunosuppressive agents: Antimetabolites
Cytotoxic agents: Alkylating agents, antimetabolites, anthracyclines, *Vinca* alkaloids, cisplatin, hydroxyurea, dactinomycin
Other agents: Recombinant interferons, allopurinol, ethanol, levamisole, penicillamine, zidovudine, streptokinase, carbamazepine, clopidogrel, ticlopidine

TABLE 81 Miscellaneous Inherited Neutropenia Disorders

Diagnosis	Genetics	Mapping	Mutant Gene	Additional Features
Hyper IgM syndrome, type 1	X-L	Xq26	*CD40L*	↓IgG, IgA, IgE, autoimmune cytopenias
Hermansky-Pudlak syndrome, type 2	AR	5q14.1	*AP3B1*	↓IgG, partial albinism, platelet dysfunction
Griscelli syndrome, type 1	AR	15q21	*MYO5A*	Neurologic dysfunction, partial albinism
Griscelli syndrome, type 2	AR	15q21	*RAB27A*	Same as type 1 plus hemophagocytosis
Chédiak-Higashi syndrome	AR	1q42.1-q42.2	*LYST (CHSI)*	Immunodeficiency, partial albinism
Poikiloderma with neutropenia	AR	16q13	*C160RF57*	Rash, short stature, dystrophic nails
P14 deficiency	AR	1q22	*MAPBPIP*	Immunodeficiency, hypopigmentation
Cohen syndrome	AR	8q22-q23	*VPS13B/COH1*	Retinopathy, retardation, skeletal anomalies
Charcot-Marie-Tooth syndrome, type 2	AD	19p13.2	*DMN2*	Axonal demyelinating neuropathy

AD, Autosomal dominant; *AR,* autosomal recessive; *Ig,* immunoglobulin; *X-L,* X-linked recessive.
Data compiled from Online Mendelian Inheritance in Man (http://ncbi.nlm.nih.gov/omim); From Hoffman R: *Hematology: basic principles and practice,* ed 6, Philadelphia, 2013, Saunders.

NEISSERIA GONORRHOEAE PCR

Test description: Test can be performed on endocervical swab, urine, and intraurethral swab
Normal: Negative

NEUTROPHIL COUNT

Normal range: 50%-70%
Subsets
22. Stabs (bands, early mature neutrophils): 2%-6%
23. Segs (mature neutrophils): 60%-70%

Elevated in: Acute bacterial infections, acute myocardial infarction, stress, neoplasms, myelocytic leukemia
Decreased in: Viral infections, aplastic anemias, immunosuppressive drugs, radiation therapy to bone marrow, agranulocytosis, drugs (antibiotics, antithyroidals, clopidogrel), lymphocytic and monocytic leukemias

Box 23 describes various drugs that can cause neutropenia. Table 81 describes miscellaneous inherited neutropenia disorders. Classification of neutropenia is covered in Table 82. Table 83 lists drugs associated with agranulocytosis. Table 84 describes causes of neutrophilia.

NOREPINEPHRINE

Normal range: 0-600 pg/ml
Elevated in: Pheochromocytomas, neuroblastomas, stress, vigorous exercise, certain foods (bananas, chocolate, coffee, tea, vanilla)

5′-NUCLEOTIDASE

Normal range: 2-16 IU/L (3-27 × 10^8 kat/L [CF: 1.67 × 10^8; SMI: 1 × 10^8 kat/L])
Elevated in: Biliary obstruction, metastatic neoplasms to liver, primary biliary cirrhosis, renal failure, pancreatic carcinoma, chronic active hepatitis

TABLE 82 Classification of Neutropenia

CONGENITAL	
Primary	Autoimmune neutropenia
	Pure white cell aplasia
	Idiopathic
	Thymoma
	Hematologic malignancies (e.g., T-LGL leukemia)
	Infections/postinfectious
	Viral
	b. Measles, mumps, roseola, rubella, RSV, influenza
	c. Hepatitis A, B, and C
	d. CMV, EBV, HIV
	e. Parvovirus
	q. Bacterial
	Tuberculosis
	Brucellosis
	Tularemia
	Typhoid fever
	Rickettsial
	Rocky Mountain spotted fever
	Ehrlichiosis
	Fungal
	Histoplasmosis
	Parasitic
	Malaria, leishmaniasis
	Autoimmune conditions (e.g., SLE, RA)
	Drugs and chemicals
	Neutropenia associated with immunodeficiency
	Severe nutritional deficiencies
	Neutropenia caused by increased margination
	Iatrogenic (e.g., hemodialysis)

CMV, Cytomegalovirus; *EBV,* Epstein-Barr virus; *HIV,* human immunodeficiency virus; *RA,* refractory anemia; *RSV,* respiratory syncytial virus; *SLE,* systemic lupus erythematosus; *T-LGL,* T-cell large granular lymphocyte.

Modified from Hoffman R: *Hematology: basic principles and practice*, ed 7, Philadelphia, 2018, Elsevier.

TABLE 83 Drugs Associated with Agranulocytosis

	ETIOLOGIC FRACTION	
	Agranulocytosis (%)	**Aplastic Anemia (%)**
Overall	64	62
IAAAS	12	27
United States	72	17
Thailand	70	2
Drugs associated with agranulocytosis (IAAAS and other drugs of interest)		
Acetyldigoxin		
ACE inhibitors		
Allopurinol		
Amodiaquine		
Bezafibrate		
β-Blockers		
β-Lactam antibiotics		
Carbamazepine		
Cinepazide		
Corticosteroids		
Cotrimoxazole, other sulfonamides		
Dipyridamole		
Deferasirox (Exjade)		
Dipyrone		
Histamine-2 receptor antagonist		
Indomethacin		
Isoniazid		
Macrolides		
Mefloquine		
Nifedipine		
Phenytoin		
Procainamide		
Salicylates		
Sulfasalazine		
Sulfonylureas		
Tetracyclines		
Thenalidine		
Thyrostatics		
Troxerutin		

ACE, Angiotensin-converting enzyme; *IAAAS,* International Agranulocytosis and Aplastic Anemia Study.

Modified from Hoffman R: *Hematology: basic principles and practice*, ed 7, Philadelphia, 2018, Elsevier.

OSMOLALITY (serum)

Normal range: 280-300 mOsm/kg (280-300 mmol/kg [CF: 1; SMI: 1 mmol/kg])

It can also be estimated by the following formula:

$$2\,([Na] + [K] + glucose/18 + BUN/2.8)$$

The relationship between plasma osmolality and plasma arginine vasopressin is illustrated in Fig. 40.

The relationships between plasma and urine osmolality are illustrated in Fig. 41.

Elevated in: Dehydration, hypernatremia, diabetes insipidus, uremia, hyperglycemia, mannitol therapy, ingestion of toxins (ethylene glycol, methanol, ethanol), hypercalcemia, diuretics

Decreased in: Syndrome of inappropriate diuretic hormone secretion, hyponatremia, overhydration, Addison disease, hypothyroidism

OSMOLALITY, URINE

Normal range: 50-1200 mOsm/kg (50-1200 mmol/kg [CF: 1; SMI: 1 mmol/kg])

Elevated in: Syndrome of inappropriate antidiuretic hormone secretion, dehydration, glycosuria, adrenal insufficiency, high-protein diet

Decreased in: Diabetes insipidus, excessive water intake, IV hydration with D_5W, acute renal insufficiency, glomerulonephritis

TABLE 84 Causes of Neutrophilia

Hematologic malignancy (CML, CNL, CMML)
Infection
Inflammation, physiologic stress, hemorrhage, hemolysis
Hereditary or congenital neutrophilias
Smoking
Drugs: Colony-stimulating factors, glucocorticoids, epinephrine, lithium
Nonhematologic malignancy
Asplenia
Obesity
Recovery from neutropenia

CML, Chronic myeloid leukemia; *CMML,* chronic myelomonocytic leukemia; *CNL,* chronic neutrophilic leukemia.

From Hoffman R: *Hematology: basic principles and practice*, ed 7, Philadelphia, 2018, Elsevier.

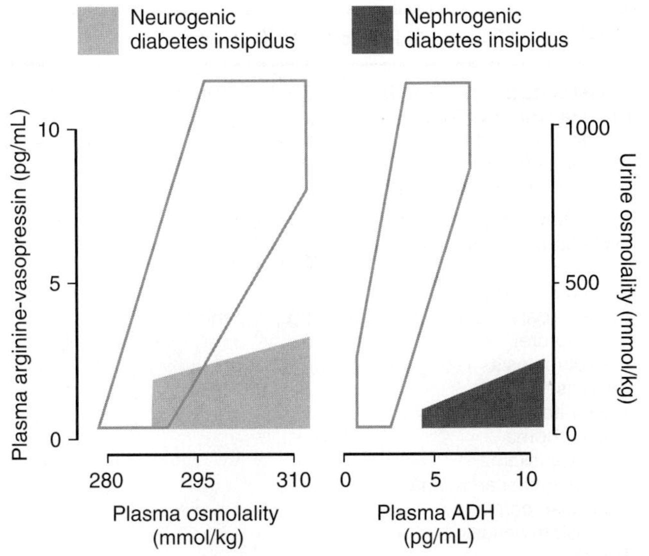

FIG. 40 *Left,* Relationship between plasma arginine vasopressin *(AVP/ADH)* and plasma osmolality during the infusion of hypertonic saline. Patients with primary polydipsia and nephrogenic diabetes insipidus *(DI)* have values within the normal range *(open area),* in contrast to patients with neurogenic DI, who show a subnormal plasma ADH response to a rise in osmolality *(pink). Right,* Relationship between urine osmolality and plasma ADH during dehydration and water loading. Patients with primary polydipsia and neurogenic DI have values within the normal range *(open area),* in contrast to patients with nephrogenic DI, who have hypotonic urine despite high plasma ADH *(green).* (Redrawn from Bichet DG: Diabetes insipidus and vasopressin. In McPherson RA, Pincus MR: *Henry's clinical diagnosis and management by laboratory methods*, ed 23, St Louis, 2017, Elsevier.)

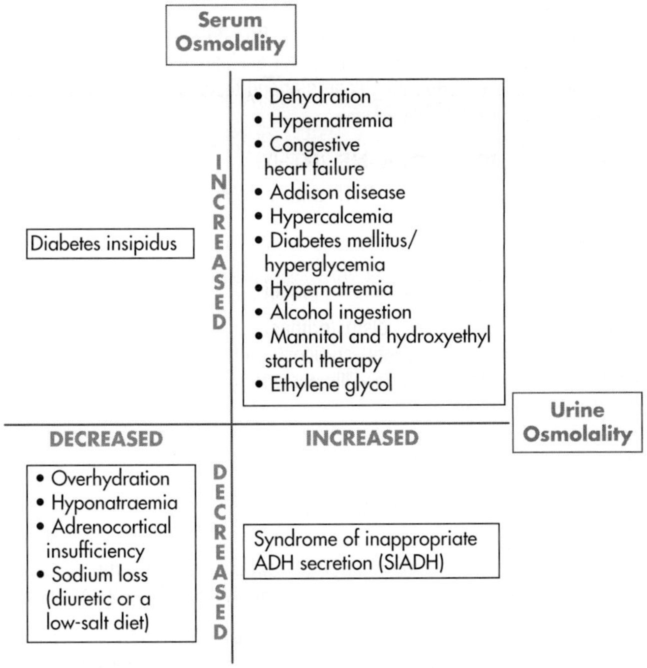

FIG. 41 Relationships between plasma and urine osmolality. *ADH,* Antidiuretic hormone. (From Vincent JL et al: *Textbook of critical care*, ed 7, Philadelphia, 2017, Elsevier.)

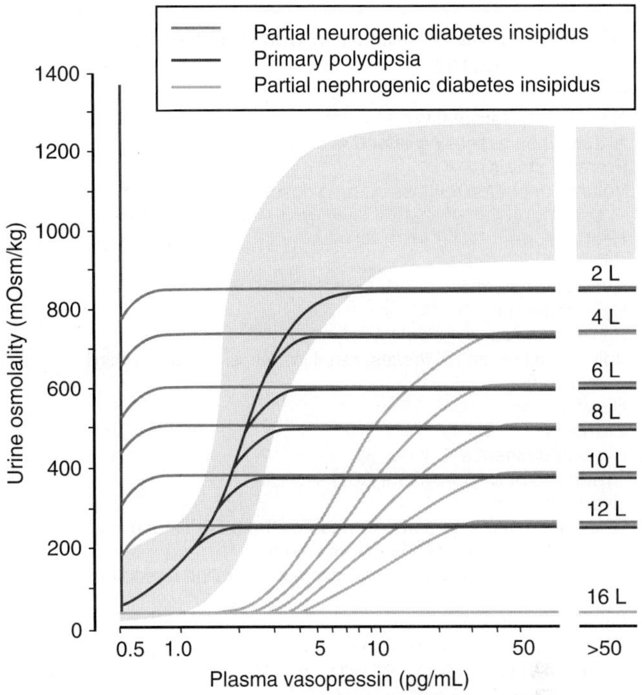

FIG. 42 The relationship between urine osmolality (Uosm) and plasma arginine vasopressin (AVP/ADH) in patients with polyuria of diverse causes and severity. Each of the three categories of polyuria is described by its own family of sigmoid curves of differing heights. Differences in height within a family reflect differences in maximum concentrating capacity caused by "washout" of the medullary concentration gradient. They are proportional to the severity of the polyuria (indicated in liters per day at the right end of each plateau). The normal response is depicted in yellow. The three categories of polyuria differ principally in the ascending portion of the dose-response curve. In patients with partial neurogenic diabetes insipidus *(DI),* the curve lies to the left of normal, reflecting increased sensitivity to the antidiuretic effects of very low concentrations of plasma ADH. In contrast, in patients with partial nephrogenic DI, the curve lies to the right of normal, reflecting decreased sensitivity to ADH. In primary polydipsia, the relationship of Uosm to ADH remains relatively normal. (In McPherson RA, Pincus MR: *Henry's clinical diagnosis and management by laboratory methods*, ed 23, St Louis, 2017, Elsevier.)

The relationship between plasma urine osmolality and plasma arginine vasopressin in patients with polyuria is illustrated in Fig. 42. Box 24 describes urine osmolality variances in common clinical situations.

OSMOTIC FRAGILITY TEST

Normal: Hemolysis begins at 0.50, w/v [5.0 g/L] and is complete at 0.30, w/v [3.0 g/L] NaCl.
Elevated in: Hereditary spherocytosis, hereditary stomatocytosis, spherocytosis associated with acquired immune hemolytic anemia
Decreased in: Iron deficiency anemia, thalassemias, liver disease, leptocytosis associated with asplenia

BOX 24 Urine Osmolality in Common Clinical Situations

High Urine Osmolality
AKI or when assessing effective circulating volume
Prerenal states
Volume depletion (GI losses, renal losses, skin losses, third spacing)
Heart failure
Cirrhosis
Hypoalbuminemia
Hyponatremia
Prerenal states
Volume depletion (GI losses, renal losses, skin losses, third spacing)
Heart failure
Cirrhosis
Hypoalbuminemia
Syndrome of inappropriate ADH secretion
Hypernatremia
GI losses (vomiting, diarrhea, nasogastric tube, fistula)
Skin losses (fever, exercise, ventilation)
Sodium overload (received excess normal saline or sodium bicarbonate)
Mineralocorticoid excess
Seizures (↑ intracellular osmoles → water shifts → transient increase in serum Na)

Low Urine Osmolality
r. *AKI or when assessing effective circulating volume*
s. Euvolemic or hypervolemic
t. Established AKI
u. Chronic kidney disease
v. *Hyponatremia*
w. In process of correcting hyponatremia
x. Primary polydipsia
y. Extremely low solute intake (tea and toast diet or beer potomania)
z. *Hypernatremia*
aa. Osmotic diuresis (glucose, mannitol, urea)
bb. Loop diuretics
cc. Nephrogenic DI
dd. Central DI

ADH, Antidiuretic hormone; *AKI,* acute kidney injury; *DI,* diabetes insipidus; *GI,* gastrointestinal.
From Ronco C: *Critical care nephrology,* ed 3, Philadelphia, 2019, Elsevier.

PARACENTESIS FLUID

Testing and evaluation of results:
Process the fluid as follows:

a. Tube 1: LDH, glucose, albumin
b. Tube 2: Protein, specific gravity
c. Tube 3: Cell count and differential
d. Tube 4: Save until further notice
e. Draw serum LDH, protein, albumin.
f. Gram stain, acid-fast bacilli stain, bacterial and fungal cultures, amylase, and triglycerides should be ordered only when clearly indicated; bedside inoculation of blood-culture bottles with ascitic fluid improves sensitivity in detecting bacterial growth.
g. If malignant ascites is suspected, consider a carcinoembryonic antigen level on the paracentesis fluid and cytologic evaluation.
h. In suspected spontaneous bacterial peritonitis (SBP) the incidence of positive cultures can be increased by injecting 10-20 ml of ascitic fluid into blood culture bottles.
i. Peritoneal effusion can be subdivided as exudative or transudative based on its characteristics (see "Section II").
j. The serum-ascites albumin gradient (serum albumin level-ascitic fluid albumin level [SAAG]) correlates directly with portal pressure and can also be used to classify ascites. Patients with gradients ≥1.1 g/dl have portal hypertension, and those with gradients ≤1.1 g/dl do not; the accuracy of this method is >95%.

BOX 25 Causes of Peritoneal Effusions

Transudates: Increased Hydrostatic Pressure or Decreased Plasma Oncotic Pressure
Congestive heart failure
Hepatic cirrhosis
Hypoproteinemia (e.g., nephrotic syndrome)

Exudates: Increased Capillary Permeability or Decreased Lymphatic Resorption
Infections
- Primary bacterial peritonitis
- Secondary bacterial peritonitis (e.g., appendicitis, bowel rupture)
- Tuberculosis

Neoplasms
- Hepatoma
- Lymphoma
- Mesothelioma
- Metastatic carcinoma
- Ovarian carcinoma
- Prostate cancer

Trauma
Pancreatitis
Bile peritonitis (e.g., ruptured gallbladder)

Chylous Effusion
Damage to or obstruction of thoracic duct (e.g., trauma, lymphoma, carcinoma, tuberculosis and other granulomas [e.g., sarcoidosis, histoplasmosis], parasitic infestation)

From McPherson RA, Pincus MR: *Henry's clinical diagnosis and management by laboratory methods*, ed 23, St Louis, 2017, Elsevier.

k. For the differential diagnosis of ascites, refer to Section II.
l. An ascitic fluid polymorphonuclear leukocyte count >500/μl is suggestive of SBP.
m. A blood-ascitic fluid albumin gradient. Box 25 summarizes causes of peritoneal effusions. Useful criteria for evaluation of peritoneal lavage is summarized in Box 26. Recommended tests in peritoneal effusions are summarized in Box 27.

PARATHYROID HORMONE (PTH)

Table 85 describes serum PTH and calcium patterns in various disorders.

Normal
Serum, intact molecule 10-65 pg/ml
Plasma 1.0-5.0 pmol/L

Elevated in: Hyperparathyroidism (primary or secondary), pseudohypoparathyroidism, anticonvulsants, corticosteroids, lithium, isoniazid (INH), rifampin, phosphates, Zollinger-Ellison syndrome, hereditary vitamin D deficiency

Decreased in: Hypoparathyroidism, sarcoidosis, cimetidine, beta-blockers, hyperthyroidism, hypomagnesemia.

PARIETAL CELL ANTIBODIES

Normal: Negative

Present in: Pernicious anemia (>90%), atrophic gastritis (up to 50%), thyroiditis (30%), Addison disease, myasthenia gravis, Sjögren syndrome, type 1 DM

PARTIAL THROMBOPLASTIN TIME (PTT), ACTIVATED PARTIAL THROMBOPLASTIN TIME (APTT)

See Table 86 for interpretation of coagulation protein screening tests.

Normal range: 25-41 sec

Elevated in: Heparin therapy, coagulation factor deficiency (I, II, V, VIII, IX, X, XI, XII), liver disease, vitamin K deficiency, disseminated intravascular coagulation, circulating anticoagulant, warfarin therapy, specific factor inhibition (penicillin [PCN] reaction, rheumatoid arthritis), thrombolytic therapy, nephrotic syndrome

NOTE: Useful to evaluate the intrinsic coagulation system.

BOX 26 Criteria for Evaluation of Peritoneal Lavage

Positive Result
Aspiration of >15 ml gross blood on catheter placement
Grossly bloody lavage fluid
RBC >100,000/μL after blunt trauma
RBC >50,000/μL after penetrating trauma
WBC >500/μL
Amylase >110 U/dl

Indeterminate Result
Small amount of gross blood on catheter placement
RBC 50,000-100,000/μL after blunt trauma
RBC 1000-50,000/μL after penetrating trauma
WBC 100-500/μL

Negative Result
RBC <50,000/μL after blunt trauma
RBC <1000/μL after penetrating trauma
WBC <100/μL

RBC, Red blood cells; *WBC,* white blood cells.
Modified from Feied CF: Diagnostic peritoneal lavage, *Postgrad Med* 85:40, 1989, with permission. In McPherson RA, Pincus MR: *Henry's clinical diagnosis and management by laboratory methods*, ed 23, St Louis, 2017, Elsevier.

BOX 27 Recommended Tests in Peritoneal Effusions

Useful in Most Patients
Gross examination
Cytology
Stains and culture for microorganisms
Serum-ascites albumin concentration gradient

Useful in Selected Disorders
Total leukocyte and differential cell counts
RBC count (lavage)
Bilirubin
Creatinine/urea nitrogen
Enzymes (ADA, ALP, amylase, LD, telomerase)
Lactate
Cholesterol (malignant ascites)
Fibronectin
Tumor markers (CEA, PSA, CA 19-9, CA 15-3, CA-125)
Immunocytology/flow cytometry
Tuberculostearic acid

ADA, Adenosine deaminase; *ALP*, alkaline phosphatase; *LD*, lactate dehydrogenase; *RBC*, red blood cell.
Modified from Kjeldsberg CR, Knight JA: *Body fluids: laboratory examination of amniotic, cerebrospinal, seminal, serous and synovial fluids*, ed 3, Chicago, 1993, American Society for Clinical Pathology, with permission. In McPherson RA, Pincus MR: *Henry's clinical diagnosis and management by laboratory methods*, ed 23, St Louis, 2017, Elsevier.

PEPSINOGEN I

Normal: 124-142 ng/ml
Elevated in: Zollinger–Ellison (ZE) syndrome, duodenal ulcer, acute gastritis
Decreased in: Atrophic gastritis, gastric carcinoma, myxedema, pernicious anemia, Addison disease

PH, BLOOD

Normal values
Arterial: 7.35-7.45
Venous: 7.32-7.42
For abnormal values, refer to ARTERIAL BLOOD GASES.

PH, URINE

See "URINE pH"

PHENOBARBITAL

Therapeutic range and general information are summarized in Table 87.
Normal therapeutic range: 15-30 mc g/ml for epilepsy control

TABLE 85 Patterns of Serum Levels of Calcium and PTH in Different Conditions

Condition*	Ionized Calcium	PTH	Cause of Disease
Normocalcemia	Normal	Normal	None
"Primary" hypocalcemia	Low	High	CHARD†
"Secondary" hypocalcemia	Low	Low	Parathyroid glands
"Primary" hypercalcemia	High	Low	CHIMPS‡
"Secondary" hypercalcemia	High	High	Parathyroid glands (e.g., adenoma, carcinoma)

*The terms *primary* and *secondary* are not usually employed for hypocalcemia and hypercalcemia.
†Mnemonic for **C**alcitonin, **H**ypoparathyroidism, **A**lkalosis, **R**enal failure, and vitamin **D** deficit.
‡Mnemonic for **C**ancer, **H**yperthyroidism, **I**atrogenic causes, **M**ultiple myeloma, hyper**P**arathyroidism, and **S**arcoidosis.

TABLE 86 Clinical Peculiarities of Coagulation Protein Screening Tests

Long aPTT, normal or long PT, no bleeding	Normal aPTT, PT, *with bleeding*
Long aPTT only	
Factor XII deficiency	Factor XIII deficiency or inhibitor
Prekallikrein deficiency	α_2-Antiplasmin deficiency or defect
High-molecular-weight kininogen	Plasminogen activator inhibitor deficiency or defect
Lupus anticoagulant	α_1-Antitrypsin Pittsburgh defect
Long aPTT and PT	
Dysfibrinogenemia with fibrinopeptide B release	
Lupus anticoagulant	

aPTT, Activated partial thromboplastin time; *PT,* prothrombin time.
From Hoffman R et al: *Hematology: basic principles and practice,* ed 5, Philadelphia, 2009, Churchill Livingstone.

PHENYTOIN (Dilantin)

Therapeutic range and general information are summarized in Table 88.
Normal therapeutic range: 10-20 mcg/ml

PHOSPHATASE, ACID

See "ACID PHOSPHATASE"

PHOSPHATASE, ALKALINE

See "ALKALINE PHOSPHATASE"

PHOSPHATE (serum)

Phosphate levels in various disorders are summarized in Table 89.
Normal range: 2.5-5 mg/dl (0.8-1.6 mmol/L [CF: 0.3229; SMI: 0.05 mmol/L])
DECREASED
Parenteral hyperalimentation
Diabetic acidosis
Alcohol withdrawal
Severe metabolic or respiratory alkalosis
Antacids that bind phosphorus
Malnutrition with refeeding using low-phosphorus nutrients
Renal tubule failure to reabsorb phosphate (Fanconi syndrome; congenital disorder; vitamin D deficiency)
Glucose administration
Nasogastric suction
Malabsorption

TABLE 87 Phenobarbital

Purpose	Treatment of Generalized Tonic-Clonic Seizures, Simple Partial Seizures, Anxiety, Insomnia
General adult dose	Oral: 100-200 mg/day for seizure control; 30-120 mg/day for anxiety; 100-320 mg for sleep induction
Usual bioavailability	Approximately 90%-100%
Half-life	Approximately 5-6 days in adults; approximately 3-4 days in children
General therapeutic range	15-30 mcg/ml for epilepsy control
General toxic level	>40 mcg/ml, although tolerance may develop
Transport	Approximately 40%-60% plasma protein bound
Metabolism	Approximately 75% hepatic: *p*-hydroxyphenobarbital, inactive
Elimination	Approximately 25% unchanged in urine
Steady state	Approximately 14-21 days
Mechanism of action	Stabilizes damaged membranes and raises threshold for neuronal membrane depolarization
Toxic effects	Drowsiness, depression, respiratory depression, coma, sedation, hypotension. Respiratory depression may be caused by rapid intravenous administration

From McPherson RA, Pincus MR: *Henry's clinical diagnosis and management by laboratory methods*, ed 23, St Louis, 2017, Elsevier.

TABLE 88 Phenytoin (Dilantin)

Purpose	Treatment of Generalized Tonic-Clonic Seizures, Simple Partial Seizures, Complex Partial Seizures
General adult dose	Oral: 300-400 mg/day maintenance dose
Usual bioavailability	Variable: 30%-95%
Half-life	24 ± 12 hours, and dose dependent
General therapeutic range	10-20 mcg/ml
General toxic level	>20 mcg/ml
Transport	Approximately 90%-95% plasma protein bound
Metabolism	Hepatic: 5-(*p*-hydroxyphenyl)5-phenylhydantoin, inactive
Elimination	Approximately 5% unchanged in urine
Steady state	Approximately 7-8 days
Mechanism of action	Appears to block sodium and calcium ion influxes into repeatedly depolarizing CNS neurons
Toxic effects	Nystagmus, ataxia, diplopia, drowsiness, coma; rapid intravenous administration may produce cardiovascular collapse and/or CNS depression

CNS, Central nervous system.
From McPherson RA, Pincus MR: *Henry's clinical diagnosis and management by laboratory methods*, ed 23, St Louis, 2017, Elsevier.

Gram-negative sepsis
Primary hyperthyroidism
Chlorothiazide diuretics
Therapy of acute severe asthma
Acute respiratory failure with mechanical ventilation
INCREASED
Renal failure
Severe muscle injury
Phosphate-containing antacids
Hypoparathyroidism
Tumor lysis syndrome
For a diagnostic algorithm of hyperphosphatemia, see Fig. 43.
For a diagnostic algorithm for hypophosphatemia, see Fig. 44.
For causes and treatment of hypophosphatemia see Tables 90 and 91.

PLASMA CELLS

Plasma cells are not normally present in circulating blood. They are increased in a variety of chronic infections, in allergic states, in the presence of neoplasms, and in other conditions in which the serum γ-globulin concentration is elevated. Plasma cells have also been recorded in the blood of patients with viral disorders, including rubella, measles, chickenpox, and mumps. They are moderately increased in cutaneous exanthemas, infectious mononucleosis, syphilis, subacute bacterial endocarditis, sarcoidosis, and collagen disease. Rarely, bacterial sepsis may show a peripheral plasmacytosis mimicking plasma cell leukemia. Their increase is usually linked with increases in lymphocytes, monocytes, and eosinophils. Causes and conditions associated with plasmacytosis include those listed in Box 28.

PLASMINOGEN

Normal: Immunoassay (antigen): <20 mg/dl
Elevated in: Infection, trauma, neoplasm, myocardial infarction (acute phase reactant), pregnancy, bilirubinemia
Decreased in: Disseminated intravascular coagulation (DIC), severe liver disease, thrombolytic therapy with streptokinase or urokinase, alteplase

PLATELET AGGREGATION

Normal: Full aggregation (generally >60%) in response to epinephrine, thrombin, ristocetin, adenosine diphosphate (ADP), collagen
Elevated in: Heparin, hemolysis, lipemia, nicotine, hereditary and acquired disorders of platelet adhesion, activation, and aggregation
Decreased in: Aspirin, some penicillins, chloroquine, chlorpromazine, clofibrate, captopril, Glanzmann thrombasthenia, Bernard-Soulier syndrome, Wiskott-Aldrich syndrome, cyclooxygenase deficiency. In von Willebrand disease there is normal aggregation with ADP, collagen, and epinephrine but abnormal agglutination with ristocetin.

PLATELET ANTIBODIES

Normal: Absent
Present in: Idiopathic thrombocytopenic purpura (ITP) (>90% of patients with chronic ITP). Patients with nonimmune thrombocytopenias may have false-positive results.

PLATELET COUNT

A classification of inherited thrombocytopenias by platelet size is described in Table 92.
See Fig. E45 for evaluation of thrombocytosis. Box E29 describes testing for thrombocytopenia. See Table 93 for differential diagnosis. Table 94 describes antibody-mediated thrombocytopenic disorders caused by autoantibodies, alloantibodies, or potentially both. Tables 95 and 96 indicate differential diagnosis of thrombocytopenia in newborns and differential diagnosis of thrombocytopenia in pregnancy, respectively. Table 97 describes laboratory tests used to investigate a patient with thrombocytopenia.
Normal range: 130 to 400 × 103/mm3 (130-400 × 109/L [CF: 1; SMI: 5 × 109/L])
Elevated in
REACTIVE THROMBOCYTOSIS
Infections or inflammatory states: Vasculitis, allergic reactions, etc.
Surgery and tissue damage: Myocardial infarction, pancreatitis, etc.
Postsplenectomy state
Malignancy: Solid tumors, lymphoma
Iron deficiency anemia, hemolytic anemia, acute blood loss
Uncertain etiology
Rebound effect after chemotherapy or immune thrombocytopenia
Renal disorders: Renal failure, nephrotic syndrome
MYELOPROLIFERATIVE DISORDERS
Chronic myeloid leukemia
Primary thrombocythemia
Polycythemia vera
Idiopathic myelofibrosis

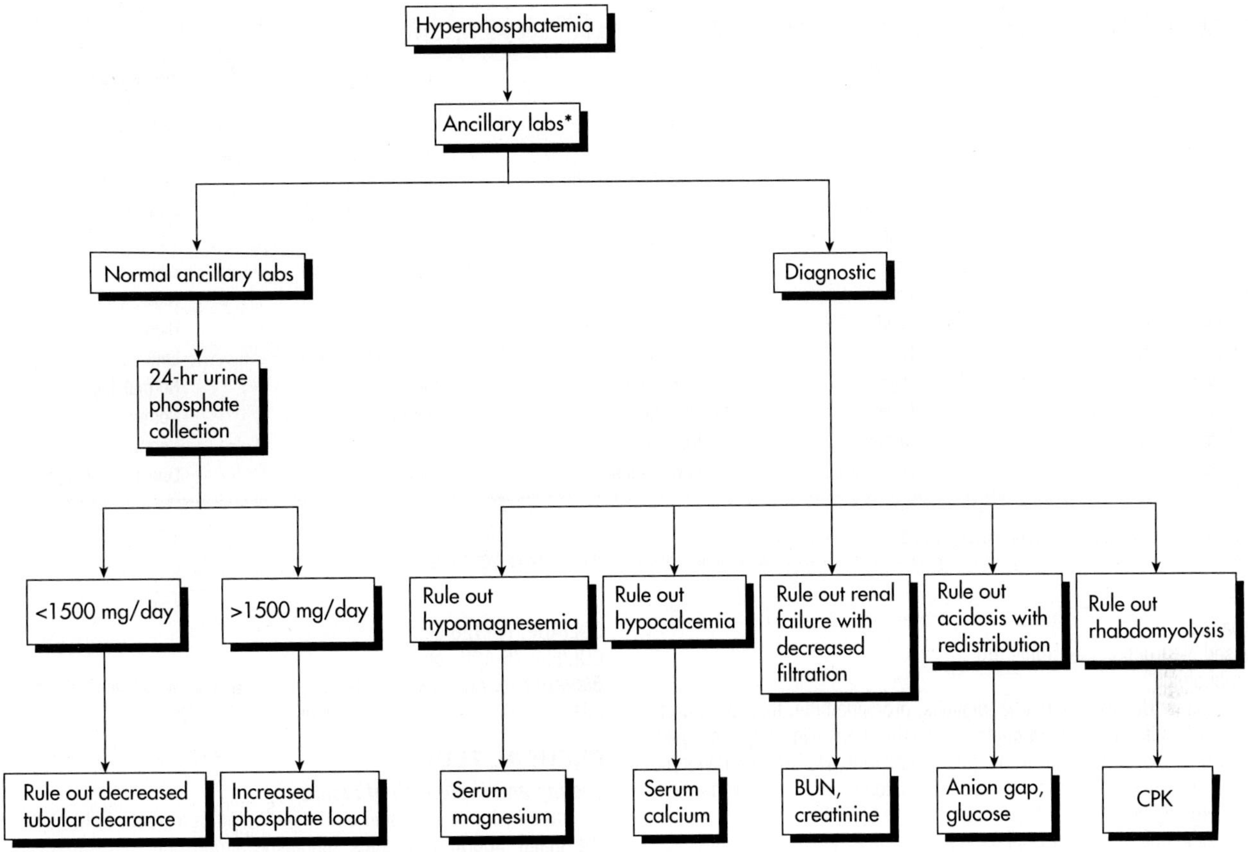

FIG. 43 Diagnostic algorithm for hyperphosphatemia. *Serum calcium, electrolytes, creatinine, glucose, arterial blood gases (ABGs), urinalysis, creatine phosphokinase (CPK), magnesium. *BUN,* Blood urea nitrogen. (From Ferri F: *Ferri's best test: a practical guide to clinical laboratory medicine and diagnostic imaging*, ed 4, Philadelphia, 2017, Saunders.)

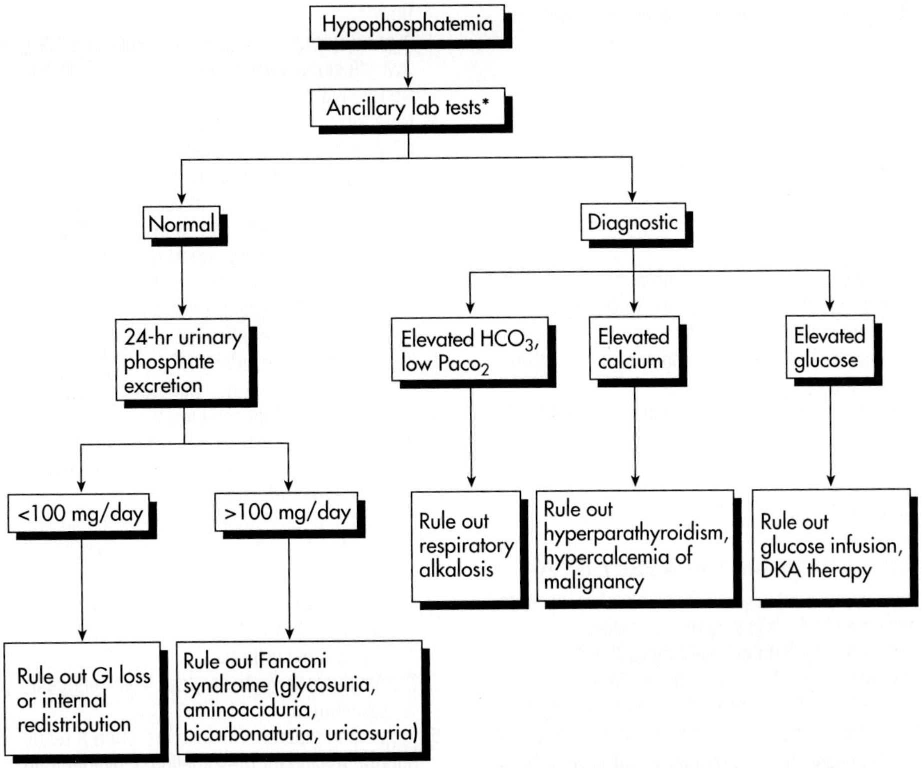

FIG. 44 Diagnostic algorithm for hypophosphatemia. *Serum creatinine, blood urea nitrogen *(BUN)*, electrolytes, magnesium, calcium, glucose, urinalysis, creatine phosphokinase *(CPK)*. *DKA,* Diabetic ketoacidosis; *GI,* gastrointestinal; *$Paco_2$,* partial pressure of carbon dioxide in the arterial blood. (From Ferri F: *Ferri's best test: a practical guide to clinical laboratory medicine and diagnostic imaging*, ed 4, Philadelphia, 2017, Saunders.)

TABLE 89 Serum Calcium, Phosphate, and Vitamin D Levels in Various Disorders

Disorder	Calcium	25(OH)D	1,25(OH)D	Phosphate
25(OH)D intoxication	High	High	Low, normal	Normal, high
Primary hyperparathyroidism	High	Normal	Normal, high	Low
Secondary hyperparathyroidism	Low	Low, normal, high	Low, normal, high	Low, normal, high
Tertiary hyperparathyroidism	Normal, high*	Low, normal, high	Low, normal, high	Low, normal, high
Malignancy	High	Normal	Low, normal	Low
Vitamin D deficiency	Low	Low	Low, normal, high	Low
Renal failure	Low	Normal	Low	High
Hyperphosphatemia	Low	Normal	Low	High
Vitamin D rickets type I, II	Low	Normal, high	Low, normal, high	Low
Granulomatous diseases (sarcoid/TB)	High	Low, normal, high	High	Normal, high
Postmenopausal osteoporosis	Normal	Normal	Normal	Normal
Senile osteoporosis	Normal	Normal	Normal	Normal
Osteomalacia	Low, normal	Low, normal	Low	Low, normal, high

TB, Tuberculosis.
*Calcium may be normal in the setting of concurrent 1,25$(OH)_2D_3$ deficiency.
From McPherson RA, Pincus MR: *Henry's clinical diagnosis and management by laboratory methods*, ed 23, St Louis, 2017, Elsevier.

Decreased

Increased destruction (see Table 98)
- Immunologic
  - a. Drugs: Quinine, quinidine, digitalis, procainamide, thiazide diuretics, sulfonamides, phenytoin, aspirin, penicillin, heparin, gold, meprobamate, sulfa drugs, phenylbutazone, NSAIDs, methyldopa, cimetidine, furosemide, INH, cephalosporins, chlorpropamide, organic arsenicals, chloroquine
  - b. Idiopathic thrombocytopenic purpura
  - c. Transfusion reaction: Transfusion of platelets with platelet antigen HPA-1a (PL^{A1}) in recipients without PL^{A1}
  - d. Fetal/maternal incompatibility
  - e. Vasculitis (e.g., systemic lupus erythematosus)
  - f. Autoimmune hemolytic anemia
  - g. Lymphoreticular disorders (e.g., chronic lymphocytic leukemia)
- Nonimmunologic
  - Prosthetic heart valves
  - Thrombotic thrombocytopenic purpura
  - Sepsis
  - Disseminated intravascular coagulation
  - Hemolytic-uremic syndrome
  - Giant cavernous hemangioma

Decreased production
- Abnormal marrow
  - Marrow infiltration (e.g., leukemia, lymphoma, fibrosis)
  - Marrow suppression (e.g., chemotherapy, alcohol, radiation)
- Hereditary disorders (see Table 99)
  - Wiskott-Aldrich syndrome: X-linked disorder characterized by thrombocytopenia, eczema, and repeated infections
  - May-Hegglin anomaly: Increased megakaryocytes but ineffective thrombopoiesis
- Vitamin deficiencies (e.g., vitamin B_{12}, folic acid)

Splenic sequestration, hypersplenism
Dilutional, secondary to massive transfusion

PLATELET FUNCTION ANALYSIS 100 ASSAY (PFA)

Normal: This test is a two-component assay where blood is aspirated through two capillary tubes, one of which is coated with collagen and ADP (COL/ADP) and the other with collagen and epinephrine (COL/EPI). The test measures the ability of platelets to occlude an aperture in a biologically active membrane treated with COL/ADP and COL/EPI. During the test, the platelets adhere to the surface of the tube and cause blood flow to cease. The closing time refers to the cessation of blood flow and is reported in conjunction with the hematocrit and platelet count. Hematocrit count must be >25% and platelet count >50 K/microliter for the test to be performed.

COL/ADP: 70-120 sec
COL/EPI: 75-120 sec

Elevated in: Acquired platelet dysfunction, von Willebrand disease, anemia, thrombocytopenia, use of aspirin and NSAIDs

PLEURAL FLUID

Testing and evaluation of results

Pleural effusion fluid should be differentiated in exudate or transudate.

The initial laboratory studies should be aimed only at distinguishing an exudate from a transudate.

Tube 1: Protein, LDH, albumin.

Tubes 2, 3, 4: Save the fluid until further notice. In selected patients with suspected empyema, a pH level may be useful (generally ≤7.0). See following for proper procedure to obtain a pH level from pleural fluid.

1. A serum/effusion albumin gradient of ≤1.2 g/dl is indicative of exudative effusions, especially in patients with congestive heart failure (CHF) treated with diuretics.
2. Note the appearance of the fluid:
   a. A grossly hemorrhagic effusion can be a result of a traumatic tap, neoplasm, or an embolus with infarction.
   b. A milky appearance indicates either of the following:
      (1) Chylous effusion: Caused by trauma or tumor invasion of the thoracic duct; lipoprotein electrophoresis of the effusion reveals chylomicrons and triglyceride levels >115 mg/dl.
      (2) Pseudochylous effusion: Often seen with chronic inflammation of the pleural space (e.g., TB, connective tissue diseases).
3. If transudate, consider CHF, cirrhosis, chronic renal failure, and other hypoproteinemic states and perform subsequent workup accordingly.
4. If exudate, consider ordering these tests on the pleural fluid:
   a. Cytologic examination for malignant cells (for suspected neoplasm).
   b. Gram stain, cultures (aerobic and anaerobic), and sensitivities (for suspected infectious process).
   c. AFB stain and cultures (for suspected TB).
   d. pH: A value <7.0 suggests parapneumonic effusion or empyema; a pleural fluid pH must be drawn anaerobically and iced immediately; the syringe should be prerinsed with 0.2 ml of 1:1000 heparin.
   e. Glucose: A low glucose level suggests parapneumonic effusions and rheumatoid arthritis.
   f. Amylase: A high amylase level suggests pancreatitis or ruptured esophagus.
5. Perplexing pleural effusions are often a result of malignancy (e.g., lymphoma, malignant mesothelioma, ovarian carcinoma), TB, subdiaphragmatic processes, prior asbestos exposure, and postcardiac injury syndrome.

TABLE 90 Causes of Hypophosphatemia

Decreased Phosphate Intake
- Starvation, inadequate phosphate intake, chronic diarrhea, chronic alcoholism
- Total parenteral nutrition with insufficient phosphate content

Increased Loss of Phosphate
- Increased renal phosphate excretion
- Primary hyperparathyroidism
- Secondary hyperparathyroidism: Vitamin D deficiency or resistance (including 1α-hydroxylase deficiency, VDR mutations, VDDR); imatinib
- Excess FGF-23 or phosphatonins: X-linked hypophosphatemia, AD hypophosphatemic rickets, tumor-induced osteomalacia, epidermal nevus, McCune-Albright syndrome
- Fanconi syndrome, cystinosis, Wilson disease, Dent disease, Lowe syndrome, multiple myeloma, amyloidosis, heavy-metal toxicity, rewarming of hyperthermia, Na/Pi-IIa and Na/Pi-IIc mutation (HHRH)
- PTHrP-dependent hypercalcemia of malignancy
- Hypomagnesemia
- Decreased intestinal absorption
  - Vitamin D deficiency or resistance (VDDR I and II)
  - Malabsorption
- Increased intestinal loss
  - Phosphate binding antacids used in treating peptic ulcers
- Increased loss from other routes
  - Skin: Severe burns
  - Vomiting

Phosphate Shifting from Extracellular Compartment to Cells and Bones
- Diabetic ketoacidosis
- Alcohol intoxication
- Acute respiratory alkalosis, salicylate intoxication, gram-negative sepsis, toxic shock syndrome, acute gout
- Refeeding syndromes from starvation, anorexia nervosa, hepatic failure: Acute intravenous glucose, fructose, glycerol
- Rapid cellular proliferation: Intensive erythropoietin therapy, GM-CSF therapy, leukemic blast crisis
- Recovery from hypothermia
- Heat stroke
- Postparathyroidectomy; "hungry bone" disease: Osteoblastic metastases, antiresorptive treatment of severe Paget disease
- Catecholamine (albuterol, dopamine, terbutaline, epinephrine)
- Thyrotoxic periodic paralysis
- Hypocalcemic periodic paralysis

Miscellaneous

Hyperaldosteronism
- Oncogenic hypophosphatemia
- Post kidney transplantation
- Post partial hepatectomy
- High-dose corticosteroids, estrogens
- Medications: Ifosfamide; toluene; calcitonin; bisphosphonate; tenofovir; paraquat, cisplatin; acetazolamide and other diuretics
- Post obstructive diuresis

AD, Autosomal dominant; *FGF-23,* fibroblast growth factor 23; *GM-CSF,* granulocyte-macrophage colony-stimulating factor; *HHRH,* hereditary hypophosphatemic rickets with hypercalciuria; *Na/Pi-II,* type II sodium-dependent phosphate cotransporter; *PTHrP,* parathyroid hormone-related peptide; *VDDR,* vitamin D-dependent rickets; *VDR,* vitamin D receptor.
From Skorecki K et al: *Brenner & Rector's the kidney,* ed 10, Philadelphia, 2016, Elsevier.

Box 30 Describes a cellular differential of pleural effusions. Features differentiating exudative from transudative pleural effusion are summarized in Table 100.

POTASSIUM (serum)

Normal range: 3.5-5 mEq/L (3.5-5 mmol/L [CF: 1; SMI: 0.1 mmol/L])

CAUSES OF HYPERKALEMIA

See Fig. E46 for evaluation and treatment of hyperkalemia, and Fig. E47 for electrocardiographic changes in hyperkalemia.
- Pseudohyperkalemia
  1. Hemolysis of sample
  2. Thrombocytosis
  3. Leukocytosis
  4. Laboratory error

TABLE 91 Treatment of Hypophosphatemia

Therapy	Dosage	Administration
Mild and Moderate Hypophosphatemia		
	Low-fat milk	Phosphate 0.9 mg/ml
	Buffered Na phosphate (Fleet enema)	1-3 g/day in 4 divided doses
	Neutra-Phos (250 mg elemental phosphorus per capsule)	1-3 g/day in 4 divided doses
	Calcitriol	30-70 ng/kg body weight per day
Asymptomatic Severe Hypophosphatemia		
Elemental phosphate	2.5 mg/kg body weight	IV over 6 hr
Symptomatic Severe Hypophosphatemia		
Elemental phosphate	5 mg/kg body weight	IV over 6 hr

IV, Intravenously.
From Skorecki et al: *Brenner & Rector's the kidney,* ed 10, Philadelphia, 2016, Elsevier.

BOX 28 Key Causes of Plasmacytosis

- Viral—infectious mononucleosis, measles, rubella, HIV
- Bacterial—tuberculosis, syphilis, streptococcus, staphylococcus
- Parasitic—malaria, trichinosis
- Inflammatory—SLE, RA, inflammatory bowel disease, alcoholic liver disease
- Neoplastic—plasma cell leukemia, myeloma
- Immune stimulation—immune complex disease (serum sickness), drug sensitivity, transfusion
- Trauma

HIV, Human immunodeficiency virus; *RA,* rheumatoid arthritis; *SLE,* systemic lupus erythematosus.
McPherson RA, Pincus MR: *Henry's clinical diagnosis and management by laboratory methods,* ed 23, St Louis, 2017, Elsevier.

TABLE 92 Classification of Inherited Thrombocytopenias by Platelet Size

Small Platelets (MPV <7 fL)	Normal-Sized Platelets (MPV 7-11 fL)	Large Platelets (MPV>11 fL)
Wiskott-Aldrich syndrome	Congenital amegakaryocytic thrombocytopenia	*MYH9*-related disorders
X-linked thrombocytopenia	Thrombocytopenia absent radius syndrome	Bernard-Soulier syndrome
	Radioulnar synostosis with amegakaryocytic thrombocytopenia	Gray platelet syndrome
	RUNX1 mutations (FPD/AML)	Velocardiofacial syndrome
	ANKRD26-related thrombocytopenia	*GATA*-1 mutations
	CYCS-related thrombocytopenia	Type 2B von Willebrand disease
		Platelet-type von Willebrand disease
		Paris-Trousseau (Jacobsen) syndrome
		TUBB1-related macrothrombocytopenia
		Thrombocytopenia associated with sitosterolemia

Modified with permission from Kumar R, Kahr WHA: Congenital thrombocytopenia: Clinical manifestations, laboratory abnormalities, and molecular defects of a heterogeneous group of conditions. In Rao AK, editor: *Hematology/oncology clinics of North America: disorders of the platelets* (vol 27), Philadelphia, 2013, Elsevier, pp 465-494. In: McPherson RA, Pincus MR: *Henry's clinical diagnosis and management by laboratory methods,* ed 23, St Louis, 2017, Elsevier.

- Increased potassium intake and absorption
  1. Potassium supplements (oral and parenteral)
  2. Dietary: Salt substitutes
  3. Stored blood
  4. Potassium-containing medications
- Impaired renal excretion
  1. Acute renal failure
  2. Chronic renal failure
  3. Tubular defect in potassium secretion
     a. Renal allograft
     b. Analgesic nephropathy
     c. Sickle cell disease
     d. Obstructive uropathy

TABLE 93 Differential Diagnosis of Thrombocytopenia in Suspected Disseminated Intravascular Coagulation

Differential Diagnosis	Additional Diagnostic Clues
DIC	Prolonged aPTT and PT, increased FDP, low levels of AT or protein C
Sepsis without DIC	Positive (blood) cultures, positive sepsis criteria, hematophagocytosis in BM aspirate
Massive blood loss	Major bleeding, low hemoglobin, prolonged aPTT and PT
Thrombotic microangiopathy	Schistocytes in blood smear, Coombs-negative hemolysis, fever, neurologic symptoms, renal insufficiency, coagulation test results usually normal, ADAMTS13 levels decreased
Heparin-induced thrombocytopenia	Use of heparin, venous or arterial thrombosis, positive HIT test (usually immunoassay for heparin-platelet factor 4 antibodies), increase in platelet count after cessation of heparin; coagulation tests usually normal
Immune thrombocytopenia	Antiplatelet antibodies, normal or increased number of megakaryocytes in BM aspirate, TPO decreased; coagulation tests usually normal
Drug-induced thrombocytopenia	Decreased number of megakaryocytes in BM aspirate or detection of drug-induced antiplatelet antibodies, increase in platelet count after cessation of drug; coagulation test results usually normal

ADAMTS13, A disintegrin and metalloproteinase with a thrombospondin type 1 motif, member 13; *aPTT*, activated partial thromboplastin time; *AT*, antithrombin; *BM*, bone marrow; *DIC*, disseminated intravascular coagulation; *FDP*, fibrin degradation product; *HIT*, heparin-induced thrombocytopenia; *PT*, prothrombin time; *TPO*, thrombopoietin.
From Hoffman R: *Hematology: basic principles and practice*, ed 6, Philadelphia, 2013, Saunders.

TABLE 95 Differential Diagnosis of Thrombocytopenia in Newborns

Perinatal Hypoxemia
Placental Insufficiency
Congenital Infection
- Sepsis
- Toxoplasmosis
- Rubella
- Cytomegalovirus

Autoimmune
- Maternal immune thrombocytopenia
- Maternal systemic lupus erythematosus

Disseminated Intravascular Coagulation
Maternal Drug Exposure
Congenital Heart Disease
Hereditary Thrombocytopenia
- MYH9 macrothrombocytopenia (including May-Hegglin anomaly)
- Thrombocytopenia absent radii syndrome
- Amegakaryocytic thrombocytopenia
- Wiskott-Aldrich syndrome
- Fanconi anemia

Hemangioma with Thrombocytopenia
- Kasabach-Merritt syndrome

Bone Marrow Infiltration
- Congenital leukemia

From Hoffman R: *Hematology: basic principles and practice*, ed 7, Philadelphia, 2018, Elsevier.

TABLE 96 Differential Diagnosis of Thrombocytopenia in Pregnancy

Incidental thrombocytopenia of pregnancy (gestational thrombocytopenia)
Preeclampsia or eclampsia[a]
DIC secondary to:
- Abruptio placentae
- Endometritis
- Amniotic fluid embolism
- Retained fetus
- Preeclampsia or eclampsia[a]

Peripartum or postpartum thrombotic microangiopathy
- TTP
- HUS

DIC, Disseminated intravascular coagulation; *HUS*, hemolytic uremic syndrome; *TTP*, thrombotic thrombocytopenic purpura.
[a]Preeclampsia or eclampsia usually is not associated with overt DIC.
From Hoffman R: *Hematology: basic principles and practice*, ed 7, Philadelphia, 2018, Elsevier.

TABLE 94 Antibody-Mediated Thrombocytopenic Disorders Caused by Autoantibodies (Immune Thrombocytopenia), Alloantibodies (Neonatal Alloimmune Thrombocytopenia), or Potentially Both (Posttransfusion Purpura)

	Immune Thrombocytopenia	Neonatal Alloimmune Thrombocytopenia	Posttransfusion Purpura
Immune reaction	Autoimmune	Alloimmune	Features of both allo- and autoimmunity
Incidence	5 per 100,000 population	40 per 100,000 births (or 1 per 2500)	1 per 100,000 blood transfusions
Principal antigenic target	GPIIb/IIIa	HPA-1a	HPA-1a plus autoantigens
Nature of the antibody	Intermittent	Persistent (past 1 yr)	Persistent often at high titers
Mode of sensitization	Autoantibody	Alloantibody	Features of allo- and autoantibodies
Sensitizing event	Mostly unknown; some viral illnesses, chronic infection	Exposure to fetal platelet antigens early in first pregnancy	Blood transfusion (RBCs or platelets) 5-10 days earlier
Bleeding frequency	Uncommon	Common	Very common
Epidemiology	Higher incidence in children and elderly adults; female predominance in early adulthood	Majority affects fetus or newborn carrying the HPA-1a antigen	Almost all are HPA-1bb women sensitized by previous transfusion or pregnancy

GP, Glycoprotein; *HPA*, human platelet antigen; *RBC*, red blood cell.
From Hoffman R: *Hematology: basic principles and practice*, ed 7, Philadelphia, 2018, Elsevier.

TABLE 97 Laboratory Tests Used to Investigate a Patient with Thrombocytopenia

Test	Rationale
Common Tests	
CBC	Isolated thrombocytopenia usually is caused by platelet destruction, but involvement of all cell lines suggests underproduction or sequestration
Examination of the blood film	Pseudothrombocytopenia (platelet clumps)
	Toxic changes and granulocyte "left shift" suggest septicemia
	Atypical lymphocytes suggest viral infection
	RBC fragments suggest TTP or HUS
	Parasites (e.g., in malaria)
	White cell inclusions suggest hereditary macrothrombocytopenia
Blood cultures	Bacteremia, fungemia
ANA test	Systemic lupus erythematosus
Direct antiglobulin test	Exclude immune hemolysis accompanying ITP (Evans syndrome)
Coagulation Assays	
aPTT, PT (INR), thrombin time, fibrinogen, d-dimer assay	DIC
LA assay (nonspecific inhibitor), anticardiolipin and anti-β_2-glycoprotein I assays	aPL antibody syndrome
Serum protein electrophoresis; IgG, IgM, IgA levels	ITP associated with lymphoproliferative disorder (monoclonal); hypersplenism associated with chronic hepatitis (polyclonal)
HIV serologic studies	HIV-associated thrombocytopenia
BM aspiration, biopsy	Assess megakaryocyte numbers and morphology; exclude primary BM disorder
Specialized Tests	
GP-specific platelet antibody assays (e.g., MAIPA)	Relatively specific assay for primary and secondary ITP
Drug-dependent increase in platelet-associated IgG	Specific assay for D-ITP
Drug-dependent platelet activation test (e.g., platelet serotonin release assay) or PF4-heparin (or PF4-polyanion) ELISA	HIT
Radionuclide platelet life span study with imaging (e.g., In platelet survival study)	Define the mechanism of thrombocytopenia; identify an "accessory" spleen postsplenectomy

ANA, Antinuclear antibody; *aPL*, antiphospholipid; *aPTT*, activated partial thromboplastin time; *BM*, bone marrow; *CBC*, complete blood count; *DIC*, disseminated intravascular coagulation; *D-ITP*, drug-induced immune thrombocytopenia; *ELISA*, enzyme-linked immunosorbent assay; *GP*, glycoprotein; *HIT*, heparin-induced thrombocytopenia; *HIV*, human immunodeficiency virus; *HUS*, hemolytic uremic syndrome; *Ig*, immunoglobulin; *INR*, international normalized ratio; *ITP*, idiopathic (immune) thrombocytopenic purpura; *LA*, lupus anticoagulant; *MAIPA*, monoclonal antibody immobilization of platelet antigens; *PF4*, platelet factor 4; *PT*, prothrombin time; *RBC*, red blood cell; *TTP*, thrombotic thrombocytopenic purpura.
From Hoffman R: *Hematology: basic principles and practice*, ed 7, Philadelphia, 2018, Elsevier.

4. Hypoaldosteronism
   a. Primary (Addison disease)
   b. Secondary
      (1) Hyporeninemic hypoaldosteronism (type IV renal tubular acidosis [RTA])
      (2) Congenital adrenal hyperplasia
      (3) Drug-induced
      (4) NSAIDs

TABLE 98 Mechanisms of Platelet Destruction

Type of Thrombocytopenia	Specific Example(s)
Immune Mediated	
Autoantibody-mediated platelet destruction by reticuloendothelial system (RES)	Primary immune thrombocytopenic purpura; secondary immune thrombocytopenia associated with lymphoproliferative disease; collagen vascular disease; infections such as infectious mononucleosis; human immunodeficiency virus syndrome
Alloantibody-mediated platelet destruction by RES	Neonatal alloimmune thrombocytopenia; posttransfusion purpura; passive alloimmune thrombocytopenia; alloimmune platelet transfusion refractoriness
Drug-dependent, antibody-mediated platelet destruction by RES	Drug-induced immune thrombocytopenic purpura (e.g., quinine)
Platelet activation by binding of immunoglobulin G (IgG) Fc of drug-dependent IgG to platelet FcγIIa receptors	Heparin-induced thrombocytopenia
Non-Immune Mediated	
Platelet activation by thrombin or proinflammatory cytokines	Disseminated intravascular coagulation; septicemia/systemic inflammatory response syndromes
Platelet destruction via ingestion by macrophages (hemophagocytosis)	Infections; certain malignant lymphoproliferative disorders
Platelet destruction through platelet interactions with altered von Willebrand factor	Thrombotic thrombocytopenic purpura; hemolytic-uremic syndrome; aortic stenosis
Platelet losses on artificial surfaces	Cardiopulmonary bypass surgery; use of intravascular catheters
Decreased platelet survival associated with cardiovascular disease	Congenital and acquired heart disease; cardiomyopathy; pulmonary embolism

Modified with permission from Warkentin TE, Kelton JG: Thrombocytopenia due to platelet destruction and hypersplenism. In Hoffman R et al (eds): *Hematology: basic principles and practice*. Philadelphia, 2005, Elsevier Churchill Livingstone, pp 2305-2325. In: McPherson RA, Pincus MR: *Henry's clinical diagnosis and management by laboratory methods*, ed 23, St Louis, 2017, Elsevier.

      (5) ACE inhibitors
      (6) Heparin
      (7) Cyclosporine
5. Transcellular shifts
   a. Acidosis
   b. Hypertonicity
   c. Insulin deficiency
   e. Drugs
      β-blockers
      Digitalis toxicity
      Succinylcholine
   Exercise
   Hyperkalemic periodic paralysis

Cellular injury
Rhabdomyolysis
Severe intravascular hemolysis
Acute tumor lysis syndrome
Burns and crush injuries

CAUSES OF HYPOKALEMIA

For the clinical approach to hypokalemia, see Fig. 48.

Decreased intake
Decreased dietary potassium
Impaired absorption of potassium
Clay ingestion
Kayexalate

TABLE 99 Classification of Inherited Thrombocytopenias by Platelet Size

Small Platelets (MPV <7 fL)	Normal-Sized Platelets (MPV 7-11 fL)	Large Platelets (MPV >11 fL)
Wiskott-Aldrich syndrome	Congenital amegakaryocytic thrombocytopenia	*MYH9*-related disorders
X-linked thrombocytopenia	Thrombocytopenia absent radius syndrome	Bernard-Soulier syndrome
	Radioulnar synostosis with amegakaryocytic thrombocytopenia	Gray platelet syndrome
	RUNX1 mutations (FPD/AML)	Velocardiofacial syndrome
	ANKRD26-related thrombocytopenia	*GATA*-1 mutations
	CYCS-related thrombocytopenia	Type 2B von Willebrand disease
		Platelet-type von Willebrand disease
		Paris-Trousseau (Jacobsen) syndrome
		TUBB1-related macrothrombocytopenia
		Thrombocytopenia associated with sitosterolemia

MPV, Mean platelet volume.

Modified with permission from Kumar R, Kahr WHA: Congenital thrombocytopenia: clinical manifestations, laboratory abnormalities, and molecular defects of a heterogeneous group of conditions. In Rao AK (ed): *Hematology/oncology clinics of North America: disorders of the platelets,* vol 27, Philadelphia, 2013, Elsevier, pp 465-494. In: McPherson RA, Pincus MR: *Henry's clinical diagnosis and management by laboratory methods*, ed 23, St Louis, 2017, Elsevier.

BOX 30 Cellular Differential of Pleural Effusions

Neutrophilia (>50%)
Bacterial pneumonia (parapneumonic effusion)
Pulmonary infarction
Pancreatitis
Subphrenic abscess
Early tuberculosis
Transudates (>10%)

Lymphocytosis (>50%)
Tuberculosis
Viral infection
Malignancy (lymphoma, other neoplasms)
True chylothorax
Rheumatoid pleuritis
Systemic lupus erythematosus
Uremic effusions
Transudates (≈30%)

Eosinophilia (>10%)
Pneumothorax (air in pleural space)
Trauma
Pulmonary infarction
Congestive heart failure
Infection (especially parasitic, fungal)
Hypersensitivity syndromes
Drug reaction
Rheumatologic diseases
Hodgkin disease
Idiopathic

From McPherson RA, Pincus MR: *Henry's clinical diagnosis and management by laboratory methods*, ed 23, St Louis, 2017, Elsevier.

TABLE 100 Features Differentiating Exudative from Transudative Pleural Effusion

Feature	Transudate	Exudate
Appearance	Serous	Cloudy
Leukocyte count	<10,000/mm^3	>50,000/mm^3
pH	>7.2	<7.2
Protein	<3.0 g/dl	>3.0 g/dl
Ratio of pleural fluid protein to serum	<0.5	>0.5
Lactate dehydrogenase (LDH)	<200 IU/L	>200 IU/L
Ratio of pleural fluid LDH to serum	<0.6	>0.6
Glucose	≥60 mg/dl	<60 mg/dl

From Bennett JE et al: *Mandell, Douglas, and Bennett's principles and practice of infectious diseases*, ed 8, Philadelphia, 2015, Saunders.

- Increased loss
  - Renal
  - Hyperaldosteronism
    - Primary
      1. Conn syndrome
      2. Adrenal hyperplasia
    - Secondary
      1. Congestive heart failure
      2. Cirrhosis
      3. Nephrotic syndrome
      4. Dehydration
      5. Bartter syndrome
  - Glycyrrhizic acid (licorice, chewing tobacco)
  - Excessive adrenal corticosteroids
    - Cushing syndrome
    - Steroid therapy
    - Adrenogenital syndrome
  - Renal tubular defects
    - Renal tubular acidosis
    - Obstructive uropathy
    - Salt-wasting nephropathy
- Drugs
  - Diuretics
  - Aminoglycosides
  - Mannitol
  - Amphotericin
  - Cisplatin
  - Carbenicillin
- Gastrointestinal
  - Vomiting
  - Nasogastric suction
  - Diarrhea
  - Malabsorption
  - Ileostomy
  - Villous adenoma
  - Laxative abuse
- Increased losses from the skin
  - Excessive sweating
  - Burns
- Transcellular shifts
  - Alkalosis
    - Vomiting
    - Diuretics
    - Hyperventilation
    - Bicarbonate therapy
  - Insulin
    - Exogenous
    - Endogenous response to glucose
  - β2-Agonists (albuterol, terbutaline, epinephrine)
  - Hypokalemia periodic paralysis
    - Familial
    - Thyrotoxic

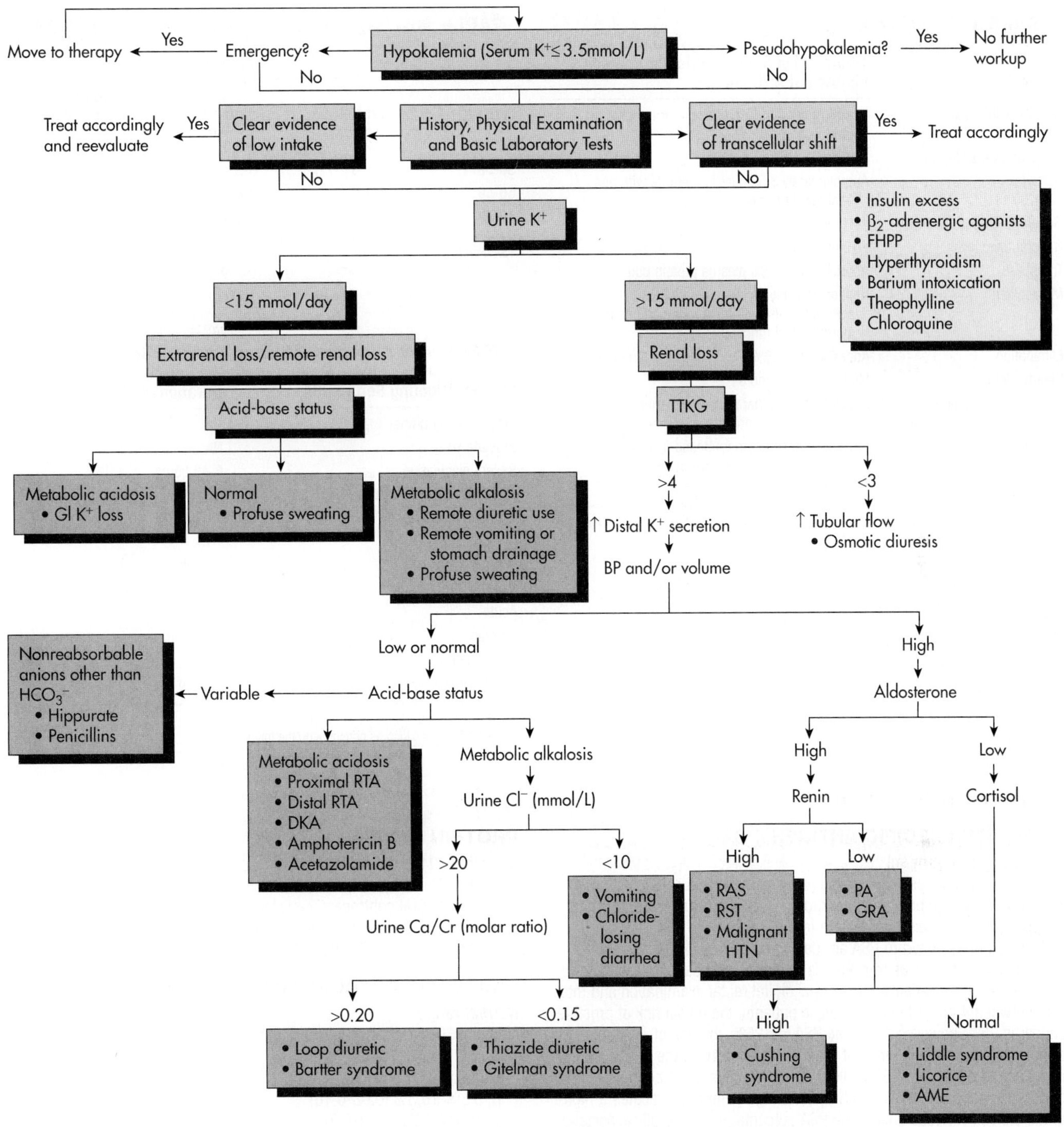

FIG. 48 Clinical approach to hypokalemia. See text for details. *AME,* Apparent mineralocorticoid excess; *BP,* blood pressure; *CCD,* cortical collecting duct; *DKA,* diabetic ketoacidosis; *FHPP,* familial hypokalemic periodic paralysis; *GI,* gastrointestinal; *GRA,* glucocorticoid-remediable aldosteronism; *HTN,* hypertension; *PA,* primary aldosteronism; *RAS,* renal artery stenosis; *RST,* renin-secreting tumor; *RTA,* renal tubular acidosis; *TTKG,* transtubular potassium gradient. (From Skorecki K et al: *Brenner & Rector's the kidney,* ed 10, Philadelphia, 2016, Elsevier.)

Miscellaneous
- Anabolic state
- Intravenous hyperalimentation
- Treatment of megaloblastic anemia
- Acute mountain sickness

POTASSIUM, URINE

See "URINE POTASSIUM"

PROCAINAMIDE

Therapeutic range and general information are summarized in Table 101.

Normal therapeutic range: 4-10 mcg/ml

PROGESTERONE (serum)

Normal

Female: Follicular phase: 15-70 ng/dl
Luteal phase: 200-2500 ng/dl
Male: 15-70 ng/dl

Elevated in: Congenital adrenal hyperplasia, clomiphene, corticosterone, 11-deoxycortisol, dihydroprogesterone, molar pregnancy, lipoid ovarian tumor

Decreased in: Primary or secondary hypogonadism, oral contraceptives, ampicillin, threatened abortion

TABLE 101 Procainamide

Purpose	Treatment of Supraventricular or Ventricular Arrhythmias
General adult dose	Oral: 4 g/day, in divided doses, for maintenance therapy
Usual bioavailability	75%-95%
Half-life	Approximately 3.5 hours in patients with normal renal function
General therapeutic range	4-10 mcg/ml
General toxic level	>12 mcg/ml
Transport	Approximately 15% plasma protein bound
Metabolism	Hepatic: *N*-acetylprocainamide (active), with approximately 7 hours in patients with normal renal function
Elimination	Approximately 50%-60% unchanged in urine
Steady state	Minimum of 12 hours
Mechanism of action	Prolongation of atrial refractory period and decreased myocardial excitability
Toxic effects	Reversible lupus erythematosus-like syndrome, irregular pulse, hypotension, rash, agranulocytosis

From McPherson RA, Pincus MR: *Henry's clinical diagnosis and management by laboratory methods*, ed 23, St Louis, 2017, Elsevier.

TABLE 102 Age-Specific Reference Ranges for PSA

	Serum PSA (ng/ml)		
Age (yr)	Whites	Japanese	African Americans
40-49	0-2.5	0-2.0	0-2.0
50-59	0-3.5	0-3.0	0-4.0
60-69	0-4.5	0-4.0	0-4.5
70-79	0-6.5	0-5.0	0-5.5

PSA, Prostate-specific antigen.

TABLE 103 Factors Affecting Serum PSA

Factors Affecting Serum PSA	Duration of Effect
Prostate cell number	NA
Prostate size	NA
Recent ejaculation	6-48 hours
Prostate manipulation	
Vigorous massage	1 wk
Cystoscopy	1 wk
Prostate biopsy	4-6 wk
Prostatitis	
Acute	3-6 mo
Chronic	Unknown
Prostate cancer	NA
Drugs: Finasteride*	3-6 mo

NA, Not applicable; *PSA,* prostate-specific antigen.
*Lowers PSA for as long as patient is on the medication.

PROLACTIN

See Fig. E49 for the evaluation of hyperprolactinemia.
Normal range: <20 ng/ml (<20 μg/L [CF: 1; SMI: 1 μg/L])
Elevated in: Prolactinomas (level >200 micrograms/L highly suggestive), drugs (phenothiazines, cimetidine, tricyclic antidepressants, metoclopramide, estrogens, antihypertensives [methyldopa], verapamil, haloperidol), postpartum, stress, hypoglycemia, hypothyroidism, chronic liver disease, end-stage renal disease, brain radiation therapy, polycystic ovary syndrome, seizures, exercise, coitus, lactation. Mild hyperprolactinemia (<100 micrograms/L) can also be caused by large sellar masses, including nonfunctioning pituitary adenoma.

PROSTATE-SPECIFIC ANTIGEN (PSA)

Normal range: 0-4 ng/ml
Table 102 describes age-specific reference ranges for PSA.
Elevated in: Benign prostatic hypertrophy, carcinoma of prostate, prostatitis, postrectal examination, prostate trauma
Factors affecting serum PSA are described in Table 103.
NOTE: Measurement of free PSA is useful to assess the probability of prostate cancer in patients with normal digital rectal examination and total PSA between 4 and 10 ng/ml. In these patients, the global risk of prostate cancer is 25%; however, if the free PSA is >25%, the risk of prostate cancer decreases to 8%, whereas if the free PSA is <10%, the risk of cancer increases to 56%. Free PSA is also useful to evaluate the aggressiveness of prostate cancer. A low free PSA percentage generally indicates a high-grade cancer, whereas a high free PSA percentage is generally associated with a slower-growing tumor.
Decreased in: 5-α reductase inhibitors (finasteride, dutasteride), saw palmetto use, antiandrogens

PROSTATIC ACID PHOSPHATASE

Normal: 0-0.8 U/L
Elevated in: Prostate cancer (especially in metastatic prostate cancer), BPH, prostatitis, postprostate surgery or manipulation, hemolysis, androgens, clofibrate
Decreased in: Ketoconazole

PROTEIN (serum)

Normal range: 6-8 g/dl (60-80 g/L [CF: 10; SMI: 1 g/L])
Elevated in: Dehydration, multiple myeloma, Waldenström macroglobulinemia, sarcoidosis, collagen vascular diseases
Decreased in: Malnutrition, low-protein diet, overhydration, malabsorption, pregnancy, severe burns, neoplasms, chronic diseases, cirrhosis, nephrosis

PROTEIN C ASSAY

See Table 104 and Fig. 50.
Normal: 70%-140%
Elevated in: Oral contraceptives, stanozolol
Decreased in: Congenital protein C deficiency, warfarin therapy, Vitamin K deficiency, renal insufficiency, consumptive coagulopathies

PROTEIN ELECTROPHORESIS (serum)

Normal range
Albumin: 60%-75% (0.6-0.75 [CF: 0.01; SMI: 0.01])
α-1: 1.7%-5% (0.02-0.05)
α-2: 6.7%-12.5% (0.07-0.13)
β: 8.3%-16.3% (0.08-0.16)
γ: 10.7%-20% (0.11-0.2)
Albumin: 3.6-5.2 g/dl (36-52 g/L [CF: 0.01; SMI: 1 g/L])
α-1: 0.1-0.4 g/dl (1-4 g/L)
α-2: 0.4-1 g/dl (4-10 g/L)
β: 0.5-1.2 g/dl (5-12 g/L)
γ: 0.6-1.6 g/dl (6-16 g/L)
Elevated in
Albumin: Dehydration
α-1: Neoplastic diseases, inflammation
α-2: Neoplasms, inflammation, infection, nephrotic syndrome
β: Hypothyroidism, biliary cirrhosis, diabetes mellitus
γ: See "IMMUNOGLOBULINS"
Decreased in
Albumin: Malnutrition, chronic liver disease, malabsorption, nephrotic syndrome, burns, systemic lupus erythematosus
α-1: Emphysema (α-1 antitrypsin deficiency), nephrosis
α-2: Hemolytic anemias (decreased haptoglobin), severe hepatocellular damage

β: Hypocholesterolemia, nephrosis
γ: See "Immunoglobulins"
Fig. 51 describes serum protein electrophoretic patterns.

PROTEIN S ASSAY

See Table 105.
Normal: 65% to 140%
Elevated in: Presence of lupus anticoagulant
Decreased in: Hereditary deficiency, acute thrombotic events, DIC, surgery, oral contraceptives, pregnancy, hormone replacement therapy, l-asparaginase treatment

PROTHROMBIN TIME (PT)

See Table 106.
Normal range: 10 to 12 sec
Elevated in: Liver disease, oral anticoagulants (warfarin), heparin, factor deficiency (I, II, V, VII, X), disseminated intravascular coagulation, vitamin K

TABLE 104 Assay Measurement in Heterozygote Protein C Deficiency

		ACTIVITY	
Type	**Antigen**	**Amidolytic**	**Coagulant**
I	Low	Low	Low
II	Normal	Low	Low
	Normal	Normal	Low

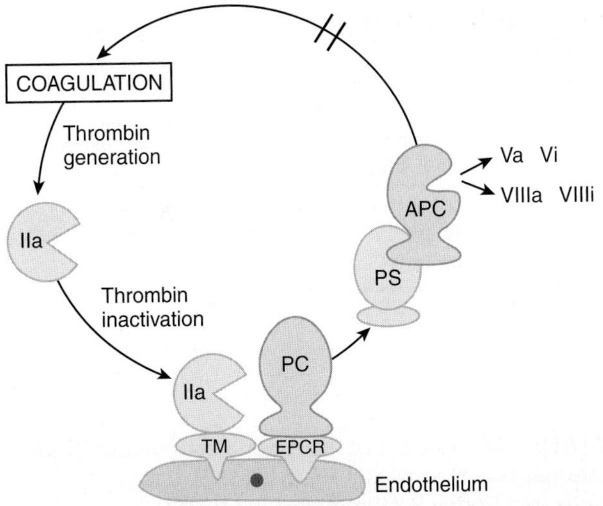

FIG. 50 Protein C pathway. Activation of coagulation triggers thrombin *(IIa)* generation. Excess thrombin binds to thrombomodulin *(TM)* on the endothelial cell surface. Once bound, the substrate specificity of thrombin is altered such that it no longer acts as a procoagulant but becomes a potent activator of protein C *(PC).* The endothelial cell protein C receptor *(EPCR)* binds protein C and presents it to thrombomodulin-bound thrombin for activation. Activated protein C *(APC),* together with its cofactor protein S *(PS),* binds to the activated platelet surface and proteolytically degrades factors Va and VIIIa into inactive fragments *(Vi* and *VIIIi).* Degradation of these activated cofactors inhibits thrombin generation *(double bar).* (From Zipes DP: *Braunwald's heart disease, a textbook of cardiovascular medicine*, ed 11, Philadelphia, 2019, Elsevier.)

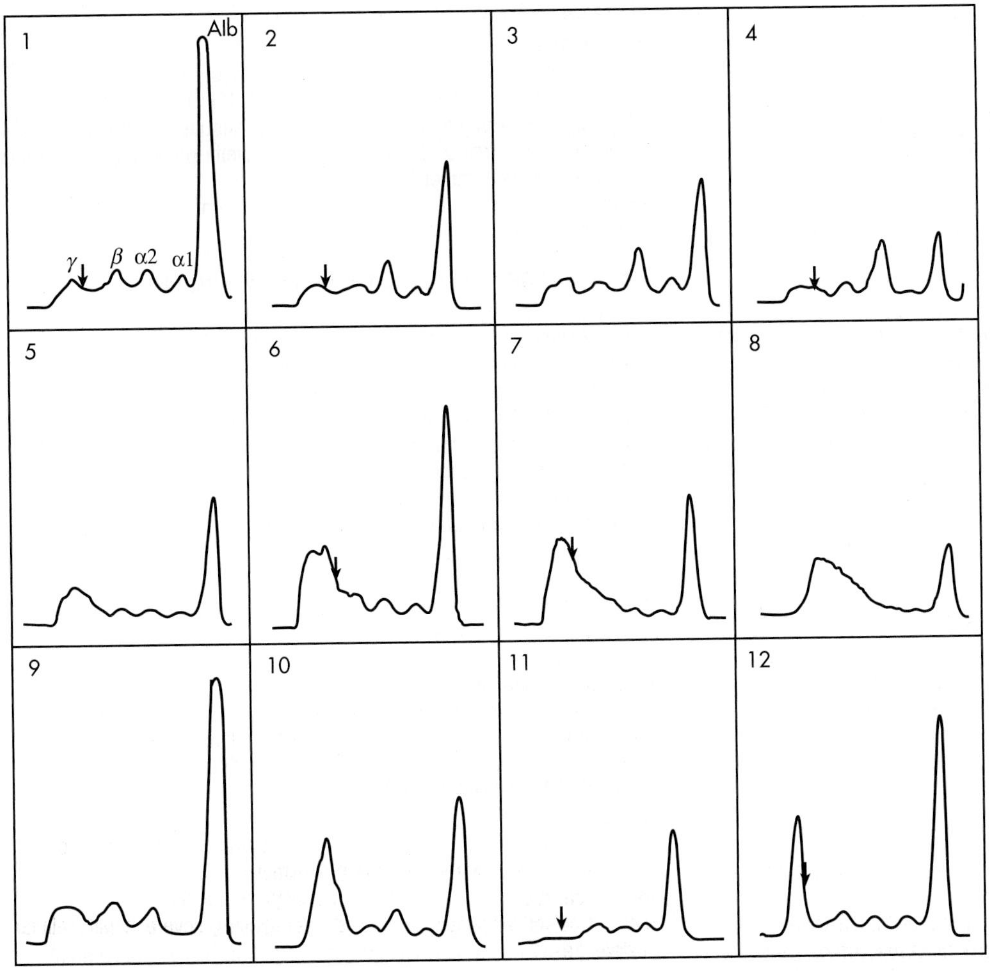

FIG. 51 Typical serum protein electrophoretic patterns. ***1,*** Normal (*arrow* near γ region indicates serum application point). ***2,*** Acute reaction pattern. ***3,*** Acute reaction or nephrotic syndrome. ***4,*** Nephrotic syndrome. ***5,*** Chronic inflammation, cirrhosis, granulomatous diseases, rheumatoid-collagen group. ***6,*** Same as 5, but γ elevation is more pronounced. There is also partial (but not complete) β-γ fusion. ***7,*** Suggestive of cirrhosis but could be found in the granulomatous diseases or the rheumatoid-collagen group. ***8,*** Characteristic pattern of cirrhosis. ***9,*** α-1 Antitrypsin deficiency with mild γ elevation suggesting concurrent chronic disease. ***10,*** Same as 5, but the γ elevation is marked. The configuration of the γ peak superficially mimics that of myeloma, but is more broad-based. There are superimposed acute reaction changes. ***11,*** Hypogammaglobulinemia or light-chain myeloma. ***12,*** Myeloma, Waldenström macroglobulinemia, idiopathic or secondary monoclonal gammopathy.

TABLE 105 Assay Measurements in Heterozygote Protein S Deficiency

	ACTIVITY		
Type	**Protein S Total Antigen**	**Protein S Free Antigen**	**Protein S Activity**
I (Classic)	Low	Low	Low
II	Normal	Normal	Low
III	Normal	Low	Low

TABLE 106 Causes of Increased Prothrombin Time/International Normalized Ratio (PT/INR) and/or Activated Partial Prothrombin Time (APTT)

Increased PT/INR—Defect in Extrinsic Pathway
- Deficiency or inhibitor of factor VII
- Early warfarin (Coumadin) therapy
- Early liver disease
- Increased APTT—Defect in intrinsic pathway

Deficiency or inhibitor of factors XII, XI, IX, or VIII
- Heparin (though usually affects PT as well)
- Liver disease (though usually affects PT as well)
- Lupus anticoagulant (may affect PT as well)

Increased PT/INR and APTT—Defect in Common Pathway or Combined Defect in Extrinsic and Intrinsic Pathways
- Heparin (all serine proteases affected, especially II and X)
- Disseminated intravascular coagulation (all factors, including pro- and anticoagulants, affected)
- Liver disease (all factors except VIII affected)
- Warfarin (factors II, VII, IX, and X affected)
- Vitamin K deficiency (factors II, VII, IX, and X affected)
- Direct thrombin inhibitors
- Lupus anticoagulant

Modified from Rizoli S, Aird WC: Coagulopathy. In: Vincent JL et al (eds): *Textbook of critical care,* ed 6, Philadelphia, 2011, Elsevier.

deficiency, afibrinogenemia, dysfibrinogenemia, drugs (salicylate, chloral hydrate, diphenylhydantoin, estrogens, antacids, phenylbutazone, quinidine, antibiotics, allopurinol, anabolic steroids). Table 107 describes a differential diagnosis of abnormal coagulation screening tests
Decreased in: Vitamin K supplementation, thrombophlebitis, drugs (glutethimide, estrogens, griseofulvin, diphenhydramine)

PROTOPORPHYRIN (Free erythrocyte)

Normal range: 16-36 μg/dl of red blood cells (0.28-0.64 μmol/L [CF: 0.0177; SMI: 0.02 μmol/L])
Elevated in: Iron deficiency, lead poisoning, sideroblastic anemias, anemia of chronic disease, hemolytic anemias, erythropoietic protoporphyria

PSA

See "PROSTATE-SPECIFIC ANTIGEN"

PT

See "PROTHROMBIN TIME"

PTH

See "PARATHYROID HORMONE"

PTT

See "PARTIAL THROMBOPLASTIN TIME"

TABLE 107 Differential Diagnosis of Abnormal Coagulation Screening Tests

Abnormal Activated Partial Thromboplastin Time (APTT) Alone
- Associated with bleeding: VIII, IX, and XI defects
- Not associated with bleeding: XII, prekallikrein (PK), high molecular weight kininogen, lupus anticoagulants
- Abnormal Prothrombin Time (PT) Alone
- Factor VII defects
- Combined Abnormal APTT and PT
- Medical conditions: Anticoagulants, disseminated intravascular coagulation (DIC), liver disease, vitamin K deficiency, massive transfusion
- Rarely dysfibrinogenemia; factor X, V, and II defects

From McPherson RA, Pincus MR: *Henry's clinical diagnosis and management by laboratory methods,* ed 23, St Louis, 2017, Elsevier.

RAPID PLASMA REAGIN (RPR)

Description: Nontreponemal test traditionally used as a screening test for syphilis. It is a quantitative test and antibody titers can be monitored to assess treatment response.
Normal: Negative
Positive: Syphilis. False-positive results may occur with pregnancy, autoimmune diseases, tuberculosis, and other inflammatory conditions. Positive results should be confirmed with treponemal serologic tests (e.g., T-pallidum enzyme immunoassay [TP-EIA]).

RDW

See "RED BLOOD CELL DISTRIBUTION WIDTH"

RED BLOOD CELL (RBC) COUNT

Normal range:
Male: 4.3 to 5.9 × 10^6/mm^3 (4.3 to 5.9 × 10^{12}/L [CF: 1; SMI: 0.1 × 10^{12}/L])
Female: 3.5 to 5 × 10^6/mm^3 (3.5 to 5 × 10^{12}/L [CF: 1; SMI: 0.1 × 10^{12}/L])
Elevated in: Polycythemia vera, smokers, high altitude, cardiovascular disease, renal cell carcinoma and other erythropoietin-producing neoplasms, stress, hemoconcentration/dehydration
Decreased in: Anemias, hemolysis, chronic renal failure, hemorrhage, failure of marrow production

RED BLOOD CELL DISTRIBUTION WIDTH (RDW)

Measures variability of red cell size (anisocytosis)
Normal range: 11.5-14.5
Normal RDW and elevated mean corpuscular volume (MCV): Aplastic anemia, preleukemia
Normal MCV: Normal, anemia of chronic disease, acute blood loss or hemolysis, chronic lymphocytic leukemia (CLL), chronic myelocytic leukemia, nonanemic enzymopathy or hemoglobinopathy
Decreased MCV: Anemia of chronic disease, heterozygous thalassemia
Elevated RDW and elevated MCV: Vitamin B_{12} deficiency, folate deficiency, immune hemolytic anemia, cold agglutinins, CLL with high count, liver disease
Normal MCV: Early iron deficiency, early vitamin B_{12} deficiency, early folate deficiency, anemic globinopathy
Decreased MCV: Iron deficiency, red blood cell fragmentation, HbH disease, thalassemia intermedia

See Table 108 for combining the reticulocyte count and RBC parameters for diagnosis.

RED BLOOD CELL FOLATE

See "FOLATE"

RED BLOOD CELL MASS (volume)

Normal range:
Male: 20-36 ml/kg body weight (1.15-1.21 L/m^2 body surface area)
Female: 19-31 ml/kg body weight (0.95-1.00 L/m^2 body surface area)

TABLE 108 Combining the Reticulocyte Count and Red Blood Cell Parameters for Diagnosis

MCV, RDW	Reticulocyte Count <100,000/µL	Reticulocyte Count ≥100,000/µL
Low, normal	Anemia of chronic disease	
Normal, normal	Anemia of chronic disease	
High, normal	Chemotherapy, antivirals, or alcohol Aplastic anemia	Chronic liver disease
Low, high	Iron-deficiency anemia	Sickle cell–β-thalassemia
Normal, high	Early iron, folate, vitamin B_{12} deficiency Myelodysplasia	Sickle cell anemia, sickle cell disease
High, high	Folate or vitamin B_{12} deficiency Myelodysplasia	Immune hemolytic anemia Chronic liver disease

MCV, Mean corpuscular volume; *RDW,* red blood cell distribution width.
From Hoffman R: *Hematology: basic principles and practice*, ed 7, Philadelphia, 2018, Elsevier.

Elevated in: Polycythemia vera, hypoxia (smokers, high altitude, cardiovascular disease), hemoglobinopathies with high oxygen affinity, erythropoietin-producing tumors (renal cell carcinoma)
Decreased in: Hemorrhage, chronic disease, failure of marrow production, anemias, hemolysis

RED BLOOD CELL MORPHOLOGY

Table 109 describes features of the peripheral blood smear. Table 110 summarizes peripheral blood film evaluation in a patient with red cell membrane disorder. See Fig. 52 for useful peripheral blood and RBC features in the evaluation of anemia.

RENIN (serum)

Blood causes of hypertension associated with high levels of plasma renin are summarized in Box 31. Low levels of renin and hypertension are listed in Box 32.
Elevated in: Drugs (thiazides, estrogen, minoxidil), chronic renal failure, Bartter syndrome, pregnancy (normal), pheochromocytoma, renal hypertension, reduced plasma volume, secondary aldosteronism
Decreased in: Adrenocortical hypertension, increased plasma volume, primary aldosteronism, drugs (propranolol, reserpine, clonidine)

Table 111 describes typical renin-aldosterone patterns in various conditions.

TABLE 109 Features of the Peripheral Blood Smear

Red Blood Cell Morphology	Definition	Interpretation
Polychromasia	Large, bluish RBCs lacking normal central pallor on peripheral blood smear; bluish stain is the result of residual ribonucleic acid	Rapid production and release of RBCs from BM; elevated reticulocyte count; most commonly seen in any hemolytic anemia and states of increased RBC turnover
Basophilic stippling	Many small bluish dots in portion of erythrocytes; comes from staining of clustered polyribosomes in young circulating RBCs	Seen in a variety of erythropoietic disorders, including acquired (e.g., myelodysplasia) and congenital hemolytic anemias and occasionally in lead poisoning
Pappenheimer bodies	Several grayish, irregularly shaped inclusions in a portion of erythrocytes visible on peripheral smear; composed of aggregates of ribosomes, ferritin, and mitochondria	Erythropoietic malfunction in congenital anemias such as hemoglobinopathies, particularly with splenic hypofunction or acquired anemias such as megaloblastic anemia
Heinz bodies	Several grayish, round inclusions visible after supravital staining with methyl crystal violet of the peripheral blood smear, often in the context of bite cells; represent aggregates of denatured hemoglobin	Indicative of oxidative injury to the erythrocyte, such as occurs in G6PD deficiency and other RBC enzymopathies or unstable hemoglobins
Howell-Jolly bodies	Usually one or at most a few purplish inclusions in the erythrocyte visible on the routine peripheral blood smear; represent residual fragments of nuclei containing chromatin	Associated with states of splenic hypofunction, splenic atrophy, splenic thrombosis, or after splenectomy
Schistocytes	RBCs that are fragmented into a variety of shapes and sizes, including helmet-shaped cells; indicative of shearing of the erythrocyte within the circulation	Associated with microangiopathic hemolytic anemias, including DIC, TTP, HUS, or aHUS, as well as other mechanical causes of hemolysis, such as prosthetic heart valves or severe cardiac valvular stenosis
Spherocytes	RBCs that have lost their central pallor and appear spherical; indicative of loss of cytoskeletal integrity from internal or external causes	Associated with hereditary spherocytosis, autoimmune hemolytic anemia; may also be observed in addition to schistocytes in the presence of microangiopathic hemolytic anemia
Teardrop cells	Pear-shaped erythrocytes visible on peripheral blood smear; indicative of mechanical stress on the RBC during release from the BM or passage through the spleen	Seen in a variety of conditions along with other poikilocytes, including severe iron deficiency anemia, congenital anemias such as thalassemias, hemoglobinopathies, and acquired disorders such as megaloblastic anemia. As isolated poikilocyte, teardrop RBCs may be initial changes of myelophthisis (BM replacement or infiltration), e.g., myelodysplastic syndrome or myelofibrosis
Burr cells (echinocytes)	RBCs that have smooth undulations present on the surface circumferentially; pathogenesis unknown	Indicative of uremia when present on a properly made peripheral blood smear
Spur cells (acanthocytes)	RBCs that have spiny points present on the surface circumferentially; reflective of abnormal lipid composition of RBC membrane	Most commonly indicative of hemolytic anemia of advanced liver disease when present in significant numbers; also seen in abetalipoproteinemia and in RBCs lacking the Kell blood group antigen

aHUS, Atypical hemolytic uremic syndrome; *BM,* bone marrow; *DIC,* disseminated intravascular coagulation; *G6PD,* glucose-6-phosphate dehydrogenase; *HUS,* hemolytic uremic syndrome; *RBC,* red blood cell; *TTP,* thrombotic thrombocytopenic purpura.
From Hoffman R: *Hematology: basic principles and practice*, ed 7, Philadelphia, 2018, Elsevier.

TABLE 110 Peripheral Blood Film Evaluation in a Patient with Red Cell Membrane Disorder

Shape	Pathobiology	Diagnosis
Microspherocytes	Loss of membrane lipids leading to a reduction of surface area resulting from deficiencies of spectrin, ankyrin, or band 3 and protein 4.2; removal of membrane material from antibody-coated red cells by macrophages; removal of membrane-associated Heinz bodies, with the adjacent membrane lipids, by the spleen	HS immunohemolytic anemias; Heinz body hemolytic anemias
Elliptocytes	Permanent red cell deformation resulting from a weakening of skeletal protein interactions (such as the spectrin dimer-dimer contact). This facilitates disruption of existing protein contacts during shear stress-induced elliptical deformation. Subsequently, new protein contacts are formed that stabilize elliptical shape; unknown	Mild common HE; iron deficiency, megaloblastic anemias, myelofibrosis, myelophthisic anemias, myelodysplastic syndrome, thalassemias
Poikilocytes/Fragments	Weakening of skeletal protein contacts resulting from skeletal protein mutations; unknown	Hemolytic HE/HPP; iron deficiency, megaloblastic anemias, myelofibrosis, myelophthisic anemias, myelodysplastic syndrome, thalassemias
Schistocytes, fragmented red cells	Red cells "torn" by mechanical trauma (fibrin strands, turbulent flow)	"Microangiopathic" hemolytic anemia associated with disseminated intravascular coagulation, thrombotic thrombocytopenic purpura, vasculitis, heart valve prostheses
Acanthocytes	Uptake of cholesterol and its preferential accumulation in the outer leaflet of the lipid bilayer; selective accumulation of sphingomyelin in the outer lipid leaflet; unknown	Spur cell hemolytic anemia in severe liver disease; abetalipoproteinemia; chorea-acanthocytosis syndrome, malnutrition, hypothyroidism; McLeod phenotype
Echinocytes	Expansion of the surface area of the outer hemileaflet of lipid bilayer relative to the inner hemileaflet; unknown	Hemolytic anemia associated with hypomagnesemia and hypophosphatemia in malnourished patients, pyruvate kinase deficiency; in vitro artifact of low blood storage (ATP depletion), contact with glass or elevated pH Hemolysis in long-distance runners, renal failure
Stomatocytes	Expansion of the surface area of the inner hemileaflet of the bilayer relative to the outer leaflet; unknown	Exposure of red cells to cationic anesthetics in vitro; in vivo the drug concentrations may not be sufficient to produce similar effect; alcoholism, inherited disorders of membrane permeability (hereditary stomatocytosis)
Target cells	Absolute excess of membrane lipids (both cholesterol and phospholipids: "Symmetric" lipid gain), followed by an increase of cell surface area; relative excess of surface area because of a decrease in cell volume	Obstructive jaundice, liver disease with intrahepatic cholestasis; thalassemias and some hemoglobinopathies (C, D, E)

ATP, Adenosine triphosphate; *HE,* hereditary elliptocytosis; *HPP,* hereditary pyropoikilocytosis; *HS,* hereditary spherocytosis.
From Hoffman R et al: *Hematology: basic principles and practice*, ed 7, Philadelphia, 2018, Saunders.

RESPIRATORY SYNCYTIAL VIRUS (RSV) SCREEN

Test description: PCR test can be performed on nasopharyngeal swab, wash, or aspirate

RETICULOCYTE COUNT

See Fig. E53, Fig. 54, and Table 112.
Normal range: 0.5%-1.5%
Elevated in: Hemolytic anemia (sickle cell crisis, thalassemia major, autoimmune hemolysis), hemorrhage, postanemia therapy (folic acid, ferrous sulfate, vitamin B_{12}), chronic renal failure
Decreased in: Aplastic anemia, marrow suppression (sepsis, chemotherapeutic agents, radiation), hepatic cirrhosis, blood transfusion, anemias of disordered maturation (iron deficiency anemia, megaloblastic anemia, sideroblastic anemia, anemia of chronic disease)

RHEUMATOID FACTOR

Normal: Negative. Present in titer >1:20
RHEUMATIC DISEASES
26. Rheumatoid arthritis
27. Sjögren syndrome
28. Systemic lupus erythematosus
29. Polymyositis/dermatomyositis
30. Mixed connective tissue disease
31. Scleroderma

INFECTIOUS DISEASES
Subacute bacterial endocarditis
Tuberculosis
Infectious mononucleosis
Hepatitis
Syphilis
Leprosy
Influenza
MALIGNANCIES
nn. Lymphoma
oo. Multiple myeloma
pp. Waldenström macroglobulinemia
qq. Postradiation or postchemotherapy
MISCELLANEOUS
Normal adults, especially the elderly
Sarcoidosis
Chronic pulmonary disease (interstitial fibrosis)
Chronic liver disease (chronic active hepatitis, cirrhosis)
Mixed essential cryoglobulinemia
Hypergammaglobulinemic purpura

RNP

See "EXTRACTABLE NUCLEAR ANTIGEN"

RPR

See "RAPID PLASMA REAGIN"

ROTAVIRUS SEROLOGY

Test description: PCR test is performed on stool specimen
Normal: Negative

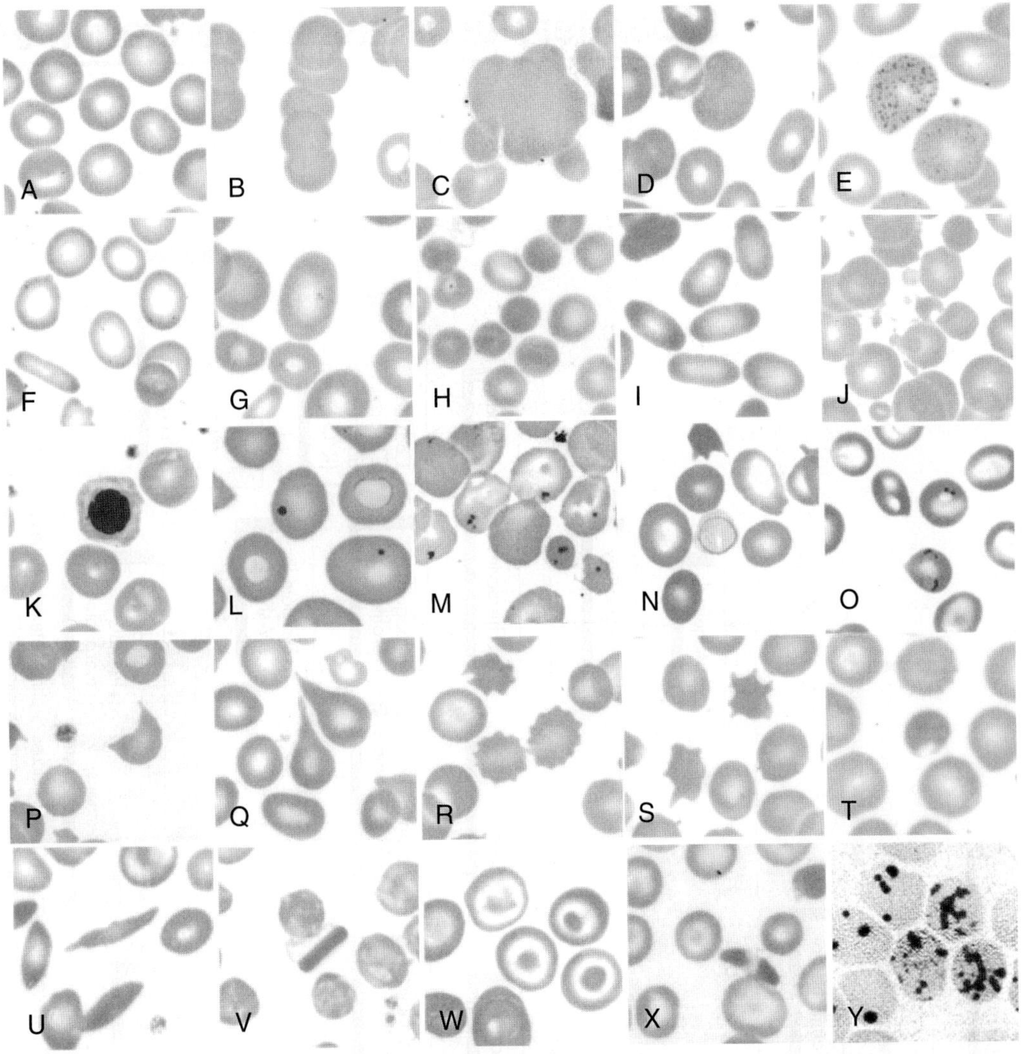

FIG. 52 Useful peripheral blood and red blood cell features in the evaluation of anemia. A, Normal red blood cells *(RBCs).* Note that the central pallor is one-third the diameter of the entire cell. **B,** Rouleaux formation is indicative of increased plasma protein. **C,** Agglutination indicates an antibody-mediated process such as cold agglutinin disease. **D,** Polychromatophilic cell. The gray-blue color is attributable to RNA and the cell is equivalent to a reticulocyte, which must be identified with a reticulocyte stain. **E,** Basophilic stippling. This also is attributable to increased RNA caused either by a left shift in erythroid cells or lead toxicity. **F,** Hypochromic microcytic cells typical of iron-deficiency anemia. Note the widened central pallor and the "pencil" cell in the *lower left.* **G,** Macroovalocyte as can be seen in either megaloblastic anemia or myelodysplastic syndrome. **H,** Microspherocytes typical of hereditary spherocytosis. **I,** Elliptocytes (ovalocytes) from a patient with hereditary elliptocytosis. **J,** RBC fragments from thermal injury (burn patient). **K,** Nucleated RBC. **L,** Howell-Jolly bodies indicative of splenic dysfunction or absence. **M,** Pappenheimer bodies from a patient with sideroblastic anemia. **N,** Cabot ring, as can be seen in megaloblastic anemia or MDS. **O,** Malarial parasites *(Plasmodium falciparum).* **P,** Schistocyte typical of a microangiopathic hemolytic anemia. **Q,** Tear-drop form indicates marrow fibrosis and extramedullary hematopoiesis. **R,** Echinocyte (Burr cell) with rounded edges. **S,** Acanthocyte (spur cell) with more irregular pointed ends. This was from a patient with neuroacanthocytosis. They can also be seen in patients with liver disease and lipid abnormalities. **T,** "Bite" cell from a patient with glucose-6-phosphate dehydrogenase *(G6PD)* deficiency. **U,** Sickle cell, from a patient with homozygous sickle cell disease. **V,** Hemoglobin C crystal. **W,** Target cells. **X,** Hemoglobin C disease. Note that the RBC in center has condensed hemoglobin at each pole. **Y,** Heinz body preparation (supravital stain) from a patient with G6PD deficiency. Note that the cells to the right have increased precipitated hemoglobin. (From Hoffman R: *Hematology: basic principles and practice*, ed 7, Philadelphia, 2018, Elsevier.)

TABLE 111 Typical Renin-Aldosterone Patterns in Various Conditions

	Plasma Renin	Aldosterone
Primary aldosteronism	Low	High
"Low-renin" essential hypertension	Low	Normal
Cushing syndrome	Low	Low-normal
Licorice ingestion syndrome	Low	Low
High-salt diet	Low	Low
Oral contraceptives	High	Normal
Cirrhosis	High	High
Malignant hypertension	High	High
Unilateral renal disease	High	High
"High-renin" essential hypertension	High	High
Pregnancy	High	High
Diuretic overuse	High	High
Juxtaglomerular tumor (Bartter syndrome)	High	High
Low-salt diet	High	High
Addison disease	High	Low
Hypokalemia	High	Low

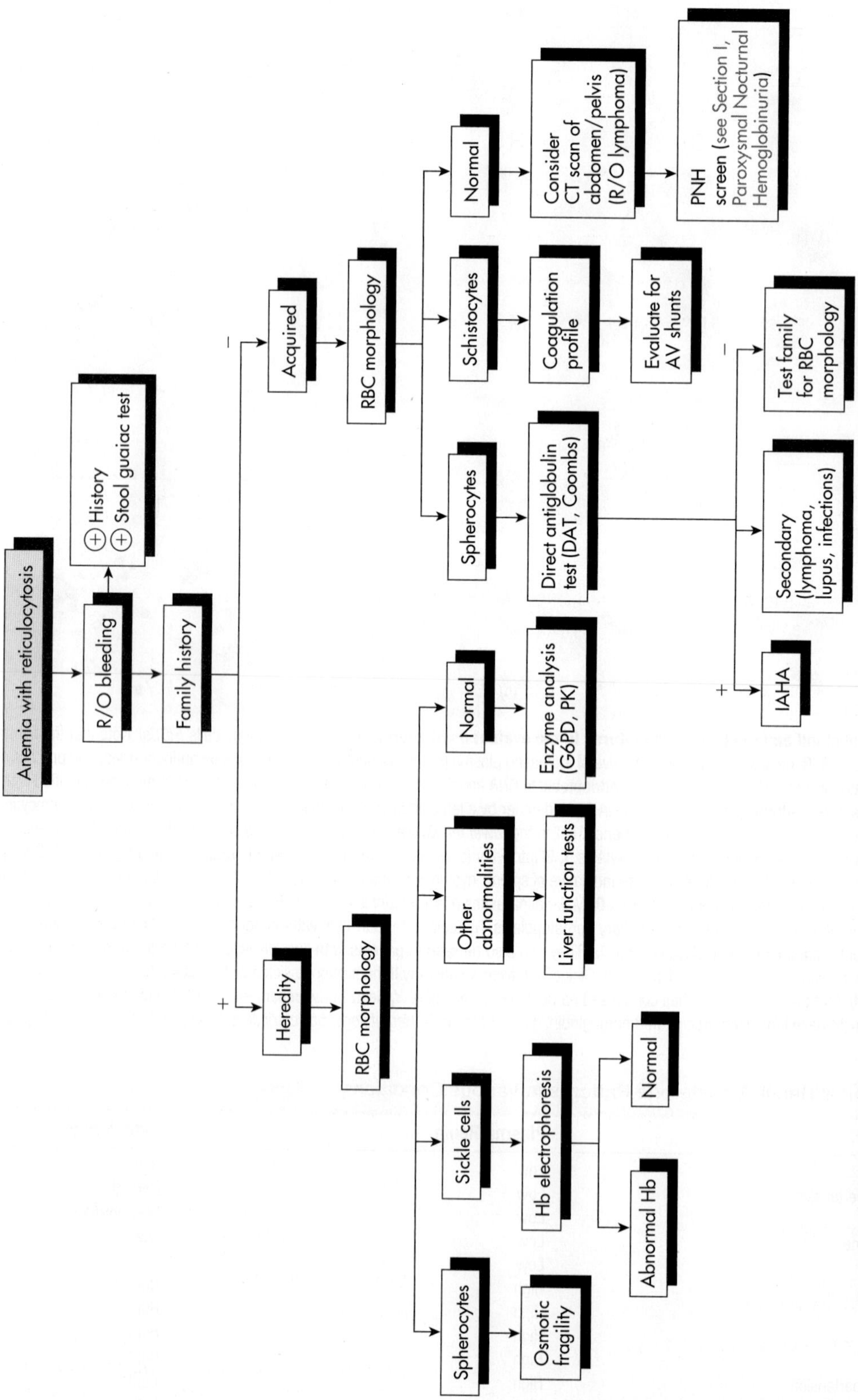

FIG. 54 Evaluation of patients with hemolytic anemia. *AV*, Arteriovenous; *CT*, computed tomography; *G6PD*, glucose-6-phosphate dehydrogenase; *Hb*, hemoglobin; *IAHA*, idiopathic autoimmune hemolytic anemia; *LS*, liver spleen; *PK*, pyruvate kinase; *PNH*, paroxysmal nocturnal hemoglobinuria; *RBC*, red blood cell; *R/O*, rule out.

TABLE 112 Combining the Reticulocyte Count and Red Blood Cell Parameters for Diagnosis

MCV, RDW	Reticulocyte Count <75,000/μL	Reticulocyte Count >100,000/μL
Low, normal	Anemia of chronic disease	
Normal, normal	Anemia of chronic disease	
High, normal	Chemotherapy/antivirals/alcohol Aplastic anemia	Chronic liver disease
Low, high	Iron deficiency anemia	Sickle cell-β-thalassemia
Normal, high	Early iron, folate, vitamin B_{12} deficiency Myelodysplasia	Sickle cell anemia, sickle cell disease
High, high	Folate or vitamin B_{12} deficiency Myelodysplasia	Immune hemolytic anemia Chronic liver disease

MCV, Mean corpuscular volume; *RDW,* red blood cell distribution width.
From Hoffman R et al: *Hematology: basic principles and practice,* ed 5, Philadelphia, 2009, Churchill Livingstone.

SARS-COV-2 ANTIBODIES

Name	Value	Reference Range
SARS-COV-2 ABS Interp.	Negative	Negative
SARS-COV-2 ABS INDEX	0.09	<1.0 (Index)

Index (COI) Value	Interpretation
<1.0	Negative for ANTI-SARS COV 2 antibodies
≥1.0	Positive for ANTI-SARS COV 2 antibodies

The ANTI-SARS-COV-2 assay is intended for the qualitative detection of antibodies to SARS-COV-2 in human serum and as an aid in identifying individuals with an adaptive immune response to SARS-COV-2, indicating recent or prior infection. At the time of this publication, it is unknown for how long antibodies persist following infection and to what degree the presence of antibodies confers protective immunity. This assay should not be used to diagnose acute SARS-COV-2 infection.

Negative results do not preclude acute SARS-COV-2 infection. If acute infection is suspected, direct PCR testing is recommended. False positive results may occur due to cross-reactivity from preexisting antibodies or other possible causes. This assay has overall sensitivity of 100% and specificity of 99.8% in patients ≥14 days post-PCR confirmation.

SED RATE

See "ERYTHROCYTE SEDIMENTATION RATE"

SEDIMENTATION RATE

See "ERYTHROCYTE SEDIMENTATION RATE"

SEMEN ANALYSIS

Table 113 describes semen analysis reference ranges.

SGOT

See "ASPARTATE AMINOTRANSFERASE"

SGPT

See "ASPARTATE AMINOTRANSFERASE"

SICKLE CELL TEST

Normal: Negative
Positive in: Sickle cell anemia, sickle cell trait, combination of *Hb S* gene with other disorders such as alpha-thalassemia, beta-thalassemia

SMOOTH MUSCLE ANTIBODY

Normal: Negative
Present in: Chronic acute hepatitis, primary sclerosing cholangitis, primary biliary cirrhosis, autoimmune hepatitis, infectious mononucleosis

TABLE 113 Semen Analysis Reference Ranges

Color	Grayish white
pH	7.3-7.8 (literature range, 7.0-7.8)
Volume	2.0-5.0 ml (literature range, 1.5-6.0 ml)
Sperm count	20-250 million/ml (literature range for upper limit varies from 100-250 million/ml)
Motility	>60% motile <3 hours after specimen is obtained (literature range, >40% to >70%)
% Normal sperm	>60% (literature range, >60% to >70%)
Viscosity	Can be poured from a pipet in droplets rather than a thick strand

SODIUM (serum)

Normal range: 135-147 mEq/L (135-147 mmol/L [CF: 1; SMI: 1 mmol/L]).
Electrolyte concentrations in extracellular and intracellular fluid are summarized in Table 114.

HYPONATREMIA
See Fig. 55.
Common causes of hyponatremia and electrolyte patterns in serum and urine with normal renal function are described in Table 115. Table E116 describes drugs associated with hyponatremia.
Sodium and water depletion (deficit hyponatremia)
- a. Loss of gastrointestinal secretions with replacement of fluid but not electrolytes
  - Vomiting
  - Diarrhea
  - Tube drainage
- Loss from skin with replacement of fluids but not electrolytes
  - Excessive sweating
  - Extensive burns
- Loss from kidney
  - Diuretics
  - Chronic renal insufficiency (uremia) with acidosis
- Metabolic loss
  - Starvation with acidosis
  - Diabetic acidosis
- Endocrine loss
  - Addison disease
  - Sudden withdrawal of long-term steroid therapy
- Iatrogenic loss from serous cavities
  - Paracentesis or thoracentesis

Excessive water (dilution hyponatremia)
- Excessive water administration
- Congestive heart failure
- Cirrhosis
- Nephrotic syndrome
- Hypoalbuminemia (severe)
- Acute renal failure with oliguria

Inappropriate antidiuretic hormone (IADH) syndrome
Intracellular loss (reset osmostat syndrome)
False hyponatremia (actually a dilutional effect)
- Marked hypertriglyceridemia
- Marked hyperproteinemia
- Severe hyperglycemia

HYPERNATREMIA
See Fig. 56.
Common causes of hypernatremia and electrolyte patterns in serum and urine with normal renal function are summarized in Table 117
Dehydration is the most frequent overall clinical finding in hypernatremia
Deficient water intake (either orally or intravenously)
Excess kidney water output (diabetes insipidus, osmotic diuresis)
Excess skin water output (excess sweating, loss from burns)
Excess gastrointestinal tract output (severe protracted vomiting or diarrhea without fluid therapy)

TABLE 114 Electrolyte Concentrations in Extracellular and Intracellular Fluids

	PLASMA		INTERSTITIAL FLUID		PLASMA WATER		CELL WATER (MUSCLE)	
	(mmol/L)	(mmol/L)	(mmol/L)	(mmol/L)	(mmol/L)	(mmol/L)	(mmol/L)	(mmol/L)
Na^+	140	140	145.3	145.3	149.8	149.8	13	13
K^+	4.5	4.5	4.7	4.7	4.8	4.8	140	140
Ca^{++}	5.0	2.5	2.8	1.4	5.3	5.3	10^{-7}	0.5×10^{-7}
Mg^{++}	1.7	0.85	1.0	0.5	1.8	0.9	7.0	3.5
Cl–	104	104	114.7	114.7	111.4	111.4	3	3
HCO_3^-	24	24	26.5	26.5	25.7	25.7	10	10
SO_4^{2-}	1.0	0.5	1.2	0.6	1.1	0.55	–	–
P	2.1	1.2+	2.1++	1.2+	2.2	1.25+	107	57+++
Protein	15	1	8	0.5	16	1	40	2.5*
Organic anion	5	5	5.6	5.6	5.3	5.3	–	–

+ The calculation is based on the assumption that the pH of the extracellular fluid is 7.4 and the pK of inorganic $H_2PO_4^-$ is 6.8.
++ The concentration of P in the interstitial fluid would be increased by the Donnan effect, but reduced by the lower protein-bound phosphate, and these two opposing effects keep interstitial phosphate concentration about equal to that of plasma.
+++ The intracellular molal concentration of phosphate is calculated with the assumption that the pK of organic phosphates in the cell is 6.1 and the intracellular pH 7.0.
*The calculation is based on the assumption that each mmol of intracellular protein has an average of 15 mEq.
From McPherson RA, Pincus MR: *Henry's clinical diagnosis and management by laboratory methods*, ed 23, St Louis, 2017, Elsevier.

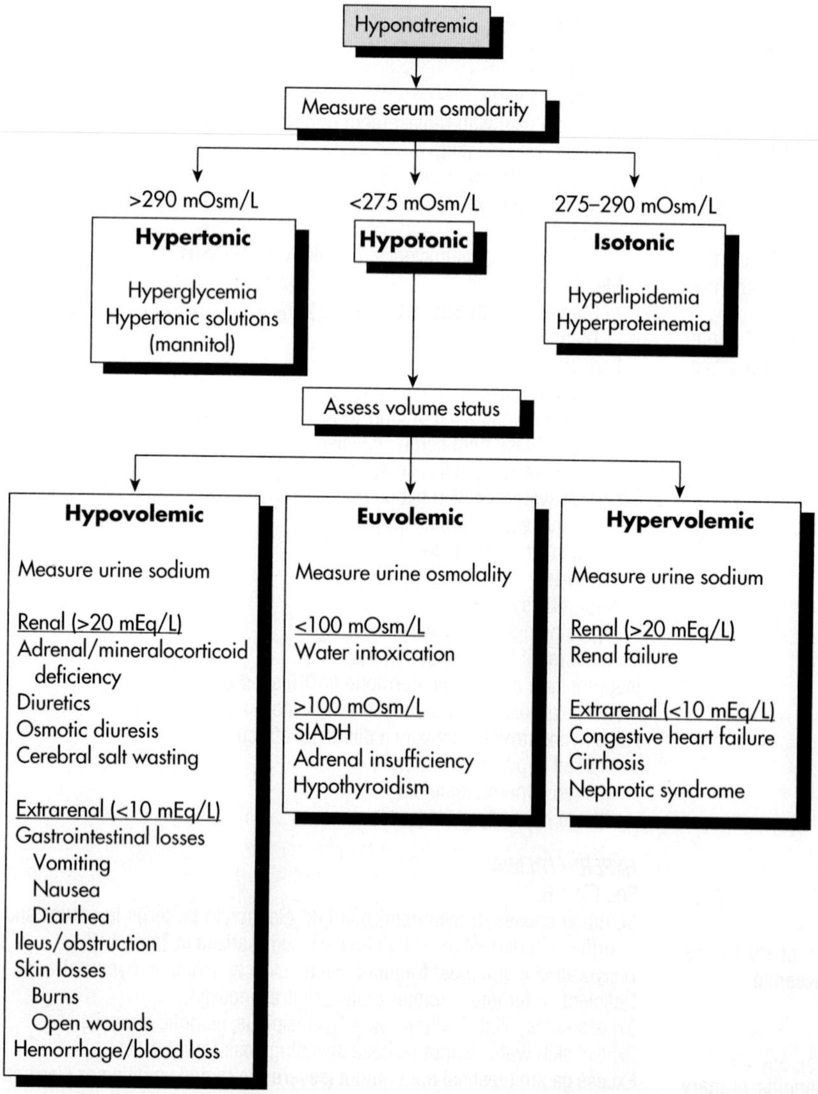

FIG. 55 Algorithm for diagnosis and treatment of hyponatremia. *SIADH,* Syndrome of inappropriate antidiuretic hormone. (From Cameron JL, Cameron AM: *Electrolyte disorders: current surgical therapy*, ed 10, Philadelphia, 2011, Saunders.)

TABLE 115 Common Causes of Hyponatremia and Electrolyte Patterns in Serum and Urine with Normal Renal Function*

Cause	Serum Na	Urine Na (UNa)	Urine Osmolality	Serum K	24-Hour UNa
Overhydration	Low	Low	Low	Normal or low	Low
Diuretics	Low	Low	Low	Low	High
• SIADH†	Low	High	High	Normal or low	High
Adrenal failure	Low	Mildly elevated	Normal	High	High
Bartter syndrome	Low	Low	Low	Low	High
Diabetic hyperosmolarity‡	Low	Normal	Normal	High	Normal

SIADH, Syndrome of inappropriate antidiuretic hormone.
*All Na and K values are concentrations, except for 24-hour UNa, which is the total number of milliequivalents of Na excreted in 24 hours in the urine.
†Secretion of inappropriate levels of antidiuretic hormone.
‡In this condition, serum glucose is markedly elevated.
From McPherson RA, Pincus MR: *Henry's clinical diagnosis and management by laboratory methods,* ed 23, St Louis, 2017, Elsevier.

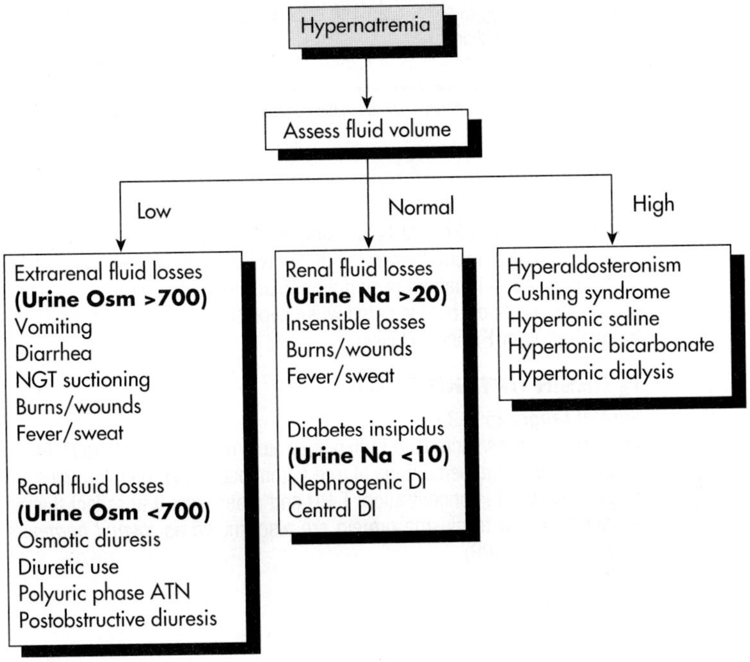

FIG. 56 Algorithm for evaluation of hypernatremia. *ATN,* Acute tubular necrosis; *DI,* diabetes insipidus; *NGT,* nasogastric tube. (From Cameron JL, Cameron AM: *Electrolyte disorders: current surgical therapy,* ed 10, Philadelphia, 2011, Saunders.)

TABLE 117 Common Causes of Hypernatremia and Electrolyte Patterns in Serum and Urine with Normal Renal Function*

Cause	Serum Na	Urine Na (UNa)	Urine Osmolality	Serum K	24-Hour UNa
Dehydration	High	High	High	Normal	Varies
15. Diabetes insipidus	High	Low	Low	Normal	Low
m. Cushing disease or syndrome	High	Low	Normal	Low	Low

*All Na and K values are concentrations, except for 24-hour UNa, which is the total number of milliequivalents of Na excreted in 24 hours in the urine.
From McPherson RA, Pincus MR: *Henry's clinical diagnosis and management by laboratory methods,* ed 23, St Louis, 2017, Elsevier.

Accidental sodium overdose
High-protein tube feedings

STREPTOZYME

See "ANTISTREPTOLYSIN O TITER"

SUCROSE HEMOLYSIS TEST (sugar water test)

Normal: Absence of hemolysis
Positive in: Paroxysmal nocturnal hemoglobinuria
False-positive: Autoimmune hemolytic anemia, megaloblastic anemias
False-negative: May occur with use of heparin or EDTA

SUDAN III STAIN (qualitative screening for fecal fat)

Normal: Negative. Test should be preceded by diet containing 100-150 g of dietary fat/day for 1 wk, avoidance of high-fiber diet, and avoidance of suppositories or oily material before specimen collection.
Positive in: Steatorrhea, use of castor oil or mineral oil droplets

SYNOVIAL FLUID ANALYSIS

Table 118 describes the classification and interpretation of synovial fluid analysis. An algorithm for analysis of joint fluid is illustrated in Fig. 57.

TABLE 118 Classification and Interpretation of Synovial Fluid Analysis

Group	Diseases	Appearance	Viscosity	Mucin Clot	WBC/mm³	% PMN	Glucose (mg/dl) (Blood-Synovial Fluid)	Protein (g/dl)
Normal	—	Clear	↑	Firm	<200	<25	<10	<2.5
I (noninflammatory)	Osteoarthritis, aseptic necrosis, traumatic arthritis, erythema nodosum, osteochondritis dissecans	Clear, yellow (may be xanthochromic if traumatic arthritis)	↑	Firm	↑ Up to 10,000	<25	<10	<2.5
II (inflammatory)	Crystal-induced arthritis, rheumatoid arthritis, Reiter syndrome, collagen vascular disease, psoriatic arthritis, serum sickness, rheumatic fever	Clear, yellow, turbid	↓	Friable	↑↑Up to 100,000	40-90	<40	<2.5
III (septic)	Bacterial (staphylococcal, gonococcal, tuberculosis)	Turbid	↓/↑	Friable	↑↑↑ Up to 5 million	40-100	20-100	>2.5

↑, Elevated; ↑↑, markedly high; ↓, decreased; *PMN*, polymorphonuclear leukocytes; *WBC*, white blood cell. Note that there is considerable overlap in the numbers listed above.

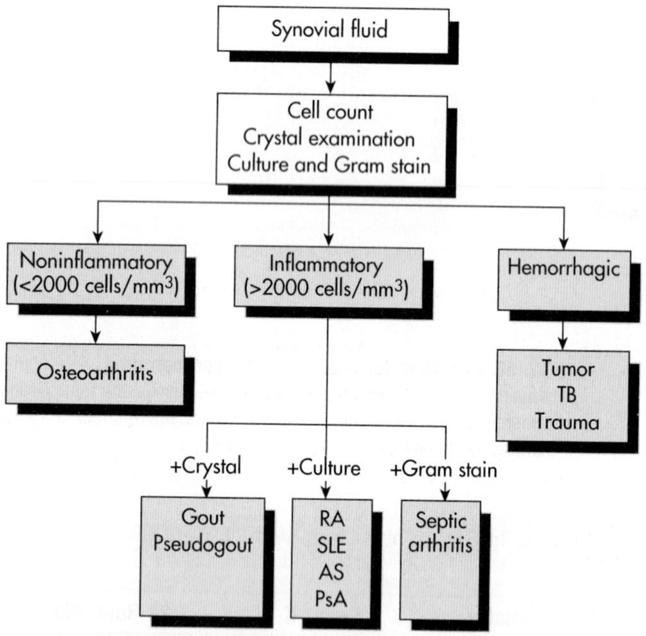

FIG. 57 Algorithm for analysis of joint fluid. Examples of inflammatory arthritis are indicated, although many conditions can produce these findings. *AS*, Ankylosing spondylitis; *PsA*, psoriatic arthritis; *RA*, rheumatoid arthritis; *SLE*, systemic lupus erythematosus; *TB*, tuberculosis. (From Goldman L, Schafer AI: *Goldman's Cecil medicine*, ed 24, Philadelphia, 2012, Saunders.)

T_3 (triiodothyronine)

See Table 119 for T_3 abnormalities.

Normal range: 75-220 ng/dl (1.2-3.4 nmol/L [CF: 0.01536; SMI: 0.1 nmol/L])

Abnormal values

32. Elevated in hyperthyroidism (usually earlier and to a greater extent than serum T_4)
33. Useful in diagnosing:
    T_3 hyperthyroidism (thyrotoxicosis): Increased T_3, normal free thyroxine index (FTI)
    Toxic nodular goiter: Increased T_3, normal or increased T_4
    Iodine deficiency: Normal T_3, possibly decreased T_4
    Thyroid replacement therapy with liothyronine (Cytomel): Normal T_4, increased T_3 if patient is symptomatically hyperthyroid

Not ordered routinely but indicated when hyperthyroidism is suspected and serum-free T_4 or FTI inconclusive

T_3 RESIN UPTAKE (T_3RU)

Normal range: 25%-35%

Abnormal values: Increased in hyperthyroidism. T_3 resin uptake (T_3RU or RT_3U) measures the percentage of free T_4 (not bound to protein); it does not measure serum T_3 concentration; T_3RU and other tests that reflect thyroid hormone binding to plasma protein are also known as *thyroid hormone-binding ratios* (THBR).

T_4, FREE (Free thyroxine)

Normal range: 0.8-2.8 ng/dl

Elevated in

rr. Graves disease, toxic multinodular goiter, toxic adenoma, iatrogenic and factitious causes, transient hyperthyroidism.

ss. Serum-free T_4 directly measures unbound thyroxine. Free T_4 can be measured by equilibrium dialysis (gold standard of free T_4 assays) or by immunometric techniques (influenced by serum levels of lipids, proteins, and certain drugs). The FTI can also be easily calculated by multiplying T_4 times T_3RU and dividing the result by 100; the FTI corrects for any abnormal T_4 values secondary to protein binding: FTI = $T_4 \times T_3RU/100$.

tt. Normal values equal 1.1-4.3.

T_4, SERUM T_4

Normal range: 0.8-2.8 ng/dl (10-36 pmol/L [CF: 12.87; SMI: 1 pmol/L])

Abnormal values: Serum thyroxine (T_4)

Elevated in:

Graves disease
Toxic multinodular goiter
Toxic adenoma
Iatrogenic and factitious
Transient hyperthyroidism
  Subacute thyroiditis
  Hashimoto thyroiditis
  Silent thyroiditis

Rare causes: Hypersecretion of TSH (e.g., pituitary neoplasms), struma ovarii, ingestion of large amounts of iodine in a patient with preexisting

TABLE 119 Findings in Thyroid Function Tests in Various Clinical Conditions

Condition	T_4	FT_4I	T_3	FT_3I	TSH	TSI	TRH Stimulation
Hyperthyroidism							
Graves disease	↑	↑	↑	↑	↓	+	↓
Toxic nodular goiter	↑	↑	↑	↑	↓	–	↓
Pituitary TSH-secreting tumors	↑	↑	↑	↑	↑	–	↓
T_3 thyrotoxicosis	N	N	↑	↑	↓	+, –	↓
T_4 thyrotoxicosis	↑	↑	N	N	↓	+, –	↓
Hypothyroidism							
Primary	↓	↓	↓	↓	↑	+, –	↑
Secondary	↓	↓	↓	↓	↓N	–	↓
Tertiary	↓	↓	↓	↓	↓, N	–	N
Peripheral unresponsiveness	↑, N	↑, N	↑, N	↑	↑, N	–	N,↑

↑, Increased; ↓, decreased; +, – variable; *FTI,* free thyroid index; *N,* normal; *T_3,* triiodothyronine; *T_4,* thyroxine; *TRH,* thyrotropin-releasing hormone; *TSH,* thyroid-stimulating hormone; *TSI,* thyroid stimulating immunoglobulin.

thyroid hyperplasia or adenoma (Jod-Basedow phenomenon), hydatidiform mole, carcinoma of thyroid, amiodarone therapy of arrhythmias

Serum thyroxine test measures both circulating thyroxine bound to protein (represents >99% of circulating T_4) and unbound (free) thyroxine. Values vary with protein binding; changes in the concentration of T_4 secondary to changes in thyroxine-binding globulin (TBG) can be caused by the following:

Increased TBG (↑T_4)	Decreased TBG (↓T_4)
Pregnancy	Androgens, glucocorticoids
Estrogens	Nephrotic syndrome, cirrhosis
Acute infectious hepatitis	Acromegaly
Oral contraceptives	Hypoproteinemia
Familial	Familial
Fluorouracil, clofibrate	Phenytoin, acetylsalicylic acid (ASA) and other NSAIDs, heroin, methadone, high-dose penicillin, asparaginase, chronic debilitating illness

To eliminate the suspected influence of protein binding on thyroxine values, two additional tests are available: T_3 resin uptake and serum free thyroxine. Table 120 summarizes the effects of pregnancy on thyroid physiology, and Table 121 describes changes in thyroid hormone levels during illness.

TEGRETOL

See "CARBAMAZEPINE"

TESTOSTERONE (total testosterone)

Normal range: Variable with age and sex. Testosterone circulates in plasma mostly bound to plasma proteins and sex hormone-binding globulin (SHBG). Approximately 2% of testosterone circulates in free form (biologically active form). Low testosterone levels in obese patients may be due to reduced levels of SHBG; therefore, it is essential to measure free testosterone when evaluating androgen deficiency in obese patients.

Serum/plasma

Males: 280-1100 ng/dl Females: 15-70 ng/dl

Urine

Males: 50-135 μg/day Females: 2-12 μg/day

TABLE 120 Effects of Pregnancy on Thyroid Physiology

Physiologic Change	Thyroid-Related Consequences
↑ Serum thyroxine-binding globulin	↑ Total T_4 and T_3; ↑ T_4 production
↑ Plasma volume	↑ T_4 and T_3 pool size; ↑ T_4 production; ↑ cardiac output
D3 expression in placenta and (?) uterus	↑ T_4 production
First-trimester ↑ in hCG	↑ Free T_4; ↓ basal thyrotropin; ↑ T_4 production
↑ Renal I– clearance	↑ Iodine requirements
↑ T_4 production; fetal T_4 synthesis during second and third trimesters	
↑ Oxygen consumption by fetoplacental unit, gravid uterus, and mother	↑ Basal metabolic rate; ↑ cardiac output

D3, Type 3 iodothyronine deiodinase; *I–,* plasma iodide; *hCG,* human chorionic gonadotropin; *T_3,* triiodothyronine; *T_4,* thyroxine.
From Melmed S et al: *Williams textbook of endocrinology,* ed 12, Philadelphia, 2011, Saunders.

TABLE 121 Changes in Thyroid Hormone Levels during Illness

Severity of Illness	Free T_3	Free T_4	Reverse T_3	TSH	Probable Cause
Mild	↓	N	↑	N	↓ D2, D1
Moderate	↓↓	N, ↑↓	↑↑	N, ↓	↓↓ D2, D1,?↑ D3
Severe	↓↓↓	↓	↑	↓↓	↓↓ D2, D1, ↑D3
Recovery	↓	↓	↑	↑	?

D1 through *D3,* iodothyronine deiodinases; *N,* no change; *T_3,* triiodothyronine; *T_4,* thyroxine; *TSH,* thyroid-stimulating hormone.
From Melmed S et al: *Williams textbook of endocrinology,* ed 12, Philadelphia, 2011, Saunders.

Elevated in: Testicular tumors, ovarian masculinizing tumors, testosterone replacement therapy
Decreased in: Hypogonadism, obesity, insulin resistance, sleep apnea. Fig. 58 illustrates testosterone level changes with age. The diagnosis of androgen deficiency should be based on at least two morning testosterone measurements (collected on separate days) in a symptomatic patient.

THEOPHYLLINE

Normal therapeutic range: 10-20 mcg/ml

THORACENTESIS FLUID

See "PLEURAL FLUID"

THROMBIN TIME (TT), Thrombin Clotting Time (TCT)

Normal range: 11.3-18.5 sec
Elevated in: Thrombolytic and heparin therapy, disseminated intravascular coagulation, hypofibrinogenemia, dysfibrinogenemia
See Table 122 for synthesizing results of PT, APTT, and TCT. Also see Fig. 59.

THYROGLOBULIN

Normal: 3-40 ng/ml. Thyroglobulin is a tumor marker for monitoring the status of patients with papillary or follicular thyroid cancer following resection.
Elevated in: Papillary or follicular thyroid cancer, Hashimoto thyroiditis, Graves disease, subacute thyroiditis

THYROID MICROSOMAL ANTIBODIES

Normal: Undetectable. Low titers may be present in 5%-10% of normal individuals.

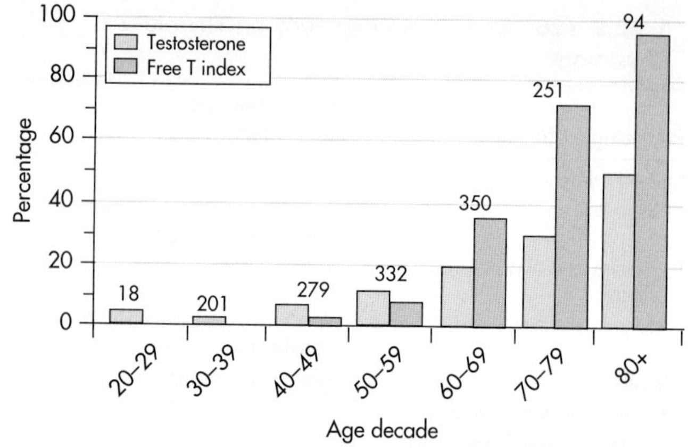

FIG. 58 Hypogonadism in aging men. Bar height indicates the percentage of men in each 10-year interval, from the third to the ninth decades, with at least one testosterone value in the hypogonadal range. The criteria used for these determinations are total testosterone less than 11.3 nmol/L (325 ng/dl) and testosterone and sex hormone-binding globulin (free T index) less than 0.153 nmol/nmol. The numbers above each pair of bars indicate the number of men studied in the corresponding decade. The fraction of men who are hypogonadal increases progressively after age 50 years by either criterion. More men are hypogonadal by free T index than by total testosterone after 50 years, and there seems to be a progressively greater difference with increasing age between the two criteria. (From Goldman L, Schafer AI: *Goldman's Cecil medicine*, ed 24, Philadelphia, 2012, Saunders.)

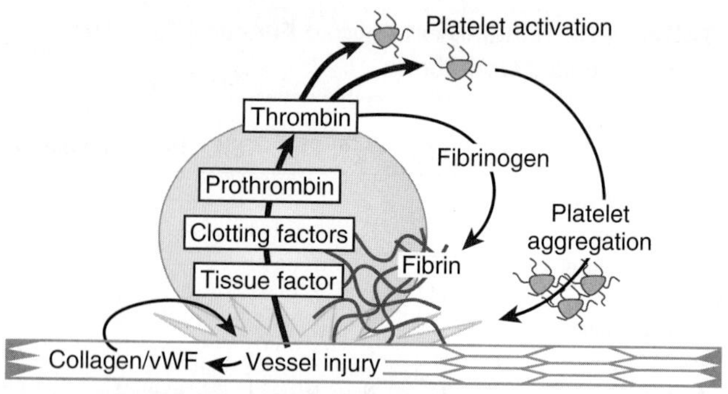

FIG. 59 Central role of thrombin in thrombogenesis. Vascular injury simultaneously triggers platelet adhesion and activation, as well as activation of the coagulation system. Platelet activation is initiated by exposure of subendothelial collagen and von Willebrand factor *(vWF)*, to which platelets adhere. Adherent platelets become activated and release ADP and thromboxane A_2, platelet agonists that activate ambient platelets and recruit them to the site of injury. Coagulation, which is triggered by tissue factor exposed at the site of injury and enhanced by assembly of clotting factor complexes on the activated platelet surface, results in thrombin generation. Thrombin not only converts fibrinogen to fibrin but also serves as a potent platelet agonist. When platelets are activated, glycoprotein *(GP)* IIb/IIIa on their surfaces undergoes a conformational change that endows it with the capacity to ligate fibrinogen and mediate platelet aggregation. Fibrin strands then weave the platelet aggregates together to form a platelet/fibrin thrombus. (From Zipes DP: *Braunwald's heart disease, a textbook of cardiovascular medicine*, ed 11, Philadelphia, 2019, Elsevier.)

TABLE 122 Synthesizing Results of PT, APTT, and TCT

TEST			
PT	**APTT**	**TCT**	**Possible Diagnoses**
Normal	Normal	Normal	Normal hemostasis, disorder of platelet function, factor XIII deficiency, disorder of vascular hemostasis, mild coagulation protein deficiency, mild vWD, disorder of fibrinolysis (α_2-antiplasmin deficiency/defect, plasminogen activator inhibitor-1 deficiency/defect)
Prolonged	Normal	Normal	Factor VII deficiency; early oral anticoagulation; lupus anticoagulant; mild factor II, V, or X deficiency; specific factor inhibitor
Normal	Prolonged	Normal	Factor VIII, IX, XI, XI, prekallikrein, or HMWK deficiency; lupus anticoagulant; amyloid-adsorbed factor IX; specific factor inhibitor
Prolonged	Prolonged	Normal	Multiple factor deficiency (e.g., liver failure, vitamin K deficiency, oral anticoagulants); factor V, X, or II deficiency; amyloid-adsorbed factor X; specific factor inhibitor
Prolonged	Prolonged	Prolonged	Anticoagulants, DIC, dilutional coagulopathy, liver disease, fibrinogen deficiency/disorder, inhibition of fibrin polymerization, hyperfibrinolysis

APTT, Activated partial thromboplastin time; *DIC,* disseminated intravascular coagulation; *HMWK,* high-molecular-weight kininogen; *PT,* prothrombin time; *TCT,* thrombin clotting time; *vWD,* von Willebrand disease.

From Hoffman R: *Hematology: basic principles and practice,* ed 7, Philadelphia, 2018, Elsevier.

Elevated in: Hashimoto disease, thyroid carcinoma, early hypothyroidism, pernicious anemia

THYROID-STIMULATING HORMONE (TSH)

Changes in TSH levels during illness are summarized in Table 123. See Fig. 60 for an algorithmic approach to thyroid testing.

TABLE 123 Changes in Thyroid Hormone Levels During Illness

Severity of Illness	Free T_3	Free T_4	Reverse T_3	TSH	Probable Cause
Mild	↓	N	↑	N	↓ D2, D1
Moderate	↓↓	N, ↑↓	↑↑	N, ↓	↓↓ D2, D1, ? ↑ D3
Severe	↓↓↓	↓	↑	↓↓	↓↓ D2, D1, ↑D3
Recovery	↓	↓	↑	↑	?

D1 through *D3,* Iodothyronine deiodinases; *N,* no change; *T_3,* triiodothyronine; *T_4,* thyroxine; *TSH,* thyroid-stimulating hormone (thyrotropin).

From Melmed S et al: *Williams textbook of endocrinology,* ed 14, Philadelphia, 2019, Elsevier.

Normal range: 2-11 μU/ml (2-11 mU/L [CF: 1; SMI: 1 mU/L])

CONDITIONS THAT INCREASE SERUM THYROID-STIMULATING HORMONE VALUES

Laboratory error
Primary hypothyroidism
Synthroid therapy with insufficient dose
Lithium or amiodarone; some patients
Hashimoto thyroiditis in later stage
Large doses of inorganic iodide (e.g., potassium iodide [SSKI])
Severe nonthyroid illness in recovery phase
Iodine deficiency (moderate or severe)
Addison disease
TSH specimen drawn in evening (peak of diurnal variation)
Pituitary TSH-secreting tumor
Therapy of hypothyroidism (3-6 wk after beginning therapy [range, 1-8 wk]; sometimes longer when pretherapy TSH is over 100 μU/ml)
Acute psychiatric illness
Peripheral resistance to T_4 syndrome
Antibodies (e.g., human antimouse antibody [HAMA]) interfering with monoclonal sandwich method of TSH assay
Telepaque (iopanoic acid) and Oragrafin (ipodate) x-ray contrast media
Amphetamines
High altitudes

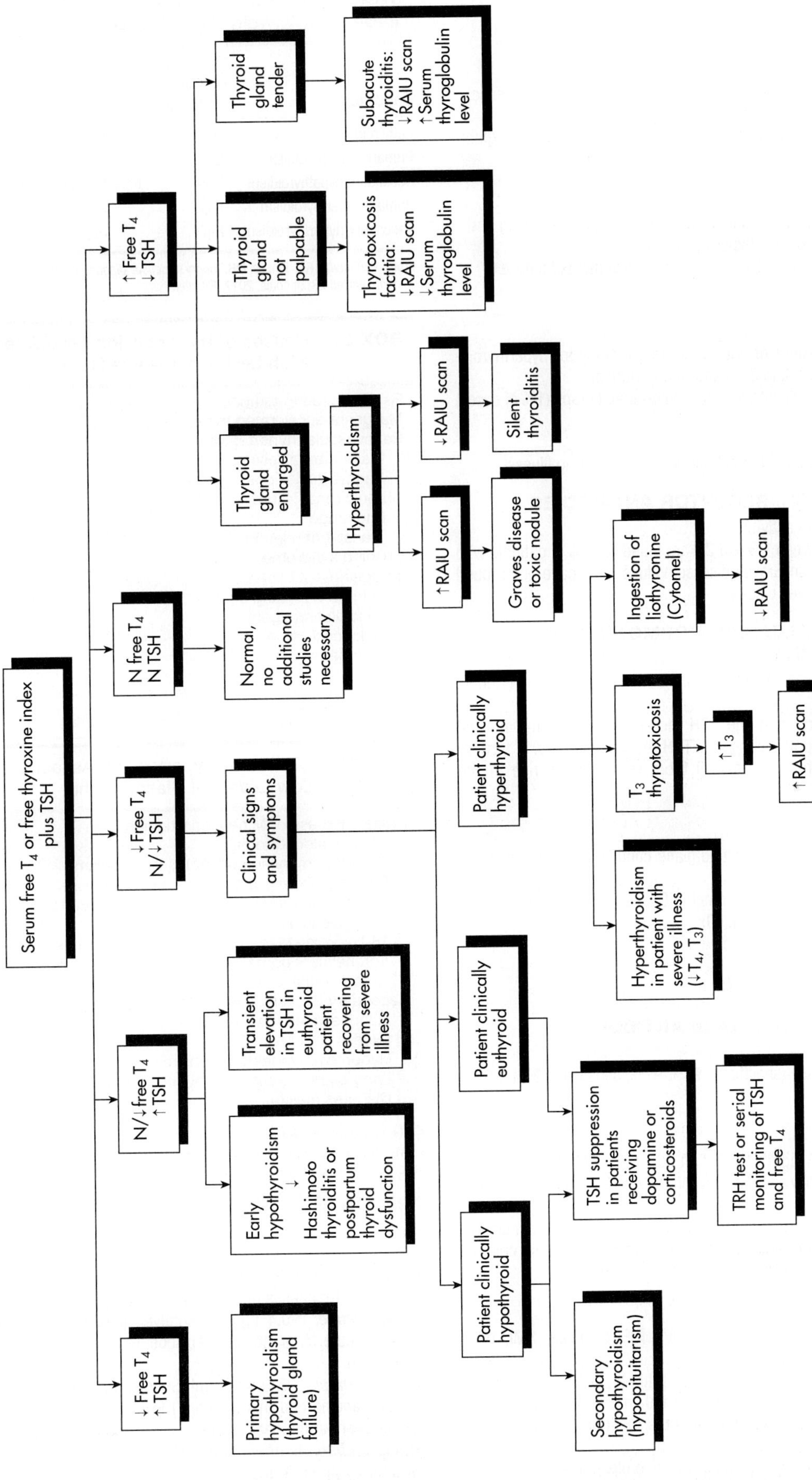

FIG. 60 Diagnostic approach to thyroid testing. *N,* Normal; *RAIU,* radioactive iodine uptake; *T_3,* triiodothyronine; *T_4,* thyroxine; *TRH,* thyrotropin-releasing hormone; *TSH,* thyroid-stimulating hormone. (From Ferri FF: *Practical guide to the care of the medical patient,* ed 9, St Louis, 2014, Mosby.)

CONDITIONS THAT DECREASE SERUM THYROID-STIMULATING HORMONE VALUES

Laboratory error
T_4/T_3 toxicosis (diffuse or nodular etiology)
Excessive therapy for hypothyroidism
Active thyroiditis (subacute, painless, or early active Hashimoto disease)
Multinodular goiter containing areas of autonomy
Severe nonthyroid illness (especially acute trauma, dopamine, or glucocorticoid)
T_3 toxicosis
Pituitary insufficiency
Cushing syndrome (and some patients on high-dose glucocorticoid)
Jod-Basedow (iodine-induced) hyperthyroidism
Thyroid-stimulating hormone drawn 2-4 hr after levothyroxine dose
Postpartum transient toxicosis
Factitious hyperthyroidism
Struma ovarii
Radioimmunoassay, surgery, or antithyroid drug therapy for hyperthyroidism 4-6 wk (range, 2 wk to 2 yr) after the treatment
Interleukin-2 drugs (3%-6% of cases) or α-interferon therapy (1% of cases)
Hyperemesis gravidarum
Amiodarone therapy
See Table 121 for changes in thyroid hormone levels during illness.

THYROTROPIN (TSH) RECEPTOR ANTIBODIES

Normal: <130% of basal activity
Elevated in: Values between 1.3 and 2.0 are found in 10% of patients with thyroid disease other than Graves disease. Values >2.8 have been found only in patients with Graves disease.

THYROTROPIN-RELEASING HORMONE (TRH) STIMULATION TEST

Normal: Baseline TSH <11 microU/ml; stimulated TSH: More than double the baseline

In primary hypothyroidism the TSH increase is 2-3× the normal result. In secondary hypothyroidism no TSH response occurs. In tertiary hypothyroidism (hypothalamic failure) there is a delayed rise in the TSH level.

THYROXINE (T_4)

Patterns in T_4 levels in different thyroid gland conditions are summarized in Table 124.
Normal range: 4-11 μg/dl (51-142 nmol/L [CF: 12.87; SMI: 1 nmol/L])
Elevated: Hyperthyroidism (see Fig. 60)

TIBC

See "IRON-BINDING CAPACITY, TOTAL"

TISSUE TRANSGLUTAMINASE ANTIBODY

Normal: Negative
Present in: Celiac disease (specificity; 94%-97%, sensitivity, 90%-98%), dermatitis herpetiformis

TRANSFERRIN

Normal range: 170-370 mg/dl (1.7-3.7 g/L [CF: 0.01; SMI: 0.01 g/L])
Elevated in: Iron deficiency anemia, oral contraceptive administration, viral hepatitis, late pregnancy
Decreased in: Nephrotic syndrome, liver disease, hereditary deficiency, protein malnutrition, neoplasms, chronic inflammatory states, chronic illness, thalassemia, hemochromatosis, hemolytic anemia

TRIGLYCERIDES

Normal range: <150 mg/dl (<1.80 mmol/L [CF: 0.01129; SMI: 0.02 mmol/L])
Elevated in: Hyperlipoproteinemias (types I, IIb, III, IV, V), hypothyroidism, pregnancy, estrogens, acute myocardial infarction, pancreatitis, alcohol intake, nephrotic syndrome, diabetes mellitus, glycogen storage disease
Decreased in: Malnutrition, congenital abetalipoproteinemias, drugs (e.g., gemfibrozil, fenofibrate, nicotinic acid, clofibrate)

TABLE 124 Patterns of Serum Levels of TSH and T_4 in Different Thyroid Gland Conditions

Condition	T_4 (Most Accurate, Free T_4)	TSH	Site of Disease
Euthyroid	Normal	Normal	None
Primary hypothyroidism	Low	High	Thyroid gland
Secondary hypothyroidism	Low	Low to normal	Pituitary
Primary hyperthyroidism	High	Low	Thyroid
Secondary hyperthyroidism	High	High	Pituitary

From McPherson RA, Pincus MR: *Henry's clinical diagnosis and management by laboratory methods*, ed 23, St Louis, 2017, Elsevier.

BOX 31 Causes of Hypertension Associated with High Levels of Plasma Renin

Renin-secreting tumor
Malignant accelerated hypertension
Renovascular hypertension
- Major arterial lesions
- Segmental lesions

Chronic renal failure
- End stage
- Transplant rejection

Cushing syndrome
Iatrogenic
- Volume-depleting agents
- Vasodilating agents
- Glucocorticoids
- Estrogens

From McPherson RA, Pincus MR: *Henry's clinical diagnosis and management by laboratory methods*, ed 23, St Louis, 2017, Elsevier.

BOX 32 Causes of Hypertension Associated with Low Levels of Plasma Renin

Primary Excess of Mineralocorticoids
- Primary aldosteronism
- Pseudoprimary (idiopathic) aldosteronism
- Glucocorticoid-suppressible aldosteronism
- 11-Deoxycorticosterone excess (CAH due to 11-β-hydroxylase deficiency)
- 18-Hydroxy-11-deoxycorticosterone excess
- Adrenal carcinoma (excess mineralocorticoids and/or glucocorticoids)

Secondary Excess of Mineralocorticoids
- Licorice ingestion
- Excess sodium intake
- Hyporenin hypoaldosteronism
- Long-standing essential hypertension
- Diabetes mellitus

CAH, Congenital adrenal hyperplasia.
From McPherson RA, Pincus MR: *Henry's clinical diagnosis and management by laboratory methods*, ed 23, St Louis, 2017, Elsevier.

TRIIODOTHYRONINE

See "T_3"

TROPONINS (serum)

See Box 33 for causes of troponin elevations.
Normal range: 0-0.4 ng/ml (negative). If there is clinical suspicion of evolving acute MI or ischemic episode, repeat testing in 5 to 6 hr is recommended.
Indeterminate: 0.05-0.49 ng/ml. Suggest further tests. In a patient with unstable angina and this troponin I level, there is an increased risk of a cardiac event in the near future.
Strong probability of acute MI: ≥0.05 ng/ml
Cardiac troponin T (cTnT) is a highly sensitive marker for myocardial injury for the first 48 hours after MI and for up to 5 to 7 days (see Fig. 20,

BOX 33 Causes of Serum Troponin T and I Elevations, Including Both Acute Coronary Syndromes, Noncoronary Cardiac Events, and Noncardiac Ailments

Acute coronary syndrome/acute myocardial infarction
Shock of any form (cardiogenic, obstructive, distributive)
Myocarditis and myopericarditis
Cardiomyopathies
Acute congestive heart failure (pulmonary edema)
Sepsis
Pulmonary embolism
Renal failure
Sympathomimetic ingestions
Polytrauma
Burns
Acute CNS event
Rhabdomyolysis
Cardiac neoplasm, inflammatory syndromes, and infiltrative diseases
Congenital coronary anomalies
Extreme physical exertion

From Vincent JL et al: *Textbook of critical care,* ed 6, Philadelphia, 2011, Saunders.

BOX 34 PPD Reaction Size Considered "Positive" (Intracutaneous 5 TU Mantoux Test at 48 hr)

5 mm or More
HIV infection or risk factors for HIV
Close recent contact with active TB case
Persons with chest x-ray consistent with healed TB

10 mm or More
Foreign-born persons from countries with high TB prevalence in Asia, Africa, and Latin America
IV drug users
Medically underserved low-income population groups (including Native Americans, Hispanics, and blacks)
Residents of long-term care facilities (nursing homes, mental institutions)
Medical conditions that increase risk for TB (silicosis, gastrectomy, undernourishment, diabetes mellitus, high-dose corticosteroids or immunosuppression Rx, leukemia or lymphoma, other malignancies)
Employees of long-term care facilities, schools, child care facilities, health care facilities

15 mm or More
All others not already listed

HIV, Human immunodeficiency virus; *IV,* intravenous; *PPD,* purified protein derivative; *Rx,* prescription; *TB,* tuberculosis; *TU,* tuberculin units.

under "Creatine Kinase Isoenzymes"). It may also be elevated in renal failure, chronic muscle disease, and trauma.

Cardiac troponin I (cTnI) is highly sensitive and specific for myocardial injury (≥CK-MB) in the initial 8 hr, peaks within 24 hr and lasts up to 7 days. With progressively higher levels of cTnI, the risk of mortality increases because the amount of necrosis increases.

TSH

See "THYROID-STIMULATING HORMONE"

TT

See "THROMBIN TIME"

TUBERCULIN TEST (PPD)

Abnormal results: See Box 34. Box 35 describes factors associated with false-negative tuberculin tests.

BOX 35 Factors Associated with False-Negative Tuberculin Tests

Technical Errors
Improper administration
Inaccurate reading
Loss of potency of antigen

Patient-Related Factors (Anergy)
Age (elderly)
Nutritional status
Medications: Corticosteroids, immunosuppressive agents
Severe tuberculosis
Coexisting diseases
- HIV infection
- Viral illness or vaccination
- Lymphoreticular malignancies
- Sarcoidosis
- Solid tumors
- Lepromatous leprosy
- Sjögren syndrome
- Ataxia telangiectasia
- Uremia
- Primary biliary cirrhosis
- Systemic lupus erythematosus

Severe systemic disease of any etiology

HIV, Human immunodeficiency virus.

BOX 36 Factors Affecting Blood Urea Nitrogen Level Independent of Renal Function

Disproportionate Increase in Blood Urea Nitrogen
Volume depletion ("prerenal azotemia")
Gastrointestinal hemorrhage
Corticosteroid or cytotoxic agents
High-protein diet
Obstructive uropathy
Sepsis
Catabolic states, tissue breakdown

Disproportionate Decrease in Blood Urea Nitrogen
Low-protein diet
Liver disease

UNCONJUGATED BILIRUBIN

See "BILIRUBIN, DIRECT"

UREA NITROGEN, BLOOD (BUN)

Normal range: 8-18 mg/dl (3-6.5 mmol/L [CF: 0.357; SMI: 0.5 mmol/L])

Box 36 describes factors affecting BUN level independent of renal function.

Elevated in: Dehydration, drugs (aminoglycosides and other antibiotics, diuretics, lithium, corticosteroids), gastrointestinal bleeding, decreased renal blood flow (shock, congestive heart failure, myocardial infarction), renal disease (glomerulonephritis, pyelonephritis, diabetic nephropathy), urinary tract obstruction (prostatic hypertrophy)

Decreased in: Liver disease, malnutrition, third trimester of pregnancy, overhydration, acromegaly, celiac disease

URIC ACID (serum)

Normal range: 2-7 mg/dl

Elevated in: Renal failure, gout, excessive cell lysis (chemotherapeutic agents, radiation therapy, leukemia, lymphoma, hemolytic anemia), hereditary enzyme deficiency (hypoxanthine-guanine-phosphoribosyl transferase), acidosis, myeloproliferative disorders, diet high in purines or protein, drugs (diuretics, low doses of ASA, ethambutol, nicotinic acid), lead poisoning, hypothyroidism, Addison disease, nephrogenic diabetes insipidus, active psoriasis, polycystic kidneys

Decreased in: Drugs (allopurinol, febuxostat, high doses of ASA, probenecid, warfarin, corticosteroid), deficiency of xanthine oxidase, syndrome of inappropriate antidiuretic hormone secretion, renal tubular deficits (Fanconi syndrome), alcoholism, liver disease, diet deficient in protein or purines, Wilson disease, hemochromatosis

URINALYSIS

Blood urinalysis abnormalities in various urinary system diseases are summarized in Table 125.

Normal range

34. Color: Light straw
35. Appearance: Clear
36. Ketones: Absent
37. pH: 4.5-8 (average, 6)
38. Protein: Absent
39. Glucose: Absent
40. Specific gravity: 1.005-1.030
41. Occult blood absent
42. Microscopic examination:
    Red blood cells: 0-5 (high-power field)
    White blood cells: 0-5 (high-power field)
    Bacteria (spun specimen): Absent
    Casts: 0-4 hyaline (low-power field)
    Abnormalities in the microscopic examination of urine are described in Table 126. Causes of abnormal appearance and color of urine are described in Table 127. Urine color changes with commonly used drugs are summarized in Table 128.

URINE AMYLASE

Normal range: 35-260 U Somogyi/hr (6.5-48.1 U/hr [CF: 0.185; SMI: 1 U/hr])

Elevated in: Pancreatitis, carcinoma of the pancreas

URINE BILE

Normal: Absent

Abnormal

uu. Urine bilirubin: Hepatitis (viral, toxic, drug-induced), biliary obstruction

TABLE 125 Various Urinary System Diseases and Corresponding Urinalysis Abnormalities

Diseases	Macroscopic Urinalysis	Microscopic Urinalysis
Acute glomerulonephritis	Gross hematuria "Smoky" turbidity Proteinuria	Erythrocyte and blood casts Epithelial casts Hyaline and granular casts Waxy casts Neutrophils Erythrocytes
Chronic glomerulonephritis	Hematuria Proteinuria	Granular and waxy casts Occasional blood casts Erythrocytes Leukocytes Epithelial casts Lipid droplets
Acute pyelonephritis	Turbid Occasional odor Occasional proteinuria	Numerous neutrophils (many in clumps) Few lymphocytes and histiocytes Leukocyte casts Epithelial casts Renal epithelial cells Erythrocytes Granular and waxy casts Bacteria
Chronic pyelonephritis	Occasional proteinuria	Leukocytes Broad waxy casts Granular and epithelial casts Occasional leukocyte casts Bacteria Erythrocytes
Nephrotic syndrome	Proteinuria Fat droplets	Fatty and waxy casts Cellular and granular casts Oval fat bodies and/or vacuolated renal epithelial cells occurring singly or as cellular clusters
Acute tubular necrosis	Hematuria Occasional proteinuria	Necrotic or degenerated renal epithelial cells Neutrophils and erythrocytes Granular and epithelial casts Waxy casts Broad casts Epithelial tissue fragments
Cystitis	Hematuria	Numerous leukocytes Erythrocytes Transitional epithelial cells occurring singly or as fragments Histiocytes and giant cells Bacteria Absence of casts
Dysuria-pyuria syndrome	Slightly turbid	Numerous leukocytes, bacteria Erythrocytes No casts
Acute renal allograft rejection (lower nephrosis)	Hematuria Occasional proteinuria	Renal epithelial cells Lymphocytes and plasma cells Neutrophils Renal epithelial casts Renal epithelial fragments Granular, bloody, and waxy casts
Urinary tract neoplasia	Hematuria	Atypical mononuclear cells with enlarged, irregular hyperchromatic nuclei and sometimes containing prominent nucleoli that occur singly or as tissue fragments Neutrophils Erythrocytes Transitional epithelial cells
Viral infection	Hematuria Occasional proteinuria	Enlarged mononuclear cells and/or multinucleated cells with prominent intranuclear and/or cytoplasmic inclusions Neutrophils Lymphocytes and plasma cells Erythrocytes

From McPherson RA, Pincus MR: *Henry's clinical diagnosis and management by laboratory methods*, ed 23, St Louis, 2017, Elsevier.

TABLE 126 Microscopic Examination of the Urine

Finding	Associations
Casts	
Red blood cell	Glomerulonephritis, vasculitis
White blood cell	Interstitial nephritis, pyelonephritis
Epithelial cell	Acute tubular necrosis, interstitial nephritis, glomerulonephritis
Granular	Renal parenchymal disease (nonspecific)
Waxy, broad	Advanced renal failure
Hyaline	Normal finding in concentrated urine
Fatty	Heavy proteinuria
Cells	
Red blood cell	Urinary tract infection, urinary tract inflammation
White blood cell	Urinary tract infection, urinary tract inflammation
Eosinophil	Acute interstitial nephritis
(Squamous) epithelial cell	Contaminants
Crystals	
Uric acid	Acid urine, acute uric acid nephropathy, hyperuricosuria
Calcium phosphate	Alkaline urine
Calcium oxalate	Acid urine, hyperoxaluria, ethylene glycol poisoning
Cystine	Cystinuria
Sulfur	Sulfa-containing antibiotics

vv. Urine urobilinogen: Hepatitis (viral, toxic, drug-induced), hemolytic jaundice, liver cell dysfunction (cirrhosis, infection, metastases)

URINE CALCIUM

Normal range: <250 mg/24 hr (<6.2 mmol/dl [CF: 0.02495; SMI: 0.1 mmol/dl])

Elevated in: Primary hyperparathyroidism, hypervitaminosis D, bone metastases, multiple myeloma, increased calcium intake, steroids, prolonged immobilization, sarcoidosis, Paget disease, idiopathic hypercalciuria, renal tubular acidosis

Decreased in: Hypoparathyroidism, pseudohypoparathyroidism, vitamin D deficiency, vitamin D-resistant rickets, diet low in calcium, drugs (thiazide diuretics, oral contraceptives), familial hypocalciuric hypercalcemia, renal osteodystrophy, potassium citrate therapy

URINE CAMP

Elevated in: Hypercalciuria, familial hypocalciuric hypercalcemia, primary hyperparathyroidism, pseudohypoparathyroidism, rickets

Decreased in: Vitamin D intoxication, sarcoidosis

URINE CATECHOLAMINES

Normal range

Norepinephrine: <100 μg/24 hr (<590 nmol/day [CF: 5.911; SMI: 10 nmol/day])

Epinephrine: <10 μg/24 hr (55 nmol/day [CF: 5.458; SMI: 5 nmol/day])

Elevated in: Pheochromocytoma, neuroblastoma, severe stress

URINE CHLORIDE

Normal range: 110-250 mEq/day (110-250 mmol/day [CF: 1; SMI: 1 mmol/day])

Elevated in: Corticosteroids, Bartter syndrome, diuretics, metabolic acidosis, severe hypokalemia

Decreased in: Chloride depletion (vomiting), colonic villous adenoma, chronic renal failure, renal tubular acidosis

URINE COPPER

Normal range: <40 μg/24 hr (<0.6 μmol/day [CF: 0.01574; SMI: 0.2 μmol/day])

TABLE 127 Appearance and Color of Urine

Appearance	Cause	Remarks
Colorless	Very dilute urine	Polyuria, diabetes insipidus
Cloudy	Phosphates, carbonates	Soluble in dilute acetic acid
	Urates, uric acid	Dissolve at 60° C (140° F) and in alkali
	Leukocytes	
	Red blood cells ("smoky")	Insoluble in dilute acetic acid
	Bacteria, yeasts	Lyse in dilute acetic acid
	Spermatozoa	Insoluble in dilute acetic acid
	Prostatic fluid	
	Mucin, mucous threads	Insoluble in dilute acetic acid
	Calculi, "gravel"	
	Clumps, pus, tissue	May be flocculent
	Fecal contamination	Phosphates, oxalates
	Radiographic dye	Rectovesical fistula
		In acid urine
Milky	Many neutrophils (pyuria)	Insoluble in dilute acetic acid
	Fat	Nephrosis, crush injury: Soluble in ether
	Lipiduria, opalescent	
	Chyluria, milky	Lymphatic obstruction: Soluble in ether
	Emulsified paraffin	Vaginal creams
Yellow	Acriflavine	Green fluorescence
Yellow-orange	Concentrated urine	Dehydration, fever
	Urobilin in excess	No yellow foam
	Bilirubin	Yellow foam if sufficient bilirubin
Yellow-green	Bilirubin-biliverdin	Yellow foam
Yellow-brown	Bilirubin-biliverdin	"Beer" brown, yellow foam
Red	Hemoglobin	Positive
	Erythrocytes	Positive
	Myoglobin	Reagent strip for blood
	Porphyrin	Positive
	Fuscin, aniline dye	May be colorless
	Beets	Foods, candy
	Menstrual contamination	Yellow alkaline, genetic
		Clots, mucus
Red-purple	Porphyrins	May be colorless
Red-brown	Erythrocytes	Acid pH
	Hemoglobin on standing	Muscle injury
	Methemoglobin	Result of unstable hemoglobin
	Myoglobin	
	Bilifuscin (dipyrrole)	
Brown-black	Methemoglobin	Blood, acid pH
	Homogentisic acid	On standing, alkaline; alkaptonuria
	Melanin	On standing, rare
Blue-green	Indicans	Small intestine infections
	Pseudomonas infections	Mouth deodorants
	Chlorophyll	

From McPherson RA, Pincus MR: *Henry's clinical diagnosis and management by laboratory methods*, ed 23, St Louis, 2017, Elsevier.

URINE CORTISOL, FREE

Normal range: 10-110 μg/24 hr (30-300 nmol/day [CF: 2.759; SMI: 10 nmol/day])

Elevated: See "CORTISOL, PLASMA"

URINE CREATININE (24 hr)

Normal range

Male: 0.8-1.8 g/day (7-16 mmol/day [CF: 8.840; SMI: 0.1 mmol/day])

Female: 0.6-1.6 g/day (5.3-14 mmol/day)

NOTE: Useful test as an indicator of completeness of 24-hr urine collection.

URINE CRYSTALS

Uric acid: Acid urine, hyperuricosuria, uric acid nephropathy

TABLE 128 Urine Color Changes with Commonly Used Drugs*

Drug	Color
Alcohol, ethyl	Pale, diuresis
Anthraquinone laxatives (senna, cascara)	Reddish, alkaline; yellow-brown, acid
Chlorzoxazone (Paraflex) (muscle relaxant)	Red
Deferoxamine mesylate (Desferal) (chelates iron)	Red
Ethoxazene (Serenium) (urinary analgesic)	Orange, red
Fluorescein sodium (given IV)	Yellow
Furazolidone (Furoxone) (Tricofuron) (an antibacterial, antiprotozoal nitrofuran)	Brown
Indigo carmine dye (renal function, cystoscopy)	Blue
Iron sorbitol (Jectofer) (possibly other iron compounds forming iron sulfide in urine)	Brown on standing
Levodopa (L-dopa) (for parkinsonism)	Red then brown, alkaline
Mepacrine (Atabrine) (antimalarial) (intestinal worms, *Giardia)*	Yellow
Methocarbamol (Robaxin) (muscle relaxant)	Green-brown
Methyldopa (Aldomet) (antihypertensive)	Darkens; if oxidizing agents present, red to brown
Methylene blue (used to delineate fistulas)	Blue, blue-green
Metronidazole (Flagyl) (for *Trichomonas* infection, amebiasis, *Giardia*)	Darkening, reddish brown
Nitrofurantoin (Furadantin) (antibacterial)	Brown-yellow
Phenazopyridine (Pyridium) (urinary analgesic), also compounded with sulfonamides (e.g., Azo Gantrisin)	Orange-red, acid pH
Phenindione (Hedulin) (anticoagulant) (important to distinguish from hematuria)	Orange, alkaline; color disappears on acidifying
Phenol poisoning	Brown; oxidized to quinones (green)
Phenolphthalein (purgative)	Red-purple, alkaline pH
Phenolsulfonphthalein (also sulfobromophthalein)	Pink-red, alkaline pH
Rifampin (Rifadin, Rimactane) (tuberculosis therapy)	Bright orange-red
Riboflavin (multivitamins)	Bright yellow
Sulfasalazine (Azulfidine) (for ulcerative colitis)	Orange-yellow, alkaline pH

*Other commonly used drugs have been noted to produce color change once or occasionally: Amitriptyline (Elavil)—blue-green; phenothiazines—red; triamterene (Dyrenium)—pale blue (blue fluorescence in acid urine).

From McPherson RA, Pincus MR: *Henry's clinical diagnosis and management by laboratory methods*, ed 23, St Louis, 2017, Elsevier.

Sulfur: Antibiotics containing sulfa
Calcium oxalate: Ethylene glycol poisoning, acid urine, hyperoxaluria
Calcium phosphate: Alkaline urine
Cystine: Cystinuria

URINE EOSINOPHILS

Normal: Absent
Present in: Interstitial nephritis, acute tubular necrosis, urinary tract infection, kidney transplant rejection, hepatorenal syndrome

URINE GLUCOSE (qualitative)

Normal: Absent

TABLE 129 Factors That Interfere with Determination of Urinary 5-HIAA

Foods	Drugs
Factors That Produce False-Positive Results	
Avocado	Acetaminophen
Banana	Acetanilid
Chocolate	Caffeine
Coffee	Fluorouracil
Eggplant	Guaifenesin
Pecan	L-Dopa
Pineapple	Melphalan
Plum	Mephenesin
Tea	Methamphetamine
Walnuts	Methocarbamol
	Methysergide maleate
	Phenmetrazine
	Reserpine
	Salicylates
Factors That Cause False-Negative Results	
None	Corticotropin
	p-Chlorophenylalanine
	Chlorpromazine
	Heparin
	Imipramine
	Isoniazid
	Methenamine mandelate
	Methyldopa
	Monoamine oxidase inhibitors
	Phenothiazine
	Promethazine

5-HIAA, 5-Hydroxyindoleacetic acid.
From Melmed S et al: *Williams textbook of endocrinology*, ed 12, Philadelphia, 2011, Saunders.

Present in: Diabetes mellitus, renal glycosuria (decreased renal threshold for glucose), glucose intolerance

URINE HEMOGLOBIN, FREE

Normal: Absent
Present in: Hemolysis (with saturation of serum haptoglobin binding capacity and renal threshold for tubular absorption of hemoglobin)

URINE HEMOSIDERIN

Normal: Absent
Present in: Paroxysmal nocturnal hemoglobinuria, chronic hemolytic anemia, hemochromatosis, blood transfusion, thalassemias

URINE 5-HYDROXYINDOLE-ACETIC ACID (urine 5-HIAA)

Normal range: 2-8 mg/24 hr (10-40 μmol/day [CF: 5.23; SMI: 5 μmol/day])
Elevated in: Carcinoid tumors, after ingestion of certain foods (bananas, plums, tomatoes, avocados, pineapples, eggplant, walnuts), drugs (monoamine oxidase inhibitors, phenacetin, methyldopa, glycerol guaiacolate, acetaminophen, salicylates, phenothiazines, imipramine, methocarbamol, reserpine, methamphetamine). See Table 129.

URINE INDICAN

Normal: Absent
Present in: Malabsorption secondary to intestinal bacterial overgrowth

URINE KETONES (semiquantitative)

Normal: Absent

TABLE 130 Medications That May Increase Measured Levels of Fractionated Catecholamines and Metanephrines

Tricyclic antidepressants (including cyclobenzaprine)
Levodopa
Drugs containing adrenergic receptor agonists (e.g., decongestants)
Amphetamines
Buspirone and antipsychotic agents
Prochlorperazine
Reserpine
Withdrawal from clonidine and other drugs (e.g., illicit drugs)
Illicit drugs (e.g., cocaine, heroin)
Ethanol

From Melmed S et al: *Williams textbook of endocrinology*, ed 12, Philadelphia, 2011, Saunders.

Present in: Diabetic ketoacidosis, alcoholic ketoacidosis, starvation, isopropanol ingestion

URINE METANEPHRINES

Normal range: 0-2.0 mg/24 hr (0-11.0 μmol/day [CF: 5.458; SMI: 0.5 μmol/day])
Elevated in: Pheochromocytoma, neuroblastoma, drugs (caffeine, phenothiazines, monoamine oxidase inhibitors), stress. Table 130 summarizes medications that may increase metanephrine levels.

URINE MYOGLOBIN

Normal: Absent
Present in: Severe trauma, hyperthermia, polymyositis/dermatomyositis, carbon monoxide poisoning, drugs (narcotic and amphetamine toxicity), hypothyroidism, muscle ischemia

Table 131 differentiates hematuria and hemoglobinuria from myoglobinuria.

URINE NITRITE

Normal: Absent
Present in: Urinary tract infections

URINE OCCULT BLOOD

Normal: Negative
Positive in: Trauma to urinary tract, renal disease (glomerulonephritis, pyelonephritis), renal or ureteral calculi, bladder lesions (carcinoma, cystitis), prostatitis, prostatic carcinoma, menstrual contamination, hematopoietic disorders (hemophilia, thrombocytopenia), anticoagulants, ASA

URINE OSMOLALITY

See "OSMOLALITY, URINE"

URINE PH

Normal range: 4.6-8 (average, 6)
Elevated in: Bacteriuria, vegetarian diet, renal failure with inability to form ammonia, drugs (antibiotics, sodium bicarbonate, acetazolamide)
Decreased in: Acidosis (metabolic, respiratory), drugs (ammonium chloride, methenamine mandelate), diabetes mellitus, starvation, diarrhea

URINE PHOSPHATE

Normal range: 0.8-2.0 g/24 hr
Elevated in: Acute tubular necrosis (diuretic phase), chronic renal disease, uncontrolled diabetes mellitus, hyperparathyroidism, hypomagnesemia, metabolic acidosis, metabolic alkalosis, neurofibromatosis, adult-onset vitamin D-resistant hypophosphatemic osteomalacia
Decreased in: Acromegaly, acute renal failure, decreased dietary intake, hypoparathyroidism, respiratory acidosis

URINE POTASSIUM

Normal range: 25-100 mEq/24 hr (25-100 mmol/day [CF: 1; SMI: 1 mmol/day])

TABLE 131 Differentiation of Hematuria, Hemoglobinuria, and Myoglobinuria

Condition	Plasma Findings	Urine Findings
Hematuria	Color—normal	Color—normal, smoky, pink, red, brown
		Erythrocytes—many
		Renal—red blood cell casts
		Protein—marked increase
		Lower urinary tract—no casts
		Protein—present or absent
Hemoglobinuria	Color—pink (early)	Color—pink, red, brown
	Haptoglobin—low	Erythrocytes—occasional
		Pigment casts—occasional
		Protein—present or absent
		Hemosiderin—late
Myoglobinuria	Color—normal	Color—red, brown
	Haptoglobin—normal	Erythrocytes—occasional
	Creatine kinase—marked increase	Dense brown casts—occasional
	Aldolase—increased	Protein—present or absent

From McPherson RA, Pincus MR: *Henry's clinical diagnosis and management by laboratory methods*, ed 23, St Louis, 2017, Elsevier.

BOX 37 Urine Potassium in Hypokalemia

Low 24-hour urinary potassium (<25 mEq/day) or low spot urine potassium (<15 mEq/L) or low potassium-to-creatinine ratio (<1.5 mEq/mmol)
GI losses: Vomiting, diarrhea, nasogastric tube
Sweat losses: Extreme heat, cystic fibrosis
Low intake

High 24-hour urinary potassium (>25 mEq/day) or high spot urine potassium (>40 mEq/L) or high potassium-to-creatinine ratio (>1.5 mEq/mmol)
- Renal potassium wasting
- Diuretics, amphotericin B
- Increased mineralocorticoid activity
- Excretion of bicarbonate (vomiting, RTA)
- Excretion of other nonreabsorbable anion (hippurate, beta-hydroxybutyrate, penicillin derivative)
- Transcellular shifts
- Hypomagnesemia
- Bartter, Gitelman, Liddle syndromes

High 24-hour urinary potassium (>25 mEq/day) and high potassium-to-creatinine ratio (>1.5 mEq/mmol) but low spot urine potassium (<15 mEq/L)
Established AKI (tubular dysfunction ± dilutional)
Primary polydipsia (dilutional)
Other polyuric states (osmotic and water diuresis)

AKI, Acute kidney injury; *GI,* gastrointestinal; *RTA,* renal tubular acidosis.
From Ronco C: *Critical care nephrology*, ed 3, Philadelphia, 2019, Elsevier.

Elevated in: Aldosteronism (primary, secondary), glucocorticoids, alkalosis, renal tubular acidosis, excessive dietary potassium intake
Decreased in: Acute renal failure, potassium-sparing diuretics, diarrhea, hypokalemia

Box 37 describes urine potassium in hypokalemia.

URINE PROTEIN (quantitative)

Normal range: <150 mg/24 hr (<0.15 g/day [CF: 0.001; SMI: 0.01 g/day])
Elevated in:
Nephrotic syndrome as a result of primary renal diseases
Malignant hypertension
Malignancies: Multiple myeloma, leukemias, Hodgkin disease
Congestive heart failure
Diabetes mellitus
Systemic lupus erythematosus, rheumatoid arthritis

Sickle cell disease
Goodpasture syndrome
Malaria
Amyloidosis, sarcoidosis
Tubular lesions: Cystinosis
Functional (after heavy exercise)
Pyelonephritis
Pregnancy
Constrictive pericarditis
Renal vein thrombosis
Toxic nephropathies: Heavy metals, drugs
Radiation nephritis
Orthostatic (postural) proteinuria
Benign proteinuria: Fever, heat or cold exposure

URINE SEDIMENT

See Fig. 61 for visual evaluation of common abnormalities. Table 132 summarizes characteristics of amorphous and crystalline urinary sediments.

URINE SODIUM (quantitative)

See Table 133 for use of urine electrolytes in the differential diagnosis of hypokalemia. Table 134 describes urine sodium findings in acute kidney injury (AKI).

Normal range: 40-220 mEq/day (40-220 mmol/day [CF: 1; SMI: 1 mmol/day])

Elevated in: Diuretic administration, high sodium intake, salt-losing nephritis, acute tubular necrosis, vomiting, Addison disease, syndrome of inappropriate antidiuretic hormone secretion, hypothyroidism, congestive heart failure, hepatic failure, chronic renal failure, Bartter syndrome, glucocorticoid deficiency, interstitial nephritis caused by analgesic abuse, mannitol, dextran, or glycerol therapy, milk-alkali syndrome, decreased renin secretion, postobstructive diuresis

Decreased In: Increased aldosterone, glucocorticoid excess, hyponatremia, prerenal azotemia, decreased salt intake

URINE SPECIFIC GRAVITY

Normal range: 1.005-1.030

Elevated in: Dehydration, excessive fluid losses (vomiting, diarrhea, fever), x-ray contrast media, diabetes mellitus, congestive heart failure, syndrome of inappropriate antidiuretic hormone secretion, adrenal insufficiency, decreased fluid intake

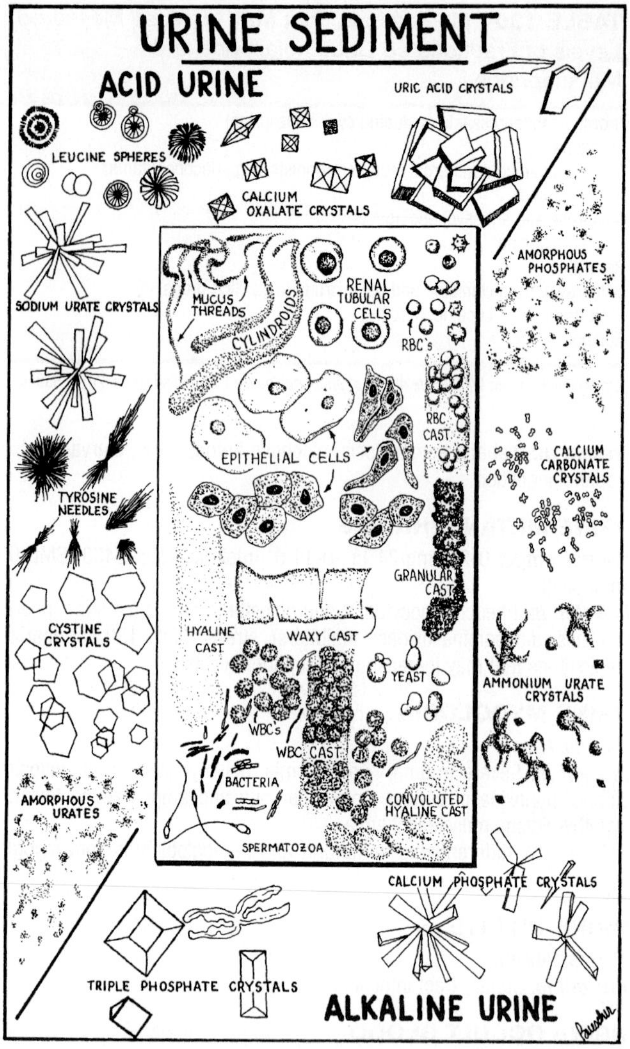

FIG. 61 Microscopic examination of urinary sediment. (From Grigorian Greene M: *The Harriet Lane handbook: a manual for pediatric house officers,* ed 17, St Louis, 2007, Mosby.)

TABLE 132 Characteristics of Amorphous and Crystalline Urinary Sediments

Substance	Description	URINE PH WHERE FOUND Acid	Neutral	Alkaline	Solubility Characteristics and Comments
Ampicillin	Uncommon: From high dose; colorless; long prisms that form clusters, sheaves	+	–	–	
Bilirubin	Reddish brown; amorphous needles, rhombic plates, or cubes; may color uric acid crystals	+	–	–	Soluble in alkali, acid, acetone, and chloroform
Cholesterol	Rare; colorless; flat plate with corner notch; accompanies fatty casts and oval fat bodies	+	+	–	Very soluble in chloroform, ether, and hot alcohol
Calcium carbonate	Colorless; small granules in pairs, fours; spheres; rarely needles	–	+	+	Soluble in acetic acid with effervescence
Calcium oxalate	Dihydrate: Common; colorless; small refractile octahedron Monohydrate: Uncommon; dumbbell and ovoid rectangle	+	+	–	Soluble in dilute HCl
Cystine	Colorless; hexagonal plates, often laminated; rapidly destroyed by bacteria; may be confused with uric acid, but cystine is soluble in dilute hydrochloric acid	+	–	–	Soluble in alkali (especially ammonia) and dilute HCl; insoluble in boiling water, acetic acid, alcohol, ether; apply cyanide-nitroprusside reaction

Continued

TABLE 132 Characteristics of Amorphous and Crystalline Urinary Sediments—cont'd

Substance	Description	URINE PH WHERE FOUND Acid	Neutral	Alkaline	Solubility Characteristics and Comments
Hematin	Small, biconvex "whetstone" seen with hemoglobinuria	+	–	–	
Hemosiderin	Golden brown; granules in clumps, in cells, casts	+	+	–	Blue with Prussian blue
Hippuric acid	Rare; colorless, needles, rhombic plates and four-sided prisms; distinguish from phosphates	+	+	+	Soluble with hot water and alkali; insoluble in acetic acid
Indigotin	Rare; blue; amorphous or small crystals; colors other crystals	+	+	+	Very soluble in chloroform; soluble in ether; insoluble in acetone
Phosphates					
Amorphous phosphate (magnesium, calcium)	Colorless; fine, granular precipitate	–	+	+	Insoluble with heat; soluble with acetic acid, dilute HCl
Calcium hydrogen phosphate	Less common; colorless, star-shaped or long, thin prisms or needles; form rosettes	sl	+	sl	Slightly soluble in dilute acetic acid, soluble in dilute HCl
Triple phosphate (ammonium, magnesium)	Common form: Colorless; three- to six-sided prisms, "coffin lids" Less often: Flat, fern leaf form, sheets, flakes	–	+	+	Soluble in dilute acetic acid
Radiographic media (meglumine diatrizoate)	Intravenous: Colorless; thin, rhombic plates, some with notch, resemble cholesterol plates; elongated crystals Retrograde: Colorless; long, pointed crystals	+	–	–	Soluble in 10% NaOH: Insoluble in ether and chloroform; high specific gravity in urine: Polarizes with interference colors
Sulfonamides					
Acetylsulfadiazine	Wheat sheaves with eccentric binding	+	–	–	
Acetylsulfamethoxazole	Brown; dense spheres or irregular divided spheres	+	–	–	
Sulfadiazine	Brown; dense globules	+	–	–	Soluble in acetone
Tyrosine	Rare; colorless or yellow, appears black with focusing; fine silky needles in sheaves or rosettes	+	–	–	Soluble in alkali, dilute mineral acid, relatively heat soluble; insoluble in alcohol, ether
Urates					
Amorphous (calcium, magnesium, sodium, potassium)	Common; colorless to yellow-brown; amorphous, granular precipitate	+	+	–	Soluble in dilute alkali; soluble at 60 °C (140 °F) or lower; change to uric acid crystal with concentrated HCl or acetic acid
Monosodium urate	Colorless; needles or amorphous precipitate	+	–	–	
Urates (sodium, potassium, ammonium)	Brown; small, spherical; clusters resemble biurates	sl	+	–	Soluble at 60 °C (140 °F); change to uric acid with glacial acetic acid
Ammonium biurate	Common in "old" urine; dark yellow or brown; spheres or "thorn apples" (spheres with horns)	–	+	+	Soluble at 60° C (140 °F) with acetic acid; soluble strong alkali; change to uric acid with concentrated hydrochloric or acetic acid
Uric acid	Common; yellow, red-brown, brown; large variety of shapes: Rhombic, four-sided plates, rosettes, "whetstones" lemon shapes; rarely, colorless hexagonals	+	–	–	Soluble in alkali: Insoluble in alcohol and acids; polarizes with interference colors
Xanthine	Rare; colorless; small, rhombic plates	+	+	–	Soluble in alkali; soluble with heat; insoluble in acetic acid

HCl, Hydrochloride; *sl,* slight.
From McPherson RA, Pincus MR: *Henry's clinical diagnosis and management by laboratory methods,* ed 23, St Louis, 2017, Elsevier.

Decreased in: Diabetes insipidus, renal disease (glomerulonephritis, pyelonephritis), excessive fluid intake or IV hydration

URINE VANILLYLMANDELIC ACID (VMA)

Normal range: <6.8 mg/24 hr (<35 μmol/day [CF: 5.046; SMI: 1 μmol/day])

Elevated in: Pheochromocytoma, neuroblastoma, ganglioblastoma, drugs (isoproterenol, methocarbamol, levodopa, sulfonamides, chlorpromazine), severe stress, after ingestion of bananas, chocolate, vanilla, tea, coffee

Decreased in: Drugs (monoamine oxidase inhibitors, reserpine, guanethidine, methyldopa)

TABLE 133 Urine Electrolytes* in the Differential Diagnosis of Hypokalemia

	URINE ELECTROLYTE	
Condition	**Na^+**	**Cl–**
Vomiting		
Recent	High†	Low‡
Remote	Low	Low
Diuretics		
Recent	High	High
Remote	Low	Low
Diarrhea or laxative abuse	Low	High
Bartter or Gitelman syndrome	High	High

*Do not use the urine electrolytes in this fashion during polyuric states.
†High = urine concentration >15 mmol/L.
‡Low = urine concentration <15 mmol/L.
From Vincent JL et al: *Textbook of critical care,* ed 6, Philadelphia, 2011, Saunders.

TABLE 134 Urinalysis Findings in Acute Kidney Injury (AKI)

Etiologic Disorder	Urine Chemistry	Urine Sediment
Prerenal	U_{Na}<20 mmol/L FE_{Na}<1% FE_{urea}<35%	Normal or nearly normal (hyaline casts and rare granular casts)
Acute tubular necrosis	U_{Na}>40 mmol/L FE_{Na}>2% FE_{urea}>60%	Renal tubular epithelial cells, epithelial cell casts, coarse pigmented (muddy brown) casts
Acute interstitial nephritis	Variable; U_{Na} may be >40 mmol/L, FE_{Na} may be >2%	Red blood cells, white blood cells, white blood cell casts, eosinophils
Acute glomerulonephritis	Variable; U_{Na} may be <20 mmol/L, FE_{Na} may be <1%	Red blood cells (dysmorphic), red blood cell casts
Acute vascular disease	Variable; U_{Na} may be <20 mmol/L, FE_{Na} may be <1%	Red blood cells, red blood cell casts in HUS/TTP, eosinophils in atheroembolic disease
Crystal-associated AKI	Variable	Crystalluria Uric acid crystals in tumor lysis syndrome Calcium oxalate crystals in ethylene glycol ingestion Drug crystals (acyclovir, methotrexate, indinavir, triamterene, sulfadiazine)
Obstructive	Variable; early U_{Na} may be <20 mmol/L, FE_{Na} may be <1%; late U_{Na} may be >40 mmol/L, FE_{Na} may be >2%	Normal or red blood cells, white blood cells and crystals

FE_{Na}, Fractional excretion of sodium; *FE_{urea},* fractional excretion of urea; *HUS,* hemolytic-uremic syndrome; *TTP,* thrombotic thrombocytopenic purpura; *U_{Na},* urine sodium concentration.
From Parrillo JE, Dellinger RP: *Critical care medicine, principles of diagnosis and management in the adult,* ed 4, Philadelphia, 2014, Elsevier.

VARICELLA-ZOSTER VIRUS (VZV) SEROLOGY

Test description: Test can be performed on whole blood, tissue, skin lesions, and CSF.

VASOACTIVE INTESTINAL PEPTIDE (VIP)

Normal: <50 pg/ml
Elevated in: Pancreatic VIP-omas, neuroblastoma, pancreatic islet cell hyperplasia, liver disease, multiple endocrine neoplasia (MEN) I, ganglioneuroma, ganglioneuroblastoma

VDRL

Normal range: Negative
Positive test: Syphilis, other treponemal diseases (yaws, pinta, bejel)
NOTE: A false-positive test may be seen in patients with systemic lupus erythematosus and other autoimmune diseases, infectious mononucleosis, HIV, atypical pneumonia, malaria, leprosy, typhus fever, rat-bite fever, relapsing fever.
NOTE: See Table 135 for interpretation of serologic tests for syphilis.

VISCOSITY (serum)

Normal range: 1.4-1.8 relative to water (1.10-1.22 centipoise)
Elevated in: Monoclonal gammopathies (Waldenström macroglobulinemia, multiple myeloma), hyperfibrinogenemia, systemic lupus erythematosus, rheumatoid arthritis, polycythemia, leukemia

VITAMIN B_{12} (cobalamin)

See Box 38 for etiopathophysiologic classification of cobalamin deficiency. Causes of false-positive and false-negative serum cobalamin levels are summarized in Table 136. Table 137 describes causes of megaloblastosis not responding to therapy with cobalamin or folate. Table 138 summarizes indications for prophylaxis with cobalamin or folate.
Normal
190-900 ng/ml
Causes of vitamin B_{12} deficiency:
a. Pernicious anemia (antibodies against intrinsic factor and gastric parietal cells)
b. Dietary (strict lacto-ovo vegetarians, food faddists)
c. Malabsorption (achlorhydria, gastrectomy, ileal resection, pancreatic insufficiency, drugs [omeprazole, cholestyramine])

Falsely low levels occur in patients with severe folate deficiency, in patients using high doses of ascorbic acid, and when cobalamin levels are measured after nuclear medicine studies (radioactivity interferes with cobalamin radioimmunoassay).
Falsely high or normal levels in patients with cobalamin deficiency can occur in severe liver disease and chronic granulocytic leukemia.
The absence of anemia or macrocytosis does not exclude the diagnosis of cobalamin deficiency.

VITAMIN D, 1,25 DIHYDROXY CALCIFEROL

Normal: 16-65 pg/ml
Elevated in: Tumor calcinosis, primary hyperparathyroidism, sarcoidosis, tuberculosis, idiopathic hypercalciuria
Decreased in: Nutritional deficiency, postmenopausal osteoporosis, chronic renal failure, hypoparathyroidism, tumor-induced osteomalacia, rickets, elevated blood lead levels. Table 139 compares vitamin D levels in various disorders. Fig. 62 illustrates vitamin D physiology.

VITAMIN K

Normal: 0.10-2.20 ng/ml
Decreased in: Primary biliary cirrhosis, anticoagulants, antibiotics, cholestyramine, GI disease, pancreatic disease, cystic fibrosis, obstructive jaundice, hypoprothrombinemia, hemorrhagic disease of the newborn

VON WILLEBRAND FACTOR

Normal: Levels vary according to blood type; blood type 0: 50-150 U/dl; blood type non-0: 90-200 U/dl
Decreased in: von Willebrand disease (however, in type II von Willebrand disease the antigen may be normal but the function is impaired)

TABLE 135 Interpretation of Serologic Tests for Syphilis*

Nontreponemal Tests	Treponemal Tests	Interpretation of Finding: Is Syphilis Present?*
Nonreactive	Nonreactive	Early primary syphilis is not ruled out by negative serologic tests. Early syphilis is present in 13%-30% of patients who have a negative microhemagglutination *Treponema pallidum* test; in about 30% of patients who present with chancre but have a nonreactive reagin test; and in about 10% of patients who have a negative FTA-ABS test. Late syphilis is present in a very small fraction of patients. Adequately treated syphilis in remote past may produce these results, but treponemal tests usually remain reactive.
	Reactive	Observed in about 10% of patients with chancre. The treponemal tests may turn positive shortly before the reagin tests. Reagin tests repeated after several days are generally positive. In adequately treated early syphilis, the reagin test may return to nonreactive within 1-2 yr, whereas the treponemal tests generally do not. Late syphilis is not ruled out by a negative reagin test. The sensitivity of the reagin tests is lower than that of treponemal tests in untreated late syphilis. In secondary syphilis, rarely, a highly reactive serum appears negative when tested undiluted with a reagin test because flocculation is inhibited by relative antibody excess. Not reported to occur with treponemal tests. Quantitative reagin tests are positive. False-positive treponemal tests occur in 40% of patients with Lyme disease.
Reactive	Nonreactive borderline (FTA-ABS)	Finding is not diagnostic of syphilis but constitutes a classic biologic false-positive reaction. Not diagnostic of syphilis; most patients (90%) with this pattern do not develop clinical or serologic evidence of syphilis. Repeat test is indicated. Chronic borderline results are associated with a variety of conditions other than syphilis.
	Beaded (FTA-ABS)	Not diagnostic of syphilis. Seen with collagen vascular disease.
	Reactive	Findings diagnostic of syphilis or other treponemal disease. In adequately treated syphilis, one would expect (1) a sustained fourfold drop in titer of reagin test, although reagin test may remain positive after adequate therapy; (2) treponemal tests remain positive after adequate therapy. Concurrent false-positive results on both nontreponemal and treponemal tests could occur in rare instances. It may be impossible to rule out syphilis in an individual with this test profile.

FTA-ABS, Fluorescent treponemal antibody, absorbed.

*Serologic data must always be interpreted in the light of a total clinical evaluation. Diagnosis based on serologic criteria alone is fraught with error. Serologic tests apparently in conflict with clinical diagnosis should be confirmed by repetition or possibly referral to a reference laboratory.

BOX 38 Etiopathophysiologic Classification of Cobalamin Deficiency

Nutritional cobalamin deficiency (insufficient cobalamin intake):
- Vegetarians, poverty-imposed near-vegetarians, breastfed infants of mothers with pernicious anemia

Abnormal intragastric events (inadequate proteolysis of food cobalamin): Atrophic gastritis, hypochlorhydria, proton pump inhibitors, H_2 blockers

Loss/atrophy of gastric oxyntic mucosa (deficient intrinsic factor [IF] molecules): Total or partial gastrectomy, adult and juvenile pernicious anemia, caustic destruction (lye)

Abnormal events in the small bowel lumen
- Inadequate pancreatic protease (R factor-cobalamin not degraded, cobalamin not transferred to IF)
- Insufficient pancreatic protease: Pancreatic insufficiency
- Inactivation of pancreatic protease: Zollinger-Ellison syndrome
- Usurping of luminal cobalamin (inadequate binding of cobalamin to IF)
- By bacteria-stasis syndromes (blind loops, pouches of diverticulosis, strictures, fistulas, anastomosis), impaired bowel motility (scleroderma), hypogammaglobulinemia
- By *Diphyllobothrium latum* (fish tapeworm)

Disorders of ileal mucosa/IF-cobalamin receptors (IF-cobalamin not bound to IF-cobalamin receptors [cubam receptors])
- Diminished or absent cubam receptors: Ileal bypass/resection/fistula
- Abnormal mucosal architecture/function: Tropical/nontropical sprue, Crohn disease, tuberculous ileitis, amyloidosis
- Cubam receptor defects: Imerslund-Gräsbeck syndrome
- Drug-effects: Metformin, cholestyramine, colchicine, neomycin

Disorders of plasma cobalamin transport (transcobalamin [TCII]-cobalamin not delivered to TCII receptors): Congenital TCII deficiency, defective binding of TCII-cobalamin to TCII receptors (rare)
- Metabolic disorders (cobalamin not used by cell)
- Inborn enzyme errors: cblA to cblG disorders
- Acquired disorders (cobalamin inactivated by irreversible oxidation): Nitrous oxide

From Hoffman R: *Hematology: basic principles and practice,* ed 6, Philadelphia, 2013, Saunders.

TABLE 136 Serum Cobalamin: False-Positive and False-Negative Test Results

Falsely Low Serum Cobalamin in the Absence of True Cobalamin Deficiency

Folate deficiency (one third of patients)
Multiple myeloma
TCI deficiency
Megadose vitamin C therapy

Falsely Raised Cobalamin Levels in the Presence of True Deficiency*

Cobalamin binders (TCI and II) increased (e.g., myeloproliferative states, hepatomas, and fibrolamellar hepatic tumors)
TCII-producing macrophages are activated (e.g., autoimmune diseases, monoblastic leukemias and lymphomas)
Release of cobalamin from hepatocytes (e.g., active liver disease)
High serum anti-IF antibody titer

IF, Intrinsic factor; *TC,* transcobalamin.

*Although a low serum cobalamin level is not synonymous with cobalamin deficiency, 5% of patients with true cobalamin deficiency have low-normal cobalamin levels, a potentially serious problem because the patient's underlying cobalamin deficiency will progress if uncorrected.

From Hoffman R et al: *Hematology: basic principles and practice,* ed 6, Philadelphia, 2013, Saunders.

TABLE 137 Causes of Megaloblastosis Not Responding to Therapy with Cobalamin or Folate

Wrong Diagnosis
Combined folate and cobalamin deficiencies being treated with only one vitamin
Associated iron deficiency
Associated hemoglobinopathy (e.g., sickle cell disease, thalassemia)
Associated anemia of chronic disease
Associated hypothyroidism

From Hoffman R: *Hematology: basic principles and practice*, ed 7, Philadelphia, 2018, Elsevier.

TABLE 138 Indications for Prophylaxis with Cobalamin or Folate

Prophylaxis with Cobalamin
Infants on specialized diets[a]
Premature infants
Infants of mothers with pernicious anemia[a]
Infants and children of mothers with nutritional cobalamin deficiency
Vegetarianism and poverty-imposed near-vegetarianism[a]
Total gastrectomy[b]

Prophylaxis with Folic Acid[c]
All women contemplating pregnancy (at least 400 μg/day)[d]
Pregnancy and lactation, premature infants
Mothers at risk for delivery of infants with neural tube defects[e,f]
Hemolytic anemias/hyperproliferative hematologic states
Patients with rheumatoid arthritis or psoriasis on therapy with methotrexate[g]
Patients on antiepileptic drugs
Patients with ulcerative colitis

[a]For vegetarians, prophylaxis with cobalamin (5- to 10-μg tablet/day) orally should suffice. In all other conditions involving any abnormality of cobalamin absorption, cobalamin tablets of 1000 μg/day should be administered orally to ensure that cobalamin transport by passive diffusion across the intestine is sufficient to meet daily needs.
[b]Consider late development of cobalamin deficiency and iron malabsorption (prophylaxis with oral cobalamin and iron).
[c]Ensure that the patient does not have a cobalamin deficiency before initiating long-term folate prophylaxis.
[d]For prevention of first occurrence of neural tube defects.
[e]Previous delivery of a child with neural tube defects (e.g., anencephaly, spina bifida, meningocele) imparts a 10-fold greater risk for subsequent delivery of infant with neural tube defects.
[f]Folic acid (4 mg/day) administered periconceptionally and throughout the first trimester.
[g]To reduce toxicity of the antifolate.
From Hoffman R: *Hematology: basic principles and practice*, ed 7, Philadelphia, 2018, Elsevier.

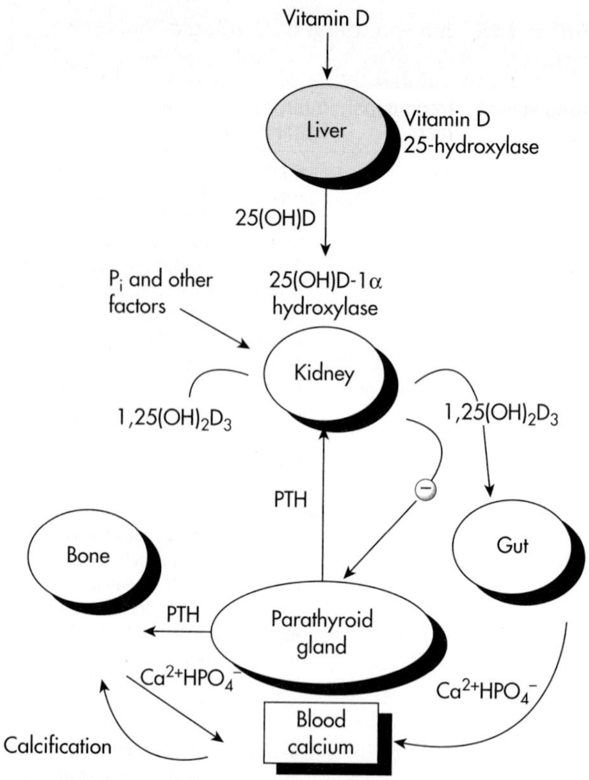

FIG. 62 Vitamin D physiology. P_i, Inorganic phosphate; *PTH*, parathyroid hormone. (From Ronco C: *Critical care nephrology*, ed 3, Philadelphia, 2019, Elsevier.)

TABLE 139 Serum Caicium, Phosphate, and Vitamin D Levels in Various Disorders

Disorder	Calcium	25(OH)D	1,25(OH)D	Phosphate
25(OH)D intoxication	High	High	Low, normal	Normal, high
Primary hyperparathyroidism	High	Normal	Normal, high	Low
Secondary hyperparathyroidism	Low	Low, normal, high	Low, normal, high	Low, normal, high
Tertiary hyperparathyroidism	Normal, high*	Low, normal, high	Low, normal, high	Low, normal, high
Malignancy	High	Normal	Low, normal	Low
Vitamin D deficiency	Low	Low	Low, normal, high	Low
Renal failure	Low	Normal	Low	High
Hyperphosphatemia	Low	Normal	Low	High
Vitamin D rickets type I, II	Low	Normal, high	Low, normal, high	Low
Granulomatous diseases (sarcoid/TB)	High	Low, normal, high	High	Normal, high
Postmenopausal osteoporosis	Normal	Normal	Normal	Normal
Senile osteoporosis	Normal	Normal	Normal	Normal
Osteomalacia	Low, normal	Low, normal	Low	Low, normal, high

TB, Tuberculosis.
*Calcium may be normal in the setting of concurrent $1,25(OH)_2D_3$ deficiency.
From McPherson RA, Pincus MR: *Henry's clinical diagnosis and management by laboratory methods*, ed 23, St Louis, 2017, Elsevier.

SECTION V

Clinical Practice Guidelines

INTRODUCTION

IMMUNIZATIONS AND CHEMOPROPHYLAXIS

Childhood and Adolescent Immunizations

TABLE 1 Recommended Immunization Schedule for Children and Adolescents Aged 18 Years or Younger—United States, 2021. (For those who fall behind or start late, see the catch-up schedule [Table 2])

These recommendations must be read with the footnotes that follow. For those who fall behind or start late, provide catch-up vaccination at the earliest opportunity as indicated by the divided bars. To determine minimum intervals between doses, see the catch-up schedule (Table 2). School entry and adolescent vaccine age groups are shaded in gray.

Vaccine	Birth	1 mo	2 mos	4 mos	6 mos	9 mos	12 mos	15 mos	18 mos	19–23 mos	2–3 yrs	4–6 yrs	7–10 yrs	11–12 yrs	13–15 yrs	16 yrs	17–18 yrs
Hepatitis B (HepB)	1st dose	◄--- 2nd dose ---►			◄--- 3rd dose ---►												
Rotavirus (RV): RV1 (2-dose series), RV5 (3-dose series)			1st dose	2nd dose	See Notes												
Diphtheria, tetanus, acellular pertussis (DTaP <7 yrs)			1st dose	2nd dose	3rd dose			◄--- 4th dose ---►				5th dose					
Haemophilus influenzae type b (Hib)			1st dose	2nd dose	See Notes		◄ 3rd or 4th dose, See Notes ►										
Pneumococcal conjugate (PCV13)			1st dose	2nd dose	3rd dose		◄--- 4th dose ---►										
Inactivated poliovirus (IPV <18 yrs)			1st dose	2nd dose	◄--- 3rd dose ---►							4th dose					
Influenza (IIV)					Annual vaccination 1 or 2 doses									Annual vaccination 1 dose only			
or																	
Influenza (LAIV4)											Annual vaccination 1 or 2 doses			Annual vaccination 1 dose only			
Measles, mumps, rubella (MMR)					See Notes		◄--- 1st dose ---►					2nd dose					
Varicella (VAR)							◄--- 1st dose ---►					2nd dose					
Hepatitis A (HepA)					See Notes		2-dose series, See Notes										
Tetanus, diphtheria, acellular pertussis (Tdap ≥7 yrs)														Tdap			
Human papillomavirus (HPV)													*	See Notes			
Meningococcal (MenACWY-D ≥9 mos, MenACWY-CRM ≥2 mos, MenACWY-TT ≥2years)			See Notes											1st dose		2nd dose	
Meningococcal B													See Notes				
Pneumococcal polysaccharide (PPSV23)											See Notes						

Legend:
- Range of recommended ages for all children
- Range of recommended ages for catch-up immunization
- Range of recommended ages for certain high-risk groups
- Recommended based on shared clinical decision-making or *can be used in this age group
- No recommendation/ not applicable

TABLE 2 Catch-up Immunization Schedule for Persons Aged 4 Months Through 18 Years Who Start Late or Who Are More Than 1 Month Behind—United States, 2021

The table below provides catch-up schedules and minimum intervals between doses for children whose vaccinations have been delayed. A vaccine series does not need to be restarted, regardless of the time that has elapsed between doses. Use the section appropriate for the child's age. Always use this table in conjunction with Table 1 and the footnotes that follow

Vaccine	Minimum Age for Dose 1	Minimum Interval Between Doses			
		Dose 1 to Dose 2	Dose 2 to Dose 3	Dose 3 to Dose 4	Dose 4 to Dose 5
Children age 4 months through 6 years					
Hepatitis B	Birth	**4 weeks**	**8 weeks *and* at least 16 weeks after first dose.** Minimum age for the final dose is 24 weeks.		
Rotavirus	6 weeks Maximum age for first dose is 14 weeks, 6 days.	**4 weeks**	**4 weeks** Maximum age for final dose is 8 months, 0 days.		
Diphtheria, tetanus, and acellular pertussis	6 weeks	**4 weeks**	**4 weeks**	**6 months**	**6 months**
Haemophilus influenzae type b	6 weeks	**No further doses needed** if first dose was administered at age 15 months or older. **4 weeks** if first dose was administered before the 1st birthday. **8 weeks (as final dose)** if first dose was administered at age 12 through 14 months.	**No further doses needed** if previous dose was administered at age 15 months or older. **4 weeks** if current age is younger than 12 months ***and*** first dose was administered at younger than age 7 months ***and*** at least 1 previous dose was PRP-T (ActHib, Pentacel, Hiberix) or unknown. **8 weeks *and* age 12 through 59 months (as final dose)** if current age is younger than 12 months ***and*** first dose was administered at age 7 through 11 months; OR if current age is 12 through 59 months ***and*** first dose was administered before the 1st birthday ***and*** second dose was administered at younger than 15 months; OR if both doses were PRP-OMP (PedvaxHIB, Comvax) ***and*** were administered before the 1st birthday.	**8 weeks (as final dose)** This dose only necessary for children age 12 through 59 months who received 3 doses before the 1st birthday.	
Pneumococcal conjugate	6 weeks	**No further doses needed** for healthy children if first dose was administered at age 24 months or older. **4 weeks** if first dose was administered before the 1st birthday. **8 weeks (as final dose for healthy children)** if first dose was administered at the 1st birthday or after.	**No further doses needed** for healthy children if previous dose was administered at age 24 months or older. **4 weeks** if current age is younger than 12 months and previous dose was administered at <7 months old. **8 weeks (as final dose for healthy children)** if previous dose was administered between 7–11 months (wait until at least 12 months old); OR if current age is 12 months or older and at least 1 dose was administered before age 12 months.	**8 weeks (as final dose)** This dose only necessary for children age 12 through 59 months who received 3 doses before age 12 months or for children at high risk who received 3 doses at any age.	
Inactivated poliovirus	6 weeks	**4 weeks**	**4 weeks** if current age is <4 years. **6 months (as final dose)** if current age is 4 years or older.	**6 months** (minimum age 4 years for final dose).	
Measles, mumps, rubella	12 months	**4 weeks**			
Varicella	12 months	**3 months**			
Hepatitis A	12 months	**6 months**			
Meningococcal ACWY	2 months MenACWY-CRM 9 months MenACWY-D 2 years MenACWY-TT	**8 weeks**	See Notes	See Notes	
Children and adolescents age 7 through 18 years					
Meningococcal ACWY	Not applicable (N/A)	**8 weeks**			
Tetanus, diphtheria; tetanus, diphtheria, and acellular pertussis	7 years	**4 weeks**	**4 weeks** if first dose of DTaP/DT was administered before the 1st birthday. **6 months (as final dose)** if first dose of DTaP/DT or Tdap/Td was administered at or after the 1st birthday.	**6 months** if first dose of DTaP/DT was administered before the 1st birthday.	
Human papillomavirus	9 years	**Routine dosing intervals are recommended.**			
Hepatitis A	N/A	**6 months**			
Hepatitis B	N/A	**4 weeks**	**8 weeks *and* at least 16 weeks after first dose.**		
Inactivated poliovirus	N/A	**4 weeks**	**6 months** A fourth dose is not necessary if the third dose was administered at age 4 years or older and at least 6 months after the previous dose.	A fourth dose of IPV is indicated if all previous doses were administered at <4 years or if the third dose was administered <6 months after the second dose.	
Measles, mumps, rubella	N/A	**4 weeks**			
Varicella	N/A	**3 months** if younger than age 13 years. **4 weeks** if age 13 years or older.			

TABLE 3 Recommended Child and Adolescent Immunization Schedule by Medical Indication, United States, 2021

Always use this table in conjunction with Table 1 and the notes that follow.

VACCINE	INDICATION									
	Pregnancy	Immunocompromised status (excluding HIV infection)	HIV infection CD4+ count[1]: <15% and total CD4 cell count of $<200/\text{mm}^3$	HIV infection CD4+ count[1]: ≥15% and total CD4 cell count of $\geq 200/\text{mm}^3$	Kidney failure, end-stage renal disease, or on hemodialysis	Heart disease or chronic lung disease	CSF leak or cochlear implant	Asplenia or persistent complement component deficiencies	Chronic liver disease	Diabetes
Hepatitis B										
Rotavirus		SCID[2]								
Diphtheria, tetanus, and acellular pertussis (DTaP)										
Haemophilus influenzae type b										
Pneumococcal conjugate										
Inactivated poliovirus										
Influenza (IIV)										
or										
Influenza (LAIV4)						Asthma, wheezing: 2–4yrs[3]				
Measles, mumps, rubella	*									
Varicella	*									
Hepatitis A										
Tetanus, diphtheria, and acellular pertussis (Tdap)										
Human papillomavirus	*									
Meningococcal ACWY										
Meningococcal B										
Pneumococcal polysaccharide										

- Vaccination according to the routine schedule recommended
- Recommended for persons with an additional risk factor for which the vaccine would be indicated
- Vaccination is recommended, and additional doses may be necessary based on medical condition. See Notes.
- Not recommended/contraindicated—vaccine should not be administered.
  *Vaccinate after pregnancy.
- Precaution—vaccine might be indicated if benefit of protection outweighs risk of adverse reaction
- No recommendation/not applicable

1 For additional information regarding HIV laboratory parameters and use of live vaccines, see the *General Best Practice Guidelines for Immunization*, "Altered Immunocompetence," at www.cdc.gov/vaccines/hcp/acip-recs/general-recs/immunocompetence.html and Table 4-1 (footnote D) at www.cdc.gov/vaccines/hcp/acip-recs/general-recs/contraindications.html.
2 Severe Combined Immunodeficiency
3 LAIV4 contraindicated for children 2–4 years of age with asthma or wheezing during the preceding 12 months

Notes Recommended Child and Adolescent Immunization Schedule for ages 18 years or younger, United States, 2021

For vaccination recommendations for persons ages 19 years or older, see the Recommended Adult Immunization Schedule, 2021.

Additional information

COVID-19 Vaccination

ACIP recommends use of COVID-19 vaccines within the scope of the Emergency Use Authorization or Biologics License Application for the particular vaccine. Interim ACIP recommendations for the use of COVID-19 vaccines can be found at www.cdc.gov/vaccines/hcp/acip-recs/.

- Consult relevant ACIP statements for detailed recommendations at www.cdc.gov/vaccines/hcp/acip-recs/index.html.
- For information on contraindications and precautions for the use of a vaccine, consult the *General Best Practice Guidelines for Immunization* at www.cdc.gov/vaccines/hcp/acip-recs/general-recs/contraindications.html and relevant ACIP statements at www.cdc.gov/vaccines/hcp/acip-recs/index.html.
- For calculating intervals between doses, 4 weeks = 28 days. Intervals of ≥4 months are determined by calendar months.
- Within a number range (e.g., 12–18), a dash (–) should be read as "through."
- Vaccine doses administered ≤4 days before the minimum age or interval are considered valid. Doses of any vaccine administered ≥5 days earlier than the minimum age or minimum interval should not be counted as valid and should be repeated as age appropriate. **The repeat dose should be spaced after the invalid dose by the recommended minimum interval.** For further details, see Table 3-1, Recommended and minimum ages and intervals between vaccine doses, in *General Best Practice Guidelines for Immunization* at www.cdc.gov/vaccines/hcp/acip-recs/general-recs/timing.html.
- Information on travel vaccination requirements and recommendations is available at www.cdc.gov/travel/.
- For vaccination of persons with immunodeficiencies, see Table 8-1, Vaccination of persons with primary and secondary immunodeficiencies, in *General Best Practice Guidelines for Immunization* at www.cdc.gov/vaccines/hcp/acip-recs/general-recs/immunocompetence.html, and Immunization in Special Clinical Circumstances (In: Kimberlin DW, Brady MT, Jackson MA, Long SS, eds. *Red Book: 2018 Report of the Committee on Infectious Diseases*. 31st ed. Itasca, IL: American Academy of Pediatrics; 2018:67–111).
- For information about vaccination in the setting of a vaccine-preventable disease outbreak, contact your state or local health department.
- The National Vaccine Injury Compensation Program (VICP) is a no-fault alternative to the traditional legal system for resolving vaccine injury claims. All routine child and adolescent vaccines are covered by VICP except for pneumococcal polysaccharide vaccine (PPSV23). For more information, see www.hrsa.gov/vaccinecompensation/index.html.

Diphtheria, tetanus, and pertussis (DTaP) vaccination (minimum age: 6 weeks [4 years for Kinrix or Quadracel])

Routine vaccination

- 5-dose series at 2, 4, 6, 15–18 months, 4–6 years
  - **Prospectively:** Dose 4 may be administered as early as age 12 months if at least 6 months have elapsed since dose 3.
  - **Retrospectively:** A 4th dose that was inadvertently administered as early as age 12 months may be counted if at least 4 months have elapsed since dose 3.

Catch-up vaccination

- Dose 5 is not necessary if dose 4 was administered at age 4 years or older and at least 6 months after dose 3.
- For other catch-up guidance, see Table 2.

Special situations

- Wound management in children less than age 7 years with history of 3 or more doses of tetanus-toxoid-containing vaccine: For all wounds except clean and minor wounds, administer DTaP if more than 5 years since last dose of tetanus-toxoid-containing vaccine. For detailed information, see www.cdc.gov/mmwr/volumes/67/rr/rr6702a1.htm.

Haemophilus influenzae type b vaccination (minimum age: 6 weeks)

Routine vaccination

- **ActHIB, Hiberix, or Pentacel:** 4-dose series at 2, 4, 6, 12–15 months
- **PedvaxHIB:** 3-dose series at 2, 4, 12–15 months

Catch-up vaccination

- **Dose 1 at age 7–11 months:** Administer dose 2 at least 4 weeks later and dose 3 (final dose) at age 12–15 months or 8 weeks after dose 2 (whichever is later).
- **Dose 1 at age 12–14 months:** Administer dose 2 (final dose) at least 8 weeks after dose 1.
- **Dose 1 before age 12 months and dose 2 before age 15 months:** Administer dose 3 (final dose) 8 weeks after dose 2.
- **2 doses of PedvaxHIB before age 12 months:** Administer dose 3 (final dose) at 12–59 months and at least 8 weeks after dose 2.
- **1 dose administered at age 15 months or older:** No further doses needed
- **Unvaccinated at age 15–59 months:** Administer 1 dose.
- **Previously unvaccinated children age 60 months or older who are not considered high risk:** Do not require catch-up vaccination
- For other catch-up guidance, see Table 2.

Special situations

- **Chemotherapy or radiation treatment:**
  12–59 months
  - Unvaccinated or only 1 dose before age 12 months: 2 doses, 8 weeks apart
  - 2 or more doses before age 12 months: 1 dose at least 8 weeks after previous dose

  Doses administered within 14 days of starting therapy or during therapy should be repeated at least 3 months after therapy completion.
- **Hematopoietic stem cell transplant (HSCT):**
  - 3-dose series 4 weeks apart starting 6 to 12 months after successful transplant, regardless of Hib vaccination history
- **Anatomic or functional asplenia (including sickle cell disease):**
  12–59 months
  - Unvaccinated or only 1 dose before age 12 months: 2 doses, 8 weeks apart
  - 2 or more doses before age 12 months: 1 dose at least 8 weeks after previous dose

  Unvaccinated persons age 5 years or older*
  - 1 dose
- **Elective splenectomy:**
  Unvaccinated persons age 15 months or older*
  - 1 dose (preferably at least 14 days before procedure)
- **HIV infection:**
  12–59 months
  - Unvaccinated or only 1 dose before age 12 months: 2 doses, 8 weeks apart
  - 2 or more doses before age 12 months: 1 dose at least 8 weeks after previous dose

  Unvaccinated persons age 5–18 years*
  - 1 dose
- **Immunoglobulin deficiency, early component complement deficiency:**
  12–59 months
  - Unvaccinated or only 1 dose before age 12 months: 2 doses, 8 weeks apart
  - 2 or more doses before age 12 months: 1 dose at least 8 weeks after previous dose

**Unvaccinated* = Less than routine series (through age 14 months) OR no doses (age 15 months or older)

Continued

Notes Recommended Child and Adolescent Immunization Schedule for ages 18 years or younger, United States, 2021

Hepatitis A vaccination
(minimum age: 12 months for routine vaccination)

Routine vaccination
- 2-dose series (minimum interval: 6 months) beginning at age 12 months

Catch-up vaccination
- Unvaccinated persons through age 18 years should complete a 2-dose series (minimum interval: 6 months).
- Persons who previously received 1 dose at age 12 months or older should receive dose 2 at least 6 months after dose 1.
- Adolescents age 18 years or older may receive the combined HepA and HepB vaccine, **Twinrix®**, as a 3-dose series (0, 1, and 6 months) or 4-dose series (3 doses at 0, 7, and 21–30 days, followed by a booster dose at 12 months).

International travel
- Persons traveling to or working in countries with high or intermediate endemic hepatitis A (www.cdc.gov/travel/):
  - **Infants age 6–11 months**: 1 dose before departure; revaccinate with 2 doses, separated by at least 6 months, between age 12–23 months.
  - **Unvaccinated age 12 months or older**: Administer dose 1 as soon as travel is considered.

Hepatitis B vaccination
(minimum age: birth)

Birth dose (monovalent HepB vaccine only)
- **Mother is HBsAg-negative:** 1 dose within 24 hours of birth for **all** medically stable infants ≥2,000 grams. Infants <2,000 grams: Administer 1 dose at chronological age 1 month or hospital discharge (whichever is earlier and even if weight is still <2,000 grams).
- **Mother is HBsAg-positive:**
  - Administer **HepB vaccine** and **hepatitis B immune globulin (HBIG)** (in separate limbs) within 12 hours of birth, regardless of birth weight. For infants <2,000 grams, administer 3 additional doses of vaccine (total of 4 doses) beginning at age 1 month.
  - Test for HBsAg and anti-HBs at age 9–12 months. If HepB series is delayed, test 1–2 months after final dose.
- **Mother's HBsAg status is unknown:**
  - Administer **HepB vaccine** within 12 hours of birth, regardless of birth weight.
  - For infants <2,000 grams, administer **HBIG** in addition to HepB vaccine (in separate limbs) within 12 hours of birth. Administer 3 additional doses of vaccine (total of 4 doses) beginning at age 1 month.
  - Determine mother's HBsAg status as soon as possible. If mother is HBsAg-positive, administer **HBIG** to infants ≥2,000 grams as soon as possible, but no later than 7 days of age.

Routine series
- 3-dose series at 0, 1–2, 6–18 months (use monovalent HepB vaccine for doses administered before age 6 weeks)
- Infants who did not receive a birth dose should begin the series as soon as feasible (see Table 2).
- Administration of **4 doses** is permitted when a combination vaccine containing HepB is used after the birth dose.
- **Minimum age** for the final (3rd or 4th) dose: 24 weeks
- **Minimum intervals:** dose 1 to dose 2: 4 weeks / dose 2 to dose 3: 8 weeks / dose 1 to dose 3: 16 weeks (when 4 doses are administered, substitute "dose 4" for "dose 3" in these calculations)

Catch-up vaccination
- Unvaccinated persons should complete a 3-dose series at 0, 1–2, 6 months.
- Adolescents age 11–15 years may use an alternative 2-dose schedule with at least 4 months between doses (adult formulation **Recombivax HB** only).
- Adolescents age 18 years or older may receive a 2-dose series of HepB (**Heplisav-B®**) at least 4 weeks apart.
- Adolescents age 18 years or older may receive the combined HepA and HepB vaccine, **Twinrix**, as a 3-dose series (0, 1, and 6 months) or 4-dose series (3 doses at 0, 7, and 21–30 days, followed by a booster dose at 12 months).
- For other catch-up guidance, see Table 2.

Special situations
- Revaccination is not generally recommended for persons with a normal immune status who were vaccinated as infants, children, adolescents, or adults.
- **Revaccination** may be recommended for certain populations, including:
  - **Infants born to HBsAg-positive mothers**
  - **Hemodialysis patients**
  - **Other immunocompromised persons**
- For detailed revaccination recommendations, see www.cdc.gov/vaccines/hcp/acip-recs/vacc-specific/hepb.html.

Human papillomavirus vaccination
(minimum age: 9 years)

Routine and catch-up vaccination
- HPV vaccination routinely recommended at **age 11–12 years (can start at age 9 years)** and catch-up HPV vaccination recommended for all persons through age 18 years if not adequately vaccinated
- 2- or 3-dose series depending on age at initial vaccination:
  - **Age 9–14 years at initial vaccination**: 2-dose series at 0, 6–12 months (minimum interval: 5 months; repeat dose if administered too soon)
  - **Age 15 years or older at initial vaccination**: 3-dose series at 0, 1–2 months, 6 months (minimum intervals: dose 1 to dose 2: 4 weeks / dose 2 to dose 3: 12 weeks / dose 1 to dose 3: 5 months; repeat dose if administered too soon)
- **Interrupted schedules:** If vaccination schedule is interrupted, the series does not need to be restarted.
- No additional dose recommended after completing series with recommended dosing intervals using any HPV vaccine.

Special situations
- **Immunocompromising conditions, including HIV infection:** 3-dose series as above
- **History of sexual abuse or assault:** Start at age 9 years.
- **Pregnancy:** HPV vaccination not recommended until after pregnancy; no intervention needed if vaccinated while pregnant; pregnancy testing not needed before vaccination

Influenza vaccination
(minimum age: 6 months [IIV], 2 years [LAIV4], 18 years [recombinant influenza vaccine, RIV4])

Routine vaccination
- Use any influenza vaccine appropriate for age and health status annually:
  - 2 doses, separated by at least 4 weeks, for **children age 6 months–8 years** who have received fewer than 2 influenza vaccine doses before July 1, 2020, or whose influenza vaccination history is unknown (administer dose 2 even if the child turns 9 between receipt of dose 1 and dose 2)
  - 1 dose for **children age 6 months–8 years** who have received at least 2 influenza vaccine doses before July 1, 2020
  - 1 dose for **all persons age 9 years or older**
- For the 2021–22 season, see the 2021–22 ACIP influenza vaccine recommendations.

Special situations
- **Egg allergy, hives only**: Any influenza vaccine appropriate for age and health status annually
- **Egg allergy with symptoms other than hives** (e.g., angioedema, respiratory distress, need for emergency medical services or epinephrine): Any influenza vaccine appropriate for age and health status annually. If using an influenza vaccine other than Flublok or Flucelvax, administer in medical setting under supervision of health care provider who can recognize and manage severe allergic reactions.
- Severe allergic reactions to vaccines can occur even in the absence of a history of previous allergic reaction. All vaccination providers should be familiar with the office emergency plan and certified in cardiopulmonary resuscitation.
- A previous severe allergic reaction to influenza vaccine is a contraindication to future receipt of any influenza vaccine.
- **LAIV4 should not be used** in persons with the following conditions or situations:
  - History of severe allergic reaction to a previous dose of any influenza vaccine or to any vaccine component (excluding egg, see details above)
  - Receiving aspirin or salicylate-containing medications
  - Age 2–4 years with history of asthma or wheezing
  - Immunocompromised due to any cause (including medications and HIV infection)
  - Anatomic or functional asplenia
  - Close contacts or caregivers of severely immunosuppressed persons who require a protected environment
  - Pregnancy
  - Cochlear implant
  - Cerebrospinal fluid-oropharyngeal communication
  - Children less than age 2 years
  - Received influenza antiviral medications oseltamivir or zanamivir within the previous 48 hours,. peramivir within the previous 5 days, or baloxavir within the previous 17 days

Notes Recommended Child and Adolescent Immunization Schedule for ages 18 years or younger, United States, 2021

Measles, mumps, and rubella vaccination (minimum age: 12 months for routine vaccination)

Routine vaccination
- 2-dose series at 12–15 months, 4–6 years
- Dose 2 may be administered as early as 4 weeks after dose 1.

Catch-up vaccination
- Unvaccinated children and adolescents: 2-dose series at least 4 weeks apart
- The maximum age for use of MMRV is 12 years.

Special situations
International travel
- **Infants age 6–11 months:** 1 dose before departure; revaccinate with 2-dose series at age 12–15 months (12 months for children in high-risk areas) and dose 2 as early as 4 weeks later.
- **Unvaccinated children age 12 months or older:** 2-dose series at least 4 weeks apart before departure

Meningococcal serogroup A,C,W,Y vaccination (minimum age: 2 months [MenACWY-CRM, Menveo], 9 months [MenACWY-D, Menactra], 2 years [MenACWY-TT, MenQuadfi])

Routine vaccination
- 2-dose series at 11–12 years, 16 years

Catch-up vaccination
- Age 13–15 years: 1 dose now and booster at age 16–18 years (minimum interval: 8 weeks)
- Age 16–18 years: 1 dose

Special situations
Anatomic or functional asplenia (including sickle cell disease), HIV infection, persistent complement component deficiency, complement inhibitor (e.g., eculizumab, ravulizumab) use:
- **Menveo**
  - Dose 1 at age 8 weeks: 4-dose series at 2, 4, 6, 12 months
  - Dose 1 at age 3–6 months: 3- or 4- dose series (dose 2 [and dose 3 if applicable] at least 8 weeks after previous dose until a dose is received at age 7 months or older, followed by an additional dose at least 12 weeks later and after age 12 months)
  - Dose 1 at age 7–23 months: 2-dose series (dose 2 at least 12 weeks after dose 1 and after age 12 months)
  - Dose 1 at age 24 months or older: 2-dose series at least 8 weeks apart
- **Menactra**
  - **Persistent complement component deficiency or complement inhibitor use:**
    - Age 9–23 months: 2-dose series at least 12 weeks apart
    - Age 24 months or older: 2-dose series at least 8 weeks apart
  - **Anatomic or functional asplenia, sickle cell disease, or HIV infection:**
    - Age 9–23 months: Not recommended
    - Age 24 months or older: 2-dose series at least 8 weeks apart
    - **Menactra** must be administered at least 4 weeks after completion of PCV13 series.
- **MenQuadfi**
  - Dose 1 at age 24 months or older: 2-dose series at least 8 weeks apart

Travel in countries with hyperendemic or epidemic meningococcal disease, including countries in the African meningitis belt or during the Hajj (www.cdc.gov/travel/)**:**
- Children less than age 24 months:
  - **Menveo (age 2–23 months)**
    - Dose 1 at age 8 weeks: 4-dose series at 2, 4, 6, 12 months
    - Dose 1 at age 3–6 months: 3- or 4- dose series (dose 2 [and dose 3 if applicable] at least 8 weeks after previous dose until a dose is received at age 7 months or older, followed by an additional dose at least 12 weeks later and after age 12 months)
    - Dose 1 at age 7–23 months: 2-dose series (dose 2 at least 12 weeks after dose 1 and after age 12 months)
  - **Menactra (age 9–23 months)**
    - 2-dose series (dose 2 at least 12 weeks after dose 1; dose 2 may be administered as early as 8 weeks after dose 1 in travelers)
- Children age 2 years or older: 1 dose Menveo, Menactra, or MenQuadfi

First-year college students who live in residential housing (if not previously vaccinated at age 16 years or older) or military recruits:
- 1 dose **Menveo, Menactra,** or **MenQuadfi**

Adolescent vaccination of children who received MenACWY prior to age 10 years:
- **Children for whom boosters are recommended** because of an ongoing increased risk of meningococcal disease (e.g., those with complement deficiency, HIV, or asplenia): Follow the booster schedule for persons at increased risk.
- **Children for whom boosters are not recommended** (e.g., a healthy child who received a single dose for travel to a country where meningococcal disease is endemic): Administer MenACWY according to the recommended adolescent schedule with dose 1 at age 11–12 years and dose 2 at age 16 years.

Note: Menactra should be administered either before or at the same time as DTaP. For MenACWY **booster dose recommendations** for groups listed under "Special situations" and in an outbreak setting and additional meningococcal vaccination information, see www.cdc.gov/mmwr/volumes/69/rr/rr6909a1.htm.

Meningococcal serogroup B vaccination (minimum age: 10 years [MenB-4C, Bexsero; MenB-FHbp, Trumenba])

Shared clinical decision-making
- **Adolescents not at increased risk** age 16–23 years (preferred age 16–18 years) based on shared clinical decision-making:
  - **Bexsero:** 2-dose series at least 1 month apart
  - **Trumenba:** 2-dose series at least 6 months apart; if dose 2 is administered earlier than 6 months, administer a 3rd dose at least 4 months after dose 2.

Special situations
Anatomic or functional asplenia (including sickle cell disease), persistent complement component deficiency, complement inhibitor (e.g., eculizumab, ravulizumab) use:
- **Bexsero:** 2-dose series at least 1 month apart
- **Trumenba:** 3-dose series at 0, 1–2, 6 months

Bexsero and **Trumenba** are not interchangeable; the same product should be used for all doses in a series.

For MenB **booster dose recommendations** for groups listed under "Special situations" and in an outbreak setting and additional meningococcal vaccination information, see www.cdc.gov/mmwr/volumes/69/rr/rr6909a1.htm.

Pneumococcal vaccination (minimum age: 6 weeks [PCV13], 2 years [PPSV23])

Routine vaccination with PCV13
- 4-dose series at 2, 4, 6, 12–15 months

Catch-up vaccination with PCV13
- 1 dose for healthy children age 24–59 months with any incomplete* PCV13 series
- For other catch-up guidance, see Table 2.

Special situations
Underlying conditions below: When both PCV13 and PPSV23 are indicated, administer PCV13 first. PCV13 and PPSV23 should not be administered during same visit.

Chronic heart disease (particularly cyanotic congenital heart disease and cardiac failure); chronic lung disease (including asthma treated with high-dose, oral corticosteroids); diabetes mellitus:

<u>Age 2–5 years</u>
- Any incomplete* series with:
  - 3 PCV13 doses: 1 dose PCV13 (at least 8 weeks after any prior PCV13 dose)
  - Less than 3 PCV13 doses: 2 doses PCV13 (8 weeks after the most recent dose and administered 8 weeks apart)
- No history of PPSV23: 1 dose PPSV23 (at least 8 weeks after completing all recommended PCV13 doses)

<u>Age 6–18 years</u>
- •No history of PPSV23: 1 dose PPSV23 (at least 8 weeks after completing all recommended PCV13 doses)

Cerebrospinal fluid leak, cochlear implant:

<u>Age 2–5 years</u>
- Any incomplete* series with:
  - 3 PCV13 doses: 1 dose PCV13 (at least 8 weeks after any prior PCV13 dose)
  - Less than 3 PCV13 doses: 2 doses PCV13 (8 weeks after the most recent dose and administered 8 weeks apart)
- No history of PPSV23: 1 dose PPSV23 (at least 8 weeks after any prior PCV13 dose)

<u>Age 6–18 years</u>
- No history of either PCV13 or PPSV23: 1 dose PCV13, 1 dose PPSV23 at least 8 weeks later
- Any PCV13 but no PPSV23: 1 dose PPSV23 at least 8 weeks after the most recent dose of PCV13
- PPSV23 but no PCV13: 1 dose PCV13 at least 8 weeks after the most recent dose of PPSV23

Notes Recommended Child and Adolescent Immunization Schedule for ages 18 years or younger, United States, 2021

Sickle cell disease and other hemoglobinopathies; anatomic or functional asplenia; congenital or acquired immunodeficiency; HIV infection; chronic renal failure; nephrotic syndrome; malignant neoplasms, leukemias, lymphomas, Hodgkin disease, and other diseases associated with treatment with immunosuppressive drugs or radiation therapy; solid organ transplantation; multiple myeloma:

Age 2–5 years

- Any incomplete* series with:
  - 3 PCV13 doses: 1 dose PCV13 (at least 8 weeks after any prior PCV13 dose)
  - Less than 3 PCV13 doses: 2 doses PCV13 (8 weeks after the most recent dose and administered 8 weeks apart)
- No history of PPSV23: 1 dose PPSV23 (at least 8 weeks after any prior PCV13 dose) and a 2nd dose of PPSV23 5 years later

Age 6–18 years

- No history of either PCV13 or PPSV23: 1 dose PCV13, 2 doses PPSV23 (dose 1 of PPSV23 administered 8 weeks after PCV13 and dose 2 of PPSV23 administered at least 5 years after dose 1 of PPSV23)
- Any PCV13 but no PPSV23: 2 doses PPSV23 (dose 1 of PPSV23 administered 8 weeks after the most recent dose of PCV13 and dose 2 of PPSV23 administered at least 5 years after dose 1 of PPSV23)
- PPSV23 but no PCV13: 1 dose PCV13 at least 8 weeks after the most recent PPSV23 dose and a 2nd dose of PPSV23 administered 5 years after dose 1 of PPSV23 and at least 8 weeks after a dose of PCV13

Chronic liver disease, alcoholism:

Age 6–18 years

- No history of PPSV23: 1 dose PPSV23 (at least 8 weeks after any prior PCV13 dose)

**Incomplete series* = Not having received all doses in either the recommended series or an age-appropriate catch-up series See Tables 8, 9, and 11 in the ACIP pneumococcal vaccine recommendations (www.cdc.gov/mmwr/pdf/rr/rr5911.pdf) for complete schedule details.

Poliovirus vaccination
(minimum age: 6 weeks)

Routine vaccination

- 4-dose series at ages 2, 4, 6–18 months, 4–6 years; administer the final dose on or after age 4 years and at least 6 months after the previous dose.
- 4 or more doses of IPV can be administered before age 4 years when a combination vaccine containing IPV is used. However, a dose is still recommended on or after age 4 years and at least 6 months after the previous dose.

Catch-up vaccination

- In the first 6 months of life, use minimum ages and intervals only for travel to a polio-endemic region or during an outbreak.
- IPV is not routinely recommended for U.S. residents age 18 years or older.

Series containing oral polio vaccine (OPV), either mixed OPV-IPV or OPV-only series:

- Total number of doses needed to complete the series is the same as that recommended for the U.S. IPV schedule. See www.cdc.gov/mmwr/volumes/66/wr/mm6601a6.htm?s_%20cid=mm6601a6_w.
- Only trivalent OPV (tOPV) counts toward the U.S. vaccination requirements.
  - Doses of OPV administered before April 1, 2016, should be counted (unless specifically noted as administered during a campaign).
  - Doses of OPV administered on or after April 1, 2016, should not be counted.
  - For guidance to assess doses documented as "OPV," see www.cdc.gov/mmwr/volumes/66/wr/mm6606a7.htm?s_cid=mm6606a7_w.
- For other catch-up guidance, see Table 2.

Rotavirus vaccination
(minimum age: 6 weeks)

Routine vaccination

- **Rotarix:** 2-dose series at 2 and 4 months
- **RotaTeq:** 3-dose series at 2, 4, and 6 months
- If any dose in the series is either **RotaTeq** or unknown, default to 3-dose series.

Catch-up vaccination

- Do not start the series on or after age 15 weeks, 0 days.
- The maximum age for the final dose is 8 months, 0 days.
- For other catch-up guidance, see Table 2.

Tetanus, diphtheria, and pertussis (Tdap) vaccination
(minimum age: 11 years for routine vaccination, 7 years for catch-up vaccination)

Routine vaccination

- **Adolescents age 11–12 years:** 1 dose Tdap
- **Pregnancy:** 1 dose Tdap during each pregnancy, preferably in early part of gestational weeks 27–36
- Tdap may be administered regardless of the interval since the last tetanus- and diphtheria-toxoid-containing vaccine.

Catch-up vaccination

- **Adolescents age 13–18 years who have not received Tdap:** 1 dose Tdap, then Td or Tdap booster every 10 years
- **Persons age 7–18 years not fully vaccinated* with DTaP:** 1 dose Tdap as part of the catch-up series (preferably the first dose); if additional doses are needed, use Td or Tdap.
- **Tdap administered at age 7–10 years:**
  - **Children age 7–9 years** who receive Tdap should receive the routine Tdap dose at age 11–12 years.
  - **Children age 10 years** who receive Tdap do not need the routine Tdap dose at age 11–12 years.
- **DTaP inadvertently administered on or after age 7 years:**
  - **Children age 7–9 years**: DTaP may count as part of catch-up series. Administer routine Tdap dose at age 11–12 years.
  - **Children age 10–18 years**: Count dose of DTaP as the adolescent Tdap booster.
- For other catch-up guidance, see Table 2.

Special situations

- **Wound management** in persons age 7 years or older with history of 3 or more doses of tetanus-toxoid-containing vaccine: For clean and minor wounds, administer Tdap or Td if more than 10 years since last dose of tetanus-toxoid-containing vaccine; for all other wounds, administer Tdap or Td if more than 5 years since last dose of tetanus-toxoid-containing vaccine. Tdap is preferred for persons age 11 years or older who have not previously received Tdap or whose Tdap history is unknown. If a tetanus-toxoid-containing vaccine is indicated for a pregnant adolescent, use Tdap.
- For detailed information, see www.cdc.gov/mmwr/volumes/69/wr/mm6903a5.htm.

**Fully vaccinated* = 5 valid doses of DTaP OR 4 valid doses of DTaP if dose 4 was administered at age 4 years or older

Varicella vaccination
(minimum age: 12 months)

Routine vaccination

- 2-dose series at 12–15 months, 4–6 years
- Dose 2 may be administered as early as 3 months after dose 1 (a dose administered after a 4-week interval may be counted).

Catch-up vaccination

- Ensure persons age 7–18 years without evidence of immunity (see *MMWR* at www.cdc.gov/mmwr/pdf/rr/rr5604.pdf) have a 2-dose series:
  - **Age 7–12 years**: routine interval: 3 months (a dose administered after a 4-week interval may be counted)
  - **Age 13 years and older**: routine interval: 4–8 weeks (minimum interval: 4 weeks)
  - The maximum age for use of MMRV is 12 years.

General Recommendations on Immunization

TABLE 3 Recommended and Minimum Ages and Intervals between Vaccine Doses*,†

Vaccine and Dose Number	Recommended Age for this Dose	Minimum Age for this Dose	Recommended Interval to Next Dose	Minimum Interval to Next Dose
HepB-1§	Birth	Birth	1-4 months	4 weeks
HepB-2	1-2 months	4 weeks	2-17 months	8 weeks
HepB-3¶	6-18 months	24 weeks	—	—
DTaP-1§	2 months	6 weeks	2 months	4 weeks
DTaP-2	4 months	10 weeks***	2 months	4 weeks
DTaP-3	6 months	14 weeks	6-12 months	6 months
DTaP-4	15-18 months	12 months	3 years	6 months
DTaP-5	4-6 years	4 years	—	—
Hib-1§§§	2 months	6 weeks	2 months	4 weeks
Hib-2	4 months	10 weeks	2 months	4 weeks
Hib-3¶¶	6 months	14 weeks	6-9 months	8 weeks
Hib-4	12-15 months	12 months	—	—
IPV-1§	2 months	6 weeks	2 months	4 weeks
IPV-2	4 months	10 weeks	2-14 months	4 weeks
IPV-3	6-18 months	14 weeks	3-5 years	6 months
IPV-4***	4-6 years	4 years	—	—
PCV-1§§	2 months	6 weeks	8 weeks	4 weeks
PCV-2	4 months	10 weeks	8 weeks	4 weeks
PCV-3	6 months	14 weeks	6 months	8 weeks
PCV-4	12-15 months	12 months	—	—
MMR-1†††	12-15 months	12 months	3-5 years	4 weeks
MMR-2†††	4-6 years	13 months	—	—
Varicella-1†††	12-15 months	12 months	3-5 years	12 weeks§§§
Varicella-2†††	4-6 years	15 months	—	—
HepA-1	12-23 months	12 months	6-18 months**	6 months**
HepA-2	≥18 months	18 months	—	—
Influenza inactivated¶¶¶	≥6 months	6 months****	1 month	4 weeks
LAIV (intranasal)¶¶¶	2-49 years	2 years	1 month	4 weeks
MCV4-1††††	11-12 years	2 years	5 years	8 weeks
MCV4-2	16 years	11 years (+8 weeks)	—	—
MPSV4-1††††	—	2 years	5 years	5 years
MPSV4-2	—	7 years	—	—
Td	11-12 years	7 years	10 years	5 years
Tdap§§§§	≥11 years	7 years	—	—
PPSV-1	—	2 years	5 years	5 years
PPSV-2¶¶¶¶	—	7 years	—	—
HPV-1*****	11-12 years	9 years	2 months	4 weeks
HPV-2	11-12 years (+2 months)	9 years (+4 weeks)	4 months	12 weeks†††††
HPV-3†††††	11-12 years (+6 months)	9 years (+24 weeks)	—	—
Rotavirus-1§§§§§	2 months	6 weeks	2 months	4 weeks
Rotavirus-2	4 months	10 weeks	2 months	4 weeks
Rotavirus-3¶¶¶¶¶	6 months	14 weeks	—	—
Herpes zoster******	≥60 years	60 years	—	—
Pneumococcal vaccine††††††	—	—	—	—

DTaP, Diphtheria and tetanus toxoids and acellular pertussis; *HepA,* hepatitis A; *HepB,* hepatitis B; *Hib, Haemophilus influenzae* type b; *HPV,* human papillomavirus; *IPV,* inactivated poliovirus; *LAIV,* live, attenuated influenza vaccine; *MCV4,* quadrivalent meningococcal conjugate vaccine; *MMR,* measles, mumps, and rubella; *MMRV,* measles, mumps, rubella, and varicella; *MPSV4,* quadrivalent meningococcal polysaccharide vaccine; *PCV,* pneumococcal conjugate vaccine; *PPSV,* pneumococcal polysaccharide vaccine; *PRP-OMB,* polyribosylribitol phosphate-meningococcal outer membrane protein conjugate; *Td,* tetanus and diphtheria toxoids; *Tdap,* tetanus toxoid, reduced diphtheria toxoid, and acellular pertussis.

†† The minimum recommended interval between DTaP-3 and DTaP-4 is 6 months. However, DTaP-4 need not be repeated if administered at least 4 months after DTaP-3.

*Combination vaccines are available. Use of licensed combination vaccines is generally preferred to separate injections of their equivalent component vaccines. When administering combination vaccines, the minimum age for administration is the oldest age for any of the individual components; the minimum interval between doses is equal to the greatest interval of any of the individual components.

†Information on travel vaccines, including typhoid, Japanese encephalitis, and yellow fever, is available at www.cdc.gov/travel. Information on other vaccines that are licensed in the United States but not distributed, including anthrax and smallpox, is available at www.cdc.gov/vaccines/hcp/vis/current-vis.html.

§Combination vaccines containing the hepatitis B component are available. These vaccines should not be administered to infants aged <6 weeks because of the other components (i.e., Hib, DTaP, HepA, and IPV).

¶HepB-3 should be administered at least 8 weeks after HepB-2 and at least 16 weeks after HepB-1 and should not be administered before age 24 weeks.

**Calendar months.

§§For Hib and PCV, children receiving the first dose of vaccine at age ≥7 months require fewer doses to complete the series.

¶¶If PRP-OMP (Pedvax-Hib, Merck Vaccine Division) was administered at ages 2 and 4 months, a dose at age 6 months is not necessary.

***A fourth dose is not needed if the third dose was administered at ≥4 years and at least 6 months after the previous dose.

†††Combination MMRV vaccine can be used for children aged 12 months to 12 years.

§§§The minimum interval from Varicella-1 to Varicella-2 for persons beginning the series at age ≥13 years is 4 weeks.

¶¶¶One dose of influenza vaccine per season is recommended for most persons. Children aged <9 years who are receiving influenza vaccine for the first time or who received only 1 dose the previous season (if it was their first vaccination season) should receive 2 doses this season.

****The minimum age for inactivated influenza vaccine varies by vaccine manufacturer. See package insert for vaccine-specific minimum ages.

††††Revaccination with meningococcal vaccine is recommended for previously vaccinated persons who remain at high risk for meningococcal disease. (Source: CDC. Updated recommendations from the Advisory Committee on Immunization Practices (ACIP) for revaccination of persons at prolonged increased risk for meningococcal disease, *MMWR* 2009;58:[1042-3]).

TABLE 3 Recommended and Minimum Ages and Intervals between Vaccine Doses*†—cont'd

§§§§Only 1 dose of Tdap is recommended. Subsequent doses should be given as Td. For one brand of Tdap, the minimum age is 11 years. For management of a tetanus-prone wound in persons who have received a primary series of tetanus–toxoid-containing vaccine, the minimum interval after a previous dose of any tetanus-containing vaccine is 5 years.

¶¶¶¶A second dose of PPSV 5 years after the first dose is recommended for persons aged ≤65 years at highest risk for serious pneumococcal infection and those who are likely to have a rapid decline in pneumococcal antibody concentration. (Source: CDC. Prevention of pneumococcal disease: recommendations of the Advisory Committee on Immunization Practices [ACIP], *MMWR* 1997;46[No. RR-8].)

*****Bivalent HPV vaccine is approved for females aged 10-25 years. Quadrivalent HPV vaccine is approved for males and females aged 9-26 years.

†††††The minimum age for HPV-3 is based on the baseline minimum age for the first dose (i.e., 108 months) and the minimum interval of 24 weeks between the first and third dose. Dose 3 need not be repeated if it is administered at least 16 weeks after the first dose.

§§§§§The first dose of rotavirus must be administered at age 6 weeks through 14 weeks and 6 days. The vaccine series should not be started for infants aged ≥15 weeks, 0 days. Rotavirus should not be administered to children older than 8 months, 0 days of age regardless of the number of doses received between 6 weeks and 8 months, 0 days of age.

¶¶¶¶¶If 2 doses of Rotarix (GlaxoSmithKline) are administered as age appropriate, a third dose is not necessary.

******Herpes zoster vaccine is recommended as a single dose for persons aged ≥60 years.

TABLE 4 Guidelines for Spacing of Live and Inactivated Antigens

Antigen Combination	Recommended Minimum Interval between Doses
Two or more inactivated*	May be administered simultaneously or at any interval between doses
Inactivated and live	May be administered simultaneously or at any interval between doses
Two or more live intranasal or injectable†	28 days minimum interval, if not administered simultaneously

*Certain experts suggest a 28-day interval between tetanus toxoid, reduced diphtheria toxoid, and acellular pertussis (Tdap) vaccine and tetravalent meningococcal conjugate vaccine if they are not administered simultaneously.

†Live oral vaccines (e.g., Ty21a typhoid vaccine and rotavirus vaccine) may be administered simultaneously or at any interval before or after inactivated or live injectable vaccines.

From Centers for Disease Control and Prevention: General recommendations on immunization: recommendations of the Advisory Committee on Immunization Practices (ACIP), *MMWR* 60(2):38, 2011.

TABLE 5 Guidelines for Administering Antibody-Containing Products* and Vaccines

Type of Administration	Products Administered		Recommended Minimum Interval between Doses
Simultaneous (during the same office visit)	Antibody-containing products and inactivated antigen		Can be administered simultaneously at different anatomic sites or at any time interval between doses
	Antibody-containing products and live antigen		Should not be administered simultaneously.† If simultaneous administration of measles-containing vaccine or varicella vaccine is unavoidable, administer at different sites and revaccinate or test for seroconversion after the recommended interval
Nonsimultaneous	**Administered First**	**Administered Second**	
	Antibody-containing products	Inactivated antigen	No interval necessary
	Inactivated antigen	Antibody-containing products	No interval necessary
	Antibody-containing products	Live antigen	Dose related
	Live antigen	Antibody-containing products	2 weeks

*Blood products containing substantial amounts of immune globulin include intramuscular and intravenous immune globulin, specific hyperimmune globulin (e.g., hepatitis B immune globulin, tetanus immune globulin, varicella zoster immune globulin, and rabies immune globulin), whole blood, packed red blood cells, plasma, and platelet products.

†Yellow fever vaccine; rotavirus vaccine; oral Ty21a typhoid vaccine; live, attenuated influenza vaccine; and zoster vaccine are exceptions to these recommendations. These live, attenuated vaccines can be administered at any time before or after or simultaneously with an antibody-containing product.

‡ The duration of interference of antibody-containing products with the immune response to the measles component of measles-containing vaccine, and possibly varicella vaccine, is dose related.

From Centers for Disease Control and Prevention: General recommendations on immunization: recommendations of the Advisory Committee on Immunization Practices (ACIP), *MMWR* 60:(RR-2), 2011.

TABLE 6 Recommended Intervals between Administration of Antibody-Containing Products and Measles- or Varicella-Containing Vaccine, by Product and Indication for Vaccination

Product/Indication	Dose (mg IgG/kg) and Route*	Recommended Interval before Measles- or Varicella-Containing Vaccine† Administration (months)
Tetanus IG	250 units (10 mg IgG/kg) IM	3
Hepatitis A IG		
Contact prophylaxis	0.02 ml/kg (33 mg IgG/kg) IM	3
International travel	0.06 ml/kg (10 mg IgG/kg) IM	3
Hepatitis B IG	0.06 ml/kg (10 mg IgG/kg) IM	3
Rabies IG	20 IU/kg (22 mg IgG/kg) IM	4
Varicella IG	125 units/10 kg (60-200 mg IgG/kg) IM, maximum 625 units	5
Measles prophylaxis IG		
Standard (i.e., nonimmunocompromised) contact	0.25 ml/kg (40 mg IgG/kg) IM	5
Immunocompromised contact	0.50 ml/kg (80 mg IgG/kg) IM	6
Blood transfusion		
RBCs, washed	10 ml/kg negligible IgG/kg IV	None
RBCs, adenine-saline added	10 ml/kg (10 mg IgG/kg) IV	3
Packed RBCs (hematocrit 65%)§	10 ml/kg (60 mg IgG/kg) IV	6
Whole blood (hematocrit 35%-50%)§	10 ml/kg (80-100 mg IgG/kg) IV	6
Plasma/platelet products	10 ml/kg (160 mg IgG/kg) IV	7
Cytomegalovirus IGIV	150 mg/kg maximum	6
IGIV		
Replacement therapy for immune deficiencies¶	300-400 mg/kg IV¶	8
Immune thrombocytopenic purpura treatment	400 mg/kg IV	8
Postexposure varicella prophylaxis**	400 mg/kg IV	8
Immune thrombocytopenic purpura treatment	1000 mg/kg IV	10
Kawasaki disease	2 g/kg IV	11
Monoclonal antibody to respiratory syncytial virus F protein (Synagis [MedImmune])††	15 mg/kg IM	None

HIV, human immunodeficiency virus; *IG,* immune globulin; *IgG,* immune globulin G; *IGIV,* intravenous immune globulin; *mg IgG/kg,* milligrams of immune globulin G per kilogram of body weight; *IM,* intramuscular; *IV,* intravenous; *RBCs,* red blood cells.

*This table is not intended for determining the correct indications and dosages for using antibody-containing products. Unvaccinated persons might not be protected fully against measles during the entire recommended interval, and additional doses of IG or measles vaccine might be indicated after measles exposure. Concentrations of measles antibody in an IG preparation can vary by manufacturer's lot. Rates of antibody clearance after receipt of an IG preparation also might vary. Recommended intervals are extrapolated from an estimated half-life of 30 days for passively acquired antibody and an observed interference with the immune response to measles vaccine for 5 months after a dose of 80 mg IgG/kg.

†Does not include zoster vaccine. Zoster vaccine may be given with antibody-containing blood products.

§Assumes a serum IgG concentration of 16 mg/ml.

¶Measles and varicella vaccinations are recommended for children with asymptomatic or mildly symptomatic HIV infection but are contraindicated for persons with severe immunosuppression from HIV or any other immunosuppressive disorder.

**The investigational VariZIG, similar to licensed varicella-zoster IG (VZIG), is a purified human IG preparation made from plasma containing high levels of antivaricella antibodies (IgG). The interval between VariZIG and varicella vaccine (Var or MMRV) is 5 months.

††Contains antibody only to respiratory syncytial virus.

From Centers for Disease Control and Prevention: General recommendations on immunization: recommendations of the Advisory Committee on Immunization Practices (ACIP), *MMWR* 60:(RR-2), 2011.

TABLE 7 Contraindications and Precautions* to Commonly Used Vaccines

Vaccine	Contraindications	Precautions
DTaP	Severe allergic reaction (e.g., anaphylaxis) after a previous dose or to a vaccine component Encephalopathy (e.g., coma, decreased level of consciousness, or prolonged seizures), not attributable to another identifiable cause, within 7 days of administration of previous dose of DTP or DTaP	Progressive neurologic disorder, including infantile spasms, uncontrolled epilepsy, progressive encephalopathy; defer DTaP until neurologic status clarified and stabilized Temperature of ≥105° F (≥40° C) within 48 hours after vaccination with a previous dose of DTP or DTaP Collapse or shocklike state (i.e., hypotonic hyporesponsive episode) within 48 hours after receiving a previous dose of DTP/DTaP Seizure ≤3 days after receiving a previous dose of DTP/DTaP Persistent, inconsolable crying lasting ≥3 hours within 48 hours after receiving a previous dose of DTP/DTaP GBS <6 weeks after previous dose of tetanus toxoid containing vaccine History of Arthus-type hypersensitivity reactions after a previous dose of tetanus toxoid containing vaccine; defer vaccination until at least 10 years have elapsed since the last tetanus toxoid containing vaccine Moderate or severe acute illness with or without fever
DT, Td	Severe allergic reaction (e.g., anaphylaxis) after a previous dose or to a vaccine component	GBS <6 weeks after previous dose of tetanus toxoid containing vaccine History of Arthus-type hypersensitivity reactions after a previous dose of tetanus toxoid containing vaccine; defer vaccination until at least 10 years have elapsed since the last tetanus toxoid containing vaccine Moderate or severe acute illness with or without fever
Tdap	Severe allergic reaction (e.g., anaphylaxis) after a previous dose or to a vaccine component Encephalopathy (e.g., coma, decreased level of consciousness, or prolonged seizures), not attributable to another identifiable cause, within 7 days of administration of previous dose of DTP, DTaP, or Tdap	GBS <6 weeks after a previous dose of tetanus toxoid containing vaccine Progressive or unstable neurologic disorder, uncontrolled seizures, or progressive encephalopathy until a treatment regimen has been established and the condition has stabilized History of Arthus-type hypersensitivity reactions after a previous dose of tetanus toxoid containing vaccine; defer vaccination until at least 10 years have elapsed since the last tetanus toxoid containing vaccine Moderate or severe acute illness with or without fever
IPV	Severe allergic reaction (e.g., anaphylaxis) after a previous dose or to a vaccine component	Pregnancy Moderate or severe acute illness with or without fever
MMR[†,§]	Severe allergic reaction (e.g., anaphylaxis) after a previous dose or to a vaccine component Pregnancy: Known severe immunodeficiency (e.g., from hematologic and solid tumors, receipt of chemotherapy, congenital immunodeficiency, or long-term immunosuppressive therapy[¶] or patients with HIV infection who are severely immunocompromised)[§]	Recent (≤11 months) receipt of antibody-containing blood product (specific interval depends on product) History of thrombocytopenia or thrombocytopenic purpura Need for tuberculin skin testing[††] Moderate or severe acute illness with or without fever
Hib	Severe allergic reaction (e.g., anaphylaxis) after a previous dose or to a vaccine component Age <6 weeks	Moderate or severe acute illness with or without fever
Hepatitis B	Severe allergic reaction (e.g., anaphylaxis) after a previous dose or to a vaccine component	Infant weight <2000 g[§§] Moderate or severe acute illness with or without fever
Hepatitis A	Severe allergic reaction (e.g., anaphylaxis) after a previous dose or to a vaccine component	Pregnancy: Moderate or severe acute illness with or without fever
Varicella	Severe allergic reaction (e.g., anaphylaxis) after a previous dose or to a vaccine component Known severe immunodeficiency (e.g., from hematologic and solid tumors, receipt of chemotherapy, congenital immunodeficiency, or long-term immunosuppressive therapy[¶] or patients with HIV infection who are severely immunocompromised)[§] Pregnancy	Recent (≤11 months) receipt of antibody-containing blood product (specific interval depends on product)[¶¶] Moderate or severe acute illness with or without fever
PCV	Severe allergic reaction (e.g., anaphylaxis) after a previous dose (of PCV7, PCV13, or any diphtheria toxoid-containing vaccine) or to a component of a vaccine (PCV7, PCV13, or any diphtheria toxoid-containing vaccine)	Moderate or severe acute illness with or without fever
TIV	Severe allergic reaction (e.g., anaphylaxis) after a previous dose or to vaccine component, including egg protein	GBS <6 weeks after a previous dose of influenza vaccine Moderate or severe acute illness with or without fever
LAIV	Severe allergic reaction (e.g., anaphylaxis) after a previous dose or to vaccine component, including egg protein Pregnancy Immunosuppression Certain chronic medical conditions***	GBS <6 weeks after a previous dose of influenza vaccine Moderate or severe acute illness with or without fever
PPSV	Severe allergic reaction (e.g., anaphylaxis) after a previous dose or to a vaccine component	Moderate or severe acute illness with or without fever
MCV4	Severe allergic reaction (e.g., anaphylaxis) after a previous dose or to a vaccine component	Moderate or severe acute illness with or without fever
MPSV4	Severe allergic reaction (e.g., anaphylaxis) after a previous dose or to a vaccine component	Moderate or severe acute illness with or without fever

Continued

TABLE 7 Contraindications and Precautions* to Commonly Used Vaccines—cont'd

Vaccine	Contraindications	Precautions
HPV	Severe allergic reaction (e.g., anaphylaxis) after a previous dose or to a vaccine component	Pregnancy: Moderate or severe acute illness with or without fever
Rotavirus	Severe allergic reaction (e.g., anaphylaxis) after a previous dose or to a vaccine component SCID	Altered immunocompetence other than SCID: History of intussusception Chronic gastrointestinal disease††† Spina bifida or bladder exstrophy††† Moderate or severe acute illness with or without fever
Zoster	Severe allergic reaction (e.g., anaphylaxis) after a previous dose or to a vaccine component Substantial suppression of cellular immunity Pregnancy	Moderate or severe acute illness with or without fever

DT, Diphtheria and tetanus toxoids; *DTaP,* diphtheria and tetanus toxoids and acellular pertussis; *GBS,* Guillain-Barré syndrome; *HBsAg,* hepatitis B surface antigen; *Hib, Haemophilus influenzae* type b; *HIV,* human immunodeficiency virus; *HPV,* human papillomavirus; *IPV,* inactivated poliovirus; *LAIV,* live, attenuated influenza vaccine; *MCV4,* quadrivalent meningococcal conjugate vaccine; *MMRV* measles, mumps, rubella; *MPSV4,* quadrivalent meningococcal polysaccharide vaccine; *PCV,* pneumococcal conjugate vaccine; *PPSV,* pneumococcal polysaccharide vaccine; *SCID,* severe combined immunodeficiency; *Td,* tetanus and diphtheria toxoids; *Tdap,* tetanus toxoid, reduced diphtheria toxoid, and acellular pertussis; *TIV,* trivalent inactivated influenza vaccine.

*Events or conditions listed as precautions should be reviewed carefully. Benefits of and risks for administering a specific vaccine to a person under these circumstances should be considered. If the risk from the vaccine is believed to outweigh the benefit, the vaccine should not be administered. If the benefit of vaccination is believed to outweigh the risk, the vaccine should be administered. Whether and when to administer DTaP to children with proven or suspected underlying neurologic disorders should be decided on a case-by-case basis.

†HIV-infected children may receive varicella and measles vaccine if CD4+ T-lymphocyte count is <15%. (Source: Adapted from American Academy of Pediatrics. Passive immunization. In: Pickering LK, ed. *Red book: 2009 report of the committee on infectious diseases.* 28th ed. Elk Grove Village.IL: American Academy of Pediatrics: 2009.)

§MMR and varicella vaccines can be administered on the same day. If not administered on the same day, these vaccines should be separated by at least 28 days.

¶Substantially immunosuppressive steroid dose is considered to be ≥2 weeks of daily receipt of 20 mg or 2 mg/kg body weight of prednisone or equivalent.

††Measles vaccination might suppress tuberculin reactivity temporarily. Measles-containing vaccine can be administered on the same day as tuberculin skin testing. If testing cannot be performed until after the day of MMR vaccination, the test should be postponed for ≥4 weeks after the vaccination. If an urgent need exists to skin test, do so with the understanding that reactivity might be reduced by the vaccine.

§§Hepatitis B vaccination should be deferred for infants weighing <2000 g if the mother is documented to be HBsAg-negative at the time of the infant's birth. Vaccination can commence at chronological age 1 month or at hospital discharge. For infants born to HBsAg-positive women, hepatitis B immune globulin and hepatitis B vaccine should be administered within 12 hours after birth, regardless of weight.

¶¶Vaccine should be deferred for the appropriate interval if replacement immune globulin products are being administered.

***Source: CDC. Prevention and control of seasonal influenza with vaccines: recommendations of the Advisory Committee on Immunization Practices (ACIP), 2010, *MMWR* 2010;59(No. RR-8).

†††For details see CDC. Prevention of rotavirus gastroenteritis among infants and children: recommendations of the Advisory Committee on Immunization Practices, *MMWR* 2009;58(No. RR-2).

From Centers for Disease Control and Prevention: General recommendations on immunization: recommendations of the Advisory Committee on Immunization Practices (ACIP), *MMWR* 60:(RR-2), 2011.

TABLE 8 Conditions Commonly Misperceived as Contraindications to Vaccination

Vaccine	Conditions Commonly Misperceived as Contraindications (i.e., Vaccination May Be Administered under These Conditions)
General for all vaccines, including DTaP, pediatric DT, adult Td, adolescent-adult Tdap, IPV, MMR, Hib, hepatitis A, hepatitis B, varicella, rotavirus, PCV, TIV, LAIV, PPSV, MCV4, MPSV4, HPV, and herpes zoster	Mild acute illness with or without fever Mild-to-moderate local reaction (i.e., swelling, redness, soreness); low-grade or moderate fever after previous dose Lack of previous physical examination in well-appearing person Current antimicrobial therapy* Convalescent phase of illness Preterm birth (hepatitis B vaccine is an exception in certain circumstances)† Recent exposure to an infectious disease History of penicillin allergy, other nonvaccine allergies, relatives with allergies, or receiving allergen extract immunotherapy
DTaP	Fever of <105° F (<40° C), fussiness or mild drowsiness after a previous dose of DTP/DTaP Family history of seizures Family history of sudden infant death syndrome Family history of an adverse event after DTP or DTaP administration Stable neurologic conditions (e.g., cerebral palsy, well-controlled seizures, or developmental delay)
Tdap	Fever of ≥105° F (≥40° C) for <48 hours after vaccination with a previous dose of DTP or DTaP Collapse or shock-like state (i.e., hypotonic hyporesponsive episode) within 48 hours after receiving a previous dose of DTaP Seizure <3 days after receiving a previous dose of DTP/DTaP Persistent, inconsolable crying lasting <3 hours within 48 hours after receiving a previous dose of DTP/DTaP History of extensive limb swelling after DTP/DTaP/Td that is not an Arthus-type reaction Stable neurologic disorder History of brachial neuritis Latex allergy that is not anaphylactic Breastfeeding Immunosuppression
IPV	Previous receipt of ≥1 dose of oral polio vaccine
MMR[§,¶]	Positive tuberculin skin test Simultaneous tuberculin skin testing** Breastfeeding Pregnancy of recipient's mother or other close or household contact Recipient is female of childbearing age Immunodeficient family member or household contact Asymptomatic or mildly symptomatic HIV infection Allergy to eggs
Hepatitis B	Pregnancy Autoimmune disease (e.g., systemic lupus erythematosus or rheumatoid arthritis)
Varicella	Pregnancy of recipient's mother or other close or household contact Immunodeficient family member or household contact†† Asymptomatic or mildly symptomatic HIV infection Humoral immunodeficiency (e.g., agammaglobulinemia)
TIV	Nonsevere (e.g., contact) allergy to latex, thimerosal, or egg Concurrent administration of Coumadin or aminophylline
LAIV	Health care providers that see patients with chronic diseases or altered immunocompetence (an exception is providers for severely immunocompromised patients requiring care in a protected environment) Breastfeeding Contacts of persons with chronic disease or altered immunocompetence (an exception is contacts of severely immunocompromised patients requiring care in a protected environment)
PPSV	History of invasive pneumococcal disease or pneumonia
HPV	Immunosuppression Previous equivocal or abnormal Papanicolaou test Known HPV infection Breastfeeding History of genital warts
Rotavirus	Prematurity Immunosuppressed household contacts Pregnant household contacts
Zoster	Therapy with low-dose methotrexate (≤0.4 mg/kg/week), azathioprine (≤3.0 mg/kg/day), or 6-mercaptopurine (≤1.5 mg/kg/day) for treatment of rheumatoid arthritis, psoriasis, polymyositis, sarcoidosis, inflammatory bowel disease, or other conditions Health care providers of patients with chronic diseases or altered immunocompetence Contacts of patients with chronic diseases or altered immunocompetence Unknown or uncertain history of varicella in a U.S.-born person

Continued

TABLE 8 Conditions Commonly Misperceived as Contraindications to Vaccination—cont'd

DT, Diphtheria and tetanus toxoids; *DTP,* diphtheria toxoid, tetanus toxoid, and pertussis; *DTaP,* diphtheria and tetanus toxoids and acellular pertussis; *HBsAg,* hepatitis B surface antigen; *Hib, Haemophilus influenzae* type b; *HPV,* human papillomavirus; *IPV,* inactivated poliovirus; *LAIV,* live, attenuated influenza vaccine; *MCV4,* quadrivalent meningococcal conjugate vaccine; *MMR,* measles, mumps, and rubella; *MPSV4,* quadrivalent meningococcal polysaccharide vaccine; *PCV,* pneumococcal conjugate vaccine; *PPSV,* pneumococcal polysaccharide vaccine; *Td,* tetanus and diphtheria toxoids; *Tdap,* tetanus toxoid, reduced diphtheria toxoid, and acellular pertussis; *TIV,* trivalent inactivated influenza vaccine.

*Antibacterial drugs might interfere with Ty21a oral typhoid vaccine, and certain antiviral drugs might interfere with varicella-containing vaccines and LAIV.

†Hepatitis B vaccination should be deferred for infants weighing <2000 g if the mother is documented to be HBsAg-negative at the time of the infant's birth. Vaccination can commence at chronologic age 1 month or at hospital discharge. For infants born to HBsAg-positive women, hepatitis B immune globulin and hepatitis B vaccine should be administered within 12 hours after birth, regardless of weight.

§MMR and varicella vaccines can be administered on the same day. If not administered on the same day, these vaccines should be separated by at least 28 days.

¶HIV-infected children should receive immune globulin after exposure to measles. HIV-infected children can receive varicella and measles vaccine if $CD4^+$ T-lymphocyte count is >15%. (Source: Adapted from American Academy of Pediatrics. Passive immunization. In: Pickering LK, ed. *Red book: 2009 report of the Committee on Infectious Diseases,* 28th ed. Elk Grove Village, IL: American Academy of Pediatrics; 2009.)

**Measles vaccination might suppress tuberculin reactivity temporarily. Measles-containing vaccine can be administered on the same day as tuberculin skin testing. If testing cannot be performed until after the day of MMR vaccination, the test should be postponed for at least 4 weeks after the vaccination. If an urgent need exists to skin test, do so with the understanding that reactivity might be reduced by the vaccine.

††If a vaccinee experiences a presumed vaccine-related rash 7 to 25 days after vaccination, the person should avoid direct contact with immunocompromised persons for the duration of the rash.

From Centers for Disease Control and Prevention: General recommendations on immunization: recommendations of the Advisory Committee on Immunization Practices (ACIP), *MMWR* 60:(RR-2), 2011.

VACCINE ADMINISTRATION*

INFECTION CONTROL AND STERILE TECHNIQUE

Persons administering vaccines should follow appropriate precautions to minimize risk for spread of disease. Hands should be cleansed with an alcohol-based, waterless antiseptic hand rub or washed with soap and water between each patient contact. Occupational Safety and Health Administration (OSHA) regulations do not require that gloves be worn when administering vaccinations unless persons administering vaccinations are likely to come into contact with potentially infectious body fluids or have open lesions on their hands. Needles used for injections must be sterile and disposable to minimize the risk for contamination. A separate needle and syringe should be used for each injection. Changing needles between drawing vaccine from a vial and injecting it into a recipient is not necessary. Different vaccines should never be mixed in the same syringe unless specifically licensed for such use, and no attempt should be made to transfer between syringes.

For all intramuscular injections, the needle should be long enough to reach the muscle mass and prevent vaccine from seeping into subcutaneous tissue, but not so long as to involve underlying nerves, blood vessels, or bone. Vaccinators should be familiar with the anatomy of the area where they are injecting vaccine. Intramuscular injections are administered at a 90-degree angle to the skin, preferably into the anterolateral aspect of the thigh or the deltoid muscle of the upper arm depending on the age of the patient.

Decision on needle size and site of injection must be made for each person on the basis of the size of the muscle, the thickness of adipose tissue at the injection site, the volume of the material to be administered, injection technique, and the depth below the muscle surface into which the material is to be injected. Aspiration before injection of vaccines or toxoids (i.e., pulling back on the syringe plunger after needle insertion before injection) is not required because no large blood vessel exists at the recommended injection sites.

INFANTS (AGED <12 MONTHS)

For the majority of infants, the anterolateral aspect of the thigh is the recommended site for injection because it provides a large muscle mass. The muscles of the buttock have not been used for administration of vaccines in infants and children because of concern about potential injury to the sciatic nerve, which is well documented after injection of antimicrobial agents into the buttock. If the gluteal muscle must be used, care should be taken to define the anatomic landmarks. Injection technique is the most important parameter to ensure efficient intramuscular vaccine delivery. If the subcutaneous and muscle tissue are bunched to minimize the chance of striking bone, a 1-inch needle is required to ensure intramuscular administration in infants. For the majority of infants, a 1-inch, 22- to 25-gauge needle is sufficient to penetrate muscle in an infant's thigh. For newborn (first 28 days of life) and premature infants, a 5/8-inch-long needle usually is adequate if the skin is stretched flat between thumb and forefinger and the needle inserted at a 90-degree angle to the skin.

TODDLERS AND OLDER CHILDREN (AGED 12 MONTHS TO 10 YEARS)

The deltoid muscle should be used if the muscle mass is adequate. The needle size for deltoid site injections can range from 22-25 gauge and from 5/8-1 inch on the basis of the size of the muscle and the thickness of adipose tissue at the injection site. A 5/8-inch needle is adequate only for the deltoid muscle and only if the skin is stretched flat between the thumb and forefinger and the needle inserted at a 90-degree angle to the skin. For toddlers, the anterolateral thigh can be used, but the needle should be at least 1 inch in length.

ADOLESCENTS AND ADULTS (AGED >11 YEARS)

For adults and adolescents, the deltoid muscle is recommended for routine intramuscular vaccinations. The anterolateral thigh also can be used. For men and women weighing <130 lb (<60 kg) a 5/8- to 1-inch needle is sufficient to ensure intramuscular injection. For women weighing 130-200 lb (60-90 kg) and men 130-260 lb (60-118 kg), a 1- to 1½-inch needle is needed. For women weighing >200 lb (>90 kg) or men weighing >260 lb (>118 kg), a 1½-inch needle is required.

SUBCUTANEOUS INJECTIONS

Subcutaneous injections are administered at a 45-degree angle, usually into the thigh for infants younger than 12 months and in the upper-outer triceps area of persons aged 12 months and older. Subcutaneous injections can be administered into the upper-outer triceps area of an infant if necessary. A 5/8-inch, 23- to 25-gauge needle should be inserted into the subcutaneous tissue.

TABLE 9 Vaccination of Persons with Primary and Secondary Immune Deficiencies

PRIMARY

Category	Specific Immunodeficiency	Contraindicated Vaccines*	Risk-Specific Recommended Vaccines*	Effectiveness and Comments
B lymphocyte (humoral)	Severe antibody deficiencies (e.g., X-linked agammaglobulinemia and common variable immunodeficiency)	OPV[a] Smallpox[b] LAIV BCG Yellow fever virus (YFV) and live-bacteria vaccinese No data for rotavirus vaccines	Annual IIV is the only vaccine given to patients receiving IG therapy; routine inactivated vaccines can be given if not receiving IGIV.	The effectiveness of any vaccine will be uncertain if it depends only on the humoral response (e.g., PPSV23). IG therapy interferes with the immune response to live vaccines MMR and VAR.
	Less severe antibody deficiencies (e.g., selective IgA deficiency and IgG subclass deficiency)	OPV[a] BCG YFV vaccine Other live vaccinesd appear to be safe.	Vaccines should be given as on the annual immunization schedule for immunocompetent people.[e] PPSV23 should be given beginning at 2 yr of age.[f]	All vaccines are probably effective. Immune response may be attenuated.
T lymphocyte (cell-mediated and humoral)	Complete defects (e.g., SCID, complete DiGeorge syndrome)	All live vaccines[c,d,g]	The only vaccine that should be given if the patient is receiving IG is annual IIV if there is some residual antibody protection.	All inactivated vaccines are probably ineffective.
	Partial defects (e.g., most patients with DiGeorge syndrome, hyper-IgM syndrome, Wiskott-Aldrich syndrome, ataxia-telangiectasia)	All live vaccines[c,d,g]	Routine inactivated vaccines should be given.[e] PPSV23 should be given beginning at 2 yr of age.[f]	Effectiveness of any vaccine depends on degree of immune suppression.
	Interferon (IFN)-γ–interleukin (IL)-12 axis deficiencies	All live vaccines for IL-12/IL-12R deficiencies, IFN-γ, IFN-α, or STAT1 deficiencies	None.	None.
Complement	Persistent complement, properdin, MBL, or factor B deficiency; secondary deficiency because taking eculizumab (Solaris)	None	PPSV23 should be given beginning at 2 yr of age.[f] MCV series beginning in infancy.[h] MenB series beginning at 10 yr of age.	All routine vaccines are probably effective.
Phagocytic function	Chronic granulomatous disease	Live-bacteria vaccines[c]	None.	All inactivated vaccines are safe and probably effective. Live-virus vaccines are probably safe and effective.
	Phagocytic deficiencies that are undefined or accompanied by defect in T-cell and NK-cell dysfunction (e.g., Chédiak-Higashi syndrome, leukocyte adhesion defects, myeloperoxidase deficiency)	MMR, MMRV, OPV,[a] smallpox, LAIV, YF, all bacteria vaccines	PPSV23 should be given beginning at 2 yr of age.[f] MCV series beginning in infancy.[h]	All inactivated vaccines are safe and probably effective.

SECONDARY

Specific Immunodeficiency	Contraindicated Vaccines*	Risk-Specific Recommended Vaccines*	Effectiveness and Comments
HIV/AIDS	OPV[a] Smallpox BCG Combined MMRV LAIV Withhold MMR, varicella, and zoster in severely immunocompromised persons. YF vaccine may have a contraindication or precaution depending on the indicators of immune function.[j]	PPSV23 should be given beginning at 2 yr of age.[f] MCV series beginning in infancy.[h] Consider Hib (if not administered in infancy).[i]	Rotavirus vaccine is recommended on standard schedule. MMR and VAR are recommended for HIV-infected children who are asymptomatic or only low-level immunocompromised.[k] All inactivated vaccines may be effective.
Generalized malignant neoplasm, transplantation, autoimmune disease, immunosuppressive or radiation therapy	Live-virus and live-bacteria vaccines, depending on immune status.[c,d,m]	PPSV23 should be given beginning at 2 yr of age.[f] Annual IIV (unless receiving intensive chemotherapy or anti-B cell antibodies). Hib vaccine may be indicated.[n]	Effectiveness of any vaccine depends on degree of immune suppression; inactivated standard vaccines are indicated if not highly immunosuppressed, but doses should be repeated after chemotherapy ends.

TABLE 9 Vaccination of Persons with Primary and Secondary Immune Deficiencies—cont'd

Specific Immunodeficiency	Contraindicated Vaccines*	Risk-Specific Recommended Vaccines*	Effectiveness and Comments
Asplenia (functional, congenital anatomic, surgical)	LAIV	PPSV23 should be given beginning at 2 yr of age.[f] MCV series beginning in infancy.[h] MenB series beginning at 10 yr of age. Hib (if not administered in infancy).[o]	All routine vaccines are probably effective.
Chronic renal disease	LAIV	PPSV23 should be given beginning at 2 yr of age.[f] HepB is indicated if not previously immunized.	All routine vaccines are probably effective.
CNS anatomic barrier defect (cochlear implant, congenital dysplasia of the inner ear, persistent CSF communication with naso-/oropharynx)	None	PPSV23 should be given beginning at 2 yr of age.[f]	All standard vaccines are indicated.

BCG, Bacille Calmette-Guérin vaccine; *CNS,* central nervous system; *Hib, Haemophilus influenzae* type b vaccine; *HIV/AIDS,* human immunodeficiency virus/acquired immunodeficiency syndrome; *IG,* immune globulin; *IIV,* inactivated influenza vaccine; *LAIV,* live-attenuated influenza vaccine; *MMR,* measles, mumps, rubella vaccine; *MMRV,* measles-mumps-rubella-varicella; *MCV,* quadrivalent meningococcal polysaccharide vaccine; *MenB,* serogroup B meningococcal vaccine; *OPV,* oral poliovirus vaccine (live); *PPSV23,* pneumococcal polysaccharide vaccine; *SCID,* severe combined immunodeficiency disease; *VAR,* varicella; *YF,* yellow fever.

*Other vaccines that are universally or routinely recommended should be given if not contraindicated.

[a]OPV is no longer available in the United States.

[b]This table refers to contraindications for nonemergency vaccination (i.e., ACIP recommendations).

[c]Live-bacteria vaccines: BCG and oral Ty21a *Salmonella typhi* vaccine.

[d]Live-virus vaccines: MMR, MMRV, VAR, OPV, LAIV, YF, zoster, rotavirus, and vaccinia (smallpox). Smallpox vaccine is not recommended for children or the general public.

[e]Children who are delayed or underimmunized should be immunized with routinely recommended vaccines, according to age and catch-up schedule.

[f]PPSV23 is begun at 2 yr or older. If PCV13 is required, PCV13 doses should be administered first, followed by PPSV23 at least 8 wk later; a 2nd dose of PPSV23 is given 5 yr after the 1st.

[g]Regarding T-lymphocyte immunodeficiency as a contraindication for rotavirus vaccine, data exist only for SCID.

[h]Age and schedule of doses depend on the product; repeated doses are required.

[i]Pneumococcal vaccine is not indicated for children with chronic granulomatous disease beyond age-based universal recommendations for PCV13. Children with chronic granulomatous disease are not at increased risk for pneumococcal disease.

[j]YF vaccine is contraindicated in HIV-infected children <6 yr old who are highly immunosuppressed. There is precaution for use of YF vaccine in asymptomatic HIV-infected children <6 yr with total lymphocyte percentage of 15%-24%, and >6 yr old with $CD4^+$ T-lymphocyte counts of 200-499 cells/mm^3.

[k]HIV-infected children should receive immune globulin after exposure to measles and may receive varicella vaccine if $CD4^+$ T-lymphocyte percentage is ≥15% for those <6 yr old, or $CD4^+$ T-lymphocyte count ≥200 cells/mm^3 for those ≥6 yr old. People with perinatal HIV infection who were vaccinated with measles, rubella, or mumps–containing vaccine before the establishment of combination antiretroviral therapy (cART) should be considered unvaccinated and should receive two appropriately spaced doses of MMR vaccine once effective cART has been established (at least 6 mo with $CD4^+$ T-lymphocytes ≥15% for children <6 yr old, or $CD4^+$ T-lymphocyte count ≥200 cells/mm^3 for children ≥6 yr old).

[l]For patients 5-18 yr old who have not received a Hib primary series and a booster dose or at least 1 Hib dose after age 14 mo.

[m]Withholding inactivated vaccines also is recommended with some forms of immunosuppressive therapy, such as anti-CD20 antibodies, induction or consolidation chemotherapy, or patients with major antibody deficiencies receiving immune globulins. Inactivated influenza vaccine is an exception, but consideration should be given to repeating doses of any inactivated vaccine administered during these therapies.

[n]For persons <60 mo old undergoing chemotherapy or radiation therapy who have not received a Hib primary series plus a booster dose or at least 1 Hib dose after age 14 mo.

[o]For persons >59 mo old who are asplenic and persons ≥15 mo who are undergoing elective splenectomy and who have not received a Hib primary series and a booster dose or at least 1 Hib dose after age 14 mo.

Data from Centers for Disease Control and Prevention: Yellow fever vaccine: Recommendations of the Advisory Committee on Immunization Practices, *MMWR Recomm Rep* 59[RR-07]; 1-27, 2010. From Kliegman RM: *Nelson textbook of pediatrics,* ed 21, Philadelphia, 2020, Elsevier.

Adapted from Immunization in special circumstances. In Kimberlin DW et al (eds): *Red Book 2018: Report of the Committee on Infectious Diseases,* ed 31, Elk Grove Village 2018, American Academy of Pediatrics.

TABLE 10A Immunizations for Pediatric Oncology Patients

Vaccine	Indications and Comments
DTaP	Indicated for incompletely immunized children <7 yr, even during active chemotherapy
Td	Indicated 1 yr after completion of therapy in children 7 yr
Hib	Indicated for incompletely immunized children if <7 yr
HBV	Indicated for incompletely immunized children
23PS	Indicated for asplenic patients
PCV13	Indicated for incompletely immunized children <5 yr
Meningococcus	Consider in asplenic patients
IPV	Indicated for incompletely immunized children; also recommended for all household contacts requiring immunization to reduce the risk of vaccine-associated polio
MMR	Contraindicated until child is in remission and finished with all chemotherapy for 3-6 mo; may need to reimmunize after chemotherapy if titers have fallen below protective levels
Influenza	Defer in active chemotherapy; may give as early as 3-4 wk after remission and off chemotherapy if during influenza season; peripheral granulocyte and lymphocyte counts should be >1000/µL; should also be given to household contact of children with cancer
Varicella	Consider immunizing children who have remained in remission and have finished chemotherapy for >1 yr; with absolute lymphocyte count of >700/µL and platelet count of >100,000/µL within 24 hr of immunization; check titers of previously immunized children to verify protective levels of antibodies

DTaP, Diphtheria, tetanus, and pertussis; *HBV,* hepatitis B virus; *Hib, Haemophilus influenzae* type b; *IPV,* inactivated polio vaccine; *MMR,* measles, mumps, rubella; *PCV13,* pneumococcal conjugate vaccine; *Td,* tetanus, diphtheria; *23PS,* 23-valent pneumococcal polysaccharide vaccine.
From *MMWR* 49(RR-10):1-147, 2000.

TABLE 10B Vaccines Recommended for Children and Adolescents with Underlying Conditions or at High Risk

Vaccines	Special Situations
PCV13 (and PPSV23 in certain conditions)	Chronic heart disease (particularly cyanotic congenital heart disease and cardiac failure), chronic lung disease (including asthma if treated with high-dose oral corticosteroid therapy), chronic liver disease, chronic renal failure
	Diabetes mellitus
	Cerebrospinal fluid leak
	Cochlear implant
	Sickle cell disease and other hemoglobinopathies
	Anatomic or functional asplenia
	HIV infection
	Nephrotic syndrome
	Diseases associated with treatment with immunosuppressive drugs or radiation therapy, including malignant neoplasms, leukemias, lymphomas, and Hodgkin disease
	Generalized malignancy
	Solid organ transplantation
	Congenital or acquired immunodeficiencies
	Multiple myeloma
Hep A	Chronic liver disease
	Clotting factor disorders
	Men who have sex with men
	Injection or noninjection drug use
	Homelessness
	Work with hepatitis A virus
	Travel in countries with high or intermediate endemic hepatitis A
	Close, personal contact with international adoptee (e.g., household or regular babysitting)
Flu	Egg allergy more severe than hives
MCV4	Anatomic or functional asplenia (including sickle cell disease)
	Persistent complement component deficiency
	Residents of or travelers to countries in African meningitis belt or pilgrims on the Hajj
	During outbreaks caused by a vaccine serogroup
	HIV infection
MenB	Anatomic or functional asplenia (including sickle cell disease)
	Children with persistent complement component deficiency
	During serogroup B outbreaks
Hib	Persons at increased risk for Hib disease, including chemotherapy recipients and those with anatomic or functional asplenia (including sickle cell disease), human immunodeficiency virus (HIV) infection, immunoglobulin deficiency, or early component complement deficiency
	Recipients of hematopoietic stem cell transplant (HSCT)
	Elective splenectomy
Hep B	Infants born to HBsAg-positive mothers or mothers whose HBsAg status is unknown (administer vaccine within 12 hr of birth)
HPV	Immunocompromising conditions, including HIV infection
	History of sexual abuse or assault

From Centers for Disease Control and Prevention: Child and adolescent schedule. www.cdc.gov/vaccines/schedules/hcp/imz/child-adolescent.html. In Kliegman RM: *Nelson textbook of pediatrics,* ed 21, Philadelphia, 2020, Elsevier.

TABLE 11 Approaches to the Evaluation and Vaccination of Persons Vaccinated Outside the United States Who Have No (or Questionable) Vaccination Records

Vaccine	Recommended Approach	Alternative Approach*
MMR	Revaccination with MMR	Serologic testing for IgG antibodies to measles, mumps, and rubella
Hib	Age-appropriate revaccination	—
Hepatitis A	Age-appropriate revaccination	Serologic testing for IgG antibodies to hepatitis A
Hepatitis B	Age-appropriate revaccination and serologic testing for HBsAg†	—
Poliovirus	Revaccinate with inactivated poliovirus vaccine	Serologic testing for neutralizing antibody to poliovirus types 1, 2, and 3 (limited availability)
DTaP	Revaccination with DTaP, with serologic testing for specific IgG antibody to tetanus and diphtheria toxins in the event of a severe local reaction	Persons whose records indicate receipt of ≥3 doses: Serologic testing for specific IgG antibody to diphtheria and tetanus toxins before administering additional doses, or administer a single booster dose of DTaP, followed by serologic testing after 1 month for specific IgG antibody to diphtheria and tetanus toxins with revaccination as appropriate
Tdap	Age-appropriate vaccination of persons who are candidates for Tdap vaccine on the basis of time since last diphtheria and tetanus toxoid containing vaccines.	—
Varicella	Age-appropriate vaccination of persons who lack evidence of varicella immunity	—
Pneumococcal conjugate	Age-appropriate vaccination	—
Rotavirus	Age-appropriate vaccination	—
HPV	Age-appropriate vaccination	—
Zoster	Age-appropriate vaccination	—

DTaP, Diphtheria and tetanus toxoids and acellular pertussis; *HBsAg,* hepatitis B surface antigen; *Hib, Haemophilus influenzae* type b; *HPV,* human papillomavirus; *IgG,* immune globulin G; *MMR,* measles, mumps, and rubella; *Tdap,* tetanus toxoid, reduced diphtheria toxoid, and acellular pertussis.

*There is a recommended approach for all vaccines and an alternative approach for some vaccines.

†In rare instances, hepatitis B vaccine can give a false-positive HBsAg result up to 18 days after vaccination; therefore, blood should be drawn to test for HBsAg before vaccinating. Source: CDC. A comprehensive immunization strategy to eliminate transmission of hepatitis B virus infection in the United States: Recommendations of the Advisory Committee on Immunization Practices [ACIP]; Part I: Immunization in infants, children, and adolescents, *MMWR* 2005;54(No. RR-16.

From Centers for Disease Control and Prevention: General recommendations on immunization: recommendations of the Advisory Committee on Immunization Practices (ACIP), *MMWR* 60:(RR-2), 2011.

Immunizations for Adults

RECOMMENDED IMMUNIZATION SCHEDULE FOR ADULTS AGED 19 YEARS OR OLDER, UNITED STATES, 2020

The *Recommended Immunization Schedule for Adults Aged 19 Years or Older, United States* became effective, as recommended by the Advisory Committee on Immunization Practices (ACIP) and approved by the Centers for Disease Control and Prevention (CDC). The adult immunization schedule was also reviewed and approved by the following professional medical organizations:

- American College of Physicians (www.acponline.org)
- American Academy of Family Physicians (www.aafp.org)
- American College of Obstetricians and Gynecologists (www.acog.org)
- American College of Nurse-Midwives (www.midwife.org)

CDC announced the availability of the 2020 adult immunization schedule at www.cdc.gov/vaccines/schedules/easy-to-read/adult.html.

The adult immunization schedule describes the age groups and medical conditions and other indications for which licensed vaccines are recommended. The 2020 adult immunization schedule consists of:

- Table 12. Recommended immunization schedule for adults by age group
- Table 13. Recommended immunization schedule for adults by medical condition and other indications
- Footnotes that accompany each vaccine containing important general information and considerations for special populations

Consider the following information when reviewing the adult immunization schedule:

- The tables in the adult immunization schedule should be read with the footnotes that contain important general information and information about vaccination of special populations.
- When indicated, administer recommended vaccines to adults whose vaccination history is incomplete or unknown.
- Increased interval between doses of a multi-dose vaccine does not diminish vaccine effectiveness; therefore, it is not necessary to restart the vaccine series or add doses to the series because of an extended interval between doses.
- Adults with immunocompromising conditions should generally avoid live vaccines, e.g., measles, mumps, and rubella vaccine. Inactivated vaccines, e.g., pneumococcal or inactivated influenza vaccines, are generally acceptable.
- Combination vaccines may be used when any component of the combination is indicated and when the other components of the combination vaccine are not contraindicated.
- The use of trade names in the adult immunization schedule is for identification purposes only and does not imply endorsement by the ACIP or CDC.

Details on vaccines recommended for adults and complete ACIP statements are available at www.cdc.gov/vaccines/hcp/acip-recs/index.html. Additional CDC resources include:

- A summary of information on vaccination recommendations, vaccination of persons with immunodeficiencies, preventing and managing adverse reactions, vaccination contraindications and precautions, and other information can be found in *General Recommendations on Immunization* at www.cdc.gov/mmwr/preview/mmwrhtml/rr6002a1.htm.
- Vaccine Information Statements that explain benefits and risks of vaccines are available at www.cdc.gov/vaccinesafety/Concerns/Index.html.
- Information and resources regarding vaccination of pregnant women are available at www.cdc.gov/vaccines/pregnancy/pregnant-women/index.html.
- Information on travel vaccine requirements and recommendations is available at www.cdc.gov/travel/destinations/list.
- *CDC Vaccine Schedules App* for clinicians and other immunization service providers to download is available at www.cdc.gov/vaccines/schedules/.
- *Recommended Immunization Schedule for Children and Adolescents Aged 18 Years or Younger* is available at www.cdc.gov/vaccines/schedules/hcp/child-adolescent.html#schedule.

Report suspected cases of reportable vaccine-preventable diseases to the local or state health department.

Report all clinically significant postvaccination reactions to the Vaccine Adverse Event Reporting System at www.vaers.hhs.gov or by telephone, 800-822-7967. All vaccines included in the 2020 adult immunization schedule except herpes zoster and 23-valent pneumococcal polysaccharide vaccines are covered by the Vaccine Injury Compensation Program. Information on how to file a vaccine injury claim is available at www.hrsa.gov/vaccinecompensation or by telephone, 800-338-2382.

The following acronyms are used for vaccines recommended for adults:

HepA	hepatitis A vaccine
HepA-HepB	hepatitis A and hepatitis B vaccines
HepB	hepatitis B vaccine
Hib	*Haemophilus influenzae* type b conjugate vaccine
HPV vaccine	human papillomavirus vaccine
HZV	herpes zoster vaccine
IIV	inactivated influenza vaccine
LAIV	live attenuated influenza vaccine
MenACWY	serogroups A, C, W, and Y meningococcal conjugate vaccine
MenB	serogroup B meningococcal vaccine
MMR	measles, mumps, and rubella vaccine
MPSV4	serogroups A, C, W, and Y meningococcal polysaccharide vaccine
PCV13	13-valent pneumococcal conjugate vaccine
PPSV23	23-valent pneumococcal polysaccharide vaccine
RIV	recombinant influenza vaccine
Td	tetanus and diphtheria toxoids
Tdap	tetanus toxoid, reduced diphtheria toxoid, and acellular pertussis vaccine
VAR	varicella vaccine

TABLE 12 Recommended Immunization Schedule for Adults Aged 19 Years or Older by Age Group, United States, 2021

These recommendations must be read with the footnotes that follow.

Table 1 Recommended Adult Immunization Schedule by Age Group, United States, 2021

Vaccine	19–26 years	27–49 years	50–64 years	≥65 years
Influenza inactivated (IIV) or **Influenza recombinant** (RIV4)	1 dose annually			
or	or			
Influenza live, attenuated (LAIV4)	1 dose annually			
Tetanus, diphtheria, pertussis (Tdap or Td)	1 dose Tdap each pregnancy; 1 dose Td/Tdap for wound management (see notes)			
	1 dose Tdap, then Td or Tdap booster every 10 years			
Measles, mumps, rubella (MMR)	1 or 2 doses depending on indication (if born in 1957 or later)			
Varicella (VAR)	2 doses (if born in 1980 or later)	2 doses		
Zoster recombinant (RZV)			2 doses	
Human papillomavirus (HPV)	2 or 3 doses depending on age at initial vaccination or condition	27 through 45 years		
Pneumococcal conjugate (PCV13)	1 dose			1 dose
Pneumococcal polysaccharide (PPSV23)	1 or 2 doses depending on indication			1 dose
Hepatitis A (HepA)	2 or 3 doses depending on vaccine			
Hepatitis B (HepB)	2 or 3 doses depending on vaccine			
Meningococcal A, C, W, Y (MenACWY)	1 or 2 doses depending on indication, see notes for booster recommendations			
Meningococcal B (MenB)	2 or 3 doses depending on vaccine and indication, see notes for booster recommendations; 19 through 23 years			
***Haemophilus influenzae* type b** (Hib)	1 or 3 doses depending on indication			

Recommended vaccination for adults who meet age requirement, lack documentation of vaccination, or lack evidence of past infection

Recommended vaccination for adults with an additional risk factor or another indication

Recommended vaccination based on shared clinical decision-making

No recommendation/ Not applicable

TABLE 13 Recommended Immunization Schedule for Adults Aged 19 Years or Older by Medical Condition and Other Indications, United States, 2021

These recommendations must be read with the footnotes that follow.

Table 2 Recommended Adult Immunization Schedule by Medical Condition and Other Indications, United States, 2021

Vaccine	Pregnancy	Immuno-compromised (excluding HIV infection)	HIV infection CD4 count <200 mm³	HIV infection CD4 count ≥200 mm³	Asplenia, complement deficiencies	End-stage renal disease; or on hemodialysis	Heart or lung disease, alcoholism[1]	Chronic liver disease	Diabetes	Health care personnel[2]	Men who have sex with men
IIV or RIV4	1 dose annually										
or										or	
LAIV4	Not Recommended					Precaution				1 dose annually	
Tdap or Td	1 dose Tdap each pregnancy	1 dose Tdap, then Td or Tdap booster every 10 years									
MMR	Not Recommended*	Not Recommended		1 or 2 doses depending on indication							
VAR	Not Recommended*	Not Recommended			2 doses						
RZV					2 doses at age ≥50 years						
HPV	Not Recommended*	3 doses through age 26 years			2 or 3 doses through age 26 years depending on age at initial vaccination or condition						
PCV13		1 dose									
PPSV23		1, 2, or 3 doses depending on age and indication									
HepA					2 or 3 doses depending on vaccine						
HepB					2, 3, or 4 doses depending on vaccine or condition				<60 years ≥60 years		
MenACWY	1 or 2 doses depending on indication, see notes for booster recommendations										
MenB	Precaution	2 or 3 doses depending on vaccine and indication, see notes for booster recommendations									
Hib		3 doses HSCT[3] recipients only			1 dose						

- Recommended vaccination for adults who meet age requirement, lack documentation of vaccination, or lack evidence of past infection
- Recommended vaccination for adults with an additional risk factor or another indication
- Precaution—vaccination might be indicated if benefit of protection outweighs risk of adverse reaction
- Recommended vaccination based on shared clinical decision-making
- Not recommended/ contraindicated—vaccine should not be administered.
- No recommendation/ Not applicable

*Vaccinate after pregnancy.

1. Precaution for LAIV4 does not apply to alcoholism. **2.** See notes for influenza; hepatitis B; measles, mumps, and rubella; and varicella vaccinations. **3.** Hematopoietic stem cell transplant.

Notes Recommended Adult Immunization Schedule for ages 19 years or older, United States, 2021

For vaccine recommendations for persons 18 years of age or younger, see the Recommended Child/Adolescent Immunization Schedule.

Additional Information

COVID-19 Vaccination

ACIP recommends use of COVID-19 vaccines within the scope of the Emergency Use Authorization or Biologics License Application for the particular vaccine. Interim ACIP recommendations for the use of COVID-19 vaccines can be found at www.cdc.gov/vaccines/hcp/acip-recs/vacc-specific/covid-19.html

Haemophilus influenzae type b vaccination

Special situations

- **Anatomical or functional asplenia (including sickle cell disease):** 1 dose if previously did not receive Hib; if elective splenectomy, 1 dose, preferably at least 14 days before splenectomy
- **Hematopoietic stem cell transplant (HSCT):** 3-dose series 4 weeks apart starting 6–12 months after successful transplant, regardless of Hib vaccination history

Hepatitis A vaccination

Routine vaccination

- **Not at risk but want protection from hepatitis A** (identification of risk factor not required): 2-dose series HepA (Havrix 6–12 months apart or Vaqta 6–18 months apart [minimum interval: 6 months]) or 3-dose series HepA-HepB (Twinrix at 0, 1, 6 months [minimum intervals: dose 1 to dose 2: 4 weeks / dose 2 to dose 3: 5 months])

Special situations

- **At risk for hepatitis A virus infection:** 2-dose series HepA or 3-dose series HepA-HepB as above
  - **Chronic liver disease** (e.g., persons with hepatitis B, hepatitis C, cirrhosis, fatty liver disease, alcoholic liver disease, autoimmune hepatitis, alanine aminotransferase [ALT] or aspartate aminotransferase [AST] level greater than twice the upper limit of normal)
  - **HIV infection**
  - **Men who have sex with men**
  - **Injection or noninjection drug use**
  - **Persons experiencing homelessness**
  - **Work with hepatitis A virus** in research laboratory or with nonhuman primates with hepatitis A virus infection
  - **Travel in countries with high or intermediate endemic hepatitis A** (HepA-HepB [Twinrix] may be administered on an accelerated schedule of 3 doses at 0, 7, and 21–30 days, followed by a booster dose at 12 months)
  - **Close, personal contact with international adoptee** (e.g., household or regular babysitting) in first 60 days after arrival from country with high or intermediate endemic hepatitis A (administer dose 1 as soon as adoption is planned, at least 2 weeks before adoptee's arrival)
  - **Pregnancy** if at risk for infection or severe outcome from infection during pregnancy
  - **Settings for exposure, including** health care settings targeting services to injection or noninjection drug users or group homes and nonresidential day care facilities for developmentally disabled persons (individual risk factor screening not required)

Hepatitis B vaccination

Routine vaccination

- **Not at risk but want protection from hepatitis B** (identification of risk factor not required): 2- or 3-dose series (2-dose series Heplisav-B at least 4 weeks apart [2-dose series HepB only applies when 2 doses of Heplisav-B are used at least 4 weeks apart] or 3-dose series Engerix-B or Recombivax HB at 0, 1, 6 months [minimum intervals: dose 1 to dose 2: 4 weeks / dose 2 to dose 3: 8 weeks / dose 1 to dose 3: 16 weeks]) or 3-dose series HepA-HepB (Twinrix at 0, 1, 6 months [minimum intervals: dose 1 to dose 2: 4 weeks / dose 2 to dose 3: 5 months])

Special situations

- **At risk for hepatitis B virus infection:** 2-dose (Heplisav-B) or 3-dose (Engerix-B, Recombivax HB) series or 3-dose series HepA-HepB (Twinrix) as above
  - **Chronic liver disease** (e.g., persons with hepatitis C, cirrhosis, fatty liver disease, alcoholic liver disease, autoimmune hepatitis, alanine aminotransferase [ALT] or aspartate aminotransferase [AST] level greater than twice upper limit of normal)
  - **HIV infection**
  - **Sexual exposure risk** (e.g., sex partners of hepatitis B surface antigen [HBsAg]-positive persons; sexually active persons not in mutually monogamous relationships; persons seeking evaluation or treatment for a sexually transmitted infection; men who have sex with men)
  - **Current or recent injection drug use**
  - **Percutaneous or mucosal risk for exposure to blood** (e.g., household contacts of HBsAg-positive persons; residents and staff of facilities for developmentally disabled persons; health care and public safety personnel with reasonably anticipated risk for exposure to blood or blood-contaminated body fluids; hemodialysis, peritoneal dialysis, home dialysis, and predialysis patients; persons with diabetes mellitus age younger than 60 years, shared clinical decision-making for persons age 60 years or older)
  - **Incarcerated persons**
  - **Travel in countries with high or intermediate endemic hepatitis B**
  - **Pregnancy** if at risk for infection or severe outcome from infection during pregnancy (Heplisav-B not currently recommended due to lack of safety data in pregnant women)

Human papillomavirus vaccination

Routine vaccination

- **HPV vaccination recommended for all persons through age 26 years:** 2- or 3-dose series depending on age at initial vaccination or condition:
  - **Age 15 years or older at initial vaccination:** 3-dose series at 0, 1–2 months, 6 months (minimum intervals: dose 1 to dose 2: 4 weeks / dose 2 to dose 3: 12 weeks / dose 1 to dose 3: 5 months; repeat dose if administered too soon)
  - **Age 9–14 years at initial vaccination and received 1 dose or 2 doses less than 5 months apart:** 1 additional dose
  - **Age 9–14 years at initial vaccination and received 2 doses at least 5 months apart:** HPV vaccination series complete, no additional dose needed
- **Interrupted schedules:** If vaccination schedule is interrupted, the series does not need to be restarted
- **No additional dose recommended after completing series with recommended dosing intervals using any HPV vaccine**

Shared clinical decision-making

- **Some adults age 27–45 years: Based on shared clinical decision-making,** 2- or 3-dose series as above

Special situations

- **Age ranges recommended above for routine and catch-up vaccination or shared clinical decision-making also apply in special situations**

Continued

Notes Recommended Adult Immunization Schedule, United States, 2021

- **Immunocompromising conditions, including HIV infection**: 3-dose series as above, regardless of age at initial vaccination
- **Pregnancy**: HPV vaccination not recommended until after pregnancy; no intervention needed if vaccinated while pregnant; pregnancy testing not needed before vaccination

Influenza vaccination

Routine vaccination

- **Persons age 6 months or older:** 1 dose any influenza vaccine appropriate for age and health status annually
- For additional guidance, see www.cdc.gov/flu/professionals/index.htm

Special situations

- **Egg allergy, hives only:** 1 dose any influenza vaccine appropriate for age and health status annually
- **Egg allergy–any symptom other than hives** (e.g., angioedema, respiratory distress): 1 dose any influenza vaccine appropriate for age and health status annually. If using an influenza vaccine other than RIV4 or ccIIV4, administer in medical setting under supervision of health care provider who can recognize and manage severe allergic reactions.
- Severe allergic reactions to any vaccine can occur even in the absence of a history of previous allergic reaction. Therefore, all vaccine providers should be familiar with the office emergency plan and certified in cardiopulmonary resuscitation.
- A previous severe allergic reaction to any influenza vaccine is a contraindication to future receipt of the vaccine.
- **LAIV4 should not be used** in persons with the following conditions or situations:
  - History of severe allergic reaction to any vaccine component (excluding egg) or to a previous dose of any influenza vaccine
  - Immunocompromised due to any cause (including medications and HIV infection)
  - Anatomic or functional asplenia
  - Close contacts or caregivers of severely immunosuppressed persons who require a protected environment
  - Pregnancy
  - Cranial CSF/oropharyngeal communications
  - Cochlear implant
  - Received influenza antiviral medications oseltamivir or zanamivir within the previous 48 hours, peramivir within the previous 5 days, or baloxavir within the previous 17 days
  - Adults 50 years or older
- **History of Guillain-Barré syndrome within 6 weeks after previous dose of influenza vaccine:** Generally, should not be vaccinated unless vaccination benefits outweigh risks for those at higher risk for severe complications from influenza

Measles, mumps, and rubella vaccination

Routine vaccination

- **No evidence of immunity to measles, mumps, or rubella:** 1 dose
  - **Evidence of immunity:** Born before 1957 (health care personnel, see below), documentation of receipt of MMR vaccine, laboratory evidence of immunity or disease (diagnosis of disease without laboratory confirmation is not evidence of immunity)

Special situations

- **Pregnancy with no evidence of immunity to rubella:** MMR contraindicated during pregnancy; after pregnancy (before discharge from health care facility), 1 dose
- **Nonpregnant women of childbearing age with no evidence of immunity to rubella:** 1 dose
- **HIV infection with CD4 count ≥200 cells/mm³ for at least 6 months and no evidence of immunity to measles, mumps, or rubella:** 2-dose series at least 4 weeks apart; MMR contraindicated for HIV infection with CD4 count <200 cells/mm³
- **Severe immunocompromising conditions:** MMR contraindicated
- **Students in postsecondary educational institutions, international travelers, and household or close, personal contacts of immunocompromised persons with no evidence of immunity to measles, mumps, or rubella:** 2-dose series at least 4 weeks apart if previously did not receive any doses of MMR or 1 dose if previously received 1 dose MMR
- **Health care personnel:**
  - **Born in 1957 or later with no evidence of immunity to measles, mumps, or rubella:** 2-dose series at least 4 weeks apart for measles or mumps or at least 1 dose for rubella
  - **Born before 1957 with no evidence of immunity to measles, mumps, or rubella:** Consider 2-dose series at least 4 weeks apart for measles or mumps or 1 dose for rubella

Meningococcal vaccination

Special situations for MenACWY

- **Anatomical or functional asplenia (including sickle cell disease), HIV infection, persistent complement component deficiency, complement inhibitor (e.g., eculizumab, ravulizumab) use:** 2-dose series MenACWY-D (Menactra, Menveo or MenQuadfi) at least 8 weeks apart and revaccinate every 5 years if risk remains
- **Travel in countries with hyperendemic or epidemic meningococcal disease, microbiologists routinely exposed to *Neisseria meningitidis*:** 1 dose MenACWY (Menactra, Menveo or MenQuadfi) and revaccinate every 5 years if risk remains
- **First-year college students who live in residential housing (if not previously vaccinated at age 16 years or older) and military recruits:** 1 dose MenACWY (Menactra, Menveo or MenQuadfi)
- For MenACWY **booster dose recommendations** for groups listed under "Special situations" and in an outbreak setting (e.g., in community or organizational settings and among men who have sex with men) and additional meningococcal vaccination information, see www.cdc.gov/mmwr/volumes/69/rr/rr6909a1.htm

Shared clinical decision-making for MenB

- **Adolescents and young adults age 16–23 years (age 16–18 years preferred) not at increased risk for meningococcal disease:** Based on shared clinical decision-making, 2-dose series MenB-4C (Bexsero) at least 1 month apart or 2-dose series MenB-FHbp (Trumenba) at 0, 6 months (if dose 2 was administered less than 6 months after dose 1, administer dose 3 at least 4 months after dose 2); MenB-4C and MenB-FHbp are not interchangeable (use same product for all doses in series)

Special situations for MenB

- **Anatomical or functional asplenia (including sickle cell disease), persistent complement component deficiency, complement inhibitor (e.g., eculizumab, ravulizumab) use, microbiologists routinely exposed to *Neisseria meningitidis*:** 2-dose primary series MenB-4C (Bexsero) at least one month apart or

Notes Recommended Adult Immunization Schedule, United States, 2021

- MenB-4C (Bexsero) at least 1 month apart or 3-dose primary series MenB-FHbp (Trumenba) at 0, 1–2, 6 months (if dose 2 was administered at least 6 months after dose 1, dose 3 not needed); MenB-4C and MenB-FHbp are not interchangeable (use same product for all doses in series); 1 dose MenB booster 1 year after primary series and revaccinate every 2–3 years if risk remains
- **Pregnancy:** Delay MenB until after pregnancy unless at increased risk and vaccination benefits outweigh potential risks
- For MenB **booster dose recommendations** for groups listed under "Special situations" and in an outbreak setting (e.g., in community or organizational settings and among men who have sex with men) and additional meningococcal vaccination information, see www.cdc.gov/mmwr/volumes/69/rr/rr6909a1.htm

Pneumococcal vaccination

Routine vaccination

- **Age 65 years or older** (immunocompetent—see www.cdc.gov/mmwr/volumes/68/wr/mm6846a5.htm?s_cid=mm6846a5_w): 1 dose PPSV23
  - If PPSV23 was administered prior to age 65 years, administer 1 dose PPSV23 at least 5 years after previous dose

Shared clinical decision-making

- **Age 65 years or older** (immunocompetent): 1 dose PCV13 based on **shared clinical decision-making** if previously not administered.
  - PCV13 and PPSV23 should not be administered during the same visit
  - If both PCV13 and PPSV23 are to be administered, PCV13 should be administered first
  - PCV13 and PPSV23 should be administered at least 1 year apart

Special situations

(www.cdc.gov/mmwr/preview/mmwrhtml/mm6140a4.htm)

- **Age 19–64 years with chronic medical conditions (chronic heart [excluding hypertension], lung, or liver disease, diabetes), alcoholism, or cigarette smoking:** 1 dose PPSV23
- **Age 19 years or older with immunocompromising conditions (congenital or acquired immunodeficiency [including B- and T-lymphocyte deficiency, complement deficiencies, phagocytic disorders, HIV infection], chronic renal failure, nephrotic syndrome, leukemia, lymphoma, Hodgkin disease, generalized malignancy, iatrogenic immunosuppression [e.g., drug or radiation therapy], solid organ transplant, multiple myeloma) or anatomical or functional asplenia (including sickle cell disease and other hemoglobinopathies):** 1 dose PCV13 followed by 1 dose PPSV23 at least 8 weeks later, then another dose PPSV23 at least 5 years after previous PPSV23; at age 65 years or older, administer 1 dose PPSV23 at least 5 years after most recent PPSV23 (note: only 1 dose PPSV23 recommended at age 65 years or older)
- **Age 19 years or older with cerebrospinal fluid leak or cochlear implant:** 1 dose PCV13 followed by 1 dose PPSV23 at least 8 weeks later; at age 65 years or older, administer another dose PPSV23 at least 5 years after PPSV23 (note: only 1 dose PPSV23 recommended at age 65 years or older)

Tetanus, diphtheria, and pertussis vaccination

Routine vaccination

- **Previously did not receive Tdap at or after age 11 years:** 1 dose Tdap, then Td or Tdap every 10 years

Special situations

- **Previously did not receive primary vaccination series for tetanus, diphtheria, or pertussis:** At least 1 dose Tdap followed by 1 dose Td or Tdap at least 4 weeks after Tdap and another dose Td or Tdap 6–12 months after last Td or Tdap (Tdap can be substituted for any Td dose, but preferred as first dose), Td or Tdap every 10 years thereafter
- **Pregnancy:** 1 dose Tdap during each pregnancy, preferably in early part of gestational weeks 27–36
- **Wound management:** Persons with 3 or more doses of tetanus-toxoid-containing vaccine: For clean and minor wounds, administer Tdap or Td if more than 10 years since last dose of tetanus-toxoid-containing vaccine; for all other wounds, administer Tdap or Td if more than 5 years since last dose of tetanus-toxoid-containing vaccine. Tdap is preferred for persons who have not previously received Tdap or whose Tdap history is unknown. If a tetanus-toxoid-containing vaccine is indicated for a pregnant woman, use Tdap. For detailed information, see www.cdc.gov/mmwr/volumes/69/wr/mm6903a5.htm

Varicella vaccination

Routine vaccination

- **No evidence of immunity to varicella:** 2-dose series 4–8 weeks apart if previously did not receive varicella-containing vaccine (VAR or MMRV [measles-mumps-rubella-varicella vaccine] for children); if previously received 1 dose varicella-containing vaccine, 1 dose at least 4 weeks after first dose
  - Evidence of immunity: U.S.-born before 1980 (except for pregnant women and health care personnel [see below]), documentation of 2 doses varicella-containing vaccine at least 4 weeks apart, diagnosis or verification of history of varicella or herpes zoster by a health care provider, laboratory evidence of immunity or disease

Special situations

- **Pregnancy with no evidence of immunity to varicella:** VAR contraindicated during pregnancy; after pregnancy (before discharge from health care facility), 1 dose if previously received 1 dose varicella-containing vaccine or dose 1 of 2-dose series (dose 2: 4–8 weeks later) if previously did not receive any varicella-containing vaccine, regardless of whether U.S.-born before 1980
- **Health care personnel with no evidence of immunity to varicella:** 1 dose if previously received 1 dose varicella-containing vaccine; 2-dose series 4–8 weeks apart if previously did not receive any varicella-containing vaccine, regardless of whether U.S.-born before 1980
- **HIV infection with CD4 count ≥200 cells/mm^3 with no evidence of immunity:** Vaccination may be considered (2 doses 3 months apart); VAR contraindicated for HIV infection with CD4 count <200 cells/mm^3
- **Severe immunocompromising conditions:** VAR contraindicated

Zoster vaccination

Routine vaccination

- **Age 50 years or older:** 2-dose series RZV (Shingrix) 2–6 months apart (minimum interval: 4 weeks; repeat dose if administered too soon), regardless of previous herpes zoster or history of zoster vaccine live (ZVL, Zostavax) vaccination (administer RZV at least 2 months after ZVL)

Special situations

- **Pregnancy:** Consider delaying RZV until after pregnancy if RZV is otherwise indicated.
- **Severe immunocompromising conditions (including HIV infection with CD4 count <200 cells/mm^3):** Recommended use of RZV under review

The Advisory Committee on Immunization Practices (ACIP) recommendations and package inserts for vaccines provide information on contraindications and precautions related to vaccines. Contraindications are conditions that increase chances of a serious adverse reaction in vaccine recipients, and the vaccine should not be administered when a contraindication is present. Precautions should be reviewed for potential risks and benefits for vaccine recipient. For a person with a severe allergy to latex, e.g., anaphylaxis, vaccines supplied in vials or syringes that contain natural rubber latex should not be administered unless the benefit of vaccination clearly outweighs the risk for a potential allergic reaction. For latex allergies other than anaphylaxis, vaccines supplied in vials or syringes that contain dry, natural rubber or natural rubber latex may be administered.

TABLE 14 Immunization and Pregnancy

Vaccine	Before Pregnancy	During Pregnancy	After Pregnancy	Type of Vaccine	Route
Hepatitis A	If at high risk for disease	If at high risk for disease	If at high risk for disease	Inactivated	IM
Hepatitis B	Yes, if at risk	Yes, if at risk	Yes, if at risk	Inactivated	IM
Human papillomavirus (HPV)	Yes, if 9-26 years of age	No, under study	Yes, if 9-26 years of age	Inactivated	IM
Influenza TIV	Yes	Yes	Yes	Inactivated	IM
Influenza LAIV	Yes, if <50 years and healthy; avoid conception for 4 weeks	No	Yes, if <50 years and healthy; avoid conception for 4 weeks	Live	Nasal spray
MMR	Yes, avoid conception for 4 weeks	No	Yes, give immediately postpartum if susceptible to rubella	Live	SC
Meningococcal	If indicated	If indicated	If indicated		
PolysaccharideConjugate				Inactivated Inactivated	SC IM
Pneumococcal polysaccharide	If indicated	If indicated	If indicated	Inactivated	IM or SC
Tetanus/diphtheria Td	Yes, Tdap preferred	If indicated	Yes, Tdap preferred	Toxoid	IM
Tdap, one dose only	Yes, preferred	If high risk of pertussis; otherwise, Td preferred	Yes, preferred	Toxoid/inactivated	IM
Varicella	Yes, avoid conception for 4 weeks	No	Yes, give immediately postpartum if susceptible	Live	SC

IM, Intramuscular; *LAIV,* live, attenuated influenza vaccine; *SC,* subcutaneous; *Tdap,* tetanus and diphtheria toxoids and acellular pertussis; *TIV,* trivalent inactivated influenza vaccine.

TABLE 15 Immunizing Agents and Immunization Schedules for Health Care Workers (HCWs)*

Generic Name	Primary Schedule and Booster(s)	Indications	Major Precautions and Contraindications	Special Considerations
Immunizing Agents Strongly Recommended for Health Care Workers				
Hepatitis B (HB) recombinant vaccine	Two doses IM 4 wk apart; third dose 5 mo after second; booster doses not necessary	**Preexposure:** HCWs at risk for exposure to blood or body fluids	Based on limited data no risk of adverse effects to developing fetuses is apparent. Pregnancy should *not* be considered a contraindication to vaccination of women. Previous anaphylactic reaction to common baker's yeast is a contraindication to vaccination	The vaccine produces neither therapeutic nor adverse effects on HB-infected persons. Prevaccination serologic screening is not indicated for persons being vaccinated because of occupational risk. HCWs who have contact with patients or blood should be tested 1-2 mo after vaccination to determine serologic response
Hepatitis B immune globulin (HBIG)	0.06 ml/kg IM as soon as possible after exposure. A second dose of HBIG should be administered 1 mo later if the HB vaccine series has not been started	**Postexposure prophylaxis:** For persons exposed to blood or body fluids containing HBsAg and who are not immune to HBV infection—0.06 ml/kg IM as soon as possible (but no later than 7 days after exposure)		
Influenza vaccine (inactivated whole-virus and split-virus vaccines)	Annual vaccination with current vaccine Administered IM	HCWs who have contact with patients at high risk for influenza or its complications; HCWs who work in long-term care facilities; HCWs with high-risk medical conditions or who are aged ≥65 yr	History of anaphylactic hypersensitivity to egg ingestion	No evidence exists of risk to mother or fetus when the vaccine is administered to a pregnant woman with an underlying high-risk condition. Influenza vaccination is recommended during second and third trimesters of pregnancy because of increased risk for hospitalization
Measles live-virus vaccine	One dose SC; second dose at least 1 mo later	HCWs† born during or after 1957 who do not have documentation of having received two doses of live vaccine on or after the first birthday **or** a history of physician-diagnosed measles or serologic evidence of immunity. Vaccination should be considered for all HCWs who lack proof of immunity, including those born before 1957	Pregnancy; immunocompromised persons,‡ including HIV-infected persons who have evidence of severe immunosuppression; anaphylaxis after gelatin ingestion or administration of neomycin; recent administration of immune globulin	MMR is the vaccine of choice if recipients are likely to be susceptible to rubella and/or mumps as well as measles. Persons vaccinated between 1963 and 1967 with a killed measles vaccine alone, killed vaccine followed by live vaccine, or with a vaccine of unknown type should be revaccinated with two doses of live measles virus vaccine
Mumps live-virus vaccine	One dose SC; second dose at least 1 mo later	HCWs† believed to be susceptible can be vaccinated. Adults born before 1957 can be considered immune	Pregnancy; immunocompromised persons,‡ history of anaphylactic reaction after gelatin ingestion or administration of neomycin	MMR is the vaccine of choice if recipients are likely to be susceptible to measles and rubella, as well as mumps
Hepatitis A virus (HAV) vaccine	Two doses of vaccine either 6-12 mo apart (HAVRIX), or 6 mo apart (VAQTA)	Not routinely indicated for HCWs in the United States. Persons who work with HAV-infected primates or with HAV in a research laboratory setting should be vaccinated	History of anaphylactic hypersensitivity to alum or, for HAVRIX, the preservative 2-phenoxyethanol. The safety of the vaccine in pregnant women has not been determined; the risk associated with vaccination should be weighed against the risk for hepatitis A in women who may be at high risk for exposure to HAV	

TABLE 15 Immunizing Agents and Immunization Schedules for Health Care Workers (HCWs)*—cont'd

Generic Name	Primary Schedule and Booster(s)	Indications	Major Precautions and Contraindications	Special Considerations
Meningococcal vaccine	One dose in volume and by route specified by manufacturer; single booster for adults 19-21 years of age if the first dose was given before age 16	Laboratory personnel and others with exposure risk	The safety of the vaccine in pregnant women has not been evaluated; it should not be administered during pregnancy unless the risk for infection is high	
Typhoid vaccine, IM, SC, and oral	IM vaccine: One 0.5-ml/dose, booster 0.5 ml every 2 yr SC vaccine: Two 0.5-ml doses, ≥4 wk apart, booster 0.5 ml SC or 0.1 ID every 3 yr if exposure continues Oral vaccine: Four doses on alternate days. The manufacturer recommends revaccination with the entire 4-dose series every 5 yr	Workers in microbiology laboratories who frequently work with *Salmonella typhi*	Severe local or systemic reaction to a previous dose. Ty21a (oral) vaccine should not be administered to immunocompromised persons† or to persons receiving antimicrobial agents	Vaccination should not be considered an alternative to the use of proper procedures when handling specimens and cultures in the laboratory
Vaccinia vaccine (smallpox)	One dose administered with a bifurcated needle; boosters administered every 10 yr	Laboratory workers who directly handle cultures with vaccinia, recombinant vaccinia viruses, or orthopox viruses that infect human beings	The vaccine is contraindicated in pregnancy, in persons with eczema or a history of eczema, and in immunocompromised persons† and their household contacts	Vaccination may be considered for HCWs who have direct contact with contaminated dressings or other infectious material from volunteers in clinical studies involving recombinant vaccinia virus
COVID-19				
Other Vaccine-Preventable Diseases				
Tetanus and diphtheria and pertussis (Tdap)	Two IM doses 4 wk apart or tetanus and diphtheria toxoid for adults with uncertain or incomplete primary vaccination; third dose 6-12 mo after second dose; booster every 10 yr. Substitute a one-time dose of Tdap for one of the doses of Td, either in the primary series or for the routine booster, whichever comes first	All adults	Except in the first trimester, pregnancy is not a precaution History of a neurologic reaction or immediate hypersensitivity reaction after a previous dose History of severe local (Arthus-type) reaction after a previous dose. Such persons should not receive further routine or emergency doses of Td for 10 yr	Tetanus prophylaxis in wound management‡
Pneumococcal polysaccharide vaccine (23 valent)	One dose, 0.5 ml, IM or SC; revaccination recommended for those at highest risk ≥5 yr after the first dose	Adults who are at increased risk of pneumococcal disease and its complications because of underlying health conditions; older adults, especially those age ≥65 who are healthy	The safety of vaccine in pregnant women has not been evaluated; it should not be administered during pregnancy unless the risk for infection is high. Previous recipients of any type of pneumococcal polysaccharide vaccine who are at highest risk for fatal infection or antibody loss may be revaccinated ≥5 yr after the first dose	

Continued

TABLE 15 Immunizing Agents and Immunization Schedules for Health Care Workers (HCWs)*—cont'd

Generic Name	Primary Schedule and Booster(s)	Indications	Major Precautions and Contraindications	Special Considerations
Rubella live-virus vaccine	One dose SC; second dose at least 1 mo later	Indicated for HCWs,† both men and women, who do not have documentation of having received live vaccine on or after their first birthday **or** laboratory evidence of immunity. Adults born before 1957, **except women who can become pregnant,** can be considered immune	Pregnancy; immunocompromised persons†; history of anaphylactic reaction after administration of neomycin	The risk for rubella vaccine-associated malformations in the offspring of women pregnant when vaccinated or who become pregnant within 3 mo after vaccination is negligible. Such women should be counseled regarding the theoretic basis of concern for the fetus. MMR is the vaccine of choice if recipients are likely to be susceptible to measles or mumps as well as rubella
Varicella-zoster live-virus vaccine	Two 0.5-ml doses SC 4-8 wk apart if ≥13 yr	Indicated for HCWs† who do not have either a reliable history of varicella or serologic evidence of immunity	Pregnancy, immunocompromised persons,‡ history of anaphylactic reaction after receipt of neomycin or gelatin. Avoid salicylate use for 6 wk after vaccination	Vaccine is available from the manufacturer for certain patients with acute lymphocytic leukemia in remission. Because 71%-93% of persons without a history of varicella are immune, serologic testing before vaccination is likely to be cost effective
Varicella-zoster immune globulin (VZIG)	Persons <50 kg: 125 μg/10 kg IM; persons ≥50 kg: 625 μg§	Persons known or likely to be susceptible (particularly those at high risk for complications, e.g., pregnant women) who have close and prolonged exposure to a contact case or to an infectious hospital staff worker or patient		Serologic testing may help in assessing whether to administer VZIG. If use of VZIG prevents varicella disease, patient should be vaccinated subsequently
BCG Vaccination				
Bacille Calmette-Guérin (BCG) vaccine (TB)	One percutaneous dose of 0.3 ml; no booster dose recommended	Should be considered only for HCWs in areas where multidrug TB is prevalent, a strong likelihood of infection exists, and where comprehensive infection control precautions have failed to prevent TB transmission to HCWs	Should not be administered to immunocompromised persons,‡ pregnant women	In the United States TB-control efforts are directed toward early identification, treatment of cases, and preventive therapy with isoniazid
Other Immunobiologics That Are or May Be Indicated for HCWs				
Immune globulin (hepatitis A)	**Postexposure**—One IM dose of 0.02 ml/kg administered ≤2 wk after exposure	Indicated for HCWs exposed to feces of infectious patients	Contraindicated in persons with IgA deficiency; do not administer within 2 wk after MMR vaccine or 3 wk after varicella vaccine. Delay administration of MMR vaccine for ≥3 mo and varicella vaccine ≥5 mo after administration of immune globulin	Administer in large muscle mass (deltoid, gluteal)

HBsAg, Hepatitis B surface antigen; *HBV,* hepatitis B virus; *HIV,* human immunodeficiency virus; *IM,* intramuscular; *MMR,* measles, mumps, rubella vaccine; *SC,* subcutaneous; *TB,* tuberculosis.

*Persons who provide health care to patients or work in institutions that provide patient care (e.g., physicians, nurses, emergency medical personnel, dental professionals and students, medical and nursing students, laboratory technicians, hospital volunteers, and administrative and support staff in health care institutions).

†All HCWs (i.e., medical or nonmedical, paid or volunteer, full time or part time, student or nonstudent, with or without patient-care responsibilities) who work in health care institutions (e.g., inpatient and outpatient, public and private) should be immune to measles, rubella, and varicella.

‡Persons immunocompromised because of immune deficiency diseases, HIV infection, leukemia, lymphoma or generalized malignancy, or immunosuppressed as a result of therapy with corticosteroids, alkylating drugs, antimetabolites, or radiation.

§Some experts recommend 125 μg/10 kg regardless of total body weight.

Modified from *MMWR* 46(RR-18), 1998.

TABLE 16 Recommendations for Persons with Medical Conditions Requiring Special Vaccination Considerations

Condition	Tdap	MMR	Varicell[a]	HBV	HAV	Pneumovax[a]	Influenza[b]	HbCV	Meningococcal	IPV	Other Live Vaccines[c]	Other Killed Vaccines[d]
HIV infection	Rou	Rou/Contr[e]	Contr[f]	Rou[g]	Rou	Rec	Rec	Cons	Rou	Rou	Contr	Rou
Severe immunocompromise[h]	Rou	Contr	Contr[f]	Rou[g]	Rou	Rec	Rec	Rou[i]	Rou	Rou	Contr	Rou
Renal failure	Rou	Rou	Rou	Rec[g]	Rou	Rec	Rec	Rou	Rou	Rou	Rou	Rou
Diabetes	Rou	Rou	Rou	Rou	Rou	Rec	Rec	Rou	Rou	Rou	Rou	Rou
Chronic liver disease	Rou	Rou	Rou	Rou	Rec	Rec	Rec	Rou	Rou	Rou	Rou	Rou
Cardiac disease	Rou	Rou	Rou	Rou	Rou	Rec	Rec	Rou	Rou	Rou	Rou	Rou
Pulmonary disease	Rou	Rou	Rou	Rou	Rou	Rec	Rec	Rou	Rou	Rou	Rou	Rou
Alcoholism	Rou	Rou	Rou	Rou	Rou	Rec	Rec	Rou	Rou	Rou	Rou	Rou
Functional/anatomic asplenia	Rou	Rou	Rou	Rou	Rou	Rec[j]	Rec	Rec[j]	Rec[j]	Rou	Rou	Rou
Terminal complement deficiency	Rou	Rou	Rou	Rou	Rou	Rou	Rou	Rou	Rec	Rou	Rou	
Clotting factor disorders	Rou	Rou	Rou	Rec	Rec	Rou	Rou	Rou	Rou	Rou	Rou	Rou

Cons, Consider vaccination; *Contr,* contraindicated; *HAV,* hepatitis A virus; *HbCV, Haemophilus influenzae* conjugate vaccine; *HBV,* hepatitis B virus; *IPV,* inactivated poliomyelitis vaccine; *MMR,* measles-mumps-rubella; *Rec,* recommended; *Rou,* routine as outlined for all adults; *Tdap,* tetanus and diphtheria toxoids and acellular pertussis.

[a]Pneumovax should be repeated in 5 yr for patients in whom vaccine is recommended. Asthma without chronic obstructive pulmonary disease is not an indication for the vaccine.

[b]Influenza vaccine should also be given to caregivers and household members.

[c]Includes bacille Calmette-Guérin, vaccinia, oral typhoid, yellow fever (if exposure cannot be avoided, persons with HIV can be given yellow fever vaccine; see text).

[d]Includes rabies (check postvaccination titers in HIV or severely immunocompromised persons), Lyme disease, inactivated typhoid, cholera, plague, and anthrax.

[e]For asymptomatic, nonseverely immunocompromised persons with HIV, MMR can be used; it is contraindicated in severely immunocompromised persons. MMR can be considered in symptomatic HIV patients without severe immunocompromise.

[f]Varicella can be given to household members and caregivers, but if varicella-like rash develops after vaccination, contact should be avoided.

[g]Recommended for persons with severe chronic renal failure approaching or already receiving dialysis, and higher doses should be given. Antibody titers should be measured after vaccination in these patients and in those with HIV or severe immunocompromise (who may require higher doses) to ensure adequate response. Yearly titers should be measured in dialysis patients.

[h]Severe immunocompromise can result from congenital immunodeficiency, leukemia, lymphoma, malignancy, organ transplant, chemotherapy, radiation therapy, or high-dose corticosteroids.

[i]Only for persons with Hodgkin's disease.

[j]Give at least 2 wk in advance of elective splenectomy.

Modified and updated from *MMWR* 42(RR-4):16, 1993.

Vaccinations for International Travel

TABLE 17 Recommended Immunizations for Travelers to Developing Countries

Immunizations	LENGTH OF TRAVEL: Brief (<2 wk)	Intermediate (2 wk-3 mo)	Long-Term Residential (>3 mo)
Review and complete age-appropriate childhood schedule	+	+	+
DTaP, poliovirus, pneumococcal, and *Haemophilus influenzae* type B vaccines may be given at 4-week intervals if necessary to complete the recommended schedule before departure. Rotavirus vaccine has maximum ages for the first and last doses; consideration should be given to the timing of an infant's travel so that the infant will be able to receive the vaccine series.			
Measles: Infants 6-11mo of age should receive 1 dose of MMR vaccine before departure. Two additional doses are given if younger than 12 mo of age at first dose.			
Varicella			
Hepatitis A*			
Hepatitis B†			
Vaccines against the following diseases should be considered depending on the geographic area and circumstances of the visit:			
Japanese encephalitis‡	±	±	+
Meningococcal disease§	±	±	±
Rabies¶	±	+	+
Typhoid fever**	±	+	+
Yellow fever††	+	+	+
COVID-19	+	+	+

DTaP, Diphtheria-tetanus-acellular pertussis.
*Indicated for travelers to areas with intermediate or high endemic rates of hepatitis A virus infection.
†If insufficient time to complete 6-month primary series, an accelerated series can be given.
‡For regions with endemic infection. For high-risk activities in areas experiencing outbreaks, vaccine is recommended, even for brief travel.
§Recommended for regions of Africa with endemic infection and during local epidemics and required for travel to Saudi Arabia for the Hajj.
¶Indicated for persons at high risk for animal exposure (especially dogs) and for travelers to countries with endemic infection.
**Indicated for travelers who will consume food and liquids in areas of poor sanitation.
††For regions with endemic infection.
From Cherry JD: *Feigin and Cherry's pediatric infectious diseases*, ed 8, Elsevier, 2019.
Modified from American Academy of Pediatrics. Immunizations in special clinical circumstances. In Kimberlin DW et al (eds) *Red book: 2015 report of the Committee on Infectious Diseases*, ed 30, Elk Grove Village, 2015, American Academy of Pediatrics, 101-107; Centers for Disease Control and Prevention. Health information for international travel, 2016: international travel with infants and young children. Available at wwwnc.cdc.gov/travel/yellowbook/2016/international-travel-with-infants-children/vaccine-recommendations-for-infants-children.

Passive Immunizations for Adults

TABLE 18 Passive Immunizations for Adults

Disease	Name of Material*	Comments and Use
Tetanus	Tetanus immune globulin, human	Management of tetanus-prone wounds in persons without adequate prior active immunization and treatment of tetanus
Cytomegalovirus	Cytomegalovirus immune globulin, intravenous	Prophylaxis for bone marrow and kidney transplant recipients
Diphtheria	Diphtheria antitoxin, equine	Treatment of established disease; high frequency of reactions to serum of nonhuman origin; in the United States, available only from CDC
Rabies	Rabies immune globulin, human	Postexposure prophylaxis of animal bites
Measles	Immune globulin, human	Prevention or modification of disease in exposed persons, not for control of outbreaks; particularly indicated for unvaccinated infants aged <12 mo, pregnant women without evidence of measles immunity, and severely immunocompromised persons
Hepatitis A	Immune globulin, human	Preexposure and postexposure prophylaxis for travelers and others who need protection before immunity can be achieved with hepatitis A vaccine
Hepatitis B	Hepatitis B immune globulin, human	Prophylaxis for needle stick or mucous membrane contact with HBsAg-positive persons, for sexual partners with acute hepatitis B or carriers of hepatitis B, for infants born to mothers who are carriers of HBsAg, for infants whose mother or primary caregiver has acute hepatitis B
Varicella	Varicella-zoster immune globulin, human	Persons with underlying disease and at risk for complications from chickenpox who have not had varicella or varicella vaccine and who are exposed to varicella; may be given up to 10 days after exposure to known susceptible adults, particularly if antibody negative
Vaccinia	Vaccinia immune globulin	Treatment of eczema vaccinatum, vaccinia necrosum, and severe inadvertent inoculations such as ocular vaccinia after vaccinia (smallpox) vaccination; available only from CDC
Erythroblastosis fetalis	Rh immune globulin	Rh-negative women who give birth to Rh-positive infants or who abort
Hypogammaglobulinemia	Immune globulin, intravenous, subcutaneous	Maintenance therapy
Idiopathic thrombocytopenic purpura	Immune globulin, intravenous	Therapy for acute episodes
Botulism	Heptavalent A, B, C, D, E, F, E, G antitoxin, equine	Treatment of botulism; available through CDC
	Botulism immune globulin for infants	Treatment of botulism in infants
Snakebite	Antivenin, equine (North American coral snake antivenin)	Specific for North American coral snake, *Micrurus fulvius*
Crotalidae, polyvalent	Effective for viper and pit viper bites, including rattlesnakes, copperheads, moccasins	
Crotalidae Immune F(ab')2 (Equine)	Equine-derived antivenin indicated for the management of adult and pediatric patients with North American rattlesnake envenomation	Specific for North American rattlesnake, *Crotalus* spp.
Spider bite	Antivenin, equine	Specific for black widow spider, *Latrodectus mactans,* and other members of the genus
Scorpion	Fab fragments, equine	Specific for *Centruroides* genus scorpions

CDC, Centers for Disease Control and Prevention; *HBsAg,* hepatitis B surface antigen.
*All products to be administered intramuscularly, unless otherwise indicated.
From Goldman L, Shafer AI: *Goldman-Cecil medicine,* ed 26, Philadelphia, 2020, Elsevier.

TABLE 19 Selected Immunizing Agents Indicated for Adults*

Disease	Immunizing Agent	Indications	Schedule	Major Contraindications (C) and Precautions (P)	Comments
Anthrax	Anthrax vaccine, adsorbed, an inactivated vaccine	Preexposure prophylaxis of persons at high risk of exposure (e.g., military, certain laboratory workers) Consider with antibiotics for postexposure prophylaxis	0.5-ml dose IM at 0, 4, and 6 wk and boosters at 12 and 18 mo, then booster annually thereafter If used after exposure, three doses at 0, 2, and 4 wk with 60 days of antimicrobial therapy; antibiotics should be continued for 14 days after third dose	C: Severe allergic reaction to a vaccine component or after a prior dose P: Moderate or severe acute illness	Effectiveness against aerosol exposure inferred primarily from animal data Limited data on the benefits of postexposure use
Cholera	Cholera vaccine, live attenuated oral cholera vaccine	Adults 18-64 yr, traveling to an area of active cholera transmission	One oral dose before travel; booster doses are not presently recommended	C: Severe allergic reaction to a vaccine component or after a prior dose P: Moderate or severe acute illness There are no data about use of this vaccine in • Pregnant women • Immunocompromised persons • Children <18 yr and adults 65 yr and older	All travelers to cholera-affected areas should follow safe food and water precautions and proper sanitation and personal hygiene measures as primary strategies to prevent cholera
Diphtheria	Tetanus and diphtheria toxoids combined	All adults	For incompletely immunized adults, three doses IM needed for primary series: Two doses IM 4 wk apart, third dose 6-12 mo after second dose; one of these doses should be Tdap Booster every 10 yr No need to repeat if schedule is interrupted	C: History of neurologic reaction after a previous dose C: Severe allergic reaction to a vaccine component or after a prior dose P: Moderate or severe acute illness	Tetanus and diphtheria toxoids combined with acellular pertussis vaccine (Tdap) preferred as one-time booster for all persons
Hepatitis A	Inactivated hepatitis A vaccine	Travelers to highly or intermediately endemic countries Men who have sex with men Illegal drug users (injection and noninjection) Persons who work with hepatitis A virus–infected primates or who do research with the virus Persons with chronic liver disease Recipients of clotting factors	Two doses at least 6 mo apart for persons aged ≥1 yr	C: Severe allergic reaction to a vaccine component or after a prior dose P: Moderate or severe acute illness	Recommended for all children Should be considered for outbreak control
Hepatitis B	Two inactivated hepatitis B virus subunit vaccines containing HBsAg; one vaccine containing HBsAg and an adjuvant	Adolescents Health care and public safety workers potentially exposed to blood Clients and staff of institutions for the developmentally disabled Hemodialysis patients Men who have sex with men Users of illicit injectable drugs Recipients of clotting factors Household and sexual contacts of HBV carriers Inmates of long-term correctional facilities Heterosexuals treated for sexually transmitted diseases or with multiple sexual partners Travelers with close contact for ≥6 mo with populations with high prevalence of HBV carriage Adults 19-59 yr with diabetes mellitus	Three doses IM at 0, 1, and 6 mo, or two doses 1 mo apart	C: Severe allergic reaction to a vaccine component or after a prior dose P: Moderate or severe acute illness	Pregnancy is not a contraindication Health care workers who have contact with patients or blood, sexual contacts of persons with chronic HBV infection, hemodialysis patients, other immunosuppressed persons, and recipients of clotting factor concentrates should be tested 1-2 mo after vaccination to determine serologic response

Human papillomavirus	L1 capsid proteins of types 6, 11, 16, 18, 31, 33, 45, 52, and 58 (nine-valent; bivalent and quadrivalent vaccines, while licensed are no longer available in the United States)	Females at 11-12 yr; catch-up vaccination of females through 26 yr Males 11-12 yr and catch-up vaccination through 21 yr; consider catch-up through 26 yr to prevent anogenital and oropharyngeal cancers and genital warts	Two 0.5-ml doses IM at 0 and 6-12 mo if initiating vaccine series before 15 yr Three 0.5-ml doses IM at 0, 1-2, and 6 mo if first dose given at 15 yr or older	C: Severe allergic reaction to a vaccine component or to a prior dose Vaccine is not recommended for pregnant women P: Moderate or severe acute illness	The vaccine will not protect against existing infections Because the types in the vaccines are not responsible for all HPV infections associated with cervical cancer, screening for cancer should occur as for unvaccinated women Approved by the FDA for 27-45 year olds
Influenza	Inactivated virus vaccine	All persons ≥6 mo of age, with greatest priority for those at higher risk for influenza complications (e.g., ≥65 yr old, persons with underlying medical conditions, pregnant women) or in contact with those at higher risk (e.g., health care workers, and persons with close contact with children <5 yr)	Annual vaccination; see annual ACIP recommendation	C: Severe allergic reaction to an influenza vaccine component (except eggs) or after a prior dose P: Moderate or severe acute illness P: GBS within 6 wk of prior dose of influenza vaccine	Optimum timing for vaccination is October. However, vaccination can occur throughout the influenza season, particularly for persons at high risk for complications and their contacts who were not vaccinated earlier Only one dose of influenza vaccine per season is recommended for adults
	Live attenuated influenza virus (LAIV)	Persons 2 through 49 yr without underlying conditions that place them at high risk of complications from influenza	Administered intranasally See annual ACIP recommendations	C: Persons <2 yr or ≥50 yr P: Persons with underlying disorders that place them at high risk of influenza complications P: History of GBS within 6 wk of prior dose of influenza vaccine C: Pregnant women C: Hypersensitivity to components of vaccine (except eggs)	Can be used for household contacts and health care workers caring for patients without severe immunocompromise
Japanese encephalitis	Inactivated Japanese encephalitis virus vaccine	Travelers to Asia spending at least 1 mo in endemic areas during transmission season	Two 0.5-ml doses IM on days 0 and 28 for persons 18 yr and older The FDA approved an alternate 0- and 7-day schedule.	C: Pregnancy	
Measles	Live virus vaccine	All adults born after 1956 without history of live vaccine on or after first birthday or detectable measles antibody Persons born before 1957 generally can be considered immune	One dose sufficient for most adults; two doses at least 1 mo apart indicated for persons entering college or medical facility employment, traveling abroad, or at risk of measles during outbreaks	C: Altered immunity (e.g., leukemia, lymphoma, generalized malignant disease, congenital immunodeficiency, immunosuppressive therapy) C: Immune globulin or other blood products within prior 3-11 mo, depending on dose of immune globulin or blood product received C: Untreated tuberculosis C: Anaphylactic hypersensitivity to neomycin or gelatin C: Pregnancy P: Thrombocytopenia	Persons with anaphylactic allergies to eggs may be vaccinated (see text) Vaccine should be administered to persons with asymptomatic HIV infection and should be considered for patients except those with severe immunocompromise
Meningococcal disease (two vaccines)	1. Meningococcal conjugate vaccines containing polysaccharide of serogroups A, C, W, and Y (age 2 mo-55 yr)	All 11- to 18-yr-old persons and all persons with persistent complement component deficiencies, HIV infection, or anatomic or functional asplenia Persons who will travel to areas with hyperendemic or epidemic diseases Microbiologists routinely exposed to isolates of *Neisseria meningitidis* May be useful during localized outbreaks	One dose with revaccination at age 16 yr of children who receive conjugate vaccine at 11-12 yr of age and every 5 yr for persons at high risk	C: Allergic reactions to a component of the vaccine, including diphtheria toxoid and latex	

Continued

TABLE 19 Selected Immunizing Agents Indicated for Adults*—cont'd

	2. Recombinant meningococcal B protein vaccines containing either two (MenB-FHbp) or three (MenB-4C) proteins (ages 10 yr and older)	All persons 10 yr and older with persistent complement component deficiencies (including inherited or chronic deficiencies in C3, C5-9, properdin, factor D, factor H, or who are taking eculizumab [Soliris]), or anatomic or functional asplenia Certain laboratory workers May be useful during localized outbreaks May be administered to adolescents and young adults aged 16-23 yr to provide short-term protection against most strains of serogroup B meningococcal disease; preferred age for MenB vaccination is 16-18 yr	Either a 2-dose series of MenB-4C at 0 and 1 mo, or a 2-dose series of MenB-FHbp at 0, and 6 mo. The two dose series of MenB-FHbp is recommended only for healthy persons who are not at increased risk for meningococcal disease. For persons at increased risk for meningococcal disease and for use during serogroup B outbreaks, MenB-FHbp should be given as 3 doses at 0, 1-2, and 6 mo. For persons at increased risk, the 2 dose series of MenB-4c at 0 and 1 mo remains in effect. The same vaccine product should be used for all doses. No revaccination recommendations at present	C: Severe allergic reaction to a vaccine component or after a prior dose C: Pregnancy P: Moderate or severe acute illness	Evidence supports use of MenB vaccines in all persons at increased risk for serogroup B meningococcal disease. Evidence for use of these vaccines in adolescents and young adults supports a recommendation for individual clinical decision making
Mumps	Live virus vaccine	All adults born after 1956 without history of live vaccine on or after first birthday or detectable mumps antibody Persons born before 1957 generally can be considered immune	One dose sufficient for most adults Two doses at least 1 mo apart indicated for persons entering college or medical facility employment or traveling abroad	C: Altered immunity (e.g., leukemia, lymphoma, generalized malignant disease, congenital immunodeficiency, immunosuppressive therapy) C: Immune globulin or other blood products within prior 3-11 mo C: Anaphylactic hypersensitivity to neomycin or gelatin C: Pregnancy P: Thrombocytopenia if administered with measles vaccine P: Moderate or severe acute illness	Although persons born after 1956 are generally immune, vaccine can be given to adults of all ages and may be particularly indicated for postpubertal males who are thought to be susceptible Persons with anaphylactic allergies to eggs may be vaccinated Persons previously vaccinated with two doses of a mumps-containing vaccine who are identified by public health as at increased risk for mumps because of a mumps outbreak should receive a third dose of a mumps-containing vaccine to improve protection against mumps disease and related complications
Pertussis	Adult preparation of pertussis antigens combined with tetanus and diphtheria toxoids (Tdap)	All 11-12 yr olds Catch-up vaccination for all persons ≥13 yr	One dose Pregnant women: One dose during each pregnancy early in the period between 27 and 36 wk of gestation	C: Severe allergic reaction to a vaccine component or after a prior dose P: Moderate or severe acute illness	Two preparations are available, one licensed for all persons ≥10 yr, one for 10- to 64-yr-olds
Pneumococcal disease	23-Valent polysaccharide vaccine (PPSV23)	All adults with cardiovascular disease, pulmonary disease (including asthma), diabetes mellitus, alcoholism, cirrhosis, cerebrospinal fluid leaks, splenic dysfunction or anatomic asplenia, Hodgkin disease, lymphoma, multiple myeloma, chronic renal failure, nephrotic syndrome, immunosuppression, HIV infection, cigarette smokers 19 yr and older High-risk populations, such as certain Native Americans, and All adults ≥65 yr	One dose IM or SC; a second dose should be considered ≥5 yr later for adults at high risk of disease (e.g., asplenic patients) and those who lose antibody rapidly (e.g., nephrotic syndrome, renal failure, transplant recipients) Revaccinate adults who received a first dose when <65 yr who are now ≥65 yr and who received their vaccine at least 5 yr earlier	C: Severe allergic reaction to a vaccine component or after a prior dose P: Moderate or severe acute illness	

	Pneumococcal conjugate vaccine (PCV13)	One dose recommended for all adults age 65 yr and older, for immunocompromised adults ≥19 yr, and those with functional/anatomic asplenia, cochlear implants, cerebrospinal fluid leaks	One dose if not previously vaccinated with PCV13) as an adult Give ≥1 yr after PPSV23; or if PPSV23-naïve, if 65 yr or older and not immunocompromised, give PPSV23 ≥1 yr after PCV13; if >19 yr old and immunocompromised, give PPSV23 ≥8 wk after PCV13	C: Severe allergic reaction (e.g., anaphylaxis) to any component of PCV13 or any diphtheria toxoid-containing vaccine P: Moderate or severe acute illness	Although licensed for use in adults ≥50 yr, it is recommended only for adults ≥19 yr with the noted medical conditions
Poliomyelitis	Inactivated poliovirus vaccine (IPV)	Certain adults who are at greater risk of exposure to wild poliovirus than the general population, including travelers to countries where poliomyelitis is epidemic or endemic or specific populations with disease caused by wild poliovirus	For unvaccinated adults, two doses IM or SC 4 wk apart and a third dose 6-12 mo after the second; if <4 wk available before protection is needed, a single dose of IPV For incompletely immunized adults, complete primary series of three doses of IPV or prior oral poliovirus vaccine (OPV); no need to restart interrupted series A single dose of IPV can be given to adults who previously received a primary series but now are at high risk, such as those traveling to an endemic area	P: On theoretical grounds, pregnant women should not receive IPV, but if immediate protection is needed, IPV can be used C: Severe allergic reaction to a vaccine component or after a prior dose P: Moderate or severe acute illness	
Rabies	Inactivated vaccine, HDCV or PCECV	High-risk persons, including animal handlers, selected laboratory and field workers, and persons traveling for ≥1 mo to areas with high risk of rabies	Preexposure prophylaxis: Three doses of 1 ml IM on days 0, 7, and 21 or 28	C: History of severe hypersensitivity reaction P: Moderate or severe acute illness	Further doses needed after exposure
Rubella	Live virus vaccine	Adults, particularly women of childbearing age, who lack history of rubella vaccine and detectable rubella-specific antibodies in serum Males and females in institutions where rubella outbreaks may occur, such as hospitals, the military, and colleges Persons born before 1957, except women who can become pregnant, generally can be considered immune	One dose SC	C: Pregnancy, altered immunity (e.g., leukemia, lymphoma, generalized malignant disease, congenital immunodeficiency, immunosuppressive therapy) C: Immune globulin or other blood products within 3-11 mo before vaccination C: Anaphylactic hypersensitivity to neomycin C: Administration of blood products should not contraindicate postpartum vaccination P: Thrombocytopenia if administered with measles vaccine P: Moderate or severe acute illness	Women should be counseled to avoid pregnancy for 1 mo after vaccination

Continued

TABLE 19 Selected Immunizing Agents Indicated for Adults*—cont'd

Smallpox	Live vaccinia virus	Persons working with orthopox viruses Members of public health and health care response teams	One dose intracutaneously with a bifurcated needle Boosters every 10 yr and perhaps every 3 yr for persons working with virulent orthopox viruses	C: History or presence of eczema or other acute, chronic, or exfoliative skin condition in patient or a close household or personal contact C: Immunosuppression or pregnancy in patient or a close household or personal contact P: History of heart disease C: Breast-feeding C: Age <1 yr C: Allergy to a vaccine component P: History of heart disease P: Moderate or severe acute illness No contraindications if exposed to smallpox	Some complications of vaccination are treatable with vaccinia immune globulin Vaccine is effective 3-4 days after exposure to variola and perhaps longer to prevent or to modify the illness Serious adverse events are rare but significant, including eczema vaccinatum, progressive vaccinia, myopericarditis, autoinoculation, and encephalitis Vaccinia is transmissible
Tetanus	Tetanus and diphtheria toxoids combined	All adults	Three doses IM needed for primary series: Two doses 4 wk apart, third dose 6-12 mo after second dose Booster every 10 yr; no need to repeat if schedule is interrupted	C: History of neurologic or severe allergic reaction after a prior dose P: Moderate or severe acute illness	Special recommendations for wound treatment (see text) Persons with GBS within the first 6 wk after immunization, particularly adults who received a prior primary series, probably should not be revaccinated in most circumstances Tetanus and diphtheria toxoids combined with acellular pertussis (Tdap) vaccine preferred for booster at age 11-12 yr One-time booster of Tdap for all adults
Typhoid fever	Vi capsular polysaccharide vaccine Live attenuated Ty21a oral vaccine	Travelers to areas where the risk of prolonged exposure to contaminated food and water is high May be considered for family and intimate contacts of carriers and laboratory workers who work with *Salmonella typhi*	Vi polysaccharide vaccine: One dose IM 0.5 ml; boosters every 2 yr Oral vaccine: Four doses on alternate days; repeat series every 5 yr if risk continues	C: Severe local or systemic reaction to a prior dose C: Ty21a vaccine should not be administered to persons with altered immunity or those receiving antimicrobial agents P: Moderate or severe acute illness	Efficacy only 50-77% Food and water precautions essential
Varicella: Chickenpox strain	Attenuated Oka strain of varicella virus	All persons without evidence of varicella immunity, especially health care personnel, childbearing-age women, and persons with household or other contact with persons at high risk of complications of varicella (e.g., susceptible immunosuppressed persons)	Two 0.5-ml doses SC 4-8 wk apart for persons ≥13 yr A second dose is recommended for all persons who previously received one dose	C: Immunocompromise C: Pregnancy C: Allergy to vaccine components P: Moderate or severe acute illness	Adults with a history of prior clinician-diagnosed or verified varicella can be considered immune Vaccine virus has rarely been transmitted to contacts from healthy vaccinees in whom rash developed Women who receive vaccine should not become pregnant for 1 mo

Varicella: Zoster	Inactivated recombinant subunit zoster vaccine with adjuvant (RZV)	1. RZV is recommended for the prevention of herpes zoster and related complications for immunocompetent adults age 50 yr and older 2. RZV is recommended for the prevention of herpes zoster and related complications for immunocompetent adults who previously received zoster vaccine live (ZVL) 3. RZV is preferred over ZVL for the prevention of herpes zoster and related complications	Two 0.5 ml doses 2-6 mo apart	C: Allergy to vaccine components P: Moderate or severe acute illness P: Pregnancy P: Active zoster disease	
	Attenuated Oka strain of varicella virus, ≥14-fold higher content than varicella vaccine (ZVL)	Persons ≥60 yr of age	One 0.65-ml dose SC	C: Immunocompromise C: Pregnancy C: Allergy to vaccine components P: Moderate or severe acute illness	May be administered regardless of a prior history of shingles
Yellow fever	Live attenuated virus (17D strain)	Persons living or traveling in areas where yellow fever exists	One dose; booster every 10 yr for at-risk laboratory personnel and certain travelers (pregnant women, hematopoietic stem cell transplant recipients vaccinated before transplant, HIV-infected persons, and travelers who will be in a higher-risk setting based on season, location, activities, and duration of their travel, such as travelers who plan to spend a prolonged period in endemic areas or those traveling to highly endemic areas such as rural West Africa during peak transmission season or an area with an ongoing outbreak)	C: Immunocompromised persons C: History of anaphylactic allergies to eggs P: Pregnancy on theoretical grounds, although may be given if risk is high P: Moderate or severe acute illness	Fever, jaundice, and multiple-organ system failure (viscerotropic disease) have been rarely reported in first-time recipients of 17D-derived yellow fever vaccinations Vaccinate only persons traveling to areas endemic to yellow fever

ACIP, Advisory Committee on Immunization Practices; *GBS,* Guillain-Barré syndrome; *HBsAg,* hepatitis B surface antigen; *HBV,* hepatitis B virus; *HDCV,* human diploid cell vaccine for rabies; *HIV,* human immunodeficiency virus; *HPV,* human papillomavirus; *IM,* intramuscularly; *IPV,* inactivated poliovirus vaccine; *MMR,* measles, mumps, and rubella vaccine; *OPV,* live trivalent oral poliovirus vaccine; *PCECV,* purified chick embryo cell culture rabies vaccine; *SC,* subcutaneously.

*See the text and package inserts for further details, particularly regarding indications, dosage, administration, side effects, and adverse reactions and contraindications.

From Goldman L, Shafer AI: *Goldman-Cecil medicine,* ed 26, Philadelphia, 2020, Elsevier.

Recommendations for Providing Sexually Transmitted Diseases Clinical Services

BOX 1 Recommendations For Obtaining A Sexual History And Conducting A Physical Examination As Part Of Sexually Transmitted Diseases Care In Primary Care And Sexually Transmitted Diseases Specialty Care Settings*

STD care in primary care settings

- A sexual history and risk assessment **should** be available as part of basic STD care services at the following patient visits:
  - Initial comprehensive or annual visit
  - Each visit concerning reproductive, genital, or urologic issues
- A physical examination **should** be available as a basic STD care service for male and female patients with STD-related symptoms, STD-related concerns, or those at high behavioral risk for incident STDs.
- A pelvic examination **should** be available as a basic STD care service.
- A sexual history and risk assessment **could** be available as basic STD care services at each visit unrelated to reproductive, genital, or urologic concerns.
- Anoscopy **could** be available as a basic STD care service.

STD care in STD specialty care settings

- A sexual history and risk assessment **should** be part of specialized STD care services at every visit for patients with STD-related symptoms, STD-related concerns, or concerns about preventing or achieving pregnancy.
- A physical examination **should** be available as a specialized STD care service for male and female patients with STD-related symptoms, STD-related concerns, or high behavioral risk for incident STDs.
- A pelvic examination **should** be available as a specialized STD care service.
- Colposcopy **should** be available as a specialized STD care service for female patients with abnormal Pap smears.
- Anoscopy **should** be available as a specialized STD care service.
- A high-resolution anoscopy **could** be available as a specialized STD care service for patients with abnormal anal Pap smears.

Pap, Papanicolaou; *STD,* sexually transmitted disease.

*Primary care setting is defined as a place where patients are evaluated for various health conditions. An STD specialty care setting is defined as a place where the focus is on providing patients with timely, comprehensive, confidential, and culturally sensitive STD care. STD care delivered in STD specialty care settings includes all care delivered in primary care settings.

Barrow RY, Ahmed F, Bolan GA, Workowski KA. Recommendations for providing quality sexually transmitted diseases clinical services, 2020, *MMWR Recomm Rep* 2020;68(No. RR-5):1-20. DOI: https://doi.org/10.15585/mmwr.rr6805a1external icon

BOX 2 Prevention Recommendations For Sexually Transmitted Diseases Care In Primary Care And Sexually Transmitted Diseases Specialty Care Settings*

STD care in primary care settings

- The following prevention services should be available as basic STD care services:
  - On-site hepatitis B vaccination or referral
  - On-site HPV vaccination or referral
  - Brief single STD/HIV prevention counseling session (up to 30 minutes)†
  - PrEP for HIV prevention and nPEP of HIV risk assessment, education, and referral or link to HIV care†
  - Emergency contraceptive pills§
  - Brief contraceptive counseling or referral
  - Referral or link to HIV care, family planning services, and behavioral health services, if indicated
- The following prevention services could be available as basic STD care services:
  - On-site condom provision¶
  - On-site hepatitis A vaccination
  - Provision of PrEP for HIV prevention**
  - Provision of nPEP of HIV††
  - Moderate-intensity STD behavioral counseling (≥30 minutes)†

STD care in STD specialty care settings

- The following prevention services should be available as specialized STD care services:
  - On-site condom provision
  - On-site hepatitis A vaccination
  - On-site hepatitis B vaccination
  - On-site HPV vaccination
  - Brief single STD/HIV prevention counseling session (up to 30 minutes)†
  - PrEP for HIV prevention and nPEP of HIV risk assessment, education, counseling, and referral or link to HIV care†
  - Provision of PrEP for HIV prevention§§
  - Provision of nPEP of HIV¶¶
  - Brief contraceptive counseling or referral
  - Emergency contraceptive pills§
  - Referral or link to HIV care, family planning services, and behavioral health services, if indicated
- The following prevention services could be available as specialized STD care services:
  - Moderate-intensity STD behavioral counseling (≥30 minutes)†
  - High-intensity STD behavioral counseling (≥2 hours)†

HIV, human immunodeficiency virus; *HPV,* human papillomavirus; *nPEP,* nonoccupational postexposure prophylaxis; *PrEP,* preexposure prophylaxis; *STD,* sexually transmitted disease.

*Primary care setting is defined as a place where patients are evaluated for various health conditions. STD specialty care setting is defined as a place where the focus is on providing patients with timely, comprehensive, confidential, and culturally sensitive STD care. STD care delivered in STD specialty care settings includes all care delivered in primary care settings.

†Provided by a clinician or other appropriately trained staff.

§If emergency contraceptive pills are not available on site or by prescription, patients can be advised that levonorgestrel emergency contraceptive pills are available over the counter and ulipristal acetate emergency contraceptive pills are only available by prescription. Emergency contraceptive pills should be taken as soon as possible within 5 days of unprotected sex.

¶Providers can partner with local organizations, such as the local health department and community-based organizations, to procure condoms. In some states, prescriptions can be written for condoms. For certain settings, such as family planning clinics, condoms should be available on site.

**PrEP could be available by starter packs or prescription with on-site follow-up care for basic STD care. If PrEP is not provided, navigator-assisted referral for PrEP should be provided with first appointment made while the patient is on site.

††nPEP starter pack (3-7 days of medication) could be available on site, with either on-site follow-up care or referral for basic STD care. nPEP starter pack or complete 28-day course could be available by prescription, with either on-site follow-up care or referral, with first appointment made while the patient is on site. Provision of the complete 28-day nPEP medication supply at the initial visit rather than a starter pack of 3-7 days has been reported to increase likelihood of adherence, especially when patients find returning for multiple follow-up visits difficult. Routinely providing starter packs or the complete 28-day course requires that health care providers stock nPEP drugs in their practice setting or have an established agreement with a pharmacy to stock, package, and urgently dispense nPEP drugs with required administration instructions (https://www.cdc.gov/hiv/pdf/programresources/cdc-hiv-npep-guidelines.pdf).

§§PrEP should be available in starter packs or by prescription with on-site follow-up care for specialized STD care. If PrEP is not provided, navigator-assisted referral for PrEP should be provided with first appointment made while the patient is on site.

¶¶nPEP starter pack (3-7 days of medication) should be available on site, with either on-site follow-up care or referral to specialized STD care. nPEP complete 28-day course should be available by prescription, with either on-site follow-up care or referral, with first appointment made while the patient is on site. Provision of the complete 28-day nPEP medication supply at the initial visit rather than a starter pack of 3-7 days has been reported to increase likelihood of adherence, especially when patients find returning for multiple follow-up visits difficult.

Barrow RY, Ahmed F, Bolan GA, Workowski KA. Recommendations for providing quality sexually transmitted diseases clinical services, 2020, *MMWR Recomm Rep* 2020;68(No. RR-5):1-20. DOI: https://doi.org/10.15585/mmwr.rr6805a1external icon

BOX 3 Screening Recommendations For Sexually Transmitted Diseases Care In Primary Care And Sexually Transmitted Diseases Specialty Care Settings*

STD care in primary care settings

- Screening and assessment for the following STDs **should** be available as basic STD care services:
  - Gonorrhea
  - Chlamydia
  - Syphilis
  - Hepatitis B
  - Hepatitis C
  - HIV
  - Cervical cancer
- Screening and assessment for the following STD **could** be available as a basic STD care service:
  - Trichomoniasis

STD care in STD specialty care settings

- Screening and assessment for the following STDs **should** be available as specialized STD care services:
  - Gonorrhea
  - Chlamydia
  - Syphilis
  - Hepatitis B
  - Hepatitis C
  - HIV
  - Cervical cancer
  - Trichomoniasis
- Screening and assessment for the following STD could be available as a specialized STD care service:
  - Anal cancer

HIV, human immunodeficiency virus; *STD,* sexually transmitted disease.

*Primary care setting is defined as a place where patients are evaluated for various health conditions. STD specialty care setting is defined as a place where the focus is on providing patients with timely, comprehensive, confidential, and culturally sensitive STD care. STD care delivered in STD specialty care settings includes all care delivered in primary care settings.

Barrow RY, Ahmed F, Bolan GA, Workowski KA. Recommendations for providing quality sexually transmitted diseases clinical services, 2020, *MMWR Recomm Rep* 2020;68(No. RR-5):1-20. DOI: https://doi.org/10.15585/mmwr.rr6805a1external icon

BOX 4 Partner Services Recommendations For Sexually Transmitted Diseases Care In Primary Care And Sexually Transmitted Diseases Specialty Care Settings*

STD care in primary care settings

- The following partner services **should** be available as basic STD care services:
  - Guidance regarding notification and care of sex partners
  - EPT (where legal and where local or state jurisdictions do not prohibit by regulation)†
- The following partner services **could** be available as a basic STD care service:
  - Interactive counseling for partner notification

STD care in STD specialty care settings

- The following partner services **should** be available as specialized STD care services:
  - Guidance regarding notification and care of sex partners
  - Interactive counseling for partner notification
  - EPT (where legal and where local or state jurisdictions do not prohibit by regulation)†
  - Health department DIS elicitation of sex partner information to identify those who might have been exposed and to identify patient follow-up needs§

DIS, disease intervention specialist; *EPT,* expedited partner therapy; *STD,* sexually transmitted disease.

*Primary care setting is defined as a place where patients are evaluated for various health conditions. STD specialty care setting is defined as a place where the focus is on providing patients with timely, comprehensive, confidential, and culturally sensitive STD care. STD care delivered in STD specialty care settings includes all care delivered in primary care settings.

†Information on legal status of EPT for each state is available at https://www.cdc.gov/std/ept/legal/default.htm.

§Partner services can be provided on site or by referral.

Barrow RY, Ahmed F, Bolan GA, Workowski KA. Recommendations for providing quality sexually transmitted diseases clinical services, 2020, *MMWR Recomm Rep* 2020;68(No. RR-5):1-20. DOI: https://doi.org/10.15585/mmwr.rr6805a1external icon

BOX 5 Evaluation Of Sexually Transmitted Disease–Related Conditions Recommendations In Primary Care And Sexually Transmitted Diseases Specialty Care Settings*

STD care in primary care settings

- Evaluation (history and examination) for the following STD-related conditions **should** be available as basic STD care services:
  - Genital ulcer disease
  - Male urethritis syndrome
  - Vaginal discharge
  - PID
  - Genital warts
  - Proctitis†
  - Ectoparasitic infections
  - Pharyngitis
  - Epididymitis
  - Systemic or dermatologic conditions compatible with or suggestive of an STD etiology

STD care in STD specialty care settings

- Evaluation (history and examination) for the following STD-related conditions **should** be available as specialized STD care services:
  - Genital ulcer disease
  - Male urethritis syndrome
  - Vaginal discharge
  - PID
  - Genital warts
  - Proctitis†
  - Ectoparasitic infections
  - Pharyngitis
  - Epididymitis
  - Systemic or dermatologic conditions compatible with or suggestive of an STD etiology

PID, pelvic inflammatory disease; *STD,* sexually transmitted disease.

*Primary care setting is defined as a place where patients are evaluated for various health conditions. STD specialty care setting is defined as a place where the focus is on providing patients with timely, comprehensive, confidential, and culturally sensitive STD care. STD care delivered in STD specialty care settings includes all care delivered in primary care settings.

†Evaluation for proctitis might include visual examination of the anus, anorectal examination with a rectal swab, digital anorectal examination, or anoscopy. For specialized STD care, high-resolution anoscopy might be included.

Barrow RY, Ahmed F, Bolan GA, Workowski KA. Recommendations for providing quality sexually transmitted diseases clinical services, 2020, *MMWR Recomm Rep* 2020;68(No. RR-5):1-20. DOI: https://doi.org/10.15585/mmwr.rr6805a1external icon

BOX 6 Laboratory Recommendations For Sexually Transmitted Diseases Care In Primary Care And Sexually Transmitted Diseases Specialty Care Settings*

STD care in primary care settings

At the time of the patient visit

- The following general services, equipment, or tests **should** be available as basic STD care services at the time of the patient visit:
  - Thermometer
  - pH paper
- The following general services, equipment, or tests **could** be available as basic STD services with test results available during the patient visit:
  - Phlebotomy
  - Test for trichomoniasis†
  - Test for bacterial vaginosis§
  - Test for vulvovaginal candidiasis¶
  - Urine dipstick
  - Urinalysis with microscopy
  - Test for pregnancy
  - Test for HIV

Clinical laboratory

- The following tests should be available through clinical laboratory as basic STD care services:
  - Urogenital NAAT for gonorrhea and chlamydia
  - Extragenital (pharynx and rectum) NAAT for gonorrhea and chlamydia
  - Quantitative nontreponemal serologic test for syphilis
  - Treponemal serologic test for syphilis
  - HSV viral culture or PCR
  - HSV serology
  - Fourth-generation antigen/antibody HIV test
  - Oncogenic HPV NAATs with Pap smear
  - nPEP and PrEP
  - Serologic tests for hepatitis A, B, and C
  - Test for pregnancy
- The following tests **could** be available through clinical laboratory as basic STD care services:
  - Gram stain, methylene blue, or gentian violet stain for urethritis
  - Gonorrhea culture
  - Gonorrhea antimicrobial susceptibility testing**
  - NAAT for trichomoniasis

STD care in STD specialty care settings

At the time of the patient visit

- The following general services, equipment, or tests **should** be available as specialized STD care services at the time of the patient visit:
  - Thermometer
  - pH paper
  - Phlebotomy
  - Test for trichomoniasis†
  - Test for bacterial vaginosis§
  - Test for vulvovaginal candidiasis¶
  - Urine dipstick
  - Urinalysis with microscopy
  - Test for pregnancy
  - Gram stain, methylene blue, or gentian violet stain for urethritis
  - On-site qualitative nontreponemal serologic test for syphilis
- The following general services, equipment, or tests **could** be available as specialized STD care services with test results available during the patient visit:
  - Dark-field microscopy for syphilis
  - Test for HIV

Clinical laboratory

- The following tests **should** be available through a clinical laboratory as specialized STD care services:
  - Urogenital NAAT for gonorrhea and chlamydia
  - Extragenital (pharynx and rectum) NAAT for gonorrhea and chlamydia
  - Quantitative nontreponemal serologic test for syphilis
  - Treponemal serologic test for syphilis
  - HSV viral culture or PCR
  - HSV serology
  - Fourth-generation antigen/antibody HIV test
  - Oncogenic HPV NAATs with Pap smear
  - nPEP and PrEP
  - Serologic tests for hepatitis A, B, and C
  - Gonorrhea culture
  - Gonorrhea antimicrobial susceptibility testing**
  - NAAT for trichomoniasis

HIV, human immunodeficiency virus; *HPV,* human papillomavirus; *HSV,* herpes simplex virus; *NAAT,* nucleic acid amplification test; *nPEP,* nonoccupational postexposure prophylaxis; *Pap,* Papanicolaou; *PCR,* polymerase chain reaction; *PrEP,* preexposure prophylaxis; *STD,* sexually transmitted disease.

*Primary care setting is defined as a place where patients are evaluated for various health conditions. STD specialty care setting is defined as a place where the focus is on providing patients with timely, comprehensive, confidential, and culturally sensitive STD care. STD care delivered in STD specialty care settings includes all care delivered in primary care settings.

†On-site test for trichomoniasis can include wet mount microscopy and OSOM Trichomonas.

§On-site test for bacterial vaginosis can include wet mount microscopy, OSOM BVBlue, and Affirm.

¶On-site test for vulvovaginal candidiasis can include wet mount microscopy.

**Access needs to be established for transport medium that adequately maintains the viability of *Neisseria gonorrhoeae* until the specimen reaches a laboratory (e.g., transport medium in transport container, transport system, or transport swab). Providers should contact their state or local health department if they have concerns about resistant *N. gonorrhoeae* infection or if assistance is required for culture and antimicrobial susceptibility testing.

Barrow RY, Ahmed F, Bolan GA, Workowski KA. Recommendations for providing quality sexually transmitted diseases clinical services, 2020, *MMWR Recomm Rep* 2020;68(No. RR-5):1-20. DOI: https://doi.org/10.15585/mmwr.rr6805a1external icon

Prevention of Hepatitis B Virus Infections in the United States

TABLE 20 Recommended Doses of Hepatitis B Vaccine, by Group and Vaccine Type

	SINGLE-ANTIGEN VACCINE				COMBINATION VACCINE			
	RECOMBIVAX		ENGERIX		PEDIARIX*		TWINRIX†	
Age Group (y)	Dose (μg)	Vol (ml)	Dose (μg)	Vol (ml)	Dose (μg)	Vol (ml)	Dose (μg)	Vol (ml)
Birth-10	5	0.5	10	0.5	10*	0.5	N/A	N/A
11-15	10§	1	N/A	N/A	N/A	N/A	N/A	N/A
16-19	5	0.5	10	0.5	N/A	N/A	N/A	N/A
≥20	10	1	20	1	N/A	N/A	20†	1
Hemodialysis Patients and Other Immune-Compromised Persons								
<20	5	0.5	10	0.5	N/A	N/A	N/A	N/A
≥20	40	1	40	2	N/A	N/A	N/A	N/A

N/A, Not applicable.
*Pediarix is approved for use in persons aged 6 weeks through 6 years (before the 7th birthday).
†Twinrix is approved for use in persons aged ≥18 years.
§Adult formulation administered on a 2-dose schedule.
From Schillie S et al: Prevention of hepatitis B virus infection in the United States: Recommendations of the Advisory Committee on Immunization Practices, *MMWR Recomm Rep* 67(No. RR-1):1-31, 2018.

TABLE 21 Hepatitis B Vaccine Schedules for Infants, by Infant Birthweight and Maternal HBsAg Status

		SINGLE-ANTIGEN VACCINE		SINGLE-ANTIGEN + COMBINATION VACCINE†	
Birthweight	Maternal HBsAg Status	Dose	Age	Dose	Age
≥2000 g	Positive	1	Birth (≤12 hr)	1	Birth (≤12 hr)
		HBIG§	Birth (≤12 hr)	HBIG	Birth (≤12 hr)
		2	1-2 mo	2	2 mo
		3	6 mo¶	3	4 mo
				4	6 mo¶
	Unknown*	1	Birth (≤12 hr)	1	Birth (≤12 hr)
		2	1-2 mo	2	2 mo
		3	6 mo¶	3	4 mo
				4	6 mo¶
	Negative	1	Birth (≤24 hr)	1	Birth (≤24 hr)
		2	1-2 mo	2	2 mo
		3	6-18 mo¶	3	4 mo
				4	6 mo¶
<2000 g	Positive	1	Birth (≤12 hr)	1	Birth (≤12 hr)
		HBIG	Birth (≤12 hr)	HBIG	Birth (≤12 hr)
		2	1 mo	2	2 mo
		3	2-3 mo	3	4 mo
		4	6 mo¶	4	6 mo¶
	Unknown	1	Birth (≤12 hr)	1	Birth (≤12 hr)
		HBIG	Birth (≤12 hr)	HBIG	Birth (≤12 hr)
		2	1 mo	2	2 mo
		3	2-3 mo	3	4 mo
		4	6 mo¶	4	6 mo¶
	Negative	1	Hospital discharge or age 1 mo	1	Hospital discharge or age 1 mo
		2	2 mo	2	2 mo
		3	6-18 mo¶	3	4 mo
				4	6 mo¶

HBIG, Hepatitis B immune globulin; *HBsAg*, hepatitis B surface antigen.
*Mothers should have blood drawn and tested for HBsAg as soon as possible after admission for delivery; if the mother is found to be HBsAg positive, the infant should receive HBIG as soon as possible but no later than age 7 days.
†Pediarix should not be administered before age 6 weeks.
§HBIG should be administered at a separate anatomical site from vaccine.
¶The final dose in the vaccine series should not be administered before age 24 weeks (164 days).
From Schillie S et al: Prevention of hepatitis B virus infection in the United States: Recommendations of the Advisory Committee on Immunization Practices, *MMWR Recomm Rep* 67(No. RR-1):1-31, 2018.

TABLE 22 Hepatitis B Vaccine Schedules for Children, Adolescents, and Adults

Age Group	Schedule* (Interval Represents Time in Months from First Dose)
Children (1-10 y)	0, 1, and 6 mo 0, 1, 2, and 12 mo
Adolescents (11-19 y)	0, 1, and 6 mo 0, 12, and 24 mo 0 and 4-6 mo† 0, 1, 2, and 12 mo0, 7 d, 21-30 d, 12 mo§
Adults (≥20 y)	0, 1, and 6 mo 0, 1, 2, and 12 mo 0, 1, 2, and 6 mo¶ 0, 7 d, 21-30 d, 12 mo§

*Refer to package inserts for further information. For all ages, when the HepB vaccine schedule is interrupted, the vaccine series does not need to be restarted. If the series is interrupted after the first dose, the second dose should be administered as soon as possible, and the second and third doses should be separated by an interval of at least 8 weeks. If only the third dose has been delayed, it should be administered as soon as possible. The final dose of vaccine must be administered at least 8 weeks after the second dose and should follow the first dose by at least 16 weeks; the minimum interval between the first and second doses is 4 weeks. Inadequate doses of hepatitis B vaccine or doses received after a shorter-than-recommended dosing interval should be re-administered, using the correct dosage or schedule. Vaccine doses administered ≤4 days before the minimum interval or age are considered valid. Because of the unique accelerated schedule for Twinrix, the 4-day guideline does not apply to the first three doses of this vaccine when administered on a 0-day, 7-day, 21-30-day, and 12-month schedule (new recommendation).

†A 2-dose schedule of Recombivax adult formulation (10 μg) is licensed for adolescents aged 11-15 years. When scheduled to receive the second dose, adolescents aged >15 years should be switched to a 3-dose series, with doses 2 and 3 consisting of the pediatric formulation administered on an appropriate schedule.

§Twinrix is approved for use in persons aged ≥18 years and is available on an accelerated schedule with doses administered at 0, 7, and 21-30 days and 12 months.

¶A 4-dose schedule of Engerix administered in two 1 ml doses (40 μg) on a 0-, 1-, 2-, and 6-month schedule is recommended for adult hemodialysis patients.

From Schillie S et al: Prevention of hepatitis B virus infection in the United States: Recommendations of the Advisory Committee on Immunization Practices, *MMWR Recomm Rep* 67(No. RR-1):1-31, 2018.

TABLE 23 Serology Testing for Needle Stick Injury Exposed Person

		TIME			
		At Exposure	**4-6 Weeks**	**3 Months**	**6 Months**
Low-risk source and negative serology		Anti-HBsAg antigen antibody		HIV and HCV antibodies testing may be offered	
High-risk source or positive serology	HBV	Anti-HBsAg antibody			
	HCV	HCV RNA PCR, Anti-HCV antibody by ELISA	HCV RNA PCR	HCV RNA PCR, Anti-HCV antibody by ELISA	HCV RNA PCR
		ALT, AST	ALT, AST	ALT, AST	
	HIV	Anti-HIV antibodies	Anti-HIV antibodies	Anti-HIV antibodies	
Unknown source, serology results not available		Anti-HBsAg, anti HCV and HIV antibodies		HIV and HCV antibodies	HIV and HCV antibodies

ALT, Alanine amino transferase; *AST*, aspartate amino transferase; *ELISA*, enzyme linked immunosorbent assay; *HBsAg*, hepatitis B surface antigen; *HCV RNA PCR*, hepatitis C virus RNA by polymerase chain reaction; *HIV*, human immunodeficiency virus; *PEP*, postexposure prophylaxis.

From Cameron P, Little M, Mitra B, Deasy C: *Textbook of adult emergency medicine*, ed 5, 2020, Elsevier.

TABLE 24 Postexposure Prophylaxis Drug Recommendations Based on Exposure

Exposure to HIV Positive Source	Estimated Transmission Risk	VL (<50 Copies/ml) Undetectable on ART	VL Unknown on ART	VL Detectable or New HIV Diagnosis Not on ART	VL Detectable on ART
Percutaneous NSI	Extremely low	No PEP or 2 drugs depending on exposure Tenofovir DPO4 + emtricitabine	2 drugs Tenofovir DPO4 + emtricitabine	3 drugs Tenofovir DPO4 + emtricitabine + dolutegravir	Presumed resistance—call HIV specialist for advice
Mucous membrane or nonintact skin	<1/1,000	No drugs	2 drugs Tenofovir DPO4 + emtricitabine	3 drugs Tenofovir DPO4 + emtricitabine + dolutegravir	Presumed resistance—call HIV specialist for advice

ART, Antiretroviral treatment; *NSI*, needle stick injury; *PEP*, postexposure prophylaxis; *VL*, viral load.

From Cameron P, Little M, Mitra B, Deasy C: *Textbook of adult emergency medicine*, ed 5, 2020, Elsevier.

TABLE 25 Postexposure Management of Health Care Personnel after Occupational Percutaneous or Mucosal Exposure to Blood or Body Fluids, by Health Care Personnel HepB Vaccination and Response Status

	POSTEXPOSURE TESTING		POSTEXPOSURE PROPHYLAXIS		
HCP Status	Source Patient (HBsAg)	HCP Testing (Anti-HBs)	HBIG	Vaccination	Postvaccination Serologic Testing
Documented responder after complete series			No action needed		
Documented nonresponder after two complete series	Positive/unknown	–*	HBIG ×2 separated by 1 month	—	N/A
	Negative			No action needed	
Response unknown after complete series	Positive/unknown	<10 mIU/ml	HBIG ×1	Initiate revaccination	Yes
	Negative	<10 mIU/ml	None	Initiate revaccination	Yes
	Any result	≥10 mIU/ml		No action needed	
Unvaccinated/incompletely vaccinated or vaccine refusers	Positive/unknown	—	HBIG ×1	Complete vaccination	Yes
	Negative	—	None	Complete vaccination	Yes

Anti-HBs, Antibody to hepatitis B surface antigen; *HBIG,* hepatitis B immune globulin; *HBsAg,* hepatitis B surface antigen; *HCP,* health care personnel; *N/A,* not applicable.
*Not indicated.
From Schillie S et al: Prevention of hepatitis B virus infection in the United States: Recommendations of the Advisory Committee on Immunization Practices, *MMWR Recomm Rep* 67(No. RR-1):1-31, 2018.

TABLE 26 Postexposure Management after Distinct Nonoccupational Percutaneous or Mucosal Exposure to Blood or Body Fluids

	MANAGEMENT	
Exposure*	Unvaccinated Person	Previously Vaccinated Person
HBsAg-positive source	HepB vaccine series and HBIG	HepB vaccine dose
HBsAg status unknown for source	Hep B vaccine series	No management

HBIG, Hepatitis B immune globulin; *HBsAg,* hepatitis B surface antigen; *HepB,* hepatitis B.
*Exposures include percutaneous (e.g., bite or needlestick) or mucosal exposure to blood or body fluids, sex or needle-sharing contact, or victim of sexual assault/abuse.
From Schillie S et al: Prevention of hepatitis B virus infection in the United States: Recommendations of the Advisory Committee on Immunization Practices, *MMWR Recomm Rep* 67(No. RR-1):1-31, 2018.

BOX 7 Persons Recommended To Receive Hepatitis B Vaccination

- All infants
- Unvaccinated children aged <19 years
- Persons at risk for infection by sexual exposure
  - Sex partners of hepatitis B surface antigen (HBsAg)-positive persons
  - Sexually active persons who are not in a long-term, mutually monogamous relationship (e.g., persons with more than one sex partner during the previous 6 months)
  - Persons seeking evaluation or treatment for a sexually transmitted infection
  - Men who have sex with men
- Persons at risk for infection by percutaneous or mucosal exposure to blood
  - Current or recent injection-drug users
  - Household contacts of HBsAg-positive persons
  - Residents and staff of facilities for developmentally disabled persons
  - Health care and public safety personnel with reasonably anticipated risk for exposure to blood or blood-contaminated body fluids
  - Hemodialysis patients and predialysis, peritoneal dialysis, and home dialysis patients
  - Persons with diabetes aged 19-59 years; persons with diabetes aged ≥60 years at the discretion of the treating clinician
- Others
  - International travelers to countries with high or intermediate levels of endemic hepatitis B virus (HBV) infection (HBsAg prevalence of ≥2%)
  - Persons with hepatitis C virus infection
  - Persons with chronic liver disease (including persons with cirrhosis, fatty liver disease, alcoholic liver disease, autoimmune hepatitis, and an alanine aminotransferase [ALT] or aspartate aminotransferase [AST] level greater than twice the upper limit of normal)
  - Persons with HIV infection
  - Incarcerated persons
- All other persons seeking protection from HBV infection

From Schillie S et al: Prevention of hepatitis B virus infection in the United States: Recommendations of the Advisory Committee on Immunization Practices, *MMWR Recomm Rep* 67(No. RR-1):1-31, 2018.

BOX 8 Testing Anti-Hbs For Health Care Personnel (Hcp) Vaccinated In The Past

The issue: An increasing number of HCP have received routine hepatitis B (HepB) vaccination during childhood. No postvaccination serologic testing is recommended after routine infant or adolescent HepB vaccination. Because vaccine-induced antibody to hepatitis B surface antigen (anti-HBs) wanes over time, testing HCP for anti-HBs years after vaccination might not distinguish vaccine nonresponders from responders.

Guidance for health care institutions: Health care institutions may measure anti-HBs upon hire or matriculation for HCP who have documentation of a complete HepB vaccine series in the past (e.g., as part of routine infant or adolescent vaccination). HCP with anti-HBs <10 mIU/ml should receive one or more additional doses of HepB vaccine and retesting (see Fig. 1). Institutions that decide to not measure anti-HBs upon hire or matriculation for HCP who have documentation of a complete HepB vaccine series in the past should ensure timely assessment and postexposure prophylaxis following an exposure (see Table 25).

Considerations: The risk for occupational HBV infection for vaccinated HCP might be low enough in certain settings so that assessment of anti-HBs status and appropriate follow-up should be done at the time of exposure to potentially infectious blood or body fluids. This approach relies on HCP recognizing and reporting blood and body fluid exposures and therefore may be applied on the basis of documented low risk, implementation, and cost considerations. Certain HCP occupations have lower risk for occupational blood and body fluid exposures (e.g., occupations involving counseling versus performing procedures), and nontrainees have lower risks for blood and body fluid exposures than trainees. Some settings also will have a lower prevalence of HBV infection in the patient population served than in other settings, which will influence the risk for HCP exposure to HBsAg-positive blood and body fluids.

From Schillie S et al: Prevention of hepatitis B virus infection in the United States: Recommendations of the Advisory Committee on Immunization Practices, *MMWR Recomm Rep* 67(No. RR-1):1-31, 2018.

BOX 9 Persons Recommended To Receive Serologic Testing Before Vaccination*

- HIV-positive persons†
- Persons with elevated alanine aminotransferase/aspartate aminotransferase of unknown etiology†
- Hemodialysis patients†
- Men who have sex with men†
- Past or current persons who inject drugs†
- Persons born in countries of high and intermediate hepatitis B virus (HBV) endemicity (HBsAg prevalence ≥2%)
- U.S.-born persons not vaccinated as infants whose parents were born in countries with high HBV endemicity (≥8%)
- Persons needing immunosuppressive therapy, including chemotherapy, immunosuppression related to organ transplantation, and immunosuppression for rheumatologic or gastroenterologic disorders
- Donors of blood, plasma, organs, tissues, or semen

*Serologic testing comprises testing for hepatitis B surface antigen (HBsAg), antibody to HBsAg, and antibody to hepatitis B core antigen.
†Denotes persons also recommended for hepatitis B vaccination. Serologic testing should occur before vaccination. Serologic testing should not be a barrier to vaccination of susceptible persons. The first dose of vaccine should typically be administered immediately after collection of the blood for serologic testing.
From Schillie S et al: Prevention of hepatitis B virus infection in the United States: Recommendations of the Advisory Committee on Immunization Practices, *MMWR Recomm Rep* 67(No. RR-1):1-31, 2018.

BOX 10 Persons Recommended To Receive Postvaccination Serologic Testing* After A Complete Series Of Hepatitis B Vaccination

- Infants born to hepatitis B surface antigen (HBsAg)-positive mothers or mothers whose HBsAg status remains unknown (e.g., when a parent or person with lawful custody safely surrenders an infant confidentially shortly after birth)†
- Health care personnel and public safety workers
- Hemodialysis patients and others who might require outpatient hemodialysis (e.g., predialysis, peritoneal dialysis, and home dialysis)
- HIV-infected persons
- Other immunocompromised persons (e.g., hematopoietic stem-cell transplant recipients or persons receiving chemotherapy)
- Sex partners of HBsAg-positive persons

*Postvaccination serologic testing for persons other than infants born to HBsAg-positive (or HBsAg-unknown) mothers consists of anti-HBs.
†Postvaccination serologic testing for infants born to HBsAg-positive (or HBsAg-unknown) mothers consists of anti-HBs and HBsAg. Persons with anti-HBs <10 mIU/ml after the primary vaccine series should be revaccinated. Infants born to HBsAg-positive mothers or mothers with an unknown HBsAg status should be revaccinated with a single dose of HepB vaccine and receive postvaccination serologic testing 1-2 months later. Infants whose anti-HBs remains <10 mIU/ml after single dose revaccination should receive two additional doses of HepB vaccine, followed by postvaccination serologic testing 1-2 months after the final dose. Based on clinical circumstances or family preference, HBsAg-negative infants with anti-HBs <10 mIU/ml may instead be revaccinated with a second, complete 3-dose series, followed by postvaccination serologic testing performed 1-2 months after the final dose of vaccine. For others with anti-HBs <10 mIU/ml after the primary series, administration of 3 additional HepB vaccine doses on an appropriate schedule, followed by anti-HBs testing 1-2 months after the final dose, is usually more practical than serologic testing after ≥1 dose of vaccine.
From Schillie S et al: Prevention of hepatitis B virus infection in the United States: Recommendations of the Advisory Committee on Immunization Practices, *MMWR Recomm Rep* 67(No. RR-1):1-31, 2018.

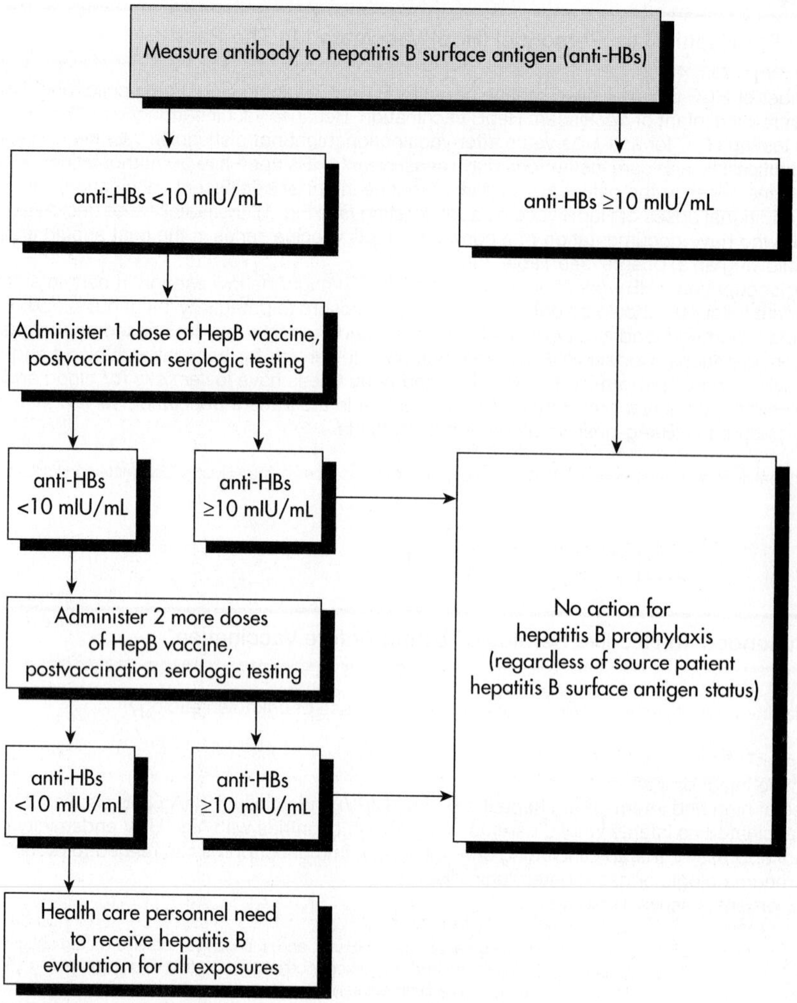

FIG. 1 Preexposure evaluation for health care personnel previously vaccinated with complete ≥3-dose HepB vaccine series who have not had post-vaccination serologic testing.*

*Should be performed 1-2 months after the last dose of vaccine using a quantitative method that allows detection of the protective concentration of anti-HBs (≥10 mIU/ml) (e.g., enzyme-linked immunosorbent assay [ELISA]). (From Schillie S et al: Prevention of hepatitis B virus infection in the United States: Recommendations of the Advisory Committee on Immunization Practices, *MMWR Recomm Rep* 67[No. RR-1]:1-31, 2018.)

(Source: Adapted from CDC: a comprehensive immunization strategy to eliminate transmission of hepatitis B virus infection in the United States: recommendations of the Advisory Committee on Immunization Practices [ACIP]. Part II: immunization of adults, *MMWR* 55 (No.RR-16), 2006.)

Hepatitis A Prophylaxis

TABLE 27 Vaccines Used to Prevent Hepatitis A Virus Infection

Vaccine	Trade Name (manufacturer)	Age group (yrs)	Dosage	Route	Schedule	Booster
HepA, inactivated (2 doses)	Havrix (GlaxoSmithKline)	1-18	0.5 ml (720 ELISA units inactivated HAV)	IM	0, 6-12 months	None
		≥19	1 ml (1,440 ELISA units inactivated HAV)	IM	0, 6-12 months	None
HepA, inactivated (2 doses)	Vaqta (Merck)	1-18	0.5 ml (25 units HAV antigen)	IM	0, 6-18 months	None
		≥19	1 ml (50 units HAV antigen)	IM	0, 6-18 months	None
Combined HepA and HepB* (3 doses)	Twinrix (GlaxoSmithKline)	≥18 (primary)	1 ml (720 ELISA units inactivated HAV + 20 µg HBsAg)	IM	0, 1, 6 months	None
		≥18 (accelerated)	1 ml (720 ELISA units inactivated HAV + 20 µg HBsAg)	IM	0, 7, 21-30 days	12 months

ELISA, enzyme-linked immunosorbent assay; *HAV,* hepatitis A virus; *HBsAg,* hepatitis B surface antigen; *HepA,* hepatitis A; *HepB,* hepatitis B; *IM,* intramuscular.
*Combined HepA and HepB vaccine (Twinrix) should not be used for postexposure prophylaxis.
From Nelson NP, Weng MK, Hofmeister MG et al: Prevention of hepatitis A virus infection in the United States: Recommendations of the Advisory Committee on Immunization Practices, 2020, *MMWR Recomm Rep* 2020;69(No. RR-5):1-38.

TABLE 28 Dosage Recommendations for GamaSTAN Human Immune Globulin for Preexposure and Postexposure Prophylaxis against Hepatitis A Infection

Indication	Time	Dose*	Route
Preexposure prophylaxis	Up to 1 month duration of travel	0.1 ml/kg	IM
Preexposure prophylaxis	Up to 2 months duration of travel	0.2 ml/kg	IM
Preexposure prophylaxis	≥2 months duration of travel	0.2 ml/kg (repeat every 2 months)	IM
Postexposure prophylaxis	Within 2 weeks of exposure	0.1 ml/kg	IM

IM, intramuscular.
*The dosage of immune globulin is based on weight for all ages and does not have a maximum dose for protection against hepatitis A.
Source: Grifols. Treating with GamaSTAN (immune globulin [human]). (https://www.hypermunes.com/en/hcp/gamastan-hepatitis-a). From Nelson NP, Weng MK, Hofmeister MG et al: Prevention of hepatitis A virus infection in the United States: Recommendations of the Advisory Committee on Immunization Practices, 2020, *MMWR Recomm Rep* 2020;69(No. RR-5):1-38.

TABLE 29 Categories of Persons with Increased Risk for Hepatitis A Virus Infection or Severe Disease from Hepatitis A Virus Infection*

Type of Risk	Risk Category	Examples
Increased risk for HAV infection	Close personal contacts of persons with HAV infection†	Household contacts Caretakers Sexual contacts Persons who anticipate close personal contact with an international adoptee
	Occupational risk	Persons working with nonhuman primates Persons working with clinical or nonclinical material containing HAV in a research laboratory
	Persons who use drugs	Persons who use injection or noninjection drugs (i.e., all those who use illegal drugs)
	Persons in settings where services to adults are provided	Group settings for persons with developmental disabilities Homeless shelters Syringe services programs Correctional facilities during outbreaks
	International travelers	Persons traveling to or working in countries with high or intermediate HAV endemicity
Increased risk for severe disease from HAV infection	Immunocompromised persons	Congenital or acquired immunodeficiency HIV infection Chronic renal failure, undergoing dialysis Solid organ, bone marrow, or stem cell transplant recipients Persons with diseases requiring treatment with immunosuppressive drugs/biologics (e.g., tumor necrosis alpha inhibitors), long-term systemic corticosteroids, radiation therapy
	Persons with chronic liver disease	Hepatitis B virus infection Hepatitis C virus infection Cirrhosis (any etiology) Fatty liver disease (hepatic steatosis) Alcoholic liver disease Autoimmune hepatitis Alanine aminotransferase or aspartate amino transferase level more than twice the upper limit of normal or persistently elevated for 6 months
	Age	Adults aged >40 years

HAV, hepatitis A virus; *HIV,* human immunodeficiency virus.
*Not all risk categories include persons recommended for routine hepatitis A vaccination. Providers should assess the risk for HAV infection or severe disease from HAV infection when making decisions regarding the provision of postexposure prophylaxis or revaccination (Table 27). Providers should consider vaccination in settings providing services to adults at risk for HAV infection (see "Implementation Strategies and Hepatitis A Vaccination During Outbreaks").
†Excludes health care personnel using appropriate personal protective equipment.
From Nelson NP, Weng MK, Hofmeister MG et al: Prevention of hepatitis A virus infection in the United States: Recommendations of the Advisory Committee on Immunization Practices, 2020, *MMWR Recomm Rep* 2020;69(No. RR-5):1-38.

TABLE 30 Recommendations for Postexposure Prophylaxis and Preexposure Protection, by Age Group and Risk Category—Advisory Committee on Immunization Practices, 2020

Indication and Age Group	Risk Category and Health Status	HepA Vaccine	IG*
Postexposure Prophylaxis			
<12 months	Healthy	No	0.1 ml/kg
12 months to 40 yrs	Healthy	1 dose†	None
>40 yrs	Healthy	1 dose†	0.1 ml/kg§
≥12 months	Immunocompromised or chronic liver disease	1 dose†	0.1 ml/kg¶
≥12 months	Vaccine contraindicated**	No	0.1 ml/kg
Preexposure Protection (e.g., travel)††			
<6 months	Healthy	No	0.1-0.2 ml/kg§§
6-11 months	Healthy	1 dose¶¶	None
12 months to 40 yrs	Healthy	1 dose***	None
>40 yrs	Healthy	1 dose***	0.1-0.2 ml/kg§§,†††
>6 months	Immunocompromised or chronic liver disease	1 dose***	0.1-0.2 ml/kg§§,†††
>6 months	Persons who elect not to receive vaccine or for whom vaccine is contraindicated**	No	0.1-0.2 ml/kg§§

HAV, hepatitis A virus; *HepA,* hepatitis A; *IG,* immune globulin.
*Measles, mumps, and rubella vaccine should not be administered for at least 2 weeks before and 6 months after administration of IG.
†A second dose of HepA vaccine is not required for postexposure prophylaxis; however, for long-term immunity, the vaccination series should be completed with a second dose at least 6 months after the first dose.
§The provider's risk assessment (Table 26) should determine the need for IG administration. If the provider's risk assessment determines that both vaccine and IG are warranted, HepA vaccine and IG should be administered simultaneously in a different anatomic site (e.g., separate limbs).
¶Vaccine and IG should be administered simultaneously in a different anatomic site (e.g., separate limbs).
**Life-threatening allergic reaction to a previous dose of HepA vaccine or allergy to any vaccine component.
††IG should be considered before travel for persons with special risk factors for either HAV infection or severe disease from HAV infection.
§§0.1 ml/kg for travel up to 1 month; 0.2 ml/kg for travel up to 2 months, 0.2ml/kg every 2 months for travel of ≥2 months' duration.
¶¶This dose should not be counted toward the routine 2-dose series, which should be initiated at age 12 months.
***For persons not previously vaccinated with HepA vaccine, administer dose as soon as travel is considered, and complete series according to routine schedule if the next dose is needed before travel.
†††May be administered based on provider's risk assessment (Table 26).
From Nelson NP, Weng MK, Hofmeister MG et al: Prevention of Hepatitis A Virus Infection in the United States: Recommendations of the Advisory Committee on Immunization Practices, 2020. MMWR Recomm Rep 2020;69(No. RR-5):1-38.

Influenza Treatment and Prophylaxis

BOX 11 Summary Of Seasonal Influenza Vaccination Recommendations

Children

All children aged 6 months to 18 years should be vaccinated annually.

Children and adolescents at higher risk for influenza complications should continue to be a focus for vaccination efforts as providers and programs transition to routinely vaccinating all children and adolescents, including those who:

- Are aged 6 months to 4 years (59 months)
- Have chronic pulmonary (including asthma), cardiovascular (except hypertension), renal, hepatic, cognitive, neurologic/neuromuscular, hematologic, or metabolic disorders (including diabetes mellitus)
- Are immunosuppressed (including immunosuppression caused by medications or by human immunodeficiency virus)
- Are receiving long-term aspirin therapy and therefore might be at risk for experiencing Reye syndrome after influenza virus infection
- Are residents of long-term care facilities
- Will be pregnant during the influenza season

NOTE: Children aged <6 months cannot receive influenza vaccination. Household and other close contacts (e.g., day-care providers) of children aged <6 months, including older children and adolescents, should be vaccinated.

Adults

Annual vaccination against influenza is recommended for any adult who wants to reduce the risk of becoming ill with influenza or of transmitting it to others. Vaccination is recommended for all adults without contraindications in the following groups, because these persons either are at higher risk for influenza complications, or are close contacts of the persons at higher risk:

- Persons aged ≥50 years
- Women who will be pregnant during the influenza season
- Persons who have chronic pulmonary (including asthma), cardiovascular (except hypertension), renal, hepatic, cognitive, neurologic/neuromuscular, hematologic, or metabolic disorders (including diabetes mellitus)
- Persons who have immunosuppression (including immunosuppression caused by medications or by human immunodeficiency virus)
- Residents of nursing homes and other long-term care facilities
- Health care personnel
- Household contacts and caregivers of children aged <5 years and adults aged ≥50 years, with particular emphasis on vaccinating contacts of children aged <6 months
- Household contacts and caregivers of persons with medical conditions that put them at higher risk for severe complications from influenza

Modified from *MMWR*58:(RR-8), 2009.

TABLE 31 Live, Attenuated Influenza Vaccine (LAIV) Compared with Inactivated Influenza Vaccine (TIV) for Seasonal Influenza, U.S. Formulations

Factor	LAIV	TIV
Route of administration	Intranasal spray	Intramuscular injection
Type of vaccine	Live virus	Noninfectious virus (i.e., inactivated)
Number of included virus strains	3 (2 influenza A, 1 influenza B)	3 (2 influenza A, 1 influenza B)
Vaccine virus strains updated	Annually	Annually
Frequency of administration	Annually*	Annually*
Approved age	Persons aged 2-49 yr	Persons aged ≥6 mo
Interval between 2 doses recommended for children aged ≥6 mo to 8 yr who are receiving influenza vaccine for the first time	4 wk	4 wk
Can be administered to persons with medical risk factors for influenza-related complications†	No	Yes
Can be administered to children with asthma or children aged 2-4 yr with wheezing during the preceding year§	No	Yes
Can be administered to family members or close contacts of immunosuppressed persons not requiring a protected environment	Yes	Yes
Can be administered to family members or close contacts of immunosuppressed persons requiring a protected environment (e.g., hematopoietic stem cell transplant recipient)	No	Yes
Can be administered to family members or close contacts of persons at high risk but not severely immunosuppressed	Yes	Yes
Can be simultaneously administered with other vaccines	Yes¶	Yes**
If not simultaneously administered, can be administered within 4 wk of another live vaccine	Prudent to space 4 wk apart	Yes
If not simultaneously administered, can be administered within 4 wk of an inactivated vaccine	Yes	Yes

*Children aged 6 months to 8 years who have never received influenza vaccine before should receive 2 doses. Those who only receive 1 dose in their first year of vaccination should receive 2 doses in the following year, spaced 4 weeks apart.

†Persons at higher risk for complications of influenza infection because of underlying medical conditions should not receive LAIV. Persons at higher risk for complications of influenza infection because of underlying medical conditions include adults and children with chronic disorders of the pulmonary or cardiovascular systems; adults and children with chronic metabolic diseases (including diabetes mellitus), renal dysfunction, hemoglobinopathies, or immunosuppression; children and adolescents receiving long-term aspirin therapy (at risk for developing Reye syndrome after wild-type influenza infection); persons who have any condition (e.g., cognitive dysfunction, spinal cord injuries, seizure disorders, or other neuromuscular disorders) that can compromise respiratory function or the handling of respiratory secretions or that can increase the risk for aspiration; pregnant women; and residents of nursing homes and other chronic-care facilities that house persons with chronic medical conditions.

§Clinicians and immunization programs should screen for possible reactive airways diseases when considering use of LAIV for children aged 2-4 years and should avoid use of this vaccine in children with asthma or a recent wheezing episode. Health care providers should consult the medical record, when available, to identify children aged 2-4 years with asthma or recurrent wheezing that might indicate asthma. In addition, to identify children who might be at greater risk for asthma and possibly at increased risk for wheezing after receiving LAIV, parents or caregivers of children aged 2-4 years should be asked: "In the past 12 months, has a health care provider ever told you that your child had wheezing or asthma?" Children whose parents or caregivers answer "yes" to this question and children who have asthma or who had a wheezing episode noted in the medical record during the preceding 12 months should not receive LAIV.

¶LAIV coadministration has been evaluated systematically only among children aged 12-15 months who received measles, mumps, and rubella vaccine or varicella vaccine.

**TIV coadministration has been evaluated systematically only among adults who received pneumococcal polysaccharide or zoster vaccine.

Modified from *MMWR* 56(RR-6), 2007.

INDICATIONS FOR USE OF ANTIVIRALS

PERSONS FOR WHOM ANTIVIRAL TREATMENT SHOULD BE CONSIDERED

If possible, antiviral treatment should be started within 48 hours of influenza illness onset. The effectiveness of initiating antiviral treatment more than 48 hours after illness onset has not been established. Persons for whom antiviral treatment should be considered include:

- Persons hospitalized with laboratory-confirmed influenza (limited data suggest benefit even for persons whose antiviral treatment is initiated more than 48 hours after illness onset)
- Persons with laboratory-confirmed influenza pneumonia
- Persons with laboratory-confirmed influenza and bacterial coinfection
- Persons with laboratory-confirmed influenza infection who are at higher risk for influenza complications
- Persons presenting to medical care with laboratory-confirmed influenza within 48 hours of influenza illness onset who want to decrease the duration or severity of their symptoms and transmission of influenza to others at higher risk for complications

PERSONS FOR WHOM ANTIVIRAL CHEMOPROPHYLAXIS SHOULD BE CONSIDERED DURING PERIODS OF INCREASED INFLUENZA ACTIVITY IN THE COMMUNITY

- Persons at high risk during the 2 weeks after influenza vaccination (after the second dose for children younger than 9 years who have not previously been vaccinated) if influenza viruses are circulating in the community
- Persons at high risk for whom influenza vaccine is contraindicated
- Family members or health care providers who are unvaccinated and are likely to have ongoing, close exposure to persons at high risk or unvaccinated persons or infants younger than 6 months
- Persons and their family members and close contacts and health care workers when circulating strains of influenza virus in the community are not matched with vaccine strains
- Persons with immune deficiencies or those who might not respond to vaccination (e.g., persons infected with HIV or other immunosuppressed conditions or who are receiving immunosuppressive medications)
- Unvaccinated staff and persons during response to an outbreak in a closed institutional setting with residents at high risk (e.g., extended-care facilities)

Modified from *MMWR* 57(RR-7), 2008.

NOTE: Recommended antiviral medications (neuraminidase inhibitors) are not licensed for chemoprophylaxis of children younger than 1 year (oseltamivir) or younger than 5 years (zanamivir). Updates or supplements to these recommendations (e.g., expanded age or risk group indications for licensed vaccines) might be required. Health care providers should be alert to announcements of recommendation updates and should check the CDC influenza website periodically for additional information (www.cdc.gov/flu).

Testing and Clinical Management of Health Care Personnel Potentially Exposed to Hepatitis C Virus

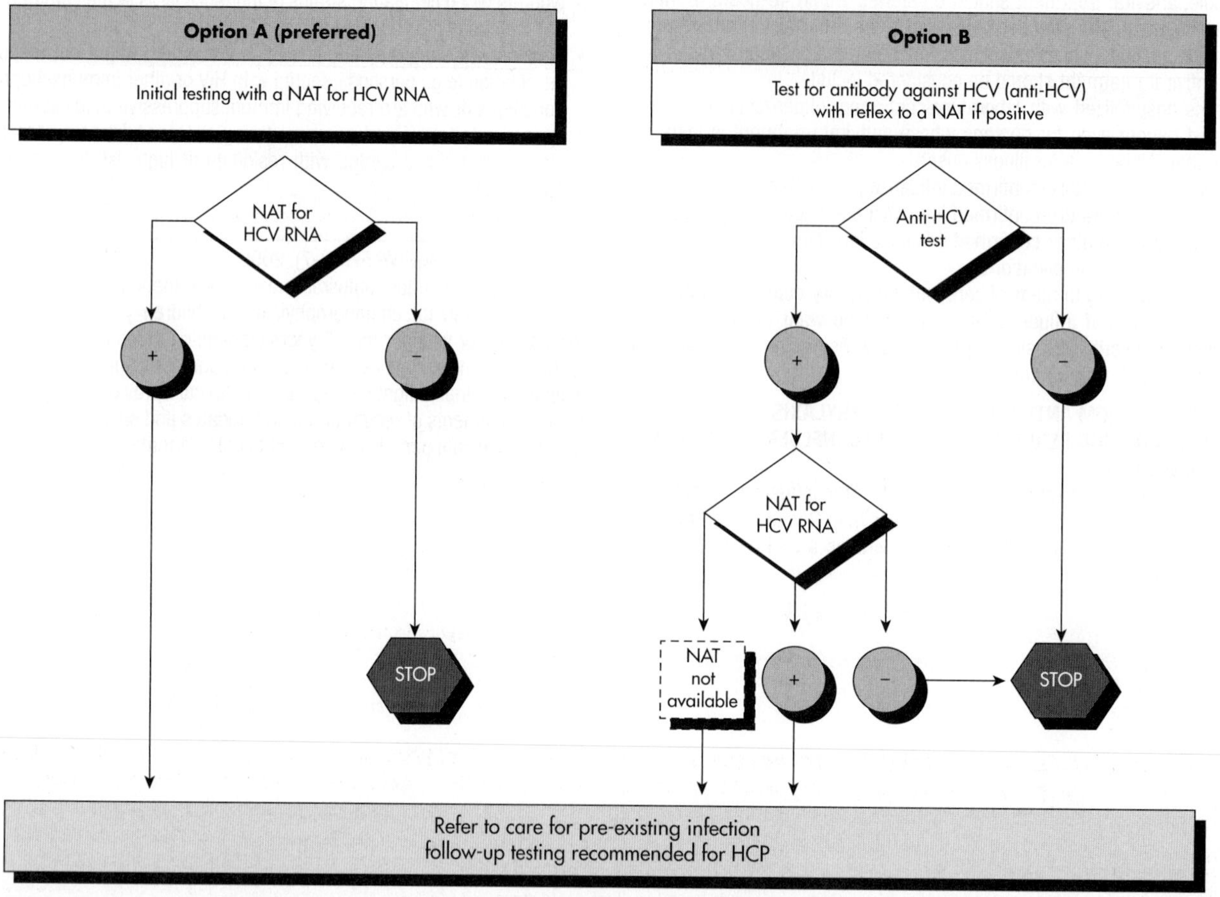

FIG. 2 Testing of source patients after potential exposure of health care personnel to hepatitis C virus—CDC guidance, United States, 2020* (From Moorman AC, de Perio MA, Goldschmidt R et al: Testing and clinical management of health care personnel potentially exposed to hepatitis C virus—CDC Guidance, United States, 2020, *MMWR Recomm Rep* 2020;69(No. RR-6):1-8.) *AASLD-IDSA,* American Association for the Study of Liver Diseases and the Infectious Diseases Society of America; *HCP,* health care personnel; *HCV,* hepatitis C virus; *NAT,* nucleic acid test. ****Testing of the source patient should be performed as soon as possible (preferably within 48 hour) after exposure.*** Testing may follow option A (preferred), which is testing with a NAT for HCV RNA, or option B, which is testing for anti-HCV with reflex to a NAT for HCV RNA if positive. If the source patient is known or suspected to have recent behaviors that increase risk for HCV acquisition (e.g., injection drug use within the previous 4 months) or if risk cannot be reliably assessed, initial testing of the source patient should include an NAT for HCV RNA. A source patient found to be positive for HCV RNA should be referred to care. Follow-up testing of HCP is recommended if the source patient is HCV RNA positive, is anti-HCV positive with HCV RNA status unknown, or cannot be tested. ***Persons with detectable HCV RNA at any point*** should be referred to care consistent with current AASLD-IDSA guidelines for evaluation and treatment of all persons with acute or chronic HCV infection. Guidance for hepatitis C treatment (https://www.hcvguidelines.org) is evolving with emerging data on treatment with direct-acting antivirals.

BOX 12 Testing Of Source Patients And Health Care Personnel Potentially Exposed To Hepatitis C Virus—Cdc Guidance, United States, 2020.

Source-patient testing

- Testing of the source patient may follow option A (preferred), which is testing with a nucleic acid test (NAT) for hepatitis C virus (HCV) RNA, **or** option B, which is testing for anti-HCV with reflex to a NAT if positive.
- If a source patient is known or suspected to have recent behaviors that increase risk for HCV acquisition (e.g., injection drug use within the previous 4 months) or if risk cannot be reliably assessed, initial testing should include a NAT.
- Follow-up testing of health care personnel (HCP) is recommended if the source patient is HCV RNA positive, is anti-HCV positive with RNA status unknown, or cannot be tested.

HCP testing*

- Baseline testing of HCP for anti-HCV with reflex to a NAT if positive should be conducted as soon as possible (preferably within 48 hours) after the exposure and may be simultaneous with source-patient testing.
- If follow-up testing of HCP is recommended based on the source-patient's status, test with an NAT at 3-6 weeks postexposure.
- If the HCP is NAT negative at 3-6 weeks postexposure, a final test for anti-HCV at 4-6 months postexposure is recommended.
- A source patient or HCP who is positive for HCV RNA should be referred to care.

*Follow-up testing of HCP is also warranted when concerns exist about specimen integrity, including handling and storage conditions that might have compromised source-patient test results, or if they exhibit any clinical signs of HCV infection.

From Moorman AC, de Perio MA, Goldschmidt R et al: Testing and clinical management of health care personnel potentially exposed to hepatitis C virus—CDC guidance, United States, 2020, *MMWR Recomm Rep* 2020;69(No. RR-6):1-8.

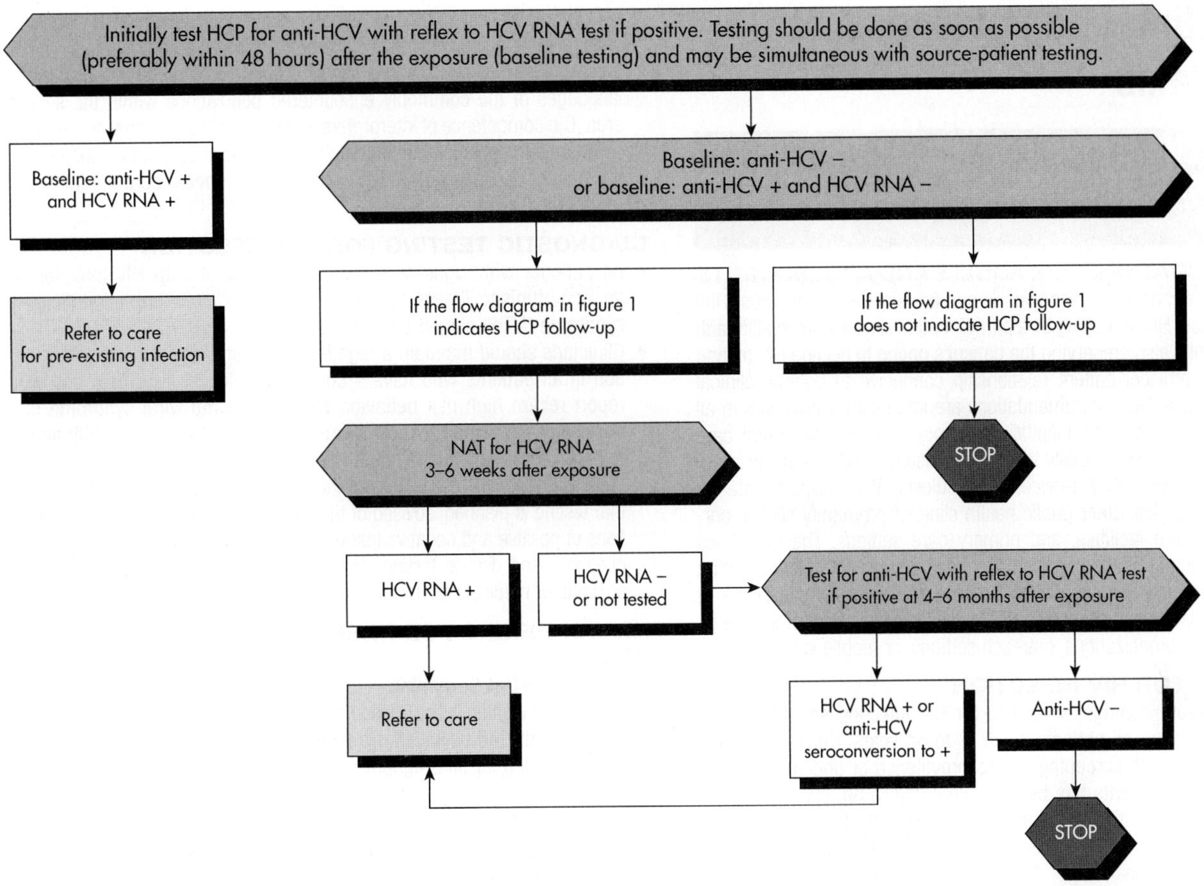

FIG. 3 Testing of health care personnel after potential exposure to hepatitis C virus—CDC guidance, United States, 2020* Abbreviations: *AASLD-IDSA,* American Association for the Study of Liver Diseases and the Infectious Diseases Society of America; *HCP,* health care personnel; *HCV,* hepatitis C virus; *NAT,* nucleic acid test. **Baseline testing of HCP for anti-HCV with reflex to a NAT for HCV RNA if positive should be done as soon as possible* (preferably within 48 hours) after the exposure and may be simultaneous with source-patient testing. ***If follow-up testing is recommended based on the source-patient's status, test for HCV RNA at 3-6 weeks post-exposure.*** Testing for HCV RNA performed at 6 weeks postexposure has the advantage of coinciding with human immunodeficiency virus (HIV) postexposure testing schedules if HIV surveillance is recommended. ***If HCV RNA is negative at 3-6 weeks postexposure, a final test for anti-HCV at 4-6 months postexposure is recommended*** due to the possibility of intermittent periods of aviremia in acute HCV infection. ***If the HCP was anti-HCV positive and HCV RNA negative at baseline, testing at this time should be conducted for HCV RNA detection, as persons successfully treated for HCV infection will remain anti-HCV positive and HCV RNA negative unless reinfected.*** Testing performed at 6 months postexposure has the advantage of coinciding wth hepatitis B virus (HBV) postexposure testing schedules if HBV testing is recommended. ***HCP with anti-HCV seroconversion and negative HCV RNA should be referred for further evaluation.*** False-positive anti-HCV results are known to occur among low-risk populations. Anti-HCV seroconversion occurs on average 8-11 weeks after exposure, although cases of delayed seroconversion have been documented among persons with immunosuppression such as in HIV infection. ***For persons who had a negative anti-HCV result and are immunocompromised, testing for HCV RNA can be considered.*** Also, for persons with a positive anti-HCV and negative HCV RNA result, HCV RNA testing should be repeated if an additional potential HCV exposure occurred within the past 6 months, clinical evidence of HCV infection is present, or concerns exist about specimen integrity, including handling and storage conditions that might have compromised test results. ***Exposed persons who develop viral syndromes suggestive of acute HCV infection at any point*** should be retested for HCV RNA. ***Persons with detectable HCV RNA at any point*** should be referred to care consistent with current AASLD-IDSA guidelines for evaluation and treatment of all persons with acute or chronic HCV infection. Those persons with acute infection should be treated on initial diagnosis without awaiting spontaneous resolution. Guidance for hepatitis C treatment (https://www.hcvguidelines.org) is evolving with emerging data on treatment with direct-acting antivirals. (From Moorman AC, de Perio MA, Goldschmidt R et al: Testing and clinical management of health care personnel potentially exposed to hepatitis C virus—CDC guidance, United States, 2020, *MMWR Recomm Rep* 2020;69(No. RR-6):1-8.)

HIV Testing and Postexposure Prophylaxis

RECOMMENDATIONS FOR HIV TESTING OF ADULTS, ADOLESCENTS, AND PREGNANT WOMEN

RECOMMENDATIONS FOR ADULTS AND ADOLESCENTS

The CDC recommends that diagnostic human immunodeficiency virus (HIV) testing and opt-out HIV screening be a part of routine clinical care in all health care settings while also preserving the patient's option to decline HIV testing and ensuring a provider-patient relationship conducive to optimal clinical and preventive care. The recommendations are intended for providers in all health care settings, including hospital emergency departments, urgent-care clinics, inpatient services, sexually transmitted disease (STD) clinics or other venues offering clinical STD services, tuberculosis (TB) clinics, substance abuse treatment clinics, other public health clinics, community clinics, correctional health care facilities, and primary care settings. The guidelines address HIV testing in health care settings only; they do not modify existing guidelines concerning HIV counseling, testing, and referral for persons at high risk for HIV who seek or receive HIV testing in nonclinical settings (e.g., community-based organizations, outreach settings, or mobile vans).[3]

SCREENING FOR HIV INFECTION

- In all health care settings, screening for HIV infection should be performed routinely for all patients aged 13 to 64 years. Health care providers should initiate screening unless prevalence of undiagnosed HIV infection in their patients has been documented to be less than 0.1%. In the absence of existing data for HIV prevalence, health care providers should initiate voluntary HIV screening until they establish that the diagnostic yield is less than 1 per 1000 patients screened, at which point such screening is no longer warranted.
- All patients initiating treatment for TB should be screened routinely for HIV infection.
- All patients seeking treatment for STDs, including all patients visiting STD clinics, should be screened routinely for HIV during each visit for a new complaint, regardless of whether the patient is known or suspected to have specific behavior risks for HIV infection.

REPEAT SCREENING

- Health care providers should subsequently test all persons likely to be at high risk for HIV at least annually. Persons likely to be at high risk include users of injection drugs and their sex partners, persons who exchange sex for money or drugs, sex partners of persons who are HIV infected, and men who have sex with men (MSM) or heterosexual persons who themselves or whose sex partners have had more than one sex partner since their most recent HIV test.
- Health care providers should encourage patients and their prospective sex partners to be tested before initiating a new sexual relationship.
- Repeat screening of persons not likely to be at high risk for HIV should be performed on the basis of clinical judgment.
- Unless recent HIV test results are immediately available, any person whose blood or body fluid is the source of an occupational exposure for a health care provider should be informed of the incident and tested for HIV infection at the time the exposure occurs.

CONSENT AND PRETEST INFORMATION

- Screening should be voluntary and undertaken only with the patient's knowledge and understanding that HIV testing is planned.
- Patients should be informed orally or in writing that HIV testing will be performed unless they decline (opt-out screening). Oral or written information should include an explanation of HIV infection and the meanings of positive and negative test results, and the patient should be offered an opportunity to ask questions and decline testing. With such notification, consent for HIV screening should be incorporated into the patient's general informed consent for medical care on the same basis as are other screening or diagnostic tests; a separate consent form for HIV testing is not recommended.
- Easily understood informational materials should be made available in the languages of the commonly encountered populations within the service area. The competence of interpreters and bilingual staff to provide language assistance to patients with limited English proficiency must be ensured.
- If a patient declines an HIV test, this decision should be documented in the medical record.

DIAGNOSTIC TESTING FOR HIV INFECTION

- All patients with signs or symptoms consistent with HIV infection or an opportunistic illness characteristic of acquired immunodeficiency syndrome (AIDS) should be tested for HIV.
- Clinicians should maintain a high level of suspicion for acute HIV infection in all patients who have a compatible clinical syndrome and who report recent high-risk behavior. When acute retroviral syndrome is a possibility, a plasma RNA test should be used in conjunction with an HIV antibody test to diagnose acute HIV infection.
- Patients or persons responsible for the patient's care should be notified orally that testing is planned, advised of the indication for testing and the implications of positive and negative test results, and offered an opportunity to ask questions and decline testing. With such notification, the patient's general consent for medical care is considered sufficient for diagnostic HIV testing.

HIV SCREENING FOR PREGNANT WOMEN AND THEIR INFANTS*

Universal Opt-Out Screening

- All pregnant women in the United States should be screened for HIV infection.
- Screening should occur after a woman is notified that HIV screening is recommended for all pregnant patients and that she will receive an HIV test as part of the routine panel of prenatal tests unless she declines (opt-out screening).
- HIV testing must be voluntary and free from coercion. No woman should be tested without her knowledge.
- Pregnant women should receive oral or written information that includes an explanation of HIV infection, a description of interventions that can reduce HIV transmission from mother to infant, and the meanings of positive and negative test results. They should be offered an opportunity to ask questions and decline testing.
- No additional process or written documentation of informed consent beyond what is required for other routine prenatal tests should be required for HIV testing.
- If a patient declines an HIV test, this decision should be documented in the medical record.

ADDRESSING REASONS FOR DECLINING TESTING

- Providers should discuss and address reasons for declining an HIV test (e.g., lack of perceived risk, fear of the disease, and concerns regarding partner violence or potential stigma or discrimination).
- Women who decline an HIV test because they have had a previous negative test result should be informed of the importance of retesting during each pregnancy.
- Logistical reasons for not testing (e.g., scheduling) should be resolved.
- Certain women who initially decline an HIV test might accept at a later date, especially if their concerns are discussed. Certain women will continue to decline testing, and their decisions should be respected and documented in the medical record.

Timing of HIV Testing

- To promote informed and timely therapeutic decisions, health care providers should test women for HIV as early as possible during each pregnancy. Women who decline the test early in prenatal care should be encouraged to be tested at a subsequent visit.
- A second HIV test during the third trimester, preferably less than 36 weeks of gestation, is cost effective even in areas of low HIV prevalence and may be considered for all pregnant women. A second HIV test during the third trimester is recommended for women who meet one or more of the following criteria:
  1. Women who receive health care in jurisdictions with elevated incidence of HIV or AIDS among women aged 15 to 45 years. In 2004, these jurisdictions included Alabama, Connecticut, Delaware, the

[3]Data from *MMWR* 57(RR-10), 2008.

District of Columbia, Florida, Georgia, Illinois, Louisiana, Maryland, Massachusetts, Mississippi, Nevada, New Jersey, New York, North Carolina, Pennsylvania, Puerto Rico, Rhode Island, South Carolina, Tennessee, Texas, and Virginia.[4]

2. Women who receive health care in facilities in which prenatal screening identifies at least one pregnant woman who is infected with HIV per 1000 women screened.
3. Women who are known to be at high risk for acquiring HIV (e.g., users of injection drugs and their sex partners, women who exchange sex for money or drugs, women who are sex partners of persons who are infected with HIV, and women who have had a new or more than one sex partner during this pregnancy).
4. Women who have signs or symptoms consistent with acute HIV infection. When acute retroviral syndrome is a possibility, a plasma RNA test should be used in conjunction with an HIV antibody test to diagnose acute HIV infection.

Rapid Testing During Labor

- Any woman with undocumented HIV status at the time of labor should be screened with a rapid HIV test unless she declines (opt-out screening).
- Reasons for declining a rapid test should be explored (see "Addressing Reasons for Declining Testing").

[4]A second HIV test in the third trimester is as cost effective as other common health interventions when HIV incidence among women of childbearing age is =17 HIV cases per 100,000 person-years. In 2004, in jurisdictions with available data on HIV case rates, a rate of 17 new HIV diagnoses per year per 100,000 women aged 15 to 45 years was associated with an AIDS case rate of at least nine AIDS diagnoses per year per 100,000 women aged 15 to 45 years (CDC, unpublished data, 2005). As of 2004, the jurisdictions listed above exceeded these thresholds. The list of specific jurisdictions where a second test in the third trimester is recommended will be updated periodically based on surveillance data.

- Immediate initiation of appropriate antiretroviral prophylaxis should be recommended to women on the basis of a reactive rapid test result without waiting for the result of a confirmatory test.

Postpartum/Newborn Testing

- When a woman's HIV status is still unknown at the time of delivery, she should be screened immediately postpartum with a rapid HIV test unless she declines (opt-out screening).
- When the mother's HIV status is unknown postpartum, rapid testing of the newborn as soon as possible after birth is recommended so that antiretroviral prophylaxis can be offered to infants exposed to HIV. Women should be informed that identifying HIV antibodies in the newborn indicates that the mother is infected.
- For infants whose HIV exposure status is unknown and who are in foster care, the person legally authorized to provide consent should be informed that rapid HIV testing is recommended for infants whose biologic mothers have not been tested.
- The benefits of neonatal antiretroviral prophylaxis are best realized when it is initiated within 12 hours after birth.

Confirmatory Testing

- Whenever possible, uncertainties regarding laboratory test results indicating HIV infection status should be resolved before final decisions are made regarding reproductive options, antiretroviral therapy, cesarean delivery, or other interventions.
- If the confirmatory test result is not available before delivery, immediate initiation of appropriate antiretroviral prophylaxis should be recommended to any pregnant patient whose HIV screening test result is reactive to reduce the risk for perinatal transmission.

TABLE 32 HIV Exposure, Estimated Per-Act Risk

Exposure Route	Risk per 10,000 Exposures to an Infected Source
Blood transfusion	9000
Needle-sharing injection drug use	67
Receptive anal intercourse	50
Percutaneous needle stick	30
Receptive penile-vaginal intercourse	10
Insertive anal intercourse	6.5
Insertive penile-vaginal intercourse	5
Receptive oral intercourse	1
Insertive oral intercourse	0.5

NOTE: Estimates of risk for transmission from sexual exposures assume no condom use. Source refers to oral intercourse performed on a man.

TABLE 33 Recommended Postexposure Prophylaxis (PEP) for All Occupational Exposures to Human Immunodeficiency Virus (HIV)

PREFERRED HIV PEP REGIMEN	
Raltegravir (Isentress) 400 mg PO (by mouth) twice daily *plus* tenofovir DF (Viread) 300 mg + emtricitabine (Emtriva) 200 mg; available as Truvada, PO once daily	
Alternative Regimens	
May combine one drug or drug pair from the left column with one pair of nucleoside/nucleotide reverse transcriptase inhibitors from the right column	
Dolutegravir (Tivicay)	Tenofovir DF (Viread) + emtricitabine (Emtriva); available as Truvada
Raltegravir (Isentress)	Tenofovir DF (Viread) + emtricitabine (Emtriva); available as Truvada
Darunavir (Prezista) + ritonavir (Norvir)	Tenofovir DF (Viread) + lamivudine (Epivir)
Etravirine (Intelence)	Zidovudine (Retrovir) + lamivudine (Epivir); available as Combivir
Rilpivirine (Edurant)	Zidovudine (Retrovir) + emtricitabine (Emtriva)
Atazanavir (Reyataz) + ritonavir (Norvir)	
Lopinavir/ritonavir (Kaletra)	
Stribild (elvitegravir, cobicistat, tenofovir DF, emtricitabine); a complete fixed-dose combination regimen with no additional antiretrovirals needed	
ALTERNATIVE ANTIRETROVIRAL AGENTS FOR USE AS PEP ONLY WITH EXPERT CONSULTATION	
Abacavir (Ziagen)	
Efavirenz (Sustiva)	
Enfuvirtide (Fuzeon)	
Fosamprenavir (Lexiva)	
Maraviroc (Selzentry)	
Saquinavir (Invirase)	
Stavudine (Zerit)	
ANTIRETROVIRAL AGENTS GENERALLY NOT RECOMMENDED FOR USE AS PEP	
Didanosine (Videx EC)	
Nelfinavir (Viracept)	
Tipranavir (Aptivus)	
ANTIRETROVIRAL AGENTS CONTRAINDICATED AS PEP	
Nevirapine (Viramune)	

Adapted from Kuhar DT et al: Updated U.S. Public Health Service guidelines for the management of occupational exposures to HIV and recommendations for postexposure prophylaxis, *Infect Control Hosp Epidemiol* 2013; 34:875-892. In Cameron JL, Cameron AM: *Current surgical therapy*, ed 12, Philadelphia, 2017, Elsevier.

TABLE 34 Antiretroviral Therapy Medications, Adult Dosage, and Side Effects

Medication	Adult Dosage*	Side Effects and Toxicities
Combination Tablets		
Lopinavir/ritonavir (Kaletra)‡	3 tablets twice daily 400 mg lopinavir/100 mg ritonavir	Diarrhea, nausea, vomiting; asthenia; elevated transaminases; hyperglycemia; fat redistribution; lipid abnormalities; possible increased bleeding in persons with hemophilia; pancreatitis
Zidovudine/lamivudine (Combivir)	1 tablet twice daily 300 mg zidovudine/150 mg lamivudine	See following individual medications
Zidovudine/lamivudine/abacavir (Trizivir)	1 tablet twice daily 300 mg zidovudine/150 mg lamivudine/300 mg abacavir	See following individual medications
Lamivudine/abacavir (Epzicom)	1 tablet once daily 300 mg lamivudine/600 mg abacavir	See following individual medications
Emtricitabine/tenofovir (Truvada)	1 tablet once daily 200 mg emtricitabine/300 mg tenofovir	See following individual medications
Single Agents		
Nucleoside and nucleotide reverse transcriptase inhibitors (side effects as a class: Lactic acidosis, severe hepatomegaly with steatosis, including some fatal cases)		
Abacavir (Ziagen, ABC)‡	300 mg twice daily or 600 mg once daily	Severe hypersensitivity reaction (can be fatal); nausea; vomiting
Didanosine (Videx, ddl)‡	>60 kg (132 lb) body weight: 200 mg twice daily or 400 mg daily; if with tenofovir, 250 mg/daily <60 kg (132 lb): 125 mg twice daily or 250 mg daily; if with tenofovir, dose not established Do not use with stavudine (d4T, Zerit) during pregnancy; avoid ddl/d4T combination in general because of increased risk for adverse events (e.g., neuropathy, pancreatitis, and hyperlactatemia)	Pancreatitis; nausea, diarrhea; peripheral neuropathy
Emtricitabine (Emtriva, FTC)	200 mg once daily	Minimal toxicity; lactic acidosis and hepatic steatosis a rare but possibly life-threatening event
Lamivudine (Epivir, 3TC)‡	150 mg twice daily or 300 mg once daily	Minimal toxicity; lactic acidosis and hepatic steatosis a rare but possibly life-threatening event
Stavudine (Zerit, d4T)‡	>60 kg (132 lb) body weight: 40 mg twice daily <60 kg (132 lb) body weight: 30 mg twice daily Do not use with didanosine (ddl, Videx) during pregnancy; avoid ddl/d4T combination in general because of increased risk of adverse events (e.g., neuropathy, pancreatitis, and hyperlactatemia)	Pancreatitis; peripheral neuropathy; rapidly progressive ascending neuromuscular weakness (rare)
Tenofovir (Viread)	300 mg daily	Nausea, vomiting, diarrhea; headache; asthenia; flatulence; renal impairment
Zidovudine (Retrovir, AZT)‡	200 mg three times daily or 300 mg twice daily	Bone marrow suppression (anemia, neutropenia); gastrointestinal intolerance; headache; insomnia; asthenia; and myopathy
Nonnucleoside reverse transcriptase inhibitors (side effects as a class: Stevens-Johnson syndrome)		
Efavirenz (Sustiva)	600 mg daily at bedtime	Rash; central nervous system symptoms (e.g., dizziness, impaired concentration, insomnia, and abnormal dreams); transaminase elevation; false-positive cannabinoid test
Protease inhibitors (side effects as a class: Gastrointestinal intolerance, hyperlipidemia, hyperglycemia, diabetes, fat redistribution, and possible increased bleeding in hemophiliacs; do not use during known or possible pregnancy)		
Atazanavir (Reyataz)	400 mg once daily; if administered with tenofovir plus ritonavir, 300 mg once daily	Indirect hyperbilirubinemia; prolonged PR interval (use caution in patients with underlying cardiac conduction defects or on concomitant medications that can cause PR prolongation)
Fosamprenavir (Lexiva)‡	1400 mg twice daily	Gastrointestinal intolerance, nausea, vomiting, diarrhea; rash; elevated transaminases; headache
Indinavir (Crixivan)	800 mg q8h With ritonavir (might increase risk for renal adverse events): 800 mg indinavir and 100 mg ritonavir q12h or 800 mg indinavir and 200 mg ritonavir q12h	Gastrointestinal intolerance, nausea; nephrolithiasis; headache; asthenia; blurred vision; metallic taste; thrombocytopenia; hemolytic anemia; indirect hyperbilirubinemia (inconsequential)
Nelfinavir (Viracept)‡	750 mg three times daily or one 250 mg twice daily	Diarrhea; elevated transaminases
Ritonavir (Norvir)‡	See doses used in combination with other specific protease inhibitors	Gastrointestinal intolerance; nausea, vomiting, diarrhea; paresthesias; hepatitis; pancreatitis; asthenia; taste perversion; many drug interactions
Saquinavir (hard-gel capsule) (Invirase)	With ritonavir: 400 mg saquinavir and 400 mg ritonavir twice daily or 1000 mg saquinavir and 100 mg ritonavir twice daily	Gastrointestinal intolerance; nausea, diarrhea; headache; elevated transaminases
Saquinavir (soft-gel capsule) (Fortovase)	With ritonavir: 400 mg saquinavir and 400 mg ritonavir twice daily or 1000 mg saquinavir and 100 mg ritonavir twice daily	Gastrointestinal intolerance; nausea, diarrhea; abdominal pain; dyspepsia; headache; elevated transaminases

*For pediatric dosing information, see *Guidelines for use of antiretroviral agents in pediatric HIV infection.* Available at aidsinfo.nih.gov/guidelines/html/2/pediatric-arv/108/role-of-therapeutic-drug-monitoring-in-management-of-pediatric-hiv-infection.

‡Pediatric formulation available.

Sources: Modified from U.S. Department of Health and Human Services and the Henry J. Kaiser Family Foundation: *Guidelines for the use of antiretroviral agents in HIV-infected adults and adolescents.* Available at aidsinfo.nih.gov/guidelines/html/1/adult-and-adolescent-arv/0 (refer to website for updated versions); Bartlett JG, Finkbeiner AK: HIV drugs: the guide to living with HIV infection, 2001. Available at www.thebody.com/content/art32314.html.

TABLE 35 Laboratory Tests Generally Recommended for Persons after Exposure to HIV*

Test	RECOMMENDED DURING TREATMENT		RECOMMENDED AT FOLLOW-UP		
	Baseline	**Symptom-Directed†**	**4-6 Wk**	**12 Wk**	**24 Wk**
ELISA for HIV antibodies	Yes	Yes	Yes	Yes	Yes
Creatinine, liver function, and complete blood count with differential count	Yes	Yes	No	No	No
HIV viral load	No	Yes	No	No	No
Anti-HBs antibodies	Yes‡	No	No	No	No
HBsAg	Yes‡,§	No	No	No	No
HCV antibodies	Yes	No	Yes	Yes	Yes
HCV RNA‖	No	Yes	Yes	Yes	Yes
Screening, including rapid plasma reagin test, for other sexually transmitted infections¶	Yes	Yes	No	Yes	No

Anti-HBs antibodies, Hepatitis B virus surface antibodies; *ELISA,* enzyme-linked immunosorbent assay; *HBsAg,* hepatitis B surface antigen; *HCV,* hepatitis C virus.
*Patients who receive zidovudine plus lamivudine–based regimens should have a complete blood count and measurement of liver-enzyme levels at 2 weeks of treatment, irrespective of the presence or absence of clinical symptoms. Tenofovir plus emtricitabine–based regimens generally involve few side effects, and symptom-directed assessment of serum creatinine or liver-enzyme levels should be considered. The addition of a ritonavir-boosted protease inhibitor should be followed by symptom-directed assessment of liver-enzyme levels, serum glucose levels, or both.
†Symptom-directed tests are for signs or symptoms of toxic effects (rash, nausea, vomiting, or abdominal pain) or HIV seroconversion (fever, fatigue, lymphadenopathy, rash, or oral or genital ulcers).
‡If tests for anti-HBs antibodies and HBsAg are both negative, a vaccination series against HBV infection should be initiated and completed.
§If the patient is HBsAg-positive, he or she should have monthly follow-up of liver function tests after discontinuation of postexposure prophylactic regimens containing tenofovir, lamivudine, or emtricitabine; referral to a specialist in viral hepatitis should be considered.
‖HCV RNA testing may identify early HCV seroconversion; early detection and treatment during acute HCV infection may avert or ameliorate chronic disease. Data are from Dienstag and McHutchison.
¶Rapid plasma reagin testing and testing of urethral-swab and rectal-swab specimens for gonorrhea and chlamydia and of pharyngeal-swab specimens for gonorrhea should be performed as appropriate, according to the patient's sexual risk-taking behaviors and the type of exposure to HIV.
From Landovitz RJ, Currier JS: Postexposure prophylaxis for HIV infection, *N Engl J Med* 361:1768-1775, 2009.

BOX 13 Situations For Which Expert Consultation For Hiv Postexposure Prophylaxis Is Advised[5]

- Delayed (i.e., later than 24-36 hours) exposure report
  1. The interval after which there is no benefit from postexposure prophylaxis (PEP) is undefined
- Unknown source (e.g., needle in sharps disposal container or laundry)
  1. Decide use of PEP on a case-by-case basis
  2. Consider the severity of the exposure and the epidemiologic likelihood of HIV exposure
  3. Do not test needles or other sharp instruments for HIV
- Known or suspected pregnancy in the exposed person
  1. Does not preclude the use of optimal PEP regimens
  2. Do not deny PEP solely on the basis of pregnancy
- Resistance of the source virus to antiretroviral agents
  1. Influence of drug resistance on transmission risk is unknown
  2. Selection of drugs to which the source person's virus is unlikely to be resistant is recommended if the source person's virus is known or suspected to be resistant to one or more of the drugs considered for the PEP regimen
  3. Resistance testing of the source person's virus at the time of the exposure is not recommended
- Toxicity of the initial PEP regimen
  1. Adverse symptoms such as nausea and diarrhea are common with PEP
  2. Symptoms often can be managed without changing the PEP regimen by prescribing antimotility and/or antiemetic agents
  3. Modification of dose intervals (i.e., administering a lower dose of drug more frequently throughout the day, as recommended by the manufacturer) in other situations might help alleviate symptoms

[5]Local experts and/or the National Clinicians' Postexposure Prophylaxis Hotline (PEPline [888-448-4911]).

BOX 14 Occupational Exposure Management Resources

National Clinicians' Postexposure Prophylaxis Hotline (PEPline) Run by University of California–San Francisco/San Francisco General Hospital staff; supported by the Health Resources and Services Administration, Ryan White CARE Act, HIV/AIDS Bureau, AIDS Education and Training Centers, and CDC	Phone: 888-448-4911 Internet: nccc.ucsf.edu/clinician-consultation;/pep-post-exposure-prophylaxis/
Hepatitis Hotline	Phone: 888-443-7232 Internet: www.cdc.gov/ncidod/diseases/hepatitis/index.htm
Reporting to CDC: Occupationally acquired HIV infections and failures of PEP	Phone: 800-893-0485
HIV Antiretroviral Pregnancy Registry	Phone: 800-258-4263 Fax: 800-800-1052 Address: 1410 Commonwealth Dr., Suite 215, Wilmington, NC 28405 Internet: www.apregistry.com/
Food and Drug Administration Report unusual or severe toxicity to antiretroviral agents	Phone: 800-332-1088 Address: MedWatch, HF-2, FDA, 5600 Fishers Lane, Rockville, MD 20857 Internet: www.fda.gov/medwatch
HIV/AIDS Treatment Information Service	Internet: www.hivatis.org

BOX 15 Management Of Occupational Blood Exposures

Provide Immediate Care to the Exposure Site
- Wash wounds and skin with soap and water
- Flush mucous membranes with water

Determine Risk Associated with Exposure
- Type of fluid (e.g., blood, visibly bloody fluid, other potentially infectious fluid or tissue, and concentrated virus)
- Type of exposure (e.g., percutaneous injury, mucous membrane or nonintact skin exposure, and bites resulting in blood exposure)

Evaluate Exposure Source
- Assess the risk of infection using available information
- Test known sources for HBsAg, anti-HCV, and HIV antibodies (consider using rapid testing)
- For unknown sources, assess risk of exposure to HBV, HCV, or HIV infection
- Do not test discarded needles or syringes for virus contamination

Evaluate the Exposed Person
- Assess immune status for HBV infection (i.e., by history of hepatitis B vaccination and vaccine response)

Give PEP for Exposures Posing Risk of Infection Transmission
- HBV: See Table 5
- HCV: PEP not recommended
- HIV: See Tables 33, 34, and 35
  1. Initiate PEP as soon as possible, preferably within hours of exposure
  2. Offer pregnancy testing to all women of childbearing age not known to be pregnant
  3. Seek expert consultation if viral resistance is suspected
  4. Administer PEP for 4 weeks if tolerated

Perform Follow-up Testing and Provide Counseling
- Advise exposed persons to seek medical evaluation for any acute illness occurring during follow-up

HBV Exposures
- Perform follow-up anti-HBs testing in persons who receive hepatitis B vaccine
  1. Test for anti-HBs 1-2 months after last dose of vaccine
  2. Anti-HBs response to vaccine cannot be ascertained if HBIG was received in the previous 3-4 months

HCV Exposures
- Perform baseline and follow-up testing for anti-HCV and alanine aminotransferase 4-6 months after exposure
- Perform HCV RNA at 4-6 weeks if earlier diagnosis of HCV infection desired
- Confirm repeatedly reactive anti-HCV enzyme immunoassays with supplemental tests

HIV Exposures
- Perform HIV-antibody testing for at least 6 months after exposure (e.g., at baseline, 6 weeks, 3 months, and 6 months)
- Perform HIV-antibody testing if illness compatible with an acute retroviral syndrome occurs
- Advise exposed persons to use precautions to prevent secondary transmission during the follow-up period
- Evaluate exposed persons taking PEP within 72 hr after exposure and monitor for drug toxicity for at least 2 weeks

HBIG, Hepatitis B immune globulin; *HBsAg,* hepatitis B surface antigen; *HBV,* hepatitis B virus; *HCV,* hepatitis C virus; *HIV,* human immunodeficiency virus; *PEP,* postexposure prophylaxis; *RNA,* ribonucleic acid.

ENDOCARDITIS PROPHYLAXIS[6]

TABLE 36 Cardiac Conditions Associated with the Highest Risk of Adverse Outcome from Endocarditis for Which Prophylaxis with Dental Procedures Is Recommended

Prosthetic cardiac valve
Previous infective endocarditis
CHD*
Unrepaired cyanotic CHD, including palliative shunts and conduits
Completely repaired congenital heart defect with prosthetic material or device, whether placed by surgery or by catheter intervention, during the first 6 mo after the procedure†
Repaired CHD with residual defects at the site or adjacent to the site of a prosthetic patch or prosthetic device (that inhibit endothelialization)
Cardiac transplant recipients who develop cardiac valvulopathy

CHD, Congenital heart disease.
*Except for the conditions listed above, antibiotic prophylaxis is no longer recommended for any other form of CHD.
†Prophylaxis is recommended because endothelialization of prosthetic material occurs within 6 mo after the procedure.

TABLE 37 Dental Procedures for Which Endocarditis Prophylaxis Is Recommended for Patients in Table 36

All dental procedures that involve manipulation of gingival tissue or the periapical region of teeth or perforation of the oral mucosa*

*The following procedures and events do not need prophylaxis: Routine anesthetic injections through noninfected tissue, taking dental radiographs, placement of removable prosthodontic or orthodontic appliances, adjustment of orthodontic appliances, placement of orthodontic brackets, shedding of deciduous teeth, and bleeding from trauma to the lips or oral mucosa.

TABLE 38 Regimens for a Dental Procedure

	REGIMEN: SINGLE DOSE 30-60 MIN BEFORE PROCEDURE		
Situation	**Agent**	**Adults**	**Children**
Oral	Amoxicillin	2 g	50 mg/kg
Unable to take oral medication	Ampicillin OR	2 g IM or IV	50 mg/kg IM or IV
	Cefazolin or ceftriaxone*	1 g IM or IV	50 mg/kg IM or IV
Allergic to penicillins or ampicillin, oral	Cephalexin OR	2 g	50 mg/kg
	Clindamycin OR	600 mg	20 mg/kg
	Azithromycin or clarithromycin	500 mg	15 mg/kg
Allergic to penicillins or ampicillin and unable to take oral medicine	Cefazolin or ceftriaxone† OR	1 g IM or IV	50 mg/kg IM or IV
	Clindamycin	600 mg IM or IV	20 mg/kg IM or IV

IM, Intramuscular; *IV,* intravenous.
*Or other first-generation or second-generation oral cephalosporin in equivalent adult or pediatric dosage.
†Cephalosporins should not be used in an individual with a history of anaphylaxis, angioedema, or urticaria with penicillins or ampicillin.

[6]From Prevention of infective endocarditis. A guideline from the American Heart Association Rheumatic Fever, Endocarditis, and Kawasaki Disease Committee, Council on Cardiovascular Disease in the Young, and the Council on Clinical Cardiology, Council on Cardiovascular Surgery and Anesthesia, and the Quality of Care and Outcomes Research Interdisciplinary Working Group. Circulation published online Apr 19, 2007, DOI: 10.1161/CIRCULATIONAHA.106.183095. Print ISSN: 0009-7322. Online ISSN: 1524-4539.

TABLE 39 Summary of Major Changes in Updated Recommendations

We concluded that bacteremia resulting from daily activities is much more likely to cause IE than bacteremia associated with a dental procedure.

We concluded that only an extremely small number of cases of IE might be prevented by antibiotic prophylaxis even if prophylaxis is 100% effective.

Antibiotic prophylaxis is not recommended based solely on an increased lifetime risk of acquisition of IE.

Limit recommendations for IE prophylaxis only to those conditions listed in Table 36.

Antibiotic prophylaxis is no longer recommended for any other form of CHD, except for the conditions listed in Table 36.

Antibiotic prophylaxis is recommended for all dental procedures that involve manipulation of gingival tissues or periapical region of teeth or perforation of oral mucosa only for patients with underlying cardiac conditions associated with the highest risk of adverse outcome from IE (see Table 36).

Antibiotic prophylaxis is recommended for procedures on respiratory tract or infected skin, skin structures, or musculoskeletal tissue only for patients with underlying cardiac conditions associated with the highest risk of adverse outcome from IE (see Table 36).

Antibiotic prophylaxis solely to prevent IE is not recommended for GU or GI tract procedures.

The writing group reaffirms the procedures noted in the 1997 prophylaxis guidelines for which endocarditis prophylaxis is not recommended and extends this to other common procedures, including ear and body piercing, tattooing, and vaginal delivery and hysterectomy.

NOTE: A guide to the clinical preventive services described is available online at www.ahrq.gov/clinic/pocketgd07/. *CHD,* Congenital heart disease; *GI,* gastrointestinal; *GU,* genitourinary; *IE,* infective endocarditis.

Recommendations for Meningococcal Vaccination

TABLE 40 Recommendations for Meningococcal Vaccination of Children at Increased Risk for Meningococcal Disease

Vaccine	Age of Primary Vaccination	Booster Doses	Indicated for Infants	Not Indicated for Infants
MenACWY-CRM (Menveo)	2, 4, 6, and 12 mo	1st booster 3 yr after primary series Additional boosters every 5 yr	Complement component deficiencies Functional or anatomic asplenia The risk groups for an outbreak for which vaccination is recommended Traveling to or residing in epidemic or hyperendemic regions	
MenACWY-D (Menactra)	9 and 12 mo	1st booster 3 yr after primary series Additional boosters every 5 yr	Complement component deficiencies The risk groups for an outbreak for which vaccination is recommended Traveling to or residing in epidemic or hyperendemic regions	Functional or anatomic asplenia
Hib-MenCY-TT (MenHibrix)	2, 4, 6, and 12-15 mo	1st booster (using MenACWY-CRM or MenACWY-D) 3 yr after primary series	1st booster 3 yr after primary series	Traveling to or residing in epidemic or hyperendemic regions
MenB-FHbp (Trumenba)	3-dose series, with 2nd and 3rd doses after 2 and 6 mo after 1st dose; 2nd dose 6 mo after 1st dose is an option	None	≥10 yr at increased risk for serogroup B disease (complement component deficiencies, functional or anatomic asplenia, the risk groups for an outbreak for which vaccination is recommended)	Children aged <10 yr Traveling to or residing in epidemic or hyperendemic regions
MenB-4C (Bexsero)	2-dose series, with doses at least 1 mo apart	None	≥10 yr at increased risk for serogroup B disease (complement component deficiencies, functional or anatomic asplenia, the risk groups for an outbreak for which vaccination is recommended)	Children aged <10 yr Traveling to or residing in epidemic or hyperendemic regions

From Cherry JD: *Feigin and Cherry's pediatric infectious diseases*, ed 8, Philadelphia, 2019, Elsevier.

Vaccine Websites and Resources

TABLE 41 Vaccine Websites and Resources

Organization	Website
Health Professional Associations	
American Academy of Family Physicians (AAFP)	www.familydoctor.org/online/famdocen/home.html
American Academy of Pediatrics (AAP)	www.aap.org/
AAP Childhood Immunization Support Program	www.aap.org/immunization/
American Association of Occupational Health Nurses (AAOHN)	www.aaohn.org/
American College Health Association (ACHA)	www.acha.org/
American College of Obstetricians and Gynecologists (ACOG)–Immunization for Women	www.immunizationforwomen.org/
American Medical Association (AMA)	www.ama-assn.org/
American Nurses Association (ANA)	www.nursingworld.org/
American Pharmacists Association (APhA)	www.pharmacist.com/
American School Health Association (ASHA)	www.ashaweb.org/
American Travel Health Nurses Association (ATHNA)	www.athna.org/
Association for Professionals in Infection Control and Epidemiology (APIC)	www.apic.org/
Association of State and Territorial Health Officials (ASTHO)	www.astho.org/
Association of Teachers of Preventive Medicine (ATPM)	www.atpm.org/
National Medical Association (NMA)	www.nmanet.org/
Society of Teachers of Family Medicine—Group on Immunization Education	www.immunizationed.org/
Nonprofit Groups and Universities	
Albert B. Sabin Vaccine Institute	www.sabin.org/
Brighton Collaboration	brightoncollaboration.org/public
Center for Vaccine Awareness and Research—Texas Children's Center	www.texaschildrens.org/departments/immunization-project
Children's Vaccine Program	www.path.org/vaccineresources/
Every Child by Two (ECBT)	www.ecbt.org/
Families Fighting Flu	www.familiesfightingflu.org/
GAVI, the Vaccine Alliance	www.gavialliance.org/
Health on the Net Foundation (HON)	www.hon.ch/
Immunization Action Coalition (IAC)	www.immunize.org/
Infectious Diseases Society of America (IDSA)	www.idsociety.org/Index.aspx
Institute for Vaccine Safety (IVS), Johns Hopkins Bloomberg School of Public Health	www.vaccinesafety.edu/
National Academies: Health and Medicine Division	www.nationalacademies.org/hmd/
National Alliance for Hispanic Health	www.hispanichealth.org/
National Foundation for Infectious Diseases (NFID)	www.nfid.org
National Foundation for Infectious Diseases (NFID)—Childhood Influenza Immunization Coalition (CIIC)	www.preventchildhoodinfluenza.com/
National Network for Immunization Information (NNii)	www.immunizationinfo.net/
Parents of Kids with Infectious Diseases (PKIDS)	www.pkids.org/
PATH Vaccine Resource Library	www.path.org/vaccineresources/
Vaccine Education Center at the Children's Hospital of Philadelphia	www.chop.edu/service/vaccine-education-center/home.html
Vaccinate Your Baby	www.vaccinateyourbaby.org/
Government Organizations	
Centers for Disease Control and Prevention (CDC)	
Advisory Committee on Immunization Practices (ACIP)	www.cdc.gov/vaccines/acip/index.html
ACIP Vaccine Recommendations	www.cdc.gov/vaccines/hcp/acip-recs/index.html
Current Vaccine Delays and Shortages	www.cdc.gov/vaccines/vac-gen/shortages/
Epidemiology and Prevention of Vaccine-Preventable Diseases (also known as the *Pink Book*)	www.cdc.gov/vaccines/pubs/pinkbook/index.html
Manual for the Surveillance of Vaccine-Preventable Diseases	www.cdc.gov/vaccines/pubs/surv-manual/index.html
Public Health Image Library	phil.cdc.gov/phil/home.asp
Travelers' Health	www.cdc.gov/travel/
CDC Health Information for International Travel (also known as the *Yellow Book*)	wwwnc.cdc.gov/travel/yellowbook/2016/table-of-contents
Vaccine Adverse Events Reporting System (VAERS)	www.cdc.gov/vaccinesafety/Activities/vaers.html
Vaccine Administration: Recommendations and Guidelines	www.cdc.gov/vaccines/recs/vac-admin/default.htm
Vaccines and Immunizations	www.cdc.gov/vaccines/
Vaccines for Children Program	www.cdc.gov/vaccines/programs/vfc/index.html
Vaccines for Children—Vaccine Price List	www.cdc.gov/vaccines/programs/vfc/awardees/vaccine-management/price-list/index.html
Vaccine Information Statements	www.cdc.gov/vaccines/hcp/vis/index.html
Vaccine Safety	www.cdc.gov/vaccinesafety/index.html
Vaccine Storage and Handling	www.cdc.gov/vaccines/recs/storage/default.htm
Department of Health and Human Services (HHS)	
National Vaccine Program Office (NVPO)	www.hhs.gov/nvpo/
Health Resources and Services Administration	
National Vaccine Injury Compensation Program	www.hrsa.gov/vaccinecompensation/
National Institute of Allergy and Infectious Diseases (NIAID)	
Vaccines	www.niaid.nih.gov/about/vrc
World Health Organization (WHO)	
Immunization, Vaccines, and Biologicals	www.who.int/immunization/en/

From Kliegman RM: *Nelson textbook of pediatrics,* ed 21, Philadelphia, 2020, Elsevier.

APPENDIX

Appendix Ia

Definitions of Complementary and Alternative Medicine Terms

Acupuncture: Thin needles are inserted superficially on the skin at locations throughout the body. These points are located along "channels" of energy. Heat can be applied by burning (moxibustion), electric current (electroacupuncture), or pressure (acupressure). Healing is proposed by the restoration of a balance of energy flow called *Qi.* Another explanation suggests that, possibly, the stimulation activates endorphin receptors.

Alexander Technique: A bodywork technique in which rebalancing of "postural sets" (i.e., physical alignment) is taught by mentally focusing on the way correct alignments should look and feel and through verbal and tactile guidance by the practitioner.

Applied Kinesiology: A form of treatment that uses nutrition, physical manipulation, vitamins, diets, and exercise to restore and energize the body. Weak muscles are proposed as a source of dysfunctional health.

Aromatherapy: A form of complementary medicine that uses various plant oils such as those from lavender. Route of administration can be through absorption in the skin or inhalation. The aromatic biochemical structures of certain plants are thought to act in areas of the brain related to past experiences and emotions (e.g., limbic system).

Ayurveda: A major health system that originated in India and incorporates the body, mind, and spirit to prevent and treat disease. Includes special types of diets, herbs, and minerals.

Biofeedback: A mind-body therapy procedure in which sensors are placed on the body to measure muscle tension, heart rate, and sweat responses or neural activity. Information is provided by visual, auditory, or body-muscle cell activation so as to teach either to increase or decrease physiologic activity, which, when reconstituted, is proposed to improve health problems (e.g., pain, anxiety, or high blood pressure). In some cases, relaxation exercises complement this procedure.

Chelation Therapy: Involves the removal—through intravenous infusion of a chelating agent (synthetic amino acid ethylenediamine tetraacetic acid [EDTA])—of heavy metals, including lead, nickel, and cadmium, as a way to treat certain diseases. Chelation therapy has been promoted for the treatment of heart disease, autism, and Alzheimer disease and as an "anti-aging" therapy. Minimal evidence supports these uses.

Cognitive Therapy: Psychological therapy in which the major focus is altering and changing irrational beliefs through a type of Socratic dialogue and self-evaluation of certain illogical thoughts. Conditioning and learning are important components of this therapy.

Craniosacral Therapy: A form of gentle manual manipulation used for diagnosis and for making corrections in a system made up of cerebrospinal fluid, cranial and dural membranes, cranial bones, and sacrum. This system is proposed to be dynamic, with its own physiologic frequency. Through touch and pressure, tension is proposed to be reduced and cranial rhythms normalized, leading to improvement in health and disease.

Diathermy: The use of high-frequency electrical currents as a form of physical therapy and in surgical procedures. The term *diathermy,* derived from the Greek words *dia* and *therma,* literally means "heating through." The three forms of diathermy used by physical therapists are short wave, ultrasound, and microwave.

Eye Movement Desensitization and Reprocessing (EMDR): A technique that proposes to remove painful memories by behavioral techniques. Rhythmic, multisaccadic eye movements are produced by allowing the patient to track and follow a moving object while imagining a stressful memory or event. By using deconditioning, including verbal interaction with the therapist, the painful memory is extinguished and health improved.

Feldenkrais Method: A bodywork technique that integrates physics, judo, and yoga. The practitioner directs sequences of movement using verbal or hands-on techniques or teaches a system of self-directed exercise to treat physical impairments through the learning of new movement patterns.

Hatha Yoga: The branch of yoga practice that involves physical exercise, breathing practices, and movement. These exercises are designed to have a salutary effect on posture, flexibility, and strength and are intended ultimately to prepare the body to remain still for long periods of meditation.

Hellerwork: A bodywork technique that treats and improves proper body alignment through the development of a more complete awareness of the physical body. The goal is to realign fascia for improvement of standing, sitting, and breathing using "body energy," verbal feedback, and changing emotions and attitudes.

Homeopathy: A form of treatment in which substances (minerals, plant extracts, chemicals, or disease-producing germs), which in sufficient doses would produce a set of illness symptoms in healthy individuals, are given in microdoses to produce a "cure" of those same symptoms. The *symptom* is not thought to be part of the illness but part of a curative process.

Hyperbaric Oxygen: A therapy in which 100% oxygen is given at or above atmospheric pressure. An increase in oxygen in the tissue is proposed to increase blood circulation and improve healing and health and influence the course of disease.

Jin Shin Jyutsu: An ancient bodywork technique to harmonize body, mind, and spirit by gentle touch that uses specific "healing points" at the body surface. The points are proposed to overlie flowing energy (Qi). The therapist's fingers are used to "redirect, balance, and provide a more efficient energy flow" to and throughout the body.

Light Therapy: Natural light or light of specified wavelengths is used to treat disease. This may include ultraviolet light, colored light, or low-intensity laser light. Generally, the eye is the initial entry point for the light because of its direct connection to the brain.

Magnetic Therapy: Magnets are placed directly on the skin, theoretically stimulating living cells and increasing blood flow by ionic currents that are created from polarities on the magnets.

Modified and updated from Spencer JW: *Complementary/alternative medicine: an evidence-based approach,* St Louis, 1999, Mosby.

Mediterranean Diet: A diet that includes 50% to 60% carbohydrates, 30% fats, and 10% proteins. The diet is derived from the eating habits of people in the Mediterranean area, who were shown to have reduced rates of cardiovascular disease. Clinical trial evidence has indicated that it may reduce the risk of cardiovascular disease in people at high risk for CVD.

Mind-Body Therapies: A group of therapies that emphasize using the mind or brain in conjunction with the body to assist healing. Mind-body therapies can involve varying degrees of levels of consciousness, including *hypnosis,* in which selective attention is used to induce a specific altered state (trance) for memory retrieval, relaxation, or suggestion; *visual imagery,* in which the focus is on a target visual stimulus; *yoga,* which involves integration of posture and controlled breathing, relaxation, and/or meditation; *relaxation,* which includes lighter levels of altered states of consciousness through indirect or direct focus; and *meditation,* in which there is an intentional use of posture, concentration, contemplation, and visualization.

Muscle Energy Technique: A manual therapy in osteopathic medicine that includes both passive mobilization and muscle reeducation. Diagnosis of somatic dysfunction is performed by the practitioner, after which the patient is guided to provide corrective muscle contraction.

Music Therapy: The use of music in an either active or passive mode. Used mainly to reduce stress, anxiety, and pain, especially in the palliative care setting.

Naturopathy: A major health system that includes practices that emphasize diet, nutrition, homeopathy, acupuncture, herbal medicine, manipulation, and various mind-body therapies. Focal points include self-healing and treatment through changes in lifestyle and emphasis on health prevention.

Ornish Diet: A life-choice program based on eating a vegetarian diet containing less than 10% fat. The diet is high in complex carbohydrates and fiber. Meat and fish are generally avoided.

Oslo Diet: An eating plan that emphasizes increased intake of fish and reduced total fat intake. Diet is combined with regular endurance exercise.

Pilates: An educational and exercise approach using the proper body mechanics, movements, truncal and pelvic stabilization, coordinated breathing, and muscle contractions to promote strengthening. Attention is paid to the entire musculoskeletal system.

Prayer: The use of prayer(s) that are offered to "some higher being" or authority to heal and/or arrest disease. May be practiced by the individual patient, by groups, or by other(s) with or without the patient's knowledge (e.g., intercessory).

Pritikin Diet: A weight management plan that is based on a vegetarian framework. Meals are low in fat, high in fiber, and high in complex carbohydrates.

Qi Gong: A form of Chinese exercise-stimulation therapy that proposes to improve health by redirecting mental focus, breathing, coordination, and relaxation. The goal is to "rebalance" the body's own healing capacities by activating proposed electrical or energetic currents that flow along meridians located throughout the body. These meridians, however, do not follow conventional nerve or muscle pathways. In Chinese medical training and practice this therapy includes "external Qi," which is energy transmitted from one person to another so as to heal.

Raja Yoga: Yoga practice that includes all of the other forms of yoga. The practitioner is instructed to follow moral directives, physical exercises, breathing exercises, meditation, devotion, and service to others to facilitate religious awakening.

Reflexology: A bodywork technique that uses reflex points on the hands and feet. Pressure is applied at points that correspond to various body parts, to eliminate blockages thought to produce pain or disease.

Reiki: Comes from the Japanese word meaning "universal life force energy." The practitioner serves as a conduit for healing energy directed into the body or energy field of the recipient without physical contact with the body.

Rolfing: A bodywork technique that involves the myofascia. The body is realigned by using the hands to apply deep pressure and friction that allow more sufficient posture, movement, and the "release" of emotions from the body.

Shiatsu: A Japanese bodywork technique involving finger pressure at specific points on the body mainly to balance "energy" in the body. The major focus is on prevention by keeping the body healthy. The therapy uses more than 600 points on the skin that are proposed to be connected to pathways through which energy flows.

T'ai Chi: A technique that uses slow, purposeful motor-physical movements of the body to control and achieve a more balanced physiologic and psychological state.

Therapeutic Touch: A body energy field technique in which hands are passed over the body without actually touching to recreate and change proposed "energy imbalances" for restoring innate healing forces. Verbal interaction between patient and therapist helps maximize effects.

Traditional Chinese Medicine: An ancient form of medicine that focuses on prevention and secondarily treats disease with an emphasis on maintaining balance through the body by stimulating a constant, smooth-flowing Qi energy. Herbs, acupuncture, massage, diet, and exercise are also used.

Trager Psychophysical Integration: A bodywork technique in which the practitioner enters a meditative state and guides the client through gentle, light, rhythmic, nonintrusive movements. "Mentastics" exercises using self-healing movements are taught to the clients.

AUTHOR: **Anne L. Hume, PharmD**

Appendix Ib

Relaxation Techniques

Relaxation Technique	Summary	Further Resources
Breathing exercise	This is the foundation of most relaxation techniques. Have patients place one hand on the chest and the other on the abdomen. Instruct them to take a slow, deep breath, as if they were sucking in all the air in the room. While doing this, the hand on the abdomen should rise higher than the hand on the chest. This promotes diaphragmatic breathing that increases alveolar expansion in the bases of the lungs. Have them hold the breath for a count of 7 and then exhale. Exhalation should take twice as long as inhalation. Repeat this for a total of five breaths, and encourage patients to do this three times a day.	*Conscious Breathing* by Gay Hendricks is one of many good resources on using breathing for relaxation and health.
Meditation		
Transcendental/the relaxation response	To prevent distracting thoughts, the subject repeats a mantra (a word or sound) over and over again while sitting in a comfortable position. If a distracting thought comes to mind, it is accepted and let go, with the mind focusing again on the mantra.	*The Relaxation Response* by Herbert Benson; www.tm.org for information on transcendental meditation.
Mindful meditation	This represents the philosophy of living in the present or in the moment. The *body scan* is one technique where the subject uses breathing to obtain a relaxed state while lying or sitting. The mind progressively focuses on different parts of the body, where it feels any and all sensations intentionally but nonjudgmentally before moving on to another part of the body. A patient with back pain may focus on the quality and characteristics of the pain as if to better understand it and bring it under control.	*Full Catastrophe Living* by Jon Kabat-Zinn describes this technique in full and the program for stress reduction at the University of Massachusetts Medical Center.
Centering prayer	This is a form similar to transcendental meditation that has a more religious foundation. The subject repeats a "sacred word" similar to a mantra. As thoughts come to mind, they are accepted and let go, clearing the mind to become more centered on the spirit within, as if the mind's preoccupied thoughts are the layers of an onion that are peeled away, allowing better understanding of the spirit at the core.	www.centeringprayer.com; look under "method of centering prayer" for a nondenominational discussion.
Progressive muscle relaxation (PMR)	A form of relaxation in which the subject is attuned to the difference in feeling when the muscles are tensed and then relaxed. In a comfortable position, start by tensing the whole body from head to toe. While doing this, notice the feelings of tightness. Take a deep breath in and as you let it out, let the tension release and the muscles relax. This is then followed by progressive tension and relaxation throughout the body. One may start by clenching the fists and then tensing the arms, shoulders, chest, abdomen, hips, legs, and so on, with each step followed by relaxation.	*You Must Relax* is a book by the founder of this technique, Edmund Jacobson. Anxiety Canada: www.anxietycanada.com/articles/how-to-do-progressive-muscle-relaxation/ Mayo Clinic: www.mayoclinic.org/healthy-lifestyle/stress-management/in-depth/relaxation-technique/art-20045368
Visualization/Self-hypnosis	The subject uses visualization to recruit images that create a relaxed state. For example, if a person is anxious, visualizing images of a place and a time that were peaceful and comforting would help induce relaxation. This is best used in conjunction with a breathing exercise.	There are many CDs, MP3s, and DVDs that can guide people through a visualization "script" that can result in relaxation. Emmett Miller is one well-known author.
Autogenic training	This induces a physiologic response by using simple phrases. For example, "My legs are heavy and warm" is meant to increase the blood flow to this area, resulting in relaxation. This is done progressively from head to toe with the use of deep breathing and repetition of the phrase. After completing this, focus attention on any body part that may still be tense, and then focus the breath and phrase to that area until the whole body is relaxed.	The British Autogenic Society at www.autogenic-therapy.org.uk/ is a good resource for more information.

Continued on following page

Relaxation Technique	Summary	Further Resources
Exercise/Movement		
Aerobic	While performing an aerobic exercise, focus attention on a phrase, sound, word, or prayer and passively disregard other thoughts that may enter the mind. Some may focus on their breathing, saying to themselves, "In" with inhalation and "Out" with exhalation, or repeating "one-two, one-two" with each step they take with jogging. Doing this will help the mind focus, preventing other thoughts that may cause tension.	*Beyond the Relaxation Response* by Herbert Benson includes discussion of his research on inducing the relaxation response while exercising.
Yoga	This has been practiced for thousands of years in India. In America, it has been divided into three aspects: Breathing (pranayama yoga), bodily postures or asanas (hatha yoga), and meditation to maintain balance and health. Regular practice induces relaxation.	For Yoga, t'ai chi, and qi gong therapies, it is best to encourage patients to take a class at a local community center or gym and to pick up an introductory book at a library or bookstore.
T'ai chi	An ancient Chinese martial art that uses slow, graceful movements combined with inner mindfulness and breathing techniques to help bring balance between the mind and body.	See above.
Qi gong	A traditional Chinese practice that uses movement, meditation, and controlled breathing to balance the body's vital energy force, Qi.	See above.

Updated from Rakel RE (ed): *Principles of family practice,* ed 6, Philadelphia, 2002, Saunders.

Appendix Ic

Overview of Selected Natural Products

This table includes a few of the common uses and side effects of selected natural products. The evidence supporting the uses and side effects of these products varies considerably and may be based on anecdotal information or theoretical concerns with the natural products.

Natural Products	Common Use(s)	Adverse Effects/Potential Concerns
African plum (Pygeum)	Benign prostatic hyperplasia	Nausea and abdominal pain have been reported, but pygeum is generally well tolerated. Pygeum does not decrease prostate size or influence PSA concentrations.
Black cohosh	Management of hot flashes in peri- and postmenopausal women	Dyspepsia, rash, weight gain, headache, and cramping have been reported. Concern exists that black cohosh causes liver toxicity, although the botanical was part of a multi-ingredient blend. The potential development of mild estrogen-like adverse effects, especially endometrial hyperplasia, is of concern.
Butterbur	Prevention of migraine headaches and supported by 2012 American Academy of Neurology; allergic rhinitis	Diarrhea, stomach upset, fatigue, belching, headache, and drowsiness may occur. Due to concern about hepatotoxicity, butterbur products should be free of pyrrolizidine alkaloids. Products should be standardized to 15% petasin and isopetasin.
Chamomile (German)	Motion sickness, anxiety, insomnia; gastrointestinal spasms; mucositis	Allergic reactions occur on rare occasion. Patients with a ragweed allergy should use chamomile with caution.
Chasteberry	Premenstrual dysphoric disorder, premenstrual syndrome, menopausal symptoms, female infertility, mastalgia	Gastrointestinal upset, headache, rash, acne, weight gain, and menstrual bleeding have been reported.
Chitosan	Weight loss, Crohn disease, hypercholesterolemia, anemia	Gastrointestinal upset, nausea, flatulence, and constipation have been reported. Patients with a shellfish allergy should avoid the use of chitosan.
Chondroitin sulfate	Osteoarthritis, osteoporosis, hyperlipidemia	Gastrointestinal upset, nausea, diarrhea, constipation, and alopecia. Concern exists that chondroitin may have anticoagulant activity due to its structural similarity to part of heparin.
Cinnamon	Type 2 diabetes mellitus, flatulence, gastrointestinal spasms, anorexia, menopausal symptoms, impotence	Cassia cinnamon is one of three types of cinnamon in commercial food products; this is the only type that may have minor effects to improve blood glucose concentrations.
Coenzyme Q10	Chronic heart failure, angina, dilated cardiomyopathy, statin-induced myopathy, Parkinson disease	Nausea, vomiting, diarrhea, anorexia, heartburn, and rash have been reported. Coenzyme Q10 is structurally similar to vitamin K; concern exists about potential interaction with warfarin.
Cranberry	Prevention and treatment of urinary tract infections; type 2 diabetes mellitus; chronic fatigue syndrome; pleurisy	Gastrointestinal upset and diarrhea have been reported with large doses of cranberry. Uric acid kidney stone formation is also possible with large doses of cranberry over prolonged periods of time.
Dehydroepiandrosterone (DHEA)	Slow or reverse aging, weight loss, metabolic syndrome, erectile dysfunction, immune stimulant, osteoporosis, systemic lupus erythematosus, multiple sclerosis, depression, schizophrenia	Acne and other androgenic effects commonly occur in women. Alopecia, insulin resistance, hepatic dysfunction, and hypertension have been reported. Ingested wild yam and soy cannot be converted into DHEA by humans.
Devil's claw	Osteoarthritis, atherosclerosis, gout, myalgias, fever, migraines	Diarrhea, nausea, and vomiting, as well as allergic reactions, have been reported.
Echinacea	Prevention and treatment of viral respiratory infections; urinary tract infections; chronic fatigue syndrome; attention deficit hyperactivity disorder	Nausea, vomiting, diarrhea, heartburn, headaches, dizziness, arthralgias, and allergic reactions have been reported with echinacea. Patients with a ragweed allergy should avoid use of echinacea.
Eleuthero (Siberian ginseng)	Maintenance of a normal blood pressure; atherosclerosis; Alzheimer disease; chronic fatigue syndrome; diabetes; herpes simplex infections	Drowsiness, anxiety, and irritability have been reported.

Continued on following page

Natural Products	Common Use(s)	Adverse Effects/Potential Concerns
Evening primrose oil (EPO)	Premenstrual syndrome, mastalgia, osteoporosis, asthma, menopausal symptoms, eczema, chronic fatigue syndrome	EPO is well tolerated.
Fenugreek	Type 2 diabetes mellitus, anorexia, atherosclerosis; also used as galactogogue	Gastrointestinal upset, flatulence, and hypoglycemia are possible side effects. Patients with a peanut allergy (and an allergy to related plants) should use fenugreek with caution. Nursing mothers who use fenugreek may notice a "maple syrup" smell in their sweat and in the urine of their infants. This may be mistaken to be maple syrup urine disease in the infant.
Feverfew	Prevention of migraines; fever; menstrual-related problems; arthritis; infertility; asthma	Gastrointestinal side effects are the most common with feverfew. A "post-feverfew syndrome" has been reported in individuals who have taken feverfew for prolonged periods of time and then have abruptly stopped the herbal.
Fish oil	Hypertriglyceridemia, coronary heart disease, hypertension, asthma, depression, rheumatoid arthritis, osteoporosis, psoriasis	Heartburn, nausea, rash, and a "fishy" aftertaste can occur. Contamination with pesticides (as well as with mercury and other heavy metals) is a potential concern, although this is unlikely.
Garlic	Hyperlipidemia, hypertension, peripheral arterial disease, type 2 diabetes mellitus	Nausea, vomiting, heartburn, and body odor are most common. "Deodorized" garlic products may lack the active ingredient, allicin.
Ginger	Nausea and vomiting secondary to pregnancy, chemotherapy, motion sickness, surgery	Heartburn, belching, and dermatitis have been reported. In overdoses, ginger has been associated with central nervous system depression and arrhythmias. Efficacy for hyperemesis gravidarum is unknown, and use is not recommended.
Ginkgo	Alzheimer disease, vascular dementias, tinnitus, acute mountain sickness, intermittent claudication	Gastrointestinal side effects, headaches, dizziness, and allergic skin reactions. Seizures have been reported in several case reports. Products should contain 24% ginkgo flavone glycosides and 6% terpenoids.
Ginseng (Panax)	Increased resistance to stress and improved well-being; increased physical stamina; depression; diabetes; erectile dysfunction	Insomnia has been reported with ginseng. Vaginal bleeding, mastalgia, and amenorrhea have also been reported.
Glucosamine sulfate	Osteoarthritis	Nausea, heartburn, skin reactions, and headache have been reported. Increased glucose concentrations have been a concern but have not been documented. Patients with a shellfish allergy should use glucosamine with caution.
Green tea	Improve cognitive performance; prevention of breast, prostate, and colon cancer; hyperlipidemia; Parkinson disease; obesity; diabetes; cardiovascular disease	Nausea, vomiting, dyspepsia, dizziness, insomnia, and nervousness have been reported. Side effects may be a result of the large amount of caffeine in green tea products. Hepatotoxicity has been a potential concern with green tea.
Hawthorn	Mild heart failure, angina, arrhythmias, hypertension	Mild gastrointestinal effects, dizziness, rash, palpitations, and nervousness have been reported.
Hoodia	Obesity	Side effects have not been reported. Many products have been adulterated and lack the actual ingredient.
Horse chestnut	Chronic venous insufficiency, including varicose veins; benign prostate hyperplasia; diarrhea	Mild nausea, vomiting, dizziness, headache, and itching. Products are standardized to 16%-20% aescin.
Huperzine	Alzheimer disease, increased alertness and energy, myasthenia gravis, memory enhancement	Nausea, vomiting, diarrhea, sweating, and blurred vision as a result of the cholinergic effects of huperzine have been reported.
Kava	Anxiety, insomnia, restlessness, seizure disorders, depression, chronic fatigue syndrome	Gastrointestinal upset, headache, dizziness, "kava" dermopathy, and allergic skin reactions. Hepatotoxicity is the primary concern with kava; some countries have banned the use of kava.
Melatonin	Jet lag, insomnia, migraine, chronic fatigue syndrome, breast cancer, gastritis/PUD, osteoporosis; also used for insomnia in children with ADHD	Daytime drowsiness, headache, and dizziness have been reported. Vaginal bleeding has occurred in perimenopausal women. Melatonin from animal sources should be avoided.
Melissa	Cold sores (topically), anxiety, insomnia, Alzheimer disease, hypertension, dyspepsia	Nausea, vomiting, dizziness, and wheezing have occurred with oral melissa.
Methylsulfonylmethane (MSM)	Chronic pain, arthritis, diabetes, osteoporosis, allergies, obesity, premenstrual syndrome	Nausea, bloating, diarrhea, fatigue, and insomnia have been associated with MSM. This substance is used frequently in combination with glucosamine and chondroitin.
Milk thistle	Protective agent against liver damage due to alcohol, acetaminophen, and carbon tetrachloride; hepatitis C	Nausea, abdominal fullness, diarrhea, and allergic reactions. Patients with a ragweed allergy should use milk thistle with caution.
Peppermint	Irritable bowel syndrome, sinusitis, morning sickness, dysmenorrhea	Heartburn has been reported, as well as laryngeal and bronchial spasm in infants and children.
Policosanol	Hyperlipidemia, intermittent claudication, atherosclerosis	Migraines, insomnia, dizziness, skin rash, and bleeding have been reported with policosanol. The product has antiplatelet effects.
Probiotics	Treatment and prevention of diarrhea including antibiotic-associated diarrhea; irritable bowel syndrome; atopic dermatitis; Crohn disease	Theoretically, probiotic products may increase risk of infections in immunocompromised individuals.
Red clover phytoestrogens	Menopausal symptoms, premenstrual syndrome, asthma	Rash, myalgias, headaches, and vaginal bleeding have been reported. Theoretically, endometrial hyperplasia is an adverse effect from the use of these compounds.
Red yeast rice	Hyperlipidemia, indigestion, diarrhea, circulatory conditions	Gastrointestinal upset and dizziness may occur. Red yeast rice may contain lovastatin-like compounds and potentially cause rhabdomyolysis.
S-adenosylmethionine (SAM-e)	Depression, anxiety, dementia, osteoarthritis, heart disease	Nausea, vomiting, diarrhea, headache, and nervousness have been reported. Concern exists that SAM-e raises homocysteine levels.

Natural Products	Common Use(s)	Adverse Effects/Potential Concerns
St. John's wort	Depression, anxiety, chronic fatigue syndrome, HIV/AIDS	Anxiety, gastrointestinal upset, vaginal bleeding, neuropathy, and rash can occur. Hypomania has been induced by St. John's wort.
Tea tree oil	Topical use for acne, fungal infections, lice, scabies	Local inflammation and contact dermatitis may occur.
Valerian	Insomnia, depression, chronic fatigue syndrome, menstrual cramps	Headaches, gastrointestinal upset, and drowsiness can occur. Hepatotoxicity is a potential concern with valerian.

ADHD, Attention deficit hyperactivity disorder; *AIDS,* acquired immune deficiency syndrome; *HIV,* human immunodeficiency virus; *PUD,* peptic ulcer disease; *PSA,* prostate-specific antigen.

AUTHOR: **Anne L. Hume, PharmD**

Appendix Id

Natural Products and Drug Interactions

This table lists interactions between selected natural products and prescription and nonprescription drugs. Many of the listed interactions are theoretical in nature and have not been documented to occur in humans. However, interactions with St. John's wort are potentially life threatening in nature. Other interactions are based on small studies of healthy volunteers and use pharmaceutical-quality natural products that may or may not be commercially available.

Natural Products	Drugs	Interactions
Black cohosh	Hepatotoxic drugs	Concern exists that the risk of hepatotoxicity with black cohosh is increased in the presence of hepatotoxic drugs.
	Cisplatin	Animal studies suggest that the efficacy of cisplatin against breast cancer cells may be decreased by black cohosh.
	CYP2D6 substrates	Black cohosh may modestly inhibit CYP2D6 enzyme activity to result in higher drug concentrations.
Butterbur	CYP3A4 inducers (rifampin, carbamazepine, etc.)	Drugs that induce the activity of CYP3A4 increase the risk of the formation of hepatotoxic metabolites from pyrrolizidine alkaloids from some butterbur products.
Chamomile	CNS depressants	Chamomile may have additive CNS depressant effects.
	CYP1A2 substrates	Chamomile may inhibit CYP1A2 enzyme activity to result in higher drug concentrations.
	CYP3A4 substrates	Chamomile may inhibit CYP3A4 enzyme activity to result in higher drug concentrations.
	Estrogens	Chamomile may compete for estrogen receptors.
	Tamoxifen	Chamomile may interfere with the effects of tamoxifen because of its estrogenic effects.
Chaste tree berry	Antipsychotic agents	Chaste tree berry may antagonize the effects of antipsychotic agents through its dopaminergic activity.
	Metoclopramide	Chaste tree berry may antagonize the effects of metoclopramide through its dopaminergic activity.
	Dopamine agonists	Chaste tree berry may possess additive effects to drugs such as levodopa through its dopaminergic activity.
	Oral contraceptives/estrogens	Chaste tree berry may possess additive hormonal effects.
Chondroitin	Warfarin	High-dose chondroitin has structural similarity to a heparinoid and may possess weak anticoagulant effects.
Cinnamon	Hypoglycemic agents	Cinnamon may possess additive effects on blood glucose to those of hypoglycemic agents.
Coenzyme Q10	Antihypertensive agents	Coenzyme Q10 may possess additive effects on blood pressure to those of antihypertensive agents.
	Warfarin	Coenzyme Q10 may lessen the anticoagulant effects of warfarin because of its structural similarity to vitamin K.
	Chemotherapy	The antioxidant effects of coenzyme Q10 may blunt the efficacy of chemotherapeutic agents that depend on the formation of free radicals.
Cranberry	CYP2C9 substrates (warfarin)	Cranberry may inhibit CYP2C9 enzyme activity to result in higher drug concentrations, although evidence with warfarin is contradictory.
Dehydroepiandrosterone (DHEA)	Tamoxifen and aromatase inhibitors such as anastrozole	DHEA may interfere with the antiestrogenic effects of these drugs.
	CYP3A4 substrates	DHEA may slightly inhibit CYP3A4 enzyme activity to result in higher drug concentrations.
Devil's claw	Antihypertensive agents	Devil's claw may possess additive effects on blood pressure to those of antihypertensive agents.
	Hypoglycemic agents	Devil's claw may possess additive effects on blood glucose to those of hypoglycemic agents.
	H_2 antagonists and PPIs	Devil's claw may raise gastric pH and blunt the efficacy of H_2 antagonists and PPIs.
	CYP3A4 substrates	Devil's claw may inhibit CYP3A4 enzyme activity to result in higher drug concentrations.
	CYP2C9 substrates	Devil's claw may inhibit CYP2C9 enzyme activity to result in higher drug concentrations.
	CYP2C19 substrates	Devil's claw may inhibit CYP2C19 enzyme activity to result in higher drug concentrations.
	Warfarin	Devil's claw may inhibit CYP2C9 enzyme activity to result in higher concentrations of warfarin; purpura has been reported.

Continued on following page

Natural Products	Drugs	Interactions
Echinacea	Immune suppressants	Echinacea may stimulate immune function, potentially decreasing the effectiveness of drugs such as cyclosporine and prednisone.
	CYP3A4 substrates	Echinacea may modestly induce hepatic CYP3A4 enzyme activity to result in lower drug concentrations.
	CYP1A2 substrates	Echinacea may inhibit CYP1A2 enzyme activity to result in higher drug concentrations.
Eleuthero (Siberian ginseng)	CNS depressants	Eleuthero may have additive CNS depressant effects.
	Antiplatelet and anticoagulant agents	Eleuthero may have antiplatelet activity, potentially increasing the risk of bleeding.
	CYP3A4 substrates	Eleuthero may inhibit CYP3A4 enzyme activity to result in higher drug concentrations.
	CYP1A2 substrates	Eleuthero may modestly inhibit CYP1A2 enzyme activity to result in higher drug concentrations.
	CYP2C9 substrates	Eleuthero may modestly inhibit CYP2C9 enzyme activity to result in higher drug concentrations.
	CYP2D6 substrates	Eleuthero may inhibit CYP2D6 enzyme activity to result in higher drug concentrations.
	Digoxin	Concentration of digoxin has been reported to increase but without evidence of toxicity.
Evening primrose oil (EPO)	Antiplatelet and anticoagulant agents	EPO may have anticoagulant activity, potentially increasing the risk of bleeding.
Fenugreek	Antiplatelet and anticoagulant agents	Fenugreek may have antiplatelet activity, potentially increasing the risk of bleeding.
	Hypoglycemic agents	Fenugreek may potentially lower blood glucose concentrations and have additive effects with hypoglycemic agents.
Feverfew	Antiplatelet and anticoagulant agents	Feverfew may have antiplatelet activity, potentially increasing the risk of bleeding.
	CYP3A4 substrates	Feverfew may inhibit CYP3A4 enzyme activity to result in higher drug concentrations.
	CYP1A2 substrates	Feverfew may inhibit CYP1A2 enzyme activity to result in higher drug concentrations.
	CYP2C9 substrates	Feverfew may inhibit CYP2C9 enzyme activity to result in higher drug concentrations.
	CYP2C19 substrates	Feverfew may inhibit CYP2C19 enzyme activity to result in higher drug concentrations.
Fish oils (omega-3 fatty acids)	Antiplatelet and anticoagulant agents	Fish oils may have antiplatelet activity, potentially increasing the risk of bleeding, although this has not been documented in humans.
	Antihypertensive agents	Fish oils may possess additive effects on blood pressure to those of antihypertensive agents.
	Oral contraceptives	Oral contraceptives may potentially interfere with the triglyceride-lowering effects of fish oil.
Garlic	Antiplatelet and anticoagulant agents	Garlic may have antiplatelet activity, potentially increasing the risk of bleeding.
	CYP3A4 substrates	Garlic may potentially induce CYP3A4 enzyme activity to result in lower drug concentrations; evidence is contradictory.
	CYP2E1 substrates	Garlic may modestly inhibit CYP2E1 enzyme activity to result in higher drug concentrations.
Ginger	Antiplatelet and anticoagulant agents	Ginger may have antiplatelet activity, potentially increasing the risk of bleeding.
	Hypoglycemic agents	Ginger may potentially lower blood glucose concentrations and have additive effects with hypoglycemic agents.
Ginkgo	Antiplatelet and anticoagulant agents	Ginkgo may have antiplatelet activity, potentially increasing the risk of bleeding.
	CYP2C19 substrates	Ginkgo may induce CYP2C19 enzyme activity to result in lower drug concentrations.
	CYP1A2 substrates	Ginkgo may modestly inhibit CYP1A2 enzyme activity to result in higher drug levels.
	CYP2C9 substrates	Ginkgo may modestly inhibit CYP2C9 enzyme activity to result in higher drug concentrations.
	CYP2D6 substrates	Ginkgo may inhibit CYP2D6 enzyme activity to result in higher drug concentrations.
Ginseng (Panax)	Antiplatelet and anticoagulant agents	Panax ginseng may have antiplatelet properties; American ginseng may decrease the effectiveness (international normalized ratio [INR]) of warfarin.
	CYP2D6 substrates	Panax ginseng may modestly inhibit CYP2D6 enzyme activity to result in higher drug concentrations.
	Immune suppressants	Panax ginseng may stimulate immune function, potentially decreasing the effectiveness of drugs such as cyclosporine and prednisone.
	Hypoglycemic agents	Panax ginseng may potentially lower blood glucose levels and have additive effects with hypoglycemic agents.
Glucosamine	Warfarin	High-dose glucosamine (along with high-dose chondroitin) may have additive effects to those of warfarin because of structural similarity to heparin. Evidence is lacking.
Green tea extract	Antiplatelet agents	Green tea possesses compounds that may have antiplatelet activity, potentially increasing the risk of bleeding.
	Amphetamines	Caffeine in green tea may increase the risk of CNS toxicity.
	Cocaine	Caffeine in green tea may increase the risk of CNS toxicity.
	Oral contraceptives	Oral contraceptives may decrease the clearance of caffeine in green tea.
	Warfarin	Small amounts of vitamin K have been reported to be present in green tea, potentially decreasing the effectiveness of warfarin.
	Theophylline	Caffeine potentially decreases theophylline clearance.
	Verapamil	Verapamil decreases caffeine clearance, resulting in increased concentrations.
	Quinolone antibiotics	Some quinolone antibiotics decrease the clearance of caffeine.
	Hepatotoxic drugs	Concern exists that the risk of hepatotoxicity with green tea is increased in the presence of hepatotoxic drugs.
Hawthorn	β-Blockers	Hawthorn and β-blockers may have additive effects on blood pressure and heart rate.
	CCBs, nitrates	Hawthorn and CCBs (or nitrates) may have additive effects due to coronary vasodilation.
	Digoxin	Hawthorn may have additive effects to those of digoxin.
	Phosphodiesterase inhibitors	Hawthorn may have additive vasodilatory and hypotensive effects with these drugs.
Horse chestnut seed extract (HCSE)	Antiplatelet and anticoagulant agents	HCSE may have antiplatelet activity, potentially increasing the risk of bleeding.
	Hypoglycemic agents	HCSE may potentially lower blood glucose concentrations and have additive effects with hypoglycemic agents.

Natural Products	Drugs	Interactions
Huperzine	AChE inhibitors (donepezil, etc.)	Huperzine may have additive effects when combined with AChE inhibitors.
	Anticholinergic drugs	The effectiveness of huperzine and/or the anticholinergic drug may be decreased by their concomitant administration.
	Cholinergic drugs (bethanechol, etc.)	Huperzine may have additive effects when combined with cholinergic drugs.
Kava	CYP3A4 substrates	Kava may inhibit CYP3A4 enzyme activity to result in higher drug concentrations.
	CYP1A2 substrates	Kava may inhibit CYP1A2 enzyme activity to result in higher drug concentrations.
	CYP2C9 substrates, CYP2C19 substrates	Kava may inhibit CYP2C9 and CYP2C19 enzyme activity to result in higher drug concentrations.
	CYP2D6 substrates	Kava may inhibit CYP2D6 enzyme activity to result in higher drug concentrations.
	P-glycoprotein substrates (digoxin; itraconazole; diltiazem, verapamil; and many other drugs)	Kava may inhibit P-glycoprotein transporter systems.
	Hepatotoxic drugs	Concern exists that the risk of hepatotoxicity from kava is increased in the presence of hepatotoxic drugs.
Melatonin	Antiplatelet and anticoagulant agents	Melatonin may potentiate the effects of antiplatelets and anticoagulants, although the mechanism is unknown.
	CNS depressants	Melatonin may have additive CNS depressant effects.
	Fluvoxamine	Fluvoxamine may increase levels of melatonin.
	Immune suppressants	Melatonin may stimulate immune function, potentially decreasing the effectiveness of drugs such as cyclosporine and prednisone.
	Hypoglycemic agents	Melatonin may impair glucose utilization and may decrease the efficacy of hypoglycemic agents.
Milk thistle	Estrogens (and other drugs that undergo glucuronidation)	Silymarin may increase the clearance of estrogens.
	CYP2C9 substrates	Milk thistle may modestly inhibit CYP2C9 enzyme activity to result in higher drug concentrations.
Peppermint oil	H_2 antagonists and proton pump inhibitors	Peppermint oil may raise gastric pH and blunt efficacy of H_2 antagonists and PPIs.
	CYP3A4 substrates	Peppermint oil may modestly inhibit CYP3A4 enzyme activity to result in higher drug concentrations.
	CYP1A2 substrates	Peppermint oil may modestly inhibit CYP1A2 enzyme activity to result in higher drug concentrations.
	CYP2C9 substrates, CYP2C19 substrates	Peppermint oil may modestly inhibit CYP2C9 and CYP2C19 enzyme activity to result in higher drug concentrations.
Policosanol	Antiplatelet and anticoagulant agents	Policosanol may have antiplatelet activity, potentially increasing the risk of bleeding.
Probiotics	Antibiotics	Antibiotics may kill the live organisms in different probiotic preparations.
	Immune suppressants	Theoretically, probiotics may cause bacterial or fungal infections in patients who are taking immune suppressants chronically.
Red clover phytoestrogens	Antiplatelet and anticoagulant agents	Theoretically, red clover may possess coumarins, which increase the risk of bleeding with antiplatelet and anticoagulants. Evidence is lacking. Red clover may inhibit CYP3A4 enzyme activity to result in higher drug concentrations.
	CYP3A4 substrates	
	CYP2C9 substrates, CYP2C19 substrates	Red clover may inhibit CYP2C9 and CYP2C19 enzyme activity to result in higher drug concentrations.
	CYP1A2 substrates	Red clover may inhibit CYP1A2 enzyme activity to result in higher drug concentrations.
Red yeast rice	CYP3A4 inhibitors	Drugs that inhibit CYP3A4 may decrease the metabolism of lovastatin in red yeast rice.
	Statins	Red yeast rice contains lovastatin and increases the risk of myopathy.
	Fibrates and niacin	Fibrates and niacin may increase concentrations of lovastatin in red yeast rice.
S-adenosylmethionine (SAM-e)	Antidepressants (including MAOIs)	Additive effects are possible, and there is potential for toxicity.
	Serotonergic drugs (triptans, SSRIs, tramadol, dextromethorphan, etc.)	SAM-e may increase the risk of development of serotonin syndrome when used concomitantly.
Soy phytoestrogens	Estrogens	Soy potentially may inhibit the effects of estrogen.
	Tamoxifen/aromatase inhibitors	Soy's estrogenic effects may antagonize the antitumor effects of tamoxifen/aromatase inhibitors.
	MAOIs	Fermented soy products may contain tyramine.
St. John's wort	CYP3A4 substrates	St. John's wort strongly induces CYP3A4 enzyme activity to result in lower drug concentrations.
	CYP1A2 substrates	St. John's wort modestly induces CYP1A2 enzyme activity to result in lower drug levels.
	CYP2C9 substrates	St. John's wort induces CYP2C9 enzyme activity to result in lower drug concentrations.
	P-glycoprotein substrates (digoxin; itraconazole; diltiazem, verapamil; and many other drugs)	St. John's wort induces P-glycoprotein transporter systems.
	Serotonergic drugs (triptans, SSRIs, tramadol, dextromethorphan, etc.)	St. John's wort may increase the risk of development of serotonin syndrome when used concomitantly.
Valerian	CNS depressants	Valerian may increase the sedative effects of CNS depressants.
	CYP3A4 substrates	Valerian may modestly inhibit the CYP3A4 enzyme activity.

AChE, Acetylcholinesterase; *CCBs,* calcium channel blockers; *CNS,* central nervous system; *MAOIs,* monoamine oxidase inhibitor; *PPIs,* proton pump inhibitors; *SSRIs,* selective serotonin reuptake inhibitors.

EXAMPLES OF DRUGS METABOLIZED BY CYP ENZYMES

The following are examples of drugs that are metabolized through the different cytochrome P450 isoenzymes:

CYP1A2 substrates: Theophylline, imipramine, clozapine, naproxen
CYP2C9 substrates: Warfarin, tamoxifen, irbesartan, ibuprofen, glipizide
CYP2C19 substrates: Omeprazole and other proton pump inhibitors, phenytoin, phenobarbital, cyclophosphamide
CYP2D6 substrates: S-metoprolol, propafenone, paroxetine, risperidone, tramadol
CYP2E1 substrates: Acetaminophen, alcohol
CYP3A4 substrates: Most statins, indinavir, amlodipine, verapamil, alprazolam, buspirone

AUTHOR: **ANNE L. HUME, PharmD**

Appendix Ie

Commonly Ingested Plants with Significant Toxic Potential

Plant	Symptoms	Management
Autumn crocus (*Colchicum autumnale*)	Vomiting Diarrhea Initial leukocytosis followed by bone marrow failure Multisystem organ failure	Activated charcoal decontamination Aggressive fluid resuscitation and supportive care
Belladonna alkaloids: Jimson weed *(Datura stramonium)* Belladonna ("deadly nightshade;" *Atropa belladonna)*	Anticholinergic toxidrome Seizures	Supportive care, benzodiazepines Consider physostigmine if patient is a threat to self or others; only use if no conduction delays on ECG
Cardiac glycoside-containing plants (foxglove, lily of the valley, oleander, yellow oleander, etc.)	Nausea Vomiting Bradycardia Dysrhythmias (AV block, ventricular ectopy) Hyperkalemia	Digoxin-specific Fab fragments
Jequirity bean and other abrin-containing species (e.g., rosary pea, precatory bean)	Oral pain Vomiting Diarrhea Shock Hemolysis Renal failure	Supportive care, including aggressive volume resuscitation and correction of electrolyte abnormalities
Monkshood (*Aconitum* species)	Numbness and tingling of lips/tongue Vomiting Bradycardia	Atropine for bradycardia Supportive care
Oxalate-containing plants: *Philodendron, Dieffenbachia, Colocasia* ("elephant ear")	Local tissue injury Oral pain Vomiting	Supportive care, pain control
Poison hemlock *(Conium maculatum)*	Vomiting Agitation followed by CNS depression Paralysis Respiratory failure	Supportive care
Pokeweed	Hemorrhagic gastroenteritis Burning of mouth and throat	Supportive care
Rhododendron	Vomiting Diarrhea Bradycardia	Atropine for symptomatic bradycardia Supportive care
Tobacco	Vomiting Agitation Diaphoresis Fasciculations Seizures	Supportive care
Water hemlock (*Cicuta* species)	Abdominal pain Vomiting Delirium Seizures	Supportive care, including benzodiazepines for seizures
Yew (*Taxus* species)	GI symptoms QRS widening Hypotension CV collapse	Supportive care Atropine for bradycardia Sodium bicarbonate does not appear to be effective

AV, Atrioventricular; *CNS,* central nervous system; *CV,* cardiovascular; *ECG,* electrocardiogram; *Fab,* fragment, antigen binding; *GI,* gastrointestinal.
From Kliegman RM et al: *Nelson textbook of pediatrics,* ed 21, Philadelphia, 2020, Elsevier.

Appendix If

Herbs Associated with Toxicity

Table 1 Clinical Toxicity of Selected Herbs

Common Name	Botanical Name	Therapeutic Uses	Potential Toxicity
Aconite (monkshood, wolfsbane)	*Aconitum* spp.	Sedative, analgesic, antihypertensive	Cardiac arrhythmias
Aloe	*Aloe* spp.	Burns, skin diseases	Nephritis, GI upset
Betel nut	*Areca catechu*	Mood elevation	Bronchoconstriction, oral cancers
Bloodroot	*Sanguinaria canadensis*	Emetic, cathartic, eczema	GI upset, vertigo, visual disturbances
Chaparral (greasewood)	*Larrea tridentata*	Aging, free radical scavenging	Hepatitis
Compound Q	*Trichosanthes kirilowii*	Anthelmintic, cathartic	Diarrhea, hypoglycemia, CNS toxicity
Dandelion	*Taraxacum officinale*	Diuretic, heartburn remedy	Anaphylaxis
Figwort (xuan shen)	*Scrophularia* spp.	Antiinflammatory, antibacterial	Cardiac stimulation
Ginseng	*Panax quinquefolium*	Antihypertensive, aphrodisiac, stimulant, mood elevation, digestive aid	Ginseng abuse syndrome
Goldenseal	*Hydrastis canadensis*	Digestive aid, mucolytic, anti-infective	Uterine, cardiac stimulation; GI upset, leukopenia
Hellebore	*Veratrum* spp.	Antihypertensive	Vomiting, bradycardia, hypotension
Hyssop	*Hyssopus officinalis*	Asthma, mucolytic	Seizures
Juniper	*Juniperus communis*	Hallucinogen	GI upset, seizures, renal injury, hypotension, bradycardia
Kava kava	*Piper methysticum*	Sedative	Inebriation
Kombucha		Stimulant	Metabolic acidosis, hepatotoxicity, death
Licorice	*Glycyrrhiza* spp.	Indigestion	Mineralocorticoid effects
Lily of the valley	*Convallaria* spp.	Cardiotonic	GI (nausea, vomiting), cardiac arrhythmias
Linn (willow)	*Salix caprea*	Purgative	Hemolysis with glucose-6-phosphate dehydrogenase deficiency
Lobelia (Indian tobacco)	*Lobelia* spp.	Stimulant	Nicotine intoxication
Ma Huang	*Ephedra sinica*	Stimulant	Sympathetic crisis, especially with monoamine oxidase inhibitors
Mandrake	*Mandragora officinarum*	Hallucinogen	Anticholinergic syndrome
Mormon tea	*Ephedra nevadensis*	Stimulant, asthma, antipyretic	Hypertension, sympathomimetic
Nutmeg	*Myristica fragrans*	Hallucinogen, abortifacient	Hallucinations, GI upset
Oleander	*Nerium oleander*	Cardiac stimulant	Cardiac arrhythmias
Passionflower	*Passiflora caeruliea*	Hallucinogen	Hallucinations, seizures, hypotension
Periwinkle	*Vinca* spp.	Antiinflammatory, diabetes	Alopecia, seizures, hepatotoxicity
Pokeweed	*Phytolacca* spp.	Arthritis, chronic pain	GI upset, seizures, death
Sabah	*Sauropus androgynus*	Weight loss, vision	Pulmonary injury
Sage	*Salvia* spp.	CNS stimulant	Seizures
Snakeroot	*Rauwolfia serpentina*	Sedative, antihypertensive	Bradycardia, coma
Squill	*Urginea maritima*	Arthritis, cardiac stimulant	Seizures, arrhythmias, death
Thorn apple (jimsonweed)	*Datura stramonium*	Hallucinations	Anticholinergic
Tonka bean	*Dipteryx odorata*	Anticoagulant	Bleeding diathesis
Valerian root	*Valeriana* spp.	Sedative	Sedation, obtundation
Wild (squirting) cucumber	*Ecballium elaterium*	Constipation, antiinflammatory, rheumatic disease	Airway obstruction
Wormwood (mugwort)	*Artemisia* spp.	Stimulant, hallucinogen	Hallucinations, seizures, uterine stimulation
Yohimbine	*Corynanthe yohimbe*	Aphrodisiac, stimulant	Hypertension, sympathetic crisis

CNS, Central nervous system; *GI,* gastrointestinal.
From Kingston RL, Foley C: Herbal, traditional, and alternative medicines. In *Haddad and Winchester's clinical management of poisoning and drug overdose,* ed 4, Philadelphia, 2007, Saunders/Elsevier, p 1081.

Table 2 Common Herbal Dietary Supplements (HDS)–Drug Interactions

HDS	Drugs	Potential Consequences/Reactions
Aloe vera	Glibenclamide (glyburide)	↑ Oral aloe vera gel can cause additive glycemic-lowering effects when taken concurrently with a hypoglycemic agent
Bitter orange	Phenelzine	↑ Risk of hypertensive crisis
Garlic	Ritonavir	↓ Effect of ritonavir
	Saquinavir	↓ Effect of saquinavir
Licorice	Warfarin	↑ Risk of bleeding
Grapefruit	Calcium channel blockers	Grapefruit juice has been found to increase bioavailability of certain drugs by inhibition of cytochrome P450 (CYP) 3A4 isozyme in liver and gut wall.
Melatonin	Zolpidem	↑ Sedative effects
Valerian	Alprazolam, phenobarbital	↑ Central nervous system depression
Goldenseal	Inhibition of CYP2D6 and CYP3A4	May affect approximately 50% of common pharmaceutical agents
St. John's wort	Cyclosporine, tacrolimus, warfarin, protease inhibitors, digoxin, theophylline, venlafaxine, oral contraceptives	May decrease drug effectiveness

↓, Decreasing; ↑, increasing.
From Kliegman RM: *Nelson textbook of pediatrics,* ed 21, Philadelphia, 2020, Elsevier.

Appendix Ig

Websites Providing Data on Herbal Therapy Hazards

Web Address	Website
www.fda.gov	On the U.S. Food and Drug Administration website under the title "MedWatch," some herb warnings can be found ("special adverse event monitoring system" link)
www.faseb.org	ASPET Herbal and Medicinal Plant Interest Group: A site for an herb discussion group with pharmacologists
www.abc.herbalgram.org	American Botanical Council
nccih.nih.gov	The National Center for Complementary and Integrative Health is 1 of 27 institutes and centers that make up the U.S. National Institutes of Health; their mission is to define, through rigorous scientific investigation, the usefulness and safety of complementary and integrative health interventions and their roles in improving health and health care
www.nlm.nih.gov/toxnet/index.html	A cluster of databases on toxicology, hazardous chemicals, and related areas

Modified from Floege J et al: *Comprehensive clinical nephrology,* ed 4, Philadelphia, 2010, Saunders.

Appendix Ih

Common Herbs in Integrated Medicine

Herb	Common Uses	Activity	Adverse Effects and Contraindications	Doses[b]	Drug Interactions[c]
Aloe *(Aloe vera, Aloe barbadensis)*	Burns and wound healing Constipation Gastritis Ulcers Psoriasis	Antiinflammatory Antiseptic	Dermatitis GI upset (PO) Diarrhea Avoid in children and pregnancy Avoid latex with inflammatory intestinal disease	Liberal application of gel topically No more than 1 qt of juice per day	Cardiac glycoside containing herbs and drugs Licorice Stimulant laxatives
Bilberry *(Vaccinium myrtillus)*	Eye disorder Antidiarrheal Circulatory disorders Diabetes	Antioxidant Collagen stabilizer Vasoprotective Astringent ↓ Platelet aggregation	May alter insulin requirements	Anthocyanosides (calculated as anthocyanidin): 20-40 mg tid *V. myrtillus* (25% extract): 80-160 mg tid Fresh berries: 55-115 g tid	Warfarin (at high doses of bilberry)
Black cohosh *(Cimicifuga racemosa)*	Menopause symptoms Menstrual problems Rattlesnake bites	Probable SSRI-like effects Possible estrogenic activity Possible luteinizing hormone suppression	GI upset ↑ BP Avoid in pregnancy and lactation Vertigo Rash Liver disease	27-Deoxyacteine: 2 mg bid Powdered rhizome: 1-2 g Tincture (1:5): 4-6 ml Fluid extract (1:1): 3-4 ml (1 tsp) Solid (dry powder) extract (4:1):	Hepatotoxic herbs and drugs
Cat's claw *(Uncaria tomentosa)*	Arthritis Cancer HIV Diverticulitis Herpes simplex and zoster	Immune stimulant Antiinflammatory Antimutagenic	Avoid in pregnancy and lactation, autoimmune illness, MS, TB, and leukemia (awaiting bone marrow transplant) Avoid in children <3 years old Headaches Dizziness Vomiting	Tea (1 g/250 ml): 1 cup tid Tincture: 1-2 ml tid Standardized dry extract: 20-60 mg qd	Avoid combining with hormone drugs, insulin, vaccines, iron, NSAIDs, and salicylates Antihypertensives Cytochrome P450 substrates Chemotherapy Hyperimmune globulin IV thymic preparations
Cayenne *(Capsicum annum)*	Arthritis Muscle pain Neuralgia Postmastectomy pain Psoriasis Diabetes Antiflatulent Diarrhea	Blocks substance P (pain peptide) ↓ Lipids ↓ Platelet aggregation	Eye irritation Burning, local and mucous membranes Gastritis Diarrhea (with internal use) Avoid in children <2 years old	Cream (0.025% or 0.075% capsaicin) topically qid	Warfarin: ↓ platelet aggregation with internal use MAOIs ACE inhibitors Aspirin Cocaine Antacids H_2 blockers Theophylline

Continued on following page

Herb	Common Uses	Activity	Adverse Effects and Contraindications	Doses[b]	Drug Interactions[c]
Chamomile *(Matricaria recutita, Matricaria chamomilla)*	GI complaints Skin and mucous membrane problems Stress and anxiety Wound healing	Antispasmodic effect Sedative effect Antiinflammatory Carminative	Avoid if allergy to member of daisy family (Asteraceae; e.g., ragweed, asters, chrysanthemums) Contact dermatitis Urticaria	Tea: 3-4 cups per day Capsules: 300-500 mg tid-qid Tincture: 4-6 ml tid Apply topically to affected area	Caution if using with tranquilizers or CNS depressants (?) Warfarin Chemotherapy Cytochrome P450 substrates
Chaste tree *(Vitex agnus-castus)*	Menstrual problems Hyperprolactinemia Acne Infertility	Hormonal modulator	Rash Headache GI upset Avoid in pregnancy and lactation	Solution (9 g in 100 ml): 40 gtts QAM Dried extract: 4.2 mg qd Must take consistently for several months to see effect	Metoclopramide (Reglan) Contraceptive agents Avoid with dopamine agonists
Cranberry *(Vaccinium macrocarpon)*	Urinary tract infections	↓ Bacterial adherence to bladder endothelium	Diarrhea May increase risk of kidney stones	Prophylaxis: 90 ml qd Treatment: 360-960 ml qd Tincture 0.5-1 tsp tid	Lansoprazole, omeprazole Warfarin Cytochrome P450 substrates
Dong quai *(Angelica sinensis)*	Dysmenorrhea Other menstrual disorders Menopause symptoms Allergies	Phytoestrogen Antimicrobial effects Smooth muscle relaxant IgE inhibition	Photodermatitis Uterine stimulant Carcinogenic constituents Hypersensitivity Excess bleeding and fever Avoid with hormone-sensitive tumors	Dried root or rhizome: 1-2 g PO or IV tid Tincture (1:5): 3-5 ml tid Fluid extract (1:1): 0.5-2 ml tid	Warfarin Heparin Ticlopidine
Echinacea (*Echinacea* spp)	Colds and flu Immunity Upper respiratory infections Urinary tract infections Wound healing (topical) Recurrent candidal vaginitis	Immunostimulant ↑ Macrophage phagocytosis Stimulates lymphocyte activity Antiinflammatory Antimicrobial properties	Avoid in HIV/AIDS, autoimmune disease, collagen vascular disease, MS, and TB Avoid if allergy to sunflower seeds or member of daisy family (Asteraceae) such as ragweed (?) Avoid during pregnancy	Dried root (or as tea): 0.5-1 g Freeze-dried plant: 325-650 mg Juice of aerial portion of *E. purpurea* stabilized in 22% ethanol: 2-3 ml (0.5-0.75 tsp) Tincture (1:5): 2-4 ml (1-2 tsp) Solid (dry powdered) extract (6.5:1 or 3.5% echinacoside): 150-300 mg	Chemotherapy agents Cytochrome P450 substrates Immunosuppressants
Eleuthero *(Eleutherococcus senticosus)*	Herpes type II Fatigue Athletic performance Influenza complications	↑ Lymphocyte count Tonifying Immunomodulator Adaptogen	Diarrhea Sleep disturbance Anxiety Alters diabetes control Caution with cardiovascular disorders Avoid during antibiotic treatment of dysentery	Dried root: 2-4 g Tincture (1:5): 10-20 ml Fluid extract (1:1): 2-4 ml Solid (dry powdered) extract (20:1): 100-200 mg	Caution with antipsychotics, barbiturates, and sedatives Anticoagulants Chemotherapy agents Digoxin Hypoglycemics Kanamycin
Ephedra *(Ephedra sinensis, ma huang)*	Asthma Bronchitis Cough Decongestant Energy Weight loss Diuretic	Sympathomimetic activating α and β_1/β_2 receptors CNS stimulant Stimulates uterine contractions	↑ BP, root ↓ BP, plant above ground Anxiety, restlessness Headaches Irritability Nausea, vomiting Urinary obstruction with BPH Addictive potential Dysrhythmias Alters diabetes control Kidney stones Glaucoma Caution in heart disease, hypertension, diabetes, or thyroid disease	Based on alkaloid content 1%-3% 12.5-25 mg bid-tid Crude herb 500-1000 mg tid	Cardiac glycosides Halothane Guanethidine MAOIs Oxytocin Diabetic medication Dexamethasone Ergot derivatives Methylxanthines Reserpine Must be protected from the light
Evening primrose oil *(Oenothera biennis)*	Fibrocystic breast Eczema Diabetic neuropathy Psoriasis Breast pain Lactation	Source of gamma-linoleic acid (GLA)	Headache GI symptoms Insomnia May exacerbate temporal lobe epilepsy and schizophrenia	Based on 8% GLA content 500-2000 mg tid-qid	Phenothiazines Tamoxifen Anesthetics Anticoagulants

Continued on following page

Herb	Common Uses	Activity	Adverse Effects and Contraindications	Doses[b]	Drug Interactions[c]
Feverfew *(Tanacetum parthenium)*	Migraine prophylaxis and treatment Dizziness Tinnitus Dysmenorrhea	↓ Platelet aggregation Smooth muscle relaxant ↓ Prostaglandin synthesis and serotonin release from platelets and WBCs Antinociceptive Inhibits serotonin release	Stop 2 weeks before major surgery Oral ulcers GI upset Rash Rebound migraine Nervousness Avoid in pregnancy and lactation, or if allergy to sunflower seeds or member of daisy family (Asteraceae) such as ragweed	Depends on adequate level of parthenolide (0.4%-0.66%) Freeze-dried, pulverized leaves: 25-50 mg bid	Warfarin: ↓ platelet aggregation NSAIDs
Flax seed *(Linumus itatissimum)*	Hyperlipidemia Constipation Cardiovascular risk reduction Systemic lupus erythematosus Breast cancer risk reduction Irritable bowel; inflammatory bowel disease	↓ Platelet aggregation Antiinflammatory	Diarrhea Allergic reaction Caution with hormone-sensitive cancers Contraindicated with bowel obstruction	Capsule (1 g): 3-6 capsules qd Oil: 1-2 tbsp qd	Mucilage may affect absorption of oral drugs Anticoagulants Antidiabetic drugs
Garlic *(Allium sativum)*	Hyperlipidemia Hypertension Cancer prevention Antimicrobial Atherosclerosis	Inhibits platelet aggregation ↑ Fibrinolysis Antioxidant ↓ Systolic and diastolic blood pressure	Stop 2 weeks before major surgery Heartburn GI upset Flatulence Body/breath odor ↓ Blood glucose	10 mg allicin or 4 g fresh garlic; equivalent to 1-2 cloves/day	May potentiate antithrombotic effect of antiinflammatories, warfarin, and aspirin Saquinavir Cyclosporin Chlorzoxazone Dipyridamole Ticlopidine Cytochrome P450 substrates
Ginger *(Zingiber officinale)*	Antiemetic Nausea Motion sickness Morning sickness Arthritis Antiinflammatory Rheumatological	Stimulates intestinal tone and peristalsis Cholagogue Antiinflammatory Antioxidant Positive inotrope Inhibits platelet aggregation	Stop 2 weeks before major surgery GI upset Caution if patient has gallstones	Dry powder ginger root: 1 g Extract (20% gingerol and shogaol): 100-200 mg tid	Warfarin: ↓ platelet aggregation Chemotherapy agents General anesthetics Heparin Antacids Antidiabetic drugs Antihypertensives Barbiturates H_2 blockers Proton pump inhibitors
Ginkgo biloba *(Ginkgo biloba)*	Cerebrovascular insufficiency Peripheral vascular disease Vascular dementia Alzheimer disease Memory Vertigo Tinnitus Macular degeneration Depression PMS Diabetic neuropathy Raynaud syndrome Retinopathy Glaucoma Sexual dysfunction associated with SSRIs	Membrane stabilizer Antiplatelet activating factor (PAF) Free radical scavenger Antioxidant ↑ Alpha brain waves ↓ Theta brain waves	Stop 2 weeks before major surgery GI upset Allergies (whole plant) Spontaneous bleeding problems Headaches Skin rashes Dizziness Palpitations Seizures Avoid in pregnancy	Based on standard extract 25% ginkgo heterosides 40 mg tid up to 80 mg bid-tid Use consistently for at least 12 weeks to determine effectiveness	Warfarin Aspirin (↓ platelet aggregation) MAOIs (↑ effect) Fluoxetine Glyburide Insulin Haloperidol Heparin Metformin Thiazide diuretics Ticlopidine Trazodone Buspirone Cytochrome P450 substrates

Continued on following page

Herb	Common Uses	Activity	Adverse Effects and Contraindications	Doses[b]	Drug Interactions[c]
Ginseng *(Panax ginseng)* *(Ginseng radix)* *(Eleutherococcus senticosus)*	Fatigue Weakness Energy Immunity Mentation Diabetes Respiratory illnesses Libido Stress-induced GI ulcers Postoperative stress	Immune enhancement Prevention of platelet aggregation Tonic effect	Stop 2 weeks before major surgery Agitation Insomnia (PM doses) BP Edema Hypertonia Caution with cardiac problems, diabetes, psychosis, and agitation	Based on ginsenoside content 4.5-6 g daily Root powder (5% ginsenoside): 100 mg qd-tid May use cyclically for 15-20 days, followed by 2-week interval without ginseng	Warfarin (↓ platelet aggregation) Corticosteroids (↑ side effects) Digoxin (↑ serum levels) MAOIs, hypoglycemics (↑ effects) Opioids, diuretics (↓ effect) Stimulants Antidiabetic drugs
Goldenseal *(Hidrastis canadensis)*	Cold Immunity Diarrhea Sore throat Ocular trachoma infections	Antimicrobial (often combined with echinacea) Immune stimulant Activates phagocytes	Avoid in pregnancy, lactation, and diabetes (may lower glucose) Mouth irritation Digestive disorders Avoid in infants	Dried root or as infusion (tea): 2-4 g Tincture (1:5): 6-12 ml (1.5-3 tsp) Fluid extract (1:1): 2-4 ml (0.5-1 tsp) Solid (powdered dry) extract (4:1 or 8%-12% alkaloid content): 250-500 mg	Antihypertensives Cytochrome P450 substrates Antacids CNS depressants Heparin H_2 blockers Proton pump inhibitors
Grape seed extract *(Vitis vinifera)*	Atherosclerosis Retinopathy Venous insufficiency Hepatic protective Dental caries	Proanthocyanidins: Powerful antioxidants Vascular renewal and stability Collagen support	None known	25-250 mg bid	Tetracycline, doxycycline Warfarin
Hawthorn *(Crataegus laeviagata)*	Congestive heart failure Hypertension Angina Cardiac function	Cardioactive glycosides Positive inotropic ACE inhibition Mild diuretic Collagen stabilizer Dilates coronary vessels ↓ Peripheral resistance ↓ Oxygen consumption	Hypotension GI distress Rash Arrhythmia Avoid in pregnancy	Berries or flowers (dried): 3-5 g or as infusion Tincture (1:5): 4-5 ml (alcohol may elicit pressor response in some individuals) Fluid extract (1:1): 1-2 ml Freeze-dried berries: 1-1.5 g Flower extract (standardized to contain 1.8% vitexin-4)	May potentiate effects of digitalis drugs Calcium channel blockers CNS depressants Nitrates
Horse chestnut *(Aesculus hippocastanum)*	Venous insufficiency Varicose veins Nocturnal leg cramps Pruritus and swelling of legs Topically for hemorrhoids, skin ulcers, varicose veins, sport injuries, trauma	Aescin component reduces lysosomal activity, improves venous tone, and inhibits capillary protein permeability Diuretic	GI irritation ↓ gastric emptying Pruritus Nausea Standardized seed extracts are safe, but whole herb may be fatal Avoid in pregnancy and lactation, liver disease, renal disease May cross-react with latex allergy	Based on aescin 90-150 mg initially, followed by 35-70 mg qd	Anticoagulants Antidiabetic drugs
Kava *(Piper methysticum)*	Anxiety Restlessness Insomnia Anticonvulsant Oral anesthetic Depression Attention-deficit/hyperactivity disorder	GABA receptor–like actions Limbic system modulation Inhibits voltage-dependent sodium channels in brain Skeletal muscle relaxant	Dermatitis Sedation May impair reflexes and judgment for driving Avoid in pregnancy and lactation, depression, and Parkinson disease. Contraindicated in endogenous depression Hepatotoxicity *Note:* Kava is nonaddictive	Anxiolytic dose: 45-70 mg kavalactones tid Sedative dose: 180-210 mg 1 hour before bedtime	Alcohol Benzodiazepines Barbiturates Anti-Parkinson drugs Other psychopharmacological agents, general anesthetics Cytochrome P450 substrates

Continued on following page

Herb	Common Uses	Activity	Adverse Effects and Contraindications	Doses[b]	Drug Interactions[c]
Licorice (*Glycyrrhiza* spp)	Upper respiratory infection Oral and gastric ulcers Infection	Antiinflammatory Expectorant Antioxidant Demulcent Adrenocorticotropin	Avoid in pregnancy Contraindicated in cholestatic liver disease, cirrhosis, hypertension, hypokalemia, and renal insufficiency	Powdered root: 1-2 g Fluid extract (1:1): 2-4 ml Solid (dry powdered) extract (4:1): 250-500 mg	Furosemide Estrogens Chlorothiazide, metolazone Isoniazid Antihypertensives Insulin Risperidone Ibuprofen Digitalis glycosides Corticosteroids Cytochrome P450 substrates
Milk thistle (*Silybum marianum*)	Cirrhosis Alcoholic and viral hepatitis Mushroom poisoning (*Amanita*) Other hepatotoxins	Cell membrane stabilizer Stimulates ribosomal protein synthesis Free radical scavenger Antioxidant Contraindicated in liver disease Inhibits leukotriene formation Choleretic and lipotropic	GI upset Laxative effect Alcohol-based extracts Contraindicated in liver disease	Based on silymarin content 70-210 mg tid Silybin bound to phosphatidylcholine: 120-240 mg bid	Acetaminophen Butyrophenones Phenothiazines Indinavir Metronidazole Nitrous oxide Chemotherapy Clofibrate General anesthetics Haloperidol Cytochrome P450 substrates
Peppermint (*Mentha piperita*)	Dyspepsia Irritable bowel syndrome Biliary dyskinesia Digestive aid Myalgia Neuralgia Nasal decongestant Tension headache (topically)	Antispasmodic Cholagogue Menthol is active ingredient Antibacterial Antiviral Stimulates gastric secretion Coolant ↓ Lower esophageal sphincter tone Carminative	Nonenteric dosage may worsen heartburn in esophageal reflux and hiatal hernia Caution in pregnancy and in small children (choking from menthol) Allergic reactions Bradycardia Muscle tremor Dermatitis, skin rash Contraindicated in gallstones, achlorhydria, and liver damage	Infusion: 1-2 tsp dried leaves per 8 oz water Enteric-coated capsule (0.2 ml oil/capsule): 1-2 capsules tid Menthol 1.26%-16% applied topically up to qid	Antacids Cisapride
Saw palmetto (*Serenoa repens*)	Benign prostatic hyperplasia (stages I and II) Prostatitis	Antiandrogenic (5α-reductase) Bladder muscle spasmolytic Antiinflammatory	GI side effects Diarrhea Avoid in pregnancy Potential risk of aggravation of estrogen-sensitive tumors Rule out advanced prostatic hypertrophy and prostate cancer	Crude berries: 10 g bid Liposterolic extract (standardized at 85%-95% fatty acids and sterols): 160 mg bid	Anticoagulants Contraceptives Estrogens
St. John's wort (*Hypericum perforatum*)	Depression: Mild to moderate Anxiety Insomnia Contusions First-degree burns Wound healing Antiinflammatory (topically) Myalgias Eczema	Affects neurotransmitters serotonin, dopamine, catecholamines, and possibly MAOIs; reduction of interleukin-6 Antiviral Antibacterial	Avoid in pregnancy (? uterotonic) GI side effects Photodermatitis Allergy Fatigue Insomnia Headache Restlessness Avoid in bipolar disorder	Dried flowers: 2-4 g tid Tincture (1:5): 3-6 ml tid Fluid extract (1:1): 1-2 ml tid Standardized fluid extract (0.14% hypericin: 1 mg hypericin/3 ml): 0.5-0.9 ml tid Standardized solid (dry powdered) extract (0.14% hypericin): 600 mg tid Standardized solid (dry powdered) extract (0.3% hypericin): 300 mg tid	Potential interaction with SSRIs, general anesthetics, and benzodiazepines Chemotherapy Cyclosporine Digoxin Indinavir Oral contraceptives Theophylline Trazadone *No longer contraindicated:* Use with MAOIs, tyramine-containing compounds, 5-L-dopa, hydroxytryptophan

Continued on following page

Herb	Common Uses	Activity	Adverse Effects and Contraindications	Doses[b]	Drug Interactions[c]
Tea tree oil (*Melaleuca alternifolia)*	Skin infections Acne Mucosal and vaginal lesions Fungal infections (skin/nails)	Antibacterial Antiviral Antifungal	Contact dermatitis Allergic reaction Orally may cause significant toxicity; confusion and ataxia	Apply topically to affected area	None known
Valerian *(Valeriana officinalis)*	Insomnia Anxiety	GABA domain effects Improves latency and quality of sleep Improves slow-wave sleep	Overdose with temporary GI, chest, and CNS symptoms (?) Use in pregnancy and lactation Caution in children <12 years old Odor Cardiac disturbances *Note:* Valerian is not habit forming	Dried root (or as tea): 1-2 g Tincture (1:5): 4-6 ml (1-1.5 tsp) Fluid extract (1:1): 1-2 ml (0.5-1 tsp) Solid (dry powdered) extract (4:1): 250-500 mg Valerian extract (1%-1.5% valtrate or 0.5% valerenic acid): 150-300 mg	Avoid with benzodiazepines, barbiturates, general anesthetics, and alcohol Cytochrome P450 substrates

↑, Increased; ↓, decreased; *ACE,* angiotensin-converting enzyme; *AIDS,* acquired immunodeficiency syndrome; *bid,* twice daily; *BP,* blood pressure; *BPH,* benign prostatic hypertrophy; *CNS,* central nervous system; *g,* gram(s); *GABA,* gamma-aminobutyric acid; *GI,* gastrointestinal; *HIV,* human immunodeficiency virus; *IgE,* immunoglobulin E; *IV,* intravenous; *MAOIs,* monoamine oxidase inhibitors; *MS,* multiple sclerosis; *NSAIDs,* nonsteroidal antiinflammatory drugs; *PMS,* premenstrual syndrome; *PO,* oral; *QAM,* every morning; *qd,* every day; *qid,* four times daily; *SSRI,* selective serotonin reuptake inhibitor; *TB,* tuberculosis; *tid,* three times daily; *WBCs,* white blood cells.

[a]The most frequent indications are shown in boldface type.

[b]Dosages vary by preparation. Consult sources listed or expert practitioner.

[c]Drug–herb interactions: Many interactions as cited are theoretical, based on mechanism of action, pharmacokinetics, or other preclinical data and have not been observed in patients. Although this type of data suggests caution, it may not contraindicate combined use. For in-depth detail on interactions, consult the Natural Medicine Comprehensive Database, other sources listed, or an expert botanical medicine practitioner.

From Micozzi MS: *Fundamentals of complementary, alternative, and integrative medicine,* ed 6, St Louis, 2019, Elsevier.

Appendix Ii

Herbal Activities Against Pain and Chronic Diseases

Herb	Common Uses	Activity	Adverse Effects and Contraindications	Doses	Drug Interactions
Aloe vera—*Aloe vera*	Orally—constipation, ulcerative colitis, gastroesophageal reflux, gastritis, peptic ulcer disease Topically—psoriasis, minor cuts and burns	Orally the anthraquinone has powerful cathartic properties Also has antibacterial, antifungal, and antioxidant properties	General pain, abdominal pain and cramps, reduces inflammation Long-term use or abuse can cause diarrhea, weight loss, albuminuria, hematuria, and potassium depletion	Orally 100-200 mg aloe or 50 mg aloe extract daily Topically 0.5% aloe extract cream applied to area tid	Caution in patients on digoxins; prolonged use can lead to hypokalemia
Bilberry—*Vaccinium myrtillus*	Diabetic and hypertensive retinopathy	Flavonoid complex (anthocyanoside)		160 mg bid for retinopathy	—
Black cohosh—*Cimicifuga racemosa*	Menopausal symptoms (hot flashes) and mood disturbances	Estrogen-like effects without estrogenic activity	GI upset, rash, headache, dizziness Avoid in patients with hepatitis, breast cancer	Remifemin 20 mg tablet bid	No well-known drug interactions
Cranberry—*Vaccinium macrocarpon*	UTI prevention, urinary deodorizer	Proanthocyanidins seem to interfere with bacterial adherence to urinary tract epithelial cells Mild antiinflammatory, antiplatelet, and antitumor effects	Excessive use (greater than 1 L/day) over a prolonged period of time could lead to uric acid kidney stone formation	One 8-ounce glass per day	Daily ingestion of 250 ml cranberry juice can increase serum and urine salicylate level
Echinacea—*Echinacea angustifolia*	Decreases symptoms of common cold, diminishes recurrence of vaginal yeast infections	Immune stimulant	Nausea, abdominal pain, diarrhea, and vomiting Caution in patients with autoimmune disorders	A tablet of 300 mg of Echinacea dosed as 1-2 tablets given 3× daily	Theoretically can interfere with immunosuppressant medications
Elderberry—*Sambucus nigra*	Influenza	Antioxidant, antiinflammatory, and immunomodulating effects	—	Adult 15 ml qid for 3-5 days, child's dose is 15 ml (1 tablespoon) twice daily	—
Evening primrose oil—*Oenothera biennis*	Mastalgia, osteoporosis, atopic dermatitis, neuropathy	Gamma-linoleic acid (GLA)—antiinflammatory properties, possible antiestrogenic effects	Avoid in patients taking phenothiazines	3-4 g daily	Can potentiate effects of antiplatelet/anticoagulant drugs

Continued on following page

Herb	Common Uses	Activity	Adverse Effects and Contraindications	Doses	Drug Interactions
Garlic—*Allium sativum*	Hypertension, atherosclerosis, prevention of stomach and colon cancer Topical treatment of dermal fungal infections (tinea corporis, tinea cruris, and tinea pedis)	Pharmacological effects attributed to allicin, ajoene, and other organosulfur constituents such as S-allyl-L-cysteine	Orally: Breath and body odor, mouth and GI burning or irritation, heartburn, flatulence, nausea, vomiting, and diarrhea Topically: Dermatitis, eczema, blisters, and scarring	Fresh garlic (1-2 cloves) per day, garlic extract (200-400 mg) 2-3× per day, topical garlic constituent ajoene at 0.4% cream, 0.6% gel, and 1.0% gel for the treatment of tinea	May potentiate effects of antiplatelet/anticoagulant drugs May decrease concentrations of HIV medications
Ginger—*Zingiber officinale*	Morning sickness, motion sickness, nausea/vomiting, arthritis	Antiemetic, antiinflammatory, antihypertensive, antiplatelet, antipyretic, and antitussive properties	Rare—abdominal discomfort, heartburn, diarrhea, and a pepper-like irritant effect in the mouth and throat	250 mg qid prn for morning sickness, 500-1000 mg 30 min before travel for motion sickness, 500-1000 mg 2-3× a day for arthritis	Theoretically ginger can potentiate the effects of antiplatelet and anticoagulant drugs
Ginkgo—*Ginkgo biloba*	Age-related memory impairment, improving cognitive function, dementia, diabetic retinopathy, glaucoma, intermittent claudication, PMS, Raynaud syndrome, vertigo, tinnitus, sexual dysfunction related to SSRIs	Antiinflammatory, reduces pain, antioxidant, free radical scavenger, inhibits platelet aggregation, protects cell membranes, erythrocytes, neurons, and retinal tissue	Mild GI upset, headache, dizziness, palpitations, constipation, and allergic skin reactions Rare cases of spontaneous bleeding and seizures	120-240 mg divided tid	Can potentiate effects of antiplatelet/anticoagulant drugs
Ginseng—*Panax ginseng*	Adaptogen, improving cognition, nourishing stimulant, aphrodisiac, treatment of diabetes, treatment of erectile dysfunction and premature ejaculation	Ginsenosides or panaxosides	Adverse effects and contraindications—generally well tolerated, most common adverse effect is insomnia	200-500 mg daily For erectile dysfunction: 900 mg tid	None known to exist, but there are several potential theoretical drug interactions
Grape seed—*Vitis vinifera*	Venous insufficiency, ocular stress, atherosclerosis, hypertension	Antioxidant, vasodilating, antilipoperoxidant, and antiplatelet effects	—	360-720 mg/day	Induces cytochrome P450 and may decrease plasma levels of common prescription drugs such as warfarin, clopidogrel, and propranolol
Kava kava—*Piper methysticum*	Anxiety, social anxiety disorder, cancer	Attributed to the kavalactones, which have anxiolytic, sedative, anticonvulsant, spasmolytic, antiinflammatory, and analgesic properties	Concern about potential hepatotoxicity has caused it to be banned from several countries, including Germany	100 mg tid (100 mg—standardized to contain 70% kavalactones)	Caution should be taken to avoid use with CNS depressants, such as benzodiazepines, alcohol, and barbiturates
Milk thistle—*Silybum marianum*	Type 2 diabetes, alcohol-induced liver damage and hepatitis B or C infection	Silymarin—antioxidant, free-radical scavenger, inhibitor of lipid peroxidation, TNF inhibitor, decreases insulin resistance	—	Silymarin 200 mg tid	Might inhibit cytochrome P450
Olive leaf—*Olea europaea*	Hyperlipidemia, hypertension, prevention of CAD, osteoarthritis, rheumatoid arthritis	Antiinflammatory, antiplatelet, antioxidant effects	—	2-3 tablespoons per day added to diet	—

Herb	Common Uses	Activity	Adverse Effects and Contraindications	Doses	Drug Interactions
Red clover—*Trifolium pretense*	Hot flashes, menopausal symptoms, hyperlipidemia	Contains isoflavones, acts as an alterative	Myalgia, headache, nausea, vaginal spotting	40-160 mg/day of standardized extract, 1-2 tsp dried flowers to make a cup of tea, or 2-4 ml of tincture 3 times a day	Theoretical interactions with birth control pills, estrogen replacement hormonal products, tamoxifen, blood thinners, and diabetes medications
Saw palmetto—*Serenoa repens*	BPH, alopecia	Antiandrogenic, antiproliferative, and antiinflammatory	Dizziness, headache, nausea, vomiting, constipation One case report of excessive bleeding during surgery (? antiplatelet effect)	160 mg twice daily or 320 mg once daily for BPH	Theoretically can potentiate effects of antiplatelet/anticoagulant drugs
Soy—*Glycine max*	Hyperlipidemia, menopausal symptoms, osteoporosis, cardiovascular disease	Contains phytoestrogens, known as isoflavones and lignans Rich in calcium, iron, potassium, amino acids, vitamins, and fiber	May cause endometrial hyperplasia	20-100 g/day of soy protein 50-120 mg/day of concentrated soy isoflavones	Tofu and soy sauce contain tyramine—avoid with MAO inhibitors Can interfere with absorption of oral thyroid hormone replacement
St. John's wort—*Hypericum perforatum*	Depression, somatization disorder, menstrual symptoms	Inhibits reuptake of serotonin, dopamine, and norepinephrine	Insomnia, vivid dreams, restlessness, anxiety, agitation, irritability, and mild GI complaints	300 mg tid	Multiple drug interactions, probably due to it being a potent inducer of cytochrome P450 Can decrease levels of common important drugs (digoxin, oral contraceptive pills, phenobarbital, phenytoin, and cyclosporine) Can also potentiate serotonin effects when taken with other SSRIs, Demerol, tramadol
Valerian—*Valeriana officinalis*	Insomnia, anxiety	GABA agonist	—	400-900 mg taken up to 2 hours before bedtime	Can theoretically potentiate effects of other CNS depressants such as benzodiazepines, alcohol, and opiates
Yohimbe—*Pausinystalia yohimbe*	Erectile dysfunction, sexual dysfunction	MAO inhibiting, calcium channel blocking, and peripheral serotonin receptor blocking effects	Excitation, tremor, insomnia, anxiety, hypertension, tachycardia, dizziness, gastric intolerance, salivation, sinusitis, irritability, headache, urinary frequency, fluid retention, rash, nausea, and vomiting Avoid in patients with CAD, hypertension, BPH, anxiety	15-30 mg daily	Can potentiate MAO inhibitors, TCAs, phenothiazines, and stimulant drugs Also antagonizing effects with antihypertensive drugs

bid, Twice daily; *BPH*, benign prostatic hypertrophy; *CAD*, coronary artery disease; *CNS*, central nervous system; *GABA*, gamma-aminobutyric acid; *GI*, gastrointestinal; *GLA*, gamma-linoleic acid; *MAO*, monoamine oxidase; *PMS*, premenstrual syndrome; *qid*, four times daily; *tid*, three times daily; *SSRI*, selective serotonin reuptake inhibitor; *TCA*, tricyclic antidepressant; *TNF*, tumor necrosis factor; *UTI*, urinary tract infection.

From Micozzi MS: *Fundamentals of complementary, alternative, and integrative medicine*, ed 6, St Louis, 2019, Elsevier.

Appendix IIa

Dietary Supplements: What Every Primary Care Provider Should Know

Primary care providers must be knowledgeable regarding the safety, efficacy, and drug interactions associated with common dietary supplements because of the following:

- An estimated 33.2% of adults ages 18 years and older reported the use of at least one form of complementary health approach, according to the National Health Interview Survey in 2012.
- 18% of adults specifically reported the use of dietary supplements, with fish oil, glucosamine, chondroitin, melatonin, and pre/probiotics the most frequently used nonvitamin, nonmineral supplement.
- In a 2010 AARP telephone survey of older adults, almost one third reported the use of herbal and other supplements, and almost half of those individuals using supplements did not tell their health care provider. www.aarp.org/health/alternative-medicine/info-04-2011/complementary-alternative-medicine-nccam.html

COMMON TERMINOLOGY

- A *dietary supplement* is defined as an oral product containing vitamins, minerals, herbs, or other botanicals; amino acids; dietary substances used to supplement the diet by increasing the total dietary intake; or a concentrate, metabolite, constituent, extract, or combination.
- *CAM* refers to the broad domain of healing practices that include diverse health systems, modalities, and practices and their accompanying theories and beliefs (see glossary of terms in Appendix Ia).
- *Complementary therapies* are those that are used *in addition to* conventional therapies, whereas *alternative therapies* are those that are used *instead of* conventional therapies. Integrative therapy is generally defined as the use of complementary medicine with conventional Western medicine in a coordinated manner. https://nccih.nih.gov/health/integrative-health#integrative

LEGISLATION

The U.S. Food and Drug Administration (FDA) is frequently criticized for not closely regulating dietary supplements and monitoring their safety. However, although the agency regulates prescription drugs and over-the-counter (OTC) products, the FDA has limited regulatory authority over dietary supplements. This is because the Dietary Supplement and Health Education Act (DSHEA) of 1994 and its resulting regulations limit the FDA's authority. As a result of DSHEA, the FDA is able to act only when a dietary supplement has been documented to contain a prescription drug, such as sildenafil and related compounds in supplements for erectile dysfunction or sibutramine in a weight-loss preparation. In addition, the FDA can act when safety issues related to a product have been clearly documented, although these cases are frequently challenged in the courts.

HEALTH CLAIMS

Dietary supplements generally are marketed under three types of health claims. The first category is the "nutrient content" claim, in which the product is identified as an excellent source of, typically, a mineral such as calcium, based on recommended daily values. The second type is the "significant scientific agreement" claim; these claims are used when some evidence of the product's efficacy exists (e.g., fish oil supplements). The third and most common type of health claim is called a "structure/function" claim; these claims state that the product has some effect on health—for example, "helps to maintain a healthy heart." However, dietary supplements are not permitted to carry claims stating that they are effective in preventing, treating, or curing diseases.

INFORMATION RESOURCES

Appendix Ic provides a brief overview of common dietary supplements. In the past, few evidence-based resources on dietary supplements were available. Clinical studies and systematic reviews on dietary supplements are now widely available through PubMed, EMBASE, and the Cochrane Database of Systematic Reviews. Although more information is available, references on specific products vary in their interpretation of the available evidence and may exhibit an unintentional bias, either pro or con, regarding the safety and efficacy of dietary supplements.

"Gold standard" evidence-based databases on dietary supplements (subscription required) include the following:

- Natural Medicines Professional Database (https://naturalmedicines.therapeuticresearch.com/) contains multiple databases including one listing many dietary supplements. Monographs include the different common and scientific names; uses and likely effectiveness for different uses; chemical constituents; interactions with drugs, diseases, foods, and laboratory tests; adverse effects; and cautions. The information is extensively referenced and is updated on a daily basis.
- ConsumerLab has a subscription-based database containing common popular dietary supplements as well as almost daily updates related to supplements in the news on its website (www.consumerlab.com). This organization is not affiliated with Consumer Reports and primarily conducts independent tests of the content of commercially available supplements.

Evidence-based free websites on dietary supplements include the following:

- National Center for Complementary and Integrative Health (NCCIH) https://nccih.nih.gov/health/providers
- Memorial Sloan-Kettering Cancer Center www.mskcc.org/cancer-care/diagnosis-treatment/symptom-management/integrative-medicine/herbs

DRUG INTERACTIONS

Clinically significant interactions have been documented between dietary supplements and prescription or OTC drugs. The challenge for primary care providers is to identify real, clinically relevant interactions versus potential or theoretical interactions. Data on interactions with dietary supplements are usually based on isolated case reports or on studies enrolling healthy volunteers. As with drug–drug interactions, the likelihood of an interaction and its severity are influenced especially by concomitant medical conditions, such as heart failure and presence or absence of impaired kidney and liver function. Data also has suggested that the individual's genetic profile may influence the potential for drug–botanical supplement interactions.

Appendix Id lists interactions between selected dietary supplements and prescription and nonprescription drugs. The following two broad interactions are particularly important in primary care practice:

- St. John's wort, commonly used for depression, is a potent inducer of cytochrome P450 3A4 isoenzymes and has been documented to increase the clearance of many drugs that are metabolized through this and other pathways. In addition, St. John's wort may induce P-glycoprotein transporter systems that are important for digoxin and some chemotherapeutic agents. St. John's wort has also been associated with the development of serotonin syndrome when used with drugs that have significant serotonergic activity.
- Dietary supplements such as garlic, ginkgo, and feverfew, as well as many others, have been purported to either have antiplatelet activity or have effects on the clotting cascade. This may be important for adults also taking aspirin and other platelet-active agents, as well as warfarin and the direct-acting oral anticoagulants (DOACs).

COUNSELING POINTS

The single most important counseling point related to dietary supplements is to ask patients about their use of these products and to do so in an open, nonjudgmental manner. The approach should emphasize that many consumers have been interested in vitamins, minerals, herbs, teas, and so on, to maintain their health or to treat illness. If the clinician is unaware of the safety, efficacy, and interactions of a specific product, several websites are available to quickly scan for information. Also, access to drug information centers at colleges of pharmacy is frequently available, and some hospitals now offer programs in integrative medicine.

Patients should be asked about their goals in using the product, as well as how long they have taken it and in what dosage. Allergies to plants should be documented because cross-allergies are common. Clinicians should appreciate that individuals who use dietary supplements may be interested in making lifestyle changes and potentially decreasing their use of prescription drugs. In addition, if an individual is also consulting an alternative medicine practitioner, clinicians should recognize that some alternative health systems discourage the use of established therapies such as vaccines.

Although problems with safety and efficacy have been identified, many dietary supplements are benign except for their cost. Some patients are at higher risk for adverse outcomes from the use of dietary supplements (e.g., those with chronic kidney and liver disease). Patients should be counseled specifically to avoid purchasing dietary supplements over the Internet.

RESEARCH ISSUES

Many clinical and observational studies of dietary supplements have been published. In the past, clinicians frequently stated either that published studies of dietary supplements did not exist or that only a few were available. The reason for this finding was that in the past the National Library of Medicine did not abstract from the peer-reviewed alternative medicine literature. As with all research, the more rigorous the study methodology, the less likely the dietary supplement is to demonstrate clinical benefit.

In evaluating published studies of dietary supplements, the following should be considered:

- Has the correct plant and part of the plant (root, stem, leaf) been used? This critical information may not be known to many clinicians. Consulting a resource such as the National Medicines database can usually provide the needed information to judge this component of the study.
- Has the content of active ingredients been verified throughout the study? In a review of 81 major randomized controlled trials of herbal products, only 12 (15%) reported performing tests to quantify actual contents, and 3 (4%) provided adequate data to compare actual with expected content values of at least one chemical constituent.
- Is the severity of the disease appropriate for study? Negative studies with dietary supplements sometimes inappropriately enroll participants who have moderate-to-severe disease (e.g., those with depression or benign prostatic hyperplasia) when only mild disease would be appropriate.
- Is the duration of the study appropriate? Early studies comparing glucosamine and nonsteroidal antiinflammatory agents (NSAIAs) demonstrated greater efficacy with the NSAIAs because of an inadequate study duration for glucosamine to show any benefit.
- Is a placebo group included? Recent studies with dietary supplements for menopausal symptoms and osteoarthritis have demonstrated placebo responses over 40% to 50%.
- Was the blinding maintained throughout the study? Some dietary supplements, such as saw palmetto, have distinctive odors and tastes that are not easily masked.
- Is the preparation commercially available? Most important, when a study with dietary supplements does show benefit, it frequently is difficult to use the product in practice because the specific formulation studied is not commercially available.

AUTHOR: **Anne L. Hume, PharmD**

Appendix IIb

Vitamins and Their Functions

	Biochemistry and Physiology	Deficiency [RDA*]	Toxicity [TUL†]	Assessment of Status
Fat-Soluble Vitamins				
Vitamin A	A family of the retinoid compounds, each member having biologic activity qualitatively similar to retinol. Carotenoids are structurally related to retinoids. Some carotenoids, most notably β-carotene, are metabolized into compounds with vitamin A activity and are therefore considered to be provitamin A compounds. Vitamin A is an integral component of rhodopsin and iodopsins, light-sensitive proteins in rod and cone cells in the retina. *Additional functions:* Induction and maintenance of cellular differentiation in certain tissues; signal for appropriate morphogenesis in the developing embryo; maintenance of cell-mediated immunity. 1 μg of retinol = 3.33 IU of vitamin A.	Follicular hyperkeratosis and night blindness are early indicators. Conjunctival xerosis, degeneration of the cornea (keratomalacia), and dedifferentiation of rapidly proliferating epithelia are later indications of deficiency. *Bitot spots* (focal areas of the conjunctiva or cornea with foamy appearance) are an indication of xerosis. Blindness, due to corneal destruction and retinal dysfunction, ensues if left uncorrected. Increased susceptibility to infection is also a consequence. [F: 700 μg; M: 900 μg]	In adults, >150,000 μg may cause *acute* toxicity: Fatal intracranial hypertension, skin exfoliation, and hepatocellular necrosis. *Chronic* toxicity may occur with habitual daily intake of >10,000 μg: Alopecia, ataxia, bone and muscle pain, dermatitis, cheilitis, conjunctivitis, pseudotumor cerebri, hepatocellular necrosis, hyperlipidemia, and hyperostosis are common. Single, large doses of vitamin A (30,000 μg) or habitual intake of >4500 μg/day in early pregnancy can be teratogenic. Excessive intake of carotenoids causes a benign condition characterized by yellowish discoloration of the skin. Habitually large doses of canthaxanthin, a carotenoid, have the additional capability of inducing a retinopathy. [3000 μg]	Retinol concentration in the plasma and vitamin A concentrations in the milk and tears are reasonably accurate measures of adequate status. Toxicity is best assessed by elevated levels of retinyl esters in plasma. A quantitative measure of dark adaptation for night vision and electroretinography are useful functional tests.
Vitamin D	A group of sterol compounds whose parent structure is cholecalciferol (vitamin D_3). Cholecalciferol is formed in the skin from 7-dehydrocholesterol (provitamin D_3) by exposure to UVB radiation. A plant sterol, ergocalciferol (provitamin D_2), can be similarly converted into vitamin D_2 and has similar vitamin D activity. The vitamin undergoes sequential hydroxylations in the liver and kidney at the 25 and 1 positions, respectively, producing the most bioactive form of the vitamin, 1,25-dihydroxy vitamin D. Vitamin D maintains intracellular and extracellular concentrations of calcium and phosphate by enhancing intestinal absorption of the two ions and, in conjunction with PTH, promoting their mobilization from bone mineral. It retards proliferation and promotes differentiation in certain epithelia. Purported actions of vitamin D as an anti-diabetes, anti-inflammatory, and cancer preventive agent remain controversial and are under investigation. 1 μg = 40 IU.	Deficiency results in decreased mineralization of newly formed bone called *rickets* in childhood and *osteomalacia* in adults. Expansion of the epiphyseal growth plates and replacement of normal bone with unmineralized bone matrix are the cardinal features of rickets; the latter feature also characterizes osteomalacia. Deformity of bone and pathologic fractures occur. Decreased serum concentrations of calcium and phosphate may occur. [15 μg, ages 19-70 yr; 20 μg, age >70 yr]	Excess amounts result in abnormally high concentrations of calcium and phosphate in the serum; metastatic calcifications, renal damage, and altered mentation may occur. [100 μg for ages ≥9 yr]	The serum concentration of the major circulating metabolite, 25-hydroxyvitamin D, is the best indicator of systemic status except in advanced kidney disease (stages 4 and 5), in which the impairment of renal 1-hydroxylation results in disassociation of the mono- and dihydroxyvitamin concentrations. Measurement of the serum concentration of 1,25-dihydroxyvitamin D is then necessary.

Continued on following page

	Biochemistry and Physiology	Deficiency [RDA*]	Toxicity [TUL†]	Assessment of Status
Vitamin E	A group of at least 8 naturally occurring compounds, some of which are tocopherols and some of which are tocotrienols. At present, the only dietary form that is thought to be biologically active in humans is α-tocopherol. Vitamin E acts as an antioxidant and free radical scavenger in lipophilic environments, most notably in cell membranes. It acts in conjunction with other antioxidants, such as selenium.	Deficiency due to dietary inadequacy is rare. It is usually seen in premature infants, individuals with fat malabsorption, and individuals with abetalipoproteinemia. Red blood cell fragility occurs and can produce a hemolytic anemia. Neuronal degeneration produces peripheral neuropathies, ophthalmoplegia, and destruction of posterior columns of spinal cord. Neurologic disease is frequently irreversible if deficiency is not corrected early enough. May contribute to the hemolytic anemia and retrolental fibroplasia seen in premature infants. Reported to suppress cell-mediated immunity. [15 mg]	Depressed levels of vitamin K–dependent procoagulants and potentiation of oral anticoagulants have been reported, as has impaired WBC function. Doses of 800 mg/day have been reported to increase slightly the incidence of hemorrhagic stroke. [1000 mg]	Plasma or serum concentration of α-tocopherol is most commonly used. Additional accuracy is obtained by expressing this value per milligram of total plasma lipid. RBC peroxide hemolysis test is not entirely specific but is a useful functional measure of the antioxidant potential of cell membranes.
Vitamin K	A family of naphthoquinone compounds with similar biologic activity. Phylloquinone (vitamin K_1) is derived from plants; a variety of menaquinones (vitamin K_2) are derived from bacterial and animal sources. Vitamin K serves as an essential cofactor in the post-translational γ-carboxylation of glutamic acid residues in many proteins. These proteins include several circulating procoagulants and anticoagulants as well as proteins in a variety of tissues.	Deficiency syndrome is uncommon except in breast-fed newborns, in whom it may cause "hemorrhagic disease of the newborn"; in adults with fat malabsorption or who are taking drugs that interfere with vitamin K metabolism (e.g., coumarin, phenytoin, broad-spectrum antibiotics); and in individuals taking large doses of vitamin E and anticoagulant drugs. Excessive hemorrhage is the usual manifestation. [F: 90 μg; M: 120 μg]	Rapid intravenous infusion of K_1 has been rarely associated with dyspnea, flushing, and cardiovascular collapse; this is likely related to the dispersing agents in the solution. Supplementation may interfere with coumarin-based anticoagulation. Pregnant women taking large amounts of the provitamin menadione may deliver infants with hemolytic anemia, hyperbilirubinemia, and kernicterus. [no TUL established]	Prothrombin time is typically used as a measure of functional K status; it is neither sensitive nor specific for vitamin K deficiency. Determination of fasting plasma vitamin K is an accurate indicator of status. Undercarboxylated plasma prothrombin is also an accurate metric, but only for detecting the deficient state, and is less widely available than plasma vitamin K.
Water-Soluble Vitamins				
Thiamin (vitamin B_1)	A water-soluble compound containing substituted pyrimidine and thiazole rings and a hydroxyethyl side chain. The coenzyme form is thiamin pyrophosphate (TPP). Thiamin serves as a coenzyme in many α-ketoacid decarboxylation and transketolation reactions. Inadequate thiamin availability leads to impairments of these reactions, resulting in inadequate adenosine triphosphate synthesis and abnormal carbohydrate metabolism, respectively. It may have an additional role in neuronal conduction independent of the aforementioned actions.	Classic deficiency syndrome (beriberi) is described in Asian populations consuming a polished rice diet. Alcoholism, chronic renal dialysis, and persistent nausea and vomiting after bariatric surgery are also common precipitants. High carbohydrate intake increases need for B_1. *Mild deficiency:* Irritability, fatigue, and headaches. *More severe deficiency:* Combinations of peripheral neuropathy, cardiovascular dysfunction, and cerebral dysfunction. Cardiovascular involvement (wet beriberi): Congestive heart failure and low peripheral vascular resistance. Cerebral disease: Nystagmus, ophthalmoplegia, and ataxia (Wernicke encephalopathy); hallucinations, impaired short-term memory, and confabulation (Korsakoff psychosis). Deficiency syndrome responds within 24 hr to parenteral thiamin but is partially or wholly irreversible after a certain stage. [F: 1.1 mg; M: 1.2 mg]	Excess intake is largely excreted in the urine, although parenteral doses of >400 mg/day are reported to cause lethargy, ataxia, and reduced tone of the gastrointestinal tract. [TUL not established]	The most effective measure of B_1 status is the erythrocyte transketolase activity coefficient, which measures enzyme activity before and after addition of exogenous TPP; RBCs from a deficient individual express a substantial increase in enzyme activity with addition of TPP. Thiamin concentrations in blood or urine are also used.

	Biochemistry and Physiology	Deficiency [RDA*]	Toxicity [TUL†]	Assessment of Status
Riboflavin (vitamin B_2)	Consists of a substituted isoalloxazine ring with a ribitol side chain. Riboflavin serves as a coenzyme for a diverse array of biochemical reactions. The primary coenzymatic forms are flavin mononucleotide and flavin adenine dinucleotide. Riboflavin holoenzymes participate in oxidation-reduction reactions in myriad metabolic pathways.	Deficiency is usually seen in conjunction with deficiencies of other B vitamins. Isolated deficiency of riboflavin produces hyperemia and edema of nasopharyngeal mucosa, cheilosis, angular stomatitis, glossitis, seborrheic dermatitis, and a normochromic, normocytic anemia. [F: 1.1; M: 1.3]	Toxicity is not reported in humans. [TUL not established]	The most common method of assessment is to determine the activity coefficient of glutathione reductase in RBCs (the test is invalid for individuals with glucose-6-phosphate dehydrogenase deficiency). Measurements of blood and urine concentrations are less desirable methods.
Niacin (vitamin B_3)	Refers to nicotinic acid and the corresponding amide, nicotinamide. The active coenzymatic forms are composed of nicotinamide affixed to adenine dinucleotide, forming NAD or NADP. More than 200 apoenzymes use these compounds as electron acceptors or hydrogen donors, either as a coenzyme or as a co-substrate. The essential amino acid tryptophan is a precursor of niacin; 60 mg of dietary tryptophan yields approximately 1 mg of niacin. Dietary requirements thus depend partly on tryptophan intake. Requirement is often determined on basis of calorie intake (i.e., niacin equivalents/1000 kcal). Large doses of nicotinic acid (1.5-3 g/day) effectively lower low-density lipoprotein cholesterol and elevate high-density lipoprotein cholesterol.	*Pellagra* is the classic deficiency syndrome and is often seen in populations in which corn is the major source of energy; it is still endemic in parts of China, Africa, and India. Diarrhea, dementia (or associated symptoms of anxiety or insomnia), and a pigmented dermatitis that develops in sun-exposed areas are typical features. Glossitis, stomatitis, vaginitis, vertigo, and burning dysesthesias are early signs. It is reported occasionally to occur in carcinoid syndrome because tryptophan is diverted to other synthetic pathways. [F: 14 mg; M: 16 mg]	Human toxicity is known largely through studies examining hypolipidemic effects. Includes vasomotor phenomenon (flushing), hyperglycemia, parenchymal liver damage, and hyperuricemia. [35 mg]	Assessment of status is problematic; blood levels of the vitamin are not reliable. Measurement of urinary excretion of the niacin metabolites *N*-methylnicotinamide and 2-pyridone is thought to be the most effective means of assessment at present.
Vitamin B_6	Refers to several derivatives of pyridine, including pyridoxine, pyridoxal, and pyridoxamine, which are interconvertible in the body. The coenzymatic forms are pyridoxal-5-phosphate (PLP) and pyridoxamine-5-phosphate. As a coenzyme, B_6 is involved in many transamination reactions (and thereby in gluconeogenesis), in the synthesis of niacin from tryptophan, in the synthesis of several neurotransmitters, and in the synthesis of δ-aminolevulinic acid (and therefore in heme synthesis). It also has functions unrelated to coenzymatic activity: Pyridoxal and PLP bind to hemoglobin and alter oxygen affinity; PLP also binds to steroid receptors, inhibiting receptor affinity to DNA and thereby modulating steroid activity.	Deficiency is usually seen in conjunction with other water-soluble vitamin deficiencies. Stomatitis, angular cheilosis, glossitis, irritability, depression, and confusion occur in moderate to severe depletion; normochromic, normocytic anemia has been reported in severe deficiency. Abnormalities on electroencephalography and, in infants, convulsions have also been observed. Some sideroblastic anemias respond to B_6 administration. Isoniazid, cycloserine, penicillamine, ethanol, and theophylline can inhibit B_6 metabolism. [Ages 19-50 yr: 1.3 mg; >50 yr: 1.5 mg for women, 1.7 mg for men]	Long-term use with doses exceeding 200 mg/day (in adults) may cause peripheral neuropathies and photosensitivity. [100 mg]	Many useful laboratory methods of assessment exist. The plasma or erythrocyte PLP levels are most common. Urinary excretion of xanthurenic acid after an oral tryptophan load and activity indices of RBC alanine or aspartate transaminase are functional measures of B_6-dependent enzyme activity.

Continued on following page

	Biochemistry and Physiology	Deficiency [RDA*]	Toxicity [TUL†]	Assessment of Status
Folate	A group of related pterin compounds. More than 35 forms of the vitamin are found naturally. The fully oxidized form, folic acid, is not found in nature but is the pharmacologic form of the vitamin. All folate functions relate to its ability to transfer one-carbon groups. It is essential in the de novo synthesis of nucleotides and in the metabolism of several amino acids; it is an integral component for the regeneration of the "universal" methyl donor, *S*-adenosylmethionine. Inhibition of bacterial and cancer cell folate metabolism is the basis for the sulfonamide antibiotics and chemotherapeutic agents, such as methotrexate and 5-fluorouracil, respectively.	Women of childbearing age are most likely to be deficient. *Classic deficiency syndrome*: Megaloblastic anemia, diarrhea. The hematopoietic cells in bone marrow become enlarged and have immature nuclei, reflecting ineffective DNA synthesis. The peripheral blood smear demonstrates macro-ovalocytes and polymorphonuclear leukocytes with an average of more than 3.5 nuclear lobes. Megaloblastic changes also occur in other epithelia that proliferate rapidly (e.g., oral mucosa and gastrointestinal tract, producing glossitis and diarrhea, respectively). Sulfasalazine and diphenytoin inhibit absorption and predispose to deficiency. [400 μg of dietary folate equivalents (DFE); 1 DFE = 1 μg food folate = 0.6 μg folic acid]	Doses >1000 μg/day may partially correct the anemia of B_{12} deficiency and may therefore mask (and perhaps exacerbate) the associated neuropathy. Large doses are also reported to lower seizure threshold in individuals prone to seizures. Parenteral administration is rarely reported to cause allergic phenomena, which is probably due to dispersion agents. [1000 μg]	Serum folate measures short-term folate balance, whereas RBC folate is a better reflection of tissue status. Serum homocysteine rises early in deficiency but is nonspecific because B_{12} or B_6 deficiency, renal insufficiency, and older age may also cause elevations.
Vitamin C (ascorbic and dehydroascorbic acid)	Ascorbic acid readily oxidizes to dehydroascorbic acid in aqueous solution. Dehydroascorbic acid can be reduced in vivo, so it possesses vitamin C activity. Total vitamin C is therefore the sum of ascorbic and dehydroascorbic acid content. Vitamin C serves primarily as a biologic antioxidant in aqueous environments. Biosyntheses of collagen, carnitine, bile acids, and norepinephrine as well as proper functioning of the hepatic mixed-function oxygenase system depend on this property. Vitamin C in foodstuffs increases the intestinal absorption of nonheme iron.	Overt deficiency is uncommon in developed countries. The classic deficiency syndrome is *scurvy:* Fatigue, depression, and widespread abnormalities in connective tissues, such as inflamed gingivae, petechiae, perifollicular hemorrhages, impaired wound healing, coiled hairs, hyperkeratosis, and bleeding into body cavities. In infants, defects in ossification and bone growth may occur. Tobacco smoking lowers plasma and leukocyte vitamin C levels. [F: 75 mg; M: 90 mg; increase requirement for cigarette smokers by 35 mg/day]	≥500 mg/day (in adults) may cause nausea and diarrhea. >1 g/day modestly increases risk for oxalate kidney stones. Supplementation may interfere with laboratory tests based on redox potential (e.g., fecal occult blood testing, serum cholesterol, and glucose). Withdrawal from chronic ingestion of high doses of vitamin C supplements should be done gradually because accommodation appears to occur, raising a concern of "rebound scurvy." [2 g]	Plasma ascorbic acid concentration reflects recent dietary intake, whereas WBC levels more closely reflect tissue stores. Women's plasma levels are approximately 20% higher than men's for any given dietary intake.
Vitamin B_{12}	A group of closely related cobalamin compounds composed of a corrin ring (with a cobalt atom in its center) connected to a ribonucleotide through an aminopropanol bridge. Microorganisms are the ultimate source of all naturally occurring B_{12}. The two active coenzyme forms are deoxyadenosylcobalamin and methylcobalamin. These coenzymes are needed for the synthesis of succinyl CoA, which is essential in lipid and carbohydrate metabolism, and for the synthesis of methionine. The synthesis of methionine is essential for amino acid metabolism, for purine and pyrimidine synthesis, for many methylation reactions, and for the intracellular retention of folates.	Dietary inadequacy is a rare cause of deficiency except in strict vegetarians. Most deficiencies arise from loss of intestinal absorption, which may occur with pernicious anemia, pancreatic insufficiency, atrophic gastritis, small bowel bacterial overgrowth, or ileal disease. Megaloblastic anemia and megaloblastic changes in other epithelia (see "Folate") are the result of sustained depletion. Demyelination of peripheral nerves, posterior and lateral columns of spinal cord, and nerves within the brain may occur. Altered mentation, depression, and psychoses occur. Hematologic and neurologic complications may occur independently. Folate supplementation, in doses of 1000 μg/day, may partly correct the anemia, thereby masking (or perhaps exacerbating) the neuropathic complication. [2.4 μg]	A few allergic reactions have been reported to crystalline B_{12} preparations and are probably due to impurities, not the vitamin. [TUL not established]	Serum or plasma concentrations are generally accurate. Subtle deficiency with neurologic complications, as described in the Deficiency column, can best be established by concurrently measuring the concentration of plasma B_{12} and serum methylmalonic acid, which is a sensitive indicator of cellular deficiency.

	Biochemistry and Physiology	Deficiency [RDA*]	Toxicity [TUL†]	Assessment of Status
Biotin	A bi-cyclic compound consisting of a ureido ring fused to a substituted tetrahydrothiophene ring. Endogenous synthesis by intestinal flora may contribute significantly to biotin nutriture. Most dietary biotin is linked to lysine, a compound called biotinyl lysine, or biocytin. The lysine must be hydrolyzed by an intestinal enzyme called biotinidase before intestinal absorption occurs. Biotin acts primarily as a coenzyme for several carboxylases; each holoenzyme catalyzes an adenosine triphosphate–dependent carbon dioxide transfer. The carboxylases are critical enzymes in carbohydrate and lipid metabolism.	Isolated deficiency is rare. Deficiency in humans has been produced by prolonged total parenteral nutrition lacking the vitamin and by ingestion of large quantities of raw egg white, which contains avidin, a protein that binds biotin with such high affinity that it renders it bio-unavailable. Alterations in mental status, myalgias, hyperesthesias, and anorexia occur. Later, a seborrheic dermatitis and alopecia develop. Deficiency is usually accompanied by lactic acidosis and organic aciduria. [30 μg]	Toxicity has not been reported in humans with doses as high as 60 mg/day in children. [TUL not established]	Plasma and urine concentrations of biotin are diminished in the deficient state. Elevated urine concentrations of methyl citrate, 3-methylcrotonylglycine, and 3-hydroxyisovalerate are also observed in deficiency.
Pantothenic acid	Consists of pantoic acid linked to β-alanine through an amide bond. Pantothenic acid is an essential component of CoA and phosphopantetheine, which are essential for synthesis and β-oxidation of fatty acids as well as for synthesis of cholesterol, steroid hormones, vitamins A and D, and other isoprenoid derivatives. CoA is also involved in the synthesis of several amino acids and δ-aminolevulinic acid, a precursor for the corrin ring of vitamin B_{12}, the porphyrin ring of heme, and of cytochromes. CoA is also necessary for the acetylation and fatty acid acylation of a variety of proteins.	Deficiency is rare; it has been reported only as a result of feeding of semisynthetic diets or an antagonist to the vitamin. Experimental, isolated deficiency in humans produces fatigue, abdominal pain, vomiting, insomnia, and paresthesias of the extremities. [5 mg]	In doses of 10 g/day, diarrhea is reported to occur. [TUL not established]	Whole blood and urine concentrations of pantothenate are indicators of status; serum levels are not thought to be accurate.

CoA, Coenzyme A; *NAD,* nicotinamide adenine dinucleotide; *NADP,* nicotinamide adenine dinucleotide phosphate; *PTH,* parathyroid hormone; *RBC,* red blood cell; *UVB,* ultraviolet B; *WBC,* white blood cell.

*Recommended daily allowance (RDA) established for female (F) and male (M) adults by the U.S. Food and Nutrition Board, 1999-2001. In some instances, insufficient data exist to establish an RDA, in which case the adequate intake (AI) established by the board is listed.

†Tolerable upper limit (TUL) established for adults by the U.S. Food and Nutrition Board, 1999-2001.

From Goldman L, Schafer AI: *Goldman-Cecil medicine,* ed 25, Philadelphia, 2016, Elsevier.

Appendix IIc

Nutritional Trace Elements and Their Clinical Implications

	Biochemistry and Physiology	Deficiency [RDA*]	Toxicity [TUL†]	Assessment of Status
Chromium	Dietary chromium consists of both inorganic and organic forms. Its primary function in humans is to potentiate insulin action. It accomplishes this function as a circulating complex called *glucose tolerance factor*, thereby affecting carbohydrate, fat, and protein metabolism.	Deficiency in humans has been described only in long-term total parenteral nutrition (TPN) patients receiving insufficient chromium. Hyperglycemia or impaired glucose tolerance occurs. Elevated plasma free fatty acid concentrations, neuropathy, encephalopathy, and abnormalities in nitrogen metabolism are also reported. Whether supplemental chromium may improve glucose tolerance in glucose-intolerant individuals remains controversial. [F: 25 μg; M: 35 μg]	Toxicity after oral ingestion is uncommon and seems confined to gastric irritation. Airborne exposure may cause contact dermatitis, eczema, skin ulcers, and bronchogenic carcinoma. [TUL not established]	Plasma or serum concentration of chromium is a crude indicator of chromium status; it appears to be meaningful when the value is markedly above or below the normal range.
Copper	Copper is absorbed by a specific intestinal transport mechanism. It is carried to the liver, where it is bound to ceruloplasmin, which circulates systemically and delivers copper to target tissues in the body. Excretion of copper is largely through bile and then into the feces. Absorptive and excretory processes vary with the levels of dietary copper, providing a means of copper homeostasis. Copper serves as a component of many enzymes, including amine oxidases, ferroxidases, cytochrome *c* oxidase, dopamine β-hydroxylase, superoxide dismutase, and tyrosinase.	Dietary deficiency is rare; it has been observed in premature and low-birth-weight infants fed exclusively a cow's milk diet and in individuals on long-term TPN lacking copper. It has also been described after gastric bypass surgery and with chronic zinc supplementation. Clinical manifestations include depigmentation of skin and hair, myelopathy and other neurologic lesions, leukopenia, anemia, and skeletal abnormalities. Anemia arises from impaired utilization of iron and therefore often is manifested as a sideroblastic anemia. The peripheral smear and bone marrow may mimic myelodysplasia. A deficiency syndrome is also observed in Menkes disease, a rare inherited condition associated with impaired copper utilization. [900 μg]	Acute copper toxicity has been described after excessive oral intake and with absorption of copper salts applied to burned skin. Milder manifestations include nausea, vomiting, epigastric pain, and diarrhea; coma and hepatic necrosis may ensue in severe cases. Toxicity may be seen with doses as low as 70 μg/kg/day. Chronic toxicity is also described. Wilson disease is a rare, inherited disease associated with abnormally low ceruloplasmin levels and accumulation of copper in the liver and brain, eventually leading to damage to these two organs. [10 mg]	Practical methods to detect marginal deficiency are not available. Marked deficiency is reliably detected by diminished serum copper and ceruloplasmin concentrations as well as by low red blood cell superoxide dismutase activity.
Fluorine	Known more commonly by its ionic form, fluoride. Fluorine is incorporated into the crystalline structure of bone, thereby altering its physical characteristics.	Intake of <0.1 mg/day in infants and <0.5 mg/day in children is associated with an increased incidence of dental caries. Optimal intake in adults is between 1.5 and 4 mg/day. [F: 3 mg; M: 4 mg]	Acute ingestion of >30 mg/kg body weight is likely to cause death. Excessive chronic intake (0.1 mg/kg/day) leads to mottling of teeth (dental fluorosis), calcification of tendons and ligaments, and exostoses and may increase the brittleness of bones. [10 mg]	Estimates of intake and clinical assessment are used because no good laboratory test exists.

Continued on following page

	Biochemistry and Physiology	Deficiency [RDA*]	Toxicity [TUL†]	Assessment of Status
Iodine	Iodine is readily absorbed from the diet, concentrated in the thyroid, and integrated into the thyroid hormones thyroxine and triiodothyronine. These hormones circulate largely bound to thyroxine-binding globulin. They modulate resting energy expenditure and, in the developing human, growth and development.	In the absence of supplementation, populations relying primarily on food from soils with low iodine content have endemic iodine deficiency. Maternal iodine deficiency leads to fetal deficiency, which produces spontaneous abortions, stillbirths, hypothyroidism, cretinism, and dwarfism. Permanent cognitive deficits may result from iodine deficiency during the first 2 years of life. In the adult, compensatory hypertrophy of the thyroid (goiter) occurs along with varying degrees of hypothyroidism. [150 μg]	Large doses (>2 mg/day in adults) may induce hypothyroidism by blocking thyroid hormone synthesis. Supplementation with >100 mg/day to an individual who was formerly deficient occasionally induces hyperthyroidism. [1.1 mg]	Iodine status of a population can be estimated by the prevalence of goiter. Urinary excretion of iodine is an effective laboratory means of assessment. Thyroid-stimulating hormone blood level is an indirect and therefore not entirely specific means of assessment.
Iron	Conveys the capacity to participate in redox reactions to a number of metalloproteins, such as hemoglobin, myoglobin, cytochrome enzymes, and many oxidases and oxygenases. The primary storage form of iron is ferritin and, to a lesser degree, hemosiderin. Intestinal absorption is 15%-20% for "heme" iron and 1%-8% for iron contained in vegetables. Absorption of the latter form is enhanced by the ascorbic acid in foodstuffs; by poultry, fish, or beef; and by an iron-deficient state. It is decreased by phytate and tannins.	Iron deficiency is the most common micronutrient deficiency in the world. Women of childbearing age are the group at highest risk because of menstrual blood losses, pregnancy, and lactation. The classic deficiency syndrome is hypochromic, microcytic anemia. Glossitis and koilonychia ("spoon" nails) are also observed. Easy fatigability often is an early symptom, before anemia appears. In children, mild deficiency of insufficient severity to cause anemia is associated with behavioral disturbances and poor school performance. [postmenopausal F and M: 8 mg; premenopausal F: 18 mg]	Iron overload typically occurs when habitual dietary intake is extremely high, intestinal absorption is excessive, repeated parenteral administration occurs, or a combination of these factors exists. Excessive iron stores usually accumulate in the reticuloendothelial tissues and cause little damage (hemosiderosis). If overload continues, iron eventually begins to accumulate in tissues such as the hepatic parenchyma, pancreas, heart, and synovium, causing hemochromatosis. Hereditary hemochromatosis results from homozygosity of a common recessive trait. Excessive intestinal absorption of iron is seen in homozygotes. [45 mg]	Negative iron balance initially leads to depletion of iron stores in the bone marrow; a bone marrow biopsy and the concentration of serum ferritin are accurate indicators of early depletion. As the severity of deficiency proceeds, serum iron (SI) decreases and total iron-binding capacity (TIBC) increases; an iron saturation (SI/TIBC) of <16% suggests iron deficiency. Microcytosis, hypochromia, and anemia ensue. Elevated levels of serum ferritin or an iron saturation of >60% suggests iron overload, although systemic inflammation elevates serum ferritin regardless of iron status.
Manganese	A component of several metalloenzymes. Most manganese is in mitochondria, where it is a component of manganese superoxide dismutase.	Manganese deficiency in the human has not been conclusively demonstrated. It is said to cause hypocholesterolemia, weight loss, hair and nail changes, dermatitis, and impaired synthesis of vitamin K–dependent proteins. [F: 1.8 mg; M: 2.3 mg]	Toxicity by oral ingestion is unknown in humans. Toxic inhalation causes hallucinations, other alterations in mentation, and extrapyramidal movement disorders. [11 mg]	Until the deficiency syndrome is better defined, an appropriate measure of status will be difficult to develop.
Molybdenum	A cofactor in several enzymes, most prominently xanthine oxidase and sulfite oxidase	A probable case of human deficiency is described as being secondary to parenteral administration of sulfite and resulted in hyperoxypurinemia, hypouricemia, and low sulfate excretion. [45 μg]	Toxicity not well described in humans, although it may interfere with copper metabolism at high doses. [2 mg]	Laboratory means of assessment are not meaningful until the deficiency syndrome is better described.

	Biochemistry and Physiology	Deficiency [RDA*]	Toxicity [TUL†]	Assessment of Status
Selenium	Most dietary selenium is in the form of an amino acid complex. Nearly complete absorption of such forms occurs. Homeostasis is largely performed by the kidney, which regulates urinary excretion as a function of selenium status. Selenium is a component of several enzymes, most notably glutathione peroxidase and superoxide dismutase. These enzymes protect against oxidative and free radical damage of various cell structures. The antioxidant protection conveyed by selenium apparently operates in conjunction with vitamin E because deficiency of one seems to potentiate damage induced by a deficiency of the other. Selenium also participates in the enzymatic conversion of thyroxine to its more active metabolite, triiodothyronine.	Deficiency is rare in North America but has been observed in individuals on long-term TPN lacking selenium. Such individuals have myalgias or cardiomyopathies. Populations in some regions of the world, most notably some parts of China, have marginal intake of selenium. In these regions *Keshan disease*, a condition characterized by cardiomyopathy, is endemic; it can be prevented (but not treated) by selenium supplementation. [55 μg]	Toxicity is associated with nausea, diarrhea, alterations in mental status, peripheral neuropathy, and loss of hair and nails; such symptoms were observed in adults who inadvertently consumed 27-2400 mg. [400 μg]	Erythrocyte glutathione peroxidase activity and plasma or whole blood selenium concentrations are the most commonly used methods of assessment. They are moderately accurate indicators of status.
Zinc	Intestinal absorption occurs by a specific process that is enhanced by pregnancy and corticosteroids and diminished by coingestion of phytates, phosphates, iron, copper, lead, or calcium. Diminished intake of zinc leads to an increased efficiency of absorption and decreased fecal excretion, providing a means of zinc homeostasis. Zinc is a component of more than 100 enzymes, among which are DNA polymerase, RNA polymerase, and transfer RNA synthetase.	Zinc deficiency has its most profound effect on rapidly proliferating tissues. *Mild deficiency:* Growth retardation in children. *More severe deficiency:* Growth arrest, teratogenicity, hypogonadism and infertility, dysgeusia, poor wound healing, diarrhea, dermatitis on the extremities and around orifices, glossitis, alopecia, corneal clouding, loss of dark adaptation, and behavioral changes. Impaired cellular immunity is observed. Excessive loss of gastrointestinal secretions through chronic diarrhea and fistulas may precipitate deficiency. *Acrodermatitis enteropathica* is a rare, recessively inherited disease in which intestinal absorption of zinc is impaired. [F: 8 mg; M: 11 mg]	Acute zinc toxicity can usually be induced by ingestion of >200 mg of zinc in a single day (in adults). It is manifested by epigastric pain, nausea, vomiting, and diarrhea. Hyperpnea, diaphoresis, and weakness may follow inhalation of zinc fumes. Copper and zinc compete for intestinal absorption: Long-term ingestion of >25 mg/day of zinc may lead to copper deficiency. Long-term ingestion of >150 mg/day has been reported to cause gastric erosions, low high-density lipoprotein cholesterol levels, and impaired cellular immunity. [40 mg]	No accurate indicators of zinc status exist for routine clinical use. Plasma, red blood cell, and hair zinc concentrations are often misleading. Acute illness, in particular, is known to diminish plasma zinc levels, in part by inducing a shift of zinc out of the plasma compartment and into the liver. Functional tests that determine dark adaptation, taste acuity, and rate of wound healing lack specificity.

*Recommended daily allowance (RDA) established for female (F) and male (M) adults by the U.S. Food and Nutrition Board, 1999–2001. In some instances, insufficient data exist to establish an RDA, in which case the adequate intake (AI) established by the board is listed.

†Tolerable upper limit (TUL) established for adults by the U.S. Food and Nutrition Board, 1999–2001.

From Goldman L, Schafer AI: *Goldman-Cecil medicine*, ed 25, Philadelphia, 2016, Elsevier.

Appendix IId

Summary of Vitamin and Mineral Deficiencies

Vitamin and Mineral Deficiencies	Neurologic Syndrome or Syndromes	Supporting Tests	Treatment	Causes (Other Than Malnutrition)
A (retinol)	Blindness from retinal or corneal damage	Visual fields, visual acuity Serum level <30-65 µg/dl	30,000 IU vitamin A daily ×1 wk	Hypothyroidism, diabetes, renal or liver failure
B_1 (thiamine)	Wernicke encephalopathy: Ataxia, nystagmus, ophthalmoparesis, confusion, delirium Korsakoff syndrome: Amnesia, confabulation Beriberi: Axonal neuropathy	MRI: Symmetric lesions of midbrain (periaqueductal area), pons, hypothalamus, thalamus, cerebellum MRI: Necrosis of mammillary bodies, dorsomedial and anterior thalamus Nerve conduction tests: Decreased amplitude Serum thiamine level <20 ng/dl Erythrocyte transketolase	Prevent by 100 mg PO daily before and 1 year after bariatric surgery, 100 mg IV before glucose administration or refeeding Treat Wernicke encephalopathy with 5 days of thiamine, 100-500 mg IV or IM daily, then PO 100 mg daily Antioxidants (*N*-acetylcysteine)	Alcoholism, bariatric or other major GI surgery, prolonged vomiting, hemodialysis, diuretic treatment of heart failure, cachexia, 5-fluorouracil, other blockers of thiamine phosphate production
B_3 (niacin)	Pellagra: Confusion, dementia, weakness, ataxia, spasticity, myoclonus, glossitis, dermatitis, photosensitivity	Erythrocyte NAD, plasma niacin, urinary N_1-methylnicotinamide	Nicotinic acid, 50 mg PO tid or 25 mg IV tid; nicotinamide, 50-100 mg IM or PO tid	Alcoholism, corn- or cereal-based diet, Hartnup syndrome, carcinoid syndrome
B_5 (pantothenic acid)	Dysesthesias, foot paresthesias	Deficient coenzyme A	5 mg PO daily	Severe malnutrition
B_6 (pyridoxine)	Neuropathy, sensory ataxia, depression Infantile pyridoxine-deficient epilepsy	Plasma PLP <27 nmol/L; urinary 4-pyridoxic acid, <3 nmol ↑ Homocysteine after methionine loading challenge ↑ α-AASA in urine, plasma, CSF	50-100 mg PO daily for neuropathy (preventive use if taking B_6 antagonist) 100-200 mg daily for adult epilepsy	Diverticulosis, isoniazid, cycloserine, other antagonists Genetic defects in antiquitin (aldehyde dehydrogenase), pyridoxal synthesis
B_{12} (cobalamin)	Myelopathy with spastic paraparesis and sensory ataxia, peripheral neuropathy, optic neuropathy, memory loss, dementia; indirect contributor to stroke	Blood level <200 pg/ml↑ Methylmalonic acid >145 nmol/L Intrinsic factor antibodies Schilling test, megaloblastic anemia Delayed somatosensory evoked potentials ↑ Homocysteine, total >12.5 µmol/L	IM B_{12}, 1000 µg daily for 1 week, then weekly for 1 month, then monthly or oral B_{12}, 1000 µg daily, or nasal B_{12}, 500 µg weekly for lifetime if abnormal absorption, 50-100 µg daily if normal absorption	Achlorhydria, gastric or ileal resection, blind loop syndrome, sprue, HIV infection, nitrous oxide anesthesia (especially abuse), fish tapeworm, vegan diet
D (calciferol)	Proximal myopathy, often painful; cognitive impairment Secondary compression of spinal cord, plexus, or peripheral nerves from rickets or osteomalacia	25-(OH) vitamin D_3 level <10 ng/ml in urine Serum calcium ↑ PTH >54 pg/ml Osteopenia/porosis on bone densitometry	Daily supplementation with 400 IU, >50,000 IU 3 times per wk if malabsorption; use blood level or urine calcium excretion to guide (should be >100 mg/day)	Lack of exposure to sunlight, including sunblock protection; chronic antiepileptic drug use

Vitamin and Mineral Deficiencies	Neurologic Syndrome or Syndromes	Supporting Tests	Treatment	Causes (Other Than Malnutrition)
E (tocopherol)	Spinal and cerebellar ataxia, Babinski sign, ophthalmoplegia, peripheral neuropathy, retinitis pigmentosa	Vitamin E level <2.5 mg/L (normal, 6-15 with normal lipid level) ↑ A-β-lipoprotein levels, antigliadin antibodies Genetic analysis to rule out other spinocerebellar ataxias such as Friedreich ataxia	Supplement with 6-800 IU, 5-10 mg/kg twice daily, for ataxia of genetic causes, water-soluble 200 mg/kg/day or IM α-tocopherol for malabsorption	Biliary atresia, celiac sprue, genetic: ↓ α-tocopherol transport protein (8q13), microsomal triglyceride transfer protein
Folate	Dementia, B_{12} deficiency, stroke	↑ Homocysteine, plasma level <2.5 μg/L	1 mg 3 times per day until normal level, then maintenance of 1 mg/day Pregnancy: Additional 0.4 mg/day if taking a folate antagonist	Malabsorption or use of antagonist (methotrexate) or antiepileptic medication
K (phytonadione)	Intracranial hemorrhage	INR or PT elevation	IM phytonadione at birth, maternal vitamin K for last month of pregnancy	Medication use that increases metabolism, such as phenytoin
Copper	Myelopathy, neuropathy	Serum Cu <75 μg/dl, ↓ urinary Cu, ceruloplasmin <23 mg/dl MRI: ↑ T_2 signal in cervical cord, dorsal column Mutation in ATP7A gene (Menkes disease)	Elemental Cu, 8 mg/day PO week 1, 6 mg/day week 2, 4 mg/day week 3, 2 mg/day ongoing malabsorption Menkes disease: 250 mg SC bid	Wilson disease, Menkes disease, alcoholism, malabsorption, gastric bypass, zinc toxicity
Magnesium	Seizures, encephalopathy	Serum magnesium <1.5 mg/ dl, correct for low albumin	Magnesium sulfate IV or PO; avoid magnesium-wasting drugs	Alcoholism, especially beer
Potassium	Muscle weakness, chronic, acute	Serum potassium <3.5 mEq/L, ECG	IV or PO KCl until normalized	Diuretic use, bulimia

AASA, Aminoadipic semialdehyde; *CSF,* cerebrospinal fluid; *ECG,* electrocardiography; *GI,* gastrointestinal; *HIV,* human immunodeficiency virus; *IM,* intramuscularly; *INR,* international normalized ratio; *IU,* international units; *IV,* intravenously; *MRI,* magnetic resonance imaging; *NAD,* nicotinamide adenine dinucleotide; *PLP,* pyridoxal-5-phosphate (active coenzyme of pyridoxine); *PO,* by mouth; *PT,* prothrombin time; *PTH,* parathyroid hormone; *tid,* three times a day.

From Goldman L, Schafer AI: *Goldman's Cecil medicine,* ed 24, Philadelphia, 2012, Saunders.

Appendix IIIa

Selected Historical and Physical Findings in Poisoning

Sign	Toxin
Odor	
Bitter almonds	Cyanide
Acetone	Isopropyl alcohol, methanol, paraldehyde, salicylates
Rotten eggs	Hydrogen sulfide, sulfur dioxide, methyl mercaptans (additive to natural gas)
Wintergreen	Methyl salicylate
Garlic	Arsenic, thallium, organophosphates, selenium
Ocular Signs	
Miosis	Opioids (except propoxyphene, meperidine, and pentazocine), organophosphates and other cholinergics, clonidine, phenothiazines, sedative-hypnotics, olanzapine
Mydriasis	Anticholinergics (e.g., antihistamines, TCAs, atropine), sympathomimetics (cocaine, amphetamines, PCP), post-anoxic encephalopathy, opiate withdrawal, cathinones, MDMA
Nystagmus	Anticonvulsants, sedative-hypnotics, alcohols, PCP, ketamine, dextromethorphan
Lacrimation	Organophosphates, irritant gas or vapors
Retinal hyperemia	Methanol
Cutaneous Signs	
Diaphoresis	Cholinergics (organophosphates), sympathomimetics, withdrawal syndromes
Alopecia	Thallium, arsenic
Erythema	Boric acid, elemental mercury, cyanide, carbon monoxide, disulfiram, scombroid, anticholinergics, vancomycin
Cyanosis (unresponsive to oxygen)	Methemoglobinemia (e.g., benzocaine, dapsone, nitrites, phenazopyridine), amiodarone, silver
Oral Signs	
Salivation	Organophosphates, salicylates, corrosives, ketamine, PCP, strychnine
Oral burns	Corrosives, oxalate-containing plants
Gum lines	Lead, mercury, arsenic, bismuth
Gastrointestinal Signs	
Diarrhea	Antimicrobials, arsenic, iron, boric acid, cholinergics, colchicine, opioid withdrawal
Hematemesis	Arsenic, iron, caustics, NSAIDs, salicylates
Constipation	Lead
Cardiac Signs	
Tachycardia	Sympathomimetics, anticholinergics, antidepressants, antipsychotics, methylxanthines (theophylline, caffeine), salicylates, cellular asphyxiants (cyanide, carbon monoxide, hydrogen sulfide), withdrawal (ethanol, sedatives, clonidine, opioids), serotonin syndrome, neuroleptic malignant syndrome, MDMA, cathinones
Bradycardia	β-blockers, calcium channel blockers, digoxin, clonidine, organophosphates, opioids, sedative-hypnotics
Hypertension	Sympathomimetics, anticholinergics, monoamine oxidase inhibitors, serotonin syndrome, neuroleptic malignant syndrome, clonidine withdrawal
Hypotension	β-blockers, calcium channel blockers, cyclic antidepressants, iron, antipsychotics, barbiturates, clonidine, opioids, arsenic, amatoxin mushrooms, cellular asphyxiants (cyanide, carbon monoxide, hydrogen sulfide), snake envenomation
Respiratory Signs	
Depressed respirations	Opioids, sedative-hypnotics, alcohol, clonidine, barbiturates
Tachypnea	Salicylates, sympathomimetics, caffeine, metabolic acidosis, carbon monoxide, hydrocarbon aspiration

Continued on following page

Sign	Toxin
Central Nervous System Signs	
Ataxia	Alcohols, anticonvulsants, sedative-hypnotics, lithium, dextromethorphan, carbon monoxide, inhalants
Coma	Opioids, sedative-hypnotics, anticonvulsants, antidepressants, antipsychotics, ethanol, anticholinergics, clonidine, GHB, alcohols, salicylates, barbiturates
Seizures	Sympathomimetics, anticholinergics, antidepressants (especially TCAs, bupropion, venlafaxine), cholinergics (organophosphates), isoniazid, camphor, lindane, salicylates, lead, nicotine, tramadol, water hemlock, withdrawal
Delirium/psychosis	Sympathomimetics, anticholinergics, LSD, PCP, hallucinogens, lithium, dextromethorphan, steroids, withdrawal, MDMA, cathinones
Peripheral neuropathy	Lead, arsenic, mercury, organophosphates, nicotine

GHB, γ-hydroxybutyrate; *LSD,* lysergic acid diethylamide; *MDMA,* 3,4-methylenedioxymethamphetamine (Ecstasy); *NSAIDs,* nonsteroidal antiinflammatory drugs; *PCP,* phencyclidine; *TCAs,* tricyclic antidepressants.

From Kliegman RM: *Nelson textbook of pediatrics,* ed 21, Philadelphia, 2020, Elsevier.

Appendix IIIb

Toxidromes

Table 1 Recognizable Poison Syndromes

Toxidrome	Signs						Possible Toxins
	Vital Signs	Mental Status	Pupils	Skin	Bowel Sounds	Other	
Sympathomimetic	Hypertension, tachycardia, hyperthermia	Agitation, psychosis, delirium, violence	Dilated	Diaphoretic	Normal to increased		Amphetamines, cocaine, PCP, bath salts (cathinones), ADHD medication
Anticholinergic	Hypertension, tachycardia, hyperthermia	Agitation, delirium, coma, seizures	Dilated	Dry, hot	Diminished	Ileus urinary retention	Antihistamines, TCAs, atropine, jimsonweed
Cholinergic	Bradycardia, BP and temp typically normal	Confusion, coma, fasciculations	Small	Diaphoretic	Hyperactive	Diarrhea, urination, bronchorrhea, bronchospasm, emesis, lacrimation, salivation	Organophosphates (insecticides, nerve agents), carbamates (physostigmine, neostigmine, pyridostigmine) Alzheimer medications, myasthenia treatments
Opioids	Respiratory depression, bradycardia, hypotension, hypothermia	Depression, coma, euphoria	Pinpoint	Normal	Normal to decreased		Methadone, buprenorphine, morphine, oxycodone, heroin, etc.
Sedative-hypnotics	Respiratory depression, HR normal to decreased, BP normal to decreased, temp normal to decreased	Somnolence, coma	Small or normal	Normal	Normal		Barbiturates, benzodiazepines, ethanol
Serotonin syndrome (similar findings with neuroleptic malignant syndrome)	Hyperthermia, tachycardia, hypertension or hypotension (autonomic instability)	Agitation, confusion, coma	Dilated	Diaphoretic	Increased	Neuromuscular hyperexcitability: Clonus, hyperreflexia (lower > upper extremities)	SSRIs, lithium, MAOIs, linezolid, tramadol, meperidine, dextromethorphan
Salicylates	Tachypnea, hyperpnea, tachycardia, hyperthermia	Agitation, confusion, coma	Normal	Diaphoretic	Normal	Nausea, vomiting, tinnitus, ABGs with primary respiratory alkalosis and primary metabolic acidosis; tinnitus or difficulty hearing	Aspirin and aspirin-containing products, methyl salicylate
Withdrawal (sedative-hypnotic)	Tachycardia, tachypnea, hyperthermia	Agitation, tremor, seizure, hallucinosis, delirium tremens	Dilated	Diaphoretic	Increased		Lack of access to ethanol, benzodiazepines, barbiturates, GHB, or excessive use of flumazenil
Withdrawal (opioid)	Tachycardia	Restlessness, anxiety	Dilated	Diaphoretic	Hyperactive	Nausea, vomiting, diarrhea	Lack of access to opioids or excessive use of naloxone

ABGs, Arterial blood gases; *ADHD,* attention-deficit/hyperactivity disorder; *BP,* blood pressure; *GHB,* γ-hydroxybutyrate; *HR,* heart rate; *MAOIs,* monoamine oxidase inhibitors; *PCP,* phencyclidine; *SSRIs,* selective serotonin reuptake inhibitors; *temp,* temperature; *TCAs,* tricyclic antidepressants.

From Kliegman RM: *Nelson textbook of pediatrics,* ed 21, Philadelphia, 2020, Elsevier.

Table 2 Laboratory Clues in Toxicologic Diagnosis

Anion Gap Metabolic Acidosis (Mnemonic = Mudpiles Cat)	*Hyperglycemia*
Methanol, metformin	Salicylates (early)
Uremia	Calcium channel blockers
Diabetic ketoacidosis	Caffeine
Propylene glycol	*Hypocalcemia*
Isoniazid, iron, massive ibuprofen	Ethylene glycol
Lactic acidosis	Fluoride
Ethylene glycol	*Rhabdomyolysis*
Salicylates	Neuroleptic malignant syndrome, serotonin syndrome
Cellular asphyxiants (cyanide, carbon monoxide, hydrogen sulfide)	Statins
Alcoholic ketoacidosis	Mushrooms (*Tricholoma equestre*)
Tylenol (clinical significance depends upon presence or absence of liver injury)	Any toxin causing prolonged immobilization (e.g., opioids, antipsychotics), excessive muscle activity or seizures (e.g., sympathomimetics)
Elevated Osmolar Gap	*Radiopaque Substance on KUB (Mnemonic = Chipped)*
Alcohols: Ethanol, isopropyl, methanol, ethylene glycol	**C**hloral hydrate, calcium carbonate
Hypoglycemia (Mnemonic = Hobbies)	**H**eavy metals (lead, zinc, barium, arsenic, lithium, bismuth)
Hypoglycemics, oral: Sulfonylureas, meglitinides	**I**ron
Other: Quinine, unripe ackee fruit	**P**henothiazines
Beta-blockers	**P**lay-Doh, potassium chloride
Insulin	**E**nteric-coated pills
Ethanol	**D**ental amalgam, drug packets
Salicylates (late)	

KUB, Kidney-ureter-bladder radiograph.
From Kliegman RM: *Nelson textbook of pediatrics,* ed 21, Philadelphia, 2020, Elsevier.

Table 3 Substances Poorly Adsorbed by Activated Charcoal

Alcohols
Caustics: Alkalis and acids
Cyanide
Heavy metals (e.g., lead)
Hydrocarbons
Iron
Lithium

From Kliegman RM: *Nelson textbook of pediatrics,* ed 21, Philadelphia, 2020, Elsevier.

Appendix IIIc

Antidotes and Indications for Use

Antidote	Indication for Use	Dose*	Treatment End Point	Comments
Antivenom, *Crotalidae* (Fab)†	Crotaline snake (e.g., rattlesnakes, copperhead)	4-6 vials; repeat for persistent or worsening clinical condition; repeated doses of 2 vials at 6, 12, and 18 hr after initial antivenom dose are recommended	Halt in progression of circumferential and proximal swelling Resolving systemic effects	Better safety profile than historical equine-derived antivenom Repetitive dosing indicated for recurrent soft tissue swelling Less effective at correcting hematologic (i.e., coagulation and platelet) disorders
Antivenom, *Latrodectus* (equine)†	Black widow spider (*Latrodectus* sp)	1 vial diluted in 50-100 ml NS, infused during 1 hr; can repeat	Resolution of symptoms, vital signs normal	Dilution and slow infusion rate are *critical* to avoid anaphylactoid reaction Indications include severe pain unresponsive to opioids and severe hypertension Serum sickness can occur IV calcium is ineffective
Atropine	Carbamates Nerve agents Organophosphorus compounds	2 mg IV; double the dose every 5 min to achieve atropinization and hemodynamic stability; then start continuous infusion of 10-20% of total stabilizing dose per hour	Cessation of excessive oral and pulmonary secretions, >80 beats/min, systolic blood pressure >80 mm Hg	Doubling of the dose every 5 min (e.g., 2, 4, 8, and 16 mg) estimated to achieve atropinization within 30 min Stop infusion when patient develops concerning signs or symptoms of anticholinergic toxidrome; restart infusion at lower rate when signs or symptoms abate
Calcium salt‡	Calcium-channel antagonists	Calcium chloride 10%, 10 ml (1 g) during 10 min; can be given in 1 min if critically ill Calcium gluconate 10%, 30 ml (3 g) during 10 min; can be given in 1 min if critically ill	Reversal of hypotension; may not reverse bradycardia	*All indications:* Monitor ionized calcium levels IV extravasation causes tissue necrosis, especially with calcium chloride Can administer at faster than stated rates for immediate life-threatening conditions (i.e., in 1 min) Calcium chloride contains three times more elemental calcium than calcium gluconate does
	Hydrofluoric acid	Systemic toxicity: calcium gluconate 10%, 1-3 g (10-30 ml) per dose IV during 10-min period; repeat as needed every 5-10 min	Reversal of life-threatening manifestations of hypocalcemia and hyperkalemia	Can dilute and give intra-arterially or IV with a Bier block for extremity exposures and burns
	Hyperkalemia (except cardiac glycosides)	Calcium gluconate 10%, 1 g (10 ml) per dose IV during 10-min period; repeat as needed every 5-10 min	Reversal of myocardial depression and conduction delays	May precipitate ventricular arrhythmias
	Hypermagnesemia	Calcium gluconate 10%, 1-2 g (10-20 ml) per dose IV during 10-min period; repeat as needed every 5-10 min	Reversal of respiratory depression, hypotension, and cardiac conduction blocks	Simultaneous therapies to increase magnesium elimination should be instituted
	Hypocalcemia (e.g., ethylene glycol)	Calcium gluconate 10%, 0.5-1.0 g (5-10 ml) per dose during 10-min period; repeat as needed every 10 min	Reversal of tetany	Correct symptomatic hypocalcemia; avoid excessive administration that may increase production of calcium oxalate crystals in ethylene glycol poisoning
L-Carnitine	Valproate-induced hyperammonemia or hepatotoxicity	100 mg/kg (maximum 6 g) IV during 30 min, then 15 mg/kg IV during 30-min period q4h (maximum 6 g/day)	Treat until clinical improvement occurs	Levocarnitine is active form Adjust dose for end-stage renal disease

Continued on following page

Antidote	Indication for Use	Dose*	Treatment End Point	Comments
Cyanide antidote kit Amyl nitrite Sodium nitrite Sodium thiosulfate [Hydroxocobalamin is preferred if available, see below]	Cyanide	Amyl nitrite: 0.3-ml pearls, crush and inhale during 30-sec period Sodium nitrite 3%: 10 ml IV during 10-min period Sodium thiosulfate 25%: 50 ml (12.5 g) IV during 10-min period	Resolution of lactic acidosis and moderate to severe clinical signs and symptoms: Seizures, coma, dyspnea, apnea, hypotension, bradycardia	Coordinate amyl nitrite with continued oxygenation and give only until sodium nitrite infusion is begun; nitrites may produce hypotension and excess methemoglobinemia Sodium nitrite dose must be adjusted if patient has hemoglobin <12 g/dl Sodium thiosulfate dosing can be repeated
Deferoxamine	Iron	Initiate at 5 mg/kg/hr, titrate to 15 mg/kg/hr IV (maximum 8 g/day) Mild to moderate: Administer for 6-12 hr Severe toxicity: Administer 24 hr	Resolution of clinical signs and symptoms Do not use urine color, which is an unreliable marker for iron clearance Laboratory testing is unreliable while antidote is being received	Indications: Symptomatic patients with lethargy, severe abdominal pain, hypovolemia, acidosis, shock; any symptomatic patient with peak serum iron level >350 g/dl Prolonged therapy can cause pulmonary toxicity
Digoxin-specific antibody fragments (Fab)	Digoxin Digitalis and related plants (e.g., oleander, lily of the valley) Other cardiac glycosides (e.g., bufadienolides [Bufo toads])	Unknown digoxin dose or serum level, or for plant or toad source: Acute toxicity—10-20 vials; chronic toxicity—3-6 vials Digoxin dose known: Number of vials = (mg ingested × 0.8) ÷ 0.5 Digoxin serum level known: Number of vials = [serum level (ng/ml) × weight (kg)] ÷ 100 Infuse dose during 30 min	Resolution of hyperkalemia, symptomatic bradydysrhythmias, ventricular arrhythmias, Mobitz II or third-degree heart block	Each vial binds 0.5 mg of digoxin or digitoxin Monitor ECG and potassium levels Digoxin serum levels unreliable after antidote administered unless test is specific for free serum digoxin
Dimercaprol (BAL)	Arsenic Lead Mercury, elemental and inorganic salts	Arsenic: 3-5 mg/kg IM q4h Lead: 75 mg/m^2 (4 mg/kg) IM q4h for 5 days Inorganic mercury: 5 mg/kg IM, then 2.5 mg/kg IM q12h for 10 days or until patient is clinically improved	Arsenic: 24-hr urinary arsenic <50 μg/L Lead: Encephalopathy resolved, blood lead level <100 μg/dl, and succimer therapy can be started Mercury, elemental and inorganic: 24-hr urinary mercury <20 μg/L	Formulated in peanut oil; painful IM injection and caution with allergy Maximum adult dose is 3 g/day BAL started 4 hr before initiation of concomitant $CaNa_2$ EDTA for lead encephalopathy Dosing not well established for arsenic and elemental or inorganic mercury toxicity; not used for organic mercury poisoning Adverse effects: Painful injections, fever, diaphoresis, agitation, headache, salivation, nausea and vomiting, hemolysis in G6PD-deficient patients, chelation of essential metals Check essential metal levels if chelation is prolonged Succimer is replacing BAL for many indications except lead encephalopathy Treatment end points for arsenic and mercury include improving clinical condition
Edetate calcium disodium ($CaNa_2$ EDTA)	Lead	1500 mg/m^2/24 hr (maximum 3 g) by continuous infusion	Treat for 5 days, followed by 2-day hiatus; repeat until encephalopathy resolved, lead level <100 μg/dl, and succimer therapy can be started	Use in patients with lead encephalopathy or lead level >100 g/dl Administer BAL 4 hr before initiating $CaNa_2$ EDTA Hydrate patient and establish good urinary output before starting therapy Avoid thrombophlebitis by diluting in NS or D_5W to a concentration ≤0.5% Substitution of Na_2 EDTA can cause fatal hypocalcemia
Flumazenil	Benzodiazepines	0.1 mg/min IV to a total dose of 1 mg	Reversal of coma	Limit use to reversal of inadequate ventilation in benzodiazepine-toxic patients Acute benzodiazepine withdrawal may occur in patients dependent on benzodiazepines Increases intracranial pressure and risk for seizures in presence of underlying seizure disorder or ingestion of seizure-producing toxicants Monitor for resedation up to 2 hr after last dose

Antidote	Indication for Use	Dose*	Treatment End Point	Comments
Folinic acid (tetrahydrofolic acid [leucovorin])	Methanol Methotrexate	Methanol: 50 mg IV q4h Methotrexate: 100 mg/m^2 IV during 15-30 min q3-6h; dosing lower when used as "rescue" in chemotherapy	Methanol: Methanol undetectable, metabolic acidosis cleared Methotrexate: Serum level <1 × 10–^{8} mol/L	Essential therapy for both toxicants Little concern with excessive dosing when used for methotrexate overdose Methotrexate: Large overdoses may require increased dose Glucarpidase administered 2-4 hr before or after folinic acid
Fomepizole	Ethylene glycol Methanol	Dose 1: 15 mg/kg IV Doses during next 48 hr: 10 mg/kg IV All subsequent doses: 15 mg/kg IV Administer q12h, except when HD performed: HD initiation: Next dose if >6 hr since last dose HD ongoing: q4h End of HD (based on time of last dose): <1 hr, no dose; 1-3 hr, next dose; >3 hr, next dose	For both: Serum level <25 mg/dl and metabolic acidosis resolved	Start immediately if toxic alcohol suspected, without waiting for confirmatory levels Dose amount is not affected by interval timing of doses
Glucagon	β-Adrenergic receptor antagonists Calcium-channel antagonists	Bolus of 3-5 mg IV; can repeat to achieve clinical effect, then infusion of 2-10 mg/hr	Reversal of hypotension and bradycardia; taper infusion	Can precipitate vomiting; be prepared to protect airway Mild hyperglycemia occurs Maximum dosing amounts unknown; bolus doses up to 30 mg reported Duration of effect is 15 min; thus infusion must be started immediately
Hydroxocobalamin	Cyanide	Initial: 5 g IV during 15-min period Second dose: 5 g IV during 15 min to 2 hr; maximum total dose is 10 g Follow each hydroxocobalamin dose with sodium thiosulfate 25%: 50 ml (12.5 g) IV during 10-min period	Resolution of lactic acidosis and moderate to severe clinical signs and symptoms: Seizures, coma, dyspnea, apnea, hypotension, bradycardia	Can be administered IV push if patient is in cardiac arrest Do not give hydroxocobalamin and sodium thiosulfate through the same IV line Adverse effects: Red discoloration of plasma, urine, mucous membranes, skin; transient hypertension Interference with laboratory colorimetric assays: Levels increased: Bilirubin; creatinine; glucose; hemoglobin; magnesium; co-oximetry total Hb, COHb%, MetHb% Levels decreased: AST, ALT, creatinine, co-oximetry O_2 Hb%
Hyperbaric oxygen (HBO)	Carbon monoxide Experimental: Carbon tetrachloride, cyanide, hydrogen sulfide	3.0 atm pressure for 60 min (25 min O_2, 5 min air, 25 min O_2, 5 min air), then 2.0 atm for 65 min (30 min O_2, 5 min air, 30 min O_2), then "surface" to 1.0 atm	One treatment Repeated treatment controversial	Carbon monoxide: Treatment protocols may vary HBO indicated for loss of consciousness; seizures; cerebellar dysfunction; impaired cognition; headache, nausea/vomiting persisting after 4 hr of O_2 therapy regardless of carboxyhemoglobin level
Insulin-glucose	Calcium-channel antagonists β-Adrenergic receptor antagonists	Regular insulin, 1 U/kg bolus, followed by 0.5-1 U/kg/hr Titrate 50% dextrose IV to avoid hypoglycemia	Reversal of myocardial depression	Initiate early to reverse myocardial depression Monitor glucose and potassium; hypoglycemia can occur during and after therapy Hyperglycemia results from calcium-channel antagonist–induced insulin resistance, and initial dextrose requirements may be less than anticipated Recovery may be heralded by normalization of glucose levels, with increased dextrose required to avoid hypoglycemia
Lipid emulsion	Cardiac toxicity from local anesthetics (e.g., bupivacaine, ropivacaine) Experimental: Verapamil, diltiazem, tricyclic antidepressants, bupropion, propranolol, and other lipophilic toxicants	Use 20% formulation Initial bolus: 1.5 ml/kg IV during 1 min, followed immediately by infusion of 0.25 ml/kg/min for 30-60 min Can repeat bolus for asystole	Return of hemodynamic stability	Use for other than bupivacaine based on animal experiments and human case reports; numerous dosing regimens have been used Use if advanced life support measures fail; continue CPR as needed during drug administration

Continued on following page

Antidote	Indication for Use	Dose*	Treatment End Point	Comments
Methylene blue	Methemoglobin-producing agents	1-2 mg/kg body weight (0.1-0.2 ml/kg of 1%) methylene blue during 5-min period; repeat dose for persistent or recurrent symptoms or signs	Resolution of dyspnea and altered mental status	Use if patient is symptomatic (i.e., dyspneic, altered mental status) Maximum dose should not exceed 7 mg/kg (0.7 ml/kg) Contraindicated in G6PD-deficient patients; may cause hemolysis Some toxicants (e.g., dapsone) may require prolonged therapy
N-Acetylcysteine (NAC)[7]	Acetaminophen Experimental: Carbon tetrachloride, chloroform, pennyroyal oil	Oral (total 72 hr) Load: 140 mg/kg Maintenance (starting 4 hr after load): 70 mg/kg q4h × 17 doses IV (total 21 hr) Load: 150 mg/kg during 1-hr period Maintenance infusion: 12.5 mg/kg/hr during 4-hr period, then 6.25 mg/kg/hr over 16 hr as continuous infusion	At the end of therapy, repeat AST and APAP levels: If AST normal and APAP not detected, treatment complete; if AST normal and APAP detected, continue NAC; if AST elevated, continue NAC After patient has received full course of NAC therapy, if INR ≥2.0 or severe hepatotoxicity present (AST >1000 U/L), continue NAC until INR <2.0 and aminotransferases normalize	Most effective if initiated within 8 hr after ingestion; may be started any time after ingestion and is beneficial in severe hepatotoxic states Longer duration of treatment may be required in patients with hepatotoxicity Treatment end points simplified for ease of use INR result not valid indicator if FFP recently administered
Naloxone	Opioids	Opioid dependence possible: 40-50 μg (0.04-0.05 mg) IV titrated upward to reversal, while avoiding withdrawal if concerns for opioid dependence Opioid dependence not likely: 0.4 mg by any route and titrate up to 10 mg Continuous infusion: Establish bolus dose required to reverse respiratory depression; begin infusing two thirds of reversal dose every hour and titrate to maintain adequate respirations; repeated bolus with half of reversal dose 15 min after reversal of respiratory depression	Initial: Reversal of respiratory depression with resolution of hypoxia and hypercapnia Final: Resolution of CNS and respiratory depression	Pre-ventilate patients with respiratory depression by bag-valve-mask or intubation before administration Use smaller doses in opioid-dependent patients Some opioids (e.g., buprenorphine) may require larger doses of naloxone Use continuous infusion for recurrent symptoms and prolonged action of some formulations (e.g., sustained-release morphine, methadone) Resedation can occur Do not use naltrexone to reverse acute toxicity
Octreotide	Sulfonylurea-induced hypoglycemia	50 mg SC q6h	Resolution of hypoglycemia and dextrose not required	Maintain dextrose infusion as needed Not for insulin-induced hypoglycemia
Physostigmine	Anticholinergic agents (e.g., diphenhydramine, jimsonweed [*Datura* sp], scopolamine)	1-2 mg IV during 5-min period; can repeat in 5 min if no effect and cholinergic effects do not occur	Reversal of anticholinergic effects	Duration of effect is 60-90 min Benzodiazepine used for subsequent treatment of agitation and seizures; additional physostigmine used rarely (e.g., refractory seizures or agitation) Adverse effects include seizures, excessive oral secretions, bradyarrhythmias; contraindicated in cyclic antidepressant toxicity
Pralidoxime chloride	Organophosphorus compounds Nerve agents: Sarin, VX	30 mg/kg IV bolus (maximum 2 g) during 30 min, followed by continuous infusion of 8-10 mg/kg/hr (maximum 650 mg/hr)	Resolution of signs and symptoms, atropine no longer required	Can give initial dose during 2-min period for life-threatening clinical effects Administer early when diagnosis known or strongly suspected Efficacy variable, depending on the organophosphate Fat-soluble organophosphates may require prolonged treatment
Pyridoxine	Ethylene glycolisoniazid Monomethylhydrazine (*Gyromitra esculenta* mushrooms)	100 mg IV 5 g IV, repeat for refractory seizures	One dose Resolution of seizures	Efficacy theoretical for ethylene glycol to enhance elimination of toxic metabolites Pyridoxine may be required even with benzodiazepines to stop seizures, but patient can remain comatose (isoniazid, *Gyromitra* mushrooms) Excessive dosing can cause neuropathy

Antidote	Indication for Use	Dose*	Treatment End Point	Comments
Sodium bicarbonate ($NaHCO_3$)	Reversal of myocardial sodium-channel blockers (e.g., cyclic antidepressants, cocaine, sodium-channel–blocking antiarrhythmics with $\tau_{recovery}$ >1 sec, piperidine phenothiazines (thioridazine, mesoridazine) Altered tissue distribution or enhanced elimination of salicylates; may be used for chlorophenoxy herbicides, formic acid, methotrexate, phenobarbital	1-2 mEq $NaHCO_3$/kg by intermittent bolus; repeat as needed 1-2 mEq $NaHCO_3$/kg, followed by 3 ampules (150 ml) $NaHCO_3$ (44 mEq per 50 ml) in 850 ml of D_5W, infused at 2-3 times normal maintenance fluid rate	Narrowing of prolonged QRS, resolution of ventricular arrhythmias, reversal of hypotension Serum salicylate <30 mg/dl and patient clinically stable	Monitor blood pH (optimal pH approximately 7.50); avoid pH >7.55 Target blood pH: 7.50-7.55 Monitor urinary pH hourly; adjust infusion to maintain urine pH of 7.5-8.0 (avoid blood pH >7.55) Monitor ABGs Maintain normokalemia
Succimer (DMSA)	Arsenic Lead Mercury, all forms	10 mg/kg/dose q8h for 5 days, followed by q12h for 14 days Drug holiday for 2 weeks; repeat if treatment end point not reached	Arsenic: 24-hr urinary arsenic <50 μg/L Lead: Resolution of encephalopathy, gastrointestinal symptoms, neuropathy, nephropathy, arthralgias, myalgias, and blood lead level <70 μg/dl Mercury, elemental and inorganic: 24-hr urinary mercury <20 μg/L Mercury, organic: End point not well established	Oral chelator; adverse effects include rash, transient AST and alkaline phosphatase elevations, and gastrointestinal distress; minimal chelation of essential metals occurs Dosing for arsenic and mercury not well established Therapeutic end point for organic mercury not established; neurotoxicity not responsive to chelation therapy; suggest chelation until blood mercury level within normal-value range for reference laboratory
Vitamin K	Vitamin K antagonist anticoagulants (e.g., warfarin, long-acting anticoagulant rodenticides [LAARs]) [note that this is not for normalizing a supratherapeutic INR in patients prescribed warfarin]	Subcutaneous: AquaMEPHYTON (K_1), 10-25 mg, repeat every 6-12 hr until oral vitamin K_1 started Oral: 25-50 mg q6h; larger doses may be required	INR is normal 48-72 hr after stopping vitamin K_1 therapy Can also monitor factor VII activity	Anaphylactoid reaction can occur with rapid IV administration Severe bleeding may also require FFP, prothrombin protein concentrate (off label), or factor concentrates Base decision to treat on finding of elevated INR; do not administer prophylactic vitamin K_1 Oral therapy may be required for months with LAAR poisoning because of lipophilicity of toxicant, with slow body clearance

ABGs, Arterial blood gases; *ALT,* alanine aminotransferase; *APAP,* acetyl-*p*-aminophenol (acetaminophen); *AST,* aspartate aminotransferase; *BAL,* British antilewisite; *CNS,* central nervous system; *COHb%,* percentage carboxyhemoglobin; *CPR,* cardiopulmonary resuscitation; *D_5W,* 5% dextrose in water; *DMSA,* 2,3-dimercaptosuccinic acid; *ECG,* electrocardiogram; *FFP,* fresh-frozen plasma; *G6PD,* glucose-6-phosphate dehydrogenase; *Hb,* hemoglobin; *HD,* hemodialysis; *INR,* international normalized ratio; *MetHb%,* percentage methemoglobinemia; *NS,* normal saline; *O_2 Hb%,* percentage oxyhemoglobin; $\tau_{recovery}$, drug blockade recovery rate.

*Dose concentrations and infusion times are not given. Drug dosages may require adjustment in patients with renal or hepatic failure.

†Administer antivenom in a monitored setting; antivenom must be reconstituted and then diluted; initially infuse at a rate of 2-5 ml/hr, and double the infusion rate every 5 min as tolerated to administer antivenom during a 1-hr period.

‡Ten percent calcium chloride solution = 100 mg/ml (27.2 mg/ml elemental calcium); 10% calcium gluconate solution = 100 mg/ml (9 mg/ml elemental calcium).

From Goldman L, Schafer AI: *Goldman-Cecil medicine,* ed 25, Philadelphia, 2016, Elsevier.

Appendix IIId

Management of Acute Poisoning

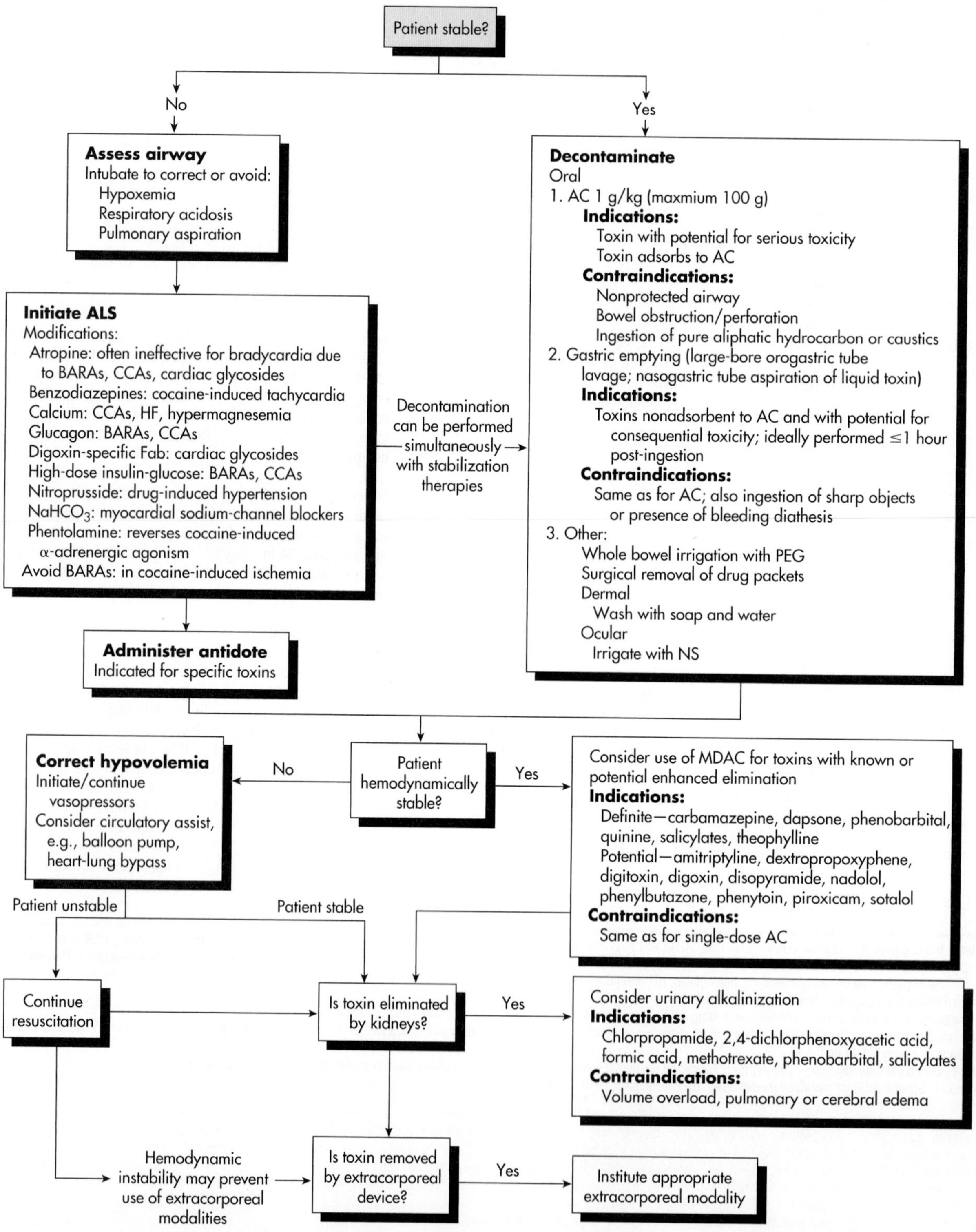

FIG 1 Algorithm for the management of acute poisoning. See also Appendix IIIe: Pathophysiology, Clinical Effects, and Management of Specific Drugs and Toxicants. *AC,* Activated charcoal; *ALS,* advanced life support; *BARAs,* β-adrenergic receptor antagonists; *CCAs,* L-type calcium-channel antagonists; *HF,* hydrofluoric acid; *MDAC,* multidose activated charcoal; *NS,* 0.9% saline solution; *PEG,* nonabsorbable polyethylene glycol solution. (Modified from Goldman L, Schafer AI: *Goldman-Cecil medicine,* ed 25, Philadelphia, 2016, Elsevier.)

TABLE 1 Qualitative Urine Drug Screens: Causes of Erroneous Results

Drug/Toxicant	Interferents/Irrelevants†	Comments
Amphetamines	Amantadine, bupropion, chlorpromazine, ephedrine, pseudoephedrine, desoxyephedrine, ephedra alkaloids (from *Ephedra* spp.), mexiletine, phenylephrine, phenylpropanolamine, selegiline, trazodone	Many false-positives from medicinal sympathomimetics; nasal inhaler (desoxyephedrine) and selegiline cause positive GC-MS findings; chiral confirmation is required; newer immunoassays have reduced false rates but also lower sensitivity for the class of amphetamines
Benzodiazepines	Oxaprozin, sertraline	Most assays directed against oxazepam; poor detection of benzodiazepines without the oxazepam metabolite (e.g., alprazolam, lorazepam, triazolam)
Cocaine	Coca leaf teas (clinical false-positive; still considered illicit use)	Few analytic false-positives; urine is reliable for detecting true positives
Opioids	Poppy seeds (contain morphine)	Assay directed against morphine; poorly detects semisynthetic opioids and does not detect synthetic opioids (e.g., fentanyls, meperidine, methadone, propoxyphene)
Phencyclidine	Dextromethorphan, diphenhydramine, doxylamine, ibuprofen, ketamine, tramadol, venlafaxine	Can be used, although not reliably, to identify dextromethorphan or ketamine
Tetrahydrocannabinol	Dronabinol, efavirenz, proton pump inhibitors	Positive result is seldom clinically relevant; synthetic cannabinomimetics (e.g., spice, K2) are not reliably detected
Tricyclic antidepressants	Carbamazepine, cyclobenzaprine, cyproheptadine, diphenhydramine, phenothiazines, quetiapine	

GC-MS, Gas chromatography–mass spectrometry.
*Advances in drug screening and variability in immunoassay results should be considered by the clinician when interpreting qualitative drug screening results. There are many marketed assays, so consultation with the testing laboratory is advised. Positive screening results are considered presumptive and should be verified by GC-MS or another advanced analytical methodology.
†*Irrelevants* are agents causing true-positive but clinically irrelevant results on laboratory screening tests; they vary, depending on the screening method.
From Goldman L, Shafer AI: *Goldman-Cecil medicine,* ed 26, Philadelphia, 2020, Elsevier.

TABLE 2 Clinically Important Quantitative Drug Levels

	Levels	
Drug or Toxicant	**Therapeutic**	**Toxic***
Source: Blood or Serum		
Acetaminophen†	10-30 µg/ml	≥150 µg/ml 4 hr after ingestion‡
Carbamazepine	4-12 µg/ml	>15 µg/ml
Carboxyhemoglobin	Nonsmoker: 0.5%-1.5% Smoker: 4%-9%	>20%§
Cholinesteraseǀ		
Serum (butyrylcholinesterase)	3100-6500 U/L	<50% of normal value
Red blood cell (acetylcholinesterase)	26.7-49.2 U/g of hemoglobin	<50% of normal value
Digoxin (≥6 hours after oral dose for long-term therapy)	0.8-2.0 ng/ml¶	>2.0 ng/ml
Ethanol	None measured	>80 mg/dl**
Ethylene glycol	None measured	>25 mg/dl
Iron	50-175 µg/dl	>350 g/dl
Lead	<10 µg/dl	>25 g/dl
Lithium	0.6-1.2 mEq/L	>1.2 mEq/L††
Methanol	None measured	>25 mg/dl
Methemoglobin	1%-2%	>15%
Phenobarbital	15-40 µg/ml	>40 g/ml
Phenytoin	10-20 µg/ml	>20 g/ml
Salicylates	≤30 mg/dl	>30 mg/dl
Theophylline	8-20 µg/ml	>20 g/ml
Valproic acid	50-100 µg/ml	>100 g/ml
	Normal	**Toxic***
Source: Urine		
Arsenic	<50 µg/day	>100 g/24-hr urine††
Mercury	<20 µg/L	>20 g/L††
Thallium	<5.0 µg/L	>200 g/L††

*The "toxic" level is provided for perspective. For many toxicants, simply being above this value does not imply a specific need for therapy or a necessarily poor prognosis. It does, however, generally suggest a need for additional evaluation, observation, or monitoring. Similarly, depending on the clinical context, levels below the "toxic" range may still be consequential.
†False-positive levels of 16-28 µg/ml have been reported in patients with bilirubin levels greater than 17 mg/dl.
‡Levels drawn more than 4 hr after ingestion should be plotted on the nomogram provided by Rumack and Matthew (Rumack BH, Matthew H: Acetaminophen poisoning and toxicity, *Pediatrics* 1975;55:871-876) to assess the potential for toxicity.
§Lower levels may be toxic in pregnant patients and in those with prolonged exposure to carbon monoxide.
ǀConsult a reference laboratory for normal values; results are assay dependent.
¶Some patients may require levels above the therapeutic range to control symptoms.
**The value of 80 mg/dl (0.08 g/dl) for ethanol is the statutory limit for operating a motor vehicle. Consequential clinical effects other than inebriation are uncommon with concentrations below 200 mg/dl.
††Lower values may indicate toxicity if appropriate clinical findings are present.
From Goldman L, Shafer AI: *Goldman-Cecil medicine,* ed 26, Philadelphia, 2020, Elsevier.

TABLE 3 Chelators for Adult Heavy Metal Poisoning

Symptoms	Chelator	Recommended Dose†	Adverse Effects
Lead			
Asymptomatic, BLL*<70	None		
Mild-moderate, BLL 70-100	DMSA	10 mg/kg tid PO × 5 days, then bid for 14 days	Nausea, vomiting, diarrhea; mild elevations in aminotransferase levels
Encephalopathy, BLL >100	BAL +	4 mg/kg deep IM q4h × 5 days	Local injection site (pain, redness, sterile abscess); nausea, vomiting, diarrhea; anxiety, hypertension, tachycardia, fever; contraindicated in peanut allergy
	$CaNa_2$ EDTA‡	1500 mg/m²/day (approximately 50-75 mg/kg/day, maximum 3 g) either continuous infusion or in 2-4 divided IV doses for 5 days, adjusted for renal insufficiency	Renal toxicity (from metal chelate), constitutional symptoms, transient hypotension
Mercury			
Acute (elemental or inorganic) with moderate/severe symptoms	BAL	5 mg/kg deep IM then 2.5 mg/kg every 12-24 hr for 10 days or until symptoms improve and patient is able to take PO	Local injection site (pain, redness, sterile abscess); nausea, vomiting, diarrhea; anxiety, hypertension, tachycardia, fever; contraindicated in peanut allergy
Chronic (elemental or inorganic) or organic with symptoms	DMSA	10 mg/kg tid PO × 5 days, then bid for 14 days	Nausea, vomiting, diarrhea; mild elevations in aminotransferase levels
Arsenic			
Acute exposure with moderate to severe symptoms	BAL	3 mg/kg deep IM q4h × 2 days, then bid for 7-10 days	Local injection site (pain, redness, sterile abscess); nausea, vomiting, diarrhea; anxiety, hypertension, tachycardia, fever; contraindicated in peanut allergy
Chronic exposure with moderate symptoms§	DMSA	10 mg/kg tid PO × 5 days, then bid for 14 days	Nausea, vomiting, diarrhea; mild elevations in aminotransferase levels
Aluminum			
Acute or chronic exposure in dialysis patient with encephalopathy	Deferoxamine	See http://www2.kidney.org/professionals/kdoqi/guidelines_bone/Guide12.htm	Hypotension, increased risk of sepsis, acute lung injury
THALLIUM			
Acute thallium poisoning with moderate to severe symptoms	Prussian Blue	3 g tid PO until the urinary thallium excretion is less than 0.5 mg/day	Constipation, blue stool

BAL, British anti-Lewisite, dimercaprol; *BLL,* blood lead level; *DMSA,* 2,3-dimercaptosuccinic acid, succimer; *EDTA,* ethylenediaminetetraacetic acid.
*Adult recommendations.
†Chelation doses in general are not well studied or validated, with the exception of lead in children. Optimal dosing is not well established, particularly for BAL. Doses listed are author's suggestions.
‡Start 4 hours after first dose of BAL is administered.
§Benefit in this setting is not established.
From Goldman L, Shafer AI: *Goldman-Cecil medicine,* ed 26, Philadelphia, 2020, Elsevier.

Appendix IIIe

Pathophysiology, Clinical Effects, and Management of Specific Drugs and Toxicants

Drug or Toxicant	Pathophysiology	Clinical Effects	Laboratory	Specific Therapy
Acetaminophen	NAPQI (toxic metabolite) binds hepatic and renal tubular cells; acetaminophen itself induces transient decrease in functional factor VII	• Initial: Nausea, vomiting, coma, lactic acidosis in severe cases • Days 1-3: Elevated INR, aminotransferase, and bilirubin levels; RUQ tenderness; increased creatinine level in severe cases • Days 4-14: Gradual recovery or continued increase in INR and creatinine, lactic acidosis, coma, cerebral edema, death	• Potentially toxic level ≥150 μg/ml 4 hr after ingestion* • INR may be transiently elevated in first 24 hr because of decrease in functional factor VII; further increases indicate hepatic necrosis; elevated aminotransferase and bilirubin levels not predictive of hepatic failure • Creatinine elevated in severe cases	NAC can increase INR but not aPTT†
Amphetamines	• Increased release of presynaptic norepinephrine and dopamine • Increased serotonin release (especially MDMA, PMA, DOB, other synthetic amphetamines)	• Mild: Euphoria, decreased appetite, repetitive behavior • Moderate: Vomiting, agitation, hypertension, tachycardia, mydriasis, bruxism, diaphoresis • Severe: Hypertension or hypotension, arrhythmias, hyperthermia, seizures, coma, hepatotoxicity, rhabdomyolysis, DIC, hyponatremia (SIADH), renal failure, cerebral infarction or hemorrhage	Not helpful; many false-positives and false-negatives on screening tests	• IV crystalloid • External cooling • Benzodiazepines or barbiturates to control agitation or seizure • Benzodiazepines or nitroprusside for hypertension • See "SSRIs/SRIs" for features and treatment of serotonin syndrome
β-Adrenergic receptor antagonists	Blocks catecholamines from β-adrenergic receptors • α- and β-adrenergic receptor antagonism: Carvedilol, labetalol • Delayed rectifier potassium-channel blockade: Sotalol	Bradyarrhythmias, decreased myocardial contractility, hypotension, respiratory depression, decreased consciousness with seizures or coma (lipophilic agents, e.g., propranolol), prolonged QT interval (sotalol)	• ECG • No specific tests	• IV glucagon, 3.5-5 mg over 2-min period; if no increase in BP or HR, can repeat up to 10 mg; if effective, immediately start continuous infusion at 2-10 mg/hr; if still unstable, options include (1) regular insulin, 1 U/kg by IV bolus, followed by 1 U/kg/hr, plus dextrose to maintain euglycemia; (2) norepinephrine or dobutamine infusion titrated to desirable BP and HR; (3) IV milrinone, 50 μg/kg over 10-min period, then 0.375-0.75 μg/kg/min based on hemodynamic status‡ • Electrical pacing and IABP in refractory cases

Drug or Toxicant	Pathophysiology	Clinical Effects	Laboratory	Specific Therapy
L-type calcium-channel antagonists	• Blocks L-type voltage-sensitive calcium channels, thereby decreasing calcium entry into myocardial and vascular smooth muscle cells • Decreases pancreatic insulin release and increases insulin resistance	Bradyarrhythmias (verapamil, diltiazem), hypotension, hyperglycemia	• ECG • No specific tests	• IV 10% calcium chloride, 10-20 mg/kg (0.1-0.2 ml/kg); can repeat once; if BP improves, continuous infusion at 0.2-0.5 ml/kg/hr (20-50 mg/kg/hr) • Ionized Ca2+ levels should not exceed 2× normal (severe cases will be refractory to calcium therapy) • Glucagon, high-dose insulin and dextrose, catecholamines, and milrinone (as for β-adrenergic antagonists)
Cardiac glycosides, including digoxin, bufadienolides (toxic toad venom), or cardenolides (e.g., oleander, lily of the valley, dogbane)	• Inhibits Na+, K+-ATPase • Decreased CNS sympathetic output • Decreased baroreceptor sensitivity • Increased vagal acetylcholine discharge	• Bradyarrhythmias, including second- and third-degree AV block and asystole • Ventricular ectopy, tachycardia, fibrillation • Junctional tachycardia, paroxysmal atrial tachycardia with block • Weakness, visual disturbances, nausea, vomiting	• Serum digoxin level • Serum potassium (hyperkalemia occurs in acute poisoning; hypokalemia may be present in chronic poisoning), magnesium, and creatinine levels	• Correct hypokalemia and hypomagnesemia; do not give calcium • Digoxin-specific antibody fragments (Fab) indicated if patient has hemodynamically significant arrhythmias, serum potassium ≥5 mg/L, Mobitz II or third-degree AV block, ingestion of bufadienolide- or cardenolide-containing agents, or renal insufficiency • Empirical dose • Chronic: 2-5 vial • Acute: 10-20 vial • Calculated dose • Chronic: Number of vials = 2 × serum digoxin level (ng/ml) × 5.6 × weight (kg)/1000 • Acute: Number of vials = 2 × oral digoxin dose (mg) × 0.8
Cyclic antidepressants	Myocardial sodium- and potassium-channel blockade Blockade of α-adrenergic and cholinergic muscarinic receptor Inhibition of norepinephrine reuptake	• Decreased level of consciousness (can develop rapidly), myoclonus, seizures, coma • Anticholinergic toxidrome • Sinus tachycardia, ventricular conduction delays, ventricular arrhythmias, asystole • Hypotension	Serum levels not helpful in management	• Intermittent IV boluses of NaHCO3 (1 mEq/kg) to maintain arterial pH at 7.5 because acidemia can worsen cardiovascular complications • Intubation and neuroparalytic drugs may be useful to ameliorate acidemia from muscular hyperactivity while seizures are being treated • Contraindicated drugs: Types IA and IC antiarrhythmic agents; physostigmine, flumazenil
Ethylene glycol, methanol (e.g., antifreeze, window cleaners, camping stove fuels)	• Ethylene glycol: Toxic metabolites produce cytotoxicity in CNS, kidneys, lungs, heart, liver, muscles; metabolic acidosis is due to glycolate accumulation; oxalate complexes with calcium, so hypocalcemia can develop • Methanol: Metabolized to formic acid, which is responsible for metabolic acidosis and inhibition of cytochrome aa3; target organs include retina, optic nerve, CNS	• Ethylene glycol: CNS depression, cerebral edema, seizures, anion gap metabolic acidosis, renal failure with acute tubular necrosis, pulmonary edema, myositis • Methanol: Nausea, vomiting; cerebral edema, hemorrhage, infarcts; necrosis of thalamus and putamen; anion gap metabolic acidosis; visual disturbances, papilledema, hyperemic optic disc, nonreactive pupils	• Serum ethylene glycol and methanol levels; levels may be low or undetectable if significant metabolism has occurred • Ethylene glycol: Serum calcium, creatinine, BUN levels; examine urine for calcium oxalate crystals; false hyperlactatemia occurs with certain analyzers using l-lactate oxidase, which cross-reacts with glycolic and glyoxylic acids	• For both: Fomepizole (which inhibits alcohol dehydrogenase and blocks formation of toxic metabolites), 15 mg/kg IV loading dose, then 10 mg/kg IV for 4 doses during the next 48 hr, then 15 mg/kg for subsequent doses; interval dosing is q12h (q4h during hemodialysis, with dosing interval adjustments at start and finish); continue until ethylene glycol or methanol is no longer detectable • Use of ethanol is no longer recommended • Hemodialysis: Initiate if level is ≥50 mg/dl or metabolic acidosis with end-organ toxicity; continue until acidosis resolves and serum level of ethylene glycol or methanol is undetectable • Monitor for cerebral edema with possible herniation • Ethylene glycol: IV calcium for symptomatic hypocalcemia • Methanol: Folinic acid, 50 mg IV q4h until methanol not detectable and acidosis cleared
γ-Hydroxybutyrate (GHB) and its precursors (γ-butyrolactone and 1,4-butanediol [1,4-BD])	Agonist effect on CNS GHB receptors; indirect action with opioid receptors (may increase proenkephalins); metabolized to GABA, interacts with $GABA_B$ receptors; decreases dopamine release	• CNS: Rapid loss of consciousness, with recovery typical within 2-4 hr; myoclonus (possible seizures) • Respiratory depression; bradycardia; nausea, vomiting	No specific tests	• Supportive care, including respiratory support as needed • Withdrawal resembles sedative-hypnotic withdrawal and can be treated with benzodiazepines or pentobarbital

Drug or Toxicant	Pathophysiology	Clinical Effects	Laboratory	Specific Therapy
Lithium	Decreases brain inositol; alters CNS serotonin, dopamine, and norepinephrine; inhibits adenylate cyclases, including those that mediate vasopressin-induced renal concentration and thyroid function	• Chronic toxicity usually more severe than acute toxicity: Tremor, hyperreflexia, drowsiness, incoordination, clonus, confusion, ataxia; in severe cases, seizures, coma, death; recovery may take weeks, and CNS deficits may persist • Sinus node dysfunction, QT prolongation, T wave abnormalities, U waves • Nephrogenic diabetes insipidus, hypothyroidism, hyperthyroidism, hypercalcemia, pseudotumor cerebri • Acute toxicity: Nausea, vomiting, diarrhea, and milder neurologic findings	• Peak serum levels: • Normal dose 2-3 hr; up to 5 hr for sustained-release lithium • Acute overdose: Peak may be delayed ≥4-12 hr	• Replenish intravascular volume, maintain urinary output at 1-2 ml/kg/hr • Consider GI decontamination with oral polyethylene glycol electrolyte solution within 1-2 hr after acute overdose of sustained-release drug • Hemodialysis§ in patients with altered mental status, ataxia, seizures, or coma or in patients with mild symptoms in the setting of acute overdose or renal insufficiency • Ineffective or contraindicated therapies include oral activated charcoal, diuretics, and aminophylline
Opioids (e.g., heroin, morphine, oxycodone, fentanyl)	Agonist effect at CNS μ, κ, and δ opioid receptors; result is cell hyperpolarization and decreased neurotransmitter release	• CNS depression, respiratory depression, miosis • Dextromethorphan increases CNS serotonin and inhibits NMDA receptors, which causes hallucinations • Propoxyphene and its metabolite norpropoxyphene block sodium channels and can cause seizures and wide-complex arrhythmias similar to cyclic antidepressants; NaHCO3 treats arrhythmias • Seizure risk with tramadol, meperidine, propoxyphene • Rapid, powerful heroin-like effect when sustained-release oxycodone is crushed before ingestion, snorting, or smoking • QTc prolongation and torsades de pointes with methadone	Rapid urine drug screens detect morphine and codeine but may not detect semisynthetic and synthetic opioids; some interferents/irrelevants	• IV naloxone, 0.4-2 mg; can repeat up to 10 mg if no response • Continuous infusion for recurrent symptoms or sustained-release opioid ingestion; give 50% of dose that produces desired effect 15 min after initial effect is obtained, then infuse two thirds of this dose every hr; infusion rate can be increased or decreased to maintain normal respiration and avoid withdrawal symptoms • Contraindicated therapies: Nalmefene and naltrexone should not be used for acute opioid reversal
Organophosphorus compounds and carbamates (e.g., diazinon, mevinphos, fenthion, aldicarb)	Inhibits acetylcholinesterase, resulting in excessive acetylcholine stimulation of nicotinic and muscarinic receptors in autonomic and somatic motor nervous systems and CNS	• Nicotinic-mediated effects: Tachycardia, mydriasis, hypertension, delirium, coma, seizures, muscle weakness, fasciculations • Muscarinic-mediated effects: Salivation, lacrimation, urination, vomiting, defecation, miosis, bronchorrhea, bronchospasm, bradycardia	• Serum (butyrylcholinesterase) or RBC (acetylcholinesterase) activity <50% of normal • Clinical recovery occurs before serum cholinesterase levels normalize	• Atropine, 1-2 mg by initial IV bolus; double the dose every 5 min (2 mg, 4 mg, 8 mg, 16 mg, etc.) until drying of bronchial secretions, adequate oxygenation, pulse >80 bpm, systolic blood pressure >80 mm Hg achieved; continuous infusion at 10%-20% of total stabilizing dose per hr; stop infusion if patient develops any signs or symptoms of anticholinergic toxidrome; restart infusion at lower rate when signs or symptoms abate • Pralidoxime‖ chloride 30 mg/kg (maximum 2 g) IV bolus over 30 min, then 8-10 mg/kg/hr (maximum 650 mg/hr) continuous infusion; administer as soon as possible after poisoning; continue 12-24 hr after atropine no longer required and symptoms resolve

Drug or Toxicant	Pathophysiology	Clinical Effects	Laboratory	Specific Therapy
Salicylates	Inhibits cyclooxygenase; decreases formation of prostaglandins and thromboxane A_2; stimulates CNS medullary respiratory receptor and chemoreceptor trigger zone; impairs platelet function; disrupts carbohydrate metabolism; uncouples oxidative phosphorylation; increases vascular permeability	• Acute toxicity • Mild: Nausea, vomiting, diaphoresis, tinnitus, decreased hearing, hyperpnea, tachypnea • Moderate–severe: Confusion, delirium, coma, seizures, hyperthermia, ALI; death can occur within hours of overdose • Chronic toxicity: Same as acute, but may not have diaphoresis or vomiting • Consider diagnosis in patients with new-onset confusion, anion gap metabolic acidosis, or ALI	• Serum salicylate level: Toxic ≥30 mg/dl; level ≥100 mg/dl indicates life-threatening toxicity with possible sudden, rapid clinical deterioration; in chronic toxicity, levels may be minimally elevated (>30 mg/dl), and clinical evaluation is more reliable for gauging degree of toxicity • Arterial blood gases: Respiratory alkalosis with metabolic acidosis • Anion gap metabolic acidosis • Prolonged PT and PTT, ketonuria, ketonemia	Multidose activated charcoal q2-3h in acute overdose with progressive symptoms or rising salicylate level
SSRIs/SRIs	• Inhibits reuptake of serotonin • SRIs have additional effects (e.g., duloxetine inhibits norepinephrine reuptake, nefazodone inhibits serotonergic 5-HT2 receptors, trazodone inhibits peripheral α-adrenergic receptors, venlafaxine inhibits norepinephrine and dopamine reuptake)	• Vomiting, blurred vision, CNS depression, tachycardia • Seizures and coma rare • Torsades de pointes reported with citalopram • Serotonin syndrome: Clonus, agitation, tremor, diaphoresis, hyperreflexia; hyperthermia and hypertonicity in severe cases	• No specific tests • If serotonin syndrome suspected: Electrolytes, BUN, glucose, liver enzymes, coagulation panel, blood gases, chest radiograph	• Respiratory support as needed • Benzodiazepines for agitation or seizures • Serotonin syndrome: Consider cyproheptadine, 12 mg PO initial dose then 2 mg PO q2h (to a maximum of 32 mg/day) until symptoms resolve • Critical care therapies for hyperthermia, rhabdomyolysis, DIC, ARDS, renal and hepatic dysfunction, torsades de pointes

ALI, Acute lung injury; *aPTT,* activated partial thromboplastin time; *ARDS,* acute respiratory distress syndrome; *AV,* atrioventricular; *BP,* blood pressure; *bpm,* beats per minute; *BUN,* blood urea nitrogen; *CNS,* central nervous system; *DIC,* disseminated intravascular coagulation; *DOB,* 4-bromo-2,5-dimethoxyamphetamine; *ECG,* electrocardiogram; *GABA,* α-aminobutyric acid; *GI,* gastrointestinal; *HR,* heart rate; *IABP,* intra-aortic balloon counterpulsation; *INR,* international normalized ratio; *IV,* intravenous; *MDMA,* 3,4-methylenedioxymethamphetamine; *Na^1,K^1-ATPase,* sodium, potassium adenosine triphosphatase; *NAC,* N-acetylcysteine; *NAPQI,* N-acetyl-p-benzoquinone imine; *NMDA,* N-methyl-D-aspartate; *PMA,* paramethoxyamphetamine; *PT,* prothrombin time; *PTT,* partial thromboplastin time; *RBC,* red blood cell; *RUQ,* upper right quadrant (abdomen); *SIADH,* syndrome of inappropriate antidiuretic secretion; *SRI,* serotonin reuptake inhibitor; *SSRI,* selective serotonin reuptake inhibitor.

[l]A double-blind, randomized, placebo-controlled trial of pralidoxime in acute organophosphorus poisoning found no significant difference in mortality rates or need for intubation.

*A nomogram to evaluate the potential toxicity of levels drawn more than 4 hours after ingestion is provided in Fig. 7, from Rumack BH, Matthew H: Acetaminophen poisoning and toxicity, *Pediatrics* 1975(55):871-876. The nomogram is valid only for levels drawn after a single acute ingestion.

†NAC can be discontinued in patients with uncomplicated disease after a loading dose plus six maintenance doses if hepatic aminotransferase levels are normal and acetaminophen is not detected; otherwise, the full regimen should be administered.

‡Adjust infusion for reduced renal function.

§Continue hemodialysis until the serum lithium level is less than 1 mEq/L. Recheck the level 8 hr after dialysis, and restart hemodialysis if the level is higher than 1 mEq/L. Repeat this cycle until the serum lithium level remains lower than 1 mEq/L.

From Goldman L, Schafer AI: *Goldman's Cecil medicine,* ed 24, Philadelphia, 2012, Elsevier.

Appendix IIIf

Accidental Poisoning by Exposure to Other Drugs Acting on the Autonomic Nervous System

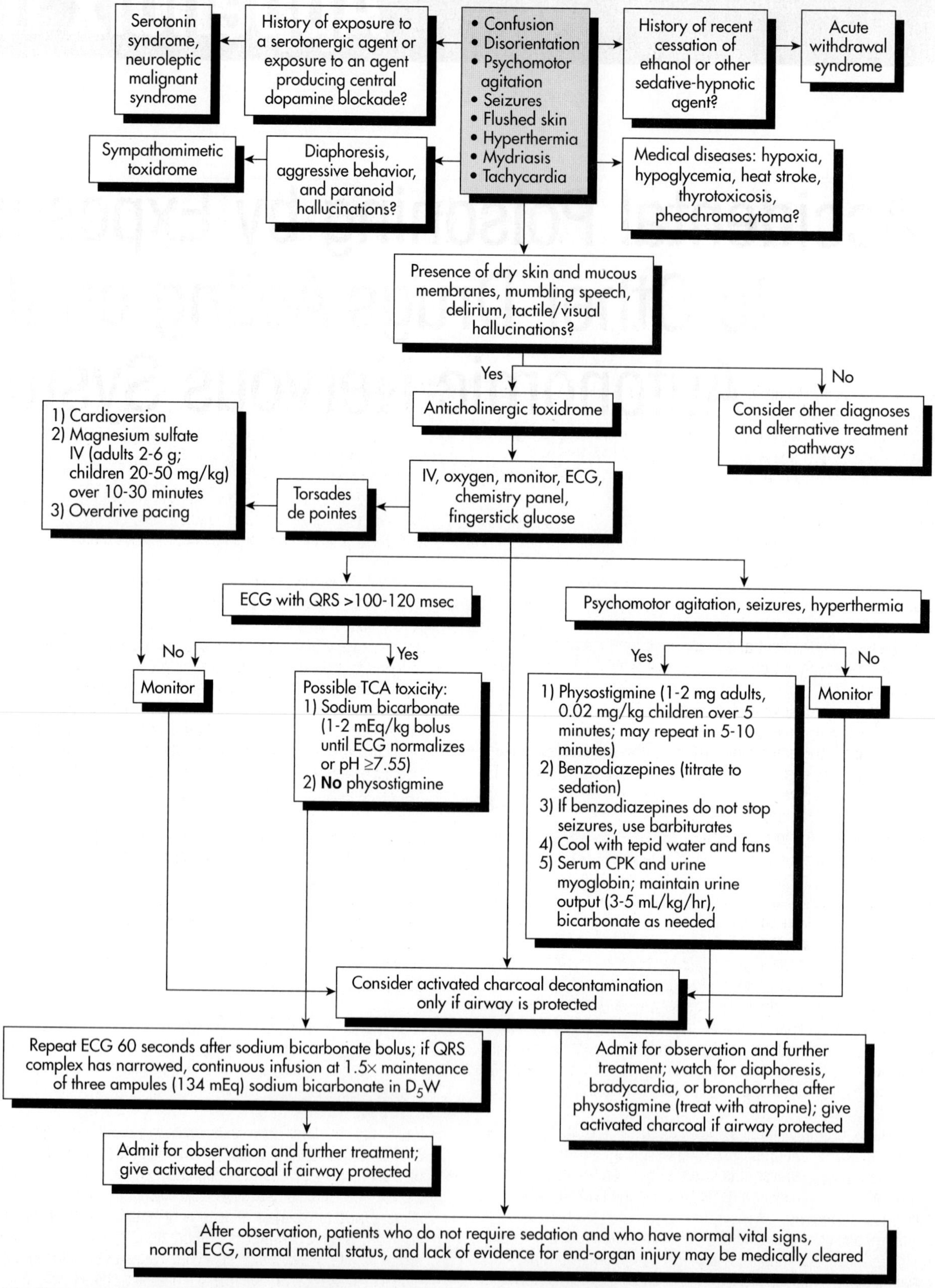

Algorithm for the recognition and treatment of anticholinergic toxicity. *CPK,* Creatine phosphokinase; *D_5W,* 5% dextrose in water; *ECG,* electrocardiogram; *IV,* intravenous line; *TCA,* tricyclic antidepressant. (From Adams JG et al: *Emergency medicine: clinical essentials,* ed 2, Philadelphia, 2013, Elsevier.)

Appendix IV

Impairment and Disability Issues

Impairment describes harm to anatomy and physiology, whereas *disability* denotes the difficulty a person has performing a function. Reporting disability for different sectors of society has its own nuances. Proper evaluation of impairment/disability starts with knowing who is asking for what. It is an area of practice in which an understanding of some basic concepts can make it rewarding rather than distressing.

- Ultimately, disability is a measure of function. Functional outcomes are becoming increasingly important in medicine, mirroring the shift toward patient-centeredness. All practitioners should have some facility with documenting the effects of an intervention on a patient's physical, psychological, and social functioning. For example, the continuation of an opioid analgesic should be predicated on meeting functional goals negotiated between the patient and physician before initiation of treatment. Even a brief comment on walking distance or work tolerance is better than nothing.
- Some concepts apply to all venues of disability. Primary care providers should rarely be in the position to determine whether a patient can be on or off a specific job. Rather, their task is to give general parameters about which physical exertions are medically dangerous. Try to be specific and use objective criteria where appropriate, but don't be intimidated by a form. Ballpark estimates can often suffice. For example, many chronic low back pain patients may conservatively and safely be described as able to lift/carry up 10 lbs, push/pull 25 lbs, and change positions as needed to keep comfortable. Have thorough medical records and be consistent; lawyers may focus on contradictions in your documentation to help their clients.
- Rehabilitation centers across the country are required to monitor function using a standardized set of criteria called the "Functional Independence Measure (FIM)," which categorizes activities of daily living into divisions such as mobility, transfers, feeding, grooming/hygiene, dressing, bathing, and toileting. In therapy notes, you may come across scores in these categories rating patients on a seven-point scale from totally dependent to moderate-assistance (mod A; patient can perform 50% of task) to modified-independent (patient requires an assistive device) to independent.
- Psychosocial contributing factors such as medicolegal issues can profoundly influence patients' presentations through somatization from secondary gain. However, it is important to differentiate this from malingering, Munchausen syndrome, or "gaming the system," which are remarkably less prevalent.
- The number of stakeholders expands in the disability system to include the employer, the government, the legal system, and the payer. Each sector has its own regulations. You may be required to fill out disability questionnaires as a condition of accepting payment for clinical services from a payer, such as in the workers' compensation system. Much more commonly, you will be seeing patients for clinical services paid for by an evaluation and management code. In these cases, you are not obligated to provide free medicolegal assessments. Settling payment issues in advance can avoid misunderstanding. Again, before assessing disability, understand who is asking and why.

GOVERNMENT-ADMINISTERED DISABILITY

State Temporary Disability Insurance (TDI) programs, the Family Medical Leave Act of 1993 (FMLA), the Social Security Administration (SSA), and the Department of Veterans Affairs offer disability benefits through the state and federal government.

- State TDI forms must be filled out for the patient to receive any income. They are generally very basic and just engage the social support network for a patient. This may not be the best venue to stipulate partial disability.
- The FMLA provides unpaid leave for qualified medical and family reasons. Because it is a federal program, the forms involved are standard across states and employers. They can be intimidating at first but are reasonably easy to complete once the basic definitions used are understood. It is recommended that you familiarize yourself with this paperwork the first few times it is encountered. Completing the form for subsequent patients should not be overly burdensome.
- The SSA and the Department of Veterans Affairs have their own internal mechanisms for quantifying disability, but they may subpoena your records or request a summary narrative as part of their processes. If you've kept good clinical notes, your existing documentation should satisfy their requirements. Many patients choose to apply for Social Security Disability Insurance (SSDI) and/or Supplemental Security Income (SSI) through a legal representative. These lawyers may send you a lengthy questionnaire to prepare their case. There are physicians whose practices perform these services and who can be hired by attorneys to facilitate patients' applications. If this nonclinical work appeals to you, consider affiliating with the SSA or contracting your time to lawyers under separate indenture. If not, you may want to recommend the law office contact a suitable practice.

WORKERS' COMPENSATION

In workers' compensation, the payer and employer join the provider in trying to rehabilitate the injured worker. Confidentiality issues are handled differently because these stakeholders may have a right to protected health information.

- Each state has their own laws regarding reporting requirements, and the U.S. Department of Labor governs injured federal employees. If you plan on accepting workers' compensation patients, you must familiarize yourself with the necessary paperwork. Typically, this is a standard, short form that includes measures of function. It may make sense to copy your state's parameters and create a "work note" to be used uniformly in your practice for cases both inside and outside of the workers' compensation system. Functional limitations should pertain to any task, not just to the employee's vocation. In general, employees should not be labeled "on" or "off."
- A notification that an employee has reached "maximal medical improvement" should be made once an employee's condition is expected to change over months/years rather than days/weeks. At this juncture they will transition from temporary disability benefits to permanent disability benefits, possibly including vocational rehabilitation. If ongoing sequelae exist, a

permanent impairment rating may be needed to resolve an employee's claim and allow them to progress to the next stage of their life. These are more sophisticated determinations, usually directed by the American Medical Association's (AMA) *Guides to the Evaluation of Permanent Impairment*, now in its sixth edition. Analysis of permanent impairment, causation, and apportionment generally fall outside of workers' compensation reporting requirements. Someone with appropriate training may be best suited to complete this task. Consider providing these more detailed services under a separate indenture, such as a consultation arrangement with the employee's attorney. Your state workers' compensation board may have specific guidelines governing these reports. In any case, the work should be done under a clear written agreement, not based on a verbal request by the employee. Very complex cases may also require a formal functional capacity evaluation through an appropriate rehabilitation resource.

PERSONAL INJURY

Patients hurt in car accidents or other personal injuries often are involved in legal cases covering medical care, personal damages, and pain and suffering. Most commonly, you will be helping these patients with their clinical issues under their regular medical insurance, although some providers agree to provide services under a legal lien on the claim. Regardless of your role in a personal injury case, it is helpful to document objective details about the injury and functional parameters. If you are asked to keep someone out of work, try to delineate functional limitations as you would in a workers' compensation employee.

- Similar to the workers' compensation system, it is helpful to state when a patient has reached maximal medical improvement. Personal injury claims can take longer to resolve than in the workers' compensation system, as the employer and insurance company are strongly incentivized to reach a resolution in those cases. In general, an ongoing legal case may hinder a patient from achieving a healthful balance of wellness. It is in the patient's best interest to move the claim toward completion.
- Quantifying permanent disability is a key component of resolving these cases. If a clinician is providing services under a legal lien, there may be a conflict of interest in having that provider quantify the permanent impairment. There may be financial implications to the degree of disability awarded, and this may influence whether or not the clinician will receive payment on their lien. These cases are almost always contentious and may be best handled by providers with special training, such as an independent medical examiner. Again, the determination typically follows the AMA's *Guides to the Evaluation of Permanent Impairment*. A clinician's role is to manage the patient's injuries, not to negotiate medicolegal issues. If you are not appropriately trained, consider deferring questions regarding disability to someone who is.

PRIVATE DISABILITY

Some patients purchase private insurance plans to provide income in addition to that offered through the government in the case of long-term disability. These forms vary by insurance carrier and change over time. They may need to be filled out periodically to maintain benefits. Many providers opt to charge a separate fee for the completion of this type of paperwork.

CONCLUSION

In summary, impairment and disability are measures of function and should be followed by all good doctors as part of patient-centered care. Providers can be most effective interacting with the various disability systems if they know when they are acting as clinicians and when they are acting as legal consultants. Understanding the principles involved with the different sectors will help you avoid confusion between obligations and opportunities when doing this work.

AUTHOR: **Matthew J. Smith, MD**

Appendix V

Protection of Travelers

TABLE 1 Structured Approach to the Pretravel Office Visit with a Traveler to the Developing World

Perform Risk Assessment

The following must always be ascertained to determine appropriate preventive medical recommendations. Preprinted medical record forms may be used to record these.

Exact itinerary, including regions within each country to be visited
Dates of travel to assess risk of seasonal diseases
Age
Past vaccination history
Underlying illness(es)
Current medications
Pregnancy status
Allergies
Purpose of trip
Risk exposures—blood, body fluids, adventure, or extensive outdoor exposures
Urban versus rural travel
Type of accommodations
Level of aversion to risk
Financial limitations that may necessitate prioritization of interventions

Administer Immunizations

Administer routine vaccinations that are not up-to-date.
Administer indicated travel vaccines.
Provide to patient legally mandated Vaccine Information Statements from the Centers for Disease Control and Prevention (www.cdc.gov/vaccines/hcp/vis/index.html).
Provide printed checklist to patient, listing vaccines administered.
Record in the clinic record vaccines administered, lot number, and date.
Document vaccines offered to but declined by patient, as well as nonrecommended vaccines administered at the patient's request.

Provide Malaria Prevention (If Indicated)

Determine whether malaria risk exists for the destination country. If yes:
Does the patient's itinerary within that country put him or her at risk? If yes:
Recommend malaria chemoprophylaxis. Several equally effective drugs of choice may be indicated. Ascertain which is best suited to the individual patient and itinerary.
Educate on personal protection against arthropods.

Educate on Traveler's Diarrhea

Recommend food and water precautions.
Prescribe and educate on standby therapy with a quinolone antibiotic or azithromycin and advise on use of loperamide and oral hydration if needed.

Teach Essential Preventive Behaviors

Most travel-related health problems, including vaccine-preventable diseases, can be avoided through simple behaviors initiated by the traveler.
Educate on appropriate strategies in the following categories (some topics are not applicable to all destinations): Blood-borne and sexually transmitted diseases, safety and crime avoidance, injury prevention, swimming safety, rabies, skin/wound care, tuberculosis, packing for healthy travel, obtaining health care abroad.

Discuss Other Applicable Heath Issues

Advise and prescribe for altitude illness, motion sickness, or jet lag.
Discuss prevention of specific travel-related infections that are of some risk to the traveler and have a possible preventive strategy not included in the strategies above.
Discuss any minimal-risk conditions (e.g., hemorrhagic fevers) that are a frequent cause of patient anxiety.

Updated from Bennett JE et al: *Mandell, Douglas, and Bennett's principles and practice of infectious diseases,* ed 8, Philadelphia, 2015, Elsevier.

TABLE 2 In-Depth Information Resources for Travel Medicine

Authoritative Websites Updated Constantly with Epidemiologic and Outbreak Information
Centers for Disease Control and Prevention (CDC) Travelers Health www.cdc.gov/travel
World Health Organization (WHO) Travelers' Health www.who.int/ith
Public Health Agency of Canada. Committee to Advise on Tropical Medicine and Travel (CATMAT) www.phac-aspc.gc.ca/tmp-pmv/catmat-ccmtmv/index-eng.php
WHO Disease Outbreak News www.who.int/csr/don/en/
WHO Weekly Epidemiological Record www.who.int/wer/en/
CDC Morbidity and Mortality Weekly Report www.cdc.gov/mmwr
WHO Disease by Disease Health Topics www.who.int/health-topics/
In-Depth References on Specialized Topics
Centers for Disease Control and Prevention. Health Information for International Travel 2018 (The "CDC Yellow Book"). U.S. Public Health Service. Atlanta. Full text and hard copy order information available at www.nc.cdc.gov/travel/page/yellowbook-home
World Health Organization. International Travel and Health (WHO "Green" Book). Published annually. Available from authorized WHO book agents. Full text online at www.who.int/ith/en/
Keystone JS et al (eds): *Travel medicine,* ed 4, Philadelphia, 2019, Elsevier (ISBN: 9780323546966)
Plotkin SA et al: *Plotkin's vaccines,* ed 7, Philadelphia, 2017, Elsevier (ISBN: 9780323393010)
Auerbach PS et al: *Wilderness medicine,* ed 7, St Louis, 2016, Elsevier (ISBN: 9780323359429)

Updated from Bennett JE et al: *Mandell, Douglas, and Bennett's principles and practice of infectious diseases,* ed 8, Philadelphia, 2015, Elsevier.

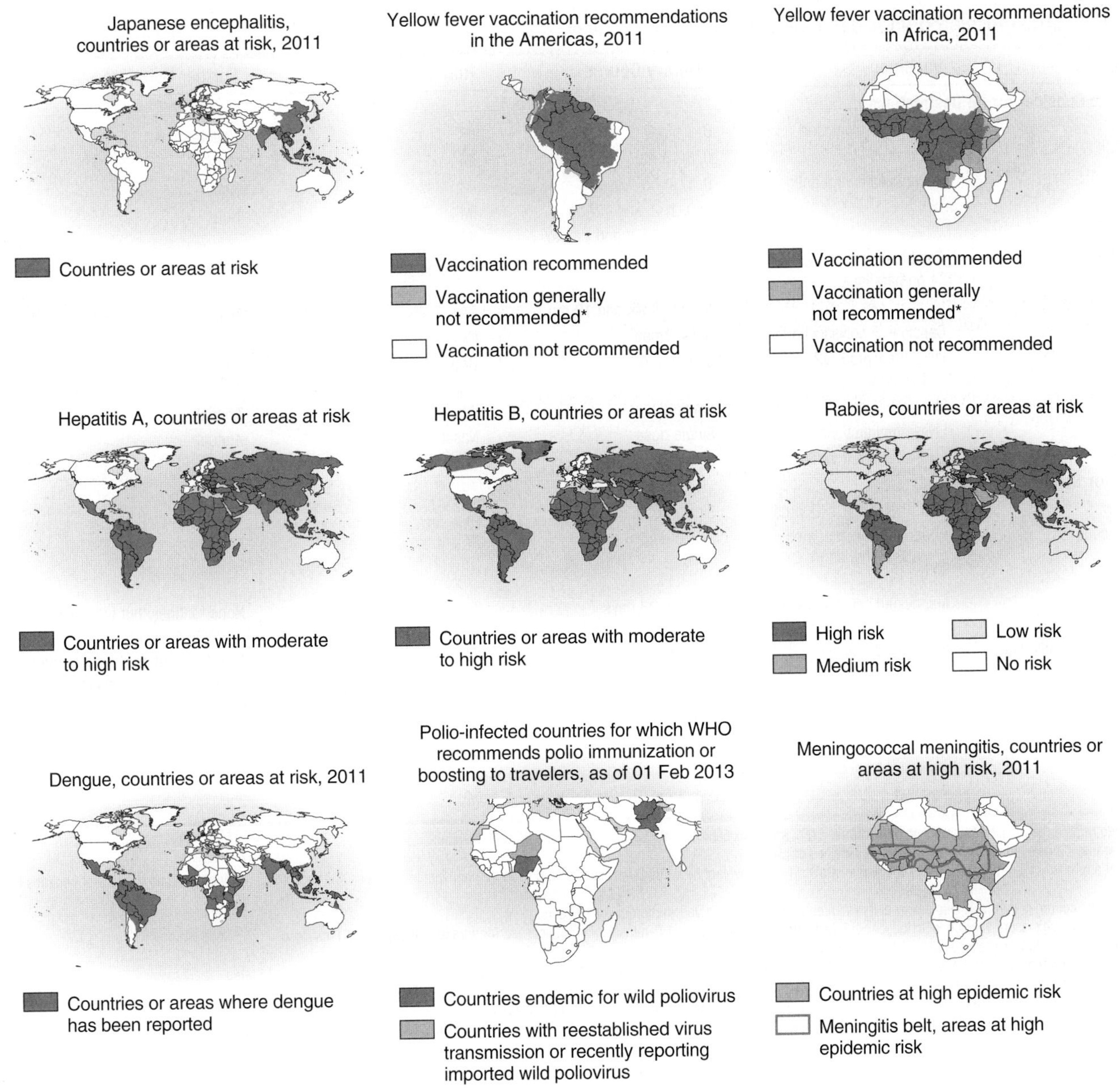

FIG. 1 Worldwide distribution of important travel-related diseases. *Yellow Fever (YF) vaccination is generally not recommended in areas where there is low-potential YF virus exposure. However, vaccination might be considered for a small subset of travelers to these areas who are at increased risk for exposure to YF virus because of prolonged travel, heavy exposure to mosquitoes, or inability to avoid mosquito bites. Consideration for vaccination of any traveler must take into account the traveler's risk of being infected with YF virus, country entry requirements, and individual risk factors for serious vaccine-associated adverse events (e.g., age, immune status). (From World Health Organization. International Travel and Health. Available at www.who.int/ith. In Bennett JE et al: *Mandell, Douglas, and Bennett's principles and practice of infectious diseases,* ed 8, Philadelphia, 2015, Elsevier.)

TABLE 3 Travel-Related Vaccines of Adults

Disease	Vaccine	Primary Course	Route	Further Boosters
Vaccines to Consider for All Destinations				
COVID-19	mRNA-based vaccine	0, 1 mo	IM	Undetermined
Hepatitis A	Killed virus	0, 6-18 mo[a]	IM	None
Hepatitis B	Recombinant viral antigen	0, 1, 6 mo	IM	None
		A: 0, 1, 2, and 12 mo	IM	None
		A: 0, 1, 3 wk and 12 mo[b]	IM	
Hepatitis A/B	Combination of monovalent preparations	0, 1, 6 mo	IM	None
		A: 0, 1, 3 wk and 12 mo	IM	None
Typhoid	Capsular Vi polysaccharide	Single dose	IM	2-3 yr
	Live-attenuated Ty21a bacteria	0, 2, 4, 6 days	Oral	5 yr
Influenza	Inactivated viral	Single dose	IM	Annual
	Live-attenuated virus	Single dose	Nasal	Annual
Varicella	Live-attenuated virus	0, 4-8 wk	SC	None
Vaccines for Selected Destinations				
Yellow fever	Live-attenuated 17D virus	Single dose	SC	Lifetime protection[c]
Meningococcus	Quadrivalent conjugated polysaccharide (A, C, Y, W135)	Single dose	IM	5 yr
Rabies	Inactivated cell culture viral	0, 7, 21-28 days	IM[d]	None routinely but two doses after each exposure
Japanese encephalitis (Vero cell)	Inactivated viral	0, 28 days	IM	1 yr if at continued risk; no data on subsequent doses
Polio[e]	Inactivated viral	Single dose if adequate childhood series	SC; IM acceptable	None
Cholera	Killed bacteria + recombinant B toxin subunit	0, 1 wk	Oral	2 yr for cholera; 3 mo for ETEC
Tick-borne encephalitis[h]	Inactivated viral[f,g]	0, 1-3 mo, 9-12 mo	IM	3 yr

A, Accelerated regimen to be used for imminent departures; *ETEC,* enterotoxigenic *E. coli; IM,* intramuscular; *SC,* subcutaneous.
[a]Second dose may be delayed up to 8 years without diminished efficacy.
[b]Regimen not approved by the U.S. Food and Drug Administration for monovalent hepatitis B vaccine but approved for combination hepatitis A/B vaccine containing the same quantity of hepatitis B antigen.
[c]Until 2016, some countries that have mandatory entry requirements may require vaccination every 10 years.
[d]Intradermal rabies preexposure vaccine is no longer produced, and the intramuscular 1.0-ml vials are not licensed for intradermal use in a 0.1-ml dose.
[e]Oral polio vaccine is no longer produced in the United States.
[f]Not available in the United States but available in Canada and most European countries. No cholera vaccine of any kind is currently available in the United States.
[g]Also licensed in some countries for traveler's diarrhea because of enterotoxigenic *Escherichia coli.*
[h]Not available in United States but available in endemic areas and in Canada and the United Kingdom by special release.
From Bennett JE et al: *Mandell, Douglas, and Bennett's principles and practice of infectious diseases,* ed 8, Philadelphia, 2015, Elsevier.

TABLE 4 Travel Vaccinations for Children

Vaccine	Formulation	Route and Dose	Schedule	Indications	Comments
Hepatitis A	Pediatric: Havrix (GlaxoSmithKline); 720 EU VAQTA (Merck); 25 U	IM; 0.5 ml	Primary series: 2 doses, 6-18 mo apart Booster: Currently not recommended	Children >6 months of age	Inactivated vaccine Lifelong protection is likely.
	Adult: Havrix (GlaxoSmithKline); 1440 EU VAQTA (Merck); 50 U	IM; 1.0 ml	Primary series: 2 doses, 6-18 mo apart Booster: Currently not recommended	Adults ≥19 yr old	Inactivated vaccine Lifelong protection is likely.
Hepatitis A and B	Twinrix (GlaxoSmithKline)	IM; 1.0 ml	Primary series: 3 doses at 0, 1, and 6 mo Accelerated schedule: 0, 7, and 21 days; 4th dose 12 mo later Boosters: Not needed	Adults ≥18 yr old	Inactivated vaccine Lifelong protection is likely. Accelerated schedule is as effective.
Immunoglobulin, human	Injectable	IM	Travel up to 1 mo duration: 0.1 ml/kg Travel up to 2 mo duration: 0.2 ml/kg Travel 2 mo or more: 0.2 ml/kg (repeat every 2 mo)	Infants <1 yr old	Passive immunizations against hepatitis A. Its use would require delay of measles and varicella vaccinations (at least 3 mo).
Japanese encephalitis virus (JEV)	Inactivated: Ixiaro (Intercell USA)	IM 2 mo to <3 yr old: 0.25 ml ≥3 yr old: 0.5 ml	Primary series: 2 doses at days 0 and 28 Booster: 1 dose 1 yr later if exposure to JEV expected	Travel to high-risk areas; prolonged stays	Booster recommendation is extrapolated from recommendation for individuals ≥17 yr old.
Meningococcal, polysaccharide	Quadrivalent: A, C, Y, W135	SC; 0.5 ml	Primary series: Single dose Booster: 5 yr in persons ≥4 yr old; 2-3 yr in children 2-4 yr old	≥2 yr old	Required for entry to Saudi Arabia during the Hajj. Recommended for travelers visiting "meningitis belt" in sub-Saharan Africa during dry months. This vaccine is rarely used in U.S. since conjugate vaccines are more immunogenic.
Meningococcal, conjugate	Quadrivalent: ACWY-D: Menactra (Sanofi Pasteur)	IM: 0.5 ml	Children 9-23 mo old: 2 doses, 3 mo apart 2-55 yr old: 1 dose	Routine vaccination in U.S. at ≥11-12 yr old with recommended booster 5 yr later	Required for entry to Saudi Arabia during the Hajj. Recommended for travelers visiting "meningitis belt" in sub-Saharan Africa during dry months. This vaccine should not be used in infants <9 mo old since it may interfere with antibody production by pneumococcal conjugate vaccine.
	Quadrivalent: ACWY-CRM: Menveo (Novartis)	IM; 0.5 ml	Children initiating vaccination at 2 mo: Doses at 2, 4, 6, and 12 mo old Children starting vaccination at 7-23 mo old: 2 doses, with 2nd dose after 2 yr old and at least 3 mo after 1st dose	Routine vaccination in U.S. at ≥11-12 yr old with recommended booster 5 yr later	Required for entry to Saudi Arabia during the Hajj. Recommended for travelers visiting "meningitis belt" in sub-Saharan Africa during dry months.
Rabies	Inactivated	IM; 1.0 ml	Preexposure series: 3 doses at days 0, 7, and 21 or 28 Booster: Depends on risk category and serologic testing. Postexposure: Rabies immune globulin; day 0; vaccines at days 0, 3, 7, and 14; 5th dose at day 28 is recommended if host is immunocompromised.		Consider for young travelers planning prolonged stays; especially away from large urban centers with adequate medical care systems and airport.

Continued

TABLE 4 Travel Vaccinations for Children—Cont'd

Vaccine	Formulation	Route and Dose	Schedule	Indications	Comments
Typhoid fever	Live-attenuated Ty21a1	Oral	1 capsule every other day for 4 doses Boosters: Every 5 yr	Persons ≥6 yr old	If series sequence not completed, all 4 doses need to be repeated. Contraindicated in immunocompromised hosts. Cannot be taken with hot beverage. Person must not be taking antibiotics.
	Injectable Polysaccharide Vi antigen	IM; 0.5 ml	Primary series: 1 dose Booster: Every 2 yr	Persons ≥2 yr old	
Yellow fever	Live injectable	SC; 0.5 ml	Primary series: 1 dose Dose must be given at least 10 days before arrival to risk area. Booster: No longer required by WHO. U.S. travelers: Recommended every 10 yr for high-risk travelers.	≥9 mo old	Contraindicated in immunocompromised hosts. Avoid in pregnancy and in breastfeeding mothers, unless high-risk travel cannot be avoided. Contraindicated in infants <4 mo old. Avoid in persons with thymus disorders. Infants 6-8 mo old: Consider vaccination with caution if risk or travel cannot be avoided; consult travel medicine specialist. Caution in persons ≥60 yr old (high risk for vaccine-related infection). Requires official certificate of vaccination.

IM, Intramuscular; *SC*, subcutaneous; *WHO*, World Health Organization.
From Kliegman RM: *Nelson textbook of pediatrics*, ed 21, Philadelphia, 2020, Elsevier. Table 200.1.

TABLE 5 Causes of Fever Associated with Geographic Areas and Specific Risk Factors[1]

Risk Factor	Common	Occasional	Rare but Important
Geographic Area			
Sub-Saharan Africa	HIV-associated infections (including seroconversion) Malaria Rickettsiae	Acute schistosomiasis (Katayama) Amebic liver abscess Brucellosis Dengue Enteric fever Meningococcus	Histoplasmosis Other arbovirus (e.g., Rift Valley, West Nile fever, yellow fever) Trypanosomiasis Viral hemorrhagic fever (Lassa, Ebola, Marburg, CCHF) Visceral leishmaniasis
North Africa, Middle East, and Mediterranean		Brucellosis Q fever Toscana (sandfly fever) MERS	Visceral leishmaniasis
Eastern Europe and Scandinavia		Lyme disease	Hantavirus Tick-borne encephalitis Tularemia
Central Asia		Q fever Rickettsia Sandfly fever	
South Asia	Dengue Enteric fever Malaria	Chikungunya Visceral leishmaniasis	CCHF Japanese encephalitis Other arbovirus (Nipah virus) Rickettsiae
Southeast Asia	Chikungunya Dengue Zika (emerging) Enteric fever Malaria	Leptospirosis Melioidosis	Hantavirus Japanese encephalitis Other arbovirus Nipah virus Paragonimiasis Penicilliosis Scrub typhus
North Australia		Dengue Murray Valley Q fever Rickettsiae Ross River fever	Barmah Forest Melioidosis
Latin America and Caribbean	Dengue Enteric fever Malaria Chikungunya Zika	Brucellosis Paracoccidioidomycosis Histoplasmosis Leptospirosis	Acute trypanosomiasis (Chagas) Hanta virus Yellow fever
North America		Coccidioidomycosis Histoplasmosis Lyme disease Rocky Mountain spotted fever	Babesiosis Anaplasmosis Ehrlichiosis West Nile fever
Specific Risk Factors			
Game parks	African tick typhus		Anthrax Trypanosomiasis
Freshwater exposure		Acute schistosomiasis Leptospirosis	
Caves		Histoplasmosis	Marburg Rabies
HIV	Amebiasis Non-typhoidal salmonella Tuberculosis	STI (e.g., syphilis) Visceral leishmaniasis	Blastomycosis Coccidioidomycosis Histoplasmosis Penicilliosis

CCHF, Crimean-Congo hemorrhagic fever; *MERS*, Middle Eastern Respiratory Syndrome; *STI*, sexually transmitted infection.

[1]Johnston V et al: Fever in returned travellers presenting in the United Kingdom: recommendations for investigation and initial management, *J Infect* 2009; 59: pp. 1-18.

Table adapted with permission from British Infection Society. Fever in returned travelers presenting in the United Kingdom: recommendations for investigation and initial management. In Ryan ET et al: *Hunter's tropical medicine and emerging infectious diseases,* ed 10, Philadelphia, 2019, Elsevier. Table 150.1.

TABLE 6 Leading Causes of Persistent Abdominal Symptoms in Returned Travelers

Infectious	Postinfectious Process	Structural or Organic Disease
Giardia spp.		
Cryptosporidium spp.		
Cyclospora		
Isospora		
Microsporidium		
Entamoeba histolytica		
Strongyloides stercoralis		
Schistosoma mansoni		
Campylobacter spp.		
Salmonella spp.		
Yersinia spp.		
Helicobacter pylori		
Blastocystis spp.	Malabsorption	
Secondary lactose intolerance		
Small intestinal bacteria overgrowth		
Irritable bowel syndrome		
Functional dyspepsia		
Functional bowel disorder, not otherwise specified		
Tropical sprue		
Brainerd's diarrhea	Celiac sprue	
Inflammatory bowel disease		
Colon cancer		
Microscopic colitis		
Peptic ulcer disease		

From Ryan ET et al: *Hunter's tropical medicine and emerging infectious diseases,* ed 10, Philadelphia, 2019, Elsevier. Table 153.1.

TABLE 7 Management Strategies for the Ill-Returning Traveler with Persistent Abdominal Symptoms

History

1. Location and duration of travel and particular features of travel that might be high risk for soil-transmitted helminths or water-borne protozoa
2. Timing of the symptom onset in relation to travel, development of acute traveler's diarrhea, and/or antibiotic use
3. Careful history of gastrointestinal symptoms preceding recent travel, which may indicate the preexisting nature of a functional bowel disorder or other organic/structural disorder
4. Quantitative and phenotypic features of stool, including spectrum from solid to liquid (Bristol Scale Chart may be useful), greasy, floating, malodorous, containing blood or mucus, etc., as well as frequency, volume, and association with any other GI symptoms
5. Association with particular food types (e.g., milk or fatty foods) and relationship in time to taking in meals
6. Any alarm features, including fever, night sweats, weight loss, and nocturnal symptoms

Diagnostics

1. Stool studies for common protozoal pathogens and bacterial causes of persistent abdominal symptoms (e.g., *Giardia, Cryptosporidium, Entamoeba hystolitica, Clostridium difficile, Campylobacter* spp., *Salmonella* spp.)
2. Serologies directed toward patient history, exposure, and clinical symptomatology, including *Strongyloides*
3. Hematology—WBC and particularly eosinophilia would be directive toward an extraintestinal protozoa
4. Additional blood chemistries—C-reactive protein, erythrocyte sedimentation rate, liver function tests
5. Other—intestinal malabsorption studies, breath testing for SIBO
6. Upper endoscopy/colonoscopy to rule out structural and organic disease as indicated

Suggested Treatments (Ideally Based on Positive Identification; Empirical Strategies Sometimes Indicated; Alternative Regimens May Be Equivalent) (Adult Doses Listed)

1. Antibacterial therapy: Azithromycin 500 mg qd × 3 days
2. Giardiasis: Metronidazole 250 mg tid 5-7 days OR tinidazole 2 g one dose OR nitazoxanide 500 mg bid × 3 days
3. Cryptosporidiosis: Nitazoxanide 500 mg bid × 3 days
4. Amebiasis: Metronidazole 750 mg tid 5-10 days followed by luminal agent (diloxanide furoate 500 mg tid × 10 days OR paromomycin 25-35 mg/kg/d tid × 7 days) OR nitazoxanide 500 mg bid for 3 days
5. Strongyloides: Ivermectin 200 µg/kg/d × 2 days
6. Empiric antiprotozoal/antihelminthic therapy: Tinidazole 1000 mg bid × 2 days followed by oral albendazole 400 mg bid × 5 days (NOTE: in locations where albendazole is cost-prohibitive, tinidazole alone may be tried) OR nitazoxanide 500 mg bid × 3 days
7. Functional bowel disorder (IBS-D most common):
   - Identify key patient characteristics
   - Educate and reassure the patient, trial of lifestyle/dietary modification
   - Optimize treatment for predominant symptoms (e.g., diarrhea, bloating, pain), preference, and availability; may include antimotility, bile acid sequestrants, rifaximin, probiotics, antispasmodics, eluxadoline, TCAs, low-FODMAP diet (bloating)
   - Follow-up: Reassess every 4-8 weeks (until stable) to assess response, tolerability, and reassurances
8. Small intestinal bacterial overgrowth/IBS-D: Rifaximin 550 mg three times daily for 2 weeks (repeat dosing may be necessary for recurrent symptoms)
9. Food-associated symptoms: Avoid and slowly reintroduce; bile-acid sequestrants if indicated

GI, Gastrointestinal; *IBS-D,* diarrhea-predominant inflammatory bowel disease; *SIBO,* small intestine bacterial overgrowth; *TCA,* tricyclic antidepressants; *WBC,* white blood cell count.
From Ryan ET et al: *Hunter's tropical medicine and emerging infectious diseases,* ed 10, Philadelphia, 2019, Elsevier. Table 153.2.

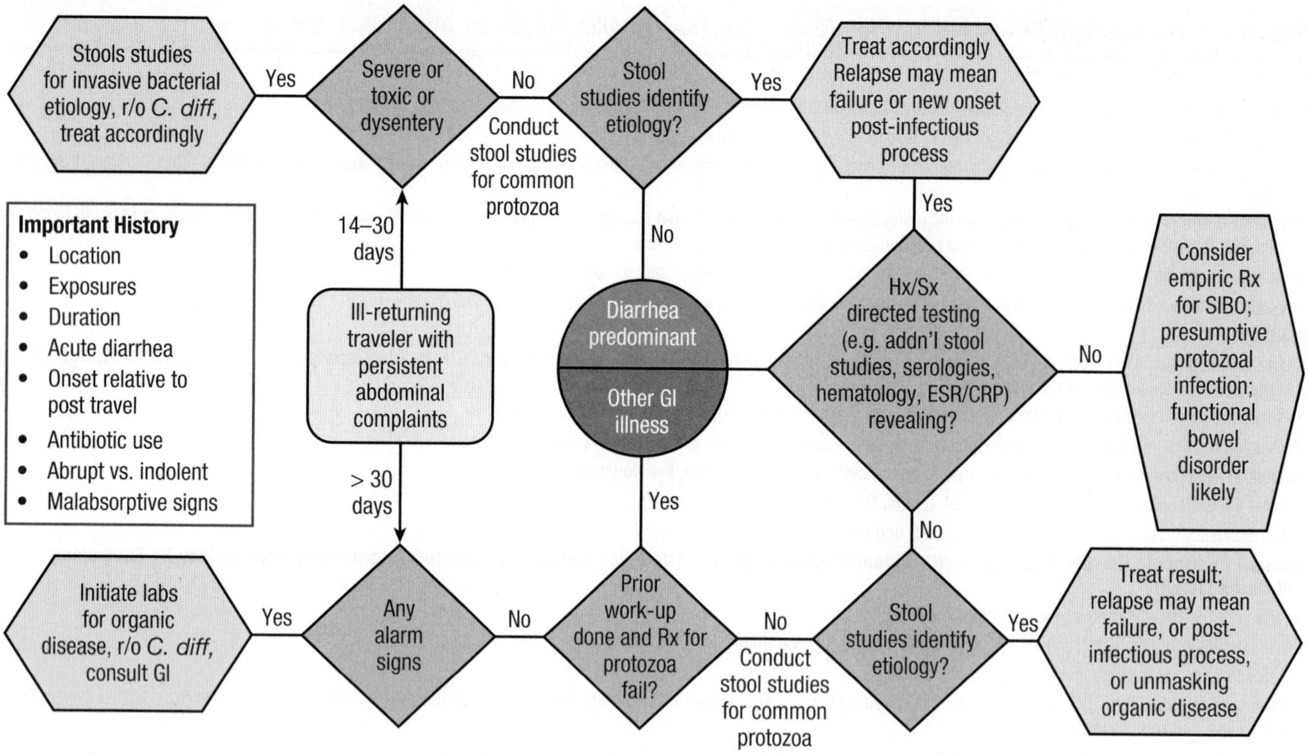

FIG. 2 Algorithmic approach to the individual returning from travel with persistent abdominal symptoms. (From Ryan ET et al: *Hunter's tropical medicine and emerging infectious diseases,* ed 10, Philadelphia, 2019, Elsevier. Fig. 153.1.)

Appendix VI

Care of the Transgender Patient

TABLE 1 DSM-5 Criteria for Gender Dysphoria in Adolescents and Adults

A. A marked incongruence between one's experienced/expressed gender and assigned gender, of at least 6 mo duration, manifested by at least two of the following:
   1. A marked incongruence between one's experienced/expressed gender and primary or secondary sex characteristics.
   2. A strong desire to be rid of primary or secondary sex characteristics.
   3. A strong desire for the primary or secondary sex characteristics of the other gender.
   4. A strong desire to be the other gender (or some alternative gender).
   5. A strong desire to be treated as the other gender (or some alternative gender).
   6. A strong conviction that one has the typical feelings and reactions of the other gender (or some alternative gender).

B. The condition is associated with clinically significant distress or impairment in social, occupational, or other important areas of functioning.

Specifiers:

With a disorder of sex development

Posttransition

DSM-5, Diagnostic and Statistical Manual of Mental Disorders, Fifth Edition.
From Ferrando CA: *Comprehensive care of the transgender patient,* Philadelphia, 2019, Elsevier. Table 2.1.

TABLE 2 ICD-11 Criteria for Gender Incongruence of Adolescence and Adulthood

Characterized by a marked and persistent incongruence between an individual's experienced gender and the assigned sex, as manifested by at least two of the following:

1. A strong dislike or discomfort with the one's primary or secondary sex characteristics (in adolescents, anticipated secondary sex characteristics) due to their incongruity with the experienced gender.
2. A strong desire to be rid of some or all of one's primary and/or secondary sex characteristics (in adolescents, anticipated secondary sex characteristics) due to their incongruity with the experienced gender.
3. A strong desire to have the primary and/or secondary sex characteristics of the experienced gender.

The individual experiences a strong desire to be treated (to live and be accepted) as a person of the experienced gender.

The experienced gender incongruence must have been continuously present for at least several months.

The diagnosis cannot be assigned prior to the onset of puberty.

Gender variant behavior and preferences alone are not a basis for assigning the diagnosis.

From Ferrando CA: *Comprehensive care of the transgender patient,* Philadelphia, 2019, Elsevier. Table 2.2.

BOX 1 Proposed Sexual Orientation and Gender Identity Questions for Incorporation into Clinical Practice

What is your current gender identity? (Check all that apply):
- ☐ Male
- ☐ Female
- ☐ Trans male/Trans man
- ☐ Trans female/Trans woman
- ☐ Gender queer/Gender nonconforming
- ☐ Additional Category (Please specify): ________
- ☐ Decline to state

What sex were you assigned at birth, on your original birth certificate?
- ☐ Male
- ☐ Female
- ☐ Decline to state

Self-identification: How one identifies one's sexual orientation (gay, lesbian bisexual, or heterosexual)

Do you think of yourself as:
- ☐ Lesbian, gay, or homosexual
- ☐ Straight or heterosexual
- ☐ Bisexual
- ☐ Something else
- ☐ Don't know
- ☐ Another (Please specify):______
- ☐ Decline to state

Additional questions to refine sexual behavior and sexual attraction:

Sexual behavior: The gender(s) of sex partners (e.g., individuals of the same gender, different gender, or multiple genders). Note: Additional information about specific sexual activities and body parts used for sex should also be assessed.

In the past (time period e.g., year) who have you had sex with?
- ☐ Men only (cisgender men and/or transgender men)
- ☐ Women only (cisgender women and/or transgender women)
- ☐ People with various gender identities: Please specify
- ☐ I have not had sex

Sexual attraction: The gender(s) of individuals that someone feels attracted to

People are different in their sexual attraction to other people. Which best describes your feelings? Are you:
- ☐ Only attracted to females?
- ☐ Mostly attracted to females?
- ☐ Equally attracted to females and males?
- ☐ Mostly attracted to males?
- ☐ Only attracted to males?
- ☐ Not sure?

Cahill S et al: Do ask, do tell: high levels of acceptability by patients of routine collection of sexual orientation and gender identity data in four diverse American community health centers, *PLoS One* 9, 2014.

Sausa LA et al: *Policy recommendations for inclusive data collection of trans people in HIV prevention, care, & services*, San Francisco, 2009, Center of Excellence for Transgender HIV Prevention, University of California.

Sexual Minority Assessment Research Team (SMART): *Best practices for asking questions about sexual orientation on surveys*, Los Angeles, CA, 2009, The Williams Institute.

The Gender Identity in U.S. Surveillance (GenIUSS) Group: Best practices for asking questions to identify transgender and other gender minority respondents on population-based surveys, Los Angeles, CA, 2014, The Williams Institute.

From Ferrando CA: *Comprehensive care of the transgender patient,* Philadelphia, 2019, Elsevier. Box 13.1.

BOX 2 Training Resources for Providers

- Association of American Medical Colleges. Diversity 3.0 Learning Series. Section: LGBT, Gender Nonconforming, and DSD Health. Includes over 20 videos on integrating LGBT health into medical education, interviewing techniques, strategies for teaching learners, development activities, curricular, and health promotion strategies. https://www.aamc.org/initiatives/diversity/learningseries/
- Deutsch MB, ed. *Guidelines for the Primary and Gender-Affirming Care of Transgender and Gender Nonbinary People.* 2nd ed. University of California, San Francisco—Center of Excellence for Transgender Health. http://transhealth.ucsf.edu/trans?page=guidelines-home. Accessed June 17, 2016.
- Pronouns Matter. http://callen-lorde.org/transhealth. Callen Lorde. June 2016.
- NYC Health and Hospitals (2011). LGBT Healthcare Training Video: To Treat Me, You Have to Know Who I Am. https://www.youtube.com/watch?v=NUhvJgxgAac&feature=kp. Accessed September 5, 2016.
- University of California Center of Excellence for Transgender Health (2014). Online Learning: Acknowledging Gender and Sex. Transgender Health Learning Center. http://transhealth.ucsf.edu/video/story.html. Accessed September 7, 2015.
- National LGBT Health Education Center (2015). Achieving Health Equity for Lesbian, Gay, Bisexual, and Transgender People. http://www.lgbthealtheducation.org/lgbt-education/continuing-education/?y=130. Accessed September 5, 2016.
- National LGBT Health Education Center (2012). Meeting the Health Care Needs of Transgender People. http://www.lgbthealtheducation.org/lgbt-education/online-courses/continuing-education/?y=13. Accessed September 5, 2016.
- National LGBT Health Education Center (2013). Providing Care and Support for Transgender Rural Latino/as and Migrant Farmworker. http://www.lgbthealtheducation.org/lgbt-education/continuing-education/?y=53. Accessed September 5, 2016.
- National LGBT Health Education Center (2015). Supporting LGBTQ Youth: Providing Affirmative and Inclusive Care Across the Spectrum of Gender and Sexual Identity. http://www.lgbthealtheducation.org/lgbt-education/continuing-education/?y=123. Accessed September 5, 2016.
- National Center for Transgender Equality (2016). An Introduction to Transgender People. https://www.facebook.com/TransEqualityNow/videos/vb.40078161989/10153582088701990/?type=2&theater. Accessed September 5, 2016.
- National Center for Transgender Equality (2016). Supporting the Transgender People in Your Life: A Guide to Being a Good Ally. http://www.transequality.org/sites/default/files/docs/resources/Ally-Guide-July-2016_0.pdf. Accessed September 5, 2016.
- National Center for Transgender Equality (2016). Understanding Non-Binary People: How to Be Respectful and Supportive. http://www.transequality.org/sites/default/files/docs/resources/Understanding-Non-Binary-July-2016_1.pdf. Accessed September 5, 2016.

From Ferrando CA: *Comprehensive care of the transgender patient,* Philadelphia, 2019, Elsevier. Box 13.2.

BOX 3 Resources on Evaluating and Enhancing Clinical Environments for the Service of Transgender People

- National LGBT Health Education Center (2015). Ten Things: Providing an Inclusive and Affirmative Health Care Environment for LGBT People. http://www.lgbthealtheducation.org/lgbt-education/continuing-education/?y=114. Accessed September 5, 2016.
- The Joint Commission (2011). Advancing Effective Communication, Cultural Competence, and Patient- and Family-Centered Care for the Lesbian, Gay, Bisexual, and Transgender (LGBT) Community. https://www.jointcommission.org/assets/1/18/LGBTFieldGuide_WEB_LINKED_VER.pdf. Accessed September 5, 2016.
- National LGBT Cancer Network (2012). Best Practices in Creating and Delivery LGBTQ Cultural Competency Trainings for Health and Social Service Agencies. http://www.cancer-network.org/downloads/best_practices.pdf. Accessed September 2016.
- Human Rights Campaign. All Children, All Families. http://hrc-assets.s3-website-us-east-1.amazonaws.com//files/assets/resources/HRC_All_Children_All_Families_Benchmarks_2016.pdf. Accessed September 5, 2016.

From Ferrando CA: *Comprehensive care of the transgender patient,* Philadelphia, 2019, Elsevier. Box 13.3.

BOX 4 Sexual History Taking and Key Questions to Add to Encounter Forms/Clinical Interviews

- Association of American Medical Colleges. Diversity 3.0 Learning Series. Section: LGBT, Gender Nonconforming, and DSD Health. Includes over 20 videos on integrating LGBT health into medical education, interviewing techniques, strategies for teaching learners, development activities, curricular, and health promotion strategies. https://www.aamc.org/initiatives/diversity/learningseries/.
- National LGBT Health Education Center (2016). Do Ask, Do Tell! Collecting Data on Sexual Orientation and Gender Identity in Health Centers http://www.lgbthealtheducation.org/lgbt-education/online-courses/continuing-education/?y=142. Accessed September 5, 2016.
- National LGBT Health Education Center (2016). Training Front-line Staff to Collect Data on Sexual Orientation and Gender Identity. http://www.lgbthealtheducation.org/lgbt-education/online-courses/continuing-education/?y=149. Accessed September 5, 2016.
- National LGBT Health Education Center (2014). Taking a History of Sexual Health: Opening the Door to Effective HIV and STI Prevention. http://www.lgbthealtheducation.org/lgbt-education/continuing-education/?y=72. Accessed September 5, 2016.
- National LGBT Health Education Center (2014). Understanding and Assessing the Sexual Health of Transgender Patient. http://www.lgbthealtheducation.org/lgbt-education/webinars/. Accessed September 5, 2016.
- The Fenway Institute (2009). Knowing Your Patients: Taking a History and Providing Risk Reduction Counseling. http://www.lgbthealtheducation.org/wp-content/uploads/Module-2-Knowing-Your-Patients.-Taking-a-History-and-Providing-Risk-Reduction-Counseling.pdf. Accessed September 5, 2016.

From Ferrando CA: *Comprehensive care of the transgender patient,* Philadelphia, 2019, Elsevier. Box 13.4.

BOX 5 Role of the Mental Health Provider in Working with Gender Nonconforming and Transgender Youth

- Diagnosing and addressing gender dysphoria
- Providing family counseling
- Helping youth explore their gender identity
- Assessing and treating any coexisting mental health concerns
- Referring for physical interventions (puberty suppression and gender-affirming hormones)
- Educating and advocating for the child and their family
- Providing or referring youth and their families to peer support resources

From Ferrando CA: *Comprehensive care of the transgender patient,* Philadelphia, 2019, Elsevier. Box 3.3.

BOX 6 Considerations for the Adolescent

Fertility	• Providers should start discussions with both the adolescent and parents around considerations for fertility preservation as medical interventions (puberty suppression or gender affirming hormones) which can impact fertility status
Assessment for Autism Spectrum Disorder (ASD)	• Studies have shown increased rates of gender variance in ASD populations • Should be considered when assessing and working with adolescents given potential difficulties with social communication, and possible intellectual or language impairments may require additional consultation with specialists that work with ASD • Mental health providers should routinely screen for ASD when doing assessments for gender dysphoria • Diagnosis of ASD does not exclude one from treatment/interventions that would otherwise be given for gender dysphoria.
Legal	• Care should be taken when parents disagree on management and support of child, team approaches may be helpful in understanding differing perspectives • Ensure confidentiality and ask adolescent about whom they have or have not disclosed their gender identity to
School	• Providers may need to serve in the role as advocate for youth who attend schools that are uninformed on how to best support their students • Adolescent should guide decisions about disclosure to peers or staff, as well as decisions on facilities/activities that are gender segregated (e.g., bathrooms, locker rooms, sports teams) • Providers should assess and monitor for bullying which can have negative mental health consequences
Advocacy	• Providers may be called upon to share their knowledge/expertise to help ensure settings the adolescent is involved in are supportive • Providers should become familiar with resources that they can refer community members and families to for support

From Ferrando CA: *Comprehensive care of the transgender patient,* Philadelphia, 2019, Elsevier. Box 3.4.

TABLE 3 Hormone Regimens for Transgender Men

Transdermal Patch 2.5-7.5 mg/day
Gel 1% 2.5-10 g/day
Subcutaneous/intramuscular testosterone enanthate, cypionate
50-200 mg/wk
100-200 mg/2 wk
Testosterone undecanoate
1000 mg/12 wk
Oral testosterone undecanoate
160-240 mg/day

From Ferrando CA: *Comprehensive care of the transgender patient,* Philadelphia, 2019, Elsevier. Table 5.1.

TABLE 4 Hormone Regimen for Transgender Women

Estrogen therapy
Transdermal
17-beta estradiol 0.1-0.4 mg 1 or 2 times/wk
Oral
Conjugated estrogens 2.5-7.5 mg/day
17-beta estradiol 2-8 mg/day
Intramuscular
Estradiol valerate 5-30 mg/2 wk
Antiandrogen therapy
Spironolactone (PO) 100-400 mg/day
Leuprolide (IM) 3.75-7.5 mg/mo
Histrelin acetate (SC implant) 50 mg/12 mo
Goserelin acetate (SC implant) 3.6 mg/mo
Cyproterone acetate (PO) 50-100 mg/day

IM, Intramuscular; *PO,* oral; *SC,* subcutaneous; *TD,* transdermal.
From Ferrando CA. *Comprehensive care of the transgender patient,* Philadelphia, 2019, Elsevier. Table 5.2.

TABLE 5 Hormone Regimens: Transfeminine Patients

Medications	How Supplied	Initial Dose	Comments
Estrogens Transdermal (once or twice weekly)	0.025, 0.0375, 0.05, 0.075, 0.1 mg/24 hr patches	0.025 mg/24 hr for induction and increase dose as tolerated	Mimics physiology closest; bypasses first-pass metabolism of the liver Several brands with various sizes/adhesives Concentration Max (Cmax) highest when applied to buttocks
Oral	0.5-, 1-, 2-mg tablets	0.5 mg/day and increase dose as tolerated	Undergoes first-pass metabolism through the liver, circulated as estrone sulfate
Antiandrogens			
Spironolactone	25-, 50-, 100-mg tablets	50 mg/day and increase dose as tolerated	Mild diuretic and may cause hyperkalemia, hyponatremia, hypomagnesemia

From Ferrando CA: *Comprehensive care of the transgender patient,* Philadelphia, 2019, Elsevier. Table 6.2.

TABLE 6 Hormone Regimens: Transmasculine Patients

Testosterone Formulation	How Supplied	Starting Dose	Comments
Testosterone cypionate	100 and 200 mg/ml in 1- and 10-ml multiuse vials	20-25 mg/wk subcutaneous or intramuscular and increase dose as tolerated	Excipient is sesame oil; allergic reaction possible
Testosterone enanthate	200 mg/ml in 1- and 10-ml multiuse vials	20-25 mg/wk subcutaneous or intramuscular and increase dose as tolerated	
Testosterone gel	1.62% (20.2 mg/pump press) or 20.25 or 40.5 mg/packet	2.5 g gel (1 packet or 1 pump)	Must be applied to upper shoulders/back. Beware of contact transfer
Testosterone gel	1% (25 or 50 mg/packet)	5 g gel (1 packet)	Must be applied to upper shoulders/back. Beware of contact transfer. Requires a large surface area

From Ferrando CA: *Comprehensive care of the transgender patient,* Philadelphia, 2019, Elsevier. Table 6.3.

TABLE 7 Effects of Testosterone and Estradiol on Metabolic and Other Parameters

Parameter	Effect	Comment
Testosterone		
Cholesterol (total)	No significant change	
High-density lipoprotein (HDL)	Decrease by 12 mg/dl	
Low-density lipoprotein (LDL)	No significant change	
Triglycerides	Increase by 35 mg/dl	
Blood pressure	Possible 3-5 mm Hg increase	Antihypertensives as needed
Erythrocytosis	4% increase in hematocrit	Adjust dose. Keep below 50%
Bone density	No increase in osteoporosis risk	
Liver function tests	2%-8% increase in enzymes	
Male pattern alopecia	May or may not be desirable	Consider low dose finasteride
Acne	Reported severe in 16%	Treat or refer if severe
Estradiol		
Cardiovascular mortality	Possible increase in risk	Intensive treatment of cardiovascular risk factors
Venous thromboembolism	Increase	Consider stopping estradiol prior to surgery, use patch in older patients and high-risk patients
Lipids	Increase in triglycerides	Patch causes less elevation
Blood pressure	No significant effect	
Bone density	No change	

From Ferrando CA: *Comprehensive care of the transgender patient,* Philadelphia, 2019, Elsevier. Table 12.1.

TABLE 8 Preventative Care and Monitoring for Patients on Testosterone (Female-to-Male)

Parameter	Recommendation
Erythrocytosis	Complete blood count every 3 mo first year, then annually
Cholesterol	Periodic screening ages 40-75
Hypertension	Usual treatment
Testosterone level	Consider yearly screen to avoid levels greater than 1000 ng/dl (check midway between shots)
Breast cancer screening	No screening mammograms after mastectomy. Routine mammography starting age 50 prior to mastectomy
Colon cancer screening	Colonoscopy or fecal occult testing starting age 50
Osteoporosis	Screen if post-oophorectomy, or has had an interruption in testosterone therapy
Liver function	Consider annual screening
Diabetes screening	Per usual guidelines for general population

From Ferrando CA: *Comprehensive care of the transgender patient,* Philadelphia, 2019, Elsevier. Table 12.2.

TABLE 9 Preventative Care and Monitoring for Patients on Feminizing Hormones (Male-to-Female)

Parameter	Recommendation
Cholesterol	Periodic screening ages 40-75
Hypertension	Treat intensively, to keep blood pressure below 140/90
Breast cancer	Screening not universally recommended; consider screening age 50-75 in patients with other risk factors, or who request screening after discussion of risks and benefits
Colon cancer	Colonoscopy or fecal occult testing starting age 50
Prostate cancer	Screening not recommended
Osteoporosis	Screen if postorchiectomy
Prolactin	Obtain baseline level and monitor for clinical signs
Hormone levels	Monitor testosterone (goal<50 ng/dl) and estradiol (goal 100-200 pg/ml) at 3, 6, and 12 mo, then annually
Creatinine, potassium	Periodically if on spironolactone to monitor for hyperkalemia and renal insufficiency
Diabetes screening	Per usual guidelines for the general population

From Ferrando CA: *Comprehensive care of the transgender patient,* Philadelphia, 2019, Elsevier. Table 12.3.

TABLE 10 Reproductive Options for Transgender Individuals and Their Partners by Index Patient Stage of Transition

Index Patient	*Partner:* Cisgender woman or person born with uterus, ovaries, and fallopian tubes who identifies as a woman	*Partner:* Cisgender man or person born with penis and testes who identifies as a man	*Partner:* Transgender woman, transfeminine person, or person born with penis and testes	*Partner:* Transgender man, transmasculine person or person born with uterus, ovaries, and fallopian tubes	No partner
Transgender man, transmasculine person or person born with uterus, ovaries, and fallopian tubes (Social Transition)	*Need:* Sperm *Decide:* Whose oocytes? Whose uterus? Source of sperm (known or unknown donor).	*Need:* None: All gametes (sperm and eggs) and uterus present *Decide:* Will use transgender man oocytes? Will transgender man carry or surrogate?	*Need:* Possibly none. Ostensibly sperm, ovaries, and uterus present. Depending on sperm availability/viability. *Decide:* Will use transgender man oocytes or egg donor? Will transgender man carry or surrogate? Does transgender woman have viable sperm?	*Need:* Sperm *Decide:* Whose eggs? Whose uterus? Source of sperm (known or unknown donor). Dependent on desires of couple and stage of transition of partner.	*Need:* Sperm *Decide:* Will transgender man use own oocytes? Will transgender man carry? Source of sperm (known or unknown donor).
Transgender woman, transfeminine person, or person born with penis and testes (Social Transition)	*Need:* None: Gametes (sperm and eggs) and uterus present. *Decide:* Timing of pregnancy and method of insemination (coital vs. ART).	*Need:* Uterus and oocytes. *Decide:* Whose sperm will be used? Surrogate to be used.	*Need:* Uterus and oocytes. *Decide:* Whose sperm will be used (dependent on viability of partner sperm). Surrogate to be used.	*Need:* Possibly none. Ostensibly gametes and uterus present depending on oocyte and uterus availability in partner. *Decide:* Will use transgender man oocytes? Will transgender man carry or surrogate?	*Need:* Oocytes and uterus. *Decide:* Whether to use a surrogate +/− egg donor versus adopting.
Transgender man, transmasculine person or person born with uterus, ovaries, and fallopian tubes (Hormonal Transition)	*Need:* Sperm *Decide:* Whose oocytes? Whose uterus? Source of sperm (known or unknown donor). *Note:* Transgender man would have to stop testosterone to produce oocytes and/or carry.	*Need:* Possible none: Ostensibly all gametes (sperm and oocytes) and uterus present. *Decide:* Will use transgender man oocytes or egg donor? Will transgender man carry or surrogate? *Note:* Transgender man would have to stop testosterone to produce oocytes and/or carry.	*Need:* Possibly none. Ostensibly all gametes (sperm and oocytes) and uterus present depending on sperm availability and transgender man's feelings about oocyte harvesting/usage and carrying. *Decide:* Will use transgender man oocytes or will use oocyte donor? Will transgender man carry or surrogate? Does transgender woman have viable sperm? Does transgender woman need to come off estrogen to produce sperm? *Note:* Transgender man would have to stop testosterone to produce oocytes and/or carry.	*Need:* Sperm (known or unknown donor). *Decide:* Whose eggs? Whose uterus?	*Need:* Sperm *Decide:* Will use transgender man oocytes? Will transgender man carry or surrogate? Source of sperm (known or unknown donor).
Transgender woman, transfeminine person, or person born with penis and testes (Hormonal Transition, assume retention of uterus, ovaries, and tubes)	*Need:* None: Gametes (sperm and oocytes) and uterus ostensibly present. *Decide:* Is there viable sperm from transgender woman? *Note:* Here transgender woman would have to go off estrogen to produce sperm if not cryopreserved. Timing of pregnancy and method of insemination (coital vs. ART).	*Need:* Uterus and oocytes. *Decide:* Whose sperm will be used. Surrogate to be used. *Note:* Here transgender woman would have to go off estrogen to produce sperm if not cryopreserved.	*Need:* Uterus and oocytes. *Decide:* Whose sperm will be used (dependent on availability and viability of both index patient and partner sperm). Surrogate to be used. *Note:* Here transgender woman may have to go off estrogen to produce sperm if not cryopreserved.	*Need:* Possibly none. Ostensibly gametes and uterus present depending on oocyte and uterus availability in partner and sperm viability and availability of index patient. *Decide:* Will use transgender man oocytes or will use an egg donor? Will transgender man carry or surrogate? *Note:* Here transgender woman may have to go off estrogen to produce sperm if not cryopreserved.	*Need:* Oocytes and uterus. *Decide:* Whether to use a surrogate +/− egg donor. *Note:* Here transgender woman may have to go off estrogen to produce sperm if not cryopreserved.

Continued on following page

TABLE 10 Reproductive Options for Transgender Individuals and Their Partners by Index Patient Stage of Transition—cont'd

Index Patient	*Partner:* Cisgender woman or person born with uterus, ovaries, and fallopian tubes who identifies as a woman	*Partner:* Cisgender man or person born with penis and testes who identifies as a man	*Partner:* Transgender woman, transfeminine person, or person born with penis and testes	*Partner:* Transgender man, transmasculine person or person born with uterus, ovaries, and fallopian tubes	No partner
Transgender man, transmasculine person or person born with uterus, ovaries, and fallopian tubes (Surgical Transition, assume removal of uterus ovaries, and tubes)	*Need:* Sperm. *Decide:* Source of sperm. Method of insemination (coital vs. ART).	*Need:* Uterus and oocytes. *Decide:* Surrogate +/− egg donor. Method of insemination (coital vs. ART).	*Need:* Uterus and oocytes, possibly sperm, depending on sperm availability and viability of partner. *Decide:* Surrogate +/− egg donor. Method of insemination (coital vs. ART). *Note:* Here transgender woman may have to go off estrogen to produce sperm if not cryopreserved.	*Need:* Sperm, possibly uterus and oocytes depending on stage of transition of partner. *Decide:* Is partner going to carry and/or be source of oocytes? Versus using a surrogate +/− egg donor? Source of sperm (known vs. donor).	Need: Sperm, uterus, and oocytes. *Decide:* Whether to use donor egg, donor sperm, and surrogate, or to adopt.
Transgender woman, transfeminine person, or person born with penis and testes (Surgical Transition, assume removal of testes)	*Need:* Sperm. *Decide:* Is there viable sperm from transgender woman cryopreserved, if not will need to use donor sperm.	*Need:* Uterus and oocytes. *Decide:* Whose sperm will be used (depending on if cryopreserved sperm from transgender woman or not). Surrogate to be used. Method of insemination of surrogate (coitus vs. ART).	*Need:* Uterus, oocytes, and possibly sperm. *Decide:* Whose sperm will be used (dependent on if cryopreserved sperm from index patient and considering availability and viability of sperm of partner. Surrogate to be used.	*Need:* Possibly none depending on oocyte and uterus availability in partner and if cryopreserved sperm availability from index patient. *Decide:* Will use transgender man oocytes or will use an egg donor? Will transgender man carry or surrogate?	*Need:* Oocytes, uterus, and possibly sperm (depending on availability of cryopreserved sperm from index patient). *Decide:* Whether to use a surrogate +/− egg donor +/− sperm donor (versus adopting.

ART, Assisted reproductive technology. This includes but is not limited to: Intracervical insemination, intrauterine insemination, in-vitro fertilization. *Social Transition:* Signifies (adult) individuals who socially identify with their affirmed gender but have not initiated hormones or surgical procedures that would affect fertility. In this table we do not consider modifications stemming from baseline fertility issues (e.g., undiagnosed infertility, or age-related fertility). *Hormonal Transition* (i.e., use of gender affirming hormones): Signifies (adult) individuals who retain natal anatomy but have undergone medical; also known as hormonal therapies for gender affirmation. *Surgical Transition* (i.e., use of gender affirming surgical procedures including gonadectomy): Signifies (adult) individuals who have undergone surgical procedures as part of gender affirmation. Note, we delineate adults here because the care and reproductive considerations of youth are handled in a separate section. Additionally, this table assumes that at baseline there is full anatomic and functional fertility. Fertility problems from any partners will augment levels of diagnostic and therapeutic interventions needed. Furthermore, we are approaching options from a functional perspective; different options may have different physiologic, emotional, fiscal, and legal implications. Finally, this table is directed towards achieving a genetically related offspring when possible. Other options for family creation are available.
From Ferrando CA: *Comprehensive care of the transgender patient,* Philadelphia, 2019, Elsevier. Table 13.2.

Appendix VIII

Palliative Care

According to the American Academy of Hospice and Palliative Medicine (AAHPM), palliative care involves "the **relieving of symptoms** of a disease or disorder while aiming to maintain the highest possible **quality of life** for patients" and their families. This entails making every day the best day possible in the setting of serious illness, often requiring **goals of care** discussions with patients and their family members. Palliative care is appropriate at any age and at any stage of serious illness, *not* only at the end of life, and can be employed at the same time as treatments and life-prolonging therapies, such as chemotherapy, radiation therapy, or hemodialysis. The World Health Organization (WHO) adds that a palliative care approach:

- Affirms life and regards dying as a normal process
- Intends neither to hasten nor to postpone death
- Integrates psychologic and spiritual aspects of patient care
- Offers a **support system** to help patients live as actively as possible until death
- Offers a support system to help the family cope during the patient's illness and after the patient's death

A palliative care team may involve chaplains, doctors, nurse practitioners, nurses, pharmacists, physician assistants, and social workers. Keys to a successful family meeting for cancer patients are summarized in Box 1.

PRIMARY PALLIATIVE CARE

According to Quill and Abernethy (2013), all medical providers, including primary care and specialists, should possess core symptom management and **communication skills** for providing primary palliative care, not necessarily requiring a palliative care specialist. These areas of proficiency should include:

- Basic discussions about patient goals, quality of life, advance care planning, and prognosis
- Recognizing the importance of social, cultural, and spiritual aspects of patient care
- Basic symptom management of pain, nausea, dyspnea, and fatigue
- Basic management of depression and anxiety

The rationale for obtaining and employing these skills is to embrace the excellent opportunity for early palliative care discussions by providers that already have a working relationship and knowledge of their patients. Key points in addressing the needs of the family are summarized in Box 2. Palliative care should be considered for any patient living with a progressive, chronic medical condition, including cancer, heart or lung disease, dementia, renal or liver failure, or stroke with significant functional impairment. Personal and external influences concerning preferred place of care are illustrated in Fig. 1. Kelley and Morrison (2015) point out that over 80% of advanced cancer patients experience pain and over 90% of advanced

BOX 1 Keys to a Successful Family Meeting

One of an oncology clinician's most difficult tasks is to conduct a successful family meeting when the burden of disease-directed therapies exceeds the benefits. Although chemotherapy or radiation might no longer offer benefit, it is never true that "there is nothing more we can do for you." The following steps increase the chance that the meeting will enhance communication among clinicians, patients, and family members; relieve concerns of abandonment; enhance trust; and provide a conversational template for the tough times to come.

1. **Schedule a Premeeting (Actual or Virtual) and Consider the Following Questions:**
   - A. Who needs to be there (which family members and which members of the clinical team)?
   - B. What is the realistic prognosis or functional goal for the patient?
   - C. Who will run the meeting? How can others help (e.g., the palliative care clinicians or the social worker)?
   - D. Who will stay with the patient and family to debrief?
2. **During the Meeting:**
   - A. Everyone must be seated.
   - B. Introduce everyone present.
   - C. ASK–tell–ask:
     - i. How do you think you (or "the patient") is/are doing?
     - ii. What changes have you seen in the last (days, weeks, months)?
     - iii. What are you hoping for? And what else?
     - iv. What are you most concerned about? What are your worst fears?
     - v. How can we help?
   - D. Ask–TELL–ask:
     - i. Answer their questions.
     - ii. Provide key medical information but AVOID giving medical details that obscure the big picture.
       - Example: The (disease) is clearly progressing despite our best efforts. In my best judgment, s/he has only (days, weeks, months) of good time left. S/he may well live longer, but this is the time when s/he will have the most energy, think the most clearly, and be most him/herself.
     - iii. STOP TALKING.
       - Counting silently to 20 helps.
     - iv. Respond to their grief.
   - E. Ask–tell–ASK:
     - i. What do you still want to accomplish during your life?
     - ii. What might be left undone if you were to die today?
     - iii. What legacy do you want to leave to your family?
     - iv. What do you want your children and grandchildren to remember about you?
     - v. How can we help NOW?
3. **After the Meeting:**
   - A. Review with your team how everyone is doing.
   - B. Make a plan for who will follow up next with the family.
   - C. Success is measured by how much they trust you and how little they feel abandoned. Feeling bad is normal and expected, both on your part and theirs; it does not mean that you were not successful.

From Niederhuber JE: *Abeloff's clinical oncology,* ed 6, Philadelphia, 2020, Elsevier.

BOX 2 Addressing the Needs of the Family

During the last weeks to months of the patient's life, office visits become impractical. Regular contact by telephone, supplemented, when possible, by one or more home visits, retains the connection that patients and families need with their primary treatment team. Clinicians also can promote continuity and minimize feelings of abandonment by collaborating with the home care or hospice nurses and, as requested, with the social workers who are part of the home care team. Praising the family caregivers for the work they are doing, helping them to anticipate upcoming problems and make contingency plans, and checking in with them at regular intervals promote timely identification and, when possible, resolution of new problems.

Many family members and medical staff, as well as trainees, have never seen anyone die an expected death outside an intensive care unit. A clinician who is familiar with the dying process can be a crucial source of information and comfort. For inpatients, the clinician works with the nursing team caring for the patient and serves as an attentive observer, striving to provide maximum comfort. Because clinical status and comfort level can change rapidly and frequently even in seemingly stable patients at the end of life, it can be helpful to make two or more visits a day to patients to monitor their comfort through reports from nursing and family, to answer questions, and to educate professional and family caregivers as to what they should expect in the last days.

Patients who were formerly alert and communicative usually become less so. They are apparently still comforted by the touch and voices of those they love and might even emerge from what seemed to be an unconscious state to greet a welcome newcomer. I tell families that to me, it is as though the patient lives in a house with many rooms, a mansion. As they come closer to dying, the patient moves farther and farther back in the house, and it is more and more effort for them to greet callers at the front of the house. But the callers are still welcome, as are their voices and conversation. I ask families to let patients know they have arrived and then to add that patients should not feel obliged to speak to them. Patients can also be asked to provide a hand squeeze or other sign of recognition. With close family, I discuss the "Five Things" (see the section of the chapter titled "Social Causes") and suggest that they find the time to share with the patient any of those sentiments they believe would be appropriate.

I reassure families that we know that dying patients are rarely hungry or thirsty and that moistening the mouth is all that is needed. If necessary, I review the burdens of hydration (see the section titled "Xerostomia"). I also explain about Cheyne-Stokes breathing and that it does not indicate that the patient is gasping for breath. I also ask them to feel free to let us know if the patient seems uncomfortable or develops noisy breathing because we want to address any source of discomfort as rapidly as possible. I offer the services of chaplaincy, and I am alert to whether a social worker would be helpful, if chaplains and social workers are not already involved. Many family members do not know that this kind of help is available to them in the hospital.

If the family has not done so already, I urge them to choose a funeral home and make all the necessary arrangements before the patient has actually died, to free themselves of that task when the death occurs. Families often ask how they will know that the patient is dying. I ask them to look for a marked decrease in urine output (in a Foley bag or diapers), cooling of the arms and legs, and new pallor or mottling of the skin. Some patients experience fecal incontinence as they die, so if hospice is not involved and the patient is at home, I alert the family to this possibility.

Supporting the Ward Personnel and the House Staff

To decrease potential feelings of guilt and anxiety, I review with all team members the history of the illness, the limits of the treatments that remain, the burdens of those treatments, and, when appropriate, the limits the patient has placed on further supportive measures. I also remind them that despite our best efforts, patients still die, and it is no one's fault. I also suggest things they can do that will enhance the patient's last days and that will further the healing process of the survivors.

During the hospitalizations that lead to death and after the death itself, I try to dispel any misconceptions they have about their "fault" for the death and to praise the work they did to make the dying person as comfortable as possible. This kind of support goes a long way toward enabling young physicians and ward staff to recover from the pain they experience when a patient dies and to allow themselves to feel a sense of satisfaction for a job well done.

From Niederhuber JE: *Abeloff's clinical oncology,* ed 6, Philadelphia, 2020, Elsevier.

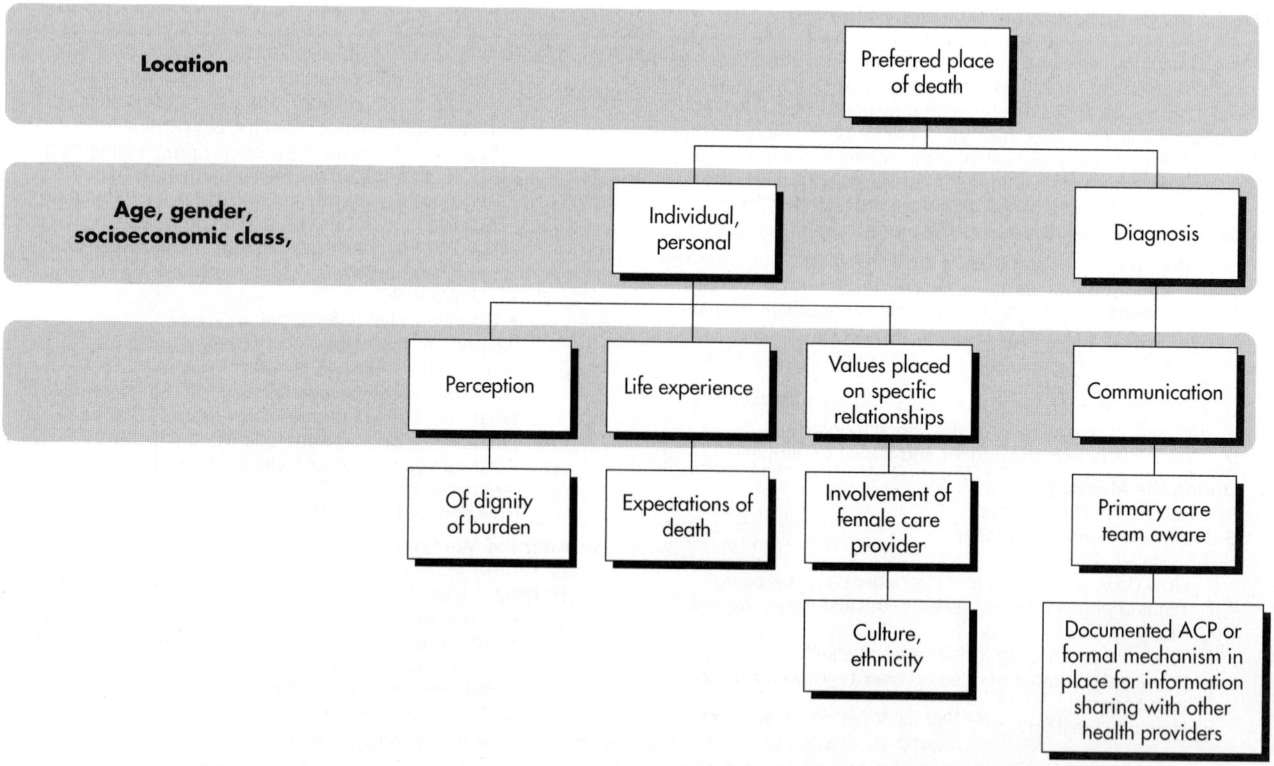

FIG. 1 Personal and external influences concerning preferred place of care. *ACP,* Advance care planning. (From Fillit HM: *Brocklehurst's textbook of geriatric medicine and gerontology,* ed 8, Philadelphia, 2017, Elsevier.)

heart failure patients experience dyspnea, so early identification and proficiency in symptom management are imperative.

SPECIALTY PALLIATIVE CARE

Involvement of a palliative care specialist with additional training or expertise may be required in more complex situations involving complicated family dynamics; ethical issues, including but not limited to medical futility, voluntary stopping of eating and drinking (VSED), and palliative sedation; uncontrolled existential distress; and refractory symptom management. Fig. 2 illustrates an algorithm for treatment of agitation in the last days of life. Palliative care specialists also work in specialty clinics alongside a patient's oncologist, cardiologist, or pulmonologist. Many of these specialists have completed fellowship training and are recognized with board certification by the American Board of Medical Specialties (ABMS).

INITIATING PRIMARY PALLIATIVE CARE

There's no perfect time to start thinking about palliative care for a patient, but if the "surprise question" of "would you be **surprised** if your patient died in the next 12 months?" answer is "no," then now may be a good time. Other situations suggesting appropriateness for a palliative care discussion may be:

- New serious diagnoses (e.g., cancer, COPD, heart failure, advanced dementia)
- Irreversible decline of a known illness
- Drastic changes in symptoms
- Changes in functional status (e.g., immobility, activities of daily living, weight loss)
- Treatment or cure failure
- Change in setting (e.g., home → hospital → home or nursing facility)

Palliative care often begins with **goals of care** discussions with the patient, family, or friends. The patient should be **asked permission** to initiate these discussions and allowed the opportunity to have his or her support system present. Ideally, the patient's **durable power of attorney for health care** (also known as a health care proxy or health care surrogate) is present for these discussions to be best informed what the patient's instructions would be if the patient were unable to verbalize with the health care providers.

GOALS OF CARE/DELIVERING SERIOUS NEWS

Good communication is one of the foundations of a palliative care approach. Practicing these skills is the only way to improve and become comfortable delivering serious news and having proficient goals of care and family meetings. There are several approaches and variations of formats for these discussions throughout the literature.

1. Ask permission to have a serious news discussion.
   a. "How do you feel about discussing your health issues at this time?"
   b. "What are you hoping to talk about today?"
   c. "What other family or friends would like here during these discussions?"
2. Get the patient's story.
   a. "What do you know about your health situation?"
   b. "Tell me more about…"
   c. "How is your illness affecting your life?"
   d. "Where do you get your strength or support?"

- Give the medical story after receiving permission to fill in any medical information gaps.

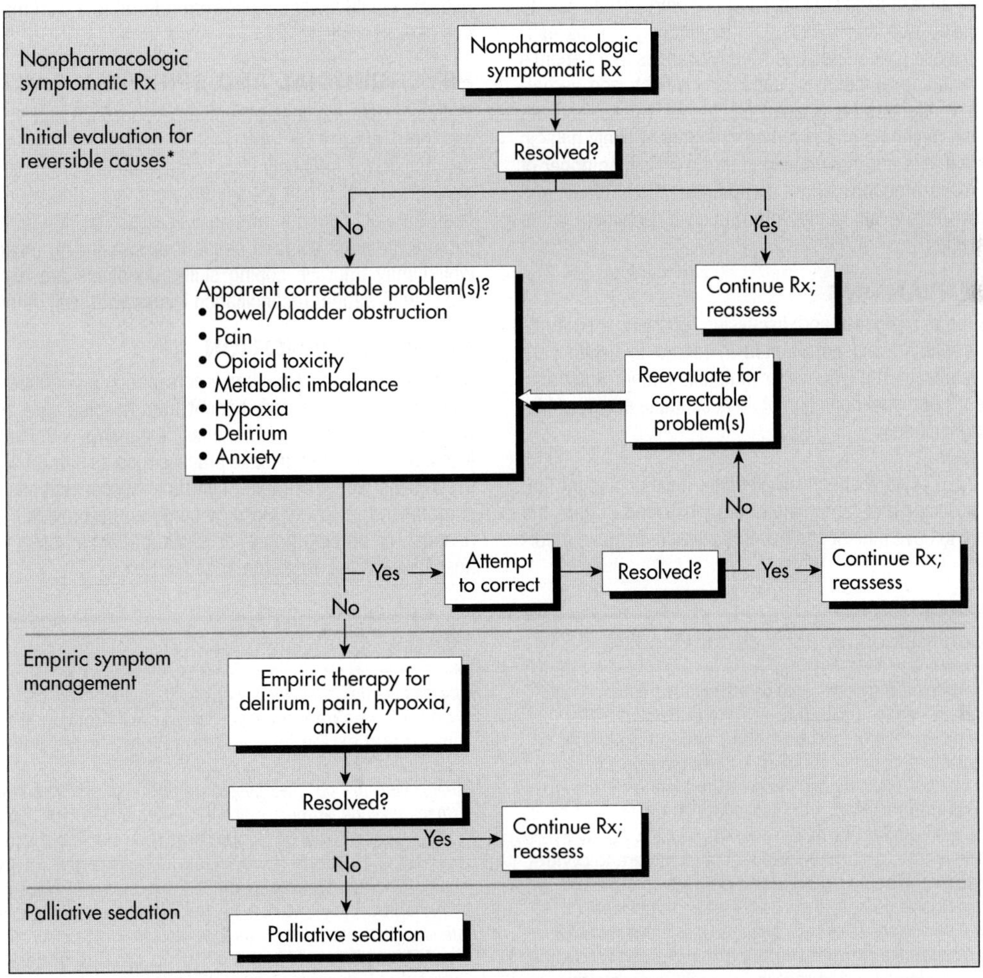

FIG. 2 Algorithm for treatment of agitation in the last days of life. *Guided by patient/family wishes and burden versus benefit. *Rx,* Prescription. (From Niederhuber JE: *Abeloff's clinical oncology,* ed 6, Philadelphia, 2020, Elsevier.)

1. Give a forewarning to prepare the patient for serious news, such as: "I wish we had better news but we're worried…"
2. Practice silence, silence, and more silence. Let the patient break the silence.
3. "Is this information surprising for you to hear?"
4. "Knowing this information, what's most important to you going forward?"
5. "What path going forward makes the most sense for you?"
6. Offer a **best case/worst case scenario.**
7. Acknowledge and validate emotions by patient and family: "I cannot imagine how difficult this must be for you."

- Ask permission to make a recommendation based on patient's priorities and goals.
  1. "Based on what you've told me is important to you, I recommend…"
  2. Consider a time trial for an intervention (e.g., dialysis, feeding tube), if necessary.
  3. Promise continued support to patient and family.

General communication pearls:

- Ask open-ended questions as often as possible.
- Use the teach back method as you go—"In your own words, what did you take away from our discussion?"
- The patient and family should spend more time talking than the provider.
- Question, reflect, and summarize back in the patient's own words.
- Obtaining substituted judgment from a health care proxy—"Given her current medical condition, what would be most important to your loved one?"

PROGNOSTICATION

Prognostication is not an exact science but can be very useful to the patient's medical decision-making process. Life expectancy can be estimated using known disease trajectories and recent changes in a patient's functional capacity, including ambulation, cognition, weight, and verbalization abilities. If these changes have taken place over weeks, and the underlying cause of the decline is not reversed, the patient likely has "in the weeks range" to live. It is not recommended that a specific number of weeks be included in the prognosis. The "surprise question" mentioned above has been shown to provide useful information to providers when attempting prognostication.

ADVANCE CARE PLANNING

Advance care planning is a process and discussion regarding a patient's wishes about what is wanted and not wanted in regard to health care under certain circumstances. The goal is to maintain patient autonomy while defining a patient's personal definition of an acceptable quality of life. Advance care planning includes:

- Code status discussion.
- Advance directives (e.g., Five Wishes) completion—legal document that tells an individual's doctor and family members what kind of care the individual would like to have if he or she becomes unable to make medical decisions.
  1. Includes living will and durable power of attorney for health care/health care proxy.
  2. No lawyer is required.
- Medical Orders for Life-Sustaining Treatment (MOLST) form completion—a physician order for end-of-life treatments for seriously ill patients that should be placed in the chart and be very visible to EMTs/paramedics who enter a patient's home.

BASIC PAIN MANAGEMENT

Primary care providers may choose to treat patients with pain associated with their serious or terminal illness, such as cancer syndromes. Chronic pain management is covered elsewhere in this text but here are a few "pearls":

- Evaluate pain in all patients using a 0 to 10 scoring scale.
- Assess the patient's goal for an acceptable pain level.
- "Total pain," caused by a combination of physical, emotional, spiritual, and psychological pain, is usually refractory to escalating opioid doses.
- When pain is chronic and opioids are required, long-acting preparations should be used after a total required daily dose is determined.
- PRN doses of short-acting opioids should be 10% to-15% of the total daily dose.
- When rotating opioids, calculate a 24-hour requirement to "oral morphine equivalents" (OMEs) and then use a standard conversion table (see the "Chronic Pain Management" chapter in this text).
- When rotating opioids, consider reducing the equianalgesic dose by 25% to 50% to account for "incomplete cross-tolerance."
- Patient-controlled analgesia (PCA) has minimal risk for overdose or respiratory depression because the patient will fall asleep before he or she can administer a toxic dose.

When considering buprenorphine, ketamine, or methadone for pain, patients would likely benefit from referral to a pain management or palliative care specialist.

PSYCHOSOCIAL AND SPIRITUAL CARE

Palliative care includes attentive psychosocial and spiritual care. Primary providers should be proficient in assessing and treating anxiety and depression for seriously ill patients. Patients often ask, "Why is this happening to me?" When asked "Where do you find your strength during difficult times?" patients may answer "God" or "My faith." It is important to explore patients' spiritual needs to assist finding meaning in their illness, which may improve coping skills. Chaplains are excellent resources to assist with patient reconciliation issues with self, others, and God.

HOSPICE TRANSITION

At some point, most palliative care patients continue to decline clinically and functionally and may benefit from hospice care. Hospice is a specific type of palliative care for seriously ill patients with likely life expectancy of less than 6 mo if the disease process runs its natural course and is deemed irreversible and incurable. Common misconceptions about hospice are summarized in Box 3. Hospice care can be provided at a hospice facility, hospital, or nursing home, or in the patient's home. Medicare-mandated hospice services are summarized in Box 4.

BOX 3 Common Misconceptions about Hospice

Patients enrolling in hospice must choose not to be resuscitated. Patients do not have to relinquish resuscitation to enroll in hospice. After they and their families fully understand the implications of the resuscitation, most patients elect not to be resuscitated.

Patients enrolled in hospice lose their primary physicians. The referring attending physician continues to direct and approve all the patient's care.

Hospice patients cannot be hospitalized and remain enrolled in hospice. Any hospice patient can be admitted to an acute, inpatient level of care to control a distressing symptom. Hospices can admit patients to contract beds in acute care hospitals or to their own inpatient facilities.

Hospice patients cannot participate in research projects while enrolled in hospice. Hospice patients have the right to participate in research studies. Hospice ethics and research committees usually evaluate the burden versus the benefit of the research for the patient, family, and hospice staff.

Hospice nursing personnel do not provide sophisticated care. Hospice personnel provide expert palliative care that requires astute assessment and expert intervention tailored to the patient and family goals.

Patients can "use up" their hospice eligibility, so it is important not to enroll them too soon. Patients are initially certified for 3 mo of service, after which their physician and the hospice medical director are asked to recertify them indefinitely, at 2-mo intervals. Patients who choose to revoke the hospice benefit to seek life-prolonging therapies may choose to reenroll if their goals change.

Patients must have a live-in caregiver to enroll in hospice. With appropriate safeguards (e.g., "lock boxes" to provide access in emergencies and daily phone contact), hospice care can be safely provided to patients who live alone.

From Niederhuber JE: *Abeloff's clinical oncology,* ed 6, Philadelphia, 2020, Elsevier.

BOX 4 Medicare-Mandated Hospice Services

Practitioners Available
Medical director, nurses, social workers, home health aides, chaplains, volunteers, administrative personnel, medical consultations, occupational therapy, physical therapy, speech therapy, bereavement counseling

Palliative Treatment of Terminal Illness
Prescription medications
Durable medical equipment and supplies
Oxygen
Radiation and chemotherapy
Laboratory and diagnostic procedures

Other Benefits
Transportation when medically necessary for changes in level of care
When needed, continuous care at home or in a skilled nursing facility or inpatient setting
Respite care (care in a nursing facility that provides a "respite" for the caregivers)

Data from Medicare Hospice Regulations: 42 Codes of Federal Regulations, Part 418, 1993. From Niederhuber JE: *Abeloff's clinical oncology,* ed 6, Philadelphia, 2020, Elsevier.

PALLIATIVE CARE RESOURCES & REFERENCES

- American Academy of Hospice and Palliative Medicine (AAHPM).
- Back A, Arnold R, Tulsky J. *Mastering communication with seriously ill patients,* 2009, Cambridge University Press.
- Center for Advancement of Palliative Care (CAPC).
- Five Wishes® (agingwithdignity.org)—living will document.
- Kelley & Morrison: Palliative care for the seriously ill, *NEJM* 373;747, 2015.
- Medicare.gov: How hospice works. Available at medicare.gov/what-medicare-covers/what-part-a-covers/how-hospice-works.
- Palliative Care Network of Wisconsin (PCNOW)—Fast Facts. Available at www.mypcnow.org/fast-facts/.
- Quill & Abernethy: Generalist plus specialist palliative care—creating a more sustainable model, *NEJM* 368;13, 2013.
- Vital Talk (vitaltalk.org): Providing trainings to teach providers communication skills for discussing serious illness.

AUTHOR: **Gregory Rachu, MD, MPH**

Appendix IX (ALG)

Preoperative Evaluation

BASIC INFORMATION

DEFINITION

Preoperative evaluation is the clinical risk evaluation for patients undergoing surgery. It is an overall assessment of the patient's health and surgery's risk. The goal of the assessment is not to "clear" the patient for the surgery, because there is always some level of risk, but to provide accurate preoperative risk stratification and implement possible risk reduction strategies. Preoperative evaluation should also include functional assessment and determining social support. It also provides an opportunity for discussion and helps to alleviate the patient's anxiety before surgery.

SYNONYMS

Preoperative evaluation and risk reduction
Risk reduction in patients undergoing invasive procedures
Preoperative clearance

ICD-10CM CODES
Z01.810 Encounter for preprocedural cardiovascular examination
Z01.811 Encounter for preprocedural respiratory examination
Z01.812 Encounter for preprocedural laboratory examination
Z01.818 Encounter for other preprocedural examination

TABLE 1 Cardiac Risk* Stratification for Noncardiac Surgical Procedures

Risk Stratification	Examples of Procedures
High (reported cardiac risk often >5%)	Aortic and other major vascular surgery Peripheral vascular surgery
Intermediate (reported cardiac risk generally 1%-5%)	Intraperitoneal and intrathoracic surgery Carotid endarterectomy Head and neck surgery Orthopedic surgery Prostate surgery
Low† (reported cardiac risk generally <1%)	Endoscopic procedures Superficial procedure Cataract surgery Breast surgery Ambulatory surgery

*Combined incidence of cardiac death and nonfatal myocardial infarction.
†These procedures do not generally require further preoperative cardiac testing.
From Fleisher LA et al: 2009 ACCF/AHA focused update on perioperative beta blockade incorporated into the ACC/AHA 2007 guidelines on perioperative cardiovascular evaluation and care for noncardiac surgery: a report of the American College of Cardiology Foundation/American Heart Association Task Force on Practice Guidelines, *J Am Coll Cardiol* 54(22):e13, 2009. In Zipes DP: *Braunwald's heart disease, a textbook of cardiovascular medicine,* ed 11, Philadelphia, 2019, Elsevier.

EPIDEMIOLOGY & DEMOGRAPHICS

The number of outpatient surgical procedures performed in the U.S. has been gradually increasing over the years.

Some studies have shown the benefits of preoperative testing whereas others have shown no added benefit. Lack of added benefit has been particularly true for otherwise healthy individuals: The prevalence of significant unrecognized disease and the predictive value of tests are both low for this population, leading to an excess of false-positive tests.

Certain risk factors do exist that may be helpful: The nature and extent of surgery appear to play a role, as do increasing age, exercise capacity, and certain medications. Additionally, patients with certain preexisting conditions such as diabetes may benefit from adjustments to their insulin preoperatively, for instance. The primary care physician may be best suited to adjust medications. Table 1 describes stratification of risk of common noncardiac surgical procedures.

Preoperative evaluation offers an excellent opportunity to reach out to patients about other preventive, screening, and routine health care issues as well. The primary care physician is uniquely poised to provide an accurate assessment and risk stratification of patients and to develop care plans for follow-up. This information can then be used to help surgeons counsel patients and guide patients' decision making.

PEAK INCIDENCE: When there are adverse consequences from surgery, cardiovascular complications account for the majority of morbidity and mortality in patients. Perioperative myocardial infarctions (PMIs) are one of the most important predictors of short- and long-term morbidity and mortality associated with surgery. The highest incidence of PMI is in the first 3 to 5 days after surgery.

PHYSICAL FINDINGS & CLINICAL PRESENTATION

The history, physical, and other studies need to assess the risks for myocardial infarction, arrhythmias, heart failure, endocarditis, stroke, venous thrombosis and pulmonary embolism, prolonged mechanical ventilation and respiratory failure, hemorrhage, diabetic acidosis, renal or hepatic failure, and infection.

Dx DIAGNOSIS

WORKUP (FIG. 1)

HISTORY: A thorough medical history is the most valuable tool. Assess the urgency of the surgical procedure. A conversation with the surgical team is helpful for urgent and emergent procedures.

Some standard screening questionnaires have been adapted to help identify patients who would benefit from formal preoperative evaluation.

- Age is important to consider because age is often associated with an increasing number of comorbidities, which are in turn associated with an increase in perioperative risk.
- All patients should be asked about their exercise capacity before surgery. One way to assess functional capacity is in metabolic equivalents (METs) (Table 2). Studies have shown that those who have a low

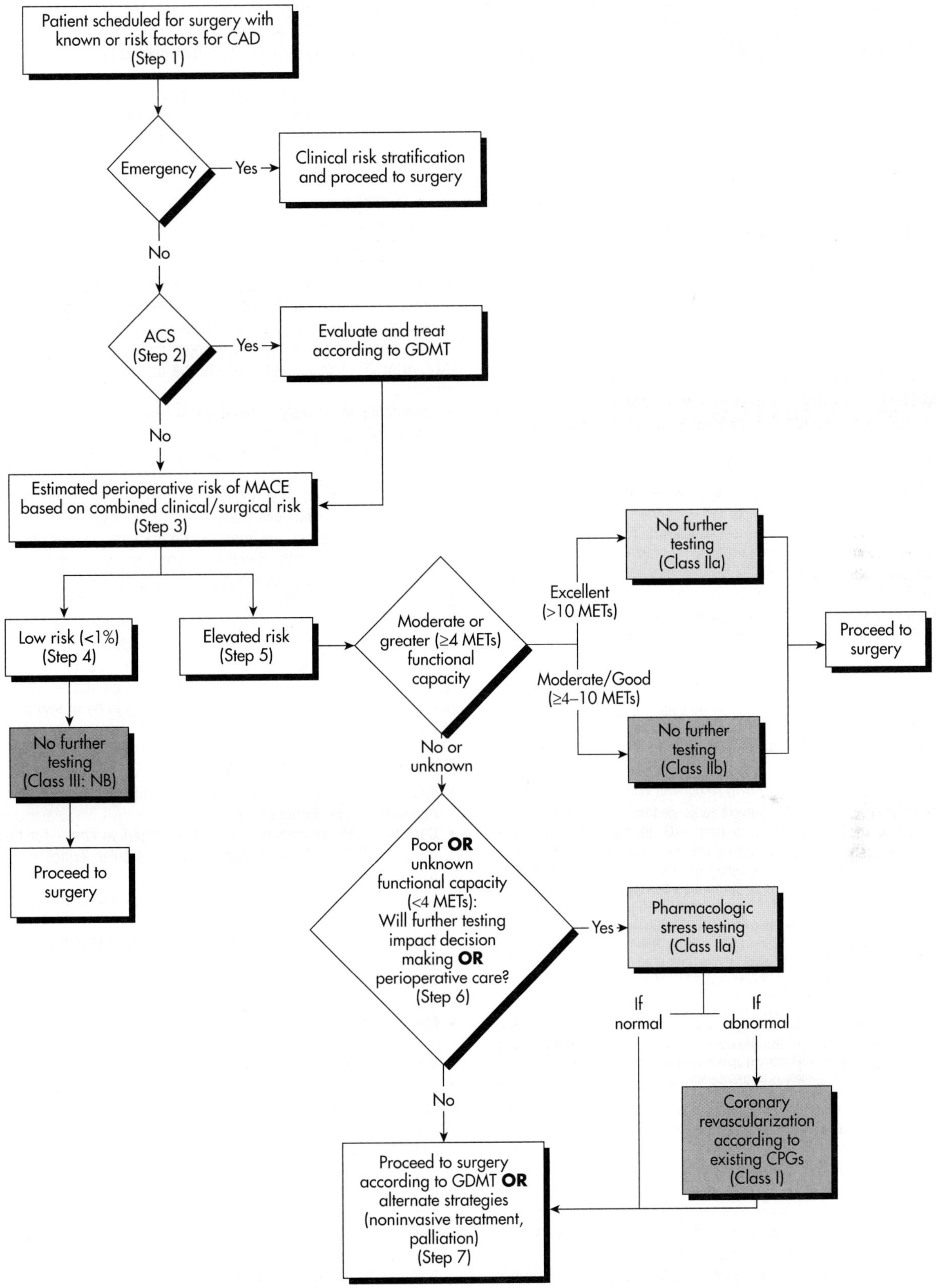

FIG. 1 The 2014 ACC/AHA guideline algorithm depicting the stepwise approach to perioperative cardiac assessment for CAD. *ACS,* Acute coronary syndrome; *CAD,* coronary artery disease; *CPG,* clinical practice guideline; *GDMT,* guideline-directed medical therapy; *MACE,* major adverse cardiac event; *MET,* metabolic equivalent. (From Fleisher LA et al: 2014 ACC/AHA guideline on perioperative cardiovascular evaluation and management of patients undergoing noncardiac surgery: a report of the American College of Cardiology/American Heart Association Task Force on Practice Guidelines, *J Am Coll Cardiol* 64:e77-137, 2014. In Zipes DP: *Braunwald's heart disease, a textbook of cardiovascular medicine,* ed 11, Philadelphia, 2019, Elsevier.)

TABLE 2 Functional Capacity (Metabolic Equivalents [METs])

<4 METs	4-10 METs	>10 METs
Daily living activities	Heavy housework	Strenuous exercise
Walking (2 mph)	Walking up a hill	Skiing
Walk 1-2 blocks	Walking (4 mph)	Tennis (single)
	Cycling	
	Golf	
	Tennis (double)	

(1 MET: Energy expenditure of 70-kg man sitting quietly)

Adapted from Fleisher LA et al: ACC/AHA 2007 Guidelines on perioperative cardiovascular evaluation and care for noncardiac surgery, *Circulation* 116:e418-e500, 2007.

TABLE 3 Active Cardiac Conditions for Which Patients Should Undergo Evaluation and Treatment Before Noncardiac Surgery (Class I; Level of Evidence: B)

Condition	Examples
Unstable coronary syndromes	Unstable or severe angina* (CCS class III or IV)† Recent myocardial infarction (MI)‡
Decompensated HF (NYHA functional class IV; worsening or new-onset HF)	
Significant arrhythmias	High-grade atrioventricular block Mobitz II atrioventricular block Third-degree atrioventricular heart block Symptomatic ventricular arrhythmias Supraventricular arrhythmias (including atrial fibrillation) with an uncontrolled ventricular rate (heart rate >100 beats/min at rest) Symptomatic bradycardia Newly recognized ventricular tachycardia
Severe valvular disease	Severe aortic stenosis (mean pressure gradient >40 mm Hg, aortic valve area <1.0 cm^2, or symptomatic) Symptomatic mitral stenosis (progressive dyspnea on exertion, exertional presyncope, or HF)

CCS, Canadian Cardiovascular Society; *HF,* heart failure; *NYHA,* New York Heart Association.
*According to Campeau L et al: Atherosclerosis and late closure of aortocoronary saphenous vein grafts: sequential angiographic studies at 2 wk, 1 yr, 5 to 7 yr, and 10 to 12 yr after surgery, *Circulation* 68(Suppl II):1, 1983.
†May include "stable" angina in patients who are unusually sedentary.
‡The American College of Cardiology National Database Library defines "recent" MI as more than 7 days but 1 mo or less (within 30 days), although the 2014 guidelines suggest 60 days.
From Fleisher LA et al: 2009 ACCF/AHA focused update on perioperative beta blockade incorporated into the ACC/AHA 2007 guidelines on perioperative cardiovascular evaluation and care for noncardiac surgery: a report of the American College of Cardiology Foundation/American Heart Association Task Force on Practice Guidelines, *J Am Coll Cardiol* 54(22):e13, 2009. In Zipes DP: *Braunwald's heart disease, a textbook of cardiovascular medicine,* ed 11, Philadelphia, 2019, Elsevier.

exercise capacity have twice as much risk for postoperative complications compared to those who have high exercise capacity.

- Evaluate for evidence of active cardiac conditions: Unstable angina, recent MI (<30 days), significant arrhythmia, decompensated CHF, and severe valvular disease. Table 3 describes active cardiac conditions for which patients should undergo evaluation and treatment before noncardiac surgery. Fig. 2 illustrates a treatment algorithm for patients with coronary stents undergoing noncardiac surgery.
- Other medical conditions and risk factors:
  1. Stable CAD, compensated CHF, HTN
  2. Chronic lung diseases
  3. Obstructive sleep apnea (preoperative screening [STOP-Bang, Berlin scores] in all patients)
  4. Other medical comorbidities: CVA, diabetes mellitus (DM), CKD, liver diseases
  5. Personal or family history of anesthetic complications
  6. Personal or family history of hypercoagulable states or bleeding disorders
  7. Medications such as anticoagulants, antiplatelets, NSAIDs, and oral hypoglycemic agents
  8. Smoking
  9. Alcohol
  10. Obesity
  11. Pregnancy
- Consider further testing based on above risk factors. The decision to order preoperative tests should be guided by the patient's clinical history, comorbidities, and physical examination findings.

The American College of Cardiology and American Heart Associated (ACC/AHA) 2014 guidelines[1] classify the urgency of surgery in four categories:

- Emergency (necessary within 6 hr)
- Urgent (necessary within 6-24 hr)
- Time-sensitive (can delay 1-6 wk)
- Elective (can delay up to 1 yr)

Surgical risk based on surgical and patient characteristics is either low (<1% risk of major adverse cardiac events) or high (≥1% risk of major adverse cardiac events). The intermediate risk category has been eliminated. Examples of high-risk procedures include vascular surgery, orthopedic surgery, intraperitoneal and intrathoracic surgery, head and neck surgery, and prostate surgery. Ambulatory surgery, endoscopic procedures, and cataract surgery are considered low risk. The Revised Cardiac Risk Index (RCRI) is based on the following six factors, each worth a point: High-risk surgery, ischemic heart disease, heart failure, stroke or TIA, diabetes requiring insulin, and renal insufficiency (serum creatinine >2.0 mg/dl). A patient with an RCRI score 0 to 1 is considered to be at low risk; a value of 2 or above is high risk.

PHYSICAL EXAMINATION

- Vital signs: Blood pressure, heart rate and rhythm, rate and ease of respirations, and temperature.
- Cardiovascular examination: Auscultate heart to check for heart murmurs, pathologic heart sounds, and ventricular systolic or diastolic dysfunction.
- Respiratory examination: Auscultate lungs for crackles, wheezes, decreased breath sounds.
- Vascular examination: Examine for carotid, abdominal, and femoral bruits.
- Integumentary examination: Check for evidence of venous stasis in lower extremities, petechiae, and unusual bruises.
- Mental status: Conduct a mini-mental status examination.

LABORATORY TESTS & IMAGING STUDIES

- Determine the patient's age, height, weight.
- Routine laboratory studies are not necessary unless there is a specific medical indication. Testing need not be repeated if results are recently available, unless there has been a change in clinical status.
  1. Low-risk procedures do not require routine basic metabolic panel, blood glucose, liver function, hemostasis evaluation, or urine analysis.
  2. For intermediate- and high-risk procedures as well as in the setting of diabetes, cardiac, or renal disease, obtain a complete blood count (CBC).
  3. A CBC is recommended for all patients older than age 65 undergoing major surgery as well as anyone undergoing a surgery with expected large amounts of blood loss.

[1] Fleisher LA et al: 2014 ACC/AHA guideline on perioperative cardiovascular evaluation and management of patients undergoing noncardiac surgery: a report of the American College of Cardiology/American Heart Association Task Force on practice guidelines, *J Am Coll Cardiol* 64:e77-e137, 2014.

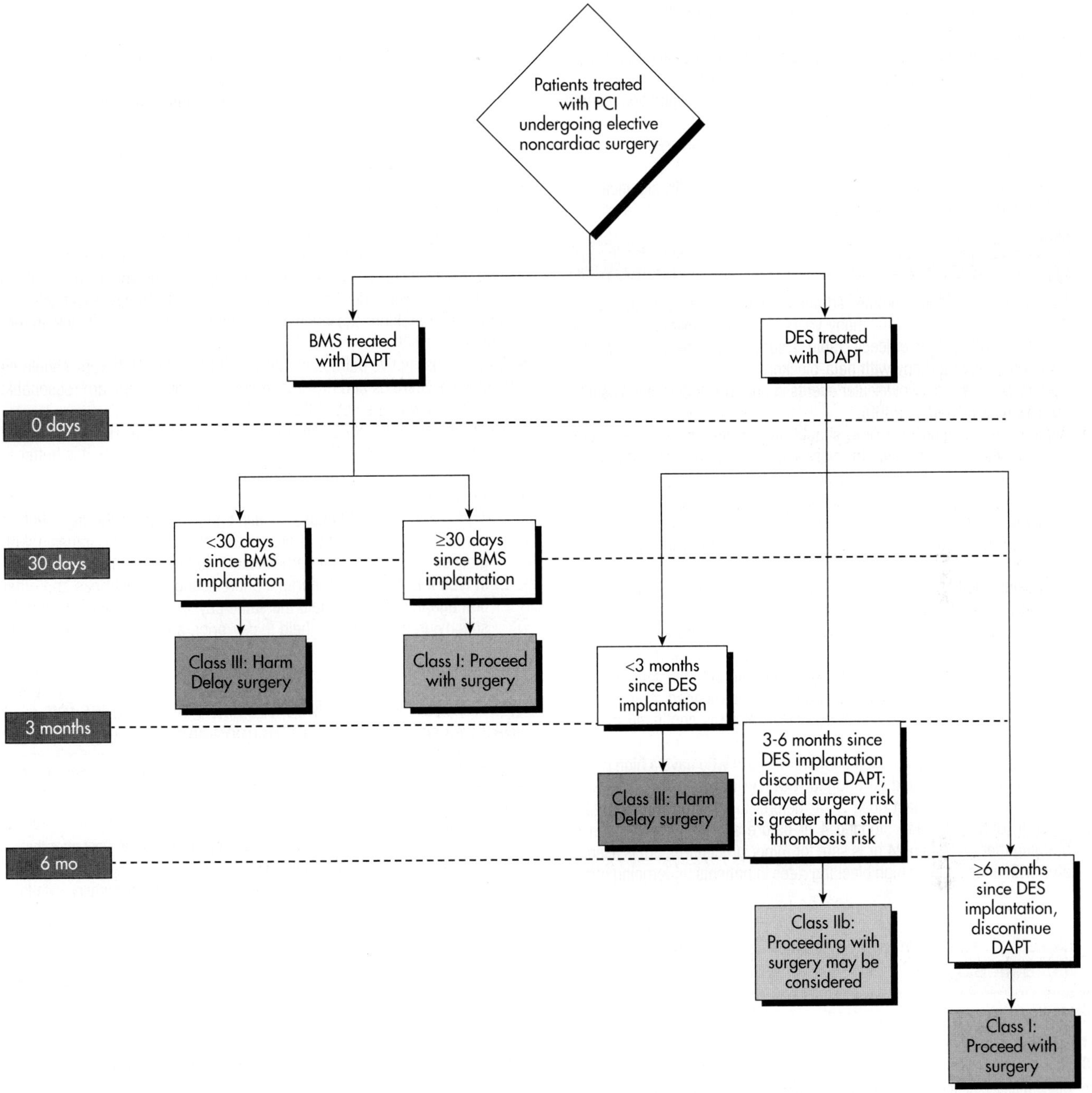

FIG. 2 Treatment algorithm for patients with coronary stents undergoing noncardiac surgery. *BMS,* Bare metal stent; *DAPT,* dual-antiplatelet therapy; *DES,* drug-eluting stent; *PCI,* percutaneous coronary intervention. (From Levine GN et al: 2016 ACC/AHA guideline focused update on duration of dual antiplatelet therapy in patients with coronary artery disease: a report of the American College of Cardiology/American Heart Association Task Force on Clinical Practice Guidelines, *J Am Coll Cardiol* 68:1082-1115, 2016. In Zipes DP: *Braunwald's heart disease, a textbook of cardiovascular medicine,* ed 11, Philadelphia, 2019, Elsevier.)

4. Fasting glucose is recommended for all patients age >45 yr. Coagulation studies are only needed for patients with personal or family history of bleeding or thrombophilia and for those taking anticoagulants.
5. Urine hCG is recommended for all women of childbearing age.

- Electrocardiogram: Routine ECG is not recommended. ACC/AHA guidelines recommend resting 12-lead ECG for patients with:
  1. At least one clinical risk factor for those who are undergoing vascular surgery (class I, level of evidence [LOE] B)
  2. Known cardiovascular disease, peripheral arterial disease, and cerebrovascular disease for patients scheduled for intermediate-risk surgery (class I, LOE C)
  3. No clinical risk factors for patients scheduled to undergo vascular surgery (class IIa, LOE B)
  4. At least one clinical risk factor for patients who are undergoing intermediate-risk surgery (class IIb LOE B)
- Echocardiography: Indicated only if new signs and symptoms of CHF or new cardiac murmurs on physical examination.
- Exercise or pharmacologic stress testing: Only indicated for evaluation of potentially high-risk patients: For patients scheduled to undergo vascular surgery with three or more clinical risk factors and poor functional capacity (<4 METs) if it will change management (class IIa). Chest x-ray: Routine CXR is not recommended. It is indicated for patients >50 yr of age undergoing high-risk procedures (American College of Physicians

[ACP] recommendations) and patients with new respiratory symptoms, suspected congestive heart failure, or valvular heart disease.
- Pulmonary function tests: It is only recommended for patients undergoing lung resection surgery but can be considered in:
  1. Patients with COPD or asthma, only if clinical evaluation cannot determine if they are at their best baseline.
  2. Patients with dyspnea or exercise intolerance that remains unexplained after clinical evaluation.
- Arterial blood gas: Should be obtained only when clinically significant (to determine if lung disease is compensated).

Rx TREATMENT

- Beta-blockers: While routine administration of perioperative beta-blockers was advocated for many years, conflicting evidence currently exists regarding their efficacy. Table 4 summarizes recommendations for perioperative therapy with beta-blockers.
- Statins: Decrease cardiovascular events in patients undergoing vascular surgery (*N Engl J Med,* 2009).
- Aspirin: Continuation of aspirin should be considered in patients who were previously taking aspirin (class IIa, LOE B). For surgeries where increased bleeding could result in significant morbidity (e.g., neurosurgery) or when the risk of stopping aspirin is minimal, aspirin should be stopped 7 days or more before surgery. Aspirin can be restarted on the first postoperative day as long as adequate hemostasis has been achieved.
- Adenosine diphosphate (ADP) antagonists (ticlopidine, clopidogrel, prasugrel): In patients with recently placed stents, elective surgical procedures should be delayed (minimum 3 wk for bare metal stents [BMSs] and 3 mo for drug-eluting stents [DESs]) while the patient is undergoing dual antiplatelet therapy. For procedures that must be performed, continuation of aspirin therapy is recommended. A short-term discontinuation of anti-ADP therapy while aspirin is continued may be relatively safe.
- Anticoagulation therapy: Patients taking warfarin who have a high risk of thromboembolism should be bridged with low-molecular-weight heparin (LMWH) (with the last dose 24 hr before surgery) or unfractionated heparin (UFH) (with drip stopped 4 hr before surgery). Resumption of bridging therapy within 24 hr is safe for minor procedures but is associated with unacceptably high bleeding rates in patients undergoing major surgery. Therefore it is recommended to wait 48 to 72 hr postoperatively to resume bridging therapy in patients who had major surgery. Another alternative regimen is to resume warfarin 12 to 24 hr postoperatively without any bridging therapy. Bridging anticoagulation is not indicated in atrial fibrillation patients when direct oral anticoagulants (e.g., edoxaban, apixaban, rivaroxaban, dabigatran) are interrupted for procedures. Table 5 summarizes perioperative management strategies for patients on chronic oral anticoagulant therapy.
- NSAIDs: NSAID therapy is almost never necessary, and it should be stopped before surgery (5-10 days prior).
- Pacemakers and defibrillators: Consultation with an electrophysiologist is recommended. Pacemaker should be reprogrammed to an asynchronous mode (VOO, DOO), and defibrillation function must be set off to avoid unintentional discharge during surgery (electrocauterization).
- Smoking: Smoking cessation is recommended at least 8 wk before surgery.
- Chronic obstructive pulmonary disease (COPD): COPD therapy should be optimized. Steroids and maximal bronchodilator therapy are reasonable for patients who are not at their best baseline.
- Hypertension: SBP <180 mm Hg and DBP <110 mm Hg are generally considered acceptable. In case of elective surgery, though, it is better to postpone it to allow for better BP control.
- Diabetes mellitus (DM):
  1. Type I DM: Scheduled basal insulin should be given the night before surgery or the morning of surgery. Continuous insulin infusion with glucose infusions might be necessary during prolonged procedures.
  2. In type II DM with oral therapy: Short-acting sulfonylureas and other oral agents should be held the same day. Metformin and long-acting sulfonylureas should be held 1 day prior, and metformin should be

TABLE 4 Recommendations for Perioperative Therapy with Beta-Blockers

Class I
- Continue beta-blockers in patients who are receiving beta-blockers chronically.

Class IIa
- Guide management of beta-blockers after surgery by clinical circumstances.

Class IIb
- In patients with intermediate- or high-risk preoperative tests, it may be reasonable to begin beta-blockers.
- In patients with ≥3 Revised Cardiac Risk Index (RCRI) factors, it may be reasonable to begin beta-blockers before surgery.
- Initiating beta-blockers in the perioperative setting as an approach to reduce perioperative risk is of uncertain benefit in those with a long-term indication but no other RCRI risk factors.*
- It may be reasonable to begin perioperative beta-blockers long enough in advance to assess safety and tolerability, preferably >1 day before surgery.

Class III
- Beta-blocker therapy should not be started on the day of surgery.

*Clinical risk factors include a history of ischemic heart disease, history of compensated or previous heart failure, history of cerebrovascular disease, diabetes mellitus, and renal insufficiency (defined in the RCRI as a preoperative serum creatinine level of 2 mg/dl).

From Fleisher LA et al: 2014 ACC/AHA guideline on perioperative cardiovascular evaluation and management of patients undergoing noncardiac surgery: a report of the American College of Cardiology/American Heart Association Task Force on Practice Guidelines, *J Am Coll Cardiol* 64:e77-137, 2014. In Zipes DP: *Braunwald's heart disease, a textbook of cardiovascular medicine,* ed 11, Philadelphia, 2019, Elsevier.

TABLE 5 Perioperative Management Strategies for Patients on Chronic Oral Anticoagulant Therapy

Clinical Situation	Suggested Anticoagulation Management
Low bleeding-risk surgery (dental, cataract, skin)	• Consider reducing dose of warfarin to achieve INR ≤2.0 • Consider holding dose of DOAC until after the procedure
Low thrombotic risk Aortic valve prosthesis without other thrombotic risk factors[a] *Or* AF with low stroke risk *Or* VTE >3 mo previously	• Stop warfarin 4-5 days before surgery, safe to operate when INR ≤1.5 • Hold DOACs for 5 half-lives—dabigatran for 3-4 days, rivaroxaban, apixaban, edoxaban for 2-3 days • Restart warfarin in evening of the day of surgery after hemostasis secured; restart DOACs on postoperative day 3 or 4 • Start prophylactic LMWH on the morning of the day after surgery and continue until INR >1.8 or full dose of DOACs resumed
Moderate thrombotic risk Mitral or multiple valve prostheses *Or* Aortic prosthesis with risk factors for thrombosis *Or* AF at high stroke risk *Or* VTE within past 3 mo	• Stop VKA 5 days before surgery • Begin twice-daily LMWH in therapeutic doses starting 3 days before surgery with last dose at least 12 hr before surgery • Hold DOACs for 5 half-lives—dabigatran for 3-4 days, rivaroxaban, apixaban, edoxaban for 2-3 days; no bridging • Restart warfarin in evening of the day of surgery after hemostasis secured; restart DOACs on postoperative day 3 or 4 • Start prophylactic LMWH on the morning of the day after surgery and continue until INR >1.8 or full dose of DOACs resumed

AF, Atrial fibrillation; *DOAC,* direct oral anticoagulant; *INR,* international normalized ratio; *LMWH,* low-molecular-weight heparin; *VKA,* vitamin K antagonist (i.e., warfarin); *VTE,* venous thromboembolism.

[a]Risk factors include caged-ball or single tilting-disk valve, AF, history of stroke/transient ischemic attack/other embolic event, left ventricular failure, and underlying hypercoagulable state, including cancer.

From Hoffman R et al: *Hematology: basic principles and practice,* ed 7, Philadelphia, 2018, Elsevier.

kept on hold for 48 hr postoperatively. Short-acting insulin sliding scale should be used for blood glucose control meanwhile.
3. In insulin-dependent type II DM: 50% to 100% of the basal insulin should be given depending on whether the patient will be able to eat postoperatively. During major procedures, patients may need an insulin drip and D5% infusion.

Currently, a blood glucose level <180 mg/dl postoperatively is considered appropriate. Aggressive blood glucose control (81-108 mg/dl vs. <180 mg/dl) showed a slight increase in risks in both surgical and medical critical care patients.

- Liver disease: Nonoperative alternative should be strongly recommended in patients with advanced cirrhosis. If surgery is deemed necessary, optimize preoperative status: Correct coagulopathy, thrombocytopenia, volume status, electrolytes, ascites, and encephalopathy.
- End-stage renal disease: Achieve euvolemia and correct electrolytes. Patients receiving hemodialysis should undergo dialysis the day before surgery. In patients with a prior history of uremic bleeding, desmopressin administration should be considered.
- Corticosteroid management and adrenal insufficiency: In patients taking exogenous steroids, continuation of the same steroid regimen is reasonable. In those with chronic adrenal insufficiency, steroid supplementation is generally recommended with the dose titrated to the level of stress of the surgical procedure.

PEARLS & CONSIDERATIONS

COMMENTS

Although most individuals will not require any significant preoperative testing, certain conditions will require further workup.

- Ischemic heart disease:
  1. If patient has angina, determine frequency, precipitating factors, and response to rest and nitroglycerin.
  2. If patient has had prior cardiac catheterizations or coronary revascularizations, obtain previous records.
- Dysrhythmias and pacemakers:
  1. Examine current and prior ECGs for high-grade atrioventricular block, symptomatic ventricular arrhythmias, and supraventricular tachycardias at uncontrolled rates.
  2. If patient has a pacemaker, establish the type and mode, date of implantation, and when it was last interrogated.
- Valvular and congenital heart disease:
  1. Look for signs of severe valvular heart disease on last echocardiographic evaluations.
- Cerebrovascular disease:
  1. Inquire about prior carotid artery ultrasounds.
- Venous thromboembolism:
  1. Determine results of studies for thrombophilia (factor V Leiden mutation, lupus anticoagulant, antithrombin III, protein C or S).

PATIENT & FAMILY EDUCATION

Advise patients that their preoperative evaluation visit with their PCP is another opportunity for them to bring up concerns or get questions answered about their upcoming procedure.

SUGGESTED READINGS

Available at ExpertConsult.com

AUTHOR: **Fred F. Ferri, MD**

Index

A

 Page numbers followed by *f* indicate figures, *b* indicate boxes, *t* indicate tables, and *e* indicate online content.

Page numbers followed by *f* indicate figures, *b* indicate boxes, *t* indicate tables, and *e* indicate online content.

Page numbers followed by *f* indicate figures, *b* indicate boxes, *t* indicate tables, and *e* indicate online content.

Page numbers followed by *f* indicate figures, *b* indicate boxes, *t* indicate tables, and *e* indicate online content.

B

C

Page numbers followed by *f* indicate figures, *b* indicate boxes, *t* indicate tables, and *e* indicate online content.

Page numbers followed by *f* indicate figures, *b* indicate boxes, *t* indicate tables, and *e* indicate online content.

Page numbers followed by *f* indicate figures, *b* indicate boxes, *t* indicate tables, and *e* indicate online content.

Page numbers followed by *f* indicate figures, *b* indicate boxes, *t* indicate tables, and *e* indicate online content.

D

Page numbers followed by *f* indicate figures, *b* indicate boxes, *t* indicate tables, and *e* indicate online content.

E

Page numbers followed by *f* indicate figures, *b* indicate boxes, *t* indicate tables, and *e* indicate online content.

F

Page numbers followed by *f* indicate figures, *b* indicate boxes, *t* indicate tables, and *e* indicate online content.

G

H

Page numbers followed by *f* indicate figures, *b* indicate boxes, *t* indicate tables, and *e* indicate online content.

I

Page numbers followed by *f* indicate figures, *b* indicate boxes, *t* indicate tables, and *e* indicate online content.

J

K

Page numbers followed by *f* indicate figures, *b* indicate boxes, *t* indicate tables, and *e* indicate online content.

Page numbers followed by *f* indicate figures, *b* indicate boxes, *t* indicate tables, and *e* indicate online content.

M

Page numbers followed by *f* indicate figures, *b* indicate boxes, *t* indicate tables, and *e* indicate online content.

O

P

Page numbers followed by *f* indicate figures, *b* indicate boxes, *t* indicate tables, and *e* indicate online content.

S

Page numbers followed by *f* indicate figures, *b* indicate boxes, *t* indicate tables, and *e* indicate online content.

Page numbers followed by *f* indicate figures, *b* indicate boxes, *t* indicate tables, and *e* indicate online content.

T

U

V

W